RUDOLPH'S PEDIATRICS

NOTICE

Medicine is an ever-changing science. As new research and clinical experience broaden our knowledge, changes in treatment and drug therapy are required. The editors and the publisher of this work have checked with sources believed to be reliable in their efforts to provide information that is complete and generally in accord with the standards accepted at the time of publication. However, in view of the possibility of human error or changes in medical sciences, neither the editors nor the publisher nor any other party who has been involved in the preparation or publication of this work warrants that the information contained herein is in every respect accurate or complete, and they disclaim all responsibility for any errors or omissions or for the results obtained from use of the information contained in this work. Readers are encouraged to confirm the information contained herein with other sources. For example and in particular, readers are advised to check the product information sheet included in the package of each drug they plan to administer to be certain that the information contained in this work is accurate and that changes have not been made in the recommended dose or in the contraindications for administration. This recommendation is of particular importance in connection with new or infrequently used drugs.

21ST EDITION

RUDOLPH'S PEDIATRICS

Editors

Colin D. Rudolph, MD, PhD

Professor and Chief, Pediatric Gastroenterology & Nutrition
Medical College of Wisconsin
Milwaukee, Wisconsin

Abraham M. Rudolph, MD

Professor Emeritus of Pediatrics
School of Medicine
University of California-San Francisco
San Francisco, California

Coeditors

Margaret K. Hostetter, MD

Professor of Pediatrics and Microbial Pathogenesis
Yale University School of Medicine
New Haven, Connecticut

George Lister, MD

Professor of Pediatrics and Anesthesiology
Yale University School of Medicine
New Haven, Connecticut

Norman J. Siegel, MD

Professor of Pediatrics and Medicine
Yale University School of Medicine
New Haven, Connecticut

McGraw-Hill
MEDICAL PUBLISHING DIVISION

New York   Chicago   San Francisco   Lisbon   London   Madrid
Mexico City   Milan   New Delhi   San Juan   Seoul   Singapore   Sydney   Toronto

McGraw-Hill

A Division of The **McGraw·Hill** *Companies*

Rudolph's Pediatrics, Twenty-First Edition

1 2 3 4 5 6 7 8 9 0   KGP/KGP   0 9 8 7 6 5 4 3 2

ISBN 0-8385-8285-0

This book was set in Galliard Regular by
  Progressive Information Technologies.
The editors were Martin J. Wonsiewicz, Sally Barhydt,
  Jim Shanahan, and Karen G. Edmonson.
The production supervisor was Richard Ruzycka.
The designer was Marsha Cohen/Parallelogram.
The index was prepared by Maria Coughlin Indexing.

Quebecor Kingsport was printer and binder.

This book is printed on acid-free paper.

Library of Congress Cataloging-in-Publication Data

Rudolph's Pediatrics / Abraham M. Rudolph ... [et al.].-- 21st ed.
      p. ; cm.
    Includes bibliographical references and index.
    ISBN 0-8385-8285-0
    1. Pediatrics. I. Title: Pediatrics. II. Rudolph, Abraham M., 1924-
    [DNLM: 1. Pediatrics. WS 200 R917 2001]
  RJ45 .R87 2001
  618.92--dc21

CONTENTS

P R E F A C E

The 21st edition of *Rudolph's Pediatrics* continues a tradition of evolving and adapting to changes in pediatric medicine. Originally published in 1897 as *Diseases of Infancy and Childhood,* written by L. Emmett Holt, the editors have consistently strived not only to provide descriptions of the clinical features and treatment of diseases of childhood but also to review the biologic principles underlying these processes. Achieving this goal is increasingly challenging during this era due to the extraordinary explosion of knowledge in all areas of pediatrics that has been spurred by our increased understanding of the molecular basis of disease and the rapid emergence of new technologies for diagnosis and treatment.

In an effort to adapt to these changes, the twenty-first edition of Rudolph's Pediatrics has been extensively revised. I have been aided in this endeavor by the previous editor, my father, Abraham M. Rudolph. The editorial expertise and perspective has been further expanded by the addition of three new co-editors, Margaret K. Hostetter, George Lister, and Norman J. Siegel. New associate editors participated in updating and reorganizing twenty of the twenty-seven chapters. A new chapter edited by Norman Siegel provides a concise overview of contemporary diagnostic techniques utilized across pediatric specialties. Other chapters were reorganized to align with emerging specialties in pediatric medicine. The chapter on toxicology and accidents has been replaced by a chapter on emergency medicine and critical care to provide more focused discussions on the management of the acutely ill child. The chapter on ethical issues in pediatrics has been expanded to include a review of terminal and palliative care and coping with the dying child. A new section on rehabilitation and care of the disabled child provides guidance on the management of this expanding population of children. The previous chapter on genetic disorders and birth defects has been expanded into two new chapters, one that discusses metabolic disorders and the other on genetics and dysmorphology.

In the previous edition, we introduced sections focused on the approach to diagnosis and management of various symptom complexes. These were often presented in algorithmic form. Because this was well received, most chapters in this edition now include sections on the approach to evaluation of relevant symptom presentations. In order to maintain the textbook as a single volume, we often needed to limit the discussion of various topics. Hopefully, the numerous changes in this edition continue the tradition of providing a balanced, comprehensive resource to aid health professionals in the care of infants and children.

I am most grateful for the collaboration of my co-editors, Abraham M. Rudolph, and Margaret K. Hostetter, George Lister, and Norman J. Siegel. Of particular importance was the guidance of my father, Abraham M. Rudolph, who shared his experience, wisdom and perspective (often humorous) during the inevitable frustrations I and the co-editors encountered as we prepared this edition of the textbook. I am also indebted to the associate editors who enlisted the aid of the 495 authors that contributed to the textbook and assured timely submission of their manuscripts. Finally, I am most thankful for the support and patience of my wife, Harriet and son, Jared.

DEDICATION

The 21st edition of Rudolph's Pediatrics
is dedicated to the memory of a great clinician
and teacher of Pediatrics.

Arnold "Jack" Rudolph
(1918–1995).

Leonard Apt, MD, Professor of Ophthalmology, Director Emeritus, Division of Pediatric Ophthalmology, University of California, Los Angeles, Jules Stein Eye Institute, School of Medicine, Special Consultant in Pediatric Ophthalmology, Los Angeles City Health Department and Bureau of Maternal and Child Health, Department of Public Health, State of California, Los Angeles, California

Chapter 26/The Eyes

Michael J. Bamshad, MD, Eccles Institute of Human Genetics, Assistant Professor of Pediatrics and Human Genetics, University of Utah School of Medicine, Salt Lake City, Utah

Chapter 10/Genetics and Dysmorphology

Richard D. Bland, MD, Formerly: Professor of Pediatrics, University of Utah School of Medicine, Salt Lake City, Utah

Chapter 2/The Newborn Infant

W. Thomas Boyce, MD, Professor of Epidemiology and Child Development, Division of Health and Medical Sciences, The School of Public Health and Institute of Human Development, University of California, Berkeley, California

Chapter 5/Developmental-Behavioral Pediatrics

John C. Carey, MD, MPH, Professor of Pediatrics, University of Utah School of Medicine, Division of Medical Genetics, Primary Children's Hospital and University of Utah Medical Center, Salt Lake City, Utah

Chapter 10/Genetics and Dysmorphology

Robin T. Cotton, MD, Professor, Otolaryngology-Head and Neck Surgery, University of Cincinnati College of Medicine, Director, Otolaryngology and Maxillofacial Surgery, Children's Hospital Medical Center, Cincinnati, Ohio

Chapter 15/Ear, Nose, Oropharynx, and Larynx

Alvin H. Crawford, MD, Professor of Pediatric Orthopedic Surgery, University of Cincinnati College of Medicine, Director of Orthopedic Surgery, Children's Hospital Medical Center, Cincinnati, Ohio

Chapter 27/Orthopedic Problems

Darryl C. De Vivo, MD, Professor of Pediatrics and Neurology, Columbia University College of Physicians and Surgeons, Director of The Neurological Institute, Division of Pediatric Neurology, Columbia Presbyterian Hospital, New York, New York

Chapter 25/The Nervous System

Murray Dock, DDS, MSD, and Robert L. Creedon, DDS, Associate Professor of Clinical Pediatrics, University of Cincinnati College of Medicine, Director of Residency Training, Pediatric Dentistry and Orthodontics, Children's Hospital Medical Center, Cincinnati, Ohio; Formerly: Director of Pediatric Dentistry, Children's Hospital Medical Center, Cincinnati, Ohio

Chapter 16/The Teeth and Supporting Structures

Jonathan D. Gitlin, MD, Helene B. Roberson Professor of Pediatrics, Professor of Pathology and Immunology, Washington University School of Medicine, Director, Division of Immunology and Rheumatology, St. Louis Children's Hospital, St. Louis, Missouri

Chapter 11/Allergy and Immunology

David N. Glass, MD, Professor of Pediatrics, University of Cincinnati College of Medicine, Director, Division of Rheumatology, Children's Hospital Medical Center, Cincinnati, Ohio

Chapter 12/Rheumatology

Thomas A. Hazinski, MD, Professor and Associate Chair of Pediatrics, Vanderbilt University School of Medicine, Director, Pediatric Pulmonary Medicine, Vanderbilt University Medical Center, Nashville, Tennessee

Chapter 23/The Respiratory System

Julien I. E. Hoffman, MD, Professor Emeritus, Department of Pediatrics, University of California School of Medicine, San Francisco, California

Chapter 22/The Circulatory System

Angela R. Holder, LLM, Professor of the Practice of Medical Ethics, Center for the Study of Medical Ethics and Humanities, Duke University Medical Center, Durham, North Carolina

Chapter 7/Ethical Issues in Pediatrics and Terminal Care

Charles E. Irwin, MD, Professor of Pediatrics, Director, Division of Adolescent Medicine, University of California School of Medicine, San Francisco, California
Chapter 3/The Adolescent Patient

Maureen M. Jonas, MD, Associate Professor of Pediatrics, Harvard Medical School, Associate in Medicine, Department of Gastroenterology and Nutrition, Children's Hospital, Boston, Massachusetts
Chapter 18/The Liver and Bile Ducts

George Lister, MD, Professor of Pediatrics and Anesthesiology, Section Chief, Pediatric Emergency Services, Department of Pediatrics, Yale University School of Medicine, New Haven, Connecticut
Chapter 4/Emergency and Critical Care

Bernard Lo, MD, Professor of Medicine and Director, Program in Medical Ethics, University of California-San Francisco, San Francisco, California
Chapter 7/Ethical Issues in Pediatrics and Terminal Care

Roderick McInnes, MD, PhD, and Joe T.R. Clarke, MD, Professor of Paediatrics and Molecular and Medical Genetics, University of Toronto, Chair, Molecular Medicine, Hospital for Sick Children, Toronto, Ontario, Canada; Department of Genetics
Chapter 9/Metabolic Disorders

Linda J. Michaud, MD, Associate Professor, Physical Medicine and Rehabilitation and Pediatrics, University of Cincinnati College of Medicine, Director, Pediatric Rehabilitation, Children's Hospital Medical Center, Cincinnati, Ohio
Chapter 6/Rehabilitation and the Child with Disability

Kevin M. Miller, MD, Associate Professor of Clinical Ophthalmology, Division of Comprehensive Ophthalmology, Los Angeles, California
Chapter 26/The Eyes

Walter L. Miller, MD, Professor of Pediatrics, the Metabolic Research Unit, and the Biomedical Sciences Graduate Program, Chief of Endocrinology, University of California School of Medicine, San Francisco, California
Chapter 24/The Endocrine System

Anna-Barbara Moscicki, MD, Professor of Pediatrics, Division of Adolescent Medicine, University of California-San Francisco, San Francisco, California
Chapter 3/The Adolescent Patient

Dennis L. Murray, MD, Professor of Pediatrics, Medical College of Georgia, Chief, Pediatric Infectious Diseases, Medical College of Georgia Children's Center, Augusta, Georgia
Chapter 13/Infectious Disorders

Kim J. Overby, MD, Pediatric Medical Care Coordinator, Child Welfare Division, Elwyn, Inc., Elwyn, Pennsylvania
Chapter 1/Pediatric Health Supervision

Amy S. Paller, MD, Professor of Pediatrics, Northwestern University Medical School, Director, Division of Dermatology, Children's Memorial Hospital, Chicago, Illinois
Chapter 14/The Skin

Howard A. Pearson, MD, Professor of Pediatrics, Yale University School of Medicine, Director, Sickle Cell and Thalassemia Programs, Yale-New Haven Medical Center, New Haven, Connecticut
Chapter 19/Blood and Blood Forming Tissues

Julio Pérez-Fontán, MD, Alumni Endowed Professor of Pediatrics, Professor of Anesthesiology, Director, Division of Critical Care Medicine, Department of Pediatrics, Washington University School of Medicine, St. Louis, Missouri
Chapter 4/Emergency and Critical Care

David Pleasure, MD, Professor of Neurology and Pediatrics, University of Pennsylvania School of Medicine, Director, Division of Neurology, Children's Hospital of Philadelphia, Philadelphia, Pennsylvania
Chapter 25/The Nervous System

Colin D. Rudolph, MD, PhD, Professor of Pediatrics, Medical College of Wisconsin, Director, Division of Gastroenterology, Children's Hospital of Wisconsin, Milwaukee, Wisconsin
Chapter 17/Gastroenterology and Nutrition

Alan L. Schwartz, MD, PhD, Department Head, Pediatrics, Professor, Molecular Biology and Pharmacology, Washington University School of Medicine, Physician-in-Chief, St. Louis Children's Hospital, St. Louis, Missouri
Chapter 20/Oncology

Mary-Ann Shafer, MD, Professor in Residence of Pediatrics, University of California-San Francisco, San Francisco, California
Chapter 3/The Adolescent Patient

Jack P. Shonkoff, MD, Dean, Florence Heller Graduate School for Advanced Studies in Social Welfare, Brandeis University, Waltham, Massachusetts
Chapter 5/Developmental-Behavioral Pediatrics

Norman J. Siegel, MD, Professor of Pediatrics and Medicine, Yale University School of Medicine, Physician-in-chief, New Haven, Connecticut
Chapter 8/Contemporary Diagnostic Techniques
Chapter 21/Kidneys

CONTRIBUTORS

Arthur R. Ablin, MD, Professor Emeritus, Clinical Pediatrics, Program Member, UCSF Comprehensive Cancer Center, University of California-San Francisco, San Francisco, California

Steven H. Abman, MD, Professor of Pediatrics, University of Colorado Health Sciences Center, Division of Pulmonary Medicine, Children's Hospital, Denver, Colorado

N. Scott Adzick, MD, C. Everett Koop Professor of Pediatric Surgery, University of Pennsylvania School of Medicine, Surgeon-in-Chief, Children's Hospital of Philadelphia, Philadelphia, Pennsylvania

Salman Ahmad, MD, University of Florida Health Science Center, Department of Pediatrics, Jacksonville, Florida

Samhar Al-Akash, MD, Consultant, Pediatric Neurology, Department of Pediatrics, Riyadh, Saudi Arabia

Abby D. Alkon, RN, PhD, Assistant Professor, Family Health Care Nursing, University of California-San Francisco, San Francisco, California

Marilee C. Allen, MD, Associate Professor of Pediatrics, Johns Hopkins University School of Medicine, Director, NICU Follow Up Clinic, Johns Hopkins Hospital, Baltimore, Maryland

Rudy Allen, MD, Cancer Institute of New Jersey, New Brunswick, New Jersey

Blanche P. Alter, MD, Visiting Professor of Pediatrics, Johns Hopkins University School of Medicine, Baltimore, Maryland

Claudine Amiel-Tison, MD, Professor Emeritus of Pediatrics, Port-Royal-Baudelocque Hospital, Paris, France

Michael Apkon, MD, PhD, Associate Professor of Pediatrics, Yale University School of Medicine, New Haven, Connecticut

Leonard Apt, MD, MPH, Professor of Ophthalmology, Director Emeritus, Pediatrics, Jules Stein Eye Institute, Los Angeles, California

Robert J. Arceci, MD, PhD, Jacob Schmidlapp Professor of Hematology/Oncology, University of Cincinnati College of Medicine, Director of Hematology/Oncology, Children's Hospital Medical Center, Cincinnati, Ohio

Susan T. Arnold, MD, Assistant Professor of Pediatrics and Neurology, Washington University School of Medicine, Co-Director, Epilepsy Center at St. Louis Children's Hospital, St. Louis, Missouri

Harvey Artsob, PhD, Zoonotic Diseases Section, Bureau of Microbiology, Winnipeg, Manitoba, Canada

Basim I. Asmar, MD, Professor of Pediatrics, Wayne State University School of Medicine, Director, Division of Pediatric Infectious Diseases, Children's Hospital of Michigan, Detroit, Michigan

Jane T. Atkins, MD, Assistant Professor of Pediatrics, University of Texas Health Sciences Center, Hermann Children's Hospital, Houston, Texas

Rita Ayangar, MD, Clinical Assistant Professor of Physical Medicine and Rehabilitation, University of Michigan School of Medicine, Attending Physician, University of Michigan Medical Center, Ann Arbor, Michigan

Richard Azizkhan, MD, Professor of Pediatric Surgery and Pediatrics, University of Cincinnati College of Medicine, Surgeon-in-Chief and Director, Pediatric Surgery, Children's Hospital Medical Center, Cincinnati, Ohio

Leonard Bacharier, MD, Instructor in Pediatrics, Washington University School of Medicine, Attending Physician, Allergy and Pulmonary Medicine, St. Louis Children's Hospital, St. Louis, Missouri

Peter Baehler, MD, Clinique de Pediatrie, Hopital Cantonal, Fribourg, Switzerland

M. Douglas Baker, MD, Professor of Pediatrics, Section Chief, Pediatric Emergency Services, Department of Pediatrics, Yale University School of Medicine, New Haven, Connecticut

Hanan H. Balkhy, MD, Jeddah, Saudi Arabia

Philip L. Ballard, MD, PhD, Professor of Pediatrics, Director of Research, Division of Neonatology, Children's Hospital of Philadelphia, Philadelphia, Pennsylvania

Michael J. Bamshad, MD, Eccles Institute of Human Genetics, Assistant Professor of Pediatrics and Human Genetics, University of Utah School of Medicine, Salt Lake City, Utah

Eduardo Bancalari, MD, Professor of Pediatrics, University of Miami School of Medicine, Director, Division of Neonatology, Jackson Children's Hospital, Miami, Florida

Stephen J. Barenkamp, MD, Professor of Pediatrics, Saint Louis University School of Medicine, Director, Pediatric Infectious Diseases, Cardinal Glennon Children's Hospital, St. Louis, Missouri

Frederic G. Barr, MD, PhD, Associate Professor, Anatomic Pathology, University of Pennsylvania School of Medicine, Philadelphia, Pennsylvania

Ronald G. Barr, MD, Professor of Pediatrics, McGill University Faculty of Medicine, Head, Child Development Programme, Montreal Children's Hospital, Montreal, Quebec, Canada

Karyl S. Barron, MD, Division of Intramural Research, NIAID-National Institutes of Health, Bethesda, Maryland

J. Bronwyn Bateman, MD, Professor and Chair, Rocky Mountain Lions Eye Institute, Aurora, Colorado

Mark L. Batshaw, MD, Chairman of Pediatrics, George Washington University School of Medicine, Chief Academic Officer, Children's National Medical Center, Washington, DC

Agatino Battaglia, MD, DPED, DNEVROL, Adjunct Professor of Child Neuro-Psychiatry, University of Pisa, Italy, Director, Center for Congenital Malformation Syndromes, Neurologist-in-Chief, Clinical Neurophysiology, Stella Maris Scientific Research Institute, Calambrone, 56018, Italy

Roberta E. Bauer, MD, Developmental Pediatrician, The Cleveland Clinic Children's Hospital for Rehabilitation, Cleveland, Ohio

Michel Baum, MD, Sara M. and Charles E. Seay, Chair of Pediatric Research, Director of Pediatric Nephrology, University of Texas Southwestern Medical School, Dallas, Texas

Laurie J. Bauman, PhD, MD, Professor of Pediatrics, Albert Einstein College of Medicine, Bronx, New York

Jacqueline A. Bello, MD, Professor of Clinical Radiology and Clinical Neurological Surgery, Albert Einstein College of Medicine, Director of Neuroradiology, Montefiore Medical Center, Bronx, New York

Kurt Benirschke, MD, Professor Emeritus of Pathology, University of California School of Medicine, San Diego, California

Robert A. Berg, MD, Professor and Associate Head, Department of Pediatrics, University of Arizona School of Medicine, Director of Critical Care, University Medical Center, Tucson, Arizona

Brad Berman, MD, Assistant Clinical Professor of Pediatrics, Division of Behavior and Development, University of California-San Francisco, San Francisco, California

Daniel Bernstein, MD, Professor of Pediatrics, Stanford University School of Medicine, Director, Division of Cardiology, Children's Hospital, Palo Alto, California

David I. Bernstein, MD, Professor of Pediatrics, University of Cincinnati College of Medicine, Director of Infectious Diseases, Children's Hospital Medical Center, Cincinnati, Ohio

Richard D. Bland, MD, Formerly: Professor of Pediatrics, University of Utah Health Sciences Center, Salt Lake City, Utah

Johan Blickman, MD, Professor of Radiology and Pediatrics, Boston University School of Medicine, Boston, Massachusetts

Eduardo Bonilla, MD, Professor of Clinical Neurology and Pathology, Columbia University College of Physicians and Surgeons, New York, New York

Margaret Bouwkamp, MA CC/SLP, Assistive Technologies Consultant, South Bend, Indiana

W. Thomas Boyce, MD, Professor of Epidemiology and Child Development, School of Public Health and Institute of Human Development, University of California, Berkeley, California

John Boyle, MD, Associate Professor of Pediatrics, University of South Carolina School of Medicine, Medical Director of Gastroenterology, Children's Hospital of Greenville, Greenville, South Carolina

Francisco Bracho, MD, Assistant Professor of Pediatrics, Division of Pediatric Hematology/Oncology, Bone and Marrow Transplant, Georgetown University Children's Medical Center, Washington, DC

Michael T. Brady, MD, Professor of Pediatrics and Preventitive Medicine, Ohio State University, Physician Director of HIV Program, Physician Director of Department of Epidemiology, Children's Hospital, Columbus, Ohio

Rebecca C. Brady, MD, Instructor of Pediatrics, University of Cincinnati College of Medicine, Division of Infectious Diseases, Cincinnati Children's Medical Center, Cincinnati, Ohio

Denise Bratcher, DO, Associate Professor, Infectious Diseases University of Louisville, Louisville, Kentucky

Philip P. Breitfeld, MD, Kligler Professor of Pediatrics and Biochemistry & Molecular Biology, Indiana University School of Medicine, Director, Pediatric Hematology/Oncology, James Whitcomb Riley Hospital for Children, Indianapolis, Indiana

David Brent, MD, Professor of Psychiatry, Pediatrics, and Epidemiology, University of Pittsburgh School of Medicine, Academic Chief, Child and Adolescent Psychiatry, University of Pittsburgh Medical Center, Pittsburgh, Pennsylvania

Kenneth R. Bridges, MD, Associate Professor of Medicine, Harvard Medical School, Director, Joint Center for Sickle Cell and Thalassemic Disorders, Brigham and Women's Hospital, Boston, Massachusetts

James D. Bristow, MD, Professor of Pediatrics, University of California-San Francisco, San Francisco, California

Michael M. Brook, MD, Associate Professor of Clinical Pediatrics, University of California at San Francisco, San Francisco, California

Garrett M. Broudeur, MD, Professor of Pediatrics and Oncology, Chief, Division of Oncology, Children's Hospital of Pennsylvania, Philadelphia, Pennsylvania

Rebecca Brown, MD, Assistant Professor of Clinical Surgery and Pediatrics, University of Cincinnati College of Medicine, Children's Hospital Medical Center, Cincinnati, Ohio

Frederick W. Bruhn, MD, Clinical Associate Professor Pediatrics, University of California-San Francisco, Hospitalist, Valley Children's Hospital, Madera, California

Jane L. Burns, MD, Associate Professor of Pediatrics, University of Washington School of Medicine, Clinic Chief, Infectious Diseases, Children's Hospital and Regional Medical Center, Seattle, Washington

Christina Butera, MD, Office Park Eye Center, Jacksonville, North Carolina

David A. Cabral, MBBS, FRCPC, British Columbia Children's Hospital, Vancouver, British Columbia, CANADA

Enrique Cacares, MD, Pediatric Infectious Disease Specialist, Rainbow Pediatric Clinic, McAllen, Texas

Mitchell S. Cairo, MD, Professor of Pediatrics, Associate Director of Pediatric Oncology, Columbia University College of Physicians and Surgeons, New York, New York

Michael Cappello, MD, Associate Professor of Pediatrics and Epidemiology, Yale University School of Medicine, New Haven, Connecticut

Michael P. Carboni, MD, Pediatric Cardiology and Electrophysiology, Nemours Cardiac Center, Wilmington, Delaware

John C. Carey, MD, MPH, Professor of Pediatrics, University of Utah Health Sciences Center, Division of Pediatric Genetics, Primary Children's Medical Center, Salt Lake City, Utah

David P. Carlton, MD, Associate Professor of Pediatrics, University of Wisconsin Medical School, Director of Neonatology, Meriter Hospital, Madison, Wisconsin

William L. Carroll, MD, Formerly: Professor of Pediatrics, University of Utah Health Sciences Center, Salt Lake City, Utah

Pranash K. Chakraborty, MD, Division of Clinical and Metabolic Genetics, Hospital for Sick Children, Toronto, Ontario, Canada

Tien-Lan Chang, MD, Instructor in Pediatrics, Harvard Medical School, Boston, Massachusetts

Valerie E. Charlton, MD, Clinical Professor of Pediatrics, University of California-San Francisco, Chief, Childhood Lead Poisoning Prevention Branch, California Department of Health Services, San Francisco, California

Talal A. Chatila, MD, Associate Professor of Pediatrics, Washington University School of Medicine, Division of Pediatric Immunology and Rheumatology, St. Louis Children's Hospital, St. Louis, Missouri

Yuan-Tsong Chen, MD, PhD, Professor of Pediatrics, Chief of Medical Genetics, Duke University Medical Center, Durham, North Carolina

Zhong Chen, MD, Associate Professor of Pediatrics, University of Utah Health Sciences Center, Co-Director Medical Cytogenetics Laboratory, Salt Lake City, Utah

Patricia J. Chesney, MD, Professor of Pediatrics, University of Tennessee School of Medicine, Department of Infectious Diseases, St. Jude's Children's Research Hospital, Memphis, Tennessee

Steven D. Chernausek, MD, Professor of Pediatrics, University of Cincinnati College of Medicine, Associate Director of Endocrinology, Children's Hospital Medical Center, Cincinnati, Ohio

Daniel R. Chernavvsky, MD, Research Fellow, Pediatric Nephrology, University of Virginia, Charlottesville, Virginia

Robert L. Chevalier, MD, Benjamin Armistead Shepard Professor and Chair, Department of Pediatrics, University of Virginia, Charlottesville, Virginia

Clifford Chin, MD, Assistant Professor of Pediatrics, Stanford University, Lucile Salter Packard Children's Hospital, Palo Alto, California

Claudia A. Chiriboga, MD, Associate Professor of Clinical Neurology, Columbia University, New York, New York

Daniel Choo, MD, Assistant Professor, Otolaryngology-Head and Neck Surgery, University of Cincinnati College of Medicine, Assistant Professor, Children's Hospital Medical Center, Cincinnati, Ohio

John C. Christenson, MD, Professor of Pediatrics, University of Utah School of Medicine, Chief, Division of Infectious Diseases and Geographic Medicine, Salt Lake City, Utah

Robin B. Churchill, MD, Assistant Professor, Pediatrics, Eastern Virginia Medical School, Attending Physician, Pediatrics, Children's Hospital of the King's Daughters, Norfolk, Virginia

Joe T.R. Clarke, MD, Division of Clinical and Metabolic Genetics, Hospital for Sick Children, Toronto, Ontario, Canada

Ronald I. Clyman, MD, Professor in Residence of Pediatrics, University of California-San Francisco, San Francisco, California

Stephen L. Cochi, MD, MPH, Division Director of Global Immunization, Centers for Disease Control and Prevention, Atlanta, Georgia

Janice L. Cockrell, MD, Clinical Associate Professor, Oregon Health Sciences University, Medical Director, Pediatric and Adolescent Rehabilitation, Emanuel Children's Hospital, Portland, Oregon

Bruce H. Cohen, MD, Director, Pediatric Neurology, The Cleveland Clinic Foundation, Cleveland, Ohio

Mitchell Cohen, MD, Professor, Pediatric Gastroenterology and Nutrition, Attending Physician, Pediatric Gastroenterology and Nutrition, Children's Hospital Medical Center, Cincinnati, Ohio

Pinchas Cohen, MD, Professor of Pediatrics, University of California-Los Angeles School of Medicine, Division of Endocrinology, Mattel Children's Hospital, Los Angeles, California

John W. Colberg, MD, Associate Professor of Surgery, Division of Urology, Yale University School of Medicine, New Haven, Connecticut

Beverly L. Connelly, MD, Associate Professor, Pediatrics, University of Cincinnati College of Medicine, Assistant Director, Infectious Diseases, Director, Infection Control Program, Children's Hospital Medical Center, Cincinnati, Ohio

Dan Michael Cooper, MD, Department of Pediatrics, University of California-Irvine School of Medicine, Division of Pulmonary Medicine, Miller Children's Hospital, Irvine, California

Michael J. Corwin, MD, Associate Professor of Pediatrics, Boston University School of Medicine, Boston, Massachusetts

Juliet M. Coscia, PhD, Neuropsychologist, Assistant Professor of Clinical Pediatrics, Children's Hospital Medical Center, Cincinnati, Ohio

C. Michael Cotten, MD, Clinical Professor of Pediatrics, Duke University Medical School, Durham, North Carolina

Robin T. Cotton, MD, Professor, Otolaryngology-Head and Neck Surgery, University of Cincinnati College of Medicine, Director, Otolarynology and Maxillofacial Surgery, Children's Hospital Medical Center, Cincinnati, Ohio

Joseph Cox, MD, Clinical Professor of Surgery & Pediatrics, University of Cincinnati College of Medicine, Division of Pediatric Surgery, Children's Hospital Medical Center, Cincinnati, Ohio

Alvin H. Crawford, MD, Professor of Pediatrics, University of Cincinnati, Director, Orthopedic Surgery, Children's Hospital Medical Center, Cincinnati, Ohio

David F. Crawford, MD, PhD, Fellow in Pediatric Hematology and Oncology, Washington University School of Medicine, St. Louis Children's Hospital, St. Louis, Missouri

Robert L. Creedon, DDS, Professor Emeritus of Pediatrics, University of Cincinnati College of Medicine, Cincinnati, Ohio

Bari B. Cunningham, MD, Assistant Professor of Pediatrics and Medicine (Dermatology), Division of Pediatric and Adolescent Dermatology, Children's Hospital, San Diego, California

Michael L. Cunningham, MD, PhD, Assistant Professor of Pediatrics, University of Washington, Director, Craniofacial Center, Children's Hospital and Regional Medical Center, Seattle, Washington

Leonna Cuttler, MD, Professor of Pediatrics and Pharmacology, Case Western Reserve University School of Medicine, Chairman, Pediatric Endocrinology and Metabolism, Cleveland, Ohio

Michael W. Dae, MD, Professor in Residence of Radiology, University of California-San Francisco, San Francisco, California

Ronald E. Dahl, MD, Associate Professor of Psychiatry and Pediatrics, University of Pittsburgh School of Medicine, Director, Child and Adolescent Sleep Evaluation Center, Western Psychiatric Institute and Clinic, Pittsburgh, Pennsylvania

Peter R. Dallman, MD, Emeritus Professor of Pediatrics, University of California-San Francisco, San Francisco, California

Toni Darville, MD, Associate Professor of Pediatrics, University of Arkansas, Associate Professor of Pediatrics, Arkansas Children's Hospital, Little Rock, Arkansas

Brian Davison, MD, Boston University Medical Center, Boston, Massachusetts

J. Michael Dean, MD, Professor of Pediatrics, University of Utah School of Medicine, Chief, Critical Care Medicine, Primary Children's Hospital, Salt Lake City, Utah

Jaime de Inocencio, MD, PhD, Pediatra EAP, Insalud Atencion Primaria Area Madrid, Madrid, Spain

William DeMeyer, MD, Professor, Neurology and Pediatrics, Indiana University, Riley Hospital for Children, Indianapolis, Indiana

A. Joseph D'Ercole, MD, Professor of Pediatrics, University of North Carolina School of Medicine, Chief, Pediatric Endocrinology, Women's and Children's Hospital, Chapel Hill, North Carolina

Robert Desnick, MD, PhD, Professor and Chairman, Department of Human Genetics, Mount Sinai School of Medicine, New York, New York

Darryl C. De Vivo, MD, Professor of Pediatrics and Neurology, Columbia University College of Physicians and Surgeons, Director of The Neurological Institute, Division of Pediatric Neurology, Columbia Presbyterian Hospital, New York, New York

William H. Dietz, MD, PhD, Director, Nutrition and Physical Activity, Centers for Disease Control and Prevention, Atlanta, Georgia

Carlo DiLorenzo, MD, Associate Professor of Pediatrics, University of Pittsburgh, Director, Motility Center, Children's Hospital of Pittsburgh, Pittsburgh, Pennsylvania

Salvatore DiMauro, MD, Professor of Neurology, Columbia University, New York, New York

Suzanne D. Dixon, MD, Associate Clinical Professor, Pediatrics, University of Washington, Behavioral and Developmental Pediatrician, Great Falls Clinic, Great Falls, Montana

Murray Dock, DDS, Associate Professor of Clinical Pediatrics, University of Cincinnati College of Medicine, Pediatric Dentistry, Children's Hospital Medical Center, Cincinnati, Ohio

Marla Dubinsky, MD, Director, Pediatric Bowel Disease Center, Cedars-Sinai Medical Center, Los Angeles, California

Peter Duric, MD, FRCP (C), Professor, Pediatrics, University of Toronto, Head, Cystic Fibrosis Research Group, The Hospital for Sick Children, Toronto, Ontario, Canada

Paul H. Dworkin, MD, Professor and Chairman, Pediatrics, University of Connecticut School of Medicine, Director and Chairman, Pediatrics, Saint Francis Hospital and Medical Center, Hartford, Connecticut

Allison A. Eddy, MD, Professor of Pediatrics, University of Washington, Head, Division of Nephrology, Children's Hospital and Regional Medical Center, Seattle, Washington

Morven S. Edwards, MD, Professor of Pediatrics, Infectious Diseases, Baylor College of Medicine, Active Staff, Infectious Diseases, Texas Children's Hospital, Houston, Texas

Lawrence F. Eichenfield, MD, Associate Clinical Professor of Medicine, Chief, Division of Pediatric and Adolescent Dermatology, Children's Hospital and Health Center, San Diego, California

Glen R. Elliott, MD, PhD, Associate Professor of Psychiatry, Langley Porter Psychiatric Institute, University of California, San Francisco, California

Cynthia Epstein, MD, Assistant Professor of Pediatrics, Virginia Commonwealth University School of Medicine, Division of Pediatric Pulmonology, VCU Health System-MCV Hospitals, Richmond, Virginia

Michele M. Estarbrook, MD, Associate Clinical Professor of Pediatrics, University of California-San Francisco, San Francisco, California

Robert Ettenger, MD, Professor of Pediatrics, University of California–Los Angeles School of Medicine, Head, Division of Pediatric Nephrology, Children's Hospital, Los Angeles, California

John Fahey, MD, Associate Professor of Pediatrics, Yale University School of Medicine, New Haven, Connecticut

Sheila Fallon-Friedlander, MD, Associate Clinical Professor of Pediatrics and Medicine (Dermatology), University of California–Los Angeles School of Medicine, Staff Physician, Children's Hospital, Los Angeles, California

Leland Fan, MD, Professor of Pediatrics, Baylor College of Medicine, Cystic Fibrosis Center, Texas Children's Hospital, Houston, Texas

Avroy A. Fanaroff, MD, Professor of Pediatrics and Reproductive Biology, Case Western Reserve University School of Medicine, Co-Director, Neonatology, Rainbow Babies and Children's Hospital, Cleveland, Ohio

Michael Farrell, MD, Professor of Pediatrics, University of Cincinnati College of Medicine, Chief of Staff, Children's Hospital Medical Center, Cincinnati, Ohio

Jeffrey A. Feinstein, MD, Lucile Salter Packard Children's Hospital, Stanford University School of Medicine, Palo Alto, California

Neil A. Feldstein, MD, Assistant Professor of Clinical Neurosurgery, Columbia University College of Physicians and Surgeons, New York, New York

Jeffrey R. Fineman, MD, Professor of Pediatrics, University of California-San Francisco, San Francisco, California

Delbert A. Fisher, MD, Professor Emeritus, University of California, Los Angeles, School of Medicine, Chief Science Officer, Quest Diagnostics-Nichols Institute, San Juan, California

Margaret C. Fisher, MD, Professor of Pediatrics, Associate Chair of Medical Education, Medical College of Pennsylvania Hahnemann School of Medicine, Section of Infectious Disease, St. Christopher's Hospital for Children, Philadelphia, Pennsylvania

Marvin A. Fishman, MD, Professor of Pediatrics and Neurology, Baylor University School of Medicine, Director, Pediatric Neurology, Texas Children's Hospital, Houston, Texas

Patricia M. Flynn, MD, Associate Professor, Pediatrics, University of Tennessee, Associate Member, Department of Infectious Diseases, St. Jude Children's Research Hospital, Memphis, Tennessee

Robert P. Foglia, MD, Surgeon-in-Chief, St. Louis Children's Hospital, St. Louis, Missouri

E. Lee Ford-Jones, MD, FRCP(C), Associate Professor, University of Toronto, Department of Infectious Diseases, Hospital for Sick Children, Toronto, Ontario, Canada

John W. Foreman, MD, Professor of Pediatrics, Duke University, Chief, Pediatric Nephrology, Duke University Medical Center, Durham, North Carolina

Melvin H. Freedman, MD, Professor of Pediatrics, University of Toronto School of Medicine, Hospital for Sick Children, Toronto, Ontario, Canada

Ilona J. Frieden, MD, Clinical Professor of Pediatrics and Dermatology, Director of Pediatric Dermatology Clinics, University of California-San Francisco, San Francisco, California

Sheila Friedlander, MD, Department of Dermatology, Children's Hospital and Health Center, San Diego, California

Philip Frykman, MD, University of Cincinnati, Children's Hospital Medical Center, Cincinnati, Ohio

Tina Gabby, MD, Assistant Clinical Professor of Pediatrics, Division of Behavioral and Developmental Pediatrics, University of California–San Francisco, San Francisco, California

Giuliana Galassi, MD, Modena, Italy

Susan A. Galel, MD, Associate Professor of Pathology, Stanford Medical School Blood Center, Associate Medical Director, Stanford Hospital Transfusion Service, Palo Alto, California

James H. Garvin, Jr., MD, Professor of Clinical Pediatrics, Columbia University, Attending Pediatrician, Babies and Children's Hospital of New York, New York Presbyterian Hospital, New York, New York

Aditya Gaur, MD, DCH, Fellow, Pediatric Infectious Diseases, University of Tennessee and St. Jude Children's Research Hospital, Memphis, Tennessee

Michael A. Gerber, MD, Medical Officer, National Institute of Allergy and Infectious Diseases, National Institutes of Health, Bethesda, Maryland

Jill P. Ginsberg, MD, Division of Oncology, Children's Hospital of Philadelphia, Philadelphia, Pennsylvania

Brett P. Giroir, MD, Division Director, Critical Care Medicine, Department of Pediatrics, University of Texas-Southwestern Medical Center, Dallas, Texas

Stephen E. Gitelman, MD, Associate Professor of Pediatrics, University of California-San Francisco, San Francisco, California

Jonathan D. Gitlin, MD, Helene B. Roberson Professor of Pediatrics, Professor of Pathology and Immunology, Washington University School of Medicine, Director, Division of Immunology and Rheumatology, St. Louis Children's Hospital, St. Louis, Missouri

David N. Glass, MD, Professor of Pediatrics, University of Cincinnati College of Medicine, Director, Pediatric Rheumatology, Children's Hospital Medical Center, Cincinnati, Ohio

Wallace Gleason, Jr., MD, Professor of Pediatrics, Assistant Dean for Admissions, The University of Texas-Houston Health Sciences Center, Chief, Gastroenterology, Hepatology and Nutrition, Hermann Children's Hospital, Houston, Texas

Maurice Godfrey, PhD, Associate Professor of Pediatrics, University of Nebraska Medical Center, Omaha, Nebraska

Ronald N. Goldberg, MD, Professor and Vice Chair of Pediatrics, Duke University School of Medicine, Chief, Neonatal and Perinatal Medicine, Duke University Medical Center, Durham, North Carolina

Lauren Heim Goldstein, PhD, Research Psychologist, University of California, Berkeley Institute of Human Development, Berkeley, California

R. Ariel Gómez, MD, Genentech Professor of Pediatrics, Associate Chair for Research, Pediatric Nephrology Division, University of Virginia, Charlottesville, Virginia

Regino P. Gonzales-Peralta, MD, Assistant Professor, Pediatric Gastroenterology and Hepatology, University of Florida, Attending Physician, Pediatric Gastroenterology and Hepatology, Shands Children's Hospital, Gainesville, Florida

Stephen Irwin Goodman, MD, Professor, Pediatrics and Cellular and Structural Biology, Chief, Section of Metabolism and Birth Defects, University of Colorado Health Sciences Center, Denver, Colorado

Ramya Gopinath, MD, National Institutes of Health, Heminth Immunology Section, Laboratory of Parasitic Diseases, Bethesda, Maryland

Ralph C. Gordon, MD, Professor of Pediatrics/Human Development, Michigan State University, Associate Director, Pediatrics, Kalamazoo Center for Medical Studies, Kalamazoo, Michigan

Stephen J. Gould, PhD, Associate Professor, Departments of Biological Chemistry, Cell Biology and Anatomy, Johns Hopkins University School of Medicine, Baltimore, Maryland

Elizabeth A. Grady, RRT, Children's Hospital Medical Center, Cincinnati, Ohio

Christopher G. Green, MD, Professor and Associate Chairman of Pediatrics, University of Wisconsin School of Medicine, Madison, Wisconsin

Daniel M. Green, MD, Professor of Pediatrics, State University of New York, Associate Chief, Pediatrics, Roswell Park Cancer Institute, Buffalo, New York

William A. Greenhill, DMD, Assistant Professor, Clinical Pediatrics, University of Cincinnati College of Medicine, Division of Pediatric Dentistry, Children's Hospital Medical Center, Cincinnati, Ohio

George A. Gregory, MD, Professor Emeritus of Anesthesia/Perioperative Care, University of California–San Francisco, San Francisco, California

Holcombe E. Grier, MD, Associate Professor of Pediatrics, Harvard Medical School, Clinical Director of Pediatric Oncology, Dana Farber Cancer Institute, Boston, Massachusetts

Markus Grompe, MD, Professor, Molecular and Medical Genetics and Pediatrics, Oregon Health and Science University, Portland, Oregon

Moses Grossman, MD, Professor Emeritus of Pediatrics, University of California-San Francisco, San Francisco, California

Jeffrey R. Gruen, MD, Associate Professor of Pediatrics, Yale Child Health Research Center, Yale University School of Medicine, New Haven, Connecticut

Melvin M. Grumbach, MD, DM Hon. causa, Edward B. Shaw Professor of Pediatrics and Emeritus Chairman, Pediatrics, University of California-San Francisco, Attending Physician, Pediatrics, Medical Center at the University of San Francisco and San Francisco General Hospital, San Francisco, California

Thomas N. Hansen, MD, Professor and Chair, Department of Pediatrics, Ohio State University School of Medicine and Children's Hospital, Columbus, Ohio

Philip J. Hashkes, MD, Clinical Lectures, Pediatrics, Technion School of Technology, Senior Physician, Consultant in Pediatric Rheumatology, Safed, Israel

David B. Haslam, MD, Assistant Professor of Pediatrics and Molecular Microbiology, Attending Physician, Division of Infectious Diseases, St. Louis Children's Hospital, St. Louis, Missouri

Eric Hassall, MB, CHB, FRCP (C), Associate Professor, Gastroenterology, University of British Columbia, British Columbia's Children's Hospital, Vancouver, British Columbia, Canada

Samuel Hawgood, MD, Professor of Pediatrics, Director, Neonatal Intensive Care Nursery, University of California-San Francisco, San Francisco, California

William W. Hay, Jr., MD, Professor of Pediatrics, University of Colorado Health Sciences Center, Director, Training Program in Neonatal-Perinatal Medicine and Neonatal Clinical Research Center, Denver, Colorado

Robert J. Hayashi, MD, Assistant Professor, Pediatric Hematology/Oncology, Washington University, Director, Pediatric Bone Marrow Transplant Program, St. Louis Children's Hospital, St. Louis, Missouri

Morey W. Haymond, MD, Professor of Pediatrics, Program Director, Child Health Research Center, Baylor College of Medicine, Houston, Texas

Arthur P. Hays, MD, Associate Professor of Clinical Neuropathology, Columbia University College of Physicians and Surgeons, New York, New York

Thomas A. Hazinski, MD, Professor and Vice Chairman, Pediatrics, Vanderbilt University, Director, Pediatric Pulmonary Medicine, Vanderbilt University Medical Center, Nashville, Tennessee

Adelaide A. Hebert, MD, Professor and Vice Chairman of Dermatology, University of Texas–Houston Medical School, Houston, Texas

Markku Heikinheimo, MD, PhD, Associate Professor, Children's Hospital, University of Helsinki, Helsinki, Finland

Leo A. Heitlinger, MD, Chief of Pediatrics, St. Luke's Hospital, Bethlehem, Pennsylvania

Melvin Heyman, MD, Professor of Pediatrics, Chief, Pediatric Gastroenterology, Hepatology & Nutrition, Director, Training Program in Pediatric GI/Nutrition, University of California-San Francisco, San Francisco, California

Lisa Jo Hicks, CTRS, Recreational Therapist, Children's Hospital Medical Center, Chattanooga, Tennessee

Charles B. Higgins, MD, Professor of Radiology, University of California–San Francisco, San Francisco, California

Friedhelm Hildebrandt, MD, Department of Pediatric Nephrology, University Children's Hospital, Freiburg, Germany

Alan Hill, MD, Professor and Head, Neurology, Pediatrics, University of British Columbia, British Columbia's Children's Hospital, Vancouver, British Columbia, Canada

Ivor D. Hill, MD, Professor of Pediatrics and Internal Medicine/Gastroenterology, Wake Forest University School of Medicine, Winston-Salem, North Carolina

Dee Hodge, III, MD, Associate Professor of Pediatrics, Washington University School of Medicine, Associate Director, Clinical Affairs for Emergency Services, St. Louis Children's Hospital, St. Louis, Missouri

W. Alan Hodson, MD, Professor of Pediatrics, University of Washington School of Medicine, Attending Physician, Division of Neonatology, Children's Hospital and Regional Medical Center, Seattle, Washington

Edward Hoffenberg, MD, Associate Professor, Pediatrics, University of Colorado School of Medicine, Director, Center for Pediatric Inflammatory Bowel Diseases, The Children's Hospital of Denver, Denver, Colorado

Julien I.E. Hoffman, MD, Professor of Pediatrics (Emeritus), University of California-San Francisco, Attending Physician, Moffitt/Long Hospitals, San Francisco, California

Angela R. Holder, LL.M, Professor of the Practice of Medical Ethics, Center for the Study of Medical Ethics and Humanities, Duke University School of Medicine, Durham, North Carolina

Allison Holm, MD, Clinical Instructor, Pediatrics and Dermatology, University of Rochester School of Medicine, Rochester, New York

Miriam Horowitz, RD, Pediatric Nutrition Support Nutritionist, Division of Pediatric Gastroenterology, Nutrition, and Liver Diseases, New York, New York

Margaret K. Hostetter, MD, Professor of Pediatric and Microbial Pathogenesis, Chief, Pediatric Immunology, Yale University School of Medicine, Attending Physician, Yale-New Haven Children's Hospital, New Haven, Connecticut

Barbara J. Howard, MD, Assistant Professor of Pediatrics, Division of Behavioral and Developmental Pediatrics, Johns Hopkins University School of Medicine, Baltimore, Maryland

Frederick Huang, MD, Research Associate, Department of Hematology/Oncology, Children's Hospital Medical Center, Cincinnati, Ohio

Melissa M. Hudson, MD, Associate Professor, Pediatrics, University of Tennessee, Associate Member, Hematology/Oncology, St. Jude Children's Research Hospital, Memphis, Tennessee

Walter T. Hughes, MD, Professor of Pediatrics and Preventive Medicine, University of Tennessee College of Medicine, Emeritus Member, Department of Infectious Diseases, St. Jude Children's Research Hospital, Memphis, Tennessee

Janellen Huttenlocher, MD, William S. Gray Professor of Psychology, Chair, Developmental Psychology, University of Chicago, Chicago, Illinois

Peter R. Huttenlocher, MD, Professor of Pediatrics and Neurology, University of Chicago School of Medicine, Division of Pediatric Neurology, University of Chicago Children's Hospital, Chicago, Illinois

Charles E. Irwin, Jr., MD, Professor of Pediatrics, Director of Adolescent Medicine, University of California-San Francisco, San Francisco, California

Richard F. Jacobs, MD, Horace C. Cabe Professor of Pediatrics, University of Arkansas for Medical Sciences, Chief, Division of Pediatric Infectious Diseases, Children's Hospital, Little Rock, Arkansas

David M. Jaffe, MD, Dana Brown Professor of Pediatrics, Washington University School of Medicine, Director, Pediatric Emergency Medicine, St. Louis Children's Hospital, St. Louis, Missouri

Julia Jaskiewicz, MD, Pediatrician, Eastgate Pediatrics, Cincinnati, Ohio

Michael Jellinek, MD, Professor of Psychiatry and Pediatrics, Harvard Medical School, Chief, Child Psychiatry Service, Massachusetts General Hospital, Boston, Massachusetts

Linda Bone Jeng, MD, PhD, Center for Human Genetics, Rainbow Babies and Children's Hospital, Cleveland, Ohio

John M. Jemerin, MD, Assistant Professor in Residence, Department of Pediatrics, University of California–San Francisco, San Francisco, California

Chandy C. John, MD, Assistant Professor, Geographic Medicine and Infectious Diseases, Case Western Reserve University, Rainbow Babies and Children's Hospital, Cleveland, Ohio

Christopher Jolley, MD, Assistant Professor of Pediatrics, University of Florida, Attending Physician, Pediatrics, Shands Children's Hospital, Gainesville, Florida

Maureen M. Jonas, MD, Associate Professor, Pediatrics, Harvard Medical School, Associate in Gastroenterology, Children's Hospital, Boston, Massachusetts

M. Douglas Jones, Jr, MD, Chairman, Department of Pediatrics, University of Colorado Health Sciences Center, Pediatrician-in-Chief, Children's Hospital, Denver, Colorado

Lynn B. Jorde, PhD, Professor of Genetics, University of Utah School of Medicine, Salt Lake City, Utah

Jill Jump, CCC-SLP, Assistant Technology Coordinator, Children's Hospital Medical Center, Cincinnati, Ohio

Stephen G. Kahler, MSD, Principal Fellow (Assoc. Professor), Pediatrics, Murdoch Children's Research Institute, Director of Genetics, Royal Children's Hospital, Parkville, Australia

Barton A. Kamen, MD, American Cancer Society, Clinical Research Professor, Professor of Pediatrics and Pharmacology, Cancer Institute of New Jersey

Clifford E. Kashtan, MD, Professor of Pediatrics, Division of Pediatric Nephrology, University of Minnesota Medical School, Minneapolis, Minnesota

Michael Katz, MD, Vice-President for Research, March of Dimes Birth Defects Foundation, White Plains, New York

Samuel L. Katz, MD, DSC, Wilburt C. Davison Professor and Chairman Emeritus, Department of Pediatrics, Division of Infectious Diseases, Duke University Medical School, Durham, North Carolina

Edward Kaye, MD, Formerly: Professor of Pediatrics, University of Pennsylvania School of Medicine, Chief, Division of Metabolism, Children's Hospital of Philadelphia, Philadelphia, Pennsylvania

Constance Helen Keefer, MD, Instructor in Pediatrics, Harvard Medical School, Child Development Unit, Children's Hospital, Boston, Massachusetts

Desmond P. Kelly, MD, Associate Professor of Pediatrics, University of South Carolina School of Medicine, Medical Director of Developmental Pediatrics, Children's Hospital, Greenville, South Carolina

Thomas Kennedy, MD, Chairman, Department of Pediatrics, Bridgeport Hospital, Bridgeport, Connecticut, Clinical Professor of Pediatrics, Yale University School of Medicine, New Haven, Connecticut

Ali S. Khan, MD, Director, Bioterrorism Division, Centers for Disease Control and Prevention, Atlanta, Georgia

Janice J. Kim, MD, Adjunct Assistant Professor of Pediatrics, University of California–San Francisco, San Francisco, California

Douglas G. Kinnett, MD, Assistant Professor of Clinical Physical Medicine and Rehabilitation and Clinical Pediatrics, University of Cincinnati College of Medicine, Children's Hospital Medical Center, Cincinnati, Ohio

John P. Kinsella, MD, Associate Professor of Pediatrics, University of Colorado Health Sciences Center, Section of Neonatology, Children's Hospital, Denver, Colorado

Joseph A. Kitterman, MD, Professor of Pediatrics in Residence, Senior Staff Member, Cardiovascular Research Institute, University of California–San Francisco, San Francisco, California

Martin B. Kleiman, MD, Ryan White Professor of Pediatrics, Indiana University School of Medicine, Indianapolis, Indiana

Teresa M. Kohlenberg, MD, Instructor in Psychiatry, Harvard Medical School, Staff Psychiatrist, Children's Hospital, Watertown, Massachusetts

E. Kent Korgenski, MS, MT(ASCP), Clinical Microbiology Laboratory, Primary Children's Medical Center, Salt Lake City, Utah

Peter J. Krause, MD, Professor of Pediatrics, University of Connecticut School of Medicine, Chief, Division of Infectious Diseases, Connecticut Children's Medical Center, Hartford, Connecticut

Beatriz D. Kuizon, MD, Assistant Professor of Pediatrics, Department of Pediatrics, University of California, Los Angeles, School of Medicine, Los Angeles, California

Ashir Kumar, MD, Professor of Pediatrics and Human Development, Division of Pediatric Infectious Diseases, Michigan State University, East Lansing, Michigan

Ann W. Kummer, PhD, Director, Speech Pathology, Children's Hospital Medical Center, Cincinnati, Ohio

Lisa A. Kurtz, M.Ed, OTR/L, FAOTA, Clinical Assistant Professor of Occupational Therapy, University of New England, Occupational Therapist, Jameson School, Scarborough, Maine

Peter O. Kwiterovich, Jr., MD, Professor of Pediatrics and Medicine, Johns Hopkins University School of Medicine, Baltimore, Maryland

Craig B. Langman, MD, Professor of Pediatrics, Northwestern University School of Medicine, Head, Nephrology and Mineral Metabolism, Children's Memorial Hospital, Chicago, Illinois

Allan S.Y. Lau, MD, Honorary Consultant, Department of Pediatrics, Queen Mary Hospital, Hong Kong

Deborah Lehman, MD, Assistant Clinical Professor, Pediatrics, UCLA School of Medicine, Los Angeles, Cedars-Sinai Medical Center, Los Angeles, California

Neal Leleiko, MD, PhD, Chief, Pediatric Gastroenterology and Nutrition, Mount Sinai Medical Center, New York, New York

Robert Lemanske, Jr., MD, Professor of Pediatrics and Medicine, University of Wisconsin School of Medicine, Madison, Wisconsin

Marsha Leen-Mitchell, MD, Pregnancy RiskLine, University of Utah Medical Center, Salt Lake City, Utah

Claire O. Leonard, MD, FAAP, Associate Professor of Pediatrics, Division of Medical Genetics, University of New Mexico School of Medicine, Albuquerque, New Mexico

Nicole M.A. LeSaux, MD, Division of Infectious Diseases, Children's Hospital of Eastern Ontario, Ottawa, Ontario, Canada

John M. Leventhal, MD, Professor of Pediatrics, Yale University School of Medicine, New Haven, Connecticut

Melvin D. Levine, MD, Professor of Pediatrics, Director, Clinical Center for Study of Development and Learning, University of North Carolina, Chapel Hill, North Carolina

Fiona Howard Levy, MD, Assistant Professor of Pediatrics, Washington University School of Medicine, Medical Director of the Pediatric Intensive Care Unit, St. Louis Children's Hospital, St. Louis, Missouri

B.U.K. Li, MD, Professor of Pediatrics, Northwestern University, Director of Gastroenterology, Children's Memorial Hospital, Chicago, Illinois

Poh-Lian Lim, MD, Fellow, Infectious Diseases, Tulane University School of Medicine, New Orleans, Louisiana

Dana Thompson Link, MD, MS, Department of Otorhinolaryngology, Head and Neck Surgery, Division of Pediatric Otolaryngology, Rochester, Minnesota

Jeffrey Michael Lipton, MD, PhD, Associate Professor, Albert Einstein College of Medicine, Director, Pediatric Hematology/Oncology and Stem Cell Transplantation, Schneider Children's Hospital, New Hyde Park, New York

George Lister, MD, Professor of Pediatrics and Anesthesiology, Yale University School of Medicine, Director, Pediatric Critical Care, Yale-New Haven Children's Hospital, New Haven, Connecticut

James H. Liu, MD, Clinical Fellow, Division of Pediatric Otolaryngology, University of Cincinnati College of Medicine, Cincinnati, Ohio

Bernard Lo, MD, Professor of Medicine and Director, Program in Medical Ethics, University of California–San Francisco, San Francisco, California

Ashima Madan, MD, Assistant Professor of Pediatrics, Stanford University School of Medicine, Palo Alto, California

Deborah Madansky, MD, Medical Director, CARE Children's Counseling Center, Sebastoplo, California

Joseph A. Majzoub, MD, Chief, Division of Endocrinology, Harvard Medical School, Children's Hospital, Boston, Massachusetts

Anthony J. Mancini, MD, Assistant Professor of Pediatrics and Dermatology, Northwestern University Medical School, Attending Physician and Clinical Practice Director, Children's Memorial Hospital, Chicago, Illinois

Marilyn J. Manco-Johnson, MD, Professor of Pediatrics, University of Colorado Health Science Center, The Children's Hospital of Denver, Denver, Colorado

Arik V. Marcell, MD, MPH, Adolescent Medicine Fellow, University of California–San Francisco, San Francisco, California

Andrew M. Margileth, MD, Clinical Professor, Pediatrics, Mercer University School of Medicine, Director, Pediatric Dermatology, Backus Children's Hospital, Savannah, Georgia

John M. Maris, MD, Assistant Professor of Pediatrics Oncology, University of Pennsylvania School of Medicine, Children's Hospital of Philadelphia, Philadelphia, Pennsylvania

Lynne P. Martinez, MD, Program Manager, Pregnancy RiskLine, Salt Lake City, Utah

Deborah Mason, RN, MSN, CPNP, Nurse Coordinator Interdisciplinary Feeding Team, Department of Pediatric Surgery, Children's Hospital Medical Center, Cincinnati, Ohio

Theresa L. Massagli, MD, Associate Professor of Rehabilitation Medicine and Pediatrics, University of Washington, Attending Physician, Children's Hospital and Regional Medical Center, Seattle, Washington

Dietrich Matern, MD, Assistant Professor of Laboratory Medicine, Co-director, Biochemical Genetics Laboratory, Mayo Clinic and Foundation, Rochester, Minnesota

John McBride, MD, Professor and Vice Chair of Pediatrics, Northeastern Ohio University College of Medicine, Director, Robert T. Stone, MD Respiratory Center, Children's Hospital Medical Center of Akron, Akron, Ohio

Roderick McInnes, MD, PhD, Professor of Pediatrics and Molecular and Medical Genetics, University of Toronto, Chair of Molecular Medicine, Hospital for Sick Children, Toronto, Ontario, Canada

Mary A. McMahon, MD, Assistant Professor of Clinical and Physical Medicine and Rehabilitation and Clinical Pediatrics, Cincinnati, Ohio

Julia A. McMillan, MD, Associate Professor of Pediatrics, Johns Hopkins University School of Medicine, Vice Chair, Pediatric Education, Johns Hopkins Hospital, Baltimore, Maryland

Charles T. Mehlman, DO, MPH, Assistant Professor of Surgery, University of Cincinnati, Director, Musculoskeletal Outcomes Research, Children's Hospital Medical Center, Cincinnati, Ohio

William C. Mentzer, Jr., MD, Professor and Director, Hematology/Oncology, University of California, San Francisco, Professor and Director, Hematology/Oncology, San Francisco General Hospital, San Francisco, California

Kathy Ann Merritt, MD, Assistant Consulting Professor, Community Programs, Duke University Medical Center, Durham, North Carolina

Denise W. Metry, MD, Assistant Professor of Pediatrics and Dermatology, Baylor College of Medicine, Houston, Texas

W. Peter Metz, MD, Associate Professor of Psychiatry and Pediatrics, University of Massachusets Medical School, Director, Division of Child and Adolescent Psychiatry, University of Massachusetts Memorial Health Care Inc., Worcester, Massachusetts

Rebecka L. Meyers, MD, Associate Clinical Professor of Surgery and Chief of Pediatric Surgery, University of Utah School of Medicine, Pediatric Surgical Director of the Liver Transplant Team, Primary Children's Hospital, Salt Lake City, Utah

Tory Meyers, MD, Pediatric Surgeon, Children's Hospital, Austin, Texas

Wayne M. Meyers, MD, PhD, D.Sc.(HON), Chief, Mycobacteriology, Armed Forces Institute of Pathology, Washington, District Columbia

Linda J. Michaud, MD, Associate Professor of Clinical Physical Medicine and Rehabilitation and Clinical Pediatrics, University of Cincinnati College of Medicine, Director, Pediatric Rehabilitation, Children's Hospital Medical Center, Cincinnati, Ohio

Peter Milla, MD, Professor of Pediatric Gastroenterology and Nutrition, University College, Honorary Consultant, Pediatric Gastroenterology, Institute of Child Health, London, WC 1, England

Kevin M. Miller, MD, Associate Professor of Clinical Ophthalmology, Division of Comprehensive Ophthalmology, Los Angeles, California

Walter L. Miller, MD, Professor of Pediatrics, The Metabolic Research Unit, and The Biomedical Sciences Graduate program, Chief of Pediatric Endocrinology, University of California–San Francisco, San Francisco, California

Marsha Leen-Mitchell, Teratology Educator, Pregnancy Risk Line, University of Utah, Salt Lake City, Utah

Christopher M. Mjaanes, MD, Pediatrics Resident, University of Wisconsin Children's Hospital, Madison, Wisconsin

James H. Moller, MD, Professor and Head of Pediatrics, Paul Dwan Professor of Pediatric Cardiology, University of Minnesota College of Medicine, Minneapolis, Minnesota

Ramon Montes, MD, Staff Gastroenterologist, Phoenix Children's Hospital, Phoenix, Arizona

Phillip Moore, MD, Associate Clinical Professor of Pediatric Cardiology, Director, Congenital Cardiac Catherization Program, University of California at San Francisco, San Francisco, California

Claire Morress, OTR/L, Aaron W. Perlman Center for Children, Children's Hospital Medical Center, Cincinnati, Ohio

Anna-Barbara Moscicki, MD, Professor of Pediatrics, Division of Adolescent Medicine, University of California-San Francisco, San Francisco, California

Mark H. Moss, MD, Assistant Professor of Medicine and Pediatrics, Section of Allergy and Immunology, University of Wisconsin Hospital and Clinics, Madison, Wisconsin

Kevin P. Murphy, MD, Associate Professor, University of Minnesota Deluth Medical School, Medical Director, Gillette Children's Northern Clinics, Deluth, Minnesota

Dennis L. Murray, MD, FAAP, Professor of Pediatrics and Chief, Pediatric Infectious Diseases, Medical College of Georgia, Atlanta, Georgia

Robert D. Murray, MD, Associate Professor of Pediatrics, Ohio State University, Children's Hospital, Columbus, Ohio

Charles M. Myer III, MD, Professor of Otolaryngology, University of Cincinnati College of Medicine, Division of Otolaryngology, Children's Hospital Medical Center, Cincinnati, Ohio

J. Lawrence Naiman, MD, Clinical Professor, Pediatrics, Stanford University School of Medicine, Chief Medical Officer, American Red Cross Blood Services, Palo Alto, California

Ran Namgung, MD, Yonsei University College of Medicine, Seoul, Korea

Ruth Nass, MD, Professor, Pediatrics, New York University Medical Center, New York, New York

Audrey M. Nelson, MD, Associate Professor of Medicine, Head, Pediatric Rheumatology, Mayo Medical School and Mayo Foundation, Rochester, Minnesota

Charles A. Nelson, MD, Professor of Child Psychology, Neuroscience, and Pediatrics, University of Minnesota, Minneapolis, Minnesota

Virginia Simson Nelson, MD, MPH, Clinical Associate Professor, Physical Medicine and Rehabilitation, Lecturer, Pediatrics, University of Michigan Medical School, Chief, Pediatrics and Adolescent Physical Medicine, C.S. Mott Children's Hospital, Ann Arbor, Michigan

Charles A. Nichter, MD, Assistant Professor of Pediatrics, Washington University School of Medicine, Division of Neurology, St. Louis Children's Hospital, St. Louis, Missouri

Donna M. Nobile, MD, Clinical Assistant Professor of Pediatrics, Indiana University, Clinical Assistant Professor/ Attending, Pediatric Infectious Diseases, Riley Hospital for Children/Wishard Memorial Hospital, Indianapolis, Indiana

Douglas R. Nordli, Jr. MD, Associate Professor of Clinical Neurology and Clinical Pediatrics, College of Physicians and Surgeons, Babies and Children's Hospital, New York, New York

Victoria F. Norwood, MD, Associate Professor of Pediatrics, Division of Pediatric Nephrology, University of Virginia School of Medicine, Charlottesville, Virginia

Thomas B. Nutman, MD, Head, Helminth Immunology Section, National Institutes of Health, Head, Clinical Parasitology Unit, National Institutes of Health, Bethesda, Maryland

Richard A. Oberhelman, MD, Associate Professor, Tulane School of Public Health and Tropical Medicine, New Orleans, Louisiana

Paul A. Offit, MD, Associate Professor, Pediatrics, University of Pennsylvania School of Medicine, Chief, Infectious Disease, Children's Hospital of Philadelphia, Philadelphia, Pennsylvania

Edward S. Ogata, MD, Professor of Pediatrics, Northwestern University School of Medicine, Chief Medical Officer, Children's Memorial Hospital, Chicago, Illinois

Bernadette A. O'Hare, MB, BS, Fellow of Infectious Diseases, Hospital for Sick Children, Toronto, Ontario

Kwaku Ohene-Frempong, MD, Professor of Pediatrics, University of Pennsylvania School of Medicine, Director of the Sickle Cell Program, Children's Hospital, Philadelphia, Pennsylvania

Greg Omlor, MD, Associate Professor, Clinical Pediatrics, Director, Division of Pulmonary Medicine, Children's Hospital Medical Center of Akron, Akron, Ohio

Deborah Orel-Bixler, PhD, OD, Associate Clinical Professor/Residency Director, University of California, School of Optometry, Berkeley, California

David M. Orenstein, MD, Professor of Pediatrics, University of Pittsburgh, Director, Antonio and Janet Columbo Cystic Fibrosis Center, Children's Hospital of Pittsburgh, Pittsburgh, Pennsylvania

Seth J. Orlow, MD, PhD, Professor of Dermatology, Cell Biology and Pediatrics, New York University School of Medicine, Director of Pediatric Dermatology, New York University/Tisch, Bellevue & Lenox Hill Hospitals, New York, New York

Eduardo Ortega-Barria, MD, Department of Parasitology, Gorgas Memorial Institute, Panama City, Panama

Joy D. Osofsky, PhD, Professor of Psychiatry, Louisiana State Medical Center, New Orleans, Louisiana

Robert Ouvrier, MD, Department of Neurology and Neurosurgery, Children's Hospital at Westmead, Sydney, Australia

Kim J. Overby, MD, Pediatric Medical Care Coordinator, Child Welfare Program, Elwyn, Inc., Elwyn, Pennsylvania

Gary D. Overturf, MD, Professor, Pediatric Infectious Diseases, University of New Mexico, Professor, Pediatric Infectious Diseases, Children's Hospital of New Mexico, Albuquerque, New Mexico

James F. Padbury, MD, Vice Chair of Pediatrics, Brown University School of Medicine, Chief of Neonatology, Women & Infants Hospital of Rhode Island, Providence, Rhode Island

Amy S. Paller, MD, Professor of Pediatrics and Dermatology, Northwestern University, Head, Division of Dermatology, Children's Memorial Hospital, Chicago, Illinois

J.T. Parer, MD, Professor of Obstetrics and Gynecology, University of California–San Francisco, San Francisco, California

Murray H. Passo, MD, Professor of Clinical Pediatrics, University of Cincinnati College of Medicine, Clinical Director, Pediatric Rheumatology, Children's Hospital Medical Center, Cincinnati, Ohio

Bonnie J. Patterson, MD, Associate Professor of Pediatrics, Developmental Pediatrician, Director of Down Syndrome Clinic, Cincinnati Center for Developmental Disorders, Cincinnati, Ohio

Maria Jevitz Patterson, MD, PhD, Professor, Infectious Disease, Michigan State University, East Lansing, Michigan

Andrew T. Pavia, MD, Associate Professor, Infectious Diseases and Geographic Medicine, University of Utah, Director for Clinical Research, University of Utah AIDS Center, Salt Lake City, Utah

Howard A. Pearson, MD, Professor of Pediatrics, Yale University School of Medicine, New Haven, Connecticut

Timothy A. Pedley, MD, Chair, Neurology, Columbia University, New York, New York

Audrey S. Penn, MD, Deputy Director, National Institute for Neurologic Disorders and Stroke, Bethesda, Maryland

Julio Pérez-Fontán, MD, Professor of Pediatrics and Anesthesiology, Director of Pediatric Intensive Care Unit Washington University School of Medicine, St. Louis, Missouri

Elizabeth Perkett, MD, Director, Pediatric Pulmonary Centers, University of New Mexico Health Sciences Center, Albuquerque, New Mexico

Ellen C. Perrin, MD, Associate Professor of Pediatrics and Child Study, Yale University School of Medicine, New Haven, Connecticut

Heidi L. Peters, MBBS, FRACP, Clinical Geneticist, Murdoch Children's Research Institute, Parkville, Australia

William A. Petri, Jr., MD, PhD, Professor of Medicine, Microbiology & Pathology, University of Virginia Health Sciences Center, Charlottesville, Virginia

Roderic H. Phibbs, MD, Professor Emeritus of Pediatrics, University of California–San Francisco, San Francisco, California

Anthony F. Philipps, MD, Professor and Department Chair, Pediatrics, University of California-Davis Medical Center, University of California-Davis Children's Hospital, Sacramento, California

Larry K. Pickering, MD, Professor of Pediatrics, Eastern Virginia Medical School, CHKD Chair in Pediatric Research, Director, Center for Pediatric Research, Children's Hospital of the King's Daughters, Norfolk, Virginia

David Pleasure, MD, Professor of Neurology and Pediatrics, University of Pennsylvania School of Medicine, Director, Division of Neurology, Children's Hospital of Philadelphia, Philadelphia, Pennsylvania

David G. Poplack, MD, Elsie C. Young Chair of Pediatric Oncology, Head, Hematology/Oncology, Baylor College of Medicine, Director, Texas Children's Cancer Center, Texas Children's Hospital, Houston, Texas

Donald E. Potter, MD, Clinical Professor of Pediatric Nephrology, University of California–San Francisco, San Francisco, California

Dwight A. Powell, MD, Professor of Pediatrics, Ohio State University, Chief, Infectious Diseases, Children's Hospital, Columbus, Ohio

Julie Prendiville, MD, Clinical Associate Professor in Pediatrics, University of British Columbia, Head, Pediatric Dermatology, British Columbia Children's Hospital, Vancouver, British Columbia, Canada

Charles G. Prober, MD, Professor of Pediatrics, Medicine, Microbiology and Immunology, Associate Chairman, Department of Pediatrics, Stanford University, Professor of Pediatrics, Medicine, Microbiology and Immunology, Lucile Salter Packard Children's Hospital, Palo Alto, California

Janice Prontnicki, MD, Division of Child Neurology, Robert Wood Johnson Medical School, New Brunswick, New Jersey

Neil S. Prose, MD, Associate Professor, Dermatology, Pediatrics and Medicine, Duke University Medical Center, Durham, North Carolina

Linda Quan, MD, Professor, University of Washington School of Medicine, Chief, Emergency Services, Children's Hospital and Regional Medical Center, Seattle, Washington

Graham E. Quinn, MD, Professor of Ophthalmology and Pediatrics, University of Pennsylvania School of Medicine, Division of Ophthalmology, Children's Hospital of Philadelphia, Philadelphia, Pennsylvania

Isabelle Rapin, MD, Professor, Neurology and Pediatrics, Albert Einstein College of Medicine, Albert Einstein College of Medicine, Bronx, New York

Mobeen H. Rathore, MD, Professor and Assistant Chair of Pediatrics, University of Florida College of Medicine, Jacksonville, Florida

Gerald V. Raymond, MD, Neurologist, Kennedy Krieger Institute, Baltimore, Maryland

Edward O. Reiter, MD, Professor, Pediatrics, Tufts University School of Medicine, Chairman, Pediatrics, Baystate Medical Center Children's Hospital, Longmeadow, Massachusetts

Judith C. Rhodes, PhD, Associate Professor, University of Cincinnati Hospital, Scientific Director, Microbiology, Health Alliance of Greater Cincinnati, Cincinnati, Ohio

Lisa G. Rider, MD, Center for Blood and Biologics Research, FDA, Bethesda, Maryland

Stephanie R. Ried, MD, MA, Medical Director for Rehabilitation, Driscoll Children's Hospital, Corpus Christi, Texas

J. Erin Riehle, RN, MSN, Co-Director Project SEARCH, Children's Hospital Medical Center, Cincinnati, Ohio

Piero Rinaldo, MD, PhD, Professor, Laboratory Medicine, Director, Biochemical Genetics Laboratory, Department of Laboratory Medicine and Pathology, Mayo Clinic and Foundation, Rochester, Minnesota

Eve Roberts, MD, Professor of Pediatrics, Medicine and Pharmacology, Division of Clinical Nutrition and Gastroenterology, Senior Scientist Hospital for Sick Children Research Institute, Toronto, Ontario, Canada

Julia Robertson, MD, Pregnancy RiskLine, Utah Department of Health, Salt Lake City, Utah

Nathaniel H. Robin, MD, Director, Medical Genetics Residency Program, Case Western Reserve University School of Medicine, Director, Prenatal Genetics Service, Rainbow Babies and Children's Hospital, Cleveland, Ohio

Nathaniel Robinson, MD, Center for Human Genetics, Case Western Reserve University, Cleveland, Ohio

Thomas N. Robinson, MD, Assistant Professor, Center for Research in Disease Prevention, Stanford University School of Medicine, Palo Alto, California

Allen W. Root, MD, Professor of Pediatrics, Biochemistry and Molecular Biology, University of South Florida, St. Petersburg, Florida

Harley A. Rotbart, MD, Associate Professor of Pediatrics, University of Colorado Health Sciences Center, Division of Pediatric Infectious Diseases, Children's Hospital, Denver, Colorado

Lorry G. Rubin, MD, Professor of Pediatrics, Albert Einstein College of Medicine, Chief, Pediatric Infectious Diseases, Schneider Children's Hospital of North Shore, New Hyde Park, New York

Abraham M. Rudolph, MD, Professor Emeritus of Pediatrics, School of Medicine, University of California–San Francisco, San Francisco, California

Colin D. Rudolph, MD, PhD, Professor of Pediatrics, Medical College of Wisconsin, Chief, Pediatric Gastroenterology, Children's Hospital, Milwaukee, Wisconsin

Guillermo Ruiz-Palacios, MD, Professor and Head, Department of Infectious Diseases, National Institute of Medical Science and Nutrition, Mexico City, Mexico

Susan Rutkowski, MEd, Director, Special Education, Great Oaks Institute of Technology and Career Development, Cincinnati, Ohio

Michael J. Rutter, MD, Associate Professor of Pediatric Otolaryngology, Head and Neck Surgery, University of Cincinnati College of Medicine, Cincinnati, Ohio

Stephen G. Ryan, MD, Assistant Professor, Neurology and Pediatrics, University of Pennsylvania, Children's Hospital of Philadelphia, Philadelphia, Pennsylvania

Frederick C. Ryckman, MD, Professor of Surgery, University of Cincinnati College of Medicine, Children's Hospital Medical Center, Cincinnati, Ohio

Isidor B. Salusky, MD, Professor of Pediatrics, UCLA School of Medicine, Los Angeles, California

Scott Santibanez, MD, MPHTM, Fellow, Infectious Diseases, Tulane University School of Medicine, New Orleans, Louisiana

David Sarraf, MD, Assistant Professor of Ophthalmology, Jules Stein Eye Institute, Los Angeles, California

Mark R. Schleiss, MD, Research Assistant Professor of Pediatrics, University of Cincinnati College of Medicine, Division of Infectious Diseases, Children's Hospital Medical Center, Cincinnati, Ohio

David J. Schonfeld, MD, Associate Professor of Pediatrics and Child Study, Yale University School of Medicine, New Haven, Connecticut

Mary K. Schroth, MD, Associate Professor, Department of Pediatrics, Division of Pulmonology, University of Wisconsin School of Medicine, Madison, Wisconsin

Gordon E. Schutze, MD, Associate Professor of Pediatrics, Pediatric Program Director, University of Arkansas for Medical Sciences, Arkansas Children's Hospital, Little Rock, Arkansas

Alan L. Schwartz, PhD, MD, Chair, Department of Pediatrics, Washington University School of Medicine, Pediatrician-in-Chief, St. Louis Children's Hospital, St. Louis, Missouri

Deborah Schwengel, MD, Department of Anesthesia and Critical Care Medicine, Johns Hopkins Hospital, Baltimore, Maryland

Alan R. Seay, MD, Professor of Pediatric Neurology, Children's Hospital of Denver, Denver, Colorado

Gunnar Sedin, MD, University Children's Hospital, Uppsala, Sweden

Ernest Seidman, MD, FRCP, Professor of Pediatrics, University of Montreal, Chief, Gastroenterology and Nutrition, Ste Justine Hospital, Montreal, Quebec, Canada

Mary-Ann Shafer, MD, Professor in Residence of Pediatrics, University of California-San Francisco, San Francisco, California

Thomas H. Shaffer, PhD, Professor of Physiology and Pediatrics, Temple University, Philadelphia, Pennsylvania

Kevin M. Shannon, MD, Professor of Pediatrics, University of California-San Francisco, San Francisco, California

Michael P. Sherman, MD, Professor of Pediatrics, Chief, Division of Neonatology, University of California-Davis, Sacramento, California

David D. Sherry, MD, Associate Professor of Pediatrics, University of Washington, Associate Professor of Pediatrics and Director of Rheumatology, Children's Hospital and Regional Medical Center, Seattle, Washington

Benjamin Shneider, MD, Associate Professor of Pediatrics, Mount Sinai School of Medicine, Associate Professor, Mount Sinai Medical Center, New York, New York

John M. Shoffner, MD, Director, Molecular Medicine Laboratory, Children's Healthcare of Atlanta, Atlanta, Georgia

Jack P. Shonkoff, MD, Florence Heller Graduate School for Advanced Studies in Social Welfare, Brandeis University, Waltham, Massachusetts

Billie Lou Short, MD, Professor of Pediatrics and Chair, Neonatology, Children's National Medical Center, Washington, District of Columbia

Sally R. Shott, MD, Associate Professor, Otolaryngology-Head and Neck Surgery, University of Cincinnati Hospital, Children's Hospital Medical Center, Cincinnati, Ohio

Stanford T. Shulman, MD, Professor of Pediatrics, Northwestern University Medical School, Head, Division of Infectious Diseases, Children's Memorial Hospital, Chicago, Illinois

Robert Sidbury, MD, Fellow, Pediatric Dermatology, Northwestern University Children's Memorial Hospital, Chicago, Illinois

Norman J. Siegel, MD, Professor of Pediatrics and Medicine, Director, Division of Pediatric Nephrology, Yale University School of Medicine, New Haven, Connecticut

Elaine C. Siegfried, MD, Associate Professor, St Louis University, Associate Professor, Cardinal Glennon Children's Hospital, St. Louis, Missouri

Earl D. Silverman, MD, Professor of Pediatrics and Immunology, Senior Scientist, University of Toronto, Hospital for Sick Children, Toronto, Ontario, Canada

Norman H. Silverman, MD, DSDc(Med), Professor of Pediatrics and Radiology, University of California-San Francisco, Former Director, Pediatric Echocardiography Laboratory, San Francisco, California

William A. Silverman, MD, Professor of Pediatrics (Retired), Columbia University, Greenbrae, California

Jean M. Silvestri, MD, Associate Professor of Pediatrics, Rush University, Director, Center for SIDS Research and Disorders of Respiratory Control in Infancy and Childhood, Rush Children's Hospital, Chicago, Illinois

William B. Slayton, MD, Associate Professor, Department of Pediatrics, University of Florida College of Medicine, Gainesville, Florida

Arnold L. Smith, MD, Professor and Chair, Molecular Microbiology and Immunology, University of Missouri-Columbia School of Medicine, Columbia, Missouri

Susan Sniderman, MD, Professor of Clinical Pediatrics, University of California-San Francisco, San Francisco, California

Augusto Sola, MD, Professor of Pediatrics, Director, Division of Neonatology and Perinatal Medicine, Emory University School of Medicine, Atlanta, Georgia

Judith Sondheimer, MD, Professor of Pediatrics, University of Colorado Health Science Center, Chief of Gastroenterology and Hepatology, The Children's Hospital, Denver, Colorado

Rachel Sparks, Yale Child Health Research Center, Yale University School of Medicine, New Haven, Connecticut

Lewis W. Sprunger, MD, Northwest Permanente, Clackamas, Oregon

Robert Squires, Jr., MD, Associate Professor, Pediatrics, University of Texas Southwestern Medical Center, Children's Medical Center, Dallas, Texas

Mary Allen Staat, MD, MPH, Assistant Professor of Pediatrics, University of Cincinnati College of Medicine, Director, International Adoption Center, Children's Hospital Medical Center, Cincinnati, Ohio

Sergio Stagno, MD, Katharine Reynolds Ireland Professor and Chair, Department of Pediatrics, University of Alabama, Birmingham, Alabama

Paul Stanger, MD, Professor of Pediatrics, University of California, San Francisco, San Francisco, California

Jeffrey R. Starke, MD, Professor of Pediatrics, Baylor College of Medicine, Infection Control Director, Division of Infectious Diseases, Texas Children's Hospital, Houston, Texas

Russell Steele, MD, Professor and Vice Chairman of Pediatrics, Lousiana State University School of Medicine, Director, Pediatric Infectious Diseases, Children's Hospital, New Orleans, Louisiana

Martin T. Stein, MD, Professor of Pediatrics, University of California-San Diego, San Diego, California

Ruth E.K. Stein, MD, Professor and Vice Chairman, Office of Academic Affairs, Albert Einstein College of Medicine, Montefiore Medical Center, Bronx, New York

Kurt R. Stenmark, MD, Professor of Pediatrics, University of Colorado Health Sciences Center, Division of Critical Care, Children's Hospital, Denver, Colorado

C. Philip Steuber, MD, Professor of Pediatrics, Baylor College of Medicine, Houston, Texas

David K. Stevenson, MD, Professor of Pediatrics, Stanford University School of Medicine, Chief of Neonatology, Lucile Packard Children's Hospital, Palo Alto, California

Richard Stevenson, MD, Associate Professor, Pediatric Surgery, University of Cincinnati, Pediatric Surgeon, Children's Hospital Medical Center, Cincinnati, Ohio

Wendy Zolter Stiles, MD, Boston University Medical Center, Boston, Massachusetts

Janet A. Stockheim, MD, MPH, Instructor, Department of Pediatrics, Northwestern University Medical School Children's Memorial Hospital, Chicago, Illinois

Robert C. Strunk, MD, Professor of Pediatrics, Washington University School of Medicine, St. Louis, Missouri

Dennis M. Styne, MD, Professor of Pediatrics, University of California-Davis, Sacramento, California

Frederick Suchy, MD, Professor and Chair, Pediatrics, Mount Sinai School of Medicine, New York, New York

Agneta L. Sunehag, MD, PhD, Instructor, Pediatrics, Baylor College of Medicine, Houston, Texas

Roland W. Sutter, MD, Chief, Technical Services Branch, Centers for Disease Control and Prevention, Atlanta, Georgia

Theresa A. Tacy, MD, Assistant Professor of Pediatrics, Division of Pediatric Cardiology, University of California-San Francisco, San Francisco, California

Lawrence Taft, MD, Professor of Pediatrics, Neurodevelopmental Assessment Program, Robert Wood Johnson Medical School, New Brunswick, New Jersey

Norman S. Talner, MD, Clinical Professor of Pediatrics, Duke University, Durham, North Carolina

J. Lane Tanner, MD, Associate Clinical Professor of Behavioral and Developmental Pediatrics, University of California, School of Medicine, San Francisco, Lucile Packard Children's Health Services, San Francisco, California

David F. Teitel, MD, Professor of Pediatrics, University of California-San Francisco, San Francisco, California

Jonathan E. Teitelbaum, MD, Assistant Professor, Monmouth Medical Center, Long Branch, New Jersey

Milton Tenenbein, MD, Professor of Pediatrics and Pharmacology and Medicine, University of Manitoba, Director, Emergency Services, Children's Hospital, Winnipeg, Manitoba, Canada

Andreas A. Theodorou, MD, Associate Professor of Clinical Pediatrics, University of Arizona, Tucson, Arizona

Michael Thomasgard, MD, Associate Professor of Pediatrics, Ohio State University, Children's Hospital, Columbus, Ohio

Susan D. Thompson, PhD, Research Assistant Professor, Division of Rheumatology, Cincinnati, Ohio

Olafur Thorarensen, MD, Associate Professor, Neurology and Pediatrics, University of Pennsylvania, Children's Hospital of Philadelphia, Philadelphia, Pennsylvania

John T. Tong, MD, Clinical Assistant Professor, Division of Orbital and Ophthalmic Plastic Surgery, Sacramento, California

Eveline Traeger, MD, Child Specialized Hospital, Mountainside, New Jersey

Werner Trojaborg, MD, Hellerup, Copenhagen, Denmark

William E. Truog, MD, Sosland Family Professor of Pediatrics, Children's Mercy Hospital and Clinics, Kansas City, Missouri

Reginald C. Tsang, MD, Professor Emeritus of Pediatrics, University of Cincinnati School of Medicine, Cincinnati, Ohio

Mendel Tuchman, MD, Children's Research Institute, Children's National Medical Center, Washington, District of Columbia

Lori B. Tucker, MD, Clinical Associate Professor of Pediatrics, University of British Columbia, Pediatric Rheumatologist, British Columbia Children's Hospital, Vancouver, British Columbia

Jay Tureen, MD, Clinical Professor of Pediatrics and Infectious Disease, University of California-San Francisco, San Francisco, California

Jerrold A. Turner, MD, DTM&H, Professor of Clinical Medicine, UCLA, Los Angeles, Chief, Section of Parasitic Diseases, Harbor-UCLA Medical Center, Torrance, California

David Valle, MD, FACMG, Professor of Pediatrics, Molecular Biology and Genetics, Howard Hughes Medical Institute, Baltimore, Maryland

George F. Van Hare, Associate Professor of Pediatrics, Stanford University College of Medicine, Lucile Packard Children's Hospital, Palo Alto, California

Jilda Vargus-Adams, MD, Research Fellow, Pediatric Rehabilitation, Instructor of Clinical Physical Medicine and Rehabilitation and Clinical Pediatrics, Children's Hospital Medical Center, Cincinnati, Ohio

David H. Viskochil, MD, PhD, Associate Professor of Pediatrics, University of Utah School of Medicine, Salt Lake City, Utah

Fred R. Volkmar, MD, Professor of Child Psychiatry, Pediatrics and Psychology, Yale University, New Haven, Connecticut

Shari L. Wade, PhD, Adjunct Associate Professor of Pediatrics, Staff Psychologist, Cincinnati Children's Hospital Medical Center, Cincinnati, Ohio

Eric J. Wall, MD, Assistant Clinical Professor of Orthopedic Surgery, University of Cincinnati College of Medicine, Cincinnati, Ohio

Carol A. Wallace, MD, Associate Professor of Pediatrics, University of Washington, Children's Hospital and Regional Medical Center, Seattle, Washington

Danielle S. Walsh, MD, Massachusetts General Hospital, Boston, Massachusetts

Elaine E.L. Wang, MD, Associate Professor, Pediatrics, University of Toronto, Clinical Director, Research and Development, Pasteur Merieux Connaught, Toronto, Ontario, Canada

Robert M. Ward, MD, Professor of Pediatrics, University of Utah School of Medicine, Salt Lake City, Utah

Sally L. Davidson Ward, MD, Department of Pulmonology, Children's Hospital of Los Angeles, Los Angeles, California

Brad Warner, MD, Associate Professor, Pediatric Surgery, University of Cincinnati, Attending Surgeon, Children's Hospital Medical Center, Cincinnati, Ohio

Sandra L. Watkins, MD, Professor of Pediatrics, Medical Director of Dialysis, Children's Hospital and Regional Medical Center, University of Washington, Seattle, Washington

Debra E. Weese-Mayer, MD, Professor of Pediatrics, Rush University, Chief, Pediatric Respiratory Medicine, Rush Children's Hospital, Chicago, Illinois

Ann E. Weidenbenner, MS, RD, LD, Nutrition Consultant, Ohio Department of Health, Columbus, Ohio

Howard J. Weinstein, MD, Professor of Pediatrics, Harvard Medical School, Chief, Pediatric Hematology and Oncology, Massachusetts General Hospital, Boston, Massachusetts

Peggy Sue Weintrub, MD, Clinical Professor, Chief, Pediatric Infectious Diseases, University of California-San Francisco, San Francisco, California

Sheila Weitzman, MB, ChB, FCP(SA), FRCP(C), Associate Professor, University of Toronto, Senior Oncologist, Associate Director-Clinical, Hematology/Oncology, Hospital for Sick Children, Toronto, Ontario, Canada

Richard J. Whitley, MD, Loeb Eminent Scholar Chair in Pediatrics, Professor of Pediatrics, Microbiology, and Medicine, University of Alabama School of Medicine, Birmingham, Alabama

Andrew R. Wilkinson, MD, Chairman of Pediatrics, John Radcliffe Hospital, Oxford, England

J. Paul Willging, MD, Associate Professor, Otolaryngology-Head and Neck Surgery, University of Cincinnati College of Medicine, Children's Hospital Medical Center, Cincinnati, Ohio

Calvin B. Williams, MD, PhD, Associate Professor of Pediatrics, Medical College of Wisconsin, Chief, Division of Pediatric Rheumatology, Milwaukee Childrens Hospital, Milwaukee, Wisconsin

David B. Wilson, MD, PhD, Associate Professor of Pediatrics, Molecular Biology and Pharmacology, Director, Hematology-Oncology, Washington University School of Medicine, St. Louis, Missouri

Harland Winter, MD, Professor of Pediatrics, Massachusetts General Hospital, Boston, Massachusetts

Sarah L. Winter, MD, Assistant Professor, University of Cincinnati College of Medicine, Developmental Pediatrics, Children's Hospital Medical Center, Cincinnati, Ohio

Marla R. Wolfson, PhD, Associate Professor of Physiology and Pediatrics, Temple University School of Medicine, Philadelphia, Pennsylvania

Jan B. Wollack, MD, PhD, Associate Professor of Pediatrics and Neurology, Robert Wood Johnson Medical School, University of Medicine and Dentistry of New Jersey, New Brunswick, New Jersey

J. Edmond Wraith, MD, Director, Wilink Biochemical Genatics Unit, Royal Manchester Children's Hospital, Manchester, England

Robert Wyllie, MD, Chair, Pediatric Gastroenterology & Nutrition, Cleveland Clinic Foundation, Cleveland, Ohio

Yvette Yachmirk, MD, PhD, Assistant Professor of Pediatrics, University of Massachusetts Medical School, Director, Infant Toddler & Preschool Clinics, University of Massachusetts Memorial Medical Center, Worcester, Massachusetts

Donald P. Younkin, MD, Associate Professor, Neurology and Pediatrics, University of Pennsylvania, Children's Hospital of Philadelphia, Philadelphia, Pennsylvania

Barry S. Zuckerman, MD, Professor and Chairman, Pediatrics, Boston University School of Medicine, Chief, Pediatrics, Boston Medical Center, Boston, Massachusetts

RUDOLPH'S PEDIATRICS

PEDIATRIC HEALTH SUPERVISION

Kim J. Overby, Associate Editor

The goal of primary-care pediatrics is to facilitate optimal health and well-being for children and their families. This is accomplished through a variety of interrelated activities, including problem surveillance and management, problem prevention, health promotion, and the coordination of care for special-needs children. The traditional focus on problem diagnosis and management has been broadened to include screening for disease and its precursors in asymptomatic populations. Pediatric providers have long recognized the value of preventive programs such as mass immunization and continue to lead the way in this area through an emphasis on regular health surveillance, anticipatory guidance, and involvement in community-based prevention strategies. Recent emphasis has also been placed on the related concept of health promotion, whereby optimal health and well-being can be positively encouraged. A by-product of the successes of modern medicine has been the creation of an increasing population of children with chronic illness, disability, and other special needs. The primary-care provider is in a unique position to coordinate the often complex care of these children and to facilitate communication among the various individuals involved. These areas form the foundation for current recommendations regarding routine child health surveillance (Tables 1-1 and 1-2). These guidelines are based largely on common sense and a consensus of experts. Much additional research is needed to help providers determine the optimal schedule for and content of the well-child visit.

Caring for children provides many unique rewards and challenges. The interplay between environmental influences and factors intrinsic to the child becomes evident in many aspects of pediatric health and development. Continuity care is based on a developmental framework that recognizes the constancy of growth and change throughout childhood. At each visit, the developmental level of the child dictates both the approach to the patient and much of the visit's content. Flexibility in performing the physical examination is essential. A focus on examining the least-threatening areas first and utilizing age-appropriate methods to minimize the child's anxiety is important. In pediatrics, the therapeutic alliance must necessarily include both the child and the family; the importance of establishing a trusting longitudinal relationship cannot be overemphasized.

This chapter is divided into five main sections (Physical Growth, Motor and Psychological Development, Screening, Counseling and Anticipatory Guidance, and Immunizations) and is intended to provide a functional overview of the major components of pediatric health supervision as well as common issues and problems frequently encountered in each of these areas. Recommendations regarding adolescent preventive services are discussed in greater detail in Chapter 3.

1.1 PHYSICAL GROWTH

1.1.1 Overview

Monitoring physical growth is fundamental to pediatric health supervision. Knowledge of both normal patterns and common individual variations gives the pediatrician a framework from which to provide reassurance and guidance to parents as well as to identify potential problems.

Changes in physical size and appearance are a visible manifestation of the complex morphologic, biochemical, and physiological changes taking place during childhood. Although such change is a continuous process, the rate of a child's growth is not constant and normally varies with both age and organ system (Fig. 1-1). Postnatally, two periods of rapid growth are observed: during infancy and at puberty. A decreased but steady rate of growth characterizes the intervening period. The growth of most body tissues and organs parallels this pattern, with several notable exceptions. Brain growth remains rapid throughout the first 6 years of life, with minimal change in head size after age 10. Lymphoid tissue volume increases rapidly before puberty and then declines steadily until adult levels are achieved. Growth of the reproductive organs remains slow until puberty.

Both normal and pathologic growth patterns are determined by a complex interaction among genetic, environmental, and hormonal factors. Parental size and patterns of growth are strongly predictive of both absolute size and the timing of growth spurts in their offspring. After the age of 3 years, a child's height correlates significantly with parental stature. Parental heights can be used to determine the consistency of a child's height at a given time with his or her genetic potential as well as to predict ultimate adult stature (Table 1-3). A variety of environmental factors are also known to affect growth. Seasonal variation has been noted, with maximal growth rates occurring in the spring and summer. The population trend toward greater physical size observed during the late 19th to mid-20th century is felt to be largely a result of improvements in nutritional, socioeconomic, and overall health conditions that occurred during the same time period. The importance of such factors is underscored by our current understanding and approach to pediatric growth problems such as failure to thrive (Sec. 1.1.2). The impact of genetic and environmental factors on growth ultimately is modulated by a complex system of hormonal regulation. Endocrine control of growth is discussed in Sec. 24.2.

Pediatric health-care providers routinely monitor weight, length, head circumference, dental development, and the appearance of secondary sexual characteristics to assess the overall adequacy of a child's growth. Consistent measurement technique is

TABLE 1-1

RECOMMENDATIONS FOR PREVENTIVE PEDIATRIC HEALTH CARE (RE9535): Committee on Practice and Ambulatory Medicine

Each child and family is unique; therefore, these Recommendations for Preventive Pediatric Health Care are designed for the care of children who are receiving competent parenting, have no manifestations of any important health problems, and are growing and developing in satisfactory fashion. Additional visits may become necessary if circumstances suggest variations from normal.

These guidelines represent a consensus by the Committee on Practice and Ambulatory Medicine in consultation with national committees and sections of the American Academy of Pediatrics. The Committee emphasizes the great importance of continuity of care in comprehensive health supervision and the need to avoid fragmentation of care.

		INFANCY[4]								EARLY CHILDHOOD[4]					MIDDLE CHILDHOOD[4]				ADOLESCENCE[4]										
AGE[5]	PRE-NATAL[1]	NEW-BORN[2]	2–4d[3]	By 1mo	2mo	4mo	6mo	9mo	12mo	15mo	18mo	24mo	3y	4y	5y	6y	8y	10y	11y	12y	13y	14y	15y	16y	17y	18y	19y	20y	21y
HISTORY Initial/Interval	•	•	•	•	•	•	•	•	•	•	•	•	•	•	•	•	•	•	•	•	•	•	•	•	•	•	•	•	•
MEASUREMENTS Height and Weight		•	•	•	•	•	•	•	•	•	•	•	•	•	•	•	•	•	•	•	•	•	•	•	•	•	•	•	•
Head Circumference		•	•	•	•	•	•	•	•	•	•	•																	
Blood Pressure													•	•	•	•	•	•	•	•	•	•	•	•	•	•	•	•	•
SENSORY SCREENING Vision		S	S	S	S	S	S	S	S	S	S	S	O[6]	O	O	O	O	O	S	O	S	S	O	S	S	O	S	S	S
Hearing		O[7]	S	S	S	S	S	S	S	S	S	S	S	O	O	O	O	O	S	O	S	S	O	S	S	O	S	S	S
DEVELOPMENTAL/ BEHAVIORAL ASSESSMENT[8]		•	•	•	•	•	•	•	•	•	•	•	•	•	•	•	•	•	•	•	•	•	•	•	•	•	•	•	•
PHYSICAL EXAMINATION[9]		•	•	•	•	•	•	•	•	•	•	•	•	•	•	•	•	•	•	•	•	•	•	•	•	•	•	•	•
PROCEDURES-GENERAL[10] Hereditary/Metabolic Screening[11]			←———•———→																										
Immunization[12]		•	•	•	•	•	•		•	•	•			•					•	•	•	•	•	•					•
Hematocrit or Hemoglobin[13]								•———→		★			•———→						←———•[14]———————————————————————————→										
Urinalysis															•				←———•[15]———————————————————————————→										
PROCEDURES-PATIENTS AT RISK Lead Screening[16]								★———→				★																	
Tuberculin Test[17]										★	★	★	★	★	★	★	★	★	★	★	★	★	★	★	★	★	★	★	★
Cholesterol Screening[18]												★	★	★	★	★	★	★	★	★	★	★	★	★	★	★	★	★	★
STD Screening[19]																			★	★	★	★	★	★	★	★	★	★	★
Pelvic Exam[20]																			★	★	★	★	★	★	★	★ ←——[20]——→ ★			★
ANTICIPATORY GUIDANCE[21]	•	•	•	•	•	•	•	•	•	•	•	•	•	•	•	•	•	•	•	•	•	•	•	•	•	•	•	•	•
Injury Prevention[22]	•	•	•	•	•	•	•	•	•	•	•	•	•	•	•	•	•	•	•	•	•	•	•	•	•	•	•	•	•
Violence Prevention[23]	•	•	•	•	•	•	•	•	•	•	•	•	•	•	•	•	•	•	•	•	•	•	•	•	•	•	•	•	•
Sleep Positioning Counseling[24]	•	•	•	•	•	•	•																						
Nutrition Counseling[25]	•	•	•	•	•	•	•	•	•	•	•	•	•	•	•	•	•	•	•	•	•	•	•	•	•	•	•	•	•
DENTAL REFERRAL[26]												←———————————•																	

(continued)

2

TABLE 1-1   Continued

1. A prenatal visit is recommended for parents who are at high risk, for first-time parents, and for those who request a conference. The prenatal visit should include anticipatory guidance, pertinent medical history, and a discussion of benefits of breastfeeding and planned method of feeding per AAP statement "The Prenatal Visit" (1996).

2. Every infant should have a newborn evaluation after birth. Breastfeeding should be encouraged and instruction and support offered. Every breastfeeding infant should have an evaluation 48–72 hours after discharge from the hospital to include weight, formal breastfeeding evaluation, encouragement, and instruction as recommended in the AAP statement "Breastfeeding and the Use of Human Milk" (1997).

3. For newborns discharged in less than 48 hours after delivery per AAP statement "Hospital Stay for Healthy Term Newborns" (1995).

4. Developmental, psychosocial, and chronic disease issues for children and adolescents may require frequent counseling and treatment visits separate from preventive care visits.

5. If a child comes under care for the first time at any point on the schedule, or if any items are not accomplished at the suggested age, the schedule should be brought up to date at the earliest possible time.

6. If the patient is uncooperative, rescreen within 6 months.

7. All newborns should be screened per the AAP Task Force on Newborn and Infant Hearing statement, "Newborn and Infant Hearing Loss: Detection and Intervention" (1999).

8. By history and appropriate physical examination: If suspicious, by specific objective developmental testing. Parenting skills should be fostered at every visit.

9. At each visit, a complete physical examination is essential, with infant totally unclothed, older child undressed and suitably draped.

10. These may be modified, depending upon entry point into schedule and individual need.

11. Metabolic screening (eg, thyroid, hemoglobinopathies, PKU, galactosemia) should be done according to state law.

12. Schedule(s) per the Committee on Infectious Diseases, published annually in the January edition of *Pediatrics*. Every visit should be an opportunity to update and complete a child's immunizations.

13. See AAP *Pediatric Nutrition Handbook* (1998) for a discussion of universal and selective screening options. Consider earlier screening for high-risk infants (eg, premature infants and low birth weight infants). See also Recommendations to Prevent and Control Iron Deficiency in the United States. *MMWR* 1998;47 (RR-3):1–29.

14. All menstruating adolescents should be screened annually.

15. Conduct dipstick urinalysis for leukocytes annually for sexually active male and female adolescents.

16. For children at risk of lead exposure consult the AAP statement "Screening for Elevated Blood Levels" (1998). Additionally, screening should be done in accordance with state law where applicable.

17. TB testing per recommendations of the Committee on Infectious Diseases, published in the current edition of *Red Book: Report of the Committee on Infectious Diseases*. Testing should be done upon recognition of high-risk factors.

18. Cholesterol screening for high-risk patients per AAP statement "Cholesterol in Childhood" (1998). If family history cannot be ascertained and other risk factors are present, screening should be at the discretion of the physician.

19. All sexually active patients should be screened for sexually transmitted diseases (STDs).

20. All sexually active females should have a pelvic examination. A pelvic examination and routine pap smear should be offered as part of preventive health maintenance between the ages of 18 and 21 years.

21. Age-appropriate discussion and counseling should be an integral part of each visit for care per the AAP *Guidelines for Health Supervision III* (1998).

22. From birth to age 12, refer to the AAP injury prevention program (TIPP) as described in *A Guide to Safety Counseling in Office Practice* (1994).

23. Violence prevention and management for all patients per AAP Statement "The Role of the Pediatrician in Youth Violence Prevention in Clinical Practice and at the Community Level" (1999).

24. Parents and caregivers should be advised to place healthy infants on their backs when putting them to sleep. Side positioning is a reasonable alternative but carries a slightly higher risk of SIDS. Consult the AAP statement "Changing Concepts of Sudden Infant Death Syndrome: Implications for Infant Sleeping Environment and Sleep Position" (2000).

25. Age-appropriate nutrition counseling should be an integral part of each visit per the AAP *Handbook of Nutrition* (1998).

26. Earlier initial dental examinations may be appropriate for some children. Subsequent examination as prescribed by dentist.

Key: ● = to be performed   ★ = to be performed for patients at risk
   S = subjective, by history   O = objective, by a standard testing method
   ◀—●—▶ = the range during which a service may be provided, with the dot indicating the preferred age.

NB: Special chemical, immunologic, and endocrine testing is usually carried out upon specific indications. Testing other than newborn (eg, inborn errors of metabolism, sickle disease, etc) is discretionary with the physician.

The recommendations in this statement do not indicate an exclusive course of treatment or standard of medical care. Variations, taking into account individual circumstances, may be appropriate. Copyright ©2000 by the American Academy of Pediatrics. No part of this statement may be reproduced in any form or by any means without prior written permission from the American Academy of Pediatrics except for one copy for personal use.

SOURCE: From: *American Academy at Pediatrics, Committee on Practice and Ambulatory Medicine. (RE9535) March 2000.*

TABLE 1-2

RECOMMENDED FREQUENCY OF GAPS PREVENTIVE SERVICES

STAGE OF ADOLESCENCE	EARLY (11-14 Y)	MIDDLE (15-17 Y)	LATE (18-21 Y)	STAGE OF ADOLESCENCE	EARLY (11-14 y)	MIDDLE (15-17 y)	LATE (18-21 y)
Health guidance				**Screening**			
Parenting	●	●	❯	Hypertension[a]	■	■	■
Adolescent development	■	■	■	Hyperlipidemia[b]	HR-1		●
Safety practices	■	■	■	Eating disorders	■	■	■
Diet and fitness	■	■	■	Obesity	■	■	■
Healthy lifestyles (sexual behavior, smoking, alcohol and drug use)	■	■	■	Tobacco use	■	■	■
				Alcohol and drug use	■	■	■
				Sexual behavior	■	■	■
Immunizations[c]				Sexually transmissible diseases (STDs)			
Measles, mumps, and rubella	HR-4	HR-4	HR-4	Gonorrhea	■[d]	■[d]	■[d]
				Chlamydia	■[d]	■[d]	■[d]
Diphtheria and tetanus		HR-5		Genital warts	■[d]	■[d]	■[d]
Hepatitis B	HR-6	HR-6	HR-6	Syphilis	HR-2	HR-2	HR-2
				HIV infection	HR-2	HR-2	HR-2
				Cervical cancer	■[d]	■[d]	■[e]
				Depression/suicide risk	■	■	■
				Physical, sexual, or emotional abuse	■	■	■
				Learning problems	■	■	■
				Tuberculosis	HR-3	HR-3	HR-3

[a] Recommendation developed by the National Heart, Lung, and Blood Institute Second Task Force on Blood Pressure in Children.
[b] Recommendation developed by the National Cholesterol Education Program: Report of the Expert Panel on Blood Cholesterol Levels in Children and Adolescents, 1991.
[c] Recommendation developed by the Advisory Committee for Immunization Practices.
[d] Screening should be performed if the adolescent is currently sexually active.
[e] Screening should be performed if the adolescent girl is sexually active or 18 years or older.
Key and notations: ●, once per time period; ■, yearly; ❯, optional.
HR, high-risk category.
HR-1: Test should be performed if there is a family history of cardiovascular disease before age 55 or parental history of high cholesterol. Physician may choose to perform test if family history is unknown or if adolescent has multiple risk factors for future cardiovascular disease.
HR-2: Syphilis test should be performed on and HIV test offered to adolescents who are at high risk for infection. This includes having had more than one sexual partner in last 6 months, having exchanged sex for drugs, being a man who has engaged in sex with other men having used intravenous drugs (HIV), having had other STDs, having lived in an area endemic for infection, and having had a sexual partner who is at risk for infection.
HR-3: Test should be performed on adolescents who have been exposed to active TB, have lived in a homeless shelter, have been incarcerated, have lived in an area endemic for TB, or currently work in a health-care setting.
HR-4: Vaccination should be provided to adolescents who have had only one previous MMR.
HR-5: Vaccination should be given 10 years following previous dT booster.
HR-6: Hepatitis B virus vaccination (HBV) should be given to susceptible adolescents at high risk for infection (see HR-2).
SOURCE: *Elster AB, Kuznets NJ Guidelines for Adolescent Preventive Services (GAPS). Baltimore: Williams & Wilkins, 1993.*

essential for both accuracy and interpretation of serial values. Infants and children should be weighed without their clothes on, using the same scale at each visit. Length generally is measured in the recumbent position until children are 2 years of age. Greatest accuracy is achieved using a device that has a stationary headboard and sliding footboard. While the infant's head is positioned against the headboard and the body and legs are held straight and flat, the footboard is brought up to meet the infant's soles at right angles to the table. Between 2 and 3 years of age, a standing height measurement is generally obtained. Using a stadiometer, the child is instructed to stand as tall as possible with his or her feet flat on the ground, heels and shoulders against the backboard, and chin parallel to the floor, while a sliding headboard is lowered to touch the top of the head. Head size is obtained by measuring the greatest occipitofrontal circumference using a flexible but nonstretchable tape measure. Common "rules of thumb" regarding physical growth patterns are given in Table 1-4. Dental development is discussed in Sec. 16.1. The normal progression of secondary sexual characteristics is discussed in Secs. 3.4.1, 3.4.2 and 24.8.

In the absence of an absolute definition of normality, the adequacy of a child's growth is determined by comparison with others of the same sex and similar age as well as by the presence or absence of concordance between growth parameters and the consistency of growth patterns over time. Plotting a child's height, weight, and head circumference on a standard National Center for Health Statistics (NCHS) cross-sectional growth chart provides a statistical definition of normality by comparing that individual to others of similar age and sex (see Appendix A). Normative growth data are also available for age- and gender-based comparison of a child's rate of height or weight gain per unit time (Appendix B1-7). Although the likelihood of a growth problem increases the further a child's growth parameters are from population norms (traditionally

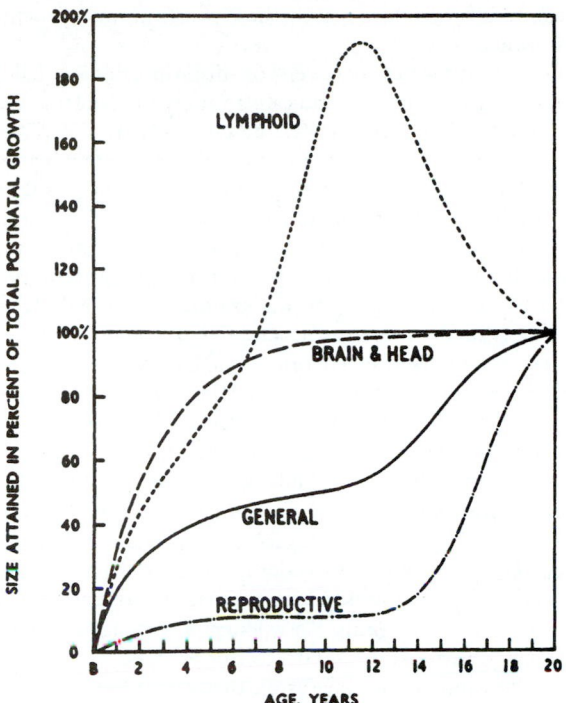

FIGURE 1-1 Postnatal growth curves of four major organ systems. All values are calculated in terms of size attained at 20 years. General type includes body as a whole, respiratory and digestive organs, kidney, spleen, musculature, and skeleton. SOURCE: *Tanner JM: Growth at Adolescence. Oxford: Blackwell, 1962, with permission.*

defined as two standard deviations above and below the mean), making assumptions about the adequacy of a child's growth on the basis of a single set of growth points can be misleading. By definition, approximately 5% of the population will fall above and below the range of growth parameters statistically defined as normal. Furthermore, the standard NCHS growth curves were generated by measuring different groups of primarily white, middle-class children at each age; extrapolating these values to children of different ethnic or racial background may erroneously label their growth as abnormal.

Of even greater importance to the overall assessment of a child's growth is the observation of growth curves over time. Serial measurements provide the most accurate indication of whether physical growth is progressing normally for a given individual. The shape and placement of growth curves provide important information (Fig. 1-2). Children who are growing normally at an average tempo

TABLE 1-3
MIDPARENTAL HEIGHT[a]

Midparental height for girls
$$\frac{(\text{father's height} - 13 \text{ cm}) + (\text{mother's height})}{2}$$
Midparental height for boys
$$\frac{(\text{mother's height} + 13 \text{ cm}) + (\text{father's height})}{2}$$

[a] Based on genetic factors alone, a child's predicted adult height should fall within 5 cm above or below the calculated midparental height.

TABLE 1-4
TYPICAL PATTERNS OF PHYSICAL GROWTH

Weight
  Birth weight (BW) is regained by 10th to 14th day
  Average weight gain/day: 0–6 mo = 20 g; 6–12 mo = 15 g
  BW doubles at ~4 mo, triples at ~12 mo, quadruples at
    ~24 mo
  During second year, average weight gain/mo = ~0.25 kg
  After age 2 y, average annual gain until adolescence = ~2.3 kg (5 lb)
Length/height
  By end of first year, birth length increases by 50%
  Birth length doubles by 4 y, triples by 13 y
  Average height gain during second year = ~12 cm (5 in.)
  After age 2 y, average annual growth until adolescence ≥ 5 cm (2 in.)
Head circumference
  Average head growth/wk: 0–2 mo = ~0.5 cm; 2–6 mo = ~0.25 cm
  Average total head growth from 0–3 mo = ~5 cm; 3–6 mo =
    ~4 cm; 6–9 mo = ~2 cm; 9 mo–1 y = ~1 cm

will parallel their genetically determined percentile on the standard NCHS growth curves. The child who is genetically small will parallel the standard curves at the low end of, or just below, the statistically defined normal range of heights and weights in the population. These children tend to be small at birth, and growth parameters are consistent with parental size. They have a normal weight for height (both equally below the third percentile), a normal skinfold thickness, and a bone age consistent with chronologic age.

The child who has suffered a significant prenatal event leading to growth failure is typically proportionally small for gestational age at birth and, with time, continues to fall further away from population means on all parameters. Postnatal onset of a growth problem is manifested by a downward trend in a previously stable growth curve. Although the downward crossing of percentiles should always provoke concern during the first 2 years after birth, this pattern can also result from two normal growth variants that may be difficult to differentiate from growth failure. A baby's

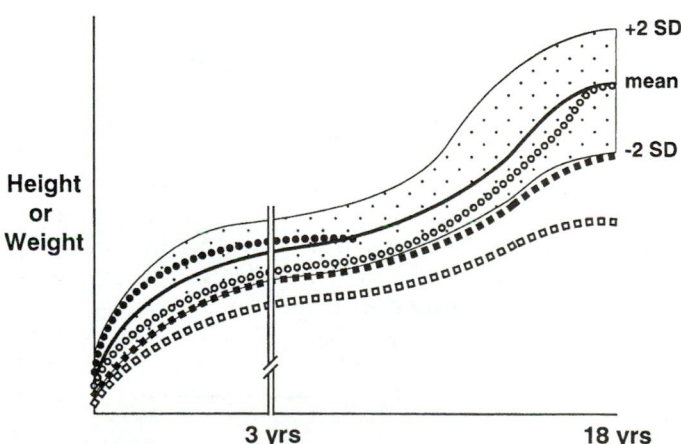

FIGURE 1-2 Growth curve patterns for children with: postnatal-onset pathologic growth (●); prenatal-onset pathologic growth (□); constitutional growth delay (○); genetic short stature (■). *Shaded area* represents mean growth curve ± 2 SD.

size at birth is influenced significantly by maternal intrauterine conditions, and some downward shifting may occur as the percentile representing the child's true genetic growth potential is achieved. Such shifting generally occurs between 6 and 12 months after birth and is associated with a steady but decreased rate of weight gain.

Downward percentile shifting also can occur as a result of normal variations in the rate and timing of growth spurts. Because NCHS growth curves were constructed using different samples of children at each age rather than by following the same cohort over time, they can not differentiate normal variations in the tempo of growth from early pathologic growth. In constitutional growth delay, a child's height and weight are normal at birth; drop off proportionally during the first 2 years, eventually to parallel NCHS growth curves at or just below the third percentile for most of middle childhood; and then cross percentiles upward to achieve a normal final adult size. The bone age is delayed for the child's chronologic age but consistent with height age (the age at which the child's height is at the 50th percentile). Although delays in early growth spurts may raise concerns regarding growth failure, constitutional growth delay is often first recognized when the shifted adolescent growth spurt results in the delayed appearance of secondary sexual characteristics. Like genetic short stature, constitutional growth delay is familial; parents frequently report delayed adolescent development in themselves ("late bloomer") and/or similar growth patterns in other offspring. The recent availability of longitudinal growth charts, which provide normative data for early-, average-, and late-tempo developing children, allows the

physician to identify more readily these constitutional growth variants as normal.

Major discrepancies between or disproportionate falloff in growth parameters may also indicate a variety of problems. Several characteristic patterns have been described (Fig. 1-3). Weight, height, and head circumference that are all significantly below that expected for the child's chronologic age suggest the possibility of an intrauterine insult or genetic abnormality. Relative sparing of the head circumference in relation to weight and height that are significantly below that predicted for chronologic age is more characteristic of the normal variants of constitutional growth delay and genetic short stature as well as structural dystrophies and endocrine causes of growth failure. Caloric insufficiency from inadequate intake, increased loss, or a hypermetabolic state is suggested when weight is significantly below that expected for chronologic age, with relative sparing of both head circumference and height.

Routine surveillance of a child's growth provides a framework for periodic discussions regarding normal growth patterns, nutritional needs, and developmental feeding behaviors of infants and children. The primary-care provider is also in a unique position to detect and orchestrate subsequent evaluation and management of a variety of growth problems. Knowledge of both normal and pathologic growth patterns is essential to this process.

The following section focuses on two areas of growth concern that frequently confront pediatricians: failure to thrive and variations in head size and shape. The approach to several other common growth concerns including obesity (Sec. 5.6.11), short stature

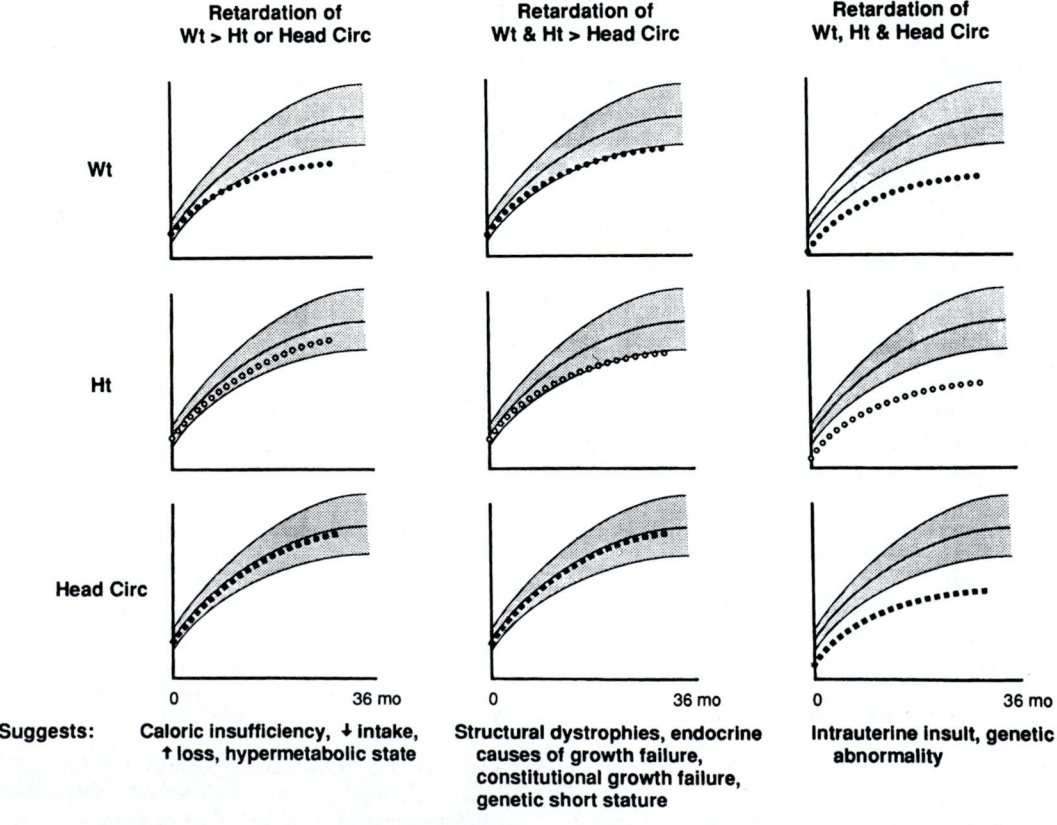

FIGURE 1-3 Characteristic patterns of growth parameters and suggested etiologies.

(Sec. 24.2), and variations in pubertal development (Sec. 24.8) are discussed in subsequent chapters.

1.1.2 Common Growth Concerns

FAILURE TO THRIVE

The term "failure to thrive" was first used to describe the malnourished and depressed condition of many institutionalized infants in the early 1900s. It remains a descriptive rather than a diagnostic label applied to children whose attained weight or rate of weight gain is significantly below that of other children of similar age and same sex. Depending on the duration and severity of malnourishment, linear growth and head circumference also may be affected. Although the adverse acute and long-term consequences of childhood malnutrition are well established, the point at which deviations from age-related norms exceed normal growth variation and place the child at risk is less certain. The lack of consensus regarding specific anthropomorphic criteria for identifying the child who is failing to thrive is reflected in the number of commonly used definitions (Table 1-5).

Growth failure in infancy and childhood can result from a wide range of factors, including serious medical disease, behavioral and neurologic feeding problems, parental misinformation, poverty, and dysfunctional and/or abusive child–caregiver interactions (Table 1-6). In the majority of cases, an underlying organic etiology is not found; when one is identified, it rarely presents with growth failure as its only manifestation. On the other hand, psychosocial and behavioral feeding problems resulting in growth failure are common and should no longer be perceived as diagnoses of exclusion. Whether the condition is primarily organic or psychosocial in origin, all children who are failing to thrive suffer the physical and psychological consequences of malnutrition and are at significant risk for long-term physical and psychodevelopmental sequelae.

In recognition of this fact, and the fact that biological, psychosocial, and behavioral problems frequently coexist, the approach to the child with apparent growth failure has shifted away from attempts to define a purely organic or nonorganic etiology toward assessment of both physical and psychosocial risk factors, the degree of malnourishment present, and the resultant physiological and psychodevelopmental consequences for that child. Key components of the evaluation include a review of past and present growth data, a thorough history and physical examination, a developmental/behavioral assessment, observation of a feeding, assessment of both situation-specific and global child–parent interactions, and selected laboratory studies based on concerns raised by the above (Table 1-7). By performing each aspect of the evaluation, the provider should attempt to answer several questions that are key to arriving at the correct diagnosis and an appropriate treatment plan (Table 1-8).

Because many parents occasionally worry about their child's growth, and several normal variants can be confused with growth failure, the first issue to be addressed is whether or not the child is truly failing to thrive. This question can best be answered by reviewing the child's past and present growth data for deviations from population norms, consistency over time, and concordance between growth parameters. Findings characteristic of the normal variants of genetic short stature and constitutional delay, as well as growth curves and relationships between growth parameters suggestive of specific problems, have been discussed previously (Sec. 1.1.1).

When review of growth data reveals inadequate growth, the physician must ascertain whether this is primarily caused by inadequate caloric intake, calorie wasting, an increased caloric requirement, or an altered growth potential (Table 1-6). Evidence should be elicited to support a specific situational, behavioral, interactional, and/or medical problem. In addition to detailed medical information, a thorough dietary/feeding, social, behavioral, and developmental history is essential. Most cases of failure to thrive result from inadequate consumption of appropriate amounts and/or kinds of food. Inadequate caloric intake is most often related to psychosocial and/or behavioral problems, including parental ignorance and misperceptions regarding appropriate feeding; variations in infant temperament, appetite, and behavioral response (both infant's and caregivers') to progressive stages of infant feeding; a dysfunctional feeding environment/interaction; more global problems with the parent–child relationship; and/or a lack of access to food. However, inadequate intake also can occur secondary to oromotor or other feeding dysfunctions and to medical problems that result in secondary anorexia or food refusal. When caloric intake appears to be adequate, evidence suggesting a condition associated with calorie wasting or an increased caloric requirement must be sought. Excessive caloric losses occur primarily with several gastrointestinal and renal disorders. Children with cardiopulmonary problems, malignancies, hyperthyroidism, and chronic or recurrent infections may have increased caloric needs. In addition to other stigmata, many genetic syndromes may present with altered growth patterns.

The physical examination of a child who is growing poorly should focus on identifying signs of an underlying organic disease or syndrome, severity of malnutrition, and important concomitant findings such as evidence of physical abuse or neglect or the presence of deprivational behaviors. The parent–child interaction should be observed throughout the visit. Watching a feeding session is an excellent way to identify specific behavioral or interactional problems that occur during feeding. A psychomotor developmental assessment should also be obtained. Children with severe psychosocial failure to thrive may manifest a variety of gaze disturbances ranging from hyperalert wary watchfulness to total avoidance of eye contact and apathetic withdrawal. Infants may resist cuddling and prefer interactions with inanimate objects, whereas toddlers may demonstrate indiscriminate affection-seeking behav-

---

TABLE 1-5

DEFINITIONS OF FAILURE TO THRIVE

Attained growth
  Weight <3rd percentile on NCHS growth chart
  Weight for height <5th percentile on NCHS growth chart
  Weight 20% or more below ideal weight for height
  Triceps skinfold thickness ≤5 mm
Rate of growth
  Depressed rate of weight gain
    <20 g/d from 0 to 3 months of age
    <15 g/d from 3 to 6 months of age
  Falloff from previously established growth curve
    Downward crossing of ≥2 major percentiles on NCHS growth chart
  Documented weight loss

SOURCE: NCHS = National Center for Health Statistics.

TABLE 1-6
CAUSES OF INADEQUATE WEIGHT GAIN

Inadequate intake
- Lack of appetite
  - Chronic disease (eg, central nervous system pathology, gastrointestinal disorders, chronic infections)
  - Anemia (eg, iron deficiency)
  - Psychosocial problems (eg, apathy)
- Difficulty with ingestion
  - Feeding disorder
  - Psychosocial problems (eg, apathy, rumination)
  - Neurologic disorders (eg, cerebral palsy, hypertonia, hypotonia, generalized muscle weakness/pathology)
  - Craniofacial anomalies (eg, choanal atresia, cleft lip and palate, micrognathia)
  - Dyspnea (eg, congenital heart disease, pulmonary diseases)
  - Generalized muscle weakness/pathology (eg, myopathies)
  - Tracheoesophageal fistula
  - Genetic syndromes
  - Congenital syndromes (eg, fetal alcohol syndrome)
- Unavailability of food
  - Inappropriate feeding technique
  - Insufficient/inadequate volume of food
  - Inappropriate food for age
  - Withholding of food (abuse, neglect)

Altered growth potential regulation
- Prenatal insult
- Chromosomal abnormality/genetic syndrome
- Endocrinopathies

Calorie wasting
- Vomiting
  - CNS pathology (increased intracranial pressure)
  - Intestinal tract obstruction (eg, pyloric stenosis, malrotation)
  - Gastrointestinal reflux
  - Metabolic problems
  - Drugs/toxins
- Malabsorption
  - Primary gastrointestinal diseases: biliary atresia/cirrhosis, celiac disease
  - Inflammatory bowel disease, enzymatic deficiencies, food (protein) sensitivity/intolerance, Hirschsprung disease
  - Cystic fibrosis
  - Immunologic deficiency
  - Infections
  - Endocrinopathies
  - Drugs/toxins
- Renal losses
  - Diabetes
  - Renal tubular acidosis

Increased caloric requirements
- Increased metabolism/increased use of calories
  - Congenital heart disease/acquired heart disease
  - Chronic respiratory disease (eg, bronchopulmonary dysplasia)
  - Neoplasms
  - Chronic/recurrent infection
  - Endocrinopathies (eg, hyperthyroidism, hyperaldosteronism)
  - Chronic anemia
  - Drugs/toxins (eg, lead, levothyroxine)
- Defective use of calories
  - Metabolic disorders (eg, aminoacidopathies, inborn errors of carbohydrate metabolism)
  - Renal tubular acidosis

SOURCE: *Adapted from Zenel JA: Failure to thrive: a general pediatrician's perspective. Pediatr Rev 1997; 18:371–378.*

iors. Many of these children also manifest developmental delays, especially in the areas of language and social adaptive behavior that are most dependent on environmental stimulation.

The diagnostic laboratory evaluation should be guided by concerns raised in the history, physical examination, and review of growth data. Organic disease presenting only with growth failure is extremely uncommon. An undirected laboratory evaluation rarely identifies an unsuspected diagnosis and is potentially harmful. Depending on the duration and severity of growth failure, additional laboratory studies may be useful to help assess nutritional status and the presence of concomitant problems such as iron-deficiency anemia. Although no laboratory studies should be considered routine, most children receive a complete blood count, serum electrolytes, serum creatinine, total protein/albumin, urinalysis, urine culture, and bone age (if height growth is also poor) as part of their evaluation.

Most children with growth failure can be evaluated and managed as outpatients, with several important exceptions. Children with psychosocial failure to thrive should be hospitalized if they manifest evidence of, or are at high risk for, physical abuse and/or severe neglect, are severely malnourished or medically unstable, or have failed a trial of outpatient management.

The approach to a child with failure to thrive requires time and sensitivity. To facilitate subsequent communication and management, it is important to understand the parents' perspective regarding their child's growth and health as well as to be cognizant of previous efforts to intervene when concerns have been present. Many parents of children who are failing to thrive experience feelings of guilt, inadequacy, and anger when behavioral and/or psychosocial problems are uncovered, and subsequent efforts to intercede are often perceived as being critical of their parenting abilities. Focusing on concern for the child's health and well-being as well as the positive goal of enhancing the parent–child relationship may help to defuse some of these feelings. Ultimately, the success of treatment often depends on the establishment of a positive and caring longitudinal alliance with the child and caretakers. Management of the child with psychosocial failure to thrive must be individualized to the specific needs of the child and family. In addition to nutritional rehabilitation, efforts are focused on correcting the dysfunctional child–parent interactions by addressing areas of parental misinformation, providing and helping to implement specific feeding guidelines, and addressing the larger psychosocial needs of the family. A multidisciplinary team approach involving the primary-care provider, nutritionist, social worker, child behavior spe-

TABLE 1-7
FAILURE TO THRIVE: COMPONENTS OF EVALUATION

Growth data
  Current growth parameters
  Growth curves over time
  Relationship of growth parameters to each other
History
  Problem context
    Parents' perception of child's growth and overall health
    When growth problem first became a concern
    Previous interventions attempted
  Medical
    Prenatal care and complications (infection, maternal nutrition, drug
      exposure)
    Gestational age and growth parameters at birth (SGA, prematurity)
    Perinatal complications (infections, CNS insults, anomalies)
    Previous hospitalizations, illnesses, and surgery
    Current medications
    Review of systems (vomiting, stooling patterns, mechanics of feed-
      ing/swallowing, anorexia, distress/tiring with feeds)
  Nutritional
    Caloric intake
      Breast-fed: schedule and length of feeds; maternal cues to prefeed-
        ing engorgement, milk let-down, and drainage postfeeding; ma-
        ternal diet, rest, stress, and medications
      Formula fed: type, method of preparation; feeding schedule;
        amount offered and consumed
      Mixed diet: 3-day diet history (food/beverage type, method of
        preparation, quantity consumed)
    Schedule and length of feedings
    Cue to infant's/child's hunger and satiety
    Daily feeding/mealtime environment
    Location/positioning during feedings
    Perceptions of suck, swallow, and grasp of nipple
    Caregivers involved with feedings
    Amount and type of mealtime supervision
    Behavior during feeding
    History of progression to solid/table foods
    Favorite/disliked foods
    Parental knowledge/beliefs regarding child/infant feeding
    Family eating practices and beliefs
    Financial constraints affecting food availability

Psychosocial
  Caregiving environment
  Family support systems
  Family finances
  Stability of parents and their relationship
  Family/household composition
  Parent–child relationship
  Attitudes toward parenting
  Content/structure of typical day for child
  Parents' perceptions of child's needs
Developmental/behavioral
  Age-related behavior problems (eg, attachment, autonomy)
  Developmental milestones: gross/fine motor, language, social/emo-
    tional, cognition
  Parents' perception of child's temperament/behavior
Physical examination
  Physician–child interaction
  Skinfold measurements
  Complete physical examination
Developmental/behavioral assessment
  Neurodevelopmental assessment of gross/fine motor, language, socioe-
    motional, cognitive skills
Observation of a feeding
  Feeding environment (home observation)
  Type and amount of food offered
  Pace and duration of feeding
  Child's oromotor and fine motor skills
  Child's cues to and parental response regarding readiness to eat and sa-
    tiation
  Parents' utilization of opportunities for positive reinforcement and so-
    cial interaction
  Parents' awareness and use of child's developmental abilities
  Overall parent–child interaction
Laboratory studies
  Diagnostic tests directed by positive findings on history, physical, and
    review of growth date
  Consider: complete blood count, serum electrolytes, serum creatinine,
    urinalysis (± culture), total protein/albumin, bone age (if height
    growth also poor)
Disposition
  Hospitalize if:
    Evidence of physical abuse and/or severe neglect
    High risk for abuse and neglect, very disturbed parent–child interac-
      tion, poor parent functioning, and/or an extremely stressful envi-
      ronment
    Severe malnutrition and/or medically unstable
    Outpatient management failure

---

cialist, and community-based outreach services is often most beneficial.

VARIATIONS IN HEAD SIZE AND SHAPE: MICROCEPHALY, MACROCEPHALY, AND PLAGIOCEPHALY

Head size is obtained by measuring the greatest occipitofrontal circumference and reflects the volume of intracranial contents, including brain, cerebrospinal fluid, and blood, as well as the thickness of the skull and scalp. Macrocephaly and microcephaly are
statistically defined as a head circumference more than two standard

deviations above and below the mean for children of similar age.
Under this definition, approximately 5% of the population will be
labeled as either macro- or microcephalic. As with other growth
parameters, the significance of a given measurement is best defined
within the context of normal variations, the pattern of past head
growth, the relationship of head size to other growth parameters,
and the presence or absence of associated historical and/or physical
findings.

Unrelated to intracranial volume, the presence of scalp edema
or a cephalhematoma may significantly increase the head circumference. The effect of head shape on circumference should also be
kept in mind. For the same intracranial volume, a round head will

TABLE 1-8
FAILURE TO THRIVE: KEY QUESTIONS

Growth data

Is the child failing to thrive, or does growth represent a normal variant?

Do growth parameters and curves suggest a specific etiology?

History (medical, nutritional, psychosocial, developmental/ behavioral)

Do caretakers perceive growth to be a problem?

Does the history suggest growth failure is caused by inadequate caloric intake, calorie wasting, increased caloric requirement, or altered growth potential?

Does the history suggest a specific situational, behavioral, interactional, and/or medical problem?

Physical examination

Is there evidence to suggest an underlying organic etiology?

Is there evidence of severe malnutrition and/or nutritional deficiency?

Is there evidence of a disturbed parent–child relationship, including the presence of derivational behaviors and/or signs of physical abuse/neglect?

Developmental/behavioral assessment

Is there global or asymmetric developmental delay?

Are global behavioral problems present?

Observation of a feeding

Is a specific situational, behavioral, interactional, and/or medical problem observed?

Laboratory studies

Are specific diagnostic studies indicated?

Does the extent of malnutrition warrant further laboratory studies?

Disposition

Is inpatient evaluation and management warranted?

have a smaller head circumference than a more oval-shaped head. Gestational age rather than chronologic age should be used when plotting the head circumference of preterm infants. Because of catch-up growth, these infants also exhibit accelerated head growth compared with full-term babies, initially exceeding gains in weight and height. The disproportionately enlarging head may raise concerns regarding hydrocephalus. The fact that many premature infants are also at increased risk for this complication emphasizes the need for close observation of these children.

When a child's head size or rate of head growth provokes concern, a thorough history, physical examination, and review of growth curves should be obtained. Knowledge of head size at birth and the pattern of prior head growth is important. A child whose head circumference consistently follows the same percentile is more likely to be normal than one whose growth channel shifts upward or downward across percentiles. Head size must also be assessed within the context of the child's overall body size. General concordance exists between growth parameters in a given individual; significant discrepancies between head circumference and body size (height and weight) increase the likelihood of a pathologic basis. The influence of benign familial factors, as well as specific syndromes and problems, can be identified by evaluating the head circumference of the child's parents and siblings. The history and physical examination should seek to identify signs and symptoms of causal and/or concomitant problems, including developmental disabilities; mental retardation; neurologic abnormalities such as cerebral palsy, seizures, and focal deficits; dysmorphology; abnormal fontanels and sutures; or skin findings suggestive of a neurocutaneous disorder. A history of prenatal, perinatal, and postnatal fac-

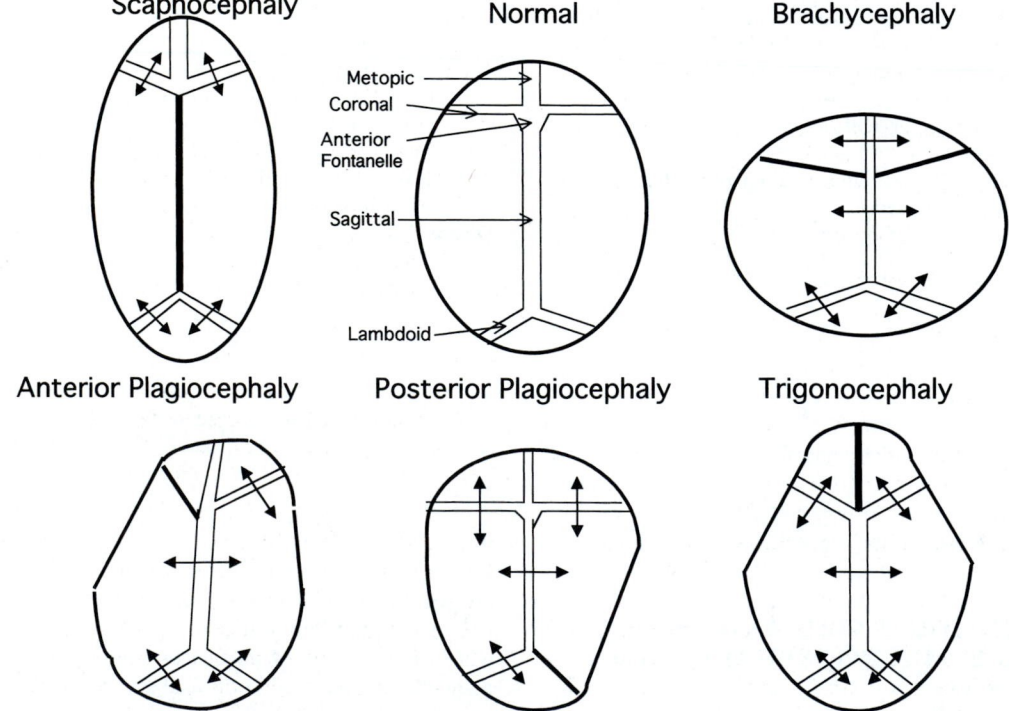

FIGURE 1-4 **Craniosynostosis and corresponding head shapes. The fused or absent sutures are shown as *solid lines,* and the *arrows* indicate compensatory growth along the open sutures, resulting in the characteristic head shape. The fused or absent sutures for different head shapes are: scaphocephaly, sagittal; brachycephaly, bilateral coronal; anterior plagiocephaly, unilateral coronal; posterior plagiocephaly, unilateral lambdoidal; trigonocephaly, metopic.**

tors and events with potential import to subsequent central nervous system growth and development should be elicited, including poor prenatal care, maternal drug use or infection during pregnancy, prematurity, perinatal asphyxia, hypoglycemia, hypotension, and central nervous system infection.

Macrocephaly can result from excess cerebrospinal fluid (hydrocephalus), excess brain tissue (macrencephaly), thickening of the skull, or hemorrhage into the subdural or epidural spaces. Each of these problems, in turn, may be secondary to a variety of inborn or acquired disorders, which rarely present exclusively with head growth abnormalities. Megalencephaly refers to the presence of excess brain tissue secondary to an increased size or number of brain cells. This may be a primary anatomic condition with or without concomitant syndromic or neurologic abnormalities or may be caused by a variety of metabolic disorders that are associated with cerebral edema and/or brain cell storage of accumulated substances. Infants with anatomic megalencephaly generally are born with large heads, whereas babies with metabolic causes of megalencephaly typically have a normal head size at birth with subsequent enlargement during the neonatal period. Metabolic megalencephaly is frequently accompanied by developmental regression or delay, signs of increased intracranial pressure, and/or concomitant neurologic problems such as seizures.

The widespread availability and use of the CT scanner has also identified several benign conditions associated with macrocephaly. Benign enlargement of the subarachnoid space is a relatively common cause of macrocephaly in otherwise normal infants. These children typically have large (but within normal range) heads at birth but provoke concern during infancy when the head circumference subsequently crosses percentiles upward to exceed and then parallel the 98th percentile for children of similar age and same sex. A head CT scan, if obtained, demonstrates an enlarged subarachnoid space, normal to slightly increased ventricular size, and widened sulci and sylvian fissure. A genetic cause is suspected because of the observed male predominance of this condition and the frequent concomitant finding of macrocephaly in the identified child's father.

Aside from the head growth abnormalities, these children are neurologically and intellectually normal. Genetic megalencephaly (large brain) is another common normal variant causing macrocephaly and may be indistinguishable from the previously described condition unless a head CT scan is performed. These children may or may not have large heads at birth but subsequently cross percentiles upward to parallel the curve above the 98th percentile. A head CT scan, if obtained, is normal. The family history is usually positive for megalencephaly and, as in children identified with benign enlargement of the subarachnoid space, neurologic and mental function are normal. A child identified as having one of these two benign conditions does not require further evaluation unless head growth subsequently deviates further from the normal curve, or a neurologic abnormality or developmental delay is detected.

Microcephaly is indicative of a small brain and is typically the result of a primary or secondary defect in brain development. Although normal intelligence can occur, microcephaly is frequently associated with mental retardation. Primary microcephaly refers to the presence of a genetic or chromosomal condition in which bulk and/or structural brain growth is intrinsically flawed. In secondary microcephaly, previously normal brain development is subsequently impaired by a variety of pre- and postnatal infections, toxins, and central nervous system injuries. Because brain expansion dictates skull growth, inadequate brain growth may result in premature fusion of the cranial bones. This cause of premature suture closure generally can be differentiated from primary craniosynostosis by the absence of both an abnormally shaped skull and palpably thickened suture lines.

The presence of microcephaly at birth establishes the antenatal timing of impaired brain growth but does not differentiate primary from secondary etiologies. With the exception of some chromosomal disorders, a normal-sized head at birth with the subsequent development of growth failure strongly suggests a secondary etiology for the microcephaly. Perinatal insults to the central nervous system rarely result in recognizably impaired head growth before the age of 3 to 6 months. When such insults cause microcephaly and mental retardation, they are also associated with motor deficits (cerebral palsy) and frequently with seizures. Cranial CT scans of children with primary microcephaly typically either are normal or reveal dysmorphology characteristic of the specific etiology, whereas CT scans of those with secondary microcephaly usually are abnormal and show a combination of nonspecific findings such as ventricular enlargement and cerebral atrophy.

Plagiocephaly, or asymmetric head growth, is caused by alterations of the normal internal and external forces that impact on skull growth as well as by inherent or acquired abnormalities in bone formation. Most infants born vaginally have some degree of head molding at birth, which resolves during the first few weeks of life unless other factors are present to perpetuate it. Deformational flattening from lack of variation in head positioning both pre- and postnatally is the most common cause of an asymmetric head shape and can be exacerbated by factors associated with delayed head control (eg, prematurity) and conditions that predispose the infant to turn to one side (torticollis, neurologic/ophthalmologic conditions). In recent years, pediatricians have seen a significant increase in the number of infants presenting with posterior plagiocephaly as a result of the success of the "Back to Sleep" campaign, which has significantly decreased the incidence of sudden infant death syndrome (SIDS) by promoting the supine sleeping position for young infants.

It is most important for clinicians to be able to differentiate this common form of deformational plagiocephaly from asymmetric growth caused by premature closure of one or more of the cranial sutures (synostotic plagiocephaly). Normally most sutures are closed by 12-24 months of age. The majority are ossified by 8 years of age, and fusion is complete by early adulthood. With craniosynostosis, premature closure or absence of one or more cranial sutures results in compensatory growth along the remaining open sutures in a direction parallel to the closed suture. The resultant head shape can be predicted based on the suture(s) involved (Fig. 1-4). Although it primarily causes problems with cosmetic appearance, craniosynostosis can be associated with ocular problems, neurologic impairment, and increased intracranial pressure. Craniosynostosis involving only one suture is usually an isolated condition, occurring with a prevalence of 1-2/1000. Eighty-five percent of cases occur in Caucasian children, with a male-to-female ratio of 3:2. The sagittal suture is involved in almost half the cases, with stenosis of the coronal (one-tenth) and metopic (one-tenth) sutures the next most commonly observed. Most importantly, premature closure of the lambdoidal suture, causing posterior plagiocephaly, occurs rarely. Craniosynostosis involving more than one suture is often associated with one of several genetic syndromes. Head shape is generally severely distorted, and ophthalmologic/neurologic problems and/or other stigmata of the syndrome are usually present.

The approach to a child with an asymmetric head should include a thorough history, physical examination, and directed laboratory/radiographic evaluation. The physician should ascertain when the asymmetry was first noted and whether it has been progressive. Risk factors for deformational (eg, favored side or position, torticollis, prematurity, neuromotor problems) and synostotic plagiocephaly (eg, ventriculoperitoneal shunting of hydrocephalus, microcephaly, metabolic bone disease) should also be explored. Evaluation of head circumference is important: children with deformational plagiocephaly and single-suture craniosynostosis have a normal head size and rate of growth. Although premature closure of multiple sutures can rarely be the cause of restricted brain growth, more often, the absence of the outward pressure of a normally growing brain causes premature closure of multiple cranial sutures. When microcephaly is the primary problem, gross skull malformation and signs of increased intracranial pressure are absent.

The physical examination can be very helpful in differentiating deformational posterior plagiocephaly from true craniosynostosis. In synostotic posterior plagiocephaly, occipital flattening may be accompanied by a thick ridge overlying the fused lambdoid suture or the absence of a palpable suture. Compensatory growth causes frontal and parietal prominence on the side opposite the occipital flattening, resulting in an overall trapezoidal head shape. The ear on the side of the fused suture is displaced downward and backward. In deformational posterior plagiocephaly, the occiput is flattened, but the sutures are open, and ridging is absent. Occipital flattening results in a prominence of the frontal and temporal areas on the same side, giving the head an overall parallelogram shape, and, in contrast to lambdoid synostosis, the ear is pushed forward and down, away from the area of flattening.

During the physical examination the provider should also focus on identifying evidence of a specific etiology (torticollis, neuromuscular and/or developmental problems, syndromic stigmata) or complications (increased intracranial pressure, ocular and neurologic problems). If the deformation observed is severe, suggestive of synostosis, progressive after several weeks of conservative treatment, and/or associated with significant parental anxiety, plain skull radiographs are warranted. In most children, skulls films interpreted within the context of clinical data will clarify the diagnosis. However, because plain radiographs will not identify all synostotic sutures, when the clinical situation is suggestive and plain films are equivocal, a head CT or three-dimensional CT reconstruction is indicated.

Mild positional posterior plagiocephaly is largely a benign self-correcting condition, as the child spends less and less time lying down and in one position. Parents should be counseled to use the supine sleeping position for infants but to try to vary head positioning during sleep. Crib toys may be moved to encourage turning to a less favored side. Babies should also be given the opportunity to spend time in the prone position when awake and observed. This "positional therapy" should be combined with physical therapy (stretching exercises to achieve normal neck mobility) in the infant with torticollis. For most children with mild to moderate positional plagiocephaly, implementation of these conservative measures will result in a normal or near-normal appearance within 2 to 3 months. For infants with severe positional plagiocephaly and those with a moderate deformity that does not respond to a period of conservative measures, use of helmet molding may be considered. In order

to be effective and to avoid potential complications, this therapy requires almost constant use of the helmet (22 h/day) and involvement of an orthotics expert. Optimal therapeutic results from helmet molding are achieved when treatment is initiated before 6 months of age. Treatment for craniosynostotic plagiocephaly is surgical. Because the cosmetic outcome is dependent on the potential for further skull growth, surgical correction of single-suture synostosis should ideally take place by 6-12 months of age. The diagnosis and treatment of craniosynostosis are discussed further in Sec. 10.3.4.

References

Bithoney WG, Dubowitz H, Egan H: Failure to thrive/growth deficiency. Pediatr Rev 13:453–460, 1992

Fenichel GM: Disorders of cranial volume and shape. In: Clinical Pediatric Neurology: A Signs and Symptoms Approach, 2nd ed. Philadelphia, WB Saunders, 1993

Frank DA, Zeisel SH: Failure to thrive. Pediatr Clin North Am 35:1187–1206, 1988

Guo SM, Roche AF, Fomon SJ, et al: Reference data on gains in weight and length during the first two years of life. J Pediatr 119:355–362, 1991

Pollack IF, Losken HW, Fasick P: Diagnosis and management of posterior plagiocephaly. Pediatrics 99:180–185, 1997

Rohan AJ, Golombek SG, Rosenthal AD: Infants with misshapen skulls: When to worry. Cont Pediatr 16:47–73, 1999

Zenel JA: Failure to thrive: A general pediatrician's perspective. Pediatr Rev 18:371–378, 1997

1.2 MOTOR AND PSYCHOLOGICAL DEVELOPMENT

1.2.1 Overview

To assess children's overall developmental progress and functioning and to counsel parents regarding a variety of developmentally based issues, the physician must have a firm understanding of both normal patterns and common variations in the developmental process. Knowing the average ages at which children achieve certain neurodevelopmental milestones and encounter specific developmental tasks helps to provide a conceptual framework for determining whether or not a child's development is age-appropriate. However, developmental normality cannot be defined in absolute terms. Although the sequence of development is similar for all children, the rate of progress may vary from child to child, and "dissociation" of performance between developmental fields can often be normal. By comparing a child's performance with others', one can only say that the further the child is from "average," the less likely he or she will be "normal." It is important to remember that a child's developmental level and progress are the end result of a variety of factors, many unrelated to the child's genetic mental endowment, such as the presence of acute or chronic illness, physical or sensory handicaps, and the quality of the nurturing environment. Current developmental thinking emphasizes the interactional contributions of both "nature" and "nurture" to the child's overall functioning. Developmental assessment should emphasize their shared importance by addressing the child's medical history, physical examination, and psychosocial history in addition to eliciting specific developmental skills and information. A longitudinal and multidimensional approach to developmental monitoring should be encouraged, and an overreliance on isolated developmental scales and tests avoided.

Table 1-9 outlines general areas of developmental observation and the average ages at which common milestones occur. Motor development tends to parallel central nervous system maturation, progressing in a cephalocaudal and proximal-to-distal direction. The disappearance of primitive reflexes must precede the appearance of volitional movements, and generalized mass activity is replaced by specific responses. Controlled use of the upper extremities precedes that of the lower extremities, and truncal coordination occurs before mastery of the extremities. In general, there is greater variation in the timing of gross motor development than in the acquisition of fine motor skills. One must remember that some of the most important aspects of developmental assessment, such as alertness, responsiveness, persistence, and concentration, defy objective scoring, whereas some of the most easily scored items, such as gross motor development in infancy, are the least reliable indicators of overall mental ability. Among objective areas of assessment, speech and language development are the best predictors of subsequent cognitive performance. However, problems in this area may also be related to a variety of factors unrelated to mental endowment.

An important aspect of the pediatric health supervision visit is the opportunity for periodic assessment of a child's overall developmental functioning. For this purpose, standardized developmental screening instruments are frequently used, such as the *Denver II*. Developmental screening implies the detection of children at high risk for otherwise unsuspected developmental problems. Screening tests are by definition not diagnostic and, when abnormal, must be followed by a thorough diagnostic evaluation. The value of a screening test lies in its ability to decrease morbidity through early detection and treatment (Sec. 1.3). Definitive diagnostic strategies and efficacious treatment programs must exist and be supported to achieve this goal. A screening test of sufficient sensitivity, specificity, and predictive value for the population in which it is to be used must be available to minimize the psychological and financial costs of identifying false positives and missing true cases. Each of these areas has provoked considerable controversy with regard to developmental screening. Most moderate to significant disabilities, rather than being identified during routine developmental screening, are suspected and diagnosed because of concerns raised by a parent, teacher, or physician in the context of an ongoing relationship with the child.

Information regarding the efficacy of intervention programs for children with a variety of developmental disabilities remains incomplete, and in many communities the availability of subsequent comprehensive diagnostic and treatment programs is limited. Much discussion has focused on the strengths and weaknesses of specific developmental screening tests. Such tests were designed to assess the likelihood of a developmental problem at one point in time. Because of the dynamic and multifactorial nature of the developmental process, it is not surprising that developmental screening tests are only weakly predictive of later developmental performance and correlate poorly with subsequent school problems or failure. The sensitivity, specificity, and predictive value of a test vary with the population to which it is applied. Considerable problems in interpretation and validity arise when a test is administered to individuals in populations significantly different from those in which the instrument was standardized. Concern has arisen especially with respect to cross-cultural applications and with the screening of developmentally "high-risk" populations, such as premature infants, not originally included in the population used to validate the screening instruments.

Despite the concerns and uncertainties, developmental screening instruments provide a measure of normative development within a given population and a useful framework on which to structure developmental observation and discussion during the health supervision visit. If a screening tool is used, one should be familiar with the specific strengths and weaknesses of the instrument chosen and consider whether its use in the intended patient population is appropriate. In evaluating developmental performance in the office, it is important to allow children to demonstrate their best effort and ability. Testing should not occur when the child is sick or frightened. Care must be taken to avoid prognosticating or labeling a child on the basis of a screening test.

The information obtained through screening tests should enhance rather than supplant broader ongoing developmental monitoring in the context of a primary-care relationship with the parents and family. Because of the limitations of developmental screening tests, the much broader, time-honored concept of developmental surveillance is receiving renewed attention and support. Surveillance, although it requires no less thorough a knowledge of normal and deviant patterns of development, relies less on developmental testing and more on continual monitoring of developmental functioning and well-being by paying attention to parental concerns and making longitudinal observations during all encounters with the child and family.

In the context of such a relationship, pediatric primary-care providers frequently face concerns regarding a child's global or selective developmental abilities. The remainder of this section addresses the initial evaluation of children with suspected developmental delay and speech/language problems. Mental retardation and specific language disorders are discussed in more depth in Secs. 5.6.3, 5.6.4 and 10.4.

1.2.2   Common Issues and Concerns

SUSPECTED DEVELOPMENTAL DELAY

Because parents more commonly overestimate rather than underestimate their child's abilities, developmental concerns should be taken seriously when expressed. Although parents of children with suspected developmental delays most often worry about the possibility of mental retardation, many factors besides inherent mental ability can affect a child's apparent developmental level. Performance can be artificially lowered if testing occurs when a child is sick, frightened, or uncooperative or if screening instruments are indiscriminately applied, as previously noted. Otherwise normal premature infants may manifest slight differences in their patterns of development, particularly with respect to gross motor skills, and may erroneously be labeled as abnormal when compared with the performance of full-term babies. Furthermore, an age correction for the extent of prematurity should be made until the child is 18 to 24 months of age. Developmental disabilities, frequently unrelated to intellectual endowment, may result from cerebral palsy, a major sensory deficit such as hearing or vision loss, specific speech

TABLE 1-9

ASPECT OF DEVELOPMENTAL ASSESSMENT AND COMMON DEVELOPMENTAL MILESTONES

Perceptions/concerns of others: parents, teachers, and other caregivers		Grasps cube against lower thumb	8–10 mo
General responsiveness and alertness		Mature cube grasp: fingertips and distal thumb	10–12 mo
Symmetry of movement		Index finger approach to small objects and finger-thumb opposition	10 mo
Use of eyes and ears		Voluntary release of objects	10 mo
Follows dangling object from midline through a range of <45°	0–1 mo	Plays pat-a-cake	9–10 mo
Follows dangling object from midline through a range of 90°	1 mo	Enjoys putting objects in and out of box	≥11 mo
		Casting objects	10–13 mo
Follows dangling object from midline through a range of 180°	3 mo	Tower of 2 cubes	13–15 mo
		Tower of 4 cubes	18 mo
Consistent conjugate gaze (binocular vision)	4 mo	Tower of 6–7 cubes	2 y
Alerts or quiets to sound	0–2 mo	Tower of 10 cubes	3 y
Lateralizes sound (turns head to sound made on level with ear)	3 mo	Good use of cup and spoon	15–18 mo
		Weight-bearing and walking	
Localizes sound well in all directions	7–10 mo	Some weight-bearing	3 mo
Tone: posture, resistance to passive movement, clonus, deep-tendon reflexes, head and truncal control		Supports most weight	6 mo
		Pulls to stand	9 mo
Primitive and postural reflexes		Walks holding onto furniture (cruising)	11 mo

	Present by	Absent by	
Moro		3–4 mo	Walks with one hand held — 12 mo
Palmar grasp		2–3 mo	Walks without help — 13 mo
Asymmetric tonic neck		2–3 mo	Walks well — 15 mo
Placing/stepping		1.5–2 mo	Runs well — 2 y
Landau	3 mo	1 y	Up and down stairs, two feet each step — 2 y
Parachute	6–9 mo		Up and down stairs, one foot per step down, two feet per step up — 3 y

Head control		Up and down stairs, one foot per step	4 y
Prone		Jumps off ground with two feet	2.5 y
Head rests on table turned to one side	1 mo	Hops on one foot	4 y
Lifts head momentarily	1 mo	Skips	5–6 y
Head up 45°	2 mo	Balances on one foot 2–3 sec	3 y
Head up 90°	3–4 mo	Balances on one foot 6–10 sec	4 y
Weight on forearms	3–5 mo	Personal/social and cognitive	
Weight on hands with arms extended	5–6 mo	Social smile	1–2 mo
Ventral suspension		Smiles at image in mirror	5 mo
Head hangs completely down	newborn	Looks after dropped toy—beginning of object permanence	6 mo
Momentarily holds head in plane of body	6 wk		
Head sustained in plane of body	2 mo	Separation anxiety/stranger awareness	6–12 mo
Maintains head beyond plane of body	3 mo	Interactive games: peek-a-boo and pat-a-cake	9–12 mo
Pull to sitting		Waves "bye-bye"	10 mo
Complete head lag, back uniformly rounded	newborn	Rolls ball to examiner	12 mo
Slight head lag	3 mo	Feeds self with cup and spoon	15–18 mo
No head lag, back straightening	5 mo	Dresses self, except for buttons in back	3 y
Lifts head off table when about to be pulled up	6 mo	Ties shoe laces	5 y
Raises head spontaneously from supine	7 mo	Autonomy and independence issues often begin	18 mo–2 y
Rolling		Parallel play	1–2 y
Rolls front to back	4–5 mo	Cooperative play	3–4 y
Rolls back to front	5–6 mo	Magical thinking and symbolic (pretend) play	18 mo–5 y
Sitting		Able to distinguish fantasy from reality	5 y
Back uniformly rounded, cannot sit unsupported	newborn	Speech and language	
Back straightening, sits with propping	5–6 mo	Cooing	2–4 mo
Back straight, sits with arms forward for support	6–7 mo	Babbles with labial consonants ("ba, ma, ga")	5–8 mo
Sits with no support	7 mo	Imitates sounds made by others	9–12 mo
Fine motor/manipulation		First words (~4–6, including "mama," "dada")	9–12 mo
Hands predominantly closed	1 mo	Understanding one-step command (with gesture)	15 mo
Hands predominantly open	3 mo	Jargon (ie, expressive, unintelligible language; recognizable words increase with age)	15–24 mo
Hand regard	3–5 mo		
Hands come together	4 mo	Vocabulary of 10–50 words	13–18 mo
Foot play	5 mo	Vocabulary of 50–75 words	18–24 mo
Voluntary grasp (no release)	5 mo	Vocabulary of 250 words	3 y
Transfers objects from hand to hand	6 mo	2-word sentences	18–24 mo
Ulnar grasp of cube	5–6 mo	3-word sentences	2–3 y
Grasps cube against thenar eminence	6–8 mo	4-word sentences	3–4 y
		5-word sentences	4–5 y

SOURCE: *Modified from Illingworth RS: The Development of the Infant and Young Child: Normal and Abnormal. New York: Churchill Livingstone, 1980, 1987. Ages are averages based primarily on data of Arnold Gesell.*

or language problems, emotional/behavioral disturbances such as autism, specific learning disabilities, a neglectful or abusive environment, or chronic illness. Many of these conditions interfere with a child's developmental performance and may present initially as developmental delay. The therapeutic and prognostic implications of differentiating these conditions are great.

When a developmental problem is suspected, a definitive diagnostic evaluation should be undertaken to determine whether a delay is truly present and, if so, whether a specific etiology can be identified with implications for prognosis, therapy, and subsequent offspring (Table 1-10). Key questions to be addressed in the evaluation are listed in Table 1-11. A comprehensive developmental assessment should be obtained by trained personnel, using a standardized age-appropriate instrument. If a developmental problem is confirmed, it is important to ascertain whether the delay is global or selective. For example, a problem primarily with language may suggest a hearing problem, inadequate environmental stimulation, or autism. An isolated motor problem may occur with neuromuscular disease, hemi- or paraplegia, or cerebral palsy. With confirmation of a delay, a complete history and physical examination are essential, as well as formal evaluation of hearing and vision. It is important to ascertain from the parents whether their child's developmental problems had a distinct age of onset, suggesting specific causal factors or etiologies, and whether any developmental regression has been noted. Slow developmental progress may be indicative of either a static or progressive process. However, developmental regression manifested by loss of previously achieved developmental milestones should always suggest a progressive neurologic disorder. The presence of prenatal, perinatal, and postnatal risk factors for subsequent developmental problems should be elicited, as well as a positive family history for similar problems.

A thorough psychosocial and behavioral assessment should also be obtained, with emphasis on exploring the caretaking environment and on the presence of any concomitant behavioral problems. Nonwillful problems such as hyperactivity, impulsivity, distractibility, and poor social interactions should be differentiated from willful behavioral problems such as tantrums, hitting, and disobedience, which may be indicative of a specific underlying behavioral etiology. Overall patterns of growth should be noted, with special emphasis on head circumference. A complete physical examination should be performed with a focus on detecting the presence of neurologic problems, dysmorphic features, congenital anomalies, and skin pigment abnormalities suggestive of neurocutaneous disorders. When congenital anomalies or dysmorphic features are identified, evaluation by a dysmorphologist skilled in the identification of specific syndromes is warranted. During the examination, the child's general alertness, curiosity, persistence, and interpersonal interactions can also be assessed.

The laboratory evaluation of a child with a confirmed developmental delay should be guided by the history and physical examination (Tables 1-10 and 1-12). Because of the deleterious effects of relatively low levels of ingested lead and its pervasive presence in our environment, children with unexplained developmental delay should be screened for lead toxicity. Thyroid studies should also be considered. A child with significant mental retardation should have chromosomal studies performed, including specific cytogenetic testing for fragile-X syndrome if clinical features are suggestive.

The routine use of neuroimaging in the evaluation of idiopathic mental retardation is controversial. The recent availability of high-

TABLE 1-10
SUSPECTED DEVELOPMENTAL DELAY: COMPONENTS OF EVALUATION

Developmental assessment
　Developmental screening/surveillance
　Definitive developmental test utilizing standardized instrument (eg, Baley Scales of Infant Development)
History
　Problem context
　　Parental concerns/problem perceptions
　　Parental expectations
　Developmental history
　　Parental recollection of milestones, problem onset
　Family history
　　Family history of developmental problems/syndromes
　Medical history
　　Prenatal care and complications: infection, toxin/drug exposure
　　Perinatal complications: problems with delivery, asphyxia, infection, CNS insults, anomalies, postpartum problems
　　Gestational age and growth parameters at birth: prematurity, SGA, microcephaly
　　Previous hospitalizations, illnesses, and surgery
　　Current medications
　Review of systems
　　Complete review of systems with emphasis on detecting symptoms of neurologic disorders (eg, seizures) and chronic illness
Psychosocial/behavioral assessment
　Caregiving environment
　Parent–child relationship
　Family stressors
　Behavioral problems: "willful," eg, tantrums, hitting, disobedience; "nonwillful," eg, hyperactivity, impulsivity, distractibility, problems with interpersonal interactions
Physical examination
　Growth parameters (esp. head circumference)
　Observations of child's interpersonal interactions, alertness, curiosity, and persistence
　Complete physical examination with emphasis on detecting neurologic abnormalities, dysmorphic features, congenital anomalies, skin pigment abnormalities
Sensory evaluation
　Hearing test
　Vision test
Laboratory evaluation
　Diagnostic tests directed by concerns raised in history and physical examination
　Newborn/infant: follow-up of state metabolic screen
　Serum lead level
　Idiopathic mental retardation:
　　Chromosomal testing (cytogenetic)
　　Testing for fragile X must be specifically requested
　　Based on clinical presentation and philosophy
　　　MRI (magnetic resonance imaging)
　　　Metabolic screen

resolution magnetic resonance imaging has increased our ability to detect varying degrees of cerebral dysgenesis and to provide parents with at least a partial explanation for their child's disability, although not necessarily the primary etiology itself. The desire to identify a specific etiology, however, must also be weighed against the cost of the test and the low likelihood of identifying specific findings with relevance to the child's subsequent treatment and prognosis. Routine screening for metabolic disorders in otherwise

TABLE 1-11

SUSPECTED DEVELOPMENTAL DELAY: KEY QUESTIONS

Developmental assessment
Is a developmental delay present?
Is the delay global or selective?
History (problem context, developmental, family, medical, review of systems)
Do caretakers perceive development to be a problem?
Was there a distinct onset to the developmental problem?
Has developmental regression been noted?
Does the history suggest a potential etiology?
Psychosocial/behavioral assessment
What is the nature of the caretaking environment?
Are significant emotional/behavioral problems present?
Physical examination
Is there physical evidence of a potential etiology?
Is growth retardation and/or microcephaly present?
Sensory evaluation
Is hearing or visual deficit present?
Laboratory evaluation
Are specific diagnostic tests warranted?

asymptomatic children with idiopathic mental retardation is generally nonproductive. Most of these conditions present with additional findings such as seizures, hypoglycemia, acidosis, vomiting, and coma. However, when the clinical situation is suggestive, appropriate metabolic screening tests should be obtained. In addition, results of state-mandated newborn metabolic screening should always be followed up in the newborn period.

While a developmental evaluation is ongoing, it is important to avoid labeling the child with terms such as "developmentally delayed," "disabled," or "mentally retarded." If an otherwise unexplained problem is confirmed by definitive testing, it should be pointed out to parents that the delay observed relates to the child's current performance and that, although the likelihood of having normal ability decreases the further a child's performance is from expected norms, present developmental tests, particularly those used during infancy and toddlerhood, are poor predictors of future performance.

Perhaps the parents' greatest concern during such an evaluation is that their child will be discovered to be mentally retarded. Mental retardation is defined as subnormal intellectual functioning statistically represented by an IQ less than 2 SD below the population mean on standardized intelligence testing and associated with co-existing delays in adaptive skills such as self-care, home living, communication, and social interactions. This corresponds to an IQ of approximately 70–75 on both the Stanford-Binet and Wechsler intelligence tests. Mild mental retardation is generally defined as an IQ of 50–70 and moderate to severe retardation as an IQ less than 50. In more recent definitions, an effort has been made to avoid categorization on the basis of IQ levels and to place greater emphasis on descriptions of functional deficits in a variety of adaptive skill areas.

Mild mental retardation occurs with an incidence of 20–30 per 1000 individuals, is often familial or polygenic, and is more frequently noted in boys and in groups of lower socioeconomic status. Identifiable chromosomal abnormalities account for only 4–8%. Although most cases of mild mental retardation are felt to be idio-

pathic, a variety of insults and pathogenic processes, such as prenatal substance exposure and postnatal lead toxicity, may be causal. By contrast, severe mental retardation occurs with an incidence of 3–4 per 1000 individuals, is typically sporadic, and although still more common in boys, shows no socioeconomic predilection. An etiology can be determined in approximately 60–70% of cases. Chromosomal abnormalities are the single largest group of etiologies detected (30%), and among these, Down syndrome, or trisomy 21, is the most frequent disorder identified. A history of central nervous system injury secondary to teratogens, infection, and prenatal, perinatal, and postnatal insults can be found in 15–20% of cases of severe mental retardation in children. Neuroradiologic imaging studies can identify another 10–15% as having significant cerebral dysgenesis. When severe mental retardation is found in the absence of other anomalies of the stigmata of a specific syndrome, this usually indicates a sporadic and nonprogressive process. Children with multiple congenital anomalies and an identifiable syndrome constitute only 4–5% of cases of severe mental retardation. However, it is important to identify these conditions through a thorough assessment of dysmorphology and family history because

TABLE 1-12

SUGGESTED INDICATIONS FOR DIAGNOSTIC OR SCREENING TESTS RECOMMENDED IN CHILDREN WITH UNEXPLAINED MENTAL RETARDATION AND SPECIFIC FINDINGS

Magnetic resonance imaging of the brain
Cerebral palsy or motor asymmetry
Abnormal head size or shape
Craniofacial malformation
Loss or plateau of developmental skills
Multiple somatic anomalies
Neurocutaneous findings
Seizures
IQ < 50
Cytogenetic studies[a]
Microcephaly
Multiple (even minor) somatic anomalies
Family history of mental retardation
Family history of fetal loss
IQ < 50
Skin pigmentary anomalies (mosaicism)
Suspected contiguous gene syndromes (eg, Prader-Willi, Angelman, Smith-Magenis)
Metabolic studies[b]
Episodic vomiting or lethargy
Poor growth
Seizures
Unusual odors
Somatic evidence of storage
Loss or plateau of developmental skills
Movement disorder (choreoathetosis, dystonia, ataxia)
Sensory loss (especially retinal abnormality)
Acquired cutaneous disorders

[a] Because of high prevalence, lack of specific clinical features, and variable developmental manifestations, some experts suggest specific cytogenetic testing for fragile X syndrome in both male and female children with otherwise unexplained mental retardation.
[b] Basic laboratory screen: fasting plasma amino acids, blood lactate, ammonia, very–long-chain fatty acids, urinary oligosaccharides/mucopolysaccharides. Further metabolic evaluation is usually directed best by a specialist.
SOURCE: *Palmer FB, Caputo AJ: Mental retardation. Pediatr Rev 1994;15:473.*

many represent single-gene disorders with important implications for parents' subsequent childbearing. Endocrine and metabolic causes of severe mental retardation account for 3–5% of cases. Mental retardation and its etiologies are discussed in more detail in Secs. 5.6.3 and 10.4.

Many physicians, as well as parents, may delay evaluation of a child for whom they have developmental concerns because they perceive that effective interventions are lacking. However, in light of the many factors that can influence developmental performance, a variety of specific treatable conditions can be detected. By performing such an evaluation, the physician also may identify conditions with important implications for the parents' future childbearing. Furthermore, although the field of developmental intervention is relatively new, and many questions remain, a growing body of data suggests that long-term, comprehensive programs that combine child-focused services with parental education and family support can effectively enhance the developmental abilities of many children with established disabilities as well as help families cope better with the varying demands of a child who is developmentally disabled. Helping parents adjust to the realization that their child has a developmental disability can be difficult. Feelings of denial, guilt, anger, and sadness are often exacerbated by the frequent underlying uncertainty regarding cause, subsequent prognosis, and risk of recurrence. Pediatric primary-care providers can provide the long-term support and coordination of care so important to these families and are in a unique position to advocate for the needs of these children and their families with schools and other outside agencies.

SUSPECTED SPEECH AND/OR LANGUAGE DELAY

Although speech and language problems frequently coexist with more global developmental delays, pediatricians are often faced with specific concerns regarding a child's progress in this area. Approximately 50% of children with delayed language development have delays in other areas. Particularly when more global problems are present, a child's language ability is highly correlated with subsequent cognitive performance. However, problems in this area can be indicative of a variety of primary language disorders and/or additional factors that are independent of intellectual endowment. The most frequent causes of inadequate language development are given in Table 1-13. These are discussed in detail in Sec. 5.6.4.

Early language development can be divided into prespeech, naming, and word-combination stages. During the prespeech pe-

TABLE 1-13
CAUSES OF INADEQUATE LANGUAGE DEVELOPMENT

Hearing problem
Mental retardation
Dysphasia (developmental language disorder)
Autistic spectrum disorder
Dysarthria
Structural problems of the oropharynx and upper respiratory tract
Elective mutism
Child abuse and neglect

riod (0–10 months), the infant learns to localize sounds, produce melodious vowel sounds (cooing), first randomly and then in a give-and-take pattern with caregivers, and, beginning around 6 months, add consonants to the vowels to make repetitive syllables (babbling). Although deaf infants will coo, progression to interactional cooing and babbling is impaired. By the end of this period, vocalizations become very interactive, and when random utterances approximate words ("dada," "mama"), positive responses from caregivers' begin to reinforce their repeated use. The naming period (10–18 months) is characterized by the rapid acquisition of names and labels for the people and objects around them as children learn the symbolic significance of language. Receptive understanding of words precedes expressive language skills. By 12 months of age, many infants understand 75-100 words, can follow simple commands (first with gestures, then without), and can vocalize several "first words." Increasingly complex babbling is interspersed with recognizable words and strung together with an intonation and cadence that resembles mature sentences (jargoning).

Pointing also becomes very important during this period as a way to obtain desired objects, gain parental attention, learn the name of a specific object, and communicate a shared experience (eg, pointing and vocalizing "Airplane!"). The word-combination period typically begins around 18 months of age. Before this time, children may use "giant word" combinations such as "Stop it" or "Let's go" and "holophrases," single words that imply a whole sentence of meaning (eg, pointing at and saying "book" to mean this book is mine). True word combinations generally occur after the child has acquired an adequate expressive vocabulary (at least 50 words). First sentences are telegraphic in nature, with prepositions, pronouns, and articles typically omitted. Vocabulary and syntax/grammar skills progress rapidly after the second year of life.

Because of the influence of individual temperament, sociocultural factors, and the child's verbal/language environment, children manifest greater variability in the acquisition of language than in other developmental areas. This is especially true with respect to expressive verbal skills. Furthermore, the pace of observable development is not constant. Parents frequently become concerned during the beginning of their child's second year of life, when the acquisition and use of new words occurs rather slowly, only to be amazed by the veritable explosion in vocabulary and comprehension that occurs during the second half of the same year. A transient and relative delay in the emergence of expressive language skills may be caused by differences in the kinds and extent of opportunities for verbal interaction encountered by children in different families. Children from bilingual families may also manifest transient delays in their expressive language and frequently combine elements of both languages in their early verbalizations. By 2 to 3 years of age, however, most of these children are able to separate the languages appropriately and use them in their respective contexts.

As children learn the patterns of their language, rules are often overgeneralized, leading to common developmental "mistakes" (eg, "sheeps" instead of sheep, "goed" instead of went), which must be differentiated from deviant language development. In general, screening instruments rely heavily on the assessment of expressive language abilities. Because of normal variability in this area, and the frequently encountered difficulties with obtaining an accurate expressive performance in an office setting, many children may be erroneously labeled as language-delayed. A longitudinal approach regarding the child's language and overall development can

TABLE 1-14

CLINICAL EVALUATION OF LANGUAGE SKILLS

AGE	RECEPTIVE SKILLS	EXPRESSIVE SKILLS	SPECIFIC INDICATION FOR REFFERRAL
0–1 mo	Recognizes sound with startle; turns to sound and looks for source; quiets motor activity to sound; "prefers" human speech with high inflection	Differentiated crying; body language of positive and negative response	No response to pleasing sound when alert; neonatal sepsis; meningitis; neonatal asphyxia; prematurity; congenital infection; familial deafness; renal abnormalities; aminoglycoside therapy
2–4 mo	Prolonged attention to sounds; responds to familiar voice; watches the speaking mouth; enjoys rattle; attempts to repeat pleasing sounds with objects; shifts gaze back and forth between sounds	"Eh, ih, uh" (hind mouth vowels); cooing, blows bubbles; enjoys using tongue and lips; reciprocal cooing; play dialogues; loudness varies	No response to pleasing sounds; does not attend to voices
5–7 mo	Seeks out speaker; localizes sounds; understands own name, familiar words; associates word with activity (e.g., bath, car)	Initiates sounds; pitch varies; babbles with labial consonants ("ba, ma, ga"); uses sounds to get attention, express feeling; sounds directed at object	Decrease or absence of vocalizations
8–12 mo	Begins word comprehension; responds to simple commands—"point to your nose," "say bye-bye"; knows names of family members; responds to a few words, those associated with specific objects	First words, five to six—"mama, dada"; inflected vocal play; repeats sounds and words made by others; "oo, ee" (foremouth vowels); intentional gestures	No babbling with consonant sounds; no response to music
13–20 mo	Single-step element commands; identifies familiar objects	Points to objects with vocalization; vocabulary of 10–50 words; pivot and open class words, rate, and content varies	No comprehension of words; does not understand simple requests
18–24 mo	Recognizes many nouns; understands simple questions	Telegraphic speech; vocabulary of 50–75 words; 20-word sentences, phrases; stuttering common	Vowel sounds, but no consonants; no words
24–36 mo	Understands prepositions; can follow story with pictures	Identifies body parts; vocabulary of 200 words; dependent on phrases, three-word sentences; uses words for expressive needs; pronouns; early grammar	No words; does not follow simple directions; no sentences
30–36 mo	Understands some syntax (difference between car hit train and train hit car); understands opposites; understands action in pictures	Sentences of four or five words, three elements; tells stories; uses "what" and "where" questions: uses negation; uses progressive and past tense, all regular form; uses plurals, regular form	Speech largely unintelligible to stranger; dropout of initial consonants; no sentences
3–4 y	Understands three-element commands	Talks about what she is doing; uses "I" with grammar by her own rules; vocabulary of 40–1500 words; speech intelligible to strangers; "why" questions; commands; uses past and present tense; passive speech in spontaneous speech; nursery rhymes; says colors, numbers 1–4, full name, sex; articulation of "m, n, p, h, and w"; four-word sentences	Speech not comprehended by strangers; still dependent on gestures; consistently holds hands over ears; speech without modulation
4–5 y	Understands four-element commands; links past and present events; decreasing ability for second language acquisition	2700-word vocabulary; defines simple words; auxiliary verbs "has" and "had"; conversation mature with "how" and "why" questions in response to others; articulation of "b, k, g, and f"; five-word sentences; "normalizes" irregular verbs and nouns; increases in accessibility of forms	Stuttering; consistently avoids loud places
5–6 y	Understand five-element commands; can follow a story without pictures; enjoys jokes and riddles; can comprehend two meanings of a single word	Correct use of all parts of speech; vocabulary 5000 words; articulation of "y, ng, and d"; six-word sentences; corrects own errors in speech, can use logic in recounting story plots	Word endings dropped; faulty sentence structure; abnormal rate, rhythm, or inflection
6–7 y	Asks for motivation and explanation of events; understands time intervals (months, seasons); right and left differences	Articulation of "l, r, t, sh, ch, dr, cl, bl, gl, and cr"; has formal adult speech patterns	Poor voice quality, articulation
7–8 y	Can use language alone to tell a story sequentially; reasons using language	Articulation of "v, th, j, s, z, tr, st, sl, sw, and sp"	
8–9 y		Articulation of "th, sc, and sh"	

SOURCE: *Dixon SD, Stein MJ: Encounters with Children. Pediatric Behavior and Development, 3rd ed. Chicago: Mosby, 2000.*

help to put concerns into perspective. Although care must be taken to avoid mislabeling normal children, the availability of effective treatments for a variety of conditions with primary or secondary effects on speech and language development makes prompt evaluation of significant and/or persistent concerns important.

Initial evaluation of a child with a suspected language delay should include direct assessment of the child's language abilities through the use of informal observation and specific language-screening instruments; a thorough developmental history and assessment; formal hearing evaluation; a complete medical, family, psychological, and behavioral history; and a thorough physical examination. Table 1-14 lists important expressive and receptive developmental language milestones as well as specific indications for further evaluation and referral.

Key findings that should prompt concern include the absence of apparent response to sound in an infant, the absence of babbling by 9-12 months of age, the absence of any words by 18 months, the absence of meaningful phrases by 24 months, speech that is largely unintelligible to strangers at 3 years, an inability to use language communicatively, and apparent difficulties with language comprehension.

To optimize the likelihood of an accurate assessment, attempts to evaluate a child's language ability should take place in a quiet, nonthreatening environment when the child is otherwise well and before other more distressing aspects of the visit are performed. Although observation of children's verbal interaction with their parents and simple toys and picture books to engage them in casual conversation can be very useful, a variety of specific language-screening instruments, such as the Early Language Milestone (ELM) scale and Clinical Linguistic Assessment Measurement (CLAM) are available for use in the office setting. These scales are designed to differentiate receptive, expressive, and mixed language disorders. It is also important to ascertain through a thorough developmental assessment whether the language delay is an isolated problem or part of more global developmental concerns.

A formal hearing assessment using behavioral or brainstem evoked response audiometry should always be performed on a child with suspected speech and language problems. Medical and familial risk factors for hearing or speech and language problems, such as prematurity, perinatal asphyxia, prolonged aminoglycoside use, known central nervous system insults, and a family history of prior syndromes or hearing and language problems should be elicited. A thorough behavioral assessment is essential, with special emphasis on detecting behaviors suggestive of autism. The nature and quality of the child's psychosocial environment should also be evaluated. Children exposed to neglectful or abusive environments frequently manifest delays in language and personal social skills disproportionate to their motor abilities. The physical examination should focus on identifying abnormal growth patterns (especially microcephaly), congenital anomalies and dysmorphism suggestive of an underlying syndrome or prenatal insult, neurologic abnormalities, ear pathology, and abnormalities of the oropharynx. The evaluation of the child with language delay and specific language disorders is discussed in greater detail in Sec. 5.6.4.

Specific therapies are available for a variety of conditions that result in inadequate speech and language development. Success in treating primary developmental language disorders depends on the type and severity of dysphasia, the age at which the diagnosis is made, and the presence of concomitant developmental, behavioral, psychosocial, and/or other medical disorders (see Sec. 5.6.4 and 25.6).

References

Bennett FC, Guralnick MJ: Effectiveness of developmental intervention in the first five years of life. Pediatr Clin North Am 38:1513–1528, 1991

Blasco PA: Pitfalls in developmental diagnosis. Pediatr Clin North Am 38:1425–1438, 1991

Colson ER, Dworkin PH. Toddler development. Pediatr Rev 18:255–259, 1997

Dixon SD, Stein MT: Encounters with Children: Pediatric Behavior and Development, 2nd ed. Chicago Year Book, 1992

Dworkin PH: British and American recommendations for developmental monitoring: The role of surveillance. Pediatrics 84:1000–1010, 1989

Dworkin PH: Developmental screening: (Still) expecting the impossible? Pediatrics 89:1253–1255, 1992

First LR, Palfrey JS: The infant or young child with developmental delay. N Engl J Med 330:478–483, 1994

Frankenburg WK, Dodds J, Archer P, Shapiro H, Bresnick B: The Denver II: A major revision and restandardization of the Denver Developmental Screening Test. Pediatrics 89:91–97, 1992

Illingworth RS: The Development of the Infant and Young Child: Normal and Abnormal. New York, Churchill-Livingstone, 1987.

Johnson CP, Blasco PA: Infant growth and development. Pediatr Rev 18:224–242, 1997

Palmer FB, Capute AJ: Mental retardation. Pediatr Rev 15:473, 1994

Sturner RA, Howard BJ: Preschool development: Part 1. Communicative and motor aspects. Pediatr Rev 18:291–301, 1997

Sturner RA, Howard BJ: Preschool development: Part 2. Psychosocial/behavioral development. Pediatr Rev 18:327–336, 1997

1.3   SCREENING

1.3.1   Overview

Much of the history and physical examination obtained at each health supervision visit is directed toward identifying undetected problems or their risk factors. Pediatricians need to be aware not only of current recommendations regarding screening and the specific tests available but also of the basic principles and concepts behind screening to evaluate whether a given program does more good than harm for their particular patients and community. Screening implies the presumptive identification of disease or its precursors in an otherwise asymptomatic individual or population and is, by definition, not diagnostic. It assumes that persons so identified will undergo definitive diagnostic testing and subsequently will benefit by earlier implementation of treatment or prevention programs. The effectiveness of a given screening program can be demonstrated by performing a randomized clinical trial in which all pertinent outcomes are evaluated. Unfortunately, such data are often lacking or difficult to obtain. In the absence of such studies, the value of a given screening program must be defined in relation to certain characteristics of the condition being screened for, the test being used, the population being evaluated, and the larger social context in which decisions regarding the value of detection and the allocation of resources are being made.

In deciding what conditions are worth screening for, one must consider both the burden of suffering caused by a particular condition, as defined by its prevalence and severity, and the availability of a specific treatment or prevention strategy that, when implemented early, results in a longer or greater benefit to the individual than would have occurred with diagnosis at the onset of symptoms. Identification of conditions for which no treatment exists, or the benefit of existing therapy is unproven, is of questionable value and potentially harmful. Even where effective interventions exist, one must weigh the potential risks and benefits of the treatment itself with that of the identified condition and consider the impact of public acceptance on compliance with screening and treatment recommendations.

The value of screening also depends on the existence of a good screening test. The accuracy of a test is defined by its sensitivity and specificity compared with gold-standard measures of the presence or absence of disease and by its positive and negative predictive value within a population with a given disease prevalence. It is important to understand how these test characteristics affect the overall value of and implementation strategies for screening programs.

The sensitivity of a test refers to the proportion of individuals with a condition who have an abnormal test result. Thus, a highly sensitive test will miss few true cases, as a high proportion of individuals with the disease will have an abnormal test. The specificity of a test refers to the proportion of individuals without disease who have a normal test result. A highly specific test will identify few false-positive results because most individuals without disease will have a normal test. Acceptable sensitivity and specificity in a screening test reflects a relative weighing of the risk of missing true cases (sensitivity) with the risk of identifying false-positive results (specificity).

The predictive value of a test is the probability of the presence or absence of disease in the presence of an abnormal or normal test result. Positive predictive value refers to the probability that, given an abnormal result, an individual actually has the condition. Negative predictive value indicates the probability of the absence of the condition in an individual whose test result is normal. Predictive value depends on the sensitivity and specificity of the screening test being used as well as on the prevalence of the disorder in the population being screened. The greater the sensitivity of a test, the greater its negative predictive value, and the greater the specificity of a test, the greater its positive predictive value. Independent of the screening test's sensitivity and specificity, diminishing population prevalence of the condition being sought diminishes the positive predictive value of the test by changing the proportion of true-to false-positive results. One should be aware of the population on which the test was standardized and whether the group to be screened is sufficiently similar that measures of predictive ability are comparable and application of the instrument is appropriate. For most screening situations, it is important to know the predictive ability of the test in a population with low disease prevalence because this is generally how screening tests are used. In many cases, selective testing of high-risk subgroups may make more sense than mass screening.

The costs associated with a screening program must be broadly defined. Costs include not only the screening itself but also the subsequent diagnostic, therapeutic, and supportive services required. The psychological impact on individuals identified as false positives and the costs involved in definitive evaluation of these individuals may be significant. Early identification through screening does not always imply a better outcome. One must question the ultimate value of the screening program if the health-care system or community is unable to provide the necessary subsequent diagnostic and therapeutic services. If persons at greatest risk do not avail themselves of the screening program, or if individuals with abnormal screening tests do not follow through with subsequent

diagnostic and therapeutic recommendations, the screening program will fail to achieve the benefits intended.

Current recommendations regarding screening during routine health supervision visits reflect an increasing awareness of the importance of these issues in deciding the value of specific screening programs. They also recognize that different strategies may be appropriate for different populations. The following section addresses specific aspects of screening during the health supervision visit. Areas of health screening unique to adolescents are discussed in Chapter 3.

1.3.2   Specific Screening Areas

NEWBORN SCREENING FOR METABOLIC DISEASES AND HEMOGLOBINOPATHIES

The number of metabolic diseases that can be diagnosed and treated in the newborn period is rapidly increasing (Chap. 9). Although all states in the United States have initiated neonatal metabolic screening programs, the absence of federal guidelines has led to considerable state-to-state variability. Currently, all states screen for congenital hypothyroidism and phenylketonuria (PKU). Two-thirds also screen for galactosemia. All of these disorders are treatable and, if not diagnosed early, lead to irreversible brain damage. To minimize the number of infants inadvertently missed by the screening program, a blood sample should be obtained on all full-term neonates just before hospital discharge. In no case should this be obtained later than 7 days of age.

Special testing arrangements must be made if birthing takes place in a nontraditional setting. Identification of some disorders, such as PKU, require sufficient build-up of metabolites to be detected. If, because of early discharge, blood was drawn before the infant was 24 hours old, a second sample should be obtained when the child is 1 to 2 weeks of age. Blood transfusions and dialysis, by introducing foreign blood cells and reducing concentrations of circulating metabolites, may result in both false-negative and false-positive results when newborns are screened for metabolic disorders and hemoglobinopathies. When feasible, samples should be obtained before these procedures. However, preterm and sick infants should be screened by 1 week of age regardless of the presence or absence of these or other factors (parenteral feeding, antibiotic use, prematurity) that may interfere with specific assays or the interpretation of test results. Where such concerns exist, a repeat sample should be obtained at a time interval appropriate to resolution of the confounding factors. It should also be remembered that, because of variability in disease presentation and the technical aspects of screening, some affected infants may test falsely normal on their initial screen. Irrespective of the results of prior screening, specific diagnostic testing should always be performed when clinical suspicions warrant.

Hemoglobinopathies occur with significant frequency and are a major cause of morbidity and mortality in this country. Sickle-cell disease alone (S, SC, and S-β-thalassemia) affects approximately 1 out of every 400 African-American newborns in the United States as well as a variety of other ethnic and racial groups. Although the technology has existed for some time, compelling support for hemoglobinopathy screening in the newborn period occurred when a significant decrease in morbidity and mortality was demonstrated for children with sickle-cell disease if diagnosis and initiation of a comprehensive treatment program, including prophylactic penicillin, was instituted before symptomatic presentation. In 1987, a National Institutes of Health (NIH) Consensus Conference on this subject recommended that each state provide universal newborn screening for hemoglobinopathies. Debate continues on the need for universal versus selective screening and on the optimal screening procedure to be used. Concern also has been raised over variability in laboratory accuracy and the adequacy of subsequent diagnostic and counseling services for individuals identified as either heterozygotes or homozygotes for these conditions. Current screening policies vary widely; both heel-stick and cord blood samples may be used. Specimens generally are examined using electrophoresis at an alkaline pH, and abnormal samples are further evaluated using acid electrophoresis.

Because of the rapid pace of change regarding newborn screening, the Committee on Genetics of the American Academy of Pediatrics periodically issues updated information for physicians regarding currently available tests and screening recommendations. Because the choice of screening test, threshold values, and implementation strategies often vary from state to state, providers should be familiar with the methodology, standards, and follow-up procedures for their regional screening program.

THE SCREENING PHYSICAL EXAMINATION

During routine health surveillance visits, a physical examination is performed for diagnostic and case-finding (screening) purposes; it also provides a useful framework for parent and child education and reassurance. Although the importance of this latter function should not be overlooked, the case-finding value of routine physical examinations, when pathology is otherwise unsuspected, is limited and may not be the most effective use of the limited time available during the well-child visit. Except in the newborn period, among high-risk populations, or in the absence of an adequate history, the primary aims of the well-child physical examination should be to assess pathology suspected by history or observation and to provide reassurance and guidance to families.

DEVELOPMENTAL SCREENING

See Secs. 1.2, 5.4.

VISION AND HEARING SCREENING

Routine vision screening is an effective way to identify otherwise unsuspected problems that are amenable to correction. Because normal visual development depends on the brain's receipt of clear binocular visual stimulation, and because the plasticity of the developing visual system is time-limited (first 6 years of life), early detection and treatment of a variety of problems impairing vision are essential to preventing permanent and irreversible visual deficits. An age-appropriate assessment should be incorporated into each health supervision visit beginning with the newborn examination. At all ages this should include a review of relevant historical information regarding visual concerns and family history, gross inspection of the eye and surrounding structures, observation of pupillary symmetry/reactivity, assessment of ocular movements, elicitation of the red reflex (to detect opacities/asymmetries in the visual axis), and age-appropriate methods to assess ocular preference and alignment and visual acuity. A successful ophthalmoscopic examination can generally be accomplished by 5 years of age.

In the infant, ocular preference and alignment and visual acuity can be grossly assessed by observing the baby's ability to visually track an object, noting any behavioral cues of an eye preference by alternately covering each eye while presenting an interesting object and observing the position and symmetry of the light reflected off the corneas when a light is held several feet in front of the eyes (corneal light reflex). Ocular alignment (conjugate gaze) should be consistently present by 4 months of age. It is especially important to assess the red reflex during infancy. Identification of an absent, defective, or asymmetric red reflex is key to the timely identification and treatment of opacities in the visual axis and many abnormalities at the back of the eye. In the toddler and preschooler, ocular preference and alignment can be additionally assessed by performing a more sophisticated unilateral cover test. This involves covering and uncovering each eye while the child is looking straight ahead at an object approximately 10 feet away. The observation of any movement of the uncovered eye when the opposite is covered or of the covered eye when the occluder is removed suggests potential ocular misalignment (strabismus) and warrants referral to an ophthalmologist for further evaluation. Regardless of the underlying etiology, strabismus that is left untreated will eventually result in cortical suppression of visual input from the nondominant eye and the absence of depth perception, making early detection and treatment critical.

By 3–5 years of age stereoscopic vision can also be assessed using the Random-dot-E stereo test or stereoscopic screening machines. Formal visual acuity testing should begin at 3 years of age using age-appropriate methods. Approximately 20% of children will have a refractive error identified, usually myopia (nearsightedness), before adulthood. Picture tests such as the LH test and Allen picture cards are most effective for screening preschoolers. By 5 years of age, most children can be successfully screened using a standard Snellen alphabet chart, the tumbling-E test, or the HOTV test. School-aged children, including adolescents, should have their acuity checked yearly. Preschoolers should be referred for further testing if the acuity in either eye is 20/40 or worse. In children 5 to 6 years of age, inability to read the majority of a 20/30 line warrants referral. At all ages, a difference of more than one line in the acuity measurements between eyes necessitates further evaluation.

Approximately 1 to 3 out of every 1000 infants are born deaf, and many children develop sensorineural hearing deficits during childhood. Timely detection of these problems allows for earlier initiation of interventions aimed at enhancing the communication, social, and educational skills of these children. Controversy has recently centered around the value of selective versus universal audiologic screening during infancy. Only half of the infants with significant hearing impairment are identified with the use of a selective screening strategy based on the presence or absence of risk factors for hearing impairment (family history of childhood hearing abnormalities; a history of congenital infection; anatomic malformations of the head, neck, or ears; birth weight less than 1500 g; a history of hyperbilirubinemia exceeding exchange levels; severe birth asphyxia; a history of bacterial meningitis; significant exposure to ototoxic medications; prolonged mechanical ventilation; and the presence of a syndrome or its stigmata associated with sensorineural hearing loss).

Currently the average age at which a child with a significant hearing problem is identified is 14 months. However, both limitations in existing screening technologies, which lead to inconsistencies in interpretation and high rates of false-positive results, and logistic problems with availability and implementation have raised concerns about the larger implications of a universal screening policy. In 1995 and again in 1999, after reviewing these issues, the American Academy of Pediatrics (AAP) endorsed a policy of universal hearing screening during infancy with the goal of identifying all infants with significant hearing impairment by 3 months of age so that intervention could be initiated by 6 months of age. Ideally, screening would take place before nursery discharge. In their 1999 statement, the AAP additionally outlined essential components of an effective universal newborn hearing-screening program. Subsequent recommendations will no doubt be influenced by prospective data addressing the overall costs and benefits of such programs.

Infants younger than 6 months of age have traditionally been screened with the use of auditory brainstem response testing (ABR). A newer physiological measure, evoked otoacoustic emissions testing (EOEA), holds promise as a simpler screening technique. However, problems with specificity (overreferral) and logistic issues with consistent use and interpretation have raised questions regarding the implementation of this method for universal screening. Some groups have advocated a two-step screening strategy whereby infants failing EOEA are referred for screening with ABR. Until a clearly superior screening method emerges, the AAP has not endorsed a specific methodology for newborn hearing screening. Children older than 6 months of age may be screened by using behavioral, auditory brainstem response, or evoked otoacoustic emissions testing. Regardless of the technique used, screening programs must be able to detect a hearing loss of 35 dB or greater in the 500-Hz to 4000-Hz region (speech frequencies), the level of deficit at which normal development of speech and language may begin to be impaired. If a hearing deficit is identified, the child should be referred in a timely manner for further evaluation and early intervention.

In addition to performing a gross hearing assessment and inquiring about hearing concerns at each well visit, the AAP endorses a policy of formal hearing screening for all children at 3, 4, and 5 years of age and every 2-3 years during adolescence. The U.S. Preventive Services Task Force does not recommend routine hearing screening for asymptomatic children beyond the age of 3 years. Risk factors warranting formal hearing screening beyond the newborn period include parental concerns regarding hearing and/or language/developmental delay; a history of bacterial meningitis; the presence of neonatal risk factors associated with progressive hearing loss; history of significant head trauma, especially involving fractures of the temporal bone; the presence of a syndrome associated with sensorineural hearing loss; significant exposure to ototoxic medications; the presence of a neurodegenerative disorder; and the diagnosis of infectious diseases such as mumps and measles that are associated with hearing loss. Because a variety of transient conditions, such as middle-ear effusion, as well as testing problems can affect the hearing evaluation of older, otherwise healthy children, the results of audiologic screening must be interpreted within the context of the child's ear-disease history and physical findings.

BLOOD PRESSURE SCREENING

Routine blood pressure screening during the well-child visit allows for the identification and potential treatment of children with persistently elevated blood pressure who are at increased risk for hypertension and its subsequent complications as adults. In a minority of patients, an underlying medical etiology may be found. Screening also provides an opportunity to evaluate and potentially modify additional cardiovascular risk factors and to provide education regarding prudent dietary and life-style choices.

In 1996, the National High Blood Pressure Education Program issued updated guidelines for pediatric blood pressure norms (Appendix C), screening, evaluation, and treatment. Blood pressure standards vary with age, gender, and body size (as reflected by height). Routine blood pressure screening at least once a year is recommended for all otherwise well children 3 years of age and older. Blood pressure measurements should also be taken in ill and potentially symptomatic children as well as in children younger than 3 years who are believed to be at increased risk for hypertension because of coexisting medical conditions.

In the child, blood pressure should be measured in the sitting position with the arm held at heart level. The width of the cuff bladder should be approximately 40% of the circumference of the upper arm at its midpoint and, when wrapped, should cover 80-100% of the circumference of the arm in order to avoid an artificially elevated reading. The cuff is inflated to approximately 20 mm Hg above the point at which the radial pulse disappears and deflated 2 to 3 mm Hg/s while the practitioner listens over the brachial artery. The level at which the first tapping sound is heard (Korotkoff sound 1, or K1) is recorded as the systolic blood pressure. The level at which all sounds disappear (K5) represents the diastolic pressure.

Normal blood pressure is defined as systolic and diastolic readings less than the 90th percentile for age and sex. High-normal and high blood pressure (hypertension) are defined, respectively, as readings between the 90th and 95th percentile and greater than or equal to the 95th percentile for age and sex, found on at least three separate occasions. Children with persistently elevated blood pressure readings (>90th percentile) warrant a thorough history and physical examination to identify underlying causal factors, end-organ damage, and concomitant cardiovascular risk factors as well as a long-term surveillance and/or treatment plan (see Sec. 22.4.5).

CHOLESTEROL AND LIPID SCREENING

Epidemiologic data support the hypothesis that atherosclerosis and coronary heart disease have their precursors in childhood and that identifiable risk factors such as hypertension, obesity, and hyperlipidemia are associated with an increased incidence of atherosclerotic disease. Serum cholesterol as well as other cardiovascular risk factors can be influenced significantly by dietary and life-style choices, and although long-term pediatric data are lacking regarding the risks and benefits of following prudent life-style recommendations during childhood, until more definitive information is available, it seems reasonable that pediatricians should provide preventive counseling to all their patients and families regarding these areas.

Controversy has centered around the value of selective versus universal cholesterol- and lipid-screening strategies for children as a part of routine pediatric health surveillance. The American Academy of Pediatrics, the American Heart Association, and the recent National Cholesterol Education Program (NCEP) report endorse a selective screening strategy for children based on the presence of a high-risk family history and, where this is unknown, the presence of additional risk factors for atherosclerotic disease. Because of the current paucity of information regarding the risks and benefits of treatment for hyperlipidemia in childhood, the costs and limitations of available screening tests, and the potential benefit of promoting healthy life-style and dietary choices to all families (see Sec. 1.4.2), these groups do not support universal cholesterol screening for children. On the basis of the NCEP report, the American Academy of Pediatrics recommends that children older than 2 years of age whose parents or grandparents have a history of early athero-

TABLE 1-15
RECOMMENDED FOLLOW-UP SERVICES, ACCORDING TO DIAGNOSTIC BLOOD LEAD LEVEL (BLL)

BLL (μg/dL)	ACTION
<10	No action required

0–14	Obtain a confirmatory venous BLL within 1 month; if still within this range,
	    Provide education to decrease blood lead exposure
	    Repeat BLL test within 3 months

15–19	Obtain a confirmatory venous BLL within 1 month; if still within this range,
	    Take a careful environmental history
	    Provide education to decrease blood lead exposure and to decrease lead absorption
	    Repeat BLL test within 2 months

20–44	Obtain a confirmatory venous BLL within 1 week; if still within this range,
	    Conduct a complete medical history (including an environmental evaluation and nutritional assessment) and physical examination
	    Provide education to decrease blood lead exposure and to decrease lead absorption
	    Either refer the patient to the local health department or provide case management that should include a detailed environmental investigation with lead hazard reduction and appropriate referrals for support services
	    If BLL is >25 μg/dL, consider chelation (not currently recommended for BLLs <45 μg/dL) after consultation with clinicians experienced in lead toxicity treatment

45–69	Obtain a confirmatory venous BLL within 2 days; if still within this range,
	    Conduct a complete medical history (including an environmental evaluation and nutritional assessment) and a physical examination
	    Provide education to decrease blood lead exposure and to decrease lead absorption
	    Either refer the patient to the local health department or provide case management that should include a detailed environmental investigation with lead hazard reduction and appropriate referrals for support services
	    Begin chelation therapy in consultation with clinicians experienced in lead toxicity therapy

≥70	Hospitalize the patient and begin medical treatment immediately in consultation with clinicians experienced in lead toxicity therapy
	    Obtain a confirmatory BLL immediately
	    The rest of the management should be as noted for management of children with BLLs between 45 and 69 μg/dL

SOURCE: *American Academy of Pediatrics, Committee on Environmental Health. Screening for elevated blood lead levels. Pediatrics 101:1075, 1998.*

sclerotic disease (a myocardial infarct, angina pectoris, positive coronary arteriogram, cerebrovascular or peripheral vascular disease, or sudden cardiac death before age 55) should be screened with a fasting (12-hour) serum lipid profile (total cholesterol, high-density lipoprotein cholesterol, triglycerides, and low-density lipoprotein cholesterol). In children whose parents have a significantly elevated blood cholesterol level (>240), a nonfasting total serum cholesterol level should be obtained, followed by the fasting lipid panel if the former is significantly elevated. When family history is unclear or unknown, or if a child presents with additional cardiovascular risk factors such as obesity, smoking, hypertension, physical inactivity, or diabetes, screening with a nonfasting total serum cholesterol may be appropriate. Selective screening, evaluation, and follow-up of children with elevated cholesterol levels, as well as familial and secondary causes of hyperlipidemia, are discussed in Sec. 9.14.

LEAD SCREENING

This country has made significant progress toward the elimination of ongoing sources of environmental lead contamination. However, lead poisoning remains a significant health problem for children in the United States. Although the use of lead-based paint was effectively banned in the 1970s, ingestion of lead-containing paint chips and dust created by the deterioration or renovation of older homes remains the primary source of lead contamination in children. Considerable attention has been focused on this issue recently because of a growing body of evidence that suggests an association between subtle neurobehavioral effects and blood lead levels previously felt to be innocuous. These studies, in combination with national data demonstrating a significant prevalence of low but po-

tentially clinically significant lead levels among U.S. children, prompted the CDC in 1991 to recommend universal blood lead screening for all children ages 6 to 72 months and to lower the intervention threshold to levels above 10 μg/dL. Since their issue, the CDC recommendations have provoked an ongoing debate regarding the risks and benefits of universal versus selective (risk-based) lead screening.

Subsequent national prevalence data have suggested that, apart from the presence of known risk factors, the likelihood of lead exposure in a given community can be predicted from local blood lead levels and housing age data. This led the CDC in 1997 to revise their screening recommendations to endorse a regional selective (risk-based) or universal screening policy based on local prevalence and housing data. Specifically, universal screening is still recommended for communities with inadequate prevalence data, for those in which ≥12% of 1- and 2-year-old children have blood lead levels ≥10μg/dL, and for those with ≥27% of their housing built before 1950. For all other communities, a targeted screening strategy based on the presence or absence of established risk factors is recommended.

Primary care providers should periodically review lead exposure risk for all children beginning at 6 months of age. Risk factors that should be assessed include (1) whether the child lives in or regularly visits a house that was built before 1950, (2) whether he or she lives in or regularly visits a house that was built before 1978 and is being or has recently been remodeled (during last 6 months), and (3) whether he or she has a sibling or playmate who has or has had an elevated blood lead level. State and local health departments may add additional questions to their routine risk assessment based on specific local conditions. Additional risk factors that have been iden-

TABLE 1-16

REVISED TUBERCULIN SKIN TEST RECOMMENDATIONS[a]

Children for whom immediate skin testing is indicated
Contacts of persons with confirmed or suspected infectious tuberculosis (contact investigation); this includes children identified as contacts of family members or associates in jail or prison in the last 5 y
Children with radiographic or clinical findings suggesting tuberculosis
Children immigrating from endemic countries (eg, Asia, Middle East, Africa, Latin America)
Children with travel histories to endemic countries and/or significant contact with indigenous persons from such countries

Children who should be tested annually for tuberculosis[b]
Children infected with HIV
Incarcerated adolescents

Children who should be tested every 2–3 y[b]
Children exposed to the following individuals: HIV infected or homeless individuals, residents of nursing homes, institutionalized adolescents or adults, users of illicit drugs, incarcerated adolescents or adults and migrant farm workers; this would include foster children with exposure to adults in the above high-risk groups

Children who should be considered for tuberculin skin testing at ages 4–6 and 11–16 y
Children whose parents immigrated (with unknown tuberculin skin test status) from regions of the world with high prevalence of tuberculosis; continued potential exposure by travel to the endemic areas and/or household contact with persons from the endemic areas (with unknown tuberculin skin test status) should be an indication for repeat tuberculin skin testing
Children without specific risk factors who reside in high-prevalence areas; in general, a high-risk neighborhood or community does not mean an entire city is at high risk; it is recognized that rates in any area of the city may vary by neighborhood, or even from block to block; physicians should be aware of these patterns in determining the likelihood of exposure; public health officials or local tuberculosis experts should help clinicians identify areas that have appreciable tuberculosis rates

Risk for progression to disease
Children with other medical risk factors, including diabetes mellitus, chronic renal failure, malnutrition, and congenital or acquired immunodeficiencies deserve special consideration; without recent exposure, these persons are not at increased risk of acquiring tuberculous infection; underlying immune deficiencies associated with these conditions theoretically would enhance the possibility for progression to severe disease; initial histories of potential exposure to tuberculosis should be included on all of these patients; if these histories or local epidemiologic factors suggest a possibility of exposure, immediate and periodic tuberculin skin testing should be considered in these patients; an initial Mantoux tuberculin skin test should be performed before initiation of immunosuppressive therapy in any child with an underlying condition that necessitates immunosuppressive therapy

[a] Bacillus Calmette-Guérin immunization is not a contraindication to tuberculin skin testing.
[b] Initial tuberculin skin testing initiated at the time of diagnosis or circumstance.
SOURCE: *Committee on Infectious Diseases, American Academy of Pediatrics: Update on tuberculosis skin testing of children. Pediatrics 97:282, 1996.*

tified include use of lead-containing folk remedies, emigration or adoption from countries with a high prevalence of lead poisoning, known exposure to lead-containing dust or soil, and parental lead exposure secondary to vocation, avocation, or remodeling. Irrespective of age or risk factors, children who exhibit pica or excessive hand-to-mouth activity or have unexplained anemia/iron deficiency, seizures, neurologic symptoms, developmental delay, abdominal pain, or other symptoms consistent with lead poisoning should also have a blood lead level drawn.

In communities where universal screening is recommended, asymptomatic children without identified risk factors should be routinely screened at 9–12 and 24 months of age. Asymptomatic children having one or more identified risk factors should be screened initially at 6 months and again at 12 months. If both of these levels are normal, the testing frequency is decreased to once a year. Recommended follow-up intervals for children whose levels are elevated are given in Table 1-15. Because of an increased potential for contamination from environmental sources, venous blood specimens are preferred over capillary (finger-stick) samples. Elevated values obtained from capillary specimens should be confirmed using venous blood testing.

SCREENING FOR IRON-DEFICIENCY ANEMIA

The recent decline in the prevalence of iron-deficiency anemia in the United States has caused a reevaluation of the standard policy of obtaining screening hematocrit or hemoglobin values on all children at 9 to 15 months, 4 to 6 years, and during adolescence. Current thinking favors a selective screening approach including infants (at 9–15 months) and adolescents (at health supervision visits) who belong to groups at increased risk for iron deficiency and any children in whom anemia is suspected by history or examination. Risk factors for iron deficiency during infancy include prematurity, low birth weight, introduction of cow's milk before 12 months of age, insufficient dietary iron intake, and low socioeconomic status. Adolescents at increased risk for iron deficiency include menstruating girls and both male and female athletes. Because of the frequent occurrence of mild transient anemia with acute illness, hemoglobin screening should not be done while the child is ill or within several weeks of a fever or infection. Hemoglobin measurements obtained by venipuncture are more accurate and reproducible than capillary hematocrits obtained by skin puncture. Abnormally low values are defined as being more than two standard deviations below the mean for children of similar age and same sex (see Sec. 19.1).

SCREENING URINALYSES AND URINE CULTURES

Although they are frequently obtained, many studies have shown that, in the absence of clinical concerns or risk factors, routine surveillance urinalyses and urine cultures are not cost-effective. The relatively frequent occurrence of minor abnormalities, such as microscopic proteinuria, are of questionable significance but, along with contaminated culture specimens, necessitate costly and inconvenient repeat urine studies. Routine screening rarely leads to detection of significant asymptomatic renal disease, and when it does, one must ask whether early detection benefits the patient more than diagnosis with the onset of symptoms. In recent years, some have stressed the benefit of establishing a normal baseline through periodic screening urinalyses or dipstick assays so that if hematuria or proteinuria subsequently develop, their duration and significance can be more easily determined. The costs associated with acquiring these background data, however, both for the individual and the population as a whole, may be quite high. In general, urine studies should be obtained when disease is suspected or when the child is at increased risk for specific renal problems.

SCREENING FOR TUBERCULOSIS

Yearly tuberculin testing is no longer recommended for all children. Although the number of cases of tuberculosis in the United States has risen in recent years, these cases continue to occur primarily within previously identified high-risk groups. In populations with a low prevalence of tuberculosis, most reactive tests reflect false-positive results, often because of cross-reactivity with nontubercular mycobacteria, leading to unnecessary treatment with isoniazid. The AAP Committee on Infectious Diseases, the American Thoracic Society, and the Centers for Disease Control currently endorse a selective screening strategy based on the presence of risk factors and/or residence in a community with a high prevalence of tuberculosis (Table 1-16).

Routine tuberculin testing is not recommended for low-risk, asymptomatic children who live in areas of low disease prevalence. Children with one or more risk factors should be screened on a regular basis, the frequency of which is determined by the degree of risk present. Children who do not have risk factors but reside in high-prevalence communities and those whose history regarding risk status is unknown or incomplete may be screened on a periodic basis at 4–6 and 11–16 years of age. In all screening situations, intradermal Mantoux testing should replace multipuncture testing, and results should be read by qualified medical personnel. Prior bacillus Calmette-Guérin vaccination is not a contraindication to tuberculin skin testing. Individuals who have received this vaccine can still acquire tuberculosis. Although some previously vaccinated individuals have a positive tuberculin skin test result, there is no reliable way to differentiate this reaction from that resulting from a natural infection with *Mycobacterium tuberculosis,* and recommendations regarding screening, test interpretation, and subsequent evaluation and treatment remain the same.

Tuberculin testing relies on the presence of skin hypersensitivity to indicate subclinical or clinical infection. Reactivity generally develops within 2 to 10 weeks of infection. Two forms of tuberculin are currently available: old tuberculin, used in the multiple-puncture tests (Tine and Mono-Vacc), and the less expensive purified protein derivative (PPD), used in intracutaneous (Mantoux) testing. Multiple-puncture tests have the advantage of easy administration but lack consistency in the amount of tuberculin delivered. Reactions cannot be accurately quantified, and the numbers of false-positive and false-negative results are significant. All positive multiple-puncture tests should be confirmed by subsequent Mantoux testing. However, some individuals may experience a booster effect when retesting occurs within 10 days to 12 months of the

previous tuberculin exposure, thereby falsely enhancing the degree of reactivity. Because of these problems, the Mantoux test should be used preferentially in tuberculosis screening, when disease is clinically suspected, and when persons known to have been exposed to tuberculosis are tested.

The intracutaneous test (Mantoux), in which a standardized dose of tuberculin (5 tuberculin units in 0.1 mL solution) is delivered intradermally using a 26-gauge needle, has the advantage of allowing quantification of the subsequent response. The Mantoux test should be read at 48 to 72 hours by tactile measurement of the margins of induration. Erythema alone does not signify a positive reaction. Test interpretation is based on the size of induration, reason for testing, and the presence or absence of other risk factors. Guidelines for interpreting test findings have been defined by the AAP, the American Thoracic Society, and the CDC (Table 1-17). This classification presumes the physician's knowledge of the child's and family's risk factors as well as the background prevalence of tuberculosis in the community. One should remember that skin testing may be negative early in the course of the disease or in the presence of anergy. A positive Mantoux test necessitates obtaining a posteroanterior and lateral chest x-ray study and investigating contacts for disease. Criteria for prophylactic and therapeutic treatment of tuberculosis are presented in Sec. 13.2.21.

TABLE 1-17

DEFINITION OF A POSITIVE MANTOUX SKIN TEST RESULT (FIVE TUBERCULIN UNITS OF PURIFIED PROTEIN DERIVATIVE) IN CHILDREN[a]

Reaction ≥5 mm
  Children in close contact with known or suspected infectious cases of tuberculosis
    Households with active or previously active cases if treatment cannot be verified as adequate before exposure, treatment was initiated after the child's contact, or reactivation is suspected
  Children suspected to have tuberculous disease
    Chest roentgenogram consistent with active or previously active tuberculosis
    Clinical evidence of tuberculosis[b]
  Children receiving immunosuppressive therapy[c] or with immunosuppressive conditions, including HIV infection
Reaction ≥10 mm
  Children at increased risk of dissemination
    Young age (<4 y)
    Other medical risk factors, including diabetes mellitus, chronic renal failure, or malnutrition
  Children with increased environmental exposure
    Born, or whose parents were born, in high-prevalence regions of the world
    Frequently exposed to adults who are HIV infected, homeless, users of illicit drugs, medically indigent city dwellers, residents of nursing homes, incarcerated or institutionalized persons, and migrant farm workers
    Travel and exposure to high-prevalence regions of the world
Reaction ≥15 mm
  Children ≥4 y of age without any risk factors

---

[a] The recommendations should be considered regardless of previous bacillus Calmette-Guérin administration.
[b] Evidence on physical examination or laboratory assessment that would include tuberculosis in the working diagnosis (ie, meningitis).
[c] Including immunosuppressive doses of corticosteroids.
SOURCE: *American Academy of Pediatrics, Committee on Infectious Diseases. Update on tuberculosis skin testing of children Pediatrics 97:282, 1996.*

References

American Academy of Pediatrics: Newborn screening for sickle cell disease and other hemoglobinopathies. Pediatrics 83:813–914, 1989

American Academy of Pediatrics, Committee on Environmental Health: Screening for elevated blood lead levels. Pediatrics 101:1072–1078,1998

American Academy of Pediatrics, Committee on Genetics: Issues in newborn screening. Pediatrics 89:345–349, 1992

American Academy of Pediatrics, Committee on Genetics: Newborn screening fact sheets. Pediatrics 98:467–472, 1996

American Academy of Pediatrics, Committee on Infectious Diseases: Screening for tuberculosis in infants and children. Pediatrics 93:131–134,1994

American Academy of Pediatrics, Committee on Infectious Disease: Update on tuberculosis skin testing of children. Pediatrics 97:282–284, 1996

American Academy of Pediatrics, Committee on Nutrition: Cholesterol in childhood. Pediatrics 101:141–147, 1998

American Academy of Pediatrics, Committee on Practice and Ambulatory Medicine, Section on Ophthalmology: Eye examination and vision screening in infants, children, and young adults. Pediatrics 98:153–157, 1996

American Academy of Pediatrics, Joint Committee on Infant Hearing: 1994 position statement. Pediatrics 95:152–156, 1995

American Academy of Pediatrics, Section on Endocrinology and Committee on Genetics, and the American Thyroid Association Committee on Public Health: Newborn screening for congenital hypothyroidism: recommended guidelines. Pediatrics 91:1203–1209, 1993

American Academy of Pediatrics, Task Force on Newborn and Infant Hearing: Newborn and infant hearing loss: Detection and intervention. Pediatrics 103:527–530, 1999

Bess FH, Paradise JL: Universal screening for infant hearing impairment: Not simple, not risk-free, not necessarily beneficial, and not presently justified. Pediatrics 93:330–334, 1994

Cadman D, Chambers L, Feldman W, Sackett D: Assessing the effectiveness of community screening programs. JAMA 251:1580–1585, 1984

Calhoun JH: Eye examinations in infants and children. Pediatr Rev 18:28–31, 1997

Centers for Disease Control and Prevention: Screening young children for lead poisoning: Guidance for state and local public health officials. Atlanta, GA: US Department of Health and Human Services, Public Health Service, 1997

Consensus Conference: Newborn screening for sickle cell disease and other hemoglobinopathies. JAMA 258:1205–1209, 1987

Dallman PR: Has routine screening of infants for anemia become obsolete in the United States? Pediatrics 80:439–441, 1987

Dodge WF, West EF, Smith EH, Bruce H III: Proteinuria and hematuria in schoolchildren: epidemiology and early natural history. J Pediatr 88:327–347, 1976

Fletcher RH, Fletcher SW, Wagner EH: Clinical Epidemiology—The Essentials. Baltimore, Baltimore: Williams & Wilkins, 1996

Kaplan RE, Springate JE, Feld LG: Screening dipstick urinalysis: A time to change. Pediatrics 100:919–921, 1997

National High Blood Pressure Education Program Working Group on Hypertension Control in Children and Adolescents: Update on the 1987 task force report on high blood pressure in children and adolescents: Pediatrics 98:649–658, 1996

National Institutes of Health: Early identification of hearing impairment in infants and young children. NIH Consensus Statement 11:1–24, 1993

Sackett DL, Haynes RB, Tugwell P, et al: Clinical Epidemiology: A Basic Science for Clinical Medicine, 2nd ed. Boston, Little, Brown, 1991.

Starc TJ, Deckelbaum RJ: Evaluation of hypercholestrolemia in children. Pediatr Rev 17:94–97, 1996

Task Force on Blood Pressure Control in Children: Report of the second task force on blood pressure control in children—1987. National Heart, Lung, and Blood Institute, Bethesda, MD. Pediatrics 79:1–25, 1987

US Preventive Services Task Force: Guide to Clinical Preventive Services, 2nd ed. Alexandria, VA, International Publishing, 1996

1.4   COUNSELING AND ANTICIPATORY GUIDANCE

1.4.1   Overview

An integral part of child health supervision is providing information, support, and anticipatory guidance to parents and children regarding a variety of age-related topics important to the health and well-being of the growing child. Parents increasingly turn to their pediatrician for the advice and support once provided by an extended family. The physician, by developing a strong long-term relationship with patients and their families, is in a unique position to respond to specific problems and concerns as they arise as well as to facilitate health promotion and disease prevention by providing and personalizing information and support.

The pediatric health surveillance visit allows for discussion of age-appropriate topics related to nutrition, daily care, behavior and development, injury prevention, family functioning, and the management of minor medical problems. Although problem prevention is an important aspect of anticipatory guidance, an equally important goal is the promotion of health and development by optimizing the parent–child relationship and encouraging positive health behaviors. Helping parents to understand the impact of the child's temperament and his or her environment on growth and development and to anticipate abilities, behaviors, and issues that typically emerge at different ages encourage an understanding of how the child is both similar to other children and unique.

Despite the potential benefits, limited and conflicting data exist regarding the optimal content, technique, and overall effectiveness of anticipatory guidance. In this era of cost containment, providers are increasingly being asked to provide tangible cost-benefit data to justify the services they provide. Further research is needed to define the most effective use of the clinician's limited time during the well-child visit and the relative roles of the physician, health educator, and other personnel in the areas of prevention and health counseling. Several general principles, however, should be kept in mind when anticipatory guidance is incorporated into child health supervision. The perceived need to cover a predetermined list of topics at each visit should not overshadow the importance of establishing a strong doctor–parent–child relationship. Advice given within the context of such a relationship can have a powerful effect on health behavior choices.

It is always important to listen to and address the immediate concerns and needs of the parent and child before going on to cover other issues. Discussion, using appropriate language and explanations, should be encouraged, and advice personalized to the resources and experience of the child and family. Emphasizing the developmental basis for age-appropriate issues, although enjoyable for some parents, is not essential to providing meaningful information and discussion. More is not always better: one should prioritize the information and not try to cover too much at each visit. It is also wise to recognize when scientific evidence regarding a particular approach or issue is limited and, therefore, to avoid being overly dogmatic or judgmental when giving advice.

One should try to learn what information and beliefs parents already have about a specific topic and to whom they turn for additional information and advice. When differences in approach or resistance to suggestions are encountered, one must decide how important the particular area is in relation to others. Making an issue over a relatively minor point may, in the long run, diminish your chances of influencing the parents on matters of importance where data are well established. Clinicians should make use of "natural" counseling moments as they occur, such as while reviewing the child's growth chart with the parents, doing the physical examination, or when a particular behavior is observed. Important information should be repeated several times during the visit. Both children and adults respond best to positive reinforcement; it is always important to recognize and acknowledge good parenting and child–parent interactions.

Primarily on the basis of a consensus of expert opinion, the American Academy of Pediatrics (Guidelines for Health Supervision III) and the National Center for Education in Maternal and Child Health (Bright Futures: Guidelines for Health Supervision of Infants, Children, and Adolescents) have issued guidelines regarding recommended anticipatory guidance content for child health supervision visits. Guidelines for Adolescent Preventive Services (GAPS) expand on issues relevant to the preventive health care needs of adolescents (Table 1-2). These areas are addressed further in Chapter 3. A condensation of suggested topics for discussion at different ages is given in Table 1-18. Selected areas of anticipatory guidance and common age-related issues are expanded on in the subsequent sections. In-depth discussions of the diagnosis and management of specific behavioral problems are addressed in Chapter 5.

1.4.2   Specific Issues and Topics

NUTRITION AND FEEDING ISSUES

Breast-Feeding

Infant feeding practices, influenced by a variety of social, cultural, scientific, and commercial factors, have varied widely over the past half-century. The availability of nutritionally sound infant formulas has given parents more flexibility and options in feeding their infant. Nevertheless, the nutritional, immunologic, and psychological advantages of breast-feeding remain compelling. The decision to breast- or bottle-feed is usually made before the baby is born and therefore is an important topic for discussion during the prenatal visit. Physicians should promote the benefits of breast-feeding by providing information, dispelling misconceptions, and helping parents to clarify their own feelings and attitudes about infant feeding. Once a decision is made, however, it is important to be supportive and nonjudgmental.

Most breast-feeding mothers who wean their infants in the first several weeks postpartum do so because of a lack of information regarding breast-feeding norms and supportive guidance in dealing with a variety of common problems. Postpartum counseling should encourage maternal confidence by providing training in correct nursing technique and anticipatory guidance regarding breast-feeding physiology, norms, and common problems. Because questions commonly arise, early follow-up counseling is especially important for parents who elect to breast-feed their infants.

The suckling newborn stimulates the mother's pituitary to release prolactin and oxytocin, which in turn stimulate the production and "let-down" of breast milk (milk ejection reflex), respectively.

Prolactin levels are maintained by adequate breast drainage and may be adversely affected by a variety of factors such as the use of certain medications, maternal fatigue, and stress. Oxytocin release and the subsequent milk ejection reflex occur in response to the infant's suckling and are facilitated by rest, warmth, a quiet conducive atmosphere, and the sight and sound of the infant. Release may be inhibited by pain, embarrassment, distraction, and fatigue. Although not all women experience a symptomatic milk ejection reflex, evidence that milk let-down has occurred include a tingling sensation in the nipples, dripping of milk before nursing or from the opposite side while nursing, relief of nipple discomfort, and uterine cramping.

During the first several days postpartum, the infant receives low-volume, antibody-rich colostrum. Suboptimal feeding routines during this time rarely interfere with ultimate breast-feeding success. However, once the mother's milk has "come in," usually 2 to 5 days after delivery, and she begins to produce a significant volume, suboptimal breast emptying or other factors that interfere with the complex hormonal balance may jeopardize the success of continued lactation. Parents who wish to supplement breast-feeding with an occasional bottle should wait several weeks until the breast-feeding pattern is well established. The mouth and tongue movements used in breast-feeding are different from, and generally more effort-intensive than, those used with an artificial nipple. Some infants may have difficulty switching back and forth or may prefer the artificial nipple once exposed to it. However, older infants who have never experienced the use of an artificial nipple also may have difficulty transitioning from the breast to the bottle if this becomes necessary or desirable.

Most women find the optimal position for nursing to be with the infant cradled at the level of the breast in front of and completely facing the mother. In this position, the mother's free hand can be used to gently squeeze the breast, making the nipple and areola more protractile. Stroking the infant's lips with the nipple stimulates the mouth to open. When this occurs, the baby should be moved gently but firmly to the breast so that the mouth covers the nipple and as much areola as possible. Once the baby is positioned, the presence of a symptomatic mild ejection reflex, slow rhythmic movements of the mandible, and audible swallowing are important indicators that the baby is getting milk. When removing the infant from the breast, the mother should gently insert a finger between the infant's mouth and the breast to break the suction and minimize nipple trauma.

Current breast-feeding philosophy discourages rigid schedules for feeding duration and timing. Nipple soreness, once believed to be caused by early prolonged suckling, is now believed to be related primarily to poor positioning and trauma when the infant is removed without suction first being broken. Over the first several days postpartum, most women work up to feedings of 10 to 15 minutes at each breast with each feed. In general, the infant will determine when the feeding is over; parents should be helped to recognize the signs of satiety. To facilitate optimal breast drainage and milk production, it is important that the infant take from both breasts at each feeding. Alternating the breast offered first, when feeding is most vigorous, is also encouraged for this reason. Intervals between demand feedings vary but average every 1.5 to 3 hours (8-12 feedings per day) during early infancy. Newborns should not go longer than 4 to 5 hours between feedings. Most infants omit one of the middle-of-the-night feedings by 2 months of age. However, because the protein composition of breast milk results in a more rapid digestion time than occurs with formula, breast-fed in-

TABLE 1-18

ANTICIPATORY GUIDANCE: SUGGESTED TOPICS AT EACH VISIT

Prenatal

Injury prevention	Safe baby furniture; car safety restraints; smoke detector; water thermostat set <120°F
Feeding/nutrition	Breast vs. bottle
Medical	Circumcision; what to expect at delivery; schedule of health supervision visits
Other	Maternal health issues; social supports; siblings

Newborn

Injury prevention	Review above. Emphasize: never leave infant unattended, use car restraints
Feeding/nutrition	Issues with breast or bottle feeding: norms, common problems
Daily care/activities	Crying, sleeping, sleep position, and SIDS; stooling patterns; bathing and skin care; hiccups, sneezing, "wet burps"
Developmental/behavioral issues	Normal reflexes (startle); individuality of infant; importance of close interaction and responding to infant's needs (cannot spoil)
Medical	Care of umbilical cord and circumcision; jaundice; how to take a baby's temperature; when and how to call the doctor: fever, vomiting, diarrhea, decreased feeding; review schedule of health supervision visits
Other	Postpartum adjustment; change in parent and family relationships; sibling reactions

2–4 Weeks

Injury prevention	Review above; bath safety; sun exposure/protection
Feeding/nutrition	Issues with breast vs bottle feeding; fluoride supplementation, if indicated
Daily care/activities	Sleep patterns; crying and "colic"; bladder and bowel habits
Developmental/behavioral issues	Emphasize infant's abilities; enjoy holding, cuddling, talking to baby (cannot spoil)
Medical	Reinforce when to call the doctor
Other	Time to themselves for parents: baby sitters; spending time with siblings; plans for substitute care if mother works outside home

2 Months

Injury prevention	Review above. Emphasize: use car restraints, protect from falls, rolling, do not leave unattended on bed or table; caution about hot liquids, burns; advise against infant walkers
Feeding/nutrition	As above; waiting to introduce solids at 4–6 mo
Daily care/activities	Sleep, crying, and bowel patterns
Developmental/behavioral issues	As above
Medical	Immunizations; URI management: bulb syringe, saline nose drops
Other	As above; child care arrangements and support

4 Months

Injury prevention	Review above. Emphasize: keep small objects out of reach
Feeding/nutrition	Introducing solid foods: iron-fortified cereal, fruits and vegetables
Daily care/activities	Sleep: night awakening; teething/drooling
Developmental/behavioral issues	As above; talk to baby; respond to vocalizations

Medical	Immunizations; management of mild gastroenteritis
Other	Parent and family functioning; child care arrangements and support

6 Months

Injury prevention	"Child-proofing" house in preparation for mobility; syrup of ipecac/Poison Control Center number; car safety; walkers and stair gates; window-guards; bathtub safety; electrical cords and outlets; burn risks
Feeding/nutrition	Issues with feeding solids; norms regarding caloric needs (volumes); introducing finger foods (7–9 mo); begin practice with cup; discourage milk or juice as pacifier or bottle to bed; discuss when to introduce cow's milk (end of first year, if possible)
Daily care/activities	Resistance to sleep: suggest favorite toy or possession (transitional objects); teething/dental care; shoes (soft, flexible)
Developmental/behavioral issues	Separation and stranger anxiety
Medical	Immunizations
Other	As above

9 Months

Injury prevention	Review above. Emphasize: toddler car restraint when ≥20 lb; ingestants, eg, small objects, peanuts, grapes, hot dogs; burns
Feeding/nutrition	Finger/table foods; self-feeding: cup and spoon practice; begin to wean from bottle; anticipate decreased food intake; introducing cow's milk
Daily care/activities	Sleep: night awakening, favorite toy or possession; shoes; dental care
Developmental/behavioral issues	Separation and stranger anxiety; vocalization, communication, imitation; social games; anticipate autonomy issues of toddler period; discipline: limit-setting, consistency, distraction
Other	Parent and family functioning; child care arrangements and support

12 Months

Injury prevention	Reinforce: syrup of ipecac/Poison Control Center number; tap water at maximum of 120°F; kitchen, stair, water, and car safety; fences, gates, and latches; burn risks
Feeding/nutrition	Table foods, weaning from bottle; decreased food intake; introducing cow's milk
Daily care/activities	As above.
Developmental/behavioral issues	Speech development; talk to baby; discuss autonomy, limit-setting, discipline; praise desired behavior (positive reinforcement); prohibitions: few but firm
Other	As above

15 Months

Injury prevention	Review above
Feeding/nutrition	Self-feeding, eats meals with family; phase out bottle use, advise against bottle in bed
Daily care/activities	As above

(continued)

TABLE 1-18   Continued

Developmental/ behavioral issues	Review indicators of toilet training readiness; discipline/temper tantrums: remove from temptation, consistency between parents, time-out, substitution, avoid reinforcing tantrum behavior, praise good behavior; read books together	**4 Years** Injury prevention	Review above. Emphasize: bicycle and pedestrian safety; water safety; car seat, booster, or seat belt; refusal of food or rides from strangers; electrical tools, fire arms, matches, and poisons; know emergency number and address; home fire safety drills
Medical	Immunizations	Feeding/nutrition	Balanced diet, social aspects of meals
Other	Parent and family functioning; child care arrangements and support; sibling rivalry	Daily care/activities	Dental care, sleep
18 Months		Developmental/ behavioral issues	Toilet training; discipline; provide interactions with other children; assign chores; limit television viewing; sexual curiosity, masturbation; nursery school, day care; issues around school, readiness assessment
Injury prevention	Review above. Emphasize: supervised play near street, in driveway; yard, pedestrian, and playground safety; dangers of climbing; never leave unattended in car or in house; unsafe toys, plastic bags and balloons	Other	Family functioning
Feeding/nutrition	Wean from bottles; good use of spoon and cup in self-feeding	**5 Years** Injury prevention	Review above
Daily care/activities	Sleep: short ritual before regular bed time, night fears, night awakening; self-comforting behaviors: thumb-sucking, masturbation, favorite toy or possession	Feeding/nutrition	Balanced diet
		Daily care/activities	Dental care, sleep
Developmental/ behavioral issues	Discipline; need for autonomy and independence; "rapproachement"—transient return to clinging behavior; may show toilet training readiness at 18–24 mo; play games: praise, show affection; read simple stories to child regularly	Developmental/ behavioral issues	School readiness: plays well with other children, normal development, endures half-day separation from home; promote interactions with other children; assign chores; discipline; sexual curiosity, masturbation
Medical	Immunizations	Medical	Immunizations
Other	As above	Other	Family functioning
24 Months		**6–8 Years**	
Injury prevention	Review above	Injury prevention	Bicycle safety; seat belts; learn to swim; child supervision when away
Feeding/nutrition	Avoid struggles about eating; discourage non-nutritious snacks; encourage social/family aspects of meals	Feeding/nutrition	Avoid junk food, maintain appropriate weight; encourage social aspects of meal time
Daily care/activities	Sleep; discuss a move to regular bed; reassure that day-napping varies; use of toothbrush	Daily care/activities	Exercise regularly; brush teeth; get adequate sleep; school and academic activities; peer interactions; family interactions
Developmental/ behavioral issues	Autonomy: do not hurry, consistent limits, present choices. Toilet learning: does child show interest and readiness, understand expectations? Curiosity about body parts; provide for play and peer contacts; imaginary friends	Developmental/ behavioral issues	Establish rules, act as role model; provide allowance; spend time with child; show interest in school; praise, encourage, show affection; limit television viewing
Other	Parent and family functioning; child care arrangements and support; sibling rivalry	Other	Library card
3 Years		**10 Years**	
Injury prevention	Review above. Emphasize: car safety restraints; street and water safety; animals and pets; teach full name, emergency number, and address	Injury prevention	Review above. Emphasize: skateboard and bicycle safety; drugs, alcohol, and tobacco; supervise potentially hazardous activities; sport safety
Feeding/nutrition	Balanced diet, avoidance of junk foods	Feeding/nutrition	As above
Daily care/activities	First dental appointment; sleep: regular bedtime and routine, napping variability	Daily care/activities	As above
Developmental/ behavioral issues	Discipline; toilet training; nursery school, day care, baby sitters: encourage out-of-home experiences, peer interactions; allow to explore, show initiative, and communicate; talk about activities with child; reserve time alone with child; limit television viewing; watch children's programs with child; masturbation; satisfy curiosity about babies, sex differences	Developmental/ behavioral issues	As above; social interactions: peers, hobbies, social skills; sex education at home, school; discuss pubertal changes; academic activities; family communications: method of resolution, limit-setting, sense of responsibility
		12 Years	
		Injury prevention	Review above
		Feeding/nutrition	Avoid junk food, maintain appropriate weight; encourage social aspects of meal time
Other	Family functioning	Daily care/activities	Exercise regularly, brush teeth, get adequate sleep; school and academic activities; sports, hobbies, and weekend jobs; peer and family interactions

(continued)

TABLE 1-18 Continued

Developmental/ behavioral issues	Discuss: rapid physical growth and sexual development, body image; sex education; establish rules, communicate with child; respect privacy, allow decision-making	**16–20 Years**	
14 Years		Injury prevention	Review above. Emphasize: responsibility for health; driving safety; substance abuse; CPR training
Injury prevention	Review above. Emphasize: risk-taking behaviors; encourage responsibility for health and health behavior choices	Feeding/nutrition	Healthy diet, maintaining appropriate weight
		Daily care/activities	School and academic activities; sports, hobbies, jobs; regular physical exercise; peer and family interactions
Feeding/nutrition	As above		
Daily care/activities	As above	Developmental/ behavioral issues	Goals and values clarification, future plans; fair rules, allow decision-making; family and peer communication; expect periods of estrangement; respect privacy; encourage independence; serve as role model; sexuality and activity, contraception and prevention of sexually transmitted diseases
Developmental/ behavioral issues	Review above. Emphasize: dating, peer pressure; sexuality		

SIDS = sudden infant death syndrome; URI = upper respiratory tract infection; CPR = cardiopulmonary resuscitation.
SOURCE: *American Academy of Pediatrics, Committee on Psychosocial Aspects of Child and Family Health. Guidelines for Health Supervision II, 2nd ed: 1988.*

fants tend to continue to feed more frequently than bottle-fed infants at this age.

Maternal pain, stress, fatigue, and anxiety can have a significant impact on the hormonal milieu necessary for effective lactation. It is important to encourage the lactating mother to get as much rest as possible and to enlist the assistance of the baby's father or other support persons in this regard. The mother's diet should be nutritious and include plenty of fluids. Suggestions to facilitate milk let-down during feedings include nursing in a quiet, comfortable place, nursing while lying down, and taking a hot shower or bath just before a feeding.

Sore nipples, engorgement, and maternal fatigue are common problems that may undermine successful breast-feeding. Nipple soreness is a frequent and almost always self-limited condition that diminishes as nipples become conditioned. It can, however, be exacerbated by improper nursing technique or factors that interfere with successful milk let-down and flow. The most frequently observed problems with technique include not using the ventral-to-ventral position, placing an insufficient amount of the surrounding areola in the mouth so that the infant grasps ineffectively and puts tension on the nipple, and forgetting to break suction before removing the baby from the breast. A warm shower or heating pad may enhance milk let-down and flow. Spreading a thin layer of breast milk on nipples and allowing them to air-dry with the help of a warm lamp facilitates healing and conditioning. Application and removal of creams and ointments with each feed may actually increase trauma and abrasion and is generally discouraged. Trying different nursing positions to vary the feeding on the less sore side and manually expressing enough milk to initiate milk let-down so that the most vigorous period of sucking is avoided may help to alleviate soreness. It is important, however, that the nursing mother not decrease feeding because of sore nipples, as this may lead, through inadequate breast drainage, to engorgement.

Engorgement refers to the uncomfortable swelling of the breasts that occurs when regular, effective breast emptying does not take place. Feedings on an engorged breast may be both painful and difficult because of decreased nipple protractility. If adequate drainage does not occur, a cycle of decreased feeding leading to increasing engorgement, involution of the milk supply, and possible mastitis can result. Engorgement can be avoided with regular, frequent nursing. If it occurs, one should counsel mothers that increasing

rather than decreasing feedings on the affected side will hasten relief. This may be facilitated initially by expressing some milk manually, or using a hand pump, until it is easier and less painful for the infant to suckle. Warm compresses to facilitate milk let-down during feeds and cool compresses between feedings may also be helpful.

Breast-feeding mothers frequently worry about whether their milk supply is adequate and whether the infant is getting enough. Not all women experience fullness or the sensation of milk let-down despite successful breast-feeding. Parents should be counseled on ways to assess indirectly whether intake is adequate, such as weight gain, signs of hydration, and satiety behavior (Table 1-19). Breast-fed infants may lose up to 10% of their birth weight before regaining it by 10 to 14 days of age. Greater or more prolonged weight loss may be a sign of feeding difficulty. During growth spurts (typically at 3, 6, and 12 weeks), the infant may transiently decrease the interval between feeds to stimulate more milk production. It is important to inform parents of this normal phenomenon so that the change is not perceived as a sign of an inadequate milk supply. The use of vitamin and fluoride supplements and the introduction of solid foods in conjunction with breast-feeding are discussed below.

The decision about when to begin weaning should take into account the needs and realities of both infant and mother. Weaning is ideally a gradual process whereby nutritive and psychological needs are increasingly provided by other sources and activities. One can begin by substituting a cup or bottle for the least-favorite

TABLE 1-19

CUES TO ASSESSING THE ADEQUACY OF BREAST-FEEDING

Nursing frequency greater than eight feeds per day
Presence of fullness before feeding and relief of fullness after feeding
Presence of symptomatic milk-ejection reflex
Audible swallowing by infant
Signs of satiation in infant after feeding
At least six wet diapers per day (normally 6-8 per day)
At least four stools per day (normally 6-10 per day)
Birth weight loss less than 10% (birth weight regained by 2 weeks of age)

breast-feeding session at the same time each day. The last feeding to be eliminated should be the one to which the child is most attached. Cuddling and holding without nursing should also be encouraged. In the somewhat older child, periods of separation from the mother and the use of distraction techniques may be helpful. A supportive bra will increase the mother's comfort during the weaning process, and maternal fluid intake should be decreased accordingly.

Formula Feeding

For parents who elect not to breast-feed, a variety of manufactured formulas are available. Parents should be informed regarding the similarities and differences between formulas, their appropriate preparation and storage, and what to expect in terms of frequency and volume of feedings.

Most common commercial formulas designed for healthy full-term infants are cow's milk–based, composed of reconstituted skim milk or skim milk with added whey protein. The source of carbohydrate is lactose (some add starch or complex carbohydrates as well). The fat content consists of a mixture of vegetable oils that are better digested and absorbed than butterfat, which is removed. The compositions of these formulas are believed to provide an adequate nutritional alternative to breast milk. Differences within this group are relatively small; in choosing among them, weight should be given to relative cost and the infant's taste preference.

Soy-protein formulas, introduced in the 1920s as hypoallergenic alternatives to cow's milk–based preparations, initially were deficient in several important nutrients. Since then they have undergone a series of refinements and are now considered to be a nutritionally satisfactory alternative to the milk-based formulas in full-term infants. Soy-based formulas have been found to contain relatively high levels of aluminum. Because of reduced renal function, use in preterm infants has raised concerns about potential aluminum toxicity and reduced skeletal mineralization because of competitive absorption with calcium. Soy-based formulas have also been associated with poorer growth rates in premature infants than that observed with cow's milk protein–based formulas. For these reasons, soy-based formulas are not recommended for preterm infants who weigh less than 1800 g. Despite their origin, soy protein–based formulas are of limited value as hypoallergenic preparations because of both the high incidence of cross-reactivity to soy protein among infants with cow's-milk protein allergy and the current availability of protein hydrolysate formulas for this purpose. The fat composition of soy formulas is similar to that of the cow's-milk group. Because the source of carbohydrate is sucrose and/or corn syrup solids, soy-protein formulas may also be useful as a transitional formula for the infant with transient lactase deficiency after a significant diarrheal illness. However, formula switching for vague constitutional and gastrointestinal symptoms, or for mild viral gastroenteritis, risks inappropriately labeling the child as sickly or allergy-prone and should be discouraged. The lack of any evidence linking gastrointestinal symptomatology with the concentration of iron in both cow's milk–and soy-based formulas should be discussed with parents and is addressed further below.

Recently, weaning formulas have been introduced designed for infants older than 6 months of age. Although these formulas provide satisfactory nutrient content, they offer no demonstrable advantage over the currently recommended combinations of breast-feeding, routine infant formula, and iron- and vitamin-containing solids for children of this age. An expanded discussion regarding the composition and rationale for the use of both routine and special infant formulas is presented in Sec. 17.3.

Most formulas can be purchased in powdered, concentrate, and ready-to-eat form. Although powdered and concentrate preparations are the least expensive, they require care in reconstituting to the appropriate concentration. Unless the family lives in an area where the water supply is potentially unsafe, sterilization of both bottle and formula is no longer necessary. Between use, bottles and nipples should be cleaned with warm, soapy water. Once opened, a can of concentrate or ready-to-eat formula should be refrigerated and used within 48 hours.

As with breast-feeding, an on-demand feeding schedule should be encouraged. Most newborns will feed 2 to 3 ounces every 2 to 3 hours and should not be allowed to go longer than 5 hours between feedings. Formula-fed infants generally lose less than 8% of their birth weight and regain birth weight by 7 to 10 days of age. After the first week, most infants take 2 to 4 ounces every 2 to 4 hours, or average approximately 150 to 200 mL/kg (2-3 oz/lb) per day. Most bottle-fed infants eliminate the middle-of-the-night feeding by 2 months of age. The 6-month-old infant should generally be taking less than 30 ounces of formula per day in combination with solids, and calories from formula should not exceed 65% of the total daily intake. It is especially important with bottle-fed infants to encourage parents to learn to distinguish the crying of hunger from that of other causes and to recognize the signs of satiety to avoid the common problem of overfeeding. Putting the older infant to sleep with a bottle should also be discouraged because of the risk of nursing-bottle caries as well as the potential for creating subsequent sleep problems, as the child is trained to associate falling asleep with feedings. Most parents begin weaning the infant from the bottle to the cup at 9 to 12 months of age.

Vitamin, Iron, and Fluoride Supplementation

The American Academy of Pediatrics does not encourage routine vitamin supplementation for otherwise healthy children who have no specific risk factors for deficiency. Because commercial formulas are fortified with vitamins and minerals, formula-fed full-term infants require no additional supplementation. Breast milk is naturally rich in vitamins A and C. Although quantitative levels of vitamin D are low, clinical rickets is uncommon in breast-fed infants. Vitamin D supplementation (400 IU/d) is recommended for the nursing infant if the mother's diet is deficient in vitamin D or the infant's sun exposure is limited because of deeply pigmented skin coloration or inadequate sunlight exposure. Vitamin B_{12} deficiency may also occur in breast-fed infants of mothers who are strict vegetarians.

If dietary iron is not provided, full-term infants begin to deplete their iron stores by 4 months of age. For all but exclusively breast-fed infants, iron supplementation from one or more sources, such as infant formula, iron-fortified cereal, or ferrous sulfate drops, should begin at 4 to 6 months of age in the full-term infant and 2 months of age in the preterm infant. Although the iron content of breast milk is lower than that of formula, full-term infants who are exclusively breast-fed require no extra source of iron because of the greater bioavailability of iron in breast milk. When solids are started and breast-milk intake is decreased, however, iron-rich foods are indicated, as with formula-fed children. Breast-fed preterm infants should receive iron-containing drops after 2 months of age. Early introduction of whole cow's milk can exacerbate iron deficiency through occult gastrointestinal blood loss and thus should be discouraged before 12 months of age. Contrary to popular belief, there is ample evidence that iron-containing formulas do not cause an increase in gastrointestinal symptoms such as constipation or gas in most children. It is wise to discuss this with parents and to explain why iron is important in their child's diet. The American Academy of Pediatrics has recently released an updated statement reaffirming the importance of iron fortification of infant formula and continues to call for the discontinued manufacture of low iron–containing preparations.

The topical and systemic use of fluoride has dramatically decreased the incidence of dental caries. Excess fluoride, however, can cause fluorosis of the enamel, a cosmetically disfiguring condition. Current recommendations regarding supplementation take into account both the age of the child and the concentration of fluoride in the local water supply (Table 1-20). Both the American Academy of Pediatrics and the American Dental Association Council on Dental Therapeutics recommend beginning fluoride supplementation, if needed, at 6 months of age. Although levels of fluoride in breast milk are low, the incidence of caries in exclusively breast-fed infants whose mothers drink fluoridated water is similar to that of formula-fed infants living in the same area. Therefore, only breast-fed infants living in areas of inadequate fluoridation need supplementation. When the toddler is assisted in brushing primary teeth, it is important to use no toothpaste or only a very small amount, as much of it is swallowed and can lead to excess fluoride intake with subsequent enamel fluorosis (see Sec. 16.3.2).

Advancing to Solids, Cow's Milk, Self-Feeding, and a Prudent Diet

Current recommendations (see Table 17-12) regarding the introduction of solid foods are based on considerations of developmental readiness, nutrient needs, and the potential for adverse reactions. In the first 4 to 6 months after birth, breast milk or infant formula provides optimal nutrition for babies, and the use of solid foods should be discouraged. Gastrointestinal enzymes are not suited to the digestion of complex carbohydrates, starches, and proteins during this time, and the immature gut, by allowing passage of macromolecules across the intestinal barrier, may predispose the infant to subsequent allergy. Although they can be force-fed, babies less than 4 months of age have a strong tongue protrusion reflex and have not yet developed the mouth and tongue movements necessary for coordinated swallowing of solid foods.

By 4 to 6 months, an infant's head and oromotor control are sufficiently developed for him or her to begin actively participating in exploring the different tastes and textures of solid food as well

as indicating hunger or satiety. Initially, the volume of food consumed is less important than the experience (usually start with a few bites to 1-2 tablespoons). Mealtimes should be safe, pleasant, relaxing, and interactive. Parents should be prepared for some fun and mess, allowing infants to explore foods with their mouth, fingers, and/or a second spoon given to them to grasp. Many begin by offering solid foods at one or two feedings each day and then advance to a schedule that gradually approaches the family's mealtimes.

The order in which foods are introduced is, to a large extent, dictated by tradition. Most parents begin with iron-fortified infant cereals and advance to strained or pureed vegetables and fruits, followed by meats and poultry. Because of concerns about the impact of gastrointestinal immaturity on the development of food allergy, it is generally recommended that substances frequently associated with allergic symptomatology, such as egg white, wheat, and fish, be introduced later. It is important to remind parents to begin new foods one at a time and to wait 3 to 5 days before adding another in order to appreciate any adverse effects. With time, a variety of foods should be offered routinely. All infants have food preferences and dislikes, which can and should be respected. However, foods previously refused should be periodically reoffered. It is important to let the infant determine when he or she has had enough and to avoid force-feeding. Among commercial baby foods, one-item foods are preferable to combination dinners. Infant preparations can also be easily and cheaply made at home by cooking foods until tender and then pureeing them with a blender, food mill, or kitchen strainer. Food can be prepared in advance and stored in meal-sized portions by freezing the puree in ice-cube trays. Babies appear to be born with a preference for sweetness, but salt is purely an acquired taste. Parents should avoid adding salt or processed sugar to their infant's food, as well as sweetened baby "desserts."

As previously mentioned, the early introduction of whole cow's milk, because of its poor iron content and potential to cause occult gastrointestinal blood loss, has been associated with iron deficiency in early infancy. Its introduction should be delayed until 12 months of age. As discussed below, when cow's milk is introduced, whole rather than low-fat or skim milk is recommended in the first 2 years of life.

By 6 to 9 months of age, most infants can sit, bring objects to their mouths, and begin holding a cup and spoon. With practice, relatively controlled use of the cup and spoon usually occurs between 15 and 18 months of age. Most infants are ready to enjoy finger foods by 7 to 9 months of age. Mature chewing skills usually are present by 18 months. In choosing what to offer, it is important to avoid large, hard, spherical, or coin-shaped items that could cause airway obstruction if aspirated. These include such foods as raw carrots, large pieces of raw apple, whole or coin-shaped slices of hot dog, whole grapes, large cookies, peanuts, and hard candy. Infants and toddlers should always be seated and observed by an adult while eating.

Ample evidence now exists that atherosclerotic disease begins in childhood. Prudent dietary practices begun early may prevent or decrease atherosclerotic morbidity in later life. However, excessive dietary fat restriction may lead to impaired growth and nutrition in the developing child. Many expert panels and groups, including the National Cholesterol Education Program, the American Academy of Pediatrics, and the American Heart Association, have issued recommendations regarding a prudent diet for children. While differing in minor detail, all emphasize the need for a varied and nutri-

TABLE 1-20
FLUORIDE SUPPLEMENTATION[a]

AGE	WATER FLUORIDE CONTENT (PPM)		
	<0.3	0.3–0.6	>0.6
Birth to 6 mo	0	0	0
6 mo to 3 y	0.25	0	0
3–6 y	0.50	0.25	0
6–16 y	1.00	0.50	0

[a] Fluoride daily doses are given in milligrams.
SOURCE: *American Association of Pediatrics, Committee on Nutrition: Fluoride supplementation for children: interim policy recommendations. Pediatrics 95:777, 1995.*

tionally balanced diet, maintaining ideal body weight, decreasing total fat intake, increasing polyunsaturated fats at the expense of saturated fats and cholesterol, and avoiding excessive salt. Children less than 1 to 2 years of age need adequate amounts of dietary fat (30-50% of daily calorie intake) for optimal growth and development. During this time, dietary fat and cholesterol should not be restricted, and whole milk should be used rather than skim or 2% milk. After age 2 years, the child should gradually be transitioned (by age 5 years) to a prudent diet containing (1) no more than 30% and no less than 20% of total calories from fat, (2) less than 10% of total calories from saturated fats, and (3) less than 300 mg per day of dietary cholesterol.

Common Toddler Feeding Issues

Parents of toddlers often become concerned about their child's dietary intake and eating habits. Worry frequently centers around the volume and variety of food consumed. It is important to inform parents that the child's rate of growth slows considerably after the first year of life, and caloric needs per pound decrease even as activity increases. Reviewing the growth chart with parents can be very reassuring. It is also important to point out that otherwise healthy (physically and psychosocially) children will not willfully starve themselves. Parents should be advised to evaluate success at meeting nutritional needs, such as sufficient intake from the various food groups, over the course of a week rather than by what is consumed at each meal. It is also important to stress to parents that normal toddler issues of autonomy and self-assertion frequently present themselves around mealtimes and that parental responses to such events often play an important role in exacerbating or preventing a subsequent feeding problem.

Several specific suggestions can be given to parents to help prevent common toddler feeding and mealtime behavior problems. Toddlers need and appreciate consistent mealtime routines and rules. However, mealtimes must not be allowed to become a battleground. Parents should strive to create a structured but pleasant and interactive atmosphere in which the social as well as the nutritional aspects of the meal can be emphasized. Families should sit down together and avoid distracting activities such as TV watching and reading during the meal. Efforts should be made to include children in table talk and to avoid long conversations between adults. The family meal is also an excellent time to find opportunities to praise the child for appropriate mealtime and/or daytime behaviors. With toddlers, it is important to give realistic portions, starting with small, achievable volumes and giving seconds rather than initially overwhelming the child with a seemingly insurmountable mountain of food. It is also helpful to provide the child with opportunities for choice while maintaining control over the more important dietary issues. Self-feeding should be allowed and encouraged, even if messy. Mealtimes should be of a finite duration (20-30 minutes): long, drawn-out battles are rarely productive. Leaving the table should not be contingent on cleaning the plate. Food not finished after the allotted time period should be removed, and except for routine between-meal snacks, parents should avoid additional feedings until the next meal. Excessive intake of liquids such as juice and milk and continual "grazing" between meals should be avoided. All toddlers will have preferred and nonpreferred foods. If a child consumes a reasonable quantity and variety of food, such preferences can be respected. However, a variety of "new" and "old" foods, including those previously rejected, should continue to be offered, and the temptation to prepare routinely a separate meal for the child should be resisted. Finally, children learn by observation: parents should model the same good eating behaviors that they wish their child to exhibit.

Such anticipatory guidance will help many parents to recognize their toddler's intake and mealtime behavior as normal and therefore to avoid inadvertently creating a subsequent feeding problem. However, the pediatric health-care provider is also frequently confronted by children for whom a significant feeding and/or mealtime behavioral problem has already arisen. The approach to the child who is failing to thrive or is obese is addressed in Sec. 1.1.2 and Secs. 5.6.11 and 24.12. The diagnosis and management of common behavioral feeding problems are discussed in Sec. 5.5.3.

SLEEP PATTERNS AND COMMON PROBLEMS

The character and patterns of sleep undergo a normal transition from infancy to adulthood that is influenced not only by neuromaturational factors but also by the child's temperament and caretaking environment. Sleep comprises two distinct states: active or REM sleep, characterized by rapid eye movements, motor movements, vocalizations, dreaming, and easy awakening; and the deeper quiet or non-REM sleep. Fifty percent of an infant's sleep time is spent in the REM state, with non-REM intervals of 50 to 60 minutes between active phases, whereas only 20% of the adult sleep cycle consists of REM sleep interspersed with 90- to 100-minute intervals of quiet sleep.

Newborns sleep approximately 18 hours per day, with sleep time distributed evenly over the day and night hours. However, sleep-wake patterns quickly become entrained to a day-night cycle because of inherent circadian rhythms and parental caregiving schedules. Between 6 and 15 months of age, most children sleep approximately 10 to 12 hours at night and take two daytime naps, each lasting more than an hour, in the midmorning and afternoon. After 15 months of age, children usually take only one nap during the day, and by 4 years of age they have discontinued napping altogether. Although there are significant individual differences, the 5-year-old requires approximately 11 hours and the 10-year-old 9.5 hours of sleep per night. Most adolescents need 8 to 9 hours of sleep each night.

By inquiring about sleep habits or problems and providing information and anticipatory guidance, pediatric primary-care providers are in a unique position to diagnose and manage as well as to prevent several common age-related sleep problems. Several excellent suggestions to help parents facilitate optimal sleep habits and prevent subsequent sleep problems in their infant and young toddler are given in Table 1-21.

Parents may inadvertently slow their early infant's entrainment to a day-night sleep schedule by providing prolonged or frequent periods of nocturnal feeding and attention. Spontaneous awakenings are normal and occur often during periods of REM sleep. The ability of infants to use internal mechanisms to return themselves to sleep usually develops around 3 to 4 months of age and is referred to as "settling." At this time an infant will begin to sleep for 6 to 8 uninterrupted hours during the night. Although the vast majority of infants "settle" by 6 months of age, some continue to have frequent and prolonged nighttime awakenings. Aside from inherent temperamental differences, several environmental factors may be involved. First, parents may misperceive the movements, vocalizations, and brief awakenings of REM sleep as indicating a

TABLE 1-21
STRATEGIES TO ENCOURAGE NIGHT SETTLING

Early infancy (birth to 4 months)
During the day, limit the duration of sleep to 3 to 4 consecutive hours
Place baby to sleep in crib in own room, if feasible
Place baby in crib sleepy but awake
Allow baby to fall asleep alone (eg, without rocking, feeding, or pacifier)
Allow baby to self-calm (eg, find his or her own thumb)
Make middle-of-the-night feedings "brief and boring"
Do not respond to normal sounds made during sleep by picking up the baby

Middle infancy (4 to 6 months)
Delay response to fussing for several minutes to allow infant opportunity to fall back asleep
Gradually reduce duration and amount of night-time feeding
Avoid unnecessary stimulation (eg, picking up) when checking on fussy infant

Later infancy (6 to 12 months)
For separation anxiety: Provide a transitional object (eg, blanket, toy) or night light; leave door to bedroom open
Provide extra reassurances and cuddling during day
Make bedtime routine pleasant, predictable, and quiet
Set firm limits after infant is put to bed (eg, "once in bed, stay in bed")
Further delay response in infant fussing, and avoid physical contact and extra stimulation
Promptly respond to nightmares and bedtime fears
Promptly reinstitute strategies after recovery from illness

SOURCE: *Algranati PS, Dworkin PH: Infancy problem behaviors. Pediatr Rev 13:16, 1992.*

need for intervention and, in attending to the infant, may inadvertently cause the child to arouse further. Frequent nighttime feedings and prolonged nocturnal attention also may encourage this pattern. Feeding at night is a learned habit after 6 to 9 months of age. Older infants who are accustomed to receiving several full feedings during the nighttime hours will be hungry and continue to awaken at these times until such feedings are gradually weaned. Infants who always fall asleep while being rocked, fed, or otherwise soothed may be unable to return themselves to sleep when normal nighttime awakening occurs and the same conditions are not present. To avoid this problem, parents should be encouraged to allow infants to fall asleep on their own in their cribs.

Toddlers frequently resist going to bed. A passion for experience and the desire for autonomy and control contribute to this behavior. At this age, transient changes in routine, such as travel or a minor illness, can frequently unravel a previously stable bedtime pattern. Normal separation issues may make going to sleep difficult for the 9- to 18-month-old child. Use of a transitional object, such as a favorite blanket or stuffed animal, that the child can take to bed may make falling and staying asleep easier. In many households, toddler bedtime struggles are the result of inconsistent, inappropriate, or nonexistent limit setting. At this age, it is especially important to have established consistent bedtime routines and rituals that provide structure and allow the child to "wind down" from more stimulating activities as well as to take charge of certain aspects of the bedtime process. Parents must also be able to assess whether expectations regarding naps, bedtime, and total sleep requirements are age-appropriate and whether illness, specific fears, or emotional stress is contributing to bedtime struggles.

During the preschool and school-age years, nighttime fears are frequent and usually transient. Potentially frightening activities, such as watching disturbing television programs or reading scary books, should be avoided, especially before bedtime. A night light or open door may also help to minimize such fears. Nightmares are also common during this period. These occur during REM sleep, typically during the latter part of the night, and frequently cause spontaneous wakening with vivid recall. Nightmares usually are easily distinguished from night terrors, which affect approximately 3- to 5% of young children (peak age 3-8 years) and occur during deepest non-REM sleep, usually in the first third of the night. During a night terror, the child appears extremely frightened and agitated and, although seemingly awake, is actually in deep sleep and difficult to arouse. On awakening, the child has no apparent memory of the event. Although frightening to parents, night terrors are believed to be self-limited and benign.

A more detailed discussion regarding the diagnosis and management of common behavioral sleep problems encountered during infancy and childhood is provided in Sec. 5.5.2.

CRYING AND COLIC

Crying is a normal physiological response to distress or discomfort and serves to alert the caretaker to the baby's needs. The quality and duration of an infant's crying may vary with the cause of distress, the temperament of the child, and the caretaking response that it elicits. According to Brazelton's study of 80 otherwise healthy middle-class infants, a 2-week-old infant cries approximately 2 hours per day. Crying tends to increase to an average of 3 hours per day at 6 weeks and then decreases to 1 hour per day by 3 months of age. Most crying occurs during the evening hours.

Many parents become concerned about what they perceive to be excessive crying in their infant. Parents' perceptions of their baby's crying may be affected by prior expectations about what is normal, the duration or character of the crying, its responsiveness to attempts at consoling, and parental functioning in the face of a variety of environmental stresses. Evaluation of such a complaint should prompt a thorough history, including a description of the character and pattern of crying, past and current attempts at management, specific parental concerns, environmental stresses, and overall parental coping. A physical examination is important to rule out any underlying medical problem and to provide reassurance to the parent.

Although there is no universally accepted definition, the term *colic* is generally used to refer to excessive, unexplained paroxysms of crying in an otherwise well-nourished, healthy infant lasting more than 3 hours per day and occurring more than 3 days per week. The crying usually occurs at the same time each day, most commonly during the evening hours, and is frequently resistant to simple soothing maneuvers. During these episodes, the infant may have excess flatus and draw the legs up to the chest, leading many parents to believe that the child is having abdominal discomfort. When present, colic typically begins during the first week of life and subsides by 3 to 4 months of age regardless of the management strategy used.

Approximately 10 to 30% of infants will be described as having colic. Although many etiologic theories have been proposed, the cause of colic is probably multifactorial. The current interactional model suggests that in most cases, excessive crying is the end result of a combination of intrinsic and extrinsic factors such as normal neuromaturational events, differences in infantile temperament, and the caretaking environment. It should be pointed out that, although evidence suggests that milk protein allergy or *lactose* intolerance may explain the symptoms in a small subset of infants diagnosed as having colic, the vast majority will not have an identifiable gastrointestinal problem. Formula switching should be discouraged without other evidence of dietary intolerance or before a variety of behavioral management techniques are tried.

Just as one etiology cannot be determined, no single intervention will be effective for all infants with colic. As described above, it is important to start with a thorough history and physical examination to reassure oneself and the parents that nothing is medically wrong and to better individualize management suggestions. Parents should also be reassured that they cannot spoil infants at this age by responding promptly to their crying and that the duration of colic is time-limited. Caretakers should be encouraged to develop a consistent set of responses to the infant's crying episodes (Table 1-22).

A variety of behavioral techniques have been proposed to help soothe the colicky baby; parents should be encouraged to find what works best for them. For some infants, decreasing stimulation by swaddling them or laying them down in a quiet, darkened room may be helpful. For others, gentle, rhythmic stimulation is most effective. This might include rocking the baby, walking while holding the baby or using a soft front carrier, offering a pacifier, putting the child in a wind-up swing, taking a ride in the car or stroller, or gently rubbing or patting the infant. Soothing sounds such as singing or other music may be helpful. Parents should be encouraged to take turns soothing their child during crying episodes and to schedule "quality time" together away from the infant.

For those infants with severe colic that appears to be unresponsive to such behavioral interventions, a trial of a non–cow's milk–based, non–lactose-containing formula (soy or protein hydrolysate formula) or a maternal milk-free diet in breast-fed infants may be

warranted. The use of pharmacologic agents, such as dicyclomine hydrochloride, remains controversial and should be avoided except in the most extreme cases, when they may be used as a temporary adjunct to behavioral techniques. Good follow-up is essential in the management of colic in order to evaluate the success of previous suggestions and to provide ongoing support. The time-limited nature of this problem is a relief to both parents and physicians. Additional discussion regarding the etiology and treatment of infantile colic is given in Sec. 5.5.1.

DISCIPLINE

Parents frequently consult pediatricians for advice regarding discipline. The health supervision visit provides an excellent opportunity to discuss age-appropriate guidelines and to help parents understand how normal developmental pressures, parenting styles, environmental factors, and individual temperamental differences interact to affect a child's behavior and socialization. Although frequently used to refer to punishment, discipline is derived from the Latin word *disciplinare,* meaning "to teach," and in its broadest definition is the structure provided by parents that helps to foster a child's sense of being a lovable and capable human being. Parents who make an effort to listen to and get to know their child and spend even a short period of uninterrupted "special" time with their child each day are conveying to them the powerful message that they are loved and important. By showing interest and caring, complimenting good behavior, providing consistent, appropriate limits, and setting a good example, parents can best shape their child's behavior and conscience according to their own values and practices. Punishment, when necessary, should be age-appropriate, close in time to the misbehavior, and not physically or psychologically destructive. Corporal punishment is not only less effective than positive reinforcement but is also potentially harmful and teaches children that physical aggression is an acceptable means of dealing with anger.

Contrary to common belief, infants less than 4 months of age cannot be "spoiled," and parents should be encouraged to respond to their child's needs with unrestricted nurturing and care. By 4 to 6 months of age, infants can begin to use crying in manipulative ways, for which behavior modification techniques may be helpful. Care must be taken not to inadvertently reinforce behaviors such as frequent nocturnal awakening or feeding by providing excessive nighttime attention. Setting limits becomes important for the older infant and beyond, and verbal or nonverbal expression of disapproval is an effective form of punishment for this and older age groups. At all ages, verbal disapproval is most effective when combined with positive instruction regarding appropriate behavior alternatives and should focus on the misbehavior rather than personally belittling the child.

Parental use of "I" statements, which express how a parent feels about or is affected by a specific observed behavior, minimizes the likelihood that the child will overgeneralize the criticism. The older infant and early toddler may respond to constructive distraction or redirecting techniques, which have the added advantage of being able to be used preventively.

As the naturally curious child develops mobility, parents must take responsibility for structuring an environment that not only is safe but also minimizes temptations for misadventure. Parents who accomodate their playing toddler's need for frequent brief verbal and nonverbal contact may prevent an escalation of negative attention-seeking behavior, which can occur when a parent is otherwise

---

TABLE 1-22
STRATEGIES TO MANAGE FUSSY PERIODS DURING EARLY INFANCY

To diminish the amount of crying and fussing
Carry and cuddle frequently during both fussy and nonfussy periods
Respond promptly to baby's cry, and do not worry about "spoiling" infant
Help baby to become a self-soother (example: help baby to find own thumb or a comfortable body position)

Develop a routine series of responses to soothe baby (examples)
Pick up baby
Change diaper if soiled
Cuddle
Offer feeding if last feeding was more than 2 hours ago
Burp
Offer a pacifier
Check to see that baby is neither too hot nor too cold and that clothing or diaper is not constricting
Place baby in a swing or crib rocker or carry in a front pack
Turn on music or heartbeat simulator
Go for a walk or ride in the car
Put baby in crib and allow to cry and fuss
Repeat routine

SOURCE: *Algranati PS, Dworkin PH: Infancy problem behaviors. Pediatr Rev 13:16, 1992.*

preoccupied. Toddlers often have difficulty with shifts in their routine or abrupt transitions from one activity to the next and, when possible, should be given advance warning of such changes. Providing the toddler with the opportunity to make choices among acceptable options (eg, clothing, food) allows the child to express positively his or her growing need for control and independence. Negativism and temper tantrums are common expressions of the toddler's struggle for autonomy and self-control. Harmless behaviors such as tantrums, sulking, and whining frequently can be averted by redirecting the child or forestalling excessive fatigue and hunger, and are most effectively extinguished by ignoring them.

A child who is engaging in harmful or potentially harmful behavior may need to be removed from the situation manually. The technique of "time-out," described below, is an effective method for dealing with harmful or disruptive behavior. From an early age, it is also important to help children recognize and verbalize their feelings rather than act them out physically. Preschoolers and older children often respond to natural and logical consequences whereby, within the bounds of safety, they learn by experiencing the negative natural or social consequences of their actions. For example, the child who is late for dinner is confronted by a plate of cold food, toys that are mishandled are removed, and the child who spills juice helps to clean it up. Family conferences that permit the child to participate in discussion and negotiation are important when rules are established for older school-aged children and adolescents. Delaying privileges until other less pleasurable tasks are completed, negotiating contracts regarding expected behavior and responsibilities, and "grounding," whereby privileges are removed as a consequence of rule infractions, are also frequently effective for the older child.

"Time-out" is an effective method for extinguishing harmful or disruptive behavior and works by temporarily withdrawing social interaction. It may be used as early as 9 to 12 months of age and should begin being phased out by 5 to 6 years of age. A time-out location, such as a chair in the corner where the child can be observed but that is devoid of interesting distractions, should be chosen in advance. Caregivers should agree on a limited number of specific behaviors that will result in a time-out and apply these rules consistently. When a preagreed behavior warranting time-out occurs, parents should give one warning, then ask the child to go to the time-out location if the behavior persists. No warning is necessary for physically aggressive behavior. The child who does not go voluntarily may need to be guided there manually. Parents should attempt to maintain a perspective of calm control and avoid engaging in angry lecturing or negotiations when applying time-out. Out-of-control behavior initially may be exacerbated by attempts to establish control. However, consistency and persistence are essential to the success of this technique. The length of time-out should be brief, approximately 1 minute for every year of life up to a maximum of 5 minutes. Use of a kitchen timer may be helpful. A child who leaves the time-out location prematurely should be calmly returned, and the clock restarted. It is not important that the child be quiet, only that he or she stay in time-out. Occasionally it may be necessary to gently restrain the child from behind in the chair or other time-out location for the prescribed duration while minimizing conversation and interaction. When the time period is over, the child should be verbally released from time-out and welcomed back into the social setting without further mention of the previous infraction. After time-out, it is important to help the child learn socially acceptable alternative behaviors and, as

TABLE 1-23

CHARACTERISTICS OF COMMON NONFATAL UNINTENTIONAL INJURIES REQUIRING EMERGENCY ROOM TREATMENT

AGE GROUP	COMMON MECHANISMS	COMMON LOCATIONS	COMMON PRODUCTS
Preschool	Falls Struck by object Cutting, piercing Burns Poisoning Foreign body Animal bites	House and yard	Home structures Home furnishings Playground equipment Home-cleaning products Pharmaceuticals House plants Cosmetics and personal care products Nursery equipment Toys
School-age	Falls Struck by object Sports[a] Cutting, piercing Bicycle (non-MV) Animal bites	School and schoolyard Playground Street and sidewalk House and yard	Home structures Bicycles Sports and recreational equipment
Adolescent	Sports[a] Cutting, piercing Struck by object Falls MV occupant Overexertion[b]	School and schoolyard Street and sidewalk Playing field House and yard	Bicycles Sports and recreational equipment Home structures

[a] Sports injuries are largely sprains and fractures.
[b] "Overexertion" includes injury from lifting, pulling, and twisting.
MV = motor vehicle.
SOURCE: *Widome MD: Pediatric injury prevention for the practitioner. Curr Probl Pediatr 21:428, 1991.*

TABLE 1-24
OFFICE-BASED COUNSELING FOR INJURY PREVENTION

All children should grow up in a safe environment.

Anticipatory guidance for injury prevention should be an integral part of the medical care provided for all infants and children.

In addition to below, all physicians caring for children should counsel parents in age-appropriate, season-appropriate, and locality-appropriate prevention strategies that reduce common serious injuries. Medical records should reflect this counsel.

Infants and preschoolers

Physicians caring for infants and preschool children should advise parents about the following issues:

- Traffic safety: appropriate use of currently approved child safety restraints (car seats); parental use of their own seat belts.
- Burn prevention: installation and maintenance of smoke detectors in home; setting of hot-water heater temperature between 120 and 130°F, or lower.
- Fall prevention: use of window and stairway guards/gates in place; use of infant walkers discouraged.
- Poison prevention: storage of medicines/household products out of sight and reach and in original childproof containers; storage of 1-oz bottle of syrup of ipecac at home for use as advised by pediatrician.
- Choking prevention: provision of age-appropriate foods; avoidance of running/playing during eating; supervision of mealtime; use of age-appropriate toys.
- Drowning prevention: supervision of infant/young child in bathtub or wading pool; emptying of all buckets, tubs, wading pools immediately after use; installation of appropriate fencing/safety guards with swimming pools; supervision of preschool-aged child while swimming (irrespective of child's swimming ability).
- Cardiopulmonary resuscitation (CPR) training: training of parents in CPR; knowledge of how to access local emergency care system.

School-aged children

Physician advice to parents of elementary school–aged children begins to be more focused on the child's behavior. The child is included in this process as well, while the parents are reminded of their need to model safe behaviors.

- Traffic safety: use of seat belts/booster seats; knowledge of safe pedestrian practices; use of approved bicycle helmets when cycling and protective equipment for in-line skating/skate boarding.
- Water safety: provision of swimming instruction for children older than 5 years of age; knowledge of appropriate rules for water play; supervision of swimming; use of personal flotation devices with boating activities.
- Sports safety for adults who supervise children participating in organized sports: importance of appropriate safety equipment and physical conditioning.
- Firearm safety: removal of any handguns in the home. (If parents choose to keep a firearm, gun must be unloaded and both gun and ammunition must be kept in separate locked cabinets.)

Adolescents

Injury prevention advice to adolescents should be included in a broader discussion of healthy life-style choices (eg, alcohol/drug use, sexual activity, diet/physical activity). Specific areas of injury prevention guidance should include the following:

- Traffic safety: use of seat belts; role of alcohol in teenage motor vehicle accidents; use of motorcycle/bicycle helmets; use of protective equipment for in-line skating and skateboarding.
- Water safety: alcohol use in water-related activities; use of approved personal flotation devices when boating.
- Sports safety: importance of proper safety equipment and physical conditioning for adolescents participating in organized sports programs.
- Firearm safety: knowledge of unique dangers of in-home firearms during adolescence—risk of impulsive, unplanned use resulting in suicide, homicide, or other serious injuries. (If parents choose to keep a firearm, unloaded gun and ammunition must be kept in separate locked cabinets.)

SOURCE: Modified and reproduced, with permission, from *American Academy of Pediatrics, Committee on Injury and Poison Prevention: Office-based counseling for injury prevention. Pediatrics 94:566, 1994.*

---

soon as possible, to recognize and compliment positive behavior. Disruptive behavior is discussed further in Sec. 5.6.1.

SAFETY AND INJURY PREVENTION

Unintentional and intentional injuries are responsible for more childhood morbidity and mortality than all other diseases and conditions combined. Perhaps not surprisingly, toddlers and adolescents are at highest risk for injury-related morbidity and mortality.

Data from the National Center for Health Statistics (1993-1995) show that more than three-fourths of all unintentional injury-related deaths among infants less than 1 year of age are caused by suffocation (44%), motor vehicle accidents (21%), fires/burns (11%), and drowning (8%). Among preschoolers, motor vehicle accidents (30%), fires (22%), drowning (21%), suffocation (7%), and pedestrian injuries (5%) account for 85% of such deaths. Over half of all unintentional injury-related deaths in the school-age years result from motor vehicle accidents (53%), with fires/burns and drowning causing 14% and 12%, respectively. Among adolescents aged 10 to 14, motor vehicle accidents (41%), homicide (16%), and suicide (12%) cause more than three fourths of all injury-related

deaths, with motor vehicle accidents alone causing 57% of those that were unintentional. Motor vehicle accidents (39%), homicide (30%), and suicide (18%) are also the leading causes of death from injury (and death overall) among 15- to 24-year-olds. Among those deaths that were unintentional, motor vehicle accidents were responsible for 75% of injury-related death in this age group. Such mortality statistics underestimate the frequency of injuries that less frequently result in death. Common nonfatal unintentional injuries for each age group are listed in Table 1-23.

Many people believe that injuries are random, unavoidable events and that children who incur them are simply "accident-prone." However, an increasing body of data suggests that with appropriate personal, community, and/or legislative action, many injuries can be either prevented or diminished in severity. Furthermore, although certain behavioral and environmental characteristics may be associated with higher rates of injury, most injuries occur to children without such risk factors.

Recent epidemiologic data suggest that prevention efforts have had a significant impact on lowering the incidence of some unintentional injuries in children. However, recent years have also witnessed an alarming increase in intentional injury and violence within the pediatric population. Homicide and suicide are currently the

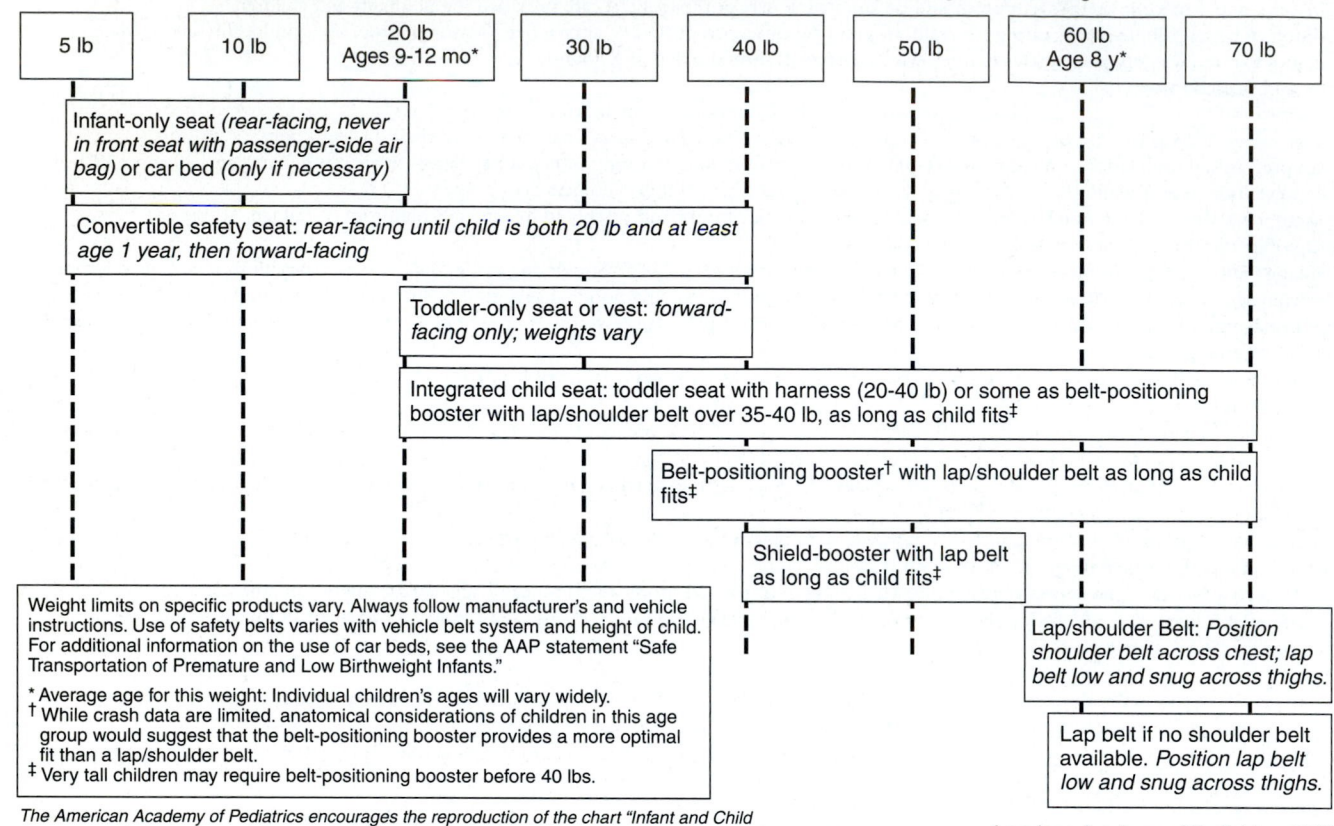

FIGURE 1-5 **Recommendations for selecting and using appropriate car safety seats for growing children.**

second and third leading causes of death among adolescents. Children and teens are increasingly confronted with violence in their homes, schools, communities, and larger society. The causes of these trends are complex and multifactorial. However, disintegration of traditional social networks and institutions, socioeconomic inequities, lack of appropriate adult role models or guidance regarding nonviolent conflict resolution and tolerance of differences, media glorification of violence as entertainment, and the availability of handguns and other weapons all contribute to the growing problem with violence.

The pediatrician is in a unique position to help prevent injuries, both as an advocate for safety legislation and as a resource and counselor for prevention strategies in which both individual families and communities can engage. Prompting parents to translate this information into preventive action and changes in behavior presents a key challenge to the primary-care provider. Individuals are much more likely to engage in preventive behaviors if they feel personally susceptible to a given problem and believe that they can decrease their risk by modifying behavior. It is easier to move people to take single actions such as buying a car seat, installing a smoke detector, or turning down the temperature on the hot water heater than to engage in regular or frequent action such as the consistent, appropriate use of car restraints. The amount of effort, decrease in com-

fort, and cost associated with a particular prevention strategy also affect how widely it is adopted. At the health surveillance visit, providing an all-inclusive list of potential safety hazards to parents is less important than focusing on the most prevalent problems at each age and attempting to facilitate preventive action by personalizing the information provided. An integrated approach to injury prevention involving both individual counseling and community-based action has a greater chance of success than either approach alone.

The American Academy of Pediatrics recommends that all parents be counseled regarding the safety measures outlined in Table 1-24, which focus on the major causes of accidental death and injury in childhood. The American Academy of Pediatrics has recently released updated recommendations regarding the selection and use of car safety seats for infants and children (Fig. 1-5). In addition to these specific topics, the AAP suggests regular discussion during the health supervision visit of age-, season-, and locality-appropriate safety issues and corresponding prevention strategies. Suggested safety topics to cover at each visit are given in Table 1-18.

A developmental approach to counseling allows the pediatrician to emphasize normal age-related variations in cognitive, motor, and perceptual skills that significantly affect the frequency and kinds of problems children encounter. It is no surprise that infants 1 to 2 years of age have the highest rates of accidental injury. At this age, the child's insatiable desire for experience and autonomy coupled with difficult impulse control may outstrip cognitive or motor abilities, increasing the risk of accidental injury. Recently acquired mobility, a pincer grasp, and an enjoyment of oral exploration also put children of this age at increased risk. With the achievement of object permanence, the infant and toddler will actively search for objects and, as they begin to learn about cause and effect, may engage in dangerous behavior in an attempt to recreate a particularly fascinating event. Children at this age cannot understand or foresee the consequences of their actions and require parents to provide a safe environment, firm limit-setting, and appropriate supervision. These remain important for preschoolers who, immersed in magical, egocentric, prelogical thinking, have difficulty understanding that cause and effect is not a function of their own desires and intentions. Three-year-olds may believe that just by not intending or wanting something to happen, they can avoid an undesirable outcome of their actions. At this age, fantasy and reality may sometimes be confused. Preschoolers are, in general, unable to empathize with others who might be hurt by their actions. An inability to generalize or learn from past experiences is also common during this period.

To the school-aged child, peer-group identification and acceptance become increasingly important. Dangerous or irresponsible behavior may arise out of a desire to be accepted by, or to not "lose face" within, a peer group. In challenging themselves to do things on their own, children at this age may overestimate their skills and competence. During this period, children develop the capacity for concrete operational thinking and understand the concept of rules, although they may often challenge them, believing that they know more than their parents. It is important to allow school-aged children to be involved in the rule-making process and, within the constraints of safety, to learn from experience and gradually increasing responsibility.

After toddlers, adolescents have the highest rate of injury-related death during childhood. Intentional (suicide, homicide, violent assault) as well as unintentional injuries (motor vehicle accidents) are responsible for the majority of morbidity and mortality in this age group. Feelings of invulnerability, susceptibility to peer pressure, a need to establish independence, and high rates of substance experimentation and use all contribute to these problems. Adolescent risk-taking behavior is discussed in more depth in Sec. 3.2.1.

References

Adair RH, Bauchner H: Sleep problems in childhood. Curr Probl Pediatr 23:147–170, 1993

Agran P, Winn D, Anderson C: Child occupant protection in motor vehicles. Pediatr Rev 18:413–423, 1997

American Academy of Pediatrics, Committee on Injury and Poison Prevention: Office-based counseling for injury prevention. Pediatrics 94:566–567, 1994

American Academy of Pediatrics, Committee on Injury and Poison Prevention and Committee on Fetus and Newborn: Safe transportation of premature and low birth weight infants. Pediatrics 97:758–760, 1996

American Academy of Pediatrics, Committee on Injury and Poison Prevention: Selecting and using the most appropriate car safety seats for growing children: Guidelines for counseling parents. Pediatrics 97:761–763, 1996

American Academy of Pediatrics, Committee on Nutrition: The use of whole cow's milk in infancy. Pediatrics 89:1105–1109, 1992

American Academy of Pediatrics, Committee on Nutrition: Fluoride supplementation for children: Interim policy recommendations. Pediatrics 95:777, 1995

American Academy of Pediatrics, Committee on Nutrition: Cholesterol in childhood. Pediatrics 101:141–147, 1998

American Academy of Pediatrics, Committee on Nutrition: Soy protein-based formulas: Recommendations for use in infant feeding. Pediatrics 101:148–153, 1998

American Academy of Pediatrics, Committee on Nutrition: Iron fortification of infant formulas. Pediatrics 104:119–123, 1999

American Academy of Pediatrics, Committee on Psychosocial Aspects of Child and Family Health: Guidance for effective discipline. Pediatrics 101:723–728, 1998

American Academy of Pediatrics, Committee on Psychosocial Aspects of Child and Family Health: Guidelines for Health Supervision III. Elk Grove Village, IL, American Academy of Pediatrics, 1994

American Academy of Pediatrics, Work Group on Breastfeeding: Breastfeeding and the use of human milk. Pediatrics 100:1035–1039, 1997

Blum NJ, Carey WB: Sleep problems among infants and young children. Pediatr Rev 17:87–93, 1996

Brazelton TB: Crying in infancy.Pediatrics 29:579–588, 1962

Green M, ed: Bright futures: Guidelines for Health Supervision of Infants, Children, and Adolescents (rev ed). Arlington, VA, National Center for Education in Maternal and Child Health, 1998

Howard BJ: Discipline in early childhood. Pediatr Clin North Am 38:1351–1369, 1991

McIntosh BJ: Spoiled child syndrome. Pediatrics 83:108–115, 1989

Neifert M: Early assessment of the breastfeeding infant. Contemp Pediatr 13:142–163, 1996

Rivara FP: Pediatric injury control in 1999: where do we go from here? Pediatrics 103:883–888, 1999

Rivara FP, Grossman DC, Cummings P: Injury prevention (first of two parts). N Engl J Med 337:543–548, 1997

Rivara FP, Grossman DC, Cummings P: Injury prevention (second of two parts). N Engl J Med 337:613–618, 1997

Slusser W, Powers NG: Breastfeeding update 1: Immunology, nutrition, and advocacy. Pediatr Rev 18:111–119, 1997

Slusser W, Powers NG: Breastfeeding update 2: Clinical lactation management. Pediatr Rev 18:147–161, 1997

US Preventive Services Task Force: Guide to Clinical Preventive Services, 2nd ed. Alexandria, VA, International Medical Publishing, 1996

1.5   IMMUNIZATIONS

1.5.1   Overview

Routine immunization has dramatically decreased morbidity and mortality from a variety of infectious diseases and has become an important aspect of pediatric preventive health care. Although the value of such programs is well established, the field is a dynamic and rapidly changing one. The number of infectious diseases against which children can be effectively immunized has grown significantly in recent years. Currently, children are routinely immunized against 11 infectious diseases (Table 1-25). All are examples of active immunization, whereby live attenuated or inactivated organisms, their components, or their products are administered to the recipient to stimulate a protective immunologic response. The Committee on Infectious Diseases of the American Academy of Pediatrics (Red Book) and the Advisory Committee on Immuni-

TABLE 1-25
ROUTINE CHILDHOOD VACCINES: ROUTE AND DOSE

VACCINE	TYPE	ROUTE	DOSE

DTaP/DT/Td/DTwP
  D = diptheria
  T = tetanus
  aP = acellular pertussis
  wP = whole-cell pertussis
  d = reduced amt. toxoid
	Toxoids (D and T)
	Bacterial components (aP)
	Inactivated whole bacteria (wP)
		Intramuscular	0.5 mL

HbCV *Hemophilus influenzae* type b conjugate vaccine	Bacterial polysaccharide conjugated to protein	Intramuscular	0.5 mL

Poliovirus vaccines
  OPV = oral
  IPV = inactivated
	Live viruses of all three serotypes
	Inactivated viruses of all three serotypes
		Oral
		Subcutaneous
			Unit dose
			0.5 mL

MMR
  M = measles
  M = mumps
  R = rubella
	Live viruses	Subcutaneous	0.5 mL

HBV (hepatitis B)	Plasmid-derived viral antigen	Intramuscular	Varies with preparation and recipient's age
Varicella	Live viruses	Subcutaneous	0.5 mL
PCV Pneumococcal conjugate vaccine	Bacterial polysaccharides conjugated to nontoxic diphtheria toxin	Intramuscular	0.5 mL

zation Practices of the US Public Health Service (MMWR) both regularly publish updated recommendations, which differ only in minor ways regarding the administration and schedule of routine immunizations. These guidelines offer a current standard of care, which is subject to change as our knowledge continues to evolve (Tables 1-26 and 1-27).

To maximize efficacy and minimize toxicity, recommendations regarding schedule, dose, route, and site of administration should be followed for each immunization. Subcutaneous and intramuscular injections are usually given in the anterolateral upper thigh in infants and, when muscle mass is sufficient, in the deltoid area in children and adults. The buttock should be avoided as a site of injection because of the potential for sciatic nerve damage and inconsistent intramuscular deposition. For intramuscular injections in infants and children, a 20- or 22-gauge $\frac{5}{8}$- to $1\frac{1}{4}$-inch needle is used, whereas in adults, the standard needle length is $1\frac{1}{2}$ inches. Subcutaneous injections are administered using a 25-gauge $\frac{5}{8}$- to $\frac{3}{4}$-inch needle for all ages. To avoid accidental intravascular injection, it is important to pull the syringe plunger back and observe for blood return before injecting any substance.

The value of a given vaccine depends on the prevalence and severity of the disease targeted, the vaccine's ability to prevent or ameliorate this disease, and the incidence and severity of vaccine-related morbidity. With the dramatic decrease in morbidity and mortality brought about by current immunization practices, attention has increasingly focused on potential adverse effects of the vaccines themselves. In addition to the active immunizing antigen(s), vaccines contain a variety of other materials, including suspending fluids such as saline or complex tissue culture, preservatives, stabilizers, antibiotics to prevent bacterial overgrowth, and adjuvants, which enhance immunogenicity.

All of these components may contribute to local and systemic side effects attributed to the vaccine. Although rare, anaphylactic

allergic reactions are most frequently caused by egg antigens in the suspending fluid of vaccines prepared in embryonated egg (influenza, yellow fever), antibiotics used to prevent bacterial overgrowth (streptomycin, neomycin, and polymixin B in IPV, OPV; neomycin in MMR, varicella, and rotavirus; amphotericin B in rotavirus), and gelatin, which is used as a stabilizer (MMR, varicella, yellow fever). Individuals with a history suggestive of an anaphylactic reaction to any of the above components should undergo skin testing to determine the safety of subsequent immunizations with these vaccines.

Several currently available preparations of childhood vaccines contain minute quantities of a mercury-containing compound called thimerosal, which has been used since the 1930s as a bactericidal agent (all DTP, several DTaP, Hib, and HB preparations). Although no clinically apparent adverse effects have been noted with recommended doses, the fact that with immunization some infants less than 6 months of age may accumulate mercury levels exceeding federal guidelines has raised recent concern regarding the potential for more subtle central nervous system toxicity. Vaccine manufacturers are currently working to eliminate mercury-containing preservatives from all vaccines. In the interim, because the adverse consequences of wild-type infections far exceed any known risk of exposure to thimerosal-containing vaccines, the American Academy of Pediatrics (AAP) and the Advisory Committee on Immunization Practices (ACIP) of the United States Public Health Service recommend that children continue to be vaccinated with thimerosal-containing preparations if mercury-free preparations are not available (see hepatitis B section for suggested minor modifications in timing of first dose).

Many side effects, such as local tenderness, low-grade fever, and allergic reactions, can be attributed directly to the vaccine because of their temporal relationship, frequency, and unique presentations. These adverse reactions, whether common or rare, are predictable

TABLE 1-26

RECOMMENDED CHILDHOOD IMMUNIZATION SCHEDULE

United States, January - December 2001

Vaccines[1] are listed under routinely recommended ages. Bars indicate range of recommended ages for immunization. Any dose not given at the recommended age should be given as a "catch-up" immunization at any subsequent visit when indicated and feasible. Ovals indicate vaccines to be given if previously recommended doses were missed or given earlier than the recommended minimum age.

Age ▶ Vaccine ▼	Birth	1 mo	2 mos	4 mos	6 mos	12 mos	15 mos	18 mos	24 mos	4-6 yrs	11-12 yrs	14-18 yrs
Hepatitis B[2]		Hep B #1										
			Hep B #2			Hep B #3					Hep B[2]	
Diphtheria, Tetanus, Pertussis[3]			DTaP	DTaP	DTaP		DTaP[3]			DTaP	Td	
H. Influenzae type b[4]			Hib	Hib	Hib	Hib						
Inactivated Polio[5]			IPV	IPV		IPV[5]				IPV[5]		
Pneumococcal Conjugate[6]			PCV	PCV	PCV	PCV						
Measles, Mumps, Rubella[7]						MMR				MMR[7]	MMR[7]	
Varicella[8]						Var					Var[8]	
Hepatitis A[9]										Hep A — in selected areas[9]		

Approved by the Advisory Committee on Immunization Practices (ACIP), the American Academy of Pediatrics (AAP), and the American Academy of Family Physicians (AAFP).

1. This schedule indicates the recommended ages for routine administration of currently licensed childhood vaccines, as of 11/1/00, for children through 18 years of age. Additional vaccines may be licensed and recommended during the year. Licensed combination vaccines may be used whenever any components of the combination are indicated and its other components are not contraindicated. Providers should consult the manufacturers' package inserts for detailed recommendations.

2. *Infants born to HBsAg-negative mothers* should receive the 1st dose of hepatitis B (Hep B) vaccine by age 2 months. The 2nd dose should be at least 1 month after the 1st dose. The 3rd dose should be administered at least 4 months after the 1st dose and at least 2 months after the 2nd dose, but not before 6 months of age for infants.

   Infants born to HBsAg-positive mothers should receive hepatitis B vaccine and 0.5 mL hepatitis B immune globulin (HBIG) within 12 hours of birth at separate sites. The 2nd dose is recommended at 1-2 months of age and the 3rd dose at 6 months of age.

   Infants born to mothers whose HBsAg status is unknown should receive hepatitis B vaccine within 12 hours of birth. Maternal blood should be drawn at the time of delivery to determine the mother's HBsAg status; if the HBsAg test is positive, the infant should receive HBIG as soon as possible (no later than 1 week of age).

   All children and adolescents who have not been immunized against hepatitis B should begin the series during any visit. Special efforts should be made to immunize children who were born in or whose parents were born in areas of the world with moderate or high endemicity of hepatitis B virus infection.

3. The 4th dose of DTaP (diphtheria and tetanus toxoids and acellular pertussis vaccine) may be administered as early as 12 months of age, provided 6 months have elapsed since the 3rd dose and the child is unlikely to return at age 15-18 months. Td (tetanus and diphtheria toxoids) is recommended at 11-12 years of age if at least 5 years have elapsed since the last dose of DTP, DTaP or DT. Subsequent routine Td boosters are recommended every 10 years.

4. Three *Haemophilus influenzae* type b (Hib) conjugate vaccines are licensed for infant use. If PRP-OMP (PedvaxHIB® or Com Vax® [Merck]) is administered at 2 and 4 months of age, a dose at 6 months is not required. Because clinical studies in infants have demonstrated that using some combination products may induce a lower immune response to the Hib vaccine component, DTaP/Hib combination products should not be used for primary immunization in infants at 2, 4 or 6 months of age, unless FDA-approved for these ages.

5. An all-IPV schedule is recommended for routine childhood polio vaccination in the United States. All children should receive four doses of IPV at 2 months, 4 months, 6-18 months, and 4-6 years of age. Oral polio vaccine (OPV) should be used only in selected circumstances. [See *MMWR. Morb Mortal Wkly Rep.* May 19, 2000/49(RR-5);1-22].

(continued)

TABLE 1-26   Continued

6. The heptavalent conjugate pneumococcal vaccine (PCV) is recommended for all children 2-23 months of age. It also is recommended for certain children 24-59 months of age. [See *MMWR. Morb Mortal Wkly Rep.* Oct. 6, 2000/49(RR-9);1-35].

7. The 2nd dose of measles, mumps, and rubella (MMR) vaccine is recommended routinely at 4-6 years of age but may be administered during any visit, provided at least 4 weeks have elapsed since receipt of the 1st dose and that both doses are administered beginning at or after 12 months of age. Those who have not previously received the second dose should complete the schedule by the 11-12 year old visit.

8. Varicella (Var) vaccine is recommended at any visit on or after the first birthday for susceptible children, i.e. those who lack a reliable history of chickenpox (as judged by a health care provider) and who have not been immunized. Susceptible persons 13 years of age or older should receive 2 doses, given at least 4 weeks apart.

9. Hepatitis A (Hep A) is shaded to indicate its recommended use in selected states and/or regions, and for certain high risk groups; consult your local public health authority. [See *MMWR. Morb Mortal Wkly Rep.* Oct. 1, 1999/48(RR-12);1-37].

For additional information about the vaccines listed above, please visit the National Immunization Program Home Page at http://www.cdc.gov/nip/ or call the National Immunization Hotline at 800-232-2522 (English) or 800-232-0233 (Spanish).

SOURCE: From: *American Academy of Pediatrics, Committee on Infectious Diseases: Recommended childhood immunization schedule–United States, January–December 2001. Pediatrics 3:202–203, 2001.*

TABLE 1-27

RECOMMENDED IMMUNIZATION SCHEDULES FOR CHILDREN NOT IMMUNIZED IN THE FIRST YEAR OF LIFE*○

RECOMMENDED TIME/AGE	IMMUNIZATION(S)[†]	COMMENTS
Younger Than 7 Years		
First visit	DTaP, Hib,[‡] HBV, MMR	If indicated, tuberculin testing may be done at same visit. If child is 5 y of age or older, Hib is not indicated in most circumstances.
Interval after first visit		
1 mo (4 wk)	DTaP, IPV, HBV, Var[§]	The second dose of IPV may be given if accelerated poliomyelitis immunization is necessary, such as for travelers to areas where polio is endemic.
2 mo	DTaP, Hib,[‡] IPV	Second dose of Hib is indicated only if the first dose was received when younger than 15 mo.
≥8 mo	DTaP, HBV, IPV	IPV and HBV are not given if the third doses were given earlier.
Age 4–6 y (at or before school entry)	DTaP, IPV, MMR[‖]	DTaP is not necessary if the fourth dose was given after the fourth birthday; IPV is not necessary if the third dose was given after the fourth birthday.
Age 11–12 y	See Table 1-26	
7–12 Years		
First visit	HBV, MMR, dT, IPV	
Interval after first visit		
2 mo (8 wk)	HBV, MMR,[‖] Var,[§] dT, IPV	IPV also may be given 1 mo after the first visit if accelerated poliomyelitis immunization is necessary.
8–14 mo	HBV,[¶] dT, IPV	IPV is not given if the third dose was given earlier.
Age 11–12 y	See Table 1-26	

* Table is not completely consistent with all package inserts. For products used, also consult manufacturer's package insert for instructions on storage, handling, dosage, and administration. Biologics prepared by different manufacturers may vary, and package inserts of the same manufacturer may change. Therefore, the physician should be aware of the contents of the current package insert. Vaccine abbreviations: HBV indicates hepatitis B virus; Var, varicella; DTaP, diphtheria and tetanus toxoids and acellular pertussis; Hib, *Haemophilus influenzae* type b conjugate; IPV, inactivated poliovirus; MMR, live measles-mumps-rubella; dT, adult tetanus toxoid (full dose) and diphtheria toxoid (reduced dose), for children 7 years of age or older and adults.

† If all needed vaccines cannot be administered simultaneously, priority should be given to protecting the child against the diseases that pose the greatest immediate risk. In the United States, these diseases for children younger than 2 years usually are measles and *Haemophilus influenzae* type b infection; for children older than 7 years, they are measles, mumps, and rubella. Before 13 years of age, immunity against hepatitis B and varicella should be ensured. DTaP, HBV, Hib, MMR, and Var can be given simultaneously at separate sites if failure of the patient to return for future immunizations is a concern. For further information on pertussis and poliomyelitis immunization, see the respective sections.

‡ See *Haemophilus influenzae* vaccine section.

§ Varicella vaccine can be administered to susceptible children any time after 12 months of age. Unimmunized children who lack a reliable history of varicella should be immunized before their 13th birthday.

‖ Minimal interval between doses of MMR is 1 month (4 wk).

¶ HBV may be given earlier in a 0-, 2-, and 4-month schedule.

○ See Pneumococcal conjugate vaccine section for recommendations regarding this vaccine.

SOURCE: From: *American Academy of Pediatrics. In Pickering LK, ed. 2000 Red Book: Report of the Committee on Infectious Diseases. 25th ed. Elk Grove Village, IL, American Academy of Pediatrics; 2000.*

and unavoidable. The relationship between vaccination and other uncommon but naturally occurring events, such as seizures, mental retardation, and encephalopathy, is much less well established. Such outcomes, if sometimes vaccine-related, occur against a background of indistinguishable idiopathic events, making differentiation between a temporal and a causal relationship difficult. Current standards regarding valid and nonvalid contraindications to specific vaccinations are given in Table 1-28.

In recognition of the fact that some persons may be adversely affected by their participation in mass immunization programs, and to provide some stability to vaccine supply and cost in the face of escalating liability litigation, the US Congress passed the National Childhood Vaccine Injury Compensation Act in 1986. This Act, which was amended in 1987 and became effective in 1988, establishes an optional no-fault system of compensation with mandatory initial approach for a predefined list of possible vaccine-related reactions. The Act also requires that all physicians and health-care workers who administer vaccines comply with new guidelines regarding record-keeping, centralized reporting of potential vaccine reactions, and distribution of standardized pamphlets describing risks and benefits to vaccine recipients and their parents. The American Academy of Pediatrics's *Red Book* should be consulted for more detailed information.

The following section provides specific information about each of the childhood vaccines routinely recommended in the United States. Many other vaccines are available and recommended for use in selected populations based on increased susceptibility or potential for morbidity (eg, influenza, pneumococcus) and/or the likelihood of exposure (eg, meningococcus, hepatitis A, yellow fever, typhoid, rabies for international travelers). The reader is referred to the American Academy of Pediatrics' *Red Book* and the Centers for Disease Control and Prevention's *Morbidity and Mortality Weekly Report* for detailed information regarding the use of these vaccines. In addition, the CDC maintains an excellent web site with up-to-date international travel information regarding regional vaccine recommendations, current infectious disease outbreaks, and other helpful travel tips (CDC Travel Home Page: *http://www.cdc.gov*).

1.5.2 Specific Vaccines

DIPHTHERIA, TETANUS, WHOLE-CELL PERTUSSIS (DTwP) AND DIPHTHERIA, TETANUS, ACELLULAR PERTUSSIS (DTaP)

The DTwP is composed of diphtheria toxoid, tetanus toxoid, and inactivated whole *Bordetella pertussis* cells. Since 1991, several vaccines substituting acellular for whole-cell pertussis (DTaP) became available. These contain one or more pertussis antigens but little or no endotoxin. Because acellular pertussis preparations are associated with fewer side effects than whole-cell vaccine, the DTaP is currently the preferred vaccine for both primary and booster doses. Single-antigen products, combinations of diphtheria and tetanus toxoids, and combined DTwP or DTaP/*Haemophilus influenzae* type b (Hib) vaccines are also available. Adults and children 7 years of age and older are not given pertussis vaccine because potential morbidity from wild-type disease is greatly diminished by this age. Because of enhanced local reactivity, these individuals also receive a booster vaccine containing 10% of the concentration of diphtheria toxoid (Td) given to younger children.

With all preparations, a dose of 0.5 mL is delivered intramuscularly using needle sizes and sites as described above. The recommended DTaP/Td immunization schedule for children vaccinated at standard and nonstandard ages is given in Tables 1-26 and 1-27. The primary series consists of three doses of DTaP separated by 4- to 8-week intervals beginning at 6 weeks to 2 months of age (usually at 2, 4, and 6 months). A fourth primary dose is given 6 to 12 months after the third (usually at 15-18 months of age), and a fifth (booster) dose between 4 and 6 years of age. The fifth dose is not necessary if the fourth dose was administered after the fourth birthday.

Several acellular products are available for use. Until data confirm the interchangeability of these products, it is recommended that the same vaccine be used for at least the first three doses. If this information is unknown, or the previous product is not available, immunization should continue with any of the licensed acellular vaccines. Additional booster doses with Td are recommended at 11-12 years of age (not later than 16 years of age) and every 10 years thereafter. If the child is 7 years or older when vaccination is instituted, a primary series is given consisting of two Td separated by 4 to 8 weeks, followed by a third dose 6 to 12 months after the second. Booster doses are required every 10 years as above. The DTP can be given concurrently (different sites) with all other routine childhood immunizations without diminishing antibody responses. Studies of the immunologic response and side effects to DTP vaccination in premature infants would support the approach of ignoring gestational age and beginning immunization at the usual chronologic age.

Common side effects of the DTwP, which are attributed primarily to the whole-cell pertussis component, include local redness, swelling, and pain at the site of injection and systemic reactions such as low to moderate fever, fretfulness, drowsiness, vomiting, and anorexia. The incidence of local reactions and fever associated with DTwP administration appears to increase with the number of doses given, whereas the likelihood of other minor systemic reactions decreases. For any given child, however, the risk of a mild systemic reaction is greater with subsequent doses if it occurred with the first. Giving prophylactic acetaminophen (15 mg/kg) at the time of DTwP administration has been shown to decrease the incidence and severity of local reactions and fever.

More serious but less frequent systemic events have also been reported in relation to administration of the whole-cell DTwP vaccine including persistent inconsolable crying for more than 3 hours, temperature greater than 40.5°C, hypotonic-hyporesponsive episodes, convulsions with or without fever, encephalopathy, and a variety of neurologic defects such as mental retardation and cerebral palsy. Considerable controversy has surrounded the relationship between pertussis vaccine and several serious neurologic conditions that, although indistinguishable from otherwise naturally occurring idiopathic events, have at times appeared temporally related to DTwP vaccination. Several recent studies using sophisticated statistical and experimental techniques have found no evidence to support a causal relationship between pertussis vaccination and some alleged reactions (eg, sudden infant death syndrome, infantile spasms, ADHD, learning disorders, autism) and, with respect to others, have suggested that vaccination may bring forward in time events otherwise destined to occur in a given individual (eg, seizures).

Although an increased incidence of seizures has been consistently observed after DTwP administration, most are associated with fever and have the clinical characteristics of benign febrile sei-

TABLE 1-28

OVERVIEW OF VALID AND NONVALID CONTRAINDICATIONS TO VACCINATION[a]

TRUE CONTRAINDICATIONS AND PRECAUTIONS	NOT TRUE (VACCINES MAY BE ADMINISTERED)
General for All Vaccines (DTwP/DTaP, OPV, IPV, MMR, Hib, HBV, Varicella)	
Contraindications Anaphylactic reaction to a vaccine contraindicates further doses of that vaccine Anaphylactic reaction to a vaccine constituent contraindicates the use of vaccines containing that substance Moderate or severe illnesses with or without a fever	Mild to moderate local reaction (soreness, redness, swelling) following a dose of an injectable antigen Mild acute illness with or without low-grade fever Current antimicrobial therapy Convalescent phase of illnesses Prematurity (same dosage and indications as for normal, full-term infants) Recent exposure to an infectious disease History of penicillin or other nonspecific allergies or family history of such
DTwP/DTaP	
Contraindications Encephalopathy within 7 days of administration of previous dose of DTwP/DTaP **Precautions[b]** Fever of ≥40.5°C (105°F) within 48 hrs after vaccination with a prior dose of DTwP/DTaP Collapse or shocklike state (hypotonic-hyporesponsive episode) within 48 hr of receiving a prior dose of DTwP/DTaP Seizures within 3 days of receiving a prior dose of DTwP/DTaP[c] Persistent, inconsolable crying lasting ≥3 hr within 48 hr of receiving a prior dose of DTwP/DTaP	Temperature of <40.5°C (105°F) following a previous dose of DTwP/DTaP Family history of convulsions[c] Family history of sudden infant death syndrome Family history of an adverse event following DTwP/DTaP administration
OPV	
Contraindications Infection with HIV or a household contact with HIV Known altered immunodeficiency (hematologic and solid tumors; congenital immunodeficiency; and long-term immunosuppressive therapy) Immunodeficient household contact **Precaution[b]** Pregnancy	Breast-feeding Current antimicrobial therapy Diarrhea
IPV	
Contraindication Anaphylactic reaction to neomycin or streptomycin **Precaution[b]** Pregnancy	
MMR	
Contraindications Anaphylactic reactions to neomycin, gelatin Pregnancy Known altered immunodeficiency (hematologic and solid tumors; congenital immunodeficiency; long-term immunosuppressive therapy), severely immunocompromised HIV-infected individuals **Precaution[b]** Recent (within 3 mo) immune globulin administration History of thrombocytopenia (see text)	Tuberculosis or positive skin test Simultaneous TB skin testing[d] Breast-feeding Pregnancy of mother of recipient Immunodeficient family member or household contact Infection with HIV (except severely immunocompromised HIV-infected individual) Nonanaphylactic reactions to neomycin Anaphylactic and nonanaphylactic reactions to egg
Hib	
None identified	
HBV	
None identified	Pregnancy
Varicella	
Contraindications History of anaphylactic reaction to neomycin, gelatin Known cellular or combined cellular and humoral immunodeficiency such as HIV infection with significant immunosuppression; congenital immunodeficiency, long-term immunosuppressive therapy (exception: asymptomatic or mildly symptomatic HIV-infected children meeting CDC criteria)	Nonanaphylactic reactions to neomycin Persons with isolated humoral immunodeficiency Pregnant household member Immunocompromised household member Breast-feeding (mother and infant) Children receiving inhaled or low-dose oral steroids (see text)

(continued)

TABLE 1-28 Continued

Persons with blood dyscrasias, leukemia, lymphomas, and other malignant neoplasms of bone marrow or lymphatic systems (exception: acute lymphocytic leukemia in remission meeting protocol criteria) Children with a family history of congenital or hereditary immunodeficiency in a first-degree relative unless recipient's immune competence has been documented Pregnancy **Precautions** Recent administration of immune globulin or other blood products Children requiring long-term salicylate therapy (see text)	

[a] This information is based on the recommendations of the Advisory Committee of Immunization Practices (ACIP) and those of the Committee on Infectious Diseases (*Red Book* Committee) of the American Academy of Pediatrics (AAP) as of Nov. 1999. Sometimes these recommendations vary from those contained in the manufacturer's package inserts. For more detailed information, providers should consult the published recommendations of the ACIP, AAP, American Association of Family Practice Physicians, and the manufacturer's package inserts.

[b] The events or conditions listed as precautions, although not contraindications, should be carefully reviewed. The benefits and risks of administering a specific vaccine to an individual under the circumstances should be considered. If the risks are believed to outweigh the benefits, the vaccination should be withheld; if the benefits are believed to outweigh the risks (eg, during an outbreak or foreign travel), the vaccination should be administered. Whether and when to administer DTP to children with proven or suspected underlying neurologic disorders should be decided on an individuals basis. It is prudent on theoretical grounds to avoid vaccinating pregnant women. However, if immediate protection against poliomyelitis is needed, OPV, not IPV, is recommended.

[c] For children with a personal or family (siblings or parents) history of convulsions, acetaminophen should be considered before DTwP/DTaP is administered and thereafter every 4 hours for 24 hours.

[d] Measles vaccination may temporarily suppress tuberculin reactivity. If testing cannot be done the day of MMR vaccination, the test should be postponed for 4 to 6 weeks.
DTwP = diphtheria-tetanus toxoid and whole cell pertussis vaccine; DTaP = diphtheria and tetanus toxoids and acellular pertussis vaccine; OPV = oral poliovirus vaccine; IPV = inactivated poliovirus vaccine; MMR = measles-mumps-rubella vaccine; Hib = *Haemophilus influenzae* type b vaccine; HBV = hepatitis B vaccine.
SOURCE: *Modified from National Vaccine Advisory Committee: Standards for pediatric immunization practices. MMWR 42:1-10, 1993.*

zures. There is no evidence that convulsions after DTwP administration cause neurologic damage or epilepsy. As an outgrowth of the National Childhood Vaccine Injury Act, the National Academy of Science's Institute of Medicine undertook an extensive analysis of all existing scientific data pertaining to potential adverse effects of the whole-cell pertussis vaccine. It found that evidence was consistent with a causal relationship between DTwP vaccination and several rare events including acute encephalopathy, hypotonic-hyporesponsive shock-like episodes, anaphylaxis, and prolonged inconsolable crying. It also found that children experiencing a severe acute neurologic illness (eg, encephalopathy) within 7 days after DTwP vaccination were at increased risk for chronic neurologic dysfunction at levels similar to those seen in children experiencing these same acute neurologic events temporally unrelated to DTwP administration. In these rare children, the committee believed that evidence was consistent with, but did not prove, a causal relationship between DTwP vaccination and some forms of chronic nervous system disorders. On the basis of their own review of the data, the National Vaccine Advisory Committee concluded that evidence was insufficient to determine whether a history of administration of DTwP before an acute neurologic event independently influenced the potential for subsequent long-term neurologic dysfunction. The ACIP and AAP both concur with this analysis.

Use of acellular vaccine results in significantly lower rates of minor local and systemic reactions, such as tenderness and fever, than does use of the whole-cell product. Prophylactic administration of acetaminophen (15 mg/kg) at the time of injection can further reduce the incidence of these side effects. Decreased frequency of several moderate to severe systemic events (compared with DTwP) has also been documented, including hypotonic-hyporeponsive episodes, fever greater than 40.5°C, and prolonged crying lasting more than 3 hours. Because of its rarity, the frequency of temporally associated encephalitis following DTaP has yet to be determined. Current contraindications to vaccination with DTwP/DTaP are given in Table 1-28.

POLIOMYELITIS

Poliovirus vaccines were introduced in the 1950s and 1960s. Their use since that time has resulted in a dramatic decrease in wild-type poliomyelitis worldwide, making global eradication of this disease an attainable goal for the near future. Two forms of trivalent polio vaccine—the enhanced-potency inactivated injected IPV (introduced at original potency by Salk in 1954) and the live attenuated oral OPV (Sabin, 1961)—are available for use. In addition to the immunizing agents, the IPV and the OPV contain various combinations of neomycin, streptomycin, and polymyxin B to prevent bacterial overgrowth.

In determining the relative advantages and disadvantages of using OPV or IPV, a number of epidemiologic and societal factors need to be considered. For a heterogeneous society with endemic disease or one that receives many immigrants from polio-endemic areas and where universal immunization can not be assured, OPV offers several advantages. First, oral vaccination with attenuated live virus is felt to induce lifelong immunity in much the same way as a natural infection, thereby avoiding the need for boosters. Second, because of the induction of mucosal immunity (pharyngeal, intestinal) as well as systemic immunity, the natural transmission of wild-type virus in the population is interrupted. Third, because of fecal shedding of the vaccine viruses for several weeks after vaccination, indirect immunization or boosting of immunity in contacts is also achieved. The lack of the need for injections, which may prevent some individuals from being vaccinated, and the lower cost of OPV compared to IPV are also added advantages.

The disadvantage of the use of OPV is its ability, although rare, to cause paralytic disease in both the recipient and his or her contacts. Approximately eight or nine cases of vaccine-associated paralytic poliomyelitis (VAPP) are reported in the United States each year. Most cases occur in immunocompetent adults. Only 10% to 15% of afflicted individuals are found to have an underlying immunodeficiency. However, immunodeficient individuals are at increased risk of vaccine-induced disease; therefore, they and their family members should not be immunized with live-virus vaccine. Household contacts are at higher risk of disease than community contacts, and the risk for both recipients and contacts is highest after exposure to a first dose.

The inactivated injectable polio vaccine offers the advantage of being unable to cause paralytic poliomyelitis. The current enhanced-potency product provides some mucosal immunity, although less than that provided by OPV. At its original potency the IPV required booster doses every 4 to 5 years. However, the current enhanced-potency injected vaccine induces significantly prolonged and possibly lifelong immunity, thereby reducing or potentially eliminating the need for subsequent boosters.

Other than the risk of vaccine-acquired polio with live-virus vaccine, side effects of both OPV and IPV are minimal and consist of rare hypersensitivity and anaphylactic reactions, primarily caused by trace amounts of neomycin, streptomycin, and polymyxin B. Although concern has been raised about a possible connection between OPV or IPV administration and Guillain-Barré syndrome, recent data do not confirm a causal relationship. Valid and nonvalid contraindications to vaccination are listed in Table 1-28.

Until recently the live attenuated oral vaccine (OPV) was the vaccine of choice for routine childhood vaccination in the United States. (In order to further the goal of global eradication, OPV remains the preferred vaccine for use in countries where wild-type poliomyelitis is or has recently been endemic and in most developing countries where relative cost issues and inadequate sanitation systems provide compelling reasons for use of OPV over IPV.) Recent changes in the epidemiology of poliomyelitis in the United States and surrounding regions has caused the ACIP and the AAP to reevaluate the relative advantages and disadvantages of using OPV versus IPV in the United States and has led them to revise their recommendations regarding the use of these products in routine childhood immunization. The last case of indigenously acquired wild-type virus poliomyelitis in the United States was reported in 1979. From 1980 to 1994, however, 125 cases VAPP were reported. Because the risk of acquiring vaccine-associated polio in the United States, although low, is currently significantly greater than the risk of acquiring the wild-type viral infection, both the ACIP and the AAP now recommend an IPV-only regimen for routine vaccination of all children in the United States. A series of four injections are given at 2 months, 4 months, 6-18 months, and 4-6 years of age (Table 1-26). A minimum of 4 weeks should separate the first two doses. If the third dose of vaccine is given after the child's fourth birthday, the fourth dose is unnecessary. OPV is still the vaccine of choice for controlling outbreaks of wild-type poliovirus and for use in polio eradication programs in countries where wild-type polio still circulates.

MEASLES, MUMPS, RUBELLA (MMR)

The MMR is a combination vaccine containing three attenuated live viruses. Single-agent preparations are also available. Vaccine strains of measles and mumps are grown in chick embryo tissue culture, whereas rubella is grown in human diploid cell culture. All of these vaccines contain minute quantities of neomycin to prevent bacterial overgrowth. A 0.5-mL dose is administered subcutaneously using needle sizes and sites described previously. The MMR can be administered concurrently (different sites) with all of the other routinely recommended childhood vaccines without diminishing antibody response. However, it is recommended that in-

jected live-virus vaccines, if not given on the same day, should be spaced 4 weeks or more apart. Measles vaccination may temporarily suppress tuberculin reactivity for 4 to 6 weeks after immunization but will not interfere with the accuracy of the test placed on the same day. Administration of immunoglobulin interferes with the immune response to MMR vaccination for a dose-dependent period of time. Ideally, MMR vaccination should be given at least 2 weeks before the administration of immunoglobulin or, if this is not possible, delayed for a period of time appropriate to the dose of immunoglobulin received (see *Red Book*).

Recommendations regarding the optimal timing and frequency of immunization against measles, mumps, and rubella (Table 1-26) reflect a balance among several factors including the duration of maternal antibody protection conferred to the infant, the seroresponse to vaccine at different ages, the rate of primary vaccine failure, the duration of vaccine-induced immunity, and the overall level of vaccination achieved within the population. During the 1980s, when it was recommended that children receive one dose of MMR at 15 months of age, several outbreaks of measles were reported. These occurred primarily among three populations: unvaccinated preschool children less than 15 months of age, unvaccinated preschool children over 15 months of age, and previously vaccinated school-aged children. Cases occurring in children less than 15 months of age were believed to be caused in part by an earlier decline in levels of protective maternal antibody among infants born to women who themselves had received measles vaccine, rather than experiencing a natural infection. A 2 to 10% primary vaccine failure rate was believed to be the primary cause of cases occurring in previously vaccinated school-aged children, although waning immunity was also a potentially important factor.

Outbreaks among unvaccinated children who had not received the MMR at the recommended age represented a failure of the vaccine delivery system to maximize access, catchment, and public acceptance. The AAP and ACIP subsequently changed their policy to recommend a two-dose MMR vaccine schedule and lowered the age for administration of the initial dose from 15 months to 12-15 months for all children. Both groups currently recommend that the second dose be routinely given at school entry, between the ages of 4 and 6 years. This dose can, however, be administered as early as 1 month after the initial vaccine as long as the first was given at 12 months of age or older. To better address problems with vaccine delivery, immunization practice guidelines for health-care providers have also been issued by the National Vaccine Advisory Committee. Since implementation of these changes, the number of cases of measles reported in the United States has decreased dramatically, with the vast majority occurring in previously unvaccinated children.

A recent increase in the number of mumps cases among adolescents and young adults has also been observed and is believed to reside primarily among a relatively underimmunized cohort of children born between 1967 and 1977, when mumps vaccine was available but not routinely recommended. Individuals should be vaccinated against mumps who were not immunized with live mumps virus vaccine on or after their first birthday or have not experienced a natural infection as diagnosed by a physician or documented by the presence of serum antibody. Most people born before 1957 are likely to have been infected naturally and generally can be considered immune even if they do not remember having had a symptomatic case.

Unlike the characteristic presentation of mumps, a clinical diagnosis of rubella is notoriously unreliable. Individuals should not be considered immune to rubella unless they have been immunized with live-virus vaccine on or after their first birthday or have evidence of serum antibody present. There is no evidence to suggest that it is harmful to immunize someone against mumps or rubella who has previously received vaccine or had a natural infection.

Contraindications to receiving the MMR are given in Table 1-28. Although the MMR is prepared in chick embryo cell culture, it does not contain significant amounts of cross-reacting egg proteins. A history of anaphylactic allergy to chicken eggs is no longer a contraindication to vaccination with MMR. Children with significant egg allergy are at low risk of an anaphylactic reaction and should be routinely vaccinated. A history of anaphylactic allergy to neomycin, however, warrants withholding this vaccine until skin testing can be obtained. Lesser degrees of allergy to antibiotics, chicken, and chicken feathers are not contraindications to vaccination.

Individuals with a history of thrombocytopenia, particularly if this was temporally related to a first dose of MMR, may be at slightly increased risk of recurrent thrombocytopenia following MMR vaccination. Because the incidence of thrombocytopenia with wild-type measles or mumps is much greater, and the natural history of vaccine-induced thrombocytopenia is generally benign and self-limited, in most instances the benefits of vaccinating a child with a previous history of thrombocytopenia outweigh the disadvantages. However, if the previous thrombocytopenia occurred following a first dose of MMR, it may be prudent to withhold the second dose.

Live-virus vaccines should not be given to individuals who are known to be or are suspected of being immunodeficient. An exception to this rule, however, is the recommendation that both asymptomatic and symptomatic HIV-infected children who are not severely immunecompromised (based on age-specific quantification of CD4 lymphocytes) should receive the MMR vaccine because of their increased risk of morbidity and mortality with the acquisition of wild-type measles infection.

Concerns about immunization during pregnancy apply to all live-virus vaccines, although the greatest attention has centered on rubella. The Centers for Disease Control reporting registry shows no evidence of defects consistent with wild-type congenital rubella syndrome among the live-born infants or aborted fetuses of women inadvertently vaccinated against rubella during or just before their pregnancies. Vaccine virus, however, has been isolated from aborted products of conception, proving that the attenuated virus can cross the placenta. Although it is to be avoided, rubella vaccination just before or during pregnancy is not by itself a reason to interrupt pregnancy.

Side effects of measles vaccination include frequent local tenderness and swelling, fever appearing 7 to 12 days after immunization (5-15%), and a morbilliform rash following the same time course (5%). Recipients of the killed measles vaccine, available from 1963 to 1967, have a higher incidence of local reactions when revaccinated with the live-virus vaccine. Because there is a greater risk of developing serious atypical measles if exposed to wild-type virus, however, these individuals should be revaccinated. As previously mentioned, thrombocytopenia presenting in the 2 months following immunization has rarely been reported in association with the MMR. This condition is generally transient and benign and occurs at a rate significantly lower than that associated with wild-type measles or mumps infection.

Encephalitis and encephalopathy have occasionally been reported to follow measles and mumps vaccination, but at an incidence lower than the "background" frequency of encephalitis from unknown etiology, suggesting a temporal relationship only. Although subacute sclerosing panencephalitis, a late complication of wild-type measles infection, has been reported to occur after measles vaccination in the absence of a known natural infection, the incidence of this devastating disease has been reduced dramatically by mass immunization. Side effects of the mumps vaccine include local tenderness, low-grade fever, and, rarely, a mild orchitis or parotitis. In addition to local tenderness and a rubella-like syndrome consisting of rash, fever, and lymphadenopathy, rubella vaccination is associated with transient arthritis and arthralgias occurring 1 to 3 weeks after vaccination, most commonly among postpubertal women (10-15%). In a recent review of all scientific data pertaining to potential adverse effects of the MMR vaccine, the National Academy of Sciences' Institute of Medicine found evidence to establish a causal relationship between this vaccine and anaphylaxis, thrombocytopenia, febrile seizures, and acute arthritis. Evidence did not support a causal link between this vaccine and other events such as neuropathies, Guillain-Barré syndrome, and thrombocytopenic purpura.

HAEMOPHILUS Influenzae TYPE b (Hib) CONJUGATE VACCINE

Vaccines against invasive *H. influenzae* type b infections have undergone significant evolution since their licensure in 1985. Four conjugate *H. influenzae* type b vaccines are currently available for use. Each of these consists of Hib capsular polysaccharide linked to a different carrier protein (Table 1-29). Only HbOC, PRP-OMP, and PRP-T are licensed by the FDA for use in infants less than 1 year of age. PRP-D is licensed for booster use at at least 12 months of age and for primary administration at 15 months of age or older. DTaP/Hib combination vaccines are also available. However, because some of these products may result in a suboptimal immune response when used at 2, 4, and 6 months of age, only those licensed for this age group should be utilized in young infants.

Conjugate vaccines offer a significant advantage over the original unconjugated polysaccharide vaccine in their ability to elicit a protective antibody response in young infants when the incidence of invasive *H. influenzae* disease is greatest. As with the original vaccine, the conjugate *H. influenzae* vaccines do not protect against nontypeable strains of *H. influenzae*, which are responsible for many recurrent upper respiratory diseases such as otitis media. Conjugate vaccine should also not be considered a protective immunizing agent against their carrier protein (eg, diphtheria, *N. meningitidis*, or tetanus). For all products, a dose of 0.5 mL is given IM using needle sizes and sites described previously. All of the Hib vaccines can be given simultaneously (at different sites unless a licensed combination vaccine is used) with other routinely recommended childhood immunizations without diminishing the immunologic response. Side effects attributed to the *H. influenzae* conjugate vaccines are minimal and include primarily local tenderness, swelling, erythema, and low-grade fever in a minority of recipients (25%). There are no specific contraindications to vaccination with Hib vaccines. Premature infants should be vaccinated in accordance with the recommended schedule based on their chronologic, not gestational, age.

The recommended schedule of administration for *H. influenzae* vaccination differs with the preparation used and the age of the child at first immunization. Recipients of HbOC or PRP-T who are immunized at the recommended times should receive a primary series of three doses at 2, 4, and 6 months of age. Use of PRP-

TABLE 1-29

LICENSED *HAEMOPHILUS influenzae* TYPE b CONJUGATE VACCINES AVAILABLE IN THE UNITED STATES[a]

MANUFACTURER	ABBREVIATION	TRADE NAME	CARRIER PROTEIN
Lederle Laboratories, Pearl River, NY (distributed by Wyeth-Lederle Vaccines, Wyeth-Ayerst Laboratories, Philadelphia, PA)	HbOC	HibTITER	CRM_{197} (a nontoxic mutant diphtheria toxin)
Merck & Co, Inc, West Point, PA[b]	PRP-OMP	PedvaxHIB	OMP (an outer membrane protein of *Neisseria meningitidis*)
Pasteur Mérieux Sérums & Vaccins, SA, Lyon, France (distributed by Connaught Laboratories, Swiftwater, PA, and by SmithKline Beecham Pharmaceuticals, Philadelphia, PA)	PRP-T	ActHIB, OmniHIB	Tetanus toxoid
Pasteur Mérieux Connaught, Swiftwater, PA	PRP-D	ProHIBiT	Diphtheria toxoid

[a] HbOC (diphtheria CRM_{197} protein conjugate), PRP-OMP (polyribosylribotol phosphate—outer membrane protein), and PRP-T are recommended for infants beginning at approximately 2 months of age. PRP-D is recommended only for children 12 months of age or older. The US Food and Drug Administration (FDA), however, has approved labeling for PRP-D for booster administration beginning at 12 months of age and for primary administration at 15 months of age. These vaccines may be given in combination products or as reconstituted products with DTaP (diphtheria and tetanus toxoids and acellular pertussis) or DTwP (diphtheria and tetanus toxoids and pertussis), provided the combination or reconstituted vaccine is approved by the FDA for the child's age and administration of the other vaccine component(s) also is justified.

[b] A combination of *H. influenzae* (PRP-OMP) and hepatitis B (Recombivax, 5 μg) vaccine is licensed for use at 2, 4, and 12 to 15 months of age (Comvax).

SOURCE: From: *American Academy of Pediatrics. In Pickering LK, ed. 2000 Red Book: Report of the Committee on Infectious Diseases. 25th ed. Elk Grove Village, IL, American Academy of Pediatrics; 2000.*

OMP requires only two primary doses, at 2 and 4 months of age. Because seroconversion following a first dose of PRP-OMP is significantly higher than that seen with the other conjugate products (60% vs 20%), when available, this preparation is preferred for use in populations and regions with an increased frequency of Hib invasive disease (eg, American Indian, Alaska Natives). When possible, the same preparation should be used to complete the primary series. However, when this is unknown, or if this product is unavailable, three doses of any of the conjugate products licensed for use in infants less than 12 months of age are considered sufficient to complete the primary series. All children should receive a booster dose at 12 to 15 months of age using any of the four available preparations.

Children not initiating vaccination at the recommended age who are between 2 and 6 months of age should receive a primary series of three HbOC or PRP-T (or two PRP-OMP), each separated by at least 2 months, and a booster dose at 12 to 15 months of age. Unvaccinated children 7 to 11 months of age require two primary doses using any of the three preparations licensed for this age group, separated by at least 2 months, and a booster dose (at least 2 months from the last) at 12 to 18 months of age. Children 12 to 14 months of age should receive two doses of vaccine (given 2 months apart).

Individuals 15 to 60 months of age who have not been previously immunized require only one dose using any of the four conjugate vaccines available. Children less than 24 months of age who have had invasive *H. influenzae* disease still should be vaccinated because many fail to develop adequate immunity following natural infection. Irrespective of age, children who are believed to be at increased risk for invasive *H. influenzae* disease, such as those with functional or anatomic asplenia, should also receive conjugate vaccine.

HEPATITIS B VACCINE (HBV)

Acute hepatitis B and its chronic sequelae are the cause of significant morbidity and mortality in this country. A plasma-derived hepatitis B vaccine, licensed in 1982, has since been replaced by two recombinant vaccines (Recombivax and Engerix B), which use synthetic HBsAg produced in yeast by plasmid gene insertion. These vaccines are highly immunogenic, conferring protection against hepatitis B infections in more than 90% of recipients, including infants. The failure of control strategies utilizing selective immunization of high-risk groups and HBsAg screening of pregnant women led both the American Academy of Pediatrics and the Advisory Committee Immunization Practices (ACIP) of the US Public Health Service to recommend universal hepatitis B immunization during infancy. These groups also recommend universal vaccination for older children and adolescents who missed vaccination during infancy as well as vaccination of adults at high risk for hepatitis B exposure (Table 1-30).

Although recombinant Hep B was felt to be one of our safest vaccines, two recent issues have caused the AAP, ACIP, and WHO to review existing data regarding potential adverse effects and to recommend several temporary modifications in their routine schedule of administration. In recent years, several cases of multiple sclerosis and other demyelinating diseases have been reported in adults who had received hepatitis B vaccines within the preceding 2-3 months. In 1998, the Viral Hepatitis Prevention Board, a part of the World Health Organization's Center for the Evaluation of Vaccination, undertook a thorough review of existing data to determine whether or not a causal relationship might exist between these two events. This group found no statistically significant association between hepatitis B vaccination and multiple sclerosis or other CNS demyelinating diseases in studies conducted to date. Furthermore, the age and gender distribution of cases of multiple sclerosis has not changed following widespread use of hepatitis B vaccine and dose not differ between groups whose diagnosis was and was not temporally related to vaccination. Although additional research is ongoing, this group concluded that current data do not demonstrate a causal association between hepatitis B vaccination and CNS demyelinating disease and therefore do not warrant a change in current recommendations regarding universal childhood vaccination. These findings have subsequently been endorsed by other recommending organizations.

TABLE 1-30

PERSONS WHO SHOULD RECEIVE PREEXPOSURE HEPATITIS B IMMUNIZATION[a]

All infants
Children at high risk for early childhood HBV infection[b]
Adolescents[c]: Hepatitis B vaccination should be given by or before 11 to 12 years of age.
  Special efforts should be made to vaccinate **all** adolescents, not only those at high risk.
Injection drug users
Sexually active heterosexual persons with more than one sex partner during the previous 6 months or who have a sexually transmitted disease
Sexually active men who have sex with men
Household contacts and sexual partners of HBsAg-positive persons
Health care personnel and others at occupational risk of exposure to blood or blood-contaminated body fluid
Residents and staff of institutions for developmentally disabled persons
Staff of nonresidential child care and school programs for developmentally disabled persons if the program is attended by a known HBsAg-positive person
Patients undergoing hemodialysis
Patients with bleeding disorders who receive clotting factor concentrates
Members of households with adoptees who are HBsAg-positive
International travelers to areas in which HBV infection is of high or intermediate endemicity
Inmates of juvenile detention and other correctional facilities

---

[a] HBV indicates hepatitis B virus; HBsAg, hepatitis B surface antigen.
[b] Alaskan Native and Asian-Pacific Islander children and children born to first-generation immigrants from HBV-endemic areas.
[c] Immunization can be initiated before children reach adolescence.
SOURCE: From: *American Academy of Pediatrics: In: Pickering LK, ed: 2000 Red Book: Report of the Committee on Infectious Diseases, 25th ed. Elk Grove Village, IL, American Academy of Pediatrics, 2000.*

As previously mentioned, Hep B and several other childhood vaccines contain minute quantities of a mercury-containing preservative called thimerosal. Although no adverse effects have been documented, some infants receiving routine vaccinations at recommended ages may cumulatively exceed FDA guidelines for mercury exposure. Manufacturers are currently working to eliminate mercury-containing preservatives from all vaccines. However, there is currently only one mercury-free hepatitis B product (COMVAX) that does not contain thimerosal, and this vaccine is combined with Hib vaccine (PRP-OMP) and not licensed for use in infants under 6 weeks of age. Until all preparations are mercury-free, the AAP and ACIP recommend continued vaccination with thimerosal-containing products but on a slightly modified schedule to minimize any theoretical risks (see below).

Current recommendations regarding the dose and volume of vaccination vary with the preparation used, the age of the child being vaccinated, the mother's HBsAg serologic status, and the presence of relevant underlying disease (Table 1-31). The vaccine is administered intramuscularly in the anterolateral thigh or upper arm and can be given simultaneously at different sites with all other routinely recommended childhood vaccines. If thimerosal-free vaccine is not available (COMVAX combined HepB/Hib vaccine can be given after 6 weeks of age), the AAP recommends delaying administration of the first hepatitis B vaccine (previously given at birth) until 6 months of age (ACIP recommends delaying until 2-6 months of age) in otherwise healthy full-term infants born to

HBsAg-negative mothers. Two subsequent doses should be given before 18 months of age with a minimum interval between the first and second doses of 1 month and between the second and third doses of 2 months. Not less than 4 months should separate the first and third doses.

Until mercury-free products are available, premature infants whose mothers are HBsAg-negative should not receive their first Hep B vaccination until they have reached a term gestational age, weigh at least 2.5 kg, and are at least 6 months of age chronologically. Recommendations regarding vaccination of babies born to HBsAg-positive mothers and those whose HBsAg status is unknown remain unchanged (Table 1-32). Infants whose mothers are HBsAg-positive should receive hepatitis B immune globulin (HBIG) and their first immunization at birth. For these infants, the second and third doses are recommended to be given at 1-2 and 6 months of age. Although routine testing for postimmunization antibody response is not recommended for all infants, babies born to HBsAg-positive women should be tested for HBsAg and anti-HBs at 9 months of age (1-3 months after completion of series) and revaccinated if measured antibody titers are below 10 mIU/mL. When the HBsAg status of the mother is unknown, the infant should receive the first immunization at birth and HBIG as close to this as possible (within 1 week) if the mother is subsequently found to be HBsAg-positive. As previously noted, the AAP and ACIP also recommend immunization for all older children and adolescents who were not immunized during infancy as well as adults

TABLE 1-31

RECOMMENDED DOSAGES OF HEPATITIS B VACCINES[a]

	VACCINE[b]	
	RECOMBIVAX HB[c] **DOSE,** μg (mL)	**ENGERIX-B**[d] **DOSE,** μg (mL)
Infants of HBsAg-negative mothers, children and adolescents younger than 20 y of age	5 (0.5)	10 (0.5)
Infants of HBsAg-positive mothers (HBIG, 0.5 mL, also is recommended)	5 (0.5)	10 (0.5)
Adults 20 y of age or older	10 (1.0)	20 (1.0)
Patients undergoing dialysis and other immunosuppressed adults	40 (1.0)[e]	40 (2.0)[f]

---

[a] HBsAg indicates hepatitis B surface antigen; HBIG, Hepatitis B immune globulin.
[b] Vaccines should be stored at 2°C to 8°C (36°F–46°F). Freezing destroys effectiveness. Both vaccines are administered in a 3-dose schedule. A 2-dose schedule, administered at 0 and 4 to 6 mo later, is available for adolescents 11–15 years of age using the adult dose of Recombivax HB (10 μg).
[c] Available from Merck and Co, Inc, West Point, Pa. A combination of hepatitis B (Recombivax, 5 μg) and *Haemophilus influenzae* b (PRP-OMP) vaccine is licensed for use at 2, 4, and 12 to 15 months of age (Comvax).
[d] Available from SmithKline Beecham Pharmaceuticals, Philadelphia, PA. The US Food and Drug Administration has approved this vaccine for use in an optional 4-dose schedule at 0, 1, 2, and 12 mo.
[e] Special formulation for dialysis patients.
[f] Two 1.0-mL doses given in 1 site in a 4-dose schedule at 0, 1, 2, and 6 to 12 mo.
SOURCE: From: *American Academy of Pediatrics: In: Pickering LK, ed: 2000 Red Book: Report of the Committee on Infectious Diseases, 25th ed. Elk Grove Village, IL, American Academy of Pediatrics, 2000.*

TABLE 1-32

RECOMMENDED SCHEDULE OF HEPATITIS B IMMUNOPROPHYLAXIS TO PREVENT PERINATAL TRANSMISSION[a]

VACCINE DOSE[b] AND HBIG	AGE
Infant born to mother known to be HBsAg-positive[c]	
First	Birth (within 12 h)
HBIG[d]	Birth (within 12 h)
Second	1–2 mo
Third	6 mo
Infant born to mother not screened for HBsAg[c]	
First	Birth (within 12 h)
HBIG[d]	If mother is HBsAg-positive, give 0.5 mL as soon as possible, not later than 1 wk after birth[e]
Second	1–2 mo
Third	6 mo[f]

[a] HBsAg indicates hepatitis B surface antigen; HBIG, hepatitis B immune globulin.
[b] See Table 1-31 for appropriate vaccine dose.
[c] See text for recommendations for subsequent serologic testing.
[d] HBIG (0.5 mL) given intramuscularly at a site different from that used for vaccine.
[e] See text for immunization recommendations for preterm infants.
[f] Infants of HBsAg-negative mothers should receive third dose at 6–18 months of age.
SOURCE: *American Academy of Pediatrics: In: Pickering LK, ed: 2000 Red Book: Report of the Committee on Infectious Diseases, 25th ed. Elk Grove Village, IL, American Academy of Pediatrics, 2000.*

at high risk of hepatitis B exposure (Table 1-30). The recommended schedule for administration in these individuals is 0, 1, and 6 months.

Adverse effects associated with hepatitis B vaccination are minimal and limited primarily to local tenderness, although several rare hypersensitivity reactions to yeast and vaccine preservative have been reported. As mentioned previously, there are no data to date that confirm a causal relationship between hepatitis B vaccination and Guillain-Barré syndrome, multiple sclerosis, or other demyelinating diseases.

VARICELLA VACCINE

Before the availability of a varicella vaccine (licensed in 1995), approximately 4 million cases of chicken pox occurred each year in the United States. Although most of these infections were self-limited, secondary complications, such as bacterial soft tissue infections, pneumonia, and encephalitis, led to more than 10,000 hospitalizations and 100 deaths annually. Although morbidity from varicella is greater in adolescents and adults, 90% of all cases, 60% of hospitalizations, and 40% of deaths occurred in children less than 10 years of age. Furthermore, the economic and social costs of this infection, which necessitates prolonged school absence and home care by a parent or other caregiver, are great. After weighing these issues with data regarding vaccine efficacy and safety, the ACIP and the AAP recommended routine varicella vaccination for all children who have not had the clinical disease.

Varicella vaccine is composed of a live attenuated virus and min-

ute quantities of neomycin and gelatin. For individuals 12 years of age or younger, a single dose of 0.5 mL is delivered subcutaneously using needle sizes and sites as described above. Routine vaccination is recommended at 12-18 months of age (Table 1-26) and can be given concurrently (using separate sites and syringes) with other routine childhood immunizations. If the MMR is not given on the same day, however, these live-virus vaccines should be administered at least 1 month apart. Teenagers and adults who lack a history of natural infection should also be vaccinated. Ninety-five percent of children 12 years of age or younger will seroconvert after one dose of vaccine. However, a diminished antibody response is observed in adolescents and adults. It is therefore recommended that individuals 13 years of age or older be given a two (0.5 mL)-dose regimen separated by 4-8 weeks. Because 70-90% of adults who do not recall an episode of varicella will have antibody evidence of prior infection, it may be cost-effective to test immune status in adults and older children (if return can be assured) before giving the vaccine. However, there are no problems associated with immunizing an individual who has previously experienced a natural varicella infection. Varicella vaccination is 85% effective in preventing all disease and more than 95% effective in preventing moderate and severe disease. On the basis of follow-up studies to date (>20 years), serologic evidence of immunity appears to be long-lasting and, like many other live-virus vaccines, is likely to be lifelong. However, the need for subsequent booster doses continues to be assessed.

The varicella vaccine is associated with few side effects. Approximately 20-30% of recipients will experience transient pain and tenderness at the site of injection. Of greater significance, a mild varicelliform skin eruption will develop in approximately 3-5% of children within 1 month of receiving the immunization. Because the vaccine virus has rarely been recovered from these lesions, a very small risk exists for exposing others to the attenuated virus. Relevant precautions are given below. A mild zoster-like disease also has been reported to occur in some vaccine recipients. This is less severe and occurs at a significantly lower rate than that observed with reactivation of the wild-type virus.

Valid and nonvalid contraindications to varicella vaccination are given in Table 1-28. Based on a review of new risk-benefit data, the ACIP has recently modified its recommendations regarding the use of this live-virus vaccine in individuals with certain primary or acquired immunodeficiencies. Individuals with selectively impaired humoral immunity, such as hypogammaglobulinemia and dysgammaglobulinemia, may now be vaccinated. Vaccination of individuals with cellular immunodeficiencies and illnesses/therapies (eg, high-dose steroids) resulting in global immunosuppression is still contraindicated with two exceptions: Although varicella vaccine is not licensed for use in individuals with neoplasms affecting the bone marrow or lymphatic systems, children with acute lymphocytic leukemia (ALL) who have been in remission for at least a year and who meet strict protocol cell count criteria can be safely and effectively immunized. Vaccine is provided free of charge to this population by the manufacturer as a part of a research protocol. Because of their increased risk for severe wild-type disease, children infected with HIV who are asymptomatic or mildly symptomatic (see ACIP recommendation) should also be considered candidates for vaccination. For these children as well as those in the ALL protocol, a two-dose regimen (irrespective of age) is recommended. Otherwise immunocompetent children with asthma or other conditions for which they are receiving inhaled steroids or <2 mg/kg of prednisone or its equivalent per day (<20 mg/d if weight >10 kg) can be vaccinated. Children living in households with immunodeficient individuals can and should receive the vaccine. If a vaccine-related skin rash develops, contact between the recipient and the immunocompromised individual should be avoided until the rash resolves.

Varicella vaccine should not be given to a pregnant woman, and pregnancy should be avoided for at least 1 month after receiving the vaccine because of the potential risk to the fetus. However, the presence of a pregnant woman is not a contraindication to vaccinating a child living in the same household. The varicella vaccine should also not be administered to individuals with a history of an anaphylactic reaction to neomycin or gelatin. Caution is advised when vaccinating children taking salicylates. Although no cases of Reye syndrome have been reported in association with the varicella vaccine, the manufacturer recommends that salicylates be avoided for 6 weeks after administration of the vaccine because of the well-established relationship between Reye syndrome and the use of salicylates during wild-type infection. The ACIP and AAP recommend that vaccination (with close monitoring) be carefully considered for children requiring chronic salicylate therapy (eg, rheumatoid arthritis) because the risk of aspirin-associated complications is likely to be greater with acquisition of wild-type virus.

PNEUMOCOCCAL CONJUGATE VACCINE

S. pneumoniae is currently the most common cause of invasive bacterial disease, including sepsis, meningitis and bacteremia, in children in the United States, with a peak incidence of disease occurring between 6 and 23 months of age. This organism is also the causative agent in many noninvasive respiratory diseases including acute otitis media, sinusitis, and pneumonia. Groups at highest risk for invasive disease include children with sickle hemoglobinopathies, functional or anatomic asplenia, primary and secondary immunodeficiencies (eg HIV infection, malignancies), and certain chronic diseases (eg cardiac and pulmonary diseases, diabetes, chronic renal failure). Children of Native American (American Indian and Alaska Native) and African-American descent have a moderately increased risk for invasive pneumococcal infection compared to other healthy children. An increased incidence of infection (two- to threefold increase) and nasopharyngeal colonization has also been documented in children attending out-of-home group childcare compared to their at-home peers. Since the 1980s, a 23-valent pneumococcal polysaccharide vaccine (23PS vaccine) has been available for use in adults and children over the age of 2 years who are at highest risk for invasive pneumococcal infections. However, this vaccine is not effective in children less than 2 years of age, and it has not been recommended for universal childhood vaccination.

In February of 2000, the FDA licensed a new 7-valent pneumococcal conjugate vaccine (PCV7) that is effective in children less than 24 months of age. It is composed of seven serotype capsular polysaccharides coupled to a nontoxic variant diphtheria toxin. (As with other vaccines using diphtheria toxin as their protein conjugate, this vaccine does not provide protection against diphtheria.) The vaccine also contains a small amount of an aluminum phosphate adjuvant. The serotypes included (out of 90 potential) are responsible for 80% of the invasive pneumococcal infections occurring in children less than 6 years of age in the United States and currently encompass the majority of those strains with the highest rates of penicillin resistance. In studies to date, the vaccine has been shown to be highly efficacious in preventing invasive pneumococcal disease. Its use has also been associated with a modest decrease in

TABLE 1-33

RECOMMENDED SCHEDULE OF DOSES FOR PCV7, INCLUDING PRIMARY SERIES AND CATCH-UP IMMUNIZATIONS, IN PREVIOUSLY UNVACCINATED CHILDREN*

AGE AT FIRST DOSE	PRIMARY SERIES	BOOSTER DOSE†
2–6 mo	3 doses, 6–8 wk apart	1 dose at 12–15 mo of age
7–11 mo	2 doses, 6–8 wk apart	1 dose at 12–15 mo of age
12–23 mo	2 doses, 6–8 wk apart	
≥24 mo	1 dose	

* Recommendations for high-risk groups are given in Table 1-35.
† Booster doses to be given at least 6 to 8 weeks after the final dose of the primary series.
SOURCE: Reproduced with permission from: *American Academy of Pediatrics, Committee on Infectious Diseases: Policy statement: Recommendations for the prevention of pneumococcal infections, including the use of pneumococcal conjugate vaccine (Prevnar), pneumococcal polysaccharide vaccine, and antibiotic prophylaxis. Pediatrics 106:363, 2000.*

the incidence of acute otitis media, pneumonia, antibiotic usage, and nasopharyngeal carriage of vaccine strains. The duration of protection following primary immunization with PCV7 is currently unknown, although immunologic memory (booster response to subsequent doses) has been documented. Whether or not addi-

TABLE 1-34

CHILDREN AT HIGH RISK OF INVASIVE PNEUMOCOCCAL INFECTION

High risk (attack rate of invasive pneumococcal disease >150/100,000 cases/y)
1. SCD, congenital or acquired asplenia, or splenic dysfunction
2. Infection with HIV

Presumed high risk (attack rate not calculated)
1. Congenital immune deficiency: some B- (humoral) or T-lymphocyte deficiencies, complement deficiencies (particularly C1, C2, C3, and C4 deficiencies), or phagocytic disorders (excluding chronic granulomatous disease)
2. Chronic cardiac disease (particularly cyanotic congenital heart disease and cardiac failure)
3. Chronic pulmonary disease (including asthma treated with high-dose oral corticosteroid therapy)
4. Cerebrospinal fluid leaks
5. Chronic renal insufficiency, including nephrotic syndrome
6. Diseases associated with immunosuppressive therapy or radiation therapy (including malignant neoplasms, leukemias, lymphomas, and Hodgkin's disease) and solid organ transplantation*
7. Diabetes mellitus

Moderate risk (attack rate of invasive pneumococcal disease >20 cases/100,000/y)
1. All children 24–35 mo old
2. Children 36–59 mo old attending out-of-home care
3. Children 36–59 mo old who are of Native American (American Indian and Alaska Native) or African American descent

* Guidelines for the use of pneumococcal vaccines for children who have received bone marrow transplants are currently undergoing revision (Centers for Disease Control and Prevention, personal communication, 2000).
SOURCE: Reproduced with permission from: *American Academy of Pediatrics, Committee on Infectious Diseases: Policy statement: Recommendations for the prevention of pneumococcal infections, including the use of pneumococcal conjugate vaccine (Prevnar), pneumococcal polysaccharide vaccine, and antibiotic prophylaxis. Pediatrics 106:364, 2000.*

TABLE 1-35

RECOMMENDATIONS FOR PNEUMOCOCCAL IMMUNIZATION WITH PCV7 OR 23PS VACCINE FOR CHILDREN AT HIGH RISK OF PNEUMOCOCCAL DISEASE, AS DEFINED IN TABLE 1-34*

AGE	PREVIOUS DOSES	RECOMMENDATIONS
≤23 mo	None	PCV7 as in Table 1-33
24–59 mo	4 doses of PCV7	1 dose of 23PS vaccine at 24 mo, at least 6–8 wk after last dose of PCV7
		1 dose of 23PS vaccine, 3–5 y after the first dose of 23PS vaccine
24–59 mo	1–3 doses of PCV7	1 dose of PCV7
		1 dose of 23PS vaccine, 6–8 wk after the last dose of PCV7
		1 dose of 23PS vaccine, 3–5 y after the first dose of 23PS vaccine
24–59 mo	1 dose of 23PS	2 doses of PCV7, 6–8 wk apart, beginning at least 6–8 wk after last dose of 23PS vaccine
		1 dose of 23PS vaccine, 3–5 y after the first dose of 23PS vaccine
24–59 mo	None	2 doses of PCV7 6–8 wk apart
		1 dose of 23PS vaccine, 6–8 wk after the last dose of PCV7
		1 dose of 23PS vaccine, 3–5 y after the first dose of 23PS vaccine

* Children with sickle cell disease (SCD), asplenia, HIV infection, and other high-risk factors.

SOURCE: Reproduced with permission from: *American Academy of Pediatrics Committee on Infectious Diseases: Policy statement: Recommendations for the prevention of pneumococcal infections, including the use of pneumococcal conjugate vaccine (Prevnar), pneumococcal polysaccharide vaccine, and antibiotic prophylaxis. Pediatrics 106:364, 2000.*

tional doses will be necessary for high-risk children remains to be determined. In studies to date, adverse effects appear to be minimal and include local erythema, induration and tenderness at the site of injection, fussiness, and low-grade to moderate fever in a minority of recipients. Contraindications to vaccination include known hypersensitivity to any of the vaccine components. Vaccination should also be deferred in children with moderate or severe illness.

The availability of the new conjugate vaccine has led both the Advisory Committee on Immunization Practices (ACIP) and the Committee on Infectious Diseases of the American Academy of Pediatrics to recommend that all children less than 24 months of age be routinely immunized during infancy. A dose of 0.5 mL is given via intramuscular injection in a four-dose series at 2, 4, 6, and 12-15 months of age. The first dose should not be given before 6 weeks of age. The PCV may be administered concurrently with other childhood vaccines using separate syringes and sites. Prema-

ture and low birth weight infants should receive the vaccine at the chronologic age of 6-8 weeks. Recommendations for "catch-up" dosing in older infants and children are given in Table 1-33. Routine vaccination of children 24-59 months of age at high risk for invasive pneumococcal infection is also recommended. Groups at highest risk and AAP guidelines regarding the use of PCV7 and 23PS vaccine in these populations are given in Tables 1-34 and 1-35, respectively. Consideration may also be given to vaccinating children 24-59 months of age who are at moderately increased risk for invasive pneumococcal disease (children 24-35 months of age children of Native Alaskan, American Indian, and African-American descent and children who attend group daycare) using one dose of PCV7. Data are limited regarding the use of PCV7 in adults and children older than 5 years of age. Those who are at high risk for pneumococcal disease (eg sickle cell disease, HIV infection) may receive either 23PS vaccine or PCV7; however, there is some rationale in this age group for using the 23PS vaccine since only 50-60% of invasive pneumococcal infections in older children and adults are covered by PCV7.

ROTAVIRUS VACCINE

In the United States, rotavirus is the most common cause of severe gastroenteritis in children and infants, accounting for 30-50% of all hospitalizations for dehydration from diarrheal disease in children less than 5 years of age.

Because of the considerable morbidity and social/economic costs associated with this illness, the AAP (December 1998) and the ACIP (March 1999) recommended that all infants be routinely immunized with a rotavirus vaccine. However, as use became more widespread, an increased number of cases of intussusception were reported in the first few weeks following vaccination. This observation led the AAP and ACIP to recommend suspension of the routine use of this vaccine.

References

American Academy of Pediatrics: Immunization of adolescents: Recommendations of the Advisory Committee on Immunization Practices, the American Academy of Pediatrics, the American Academy of Family Physicians, and the American Medical Association. Pediatrics 99:479–488, 1997

American Academy of Pediatrics: Combination vaccines for childhood immunization: Recommendations of the Advisory Committee on Immunization Practices (ACIP), the American Academy of Pediatrics (AAP), and the American Academy of Family Physicians (AAFP). Pediatrics 103:1064–1077, 1999

American Academy of Pediatrics, Committee on Infectious Diseases: The relationship between pertussis vaccine and central nervous system sequelae: Continuing assessment. Pediatrics 97:279–281, 1996

American Academy of Pediatrics, Committee on Infectious Diseases: 1997 Red Book. Report of the Committee on Infectious Diseases, 24th ed. Elk Grove Village IL, American Academy of Pediatrics, 1997

American Academy of Pediatrics, Committee on Infectious Diseases: Poliomyelitis prevention: Recommendations for use of inactivated poliovirus vaccine and live oral poliovirus vaccine. Pediatrics 99:300–305, 1997

American Academy of Pediatrics, Committee on Infectious Diseases: Age for routine administration of the second dose of measles-mumps-rubella vaccine. Pediatrics 101:129–133, 1998

American Academy of Pediatrics, Committee on Infectious Diseases: Policy Statement: Recommendations for the prevention of pneumococcal infections, including the use of pneumococcal conjugate vaccine (Prevnar), pneumoncoccal polysaccharide vaccine, and antibiotic prophylaxis. Pediatrics 106:362–366, 2000

American Academy of Pediatrics, Committee on Infectious Diseases: Possible association of intussusception with rotavirus vaccination. Pediatrics 104:575–576, 1999

American Academy of Pediatrics, Committee on Infectious Diseases: Poliomyelitis prevention: Revised recommendations for use of inactivated and live oral poliovirus vaccines. Pediatrics 103:171–172, 1999

American Academy of Pediatrics, Committee on Infectious Diseases: Prevention of poliomyelitis: Recommendations for use of only inactivated poliovirus vaccine for routine immunization. Pediatrics 104:1404–1406, 1999

American Academy of Pediatrics, Committee on Infectious Diseases: Recommended childhood immunization schedule—United States, January-December 1999. Pediatrics 103:182–185, 1999

American Academy of Pediatrics, Committee on Infectious Diseases and Committee on Environmental Health: Thimerosal in vaccines—an interim report to clinicians. Pediatrics 104:570–574, 1999

American Academy of Pediatrics, Committee on Infectious Diseases and Committee on Pediatric AIDS: Measles immunization in HIV-infected children. Pediatrics 104:1057–1060, 1999

American Academy of Pediatrics, Committee on Native American Child Health and Committee on Infectious Diseases: Immunizations for Native American children. Pediatrics 104:564–567, 1999

American Academy of Pediatrics, Overturf GD and the Committee on Infectious Diseases: Technical report: Prevention of pneumococcal infections, including the use of pneumococcal conjugate and polysaccharide vaccines and antibiotic prophylaxis. Pediatrics 106;367–376, 2000

Advisory Committee on Immunization Practices, Centers for Disease Control: Measles, mumps, and rubella—vaccine use and strategies for elimination of measles, rubella, and congenital rubella syndrome and control of mumps: Recommendations of the Advisory Committee on Immunization Practices (ACIP). MMWR 47(RR-8):1–57, 1998

Advisory Committee on Immunization Practices, Centers for Disease Control: Poliomyelitis prevention in the United States: introduction of a sequential vaccination schedule of inactivated poliovirus vaccine followed by oral poliovirus vaccine. MMWR 46(RR-3):1–25, 1997

Advisory Committee on Immunization Practices, Centers for Disease Control: Prevention of varicella: Recommendations of the Advisory Committee on Immunization Practices (ACIP). MMWR 45(RR-11):1–35, 1996

Advisory Committee on Immunization Practices, Centers for Disease Control: Prevention of varicella: updated recommendations of the Advisory Committee on Immunization Practices (ACIP). MMWR 48(RR06):1–5, 1999

Advisory Committee on Immunization Practices, Centers for Disease Control: Revised recommendations for routine poliomyelitis vaccination. MMWR 48:590, 1999

Advisory Committee on Immunization Practices, Centers for Disease Control: Update: Vaccine side effects, adverse reactions, contraindications, and precautions. MMWR 45(RR-12):1–35, 1996

Advisory Committee on Immunization Practices, Centers for Disease Control: Rotavirus vaccine for the prevention of rotavirus gastroenteritis among children—recommendations of the Advisory Committee on Immunization Practices (ACIP). MMWR 48(RR-2):20, 1999

Advisory Committee on Immunization Practices, Centers for Disease Control: Preventing pneumococcal diseases among infants and young children: Recommendations of the Advisory Committee on Immunization Practices (ACIP). MMWR 49(RR09):1–38, 2000

Halsey NA, Duclos P, Van Damme P, et al: Hepatitis B vaccine and central nervous system demyelinating diseases. Pediatr Infect Dis J 18:23–24, 1999

THE NEWBORN INFANT

Associate Editor, Richard D. Bland

2.1 A HISTORICAL PERSPECTIVE ON NEWBORN CARE

William A. Silverman

Human reproduction has always been a remarkably inefficient process. As in all animal species, and for all of the eons of human existence, most offspring launched at conception died early in embryonic life or soon after birth. The care taken at birth to improve the chances of survival of a newly born baby has been, until very recent times, strongly influenced by a family's means of subsistence and also by a neonate's state of health in the first hours of extrauterine life.

Almost two millennia ago, Soranus of Ephesus (ca AD 98–138), in his book *Gynaecia,* gave meticulous instructions to midwives about the management of labor and delivery and about care of the newborn. Several chapters dealt with the latter topic, and the first of these was entitled "How to recognize the newborn that is worth rearing" (notably, this advice preceded his chapters on "How to sever the navel cord," and "How to cleanse"). Only healthy infants were deemed acceptable (eg, among other characteristics, "the infant suited by nature for rearing . . . has been born at the due time . . . and is perfect in all its parts . . . "). The fate of babies who failed to come up to his high standard was not specified by Soranus, but exposure was the well-known means of disposing of flawed offspring in the ancient Greco-Roman cultures. In Roman society, the newly born infant was examined by the midwife for signs of imperfection, and the baby was placed on the ground to await the father's judgment. If he then "raised the infant up" in his arms (origin of the phase "to raise a child"), this gesture indicated the father's acceptance of the child as his own. If he turned his back, the infant was exposed in a public place to be picked up by strangers or to die of cold and starvation. Infanticide was sanctioned in many societies throughout the world, and the practice persisted well into the modern era despite religious and legal proscriptions.

In the last third of the 18th century, British obstetricians began to take aggressive measures to resuscitate infants who did not breathe spontaneously at birth. (Baker wrote that this "surge of interest in the treatment of 'apparent death' emerged as a part of a broader current of enthusiasm for resuscitation . . . of victims of drowning and other accidents.") But the period of heroic intervention was relatively short-lived, and a pessimistic attitude returned. Given the very high mortality in the first year of life, doctors questioned whether the rescue of marginally viable neonates at birth made any important difference in eventual outcome. Additionally, as noted by Baker, before late in the 19th century, obstetricians did not distinguish premature infants (the largest category of "feeble" neonates) as a specific class of patients, "much less a medical problem that demanded a solution."

Organized efforts to save less-than-robust newborn infants began in France in the last quarter of the 19th century. The attempts began as an extension of a successful campaign of hospital reform to prevent puerperal fever in mothers, carried out at the Maternité Hospital in Paris by a prominent obstetrician, Etienne Stéphane Tarnier. Tarnier was disturbed by the sight of so many small infants dying on the hospital wards. He observed that their bodies were "rigid with cold even though wrapped in fleece." According to Baker, Tarnier in 1880, following his "discovery of premature infants," asked Odile Martin, a technician at the Paris Zoo, to build an incubator for small babies (a closed design, warmed by a large reservoir of heated water and ventilated by convective currents of warm air, similar to an incubator used at the zoo for poultry). Following introduction of the Tarnier-Martin incubator for small infants (below 2 kg), mortality fell "from 66 percent to 38 percent."

The success of the hospital campaign to rescue premature infants took on additional significance when it was viewed in the context of French anxieties about depopulation (brought about by the immense loss of life from military action and months of starvation during the Franco-Prussian War in 1870–1871 and by a steady decline in the birth rate). Because most births took place at home, the gains in survival associated with incubator care in the maternity hospital had very little influence on the national decrease in population. In the 1890s Tarnier's pupil, obstetrician Pierre Constant Budin, extended the "incubator revolution" to the city at large by promoting the establishment of in-hospital departments of special services for weaklings. Here "feeble" infants were admitted to special wards without their mothers, placed in incubators, cared for by expert nurses, and fed by wet nurses. Budin extended the supervision of care after discharge from the hospital by establishing a system of "consultation clinics" throughout the city. These "schools for mothers," he emphasized, involved the mother in her baby's care and helped to preserve an infant's favorable course in the hospital. The organized program of rescue designed by French obstetricians (to provide favorable conditions for survival, so that those infants "meant to survive" will do so) was very successful, but they recognized a practical limit. Budin wrote, "We shall not discuss infants of less than 1000 grams. They are seldom saved . . . " This judgment was widely accepted for many decades: infants who weighed less than 1 kg at birth were labeled as "previable."

Curiously, the passive approach in France (essentially a farm-like screening process to identify infants who were "meant" to live) was not copied widely. American obstetricians were more concerned with the mother than with her newborn. And there was little enthusiasm for saving the lives of feeble infants in impoverished families living in wretched tenements, when "scarcely one-half [of these babies] live five years." Moreover, depopulation was not an important issue in the United States, where immigration more than compensated for the large loss of infant life.

In 1899, the first organized effort to rescue premature infants in the United States was made in Chicago by Joseph B. DeLee, an idealistic obstetrician. He opened an incubator station at the Chicago Lying-In Hospital and wrote, "[This is] the only attempt in this country to make a [specialized service for debilitated infants] similar to those in Paris." However, DeLee's program was short-lived, and subsequent interest in the rescue of prematurely born infants waxed and waned in the first half of the 20th century (despite the fact that the practical success of the French approach was widely known, as demonstrated in bizarre incubator-baby side shows at fairs and expositions throughout the world during this era). A notable pediatrician-led premature infant station was established in Chicago by Julius Hess in 1922. The program was based on Budin's plan. In this nursery dominated by expert nurses, doctors were discouraged from disturbing the "weak," easily exhausted babies. And the dogmatic "hands-off" approach, Baker noted, acted as a bridge between the older techniques originating in Paris and a new style of "hands-on" intervention that appeared, haltingly, following world War II.

One of the earliest of the "slight" modifications was the routine use of high concentrations of oxygen in the incubators of small infants. This alteration was made to convert the usual pattern of respirations (periodic breathing) in the most immature infants to the regular rhythm seen in normal term infants. The new and untested practice was introduced in 1942 in the hope of improving survival and reducing the risk of brain damage in prematurely born babies, and the policy was adopted widely before it came under a cloud of suspicion in Britain and in Australia in 1951. The latter conjectures ignited fierce arguments about the possible link between routine high-oxygen exposure and the increased risk of a newly recognized form of blindness (retinopathy of prematurity, then called retrolental fibroplasia). The paralyzing confusion was resolved when a multicenter randomized trial was carried out in the United States in 1953–1954. The trial demonstrated that curtailment of supplement oxygen reduced the risk of eye damage in small premature infants by two-thirds. About 10,000 children were blinded as the result of what seemed to be a rational application in the use of oxygen—a life-saving gas! This disaster made it painfully clear that none of the time-honored routines to provide "favorable conditions for survival" had ever been tested rigorously. And it was soon found that other "bombs" were ticking away in the premature infant nurseries. For example, controlled trials of prophylactic use of antibacterial drugs (sulfisoxazole and chloramphenicol) revealed unsuspected lethal effects.

These humbling experiences served as powerful reminders of how little was known about the life-threatening problems affecting neonatal patients. The innovative field of activity set out to alter the expected course of any and all biological circumstances that had heretofore limited survival. The net results were dramatic. There was concrete evidence of a striking increase in survival of infants who were abandoned previously as previable. The momentum of this revolution has continued to the present day.

References

Baker JP: The Machine in the Nursery. Incubator Technology and the Origins of Newborn Intensive Care. Baltimore, Johns Hopkins University Press, 1998

Budin P (Malony WJ, transl): The Nursling: The Feeding and Hygiene of Premature and Full-Term Infants. London, Caxton Publishing Co, 1907

Cone TE JR: History of the Care and Feeding of the Premature Infant. Boston, Little, Brown, 1985

Desmond MM: Newborn Medicine and Society. European Background and American Practice (1750–1975). Austin, TX, Eakin Press, 1998

Galanakis E. Apgar score and Soranus of Ephesus. Lancet 352:2012–2013, 1998

Grudzinskas J, Nysenbaum A: Failure of human pregnancy after implantation. Ann NY Acad Sci 442:39–44, 1985

Jameton AL: Pediatric nursing ethics. In: Goldworth A, Silverman WA, Stevenson DK, et al, eds: Ethics and Perinatology. Oxford, Oxford University Press, 1995

Silverman WA: Mismatched attitudes about neonatal death. Hastings Center Rep 11(6):12–16, 1981

Silverman WA: Incubator-baby side shows. Pediatrics 64:127–141, 1979

Silverman WA: Retrolental Fibroplasia. A Modern Parable. New York, Grune & Stratton, 1961

2.2 NEONATAL MORTALITY AND MORBIDITY

Avroy A. Fanaroff

Infant mortality is an important outcome measure of the health services of a population. In the United States, where there are approximately four million births each year, the infant mortality hovers around seven per 1000 live births. The highest risk of infant death is within 24 hours of birth, but mortality and morbidity remain high during the neonatal period, from birth to the 28th day of life. In the United States each year nearly 1% of pregnancies are complicated by fetal death, and about 0.5% by neonatal mortality. The fetus and newborn are most vulnerable during labor, delivery, and the neonatal period, as central nervous system injury, at this time, may result in lifelong morbidity and neurodevelopmental impairment. The perinatal period, from "28 weeks of gestation to the 28th day of life," is the period of greatest mortality. In the modern era with survival of extremely low-birth-weight infants, postneonatal mortality also contributes significantly to the infant mortality rate.

DEFINITIONS

The reduction of maternal and infant mortality and the improvement of the health of mothers and infants in the United States are high priorities. Statistical comparisons among countries, states, regions, and individual centers have been hampered by differences in definitions. In order to compare outcomes and plan interventions, it is imperative that standard definitions be utilized. These include terms such as live birth, fetal death, low birth weight, preterm, term, and postterm *(modified from Guidelines for Perinatal Care, 4th ed, AAP, ACOG)*.

Live birth: The complete expulsion or extraction from the mother of a product of human conception, irrespective of the duration of pregnancy, which, after such expulsion or extraction, breathes or shows any other evidence of life, such as beating of the heart, pulsation of the umbilical cord, or definite movement of voluntary muscles, whether or not the umbilical cord has been cut or the placenta is attached. Heartbeats are to be distinguished from transient cardiac contractions; respirations are to be distinguished from fleeting respiratory efforts or gasps.

Birth weight: The weight of a neonate determined immediately after delivery or as soon thereafter as feasible. It should be expressed as to the nearest gram.

Gestational age: The number of weeks that have elapsed between the first day of the last normal menstrual period (not the presumed time of conception) and the date of delivery, irrespective of whether the gestation results in a live birth or a fetal death.

Appropriate for gestational age (AGA): An infant with a birth weight between the 10th and 90th percentiles for that gestational age. Those below the 10th percentile are regarded as small for gestational age (SGA), whereas those above the 90th percentile are considered large for gestational age (LGA).

Low birth weight: Any neonate, regardless of gestational age, whose weight at birth is less than 2500 g.

Preterm: Any neonate whose birth occurs through the end of the last day of the 37th week (259th day) following the onset of the last menstrual period.

Term: Any neonate whose birth occurs from the beginning of the first day (260th day) of the 38th week through the end of the last day of the 42nd week (294th day) following the onset of the last menstrual period.

Postterm: Any neonate whose birth occurs from the beginning of the first day (295th day) of the 43rd week following the onset of the last menstrual period.

Fetal death: Death before the complete expulsion or extraction from the mother of a product of human conception, fetus and placenta, irrespective of the duration of pregnancy; the death is indicated by the fact that, after such expulsion or extraction, the fetus does not breathe or show any other evidence of life, such as beating of the heart, pulsation of the umbilical cord, or definite movement of voluntary muscles. Heartbeats are to be distinguished from transient cardiac contractions; respirations are to be distinguished from fleeting respiratory efforts or gasps. This definition excludes induced termination of pregnancy.

Neonatal death: Death of a liveborn neonate before the neonate becomes 28 days old (up to and including 27 days, 23 hours, and 59 minutes from the moment of birth).

Infant death: Any death at any time from birth up to, but not including, 1 year of age (364 days, 23 hours, and 59 minutes from the moment of birth).

Perinatal death: Death from the 28th week of gestation to the 28th day of life.

REGIONALIZATION

Regionalization of perinatal care to various levels (see Table 2-1), first introduced in the 1970s, was cost effective and reduced morbidity and mortality. Market forces and economics have disrupted regionalization in the 1990s. Nonetheless, the evidence clearly demonstrates that the best outcomes for low-birth-weight infants are achieved when they are delivered at the larger subspecialty centers (formerly known as level III), those with an average neonatal intensive care unit (NICU) daily census in excess of 15. Risk-adjusted neonatal mortality for infants born in smaller level III NICUs, and in level II+ and level II NICUs (specialty), regardless of size, was not significantly different from that in hospitals without an NICU and was significantly higher than in hospitals with large subspecialty NICUs. Despite the differences in outcomes, costs for the birth of infants born at hospitals with large subspecialty NICUs were not more than those for infants born at other hospitals with NICUs. Concentration of high-risk subspecialty NICU care has the potential to decrease neonatal mortality without increasing costs.

NEONATAL MORTALITY

Infant and neonatal mortality rates are presented in Table 2-2 and Fig. 2-1. Advances in perinatal care have improved the chances for survival of infants with major congenital anomalies in addition to

TABLE 2-1
LEVELS OF IN-HOSPITAL PERINATAL CARE

MATERNAL	NEONATE
Basic Care	
Monitor and care for low-risk patients	Examination and care of healthy neonate
Identify high risk for transfer	Resuscitation and stabilization
Detection and care of unanticipated labor/delivery problems	Consultation and transfer protocols
Emergency cesarean delivery within 30 minutes	Nursery care
Blood bank, anesthesia, radiology, ultrasound, and laboratory support	Parent/sibling visitation
Care of postpartum problems	General pediatrician staff (capable of neonatal resuscitation)
Obstetrician, nurse, midwife staff	
Special Care	
Basic services plus	*Basic services plus*
Care of high-risk pregnancies	Care of high-risk neonate with short-term problems
Triage, transfer of high-risk pregnancies (<32 weeks, IUGR, preeclampsia, severe anomalies, chorioamnionitis, severe maternal medical illness)	Stabilization before transfer (<1500 g, <32 weeks, critically ill)
	Accept convalescing back (reverse) transfers
Subspecialty Care	
Basic plus speciality care plus	*Basic plus speciality care plus*
Experienced perinatologist (24-hour coverage)	Experienced neonatologist (24-hour coverage)
Evaluation of high-risk therapies	Inborn plus tranferred patients
Care for severe maternal medical or obstetric illnesses	Evaluation of high-risk therapies
High-risk fetal care (Rh disease, nonimmune hydrops, life-threatening anomalies) and surgical capabilities	All pediatric medical, radiologic, and surgical subspecialties
	NICU with operating room capabilities
Research	High-risk follow-up
Community education	Outcomes research
	Community education

IUGR = intrauterine growth restriction; NICU = neonatal intensive care unit.
SOURCE: *Perinatal Guidelines, 4th ed. Carol Stream, IL, AAP, 1997.*

those with cardiorespiratory disorders and other major organ system failure. The outlook for extremely low-birth-weight and low-gestational-age infants has also improved remarkably. Many factors influence neonatal mortality. In addition to race, birth weight, gestational age, gender, place of delivery, and intrauterine growth, there are wide variations in population descriptions, in the criteria used for starting or withdrawing treatment, in the reported duration of survival, and in care.

RACE Factors that increase mortality rates severalfold include prematurity, no prenatal care, inadequate weight gain in pregnancy, African-American ethnicity, and inadequate prenatal care. The importance of race as a determinant of neonatal mortality is shown by the 1997 mortality rates in the United States for infants born to Asian and Pacific Islander mothers (5/1000 live births) followed by White (6.0), American Indian (8.7), and black (13.7) mothers. African-American women have many more preterm and very early preterm births, which, in part, explains the doubling of their fetal and infant mortality rates. In general, however, the racial discrepancies in preterm birth and other pregnancy outcomes remain unexplained. Although there has been a noticeable decline in the peri-

TABLE 2-2

INFANT AND NEONATAL MORTALITY RATES BY BIRTH WEIGHT AND RACE OF MOTHER, UNITED STATES, 1997, LINKED FILE

BIRTH WEIGHT (g)	INFANT MORTALITY RATE[a]				NEONATAL MORTALITY RATE[a]			
	ALL RACES[b]	NONHISPANIC WHITE	BLACK	HISPANIC	ALL RACES[b]	NONHISPANIC WHITE	BLACK	HISPANIC
Total	7.2	6.0	13.7	6.0	4.8	3.9	9.2	4.0
<2500	61.7	56.0	75.8	58.4	50.3	46.0	61.3	47.6
<1500	252.8	240.7	270.1	250.1	223.8	215.7	236.1	218.3
<500	883.9	899.7	875.2	864.1	869.2	886.0	861.1	838.9
500–749	492.7	510.7	456.9	506.3	437.5	461.0	396.2	446.5
750–999	161.3	172.5	140.4	174.6	122.4	136.6	96.8	137.4
1000–1249	75.9	75.8	72.3	84.9	53.7	58.4	42.5	61.7
1250–1499	48.6	51.7	38.9	56.0	34.3	39.3	22.6	38.2
1500–1999	30.2	31.1	26.6	33.4	18.8	20.2	14.0	22.2
2000–2499	12.4	12.5	12.3	12.0	6.5	7.0	5.2	7.1
≥2500	2.7	2.5	4.1	2.3	1.0	1.0	1.1	0.9
2500–2999	4.9	5.0	5.8	4.3	2.0	2.1	1.8	2.0
3000–3499	2.6	2.5	3.7	2.1	0.9	.09	0.9	0.8
3500–3999	1.9	1.8	2.9	1.6	0.6	0.6	0.7	0.5
4000–4499	1.7	1.5	3.0	1.6	0.7	.06	1.0	0.7
≥4500	2.2	1.9	5.1	2.1	1.0	0.8	c	c

[a] Mortality per 1000 births.
[b] Includes races other than black and white.
[c] Figure does not meet standards of reliability or precision.

Note: Infant and neonatal mortality rates by race from the linked file differ slightly from those based on unlinked data because the linked file uses the self-reported race of mother from the birth certificate, whereas the unlinked data uses the race of child as reported by the funeral director on the death certificate. Births are tabulated separately by race and Hispanic origin; persons of Hispanic origin may be of any race.

SOURCE: *MacDorman MF, Atkinson JO: Infant mortality statistics from the 1997 period linked birth/infant death data set. Natl Vital Stat Rep 47:1, 1999.*

natal mortality rates for the past few decades, the prematurity rate has remained fairly constant, and African-American infants continue to have a higher mortality rate than their white counterparts. Although for the total birth cohort blacks have a higher mortality risk than whites, the reverse is noted at the lower weight group/ gestational age distributions.

MATERNAL FACTORS Infant mortality rates are higher for pregnancies in which prenatal care is initiated after the first trimester of pregnancy and in infants born to teenagers or to women 40 years

of age or older who did not complete high school, were unmarried, or smoked during pregnancy. Infant mortality is also higher for male infants, multiple births, and infants born preterm or at low birth weight. In many instances the precipitating cause of preterm delivery remains undetected, but risk factors for premature birth include uterine abnormalities, placental bleeding including abruptio placenta associated with cocaine use, maternal chronic illnesses, multifetal gestation, premature rupture of the membranes, chorioamnionitis, and bacterial vaginosis. Bacterial vaginosis, a short cervix, and the presence of fetal fibronectin in the vaginal tract are predictors of preterm delivery, but treatment of the bacterial vaginosis has been ineffective in preventing prematurity. Premature delivery complicates almost 10% of births but contributes disproportionately to at least two-thirds of the infant deaths and to a significant amount of neonatal and long-term morbidity, which may include cerebral palsy, mental restriction, physical handicap, blindness, and deafness in addition to major and minor school adaptive and learning problems. Although there has been a substantial decline in the number of medically preventable deaths and deaths from respiratory distress syndrome, the number of deaths from extremely low birth weight has increased relative to other causes; asphyxia, birth trauma, early-onset sepsis, and meconium aspiration syndrome have been reduced to a minimum. Nonetheless, congenital malformation is the leading cause of infant death in the United States and accounts for a much greater proportion of infant mortality than does premature birth. To further reduce neonatal mortality the incidence of lethal congenital malformations and very low birth weight infants must be addressed; congenital anomalies cause ~23% of infant mortality, and short gestation and low birth weight ~15%.

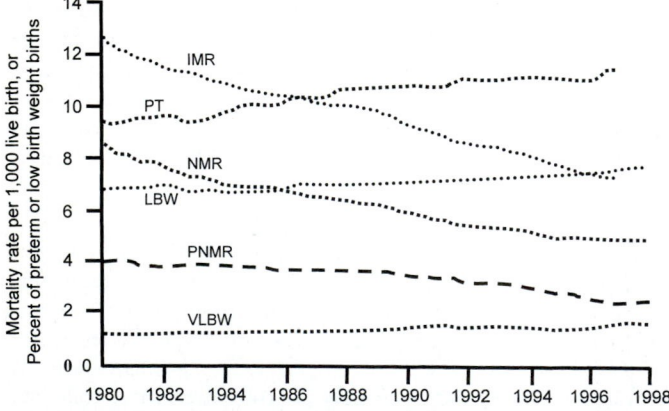

FIGURE 2-1   Mortality rate and percentage of preterm birth or low birth weight from 1980 to 1998 in the United States. IMR, NMR, PNMR = infant, neonatal and perinatal mortality rates; PT = preterm (<37 weeks of gestation); LBW and VLBW = low (<2500 g) and very low (<1500 g) birth weight.

MULTIPLE GESTATION Perinatal morbidity and mortality are significantly increased in multiple gestation, and the incidence of severe handicap is increased in survivors of multiple gestation, predominantly because of preterm delivery. In the United States, the number and rate of multiple births have risen dramatically. An ever-increasing number of multiple births are related to infertility treatments; the number of triplet and higher-order multiple births jumped 16% between 1996 and 1997, contributing to the increase in the percentage of low-birth-weight infants. Multiple gestation accounts for 26% of deliveries with birth weight below 1500 g. In addition to multiple gestation, aggressive interventions for fetal compromise identified in extremely immature infants contribute to the continuing toll of preterm birth.

CAUSES OF DEATH Congenital anomalies, disorders relating to short gestation and low birth weight, and sudden infant death syndrome accounted for nearly one-half of all infant deaths in the United States in 1997. Other leading causes of death in the neonatal period include respiratory distress syndrome (RDS), newborn complications of pregnancy, newborn complications related to placental disorders, cord accidents, and membrane disorders, neonatal infections, intrauterine hypoxia, and birth asphyxia. Advances in neonatal and perinatal care have reduced the infant mortality rate from RDS, which was 156.2 per 100,000 live births and 12% of infant deaths in 1979, to 33.7 per 100,000 live births and only 4.7% of infant deaths in 1998.

PRETERM BIRTH "In the United States in the last 2 decades, despite increasing availability of prenatal care, nutrition supplementation programs, and drugs to stop preterm contractions, the preterm birth rate has increased from 9.5% in 1980 to 11% in 1998. Part of this increase is due to multiple births associated with infertility treatments, but many preterm births occur spontaneously. None of the medical or public health strategies used to reduce preterm birth have succeeded (from Goldenberg RL, Jobe AH: JAMA 285, p 635, 2001)." Because of their high risk of mortality and serious morbidity, most studies on prematurity (defined as birth at less than 37 weeks) have focused on very preterm infants (birth at <32 weeks). However, risks for infant death from all causes among singletons born at 32 through 33 gestational weeks were increased over sixfold in the United States and 15-fold in Canada, whereas among singletons born at 34 through 36 gestational weeks, the relative risks were increased at least threefold. Mildly and moder-

ately preterm-birth infants are more numerous than extremely low-birth-weight infants and so are responsible for an important fraction of infant deaths.

There has been little to no success at reducing the incidence of preterm birth, intrauterine growth restriction, and congenital malformations. However, over the past 15 years the survival of extremely low-birth-weight infants (<1500 g) has increased from 74% to 84%. Mortality for 195 infants weighing 401 to 500 g was 89%; mortality in infants weighing 501 to 600 g was 71%; among survivors at this birth weight, 62% had chronic lung disease (CLD), 35% had severe intracranial hemorrhage (ICH), and 15% had proven necrotizing enterocolitis (NEC). These numbers are very comparable to those in the Oxford-Vermont Network, which accumulates data on more than 20,000 low-birth-weight infants each year (Fig. 2-2). Similar improvements are noted when the data are analyzed by gestational age. A comprehensive prospective geographically based study of all births between 20 and 25 weeks of gestation from the United Kingdom and Ireland documented mortality, neonatal morbidity, and early neurodevelopmental outcomes consistent with the data from the United States.

Although the validity of the Apgar scoring system continues to be challenged, a 5-minute Apgar score below 4 remains a better predictor of mortality than severe metabolic acidosis (pH < 7.0) measured from the cord blood. Male sex, failure to receive antenatal steroids, persistent bradycardia at 5 minutes, hypothermia, and poor intrauterine growth all independently increase the risk for death.

FETAL GROWTH RESTRICTION The most common causes of inadequate fetal growth relate to maternal hypertension, malnutrition, and smoking. These disorders may be associated with intrauterine fetal demise, neonatal adaptive problems including severe hypoglycemia or long-term abnormalities of growth and neurodevelopment. Cigarette smoking remains a major cause of intrauterine growth restriction, preterm birth, fetal and neonatal deaths, and sudden infant death syndrome. Alcohol and drug use may also affect pregnancy outcome. Prenatal alcohol exposure is an important cause of fetal growth restriction, including microcephaly, which results in long-term growth failure in addition to substantial neurodevelopmental delay and mental restriction. Mortality and morbidity are increased among infants born at term whose birth weights are at or below the third percentile for their gestational age. The incidence of intubation at birth, seizures during the first day of life,

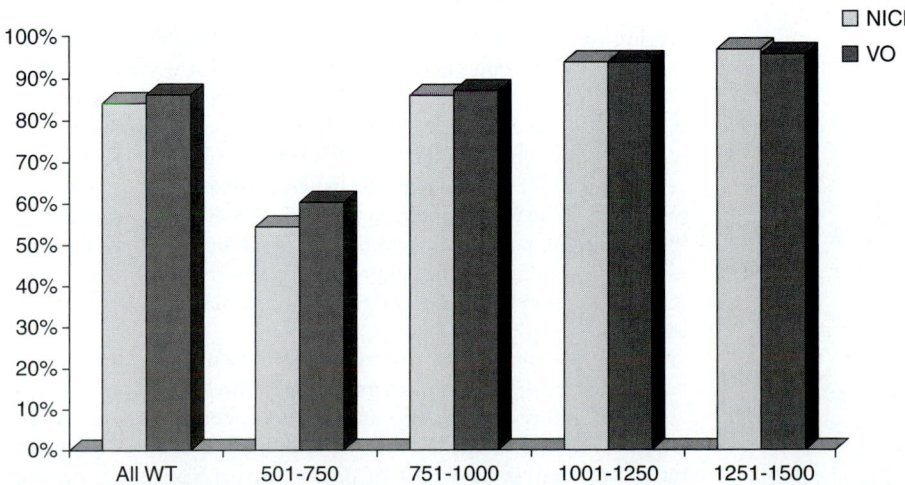

FIGURE 2-2 Survival by birth weight from 1995 to 1996. NICHD = National Institute of Child Health and Human Development Neonatal Research Network Centers; VO = Oxford-Vermont Network.

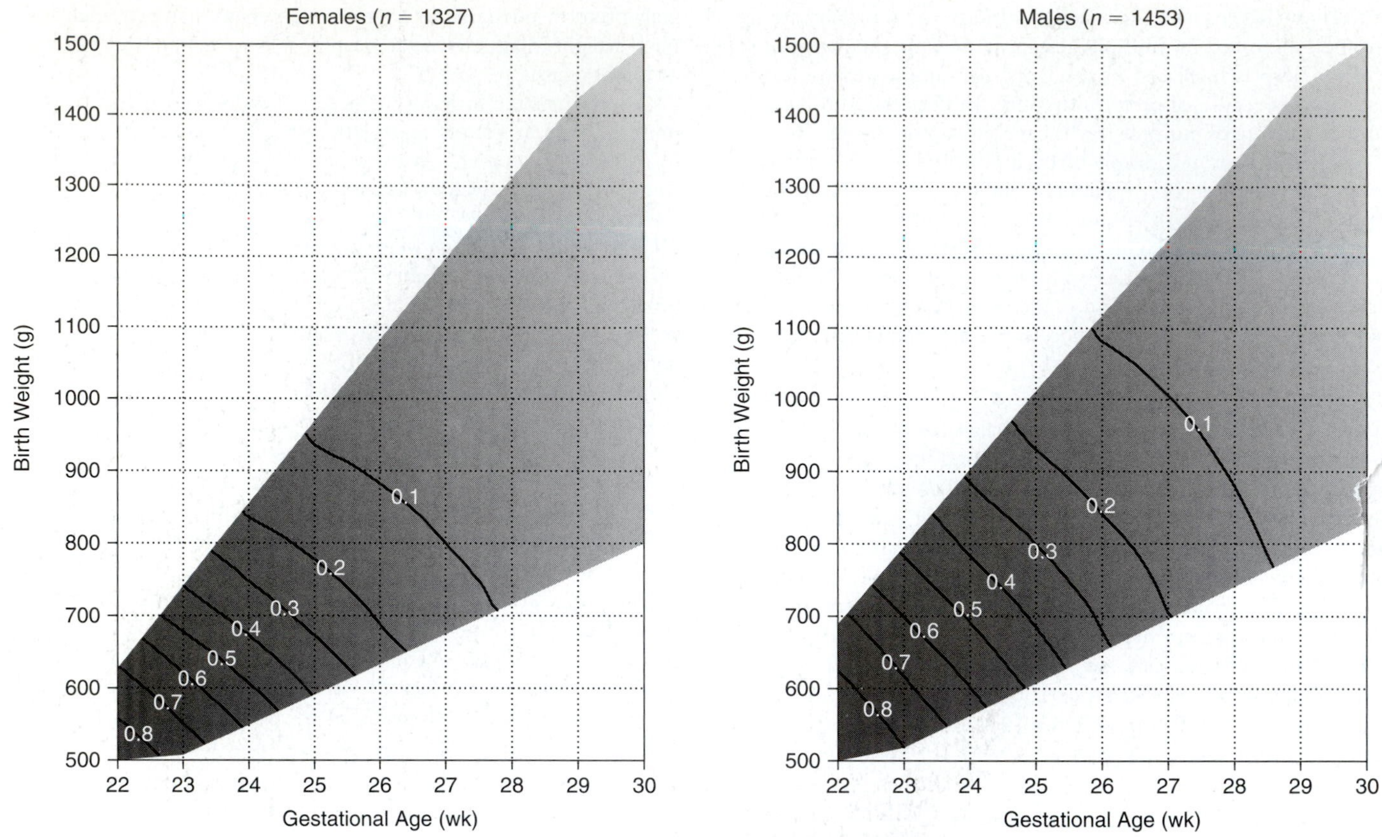

Females (*n* = 1327)

Males (*n* = 1453)

FIGURE 2-3   **Estimated mortality risk by birth weight and gestational age based on singleton infants born in NICHD Neonatal Research Network Centers between January 1, 1995 and December 31, 1996.**

and sepsis were also significantly increased among term infants with birth weights at or below the third percentile.

GENDER   Gender is a major determinant of survival with the female advantage most noticeable at the youngest gestational ages (Fig. 2-3). For example, the mortality rate of a girl who weighs 700 g at 24 weeks 2 of gestation is 30 to 40%, whereas a boy of equal weight and gestational age has a mortality risk of 50%. In addition to a higher mortality than girls, boys are more likely to need cardiopulmonary resuscitation at delivery and are at greater risk for most

adverse neonatal outcomes including chronic lung disease, intracranial hemorrhage, and nosocomial infections.

Inspection of Fig. 2-3 makes it apparent that there is a wide spread in the mortality risk at a given gestation and that the larger infants at each gestational age have a greater chance of surviving. Similarly, there is variability in the morbidity at each gestational age, and babies in the bottom percentiles for weight are more likely to be acidotic, require admission to the intensive care unit, develop major morbidities including respiratory failure, or die (Fig. 2-4).

FACTORS REDUCING MORBIDITY

During the past decade mortality has been reduced by the introduction of surfactant therapy for respiratory distress syndrome in 1990 and the widespread use of antenatal steroids that followed the NIH consensus conference in 1994. Before that time only 20% of women who delivered infants with a birth weight of ≤1500 g received antenatal corticosteroids, whereas that number now approaches 80% in most centers in the United States and may be even higher in other parts of the world. Care of infants with birth weights ≤750 g has become more aggressive so that the rate of cesarean section has increased from 17 to 44%, and that of delivery room intubation from 54 to 82%.

Some reports indicate that the survival chances for infants between 501 and 1500 g at birth improved in the 1990s, but concerns about morbidity and the high rates of neurodevelopmental handicap persist. The incidence of CLD (defined as receiving supplemental oxygen at 36 weeks of postmenstrual age; 23%), proven NEC (7%), and severe ICH (grade III or IV; 11%), and retinopathy

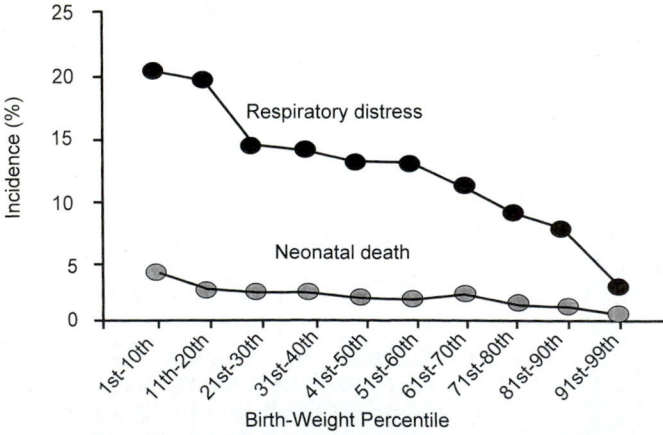

FIGURE 2-4   **Incidence of respiratory distress and neonatal death in infants born at 24 to 36 weeks of gestation.**

of prematurity (76%) among infants with birth weights between 501 and 1500 g fluctuated only slightly between 1991 and 1996. Lemons noted that 97% of all very low-birth-weight (VLBW) infants and 99% of infants weighing <1000 g at birth had weights less than the 10th percentile at 36 weeks of postmenstrual age.

Although infant mortality rates continue to decrease, specific factors, including prematurity, lack of or inadequate prenatal care, inadequate weight gain in pregnancy, and African-American ethnicity increase mortality rates severalfold.

NEURODEVELOPMENTAL OUTCOMES

Advances in perinatal care have led to increased survival of children born at the lower limits of viability. Children with VLBWs have poorer outcomes relative to normal-birth-weight term-born controls in neurologic and health status, cognitive-neuropsychological skills, school performance, academic achievement, and behavior. Outcomes are highly variable but are related to neonatal medical complications of prematurity and social risk factors.

Factors predictive of poor neurodevelopmental outcome include low birth weight, male gender, the severity of cerebral ultrasound abnormality including periventricular leukomalacia and persistent ventriculomegaly, bronchopulmonary dysplasia, and growth failure. In addition to gross neurologic deficits including cerebral palsy, hydrocephalus, and hemiplegia, these infants are susceptible to growth failure, deafness, and blindness.

Major neonatal mortality increases with decreasing gestational age and birth weight: survival at 23 weeks of gestation ranges from 2 to 35%, at 24 weeks of gestation 17 to 62%, and at 25 weeks of gestation 35–72% (Fig. 2-4). Major neonatal morbidity also increases with decreasing gestational age and birth weight. At 23 weeks of gestation, chronic lung disease occurs in 57 to 86% of survivors, at 24 weeks in 33 to 89%, and at 25 weeks of gestation in 16 to 71% of survivors. The rates of severe cerebral ultrasound abnormality range from 10 to 83% at 23 weeks of gestation, 9 to 64% at 24 weeks, and 7 to 22% at 25 weeks' gestation. Of 77 survivors at 23 weeks of gestation, 26 (34%) have severe disability (defined as subnormal cognitive function, cerebral palsy, blindness, and/or deafness). At 24 weeks of gestation, the rates of severe neurodevelopmental disability range from 22 to 45%, and, at 25 weeks of gestation, 12 to 35%. The continuing toll of major neonatal morbidity and neurodevelopmental handicap is of serious concern.

In Cleveland, Ohio, we compared the outcomes of 114 children with birth weight 500 to 749 g born in 1990 to 1992 to 112 infants born in 1993 to 1995. Twenty-month survival was similar (43% vs 38%). Although the use of antenatal and postnatal steroids increased, the rates of chronic lung disease, subnormal cognitive function at 20 months corrected age, and rate of cerebral palsy also increased. Similar findings have been reported elsewhere. Vohr, on the basis of evaluation of a multicenter cohort at 18 to 22 months corrected age, noted that extremely low-birth-weight (ELBW) infants (<1 kg) are at significant risk of neurologic abnormalities, developmental delays, and functional delays. Twenty-five percent of the children had an abnormal neurologic examination; 37% had a Bayley II Mental Developmental Index <70; 29% had a Psychomotor Developmental Index <70; 9% had vision impairment; and 11% had hearing impairment. Neurologic, developmental, neurosensory, and functional morbidities increased with decreasing birth weight. Factors significantly associated with increased neurodevelopmental morbidity included CLD, grades III to IV intraventricular hemorrhage (IVH)/periventricular leukomalacia (PVL), the use of steroids for CLD, NEC, and male gender. Factors significantly associated with decreased morbidity include increased birth weight, female gender, higher maternal education, antenatal corticosteroids, and white race.

Wood evaluated all children who were born at 25 or fewer completed weeks of gestation in the United Kingdom and Ireland from March through December 1995, at the time when they reached a median age of 30 months. Two hundred eighty-three (92%) of the 308 surviving children were formally assessed. The mean ($\pm$SD) scores on the Bayley Mental and Psychomotor Developmental Indices, referenced to a population mean of 100, were 84 $\pm$ 12 and 87 $\pm$ 13, respectively. Nineteen percent had severely delayed development (with scores more than 3 SD below the mean), and 11% had scores from 2 SD to 3 SD below the mean. Twenty-eight children (10%) had severe neuromotor disability, seven (2%) were blind or perceived light only, and eight (3%) had hearing loss that was uncorrectable or required aids. This cohort included 49% of survivors with no disability. Physicians and parents anticipating the delivery of ELBW infants must be aware of these outcomes to make informed decisions as to the advisability of aggressive care at birth and thereafter.

In summary, there have been marked improvements in the perinatal outcomes so that in the United States in 1997 the expectation of life at birth is 76.7 years for all gender and race groups combined. However, our national perinatal mortality rates still lag behind those of other industrialized countries, especially for minority groups.

References

American Academy of Pediatrics, The American College of Obstetricians and Gynecologists: Guidelines for Perinatal Care 4th ed. AAP, ACOG, 1997.

Casey BM, Mcintire DD, Leveno KJ: The continuing value of the Apgar score for the assessment of newborn infants. N Engl J Med 344:467–471, 2001

Costeloe K, Hennessy E, Gibson AT, Marlow N, Wilkinson AR: The EPICure study: outcomes to discharge from hospital for infants born at the threshold of viability. Pediatrics 106:659–661, 2000

Goldenberg RL, Hauth JC, Andrews WW: Intrauterine infection and preterm delivery. N Engl J Med 342:1500–1507, 2000

Goldenberg RL, Jobe AH: Prospects for research in reproductive health and birth outcomes. JAMA 285:633–639, 2001

Goldenberg RL, Rouse DJ: Prevention of premature birth. N Engl J Med 339:313–320, 1998

Guyer B, Freedman MA, Strobino DM, Sondik EJ: Annual summary of vital statistics: Trends in the health of Americans during the 20th century. Pediatrics 106:1307–1317, 2000

Guyer B, Hoyert D, Martin J, et al: Annual summary of vital statistics. Pediatrics 104:1229–1246, 1999

Guyer B, Macdorman M, Martin I, et al: Annual summary of vital statistics—1997. Pediatrics 102:1333, 1998

Hack M, Fanaroff AA: Outcomes of children of extremely low birthweight and gestational age in the 1990s. Semin Neonatal 5:89–106, 2000

Kramer MS, Demissie K, Yang H, et al: The contribution of mild and moderate preterm birth to infant mortality. Fetal and Infant Health Study Group of the Canadian Perinatal Surveillance System. JAMA 284:843–849, 2000

Lemons JA, Bauer CR, Oh W, et al: Very low birth weight outcomes of the National Institute of Child health and Human Development Neonatal Research Network, January 1995 through December 1996. NICHD Neonatal Research Network. Pediatrics 107:E1, 2001

McDorman MF, Atkinson JO: Infant mortality statistics from the 1997 period linked birth/infant death data set. Natl Vital Stat Rep 47:1–23, 1999

McIntire DD, Bloom SL, Casey BM, Leveno KJ: Birth weight in relation to morbidity among newborn infants. N Engl J Med 340:1234–1238, 1999

Phibbs CS, Bronstein JM, Buxton E, Phibbs RH: The effects of patient volume and level of care at the hospital of birth on neonatal mortality. JAMA 276:1054–1059, 1996

Vohr BR, Wright LL, Dusick AM, et al: Neurodevelopmental and functional outcomes of extremely low birth weight infants in the National Institute of Child Health and Human Development Neonatal Research Network, 1993–1994. Pediatrics 105:1216–1226, 2000

Wood NS, Marlow N, Costeloe K, et al: Neurologic and developmental disability after extremely preterm birth. EPICure Study Group. N Engl J Med 343:378–384, 2000

2.3 PLACENTA STRUCTURE AND FUNCTION

Kurt Benirschke

The human placenta is a discoid hemochorial organ that connects to the mother by interstitial implantation into the endometrium, which has changed into decidua because of the pregnancy's progesterone dominance. When the early blastocyst implants after its journey through the fallopian tube, approximately 6 days after fertilization, its shell is the trophoblast that deeply invades the endometrium and continues to cover the entire placenta. This tissue is composed largely of the placental villi and membranes. The trophoblast invades the maternal blood vessels to ensure the maternal intervillous circulation. It also functions as the barrier between mother and fetus and produces hormones, including human chorionic gonadotropin. The outermost trophoblast, the syncytium, makes the contact with the mother and is not "recognized" by her because it lacks the major histocompatibility antigens. Through its microvillous surface and an extensive cytoplasmic microvesicular system, the syncytium serves to transport nutrients, oxygen, and water from mother to fetus and to excrete fetal wastes into the maternal bloodstream. The villi at term are finely branched and provide about 10 m² of diffusional surface.

The normal term placenta weighs about 450 g and has membranes (the chorion laeve) attached to its edges. The innermost surface is the amnion, an epithelial layer on a thin strip of connective tissue. It is an avascular membrane that is only passively attached to the chorionic membrane. The amnion subsists on oxygen and nutrients contained in the amnionic fluid, and, when there is none, as in renal agenesis, it degenerates to form amnion nodosum. The chorion is a tougher membrane that carries the fetal blood vessels from the umbilical cord insertion to the villous ramifications. Generally, one artery supplies a single villous cotyledon, which is drained by a vein. The cotyledon has a central maternal arterial vessel that injects blood into the center of this villous district. The fetal arteries cross over the veins on the placental surface and thus are easily recognized.

The umbilical cord contains two arteries and one vein that lie within the very compressible Wharton jelly. This mucopolysaccharide-rich connective contains some mast cells and macrophages and is covered with a single layer of amnionic epithelium. The two umbilical arteries connect through "Hyrtl anastomosis" within the last inch before the cord inserts on the placental surface, usually near the center and less commonly at the margin. Insertion onto the membranes (velamentous insertion) occurs in about 1% of fetuses and is often associated with growth restriction and frequently with absence of one artery. Also, because the membranous vessels are not supported by Wharton jelly, they are more prone to undergo thrombosis or rupture during delivery, sometimes leading to severe, acute fetal blood loss. The umbilical cord at term normally measures 55 cm in length. Cords shorter than 40 cm are uncommon and correlate with reduced fetal mobility (amnionic bands, muscular disorders, trisomy, multiple gestation). Longer cords are much more frequent and are prone to form knots, prolapse, or encircle the fetus. They are also more often associated with fetal venous thromboses that occur on the surface of the placenta. These are recognized as white streaks that may calcify after several days.

The cord is always spiraled, most often with the spiral to the left, rarely to the right. The reason for this twisting is unknown. Absence of one umbilical artery (SUA, single umbilical artery) is the most common anomaly of development. In about 40% of SUA, the neonate dies or has a significant congenital anomaly. In the remainder, however, there are no adverse findings; the presence of SUA should prompt a careful search for other fetal anomalies. Multiple pregnancy and velamentous cord insertion are more frequent in placentas with SUA.

The fetal surface of the placenta is normally blue, translucent, and shiny. When it is opacified or white, with variable degrees of visual obliteration of underlying fetal vessels, a microscopic evaluation for chorioamnionitis should be performed. Chorioamnionitis, infection of the amnionic fluid, is most common between 20 and 30 weeks of gestation and is always the result of an ascending infection. The release of phospholipases, and subsequently prostaglandins, in the endocervical canal leads to cervical dilation and premature delivery. Green discoloration of the amnion, sometimes with a slimy quality, is the common result of meconium discharge before birth. The meconium pigment is engulfed by surface macrophages and transported from amnion to chorion and then disseminated into the mother. In the umbilical cord, meconium often injures the arterial wall and interferes with perfusion of arterial blood.

The maternal surface of the placenta may or may not show the subdivisions of cotyledons. When the placenta has been delivered gently, the maternal surface is intact and smooth and covered with a thin layer of decidua basalis and often fresh blood. A firm layer of blood may be associated with compression of villous tissue as a result of retroplacental hemorrhage (abruptio placentae). The placenta is pale if the fetus is anemic as with erythroblastosis, parvovirus infection, or transplacental bleeding. In diabetic pregnancies, the villous tissue is generally darker, softer, and plethoric, and the placenta is also often larger than normal and microscopically may show chorangiosis, a proliferation of capillaries. Careful examination may reveal whether a placenta previa had been present because the membranes rupture at the placental margin. Placenta accreta develops when the uterus lacks normal decidua because of previous curettage, myomectomy, or antecedent cesarean section that has left scars in the uterus. The placenta may penetrate such scars (placenta percreta), sometimes resulting in serious hemorrhage.

Areas of firmness in the villous tissue may represent either infarcted tissue, as often is found with preeclampsia, or, more rarely, chorangiomas. Infarcts are usually at the placental margin and result from obstruction of maternal blood flow by atherosis and thrombosis in spiral arteries; they become white over time. Severe villous infarction may result in fetal growth restriction. Maternal floor infarction is a different type of infarction that is not associated with maternal disease and has no known cause. It is associated with deposition of excessive amounts of fibrinoid (basement membrane substances) by the trophoblast. It severely affects fetal growth and may cause recurrent fetal demise.

Chorangiomas arise from the fetal villous circulation. When large, they may interfere with the fetal circulation and cause heart failure and hydrops. They may also undergo thrombosis and atrophy. Occasionally, chorangiomas are associated with angiomas in the fetus, and, when they are massive, they may lead to thrombocytopenia.

Infection of the villi is commonly recognized on microscopic examination of the placenta. This is often referred to as villitis of unknown etiology (VUE), but rarely an infectious agent can be identified (cytomegalovirus, syphilitic spirochetes, rubella virus). VUE is associated with fetal growth restriction and can lead to fetal demise when extensive.

The placentas of multiple pregnancies should be examined carefully because they can provide substantial information about the genetic relationship of the fetuses. The placentas may be fused or separate, and it is important to decide whether the membrane relationship is monochorionic or dichorionic. This can be ascertained by examining the dividing membranes separating the fetal sacs. Monochorionic membranes are present when the dividing membranes are thin and translucent (Fig. 2-5). The membranes can be easily separated, yielding a single chorionic surface that covers the villous tissue. These placentas are referred to as diamnionic, monochorionic twin placentas ("DiMo") and are absolutely diagnostic for monozygotic (MZ), single-ovum-derived ("identical") twins. The membranes of dichorionic twins are generally opaque and are composed of two amnionic and two chorionic layers. It is usually difficult to separate the membranes, and in the process, the placental surface often becomes disrupted at the base. Such diamnionic, dichorionic ("DiDi") twin placentas are usually associated with fraternal twins, but some identical twins have such membranes. These twins would have separated early in embryogenesis, before formation of the chorionic cavity, which occurs on day 3 after fertilization. Interference with implantation may account for the higher incidence of velamentous insertion (Fig. 2-5) and SUA in multiple

pregnancies. Monochorionic twin placentas of identical twins always have some anastomoses between their circulations. Artery-to-artery communication is most frequent, and this has few sequelae. When an artery from one twin supplies a cotyledon that is then drained by a vein into the other twin, this provides the basis of the twin-to-twin transfusions syndrome (TTTS). Polycythemia develops in one twin and anemia in the other, often resulting in heart failure, hydramnios, hydrops, and fetal demise or injury. It is important to recognize this syndrome prenatally because it is now treatable by laser obliteration of the connecting blood umbilical vessels. Various vascular connections are common in DiMo twin placentas, and the extent and type of anastomosis determine fetal outcome. If one twin dies in utero, the surviving twin may lose blood rapidly through these anastomoses into the dead twin, resulting in fetal hypoxia and possible brain injury.

Monoamnionic twin placentas may occur when embryonic splitting occurs after the amnion has already formed. This is uncommon (1% of twins) but often has serious consequences. Entangling or knotting of cords often results in fetal demise.

References

Baldwin VJ: Pathology of Multiple Pregnancy. New York, Springer-Verlag, 1994

Benirschke K, Kaufmann P: The Pathology of the Human Placenta, 4th ed. New York, Springer-Verlag, 2000

Fox H: Pathology of the Placenta, 2nd ed. Philadelphia, WB Saunders, 1997

Kaplan CG: Color Atlas of Gross Placental Pathology. New York, Igaku-Shoin, 1994

Langston C, Kaplan C, MacPherson T, et al: Practice guidelines for examination of the placenta. Developed by the placental pathology practice guideline development task force of the College of American Pathologists. Arch Pathol Lab Med 121:449–476, 1997

Lewis SH, Perrin VDK, eds: Pathology of the Placenta. New York, Churchill Livingstone, 1999

Naeye RL: Disorders of the Placenta, Fetus, and Neonate. St Louis, Mosby Year-Book, 1992

2.4   FACTORS INFLUENCING FETAL GROWTH

Dennis M. Styne

Growth of a fetus is a remarkable event; in the human the process encompasses multiplication of a single fertilized ovum into more than 200 cell types, an increase in length of 5000-fold, an increase in surface area by 61×10^6 and an increase in weight by 6×10^{12}. Fetal growth requires availability of adequate oxygen and nutrition in concert with the effects of growth factors and oncogenes, all operating according to a basic plan dictated by genetics, especially important early in gestation, and influenced by the maternal environment, of greatest importance late in gestation.

INTRAUTERINE GROWTH RESTRICTION

Disorders of intrauterine growth offer insight into the control of normal fetal growth. Intrauterine growth restriction (IUGR; intra-

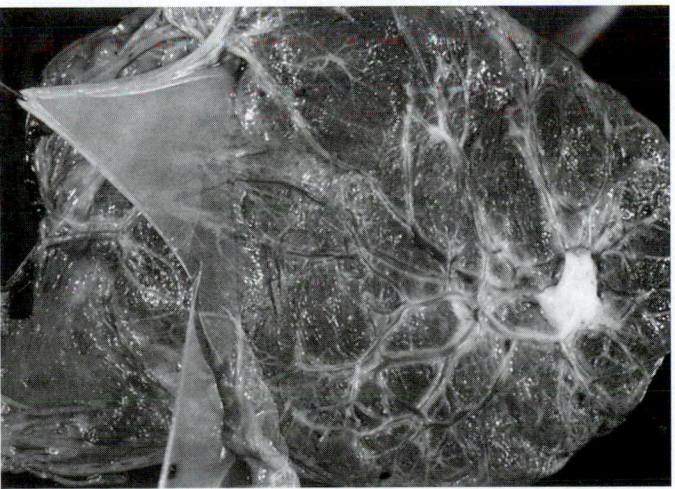

FIGURE 2-5 Diamnionic, monochorionic twin placenta from "identical" twins. Note the translucent membrane that divides the two amnionic cavities. Beneath, a single stretched-out chorion carries the fetal blood vessels. The umbilical cord of the twin on the left has a velamentous (membranous) insertion. It is easy to identify these surface blood vessels as arteries because they cross over the veins.

uterine growth restriction, fetal growth restriction, or small for gestational age) is the final pathway of a wide range of factors including maternal nutrition and vascular, genetic, and endocrine effects. IUGR is discussed in Sec. 2.14. This section focuses predominantly on endocrine factors affecting fetal growth.

THE PLACENTA

Embryonic growth during the first trimester is controlled by nutrient supply and locally active growth factors, whereas fetal growth later in gestation depends largely on the delivery of nutrients to the fetus. The placenta influences all these aspects, and placeta is an active endocrine organ that produces numerous hormones normally associated with hypothalamic and pituitary hormones and gonadal and adrenal function. The structure and function of placental hormones may mimic those of the hormones produced in the other endocrine organs (eg, the hypothalamus or pituitary gland) or may differ substantially. Human chorionic gonadotropin (hCG), human chorionic somatomammotropin (hCS), placental gonadotropin-releasing factor (GnRH), somatostatin (SRIF), corticotropin-releasing factor (CRH), adrenocortical stimulating hormone (ACTH), β-endorphin, enkephalin, inhibin, and neurotpeptide Y (NPY), among other peptides, are found in the placenta. These hormones are regulated and active; eg, (1) placental GnRH stimulates the release of placental hCG, and serum levels of GnRH are highest in the first trimester; (2) placental SRIF is higher early in gestation and decreases as hCS rises during pregnancy; and (3) placental CRH stimulates the release of ACTH and β-endorphin, and their plasma concentrations increase in the last 5 weeks of pregnancy. Several growth factors such as transforming growth factor β (TGF-β), insulin-like growth factor (IGFs), epidermal growth factor (EGFs), platelet-derived growth factor (PDGF), fibroblast growth factor (FGF), and many of their receptors are produced in the placenta.

Differences between placental hormones and those produced in the hypothalamus and pituitary are demonstrated by the biology of placental growth hormone, a maternal hormone. Placental growth hormone (from the GH-v gene) is released continuously, in contrast to the pulsatile release of pituitary growth hormone (produced from the GH-n gene). Placental growth hormone structure differs from that of pituitary growth hormone by 13 amino acids, and placental growth hormone has a greater anabolic than lactogenic effect, as compared with pituitary growth hormone. The concentration of placental growth hormone is significantly decreased in sera of pregnant women bearing a fetus with intrauterine growth restriction.

GROWTH FACTORS AND ONCONGENES

Growth factors and oncogenes exert important effects on fetal growth. Oncogenes contain sequences of a viral genome that, when transfected by a retrovirus into a host, produces neoplasia; protooncogenes are similar in structure to viral oncogenes but are normal cell constituents. Some oncogenes may code for growth factors or growth factor receptors; for example, *src* and *abl* code for tyrosine-specific protein kinase; *erb B* codes for a truncated EGF receptor; *myc, myb, fos,* and *jun* code for phosphoproteins that regulate gene transcription. Growth factors may act independently, or they may stimulate or inhibit the expression of oncogenes. Several oncogenes (eg, *c-fos*) are expressed in human placenta in an age-related manner. It is noteworthy that some of the same oncogenes

that cause postnatal neoplasia do not cause tumors in the normally differentiating fetus; rather, expression of these oncogenes is important in the normal development of many fetal organs.

Polypeptide growth factors, their membrane-bound receptors, and some of their binding proteins have prime importance in fetal growth. Although these peptides are named "growth factors," some actually inhibit growth and development and are therefore critically important in reorganization of the fetus. Growth factors control the essential aspects of fetal growth: (1) cellular hyperplasia and (2) cellular differentiation including hypertrophy, migration, and apoptosis (programmed cell death) leading to organ formation. Early in fetal development, cell-to-cell interactions mediate growth by autocrine (the effect of a growth factor on the cell of origin) and paracrine (the effect of a growth factor on a neighboring cell) action of growth factors. Later in gestation, after development of the fetal circulation, endocrine action (exerting effects at a distance) becomes prominent.

INSULIN-LIKE GROWTH FACTORS

IGFs have been studied extensively. IGF-1 is regulated postnatally by growth hormone (GH), nutrition, sex steroids, and thyroid hormone as well as other agents and is primarily responsible for postnatal linear growth. IGF-1 exerts effects through the type 1 cell membrane receptor that structurally resembles the insulin receptor. IGFs can be demonstrated by 12 weeks in human fetal tissue, and IGF-1 and IGF-2 are measurable in plasma by 15 weeks of gestation. Fetal IGF-1 concentrations increase with advancing gestation, but even by term, they are lower than maternal plasma concentrations.

Serum IGF-2 concentrations are higher in the human fetus than in the adult. In fetal life, IGF-2 interacts with the type 1 receptor and the insulin receptor, whereas postnatally it interacts with the type 2 receptor (identical to the mannose-6-phosphate receptor). A soluble form of the type 2 receptor is present in the fetal circulation and in amniotic fluid; concentrations of this protein decrease with advancing gestation and fall even further after birth.

IGFs exert effects on fetal growth mainly by reducing placental uptake of nutrients, preferentially shunting them to the fetus and thus leading to anabolism. IGF-1 has the ability to stimulate the growth of human fetal fibroblasts, myoblasts, chondrocytes, osteoblasts, hepatocytes, glial cells, and adrenal cells. IGFs also affect the differentiation of fetal cells in muscle, cartilage, and the nervous system.

IGFs are associated with six IGF-binding proteins (IGFBPs), some of which decrease and some increase the IGF effect. IGFBP-1 is identical to placental protein 12, a product of the decidua; amniotic fluid concentrations of IGFBP-1 are higher in early than in late gestation. Fetal serum IGF-1 and IGFBP-3 concentrations have a strong positive relationship to birth weight, ponderal index, and placental weight; they are decreased in fetal growth retardation. This is accompanied by a concurrent elevation of fetal IGFBP-1 and IGFBP-2. Fetal IGFBP-2 concentrations are also decreased in fetal malnutrition and hypoxia. Conversely, IGFBP-1 concentrations are decreased in fetuses that are large for gestational age. intrauterine growth rate (IUGR) is associated with a decrease in IGF-1 and elevation of IGFBP-2 concentrations in maternal serum; IGFBP-3 does not relate to birth weight. These findings suggest that IGF-1 has a role in regulating fetal growth, with IGFBP-3 serving to regulate the reservoir of available IGF-1. IGFBP-1 inhibits IGF-1 action, thereby exaggerating the effects of these changes on fetal growth. Another level of control of the IGFs in fetal growth is furnished by the specific IGFBP proteases produced in the placental decidua that degrade IGFBPs in maternal serum.

Gene manipulation and infusion of growth factors in animals have been used to demonstrate the influence that these factors may have on fetal growth. IGF-1 knockout mice, which produce no IGF-1, exhibit poor late fetal and postnatal development with organ hypoplasia and delayed ossification of cartilage. They die as a result of diaphragmatic muscular hypoplasia. IGF-2 knockout mice show reduced growth in early gestation but a normal growth rate later in gestation. Thus, IGF-2 appears to be important in promoting fetal growth in early gestation, whereas IGF-1 is more important in later gestation. Elimination of type 1 receptors by gene knockout leads to more profound growth failure than in mice with IGF-1 knockout alone, indicating that factors other than IGF-1, such as IGF-2, affect fetal growth through the type 1 receptor. Artificial elevation of maternal IGF-1 concentrations can increase growth in mouse and rat fetuses and overcome the growth restriction imposed by uterine limitations associated with large litter size. Knockout of the maternal gene for the type 2 receptor leads to high birth weight, generalized organomegaly, and various lethal anomalies. Thus, the type 2 receptor appears to be essential for postnatal life. Transgenic mice that overexpress IGFBP-1 are smaller at birth, grow poorly after birth, and have small organs; the brain is particularly small. They also have fasting hyperglycemia and impaired glucose tolerance and frequently die postnatally. Overexpression of IGFBP-1 in mice is associated with impaired postnatal growth, suggesting an inhibitory role for IGFBP-1 in late gestation and after birth. Overexpression of IGFBP-3 in mice results in enlargement of the spleen, liver, and heart; birth weight is normal. Thus, excess IGFBP-1 stunts fetal growth, whereas excess IGFBP-3 leads to selective organomegaly. Administration of synthetic IGF-1 to fetal rhesus macaques resulted in an increase in weight of the spleen, thymus, and kidney and an increase in small intestinal length.

INSULIN

Insulin, a key regulatory factor in carbohydrate metabolism, also has a major role in fetal growth. The ability of insulin either to signal metabolic processes or to stimulate growth seems to relate to its ability to cause phosphorylation of IRS-1. Knockout of the IRS-1 gene leads to a growth-retarded fetal mouse that is born viable but has fetal and postnatal growth deficiency and hyperglycemia. Knockout of the IRS-2 gene leads to diabetes. Membrane-bound insulin receptors are expressed in greater numbers and with higher affinity in fetal tissues such as lung, liver, erythrocytes, and monocytes than in the adult. Insulin receptors are similar to type 1 IGF-1 receptors, and IGFs can bind to insulin receptors just as insulin can bind to IGF-1 receptors. Fetal insulin deficiency, which is characteristic of congenital diabetes mellitus and pancreatic dysgenesis, results in IUGR. Similarly, a deficiency of the insulin receptor in the leprechaun syndrome is associated with extreme elevation of serum insulin and low glucose concentrations, hypotrophic adipose tissue, transient ketoacidosis, virilization, and intrauterine growth restriction.

Macrosomia is usually denoted as a birth weight over 4 kg in the term infant. Symmetric macrosomia is denoted by a ponderal index between the 10th and 90th percentiles, whereas with asymmetric macrosomia the ponderal index is higher. Asymmetric macrosomia is a well-known effect of fetal hyperinsulinism. It is discussed in Sec 2.15.

EPIDERMAL GROWTH FACTOR

EGF and TGF-α differ by the chromosome locations for the genes that code for the proteins as well as by their different amino acid sequences. EGF and TGF-α utilize the same receptor, the EGF receptor (EGF-R), which has tyrosine phosphorylase activity, and they have biological actions. In the fetus, there is virtually no detectable EGF, but TGF-α is plentiful early in gestation as a result of production by the maternal decidua and transfer to the fetus.

EGF plays a major role in placental implantation, growth, and differentiation. The first fetal cell type to arise during embryogenesis is the cytotrophoblast, and EGF and TGF-α are responsible for cytotrophoblast cell division. The cytotrophoblast then differentiates into the invasive extravillous and noninvasive villous populations of cells. The villous trophoblast cells of the cytotrophoblast express the EGF-R located primarily at the fetomaternal interface. EGF-R ligands play an important role in the regulatory pathway of placental and fetal growth. Microvilli purified from placentas of infants with IUGR have decreased or absent placental EGF-R phosphorylation and tyrosine kinase activity. There are decreased numbers of EGF receptors and reduced affinity for EGF receptors in placentas of women with a history of heavy smoking and in hypertensive women. This suggests that EGF may contribute to the impaired fetal growth associated with smoking and hypertension. EGF is plentiful in amniotic fluid and in fetal urine, whereas the fetal intestinal tract contains only TGF-α. EGF concentrations in amniotic fluid increase toward term. Levels are decreased in pregnancies associated with IUGR, but they are not increased in infants who are large for gestational age.

EGF stimulates production of ornithine decarboxylase, fibronectin, prolactin, and prostaglandin E_2. Effects of EGF and TGF-α on normal development include stimulation of growth and development of the craniofacial region, the intestine, the brain, and some regions of the skin. TGF-α, EGF, and their common EGF-R are present throughout gestation in the mesenchymal cells of the fetal lung, but the immunoreactivity migrates to the airway epithelium as gestation progresses. EGF-R are found throughout the fetal intestinal tract. Thus, EGF and its receptor may have a role in growth of the lung and gastrointestinal tract as well as in development of the fetus.

EGF has potential as a therapeutic agent for premature infants based on effects reported in the nonhuman primate. EGF administered to fetal monkeys resulted in histologic and biochemical maturation of the lungs, leading to improved air exchange and a reduced requirement for respiratory support in the prematurely delivered rhesus infant.

FIBROBLAST GROWTH FACTOR

FGF plays an important role in embryonic growth and morphogenesis by regulating cellular proliferation, differentiation, and tissue patterning during vertebrate embryogenesis. Both FGF-2 and FGF-receptor-1 messenger RNA and proteins are found in every organ but have defined cellular localization in the midtrimester human fetus. FGF-2 immunoreactivity peaks in cord serum at 18 to 20 weeks of gestation, then slowly decreases to term. Amniotic fluid also contains immunoreactive FGF-2 at term. FGF-2 is present in maternal serum from at least 18 weeks of gestation, rises to maximum values at the end of the second trimester, and decreases progressively to term.

Aberrant FGF signaling during limb and skeletal development can lead to dysmorphic syndromes. Achondroplasia results from mutations in the transmembrane domain of the type 3 fibroblast growth factor receptor (FGF-R3; gene at 4p16.3); other mutations of this gene lead to abnormalities ranging from lethal thanatropic dwarfism to hypochondroplasia.

SUBSTANCE EXPOSURES AND FETAL GROWTH

Fetal alcohol syndrome (FAS) is characterized by IUGR, short stature throughout childhood, dysmorphic facial features, abnormality of brain development, behavior abnormalities, and developmental delay (see Sec. 10.3.8 and 26.17.2, and Fig. 10-24). Fetal cocaine exposure causes decreased growth rate and decreased head growth (See Sec 25.0). Heavy maternal smoking is associated with a reduction of birth weight averaging 200 g, with the major effect occurring in late pregnancy. This decrease in birth weight is thought to be dose related.

OTHER IMPORTANT CAUSES OF ABERRANT FETAL GROWTH

Numerous other conditions impair fetal growth despite adequate maternal nutrition. Notable examples are maternal infection, as with toxoplasmosis, rubella, cytomegalovirus, and herpes simplex (TORCH), chromosome abnormalities such as trisomy 21 (Down syndrome), gonadal dysgenesis (Turner syndrome), and various dysmorphic syndromes. Anatomic malformations of the uterus may also impair fetal growth.

FETAL ORIGINS OF ADULT DISEASE

The effects of abnormalities of the fetal environment may extend well beyond infancy. Considerable evidence has now been accumulated indicating that interference with fetal nutrition may have an effect on postnatal development and also increase the likelihood of the occurrence of certain diseases in adult life. This has been referred to as the "Barker hypothesis."

The differential effects of maternal starvation early and late in pregnancy on human fetal growth have been reported in survivors of famine. Infants of mothers who experienced famine during the last two trimesters of pregnancy during World War II in Holland had birth weights 8 to 9% lower than those born in the same location before the famine. In contrast, birth weight appeared to be unaffected by nutritional deprivation that occurred during the first trimester in pregnant women in the Leningrad and Holland famines. However, women who were born during the famine subsequently gave birth to infants of lower weight.

In addition to the effects on postnatal weight, there is increasing evidence that interference in fetal nutrition may program the individual to be subject to development of diseases in adult life. It has been reported that individuals with reduced weight at birth are prone to develop insulin resistance and type 2 diabetes, hypertension, hyperlipidemia, and coronary artery disease in later life. The suggestion that these far-ranging consequences are associated with low birth weight has been criticized on several grounds. It has been stated that it is very hard to establish the relationship as long as five decades after birth. More detailed studies are necessary to determine the strength of these possible relationships.

References

Ashworth A: Effects of intrauterine growth restriction on mortality and morbidity in infants and young children. Eur Clin Nutr 52:S34–S41, 1998

Baker J, Liu JP, Robertson EJ, Efstratiadis A: Role of insulin-like growth factors in embryonic and postnatal growth. Cell 75:73–82, 1993

Barker DJ: The fetal origins of coronary heart disease. Acta Paediatr 422(Suppl):78–82, 1997

Bauer MK, Harding JE, Bassett NS, et al: Fetal growth and placental function. Mol Cell Endocrinol 140:115–120, 1998

Cheatham B, Kahn CR: Insulin action and the insulin signaling network. Endocrinol Rev 16:117–142, 1995

Evain-Brion D: Hormonal regulation of fetal growth. Horm Res 42:207–214, 1994

Fondacci C, Alsat E, Gabriel R, Blot P, Nessmann C, Evain-Brion D: Alterations of human placental epidermal growth factor receptor in intrauterine growth restriction. J Clin Invest 93:1149–1155, 1994

Garnica AD, Chan WY: The role of the placenta in fetal nutrition and growth. J Am Coll Nutr 15:206–222, 1996

Giudice LC, de Zegher F, Gargosky SE, et al: Insulin-like growth factors and their binding proteins in the term and preterm human fetus and neonate with normal and extremes of intrauterine growth. J Clin Endocrinol Metab 80:1548–1555, 1995

Gluckman PD, Harding JE: Fetal growth retardation: underlying endocrine mechanisms and postnatal consequences. Acta Paediatr 422(Suppl):69–72, 1997

Hills FA, English J, Chard T: Circulating levels of IGF-I and IGF-binding protein-1 throughout pregnancy: relation to birthweight and maternal weight. J Endocrinol 148:303–309, 1996

Joseph KS, Kramer MS: Review of the evidence on fetal and early childhood antecedents of adult chronic disease. Epidemiol Rev 18:158–174, 1996

Menon RK, Sperling MA: Insulin as a growth factor. Endocrinol Metab Clin North Am 25:633–647, 1996

Mirlesse V, Frankenne F, Alsat E, Poncelet M, Hennen G, Evain-Brion D: Placental growth hormone levels in normal pregnancy and in pregnancies with intrauterine growth restriction. Pediatr Res 34:439–442, 1993

Pirazzoli P, Cacciari E, De Lasio R, et al: Developmental pattern of fetal growth hormone, insulin-like growth factor I, growth hormone binding protein and insulin-like growth factor binding protein-3. Arch Dis Child Fetal Neonat Ed 77:F100–F104, 1997

Stein AD, Ravelli AC, Lumey LH: Famine, third-trimester pregnancy weight gain, and intrauterine growth: the Dutch Famine Birth Cohort Study. Hum Biol 67:135–150, 1995

Styne DM: Fetal growth. Clin Perinatol 25:917–938, 1998

2.5   PRENATAL CARE AND THE AT-RISK PREGNANCY

J. T. Parer

2.5.1   Routine Prenatal Care

The objective of prenatal care is to optimize the outcome for both mother and baby. This is achieved through a series of visits with the mother during which history, physical examination, laboratory and other measurements, and patient education all are essential parts.

On the first visit, the last menstrual period is ascertained to date the current pregnancy. In addition, the patient is questioned about previous pregnancies, ethnic background, current problems, current medications, and medical, social, psychosocial, nutritional, and family history. Also on the first (or an early) visit, the mother is given a screening physical examination and a full pelvic examination including estimation of uterine size and clinical pelvimetry. Her weight and height are recorded, and blood pressure measured. Urine is examined for protein and glucose and may also be screened for bacteriuria. Standard blood studies include complete blood count, Venereal Disease Research Laboratory test (VDRL) for syphilis, rubella antibodies, hepatitis B surface antigen, blood type and Rh, and red cell antibodies.

During these early visits, education of the mother continues on such topics as promoting healthy behaviors, general knowledge of pregnancy, nutritional information, and information on the structure of prenatal care. This educational portion of the visit is supplemented by written materials appropriate to individual needs.

Referral to medical, social, or financial resources may begin at this time.

The frequency of prenatal visits is tailored to individual requirements. The first visit is generally between 6 and 8 weeks of gestation. The second visit, 6 weeks later, is at gestation greater than 10 weeks, when fetal heart tones can be detected. The next visit, approximately 6 weeks later, is when the mother is offered expanded maternal serum screening for neural tube defects and some chromosomal anomalies. At 18 to 20 weeks of gestation a fetal and obstetric ultrasound study is done. The mother will be seen again approximately 4 to 6 weeks later, and again at 28 weeks of gestation, when blood glucose concentration is measured 1 hour after a standard dose of oral glucose, a CBC is repeated, and the mother is evaluated for the need for Rh immune globulin. Visits continue at 4-week intervals until 36 weeks of gestation, then at 38 weeks, and weekly thereafter.

2.5.2   The Concept of Risk Assessment

Risk assessment in obstetrics was introduced before more specific tests of fetal evaluation were developed. The concept is that certain maternal or fetal conditions make it more likely that the pregnancy outcome will be worse than in the average mother. It is still used as an indication for screening and for deciding which mothers are more likely to benefit from specific tests such as fetal heart rate monitoring, ultrasound imaging, amniotic fluid volume, amniocentesis, etc. The combination of a number of tests of fetal condition and pulmonary maturity has lead to the important concept of optimal timing of delivery in the at-risk pregnancy.

2.5.3   Important Risk Factors and Conditions

PRETERM DELIVERY

Preterm delivery assumes an overwhelming importance in obstetrics because of the mortality and morbidity statistics (Sec. 2.2). Although great efforts have been made to reduce preterm delivery, success rates are unimpressive. Greater success has been achieved in ameliorating the consequences of preterm delivery by developments such as tertiary referral centers, neonatal intensive care units, tests of fetal pulmonary maturity, glucocorticoid treatment for accelerating fetal pulmonary maturity, and neonatal surfactant administration.

PRETERM LABOR Preterm labor is defined as the onset of regular uterine contractions producing cervical change before 37 weeks of gestation, indicating a risk for preterm delivery. Great efforts have gone into the study of this condition, and even greater efforts have gone into attempting to abort the preterm contractions in order to continue the pregnancy. This intervention has proved less successful than at first hoped. There is a high incidence of overdiagnosis

of "preterm labor," and the consequences of its treatment are not always benign.

Attempts have been made to identify mothers at risk for preterm labor by scoring systems. The most powerful risk factor for preterm delivery is a history of an infant being delivered prematurely previously. Women with this history have as much as a 25% risk of producing a second preterm baby, and if they have had two preterm deliveries, the risk rises to 75%. Risk scoring of nulliparas is neither sensitive nor specific.

Intervention generally takes the form of bed rest plus tocolytic agents. Tocolytic drugs, such as β-adrenoreceptor stimulants, magnesium sulfate, calcium channel blockers, and prostaglandin synthetase inhibitors, reduce the incidence of uterine contractions. However, there is little sound evidence that either one agent or a combination is effective in prolonging pregnancy much more than 48 hours. In early studies, the placebo effect of tocolytic therapy was shown to be up to 50% effective; few recent studies have used placebo groups but rather compare effects of different tocolytic agents. The apparent success rates of tocolytics are further enhanced by incorrect diagnosis and treatment of mothers who are not, in fact, in preterm labor.

A subgroup of the preterm labor group includes those individuals diagnosed with incompetent cervix (inappropriately maturing cervical tissue before term). This condition is rarely identified in nulliparas and requires a history consistent with incompetent cervix for appropriate treatment in subsequent pregnancies by early placement of a cerclage or a stitch around the cervix, either vaginally or transabdominally.

The diagnosis of incompetent cervix is improved considerably by use of transvaginal ultrasound to detect cervical funneling of the internal os. This allows a better selection of those who are likely benefit from a cerclage.

PRETERM PREMATURE RUPTURE OF MEMBRANES This refers to rupture of membranes before 37 weeks of gestation. It is believed that either infection or premature opening of the internal cervical os is often responsible, but a reason for premature rupture is rarely found.

At term, the mother is evaluated by a sterile speculum exam to confirm rupture and exclude advanced dilatation, a fetal heart rate recording to rule out fetal acidemia, and determination of fetal presentation. Many practitioners proceed to induction, but others allow selected patients to return home for 24 to 48 hours to await the onset of labor, with precautions regarding infections and group B *Streptococcus* prophylaxis.

If membranes rupture prematurely at 36 weeks of gestation, the fetus is usually managed as at term. Between 34 and 36 weeks of gestation, when newborn morbidity is extremely low except for respiratory distress syndrome, the fetus can be treated as at term, if pulmonary maturity can be demonstrated. Before 34 weeks, when pulmonary maturity is less likely, management diverges. Some physicians perform an amniocentesis to test for pulmonary maturity, but others simply allow the mother to stay in hospital at bed rest, with glucocorticoid treatment to accelerate pulmonary maturity. Such a policy generally is adopted down to age 28 weeks of gestation. Before 28 weeks, when mortality from immaturity tends to rise, some would institute tocolysis to prolong pregnancy even in the face of contractions after the betamethasone treatment has been instituted.

All of the above approaches are subservient to the onset of infection. If infection is diagnosed clinically, either by fever, elevated white blood cell count, and fetal tachycardia or by laboratory demonstration of bacteria in the amniotic fluid, the current consensus is that such patients should be delivered. There is reasonably good evidence that treatment of preterm rupture of membranes with antibiotics will prolong the latency period before delivery in the absence of infection.

CLINICALLY INDICATED PRETERM DELIVERY   Preterm delivery may be indicated in several conditions such as severe fetal intrauterine growth restriction and severe maternal disease such as preeclampsia with HELLP (hemolysis, elevated liver enzymes, low platelets) syndrome.

MULTIPLE BIRTHS

Multiple births pose a problem for obstetric and neonatal outcome because of the relatively high incidence of preterm delivery, and of congenital defects, including both structural anomalies and those caused by discordance of the twins. The mean gestational age of delivery of twins is 37 weeks. The mortality and morbidity of twin pregnancies are much higher than for singletons.

The important obstetric observations in multiple pregnancies are early diagnosis, particularly to determine chorionicity, and ultrasound biometry to determine the differential growth of each twin. Fetal anomalies are more common among monochorionic, diamnionic twins. In such twins sharing a placenta, the possibility of twin-twin transfusion is real and can be determined by evaluation of each twin's continued appropriate growth and amniotic fluid volume. If both twins show appropriate growth, no intervention is necessary. However, when one twin is growing faster than the other, and there is evidence of compromise or extremely decreased head growth in one, intervention may be recommended to optimize the outcome of the pair. A further consideration with twins is the higher incidence of preeclampsia, which may require early delivery.

Recommendations for mode of delivery vary. In a number of centers, cesarean section is recommended for twins when one has a malpresentation. In other centers, a twin pregnancy is treated much the same as a singleton pregnancy: if the weight is appropriate (neither too small nor too large), the first twin is delivered vaginally with either spontaneous delivery of the second twin or breech extraction if it presents in anything but vertex presentation. The evidence points to neither approach as being superior (see Sec 2.13 for other aspects of multiple births).

DIABETES MELLITUS

The outcome of pregnancy in diabetes mellitus is now excellent, except for the persistent higher incidence of congenital anomalies. Diabetes mellitus also brings an increased incidence of macrosomia, thought to be caused by fetal hyperinsulinemia (Sec. 2.15). The obstetric goal in diabetics is prevention of complications by continuous maintenance of normal glycemia, especially beginning before conception, to decrease the incidence of congenital anomalies.

The target is for fasting blood glucose concentrations of 60 to 100 mg/dL during pregnancy, with 1-hour postmeal values 100 to 140 mg/dL. A further target is prepregnancy or early pregnancy glycosolated hemoglobin (HbA$_{1C}$ of less than 6%, indicating near normoglycemia over the previous several months. These targets are achieved by careful attention to diet, including content, quantity, and frequency of eating, and frequent (at least four times per day) blood glucose measurements. If required, insulin generally is administered twice daily, using a combination of neutral protamine Hagedorn (NPH) and regular insulin. During the intrapartum period, insulin-dependent diabetics are generally treated with an insulin infusion, and blood glucose may be measured up to every hour.

Under the above conditions, the outcome for pregnant diabetics is usually excellent, with an extremely low incidence of third-trimester stillbirth and diabetic ketoacidosis. There is also a reduction in neonatal hypoglycemia. Unfortunately, in a small proportion of patients, macrosomia persists despite good glucose control. The reduction in the incidence of congenital anomalies will be greater if patients are controlled before conception. Diagnosis of anomalies in fetuses of diabetic mothers is improved by biochemical screening, a level II ultrasound study at approximately 20 weeks, and fetal echocardiogram if indicated.

PREECLAMPSIA

Preeclampsia occurs in approximately 7 to 10% of pregnant women in the United States. The etiology of the disorder is still unknown, but recognition and treatment of complications have improved recently. This is largely a result of recognizing the multiorgan involvement, aggressive intensive-care management of intrapartum preeclamptics and eclamptics, and rational timing of delivery when preeclampsia is recognized. Preeclampsia is recognized by late second- or third-trimester elevations in blood pressure and proteinuria. Although edema is still part of the definition of preeclampsia, it occurs in normal pregnant women and thus, by itself, is not a useful sign.

Women with preeclampsia should be evaluated frequently for the development of severe preeclampsia, which has the following characteristics: (1) blood pressure $\geq$160 mm Hg systolic or $\geq$110 mm Hg diastolic on two measurements 6 hours apart at bed rest; (2) proteinuria >5 g in a 24-hour collection or $\geq$3-plus persistently by dipstick; (3) oliguria <500 mL in 24 hours; (4) cerebral or visual disturbances; (5) pulmonary edema or cyanosis; (6) epigastric or upper abdominal pain; (7) impaired liver function without other apparent cause; and (8) thrombocytopenia (<100,000 platelets/mm^3).

The onset of severe preeclampsia generally mandates that delivery must occur within a short period of time, either by induction or by cesarean section. Ancillary management will depend on the condition occurring: oliguria unresponsive to fluid administration generally requires central cardiac monitoring, and severe coagulopathy may require blood product replacement. Most patients have blood pressure controlled either by apresoline or labetalol. In addition, magnesium sulfate is administered for suppression of eclamptic seizure activity. Obstetric outcome in preeclampsia is generally favorable provided the patient is undergoing in-hospital care. The major newborn adverse outcomes with preeclampsia are either the result of prematurity, because of the need for early delivery, or the consequences of growth restriction in utero.

THIRD-TRIMESTER HEMORRHAGE

Third-trimester hemorrhage is primarily caused by placenta previa and abruptio placentae. These need to be distinguished for appropriate obstetric management. Fortunately, the wide availability of ultrasound imaging makes the diagnosis of placenta previa rapid and usually certain.

Bleeding from a placenta previa is usually painless, and this remains the prime means of distinguishing placenta previa from abruptio placentae. Placenta previa is generally managed conservatively until the third trimester, although this can be modified by the degree of bleeding and the gestational age. In patients who have a known placenta previa but no vaginal bleeding, management may be simply bed rest at home with delivery at or about 37 weeks, after demonstration of pulmonary maturity. Patients who have had bleeding from the placenta previa may be delivered prematurely in order to avoid potential hazard to the mother with a further bleed and to minimize the need for blood transfusions.

Abruptio placentae, representing a premature separation of part or all of the placenta, is generally accompanied by pain and uterine contractions. The diagnosis is supported by ruling out placenta previa by ultrasonography. The management of abruptio placentae depends on the size of the abruption, which usually determines the maternal symptoms and the degree of uterine activity. The management will also be determined by the fetal response. If a sufficient area of the placenta is lost, oxygen transport to the fetus may be compromised; this will be detected by fetal heart rate monitoring. The occurrence of abruptio placentae is generally unpredictable but correlates with hypertension and preeclampsia as well as with cocaine abuse.

The consequences for the fetus of both placenta previa and abruptio placentae are related to gestational age at delivery and the possible development of fetal asphyxia from either excessive bleeding or maternal cardiovascular instability. Both of these conditions may be accompanied by fetal anemia, presumably caused by disruption of fetal villi.

The differential diagnosis of third-trimester hemorrhage must also include the possibility of vasa previa. Bleeding from vasa previa will occur painlessly and will often be accompanied by signs of fetal compromise, as noted on the fetal heart rate monitor.

2.5.4   Assessment of Fetal Growth

FUNDAL HEIGHT

Measurement of the curved fundal height (ie, the distance from the top of the uterine fundus to the symphysis pubis) remains the basic screening technique for suspected macrosomia or intrauterine growth restriction (IUGR). Up to two-thirds of IUGR fetuses can be detected by noting a deceleration of this growth over a period of 3 to 4 weeks. Estimates of fetal weight are less useful because the standard deviation in general is at least 10% of the actual weight. However, extremes of fetal weight are generally determined with a fair degree of accuracy by clinical evaluation. Babies with suspected growth restriction should be evaluated by ultrasound imaging and biometry.

ULTRASOUND IMAGING AND BIOMETRY

This has become the standard method by which fetal size, and at times gestational age, are determined. Until approximately 20 weeks, fetuses tend to grow at a reasonably standard rate; therefore, determining gestational age by size is accurate in the majority of cases. After 20 weeks, fetuses grow at different rates, and the accuracy of gestational age from the measurements is less certain. Gestational age must be known to assess growth accurately during this period. In cases of uncertain dating, many authorities now recommend an ultrasound study at 18–20 weeks to determine gestational age because the accuracy is almost equal to that of earlier measurements, and much more information is gained about fetal morphology from the study.

In determining adequacy of growth, a number of measurements of the fetus are made and related to the equivalent gestational age. These include biparietal diameter of the head, head circumference, abdominal circumference, and femur length. An examination of the consistency of these four measurements gives an idea of the internal accuracy of the measurements. It may also show asymmetric growth restriction because generally the fetus's abdominal girth will fall off before head circumference and before restriction of growth of the long bones. However, such measurements, if symmetric, may still be consistent with early-onset symmetric growth retardation, so accurate determination of gestational age is important. As part of the ultrasound report, the clinician receives an estimated fetal weight and an estimate of the growth percentile of the baby for its gestational age. Growth restriction is defined as less than the 10th percentile.

The level 1 ultrasound study includes the measurements just mentioned and also a number of other observations. Of importance to growth restriction is an assessment of the volume of amniotic fluid. Obstetric ultrasonographers tend to favor the application of the amniotic fluid index, a semiquantitative measure of the amount of amniotic fluid (see below).

Other aspects of the level 1 ultrasound report include number of fetuses, presence of fetal cardiac motion, presentation, placental location, evaluation of the uterus and adnexal structures, and several aspects of fetal anatomy. These currently include cerebral ventricles, four-chamber view of the heart, spine, stomach, renal region, urinary bladder, and umbilical cord insertion site on the anterior abdominal wall. Suspected abnormalities in any of the above generally require a more specialized (level 2) study. This can define many congenital anomalies of the central nervous system, heart, gastrointestinal tract, genitourinary system, and skeleton. Many of these are associated with abnormal fetal growth or poly- or oligohydramnios, which leads to the initial sonogram. Because many detectable anomalies are associated with chromosomal disorders, amniocentesis for karyotyping is often indicated.

2.5.5   Antepartum Testing

An approach to antepartum surveillance has evolved that includes the following steps:

- Basic screening with fetal movement counting.
- Nonstress testing in cases of suspicious kick counts or in certain high-risk situations.
- Biophysical profile (BPP) or contraction stress testing (CST) in the presence of nonreactive or suspicious nonstress tests.
- In the case of a suspicious or positive CST, a biophysical profile for an infants so premature that delivery seems unwarranted.

Controversy continues regarding the relative merits and efficacy of these approaches.

NONSTRESS TESTING

Nonstress testing (NST) consists of detecting the fetal heart rate, fetal movement, and uterine activity by external means and noting the presence of fetal heart rate variability with fetal movement. The presence of these features predicts a normal fetal outcome.

Fetal movements may be detected by maternal sensation, attendant's observation or palpation of maternal abdomen, and sharp, upward marks on the tocodynamometer tracing. Fetuses have been observed to have sleep or inactive cycles that often last 20 to 40 minutes and can last up to twice that time. If the fetus is initially inactive, it may be stimulated manually, or the mother may be given appropriate liquid to ensure adequate glucose level. A variant of this test is the fetal vibroacoustic stimulation test. This test depends on fetal response to an acoustic stimulation (generally produced by an artificial larynx) applied to the maternal abdomen.

A *reactive* test, two accelerations of the fetal heart rate in 20 minutes, is associated with survival of the fetus for 1 week or more in more than 99% of cases. A *nonreactive* test is associated with poor fetal outcome (ie, perinatal death, low 5-minute Apgar score, late decelerations in labor) in approximately 20% of cases. Because of the high false-positive rate in clinical application of this test, a nonreactive fetus requires further evaluation by means of the biophysical profile or a contraction stress test unless contraindicated.

BIOPHYSICAL PROFILE

The biophysical profile (BPP) is the combined observation of five separate fetal biophysical variables: movement, tone, reactivity, breathing, and amniotic fluid volume. Fetal reactivity is assessed by the nonstress test (NST). The remaining four variables are assessed with the use of real-time ultrasound for a maximum of 30 minutes or less if the fetus achieves a perfect score.

The biophysical profile is sometimes used as the primary surveillance technique, but others use it to follow a nonreactive NST or to clarify the significance of a suspicious or positive CST. The biophysical profile has been reported to have a lower false-abnormal rate than either the NST or CST. However, it has not generally been accepted as a prime means of fetal surveillance.

The requirements for maximum scoring, and therefore a well-oxygenated fetus, are a reactive nonstress test, presence of fetal breathing movements, presence of fetal body movements, fetal tone, including an episode of extension of extremities and return to the flexed position, and adequate amniotic fluid volume.

Points from 0 to 2 are given for each factor. The lower the score, the more likely the fetus is to be compromised. The following is a guideline for acting on the BPP score:

- 8–10: Repeat NST/AFI per schedule
- 6: Repeat, usually in 24 hours or less
- 0–4: Consider for delivery

A number of perinatologists are now using the *modified biophysical profile,* which includes the NST and amniotic fluid index (AFI), the latter being a semiquantitative measure of amniotic fluid volume (see below). When normal, this test is probably as predictive of good outcome as the full BPP and is far less time-consuming.

AMNIOTIC FLUID INDEX

The AFI is a semiquantitative technique used for evaluating amniotic fluid volume. The uterus is divided into four quadrants with the linea nigra and the umbilicus serving as the dividing points. Each quadrant is scanned using ultrasound, and the vertical dimension of the largest pocket in each quadrant is measured in centimeters. (A pocket is excluded from the analysis if more than 50% of it is occupied by umbilical cord.) The sum of the numbers represents the total AFI.

Results are defined as ≤ 5 cm, oligohydramnios; 5.1 to 24 cm, normal; ≥ 24 cm, polyhydramnios.

CONTRACTION STRESS TEST

This test consists of noting the fetal heart rate response to uterine contractions induced by breast stimulation or oxytocin. Interpretation requires three recorded contractions in a 10-minute period,

each with a duration of at least 1 minute (see Sec. 2.5.6). The following are criteria used for interpretation of the CST.

NEGATIVE CST RESULT   No late decelerations and normal baseline fetal heart rate.

POSITIVE CST RESULTS   Persistent late decelerations with an adequate challenge; persistent late decelerations even with less than three uterine contractions per 10 minutes; possible absence of fetal heart rate (FHR) variability.

SUSPICIOUS CST RESULT   Intermittent late decelerations with an adequate challenge; variable decelerations (as occurs in the growth-restricted fetuses with oligohydramnios and may result from the cord being compressed during contractions because it is unprotected by amniotic fluid); abnormal baseline fetal heart rate (ie, less than 110 or more than 160 beats per minute). A negative CST result is associated with fetal survival for 1 week in more than 99% of cases. A positive CST result (ie, late decelerations following contractions) has been associated with poor fetal outcome and perinatal death, low 5-minute Apgar score, or late decelerations in labor in approximately 50% of cases. However, because of the high false-positive rate, it is recommended that if delivery is chosen, such patients be given a trial of labor with optimal fetal heart rate monitoring. A positive CST result is prognostically worse if it is accompanied by a nonreactive NST result with absence of FHR variability.

PROTOCOL FOR TESTING

The basic formal testing scheme is NST/AFI. On occasion an NST alone may suffice. Antenatal testing begins at different gestational ages depending on the maternal and/or fetal condition. It is started either when the condition is recognized (eg, suspected or actual intrauterine growth restriction) or at specific times (eg, the post-dates pregnancy). For other conditions it usually begins in mid–third trimester, about 34 weeks (eg, history of late unexplained intrauterine fetal demise).

Some of the conditions used to determine testing are as follows: postdates ($41\frac{1}{2}$ weeks); decreased fetal movement; hypertensive diseases; diabetes mellitus; intrauterine growth restriction; previous unexplained third-trimester intrauterine fetal demise; active substance abuse weekly (often these patients have other problems warranting surveillance, and testing may improve compliance); increased maternal serum α-fetoprotein or elevated hCG with normal amniocentesis; twins with discordant growth; preterm premature rupture of membranes: systemic lupus erythematosus; oligohydramnios; Rh alloimmunization in the presence of erythroblastosis; hyperthyroidism, if uncontrolled; cholestasis of pregnancy. There are many conditions that may not necessitate antepartum testing if seen alone. Some examples include hydramnios, well-controlled asthma, advanced maternal age, simple scleroderma, smoking, inactive substance abuse, seizure disorders, Raynaud disease, noncyanotic maternal heart or lung disease, fetal cardiac problems, omphalocele, etc.

2.5.6   Intrapartum Evaluation and Management

FETAL HEART RATE MONITOR

The fetal heart rate monitor is a device with two components, one to recognize and process heart rate and the other to recognize uter-

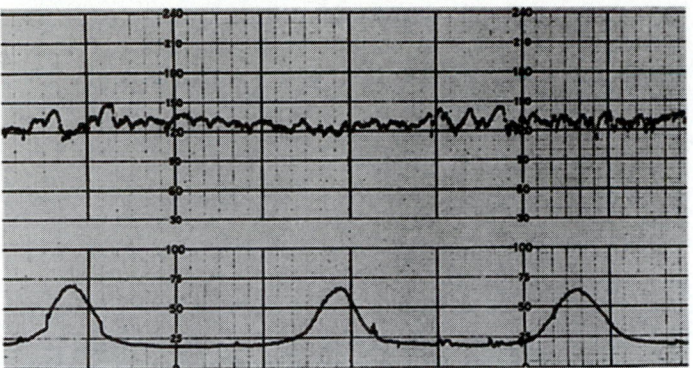

FIGURE 2-6 Normal FHR pattern with normal rate (about 130 beats/minute) and normal short-term and long-term variability (amplitude range about 15 beats/minute) and absence of periodic changes. This pattern represents a normally oxygenated fetus without evidence of asphyxial stress. Uterine contractions are 2 to 3 minutes apart, and about 60 mm Hg in intensity. SOURCE: *Parer JT: Fetal heart rate. In: Creasy R, Resnick R: Maternal-Fetal Medicine: Principles and Practice, 3rd ed. Philadelphia, Saunders, 1994:298–325.*

ine contractions. The monitor uses the R wave of the fetal electrocardiogram complex (the most accurate device) or a signal generated by the movement of a cardiovascular structure using ultrasound and the Doppler principle. Uterine contractions are detected either by an open-ended or balloon-tipped catheter inserted transcervically into the amniotic cavity and attached to a strain gauge transducer, or an external device called a tocodynamometer, which is placed on the maternal abdomen and recognizes the tightening of the maternal abdomen during a contraction.

Monitoring with devices attached directly to the fetus or placed within the uterine cavity is called *direct*, *internal*, or *invasive*. Devices that do not require direct connection with the fetus are called *noninvasive* or *external*.

CHARACTERISTICS OF FETAL HEART RATE PATTERNS

BASIC PATTERNS The characteristics of the fetal heart rate pattern are classified as baseline, periodic, or episodic. The baseline features are heart rate and variability recorded between uterine contractions; periodic changes occur in association with uterine contractions; and episodic patterns are those not associated with uterine contractions.

BASELINE RATE Baseline FHR is the appropriate mean FHR rounded to increments of 5 bpm during a 10-minute segment, excluding

1. Periodic or episodic changes.
2. Periods of marked FHR variability.
3. Segments of the baseline that differ by 25 bpm.

In any 10-minute window, the minimum baseline duration must be at least 2 minutes or the baseline for that period would be indeterminate. In this case, one may need to refer to the previous 10-minute segment(s) to determine the baseline.

The normal baseline fetal heart rate is 110 to 160 beats per minute (bpm). Values below 110 bpm are termed bradycardia, and those above 160 bpm tachycardia.

FETAL HEART RATE VARIABILITY Baseline FHR variability is defined as fluctuations in the baseline FHR of two cycles per minute or greater. These fluctuations are irregular in amplitude and frequency and are visually quantified as the amplitude of the peak to trough in beats per minute as follows:

1. Amplitude range undetectable: absent FHR variability.
2. Amplitude range >undetectable, ≤5 bpm; minimal FHR variability.
3. Amplitude range 6 to 25 bpm; moderate FHR variability.
4. Amplitude range >25 bpm; marked FHR variability.

The sinusoidal pattern differs from variability in that it has a smooth, sine wave–like pattern of regular frequency and amplitude and is excluded in the definitio of FHR variability.

PERIODIC PATTERNS Periodic patterns are the alterations in fetal heart rate that are associated with uterine contractions. These consist of (1) late decelerations, (2) variable decelerations, and (3) accelerations.

THE NORMAL PATTERN

The normal fetal heart rate pattern (Fig. 2-6) has a predominant heart rate of 110 to 160 bpm. The FHR variability has an amplitude range of 6 to 25 bpm. There are no decelerative periodic changes, but there may be periodic accelerations. The fetus born with this normal heart rate pattern is virtually always vigorous and nonacidemic if it is delivered at the time when the normal heart rate pattern is traced. This, of course will not hold true if there is a subsequent traumatic delivery or a congenital anomaly inconsistent with extrauterine life. In contrast to this high predictability of fetal normal acid-base state and vigor in the presence of the normal pattern, a number of variant patterns are not so accurately predictive of fetal acidemia. However, in the context of the clinical case, the progressive change in the patterns, and the duration of the variant patterns, reasonable judgments can be made about the likelihood of development of fetal acidemia. By using this FHR interpretation as a screening approach, impending intolerable fetal acidemia can be presumed or, in certain cases, ruled out by the use of ancillary techniques such as the fetal stimulation test, vibroacoustic stimulation, or fetal blood sampling.

VARIANT FETAL HEART RATE PATTERNS

BASELINE RATE *Bradycardia* differs from a deceleration, which is transient. Bradycardia is a decrease in heart rate below 110 bpm for 10 minutes or longer. The initial response of the normal fetus to acute hypoxia or asphyxia is bradycardia. Bradycardia occurs because initially the vagal nerve activity is greater than sympathetic activity. There are a number of nonasphyxial causes of bradycardia. These include the bradyarrhythmias (eg, complete heart block), certain drugs (eg, β-adrenergic blockers or local anesthetic drugs), or hypothermia. Some fetuses have a heart rate below 110 bpm but are otherwise totally normal and simply represent a normal variation outside arbitarily set limits.

Prolonged deceleration (>2 minutes duration) or bradycardia is considered to represent a prolonged stepwise decrease in fetal oxygenation. The bradycardia may be a consequence of fetal hypoxia stimulating vagal activity or, later, hypoxic myocardial decompensation, or the bradycardia may eventually result in fetal hypoxia because of the inability of the fetus to maintain a compensatory increase in stroke volume. The hypoxic fetus has some ability to increase stroke volume in response to bradycardia, but this compensation fails at severe decreases in heart rate, probably below 60 bpm. Under these conditions, fetal cardiac output cannot be maintained; therefore, umbilical blood *flow* decreases. This results in insufficient oxygen transport from the fetal placenta to the fetal body, eventually leading to fetal hypoxic decompensation.

Tachycardia may occur with fetal asphyxia, but never as an isolated finding. That is, in the presence of normal FHR variability and absent periodic changes, the tachycardia must be assumed to be caused by some other cause besides hypoxia. Tachycardia is sometimes seen on recovery from asphyxia; this probably represents catecholamine release following sympathetic nervous or adrenal medullary activity in response to hypoxic stress and withdrawal of vagal activity when the hypoxia is relieved.

Nonasphyxial causes of tachycardia include maternal or fetal infection, especially chorioamnionitis; drugs such as β-adrenoreceptor stimulants or parasympathetic blockers. Tachyarrhythmias occasionally occur; at severe elevations of rate (eg, >240 bpm), these may cause fetal cardiac failure and result in fetal hydrops.

BASELINE VARIABILITY As noted above, there are four gradations of heart rate variability. Moderate variability, in which the amplitude range of the variability is 6 to 25 bpm, is considered to represent the "normal" type.

Although the physiological origin and significance of FHR variability are not yet known for certain, there is a good deal of evidence to support the clinical belief that moderate FHR variability represents an intact nervous pathway through cerebral cortex, midbrain, vagus nerve, and cardiac conduction system. Thus, the integrity of this pathway is intact in the presence of normal FHR variability.

The most important aspect of these clinical correlates is that in the presence of normal FHR variability, no matter what other FHR patterns may be present, the fetus is unlikely to be suffering serious cerebral tissue acidemia because it has been able successfully to centralize the available oxygen and is thus physiologically compensated. In the presence of excessive hypoxic stress, however, as evidenced by severe periodic changes or prolonged bradycardia, this compensation may break down, and the fetus may have progressive central tissue asphyxia (ie, asphyxia in cerebral and myocardial tissues). In this case, FHR variability decreases and eventually is lost.

Nonasphyxial causes of decreased or absent FHR variability include absence of cortex (anencephaly); narcotized or drugged higher centers (eg, by morphine, meperidine, diazepam, magnesium sulfate); vagal blockade (eg, by atropine or scopolamine); and defective cardiac conduction system (eg, complete heart block).

Fetuses with unexplained virtual absence of FHR variability and no periodic changes fall into three categories: deep asphyxia with

inability of the heart to manifest periodic changes; congenital neurologic damage either caused by a developmental CNS defect or acquired from an in utero infection or asphyxial event; or idiopathic reduced FHR variability with no obvious explanation but no evidence of asphyxia or compromised CNS.

Fortunately, the vast majority of fetuses begin labor with normal FHR variability, so changes can be followed. If the FHR variability is minimal or absent on initial placement of the monitor, it is much more difficult, or even impossible, for the clinician to determine whether progressive asphyxia has occurring; therefore, ancillary testing will be necessary to determine whether acidemia is present.

PERIODIC CHANGES IN FETAL HEART RATE Late deceleration of the FHR is a visually apparent gradual decrease (defined as onset of deceleration to nadir $\geq$30 seconds) in FHR and return to baseline associated with a uterine contraction. The decrease is calculated from the most recently determined portion of the baseline. The deceleration is delayed in timing, with the nadir of the deceleration occurring after the peak of the contraction.

In most cases, the onset, nadir, and recovery of the deceleration occur after the beginning, peak, and ending of the contraction, respectively. The depth of the dip is related to the intensity of the contraction.

Late decelerations are of two varieties. The first type, *reflex late deceleration,* is seen when a sudden acute insult (eg, reduced uterine blood flow because of maternal hypotension) is superimposed on a previously normally oxygenated fetus. These late decelerations are caused by a decrease in uterine blood flow (with the uterine contraction) beyond the capacity of the fetus to extract sufficient oxygen. The deoxygenated blood is carried from the fetal placenta through the umbilical arteries to the heart and is distributed to the aorta, neck vessels, and head. Here, the low oxygen tension is sensed by chemoreceptors, and neuronal activity results in a vagal discharge, which causes the transient deceleration. The deceleration is presumed to be "late" because of the circulation time from the fetal placental site to the chemoreceptors and also because the progressively decreasing PO_2 must reach a certain threshold before vagal activity occurs. There also may be baroreceptor activity causing the vagal discharge. Between contractions, oxygen delivery is adequate, and there is no additional vagal activity, so the heart rate is normal. These late decelerations are accompanied by normal fetal heart rate variability and thus signify normal central nervous system integrity (ie, the fetus is physiologically "compensated" in the vital organs) (Fig. 2-7).

The periodic change previously called *early deceleration* appears simply to be a variant of the reflex late deceleration.

The second type of late deceleration is a result of the same initial mechanism, except that the deoxygenated bolus of blood from the placenta is presumed to be sufficient to interfere with myocardial action, so for the period of the contraction, there is direct myocardial hypoxic depression as well as vagal activity. Variability is lost (Fig. 2-8), signifying fetal "decompensation" (ie, inadequate fetal

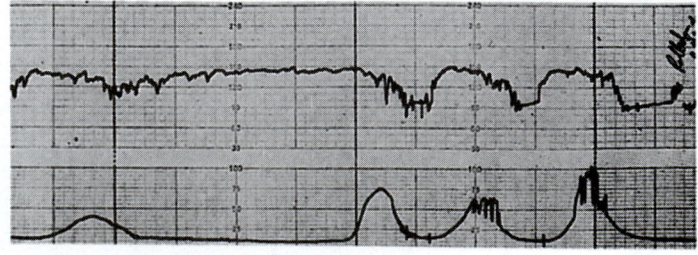

FIGURE 2-7 Reflex late decelerations. The FHR pattern was previously normal, but late decelerations appeared following severe maternal hypotension (70/30 mm Hg) after sympathetic blockade caused by a caudal anesthesia. SOURCE: *Parer JT: Fetal heart rate. In: Creasy R, Resnick R: Maternal-Fetal Medicine: Principles and Practice, 3rd ed. Philadelphia, Saunders, 1994:298–325.*

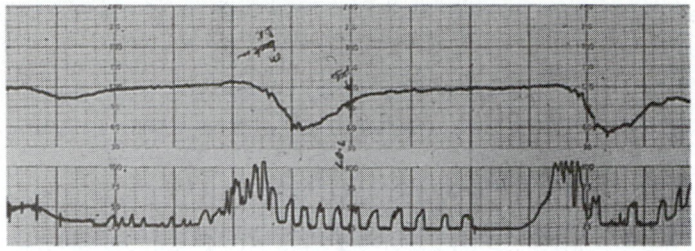

FIGURE 2-8 Nonreflex late decelerations with virtual absence of FHR variability. The decelerations represent transient asphyxial myocardial failure as well as intermittent vagal decreases in heart rate. The lack of FHR variability also signifies decreased cerebral oxygenation. Note the acidemia in fetal scalp blood (7.07). The baby, a 3340-g female with Apgar scores of 3 (1 min) and 4 (5 min), was delivered soon after this tracing. Cesarean section was considered to be contraindicated owing to a severe pre-eclamptic coagulopathy. SOURCE: *Parer JT: Fetal heart rate. In: Creasy R, Resnick R: Maternal-Fetal Medicine: Principles and Practice, 3rd ed. Philadelphia, Saunders, 1994:298–325.*

cerebral and myocardial oxygenation). It is seen most commonly in states of decreased placental reserve, such as preeclampsia or intrauterine growth restriction, or following prolonged hypoxic stresses such as a long period of severe reflex late decelerations.

The distinguishing feature between reflex and nonreflex decelerations, therefore, is the presence of FHR variability in the former. Each category has been shown to dichotomize into two groups based on fetal pH, the reflex late deceleration group being in the normal range, and the nonreflex late deceleration group being acidemic.

Severe late decelerations are those with a drop of more than 45 bpm below the baseline and may be seen with reflex or nonreflex late decelerations. There are heart rate and duration criteria for identifying mild and moderate late decelerations, with the cutoff being 15 bpm below the baseline.

When late decelerations are present, efforts should be made to eliminate them by optimizing placental blood flows and maternal hypoxia (see below). Vagal late decelerations, which in most cases are a result of an acute asphyxial episode, generally can be abolished. However, those caused by transient myocardial failure usually are seen when placental reserve is surpassed and the intermittent decreases in uterine blood flow with each contraction can no longer be tolerated. Abolishing such late decelerations is unlikely.

Variable deceleration of the FHR is defined as a visually apparent abrupt decrease (defined as onset of deceleration to the beginning of nadir <30 seconds) in FHR below the baseline. The decrease is calculated from the most recently determined portion of the baseline. The decrease in FHR below the baseline is ≥15 bpm, lasting ≥15 seconds, and <2 minutes from the onset to return to baseline (Fig. 2-9).

When variable decelerations are associated with uterine contractions, their onset, depth, and duration commonly vary with successive uterine contractions.

These abrupt decelerations in heart rate represent the firing of the vagus nerve in response to certain stimuli, either umbilical cord compression, generally in the first stage of labor, or substantial head compression (eg, during pushing) late in the second stage of labor.

Whether the fetus is still normoxic in the central tissues (ie, physiologically compensated) can be determined by observations of the maintenance of FHR variability.

The clinical significance of variable decelerations is that they represent insufficiency of umbilical blood flow. It is obvious why this is so if they are caused by compression of the umbilical cord. If they are caused by intensed vagal activity, then the associated decrease in umbilical blood *flow* results from a drop in fetal cardiac output because of the relative inability of the fetus to maintain cardiac output at very low heart rates (eg, below about 60 bpm).

When severe variable decelerations are present (ie, below 60 bpm for 60 seconds), efforts should be made to abolish them because it is likely that even the normally grown fetus with normal placental function eventually will decompensate, although usually not before 30 minutes. The normal fetus has a much greater ability to tolerate mild or moderate variable decelerations for a prolonged period.

The idea that variable decelerations are caused by cord compression has given rise to the technique of amnioinfusion. In this straightforward technique, sterile crystalloid is infused into the amniotic cavity through an intrauterine catheter, with an initial bolus of 250 to 1000 cc and maintenance of about 2 to 3 cc/min. This has been shown to result in a lowered incidence of severe variable decelerations and may allow a vaginal delivery instead of a cesarean section for presumed fetal acidemia. It may also decrease the incidence of meconium aspiration when the meconium is thick. It appears to be more efficacious in premature fetuses than term fetuses and is not as effective in the second stage of labor, lending support to the theory that second-stage variable decelerations are caused by head and not cord compression.

Acceleration is defined as a visually apparent abrupt increase (defined as onset of acceleration to peak in <30 seconds) in FHR above the baseline. The increase is calculated from the most recently determined portion of the baseline. The acme is ≥15 bpm above the baseline, and the acceleration lasts ≥15 seconds and <2 minutes from the onset to return to the baseline. Before 32 weeks of gestation, accelerations are defined as having an acme ≥10 bpm

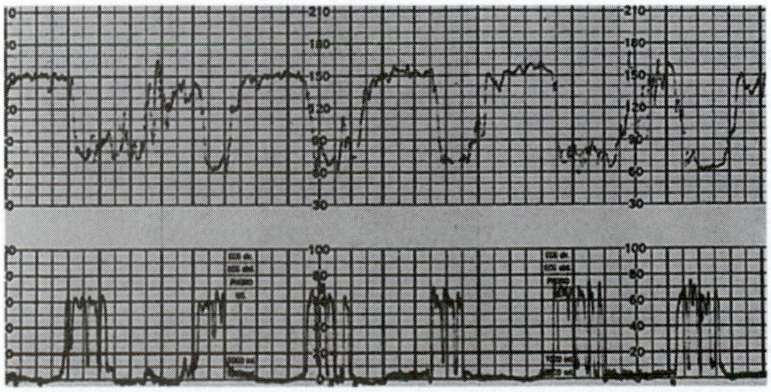

FIGURE 2-9 Variable decelerations. Intrapartum recording using fetal scalp electrode and tocodynamometer. The spikes in the uterine activity channel represent maternal pushing efforts in the second stage of labor. Note normal baseline variability between contractions, signifying normal central oxygenation despite the intermittent asphyxial stress represented by the severe variable decelerations. SOURCE: *Parer JT: Fetal heart rate. In: Creasy R, Resnick R: Maternal-Fetal Medicine: Principles and Practice, 3rd ed. Philadelphia, Saunders, 1994:298–325.*

above the baseline and a duration of ≥10 seconds. Prolonged acceleration is ≥2 minutes and <10 minutes in duration. Acceleration of ≥10 minutes is a baseline change.

Accelerations with uterine contractions sometimes occur and have no adverse prognostic significance. They are probably similar to the accelerations that are seen with fetal movement in the antepartum period and thus are indicative of a reactive and healthy fetus. Accelerations with contractions probably represent the net result of greater sympathetic activity than parasympathetic activity during contractions in the case of a particular fetus.

OTHER PATTERNS A number of patterns do not simply fit into the category of basic patterns. They are less common, and their significance is generally more controversial. They generally may be classified as various types of bradycardias, sinusoidal patterns, overshoot patterns, saltatory patterns, arrhythmia patterns, and those associated with congenital anomalies and the premature fetus.

INFLUENCE OF IN UTERO TREATMENT

Fetal oxygenation can be improved, acidemia relieved, and abnormal FHR patterns abolished by certain modes of treatment. The events that may result in fetal acidemia (recognized by FHR patterns) are presented in Table 2-3 together with the recommended treatment maneuvers and presumed mechanisms for improving fetal oxygenation. If the hypoxic insult is acute and the fetus was previously normoxic, there is an excellent chance that the variant FHR pattern will be abolished. Late decelerations, if present, are most likely of the reflex type rather than caused by myocardial failure.

During labor an FHR pattern with decreasing variability from asphyxia is virtually always preceded by a heart rate pattern signifying hypoxic stress (eg, late decelerations, severe variable decelerations, or a prolonged bradycardia). In the antepartum period, however, before the onset of uterine contractions, this does not necessarily hold, and a fetus may develop decreasing or absent vari-

ability *without* periodic or baseline FHR changes. In addition, the normal evolution to decreased or absent variability sometimes occurs with relatively minor decelerations in the presence of chorioamnionitis and dysmaturity. If the FHR patterns cannot be improved, ie, if the patterns indicative of peripheral tissue or central tissue hypoxia persist for a significant period, further diagnosis or delivery may be indicated.

Certain patterns are of such a severe character that immediate delivery without ancillary testing, such as fetal scalp sampling, is warranted if they cannot rapidly be relieved. They include patterns with undetectable FHR variability and severe uncorrectable late or variable decelerations or a prolonged bradycardia below 60 bpm. Fetuses exhibiting these patterns may already be acidemic or soon will become so. It is appropriate to diagnose presumed fetal acidemia in these cases and manage the case accordingly.

2.5.7 Current Intrapartum Management Recommendations

The clinical approach currently used is that in the presence of bradycardias, or a prolonged series of late or variable decelerations when fetal heart rate variability decreases or is intermittently lost, one must assume that the fetus is becoming centrally acidemic unless one can demonstrate otherwise by other techniques.

The evolution of intrapartum fetal heart rate patterns during hypoxia has been established, and it is known that fetal heart rate variability decreases and then disappears before substantial fetal depression or fetal death in utero. This decrease in fetal heart rate variability is considered to correlate clinically with decreased central nervous system (CNS) function, which is presumed to precede CNS damage.

In terms of clinical management, this approach is an important one. It suggests that there is time for conservative management to alleviate the stress patterns before operative delivery is warranted. Thus, with uncorrectable absent fetal heart rate variability in the

TABLE 2-3
INTRAUTERINE TREATMENT FOR VARIANT FHR PATTERNS

CAUSES	POSSIBLE RESULTING FHR PATTERNS	CORRECTIVE MANEUVER	MECHANISM
Hypotension, eg, supine hypotension, conduction anesthesia	Bradycardia, late decelerations	Intravenous fluids, position change, ephedrine	Return of uterine blood flow toward normal
Excessive uterine activity	Bradycardia, late decelerations	Decrease in oxytocin, lateral position	Same as above
Transient umbilical cord compression	Variable decelerations	Change in maternal position, eg, left or right lateral	Same as above
		Trendelenburg position Amnioinfusion	"Pads" the cord, protecting it from compression
Head compression, usually second stage	Variable decelerations	Push only with alternate contractions	Same as above
Decreased uterine blood flow associated with uterine contraction below limits of fetal basal O₂ needs	Late decelerations	Change in maternal position, eg, left lateral or Trendelenburg; establishment of maternal hyperoxia	Enhancement of uterine blood flow toward optimum; increase in maternal-fetal O₂ gradient
		Tocolytic agents, eg, ritodrine or terbutaline	Decrease in contractions or uterine tonus, thus abolishing associated decrease in uterine blood flow
Prolonged asphyxia	Decreasing FHR variability[a]	Change in maternal position (eg, left lateral or Trendelenburg); establishment of maternal hyperoxia	Enhancement of uterine blood flow to optimum; Increase in maternal-fetal O₂ gradient

[a] During labor this is virtually always preceded by a heart rate pattern signifying asphyxial stress (eg, late decelerations, usually severe), severe variable decelerations, or a prolonged bradycardia. This is not necessarily so in the antepartum period, before the onset of uterine contractions.

presence of persistent hypoxic stress patterns, delivery should be carried out as soon as possible. In the presence of continued normal fetal heart rate variability with those stress patterns, one can conservatively await vaginal delivery in selected cases. Fetal stimulation testing or fetal blood sampling for acid-base measurement may be of value in uncertain cases. This approach does depend on the ability to rescue the fetus rapidly if variability decreases persistently, so decision-delivery times may need to be relatively short.

2.5.8   Recommendations for Usage of FHR Monitoring

The incidence of intrapartum fetal asphyxia and subsequent morbidity is relatively low. Subtle deleterious effects of intrapartum asphyxia may occur and not manifest as cerebral palsy, but their incidence is not known. The incidence of cerebral palsy from all causes is two to three per 1000, but intrapartum asphyxia is only a relatively small part of this, possibly 10%. Thus, the number of fetuses who can benefit from electronic FHR monitoring, especially in the normal population, is probably less than 1%, although in a high-risk group, such as premature or postdate fetuses, the proportion may well be higher.

Typical guidelines for monitoring are as follows. On admission to rule out labor, or in a patient in actual labor, an FHR record with either external or internal monitoring should be documented for approximately 20 minutes. In the case of an at-risk patient, the monitoring should continue throughout labor. Should the contractions be obvious, cervical dilatation progressive, and the FHR pattern "normal" (normal rate, normal FHR variability, and absence of periodic changes except accelerations), the tocodynamometer need not be placed. The need for the tocodynamometer to measure contraction frequency or for the intrauterine pressure catheter to measure intrauterine pressure arises when cervical change is inappropriate.

For a low-risk patient who continues to be at low risk, in that she does not develop any abnormality of labor or have risk factors appearing subsequently, electronic FHR monitoring may be intermittent. A short strip recorded for about 5 minutes every 30 minutes, or in accordance with the hospital's policy or American College of Obstetrics and Gynecology (ACOG) recommendation for frequency of auscultation, should be sufficient. Should equivocal changes in these short strips occur, continuous electronic FHR monitoring should be instituted until the condition of the fetus is resolved. During the second stage of labor, the frequency of recording needs to be increased in accordance with the hospital's protocol. When the second stage exceeds about 60 minutes, the institution of continuous monitoring is advisable.

2.5.9   Operative Delivery

CESAREAN SECTION

Approximately one in four babies in North America are delivered by cesarean section. The indications for cesarean section fall into five broad categories: dystocia, previous cesarean section or uterine scar, "fetal distress," meaning presumed impending or actual fetal asphyxia, malpresentation, generally breech, and miscellaneous indications.

The rise in cesarean section rate in the past several decades is inversely correlated with the improvement in neonatal mortality. However, there are many reasons to believe the relationship is not necessarily causative. Various surveys have shown a wide variation in cesarean section rate among hospitals with similar populations but little variation in neonatal mortality. In addition, in some institutions, neonatal mortality has decreased despite relatively stable cesarean section rates, no doubt because of improvements in neonatal care and the improved ability to recognize the fetus requiring early delivery by the means outlined above in Sec. 2.5.4.

There is a widespread opinion that the cesarean section rate is excessive, and numerous attempts have been made to decrease the rate to acceptable levels because the morbidity and mortality for the mother are increased. It is likely that the mortality rate is twice that of a vaginal delivery, all other things being equal, although the rate is still extremely low, about 20 versus 10 per 100,000 births. In addition, the morbidity stemming from infection, blood loss, and damage to internal organs is higher with cesarean section.

A major improvement in cesarean section rate has been shown when each cesarean section done in an institution is subject to peer review. There are further ways in which the rate can be decreased.

Dystocia needs to be firmly defined by reference to known progress in cervical effacement and dilation. This is often noted by graphic representation of the progress in labor on a labor curve. Appropriate evaluation of uterine activity by appropriate recording of frequency and/or intrauterine pressure, and use of oxytocin when it is inadequate, are further means of decreasing the cesarean section rate.

In individual series, approximately 70% of women with previous cesarean sections (low transverse uterine incisions) are candidates for a trial of labor in a subsequent pregnancy. Of these women, approximately 70% achieve a vaginal delivery. Uterine rupture rate is approximately 0.6% during labor, and if emergency delivery occurs quickly enough, consequences for the fetus are minimal. There is much discussion at present about the appropriate facilities needed to safely achieve vaginal birth after cesarean. In our institution, with an obstetrician and anesthesiologist on the labor and delivery floor at all times, our current recommendations are that every person with a uterine scar be evaluated for a trial of labor and encouraged to do so if she is an appropriate candidate.

The number of cesarean sections for fetal distress can be decreased considerably by knowledgeable and timely interpretation of fetal heart rate patterns. Much of the excessive cesarean section rate stems from a poor knowledge of fetal heart rate pattern analysis.

A trial of vaginal delivery may safely be attempted with certain malpresentations. In moderately sized term breech presentations where pelvic size is adequate by pelvimetry and there is normal progress in labor, the outcome for the fetus equals that with cesarean section. It is likely that approximately 50% of term breeches could successfully deliver vaginally.

OPERATIVE VAGINAL DELIVERY

Operative vaginal delivery is carried out on specific indications with either forceps or the vacuum extractor. Both forms are safe with the exercise of appropriate skill and precautions. In the past two decades in particular, there has been a reduction in the number of deliveries done with forceps and an increase in the number done with a vacuum extractor. The reasons for the changing incidence of operative vaginal delivery are many, but they include fear of medicolegal repercussions, patient preference, increasing popularity of cesarean section in place of operative vaginal delivery, decrease in training opportunities for obstetrics and gynecology residents, and decreasing skill among resident teachers. There is little doubt that traumatic deliveries are possible with either instrument, although the early literature suggests that many of these were forced deliveries at a time when the safety of cesarean section was in doubt. However, sufficient information is now available to show that with appropriate skill, restricted traction, and appropriate indications, such vaginal deliveries can be carried out safely.

The indications for operative vaginal delivery include either fetal indication (as noted on the fetal heart rate monitor) or maternal indication, primarily related to a prolonged second stage. On rare occasions a mother would be advised not to use prolonged Valsalva and pushing efforts in the second stage because of a medical condition, eg, maternal cardiac disease, so she will have her second stage shortened by the operative approach.

Fetal indications for operative vaginal delivery are presumed fetal intolerance of labor as noted by specific patterns on the fetal heart rate monitor. In such cases the obstetrician may interpret the pattern as indicating hypoxic stresses in the fetus, which is cumulative and may result in fetal acidemia. On other occasions there is a substantial bradycardia, or loss of variability in the presence of decelerations, which suggest to the obstetrician that the baby is acidemic and needs rapid delivery. The physician then makes a judgment regarding the most rapid route of delivery of the fetus, and if this is in the second stage of labor, the obstetrician may make the decision that he can more rapidly deliver the fetus more safely by the operative vaginal route.

The choice between the vacuum extractor and forceps is dependent on factors such as physician skill, physician choice, presentation of the fetus, and at times maternal choice. The use of either forceps or vacuum is subject to a restriction in the amount of force and number of tractions used. For example, the fetal head is expected to descend with each traction with either technique, and in the absence of descent, the procedure should be abandoned. From the point of view of number of tractions, the vacuum is safe if used for three (occasionally four) tractions and no more. Under these conditions fetal trauma is restricted in the vast majority of cases to temporary bruising or skin lacerations.

The widespread use of epidural anesthesia in many institutions has changed the length of the average second stage of labor. The outer limits of normal for the second stage with epidural anesthesia is 2 hours for multiparas and 3 hours for primiparas. Few women retain the strength to push beyond 3 hours, so many are delivered operatively for the indication of "maternal exhaustion."

The station of the presenting part of the fetus is defined by centimeters below or above the ischial spines, and the virtually delivered head is represented by +5 station. The head at this time is said to be "crowning." Forceps or vacuum extraction deliveries are defined as mid if the presenting part at the beginning of the operation is higher than +2 station, low if the presenting part is station +2 to +4, and outlet if the head is on the pelvic floor. High forceps, above 0 station, are rarely justified. An important concept that is widely accepted with the use of operative vaginal delivery is that all operative deliveries should be considered a trial, and the attempt should be abandoned if the likelihood of fetal trauma arises.

2.5.10   Management of the Marginally Viable Fetus

Recommendations for management of the marginally viable fetus should depend on individual hospital and neonatal mortality and morbidity figures. Decisions regarding management of extremely premature infants need to be made and discussed with the parents before situations arise. The reason for this is that many midtrimester

fetuses are admitted for reasons such as preterm premature rupture of the membranes, and many will have malpresentations, particularly breech presentation. It is advisable for delivery services to have a formal plan of action based on their recent experience. An example of such an approach follows.

If the gestational age is under 24 weeks, the parents are informed that survival is extremely unlikely, and morbidity is likely to be very high. There is no recommendation for cesarean section for fetal indications in such cases, and neonatologists generally are not expected to be present at the delivery. This guideline, of course, applies only where there are excellent data on the gestational age of the fetus.

At gestational ages of 24 weeks up to but not including 25 weeks, cesarean section is not recommended but would be done for fetal indications if the parents, after knowledgeably considering the mortality and morbidity figures of such fetuses, strongly wish such an intervention should it arise. The mortality rate is usually ~50%, and severe morbidity in survivors is high. Neonatologists are present at delivery and will begin resuscitation. Decisions are made at a later time whether the resuscitation and support should be continued. In such cases, it is important that the parents should meet with both obstetrician and neonatalogist in order to make a plan beforehand.

If the gestational age is 25 weeks or greater, a cesarean section for fetal indications is advised, and neonatologists are present at delivery.

2.5.11   Management of Group B *Streptococcus* Infection in Pregnancy

Because group B streptococci (GBS) are an important cause of perinatal morbidity and mortality, strategies have been devised for prevention of early-onset GBS disease in newborns. Currently two different strategies are recommended by the Centers for Disease Control and Prevention. The strategies are broadly based on either late prenatal maternal cultures at 35 to 37 weeks or the use of risk-based indications during labor for treatment of the mother. Relatively large observational surveys show that both of these strategies are valuable in minimizing the incidence of early-onset GBS disease in newborns. With these strategies, approximately 18 to 27% of women will be treated with antibiotics, and this will prevent 69 to 86% of early-onset disease in newborns. The incidence of disease is expected to be 0.5% of neonates born to women who are carriers of the disease but have no risk factors.

The screening recommendations include an anogenital GBS culture at 35 to 37 weeks of gestation. Intrapartum chemoprophylaxis is offered to all women who are identified as carriers.

For the protocol using risk factors, those requiring treatment include gestation of less than 37 weeks, duration of membrane rupture greater than or equal to 18 hours, or temperature greater than 38°C during labor.

In addition to these strategies, women who are found to have asymptomatic GBS bacteriuria during pregnancy are treated both at the time of diagnosis and during the intrapartum period. Also, women with a history of previously giving birth to an infant with GBS disease would be treated during labor. The rationale for this treatment is they will usually be heavily colonized with GBS.

The treatment recommended by the CDC is intravenous penicillin G, 5 million units initially and 2.5 million units every 4 hours until delivery. Intravenous ampicillin, 2 g initially and 1 g every 4 hours until delivery, is considered an acceptable alternative to penicillin G. Penicillin G is preferred because it has a narrow spectrum and is therefore less likely to select antibiotic-resistant organisms and result in an increase in gram-negative infection in newborns. Where there is allergy to penicillin use, clindamycin or erythromycin may be used for treatment.

References

Centers for Disease Control and Prevention: Prevention of perinatal group B streptococcal disease: a public health perspective. MMWR 45(RR-7): 1–24, 1996

Creasy RK, Resnick R: Maternal-Fetal Medicine: Principles and Practice, 4th ed. Philadelphia, WB Saunders, 1999

Goldenberg RL, Iams JD, Das A, et al: The preterm prediction study: sequential cervical length and fibronectin testing for the prediction of spontaneous preterm birth. National Institute of Child Health and Human Development Maternal-Fetal Medicine Units Network. Am J Obstet Gynecol 182(3):636–643, 2000

Goodwin TM, Belai I, Hernandez P, Durand M, Paul RH: Asphyxial complications in the term newborn with severe umbilical acidemia. Am J Obstet Gynecol 167:1506–1512, 1992

Kilpatrick SJ, Schlueter MA, Piecuch R, Leonard CH, Rogido M, Sola A: Outcome of infants born at 24–26 weeks' gestation: I. Survival and cost. Obstet Gynecol 90(5):803–808, 1997

Parer JT: Handbook of Fetal Heart Rate Monitoring, 2nd ed. Philadelphia, WB Saunders, 1997

Piecuch RE, Leonard CH, Cooper BA, Kilpatrick SJ, Schlueter MA, Sola A: Outcome of infants born at 24–26 weeks' gestation: II. Neurodevelopmental outcome. Obstet Gynecol 90(5):809–814, 1997

Rouse DJ, Goldenberg RL, Cliver SP, Cutter GR, Mennemeyer ST, Fargason CA JR: Strategies for the prevention of early-onset neonatal group B *Streptococcus* sepsis: a decision analysis. Obstet Gynecol 83:483–494, 1994

2.6   FETAL DISORDERS AND THEIR PRENATAL MANAGEMENT

Danielle S. Walsh and N. Scott Adzick

Advances in prenatal testing and imaging techniques now permit diagnosis of many congenital defects during pregnancy. Anomalies readily imaged by ultrasound and ultrafast fetal magnetic resonance imaging include diaphragmatic hernia, lung lesions, sacrococcygeal teratoma, neural tube defects, obstructive uropathy, abdominal wall defects, bowel obstruction, neck masses, and abnormal hemodynamics in twin pregnancies. Other prenatal conditions, such as hemoglobinopathies and inborn errors of metabolism, may be diagnosed by genetic testing.

Fetal intervention has developed as our understanding of fetal pathology, technical ability, and postoperative care have improved. Previously, care of most congenital disorders was limited to postnatal management, but some fetuses do not survive to term. In utero intervention through both medical and surgical techniques has been introduced for select life-threatening and highly debilitating birth defects; with some conditions, this practice has led to improved outcomes. By addressing disorders during fetal development, the natural history may be altered in ways not possible postnatally. In other conditions, prenatal diagnosis may lead to consideration of the elective termination of pregnancy.

SURGICAL INTERVENTION

Congenital diaphragmatic hernia (CDH) occurs in approximately one in 2000–3000 live births, and despite improvements in postnatal management, overall mortality remains about 50% (Section 2.17.13). Consequently, fetal intervention has been advocated for fetuses with less than 10% chance of postnatal survival (Fig. 2-10). Early attempts to repair the diaphragmatic defect in the fetus did not meet with much success, but temporary tracheal occlusion has proven a more promising approach. Fetal tracheal occlusion induces pulmonary growth through retention of lung fluid and expansion of lung volume and can be accomplished by both open and fetoscopic techniques. Definitive repair of the diaphragmatic defect is deferred until the postnatal period.

Large mass lesions of the lungs can cause mediastinal shift, hypoplasia of normal lung tissue, polyhydramnios, and cardiovascular compromise, leading to fetal hydrops and death. *Congenital cystic adenomatoid malformation* (CCAM) is a benign cystic mass of the lung formed by overgrowth of the terminal respiratory bronchioles. About 20% of these lesions may diminish in size with advancing gestation, but others continue to enlarge and may require intervention if hydrops develops. CCAMs with a single large cyst may be treated in utero by percutaneous placement of a thora-

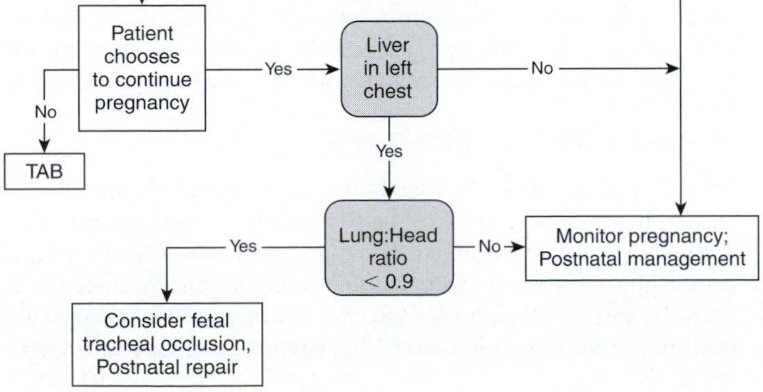

FIGURE 2-10   An algorithm for management of a fetus with a left-sided congenital diaphragmatic hernia. Amnio = amniocentesis; PUBS = percutaneous umbilical blood sampling; TAB = therapeutic abortion.

coamniotic shunt. If cardiac function improves and signs of hydrops resolve, resection can be delayed until the postnatal period. Multiloculated and microcystic CCAMs that are associated with fetal hydrops require a timely fetal thoracotomy with resection of the involved lobe(s) to maintain viability. Large collections of fluid in the pleural space (*fetal hydrothorax,* often the result of a chylothorax) also may result in mediastinal compression and can be alleviated with a percutaneously placed thoracoamniotic shunt. *Bronchopulmonary sequestrations* (BPS) are nonfunctional segments of lung with a systemic vascular supply; most fetal BPSs regress spontaneously. They may, however, be associated with hydrops and threaten fetal survival unless they are resected. Possibly thoracic masses may be treated by less invasive procedures such as laser cryo- or laser therapy or radiofrequency thermal ablation in the future.

Sacrococcygeal teratoma (SCT), the most common tumor of the newborn infant, has a mortality of 30 to 50% when diagnosed prenatally. Tumor mass effect can result in polyhydramnios and premature birth. Lethal hemorrhage from these highly vascular tumors may result from rupture either spontaneously or during delivery. SCTs occasionally reach massive proportions, resulting in high-output cardiac failure, hydrops, and fetal death. Resection of massive tumors before birth has been reported to improve fetal hemodynamics and allow fetal survival.

Myelomeningocele (MMC), the most common and severe form of spina bifida, is characterized by protrusion of the meninges and spinal cord through open vertebral arches. Although folic acid supplementation has greatly reduced the incidence of this disorder, it still affects about one in 2000 live births. MMC is the first nonlethal disorder in which fetal surgery was performed. Reports indicate that in selected patients fetal repair may improve neurologic function and reduce morbidity and mortality from hydrocephalus and the Arnold-Chiari II malformation by reversing hindbrain herniation and diminishing the need for postnatal ventriculoperitoneal shunting. The long-term effectiveness of fetal intervention is still to be assessed.

Fetal obstructive uropathy is a relatively common cause of dilation of the urinary tract in utero. Prenatal sonographic studies typically show unilateral hydronephrosis with upper tract disease, whereas lower tract obstruction is associated with bladder distension, bilateral hydronephrosis, and decreased amniotic fluid volume. Urethral obstruction can lead to bladder wall hypertrophy and hyperplasia, loss of bladder compliance, and progressive compression of the renal parenchyma with dysplasia and dysfunction. Mortality in prenatally diagnosed obstructive uropathy is not, however, caused by the renal disease but is the result of pulmonary hypoplasia. Failure of urine to drain into the amniotic space leads to progressive oligohydramnios and fetal compression, resulting in diminished lung growth, limb deformities, abnormal abdominal wall development, and distorted facial features. Criteria for fetal treatment have been developed, based on the ability to predict fetal renal function from fetal urine electrolyte concentrations and the sonographic appearance of the fetal kidneys (Fig. 2-11). Prenatal therapy is aimed at relieving the obstruction by means of a vesicoamniotic shunt placed percutaneously under sonographic guidance. This should prevent further renal damage and correct the oligohydramnios. Posterior urethral valves may be treated by cystoscopic ablation of the obstruction.

Fetoscopic procedures also have been applied successfully to manage two complications of twin pregnancies, *twin-twin transfusion syndrome* (TTTS) and *twin reversed arterial perfusion* (TRAP) sequence. In TTTS, abnormal placental vascular connec-

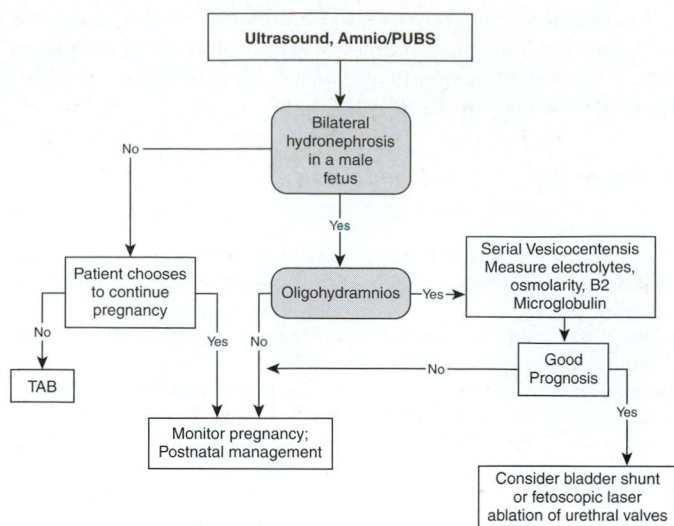

FIGURE 2-11   An algorithm for managing a fetus with obstructive uropathy. Amnio = amniocentesis; PUBS = percutaneous umbilical blood sampling; TAB = therapeutic abortion.

tions between monozygotic, monochorionic twins can lead to severe growth discordance, hydrops, and fetal demise (Sec. 2.13). When this is diagnosed before 26 weeks of gestation, mortality is greater than 50% for both twins, and survivors have a high incidence of neurologic injury. Serial amniocentesis, with or without a microseptostomy between the amniotic membranes, is usually successful, but in some instances laser ablation of placental vessels is necessary to reverse the pathophysiology and salvage both fetuses. If TTTS is advanced, selective fetocide by ligation of the umbilical cord may be necessary to salvage the less compromised twin. In TRAP sequence, an acardiac recipient twin is perfused by the heart of the normal twin, which develops cardiac failure as a result. When this condition is severe, ligation of the umbilical cord to the acardiac twin by bipolar cauterization or ligatures may salvage the normal twin.

Cutting and cauterization by fetoscopy has been used to treat severe *amniotic band syndrome,* an uncommon disorder in which constricting bands of amnion wrap around the fetus and may cause vascular and lymphatic occlusion. Tight constrictions may result in amputation of the affected digit or extremity (see Fig 2-17, p. 91, in Sec. 2.8.1). Fetoscopic release may be warranted in the second trimester if the bands threaten life or limb.

As an outgrowth of fetal intervention, the concept of ex utero intrapartum therapy (EXIT) was developed, in which the fetus is maintained on its placental circulation while a secure airway is established. EXIT procedures may be used to establish an airway in infants with massive *cervical teratomas, cystic hygromas,* and *congenital high airway obstruction syndrome* (CHAOS). When a secure airway and ventilation are established, the umbilical cord is cut. The mother is then treated as with the usual cesarean section.

NONSURGICAL THERAPY

Several inborn errors of metabolism have been diagnosed and treated medically prenatally. The presentation of *congenital adrenal hyperplasia* ranges from ambiguous genitalia in girls or virilization in boys to life-threatening adrenal insufficiency (Sec. 24.4.7). The most common enzyme defect is in 21-hydroxylase, resulting in accumulation of 17-hydroxyprogesterone in the amniotic fluid. The purpose of prenatal therapy is to prevent masculinization of female fetuses by administering dexamethasone to the mother to produce adrenal supression in the fetus. Because masculinization may occur early in the first trimester, chorionic villus sampling and measurement of molecular markers should be undertaken early in pregnancy in at-risk mothers to identify the need for steroid treatment.

Several inborn errors of metabolism may be diagnosed prenatally. In some of these disorders, prenatal supplementation may be beneficial to the fetus or newborn infant. A number of genetic disorders are associated with irreversible damage to the fetus in utero, making postnatal therapies ineffective. The potential benefit of fetal gene therapy for many these is being considered. Success with treatment of X-linked, recessive combined immune deficiency syndrome (X-SCID) has been achieved with second-trimester transplantation of paternal T cells. Similarly, injections of bone marrow into fetuses with hemoglobinopathies early in the second trimester is now under investigation.

References

Adzick NS, Crombleholme TM, Morgan MA, Quinn TM: A rapidly growing fetal teratoma. Lancet 349:538, 1997

Adzick NS, Harrison MR, Crombleholme TM, Flake AW, Howell LJ: Fetal lung lesions: management and outcome. Am J Obstet Gynecol 179: 884–889, 1998

Bruner JP, Tulipan M, Paschall RL, et al: Intrauterine repair of myelomeningocele, "hindbrain restoration" and the incidence of shunt-dependent hydrocephalus. JAMA 282:1819–1825, 1999

Johnson MP, Freedman AL: Fetal uropathy. Curr Opin Obstet Gynecol 11: 185–194, 1999

Sutton LN, Adzick NS, Bilaniuk LT, Johnson MP, Crombleholme TM, Flake AW: Improvement in hindbrain herniation demonstrated by serial fetal MRI following fetal surgery for myelomeningocele. JAMA 282: 1826–1831, 1999

Zanjani ED, Anderson WF: Prospects for in utero human gene therapy. Science 285:2084–2088, 1999

2.7 TRANSITIONAL CHANGES IN THE NEWBORN INFANT AROUND THE TIME OF BIRTH

David P. Carlton

Birth involves changes in numerous organ systems in the infant, but only a few require relatively rapid postnatal adjustment. The most important of these birth-related changes involve transitional function in the respiratory, cardiovascular, thermoregulatory, and metabolic systems.

2.7.1 Respiratory Transition

Within minutes after birth, regular breathing efforts are sustained, lung compliance begins to improve, airway resistance begins to diminish, and a functional residual capacity is established. With these changes, blood tensions of both oxygen and carbon dioxide approach those expected in the mature postnatal infant.

One factor that facilitates pulmonary adaptation after birth is surfactant. Surfactant is synthesized in the type II cells that line the distal air spaces. It is composed primarily of lipids, but a small fraction of surfactant is composed of proteins that are necessary for normal surfactant function. Disaturated phospholipids are primarily responsible for the relevant biophysical properties of surfactant. The protein fraction is composed of the surfactant-associated proteins A, B, C, and D. Proteins B and C are water-insoluble, hydrophobic proteins that are closely associated with the lipid component of surfactant. In the absence of surfactant proteins B or C, the newborn infant suffers severe respiratory distress.

Surfactant derives its importance from its ability to lower the surface tension of the alveolar lining layer, the shallow pool of liquid that overlies the cells of the distal air spaces. Without a very low surface tension at end-expiration, the air spaces would collapse with each exhalation. It is a deficiency of surfactant that underlies the pathophysiology of the respiratory distress observed after premature birth (Sec. 2.16.1).

During the later stages of intrauterine development, the enzymes important in surfactant production increase, resulting in an increase in intracellular surfactant content. At the time of birth, much of this stored surfactant is released into the alveolar space. Surfactant release is stimulated by lung inflation and the increase in circulating catecholamine concentration that accompanies birth. The premature infant has less surfactant available for extrusion into the air space at the time of birth than does a term infant.

In addition to surfactant, postnatal lung adaptation also depends on clearance of fluid from the lumen of the lung. Before birth the potential air spaces are filled with liquid, and failure to remove this liquid after birth results in respiratory difficulty and hypoxemia (Sec. 2.17.10).

The composition of the liquid that fills the lumen of the lung during fetal life is different from amniotic fluid or lung interstitial fluid, indicating that lung liquid is not simply an extension of one of these compartments. Fetal lung liquid is produced by a process that is dependent on the secretion of Cl ions across the respiratory epithelium into the lung lumen. The importance of fetal lung liquid derives from its ability to act as a dynamic template around which the lung develops *in utero*. If the fetal lung is inadequately distended with liquid, lung growth and differentiation are stunted.

Clearance of fetal lung liquid at the time of birth does not occur primarily by expectoration, that is, by egress of fluid from the lungs by way of the trachea into the mouth. At one time this process was thought to be important, presumably aided by compression of the chest and abdomen during vaginal birth. Our understanding now is that liquid contained within the lung lumen at the time of birth is reabsorbed across the respiratory epithelium, a process that is driven by transcellular movement of Na ions from the lung liquid into the interstitium. The complete characterization of events that initiate and maintain Na and liquid reabsorption from the lung is not clear, but they likely involve changes in oxygen tension and circulating catecholamines associated with delivery.

2.7.2 Circulatory Transition

Profound changes in central circulatory patterns occur after birth and are necessary for the successful transition to extrauterine life as discussed in Sec. 22.1.2, 2.16.2 and 2.17.11. The extent to which this transition fails to take place influences not only the clinical condition of patients who have structural heart disease but also infants whose primary illness may appear to have little, if any, relationship to the circulation.

2.7.3 Thermoregulatory Transition

In utero the fetus consumes oxygen to maintain normal cellular respiration and produce energy. Heat is generated as an expected by-product of these reactions. Normalized per kilogram body weight, the fetus generates about twice as much heat as an adult of that species. Most of the heat generated by the fetus is dissipated in the placenta as fetal blood is cooled by the maternal circulation. The balance, perhaps 10 to 20% of the total fetal heat production, is dissipated through the fetal skin, amniotic fluid, and uterine wall. Under conditions in which the efficiency of heat transfer in the placental circulation is diminished, the fetal skin and amniotic fluid can assume a greater role in heat removal. The uterus and placenta are metabolically active, but most of the heat generated in the uterus is a result of fetal metabolism.

At equilibrium the sum of fetal heat generation and dissipation results in a fetal temperature that is about 0.5°C greater than maternal temperature. An increase in maternal temperature will result in an increase in fetal temperature, and this observation highlights the disadvantage the fetus has to overcome in regulating body temperature. This disadvantage extends to hypothermic situations as well, although this condition is encountered much less frequently than maternal fever.

Unlike the newborn, the fetus has a limited capacity for thermogenesis, and the biological basis for this limitation is unclear. Replicating in utero those events that occur after birth, including inflating the lungs, exposure to oxygen, body cooling, and thyroid hormone infusion, does not induce a substantial thermogenic response, whereas cord occlusion does so.

After delivery the relatively low ambient environmental temperature and evaporation of the residual amniotic fluid from the skin combine to increase heat loss from the newborn infant. In addition to these environmental challenges, the newborn is intrinsically disadvantaged compared to the adult by virtue of the high surface area to mass ration. Thus, heat production, relative to body weight, must be greater in the newborn to maintain a normal body temperature to overcome this relative increase in surface area. Measurements of perinatal thermal balance suggest that heat production increases by about twofold shortly after birth.

Heat production postnatally is the result of shivering and nonshivering thermogenesis. In adults heat production from shivering thermogenesis contributes significantly to maintenance of body temperature under conditions of cold stress. In general, nonshivering thermogenesis is thought to be more important than shivering thermogenesis soon after birth. However, some experimental observations suggest that the newborn may have some capacity for shivering even though it is not a common response.

The immediate control of thermogenesis, both shivering and nonshivering, is by way of the CNS. Cutaneous receptors responsive to thermal stimuli are present on the skin, and such receptors can be shown to respond independently to cold and warm stimuli. Nearly all skin surfaces have receptors for both cold and warm stimuli, but receptors responsive to cold are more abundant than are receptors responsive to heat. The thermoreceptive afferent signals are ultimately processed in several areas of the brain, including the midbrain and hypothalamus. Efferent signaling responsible for initiating shivering thermogenesis is by way of the motor neurons.

Nonshivering thermogenesis is also mediated by efferents from the CNS.

Brown adipose tissue is responsible for the generation of heat associated with nonshivering thermogenesis. Although brown adipose tissue can be found in a variety of locations with the body, the upper back and neck, mediastinum, and perinephric areas are major sites of brown fat storage in the newborn. Brown adipose tissue is present in the adult, but it is relatively more abundant in the newborn. Brown fat increases in abundance postnatally, at least for some period of time. The degree to which brown fat supplies significant amounts of heat in the premature infant is less clear than it is in the term newborn.

The thermogenic response attributed to brown adipose tissue is the result of both neurogenic and biochemical responses. Sites within the hypothalamus coordinate input from thermoreceptive afferents and also regulate sympathetic output to the brown fat stores in the body. Sympathetic stimulation of nerves in the brown adipose tissue results in the release of norepinephrine. Subsequent binding of norepinephrine to β-adrenergic receptors on the fat cell triggers an increase in adenosine 3,5′-cyclic phosphate (cyclic AMP) through the action of adenylate cyclase. An intracellular lipase then liberates fatty acids from cytoplasmic stores of triglycerides, making them available for mitochondrial processing, oxidation, and heat generation.

An important finding in the study of thermogenesis was the discovery of uncoupling protein 1 (UCP-1). UCP-1 represents a critical factor in the mechanism of heat generation in nonshivering thermogenesis, exemplified by the observation that genetically altered mice that lack UCP-1 are unable to produce heat efficiently when exposed to cold and therefore become hypothermic.

During mitochondrial respiration, protons are generated outside of the inner mitochondrial membrane and contribute to the electrochemical gradient for protons across this barrier. Under conditions in which adenosine 5′-diphosphate (ADP) is plentiful, the adenosine 5′-triphosphate (ATP) synthase present on the inner mitochondrial membrane uses protons as the driving force for ATP synthesis. In the absence of this pathway for proton entry, mitochondrial respiration slows. UCP-1 acts as an ion transport protein allowing the entry of protons so that respiration can continue, albeit generating heat instead of ATP in the process. There are at least two other uncoupling proteins, UCP-2 and UCP-3, but their role in thermogenesis by brown adipose tissue is unclear. UCP-1 is activated by free fatty acids and inhibited by purine nucleotides. Long-term regulation of UCP-1 is not well characterized.

An important intracellular source of energy for thermogenesis is the generation of free fatty acids from triglycerides. The glycerol produced as part of this reaction is released into the circulation and is one means by which thermogenesis is measured indirectly in experimental studies. Lipoprotein lipase is developmentally regulated, and its activity is increased after birth. Free fatty acids generated by lipoprotein lipase may contribute to intracellular sources of energy for heat production. Circulating free fatty acids probably do not serve as an acute source of energy during periods of cold stress but rather act to replenish depleted intracellular fat stores.

There exists an ambient temperature range in which the infant's body temperature is normal and its metabolic rate at a minimum. The ambient temperature around this point is designated the *neutral thermal environment*. In this temperature range, no extra metabolic energy is used to produce heat, and the infant has no need to dissipate any extra heat. If heat loss occurs (commonly by exposure to a lower ambient temperature or by evaporative heat loss) the infant must resort to thermogenesis in an effort to maintain body temperature. This results in an increase in energy consumption and oxygen demand.

As heat loss continues, body temperature will begin to decrease if the increase in metabolic rate can not keep pace with heat loss. Although the newborn infant has the capacity to respond to a cold stress by increasing heat production, the absolute extent to which the newborn can sustain a cold stress and maintain a normal temperature is limited when compared to the adult. In infants and adults, the length of time that such a stress may be tolerated without hypothermia is short. Thermal insulation with clothing can lower the neutral thermal environmental temperature, as will maneuvers that reduce radiative, conductive, and convective heat losses.

As the ambient temperature increases above the neutral thermal environment, body temperature will increase unless heat loss can be increased by sweating or changes in the environment. Vasomotor responses will have already been recruited maximally by the time an increase in ambient temperature causes the infant's body temperature to increase. Thus, if sweating is limited, neutral thermal environment is likely near that ambient temperature at which the infant's body temperature begins to increase.

2.7.4   Endocrinologic Transition

The endocrinologic regulation of the fetus is determined to a great extent by the fetus itself, although placental and maternal hormones are not unimportant. The capacity for self-regulation occurs early in development. The fetal hypothalamus has demonstrable concentrations of releasing hormones by the late first or early second trimester, and hormone appearance in the pituitary occurs during a similar time frame. Placentally derived hormones include estrogens, progesterone, hCG, and human placental lactogen, but the importance to the fetus of many of the placental hormones is uncertain. Although the placenta restricts the movement of many maternal hormones into the fetus, important maternal hormones that cross the placenta directly or do so after modification in the placenta include steroid hormones and thyrotropin-releasing hormone (TRH). Cortisol and thyroid hormone are two hormones involved indirectly in postnatal adaptation.

The fetal adrenal gland develops early in the first trimester and contains the full spectrum of enzymes important in steroidogenesis in the mature adrenal gland. Corticotropin-releasing factor is present in the fetal hypothalamus during early development, and ACTH is present at the same time in the pituitary. ACTH has the dual effect of not only increasing steroid synthesis in the adrenal gland but also promoting growth and maturation of the gland. Most of the circulating fetal cortisol derives from the fetal adrenal gland, with the remainder being transplacental. The synthetic capability of the fetal adrenal gland, at least for cortisol, is at least as great as in the adult.

Circulating cortisol concentrations increase through development, beginning near the end of the first trimester and increasing more rapidly during the final weeks of gestation. The increase in cortisol during the third trimester appears to have at least a permissive effect on the development of several major organ systems, including the lung, in which the molecular processes important in surfactant homeostasis and in lung water removal are favorably influenced by circulating cortisol. Although the fetal adrenal gland provides the cortisol needed by the fetus for normal development,

under conditions in which sufficient fetal cortisol is unavailable, placental or maternal steroids appear adequate for normal development. At the time of birth, both ACTH and cortisol concentrations are increased, at least relative to their values several days after delivery.

Similar to cortisol, thyroid hormone also plays a permissive role in postnatal adaptation. In utero, thyroid hormone concentrations begin to increase near midgestation, increasing more rapidly during the last few weeks before birth and then decreasing during the days to weeks after delivery. At the time of birth there is an increase in thyroid-stimulating hormone (TSH) and a severalfold increase in circulating thyroid hormone concentration. The increase in TSH at birth appears to be a result of the thermal stress associated with delivery.

Transplacental passage of maternal TRH occurs readily, but maternal TSH and thyroid hormone transfer less well. Despite this inefficiency, adequate maternal thyroid hormone is now known to be important for optimal childhood neurologic development. This observation provides an important impetus for treatment of maternal hypothyroidism during pregnancy.

Thyroid hormone appears to play a role in regulating nonshivering thermogenesis and postnatal cardiovascular function, but the absolute necessity of thyroid hormone to the successful extrauterine transition of the newborn infant is unclear. Patients who are diagnosed with congenital hypothyroidism rarely have clinical abnormalities that bring them to medical attention immediately after birth. This empiric observation highlights the importance of newborn-screening programs in the detection of these infants.

2.7.5   Glucose Balance After Birth

Glucose concentration in the fetal blood during the third trimester of pregnancy is approximately 80% of the maternal concentration. In the fetus, glucose is supplied transplacentally, and most of this glucose is metabolized by the fetus for energy. There is little, if any, glucose synthesized by the fetus under normal conditions. The small portion of transplacental glucose that is not used immediately as energy is stored as glycogen in the fetal liver. Energy sources other than glucose are available to the fetus, including lactate, free fatty acids, ketones, and amino acids, but glucose is the major metabolic fuel during intrauterine development.

At the time of delivery, glucose transport ceases with clamping of the umbilical cord. Circulating glucose concentrations in the infant must then be maintained by a combination of glycogenolysis and gluconeogenesis. During the initial hours after birth, glucose concentration in the newborn decreases substantially and then increases over the next several hours to days to plateau near a value of 70 mg/dL. The production of glucose in the newborn averages 4 to 8 mg/kg body weight/min and exceeds by two- to threefold the basal synthetic rate in adults. The brain consumes a significant amount of the circulating glucose in the newborn because of the disproportionate size of the brain in relation to body weight compared to the adult. The usual postnatal increase in circulating catecholamine and glucagon concentrations, and the simultaneous decrease in insulin concentration, are important factors in the modulation of glucose concentrations in the newborn shortly after birth.

Hepatic glycogen stores increase significantly only during the latter part of gestation; this places premature infants at risk for hypoglycemia after birth if a source of exogenous glucose is not readily available soon after delivery. Hepatic stores of glycogen decrease in abundance soon after birth as they are metabolized for energy. They are sufficient to maintain adequate circulating glucose concentration for only a limited number of hours. Gluconeogenesis and enteral sources of glucose are then necessary to maintain glucose concentrations in an acceptable range. Glycogen stores in the liver release glucose in response to changes in glucagon and circulating catecholamines, changes that are associated with the mechanical event of cord clamping. The normal decrease in insulin concentration after birth also participates in the maintenance of normal circulating concentrations of glucose, although the decline in insulin concentration is not a result of the decrease in glucose concentration after delivery. The relative contributions of epinephrine, norepinephrine, and glucagon in the regulation of hepatic glycogenolysis postnatally in human infants is incompletely understood because the circulating concentrations of each of these are not independent of one another. Receptor-mediated stimulation of glycogenolysis occurs with both glucagon and catecholamines.

One of the enzymes important in liberating glucose from glycogen is glycogen phosphorylase, an enzyme regulated in part by catecholamines, glucagon, and thermal stress. As a result of the action of this enzyme, glucose-1-phosphate is generated and is itself converted to glucose-6-phosphate. Tissues containing glucose-6-phosphatase can then use this substrate to synthesize glucose and subsequently release it into the circulation. There are, however, a number of tissues that lack glucose-6-phosphatase, and in these tissues, glucose can not be produced, necessitating that glucose-6-phosphate be metabolized intracellularly.

Because glycogen stores are limited, gluconeogenesis also plays an important role in regulating glucose concentration in the newborn. In animal studies inhibition of gluconeogenesis after birth results in a profound decrease in circulating glucose concentrations. Lactate, pyruvate, and certain amino acids are substrates from which glucose can be synthesized. The enzymes responsible for the conversion of these compounds include glucose-6-phosphatase, fructose-1,6-diphosphatase, pyruvate carboxylase, and phosphoenolpyruvate carboxykinase. The cytosolic form of phosphoenolpyruvate carboxykinase is the rate-limiting enzyme in gluconeogenesis during development. It increases in concentration rapidly after birth as a result of an increase in transcription. Events associated with birth are considered the physiological trigger for the increase in cytosolic activity of phosphoenolpyruvate carboxykinase, but the specific downstream effector molecules associated with birth that increase enzyme activity are unknown.

Although gluconeogenic precursors are essential to hepatic glucose production postnatally, fatty acid oxidation also influences gluconeogenesis. Energy stored as fat exceeds the energy stored as glycogen by five- to 10-fold in the term infant at birth. Medium-chain triglycerides increase gluconeogenesis and circulating glucose concentrations even in the absence of exogenous gluconeogenic precursors. Conversely, inhibition of long-chain fatty acid oxidation results in a significant decrease in circulating glucose concentration.

Disturbances of glucose homeostasis are common in patients with problems specific to the neonatal period. Prominent in this group of patients are premature infants, infants who are small for gestational age, and infants born to mothers with diabetes mellitus (Sec. 2.15). Hypoglycemia is associated with premature birth as a result of diminished activity of gluconeogenic enzymes and reduced hepatic glycogen stores. Similar explanations are relevant for the small-for-gestational-age infant, whether term or preterm, but the data regarding a reduction in gluconeogenic potential are contro-

versial. Most patients who have hypoglycemia after birth are easily treated simply with exogenous glucose, but monitoring circulating glucose concentration is essential to confirm the resolution of the problem.

2.7.6   Water Balance After Birth

During fetal development, the proportion of body weight comprised of water decreases from 80 to 85% at 24 weeks of gestation to 75 to 80% at term. In term infants at birth, intracellular water accounts for two-thirds of total body water, and extracellular water accounts for the remaining one-third. During the first week after birth, body weight decreases, an effect that is the result of water loss.

The changes in water balance associated with birth appear to begin shortly before delivery. The biological basis of these changes is not completely understood, but they likely arise from perinatal changes in circulating hormone concentrations, which result in a loss of fluid from the circulation into the interstitial space and a simultaneous increase in hematocrit. Longer-term changes in body water balance occur after birth as well. During the first week after delivery, infants born at term tend to lose about 5% of their birth weight, probably as a result of decreases in intracellular and interstitial fluid.

In the preterm infant, body weight decreases after birth in a fashion similar to that seen in term infants, but in an exaggerated fashion. Infants born moderately preterm may lose 5 to 10% of their birth weight, whereas the youngest of premature infants may lose 15 to 20% of their birth weight with no apparent ill effects. Their weight loss is a result of salt and water loss over the first week after birth, and the fluid is lost primarily from the interstitial space. Whether this weight loss is "normal" is a matter of definition. The spontaneous feeding and apparent health of term newborns suggest that the observed weight loss in term infants is normal. However, because fluid intake in small premature infants is often determined by rates of intravenous fluid infusions, these smallest of preterm infants can not be considered to regulate fluid intake in the same manner as term infants. Thus, the range of "normal" for variables such as weight loss in this population is somewhat arbitrary and probably should be abandoned in favor of what is most desirable for optimal health. In this regard, the interpretation of epidemiologic and prospective intervention studies suggests that there is a direct relationship between morbidity and the abundance of salt and water intake, at least in the early newborn period. Thus, the most prudent extrapolation of this information would lead to a strategy in which fluid intake is adjusted to allow a gradual loss of body weight over the first postnatal week, with restriction of sodium intake until near the time when the target weight loss has occurred. Frequent measurement of body weight, urine output, and serum concentrations of electrolytes help to assure this gradual transition.

References

Bauer K, Bovermann G, Roithmaier A, Gotz M, Proiss A, Versmold HT: Body composition, nutrition, and fluid balance during the first two weeks of life in preterm neonates weighing less than 1500 grams. J Pediatr 118:615–20, 1991

Costarino AT, Baumgart S: Controversies in fluid and electrolyte therapy for the premature infant. Clin Perinatol 15:863–878, 1988

Farrag HM, Cowett RM: Glucose homeostasis in the micropremie. Clin Perinatol 27:1–22, 2000

Kalhan S, Parimi P: Gluconeogenesis in the fetus and neonate. Semin Perinatol 24:94–106, 2000

Lakshminrusimha S, Steinhorn RH: Pulmonary vascular biology during neonatal transition. Clin Perinatol 26:601–619, 1999

Ng PC: The fetal and neonatal hypothalamic-pituitary-adrenal axis. Arch Dis Child Fetal Neonatal Ed 82:F250–254, 2000

Perlstein PH: Thermoregulation. Pediatr Ann 24:531–537, 1995

Polk DH: Thyroid hormone metabolism during development. Reprod Fertil Dev 7:469–477, 1995

Teitel DF, Iwamoto HS, Rudolph AM: Effects of birth-related events on central blood flow patterns. Pediatr Res 22:557–566, 1987

2.8 EXAMINATION OF THE NEWBORN INFANT

Andrew R. Wilkinson, Valerie E. Charlton, Roderic H. Phibbs and Claudine Amiel-Tison

"Newborn infants should be accorded the best quality of health-care available . . . It should be the right of every newborn infant to be thoroughly examined at birth in order to detect disease or potential disorders that may be either treated or prevented"
FIGO Committee for the Study of Ethical Aspects of Human Reproduction (Cairo, December 1991)

2.8.1 General Examination

INITIAL AND SUBSEQUENT ASSESSMENTS

All babies should be briefly examined immediately after birth for major congenital abnormalities and to detect the presence of any serious illness. Any discrepancy between the expected gestational age and weight for gestation should be noted. After this the mother and her partner should have a period of privacy to enjoy their baby. How many nursing evaluations and how frequently they are carried out in the next few hours will depend on whether any problems are anticipated, but should include notation of heart rate, respiratory rate and effort, temperature, skin perfusion, skin color, and neuromuscular activity. The first feeding normally occurs within the first 6 hours, and any difficulty with sucking and swallowing should be noted. Further observation of a normal infant should be carried out at least every 8 hours. If any abnormalities are detected at any time, more frequent examination should occur, and a plan made for investigation and initial therapy.

A more detailed medical examination should be performed on all infants within 24 hours of birth so that investigations and treatment or preventive management, when indicated, may be implemented as soon as possible. This is also an opportunity to listen to concerns that the mother may have about her baby, which often have not been raised before the delivery. Reassurance given to the mother at this stage is immensely important whether this is her first baby or she has other children. Further examinations should be carried out if any neonatal problems have been detected; infants discharged early, before 24 hours, should be reexamined by 3 to 4 days of age.

PRINCIPLES OF THE NEWBORN EXAMINATION

The neonatal examination should be carried out in a warm, draft-free room specifically equipped for this procedure, and preferably with the mother present. If a satisfactory ambient temperature cannot be guaranteed, examining the infant under a servocontrolled radiant warmer is an alternative. Thorough hand-washing before and after handling each infant is essential to prevent the spread of pathogenic organisms. It is also important to clean the stethoscope and all other instruments between infants. Introduce yourself to the mother and inquire whether she has any specific concerns or questions. These should then be incorporated into your evaluation of mother and baby. Allow the mother to undress her baby if she wishes. Take this opportunity to notice how she handles her baby. Observe the infant's appearance, posture, and state of consciousness before proceeding with the formal aspects of palpation and auscultation. If any anomaly is found, look carefully for others, because they often coexist. Constellations of physical findings may indicate the presence of a syndrome. For example, if the physical features of Down syndrome are found, confirmatory chromosomal analysis is required. In addition, the infant, who later will show some degree of mental retardation, may have polycythemia, congenital heart disease, and congenital bowel obstruction, which need to be excluded. Signs of trauma that occurred during the birth should be noted. This is particularly common in large infants or after difficult deliveries by the breech or when forceps have been used. Evidence of trauma in one part of the baby should lead to a search for trauma in other areas.

The obstetric history of the pregnancy and delivery can provide clues to some neonatal problems. For example, polyhydramnios may be a sign of obstruction at some level in the bowel, and oligohydramnios may result from renal anomalies and give rise to serious life-threatening pulmonary insufficiency. Small-for-gestational-age and postmature infants may have hypoglycemia and polycythemia. Prolonged rupture of the membranes, maternal fever, and fetal tachycardia all raise the serious possibility of neonatal sepsis. The neonatal consequences of intrauterine growth restriction, prematurity, multiple births, maternal diabetes, and meconium-stained amniotic fluid are discussed in detail in other sections.

GESTATIONAL AGE AND SIZE

The infant's gestational age should be estimated and body size compared with appropriate normal standards.

There are several ways to estimate *gestational age*. The maternal history is reliable provided the first day of the last menstrual period is known and the pattern of menstruation has been regular before conception. Otherwise the measurements made by an experienced ultrasonographer on a scan taken before 20 weeks of gestation can be used. Gestation can also be assessed from the physical characteristics of the skin, external genitalia, ears, breasts, and from neuromuscular behavior. Physical development over the third trimester is shown in Fig. 2-12. Infants who are born after completing less than 37 completed weeks of gestation are considered to be *preterm* (or premature). *Term* infants have completed 37 to 42 weeks, and infants past 42 weeks of gestation are *postterm* (or postmature).

Birth weight, occipitofrontal head circumference, and crown-to-heel length should be measured and recorded. Length is measured from vertex to heel with the infant's legs fully extended. These measurements are then compared for gestational age against standard growth charts (Fig. 2-13). Ideally, growth charts for the

Physical Findings		Gestation (wk)																											
		20	21	22	23	24	25	26	27	28	29	30	31	32	33	34	35	36	37	38	39	40	41	42	43	44	45	46 47 48
Vernix		Appears			Covers body, thick layer															On back, scalp, in the creases	Scant, in the creases	No vernix						
Breast tissue and areola		Areola and nipple barely visible. No palpable breast tissue																Areola raised	1–2 mm nodule	3–5 mm	5–6 mm	7–10 mm						
Ear	Form	Flat, shapeless																Beginning incurving superior	Incurving upper ⅔ pinnae	Well-defined incurving to lobe								
	Cartilage	Pinna soft, stays folded													Cartilage scant, returns slowly from folding			Thin cartilage, springs back from folding		Pinna firm, remains erect from head								
Sole creases		Smooth soles without creases													1–2 anterior creases	2–3 anterior creases		Creases anterior ⅔ sole	Creases involving heel		Deeper creases over entire sole							
Skin	Thickness and appearance	Thin, translucent skin, plethoric, venules over abdomen, edema												Smooth, thicker, no edema				Pink	Few vessels	Some desquamation, pale pink	Thick, pale, desquamation over entire body							
	Nail plates	Appear												Nails to finger tips							Nails extend well beyond finger tips							
Hair		Appears on head		Eyebrows and lashes			Fine, woolly; bunches out from head										Silky, single strands, lays flat			Receding hairline or loss of baby hair, short/fine underneath								
Lanugo		Appears		Covers entire body											Vanishes from face				Present on shoulders		No lanugo							
Genitalia	Testes								Testes palpable in inguinal canal							In upper scrotum			In lower scrotum									
	Scrotum								Few rugae							Rugae, anterior portion			Rugae cover	Pendulous								
	Labia and clitoris										Prominent clitoris; labia majora small, widely separated				Labia majora larger, nearly covers clitoris			Labia minora and clitoris covered									
Skull firmness		Bones are soft						Soft to 1 inch from anterior fontanelle							Spongy at edges of fontanelle, center firm			Bones hard, sutures easily displaced		Bones hard, cannot be displaced								

FIGURE 2-12   Examination: First hours of life. SOURCE: *Adapted from Kempe C, Silver H, O'Brien D, eds: Current Pediatric Diagnosis and Treatment, 3rd ed. Lange, Los Altos, CA, 1974.*

specific population should be used. Babies born to mothers living at high altitude are smaller than babies born at or near sea level. An infant is considered to be appropriate for gestational age (AGA) if it falls within ±2 standard deviations (SD) of the mean on these charts. Infants who are more than 2 SD below the mean are small for gestational age (SGA), and those more than 2 SD above the mean are large for gestational age (LGA). Both groups need special observation (see Secs. 2.14 and 2.15). Twenty percent of infants with serious congenital malformations are SGA.

GENERAL INSPECTION

Most babies born at term cry at birth and then establish normal regular breathing. They may then remain awake and can be quite active for a half-hour or more. Their eyes are often open, and they make sucking, chewing, and swallowing movements. They may have bursts of flexion and extension of the arms and legs and make facial grimaces. This activity may be continuous or interspersed with quiet periods, during which the eyes are open.

Following the first few hours after birth, the normal term baby spends approximately 80% of time in active or quiet sleep. The remaining 20% of the time is spent awake in varying states of activity with or without crying.

When the infant cries, the cry is vigorous. A *weak or wimpering cry* is abnormal and warrants closer examination of the baby, as is a *high-pitched* or *shrieking cry,* which suggests a neurologic problem. A *hoarse cry* may result from vocal cord paralysis, hypothyroidism, or trauma to the hypopharynx.

Initially infants often adopt a position similar to that assumed in utero. If the examiner gently flexes the shoulders, knees, and hips, the limbs will move into a position that reproduces the intrauterine position (Fig. 2-14). A crying infant often can be calmed by assuming this posture. About 2% of infants have significant deformities caused by mechanical forces that acted in utero to restrict motion or to create pressure on the limbs, spine, thorax, or skull. This can occur with oligohydramnios, uterine malformations, or in multiple pregnancies.

TEMPERATURE

The normal infant is pink and feels warm to the touch, but exposure to even a moderately cold environment leads to the hands and feet quickly becoming cool and slightly cyanotic. The *normal axillary temperature* is between 36.5 and 37.4°C. The most common reasons for a low or high temperature are exposure to a cool environment and overheating. However, persistence of an abnormal tem-

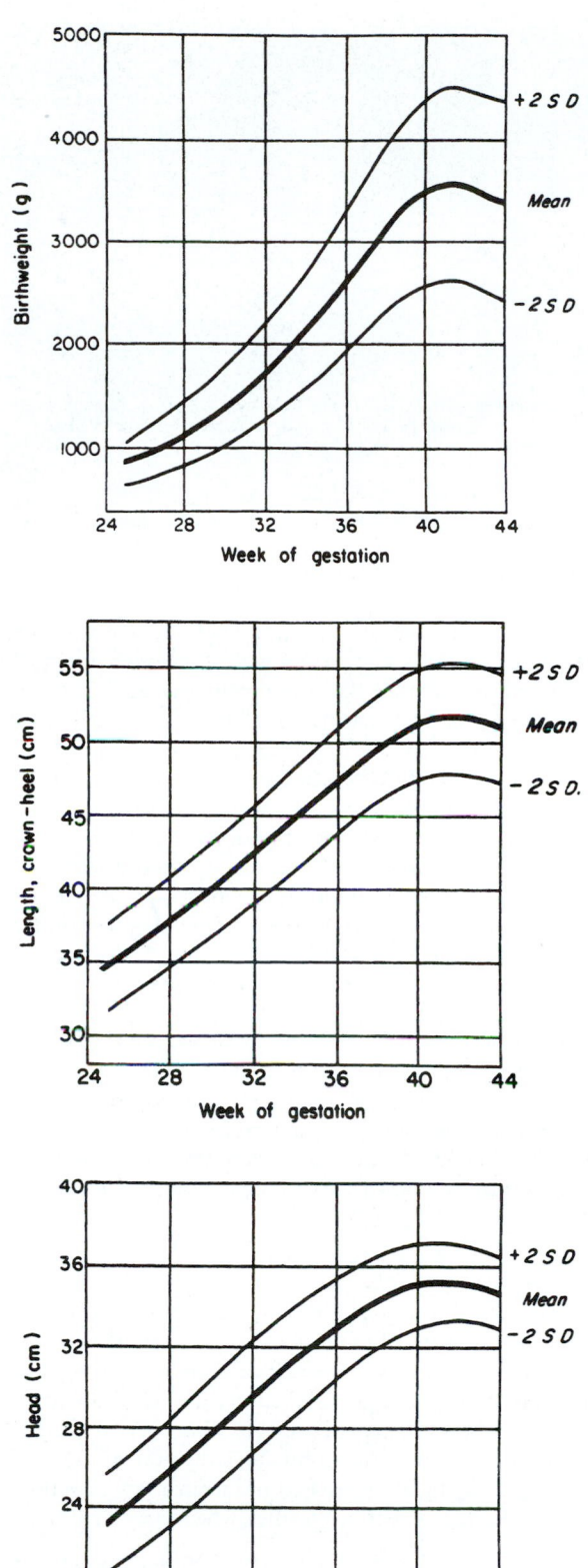

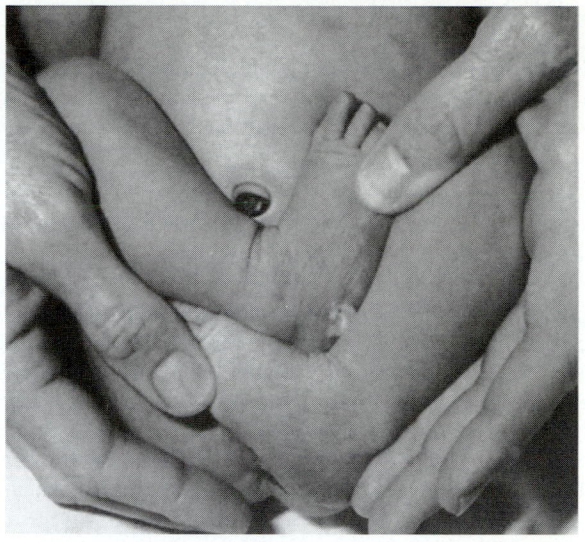

FIGURE 2-14 Position of comfort in a 20-hour-old infant. When placed in this position, the infant, who had been crying, was quiet. The ankles and metatarsals appear to be deformed but all these apparent deformities can be easily corrected with gentle pressure.

perature in a normal thermal environment indicates a pathologic problem. Sepsis may present with either fever, hypothermia, or an unstable temperature. *Hypothermia* may also occur with hypoglycemia, hypoxia, or hypothyroidism. *Hyperthermia* can be seen during drug withdrawal and with intracranial or adrenal hemorrhage.

SKIN

GESTATIONAL CHANGES Fine, soft, *lanugo hair* covers the entire body in very preterm infants and disappears from the face and lower back between 32 and 37 weeks. The term infant has lanugo hair on the upper back and dorsal aspects of the limbs. *Vernix caseosa,* a thick white material with the consistency of soft cheese, covers the skin of the entire body until 35 to 37 weeks. By term the amount of vernix has decreased so that it is present mainly in the flexor creases. Also by term, the subcutaneous tissue is relatively thick, and the fingernails and toenails are fully formed and extend slightly beyond the ends of the digits. If fetal hypoxia occurs at term, *meconium* may be passed into the amniotic fluid. If meconium has been in the amniotic fluid for several hours, it will also stain the skin, fingernails, toenails, and umbilical cord with a greenish hue. Fetuses at less than 34 weeks of gestation rarely pass meconium in response to hypoxia. The postmature infant (beyond 42 weeks) may have a somewhat wasted appearance with dry, peeling skin, a decreased amount of subcutaneous tissue, long fingernails, and an alert appearance.

UNUSUAL AND RARE SKIN ABNORMALITIES Discolored skin that looks like a cracking layer of thin yellow plastic is called *collodion skin*. Infants with this appearance often develop forms of ichthyosis later. Blistering or easily eroded skin may be caused by **epidermolysis bullosa,** but the blistering lesions of staphylococcal skin infection should be suspected first, as this will need urgent treatment (see Sec. 13.2.31).

Aplasia cutis is a congenital absence of skin that usually occurs in a small, localized area. Multiple defects on the vertex of the scalp

FIGURE 2-13 Intrauterine growth charts showing the normal values of body weight, length, and head circumference for infants born at different gestational ages at sea level (Montreal). **SOURCE:** *From the data of Usher, McLean: J Pediatr 74:901, 1969.*

occur in trisomy 13, and a midline defect over the back suggests spinal dysraphia.

Sclerema neonatorum is a diffuse hardening of subcutaneous tissue seen in severely ill newborns with systemic infections or hypothermia. The skin is hard and cold and may tighten around joints.

COLOR The skin of the normal white newborn is pink. *Pallor* may result from anemia or poor perfusion. With *poor perfusion* from vasoconstriction or low cardiac output, capillary filling after blanching of the skin over the tibia is delayed (more than 3 seconds). In pigmented babies, poor perfusion is more readily detected by delayed capillary filling after blanching of the toes or fingers. Anemia in these infants is recognized by pallor of mucous membranes. A generalized *gray* hue may indicate acidosis. *Pale, mottled skin* occurs with sepsis or hypothermia. There may be cyanosis of the hands and feet (*acrocyanosis*), which is normal immediately after birth or if the infant has been exposed to a cold environment. Generalized *cyanosis* occurs with significant arterial hypoxemia as well as with methemoglobinemia. *Plethora* may indicate polycythemia. *Harlequin skin* is a transient change in the skin color in which one side of the body turns pale while the other side remains pink with a sharp line of demarcation in the midline. Harlequin change can last for seconds or a few minutes and may recur but is of no known pathologic significance.

Ecchymoses generally result from birth trauma and are often present over the head after vertex delivery or on the feet, lower limbs, and buttocks following breech delivery. With severe birth trauma, there can be extensive hemorrhage into the muscles underlying areas of bruised skin. Localized *petechiae* are usually found in areas of vascular stasis or compression that occurred during delivery, on the face after a vertex delivery, or on the lower limbs after a breech delivery. More generalized petechiae suggest thrombocytopenia.

The skin overlying an area of *subcutaneous fat necrosis* often appears red. The subcutaneous tissue is hard and sharply demarcated, with lesions most common on the cheeks, buttocks, limbs, or back.

Neonatal *jaundice,* with a yellow skin color, is caused by an elevation in indirect-reacting bilirubin. Elevation of direct-reacting bilirubin gives a yellow-to-green discoloration. It is easier to assess the degree of jaundice in a newborn by briefly pressing on the infant's skin with a finger and observing the color in the blanched area. This is of particular value in pigmented infants. The normal newborn commonly develops mild physiological jaundice between days 2 and 4 after birth. Jaundice in the first day warrants prompt investigation; it is usually from sepsis or hemolytic anemia. The differential diagnosis of neonatal jaundice is discussed in Secs. 2.17.6

RASHES The normal newborn often has some form of benign skin rash. *Milia* are tiny white papules formed at the surface of sebaceous glands; they commonly appear over the nose. *Milaria* are lesions that develop over obstructed sweat glands and are usually a result of overheating. The *crystallina* form of milaria are superficial clear vesicles, whereas the *rubra* type are inflamed and lie deeper in the epidermis. *Erythema toxicum* (Fig. 2-15) consists of small pustules filled with eosinophils surrounded by patchy erythema. This is benign, fades, and reappears in other sites rapidly. It usually has less erythema than the more serious pustules of staphylococcal infection. *Pustular melanosis* are small vesicles that leave a scaly ring and pigmented macule when they open; they can be present at birth and are not associated with any known infection.

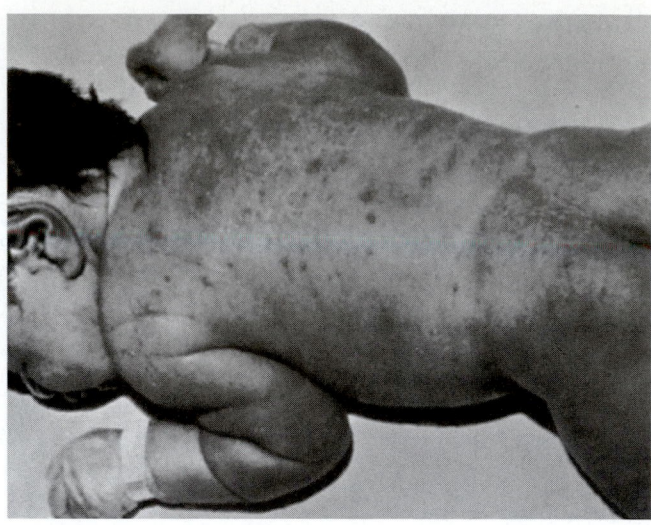

FIGURE 2-15 Erythema toxicum.

A neonatal rash may also indicate a serious systemic infection. Intrauterine infections may present with *thrombocytopenic purpura.* A red maculopapular rash may occur with *toxoplasmosis. Congenital rubella* often produces macular or slightly raised purple lesions, called a "blueberry muffin" rash. *Herpes simplex* can cause a few vesicles or a generalized vesicobullous eruption with an erythematous base; these cutaneous lesions may precede disseminated disease or may appear following the onset of disease in other organs. *Congenital syphilis* may cause a pink, maculopapular rash that later turns brown or becomes vesicobullous and hemorrhagic. Syphilitic rashes commonly involve the palms or soles. *Staphylococcal infection* may appear as pustules, generalized erythema, or extensive bullous eruptions (termed *scalded skin syndrome, toxic epidermal necrolysis,* or *Ritter disease*). *Listeria monocytogenes* can produce purple, miliary granulomas of the skin. Cutaneous *moniliasis* often produces macerated, erythematous skin, usually in the diaper area, and often occurs in infants treated with antibiotics. Many of these skin lesions contain viable organisms (eg, syphilis, herpes, *Staphylococcus*) and are highly infectious. Some generalized viral infections are characterized by small red papules that contain infiltrations of erythroid cells.

VASCULAR LESIONS *Macular* or *salmon patch hemangiomas* occur in over 30% of newborn infants, most often on the forehead, upper eyelids, or nape of the neck. They are deep pink and tend to fade later in infancy. *Port-wine stain* or *nevus flammeus* is less common; it can be red, purple, or even black in dark-skinned babies and has a leathery, thickened surface. When a port-wine stain is found on the face, over the ophthalmic division of the trigeminal nerve, there may be an associated intracranial arteriovenous malformation (Sturge-Weber syndrome) which may give rise to seizures.

Strawberry hemangiomas may appear as small pale areas of discoloration; these develop into full hemangiomas later in infancy. *Cavernous hemangiomas* are subcutaneous and give a faint red or purple discoloration to the overlying skin. Spinal dysraphism with a tethered cord may be accompanied by a hemangioma in the midline over the back, sometimes with a central area of cutis dysplasia.

PIGMENTED LESIONS AND NEVI *Mongolian spots* are gray-blue in color. They occur on the lower back, buttocks, and extensor surfaces. *Café-au-lait spots* are flat and usually uniform in color; these vary from light to dark brown. One or two café-au-lait spots may occur in normal infants, but large lesions (>3 cm) or multiple lesions may indicate a neurocutaneous syndrome (eg, neurofibromatosis, Albright syndrome). *Small, flat melanocytic nevi* are found in 3% of white and 16% of African-American neonates. The much larger *giant hairy pigmented nevus* can occupy up to one-third of the body surface and has a 10% chance of malignant degeneration. *Sebaceous nevi* usually appear on the face or head and are hairless, yellow-orange in color, and appear verrucose. Lesions that are raised, large, linearly streaked, or irregularly pigmented should usually be referred for a dermatologic evaluation. *Depigmented nevi* are a feature of tuberous sclerosis but may be absent at birth.

HEAD

Scalp hair of the infant is fine and silky. The *head shape* differs in infants who were in vertex or breech positions. After vertex presentation and vaginal delivery, there can be pronounced vertical elongation of the head. Breech infants often have occipital-frontal head elongation, with a prominent occipital shelf.

The cranial sutures should be palpably open and may be separated by up to several millimeters. Temporary overlap of bones, from molding, needs to be distinguished from *craniosynostosis* (premature closure of a suture). If a suture closes in utero, it prevents growth of the skull perpendicular to the fused suture line. This results in a sustained, abnormal skull configuration. In contrast, after molding occurs, the bones return to their normal positions in a few days. There may be a small concomitant decrease in head circumference.

Normally the *anterior fontanelle* is open, soft, and flat; mean diameter is less than 3.5 cm. The *posterior fontanelle* is often only fingertip size or just palpably open. A *bulging* or *tense fontanelle*, with separation of the bony sutures, indicates increased intracranial pressure.

Caput succedaneum is edema of the scalp caused by local pressure and trauma during labor. With severe trauma (see Sec. 2.17.12), there may be extensive *subgaleal hemorrhage* under the galea aponeurotica. The scalp feels tensely distended, and the swelling may extend to the suboccipital region and push the ears laterally. Hemorrhage can be massive and produce shock. *Cephalohematomas* are subperiosteal hemorrhages caused by the trauma of labor and usually involve the parietal or occipital bones. Cephalohematomas are fairly firm, fluctuant masses with a palpable rim that gives the impression of a shallow crater in the bone under the mass. They are distinguished from caput succedaneum because they do not extend beyond the suture lines of the affected bone. Parietal bone cephalohematomas may be bilateral but are palpably distinct from one another. Cephalohematomas should not be aspirated; they gradually resorb but can calcify before disappearing. Trauma to the head may also be accompanied by more serious intracranial hemorrhage. Other common traumatic scalp lesions include *puncture wounds* from fetal monitor electrodes and fetal scalp blood gas sampling. A *circular hematoma* may be seen at the site of application of a vacuum extractor.

FACE

The newborn's face often gives the first clue to the presence of a dysmorphic syndrome. There may be obvious malformations, such as cleft lip or the characteristics of the *Pierre Robin sequence* with a small mandible (micrognathia), a high-arched or cleft palate, and a tongue that falls back into the hypopharynx (glossoptosis); this

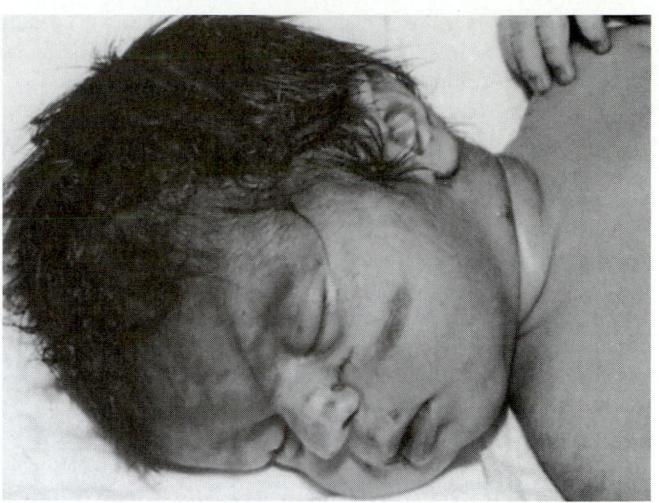

FIGURE 2-16　Forceps marks.

causes *airway obstruction*, which must be recognized promptly. The obstruction can be relieved with an oral airway and by pulling the tongue or the mandible forward. Infants with *fetal alcohol* exposure may be more difficult to identify but may have growth deficiency, microcephaly, maxilla hypoplasia and short palpebral fissures.

Intrauterine position may cause asymmetry of the face. Pressure over the stylomastoid foramen during labor and delivery may cause a peripheral *facial paralysis*, which is most obvious during crying. The paralysis usually resolves and should be distinguished from congenital absence of the depressor anguli oris muscle, which also results in an *asymmetric crying facies*.

Fracture of the zygomatic arch can occur during labor and delivery; this is detectable by palpation. *Forceps* often leave bruises on the face, usually in the shape of the forceps blade (Fig. 2-16).

EYES

Newborns generally open their eyes to permit inspection when they are awake, held upright, and shaded from bright light. An infant who is quiet and alert during the examination will fix on the examiner's face and follow it, at least part way, as the examiner moves slowly from side to side.

Congenital lid ptosis will manifest itself as a drooping lid, and *failure to close the eye fully* can occur with facial paralysis. *Horner syndrome*, caused by lower brachial plexus injury, appears as ptosis, miosis, and enophthalmos. *Congenital microphthalmia* is usually obvious on inspection and palpation. Mass lesions, such as orbital tumors, hemangiomas, and encephaloceles, may be immediately apparent. *Proptosis* may be caused by mass lesions or retrobulbar hemorrhage.

Birth trauma may also cause *subconjunctival hemorrhages* or hemorrhages in the *anterior chamber, vitreous,* and *retina*. Forceps deliveries can result in *lacerations* of the lid or globe. A rupture of the Descemet membrane in the cornea may become apparent because of corneal clouding.

Congenital glaucoma initially appears as an enlarged cornea that becomes progressively cloudy. A corneal diameter of 11 mm or more is suspect and warrants further investigation, as early detection is important in preventing eye damage (see Sec. 26.12.6).

Ophthalmoscopic examination should begin by focusing on the anterior portion of the eye and then progressing back to the retina. This allows detection of anterior lesions, such as cataracts and *co-*

lobomas (defects) of the iris, which may occur alone but are often components of various dysmorphic syndromes. The iris is blue or blue-gray in fair-skinned babies but is dark gray to brown in darker infants. In fair babies, a *red reflex* is transmitted back through the lens, whereas in darker infants a *paler orange-tan* color may be seen. Focusing down to the retina and visualizing retinal vessels will verify that a normal retina is being seen. A *cataract* will appear as a *black opacity* that interferes with light transmission through the lens. A *white pupillary reflex* is abnormal and may occur with a large retinoblastoma or developmental abnormalities such as retinal coloboma, retinopathy of prematurity, and persistent hypoplastic primary vitreous. A family history of retinoblastoma warrants a thorough ophthalmologic examination to exclude small or peripheral tumors.

Conjunctivitis usually becomes apparent after the second day; common pathogens include *Staphylococcus aureus*, streptococci, and coliform bacteria. *Gonococcal conjunctivitis* is acquired from the birth canal and can progress rapidly to a panophthalmitis with eye destruction. *Inclusion blennorrhea* is also acquired from the mother's birth canal; it is caused by *Chlamydia trachomatis* and typically appears toward the end of the first week of life. The various causes of conjunctivitis must be distinguished from one another by Gram stain and appropriate cultures (see Sec. 26.6.2).

EARS

At term, the ears are well formed and contain sufficient cartilage to retain a normal shape and resist deformation. *Preauricular pits* are common and inherited in an autosomal dominant pattern; *preauricular skin appendages* also may be seen. When these are hereditary they may be associated with deafness. *Malformed auricles* or *low-set-ears* are found in many dysmorphic syndromes and are associated with urogenital malformations.

To examine the *ear canal* and *tympanic membrane*, gently pull the pinna back and down. The tympanic membrane angles back more sharply in an infant than in an older child and is located more superiorly in relation to the external canal. Otitis media is uncommon but should be considered in an infant suspected of having an infection in the first days after birth. A crude estimate of *hearing* can be obtained if the infant is quiet and the examination is done in an environment without distracting noise. The alert, normal newborn will turn toward human speech, react and turn toward a ringing bell, and startle to a loud noise.

NOSE

Most newborn infants are nose breathers; rarely, obstructive lesions or foreign bodies in the nose can be lethal. Initially an infant will become cyanotic and have respiratory difficulty but, if stimulated to cry, will breathe through the mouth. Occasional sneezing is the normal mechanism infants use to clear the nose. Nasal patency can be verified by checking each naris for a good airstream with a thin strip of tissue or cotton. To avoid confusion, the mouth may need to be occluded transiently. Unilateral or bilateral anatomic obstruction from *choanal atresia* is rare. When there is doubt, a thin catheter should be passed gently through each nostril into the hypopharynx. Masses, such as an encephalocele protruding into the nasopharynx, can also cause obstruction. *Nasal stuffiness* can occur as a result of retained mucus or trauma. Nasal stuffiness may be a sign of drug withdrawal.

MOUTH

Examine the mouth of the newborn infant by inspection and palpation. A *cleft palate* may not be seen but may be detectable by palpation; a *cleft uvula* should raise suspicion of a palatal defect. Small, shiny white masses on the gums (*epithelial pearls*) are common. White *Epstein pearls* are found in the midline on the roof of the mouth, at the junction of the hard and soft palate. A *ranula* is a small benign mass that arises from the floor of the mouth. A *high-arched* or *narrow palate* is found in many dysmorphic syndromes.

The tongue may be attached to a short central *frenulum;* this rarely interferes with feeding or future function. An enlarged or *protruding tongue* can be seen with hemangiomas, isolated macroglossia, hypothyroidism, or in Down and Beckwith syndromes. Relative macroglossia because of a small mandible is found in the Pierre Robin sequence.

The normal, awake newborn will usually suck vigorously on a finger placed in the mouth. With *normal effective sucking,* the finger is actively drawn into the mouth by the movement of the tongue against the palate in a forward-to-backward motion. This coordinated function is easily distinguished from disorganized biting movements, which are ineffective in feeding from the nipple.

Natal teeth, if present, usually erupt in the lower incisor position. These can either be supernumerary teeth or true, deciduous "milk" teeth. If very loose or painful for breast feeding, they may be removed. However, removal of deciduous teeth will leave a defect for 7 years, until the permanent teeth appear, and may alter positioning of the 6-year molars and dental arch.

NECK

The neck of the newborn should have a full range of motion; limitation may indicate an abnormality of the cervical spine. Cervical masses, such as a *goiter, cavernous hemangioma,* or *cystic hygroma,* may compress the trachea and cause inspiratory obstruction. This may require tracheal intubation beyond the site of obstruction to establish an airway. *Brachial cleft anomalies* include cysts or sinuses along the anterior edge of the sternocleidomastoid muscle. *Thyroglossal duct cysts* usually occur in the ventral midline. *Torticollis* is seen with a tightened sternocleidomastoid muscle on one side and an atretic sternocleidomastoid muscle on the side toward which the head is turned; facial asymmetry is a common accompaniment.

Lateral traction during delivery may damage the upper root of the brachial plexus involving the fifth and sixth cervical roots, resulting in paralysis of the shoulder and arm. The arm is held alongside the body in internal rotation (Erb-Duchenne paralysis). The lower root of the brachial plexus, involving the eighth cervical and first thoracic roots, may be damaged, particularly during breech delivery. The small muscles of the hand are paralyzed, resulting in a clawlike posture (Klumpke paralysis). When there is neck trauma, the cervical sympathetic nerves may be damaged, resulting in an associated Horner syndrome, and the phrenic nerve may be injured, causing diaphragmatic paralysis.

CHEST

The chest of the normal newborn is barrel-shaped, and the xiphoid is often prominent. The most frequent birth injury to the thoracic region is *fracture of the clavicles,* identified by crepitation when the clavicle is palpated. *Supernumerary nipples* are a common minor anomaly; *wide spacing* of the nipple is seen in Turner syndrome.

Breast engorgement may occur in boys or girls and increases over the first few days.

LUNGS The *normal respiratory rate* is 35 to 60 breaths per minute. *Respiratory excursion* is most easily judged in the lateral view. Excursion of the abdomen is quite prominent, as infants breathe principally with their diaphragms. With normal breathing, chest and abdomen move together. When the airway is obstructed or the lungs are stiff, the abdomen appears to enlarge and the chest cage to get smaller with inspiration (*thoracoabdominal asynchrony*). The tissue between the ribs may be pulled in during inspiration; these *retractions* are normal during the first few minutes after birth. Thereafter, they are usually a sign of increased inspiratory effort from noncompliant lungs or airway obstruction. Inspiratory retractions of the ribs and sternum occur in severe lung disease or occasionally with an abnormal chest wall. Mild *expiratory grunting, nasal flaring,* and *tachypnea* occur during the first few minutes after birth. There may also be scattered rales caused by residual intraalveolar lung fluid that clears rapidly. These signs, attributable to retained lung fluid, are more noticeable after cesarean section. Persistence or worsening of respiratory symptoms may indicate more serious problems, such as *respiratory distress syndrome, bacterial pneumonia, meconium aspiration,* or *cardiac disease.*

Chest wall respiratory movement should be symmetric. One side moving less or lagging behind the other suggests an elevated paralyzed diaphragm from *phrenic nerve palsy* or an *intrathoracic mass* such as herniation of bowel through a *diaphragmatic hernia*. However, the absence of such findings does not rule out these lesions. Breath sounds may be heard even when a *pneumothorax* is present. *Coughing* in the newborn period is abnormal and usually accompanies interstitial lung disease such as viral pneumonia.

HEART AND VASCULATURE The point of *maximal cardiac impulse* is along the left side of the sternum at the fourth to fifth interspace and medial to the midclavicular line. The heart may be displaced if there is a pneumothorax or space-occupying lesion.

The heart rate may be 160 to 180 bpm during the first few hours after birth. Thereafter, the normal *awake heart rate* averages 120 to 130 bpm. Occasionally a normal newborn infant may have heart rates of 80 bpm, which may fall transiently to 60 bpm for short periods. A persistent heart rate below 80 bpm raises concern and warrants investigation. Conditions associated with *bradycardia* include birth asphyxia, increased intracranial pressure, hypothyroidism, congenital heart disease, and heart block. *Tachycardia* occurs with hypovolemia, fever, drug withdrawal, congenital heart disease, tachyarrhythmias, anemia, and hyperthyroidism. Cardiac rhythm should be checked; premature atrial contractions are not uncommon.

Despite the rapid heart rate, *heart sounds* can be clearly distinguished. The pulmonic component of S_2 may be prominent on the first day. Splitting of the second sound is audible along the left upper and midsternum. While postnatal circulatory adjustments are occurring, transient benign *murmurs* can be heard over the pulmonic area or cardiac apex. Murmurs accompanied by other symptoms, such as cyanosis, poor perfusion, or tachypnea, and murmurs that persist past the first day require further evaluation.

Over the first 12 hours, the *mean blood pressure* averages 50 to 55 mm Hg in term infants. Pulses should be palpable in all four extremities, and there should be no delay between brachial and femoral pulses. (For further discussion of postnatal circulatory and respiratory changes, see Sec. 2.7).

ABDOMEN

An extremely hollow abdomen suggests absence of some of the normal contents, such as *diaphragmatic herniation* of the bowel into the chest. *Distension* occurs with dilatation of the bowel from functional or anatomic obstruction, ascites, intraabdominal blood, or a large mass. If abdominal distension is noted, an oral catheter should be advanced into the stomach for decompression.

Signs of obstruction of the upper gastrointestinal tract include polyhydramnios (excess amniotic fluid), regurgitation, and pooling of secretions in the hypopharynx. When obstruction is suspected, pass a soft catheter into the stomach and aspirate the gastric contents. Bile-stained fluid suggests a high intestinal obstruction. In the most common form of *tracheoesophageal fistula*, proximal esophageal atresia prevents passage of the tube into the stomach. Pass a radiopaque orogastric catheter and check its course by radiography.

Examine the structures of the abdominal wall. A gap between the abdominal rectus muscles in the midline (*diastasis recti*), most noticeable with crying, is quite common. There is also often a small defect in the periumbilical musculature of the anterior abdominal wall, which may allow an *umbilical hernia;* this usually closes as the muscles develop toward the end of the first year. There are several serious possible defects of the anterior abdominal wall. In an *omphalocele*, some of the abdominal contents pass out through a periumbilical defect and are in close approximation with the umbilical cord; in this lesion the extraabdominal viscera are covered with a membrane that will form an enclosing sac unless it has ruptured (Sec. 2.18.1). The extent of the lesion varies greatly. In severe defects, the liver and spleen, as well as most of the intestines, are included in the extraabdominal mass. The most severe ventral defects involve the chest so that the heart is external (ectopia cordis). At the other extreme, a small piece of peritoneum may extend into the umbilical cord; it may not be recognized at birth and can be severed accidentally if the umbilical cord is cut too close to the abdominal wall. *Gastroschisis* results from primary failure of closure of the lateral ventral folds of the developing abdominal wall, so that small and large bowel pass out of the abdominal cavity through the defect. Unlike an omphalocele, the herniated bowel is not associated with the umbilical cord and has no covering membrane. Absence of the musculature of the anterior abdominal wall (the so-called *prune belly infant*) is an anomaly associated with urinary tract abnormalities (Sec. 21.16.2).

The *umbilical cord* normally contains two arteries and one vein, with the vein being larger than the arteries. Approximately 1% of newborns have a *single umbilical artery,* and 15% of these have one or more congenital anomalies, usually involving the nervous, gastrointestinal, genitourinary, pulmonary, or cardiovascular system. Otherwise normal infants with a single umbilical artery rarely have a serious anomaly. Remnants of the vitelline (*omphalomesenteric*) duct may persist and communicate with the umbilicus. If the remnant is a mucosal cyst, there may be umbilical mucus discharge. Persistence of the entire duct will create a fistula with the ileum, and some meconium may exit through the umbilicus. Persistent patency of the *urachus* results in a sinus extending from the bladder to the umbilicus, with urinary discharge from the umbilicus. A noncommunicating urachal cyst may also develop along the line of the urachus.

Palpate the abdomen to define the size and shape of the internal organs. To avoid aspiration of gastric contents into the lungs, palpation should not be done immediately after a feeding. The examination will be most successful if the examiner is gentle and rests the fingers on the abdominal wall and allows respiration to move the organs. The edge of the *liver* is normally felt 1 to 2 cm below the right costal margin. The *spleen* tip may be palpable but usually no more than 1 cm below the rib margin. In some pathologic conditions, the liver and spleen may be so massively enlarged that their edges are in the pelvis and not initially identified. Renal examination is easiest on the first day, before the bowel is filled with gas. The lower portion of each *kidney* is normally palpable on each side; the lateral and lower edges can be felt above the level of the umbilicus and lateral to the midclavicular line. The right kidney is situated slightly lower than the left kidney, and the palpable portion of the kidney normally feels about 2 cm wide. Enlarged kidneys may result from hydronephrosis, cystic malformation, a neoplasm, or renal vein thrombosis. Over 50% of all *abdominal masses* in the newborn arise from the genitourinary system. Mass lesions may also be caused by gastrointestinal malformation, neoplasms, or, rarely, neural lesions such as an anterior meningomyelocele.

Traumatic lesions to the abdomen at birth include subcapsular hematoma of the liver, which appears as an enlarging liver, an elevated right diaphragm, and shock when the hematoma ruptures; adrenal hemorrhage, which appears as a discrete palpable mass above the kidney and associated fever; and rupture of the spleen, when splenomegaly has been present in utero, with free blood in the peritoneum.

During the first few postnatal days the umbilical cord stump dries and then turns brown and brittle. The cord usually falls off between 10 and 14 days, releasing a small amount of opaque, yellowish discharge. Separation after 3 weeks, however, is not uncommon. Delayed separation of the cord occurs in infants who develop recurrent bacterial infections because of defective phagocyte function. A small, raw-appearing granuloma at the site of cord separation is termed an *umbilical polyp*. During the first week, a small amount of erythema at the rim of the umbilical stump is common and of no consequence, but more extensive erythema, a deeper red color, or associated edema may indicate the onset of *omphalitis*. Omphalitis is a serious infection requiring intravenous antibiotic therapy because of possible spread along the umbilical vein into the portal venous sinus of the liver. Omphalitis may progress to peritonitis or necrotizing fasciitis of the abdominal wall, which often proves fatal despite antibiotic therapy.

EXTERNAL GENITALIA

In preterm female infants, separation of the labia majora may give the illusion that the *clitoris* is enlarged. In term female infants, the labia majora meet in the midline, covering the rest of the genitalia. It is important to identify the *urethra*, which is just below the clitoris, and the vagina as distinct orifices; a single orifice or urogenital sinus is abnormal. Normally, the vagina has white secretions secondary to fetal stimulation by maternal hormones. These persist for a week or more and occasionally become tinged with blood several days after birth. *Hydrometrocolpos* results from an imperforate hymen or from vaginal atresia. It can present as a lower abdominal mass or as a bulging mass protruding through the labia and requires decompression.

The term male newborn has a *penis* approximately 3 to 4 cm long and a scrotum that is pigmented and has extensive rugae. Penile length less than 2.5 cm is abnormal and requires endocrinologic evaluation. The foreskin should not be forcibly retracted. *Penile hypospadias* is a common anomaly that can vary from a small

ventral cleft at the distal end of the penile urethra to a major ventral defect along the length of the penis. *Chordee,* a ventral bend in the penis, commonly accompanies hypospadias. *Epispadias,* a similar defect on the dorsum of the penis, is much less common and is a variant of *exstrophy of the bladder.*

The *testes* are usually in the scrotum but, if not fully descended, are often palpable in the upper scrotum or inguinal canal. Unilateral *undescended testes* cause an asymmetry in the scrotum, with an immature appearance on the affected side. *Hydroceles* or fluid collections in the remnants of the processus vaginalis cause a swelling of the scrotum. They are common, usually do not communicate with the peritoneal cavity, and disappear gradually. Hydroceles that fluctuate in size, or persist, are in communication with the peritoneal cavity and indicate a potential indirect *inguinal hernia.* Intestinal herniation can occur in the newborn period. Testicular enlargement, with discoloration of the overlying scrotum, suggests a *testicular torsion* that is a surgical emergency.

Ambiguous genitalia is a problem that requires investigation. Mild masculinization of the female newborn, with some enlargement of the clitoris, usually can be distinguished from mild feminization of the male neonate, with a small penis and hypospadias. When the processes are more extensive, however, the distinction between a girl with a very enlarged clitoris and a partially fused and pigmented labium and a boy with a very small penis and extensive hypospadias and bifid scrotum is much less clear (see Sec. 24.7).

Trauma to the external genitalia may occur during breech delivery. In addition to ecchymoses, there may be hemorrhage into the testes, scrotum, and pelvic muscles. This generally resolves in a few weeks.

ANUS

Imperforate anus is not always obvious on inspection. The imperforate anus may be accompanied by a fistula that opens onto the perineum, ventral to the normal anus. However, this fistula will not have the radiating skin creases of a normal anus. There can also be a normal-appearing anal dimple with no opening. Presence of meconium on the perineum and perianal area does not rule out imperforate anus; meconium in the anal area may have been passed by way of the skin fistula or, in a girl, a fistula from the rectum to the vagina.

SPINE

The spine of the newborn is quite flexible in both the dorsoventral and lateral axes; restricted movement suggests vertebral anomalies. The entire length of the spine, including the sacrum, should be palpated for bony defects and asymmetries. A *midline abnormality* of the skin over the spine, such as a small dimple, tufts of hair, or a pilonidal sinus, warrants close inspection, for any fluid extruding may indicate a tract that can allow bacteria on the skin to reach the cerebrospinal fluid. Midline cutaneous abnormalities may also indicate an occult spina bifida or a *diastematomyelia* (division of the spinal cord into two parts, which may become tethered as the child grows). Neural crest defects of the spine include *meningocele, myelomeningocele,* and *rachischisis.* Tumors of the spine, presenting at birth, are usually *teratomas* (see Sec. 20.15 and Table 20-20).

LIMBS

Trauma and positional deformities secondary to intrauterine position can occur in the newborn. The most common forms of *trauma of the limbs* include fractures in the shaft of the femur, humerus, or

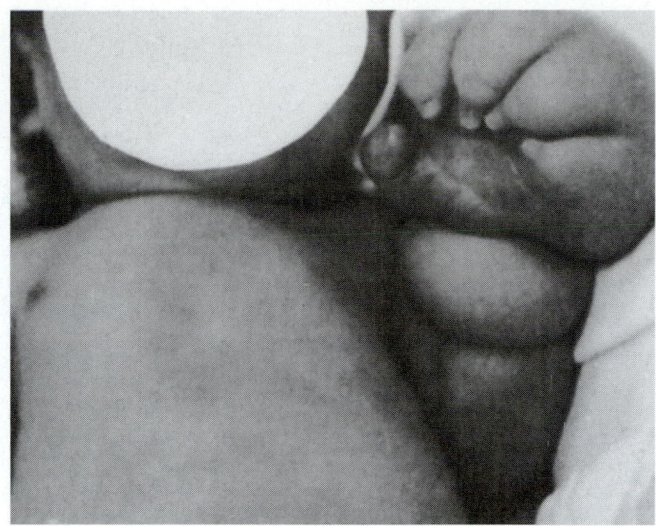

FIGURE 2-17   Circumferential amniotic constriction bands causing localized edema with a "lobster claw" deformity of the hand. There were also amputations of the distal phalanges of several fingers on the other hand.

clavicles and injury to the brachial plexus, causing paralysis of the hand and arm (discussed previously under examination of the neck).

It is important to distinguish between joints in one extreme of their normal position and joints that are deformed. As a rule, if simple manual pressure will correct a deformed joint back to its neutral position and a bit beyond, corrective positioning or simple exercise and stretching will correct the deformity. If the deformity cannot be corrected by gentle pressure, orthopedic evaluation is needed.

If the hips are flexed to 90°, the legs normally can be abducted until the knees touch the table the infant is lying upon. If this cannot be done, or if the maneuver can be done on one side only, there may be *congenital dislocation of the hip*. In this condition, the head of the femur is displaced posteriorly, out of the acetabular fossa. The affected leg may appear shorter. The examiner will feel a click when abducting and adducting the hips in about 10% of all infants. However, only 10% of infants with hip clicks have congenital hip dislocation. Two diagnostic manipulations of the hip joint can test for a dislocatable hip: the Ortolani and the subluxation maneuvers (see Sec. 27.6.1). Infants constrained in a breech position in utero tend to keep their hips flexed after birth and resist full hip extension. These infants, particularly girls, also have an increased incidence of dislocatable hips.

Malformations of the limbs include *hemihypertrophy* and *hemiatrophy;* in both conditions, the limbs on each side of the body are noticeably different in size but normally proportioned. With *phocomelia*, there is underdevelopment and abnormal shape of the limbs to a variable degree. The arms may be flipper-like with small digits projecting from the ends, or there may be only a nubbin of tissue at the site of origin of the limb. This malformation was particularly common among infants whose mothers took the drug thalidomide during pregnancy, but it also occurs spontaneously. The short limbs with *achondroplastic* and *thanatophoric* dysplasia are evident at birth (see Sec. 10.3.5). Newborns with *arthrogryposis multiplex congenita* have severe contractions of multiple joints that cannot be corrected by simple manual pressure.

The most obvious anomalies of the hands and feet are fusions of digits (*syndactyly*) and extra digits (*polydactyly*). The latter may be well-formed digits or merely small tags of tissue. Some minor malformations of hands and feet occur in many of the dysmorphic syndromes. For example, widely spaced first and second toes, hands with simian creases, downward displaced origin of the thumbs, and incurved little fingers are found in trisomy 21 (Down syndrome). A *clenched hand* with overriding index finger and a convex or *rocker-bottom* foot are seen in trisomy 18. *Bands originating from the amnion* may wrap tightly about a limb and cause a sharp, deep, circumferential depression. These intrauterine constriction bands may amputate the digits or cause localized edema by obstructing lymphatic drainage (Fig. 2-17).

References

Alper J, Holmes LB, Mihm MC JR: Birthmarks with serious medical significance: nevocellular nevi, sebaceous nevi, and multiple café au lait spots. J Pediatr 95:696–700, 1979

Ballard JL, Khoury JC, Wedig K, et al: New Ballard score, expanded to include extremely premature infants. J Pediatr 119:417–423, 1991

Dubowitz LM, Dubowitz V, Goldberg C: Clinical assessment of gestational age in the newborn infant. J Pediatr 77:1–10, 1970

Enjolras O, Riche MC, Merland JJ: Facial port-wine stains and Sturge-Weber syndrome. Pediatrics 76:48–51, 1985

FIGO International Federation of Gynecologists and Obstetricians Committee for the Ethical Aspects of Human Reproduction and Women's Health: Ethical aspects of newborn care. In: Recommendations on Ethical Issues in Obstetrics and Gynecology. London, FIGO, 2000:43–44

Froehlich LA, Fujikura T: Follow-up of infants with single umbilical artery. Pediatrics 52:6–13, 1973

Gardosi J, Mul T, Mongelli M, Wilcox M: Ultrasound dating and birth weight at term. Lancet 308:1635, 1994

Jones DA: Importance of the clicking hip in screening for congenital dislocation of the hip. Lancet 1:599–601, 1989

Khoury MJ, Erickson JD, Cordero JF, McCarthy BJ: Congenital malformations and intrauterine growth restriction: a population study. Pediatrics 82:83–90, 1988

Popich GA, Smith DW: Fontanels: range of normal size. J Pediatr 80:749–752, 1972

Stern E, Parmelee AH, Akiyama Y, Schultz MA, Wenner WH: Sleep cycle characteristics in infants. Pediatrics 43:65–70, 1969

Usher R, McLean F, Scott KE: Judgment of fetal age. II. Clinical significance of gestational age and an objective method for its assessment. Pediatr Clin North Am 13:835–862, 1966

Yip R: Altitude and birth weight. J Pediatr 111:869–876, 1987

Yudkin PL, Aboualfa M, Eyre JA, Redman CW, Wilkinson AR: New birth-weight and head circumference centiles for gestational ages 24 to 42 weeks. Early Hum Dev 15:45–52, 1987

2.8.2   Neurologic Examination

During the third trimester of gestation a very rapid maturation of the CNS takes place. Interpretation of neurologic signs in a newborn infant requires knowledge of normal development because these maturational changes are paralleled by an increase in the level and complexity of neurologic function. Examination of a baby differs from that of the older child or adult, but it is useful to retain the same basic approach in evaluating neurologic function. This includes a systematic assessment of mental status (level of alertness), cranial nerve function, the motor and sensory systems, and the evoked reflexes.

MENTAL STATUS

The examination of mental status includes observation of spontaneous eye opening and movements of the eyes, face, and extremities as well as the response to stimulation. A preterm infant born before 32 weeks of gestation spends much of the time *sleeping* but can be aroused by gentle stimulation. Arousal is marked by transient eye opening and movement of the face and extremities. After 32 weeks of gestation, there are periods of spontaneous eye opening with roving eye movements and movements of the face and extremities. More mature babies show an increase in the frequency, duration, and quality of alertness, so that by term there are periods in which the infant may attend to auditory and visual stimuli. The state of *quiet alertness* (State 3 of Prechtl, Table 2-4) is ideal for eliciting optimal responses. Subtle abnormalities are marked by irritability or lethargy. The irritable and agitated infant cries spontaneously with minimal stimulation and cannot be calmed. Lethargy is revealed by a delayed or poorly maintained response to stimulation. In coma, arousal is impossible. The depth of coma is identified by the level of reflex response to stimulation.

CRANIAL NERVE EXAMINATION

At 28 weeks of gestation a baby will blink when a bright light is shone in the eyes (cranial nerves II and VII). A term infant retains this reflex and, in addition, when alert, may fixate on a face or large object and track it (cranial nerves II, III, IV, and VI). From 34 weeks of gestation onward, the demonstration of "fix and track" abilities is an essential part of routine examination. The "bull's eye," a round piece of cardboard printed with glossy black and white concentric circles, makes visual pursuit testing easy to perform (Fig. 2-18). The pupillary reaction to light appears between 28 and 32 weeks of gestation (cranial nerves II and III). Funduscopic examination may reveal atrophy or hypoplasia of the optic disc or defects of the retina, indicating congenital malformations involving the optic nerve or retina. Retinitis suggests an intrauterine infection. Retinal hemorrhages are not uncommon and do not necessarily indicate clinically significant intracranial hemorrhage. Extraocular movements (cranial nerves III, IV, and VI) can be assessed by observing spontaneous or reflex eye movements.

Disconjugate gaze is common in normal newborn infants when they are not fixating. The corneal reflex and withdrawal to gentle pinprick on the face (cranial nerve V) are intact in the term infant. The symmetry and amplitude of facial movements (cranial nerve VII) are observed during spontaneous and evoked facial movements, including crying. Subtle facial weakness may be marked by mild ptosis and asymmetry of spontaneous movements only. Hearing (cranial nerve VIII) is assessed by eliciting a blink to a loud sound such as a hand clap. The alert term infant will often become quiet to a soft, high tone. Sucking reflexes are used to evaluate the function of cranial nerves V, VII, and XII, and swallowing reflexes to evaluate cranial nerves IX and X. The strength of the suck and

TABLE 2-4

PRECHTL STATES OF SLEEP AND WAKEFULNESS IN THE NEWBORN

State 1: Eyes closed, regular respiration, no movements
State 2: Eyes closed, irregular respiration, no gross movement
State 3: Eyes open, no gross movements
State 4: Eyes open, gross movements, no crying
State 5: Eyes open or closed, crying

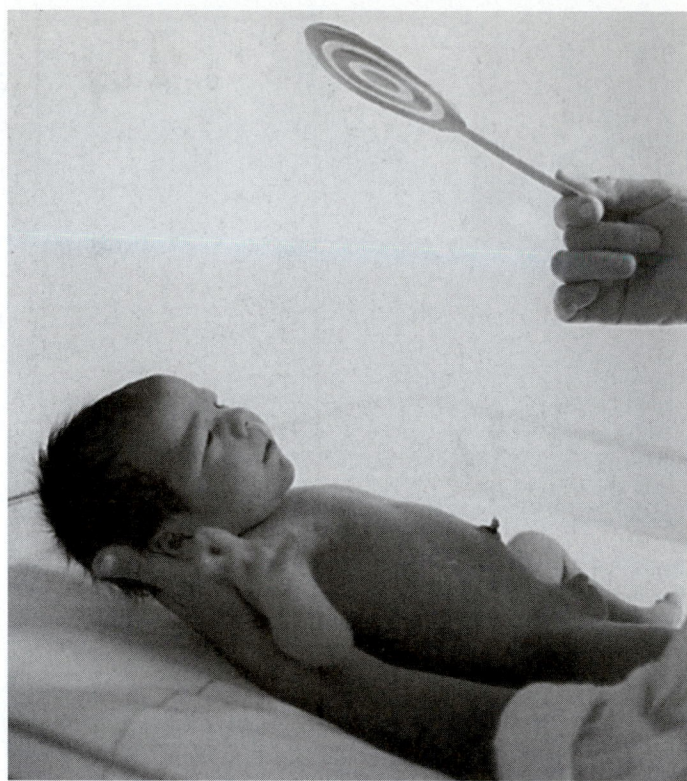

FIGURE 2-18   Testing for fixing and tracking with the "bull's eye." Note the testing position.

coordination of sucking and swallowing increase with increasing gestational age. Abnormalities of sucking and swallowing are shown by an inability to feed and an excess of oral secretions. Severe gastroesophageal reflux leading to aspiration may also occur. The tongue (cranial nerve XII) is examined for atrophy or fasciculations, and the sternocleidomastoid muscle (cranial nerve XI) for atrophy or contracture. The quality of the cry is assessed, as it is altered in many neurologic disorders in infancy.

MOTOR EXAMINATION

The motor examination includes an assessment of spontaneous movements and muscle tone. Posture and resistance of muscles to passive movement are used to assess resting or passive tone. Evoked changes in extremity tone and evoked postures of the head, trunk, and extremities are used to assess active tone.

To understand the transitional stage of motor function seen in the term newborn infant, the clinician needs a simplified description of the motor pathways, the timing and direction of their myelination, and their roles in determining motor function (Fig. 2-19). Under 34 weeks of gestation, brainstem motor control is progressing upward. After a transitional period, cortical motor control is progressing downward and gradually takes over.

SPONTANEOUS MOVEMENTS Before the infant is disturbed, observe the frequency and symmetry of spontaneous movements, with particular attention to their amplitude and duration. This will vary with the infant's level of arousal; spontaneous movements of the extremities in the term infant are organized and smooth. Movements of the fingers become independent and controlled as term is approached. The ability to abduct the thumb is particularly mean-

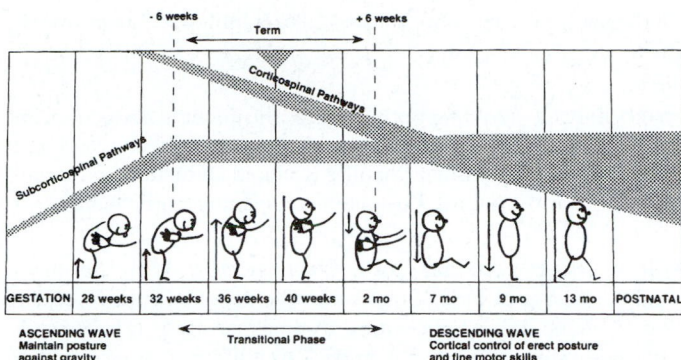

FIGURE 2-19 Maturation in motor control from fetal life through infancy. The *subcorticospinal pathways* derive from the brain stem with myelination taking place between 24 and 32 weeks of gestation and proceeding upward, starting in the spinal cord. Their essential role is to maintain posture against gravity. The *corticospinal pathways* originate in the motor and the premotor cortex; 80% of the descending fibers cross the midline in the medulla (pyramidal tract). Their myelination starts around 32 weeks of gestation, proceeds downward from the pons to the spinal cord very slowly, reaching completion at about 12 years of age. They are responsible for control of erect posture and for movements of the extremities including fine motor skills. From term onward, corticospinal control takes over, allowing development of mature head control, sitting, and walking.

ingful, as persistent adduction suggests a lesion involving the corticospinal tract.

POSTURE AND PASSIVE TONE The symmetry and maturity of passive tone are evaluated by observing the resting posture of the infant and by moving the extremities while the infant is awake and quiet. The movements are performed slowly and gently while the examiner ascertains the degree of resistance to movement. The angles through which each extremity can be moved provide an objective evaluation of passive tone. It is important to keep the infant's head in the midline position during the motor examination to avoid eliciting asymmetries in tone relating to the asymmetric tonic neck reflex. Six maneuvers are described:

1. *Popliteal angle:* Flex the infant's thighs laterally beside the abdomen, and then extend the knee to its limit. Measure the angle formed at the knee, which is the popliteal angle.
2. *Foot dorsiflexion angle:* With the knee extended, dorsiflex the ankle by applying pressure with a finger on the sole of the foot. Measure the angle between the dorsum of the foot and the anterior aspect of the leg (Fig. 2-20) Foot dorsiflexion angle is

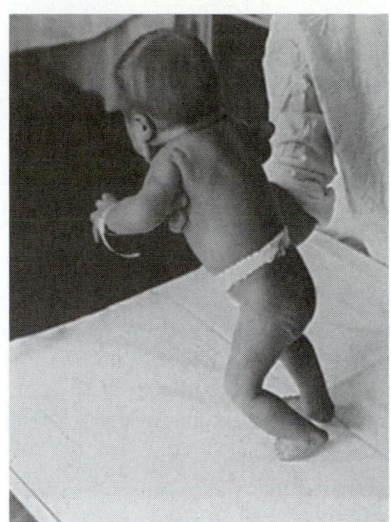

FIGURE 2-21 Righting reaction.

a physical criterion of gestational age because the result depends on the progressive restriction of space in utero up to term.

3. *Scarf sign:* With one hand support the infant in a semireclining supine position keeping the head straight. Pull one of the infant's hands across the chest toward the opposite shoulder and note the position of the elbow.
4. *Forearm recoil:* This can be elicited only when the infant is in a spontaneously flexed position. Extend the arm passively at the elbow by pulling on the hand. Then immediately release the hand and observe the speed of recoil of the forearm to its former position. If the forearm recoils normally, the test can be repeated after the forearm has been held in extension for 20 to 30 seconds.
5. *Ventral flexion in the axis:* With the child supine, grasp the lower limbs and push both legs and pelvis toward the head in order to achieve the maximum curvature of the spine. Some passive flexion of the trunk is normally present.
6. *Dorsal extension in the axis:* With the infant lying on his or her side, place the flat of the palm of one hand on the lumbar region and pull both legs backward with the other hand. Extension is normally minimal or absent.

There is much individual variation in the extent of flexion and extension at all ages, but in a normal baby, *flexion always exceeds extension.*

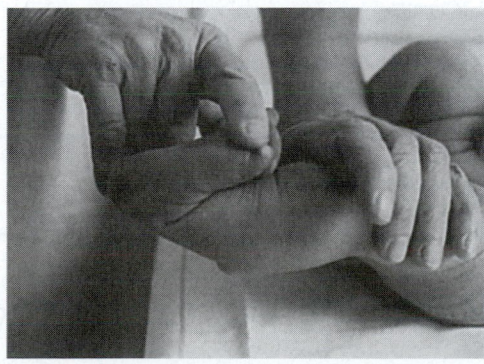

FIGURE 2-20 Foot dorsiflexion.

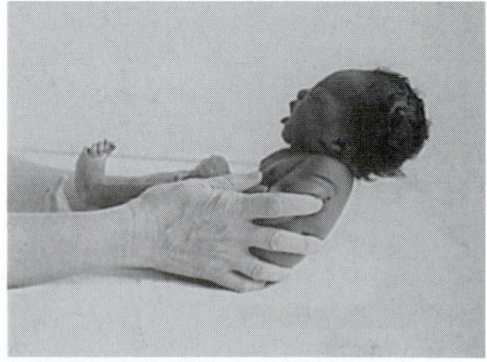

FIGURE 2-22 Raise-to-sit maneuver.

ACTIVE TONE This term refers to the tone observable when the infant makes an active movement in reaction to certain situations.

RIGHTING REACTION To elicit this reaction, place the infant in the standing position with the feet on a horizontal surface while supporting the trunk. A normal mature response consists of extension of the legs and trunk so that the infant supports his or her own weight (Fig. 2-21).

NECK FLEXOR TONE TESTED BY THE RAISE-TO-SIT MANEUVER Hold the infant's shoulders and pull the infant from the lying to the sitting position, noting the relationship between the head and the trunk. The forward movement elicits active contraction of the neck flexor muscles in an attempt to raise the head to a vertical position (Fig. 2-22).

NECK EXTENSOR TONE TESTED BY THE BACK-TO-LYING MANEUVER With the infant held in the sitting position and the head hanging forward on the chest, move the trunk gently backward while observing the reaction of the head extensor muscles. A normal reaction consists of a contraction of the extensors, tending to lift the head before the trunk reaches the vertical position (Fig. 2-23).

PRIMARY REFLEXES Primary reflexes normally are present in the preterm infant as well as in the term infant. They are not inhibited until the infant reaches several months of age; when they cannot be elicited in the newborn infant, this is a sign of CNS depression.

Of the many primary (or primitive) reflexes, only a few are routinely used.

MORO REFLEX Holding both hands of the infant in abduction, lift the infant's shoulders a few inches off the bed and then release the hands briskly. The normal response is a rapid abduction and extension of the arms, followed by complete opening of the hands.

FINGER GRASP AND RESPONSE TO TRACTION With the infant supine, insert your index fingers into the infant's hands to obtain flexion of the fingers amounting to a palmar grasp. The grasp is sufficiently strong to take the infant's weight when you raise your index fingers. This "response to traction" provides a very good estimate of the strength of active tone (Fig. 2-24).

AUTOMATIC WALKING Hold the infant upright with the feet on a table in a standing position to obtain a supporting reaction by the infant. Then tilt the infant forward slightly, and he or she should make a step forward.

CROSSED EXTENSION Hold one leg in extension and gently stroke the plantar surface of the foot. This produces a sequence of three movements of the opposite leg (Fig. 2-25): (1) a rapid movement of withdrawal followed by extension of the leg, (2) fanning of the toes, and (3) adduction of the leg toward the stimulated side. The third component shows a distinct maturational change, first appearing at 26 weeks and becoming fully developed at 40 weeks (Fig. 2-25).

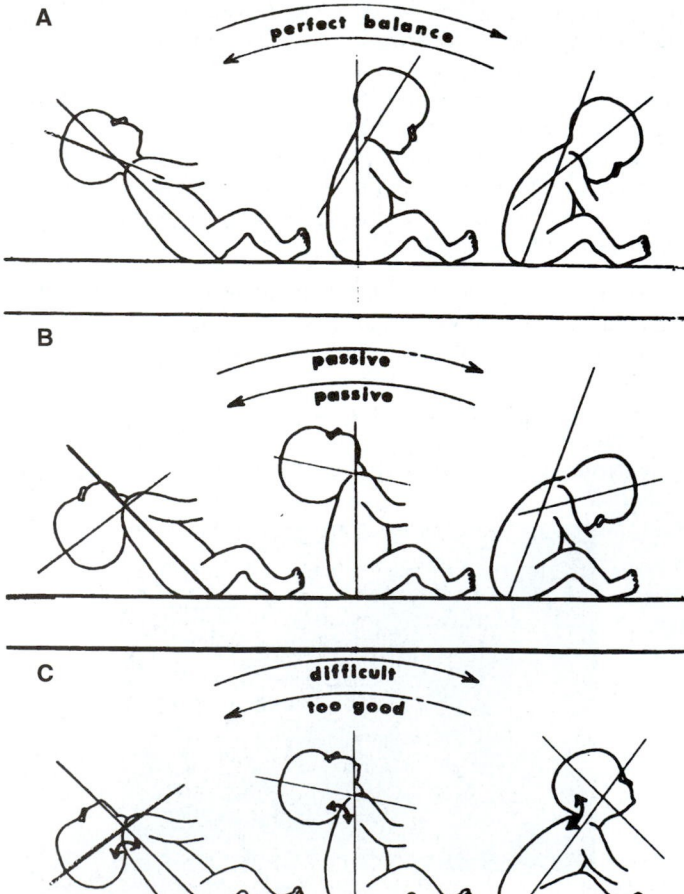

FIGURE 2-23 Responses to raise-to-sit and back-to-lying maneuvers. (A) Normal. (B) Absent passive and active tone in axis and limbs. (C) Imbalance between extensor and flexor tone in the axis.

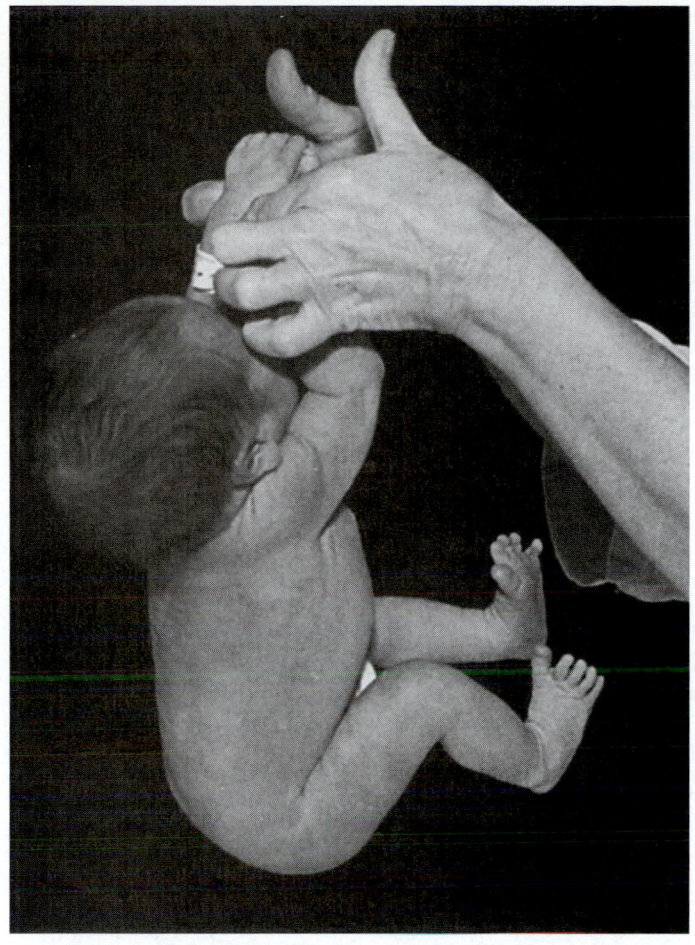

FIGURE 2-24   Finger grasp and response to traction.

SUCK-SWALLOW REFLEX Place a clean finger in the infant's mouth and note the strength and rhythm of sucking and its synchrony with swallowing. One can roughly estimate the number of movements in a burst, the rate, the negative pressure perceived, and the interburst time (Fig. 2-26).

MATURATIONAL CHANGES IN TONE AND REFLEXES During the second half of gestation, changes occur in the quality of passive and active tone. Up to term, there is an ascending wave of increased flexor tone in the limbs and of extensor, postural reactions in the body axis (spine and lower limbs). This was described by Saint-Anne Dargassies in the 1950s and was the basis for a system of neurologic evaluation to determine gestational age. However, by the 1970s, the introduction of intensive care made it progressively more difficult to perform a neurologic examination correctly in the smallest and sickest infants. As a consequence, physical, nonneurologic criteria have been developed to estimate the stage of maturation at birth when the gestation by maternal history is uncertain.

Maternal menstrual history or early fetal sonography have been shown to provide the best possible dating before 32 weeks of gestation; from 32 weeks on, it appears reasonable to confirm gestational age by the physical criteria and to assess CNS function of the infant according to the normal steps of development described in Fig. 2-25.

Ten signs have been selected, consisting of four passive tone items (popliteal angle, scarf sign, forearm recoil, dorsiflexion angle of the foot), three active tone items (righting reaction, neck flexor tone, neck extensor tone), and three primary reflexes (finger grasp and response to traction, crossed extension, sucking-swallowing). The selected items are grouped in 2-week stages, and the estimated stage of maturation of each item is recorded by identifying the 2-week period to which the observed finding corresponds. A chart is used in which the time between 32 and 40 weeks is divided into 2-week periods, and the result for each neurologic sign is recorded by circling the result obtained.

A definite conclusion on neurologic maturation is reached from this assessment only if seven of the 10 responses correspond to the same 2-week gestation period (ie, are arranged in line on the chart of 2-week gestation groups). When more than three responses are out of line, which happens in some 10% of cases, it is wisest to reach no firm conclusion on neurologic maturation. A discordant result of this kind also raises the probability that some neurologic abnormality is present. The pattern of progressive equalization of flexor and extensor muscle activity with maturation by comparison of the responses obtained by the raise-to-sit and back-to-lying maneuvers (Figs. 2-24 and 2-25) must be taken into account to identify abnormal responses in the preterm infant.

ACTIVE TONE AND PRIMITIVE REFLEXES Active tone and evoked reflexes are evaluated by observing changes in the infant's posture in response to changes in position with respect to gravity (Fig. 2-23) or by observing the infant's responses to other stimuli, such as touch, pressure, and pinprick. A number of primitive reflexes have been described in the neonate, but many are redundant in the information they yield about the integrity of the nervous system. It is far better for the beginner to become familiar with a few reflexes and the changes in these reflexes that occur with maturation.

MATURATIONAL CHANGES IN THE MOTOR EXAMINATION During the last trimester of gestation, changes occur in the frequency and amplitude of spontaneous movements, in the quality of passive and active tone, and in the strength and duration of primitive reflexes. As a general rule, an increase in flexor tone begins in the lower extremities and progresses cephalad between 28 and 40 weeks of gestation. This progression correlates with increasing myelination of subcortical motor pathways originating in the brainstem. After 40 weeks of gestation, maturation of tone and coordination, which begins rostrally and progress caudally, is linked to

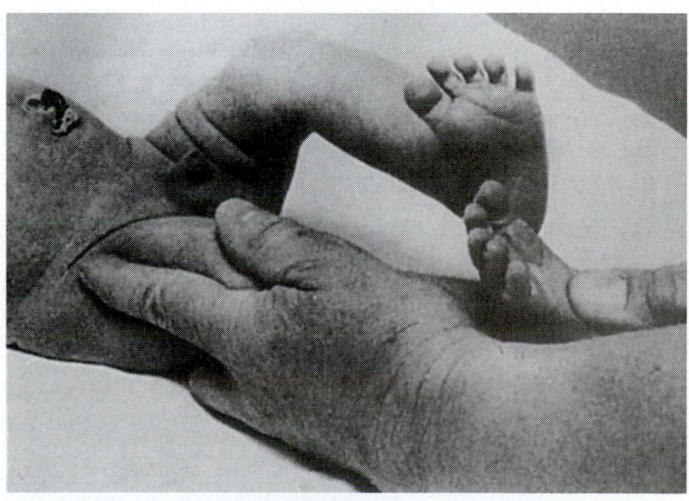

FIGURE 2-25   Crossed extension.

Weeks gestation	Below 32	32–33	34–35	36–37	38–39	40–41
POPLITEAL ANGLE	130° or more	120°-110°	110°-100°	100°-90°	90°	90° or less
SCARF-SIGN	no resistance	very weak resistance	largely passes midline	slightly passes midline	does not reach midline	very tight
RETURN TO FLEXION OF FOREARMS	posture in extension most of the time		weak or absent	present, less than 4 times	4 times or more brisk but inhibited	4 times or more very strong & not inhibited
FINGER GRASP AND RESPONSE TO TRACTION	absent		very weak or absent	able to lift part of the body weight	able to lift all body weight for 1 sec.	maintains 2 to 3 sec with head passing forwards
RIGHTING REACTION lower limbs and trunk	no support	brief support lower limbs only	begins to maintain trunk	trunk more firm	begins to raise head	complete righting for a few secs.
RAISE-to-SIT (neck flexor muscles)	no movement of the head forwards		head rolls on the shoulder (BETTER BACKWARDS)	passes briskly in the axis (PROGRESSIVE EQUALISATION)	more powerful	perfect, minimal lag (SYMMETRICAL)
BACK- to-LYING (neck extensor muscles)	no movement of the head backwards	head begins to lift but cannot pass backwards	passes briskly in the axis	powerful movement backwards		perfect, minimal lag
CROSSED EXTENSION		good extension but no adduction		tendency to adduction	reaches the stimulated foot	crosses immediately
SUCKING	n° mvts in a burst rate of mvts negative pressure interburst time	3 or less 1/sec. weak or none 15–20 sec.	4 to 7 1, 5/sec. intermediate 5 to 10 sec.	8 or more 2/sec. high 5 to 10 sec.	idem	idem
FOOT-DORSIFLEXION ANGLE	≥ 50°	40°-30°		20°-1 0°		nul

FIGURE 2-26 Neurologic criteria described at 2-week intervals, from 32 to 40 weeks' gestation. Periods of rapid modifications are enclosed by heavy borders, indicating the most discriminative period for each observation. idem = refer to same response as 36-37 weeks; nul = no flexion. *From Amiel-Tison C. Clinical assessment of the infant nervous system (Chapter 5). In: Levene MI, Bennett MJ, Puni J, eds: Fetal and Neonatal Neurology and Neurosurgery, 2nd ed. London, Churchill Livingstone, 1995:83–104, with permission.*

myelination of corticospinal motor pathways. For example, the infant at 28 weeks of gestation lies with both upper and lower extremities fully extended, and there is little or no resistance to passive movement of the extremities. As the infant matures, there is an increase in the muscle tone of the flexors in the lower extremities, so that by 34 weeks, the lower extremities are flexed at the knees and the hips. Flexion of the upper extremities is present at 36 weeks. In the term infant, both lower extremities are flexed at the knees and the hips, and both upper extremities are flexed at the elbows. After 40 weeks, there is a gradual loss of the resting flexor posture, beginning in the upper extremities. The active tone of neck muscles increases with maturation, as shown in Fig. 2-25. At term both neck flexors and extensors can maintain the head in the axis of the trunk for more than a few seconds. Primitive reflexes such as the Moro and grasp reflex are present very early in fetal life; however, they become stronger, easier to elicit, and more complete as gestation increases.

SENSORY EXAMINATION

In the neonate, the sensory examination usually is limited to the evaluation of touch and pinprick appreciation. A positive response to pinprick is identified by a change in facial expression or in level of alertness. The response to stimulation of individual dermatomes, including the sacral area (anal wink), may be necessary to localize the level of a spinal lesion.

TENDON REFLEXES

Biceps, knee, and ankle jerks can be elicited readily in the term infant. Some ankle clonus is common in the normal newborn. Asymmetry or absence of reflexes may indicate a significant central or peripheral nervous system abnormality.

HEAD CIRCUMFERENCE, SKULL, AND SUTURES

Evaluation of the head includes observation of the shape and size with measurement of the occipitofrontal circumference. Cephalhematoma and caput succedaneum are described in Sec. 2.17.12. The head is palpated to examine the sutures and fontanelles and to detect defects in the skull as well as evidence of trauma such as fracture or cephalhematoma. A full, pulsating or bulging, tense fontanelle is an important sign of increased intracranial pressure. Careful examination of the spine for vascular malformations or dermal sinus tracts may lead to the identification of an underlying spinal defect.

VALUE OF A NORMAL NEUROSENSORIAL ASSESSMENT

A normal neurologic assessment within the first week of life of the term neonate is a good predictor of later development. Similarly, for a premature newborn who has reached 40 weeks (conceptual age), a normal neurologic assessment correlates better with a normal outcome than does absence of visible damage on brain imaging.

References

Amiel-Tison C: Clinical assessment of the infant nervous system. In: Levene MI, Lilford RJ, eds: Fetal and Neonatal Neurology and Neurosurgery, 2nd ed. London, Churchill Livingstone, 1988:83–104

Amiel-Tison C, Stewart A, eds: The Newborn Infant: One Brain for Life. Paris, Editions INSERM, 1994

Dubowitz LM, Dubowitz V, Goldberg C: Clinical assessment of gestational age in the newborn infant. J Pediatr 77:1–10, 1970

Saint-Anne Dargassies S: Neurological Development in the Full-Term and Premature Neonate. Amsterdam, Elsevier/North-Holland Excerpta Medica, 1977

Stewart A, Hope PL, Hamilton PA, et al: Prediction in very preterm infants of satisfactory neurolodevelopmental progress at 12 months. Dev Med Child Neurol 30:53–63, 1988

Volpe JJ: Neurology of the Newborn. Philadelphia, WB Saunders, 1995

2.9 DELIVERY ROOM EMERGENCIES AND NEWBORN RESUSCITATION

Augusto Sola and George A. Gregory

2.9.1 Need for Newborn Resuscitation

Close to 10% of newborn infants experience difficulty with extrauterine adaptation immediately after delivery and require some degree of resuscitative support. The incidence of serious cardiovascular or respiratory problems occurring around the time of birth is much greater among premature infants of very low birth weight (less than 1500 g) than it is among infants who are born near term. Conditions that require emergency treatment of newborn infants in the delivery room are among the most frequent problems encountered in neonatal medicine. The most serious of these conditions is asphyxia, in which oxygen delivery to vital organs and carbon dioxide elimination from the body are impaired. Failure to reverse this condition rapidly results in multiorgan failure and death or permanent disability. Although perinatal asphyxia cannot always be prevented, nor can the need for life support measures always be predicted, prompt effective resuscitation of severely depressed neonates can facilitate successful transition from fetal to neonatal life and prevent or minimize organ damage and adverse outcome. This section describes the organization needed to ensure adequate anticipation of problems in the delivery room, the most frequent neonatal conditions that require emergency treatment at birth, and the necessary steps required to achieve optimal resuscitation.

2.9.2 Preparation and Resuscitation for Delivery

Anticipation and planning for unexpected emergencies are the most important requirements for successful resuscitation of the neonate. The antepartum and intrapartum history often helps to identify in advance the infant who will be critically ill at birth. In such instances, the birth should occur in a hospital that has a neonatal intensive care unit (NICU). The NICU should be staffed with skilled personnel and have specialized equipment kept in a designated resuscitation room immediately adjacent to the delivery suite where the patient can be effectively resuscitated and stabilized. Because it is impossible to identify every infant who will require assistance at birth, someone skilled in neonatal resuscitation must be available for every delivery, wherever it occurs. Other important issues to facilitate successful resuscitation include establishment of detailed plans of exactly how to proceed when an unexpected emergency occurs and fail-safe measures to provide accurate neonatal evaluation and prompt implementations of appropriate resuscitative measures.

At least one person skilled in newborn resuscitation should attend every birth. Those involved in neonatal resuscitation should receive intensive practical training by people who are experienced in the relevant procedures. Two or more people are needed to carry out a complex resuscitation in a timely matter. The tasks that must be performed should be assigned in advance among the personnel who will attend the infant, and one member of the team should be selected to supervise the resuscitation. One team member should be assigned to perform tracheal intubation, provide assisted ventilation, secure the endotracheal tube, and administer surfactant when necessary. Others should be assigned to monitor the infant's condition and to keep an accurate written record, to perform external cardiac massage if needed, to establish vascular access, to sample blood for relevant tests, to administer drugs, and to perform other emergency procedures as indicated by the infant's condition, such as thoracentesis or paracentesis.

Immediately after birth, the skin should be dried with warm, sterile blankets or towels, electrocardiographic leads and pulse oximeter should be applied for measuring heart rate and oxygen saturation, and there should be accurate documentation and recording of all events, including times, specific treatments, and blood volumes sampled. Equipment and personnel to measure essential blood values, such as pH, oxygen, and carbon dioxide tensions, hematocrit, blood glucose concentration, and serum electrolytes, should be available throughout the resuscitation.

Essential equipment and supplies for resuscitation must be available and operative at all times. A vacuum device or wall suction is required to remove secretions from the airway, and a pressure manometer is needed to measure the amount of negative pressure generated by this suction. Sufficient electrical outlets must be available for all of the electrical devices. An electronic scale is needed to obtain the birth weight so that correct medication doses and fluid volumes can be administered. A ventilation system must be available that allows delivery of positive-pressure breathing. There should be at least two sources of oxygen and air, and blenders to mix the gases, as well as a flowmeter and tubing to deliver the gas, which should be humidified and warmed to near body temperature. A bulb syringe, meconium aspirator, suction catheters of various sizes, cushioned face masks, oral airways, and endotracheal tubes of various sizes should be at hand. In addition, there must be a functioning laryngoscope and multiple blades of different size, ranging from 00 to 1, and a stethoscope should be at the bedside. Sterile packs of instruments and supplies should be nearby in the event that vascular catheterization or sterile procedures need to be carried out.

2.9.3 Indications for and Goals of Resuscitation

Newborn infants may exhibit cyanosis, apnea, bradycardia, hypotonia, unresponsiveness, or evidence of respiratory distress in the delivery room because of prior intrauterine problems or because of problems that arise during labor or immediately after birth. In utero events that require neonatal resuscitation may be of maternal, placental, or fetal origin. Problems that arise from any of these sources may compromise vital functions immediately after birth. When cardiovascular or respiratory failure develops as a result of postnatal,

rather than antenatal, events, the infant may initially appear well, with subsequent deterioration leading to multiorgan failure. Table 2-5 lists antepartum, intrapartum, and postpartum risk factors that may be associated with asphyxia and require immediate treatment in the delivery room.

Whether the process that causes asphyxia is initiated during intrauterine or extrauterine life, the objective of resuscitation is to establish effective respiratory gas exchange and cardiovascular function and thereby prevent death or serious injury to vital organs, most notably the brain. In the perinatal period, asphyxia causes redistribution of blood flow from the skin, muscle, and splanchnic circulation to the heart, brain, and adrenal glands. This redistribution of blood flow occurs because asphyxia and associated release of catecholamines cause constriction of most peripheral blood vessels. Early in the asphyxial process the arterial blood pressure increases, and it remains elevated as long as the cardiac output is relatively normal. During this immediate postnatal phase, oxygen delivery to the brain and heart is normal. When severe hypoxia and acidosis occur, cardiac output and arterial blood pressure generally decrease, oxygen delivery to vital organs plummets, and organ failure follows. The most devastating result is severe hypoxic-ischemic encephalopathy, often accompanied by cardiac, pulmonary, renal, hepatic, gastrointestinal, and hematologic dysfunction (Table 2-6).

TABLE 2-5

FACTORS ASSOCIATED WITH NEED FOR EMERGENCY TREATMENT IN THE DELIVERY ROOM

ANTEPARTUM FACTORS	INTRAPARTUM FACTORS	POSTPARTUM FACTORS
Maternal age greater than 35 years	Abnormal presentation (breech, transverse)	Drug induced depression
Maternal hypertension	Placental abruption	CNS anomalies
Maternal anemia	Placenta previa	CNS injury
Maternal infection	Cord compression	Spinal cord injury
Maternal drug abuse	Precipitous labor	Airway obstruction
Maternal illnesses	Prolonged labor	Immaturity
Maternal drug therapy	Prolonged second stage of labor greater than 2 hours	Severe lung disease
Magnesium		Sepsis infection
Adrenergic blockade	Narcotics given to the mother less than 4 hours before delivery	Diaphragmatic hernia
Lithium carbonate		Pneumothorax
No prenatal care		Deformities
Vaginal bleeding	Foul-smelling amniotic fluid	Abdominal anomalies
Polyhydramnios		Heart anomalies
Oligohydramnios	Meconium stained amniotic fluid	
Postterm gestation		
Multiple fetuses	Emergency cesarean section	
Size-dates discrepancy		
Lung immaturity	Abnormal fetal heart rate	
Diminished fetal activity		
Fetal malformations	Uterine tetany	
	Preterm labor and delivery	
	Ruptured membranes greater than 24 hours	
	Regional anesthesia	
	Maternal hypotension	
	Mid- or high-forceps application	

TABLE 2-6

NEONATAL SIGNS AND CONSEQUENCES OF PERINATAL ASPHYXIA

Central nervous system: cerebral edema, intracranial hemorrhage, hypoxic-ischemic encephalopathy, seizures, brain infarcts

Respiratory: apnea, retained fetal lung fluid, respiratory distress syndrome, meconium aspiration syndrome, tachypnea

Cardiovascular: systemic hypertension or hypotension, myocardial failure, shock, persistent pulmonary hypertension, tricuspid regurgitation, myocardial infarct, papillary muscle necrosis

Hematologic: increased erythroblasts, leukocytosis, lymphopenia, thrombocytopenia, disseminated intravascular coagulation

Renal: oliguria, anuria, urinary retention, renal failure, cortico-tubular-medullary necrosis

Gastrointestinal: delayed gastric emptying, feeding intolerance, gastric ulcers, intestinal ischemia and necrotizing enterocolitis

---

There are characteristic respiratory patterns that develop in response to asphyxia. Initially, inspirations are deep and gasping in nature. If this breathing pattern occurs in utero, it can lead to inhalation of amniotic liquid that sometimes contains meconium or other noxious substances. If the asphyxial process continues without effective resuscitation, gasping becomes more irregular and eventually progresses to terminal apnea. Following successful resuscitation with positive-pressure ventilation and oxygen, spontaneous rhythmic breathing usually resumes. The delay in onset of rhythmic breathing is directly related to the length of time between onset of apnea and effective resuscitation. If the duration of apnea has been brief, spontaneous ventilation usually returns rapidly. Recovery of organ function and long-term outcome depend to a large extent on the severity and duration of the asphyxial episode as well as the speed and effectiveness of resuscitation. Because it is difficult, if not impossible, to determine at birth if brain injury has occurred, it is essential to provide effective resuscitation immediately after birth.

2.9.4 Essential Elements of Initial Stabilization and Evaluation

Both hypothermia and hyperthermia should be avoided in all newborns by preventing evaporative and conductive heat loss and by avoiding excessive radiant heat in the resuscitation area. This is readily accomplished by maintaining a warm delivery room, placing the infant under a preheated, temperature-controlled radiant warmer, and quickly drying the infant with warm blankets or towels. These steps are particularly important for small, preterm infants and for newborns who have experienced asphyxia, as these infants have ineffective thermoregulation and quickly become cold, oxygen-deficient, and acidotic. Both cold stress and hyperthermia may delay recovery from acidosis and may increase oxygen consumption.

A critical aspect of successful adaptation at birth is maintenance of a patent airway. This often can be accomplished by the delivery physician, who should gently suction the nose and mouth with a bulb syringe before the infant's thorax is delivered. The infant then should be placed on a firm supporting mattress, preferably situated on top of a calibrated electronic bed scale, beneath a radiant warmer that is regulated by a servocontrol system through a wire lead attached to the baby's skin. The skin should be dried, as noted above, to reduce evaporation and heat loss and to stimulate breathing.

Placing a 1-inch-thick cloth roll under the infant's shoulders may help to maintain the head and neck in a neutral position and thereby prevent airway obstruction caused by flexion or overextension of the neck. Some newborns have large quantities of upper airway secretions that require removal at birth. This usually can be achieved with a bulb syringe or with a soft rubber or polyethylene catheter connected to regulated wall suction. Repeated deep suctioning of the oropharynx should be avoided soon after birth because this can cause vagal stimulation, bradycardia, and apnea. If bradycardia occurs during airway suctioning, the procedure should be discontinued, and oxygen should be given to reverse any cyanosis. Treatment of infants who have passed meconium into the amniotic fluid is described elsewhere in this chapter.

The above sequence of events usually is sufficient to induce effective spontaneous breathing, such that the baby becomes pink and active. If, however, spontaneous and effective respiration is not established after 10 to 15 seconds of tactile stimulation and airway suctioning, positive-pressure ventilation should be initiated with a bag and mask device. If this procedure does not improve respiratory gas exchange, as assessed by skin color, auscultation of the lungs and heart, and chest rise, a tube should be inserted into the trachea immediately so that positive-pressure ventilation can be delivered.

IMPORTANCE OF THE APGAR SCORING

Dr. Virginia Apgar devised a simple scoring system for assessing an infant's physiological status soon after birth. A score of 0, 1, or 2 is assigned for each of five variables: respiratory effort, heart rate, skin color, muscle tone, and reflex responsiveness (Table 2-7). The sum of these scores is determined at 1 and 5 minutes after birth. The maximum score is 10. If the 5-minute score is less than 7, scoring should be repeated every five minutes thereafter until the score is 7 or greater or until the infant is at least 20 minutes old. Careful, objective, and timely observations are critical for obtaining an accurate and meaningful score. If the score is less than or equal to 3 within the first minute or at any time thereafter, prompt resuscitative measures are indicated. Because many causes of asphyxia begin in utero, resuscitation sometimes must begin immediately at birth in order to reverse hypoxia before the 1-minute Apgar score is ascribed. In such instances, the 1-minute Apgar score often reflects the impact of resuscitation on the infant's physiological status. The Apgar score at 1 and 5 minutes after birth does not correlate especially well with long-term neurobehavioral outcome, but a score of 3 or less at 15 minutes after birth has been associated with

TABLE 2-7

APGAR SCORING SYSTEM

SCORE	0	1	2
Heart rate	Absent	Less than 100/min	Greater than 100/min
Respirations	Absent	Slow, irregular	Good, crying
Muscle tone	Limp	Some flexion	Active motion
Reflex irritability (in response to catheter in nose)	No response	Grimace	Cough, sneeze, cry
Color	Blue, pale	Body pink, blue limbs	Completely pink

high mortality (more than 50%) and severe, permanent neurologic sequelae (about 60%) among survivors.

2.9.5 Oxygen Administration

If the neonate remains cyanotic or has an oxygen saturation (pulse oximeter reading) of less than 85% despite breathing regularly and having a heart rate above 100 beats per minute, oxygen should be administered through a free-flowing system. A self-inflating bag with an open reservoir should not be used, as gas flows in such a system only when the bag is squeezed. It is best to deliver oxygen through an oxygen-air blender and to warm and humidify the gas mixture to near body temperature. If the infant simply gasps for air, or if breathing efforts are insufficient to sustain a heart rate of 100 or more beats per minute, positive-pressure ventilation should be initiated.

Although it is important to avoid or to reverse cyanosis during resuscitation, it also is important to avoid hyperoxia, which, following a period of asphyxia, may result in hypotension and suppression of spontaneous breathing. Recent reports have indicated that resuscitation with pure oxygen sometimes may be detrimental and that positive-pressure ventilation with lower concentrations of oxygen, or even room air, may be more suitable for neonatal resuscitation as soon as adequate ventilation and oxygenation occur. Excessive oxygen in the blood may yield toxic metabolites such as superoxide anion, hydroxyl radicals, and hydrogen peroxide that can injure tissues and lead to multiorgan failure. Thus, reperfusion with hyperoxic blood of a previously ischemic, hypoxic vital organ, such as the brain, may enhance neuronal injury and lead to permanent neurologic impairment. An appropriate strategy for resuscitation, therefore, is to rapidly reduce the inspired oxygen concentration in order to keep the partial pressure of oxygen in arterial blood (PaO_2) between 50 and 70 mm Hg and the oxygen saturation between 90 and 95%. These oxygen levels should be sufficient to meet tissue oxygen demands in the presence of adequate cardiac output, tissue perfusion, and blood hemoglobin concentration. In preterm infants, blood oxygen saturation levels greater than 95% for more than a few minutes may increase the risk of subsequent retinopathy.

2.9.6 Assisted Ventilation Techniques in Resuscitation

Positive-pressure ventilation can be achieved in the delivery room with an inflatable bag connected to either a face mask or an endotracheal tube. Ineffective breathing efforts or apnea, usually associated with bradycardia and cyanosis, signals the immediate need for assisted ventilation. Usually this can be initiated with a bag-and-mask device. In most infants, effective ventilation and oxygenation can be achieved using inflation pressures less than 25 cm H_2O at rates of between 20 and 40 breaths/min. The chest should rise with each breath, and breath sounds should be heard bilaterally. Oxygenation should improve quickly, and the heart rate should increase to normal values. Giving excess tidal volumes may cause abdominal distension and thereby hinder lung inflation. To reduce this risk, it is often useful to place a small catheter in the stomach to withdraw gas that accumulates there during bag-and-mask ventilation. If the infant remains cyanotic, or if there is persistent bradycardia, an endotracheal tube should be inserted immediately to facilitate lung inflation, oxygenation, and ventilation. When a congenital diaphragmatic hernia is suspected or has been diagnosed

by fetal ultrasound, assisted ventilation should be administered directly through an endotracheal tube in order to avoid gaseous distension of the intrathoracic stomach and intestine.

Endotracheal intubation is a skill that is easily learned and maintained with periodic practice. The newborn larynx is considerably more anterior than is the larynx of an adult, and extension of the neck places the larynx even more anterior, making tube insertion into the trachea more difficult. Therefore, the head should be placed in a neutral ("sniffing") position during bag-and-mask ventilation and during tracheal intubation. The laryngoscope should be held with the thumb and index finger as the chin is grasped with the ring and middle fingers of the left hand. This tends to fix the hand against the infant's head and thereby reduces the likelihood of pharyngeal lacerations from head movement during the procedure. To improve the view of the larynx pressure should be applied over the hyoid bone with the small finger of the left hand (Fig. 2-27). An endotracheal tube of appropriate size should be inserted, and the tip of the tube should be placed 1 to 2 cm below the vocal cords, depending on the infant's size. A proper size tube should allow a small amount of gas to leak from between the tube and the surrounding trachea when an airway pressure of about 20 cm H_2O is generated. This usually is achieved with tubes measuring 2.5 mm in external diameter for infants who weigh less than 1.5 kg; 3 mm for infants who weight 1.5–2.5 kg; and 3.5 mm for infants who weigh more than 2.5 kg. The distance from the distal (intratracheal) end of the tube to the gingiva usually is 7 cm for 1-kg infants, 8 cm for 2-kg infants, 9 cm for 3-kg infants, and 10 cm for 4-kg infants. These distances should place the tip of the tube in the middle portion of the trachea, at least 1 cm above the bifurcation. The chest should be examined soon after the tube is inserted in the trachea to be sure that both sides of the chest rise equally with each inspiration and that breath sounds are present bilaterally. If breath sounds are absent or decreased on one side, the tip of the tube may be beyond the tracheal bifurcation, or there may be a pneumothorax. The first of these conditions usually can be corrected by withdrawing the tube a short distance; the latter condition usually

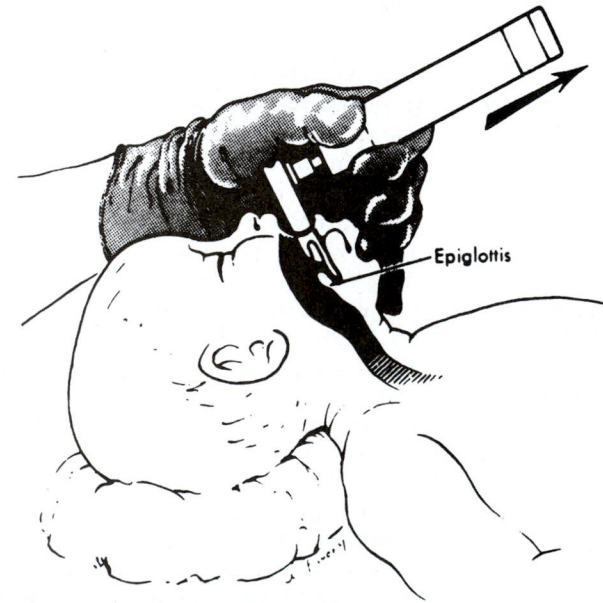

FIGURE 2-27 Laryngoscopy technique. *From Gregory: In Schnider, Moya, eds: The Anesthesiologist, the Mother and the Newborn. Williams & Wilkins, 1974.*

can be diagnosed by transillumination of the chest or by obtaining a radiograph.

The primary goal of positive-pressure ventilation in the immediate postnatal period is to gently expand the lungs without injuring them and to facilitate effective exchange of respiratory gases. Delivery of oxygen to the circulating blood and elimination of carbon dioxide rapidly improves cardiac function and increases the heart rate of a previously asphyxiated infant. Inadequate lung expansion sometimes occurs during resuscitation because insufficient inspiratory pressures are used to inflate the lungs for fear of causing extrapulmonary air leak. In the absence of lung abnormalities, iatrogenic pneumothorax is uncommon. An initial inflation pressure of 20 to 25 cm H_2O is a good place to start, but occasionally an inflation pressure in excess of 50 cm H_2O may be needed to achieve adequate lung expansion. Use of high inflation pressures and large tidal volumes in premature infants, however, may cause lung injury and impair surfactant function. Application of modest (3–5 cm H_2O) positive end-expiratory pressure (PEEP) during resuscitation can help to establish and maintain an adequate volume of gas within the lungs, which is essential for delivering oxygen to the blood. Effective lung inflation soon after birth may require several prolonged breaths to overcome atelectasis, after which a rate of 30 to 60 breaths/min and an inspiratory time of 0.3 to 0.5 seconds usually suffices. When the lungs are adequately inflated, peak airway pressures in excess of 25 cm H_2O are seldom needed to maintain normal oxygenation and ventilation. Thereafter, in order to avoid lung overdistension, inflation pressure and inspiratory time should be reduced to the minimum settings needed to allow adequate oxygenation and ventilation. Care should be taken to prevent excessive ventilation ($PaCO_2$ less than 40 cm H_2O), which can have adverse effects not only on the lungs but on cerebral blood flow as well. If adequate lung inflation and ventilation fail to reverse bradycardia quickly, external cardiac compression should be initiated.

2.9.7   External Cardiac Compression

If the heart rate remains less than 100 beats/min soon after birth, the lungs should be ventilated with oxygen delivered through an endotracheal tube, and external cardiac compressions should be applied. Closed-chest massage is easily accomplished in neonates by placing both thumbs on the midportion of the sternum and by gently encircling the chest with the fingers of both hands to support the back (Fig. 2-28). The sternum is compressed 1 to 2 cm at a rate of 100 to 150 times per minute. It is not necessary to interrupt either lung inflations or external cardiac compressions during resuscitation. Experimental work has shown that cardiac function is enhanced when external cardiac massage and positive-pressure ventilation are performed simultaneously without interruption in infants. The effectiveness of external chest compressions is determined by feeling the arterial pulse and measuring arterial blood pressure, pH, and partial pressures of oxygen and carbon dioxide in arterial blood. Examination of the eyes for pupillary size (not dilated) also can be useful for accessing the efficacy of external cardiac massage and ventilation. External chest compressions should generate a systolic pressure of 80 mm Hg in a term infant and 50 mm Hg in a preterm infant. This pressure, plus a cardiac compression rate of about 120 per minute, usually maintains a diastolic pressure of 20 to 25 mm Hg, which is sufficient to provide coronary artery perfusion during diastole in neonates. Failure to generate these pressures and rates allows the diastolic pressure to fall below 20 mm Hg, such that coronary artery perfusion is inadequate.

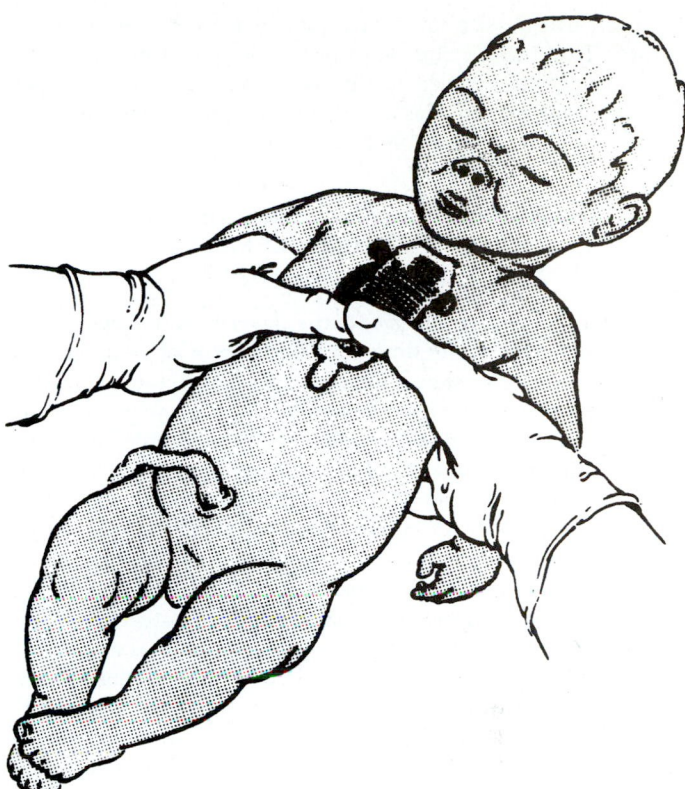

FIGURE 2-28   Closed chest cardiac massage. For simplification, ventilation of the infant is not shown. *From Gregory: In: Schnider, Moya, eds: The Anesthesiologist, the Mother and the Newborn. Williams & Wilkins, 1974.*

2.9.8   Treatment of Cardiac Arrest

If cardiac arrest occurs, external cardiac compressions and positive-pressure ventilation of the lungs should be started immediately. If there is no response, it may be necessary to administer drugs to restart the heart, increase the heart rate, and support the circulation. The drug most commonly used to treat cardiac arrest or persistent bradycardia is epinephrine. This drug is effective because it stimulates α-adrenergic receptors, enhances cardiac contractility, and constricts the peripheral circulation, thereby distributing blood preferentially to the brain and heart. Epinephrine also has chronotropic and inotropic effects through its actions on β-adrenergic receptors in the heart. For neonates, the recommended dilution of epinephrine is 1:10,000, and the prescribed dose is 0.01 to 0.03 mg/kg (0.1–0.3 mL/kg). This dose was extrapolated from the dose that has been recommended for adults. In newborn animals, however, higher doses of epinephrine have been shown to increase arterial blood pressure and heart rate more rapidly. Doses greater than 0.1 mg/kg (1 mL/kg) can have detrimental effects on stroke volume and cardiac output.

Epinephrine can be administered directly into the trachea with good transpulmonary absorption. If heart rate and blood pressure remain low, the dose may be repeated as needed. Bradycardia that is associated with abnormal vagal tone often responds to parenteral atropine (0.01–0.1 mg/kg). The most common reason for persistent bradycardia in an apneic infant, however, is insufficient lung inflation, most often from ineffective bag-mask ventilation, esophageal intubation, or airway obstruction.

Ventricular fibrillation is rare during cardiac arrest in newborn infants. If ventricular fibrillation occurs, it should be treated by electrical impulses applied to the chest, using 2 J of energy per kilogram body weight. This dose can be repeated and the intensity doubled (4 J/kg) to stop fibrillation.

2.9.9 Establishing Vascular Access for Treatment with Drugs and Fluid

Intravascular access is often needed during resuscitation of the newborn infant to administer drugs and fluids. In most instances, this can be achieved by passing a narrow-gauge catheter into a peripheral vein. If an infant is hypovolemic without visible veins, however, a catheter can be placed in the umbilical vein to deliver emergency drugs and solutions. The tip of this catheter should be situated in the inferior vena cava above the diaphragm to reduce the risk of liver damage from direct injection into the portal circulation. To determine if the catheter tip is above or below the diaphragm, the catheter can be connected to a pressure transducer so that the venous pressure waveform can be observed as the catheter is being inserted. If the catheter is in the thorax during spontaneous breathing, the pressure should decrease during inspiration; during positive-pressure ventilation, however, the vascular pressure in the chest should increase during lung inflation. If the catheter tip cannot be passed through the ductus venosus into the inferior vena cava, it should be inserted so that the tip of the catheter is in the umbilical vein just beneath the abdominal wall (approximately 1–2 cm). Extreme caution should be taken to assure that no air enters the bloodstream, as air emboli can flow across the foramen ovale into the cerebral or coronary microcirculation. If the position of the umbilical venous catheter tip is uncertain, it is best to inject drugs that are well mixed in isotonic solutions and to avoid hyperosmolar solutions for treating acidosis and for restoring intravascular volume. If venous access is unobtainable, drugs such as epinephrine or atropine can be given through an endotracheal tube. For monitoring arterial pH, PaO_2, $PaCO_2$, and blood pressure during resuscitation, a catheter can be inserted into the umbilical artery.

Various drugs and intravenous fluids are often needed to correct metabolic abnormalities and to support the circulation during resuscitation. Severe acidemia and hypoxia can impair pharmacologic responses to epinephrine and adversely affect both pulmonary and systemic blood flow. If severe metabolic acidosis occurs, sodium bicarbonate ($NaHCO_3$) administration may be required. Wherever possible, pH and $PaCO_2$ should be measured before $NaHCO_3$ is given to ascertain the extent and metabolic nature of the acidosis and to be sure that the $PaCO_2$ is not markedly elevated. Adequate lung inflation and ventilation must be maintained when $NaHCO_3$ is administered in the delivery room, as alkali administration often increases CO_2 in the blood. Rapid increases of $PaCO_2$ may dilate the cerebral circulation and increase blood flow to the brain, induce dysrhythmias, and even lead to cardiac arrest. The concentration of $NaHCO_3$ should not exceed 0.5 mEq/mL, and in most instances it can be mixed with sterile water to render it iso-osmolar. The initial dose of $NaHCO_3$ is usually 2 mEq/kg, and the rate of administration should not exceed 0.5 to 1 mEq/kg per minute. In the unusual situation wherein $PaCO_2$ remains elevated despite assisted ventilation, tromethamine (THAM) at a concentration of 0.3 mol/L can be administered at a dose of 3 mL/kg. The possible advantage of THAM over $NaHCO_3$ is that THAM binds CO_2 in

addition to hydrogen ions, and it enters cells, thereby raising intracellular pH.

Calcium gluconate or calcium chloride should be not be administered routinely during resuscitation of the neonate because calcium may contribute to cellular damage associated with hypoxia and ischemia, notably in the brain. When cardiac arrest occurs, however, it may be necessary to infuse calcium gluconate (10% solution), 100 to 200 mg/kg over 3 to 5 minutes, in order to improve cardiac function.

If hypoglycemia is documented during resuscitation, intravenous glucose should be given by slow infusion of a 10% solution, 2 to 3 mL/kg, and a continuous infusion of glucose should be maintained thereafter. The blood glucose concentration should be measured frequently to assure that it is within the normal range. In the absence of hypoglycemia, however, excess glucose should not be given, as hyperglycemia during and after episodes of hypoxia and ischemia may increase the severity of postasphyxial brain damage.

When a newborn infant is apneic or has respiratory depression, and there is a history of narcotic administration to the mother during the 4 hours before delivery, naloxone, IM or IV, 0.1 mg/kg, may reverse the apnea. Depending on the infant's response to this drug, the dose can be repeated every 2 to 3 minutes up to four times in order to reverse the effects of prior narcotic administration.

Some infants who have experienced asphyxia, either antenatally or postnatally, may exhibit evidence of myocardiopathy with resultant hypotension. This condition often responds favorably to a continuous intravenous infusion of dopamine, usually beginning at a dose of 5 to 10 $\mu g/kg/min$. Sometimes higher doses of the drug may be required to increase systemic arterial pressure, improve tissue perfusion, and increase urine output.

Newborn infants with acute asphyxia usually have a normal circulating blood volume immediately after birth, though it may decrease later if central venous pressure is elevated or if microvascular permeability is increased, as in sepsis or prolonged anoxia. If shock complicates asphyxia, it often reflects myocardial ischemia, impaired myocardial function, and decreased cardiac output. Such infants usually respond well to effective oxygenation and ventilation, but inotropic drugs, such as dopamine, dobutamine, or in rare instances epinephrine, may be useful for improving blood pressure and tissue perfusion.

The causes of postnatal shock from hypovolemia are summarized in Table 2-8. Most often it stems from antenatal or early

TABLE 2-8
CAUSE OF PERINATAL HYPOVOLEMIA

Fetal placental hemorrhage
  Twin-twin transfusion
  Fetal-placental/maternal transfusion
  Placental incision
  Abruptio (hemorrhage from fetal side of placenta)
Decreased blood return from placenta
  Maternal hypotension
  Abruptio (with decreased placental return to fetus)
  Umbilical vein occlusion (cord compression by after-coming head in breech presentation)
Neonatal hemorrhage (trauma)
  Subgaleal
  Intrahepatic
  Intraperitoneal
  Adrenal

postnatal blood loss, which usually is heralded by a large amount of vaginal bleeding before and during delivery. In some cases this is associated with extreme pallor of the newborn, but in many instances the infant may be cyanotic and have a normal hematocrit initially despite a very large blood loss. In such instances, the hematocrit may not be useful as a guide for volume repletion. Only after "reequilibration" has occurred, or after isotonic saline has been administered to replenish the blood volume loss, will the hematocrit decrease.

Blood volume expanders should be administered when the cause of hypotension is thought to be related to decreased intravascular fluid volume. Tachycardia, when associated with hypotension, is often a sign of hypovolemia that requires intravascular infusion of either isotonic saline or blood products. Metabolic acidosis is another possible indicator that hypotension may be secondary to diminished intravascular volume, which may benefit from fluid administration. Poor peripheral perfusion, usually detected by slow return of color to an area of skin that has been blanched by local finger compression, is sometimes a useful sign that intravascular volume is diminished. Restoring blood volume generally lowers heart rate, increases urine output, and corrects any prevailing metabolic acidosis.

Blood volume expanders can be infused over a period of 30 to 60 minutes, usually 10 to 20 mL/kg body weight, to increase blood pressure and improve renal, splanchnic, and peripheral perfusion. The rate and amount of fluid, as well as the type of fluid given, depend on the clinical situation. If there is strong clinical evidence of prior blood loss, the most effective intravascular volume expander is whole blood or packed red blood cells mixed with either saline or plasma. In an emergency, blood type O-negative packed red blood cells can be given. If blood is not available immediately after birth in the setting of known blood loss, isotonic saline can be used to increase the blood volume transiently as blood is procured from the blood bank. If bleeding is ongoing, coagulation studies should be performed to determine if specific blood products are needed to correct a coagulopathy.

Other conditions that may lead to severe depression or distress at birth and that require early resuscitation include bacterial or viral sepsis, pneumothorax, airway obstruction associated with micrognathia (Pierre Robin constellation), choanal atresia, upper airway tumors or webs, massive cardiomegaly associated with pulmonary hypoplasia, pleural effusions, ascites, and anasarca. Many of these conditions interfere with effective ventilation and oxygenation and therefore may require specific interventions, such as fluid removal from the chest or abdomen, or specific surgical intervention. These conditions are described in more detail elsewhere in this volume and therefore are not within the scope of this section on resuscitation. Emergency measures, as described above, are needed to manage these infants if the underlying problem interferes with effective ventilation or oxygenation.

References

American Heart Association/American Academy of Pediatrics: Textbook of Neonatal Resuscitation. Dallas, AHA/AAP, 1995

Apgar V, James LS: Further observations of the newborn scoring system. Am J Dis Child 104:419–428, 1962

Bjorklund LJ, Ingimarsson J, Curstedt T, et al: Manual ventilation with a few large breaths at birth compromises the therapeutic effect if subsequent surfactant replacement in immature lambs. Pediatr Res 42:348, 1997

Burchfield DJ, Preziosi MP, Lucas VW, et al: Effects of graded doses of epinephrine during asphyxia-induced bradycardia in newborn lambs. Resuscitation 25:235, 1993

Byrne PJ, Tyebkhan JM, Laing LM, et al: Ethical decision-making and neonatal resuscitation. Semin Perinatol 18:36–41, 1994

Graf H, Leach W, Arieff AI, et al: Evidence for a detrimental effect of bicarbonate therapy in hypoxic lactic acidosis. Science 227:754, 1985

Gregory GA: Laryngoscopy. In: Schnider SM, Moya F, eds: The Anesthesiologist, the Mother and the Newborn. Baltimore, Williams & Wilkins, 1974

Gunn AJ, Gunn TR, de Haan HH, et al: Dramatic neuronal rescue with prolonged selective head cooling after ischemia in fetal lambs. J Clin Invest 99:248, 1997

Houri PK, Frank LR, Menegazzi JJ, et al: A randomized controlled trial of two-thumb vs two-finger chest compression in a swine infant model of cardiac arrest. Prehosp Emerg Care 1:65–67, 1997

Jonmarker C, Olsson AK, Jogi P, et al: Hemodynamic effects of tracheal and intravenous adrenaline in infants with congenital heart anomalies. Acta Anaesthesiol Scand 40:927–931, 1996

Kattwinkel J, Niermeyer S, Nadkarni V, et al: ILCOR Advisory statement: resuscitation of the newly born infant: an advisory statement from the Pediatric Working Group of the International Liaison Committee on Resuscitation. Circulation 99:1927–1938, 1999

Nelson KB, Ellenberg JH: Apgar scores as predictors of chronic neurologic disability. Pediatrics 68:36, 1981

Paterson SJ, Byrne PJ, Molesky MG, et al: Neonatal resuscitation using the laryngeal mask airway. Anesthesiology 80:1248–1253, 1994

Preziosi MP, Roig JC, Hargrove N, et al: Metabolic acidemia with hypoxia attenuates the hemodynamic responses to epinephrine during resuscitation in lambs. Crit Care Med 21:1901, 1993

Ramji S, Anuja S, Thirupuram S, et al: Resuscitation of asphyxtic newborn infants with room air or 100% oxygen. Pediatr Res 34:809–812, 1993

Sameshima H, Ota A, Ikenove T, et al: Pretreatment with magnesium sulfate protects against hypoxic-ischemic brain injury but postasphyxial treatment worsens brain damage in seven day old rats. Am J Obstet Gynecol 180:725, 1999

Saugstad OD, Rootwelt T, Aalen O, et al: Resuscitation of asphyxiated newborn infants with room air or oxygen: an international controlled trial: the Resair 2 Study. Pediatrics (electronic pages) 102(1):e1, 1998

2.10   ROUTINE POSTNATAL CARE AND OBSERVATION

Susan Sniderman and Valerie E. Charlton

2.10.1   General

Newborn nurseries follow a set of established routines to promote a healthy transition from intrauterine to extrauterine life. Routines vary from one nursery to another in details but follow the principles given in *Guidelines for Perinatal Care* (AAP/ACOG 1997). Every nursery should have written criteria for routine well-baby nursery admission and for admission to a high-observation, special care, or intensive care nursery.

BODY TEMPERATURE

The newborn is likely to lose much body heat after birth. At delivery the skin is covered with amniotic fluid; the infant is usually exposed to low ambient temperature in the delivery room and frequently is kept unclothed to allow adequate initial observation. Therefore, heat is lost by evaporation, radiation, and convection. The infant responds to this cooling by sympathetic stimulation of metabolism, which increases heat production. Heat is also conserved by decreasing skin blood flow. The metabolic demands of these responses may double the infant's oxygen consumption, but hypoxic infants are unable to respond with an increase in heat production. Thermogenesis also can be blocked by warming the skin, even though the central body temperature remains subnormal.

If measures are not taken to prevent heat loss, body temperature can fall precipitously. Drying with an absorbent towel immediately after birth and keeping the infant wrapped in a warm, dry towel or blanket between examinations in the delivery room reduce heat loss. Delivery room assessments and resuscitation should be performed under a radiant warmer. Care must be taken to avoid overheating and burns from radiant warmers. This is best achieved with a servo-controlled feedback device that attaches to the infant's skin. It is important to prevent hyperthermia, as it increases metabolic demands and oxygen consumption.

An infant who needs frequent or continuous observation can be nursed unclothed in an incubator set to maintain a neutral thermal environment. This is the range of ambient temperature and humidity at which heat loss, metabolic demands, and oxygen consumption are lowest. For an undressed, normal term newborn, a neutral thermal environment is in the range of 31 to 34°C at 50% humidity. Use of a radiant warmer to maintain body temperature increases evaporative water loss.

In the first few hours after birth, body temperature should be measured and recorded repeatedly. Skin temperature is usually lower than central body or core temperature, particularly in a chilled infant, in whom skin blood flow is reduced. Rectal temperature is a good indicator of core temperature, but a firm temperature probe left in the rectum without constant attention can perforate the large bowel. Measurement of axillary temperature is generally a suitable and safe alternative. The range of normal axillary temperature is 36.5 to 37.4°C. When an infant is in an incubator, both the infant's temperature and that of the environment inside the incubator should be monitored and recorded. Although a rise in body temperature can reflect excessive environmental temperature, abnormal body temperature, either above or below the normal range, or an acute change in body temperature may be an important indication of illness and, in particular, of infection. Thus, abnormal thermoregulation of a newborn infant warrants careful evaluation for possible sepsis.

An infant who is hypothemic soon after birth should be warmed in an incubator or beneath a radiant warmer at a moderate rate to avoid both the adverse consequences of cold stress and of excessive application of external heat. When an infant achieves a stable normal temperature, care can be provided in an open crib with adequate clothing and a blanket to prevent cooling. The nursery should be free of drafts at a temperature of 24 to 26°C to assure a proper thermal environment for the healthy term infant.

CARDIOPULMONARY FUNCTION

The newborn's heart rate, blood pressure, respiratory rate, quality of respirations, and color of skin and mucous membranes should be monitored and recorded frequently during the first 6 hours after birth. This is the period during which the majority of life-threatening cardiopulmonary conditions appear. Thereafter, observations can be less frequent if the infant appears well.

In the first 10 minutes after birth, the average heart rate is 160 beats per minute but may vary from 120 to 180 bpm. Thereafter, the average is 120 to 130 bpm (range 90 to 175). Consistently low or high heart rates suggest a pathologic condition. Tachycardia may

be a sign of low intravascular volume, cardiovascular or respiratory disease, drug withdrawal, pain, or hyperthyroidism. Bradycardia is often seen after perinatal asphyxia and also may occur in association with apnea.

When asleep, newborn infants normally have brief pauses in respiration. These are usually 5 seconds or less in duration but occasionally last as long as 10 to 15 seconds. Prolonged apnea or apnea with associated bradycardia is abnormal and requires investigation. It is a nonspecific sign; it may be caused by such diverse conditions as sepsis, cardiac disease, hypoglycemia, polycythemia, and intracranial hemorrhage.

The normal range of blood pressure measured with a properly fitting limb cuff is 65 to 95 mm Hg systolic and 30 to 60 mm Hg diastolic in term infants. Arterial blood pressure varies directly with birth weight and gestational age. In the first 12 hours after birth, mean blood pressure averages 50 to 55 mm Hg in infants over 3 kg and 40 to 45 mm Hg in infants weighing between 2 and 3 kg.

GASTROINTESTINAL FUNCTION

Feeding can be initiated once the infant has been assessed and is stable. Choanal and esophageal atresia should be excluded before feeding is attempted. A soft catheter can be passed through the nares into the stomach and nasal airstreams can be assessed with a strip of cotton. Careful observation during the first one or two feedings may yield valuable information regarding coordination of suck and swallow, possible presence of gastrointestinal obstruction, and the potential for aspiration of gastric contents. Newborns commonly regurgitate a few milliliters of milk with each feeding, especially when they burp. Vomiting larger amounts or bile-stained material may reflect intestinal obstruction that requires immediate diagnostic evaluation. During the first day, infants who have large amounts of mucus or swallowed blood in the stomach may repeatedly regurgitate small amounts of material or have difficulty in feeding. Orogastric lavage with saline is sometimes used to remove this material and may improve feeding. If vomiting persists, further assessment, including abdominal radiographs, should be pursued.

In infants who are breast-fed, feeding behavior, frequency of feeding, stool characteristics, and initiation of maternal milk production should be noted and recorded. To determine nutritional intake, the change in weight before and after feeding can be measured. However, it is not necessary or appropriate to weigh a healthy term newborn with each breast-feeding. In babies who are fed milk formula, nutritional intake can be judged by the volume of formula taken.

Breast-feeding should be encouraged except in those few circumstances where the risks to the infant outweigh the benefits. Breast-feeding is contraindicated in maternal conditions that may result in transmission of infection to the infant, such as active pulmonary tuberculosis (until treatment is started and the mother considered to be noncontagious), herpetic breast lesions, or infection with HIV. Possible effects on the infant of maternal medications and chemical exposures also should be considered, as many drugs and other chemicals can pass from mother to infant in breast milk.

Approximately 70% of normal newborn infants excrete meconium during the first 12 hours, and 95% of infants pass at least one stool within 24 hours. Passage of meconium may be delayed in infants with distal intestinal obstruction, as in meconium plug syndrome or in infants with aganglionic colon (Hirschsprung disease). Other causes of abnormal gastrointestinal motility and delayed stool excretion are premature birth, sepsis, hypothyroidism, and various drugs, including narcotics.

Babies with high gastrointestinal obstruction usually present with vomiting but may not have abdominal distension or abnormal stool frequency during the first 24 hours after birth. Infants with lower intestinal obstruction are less likely to exhibit vomiting early but often exhibit abdominal distension and absent stools.

The color and consistency of stools change from green-black and very viscous on the first day to green-yellow and paste-like by the third or fourth postnatal day. Normal stools are not watery, but those of breast-fed infants are often softer and less formed than are the stools of formula-fed infants. During the first week, the normal frequency of stool output varies from one to 10 per day, usually averaging three to five stools daily. Stools that are dark red and tar-like in consistency are indicative of old blood, usually maternal in origin, that was swallowed at the time of delivery. This can be distinguished from the infant's blood by a test that differentiates between adult and fetal hemoglobin (Apt test for alkali resistance of fetal hemoglobin). Small streaks of bright red blood in the stools often reflect the presence of a rectal fissure. If no fissure is found, or if there are large quantities of blood in the stools, further evaluation is indicated. Diarrhea is a common sign of systemic or gastrointestinal infection, feeding intolerance, or drug withdrawal.

URINARY FUNCTION

Approximately two-thirds of newborn infants urinate within 12 hours of birth, and virtually all normal infants have voided at least once within 24 hours. Absence of urine output may be of prerenal origin (severe hypovolemia and hypotension, myocardial failure, dehydration), or it may reflect renal anomalies, such as absent kidneys, acute tubular necrosis from ischemia, or renal vein thrombosis, or it may signal obstruction to urinary outflow, possibly from posterior urethral valves or from a blocked urethra.

Neonatal urine is normally yellow or light brown. Urate crystals, which vary from deep pink to tan in color, are a common source of diaper stain in the newborn period. Hematuria is pathologic and requires urgent evaluation.

BODY SIZE

The newborn infant should be weighed daily in the hospital and at postnatal follow-up examinations. The normal newborn loses approximately 5 to 10% of its birth weight during the first few days after birth and usually begins to regain weight by the second half of the first week. Weight loss of more than 10% in a term infant is considered abnormal. Body length does not change measurably during this period. Head circumference may decrease by up to 1 cm as tissue edema abates during the week after birth. In some infants, head circumference may increase by up to 1 cm as the cranial molding that occurred during labor resolves. Rapid expansion of the head size in the first week may be a sign of ventricular enlargement and merits evaluation by cranial imaging studies.

2.10.2 Prophylaxis

EYE PROPHYLAXIS

To prevent gonococcal ophthalmia, all newborn infants should have two drops of a solution of 1% silver nitrate or a 1- to 2-cm ribbon of ophthalmic ointment, containing either 1% tetracycline or 0.5% erythromycin, placed in each eye within 1 hour after birth. The solution or ointment should reach all parts of the conjunctival sac and should be dispensed from a single-use container. The eyes should not be rinsed after treatment, as this decreases effectiveness.

VITAMIN K

All newborns should receive a single dose of vitamin K_1 (1 mg, intramuscularly) during the first few hours after birth to prevent the development of hemorrhagic disease of the newborn. This condition can cause gastrointestinal, intracranial, or generalized bleeding either soon after birth or even several weeks later. The late form of hemorrhagic disease occurs mainly in babies who are breast-fed exclusively. A 2-mg oral dose of vitamin K maintains normal coagulation status in the first few days, but the effect may be transient and the dose should be repeated.

HEPATITIS B PROPHYLAXIS

It is now public policy in the United States to immunize all infants against hepatitis B. In infants born to mothers who are negative for hepatitis B surface antigen (HBsAg), the first dose of recombinant vaccine should be administered before 2 months of age. If the vaccine is given prior to discharge from the nursery, an immunization record should be filled out and given to the parents.

Infants born to mothers who are positive for HBsAg or to mothers of unknown hepatitis status need special management. If the mother is positive for HBsAg, the infant should be bathed soon after birth to remove infectious bloody material, and the skin should be swabbed with disinfectant before any drug injection or blood drawing. In addition, the infant should receive hepatitis B immune globulin (0.5 mL) intramuscularly at one site, and recombinant hepatitis vaccine concurrently in another site within the first 12 h after birth.

If the mother is of unknown hepatitis status, her blood should be sent for immediate testing, and the infant should receive vaccine within 12 hours as described above for the infant of a mother who is positive for HBsAg. If the mother is proven to be positive for HBsAg, the infant should receive hepatitis B immune globulin as soon as possible and no later than 7 days postnatally. If the mother is HBsAg negative, the regular schedule of immunizations should be followed.

Babies whose mothers are positive for HBsAg should be immunized on an accelerated schedule, with the second dose at 1 month and the third at 6 months after birth. The manufacturer's guidelines should be checked for appropriate vaccine dose.

UMBILICAL CORD CARE

Care of the umbilicus is necessary to prevent infection. Cord care is best accomplished by leaving the umbilicus exposed to air and swabbing it daily with alcohol. The umbilicus should not be covered with a moist or air-tight dressing. Topical application of antiseptic agents to the cord may reduce colonization, but unless there is an increase in staphylococcal infection in the nursery, antiseptics usually are not necessary.

CARE OF THE PENIS AND CIRCUMCISION

Parents should receive instruction soon after delivery and at subsequent physician office visits regarding proper hygiene for the uncircumcised penis. Circumcision, or removal of the penile foreskin to near the coronal sulcus, is frequently performed to prevent late inflammatory diseases of the penis (eg, balanoposthitis) and stenotic or constrictual foreskin problems (phimosis and paraphimosis). Circumcision has been associated with decreased incidence of penile cancer, urinary tract infections, and sexually transmitted diseases. A recent policy statement of the American Academy of Pediatrics, however, states that the potential medical benefits of circumcision are not sufficient to warrant its recommendation as a routine procedure.

Circumcision is performed by either a surgical clamp technique (eg, Gomco or Mogen) or use of a plastic bell. With the former, diaper adhesion to the surgical site is prevented postoperatively by a petrolatum gauze dressing or petrolatum (vaseline) applied to the diaper or penis. With the plastic bell technique, the underlying tissue is normally healed by the time the bell falls off. Circumcision should be performed using local anesthesia.

2.10.3   Screening

BLOOD GLUCOSE

Blood glucose concentration should be measured with a rapid bedside screening method within 2 to 4 hours after birth to detect possible hypoglycemia. Special protocols, with multiple glucose measurements and early feedings, should be developed for infants at risk for hypoglycemia (infants of diabetic mothers, undergrown infants, very large infants, infants who have experienced intrapartum asphyxia, premature and postmature infants). Blood glucose measurement of <40 mg/dL by the screening technique should be evaluated by a specific assay for serum or plasma glucose, and treatment for hypoglycemia should be initiated while the result is pending.

Until recent years, hypoglycemia was defined as a blood glucose concentration less than 30 mg/dL in term infants, but more current information indicates that most normal term infants have a serum or plasma glucose concentration higher than 40 mg/dL on the first day of life and over 45 to 50 mg/dL thereafter. In one study, however, 16% of term newborns who had multiple serum glucose measurements had at least one glucose measurement at or below 40 mg/dL between 3 and 52 hours after birth, and almost one-third of term newborns had a glucose concentration at or below 40 mg/dL when glucose measurements obtained before the first feeding were included.

HEMATOCRIT

The hematocrit can be measured to exclude possible anemia or polycythemia at the same time that the blood glucose concentration is measured. Anemia may result from hemolysis or blood loss, whereas polycythemia is often associated with delayed cord clamping at birth (placental-to-infant transfusion), postmaturity, severe intrauterine growth restriction, monozygotic twins, or infants born to diabetic or hypertensive mothers.

ISOIMMUNE HEMOLYTIC DISEASE

If a mother's blood type is either O or Rh-negative, her infant's blood type should be determined, and a direct Coombs test should be performed. Blood type and Coombs test also should be determined if the mother has a positive antibody titer.

INBORN ERRORS OF METABOLISM AND HEMOGLOBINOPATHIES

Before hospital discharge, all newborns should be screened for at least primary hypothyroidism, galactosemia, phenylketonuria, and

sickle cell disease (along with the other hemoglobinopathies that are detected with sickle cell testing). In the United States, screening tests are usually performed under the auspices of a mandated statewide program. Additional tests may be included depending on their availability in the region. In some states, neonatal screening tests for cystic fibrosis, congenital adrenal hyperplasia, maple syrup urine disease, additional hemoglobinopathies, and other infectious and metabolic diseases are routinely performed.

AUDIOLOGIC TESTING

Screening newborn infants for deafness and auditory abnormalities has been recommended by the American Academy of Pediatrics, so that infants with sensorineural or conductive hearing loss can be diagnosed by 3 months of age, and early intervention initiated. Currently there are two methods of automated testing: the auditory brainstem response (ABR) and the otoacoustic emissions (OAE) test. Both of these tests can be performed by nursery personnel trained in their use. Infants who fail these screening tests in one or both ears should be referred for formal diagnostic studies at an audiology center that is capable of testing young infants.

SCREENING FOR TOXIC SUBSTANCES

Infants who have been exposed in utero to drugs of abuse should be identified in the neonatal period so that they can be monitored carefully for signs of neonatal abstinence syndrome. Every nursery should have a protocol that defines specific criteria based on maternal risk factors and on infant symptoms to determine those patients for whom a urine sample should be sent for detection of illicit drugs. If toxicology testing is positive, a social service evaluation should be performed, and arrangements should be made for appropriate care and follow-up evaluation of the infant.

2.10.4   Infections

Acute infections acquired during the perinatal period are common. Progression is often rapid and potentially lethal if detection and treatment are delayed. Sepsis and pneumonia commonly coexist, and spread of the infection to the central nervous system can lead to long-term disability or death. Many of the warning signs from intrapartum events and neonatal findings are nonspecific. Consequently, many infants must be evaluated for infection and treated presumptively with antimicrobial agents at least until diagnostic test results are known.

Prolonged (>18 hours) rupture of membranes increases the risk of neonatal infection. The risk of sepsis increases when delivery occurs prematurely or if there is evidence of clinical chorioamnionitis or signs of fetal infection such as tachycardia or birth depression. The presence of several risk factors together further increases the likelihood of neonatal sepsis.

Signs and symptoms of neonatal sepsis include abnormal body temperature, poor feeding, abdominal distension, lethargy, hypoglycemia or glucose intolerance, hypotension, cyanosis, respiratory distress, petechiae, apnea, and irritability or seizures. Sepsis is often associated with poor peripheral perfusion, pallor or cyanosis, and mottled skin. Umbilical erythema, sometimes accompanied by a generalized rash, is indicative of serious infection and merits prompt evaluation and treatment with antibiotics. Jaundice in the first 24 hours after birth also may indicate the presence of infection. Often serious neonatal infections are associated with either very low or very high white blood cell counts (<5000/mm³ or >20,000/mm³ of blood) with a high percentage of immature cells (bands, myelocytes, metamyelocytes). The subtleties of presentation and potential gravity of neonatal sepsis are cause for a high index of suspicion and low threshold for conducting a careful diagnostic evaluation. The response to multiple risk factors or to one factor that carries a very high risk is to perform diagnostic tests for infection, including a white blood cell count and bacterial cultures, and to begin antibiotic treatment immediately. The response to a condition that carries a modest risk of sepsis (eg, prolonged rupture of membranes) is to obtain a white blood cell count and bacterial cultures and to observe the infant carefully for any other abnormalities. Cultures of blood, urine, and cerebrospinal fluid should be obtained and antibiotic treatment begun immediately if there are clear-cut signs and symptoms of sepsis. When sepsis is suspected, it is also important to consider the possibility of infection with herpes simplex as well as the usual neonatal pathogenic bacteria, such as group B *Streptococcus, Escherichia coli,* and *Listeria,* and antimicrobial treatment should be prescribed accordingly.

2.10.5   Maternal Education and Discharge

The time that a newborn infant spends in the hospital nursery provides an important opportunity for maternal education as well as for critical infant evaluation. Before the infant is discharged from the hospital, the mother should have received sufficient practical instruction to assure appropriate home management of feeding, bathing, and general care of the infant, including recognition of well-being and illness.

The discharge examination of the infant should be done, if possible, in the mother's presence to allow her ample opportunity to express her concerns and ask questions about the findings she may think are abnormal. Plans for subsequent well-baby care of the infant should be established, and instructions given for communicating concerns to the appropriate medical provider. Babies who are discharged within 48 hours after birth should be seen again in 2 to 3 days. The mother also should be advised that if her infant becomes sick in the neonatal period and receives treatment elsewhere, the relevant information should be transmitted to the nursery that provided early postnatal care. Contagious infections, such as diarrhea or staphylococcal disease, often manifest symptoms after discharge from the nursery, and failure of communication may lead to delay in identifying the problem and in taking corrective measures.

Before discharge, anticipatory counseling should be done to promote infant safety and to prevent exposure to potential infections and toxins such as tobacco smoke. If the baby is going home in an automobile, the mother should have an infant car seat and know how to use it properly. The adequacy of the home situation for the newborn infant should be evaluated, as well as the presence of particular stresses, such as domestic violence, isolation, depression, and homelessness. Social service and public health nurse referrals may be very helpful in ensuring a safe and nurturing environment for the baby after discharge.

References

American Academy of Pediatrics: 2000 Red Book: Report of the Committee on Infectious Diseases, 25th ed. Elk Grove Village, IL, AAP, 2000

American Academy of Pediatrics and American College of Obstetricians and Gynecologists: Guidelines for Perinatal Care, 4th ed. Elk Grove Village, IL, AAP, 1997

American Academy of Pediatrics, Committee on Drugs: The transfer of drugs and other chemicals into human milk. Pediatrics 93:137, 1994

American Academy of Pediatrics, Joint Committee on Infant Hearing. 1994 Position Statement. Pediatrics 95:152, 1995

American Academy of Pediatrics, Task Force on Circumcision: Circumcision policy statement. Pediatrics 103:686, 1999

American Academy of Pediatrics, Vitamin K Ad Hoc Task Force: Controversies concerning vitamin K and the newborn. Pediatrics 84:388, 1989

American Academy of Pediatrics, Work Group on Breastfeeding: Breastfeeding and the use of human milk. Pediatrics 100:1035, 1997

Bell TA, Grayston JT, Krohn MA, Kronmal RA: Randomized trial of silver nitrate, erythromycin, and no prophylaxis for the prevention of conjunctivitis among newborns not at risk for gonococcal ophthalmitis. Eye Prophylaxis Study Group. Pediatrics 92:755, 1993

Chaou WT, Chou ML, Eitzmann DV: Intracranial hemorrhage and vitamin K deficiency in early infancy. J Pediatr 105:888, 1984

Dahm LS, James LS: Newborn temperature and calculated heat loss in the delivery room. Pediatrics 49:504, 1972

Fielkow S, Reuter S, Gotoff SP: Cerebrospinal fluid examination in symptom-free infants with risk factors for infection. J Pediatr 119:971, 1991

Heck L, Erenberg A: Serum glucose levels in term neonates during the first 48 hours of life. J Pediatr 110:119, 1987

Kramer I, Sherry S: The time of passage of the first stool and urine by the premature infant. J Pediatr 51:373, 1957

Motil KJ, Blackburn MG, Pleasure JR: The effects of four different radiant warmer temperature set-points used for rewarming neonates. J Pediatr 85:546, 1974

Schwartz R: Neonatal hypoglycemia: how low is too low? J Pediatr 131:171, 1997

Sexson WR: Incidence of neonatal hypoglycemia: a matter of definition. J Pediatr 105:149, 1984

Sherry S, Kramer I: The time of passage of the first stool and first urine by the newborn infant. J Pediatr 46:158, 1955

Sinclair J: Temperature Regulation and Energy. Metabolism in the Newborn. New York, Grune & Stratton, 1978

Sutor AH, Von Kries R, Cornelissen EA, McNinch AW, Andrew M: Vitamin K deficiency bleeding in infancy. Pediatric/Perinatal Subcommittee, International Society on Thrombosis and Hemostasis. Thromb Hemostas 81:456, 1999

Versmold H, Kitterman J, Phibbs R, et al: Aortic blood pressure during the first 12 hours of life in infants with birth weight 610 to 4220 grams. Pediatrics 67:607, 1981

2.11   NEONATAL NUTRITION AND GASTROINTESTINAL FUNCTION

Anthony F. Philipps and Michael P. Sherman

Nutritional sufficiency of the newborn is a topic that continues to engage great debate. Delivery of the fetus is marked by the abrupt transition from the fetal nutritional state. This state is marked by a relatively constant supply of nutrients via the maternoplacental circulation, supplemented to a minor degree by enteral absorption of nutrients derived from swallowed amniotic fluid. The transition to an intermittent and wholly enteral route for neonatal nutritional needs is a critical aspect of successful adaptation at birth.

Although suspected previously, data continue to accumulate that nutritional intake and growth in the perinatal period may be important predictors of risk factors for a variety of adult ills including cardiovascular disease, diabetes, hypertension, stroke, and obesity. Other potential long-term sequelae that have been less well studied include the effects of undernutrition on cognitive function, changes in bone density, and incidence of cancer.

BREAST-FEEDING AND HUMAN MILK

During the last century, the almost exclusive use of human milk was abandoned for a time by some in favor of the fashionable (and occasionally truly necessary) use of cow milk–based formula fed by bottle in "developed" countries. Over the past 50 years, however, most authorities on infant nutrition the (the American Academy of Pediatrics, among others) have advocated human milk for healthy term babies. This recommendation reflects the results of the vast literature supporting breast-feeding and the use of human milk as a superior form of nutrition for infants. The psychological, nutritional, hormonal, immunologic, and economic benefits of human milk are now well established. Some of these are briefly detailed below. Despite these widely acknowledged benefits, however, a recent survey showed that the proportion of women breast-feeding their babies at time of hospital discharge was only 59% even when those partially using formula were included. Only 22% were found to be nursing by 6 months postnatally.

Many obstacles to successful breast-feeding have been identified (Table 2-9), as well as potential remedies for each. In some situations, such as prematurity, intestinal or metabolic illness, or maternal use of drugs that may be incompatible with the health of the newborn (ie, chemotherapy), artificial formulas are clearly useful and, in selected instances, essential. Intravenous nutrition is a valuable and, in some cases, life-saving adjunct form of therapy for infants unable to receive enteral feedings.

As noted above, breast milk is the ideal food for the newborn. In addition to strictly nutritional issues, there are a number of other advantages to breast-feeding over the use of artificial formulas, including psychosocial, maternal, and immunologic benefits.

Successful breast-feeding promotes and strengthens maternal–infant bonding and is generally considered a satisfying experience for both mother and baby. Maternal benefits include stimulation of uterine involution, reduction in the incidence of postpartum hemorrhage, reduction in menses and ovulation leading to diminished postpartum iron loss and increased intervals between pregnancies, and decreased incidences of premenopausal breast and ovarian cancer.

From the standpoint of prevention of infections in the newborn, breast milk is less likely to be contaminated by bacterial pathogens, particularly in women who reside in countries where sanitation and access to clean water are problematic. Fresh human milk contains maternal cellular elements, including lymphocytes, macrophages, and neutrophils, particularly in early colostral milk. These, as well as pathogen-specific milk-borne secretory IgA, may help to inhibit the development of neonatal infections, particularly of the respiratory and gastrointestinal systems. In certain high-risk groups, however, viral pathogens such as human immunodeficiency virus (HIV), cytomegalovirus (CMV), or hepatitis B virus (HBV) may be transmitted in human milk.

OPTIMAL NEWBORN NUTRITION

Because breast-feeding and ingestion of human milk provide optimal intakes of water and nutrients for growth of healthy term newborns over the first months of postnatal life, growth and developmental patterns of infants reared exclusively on human milk have become the benchmarks by which alternative forms of enteral and parenteral nutritional programs are assessed. Guidelines for optimal intakes of energy, major nutrients, minerals, and water in infancy derive from a variety of sources, including direct experimental observations, such as those involving studies of nutrient balance (ie, protein, fat, calcium), energy expenditure, and metabolic rate as

TABLE 2-9

OBSTACLES TO BREAST MILK FEEDING

Insufficient prenatal education
Inappropriate interruption of feeding
Maternal employment and workplace issues
Lack of family and societal support
Commercial promotion of infant formulas via variety of routes
Physician misinformation and apathy
Lack of routine follow-up or access to pre- and postnatal care
Home stresses

well as those involving more indirect estimates based on measurements of known intakes in healthy term infants (ie, trace minerals, vitamins). Specific references may be found at the end of this section.

ENERGY   Estimates for neonatal energy needs (Table 2-10) derive in part from indirect estimates of human fetal oxygen consumption in late gestation as well as postnatal assessment of metabolic rate using direct and indirect calorimetry and measurement of respiratory gas exchange. In general, most estimates suggest a basal consumption rate of 7 to 8 mL of O_2/kg/min, which translates into approximately 50 kcal/kg body weight/d.

In the first month of postnatal life, total energy intake in breast-fed babies (100 kcal/kg/d) is somewhat lower than it is in bottle-fed babies (110–120 kcal/kg/d), possibly because of measured differences in activity level and sleep state between these two groups. Estimates of total energy expenditure (TEE, or basal metabolic needs plus those for metabolic "work," physical activity, growth, and thermoregulation purposes) have more recently been measured in babies. With use of stable nonradioactive isotopes (doubly labeled water method), TEE is approximately 60 to 70 kcal/kg/d in breast-fed babies, with somewhat higher values in bottle-fed babies, corresponding to the previously noted differences in energy intake. Thus, caloric intakes below 80 kcal/kg/d are clearly inadequate to provide for accretion of fat and protein (see below). Whether or not excessive caloric intake leads to later obesity or other problems is an unresolved question, and currently no information is available to properly address this issue. Energy needs and expenditures for infants who are small for gestational age are generally higher than for infants of normal size.

PROTEIN AND PROTEIN DIGESTION   Rates of protein synthesis in the fetus and infant are considerably greater than the respective rates of protein accretion. Moreover, the rate of protein synthesis is greater before and soon after birth than it is later in life. Excessive

TABLE 2-10

NUTRIENT INTAKE: NEWBORN

Energy		
	100–120 kcal/kg/d	
Protein		
	Intake:	1.8–2.0 g/100 kcal/d
	Deposition:	3.5 g/d
Fat		
	Intake:	3–5 g/100 kcal/d
	Deposition:	6 g/d
Carbohydrate		
	Intake:	10–12 g/100 kcal/d
	Deposition:	—

protein breakdown and turnover presumably allow for significant remodeling during a period of rapid growth and cell differentiation. Thus, protein intakes are also considerably higher than measured accretion rates, even in healthy term babies (Table 2-10). In the first months of postnatal life, protein intake in breast-fed babies averages 2 g/kg/d, with an estimated protein accretion rate of 1 g/kg/d. Because breast milk contains less protein (9 g/L) than current infant formulas (15 g/L) or cow milk (33 g/L), breast-fed babies receive less protein than do bottle-fed babies, provided that fluid intakes are equivalent. The protein constituents of human milk (whey: α-lactalbumin, serum albumin, IgA, lactoferrin; casein: α- and β-caseins), however, are somewhat different from those of cow milk, as are the whey:casein ratios (50-60:50-40 for human, 20:80 for cow). Protein intake and plasma amino acid concentrations in breast-fed babies are currently utilized as the standard for development of artificial milk formula, including formula produced for consumption by premature babies.

Proteolytic activity in the fetal gastrointestinal tract has been described as early as 16 weeks of gestation. Proteolytic enzymes are produced in the stomach (pepsinogen, cathepsin), but relatively little functional protein digestion occurs here, particularly in the first few weeks of postnatal life. Gastric acid secretion is low in preterm infants and also in term infants shortly after delivery. Thus, there is relatively little gastric and duodenal protein denaturation at this early stage of development. Protein denaturation in the stomach contributes to the rate of proteolysis but is less important functionally than those processes that occur in the duodenum and proximal jejunum. Gastric acid secretion increases to adult levels by approximately 2 years of age.

Pancreatic enzymes (trypsin, chymotrypsin, carboxypeptidase, elastase, phospholipase) and intestinal enzymes (enterokinase, intestinal di- and tripeptidases) account for the majority of protein digestion in the newborn. Protein digestion is relatively well developed in infancy, although trypsin and chymotrypsin activities increase over the first 4 months of postnatal life. It is noteworthy that fecal excretion of several pancreatic enzymes is greater in bottle-fed infants than in breast-fed babies, and there is some evidence that increased enteral protein intake may lead to enhanced trypsin production.

Absorption of oligopeptides and amino acids across the intestinal epithelium is mediated by specific amino acid transport carrier proteins, some of which are sodium dependent. Several of these carrier proteins have been identified and their abundance noted in infancy. Studies have shown that as much as 80 to 85% of dietary protein is absorbed in infancy, as assessed by nitrogen retention. There is also evidence that some proteins, such as β-lactoglobulin, milk-derived growth factors, and some cow milk proteins, may be absorbed intact into the circulation. It is likely that absorption of some macromolecules also may be increased in states of intestinal injury, potentially inducing sensitization to foreign proteins.

FAT AND FAT DIGESTION Lipids provide the predominant source of energy in infancy. Approximately 40 to 50% of the calories provided by human milk and artificial formulas derive from fat. In human milk, triglycerides (Tg) constitute the vast majority (98%) of lipid, with small amounts of mono- and diglycerides, phospholipids and cholesterol making up the remainder. The fat content of human milk (approximately 4% by weight) increases over the first month of lactation; the last portion of a feed ("hind milk") has a greater fat content than does the earlier portion of the feeding ("fore milk"). Although the exact constituents and degree of unsaturation of the Tg-related fatty acids (FAs) vary among women

and between populations (in part, because of dietary differences), concentrations of essential FAs do not differ appreciably. In infant formulas derived from cow milk, the fat (also mostly Tg) originates from vegetable oils (soy, coconut, corn). Fat deposition in the first postnatal month is approximately 6 g/d (1.5 g/kg/d) (Table 2-10), most of which is derived from dietary fat. Because the caloric value of lipid (9 kcal/g) is 2.25 times that of carbohydrate or protein, it is not surprising that dietary lipids from milk account for approximately 35% of early postnatal weight gain. Oxidation of fat in the fetus is limited but postnatally takes on great importance, such that some dietary lipid is also used for energy purposes.

In contrast to the digestion of protein, the processes of lipolysis and fatty acid absorption are less well developed in early infancy. This is particularly true for very premature babies. Absorption is dependent on fatty acid chain length and the degree of saturation. Babies absorb the lipid in human milk somewhat better than the lipid in cow milk, partly because human milk fat requires less emulsification by bile acids. Modern infant formulas and use of vegetable oil supplements have obviated this problem to some extent, but fat malabsorption continues to be a problem for very premature babies who are fed enterally. Lipolysis occurs from the action of various lipases. In addition to pancreatic lipases, which are in relatively low concentration in the term newborn and even lower in premature babies, several other lipases contribute to neonatal fat digestion. A bile salt–dependent lipase that is present in human colostrum and mature milk remains intact in the stomach and helps to hydrolyze long-chain fats in human newborns. Human milk also contains a lipoprotein lipase (LPL), but its contribution to intestinal lipolysis is unclear because bile salts inhibit its action. Lipases produced in the tongue (lingual lipase) and stomach (gastric lipase) also have been noted to cause significant hydrolysis of triglycerides before they reach the duodenum and are currently thought to play major roles in neonatal fat absorption. Globules of human milk fat are also more available to the actions of lingual and gastric lipases than to pancreatic or intestinal lipases. Other intestinally derived lipases, such as colipase, appear to have more action after infancy.

Bile acids are necessary for efficient absorption of dietary lipids. Bile flow increases rapidly after birth, with increased delivery of bile acids to the small intestine. Cholic and chenoxycholic acids make up the majority of active bile acids and are conjugated with taurine more than with glycine, as is found later in infancy.

CARBOHYDRATES AND CARBOHYDRATE DIGESTION Lactose is the principal carbohydrate in human milk and in many infant formulas. Intake of lactose is estimated at 10 to 12 g/100 kcal/d for term babies (Table 2-10). In general, digestion of disaccharides, such as lactose and sucrose, or of glucose polymers is initiated by hydrolysis to monosaccharides. This process usually occurs at the brush border of intestinal epithelial cells and in the luminal fluid as well. The brush border enzymes lactase and sucrase—isomaltase, the concentrations of which are developmentally regulated, mediate the process. Sucrase activity appears earlier in fetal life (3–4 months) than does lactase activity (5 months). High intestinal lactase activity is a distinct characteristic of the term newborn, but this activity declines later in childhood. Lactase concentrations decrease by 75% over the first year of life. In addition to the lactose that is hydrolyzed in the small intestine, some nonhydrolyzed lactose is also metabolized via bacterial fermentation in the colon. Such fermentation produces hydrogen as well as short-chain fatty acids, such as acetate and propionate. Although lactose absorption may be inefficient in premature infants and in infants with intrauterine growth restriction, recent studies indicate that between 80 and

100% of ingested lactose is absorbed in the intestine of the term newborn.

The protein moiety responsible for sucrase activity differs between the fetus and infant and the adult, in both molecular weight and degree of glycosylation. Before 30 weeks of gestation, a single molecule possesses both sucrase and isomaltase activity; after 30 weeks of gestation, the activities of these two enzymes become distinct. The parent molecule, in the adult, and presumably in the infant as well, is cleaved by pancreatic proteases into individual sucrase and isomaltase molecules. Sucrase activity in the intestine of the term baby is higher than that of the adult and is, even at 34 weeks, at least 70% of that in the term baby. Salivary and pancreatic amylases are responsible for hydrolysis of glucose polymers and complex carbohydrates (starches). These enzymes, in addition to the brush border enzyme glucoamylase, probably function in the hydrolysis of glucose polymers, which commonly are present in premature infant formulas.

Digestion of carbohydrates yields monosaccharides such as glucose, galactose, and fructose that are then transported through the enterocyte to the portal venous system via passive and active transport mechanisms. In the case of glucose, intestinal expression of specific glucose transporter proteins, such as SGLT-1, or the sodium-dependent glucose transporter, and GLUT-1, 2, and 5, have been demonstrated in the fetus and newborn. Direct absorption of monosaccharides, such as glucose, has been studied in human infants and is less well developed than it is later in life. Monosaccharides derived from enzymatic digestion of disaccharides are better absorbed than monosaccharides that are presented directly to the intestinal lumen, but the reasons for this observation are unclear.

MINERALS AND VITAMINS   In general, most minerals are present in human milk in quantities sufficient for growth and metabolism in infancy, with certain exceptions. Newborn dietary requirements for these are presented in a variety of source texts that are listed at the end of this section. In both human and artificial milks, the amounts of the minerals sodium, potassium, chloride, magnesium, calcium, and phosphorus are adequate for term babies, assuming adequate fluid intake. However, because calcium is bound with phosphates and casein into a variety of complex forms, and because of the aforementioned malabsorption of fat in premature infants, calcium absorption in very premature babies is often inadequate for normal skeletal growth. The demonstration that human milk is relatively low in available calcium and even lower in phosphorus prompted the development of human milk fortifiers in addition to milk formulas specifically designed to provide extra calcium and phosphorus for bone mineralization. Magnesium absorption ranges from 60 to 90% in term newborns and increases in premature infants with advancing gestational age. Some studies in very premature infants have shown that magnesium absorption and retention may fall when the milk is supplemented with high concentrations of calcium and phosphorus. This, however, is rarely a clinically significant problem in the term infant.

Microminerals, such as zinc, copper, molybdenum, manganese, selenium, and iron, make up less than 0.01% of body mass but are important for nutritional needs in infancy, partly because they act as enzymatic cofactors in a variety of metabolic pathways. Provision of microminerals in infant formulas derives from their concentrations in human milk. For some, such as iron, specific carrier proteins in human milk (ie, lactoferrin) facilitate enhanced intestinal absorption and transit. In the case of zinc, absorption is enhanced in human milk compared with cow milk formula, as zinc binds more tightly to casein, which is a major constituent of cow milk protein.

Intake of other microminerals, such as fluoride and iodine, is more dependent on regional differences in diet and the concentration of these minerals in water. Recently, chromium has been identified as an element that is necessary for normal glucose tolerance.

Water-soluble vitamins, such as thiamin, riboflavin, pantothenic acid, niacin, vitamins B_6 and B_{12}, vitamin C, biotin, and folate, function as necessary cofactors for a variety of metabolically important enzymes. These vitamins are normally present in human milk and in infant formulas. Most of the vitamins listed above are transported efficiently across the placenta against a concentration gradient. Thus, at birth, the whole-body concentrations of these vitamins are greater in the fetus than in the mother, but vitamin deficiency can occur if dietary vitamin supplements are not utilized during pregnancy and lactation, or if the mother is severely malnourished. Human milk and infant formulas generally contain sufficient concentrations of these vitamins to prevent overt vitamin deficiency. Thus, water-soluble vitamin supplements are not usually necessary for healthy term infants who are either breast- or bottle fed.

In contrast, the fat-soluble vitamins A (all-*trans*-retinol and its plant precursor carotene), D (cholecalciferol from animals and endogenous synthesis and ergocalciferol from plants), E (tocopherol), and K (K_1, or phylloquinone, and menaquinone) are poorly transported across the placenta to the fetus; the marginal amounts of transplacentally derived vitamin K_1 are particularly noteworthy in this respect. Vitamin D is transferred somewhat better transplacentally than the others noted above, but transfer is enhanced predominantly beyond 34 weeks of gestation. In postnatal life these vitamins are absorbed from the small intestine and require the presence of bile salts, pancreatic enzymes, and micelle formation for uptake into lymphatic chyle and subsequently into blood. In general, the absorption of these vitamins is between 50 and 75%, but this is significantly diminished in premature babies because of malabsorption of enteral fats. The major storage sites of vitamin D are liver and, to a lesser extent, adipose tissue. Vitamin K, among its other functions, is an important cofactor for the carboxylase enzyme that activates prothrombin. Because of poor transplacental uptake by the fetus, coupled with the low levels of vitamin K in human milk, it is recommended that newborns receive parenteral vitamin K in the immediate postnatal period to prevent hemorrhagic disease. Vitamin E is an important antioxidant and acts as a free radical scavenger to help protect cell membranes from oxidation. Vitamins A and D also have a role in regulation of gene expression. Vitamin A helps to regulate gene transcription, cell differentiation, and immune function, and vitamin D is converted in the liver and kidneys to active forms that regulate calcium and phosphorus balance.

Human milk normally contains sufficient concentrations of vitamins A and E to meet the needs of the newborn. This is not the case for vitamins K and D, however, and infants who are fed breast milk exclusively should receive supplemental vitamin D. There are no current recommendations for vitamin K supplementation beyond the immediate postnatal period. Infant formulas contain sufficient concentrations of the essential fat-soluble vitamins noted above. Because premature babies have a significant degree of fat malabsorption, including fat-soluble vitamins, vitamin supplements are recommended for such infants, especially those who are fed human milk without fortifier.

GASTROINTESTINAL MOTILITY

Gastric and intestinal propulsive motility allows for effective proximal-to-distal passage of nutrients and also facilitates their efficient

TABLE 2-11

NEWBORN GASTROINTESTINAL MOTILITY (COMPARED TO ADULT)

	PRETERM	TERM
Upper esophageal sphincter tone	nl	nl
Esophageal peristalsis	↑	nl
Uncoordinated esophageal peristalsis	+	−
Lower esophageal sphincter tone	↓	nl
Gastric emptying	↓	nl
Intestinal transit	9 hours (at 32 weeks)	4–7 hours
Intestinal migrating motor complexes		
Amplitude	↓	nl
Cycle length	↑	nl

absorption. The myenteric (Auerbach) and submucosal (Meissner) neural plexuses serve to initiate, coordinate, and transmit electrical impulses to intestinal smooth muscle in order to promote rhythmic intestinal peristalsis. The process is inhibited by a variety of ingested nutrients, particularly dietary fat, and stimulated by at least several important hormones (motilin, somatostatin, pancreatic polypeptide, and gastrin, to name a few). Coordination of electrical activity ("motor complexes") is also developmentally regulated, with premature infants (particularly those less than 32 weeks of gestational age) having intestinal contractions of low amplitude and with ineffective distal migration. The coordination that characterizes sequential contractions of the gastric antrum and duodenum in the term newborn infant is not as well developed in the premature infant. Likewise, esophageal peristalsis is less effective in the premature than in the term infant. Whether or not the poorly developed lower esophageal sphincter tone in premature babies contributes to their propensity toward significant gastroesophageal reflux is unclear. Birth asphyxia and other types of central nervous system injury, such as meningitis and intracranial hemorrhage, also are associated with decreased gastrointestinal motility. Some of the features regarding esophageal and intestinal motility in the newborn are summarized in Table 2-11.

Colonic motility in newborns has received relatively little attention. The aforementioned neural plexuses innervate the large intestine by 24 weeks of gestation. Meconium is present in the fetal colon after 4 to 6 months of gestation and becomes increasingly firm and dark as gestation progresses. It is composed of sloughed intestinal epithelial cells, lanugo hair, digested vernix, and pancreatic secretions. More than 98% of term babies pass a meconium stool by 36 to 48 hours of postnatal life. By 4 to 5 days, meconium is no longer present, and the stool becomes yellow and seedy.

Because of the well-identified intestinal motility problems of very low-birth-weight babies, a number of relevant studies have been performed in this unique population of infants. Recent observations indicate that postnatal delay of enteral feeding slows the rate of maturation of gastrointestinal motility in infants who are born prematurely. As in the adult, composition, rate of feeding, and feed volume all are important in affecting intestinal motor responses of premature babies. Thus, early postnatal feedings of very small volumes of milk ("trophic feedings") are considered useful in hastening and facilitating gastric emptying and intestinal peristalsis. Feeding practices for very premature infants continue to be a major source of controversy and often present a formidable challenge for those who work in neonatal intensive care.

References

American Academy of Pediatrics and American College of Obstetricians and Gynecologists: Guidelines for Perinatal Care, 4th ed. Elk Grove Village, IL, AAP, 1997

American Academy of Pediatrics Work Group on Breastfeeding: Breast-feeding and the use of human milk. Pediatrics 100:1035, 1997

Berseth CL: Feeding and maturation of gut motility. In: Nutrition of the Very Low Birthweight Infant, Nestlé Nutritional Workshop Series Paediatric Programme, 43:211, 1999

Fomon SJ: Nutrition of Normal Infants. St Louis: CV Mosby, 1993

Koldovsk O: Digestive-absorption functions of fetuses, infants, and children. In: Fetal and Neonatal Physiology, 2nd ed, vol 2. Philadelphia, WB Saunders, 1998:1400

Kunz C, Rodriquez-Palmero M, Koletzko B, Jensen R: Nutritional and biochemical properties of human milk, part I: general aspects, proteins, and carbohydrates. Clin Perinatol 26:307, 1999

Lucas A: Programming by early nutrition: an experimental approach. J Nutr 128:401S, 1998

National Research Council: Recommended dietary allowances, 10th ed. Washington, DC, National Academy Press, 1990

Philipps AF: Carbohydrate metabolism in the fetus. In: Polin R, Fox W, eds: Fetal and Neonatal Physiology, 2nd ed. Philadelphia, WB Saunders, 1998:560

Rodriguez-Palmero M, Koletzko B, Kunz C, Jensen R: Nutritional and biochemical properties of human milk: II. lipids, micronutrients, and bioactive factors. Clin Perinatol 26:335, 1999

Tsang RC, Zlotkin SH, Nichols BL, Hansen JW, eds: Nutrition during Infancy, Principles and Practice, 2nd ed. Cincinnati Digital Educational Publishing, 1997

2.12   SUPPORTIVE CARE OF THE PRETERM INFANT

Gunnar Sedin and Richard D. Bland

After initial resuscitation and stabilization in the delivery room, the primary goal of newborn intensive care for preterm infants, particularly those who are born at less than 28 weeks of gestation and less than 1000 g birth weight, is to provide supportive measures that facilitate normal respiratory gas exchange and cardiovascular function as well as appropriate fluid balance, nutrition, and growth while minimizing the risk for iatrogenic complications. This section focuses on issues that are important in the routine management of infants who are born too small too soon, with special attention to early postnatal care and monitoring of critical variables, consideration of conditions that impact fluid and electrolyte balance and nutrient needs, and specific concerns regarding transport and handling of preterm infants.

2.12.1   Early Postnatal Management and Monitoring

Infants who are born prematurely commonly lack regulatory mechanisms to control essential life functions, such as regular breathing, thermal homeostasis, and enteral intake of nutrients. They often require assisted ventilation and supplemental oxygen beginning at birth, and an immature heart and circulation sometimes leads to systemic hypotension, inadequate organ perfusion with resultant oliguria, and metabolic acidosis. Thus, frequent or continuous monitoring of vital signs, namely temperature, blood pressure,

TABLE 2-12
ESTIMATES OF BODY COMPOSITION IN HUMAN FETUSES

Gestation (wks)	24–27	28–31	32–36	37–40
Body Weight (g)	<1000	1100–1700	1800–2700	>2700
Body Fat (g/100 g BW)	0.1–2.4	3.3–5.6	6.3–8.7	9.3–16.2
Total Body Water (g/100 g BW)	86–89	82–85	77–81	71–76
(g/100g fat-free BW)	88–89	87–88	85–86	82–84
Extracellular Water (g/100g BW)	55–60	—	—	35–45
Sodium (mmol/100g fat-free BW)	9.5–10	9.1–9.4	8.8–9.1	8.7–8.8
Potassium (mmol/100g fat-free BW)	4.0–4.1	4.2–4.3	4.3–4.5	4.5–4.6
Chloride (mmol/100g fat-free BW)	6.9–7.0	6.7–6.9	6.1–6.5	5.7–6.0

SOURCE: Adapted from: Brans, Clin Perinatol 13: 403–417, 1986; Widdowson and Spray, Arch Dis Child 26: 205–214, 1951, Ziegler et al, Growth 40:329–341, 1976.

heart rate, breathing pattern, and oxygen saturation, is an extremely important aspect of intensive care for very immature infants. Monitoring of these critical variables should begin immediately after birth, with appropriate provision of an adequate heat source to prevent hypothermia in the delivery room and during transport to the intensive care nursery; assisted ventilation with sufficient supplemental oxygen to prevent hypoxia and hypercapnia; and early intravenous access to allow delivery of glucose-containing solutions and emergency drugs if needed.

In the intensive care nursery, a more thorough assessment of the infant's condition should include accurate baseline measurements of body weight, length, and head circumference to identify possible discordance between gestational age and prior intrauterine growth. For management of extremely small, immature, and sick newborns, it is often useful to care for the infant on a platform balance beneath the bedding to allow frequent weight determination with minimal disturbance of the infant. The infant should remain in a warm environment, with continuous monitoring of heart and respiratory rates, oxygen saturation (SaO$_2$; pulse oximetry), and temperature. If extra oxygen is needed, with or without mechanical ventilation, partial pressures of oxygen (PaO$_2$) and carbon dioxide (PaCO$_2$) should be measured at frequent intervals or monitored continuously with transcutaneous electrodes. The target for PaO$_2$ should be 50 to 80 mm Hg (SaO$_2$ 90–95%), and the target for PaCO$_2$ should be 40 to 50 mm Hg, although higher values for PaCO$_2$ may be tolerated to reduce the risk of lung injury if the infant is being managed on mechanical ventilation.

In all seriously ill preterm infants, and in those who have evidence of poor peripheral circulation, the arterial blood pressure should be monitored either through an indwelling catheter placed in the umbilical artery or through a catheter inserted percutaneously in a peripheral artery, or noninvasively with a limb cuff and oscillometric recording device. The arterial catheter also can be used for blood sampling, including measurements of arterial pH, PaO$_2$, and PaCO$_2$. Indwelling catheters should be removed when the infant becomes stable and does not require continuous monitoring of blood pressure or frequent measurements of arterial blood gas values. For infants who are born prematurely, or for those with suspected infection, a sample of blood for culture, complete blood count, and glucose concentration should be obtained soon after birth in advance of antibiotic therapy and intravenous nutrient delivery.

Infants with mild to moderate respiratory distress who require supplemental oxygen often can be treated effectively with nasal application of continuous positive airway pressure (CPAP) of between 5 and 8 cm H$_2$O. The device used for nasal CPAP should be lightly attached to the nose to avoid damage to the skin and nasal septum.

Infants with more severe respiratory distress usually require endotracheal intubation and mechanical ventilation with PEEP of 3 to 5 cm H$_2$O, with ventilation settings adjusted to maintain modest chest rise and adequate oxygenation and ventilation. Specifics of assisted breathing are discussed elsewhere in this chapter.

2.12.2   Fluid and Electrolyte Balance

In order to define water and salt needs for very small preterm infants, several issues should be considered, including body composition; prevailing water losses through the skin, lungs, and urinary and intestinal tracts; environmental conditions; and postnatal changes in renal function and related salt loss.

DEVELOPMENTAL DIFFERENCES IN BODY COMPOSITION

As shown in Table 2-12 Very small preterm infants have considerably less body fat and relatively more water, most of which is extracellular, than do infants who are born at term. In addition, sodium and chloride content are relatively greater in preterm infants because of their proportionally greater extracellular fluid compartment. Loss of extracellular fluid during the first week after birth is a normal developmental adaptation that facilitates appropriate function of vital organs, including the lungs, heart, and gastrointestinal tract. Expected weight loss in the first postnatal week averages 5 to 10% in healthy term infants and 8 to 15% in small (<1500 g) preterm infants. In some cases, "micropremies" (<750 g) may lose as much as 20% of their weight during the first 7 to 10 days. This loss is mostly extracellular water and should be accompanied by a corresponding loss of sodium to maintain normal osmolality. Extremely premature infants are unable to manage their own intake, and feedback mechanisms, such as hunger and thirst, are poorly developed. It is therefore difficult to determine what degree of weight reduction is "physiological" in these infants.

WATER LOSS THROUGH THE SKIN, LUNGS, AND GUT

Very immature infants have a thin, extremely permeable epidermal layer, with little or no effective barrier to the diffusion of water. On the first postnatal day, there is a very high transepidermal water loss (TEWL) from the skin surface. Evaporative water loss is influenced by skin surface area (relatively greater in small infants than in larger infants); skin blood flow (increased by exposure to radiant heat), surrounding air currents, water vapor pressure (relative humidity) at the skin surface (Table 2-13), and radiant heat sources. Evaporative water loss is costly in terms of energy balance: vaporization

TABLE 2-13

MEAN INSENSIBLE WATER LOSS FROM THE SKIN IN 68 NEWBORN APPROPRIATE-FOR-GESTATIONAL-AGE INFANTS AT AN AMBIENT HUMIDITY OF 50%

GESTATIONAL AGE (WEEKS)	INFANTS NO.	MEAN BIRTH WEIGHT (kg)	POSTNATAL AGE (DAYS)					
			<1	3	7	14	21	28
25–27	9	860	129	71	43	32	28	24
28–30	13	1340	42	32	24	18	15	15
31–36	22	2110	12	12	12	9	8	7
37–41	24	3600	7	6	6	6	6	7

Data for Insensible Water Loss from <1 to 28 days is expressed as g/kg body wt/day.

SOURCE: *Hammarlund K, Sedin G, Strömberg B: Transendermal water loss in newborn infants, VIII. Relation to gestational age and post-natal age in appropriate and small for gestational age infants. Acta Paediatr Scand 72:721–728, 1983.*

of 1 g of water causes the body to lose about 0.6 kcal of heat. Evaporative water loss and related heat loss are inversely related to the relative humidity (Fig. 2-29). There is considerable variability in evaporative water loss among infants, but in general it is inversely related to gestational and postnatal age (Fig. 2-30). In a population of infants born after 24 to 25 weeks of gestation and nursed at 50% relative humidity, daily insensible water loss from the skin averaged 114 ± 27 g/kg on the first day after birth and 51 ± 15 g/kg at postnatal day 28. In general, infants with intrauterine growth restriction (IUGR) lose water across their skin at a greater rate than infants of the same gestational age who are appropriately grown. It is noteworthy that radiant warmers and phototherapy may cause as much as a threefold increase in evaporative water loss. Plastic shields have been shown to reduce water and heat losses through the skin. Because of the extreme vulnerability of the very immature infant to acute dehydration from water loss across the skin, it is critical that in the immediate postnatal period (3–4 days), such infants be managed in an environment with high humidity and absent air currents and that serum Na concentrations be monitored closely to avoid hypernatremia.

Antenatal glucocorticoid exposure has been shown to have a significant effect on water loss across the skin. In a recent study of infants who were born at about 26 weeks of gestation with a birth weight that averaged about 1000 g, insensible water loss was reduced by about 50% in infants whose mothers received glucocorticoids. In addition, diuresis and urinary sodium loss occurred earlier, with lower serum sodium concentrations in the first few postnatal days despite a smaller water intake.

Water loss through the respiratory tract is directly related to minute ventilation and inversely related to the water vapor pressure of the inspired gas. In a neutral thermal environment, infants at 26 to 28 weeks gestation lose through their lungs about 5 to 10 mL of water/kg body weight each day if they are not receiving assisted ventilation. At high breathing rates, respiratory water loss in extremely preterm infants may be as great as 20 mL/kg/d. Assisted ventilation with dry gas can increase this water loss up to threefold. In healthy term infants, daily respiratory water loss averages about 9 g/kg at an ambient humidity of 20%; 7 g/kg at 50% humidity; and 5 g/kg at 80% humidity. This loss may double if metabolic rate and minute ventilation increase. During positive-pressure mechanical ventilation, the lungs may absorb water from the inspired gas if the gas is warm and fully saturated with water.

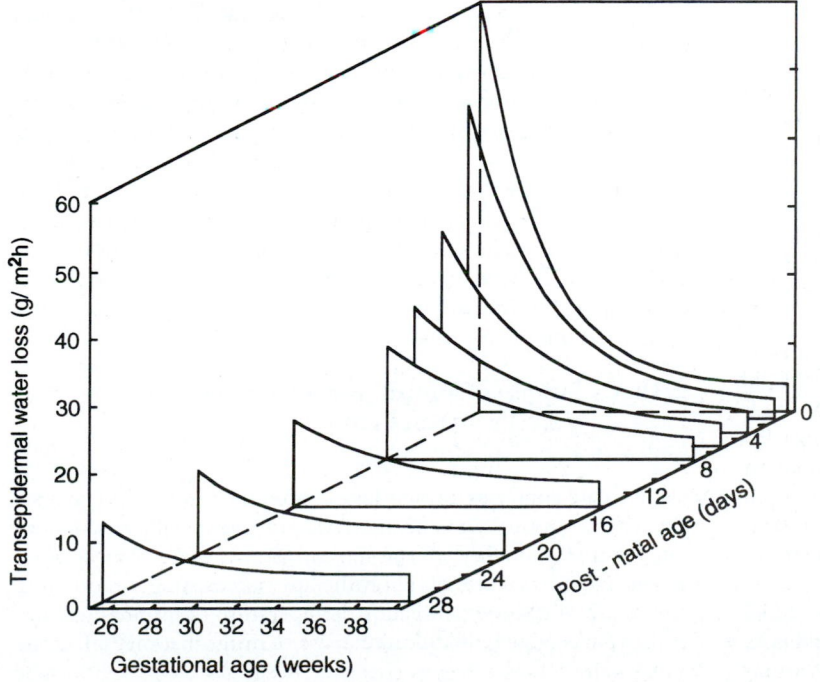

FIGURE 2-29 The relationship of transepidermal water loss (g/m²/h, *vertical axis*) to gestational age at birth (weeks, *horizontal axis*) at different postnatal ages (days, *third dimension axis*). The data are for infants appropriate for gestational age, unclothed, in an incubator at 50% humidity with the ambient temperature adjusted to keep the core temperature at 36 to 37°C. SOURCE: *Hammarlund K, Sedin G, Strömberg B: Transepidermal water loss in newborn infants. VIII. Relation to gestational age and post-natal age in appropriate and small for gestational age infants. Acta Paediatr Scand 72:721, 1983.*

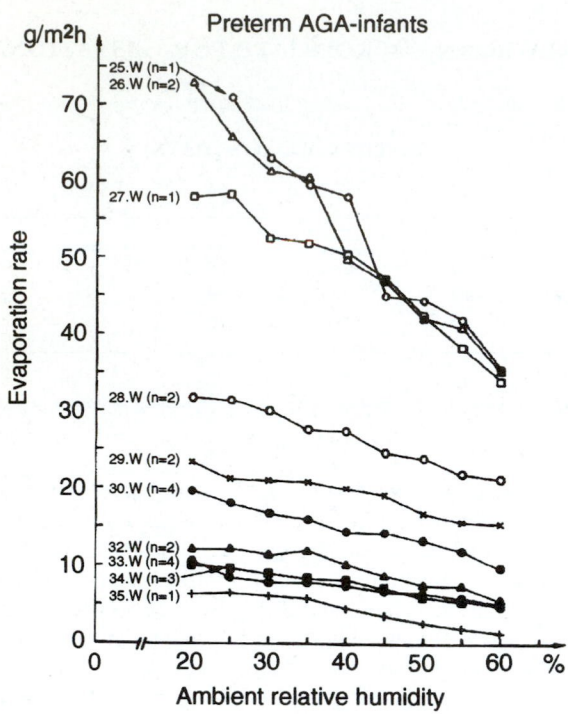

FIGURE 2-30 **The relation between evaporation rate and ambient relative humidity in preterm appropriate-for-gestational-age, newborn infants in different gestational age groups on first day after birth. w = completed weeks of gestation.** SOURCE: *Hammarlund K, Sedin G: Transepidermal water loss in newborn infants. III. Relation to gestational age. Acta Paediatr Scand 68:795, 1979.*

Water losses through the gastrointestinal tract are usually minimal during the first 1 to 2 days after birth. When enteral feedings begin, stool output may increase considerably, especially in preterm infants who receive their mother's breast milk, in which case fluid losses per rectum must be considered in assessing daily water and electrolyte needs.

KIDNEY FUNCTION AND EXCRETION OF WATER AND SALT

Renal blood flow and glomerular filtration rate (GFR) are considerably less in small preterm infants than they are in term infants. Thus, plasma creatinine concentrations are greater in preterm than term infants. GFR correlates better with postconceptional age than with postnatal age in preterm infants who are born at less than 34 weeks of gestation. Beyond 34 weeks of gestation, GFR increases rapidly in the first week (nephrogenesis is complete at about 34 weeks of gestation), whereas the postnatal increase of GFR is less in infants who were born earlier than 34 weeks of gestation. At 26 to 28 weeks of gestation, urine output averages about 1 mL/kg body weight on the first day and increases to about 3 to 4 mL/kg body weight by the third to fourth day after birth. Several conditions reduce urine output: hypoxia, hypercapnia, hypovolemia, low renal perfusion (a large patent ductus arteriosus, sepsis), indomethacin treatment, and mechanical ventilation. Plasma concentrations of vasopressin, renin, and aldosterone are high in newborn infants, especially in those who are stressed by asphyxia or severe lung disease, and this may contribute to a low urine output.

The concentration of sodium in urine of preterm infants is high during the first week after birth, as excess extracellular fluid is ex-

creted. Thereafter, urine sodium concentration reflects intake and averages 1 to 2 mEq/100 mL of urine at a daily sodium intake of about 2 mEq/kg body weight. Fractional excretion of sodium is greater in preterm than in term infants, as there is more extracellular water and sodium to be excreted postnatally in the preterm infant.

Preterm infants generally have difficulty excreting excess salt, as salt-containing solutions tend to leave the circulation quickly and cause edema. Small preterm infants, however, are sometimes unable to conserve sodium despite a low serum sodium concentration. This situation may develop after asphyxia or in the presence of a large patent ductus arteriosus with resultant reduction of renal blood flow and diminished tubular reabsorption of sodium. High concentrations of circulating atrial natriuretic factor in preterm infants also may contribute to salt loss. Preterm infants have higher fractional sodium excretion rates than term infants have. Urinary sodium excretion generally decreases after the first week in both preterm and term infants. High urine sodium losses may lead to hyponatremia if water intake is high.

The newborn kidney is better equipped to excrete a water load than a salt load; that is, it dilutes more effectively than it concentrates. The maximum concentrating capacity of the preterm kidney is such that urine osmolality does not exceed 400 mOsm/L in the first week, increasing to 600 to 700 mOsm/L by 4 to 6 weeks after birth (adults can achieve a urine osmolality of 1200 mOsm/L). Diluting capacity of the preterm kidney is at least equivalent to that of the adult kidney, such that urine osmolality may decrease to 30 to 50 mOsm/L.

2.12.3 Assessment of Water and Salt Balance in Preterm Infants

The most reliable means of assessing water balance in babies is frequent, accurate measurement of body weight on a platform balance kept beneath the infant's mattress. Less sensitive methods for evaluating fluid balance include measurement of hematocrit, plasma protein concentration, urine output, urine specific gravity, and serum concentrations of sodium, creatinine, and urea nitrogen. The most reliable means for assessing sodium balance is frequent measurement of body weight coupled with periodic (every 6–24 hours if the infant is sick, every 3–7 days if the infant seems well) measurements of serum sodium, in addition to monitoring urine volume and urine concentrations of sodium. Some of the problems that have been associated with excessive intake of water and salt include respiratory distress from pulmonary edema, patent ductus arteriosus, chronic lung disease, necrotizing enterocolitis and abnormal serum concentrations of electrolytes. Problems associated with too little intake of water and salt include hypotension, poor perfusion of the kidneys and intestinal tract, sometimes leading to renal failure or bowel ischemia, growth failure, and abnormal serum concentrations of electrolytes.

2.12.4 Supply of Fluids and Electrolytes to Very Premature Infants

To estimate anticipated water losses, several items need to be considered: gestational age and body weight; postnatal age; ambient temperature, humidity, and air movement; use of a radiant warmer versus incubator; use of phototherapy; preexisting or ongoing stress; use of assisted ventilation (temperature of inspired gas and effectiveness of its humidification); use of drugs that may affect the circulation and kidney function; caloric intake (oxidative metabolism produces water, 5–10 g/kg body weight); and growth status (approximately 20–30 g of water and 0.5 mEq of NaCl are needed daily for growth).

The need for fluids and electrolytes in very premature infants depends greatly on the environment in which the infant is nursed. In a humid environment, the insensible water loss is low, and the supply of fluid can be adjusted accordingly. In most preterm infants, approximately 65 to 90 mL/kg intake usually suffices during the first few days after birth. As noted above, body weight normally decreases during this period. Infants who are extremely premature and who are nursed in an environment with low humidity have a much higher insensible water loss that needs to be compensated by a larger fluid intake. Such management may result in complications, such as a patent ductus arteriosus, necrotizing enterocolitis, and pulmonary and generalized edema. It is usually not necessary to add either sodium or potassium to the fluids that are administered to the very premature infant during the first few days after birth. Thereafter, sodium and potassium intake need to be adjusted according to urinary losses of these electrolytes plus a small additional amount to provide for normal growth. The usual requirements for sodium and potassium after the first week are 2 to 3 mmol/kg/d.

EARLY POSTNATAL HYPERKALEMIA IN EXTREMELY PRETERM INFANTS

With the recent increase in survival of extremely immature (<26 weeks of gestation) infants, hyperkalemia has become a frequent, life-threatening condition, especially among infants who are nursed in a non-humidified environment. Recent reports indicate that between one-third and one-half of these extremely premature, low birthweight infants have serum potassium concentrations greater than 6.7 mmol/L, often associated with electrocardiographic dysrhythmias. Serum potassium concentrations in these infants generally peak between 12 and 72 hours after birth. The disorder, which can be lethal, reflects both a shift of potassium from the intracellular to the extracellular space and a very low GFR, which limits urinary potassium excretion.

Conditions that may affect extracellular potassium concentration include hypocalcemia, acidosis, hemolysis, blood transfusions, hemorrhage, tissue injury and adrenal insufficiency, all of which are associated with extreme preterm birth and perinatal asphyxia. One study showed that erythrocyte Na,K-ATPase activity and intracellular potassium concentrations were less in extremely preterm infants with hyperkalemia compared to infants without hyperkalemia. If this finding reflects a generalized decrease in cell Na,K-ATPase activity in such infants, this could contribute to the development of postnatal hyperkalemia.

Several treatment strategies have been advocated to manage this condition, including correction of existing acidosis or hypocalcemia, intravenous infusion of glucose and insulin to drive potassium into cells, and administration of either cortisol or β2-adrenergic agents, such as salbutamol, which have been shown to increase Na,K-ATPase activity under a variety of experimental conditions.

2.12.5   Types of Fluid for Intravenous and Enteral Nutrition

In order to provide sufficient energy for normal body function of very premature infants, it is necessary to administer glucose soon after birth, with addition of amino acids and lipid thereafter. In some instances, glucose infusion may lead to glucosuria and osmotic diuresis, in which case the glucose concentration of the intravenous fluids being administered should be reduced. In most infants who are born very prematurely but who are not sick, small feedings of breast milk (0.5–1.5 mL/kg every 2 to 3 hours) can be initiated through a gastric tube within a few hours after birth. The volume of breast milk that is given every 2 to 3 hours can be increased to 1 to 2 mL/kg on the second day and 2 to 4 mL/kg on the third day, provided that there is no gastric retention of feedings. The volume of feedings should gradually be increased until sufficient nutrients and energy are supplied. The target for caloric intake is approximately 60 to 80 kcal/kg/d by the fifth postnatal day and approximately 100 to 120 kcal/kg by 7 to 10 days.

In addition to the gradual increase of enteral feedings, intravenous infusion of increasing amounts of amino acids and lipid emulsion can be started within the first 24 hours after birth, with careful monitoring of blood glucose concentration, plasma turbidity, and acid-base status. If an infant has been on assisted ventilation, feedings are often withheld for several hours after extubation to lessen the possibility of aspiration, and during this time the entire supply of fluid and nutrients must be given intravenously. In the very tiny preterm infant, this is often achieved by insertion of a central venous catheter through a peripheral venous site. It is important to provide adequate nutrition to very premature infants and to avoid unnecessary heat loss from the body surface. When partial or total parenteral nutrition is given, it is essential to include not only glucose, amino acids, and fat emulsion, but also trace minerals and vitamins.

2.12.6   Appropriate Environment for Very Premature Infants

Because evaporation of fluid from the body surface results in heat loss, which in turn may cause hypothermia and increase caloric needs, it is important to gently remove amniotic fluid from the infant's skin with a warm towel soon after birth. Thereafter, the infant should be nursed in an incubator or under a radiant warmer beneath a plastic shield to maintain a neutral thermal environment and thereby minimize energy requirements and facilitate growth.

Heat exchange between the preterm infant and the environment occurs primarily through the skin and to a lesser degree through the respiratory tract. Heat exchange through the skin takes place through conduction, evaporation, radiation, and convection. The magnitude of heat exchange depends on the body surface area of the infant, and the temperature of nearby surfaces (radiant heat exchange), environmental air (convective heat exchange), and in direct contact with the skin (conductive heat exchange). During the first day after birth, evaporative loss of heat is high in very premature infants who are not nursed in a humid environment. Evaporative heat loss is inversely related to the ambient relative humidity. In an incubator, the radiant heat exchange is low because of the warm inner surface of the incubator walls, such that preterm infants may gain heat through convection within an incubator.

2.12.7   Stress Reduction in the Care of Very Preterm Infant

In the past decade or so, considerable effort has been directed at stress reduction in the management of infants who are born very prematurely. There is considerable interest in avoiding procedures that are uncomfortable or painful, and methods have been developed for controlling or modifying external stimuli such as bright light and loud noise. In addition, care activities are clustered to minimize sleep disturbance, and tiny infants are positioned and swaddled for comfort. These approaches have made it possible to provide a more nurturing environment for the infant, with the expectation that less stress will facilitate well-being and better growth.

Involvement of parents in the care of their infant is important for the family, particularly with respect to bonding and preparation for home care. Parents should be well informed about the condition of their infant and about the ongoing care and expectations for the future. Parents need to be familiar with their infant's behavioral states and reactions when they approach, touch, or talk to their infant. If the infant is stable, most caregivers agree that skin-to-skin contact between infant and parent is beneficial. If an infant does not require assisted ventilation, it is often recommended that contact with the mother's breast and taste of the mother's milk may improve subsequent nursing. Even some of the smallest infants show rooting and suckling behavior, and spontaneous intake of small amounts of breast milk may be possible as early as 30 weeks postconception.

2.12.8   Transport and Handling of Preterm Infants

The outcome of a preterm delivery is greatly dependent on the quality of the care that the infant receives soon after birth. Thus, in utero transport of the fetus to a tertiary perinatal unit that can offer the most comprehensive and evidence-based neonatal intensive care for every preterm infant and other infants at risk offers the best chance for an excellent outcome. There are many situations, however, that preclude in utero fetal transport, and therefore, it is essential to provide optimal management at the referring hospital and during transport to the neonatal intensive care unit.

Communication between referring physician and the admitting physician at the NICU is extremely important in order to assure proper attention to potential problems at the referring institution. Transport personnel should have considerable experience in neonatal intensive care and be able to monitor the health condition of the infant and adjust mechanical ventilation, administration of fluids, nutrients, and drugs as deemed appropriate during the journey. Parents should be well informed about the infant's condition and understand why the infant needs care that can be provided only at a different hospital.

Stabilization of the infant before transport from the referring hospital to the NICU should include maintenance of a neutral thermal environment, close monitoring of vital signs and oxygenation, and if respiration is insufficient, the infant should receive mechanical ventilation through an endotracheal tube during transport. If possible, the infant should have a normal arterial pH, PaO_2, and $PaCO_2$ and be in stable condition when the transport begins. Before transport, the infant should be moved to a preheated incubator equipped with a respirator, humidifier, oxygen, and compressed air. Devices for suction and monitoring of vital functions, preparation of drugs that might be needed during transport, and equipment for manual ventilation should accompany the infant. During transport, the infant must be securely positioned away from the incubator walls, and equipment must be available for monitoring heart rate, respiratory rate, ECG tracing, oxygen saturation, and blood

pressure. Careful attention to the fluid volume administered during transport is essential.

2.12.9   Nosocomial Infections and Hygienic Measures

Infections that occur at a postnatal age of 3 days or more are considered to be acquired in the nursery and are termed nosocomial. The incidence of nosocomial infections is much higher in extremely preterm infants than in more mature infants. Progression of disease is often more rapid and life-threatening in the very premature infant. Whereas infections often appear first on the skin or around the umbilicus in more mature infants, infections in extremely preterm infants commonly present as respiratory failure or as generalized sepsis with shock.

Nosocomial infections in a nursery are a major cause of morbidity and mortality. They prolong the duration and cost of care and result in frequent use of antibiotics, which increases the risk of later colonization with bacteria that are resistant to many of the usual antimicrobial therapies. At present, colonization with methicillin-resistant *Staphylococcus aureus* poses a major threat in many NICUs. Previously published studies on the variables that influence the incidence of nosocomial infection indicate that basic care of the skin and umbilicus is critical in controlling neonatal infection. Most nosocomial infections derive from transmission of bacteria via the hands of hospital staff or parents. Understaffing, overcrowding, and poor hygienic practices are also considered to increase the risk of nosocomial infections. To reduce the risk of such infections, strict routines regarding hand-washing, invasive procedures, and sterilization of equipment should be an important aspect of the NICU policy. The infant and materials close to the infant, such as electrodes, catheters, endotracheal tubes, diapers, and blankets, should be touched only with hands that are clean or covered with protective gloves. Before entering the NICU, jewelry should be removed from the hands and arms, which should then be carefully washed with soap and water and disinfected with an appropriate antiseptic agent.

The use of gowns is controversial. A gown is worn to prevent soiling of clothing and thus to reduce the likelihood of transferring organisms from patient to patient. Therefore, each gown should be restricted to use with a specific patient. Sterile technique is essential for all invasive procedures, and indwelling vascular catheters must be properly dressed with antiseptic technique daily. In order to prevent or decrease communicable infections, visitors other than parents and grandparents should be discouraged.

References

Ågren J, Sjörs G, Sedin G: Transepidermal water loss in infants born at 24 and 25 weeks of gestation. Acta Paediatr 87:1185–1190, 1998

Baley JE, Fanaroff AA: Neonatal infections, Part 1: Infection related to nursery care practices. In: Sinclair JC, Bracken MB, eds: Effective Care of the Newborn Infant. Oxford University Press, 1992:474–476

Bauer K, Bovermann G, Roithmaier A, et al: Body composition, nutrition, and fluid balance during the first two weeks of life in preterm neonates weighing less than 1500 grams. J Pediatr 118(4):615–620, 1991

Beckwith JB: Extreme cytomegaly of the adrenal fetal cortex, omphalocele, hyperplasia of kidneys and pancreas and Leydig cell hyperplasiac. Another syndrome? Proc West Soc Pediatr Res Los Angeles, Western Society for Pediatric Research, 1963

Bell EF, Warburton D, Stonestreet BS, et al: Effect of fluid administration on the development of symptomatic patent arteriosus and congestive heart failure in premature infants. N Engl J Med 302:598–604, 1980

Boyce JM, Kelliher S, Vallande N: Skin irritation and dryness associated with two hand-hygiene regimes: soap-and-water hand washing versus hand antisepsis with an alcoholic hand gel. Infect Control Hosp Epidemiol 21:442–448, 2000

Fisher DA: Thyroid function in premature infants. The hypothyroxinemia of prematurity. Clin Perinatol 25:999–1014, 1998

Fries-Hansen B: Changes in body water compartments during growth. Acta Paediatr Scand [Suppl] 110, 1956

Hammarlund K, Sedin G: Transepidermal water loss in newborn infants. III. Relation to gestational age. Acta Paediatr Scand 68:795–801, 1979

Hammarlund K, Sedin G, Strömberg B: Transepidermal water loss in newborn infants. VIII. Relation to gestational age and post-natal age in appropriate and small for gestational age infants. Acta Paediatr Scand 72:721–728, 1983

Harpin VA, Rutter N: Development of emotional sweating in the newborn infant. Arch Dis Child 57:691–695, 1982

Hawdon JM, Ward Platt MP, Aynsley-Green A: Patterns of metabolic adaptation for preterm and term infants in the first neonatal week. Arch Dis Child 67:357–365, 1992

Hedberg Nyqvist K, Sjödén P-O, Ewald U: The development of preterm infant's breast feeding behavior. Early Hum Dev 55:247–264, 1999

Herin P, Aperia A: Neonatal kidney, fluids, and electrolytes. Curr Opin Pediatr 6:154–157, 1994

Meetze W, Bowsher R, Compton J, et al: Hyperglycemia in extremely-low-birth-weight infants. Biol Neonate 74:214–221, 1998

Sedin G: Fluid management in the extremely preterm infant. In: Hansen TN, McIntosh N, eds: Current Topics In Neonatology, No. 1. London, WB Saunders, 1996

Sedin G: Physics and physiology of human neonatal incubation. In: Polim R, Fox W, eds: Fetal and Neonatal Physiology. Chapter 69, p 702–715. Philadelphia, WB Saunders, 1997:702–715

Sedin G, Agostino R, Chabernaud J-L, et al: Technical aspects of neonatal transport in Europe. Prenat Neonat Med 4(Suppl 1):35–45, 1999

Sedin G, Hammarlund K, Nilsson GE, et al: Measurements of transepidermal water loss in newborn infants. Clin Perinatol 12:79–99, 1985

Symington A, Pinelli J: Developmental care for promoting development and preventing morbidity in preterm infants (Cochrane Review). In: The Cochrane Library, Issue 4, 2000

Thornton PS, Satin-Smith MS, Herold K, et al: Familial hyperinsulinism with apparent autosomal dominant inheritance: clinical and genetic differences from the autosomal recessive variant. J Pediatr 132:9–14, 1998

Zimmerman D: Fetal and neonatal hyperthyroidism. Thyroid 9:727–733, 1999

2.13 MULTIPLE BIRTHS

W. Alan Hodson

In recent years there has been a marked increase in the incidence of multiple births, and this has contributed significantly to the risk of prematurity and its associated medical problems. Multiple births account for a disproportionate number of newborn infants who require special care. The risk of abnormality is increased in proportion to the number of multiple births. The major risk is prematurity, although there is an increased chance of misadventure during delivery. Other serious problems may arise before delivery as a result of the increased incidence of congenital malformations, twin-to-twin transfusions, and intrauterine growth restriction (IUGR), with one twin usually affected more than the other. The neonatal mortality is increased by five- to sixfold, and fetal mortality rises with the increase in number of fetuses. A common issue with twins is whether they are identical or fraternal. This determination, although not always easy, is of intense interest to the parents and important for medical management of the infants if one or both have an abnormality and to possible organ transplantation in the future.

Fortunately, multiple births are rarely a surprise, as 90% are diagnosed prenatally. Prenatal information is of immense benefit in anticipating delivery room or subsequent neonatal problems. The antenatal diagnosis of multiple births should be communicated to the pediatrician, and any prenatal concerns should dictate the presence of a pediatrician or neonatologist at the delivery. The ultrasound detection of two separate placental masses or the presence of different sexes indicates dichorionic placentation. If the placentas are joined and the twins are the same sex, determination is more difficult. It is possible to determine the thickness and number of layers of the dividing membrane by ultrasound examination. Postnatal study of the placenta and blood group typing are useful in determining zygocity. It is helpful if zygosity is determined prenatally as either monochorionic or dichorionic (separate or fused), diamnionic monochorionic or monoamnionic monochorionic (Fig. 2-31). Absolute confirmation of zygocity requires DNA analysis.

EPIDEMIOLOGY

The incidence of twin births has increased significantly over the past three decades in the United States from approximately one in 80 pregnancies to one in 43, with a threefold increase in higher-order multiple births. Triplets occur at a rate of one in 13,410 pregnancies. Assisted reproduction and advanced maternal age have resulted in an increase in multiple pregnancies. Over the past decade the twinning rate, primarily in dizygous twins, has increased approximately 63% for women between 40 and 44 years and 100% for women between 45 and 49 years of age. The rate of monozygous twinning has remained constant around the world and has not changed with advancing age or parity. Of relevance to the pediatrician is that 3% of all births are multiple, and the majority of these are born preterm or low birth weight. Multiple births account for approximately one-third of all admissions to a neonatal special care unit and 16% of all neonatal deaths.

PRENATAL ASSESSMENT

The pediatrician should be aware of the increased incidence of complications of pregnancy, particularly as they affect the newborn infant. These complications include a 20 to 50% incidence of premature labor, a slight increase in premature rupture of the membranes, pregnancy-induced hypertension, placenta previa, and polyhydramnios. Polyhydramnios is associated with increased perinatal mortality and fetal abnormalities and often leads to premature delivery.

Assessment of fetal growth by ultrasound should begin at about 18 to 20 weeks and should occur every 3 to 4 weeks thereafter. The ultrasound evaluations will also determine growth discordances between twins, abnormal amniotic fluid volume, and structural abnormalities. Estimated fetal weight and abdominal circumference continue to be the most reliable predictors of discordant growth. Discordance of twin size, which may indicate an abnormality such as congenital malformation or twin-to-twin transfusion, requires frequent ultrasound monitoring throughout pregnancy.

NEONATAL PROBLEMS

Multiple births increase the risk for delivery room complications; hence, the possibility for resuscitation should be anticipated with

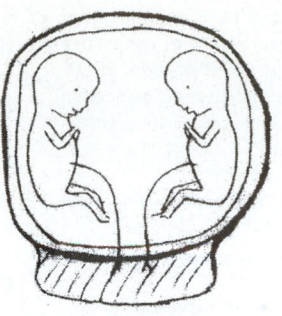
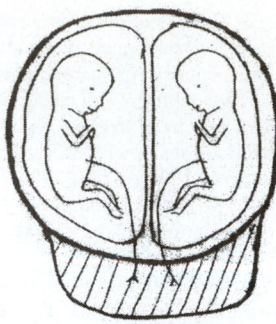

monochorionic
monoamniotic

monochorionic
diamniotic

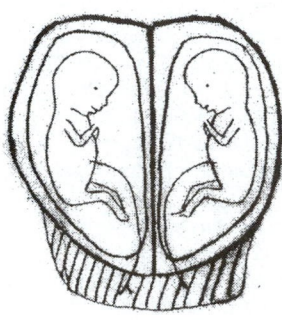
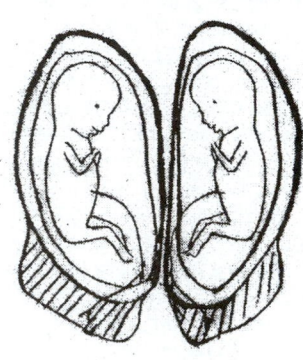

dichorionic
diamniotic

dichorionic
diamniotic
diplacentae

FIGURE 2-31 **Possible twin placentations.**

the presence of appropriate personnel. Delivery room complications include malpresentation, umbilical cord compression, placental abruption, congenital malformations, and prematurity. Approximately 80% of twin pregnancies will result in a vertex position of twin A; however, approximately 50% of twins and 75% of triplets are delivered by cesarean section, with malpresentation the major reason. Fetal lung maturity is tested from amniotic fluid obtained from the nonpresenting or least stressed fetus and should aid in the timing of elective cesarean section. If neither twin is stressed, lung maturation is comparable to that in singleton fetuses at the same gestational age. The risk for respiratory distress, necrotizing enterocolitis, and other problems of prematurity are the same as gestational age–matched controls for singletons. Although problems at birth are decreased by cesarean section, the high incidence of prematurity accounts for the increased risk of delivery room problems in twins. Monoamniotic twins are at extremely high risk for cord entanglement, require intense fetal surveillance, and often must be delivered prematurely to avoid fatal cord occlusion.

CONGENITAL MALFORMATIONS

Both congenital malformations and deformations are more common in twins than in singletons. Almost all twins will have some deformational or positional deformity associated with in utero crowding; the lower extremities are most often affected, and plagiocephaly is also common among twins. Monozygous twins have an estimated risk of 6 to 10% for congenital malformations compared to approximately 2% for singletons. The perinatal mortality rate is markedly higher in the structurally abnormal twin than in the unaffected twin. Malformation should be suspected in the

presence of polyhydramnios or fetal growth retardation. Monochorionic twinning is associated with an increased incidence of anencephaly, hydranencephaly, omphalocele, gastrointestinal abnormalities, congenital heart disease, and associated multiple organ (vertebral, cardiac, esophageal, renal) anomalies. Thromboembolic events in monozygous twins may be responsible for CNS abnormalities, limb amputations, intestinal atresia, cardiac malformations, and aplasia cutis, raising an important question of genetic versus environmental causation of the increased incidence of anomalies.

CONJOINED TWINS

Conjoined twins occur in about one in 50,000 births. This abnormality occurs in monoamniotic, monochorionic twins during the third week of gestation as a result of failure of separation in a monozygous twin. The most common fusion sites are the chest and abdomen and, more rarely, the pelvis or the head. Serial ultrasound or MRI studies of the fetus are useful for predicting viability after birth and for determining the feasibility of surgical separation to save one or both twins. Viability and long-term outcome depend largely on the number and extent of shared organs and anomalies.

TWIN-TO-TWIN TRANSFUSION

Transfer of blood between twins occurs through arterial-to-venous connections within a monochorionic placenta. Unidirectional flow may lead to polycythemia, heart failure, hydrops, and polyhydramnios in the recipient twin and anemia, hypovolemia, growth retardation, and oligohydramnios in the donor twin. The diagnosis should be suspected prenatally by ultrasound detection in monochorionic twinning of growth discordance and difference in amniotic fluid volume. Twin-to-twin transfusion syndrome (TTTS) accounts for some cases of a "trapped" or "stuck" twin wherein one twin has a small volume of amniotic fluid, restricted growth and mobility, and often a congenital malformation. There is a poor prognosis if one twin has oligohydramnios detected before 26 weeks of gestation. Efforts to ablate the cross circulation by laser photocoagulation or vascular clipping under fiberoptic vision are under investigation at a number of perinatal centers. The efficacy of these procedures remains unproven. The pediatrician should be involved at delivery regarding the immediate management of hemodynamic problems, including hydrops or severe anemia and hypovolemia. Preterm delivery is almost always necessary to increase neonatal survival of twins with this condition. Oligohydramnios may indicate decreased urine output, ruptured amnion, or growth retardation. Polyhydramnios may also be associated with a neural tube defect, upper gastrointestinal obstruction, or hydrops.

FETAL GROWTH RESTRICTION

There is an increased incidence of fetal growth restriction among twins, and this may be associated with increased neonatal mortality. The growth rate of twins diverges from that of singletons after 30 weeks and becomes linear in contrast to the accelerated pattern of singletons. Triplets also maintain a linear growth pattern throughout the third trimester. The average gestational age is approximately 37 weeks for twins with a birth weight of 2,400 g. Significant intrauterine growth restriction (IUGR) in twins usually affects only one infant. IUGR in twins is generally defined as a birth weight more than 10% below that of a similar gestation singleton. Discordance of growth, which is more common in monochorionic twins, has been defined as a difference greater than 20% in weight at birth. Discordance greater than 20% is not a risk factor if the smaller twin is above 2500 g at birth. Serial measurements of femur length, biparietal diameter, head circumference, abdominal circumference, and amniotic fluid volume of each fetus are more helpful than differences between them. The causes of growth restriction or discordance include limited or abnormal placentation (decreased vascular supply), crowding, twin-to-twin transfusion, and congenital anomalies. Growth retardation is associated with a number of neonatal and possibly longer-term problems (see Sec. 2.14).

PREMATURITY

Prematurity is the most common complication of multiple births; morbidity is similar to that for singletons born prematurely. If twins with known fetal anomalies or twin-to-twin transfusion are excluded, there are no differences in Apgar scores, perinatal mortality, respiratory distress syndrome, intracranial hemorrhage, or necrotizing enterocolitis between twins and singletons of the same gestation. Respiratory distress syndrome occurs more frequently and with greater severity in the second twin. Twin pregnancies have an increased maternal risk of premature rupture of membranes (PROM), which is associated with an increased risk of neonatal sepsis. The risk for hypoglycemia is also increased in twins and is unrelated to growth restriction. There is no evidence that the in utero maturation of twins is different from that of singletons.

TRIPLETS

Triplets have about an 85% risk of premature birth with a mean birth weight of 1700 g. Intrauterine growth restriction in one fetus is more likely in triplets than in twins (67% vs 13%). Discordance in growth also occurs in about two-thirds of triplet pregnancies. Maternal complications are also increased, most notably premature labor and toxemia. Lethal congenital anomalies are more common in triplets delivered between 24 and 34 weeks of gestation than in twins or singletons. There is an increased incidence of retinopathy of prematurity among triplets compared to twins and singletons born at the same gestational age.

References

Benirschke K: The biology of the twinning process: how placentation influences outcome. Semin Perinatol 19:342, 1995

Gardner MO, Goldenberg RL, Cliver SP, Tucker JM, Nelson KG, Copper RL: The origin and outcome of preterm twin pregnancies. Obstet Gynecol 85:553, 1995

Guyer B, Hoyert DL, Martin JA, Ventura SJ, MacDorman MF, Strobino DM: Annual summary of vital statistics—1998. Pediatrics 104:1229, 1999

Jewell SE, Yip R: Increasing trends in plural births in the United States. Obstet Gynecol 85:229, 1995

Jones JS, Newman RB, Miller MC: Cross-sectional analysis of triplet birth weight. Am J Obstet Gynecol 164:135, 1991

Kaufman GE, Malone FD, Harvey-Wilkes KB, Chelmow D, Penzias AS, D'Alton ME: Neonatal morbidity and mortality associated with triplet pregnancy. Obstet Gynecol 91:342, 1998

Kilpatrick SJ, Jackson R, Croughan-Minihane MS: Perinatal mortality in twins and singletons matched for gestational age at delivery at > or = 30 weeks. Am J Obstet Gynecol 174:66, 1996

Luke B, Keith LG: Monozygotic twinning as a congenital defect and congenital defects in monozygotic twins. Fetal Diagn Ther 5:61, 1990

Martin JA, Park MM: Trends in twin and triplet births: 1980–97. Natl Vital Stat Rep 47, 1999

Milner R, Crombleholme TM: Troubles with twins: fetoscopic therapy. Semin Perinatol 23:474, 1999

Moise J, Laor A, Armon Y, Gur I, Gale R: The outcome of twin pregnancies after IVF. Hum Reprod 13:1702, 1998

Sassoon DA, Castro LC, Davis JL, Hobel CJ: Perinatal outcome in triplet versus twin gestations. Obstet Gynecol 75:817, 1990

Wennerholm UB, Hamberger L, Nilsson L, Wennergren M, Wikland M, Bergh C: Obstetric and perinatal outcome of children received from cryopreserved embryos. Hum Reprod 12:1819, 1997

Wolf EJ, Vintzileos AM, Rosenkrantz TS, Rodis JF, Lettieri L, Mallozzi A: A comparison of pre-discharge survival and morbidity in singleton and twin very low birth weight infants. Obstet Gynecol 80:436, 1992

2.14   THE SMALL-FOR-GESTATIONAL-AGE INFANT

William W. Hay, Jr.

DEFINITIONS AND INCIDENCE

SMALL FOR GESTATIONAL AGE Newborn infants are classified according to birth weight as small, average, or large for gestational age (Table 2-14). Small-for-gestational-age (SGA) infants are a heterogeneous group of infants who are smaller than normal at birth because of genetic or constitutional conditions, diseases, or nutrient insufficiency. SGA infants have a birth weight less than the 10th percentile of a population-specific birth weight versus gestational age relationship. Broader definitions include less-than-normal

TABLE 2-14

CLASSIFICATION OF FETAL GROWTH

SGA. small for gestational age; birth weight <10th percentile for gestational age

AGA. average for gestational age; birth weight >10th, <90th percentile for gestational age

LGA. large for gestational age; birth weight >90th percentile for gestational age

IUGR (intrauterine growth restriction). slower than normal rate of fetal growth

Normal birth weight. greater than 2500 at term

Low birth weight. LBW, less than 2500 at birth

Very low birth weight. VLBW, less than 1500 g at birth

Extremely low birth weight. ELBW, less than 1000 at birth

---

lengths and head circumferences and marked discrepancies between different growth parameters even within the normal range, eg, weight at 25th percentile but length and head circumference at 75th percentile. In the latter case, the weight/length ratio [or the ponderal index = (weight, g) / (length, cm)^3] is less than normal, indicating that growth rates of visceral organs, adipose tissue, and skeletal muscle, the principal determinants of weight, are less than that of length. A low weight/length ratio is important in defining those infants with late gestation nutritional deficiency, which is usually a result of placental insufficiency.

INTRAUTERINE GROWTH RESTRICTION   Intrauterine growth restriction (IUGR) is defined as a rate of fetal growth that is less than normal for the population and for the growth potential of a specific infant. IUGR, therefore, produces infants who are SGA. Constitutionally small SGA infants are normal infants who are born after slower than average rates of fetal growth; such infants usually have small parents, particularly a small mother. SGA infants also are born after abnormally slow fetal growth that is caused by pathophysiological conditions. Nearly any aberration of biological activity in the placenta and/or fetus can lead to fetal growth failure. Moderately and severely IUGR infants tend to have asymmetric growth restriction; ie, body growth restriction is greater than brain growth restriction, though to varying degrees depending on the duration and severity of the growth inhibition. Constitutionally small infants tend to have symmetrically restricted brain and body growth. Asymmetric and symmetric growth restriction therefore represent extreme patterns of abnormally slow fetal growth rates.

LOW BIRTH WEIGHT   Most infants with low birth weights (see Table 2-14 for definitions) are the result of a shorter than normal gestation; ie, they are preterm. Also, a large fraction of preterm infants are growth restricted. Thus, low birth weight does not determine gestational age at any stage of prenatal development.

ETIOLOGY

Intrinsic abnormalities in the fetus usually cause symmetric growth restriction and begin early in fetal life, whereas the onset of extrinsic adverse factors, such as undernutrition or hypoxia from placental insufficiency, which usually cause asymmetric growth, develop at variable times during gestation. Abnormalities that limit the growth of both the fetal brain and body include chromosomal anomalies (particularly trisomy conditions), congenital infections (eg, toxoplasmosis, rubella, and cytomegalovirus), dwarf syndromes, some inborn errors of metabolism, and some drugs (maternal smoking

and excessive alcohol consumption). The mechanisms by which these abnormalities limit fetal growth are multifactoral. Most other cases of fetal growth restriction are the result of a small or poorly functioning placenta (Table 2-15). Small placentas can result from natural conditions such as a small mother with a small uterus or multiple fetuses or abnormal conditions such as uterine structural abnormalities or preeclampsia.

EPIDEMIOLOGY AND INTERPRETATION OF GROWTH CURVES

NEONATAL GROWTH CURVES   Cross-sectional growth curves have been developed from anthropometric measurements in populations of infants born at different gestational ages. Such curves have been used to demonstrate whether an infant's weight is within the normal range for a given gestational age and thus to estimate whether that infant's in utero growth was greater or less than normal. Each curve is based on local populations with variable composition of maternal age, parity, socioeconomic status, race, ethnic background, body size, degree of obesity or thinness, health, pregnancy-related problems, and nutrition as well as the number of fetuses per mother, the number of infants included in the study, and by what methods and how accurately measurements of body size and gestational age are made. Estimating gestational age has considerable error, derived from variability in dating conception, the physical features of maturation in the infant, and interobserver differences in assessment of an infant's developmental stage.

FETAL GROWTH CURVES

Fetal growth curves have been developed from serial ultrasound measurements of fetuses who subsequently were born at term in healthy condition and with normal anthropometric measurements, providing longitudinal indices of fetal growth. Serial ultrasound measurements of fetal growth more accurately determine how environmental factors, such as severe maternal illness and undernutrition, inhibit fetal growth and are useful as a clinical tool to assess ongoing fetal growth.

TABLE 2-15

PLACENTAL GROWTH DISORDERS THAT LEAD TO OR ARE ASSOCIATED WITH IUGR

Abnormal umbilical vascular insertions (circumvallate, velamentous)

Abruption (chronic, partial)

Avascular villi

Decidual arteritis

Fibrinosis, atheromatous changes

Cytotrophoblast hyperplasia, basement membrane thickening

Infectious villitis

Ischemic villous necrosis and umbilical vascular thromboses; multiple infarcts

Multiple gestation (limited endometrial surface area, vascular anastomoses)

Partial molar pregnancy

Placenta previa

Single umbilical artery

Spiral artery vasculitis, failed or limited erosion into intervillous space

Syncytial knots

Tumors including chorioangioma and hemangiomas

IUGR = intrauterine growth restriction.

PATHOPHYSIOLOGY: GROWTH OF BODY COMPONENTS IN THE FETUS

NITROGEN AND PROTEIN ACCRETION IN SGA INFANTS Nitrogen and protein contents are reduced for body weight in SGA infants, primarily from deficient production of muscle mass. In fact, they often are reduced below that of fat as a fraction of body weight, even when growth restriction is moderate.

GLYCOGEN DEFICIENCY IN SGA INFANTS Glycogen content is markedly reduced, particularly in the liver and in skeletal muscle, in SGA infants who have had IUGR. Glycogen deficiency in IUGR fetuses results from low fetal glucose and insulin concentrations, which are the principal regulators of glycogen synthesis. Repeated episodes of hypoxemia that increase epinephrine secretion deplete glycogen further by activating glycogen phosphorylase and increasing glycogenolysis.

ADIPOSE TISSUE DEFICIENCY IN SGA INFANTS Fat content in human fetuses with IUGR may be less than 10% of body weight at term gestation or 30 to 40% less than normal. This usually results from a smaller than normal placenta, which limits fetal fatty acid and triglyceride supply to the fetus and decreases fetal glucose and insulin concentrations. These deficiencies reduce glycerol production, triglyceride synthesis, and fat production. Growth of fat and of nonfat (primarily muscle) tissues are metabolically linked through energy supply, which is necessary for protein synthesis, and production of anabolic hormones as well as fat production. Thus, restriction of nutrient supply restricts growth of all tissues, not just fat.

2.14.1 Antenatal Evaluation of the IUGR Fetus

Serial ultrasound evaluation of growth of fetal body proportions and Doppler velocimetry assessment of uterine, placental, and fetal circulations are the standard diagnostic approaches used to determine the severity of IUGR, detect deteriorating fetal physical condition, and predict impending fetal death. Chronic fetal distress resulting from placental insufficiency, hypoxia, and ischemia, with or without acidosis, is associated with increased Doppler arterial waveform amplitudes in the fetal peripheral vasculature that indicate increased vascular resistance and reduced blood flow to fetal tissues and the placenta. Various ratios of systolic to diastolic flow velocity (amplitude) waveforms have been used to detect decreased peripheral blood flow in the fetus, including the systolic-to-diastolic ratio, (systolic − diastolic)/systolic ratio (resistance index), or (systolic − diastolic)/mean ratio (pulsatility index). The most severely affected IUGR fetuses with the greatest risk of death demonstrate absent or reversed diastolic flow in their systemic arteries, with increased umbilical venous pulsation and reversed flow in the abdominal vena cava. Because of associated fetal hypoxemia, which causes vasodilation of certain vital organs such as the brain, some of these fetuses can have increased cerebral or internal carotid artery flow velocities and cerebral blood flow rates. Such conditions have been hypothesized to help maintain brain growth. Doppler waveform abnormalities usually precede less specific signs of fetal distress such as abnormal changes in fetal heart rate that occur spontaneously under basal conditions or in response to increased uterine contractions during oxytocin challenge testing.

2.14.2 Clinical Evaluation and Treatment of the SGA Infant

GENERAL EVALUATION AND TREATMENT IN THE DELIVERY ROOM

SGA infants lose heat rapidly because of their large surface area relative to body weight and their scant subcutaneous insulation. To prevent hypothermia, they should be dried quickly and completely, placed under a radiant warmer, and protected from drafts with warmed blankets. Hypoglycemia and hypoxia are common in SGA infants and also can impair heat production. Severely undergrown SGA infants often experience marked oxygen and substrate deprivation in utero, which can lead to cardiopulmonary failure at birth. Close to term they can present with meconium aspiration syndrome and exhibit signs of acute and chronic hypoxia, including hypotension, metabolic and respiratory acidosis, and persistent pulmonary hypertension.

PHYSICAL EXAM

Markedly SGA infants who have had severe IUGR usually have disproportionately large heads relative to their undergrown trunks and extremities. Their abdomen can appear shrunken or "scaphoid," and they must be distinguished from infants with diaphragmatic hernias, who also present with respiratory distress. Their extremities often appear scrawny, with thin skinfolds and decreased amounts of subcutaneous fat and skeletal muscle. The skin is loose and often rough, dry, and peeling. In term and postterm infants who are markedly SGA, the fingernails can be long, and the hands and feet tend to look large for the size of the body. The face often appears shrunken or "wizened." Cranial sutures can be widened or overriding. The anterior fontanel often is larger than expected, representing diminished membranous bone formation. The umbilical cord often is thinner than usual, and when meconium has been passed in utero, the cord, nails, and skin may have a yellow or green discoloration. SGA infants also have an increased incidence of severe malformations and chromosomal abnormalities accompanied by dysmorphic features and congenital anomalies, "funny-looking facies," abnormal hands and feet, and the presence of palmar creases. SGA infants with congenital infections can have ocular disorders such as chorioretinitis, cataracts, glaucoma, and cloudy cornea plus hepatosplenomegaly, jaundice, and a "blueberry-muffin" rash, which represents subcutaneous accumulations of blood.

GESTATIONAL AGE ASSESSMENT

Gestational age assessment using physical criteria often is erroneous in infants who are SGA. Vernix caseosa frequently is reduced or absent; thus, the skin more readily desquamates, and sole creases appear more prominent and thus more mature because of increased wrinkling from greater exposure to amniotic fluid. Breast tissue formation also is reduced, and the female external genitalia appear less prominent because of decreased perineal adipose tissue covering the labia. Specific organ maturity often continues at normal developmental rates despite diminished somatic growth; thus, cerebral cortical convolutions, renal glomerular development, and alveolar maturation correlate better with gestational age than with body size.

NEUROLOGIC AND BEHAVIORAL EXAMINATION

SGA infants often appear to have advanced neurologic maturity, although this observation is derived primarily from comparisons with infants of similar birth weight rather than similar gestational age. Active and passive tone and posture are usually normal in SGA infants and are reliable guides to gestational age unless there are other factors, eg, serious central nervous system disorders, that could alter tone. SGA infants often have a "hyperalert" appearance, generally look "starved and hungry," and often are described as jittery and hypertonic, even without simultaneous hypoglycemia. They can be hyperexcitable but show mixed aberrations in tone, from hypotonia to hypertonia. When IUGR is severe, SGA infants tend to show abnormal sleep cycles and diminished muscle tone, decreased deep tendon and facial tactile reflexes, and general physical inactivity and apathy. These neurologic abnormalities usually reflect brain injury during fetal development.

2.14.3   Clinical Problems of the SGA Neonate

SGA infants frequently have problems of perinatal depression ("asphyxia"), hypothermia, hypoglycemia, polycythemia, long-term growth failure, neurodevelopmental handicaps, and relatively high mortality rates (Table 2-16).

IUGR/SGA STATUS VERSUS PRETERM BIRTH AND EFFECTS ON MORTALITY AND MORBIDITY

Constitutionally small infants are not likely to have increased risks of mortality or morbidity. At very early gestational ages, the problems that are associated with prematurity have an especially great impact on the outcome of both SGA and AGA infants. In contrast, the more mature infant may suffer more from the impact of growth restriction. The perinatal mortality rate for SGA infants with relatively severe IUGR is 5 to 20 times that of AGA infants of the same gestational age. This heightened mortality rate is related to intrauterine death from chronic fetal hypoxia, immediate birth asphyxia, multisystem disorders associated with asphyxia (hypoxic-ischemic encephalopathy, persistent pulmonary hypertension, cardiomyopathy, meconium aspiration), and lethal congenital anomalies.

ASPHYXIA

Severely IUGR fetuses frequently show signs of distress (fetal bradycardic arrhythmias and decreased movement) and often do not tolerate labor and vaginal delivery. In such cases, the already stressed, chronically hypoxic fetus is exposed to the acute stress of diminished blood flow during uterine contractions. SGA infants with IUGR tend to have low Apgar scores and frequently need resuscitation.

HYPOGLYCEMIA

Hypoglycemia is extremely common in SGA infants, increasing with the severity of IUGR. The risk of hypoglycemia is greatest during the first 3 postnatal days, but fasting hypoglycemia can occur repeatedly for several days after birth. Early hypoglycemia usually results from diminished hepatic and skeletal muscle glycogen content and is aggravated by diminished alternative energy substrates, including reduced concentrations of fatty acids from the

scant adipose tissue and decreased concentrations of lactate from hypoglycemia. Less commonly, hyperinsulinemia, increased sensitivity to insulin, or both may contribute to a greater incidence of hypoglycemia. Gluconeogenesis usually is decreased, and resolution of persistent hypoglycemia is coincident with improved gluconeogenic capacity and rate. Deficient counterregulatory hormones, particularly catecholamines, also can contribute to the pathogenesis of hypoglycemia. All SGA infants should have early and frequent measurements of blood or plasma glucose concentrations. Blood glucose concentrations should be kept greater than 50 mg/dL (plasma or serum glucose concentrations greater than 55–60 mg/dL). Early enteral feeding usually can prevent hypoglycemia. In less mature infants or those who have other clinical problems, intravenous glucose should be started at 6 to 8 mg/min per kg body weight as soon after birth as possible, preferably within the first 30 minutes. This relatively high rate of glucose infusion is indicated because of the high brain-to-body weight ratio in SGA infants. SGA infants with asphyxia and those who are extremely thin and therefore possess the least amount of body glycogen are at greatest risk of severe hypoglycemia.

HYPERGLYCEMIA

SGA infants who are born very prematurely have low insulin secretion rates and plasma insulin concentrations, leading to the relatively common problem of hyperglycemia that is principally caused by excessive rates of glucose infusion (usually greater than 14 mg/min/kg). Higher concentrations of stress-induced hormones, such as epinephrine, glucagon, and cortisol, also contribute to hyperglycemia. Insulin treatment of these infants usually decreases glucose concentrations promptly, indicating that they have appropriate insulin sensitivity.

LIPID METABOLISM

SGA infants have low plasma free fatty acid concentrations. Fasting glucose concentrations in SGA infants directly correlate with plasma concentrations of free fatty acids and ketoacids. When fed intravenously, however, SGA infants often have deficient cellular uptake and metabolism of intravenous triglycerides, which produces high plasma concentrations of fatty acids and triglycerides but reduced concentrations of ketoacids.

ENERGY METABOLISM

Basal oxygen consumption often decreases immediately after birth in SGA infants but then increases markedly with early feeding. SGA infants have higher oxygen consumption and total energy expenditure rates than normally grown infants at the same gestational age, primarily because their resting energy expenditure rate also is higher. This reflects an increase in cell number relative to body mass and greater heat production in response to increased heat loss.

AMINO ACID AND PROTEIN METABOLISM

Because SGA infants are particularly deficient in muscle mass, providing adequate nutrition for accretion of skeletal muscle, as well as total body protein, is a priority in these infants. There is conflicting information, however, about how well SGA infants tolerate high rates of amino acid and protein nutrition. SGA infants who are born very prematurely often have greater than normal protein and lipid loss in stools. Higher intakes of these nutrients can partly compensate for these losses. It is unclear, however, whether in-

TABLE 2-16

CLINICAL PROBLEMS OF THE SGA NEONATE

PROBLEM	PATHOGENESIS/ PATHOPHYSIOLOGY	PREVENTION/TREATMENT
Intrauterine death	Chronic hypoxia	Antenatal surveillance
	Placental insufficiency	Fetal growth by ultrasound
	Growth failure	Doppler velocimetry
	Malformation	Maternal treatment: ? bed rest, ?O_2
	Infection	Delivery for severe or worsening fetal distress
	Infarction/abruption	
	Preeclampsia	
Asphyxia	Acute hypoxia/abruption	Antepartum/intrapartum monitoring
	Chronic hypoxia	Adequate neonatal resuscitation
	Placental insufficiency/preeclampsia	
	Acidosis	
	Glycogen depletion	
Meconium aspiration	Hypoxia	Resuscitation including tracheal suctioning for definite, severe aspiration
Hypothermia	Cold stress	Protect against increased heat loss
	Hypoxia	Dry infant
	Hypoglycemia	Radiant warmer
	Decreased fat stores	Hat
	Decreased subcutaneous insulation	Thermoneutral environment
	Increased surface area	Nutritional support
	Catecholamine depletion	
Persistent pulmonary hypertension	Chronic hypoxia	Cardiovascular support
		Mechanical ventilation, nitric oxide
Hypoglycemia	Decreased hepatic/muscle glycogen	Frequent measurement of blood glucose
	Decreased alternative energy sources	Early intravenous glucose support
	Heat loss	
	Hypoxia	
	Decreased gluconeogenesis	
	Decreased counterregulatory hormones	
	Increased insulin sensitivity	
Hyperglycemia	Low insulin secretion rate	Glucose monitoring
	Excessive glucose delivery	Decrease glucose infusion to <8 mg/min/kg
	Increased catecholamine and glucagon effects	Intravenous insulin administration for severe cases
Polycythemia-hyperviscosity	Chronic hypoxia	Intravenous glucose, oxygen
	Maternal-fetal transfusion	Partial volume exchange transfusion for severe, symptomatic cases
	Increased erythropoiesis	
Gastrointestinal perforation	Focal ischemia	Cautious enteral feeding
	Hypoperistalsis	
Acute renal failure	Hypoxia/ischemia	Cardiovascular support
Immunodeficiency	Malnutrition	Early, optimal nutrition
	Congenital infection	Specific antibiotic and immune therapy

SGA = small for gestational age.

creasing protein and nonprotein calorie intakes can increase growth rates in SGA infants. Also, pancreatic development and intestinal size often are decreased in SGA infants, which can limit protein and lipid digestion, attenuate insulin production, and cause feeding tolerance.

POLYCYTHEMIA-HYPERVISCOSITY SYNDROME

SGA infants have an increased incidence of polycythemia, probably because of chronic intrauterine hypoxia, which induces increased rates of erythropoiesis. About one-half of all SGA infants have a central hematocrit greater than 60%, and approximately 15 to 20% of term SGA infants have a central hematocrit greater than 65%. In contrast, only about 5% of term AGA infants have a central hematocrit greater than 65% (see Section 2.17.14 for management).

IMMUNE FUNCTION AND INFECTIOUS DISEASE RISK

Immunologic function of SGA infants can be impaired at birth and even in childhood. SGA infants often have deficiencies in lymphocyte number and function, low immunoglobulin levels during infancy, and attenuated antibody response to vaccines.

POSTNATAL PHYSICAL GROWTH OF SGA INFANTS

SGA infants who have had severe IUGR continue to be smaller and relatively underweight for age as they age. These infants more commonly have short stature as young adults, indicating lifelong growth deficits. SGA infants who have had mild to moderate IUGR tend to have accelerated growth velocity during the first six months, and some achieve a growth rate and body size similar to those of AGA infants.

POSTNATAL NEURODEVELOPMENTAL OUTCOME

Neurologic disorders occur 5 to 10 times more often in SGA than in AGA infants. Such disorders include hyperactivity, short attention span, and learning disabilities associated with substandard school performance. Many of these infants even those with normal intelligence, also have subtle neurologic and behavioral problems, including fine motor incoordination hyperreflexia, speech problems, and diffuse electroencephalographic abnormalities. Relative microcephaly at birth is especially to be associated with poor developmental outcome in severely SGA infants.

ADULT DISORDERS RESULTING FROM IUGR

Recent epidemiologic evidence indicates that insulin resistance, glucose intolerance, obesity, diabetes, and cardiovascular disease are more common among adults who were SGA secondary to IUGR compared to those who were AGA at birth. Thus, certain adult pathologies may be unavoidable consequences of environmentally imposed conditions, such as severe and prolonged fetal undernutrition, that allow fetal survival at the expense of normal rates of fetal growth. IUGR, therefore, is increasingly seen as a successful adaptive physiological process for short-term survival, even though it produces pathology in early and later life.

References

Anderson MS, Hay WW JR: Intrauterine growth restriction and the small-for-gestational-age infant. In: Avery GB, Fletcher MA, MacDonald MG, eds: Neonatology, 5th ed. Philadelphia, Lippincott Williams & Wilkins, 1999:411–444

Barker DJ: Fetal and infant origins of adult disease. BJ 301:1111, 1990

Fitzharding PM, Steven EM: The small-for-date infant. II. Neurologic and intellectual sequelae. Pediatrics 50:50–57, 1972

Hawdon JM, Platt MPW: Metabolic adaptation in small for gestational age infants. Arch Dis Child 68:262–268, 1993

Hay WW JR, Catz CS, Grave GD, Yaffe SJ: Workshop summary: fetal growth: its regulation and disorders. Pediatrics 99:585–591, 1997

Lubchenco LO: The High Risk Infant. Philadelphia, WB Saunders, 1976

Lubchenco LO, Searls DT, Brazie JV: Neonatal mortality rate: relationship to birth weight and gestational age. J Pediatr 81:814–822, 1972

Milner RDG, Gluckman PD: Regulation of intrauterine growth. In: Gluckman PD, Heymann MA, eds: Pediatrics & Perinatology, The Scientific Basis, 2nd ed. London, Edward Arnold, 1993:284–289

Sinclair J: Heat production and thermoregulation in the small for date infant. Pediatr Clin North Am 17:147–158, 1970

Sparks JW, Ross JR, Cetin I: Intrauterine growth and nutrition. In: Polin RA, Fox WW, eds: Fetal and Neonatal Physiology, 2nd ed. Philadelphia, WB Saunders, 1998:267–289

2.15   INFANT OF THE DIABETIC MOTHER

Edward S. Ogata

Before the availability of insulin, the diabetic woman rarely became pregnant. Diabetes reduced her life expectancy and fertility. If she did become pregnant, the prognosis for mother and infant was poor. Before 1930, maternal mortality rates for diabetics ranged from 6 to 60%, and perinatal mortality from 25 to 73%. The availability of insulin dramatically improved the diabetic woman's life expectancy, fertility, and well-being during pregnancy. However, neonatal outcome was still poor until the establishment of a team approach by obstetricians, diabetologists, and neonatologists focused on achieving optimal maternal diabetes control to achieve a normal metabolic environment for the fetus. With this effort, perinatal mortality rates of less than 2% have been achieved.

The altered metabolic state of the pregnant diabetic is the critical factor responsible for the problems of the infant of the diabetic mother (IDM). Maternal hyperglycemia causes fetal hyperglycemia, subsequent fetal pancreatic β-cell stimulation, and hyperinsulinism. Hypertrophied β cells, seen at autopsy in IDMs, and elevated plasma insulin concentrations in newborn IDMs confirm the existence of the fetal hyperinsulinemic state.

Pregnancy in the insulin-dependent diabetic is commonly complicated by one or more of a wide variety of problems in the fetus and newborn. These include:

- Sudden fetal death late in the third trimester
- Premature birth from early induction of labor to avoid third-trimester fetal death
- Macrosomia
- Birth trauma as a result of macrosomia
- Intrapartum asphyxia
- Cesarean section delivery to avoid birth trauma and intrapartum asphyxia
- Intrauterine growth restriction
- Neonatal respiratory distress
- Hypoglycemia
- Hypocalcemia
- Hyperbilirubinemia
- Hyperviscosity (polycythemia) syndrome
- Cardiomyopathy
- Congenital anomalies
- Increased risk of obesity and of diabetes mellitus in later life

In general, the risk of neonatal problems is greater when there is a history of poor metabolic control of the mother. Many of these complications coexist: the combination of hypocalcemia, hypoglycemia, jaundice, and macrosomia is particularly common.

Gestational diabetes mellitus, the mildest form of maternal diabetes that has its onset during the pregnancy, also increases the risk of perinatal loss. Although improved maternal care has reduced the incidence of this complication, infants of women with gestational diabetes remain at increased risk of all of the morbidities except for congenital anomalies, subsequent obesity, and diabetes mellitus late in life.

BODY SIZE

Macrosomia is a well-known characteristic of the offspring of diabetic women. Their large size increases their risk of birth trauma and the incidence of cesarean delivery. The rate of delivery by cesarean section in diabetic women is four to five times greater than that in nondiabetic women. Much of the increased mass in macrosomic IDMs consists of fat. Measurement of fat-cell size and skinfold thickness in IDMs, as well as postmortem analyses of IDMs who died during the neonatal period, suggest that the IDM has almost twice as much fat as an infant of comparable gestational age born to a nondiabetic mother. In addition, the IDM has an excessive amount of nonfatty tissue. The liver and heart are often enlarged, and skeletal length is increased in proportion to weight. The macrosomic IDM head may appear disproportionately small because brain size is not increased relative to gestational age. Much of this excess tissue in IDMs is distributed in the shoulders and intrascapular area. This increases the risk of shoulder dystocia in IDMs compared with infants who are constitutionally large and have a more uniform distribution of tissue.

Because insulin is an anabolic hormone, the hyperinsulinemic state of the IDM fetus plays a major role in the development of macrosomia. The augmented insulin production by the fetus, plus excessive maternal glucose and amino acids, stimulates protein, lipid, and glycogen synthesis to cause macrosomia. Insulin-like growth factors also are increased in macrosomic IDMs and probably contribute to their large size. The excess fat in IDMs appears to accumulate during the third trimester, as IDMs who are delivered before 30 weeks of gestation are rarely large for gestational age, and serial ultrasound measurements of the fetus show that the fetal IDM does not exceed normal growth limits until 28 to 30 weeks of gestation.

Metabolic fuels other than maternal glucose may also contribute to the macrosomia of IDMs. There is a positive correlation between the body size of the IDM and the concentration of amino acids and free fatty acids in maternal plasma when measured after an overnight fast.

Because fetal macrosomia increases the risk of birth trauma, asphyxia, and delivery by cesarean section, one major goal in caring for the pregnant diabetic is to reduce accelerated fetal growth by reducing fetal hyperinsulinemia. This usually can be achieved by frequent administration of short-acting insulin, to regulate maternal blood glucose concentration and by careful attention to diet and weight gain.

Despite intensive treatment, macrosomia develops in fetuses of 20 to 30% of insulin-dependent diabetic women. Women with gestational diabetes, the mildest form of carbohydrate intolerance, have an equally high incidence of macrosomia. These observations indicate that present insulin therapy cannot completely normalize metabolic fuel availability to the fetus. In the case of gestational diabetes, the present regimen of maternal diet regulation is not always successful because of poor compliance.

Some IDMs are small for gestational age. In general, the risk of intrauterine growth restriction is directly related to the severity of maternal diabetes. The most likely explanation for fetal growth restriction in the face of maternal diabetes is the presence of maternal vascular disease with resultant fetal deficiency of nutrients, including oxygen.

HYPOGLYCEMIA

Hypoglycemia in the neonate is usually defined as a blood glucose concentration less than 40 mg/dL. Hypoglycemia occurs in 25 to 50% of IDMs within the first 24 hours after birth. This is particularly likely in those who are macrosomic. The mechanism for development of hypoglycemia in the IDM includes both diminished production and increased clearance of glucose.

Most IDMs, unlike infants of normal women, have elevated plasma C-peptide or insulin concentrations. In addition, many IDMs have pancreatic β cells that respond to glucose challenge with a brisk outpouring of insulin, as compared with the sluggish response of the normal neonate. Maintaining maternal glucose concentrations within the normal range is, therefore, an important objective for reducing the risk of hypoglycemia. Several studies also suggest that the IDM fails to release glucagon or catecholamines

in response to hypoglycemia. Thus, because insulin clears glucose from the intravascular space, and glucagon and catecholamines normally stimulate glycogen breakdown and gluconeogenesis, the IDM has both increased glucose clearance and diminished glucose production, resulting in hypoglycemia.

Infants with hypoglycemia may present with lethargy, hypotonia, tremulousness, excessive sweating or cyanosis. They also may present with seizures. If the period of hypoglycemia is prolonged, myocardial contractility diminishes, and congestive heart failure may develop. IDMs are sometimes asymptomatic despite having blood glucose concentrations less than 30 mg/dL. Because hypoglycemia, even in the absence of symptoms, may cause brain damage and lead to long-term rhonologic impairment, it is recommended that blood glucose concentrations be maintained above 40 mg/dL for all IDMs see Section 2.17.4).

HYPOCALCEMIA AND HYPOMAGNESEMIA

Hypocalcemia occurs in 10 to 20% of IDMs during the neonatal period. Hypocalcemia usually is associated with hyperphosphatemia and sometimes with hypomagnesemia. The mechanism responsible for hypocalcemia is unclear, although plasma parathormone concentrations in IDMs have been reported to be significantly less than in infants of normal mothers during the first 4 days after birth. This may result from hypomagnesemia, which limits parathormone secretion even in the presence of hypocalcemia. Maternal hypomagnesemia, perhaps caused by increased renal losses with diabetes, is believed responsible for the fetal and neonatal hypomagnesemia. Administering $MgSO_4$ to the IDM, however, does not prevent hypocalcemia. The active transport of calcium and magnesium by the placenta may be impaired in maternal diabetes. Birth asphyxia, which frequently occurs in IDMs, also may lead to hypocalcemia.

The clinical signs of hypocalcemia include tremulousness, twitching movements, or generalized convulsions. Arrhythmias also may occur, but the characteristic prolongation of the Q-T interval does not occur consistently in neonates with hypocalcemia.

Total or ionized plasma calcium concentrations should be measured 1 to 2 hours after birth and during the first several days in IDMs. Because birth asphyxia and respiratory distress syndrome increase the risk of hypocalcemia, IDMs with these disorders should receive calcium gluconate with their daily parenteral fluids in the first postnatal days. Although in neonates the daily maintenance dose of elemental calcium is usually 75 to 100 mg per kilogram body weight, at least 100 to 200 mg/kg is needed daily, and many IDMs require two to three times that dose. Symptomatic hypocalcemia should be treated with an infusion of 10% calcium gluconate at 2 mL/kg body weight given over 5 minutes. This dose provides 18 mg/kg of elemental calcium. During infusion, continuous electrocardiographic monitoring of heart rate is important because a rapid intravenous infusion of concentrated calcium may cause arrhythmias. Daily maintenance of calcium should be initiated following this initial therapy.

Infants who are hypocalcemic with associated hypomagnesemia will not become normocalcemic until their serum magnesium concentration is corrected. A 50% solution of magnesium at a dose of 0.25 mg/kg may be administered intramuscularly to correct hypomagnesemia.

HYPERBILIRUBINEMIA

Up to 30% of IDMs have jaundice with elevated indirect bilirubin concentrations within 3 days after birth. Their carbon monoxide production is increased, which is an indicator of hemoglobin catabolism and increased production of bilirubin. Hyperbilirubinemia in these infants may be related to their large size, which increases the risk of birth trauma. Resorption of blood from resulting hematomas or bruises causes hyperbilirubinemia. In addition, polycythemia frequently occurs in the IDM, and the normal rate of breakdown of the increased red cell mass results in a larger bilirubin load for the liver to conjugate than in normal infants. Therapy is the same as for neonatal jaundice from other causes (see Sec. 2.17.6).

HYPERVISCOSITY

Up to 20% of IDMs are polycythemic, which may account for their increased risk for the neonatal hyperviscosity syndrome (see Sec. 2.17.14). Several factors appear to contribute: the hematocrit of umbilical cord blood at birth tends to be elevated, probably because of increased erythropoiesis; IDMs often have enhanced placental transfusion at delivery; and elevated plasma fibrinogen concentration increases blood viscosity. The increased incidence of renal vein thrombosis reported in IDMs is probably related to hyperviscosity, although this disorder does occur in IDMs with normal hematocrits.

RESPIRATORY DISTRESS

The IDM is at risk for several forms of neonatal respiratory distress. The most important of these is hyaline membrane disease from insufficient pulmonary surfactant (see Sec. 2.16.1 and 2.17.10). The high risk of hyaline membrane disease is related to premature delivery as well as to retarded maturation of the pulmonary surfactant system. In cultured fetal lung tissue, insulin blocks the development of enzymes necessary for the synthesis of lecithin, a principal ingredient of surfactant. Even with the use of methods to detect maturation of surfactant by amniotic fluid analysis, there is a 10% incidence of hyaline membrane disease in IDMs.

CARDIOMYOPATHY

IDMs have an increased incidence of cardiomyopathy, in which there is often thickening of the interventricular septum and one or both ventricular walls (Sec. 22.3.4 and 22.4.1). This likely results from the fetal hyperinsulinemic state. The majority of these infants are asymptomatic, and the thickening is detected only by an electrocardiogram or echocardiogram. In some infants, an ejection systolic murmur is heard at the mid- to upper left sternal border. In a few with very marked septal thickening, left ventricular outflow obstruction may lead to left ventricular failure in the first few days after birth. The electrocardiographic and echocardiographic abnormalities generally regress over 3 to 6 months, and the condition appears to leave no permanent effects on the myocardium.

IDMs, especially those who experience intrapartum asphyxia, may present with severe congestive heart failure soon after birth. Respiratory distress and cardiomegaly may persist in such infants, and often they are hypoglycemic and hypocalcemic. If the left ventricle becomes dilated, a murmur of mitral valve insufficiency also may be heard. Such infants usually improved with application of assisted ventilation and correction of their metabolic abnormalities. They usually recover fully in a few days, although their hearts remain enlarged longer.

CONGENITAL ANOMALIES

Major congenital malformations occur two to four times more frequently in IDMs than in infants born to nondiabetic women. Congenital heart defects, notably ventricular septal defects, are espe-

cially common in IDMs. The incidence of neural tube defects, gastrointestinal atresia, and urinary tract malformations also is greater in IDMs than in infants born to nondiabetic women. Spinal agenesis associated with caudal regression syndrome is a malformation that occurs almost exclusively in IDMs.

A transient anomaly, unique to the IDM, is known as neonatal small left colon syndrome, or microcolon. This condition presents as gastrointestinal obstruction and may mimic congenital aganlionic megacolon or Hirshprung disease. Unlike infants with Hirschprung disease, however, these infants have normal innervation of the bowel and ultimately have normal intestinal function.

A considerable number of clinical observations indicate that poor control of maternal diabetes during the first trimester, the key period for fetal organogenesis, is a major factor in causing congenital anomalies. Alterations in the availability of numerous metabolic substances resulting from maternal diabetes have been suggested to cause these anomalies. Because the period of critical organogenesis is relatively long in the human, the day-to-day fluctuations in diabetes control may account for the frequent occurrence of multiple birth defects in a single infant and for the failure of the lesions to conform to one particular pattern. Assuring optimal metabolic control before conception and during the first trimester is an important clinical and cost-effective strategy to reduce the incidence of congenital anomalies.

OUTCOME

Infants of diabetic mothers, particularly those who are macrosomic at birth, have an increased risk of obesity later in life. Because childhood obesity of IDMs correlates with amniotic fluid insulin concentration during fetal life, insulin secretion from fetal pancreatic β cells may be an important factor in the development of obesity.

Offspring of women with insulin-dependent diabetes have an increased risk of acquiring diabetes in later life. The mechanisms responsible for this are not understood. IDMs also are at risk for subsequent development of impaired insulin responsiveness during adolescence, as assessed by insulin secretion in response to a glucose challenge. A number of studies also suggest a unique gender risk. Offspring of fathers with insulin-dependent diabetes are at significantly greater risk of acquiring diabetes than offspring of insulin-dependent diabetic mothers.

In the past, IDMs were at great risk for brain damage, with impaired motor and intellectual development. This was attributed, at least in part, to birth trauma, asphyxia, hypoglycemia, and other neonatal morbidities. Careful medical and obstetric care of the mother and appropriate neonatal care greatly reduce the risk of these complications. Maintaining excellent treatment of maternal diabetes during pregnancy is equally important for long-term cognitive and psychomotor development. Poor maternal control during the second and third trimesters, particularly alterations in ketone metabolism, can be directly correlated with abnormal neonatal behavior and with poor indices of infant development at age 2 years and of intelligence at age 4 years.

References

Barker DTP, Gluckman PD, Godfrey KM, et al: Fetal nutrition and cardiovascular disease in adult life. Lancet 341:938, 1990

Curet LB, Izquierdo LA, Gilson GJ, et al: Relative effects of antepartum and intrapartum maternal blood glucose levels on the incidence of neonatal hypoglycemia. J Perinatol 17:113, 1997

Eriksson UJ, Lewis NJ, Freinkel N: Growth retardation during early organogenesis in embryos of experimentally diabetic rats. Diabetes 33: 281–284, 1984

Freinkel N: The Banting Lecture 1980: Of pregnancy and progeny. Diabetes 29:1023, 1980

Fuhrmann K, Reiher H, Semmler K, et al: Prevention of congenital malformations in infants of insulin-dependent diabetic mothers. Diabetes Care 6:219, 1983

Husain SM, Birdsey TJ, Glazier JD, et al: Effect of diabetes mellitus on maternofetal flux of calcium and magnesium and calbindin9K mRNA expression in rat placenta. Pediatr Res 35:376, 1994

Kolderup LB, Laros RB, Musci TJ: Incidence of persistent birth injury in macrosomic infants: association with mode of delivery. Am J Obstet Gynecol 178:195, 1998

Mehta KC, Kalkwarf HO, Mimouni F, et al: Randomized trial of magnesium administered to prevent hypocalcemia in infants of diabetic mothers. J Perinatol 18:352, 1998

Meyer-Wittkopt LB, Simpson JL, Sharkind GK: Incidence of congenital heart defects in fetuses of diabetic mothers: a retrospective study of 326 cases. Ultrasound Obstet Gynecol 8:8, 1996

Mills JL, Knopp RH, Simpson JL, et al: Lack of relation of increased malformation rates in infants of diabetic mothers to glycemic control during organogenesis. N Engl J Med 318:671, 1988

Naeye R: Infants of diabetic mothers: a quantitative morphologic study. Pediatrics 28:980, 1965

Ogata ES, Sabbagha R, Metzger BE: Serial ultrasonography to assess evolving fetal macrosomia. Studies in 23 pregnant diabetic women. JAMA 243:2405, 1980

Peterson MB, Pedersen SA, Greisen G, et al: Early growth delay in diabetic pregnancy: relation to psychomotor development at age 4. Br Med J Clin Res Ed 296:598, 1988

Pettitt DJ, Aleck KA, Baird HR: Congenital susceptibility to NIDDM. Role of intrauterine environment. Diabetes 37:622, 1988

Reece EA, Quintek PA, Homko CJ: Early fetal growth delay: is it really predictive of congenital anomalies in infants of diabetic women. J Maternal Fetal Med 6:168, 1997

Rizzo T, Metzger BE, Burns WJ, et al: Correlations between antepartum maternal metabolism and child intelligence. N Engl J Med 325:911, 1991

Rizzo TA, Ogata ES, Dooley SL: Perinatal complications and cognitive development in 2 to 5 year old children of diabetic mothers. Am J Obstet Gynecol 171:706, 1994

Robert MF, Neff RK, Hubbell JP: Association between maternal diabetes and the respiratory-distress syndrome in the newborn. N Engl J Med 294:357, 1976

Silverman BL, Cho NH, Metzger BE: Impaired glucose tolerance in adolescent offspring of diabetic mothers: relationship to fetal hyperinsulinism. Diabetes Care 18:611, 1995

Sosenko IR, Kitzmiller JL, Loo SW, et al: The infant of the diabetic mother. Correlation of increased cord C-peptide levels with macrosomia and hypoglycemia. N Engl J Med 30:859, 1979

Tuomilehto J, Podeer T, Tuomilehto-Wolf E: Evidence for importance of gender and birth cohort for risk of IDDM in offspring of IDDM parents. Diabetologia 38:975, 1995

Vohr BR, Lipsitt LP, Oh W: Somatic growth of children of diabetic mothers with reference to birth size. J Pediatr 97:196, 1980

2.16 DISORDERS SPECIFICALLY RELATED TO PREMATURE BIRTH

2.16.1 Hyaline Membrane Disease

Thomas N. Hansen and Samuel Hawgood

Hyaline membrane disease (HMD) or the neonatal respiratory distress syndrome is the most common cause of respiratory failure in the first days after birth, occurring in 1 to 2% of newborn infants. Until about 30 years ago approximately 50% of infants with this condition died. In recent years improved methods of treatment have markedly reduced mortality, and in most newborn infant care centers, 85 to 95% survive.

Hyaline membrane disease results from the tendency of the alveoli and terminal bronchioles to collapse because of the absence of adequate amounts of surface-active material (lung surfactant) and the immature state of alveolarization of the lung acini. These two developmental conditions render the alveolar structure of the lung unstable. Alveoli may never open or may collapse during expiration, increasing greatly the effort needed to ventilate the lungs and creating increased venous admixture and hypoxemia.

Hyaline membrane disease is a disease of development and therefore is self-limited, provided that the patient survives. In most instances, the surge of glucocorticoids and catecholamines released around the time of birth induces surfactant synthesis and secretion in amounts sufficient to stabilize lung function. Moreover, these events and the rapid process of lung growth that takes place at that time can also promote septation of the lung saccules and capillary growth. As these changes occur, the signs and symptoms of respiratory distress subside quickly. However, during this brief interval, lung damage may occur from the combined effects of pulmonary edema, ischemia, pulmonary air leaks, oxygen toxicity, and tissue stretch and strain if positive-pressure ventilation is used. As a consequence, HMD can result in chronic lung disease that may persist for weeks or months.

PATHOLOGY

At postmortem examination, the lungs from infants with neonatal respiratory distress are firm and airless. Atelectasis (failure of aeration of the lung spaces) is striking on gross inspection; when the lungs are fixed in inflation, only the airways and a few alveolar ducts are air filled (Fig. 2-32). Diffuse atelectasis and dilated terminal bronchioles and alveolar ducts lined with a homogeneous hyaline-staining material characterize the microscopic picture (Fig. 2-33). The hyaline membranes are plasma clots containing fibrin, other plasma constituents, and cellular debris. There is congestion of pulmonary capillaries and veins and an increase in pulmonary water with dilation of the lymphatics.

Interstitial air leaks are common, and collections of air are often seen around small airways and vessels (Fig. 2-34). In some cases the alveoli contain red cells. Electron microscopic examination shows necrosis of epithelial and endothelial cells and rupture of the basement membranes. If death occurs after 3 or 4 days of respiratory distress, the hyaline membranes are fragmented, and numerous macrophages appear in the intraalveolar spaces. The pulmonary interstitium is widened and filled with round cells and fibroblasts. After the first week, there is a proliferation of alveolar epithelial type II cells and capillaries. In severe cases, chronic changes occur including metaplasia of the bronchiolar epithelium and interstitial fibrosis. These changes are discussed more completely in Sec. 23.9.

When inflated with air, the affected lungs accept only 10 to 20% of the gas accommodated by normal lungs at the same distending pressure. If after full expansion the distending pressure is lowered, the amount of gas retained at each pressure is a smaller proportion of the maximum gas volume than would be present in the lung from an infant without neonatal respiratory distress. When the lung is distended with liquid, there is less difference in the pressure-volume relationships between the normal lung and the lung with HMD. This behavior was explained when Avery and Mead showed that extracts of lungs of infants dying with the disease did not have a low surface tension when studied with a modified Wilhelmy balance. The surface tension–surface area characteristics of extracts of lung with and without neonatal respiratory distress are shown in Fig. 2-35. The immature lung with an inadequate amount of surfactant in the alveoli tends to become atelectatic, producing increasing respiratory failure.

CLINICAL FEATURES

The cardinal physical manifestions of respiratory distress (see Sec. 4.1.1) are signs of increased inspiratory effort (because of the non-compliant lungs) and hypoxemia (from the impaired gas exchange). Increased inspiratory effort is demonstrated by the use of accessory respiratory muscles and development of chest wall retractions. The large negative intrathoracic pressures generated as the infant attempts to inflate its lungs cause the chest wall to cave in. This results in visible retractions, which are particularly notable in very small preterm infants with compliant chest walls. Despite these efforts, tidal volume is reduced, and therefore the infant also breathes rapidly and shallowly (tachypnea) to systain minute ventilation. As noted above, there is a marked tendency for alveoli and terminal bronchioles to collapse at the end of expiration; in response, infants usually have grunting respiration, a maneuver that keeps airway pressure positive at the end of a breath and minimizes (but does not necessarily eliminate) closure of airways and alveoli. Infants do not grunt with every breath, and those with severe disease grunt most frequently. Apneic periods and irregularities of respiratory rhythm are common as the work of breathing increases and the infants become fatigued.

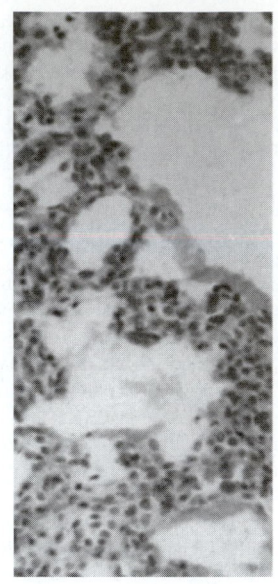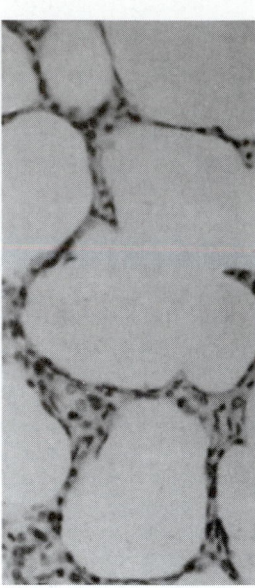

FIGURE 2-33   Left portion of the lung shown in Figure 2-32A (×100). Some of the alveolar ducts are inflated, but there are no true alveoli. The cells of the interstitial tissue appear to be crowded, but no inflammatory cells are present. The homogenous staining material lining the walls of the alveolar ducts are plasma clots (ie, hyaline membranes). Right lung shown in Figure 2-32B (×100). The interstitial tissue is thin. Although there are no true alveoli in this section, the total internal surface area is large, particularly compared with the lung in the left panel.

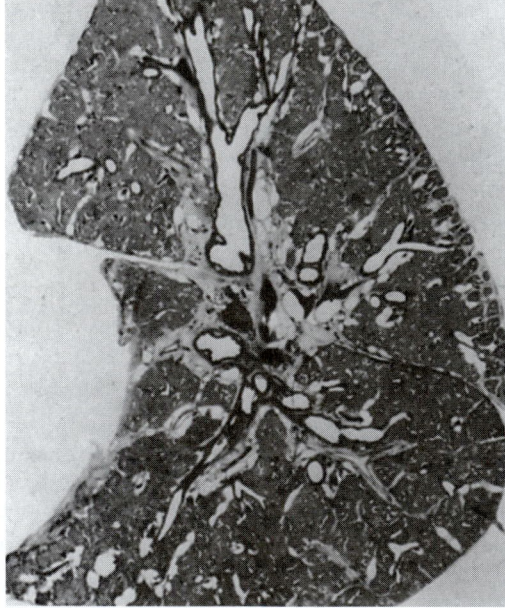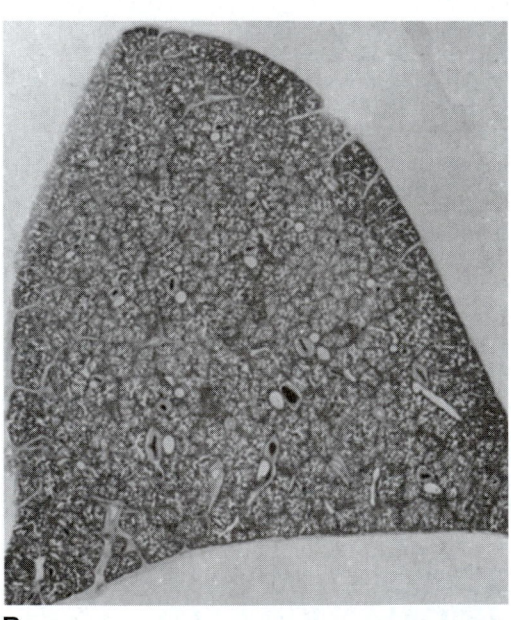

A   B

FIGURE 2-32   A. Longitudinal section of the left lung of a 1560-g infant, born at 30 weeks' gestation, who died at 2.5 days of age from neonatal respiratory distress syndrome. The lung was expanded with air to a pressure of 40 cm H_2O, then deflated to 10 cm H_2O and fixed with the bronchus clamped. The airways are distended, and a few of the respiratory bronchioles are over-inflated. Most of the alveolar ducts and alveoli are airless. B. Cross-section of the left upper lobe of a 1220-g infant, born at 29 weeks' gestation without lung disease, who died at 1 week of age with a sudden, massive intraventricular hemorrhage. Inflation and fixation were identical to those used for the lung in A. Almost all of the alveolar ducts are filled with air, and the airways are not overdistended.

Because the rib cage is so compliant in small infants, diaphragmatic contractions can decrease the volume of the rib cage during inspiration; this creates thoracoabdominal asynchrony in which the ribs and sternum move inward while the abdominal wall moves outward. Breath sounds are usually diminished in intensity and have a harsh, tubular quality. Occasionally, there are fine rales, particularly in those infants born by cesarean section, who may have excessive lung liquid. As the lungs become more difficult to ventilate, the work of breathing increases, the infant tires, and arterial carbon dioxide tension rises. At the same time the hypoxemia (see below) may worsen, and diversion of blood flow to the respiratory muscles, which are working excessively, can diminish peripheral blood flow; these problems with oxygenation and circulation can contribute to a metabolic acidosis as well as a respiratory acidosis. Urine output is usually diminished early in the course of the disease, and the infants may become progressively edematous. Some infants, especially very low-birth-weight infants, have systemic hypotension, peripheral pallor, slow capillary filling, and hypothermia.

In mild to moderate disease, respirations become increasingly labored for about 48 hours, and then, after 72 hours of age, there is rapid improvement. Recovery is usually heralded by diuresis, which is thought to relate to the clearance of fluid that accumulated in the interstitium of the lungs and possibly other tissues during the height of the illness. Clinical improvement is accompanied by a rapid fall in pulmonary vascular resistance and a rise in systemic arterial pressure. In some infants, particularly the least mature with birth weights less than 1500 g, this may permit development of a large shunt from the aorta through a patent ductus arteriosus to the pulmonary artery. In these infants, recovery may be interrupted by the development of pulmonary edema. The symptomatic ductus arteriosus will usually require treatment with the prostaglandin inhibitors or operative ligation (see Sec. 2.16.2).

PULMONARY FUNCTION

The increased surface tension increases lung recoil (decreases lung compliance), and, as a result, lung volume decreases (see Sec. 4.1.1). Minute ventilation is usually increased, but dead space ven-

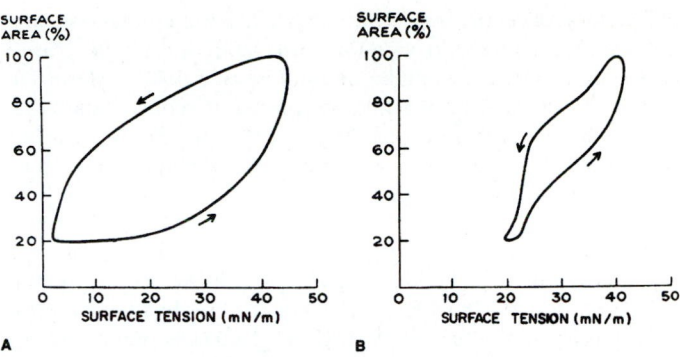

A   B

FIGURE 2-35 Surface tension–surface area diagrams of extracts of lung from an infant with neonatal respiratory distress **(A)** and a lung from an infant with normal lungs **(B)**. These were obtained from a modified Wilhelmy surface-tension balance, in which surface tension is continuously recorded as the surface area of the lung extract is reduced and increased. When the surface area is reduced to 20% (ie, equivalent to a lung changing from total lung capacity to residual volume), the surface tension of the extract from the lung with neonatal respiratory distress **(B)** is 20 mN/m, a high tension that if present at the surface of the alveolus, would favor atelectasis. The surface tension at 20% surface area for the extract of normal lung is 3 mN/m **(A)**.

tilation is also increased, such that alveolar ventilation is decreased. Lung volume may decrease during the first 48 hours after birth in infants who are not being treated with positive end-respiratory pressure; these changes likely relate to the further decrease in lung compliance as some alveoli collapse and possibly from fatigue in the patients with most severe respiratory distress syndrome (RDS). The decrease in lung volume also increases airway resistance. Furthermore, airway resistance is increased because the total number of expanded alveoli is reduced, thereby decreasing the number of patent small airways, and there can be interstitial edema from injury to the airways.

Evidence from nitrogen washout curves and expiratory flow-volume curves suggests that infants with HMD have a marked mal-

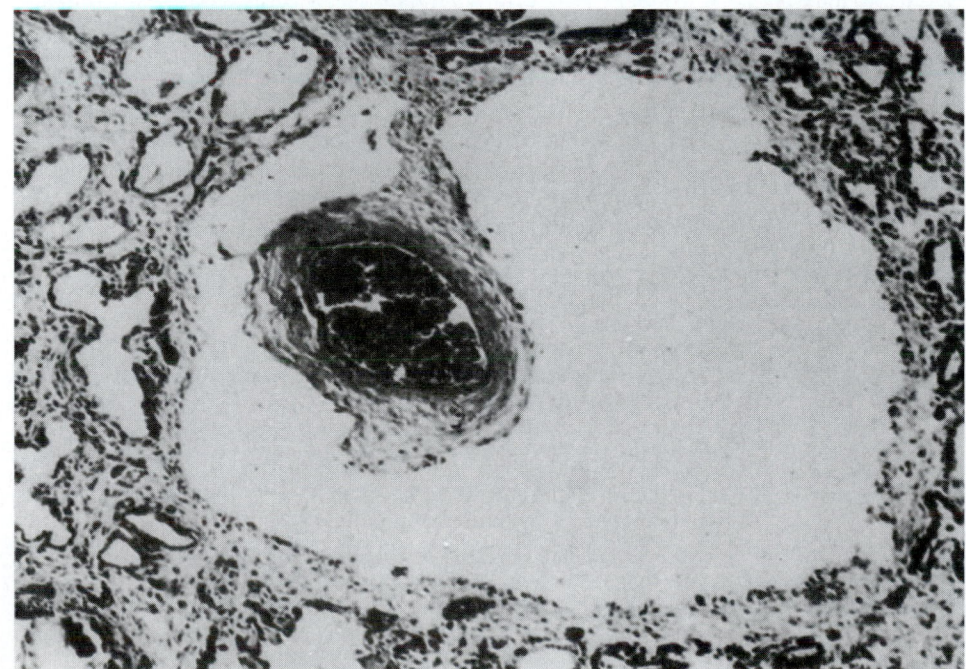

FIGURE 2-34 Lung from an infant born after 25 weeks' gestation weighing 650 g who died at 40 hours of age. Note the immature respiratory units, some of which are lined with hyaline membranes. There is a large collection of interstitial air surrounding a small vessel (×100).

distribution of ventilation. Surfactant deficiency is not uniform, and regions of the lung with adequate surfactant coexist with areas of surfactant deficiency. Compliance and resistance may be normal in surfactant-sufficient areas while compliance is reduced and resistance is increased in areas of surfactant deficiency. During inspiration, most of the gas flow into the lung is distributed to the relatively normal lung units, with very little going to the abnormal lung units. In lung units with low ventilation relative to capillary perfusion, the alveolar and pulmonary capillary PO_2, that results from equilibrium between blood and gas, is very low and potentially contributes to systemic hypoxemia that is not offset by excess ventilation of other lung units. Thus, the low ventilation:perfusion areas contribute to heterogeneous gas exchange and can cause severe hypoxemia or an apparent "right-to-left shunt," particularly at low inspired O_2 concentrations. If pulmonary vasoregulation is intact, the reduced alveolar PO_2 tends to constrict blood vessels supplying those poorly ventilated lung units and diverts blood away from this part of the lung, thereby reducing, but not eliminating, some of this "shunt-like" effect. In areas with no ventilation (eg, from collapse or consolidation), any capillary perfusion contributes to right-to-left shunt because blood exits the capillaries with the same PO_2 as in mixed venous blood. Other right-to-left shunts can contribute substantially to systemic hypoxemia in HMD. The vasoconstriction from alveolar hypoxia and possibly from other factors released during lung injury (see Sec. 2.17.11) can cause pulmonary hypertension. This, in turn, may promote right-to-left shunting across the foramen ovale and through the ductus arteriosus. Because so many factors contribute to the hypoxemia in HMD, the degree of hypoxemia may be highly variable and unpredictable, although certain measures (increasing inspired O_2 concentration, application of positive airway pressure) generally improve oxygenation.

RADIOLOGIC FEATURES

The radiographic appearance of the lungs in infants with neonatal respiratory distress is characterized by a diffuse reticulogranular pattern of increased density, usually uniform in distribution (Fig. 2-36) but occasionally more marked in the bases or on one side. The densities result from atelectasis and interstital edema. Lung volume is small, and even radiographs taken after a maximal inspiration rarely show the diaphragm to be below the eighth to ninth intercostal spaces. The bronchial tree is clearly outlined by air against the poorly aerated lung, creating an air bronchogram. The heart is usually normal in size, although it often appears large because of the large thymic shadow and decreased lung volume. Often diffuse atelectasis is not seen because the radiographic appearance of the lung can be markedly altered by treatment. Infants breathing against a positive pressure or being ventilated with intermittent positive pressure with positive end-expiratory pressure may have well-aerated lungs without air bronchograms. On the other hand, some infants with very severe disease may be unable to expand their lungs and have totally opaque radiographs in which even the heart borders are obscured. Later in the course of the disease, pulmonary edema, air leaks, or pulmonary hemorrhage can also affect the radiographic appearance.

PATHOGENESIS

HMD is caused by atelectasis, which develops from three interrelated factors: small respiratory units, a highly compliant chest wall, and an amount of pulmonary surfactant that is inadequate to cover the internal surface of the lung.

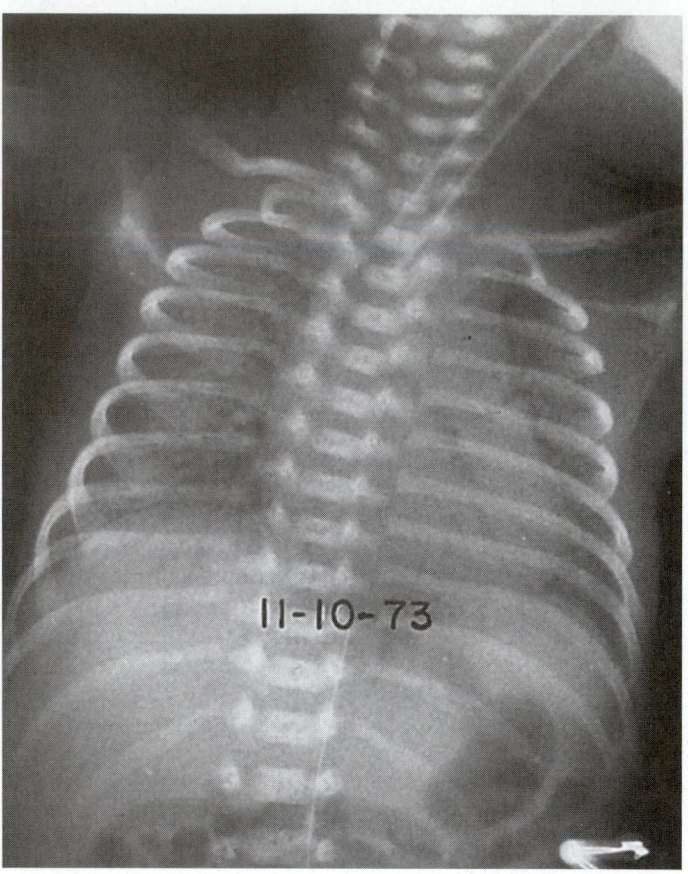

FIGURE 2-36 Chest radiograph of an infant with hyaline membrane disease. An endotracheal tube is present. Despite the application of positive pressure, the lung volume is reduced with the diaphragm at the eighth interspace. The lung parenchyma has a diffuce reticular granular pattern, and air bronchograms are present.

In the adult, the alveolar diameter is about 200 μm, and in the term infant 100 μm. In the prematurely born infant, the alveolar ducts or acini are about 80 μm in diameter—there are no true alveoli. The diameter of the respiratory bronchioles of the prematurely born infant is also smaller relative to that of infants born at term. Because the respiratory units are curved in shape, the relationship between the tension that develops in their walls and the pressure inside of them is governed by the Laplace law, which states that the pressure difference (P) needed to maintain a given radius (r) is inversely proportional to the radius and directly related to twice the surface tension (T):

$$P = 2T/r$$

Accordingly, the small respiratory units of the preterm infant require a greater pressure both to inflate and to prevent deflation than those of infants born at term. Infants born prematurely may not be able to create these pressures because their chest walls are weak and compliant. Tension is a property of the wall (determined by surface tension and the constituents of the interstitium); pressure is determined by tension and radius.

The chest wall of the infant is poorly ossified, a clear advantage during birth, when the chest needs to be squeezed through the birth canal. This advantage, however, turns into disadvantage when lung recoil is increased because it allows lung volume to decrease.

The overall decrease in lung volume is compounded by the excessive load that chest wall retractions place on the diaphragm, leading more easily to diaphragmatic fatigue, decreased tidal volume, and alveolar collapse.

Surprisingly, despite these handicaps, most prematurely born infants can inflate their lungs and develop a stable surface area sufficient for the gas transfer required to meet their metabolic needs. The success of their adaptation to extrauterine life depends on the structural development of the lung at the time of birth and on a mature surfactant system.

Pulmonary surfactant is a complex mixture of lipids and proteins synthesized in alveolar epithelial type II cells. Type II cells are one of the two epithelial cell types that line the alveolus. The surfactant component most responsible for lowering surface tension is the phospholipid dipalmitoylphosphatidylcholine (DPPC). DPPC makes up about 45 to 50% of the mass of surfactant stored and secreted by the type II cell. Other phospholipids, neutral lipids, and specific apoproteins are needed to give surfactant the biophysical properties needed to form a film at the alveolar air-liquid interface and to regulate surfactant turnover. A rare congenital deficiency of surfactant protein-B gene leads to fatal respiratory distress in affected term infants. The similarity of the clinical, radiologic, and pathologic features of this autosomal recessive disorder to HMD underscores the importance of a functional surfactant in perinatal lung adaption.

Synthesis and storage of surfactant begins at about 16 weeks of gestation, and lung homogenates have high concentrations of surfactant by 20 weeks. However, surfactant is not secreted until later, appearing in amniotic fluid between 28 and 38 weeks of gestation (Fig. 2-37) (see below). Secretion of surfactant starts at about the same time that alveolar development begins, but the timing of these events varies greatly among individuals. This explains why some infants with a gestational age less than 30 weeks do not develop neonatal respiratory distress while other infants, with a longer gestation, do.

PREDISPOSING FACTORS

In addition to premature birth, there are several factors that predispose newborn infants to neonatal respiratory distress. It is twice as common in boys as in girls at every gestational age and more common in white infants. It frequently follows delivery by cesarean section, particularly if this is done before labor has begun. Infants of diabetic mothers are five times more likely to develop HMD than infants of nondiabetic mothers with the same gestational age, sex, and mode of delivery. The second-born twin is more likely to be affected, and a family history of HMD increases the risk for any given premature infant.

On the other hand, complications of pregnancy such as pregnancy-induced hypertension, chronic maternal hypertension, premature rupture of membranes, and subacute placental abruption all decrease the incidence of HMD. Infants born to mothers addicted to narcotics are also at less risk for developing HMD.

PREDICTION

Once surfactant begins to be secreted by the alveolar epithelial type II cells in the fetus, lung fluid moves from the fetal lung into the amniotic cavity and transports suspended surfactant from the alveoli to the amniotic fluid. The concentration of surfactant in amniotic fluid reflects the amount of surfactant available at the alveolar surfaces and thus the potential stability of the respiratory units and risk of HMD. Gluck and associates showed that the concentrations of the phospholipids lecithin and sphingomyelin are equal in amniotic fluid in midgestation, but after 34 weeks there is twice as much lecithin as sphingomyelin; this change parallels the maturation of the lung. Their work led to the widespread use of the lecithin-sphingomyelin (L/S) ratio for predicting which fetuses will develop HMD when delivered.

Several other amniotic fluid tests for assessing lung maturity are now widely available, including the measurement of phsophatidyl-glycerol (PG), a relatively surfactant-specific phospholipid, and the simple and rapid foam stability or shake test. Although these tests can provide very useful clinical guidance in certain situations, they are all limited by a high false-negative rate secondary to the accumulation of normal intracellular surfactant stores well before amniotic fluid levels of surfactant change.

PREVENTION

Because neonatal respiratory distress is associated with incomplete development of the lung at the time of birth, premature delivery should be delayed, where possible, at least until the lung is mature, as judged by analysis of amniotic fluid for surfactant. When premature delivery cannot be avoided, additional efforts should be made to accelerate lung maturation. In 1972, Liggins and Howie reported that administration of betamethasone to women in premature labor at least 2 days before delivery significantly reduced the incidence of respiratory distress in infants born at a gestation of less than 34 weeks. This observation is consistent with experimental studies that have shown that glucocorticoids accelerate lung maturation in fetal rabbits and lambs (Fig. 2-38). These benefits

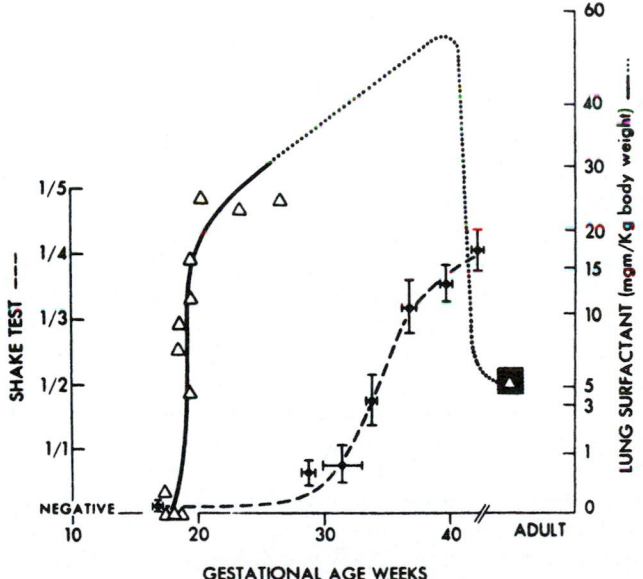

FIGURE 2-37   The relation between gestational age and surfactant in homogenates of whole lung (*open triangles and solid line*) **and surfactant in amniotic fluid as judged by the dilutions 1/1 to 1/5 of amniotic fluid in which there are stable bubbles (the shake test;** *broken line and solid dots*)**. By 22 weeks' gestation, there is more than 10 times as much surfactant per gram of fetal lung than in the adult lung. Note the lung surfactant concentration is a log scale. Surfactant usually is not detected in amniotic fluid until after 30 weeks' gestation, however, and it cannot be demonstrated in dilute amniotic fluid until 35 to 36 weeks' gestation.**

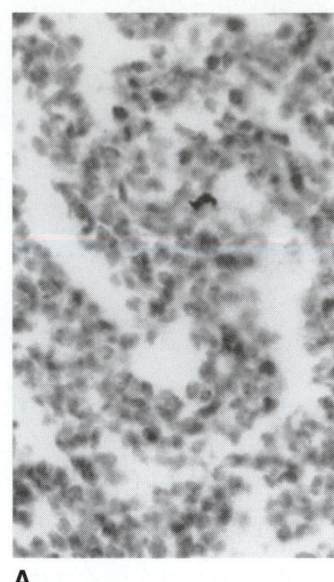 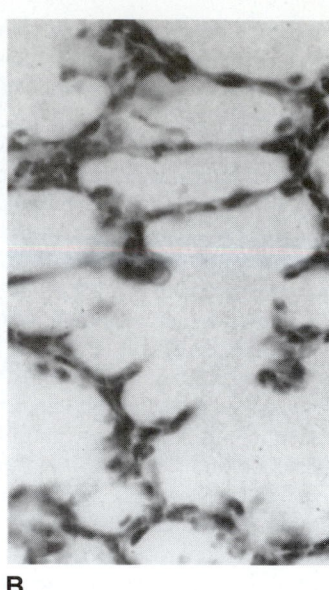

A   **B**

FIGURE 2-38 **Lungs from a pair of twin lambs delivered by cesarean section after 128 days' gestation and killed at birth. The lungs were distended with formalin at 10 cm H$_2$O pressure and fixed. A. Untreated twin. B. This twin received 10 mg betamethasone 48 hours before delivery.**

include not only a reduction in the risk of RDS but also a substantial reduction in mortality and IVH. Based on a review of the available data, a National Institutes of Health–sponsored panel of scientific advisors developed the following recommendations for the use of antenatal corticosteroids:

1. The benefits of antenatal administration of corticosteroids to fetuses at risk of preterm delivery vastly outweigh the potential risks.
2. All fetuses between 24 and 34 weeks of gestation at risk of preterm delivery should be considered candidates for antenatal treatment with corticosteroids.
3. The decision to use antenatal corticosteroids should not be altered by fetal race or gender or by the availability of surfactant replacement therapy.
4. Patients eligible for therapy with tocolytics should also be eligible for treatment with antenatal corticosteroids.
5. Treatment consists of two doses of 12 mg of betamethasone given IM 24 hours apart or four doses of 6 mg of dexamethasone given IM 12 hours apart. Optimal benefit begins 24 hours after initiation of therapy and lasts 7 days.
6. Because treatment with corticosteroids for less than 24 hours is still associated with significant reductions in neonatal mortality, RDS, and IVH, antenatal corticosteroids should be given unless immediate delivery is anticipated.
7. In preterm premature rupture of membranes at less than 30 to 32 weeks of gestation, in the absence of clinical chorioamnionitis, antenatal corticosteroid use is recommended because of the high risk of IVH at these early gestational ages.
8. In complicated pregnancies where delivery before 34 weeks of gestation is likely, antenatal corticosteroid use is recommended unless there is evidence that corticosteroids will have an adverse effect on the mother or that delivery is imminent.

Widespread acceptance of these recommendations has greatly increased the number of preterm infants exposed to prenatal steroids and contributed to the steadily improving outcomes reported. Although no long-term negative effects have been detected in infants treated by the guidelines above, valid concerns remain about potential deleterious developmental effects of repeated prenatal steroid exposures from early in gestation. For this reason, treatment

with more than two prenatal steroid courses requires further evaluation.

TREATMENT

ADEQUATE RESUSCITATION Infants born prematurely, infants of diabetic mothers, or infants subjected to marked asphyxia during delivery are at high risk of developing HMD and should be resuscitated immediately at birth. This should include expansion of the lungs with positive pressure if the infant's initial spontaneous respiratory efforts do not completely expand the lung and continued ventilatory support with intermittent positive-pressure breaths or continuous positive end-expiratory pressure (CPAP) to maintain the arterial PO$_2$ between 50 and 70 mm Hg. Assisted ventilation or CPAP should be continued until the infant can keep the PO$_2$ in these ranges while breathing spontaneously and without extraordinary effort.

GENERAL SUPPORT The infant should be cared for in a warm, neutral thermal environment. Fluid intake should be restricted until lung fluid is absorbed and diuresis is complete, usually on the third day of life. Usually 60 to 80 mL/kg/d of 10% glucose solution is adequate. The amount should be increased if the sodium concentration rises. No sodium should be given because newborn infants have a large extracellular fluid volume and hence have a relative excess of total body sodium. After any initial asphyxia is corrected, hypokalemia and hypocalcemia may occur, so that both potassium (2 mEq/kg/d) and calcium (calcium gluconate, 200 mg/kg/d) should be added to the intravascular infusion. If the arterial pressure remains low in the early course of the disease, and if peripheral circulation is inadequate, as judged by poor capillary filling, the circulating volume may be increased with normal saline or colloid solutions. Infusion of dopamine (5 to 20 μg/kg/min) may be used to support blood pressure and minimize fluid administration, especially in the very low-birth-weight infant.

RESPIRATORY SUPPORT The only way to increase the arterial PO$_2$ in infants with HMD is to increase the alveolar PO$_2$ in poorly ventilated lung units. This can be accomplished by increasing the in-

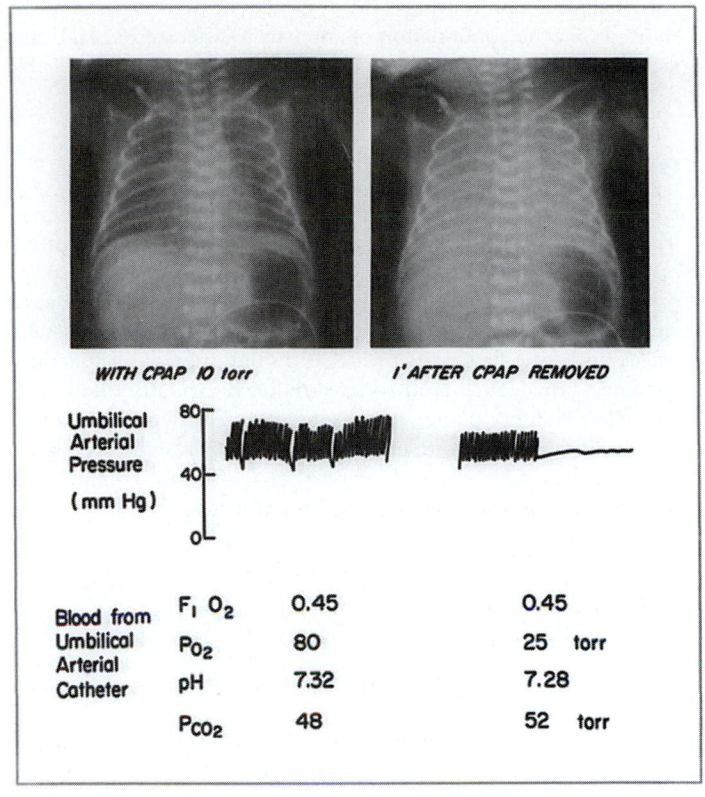

FIGURE 2-39 Chest radiographs, aortic blood pressure, pH, and blood gases in an infant with neonatal respiratory distress during spontaneous breathing *(left)* and 1 minute after constant positive airway pressure (CPAP) was temporarily removed *(right)*. The marked fall in arterial oxygen tension from 80 to 25 mm Hg parallels the rapid development of atelectasis shown in the radiograph.

spired oxygen tension or by applying positive pressure to the lung and improving ventilation in poorly ventilated lung units.

Oxygen may be administered by hood initially. The inspired oxygen tension should be kept just high enough to maintain the arterial oxygen tension between 50 and 70 mm Hg.

Because progressive atelectasis is the central characteristic of neonatal respiratory distress, distension of the collapsed lung units is the most direct treatment. If the infant is reasonably vigorous, this can be achieved by providing a continuous positive pressure by nasal prongs or an endotracheal tube. We usually institute CPAP when the infant requires more than 50% oxygen to maintain a PaO_2 >50 mm Hg. A continuous positive pressure of up to 6 to 10 cm

H_2O can be efficiently sustained by the nasal route. If nasal CPAP is not effective in maintaining oxygenation, we will intubate the infant's trachea and attempt CPAP by the endotracheal route. The increase in aeration of the lung with positive pressure is shown dramatically in Fig. 2-39. If the infant becomes apneic, or if CPAP alone is not sufficient to maintain oxygenation, positive-pressure ventilation will be needed. Recent data have suggested that strategies that are based on keeping the inspiratory time short and synchronizing the ventilator with the patient's own efforts result in the least risk of pulmonary air leak. Therefore, we ventilate infants with relative rapid rates, 60 to 80 breaths/min, with very short inspiratory times, 0.2 to 0.3 seconds, using a ventilator capable of syn-

TABLE 2-17

EFFECT OF ANTENATAL CORTICOSTEROIDS AND SURFACTANT ON MORTALITY AND MORBIDITY IN INFANTS WEIGHING 600 TO 1750 g AT BIRTH

	STEROIDS		NO STEROIDS	
	SURFACTANT (N = 58)	**NO SURFACTANT (N = 46)**	**SURFACTANT (N = 557)**	**NO SURFACTANT (N = 567)**
Birth weight	992 ± 200	1013 ± 226	1012 ± 284	1021 ± 281
Gest age	27.4 ± 1.8	27.5 ± 1.8	27.2 ± 2.6	27.1 ± 2.6
% male	62%	63%	57%	53%
RDS deaths	0	6.5%	7.2%	19.6%
All deaths	0	15.2%	17.7%	24.9%
Air leaks	1.7%	13%	11%	23%
BPD	48%	55%	61%	62%
PDA	27%	22%	47%	44%
IVH grade 3/4	8%	9%	22%	21%

BPD = bronchopulmonary dysplasia; PDA = patent ductus arteriosus; IVH = intraventricular hemorrhage.
SOURCE: *Jobe AH, Mitchell BR, Gunkel JH: Beneficial effects of the combined use of prenatal corticosteroids and postnatal surfactant on preterm infants. Am J Obstet Gynecol 168: 508, 1993.*

chronized ventilation. We try to maintain the arterial P_{O_2} between 50 and 70 mm Hg by increasing the inspired oxygen tension or positive end-expiratory pressure. Occasionally, even infants receiving synchronized intermittent mandatory ventilation (SIMV) fight the respirator and must be sedated or paralyzed. Because of data suggesting that the incidence of chronic lung disease can be decreased by not attempting to control the arterial P_{CO_2} too closely, we often allow the P_{CO_2} to increase above 50 mm Hg, especially in infants with severe HMD.

Some centers have advocated using high-frequency oscillatory ventilation for management of infants with HMD. The oscillator ventilates the infants at very rapid rates (3000 breaths/min) at very low tidal volumes. Theoretically, low-tidal-volume ventilation might lead to less barotrauma to the lung and fewer complications. Controlled trials of oscillatory ventilation for infants with HMD have not shown any consistent benefit over conventional ventilation, and two of the trials found an increased incidence of severe intraventricular hemorrhage in infants who received oscillatory ventilation. At the present time this therapy for HMD must be considered experimental (see Sec. 2.19.2)

SURFACTANT REPLACEMENT The causes of neonatal respiratory distress can be favorably altered by instilling pulmonary surfactant at birth into the lungs of infants born at high risk of having immature lungs. Since the mid 1980s, a large number of carefully controlled clinical trials have been published showing that therapy with surfactant is safe, that it clearly reduces mortality from HMD, that it decreases the incidence of air leaks, and that in small infants it decreases the incidence of intracranial hemorrhage.

There are currently three types of surfactant preparations commercially available in the United States: (1) an artificial surfactant derived from minced cow lung with added synthetic disaturated phosphatidylcholine (Survanta), (2) an artificial surfactant derived from calf lung lavage fluid (Infrasurf), and (3) a synthetic surfactant that consists primarily of disaturated phosphatidylcholine plus the alcohol of palmitic acid (Exosurf). In Europe alternative but similar surfactants derived from cow (Alveofact) or pig lungs (Curosurf) are also available. These preparations appear to be equally effective in treating and preventing HMD as measured by mortality and incidence of chronic lung disease. There is accumulating evidence that the animal-derived surfactants containing surfactant proteins B and C have a faster onset of action and prevent more air leaks.

In addition, there are now two clearly defined treatment strategies for administration of surfactant: (1) prophylactic therapy, which requires that the surfactant preparation be instilled into the infant's trachea shortly after birth, preferably in the delivery room; and (2) rescue therapy, which is designed to treat infants with established hyaline membrane disease. Although both therapies are probably efficacious for larger infants, prophylactic therapy is superior for very low-birth-weight infants (<30 weeks of gestation).

In our institution all infants under 28 weeks of gestation undergo tracheal intubation and artificial ventilation in the delivery room and receive prophylactic surfactant. They receive a second dose if there is ongoing evidence of HMD 12 hours after birth. Older infants are treated when they meet criteria for rescue therapy. The infant must be intubated and must have an arterial-to-alveolar oxygen tension ratio <0.22. We consider all infants who require F_IO_2 >0.5 to maintain P_aO_2 >50 mm Hg candidates for intubation and treatment with surfactant. Surfactant can be administered to infants who are being supported by CPAP only.

Although surfactant replacement therapy has had a major impact on the outcome for premature infants, the important role of glu-

cocorticoids in preventing HMD should be remembered. Jobe showed that the combination of antenatal corticosteroids and surfactant replacement therapy synergistically reduce mortality (Table 2-17).

OUTCOME

Of infants with HMD, 80 to 90% survive, and most of the survivors have normal lungs by 1 month of age. A few develop persistent respiratory distress, however, and may require an increased inspired oxygen concentration for many weeks. Those with a protracted chronic course have a high incidence of respiratory illness with wheezing in the first years of life. Although most lung functions become normal, they tend to have reduced expiratory flow rates and in late childhood often have exercise- or methacholine-induced bronchospasm. Premature infants with neonatal respiratory distress are more likely to have developmental disabilities than prematurely born infants without neonatal respiratory distress.

References

Avery ME, Mead J: Surface properties in relation to atelectasis and hyaline membrane disease. Am J Dis Child 97:517, 1959

Bose C, Corbet A, Bose G, et al: Improved outcome at 28 days of age for very low birth weight infants treated with a single dose of a synthetic surfactant. J Pediatr 117:947, 1990

Chu J, Clements JA, Cotton EK, et al: Neonatal pulmonary ischemia. Pediatrics 40(Suppl):709, 1967

Clements JA: Surface phenomena in relation to pulmonary function (Sixth Bowditch Lecture). Physiologist 5:11, 1962

Clements JA, Platzker AC, Tierney DF, et al: Assessment of the risk of the respiratory distress syndrome by a rapid test for surfactant in amniotic fluid. N Engl J Med 286:1077, 1972

Collaborative Group on Antenatal Steroid Treatment: Effect of antenatal dexamethasone administration on the prevention of respiratory distress syndrome. Am J Obstet Gynecol 141:276, 1981

deLemos RA, Shermeta DW, Knelson JH, et al: Acceleration of appearance of pulmonary surfactant in the fetal lamb by administration of corticosteroids. Am Rev Respir Dis 102:459, 1970

Dunn MS, Shennan AT, Possmayer F: Single- versus multiple-dose surfactant replacement therapy in neonates of 30 to 36 weeks' gestation with respiratory distress syndrome. Pediatrics 86:564, 1990

Farrell PM, Avery ME: Hyaline membrane disease. Am Rev Respir Dis 111: 657, 1975

Ferrara TB, Hoekstra RE, Couser RJ, et al: Effects of surfactant therapy on outcome of infants with birth weights of 600 to 750 grams. J Pediatr 119:455, 1991

Finlay-Jones JM, Papadimitriou JM, Barter RA: Pulmonary hyaline membrane: light and election microscopic study of the early stage. J Pathol 112:117, 1974

Fujiwara T, Chida S, Watabe Y, et al: Artificial surfactant therapy in hyaline membrane disease. Lancet 1:55, 1980

Anonymous et al: Effect of corticosteroids for fetal maturation on perinatal out: NIH Consensus Development Panel on the effect of corticosteroids for fetal maturation on perinatal duct. JAMA 273:413, 1995 (in press)

Gluck L, Kulovich MV, Borer RC, et al: Diagnosis of the respiratory distress syndrome by amniocentesis. Am J Obstet Gynecol 109:440, 1971

Gregory GA, Kitterman JA, Phibbs RH, et al: Treatment of idiopathic respiratory distress syndrome with continuous airway pressure. N Engl J Med 284:1333, 1971

Gribetz I, Frank NR, Avery ME: Static volume pressure relations of excised lungs of infants with hyaline membrane disease, newborn and stillborn infants. J Clin Invest 38:2168, 1959

HIFI Study Group: High frequency oscillatory ventilation compared with conventional mechanical ventilation in the treatment of respiratory failure in preterm infants. N Engl J Med 320:320, 1989

Horbar JD, Soll RF, Sutherland JM, et al: A multicenter randomized, placebo-controlled trial of surfactant therapy for respiratory distress syndrome. N Eng J Med 320:959, 1989

Horbar JD, Wright LL, Soll R, et al: A multicenter randomized trial comparing two surfactants for the treatment of neonatal respiratory distress syndrome. J Pediatr 123:757, 1993

James LS: Perinatal events and respiratory distress syndrome. N Engl J Med 292:1291, 1975

Jobe AH: Pulmonary surfactant therapy. N Engl J Med 328:861, 1993

Kari MA, Hallman M, Eronen M, et al: Prenatal dexamethasone treatment in conjunction with rescue therapy of human surfactant: a randomized placebo-controlled multicenter study. Pediatrics 93:730, 1994

Karlberg P, Cook CD, O'Brien D, et al: Studies of respiratory physiology in the newborn infant: observations during and after respiratory distress. Acta Paediatr 43(Suppl 100):397, 1954

Kendig JW, Notter RH, Cox C, et al: A comparison of surfactant as immediate prophylaxis and as rescue therapy in newborns of less than 30 weeks' gestation. N Engl J Med 324:865, 1991

Liggins GC: Premature deliery of fectal lambs infused with glucocorticoids. J Endocrinol 45:515, 1969

Liggins GC, Howie RN: A controlled trial of antepartum glucocorticoid treatment for prevention of the respiratory distress syndrome in premature infants. Pediatrics 50:515, 1972

Long W, Corbet A, Cotton R, et al: A controlled trial of synthetic surfactant in infants weighing 1250 g or more with respiratory distress syndrome. N Engl J Med 325:1696, 1991

Long W, Thompson T, Sundell H, et al: Effects of two rescue doses of a synthetic surfactant on mortality rate and survival without bronchopulmonary dysplasia in 700- to 1350-gram infants with respiratory distress syndrome. J Pediatr 118:595, 1991

MacArthur BA, Howie RN, Dezoete JA, Elkins J: School progress and cognitive development of 6 year old children whose mothers were treated antenatally with betamethasone. Pediatrics 70:99, 1982

Nelson NM, Prod'hom LS, Cherry RB, Lipsitz PJ, Smith CA: Pulmonary function in the newborn infant. Perfusion, estimation by analysis of the arterial-alveolar carbon dioxide difference. Pediatrics 30:975, 1962

Nogee L, de Mello DE, Dehner L, Colten H: Brief report: deficiency of pulmonary surfactant protein B in congenital alveolar proteinosis. N Engl J Med 328:406–410, 1993

OSIRIS Collaborative Group: Early versus delayed neonatal administration of a synthetic surfactant—the judgment of OSIRIS. Lancet 340:1363, 1992

Oxford Region Controlled Trial of Artificial Ventilation Study Group: Multicentre randomised controlled trial of high against low frequency positive pressure ventilation. Arch Dis Child 66:770, 1991

Sedin G: Positive pressure ventilation at moderately high frequency in newborn infants with respiratory distress syndrome (IRDS). Acta Anaesthesiol Scand 30:515, 1986

Shapiro DL, Notter RH, Morin III, et al: Double-blind, randomized trial of a calf lung surfactant extract administered at birth to very premature infants for prevention of respiratory distress syndrome. Pediatrics 76:593, 1985

Soll RF, Hoekstra RE, Fangman JJ, et al: Multicenter trial of single-dose modified bovine surfactant extract (Survanta) for prevention of respiratory distress syndrome. Pediatrics 85:1092, 1990

2.16.2   Patent Ductus Arteriosus in the Preterm Infant

Ronald I. Clyman

During fetal life the ductus arteriosus (DA) serves to divert blood away from the fluid-filled lungs toward the descending aorta and placenta. In term infants, obliteration of the DA takes place after birth through a process of vasoconstriction and anatomic remodeling. In infants who are born prematurely, the DA frequently fails to close. The clinical consequences of a patent DA (PDA) are related to the magnitude of blood flow from the systemic to the pulmonary circulation through the PDA and associated changes in perfusion of the lungs, kidneys, and intestine.

REGULATION OF PATENCY

Closure of the DA depends on an alteration in the balance between dilating and contracting forces. The DA normally has a high level of intrinsic tone during fetal life. After delivery, an increase in arterial oxygen tension plays an additional important role in DA constriction. Oxygen's mechanism of action remains unknown. The DA also produces several vasodilator substances that inhibit the ability of the intrinsic tone and oxygen to constrict the ductus. Vasodilator prostaglandins, especially PGE_2 play a significant role in maintaining ductus patency during fetal and neonatal life. By inhibiting the enzyme cyclooxygenase, blockade of prostaglandin synthesis produces constriction of the ductus. Both isoforms of cyclooxygenase (COX1 and COX2) are expressed in the DA, and both nonselective (eg, indomethacin) and selective cyclooxygenase inhibitors constrict the DA. The DA also produces a nitric oxide (NO)-like vasodilator; competitive inhibitors of nitric oxide synthase constrict the newborn ductus. Following delivery, arterial PO_2 increases, the concentration of PGE_2 in the circulation decreases, and blood pressure within the ductus lumen falls as pulmonary vascular resistance decreases. All of these events promote DA constriction in the term newborn.

The immature ductus is less likely to constrict after birth; the DA of extremely immature infants (<0.7 term gestation) has decreased intrinsic tone. In addition, there is an increased sensitivity of the immature ductus to the vasodilating effects of PGE_2 and NO. The endogenous factors that alter the sensitivity of the DA to locally produced PGE_2 and NO are unknown, although prenatal administration of glucocorticoids decreases the sensitivity of the DA to PGE_2 and thereby decreases the incidence of PDA.

In the full-term newborn, ductus constriction causes hypoxia in the muscle media of the DA. Vessel wall hypoxia is responsible for the events that prevent DA reopening and promote permanent closure by inhibiting PGE_2 and NO production and initiating the anatomic remodeling that obliterates the vessel's lumen. In preterm infants, the DA frequently remains open for many days after birth. Even when it does constrict, profound hypoxia and anatomic remodeling often fail to occur in the premature infant, which makes them susceptible to reopening of the DA.

HEMODYNAMIC AND PULMONARY ALTERATIONS

The DA in the preterm infant shunts blood predominantly from the aorta to the pulmonary artery (left-to-right shunt). The pathophysiological features of a PDA depend both on the magnitude of the left-to-right shunt and on the cardiac and pulmonary responses to the shunt. Preterm infants are capable of increasing their left ventricular output and maintaining their "effective" systemic blood flow even with left-to-right PDA shunts equal to 50% of left ventricular output. With shunts greater than 50% of left ventricular output, "effective" systemic blood flow decreases despite a continued increase in left ventricular output. The increase in left ventricular output associated with a PDA is accomplished by an increase in stroke volume. Stroke volume increases primarily as a result of the simultaneous decrease in afterload on the heart and the increase in left ventricular preload. Despite the ability of the left ventricle to increase its output in the face of a left-to-right DA shunt, blood flow is significantly redistributed. This redistribution of systemic blood flow occurs even with small shunts. Blood flow to the skin, bone, and skeletal muscle is most likely to be affected by the DA left-to-right shunt. The organs next most likely to be affected are the gastrointestinal tract and kidneys. These organs receive decreased blood flow as a result of decreased mean perfusion pressure (from a drop in diastolic pressure) as well as local vasoconstriction; they may experience significant hypoperfusion before there are any signs of left ventricular compromise. The decrease in organ perfusion contributes to some of the morbidities caused by a PDA: feeding intolerance that sometimes progresses to necrotizing enterocolitis and decreased glomerular filtration rate that often leads to oliguria and renal dysfunction.

Sometimes therapeutic interventions, such as surfactant replacement, can exacerbate the left-to-right PDA shunt in preterm infants by improving lung expansion and reducing pulmonary vascular resistance. Excessive fluid administration also has been shown to contribute to the adverse effects of a PDA. The presence of a very large PDA exposes the pulmonary microvasculature to systemic blood pressure and increased pulmonary blood flow. A rapid increase in pulmonary blood flow through a PDA can lead to pulmonary hemorrhage. Because the premature infant with RDS frequently has low plasma oncotic pressure and increased capillary permeability, any increase in pulmonary microvascular pressure can lead to an increase in lung interstitial and alveolar fluid with resultant reduction of pulmonary compliance. The increased concentrations of inspired oxygen and lung inflation pressures that are required to overcome these early changes in compliance may explain why a persistent PDA increases the risk of subsequent chronic lung disease.

In the preterm infant, there is a delicate balance between PDA-induced fluid filtration and lung lymphatic fluid reabsorption. A PDA that closes by 72 hours after birth usually has no effect on the newborn's respiratory condition. If the PDA persists for longer than 72 hours, however, or if lymphatic drainage is impaired (as it is in the presence of pulmonary interstitial emphysema or fibrosis), the likelihood of edema increases. Infants with a persistent PDA usually develop pulmonary edema and decrease in pulmonary compliance between 5 and 10 days after birth. In these infants, an increase in lung compliance occurs following closure of the PDA.

DIAGNOSIS

Two-dimensional echocardiography with color Doppler flow mapping is diagnostic and helpful in assessing the magnitude and direction of blood flow through a PDA. In normal infants, descending aortic blood flow is forward throughout both systole and diastole; in infants with a large left-to-right shunt through the PDA, there is often a reversal of aortic blood flow during diastole.

Although the magnitude of shunt flow is a significant determinant of neonatal morbidity, equally important factors are the duration of exposure to the shunt and the infant's ability to compensate for the shunt. For example, the same magnitude left-to-right PDA shunt may be clinically "silent" when present within the first 24 hours after delivery, whereas it may be associated with significant respiratory distress and signs of circulatory congestion if it persists for several days.

Clinical signs usually lag behind the echocardiographic signs but have a higher correlation with the development of PDA-associated morbidity. Certain signs, such as a continuous murmur or hyper-

active left ventricular impulse, are relatively specific for a PDA but lack sensitivity; conversely, worsening respiratory status, although a sensitive indicator, is relatively nonspecific for a PDA. Tachycardia is not a useful or reliable indicator of a PDA in preterm infants. The presence of three or more of the following clinical signs has been found to correlate well with the subsequent development of PDA-related morbidity: systolic heart murmur, hyperdynamic precordial impulse, bounding peripheral pulses, a wide pulse pressure, and worsening respiratory status. The electrocardiogram and chest roentgenogram may not be useful in making a diagnosis. Some infants with large left-to-right shunts do not have evidence of cardiomegaly and increased pulmonary vascular markings on the chest roentgenogram.

INCIDENCE

Pulsed Doppler echocardiography assessments of term infants indicate that functional closure of the DA occurs in almost 50% of infants by 24 hours, in 90% by 48 hours, and in all by 72 hours. The rate of closure is delayed in preterm infants, but complete closing usually occurs by postnatal day 4 in otherwise healthy preterm infants. RDS is associated with delayed DA closure. In infants who have had 30 weeks of gestation or more, however, the incidence of PDA beyond 4 days is only 11%, compared to 65% for preterm infants born at less than 30 weeks of gestation, who have severe RDS. Infants who have had perinatal asphyxia or excessive fluid administration during the first days of life also are more likely to develop PDA. Treatment with surfactant is often associated with an earlier clinical presentation because of surfactant's effects on improving oxygenation and lowering pulmonary vascular resistance.

TREATMENT

In some centers, conservative measures have been advocated to treat the symptoms associated with a PDA (eg, fluid restriction, diuretics, and digitalis). Although excessive fluid administration has been associated with an increased incidence of PDA, fluid restriction is unlikely to cause PDA closure. In addition, the combination of fluid restriction and diuretics frequently leads to electrolyte abnormalities and dehydration as well as caloric deprivation, which impairs growth. Digitalis usually is of no use in treating a PDA, as myocardial contractility is increased rather than reduced in infants with PDA. Application of positive end-expiratory pressure has been found useful in managing infants with a PDA. When end-expiratory pressure is added, the amount of left-to-right shunt through the ductus arteriosus decreases, and effective systemic blood flow increases. Anemia has been shown to aggravate left-to-right shunting by lowering the resistance to blood flow through the pulmonary vascular bed. Raising the hematocrit with blood transfusions may reduce blood flow through PDA and help ensure systemic oxygen delivery when perfusion is limited.

A symptomatic PDA in premature infants can often be ligated in the neonatal intensive care unit. In skilled hands, this procedure has little morbidity and a very low mortality. Indomethacin provides an effective alternative to surgery for treatment of a PDA. Its efficacy and toxicity have been explored extensively, and it appears comparable to surgical ligation in preventing the complications associated with a PDA: bronchopulmonary dysplasia (BPD), necrotizing enterocolitis (NEC), and intolerance of enteral feelings. In most intensive care nurseries, indomethacin has replaced surgery as the preferred therapy for a persistent PDA, though questions remain regarding potential adverse side effects (diminished mesenteric, renal, and cerebral blood flow), proper dosage, optimal timing, and duration of treatment. Many variations in dosage regimens have been reported. Table 2-18 outlines one successful approach. Serious toxicity is uncommon with these doses. Oliguria and dilutional hyponatremia, however, are frequent and may require interruption of treatment. Isolated intestinal perforation, usually in the distal ileum, is a well-recognized complication, the incidence of which appears to increase when indomethacin is combined with postnatal glucocorticoid treatment. The relationship between indomethacin treatment and development of necrotizing enterocolitis remains uncertain.

Conditions under which indomethacin should not be used include necrotizing enterocolitis, renal failure (serum creatinine greater than 1.6 mg/dL), severe oliguria (hourly urine output less than 1 mL/kg), bleeding disorders, and low platelets (<50,000/mm³). Intracranial hemorrhage, however, is not a contraindication to the use of indomethacin; indomethacin does not appear to increase the extent of a preexisting intracranial hemorrhage. The postnatal age at which indomethacin is administered plays an important role in determining its effectiveness. Indomethacin becomes less effective in producing PDA closure with advancing postnatal age, as prostaglandins play less of a role in maintaining ductus patency several days after birth compared to the first postnatal days. Although indomethacin treatment is most effective when given in the first 24 to 48 hours after delivery, early postnatal treatment with indomethacin remains controversial. Among infants born beyond 32 weeks of gestation, 90% of those with severe RDS have echocardiographic evidence of a PDA during the first 24 hours, yet only 40% of such infants will manifest subsequent symptoms related to a large left-to-right shunt that will require later therapeutic intervention. If this group of infants were treated during the first 24 hours after delivery, approximately 60% of the infants would have been treated unnecessarily, and some may have experienced one or more complications of therapy. Therefore, such an aggressive approach to therapy can be justified only if early treatment can be demonstrated to significantly alter outcome in these infants.

Although prophylactic indomethacin may reduce the risk of a subsequent symptomatic PDA, this approach does not appear to offer any additional advantage in reducing pulmonary morbidity or necrotizing enterocolitis when compared with an approach that waits for the first symptoms of a PDA to appear (around day 3) before initiating treatment.

TABLE 2-18

DOSAGE SCHEDULE OF INDOMETHACIN FOR PREMATURE INFANTS WITH A PDA

AGE OF ONSET OF TREATMENT	IV DOSE (mg/kg)[a]				
	TIME AFTER FIRST DOSE (IN HOURS)				
	0	12	24	36	48
Infants <1200 g					
<24 hours	0.2		0.1		0.1
>48 hours	0.2	0.1		0.1	
Infants ≥1200 g					
>48 hours	0.2	0.2		0.2	

[a] Three doses of indomethacin are usually given by intravenous (*never* intraarterial) administration over 20–30 minutes.

PDA = patent ductus arteriosus.

Ibuprofen is another nonselective cyclooxygenase inhibitor that may have fewer and less severe side effects than indomethacin. Its relative efficacy in closing the PDA in extremely low-birth-weight infants has yet to be compared with indomethacin.

Reference

Clyman RI, Narayanan M: Patent ductus arteriosus: a physiologic basis for current treatment practices. In: Hansen T, McIntosh N, ed: Current Topics in Neonatology, No. 4. Philadelphia WB Saunders, 2000 (in press)

2.16.3   Neonatal Hypotension and Hypovolemia

James F. Padbury

HEMODYNAMIC ADAPTATION AT BIRTH

Regulation of blood pressure and control of cardiac output and the distribution of blood flow are critical for successful postnatal adaptation. Major physiological adjustments to postnatal life begin in utero and continue over the first hours and days postnatally.

With the onset of labor, there are increases in the circulating concentrations of many vasoactive mediators, including catecholamines, renin, angiotensin, and posterior pituitary peptides. These changes reflect increases in the activity of the sympathetic nervous system and hypothalamic-pituitary hormone release. The concentration of catecholamines rises progressively until the time of cord clamping and delivery and increases further after birth.

The importance of this increase in circulating vasoactive mediators during postnatal adaptation, specifically in the regulation of blood pressure and cardiac output, is well established. At birth, mean arterial blood pressure and left ventricular output increase significantly. In animals in which the adrenal gland has been surgically removed several days before delivery, an absence of the increase in circulating epinephrine prevents the increase in cardiac output, blood pressure, and other physiological adjustments. In the otherwise healthy fetus in whom cardiovascular function is normal, β-adrenergic receptor blockade in utero is relatively well tolerated. In the presence of abnormal uteroplacental function and intrauterine fetal distress or asphyxia, however, β-adrenergic blockade can impair cardiovascular adaptation at near birth and may lead to intrauterine demise or poor physiological adaptation postnatally. The preterm infant is more vulnerable to aberrations in these adaptive changes because of immaturity of cardiorespiratory reflex systems, limited cardiorespiratory reserve, and complications related to prematurity.

FETAL-PLACENTAL CIRCULATION

The fetal-placental blood volume is approximately 110 to 120 mL/kg throughout the latter half of human pregnancy. Under normal physiological circumstances, two-thirds of the fetal placental blood volume, ~80 mL/kg, resides in the fetus. The remaining 40 mL/kg is contained in the placenta. The umbilical-placental circulation is responsive to physiological changes and is well adapted to the developmental and physiological state of the fetus in utero. The high circulating blood volume that is shared by the fetus and placenta maintains blood flow to vital organs and to the whole body for somatic growth. Furthermore, the large blood volume can be viewed as a buffer that confers the fetal circulation with some stability if there should be a transient reduction in blood volume.

PLACENTAL TRANSFUSION

After birth, the timing of cord clamping has a significant effect on the amount of blood "transfused" from the placenta into the newborn (Fig. 2-40). Over the first 5 to 15 seconds after delivery, blood volume increases by 5 to 15 mL/kg as a result of uterine contraction. This early "placental transfusion" does not occur if the cord is cut immediately after birth or if there is a low intrauterine pressure, a low uteroplacental perfusion pressure, or if the infant is held high above the uterus. If cord clamping is delayed for 60 to 90 seconds, or if the infant is held below the uterus, a placental transfusion of more than 25 to 30 mL/kg into the infant may occur. The majority of studies on placental transfusion have been carried out on full-term infants, though recent evidence suggests that delivery of preterm infants is associated with similar hemodynamic changes in the placenta.

NEWBORN BLOOD VOLUME

It was once assumed that "fetal distress" and associated systemic vasoconstriction would reduce fetal blood volume and shift the balance of residual blood into the placenta. Studies have shown, how-

ever, that the majority of newborns who are delivered after fetal distress actually have augmented blood volumes (Fig. 2-41). There are specific conditions in which placental blood volume is increased at the expense of the fetus. Maternal hypotension resulting from hemorrhagic shock, placental separation, or placenta previa accompanied by substantial blood loss leads to a reduction in uteroplacental perfusion pressure, "pooling" of blood in the placenta, and a shift in the balance of fetal-placental blood toward the placenta. Thus, infants delivered in the presence of maternal hypotension are often hypovolemic from redistribution of fetal-placental blood. In contrast, infants delivered rapidly because of fetal distress usually have normal or slightly increased blood volume.

BLOOD PRESSURE IN THE NEWBORN

It is now widely appreciated that accurate measurement of blood pressure in the newborn infant is an important component of the assessment of cardiovascular adaptation after birth. Normal standards for newborn blood pressure and appropriate techniques for measuring it have been well described for healthy term infants. Similar data for extremely premature infants are not as well defined.

There is a gradual increase in blood pressure over the first several days of life at each gestational age. There is also a direct relationship between gestational age and mean arterial blood pressure at any time point, as shown in Table 2-19.

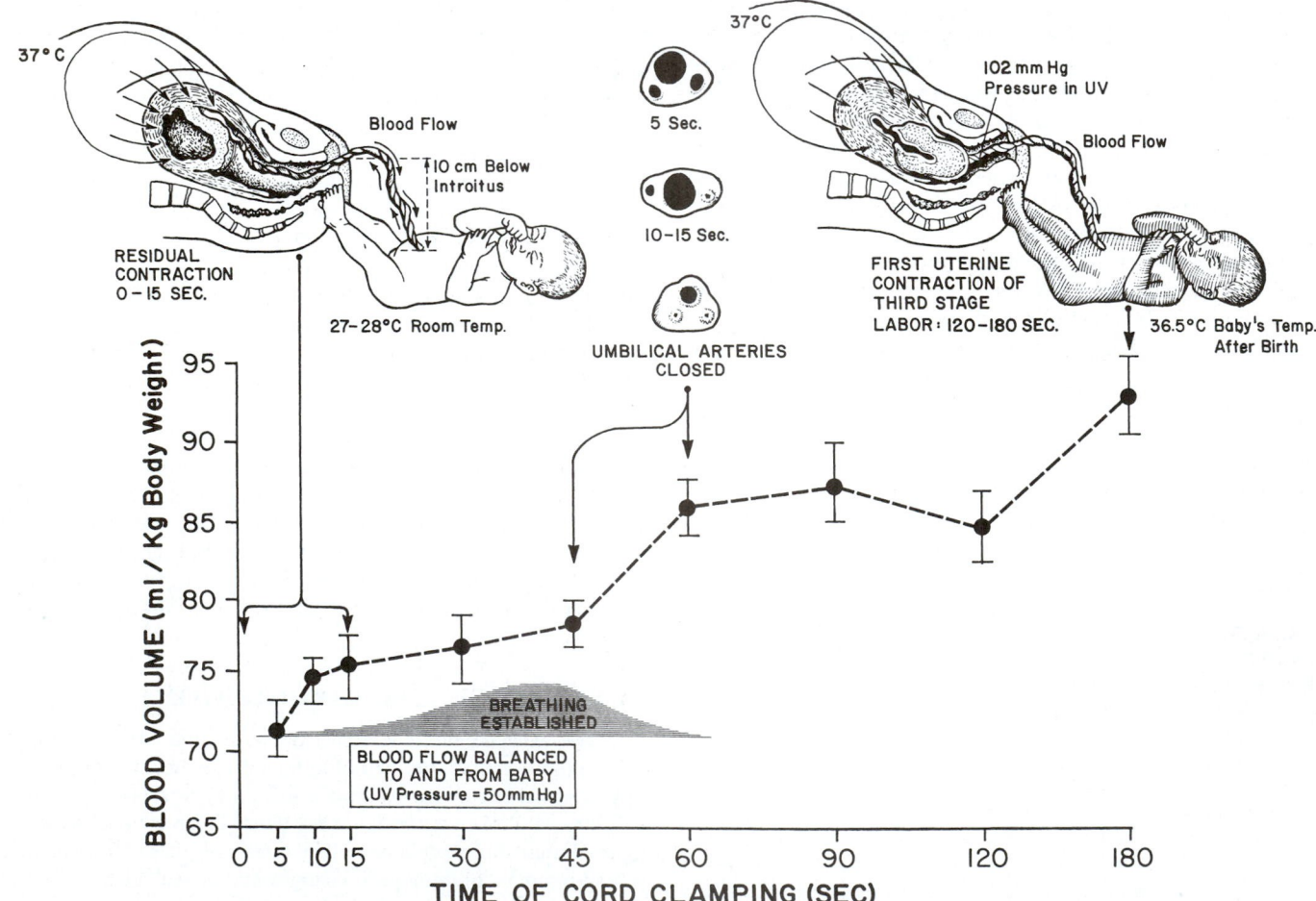

FIGURE 2-40   Change in blood volume of neonate as a function of the time of umbilical cord clamping.

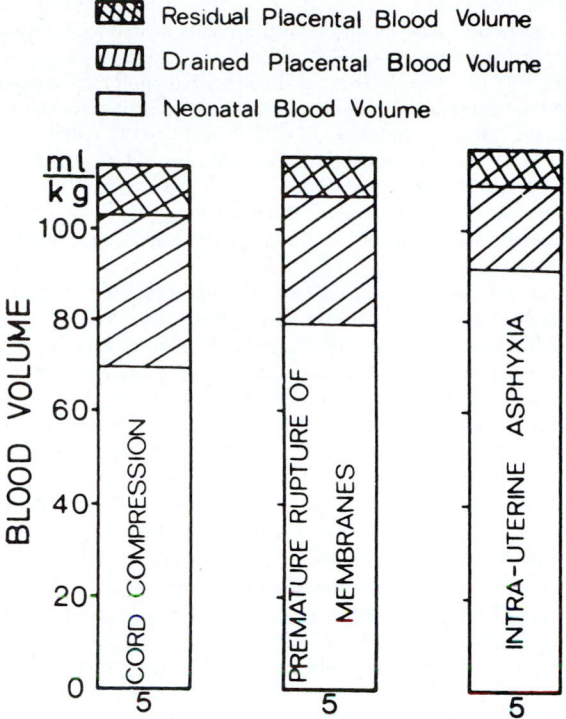

☒ Residual Placental Blood Volume
▨ Drained Placental Blood Volume
▢ Neonatal Blood Volume

FIGURE 2-41   Distribution of blood between neonate and placenta after birth. Cord-clamping times were less than 5 seconds for the infants with cord compression and 15 seconds for the other infants. In each group, five infants were studied.

Although there is no "normal blood pressure" for the extremely preterm infant, it is widely accepted that for a blood pressure to be "adequate" it must provide normal blood pH and sufficient vital organ perfusion to maintain physiological function (see Sec. 4.1.2). End organ function is usually assessed clinically by examining perfusion to the skin and somatic organs, using measures such as urine output to draw inference. Urine flow may be <1 mL/kg/h during the first day after birth and then usually increases to >2 mL/kg/h after that. However, because of birth-related and postnatal effects on hormone release and the influence of immaturity and asphyxia on renal function, urine output is not always a reliable index of renal perfusion.

CLINICAL MANAGEMENT

VOLUME EXPANSION   For hypotensive infants, intravascular volume expansion with judicious fluid usually is effective in raising blood pressure, improving tissue perfusion, and increasing urine flow. For these purposes, either isotonic saline or solutions containing 5% albumin can be given at a rate of 10 to 20 mL/kg over 30 to 60 minutes. Excessive infusion or rapid administration of fluid, however, can increase intravascular pressure abruptly and lead to serious complications, including pulmonary edema and hemorrhage in the lungs or brain.

INOTROPIC AGENTS   If fluid and electrolyte therapy and judicious volume expansion are not satisfactory in correcting disorders in blood pressure regulation and acid-base derangements, inotropic support is often effective in reversing hypotension and improving organ perfusion. It was once assumed that newborn infants were quantitatively different in their responsiveness to inotropic agents such as dopamine and needed substantially higher infusion rates to produce cardiovascular effects. Studies in both newborn animals and human infants, however, have provided strong evidence that both preterm and term infants have qualitative and quantitative responses to inotropic drugs that are similar to those of older infants and children. Dose-response studies conducted in a variety of clinical settings have examined responses in blood pressure, cardiac output, and selective organ perfusion to inotropic agents. These studies have shown that doses as low as 2 μg/kg/min of dopamine are associated with significant increases in blood pressure in infants under 1500 g and in infants with respiratory distress syndrome.

The precise pharmacodynamic (dose-response) and pharmacokinetic effects of dopamine and dobutamine have been studied in term and preterm infants. Preterm infants, like older infants and children, exhibit a threshold in their response to agents such as dopamine and dobutamine. Thus, doses as low as 2 to 5 μg/kg/min of these agents cause significant increases in blood pressure, cardiac output, renal perfusion, and urine output. The clinical threshold for a specific infant is not predictable. The relationship

TABLE 2-19

ARTERIAL PRESSURE, MEAN/10TH PERCENTILES, BY BIRTH WEIGHT AND POSTNATAL AGE

BW (g)	POSTNATAL AGE (HOURS)								
	3	12	24	36	48	60	72	84	96
500	35/23	36/24	37/25	38/26	39/28	41/29	42/30	43/31	44/33
600	35/24	36/25	37/26	39/27	40/28	41/29	42/31	44/32	45/33
700	36/24	37/25	38/26	39/28	42/29	42/30	43/31	44/32	45/34
800	36/25	37/26	39/27	40/28	41/29	42/31	44/32	45/33	46/34
900	37/25	38/26	39/27	40/29	42/30	43/31	44/32	45/34	47/35
1000	38/26	39/27	40/28	41/29	42/31	43/32	45/33	46/34	47/35
1100	38/27	39/27	40/29	42/30	43/31	44/32	45/34	46/35	48/36
1200	39/27	40/28	41/29	42/30	43/32	45/33	46/34	47/35	48/37
1300	39/28	40/29	41/30	43/31	44/32	45/33	46/35	48/36	49/37
1400	40/28	41/29	42/30	43/32	44/33	46/34	47/35	48/36	49/38
1500	40/29	42/30	43/31	44/32	45/33	46/35	48/36	49/37	50/38

Blood pressure in mmHg.

SOURCE: *Warkins AMC, West CR Cooke RWL: Blood pressure and cerebral hemorrhage and ischemia in very low-birth-weight infants. Early Hum Dev 19:103–110, 1989; with permission.*

between administered dose and effect is log-linear; that is, an exponential increase in dose is required for a linear increase in end-organ response. The choice between dopamine and dobutamine is usually dictated by current practice in a given setting, clinical judgment, and familiarity with these agents. There are, however, randomized controlled trials comparing dopamine and dobutamine for treatment of hypotension in preterm infants with respiratory distress syndrome; these suggest that the beneficial clinical response to dopamine occurs at relatively low doses (more than 90% responded to 5 $\mu g/kg/min$) and that dopamine is more effective than dobutamine for reversing hypotension.

Titration to the desired clinical response(s) is the most appropriate way to administer and monitor the effects of these agents. The recommended starting dose is 2.5 to 5 $\mu g/kg/min$ of either dopamine or dobutamine, followed by continuous monitoring of the physiologic response during the succeeding 15 to 30 minutes. The dose is doubled until the appropriate response is produced. Adverse effects, such as tachycardia and arrhythmias, are dose dependent. The goal should be to use the lowest dose possible that produces the desired effects on blood pressure, perfusion, and urine output and to reduce the dose once cardiovascular stability has been achieved.

GLUCOCORTICOIDS Use of glucocorticoids for hypotension in preterm newborns is a controversial practice that has received considerable attention recently. Antenatal glucocorticoid administration has been shown to enhance postnatal cardiovascular adaptation. In preterm animals, antenatal steroids increase blood pressure, cardiac output, and left ventricular contractility. Similar observations have been made in preterm infants who were born to mothers who received antenatal glucocorticoids, when compared with infants whose mothers did not receive these drugs. These observations have been extrapolated to the newborn, to whom low doses of glucocorticoids may be administered to improve "cardiovascular stability." Although transient adrenal insufficiency might occur in preterm infants and contribute to hypotension, documentation of this condition is important to avoid unnecessary and potentially risky treatment. Administration of adrenocorticotropin to a patient with suspected impairment of hypothalamic-pituitary-adrenal function is a simple tool for assessment of this function.

Some published reports have suggested that glucocorticoid administration may reverse hypotension in infants who are unresponsive to volume expansion and inotropic support. These reports were followed by a small series of patients who were given hydrocortisone in a wide range of doses. Glucocorticoid administration was followed by a significant increase in blood pressure and a reduction in the requirement for inotropic support. Subsequent investigators have demonstrated that dexamethasone is also efficacious in low-birth-weight infants with refractory hypotension. The potential risks of dexamethasone treatment are well documented, however, and consequently, such therapy for hypotension cannot be recommended.

References

Agata Y, Hiraishi A, Misawa H, et al: Hemodynamic adaptations at birth in neonates delivered vaginally and by cesarean section. Biol Neonate 68(6):404–411, 1995

Ambrosi B, Barbetta L, Re T, et al: The one microgram adrenocorticotropin test in the assessment of hypothalamic-pituitary-adrenal function. Eur J Endocrinol 139(6):575–579, 1998

Alkalay AL, Pomerance JJ, Puri AR, et al: Hypothalamic-pituitary-adrenal axis function in very low birth weight infants treated with dexamethasone. Pediatrics 86(2):204–212, 1990

Klarr JM, Faiz RG, Pryce CJE, et al: Randomized blind trial of dopamine versus dobutamine for treatment of hypotension in preterm infants with respiratory distress syndrome. J Pediatr 125:117–122, 1994

Linderkamp O: Placental transfusion: Determinants and effects. Clin in Perinatol 9(3):559–592, 1982

McDonnell M, Henderson-Smart DJ: Delayed umbilical cord clamping in preterm infants: a feasibility study. J Paediatr Child Health 33:308–310, 1997

Nuntnarumit P, Yang W, Bada-Ellzey HS: Blood pressure measurements in the newborn. Clin in Perinatol 26(4):981–996, 1999

Padbury JF, Agata Y, Ludlow JK, Ikegami M., Jobe A, Humme J: Effect of fetal adrenalectomy on catecholamine release and physiologic adaptation at birth in sheep. J Clin Invest 80:1096–1103, 1987

Padbury JF, Berg RA: Developmental Pharmacology of Adrenergic Agents. In: Polin R, Fox W, eds. Fetal and Neonatal Physiology, 2nd ed. Philadelphia, WB Saunders, 1996:194–202.

Padbury JF, Ervin MG, Polk DH: Extrapulmonary effects of antenatally administered steroids. J Pediatr 128:167–72, 1996

Padbury JF, Martinez AM: Sympathoadrenal system activity at birth: integration of postnatal adaptation. Semin Perinatol 12:163–172, 1988

Sasidharan P: Role of corticosteroids in neonatal blood pressure homeostasis. Clin in Perinatol 25(3):723–740, 1998

Versmold HT, Kitterman JA, Phibbs RH, et al: Aortic blood pressure during the first 12 hours of life in infants with birth weight 610 to 4220 grams. Pediatrics 67:607, 1981

Watkins AMC, West CR, Cooke RWT: Blood pressure and cerebral hemorrhage and ischemia in very low birth weight infants. Early Hum Dev 19:103, 1989

2.16.4 Necrotizing Enterocolitis

Joseph A. Kitterman

Necrotizing enterocolitis (NEC), a serious acute disease, is the most common acquired gastrointestinal illness in newborn infants. It rarely occurs in infants who have had no enteric feedings, and it mainly affects preterm infants, especially very immature, extremely low-birth-weight infants (ie, <1000 g). NEC is characterized by feeding intolerance, blood in the stools, and typical radiographic features. The disease can be relatively mild or, in more severely affected infants, may progress rapidly to shock, acidosis, clotting abnormalities, bowel perforation, sepsis, and death. The incidence of NEC, which is estimated to be between 2 and 5% of infants whose birth weight is less than 1500 g, has increased in the last several years, probably because of increased survival of very premature infants. Mortality rates range from 5% in term infants to more than 50% in infants <1000. Both the incidence and mortality from NEC vary in different centers. Conditions that are associated with an increased risk of NEC include a history of pregnancy-induced hypertension, maternal age <25 years, prolonged rupture of membranes, antepartum hemorrhage, birth weight <1000 g, and a 5-minute Apgar score <7. In a study of infants <1500 g in several centers, the incidence of NEC correlated inversely with the age at which infants regained their birth weight, suggesting that feeding practices may contribute to the development of NEC. The incidence of NEC is less among preterm infants whose mothers received antenatal steroids to accelerate lung maturity.

The etiology of NEC is unknown. It is likely that several factors are involved, including intestinal ischemia associated with hypoxia, hypothermia, or cardiovascular abnormalities and immaturity of the bowel mucosa, which in turn may adversely affect the digestive and immunologic functions of the intestine. Pathologic findings are mainly necrosis of the small bowel mucosa and submucosa. Inflammation is usually a relatively late finding. The area most commonly involved is distal ileum, often with sparing of the rest of the bowel, but in severe cases extensive areas of small and large intestine may be affected.

CLINICAL AND LABORATORY FEATURES

Clinical manifestations relate primarily to the gastrointestinal tract and include the following.

- Abdominal distension is almost always the presenting sign. In the absence of distension, NEC is rare. Frequent measurements of abdominal girth should be a routine practice during the first several weeks of feedings in preterm infants.
- Gastric residuals indicate feeding intolerance and are especially worrisome if they progressively increase in volume or are bilious.
- Blood in the stool is common and may be detectable only by chemical testing. In more fulminant cases of NEC, grossly bloody stools occur.
- Erythema of the abdominal wall indicates peritonitis and may be seen in infants who initially do not appear severely ill, especially very premature infants with thin abdominal walls.
- Lethargy may be an early sign.

Radiographic findings include the following (in increasing order of severity).

- Focal, nonspecific gaseous distension of bowel loops.
- Thickening of bowel wall from edema.
- Pneumatosis intestinalis (ie, small gas bubbles in the bowel wall; Figs. 2-42 and 2-43, the radiographic hallmark of NEC, may not be seen because of timing of the radiographs or rapid progression of disease.
- A fixed dilated loop present on more than one radiograph indicates lack of peristalsis and suggests the presence of necrotic bowel.
- Portal venous gas presents as linear radiolucent streaks over the liver.
- Free intraperitoneal gas indicates intestinal perforation (Fig. 2-44). In some cases of perforation, pneumoperitoneum is not seen because of localized abscess formation.

Laboratory findings include the following.

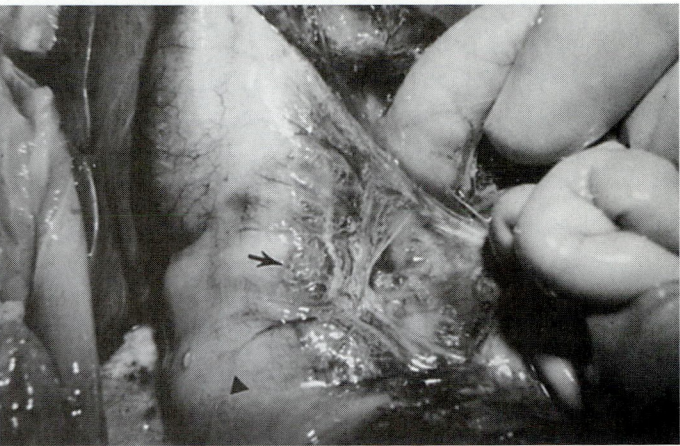

FIGURE 2-43   Gross appearance of pneumatosis intestinalis in an area of small bowel of an infant who died with necrotizing enterocolitis. Note that there are small gas bubbles in both the bowel wall and mesentery.

- Carbohydrate intolerance, manifested by reducing substances in the stool, although small amounts of reducing substances can be normal in infants who are fed breast milk.
- Thrombocytopenia may indicate necrotic bowel.
- Metabolic acidosis and evidence of consumptive coagulopathy indicate severe disease.

The differential diagnosis of pneumatosis intestinalis includes Hirschsprung disease with enterocolitis, midgut volvulus, and intestinal atresia. Conditions to be considered with pneumoperitoneum are incarcerated hernia, intussusception, perforated gastric or duodenal ulcer, pulmonary air leak (usually with pneumomediastinum), and iatrogenic perforations (eg, from an orogastric tube or rectal thermometer). Differentiation from NEC can usually be made from age of onset and other features, but diagnostic laparotomy may be necessary in some cases.

ETIOLOGY AND PATHOGENESIS

The etiology of NEC has not been fully defined and is probably multifactorial. The most likely precipitating event is an ischemic insult to the intestine with resultant necrosis. The earliest pathologic findings are ischemic necrosis of mucosa and underlying tissue, which in severe cases involves the entire thickness of bowel

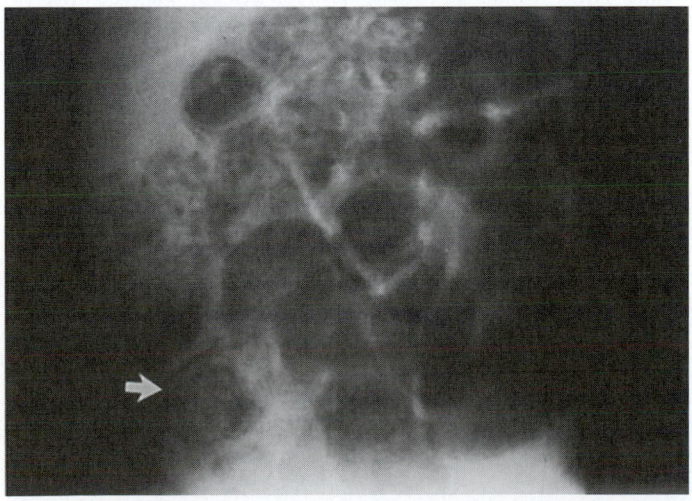

FIGURE 2-42   Abdominal radiograph of an infant with necrotizing enterocolitis. Pneumatosis intestinalis is apparent in a loop of bowel in the right lower quadrant.

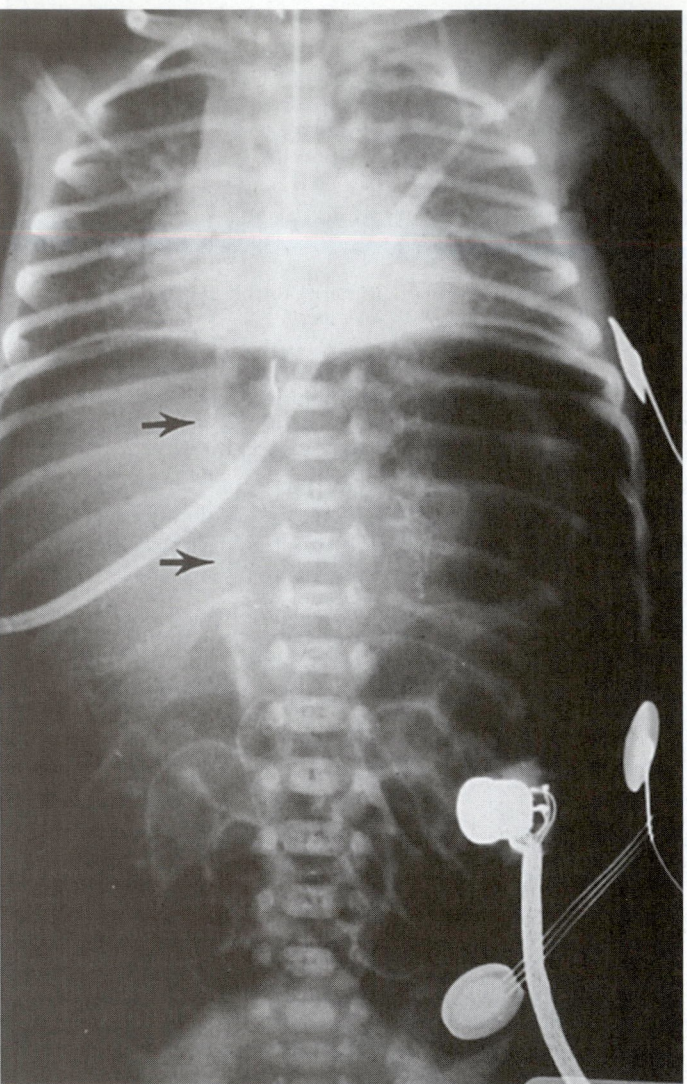

FIGURE 2-44 Free intraperitoneal gas caused by bowel perfora-tion in an infant with necrotizing enterocolitis. Signs of free intra-peritoneal gas include (a) elevation of the diaphragm above the su-perior surface of the liver, (b) the ligamentum teres visible to the left of the midline over the liver, and (c) gas visible on both the luminal and peritoneal borders of stomach and small bowel.

wall. Inflammatory changes occur later, suggesting that infection is a secondary event. Abdominal distension in NEC derives from gas that is formed by bacteria in the intestinal lumen. The gas associated with distension and pneumatosis intestinalis contains large amounts of hydrogen. Bacteria from the bowel lumen of these infants pro-duce very little hydrogen in ordinary culture media but produce large amounts of hydrogen after addition of milk or concentrated glucose. From these findings, it has been suggested that bowel is-chemia leads to decreased peristalsis and ischemic damage to the mucosa. Intestinal bacteria produce gas that leads to distension, which further decreases mesenteric blood flow and causes more tissue damage.

With mucosal necrosis, local bacterial invasion occurs and may progress to systemic infection. Pneumatosis intestinalis results from gas dissecting into the damaged bowel wall or gas production by organisms that have invaded the bowel wall. In severe cases of NEC, gas may enter the portal venous system. Perforation results from necrosis of the entire thickness of bowel wall.

Experimental studies indicate that ischemia-reperfusion injury can produce bowel damage that resembles NEC. Ischemia-reper-fusion injury, which is accentuated by previous formula feedings, increases the intestinal content of xanthine oxidase, a potent source of reactive oxygen metabolites (eg, superoxide, hydrogen peroxide

and hydroxyl free radicals), which may contribute to the tissue in-jury. In addition, the intestinal content of superoxide dismutase (SOD), a scavenger of free oxygen radicals, is decreased in ischemia-reperfusion injury, and retreatment with SOD or allopurinal, an inhibitor of xanthine oxidase, reduces the extent of tissue damage.

Various conditions can lead to bowel ischemia in newborn in-fants. These include asphyxia, cold stress, hypotension, shock, a patent ductus arteriosus (PDA), polycythemia, cocaine exposure in utero, an umbilical arterial catheter with the tip above the origin of the mesenteric arteries, and exchange transfusion through an um-bilical venous catheter with the tip in the portal circulation.

Indomethacin, used as treatment for a PDA, has been associated with bowel perforation, but other clinical and radiographic features of NEC may not be present. In almost all of these cases, the bowel perforation was in the distal ileum, the region most often affected by NEC. In experimental animals, ileal blood flow is decreased both by PDA and by indomethacin. Also, indomethacin causes bowel necrosis in mice that previously had intestinal ischemia. The inci-dence of NEC appears to be increased in preterm infants who are born at or before 30 weeks of gestation and whose mothers had received indomethacin to inhibit preterm labor. Thus, both pre-natal and postnatal exposure to indomethacin can increase the risk of NEC in preterm infants, probably by decreasing intestinal blood flow. Recently, it was reported that early postnatal administration of glucocorticoids is associated with an increased risk of localized intestinal perforation.

Other conditions that are associated with prematurity may also contribute to the pathogenesis of NEC. The immature newborn has limited ability to regulate regional distribution of blood flow and may not be able to increase mesenteric blood flow adequately after a meal. Immunologic function is decreased in preterm infants compared to term infants. Animal studies have shown that fresh breast milk protects against bowel disease caused by the combination of hypoxia, ischemia, and infection. NEC is uncommon but does occur in infants who receive only breast milk feedings; thus, breast milk does not fully protect against NEC.

Immaturity of intestinal mucosal function, including deficiency of certain enzymes, may predispose infants to NEC. Administration of TNF and PAF in experimental animals can produce NEC suggesting that they may participate in its pathogenesis.

Bacterial invasion of the bowel wall is a late event in NEC, suggesting that infection is a secondary phenomenon. Some reports link outbreaks of NEC to increased nursery colonization rates with certian enteric organisms. Prospective studies, however, have failed to show either an association of NEC with specific pathogens or a different pattern of intestinal colonization between patients with NEC and their controls.

PREVENTION AND TREATMENT

Although NEC typically occurs in the first few weeks of life, it may present considerably later, sometimes as late as 2 to 3 months after birth in extremely immature infants, possibly because the onset of feeding is later in these infants and they are older when they receive all feedings enterally. A high index of suspicion should be maintained when feeds are initiated and advanced in preterm infants, particularly in those infants who are small for gestation, in whom intestinal blood vessels may be very small. Conditions that increase the risk of intestinal ischemia should be avoided. It is prudent to postpone enteral feedings in infants who have indwelling umbilical arterial or venous catheters and in those who have clinically significant shunts through a PDA as well as those who are being treated with indomethacin for a PDA. Feedings should be advanced slowly and cautiously in all preterm infants in order to minimize the risk of NEC.

SUSPECTED NEC Enteral feedings should be withheld in preterm infants who manifest abdominal distension or significant gastric contents before feeding. In such instances an abdominal radiograph also may be helpful to establish the presence or absence of normal bowel gas patterns. If distension subsides and the radiograph is normal, feedings can be resumed with caution, but the volume and concentration of feedings should not be advanced until after the infant has taken several feedings without evidence of bowel dysfunction. If distension persists, if there is blood in the stool, or if the radiograph is abnormal, feedings should be discontinued for at least 7 days, gastric suction, should be initiated, a blood culture and complete blood count should be obtained, and broad-spectrum antibiotic therapy should be started. When NEC is suspected, a pediatric surgeon should be consulted in the event that the disease progresses and requires surgical intervention.

DEFINITE NEC In the presence of abdominal distension that is accompanied by blood in the stools and pneumatosis intestinalis or portal venous gas, the aforementioned treatment should begin immediately. In addition, blood pressure, serum electrolytes, platelets, and arterial pH and blood gas tensions should be measured at frequent intervals. Hypotension and hypovolemia should be treated promptly with intravenous fluids and inotropic agents. With NEC, fluid requirements may increase markedly because of fluid loss into the damaged bowel. To monitor for perforation, abdominal radiographs should be taken frequently, as often as every 4 to 6 hours during the acute episode. Parenteral nutrition should commence as soon as the infant's cardiovascular status becomes stable.

SURGICAL CONSIDERATIONS Operative intervention is indicated for intestinal perforation, evidence of necrotic tissue (ie, radiograph showing a fixed, dilated loop of bowel, often associated with metabolic acidosis, coagulopathy, or shock) or a progressively worsening clinical condition that fails to respond to intensive medical management. In some centers, perforation in very small infants is treated with a peritoneal drain rather than laparotomy for the acute episode. However, there have been no reports of controlled trials to compare this method with the more conventional abdominal surgery. If NEC occurs in an infant with a PDA, medical management should begin as above, and operative closure of the PDA to reestablish adequate blood flow to the bowel should be considered. Indomethacin should not be used to treat a PDA in a patient with suspected or definite NEC. **Outcome** of infants with NEC is variable. Most infants will recover without sequelae. In severe cases, bowel necrosis may be extensive, with resultant secondary infection and sepsis (usually with enteric organisms). Long-term complications include intestinal stricture with obstruction and short bowel syndrome (after extensive bowel resection). With NEC, the risk of chronic lung disease is increased, and neurodevelopmental outcome at school age may be adversely affected.

References

Azarow KS, Ein SH, Shandling D, et al: Laparotomy or drain for necrotizing enterocolitis: who gets what and why? Pediatr Surg Int 12:137, 1997

Crissinger KD, Granger DN: Mucosal injury induced by ischemia and reperfusion of the pig intestine. Gastroenterology 97:920, 1989

Crowley P: Corticosteroids after preterm premature rupture of membranes. Obstet Gynecol Clin North Am 19:317, 1992

Eronen M, Pesonen E, Kurki T, et al: Increased incidence of bronchopulmonary dysplasia after antenatal administration of indomethacin to prevent preterm labor. J Pediatr 124:782, 1994

Fanaroff AA, Wright LL, Stevenson DK, et al: Very-low-birth-weight outcomes of the National Institute of Child Health and Human Development Neonatal Research Network, May 1991 through December 1992. Am J Obstet Gynecol 173:1423, 1995

Finnstreom O, Olausson PO, Sedin G, et al: The Swedish national prospective study on extremely low birth weight infants. Incidence, mortality, morbidity and survival in relation to level of care. Acta Paediatr 86:503, 1997

Hseuh W, Caplan MS, Tan XD, et al: Necrotizing enterocolitis of the newborn: pathogenetic concepts in perspective. Pediatr Dev Pathol 1:2, 1998

McKeown RE, Marsh TD, Amarnath U, et al: Role of delayed feeding and feeding increments in necrotizing enterocolitis. J Pediatr 121:764, 1992

Meyers RL, Alpan G, Lin E, Clyman RI: Patent ductus arteriosus, indomethacin and intestinal distenson: effects on intestinal blood flow and oxygen consumption. Pediatr Res 29:569, 1991

Miller MJS, McNeill H, Mullane KM, et al: SOD prevents damage and attenuates eicosanoid release in a rabbit model of necrotizing enterocolitis. Am J Physiol 255:G556, 1988

Peter CS, Feuerhahn M, Bohnhorst B, et al: Necrotising enterocolitis: is there a relationship to specific pathogens? Eur J Pediatr 158:67, 1999

Powell RW, Dyess DL, Collins JN, et al: Regional blood flow response to hypothermia in premature, newborn and neonatal piglets. J Pediatr Surg 34:193, 1999

Uauy RD, Fanaroff AA, Korones SB, et al: Necrotizing enterocolitis in very low birth weight infants: biodemographic and clinical correlates. J Pediatr 119:630, 1991

2.16.5 Intraventricular Hemorrhage

M. Douglas Jones, Jr

Intraventricular hemorrhage arising from the periventricular germinal matrix occurs in up to 80% of infants born at 23 to 24 weeks of gestation. The periventricular germinal matrix is established early in brain development as the densely cellular and densely vascular site of differentiation of neurons and glia, after which outward migration produces discrete brain structures. By the time the fetus is viable, the intraventricular germinal matrix has been reduced to the ventrolateral aspect of the lateral ventricles along the caudate nucleus; by 35 to 36 weeks of gestation it has practically disappeared. The incidence of germinal matrix hemorrhage decreases correspondingly. Intraventricular hemorrhage in full-term infants is rare; the source of bleeding is the choroid plexus (see Sec 25.8.8).

The factors that lead to germinal matrix hemorrhage may be grouped into two general categories: an intrinsic susceptibility of delicate germinal matrix blood vessels to disruption and clinical conditions likely to produce hemodynamic stress on the vessel wall. Although studies in human infants and experimental animals suggest that the vessels of the involuting germinal matrix are both poorly supported by surrounding structures and intrinsically fragile, several observations suggest that susceptibility to rupture and bleeding is not a constant property. The incidence of hemorrhage decreases sharply during the first 72 hours after birth; interestingly, this occurs independently of initial gestational age. The incidence is lower at all ages if the mother is given antenatal corticosteroids. A positive association between hemorrhage and the presence of chorioamnionitis suggests that intrinsic susceptibility to hemorrhage may also be increased.

Experimental and clinical evidence suggests that physical stress on the vessel wall is also important. Sudden changes in arterial and cerebral venous pressure produce germinal matrix hemorrhage in experimental animals. Clinical situations that would be expected to increase cerebral blood flow and intravascular pressures have been epidemiologically, and in some cases temporally, associated with germinal matrix hemorrhage. These include asphyxia, respiratory distress syndrome (perhaps in part because of associated asphyxia and in part because variations in intrathoracic pressure cause fluctuations in arterial and cerebral venous pressure), pneumothorax, and rapid blood volume expansion. Histologic studies showing initial bleeding from small veins suggests that increases in cerebral venous pressure may be the most important event.

Hemorrhage may be confined to the germinal matrix (grade I) or break through the ependyma into the ventricle (grade II). More extensive intraventricular hemorrhages may be associated with transient ventricular dilation secondary to interference with cerebrospinal fluid circulation (grade III); in approximately a third of these infants, permanent impairment of cerebrospinal fluid circulation results in posthemorrhagic hydrocephalus.

White matter injury in the setting of intraventricular hemorrhage presents as an intraparenchymal echo-dense lesion on cranial ultrasound examination (so-called grade IV hemorrhage). This usually occurs in association with a large intraventricular hemorrhage. If the hemorrhage is unilateral, the white matter lesion tends to be on the same side. Pathologic examination shows the echo-dense lesion to be a hemorrhagic infarction. The association of infarction of white matter with a large intraventricular hemorrhage may reflect simultaneous ischemia of the germinal matrix and white matter. The more likely possibility is that the infarction is secondary to obstruction of local veins coursing through brain tissue distorted by a large germinal matrix hemorrhage.

Massive hemorrhage may be associated with apnea, stupor, decerebrate posturing, seizures, a bulging anterior fontanel, and signs and symptoms of hypovolemia and anemia. More commonly, hemorrhage is associated with little or no clinical abnormality and is identified on a routine cranial ultrasound examination. In the absence of clinical indications for an earlier examination, an ultrasound examination is usually done on postnatal day 4 to 7 in the very premature infant and repeated as indicated. White matter damage is best identified by ultrasound at 4 to 6 weeks of age.

Prevention of germinal matrix/intraventricular hemorrhage depends principally on avoidance of premature birth and its complications. The role of the route of delivery and the use of forceps to decrease cephalic compression is not clear. The incidence of hemorrhage is decreased by administration of dexamethasone or betamethasone to the mother before delivery and by administration of indomethacin to the infant after birth. Corticosteroids may affect the intrinsic susceptibility of the vessels to hemorrhage. Indomethacin causes cerebral vasoconstriction and may attenuate the effect of sudden changes in intravascular pressures. Experimental evidence suggests that it may also promote maturation and strengthening of germinal matrix vascular structure.

Prematurely born infants have a generally higher incidence of motor and cognitive problems and a higher incidence of school failure as compared to infants born at term. Most studies have failed to identify additional neurologic disability associated with isolated germinal matrix and intraventricular hemorrhage. Outcome is far worse if intraventricular hemorrhage is complicated by posthemorrhagic hydrocephalus requiring shunt placement. It is also much worse if hemorrhage is accompanied by white matter injury. The likelihood of sequelae in the case of isolated echodensities is related to size and location; large lesions are invariably associated with disability. Because white matter injury is rare in the absence of large intraventricular hemorrhages, preventive measures are the same as for hemorrhage. Diffuse loss of white matter resulting in atrophic ventricular dilatation is associated with poor outcome. The causes and prevention of diffuse white matter damage are poorly understood.

References

Perlman JF: White matter injury in the preterm infant: an important determination of abnormal neurodevelopment outcome. Early Hum Dev 53: 99–120, 1998

Volpe JJ: Neurology of the Newborn, 3rd ed. Philadelphia, WB Saunders, 1995:403–466

2.16.6   Retinopathy of Prematurity

Graham E. Quinn

INCIDENCE AND RISK FACTORS

Retinopathy of prematurity (ROP) is a disease of the developing retina and its vasculature that occurs largely in prematurely born infants. The main risk factor is extreme prematurity and the associated incomplete development of retinal vessels at the time of birth. In addition, several studies have provided compelling evidence that excessive oxygenation of arterial blood in the premature infant with incomplete retinal vascularization greatly increases the risk of ROP. Thus, careful monitoring of inspired oxygen concentration and arterial oxygen tension are crucial in the management of preterm infants. The largest report documenting the natural history of acute-phase ROP is from the Cryotherapy for Retinopathy of Prematurity study (CRYO-ROP), which included serial examinations of 4099 infants with birth weights of less than 1251 g and who were born between January 1, 1986 and November 30, 1987. Ophthalmoscopic examinations were first performed in the infants at 4 to 6 weeks after birth and subsequently every 2 weeks or less until approximately their term due date. The overall incidence of ROP was 66%, with an incidence of 90% in infants with birth weights less than 750 g, 78% in those with birth weights 751–1000 g, and 47% in infants with birth weights 1001–1250 g. In general, there was an inverse relationship between the severity of retinopathy and the birth weight; the lower the birth weight, the more likely the development of severe retinopathy.

Among 2759 infants examined 1 year after birth, about 4% developed long-term scarring (cicatricial phase) involving the posterior pole of the eye. Slightly more than 2% developed extensive posterior pole scarring or detachment, considered likely to cause serious visual handicap. No infant had been subjected to surgery at the time of the 1-year examination.

CLASSIFICATION

The International Classification of ROP of 1984 has greatly enhanced the study of the course and the treatment of both the acute and cicatricial phases of the disease. The four basic components of the classification include location, stage, extent, and vascular engorgement of the posterior pole.

1. *Location.* The anterior-posterior distribution of the retinopathy is described by dividing the retina into three concentric *zones,* each centered on the optic disc. Zone 1 includes the most posterior portion of the retina and encompasses a circle that has a radius of twice the disc-foveal distance. Zone 2 is doughnut shaped and extends from the edge of zone 1 to a circle with a radius of the distance from the disc to the nasal ora serrata. Zone 3 is the most peripheral and consists of the remaining crescent of peripheral retina anterior to Zone 2.
2. *Stage.* This describes the severity of the retinopathy manifest at the junction between the vascularized and avascular retina; the five stages range from early vascular changes to retinal detachment (Table 2-20).
3. *Extent.* This defines the distribution of the lesion in terms of 30° sectors or clock hours along the circumference of the eye.
4. *Vascular engorgement of the posterior pole.* The presence of engorged and/or tortuous vessels in the posterior pole is termed

TABLE 2-20

STAGES OF RETINOPATHY OF PREMATURITY USING THE INTERNATIONAL CLASSIFICATION[a]

Stage 1	Demarcation line: a thin, flat, white line separating the vascularized posterior retina from the gray avascular peripheral retina
Stage 2	Ridge: a thickening of the retina in the region of the demarcation line
Stage 3	Fibrovascular proliferation from area of the ridge extending into the vitreous cavity
Stage 4	Partial retinal detachment: stage 4A is a partial detachment that spares the macular area (the area of sharpest central vision), and stage 4B is a partial detachment that involves the macular area
Stage 5	Complete retinal detachment

[a] Based on International Classification for Retinopathy of Prematurity, 1984 and 1987.

"*plus disease.*" In severe forms, the designation of plus disease signifies of poor prognosis.

CLINICAL COURSE

The acute phases of ROP progress over several weeks, reaching a peak severity just before term, after which there is either regression with remodeling of the retinal vasculature or scar formation (cicatrization) that may progress to retinal detachment. Table 2-21 shows the median and fifth and 95th percentiles for postconceptional ages at onset of various stages of ROP, as observed in the CRYO-ROP study. The data show that most serious retinopathy does not occur before 32 weeks postconception and that almost all severe retinopathy will have occurred by term or shortly thereafter.

SCREENING FOR ROP

A joint statement issued by the American Academy of Pediatrics, the American Academy of Ophthalmology, and the American Association of Pediatric Ophthalmology and Strabismus in 1997 specified guidelines for selecting infants who should be screened for ROP:

1. Infants with birth weight <1500 g or gestational age of 28 weeks or less, and
2. Premature infants with birth weights >1500 g whose course has been unstable and who are judged by their primary physician to be at high risk for developing ROP.

TABLE 2-21

ONSET OF ACUTE-PHASE RETINOPATHY OF PREMATURITY BY POSTCONCEPTIONAL AGE (WEEKS)

	MEDIAN	5TH PERCENTILE	95TH PERCENTILE
Stage 1 ROP	34.3	—	39.1
Stage 2 ROP	35.4	32.0	40.7
Stage 3 ROP	36.6	32.6	42.9
Threshold ROP	36.9	33.6	42.0

SOURCE: *Palmer EA, Flynn JT, Hardy RJ, et al: Incidence and early course of retinopathy of prematurity. Ophthalmology 98:1628–1640, 1991. Courtesy of Ophthalmology.*

Surveillance for ROP should begin in the neonatal intensive care nursery 4 to 6 weeks after birth or at about 31 to 32 weeks postconception. An indirect ophthalmoscope is used for best visualization of the peripheral retina; scleral depression may sometimes be used to facilitate viewing of the extreme periphery of the retina. Examinations should be done every 1 to 2 weeks until (1) vascularization has proceeded to the outer limit of zone 3 and the infant is therefore not at risk for developing severe retinopathy; (2) successive examinations have documented low-grade nonprogressive ROP in zone 3; (3) retinopathy is definitely regressing; or (4) severe ROP that threatens vision is observed, in which case more frequent examinations, at least weekly, are indicated.

TREATMENT

Treatment depends on the severity of the acute-phase retinopathy. No treatment is needed for stages 1 or 2 or low-grade stage 3. When stage 3 in zone 1 or zone 2 involves at least five continuous or eight cumulative clock hours of fibrovascular proliferation and plus disease is present (termed "threshold" ROP in the CRYO-ROP study), ablation of the entire avascular peripheral retina, within 72 hours, should be considered. Two modalities may be considered. Cryotherapy, which was tested in the nationwide randomized CRYO-ROP clinical trial, involves freezing the avascular retina: a probe on the surface of the eye that penetrates through the conjunctiva, sclera, choroid, and outer retina is used to freeze the region of abnormal vascularization. Recent technological advances with laser photocoagulation have made it possible to ablate the abnormal retinal tissue in ROP. Laser treatment is administered through the dilated pupil directly to the avascular retina. Both techniques can be performed under local or general anesthesia and require continuing postoperative care. Cryotherapy usually leads to swelling and redness in and around the eye that resolves over about a week. Laser photocoagulation appears to have fewer short-term complications, but both techniques are usually effective in preventing progression of the acute retinopathy.

Despite appropriate treatment, retinal detachments occasionally occur. Some detachments may be treated effectively by scleral buckling procedures, in which a small band-like buckle is placed on the sclera and the eye is indented in the region of the detachment. The sclera is brought close enough to the retina to allow the retina to reattach. Despite appropriately timed retinal ablation or scleral buckling, progression to more severe detachment sometimes occurs. With such failures a vitrectomy procedure, in which some or all of the vitreous is removed, may be indicated. However, in these infants outlook for functional vision is poor.

In most infants, ROP regresses without retinal scarring. However, even in the absence of obvious retinal abnormalities, ocular complications may develop later in life, including amblyopia, myopia, and retinal detachment. Thus, infants who have had ROP merit long-term periodic evaluation by an ophthalmologist.

References

Cryotherapy for Retinopathy of Prematurity Cooperative Group: Multicenter Trial of Cryotherapy for Retinopathy of Prematurity: One year outcome—structure and function. Arch Ophthalmol 108:1408–1416, 1990

Cryotherapy for Retinopathy of Prematurity Cooperative Group: Natural history of retinopathy of prematurity (ROP): the natural ocular outcome of premature birth and retinopathy: status at one year. Arch Ophthalmol 12:903–912, 1994

Fierson WM, Palmer EA, Bigham AW, et al: Screening examination of premature infants for retinopathy of prematurity. Pediatrics 100:273, 1997

ICROP Committee: International classification of retinopathy of prematurity. Arch Ophthalmol 102:1130–1134, 1984

ICROP Committee for Classification of Late Stages of ROP: An international classification of retinopathy of prematurity: II. The classification of retinal detachment. Arch Ophthalmol 105:906–912, 1987

Palmer EA, Flynn JT, Hardy RJ, et al: Incidence and early course of retinopathy of prematurity. Ophthalmology 98:1628–1640, 1991

McNamara JA, Tasman W, Brown GC, et al: Laser photocoagulation for stage 3+ retinopathy of prematurity. Ophthalmology 98:576, 1991

Quinn GE, Dobson V, Kivlin J, et al: Prevalence of myopia between three months and $5\frac{1}{2}$ years in preterm infants with and without retinopathy of prematurity. Ophthalmology 105:1292–1300, 1998

2.16.7   Adverse Effects of Drugs in the Newborn

Robert M. Ward

The history of drug therapy for newborns is one of enormous benefits, especially through vaccines, antibiotics, and surfactant, but these are coupled with significant harm through adverse effects of drugs. Both aspects of drug therapy teach important lessons about our limited understanding of developmental physiology, which may create unique susceptibility for newborns to experience adverse effects of drugs. A reduced capacity for drug metabolism and elimination in newborns may require adjustment of dosing schedules that have not been adequately determined through prior systematic study. Variation in the rates at which different organs mature prevents broad generalizations about appropriate drug dosing during the rapidly changing development of the neonatal period.

Pediatric patients, especially newborns, have been left out of the study of most new drugs. In 1968, when 80% of new drugs included no information about effectiveness or dosing for pediatric patients, Dr. Harry Shirkey described these patients as "therapeutic orphans." Children continue to be excluded from studies of most new drugs, so that drug therapy of those patients is seldom guided by large controlled trials. Important lessons from previous adverse neonatal drug effects should serve as reminders about the importance of optimal study and cautious use of drugs today.

The newborn, however, is not always more susceptible to the toxic effects of drugs than older children and adults. Immaturity sometimes bestows greater resistance to drug toxicity. For example, immature renal epithelial transport in newborns reduces the amount of gentamicin that enters the tubular cells and thereby protects the newborn from toxicity.

Although most adverse drug effects that occur in adults and older children also occur in newborns, some effects are unique to the newborn. Toxicity related both to the active drug and to excipients in newborns have revealed unanticipated differences in their physiology and resultant drug pharmacokinetics that underscore the need for proper drug testing in this population. Although more extensive reviews of adverse drug effects in newborns are available, this brief section considers selected drugs in order to illustrate principles about newborn physiology and precautions that can help to avoid adverse outcomes with drug therapy.

TOXICITY FROM DRUG PREPARATIONS

PROPYLENE GLYCOL   Propylene glycol is an excipient, a more or less inert ingredient used as a solvent and stabilizer in many medications that are administered orally, topically (eg, nystatin and Eucerin Cream), and parenterally (eg, diazepam, digoxin, phenobarbital, and phenytoin). Hyperosmolality from propylene glycol has been used in topical treatment of burns with silver sulfadiazine in adults and infants. Consistent with its alcohol structure, propylene glycol may cause intoxication, hypoglycemia, and seizures. In premature infants, propylene glycol has induced renal failure and hyperosmolality when it was administered with multivitamins in parenteral alimentation solutions. It also has been associated with an increased frequency of seizures. Until recently, there was no requirement to identify the presence of propylene glycol as an ingredient of nonprescription drugs or cosmetics. The 1997 FDA Modernization Act now allows this agency to require that alcohol and inactive ingredients be identified in prescription and nonprescription drugs.

BENZYL ALCOHOL Benzyl alcohol is widely used as an antibacterial solvent for liquid medications that is reported to relax smooth muscle and induce hypotension when administered intravenously. It is metabolized to benzoic acid and then conjugated with glycine to form hippuric acid. Concerns raised about its toxicity in the 1970s triggered a series of animal experiments that showed 0.9% benzyl alcohol to be more toxic than ethanol even though large doses were tolerated by rats.

Reports of severe metabolic acidosis, gasping respiration, progressive hypotension, seizures, CNS depression, intraventricular hemorrhage, and death occurring in low-birth-weight (400–1400) infants prompted investigations to search for inborn errors of metabolism only to discover that urine concentrations of benzoic and hippuric acid were increased, as were serum concentrations of benzoic acid in these infants. The benzyl alcohol preservative in saline flush solutions and some dextrose solutions was identified as the cause of demise. Doses that could produce "the gasping syndrome," as it was described, were estimated at 11 to 26 mL of 0.9% benzyl alcohol/kg/d, representing about 100 to 200 mg of benzyl alcohol/kg/d.

This tragic development in newborn therapeutics led the American Academy of Pediatrics to recommend that saline and dextrose solutions free of preservatives must be used in the care of newborn infants. The FDA subsequently ordered that no medications containing benzyl alcohol as a preservative be administered to premature infants.

TOXICITY FROM REDUCED CLEARANCE: CHLORAMPHENICOL
Chloramphenicol became available commercially in the United States in 1949 and soon was used widely for its broad spectrum of antibacterial effects. Chloramphenicol inhibits microbial growth by binding to the 50S ribosome subunit to prevent protein synthesis. The drug also inhibits protein synthesis in rapidly dividing mammalian cells, such as the bone marrow, where high concentrations (>100 μg/ml) can cause aplastic anemia as it did in one of 25,000 to 30,000 patients. Other adverse effects might have been anticipated because chloramphenicol also inhibits mitochondrial protein synthesis at therapeutic concentrations as low as 10 μg/mL

Sepsis in premature newborns has always been a significant cause of mortality and morbidity. The efficacy of chloramphenicol in adults and older children set the stage for its entry into newborn therapeutics. This entry, as for many drugs, was not accompanied by pharmacokinetic or dose-ranging studies. Initial reports of unexplained deaths in newborn infants who had received chloramphenicol led to the definitive identification of chloramphenicol toxicity in a randomized comparison of four treatment strategies to prevent sepsis in premature newborns born after prolonged rupture of the membranes. Mortality for treatment with chloramphenicol alone (100–165 mg/kg/d administered IM q12h) or in combination with penicillin and streptomycin was 60 to 68% compared to 19% with no treatment and 18% for treatment with penicillin and streptomycin without chloramphenicol. The pattern of death in these premature newborns was designated the "gray baby syndrome" because of the appearance of poor perfusion and cardiovascular collapse. The gray baby syndrome developed in infants who received chloramphenicol doses that exceeded the relatively low clearance rate of the drug in the newborn; the immature liver has limited capacity to conjugate chloramphenicol by UDP-glucuronosyl transferase, and there is reduced glomerular excretion of the active (unconjugated) drug. Dose adjustments of chloramphenicol based on neonatal kinetics and careful monitoring of concentration have now provided for its safe, albeit rare, use in newborns.

INADVERTENT PERCUTANEOUS DRUG ABSORPTION: HEXA-CHLOROPHENE The skin of premature newborns at 23 to 33 weeks of gestation is immature enough to allow percutaneous drug absorption as well as increased water loss. Thus, topical application of phenylephrine blanches the skin of premature newborns with less than 30 weeks of gestation during the first few days after birth; the skin matures enough by 2 weeks of age to attenuate this response. In general, the epidermis of premature newborns matures to resemble that of term newborns by 2 to 3 weeks after birth.

Outbreaks of staphylococcal infections in newborn nurseries during the 1950s caused significant morbidity and mortality among neonates. Topical antiseptic bathing of newborns with hexachlorophene reduced colonization and infection with coagulase-positive *Staphylococcus*. A 3% hexachlorophene solution was widely used in a variety of products from surgical scrub to shaving creams. Concerns about toxicity were raised after rare ingestions of hexachlorophene caused lethargy, fever, convulsions, paralysis, coma, and death. Animal studies indicated that hexachlorophene is toxic to the CNS and causes cerebral edema and extensive vacuolization of myelin. When newborns were bathed daily with hexachlorophene, blood levels were shown to achieve toxic concentrations. Widespread use of topical hexachlorophene persisted worldwide until 1972, when talcum powder that was manufactured in France poisoned 204 infants, of whom 36 died. The powder was contaminated with 63% hexachlorophene. Clinical signs of local skin irritation were accompanied by symptoms of cerebral and spinal cord edema, which were consistent with the white matter vacuolization termed "status spongiosus" seen at autopsy. A review of autopsies from perinatal deaths at two US children's hospitals during the previous 4 to 7 years revealed spongiosus changes (vacuolization) in myelinated tracts, mostly in infants who weighed less than 1400 g and who were born at less than 32 weeks of gestation. All had been bathed with hexachlorophene at least four times. The extent of vacuolization was directly proportional to the extent of hexachlorophene exposure. During a later outbreak of staphylococcal infections treated with hexachlorophene, the absorption and kinetics of hexachlorophene were studied. Hexachlorophene concentrations showed a significant inverse relationship to birth weight and to postconceptional age consistent with greater absorption through more immature skin. The half-lives ranged from 6 to 44 hours and were longer in those infants who were premature or had liver disease.

The FDA issued a warning about the toxicity of hexachlorophene in 1971 and then restricted 3% hexachlorophene to prescription status in 1972. Hexachlorophene still provided an effective treatment for newborn staphylococcal infections, a severe problem. On the other hand, increasing survival of more premature newborns with permeable skin created a new risk that had not been suspected until an inadvertent overdose confirmed its toxicity. Previously observed neuropathologic changes in newborns were explained by hexachlorophene treatment.

EPILOGUE

Drug treatment can be essential to the survival of newborns, but immaturity of organ functions from the skin to the liver increases the risk to newborns for adverse effects from drugs. Introduction of untested medications into the treatment of newborns must be done with caution and, whenever possible, as part of a controlled trial. "Common sense" impressions about the effectiveness of specific treatments may not be accurate, such as empiric treatment to prevent sepsis in preterm newborns with prolonged rupture of membranes. At times, clinicians will have to treat empirically based on physiological principles. At the very least, data about dosing, kinetics, and safety should be obtained and reported. All clinicians should guard against the impression that a treatment is so obviously beneficial that it is "unethical" to conduct a well-controlled trial. Such trials are essential to provide a sound scientific basis on which to establish treatment and confirm or deny associations with adverse effects.

References

American Academy of Pediatrics Committee on Drugs: "Inactive" ingredients in pharmaceutical products: update (subject review). Pediatrics 99:268, 1997

American Academy of Pediatrics Committee on Fetus and Newborn and Committee on Drugs: Benzyl alcohol: toxic agent in neonatal units. Pediatrics 72:356, 1983

Brown WJ, Buist NRM, Gipson HT, Huston RK, Kennaway NG: Fatal benzyl alcohol poisoning in a neonatal intensive care unit. Lancet 1: 1250, 1982

Burns LE, Hodgeman JE, Cass AB: Fatal circulatory collapse in premature infants receiving chloramphenicol. N Engl J Med 261:1318, 1959

Craft AW, Brocklebank JT, Hey EN, Jackson RH: The 'grey toddler.' Chloramphenicol toxicity. Arch Dis Child 49:235, 1974

FDA Modernization Act of 1997: National uniformity for nonprescription drugs. Public Law 105–115, 111 Stat 2296, Title IV

Fligner CL, Jack R, Twiggs GA, Raisys VA: Hyperosmolality induced by propylene glycol, a complication of silver sulfadiazine therapy. JAMA 253:1606, 1985

Gershanik J, Boecler B, Ensley H, McCloskey S, George W: The gasping syndrome and benzyl alcohol poisoning. N Engl J Med 307:1384, 1982

Gezon HM, Thompson DJ, Rogers KD, Hatch TF, Taylor PM: Hexachlorophene bathing in early infancy: effect on staphylococcal disease and infection. N Engl J Med 270:379, 1964

Gluck L, Wood HF: Effect of an antiseptic skin-care regimen in reducing staphylococcal colonization in newborn infants. N Engl J Med 265:1177, 1961

Gupta A, Waldhauser LK: Adverse drug reactions from birth to early childhood. Pediatr Clin North Am 44:79, 1997

Harpin VA, Rutter N: Barrier properties of the newborn infant's skin. J Pediatr 102:419, 1983

Kimura ET, Darby TD, Krause RA, Brondyk HD: Parenteral toxicity studies with benzyl alcohol. Toxicol Appl Pharmacol 18:60, 1971

Laferriere CI, Marks MI: Chloramphenicol: properties and clinical use. Pediatr Infect Dis 1:257, 1982

Lapert P, O'Brien J, Garrett R: Hexachlorophene encephalopathy. Acta Neuropathol 23:326, 1973

Lovejoy FH JR: Fatal benzyl alcohol poisoning in neonatal intensive care units. A new concern for pediatricians. Am J Dis Child 136:974, 1982

Lustig FW: A fatal case of hexachlorophane ("pHISOHEX") poisoning. Med J Aust 1:737, 1963

MacDonald MG, Getson PR, Glasgow AM, Miller MK, Boeckx RL, Johnson EL: Propylene glycol: Increased incidence of seizures in low birth weight infants. Pediatrics 79:622, 1987

Macht DI: On the relation between the chemical structure of the opium alkaloids and their physiological action on smooth muscle with a pharmacological and therapeutic study of some benzyl esters. II. A pharmacological and therapeutic study of some benzyl esters. J Pharmacol Exp Ther 11:419, 1918

Martin-Bouyer G, Lebreton R, Toga M, Stolley PD, Lockhart J: Outbreak of accidental hexachlorophene poisoning in France. Lancet 1:91, 1982

McCracken GH JR: Aminoglycoside toxicity in infants and children. Am J Med 80(Suppl 6B):172, 1986

Mitchell AA, Goldman P, Shapiro S, Slone D: Drug utilization and reported adverse reactions in hospitalized children. Am J Epidemiol 110:196, 1979

Shirley H: Therapeutic orphans. J Pediatr 72:119, 1968

Wallerstein RO, Condit PK, Kasper CK, Brown JW, Morrison FR: Statewide study of chloramphenicol therapy and fatal aplastic anemia. JAMA 208:2045, 1969

Ward RM, Lugo RA: Drug therapy in the newborn. In: Avery GB, Fletcher MA, MacDonald MG, eds: Neonatology Pathophysiology and Management of the Newborn, 5th ed. Philadelphia, Lippincott Williams & Wilkins, 1999:1363

Weiss CF, Glazko AJ, Weston JK: Chloramphenicol in the newborn infant: a physiologic explanation of its toxicity when given in excessive doses. N Engl J Med 262:787, 1960

2.17 SPECIFIC NEONATAL CONDITIONS

2.17.1 Pulmonary Gas Leaks

George A. Gregory

Extrapulmonary gas can collect within the interstitial space of the lung (pulmonary interstitial emphysema), mediastinal space (pneumomediastinum), pericardial sac (pneumopericardium), or intrapleural space (pneumothorax), or it can extend into the peritoneal cavity (pneumoperitoneum). Pulmonary gas leaks are common sequelae of lung disease in newborn infants and can be fatal if the gas leak is undetected and untreated.

INCIDENCE

Spontaneous pneumothorax occurs in approximately 1% of infants who are born vaginally at term and in approximately 2% of those delivered by cesarean section; the incidence is higher among premature infants. Pneumomediastinum occurs in approximately 0.25% of newborn infants. All gas leaks occur more commonly in infants with lung disease; for example, a pneumothorax occurs in approximately 10% of infants who are born following meconium staining of the amniotic fluid. Pneumothorax occurs in approximately 5% of patients with mild neonatal respiratory distress and approximately 10% of infants with respiratory distress who require ventilatory assistance.

CLINICAL FEATURES

The clinical signs of a pulmonary gas leak depend on the size and location of the gas accumulation. Interstitial gas leaks cause progressive overexpansion of the lung, decreased movement of the chest cage, and diminished breath sounds on the affected side. Trapped gas in the peribronchial spaces compresses small airways, increases airways resistance, causes wheezing, and overdistends distal alveolar ducts. Unilateral gas leaks displace mediastinal structures to the contralateral side.

Pneumomediastinum can cause severe distress when gas within the mediastinum impedes venous return and decreases cardiac output. Often, however, pneumomediastinum is an unexpected radiographic finding and causes no symptoms. Subcutaneous air in the neck, face, and chest is often the first clue to the presence of pneumomediastinum. Subcutaneous gas in the neck may impinge on the airway and cause acute airway obstruction and respiratory distress. The Herman sign (a crunching or sandpaper-on-sandpaper sound with each heart beat) can accompany pneumomediastinum but is seldom heard in infants and children. If gas extends below the diaphragm (*pneumoperitoneum*), the abdomen distends and becomes tympanitic. This may be confused with signs of a perforated abdominal viscus; usually, however, a perforated viscus causes edema of the skin overlying the abdomen. Fingerprints can be seen on the abdominal wall when the skin is indented with a finger if the patient has peritonitis, but not when the free gas in the peritoneum is from a pneumoperitoneum. A large amount of gas in the peritoneum can reduce venous return and decrease cardiac output. It also can impede movement of the diaphragm and cause respiratory failure.

A small *pneumothorax* may be asymptomatic, or it may cause only slight tachypnea and mild retractions of the chest wall. A large pneumothorax usually causes severe respiratory distress, agitation, tachypnea, intercostal and substernal retractions, and cyanosis. Atelectasis of the ipsilateral lung and compression of the contralateral lung lead to hypoxemia, and decreased ventilation leads to hypercarbia. Hypotension often ensues because of reduced venous return. Apnea and cardiac arrest can occur with large tension pneumothoraces.

The amount of atelectasis caused by a pneumothorax depends on the compliance of the lung involved. Lungs with interstitial air leaks and pulmonary edema have poor compliance and will change little in size, even when the pneumothorax causes high intrapleural pressures (Fig. 2-45A). The affected side of the chest cage expands and bulges outward, and the breath sounds on the involved side may be decreased. Breath sounds, however, also may be normal. This is especially true in small infants because breath sounds are easily transmitted from the nonaffected to the affected side. The trachea, cardiac impulse, and heart sounds all shift toward the nonaffected side, which decreases the effectiveness of ventilation on the side without the pneumothorax. As the pneumothorax increases in size, intrathoracic pressure rises and impedes venous return, cardiac output decreases, and there is peripheral venous congestion. The decrease in cardiac output causes arterial hypotension, a narrow pulse pressure, shock, and metabolic acidosis.

RADIOGRAPHIC FEATURES

The characteristic radiograph of an interstitial gas leak is a coarse, reticular pattern with fine lines of radiolucency extending out from the hilum and running parallel to blood vessels and airways. With

a pneumomediastinum, air may elevate the thymus, producing a striking silhouette (ie, sail sign) (Fig. 2-46B).

Radiologic diagnosis of pneumothorax is easy unless the gas leak is small or the lung is very stiff. The diagnosis is best made during expiration, when the quantity of air within the lung is decreased and the lung parenchyma is more radiodense. This increases contrast between the lung and the air-filled pleural space. A pneumothorax is seen as a uniformly translucent area without lung markings. With a tension pneumothorax, the diaphragm is flattened or inverted, and the heart and trachea deviate to the nonaffected side. With bilateral tension pneumothoraces or with a severe pneumopericardium, the heart is small radiographically.

PATHOPHYSIOLOGY

Air enters the interstitial spaces of the lung through tears in the walls of alveoli or respiratory bronchioles, and it moves toward the hilum through peribronchial and perivascular tissue. Because premature infants have a particularly loose pulmonary interstitium, they are more likely than term infants to have interstitial gas leaks. When gas enters the interstitial space and cannot escape, the lung expands, alveolar volume decreases, and the lungs become difficult to ventilate. In some infants, gas moves along the peribronchial and perivascular tissues to the mediastinum and then up into the neck or down into the peritoneal cavity (Fig. 2-46B). Gas enters the intrapleural space through a pleural tear to form a pneumothorax.

DIAGNOSIS

Definitive diagnosis of a pulmonary gas leak is made radiologically. Free air is detected in the mediastinal, pericardial, interstitial, or pleural space, or in severe cases, free air seen in all of these extrapulmonary spaces. In infants the diagnosis can often be made by placing a focused, cold, intense light directly on the chest. If a pneumothorax is present, the chest will "light up." If there is no pneumothorax, there will be a small area of light surrounding the light source. Examination of the child is important in making the diagnosis. As stated above, breath sounds are not helpful unless they are absent or diminished. On the other hand, watching the chest move during the respiratory cycle may be very helpful. Infants with a pneumothorax often have hyperexpansion of the overlying chest, with diminished or absent movement compared to the nonaffected side, during inspiration. The involved side of the chest also is tympanitic to percussion.

TREATMENT

A spontaneous pneumothorax that occurs in an otherwise healthy infant and does not cause respiratory distress or significant changes of vital signs or arterial blood gas tension usually does not require active intervention. Most of these gas leaks will resolve spontaneously. Although resorption of gas can be accelerated by breathing 100% oxygen, this therapy is not recommended in premature infants because consequent hyperoxia may contribute to the development of retinopathy.

If a pneumothorax causes respiratory distress, hypoxemia, hypercarbia, or hypotension, immediate decompression of the pneumothorax is mandatory. A 22- or 20-gauge angiocath is connected to a three-way stopcock and a large syringe. The needle is advanced through the second intercostal space at the midclavicular line until it enters the pleural space. Negative pressure is maintained in the syringe while the needle is being advanced. If gas can be withdrawn

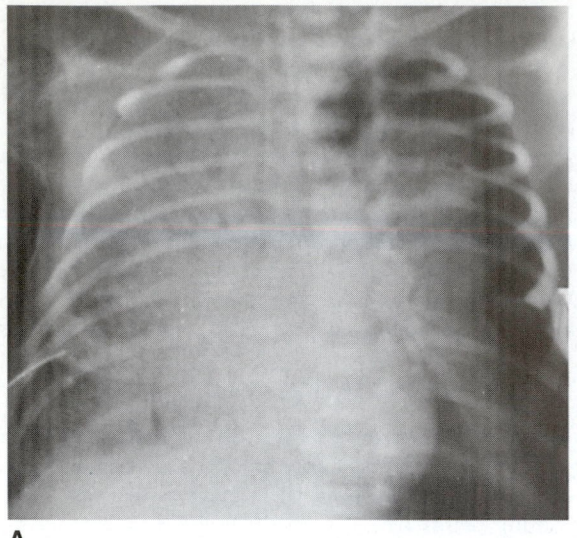

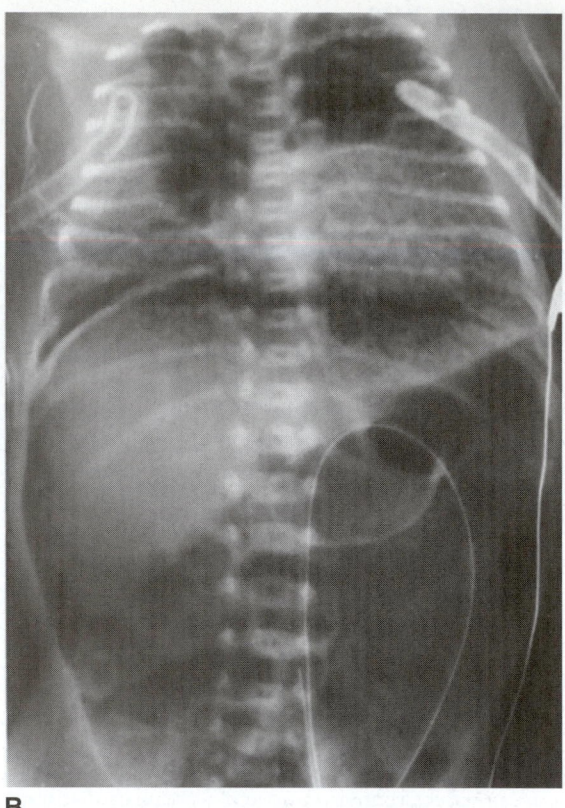

FIGURE 2-45 **A.** Neonatal respiratory distress in a 1500-g infant at 31 weeks' gestation. There is a left pneumothorax. Note that the left lung is not collapsed; this is typical of the stiff lung of hyaline membrane disease, particularly when complicated by interstitial air. There is air in the mediastinum, probably in the pericardial sac, and an interstitial air leak in the right lung. **B.** The same infant 24 hours later. There are two chest tubes decompressing bilateral pneumothoraces and interstitial air in both lungs. The mediastinal air has lifted the thymus off the heart, a typical "sail sign," and has advanced into the neck (ie, subcutaneous emphysema) and the peritoneum, producing a pneumoperitoneum. Note the sharply outlined peritoneal cavity (ie, football sign) and liver. There also is a subpleural collection of air at the base of the right lung. An umbilical arterial catheter is present with its tip at T4-5. Ventilation pressure was lowered in this infant, after which the air absorbed. The child survived and at 15 years of age is normal.

from the pleural space, the catheter is then advanced into the pleural space, the needle is withdrawn, and the stopcock and syringe are detached from the needle and immediately attached to the catheter. This method of relieving a pneumothorax may be lifesaving, but it seldom constitutes definitive treatment. Inserting the needle into the pleura may *cause* a pneumothorax if one did not exist beforehand.

After emergency decompression of a pneumothorax with a needle and syringe (which should restore venous return), a chest radiograph should be obtained to detect the persistence of or reaccumulation of the pneumothorax. Intrapleural gas collections that occupy more than 20% of the thoracic cavity, or those associated with decreased arterial blood pressure and oxygenation, should be treated by tube thoracostomy. It has been traditional to insert a chest tube into the pleural space through the second intercostal space at the midclavicular line. However, doing so is associated with more lung injury and with less success in draining gas and fluids completely than occurs with inserting a catheter into the sixth intercostal space at the midaxillary line. The chest tube should be connected to an underwater suction of 10 to 20 cm H_2O below atmospheric pressure. When no further gas leak has been observed for 8 hours, suction can be discontinued, and the chest tube can

be left unclamped and connected to the underwater seal for an additional 8 hours. If there is no further evidence of pneumothorax, the chest tube can be removed.

A pneumomediastinum seldom requires active treatment. If it obstructs venous return, a catheter should be inserted substernally, and the gas evacuated with a syringe. Similarly, pneumopericardium seldom requires evacuation. In the rare instance when a pneumopericardium obstructs venous return, the gas can be evacuated from the pericardium by inserting a needle below the xiphoid process and directing the needle tip toward the heart while observing the ECG for evidence of dysrhythmias or myocardial injury. Echocardiography is useful for guiding needle aspiration of the pericardial space.

An interstitial gas leak usually disappears if the positive pressure used to ventilate the lungs is decreased and the expiratory time is prolonged. A slowly developing respiratory acidosis is usually well tolerated by the infant and will be much less damaging than persistent interstitial air. If the air leak is unilateral, the gas often will disappear when the infant is placed on the affected side. High-frequency ventilation also may be useful in the treatment of interstitial emphysema or in the treatment of a bronchopleural fistula. If the interstitial emphysema is unilateral, inserting an endotracheal tube into the bronchus of the nonaffected lung and ventilating that lung for several days may allow the other lung to heal. After several days the endotracheal tube can be withdrawn into the trachea, and both lungs can be ventilated.

Pneumoperitoneum usually requires no direct intervention; gas will be absorbed quickly once it stops leaking into the mediastinum. However, if the amount of gas in the abdomen prevents adequate ventilation, a catheter can be inserted into the peritoneum, and the gas can be evacuated.

References

Alter SJ: Spontaneous pneumothroax in infants: a 10-year review. Pediatr Emerg Care 13(6):401–403, 1997

Booth TN, Allen BA, Royal SA: Lymphatic air embolism: a new hypothesis regarding the pathogenesis of neonatal systemic air embolism. Pediatr Radiol 25(Suppl 1):S220–227, 1995

Bratton SL, Roberts JS, Brogan TV: Efficacy and complications of percutaneous pigtail catheters for thoracostomy in pediatric patients. Chest 114(4):1116–1121, 1998

Genc A, Ozcan C, Erdener A, Mutaf O: Management of pneumothorax in children. J Cardiovasc Surg (Torino) 39(6):849–851, 1998

Ogata ES, Gregory GA, Kitterman JA, Phibbs RH, Tooley WH: Pneumothorax in respiratory distress syndrome: incidence and effect on vital signs, blood gases and pH. Pediatrics 58:177–183, 1976

Wipperman CF, Schrantz D, Baum V, Huth R: Independent right lung high frequency and left lung conventional ventilation in the management of severe air leak during ARDS. Paediatr Anaesth 5(3):189–192, 1995

2.17.2 Pulmonary Hemorrhage in the Newborn Infant

Joseph A. Kitterman

Pulmonary hemorrhage has an overall incidence of about one in 1000 live births and is present in 7 to 10% of neonatal autopsies. However, autopsy studies of very preterm infants show a very high incidence of up to 80%. When evident clinically, pulmonary hemorrhage is usually massive and associated with bleeding in other sites, involves more than one-third of the lungs with both interstitial and alveolar bleeding, and has a high mortality rate.

CLINICAL FEATURES

The factor most commonly associated with pulmonary hemorrhage is prematurity. Other related factors are those likely to cause perinatal asphyxia or bleeding disorders. Associated perinatal conditions include toxemia of pregnancy, erythroblastosis fetalis, and breech delivery. Related neonatal factors include asphyxia, clotting abnormalities, cold injury, maternal cocaine use, infection, and respiratory distress syndrome. Infants being treated with extracorporeal membrane oxygenation (ECMO) are more likely to have pulmonary hemorrhage because of their severe underlying disease and the use of anticoagulants. Surviving preterm infants who have been treated with exogenous surfactant have a slightly increased risk of pulmonary hemorrhage compared to infants who did not receive surfactant, but there is no difference between the groups in the incidence of pulmonary hemorrhage at autopsy.

When pulmonary hemorrhage occurs, there is rapid onset of respiratory distress and cyanosis. Bloody fluid oozes from the nose and mouth or the endotracheal tube. Depending on the severity of the hemorrhage, radiographic findings range from patchy infiltrates to complete opacification of the lung fields.

PATHOPHYSIOLOGY

Although the pathogenesis of pulmonary hemorrhage is uncertain, it is likely that the bloody fluid is hemorrhagic pulmonary edema. Cole and associates showed that the hemorrhagic fluid has a lower hematocrit than blood and a higher concentration of small proteins than plasma. They postulated that these infants have severe asphyxia and resultant myocardial failure, which raises the pressure in the pulmonary microcirculation. The increased filtration of plasma leads to pulmonary edema. Subsequently, there is frank bleeding into the interstitial and alveolar spaces. Contributing factors probably include clotting disorders, lung damage, and other disorders that favor increased filtration of fluid from pulmonary capillaries (eg, low concentration of plasma proteins, high alveolar surface tension, hypervolemia). Possible reasons for the slight increase in pulmonary hemorrhage with surfactant administration include overdistension of the lung with assisted ventilation as a result of a rapid increase in lung compliance, increased perfusion of the pulmonary microcirculation through a patent ductus arterious (PDA), and increased survival of severely ill, very immature infants who are at greatest risk for pulmonary hemorrhage.

TREATMENT AND OUTCOME

Immediate treatment of pulmonary hemorrhage should include tracheal suction, oxygen, and positive-pressure ventilation. To control bleeding, it is particularly important to maintain a relatively high positive expiratory pressure (ie, 6–10 cm H_2O). Underlying abnormalities such as coagulopathy, PDA, and hypoxia that constrict the pulmonary circulation should be corrected. When blood loss is large, prompt transfusion of blood may be necessary to maintain an adequate circulating blood volume.

Mortality is high among infants who experience pulmonary hemorrhage, and many are extremely premature and have severe underlying respiratory, diseases, infections, and coagulopathies. Except for a higher incidence of seizures, there are no recognized long-term pulmonary or neurodevelopmental sequelae among survivors.

References

Coffin CM, Schectman K, Cole FS, et al: Neonatal and infantile pulmonary hemorrhage: an autopsy study with clinical correlation. Pediatr Pathol 13:583, 1993

Cole VA, Normand ICS, Reynold EOR, et al: Pathogenesis of hemorrhagic pulmonary edema and massive pulmonary hemorrhage in the newborn. Pediatrics 51:175, 1973

Raju TN, Langenberg P: Pulmonary hemorrhage and exogenous surfactant therapy: a metaanalysis. J Pediatr 123:603, 1993

Tomaszewska M, Stork E, Minich MN, et al: Pulmonary hemorrhage: clinical course and outcomes among very low-birth-weight infants. Arch Pediatr Adolesc Med 153:715, 1999

2.17.3 Neonatal Pneumonia Caused by β-Hemolytic *Streptococcus* Group B

Thomas N. Hansen

Group B streptococci (GBS) remain a major cause of infectious complications in the newborn infant (Sec. 13.0). Early-onset infections occur within the first 7 days after birth and constitute over 80% of all GBS infections. They are characterized by respiratory distress from pneumonia, sepsis, and occasionally meningitis. Late-onset infections occur between 3 and 4 weeks of age and are usually characterized by sepsis and meningitis with occasional focal infections. GBS colonize the genitourinary tracts of 15 to 30% of pregnant women. Early-onset infection is vertically transmitted from the maternal genital tract to the infant either by ascending infection in utero or by inoculation during passage through the birth canal at the time of delivery. Although ascending infection can occur in the presence of intact membranes, it is much more likely when membranes are ruptured. The incidence of early-onset infection in the neonate ranges from two to four cases per 1000 live births and increases 10-fold in the face of maternal colonization. The mortality from early-onset GBS sepsis has decreased from a high of 50% in the 1970s to roughly 5% at present. Premature birth increases the risk of early-onset disease and mortality from it. Other important risk factors for early-onset disease include a history of a previously affected infant, maternal GBS bacteriuria, maternal fever, and premature rupture of membranes.

CLINICAL FEATURES

In about three-fourths of early-onset GBS infections there are one or more maternal risk factors, including ruptured membranes, fever, or chorioamnionitis. The mean age of onset of symptoms in the neonate is 8 to 12 hours. Respiratory distress is the most common presenting sign, followed by cyanosis, apnea, poor perfusion, hypotension, and lethargy. This early-onset progressive respiratory distress cannot be distinguished from that associated with other causes of neonatal respiratory distress, especially hyaline membrane disease. As the disease progresses, systemic blood pressure falls, peripheral circulation decreases, and metabolic acidosis develops. These are the clinical signs of shock and may help to differentiate the process from the other causes of neonatal respiratory distress. In some infants, release of thromboxanes and other vasoactive substances causes pulmonary vasoconstriction. The resulting persistent pulmonary hypertension causes right-to-left shunting at the level

of the ductus and foramen ovale. Death is usually the result of progressive hypoxemia and shock.

In addition to the cardiorespiratory symptoms, infected infants frequently have a marked peripheral leukopenia and thrombocytopenia. Prolonged prothrombin and partial thromboplastin times and decreased plasma fibrinogen concentrations are common.

β-Hemolytic *Streptococcus* group B is easily cultured from tracheal secretions and blood. Rapid diagnostic tests, such as latex particle agglutination, may allow for detection of GBS antigen in biological fluids (urine, cerebrospinal fluid, joint or pleural fluid). False-positive antigen detection may occur in urine samples that are contaminated with organisms from the skin or from enteral antigen absorption and excretion in the urine. Clinicians must recognize that a positive test in an asymptomatic infant is not diagnostic of invasive infection.

RADIOGRAPHIC FEATURES

Two types of radiographs are seen in group B streptococcal pneumonias. About half of the affected infants, usually those with lowest birth weight, display findings similar to those of infants with neonatal respiratory distress syndrome. Their lungs have a fine, diffuse, granular opacification against which the bronchi are sharply outlined. The edge of the diaphragm and the heart border are hazy, and the volume of the lungs appears slightly reduced. The thymus is usually small. The uniformity of the process suggests that the lungs were infected in utero by blood-borne organisms or that the organisms were inhaled when the lungs were still fluid filled. A second type of radiographic appearance is one of patchy lung infiltrates, most often in the lower lobes. Occasionally, there is fluid in the fissures and at the costophrenic angle.

PATHOLOGY

The lungs of infants who die from β-hemolytic *Streptococcus* group B pneumonia are filled with organisms, particularly if death occurs in the first day of life. The lungs are heavy, and only some of the alveolar ducts are filled with air. There are sheets of intraalveolar

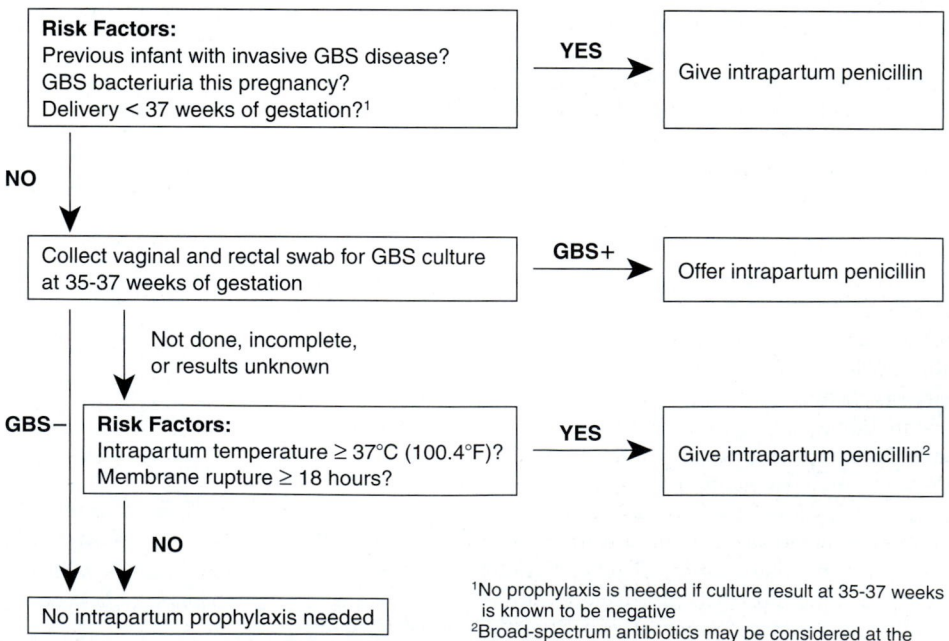

FIGURE 2-46 Prevention strategy for early-onset GBS disease using prenatal culture screening at 35 to 37 weeks of gestation. SOURCE: *Committee on Infectious Disease and Committee on Fetus and Newborn: Revised guidelines for prevention of early-onset group B streptococcal (GBS) infection. Pediatrics 99:489–496, 1997, with permission.*

Risk Factors:
Previous infant with invasive GBS disease?
GBS bacteriuria this pregnancy?
Delivery < 37 weeks of gestation?[1]

YES → Give intrapartum penicillin

NO

Collect vaginal and rectal swab for GBS culture at 35-37 weeks of gestation

GBS+ → Offer intrapartum penicillin

Not done, incomplete, or results unknown

GBS−

Risk Factors:
Intrapartum temperature ≥ 37°C (100.4°F)?
Membrane rupture ≥ 18 hours?

YES → Give intrapartum penicillin[2]

NO

No intrapartum prophylaxis needed

[1]No prophylaxis is needed if culture result at 35-37 weeks is known to be negative
[2]Broad-spectrum antibiotics may be considered at the discretion of the physician based on clinical indications

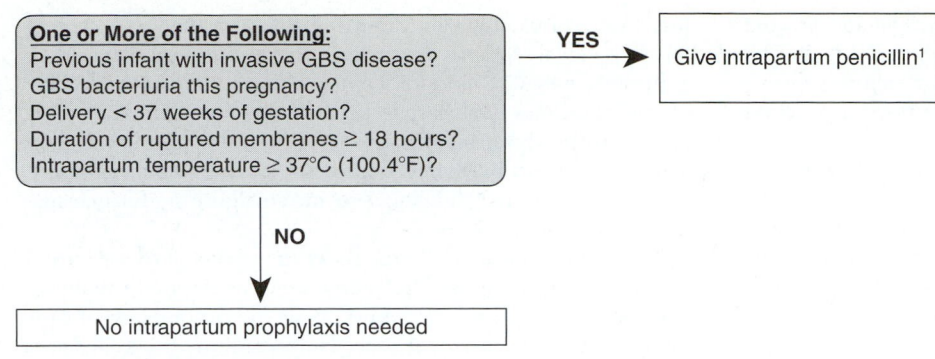

Broad-spectrum antibiotics may be considered at the discretion of the physician based on clinical indications

FIGURE 2-47 Prevention strategy for early-onset GBS disease using risk factors without prenatal culture screening. SOURCE: *Committee on Infectious Disease and Committee on Fetus and Newborn: Revised guidelines for prevention of early-onset group B streptococcal (GBS) infection. Pediatrics 99:489–496, 1997, with permission.*

and interstitial polymorphonuclear leukocytes. These sequestered white cells may account for some of the peripheral leukopenia. The small pulmonary arterioles are constricted, consistent with the clinical findings of persistent pulmonary hypertension. Hyaline membranes are prominent and line the dilated alveolar ducts. There is often diffuse interstitial hemorrhage. Except for those sections in which there are bacteria and leukocytes, the lungs resemble those of infants who die from neonatal respiratory distress syndrome.

TREATMENT

ANTIBIOTICS Penicillin or ampicillin plus an aminoglycoside is the initial treatment of choice for a newborn infant with GBS pneumonia. Penicillin G or ampicillin alone can be given when GBS is identified, susceptibility of the organism is determined, and clinical and microbiological response has been documented.

The recommended daily dose of intravenous penicillin G for treating meningitis in infants less than a week old is 250,000 to 450,000 U/kg, one-third of which is given every 8 hours; for infants beyond a week of age, the daily dose is 450,000 U/kg, one-

quarter of which is given every 6 hours. For ampicillin, the recommended daily intravenous dose for infants age 7 days or younger with meningitis is 200 mg/kg in three divided doses; infants with meningitis who are more than 7 days old should receive 300 mg/kg/d in four to six divided doses. For infants with bacteremia without a defined focus, treatment should be continued for at least 10 days. For infants with uncomplicated meningitis, 14 to 21 days of treatment is usually sufficient. Some experts recommend that a second lumbar puncture be done at approximately 24 hours after initiation of therapy to document therapeutic efficacy.

Treatment duration for infants with pneumonia should be guided by the patient's clinical and bacteriologic responses. A 10- to 14-day course of treatment is usually sufficient.

SUPPORTIVE Mechanical ventilation with supplemental oxygen remains the mainstay for treatment of respiratory failure in infants with GBS pneumonia. Plasma proteins leaking from the vascular space into the alveoli may inactivate pulmonary surfactant, and surfactant replacement therapy may help to improve lung function. Often infants with pneumonia from GBS have pulmonary vasocon-

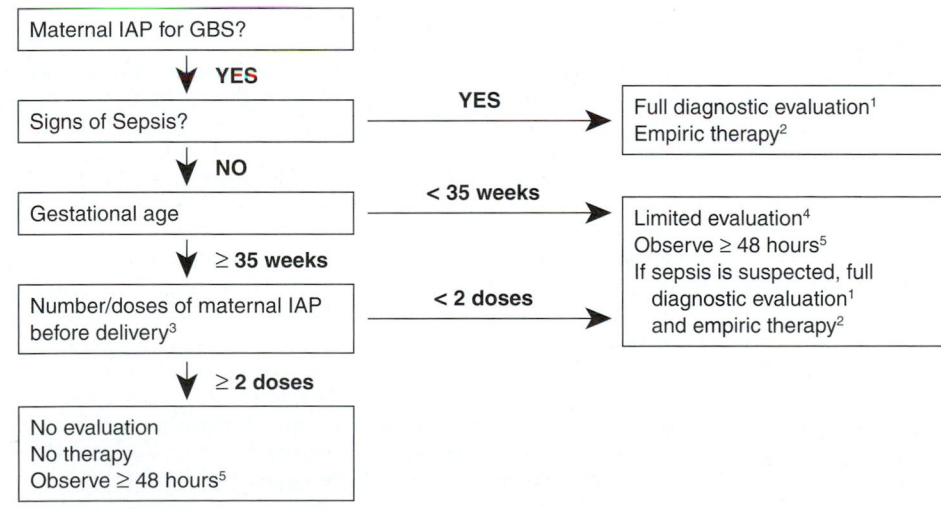

¹Includes CBC and differential, blood culture, and chest radiograph if respiratory symptoms. A lumbar puncture is performed at the discretion of the physician.
²Duration of therapy will vary depending on results of blood culture and CSF findings (if obtained) as well as the clinical course of the infant. If laboratory results and clinical course are unremarkable, duration may be as short as 48-72 hours.
³Applies to penicillin or ampicillin chemoprophylaxis
⁴CBC and differential, blood culture
⁵Does not allow early discharge

FIGURE 2-48 Algorithm for management of an infant born to a mother who has received intrapartum chemoprophylaxis. IAP = intrapartum antimicrobial prophylaxis. SOURCE: *Committee on Infectious Disease and Committee on Fetus and Newborn: Revised guidelines for prevention of early-onset group B streptococcal (GBS) infection. Pediatrics 99:489–496, 1997, with permission.*

striction and persistent pulmonary hypertension. Therapy directed at relieving this vasoconstriction is detailed in Sec. 2.17.11. The circulation must be supported with intravascular volume replacement and vasopressor drugs to maintain adequate systemic blood pressure and tissue perfusion.

Transfusion of leukocytes has been advocated by some investigators for severely neutropenic infants with GBS sepsis. A metaanalysis supports this contention, but only when the leukocytes are obtained by leukapheresis. However, granulocyte transfusions must be given early, and few centers have the ability to provide the product at all times. Granulocyte transfusions also carry the risk of graft-versus-host disease.

Several trials have investigated the role of intravenous immunoglobulin in the treatment of infants with sepsis. A metaanalysis of these trials showed a significant reduction in mortality when intravenous immunoglobulin is given in conjunction with antibiotics.

The administration of recombinant granulocyte colony-stimulating factor improves survival from group B streptococcal sepsis in rats. However, administration of recombinant granulocyte colony-stimulating factor to infants with neutropenia and clinical signs of early-onset sepsis did not increase circulating neutrophil counts, nor did this treatment affect morbidity or mortality.

PREVENTION Intrapartum chemoprophylaxis of GBS carriers has been shown to be a highly effective method of preventing neonatal GBS disease. Consensus guidelines developed for the Centers for Disease Control and Prevention provide two strategies for intrapartum chemoprophylaxis: one based on screening cultures and risk factors (Fig. 2-46) and the other on identifiable risk factors without screening cultures (Fig. 2-47).

These recommendations state that obstetric care providers should adopt a strategy for GBS disease prevention, communicate available prevention options to their patients, and respect individual patient requests regarding chemoprophylaxis. Both strategies agree that women who have symptomatic or asymptomatic bacteriuria during pregnancy, and women who previously have given birth to an infant with GBS disease, should receive intrapartum chemoprophylaxis.

The culture and risk factor approach (Fig. 2-46) requires that pregnant women be screened for anogenital colonization with GBS at 35 to 37 weeks of gestation and that all GBS carriers be offered intrapartum chemoprophylaxis, even if a risk factor is not present. If GBS status is not known at onset of labor or rupture of membranes, intrapartum chemoprophylaxis should be administered if gestation is less than 37 weeks, membranes are ruptured for longer than 18 hours, or if the mother has a temperature greater than 38°C (100.4°F). Culture techniques that maximize the likelihood of GBS recovery should be used. Oral antimicrobial agents are not effective in eliminating colonization or preventing neonatal disease and should not be used to treat women who are found to have GBS colonization during prenatal screening.

The risk factor approach (Fig. 2-47) recommends intrapartum chemoprophylaxis if the mother has symptomatic or asymptomatic bacteriuria during pregnancy, a previous infant with GBS disease, gestation is less than 37 weeks, membranes are ruptured more than 18 hours, or maternal temperature is greater than 38°C (100.4°F). Screening cultures are not recommended.

Intravenous penicillin (5 million units initially, followed by 2.5 million units every 4 hours) is the recommended treatment for intrapartum chemoprophylaxis because penicillin specifically kills GBS and, in contrast to broad-spectrum antibiotic treatment, is less likely to yield emergence of organisms that are resistant to antibi-

otic. Intravenous ampicillin (2 g initially, and then 1 g every 4 hours) is an acceptable alternative. Intravenous clindamycin or erythromycin may be used for women who are allergic to penicillin.

The guidelines further state that routine administration of antibiotics to newborn infants who are born to mothers who have received intrapartum chemoprophylaxis is *not recommended*. Instead, the consensus guidelines provide an algorithm for management of these infants (Fig. 2-48).

There remain some concerns about the effects of routine intrapartum chemoprophylaxis on emergence of antibiotic-resistant organisms, or simply shifting from GBS as the major cause of early onset sepsis to another organism. Thus, continued surveillance is warranted. In addition, widespread use of penicillin carries a risk of increased numbers of anaphylactic reactions that must be considered in assessing the benefit of this prevention strategy.

It is clear, however, that since the development of the intrapartum chemoprophylaxis strategies, the incidence of invasive GBS disease has decreased greatly. A recent multicenter study showed that in 1993 (before routine intrapartum chemoprophylaxis), the incidence of early-onset neonatal infection was 1.7 per 1000 live births, whereas in 1998 (after introduction of routine intrapartum chemoprophylaxis), the incidence of early-onset infection was 0.6 per 1000 live births. This 65% reduction in early-onset infection, when extrapolated to the entire United States, suggests that in 1998 intrapartum chemoprophylaxis resulted in 3900 fewer cases of early-onset GBS disease and 200 fewer newborn deaths.

References

Ablow RC, Driscoll SG, Effmann EL, et al: A comparison of early-onset group B streptococcal neonatal infection and the respiratory-distress syndrome of the newborn. N Engl J Med 294:65–70, 1976

Ascher DP, Wilson S, Mendiola J, Fischer GW: Group B streptococcal latex agglutination testing in neonates. J Pediatr 119:458–461, 1991

Auten RL, Notter RH, Kendig JW, Davis JM, Shapiro DL: Surfactant treatment of full-term newborns with respiratory failure. Pediatrics 87:101–107, 1991

Baley JE, Fanaroff AA: Neonatal infections, part 2: specific infectious diseases and therapies. In: Sinclair JC, Bracken MB, eds: Effective Care of the Newborn Infant. New York, Oxford University Press, 1992:477–506

Brumund TT, White CB: An update on group B streptococcal infections in the newborn: prevention, evaluation, and treatment. Pediatr Ann 27: 495–501, 1988

Committee on Infectious Disease: 1997 Red Book: Report of the Committee on Infectious Diseases, 24th ed. Elk Grove Village, IL, American Academy of Pediatrics, 1997:494–501

Committee on Infectious Disease, Committee on Fetus and Newborn: Revised guidelines for prevention of early-onset group B streptococcal (GBS) infection. Pediatrics 99:489–496, 1997

Givner LB, Nagaraj SK: Hyperimmune human IgG or recombinant human granulocyte-macrophage colony-stimulating factor as adjunctive therapy for group B streptococcal sepsis in newborn rats. J Pediatr 122:774–779, 1993

Payne NR, Burke BA, Day DL, Christenson PD, Thompson TR, Ferrieri P: Correlation of clinical and pathologic findings in early onset neonatal group B streptococcal infection with disease severity and prediction of outcome. Pediatr Infect Dis J 7:836–847, 1988

Schibler KR, Osborne KA, Leung LY, Le TV, Baker S, Thompson DD: A randomized, placebo-controlled trial of granulocyte colony-stimulating factor administration to newborn infants with neutropenia and clinical signs of early-onset sepsis. Pediatrics 102:6–13, 1998

Schrag SJ, Zwicki S, Farley MM, et al: Group B streptococcal disease in the era of intrapartum antibiotic prophylaxis. N Engl J Med 342:15–20, 2000

Schuchat A, Deaver-Robinson K, Plikaytis BD, Zangwill KM, Mohle-Boetani J, Wenger JD, The Active Surveillance Study Group: Multistate case-control study of maternal risk factors for neonatal Group B streptococcal disease. Pediatr Infect Dis J 13:623–629, 1994

Weisman LE, Stoll BJ, Cruess DF, et al: Early-onset group B streptococcal sepsis: a current assessment. J Pediatr 121:428–433, 1992

2.17.4   Disorders of Glucose Metabolism

William W. Hay, Jr

Normal postnatal glucose homeostasis is established by increased glucose production and glucose utilization. Factors that promote glucose production and release into the circulation include catecholamines and glucagon, which activate glycogenolysis, and a high glucagon:insulin ratio, which induces synthesis and activity of the enzymes required for gluconeogenesis. Once normal feedings are established, dietary fatty acids, glycerol, and amino acids continue to fuel gluconeogenesis, and galactose derived from hydrolysis of milk sugar (lactose) in the gut increases hepatic glycogen production. Feedings also induce production of intestinal peptides, or incretins, that promote insulin secretion. Insulin decreases glucose production and increases glucose utilization for energy production and storage as glycogen. These opposing conditions of glucose production and utilization continue in response to normal feed-fast cycles, regulating normal plasma glucose concentrations.

HYPOGLYCEMIA

Glucose is the major source of energy for organ function. All organs use glucose, and glucose deficiency leads to impaired cardiac performance, cerebral energy failure, hepatic glycogen depletion, and muscle weakness. Cerebral glucose metabolism accounts for as much as 90% of total glucose consumption. Thus, maintenance of glucose delivery to all organs, but particularly the brain, is an essential physiological function. Although alternate fuels can substitute for glucose metabolism, concentrations of these substances often are low in newborn infants, especially preterm infants. Newborns, therefore, are especially susceptible to hypoglycemia when they are exposed to conditions that impair glucose homeostasis during the transition from intrauterine to extrauterine life.

DEFINITION Hypoglycemia ought to be defined as any glucose concentration below the lower limit of the normal range of blood or plasma/serum glucose concentrations. This concentration, however, is uncertain, controversial, and variably defined by clinicians or in the literature. Early statistical evaluations in term infants defined hypoglycemia as a blood glucose concentration <35 mg/dL, or a plasma glucose value <40 mg/dL; even lower concentrations were used to define hypoglycemia in preterm infants. Such statistical definitions, however, have limited biological or clinical significance, as physiologically hypoglycemia is present when the concentration of glucose in the plasma produces glucose delivery rates that are inadequate to meet essential requirements for glucose utilization. Such requirements vary considerably among infants and over a broad range of glucose concentrations. Definitions of normal and hypoglycemic glucose concentrations also depend on postnatal feeding practices and when after birth glucose concentrations are measured. Glucose concentrations are higher, for example, when feedings are initiated soon after birth than when feedings are de-

layed for several hours. Postnatally, the blood glucose concentration normally decreases to a variable nadir value between 1 and 3 hours after birth, followed by a progressive increase to >50 to 60 mg/dL by 12 to 24 hours (Fig. 2-49).

The absolute glucose concentration at or below which short- or long-term organ dysfunction invariably occurs remains undefined, although animal studies suggest that concentrations <20 mg/dL, when sustained over several hours, can be associated with brain injury. Without specific evidence to support an absolute threshold value, no single value can be used to define physiological hypoglycemia. Nevertheless, most clinicians today are using higher values than previously accepted to define hypoglycemia. Several recent studies support this practice. One study reported that repeated blood glucose concentrations <48 mg/dL in preterm infants were associated with an adverse neurodevelopmental outcome. Another study reported that among a group of normal preterm infants, most achieved a serum glucose concentration >50 mg/dL by 12 to 24 hours after birth. Another report showed that human fetuses have a blood glucose concentration >50 mg/dL during normal development. These observations indicate that blood glucose concentrations of 45 to 50 mg/dL (50–60 mg/dL plasma or serum) should represent the approximate lower limit of normal neonatal glucose concentrations.

LABORATORY DIAGNOSIS The "gold standard" to measure blood or plasma/serum glucose concentration is the hexokinase method used by most diagnostic laboratories. Colorimetric reagent strip methods are commonly used at the bedside to screen for hypoglycemia, but such measurements are often inaccurate, ranging from ±10 to 30% of the true value. Because of their relative inaccuracy,

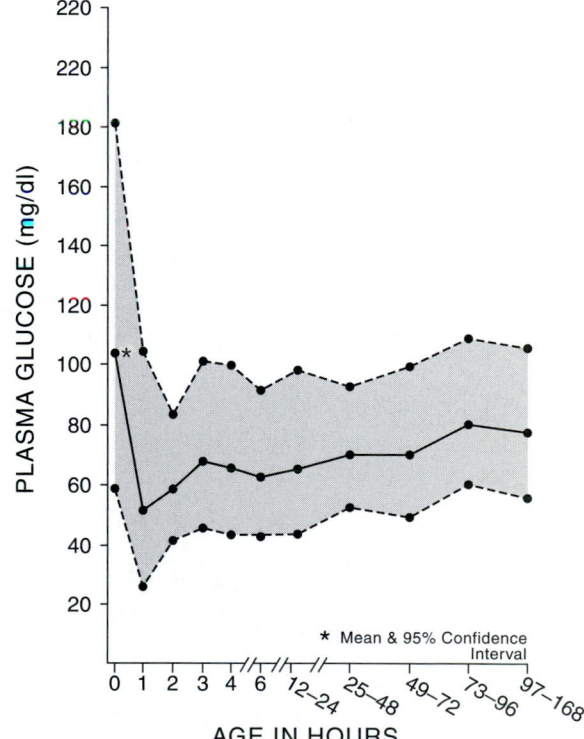

FIGURE 2-49   Plasma glucose concentrations during the first week of life in healthy appropriate-for-gestational-age (AGA) term infants. SOURCE: Modified from *Srinivasan G. Pildes RS. Cattamanchi G. Voora S. Lilien LD: Plasma glucose values in normal neonates: a new look. Journal of Pediatrics 109(1):114–7, 1986.*

any low blood glucose concentration detected by one of these colorimetric methods must be confirmed by a standard laboratory method as soon as possible.

INCIDENCE   The overall incidence of neonatal hypoglycemia has been estimated at one to five per 1000 live births; the incidence is higher in infants at increased risk of hypoglycemia (Fig. 2-50). The reported incidence varies depending on the definition of hypoglycemia, the time after birth when the concentration of glucose is measured, and the method used to measure the blood, plasma or serum glucose concentration.

CLINICAL PRESENTATION   Hypoglycemia is classified as "symptomatic" or "asymptomatic," terms that indicate the presence or absence of physical signs that accompany a low glucose concentration. Most signs are nonspecific and result from disturbances in central nervous system function. These include abnormal respiratory patterns, such as tachypnea or apnea; cardiovascular signs, such as tachycardia or bradycardia; and neurologic signs, such as jitteriness, lethargy, weak suck, temperature instability, and seizures. Many of these signs occur with other common neonatal disorders, including sepsis, hypocalcemia, and intracranial hemorrhage. Hypoglycemia must be considered in any infant who exhibits one or more of these signs, as untreated hypoglycemia can seriously impair the function of many organs, especially the brain, which may be permanently damaged by untreated hypoglycemia. Infants at risk for hypoglycemia, whether or not they exhibit clinical signs, require careful observation and random screening for repeated low glucose concentrations because asymptomatic hypoglycemia can lead to neurologic injury.

ETIOLOGY   Hepatic glycogen stores are diminished in preterm infants who have not had time or developmental capacity to accumulate sufficient glycogen in utero, and in small gestational age (SGA) infants who are hypoglycemic in utero (Table 2-22). These two groups of infants also have a relatively increased brain-to-body weight ratio, which increases glucose demand relative to the capacity for glucose production. Infants with stressful conditions, such as asphyxia, hypothermia, or respiratory distress, can break down their glycogen stores more rapidly in response to increased secretion of catecholamines and glucagon. Even normal body stores of glycogen, however, may be inadequate to meet the increased rates of glucose utilization imposed by such conditions. Gluconeogenic and ketogenic enzymes also can be low in preterm and SGA infants, preventing normal rates of new glucose production or the production of alternate fuel substrates from fatty acids. Infants of diabetic mothers (IDMs) are predisposed to hypoglycemia because of persistent hyperinsulinemia following excessive intrauterine glucose stimulation of their pancreas by maternal hyperglycemia. This leads to a persistently high insulin:glucagon ratio after birth, when placental glucose supply is interrupted. The high insulin:glucagon ratio inhibits the regulatory enzymes for glycogenolysis (glycogen phosphorylase), gluconeogenesis (phosphoenolpyruvate carboxykinase), and hepatic glucose release (glucose-6-phosphatase). Insulin also increases peripheral glucose utilization in insulin-sensitive tissues such as skeletal muscle, myocardium, and adipose tissue. Infants with erythroblastosis fetalis have increased levels of insulin and an increase in the number of pancreatic β cells, possibly a result of increased glutathione release from hemolyzed red cells. Glutathione can inactivate insulin in the circulation, leading to increased insulin secretion. Exchange transfusions exacerbate the problem because transfused blood usually is preserved in a solution that contains high concentrations of dextrose. As a result, the infant receives a relatively high glucose load during the exchange, which then induces an exaggerated insulin response from the already hyperplastic pancreas. At the end of the exchange transfusion, the rate of dextrose administration decreases abruptly to a more normal rate, but insulin concentrations remain elevated, leading to further hypogly-

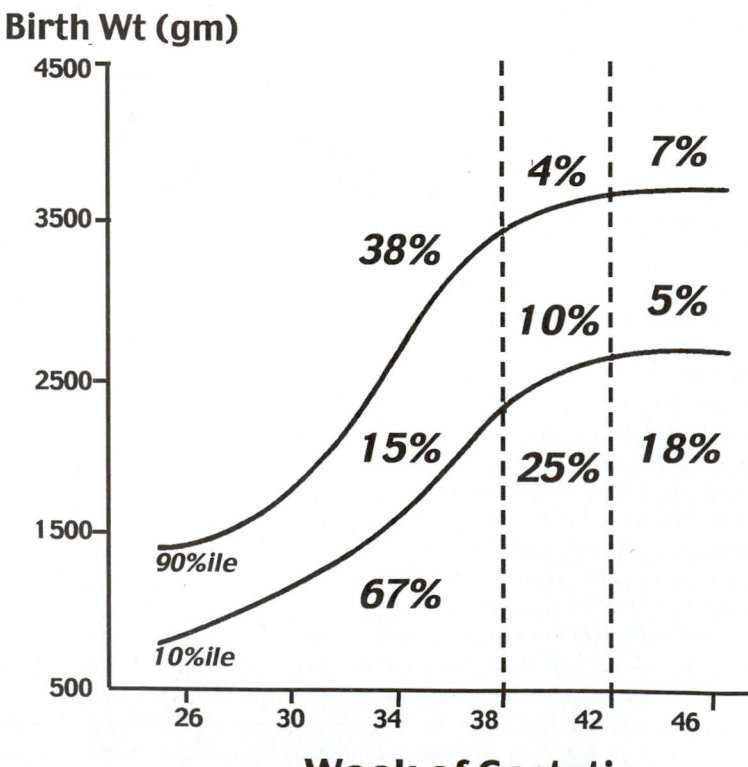

FIGURE 2-50   **Incidence of neonatal hypoglycemia by birth weight and gestational age. SOURCE: Modified from** *Lubchenco LO, Bard H: Incidence of hypoglycemia in newborn infants classified by birth weight and gestational age. Pediatrics 47(5):831–8, 1971.*

TABLE 2-22

NEONATAL HYPOGLYCEMIA: ETIOLOGIES AND TIME COURSE

MECHANISM	CLINICAL SETTING	EXPECTED DURATION
Decreased substrate availability	Intrauterine growth restriction	Transient
	Prematurity	Transient
	Glycogen storage disease	Prolonged
	Inborn errors (eg, fructose intolerance)	Prolonged
Endocrine disturbances		
Hyperinsulinemia	Infant of diabetic mother	Transient
	Beckwith-Wiedemann syndrome	Prolonged
	Erythroblastosis fetails	Transient
	Exchange transfusion	Prolonged
	Islet cell dysplasias	Transient
	Maternal β-agonist tocolytics	Transient
	Improperly placed umbilical artery catheter	
Other endocrine disorders	Hypopituitarism	Prolonged
	Hypothyroidism	Prolonged
	Adrenal insufficiency	Prolonged
Increased utilization	Perinatal asphyxia	Transient
	Hypothermia	Transient
Miscellaneous/ multiple mechanisms	Sepsis	Transient
	Congenital heart disease	Transient
	CNS abnormalities	Prolonged

SOURCE: *McGowan JE, Hagedorn MIE, Hay WW Jr: Glucose homeostasis. In: Merenstein GB, Gardner, SL, eds: Handbook of Neonatal Intensive Care, 4th ed. St. Louis, Mosby, 1998:259–274.*

cemia. Use of β-adrenergic drugs, such as terbutaline, to inhibit preterm uterine contractions and labor also is associated with hyperinsulinemia and reduced glycogen stores.

Hypoglycemia that persists for more than 5 to 7 days most often results from several types of congenital hyperinsulinism. Although uncommon, these are serious metabolic disorders and are associated with a markedly increased risk of neurologic complications. Several of these disorders are genetic, including diffuse β-cell/islet hyperplasia or nesidioblastosis and an autosomal recessive form of congenital hyperinsulinism that has been linked to a defect in the sulfonylurea receptor or K ATP channel. A single mutation on the short arm of chromosome 11 also has been described in the Ashkenazi Jewish population that produces this defect. Cases in other ethnic groups have been associated with a number of other mutations in the same region. Mutations responsible for an autosomal dominant form of hyperinsulinism remain unknown. Unlike the recessive form, the autosomal dominant form of hyperinsulinism does not appear to result from abnormal sulfonylurea receptor function. A syndrome of congenital hyperinsulinemia and asymptomatic hyperammonemia associated with mutations in the glutamate dehydrogenase gene also has been described. Beckwith-Weidemann syndrome is associated with hyperplasia of multiple organs, including the pancreas, with increased insulin secretion. Rarely, hyperinsulinemia results from localized β-cell/islet adenomas within an otherwise normal pancreas.

Inborn errors of metabolism can limit availability of gluconeogenic precursors or the function of the enzymes required for hepatic glucose production. Metabolic defects that present with hypogly-

cemia include some forms of glycogen storage disease, galactosemia, fatty acid oxidation defects, carnitine deficiency, several of the amino acidemias, hereditary fructose intolerance (fructose-1,6-diphosphatase deficiency), and defects of other gluconeogenic enzymes. Endocrine disorders, such as hypopituitarism and adrenal failure, also lead to hypoglycemia because of inadequate hormonal responses, including inadequate growth hormone and adrenal corticosteroid secretion, resulting in failure to activate hepatic glucose production. These conditions are very rare and should be considered only after common etiologies are excluded.

CLINICAL DIAGNOSIS Risk factors for hypoglycemia should be identified, such as persistent hyperglycemia on a maternal glucose tolerance test or overt maternal diabetes, maternal administration of drugs associated with neonatal hypoglycemia, ultrasound evidence of intrauterine growth restriction, or prematurity (Table 2-23). Growth parameters should be plotted to establish if the infant is SGA or large for gestational age (LGA). Sepsis should be suspected if the infant has no apparent risk factors for hypoglycemia. If hypoglycemia persists for more than 1 week, hyperinsulinism, other endocrine disorders, and inborn errors of metabolism should be investigated, especially if the hypoglycemia is refractory to standard treatment. Hyperinsulinemia is diagnosed by demonstrating normal to high concentrations of insulin during episodes of hypoglycemia. Concentrations of insulin-like growth factor 1 binding protein (IGFBP-1) also are decreased in the presence of hyperinsulinemia. Serum and urine tests for specific metabolic and endocrine disorders, such as serum amino acid profiles and cortisol and growth hormone concentrations, also may help to determine the etiology of hypoglycemia.

PATHOPHYSIOLOGY Severe hypoglycemia in the newborn is associated with selective neuronal necrosis in multiple brain regions, including the superficial cortex, dentate gyrus, hippocampus, and caudate-putamen. Brain injury appears to result from a number of processes that are initiated when blood glucose concentrations decrease (see Fig. 2-51). Energy failure leads to decreased cerebral electrical activity followed by neuronal cell membrane breakdown. Energy failure also prevents postsynaptic uptake of the principal neurotransmitter glutamate. Excess glutamate concentrations then activate NMDA (N-methyl D-aspartate) receptors in the neuronal membranes, which increases cellular entry and cytoplasmic concentrations of sodium and calcium to levels that cause osmotic swelling and acute neuronal necrosis. The high calcium concentrations also activate cellular phospholipases and proteases and prevent normal mitochondrial metabolism, which leads to increased toxic free radical formation. These processes disrupt synaptic transmission and eventually lead to delayed neuronal necrosis. Hypoglycemia also

TABLE 2-23

NEONATAL HYPOGLYCEMIA: MATERNAL RISK FACTORS

Diabetes or abnormal glucose tolerance test
Pregnancy-induced or essential hypertension
Previous macrosomic infants
Substance abuse
Treatment with β-agonist tocolytics
Antepartum administration of IV glucose

SOURCE: *McGowan JE, Hagedorn MIE, Hay WW Jr. Glucose homeostasis. In: Merenstein GB, Gardner SL, eds: Handbook of Neonatal Intensive Care, 4th ed. St. Louis Mosby, 1998:259–274.*

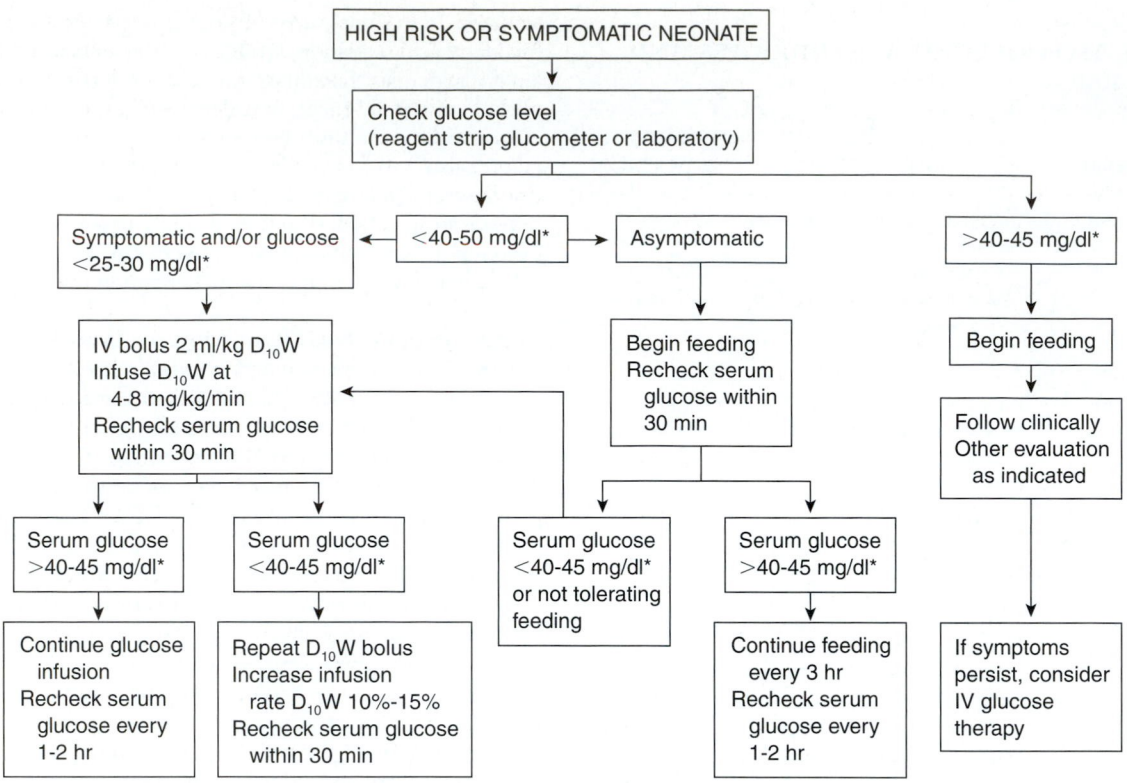

FIGURE 2-51   Algorithm for management of the neonate with hypoglycemia. SOURCE: Modified from *McGowan JE, Hagedorn MIE, Hay WW Jr: Glucose homeostasis. In: Merenstein GB, Gardner SL, eds: Handbook of Neonatal Intensive Care, 4th ed. St Louis, Mosby, 1998:259–274.*

can exacerbate brain injury during periods of cerebral hypoxia. As in hypoglycemia, cerebral hypoxia is associated with depletion of high-energy phosphates, increased extracellular glutamate concentrations, activation of ionotropic glutamate receptors, and increased intracellular sodium and calcium. In addition, anaerobic glycolysis during hypoxia accelerates depletion of glucose in the brain. Hypoglycemia also abolishes hypoxic vasodilation of cerebral blood vessels, impairing compensatory mechanisms to improve oxygen delivery to the brain during periods of hypoxemia.

MANAGEMENT   Neonatal hypoglycemia must be corrected rapidly, and further episodes of hypoglycemia must be prevented by providing adequate substrate until normal glucose homeostasis is established (Fig. 2-51). Early enteral feeding usually is successful in treating mild hypoglycemia in asymptomatic infants. Feedings with 5% dextrose solution should be avoided because the dextrose is metabolized rapidly, and hypoglycemia frequently recurs. Human milk or standard infant formulas provide carbohydrate in the form of lactose without excessively stimulating insulin secretion. Milk also includes protein and fat, which provide a sustained supply of substrates for gluconeogenesis and alternative fuels. Fat intake also decreases cellular glucose uptake. Blood glucose concentrations should increase by 20 to 30 mg/dL within the first hour after a feeding of 30 to 60 mL of milk or formula.

Intravenous glucose infusion should be used when infants are symptomatic or are unable to tolerate enteral feedings and when hypoglycemia does not respond to enteral feeding treatment. Intravenous glucose also should be used early after birth in those high-risk infants who are likely to experience severe disturbances in

glucose homeostasis that are expected to last more than a few hours. Such infants include preterm infants, SGA infants with intrauterine growth restriction (IUGR), IDMs, and infants who have underlying etiologies for hypoglycemia, such as sepsis, known or suspected inborn errors of metabolism, endocrine defects, or erythroblastosis. An initial rapid intravenous infusion of 200 mg/kg (2 mL/kg) of 10% dextrose solution should be followed by continuous infusion of 5 to 8 mg/min/kg of glucose (Fig. 2-52), ie, the glucose utilization rate of a healthy term to preterm infant. The blood glucose concentration should be measured approximately 30 minutes after the initial rapid infusion and then every 1 to 2 hours until it is stable within the normal range. If a subsequent value falls in the hypoglycemic range, the rapid infusion should be repeated, and the infusion rate increased by 10 to 15%. Infants with hyperinsulinemia often require as much as 12 to 15 mg/min/kg of IV glucose to maintain normoglycemia; these rates usually require a central venous catheter to allow infusion of dextrose concentrations >12.5%. Infants requiring intravenous therapy for hypoglycemia should continue feedings as long as there is no evidence of feeding intolerance, such as abdominal distension, persistent and large residual volumes of milk in the stomach, or emesis. Providing some carbohydrate as galactose, one of the sugars that comprise lactose, is useful in IDMs and other infants with hyperinsulinism because pancreatic insulin response to galactose is less than the response to an equivalent amount of glucose. When a normal blood glucose concentration has been established, and the requirement for IV glucose has been stable for 12 to 24 hours, the infant can be weaned from this therapy by measuring prepandial blood glucose concentrations and decreasing the infusion rate by 10 to 20% each time the blood

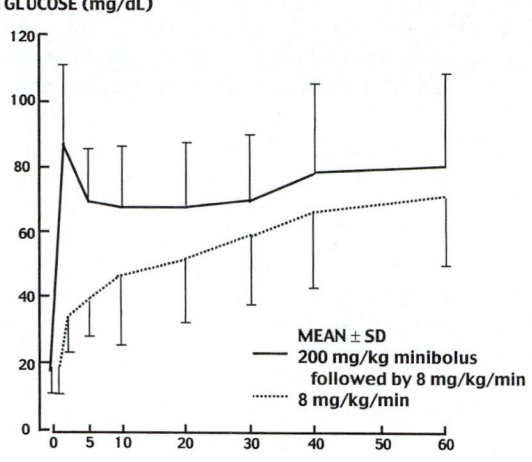

PLASMA GLUCOSE (mg/dL)

FIGURE 2-52   Plasma glucose response to glucose "minibolus" followed by continuous glucose infusion of 8 mg/min/kg as therapy for severe neonatal hypoglycemia. SOURCE: Modified from *Lilien LD, et al. J Pediatr 97:295, 1980.*

glucose is >50 to 60 mg/dL. Failure to tolerate weaning from IV glucose indicates the presence of a pervasive disorder, such as a metabolic defect or idiopathic hyperinsulinemia. Several other agents have been used to treat infants with refractory hypoglycemia, usually with coexisting hyperinsulinism (Table 2-24).

OUTCOME   Acute, severe hypoglycemia stimulates release of catecholamines and glucagon and subsequent lipolysis and glycogenolysis. The stress imposed by hypoglycemia can precipitate cardiorespiratory instability in a previously ill infant. Long-term effects of severe neonatal hypoglycemia remain controversial. Repeated episodes of symptomatic hypoglycemia, particularly in infants with persistent hyperinsulinism, have been associated with selective neuronal necrosis and impaired cognitive and motor function. Hypoglycemia alone does not alter long-term outcome in IDMs; rather, adverse outcomes are related to the presence of congenital anomalies. There is little evidence of long-term sequelae in term infants who have experienced relatively few, brief episodes of hypoglycemia. In preterm infants, however, repeated daily glucose concentrations below ~46 mg/dL have been associated with significantly lower mental and motor development and a higher incidence of cerebral palsy. Thus, mild to moderate hypoglycemia might affect outcome in high-risk infants, particularly those who cannot respond adequately to hypoglycemia, although such infants have many other confounding problems that independently or interactively lead to abnormal neurodevelopment.

HYPERGLYCEMIA

Hyperglycemia is relatively common in infants who are born extremely preterm (<26 weeks of gestation). Hyperglycemia is caused by excessive rates of IV glucose infusion in the presence of physiological and biochemical mechanisms that lead to excess glucose production, insulin resistance, and glucose intolerance.

DEFINITION   Hyperglycemia is defined as a blood glucose concentration >120 to 125 mg/dL (plasma concentration >145–150 mg/dL), regardless of gestational age, weight, or postnatal age.

DIAGNOSIS   Affected neonates usually are extremely preterm (<26 weeks of gestation) and of extremely low-birth-weight (ELBW) (<1000 g). They often are receiving relatively high rates of IV glucose. They usually are asymptomatic or have signs of associated disease processes. Recognizable signs associated with hyperglycemia include dehydration from osmotic diuresis, weight loss, fever, glycosuria, ketosis, and metabolic acidosis. The latter three signs are common among infants who have transient or permanent neonatal diabetes mellitus.

EPIDEMIOLOGY   The incidence of hyperglycemia is inversely related to birth weight in the preterm infant, ranging from about 2% in infants who weigh >2000 g to about 45% in those who weigh <1000 g, and up to 80% in ELBW infants weighing <750 g.

ETIOLOGY   Hyperglycemia occurs in about half of preterm infants receiving continuous intravenous dextrose infusions that provide glucose at rates >10 to 11 mg/min/kg and in nearly all infants at rates >14 mg/min/kg. Even after dextrose infusion rates are decreased to treat hyperglycemia, infusion rates as low as 3 to 4 mg/min/kg have been associated with persistent hyperglycemia, especially during prolonged periods of stress. Positive relationships also have been found between hyperglycemia and the severity of clinical problems in the neonate, as estimated by lower Apgar scores, higher fractional concentrations of inspired oxygen, and worse respiratory distress scores. Intravenous lipid infusion also increases the incidence and degree of hyperglycemia, as increased plasma concentrations of free fatty acids decrease peripheral glucose utilization by competing with glucose for oxidation and by stimulating the activity of enzymes that specifically promote fatty acid oxidation. Fatty acids also promote glucose production by providing substrate and cofactors, such as nicotinamide adenine dinucleotide phosphate (NADPH), for gluconeogenesis, and they inhibit the suppressive effect of insulin on hepatic glucose production. Stress, as measured by increased plasma cortisol concentrations, also is an important risk factor for the development of hyperglycemia. Stress occurs more commonly among infants who are sick, receiving catecholamine infusions, or undergoing painful procedures without ade-

TABLE 2-24

ADJUNCT THERAPIES FOR PERSISTENT NEONATAL HYPOGLYCEMIA

THERAPY	EFFECT	DOSE
Corticosteroids	Decreases peripheral glucose utilization	Hydrocortisone 5–15 mg/kg/d or prednisone 2 mg/kg/d
Glucagon	Stimulates glycogenolysis	30 μg/kg with normal insulin, 300 μg/kg with hyperinsulinemia
Diazoxide	Inhibits insulin secretion	15 μg/kg/d
Somatostatin (long-acting: octreatide acetate)	Inhibits insulin and growth hormone release	5–10 μg/kg every 6–8 hour
Pancreatectomy	Decreases insulin secretion / Causes diabetes and pancreatic insufficiency	

SOURCE: *McGowan JE, Hagedorn MIE, Hay WW Jr: Glucose homeostasis. In: Merenstein GB, Gardner SL, eds: Handbook of Neonatal Intensive Care, 4th ed. St. Louis, Mosby, 1998:259–274.*

quate anesthesia or analgesia, including surgery, venipuncture, vascular cutdowns, and endotracheal tube insertion and maintenance during ventilator treatment. Recent observations indicate that postsurgical hyperglycemia more likely is caused by increased cortisol secretion during surgery, whereas hyperglycemia immediately after the induction of anesthesia more likely is related to increased catecholamine secretion. Thus, narcotic treatment with fentanyl or morphine during and after surgery has been associated with lower circulating concentrations of catecholamines, glucocorticoids, and glucagon as well as a lower incidence of hyperglycemia. Catecholamines decrease insulin secretion and interfere with peripheral insulin action. Glucagon promotes glycogenolysis and release of hepatic glucose. Glucocorticoids promote gluconeogenesis by increasing protein breakdown and the supply of amino acids. Glucocorticoids also enhance hepatic enzyme activity in the gluconeogenic pathway, particularly phosphoenolpyruvate carboxykinase, the rate-limiting enzyme for gluconeogenesis, and glucose-6-phosphatase, which releases glucose into the circulation. Hyperglycemia also occurs more commonly among preterm and SGA infants, who have increased plasma concentrations of counterregulatory (antiinsulin) hormones. Other more common causes of neonatal hyperglycemia include the use of medications such as theophylline and dexamethasone, and sepsis. Hyperglycemia has also been associated with prostaglandin E_1 infusions.

Insulin-dependent diabetes mellitus, either transient or permanent, is an unusual but important cause of hyperglycemia in newborn infants. Neonatal diabetes mellitus usually presents early in postnatal life with weight loss, polyuria, dehydration, glycosuria, and hyperglycemia. It usually does not resolve for several weeks or even months, and sometimes is permanent. Pathogenic mechanisms are not known. Hyperglycemia has been associated with specific chromosome deletions (eg, 46,XXDq− on number 13).

PATHOPHYSIOLOGY The principal mechanism responsible for hyperglycemia in preterm infants is intravenous infusion of dextrose at rates that exceed the capacity for glucose utilization. Glucose utilization is limited by relatively inadequate insulin secretion rates as well as by decreased peripheral insulin sensitivity (primarily in skeletal muscle) in infants who experience stress and relatively increased secretion rates of catecholamines, glucocorticoids, and glucagon. Some of these stressed preterm infants also appear to maintain glucose production during insulin, glucose, and lipid infusions, indicating central (hepatic) insulin resistance. Excessive or inappropriate (for insulin secretion rates and plasma insulin concentrations) glucose production rates also can promote or prolong hyperglycemia. Even extremely low-birth-weight infants can have high rates of glucose production (4−8 mg/min/kg), primarily from gluconeogenesis, relatively soon after preterm birth.

COMPLICATIONS There are few serious consequences of neonatal hyperglycemia, although this condition has been associated with a wide spectrum of sequelae that most likely are the result of pathologic conditions that also produce hyperglycemia. Hyperglycemia in newborn infants is seldom if ever so severe as to cause osmotic injury to tissues, particularly the brain, unlike the well-known brain damage caused by salt poisoning. Another potential effect of aggressive glucose administration is steatosis, with associated impaired secretion of hepatic triglycerides. Steatosis rarely causes clinical signs in the neonate, but it can be detected by modest elevations of liver transaminases. Another complication of hyperglycemia is electrolyte imbalance in neonates who have glycosuria and increased sodium excretion. Hyperglycemia in older, more mature infants may jeopardize respiratory function by increasing lipogenesis, producing increased amounts of CO_2. This requires an increase in minute ventilation that, theoretically, might compromise infants who already have significant respiratory distress.

MANAGEMENT Treatment of hyperglycemia must include simultaneous treatment of underlying conditions. With modest hyperglycemia (plasma glucose concentration <300 mg/dL), reducing exogenous glucose (dextrose) infusion rates usually is sufficient to ameliorate or resolve the hyperglycemia. The rate of infusion should be decreased gradually by 1 to 2 mg/min/kg every 2 to 4 hours, with frequent measurement of glucose concentrations until normoglycemia is achieved.

Intravenous infusion of short-acting, regular insulin should be reserved for infants who have severe hyperglycemia (>300 mg/dL) that persists despite reducing the glucose infusion rate to less than 3 to 4 mg/min/kg. These infants also may have hyperlactatemia, metabolic acidosis, hyperkalemia, and osmotic diuresis. Insulin is given by continuous intravenous infusion, beginning at 0.02 to 0.05 U/h/kg. Higher infusion rates are not necessary and increase the risks of hypokalemia and subsequent hypoglycemia. Hypokalemia can be prevented by addition of potassium to IV solutions during the insulin infusion. Small intravenous infusions of potassium (0.1 mEq/kg potassium as potassium chloride or potassium acetate) can be added every 1 to 2 hours if hypokalemia is significant and persistent. Dextrose solutions should be infused through a very secure IV line such as an umbilical venous catheter or a peripherally placed central venous line to prevent hypoglycemia that can occur when glucose infusion is interrupted. Blood glucose concentrations should be measured frequently, every 1 to 2 hours, or whenever signs of possible hypoglycemia develop.

Early intravenous amino acid infusion has been associated with decreased incidence and severity of hyperglycemia and hyperkalemia. The rationale for this approach is that certain amino acids, such as leucine, valine, isoleucine, glutamine, and arginine, are known insulin secretagogues and are important for normal growth and development of the pancreas and the pancreatic islets and β cells. Glutamine and leucine also may promote insulin action and the disposal of glucose in skeletal muscle. Enteral feeding—even a minimal enteral feeding regimen—also promotes the secretion of insulin by inducing gut production of "enteroinsular hormones," also known as "incretins," including gastric inhibitory polypeptide and pancreatic polypeptide. These hormones increase insulin secretion by direct actions on the pancreatic β cells. Thus, enteral feeding is appropriate to prevent or ameliorate hyperglycemia unless the infant is very ill or there are clear signs of feeding intolerance.

References

Hypoglycemia

Aynsley-Green A: Glucose, the brain, and the pediatric endocrinologist. Horm Res 46:8−25, 1996

Kalhan S, Saker F: Metabolic and endocrine disorders, part one: disorders of carbohydrate metabolism. In: Fanaroff AA, Martin RJ, eds: Neonatal-Perinatal Medicine: Diseases of the Fetus and Newborn, 6th ed. St Louis, Mosby-Year Book, 1997

McGowan JE: Neonatal hypoglycemia. Pediatr Rev 20(NeoReviews 1):e6−e15, 1999

McGowan JE, Hagedorn MIE, Hay WW JR: Glucose homeostasis. In: Merenstein GB, Gardner SL, eds: Handbook of Neonatal Intensive Care, 4th ed. St Louis, CV Mosby, 1998:259–274

Stanley CA: Hyperinsulinism in infants and children. Pediatr Clin North Am 44:363–374, 1997

Williams AF: Hypoglycemia in the Newborn: A Review. WHO Publications 5778. Geneva, WHO, 1997

Hyperglycemia

Anand KJS, Sippell WG, Aynsley-green A: Randomised trial of fentanyl anesthesia in preterm babies undergoing surgery: effects on the stress response. Lancet. 1:243–248, 1987

Binder ND, Raschko PK, Benda GI, Reynolds JW: Insulin infusion with parenteral nutrition in extremely low birth weight infants with hyperglycemia. J Pediatr 114:273–280, 1989

Cowett RM, Farrag HM,: Neonatal glucose metabolism. In: Cowett RM, ed: Principles of Perinatal-Neonatal Metabolism, 2nd ed. New York, Springer-Verlag, 1998:683–672

Fosel S: Transient and permanent neonatal diabetes. Eur J Pediatr 154:944–948, 1995

Hemachandra AH, Cowett RA: Neonatal hyperglycemia. Pediatr Rev 20(NeoReviews 1):e16–e24, 1999

Lilien LD, Rosenfield RL, Baccaro MM, Pildes RS: Hyperglycemia in stressed small premature neonates. J Pediatr 94:454–459, 1979

Tyrala EE, Chen X, Boden G: Glucose metabolism in the infant weighing less than 1100 grams. J Pediatr 125:283–287, 1994

Vileisis RA, Cowett RM, Oh W: Glycemic response to lipid infusion in the premature neonate. J Pediatr 100:108–112, 1982

2.17.5   Disorders of Calcium Regulation

Ran Namgung and Reginald C. Tsang

HYPOCALCEMIA

DEFINITION Neonatal hypocalcemia is generally defined as a serum total Ca concentration below 2 mmol/L (<8 mg/dL) in term infants and 1.75 mmol/L (<7 mg/dL) in preterm infants or an ionized Ca below 0.75 to 1.1 mmol/L ($<3.0–4.4$ mg/dL), depending on the use of particular ion-selective electrode. Based on onset, hypocalcemia has been classified as either early or late, although the distinction may not be clear-cut. Early neonatal hypocalcemia typically occurs during the first few days of life, with the lowest concentrations of serum Ca being reached at 24 to 48 hours of age, whereas late neonatal hypocalcemia occurs toward the end of the first week of life.

ETIOLOGY Early-onset hypocalcemia is most commonly associated with prematurity, birth asphyxia, maternal insulin-dependant diabetes, gestational exposure to anticonvulsants, and maternal hyperparathyroidism. Hypocalcemia occurs in about 30% of all preterm infants; less mature infants have a greater chance to develop hypocalcemia (up to 90% in very low-birth-weight infants). About 25 to 50% of infants of insulin-dependant diabetic mothers develop early hypocalcemia. About 30% of infants who have an Apgar score below 5 at 1 minute of age develop early hypocalcemia. Late-onset hypocalcemia, which is less frequent than early-onset hypocalcemia, is most commonly associated with administration of relatively high phosphate-containing diets, disturbed maternal vitamin D metabolism, intestinal malabsorption of Ca, hypomagnesemia, and hypoparathyroidism.

PATHOPHYSIOLOGY Early neonatal hypocalcemia occurs as a result of the inability of the neonate to compensate for the sudden loss of placental Ca supply at birth. The usual protective changes observed in calciotropic hormone secretion may be blunted. Preterm infants may or may not exhibit the surge in parathyroid hormone (PTH) secretion observed in term infants at birth, and their restricted oral Ca intake may aggravate the problem; end-organ resistance to 1,25-dihydroxyvitamin D [1,25-$(OH)_2$D] in very low-birth-weight infants and increased serum calcitonin may contribute to hypocalcemia of prematurity. In asphyxiated infants, decreased Ca intake as a result of delayed feedings, increased endogenous P load, bicarbonate alkali therapy, and increased serum calcitonin concentration may contribute to early hypocalcemia. Hypocalcemia in infants of insulin-dependant diabetic mothers appears to be related to Mg insufficiency and consequently to impaired PTH secretion.

Late neonatal hypocalcemia commonly results from dietary Ca and P imbalance; high phosphate loads, usually dietary (cow milk–derived formula or rice cereals), lead to hyperphosphatemia and secondary hypocalcemia. The normally low neonatal glomerular filtration rate may also limit P excretion. Infants receiving currently adapted infant formulas have lower serum ionized Ca and higher serum P in the first week of life compared to breast-fed infants, related to the higher absolute P amount of formula.

Congenital hypoparathyroidism is the most significant cause of late-onset hypocalcemia that has to be treated early in life. Congenital hypoparathyroidism also occurs as part of the DiGeorge anomaly, which classically consists of the triad hypoparathyroidism, T-cell incompetence caused by partial or absent thymus, and conotruncal heart defects or aortic arch abnormalities.

Insufficiency of vitamin D arises from maternal vitamin D deficiency, sunshine deprivation coupled with insufficient dietary vitamin D intake, reduced production of vitamin D or its active metabolites caused by liver or renal disease, congenital deficiency of renal 1α-hydroxylase, and 1,25-$(OH)_2$D resistance. Deficiency of vitamin D or its metabolites causes decreased intestinal Ca absorption and renal Ca reabsorption. Most infant vitamin D disturbances do not manifest until several months of age.

When there is Ca deficiency, it is important to determine whether there is also hypomagnesemia because hypocalcemia generally cannot be corrected until hypomagnesemia is alleviated. The relationship between hypocalcemia and hypomagnesemia may arise from the important role of Mg in PTH secretion and action; chronic magnesium deficiency causes impaired secretion of PTH and PTH resistance at target organs.

CLINICAL PRESENTATION The neonate with hypocalcemia may be asymptomatic; the less mature the infant, the more subtle and varied are the clinical manifestations. In the neonatal period, the main clinical signs are jitteriness (increased neuromuscular irritability and activity), tremors, and generalized or focal convulsions; infants also may be lethargic, feed poorly, vomit, and have abdominal distension. Frank convulsions are seen more commonly with late neonatal hypocalcemia. The degree of irritability of the infants does not appear to correlate with serum Ca values. The classic signs of peripheral hyperexcitability of motor nerves (carpopedal spasm and laryngospasm) are uncommon in newborn infants.

DIAGNOSIS The diagnosis of hypocalcemia is based on the determination of ionized or total Ca. In addition to a history and physical examination, certain data are useful when there is not a clear cause for hypocalcemia: serum total Ca, ionized Ca, P, Mg, and glucose concentrations, and serum pH. Electrocardiographic determination of prolonged QTc (>0.40 second) suggests hypocalcemia. Although the QTc cannot precisely predict the ionized Ca concentration, it may be useful to monitor the response to Ca therapy.

When the infant is refractory to therapy or there are unusual findings in the initial evaluation, additional data may be of value to diagnose the less common causes of neonatal hypocalcemia (eg, primary hypoparathyroidism, malabsorption, and disorders of vitamin D metabolism). Based on the factors that can contribute to hypocalcemia, the etiology can be determined from the laboratory findings. Elevated serum P concentration (>8 mg/dL) suggests P loading (a clue to high dietary P intake), renal insufficiency, or hypoparathyroidism. Absence of thymic shadows on chest radiograph may suggest DiGeorge sequence. Hypercalciuria associated with hypocalcemia supports a deficiency of PTH. Low serum 25-hydroxyvitamin D concentration (<11 ng/mL) indicates vitamin D deficiency.

TREATMENT APPROACHES Treatment for symptomatic hypocalcemia is the administration of Ca salts. Ca supplementation at doses of 30 to 75 mg elemental Ca/kg/d is titrated to the response of the patient. The clinical signs of hypocalcemia are usually reversed rapidly by correcting serum Ca concentrations, which helps confirm the validity of the diagnosis.

When there are seizures (usually Ca <6 mg/dL), Ca can be replaced rapidly with 1 to 2 mL of Ca gluconate 10% per kg (≈9 to 18 mg elemental Ca per kilogram) given intravenously over 10 minutes; heart rate should be measured continuously during the infusion because there is often bradycardia, for which the infusion should be stopped temporarily. Calcium can cause considerable tissue injury if it extravasates from the vein, so the infusion site should be monitored. For less urgent purposes, continuous intravenous Ca supplementation at a rate of 75 mg/kg/d is generally sufficient to restore normocalcemia. After normocalcemia is achieved, a stepwise reduction of intravenous Ca may help to prevent rebound hypocalcemia: 75 mg/kg/d for the first day, half the dose next day, half again, and discontinue. Alternatively, if infants can tolerate oral fluids, Ca gluconate can be given orally at the same doses (divided into four to six doses) after initial correction. Oral Ca administration may not be practical in sick infants because oral calcium can stimulate bowel movements. The intravenous form of calcium given enterally causes less gut stimulation than syrup-based (high osmolar) preparations. Vitamin D metabolites are not recommended for clinical management of early hypocalcemia because of their variable response and potential side effects.

Because most causes of hypocalcemia in the neonate are transient, the duration of supplemental Ca therapy varies with the cause of hypocalcemia; commonly as little as 2 to 3 days of treatment is needed. Calcium supplementation is usually required for long periods in the case of hypocalcemia caused by malabsorption or hypoparathyroidism. If hypocalcemia is associated with hypomagnesemia, defined as a serum Mg concentration below 0.6 mmol/L (1.5 mg/dL), Mg sulfate 50% solution (500 mg or 4 mEq/mL), 0.1 to 0.2 mL/kg IV or IM (may cause local tissue necrosis), should be given and repeated after 12 to 24 hours. Serum Mg should be obtained before each dose (one or two doses may resolve transient hypomagnesemia).

In asymptomatic neonates with hypocalcemia, opinions vary as to the need for therapy. Most hypocalcemia of this nature resolves spontaneously, but the hypocalcemia has potential adverse effects on both the cardiovascular and central nervous systems, so others will commence treatment. For asymptomatic ill infants, or infants with severe hypocalcemia [serum total Ca <1.5 mmol/L (6.0 mg/dL) or ionized Ca <0.75 mmol/L (3 mg/dL)], therapy is usually required. Either intravenous or oral therapy, as described above, can be given.

Because late hypocalcemia is usually symptomatic, there is little debate on the treatment of late hypocalcemia. The goals of therapy are to reduce the P load and to increase Ca absorption by using feedings with a Ca/P ratio $\geq4:1$. This can be accomplished by the use of low-P feedings, such as human milk or low-P formula, in conjunction with an oral Ca supplement. Phosphate binders are generally not necessary. Hypoparathyroidism requires therapy with vitamin D or preferably one of its metabolites: 1,25-dihydroxyvitamin D (or 1α-hydroxyvitamin D_3, a synthetic analog) and lifelong Ca supplementation.

PREVENTION Prophylactic use of Ca salts or the vitamin D metabolites has been the major means to prevent neonatal hypocalcemia. Early hypocalcemia can be prevented in neonates by oral or parenteral Ca supplementation (75 mg elemental Ca/kg/d). Early feeding and provision of Ca to the gut is also important in preventing hypocalcemia. Use of continuous Ca infusion by central catheter to maintain a total Ca higher than 8.0 mg/dL and an ionized Ca level higher than 4.0 mg/dL may be helpful to prevent hypocalcemia in sick newborns who exhibit cardiovascular compromise and require cardiotonic drugs or pressure support and maintenance of normal maternal vitamin D status with exogenous vitamin D supplement, if needed, may be helpful in maintaining adequate amounts of fetal vitamin D, which, in turn, may prevent late hypocalcemia in some neonates. Vitamin D metabolites have been used in attempts to prevent neonatal hypocalcemia with variable degrees of success. In preterm infants (<1500 g), serum Ca could be normalized only at pharmacologic doses of $1,25-(OH)_2D$, the active metabolite of vitamin D. In addition to the measures just described, judicious use of bicarbonate administration and avoidance of respiratory alkalosis both reduce the risk of developing symptomatic hypocalcemia in ill infants.

Regular follow-up monitoring of serum Ca concentration and appropriate monitoring of underlying disease (eg, PTH concentration) are necessary in those infants who continue to have hypocalcemia (some of these infants may have permanent hypoparathyroidism, or "transient" hypoparathyroidism that may last for several years); these latter infants may still be at risk for "recurrence" of hypoparathyroidism and hypocalcemia, which has been reported to recur as late as adolescence.

References

Bushinsky DA, Monk RD: Calcium. Lancet 352:306–311, 1998

Itani O, Tsang RC: Calcium, phosphorus, and magnesium in the newborn: pathophysiology and management. In: Hay WW ed: Neonatal Nutrition and Metabolism, 1st ed. St Louis, Mosby Year Book, 1991:171–180

Koo WWK, Tsang RC: Building better bones: calcium, magnesium, phosphorus, and vitamin D. In: Tsang RC, Zlotkin SH, Nichols BL, Hansen JW, eds: Nutrition During Infancy: Principles and Practice, 2nd ed. Cincinnati, Digital Educational Publishing, 1997:175–207

Marks KH, Kilav R, Naveh-Many T, Silver J: Calcium, phosphate, vitamin D, and the parathyroid. Pediatr Nephrol 10:364–367, 1996

Mundy GR, Guise TA: Hormonal control of calcium homeostasis. Clin Chem 45:1347–1352, 1999

Tsang RC, Light IJ, Sutherland JM, Kleinman LI, et al: Possible pathogenetic factors in neonatal hypocalcemia of prematurity: the role of gestation, hyperphosphatemia, hypomagnesemia, urinary calcium loss and parathormone responsiveness. J Pediatr 82:423–429, 1973

HYPERCALCEMIA

DEFINITION Neonatal hypercalcemia is defined as a serum total Ca concentration above 2.75 mmol/L (11 mg/dL) or an ionized Ca concentration above 1.4 mmol/L (5.6 mg/dL). In pathologic hypercalcemia, elevation of serum ionized Ca usually occurs simultaneously with elevation of total Ca; however, elevated total Ca may occur without elevation of ionized Ca.

ETIOLOGY Hypercalcemia in infancy is uncommon in term infants but relatively more common in preterm infants. The most common cause of hypercalcemia in infants is a relative deficiency in phosphate supply and hypophosphatemia caused by use of parenteral nutrition with insufficient phosphate administration (with or without excessive Ca) or enteral human milk in preterm infants (low P content relative to preterm needs). Hypercalcemia also results from excessive administration of Ca or vitamin D; examples of this include overzealous use of Ca to treat hypocalcemia or to prevent it during exchange transfusion. Hypercalcemia of the mother and the neonate may result from chronic maternal exposure to excess vitamin D or its metabolites during treatment of maternal hypocalcemia or by maternal self-medication. Chronic diuretic therapy with thiazides during pregnancy can also cause maternal and fetal hypercalcemia and subsequently neonatal hypercalcemia.

There are rarer causes of hypercalcemia in the newborn, which may have a metabolic or familial basis. These include hyperparathyroidism (primary, which is very rare with fewer than 100 cases reported and only 20% of cases in children younger than 10 years, or secondary to maternal hypoparathyroidism), familial hypocalciuric hypercalcemia, hypercalcemia associated with subcutaneous fat necrosis, idiopathic infantile hypercalcemia (which may be part of Williams syndrome), severe infantile hypophosphatasia, and Bartter syndrome variant.

PATHOPHYSIOLOGY Normally an increase in serum Ca inhibits PTH and 1,25-dihydroxyvitamin D synthesis and thereby prevents or reduces hypercalcemia by decreasing calcium mobilization from bone, absorption from intestine, and reabsorption from kidney. A sustained elevation in serum Ca concentration implies an inappropriately increased calcium efflux from one of these pools into the extracellular fluid.

Hypophosphatemia can cause elevated circulating $1,25$-$(OH)_2D$ with attendant increased intestinal absorption of Ca and increased bone resorption; Ca cannot be deposited in bone in the absence of phosphate and thereby contributes to hypercalcemia. Pathologic conditions associated with PTH or vitamin D overactivity increase bone turnover, intestinal Ca absorption, and renal Ca absorption and can result in hypercalcemia.

Neonatal severe primary hyperparathyroidism is known to result from inheritance of two mutant alleles associated with the Ca^{2+}-sensing receptor gene on chromosome 3; homozygosity for activating Ca^{2+}-sensing receptor mutations causes neonatal severe primary hyperparathyroidism, whereas heterozygosity at these loci results in familial hypocalciuric hypercalcemia. In "benign" familial hypocalciuric hypercalcemia, the infant may have signs of hyperparathyroidism (PTH is usually in the normal range but inappro-

priately high for hypercalcemia); the condition is inherited as an autosomal dominant trait with high penetrance. Mutations in the Ca^{2+}-sensor lead to a dual defect in parathyroid cells (causing parathyroid hyperplasia) and renal tubules (causing hypocalciuria). Hypercalcemia associated with subcutaneous fat necrosis usually occurs in asphyxiated, large-for-gestational-age infants; increased prostaglandin E activity, increased release of Ca from fat and tissues, and unregulated production of $1,25$-$(OH)_2D$ from macrophages infiltrating fat necrotic lesions have been postulated to be responsible for the hypercalcemia.

Idiopathic infantile hypercalcemia (which may be associated with Williams syndrome) is associated with mutations in the elastin gene on the long arm of chromosome 7; there may be a vitamin D hyperresponsive state, and a blunted calcitonin response to Ca loading may contribute. Infantile hypophosphatasia is a rare autosomal recessive disorder and may be lethal in utero or shortly after birth because of inadequate bony support of the thorax and skull. The Bartter variant–related hypercalcemia is associated with polyhydramnios and prematurity; presumably hypercalcemia occurs in utero and results in fetal hypercalciuria and polyuria, which may in theory, contribute to early delivery and prematurity; increased serum $1,25$-$(OH)_2D$, normal serum PTH, and increased urinary prostaglandin E_2 (PGE2) are associated with the condition.

CLINICAL PRESENTATION Hypercalcemia may be asymptomatic, or the infants may have serious clinical signs (especially in hyperparathyroidism) requiring urgent treatment. Its onset may be at birth or delayed for weeks or months. The findings are frequently nonspecific, such as lethargy, irritability, poor feeding, vomiting, constipation, polyuria, dehydration, and failure to thrive (poor growth). Seizures, hypertension, respiratory distress (from hypotonia, demineralization, and deformation of the rib cage), nephrocalcinosis, and band keratopathy of the limbus of the eye (rare) may be present in severely affected infants. Long-standing hypercalcemia can lead to metastatic calcifications and primary nephrocalcinosis. Associated features, eg, elfin faces, cardiac murmur, and mental retardation (in Williams syndrome), and indurated, bluish-red skin lesions (in subcutaneous fat necrosis) may be present on physical examination. Mild hypercalcemia may present as feeding difficulties or poor linear growth.

DIAGNOSIS Diagnosis may be made incidentally or from chemistry tests. A maternal dietary and drug history (eg, excessive vitamin A or D, thiazides) or history of possible Ca-P imbalance or polyhydramnios during pregnancy, or a family history of disturbed Ca metabolism, should prompt further evaluation. If there is hypercalcemia without an obvious cause, the following approaches data are useful in deriving a diagnosis.

Very elevated serum Ca level (>15 mg/dL) usually indicates primary hyperparathyroidism or, in very-low-birth-weight infants, phosphate depletion. To differentiate hypercalcemia associated with parathyroid disorders from nonparathyroid conditions, the following measurements may be helpful: serum P concentration (low in hyperparathyroidism, familial hypocalciuric hypercalcemia, and rickets of prematurity); percentage renal tubular P reabsorption (usually lower than 85% in hyperparathyroidism; high in rickets of prematurity associated with hypophosphatemia); and serum PTH concentration (elevated in hyperparathyroidism). Very low urinary Ca/urinary creatinine ratio (U_{ca}/U_{cr}) in the face of hypercalcemia suggests familial hypocalciuric hypercalcemia. Very low serum alkaline phosphatase concentration suggests hypophosphatasia. Serum 25-hydroxyvitamin D determination may be useful when vitamin D excess is suspected. Bone x-ray films will identify demineralization and/or osteolytic lesions (hyperparathyroidism) or osteosclerotic lesions (occasionally with vitamin D excess) consistent with the etiology of the hypercalcemia.

TREATMENT APPROACHES Therapy of neonatal hypercalcemia consists of correction of specific underlying causes and removal of iatrogenic or external causes, for example, surgical removal of hyperparathyroid glands, stopping of excessive vitamin D intake, and phosphate (and Ca) supplementation of human milk given to preterm infants. In mild cases in which patients are asymptomatic, maintenance of hydration may suffice. For a moderately to severely hypercalcemic infant, prompt investigation and therapy must be instituted with the following goals: correction of dehydration, enhancement of renal excretion of Ca, inhibition of intestinal absorption or bone resorption, restriction of dietary Ca intake, and treatment of the underlying disorder. Treatment of severe hypercalcemia associated with subcutaneous fat necrosis and idiopathic infantile hypercalcemia consists of restriction of dietary intakes of Ca and vitamin D as well as minimizing exposure to sunlight; a low-Ca, low-vitamin D_3 infant formula, which contains trace amounts of Ca (<10 mg/100 kcal) and no vitamin D, is available for the short- to medium-term management of hypercalcemia in infants (CalciloXD, Ross Laboratories, Columbus, OH); note that this formula is also low in iron, so iron supplementation will be usually needed. As the hypercalcemia resolves, the usual infant formula or human milk can be mixed with the CalciloXD to ensure increasing amounts of Ca, and close follow-up is required to prevent rickets or hypocalcemia.

For short-term treatment of acute symptomatic hypercalcemic episodes (or serum Ca >14 mg/dL), expansion of the extracellular fluid compartment with 10 to 20 mL/kg of 0.9% sodium chloride intravenously, followed by an intravenous injection of a potent loop diuretic such as 1 mg/kg of furosemide every 6 to 8 hours intravenously, may increase urinary Ca excretion and decrease serum Ca; however, electrolyte balance should be monitored during this treatment. In hypercalcemic patients with low serum phosphorus concentrations, phosphate supplements of 0.5 to 1.0 mmol (16 to 31 mg) of elemental phosphorus per kilogram per day in divided oral doses may normalize the serum P concentration and lower serum Ca concentration; parenteral phosphate, however, should be avoided in severely hypercalcemic patients (serum total Ca >12 mg/dL) unless hypophosphatemia is severe (<1.5 mg/dL) because extraskeletal calcification theoretically may occur.

Calcitonin, glucocorticoids, bisphosphonate, and dialysis have also been used for severe hypercalcemia. Minimal information is available on the use of hormonal and other drug therapy for neonatal hypercalcemia. Short-term treatment with salmon calcitonin (at a dose of 4–8 IU/kg every 6 to 12 hours subcutaneously or intramuscularly), prednisone (1–2 mg/kg per day), or a combination may be useful. The hypocalcemic effect of calcitonin (a potent inhibitor of bone resorption) may be transient and abates after a few days (not ideal for chronic therapy); its effects may be prolonged if glucocorticoids are used concomitantly. There is, however, limited experience in neonates. High-dose glucocorticoids reduce the absorption of Ca in the gut and may decrease bone resorption and liberation of Ca; methylprednisolone (1–2 mg/kg per day, intravenously), hydrocortisone (10 mg/kg per day, intravenously) or its equivalent is effective but is not recommended for long-term use because of many undesirable side effects. Although

effective in several types of hypercalcemic states, glucocorticoids are relatively ineffective in the treatment of hypercalcemia associated with primary hyperparathyroidism. Bisphosphonate (an anti–bone resorptive agent) may be useful for the treatment of PTH-mediated hypercalcemia in children or for hypercalcemia in subcutaneous fat necrosis of a newborn infant, although there is scant information available.

For severe and unremitting hypercalcemia, either hemodialysis using a suitable neonatal, acute dual-lumen hemodialysis catheter (Med Comp., Harleysville, PA) if the infant is hemodynamically stable, or peritoneal dialysis may be helpful and should be prescribed with a low-Ca dialysate (1.25 mmol/L); for both hemodialysis or peritoneal dialysis, attention to serum P and Mg is essential to avoid iatrogenic depletion in patients with normal renal function; supplemental P can be given to patients treated with peritoneal dialysis either orally or intravenously, or sodium phosphate can be added to the peritoneal dialysate solution (should not exceed 0.75 mM); in this case, the bags should be inspected hourly for evidence of crystals, and fresh solutions should be prepared every 8 hours.

Virtually all cases of primary hyperparathyroidism require subtotal or total parathyroidectomy because the hypercalcemia may be life-threatening and does not respond to medical management. The need for treatment should be reassessed at regular intervals because some instances of neonatal hypercalcemia may resolve spontaneously.

References

Ghirri P, Bottone U, Coccoli L, et al: Symptomatic hypercalcemia in the first month of life: calcium-regulating hormones and treatment. J Endocrinol Invest 22:349–353, 1999

Lteif AN, Zimmernan D: Bisphosphonates for treatment of childhood hypercalcemia. Pediatrics 102:990–993, 1998

Nishiyama S: Hypercalcemia in children: an overview. Acta Pediatr Jpn 39: 479–484, 1997

Rice AM, Rivkees SA: Etidronate therapy for hypercalcemia in subcutaneous fat necrosis of the newborn. J Pediatr 134:349–351 1999

Rodd C, Goodyer P: Hypercalcemia of the newborn: etiology, evaluation, and management. Pediatr Nephrol 13:542–547, 1999

Singer FR: Medical management of nonparathyroid hypercalcemia and hypocalcemia. Otolaryngol Clin North Am 29:701–710, 1996

2.17.6 Jaundice in the Newborn

David K. Stevenson and Ashima Madan

INTRODUCTION

Jaundice, which is one of the most common conditions encountered in the care of newborn infants, refers to the yellow color of the skin and sclerae resulting from the deposition of bilirubin in these easily observable tissues. The condition arises when the rate of bilirubin production exceeds the rate at which bilirubin is eliminated. Newborn infants have an increased bilirubin formation rate which is approximately two to three times higher on a per kilogram body weight basis, compared to that of adults and is attributable mainly to the shorter life span of the newborn's red blood cells. The decrease in bilirubin elimination relates to a transiently limited ability of the newborn liver to conjugate bilirubin. Although not all full-term infants become visibly jaundiced, nearly all have a high serum total bilirubin (STB) concentration (hyperbilirubinemia) compared to adults.

In full-term formula-fed newborns, peak STB concentrations average approximately 6 mg/dL (103 μmol/L) by the third day. With more than half of the U.S. newborn population now breast-feeding (double that observed in the 1960s) and with an increase in the proportion of East Asian infants born in some U.S. regions, the 95th percentile for peak STB concentrations now probably ranges between 15 mg/dL (257 μmol/L) and 18 mg/dL (308 μmol/L) compared with 12 mg/dL (205 μmol/L) to 13 mg/dL (222 μmol/L) several decades ago. The peak now also occurs nearer to 4 days after birth rather than 3, and may not decline before the sixth or seventh day. Moreover, premature infants (including those from 35 to 37 weeks in gestation), who are often cared for in well-baby nurseries, as well as some East Asian infants, may not reach peak STB concentrations until the end of the first week of life and show an even more protracted decline.

Because most infants are discharged from the hospital within the first 2 days of life and thus before STB levels have reached a maximum, hyperbilirubinemia requiring phototherapy is the most common readmission diagnosis. The physician's intent to return the mother and child to the home environment, decreasing inappropriate use of laboratory tests, and decreasing health care costs has led to the practice of early newborn discharge in recent years. However, these good intentions have inadvertently increased the risk for missing pathologic jaundice (>18 mg/dL or 308 μmol/L). This has placed the burden for safe practice with respect to newborn jaundice on the physician in the outpatient setting.

Although there has been no uniform surveillance for the reporting of kernicterus over the last several decades, there is no doubt that kernicterus still occurs, and unfortunately can occur in some apparently healthy full-term infants. Notably, the reported kernicteric infants can be characterized as mostly male, breastfed, less than 38 weeks gestation, and discharged before 72 hours of age. In an effort to avoid such individual tragedies, there needs to be a shift from thinking about STB concentrations in terms of days of life or time epochs after birth to thinking about STB concentrations in terms of age in hours. The rate of rise of STB concentrations is an important factor when considering the need for intervention. The use of hour-specific STB concentrations represents a fundamental change in the approach to assessing the need for diagnostic evaluation or treatment of jaundiced newborns.

Compliance with the Practice Guideline of the American Academy Pediatrics (AAP) for Management of Hyperbilirubinemia in a Healthy Term Newborn, combined with its Appendix on Phototherapy, can serve as the basis for safe practice (see American Academy of Pediatrics Practice Guideline, http://www.aap.org/policy/hyperb.htm). However, the clinician must be aware of the exclusion of infants less than 38 weeks gestation and those with hemolytic disease. Moreover, a shift towards the use of hour-specific STB concentrations would avoid the arbitrariness suggested by the Practice Guideline's table of treatment recommendations, which relates specific therapeutic interventions according to different "time zones". In the absence of jaundice, the need for obtaining a STB concentration can be disputed. However, estimation of the degree of hyperbilirubinemia in the presence of jaundice is unreliable when based solely on visual inspection, even considering the cephalocaudal progression of jaundice. At a minimum, a transcutaneous bilirubin (TcB) or STB measurement should be performed on every infant who is jaundiced in the first 24 hours of life and seriously considered on any jaundiced infant discharged before the maximum STB level has been reached. If the values are plotted according to the infant's age in hours, this will provide a more accurate assessment of risk for subsequent hyperbilirubinemia greater than the 95th percentile at any subsequent time point. This will also reduce the risk of failing to: 1) identify high risk infants, such as those that present with jaundice in the first 24 hours (who are very likely to have hemolysis) or those who are less than 38 weeks gestation; 2) provide timely follow-up or measure STB concentrations in a jaundiced infant at follow-up; 3) recognize that intervention is urgent in infants with STB concentrations greater than 25 to 30 mg/dL (428 to 513 μmol/L); and 4) recognize the need for exchange transfusion in infants with STB concentrations greater than 30 mg/dL (513 μmol/L) or who show signs of kernicterus. Kernicterus is largely a preventable condition with vigilance and currently available therapies. Despite compliance with the AAP Practice Guideline, some cases of kernicterus may not be preventable because of sudden, unpredictable, and marked increases in STB concentrations (for example, in infants with glucose-6-phosphate dehydrogenase (G6PD) deficiency exposed to an environmental oxidant) or in those who have co-morbidities, which increase the likelihood that bilirubin will be toxic.

BILIRUBIN FORMATION   Bilirubin is derived exclusively from the catabolism of heme. Approximately 80% of the bilirubin produced is derived from the breakdown of hemoglobin from senescent red blood cells. Another 10% arises from ineffective erythropoiesis. The remaining 10% is derived from the breakdown of hemoproteins, such as cytochromes, myoglobin, nitric oxide synthase, glutathione peroxidase, catalase, etc. Under hemolytic conditions, the proportion of bilirubin derived from the red cells is, of course, greatly increased.

Heme is degraded in a two-step process, which can take place in all nucleated cells. In this process bilirubin and CO are produced in equimolar amounts. Carbon monoxide, which diffuses from the cell, binds to hemoglobin in circulating red blood cells to form carboxyhemoglobin (COHb), and is eventually excreted in breath (measurable as end tidal CO, ETCO). The COHb level corrected for inhaled CO (COHbc), the ETCO level corrected for inhaled CO (ETCOc), and the total body excretion rate of CO (VeCO), can serve as indices of total bilirubin formation, and thus as estimates of the hemolytic rate. When bilirubin enters the circulation, it distributes variably into tissues depending upon its binding to albumin and the pH. The greater the binding to albumin and the more alkaline the pH, the more likely bilirubin will remain in circulation until it enters the liver and is modified to an excretable conjugated form. Conjugated bilirubin is excreted into the intestine via the bile, where it can be deconjugated by β-glucuronidase and reabsorbed into the circulation (enterohepatic circulation) or converted by bacteria to nonabsorbable breakdown products (Figure 2-53).

CAUSES AND RISK FACTORS   The enterohepatic circulation of bilirubin is a normal process, which can contribute to the transitional neonatal hyperbilirubinemia observed after birth. The 2 to 3 mg/dL difference in STB concentrations by 5 days of age in exclusively breastfed versus formula-fed infants is most likely related to a comparative lack of decrease in the enterohepatic circulation of bilirubin. However, breastfeeding failure, often characterized by a decreased feeding frequency, weight loss, and dehydration, may contribute to hyperbilirubinemia in the first week of life. This phenomenon may be caused not only by an increased enterohepatic

FIGURE 2-53 Metabolic Pathway of the Heme Degradation and Bilirubin Formation. Heme released from the hemoglobin of red cells or from other hemoproteins is degraded by an enzymatic process involving heme oxygenase, the first and rate-limiting enzyme in a two-step reaction requiring NADPH and oxygen, and resulting in the release of iron and the formation of carbon monoxide (CO), a trace volatile gas, and biliverdin, a green-colored intermediate, in equimolar quantities. Metalloporphyrins, synthetic heme analogs, can competitively inhibit heme oxygenase activity (indicated by the X). Biliverdin is rapidly reduced to bilirubin by the enzyme biliverdin reductase. Carbon monoxide can activate guanylyl cyclase (GC) and lead to the formation of cyclic guanosine 3′,5′-monophosphate (cGMP). It can also displace oxygen from oxyhemoglobin and from carboxyhemoglobin (COHb) or be exhaled. The bilirubin that is formed is taken up by the liver and conjugated with glucuronides to form bilirubin monoglucuronide or diglucuronide (BMG and BDG, respectively), in reactions catalyzed by uridine diphosphate- and monophosphate glucuronosyl transferase. The bilirubin glucuronides are then excreted into the intestinal lumen but can be deconjugated by bacteria so that the bilirubin is reabsorbed into the circulation, as shown. SOURCE: Modified from *Dennery PA, Seidman DS, Stevenson DK: Neonatal hyperbilirubinemia: Pathophysiology, prevention, and treatment. N Eng J Med 344;581–590, 2001.*

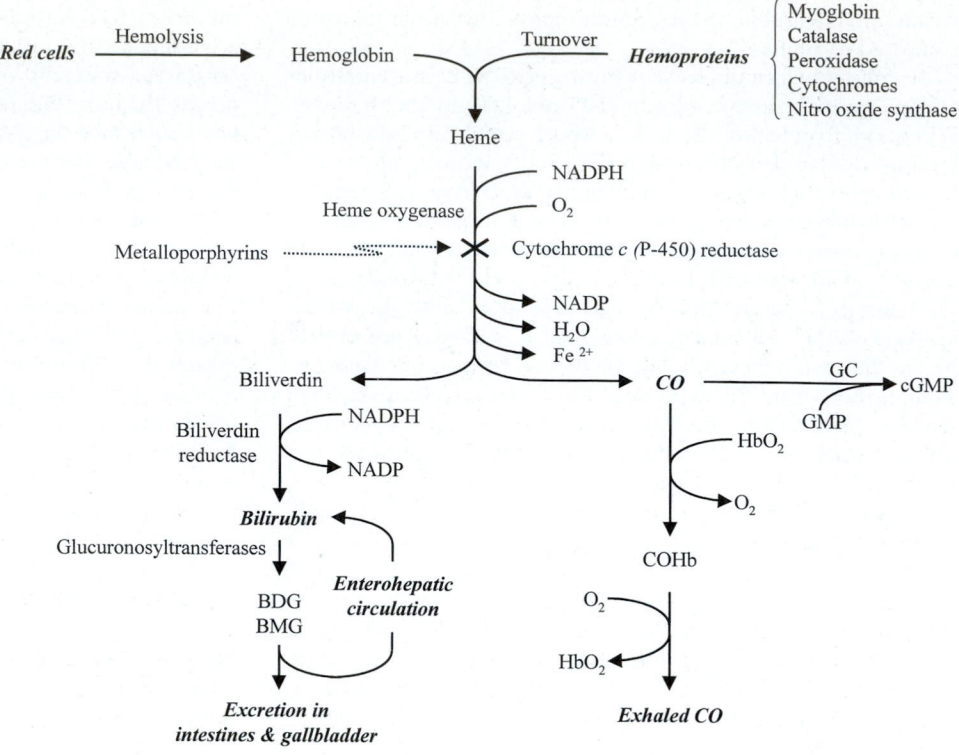

circulation but also by a lack of a normal decrease in bilirubin formation over the first week, which could be accounted for by caloric deprivation.

Jaundice from failed breastfeeding should be distinguished from true breast milk jaundice syndrome, which develops more gradually and presents typically in the second week of life, and requires the exclusion of other causes of unconjugated hyperbilirubinemia. In severe cases, cessation of breastfeeding may help confirm the diagnosis and avoid attaining elevated STB concentrations, which would require intervention based upon the AAP Practice Guideline. Although, the etiology of breast milk jaundice syndrome remains uncertain, it is most likely due to an exaggerated enterohepatic circulation and possibly to the presence of β-glucuronidase or some other substance in the breast milk, but not to an increase in bilirubin formation. The syndrome is time limited, but occasionally can persist for several months.

All of the pathologic causes of newborn jaundice can be understood in terms of an imbalance between increased bilirubin production and decreased elimination. The latter can be related to a deficiency in hepatic uptake, impaired conjugation of bilirubin, or increased enterohepatic circulation of bilirubin. Most of the common pathologic causes of neonatal hyperbilirubinemia reflect increased production of the pigment, as occurs with hemolysis arising from blood group incompatibilities, erythrocyte enzyme deficiencies, or structural defects of the erythrocytes. Increased bilirubin production also occurs in premature infants because of the shortened red cell life span; in infants of diabetic mothers because of polycythemia or ineffective erythropoiesis; in infants with closed space bleeding, such as bruising, hematoma formation, and hem-

orrhage into internal organs due to the breakdown of extruded blood; in infants with polycythemia; and in infants with sepsis.

Deficiencies of bilirubin elimination are often genetic in nature. Some patients with Gilbert's syndrome may have deficient hepatic uptake of bilirubin. More recently, infants with Gilbert's syndrome have been shown to have mildly decreased uridine diphosphate glucuronyl transferase (UDPGT) activity related to an increased number of the thymine-adenine (TA) repeats in the promoter region of the UG1TA gene, the principal gene encoding for this enzyme. Such polymorphisms may contribute to the variations in conjugating capacity observed in infants independent of their maturity. In addition, a DNA sequence variant (Gly71Arg), resulting in an amino acid change in the UDPGT protein has also been associated with neonatal hyperbilirubinemia in infants of Asian ethnicity. Hyperbilirubinemia from Crigler-Najjar syndrome type I (severe deficiency of UDPGT enzyme) and type II (the less severe form of UDPGT deficiency) is rare.

The most dangerous clinical situation occurs when increased bilirubin production is combined with impaired bilirubin elimination. Because bilirubin conjugation is transiently impaired in all newborns, increased bilirubin production, such as occurs in hemolysis, remains the most serious threat to newborn infants in terms of developing hyperbilirubinemia. Intestinal obstruction probably contributes to neonatal hyperbilirubinemia through the persistence of the enterohepatic circulation. Hypothyroidism is associated with decreased metabolism and excretion of bilirubin.

Hemolytic disease has been a common factor identified among those infants with reported kernicterus and appears to confer greater risk for the development of bilirubin encephalopathy, but the reasons are not known. Hemolysis is also an exclusion criterion for the AAP Practice Guideline, and therefore the diagnosis of hemolysis becomes paramount for planning the approach to treatment. ABO hemolytic disease is the most common form of hemolysis diagnosed in the newborn. However, only half of those infants with a positive direct antibody (Coombs') test are likely to have significant hemolysis. On the other hand, some infants with a negative direct Coombs' test have increased hemolytic rates. Therefore, depending upon their conjugating capacity, infants may develop hyperbilirubinemia. Reticulocytosis and the presence of microspherocytes on a peripheral blood smear may help confirm the diagnosis but are not pathognomonic. The recent development of a noninvasive technique for the measurement of ETCOc can provide a better index of hemolysis. An elevated ETCOc suggests increased bilirubin production, without specifically identifying the cause; whereas, hyperbilirubinemia in the presence of a normal ETCOc suggests a conjugating defect.

Besides hemolysis, which requires diagnostic testing, various epidemiologic or clinical conditions can help identify infants at risk for hyperbilirubinemia. These include a previous jaundiced sibling, East Asian race, a macrosomic infant of a diabetic mother, male sex, bruising, cephalhematoma, gestational age less than 38 weeks gestation, breastfeeding, excessive postnatal weight loss, visible jaundice before discharge, serum or transcutaneous bilirubin level above the 75th percentile for age in hours, G6PD deficiency, and short hospital stay.

BILIRUBIN TOXICITY AND KERNICTERUS There is no dispute about the toxicity of bilirubin to the central nervous system. However, there is no specific STB concentration that is unequivocally linked to neurotoxicity. Although it is very unlikely that a healthy term infant with a STB concentration less than 30 mg/dL (513 μmol/L) will suffer neurologic damage, there is also no certainty that lower STB levels under some circumstances eliminates the possibility of permanent injury, in particular with respect to auditory function. Likewise, the neurologic consequences of prolonged exposure to moderate hyperbilirubinemia is uncertain. There are few data to alleviate this concern. In addition to the STB concentration, the other major factor determining risk is the albumin binding of bilirubin. Bilirubin is bound to albumin up to a molar ratio of 1, meaning that 8.2 mg of bilirubin can be bound by 1 gram of albumin. Assuming a "perfect" binding circumstance (binding affinity is often less in premature or sick neonates), an infant with a serum albumin concentration of 3 g/dL could theoretically bind approximately 25 mg/dL of bilirubin. That the binding of bilirubin to albumin is protective is clear from the adverse consequences of bilirubin-albumin dissociation caused by sulfisoxazole and benzyl alcohol. Because bilirubin is a weak acid, an increase in blood acidity may render unbound ("free") bilirubin lipophilic, thereby enhancing tissue uptake. Avoidance of acidosis, metabolic or respiratory, is thus important clinically. Albumin-bound bilirubin and conjugated bilirubin normally do not cross the blood-brain barrier, however, conditions that alter the blood-brain barrier, such as prematurity and sepsis may facilitate bilirubin entry into vulnerable parts of the developing brain. In fact, prematurity may predispose infants to bilirubin encephalopathy because of low serum albumin concentrations and frequency of acidosis, in addition to relatively high metabolism of the brain.

Kernicterus is characterized pathologically by staining and necrosis of neurons in the basal ganglia, hippocampus, and subthalamic nuclei of the brain. Clinically, bilirubin-induced encephalop-

athy in the infant presents with poor sucking, stupor, hypotonia, and seizures in the first one to two days followed by hypertonia of extensor muscles, opisthotonus, retrocollis, and fever in the middle of the first week and hypertonia after the first week (Table 2-25). Survivors often are afflicted with hypotonia, active deep tendon reflexes, obligatory tonic neck reflexes, delayed motor skills, and after the first year, movement disorder (choreoathetosis, ballismus, tremor), upward gaze, paralytic palsies, intellectual deficits, and sensorineural hearing loss. Bilirubin encephalopathy can also be more subtle and associated with diminished cognitive function, changes in brain stem evoked responses, and auditory neuropathy. Changes in brainstem-auditory evoked responses (BAER) have been linked to elevations in "free" or unbound bilirubin levels, but their relationship to long-term permanent injury remains uncertain. Sensorineural hearing loss has been described in high-risk very low-birth-weight infants whose STB is less than 15 mg/dL (257 μmol/L). The combination of a normal otoacoustic emission test and an abnormal brainstem auditory evoked response is pathognomonic of auditory neuropathy, which may contribute to learning disabilities in some infants, especially those who are born prematurely and develop jaundice.

PREDICTION OF HYPERBILIRUBINEMIA Most newborns are discharged from the hospital before they have reached their maximum STB concentration. The use of an hour-specific STB concentration nomogram has been suggested as a means of predicting the risk of developing hyperbilirubinemia, with infants in the higher percentiles being more at risk. Conversely, infants with hour-specific STB concentrations less than the 40th percentile are probably at very low risk for subsequent hyperbilirubinemia (>95th percentile). A recent multicenter prospective study showed that measurements of ETCOc (an index of bilirubin production) alone or in combination with STB concentration are *not reliable* predictors of hyperbilirubinemia. However, this study did show that infants with STB concentrations greater than or equal to 95th percentile in general had increased bilirubin production, which was an important contributing cause of their hyperbilirubinemia. Also, a positive direct Coombs' test was not always associated with an elevated ETCOc, while a negative direct Coombs' test did not exclude hemolysis and associated hyperbilirubinemia. The combination of screening infants with hour-specific STB concentrations and ETCOc can identify infants with increased bilirubin production who need additional diagnostic work-up, follow-up for jaundice after discharge, or early intervention because of identified co-morbidities. Moreover, the study showed that some infants with increased bilirubin production handle the bilirubin load well. The presence of normal bilirubin

TABLE 2-25
CLINICAL FEATURES OF KERNICTERUS

Acute form
 Phase 1 (first 1 to 2 days): poor suckling, stupor, hypotonia, seizures
 Phase 2 (middle of first week): hypertonia of extensor muscles, opisthotonus, retrocollis, fever
 Phase 3 (after first week): hypertonia
Chronic form
 First year: hypotonia, active deep-tendon reflexes, obligatory tonic neck reflexes, delayed motor skills
 After first year: movement disorders (choreoathetosis, ballismus, tremor), upward gaze, sensorineural hearing loss

SOURCE: *Modified from Dennery et al., N Eng J Med 344;8:584, 2001.*

production and hyperbilirubinemia suggests a conjugating deficiency.

Finally, in a jaundiced infant, visual estimates of the STB concentration are not reliable. An alternative to blood sampling to determine the STB concentration is the use of a TcB measurement. Although older devices were confounded by differences in skin pigmentation, newer devices have means for adjusting for this factor. Therefore, a TcB can be used as a reliable surrogate for the STB measurement.

APPROACH TO EVALUATION, DIAGNOSIS, AND TREATMENT
In general, the AAP Practice Guideline sets the framework for management of hyperbilirubinemia in the healthy term newborn (Table 2-26). Some additional considerations are complementary to good practice. Each nursery should have a written policy outlining the criteria for the evaluation and diagnosis of hyperbilirubinemia, including those for discharge and follow-up. Because of the need to diagnose hemolytic disease, maternal blood typing and isoimmune antibody screening combined with blood typing and direct Coombs' testing are often routine. An ETCOc can be used as a more direct estimate of the hemolytic rate. Because doctors are not always present, nursing staff should routinely assess jaundice at least once a shift in a newborn nursery. There should be a low threshold for determining the STB concentration because clinical assessment is not reliable in the jaundiced infant. A TcB can be used as a surrogate for the STB concentration.

If jaundice is evident within the first 24 hours, a TcB or STB measurement should be performed. The TcB or STB concentration should be referenced to an hour-specific nomogram of STB concentrations for a relevant newborn population and serial TcB or STB concentration measurements may be indicated based on the hour-specific STB concentration percentile ranking. Before discharge, any jaundiced infant should have a TcB or STB concentration measured.

For any infant whose TcB or STB concentration exceeds the 95th percentile or might exceed it based on the rate of rise, a diagnostic evaluation is indicated, including history and physical examination and laboratory testing. The usual laboratory testing should include a hematocrit, CBC, reticulocyte count and blood smear (to assess red cell morphology) along with blood typing and a direct Coombs' test as part of the initial evaluation routine.

Routine testing for G6PD deficiency is more controversial. Testing certainly is indicated when family history or ethnic or geographic origin suggests the likelihood of G6PD deficiency. However, not all infants with G6PD deficiency have hemolysis. Some may have Gilbert's syndrome with a decreased conjugating capacity contributing to their jaundice. Although, an argument can be made for more generalized G6PD deficiency testing, such testing is not available currently in all institutions and when the testing is done, the results are usually not timely enough for immediate decision-making. Careful follow-up, which should include attention to weight loss, hydration status, voiding, and stooling patterns, is required for all discharged newborn infants who have hemolysis.

The standard procedures for treatment of hyperbilirubinemia are phototherapy and exchange transfusion. The criteria for application of phototherapy in healthy-term newborns are described in the AAP Practice Guideline. Phototherapy is effective because the yellow pigment, bilirubin, absorbs blue light mainly at the wavelength of 450 nm, and is converted to lumirubin, a water-soluble compound. The efficacy of phototherapy is determined by the dose (irradiance) and the amount of body surface area exposed. The irradiance is determined by the type of light source and the distance from the infant. Standard phototherapy using white fluorescent lights is applied at a distance of 15 to 20 cm above the infant. Intensive phototherapy can be achieved by placing a bank of fluorescent special blue lights at a distance of approximately 10 to 12 cm from the infant. A fiberoptic blanket also can be placed under the infant to increase the exposed surface area. Irradiance in the range of 30 $\mu W/cm^2/nm$ at the effective wavelength range can usually be achieved. New devices being developed using high-intensity gallium nitride light-emitting diodes (LEDs), which can generate high irradiance. These devices may be adaptable for use in home phototherapy, which has been suboptimal because of the relatively small light-emitting surface of fiberoptic blankets. When phototherapy is applied, temperature and hydration status must be monitored. Increased oral intake is usually sufficient, but intravenous fluids may be necessary when there is dehydration. Phototherapy can be interrupted for breastfeeding or for other brief periods of time in order to attend to the infant without compromising the effectiveness of phototherapy. Although the AAP Practice Guideline provides criteria for the application of phototherapy to full-term infants, there are no published AAP guidelines for preterm infants.

Phototherapy can be discontinued once the STB concentration has dropped below the 95th percentile, or by about 4 to 5 mg/dL (68 to 86 $\mu mol/L$). Except in the context of hemolytic disease,

TABLE 2-26
MANAGEMENT OF HYPERBILIRUBINEMIA IN THE HEALTHY TERM NEWBORN

AGE, HOURS	SERUM TOTAL BILIRUBIN, (mg/dL (μmol/L))			
	CONSIDER PHOTOTHERAPY*	PHOTOTHERAPY	EXCHANGE TRANSFUSION, IF INTENSIVE PHOTOTHERAPY FAILS†	EXCHANGE TRANSFUSION AND INTENSIVE PHOTOTHERAPY
≤24§	—	—	—	—
25 to 48	≥12 (170)	≥15 (260)	≥20 (340)	≥25 (430)
49 to 72	≥15 (260)	≥18 (310)	≥25 (430)	>30 (510)
>72	≥17 (290)	≥20 (430)	≥25 (430)	>30 (510)

* Phototherapy at these serum total bilirubin levels is a clinical option, meaning that the intervention is available and may be used on the basis of individual clinical judgment.
† Intensive phototherapy should produce a decline of serum total bilirubin of 1 to 2 mg/dL within 4 to 6 hours and the serum total bilirubin level should continue to fall and remain below the threshold level for exchange transfusion. If this does not occur, it is considered a failure of phototherapy.
§ Term infants who are clinically jaundiced at ≤24 hours are not considered healthy and require further evaluation.
SOURCE: *Modified from 1994 AAP Practice Guideline.*

rebound hyperbilirubinemia after phototherapy is unusual. The infant's eyes must be shielded during light exposure except when the phototherapy is applied with a fiberoptic or LED blanket or other apparel, thus avoiding direct exposure of the eyes.

If a significant proportion of elevated STB concentrations are contributed by the conjugated component, phototherapy may result in a grayish-brown discoloration of the infant's skin, which may last for weeks to months. This phenomenon has been referred to as "bronze baby syndrome". It is essential that infants with elevated direct hyperbilirubinemia be identified prior to the institution of phototherapy in order to initiate proper diagnostic work-up and to avoid a potentially harmful intervention.

Occasionally infants develop cholestatic jaundice after the application of phototherapy. In such instances, phototherapy should be discontinued. Anemia may develop as a consequence of hemolytic disease; therefore hematocrit should be monitored for several weeks in infants with ABO hemolytic disease that is successfully treated with phototherapy. A blood transfusion will sometimes be required.

Exchange transfusion was the first therapy developed for jaundice of the newborn, particularly in the context of Rh hemolytic disease (see Sec 2.17.8). Exchange transfusion removes not only bilirubin, but also circulating antibodies that can target the erythrocytes and the erythrocytes themselves, which might be hemolyzed later. The procedure can be conducted using one central catheter, removing small aliquots of blood from the infant and replacing it with similar aliquots of red cells from a donor mixed with plasma, or with two central catheters in a more continuous manner. A complete exchange transfusion involves removing and replacing twice the infants' blood volume. Sometimes a second exchange transfusion can be avoided by using immune globulin therapy (500 mg/kg). Infusion of salt-poor albumin at a dose of 1 g/kg before the exchange transfusion increases the removal of bilirubin. The complications associated with exchange transfusion are well known to most pediatricians and include thrombocytopenia, portal vein thrombosis, necrotizing enterocolitis, electrolyte imbalance, and infection. Mortality is probably less than 2% but the complication rate may be as high as 12%. Anticipatory management of hyperbilirubinemia and intense phototherapy can avoid exchange transfusion in most cases. The AAP Practice Guideline should be followed in terms of the criteria for exchange transfusion.

References

American Academy of Pediatrics: Practice parameter: Management of hyperbilirubinemia in the healthy term newborn. American Academy of Pediatrics. Provisional Committee for Quality Improvement and Subcommittee on Hyperbilirubinemia [published erratum appears in Pediatrics Mar; 95(3):458–61, 1995] [see comments]. Pediatrics 94:558–565, 1994

Bhutani VK, Johnson L, Sivieri EM: Predictive ability of a predischarge hour-specific serum bilirubin for subsequent significant hyperbilirubinemia in healthy term and near-term newborns. Pediatrics 103:6–14, 1999

Dennery PA, Seidman DS, Stevenson DK: Neonatal hyperbilirubinemia: Pathophysiology, prevention, and treatment. N Eng J Med 344;581–590, 2001

Ennever JF, Costarino AT, Polin RA, Speck WT: Rapid clearance of a structural isomer of bilirubin during phototherapy. J Clin Invest 79:1674–1678, 1987

Gourley GR, Arend RA: Beta-glucuronidase and hyperbilirubinaemia in breast-fed and formula-fed babies. Lancet 1:644–646, 1986

Kaplan M, Renbaum P, Levy-lahad E, Hammerman C, Lahad A, Beutler E: Gilbert syndrome and glucose-6-phosphate dehydrogenase deficiency: A dose-dependent genetic interaction crucial to neonatal hyperbilirubinemia. Proc Natl Acad Sci U S A 94:12128–12132, 1997

Maisels MJ, Newman TB: Kernicterus in otherwise healthy, breast-fed term newborns. Pediatrics 96:730–733, 1995

Maisels MJ, Kring E: Transcutaneous bilirubinometry decreases the need for serum bilirubin measurements and saves money. Pediatrics 99:599–601, 1997

Stevenson DK, Fanaroff AA, Maisels MJN, et al: Prediction of hyperbilirubinemia in near-term and term infants. Pediatrics 108:31–39, 2001

Valaes T: Problems with prediction of neonatal hyperbilirubinemia. Pediatrics 108:175–177, 2001

ACKNOWLEDGMENTS

This work was supported by the H. M. Lui Research Fund, the Hess Research Fund, and the Mary L. Johnson Research Fund.

2.17.7   Herpes Virus Infections in the Neonate and Children

Richard J. Whitley and Sergio Stagno

CONGENITAL AND PERINATAL CYTOMEGALOVIRUS INFECTIONS

Cytomegaloviruses (CMV) comprise a group of agents in the herpes virus family known for their ubiquitous distribution in humans. The natural history of human CMV infection is complex. Following a primary infection, viral excretion (occasionally from several sites) persists for weeks, months, or years before becoming latent. Asymptomatic episodes of recurrent infection with renewed viral shedding are common, even years after primary infection. Most maternal CMV infections are subclinical. Although infection may be without consequences for the mother, there can be serious repercussions for the fetus.

Humans are the only reservoir for CMV, and there are no known vectors in the natural transmission cycle. Transmission occurs by direct or indirect person-to-person contact. Sources of virus include urine, oropharyngeal secretions, cervical and vaginal secretions, semen, milk, tears, blood, and transplanted organs. The spread of infection requires close or intimate contact with infected secretions. Sexual contact contributes to the spread of CMV.

Congenital infection is assumed to be the result of transplacental transmission from an infected mother (vertical transmission). In contrast to the poor correlation that exists between CMV excretion during pregnancy and congenital infection, there is a good correlation between maternal shedding in the genital tract and milk and perinatal acquisition. The pathogenesis, clinical manifestations, and management of congenital and perinatal acquisition of cytomegovirus are discussed in Sec. 13.4.7.

NEONATAL HERPES SIMPLEX VIRUS INFECTIONS: HISTORY

Only 50 years ago, the first written descriptions of neonatal herpes simplex virus (HSV) infections were attributed nearly simultaneously to Hass, when he described the histopathologic findings of a fatal case, and to Batignani, who described a newborn child with HSV keratitis. Subsequently, histopathologic descriptions of the disease demonstrated a broad spectrum of involvement in infants.

In the mid-1960s, Nahmias and Dowdle demonstrated two antigenic types of HSV. The differentiation of HSV into two types resulted in the development of viral typing methods, which were critical in clarifying the epidemiology of these infections. Herpes simplex virus infections "above the belt," primarily of the lip and oropharynx, were found in most cases to be caused by HSV-1. Those infections "below the belt," particularly genital infections, were usually caused by HSV-2. With the finding that both genital herpes infections and neonatal HSV infections were most often caused by HSV-2, a natural cause-and-effect relationship developed between these two disease entities. This causal relationship was strengthened by the finding of viral excretion in the maternal genital tract at the time of delivery, suggesting that acquisition of the virus by the infant occurs by contact with infected genital secretions during birth.

EPIDEMIOLOGY OF NEONATAL HSV INFECTION

MATERNAL INFECTION   The epidemiology and clinical nature of genital HSV infection do not appear to be greatly influenced by pregnancy. Infection during gestation can manifest in a variety of ways. The most serious but fortunately uncommon problem encountered with HSV infections during pregnancy is that of widely disseminated disease. Infection has been documented to involve multiple visceral sites in addition to cutaneous dissemination. The mortality among these pregnant women is reported to be greater than 50%. Fetal deaths have also occurred in more than 50% of cases, although mortality did not necessarily correlate with the death of the mother. Surviving fetuses were delivered by cesarean section either during the acute illness or at term, and none had evidence of neonatal HSV infection.

FACTORS THAT INFLUENCE TRANSMISSION OF INFECTION TO THE FETUS   The type of maternal genital infection at the time of delivery influences the incidence of neonatal herpes. The duration and quantity of viral excretion and the time to total healing vary with primary, initial (first episode at the nonprimary site), and recurrent (HSV-1 and -2) maternal genital infection. Primary infection is associated with larger quantities of virus replicating in the genital tract and a period of viral excretion, which may persist for an average of 3 weeks. In contrast, virus is shed for an average of only 2 to 5 days and at lower concentrations (approximately 10^2 to 10^3 per 0.2 mL of inoculum) in women with recurrent genital infection.

Paralleling the type of maternal infection, the mother's antibody status to HSV at delivery appears to be an additional factor that also influences the severity of infection as well as the likelihood of transmission. Transplacental maternal neutralizing antibodies appear to have a protective, or at least an ameliorative, effect on acquisition of infection for babies inadvertently exposed to virus.

The duration of ruptured membranes is a risk factor for acquisition of neonatal infection. Observations by Nahmias and colleagues indicate that prolonged rupture of membranes (longer than 6 hours) increases the risk of acquisition of virus, probably the consequence of ascending infection from the cervix.

Fetal scalp monitors can be a site of inoculation of virus and may increase the risk of neonatal HSV infection. Such devices are contraindicated in women with a history of recurrent genital HSV infections.

INCIDENCE OF NEWBORN INFECTION   The estimated incidence of neonatal HSV infection is approximately one in 2000 to 5000 deliveries per year. Herpes simplex virus infection of the newborn can be acquired at one of three times: in utero, intrapartum, or postnatally. The mother is the source of infection for the first two routes of transmission. For postnatal acquisition of HSV infection, the mother may be the source of infection from a genital or nongenital site, or other environmental or patient sources of virus can lead to infection of the child.

Risk factors associated with intrauterine transmission are not known. However, both primary and recurrent maternal infection can result in infection of the fetus in utero.

The second, and most common, route of infection is that of intrapartum contact of the fetus with infected maternal genital secretions. Approximately 80 to 90% of infected babies acquire HSV infection by this route. Those factors that favor intrapartum transmission of infection have been described above.

The third route of transmission is postnatal acquisition. Even though HSV-1 has been associated with genital lesions, postnatal transmission of HSV has been increasingly suggested because 15 to 20% of neonatal HSV infections are caused by this virus type.

Relatives and hospital personnel with orolabial herpes may be a reservoir of virus for infection of the newborn. The recent documentation of postnatal transmission of HSV has focused attention on such sources of virus for neonatal infection. Postnatal transmission from mother to child has been documented. Maternal–infant postpartum transmission has been reported as a consequence of nursing on an infected breast. Furthermore, father-to-baby transmission has been documented.

NEONATAL INFECTION

PATHOGENESIS   Following direct exposure, either the newborn will limit viral replication to the portal of entry (the skin, eye, or mouth), or viral replication will progress and cause more serious disease, including involvement of the brain (causing encephalitis) or multiple other organs. Host mechanisms responsible for control of progression of viral replication at the site of entry are unknown. For central nervous system disease, intraneuronal transmission of viral particles provides a privileged route that may be immune to circulating humoral and cell-mediated defense mechanisms. Thus, transplacental maternal antibodies may be of less value under such circumstances. In contrast, disseminated infection may be the consequence of viremia or secondary to extensive cell-to-cell spread as occurs with pneumonitis following aspiration of infected secretions.

CLINICAL PRESENTATION   The clinical presentation of babies with neonatal HSV infection is a direct reflection of the site and extent of viral replication. Neonatal HSV infection is almost invariably symptomatic and frequently lethal. Although reported cases of asymptomatic infection in the newborn exist, they are most uncommon, and long-term follow-up of these children to document absence of subtle disease or sequelae has not been carefully performed. Classification of newborns with HSV infection is mandatory for prognostic and therapeutic considerations. Babies who are infected intrapartum or postnatally can be divided into three categories: (1) disease localized to the skin, eye, or mouth; (2) encephalitis with or without skin, eye, and/or mouth involvement; and (3) disseminated infection, which involves multiple organs, including central nervous system, lung, liver, adrenals, skin, eye, and/or mouth.

INTRAUTERINE INFECTION   In the most severely afflicted group of babies, intrauterine infection is apparent at birth and is characterized by a triad of findings, including skin vesicles or skin scarring, eye disease, and the far more severe manifestations of microcephaly or hydranencephaly. Often chorioretinitis alone or in combination with other eye findings, such as keratoconjunctivitis, is a component of the clinical presentation. Chorioretinitis alone can be a presenting sign and should alert the pediatrician to the possibility of this diagnosis, even though HSV infection is a less common cause than other congenital infections.

DISSEMINATED INFECTION Table 2-27 summarizes the disease classification of 291 babies assessed prospectively with neonatal HSV. Babies with disseminated infection have the worst prognosis in terms of both mortality and morbidity. Children with disseminated infection usually present to tertiary care centers for therapy between 9 and 11 days after birth. However, signs of infection are usually present 4 to 5 days earlier. Before antiviral therapy, this group of babies accounted for approximately one-half to two-thirds of all children with neonatal HSV infection. The principal organs involved following disseminated infection are the liver and adrenals. However, infection can involve multiple other organs including the larynx, trachea, lungs, esophagus, stomach, lower gastrointestinal tract, spleen, kidneys, pancreas, and heart. Encephalitis appears to be a common component of this form of infection, occurring in about 60 to 75% of children. Constitutional signs and symptoms include irritability, seizures, respiratory distress, jaundice, bleeding diatheses, shock, and frequently the characteristic vesicular exanthem that is often considered pathognomonic for infection. The vesicular rash, as described below, is particularly important in the diagnosis of HSV infection. However, over 20% of children with disseminated infection never develop skin vesicles during the course of illness. In the absence of skin vesicles, the diagnosis becomes exceedingly difficult because other clinical signs are often vague and nonspecific, mimicking those of other causes of neonatal sepsis. Mortality in the absence of therapy exceeds 80%; all but a few survivors are impaired. The most common cause of death in babies with disseminated disease is either HSV pneumonitis or disseminated intravascular coagulopathy.

Evaluation of the extent of disease is imperative, as with all cases of neonatal HSV infection. Laboratory data are often useful to determine which systems are involved: liver (serum glutamic-oxaloacetic transamine (aspartate aminotransferase), γ-glutamyltransferase, and bilirubin), hematologic (WBC, platelets, and blood clotting), CNS (cerebrospinal fluid, imaging, and electroencephalogram), and the lungs (chest x-ray). The radiographic picture of HSV lung disease is characterized by a diffuse interstitial pattern that progresses to a hemorrhagic pneumonitis. Not infrequently, pneumatosis intestinalis can be detected when gastrointestinal disease is present.

ENCEPHALITIS Infection of the central nervous system occurs alone or in combination with disseminated disease and presents with findings indicative of encephalitis in the newborn. Overall, nearly 90% of babies with dissemination or encephalitis have evidence of acute brain infection. Brain infection can occur either as a component of multiorgan disseminated infection or as encephalitis with or without skin, eye, or mouth involvement. Nearly one-third of all babies with neonatal HSV infection only have encephalitis.

The clinical manifestations of encephalitis include seizures (both focal and generalized), lethargy, irritability, tremors, poor feeding, temperature instability, bulging fontanelle, and pyramidal tract signs. Although babies with disseminated infection often have skin vesicles in association with brain infection, the same is not true for the baby with encephalitis alone. The latter group of children have skin vesicles in only 60% of cases at any time in the disease course. Cultures of cerebrospinal fluid (CSF) yield HSV in 25 to 40% of cases. Anticipated findings on CSF examination include pleocytosis and proteinosis (as high as 500 to 1000 mg/dL). A few babies with central nervous system infection proven by brain biopsy have been reported to have no abnormalities of their CSF, but this occurs very rarely. Serial CSF examination is useful for diagnosis because the infected child with brain disease will demonstrate progressive increases in CSF protein content. The importance of CSF examinations in all infants is underscored by the finding that even subtle changes have been associated with significant developmental abnormalities. Furthermore, as discussed below under Diagnosis, CSF provides an essential biological specimen for diagnostic evaluation by polymerase chain reaction (PCR).

Electroencephalography and computed tomography can be very useful in defining the presence of central nervous system abnormalities. Death occurs in 50% of babies with localized central nervous system disease who are not treated and is usually related to brainstem involvement. With rare exceptions, survivors are left with severe neurologic impairment.

The long-term prognosis, following either disseminated infection or encephalitis, is poor. As many as 50% of surviving children have some degree of psychomotor retardation, often in association with microcephaly, hydranencephaly, porencephalic cysts, spasticity, blindness, chorioretinitis, or learning disabilities.

SKIN, EYE, AND/OR MOUTH INFECTION Infection localized to the skin, eye, and/or mouth is associated with lower mortality but still has significant morbidity. When infection is localized to the skin, the presence of discrete vesicles remains the hallmark of disease. Clusters of vesicles often appear initially on the presenting part of the body that was in direct contact with the virus during birth.

TABLE 2-27

DEMOGRAPHIC AND CLINICAL CHARACTERISTICS OF INFANTS ENROLLED IN NIAID COLLABORATIVE ANTIVIRAL STUDY

	DISEASE CLASSIFICATION		
	DISSEMINATED	CNS	SEM
No. babies (%)	93 (32)	96 (33)	102 (35)
Male/female	54/39	0/46	51/51
Race: white/other	60/33	73/23	76/26
Premature (<36 weeks)	33 (35)	20 (21)	24 (24)
Gestational age	36.5 ± 0.4	37.9 ± 0.4	37.8 ± 0.3
Enrollment age	11.6 ± 0.7	17.4 ± 0.8	12.1 ± 1.1
Maternal age	21.7 ± 0.5	23.1 ± 0.5	22.8 ± 0.5
Clinical findings:			
Skin lesions	72 (77)	60 (63)	86 (84)
Brain involvement	69 (74)	96 (100)	0 (0)
Pneumonia	46 (49)	(4)	3 (3)
Mortality: 1 year	56 (60)	13 (14)	0 (0)
Neurologic impairment of survivors:			
Total	15/34[a] (44)	45/81[b] (56)	10/93[b] (11)
Ara-A	13/26[b] (50)	25/15[b] (49)	3/34[b] (9)
Acyclovir	1/6[b] (17)	18/27[b] (67)	4/5[b] (8)
Placebo	1/2[b] (50)	2/3[b] (67)	3/8[b] (38)

[a] Irrespective of therapy.
[b] Denominators vary according to number with follow-up available.
SEM = Skin, Eyes, Mouth

With time, the rash can progress to involve other areas of the body as well. Vesicles occur in 90% of children with skin, eye, and/or mouth infection. Children with disease localized to the skin, eye, or mouth generally present at about 10 days of life. Those babies with skin lesions invariably will suffer from recurrences over the first 6 months (and longer) after birth, regardless of whether therapy was administered or not. Although death is not associated with disease localized to the skin, eye, or mouth, approximately 30% of these children eventually develop evidence of neurologic impairment. Localized infection of the oropharyngeal cavity is found in approximately 10% of neonates with HSV infection.

Vesicles usually erupt from an erythematous base and are usually 1 to 2 mm in diameter. They can progress to larger bullous lesions greater than 1 cm in diameter. Although discrete vesicles on various parts of the body are usually encountered, crops and clusters of vesicles have also been described.

Infections involving the eye may manifest as keratoconjunctivitis or, later, chorioretinitis. The eye can be the only site of HSV involvement in the newborn. These children present with keratoconjunctivitis or, surprisingly, evidence of microphthalmia and retinal dysplasia. In the presence of persistent disease and no therapy, chorioretinitis can result, caused by either HSV-1 or -2. Keratoconjunctivitis, even in the presence of therapy, can progress to chorioretinitis, cataracts, and retinal detachment. Cataracts have been detected on long-term follow-up in three infants with proved perinatally acquired HSV infections.

Long-term neurologic impairment including spastic quadriplegia, microcephaly, and blindness has been encountered in children whose disease appeared localized to the skin, eye, and/or mouth. Important questions regarding the pathogenesis of delayed-onset neurologic debility are raised by such clinical observations. Despite normal clinical examinations, neurologic impairment develops between 6 months and 1 year of life. The clinical presentation occurs in a manner similar to that associated with congenitally acquired toxoplasmosis or syphilis. As noted below, two factors appear to predict neurologic outcome in babies with disease localized to the skin, eye, or mouth: (1) frequency of recurrent skin lesions over the first 3 months of life and (2) detection of HSV DNA by PCR in the CSF at the end of therapy.

DIAGNOSIS

CLINICAL EVALUATION The clinical diagnosis of neonatal HSV infection has become increasingly difficult because of the apparent decrease in the incidence of skin vesicles as an initial component of disease presentation. A variety of other infections of the newborn can masquerade as neonatal HSV infections, including hyaline membrane disease, intraventricular hemorrhage, necrotizing enterocolitis, and various ocular or cutaneous disorders. Bacterial infections of newborns can mimic neonatal HSV infection. It is not uncommon for some babies infected by HSV to experience a concomitant bacterial infection, particularly those caused by the group B *Streptococcus, Staphylococcus aureus, Listeria monocytogenes,* and gram-negative bacterial infections.

The most difficult clinical diagnosis to make is that of HSV encephalitis, as nearly 40% of children with central nervous system infection will not have a vesicular rash at the time of clinical presentation. Herpes simplex virus infection of the central nervous system should be suspected in the child who has evidence of acute neurologic deterioration with the onset of seizures and in the absence of intraventricular hemorrhage and metabolic causes. Serial increases in CSF fluid cell counts and protein concentrations, neg-

ative bacterial cultures of the CSF, and negative CSF antigen studies help suggest the diagnosis of HSV infection of the central nervous system. A maternal genital culture or history of genital herpes in either the mother or a sexual partner reinforces the suspicion of neonatal HSV infection. As noted previously, noninvasive neurodiagnostic studies can be used to define the sites of involvement.

LABORATORY ASSESSMENT Every effort should be made to confirm infection by viral isolation, the definitive diagnostic method. If skin lesions are present, a scraping of skin vesicles should be transferred in appropriate virus transport medium to a diagnostic virology laboratory. Clinical specimens should be shipped on ice for inoculation into appropriate cell culture systems. Shipping of specimens and their processing should be expedited. In addition to skin vesicles, other sites from which virus may be isolated include the cerebrospinal fluid, stool, urine, throat, nasopharynx, and conjunctivae.

Over the past several years, PCR detection of HSV DNA has become the diagnostic method of choice for central nervous system disease, replacing brain biopsy. It has proved both sensitive and specific when properly performed on CSF specimen.

The serologic diagnosis of HSV infection is not of great clinical value. Therapeutic decisions can not await the results of serologic studies. Further, the inability of the commonly available serologic assays to distinguish between antibodies to HSV-1 and -2 as well as to denote the presence of transplacentally acquired maternal immunoglobulin G (IgG), as opposed to endogenously produced antibodies, makes the assessment of the neonate's antibody status difficult during acute infection. Serial antibody assessment may be useful if a mother without a prior history of HSV infection has a primary infection late in gestation and transfers very little or no antibody to the fetus.

TREATMENT

ANTIVIRAL THERAPY Acyclovir is the treatment of choice for neonatal HSV infections of the central nervous system. It is a selective inhibitor of HSV replication, representing one of the most important advances in antiviral therapy. Acyclovir is a synthetic acyclic purine nucleoside analog that selectively inhibits HSV-1 and HSV-2. Acyclovir is converted to its monophosphate derivative by virus-encoded thymidine kinase, an event that does not occur to any significant extent in uninfected cells. Subsequent di- and triphosphorylation is catalyzed by cellular enzymes and result in acyclovir triphosphate concentrations 40- to 100-fold higher in HSV-infected cells than in uninfected cells. Acyclovir triphosphate inhibits viral DNA synthesis by competing with deoxyguanosine triphosphate as a substrate for viral DNA polymerase. DNA synthesis is then terminated because acyclovir triphosphate lacks the three hydroxyls required for DNA chain elongation. The viral polymerase has greater affinity for acyclovir triphosphate than cellular DNA polymerase, resulting in little incorporation of acyclovir into cellular DNA. In vitro, acyclovir is active against HSV-1 (average $ED_{50} = 0.04$ $\mu g/mL$), HSV-2 (0.10 $\mu g/mL$), and varicella-zoster virus (0.50 $\mu g/mL$).

Acyclovir has been established as efficacious for the treatment of primary genital HSV when administered by intravenous, oral, and topical routes. Furthermore, the oral and intravenous administration of acyclovir to the immunocompromised host decreases both the frequency of reactivation following immunosuppression and disease duration. Acyclovir is administered at a dosage of 20 mg/kg every 8 hours intravenously for 21 days.

TABLE 2-28

PROGNOSTIC FACTORS IDENTIFIED BY MULTIVARIATE ANALYSES FOR NEONATES WITH HSV INFECTION[a]

	RELATIVE RISK	
	MORTALITY	**MORBIDITY**
Total group (n=202)		
Extent of disease		
Skin, eyes, or mouth	1	1
CNS	5.8†	4.4†
Disseminated	33†	2.1†
Level of consciousness		
Alert or lethargic	1	NS
Semicomatose or comatose	5.2†	NS
Disseminated intravascular coagulopathy	3.8†	NS
Prematurity	3.7†	NS
Virus type		
HSV-1	2.3†	1
HSV-2	1	4.9†
Seizures	NS	3.0†
Infants with disseminated disease (n=46)		
Disseminated intravascular coagulopathy	3.5†	NS
Level of consciousness		
Alert or lethargic	1	1
Semicomatose or comatose	3.9†	4.0†
Pneumonia	3.6†	NS
Infants with CNS involvement (n=71)		
Level of consciousness		
Alert or lethargic	1	NS
Semicomatose or comatose	6.1†	NS
Prematurity	5.2†	NS
Seizures	NS	3.4†
Infants with infection of the skin, eyes, or mouth (n=85)		
No. of skin-vesicle recurrences		
<3	NA	1
≥3	NA	21†
Virus type		
HSV-1	NA	1
HSV-2	NA	14‡[b]

[a] CNS = central nervous system; NS = not statistically significant ($p > .05$); NA = not applicable (no baby with disease confined to the skin, eyes, or mouth died).
† $p < .01$; ‡ $p < .05$.
[b] Because of the correlation between virus type and skin-vesicle recurrence, virus type was not significant in the multivariate model; however, it was significant as a single factor.
SOURCE: *Whitley RJ, Arvin A, Prober C, et al, the National Institute of Allergy and Infectious Diseases Collaborative Antiviral Study Group: Predictors of morbidity and mortality in neonates with herpes simplex virus infections. N Engl J Med 324:450–454, 1991.*

Infants with ocular involvement caused by HSV should receive topical antiviral medication in addition to parenteral therapy. At the present time, few safety and tolerance data are available for topical ophthalmic antiviral drugs. In older patients, (trifluorothymidine Viroptic) has the greatest antiviral activity and is the treatment of choice for HSV infection of the eyes. Vidarabine ophthalmic and idoxuridine have been utilized for a longer period of time. There is more experience regarding their safety in both adults and children, but they are less active.

Table 2-28 summarizes the risk factors for mortality and morbidity even with therapy of neonatal HSV infection.

PREVENTION

Identifying the woman who excretes HSV at delivery and then optimizing either prophylactic protocols with safe and acceptable antiviral drugs or delivery by cesarean section is the optimal way to manage genital infection at the time of delivery. The administration of acyclovir during the last 6 weeks of gestation has resulted in a lower frequency of cesarean sections and viral shedding. However, the safety of this approach for the fetus has not been established. Specifically, the pharmacokinetics and metabolism of acyclovir in the human fetus are unknown at present. The possibility of acyclovir fetal nephrotoxicity creates a potential risk of drug administration that must be considered. In addition, it must be recognized that the women who are at greatest risk for delivering babies who acquire neonatal HSV infection are those least likely to have a history of recurrent genital HSV infection.

References

Aurelius E, Johansson B, Skoldenberg B, Forsgren M: Encephalitis in immunocompetent patients due to herpes simplex virus type 1 or 2 as determined by type-specific polymerase chain reaction and antibody assays of cerebrospinal fluid. J Med Virol 39:179–186, 1993

Batignani A: Conjunctivite da virus erpetico in neonato. Boll Ocul 13:1217, 1934

Brown ZA, Benedetti J, Ashley R, et al: Neonatal herpes simplex virus infection in relation to asymptomatic maternal infection at the time of labor. N Engl J Med 324:1247–1252, 1991

Bryson YJ, Dillon M, Lovett M, et al: Treatment of first episodes of genital herpes simplex virus infection with oral acyclovir: a randomized double-blind controlled trial in normal subjects. N Engl J Med 308:916–921, 1983

Cibis A, Burde RM: Herpes simplex virus induced congenital cataracts. Arch Ophthalmol 85:220–223, 1971

Corey L. The diagnosis and treatment of genital herpes. JAMA 248:1041–1049, 1982

Corey L, Adams H, Brown A, Holmes K: Genital herpes simplex virus infections: clinical manifestations, course and complications. Ann Intern Med 98:958–972, 1983

Corey L, Benedetti J, Critchlow C, et al: Treatment of primary first episode genital herpes simplex virus infections with acyclovir: results of topical, intravenous, and oral therapy. J Antimicrob Chemother 12:79–88, 1983

Corey L, Nahmias AJ, Guinan ME, Benedetti JK, Critchlow CW, Holmes KK: A trial of topical acyclovir in genital herpes simplex virus infections. N Engl J Med 306:1313–1319, 1982

Derse D, Chang Y-C, Furman PA, Elion GB: Inhibition of purified human and herpes simplex virus-induced DNA polymerase by 9-(2-hydroxyethoxy methyl)guanine [acyclovir] triphosphate: effect on primer-template function. J Biol Chem 256:11447–11451, 1981

Douglas J, Schmidt O, Corey L: Acquisition of neonatal HSV-1 infection from a paternal source contact. J Pediatr 103:908–910, 1983

Dunkle LM, Schmidt RR, O'Connor DM: Neonatal herpes simplex infection possibly acquired via maternal breast milk. Pediatrics 63:250–251, 1979

Elion GB, Furman PA, Fyfe JA, de Miranda P, Beauchamp L, Schaffer HJ: Selectivity of action of an antiherpetic agent, 9-(2-hydroxyethoxymethyl)guanine. Proc Natl Acad Sci USA 74:5716–5720, 1977

Field JH, Darby G, Wildy P: Isolation and characterization of acyclovir-resistant mutants of herpes simplex virus. J Gen Virol 49:115–124, 1980

Fyfe JA, Keller PM, Furman PA, Miller RA, Elion GB: Thymidine kinase from herpes simplex virus phosphorylates the new antiviral compound, 9-(2-hydroxyethoxymethyl)guanine. J Biol Chem 253:8721–8727, 1978

Hass M: Hepatoadrenal necrosis with intranuclear inclusion bodies: report of a case. Am J Pathol 11:127, 1935

Kaye EM, Dooling EC: Neonatal herpes simplex meningoencephalitis associated with fetal monitor scalp electrodes. Neurology 31:1045–1047, 1981

Lakeman FD, Whitley RJ, the National Institute of Allergy and Infectious Diseases Collaborative Antiviral Study Group: Diagnosis of herpes simplex encephalitis: application of polymerase chain reaction to cerebrospinal fluid from brain biopsied patients and correlation with disease. J Infect Dis 171:857–863, 1995

Light IJ: Postnatal acquisition of herpes simplex virus by the newborn infant: a review of the literature. Pediatrics 63:480–482, 1979

Meyers JD, Wade JC, Mitchell CD, et al: Multicenter collaborative trial of intravenous acyclovir for treatment of mucocutaneous herpes simplex virus infection in immunocompromised host. Am J Med 73:229–235, 1982

Mizrahi EM, Tharp BR: A unique electroencephalogram pattern in neonatal herpes simplex virus encephalitis. Neurology 31:164, 1981

Nahmias AJ, Dowdle WR: Antigenic and biologic differences in herpesvirus hominis. Prog Med Virol 10:110–159, 1968

Nahmias AJ, Josey WE, Naib ZM, Freeman MG, Fernandez RJ, Wheeler JH: Perinatal risk associated with maternal genital herpes simplex virus infection. Am J Obstet Gynecol 110:825–836, 1971

Nahmias AJ, Visitine A, Caldwell A, Wilson C: Eye infections with herpes simplex viruses in neonates. Surv Ophthalmol 21:100–105, 1976

Parvey LS, Chien LT: Neonatal herpes simplex virus infection introduced by fetal monitor scalp electrode. Pediatrics 65:1150–1153, 1980

Prober CG, Sullender WM, Yasukawa LL, Au DS, Yeager AS, Arvin AM: Low risk of herpes simplex virus infections in neonates exposed to the virus at the time of vaginal delivery to mothers with recurrent genital herpes simplex virus infections. N Engl J Med 316:240–244, 1987

Rowley A, Lakeman F, Whitley R, Wolinsky S: Rapid detection of herpes simplex virus DNA in cerebrospinal fluid of patients with herpes simplex encephalitis. Lancet 335:440–441, 1990

Saral R, Burns WH, Laskin OL, Santos GW, Leitman PS. Acyclovir prophylaxis of herpes simplex virus infections: a randomized, double-blind, controlled trial in bone-marrow-transplant recipients. N Engl J Med 305:63–67, 1981

Schaeffer HJ, Beauchamp L, de Miranda P, Elion GB, Bauer DJ, Collins P: 9-(2-hydroxyethoxymethyl)guanine activity against viruses of the herpes group. Nature 272:583–585, 1978

Scott LL, Sanchez PJ, Jackson GL, Zeray F, Wendel GD JR: Acyclovir suppression to prevent cesarean delivery after first-episode genital herpes. Obstet Gynecol 87:69–73, 1996

Whitley RJ, Arvin A, Prober C, et al: the National Institute of Allergy and Infectious Diseases Collaborative Antiviral Study Group: Predictors of morbidity and mortality in neonates with herpes simplex virus infections. N Engl J Med 324:450–454, 1991

Whitley RJ, Corey L, Arvin A, et al, the National Institute of Allergy and Infectious Diseases Collaborative Antiviral Study Group: Changing presentation of herpes simplex virus infection in neonates. J Infect Dis 158:109–116, 1988

Whitley RJ, Hutto C: Neonatal herpes simplex virus infections. Pediatr Rev 7:119–126, 1985

Yeager AS, Arvin AM: Reasons for the absence of a history of recurrent genital infections in mothers of neonates infected with herpes simplex virus. Pediatrics 73:188–193, 1984

Yeager AS, Ashley RL, Corey L: Transmission of herpes simplex virus from father to neonate. J Pediatr 103:905–907, 1983

2.17.8 Hemolytic Disease of the Newborn (Erythroblastosis Fetalis)

Roderic H. Phibbs

The history of erythroblastosis describes one of the most impressive successes in obstetrics and pediatrics. Erythroblastosis was a common cause of neonatal death, recurrent stillbirth, and permanent brain damage. Now, prevention has made it an increasingly rare disease, and when it does occur there is effective treatment, including fetal therapy for the most severe cases. In 1932, Diamond and co-workers suggested that three clinical syndromes, anemia of the newborn, universal edema of the fetus (hydrops fetalis), and icterus gravis neonatorum, were all part of the spectrum of a single disease. They named the disease erythroblastosis fetalis because of the high concentration of erythroblasts in the peripheral blood of the affected infant at birth. A decade later, the mechanism of the disease was identified as alloimmune hemolytic anemia caused by transplacental passage of maternal antibodies into the fetus. In the following decade, exchange transfusion was introduced to prevent brain damage from hyperbilirubinemia, and maternal antibody testing was used to identify potentially affected pregnancies. Fetal death was common when severely affected pregnancies went to term; hence, fetuses thought to be severely affected were delivered prematurely. This practice often produced an unaffected preterm infant who then died of hyaline membrane disease.

Amniotic fluid analysis of fetal bilirubin production was probably the first example of direct testing of the human fetus. It was introduced in the early 1960s and led to three advances: identification of the unaffected fetus, better timing of delivery of the affected fetus, and identification of fetuses so severely affected that they would die before they were mature enough to be delivered. That, in turn, led to development of intrauterine transfusion of the fetus, the first example of effective fetal therapy. At the same time prophylactic therapy was being developed to prevent maternal sensitization to the antigen responsible for most of the cases. With broad application of prophylaxis, few mothers have been sensitized, and more mothers who were sensitized in the past are passing beyond childbearing age. Because of these trends, the disease is now uncommon, and the incidence should continue to decline in the future.

MATERNAL SENSITIZATION

Maternal sensitization to the D antigen in the Rh system has caused most of the significant disease.[1] A woman who is D-negative can become sensitized during a pregnancy with a D-positive fetus when fetal erythrocytes cross the placenta in the second and third trimester and during delivery. Usually antibodies appear in the mother within the first 6 months after the sensitizing pregnancy, but occasionally they appear during the first pregnancy. If the father is homozygous for the D antigen, all fetuses will be heterozygous and capable of sensitizing the mother. Sensitization, however, does not occur in every potential case. If the father is heterozygous, the chance of a fetus having the antigen is 50%. With successive pregnancies bearing D-positive fetuses, the mother's antibody titer increases, causing more severe disease. The same process can cause sensitization to any of the other Rh antigens or to several other red cell antigen systems, including Kell, Duffy, Kidd, and Ss. At present anti-D is still the most common cause of severe disease, but significant numbers of cases are caused by anti-c, anti-e, anti-C, and anti-Kell.

---

[1]There are three sets of allelic antigens in the Rh system: C and c, E and e, and D and absence of D (no allelic "d" antigen has been identified). A person can be homozygous or heterozygous for each set of alleles (eg, CC, Cc, or cc). The commonly used terms "Rh positive" and "Rh negative" are confusing because they only refer to the presence or absence of the D antigen.

Prophylaxis prevents sensitization to the D antigen. If a non-sensitized D-negative mother is given anti-D globulin in the third trimester and again immediately after the birth of her D-positive infant, she will not become sensitized. This must be repeated with each pregnancy. If a mother already has been sensitized, she cannot be "desensitized" by this treatment. Prophylaxis only prevents sensitization to the D antigen.

A sensitized mother produces IgG antibodies against the antigen. Unlike IgM, IgG crosses the placenta. This occurs by active transport involving the Fc receptors in the placenta, a process that increases in the third trimester, causing hemolytic anemia in the fetus to worsen.

Pregnant mothers should have their red blood cells grouped and typed and their serum screened for all antibodies capable of causing erythroblastosis. When an antibody is detected, the corresponding red cell antigen must be identified.

When a mother develops a significant antibody titer ("significant" may vary between laboratories), the fetus is evaluated. Amniocentesis and analysis of the fluid for bilirubin is a sensitive method of assessment later in pregnancy. When there is a possibility of severe disease earlier in pregnancy, fetal blood sampling to measure fetal hematocrit is a more sensitive method. If a mother has had a pregnancy with an affected fetus, the next pregnancy with a fetus that is also positive for the antigen will result in disease that is at least as severe as the previous case.

The course of disease is variable. Hemolysis can be mild initially, then quickly become severe. Repeated evaluation of the fetus defines the course of disease and dictates the intervention when necessary. The mildest cases can deliver at term. Moderate disease requires preterm delivery. Severe cases need one or more intrauterine transfusions of the fetus to prevent the development of hydrops fetalis, which will be followed soon by fetal death.

PATHOPHYSIOLOGY IN FETUS AND NEWBORN INFANT

Fetal erythrocytes with maternal antibodies attached to the antigen sites are hemolyzed in the reticuloendothelial system. The fetus responds to the anemia with a striking increase in erythropoiesis. The erythroblast count in the peripheral blood is often 50,000 to 100,000/dL. The intense erythropoiesis can consume so much of the pool of pluripotential hematopoietic stem cells that thrombocytopenia and granulopenia result. Anti-Kell disease is a special case. The antibodies attack the red cell precursors as well as the mature red cells, leading to more severe anemia with lower nucleated red blood cell counts and less bilirubin production.

Many organ systems are affected by this fetal hemolysis. There is extensive proliferation of erythroid precursors in the liver, spleen, and bone marrow. With severe disease, these precursors become the predominant cell line, causing massive organomegaly; the enlarged spleen is vulnerable to rupture during delivery. Most of the unconjugated bilirubin from the hemolysis crosses the placenta and is conjugated and excreted by the mother. At birth the unconjugated bilirubin will be elevated only modestly but can then rise rapidly, reaching a peak during the first week after birth and declining thereafter as the infant's ability to metabolize bilirubin increases. If the erythroid proliferation in the liver has caused sufficient damage, the conjugated bilirubin will be elevated at birth and may transiently reach very high levels during the first week. Infants with hydrops (see below) have hypoalbuminemia, which may increase the likelihood of free bilirubin entering the central nervous system to cause brain injury.

Elevated levels of plasma hemoglobin from hemolysis interfere with insulin function, leading to pancreatic islet cell hyperplasia and hyperinsulinism in the fetus. This can cause hypoglycemia, which can begin within minutes after birth and continue for several days.

As anemia worsens, there is a compensatory increase in blood flow to vital organs Progressive fluid retention results in ascites, pleural effusions, and placental and generalized edema that is detectable by sonography. The course of this progression is variable, but in extreme cases it can occur over just a few days. This progression can be prevented by close fetal surveillance and intrauterine transfusion.

MANAGEMENT OF THE NEWBORN INFANT

Effective management of the newborn infant requires an accurate assessment of the status of the fetus and thorough preparations before birth. Coordination between obstetrician and pediatrician is essential. The approach to the term or near-term fetus with mild or moderately severe disease differs from that for the infant with severe disease or prematurity and is most complex in the infant who has hydrops.

THE INFANT WITH MILD OR MODERATELY SEVERE DISEASE

The major concerns in dealing with mild or moderately severe disease are to keep the bilirubin at a safe level and to prevent hypoglycemia. Laboratory studies to be done immediately after birth include (1) blood group, type, crossmatch with the donor blood, and direct antiglobulin test (if the last is less than 4+, significant disease is unlikely)[2], (2) hematocrit, white blood count, platelet and reticulocyte count, and examination of peripheral blood smear; (3) serum direct and total bilirubin and albumin concentrations; and (4) blood glucose concentration. Although bilirubin usually can be controlled by phototherapy, donor blood compatible with the mother's serum should be available at birth for possible exchange transfusion. The key to management is anticipating the need for an exchange transfusion so it can be done before the bilirubin reaches the level at which the risk of brain damage is great (see Sec 2.17.6)

Allen and Diamond developed a system for defining the course of bilirubinemia and predicting the need for exchange transfusion. Figure 2-54 illustrates this for term newborn infants. Those with bilirubin levels below the shaded area are unlikely to need an exchange transfusion. Those with a level above the shaded area will need an exchange transfusion. The shaded area is an indefinite zone. Phototherapy alters this paradigm. Some infants with moderate disease whose bilirubin exceeds the indefinite zone but has not reached the toxic level can be controlled by phototherapy. Others with severe disease will need multiple exchange transfusions. Figure 2-54 illustrates this variability in clinical course. Bilirubin measured at birth and again 2 hours later will define the initial rate of rise. Thereafter, the frequency of measurements depends on the prior values. The rate of rise will give some idea of when the bilirubin will approach the level needing exchange transfusions. In moderately severe disease it will rise at 0.5 (mg/dL)/h or less; in severe disease, at 1 mg/dL/h, and in the most extreme cases, at 2 (mg/dL)/h.

Exchange transfusion reduces the plasma bilirubin concentration, but this reduction is mitigated by the rapid shift of bilirubin

---

[2]When an unsensitized Rh (D)-negative mother has received immunoglobulin prophylaxis and has a D-positive infant, that infant may have a weakly positive direct antiglobulin test from the prophylaxis. This will not cause significant jaundice and does not mean that the mother has been sensitized.

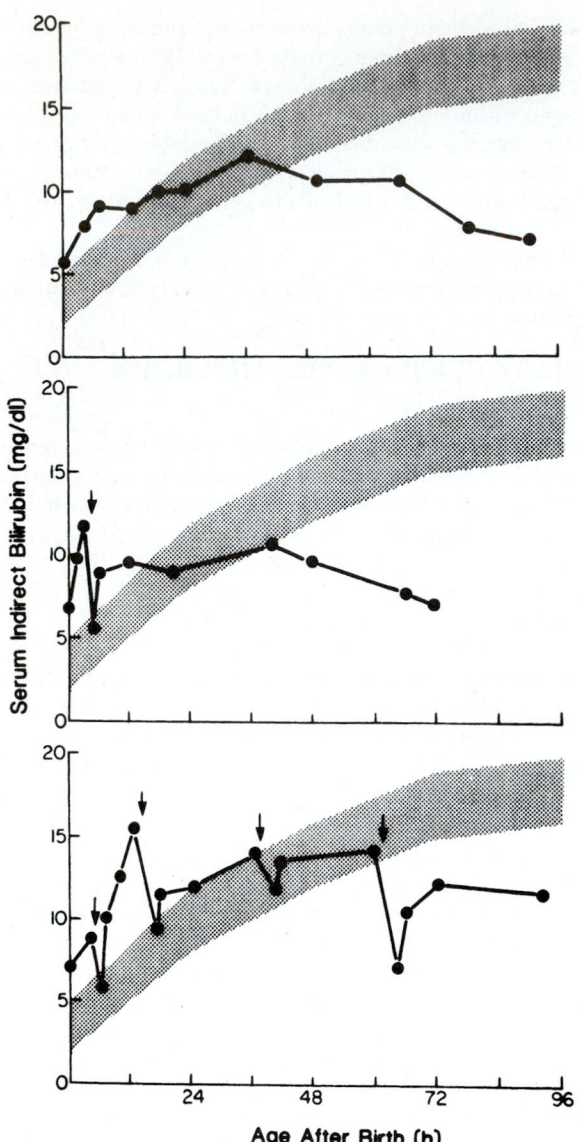

FIGURE 2-54 **Course of hyperbilirubinemia in three infants with erythroblastosis fetalis. The vertical axis is the concentration of indirect-reacting bilirubin in the serum; the horizontal axis shows hours after birth. The shaded area is the indefinite zone from Allen and Diamond's system for predicting the need for exchange transfusion (see text). Bilirubin levels above that zone indicate that the bilirubin will definitely reach toxic levels and justify an exchange transfusion. The arrows indicate exchange transfusions. In all three patients the initial value of bilirubin was very high and the subsequent rise was rapid.** *Top:* **The concentration of bilirubin reached a plateau without exchange transfusion.** *Middle:* **Only one exchange transfusion was needed despite a very rapid rise over the first 4 hours.** *Bottom:* **Two full exchange transfusions were needed because of the rapid rise over the first 18 hours. Subsequent exchange transfusions were done to keep the bilirubin below 15 mg/dL because the infant was premature and had severe respiratory distress. These patients illustrate how varied the course of bilirubinemia can be when erythroblastotic infants receive phototherapy.**

from the extravascular space into the plasma during the procedure. The total amount of bilirubin removed by a double-volume exchange transfusion is twice that which was present in the circulating plasma at the start of the procedure. The continuing shift of bili-

rubin from the tissues into the circulation accounts for the postexchange rebound of plasma bilirubin concentration.

Complications of exchange transfusion include (1) hypothermia if the blood is not warmed to body temperature, (2) hypocalcemia from the anticoagulant in the donor blood, (3) metabolic acidosis if unbuffered anticoagulant is used in the donor blood, (4) thrombocytopenia if platelet-poor donor blood is used, (5) hyperglycemia from the donor blood followed by reactive hypoglycemia, and (6) graft-versus-host disease if the exchange transfusion is done with nonirradiated donor blood.

INFANTS WHO HAVE RECEIVED INTRAUTERINE TRANSFUSIONS These babies have a different course because most of their circulating red cells are D-negative donor cells from the transfusions, and their reticulocyte counts are rarely elevated. The direct antiglobulin test is negative or weakly positive, but the indirect antiglobulin test is strongly positive. There is little hemolysis, so severe jaundice is rare. In the first or second month after birth they often become anemic from a combination of decreased marrow stimulation because of low erythropoietin levels and an increased rate of hemolysis as they begin to synthesize their own Rh-positive cells, which are then attacked by residual maternal antibodies. The direct antiglobulin test becomes positive and can remain so for months. These infants need supplemental folic acid to meet the demands of increased erythropoiesis and may benefit from a short course of treatment with recombinant human erythropoietin.

INFANTS WITH SEVERE DISEASE AND HYDROPS In addition to the management issues discussed above, infants with severe hemolysis and hydrops often require complex care at birth. Most are delivered prematurely and often have immature lungs. Anemic infants do not tolerate the stress of labor and delivery and often are asphyxiated. Severe edema may interfere with ventilation and gas exchange. An experienced properly equipped team must be present at birth to manage these problems, and whole blood or packed erythrocytes that are crossmatched against the mother must be available at birth.

Lung inflation and ventilation often are difficult in hydropic infants because of associated ascites and pleural effusions. Thus, these patients may require urgent removal of fluid by paracentesis and thoracentesis. Even after fluid is removed from the abdomen and chest, many of these babies continue to require high lung inflation pressures to provide adequate ventilation because of excess lung water and deficient surfactant if they are born prematurely.

The hematocrit or hemoglobin concentration of the blood must be measured immediately. While the baby is being ventilated and effusions are removed, the umbilical artery and vein should be catheterized to allow for physiological measurements, transfusions, and resuscitation drugs. Anemic infants usually do not respond well to resuscitative measures until their hematocrit is at least 25%. How the anemia is corrected depends on the state of the circulation. Anemic infants without hydrops tend to have a low circulating blood volume, as do most infants with hydrops. If intravascular pressures indicate that blood volume is adequate, a small exchange transfusion with packed red blood cells, keeping blood volume constant, is the appropriate treatment. If there is evidence of hypovolemia, infusion of red blood cells should help to correct both the hypovolemia and the anemia. The usual approach is to perform a partial-exchange transfusion that keeps blood volume constant while increasing the hematocrit, after which repeated small infusions of erythrocytes are given. In some instances, fresh frozen plasma also is given to support the circulation and to correct coagulation abnormalities that often exist in these infants. In cases of severe metabolic acidosis, alkali therapy may be useful as long as ventilation is sufficient to avoid CO_2 retention associated with alkali infusion. After resuscitation is complete, there usually is residual lung disease that requires assisted ventilation. In hydropic infants, diuresis often improves lung function, and therapy with furosemide may be useful.

ABO DISEASE

Group O individuals have naturally occurring anti-A and anti-B IgM antibodies. Some also have IgG anti-A and anti-B antibodies. When this occurs in a blood group O mother with a fetus that is heterozygous group A or B, hemolysis can occur. This almost never occurs when the mother is group B with a group A fetus or group A with a group B fetus. This type of hemolytic disease may occur in the first pregnancy. The resulting jaundice is milder than that in Rh disease and can usually be controlled with phototherapy.

References

Adams MM, Marks JS, Gustofsen J, Oakley GP: Rh hemolytic disease of the newborn: using incidence observations to evaluate the use of Rh immune globulin. Am J Public Health 71:1031, 1981

Allen FH JR. Diamond LK: Erythroblastosis fetalis including exchange transfusion technique. N Engl J Med 257:659, 1957

Caine ME, Mueller-Heubach E: Kell sensitization and pregnancy. Am J Obstet Gynecol 154:85, 1986

Dallacase P, Ancora G, Miniero R: Erythropoietin course in newborns with Rh hemolytic disease transfused and not transfused in utero. Pediatr Res 40:357–360, 1996

Diamond LK, Blackfan KD, Baty JM: Erythroblastosis and its association with universal edema of the fetus, icterus gravis neonatorum and anemia of the newborn. J Pediatr 1:269, 1932

Frigoletti FD, Greene MF, Benacerraf BR, et al: Ultrasonographic fetal surveillance in the management of the isoimmunized pregnancy. N Engl J Med 315:430, 1986

Gottvall T, Selbing A: Alloimmunization during pregnancy treated with high dose intravenous immunoglobulin. Effects on fetal hemoglobin concentration and anti-D concentration in the mother. Acta Obstet Gynecol Scand 71:777–783, 1995

Harman CR, Bowman JM, Manning FA, et al: Intrauterine transfusion— intraperitoneal versus intravascular approach: a case-control comparison. Am J Obstet Gynecol 162:1053, 1990

Hey E, Jones P: Coagulation failure in babies with rhesus isoimmunization. Br J Haematol 42:441, 1979

Koenig JM, Christensen RD: Neutropenia and thrombocytopenia in infants with Rh hemolytic disease. J Pediatr 114:625, 1989

Hudson L, Moise KJ JR, Hegemier SE, et al: Long-term neurodevelopmental outcome after intrauterine transfusion treatment of fetal hemolyic anemia. Am J Obstet Genecol 179:858–863, 1998

Jackson JC: Adverse events associated with exchange transfusion in healthy and ill newborns. Pediatrics 99:5e7, 1997

MacGregor SN, Socol ML, Pielet BW, Sholl JT, Minague JP: Prediction of fetoplacental blood volume in isoimmunized pregnancy. Am J Obstet Gynecol 159:1495, 1988

Mari G: Noninvasive diagnosis by Doppler ultrasonography of fetal anemia due to maternal red-cell immunization. N Engl J Med 342:9–14, 2000

Milliard DD, Gidding SS, Socol ML, et al: Effects of intravascular intrauterine transfusion of prenatal and postnatal hemolysis and erythropoiesis in severe fetal isoimmunization. J Pediatr 117:447, 1990

Nicolaides KH, Thilaganathan B, Rodeck CH, Mibashan RS: Erythroblastosis and reticulocytosis in anemic fetuses. Am J Obstet Gynecol 159:1063, 1988

Nicolaides KH, Warenski JC, Rodeck CH: The relationship of fetal plasma protein concentration and hemoglobin level to the development of hydrops in rhesus isoimmunization. Am J Obstet Gynecol 152:341, 1985

Ovali F, Samanci N, Dagoglu T: Management of late anemia in rhesus hemolytic disease: use of recombinant human erythropoietin. Pediatr Res 39:831–834, 1996

Parkman R, Mosier D, Umansky I, et al: Graft vs host disease after intrauterine and exchange transfusions for hemolytic disease of the newborn. N Engl J Med 290:359, 1974

Phibbs RH, Johnson P, Kitterman JA, et al: Cardiorespiratory status of erythroblastotic newborn infants. III. Intravascular pressures during the first hours of life. Pediatrics 58:484, 1976

Phibbs RH, Johnson P, Tooley WH: Cardiorespiratory status of erythroblastic newborn infants. II. Blood volume, hematocrit and serum albumin concentration in relation to hydrops fetalis. Pediatrics 53:13, 1974

Poissonnier MH, Brossard Y, Demedeiros N, et al: Two hundred intrauterine exchange transfusions in severe blood incompatibilities. Am J Obstet Gynecol 161:709, 1989

Schumaker B, Moise KJ JR: Fetal transfusions for red cell alloimmunization in pregnancy. Obstet Gynecol 88:137–150, 1996

Weiner CP, Widness JA: Decreased fetal erythropoiesis and hemolysis in Kell hemolytic anemia. Am J Obstet Gynecol 174:547–551, 1996

Wennberg RP, Depp R, Heinrichs WL: Indications for early exchange transfusion in patients with erythroblastosis fetalis. J Pediatr 92:789, 1978

Wible-Kant J, Beer AE: Antepartum Rh immune globulin. Clin Perinatol 10:343, 1983

2.17.9   Nonimmune Hydrops Fetalis

Thomas N. Hansen

Hydrops fetalis is a term used to describe generalized and severe fluid retention in the fetus. The condition is characterized by excessive accumulation of fluid in tissues and body cavities (abdominal, pleural, and pericardial). Nonimmune hydrops fetalis (NIHF) refers to those cases of generalized edema that are not related to Rh isoimmunization. With the reduction in the incidence of immune hydrops, nonimmune causes now account for the majority of cases of hydrops fetalis. The incidence of NIHF is roughly one in 2000 pregnancies.

PATHOPHYSIOLOGY

The fetus, placenta, membranes, and amniotic fluid comprise the fetal fluid compartment. Throughout gestation this compartment accumulates nearly 4 L of water. Fetal catabolism contributes only 20% of fetal water, so the majority of the fluid in the fetal compartment comes from the mother. With hydrops fetalis all components of the fetal fluid compartment can be affected, with marked edema of the fetus and placenta and polyhydramnios.

Fluid in fetal tissues and body cavities, the placenta, and the amniotic cavity is in equilibrium with the intravascular space of the fetus and placenta. Interstitial fluid volume in the fetus is determined by the balance between the rate of fluid filtration from the microcirculation and the rate of fluid return to the vascular space by the lymphatics. The rate of fluid filtration out of the microcirculation is determined by the vascular permeability to water and protein, the plasma protein concentration, and the microvascular hydrostatic pressure. The rate of return of fluid to the circulation by the lymphatics can be reduced by lymphatic obstruction, either mechanical obstruction or by elevated venous pressure. Amniotic fluid volume is affected by the rate of fluid filtration across the placenta and membranes, production of fetal lung fluid, and fetal swallowing and urination.

The fetus becomes edematous when the rate of fluid filtration exceeds the capacity of the lymphatics to return filtered fluid to the intravascular compartment. Increased fluid filtration can result from increased permeability of vessels to protein, or "capillary leak" decreased plasma protein concentration; or increased microvascular hydrostatic pressure. NIHF may result from capillary leak secondary to tissue hypoxia. However, the relationship between hypoxia and capillary injury is not well established, and in experimental hydrops in lambs, edema occurs without evidence of hypoxia or changes in the transcapillary escape rate for albumin, making "capillary leak" an unlikely mechanism for hydrops except in the presence of severe infection. Because hypoproteinemia almost always accompanies hydrops, it is possible that edema is the result of a reduced protein osmotic pressure. However, infants born with low plasma protein concentrations secondary to congenital nephrosis or analbuminemia usually do not develop hydrops, and fetal lambs made hypoproteinemic by partial exchange transfusions do not become edematous. In addition, in fetal lambs made hydropic by atrial pacing, protein concentrations decrease after the onset of edema and ascites, making this explanation also unlikely. The most likely mechanism for the increased rate of transvascular fluid filtration in the fetus with hydrops is increased microvascular hydrostatic pressure. Many of the known causes of hydrops are associated with increased venous pressure (Table 2-29). The protein content of ascitic fluid from hydropic infants is compatible with hydrostatic edema, and in experimental models of hydrops secondary to atrial pacing or anemia, edema does not develop unless systemic venous pressure increases.

Delays in establishing communication between the jugular lymphatic sacs and the jugular venous system may also result in fetal hydrops as well as cystic hygromas, webbing of the neck, positional deformities, or one of the multiple pterygium syndromes (jugular lymphatic obstruction sequence, JLOS). JLOS occurs more commonly in fetuses with chromosomal abnormalities, such as Turner syndrome, and probably accounts for most of the cases of hydrops that are associated with genetic disorders. Partial lymphatic obstruction can result from mechanical blockage by intrathoracic anomalies or from increases in outflow pressure secondary to increased venous pressure.

DIAGNOSIS

A careful maternal history may be helpful in determining the cause of NIHF (Table 2-30). Most cases, however, are diagnosed antenatally by ultrasound exam, with mothers typically referred because of polyhydramnios, preeclampsia, or fetal tachycardia. Ultrasound criteria for the diagnosis of hydrops include more than 5 mm of skin thickening and two or more of the following: placental enlargement, ascites, and pleural or pericardial effusions. Once isoimmunization has been excluded, a high-resolution fetal ultrasound study that includes echocardiography should be performed. A review of Table 2-27 suggests that this test alone should be effective in determining an etiology in nearly 50% of cases of NIHF. Ultrasound-directed fetal blood sampling now allows detection of anemia as a cause of NIHF, and it also permits determination of the etiology of the anemia (red cell morphology, hemoglobin electrophoresis, red cell enzyme assay). Genetic evaluation on fetal blood should include karyotyping and assays for metabolic disorders. Measurement of specific antibodies and more recently PCR analysis may help to detect infectious causes of hydrops. This combination approach (Table 2-28) allows for identification of the cause of NIHF in roughly 50 to 60% of cases.

TABLE 2-29
CAUSES OF NONIMMUNE HYDROPS

Cardiovascular (26%)
Tachyarrhythmias
Bradyarrhythmias
Hypoplastic left heart
Atrioventricular canal
Right heart hypoplasia
Primary closure of foramen ovale
Single ventricle
Transposition
Premature closure of the ductus arteriosus
Ventricular septal defect
Atrial septal defect
Tetralogy of Fallot
Ebstein anomaly
Truncus arteriosus
High-output heart failure
  Hemangioma
  Sacrococcygeal teratoma
  Chorangioma
Cardiac rhabdomyoma
Restrictive cardiomyopathy
Cardiomyopathy, other
Generalized arterial calcifications

Chromosome abnormality (10%)
45,X
Trisomy 21
Trisomy 18
Other

Thoracic abnormalities (9%)
Cystic adenomatoid malformation
Chondrodysplasia
Diaphragmatic hernia
Intrathoracic mass
Pulmonary sequestration
Airway obstruction
Pulmonary neoplasia
Bronchogenic cyst

Twin-twin transfusion (8%)

Anemia (5%)
α-Thalassemia
Parvovirus B19
Fetomaternal transfusion
Malignant osteopetrosis
Hemorrhage into neoplasm
Glucose-6 phosphate dehydrogenase deficiency
Erythroleukemia

Infection (4%)
Cytomegalovirus
Bacterial
Toxoplasmosis
Rubella
Herpes
Other

Primary lymphatic obstruction (3%)
Cystic hygroma
Multiple pterygium syndromes
Pulmonary lymphangiectasia
Congenital chylothorax

Urinary tract malformation (3%)
Urethral obstruction
Prune belly
Upper tract obstruction
Cloacal malformation

Fetal hypomobility (2%)
Arthrogryposis
Neu-Laxova syndrome
Pena-Shokeri syndrome
Myotonic dystrophy
Neuronal degeneration

Genetic metabolic disease (1%)
Gaucher disease
GM I gangliosidosis
Infantile sialidosis
β-Glucuronidase deficiency (mucopolysaccharidosis VII)
Iron storage disease
I-cell disease
mucopolysaccharidosis IVa

Other (7%) including
Peritonitis
Hepatic
Noonan syndrome

Undetermined (22%)

THERAPY

Most of the causes of NIHF, a large proportion of which are lethal disorders, respond poorly to therapy. A recent study of 100 infants with NIHF showed that only 26 were suitable for in utero therapy. The most successful treatments have been in infants with hydrops fetalis secondary to atrial arrhythmias. In a series of 18 fetuses, most with supraventricular tachycardia, 15 were managed in utero using digoxin alone or in combination with propranolol or verapamil, and most survived.

With the advent of intravascular transfusions for fetal anemias, hydrops secondary to anemia became amenable to therapy. In addition, there are reports in the literature of resolution of hydrops

TABLE 2-30

DIAGNOSTIC EVALUATION OF FETUS WITH NONIMMUNE HYDROPS

Maternal history
  Ethnicity: α-thalassemia, storage
    diseases
  Diabetes, lupus, preeclampsia/
    hypertension
  Consanguinity
Past obstetric history
  Previously affected sibling
  Spontaneous abortions
Pregnancy history
  Gravida/parity
  Gestational age
  Multiple gestations
  Size-date discrepancy
  Polyhydramnios
  Infections: erythema infec-
    tiousum, syphilis
Maternal blood samples
  Blood type and antibody screen
  Complete blood cell count and
    indices
  Hemoglobin electrophoresis
  Kleihauer-Betke stain
  VDRL and other antibody
    screens for infection
  G6PD
  Glucose

Fetal blood samples
  Anemia
    Complete blood count
    Hemoglobin electrophoresis
    Red blood cell enzymes
      (G6PD)
  Protein and albumin concentra-
    tions
  Karyotype
  Metabolic screens
  Antibody/PCR screens for in-
    fections
  Blood gases
  Lactate
  Blood type and Coombs test
Ultrasound
  Morphologic survey for anoma-
    lies
  Specific echocardiographic exam
    Cardiac morphology
    Heart rate and rhythm
Amniotic fluid
  Culture (viral and bacterial)
  α-Fetoprotein
  Karyotype
  L/S ratio

G6PD = glucose-6 phosphate dehydrogenase; L/S = lecithin:sphingomyelin; PCR = polymerase chain reaction.

following successful drainage of chest fluid from chylothoraces, lung cysts, or even diaphragmatic hernia.

Therapy for the newborn infant with hydrops begins with vigorous resuscitation, including thoracentesis and/or paracentesis, in order to establish adequate lung expansion, followed by efforts to define the cause and correct the condition responsible for the edema. Table 2-29 reveals that most of the treatable causes of NIHF are related to increased intravascular pressure secondary to heart failure caused by arrhythmias or anemia or increased venous pressure from an intrathoracic mass. In these cases, therapy is directed at reversing the rhythm disturbance, transfusion for anemia, or surgery to reduce intrathoracic pressure. Although it is tempting to treat the edema with diuretics, available evidence suggests that blood volume may not be abnormal in these infants, so that attempts to alter intravascular volume should be undertaken only after adequate resuscitation and with careful monitoring of vascular pressures.

PROGNOSIS

Historically, the mortality for infants with NIHF has remained high (80 to 100%) because of the frequent association of NIHF with severe genetic disorders and other lethal malformations. More recently, intrauterine management has improved the prognosis somewhat, with reported survival as great as 40%. One recent study showed that survival rates are dependent on gestational age at diagnosis. Survival rates for infants with hydrops detected before 24 weeks of gestation was less that 5%, whereas survival for infants diagnosed after 24 weeks of gestation was 20%. This difference is related to the greater incidence of chromosomal abnormalities in the shorter gestation group. The prognosis for the infant with

NIHF is best when hydrops is the result of intrauterine supraventricular tachycardia or anemia. Among those infants suitable for intrauterine therapy, survival is 60%.

References

Anandakumar C, Biswas A, Wong YC, et al: Management of non-immune hydrops: 8 years' experience. Ultrasound Obstet Gynecol 8:196–200, 1996

Andres RL, Brace RA: The development of hydrops fetalis in the ovine fetus after lymphatic ligation or lymphatic excision. Am J Obstet Gynecol 162:1331–1334, 1990

Blair DK, Vander Straten MC, Gest AL: Hydrops in fetal sheep from rapid induction of anemia. Pediatr Res 35:560–564, 1994

Chervenak FA, Isaacson G, Blakemore KJ, et al: Fetal cystic hygroma. Cause and natural history. N Engl J Med 309:822–825, 1983

Gest AL, Bair DK, Vander Straten MC: Thoracic duct lymph flow in fetal sheep with increased venous pressure from electrically induced tachycardia. Biol Neonate 64:325–330, 1993

Gest AL, Hansen TN, Moise AA, Hartley CJ: Atrial tachycardia causes hydrops in fetal lambs. Am J Physiol 258:H1159–H1163, 1990

Hansen TN, Gest AL: Hydrops fetalis. In: Brace RA, Ross MG, Robillard JE, eds: Fetal and Neonatal Body Fluids. Ithaca, Perinatology Press, 1989:85–116

Im SS, Rizos N, Joutsi P, Shime J, Benziel RJ: Nonimmunologic hydrops fetalis. Am J Obstet Gynecol 148:566–569, 1984

Machin GA: Hydrops revisited: literature review of 1,414 cases published in the 1980s. Am J Med Genet 34:366–390, 1989

McCoy MC, Katz VL, Gould N, Kuller JA: Non-immune hydrops after 20 weeks' gestation: review of 10 years' experience with suggestions for management. Obstet Gynecol 85:578–582, 1995

McMahan MJ, Donovan EF: The delivery room resuscitation of the hydropic neonate. Semin Perinatol 19:474–482, 1995

Wafelman LS, Pollock BH, Kreutzer J, Richards DS, Hutchison AA: Non-immune hydrops fetalis: fetal and neonatal outcome during 1983–1992. Biol Neonate 75:73–81, 1999

2.17.10   Persistent Postnatal Pulmonary Edema (Transient Tachypnea of the Newborn)

Richard D. Bland

Liquid that fills the lung lumen during normal fetal development must be absorbed into the vascular system soon after birth to permit successful pulmonary gas exchange. This transition occurs rapidly in most infants, but sometimes the process is delayed, producing the clinical and radiographic features of a condition that has been called *transient tachypnea of the newborn* or the syndrome of *retained fetal lung liquid*. However, *persistent postnatal pulmonary edema* is a more apt description because tachypnea is not a consistent finding, and some of the liquid may enter the lungs postnatally from the pulmonary circulation.

CLINICAL FEATURES

In 1966, Avery and associates described the clinical and radiographic features of eight babies with transient neonatal tachypnea, a condition that the authors attributed to delayed absorption of fetal lung liquid. All of the infants were born at term gestation, and only one was delivered by cesarean section. Subsequent reports have noted an association with premature birth, operative delivery, and excessive intravenous fluids administered to the mother during labor. Persistent postnatal pulmonary edema is more common in boys than it is in girls. The disorder typically begins soon after birth with a rapid respiratory rate, ranging from 60 to 160 per minute, sometimes with sternal and subcostal retractions of the chest wall, grunting during expiration, and occasionally mild cyanosis that disappears with delivery of supplemental oxygen. In some cases, postnatal depression from birth asphyxia or from drugs administered to the mother during labor may obscure the underlying pathology, causing hypoventilation and even apnea rather than rapid breathing.

Physical examination usually reveals clear breath sounds, without rales or rhonchi, except during the initial hour after birth, when there is still some residual liquid within the air spaces. Signs and symptoms usually resolve by 3 to 4 days after birth. Many infants with this condition have generalized edema and hypoproteinemia, supporting the view that low intravascular protein osmotic pressure may contribute to the delay in absorption of lung liquid after birth.

Studies of lung function in babies with this type of mild respiratory distress have shown increased total ventilation, low tidal volumes, normal or increased functional residual capacity, reduced dynamic compliance, and relatively uniform gas distribution in the lungs. Alveolar ventilation and pulmonary resistance have been similar to corresponding measurements in healthy infants. Echocardiographic assessment may show evidence of mild left ventricular dysfunction in babies presumed to have persistent postnatal pulmonary edema.

The differential diagnosis includes hyaline membrane disease, extrapulmonary air leaks (pneumomediastinum and pneumothorax), congestive heart failure, meconium aspiration, bacterial or viral pneumonia, airway obstruction, and diaphragmatic hernia with associated pulmonary hypoplasia. The radiographic features and greater severity of respiratory distress usually distinguish these conditions from persistent postnatal pulmonary edema.

RADIOGRAPHIC APPEARANCE

Figure 2-55 shows the characteristic radiographic features: prominent pulmonary vascular markings, particularly around the hila; hyperaeration; flattening and depression of the diaphragm; widening of the interlobar fissures; and a cardiac silhouette slightly larger than normal. In addition, there may be fluid in the pleural spaces. Rapid

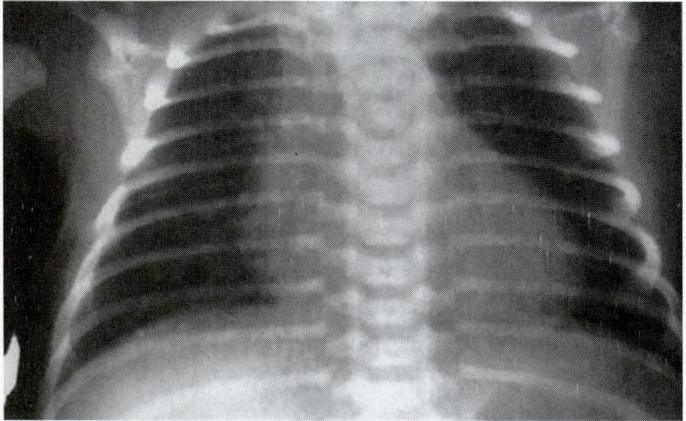

FIGURE 2-55 Chest radiograph of an infant with persistent pulmonary edema (ie, transient tachypnea of the newborn). Note the thickened interlobar fissure on the right, bilateral pleural densities, and prominent perihilar vascular markings, all of which suggest excessive fluid in the lungs. The cardiac shadow is slightly enlarged.

clinical improvement usually parallels resolution of these radiographic abnormalities.

PATHOPHYSIOLOGY

Interpretation of the underlying pathophysiology of this condition derives mainly from studies performed with fetal and newborn animals. During fetal life, the respiratory tract epithelium secretes chloride, which draws liquid from the pulmonary circulation into the lung lumen, with subsequent outflow through the trachea into the oropharynx. The upper airway functions as a low-resistance one-way valve, preventing entry of amniotic liquid into the lungs but allowing egress of lung liquid into the mouth, from which the liquid is either swallowed or expelled into the amniotic sac. This process maintains modest expansion of potential air spaces and facilitates normal intrauterine lung growth and development.

The volume of liquid within the lung lumen begins to decrease 2 to 3 days before birth, often followed by absorption during labor. Around the time of birth, the lung epithelium switches from a predominantly Cl^--secreting membrane to a predominantly Na^+-absorbing membrane, with resultant reversal of the direction of liquid flow. Several studies have shown that as birth approaches near term gestation, pulmonary expression of epithelial sodium channels and sodium pumps (Na,K ATPase) as well as sodium pump activity increase. Cells obtained from rabbits that were born prematurely or without prior labor did not exhibit increased Na,K ATPase activity, an observation that may help to explain the lung fluid retention often associated with premature birth. The stimulus for these changes at birth remains unclear, but several studies have shown that various hormones that increase in concentration in fetal plasma near birth might be important in initiating this process. Studies with fetal sheep and guinea pigs have provided evidence that epinephrine, vasopressin, aldosterone, and prostaglandin E_2 may slow secretion of lung liquid or cause its absorption late in gestation. Several reports also indicate that adrenocortical and thyroid hormones may help to induce liquid absorption from the fetal lung. Thus, the interaction of several hormones appears to have a major regulatory role in converting the respiratory epithelium from a predominantly chloride-secreting membrane during fetal development to a predominantly sodium-absorbing membrane after birth. It is noteworthy that absence of functional epithelial sodium channels in transgenic animals is associated with early neonatal death from respiratory failure. This observation underscores the pivotal role of lung epithelial sodium transport in adaptation at birth.

During delivery, a small amount of liquid may drain through the mouth as a result of chest wall compression, but most of the liquid that is absorbed during labor and after birth flows directly into the pulmonary circulation. After breathing begins, blood flow to the lungs increases, and epithelial sodium pumps and transpulmonary pressure associated with lung inflation drive residual liquid from the air spaces into the pulmonary interstitium. This liquid distends the loose connective tissue spaces beneath the pleura, between lobules, and around large pulmonary blood vessels and airways. Puddling of fluid in these connective tissue spaces, which are distant from sites of respiratory gas exchange, allows time for smaller blood vessels and pulmonary lymphatics to expel the remaining water without serious impairment of lung function. Beginning 30 to 60 minutes after birth, lung water content progressively decreases for several hours. Studies of lung liquid clearance in healthy lambs delivered vaginally after spontaneous labor indicate that the pulmonary lymphatics have a relatively small role in removal of fetal lung liquid after birth. Most of the liquid is absorbed directly into the pulmonary microcirculation, as lung vascular resistance decreases after breathing begins. Some liquid also may leave the lungs by way of the mediastinum or through the pleura, with subsequent uptake by extrapulmonary lymphatics.

The large difference in protein osmotic pressure between plasma and lung liquid (plasma contains 5 to 6 g/dL of protein, whereas lung liquid contains only 30 mg/dL) facilitates the process of liquid removal. Conditions that are associated with a low plasma protein osmotic pressure, such as premature birth, may slow the rate of liquid clearance from the interstitium into the pulmonary microcirculation. Likewise, disorders that are associated with elevated left atrial pressure, such as asphyxia, myocardial failure, and rapid intravascular infusions of protein-containing or crystalloid solutions, inhibit escape of liquid from the lungs.

TREATMENT

Unless the lungs are immature, with resultant atelectasis and respiratory distress, absorption of fetal lung liquid is usually complete within 24 hours of birth, and symptoms disappear accordingly. An increased concentration of inspired oxygen may be required to maintain a normal partial pressure of oxygen in arterial blood. Usually no other therapy is required. Infants with respiratory distress sometimes benefit from being managed in the prone, head-up position. Until symptoms subside, the fluid and salt intake of infants with persistent postnatal pulmonary edema should not exceed their insensible losses. Diuretics offer little or no benefit and may produce serious electrolyte imbalance.

References

Avery ME, Gatewood OB, Brumley G: Transient tachypnea of newborn. Possible delayed resorption of fluid at birth. Am J Dis Child 111:380, 1966

Baines DL, Folkesson HG, Norlin A, Bingle CD, Yuan HT, Olver RE: The influence of mode of delivery, hormonal status and postnatal O_2 environment on epithelial sodium channel (ENaC) expression in perinatal guinea-pig lung. J Physiol (Lond) 522:147–157, 2000

Barker PM, Markiewicz M, Parker KA, Walters DV, Strang LB: Synergistic action of triiodothyronine and hydrocortisone on epinephrine-induced reabsorption of fetal lung liquid. Pediatr Res 27:588–591, 1990

Bland RD: Lung epithelial ion transport and fluid movement during the perinatal period. Am J Physiol 259:L30, 1990

Bland RD, Nielson DW: Development changes in lung epithelial ion transport and liquid movement. Annu Rev Physiol 54:373, 1992

Chapman DL, Carlton DP, Nielson DW, Cummings JJ, Poulain FR, Bland RD: Changes in lung liquid during spontaneous labor in fetal sheep. J Appl Physiol 76:523, 1994

Chapman DL, Widdicombe JH, Bland RD: Development differences in rabbit lung epithelial cell Na-K-ATPase. Am J Physiol 259:L481, 1990

Finley N, Norlin A, Baines DL, Folkesson HG: Alveolar epithelial fluid clearance is mediated by endogenous catecholamines at birth in guinea pigs. J Clin Invest 101:972–981, 1998

Gowen CW JR, Lawson EE, Gingras J, Boucher RC, Gatzy JJ, Knowles MR: Electrical potential difference and ion transport across nasal epithelium of term neonates: correlation with mode of delivery, transient tachypnea of the newborn, and respiratory rate. J Pediatr 113:121, 1988

Hummler E, Barker P, Gatzy J, et al: Early death due to defective neonatal lung liquid clearance in a ENaC-deficient mice. Nature Genet 12:325–328, 1996

Olver RE, Ramsden CA, Strang LB, Walters DV: The role of amiloride-blockable sodium transport in adrenaline-induced lung liquid reabsorption in the fetal lamb. J Physiol (Lond) 376:321–340, 1986

Sandberg K, Sjogvist BA, Hjalmarson O, Olsson T: Lung function in newborn infants with tachypnea of unknown cause. Pediatr Res 22:581, 1987

2.17.11 Persistent Pulmonary Hypertension of the Newborn

Kurt R. Stenmark

Successful adaptation of the fetus to postnatal conditions requires a dramatic transition of the pulmonary circulation from a high-resistance state in utero to a low-resistance state within minutes after birth. The drop in pulmonary vascular resistance at birth is essential to allow a nearly 8- to 10-fold rise in pulmonary blood flow, which ensures that the lung can assume its postnatal role in gas exchange. Some infants, however, fail to achieve the normal decrease in pulmonary vascular resistance at birth, which causes a postnatal persistence of right-to-left ductal shunting or right-to-left atrial shunting. These extrapulmonary right-to-left shunts result in severe hypoxemia, which often proves refractory to treatment with supplemental oxygen. This clinical picture is referred to as persistent pulmonary hypertension of the newborn (PPHN). PPHN is not a unique disease but rather a clinical syndrome that can occur in association with many diverse neonatal cardiorespiratory disorders (Table 2-31). PPHN represents an important cause of respiratory failure and occurs at rates of one in 600 to one in 1500 live births, occurring most commonly in full-term infants without congenital anomalies. Before the newer treatments discussed below, mortality ranged from 20 to 50%, although even now there is significant morbidity and mortality with this disorder.

Because the circulatory shunts in affected infants resemble those of the fetus, PPHN is considered to represent a failure of adaptation of the fetal pulmonary circulation to postnatal conditions (and has been called *persistent fetal circulation* by some authors). The syndrome is often apparent within the first hours of life. Because significant vascular abnormalities are present in the lungs of infants dying within the first days of life, it is believed that intrauterine events are often important in the pathogenesis of PPHN. This hypothesis is supported by experimental studies that demonstrate that a variety of intrauterine stimuli, such as chronic fetal hypertension or elevations in pulmonary blood flow, can alter both pulmonary vascular reactivity and structure, causing the pulmonary vascular resistance to remain high after birth (Fig. 2-56). Structural changes associated with fatal human PPHN include increased muscularization of small pulmonary arteries and extension of smooth muscle

TABLE 2-31

DISORDERS ASSOCIATED WITH PERSISTENT PULMONARY HYPERTENSION OF THE NEWBORN

Pulmonary	Cardiac
Meconium aspiration	Myocardiopathy/myocarditis
Pulmonary infections	Obstructed pulmonary venous drainage
Neonatal respiratory distress syndrome	Transposition of great vessels
Diaphragmatic hernia	**Other**
Pulmonary hypoplasia	Idiopathic
Other aspirations	Perinatal hypoxia
Alveolar capillary dysplasia	Sepsis/infections
Misalignment of pulmonary vessels	Maternal diabetes
	Maternal ingestion (indomethacin, aspirin)

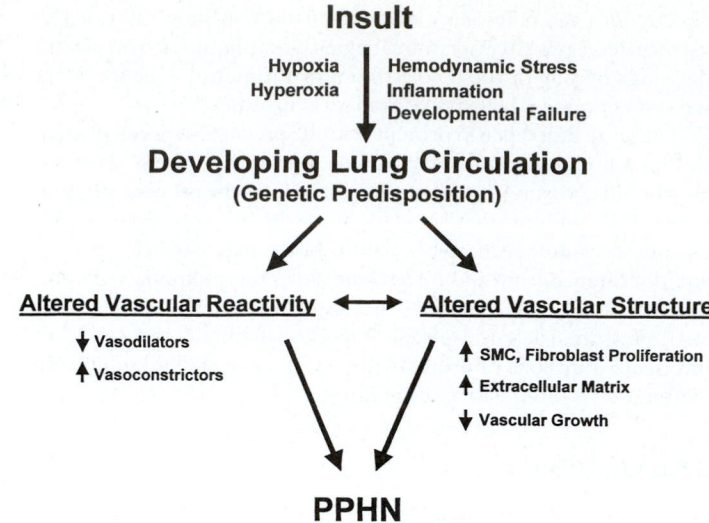

FIGURE 2-56   Potential mechanisms for the development of persistent pulmonary hypertension.

into arteries that are normally nonmuscular. Marked adventitial thickening is often observed. Neonatal disorders characterized by underdevelopment of the airways and alveoli, eg, congenital diaphragmatic hernia and lung hypoplasia associated with oligohydramnios, are also associated with PPHN, suggesting a close association between airway and vascular development in the lung. In addition to alterations in vascular structure, infants with PPHN are characterized almost uniformly by abnormalities in pulmonary vasoreactivity. The mechanisms contributing to this abnormal regulation of tone in the perinatal period are poorly understood, but possibilities include enhanced release of vasoconstrictors, decreased production of vasodilators, or altered vascular responsiveness to environmental and pharmacologic stimuli. Some infants may be exquisitely sensitive to stimuli causing pulmonary hypertension (eg, genetic predisposition). From these observations, it is clear that alterations in tone and structure of the pulmonary circulation play a central role in this clinical syndrome.

PATHOPHYSIOLOGY

Because PPHN represents a failure of the postnatal adaptation of the lung circulation at birth, understanding the basic mechanisms that contribute to the normal functional and structural development of the pulmonary circulation in utero and the mechanisms that contribute to pulmonary vasodilation and structural remodeling at birth are liiely to provide insight into the pathogenesis and treatment.

VASOREGULATION OF THE NORMAL FETAL PULMONARY CIRCULATION   The pulmonary circulation of the fetus receives less than 10% of the combined ventricular output, with most of the ventricular output crossing the ductus arteriosus to the aorta. As gestation progresses, the number of small blood vessels in the lung increases nearly 40-fold. This increase prepares the lung to accept the nearly 10-fold increase in blood flow per unit of lung that occurs at birth. However, in the fetus pulmonary vasoconstriction causes most of the pulmonary arterial blood to be diverted to the systemic circulation (see Sec. 22.1.2). The mechanisms that contribute to this high pulmonary vascular resistance in the fetus are not completely understood but include low oxygen tension, low basal production of vasodilator products [such as prostacyclin (PGI_2) and nitric oxide (NO)], production of vasoconstrictors, alterations of smooth muscle cell (SMC) reactivity, and perhaps increased sym-

pathetic tone. The relative contribution of these factors to the control of vascular smooth muscle tone and blood flow in the fetal lung naturally changes during development.

Active production of vasoconstrictors is considered to play a key role in maintaining high pulmonary vascular resistance in utero. Several candidate products, including lipid mediators (thromboxane A_2, leukotriene C_4 and D_4, and platelet-activating factor) and endothelin 1, have been studied extensively, but data demonstrating specific roles for each of these is lacking. Thromboxane A_2 has been shown to be a potent pulmonary vasoconstrictor in both neonatal and adult animals, but there is no convincing evidence that it normally plays an important role in influencing or maintaining high pulmonary vascular resistance in the fetus. Although inhibition of leukotriene production with pharmacologic agents causes fetal pulmonary vasodilation, questions regarding its specific role in maintaining high pulmonary vascular resistance have been raised because of the lack of specificity of the agents used to test its role in the fetal circulation. Similar problems are encountered in trying to interpret the role of platelet-activating factor in maintaining high pulmonary vascular resistance in the fetus.

More convincing are the data demonstrating a role for endothelin-1 (ET-1) in regulating fetal pulmonary vascular tone. Pre-pro-ET-1 transcripts have been identified in the fetal lung early in gestation, and high circulating ET-1 levels are present in umbilical cord blood. Although ET-1 causes intense vasoconstriction in vitro, its effects on the intact pulmonary circulation, particularly in the fetus, are complex. Brief infusions of ET-1 cause transient vasodilation, but pulmonary vascular resistance progressively increases during prolonged treatment. The biphasic effects of infused ET-1 on the pulmonary circulation are explained in part by stimulation of two different receptors, one on the endothelium (producing transient dilation) and the other on the SMC (producing constriction). The critical importance of the endothelin system is demonstrated by studies showing that inhibition of the SMC receptor significantly decreases fetal pulmonary vascular resistance and augments the vasodilator response to the flow-induced pulmonary vasodilation that occurs at birth. Thus, a preponderance of evidence suggests that ET-1 is important in contributing to high pulmonary vascular resistance in the fetus.

Developmental changes in endothelial and smooth muscle cell functions, especially with regard to the nitric oxide (NO)–cyclic guanosine-$3'$, $5'$ monophosphate (cGMP) system, are also thought to be critical for the ultimate changes in resistance that are necessary for normal adaptation at birth. NO is produced by the endothelial cell during the conversion of L-arginine to citrulline by the enzyme NO synthase (NOS). Once produced, NO diffuses to the underlying SMC and stimulates soluble guanylate cyclase, which increases cGMP production. Elevated cGMP stimulates cGMP kinase, which then opens calcium-activated potassium channels moving K^+ out of the cell and causing membrane hyperpolarization. This lowers intracellular calcium in the SMC by decreasing calcium entry through L-type channels and causes vasodilation. NO may also stimulate K^+ channels or voltage-gated calcium (Ca^{2+}) directly, independent of increased cGMP. Vascular responsiveness to NO thus depends on several SMC enzymes, including soluble guanylate cyclase, cGMP-specific phosphodiesterase (PDE-5), and cGMP kinase. Several studies have shown that soluble guanylate cyclase, which produces cGMP in response to NO activation, is active in the fetal lung. Similarly, PDE-5, which limits cGMP-mediated vasodilation by hydrolysis and inactivation of cGMP, is also active in utero, though the exact balance between production of cGMP and degradation via PDE is presently unclear. It has been reported that PDE-5 activity is high in the fetus compared with the postnatal lung. Thus, PDE-5 could play a critical role in pulmonary vasoregulation in the perinatal period. The importance of the NOS system in modulating pulmonary vascular resistance in the fetus is demonstrated by the fact that inhibitors of NOS increase pulmonary vascular resistance in the fetus by at least 35%.

Other important vasodilator products, especially members of the cyclooxygenase family, are also produced and released by fetal lung endothelial cells. However, their basal release appears to play a less important role than NO in modulating fetal pulmonary vascular tone.

TRANSITION OF THE PULMONARY CIRCULATION AT BIRTH
In response to birth-related stimuli, such as ventilation, increased PO_2, and sheer stress, pulmonary artery pressure falls, and blood flow increases, in the neonatal lung. These physical stimuli, which are associated with the transition, cause pulmonary vasodilation in part by increasing production of the vasodilators NO and PGI_2. Most evidence suggests that NO is more important than PGI_2 for

dilating the pulmonary circulation at birth. For instance, pretreatment of animals with NOS inhibitors attenuates pulmonary vasodilation after delivery by nearly 50%. Each of the birth-related stimuli (ie, changes in oxygen concentration, sheer stress, rhythmic breathing) can independently stimulate NO release, which is followed by vasodilation through the cGMP kinase-mediated stimulation of potassium channels. On the other hand, indomethacin, which inhibits the cyclooxygenase pathway and thus PGI_2 production, only modestly attenuates the decrease in pulmonary vascular resistance that occurs in the intact lamb at birth. It seems likely that there are important interactions between prostaglandin-mediated increases in cAMP- and NO-mediated increases in cGMP that are necessary for the normal transition.

EXPERIMENTAL PPHN, ABNORMAL VASOREACTIVITY In models of PPHN, decreased abundance of endothelial NO synthase mRNA and protein, the α_1 and β_1 subunits of soluble guanylate cyclase protein, and increased expression of phosphodiesterase-5 mRNA have been reported. In the same models, increases in the expression of prepro-ET-1 mRNA and decreased expression of the ET-B receptor have been observed. These results suggest that there is coordinated regulation of genes of the NO pathway, which act in concert to decrease NO and cGMP concentration, thereby decreasing pulmonary vasodilator activity (Fig. 2-57). There also appears to be a coordinated regulation of the genes of the ET-1 pathway that leads to increases in ET-1 concentration, increased ET-A receptor activity, and limited ET-B receptor activation, thereby increasing pulmonary vasoconstrictor activity. These alterations in gene expression act to increase fetal pulmonary vascular resistance and to inhibit the normal responses to vasodilator stimuli at birth, contributing to the development of PPHN.

EXPERIMENTAL PPHN, ABNORMAL STRUCTURE Excessive cell proliferation and matrix protein synthesis in vessel walls also contribute to severe functional abnormalities and death in PPHN. Reciprocal relationships between abnormalities of tone and structure contribute to the pulmonary hypertension. Infants dying with persistent pulmonary hypertension often exhibit striking distal exten-

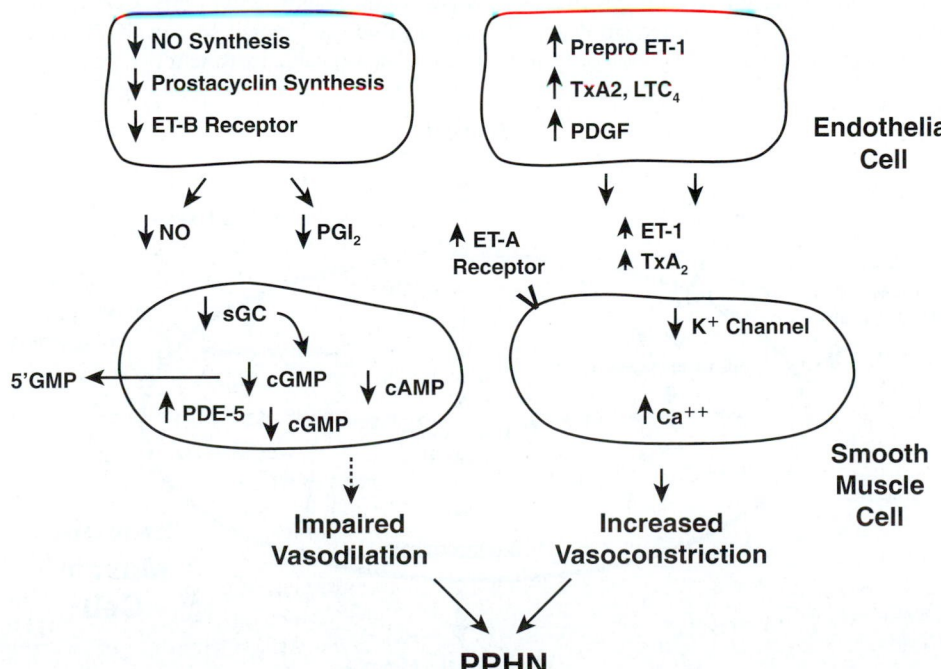

FIGURE 2-57 Alterations in the endothelial and smooth muscle cell that contribute to abnormal vascular tone in persistent pulmonary hypertension. ET = endothelin; PGI_2 = prostacyclin; sGC = soluble guanylate cyclase; PDE = phosphodiesterase; TxA_2 = thromboxane A_2; cGMP = cyclic guanosine-3',5' monophosphate; cAMP = cyclic adenosine-3',5' monophosphate; LTC_4 = leukotriene CA.

sion of smooth muscle, thickening of the media and adventitia, and excessive accumulation of matrix protein in the pulmonary vessel walls. The large numbers of SMC and adventitial fibroblasts, and the dense extracellular matrix likely raise pulmonary vascular resistance. The importance of abnormal proliferation and excessive matrix protein synthesis by pulmonary vascular wall cells is demonstrated by studies showing that inhibition of proliferation with heparin or prevention of collagen or elastin crosslinking with *cis*-hydroxyproline significantly attenuates the pulmonary hypertensive process. Therefore, there is an association between the development of significant structural change in the media and adventitia and the progressive loss of the ability to respond to vasodilating agents.

Blood vessels in the lung undergo profound structural remodeling as chronic pulmonary hypertension develops; changes include cellular hypertrophy, hyperplasia, and increased deposition of structural matrix proteins, such as collagen and elastin, in the vessel wall. The phenotype of cell populations that comprise the vessel wall (endothelial, smooth muscle, and fibroblast cells) change markedly with time and are responsible for the alterations in structure and function observed. However, the cellular and structural changes observed in pulmonary hypertension vary significantly, depending on age or state of development at the time of insult, duration and degree of the inciting event (eg, hypoxia, infection, etc), and the presence of associated abnormalities, such as chronic inflammation or high pulmonary blood flow. Studies demonstrate heightened proliferative and matrix synthetic responses in fetal and neonatal versus adult cells in response to a variety of stimuli.

Neonatal pulmonary hypertension syndromes represent injury to cells at a crucial and unique time in life. It has been proposed that if the fetal-to-neonatal transition is disrupted and persistent hypertension results, cells in the pulmonary vasculature would fail to undergo the phenotypic alterations characteristic of the normal neonate and would instead maintain a fetal pattern of gene expression. It has been shown, for example, that neonatal pulmonary hypertension is associated with a persistence of the fetal levels of genes such as tropoelastin, fibronectin, and insulin-like growth factor II, suggesting that the signals normally responsible for turning off these genes were not received. On the other hand, it was observed that some genes that are normally turned on in the vessel wall shortly after birth, eg, TGF-β (transforming growth factor β),

which can act to stop proliferation and induce hypertrophy in medial vascular wall cells) failed to be expressed in the hypertensive animals. Thus, neonatal pulmonary hypertension is associated with multiple alterations in the pattern of gene expression in SMC and fibroblasts including persistence of fetal patterns, rapid induction of new genes, reexpression of other genes that were expressed in earlier embryonic or fetal life and then down-regulated, and failure to induce new genes.

CLINICAL PRESENTATION AND TREATMENT

PPHN is characterized by postnatal persistance of right-to-left ductal shunting or right-to-left atrial shunting or both. The result of the extrapulmonary right-to-left shunts is cyanosis, which is often refractory to supplemental oxygen. These infants are often recognized shortly after birth because of their respiratory distress or cyanosis. There can be marked intercostal and sternal retractions and usually grunting respirations. Differential cyanosis, with greater oxygen saturation in the upper body than in the lower body, is pathognomonic of PPHN; this is caused by right-to-left shunting of deoxygenated pulmonary arterial blood through the ductus arteriosus. With a right-to-left ductus shunt, there will also be a positive PO_2 difference between the right radial artery and the descending aorta; a difference in PO_2 of >10 to 15 mm Hg may be considered indicative of PPHN. Many patients, however, do not have differential cyanosis because there may be limited flow via the ductus arteriosus, or most of the right-to-left shunting is intrapulmonary or across the foramen ovale.

On cardiac exam, a precordial systolic murmur (tricuspid regurgitation) is often heard in conjunction with a loud pulmonic valve closure. The loud and sometimes palpable second heart sound is the result of the pulmonary valve closing more forcefully than normal because of the pulmonary hypertension. In addition to systemic arterial hypoxemia, hypercarbia and acidemia can develop rapidly. At the current time, echocardiography provides the least invasive and perhaps most useful means to diagnose PPHN. In the absence of congenital heart defects, bowing of the atrial septum from right to left, and right-to-left shunting of blood at the ductal and atrial levels are highly supportive of the diagnosis of PPHN. Cardiac catheterization may be useful in selected patients to establish the diagnosis or to test the utility of a specific treatment.

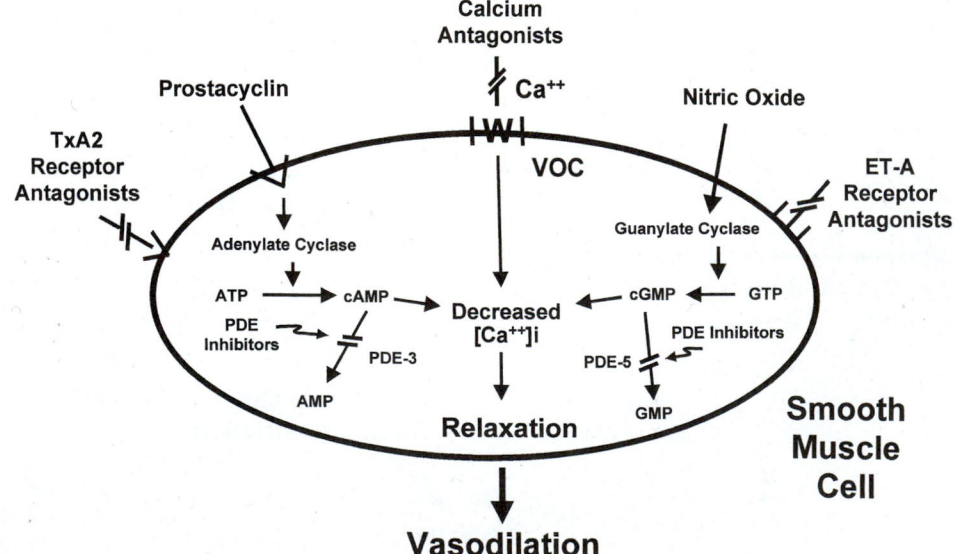

FIGURE 2-58 Pharmacologic approaches that are potentially useful in the treatment of PPHN. TxA_2 = thromboxane A_2; PDE = phosphodiesterase; cAMP = cyclic adenosine-3′,5′ monophosphate; cGMP = cyclic guanosine-3′,5′ monophosphate; GTP = guanosine triphosphate; ET = endothelin; VOL = voltage operated channel.

Initial therapies are directed toward correcting alveolar hypoxia, acidosis, and hypercarbia with administration of oxygen and buffer usually coupled with and assisted ventilation. These measures often restore normal pulmonary vasodilation and allow for alveolar recruitment. However, excessive mean airway pressures have adverse effects that can perpetuate lung injury (see Sec. 23.9). It is also important to note that although hyperventilation has become perhaps the most commonly used treatment of PPHN, it has never been prospectively demonstrated to reduce the morbidity or mortality of PPHN. Hyperventilation with 100% oxygen may, indeed, worsen pulmonary, neurologic, and ophthalmologic morbidity. In some infants with hypoplastic lungs or especially severe parenchymal lung disease, high-frequency oscillatory ventilation may permit adequate gas exchange with smaller tidal volumes and lower airway pressures. This "lung recruitment" ventilation strategy has been successful in the treatment of some infants with PPHN. If the heart and lungs cannot support gas exchange, use of extracorporeal membrane oxygenation may allow time for the lungs to recover and pulmonary hypertension to resolve. Although this technique has been successful in the treatment of a large number of infants, it remains an extremely expensive and invasive method of supportive care and has many complications (see Secs. 2.19.3 and 4.2.3). If the cause of PPHN is respiratory distress syndrome (RDS) from lack of endogenous surfactant in the near-term child, exogenous surfactant is now available to reverse atelectasis and the attendant alveolar hypoxia (see Sec. 2.16.1). Many other experimental therapies have been proposed to provide adequate gas exchange (see Sec. 2.19.1 and 2.19.5).

If treatment of the underlying lung disease is ineffective, or if there is PPHN with no underlying parenchymal disease, then direct attempts to dilate the pulmonary circulation should be made. Numerous vasodilators have been utilized in the setting of persistent pulmonary hypertension of the newborn. In the past, tolazoline was the most extensively used drug for this purpose. Many other vasodilators including nitroprusside, prostacyclin, isoproterenol, and chlorpromazine have also been given to neonates with PPHN. Unfortunately, none of these agents is a selective pulmonary vasodilator. They all decrease both pulmonary and systemic vascular resistance, and thus none of them can be expected to selectively restore the normal transition to gas exchange by the lungs. For this reason, the discovery that inhaled NO (iNO) was a potent and selective pulmonary vasodilator effective in patients with PPHN was a clinical breakthrough, and this is the current treatment of choice (see Sec. 2.19.4).

There are patients in whom PPHN persists, despite treatment with iNO, because of abnormalities of vascular development or function. In some of these patients there may be alterations in the content or activity of soluble guanylate cyclase in the lung, or there may be high concentrations of the cGMP-specific phosphodiesterase PDE-5. Therefore, inhibitors of PDE-5 such as zaprinast or dipyrimidole may prove to be useful with PPHN. Figure 2-58 demonstrates other therapeutic targets that have been tried or will be tried in the future. These include inhaled prostacyclin, calcium channel inhibitors, and even antagonists of endothelin and thromboxane receptors.

References

Abman SH: Abnormal vasoreactivity in the pathophysiology of persistent pulmonary hypertension of the newborn. Pediatr Rev (Online) 11:103, 1999

Durmowicz AG, Stenmark KR: Mechanisms of structural remodeling in chronic pulmonary hypertension. Pediatr Rev (Online) 20:e91, 1999

Mercier JC, Lacaze T, Storme L, Roze JC, Dinh-Xuan AT, Dehan M: Disease-related response to inhaled nitric oxide in newborns with severe hypoxaemic respiratory failure. French Paediatric Study Group of Inhaled NO. Eur J Pediatr 157:747, 1998

Morin FC III, Stenmark KR: Persistent pulmonary hypertension of the newborn. Am J Respir Crit Care Med 151:2010, 1995

Roberts JD JR, Fineman JR, Morin FC 3rd, et al: Inhaled nitric oxide and persistent pulmonary hypertension of the newborn. The inhaled nitric oxide study group. N Engl J Med 336:605, 1997

Steinhorn RH, Morin FC 3RD, Fineman JR: Models of persistent pulmonary hypertension of the newborn (PPHN) and the role of cyclic guanosine monophosphate (cGMP) in pulmonary vasorelaxation. Semin Perinatol 21:393, 1997

Stenmark KR, Mecham RP: Cellular and molecular mechanisms of pulmonary vascular remodeling. Annu Rev Physiol 59:89, 1997

Tulloh RM, Hislop AA, Boels PJ, Deutsch J, Haworth SG: Chronic hypoxia inhibits postnatal maturation of porcine intrapulmonary artery relaxation. Am J Physiol 272:H2436, 1997

Van Marter LJ, Leviton A, Allred EN, et al: Persistent pulmonary hypertension of the newborn and smoking and aspirin and nonsteroidal antiinflammatory drug consumption during pregnancy. Pediatrics 97:658, 1996

2.17.12   Birth-Related Injury, Including Perinatal Asphyxia

M. Douglas Jones, Jr.

PETECHIAE, ECCHYMOSES, AND SUBCUTANEOUS FAT NECROSIS

Occasional petechiae are common after an uneventful labor and delivery. Densely grouped petechiae may occur on the head and neck above a tight nuchal cord or on the presenting part with breech, face, and other unusual fetal presentations. In each case, petechiae represent capillary bleeding secondary to venous congestion. Although the possibility of thrombocytopenia or platelet dysfunction should be considered, perinatal petechiae often occur in the absence of platelet or coagulation abnormalities. Occasionally, especially in small, preterm infants, bleeding may progress to form ecchymoses, which in turn may lead to early jaundice. Venous congestion or direct pressure from the cervix or maternal bony structures is the usual cause.

Subcutaneous fat necrosis is characterized by a localized area of induration. Necrosis is the result of local ischemia, usually secondary to trauma. It may be seen at the site of forceps application. It also may occur in noninstrumented deliveries when fatty tissue is squeezed between underlying bone and the cervix or maternal pelvis, for example, over the zygoma after a face presentation. Fat necrosis also has been reported after cold injury.

Although subcutaneous induration may be noticed in the first few days, it is more likely to be noted at the end of the first week or later. Induration may be severe and sometimes is associated with red or purple skin discoloration. There may be a visible lump, and induration may increase as calcification occurs. It then resolves slowly over the next several months. Occasionally a calcified nodule remains. Extensive subcutaneous fat necrosis may be accompanied by elevated serum calcium concentrations.

CLAVICLE FRACTURES

The clavicle is the bone most often fractured during delivery. The midrange of the reported incidence lies between 0.5 and 1.5% of live births. Incidence varies somewhat with the method of ascertainment; because fractures are often of the "greenstick" variety, the incidence is highest when the fracture is identified radiographically. Fractures may not be diagnosed clinically until callus formation is detected at several weeks of age.

Although most clavicle fractures occur during normal, spontaneous vaginal delivery, the incidence is increased with shoulder dystocia and its interrelated correlates: macrosomia, prolonged pregnancy, prolonged second stage of labor, and instrument-assisted delivery. Fracture also has been associated with vaginal breech delivery. It is rare after cesarean section. Possible causes are pressure on the anterior shoulder by the maternal symphysis pubis, torsion during delivery, digital pressure by the obstetrician or midwife, or, uncommonly, deliberate fracture to facilitate delivery.

Nondisplaced fractures are often asymptomatic. Complicated fractures may be painful enough to cause a pseudoparalysis of the arm, mimicking injury to the brachial plexus. Because brachial plexus injuries occur in the same clinical settings, this may be confusing. Even complicated fractures heal with no deformity. Therapy is therefore symptomatic. Infants with painful fractures are more comfortable if the arm is gently immobilized, and periods of irritability may be treated with an oral analgesic.

BRACHIAL PLEXUS AND ASSOCIATED INJURIES

Brachial plexus injury causes paralysis of the upper limb. It is relatively infrequent, with an overall incidence of 0.3 to 2 per 1000 live births. The cause is traction on the nerves and roots of the brachial plexus during labor and delivery. Four types of injury result. Neurapraxia (a mild focal lesion secondary to stretching) is the most frequent and is almost always associated with complete recovery. Neuroma in continuity (neuroma secondary to injury) is less frequently associated with recovery. Other injury types are axonotmesis (nerve rupture) and nerve root avulsion. Injury occurs most frequently in vertex deliveries complicated by shoulder dystocia and is thus more common with fetal macrosomia. In a large series with an overall incidence of 1.03/1000, the incidence increased from 0.5/1000 in infants with birth weights <4000 g, to 3.29, 10.69, and 26.79 with weights of 4000–4499, 4500–4999, and >5000 g, respectively. The incidence is less if dystocia is managed with cesarean section.

The most common injury (Erb-Duchenne paralysis) involves damage to the fifth and sixth cervical nerve roots, causing paralysis of the deltoid, supraspinatus, infraspinatus, and biceps. Injury to the seventh cervical nerve causes paralysis of wrist and finger extensors. Together, these result in the classic "head waiter's tip" position, with the arm limp at the side and internally rotated (lack of abductor function at the shoulder and supinator function in the lower arm) and the wrist and fingers flexed (lack of extensor function). Paralysis of finger and wrist extensors can be confirmed by failure of extension in response to gentle stroking of the back of the hand. An early sign will be an asymmetric Moro reflex.

Injuries involving the entire plexus or multiroot avulsions (C5-7) lead to major sensory and motor impairment. Isolated injury to C7-T1 nerve roots or the lower trunk of the plexus (Klumpke paralysis) is exceptionally rare. It presents with normal shoulder position, flexion at the elbow, supination of the forearm, and a flaccid wrist and hand.

Brachial plexus injury raises the possibility of associated spinal nerve lesions. Respiratory distress suggests diaphragmatic paralysis from damage at C3-4. This is confirmed by asymmetric motion of the chest during respiration, and by asymmetric breath sounds. A chest radiograph during active inspiration will show elevation of the affected diaphragm, usually on the same side as the paralyzed arm. Bilateral diaphragmatic paralysis produces symmetric elevation and may be less obvious. Chest radiographs during passive inflation by positive-pressure ventilation will not demonstrate an abnormality. Because diaphragmatic paralysis usually resolves spontaneously during the first few weeks to months, management consists of mechanical ventilation as needed. Persisting paralysis may require surgical plication of the diaphragm.

A constricted pupil (meiosis) that reacts to light, accompanied by mild drooping of the eyelid (ptosis) and anhidrosis are indicative of Horner syndrome, which reflects damage to the stellate ganglion adjacent to T1. The examiner should look for associated fractures of the clavicle and humerus.

Although an association between brachial plexus injury and macrosomia is clear, most cases occur in infants with normal birth weights. Furthermore, most large infants have no injury. An association with shoulder dystocia is even stronger, but not only does injury occur in the absence of dystocia, there is evidence that paralysis is more likely to be permanent when it occurs without dystocia. Although the nerves of the brachial plexus are most often injured by excessive lateral traction on the neck during delivery of an infant with shoulder dystocia, injury also occurs after seemingly normal deliveries. Because of this, the limited ability to identify a macrosomic fetus, and the even greater difficulty in predicting shoulder dystocia, there is little support for "prophylactic" cesarean section.

Approximately 95% of brachial plexus palsies resolve spontaneously. Physical therapy is important in preserving joint mobility until function returns. Electrodiagnostic studies obtained after about 1 month of age are helpful in determining the location and severity of the injury. If recovery does not occur, joint contractures and shoulder deformity may result. Some have suggested that the incidence of permanent paralysis may be reduced by microsurgical reconstruction of damaged nerves at 4 to 6 months of age. Although this is routine in some centers, its proper place awaits prospective, controlled clinical trials. Tendon and muscle transfers are used to enhance function in older children.

ABNORMALITIES OF THE SCALP

Abnormalities following injury to tissues of the scalp, beginning with the most superficial, are caput succedaneum, subaponeurotic hemorrhage, and cephalohematoma (Fig. 2-59).

CAPUT SUCCEDANEUM Caput succedaneum represents localized, often serosanguinous, edema of the scalp. This is usually the result of pressure applied by the uterus, pelvis, or vagina during delivery. The roughly circular configuration suggests that the most frequent cause is local venous congestion and edema from cervical pressure. Vacuum extraction combines venous congestion with a forceful negative pressure applied to the scalp that can cause a particularly prominent caput succedaneum.

Physical examination shows a boggy mass with poorly defined edges. It is generally no more than a few centimeters in diameter but may be substantially larger. Regardless of the initial size, caput succedaneum resolves rapidly and has usually disappeared by 48 hours of age. A caput is occasionally defined rather sharply by a contused "halo scalp ring." Transient hair loss may occur within the ring over the next several months.

SUBAPONEUROTIC (SUBGALEAL) HEMORRHAGE Hemorrhage into the subaponeurotic, or subgaleal, space is rare but can be extremely serious. The galea aponeurotica extends from the occiput to the eyebrows and laterally to the insertion of the temporalis fascia. Although the subaponeurotic space is limited inferiorly and circumferentially, the circumference is large, and only the tissues of the scalp limit superior expansion. Subaponeurotic hemorrhage can therefore result in enormous blood loss.

Bleeding rarely results from disruption of an interosseus synchondrosis with a tear in the underlying dural sinus. The more frequent cause is traction on the scalp with shearing of emissary veins between the scalp and intracranial venous sinuses (Fig. 2-59). A coagulation defect may complicate the picture. Massive bleeding has been documented in the hemophilias and in hemorrhagic disease of the newborn, including early hemorrhagic disease in infants born to mothers who are taking anticonvulsants. Traction on the scalp is more severe in deliveries assisted by forceps, particularly midforceps, and vacuum extraction. In the latter, injury correlates with the length of time the vacuum is applied and with the type of cup (plastic or metal).

Key to diagnosis is a high index of suspicion. A subaponeurotic hemorrhage may occur together with a caput succedaneum and cephalohematoma. A caput succedaneum is limited to edema of the skin and subcutaneous tissue; a subaponeurotic hemorrhage lies beneath the scalp and can often be balloted, with an obvious fluid wave. A cephalohematoma is strictly limited by the margins of the individual bones of the skull, whereas a subaponeurotic hemorrhage extends across suture lines. With massive subaponeurotic bleeding, the head circumference is symmetrically increased.

Blood loss can be life threatening. Calculations suggest that an infant can lose approximately 38 mL of blood for each centimeter increase in head circumference. Thus, an increase of just 2 cm in head circumference might represent 30% of the blood volume of a 3–Kg infant (240–300 mL) and cause irreversible shock. Smaller hemorrhages can cause anemia and increase the likelihood of jaundice.

Identification of the site of bleeding is impossible. Management consists of recognition and prompt blood volume replacement according to the state of consciousness, skin perfusion, vital signs, urine output, and hematocrit. (It is important to recognize that acute hemorrhage need not cause an immediate change in hematocrit.) Congenital coagulation defects must be treated. Extra vitamin K is necessary in hemorrhagic disease associated with maternal anticonvulsants. The infant may also have an acquired coagulation defect from shock and disseminated intravascular coagulation.

CEPHALOHEMATOMA A cephalohematoma is a subperiosteal hematoma of the bones of the skull secondary to shearing of the periosteum over the surface of the bone. One representative study found an incidence of 3.2/1000. It is more common after prolonged labor, with abnormal presentations, and after instrument-assisted deliveries. Cephalohematomas are also found after uneventful labors and vaginal deliveries and after cesarean section; they have even been identified on prenatal ultrasound.

A cephalohematoma is characterized by a firm bulge deep underneath the scalp. Because it is a subperiosteal hemorrhage, it stops at the edge of the bone and, except in the rare situation of craniosynostosis, does not cross a suture line. Resolution over succeeding weeks and months is often accompanied by a rim of calcification around the margin, giving the mistaken impression of an underlying depressed skull fracture. Linear fractures have been identified

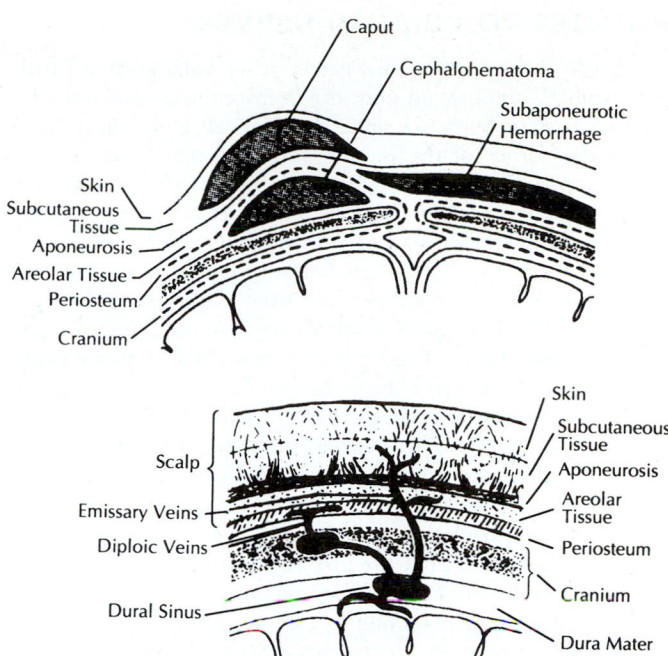

FIGURE 2-59   Top: Sites of epicranial hemorrhage in the newborn. Subaponeurotic hemorrhage occurs in the areolar tissue between the aponeurosis and the periosteum. Bottom: Emissary veins traverse the potential subaponeurotic space. SOURCE: *Levkoff AH, Macpherson RI: Unrecognized subaponeurotic hemorrhage. Am J Dis Child 146:833–834, 1992, after Goss CM: Gray's Anatomy of the Human Body. Philadelphia, Lea & Febiger, 1966:49, and Plauche WC: Fetal cranial injuries related to delivery with Malstrom vacuum extractor. Obstet Gynecol 53:750–757, 1979. Copyright 1992, American Medical Association.*

radiographically in association with about 5% of unilateral cephalohematomas. Comminuted fractures are rare.

Cephalohematomas resolve spontaneously over several months and should not be aspirated or drained. Residual calcification occasionally persists.

SKULL FRACTURES

Comminuted skull fractures are almost always associated with instrument-assisted deliveries and are rare. Linear fractures are relatively common and may occur with cephalohematomas. They are usually noted as an incidental finding on a diagnostic image of the skull. Although simple linear fractures require no therapy, they should be monitored over time for possible development of a leptomeningeal cyst. This is indicated by a widening fracture accompanied by an extracranial fluid-filled mass and requires neurosurgical management.

Congenital depressions of the skull occur with an incidence of approximately 1/10,000. They may represent a complicated fracture, with bone fragments, or a "ping pong" deformation without discontinuity, similar to a greenstick fracture of a long bone. Depressions may be secondary to pressure from forceps, the maternal spine or pelvis, uterine tumors, fetal extremities, or the obstetrician's or midwife's hand.

If physical examination or diagnostic imaging shows bone fragments, neurosurgical exploration may be required. If abnormal neurologic signs are absent, and findings are consistent with a deformation, the depression may be elevated using the vacuum of a breast pump or an obstetric vacuum extractor.

INJURIES TO CRANIAL NERVES

Trauma to the seventh cranial nerve causes facial paralysis. If the nerve trunk is compressed near its exit from the skull, the result is paralysis, with inability to wrinkle the forehead, close the eyelid, or retract the corner of the mouth. Injury to peripheral branches causes local weakness. Bilateral paralysis, isolated absence of lip depressors, deficits in other cranial nerves, or facial anomalies suggests a developmental rather than a traumatic cause.

Traumatic facial paralysis may follow spontaneous vaginal delivery, presumably caused by pressure from bones of the maternal pelvis. More commonly, obstetric forceps are the cause of injury. Paralysis is noted at birth or on the first day of life. Although complete resolution may take weeks to months, substantial improvement usually occurs over the next several days. Rarely, no recovery occurs within the first 7 to 10 days, suggesting that the nerve has been interrupted or crushed. Electromyography is useful in detecting this complication. Early identification is important because the outlook for eventual recovery remains good if the nerve is decompressed or repaired within the first several months. With rare exceptions, traumatic facial paralysis is transient. Permanent paralysis suggests a developmental cause.

Absence of lateral eye movements suggests damage to the sixth cranial nerve. The incidence of this condition varies from 0% after delivery by cesarean section to 0.1% with spontaneous vaginal delivery to 2.4% for forceps delivery, to 3.2% after vacuum extraction. Resolution is spontaneous and occurs by 6 weeks of age.

SPINAL CORD INJURIES

Injuries to the spinal cord have been associated with midforceps rotations and difficult breech deliveries and are rare in contemporary practice. Labor with a fetus presenting in the breech position with a hyperextended neck, the so-called "flying fetus," can result in damage to the cervical spinal cord. Elective delivery by cesarean section usually avoids this complication.

PERINATAL ASPHYXIA

The fetal circulatory response to acute hypoxemia (decreased arterial PO_2) or asphyxia (decreased arterial PO_2 and increased PCO_2) has been well described in experimental animals and humans. Blood flow to kidneys, gastrointestinal tract, liver, muscle, and lungs decreases, while blood flow to the heart, brain, and adrenal glands, and to a lesser extent the placenta, increases. Blood flow through the umbilical vein, is redistributed within the right atrium to favor perfusion of the heart and brain. The net result is preservation of oxygen flow (the product of blood flow and arterial O_2 content) to the heart and brain at the expense of other organs, until hypoxemia is severe enough to cause circulatory collapse. The pattern of organ damage after acute asphyxia is a consequence of the severity of the insult, the pattern of oxygen flow, and the oxygen requirements of each organ.

Oxygen flow to the brain is relatively well preserved in asphyxia, but the oxygen requirement is also high. Approximately 70% of infants with birth asphyxia (defined by a 5-minute Apgar score of 5 or less, or fetal acidosis with a scalp or umbilical arterial pH <7.2) have signs of central nervous system dysfunction. This may range from mild (hyperexcitability or hypotonia persisting for up to 72 hours) to severe (coma or stupor). In most infants the abnormality is transient, with no sequelae. Approximately 15% fall into the severe category and have a poor long-term outlook. Treatment to improve outcome is the subject of intense research. At the present time, only supportive therapy and treatment of seizures are indicated.

Some degree of myocardial dysfunction occurs in approximately 25% of infants with asphyxia, as defined above. A holosystolic murmur, heard best in the area of the xiphoid, indicates tricuspid insufficiency. This represents a combination of pulmonary hypertension and right ventricular dilation, with dilation of the annulus of the tricuspid valve and papillary muscle dysfunction (see Sec. 22.3.3) These conditions usually resolve spontaneously. Severely affected infants will be hypotensive with echocardiographic evidence of poor ventricular function and electrocardiographic signs of myocardial ischemia. Treatment of hypotension with intravascular volume and vasopressors is often beneficial.

Oliguria persisting for 24 hours has been reported in up to 40% of asphyxiated infants as defined above. Oliguria lasting for 36 to 48 hours is seen in 5 to 10%. Hematuria is common, and elevated levels of β_2-microglobulin suggest proximal tubular injury. In a small number of infants, prolonged oliguria is followed by high urine volumes, transient sodium wasting, and transient renal tubular acidosis. Management should include close attention to fluid and electrolyte balance. Irreversible renal failure is rare.

Although gastrointestinal blood flow falls during fetal asphyxia, intestinal oxygen consumption is low in the absence of feeding, and severe gastrointestinal damage is uncommon. Although transient ileus occurs in about 25% of infants, severe gastrointestinal bleeding is rare. Oral feeding should be withheld until ileus resolves.

Pulmonary dysfunction occurs in approximately 25% of term infants with asphyxia of this degree. This may be caused by meconium aspiration syndrome, pulmonary hemorrhage, or persistent pulmonary hypertension. Hypoxemia associated with persistent pulmonary hypertension may require only administration of supplemental oxygen for 24 to 48 hours. In some infants it progresses to a clinical picture of respiratory failure, a hyperreactive pulmonary vascular bed, severe pulmonary hypertension, and right ventricular failure requiring neonatal intensive care (see Sec. 2.17.11).

Metabolic consequences of asphyxia include hypoglycemia and hypocalcemia. Skeletal muscle damage, indicated by elevated serum creatinine phosphokinase concentrations and myoglobinuria, is common in severe asphyxia. Asphyxiated infants may be hypercoagulable, with thrombosis in large veins. They are prone to hemorrhage secondary to liver damage and disseminated intravascular coagulation.

Perinatal asphyxia is a global insult. Thus, severe dysfunction of any one organ in the absence of injury to others points to causes other than asphyxia. This is especially important to consider when speculating about a link between neonatal encephalopathy and later neurologic disability. One should also consider that although approximately 20% of cases of cerebral palsy are associated with adverse events around the time of birth, the percentage of cases where the relationship is causal is far less. In some cases the association is coincidental. In others the prenatal condition that led to brain dysgenesis or damage also decreases the ability of the fetus to tolerate labor. Thus, fewer than 10% of cases of cerebral palsy can be attributed to perinatal events in a previously normal fetus.

References

Ecker JL, Greeberg JA, Norwitz ER, Nadel A, Repke J: Birth weight as a predictor of brachial plexus injury. Obstet Gynecol 89:643–647, 1997

Galbraith RS: Incidence of neonatal sixth nerve palsy in relation to mode of delivery. Am J Obstet Gynecol 170:1158–1159, 1994

Kaplan B, Rabinerson D, Avrech OM, Carmi N, Steinberg DM, Merlob P: Fracture of the clavicle in the newborn following normal labor and delivery. Int J Gynaecol Obstet 63:15–20, 1998

Laing JHE, Harrison DH, Jones BM, Laing GJ: Is permanent facial palsy caused by birth trauma? Arch Dis Child 74:56–58, 1996

Laurent JP: Brachial plexus trauma and other peripheral nerve injuries of childhood. In: Albright AL, Pollack IF, Adelson PD, eds: Principles and Practice of Pediatric Neurosurgery. New York, Georg Thieme, 1999: 897–913

Martín-Ancel A, García-Alix A, Gayá F, Cabañas F, Burgueros M, Quero J: Multiple organ involvement in perinatal asphyxia. J Pediatr 127:786–793, 1995

Nelson KB: What proportion of cerebral palsy is related to birth asphyxia? J Pediatr 112:572–574, 1988

Shullinger JN: Birth trauma. Pediatr Clin North Am 40:1351–1358, 1993

Yasunaga S, Rivera R: Cephalohematoma in the newborn. Clin Pediatr 13: 256–260, 1974

Yosef B-A, Merlob P, Hirsch M, Reisner SH: Congenital depression of the neonatal skull. Eur J Obstet Gynecol Reprod Biol 22:249–255, 1986

Zelson C, Lee SJ, Pearl M: The incidence of skull fractures underlying cephalhematoma in newborn infants. J Pediatr 85:371–373, 1974

2.17.13   Pulmonary Hypoplasia and Congenital Diaphragmatic Hernia

William E. Truog

Pulmonary hypoplasia is an important cause of clinical respiratory distress and failure of pulmonary gas exchange that is manifest at or just after birth. Pulmonary hypoplasia results from disruptions in the normal sequence of pulmonary fetal developmental milestones, disruptions that can occur at various points during fetal life. Its cause can be idiopathic, secondary to premature and prolonged rupture of amniotic membranes, associated with concurrent renal aplasia or dysplasia, or secondary to thoracic space-occupying masses. The most common of these masses is congenital diaphragmatic hernia. Severe pulmonary hypoplasia commonly causes respiratory failure and and is often fatal despite timely application of assisted ventilation.

CONGENITAL DIAPHRAGMATIC HERNIA

DEFINITION Congenital diaphragmatic hernia occurs with failure of development of either the left (85%), right (13%), or both (2%) hemidiaphragms, the dome-shaped fibromuscular sheets that separate the thoracic and abdominal cavities. Typically, this defect is posterolateral in location. The diaphragmatic defect allows displacement of some or most of the abdominal contents into the corresponding hemithorax. Both ipsilateral and contralateral pulmonary hypoplasia are usually present. There are a reduced number of bronchial branches and reduced alveolar space. These anatomic abnormalities result in failure of normal transition from fetal to neonatal cardiopulmonary circulation and pulmonary gas exchange. Immediate postnatal onset of respiratory distress usually ensues, leading to respiratory failure.

INCIDENCE A reasonable estimate of incidence of congenital diaphragmatic hernia (CDH) is one per 2000–3000 live births. The incidence of CDH has remained about the same during the last 20 years. Antenatal diagnosis by fetal ultrasonography is made in approximately 50% of cases of CDH. The average fetal age at diagnosis is 26 weeks gestation. Antenatal diagnosis has not altered the number of live-born infants with this disorder.

ETIOLOGY The etiology of CDH is unknown. There have been long-held assumptions that there was a primary failure of formation of the diaphragm. Others have suggested that the primary defect may be pulmonary hypoplasia with secondary unilateral diaphragmatic underdevelopment.

The associated anomalies that occur in 10 to 15% of patients with CDH have provided no clues to etiology. Genetic analysis of families in which CDH has occurred in more than one sibling has failed to demonstrate a single gene defect.

CLINICAL PRESENTATION

CDH that is associated with severe lung hypoplasia typically leads to immediate postnatal respiratory distress, with tachypnea and labored breathing that progresses to gasping respirations and cyanosis. Auscultation reveals diminished or absent breath sounds on the affected side. The cardiac impulse is displaced to the contralateral side of the chest. Severe arterial oxygen desaturation leads to cyanosis. Instead of the normally rounded abdominal appearance, there is often a scaphoid or flattened abdomen because of dimished intraabdominal contents. The chest cavity on the side of the hernia may contain stomach, variable amounts of small intestine, and the left lobe of the liver. Absence of a scaphoid abdomen does not exclude a diagnosis of CDH. Most infants with CDH are delivered at 36 to 39 weeks gestation. Therefore, immaturity of the pulmonary surfactant system and lung architecture may coexist in infants with CDH. Biochemical immaturity of the lung exacerbates the effects of the structural hypoplasia.

Occasionally, infants with CDH appear normal immediately after birth and exhibit respiratory distress later, usually on the first day. Rarely, the radiographic appearance of CDH is noted unexpectedly weeks or months later in an infant who presents with respiratory distress from suspected pneumonia.

The severity of respiratory distress at birth can worsen as the intrathoracic stomach and intestine fill with air during spontaneous breathing. The mediastinal shift that occurs in severe CDH compromises both systemic venous and pulmonary venous return of blood to the heart and impairs cardiac function. Pulmonary microvascular hypoplasia, with reduced vascular cross-sectional area, typically presents in infants with CDH and produces an anatomic basis for pulmonary hypertension, as the entire right ventricular output must traverse a noncompliant vascular bed with a cross-sectional area that is smaller than normal. Increased pulmonary vascular resistance promotes right-to-left shunting of blood between right and left atria through the foramen ovale, and between proximal pulmonary artery and aorta through the ductus arteriosus. Intrapulmonary shunts also may be present. These shunts exacerbate hypoxemia and thereby aggravate the underlying pulmonary hypertension. Typical laboratory data include severe hypoxemia, even with 100% inspired oxygen, and carbon dioxide retention leading to severe respiratory acidosis, despite intense spontaneous respiratory effort and superimposed assisted ventilation.

Early detection of associated malformations is important in the evaluation of infants with CDH. Such malformations may include congenital heart disease and structural disorders of the central nervous system, gastrointestinal system, and genitourinary system. The finding of clinically significant malformations may influence the course of treatment and prompt discussion about the utility of initiating or continuing prolonged and invasive modes of support. Findings compatible with trisomy 18 or other major chromosomal abnormalities must be recognized. There is no other discernible congenital defect in 80 to 90% of infants with CDH.

RADIOGRAPHIC APPEARANCE

The diagnosis of CDH is readily confirmed by chest radiography (Fig. 2-60). Placement of a gastric tube into the infant's stomach before chest radiography not only helps to prevent distension of the stomach and intestine but also helps to confirm the diagnosis of CDH by demonstrating that the stomach is in the chest. Congenital cystic adenomatoid malformation (CCAM) in some instances can mimic the initial clinical and radiographic appearance of diaphragmatic hernia. In this condition, the stomach is situated below the diaphragm. Ultrasonography and additional chest radiographic procedures should differentiate the two conditions.

IN UTERO TREATMENT

During the last 20 years, attempts have been made to treat CDH in fetuses diagnosed with this condition between 24 and 28 weeks of gestation (see Section 2.6). Fetal intervention for this condition is limited to a few specialized centers, and such therapy remains experimental, with considerable variability of outcome.

NEONATAL TREATMENT

Stabilization of the respiratory system is the first and most important goal in the treatment of infants with CDH. This is accomplished by immediate postnatal endotracheal intubation and assisted ventilation. Sedation and muscle relaxation may help to inhibit spontaneous respiratory effort, thereby lessening the risk of pneumothorax. Recent experience in the medical management of this condition indicates that intentional hypoventilation of infants with pulmonary hypoplasia may help to prevent air leaks and reduce the severity of secondary lung injury. Surgical intervention to repair the diaphragmatic defect is often delayed for up to several days to allow improvement in lung and cardiovascular function.

Maintaining normal systemic blood pressure and organ perfusion is an important element in the management of infants with CDH and lung hypoplasia. Although intravascular hypovolemia is not present at the moment of birth, affected infants may exhibit systemic hypotension because of diminished cardiac output associated with diminished venous return of blood to the heart. Intravenous infusion of dopamine or other vasopressor agents may help to improve pulmonary blood flow and thereby increase arterial oxygenation. Albumin infusions are not recommended, as albumin leaks into the lung interstitium and aggravates the underlying pulmonary edema.

Infants with CDH may have superimposed pulmonary surfactant dysfunction at birth, even at 35 to 37 weeks of gestation. Thus, some physicians advocate routine administration of surfactant by endotracheal tube immediately after birth. The more immature the infant, the more likely that surfactant will help pulmonary function. After 37 weeks gestation, however, there is little or no rationale to support supplemental surfactant treatment.

ROLE OF ASSISTED VENTILATION

The goal of assisted ventilation in infants with CDH is to maintain adequate arterial oxygenation and ventilation without injuring the limited complement of functioning lung tissue. This is generally

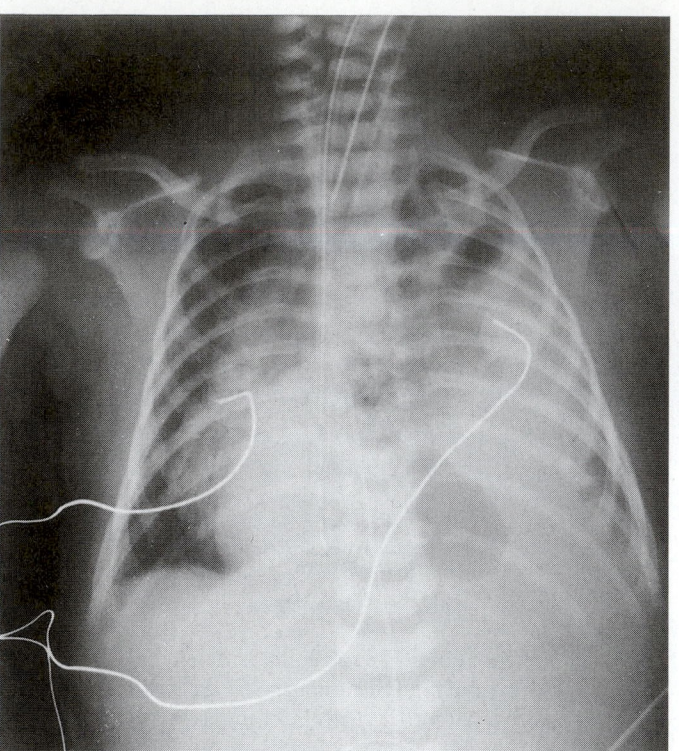

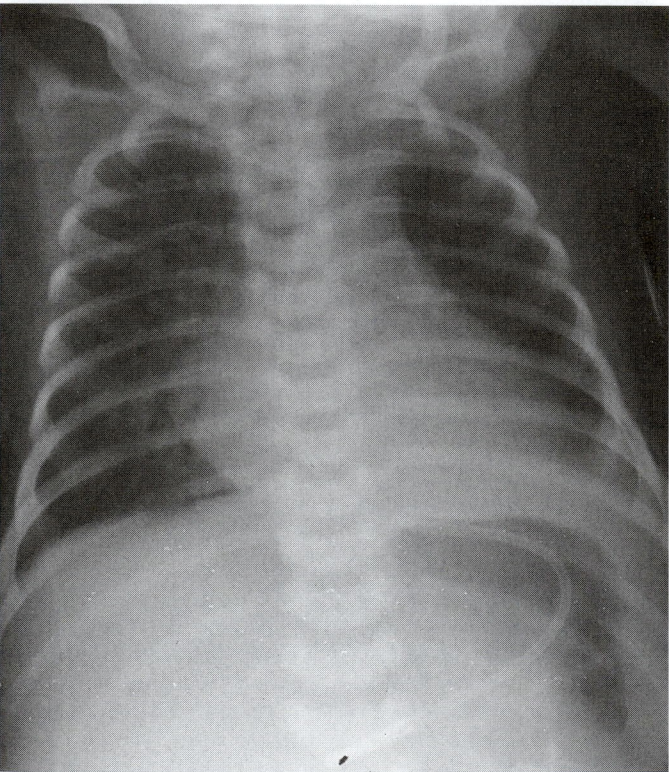

FIGURE 2-60 Term infant with congenital diaphragmatic hernia. **A: Radiograph appearance at birth. Note the air filled loop of small intestine in the left hemithorax. B: Same infant 3 weeks later following surgical repair.**

accomplished by using very small inflation volumes at very high frequencies. Although it is difficult to recommend specific limits for peak inspiratory pressure, gas flow rate, inspiratory time, or respiratory rate, the application of one of the several available forms of high-frequency ventilation, especially high-frequency oscillatory ventilation, minimizes phasic changes in lung volume and allows for adequate arterial oxygenation or CO_2 elimination. Thus, early initiation of high-frequency mechanical ventilation (Sec. 2.19.2) is now the mainstay of respiratory support of infants with CDH both before and after surgical intervention.

TIMING OF SURGERY

For many years the recommended approach for treating CDH was immediate surgical repair of the diaphragm and transfer of abdominal organs from above to below the diaphragm. The rationale for immediate surgery was to reposition the heart and mediastinal structures and allow expansion of both lungs. Only one randomized, prospective, controlled clinical trial aimed at defining the optimal time for postnatal surgery has ever been conducted. This study failed to demonstrate any difference in survival between infants operated urgently following delivery (mean age 10 hours) and those treated with deferred surgery (mean age 173 hours).

The current approach at most institutions is to undertake surgery at a time when (1) pulmonary hypertension has abated substantially; (2) arterial pH is greater than 7.30 and PCO_2 is 45 to 55 mm Hg with peak inflation pressures at less than 20 cm H_2O; and (3) physiological abnormalities, such as hypoglycemia, oliguria, bleeding disorders, and electrolyte abnormalities, have been corrected. Hemodynamic disturbances and pulmonary edema often complicate the postoperative course of infants who have undergone surgical repair of CDH.

ROLE OF INHALED NITRIC OXIDE

Inhaled nitric oxide, effective in the treatment of neonatal pulmonary hypertension, generally has not proven useful in the treatment of CDH. The diminished pulmonary vascular cross-sectional area may account for the lack of response to inhaled nitric oxide. Its use may benefit infants postoperatively who preoperatively had evidence of low pulmonary vascular resistance and excellent pulmonary gas exchange, but who postoperatively became hypoxemic.

ROLE OF EXTRACORPOREAL MEMBRANE OXYGENATION

The role of extracorporeal membrane oxygenation (ECMO) in the management of CDH has been controversial. The controversy arises over whether long-term survival is likely in infants with severe CDH who have failed conventional therapy. A multicenter trial of ECMO in Great Britain failed to demonstrate increased survival of infants with CDH. In the United States, however, 59% of infants with CDH who are treated with ECMO survive to home discharge (extracorporeal life support organization registry 1997–1998 data). In the absence of relevant control infants, however, the value of ECMO in the management of infants with CDH remains unclear.

PROGNOSIS

Infants with CDH who demonstrate no associated congenital malformations, who are ≥34 weeks of gestational age and weigh 2 kg or more body weight at birth, and who are treated in centers with the necessary medical and technical infrastructure have a reported survival to discharge of 60 to 80%. Life beyond discharge for infants with CDH often includes complications referable to the respiratory and gastrointestinal systems. Some problems identified in follow-up studies of infants with CDH during and after infancy are as follows: failure to thrive, gastroesophageal reflux, chronic lung disease, chest wall deformity, scoliosis, and recurrence of herniation, which requires surgery.

OTHER CONDITIONS ASSOCIATED WITH PULMONARY HYPOPLASIA

LUNG HYPOPLASIA ASSOCIATED WITH RUPTURE OF AMNIOTIC MEMBRANES Integrity of the fetal membranes and maintenance of a normal volume of both intrapulmonary and amniotic fluid are critical for normal fetal lung growth and development. Any disruption of the integrity of the amniotic cavity can interrupt normal pulmonary development, producing pulmonary hypoplasia. Premature rupture of membranes and loss of amniotic fluid occur frequently with preterm birth. Identifying the fetus at high risk for pulmonary hypoplasia following prolonged premature rupture of membranes (PPROM) has important clinical implications. Prolongation of a pregnancy that could be predicted to yield an infant with lethal pulmonary hypoplasia would be futile. Thus, efforts to identify predictive factors for postnatal survival have considerable importance in guiding the management of this difficult condition. Studies have been descriptive and not experimental, but there are prospectively obtained data to guide management. Factors identified as influencing outcome include the gestational age at which the rupture of membranes occurred and the development of, duration of, and severity of oligohydramnios.

LUNG HYPOPLASIA AND DEVELOPMENTAL DISORDERS IN OTHER ORGANS Renal agenesis with oligohydramnios has been associated with pulmonary hypoplasia. Because of the widespread use of antenatal ultrasonography, the incidence of cases of renal agenesis appears to be diminishing. Therefore, this particular cause of lethal pulmonary hypoplasia is also diminishing. Developmental defects in growth of spinal cord and rib cage may prevent the development of a normal thoracic volume. Thus, fetal lung growth is restricted, and gas exchange surface area available at birth is limited.

Experimental phrenic nerve denervation in sheep fetuses has demonstrated the importance of regular fetal breathing movements to normal lung development. Primary central nervous system disorders, including anencephaly or hydranencephaly, are associated with pulmonary hypoplasia. In these conditions, the paucity of mechanical forces associated with inadequate fetal breathing inhibits normal development of the fetal lung, especially during the second half of gestation. The result is variable hypoplasia. Additional rare causes of pulmonary hypoplasia are the skeletal dysplasias. These syndromes need to be considered in the management of patients presenting with unexpected respiratory difficulties.

Clinical features of infants with pulmonary hypoplasia include small chest circumference and severe respiratory embarrassment. Positive-pressure ventilation may not produce significant improvement. Pulmonary air-leak complications, including pulmonary interstitial emphysema and unilateral pneumothorax, often develop. Chest radiographs show the variable appearance of the thoracic cavity and lungs in pulmonary hypoplasia. Sublethal forms of this problem can result in development of lifelong lung dysfunction.

References

Broughton AR, Thibeault DW, Mabry SM, Truog WE: Airway muscle in infants with congenital diaphragmatic hernia: response to treatment. J Pediatr Surg 33:1471, 1998

Karamanoukian HL, Glick PL, Zayek M, et al: Inhaled nitric oxide in congenital hypoplasia of the lungs due to diaphragmatic hernia or oligohydramnios. Pediatr 94:715, 1994

Langham, MR, Kays DW, Ledbetter DJ, et al: Congenital diaphragmatic hernia: epidemiology and outcome. New insights into the pathophysiology of congenital diaphragmatic hernia. Clin Perinatol 23:671–688, 1996

Nio M, Haase G, Kennaugh J, et al: A prospective randomized trial of delayed versus immediate repair of congenital diaphragmatic hernia. J Pediatr Surg 29:618, 1994

Thibeault DW, Haney B: Lung volume, pulmonary vasculature, and factors affecting survival in congenital diaphragmatic hernia. Pediatrics 101:289, 1998.

2.17.14   Polycythemia (Hyperviscosity Syndrome)

Joseph A. Kitterman

Polycythemia in newborn infants is usually defined as a venous hematocrit >65%. With a high hematocrit, viscosity is increased, which impedes blood flow to tissues and may lead to serious organ dysfunction. This is referred to as *neonatal polycythemia* or the *hyperviscosity syndrome*. The reported incidence of neonatal polycythemia varies from 1 to 5%, although only a minority of these infants exhibits clinical signs related to hyperviscosity.

PATHOPHYSIOLOGY

Blood flow through a vessel depends on several variables, as defined by Poiseuille's law:

$$\dot{Q} = \frac{\Delta P \pi r^4}{8 l \eta}$$

where $\dot{Q}$ = blood flow, ΔP = arteriovenous pressure difference, r = radius, l = length of the blood vessel, and η = blood viscosity. Resistance to flow (R) in a blood vessel is defined as $\Delta P / \dot{Q}$. Therefore, if this is applied to Poiseuille's law, resistance to blood flow can be defined as:

$$R = \frac{8 l \eta}{\pi r^4}$$

Because resistance is inversely proportional to the fourth power of the radius but only directly proportional to viscosity and to blood vessel length, the main determinant of vascular resistance is the radius of the blood vessel. However, viscosity increases with increasing hematocrit and rises markedly as hematocrit approaches 70% (Fig. 2-61), possibly because of rouleaux formation. Therefore, polycythemia raises both systemic and pulmonary vascular resistance. Acidosis decreases deformability of red blood cells and thereby increases blood viscosity. Viscosity is also directly proportional to the concentration of plasma proteins, especially fibrinogen. Because the concentration of plasma proteins increases with gestational age and after birth, for any given hematocrit blood viscosity is generally higher in term than in preterm infants.

Hypoglycemia often accompanies polycythemia. With increased hematocrit, there is decreased plasma volume, and thus decreased glucose in whole blood. Also, as blood flow decreases because of hyperviscosity, less glucose is delivered to tissues. As discussed below, this process can be aggravated in certain conditions that are associated with a high incidence of polycythemia, such as maternal diabetes mellitus and fetal growth restriction from placental insufficiency.

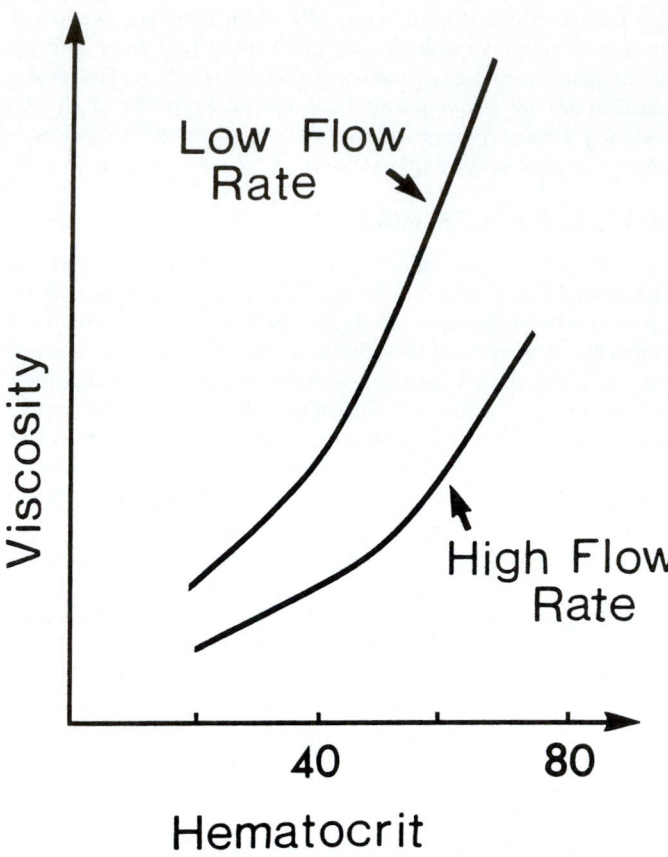

FIGURE 2-61   **Effects of hematocrit and shear rate on blood viscosity. Note that at any hematocrit, viscosity is higher at low shear rates. (Courtesy of R. H. Phibbs.)**

ETIOLOGY

In the near-term fetus, hematocrit is relatively high, about 55%, and is increased by chronic fetal hypoxemia (eg, placental insufficiency, altitude, maternal smoking). Total blood volume in the fetoplacental circulation is about 120 mL/kg, of which 30 mL/kg is in the placenta and the rest in the fetus. At birth, some placental blood moves into the fetus. Factors that increase this placental transfusion include increased duration of time between birth and cord clamping in vaginal births, holding the infant below the level of the uterus, and stripping or milking the cord toward the infant before cord clamping. With cesarean section, placental transfusion is relatively small and does not increase if cord clamping is delayed. When placental transfusion is large, the newborn will be hypervolemic. Extravasation of fluid from the circulation is a homeostatic mechanism by which blood volume can be reduced toward normal. Because red blood cell mass remains constant, hematocrit rises. This equilibration of blood volume begins immediately after birth and usually is complete within 4 hours.

Clinical conditions that are associated with a high incidence of neonatal polycythemia include, as noted above, chronic fetal hypoxemia and placental transfusion, as well as maternal diabetes mellitus, maternal hypertension, twin-to-twin transfusion, maternal–fetal transfusion, trisomy 21, hyperthyroidism, and congenital adrenal hyperplasia.

CLINICAL SIGNS

With excessive placental transfusion, the resultant hypervolemia may lead to very early evidence of respiratory distress. Signs attributable to polycythemia (ie, hyperviscosity) are usually apparent in the first few hours after birth. High blood viscosity slows flow and may lead to rouleaux formation, sludging, formation of microthrombi, platelet consumption, and, in severe cases, tissue infarction. The clinical signs depend on the organ systems that are most affected by polycythemia (Table 2-32). Studies in experimental animals indicate that as hematocrit approaches 70%, pulmonary vascular resistance exceeds systemic vascular resistance. Some polycythemic infants present with persistent pulmonary hypertension and findings that mimic cyanotic congenital heart disease.

LABORATORY FINDINGS

Infants with hyperviscosity are polycythemic, and in the vast majority, the venous hematocrit is >65%. Occasionally, hyperviscosity is present when the venous hematocrit is between 60 and 65%. Thrombocytopenia is thought to result from consumption of platelets in microthrombi and is indicative of obstruction in the microcirculation. Arterial oxygen saturation may be decreased from right-to-left shunting of blood through the foramen ovale and ductus arteriosus or from intrapulmonary shunting. Jaundice is common and results from sludging and breakdown of red blood cells. As noted above, hypoglycemia is common and may contribute to CNS injury. Pulmonary radiographic findings in polycythemic infants may include an enlarged cardiac shadow, apparently increased pulmonary vasculature, and pulmonary edema.

MANAGEMENT

Although hyperviscosity is the abnormality that leads to clinical disease, viscosity measurements are not usually available in the clinical setting. Therefore, the best screening tool for hyperviscosity in newborn infants is hematocrit. Hematocrit should be measured at age 2 to 4 hours in all infants at risk for polycythemia. These include infants of diabetic mothers, infants of hypertensive mothers, infants who are either abnormally small or abnormally large for their gestational age, and those with trisomy 21. Ideally, all infants should have hematocrit measured to detect unsuspected anemia as well as polycythemia. Because hematocrit calculated from hemoglobin concentration and red blood cell count may give falsely low values, hematocrit should be measured by microcentrifugation. A capillary blood hematocrit can be used for screening. If it is greater than 65%, venous hematocrit should be measured.

For infants with signs consistent with hyperviscosity and he-

TABLE 2-32

CLINICAL SIGNS ASSOCIATED WITH NEONATAL POLYCYTHEMIA

ORGAN SYSTEM	CLINICAL SIGNS
Pulmonary	Tachypnea, grunting, retractions, cyanosis, persistent pulmonary hypertension
Central nervous system	
Mild	Lethargy, irritability, tremors, abnormal cry
Severe	Apnea, hypotonia, seizures
Hematologic	Thrombocytopenia, jaundice
Renal	Oliguria, hematuria, renal vein thrombosis
Metabolic	Hypoglycemia
Gastrointestinal	Abdominal distension, blood in stools, pneumatosis intestinalis
Skin	Plethora, acrocyanosis, prolonged capillary filling time

matocrit >65%, the hematocrit should be reduced (see below). For those with clinical signs and hematocrit of 60 to 65%, serious consideration should be given to reducing the hematocrit.

For polycythemic infants without clinical signs of hyperviscosity, most clinicians recommend reduction of hematocrit if it exceeds 70%. There is less agreement regarding management of asymptomatic infants with hematocrit values of 65 to 70%. Neurologic outcome is an important factor that has led many to reduce hematocrit in asymptomatic polycythemic infants. Once neurologic signs related to hyperviscosity become present, 30 to 40% of infants will have abnormal neurologic findings on follow-up. Therefore, the aim of reducing hematocrit in asymptomatic polycythemic infants is to prevent neurologic injury.

REDUCTION OF HEMATOCRIT

Reduction of hematocrit should be by partial exchange transfusion with a plasma substitute. Simple phlebotomy is contraindicated because it decreases arterial blood pressure as well as blood volume. The decrease in systemic arterial pressure will decrease blood flow (see Poiseuille's equation above) and thus increase viscosity and its effects. The fluid used for the reduction exchange transfusion should be 0.9% NaCl or Ringer lactate solution, either of which is as effective as 5% albumin for reducing hematocrit. The volume to be exchanged can be calculated from the equation:

$$\text{volume (mL)} = \frac{\text{Hct}_I - \text{Hct}_D}{\text{Hct}_I} \times \text{body weight (kg)} \times 90 \text{ mL/kg}$$

Where volume is the total volume to be exchanged (mL), Hct_I = current hematocrit, Hct_D = desired hematocrit (usually 55%), and 90 mL/kg is the infant's estimated blood volume. In some cases where there is hypervolemia as well as polycythemia, the procedure may have to be repeated if the hematocrit rises again in the first few hours after completion of the reduction exchange transfusion.

The reduction exchange transfusion can be performed through an umbilical arterial or venous catheter. If the umbilical artery is used, care should be taken to maintain the tip of the catheter below the third lumbar vertebra, (ie, below the origins of the renal and inferior mesenteric arteries). If the umbilical vein is used, the tip of the catheter should be in the right atrium or inferior vena cava and not in the portal circulation. This is to avoid the decrease in intestinal blood flow that occurs when exchange transfusions are performed with the catheter tip in the portal venous circulation. If the catheter tip cannot be advanced through the ductus venosus and remains in the portal system, the procedure can be done safely by withdrawing blood from the venous catheter and infusing the exchange fluid into a peripheral vein.

It is important to prevent hypoglycemia and hypocalcemia, conditions that frequently accompany polycythemia and that may reduce cardiac output, thus worsening the effects of polycythemia. The platelet count should be measured. Thrombocytopenia may be indicative of microthrombi with tissue ischemia. Because of the association of necrotizing enterocolitis with polycythemia, infants with polycythemia who are thrombocytopenic should not be given enteral feedings until the platelet count increases to normal.

References

Aperia A, Berqvist G, Broberger O, et al: Renal function in infants with high hematocrit values before and after isovolemic haemodilution. Acta Paediatr Scand 63:878, 1974

Arendar G, Samara E, Palmas C: Neonatal acquired paraplegia: retrospective review of 30 patients. J Pediatr Orthoped [Part B] 8:80, 1999

Black VD, Lubchenco LO, Koops BL, et al: Neonatal hyperviscosity: randomized study of effect of partial plasma exchange transfusion on long term outcome. Pediatrics 75:1048.

Bonillo A, Martainez S, Uberos J, et al: Repercussions of acidosis on postnatal erythrocyte deformability in term and preterm newborns. Am J Perinatol 15:115, 1998

Brans YW, Shannon DL, Ramamurthy RS: Neonatal polycythemia: II. Plasma, blood and red cell volume estimates in relation to hematocrit levels and quality of intrauterine growth. Pediatrics 68:175, 1981

Delaney-Black V, Camp BW, Lubchenco LO, et al: Neonatal hyperviscosity association with lower achievement and IQ scores at school age. Pediatrics 83:662, 1989

Drew JH, Guaran RL, Cichello M, Hobbs J: Neonatal whole blood hyperviscosity: the important factor influencing later neurologic function is viscosity and not the polycythemia. Clin Hemorheol Microcirc 17:67, 1997

Fouron JC, Hebert F: The circulatory effects of hematocrit variations in normovolemic newborn lambs. J Pediatr 82:995, 1973

Gatti RA, Muster AJ, Cole RB, Paul MH: Neonatal polycythemia with transient cyanosis and cardiorespiratory abnormalities. J Pediatr 69:1063, 1966

Gross GP, Hathaway WE, McGaughey HR: Hyperviscosity in the neonate. J Pediatr 82:1004, 1973

Hein HA, Lathrop SS: Partial exchange transfusion in term, polycythemic neonates: absence of association with severe gastrointestinal injury. Pediatrics 80:75, 1987

Kleinberg F, Dong L, Phibbs RH: Cesarean section delivery prevents placenta-to-infant transfusion despite delayed cord clamping. Am J Obstet Gynecol 121:66, 1975

Kurlat I, Sola A: Neonatal polycythemia in appropriately grown infants of hypertensive mothers. Acta Paediatr Scand 81:662, 1992

Leibson C, Brown M, Thibodeau, et al: neonatal hyperbilirubinemia at high altitude. Am J Dis Child 143:983, 1989

Ramamurthy RS, Brans YW: Neonatal polycythemia: I. Criteria for diagnosis and treatment. J Pediatr 68:168, 1981

Roithmaier A, Arlettaz R, Bauer K, et al: Randomized controlled trial of Ringer solution versus serum for partial exchange transfusion in neonatal polycythaemia. Eur J Pediatr 154:53, 1995

Shohat M, Merlob P, Reisner SH: Neonatal polycythemia: I. Early diagnosis and incidence related to time of sampling. Pediatrics 73:7, 1984

Stevens K, Wirth FH: Incidence of neonatal hyperviscosity at sea level. J Pediatr 97:118, 1980

Surjadhana A, Rouleau J, Boerboom L, Hoffman JIE: Myocardial blood flow and its distribution in anesthetized polycythemic dogs. Circ Res 43:619, 1978

Werner EJ: Neonatal polycythemia and hyperviscosity. Clin Perinatol 22:693, 1995

Wong W, Fok TF, Lee CH, et al: Randomised controlled trial: comparison of colloid or crystalloid for partial exchange transfusion for treatment of neonatal polycythaemia. Arch Dis Child, Fetal Neonat Ed 77:F115, 1997

Wood JL: Plethora in the newborn associated with cyanosis and convulsions. J Pediatr 54:143, 1959

Yao AC, Lind J: Placental transfusion. Am J Dis Child 127:128, 1974

Zimmerman D: Fetal and neonatal hyperthyroidism. Thyroid 9:727, 1999

2.17.15 Meconium Aspiration Syndrome

Eduardo Bancalari

Meconium aspiration syndrome (MAS) is one of the most common causes of severe respiratory failure in infants born at term or postterm gestation. Meconium is present in the amniotic fluid in approximately 10 to 20% of all term deliveries, but MAS occurs in fewer than one-third of these infants. The presence of meconium in the amniotic fluid is very uncommon in preterm deliveries. The risk for MAS and associated respiratory failure is considerably increased when the meconium is thick or particulate and when it is associated with perinatal asphyxia. Some infants are born through meconium-stained amniotic fluid and exhibit respiratory distress even when no meconium is visualized below the vocal cords at birth. In such infants, aspiration may have occurred in utero before the delivery.

PATHOGENESIS

The passage of intestinal contents into the amniotic fluid is frequently associated with evidence of fetal distress, but it also may occur with normal or breech deliveries in which there is no evidence of fetal asphyxia. Prior fetal hypoxia and acidosis can induce deep respiratory efforts that draw meconium-contaminated fluid into the airways (Fig. 2-62).

At birth, a negative intrathoracic pressure is generated that facilitates aspiration of material in the nasopharynx. For this reason it has been proposed that the risk of massive aspiration of meconium can be reduced by effective nasopharyngeal suction performed at the time of birth, preferably before the chest emerges from the birth canal.

CLINICAL PRESENTATION

MAS occurs most often in term or postmature infants who have a history of fetal distress, low Apgar scores, and meconium-stained amniotic fluid. Such infants often have meconium-stained skin, nails, and umbilical cord and present with signs of respiratory distress shortly after birth, with tachypnea, intercostal retractions, and cyanosis. The chest appears overdistended, frequently barrel-shaped, with a protruding sternum. The breath sounds are usually obscured by coarse bronchial sounds, and expiration can be prolonged when there is small airway obstruction. The chest roentgenogram shows bilateral patchy areas of increased density, sometimes confluent and alternating with hyperlucent areas. (Fig. 2-63). The diaphragm is occasionally depressed, and air leaks are common in severe cases (Fig. 2-64).

Arterial blood during the first hour after birth usually reveals hypoxemia and some degree of metabolic acidosis that reflects peri-

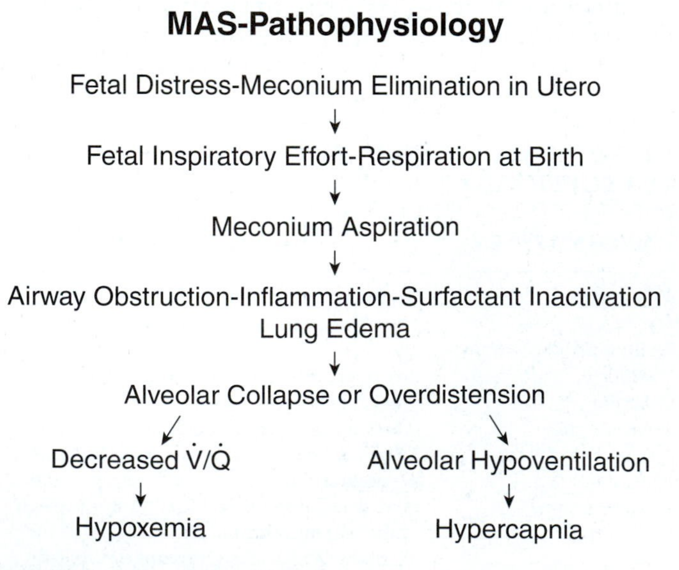

MAS-Pathophysiology

Fetal Distress-Meconium Elimination in Utero

↓

Fetal Inspiratory Effort-Respiration at Birth

↓

Meconium Aspiration

↓

Airway Obstruction-Inflammation-Surfactant Inactivation
Lung Edema

↓

Alveolar Collapse or Overdistension

↙ ↘

Decreased $\dot{V}/\dot{Q}$ Alveolar Hypoventilation

↓   ↓

Hypoxemia   Hypercapnia

FIGURE 2-62 Pathophysiology of meconium aspiration syndrome.

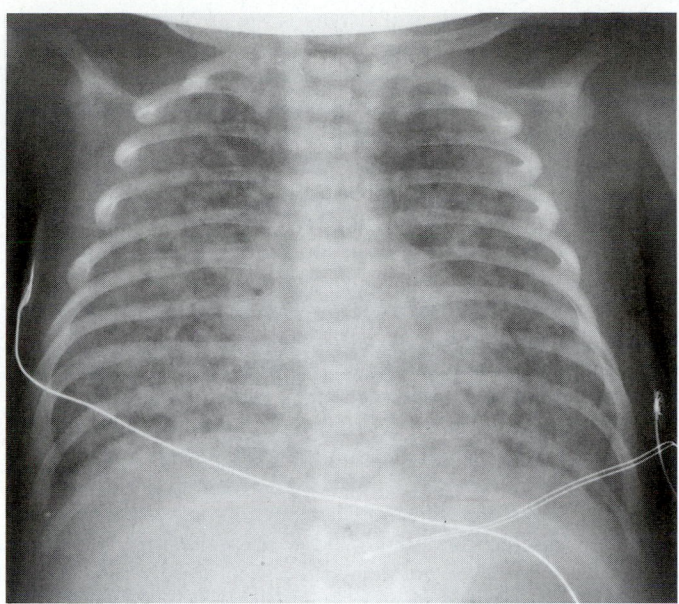

FIGURE 2-63   Chest radiograph from an infant with severe meconium aspiration syndrome showing bilateral patchy areas of increased density.

natal asphyxia. Most infants with MAS require supplemental inspired oxygen to maintain normal oxygenation. The severity of the hypoxemia depends on the degree of the pulmonary damage and is more severe in infants with pulmonary hypertension who have right-to-left shunting through the foramen ovale and ductus arteriosus. The $PaCO_2$ may be normal or even low soon after birth but subsequently may increase as the lung disease worsens, signaling the need for mechanical ventilation.

Infants with severe MAS have frequent complications, many of which may be life threatening. Pulmonary overdistension, often leading to a pneumomediastinum and/or pneumothorax, occurs in 10 to 15% of infants with MAS who require mechanical ventilation. Air leaks result from small airway obstruction that leads to uneven distribution of the inspired gas and trapping of gas in some

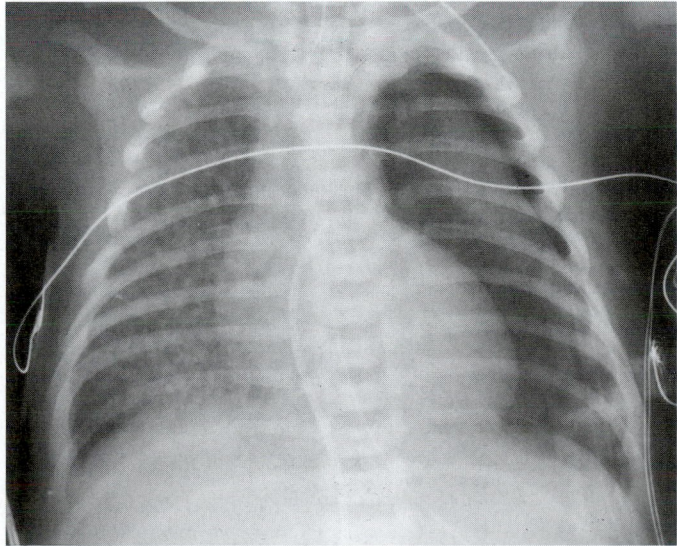

FIGURE 2-64   Same infant as in Fig. 2-63 after development of a left tension pneumothorax.

of the terminal air sacs. The risk of an air leak is increased by the high transpulmonary pressure generated by the infant or that is delivered by the mechanical ventilator to maintain adequate ventilation. Meconium also induces inflammation of lung tissue, which may contribute to the increased susceptibility to alveolar rupture.

Persistent pulmonary hypertension with right-to-left shunting of blood across the foramen ovule and ductus arteriosus with resultant hypoxemia is a frequent and severe complication of MAS that is discussed elsewhere in this chapter (see Sec. 2.17.11).

Secondary bacterial infection of the lungs is another complication of MAS. In experimental animals meconium instillation enhances bacterial growth and proliferation in the lung. Because of the similarities in the clinical and radiographic manifestations of meconium aspiration and bacterial pneumonia, it is very difficult to diagnose a superimposed bacterial infection during the acute phase of MAS; therefore, one must have a high index of suspicion. Also, infants who are infected in utero have a higher incidence of perinatal asphyxia and meconium aspiration, and therefore, MAS may be superimposed on a congenital pneumonia. Upper airway damage can occur in infants with MAS during the airway suction performed immediately after delivery. Infants with severe MAS who require prolonged mechanical ventilation also may acquire airway damage and subglottic stenosis secondary to the extended presence of the endotracheal tube.

The clinical course of MAS depends on the severity of the initial pulmonary involvement and on the occurrence of complications such as persistent pulmonary hypertension (Sec. 2.17.11), infection, or pneumothorax that can delay recovery. Whereas mild cases may require only oxygen supplementation for a few hours or days, infants with severe respiratory failure require mechanical ventilation for several days or even weeks and have a high mortality rate. In a series of infants with MAS, approximately 30% required mechanical ventilation with an overall mortality of about 4%.

Initially it is difficult to predict the clinical course that an infant with MAS will follow, and outcome is determined mainly by the presence of complications. In general, infants who have large amounts of thick meconium in the trachea and grossly abnormal chest radiographs have a more severe subsequent course, but this is not always the case.

PULMONARY FUNCTION

Few studies describing changes in pulmonary function associated with aspiration of meconium have been reported. When thick particulate meconium is aspirated into the small airways, these become partially obstructed, resulting in gas trapping and alveolar overinflation distal to the obstruction. The small airways obstruction also can result in ventilation-perfusion mismatching that manifests as hypoxemia. The increased airway resistance, combined with reduced lung compliance, often leads to increased work of breathing and resultant alveolar hypoventilation and CO_2 retention characteristic of the more severe cases of meconium aspiration. When the small airways are completely obstructed, the alveolar gas distal to the obstruction is absorbed. Resultant alveolar collapse increases intrapulmonary shunting and causes more severe arterial hypoxemia. The presence of meconium in the airways also can trigger an inflammatory reaction, resulting in a diffuse chemical pneumonitis. This can reduce the diffusing capacity and futher contribute to the hypoxemia observed in these patients.

Neonates with severe MAS have a marked reduction in dynamic lung compliance, perhaps secondary to the inflammatory reaction produced by the meconium or to inactivation of alveolar surfactant by meconium within alveoli. Increased airway resistance also may contribute to abnormal dynamic compliance. Minute ventilation is usually increased as a consequence of an increased respiratory rate, but because the tidal volume is reduced, there is an increase in dead space ventilation, and alveolar ventilation is decreased.

MANAGEMENT

Many infants with MAS have suffered some degree of perinatal asphyxia, and for this reason their respiratory course can be complicated by dysfunction of other organ systems, notably the brain, heart, liver, and kidneys.

In infants with clinical signs of respiratory failure, oxygen saturation by pulse oximetry, arterial blood gases, and a chest radiograph should be obtained as soon as possible. An increased inspired oxygen concentration must be provided to maintain the PaO_2 above 70 to 80 mm Hg or the oxygen saturation above 95%.

Some degree of metabolic acidosis is frequently observed as a result of perinatal asphyxia. If persistent, this must be corrected to decrease the risk of pulmonary vasoconstriction and hypertension. In infants who remain hypoxemic despite the use of high inspired oxygen concentration, or when their $PaCO_2$ increases rapidly to greater than 50 to 60 mm Hg, it becomes necessary to apply mechanical ventilation. Because of the reduced lung compliance and increased airways resistance, these infants often require high peak inspiratory pressures to maintain adequate ventilation and oxygenation. This, plus the meconium-induced lung damage, makes the occurrence of pneumothorax a relatively frequent complication. Because most of these infants are hyperactive and restless, it is often necessary to use sedation or even neuromuscular blockade, at least during the first 24 to 48 hours of mechanical ventilation, until the infant is stable and the peak airway pressure can be reduced.

In infants with severe respiratory failure who do not respond to conventional mechanical ventilation, the use of high-frequency ventilation may improve gas exchange. This is usually indicated when pulmonary hypertension occurs with associated right-to-left shunting of blood and severe hypoxemia, or when excessive peak inspiratory pressures are required to achieve adequate ventilation. Because meconium aspiration can inactivate alveolar surfactant, the administration of exogenous surfactant or even pulmonary lavage with a surfactant solution sometimes can be beneficial.

Because the risk of bacterial infection is increased in infants with MAS, bacterial pneumonia should be suspected when there is fever, an abnormal white blood count, or a deterioration in respiratory function and radiographic picture. Accordingly, cultures of blood and tracheal secretions should be obtained, and antibiotic therapy initiated. There is no clear evidence to justify the use of prophylactic antibiotics in meconium aspiration, but because of the difficulty in diagnosing a superimposed infection, many clinicians elect to treat these infants with antibiotics until the acute respiratory failure subsides.

PREVENTION

When meconium appears in the amniotic fluid or is present in the upper airway at the time of birth, the first concern should be to reduce the risk of aspiration of the meconium into the more distal air spaces and thereby prevent the subsequent pulmonary involvement. The recommended approach has been to suction the nasopharynx with a large catheter or a suction bulb, if possible, before the chest emerges from the birth canal. If thick meconium is present in the nasopharynx, this procedure is followed by direct visualiza-

tion of the vocal cords with laryngoscopy. When meconium is present below the vocal cords, tracheal suctioning is accomplished using the endotracheal tube until the airway is clear of meconium. The aspiration must be repeated until all meconium is removed from the larger airways. The suction of the endotracheal tube can be accomplished utilizing a number of available mechanical suction devices. Mouth suction should be avoided to prevent aspiration of contaminated material by the operator. Infants with previous intrapartum asphyxia and meconium aspiration should receive 100% oxygen immediately after birth in order to increase arterial oxygenation and reverse the pulmonary hypertension that accompanies hypoxemia and acidosis.

Recently, there has been controversy on the delivery room approach to the meconium-stained infant. Several studies have suggested that infants who are vigorous at birth should not be exposed to the risk of endotracheal suctioning because the incidence of MAS in these infants is extremely low. Based on these studies it has been recommended to limit direct tracheal suction only to those infants who are exposed to meconium and are depressed at birth. Some investigators have even questioned the need of early nasopharyngeal suction before the infant emerges from the birth canal. As this is a relatively simple and low-risk procedure, most clinicians still recommend early suctioning of the nasopharynx when there is any evidence of meconium in the amniotic fluid with the purpose of reducing the risk of aspiration of this material into the lower airways.

Although most infants with MAS survive without sequelae, long-term follow-up studies have demonstrated an increased prevalence of neurologic sequelae most likely associated with perinatal asphyxia. Hyperreactive airway disease, similar to that observed in premature infants who require prolonged mechanical ventilation, has also been described in infants who have recovered from severe MAS.

References

Bancalari E, Berlin JA: Meconium aspiration and other asphyxial disorders. Clin Perinatol 5:317–334, 1978

Bent RC, Wiswell TE, Chang A: Removing meconium from infant trachea. What works best? Am J Dis Child 146:1085–1089, 1992

Carson BS, Losey RW, Bowes WA JR, et al: Combined obstetric and pediatric approach to prevent meconium aspiration syndrome. Am J Obstet Gynecol 126:712–715, 1976

Cochrane CG, Revak SD, Merritt TA, et al: Bronchoalveolar lavage with KL_4-surfactant in models of meconium aspiration syndrome. Pediatr Res 44:705–715, 1998

Dye T, Aubry R, Gross S, et al: Amnioinfusion and the intrauterine prevention of meconium aspiration. Am J Obstet Gynecol 171:1601–1605, 1994

Falciglia HS, Henderschott C, Potter P, et al: Does DeLee suction at the perineum prevent meconium aspiration syndrome? Am J Obstet Gynecol 167:1243–1249, 1992

Fuloria M, Wiswell TE: Resuscitation of the meconium-stained infant and prevention of meconium aspiration syndrome. J Perinatol 19:234–241, 1999

Greenough A: Meconium aspiration syndrome—prevention and treatment. Early Hum Dev 41:183–192, 1995

Gregory GA, Gooding CA, Phibbs RH, et al: Meconium aspiration in infants—a prospective study. J Pediatr 85:848–852, 1974

Holopainen R, Aho H, Laine J, et al: Human meconium has high phospholipase A_2 activity and induces cellular injury and apoptosis in piglet lungs. Pediatr Res 46:626–632, 1999

Holtzman RB, Banzhaf WC, Silver RK, et al: Perinatal management of meconium staining of the amniotic fluid. Clin Perinatol 16:825–838, 1989

Lam BCC, Yeung CY: Surfactant lavage for meconium aspiration syndrome: a pilot study. Pediatrics 103:1014–1018, 1999

Linder N, Aranda JV, Tsur M, et al: Need for endotracheal intubation and suction in meconium-stained neonates. J Pediatr 112:613–615, 1988

MacFarlane PI, Heaf DP: Pulmonary function in children after neonatal meconium aspiration syndrome. Arch Dis Child 63:368–372, 1988

Peng TCC, Gutcher GR, Van Dorsten P: A selective aggressive approach to the neonate exposed to meconium-stained amniotic fluid. Am J Obstet Gynecol 175:296–303, 1996

Rossi EM, Philipson EH, Williams TG, et al: Meconium aspiration syndrome: intrapartum and neonatal attributes. Am J Obstet Gynecol 161:1106–1110, 1989

Spong CY, Ogundipe OA, Ross MG: Prophylactic amnioinfusion for meconium-stained amniotic fluid. Am J Obstet Gynecol 171:931–935, 1994

Sun BO, Curstedt T, Robertson B: Exogenous surfactant improves ventilation efficiency and alveolar expansion in rats with meconium aspiration. Am J Respir Crit Care Med 154:764–770, 1996

Swaminathan S, Quinn J, Stabile MW, et al: Long-term pulmonary sequelae of meconium aspiration syndrome. J Pediatr 114:356–361, 1989

Ting P, Brady JP: Tracheal suction in meconium aspiration. Am J Obstet Gynecol 122:767–771, 1975

Wiswell TE, Fuloria M: Management of meconium-stained amniotic fluid. Clin Perinatol 26:659–668, 1999

Wiswell TE, Henley MA: Intratracheal suctioning, systemic infection, and the meconium aspiration syndrome. Pediatrics 89:203–206, 1992

Wiswell TE, Tuggle JM, Turner BS: Meconium aspiration syndrome: have we made a difference? Pediatrics 85:715–721, 1990

Yeh TF, Lilien LD, Barathi A, et al: Lung volume, dynamic lung compliance, and blood gases during the first 3 days of postnatal life in infants with meconium aspiration syndrome. Crit Care Med 10:588–592, 1982

2.17.16   Hematologic Disorders of the Newborn

William B. Slayton and William L. Carroll

FETAL/NEONATAL HEMATOPOIESIS

During fetal development, blood formation occurs first in the yolk sac, where erythrocytes and macrophages are observed by 16 to 29 days postconception. By 4 to 5 weeks of gestation, the liver becomes the primary organ of hematopoiesis and continues to be the major site of production from the third to the sixth fetal month. All hematopoietic lineages are produced in the liver. The bone marrow does not assume a major role in hematopoiesis until the last trimester. Extramedullary hematopoiesis can occur in many organs, including the liver, spleen, and skin, in the setting of congenital infection, hemolysis, or bone marrow failure.

Fetal erythropoiesis is associated with a stepwise evolution of hemoglobin production that continues through the first 6 months of postnatal life. Eight genes encode six different hemoglobins. The ξ and α genes are located on chromosome 16 and are duplicated, resulting in four transcribed genes. The β locus is comprised of a succession of genes, ϵ, γ_1, γ_2, δ and β, residing on chromosome 11. Embryonic hemoglobin, comprised of ξ joined with ϵ or λ, is produced in erythrocytes in the yolk sac. Subsequently, fetal hemoglobin ($\alpha_2\gamma_2$) becomes the predominant hemoglobin during the second gestational month. Production of hemoglobin A (HbA) (α_2,β_2) starts at week 6 and increases rapidly during the third trimester. At term birth, HbA makes up less than 30% of the total hemoglobin, which explains why structural defects of the β chain, such as sickle cell disease and β-thalassemia, rarely are apparent during the newborn period. HbF has a higher affinity for oxygen than HbA. This higher affinity allows maternal erythrocytes to deliver oxygen to the fetus via the placental circulation (Fig. 2-65).

NEONATAL ANEMIA

Adaptation to the hypoxia of the intrauterine environment includes increased production of erythrocytes and hemoglobin. As a result, newborns have a relatively high hemoglobin concentration, averaging 16.5 g/dL. Improved oxygenation at birth results in an abrupt decrease in the production of erythropoietin (Epo), the primary growth factor that stimulates red blood cell production. During the 2 months after birth, red cell production decreases precipitously. During the "physiological nadir," the hemoglobin averages 9.5 g/dL (see Sec. 19.1.2). The hematocrit gradually rises at approximately 4 months. Preterm infants experience a lower nadir, with hemoglobin concentrations approaching 7 to 8 g/dL (see Fig. 2-65).

Another variable that influences hemoglobin concentration after birth is blood transfer from the placenta to the neonate before the umbilical cord is clamped. The placenta contains 75 to 100 mL of blood. This blood can flow to the infant through the umbilical vein, depending on the level of the infant relative to the placenta. Approximately one-half of the placental transfusion normally takes place within the first minute after birth, and delayed clamping may increase hemoglobin concentration by up to 3 g/dL postnatally.

Neonatal anemia can be classified according to the cause, such as hemorrhage, decreased erythrocyte production (hypoplastic anemia), or increased destruction (hemolytic anemia).

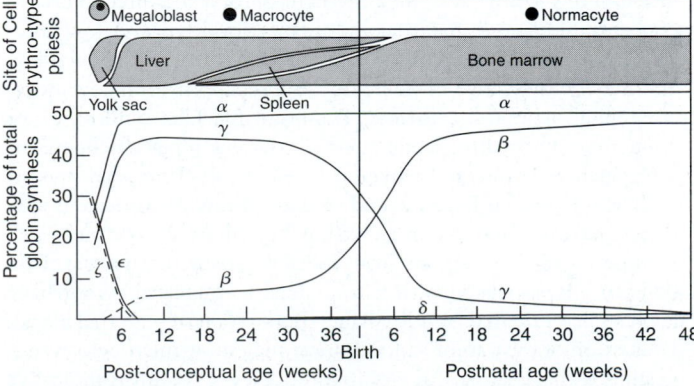

FIGURE 2-65   A depiction of the contributions of the various types of hemoglobin during human fetal development. SOURCE: *Weatherall and Clegg, The Thalassemia Syndromes, London, Blackwell, 1981.*

HEMORRHAGE Blood loss can occur before birth, at delivery, or after birth. Half of all pregnancies are associated with trivial (less than 2 mL) fetal-to-maternal hemorrhage. Risk factors for clinically significant fetal-to-maternal hemorrhage include third-trimester amniocentesis and trauma. Evidence of fetal-to-maternal hemorrhage relies on the demonstration of fetal cells within the maternal circulation.

Disorders of the placenta also can lead to hemorrhage, and include placental abruption, resulting from premature separation of the placenta from the uterus; placenta previa, wherein the placenta implants directly over the cervical opening; and rupture of the umbilical cord. Fetal-to-fetal hemorrhage occurs in the 30% of monozygotic twins who have monochorial placentas.

Anemia can result from bleeding within the neonate. Subgaleal hemorrhage can occur during difficult deliveries. Substantial bleeding can occur into the subaponeurotic space, which is not limited by periosteal attachments. Cephalohematomas, which are limited by periosteal attachments, usually lead to jaundice without anemia. Traumatic delivery, as associated with breech presentation, may result in bleeding within the retroperitoneum, liver, kidneys, spleen, or adrenal glands. Such hemorrhage can induce shock. Infants with a liver laceration may appear well for 24 to 48 hours until rupture of the capsule occurs. Abdominal distension and a palpable mass suggest subcapsular hemorrhage. Liver hemorrhage has a high associated mortality.

A major cause of anemia in the neonatal intensive care unit is red cell depletion from repeated phlebotomy. Efforts minimizing blood withdrawal by using "micromethodology," by reinfusing withdrawn blood, and by transcutaneous monitoring of hemoglobin saturation, PO_2 and PCO_2 have decreased the incidence of anemia in newborns receiving intensive care.

PREMATURITY The anticipated postnatal decrease in hemoglobin concentration is more pronounced for preterm infants less than 32 weeks of gestation than it is for term infants. The etiology of anemia of prematurity is uncertain but may be related to low levels of the erythrocyte cytokine Epo. Erythroid progenitor cells from preterm infants are highly sensitive to Epo, indicating that the mechanism of anemia may relate to a deficient growth factor stimulus. Given the low Epo levels in these patients, it is not surprising that many clinical trials have evaluated the effectiveness of Epo for improving hemoglobin concentrations and decreasing the need for blood transfusions. Most randomized studies have shown that Epo decreases both the number of transfusions and the volume of blood transfused. Supplemental iron is necessary to provide maximum benefit from Epo. Infants who received a placebo in these trials were transfused less, suggesting that adoption of transfusion guidelines also may reduce the need for transfusions.

HEMOLYSIS Hemolysis usually presents as unconjugated hyperbilirubinemia at birth or within the first 24 hours after delivery. Hemolysis can result from several mechanisms (see Sec. 19.5), including RBC membrane defects such as spherocytosis and elliptocytosis, enzyme defects including glucose-6-phosphate dehydrogenase (G6PD) deficiency, production defects such as α-thalassemia, and structural defects of the α or γ globin chains. These conditions can cause severe neonatal jaundice that peaks between the second and third day of life. Severe cases of neonatal hemolytic anemia caused by G6PD deficiency can occur after maternal ingestion of oxidant compounds such as sulfa drugs and fava beans.

Vitamin E deficiency can lead to hemolysis because of tocopherol's role in preventing oxidation of components of the erythrocyte membrane. Most vitamin E is transported to the fetus during the third trimester, and preterm infants are at greatest risk for deficiency. Infant formulas containing supplemental vitamin E have substantially reduced the incidence of this condition.

Hemolytic anemia also may occur as a complication of bacterial or viral infection. Bacterial sepsis from *Escherichia coli* or group B streptococcal disease can lead to disseminated intravascular coagulation with profound erythrocyte destruction. Hepatosplenomegaly and jaundice may occur. In contrast to immune hemolytic anemia, conjugated hyperbilirubinemia predominates in infection-mediated hemolysis. Congenital infections from cytomegalovirus, toxoplasmosis, herpes simplex, syphilis, rubella, and human immunodeficiency virus also are associated with hemolysis.

Hemolytic disorders may result from an immune response between mother and baby. Isoimmune hemolytic anemia was first described in infants born with generalized edema (hydrops), severe anemia, hyperbilirubinemia, and abundant circulating erythroblasts; thus, this disease was named erythroblastosis fetalis, a condition that is described elsewhere in this chapter (see Sec. 2.17.8).

EVALUATION OF ANEMIA IN NEWBORNS Some infants tolerate anemia. Others, especially those with concurrent disease, develop signs and symptoms. These include tachycardia, poor weight gain, supplemental oxygen need, apnea, and bradycardia. A detailed family and maternal obstetric history often provides clues to the etiology of anemia in newborns. A family history of anemia, transfusions, jaundice, or splenectomy would favor an inherited hemolytic process. Certain ethnic groups have a higher prevalence of specific anemias, such as thalassemia, sickle cell disease, and G6PD deficiency. A detailed maternal history is valuable in helping to establish a diagnosis. Practitioners should inquire about possible drug exposure, infection, and vaginal bleeding. The obstetric record should be reviewed for evidence of blood loss, maternal blood type, Coombs test, and serology for congenital infections.

The timing of signs of anemia may be helpful in establishing the cause. Neonates with acute hemorrhage are pale, tachypneic, and tachycardic. The hematocrit may be normal after delivery but gradually declines during the first day as fluid equilibrates. Neonates with chronic hemorrhage have a low hematocrit at birth but usually appear well compensated, although some infants may have signs of congestive heart failure. Chronic intrauterine hemolysis is associated with anemia, jaundice, and hepatosplenomegaly that are present at birth.

The laboratory evaluation of anemia includes a complete blood count, reticulocyte count, peripheral blood cell smear, direct antiglobulin or Coombs test, measurement of total and direct bilirubin concentrations, and maternal and infant blood types. A low reticulocyte count of less than 2% suggests direct marrow suppression and may be indicative of infection, suppression from medications, congenital hypoplastic anemia (Diamond-Blackfan syndrome), or congenital dyserythropoietic anemia. Marrow replacement by tumor, such as congenital leukemia or neuroblastoma, can present with pancytopenia. Bacterial and viral infections are associated with direct marrow suppression as well as hemolysis. A low mean cell volume (<95 fL) suggests iron deficiency or α-thalassemia. Iron deficiency is associated with chronic fetal-to-maternal hemorrhage and can be evaluated by a Kleihauer-Betke stain of maternal blood. Evaluation of the parent's blood smear may show microcytosis suggesting α-thalassemia. An elevated reticulocyte count is indicative of erythrocyte destruction, and a positive neonatal direct and maternal indirect Coombs test is evidence of isoimmune hemolytic anemia. However, a negative direct Coombs test does not rule out immune-mediated destruction, particularly in the case of ABO or minor blood group incompatibility, where antigen expression is low.

Hemolytic anemias are associated with jaundice. Erythrocyte membrane defects, such as hereditary spherocytosis and elliptocytosis, may be detected by examination of the peripheral smear, although this is especially difficult in newborns because the erythrocyte morphology is particularly heterogeneous. Anemia without jaundice is often seen with acute blood loss or disseminated intravascular coagulation.

TRANSFUSION PRACTICES   The decision to transfuse erythrocytes should be based on the clinical condition of the infant. Infants suffering from moderate cardiopulmonary disease, undergoing anesthesia, or experiencing extensive surgery may benefit from a hematocrit above 30%. Transfusion may also benefit symptomatic infants, those with unexplained metabolic acidosis, apnea and bradycardia, poor weight gain, and diminished activity. Recent studies have shown that packed red blood cells (pRBCs) from units that have undergone extended storage can be administered safely to neonates (see Sec. 19.11.1). If transfusions are large (>25 mL/kg), however, fresh pRBCs should be administered because of the increase in potassium and reduction in 2,3-diphosphoglycerate that occur with extended storage. Infants at greatest risk for transfusion-related cytomegalovirus (CMV) infection are low-birth-weight infants, infants born to CMV-negative mothers, and infants with immunodeficiency. In these circumstances, transfusion of blood products from a CMV-seronegative or leukodepleted unit would be appropriate. Finally, transfusion-related graft-versus-host disease (GVHD) has occurred in newborns. This condition is caused by lymphocytes in the transfused product proliferating in an immunodeficient recipient. GVHD occurs in association with prematurity, congenital immunodeficiency, intrauterine transfusion, and transfusion from a first-degree relative. Irradiation of the transfused blood prevents GVHD.

NEONATAL NEUTROPENIA

Neutropenia is relatively common in the immediate postnatal period, occuring in up to 8% of all infants admitted to newborn intensive care units. Like many hematologic disorders, neutropenia can be classified physiologically on the basis of the rate of neutrophil production or destruction (see Sec. 19.6.1).

DECREASED PRODUCTION   Maternal hypertension is a common cause of neutropenia that stems from diminished neutrophil production. These infants have a high rate of infection. Neutropenia is especially prevalent in infants born to mothers with HELLP syndrome (ie, hemolysis, elevated liver enzymes, and thrombocytopenia). Diminished neutrophil production is frequently associated with accelerated erythropoiesis, as occurs with Rh hemolytic disease and in donors of twin-to-twin transfusions. In all of these conditions, neutropenia usually resolves in 3 to 7 days. In contrast, infants with severe congenital neutropenia, or Kostmann syndrome (see Sec. 19.6.1), display profound neutropenia, with typical absolute neutrophil counts (ANC) less than 200 cells/μL. Patients with congenital neutropenia are at risk for the development of leukemia later in life. Other rare conditions that are characterized by

decreased neutrophil production include exocrine pancreatic insufficiency (Schwachman syndrome), reticular dysgenesis, cartilage hair hypoplasia, and cyclic neutropenia (see Sec. 19.6.1).

INCREASED DESTRUCTION   Sepsis is a common cause of increased neutrophil destruction and requires prompt medical attention. Neutropenic infants with overwhelming infections have a high mortality rate, but if they survive, neutropenia usually resolves in 72 hours. Studies have shown that granulocyte colony-stimulating factor (G-CSF) and granulocyte-monocyte colony-stimulating factor (GM-CSF) increase circulating neutrophil counts, but their impact on reducing sepsis-related morbidity and mortality remains questionable.

Neonatal isoimmune neutropenia results from incompatibility between maternal and fetal neutrophil antigens, commonly NA1, NA2, NB1, and NC1 (see Sec. 19.6.1). Sensitization can occur with the first pregnancy, and infants typically have neutropenia that persists for weeks, in contrast to the conditions discussed previously. These children are at risk for infection. Treatment with IVIG to prevent destruction of antibody-targeted neutrophils by the reticuloendothelial system yields inconsistent results. The results of recent trials with G-CSF are more promising, with a consistent elevation of the ANC. Primary autoimmune neutropenia caused by the generation of self-reactive antibodies rarely presents in the newborn period. Immunoglobulin (IgG) antibodies, however, can cross the placenta into the fetal circulation in mothers who have autoimmune neutropenia, with or without associated autoimmune disorders such as systemic lupus erythematosus.

EVALUATION OF NEONATAL NEUTROPENIA   The mechanism of neutropenia in most newborns is obvious and short-lived, so that additional tests are rarely needed. Clues to the pathophysiology of neutropenia may be provided by the peripheral blood smear. A "left shift," or ratio of immature to total neutrophils greater than 0.3, usually indicates compensation for increased destruction. If the diagnosis is not clear, a complete blood count on the mother should be performed to rule out autoimmune neutropenia. If normal, maternal neutrophil antigen typing and assays for antineutrophil antibodies are indicated. A bone marrow aspiration and biopsy is rarely needed but should be performed in cases of severe (<500/μL), prolonged neutropenia without an obvious cause.

NEONATAL PLATELET DISORDERS

Thrombocytopenia is common in the newborn period (see Sec. 19.7.1). Up to 1% of term infants and up to 35% of infants admitted to neonatal intensive care units have decreased platelet counts.

INFECTION   Infections remain a leading cause of thrombocytopenia in newborns, and often, a falling platelet count may herald the onset of systemic infection. Any viral, bacterial, or fungal pathogen is capable of inducing thrombocytopenia. In these circumstances, thrombocytopenia may be caused by both increased destruction and decreased production of platelets.

MEDICATIONS   Medications administered to mothers have been reported to cause thrombocytopenia in both mother and infant. These medications include thiazide diuretics, tolbutamide, and hydralazine. Drug-associated thrombocytopenia is often immune-mediated. With thiazide diuretics, direct suppression of megakaryopoiesis is also suspected. Drugs that affect platelet function such as aspirin can cross the placenta and cause bleeding in infants. Indomethacin, when used as therapy for closure of a patent ductus arterious, also can cause hemorrhage.

CONGENITAL THROMBOCYTOPENIA Various genetic syndromes, including trisomy 13, 18, and 21 and Turner syndrome, can be associated with thrombocytopenia. Thrombocytopenia with absent radii (TAR) syndrome is an autosomal recessive disorder characterized by bilateral absent radii and severe thrombocytopenia that is usually noted at birth (see Sec. 19.7.1).

NEONATAL IMMUNE-MEDIATED THROMBOCYTOPENIA Thrombocytopenia from platelet antigen incompatibility between the mother and fetus, a condition referred to as alloimmune thrombocytopenia, occurs in one in 2000 births (see Sec. 19.7). Unlike the analogous Rh disease, an infant can be affected in the first pregnancy. Approximately 90% of cases involve HPA-1 (P1A-1). Nearly 15% of infants with this condition experience intracranial hemorrhage, and approximately 50% of these events occur in utero. Administration of intravenous immunoglobulin (IVIG) and corticosteroids to the mother has been shown to significantly increase the platelet count of fetuses with immune-mediated thrombocytopenia. Washed maternal platelets can be transfused postnatally.

Mothers with autoimmune thrombocytopenia (ITP) have circulating antibodies that are directed against platelet antigens. Transplacental transit of antiplatelet IgG can result in increased destruction of fetal platelets (see Sec. 19.7). In contrast to alloimmune thrombocytopenia, the risk of severe thrombocytopenia, defined as a platelet count $<50,000/\mu L$, is much lower (5–20%), and serious hemorrhage is unusual. The maternal platelet count is low in autoimmune thrombocytopenia, in contrast to alloimmune thrombocytopenia. Autoimmune thrombocytopenia must be distinguished from gestational thrombocytopenia, a common condition of unknown etiology that is associated with a very mild decrease in the platelet count. Mothers with gestational thrombocytopenia rarely, if ever, deliver an infant with severe thrombocytopenia. Infants with autoimmune thrombocytopenia have an excellent response to intravenous immunoglobulin and corticosteroids.

EVALUATION OF THE THROMBOCYTOPENIA AND TRANSFUSION GUIDELINES The platelet count increases throughout development, reaching adult values at term. A platelet count below $150,000/\mu L$ is abnormal, but only when the count falls below $100,000/\mu L$ should a comprehensive evaluation be considered. Thrombocytopenic infants can be classified as "sick" or "well." "Sick" infants should be evaluated for infection and disseminated intravascular coagulation, and the underlying condition treated appropriately. A head ultrasound study may be performed to evaluate for central nervous system hemorrhage. Genetic causes may be obvious. A thorough maternal history may indicate medications or an infectious cause. "Well" infants are best evaluated by measuring a maternal platelet count. If low, maternal ITP should be considered. If the maternal platelet count is normal, maternal alloantibodies and paternal platelet antigen testing can be performed. A sustained rise in the platelet count after transfusion with maternal platelets supports the diagnosis of alloimmune thrombocytopenia, whereas a transient rise is more suggestive of other causes of platelet destruction.

Guidelines for the use of prophylactic platelet transfusions, like red cell transfusions, are controversial. Preterm infants are particularly vulnerable to serious hemorrhage, such as intracranial bleed-

ing. Thus, it is appropriate to transfuse platelets for a platelet count $<30,000/\mu L$ at term and for a platelet count $<50,000/\mu L$ in a stable preterm infant. In associated conditions that influence effective hemostasis, platelet transfusions may be warranted for counts that fall below $100,000/\mu L$. In the absence of accelerated destruction, the infusion of 10 mL/kg of a platelet suspension is usually sufficient to raise the platelet count to $>100,000/\mu L$. Transfusion guidelines that relate to CMV status and graft-versus-host disease, as discussed above for RBC transfusions, are applicable to platelets.

NEONATAL COAGULATION DISORDERS

The overall structure and function of the neonatal coagulation and fibrinolytic systems are identical to those of older children and adults (see Sec. 19.10 and Fig. 19-12). Coagulation proteins do not cross the placenta, and levels of the individual coagulation proteins rise steadily throughout gestation. Only plasma levels of fibrinogen and factor VIII are normal compared with adults at term. Levels of factors II, VII, IX, and X (vitamin K–dependent factors) and factors XI, XII, prekallekrein, and high-molecular-weight kininogen, are low relative to adult values, whereas von Willebrand factor concentration is high compared to that in adults. The primary laboratory measurements of the integrity of the coagulation system, the prothrombin time (PT) and activated partial thromboplastin time (aPTT), must be interpreted relative to gestational age (see Table 19-17). As expected, the PT and aPTT are significantly prolonged in healthy preterm infants compared to term newborns. In spite of these relative differences compared to adults, healthy infants are not in danger of spontaneous or unusual bleeding or thrombosis unless stressed by associated pathologic processes.

INHERITED FACTOR DEFICIENCIES Inherited coagulation deficiencies can present in the newborn period. In contrast to defects involving platelets and vessel walls, infants with coagulation defects do not usually display petechiae or mucous membrane bleeding. Infants with coagulation defects are more likely to present with severe cephalohematomas, prolonged bleeding from venipuncture sites, and postsurgical bleeding, notably after circumcision. Approximately 1% of hemophiliac infants will suffer an intracranial hemorrhage. A positive family history of hemophilia may be lacking when the disorder arises from a de novo mutation. The diagnosis of hemophilia A is readily made by a markedly prolonged aPTT and low factor VIII level (see Sec. 19.10). Factor IX deficiency, or hemophilia B, is another X-linked recessive disorder that presents in a similar fashion. Von Willebrand disease, the most common inherited coagulation disorder, rarely affects newborns, as factor levels are relatively high at birth. Inherited deficiencies of factors II, V, VII, X, XI, XIII, and fibrinogen have all been reported to present with hemorrhage in the newborn period.

VITAMIN K DEFICIENCY Vitamin K is a necessary cofactor for procoagulant factors II, VII, IX, and X and for anticoagulant proteins C and S. In utero, vitamin K is provided to the developing fetus, but shortly after birth, plasma concentrations decrease. Levels return to adult values by day 7, but during this critical postnatal window, infants are at risk for spontaneous hemorrhage. Bleeding may occur from venipuncture sites, the gastrointestinal tract, or circumcision. Three different clinical presentations of vitamin K deficiency may occur (see Sec. 19.10).

A prolonged PT and aPTT and a normal platelet count and fibrinogen suggest the diagnosis of vitamin K deficiency. If vitamin K deficiency is suspected, treatment should include administration of parenteral vitamin K. Quick correction of hemostasis and coagulation abnormalities supports the diagnosis of vitamin K deficiency.

DISSEMINATED INTRAVASCULAR COAGULATION Disseminated intravascular coagulation (DIC) results from the simultaneous unregulated activation of both the coagulation and fibrinolytic systems. Endothelial damage is a common feature of this condition and leads to release of tissue factor and cytokines that result in thrombin formation. The condition always occurs as a result of a primary medical disorder such as obstetric complications, infection, respiratory distress syndrome, renal vein thrombobosis, or giant hemangioma. Approximately 10% of infants admitted to the newborn intensive care unit have DIC. The clinical signs of DIC in newborns include oozing from venipuncture sites, gastrointestinal bleeding, petechiae, severe ecchymosis, and pulmonary hemorrhage. These infants usually have prolongation of the PT and aPTT, low fibrinogen concentrations, and thrombocytopenia. Enhanced fibrinolytic activity is reflected by an increase in the levels of the proteolytic fragments of fibrinogen and fibrin. Therapy for DIC should focus on the underlying cause. Blood products are used judiciously to control and prevent bleeding and to maintain hemostasis.

NEONATAL THROMBOTIC DISORDERS

The risk of thromboembolic events may be affected by the presence of maternal conditions, such as maternal diabetes mellitus, systemic lupus erythematosus, and antiphospholipid syndrome. In these disorders, antibodies are transported across the placenta and react with phospholipids, causing thrombosis.

INDWELLING CATHETERS The greatest risk factor for thromboembolic events (TEs) in the newborn infant is the presence of indwelling venous and arterial catheters. Thrombosis occurs in up to 30% of infants with indwelling vascular catheters. The prophylactic use of unfractionated heparin prolongs the patency of umbilical artery catheters and decreases the incidence of TEs.

RENAL VEIN THROMBOSIS Risk factors for renal vein thrombosis include maternal diabetes, neonatal sepsis, dehydration, cyanotic heart disease, asphyxia, and polycythemia. The presenting features are a flank mass, hematuria, and thrombocytopenia.

CONGENITAL FACTOR DEFICIENCIES Homozygous protein C and S deficiency present with extensive dermal thrombosis, purpura fulminans, and deep vein thrombosis. Heterozygous deficiency of antithrombin III rarely may cause vascular thromboses. The most common thrombophilic condition is factor V Leiden (see Sec. 19.10). Homocysteinemia is another risk factor for venous and arterial thrombotic events.

EVALUATION AND THERAPY OF NEONATAL THROMBOSIS Newborns with documented thromboembolism should have an evaluation for inherited risk factors. Laboratory evaluation may include assays for antithrombin, protein C, protein S, and homocysteine concentration, mutational analysis to detect the factor V Leiden and the prothrombin mutations, and a screening test for antiphospholipid antibodies.

The appropriate therapy for newborns with TEs depends on thrombus site, degree of vascular occlusion, and whether organ function is impaired. Catheters associated with clots should be removed. Unfractionated heparin is currently the most widely used anticoagulant (see Sec. 19.10). In general, neonates require increased doses of heparin to achieve equivalent biological effects compared to adults. Low-molecular-weight heparin (LMWH) has advantages for the treatment of TEs in newborns. LMWH is more bioavailable and has a more reproducible pharmacokinetic profile than unfractionated heparin. The use of the oral anticoagulant warfarin is difficult because levels of vitamin K–dependent factors are widely variable in newborns. In general, the use of short courses of LMWH (3 to 6 months) is preferred over oral anticoagulant therapy. Thrombolytic agents that convert plasminogen to plasmin are difficult to use in newborns because of decreased levels of plasminogen in the neonatal period. Indications for the use of thrombolytic therapy include pulmonary embolus not responding to heparin therapy, arterial occlusion, and possibly extensive venous occlusion, especially with impending organ damage.

References

Andrews M, Paes B, Johnston M: Development of the hemostatic system in the neonate and young infant. Am J Pediatr Hematol Oncol 12:95–104, 1990

Andrews M, Michelson AD, Bovill E, Leaker M, Massicotte MP: Guidelines for antithrombotic therapy in pediatric patients. J Pediatr 132:575–588, 1998

Bowman J: The management of hemolytic disease in the fetus and newborn. Semin Perinatol 21:39–44, 1997

Bussel JB, Zabusky MR, Berkowitz RL, MaFarland JG: Fetal alloimmune thrombocytopenia. N Engl J Med 337:22–26, 1997

Castle V, Andrew M, Kelton J, Giron D, Johnston M, Carter C: Frequency and mechanism of neonatal thrombocytopenia. J Pediatr 108:749–755, 1986

Christensen RD: Hematologic Problems of the Neonate. Philadelphia, WB Saunders, 2000

Forestier F, Daffos F, Catherine N, Renard M, Andreux JP: Developmental hematopoiesis in normal fetal blood. Blood 77:2360–2363, 1991

Kodish E, Potter C, Kirschbaum NE, Foster PA: Activated protein C resistance in a neonate with venous thrombosis. J Pediatr 127:645–648, 1995

Krafte-Jacobs B, Sivit CJ, Mejia R, Pollack MM: Catheter-related thrombosis in critically ill children: comparison of catheters with and without heparin bonding. J Pediatr 126:50–54, 1995

Ohls RK, Li Y, Trautman MS, Christensen RD: Erythropoietin production by macrophages from preterm infants: implications regarding the cause of the anemia of prematurity. Pediatr Res 35:169–170, 1995

Samuels P, Bussel JB, Braitman LE, et al: Estimation of the risk of thrombocytopenia in the offspring of pregnant women with presumed immune thrombocytopenic purpura. N Engl J Med 323:229–235, 1990

Schibler KR, Osborne KA, Leung LY, LeTV, Baker SI, Thompson DD: A randomized placebo controlled trial of granulocyte colony-stimulating factor administration to newborn infants with neutropenia and clinical signs of early onset sepsis. Pediatrics 102:6–13, 1998

Shannon K, Keith JF, Mentzer WC, et al: Recombinant human erythropoietin stimulates erythropoiesis and reduces erythrocyte transfusions in very low birth weight preterm infants. Pediatrics 95:1–8, 1995

Shirahata A, Shirakawa Y, Murakami C: Diagnosis of DIC in very low birth weight infants. Semin Thromb Hemostas 98:467–471, 1998

Strauss RG: Red blood cell transfusion practices in the neonate. Clin Perinatol 22:641–655, 1995

Sutor AH: Vitamin K deficiency bleeding in infants and children. Semin Thromb Hemostas 21:317–329, 1995

2.18 NEONATAL EMERGENCIES

2.18.1 Newborn Surgical Emergencies

Rebecka L. Meyers

As advances in neonatal intensive care have decreased the morbidity of newborn surgery, surgical techniques to repair congenital abnormalities of the digestive tract have improved. Knowing the signs and symptoms of these surgically repairable congenital abnormalities will result in earlier diagnosis and appropriate timely intervention. For example, congenital abdominal wall defects mandate prompt surgical attention to prevent additional injury to the herniated abdominal viscera, and some tumors, unique to newborn infants, may mandate prompt surgical intervention.

SURGICALLY CORRECTABLE CAUSES OF RESPIRATORY DISTRESS

The precise manifestation of a congenital obstructive airway lesion depends on the location and severity of the obstruction. Conditions affecting the patency of the nasal airway, pharynx, and larynx produce inspiratory obstruction, sometimes associated with stridor, whereas those that narrow the trachea often result in both inspiratory and expiratory obstruction. Lesions of the lung may present with air trapping and secondary airway compression. Congenital diaphragmatic hernia results in pulmonary hypoplasia, variable degrees of pulmonary hypertension, and extrinsic compression from the herniated abdominal viscera. Physical examination and chest x-ray help localize the obstruction to the upper airway or to the thoracic cavity, whereas specific diagnoses can be made using imaging techniques or occasionally laryngobronchoscopy.

EXTRINSIC COMPRESSION OF THE AIRWAY

Congenital cervical masses such as cystic hygroma or hemangioma may cause extrinsic compression of the trachea. Masses that cause respiratory distress are typically large and clearly evident on physical examination, and infants with severe respiratory distress require prompt tracheal intubation. Ultrasonography may help to define the lesion, revealing cystic, solid, and vascular components. Surgery is indicated for those infants with respiratory compromise. Asymptomatic or mildly symptomatic infants should be observed closely for signs of airway compromise caused by enlargement of the mass.

Craniofacial anomalies in Treacher-Collin, Crouzon, and Apert syndromes may cause abnormal maxillary development with occasional nasopharyngeal obstruction (see Sec. 10.3.4). Airway obstruction in Pierre Robin syndrome (micrognathia, posterior displacement of the tongue, and cleft palate) usually responds to forward displacement of the tongue and placement of a nasal airway. The most severe cases of micrognathia may require tracheotomy. The macroglossia seen with hypothyroidism or Beckwith Weideman may occasionally require surgical reduction of the tongue.

Vascular ring refers to congenital anomalies of the aortic arch that compress the airway or esophagus and, in the process, cause stridor, cyanosis, repeated upper respiratory infection, or dysphagia. These are discussed in Sec. 22.3.7.

Mediastinal masses such as mediastinal neuroblastoma, mediastinal teratoma, and esophageal duplication most often present in the first months or years of life with signs and symptoms of cough, dysphagia, hemoptysis, or repeated pulmonary infection. Occasionally such a mass will present in the neonatal period with life-threatening airway compression. Bronchogenic cysts are extrapulmonary anomalies without connection to the airway. Respiratory distress occurs in the neonate if the cyst compresses an adjacent bronchus causing expiratory obstruction and resultant hyperinflation of the distal lung.

Congenital cystic adenomatoid malformation is an intrinsic pulmonary lesion with cystic spaces that may communicate with the airway. Positive-pressure ventilation may cause acute air trapping and expansion of the lesion, thereby producing rapid worsening of the infant's hemodynamic and respiratory function. Some infants are diagnosed in utero and may develop hydrops fetalis, necessitating referral to a fetal treatment center. *Congenital lobar emphysema* involves a collapsible weakness in a major airway such that inspired air is not efficiently expelled from the lungs. The involved lobe becomes grossly hyperinflated, causing a vicious cycle of increasing mass effect, airway compression, and progressively severe respiratory distress. *Pulmonary sequestration* may be intralobar or extralobar and typically presents in the first years of life as a recurrent localized pneumonia. Diagnosis in a newborn is often the result of an incidental finding on prenatal ultrasound. Surgical treatment of neonatal pulmonary masses involves thoracotomy and surgical resection of the lesion or involved lobe of lung.

INTRINSIC OBSTRUCTION OF THE AIRWAY

Choanal atresia is a congenital obstruction of the nares at the posterior border of the nasal septum. The obstruction may be unilateral or bilateral, membranous or bony. The diagnosis is suggested by failure to pass a suction catheter beyond the septum, and symptoms may be worse during feeding, when mouth breathing is not possible. If the atresia is membranous, simple perforation and dilation under general anesthesia may suffice. A bony obstruction will require endoscopic visualization, resection of the bone, and placement of stents to prevent postoperative stenosis.

Laryngomalacia is the most common cause of neonatal inspiratory stridor. Usually classically the condition does not cause significant respiratory distress despite the sometimes dramatic stridor. *Vocal cord palsy* may be unilateral and cause minimal symptoms, or bilateral and require tracheotomy. *Subglottic stenosis,* once a common complication of prolonged intubation, has become progressively rare with advances in neonatal airway management. *Laryngeal cleft* may occur alone or in combination with other anomalies such as esophageal atresia. Mild clefts result in recurrent aspiration and may be self-limiting; complete stage IV clefting will result in tracheal collapse, requiring intubation from birth and eventually an extensive airway reconstruction.

Congenital *tracheal stenosis* is generally amenable to surgical repair, whereas tracheal atresia is not. Short stenotic segments are usually resected with primary reanastomosis performed by a variety of techniques designed to prevent postoperative stricture. Long stenotic segments may require more complex reconstruction and perhaps stenting. In the rare case of congenital *tracheal atresia,* the infant is usually born alive with profound perinatal respiratory distress. No long-term survivors have been reported.

CONGENITAL DIAPHRAGMATIC HERNIA

See Sec. 2.6 and 2.17.13

ALIMENTARY TRACT OBSTRUCTION

Neonatal gastrointestinal obstruction may be heralded by a number of signs including maternal polyhydramnios, bilious vomiting, abdominal distension, and failure to pass meconium. Twenty-five to 40% of the amniotic fluid is swallowed by the fetus, and instances of high obstruction such as esophageal atresia, duodenal atresia, and high jejunal atresia may result in an amniotic fluid volume of >2 L. Bilious vomiting is always pathologic, and the presence of bile in the stomach at birth should be carefully investigated. The newborn infant stomach usually contains <15 mL of clear gastric liquid at birth, and volumes in excess of 20 to 25 mL, particularly if they contain bile, may signify an intestinal obstruction. Abdominal distension is a sign of distal intestinal obstruction and may be associated with visible loops of intestine (intestinal patterning) and occasionally respiratory distress caused by thoracic restriction from elevation of the diaphragm. Abdominal radiographs may differentiate among several possible causes of abdominal distension such as free air (perforated viscus), peritoneal fluid (from ascites, blood, chyle, urine, or pus), and distended bowel (from intestinal obstruction or adynamic ileus). Meconium is dark green or black in color, sticky in consistency, and composed of amniotic fluid, amniotic debris, intestinal succus entericus, and mucus. Normal term infants should pass meconium within the first 48 hours after birth, and failure to do so may reflect a congenital intestinal obstruction or motility disorder.

PROXIMAL INTESTINAL OBSTRUCTION

Esophageal atresia/tracheoesophageal fistula typically presents shortly after birth with excess salivation, feeding intolerance, respiratory distress, and inability to pass a NG tube. When the tube cannot be advanced through the esophagus, a chest x-ray will show the tip of the tube within an air-filled pouch in the upper mediastinum. A distal tracheoesophageal fistula is associated with esophageal atresia in 85% of cases and is recognized by the finding of intestinal gas on abdominal radiograph. Less common variants of this anomaly include esophageal atresia without tracheoesophageal fistula, H-type tracheoesophageal fistula without esophageal atresia, and esophageal atresia with a proximal fistula. Additional perioperative evaluation is directed at identifying possible associated anomalies of the VACTERL association (vertebral, imperforate anus, cardiac, tracheal/esophageal, renal, limb).

The danger of esophageal atresia lies in the potential for pulmonary complications. Aspiration of saliva or milk from the proximal esophageal pouch or aspiration of refluxed gastric contents via the distal fistula will lead to pneumonitis and possible infection. A sump tube should be placed in the proximal esophageal pouch, and the baby should be placed in an antireflux position. Antibiotics and an H_2 blocker should be given, and an echocardiogram should be obtained because of the association between esophageal atresia and congenital cardiac anomalies and because the orientation of the aortic arch is important to plan for repair by thoracotomy, which should be performed on the side opposite the arch.

Preoperative positive-pressure mechanical ventilation should be avoided, if possible, to prevent massive gastric distension caused by forced insufflation of the stomach through the tracheoesophageal fistula. If the infant is stable, the proximal and distal ends of the esophagus are exposed by an extrapleural thoracotomy, the fistula ligated, and a primary esophageal repair performed. Infants with cardiovascular instability from prematurity or congenital heart disease should have a transpleural fistula ligation and placement of a gastrostomy tube. Infants with long-gap atresia (more than four vertebral bodies) often do not have a tracheoesophageal fistula and initially require only a gastrostomy tube.

Duodenal atresia results in bilious vomiting, a copious bilious gastric aspirate at birth, and a nondistended abdomen (indicating a very proximal obstruction). The radiographic finding of a "double bubble" (representing air in the distended stomach and proximal duodenum), in the absence of distal intestinal gas, is diagnostic of congenital duodenal obstruction. The presence of any air distal to the duodenum is an indication for an upper gastrointestinal series to exclude duodenal obstruction from a midgut volvulus and to establish the diagnosis. Because of the high incidence of associated trisomy 21 and congenital heart disease, a karyotype and an echocardiogram should be obtained. Once the infant is medically stable, surgical repair bypasses the site of obstruction by anastomosis between the proximal and distal duodenum.

Intestinal malrotation and midgut volvulus is a potentially life-threatening condition that usually presents with bilious vomiting often associated with abdominal distension, pain, passage of bloody stool, and a relatively gasless abdominal film. Plain abdominal radiographs, although classically described as relatively gasless, are frequently nonspecific. However, unexplained bilious vomiting in a newborn requires urgent assessment that should include contrast radiography of the gastrointestinal tract. If an upper gastrointestinal series or barium enema reveals intestinal malrotation in an infant with bilious vomiting, volvulus is assumed, and emergency surgical exploration is indicated. In intestinal malrotation the duodenum and cecum lie adjacent to each other in the epigastrium, forming a narrow, poorly fixed mesenteric stalk with the superior mesenteric vessels at its center. Volvulus around this narrow mesenteric stalk will cause obstruction of the duodenum and the mesenteric artery and vein. Surgical reduction of the volvulus restores bowel perfusion, and, unless the bowel is already necrotic, its color should improve within minutes. Ladd bands are divided, and to prevent recurrent volvulus, the base of the mesentery is broadened, placing proximal small bowel to the right and colon to the left. An appendectomy prevents future confusion caused by the abnormal left-sided location of the appendix.

DISTAL INTESTINAL OBSTRUCTION

Jejunal and ileal atresia present with varying degrees of abdominal distension proportional to the amount of time since birth and the site of the atresia (more distal obstruction usually results in more distension). Intestinal atresias may occur throughout the intestinal tract, but are far less common in the large than in the small intestine. The stool is characteristically acholic, but some bile staining may be present if the atresia occurred late in gestation. The etiology of intestinal atresia is thought to be related to an in utero vascular accident. The proximal bowel is often noted at surgery to be grossly dilated with muscular hypertrophy, which is associated with blunted villi and ineffective peristalsis. If the intestinal length is too short to permit limited intestinal resection, the dilated abnormal bowel may be plicated or tapered before an end-to-oblique anastomosis is performed to restore intestinal continuity.

Meconium ileus is the initial manifestation in 10 to 20% of neonates with cystic fibrosis. Pellets of inspissated meconium typically obstruct the terminal ileum, causing progressive abdominal distension and bilious vomiting. The abdominal radiograph may be diagnostic and reveal dilated intestinal loops with the distinctive appearance of ground glass. The presence of intraabdominal calcification is indicative of in utero intestinal perforation. Occasionally the in utero perforation is so remote that healing results in an atresia. Occasionally the perforation is recent, and the baby is acutely ill with massive abdominal distension, abdominal wall erythema, and peritonitis. In the absence of peritonitis, primary therapy entails a hyperosmolar water-soluble enema, which also usually confirms the diagnosis. The hyperosmolar contrast material draws fluid into the intestinal lumen and helps to liquefy the thickened meconium. Evidence of perforation or failure of the enemas to evacuate the meconium are indications for surgical intervention.

Meconium plug is a sticky abnormal meconium obstruction of the colon or rectum. It may result from diminished colonic motility with prematurity or maternal drugs, such as magnesium sulfate. Maternal diabetes mellitus is sometimes associated with meconium retention in the proximal large intestine resulting from congenital microcolon. Meconium retention may represent Hirschsprung disease or cystic fibrosis, and rectal biopsy and sweat chloride may be needed to diagnose these conditions.

Hirschsprung disease in the newborn is characterized by a delayed passage of meconium with subsequent abdominal distension and bilious vomiting. Rectal examination may reveal spasm of the anal sphincter, and, as the examining finger dilates the rectal musculature, there may be an explosive passage of loose stool. Infants with enterocolitis caused by intestinal stasis and bacterial overgrowth may develop fever, abdominal tenderness, and foul or bloody stool. Abdominal radiographs show dilated loops of bowel suggestive of a distal intestinal obstruction. Diagnosis and management are discussed in Sec. 17.23.3.

Imperforate anus is identified during routine examination of the anus after birth, and if it is left untreated, signs of intestinal obstruction develop within 24 to 48 hours. Anorectal anomalies occur as a result of abnormal formation of the urogenital or urorectal septum or failure of dissolution of the anal membrane. In a low imperforate anus, a perineal fistula is often present. If in doubt, a waiting period of 24 hours to allow air to reach the rectum can be followed by a cross-table prone x-ray of the rectum. In a low lesion, the air column will pass below an imaginary line from pubis to coccyx. A perineal anoplasty, or dilation of the fistula, can be performed. In a high imperforate anus, no fistula is identified, and a diverting colostomy is necessary. An intermediate-level lesion in a girl with a vaginal vestibular fistula may require colostomy to facilitate the more intricate procedure required to separate the common vaginal and rectal walls. The posterior sagittal anorectoplasty has gained favor in the treatment of most intermediate and high anomalies and can be performed when the infant is 3 to 6 months old.

Persistent cloaca presents as a single perineal opening, the urogenital sinus, into which the urethra, vagina, and rectum all empty. There are many anatomic variations of this complex anomaly, and initial treatment is directed primarily at decompression. Cystoscopy and vesicostomy and sometimes vaginostomy may appropriately be combined with the initial operation for diverting colostomy.

ABDOMINAL WALL DEFECTS

Omphalocele and gastroschisis present immediately at birth or as herniated bowel on a prenatal ultrasound. Omphalocele is an abnormally dilated umbilical ring caused by a failure of fusion of the embryologic lateral, cephalic, and caudal abdominal wall folds. The defect may be epigastric, umbilical, or hypogastric, and a sac, which protects the bowel from caustic exposure to amniotic fluid, covers the herniated bowel. Infants with omphalocele have a high incidence of associated congenital anomalies. Gastroschisis is caused by

an in utero rupture of the umbilical cord at the site of the absorbed right umbilical vein. The fascial defect consistently lies to the right of the otherwise normal umbilical cord, and there is no sac to cover the exposed, eviscerated bowel, which is usually thickened and inflamed from direct contact with amniotic fluid. Following delivery, the herniated viscera must be carefully positioned to prevent obstruction of the mesenteric blood supply, and covered with warm, sterile, saline-soaked gauze and an outer layer of plastic wrap to prevent contamination and heat loss. The timing of surgery is determined primarily by the presence or absence of an intact sac. In general, an omphalocele with an intact sac is operated on within 48 hours of delivery, whereas a gastroschisis or ruptured omphalocele requires immediate surgical attention to cover the exposed bowel and isolate the peritoneal cavity from the external environment. Complete surgical reduction of the herniated viscera may not be possible at first because of increased abdominal pressure that will impair ventilation and perfusion of the lower body and kidneys. If primary closure cannot be accomplished, staged closure is performed with the aid of a silastic silo. Reduction of the herniated bowel into the abdominal cavity is then achieved gradually over several days as the peritoneal cavity slowly expands.

Bladder extrophy is a congenital malformation of the caudal abdominal wall and pelvis with exteriorization of the urinary bladder. The fragile, exposed bladder mucosa must be carefully protected with sterile, moist gauze until primary surgical closure of the bladder and reapproximation of the pelvic pubic rami is attempted, sometime in the first 2 to 3 days after birth. *Cloacal extrophy* is a rare combination of anomalies that includes imperforate anus, bladder extrophy, omphalocele, and communication of the rudimentary bladder and intestinal tract. Definitive repair requires multiple staged procedures over months and sometimes years, whereas emergency surgical intervention in the newborn is directed toward closure of the abdominal wall defect and separation of the fecal and urinary streams.

Inguinal hernias are common congenital abdominal wall defects identified in the neonatal period. Unlike umbilical hernias, these hernias do not resolve spontaneously, and there is a high risk of incarceration in premature infants with inguinal hernia. If there has been a history of incarceration, the hernia should be repaired as soon as it is medically feasible.

SURGICAL CONDITIONS OF EXTREME PREMATURITY

Necrotizing enterocolitis (NEC) is an acquired intestinal infection usually affecting premature infants with feeding intolerance, bilious vomiting, and abdominal distension (see Sec. 2.16.4 for detailed discussion).

TUMORS OF INFANCY

Sacrococcygeal teratoma is the most common neonatal tumor and is usually benign but often reaches gigantic size. This tumor can be life threatening because its rich arterial blood supply may cause antenatal high-output cardiac failure and hydrops fetalis, or tumor rupture and hemorrhage during delivery. During transport to the intensive care unit or operating room, the baby and the tumor must be positioned carefully. The baby should usually be prone to protect the tumor from external trauma and excoriation. If there is a high risk of ongoing hemorrhage, blood should be readily available. Ultrasound and occasionally CT scan or MRI can be used to evaluate the extent of internal tumor and to detect urinary tract obstruction. The treatment of choice is complete surgical excision shortly after birth. In the absence of perinatal hydrops fetalis or malignancy, the prognosis is excellent.

Hepatic hemangioendothelioma is a benign liver tumor of infancy that may cause life-threatening high-output heart failure, anemia, and thrombocytopenia. Initial medical treatment includes appropriate blood product replacement, corticosteroids, and treatment of the circulatory congestion. The rare infant with refractory disease may require emergency hepatic arterial embolization or hepatic arterial ligation.

Malignant retroperitoneal tumors such as *neuroblastoma, Wilms tumor,* and *teratoma* may present in infancy as a palpable abdominal mass. Treatment is directed toward definitive diagnosis and complete tumor resection where possible.

References

Adzick NS, Harrison MR: Fetal surgery for cystic adenomatoid malformation of the lung. J Pediatr Surg 40:315, 1993

Delpin CA, Czyrko C, Ziegler MM, et al: Management and survival of meconium ileus, a 30 year review. Ann Surg 215:179, 1992

Frenckner B, Ehren H, Graholm T, et al: Improved results in patients with congenital diaphragmatic hernia using preoperative stabilization, extracorporeal membrane oxygenation, and delayed surgery. J Pediatr Surg 32:1185, 1997

Georgeson KE, Cohen RD, Hebra A, et al: Primary laparoscopic-assisted endorectal colon pull-through for Hirschsprung's disease. A new gold standard. Ann Surg 229:678, 1999

Grosfeld JL, Rescorla FJ: Duodenal atresia and stenosis: reassessment of treatment and outcome based on antenatal diagnosis, pathologic variance, and long-term follow-up. World J Surg 17:301, 1993

Langer JC: Gastrochisis and omphalocele. Semin Pediatr Surg 5:124, 1996

Mychaliska GB, Bullard KM, Harrison MR: In-utero management of congenital diaphragmatic hernia. Clin Perinatol 23:823, 1996

Pena A: Posterior sagittal anorectoplasty: results in the management of 332 cases of anorectal malformations. Pediatr Surg Int 3:94, 1988

Rajput A, Gauderer MV, Hack M: Inguinal hernia in low birth weight infant: incidence and timing of repair. J Pediatr Surg 27:1322, 1992

Ricketts RR: Surgical treatment of necrotizing enterocolitis and the short bowel syndrome. Clin Perinatol 21:365, 1994

Torres AM, Ziegler MM: Malrotation of the intestine. World J Surg 17:326, 1993

2.18.2 Neonatal Medical Emergencies

C. Michael Cotten and Ronald N. Goldberg

The vast majority of newborn infants have an uneventful hospital stay and require no intensive care. Some infants, however, experience considerable difficulty in making the transition from fetal to extrauterine life and require varying degrees of resuscitation in the delivery room (Sec. 2.9), while other infants exhibit major disturbances of vital organ function during their neonatal course and therefore need urgent measures to avoid a catastrophic outcome, followed by timely evaluation to determine the cause and to correct the underlying organ dysfunction. Most of these medical emergencies occur as a result of specific congenital malformations or because of premature birth and its associated complications, such as respiratory failure, intracranial bleeding, intestinal ischemia and infection. This section draws attention to the most common signs and symptoms of life-threatening disorders that develop in newborn infants, some of the underlying conditions that need to be considered, and reasonable approaches for assessing the cause and effectively treating these emergencies.

SIGNS OF ILLNESS

Although these signs might initially signal attention to a specific organ system, commonly they represent final pathways for dysfunction of a variety of systems. For example, cyanosis is caused by deoxygenated arterial or capillary blood. Thus, it can be produced by right-to-left intracardiac shunting, inadequate gas exchange within the lung, impaired ventilatory drive, or simply the result of poor perfusion to the skin. Thus, it is not possible to provide an exhaustive account of all causes for each sign. Table 2-33 contains a broad list of frequent signs of serious illness and examples of processes that cause them. The text describes the pathogenesis of these signs in some detail and suggests initial management approaches.

APNEA (AND DECREASED BREATHING EFFORT) Failure to breathe for a prolonged period (15 to 30 seconds) usually leads to bradycardia and cyanosis, and if it persists or becomes recurrent, the associated hypoxia and hypercapnia can cause permanent brain injury or death. Thus, apnea, or even a very slow or shallow breathing pattern, is a condition that warrants immediate attention and treatment, followed by rapid diagnostic evaluation and steps to prevent recurrence. Apnea is common in premature infants, in whom it usually reflects abnormal central nervous system regulation of respiratory rhythmicity and an absent or dampened response to hypoxia. Apnea also can reflect central nervous system depression from intracranial bleeding, hypoxic-ischemic encephalopathy, infection or drugs, such as narcotics or barbiturates. Proper evaluation of apnea usually includes a careful review of recently administered drugs, blood tests to rule out metabolic disturbances, such as hypoglycemia or severe acidosis, an imaging study of the brain to look for structural abnormalities or hemorrhage, tests to exclude possible sepsis or central nervous system infection, and a chest radiograph to assess the heart and lungs. This evaluation, however, should not delay therapeutic intervention for apnea and its associated adverse effects.

While brief respiratory pauses may be normal in neonates, especially in premature infants and in infants who are born at high altitude and who exhibit periodic breathing from exposure to reduced atmospheric oxygen, the implication is much more serious when the breathing pauses are protracted, or coupled with signs of either respiratory distress or other neurologic dysfunction, or when apnea causes hypoxemia or bradycardia. Although tactile stimulation is sometimes sufficient to restore regular breathing in a previously apneic infant, the response is often temporary. Thus, positive pressure ventilation with sufficient oxygen to eliminate cyanosis should be initiated, at least until the success of other strategies, such as respiratory stimulants or nasal application of continuous positive airway pressure, can be evaluated and the underlying cause of the apnea is determined.

INCREASED RESPIRATORY EFFORT (AND TACHYPNEA)

As discussed in Sec. 4.1.1, increased respiratory effort (respiratory distress) and tachypnea represent a physiological adaptation to restore gas exchange when there are mechanical abnormalities of the lung or chest wall. These impairments can be restrictive or obstructive in nature and may arise from parenchymal lung disease or processes extrinsic to the lungs. The concerns raised by these signs are that they create increased work of breathing, which may rapidly lead to fatigue, or that they are frequently associated with significantly impaired gas exchange. The development of respiratory distress soon after birth should alert the clinician to the possibility of

TABLE 2-33
SIGNS OF EMERGENCIES IN NEONATES

SIGNS	CAUSES/IMPLICATIONS	COMMON EXAMPLES OF SERIOUS CAUSES
Apnea (and decreased breathing effort)	CNS depression	Intra-ventricular hemorrhage, excess narcotic administration
Increased respiratory effort (and tachypnea)	Airway obstruction, restrictive lung, or chest wall disease	Choanal atresia, hyaline membrane disease, or diaphragmatic hernia
Cyanosis	Deoxygenated arterial or capillary blood	Aortopulmonary transposition, right heart obstruction, pneumothorax, poor peripheral perfusion
Hypotension, mottling, poor peripheral perfusion	Inadequate heart function, decreased vascular tone, vasoconstriction of the skin	Left heart obstruction, sepsis, hypovolemic shock
Tachycardia or bradycardia	Decreased cardiac output (sinus tachycardia) or tachyarrhythmia; autonomic dysfunction or bradyarrhythmia	Hypovolemic shock, supraventricular tachycardia; asphyxia
Abnormal repetitive movements	Seizures	Hypoglycemia, hypoxic-ischemic encephalopathy, meningitis
Abdominal distension ± bilious vomiting	Bowel obstruction or ileus	Volvulus, peritonitis, perforation of viscus
Bleeding	Reduced clotting factors, trauma	Disseminated intravascular coagulation, throbocytopenia, vascular laceration
Impaired temperature regulation	Diminished hypothalamic function, nonneutral thermal environment	Infection

congenital anomalies that obstruct the airway or restrict the expansion of the lungs and thorax. These invariably require immediate action, often involving support of ventilation and attempts to correct the anomalies surgically (Sec. 2.9 and 2.18.1). In the premature infant, the most common cause of restrictive lung dysfunction is hyaline membrane disease (HMD) (Sec. 2.16.1). In contrast, restrictive disease of the term infant is commonly caused by pulmonary edema, which arises from obstruction to the inflow or outflow of the systemic ventricle, infection or aspiration, or delayed clearance of interstitial or alveolar fluid (Sec. 2.17.10). These conditions may also require assisted ventilation. Furthermore, other signs or laboratory data may quickly clarify the underlying cause and provide guidance for more specific therapy.

Sometimes respiratory distress arises acutely in an infant already supported with positive-pressure ventilation. Under these circumstances, processes that cause acute obstruction (eg, blockage of a tracheal tube by malposition or mucus) or that cause acute restriction (eg, pneumothorax) must be considered and treated urgently because they are unlikely to be tolerated very long.

CYANOSIS

Cyanosis is reflective of the hemoglobin oxygen saturation in the relatively superficial capillaries of the skin. Thus, it can indicate either arterial hypoxemia or high extraction of oxygen, which usually occurs when circulation is slowed. Less commonly, cyanosis can result from the presence of reduced hemoglobin when there is an abnormal hemoglobin, eg, MetHb. Commonly, poor arterial blood oxygenation produces generalized cyanosis, whereas poor perfusion produces more cyanosis in the distal extremities (which is also associated with other signs of reduced periopheral circulation). The cyanotic infant should immediately be evaluated for signs of respiratory distress, inadequate respiratory effort, or diminished perfusion. Any of these conditions should prompt administration of supplemental O_2. However, it is very important to recognize that some causes for poor perfusion, eg, left heart obstruction, can actually be worsened by inhalation of oxygen. Thus, assessment of response to oxygen should include evaluation of perfusion as well as arterial oxygenation.

HYPOTENSION, MOTTLING, AND POOR PERIPHERAL PERFUSION

Blood pressure changes substantially during development, and it is thus important to be cognizant of the normal values for age and size. Hypotension occurs when the normal mechanisms for preserving arterial blood pressure are disrupted (eg, sepsis) or are insufficient to counterbalance severe decreases in cardiac output. Because of the importance of blood volume in maintenance of cardiac output, shift of blood from the fetus to the placenta during birth can lead to hypotension in the immediate newborn period. Hypotension is usually accompanied by signs of decreased skin perfusion, such as mottling, which occurs when there are areas of superficial vasoconstriction. Usually this occurs as part of the autonomic and humoral response to an inadequate cardiac output (Sec. 4.1.2), which manifests as cool or cold extremities, acrocyanosis, and prolonged capillary refill time. As with hypotension, it requires immediate attention and a search for other signs of circulatory dysfunction (eg, gallop rhythm, reduced peripheral pulses, venous congestion), and initiation of means to improve the circulation with volume infusion or inotropic support.

TACHYCARDIA OR BRADYCARDIA

Sinus tachycardia represents the most effective mechanism for increasing cardiac output, especially during the early stages of postnatal development, when the stroke volume cannot be raised as efficiently. Similar to blood pressure, heart rate varies substantially depending on age, body temperature, and state of alertness or activity. A heart rate of 160 beats/min is normal in a newborn but is abnormally high in a sleeping 2-month-old infant. Conversely, a heart rate of 90 beats/min is normal in a sleeping 2-month old infant but may be inadequate in a crying or febrile newborn. The finding of a rapid pulse rate is often the first indication of a circulatory derangement and thus should be followed by a rapid search for signs of decreased perfusion or respiratory distress. If available, an electrocardiographic recording may establish whether the increased heart rate reflects sinus tachycardia or a tachyarrhythmia. The differentiation of these two conditions is not always obvious, however, and expert advice may be necessary.

Bradycardia usually results from extreme disturbances in autonomic regulation of the heart. It is often a sign of brainstem abnormalities (eg, asphyxia), severe myocardial dysfunction, or defective intracardiac conduction. Complete heart block may be present prenatally, sometimes causing hydrops fetalis. Its diagnosis is usually evident from the surface electrocardiogram. When bradycardia is associated with poor perfusion, treatment by administration of oxygen, chronotropic medications, or external pacing is an emergency.

ABNORMAL REPETITIVE MOVEMENTS

Abnormal repetitive movements can signal an imbalance between activating and inhibitory influences of the central nervous system. Sometimes the distinction between a seizure and the lack of modulation of a motor response to stimulation can be difficult to establish in newborn infants. Typically a seizure is repetitive and stereotypic and usually not abated with external restraint. However, seizures in newborns are frequently subtle, limited in their spread, and may affect only the face, simulating normal movements such as sucking or swallowing. Therefore, one may be certain of their presence only by observing multiple episodes with similar activity. In these cases, a high index of suspicion is needed under conditions when such dysfunction is likely. Moreover, it is essential to search for possible inciting and treatable factors, eg, hypoglycemia, other metabolic disturbances, meningitis, or an unsuspected neurologic injury, when the concern for seizures is raised.

ABDOMINAL DISTENSION (OFTEN WITH BILIOUS VOMITING)

Abdominal distension with vomiting is always abnormal and implies loss of normal peristalsis, which can be caused by obstruction or severe injury to the bowel. Because there is normally continuous production of digestive fluids and swallowing in utero, abdominal distension is an early sign of obstruction of the gastrointestinal tract or failure for it to have normal motility. Furthermore, inflammation or infected fluid outside of the bowel can produce very similar signs as ileus. The distinction between solid masses and enlargement of a hollow viscus can sometimes be made by careful palpation, but ultrasound is such a readily available diagnostic and discriminative tool that it is imperative to use imaging to supplement the physical examination. Often the plain radiograph of the abdomen, which may be more readily available than ultrasound, can also provide a diagnosis or reduce the possibilities. The surgically remediable causes for abdominal distension are addressed in Sec. 2.18.1. Whatever the cause, abdominal distension can impair diaphragmatic excursion, interfere with breathing, and decrease perfusion. With distension and vomiting, feedings should be stopped, and the gastrointestinal tract decompressed by inserting a gastric tube that is open to atmosphere or connected to suction to evaluate fluid and air.

BLEEDING

Bleeding has important implications because it signals the loss of vascular integrity, it can be a sign of impaired clotting, and, when uncontrolled, will progress to shock. Accordingly, initiation of treatment and assessment is urgent. Bleeding at sites, such the um-

bilical cord, where blood vessels are interrupted is obvious and generally can be managed by compressing the site until vasoconstriction or clot formation stops the hemorrhage. Gastrointestinal bleeding is rare in newborns. It must be distinguished from regurgitation or vomiting of maternal blood aspirated during birth or nursing. Cephalohematoma is commonly caused by birth trauma, often during forceps delivery (Sec. 2.17.12). Rarer and more serious forms of trauma-induced hemorrhage may result from liver or adrenal gland lacerations. Although intraabdominal bleeding may produce shock, its origin may be difficult to detect unless a mass is felt during palpation of the abdominal wall or visualized during ultrasound or computerized tomography of the abdomen. Unless a clear mechanism of trauma is identified, all bleeding in a newborn constitutes an indication to examine the integrity of the clotting to assess for possible disorders of coagulation (see Sec. 2.17.16).

IMPAIRED TEMPERATURE REGULATION

The ability to regulate body temperature in response to wide changes in environmental conditions does not develop until late in infancy (Sec. 2.7). Thus, it is not surprising that term and especially premature newborns become hypothermic or febrile in response to excessive environmental cold or heat, respectively. Variations in body temperature are exaggerated by a relatively large body surface-to-body-weight ratio that is characteristic of newborn infants, especially those who are born prematurely. The cardiovascular dysfunction that accompanies neonatal sepsis or certain types of congenital heart disease contributes to the hypothermia that sometimes develops in these conditions. The finding of hypothermia or hyperthermia in a newborn infant requires immediate investigation, including the performance of blood cultures and other laboratory studies, as well as continued observation for the development of additional circulatory, respiratory, or neurologic manifestations.

INFECTION

Neonatal infections can present with non-specific, and often subtle, signs of illness, including apnea, temperature instability, cyanosis, hypotension, hypoglycemia, abdominal distension, poor feeding, irritability, and lethargy. Infections can progress rapidly into septic shock and result in significant morbidity and mortality. Hence, immediate diagnostic evaluation and treatment are crucial to successful outcome. White blood cell counts and measures of various acute-phase reactants and inflammatory markers have been used to try to identify those infants with subtle findings of infection. There is, however, no reliable means to detect most infections. Therefore, appropriate broad-spectrum antimicrobial therapy and continuous monitoring of vital signs is recommended as soon as the relevant laboratory studies and cultures have been obtained.

2.19 SPECIAL INTENSIVE CARE PROCEDURES FOR NEWBORNS

2.19.1 Mechanical Ventilation

Eduardo Bancalari

A large proportion of the neonates who require intensive care depend on mechanical ventilatory support for their survival. Preterm infants born before the 28th to 30th week of gestation are frequently ventilator dependent for many weeks or even months. Most infants who require mechanical ventilation have pulmonary disorders, but infants with severe neurologic, cardiac, metabolic, surgical, and infectious conditions also may require ventilatory support.

The introduction of continuous positive airway pressure (CPAP) in the treatment of infants with respiratory distress of the newborn represented the first use of a therapeutic measure that counteracted the main mechanism by which surfactant deficiency impairs gas exchange and increases respiratory work: the decrease in lung volume. Understanding how CPAP accomplishes this can clarify how more complex forms of ventilatory support are effective in the treatment of a variety of lung diseases. Preterm infants with mild or moderate hyaline membrane disease (HMD) or with mild apnea of prematurity can be managed with CPAP, but the smallest and sickest premature infants with severe respiratory failure often require intermittent positive-pressure ventilation (IPPV) in order to maintain their ventilation and oxygenation within acceptable limits.

CONTINUOUS POSITIVE AIRWAY PRESSURE

PHYSIOLOGICAL PRINCIPLES The volume of air remaining in the lungs at the end of each expiration is determined primarily by the balance of forces acting in opposite directions: the retractive forces of the lungs produced by the elastic properties of the tissue and the surface tension at the alveolar surface tend to decrease lung volume; the outward recoil of the chest wall tends to increase the volume of the lungs. In prematures with HMD, the increased surface tension tends to collapse the alveoli, whereas the highly compliant chest wall cannot counterbalance these forces. This results in a decreased lung volume and a tendency for airway and alveolar closure at the end of expiration, which results in pulmonary shunt and hypoxemia. An increase in transpulmonary pressure at the end of each expiration keeps the lungs more distended and avoids airway and alveolar closure. This can be accomplished by applying CPAP or by using continuous negative pressure around the chest. The result with either of these two methods is an increased functional residual capacity (FRC), reduced airways resistance, and improved gas exchange.

INDICATIONS The best results with CPAP in infants with HMD are obtained when CPAP is used early in the course of the disease. When CPAP is used before the oxygen requirement is high, it is possible to reduce the need for mechanical ventilation and its complications. In extremely small premature infants, the results with CPAP are less favorable because most of these babies have moderate or severe HMD and do not have sufficient respiratory effort to maintain ventilation without the use of IPPV.

CPAP is also used in infants with apnea of prematurity. In these patients, CPAP decreases the incidence of apnea, probably by stabilizing and reducing distortion of the chest wall and by distending the upper airway and preventing obstruction. Because these infants usually have normal lung compliance, only low pressures (4–5 cm H_2O) are needed, which helps to avoid side effects. Nasal CPAP is also used frequently after weaning from mechanical ventilation and is effective in reducing the need for reinstitution of mechanical ventilation.

The most common method to apply continuous positive airway pressure in infants with effective spontaneous respiration is the nasal route. Because the newborn breathes preferentially through the nose, it is possible to connect any of the CPAP systems to the nose using small nasal prongs or a shortened endotracheal tube passed into the nasopharynx. A limitation of this approach is the difficulty of securing the nasal prongs in place for long periods of time in infants who are very active.

The amount of pressure required usually varies between 2 and 8 cm H_2O, depending on the severity of the lung disease. The less compliant the lungs are, the higher is the pressure required to stabilize the lung volume. To the extent that lung volume is increased with CPAP, pleural pressure will also increase, which in turn can decrease venous return and cardiac output. The persistence of sternal retractions and grunting usually indicates the need for higher airway pressures. On the other hand, a decrease in blood pressure and peripheral perfusion, an increase in $PaCO_2$, or the activation of the abdominal muscles to accelerate expiration might indicate that excessive CPAP is being applied. The chest radiograph may also be helpful and show pulmonary overdistension with a lower diaphragm when excessive CPAP is used. There are a few controlled studies with small numbers of patients that suggest that CPAP reduces the severity of HMD and shortens the course of the disease. They also suggest that CPAP reduces the number of infants who require IPPV and therefore will reduce the complications associated with this therapy. These observations apply mainly to larger infants when CPAP is used early in the course of the disease. In premature infants under 700 to 800 g, most clinicians prefer to use IPPV initially without attempting the use of CPAP because of their tendency to develop severe apnea and respiratory acidosis. The occurrence of CLD is extremely uncommon in infants treated with CPAP alone.

INTERMITTENT POSITIVE-PRESSURE VENTILATION

PHYSIOLOGICAL PRINCIPLES During mechanical ventilation the activity of the respiratory muscles is replaced or supplemented by an intermittent increase in tracheal pressure that creates a pressure gradient between the proximal airway and the distal airspaces. This produces movement of gas into the lung during inspiration. During expiration, airway pressure decreases below alveolar pressure, and exhalation occurs passively because of the elastic recoil of the respiratory system. Lung compliance describes the relationship between lung volume and the distending pressure in the alveoli. Thus, the tidal volume (V_T), the volume of gas moved with each cycle, is mainly determined by the difference between peak inspiratory pressure (PIP) and positive end-expiratory pressure (PEEP) and by the compliance of the respiratory system. However, when there is continuous airflow throughout expiration, as is the case with many time-cycled infant ventilators, then PEEP exceeds alveolar pressure. The lung volume at the end of expiration, or FRC, is determined primarily by lung and chest wall compliance and the alveolar pressure (which, depending on conditions, may differ from the PEEP). For any given compliance in an unstable or in a healthy lung, mean airway pressure (MAP), the area under the positive pressure curve of an entire respiratory cycle, is a major determinant of average lung volume; because of this, arterial oxygenation is also highly influenced by the MAP. Mean airway pressure is determined primarily by the PIP, the PEEP, and the duration of inspiration and expiration. These relationships are particularly relevant for care of the patient with a surfactant-deficient lung in which the distal air spaces tend to collapse at end expiration, when transpulmonary pressure is lowest. Minute ventilation, which is the product of tidal volume and the respiratory rate, generally influences the arterial PCO_2 because it affects the rate of alveolar ventilation and CO_2 elimination.

During ventilation at high respiratory rates there is a particular risk of gas trapping in respiratory segments where airway resistance or lung compliance is high because these factors increase the time it takes for most of the breath to enter or exit the lungs. The propensity for gas trapping can be quantified by the time constant, which is determined by the product of compliance and resistance and is the time taken for about two-thirds of a breath to be expelled. An infant with a compliance of 1 mL/cm H_2O and a resistance of 120 cm H_2O/L × has a time constant of 0.12 seconds. Generally it is desirable to permit an expiratory time of at least three time constants to minimize gas trapping. When the expiratory time is not long enough, alveolar pressure is higher than the proximal airway pressure at the end of expiration, and this is known as inadvertent PEEP. The consequences of this depend on the type of underlying pulmonary pathology. In a patient with airway obstruction, inadvertent PEEP will result in lung overdistension, increased risk of alveolar rupture, and diminished venous return.

Generally, improvement in alveolar ventilation and lower $PaCO_2$ can be achieved by increasing V_T (increasing PIP or lowering PEEP) or increasing respiratory rate. Arterial oxygen tension can be improved by increasing MAP (increasing PEEP, PIP, or inspiratory time) or by using higher inspired oxygen concentrations. However, it is important to keep in mind that higher PIPs and longer inspiratory times are associated with increased risk of alveolar rupture and pneumothorax. A significant advantage of the newer ventilators is that they are equipped with flow sensors that allow the continuous monitoring of the flow and tidal volume delivered to the infant. With this it is possible to make the necessary adjustments in the ventilator settings to maintain a tidal volume that is as close as possible to the normal expected for infants, (5–7 mL per kg body weight). In infants with very low lung compliance, very high airway pressures may be required to achieve normal tidal volumes, and therefore, it is often advisable to accept lower tidal volumes to avoid further lung damage.

INDICATIONS FOR MECHANICAL VENTILATION

The strategy to provide optimal gas exchange with minimal risk varies with the type of process causing respiratory failure. In infants with processes that cause severe restrictive lung disease, eg, HMD, pneumonia, meconium aspiration, pulmonary edema, and diaphragmatic hernia, the main functional alterations are heterogeneous ventilation:perfusion ratios and alveolar collapse and consolidation. These reduce lung compliance and cause hypoxemia. The use of positive end-expiratory pressure and relatively high peak inspiratory pressures is often necessary to maintain ventilation and oxygenation. In contrast, infants with central hypoventilation and normal lung function may need relatively low airway pressures to maintain alveolar ventilation and arterial blood gases within an acceptable range.

Although there are no specific criteria for initiating mechanical ventilation in neonates, most infants are started on ventilatory assistance because of one of the following: severe apnea that does not respond to stimulation, progressive hypoxemia with increasing inspired oxygen requirement unresponsive to nasal CPAP, or progressive hypercapnia.

MODALITIES OF MECHANICAL VENTILATION

There are many different modes for mechanical ventilatory support in the neonate (see Sec. 4.2.2), but little scientific data demonstrating the advantage of one approach over the others. Most ventilators used on neonates are time cycled, pressure limited, and provide continuous flow through the respiratory circuit to allow spontaneous respiration and the generation of PEEP. This allows the operator to set the peak inspiratory and expiratory pressures and the duration of inspiration and expiration (thereby controlling the ventilatory rate).

In *controlled IPPV*, all breaths are mechanical, and the patient has no effective spontaneous respiration.

Intermittent mandatory ventilation (**IMV**) provides a mechanical rate that is less than the patient's spontaneous rate, allowing the infant to contribute to the total minute ventilation. This is the most common modality of ventilation currently utilized for neonates.

One of the major problems with IMV is the lack of synchronization between the infant's spontaneous respiratory activity and the ventilator. This lack of synchronization leads to a poorly coordinated interaction between patient and ventilator with the consequent deterioration in respiratory gas exchange and the possibility of increased risk of a pneumothorax and central nervous system hemorrhage. In some patients, it may be necessary to use sedation and even muscle relaxation to suppress spontaneous respiratory efforts and avoid those complications. However, to alleviate this problem most ventilators are equipped with triggering devices that allow synchronization between the subject's inspiratory effort and the mechanical breaths. This approach provides *synchronized IMV* (**S-IMV**), in which the infant receives a predetermined number of mechanical breaths that are initiated (triggered) by spontaneous efforts; there is continuous airflow between these mechanical breaths so that their can be air entry with any additional spontaneous breaths (just as might occur on CPAP).

Assist-control (**A-C**) supports each spontaneous inspiratory effort with a triggered mechanical breath from the ventilator, and therefore the mechanical rate is the same as that of the infant. In order to prevent an insufficient expiratory time when the patient's respiratory rate is too high, some ventilators include the possibility of terminating the inspiration when the respiratory flow decreases to a predetermined level. This shortens the inspiratory-expiratory time and the reduces the risk of gas trapping.

Pressure support ventilation (**PSV**) is similar to A-C in that each inspiratory effort triggers a mechanical breath, and all breaths are terminated when the inspiratory flow decreases to a preset level. This modality is used more frequently in older pediatric and adult patients for weaning from mechanical support. All the modalities mentioned above are available in most commercial neonatal ventilators. There are some other approaches that are less widely used or still in experimental stages but are being incorporated in some newer ventilators.

Proportional assist ventilation (**PAV**) is provided in some of the newer models of ventilators. In this mode, the ventilator increases airway pressure in proportion to the volume or flow that the subject generates during inspiration, thus reducing the elastic and or resistive load imposed by the lung disease. The airway pressure gain or degree of unloading of work is adjusted by the operator, but the timing and volume of each breath is determined by the patient. The ventilator reduces the respiratory load or effort necessary for each breath, and the magnitude of the unloading and PEEP are the only parameters set by the operator. The advantage of this mode is that the patient retains complete control of each breath, but ventilation can be supported to a degree that varies according to the severity of the alteration in lung compliance or resistance.

With *mandatory minute ventilation* (**MMV**), the ventilator continuously adjusts the mechanical rate to maintain a preset minimal minute ventilation. If the patient is able to generate minute ventilation equal to or higher than the preset number, the frequency of the ventilator decreases to a minimum background rate. When the patient is unable to maintain the preset minute ventilation, the mechanical rate increases to reach this ventilation. This mode may be beneficial in infants with variable respiratory center output.

With *volume guarantee ventilation* (**VGV**), the ventilator continuously adjusts PIP to maintain a preset exhaled tidal volume. The advantage of this mode is that it assures a minimal preset tidal volume but decreases PIP to a minimum when the patient is able to generate a normal spontaneous tidal volume. For this reason this mode can also be useful during weaning from IPPV or when there are rapid fluctuations in compliance of the respiratory system.

Intratracheal pulmonary ventilation (**ITPV**) provides an intermittent or a constant flow of gas in the distal end of the endotracheal tube. The purpose of this is to wash out the exhaled gas from the endotracheal tube, reducing the dead space volume. This allows the use of smaller tidal volumes to achieve a similar alveolar ventilation and $PaCO_2$. This method requires special ventilators and endotracheal tubes that at present are not available for clinical use in neonates.

SPECIFIC VENTILATION STRATEGIES

A number of different strategies have been proposed to ventilate preterm neonates, but few have been properly tested in controlled trials.

INTERMITTENT MANDATORY VENTILATION VERSUS CONTROLLED VENTILATION Intermittent mandatory ventilation is the preferred mode of respiratory assistance today, but there is no clear evidence that it is associated with better outcomes than controlled ventilation. The advantage of IMV is that the ventilator is weaned by a gradual reduction in the peak inflation pressure and respiratory rate while the infant increases its own respiratory effort, whereas controlled ventilation is not a mode designed for weaning.

SLOW RESPIRATORY RATE WITH LONG INSPIRATORY TIME VERSUS FAST RESPIRATORY RATE WITH SHORT INSPIRATORY TIME This is another long-standing controversy that has been explored in few clinical trials. The results suggest that although the use of long inspiratory times produces better oxygenation, it is associated with increased risk of alveolar rupture, pulmonary interstitial emphysema, and pneumothorax. For this reason, most clinicians use inspiratory times 0.25 to 0.4 seconds at respiratory rates of 10 to 60/min (the higher the rate, the shorter the inspiratory time).

HIGH VERSUS LOW TIDAL VOLUME Increasing evidence from animal and human studies suggests that the use of large tidal volumes, especially in surfactant-deficient lungs, produces a disruption of the alveolar epithelium and vascular endothelium that leads to increased interstitial lung fluid and decreased lung compliance. In view of this author, the preferred approach is use of the smallest tidal volume that achieves adequate ventilation and oxygenation. In fact, accumulating clinical evidence suggests that allowing some degree of hypoventilation and mild hypercapnia in infants with HMD may be associated with better respiratory outcome.

WEANING FROM MECHANICAL VENTILATION

It is often very difficult to wean the very small preterm infant from mechanical ventilation. Successful weaning generally requires improved lung mechanics and gas exchange, adequate central respiratory output, and an effective respiratory pump. The long process of weaning frequently starts shortly after mechanical ventilation is initiated. Ventilator settings are gradually reduced to allow the patient to assume a larger portion of the respiratory work while avoiding excessive hypoxemia or hypercapnia. The initial settings in the ventilator are determined by the type and severity of the pulmonary disease. In general, as the pulmonary function improves, PIP is often reduced to avoid excessive lung expansion and tissue damage. When modest inflation pressures have been achieved ($<20-25$ cm H_2O) the ventilator rate is reduced. Changes in ventilatory settings are facilitated by measuring tidal volume and adjusting the pressures to keep tidal volume between 5 and 7 mL/kg body weight. It is important to stress that there is no reason to keep the pH and $PaCO_2$ below normal range because this will most likely result in suppression of the spontaneous respiration. The current practice is to permit $PaCO_2$ to rise to ranges between 50 and 60 mm Hg as long as pH is >7.25. As oxygenation improves, the inspired oxygen concentration and MAP can be reduced.

Extubation is usually attempted when the infant is able to maintain acceptable blood gases for several hours on minimal setting such as an IMV rate of 10 to 15 per minute, a PIP below 15 to 18 cm H_2O, and a fraction of inspired oxygen (FiO_2) ≤ 0.3.

COMPLICATIONS

Complications occur frequently in infants who are mechanically ventilated. Many times it is difficult to determine whether the complications are caused by the mechanical ventilation or whether they are a consequence of the primary disease. Complications may be related to the use of endotracheal tubes, high positive airway pressure and inspired oxygen concentration, and infections. Common complications associated with the use of endotracheal tubes include accidental extubation, dislodgement, movement into a main stem bronchus (usually the right), and obstruction. Proper fixation of the tube and regular attention to its position with respect to the nares or mouth reduce but do not eliminate the risk of displaced or dislodged tube. Adequate heating and humidification of the inspired gas and frequent suctioning technique may help to prevent obstruction of the tube by secretions. Local trauma to the nose, larynx, and trachea may occur if the tube fits too tightly. The tube should be as large as possible but still allow for a small leak around it to prevent tracheal damage. Even with proper precautions, upper airway obstruction from subglottic stenosis may occur in some patients requiring long-term or repeated intubations.

Some reports have described pneumothoraces caused by suction catheters perforating the airway while being passed beyond the tip of the endotracheal tube. Airway suctioning must be performed using sterile technique to prevent colonization of the respiratory tract. There is a significant risk for development of pneumonia or systemic infections following airway colonization, especially in the immunocompromised preterm infant. A high proportion of infants ventilated for more than a few days become colonized with bacteria in their airways, predisposing them to serious nosocomial infections.

CARDIOVASCULAR EFFECTS When the volume of the lungs increases, pleural pressure also increases (because the chest wall compliance is not infinite). The increase in pleural pressure can, in turn, impede venous return. During application of any given airway pressure, the increase in pleural pressure depends directly on the lung compliance (because it determines how much lung volume increases) and inversely on chest wall compliance (because it determines how much pleural pressure rises for an increase in lung volume). Therefore, for any given airway pressure, pleural pressure rises less when there is low lung compliance or high chest wall compliance, as is often the case in very premature infants with respiratory distress syndrome (RDS).

The increased pleural pressure interferes with the venous return to the right heart. Alveolar overdistension can also increase pulmonary vascular resistance and impair pulmonary blood flow. The increase in pulmonary artery pressure can produce or increase an already existing right-to-left shunt through the foramen ovale or ductus arteriosus, aggravating the arterial hypoxemia. A falling PaO_2 should, therefore, suggest the possibility of an excessive positive airway pressure and raise this as a consideration for adjusting the ventilator.

One of the major complications in critically ill preterm infants is the development of intracranial hemorrhage. Although it is not clear what the role is of positive-pressure ventilation in the pathogenesis of this complication, it seems that the hemodynamic effects of excessive airway pressure or a tension pneumothorax may increase the risk of CNS hemorrhage. There is also some evidence that persistent hyperventilation is associated with an increased risk of periventricular parenchymal lesions. These may develop as a result of ischemia secondary to the cerebrovascular constriction induced by hypocapnia.

One of the major and more frequent complications associated with IPPV is alveolar rupture potentially leading to pulmonary interstitial emphysema, pneumomediastinum, pneumothorax, or pneumopericardium. Pneumothorax occurs in fewer than 10% of infants with severe HMD who require IPPV but is associated with a significant increase in morbidity and mortality.

PULMONARY SEQUELAE A significant number of small premature infants who require prolonged IPPV survive with abnormal lung function that may persist for years. The most severe form of chronic lung disease occurs in 5 to 15% of all HMD survivors who require IPPV for more than a few days. The pathogenesis of this process is not fully understood, but most likely it is the result of multiple factors including immaturity of the lung, damage produced by the HMD or infection, persistence of a ductus arteriosus, oxygen toxicity, and use of excessive positive airway pressures. Chronic lung disease (CLD) occurs frequently in infants born before 28 weeks of gestation; it is uncommon in infants between 28 and 32 weeks and extremely rare in those over 32 weeks of gestation. Most preterm infants who survive after IPPV do not have the severe alterations in lung structure and function observed in CLD but still have milder abnormalities in lung function that may predispose them to respiratory illness later in life.

References

Bernstein G, Mannino FL, Heldt GP, et al: Randomized multicenter trial comparing synchronized and conventional intermittent mandatory ventilation in neonates. J Pediatr 128:453–463, 1996

Bjorklund LJ, Ingimarsson J, Curstedt T, et al: Manual ventilation with a few large breaths at birth compromises the therapeutic effect of subsequent surfactant replacement in immature lambs. Pediatr Res 42:348–355, 1997

Bohin S, Fenton AC, Thompson JR, et al: Circulatory effects of ventilator rate and end-expiratory pressure in unparalysed preterm infants. Acta Paediatr 84:1300–1304, 1995

Boros SJ, Matalon SV, Ewald R, et al: The effect of independent variations in inspiratory expiratory ratio and end expiratory pressure during mechanical ventilation in hyaline membrane disease: the significance of mean airway pressure. J Pediatr 91:794–798, 1977

Carlton DP, Cummings JJ, Scheerer RG, et al: Lung overexpansion increases pulmonary microvascular protein permeability in young lambs. J Appl Physiol 69:577–583, 1990

Cartwright DW, Willis MM, Gregory GA: Functional residual capacity and lung mechanics at different levels of mechanical ventilation. Crit Care Med 12:422–427, 1984

Claure N, Gerhardt T, Hummler H, et al: Computer-controlled minute ventilation in preterm infants undergoing mechanical ventilation. J Pediatr 131:910–913, 1997

Da Silva WJ, Abbasi S, Pereira G, et al: Role of positive end-expiratory pressure changes on functional residual capacity in surfactant treated preterm infants. Pediatr Pulmonol 18:89–92, 1994

Dreyfuss D, Saumon G: Ventilator-induced lung injury. Lessons from experimental studies. Am J Respir Crit Care Med 157:294–323, 1998

Hausdorf G, Hellwege HH: Influence of positive end-expiratory pressure on cardiac performance in premature infants: a Doppler-echocardiographic study. Crit Care Med 15:661–664, 1987

Heicher DA, Kasting DS, Harrod JR: Prospective clinical comparison of two methods for mechanical ventilation of neonates: rapid rate and short inspiratory time versus slow rate and long inspiratory time. J Pediatr 98:957–961, 1981

Higgins RD, Richter SE, Davis JM: Nasal continuous positive airway pressure facilitates extubation of very low birth weight neonates. Pediatrics 88:999–1003, 1991

Hird M, Greenough A, Gamsu H: Gas trapping during high frequency positive pressure ventilation using conventional ventilators. Early Hum Dev 22:51–56, 1990

Hummler HD, Gerhardt T, Gonzalez A, et al: Patient-triggered ventilation in neonates: comparison of a flow- and an impedance-triggered system. Am J Respir Crit Care Med 154:1049–1054, 1996

Hummler H, Gerhardt T, Gonzalez A, et al: Influence of different methods of synchronized mechanical ventilation on ventilation, gas exchange, patient effort, and blood pressure fluctuations in premature neonates. Pediatr Pulmonol 22:305–313, 1996

Jonson B: Ventilation patterns, surfactant and lung injury. Biol Neonate 71:13–17, 1997

Kano S, Lanteri CJ, Pemberton PJ, et al: Fast versus slow ventilation for neonates. Am Rev Respir Dis 148:578–584, 1993

Kim EH, Boutwell WC: Successful direct extubation of very low birth weight infants from low intermittent mandatory ventilation rate. Pediatrics 80:409–414, 1987

Klopping-Ketelaars WAA, Maertzdorf WJ, Blanco CE: Cardiovascular changes during sustained lung inflations in premature newborn lambs. Acta Paediatr 83:897–902, 1994

Mariani G, Cifuentes J, Carlo WA: Randomized trial of permissive hypercapnia in preterm infants. Pediatrics 104:1082–1088, 1999

Michna J, Jobe AH, Ikegami M: Positive end-expiratory pressure preserves surfactant function in preterm lamb. Am J Respir Crit Care Med 160:634–639, 1999

Mirro R, Busija D, Green R, et al: Relationship between mean airway pressure, cardiac output, and organ blood flow with normal and decreased respiratory compliance. J Pediatr 111:101–106, 1987

Mitchell A, Greenough A, Hird M: Limitations of patient triggered ventilation in neonates. Arch Dis Child 64:924–929, 1989

Nilsson R, Grossmann G, Robertson B: Artificial ventilation of premature newborn rabbits: effects of positive end-espiratory pressure on lung mechanics and lung morphology. Acta Paediatr Scand 69:597–602, 1980

Schulze A, Gerhardt T, Musante G, et al: Proportional assist ventilation in low birth weight infants with acute respiratory disease. A comparison to assist/control and conventional mechanical ventilation J Pediatr 135: 339–44, 1999

Simbruner G: Inadvertent positive end-expiratory pressure in mechanically ventilated newborn infants: detection and effect on lung mechanics and gas exchange. J Pediatr 108:589–595, 1986

Tarnow-Mordi WO, Reid E, Griffiths P, et al: Low inspired gas temperature and respiratory complications in very low birth weight infants. J Pediatr 114:438–442, 1989

Taskar V, John J, Evander E, et al. Surfactant dysfunction makes lungs vulnerable to repetitive collapse and reexpansion. Am J Respir Crit Care Med 155:313–320, 1997

Wada K, Jobe AH, Ikegami M: Tidal volume effects on surfactant treatment responses with the initiation of ventilation in preterm lambs. J Appl Physiol 83:1054–1061, 1997

Wiswell TE, Graziani LJ, Kornhauser MS, et al: Effects of hypocarbia on the development of cystic periventricular leukomalacia in premature infants treated with high-frequency jet ventilation. Pediatrics 98:918–924, 1996

2.19.2   High-Frequency Mechanical Ventilation

John P. Kinsella

High-frequency ventilation (HFV) is a technique that delivers small tidal volumes with low phasic pressure changes at supraphysiological frequencies (see Sec. 4.2.2). Conventional mechanical ventilation is operated at frequencies less than 150 breaths per minute, whereas, high-frequency devices for newborn respiratory failure are typically operated at frequencies between 300 and 900 breaths per minute.

HFV can be administered by a few types of devices. High-frequency oscillatory ventilation (HFOV) generates a sinusoidal (biphasic) pressure waveform through oscillation of a piston or piston-diaphragm configuration, which is superimposed on an adjustable mean airway pressure. The hallmark of HFOV (in contrast to other forms of high-frequency ventilation) is the incorporation of an *active* phase of exhalation. High-frequency jet ventilation (HFJV) delivers rapid bursts of inspiratory gas via a cannula attached to a specially adapted endotracheal tube. The third type of device employs interruption of a high-flow gas source using solenoids and is referred to as high-frequency flow interruption (HFFI). Both HFJV and HFFI are configured with a conventional neonatal ventilator and allow the addition of tidal volume breaths during the high-frequency mode. Moreover, the design differences that determine adjustment of mean airway pressure and pressure amplitude are sufficiently different among HFV models that direct comparisons of clinical performance are problematic.

Gas exchange during HFV has been most carefully studied for the oscillatory technique. During HFOV, gas transport occurs through direct alveolar ventilation, Taylor-type dispersion, convective dispersion caused by asymmetric velocity profiles, out-of-phase oscillation (pendelluft), and molecular diffusion. Bulk convection (just as in conventional ventilation) likely remains the most important mechanism for gas exchange in the lung during HFOV.

HFV has been studied extensively in the newborn intensive care setting. Applications of HFV have included efforts to prevent or reduce the severity of chronic lung disease in premature infants with hyaline membrane disease, "rescue" treatment of preterm newborns with pulmonary interstitial emphysema, and mangagement of term newborns with severe hypoxemic respiratory failure. Differences in ventilator strategies employed in various studies have produced disparities in conclusions.

Despite the promise of early laboratory and clinical studies of HFV in premature newborns, the results of recent controlled trials have challenged the hypothesis that early HFV intervention confers substantial short- or long-term clinical benefits. Improvements in conventional mechanical ventilation strategies, increased use of prenatal corticosteroids, and the use of exogenous surfactant therapy have all contributed to a reduced risk of acute and chronic lung injury. Thus, currently available evidence from recently conducted randomized, controlled trials suggests that HFV is not essential in the early management of most premature newborns with respiratory failure. However, many practitioners believe that HFV provides a critically important tool in the management of infants with hypoxemic respiratory failure refractory to conventional ventilation.

HFV has also been studied in the term infant with hypoxemic respiratory failure and persistent pulmonary hypertension of the newborn (see Sec. 2.17.11). Clark and colleaques showed that HFOV was often effective in term newborns who failed management with conventional ventilation. In another recent study, HFOV combined with inhaled nitric oxide was compared to HFOV or nitric oxide alone during conventional ventilation infants with persistent pulmonary hypertension of newborn (PPHN). For patients with PPHN complicated by severe parenchymal lung disease, response rates for HFOV + iNO (inhaled nitric oxide) were better than for HFOV alone or iNO with conventional ventilation. In contrast, for patients without significant parenchymal lung disease, both iNO and HFOV + iNO were more effective than HFOV alone. Therefore, effective lung recruitment using HFV may be useful in neonatal hypoxemic respiratory failure or PPHN, but it is not possible to derive conclusions about mechanisms.

There are certain risks associated with HFV that require particular vigilance. Initiation of HFV can cause striking reductions in $PaCO_2$ and possibly cerebral blood flow, potentially increasing the risk of cerebral ischemic injury and periventricular leukomalacia. As in all forms of positive-pressure ventilation, failure to reduce mean airway pressure after lung volume improves may be associated with adverse hemodynamic effects and air leak. Similarly, some patients with airways disease and prolonged expiratory time constants (eg, established chronic lung disease, meconium aspiration syndrome) may be at particular risk for air trapping, and HFV should be used with caution in this setting.

References

Chang HK: Mechanisms of gas transport during ventilation by high-frequency oscillation. J Appl Physiol 56:553–563, 1984

Clark RH, Gerstmann DR, Null DM JR, Delemos RA: Prospective randomized comparison of high frequency oscillatory and conventional ventilation in respiratory distress syndrome. Pediatrics 89:5–12, 1992

Clark RH: High frequency ventilation. J Pediatr 124:661–670, 1994

Clark RH, Gerstmann DR: Controversies in high-frequency ventilation. Clin Perinatol 25:113–122, 1998

Gerstmann DR, Minton SD, Stoddard RA, et al: The Provo multicenter early high-frequency oscillatory ventilation trial: improved pulmonary and clinical outcome in respiratory distress syndrome. Pediatrics 98: 1044–1057, 1996

HIFI Study Group: High-frequency oscillatory ventilation compared with conventional ventilation in the treatment of respiratory failure in preterm infants. N Engl J Med 320:88–93, 1989

Kinsella JP, Truog WE, Walsh WF, et al: Randomized, multicenter trial of inhaled nitric oxide and high-frequency oscillatory ventilation in severe, persistent pulmonary hypertension of the newborn. J Pediatr 131:55–62, 1997

McCulloch PR, Forkert PG, Froese AB: Lung volume maintenance prevents lung injury during high frequency oscillatory ventilation in surfactant-deficient rabbits. Am Rev Respir Dis 137:1185–1192, 1988

Rettwitz-Volk W, Veldman A, Roth B, et al: A prospective, randomized, multicenter trial of high-frequency oscillatory ventilation compared with conventional ventilation in preterm infants with respiratory distress syndrome receiving surfactant. J Pediatr 132:249–254, 1998

Thome U, Kossel H, Lipowsky G, et al: Randomized comparison of high-frequency ventilation with high-rate intermittent positive pressure ventilation in preterm infants with respiratory failure. J Pediatr 135:39–46, 1999

Wiswell TE, Graziani LJ, Kornhauser MS, et al: High-frequency jet ventilation in the early management of respiratory distress syndrome is associated with a greater risk for adverse outcomes. Pediatrics 98:1035–1043, 1996

2.19.3   Extracorporeal Membrane Oxygenation

Billie Lou Short

Extracorporeal membrane oxygenation (ECMO) is the use of a modified cardiopulmonary bypass circuit to support oxygenation and removal of carbon dioxide for a prolonged period of time (days to weeks) until the underlying disease resolves (see Sec. 4.2.3). The ECMO circuit includes a membrane oxygenator and nonpulsatile roller occlusion pumping system, similar to those used to support cardiac function during heart surgery (see Fig. 2-66). Because of the invasive nature of this procedure, use of ECMO is limited to those patients with a high mortality risk. This section addresses the use of ECMO in the neonatal patient with respiratory failure.

PATIENT POPULATION AND CRITERIA

The concept of the use of ECMO therapy as an artificial placenta began in the 1960s when numerous investigators used ECMO to treat the premature infant in respiratory failure. In 1976, Bartlett and his associates reported the first neonatal ECMO survivor, a term infant with severe meconium aspiration syndrome (MAS), thus opening the door to this new therapy. Present-day ECMO therapy is used in the term or near-term infant with respiratory

failure from either MAS or other aspiration syndromes, such as blood or amniotic fluid, sepsis/pneumonia, severe hyaline membrane disease, primary pulmonary hypertension of the newborn (PPHN), both idiopathic and secondary to other underlying lung diseases, or pulmonary hypoplasia associated with congenital diaphragmatic hernia.

The systemic heparinization and the physiological changes caused by the pumping system resulted in a significant intracranial hemorrhage rate when ECMO was first used. This complication remains such a critical factor that most centers do not use ECMO for infants whose gestation is <34 weeks of gestation or birth weight <2000 g. Because infants on ECMO require heparinization to prevent clotting in the circuit, any major uncontrolled bleeding disorder is a contraindication for ECMO. Any significant intracranial hemorrhage is also a contraindication for ECMO. Selection criteria for infants to receive ECMO usually includes a risk of mortality >80%. ECMO centers vary in their determination of this mortality risk, but the most commonly used criteria today is the oxygen index (OI-mean airway pressure $\times$ F_IO_2 $\times$ 100 $\div$ PaO_2). An OI greater than 40 for at least three blood gas determinations 30 minutes apart while on maximal ventilatory support predicts a high mortality and is used by many centers to determine when to place an infant on ECMO.

THE ECMO PROCEDURE

The infant must be heparinized during the operative cannulation and remain so throughout the procedure. Activated clotting time is usually measured hourly to assess heparinization, to avoid clot formation in the circuit or bleeding in the patient. Platelet and fibrinogen levels are also monitored and maintained in a relatively normal range to reduce the risk of patient bleeding.

ECMO can be provided through a venoarterial or a venovenous approach. Although the catheters differ and cannulation vessels are different, the ECMO circuit is the same for both types of ECMO.

Venoarterial ECMO provides both pulmonary and cardiac support and can therefore be used in patients with either pulmonary or cardiac failure. To initiate venoarterial ECMO, the right common carotid artery and jugular vein are cannulated, with the jugular vein catheter advanced to the midatrial level and the carotid artery

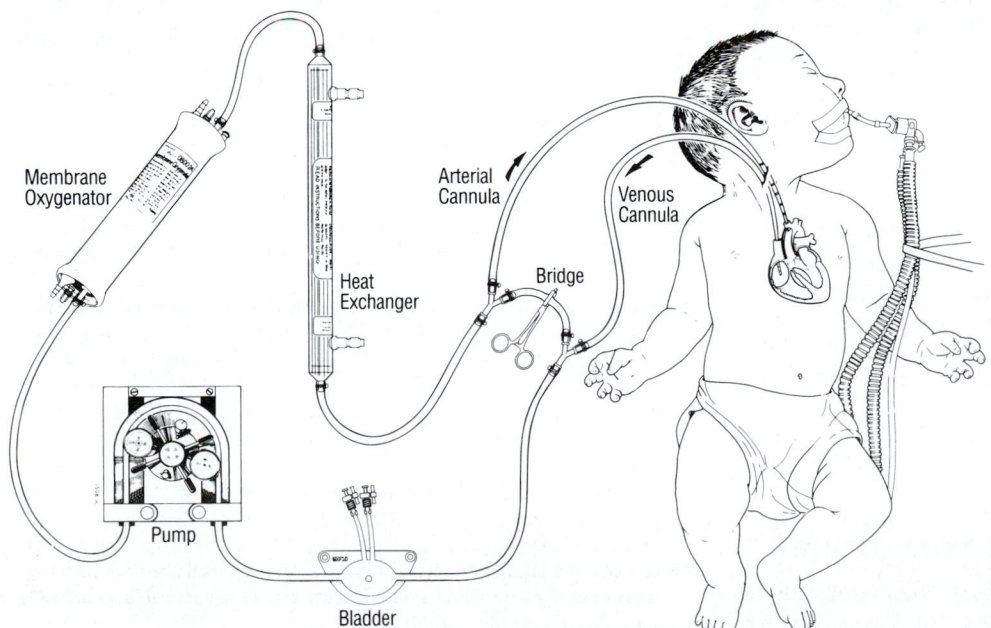

Membrane Oxygenator

Arterial Cannula

Venous Cannula

Heat Exchanger

Bridge

Pump

Bladder

FIGURE 2-66   **Schematic of the venoarterial ECMO circuit** SOURCE: *CNMC ECMO Training Manual, Washington, DC, Children's National Medical Center, with permission*). **The venous catheter enters the jugular vein and is advanced so that it rests in the right atrium. The arterial catheter enters the right common carotid artery and is advanced so that it is just entering the aortic arch. The circuit is the same for venovenous ECMO, but the two ports on the venovenous catheter hook into the arterial (inflow) and venous (outflow) tubing on the circuit.**

catheter advanced to the arch of the aorta. The ECMO circuit is primed with blood products, which allows the catheters to be connected into the system while maintaining an isovolemic status. As the pump is initiated, blood is drained via gravity from the right atrium into the circuit. Blood is then pulled out of the venous reservoir by a roller occlusion pump and pushed through the membrane lung, where gas exchange occurs. A 0.8-m² membrane (Avecor, Minneapolis) is most commonly used for neonates. Carbon dioxide transfer is so efficient with this membrane that CO_2 must be added to the gases flowing into the membrane. Gas transfers across the silicone membrane lung into the blood because of pressure gradients, increasing the oxygen level and removing carbon dioxide. Blood leaves the membrane lung and enters the heat exchanger, where it is warmed to body temperature and returned to the infant through the arterial catheter. On the first few days of ECMO therapy, most infants require 60% of their cardiac output (estimated at 120 mL/kg) to go through the circuit to allow the membrane lung to maintain good oxygenation. Because venoarterial ECMO bypasses the heart, it can supply both cardiac and pulmonary support. This form of ECMO is used in infants who have a degree of cardiac dysfunction in addition to their underlying lung disease. Many infants with respiratory failure also have cardiac dysfunction from severe hypoxia. These infants are usually candidates for venoarterial ECMO.

Venovenous ECMO can be achieved either using a double-lumen venovenous catheter placed in the right jugular vein and advanced into the right atrium or by two catheters, usually a jugular vein catheter and femoral vein catheter. For appropriate flow rates to be achieved, the jugular vein catheter is the drainage catheter, and the femoral vein catheter is the return catheter. The latter is routinely used in older patients but not in the newborns because of difficulty cannulating the femoral vein. The double-lumen catheters allow blood to be removed from and returned to the right atrium using the same catheter. This approach eliminates the risk of carotid artery ligation. The heart serves as the pumping chamber for the body with this approach. Therefore, venovenous ECMO does not provide any cardiac support. Those infants requiring high flow rates or those with unstable blood pressure are not good candidates for venovenous ECMO. ECMO centers must be experienced in venoarterial ECMO before attempting venovenous ECMO because of the added technical difficulties with venovenous ECMO. Although the rate varies from center to center, 5 to 10% of venovenous patients will need to be converted to venoarterial ECMO because of inability to oxygenate or to maintain stable blood pressures.

Most neonatal patients, with the exception of those with congenital diaphragmatic hernia (CDH), require ECMO support for 5 days. As the lungs improve, less blood flow is required to pass through the artificial lung, and the ECMO blood flow can be reduced. Weaning usually does not occur in the first 1 to 2 days, but generally is marked over the next 2 to 3 days. While on ECMO the infant is kept on *lung-rest* settings on the ventilator and allowed to breathe spontaneously. ECMO flows are weaned based on arterial blood gases until 10% of the cardiac output is reached. This level of support is called *idling*. The infant is maintained on idle flows for 4 to 8 hours. If stable after this period, the infant is ready for decannulation. Most infants treated in this fashion can be extubated from the ventilator within 24 to 48 hours after ECMO decannulation.

OUTCOME AND LONG-TERM FOLLOW-UP

Although overall survival is 80% nationally, the best results are for infants with MAS (94%) and PPHN (82%). The survival rate for infants with CDH requiring ECMO has not improved and remains at 60% nationally.

The primary cause of death in the ECMO population is intracranial hemorrhage. The risk factors associated with the development of intracranial hemorrhage include significant hypoxic or ischemic cerebral insult before ECMO, sepsis with coagulopathy, or gestational age less than 37 weeks. Because not all intracranial abnormalities are detected by ultrasound, computerized tomography or magnetic resonance imaging is recommended before discharge. A baseline hearing test and a neurologic assessment are also recommended before discharge. All infants should be followed in a neonatal high-risk follow-up program.

Developmental outcome is encouraging, with most centers reporting that 60 to 70% of ECMO survivors are normal at 1 to 2 years of age. Risk factors associated with poor outcome include severe neuroimaging abnormality, chronic lung disease, prematurity, and group B streptococcal sepsis. The 10 to 15% of ECMO-treated infants who are considered suspect for abnormalities at 1 to 2 years of age require close follow-up because a large percentage of these infants have learning disabilities by 5 years of age.

Although the need for carotid artery ligation for VA ECMO has caused concern that right-sided central nervous system lesions would occur, neuroimaging studies have not corroborated this concern. No major right-left differences have been noted in neuroimaging studies in these infants, although there is a higher incidence of posterior fossa hemorrhages. This finding raises concerns for venous congestion caused by the venous catheter. Outcome studies to date have followed these children out to 10 years of age with no abnormal findings attributed to carotid artery ligation. These patients will need to be followed into adulthood before the full effects of vessel ligation can be determined.

ECMO care requires highly trained nurses, respiratory therapists, perfusionists, and physicians. It has been estimated that only 1000 to 2500 term infants require ECMO each year in the United States. Therefore, programs should be regionalized based on need because adequate numbers of patients are required for providers of ECMO to maintain their expertise.

References

Bulas DI, Taylor GA, O'Donnell, Short BL, Fitz CR, Vezina G: Intracranial abnormalities in infants treated with extracorporeal membrane oxygenation: update on sonographic and CT findings. Am J Neuroradiol 17: 287–290, 1996

Giles JP, Firmin RK: The inflammatory coagulative response to prolonged extracorporeal membrane oxygenation, scholarly review. ASAIO J 45: 250–263, 1999

Glass P, Bulas DI, Wagner AE, et al: Severity of brain injury following neonatal ECMO and outcome at age 5. Dev Med Child Neurol 39(7): 441–448, 1997

Short BL: Extracorporeal membrane oxygenation. In: Avery GB, Fletcher MA, MacDonald MG, eds: Neonatology, the Pathophysiology and Management of the Newborn, 5th ed. Baltimore, Lippicott, Williams & Wilkins, 1999:557–568

UK Collaborative ECMO Trial Group: UK collaborative randomized trial of neonatal extracorporeal membrane oxygenation. Lancet 348:75–82, 1996

Van Meurs K, Short BL: Congenital diaphragmatic hernia: the neonatologist's perspective. Pediatr Rev 20:e79–e87, 1999 [available at www.pedsinreview.org]

Zwischenberger JB, Bartlett RH: ECMO, Extracorporeal Cardiopulmonary Support in Critical Care, 2nd ed. Ann Arbor, MI Extracorporeal Life Support Organization, 2000

2.19.4   Inhaled Nitric Oxide Therapy

Steven H. Abman

NITRIC OXIDE IN THE PERINATAL PULMONARY CIRCULATION

Endothelium-derived products, especially nitric oxide (NO), play important roles in the regulation of vascular tone and structure in the perinatal pulmonary circulation. Furchgott first recognized that vascular endothelium produces a labile but potent vasodilator substance known as "endothelium-derived relaxing factor" (EDRF), which was subsequently identified as NO or a NO-containing product. NO is formed during the conversion of L-arginine to L-citrulline by the enzyme NO synthase (NOS). Once produced, NO rapidly diffuses to neighboring smooth muscle cells, where it stimulates soluble guanylate cyclase (sGC) activity, increases intracellular cyclic guanosine 3,′5′-monophosphate (cGMP) content, and causes vasodilation (Fig. 2-67). Vascular smooth muscle also contains a cGMP-specific phosphodiesterase (PDE5) that limits NO-mediated vasodilation through the hydrolysis of cGMP. PDE5 is present in lung vascular smooth muscle and appears especially active in the normal fetal lung, as well as in experimental models of pulmonary hypertension. Thus, net "NO activity" in the pulmonary circulation depends on several factors, including the regulation of expression, activities, and availability of several components of the NO-cGMP cascade, including enzymes (NOS, sGC, and PDE5), substrate (L-arginine), and cofactors.

The NO-cGMP cascade plays an important role in vasoregulation of the perinatal lung. Experimental studies have demonstrated that NO modulates pulmonary vascular tone and reactivity during fetal life, contributes to the dramatic fall in PVR at birth, and maintains low pulmonary vascular tone in the normal newborn. Physiological stimuli, including shear stress, ventilation (or rhythmic lung distension), and increased oxygen tension, independently increase NOS activity, contributing to pulmonary vasodilation at birth. Lung endothelial NOS mRNA, protein, and activity are down-regulated in several perinatal models of PPHN, including pulmonary hypertension from chronic compression of the ductus arteriosus in fetal lambs, congenital diaphragmatic hernia in newborn rats, and chronically hypoxic newborn piglets. In addition to altered NO production, vascular smooth muscle cell function may be impaired in pulmonary hypertension, causing decreased sGC and increased PDE5 activities.

PHYSIOLOGICAL RATIONALE FOR INHALED NO THERAPY

Once it was recognized that the gas NO is an EDRF, several investigators demonstrated that NO could be inhaled (iNO) and cause selective pulmonary vasodilation in animal models or in patients with primary pulmonary hypertension. The physiological rationale for iNO therapy in the treatment of hypoxemic respiratory failure in the newborn is primarily based on the ability of iNO to reach the pulmonary vascular bed and achieve potent and sustained pulmonary vasodilation without decreasing systemic vascular tone (Fig. 2-68); the selectivity occurs because NO is rapidly bound to hemoglobin in the pulmonary circulation, thereby preventing it from reaching the systemic vasculature. Persistent pulmonary hypertension of the newborn (PPHN) is a syndrome that is associated with diverse neonatal cardiopulmonary disorders that are characterized by high pulmonary vascular resistance (PVR), causing extrapulmonary right-to-left shunting across the ductus arteriosus (DA) and foramen ovale (FO). *Extrapulmonary shunting* associated with high PVR can cause severe hypoxemia that often responds poorly to high levels of supplemental oxygen, alkalosis, or pharmacologic vasodilators. The use of vasodilator drugs that are administered intravenously, such as tolazoline and sodium nitroprusside, is often unsuccessful because of concomitant systemic hypotension, an inability to achieve or sustain pulmonary vasodilation, or adverse side effects. Thus, the ability of iNO therapy to selectively lower PVR and decrease right-to-left shunting of blood

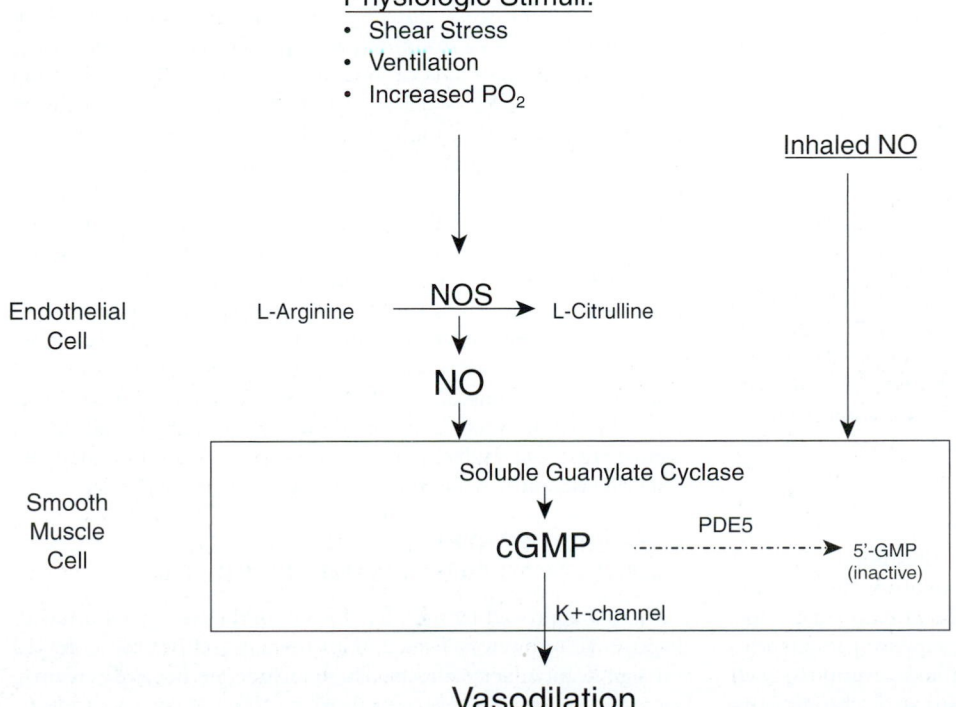

FIGURE 2-67 NO-cGMP cascade in the pulmonary circulation. Abbreviations: cGMP = cyclic guanosine 3′,5′-monophosphate; NO = nitric oxide; NOS = nitric oxide synthase; PDE5 = type V phosphodiesterase.

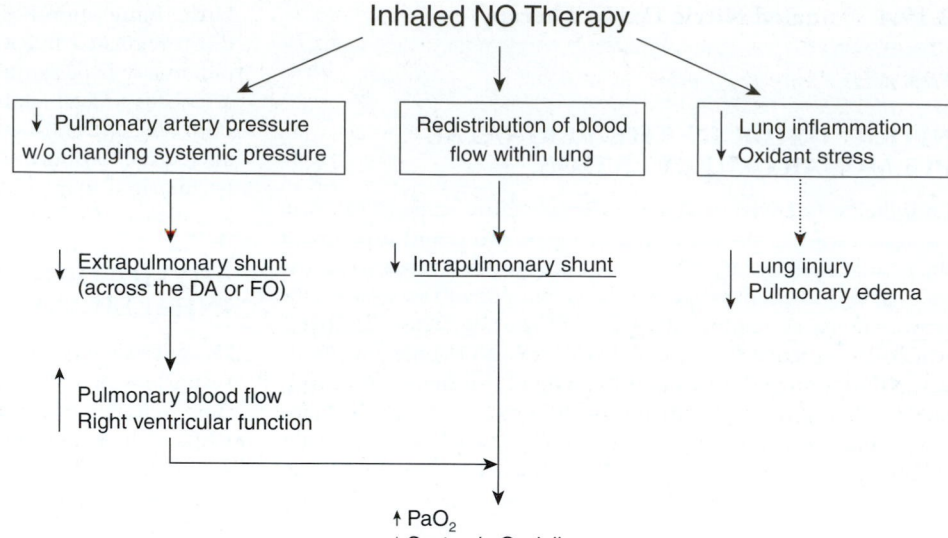

FIGURE 2-68 Physiological roles of inhaled NO therapy in the newborn with hypoxemic respiratory failure. Inhaled NO can improve oxygenation by decreasing extrapulmonary or intrapulmonary shunting of blood. The effects of inhaled NO on lung inflammation and oxidant stress is speculative and is primarily based on animal experiments. Abbreviations: DA = ductus arteriosus; FO = foramen ovale; w/o = without.

across the DA or FO accounts for the acute improvement in oxygenation observed in most newborns with PPHN.

Oxygenation also can improve during iNO therapy in some newborns who do not have extrapulmonary right-to-left shunting, suggesting that iNO could improve oxygenation in some cases of neonatal hypoxemic respiratory failure without PPHN physiology. Hypoxemia in these cases is primarily caused by *intrapulmonary shunting* or severe mismatching of ventilation and perfusion (from atelectasis, airways obstruction, hemorrhage, edema, or abnormal vasoreactivity). Distinct from its effects on improving pulmonary blood flow by lowering PVR, low-dose iNO therapy can also improve oxygenation by redirecting blood from poorly aerated or diseased lung regions to better aerated distal air spaces ("microselective effect"). In addition to the effects of iNO on vascular tone and reactivity, experimental studies have demonstrated that iNO treatment can have other physiological and biochemical effects in the lung as well, including attenuation of lung inflammation, vascular permeability, and thrombosis in situ. In contrast with the use of iNO as a selective pulmonary vasodilator, less clinical data are currently available to support its use as a part of a "lung protective" strategy to decrease acute lung injury.

CLINICAL STUDIES OF INHALED NITRIC OXIDE IN NEWBORNS

In 1992, iNO was shown to improve oxygenation and lower PVR acutely in term newborns with severe hypoxemia and PPHN that met institutional criteria for ECMO therapy. In these early studies, prolonged treatment with continuous low doses of iNO ($\leq$6 ppm) caused sustained increases in oxygenation and contributed to the successful management of PPHN without the need for ECMO. Patients included in these studies had echocardiographic evidence of PPHN with meconium aspiration syndrome (MAS), respiratory distress syndrome (of newborn) (RDS), sepsis, and congenital diaphragmatic hernia or without lung disease ("idiopathic" PPHN). In two large multicenter randomized clinical trials, iNO therapy was subsequently shown to decrease ECMO utilization by 29% and 40% in newborns with severe hypoxemic respiratory failure. Mortality was no different between placebo and iNO treatment groups, likely reflecting the availability of ECMO therapy for patients who failed medical management. The incidence and severity of such complications as seizures, neurologic morbidity, or chronic lung

disease were also not different between study groups. Differences in neurologic, developmental, cardiac, or pulmonary sequelae between treated and control patients have not been observed in infants during follow-up, but data on long-term outcomes remain limited. Based on the results of these two randomized trials, iNO therapy was recently approved by the US Food and Drug Administration for the treatment of term and near-term neonates with hypoxemic respiratory failure.

Although multicenter randomized studies have demonstrated the overall efficacy and safety of low-dose iNO therapy in reducing the need for ECMO therapy, not all hypoxemic newborns respond to iNO therapy. Factors that determine responsiveness to iNO therapy are incompletely understood but include the severity of the primary lung disease associated with hypoxemia, the presence of echocardiographic evidence of *extrapulmonary* right-to-left shunt, ventilator strategies to optimize lung recruitment, the presence of myocardial dysfunction or multiorgan disease, the severity of pulmonary vascular disease, unrecognized structural cardiac disease or pulmonary venous obstruction, diseases of abnormal lung development, among others. Poor lung inflation, especially in the setting of pneumonia, MAS, or RDS, may decrease the effective delivery of iNO to its site of action in the pulmonary circulation. In addition, low lung volumes with severe lung disease can worsen pulmonary hypertension through mechanical effects on PVR and regional hypoxia. Alternatively, hyperinflation or regional gas trapping from overaggressive mechanical ventilation can also increase PVR. The importance of interactions between lung recruitment and responsiveness to iNO therapy was supported by observations that combined treatment of HFOV with iNO was more successful than either treatment alone in some patients in a randomized study. Thus, although iNO may be an effective treatment for PPHN, it should be considered only as part of an overall clinical strategy that is carefully integrated into management of underlying lung disease, cardiac function, and systemic hemodynamics.

CONTROVERSIES IN THE USE OF INHALED NITRIC OXIDE THERAPY

Although approved by the FDA for use in the term newborn with hypoxemic respiratory failure, iNO therapy still has the potential for significant adverse effects. These include methemoglobinemia, increased exposure to nitrogen dioxide (NO_2) or peroxynitrite, rebound hypoxemia and pulmonary hypertension after rapid withdrawal of iNO therapy, and bleeding complications. Clinically significant elevations of blood methemoglobin levels and airway NO_2 production are rare during treatment with low doses (<20 ppm) of iNO but must be closely monitored. Peroxynitrite, generated by the reaction of NO with superoxide anion, cannot be directly measured in the clinical setting and can potentially cause acute lung injury with pulmonary edema. However, lung injury by peroxynitrite has generally been observed only in laboratory settings and with higher doses of iNO than are recommended for clinical use. Rapid and sometimes dramatic decreases in oxygenation and increases in PVR can occur after abrupt withdrawal of iNO. These responses are often mild and transient, and many patients with decreased oxygenation after iNO withdrawal will respond to brief elevations of inspired O_2. In general, this so-called "rebound" response appears to decrease after more prolonged therapy over time. However, iNO withdrawal can be associated with life-threatening elevations of PVR, profound desaturation, and systemic hypotension caused by decreased cardiac output. This response must be anticipated in every patient treated with iNO; discontinuation of iNO therapy, even in patients with partial or no apparent response to treatment, must be done with caution. The use of iNO in non-ECMO centers potentially can delay the initiation of transport to an ECMO center, increase risks during transport, or significantly delay ECMO. In such cases, the ability to continue iNO therapy during transport is critical to provide hemodynamic stability for safe transport.

FDA approval for the use of iNO is currently limited to term and near-term (>34 weeks) newborns with hypoxemic respiratory failure. Despite promising clinical observations, the use of iNO in premature infants (<34 weeks) remains investigational, especially in light of its potential effects on decreasing platelet aggregation. Similarly, the efficacy and therapeutic roles of iNO therapy in infants with congenital diaphragmatic hernia, chronic lung disease, and congenital heart disease with postoperative pulmonary hypertension requires more study.

References

Abman SH, Kinsella JP, Parker TA, et al: Physiologic roles of NO in the perinatal pulmonary circulation. In: Weir EK, Archer SL, Reeves JT, eds: The fetal and neonatal pulmonary circulation. New York, Futura, 1999:239–260

Clark RH, Kueser TJ, Walker MW, et al; Low-dose nitric oxide therapy for persistent pulmonary hypertension of the newborn. Clinical Inhaled Nitric Oxide Research Group. New Engl J Med 342(7):469–474, 2000

Furchgott RF: Role of endothelium in the responses of vascular smooth muscle to drugs. Annu Rev Pharmacol 24:175–197, 1984

Hobbs AJ, Ignarro LJ: NO-cGMP signal transduction system. In: Zapol WM, Bloch K, eds: Nitric Oxide and the Lung. New York, Marcel-Dekker, 1996:1–57

Kinsella JP, Neith S, Shaffer E, et al: Low dose inhalational NO in PPHN. Lancet 340:819–820, 1992

Kinsella JP, Troug W, Walsh W, et al: Randomized multicenter trial of inhaled NO and HFOV in severe PPHN. J Pediatr 131:55–62, 1997

NINOS. Inhaled NO in full term and near term infants with hypoxic respiratory failure. N Engl J Med. 336:597–604, 1997

Pepke-Aaba J, Higenbottam T, Dinh-Xuan T, et al: Inhaled NO as a cause of selective pulmonary vasodilation in pulmonary hypertension. Lancet 338:1173–1194, 1991

Roberts JD, Polaner DM, Lang P, et al: Inhaled NO in PPHN. Lancet 340:818–819, 1992

2.19.5   Liquid Ventilation

Marla R. Wolfson and Thomas H. Shaffer

Despite significant advances in respiratory care and reduction in mortality of patients with respiratory failure, there is still substantial morbidity. For this reason, many alternative means to support pulmonary gas exchange have been pursued. Liquid-assisted ventilation (LAV) with perfluorochemicals has been investigated for over 30 years as one such alternative to positive-pressure ventilation, although this remains an experimental technique. The biomedical application of perfluorochemical liquids has been incorporated in clinical medicine for a number of different organ systems (ie, intravascular PFC emulsions for volume expansion or oxygen carriage, and intracavitary PFC liquid for vitreous fluid replacement). As a result, pure medical-grade PFC liquids currently exist for LAV purposes. Simplistically, LAV utilizes a liquid as the carrier for oxygen and carbon dioxide in order to provide pulmonary gas exchange following tracheal instillation of perfluorochemical (PFC) liquid. PFC, when instilled in the airway, replaces the gas-liquid interface with a liquid-liquid interface and supports an adequate alveolar reservoir for pulmonary gas exchange because of its relatively low surface tension, high respiratory gas solubility, and high spreading coefficients. Because transmural pressures across the alveolar-capillary membrane are more evenly distributed than in the normal or injured lung, pulmonary blood flow is more homogeneous in the fluid- as compared to gas-filled lung. As a result, LAV presents a promising approach in the treatment of respiratory distress of the immature or mature injured lung.

The mechanisms through which LAV may improve gas exchange and lung mechanics are shown in Fig. 2-69. The degree to which collapsing tensions are reduced, compliance increased, inflation pressures decreased, and ventilation-to-perfusion matching and gas exchange improved depends on the distribution of the PFC liquid. Surfactant pretreatment further reduces collapsing pressures in the PFC-treated lung by decreasing tension at the PFC-lung interface. More recent studies have suggested that this form of ventilation may confer a protective benefit to the lung, either by serving as a mechanical barrier or by a direct cytoprotective action. In this regard, LAV has been associated with a reduction in the number of, as well as amount of, mediators released by pulmonary inflammatory cells.

LAV techniques for the support of respiratory gas exchange in the neonate have included tidal liquid ventilation (TLV), PFC lavage, and partial liquid ventilation (PLV). These techniques differ with respect to methodology, as well as the impact of the physicochemical profile of the PFC liquid. In the purest form, liquid breathing is the transport of respiratory gases solely in the dissolved form through tidal volume exchange of PFC to and from the lung. This constitutes tidal liquid ventilation (TLV). As such, all gas-liquid interfacial tension is eliminated, and the lung is provided maximal protection from inflation pressures, as lung volume is recruited, compliance is increased, and inflation pressures and pulmonary barotrauma are reduced. The TLV process is initiated by instilling PFC fluid into the gas-filled lung while gently manipulating the thorax to assist removal of resident gas volumes into the expiratory line. Because gas is transported in dissolved form, the gas-liquid interface at the alveolar surface is eliminated, there are no audible breath sounds, and inflation pressures are minimized. There is no free gas in the lung, and the liquid volumes in the lung and ventilator are monitored and controlled to maintain effective gas exchange. TLV is achieved by cycling fluid from a reservoir to

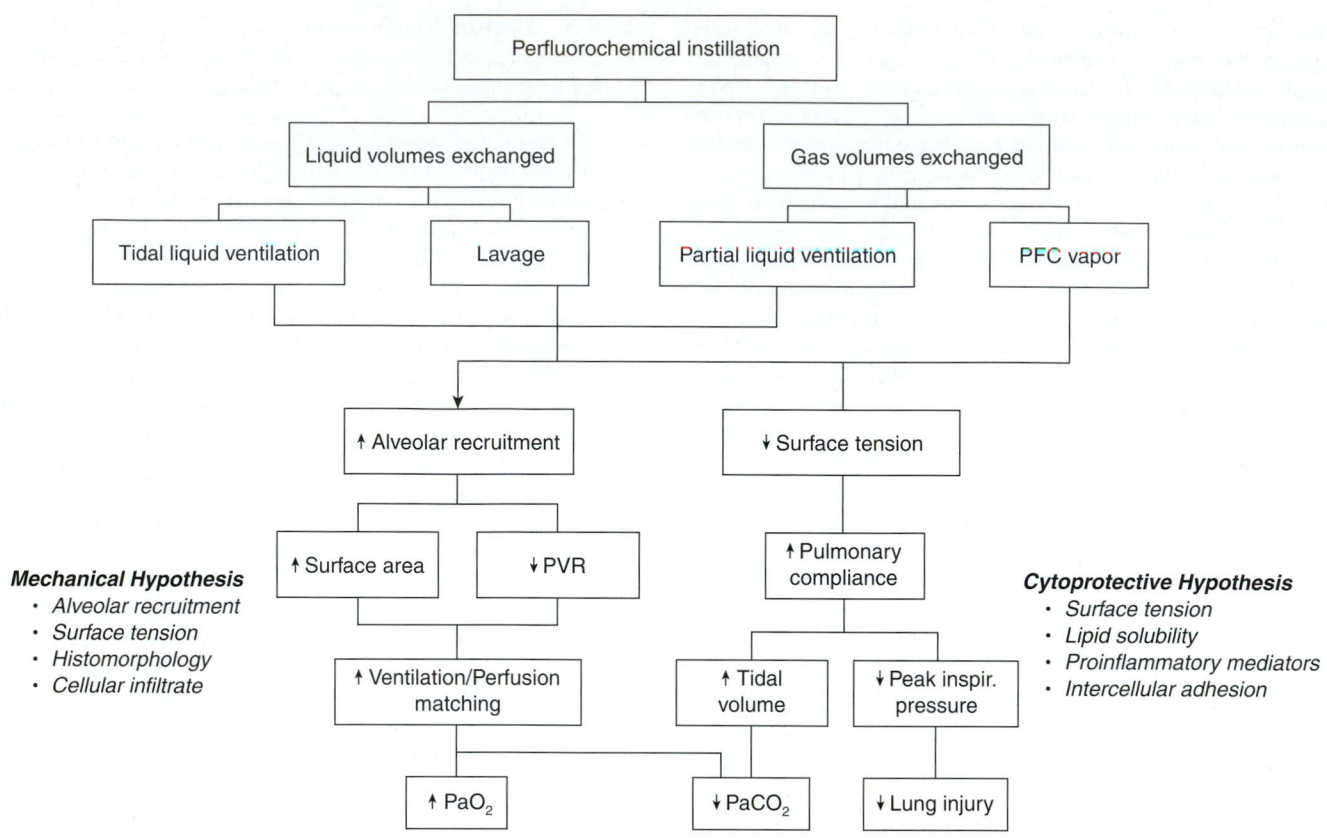

FIGURE 2-69   **Potential mechanisms of action of liquid ventilation.**

and from the lung by a mechanical ventilator that has evolved over the years to include manually controlled flow-assist pneumatic systems, roller pumps with pneumatic/fluidic/electronic controls, modified ECMO circuits, and microprocessor-based feedback control.

During inspiration, warmed and oxygenated PFC liquid is pumped from a fluid reservoir into the lung. Expiration is accomplished by actively pumping liquid from the lung with passive assist of the lung recoil. The fluid is then filtered, returned to a gas exchanger for desired levels of oxygenation and CO_2 scrubbing, and returned to the fluid reservoir. Tidal liquid ventilation algorithms that address optimum frequency (3–8 breaths/min), tidal volume (approx 15 mL/kg), and inspiratory:expiratory timing (1:2 or 1:3) have been developed to maintain adequate CO_2 elimination (up to four times steady-state values), minimize resistive pressures and expiratory flow limitations associated with moving the relatively more dense and viscous respiratory medium, and overcoming diffusional dead space associated with CO_2 diffusivity in a liquid respiratory medium. Proximal airway pressures are rapidly dissipated through the bronchopulmonary tree during TLV, such that alveolar pressures are much lower than airway pressures. Pulmonary debris (ie, exudate, meconium, mucus) is readily moved by tidal PFC volumes and cleared by the TLV filtering systems. There is no known physiological limitation on the duration of TLV.

PLV is performed by filling and maintaining the lung with a functional residual capacity (FRC) of PFC liquid while mechanical gas ventilation is performed. In this way PLV is similar to TLV, as it utilizes the alveolar recruitment capabilities of a low-surface-tension fluid to establish an adequate FRC in a surfactant-deficient or impaired lung. The PFC liquid is oxygenated, and CO_2 is exchanged in the lung through mechanical gas ventilation. The op-

timum PFC filling strategy and subsequent gas ventilation scheme are still under investigation. Effective ventilation of a lung that is partly filled with liquid and partly filled with gas is more challenging than TLV because there are many unknowns with respect to the distribution of PFC fluid in the lung, oxygen and carbon dioxide saturation of resident PFC, continually changing lung mechanics, evaporative loss of PFC, and changing volumes of gas and PFC lung volumes. Maintenance of a therapeutic PFC liquid volume following initial instillation in the lungs is dependent on a number of factors related to the PFC that include the physicochemical properties (vapor pressure, density, viscosity, spreading coefficient, and gas solubility) and physiological factors (alveolar ventilation, respective volumes and distributions of the PFC and inspired gas, nature of the impaired lung function, and the position of the patient). The importance of maintaining PFC lung volume during PLV has necessitated the development of adjunctive instrumentation to quantify evaporative loss, guide and sustain dosing levels, and reduce dose consumption, and cost. Pulmonary debris has been found to migrate from the distal to proximal lung and requires frequent and often aggressive suctioning.

PLV has also been combined with various forms of assisted ventilation, including conventional high-frequency oscillatory ventilation (HFOV). HFOV and PLV resulted in similar improvements in gas exchange and lung inflammation in preterm lambs with severe RDS.

To date, only a few phase I/II clinical trials of liquid ventilation in human neonates have been published. In an uncontrolled clinical trial of human premature newborns with severe respiratory distress syndrome, PLV was shown to be associated with improvements in arterial oxygenation and dynamic respiratory system compliance. PLV for up to 7 days, as an adjunct to extracorporeal life support in full-term neonates, has been shown to improve gas exchange and pulmonary compliance without adverse events related to the technique. Experience to date has indicated that the response to PLV of the sick term infant is more gradual than observed in the preterm infant with RDS. Whereas the majority of preclinical studies of liquid ventilation have been performed in neonatal animals, only adult clinical trials with PLV were under way by the end of 1999. Thus, PLV remains an experimental technique with intriguing potential but unproven clinical benefit.

References

Greenspan JS, Wolfson MR, Rubenstein SD, et al: Liquid ventilation of human preterm neonates. J Pediatr 117:106–111, 1990

Leach CL, Greenspan JS, Rubenstein SD, et al: Partial liquid ventilation with perflubron in premature infants with severe respiratory distress syndrome. N Engl J Med 335:761–767, 1996

Shaffer TH, Foust R, Wolfson MR, et al: Analysis of perfluorochemical elimination from the respiratory system. J Appl Physiol 83:1033–1040, 1997

Shaffer TH, Wolfson MR, Greenspan JS: Liquid ventilation: current status. Pediatr Rev 20:e134–142, 1999

Stavis RL, Wolfson MR, Cox C, et al: Physiologic, biochemical, and histologic correlates associated with tidal liquid ventilation. Pediatr Res 43:132–138, 1998

Wolfson MR, Greenspan JS, Deoras KS, et al: Comparison of gas and liquid ventilation: clinical, physiological, and histological correlates. J Appl Physiol 72:1024–1031, 1992

Wolfson MR, Greenspan JS, Shaffer TH: Liquid-assisted ventilation: an alternative respiratory modality. Pediatr Pulmonol 26:42–63, 1998

2.20   AFTER INTENSIVE CARE: FOLLOW-UP AND OUTCOME

Marilee C. Allen

RISK FACTORS IN INTENSIVE CARE NURSERY GRADUATES

Most of the conditions that place a neonate at risk of dying also increase the risk of subsequent health and neurodevelopmental problems. Over the last few decades, major advances in high-risk obstetrics and neonatal intensive care have yielded dramatic reductions in neonatal mortality. Although there is evidence that antenatal steroid and surfactant administration have improved both survival and outcomes of preterm infants, these changes have been neither dramatic nor universal. The few specific neuroprotective strategies that have been developed have not yet had a major impact on the incidence of neurodevelopmental disability in intensive care nursery (ICN) graduates.

Despite its importance, long-term function is rarely the designated outcome of multicenter randomized controlled trials (RCT) of ICN interventions. Complications, such as chronic lung disease (CLD) and intraventricular hemorrhage (IVH), have been used as proxies for long-term outcome in many trials, but they are imperfect predictors of outcome. One recent RCT follow-up study has demonstrated the importance of assessing development: the immediate improvement in CLD seen in preterm infants treated with a 42-day course of dexamethasone was associated with a higher incidence of neurologic impairment, including cerebral palsy (CP), even when cranial ultrasound abnormalities were considered.

For the individual infant, neurodevelopmental disability cannot be diagnosed during the neonatal period. Infants with complicating conditions (eg, CLD, IVH) have an increased risk of CP and mental retardation (MR), but many will have either a normal outcome or much milder disabilities. Early diagnosis of disability requires careful neurodevelopmental follow-up during infancy and childhood. The major disabilities generally can be diagnosed in the first few years, but learning disability, attention deficit, and minor neuromotor dysfunction generally require follow-up to the preschool and school years.

The absence of risk factors does not guarantee a normal outcome. The incidence of CP in the general population is 0.2 to 0.3%; that of MR is 1 to 3%. Up to 50% of children with CP or MR have no known etiology. Neurodevelopmental disability has been associated with a number of risk factors, which vary widely in their predictive value (eg, in preterm infants, IVH is more predictive than is a low Apgar score). Very strong predictors are relatively uncommon (eg, 90% of infants with bilateral cystic periventricular leukomalacia have major disability, but this condition occurs in only 3% of infants with a birth weight below 1500 g). Some risk factors are predictive of specific disabilities. For example, low socioeconomic status (SES) is strongly associated with abnormal cognitive testing but not with neurologic disability. Multiple risk factors together increase the likelihood of long-term disability.

Although there are many reasons why neonates require intensive care, there is no doubt that ICN graduates require greater attention to subsequent growth, health, and developmental progress than do healthy neonates. Risk factors can determine which infants are most likely to manifest subsequent neurodevelopmental disability and therefore might benefit from focused developmental follow-up and early intervention efforts.

FOLLOW-UP OF HIGH-RISK INFANTS

Changes in health care funding, increased reliance on managed care, and cost-cutting measures have tried to shift the burden of high-risk infant follow-up from comprehensive multidisciplinary ICN follow-up clinics to primary care providers. Because there is a continuum of risk, the ideal followup environment provides a continuum of followup, support and intervention services tailored to individual ICN graduates and families. The highest risk infants should be seen in comprehensive followup clinics whenever possible, and referred for early intervention and developmental support services as appropriate.

HEALTH AND GROWTH   ICN graduates, especially during their first year, are more vulnerable to infections, poor growth and other health problems than healthy neonates. They are more likely to require rehospitalization, surgery, home equipment, home nursing and medications. Infants with extreme prematurity, persistent pulmonary hypertension (PPHN), primary pulmonary disorders and congenital heart disease are especially vulnerable to respiratory infections, poor growth and reactive airway disease. Our current definitions of CLD, requiring oxygen beyond 28 days or 36 weeks postmenstrual age, do not adequately predict which infants will be the sickest or require the most resources. Although extremely preterm infants with CLD have the highest risk of respiratory infections, even moderately preterm infants (with birthweights 1500–2500 grams) are more vulnerable to infection than fullterm healthy infants.

After ICN discharge, growth in weight, length and head circumference should be followed carefully. Some infants with extreme prematurity or severe intrauterine growth restriction (IUGR) remain small compared to peers, but they continue to grow along their own curve, parallel to the normal growth curve, throughout childhood. Nutrition should be carefully assessed, with focus on quantity and quality of food intake. Some infants with oromotor dysfunction, gastrointestinal problems (e.g. short gut from necrotizing enterocolitis, NEC) or exercise intolerance that interferes with nippling benefit from gastrostomy with tube feedings. Good nutrition, which is often difficult to achieve in an intensive care setting, is especially important for infants with CLD and for those recovering from surgery.

ASSESSMENT OF SENSORY ABILITIES ICN graduates have a higher risk of hearing impairment than healthy fullterm neonates. Because hearing is essential for the normal development of language, many states now mandate hearing tests in all neonates. ICN graduates should have assessments with either auditory brainstem response or transient otoacoustic evoked emission studies, before discharge. Infants with suspect or abnormal tests should be reassessed within several weeks. Hearing impaired infants may coo and babble on time. Their impairment may go unrecognized for one or more years. Early diagnosis and intervention facilitate their acquisition of language. Any child who presents with language delay should have an auditory evaluation. Infants with congenital cytomegalovirus (CMV) infection and infants with PPHN should have serial auditory evaluations through infancy and early childhood, because they have a high incidence of hearing impairment, and it may be progressive.

Prior to discharge, an experienced ophthalmologist should examine the eyes of infants with birthweight <1500 grams, gestational age <28 weeks, unstable clinical course, significant perinatal asphyxia or suspected congenital cytomegalovirus, toxoplasmosis or rubella infection. In addition, all ICN graduates should have their vision screened in late infancy or during the preschool years. Myopia and strabismus are common findings in preterm and other high risk infants and children.

ASSESSMENT OF DEVELOPMENT A careful history of developmental milestone acquisition taken at each primary care visit is a quick, effective method of monitoring developmental progress. The age of milestone acquisition can be compared to published norms in order to determine delay. For preterm infants, using age corrected for degree of prematurity most accurately determines motor progress and minimizes excessive referrals. Viewing each stream of development separately allows assessment of the significance of delay. Persistent delay within a stream of development suggests major disability. Delay in motor milestones suggests CP, which can be confirmed by a detailed neurodevelopmental examination. Delay in language milestones suggests MR, language disorder or hearing impairment. Mild delays or deviations in achieving milestones suggest mild functional impairment (e.g. minor neuromotor dysfunction, learning disability).

The neurodevelopmental examination is an additional tool for assessing infant development. The examination of the normal neonate typically shows flexor hypertonia, mild neck hypotonia, hyperreflexia, primitive and pathologic reflexes, strong oromotor reflexes and poorly coordinated voluntary movements. The infant's examination changes dramatically during the first year: 1) flexor hypertonia diminishes, 2) neck control improves, 3) primitive re-

flexes and pathologic reflexes become difficult to elicit with suppression by higher cortical function, 4) the primitive suckle matures into a strong, coordinated suck, 5) postural responses and equilibrium reactions (e.g. protective responses, parachute) emerge as 6) voluntary movements become better directed and coordinated. Common neuromotor abnormalities found in ICN graduates include neck and trunk extensor hypertonia with increased shoulder retraction, asymmetries, axial or generalized hypotonia and lower extremity spasticity (especially tight heel cords).

Infants with delay and/or persistent neuromotor abnormalities should be referred for evaluation and intervention. Brain injury tends to be diffuse, not focal, so that delay in one area of development may be associated with other developmental abnormalities. Other delays or abnormalities that benefit from early intervention may emerge from a comprehensive developmental assessment. The goal of the evaluation is to provide as complete a picture as possible of a child's strengths and weaknesses for both parent counseling and devising an early intervention strategy tailored to the needs of the child and family.

Both in the ICN and after discharge home, parents of critically ill children have anxieties about their child's functional outcome. Comprehensive ICN follow-up clinics allow parents to receive answers to important questions and provide them emotional support for dealing with diagnoses of disability or impairment. The highest-risk infants and their families may be referred for early intervention and developmental supportive services, even before definitive diagnosis of disability. The goal of this early intervention is to minimize secondary complications, provide parental and developmental support and optimize the child's ability to function in the home and community.

LONG-TERM OUTCOME OF ICN GRADUATES

PREMATURITY The survival and outcome of preterm infants has generally been reported in terms of birth weight (BW) criteria: BW <1500 g (very low BW, VLBW), BW <1000 g (extremely low BW, ELBW), and, most recently, BW <750 g (incredibly low BW, ILBW). Preterm infants of all BW have a higher incidence of both CP and MR than term infants do. Nevertheless, the majority (86–95%) of preterm infants have no major disability. The most common type of CP in preterm infants is spastic diplegia, with greater spasticity in the lower than upper extremities. This spasticity is often mild. Preterm infants with asymmetric brain injury often have an associated hemiplegia. Retinopathy of prematurity (ROP) remains a major complication, developing in 1 to 6% of VLBW and 4 to 25% of ILBW infants.

The remarkable progress that has characterized the last 30 years of newborn intensive care has lowered the limit of viability to less than 500 g and less than 24 weeks of gestation. The very immature micropremies that survive, as expected, have a higher incidence of CP, MR, and severe ROP than larger preterm infants do (as high as 50% of ILBW infants and up to 70% of infants with BW <500 g have such abnormalities). Because BW is unknown when parents are counseled in the labor room, most reports try to predict outcome based on the estimated GA; at least one major disability occurs in up to almost half of infants born at 23 to 24 weeks of gestational age (GA) and in up to one-third of infants born at 25 weeks of GA. More severe CP (spastic quadriplegia or mixed CP) tends to occur in the smallest, sickest preterm infants.

Although populations of children who were born prematurely have a wide range of intelligence quotients (IQ), a metaanalysis of studies published between 1979 and 1989 found that low-birth-weight children (with BW < 2500 g) had a lower mean IQ than term infants had (98 ± 6 vs 104 ± 8). In addition, more children with a history of prematurity suffer from MR and borderline intelligence. Of the VLBW infants who subsequently had a normal IQ, many had a learning disability that required special education. Studies of VLBW, ELBW, and ILBW infants who had normal intelligence showed higher incidences of language delay, visual-perceptual problems, reading disability, and difficulty with arithmetic when compared to children who were born at term. The frequency of these abnormalities is greater in ILBW children than in children who were larger and more mature at birth. Minor neuromotor dysfunction, sensorimotor deficits, and visual-perceptual problems are common findings in preschool children with a history of prematurity. These less severe handicaps can have a devastating impact on fine motor function, adaptive skills, peer relationships, and self-esteem. By providing emotional and developmental support, early recognition and intervention can improve function and prevent secondary social and emotional problems.

The best predictors of major disability in preterm infants are significant abnormalities noted on cranial ultrasound studies (eg, severe IVH, cystic PVL, moderate to severe ventricular dilation) and abnormal findings noted on neonatal neurodevelopmental examination. Preterm infants who demonstrate neuromotor abnormalities in the first year without subsequent CP have a high incidence of learning and behavioral abnormalities. Infants with a history of prematurity and CLD have a higher incidence of respiratory infections, slow growth, CP, MR, language delay, and ROP than those without CLD.

INTRAUTERINE GROWTH RESTRICTION   Children with a history of IUGR have considerable variability in long-term outcome, perhaps related to the variability of conditions that led to IUGR as well as the wide range of perinatal complications. IUGR may result from small parental size, fetal maldevelopment from chromosomal disorders, dysmorphic syndromes, or teratogens, fetal injury, or inadequate nutrition related to maternal illness, placental insufficiency, or multiple births. IUGR infants are more likely to have experienced fetal distress, perinatal asphyxia, polycythemia, hypoglycemia, and pulmonary hemorrhage. Their outcome is determined primarily by etiology but also by timing and duration of insult, the underlying cause, and the associated perinatal complications.

Abnormalities of muscle tone and jitteriness are common in infants with IUGR, yet prospective studies of IUGR infants who were born at term but without congenital infections, anomalies, or syndromes have not shown any greater incidences of CP, MR, or sensory impairment than term infants who were of appropriate size for gestational age (AGA). Children who were born at term with a history of IUGR do have higher incidences of more subtle central nervous system (CNS) dysfunction, such as speech and language disorders, hyperactivity, attention deficit, learning disability, and minor neuromotor dysfunction. Learning disabilities and school failure are common among children who were born at term with IUGR.

Children with a history of both prematurity and IUGR are more likely to manifest developmental abnormalities and disability than are term IUGR and preterm AGA infants. Preterm infants with IUGR have a high incidence of major disability (7–23%), especially

learning disability (36–50%). Like term IUGR and preterm AGA children, those with normal intelligence demonstrate a high incidence of subtle CNS dysfunction at school and at home. More preterm IUGR children have neurologic impairment and lower developmental quotients when compared to preterm AGA infants matched for GA and socio-economic status (SES). When compared with preterm AGA infants with the same BW and SES, however, preterm IUGR infants had similar outcomes. This has important implications regarding advice given to parents in the delivery room, especially at the limit of viability: that is, the very small but mature infant with IUGR is unlikely to function any better than the less mature AGA infant, although survival and complication rates may differ.

HYPOXIC-ISCHEMIC ENCEPHALOPATHY   Two difficulties in determining the outcome of perinatal asphyxia are those of defining the type and duration of insult, and defining the population to be studied. A number of studies define asphyxia in terms of effect on the fetus or neonate, ie, very low sequential Apgar scores over a prolonged period of time, low cord pH, and extent of resuscitative efforts needed in the delivery room. With these signs of severe perinatal asphyxia, major disability (CP or MR) occurs in up to 25% of survivors. When disability occurs, it tends to be severe, including spastic quadriplegia or mixed CP, severe to profound MR, microcephaly, seizure disorder, cortical blindness, and hearing impairment.

Severity of the clinical syndrome of hypoxic-ischemic encephalopathy (HIE) and of neuroimaging abnormalities are the best predictors of neurodevelopmental outcome. All infants with severe HIE either die or acquire multiple severe disabilities. Major disability occurs in about one-fifth of children with moderate HIE. Those without major disability tend to have difficulties with visual-motor integration, reading, spelling, arithmetic, and vocabulary when compared to children with a history of mild HIE or to healthy controls.

EXTRACORPOREAL MEMBRANE OXYGENATION AND PERSISTENT PULMONARY HYPERTENSION   Critically ill term infants with compromised cardiopulmonary status may require extracorporeal membrane oxygenation (ECMO). Because of either their underlying disease or the ECMO procedure or both, they have an increased risk of neurodevelopmental disability. Major disability occurs in up to 26% of such infants, and mild disability, including borderline intelligence, sensory impairment, language delay, and minor neuromotor dysfunction, occurs up to 50% of such infants. The incidence of major disability is similar (13–24%) in term infants with PPHN, whether or not they require ECMO. Lower BW, sepsis, congenital diaphragmatic hernia, abnormalities seen in neuroimaging studies, and the need for cardiopulmonary resuscitation before ECMO were associated with adverse neurodevelopmental outcome.

CLD occurs in up to 40% of infants who have been treated with ECMO for respiratory failure, in 63% of infants with congenital diaphragmatic hernia treated with ECMO, and in up to one-third of infants with PPHN regardless of treatment strategy. Infants treated with ECMO continue with health sequelae related to CLD, often requiring rehospitalization (24–47% the first year, 17% the second year). Slow growth occurs in as many as one-fifth of these infants. Hearing impairment is common and may be progressive in infants who have been treated with ECMO (3–21%) and in infants who have had PPHN (20–53%).

References

Allen MC, Alexander GR: Using gross motor milestones to identify very preterm infants at risk for cerebral palsy. Dev Med Child Neurol 34: 226–232, 1992

Allen MC: Outcome and follow-up of high risk infants. In: Taeusch HW, Ballard RA, eds: Avery's Diseases of the Newborn. Philadelphia, WB Saunders, 1998:413–428

Aylward GP, Pfeiffer SI, Wright A, Verhulst SJ: Outcome studies of low-birth-weight infants published in the last decade: a meta-analysis. J Pediatr 115:515–520, 1989

Finnstrom O, Olausson PO, Sedin G, et al: Neurosensory outcome and growth at three years in extremely low birthweight infants: follow-up results from the Swedish national prospective study. Acta Pediatr 87: 1055–1060, 1998

Glass P, Wagner AE, Papero PH, et al: Neurodevelopmental status at age five years of neonates treated with extracorporeal membrane oxygenation. J Pediatr 127:447–457, 1995

Hack M, Fanaroff AA: Outcomes of children of extremely low birthweight and gestational age in the 1990's. Early Hum Dev 53:193–218, 1999

Lorenz JM, Wooliever DE, Jetton JR, Paneth N: A quantitative review of mortality and developmental disability in extremely premature newborns. Arch Pediatr Adolesc Med 152:425–435, 1998

O'Shea TM, Kothadia JM, Klinepeter KL, et al: Randomized placebo-controlled trial of a 42-day tapering course of dexamethasone to reduce the duration of ventilator dependency in very low birth weight infants: outcome of study participants at 1-year adjusted age. Pediatrics 104:15–21, 1999

Robertson C, Finer N: Term infants with hypoxic-ischemic encephalopathy: outcome at 3.5 years. Dev Med Child Neurol 27:473–484, 1985

Vohr B, Msall ME: Neuropsychological and functional outcomes of very low birth weight infants. Semin Perinatol 21:202–220, 1997

Walsh-sukys MC, Bauer RE, Cornell DJ, et al: Severe respiratory failure in neonates: mortality and morbidity rates and neurodevelopmental outcomes. J Pediatr 125:104–110, 1994

Yeo CL, Tudehope DI: Outcome of resuscitated apparently stillborn infants: a ten year review. J Pediatr Child Health 30:129–133, 1994

THE ADOLESCENT PATIENT

Charles E. Irwin, Jr. and Mary-Ann Shafer and Anna-Barbara Moscicki, Associate Editors

3.1 GROWTH AND DEVELOPMENT

Charles E. Irwin, Jr.

3.1.1 Somatic Growth and Development during Adolescence

Adolescence comprises a period in the life cycle between childhood and adulthood. Biological, psychological, social, environmental, and legal changes influence the definitive onset and termination of adolescence. Pubescence is often described as the onset of adolescence; however, the mean age of onset of puberty in girls in the United States varies by race and is earlier than in previous generations, with the mean age of onset for white girls being 9.7 years with a range of onset from 7.8 years to 11.6 years, and for black girls 8.1 years with a range of onset from 6.1 years to 10.1 years. In boys the onset of puberty has remained stable at 11.4 years of age with a range of 9.5 to 13.5. (Sec. 24.8). For purposes of discussion in this section, adolescence in chronologic years is defined as the period from 10 to 21 years.

All bodily tissues are affected by the biological changes of puberty. Growth of the reproductive, cardiovascular, and musculoskeletal systems is closely correlated during this period. The major biological changes occurring during puberty can be classified into six groups: skeletal growth, alterations in body composition, cardiorespiratory, hematologic, neuroendocrine development, and reproductive maturation. Chronologic age does not always correlate with biological maturity. Sexual maturation rating (SMR) stages, as described by Tanner and Marshall, provide a more accurate assessment of the biological developmental stage of the adolescent.

SKELETAL GROWTH

The secondary growth spurt at pubescence accounts for approximately 25% of final adult height. As outlined in Table 3-1, the growth spurt for girls occurs at an earlier sexual maturity rating (SMR 2–3) than for boys (SMR 4). Girls reach a final mean adult height of 163.8 cm at a mean age of 16 years compared with 176.8 cm for boys at a mean age of 18 years. Assessment of skeletal growth during adolescence is done through the use of a height-velocity curve with consideration of the gender-specific sexual maturity rating. Bone age can be determined through the use of a hand roentgenogram.

ALTERATIONS IN BODY COMPOSITION

Significant body composition changes occur during adolescence. Weight gain peaks during the growth spurt and accounts for over 40% of the ideal body weight. Weight gain differs by gender, with lean body mass increasing in boys from 80% to 90% and decreasing in girls from 80% to 75%. The mean body fat in girls increases throughout puberty from 15.7% to 26.7%. The mean body fat in boys increases from 4.3% to 11.2% early in puberty (usually SMR 1–2) and remains constant through adulthood. Girls characteristically have more subcutaneous adipose tissue in the pelvic, breast, upper back, and arm areas. Shortly after the growth spurt is completed, muscle mass peaks: for girls at SMR 3–4 and for boys at SMR 5. This increase in muscle mass can be measured by monitoring increases in creatinine excretion.

HEMATOLOGIC DEVELOPMENT

Blood volume, red blood cell mass, and hematocrit increase throughout pubescence in boys (Table 3-1). These same parameters remain constant for girls.

CARDIORESPIRATORY CHANGES

There are significant changes within the cardiovascular system during adolescence: the weight of the heart doubles, and systolic blood pressure increases for boys and plateaus in girls. The decreased heart rate seen in late childhood stabilizes in adolescence after growth of the heart. Within the respiratory system, the lung size increases with a parallel drop in respiratory rate and a significant increase in vital capacity.

NEUROENDOCRINE DEVELOPMENT

Within the central nervous system, there are no gross changes in the structure or mass of the brain. Recently, there have been documented changes in electrical activity of the brain during adolescence to predominantly the α rhythm of adulthood and MRI evidence of gray-matter spike shifts to the temporal and parietal lobe. The neuroendocrinologic control of puberty through the hypothalamic-pituitary-gonadal axis is discussed in detail in Sec. 24.8.

MATURATION OF THE REPRODUCTIVE SYSTEM

The maturation of the reproductive system and the appearance of the secondary sex characteristics are definitive changes unique to puberty. The sexual maturity ratings (SMR) of Marshall and Tanner provide a classification to monitor the normal events of puberty from prepubertal (SMR 1) to adult (SMR 5). The ratings for girls are based on breast (B1 to B5) and pubic hair (P1 to P5) development. The ratings for boys are based on pubic hair (P1 to P5) and genitalia (G1 to G5) development.

Visible sexual maturation in the girl usually begins with thelarche between 6.1 and 11.6 years. The mean age of menarche in the United States is 12.7 years (at SMR 3 or 4) with a normal range of

TABLE 3-1
CLINICAL CORRELATES OF PUBERTAL MATURATION

	SEXUAL MATURITY RATING (SMR)				
	1	2	3	4	5
Girls					
Hematocrit (%)					
White (Mean)	39.1	39.2	39.6	39.2	39.2
Range	36.1–42.1	37.1–41.3	37.0–42.2	36.9–41.6	36.2–42.2
Black (Mean)	37.3	38.9	39.0	38.4	38.7
Range	34.6–39.9	35.7–42.1	35.2–42.6	34.9–42.8	35.9–41.5
Alkaline phosphatase (IU/L) (serum)					
White (Mean)	70	89	76	33	38
Range	51–90	49–134	36–108	16–60	23–76
Black (Mean)	84	95	86	44	31
Range	69–108	65–138	26–148	18–144	13–70
Slipped capital femoral epiphysis		+	++		
Acute worsening of scoliosis		+	++	+	
Osgood-Schlatter disease		+	++		
Acne vulgaris		+	++	++	
Physiological leukorrhea		+	++		
Peak height velocity		+	++	+	
Menarche		+	++	++	+
Boys					
Hematocrit (%)					
White (Mean)	39.5	39.8	40.9	42.3	43.8
Range	37.1–41.8	36.7–42.8	38.2–43.5	39.7–44.8	41.1–46.4
Black (Mean)	37.7	38.4	39.7	41.1	42.7
Range	35.2–40.2	36.0–40.9	37.3–42.0	38.3–43.8	39.6–45.9
Alkaline phosphatase (IU/L) (serum)					
White (Mean)	72	77	101	75	58
Range	54–110	42–106	53–141	41–158	21–120
Black (Mean)	77	94	122	116	75
Range	43–130	53–204	46–240	32–228	23–228
Peak height velocity			+	++	+
Slipped capital femoral epiphysis		+	++		
Acute worsening of scoliosis		+	++	++	+
Osgood-Schlatter disease		+	++	++	
Gynecomastia		+	++	+	
Acne vulgaris		+	++	++	
Ejaculation onset		+	++	++	
Ejaculation with fertility			+	++	++

+ = May occur during this stage but less likely than ++.
++ = Occurs most often during this Sexual Maturity Rating.
SOURCE: Adapted and modified from *Daniel WA: Growth at adolescence: Clinical correlates. Semin Adolesc Med 1:15–24, 1985;* and *Copeland KC, Brookman RR, Rauh JL: Assessment of Pubertal Development. Columbus, Ross Laboratories, 1986.*

10 to 16.5 years. The average duration of puberty for girls is 4 years with a range of 1.5 to 8 years. Visible sexual maturation in the boy usually begins with testicular enlargement between 9.5 and 13.5 years of age. The average duration of puberty for boys is 3 years with a range of 2 to 5 years. Clinical correlates of male and female pubertal maturation are discussed in Table 3-1.

3.1.2 Psychological Development

PSYCHOLOGICAL CHANGES ASSOCIATED WITH PUBESCENCE

Recent evidence supports some of the general behavioral changes of adolescence. Specific behavioral changes are associated with pu-berty and its timing. Androgens have been implicated as the cause of many of the changes associated with adolescence. Family relationships undergo a transformation during puberty. During peak height velocity (SMR 3–4), boys experience more conflict with their parents, especially their mothers. This conflict tends to subside after completion of puberty, with mothers deferring more to their sons. Girls experience conflict with their mothers, and girls report decreased contact with their fathers. Hormones have been implicated as the cause of many of the behavior changes associated with normal and abnormal adolescence. Sexual behavior is associated with changes in androgens. Boys, with rising levels of testosterone, initiate coitus, and they are reported to be more impatient, aggressive, and irritable. For girls, an increase in masturbatory activity is associated with rising levels of androgens.

Specific psychosocial effects have been correlated with timing of pubertal maturation. Earlier maturation for girls is associated with greater dissatisfaction with physical characteristics, lower self-esteem, and general unhappiness. Early-developing girls receive less recognition from same-sex peers and tend to associate with older adolescents. The early-maturing girl shows increased interest in sexuality, early identity crises, greater interest in independence and decision making, and more problem behavior in school with decreased interest in academic activities.

For boys, early physical development is also associated with an increased tendency to initiate sexual intercourse. Late physical development in boys is also associated with adverse psychological effects. The late-developing boy exhibits a more negative self-concept and body image with an increased frequency of identity crises than other same-aged boys.

For both girls and boys, late physical maturation appears to be protective for initiation of most risky behaviors. The social environment tends to provide more guidance and support for these physically immature adolescents.

PSYCHOLOGICAL CHANGES THROUGHOUT ADOLESCENCE

The psychological changes of adolescence are often described as tumultuous. In reality, most adolescents traverse the second decade of life with minimal difficulty. The clinician often needs to assess whether psychosocial development of the adolescent is normal.

Normal developmental characteristics of each stage of adolescence and their associated impact on the adolescent are presented in Table 3-2. The adolescent is confronted with a series of psychological changes that, if mastered, allow for functioning as an optimal adult. These changes include individuation, sexual identity maturation, educational planning for career, and the capacity for intimacy, with functional and cognitive changes not corresponding exactly with physical maturation.

During early adolescence (ages 10 to 13 years), there is an emergence of impulsive behavior without the cognitive ability to understand the etiology of the behavior. Middle adolescence (ages 14 to 16 years) is characterized by the rapid growth in cognition along with the emergence of formal operational thinking. Adolescents are now able to understand complex concepts, which often leads to a questioning of the thinking and behavior of adults. With the onset of cognitive formal operations during middle adolescence, there begins to be a shift from the egocentric world of the early adolescent to the more sociocentric world of the middle and late adolescent. These associated new thought processes begin to modulate impulsive behavior. Late adolescence (ages 17 to 21 years) is characterized by the establishment of personal identity, the initiation and maintenance of an intimate relationship, and the beginning development of a functional role in society. The new emergence of a sociocentric view of the world with a strong sense of altruism often leads to conflict with family and society around moral and ethical issues rather than the egocentric issues of early adolescence.

TABLE 3-2
BIOPSYCHOSOCIAL DEVELOPMENT DURING ADOLESCENCE

Early Adolescence (Age 10–13 Years)	
Characteristics	Impact
Onset of puberty, becomes concerned with developing body	Major questions concerning normality of physical maturation; often concerned about the stages of sexual development and how the process relates to peers of same gender.
	Occasional masturbation.
Begins to expand social radius beyond family and concentrate on relationships with peers	Encourage some external responsibilities alone in consultation with parents, ie, visit with health care provider, contacts with school counselors.
Cognition is usually concrete	Concrete thinking requires dealing with most health situations in a simple, explicit manner using visual and verbal cues.
Middle Adolescence (Age 14–16 Years)	
Characteristics	Impact
Pubertal development usually complete, and sexual drives emerge	Explores ability to attract opposites. Sexual behavior and experimentation (same and opposite sex) begin. Masturbation increases.
Peer group sets behavioral standards, although family values usually persist	Peer group affects compliance; peers rather than parents may offer key support.
Conflicts over independence	Increased assumption of independent action, together with continued need for parental support and guidance; able to discuss and negotiate changes in rules; ambivalence on part of adolescent in discussion and negotiation.
Cognition begins to be abstract	Begins to consider full range of possibilities with poor ability to integrate into real life because of immaturity and incomplete development.
Late Adolescence (Age 17–21 Years)	
Characteristics	Impact
Physical maturation complete. Body image and gender role definition are secured	Begins to feel comfortable with relationships and decisions regarding sexuality and preference. Individual relationships being more important than peer group.
Narcissism declines; there is a process of giving and sharing	More open to specific questioning regarding behavior.
Idealistic	Idealism may lead to conflicts with family and other authority figures.
Emancipation is nearly secured	With emancipation, awareness about consequences of personal actions.
Cognitive development is complete	Most are capable of understanding a full range of options for health issues.
Functional role begins to be defined	Often interested in significant discussion of life goals because this is the primary function of this stage.

Families play a critical role in optimal development during adolescence by facilitating a graduated increase in independence and the associated responsibilities. Adolescents need to experience both individuation and involvement with their family and society to develop a positive identity and rational competence. Clinicians can assist with this process through encouraging adolescents to assume more responsibility for their own health care and encouraging parents to decrease their monitoring of clinical management issues.

ENVIRONMENTAL CHANGES DURING ADOLESCENCE

The supportive social environment of the child undergoes significant changes during adolescence, with the family providing less supervision and more freedom of choices, which increases the opportunity for initiation of health-damaging habits. Schools at the secondary level are unstructured and impersonal, thereby providing less supervision and support than was provided in the elementary school setting. Work environments for older adolescents provide less supervision than schools and little guidance about career choices. The changing socioeconomic context of families has consistently resulted in a small group of adolescents being raised in extreme poverty and most adolescents being raised in families with two working parents. Adolescents continue to represent the largest cohort of children without health insurance, thereby further limiting access to health care.

The law may further restrict access to health care, with most states requiring parental consent for medical care for children younger than 18 years of age. The Mature Minor Doctrine generally allows adolescents to seek health care independently if they are able to understand the risks and benefits of the proposed diagnostic assessment and treatment. This doctrine may also be used when adolescents present with an emergency and a delay in treatment would be detrimental to their well-being. Emancipated minors (as defined by living away from home, no longer subject to parental authority, economically self-sufficient, married, or members of the military service) may consent to their own health care. In most states adolescents may seek care without parental permission for diagnosis and treatment of sexually transmitted diseases. Also, many states allow adolescents to seek care and receive treatment without parental permission for other sensitive issues such as pregnancy, contraception, substance abuse, and some mental health problems.

3.2   HEALTH PROBLEMS OF ADOLESCENTS

Charles E. Irwin, Jr.

MORTALITY

Mortality rates in 1997 for the second decade of life continue to decline but remain high: 23.2 per 100,000 population for early adolescents (10 to 14 years) and 74.8 per 100,000 population for late adolescents (15 to 19 years). The more than 300% increase in mortality with age from early to late adolescence reflects the violent etiology of most deaths with increased access to motor vehicles and firearms. The mortality rate in male teenagers is nearly twice that of females. Race is an important determinant of life expectancy, with black male adolescents showing the lowest life expectancy.

Accidents, suicide, and homicide account for 75% of the mortality during the second decade of life. These three causes of death remain preeminent through the fourth decade of life in the United States.

Risky driving habits, including driving under the influence of alcohol or other substances, account for approximately half of fatal crashes. There is increasing evidence supporting the role of alcohol in other fatal recreation-related accidental injuries, including bicycling, skateboarding, boating, and swimming.

Suicide accounts for 6.9% (1.6 per 100,000 in 1997) of deaths in 10- to 14-year-olds. Among 15- to 19-year-olds, suicide accounts for 12.7% (9.5 per 100,000) of the deaths. Suicide is highest among white and Native American adolescents. Among black adolescents, suicide now ranks as the third leading cause of death. A further discussion of the etiology and management of suicide is provided in Sec. 5.7.2.

Homicide accounts for 6.8% (1.5 per 100,000) of the deaths in the 10- to 14-year-old age group. Among 15- to 19-year-olds, homicide accounts for 14% (13.7 per 100,000) of deaths. Among older black males, homicide remains the leading cause of death, accounting for 45.1% (92.7 per 100,000) of deaths. Adolescents who live in impoverished metropolitan areas are more likely to be victims of homicide than those who live in suburban or rural areas. Homicides often occur during fights between males of the same age and race.

The most frequent nonviolent causes of mortality during adolescence are cardiovascular diseases (1.0 per 100,000 for 10- to 14-year-olds and 2.1 per 100,000 for 15- to 19-year-olds) and malignant neoplasms (2.5 per 100,000 for 10- to 14-year-olds and 3.7 per 100,000 for 15- to 19-year-olds).

MORBIDITY

Most morbidity during the second decade results from three risky behaviors initiated in early to middle adolescence: substance abuse, sexual activity, and motor/recreational vehicle use. These three behaviors tend to covary. Additional causes of morbidity include reproductive health problems associated with sexual activity and variants of normal physiological maturation; orthopedic problems associated with skeletal growth and maturation and injuries; and mental health disorders.

3.2.1   Risk-taking Behaviors

SUBSTANCE USE AND ABUSE
Arik V. Marcell and Charles E. Irwin, Jr.

Although the prevalence for substance use over the past decade has decreased from the high rates in the late 1970s, the 1998 lifetime prevalence rates of alcohol use and cigarette smoking remain high at 81.4% and 65.3%, respectively. The initiation of alcohol and tobacco use during adolescence represents the beginning of lifetime substance use patterns with major negative health consequences throughout the life span. The 1998 high school senior survey reported that 31.5% of high school seniors (approximately 17 years old) reported at least one episode of binge drinking, or consuming more than five drinks at one time, in the 2 weeks before the survey. Both cigarette use and alcohol use begin early in adolescence, with a mean age of onset of 12 years for cigarettes and 12.6 years for alcohol. Girls consistently report greater daily use of cigarettes than boys, whereas boys report greater use of alcohol than girls. Alcohol use is almost twice as common in boys. The lower rates of cigarette smoking in boys may be due to the use of smokeless tobacco or chewing tobacco, an uncommon practice in girls.

In 1998, the reported lifetime prevalence of marijuana use during adolescence was 49%, with 22.8% of the high school seniors reporting use in the past 30 days. For the past 2 years, there has been a gradual increase in marijuana use in high school seniors, which may reflect the decreasing risk that adolescents ascribe to marijuana use. The mean age of onset of marijuana use is 14.4 years.

The lifetime prevalence of cocaine use in high school seniors in 1997 was 9.3%. The use of crack was reported to be 4.4%. These rates also reflect increases in substance abuse over the past 2 years.

The data on substance use come from high school surveys or national household surveys; both probably underestimate the actual prevalence rates of substance use in the adolescent population. Clinicians need to establish the base rates for substance use in their respective communities to develop effective prevention and intervention programs.

The criteria for substance abuse and dependence as outlined by the *Diagnostic and Statistical Manual for Mental Disorders* (DSM IV-TR) do not distinguish between abuse in adulthood or adolescence, but adolescent drug users differ in many ways from adult users. Substance abuse progresses in predictable stages from use of legal drugs to illegal drugs and from less to more serious substances, each stage serving as a "gateway" to the next. In this section, a *drug* refers to alcohol, legal and illicit drugs, chemicals, and substances. *Abuse* is defined as the use of any drugs that causes a maladaptive pattern resulting in physical, psychological, economic, legal, or social harm to the user or to others. *Dependence* is defined as use of a drug that leads to tolerance (need for increased amounts to achieve intoxication, or diminished effect with continued use of the same amount); withdrawal (physical symptoms due to drug removal); and often uncontrollable craving, seeking, and use, even in the face of negative health and social consequences. For common substances of abuse, physicians need to be familiar with national and local trends; be able to detect manifestations; understand basic principles regarding screening, counseling, and management for substance use and abuse; and be knowledgeable about appropriate referral.

There is no pathognomonic clinical presentation of drug abuse. Signs of drug abuse in an adolescent include an increasing degree of emotional and physical isolation from the family, absent or hostile communication, deteriorating school attendance and/or performance, decrease in athletic performance, a change in peer group, involvement in theft or burglary, and the initiation of other risk behaviors including sex. Known risk factors for the development of substance abuse and dependence are multifold and include household drug abuse, specifically by parents; substance abuse in the peer group; earlier age of onset; cognitive disability; attention deficit hyperactivity disorder; and mood disorders including depression, anxiety disorders, and problems of impulse control and aggression. Substance use should be considered in any older adolescent who has a sudden change in school performance.

SCREENING AND COUNSELING The adolescent patient should be interviewed alone (Sec. 3.3) and assessed regarding the type of substances used, frequency, quantity, pattern of use, time of last use, route of administration, circumstances of use, reasons for use, age of first onset, medical consequences, unreported acute intoxication or other related injury, and related legal problems. The family also should be assessed regarding substance abuse and psychiatric and legal history. Diagnoses and recommendations should be clear, unequivocal, and nonjudgmental. It is helpful to recognize the patient's state or readiness for change using a framework such as Prochaska's Theoretical Model for Change (or "Stages of Change") that identifies the individual as being in a precontemplative, contemplative, determination, action, or maintenance stage. Depending on the stage, the physician can tailor counseling accordingly. Relapse is common, should be anticipated, and should not be considered as failure.

TREATMENT This must address the adolescent's experience including cognitive, emotional, physical, social, and moral development. Age, gender, ethnicity, disability status, stage of readiness to change, and cultural background must all be considered. Every effort must be made to involve the adolescent's family and to use adolescent-specific treatment programs. Coercive pressure to seek treatment is generally not conducive to behavior change. The emergency room is not an appropriate place for an intervention, but it can be appropriate for performing a screening evaluation and to arrange follow-up evaluation and intervention once stabilization has occurred. Treatment interventions range from minimal outpatient contacts to long-term residential therapy. Treatment or placement should depend on where the adolescent falls on the substance use continuum. Programs can include but are not limited to: brief office-based interventions, 12-step-based programs, therapeutic communities, and family therapy.

Alcohol

The ethanol content of brewed alcoholic beverages is measured as "percent" (weight to volume) and of distilled beverages as "proof" units [In the United States, 1 proof 0.5% alcohol, or twice the "percent " (ie 80 proof is 40% alcohol)]. The ethanol content of beverages is variable; beer has 3 to 6%, wine has 12 to 14%, and distilled spirit has 40 to 60%. Mouthwashes may contain up to 75% ethanol and colognes and aftershave lotions 40 to 80%. The following drinks contain equivalent amounts of ethanol: 12 to 14 oz beer; 6 oz unfortified wine; 4 oz sherry; 1.5 oz whiskey. Blood alcohol level (BAL) is measured as mg percent (mg ethanol in 100 mL blood, or mg/dL). The legal intoxication BAL is 0.05 to 0.10%.

SCREENING AND COUNSELING Prevention counseling needs to start in preteen years with assessment for alcohol use at every visit. Screening should include questions regarding patterns of use, such as social versus binge drinking and for the experience of injury and drinking, and driving. Counseling should include the consequences of drinking particularly drinking and driving. Physicians should also practice using refusal skills with their adolescent patients.

CLINICAL PHARMACOLOGY AND TOXICOLOGY Ethanol acts as a central nervous system depressant with local and general anesthetic properties. The first structures to be affected include the reticular activating system and certain cortical areas (eg the frontal lobes). Ethanol competes with antidiuretic hormone and acute intoxication can result in considerable fluid loss. In children less than 7 years, ethanol metabolism may deplete the nicotinamide-adenine dinucleotide (NAD) stores needed for gluconeogenesis, resulting in hypoglycemia.

Administration is mainly oral. Absorption is rapid from the stomach (20%) and small intestine (80%). Onset of action is usually within 10 min, with peak blood ethanol levels occurring within 40 to 60 min. The duration of action depends on the quantity consumed, drinking rate, and food intake. Metabolism occurs almost exclusively in the liver by alcohol dehydrogenase, a small amount isexcreted in the urine. This hepatic enzyme does not reach adult activity levels until the age of 5 years. Blood ethanol level decreases at a fixed rate of about 28 mg/dL/h or 6 mmol/L/h.

CONSEQUENCES OF USE Addiction and tolerance to, and physical dependence on, alcohol can develop. Mental status changes depend on the blood alcohol level. Mild intoxication (BAL < 100 mg/dL) causes altered cognition, mild sedation, disinhibition, euphoria, giddiness, and talkativeness. Moderate intoxication (BAL 100 to 200 mg/dL) causes sedation, impaired mentation, mood swings, slurred speech, sensory loss, and moderate incoordination. Severe intoxication (BAL > 200 mg/dL) causes dehydration, hypothermia, hypoglycemia, lactic acidosis, insomnia, headaches, gastritis, pancreatitis, confusion, stupor, cardiorespiratory compromise, coma, and death. Eye findings include nystagmus with normal pupil size. Alcohol use during pregnancy is responsible for fetal alcohol syndrome and fetal alcohol effects in the fetus. Behavioral side effects include school failure, unprotected sex, use of other illicit drugs, and risk for injury, including motor vehicle accidents, assaults, violence, and suicide. Unlike in adults, chronic ethanol abuse in adolescents is rarely associated with medical complications.

Laboratory findings include elevated blood ethanol concentration, elevated osmolar gap, hypokalemia, and metabolic (lactic) acidosis. Hypoglycemia may present as coma or convulsions more than 3 hours postingestion and can occur with blood ethanol levels as low as 50 mg/dL. The differential diagnosis of acute ethanol intoxication includes diabetes mellitus, diabetes insipidus, infectious gastroenteritis, and central nervous system hemorrhage, infection, or trauma. Toxins producing similar effects include akee fruit, anticonvulsants, antihistamines, diuretics, ethylene glycol, hypoglycemic agents, isopropyl alcohol, methanol, psychotherapeutic agents, and sedative-hypnotic drugs.

Early withdrawal symptoms ("hangover ") include anxiety, insomnia, confusion, hallucinations, irritability, headaches, tremulousness, hyperreflexia, mydriasis, tachycardia, hypertension, nausea/vomiting, hyperthermia, and diaphoresis. Late withdrawal is manifested by delirium tremens (rare in adolescents), profound confusion, marked psychomotor agitation, seizures, respiratory depression, and hypothermia. Alcohol hallucinosis can occur in the first 48 hours of nonuse and may be life-threatening.

TREATMENT Early intervention in the outpatient setting depends on the severity of the alcohol problem; options range from brief office-based interventions to outpatient treatment programs to residential treatment programs. Anatabuse, a specific ethanol antagonist that causes unpleasant side effects when consumed with alcohol, may be used as an adjunct to other therapy in selected motivated teenagers but has not been specifically approved for use in adolescents.

In the acutely intoxicated patient, management depends on severity of symptoms. Mild intoxication (<350 mg/kg of ethanol) can be managed at home with close observation, hydration, and analgesics. Moderate to severe intoxication (>350 mg/kg of ethanol or BAL >300 mg/dL) requires appropriate airway management and supportive care. Because it is rapidly absorbed, removal of alcohol from the stomach should be attempted only within 1 hour after ingestion. Normal doses of activated charcoal do not effectively adsorb ethanol. Blood glucose and electrolyte levels should be assessed and corrected if abnormal. In patients with BAL >500 mg/dL or deterioration despite conservative support, use of hemodialysis should be considered.

Treatment of mild withdrawal symptoms include rest and hydration. For severe symptoms, benzodiazepines may be helpful. Seizures can be treated with diazepam or phenytoin. Hallucinosis and/or delirium can be treated with haloperidol.

Nicotine: Cigarettes and Other Products

The average age of first cigarette use is 12. Thus, dependence should be viewed as a pediatric disorder because the majority of chronically addicted adults begin smoking before age 18. Smoking is a major cause of stroke and death in adults in the United States. Also, more than 10% of high school students (male predominance) report use of smokeless tobacco products. Users of smokeless tobacco are more likely than nonusers to become cigarette smokers.

SCREENING AND COUNSELING Physicians should start prevention counseling in the preteen years regarding use of all tobacco products. All smokers should be advised to quit. Parents who smoke should be advised to see their own physicians for help in quitting.

CLINICAL PHARMACOLOGY AND TOXICOLOGY Nicotine comes in a variety of forms and routes of administration; cigarettes, cigars, and pipes are smoked; snuff is sniffed nasally; and tobacco is chewed orally. Derived from the tobacco plant, nicotine is a natural alkaloid and acts as a central nervous system stimulant. It also blocks cholinergic synapses in the peripheral nervous system causing sympathomimetic effects. Onset after use is immediate, with direct effects on the body for 30 minutes to about 2 hours after inhalation. Metabolism occurs in the liver and excretion by the kidneys. A single cigarette contains 8 to 9 mg of nicotine, and about 1mg is delivered to the user while smoking. In addition to nicotine, tars and other carcinogens in tobacco products are known to be associated with malignancies, and carbon monoxide in smoke is known to increase the risk of cardiovascular disease.

CONSEQUENCES OF USE Nicotine is highly addictive and toxic, and tolerance and dependence can develop quickly. Symptoms include euphoria, changes in memory, and decreased aggression. Tachycardia and/or bradycardia can occur. Respiratory symptoms include cough, sputum production, bronchitis, and dyspnea on exertion. Use during pregnancy can result in increased risk of stillborn, premature, and low birth weight infants. Long-term risks include coronary artery disease, cardiomyopathy, stroke, chronic obstructive pulmonary disease, peptic ulcer disease, and cancer of the lung, mouth, larynx, pharynx, esophagus, stomach, pancreas, uterine, cervix, kidneys, ureter, and bladder. Withdrawal symptoms include increased aggression, loss of social cooperation, and impaired psychomotor and cognitive functions, such as language comprehension. Secondhand smoke causes lung cancer in adults and greatly increases the risks of respiratory illnesses in children and sudden infant death.

TREATMENT Withdrawal symptoms are less severe in those who quit smoking gradually. Success is not usually achieved before five to seven attempts. Relapses are frequent, especially in the first few weeks, but diminish considerably after 3 months. Brief, office-based counseling has been shown to be effective in helping individuals to consider quitting. Pharmacologic, combined with psychological, treatment results in the highest long-term abstinence rates. Nicotine replacement therapy is available in many forms. Nicotine chewing gum doses range from 2 to 4 mg per piece; maximum use is 20 pieces per day. The nicotine transdermal patch delivers a relatively constant amount of nicotine of 15 to 22 mg per day; it is used for 4 to 6 weeks and then tapered. Other replacements include nasal sprays and inhalers. The FDA approves only nicotine chewing gum and transdermal patches for use in adolescents. Zyban (Bupropion) helps to control craving for nicotine. It is contraindicated in persons with depression and seizure disorders and has not been specifically approved for use in adolescents.

Cannabis

Cannabis is not an innocuous drug. Its use often precedes use of other more dangerous drugs, and it should be considered a gateway drug. Potency of street samples has increased over the past two decades. It is the illicit drug used most commonly in the United States. *Cannabis* is a collective term for various preparations of the hemp plant *Cannabis sativa*. Street names include pot, herb, weed, boom, Mary Jane, gangster, chronic, hashish, hash, cannabis, ganja, grass, and roach.

CLINICAL PHARMACOLOGY AND TOXICOLOGY *Marijuana* can be smoked as cigarettes (joints), in a pipe or bong, and as "blunts" (cigars emptied of tobacco and refilled with marijuana, often in combination with other drugs such as crack). *Cannabis* can be ingested in foods as marijuana or in liquids as hashish or hashish oil. The active ingredient, Δ-9-tetrahydrocannibol (THC), binds central nervous system receptors in the cortex, hippocampus, striatum, and cerebellum. The mechanisms by which it produces clinical effects are unknown. Onset of action with smoking is approximately 5 to 10 minutes and duration of action is about 3 hours. When taken orally, onset of action is 30 to 60 minutes with a duration of 5 to 7 hours. The liver metabolizes THC, but about 20% is excreted unchanged in the urine and feces. Approximately 20% of an inhaled dose is absorbed, compared to less than 10% after ingestion. THC is highly lipid-soluble and almost 100% is bound to plasma proteins. Regardless of THC content, the amount of tar inhaled and level of carbon monoxide absorbed are three to five times greater than among tobacco smokers.

CONSEQUENCES OF USE *Cannabis* is an addictive drug. Physical dependence and withdrawal symptoms have been reported in animal studies. Symptoms include euphoria, disinhibition, intoxication, dream-like fantasy state, hallucinations, time-space distortions, anxiety, confusion, depersonalization, and panic reactions. Central nervous system effects include impaired motor ability, visual tracking, signal detection, and visual glare recovery time and loss of coordination. These features contribute to impaired ability to operate a motor vehicle, bicycle, or mechanical equipment. The pupils may be dilated and the conjunctiva injected; tear production is reduced and intraocular pressure is low. Tachycardia and postural hypotension can occur. Respiratory effects include bronchodilation, followed by bronchoconstriction, cough, and increased respiratory infections such as sinusitis and bronchitis. Appetite is often increased. Reproductive effects include gynecomastia (reversible), decreased sperm count and motility (reversible), decreased testos-

terone levels, and pubertal arrest. Use during pregnancy may be associated with small-for-gestational-age infants. *Cannabis* is passed in breast milk and is associated with impaired motor development and muscle control in the infant. Marijuana has anti-emetic properties. It also has an adverse impact on short-term memory and causes problems with learning, thinking, and problem-solving. "Amotivational syndrome" in chronic users causes a loss of goal-directed activity. Use of *cannabis* potentiates sedation when used with alcohol and other sedatives. Symptoms of acute intoxication include anxiety, delusions, hallucinations, paranoia, and psychosis. Symptoms of withdrawal are relatively mild and rare, occurring with chronic users only and include depression, restlessness, sleep disturbances, tremor, nystagmus, nausea, vomiting, diarrhea, and anorexia.

TREATMENT Therapeutic treatment programs may be indicated for chronic users. For acute intoxication, anxiety and panic attacks can be treated with benzodiazepines and a calm environment. Gastric emptying and activated charcoal ingestion may be considered for accidental ingestion. No treatment is necessary for withdrawal symptoms.

Other Drugs

Adolescents use a variety of other illicit drugs. Drugs commonly used as part of nightclub, bar, rave and/or trance scenes include ecstasy, herbal ecstasy, and the date-rape drugs rohypnol, γ-hydroxybutyrate (GHB), and ketamine. Ecstasy is an amphetamine and a stimulant. The "date-rape drugs" are depressants and have sedative-hypnotic effects. Although use of cocaine and crack cocaine declined in the early 1990s, it has gradually increased in recent years. Heroin use by adolescents is relatively infrequent. Although injection is the most common method, use by sniffing and smoking has increased recently.

Substance Testing

The vast majority of abused substances can be detected in the blood or urine for days to weeks after use. Although mandatory drug screening is a routine part of many substance abuse treatment programs, involuntary (nonconsensual) testing of adolescents in routine practice settings remains controversial. The published policy of the American Academy of Pediatrics states that drug testing of the older, competent adolescent should be voluntary. Reasons to screen patients include history of trauma, unexplained accident, psychiatric symptoms, significant change in performance or behaviors in daily activities or school, unexplained chronic illness, suicide attempt, altered mental status, and to monitor of compliance during drug recovery programs. The physician should employ reliable test methods and, in order to ensure test accuracy, should prevent adulteration of the obtained sample by the adolescent. Less expensive and sensitive tests should be chosen initially. These, including radioimmunoassay (RIA), enzyme-multiplied immunoassay test (EMIT), fluorescent polarization immunoassay (FPIA), and latex agglutination (ONTRAK), are subject to false-negative and false-positive results. More sensitive and expensive confirmatory tests that are less subject to false-negative and false-positive results include gas chromatography, thin-layer chromatography, high-performance liquid chromatography (rarely used), and gas chromatography/mass spectrometry (most commonly used). Duration of positivity on urine testing varies greatly with different substances (Table 3-3).

TABLE 3-3

URINE DRUG TESTING AND DURATION OF POSITIVITY

SUBSTANCE	DURATION
Amphetamines	48 h
Barbiturates	24–72 h
Benzodiazepines	72 h
Cocaine	48–72 h
Ethanol	<12 h
Heroin	24 h
Methadone	3 days
Phencyclidine (PCP)	8 days
Marijuana	
One dose	48 h
Four times/week	5 days
Daily use	10 days
Chronic use	21–30 days
LSD*	—

* Lysergic acid diethylamide (LSD) is not detected in standard urinary screening.

Common false-positive test results may be obtained with poppy seeds, dextromethorphan, and chlorpromazine when testing or opiates; with ephedrine, phenylephrine, and pseudoephedrine when testing for amphetamines; and with dextromethorphan and diphenhydramine when testing for phencyclidine (PCP). Common reasons for false-negative test results include fluid substitution, water loading, and providing a sample that is not urine. Certain drugs may not be on standard drug screens. Thus, being familiar with an institution's drug screens and/or making special requests if testing is indicated may be necessary.

UNINTENTIONAL INJURIES

Unintentional injuries are the primary cause of premature mortality in adolescents, accounting for over 41% of deaths in 10- to 14-year-olds and 46.3% of deaths in 15- to 19-year-olds. Males outnumber females by more than two to one for all injuries. Motor vehicle accidents account for over 80% of the mortality in the 15- to 19-year- old category. Acute traumatic injuries resulting from nonfatal accidents account for the largest number of hospital days for both adolescent boys and girls and 16% of outpatient physician visits. Motor and recreational vehicle use are the most common etiologic agents in these injuries. Often, the primary care physician will not see the adolescent at these visits because the initial visit generally occurs in an emergency room or the office of a surgical subspecialist.

The peak time for vehicular accidents among 15- to 19-year-olds occurs on weekends between 11 p.m. and 5 a.m., when such factors as lack of experience, lethargy, substance use, high speed, and recklessness contribute to the injury situation. Increasingly, alcohol is a cofactor in injuries associated with bicycles, skateboards, boating, and swimming. Other substances may also play a role in injuries.

SEXUAL BEHAVIOR

Sexual behavior during adolescence has decreased over the past decade, with fewer adolescents initiating sexual intercourse and more adolescents using effective contraception when they initiate coitus.

The most recent 1995 survey on sexual behavior of youth between the ages of 15 and 19 shows that 55% of boys and 50% of girls had experienced coitus at least once. The percentages are somewhat different by race and ethnicity: for blacks, 66% for female and 80% for male teenagers; for Hispanics, 46% for female and 58% for male teenagers; and for whites, 44% for female and 43% for male teenagers. Currently, about three-quarters of adolescents report using some form of contraception at first intercourse. Age of menarche is an important determinant of initiation of sexual activity, with earlier-maturing girls beginning sexual intercourse earlier than age-related but later-maturing girls. Sexually transmitted diseases are higher among sexually active adolescents than in any other sexually active age group (see Sec. 3.6). Sexually active black adolescents have much higher rates of sexually transmitted diseases than do white adolescents. In 1997, there were 493,006 births to female adolescents under 20 years of age in the United States. By most estimates there are at least an equal number of spontaneous and therapeutic abortions.

COVARIATION OF RISK BEHAVIORS

Risk behaviors tend to be associated with each other in predictable ways. The onset of one behavior may indicate that another behavior has a greater likelihood of being initiated in the near future. The close association of alcohol and unintentional injury is well established. Alcohol-related motor vehicle injuries are the leading cause of mortality in late adolescence. Alcohol is also associated with other injuries including those resulting from nonmotorized recreational vehicle use and aquatic sports. The role of other substances in unintentional injury is not clear. Substance use is positively correlated with early initiation of sexual behavior. Female adolescents who report the use of illicit substances and cigarette smoking are more likely not to use effective contraception and thus to have an unintended pregnancy.

Within the area of substance use, the use patterns are associated in predictable ways. Early initiation of alcohol and tobacco predict the use of illicit substances. The sequence of progression is as follows: alcohol or cigarettes precede marijuana use; alcohol, cigarettes, and marijuana precede other illicit drugs (including psychedelics, cocaine, heroin, and nonprescribed stimulants, sedatives, and tranquilizers), and the use of prescribed psychoactive drugs follows all other substances. In girls, cigarettes are often more important than alcohol in predicting subsequent substance use. The use of a substance farther along the trajectory generally implies ongoing use of the preceding substance, leading to a cumulative effect of all the substances.

MEDICAL CONSEQUENCES OF RISK BEHAVIORS

The short-term and long-term effects of risk behaviors are listed in Table 3-4. Short-term effects are seen within a few weeks or months, that is, during adolescence; long-term effects will generally appear after adolescence.

The short-term consequences of alcohol use are generally seen in the emergency room associated with injuries. The psychoactive ingredient Δ^9-tetrahydrocannabinol in marijuana causes a mood alteration. The long-term risk of lung cancer is beginning to be documented.

Generalized psychological dysfunction is often reported in the area of substance use. Important clues to dysfunction include a general lack of motivation and a developmental lag in school. Attempting to identify the experimental user from the habitual user

TABLE 3-4
MEDICAL CONSEQUENCE OF RISK BEHAVIORS

RISK BEHAVIOR	SHORT-TERM	LONG-TERM
Cigarettes	Nicotine addiction, elevated WBC count, chronic bronchitis, decline in pulmonary function test results	Increase in cancer of lungs, larynx, esophagus, oral cavity; heart disease; chronic pulmonary disease; increased overall mortality
Smokeless tobacco	Nicotine addiction, periodontal disease (leukoplakia, gingival recession, dental caries)	Oral-pharyngeal cancer
Alcohol	Abnormal liver function test results, hepatitis, gastritis	Chronic liver disease, protein malnutrition, global dementia, peripheral neuropathy, chronic pancreatitis
Marijuana	Decreased pulmonary function, chronic bronchitis, decreased testosterone levels, gynecomastia	Increased risk of lung cancer, amotivational syndrome
Motor/recreational vehicle use	Trauma, acute disability, accidental death	Chronic disability, accidental death
Sexual activity	Sexually transmitted diseases, pregnancy	Infertility, ectopic pregnancy, AIDS/HIV infection, chronic pelvic pain, congenital STD in offspring, cervical intraepithelial neoplasia

AIDS/HIV = acquired immunodeficiency syndrome/human immunodeficiency virus; STD = sexually transmitted disease; WBC = white blood cell.
SOURCE: *Irwin CE Jr, Ryan SA: Problem behavior of adolescents. Pediatr Rev 10:235–246, 1989.*

is difficult because it is not often possible to identify where the adolescent is on the trajectory of use curve.

OTHER MEDICAL PROBLEMS ASSOCIATED WITH MORBIDITY

Approximately 6% of adolescents have a chronic disease that interferes with general functioning. The most common causes of chronic illness include mental health disorders and diseases of the respiratory and musculoskeletal systems. Younger male adolescents living in poverty are the group most impaired by chronic disease. Most adolescents suffer no major problem in their psychosocial functioning as a result of chronic disease.

Common medical problems for which adolescents seek medical care include acne, reproductive health problems, specific disorders of the skeletal system such as Osgood-Schlatter disease, idiopathic scoliosis, and common sports injuries. Reproductive health problems are discussed in Sec. 3.4; skeletal disorders are discussed in Chap. 27; and acne in Sec. 14.9.

References

Risk-Taking Behaviors

American Academy of Pediatrics Policy Statements. Committee on Substance Abuse: Alcohol. Pediatrics 95(3):439–442, 1995; Marijuana. Pediatrics 104(4):982–985, 1999; Tobacco, alcohol, and other drugs. Pediatrics 101(1):125–128, 1998; Indications for management and referral of patients involved in substance abuse. Pediatrics 106(1):143–148, 2000; Testing for drugs of abuse in children and adolescents. Pediatrics 98(2):305–307, 1996; *www-arp.org* (publications).

Diagnostic and Statistical Manual of Mental Disorders: DSM-IV, 4th ed. Washington, DC, American Psychiatric Association, 1994

Fishman M, Bruner A, Adger H: Substance abuse among children and adolescents. Pediatr Rev 18(11): 394–408, 1997

Inaba DS: Uppers, downers, all arounders. Physical and Mental Effects of Psychoactive Drugs, 4th ed. CNS Productions, Ashland, OR, 2000

NIDA Infofax. U.S. Department of Health and Human Services • National Institutes of Health. www.nida.nih.gov; Marijuana (updated March 2000); Nicotine (updated Jan 2000)

NIDA Research Reports. U.S. Department of Health and Human Services • National Institutes of Health. www.nida.nih.gov; Nicotine (updated July 1998)

Prochaska J, DiClemente C: Stages and processes of self-change of smoking: Toward an integrative model of change. J Consult Clin Psychol 51:390–395, 1983

Takahashi A, Franklin J: Alcohol abuse. Pediatr Rev 17(2):39–45, 1996

3.2.2 Mental Health Problems during Adolescence

Nearly 10% of adolescents have symptoms of psychological distress. Psychiatric disorders that appear during late childhood and throughout adolescence include anxiety and panic disorders, personality disorders, affective disorders, attention deficit disorders, conduct disorders, schizophrenia, and eating disorders. The clinician caring for adolescents will frequently encounter patients with depression, suicidal ideation, and eating disorders.

DEPRESSION

The prevalence of major depressive disorders in adolescents is about 5%. Depression is the most common feature in patients who attempt suicide. To establish the diagnosis of depression in an adolescent, the clinician uses the same criteria that are used in adulthood (see Table 3-5).

These diagnostic criteria include changes in bodily functioning, cognition, interpersonal relationships, and affect. Depressive equivalents in adolescents include decrements in academic functioning, hypochondriasis, family conflicts, problems with the law, and substance use and abuse (see Sec. 5.7.2).

SUICIDE IN ADOLESCENTS

Suicide is one of the leading causes of death in adolescents. It is discussed in Sec. 5.7.2.

EATING DISORDERS

Eating disorders usually have their onset following puberty. Seventy-five percent of eating disorders in adults had their onset during adolescence. There has been an increase in prepubertal adolescents

TABLE 3-5

CRITERIA FOR DIAGNOSIS OF MAJOR DEPRESSION

Diagnosis requires symptom 1 or 2 and at least four other symptoms for a 2-week period
1. Depressed or irritable mood
2. Diminished interest or pleasure
3. Weight loss or weight gain
4. Insomnia or hypersomnia
5. Psychomotor agitation or retardation
6. Fatigue or loss of energy
7. Feelings of worthlessness or excessive guilt
8. Decreased concentration or indecisiveness
9. Thoughts of death, suicidal ideation, or suicide attempt

SOURCE: *American Psychiatric Association: Diagnostic and Statistical Manual of Mental Disorders, 4th ed., Washington DC: American Psychiatric Association, 1994: 327.*

who fit the criteria for anorexia nervosa or bulimia nervosa; these criteria are outlined in Table 3-6. Adolescents with some of the criteria for anorexia nervosa and bulimia nervosa may need the same treatment intervention as those who meet the established criteria in the *DSM-IV*. The eating patterns in many adolescents appear abnormal, and adolescent girls frequently have dissatisfaction with body size and shape, including the fear of gaining weight. These patterns and fears are extreme in the adolescent with an eating disorder.

Genetic studies appear to be converging on the conclusion that there is an underlying biological predisposition to eating disorders. Psychosocial factors play a role, but the majority of adolescents exposed to adverse psychosocial factors do not develop eating disorders. Neurotransmitters have been implicated in the etiology of eating disorders. Preliminary studies have documented the critical importance of a disturbance of serotonin activity, which may create a vulnerability for the expression of a cluster of symptoms associated with both anorexia nervosa and bulimia nervosa.

ANOREXIA NERVOSA The prevalence of anorexia nervosa is approximately 1% in the population of white females of middle to upper socioeconomic level between the ages of 14 and 24. The disorder also occurs in other racial and socioeconomic groups. Approximately 5 to 10% are male, many of whom have gender identity issues.

Clinical reports support the observation that onset often occurs after puberty, when adipose tissue deposition increases and family and friends comment about changes in body habitus. Hypothalamic abnormalities have been documented before the onset of weight loss; a significant number of girls report secondary amenorrhea before the onset of weight loss. The psychological profile of these girls includes low self-esteem, high anxiety, and normal cognition. Often the girls are overachievers and perfectionists. There are associated psychiatric disorders that include affective disorders and obsessive-compulsive disorders. Critical risk periods appear to be developmental transition (eg, a transition to middle/junior high school, high school, or college) and a decision to embark on diets. Excessive dieting leading to starvation can trigger an obsessive focus on food, resulting in further restriction or excessive intake. Gymnasts and ballet dancers are particularly at risk.

The physical findings depend on the degree of starvation and methods used to lose weight or restrict intake. Weight and height measurements need to be made after voiding, with the adolescent

undressed and in a gown. Body mass index (BMI) needs to be calculated. Vital signs including orthostatic measurements need to be done. Laboratory data are generally of little use except when the patient has been vomiting or ingesting laxatives or diuretics, which may result in hypokalemia and metabolic alkalosis. The LH and FSH levels are often prepubertal, and serum estradiol levels are low. In males, serum testosterone concentration is usually low. Triiodothyronine levels are low. Cortisol, endorphins, and cholesterol concentrations are elevated with an increase in high-density lipoproteins. The ECG changes include ST-segment depression on exercise stress testing and prolonged QT intervals. These ECG findings have been associated with ventricular tachycardia in adults with anorexia nervosa.

Successful treatment begins with early diagnosis and the development of a comprehensive medical, nutritional, and mental health regimen. When patients have returned to a stable weight, SSR

TABLE 3-6

DIAGNOSTIC CRITERIA FOR ANOREXIA NERVOSA AND BULIMIA NERVOSA

Anorexia nervosa
Refusal to maintain body weight over a minimal normal weight for age and height, eg, weight loss leading to maintenance of body weight 85% of that expected; or failure to make expected weight gain during period of growth, leading to body weight less than 85% of that expected.
Intense fear of gaining weight or becoming fat, even though underweight
Disturbance in the way in which one's body weight or shape is experienced; undue influence of body weight or shape on self-evaluation, or denial of seriousness of current low body weight.
In postmenarcheal girls, absence of at least three consecutive menstrual cycles, ie, amenorrhea.
Specific type:
  Restricting type: during the current episode of anorexia nervosa, the person has not regularly engaged in binge-eating or purging behavior.
  Binge-eating/purging type: during the current episode of anorexia nervosa, the person has regularly engaged in binge-eating or purging behavior.
Bulimia nervosa
Recurrent episodes of binge eating (rapid consumption of a large amount of food in a discrete period of time)
A feeling of lack of control over eating behavior during the eating binges
The person regularly engages in self-induced vomiting, use of laxatives or diuretics, strict dieting or fasting, or vigorous exercise in order to prevent weight gain
A minimum average of two binge-eating episodes a week for at least 3 months
Persistent overconcern with body shape and weight
Specific type:
  Purging type: during the current episode of bulimia nervosa, the person has regularly engaged in self-induced vomiting or the misuse of laxatives, diuretics, or enemas.
  Nonpurging type: during the current episode of bulimia nervosa, the person has used other inappropriate compensatory behaviors, such as fasting or excessive exercise, but has not regularly engaged in self-induced vomiting or the misuse of laxatives, diuretics, or enemas.

SOURCE: *American Psychiatric Association, Diagnostic and Statistical Manual of Mental Disorders, 4th ed. Washington, DC, American Psychiatric Association, 1994:544–550.*

agents may be helpful to prevent relapse. Mortality rates are as high as 10% in the 10 years following diagnosis with high rates of suicide.

The clinician needs to focus on early identification of the at-risk adolescent. Adolescents with unexplained weight loss, fatigue, depression, obsessive-compulsive disorder, delayed or arrested puberty, and parental concerns about their eating behavior need to be evaluated in a comprehensive manner (see also Sec. 5.5).

BULIMIA NERVOSA The diagnosis of bulimia nervosa is made using the criteria listed in Table 3-6. Prevalence is 2 to 5% in females and less than 1% in males. The individual adolescent patient may have both anorexia nervosa and bulimia nervosa concurrently, or may alternate between the two disorders. The etiology is not clear. The adolescent with bulimia nervosa may have mild disease and be functional, or she may be severely disabled with repeated bingeing, purging, substance abuse, and suicide attempts. Typically, the patient is in middle to late adolescence, as compared with the typical anorexia nervosa patient, who is usually in early to middle adolescence. The adolescent generally begins bulimic behavior to lose weight. Symptoms often include fatigue, bloating, irregular menses, and sore throat secondary to vomiting. Patients generally do not disclose their bingeing or purging behavior unless they are specifically asked. Findings on physical examination include bilateral swelling of the parotid glands, calluses on the dorsum of the fingers used to induce vomiting, and loss of tooth enamel from the acidic nature of vomitus. Reflux esophagitis and aspiration pneumonia can occur. Use of syrup of ipecac to induce vomiting and hypokalemia can cause cardiac toxicity. Laboratory abnormalities may include an elevated serum amylase concentration and metabolic alkalosis.

After the diagnosis is established, intervention must address the bingeing and purging behavior before or at the same time as the underlying psychopathology is addressed. An affective disorder or an obsessive-compulsive disorder is often present. Pharmacotherapy with an SSRI can be helpful in the management of the patient.

References

Somatic Growth and Development During Adolescence

Biro FM, Lucky AW, Huster GA, et al: Pubertal staging in boys. Pediatr 127:100–102, 1995

Daniel WA: Growth at adolescence: Clinical correlates. Semin Adolesc Med 1:15–24, 1985

Herman-Giddens ME, Slora EJ, Wasserman RC, et al: Secondary sexual characteristics and menses in young girls seen in office practice: a study from the Pediatric Research in Office Settings Network. Pediatrics 99:505–512, 1997

Marshall WA, Tanner JM: Variation in the pattern of pubertal changes in girls. Arch Dis Child 44:291–303, 1969

Marshall WA, Tanner JM: Variation in the pattern of pubertal changes in boys. Arch Dis Child 45:13–23, 1970

Slap GB: Normal physiological and psychological growth in the adolescent. J Adolesc Health Care 7:135–235, 1986

Styne DM, Grumbach MM: Puberty: Ontogeny, neuroendocrinology, physiology, and disorder. In: Wilson J, Foster DW, Kronenberg HM, Larsen PR, eds. Williams Textbook of Endocrinology, 9th ed. Philadelphia, WB Saunders, 1999, 1509–1625

Tanner JM, Davies PSW: Clinical longitudinal standards for height and weight velocity for North American children. J Pediatr 107:317–329, 1985

Thompson PM, Giedd JN, Woods RP, et al: Growth patterns in the developing brain detected by using continuum mechanical tensor maps. Nature 404:190–193, 2000

Psychological Development

Adams GR, Montemayor R, Gullotta TP: Biology of adolescent behavior and development. Newbury Park, CA, Sage Publications, 1989

Irwin CE Jr, ed: Adolescent social behavior and new health directions for child development, no. 37. San Francisco, Jossey Bass, 1987

Jessor R: Risk behavior in adolescence: A psychological framework for understanding and action. J Adolesc Health 12:597–605, 1991

Lerner RM, ed: Early Adolescence: Perspectives on Policy, Research and Intervention. Hillsdale, NJ, Lawrence Erlbaum Associates, 1993

Orr DP, Ingersoll GM: Adolescent development: A biopsychosocial review. Curr Probl Pediatr 18:441–499, 1988

Resnick MD, Bearman PS, Blum RW, et al: Protecting adolescents from harm. Findings from the National Longitudinal Study on Adolescent Health. JAMA 278:823–832, 1997

Steinberg LD: The impact of puberty on family relations: Effects of pubertal status and puberty timing. Dev Psychol 23:451–456, 1987

Susman EJ, Nottelman ED, Inoff-Germain G: Hormonal influences on aspects of psychological development during adolescence. J Adolesc Health Care 8:492–504, 1987

Udry JR: Biological predispositions and social control in adolescent sexual behavior. Am Soc Rev 53:709–730, 1988

The Health Problems of Adolescents and Risk-Taking Behaviors

Abma JC, Chandra A, Mosher W, et al: Fertility, family planning, and women's health: new data from the 1995 National Survey of Family Growth. *Vital and Health Statistics, 23* (DHHS Pub. No. PHS 97-1995). Hyattsville, MD: National Center for Health Statistics, 1997 Centers for Disease Control and Prevention, National Center for Health Statistics, CDC wonder, mortality (compressed) data set *(http://wonder.cdc.gov)*. Atlanta, Centers for Disease Control and Prevention, 2000

Diclemente RJ, Hansen WB, Ponton LE: Handbook of Adolescent Health Risk Behavior. New York, Plenum Press, 1996

Friedman SB, Fisher MM, Schonberg SK, Alderman EM, eds: Comprehensive Adolescent Health Care, 2nd ed. St Louis, CV Mosby, 1998

Hauser ST, Powers SI, Noam GG: Adolescents and Their Families. New York, The Free Press, 1991

Hofmann AD, Greydanus DE, eds: Adolescent Medicine. Stamford, CT: Appleton & Lange, 1997

Irwin CE JR, Igra V, Eyre S, Millstein SG: Risk-taking Behavior in Adolescents: The Paradigm. In: Jacobson MS, Rees JM, Golden NH, Irwin CE Jr, eds: Adolescent Nutritional Disorders: Prevention and Treatment. New York, The New York Academy Press, 1997:1–35

Irwin CE JR, Millstein SG: Biopsychosocial correlates of risk taking behaviors during adolescence. J Adolesc Health Care 7:82S–96S, 1986

Johnston LD, O'Malley PM, Bachman JG: National Survey Results from the Monitoring the Future Study, 1975–1998: Vol I. Secondary School Students. Bethesda, MD: National Institute on Drug Abuse, 1999

Kann L, Kinchen SA, Williams BI, et al: Youth Risk Behavior Surveillance. Surveillance and Evaluation Research Branch, Division of Adolescent and School Health. Atlanta, Centers for Disease Control and Prevention, 1997

Millstein SG, Irwin CE Jr, Adler NE, et al: Health risk behaviors among young adolescents. Pediatrics 89:422–431, 1992

Newacheck PW, Brindis CD, Cart C, et al: Adolescent health insurance coverage: Recent changes and access to care. Pediatrics 104:195–202, 1999

US Congress, Office of Technology Assessment: Adolescent health—Vol I, Summary and Policy Options, OTA-H-468. Washington, DC, US Government Printing Office, 1991

Mental Health Problems

Becker AE, Grinspoon SK, Klibanski A, Herzog DB: Eating disorders. N Engl J Med 340:1092–1098, 1999

Kaye W, Gendall K, Strober M: Serotonin neuronal function and selective serotonin reuptake inhibitor treatment in anorexia and bulimia nervosa. Biol Psychiatry 44:825–838, 1998

Kreipe RE, Dukarm CP: Eating disorders in adolescents and older children. Pediatr Rev 20:410–420, 1999

Lewinsohn PM, Rohde P, Seeley JR: Major depressive disorder in older adolescents: Prevalence, risk factors, and clinical implications. Clin Psychol Rev 18:765–794, 1998.

Singer MI, Singer LT, Anglin TM, eds: Handbook for Screening Adolescents at Psychosocial Risk. New York, Lexington, 1993

Steiner H, Lock J: Anorexia nervosa and bulimia nervosa in children and adolescents: a review of the past 10 years. J Am Acad Child Adolesc Psychiatry 37:352–359, 1998

Strasburger VC, Greydanus DE. At risk adolescents: an update for the new century. Adolesc Med State Art Rev 11:1, 2000

3.3   THE ADOLESCENT VISIT

Charles E. Irwin, Jr.

Establishing him- or herself as the primary care physician for an adolescent patient is a formidable task for a pediatrician. A transition interview with adolescent patients and their families at approximately 10 years of age is an effective approach for developing a new relationship. During this interview the pediatrician will need to inform the parents and the patient about the changing nature of the relationship with the doctor: the need for the doctor to query the young person directly, the need for the patient to be examined alone, and the need of the patient to be able to generate his or her own questions for the doctor. Explaining the changes in the manner in which clinical care is provided is best done through a discussion of normal adolescence and the need for adolescents to begin to make some decisions with guidance and support from their families. During this transition interview, the clinician should provide the adolescent and family with some general information regarding the normal physiological and psychosocial changes of adolescence. Depending on the age and psychosocial functioning of the adolescent, the clinician may want to encourage the young person to come to the next clinical visit alone. As the adolescent completes the second decade of life, the pediatrician wants the young adult to be capable of assuming responsibility for his or her own health care.

Confidentiality issues are fundamental to the delivery of health care to adolescents; they need to be able to discuss all matters with the physician openly and honestly. Some physicians may feel uncomfortable with these principles and may want to clarify their position. From the first visit, the physician must assure the young person of the confidentiality of all information. The physician may need to restate this position on confidentiality during the gathering of information in such sensitive areas as sexuality and drug use. In the areas of life-threatening disease or behavior (eg, suicide, management of chronic disease), the physician always has the right to intervene on behalf of the patient's well-being, which generally involves identifying a parent, guardian, or supportive adult who can assist the young person with the problem.

3.3.1   The History

THE CLINICAL INTERVIEW

It is important to create an environment in which the adolescent is able to disclose information regarding his or her health habits. History taking should be guided by the developmental stage of the adolescent (Table 3-2). The physician also needs to recognize that many of the adolescent's concerns may not be disclosed on the first visit and may unfold after a relationship has been established. A follow-up visit for a rather minor problem may be the visit at which other health-damaging behaviors are disclosed.

SCREENING HISTORY

The screening history needs to focus on risk-taking behaviors (substance use, sexuality, recreational/motor vehicle use) and their as-

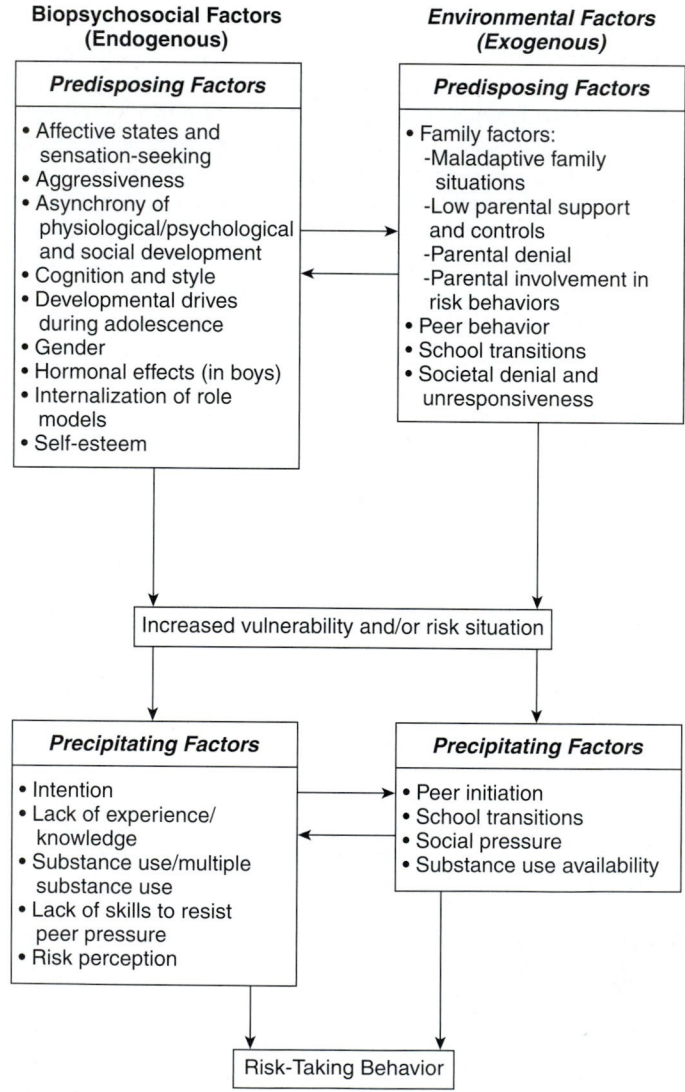

FIGURE 3-1   Principal factors in risk-taking behaviors. SOURCE: *Igra V, Irwin CE Jr: Risk and risk-taking in adolescents. In: Lindstrom B, Spencer N, eds: Social Pediatrics, New York, Oxford University Press, 1995:228.*

TABLE 3-7
PHYSICAL SIGNS WITH RISK BEHAVIORS

Recreational/motor vehicle use
  Skin
    Abrasions
    Ecchymoses
    Lacerations
  Musculoskeletal—fractures, sprains (acute and chronic)
Sexual activity
  Reproductive skin rash consistent with disease process
    Adenopathy
    Amenorrhea
    Genital lesions
    Vaginal/penile discharge
    Cervical discharge, edema, friability
    Uterine/adnexal tenderness
    Enlarged uterus (pregnant)
Substance use
  General
    Agitation, anxiety
    Decreased general functional status—sleep disturbances, anorexia
    Infection with HIV, hepatitis B, other STDs
  Skin
    Multiple bruises
    Track marks
    Abscesses
  Central nervous system/mental status
    Altered mental status
    Decreased short-term memory
    Decreased fine motor movements
    Diminished coordination
  Head, eyes, ears, nose, oropharynx
    Injected conjunctivae
    Chronic nasal discharge, nasal mucosal irritation
    Recurrent nosebleeds
    Leukoplakia, gingival recession, dental caries
    Mucosal inflammation (nasal passages, oropharynx)
    Malodorous breath
  Breast
    Gynecomastia (males)
  Cardiorespiratory
    Tachycardia
    Hypertension
    Evidence of deconditioning
    Chronic cough, recurrent bronchitis
  Gastrointestinal
    Abdominal pain and dyspepsia
    Weight loss
    Liver tenderness or enlargement
  Musculoskeletal
    Poor muscle tone/strength

HIV = human immuodeficiency virus, STD = sexually transmitted disease.
SOURCE: *Irwin CE Jr, Ryan SA. Problem behavior of adolescents. Pediatr Rev 10:235–246, 1989.*

sociated risk factors, depression and its equivalents, and dietary intake. The clinician needs to distinguish between risk-taking behaviors that are developmentally adaptive, although often dangerous, and those that are pathologic. Figure 3-1 identifies the principal factors involved in the etiologic mechanisms of the onset of risk behaviors and divides the factors into predisposing and precipitating factors. Behaviors that reflect possible involvement in risk behaviors include problems in family and peer relationships, a decrement in school functioning, legal problems, and behavioral prob-

lems reflective of substance use, including unusual or dramatic mood swings, changes in personal habits, runaway behavior, depressive symptoms, and preoccupation with generating money. Because many youths engage in risk behaviors, a checklist using Fig. 3-1 as a guide may be helpful as a screening tool to identify adolescents who are prone to engage in risk behaviors. In addition to the risk behaviors, the clinician needs to query the adolescent about general mood and dietary behaviors. A 24-hour recall of dietary intake for a weekday and weekend day provides a general assessment of nutrient and caloric intake.

MEDICAL HISTORY

The critical components of the medical history include the current concern or presenting complaint of the adolescent and family and a need to determine the risk for engaging in health-damaging behaviors through querying about the index or specific behavior and then other related problem activities or risky behaviors. For example, the female adolescent who is smoking cigarettes needs to be queried about sexual activity. Confining the evaluation to the most obvious behavior (eg, cigarette smoking) and ignoring the other highly related behavior may place the adolescent at risk for a more immediate negative outcome. After identifying the behavior that the adolescent is participating in, the clinician needs to evaluate the extent of the involvement and if the behavior has affected the health of the adolescent. The most common physical signs associated with risk behaviors on examination are outlined in Table 3-7. In adolescence, the behavioral consequences of risk behaviors often have a greater impact than the physical consequences. The components of the psychosocial inventory helpful with risk behaviors include an assessment of the intrafamily dynamics identifying major points of family support and conflict, including the parenting style of the family, and assessment of school functioning, including performance and motivation toward school, peer relationships and changes, extracurricular activities, and sexual behavior including sexual orientation.

3.3.2   Physical Assessment

PHYSICAL EXAMINATION

The extent to which each organ system is evaluated depends on the complaint. In general, the physical examination of the adolescent should include all aspects of the examination of the younger child. Features related to risk behaviors (substance use, sexuality, motor/recreational vehicle use) are outlined in Table 3-7. The following section identifies areas of the general adolescent examination that differ from that for the child.

GENERAL APPEARANCE   Particular attention should be directed to body posture, eye contact, dress, affect, mood, and energy level. Changes in weight may indicate the onset of an eating disorder, depression, or substance abuse.

SKIN   Distribution of acne, hair, striae, ecchymoses, "needle tracks," and scars should be noted. The pubertal changes should be correlated with the appropriate stages of sexual development as described by Tanner (see Sec. 24.8.1.). Striae are common in areas of rapid growth, especially where subcutaneous fat is increasing (hips, breasts, buttocks, and lower abdomen). Longitudinal scars on wrists may indicate suicide gestures or attempts. Major scars or ecchymoses may indicate a history of unintentional injuries.

EYES Conjunctival injection and alterations in pupil reactivity may indicate substance use. Visual acuity commonly changes and astigmatism can appear during adolescence. If the adolescent cannot identify more than half the letters on the 20/40 line of the Snellen chart, a referral to an ophthalmologist is indicated.

EARS Hearing is best checked by a pure-tone audiogram in early adolescence. The most common problem is high-tone sensorineural defects that may be related to listening to highly amplified music.

NOSE Constant erythema, trauma of the nose, or epistaxis may indicate substance use by inhalation. Trauma may also lead to a deviated septum.

TEETH Periodontal disease begins in adolescence. Malocclusion occurs in approximately 50% of adolescents. Referral for dental services is often indicated.

GLANDS Lymph nodes are generally palpable in the cervical, axillary, and inguinal areas. Lymph nodes greater than 1 cm and those that persist longer than 2 to 3 weeks should be investigated for infection or malignancy. Common infections associated with lymph node enlargement include infectious mononucleosis, pharyngitis, vaginitis, salpingitis, urethritis, and prostatitis. Examination of the breasts is discussed in Sec. 3.5.1.

CARDIOVASCULAR SYSTEM The examination of the cardiovascular system is standard. Precordial activity may be somewhat increased because of a hyperdynamic state secondary to anemia, anxiety, pregnancy, or substance use. Congenital cardiac abnormalities will usually be diagnosed before adolescence. Prolapsed mitral valve and lesions secondary to rheumatic fever may first be diagnosed during adolescence. Increases in blood pressure can result from anxiety or substance use.

RECTAL EXAMINATION Rectal examinations of the adolescent are indicated with symptomatic genitourinary and gastrointestinal complaints including a history of anal coitus.

MUSCULOSKELETAL SYSTEM Examination of the spine is undertaken to exclude scoliosis (see Sec. 27.7.4). Muscle strength and joint flexibility should be checked.

MENTAL STATUS Reading ability, comprehension, writing skills, and cognitive ability should be evaluated. Marked alterations in mood and energy are not consistent with normal adolescence. If the adolescent appears to have marked mood swings, the clinician needs to consider psychopathology including substance use. Higher cognitive functioning may be measured through tasks that require sequencing, memory, spatial relationships, and organizational skills.

LABORATORY SCREENING

Routine laboratory screening should include tuberculin skin tests, the frequency being determined by the risk status of the population, including environmental exposure risk. Current practice includes screening every 2 years. Table 3-8 lists screening laboratory tests for specific risk behaviors. The role of substance use screening for comatose or combative youth in the emergency setting and with

TABLE 3-8

SCREENING LABORATORY TESTS IN RISK BEHAVIORS

Substance use
  Substance use screen of urine, serum, gastric contents in acute intoxication, psychiatric symptoms, acute behavior changes
  Liver function test-ALT, AST, γ-glutaryl transpeptidase (alcohol use)
  Hepatitis B—HbsAg, HbsAb, HbcAg (parenteral drug use)
  Human immunodeficiency virus antibody (parenteral drug use)
Sexual activity
  First-voided urine in boys
  Cultures and vaginal smears for sexually transmitted diseases
  Papanicolaou smear
  Pregnancy tests
  RPR (syphilis)
  Hepatitis B antibody/antigen
  Human immunodeficiency virus antibody (consider in high-risk group)
Motor vehicle/recreational vehicle
  Substance use screen of urine and blood

SOURCE: *Irwin CE Jr, Ryan SA: Problem behavior of adolescents. Pediatr Rev 10:235–246, 1989.*

the onset of psychiatric symptoms is clear. There is considerable controversy regarding screening to confirm a suspicion of substance use in the routine office visit. There is little to be gained by screening adolescents who use substances unless they are engaged in a treatment program. Considerable problems exist with the sensitivity and specificity of urine screening for substance use. Testing indicates the presence or absence of use in the preceding few days and does not provide information about frequency, intensity, or chronicity of use. Ethical and legal issues must be addressed in obtaining the adolescent's consent in a nonemergency situation. Drug testing to confirm a history also conveys a message to the patient: the clinician does not believe the history. This statement may interfere with development of a long-term therapeutic relationship with the adolescent. Drug testing is critical in the ongoing management of an adolescent in a drug treatment program (See also Sec. 3.2.1). Screening for sexually transmitted disease is discussed in Sec. 3.6.

IMMUNIZATIONS

The clinician needs to review the adolescent's immunization status and consider whether the patient has completed his or her primary series of general immunizations (see Sec. 1.5). Adolescents should receive a bivalent Td vaccine 10 years after their previous DTP vaccination. All adolescents should receive a trivalent MMR vaccine unless there is documentation of two MMR vaccinations earlier in childhood. An MMR should not be given to an adolescent who is pregnant. All adolescents should receive vaccination against hepatitis B.

PREVENTION

Over the past decade a series of recommendations have been developed and modified (Guidelines for Adolescent Preventive Services, Bright Futures, Guidelines for Health Supervision) for preventive services and screening during adolescence. These recommendations include guidelines to assist the clinician in providing preventive services to adolescents. In Table 3-9, the recommendations from the three groups are highlighted. Many of the recommendations focus on health-promoting and health-damaging behaviors initiated during early adolescence. Sexual behavior, substance use, and vehicle use are often initiated during adolescence

TABLE 3-9

RECOMMENDATIONS FOR ADOLESCENT PREVENTIVE HEALTH CARE

AGE	11 YR	12 YR	13 YR	14 YR	15 YR	16 YR	17 YR	18 YR	19 YR	20 YR	21 YR
History (initial/interval)	●	●	●	●	●	●	●	●	●	●	●
Measurements											
Height and weight	●	●	●	●	●	●	●	●	●	●	●
Blood pressure	●	●	●	●	●	●	●	●	●	●	●
Sensory screening											
Vision	S	O	S	S	O	S	S	O	S	S	S
Hearing	S	O	S	S	O	S	S	O	S	S	S
Developmental/behavioral assessment[1]	●	●	●	●	●	●	●	●	●	●	●
Physical examination[2]	●	●	●	●	●	●	●	●	●	●	●
Procedures—general[3]											
Immunization[4]	●	●	●	●	●	●	●	●	●	●	●
Hematocrit or hemoglobin[5]	←————————————— ● —————————————————————————————→										
Urinalysis	←————————————————————————— ●[6] ——————————————→										
Procedures—patients at risk											
Tuberculin test[7]	★	★	★	★	★	★	★	★	★	★	★
Cholesterol screening[8]	★	★	★	★	★	★	★	★	★	★	★
STD screening[9]	★	★	★	★	★	★	★	★	★	★	★
Pelvic exam[10]	★	★	★	★	★	★	★	★	★	★	★
Anticipatory guidance	●	●	●	●	●	●	●	●	●	●	●
Injury prevention	●	●	●	●	●	●	●	●	●	●	●
Violence prevention	●	●	●	●	●	●	●	●	●	●	●
Nutrition counseling	●	●	●	●	●	●	●	●	●	●	●

1. By history and appropriate physical examination: if suspicious, by specific objective developmental testing. Parenting skills should be fostered at every visit.
2. At each visit, a complete physical examination is essential, with adolescent undressed and suitably draped.
3. These may be modified, depending on entry point into schedule and individual need.
4. Schedule(s) per the Committee on Infectious Diseases, published annually in the January edition of *Pediatrics*. Every visit should be an opportunity to update and complete an adolescent's immunizations.
5. All menstruating adolescents should be considered for screening.
6. Conduct dipstick urinalysis for leukocytes annually for sexually active male and female adolescents.
7. TB testing per recommendations of the Committee on Infectious Diseases, published in the current edition of *Red Book: Report of the Committee on Infectious Diseases*. Testing should be done on recognition of high-risk factors.
8. Cholesterol screening for at-risk adolescents.
9. All sexually active adolescents should be screened for sexually transmitted diseases (STDs).
10. All sexually active girls should have a pelvic examination.

Key:
● = to be performed
S = subjective
←——— ● ———→ = the range during which a service may be provided, with the dot indicating the preferred age.
★ = to be performed for patients at risk
O = objective, by a standard testing method
SOURCE: *American Academy of Pediatrics (AAP): Recommendations for Preventive Pediatric Health Care. Pediatrics 105:645, 2000.*

and continue to account for the major causes of morbidity and mortality through the fourth decade of life. Because intention to engage in a behavior is one of the most powerful predictors of initiation of a behavior, simple questions regarding intention need to become a routine part of each clinical encounter beginning in late childhood. The identification of one risk behavior should alert the clinician to inquire about other risk behaviors. In addition, the clinician needs to query every adolescent about depressive symptomatology, eating behaviors, school functioning, and family interaction.

References

American Academy of Pediatrics: Guidelines for Health Supervision. Elk Grove Village, IL, American Academy of Pediatrics, 1997

The Adolescent Visit: History, Physical Assessment

American Academy of Pediatrics: Recommendations for preventive pediatric health care. Pediatrics 105:645, 2000

Elster AB, Kuznets NJ: AMA Guidelines for Adolescent Preventive Services (GAPS): Recommendations and Rationale. Baltimore: Williams & Wilkins, 1993

English A: Treating adolescents: Legal and ethical considerations. Med Clin North Am 74:1097–1112, 1990

Ford CA, Millstein SG, Halpern-Felsher BL, Irwin CE Jr: Influence of physician confidentiality assurances on adolescents' willingness to disclose information and seek future health care: a controlled clinical trial. JAMA 278:1029–1034, 1997

Green M, Palfrey JS, eds: Bright Futures, 2nd ed. Arlington, VA: National Center for Education in Maternal and Child Health 2000

Irwin CE JR, Igra V: Risk and risk-taking in adolescents. In: Lindstrom B, Spencer N, eds Social Pediatrics. New York, Oxford University Press, 1995, 225–258

Millstein SG, Petersen AC, Nightingale EO: Promoting the health of adolescents. New York, Oxford University Press, 1993

Neinstein LS: Adolescent Health Care: A Practical Guide, 3rd ed. Baltimore, Williams & Wilkins, 1996

Sigman G, Silber TJ, English A, Epner JE: Confidential health care for adolescents: a position paper of the Society for Adolescent Medicine. Adolesc Health 21:408–415, 1997

US Preventive Services Task Force: Guide to Clinical Preventive Services, 2nd ed. Alexandria, VA, International Medical Publishers, 1996

3.4 REPRODUCTIVE HEALTH IN THE ADOLESCENT

Mary-Ann Shafer and Anna-Barbara Moscicki

Comprehension of normal reproductive physiological development in the adolescent permits the identification of pathologic conditions that deviate from the predictable sequence of hormonal, anatomic, and histologic changes of puberty.

A comprehensive overview of the hypothalamic-pituitary-gonadal axis with the associated hormonal changes of puberty is presented in Sec. 24.8. This section focuses on the anatomic and histologic changes in the major reproductive organs of female and male adolescents during puberty with specific reference to hormonal influences.

3.4.1 Reproductive Growth and Development in the Female Adolescent

Anna-Barbara Moscicki

BREAST

Major breast changes occur during two stages of reproductive development: puberty and pregnancy. The onset of breast development or thelarche heralds both anatomic and histologic changes in the breast. Estrogen is the most influential hormone affecting breast development during puberty. It binds to breast tissue, resulting in stimulation of growth of the glandular ductal system, whereas progesterone is linked to alveolar growth. Other hormones, including insulin, growth hormone, thyroxine, prolactin, cortisol, and their interactions with estrogen, also play important roles in pubertal breast development. For example, estrogen requires the presence of insulin to stimulate epithelial growth and of growth hormone to affect ductal proliferation.

DEVELOPMENTAL ANATOMY AND HISTOLOGY There are four stages of breast development during the life cycle: prepuberty (atrophic ducts); puberty (lobuloalveolar and ductal growth); lactation (milk secretion); and finally, senescence (regression to atrophic ducts). The first histologic changes at the onset of pubertal breast development consist of proliferation of ductal and stromal tissue and fat deposition resulting in increased volume and the visible "breast bud." Lobuloalveolar growth during puberty is influenced by estrogen, progesterone, prolactin, growth hormone, and adrenal steroids. Ductal growth is primarily influenced by estrogen, growth hormone, and adrenal steroids. Maturation to the stage of lactation is mainly stimulated by prolactin and adrenal steroids. The rate of growth and size of the breasts may differ, but major inequities usually disappear with maturity. Abnormalities in development and breast masses are described in Sec. 3.5.1.

VAGINA

The vaginal epithelium is very sensitive to hormonal influence. Sequential changes occur throughout a life cycle, including birth, childhood, puberty, menstrual cycles, pregnancy, and finally menopause.

DEVELOPMENTAL ANATOMY AND HISTOLOGY The embryonic development of the female reproductive tract is outlined in Fig. 3-2. At birth, the vagina is 4 cm long, lengthens approximately 1 cm during early childhood and 8 cm during late childhood, and reaches mature length of 10 to 12 cm by menarche. The vagina at birth resembles the mature vagina with its deep cryptic rugae and folds secondary to maternal estrogenic effect. As maternal estrogen levels fall in the infant within the first few weeks after birth, the vaginal wall becomes dry, thin, nonelastic, and nonrugated. The vagina remains in this quiescent state until the onset of puberty. During early puberty, increased estrogen levels affect the vaginal epithelia. Such pubertal changes can be noted on examination by identification of the more mature dull pink color of the vaginal mucosa, increased vaginal secretions, and increased vaginal wall flexibility compared with the prepubertal findings of the red translucent mucosa, sparse secretions, and a relatively rigid vaginal wall.

The distal third of the vagina is one of the first sites to be affected by estrogen during puberty. The vaginal epithelium is made of four different cell layers: basal (a single layer of cuboidal cells juxtaposed on the basement membrane), parabasal (several layers of polyhedral-shaped cells with distinct nuclei), intermediate (larger, flatter nucleated cells), and superficial (several layers of large, flat cells with pyknotic nuclei). The histology of the infant shows vaginal epithelium with a predominance of basal cells. In early childhood, the epithelium is two to eight layers thick and consists of a definitive basal layer and parabasilar intermediate cells. With the small increases of estrogen in late childhood, the intermediate cell layer proliferates, and the superficial cells undergo maturation. In the middle of puberty, the rise in estrogens results in the cornification of the epithelium and development of a tissue layer 65 to 85 cells thick, which consists of predominantly mature squamous superficial cells. Up to 12 months before menarche, an increase in vaginal secretions may be noted, resulting from desquamated superficial and intermediate cells and mucoid secretions from maturing cervical and vestibular glands.

After birth, the neonatal vagina is temporarily colonized with lactobacilli that produce lactic acid, resulting in an acidic milieu. Within several weeks after birth, the microbiological vaginal flora changes and becomes predominantly colonized with enterococci and diphtheroids, and the pH becomes alkaline. This environment persists through childhood until puberty, when lactobacilli reappear in greater concentrations and again produce an acidic vaginal milieu. More specifically, colonization with H_2O_2-producing lactobacilli seems to be important for vaginal microbiological health. With the maturation of the vagina after menarche, cyclic changes in the vaginal histology occur with the menstrual cycle. Vaginal cytology (Papanicolaou smears) can be helpful in evaluating the estrogen effect. The estrogen-induced vaginal changes provide a primary barrier to local trauma and infection. Another protective barrier to infection is the acidic pH of the mature vagina (4.5 to 5.5). Cyclic changes linked to both estrogen and progesterone are not completed until the ovarian cycle matures with establishment of monthly cycles 1 to 2 years postmenarche.

UTERINE CERVIX

The growth and maturation of the cervix result from the effects of estrogen stimulation.

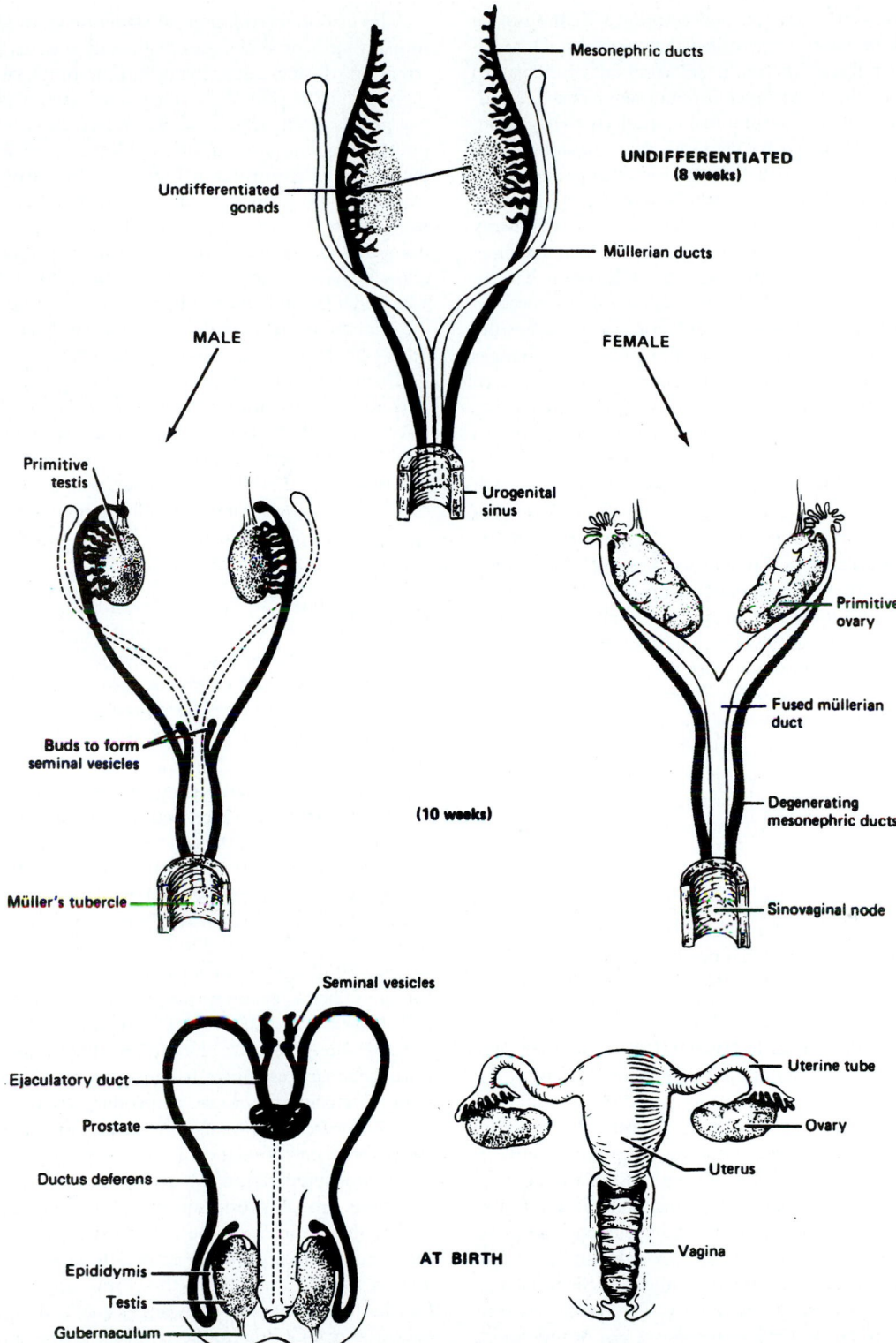

FIGURE 3-2   Transformation of the undifferentiated genital system into the definitive male and female systems. SOURCE: *Embryology of the Genitourinary System. Tanagho EA, McAnich JW, eds: Smith's General Urology, Appleton & Lange, Norwalk, CT 1988, 20.*

DEVELOPMENTAL ANATOMY AND HISTOLOGY In infancy and early childhood, the cervix appears as a two-dimensional structure. The cervical os presents as a narrow slit in the posterior vaginal wall. With puberty, the cervix enlarges to a three-dimensional knob-like structure that protrudes from the posterior vaginal wall. The nul-

liparous os is usually small, round in shape, and readily seen. During embryonic development, the cervix and vagina are initially lined with müllerian-type columnar cells, which are replaced by squamous epithelium from urogenital cells during fetal development. This replacement is usually incomplete, and an area of columnar cells remains on the ectocervix (termed ectopy) with the border between the two different epithelia called the original squamocolumnar junction. At puberty, the acidic environment of the vagina and other hormonal influences trigger developmental changes leading to further replacement of the columnar epithelia with squamous epithelia. This process of change is called squamous metaplasia, and the area of change is referred to as the transformation zone.

Adolescents, in general, have greater areas of ectopy (and active transformation zones) than adult women. The areas of immaturity appear to be particularly vulnerable to sexually transmitted infections (STI) including human papillomavirus, *Chlamydia trachomatis*, and *Neisseria gonorhoeae*. It has been shown that most cervical neoplasias arise within the transformation zone, suggesting that this area is particularly vulnerable to the pathologic changes associated with human papillomavirus infections (ie, cervical neoplasia). Therefore, adolescents with large areas of active metaplasia may be at increased risk for the development of neoplasia when exposed to human papillomavirus and other carcinogens. *Chlamydia trachomatis* and *N. gonorrhoeae* are also known to attach preferentially to columnar cells, which may be one of the factors associated with the epidemic rates of these STIs among female adolescents. Changes in the cervical mucus itself parallel those in epithelial cells during puberty. Premenarchial mucus is characteristically low in volume, viscous, and sticky and is characteristically alkaline. Just before menarche, the cervical mucus may become copious, and as the estrogen level increases further, the mucus becomes elastic, translucent, and capable of producing a fern pattern on a glass slide. Such characteristics of the mucus can be used to measure estrogen stimulation. Recent studies have shown the importance of immunoglobulin and cytokine secretions in providing protection for vaginal cervical epithelium. Disorders of immune function are commonly associated with increased rates of STIs.

UTERUS

Estrogen is the main stimulus for the remarkable growth of the uterus in both volume and weight that occurs during puberty, with the uterus increasing over 30-fold in volume.

DEVELOPMENTAL ANATOMY AND HISTOLOGY The embryonic development of the uterus is outlined in Fig. 3-2. At infancy, the uterus measures approximately 2.5 cm long and 1 cm wide and remains in this latent stage until about age 7 years. At this time, uterine growth resumes at an accelerated rate that peaks between ages 10 and 13 years. During childhood the ratio of the body of the uterus to the cervix is less than 1:1; at menarche it is 1:1; and the postmenarcheal ratio is 3:1. Histologically, the endometrium changes little until puberty. From infancy through childhood, the endometrium consists of a thin layer of low cuboidal cells and sparse stroma with no evidence of secretory activity. The rise of estrogen at the beginning of puberty stimulates endometrial proliferation. Adequate rhythmic stimuli from the hypothalamic-pituitary-gonadal axis results in physiological rises and falls in estrogen. A sudden fall of estrogen in an estrogen-primed uterus will result in withdrawal bleed; menarche may occur even without ovulation (see Sec. 24.8). The mean age of menarche in the United States is currently 12.8 years for white adolescents and slightly lower, 12.6 years, for black adolescents, with a normal range from 9 to 16 years. Anovulatory bleeds or "breakthrough" bleeds associated with a proliferative endometrium are common within the first 4 years after menarche.

The elaborate endometrial structure undergoes dramatic hormonally influenced changes that result in either pregnancy or menstruation during each hypothalamic-pituitary-ovarian–mediated menstrual cycle (Fig. 3-3). These endometrial changes include the five phases: proliferation, secretion (secretory phase), implantation preparation, endometrial breakdown, and menstruation. The proliferation phase is primarily influenced by estrogen, runs parallel to ovarian follicle growth, results in the endometrial lining increasing from about 0.5 mm to 3.5 to 5.0 mm in height, and causes endometrial glands to become tortuous and dilated. The secretory phase is characterized by further maturation of the endometrial tissues under the influence of both estrogen and progesterone, which includes progressive tortuosity of the glands and coiling of the spiral arteries with no increase in endometrial height.

During the implantation preparation phase, from the 8th to the 14th day postovulation, the endometrium develops into three distinct layers: the basal layer, the stratum spongiosum, and a superficial layer. The corpus luteum reaches its maximal activity during this time (day 22). When implantation does not take place, the corpus luteum deteriorates, resulting in rapidly decreasing levels of estrogen and progesterone, which leads to the breakdown of the endometrium and menses.

OVARY

Ovarian growth is stimulated in large part by follicle-stimulating hormone (FSH) and luteinizing hormone (LH). The ovaries themselves produce hormones for reproductive growth including estrogen and progesterone.

ANATOMY AND HISTOLOGY The ovary weighs 1 g at birth and 6 g by menarche. Located within the abdomen during their embryonic development, the ovaries descend into the true pelvic cavity with early puberty. At birth, the development of the oocytes and the primordial follicles is complete. The oocytes peak in numbers at the fifth fetal month with about 6 million oocytes present. By puberty, approximately 300,000 remain intact. For every mature follicle, 1000 have aborted during the maturation process. Maturing follicles become progressively larger before menarche and account for the rise in estrogen levels (Fig. 3-3). The follicles then begin to mature to the point required to produce adequate estrogen to promote menarche. At the critical level of estrogen necessary to produce an LH surge, the ovarian follicle matures, and ovulation ensues. Ten to 12 days of preovulatory estrogen stimulation is needed to trigger the maturation of a follicle in preparation for ovulation. Ovulation, or expulsion of the ovum, probably results from a proteolytic enzyme acting locally to free the ovum from the encapsulated follicle. After ovulation, the disrupted ovarian tissue returns to normal, and changes occur leading to the formation of the corpus luteum from the ruptured follicle. If implantation does not occur, and human chorionic gonadotropin (hCG) is not secreted by a conceptus, the corpus luteum rapidly recedes. Figure 3-3 shows the sequence of development of the primary follicle and its transformation into a corpus luteum during an ovarian cycle.

OVARIAN HORMONAL CYCLE AND PHYSIOLOGY Complete maturation of the ovarian follicle requires FSH, estradiol, and LH. The main role of FSH in women is to stimulate follicular maturation and acquisition of follicular FSH and LH receptors. In women, LH stimulates production of ovarian estrogen, progesterone, and androgens and induces luteinization. In addition to the presence

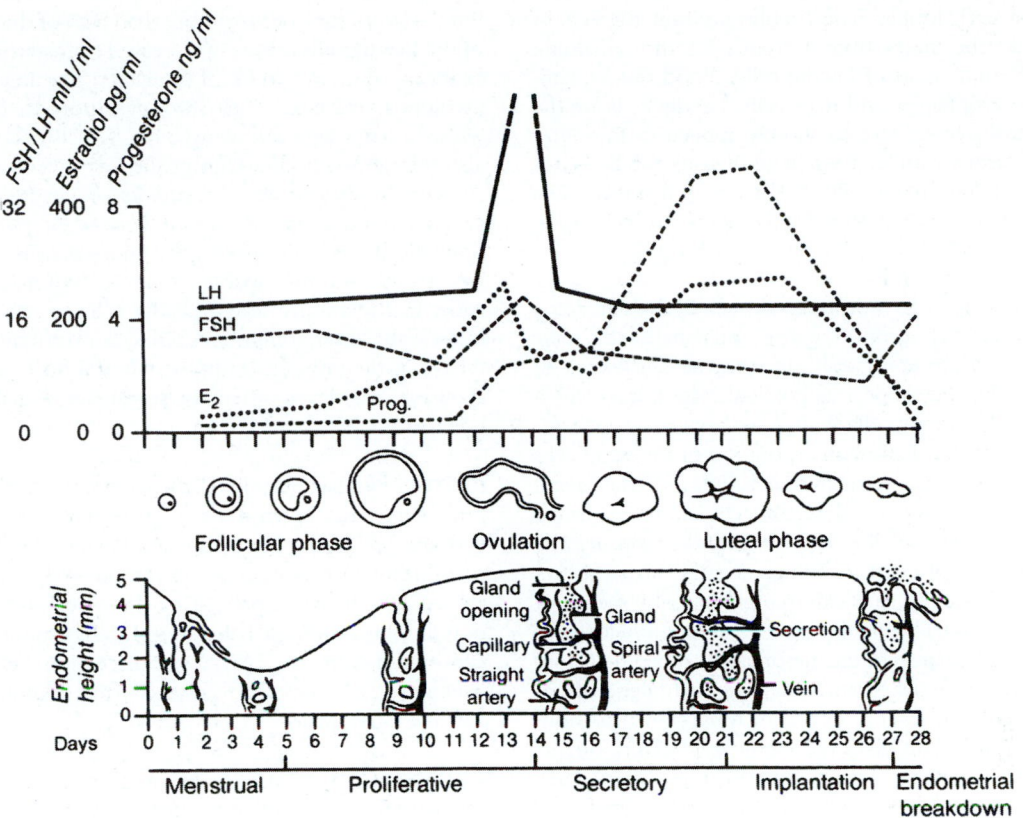

FIGURE 3-3   The menstrual cycle. Cyclic changes are outlined. LH, FSH, E$_2$, and progesterone (Prog.); follicle development to ovulation; formation of the corpus luteum; and endometrial development. SOURCE: *Speroff L, Glass RH, Kase NG, eds: Clinical Gynecologic Endocrinology and Infertility. Baltimore, Williams & Wilkins, 1989, 220; Moscicki AB, Shafer MA: Normal reproductive development in the adolescent female. J Adolesc Health Care 7(6):41S–64S, 1986.*

of the gonadotropins LH and FSH, the actual sequence of hormonal stimulation may be critical to follicle development. For example, FSH appears to stimulate initial follicle growth, resulting in estrogen production. The subsequent FSH–estrogen interaction induces further maturation and the development of LH receptors. The binding of LH to these receptors promotes progesterone secretion and complete maturation of the follicle. The midcycle LH surge appears to be responsible for ovulation (Fig. 3-3). Estradiol is the main product of the ovarian follicular granulosa cells, whereas progesterone is the main product of the corpus luteal granulosa cells.

The complex hormonal secretion by the ovarian follicle in the mature ovary is reviewed briefly. Rises in FSH levels stimulate follicular estradiol production, which in turn further stimulates follicular growth and production of progressively higher levels of estrogen. The increase in both FSH and estrogen levels promotes development of LH receptors on follicular cells and induces the limited but important production of progesterone. The pituitary detects the increasing estradiol amount and at a critical level releases a surge of LH. The FSH negative feedback appears to be more sensitive than LH secretion, resulting in a decrease of FSH immediately before ovulation. The rupture of the follicle and formation of the corpus luteum occurs approximately 16 to 24 hours after LH reaches its peak. Estradiol levels then drop and progesterone levels increase. It appears that the rupture of the follicle is the actual trigger for luteinization. During this luteal phase, progesterone levels increase with a concurrent smaller increase in estradiol and es-

trone levels. Responding to the rising estrogen and progesterone, the LH and FSH levels begin to fall. The FSH levels begin to rise just before menstruation to induce follicular growth for the subsequent cycle.

3.4.2   Reproductive Growth and Development in the Male Adolescent

Mary-Ann Shafer

TESTIS

Testicular growth and maturation are influenced in large part by testosterone, which is produced by the testicle both before and after birth. Testosterone production is regulated centrally by the hypothalamic-pituitary-testicular axis as well as intragonadally. The effects of testosterone include embryologic male genital differentiation, maturation of the internal and external male genitalia at puberty, skeletal muscle growth, deepening of the voice from laryngeal growth, epiphyseal cartilage growth during puberty, male hair growth and distribution, erythropoiesis, stimulation of sebaceous glands, and male social behavior.

DEVELOPMENTAL ANATOMY AND HISTOLOGY   The adult testicle is ovoid in shape, with an average length of 4.6 cm (range 3.6–5.5 cm) and width of 2.6 cm (range 2.1–3.2 cm). Each testis is divided into 250 lobules by fibrous septae, with one to four seminiferous tubules in each lobule. The tubules account for 90% of testicular mass, and the interstitium accounts for the remaining 10%. The interstitium consists of Leydig cells, blood vessels, lymphatic channels, macrophages, and mast cells. Leydig cells are the major source of testosterone and are closely applied to the outer wall of the seminiferous tubule. Each seminiferous tubule is approximately 60 cm in length and 150 to 175 μm in diameter. The tubule is the site of spermatogenesis and contains two cell types, Sertoli cells and germ cells.

GONADAL DIFFERENTIATION Although the sex of the embryo is genetically determined at conception, the potential male and female gonads do not differ morphologically until the seventh week of development. Initially, they appear as gonadal ridges, into which migrate the primordial germ cells in the sixth week of growth. Primitive sex cords develop before incorporation of the germ cells and are the progenitors of the seminiferous tubules. By the fourth month, the primitive germ cells and Sertoli cells can be identified in the tubules (Fig. 3-4). Leydig cells are abundant during the fourth to sixth month and assist in influencing the sexual differentiation of the genital ducts and external genitalia by means of testosterone production. The fetal testes produce inducer substances, which promote growth of the mesonephric or wolffian duct and inhibit development of the paramesonephric or müllerian duct. The mesonephric duct persists (except for the most cranial portion, the appendix epididymis) and gives rise to the epididymis, ductus deferens, and seminal vesicle. The paramesonephric duct completely degenerates except for a small portion at the cranial end, which persists as the appendix testis. Descent of the testes from their abdominal origin to their final location in the scrotal sac begins in the seventh or eighth month and is typically complete shortly before birth but is sometimes completed postnatally. From birth until puberty, the testis remains rather static, although histologic and ultrastructural changes do occur, as outlined below. The prepubertal testis demonstrates tubules of small diameter and is populated by two cell types, progenitors of Sertoli cells and primary spermatogenic cells.

LEYDIG CELLS Leydig cells are situated between the testicular cords and can first be recognized during the eighth week of gestation. They differentiate, multiply, and increase in size from weeks 9 to 14, until they occupy more than 50% of the testicle. Activation of the Leydig cells results in increased testosterone secretion, which peaks at about week 14 of fetal life. The Leydig cells gradually involute after weeks 17 to 18 of gestation. Involution is complete within a few weeks following birth. Levels of free testosterone are also thought to decline during the first several months after birth. At 4 to 8 years of age, precursors of Leydig cells reappear and can be found grouped around vessels. At puberty, Leydig cells dramatically increase in number and size. They become well differentiated and are capable of steroid synthesis, mainly testosterone. In the mature testis, Leydig cells are closely applied to the outer walls of seminiferous tubules, are the major source of testosterone in the pubertal and postpubertal male, and thereby are responsible for development of secondary sexual characteristics of puberty.

SERTOLI CELLS Sertoli cells first appear in the fetal testis at approximately the seventh week of gestation and quickly associate with the developing germ cells (gonocytes). They play an important role during spermatogenesis in the postpubertal testis by forming an occlusive barrier representing the blood–testis barrier. In addition to their histologic roles, Sertoli cells produce estrogen, androgen-binding protein (ABP, see discussion below), and inhibin, which are all essential to germ cell maturation, and phagocytize damaged germ cells.

SEMINIFEROUS TUBULES As mentioned above, primordial germ cells invade the primitive sex cords during the sixth week of gestation. They continue to divide and are known as gonocytes. The number of germ cells in the cords increases up to the 17th week with marked mitotic activity. By week 20, however, mitoses cease. At birth, the seminiferous tubules appear as solid cords, with cellular debris (degenerated spermatogonia) in the potential lumen. The primary germ cells in the neonatal testis are the gonocytes, which transform to the reserve stem cells and spermatogonia by age 6 months. Spermatogonia evolve into primary spermatocytes at 3 years of age, with no further progression until puberty. Such early transformations involve mitosis only, with meiotic transformation beginning only with puberty.

During childhood, the tubules become long and sinuous, with no increase in diameter. At puberty, the tubules begin to increase

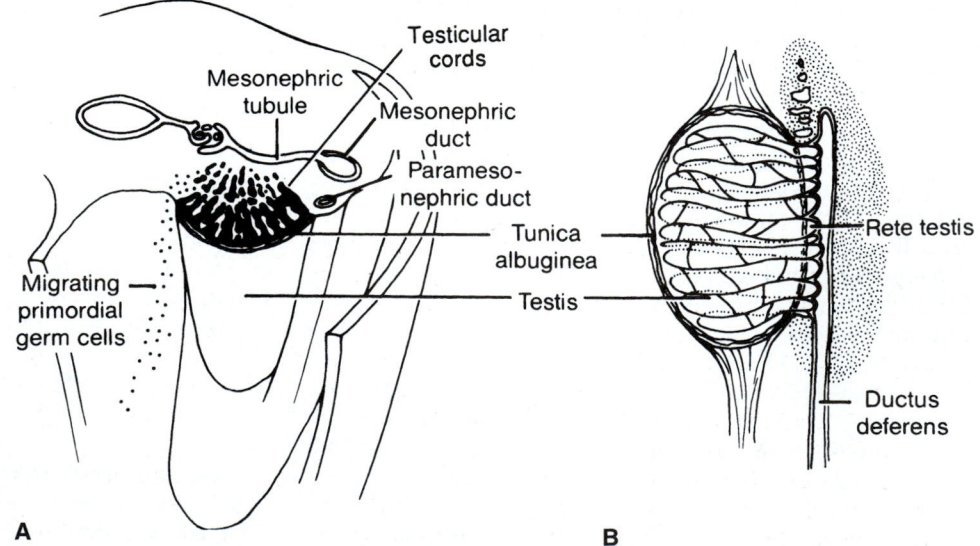

FIGURE 3-4 Fetal testicular development. A: Transverse section through the lumbar section of a 6-week embryo. Note the primordial germ cells migrating to the primitive sex cords of the indifferent gonad. B: Testis and evolving ductus deferens in the fourth month of development. SOURCE: *Langman J: Medical Embryology, Baltimore, Williams & Wilkins, 1981.*

in diameter, doubling from an average of 72 μm in the prepubertal child to that of 150 μm in the adult, resulting in the development of a lumen. In addition, cellular differentiation of the spermatogonia can be seen, and meiotic processes begin to yield true spermatogenesis. In the mature testis, the tubules are distinguished by their large cell diameter, a thin but identifiable basement membrane, a tubular wall two to three cell layers thick, and complete spermatogenic activity from basal spermatogonium, primary spermatocyte, secondary spermatocyte, and spermatid to terminal spermatozoa.

HYPOTHALAMIC-PITUITARY-TESTICULAR AXIS   To comprehend spermatogenesis fully, knowledge of the hypothalamic-pituitary-testicular axis is necessary (see Sec. 24.8). Spermatogenesis is also influenced by local hormonal control within the testicle itself. The LH produced by the pituitary binds to receptors on the Leydig cells and, by means of cyclic AMP, induces the synthesis of testosterone. Testosterone then follows one of three paths: absorption by venous channels in the testicle and subsequent systemic distribution; diffusion locally in the interstitial tissue of the testicle and into the seminiferous tubule; or binding to Sertoli cells, resulting in stimulation of the cell to produce androgen binding protein (ABP) and other proteins vital to spermatogenesis. Testosterone binds with ABP and is transported in the seminal tubule and duct system. This bound testosterone maintains the androgen milieu of the seminiferous tubule.

Control of the hypothalamic-pituitary–Leydig cells axis depends on a negative feedback system. The control mechanism results in a rather constant level of testosterone, although minute-to-minute oscillations and a circadian rhythm exist with higher levels on waking in the morning. Testosterone released into the general circulation exerts a negative feedback on the anterior pituitary to decrease LH production, although some impact on the hypothalamus may also be present.

Follicle-stimulating hormone also plays an important role in testicular function. This tropin stimulates Leydig cells to increase the number of LH receptors. In addition, FSH stimulates the Sertoli cell to produce ABP as well as inhibin. Inhibin in turn exerts a negative feedback effect on the anterior pituitary. An outline of the hormonal control of the hypothalamic-pituitary-testicular axis is presented in Fig. 3-5.

SPERMATOGENESIS

The process of spermatogenesis can be histologically identified between ages 11 and 15 years with a mean age of spermaturia of 13.3 years. As noted above, mature seminiferous tubules are lined by spermatogonia, which undergo mitotic division to give rise to primary spermatocytes. Subsequently, these cells mature and undergo meiosis so that the resultant secondary spermatocyte contains 23 chromosomes. These haploid cells then evolve into spermatids and spermatozoa. The cells are arranged in an orderly sequence in the tubule, according to their developmental stage. The complete cycle includes six stages and requires 74 days for completion, and 45 to 205 million sperm are produced by the testes each day.

Both FSH and testosterone are required for the initiation of spermatogenesis. Once spermatogenesis has started, however, testosterone alone is sufficient to maintain the process. In the normal man, LH acts on the Leydig cells to produce testosterone, which in turn acts directly on the tubule to promote spermatogenesis,

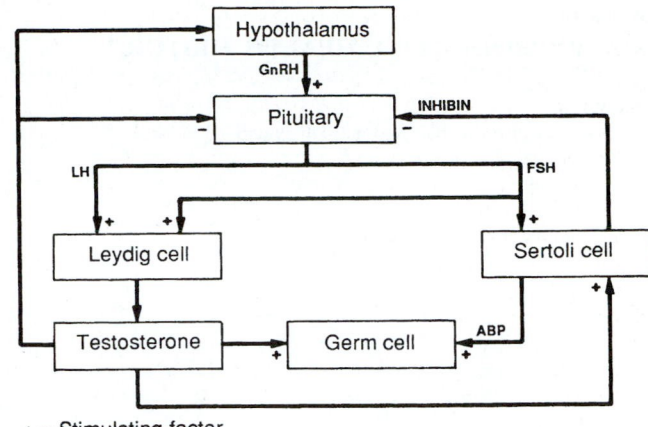

+ = Stimulating factor
− = Inhibiting factor

FIGURE 3-5   The hypothalamic-pituitary-testicular axis. SOURCE: *Fitzgerald PA, ed: Handbook of Clinical Endocrinology, 2nd ed. Norwalk, CT, Appleton & Lange, 1992, 354.*

whereas FSH acts on the Sertoli cells as outlined above. A negative feedback loop exists to prevent overstimulation of the tubules. Although testosterone and estradiol can inhibit the anterior pituitary's production of FSH, inhibin produced by the Sertoli cell has the major inhibitory role.

The onset of spermatogenesis ("spermarche") corresponds with a time of rapid increase in testicular weight as well as increases in tubular diameter, length, and relative volume. In addition, the onset of activity is more closely related to the pubertal development of the individual than to age and is progressive in nature. It occurs early in puberty and corresponds to a mean pubic hair stage of Tanner 2.5. Mean age of first reported ejaculation is 13.5 years. Apparently fertility in young males may be possible when the only sign of pubertal maturation is testicular enlargement greater than 3 cm.

MALE URETHRA

The embryologic development of the male urogenital system including the urethra is outlined in Fig. 3-2. Little data are available on the normal microflora of the adolescent male urethra. However, among adolescent males with no symptoms or signs (no pyuria in the first-voided urine specimen) of urethritis, there was a difference noted in the flora between never sexually active males and those who were sexually experienced. *Mycoplasma* species and *Ureaplasma urealyticum* were isolated only from the sexually experienced young men.

3.4.3   Clinical Assessment of Reproductive Health in the Adolescent

Anna-Barbara Moscicki

REPRODUCTIVE HEALTH HISTORY

Obtaining a sexual history is an essential component of routine adolescent health care. Discussing sexuality is valuable for adolescents who have questions about their own "normality" or who are contemplating initiating sexual activity. When discussing sexuality with the adolescent, the pediatrician needs to remain nonjudgmental and sensitive to the needs of the patient. Confidentiality en-

TABLE 3-10
MALE REPRODUCTIVE HEALTH HISTORY

Puberty
Age of onset of pubic hair and genital growth
Spontaneous ejaculation
Masturbation
Foreskin status—hygiene
Genital-urinary system problem
History of congenital anomalies
History of mumps
History of trauma
Scrotal mass, ± pain
Genitourinary surgery
Problem with erections
Sexual activity
Age of sexual debut
Sexual orientation
Frequency of coitus
Number of sexual partners
Sexual practices
History of sexual abuse
History of prostitution
Contraceptive history
Present method(s): main, other partner
Methods utilized in past
Problems: current or past methods
STD history
Current symptoms (urethritis, prostatitis, proctitis)
Type, in past
Treatment, self and partner
Associated risk behavior
Drug use before and during sex by type, amount
Partner history
Partner(s) STD symptoms
Contraceptive and drug history (IV, other)

---

courages honest and productive discussion. The language used with the adolescent must be unambiguous and appropriate to the patient's cognitive level and social experience. A suggested format for the reproductive health history for male and female adolescents is included in Tables 3-10 and 3-11.

For male adolescents, questions addressing the patient's concerns over the normality of his genital development, masturbation, and onset of spontaneous ejaculation can initiate discussion of symptoms and signs of urethritis, pregnancy prevention, STD prevention, and proper use of contraception, especially condoms.

For female adolescents, questions about menses are an excellent tool to initiate a discussion about sexuality. It is imperative to determine the date and normality of the last menses in a confidential setting. Although spotting or irregular menses are common within 2 years of menarche, this may reflect either pregnancy or a sexually transmitted infection (STI). Pregnant patients may report lighter than usual "periods" during their first trimester. Unusual cramping or intermenstrual bleeding may be associated with an STI.

Querying about dysmenorrhea provides several possible benefits to the adolescent. Many female adolescents believe that severe dysmenorrhea is "normal," when in fact medical intervention is indicated. In addition, dysmenorrhea may be a symptom of an underlying problem, such as an STD or endometriosis. A more detailed reproductive sexual health history by reproductive organ anatomic site is outlined in Table 3-11.

The physician needs to know what forms of sexual behavior other than vaginal intercourse are being anticipated or experienced by the adolescent to determine the full range of STDs and sites of infection for which the patient is at risk. Questions regarding age at sexual debut, number of partners, frequency of intercourse, use of condoms and other contraceptives, and sexual practices are vital in assessing the patient's STD risk. Information regarding drug use in the patient and the patient's partner is an important indicator of risk for STIs, including human immunodeficiency virus (HIV) infection, and alerts the clinician to risky sexual behaviors (poor decision making, inability to use condoms, etc.) when drugs are used before or during vaginal or anal intercourse. Such information forms a basis to focus counseling on risk behavior reduction.

Inquiry about same-sex behavior should be routinely obtained. Such activity may represent early adolescent exploration or may be indicative of an evolving homosexual identity.

REPRODUCTIVE HEALTH EXAMINATION OF THE MALE ADOLESCENT

Examination of the genitalia can be an uncomfortable process for the patient as well as the physician. The examination is necessary to assess sexual maturity, teach normality to the adolescent, and detect existing pathology. While respecting the patient's privacy, the physician must inform the patient that genital examination is as vital a part of physical assessment as is cardiac examination. The patient should be standing, attired in a gown, and without undergarments. Examination begins by inspecting the size and shape of the penis, circumcision status, the color and texture of penile and scrotal skin, and distribution and quality of the pubic hair to evaluate sexual maturity. Measurement of testicular size is sometimes necessary to accomplish this. For a full description of the sexual maturity scale, see Sec. 24.8. The penis should be inspected for ulcers, scars, papilloma, excoriations, or nodules. If the patient is not circumcised, the foreskin should be fully retracted, although this may not be possible until pubertal maturation is complete. The urethral meatus is assessed by compressing the glans between the thumb and forefinger to open the meatus, thereby allowing the physician to visualize the presence of erythema, discharge, papilloma, or adhesions.

The scrotum and testes are inspected for any masses, swelling, or signs of inflammation. Bilateral descent of the testes is confirmed by palpation, and the size and consistency of the testes, epididymis, and spermatic cords are assessed. Intrascrotal masses need to be transilluminated; a red glow indicates a fluid mass, probably a hydrocele. The inguinal ring must be assessed for presence of hernia by palpation of the ring while the subject is standing and performing a Valsava maneuver (eg, coughing). The common reproductive health problems of the male adolescent are discussed below, including gynecomastia, scrotal masses, contraception, and sexually transmitted diseases.

REPRODUCTIVE HEALTH EXAMINATION OF THE FEMALE ADOLESCENT

The reproductive health examination for the female adolescent by anatomic site is outlined in Table 3-12. Common reproductive health problems in the female adolescent are discussed in Sec. 3.5.

TABLE 3-11
FEMALE REPRODUCTIVE HEALTH HISTORY

QUESTION/ FOCUS	BREAST	VULVA/VAGINA	CERVIX/UTERUS	TUBES/OVARIES
Normal development	Thelarche (age of onset) Breast self-examination	Hygiene (frequency of washing, douching, avoidance of perfume/soaps, and douches) Physiological discharge Adrenarche (age of onset)	Physiological discharge Menarche Menstruation: duration, frequency, date of last period	Ovulation
Nonsexual-related problems	Delayed thelarche (> 14 yr) Mammary hyperplasia Mammary hypoplasia Tumors (nonmalignant) Tumors (malignant, including family history) Galactorrhea (hormones, tumors, drug induced) Rare congenital anomalies Atrophy Infection	Congenital anomalies Vulvovaginitis: (abnormal D/C, pain, itching; check history for irritants, douching, and poor hygiene) *Candida* (check for predisposing factors such as antibiotics, diabetes) Foreign bodies Systemic conditions: Crohn-related; dermatologic; infections (varicella, measles); and ulcers (eg, TB, amebiasis) DES exposure Tumors: carcinoma, sarcoma, vaginal polyps	Congenital anomalies Delayed menses > 16 yr: (associated with or without delayed thelarche and adrenarche) Dysmenorrhea Abnormal uterine bleeding (include frequency, duration, and intensity) Endometriosis Tumors (malignant and benign) Systemic causes of cervicitis/ endometritis (eg, SLE, TB, sarcoidosis, radiation) PCO (with or without hirsutism)	Tumors (benign and malignant) Adnexal torsion Mittelschmerz
Presexual activity[a]	As above Galactorrhea: self-stimulation	As above Discuss signs and symptoms of vaginitis, use of condoms, and importance of talking with sexual partners about symptoms and history of STD before the onset of sexual activity	As above Discuss signs and symptoms of cervicitis/endometritis, use of condoms when initiates sex Discuss need for annual pelvic exam[b]: Pap smears, cultures, and bimanual palpation	Preparation for pelvic examination Need for contraception Discuss signs and symptoms of PID and ectopic pregnancy
Sexual activity[a]–related problems	Galactorrhea: differential diagnosis includes pregnancy (LMP), sexual stimulation, lactational mastitis Trauma	STD-related vulvovaginal disease, ulcerative/nonulcerative lesions, bartholomitis or skenitis (pain), vaginitis (discharge, pain, burning) Foreign bodies Discuss protection with condoms Use of lubricant and reactions to lubricants Encourage sexual communication: partners	Abnormal discharge: (STD cause of cervicitis/PID) Unusual uterine bleeding: (PID/pregnancy) Discuss use of condoms and sexual communication	Pelvic/abdominal pain (PID, ectopic pregnancy) Pregnancy prevention: need for contraception; explore specific methods and contraindications LMP date

[a] Sexual history should include: LMP, sexual preference (male or female), sexual orientation (heterosexual, homosexual, or bisexual), and sexual behaviors that place adolescent at risk for STD (multiple partners, contraception, anal intercourse, drug use).
[b] Annual pelvic examinations should include *Chlamydia* and gonococcal cultures, Pap, and bimanual palpation.
D/C = discharge, TB = tuberculosis, DES = diethylstilbestrol, STD = sexually transmitted disease, SLE = systemic lupus erythematosus, PCO = polycystic ovaries, PID = pelvic inflammatory disease, LMP = last menstrual period.

References

General Puberty

Gupta D: Changes in the gonadal and adrenal steroid patterns during puberty. Clin Endocrinol Metab 4:27–46, 1975

Kaplan SL, Grumbach MM, Aubert MI: The ontogenesis of pituitary hormones and hypothalamic factors in the human fetus: Maturation of central nervous system regulation of anterior pituitary function. Recent Prog Horm Res 31:161–243, 1976

Penington GW: The reproductive endocrinology of childhood and adolescence. Clin Obstet Gynecol 1:509–531, 1974

Styne DM, Grumbach MM: Disorder of puberty in males and females. In: Yen SS, Jaffee RB, eds: Reproductive Endocrinology. Philadelphia, WB Saunders, 1991, 511–554

Female Reproductive Development

Crowley-Nowick PA, Bell M, Edwards RP, et al: Normal uterine cervix: Characterization of isolated lymphocyte phenotypes and immunoglobulin secretion. Am J Reprod Immunol 34:241–247, 1995

TABLE 3-12
FEMALE REPRODUCTIVE EXAMINATION BY ANATOMIC SITE

RELATED ANATOMY	BREAST	VULVA/VAGINA	CERVIX/UTERUS	FALLOPIAN TUBES/OVARIES	RECTAL
Normal	Visual and manual examination Define anatomy	Visual and manual examination Define anatomy Tanner stage	Pelvic examination Define anatomy Define cytology (Pap)	Pelvic examination Define anatomy	As indicated, not routine
Abnormal	Visual and manual examination Masses/tumors (mobility, tenderness, size, location) Galactorrhea Infection Hyperplasia Hypoplasia Nipple (anatomy, discharge) Trauma	Vulva Visual and manual examination Anatomy, imperforate hymen, clitoromegaly Infection[a] Trauma Vagina Visual and manual examination Anatomy: agenesis, septa Infection Foreign body Mass, tumor	Cervix Visual examination by speculum Anatomy: polyps, ectopy Infection: friable, mucopus,[a] cervical motion tenderness (bimanual)[a] Uterus Manual examination Presence Position Size/shape Masses, position Tenderness[a]	Tubes Manual examination Masses[a] Enlargement[a] Tenderness[a] Ovaries Manual examination Masses (torsion, cyst, abscess)[a] Tenderness[a]	Assist in evaluation of young presexually active adolescents and/or when vaginal exam not possible Vaginal cyst (hematocolpesis) Vaginal/rectal wall tumors Rectal—bimanual (presence or absence of normal anatomy) Define retroverted uterus, uterine and adnexal mass, endometriosis

[a] See STDs, Section 3.6.

Hatcher RA, Trussel J, Guest F, et al: Sexuality and reproductive health. In: Contraceptive Technology, 17th rev ed. New York, Ardent Media, 1998, 13–42.

Kieff E: Current perspectives on the molecular pathogenesis of virus-induced cancers in human immunodeficiency virus infection and acquired immunodeficiency syndrome. J Natl Cancer Inst Monogr 23:7–14, 1998

Kutteh WH, Moldoveanu Z, Mestecky J: Mucosal immunity in the female reproductive tract: Correlation of immunoglobulins, cytokines, and reproductive hormones in human cervical mucus around the time of ovulation. AIDS Res Hum Retroviruses 14 (Suppl):51–55, 1998

McNatty KP, Hunter WM, McNeilly AS, et al: Changes in the concentration of pituitary and steroid hormones in the follicular fluid of human graafian follicles throughout the menstrual cycle. J Endocrinol 64:555– 571, 1975

Mersels A, Morin C: Human papillomavirus and cancer of the uterine cervix. Gynecol Oncol 12:S111–S123, 1981

Moscicki AB, Grubbs-Burt V, Kanowitz S, et al: The significance of squamous metaplasia in the development of low grade squamous intraepithelial lesions in young women. Cancer 85:1139–1144, 1999

Moscicki AB, Shafer MA: Normal reproductive development in the adolescent female. J Adolesc Health Care 7:41S–65S, 1986

Reiter EO: Neuroendocrine control process: Pubertal onset and progression. J Adolesc Health Care 8:479–491, 1987

Shafer MA, Sweet RL, Ohm-Smith MS, et al: Microbiology of the lower genital tract in post-menarchal girls: Differences by sexual activity, contraception, and presence of nonspecific vaginitis. J Pediatr 107:974–981, 1985

Speroff L, Glass RH, Kase NG, eds: Dysfunctional uterine bleeding. In: Clinical Gynecologic Endocrinology and Infertility, 6th ed. Baltimore: Lippincott Williams & Wilkins, 1999, 575–594

Yen SS, Jaffee RB: Reproductive Endocrinology, 3rd ed. Philadelphia, WB Saunders, 1991

Male Reproductive Development

Bardin CW: Pituitary-testicular axis. In: Yen SS, Jaffee RB, eds: Reproductive Endocrinology, 3rd ed. Philadelphia: WB Saunders, 1991

Chambers CV, Shafer MA, Adger H, et al: Microflora of the urethra in adolescent boys: relationships to sexual activity and nongonococcal urethritis. J Ped 110:314–321, 1987

Czyba JC, Girod C: Development of normal testis. In: Hafez ESE, ed: Descended and Cryptorchid Testis. The Hague, Martinus Nijhoff, 1980.

Grumbach MM, Styne DM: Puberty: Ontogeny, neuroendocrinology, physiology, and disorders. In: Wilson JD, Foster DW, eds: Williams' Textbook of Endocrinology. Philadelphia, WB Saunders, 1998, 1509–1625

Jungueira LC, Carneiro J, Kelly RO: The Male Reproductive System. Basic Histology, 6th ed. San Mateo, CA, Appleton & Lange, 1989

Sharlip ID: Male reproductive disorders. In: Fitzgerald PA, ed: Handbook of Clinical Endocrinology. East Norwalk, CT, Appleton & Lange, 1992

3.5   COMMON REPRODUCTIVE HEALTH PROBLEMS

3.5.1   Breast Problems

Mary-Ann Shafer

BREAST MASSES

A variety of benign breast lesions occur in the female adolescent. The most typical presentation is a self-detected asymptomatic mass. Complaints such as bloody discharge, nipple retraction, or skin dimpling are rare.

Anatomic changes and congenital abnormalities can present during adolescence. Breast asymmetry, a benign condition in which one breast develops earlier or grows at a more rapid rate than the other, is common. This usually occurs between Tanner 2 and 4, persisting into adulthood in 25% of women. Rare congenital abnormalities of the breast include amastia (absent breast) and athelia (absent nipple). Breast atrophy during or after puberty in the adolescent is a sign of a restrictive eating disorder with the associated loss of both fat and glandular tissue in the breast during significant weight loss. Polymastia (accessory breast tissue) and polythelia (accessory nipples) occur along the mammalian nipple line in 1% to 2% of girls. Virginal (juvenile) hypertrophy, the massive enlargement of one or both breasts caused by either increased tissue sensitivity to pubertal hormones or endogenous production of hormones from within breast cells, can be associated with a variety of problems including headache, back pain, dermatitis, embarrassment, and psychological difficulties. Reduction mammoplasty after completion of breast maturation may be indicated in female adolescents with severe virginal hypertrophy.

The most common breast masses in adolescents are solitary cysts, fibrocystic change, and fibroadenomas. Masses resulting from inflammation and trauma are less frequent, and cancer is rare among female adolescents. A *solitary cyst* is the most common breast mass in the adolescent. Because over half resolve spontaneously within 2 to 3 months, biopsy is often unnecessary. Recurrent or multiple cysts in the adolescent may represent early fibrocystic change. *Fibrocystic change*, more correctly termed *benign proliferative breast change,* is a physiological response of breast tissue to cyclic hormonal activity. The result is a dilation and proliferation of duct epithelium to form gross cysts and microcysts. This benign condition is most common in women in the third and fourth decades but does occur during adolescence. Bilateral breast pain located in the upper outer quadrants is the usual symptom. The pain typically begins in the premenstrual phase of the menstrual cycle and subsides thereafter. Physical examination reveals areas of diffuse, cord-like thickening as well as discrete mobile lesions, which often increase in size during the premenstrual period. Early studies suggesting that methylxanthines (coffee, chocolate, tea, cola) were factors in the development or exacerbation of fibrocystic change have not been substantiated. Supportive care using nonsteroidal anti-inflammatory agents for pain is the most common approach to treatment. Oral contraceptives have also been shown to be efficacious in 70 to 90% of cases.

The majority (70% or more) of adolescent breast masses that undergo biopsy are identified as *fibroadenomas*. Four types of fibroadenomas have been described: common fibroadenomas, juvenile fibroadenomas, giant fibroadenomas, and cystosarcoma phyllodes. A fibroadenoma is a benign proliferation of stromal elements, ducts, and acini. The physical examination reveals a rubbery, painless, well-demarcated mass, 1 to 3 cm in size, usually located in the upper outer quadrant of the breast. Fibroadenomas can regress spontaneously but usually persist and may require excisional biopsy. The peak incidence occurs in late adolescence, but fibroadenomas have been described in premenarcheal girls. Multiple and recurrent fibroadenomas occur, but no malignant potential has been found. *Juvenile fibroadenoma*, a histologically similar lesion with less well-defined edges, presents as a rapidly enlarging breast mass that can reach immense proportions (>5 cm). Giant fibroadenomas are found most commonly in young black women, and complete excision is curative. *Cystosarcoma phyllodes* is a rare, rapidly growing lesion that is usually large, well-demarcated, and has a small potential for malignancy. *Intraductal papilloma*, a slow- growing benign tumor located under the areola, often presents with a serous or bloody nipple discharge.

A *contusion* can present as a poorly defined tender mass, with or without an overlying hematoma. Less than half of patients will give a history of trauma. The contusion usually resolves over several weeks, but if severe, a mass may persist several months. Occasionally *scar tissue* remains palpable indefinitely, or *fat necrosis* can develop, resulting in small areas of calcification. In either case, treatment consists of local excision. Trauma, however, can also draw attention to a preexisting lesion unrelated to the injury.

Mastitis, or breast infection, presents with the rapid onset of unilateral pain and localized inflammation. Infection is more common in newborns and lactating women but can occur in adolescents, unrelated to pregnancy. *Staphylococcus aureus* is the most common etiologic organism. The initial management of mastitis includes systemic antibiotics, heat, and analgesia. On occasion, acute mastitis can lead to abscess formation. Incision and drainage is then indicated and must also be considered with persistent, unresponsive mastitis.

Primary *breast cancer* is rare in teenagers. Only 0.2 to 3% of all breast cancers occur before 25 years of age. More than 60% of breast cancers are not primary breast tumors but arise metastatically from distant sites or locally from nonbreast tissue such as lymphomas or angiosarcomas. Breast cancers present very differently from benign breast diseases. It is recognized as a hard fixed mass beneath the nipple. Approximately one-third of cases have positive family histories. Breast cancer–associated genes have recently been identified but account for only a small fraction of all breast cancers (6%). Risk factors identified in adult breast cancer that were established during adolescence include menarche before age 12 years and cancer treatment–related radiation in the breast area (eg, for lymphoma).

ASSESSMENT   In assessing a breast mass, the history should identify previous trauma, fever, weight loss, and nipple discharge. A family history of breast disease and the nature of any previous lesions should be obtained. A menstrual history of cyclic pain can be helpful in diagnosing pregnancy or fibrocystic change. The history should also elicit the use of oral contraceptive pills or other hormonal agents, use of which can alter the breast. The physical examination must include an assessment of the Tanner stage to avoid confusing the normal breast bud (especially when unilateral) with a mass. The size, location, and characteristics of the lesion should be described. Tenderness, warmth, and lymphadenopathy are consistent with infection; a hard, fixed lesion with overlying skin changes must be evaluated for cancer.

Management of a benign breast mass in an adolescent begins with reassurance and an observation period of 1 to 3 months. During this time, any change that occurs with the menstrual cycle should be noted. Masses that persist beyond this time are referred for further evaluation. A fine needle aspiration can distinguish a cystic from a solid lesion. A cyst will collapse after aspiration, yielding a clear-yellow fluid, and the breast should be reexamined in 3 months. Excisional biopsy is indicated for a large solid or growing mass or one that yields an abnormal aspirate; any aspirate obtained should undergo cytologic evaluation. The purpose of excision is to obtain a definitive diagnosis, avoid a cosmetic deformity, and alleviate patient anxiety. Most of the normal breast tissue can be spared, as there is no need to remove a wide margin.

Mammography is only rarely indicated in the evaluation of a palpable mass in an adolescent. The dense parenchymal tissue in the adolescent breast makes interpretation difficult. Mammography is not indicated for screening in this age group because the incidence of malignancy is insignificant and the dose of radiation required is relatively high.

The value of teaching breast self-examination to adolescents remains controversial. Some professionals argue that routine breast self-examination in adolescents creates unnecessary anxiety and serves only to identify a greater number of benign lesions. Teaching a modified breast self-examination, however, can be a valuable educational component in the routine physical examination of the adolescent by leading to a discussion of normal development and important future health-promoting skills.

ADOLESCENT GYNECOMASTIA

Pubertal gynecomastia, the glandular enlargement of male breast tissue, is a common complaint of male adolescents. Gynecomastia occurs transiently in 40% of 10- to 16-year-old boys and peaks in incidence at SMR 2–4 or age 14 years. It results from a decreased ratio of androgen to estrogen and a change in receptor sensitivity. The breast tissue is frequently tender and often asymmetric. Spontaneous resolution occurs in 90% of boys within 3 years.

Pseudogynecomastia (fat), frequently confused with true gynecomastia (glandular), can be distinguished by comparing the consistency of the breast tissue with that of adipose tissue in the anterior axillary fold. Although the exact mechanism remains uncertain, the development of pubertal gynecomastia is related to the hormonal changes during puberty. Other rare causes of gynecomastia include endogenous states of estrogen excess such as testicular, adrenal, or pituitary tumors; hyperthyroidism; hepatic disorders; refeeding poststarvation; endogenous androgen deficiency states such as hypogonadism, Klinefelter syndrome, renal hemodialysis, and congenital adrenal hyperplasia; and specific drugs including estrogen, testosterone, anabolic steroids, human chorionic gonadotropins, tricyclic antidepressants, insulin, alcohol, marijuana, amphetamines, methadone, cimetidine, and digitalis; and cytotoxic agents.

Diagnosis is based on the typical history and examination and the exclusion of other causes of gynecomastia. The history must include current medications and illicit drug use. Physical assessment should describe the Tanner stage and findings of the testicular examination as well as the amount and quality of breast tissue present. Pubertal gynecomastia glandular tissue is usually less than 4 cm (similar to SMR 2–3 female breast). Reassurance is the most appropriate treatment. In contrast, pubertal macrogynecomastia resembles female SMR stage 3–5 breast, extends more than 5 cm, and usually does not regress spontaneously; thus, it requires treatment. A surgical referral is indicated when pubertal gynecomastia has a prolonged course or causes psychological impairment, or when macrogynecomastia is being considered. Recently two breast-cancer drugs have been used to treat gynecomastia: tamoxifen and testolactone.

3.5.2 Scrotal Masses

Mary-Ann Shafer

The discovery of a scrotal mass in a male adolescent presents a diagnostic dilemma for the clinician. Anxiety about the cause of such a lesion or embarrassment about the location of the mass can cause the adolescent to delay seeking treatment for weeks to months. Scrotal masses can represent congenital, acquired, or infectious processes. Table 3-13 outlines the etiologies and clinical management of scrotal masses. The more emergent causes of a scro-

tal mass, that is, torsion, neoplasm, and epididymitis, are discussed in more detail below.

TORSION OF THE SPERMATIC CORD

Torsion of the spermatic cord is a urologic emergency and must be considered in any patient presenting with an "acute scrotum," ie, sudden onset of pain and swelling in the scrotum. In adolescents, the most common cause of this syndrome is torsion of the spermatic cord, occurring in 1 per 4000 male adolescents. The condition is discussed in detail in Sec. 21.16.4.

TESTICULAR NEOPLASMS

Testicular cancer is becoming increasingly frequent and may be the most common malignancy in young men. Of all testicular tumors, 95% arise from malignant germ cells (germ cell tumors), whereas 5% originate from the supporting tissues (stromal tissues). Histologic types that tend to occur most frequently during adolescence are germ cell tumors and include seminoma, embryonal carcinoma, teratoma, and choriocarcinoma. Leydig and Sertoli cell tumors are of stromal origin and may occur at any age, including adolescence. Patients often present to the physician with painless scrotal swelling of gradual onset. Adolescents with testicular cancer are more likely than other adolescents to have had cryptorchism or testicular atrophy. Pain may be present if the tumor has hemorrhaged or has become necrotic. When pain accompanies a tumor, it can lead to an erroneous diagnosis of an infectious or inflammatory process.

Physical examination usually reveals a firm, irregular mass that is opaque to transillumination, but cystic or necrotic areas of the tumor can be soft on palpation. A hydrocele or varicocele may also be detected. The contralateral testis must be examined, not only for comparison but also to rule out the presence of bilateral disease. The detection of cervical or supraclavicular lymph nodes may indicate an advanced stage of disease (ie, metastases). Other possible findings include gynecomastia, breast tenderness, lymphatic or venous stasis in the genitalia or legs, pubic hair changes, prostatitis, and epididymitis. Because stromal tumors tend to produce androgens and/or estrogens, the prepubertal boy may present with early virilization, whereas the pubertal boy may present with feminization. Differential diagnosis includes orchitis, tuberculous infection of the testis, spermatocele, inguinal hernia, simple (benign) testicular cysts, and benign hydrocele, but a testicular mass is considered malignant until proven otherwise.

Laboratory examination is outlined in Table 3-13. Testicular tumor markers, most commonly human chorionic gonadotropin (hCG) and α-fetoprotein (AFP), are useful tests for certain histologic types and should be obtained before orchiectomy. The hCG is elevated in choriocarcinoma, nonseminomatous mixed germ-cell tumors, and seminoma with syncytiotrophoblasts. The AFP is elevated in nonseminomatous germ cell tumors, especially yolk sac tumors and embryonal carcinoma. Of note, 92% of pure seminomas usually produce no tumor markers.

Imaging of a scrotal mass is done using ultrasound or MRI. Staging of a proven tumor requires chest and abdominal CT. Therapy is determined by staging and definitive histology and includes orchiectomy, retroperitoneal lymph node dissection, radiation, and chemotherapy. This results in an overall survival rate of more than 70%, with 95% of patients with stage I or II tumors achieving cure.

EPIDIDYMITIS Epididymitis is an inflammatory disease of the epididymis that is largely due to STD infection in youth and must be included in the differential of any painful scrotal mass in the male adolescent. However, it remains uncommon relative to spermatic cord torsion and should not be diagnosed in adolescents without strong physical, laboratory, and radiographic evidence. It is discussed in more detail with sexually transmitted diseases (see Sec. 3.6).

3.5.3 Common Menstrual Problems

Anna-Barbara Moscicki

The establishment of regular ovulatory menstrual cycles is one of the primary clinical features that reflect the completion of puberty for girls with the maturation and synchronization of the entire hypothalamic-pituitary-gonadal (HPG) axis. Disorders in the development or maintenance of HPG axis function or anatomic abnormalities may result in abnormal menstrual bleeding. The most common menstrual disorders are amenorrhea, dysfunctional uterine bleeding (DUB), and dysmenorrhea, which are discussed in this section.

AMENORRHEA

Amenorrhea traditionally has been divided into two categories: primary and secondary. Primary amenorrhea is the absence of any menstruation by the age of expected menarche (16 to 17 years in the United States) in the presence of breast development or by age 14 to 15 years in the absence of any breast maturation or by 2 years after complete sexual maturation. Secondary amenorrhea is postmenarcheal cessation of menses for more than 6 consecutive months in females with previous regular menses or for more than 12 months in females with previous irregular menses. For purposes of discussion of the differential diagnosis, the categorization of primary and secondary amenorrhea will be retained. However, the clinical approach to primary and secondary amenorrhea in the female adolescent and young adult is similar. Oligomenorrhea, or infrequent menses, will be considered as amenorrhea in the discussion. Amenorrhea is also discussed with delayed puberty in Sec. 24.8.

Differential Diagnosis

Pregnancy is the most common cause of secondary amenorrhea and an important cause of primary amenorrhea. The diagnosis of pregnancy is reviewed in Sec. 3.5.5. Beyond pregnancy, the etiology of primary and secondary amenorrhea can be considered as central (hypothalamic, pituitary), gonadal (ovarian), or anatomic (uterine, cervical, vaginal).

Etiology

Central Causes Hypothalamic amenorrhea is thought to result from partial or complete inhibition of gonadotropin-releasing hormone (GnRH) release. It may be associated with nutritional deficiencies secondary to such diseases as regional enteritis, cystic fibrosis, and anorexia nervosa; excessive exercise and alterations in body fat and weight as found in professional athletes; stress; isolated GnRH deficiency; endocrinopathies; and specific drugs. Local lesions in the hypothalamus, such as infiltration processes, calcifications, gliomas, germinomas, and CNS radiation, are rare causes of GnRH deficiency. Occasionally isolated GnRH deficiency has been associated with the absence (anosmia) or impairment (hyposmia)

of the ability to smell (Kallman syndrome). In addition, certain medications, such as phenothiazine derivatives, can cause catecholamine depletion, resulting in amenorrhea.

Pituitary deficiencies or the inability to synthesize adequate amounts of gonadotropins may result from tumors, infiltrative processes (tuberculosis, sarcoidosis, or histiocytosis), or infarction. The most common tumor is the craniopharyngioma. Isolated gonadotropin deficiency is rare. More commonly, hypogonadotropism is a component of panhypopituitarism. A gonadotropin deficiency may be detected before the development of changes in thyroid and adrenal function. The most common pituitary cause of amenorrhea in reproductive-aged females is the prolactin-secreting adenoma. Unlike space-occupying lesions, these tumors cause inhibition of the HPG axis by secreting abnormally high levels of prolactin. Galactorrhea is found in only 50 to 60% of females with adenomas. Therefore, the absence of this sign does not eliminate the presence of this tumor in young women presenting with amenorrhea. Rarely, adenomas increase in size, causing symptoms associated with space-occupying lesions. Other causes of hyperprolactinemia include several psychoactive drugs (eg, haloperidol, phenothiazines, amitriptyline, benzodiazepine, and cocaine), breast-feeding, and renal failure.

Gonadal Causes Ovarian failure resulting in inadequate estrogen and progesterone production despite adequate gonadotropin stimulation will manifest clinically with menstrual irregularities. Such disorders include gonadal dysgenesis (abnormal ovarian development), premature ovarian failure, infection, hemorrhage or compromised blood supply, autoimmune oophoritis, and past radiation or chemotherapy in survivors of childhood cancer. Over 10% of cases of primary amenorrhea are caused by gonadal dysgenesis, including dysgenesis in Turner (XO) syndrome, mosaic Turner syndrome, and women with normal karyotype. Secondary amenorrhea can also be associated with gonadal dysgenesis, specifically mosaic Turner syndromes.

Several hormonal disorders can result in anovulation. Polycystic ovarian syndrome (PCO) and chronic hyperandrogenic anovulation are common causes of secondary amenorrhea and less common causes of primary amenorrhea in adolescents. The mechanism that produces this syndrome remains ill-defined. The hallmarks of this syndrome include menstrual dysfunction, hyperandrogenism, hypothalamic dysfunction, inappropriate gonadotropin secretion, enlarged ovaries, and metabolic defects, which include insulin resistance. The ovary and adrenal glands both contribute to the hyperandrogenism. Peripheral insulin resistance, which is common during adolescence, and excessive LH levels stimulate androgen production. The enlarged ovaries have multiple developing follicles and thickened stroma, which produce increased amounts of androgens. Classic findings of hirsutism, virilization, obesity, and amenorrhea may not be present in young adolescents. An important laboratory indicator of PCO is an LH:FSH ratio greater than 2.5:1, which reflects chronic hypothalamic dysfunction but is present in only 50% of patients with PCO.

Other causes of amenorrhea, hirsutism, and virilization are abnormal circulating androgenic hormones, which may result from Cushing syndrome; the use of anabolic steroids; virilizing ovarian tumors; adrenal adenomas; carcinomas; and adult-onset congenital adrenal hyperplasia. Specific drugs, both licit (eg, phenytoin and oral contraceptives) and illicit (eg, cocaine), are associated with the development of secondary amenorrhea and hirsutism. Other additional hormonally related causes of amenorrhea include hypothy-

TABLE 3-13

SCROTAL MASSES: ETIOLOGIES AND CLINICAL MANAGEMENT

LESION	LOCATION	ETIOLOGY	SYMPTOMS	PHYSICAL EXAM	WORKUP	TREATMENT	COMMENTS
I. Congenital							
A. Scrotal dermoid	Scrotal raphe	Embryologic	Mass at scrotal raphe	Mass at scrotal raphe	Ultrasound	Surgery	Can develop calculi/infection
B. Polyorchism	Intrascrotal	Embryologic	Scrotal mass	Duplicated testes—smaller than normal	Nuclear scan if Dx doubtful	Orchiectomy if no ductus deferens	Torsion risk
C. Scrotal rests (splenic, adrenocortical)	Upper pole Spermatic cord Tunica vaginalis	Embryologic	Scrotal mass	Scrotal mass	Liver-spleen scan	Surgery for associated cryptorchidism, hernia	Other congenital abnormalities are associated
II. Acquired							
A. Hydrocele (noncommunicating)	Fluid in tunica vaginalis	Idiopathic, or secondary to infection, torsion, lymphatic blockage	Painless enlargement	Nontender, fluid-filled mass, transillumination (+)	Ultrasound if tumor suspected	Surgery or aspiration/sclerotherapy	Rx reserved for large hydroceles or if painful
B. Spermatocele	Efferent ductal system	Painless cystic nodule	Nodule above and posterior to testes	No change with Valsalva, transillumination (+)	N/A	Surgery only if painful	Does not affect fertility
C. Varicocele	Pampiniform plexus	Idiopathic, or secondary to intraabdominal mass, hepatosplenomegaly, hydronephrosis	Usually none Pain rarely, if thrombosis present	"Bag of worms" appearance Usually left-sided ↓ Supine position ↑ Valsalva	N/A	Surgery if ipsilateral testes is hypotrophic	Depression of spermatogenesis with prolonged presence of lesion
D. Torsion of spermatic cord	Hemiscrotum	Associated with anomaly of suspension of testes	Acute onset of pain, swelling in testis, inguinal area, lower abdomen Nausea and vomiting	Diffusely swollen and tender testicle Cremasteric reflex absent	Radionuclide scan: scrotal imaging (↓ uptake except late, or large hydrocele) Doppler (no flow)	Attempt manual detorsion Emergent surgery: orchiectomy if necrotic; orchiopexy Analgesics	Emergency: salvage rate related to time torsion present
E. Torsion of testicular appendage	Hemiscrotum	Torsion of vestigial structure (appendix testis or appendix epididymis)	Sudden or gradual pain onset: upper pole of testis	Tender, pea-sized swelling at upper pole "Blue dot" sign	Doppler: normal to increased flow Radionuclide scan: normal to increased uptake	Analgesics Anti-inflammatories	Resolves spontaneously in 2–12 days

(continued)

TABLE 3-13 Continued

LESION	LOCATION	ETIOLOGY	SYMPTOMS	PHYSICAL EXAM	WORKUP	TREATMENT	COMMENTS
F. Trauma/ hematocele	Blood in tunica vaginalis	Trauma	Pain +/− swelling	Fluid-filled mass if hematocele present	Ultrasound if expanding hematocele suspected	Analgesia, ice, scrotal elevation Expanding hematocele requires drainage	
G. Neoplasms	Testicle or paratesticular structures	Unknown	Painless swelling Pain present if hemorrhage/necrosis Back pain with retroperitoneal lymph node involvement	Firm irregular mass Transillumination Hydrocele/varicocele may be present	Physical examination, CBC, LFTs, electrolytes, BUN, Ca, renal function tests, sperm analysis, hCG, AFP, testicular ultrasound, CT of chest and abdomen	Surgery (orchiectomy and peritoneal lymph node dissection) Radiation Chemotherapy Presurgery sperm banking	May be the most common malignancy in young men
III. Infectious A. Epididymitis	Epididymis	C. trachomatis N. gonorrhoeae Coliforms Pseudomonas Gram (+) cocci	Acute onset of pain and swelling Frequency, dysuria, urethral discharge, fever	Swollen and tender epididymis Testicle may be tender Cremasteric reflex (+/−)	U/A, Gram stain of discharge, Urethral culture Dx epididymitis from torsion: Radionuclide scan: ↓ uptake = torsion ↑ uptake = epididymitis Doppler ultrasound: ↓ absent flow = torsion ↑ flow = epididymitis	Antibiotics See Table 3-17	Must R/O torsion Can result in azoospermia
B. Orchitis	Testicle (unilateral or bilateral)	Usually secondary to epididymitis (viral mumps)	Swollen and tender testicle Fever Parotitis history	Swollen and tender testicle Fever	None if mumps orchitis probable	Analgesia, bed rest, scrotal support	If bilateral atrophy, infertility likely Any atrophy-cancer risk 60× ↑

roidism or hyperthyroidism, hypercortisolism, and adrenal insufficiency. Both hypercortisolism and hypothyroidism have been associated with prolactinemia and amenorrhea.

Defects in the development of the müllerian duct system are associated with primary amenorrhea. Such defects may occur anywhere along the ductal system (see Fig. 3-2), resulting in imperforate hymen, vaginal atresia, or absence or malformations of the cervix and the uterus. The uterine cavity and the endometrium may fail to develop as well. Except where there is no uterine cavity or endometrium, developmental genital tract obstructions usually present with painful swelling of the reproductive tract above the area of the blockage: hematocolpos (vaginal), hematometra (uterus), and hematoperitoneum (leakage of menstrual blood into peritoneal cavity). The pain may be cyclic and coincide with a normal menstrual cycle. Rokitansky syndrome is müllerian agenesis with primary amenorrhea and absence or hypoplasia of the vagina, cervix, and/or uterus. Uterine synechiae (Asherman syndrome) occurring after endometrial manipulation and/or infection (eg, pregnancy, dilation and curettage) can lead to secondary amenorrhea with partial or total obliteration of the endometrial cavity.

Rare causes of amenorrhea include gonadotropin-resistant ovary syndrome (an abnormality of ovarian hormone receptors), defects in estrogen biosynthesis including 17-hydroxylase deficiency and 17-ketosteroid reductase deficiency, and androgen insensitivity. In an XY male patient these latter two causes result in a female phenotype with primary amenorrhea.

Evaluation of Amenorrhea The evaluation is accomplished by doing a thorough history and physical assessment, including the onset and staging of secondary sexual characteristics as indicators of the stage of development of the HPG axis: pubic, axillary, and facial hair development and distribution as a sign of androgen effect; and breast and vulvar vaginal mucosal maturation as a sign of the estrogenic effect. The possibility of pregnancy should always be evaluated by a urine pregnancy test before an extensive workup for primary or secondary amenorrhea in the presence of secondary sexual characteristics is carried further. Factors associated with central causes of amenorrhea should be queried, including body image, weight loss, nutritional intake, excessive exercise, and stress. Physical examination should include height, weight, blood pressure, pulse rate, and signs and stages of secondary sexual characteristics. Physical signs of genetic syndromes associated with amenorrhea such as Turner's syndrome are noted. The thyroid gland is examined, and the breast is examined for estrogen effect. The areola and nipple are gently compressed to elicit galactorrhea if present. A full neurologic examination is required to assess for increased intracranial pressure or an expanding mass including evidence of bilateral temporal hemianopsia common to pituitary tumors. Signs of androgen excess include hirsutism, acne, voice changes, and clitoromegaly. The abdomen is palpated to assess the size of the uterus (hematocolpos, pregnancy, tumor) and presence of tenderness. The vulva, introitus, and vaginal mucosa are evaluated for clitoromegaly, hymenal patency, and estrogen effect. A pelvic examination is helpful to determine vaginal patency and presence or absence of the reproductive organs. If a complete pelvic examination is not possible for anatomic, cultural, or psychosocial reasons, a rectal abdominal examination can be done. Patency and depth of the vagina can be determined by passing a lubricated cotton swab through the vaginal opening. If a pelvic examination cannot be completed, or anatomic abnormalities are noted, a pelvic ultrasound or computerized tomography should be performed.

Without specific symptoms and signs, screening laboratory tests should include urine β-hCG pregnancy test, LH and FSH to differentiate between a hypothalamic-pituitary and an ovarian etiology for the amenorrhea, prolactin concentration to determine the presence of a pituitary microadenoma, and thyroid function tests. If excess androgen is suspected on physical examination, then serum testosterone and dehydroepiandrosterone levels are indicated. Further workup for adrenal dysfunction is discussed in Secs. 24.4.5 and 24.4.8. Estrogen effects can be evaluated from vaginal cytology (presence of mature superficial epithelial cells) and by examination of cervical mucus for the presence of ferning patterns. High levels of LH and FSH warrant a chromosomal evaluation.

A simple progesterone challenge will indirectly evaluate the presence of endogenous estrogen as well as the competence of the reproductive outflow tract from uterus to vaginal opening. The test dose includes 10 mg oral medroxyprogesterone acetate per day for 7 days. Within 2 to 7 days after completion of the course of progesterone, bleeding should occur. Uterine bleeding confirms minimal competence of the HPG axis and patency of the outflow tract. If no bleeding occurs after progesterone, either the reproductive outflow tract is abnormal or endogenous estrogen is inadequate or absent. The second step of a hormonal challenge test is to prime the endometrium with exogenous estrogen followed by progesterone to induce bleeding: 2.5 mg oral conjugated estrogen (Premarin) for 25 days with 10 mg oral medroxyprogesterone acetate added from day 16 to day 25. It may be necessary to repeat this combination challenge a second time if no bleeding is elicited. If bleeding occurs, minimal competence of the uterus, endometrium, and cervicovaginal outflow tracts is confirmed. If no bleeding occurs, pelvic sonography or computerized tomography and appropriate hormonal assays, including a serum estradiol level, should be obtained.

If an outflow obstruction of the reproductive tract is diagnosed, treatment depends on the type and location of the problem. Obstructions leading to painful menstrual flow blockage require urgent surgical intervention after appropriate ultrasound and computerized tomographic studies define the existing anatomy. Surgical correction of vaginal agenesis is appropriate when menstrual outflow is obstructed and, in the absence of the uterus, before sexual debut.

The complete evaluation and treatment of hypothalamic-pituitary failure is reviewed in Sec. 24.2. Specific treatment for PCO includes cycling with estrogen and progesterone. The PCO-associated hirsutism may be treated with estrogen-dominant oral contraceptive steroids and spironolactone, with equivocal results. Electrolysis is often needed. Infertility can occasionally be treated with clomiphene citrate, among other gynecologic interventions. Symptoms of hyperglycemia should prompt a glucose tolerance test in women with PCO to rule out insulin resistance. If an asymptomatic pituitary microadenoma is suspected in the presence of elevated prolactin levels, bromocriptine (a dopamine agonist) therapy should be considered. True ovarian failure is treated with replacement hormone therapy, 0.3 to 0.625 mg or more of conjugated estrogen (lowest amount to achieve desired estrogen effect) on days 1 to 25 and medroxyprogesterone acetate 10 mg on days 16 to 25, to provide estrogen stimulation and avoid the effect of unopposed estrogen on the endometrium, which has been linked to endometrial cancer in women. Anatomic abnormalities should be referred for reconstructive surgery, as indicated. When irreversible infertility of any cause is determined, counseling should be done.

DYSFUNCTIONAL UTERINE BLEEDING

Although the term *dysfunctional uterine bleeding* (DUB) has been used to denote any abnormal vaginal bleeding, DUB is defined here as vaginal bleeding that occurs in cycles less than 20 days or longer than 40 days, lasts longer than 8 days, results in blood loss greater than 80 mL, and/or is associated with anemia. Dysfunctional uterine bleeding has been divided into two categories, primary and secondary DUB, with the vast majority being of the primary type. Because primary DUB is a diagnosis of exclusion, it is made only after a careful evaluation to eliminate other serious causes.

PRIMARY DYSFUNCTIONAL UTERINE BLEEDING Primary DUB in adolescents is a disorder that results from the immaturity or dysfunction of the HPG axis. Rhythmic fluctuations of estrogen levels normally are initiated early in puberty, increase in amplitude as puberty progresses, and reach peak estrogen levels sufficient to stimulate endometrial proliferation, menstruation, and eventually ovulation. Anovulatory cycles are common 1 to 2 years after menarche and are characterized by oscillations in estrogen levels and lack of progesterone production (see Sec. 3.4). Prolonged absence of progesterone results in an abnormally thick and fragile endometrial lining that, if exposed to estrogen, may slough in a disorderly and irregular fashion, leading to irregular and excessive menstrual bleeding.

SECONDARY DYSFUNCTIONAL UTERINE BLEEDING Secondary DUB is caused by disorders of coagulation and underlying diseases and abnormalities of the reproductive organs including vagina, cervix, uterus, and ovary. The most common cause of excessive bleeding requiring hospitalization is a bleeding disorder. Abnormal vaginal bleeding at the time of menarche or thereafter may be the initial manifestation. The most common cause is von Willebrand disease. Factor VIII or IX deficiency, hereditary or acquired thrombocytopenia (including chemotherapy-induced), platelet disorders, thalassemia major, Fanconi anemia, aplastic anemia, and leukemia should also be considered.

Vaginal causes of abnormal bleeding include foreign bodies (eg, forgotten tampons or condoms), lacerations from either sexual abuse or intravaginal insertion of objects, hymenal tears, and, rarely, tumors such as sarcomas. Diethylstilbestrol (DES), an estrogen used until the early 1970s to suppress spontaneous abortion, has been known to cause reproductive tract fetal abnormalities such as adenosis of the vaginal mucosa and the rare DES-related clear-cell adenocarcinoma (incidence of 0.14 to 1.4 out of 10,000 daughters exposed to DES in utero). The DES-related clear-cell carcinoma can present with vaginal bleeding. Cervical factors associated with bleeding include sexually transmitted infectious cervicitis, hemangiomas, cervical polyps, and large fragile condylomas. Cervical as well as vaginal causes are usually associated with complaints of light spotting or postcoital bleeding rather than frank vaginal bleeding.

Complications of pregnancy are common causes of abnormal bleeding: spontaneous abortion, incomplete abortion, threatened abortion, ectopic pregnancy, molar pregnancy, and complications from legal or illegal therapeutic abortions. Additional uterine causes for unusual bleeding include endometritis with or without salpingitis. Endometritis most commonly results from endometrial infections with sexually transmitted organisms such as *C. trachomatis* and *N. gonorrhoeae*. Endometritis can also occur after gynecologic procedures such as therapeutic abortions and delivery (postpartum

infections). Submucosal myomas, endometriosis, arteriovenous malformations, and, rarely, uterine cancers have also been associated with irregular bleeding.

Ovarian cysts and malignant and benign tumors may be related to abnormal bleeding. Although characteristically associated with amenorrhea or oligomenorrhea, polycystic ovary disease, hyperthyroidism, hypothyroidism, Addison disease, and congenital adrenal hyperplasia can present with DUB. Patients with chronic illness, specifically patients receiving hemodialysis or chemotherapy, may have uterine bleeding problems leading to excessive blood loss. Last, medications such as warfarin and hormonal contraceptives (Depo-Provera, OCPs) can result in abnormal bleeding.

The evaluation of a patient with abnormal vaginal bleeding should be performed systematically; those causes requiring immediate intervention must be excluded first. The goals of the clinical assessment are to determine the acuity and volume of blood loss and the need for hospitalization, surgical intervention, and transfusion. Physical examination should include orthostatic blood pressures and pulse, neurologic examination, and pelvic examination with appropriate STD cultures. Laboratory evaluation should include a complete blood and platelet count and a β-hCG pregnancy test. Patients with vaginal bleeding with an acute abdominal complaint and/or positive pregnancy test should have immediate gynecologic consultation for possible ectopic pregnancy. Patients with significant blood loss resulting in anemia should be evaluated for a bleeding disorder and thyroid disorders. Because both PCO and prolactinomas can occasionally present with irregular bleeding, LH, FSH, and prolactin levels should be considered.

A complete description of the management of all of the causes of vaginal bleeding is beyond the scope of this section. Patients with significant orthostatic blood pressure or heart rate changes or who present with an acute abdomen should have appropriate fluid, electrolyte, and hemostatic stabilization, abdominal and pelvic evaluation (pelvic examination, sonography, and other radiographic techniques), and gynecologic and surgical consultation as indicated. Brisk uterine bleeding should be stopped with administration of Premarin, 20 to 40 mg IV every 2 to 4 hours for a total of up to six doses. Combination low-dose estrogen-progesterone pills (common oral contraceptive pill formulations) should be started with the intravenous Premarin. If the patient is stable but only mildly anemic with bleeding, the bleeding can be stopped by initiating an estrogen-dominant contraceptive (eg, low-dose fixed estrogen-progesterone combinations or Demulen), 1 pill every 4 to 8 hours until bleeding stops. The dose is tapered over the following 3 to 4 weeks, at which time a withdrawal bleed of 3 to 5 days is permitted, and cyclic combination oral contraceptive pill therapy is initiated. Antiemetics may be necessary with the high-dose estrogen therapy. After 4 to 6 months an attempt to discontinue medication can be evaluated under close medical follow-up. Other regimens include cyclic progesterone therapy; however, this regimen appears to be less efficacious in patients with primary DUB. Iron replacement may be necessary in anemic patients (Hb <12 g/dL). For patients with bleeding disorders, combination estrogen-progesterone pill therapy with or without short withdrawal periods may be indicated. For patients who are undergoing chemotherapy and have a history of severe excessive bleeding, a trial of a gonadotropin-releasing hormone agonist Synarel (naferelin) can be started 2 to 4 weeks before the chemotherapy. Synarel, 400 mg daily (200 mg intranasally BID) is begun simultaneously with low-dose estrogen-progesterone pills every day for 6 continous weeks. If a patient continues immunosuppression, longer therapy may be needed. Dilation and curettage (D&C) is no longer indicated in treatment of DUB and is contraindicated in patients with bleeding disorders. However, in the rare case, D&C may be recommended diagnostically because of the possibility of endometrial cancer.

DYSMENORRHEA

Dysmenorrhea, both primary and secondary, remains one of the leading reproductive system complaints of menstruating female adolescents and is a leading cause of school absenteeism, with a prevalence of up to 60% in postmenarcheal adolescents. Primary dysmenorrhea is thought to reflect painful prostaglandin-stimulated vasoconstriction and myometrial contractions through two pathways. The cyclooxygenase pathway of arachidonic acid produces PGE_2, PGD_2, and $PGF_{2\alpha}$, which induce opposing activities (vasoconstriction and vasodilation, and muscle contraction and relaxation). A major increase of prostaglandins is seen within the endometrium within the first 36 to 48 hours of menses, which parallels the time of greatest discomfort. In the second, lipoxygenase, pathway, leukotrienes are the primary end product; these are also potent smooth muscle–stimulating substances. The 30 to 40% of females who do not respond to cyclooxygenase inhibitors (eg, ibuprofen, naproxen sodium) are thought to have dysmenorrhea through this second pathway. Because it is linked to ovulatory cycles, primary dysmenorrhea may not become problematic until 1 year or more after menarche.

Secondary dysmenorrhea is associated with specific physiological and pathologic conditions including pelvic infections (eg, endometritis, PID), ectopic pregnancy, intrauterine pregnancy, endometriosis, intrauterine contraceptive device, uterine leiomyomas, cervical stenosis, and anatomic abnormalities.

Evaluation for dysmenorrhea includes distinguishing between primary and secondary dysmenorrhea and assessing the last menstrual period, previous pregnancies with outcomes, use of contraceptives, STD history and current symptoms, date of onset of pain, relationship of onset and duration of pain to menses, and impact of previous pain medications by type. Associated symptoms may include nausea, vomiting, diarrhea, fatigue, headache, low back pain, thigh pain, dizziness, and syncope. Assessment includes a complete physical examination and pelvic examination with STD screening in a postmenarcheal woman. Therapy for primary dysmenorrhea focuses on inhibiting the synthesis or action of prostaglandins: standard therapy includes ibuprofen, 400 to 800 mg PO TID to QID, beginning at least 24 hours before the onset of expected menses and continuing for 3 to 4 days. Naproxen sodium, 550 mg PO initially, followed by 275 mg TID to QID can be used as an alternative. Combination oral contraceptive pills are often as effective as the above regimens and have the added benefit of birth control. Combined oral contraceptives and antiprostaglandin treatment should be reserved for severe cramping pain unresponsive to a single therapeutic regimen. Patients diagnosed with primary dysmenorrhea who do not improve with adequate therapy should be evaluated for causes related to secondary dysmenorrhea.

3.5.4   Squamous Intraepithelial Lesion

Anna-Barbara Moscicki

Recent reforms in cytologic terminology combine the cytologic changes previously termed *condyloma* (or koilocytic atypia) and CIN I, resulting in a new term, *low-grade squamous intraepithelial lesion* (LSIL). Similarly, CIN II and III are now collectively referred

to as *high-grade squamous intraepithelial lesion* (HSIL). Squamous intraepithelial lesions (SIL) are considered to be a precancerous stage of cervical cancer and result from pathologic changes caused by human papillomavirus. Although cervical cancer is rare among adolescents, SIL, predominantly LSIL, affects approximately 5 to 10% of sexually active female adolescents. Although human papillomavirus (HPV) is strongly associated with anogenital cancer, it does not appear to be sufficient by itself to cause cancer. Most SILs do not progress, and cervical cancer prevention is best attained by the identification and treatment of these lesions. The Papanicolaou (Pap) smear remains the most cost-effective method of screening adolescents for SIL and cancer, even though the test is somewhat insensitive.

Sexually active adolescents need annual Pap smears performed, more frequently when indicated by abnormal cytologic findings. Adolescents with a single HSIL Pap smear or two consecutive atypical smears unrelated to inflammation or two LSILs should be referred for colposcopic evaluation. The importance of differentiating low- and high-grade SIL is related to prognosis and management: LSIL is thought to be a relatively benign expression of HPV, with fewer than 5% of lesions progressing in adolescents, and therefore can be observed if compliance is assured. In contrast, 10 to 40% of HSIL may progress. Treatment of all HSILs is currently recommended in the United States.

3.5.5   Pregnancy: Intrauterine and Ectopic

Mary-Ann Shafer

One million adolescents in the United States experience a pregnancy each year, with 50% of these pregnancies terminated by therapeutic abortion. Of those who maintain the pregnancy to term, about 95% of adolescents decide to parent the child, and about half such teen mothers are unmarried. The factors that place young women at risk for an unintended pregnancy and the interactions among these factors are complex. Lack of appropriate knowledge regarding sexual intercourse and contraception plays a role in the perpetuation of myths regarding risk for pregnancy, especially among younger teenagers. Cognitive immaturity results in adolescents' difficulty in linking the act of sexual intercourse with the possible outcome of pregnancy and therefore assessing their true personal risk for pregnancy. Environmental factors including poverty make teenage parenthood an attractive alternative role for many young women. Also, society's ambivalence regarding adolescent sexual activity, contraception, pregnancy, and teenage parenthood acts as a barrier to the development and maintenance of interventions.

INTRAUTERINE PREGNANCY

Diagnosis

During any assessment of a female adolescent, it is advisable to record the date and normality of the last menstrual period. A history of unprotected intercourse since the last menses with or without amenorrhea or unusual vaginal bleeding should alert the physician to the possibility of pregnancy. The absence of historical information does not preclude pregnancy because often the adolescent is unwilling to communicate sexual information to the clinician. In addition to amenorrhea or a "missed period," the typical symptoms associated with pregnancy (nausea, vomiting, intermenstrual spotting, breast tenderness, unexplained weight gain, urinary frequency, and fatigue, among others) may be present in any combination or may be absent early in pregnancy. A physical assessment including a pelvic examination is critical to the evaluation of a possible pregnancy.

The pregnancy test confirms the presence of an early pregnancy, using detection of serum β-hCG. Within 24 hours of implantation, the placenta initiates production of hCG ($\leq$5 mIU/mL), and concentrations double every 48 to 72 hours. By 2 weeks, the level rises to >200 mIU/mL in a normal pregnancy, and concentration peaks at approximately 100,000 mIU/mL at 6 to 8 weeks. Thereafter, the level drops to below 10,000 mIU/mL by 14 weeks. Currently, urine testing using monoclonal antibodies to β-hCG provides an accurate, sensitive, easy, and inexpensive screening tool to detect early pregnancy with sensitivities to levels less than 50 mIU/mL. Thus, testing can be performed as early as 1 week postimplantation or 5 days before the onset of the next anticipated menstruation. The recognition and management of ectopic pregnancy are discussed below.

Once the presence and gestation of an intrauterine pregnancy are established by pelvic examination (include STD screening) and pregnancy testing, counseling with the adolescent (and, when appropriate, with the parent or parents, other responsible adult, and partner) should explore options for pregnancy management. These include continuance of pregnancy, parenting, adoption, and termination of pregnancy. Such counseling can begin in the office setting and can continue at an appropriate referral agency. Confidentiality should be maintained at the request of the adolescent as appropriate.

ECTOPIC PREGNANCY

Ectopic pregnancy is an expanding problem for young sexually active women as reflected by a fourfold increase in incidence of the problem between 1970 and 1992, with 20 ectopic pregnancies reported per 1000 pregnancies in 1992. It is the leading cause of maternal death in the first trimester of pregnancy and the second leading cause of overall maternal death and occurs in 1.5% of all pregnancies. Approximately 98% of ectopic pregnancies conceived naturally occur in the fallopian tube itself. The most common factor that predisposes the young woman to tubal damage and therefore ectopic pregnancy is acute salpingitis, especially chlamydial infection. Other predisposing factors include congenital anomalies, previous pelvic or abdominal surgery, prior ectopic pregnancy, and intrauterine device (IUD) use. Less common factors linked to ectopic pregnancy include ectopic endometrial tissue within the tube (endometriosis), multiple sexual partners, cigarette smoking, vaginal douching, and early sexual debut. Although young women aged 15 to 24 years have the lowest incidence of ectopic pregnancy, they have the highest ectopic pregnancy–related death rate, especially among nonwhite teenagers.

The outcome of an ectopic pregnancy depends on the location of implantation. A spontaneous "tubal abortion" is most likely to occur when the site of implantation is in the ampulla of the tube, whereas the more dangerous tubal rupture is most likely with implantation within the tube's isthmus. When acute rupture into the peritoneum occurs, it is usually accompanied by acute hemorrhage, hypovolemia, and shock, resulting in a life-threatening situation.

Diagnosis

Recent advances in determining early pregnancy coupled with the successful conservative management of early ectopic pregnancies

have decreased mortality and morbidity while preserving fertility. The common clinical presentation of an ectopic pregnancy includes (prevalence rates in parentheses) lower abdominal pain (100%), amenorrhea (75%), intermenstrual spotting (75%), abdominal tenderness (90%), adnexal tenderness (85%), adnexal/pelvic mass (50%), and uterine enlargement mimicking early changes of pregnancy (most). Women with ectopic pregnancies have normal vital signs unless rupture occurs.

The quantitative pregnancy test is the most important factor in diagnosing of ectopic pregnancy. The quantitative β-hCG determines whether a pregnancy is present and, with serial hCG measurements, whether it is normal and intrauterine. Ectopic pregnancy often produces hCG at a slower rate, although there is considerable overlap of concentrations in normal intrauterine and ectopic pregnancies early in gestation. With current sensitive urine tests for pregnancy, urinary testing is acceptable for screening. If ectopic pregnancy is suspected, however, a blood sample should be obtained for quantitative β-hCG.

The differential diagnosis of the young woman presenting with abdominal pain, amenorrhea, or spotting includes a normal intrauterine pregnancy (IUP), a failing IUP (spontaneous abortion), and an ectopic pregnancy (must rule out PID: see Sec. 3.6). Four clinical laboratory tests and procedures will differentiate among these diagnoses: quantitative hCG, serum progesterone, transvaginal ultrasound, and uterine curettage. A viable IUP is characterized by doubling of the serum β-hCG every 48 to 72 hours or a β-hCG level greater than 25 IU/L, a progesterone level 25 ng/mL or more, and an ultrasound consistent with an intrauterine gestational sac. A failing IUP (spontaneous abortion) is characterized by an abnormally rising (plateau or decreasing level) β-hCG on serial measures, a progesterone level less than 5 ng/mL, and villi obtained by curettage. In contrast, an ectopic pregnancy is defined by a progesterone less than 5 ng/mL, an abnormally rising β-hCG, no villi on curettage, and a transvaginal ultrasound consistent with an extrauterine pregnancy.

The differential diagnosis of a suspected ectopic pregnancy includes acute or chronic salpingitis, threatened or incomplete intrauterine abortion, torsion or ruptured ovarian cyst, appendicitis, rupture of an IUD through the uterine wall, and acute gastroenteritis. Management of ectopic pregnancy frequently requires emergent surgical intervention such as laparotomy and salpingectomy on the affected side because of delayed diagnosis and rupture, with subsequent poor fertility prospects. More recently, with earlier recognition of the ectopic pregnancy before rupture, newer, more conservative management is being employed, including salpingostomies by laparoscopy and medical management with methotrexate, with comparable resolution of ectopic pregnancies and preservation of subsequent fertility. Candidates for medical management include hemodynamically stable women with an intact ectopic pregnancy mass less than 4 cm by sonography. Multiple-dose methotrexate is given alternate days (1 mg/kg IM on days 1, 3, 5, 7) with leukovarin "rescue" added in some protocols on alternative days (0.1 mg/kg IM days 2, 4, 6, 8) until β-hCG decreases by 15% or more in 48 hours or four doses of methotrexate are completed. Careful weekly follow-up is essential with β-hCG until the titer is less than 5 mIU/mL.

In addition to pregnancy, the differential to consider when abdominal pain is coupled with menstrual irregularities includes acute (see Sec. 3.6.1) or chronic salpingitis, torsion or ruptured ovarian cyst, appendicitis, IUP complication, and acute gastroenteritis.

TABLE 3-14
METHODS OF CONTRACEPTION[a]

METHOD	MECHANISM OF ACTION	EFFICACY: RATE OF PREGNANCY FIRST YEAR OF USE[b]		COITAL DEPENDENCE[c]	COST	PRESCRIPTION REQUIRED	PROTECTION FROM STDs/HIV	COMPLICATIONS	COMMENTS
		PERFECT USE	ACTUAL						
Abstinence	No intercourse	0%	0%	No	None	No	+++	None	
Oral combined contraceptive pill	Inhibits ovulation Alters cervical mucus and endometrium	0.1%	–	No	$25 per month	Yes	Some protection against PID	Side effects, STDs (See text)	See text
Oral progestin-only contraceptive pill	Same as oral combined pill	0.5%	5%	No	$25 per month	Yes	No	Side effects, STDs (See text)	See text
Intrauterine device (IUD)	Probably prevents implantation	1–2%	–	No	$200–300	Yes	No	Bleeding, cramping, pain, expulsion, increased risk of PID, ectopic pregnancy	Not recommended for teenagers
Condom (female)	Barrier	5%	21%	Yes	$3 each			Slippage	Expensive, difficult
Condom (male)	Barrier	3%	14%	Yes	$6–12/doz	No	++	Reaction to latex	Some dislike
Vaginal spermicides (foam, jelly, film, suppositories)	Spermicidal agent	6%	26%	Yes	$10–12 per container (18 uses)	No	+/–	Reaction to spermicide	Some describe as "messy" to use
Condom and foam[d]	Barrier with spermicidal agent	3%	14%	Yes	See above	No	++	Reaction to latex or spermicide	Requires using two methods
Diaphragm with spermicide[d]	Barrier with spermicidal agent	6%	20%	Can be inserted up to 6 hours before intercourse	$30–40+ spermicide	Yes	+	Reaction to spermicide, pelvic discomfort, recurrent UTIs, ↑ risk of toxic shock syndrome	Requires comfort with body

(continued)

TABLE 3-14 Continued

METHOD	MECHANISM OF ACTION	EFFICACY: RATE OF PREGNANCY FIRST YEAR OF USE[b]		COITAL DEPENDENCE[c]	COST	PRESCRIPTION REQUIRED	PROTECTION FROM STDs/HIV	COMPLICATIONS	COMMENTS
		PERFECT USE	ACTUAL						
Coitus interruptus	Withdrawal prior to ejaculation	4%	19%	Yes	None	No	No	None	Requires self-control; Preejaculatory semen contains sperm
Cervical cap with spermicide[d]	Barrier with spermicidal agent	20–40%	9–26%	Can remain in place 2–3 days	$35–40 + spermicide	Yes	?	Recurrent UTI, ↑ risk of cervical dysplasia and toxic shock syndrome	Difficult to insert/remove
Periodic abstinence	During peak fertility; Abstinence during times of peak fertility	6–10%	20%	No	None	No	No	None	Requires monitoring menstrual cycle
Chance	Chance	89%	89%	Yes	None	No	No	Pregnancy	
Depo-medroxy progesterone	Suppresses ovulation, thickens cervical mucus	<1%	<1%	No	$45/3 mo	Yes	No	(See text)	Requires q 3 mo IM injections; must comply with F/U visits
L-Norgestrel implant	Suppresses ovulation, thickens cervical mucus	<1%	<1%	No	$600 with insertion	Yes	No	(See text)	Requires surgical implantation removal q 5 yr
Emergency contraceptive pills	Suppresses ovulation/implantation	N/A	25%	No	$28	Yes	No	Nausea, bleeding	Use within 72 hr of intercourse

[a] In approximate order of decreasing theoretical efficacy.
[b] Adapted from Hatcher RA, et al, 1998 and Trussel J, et al, 1987: *theoretical efficacy* is defined as the best *estimate* of the accidental pregnancy rate during the first year of use among couples who initiated the use of a method (not necessarily for the first time) and who used it consistently and correctly. *Actual efficacy* is defined as a measure of the accidental pregnancy rate during the first year among "typical couples" who initiated the use of a method (not necessarily for the first time) if they did not stop use for any other reason.
[c] Cost exclusive of clinician visit.
[d] Efficacy rates based on use of specific method without addition of a spermicide.

257

3.5.6   Contraception

Mary-Ann Shafer

Contraception is a health behavior that often begins during adolescence and evolves throughout reproductive life. On initiation of sexual activity, most adolescents use either no contraception or nonprescriptive methods such as condoms. The first contact by a female adolescent with a clinician regarding contraception usually occurs 6 to 12 months after sexual debut and often follows a "missed period." Discussions of sexual activity, abstinence, reproduction, and contraception occur frequently as a normal part of the well-adolescent visit for female adolescents. In contrast, male adolescents, who are not at risk for pregnancy and do not require prescriptive contraceptives, may have clinician contact only during a sports physical or treatment of an injury or acute illness. Although sexuality and contraceptives are not traditionally discussed during "the sports check" for male adolescents, clinicians should emphasize the need for such discussions because this visit may be the only contact between the male adolescent and a clinician.

TYPE OF CONTRACEPTIVE

Common methods of contraception for male and female adolescents are reviewed in Table 3-14. The combination of condom and spermicidal agent is recommended for the adolescent engaging in intermittent sexual activity. This combination is relatively inexpensive, easily obtained, and highly effective for protection from pregnancy and sexually transmitted diseases.

Oral contraceptive pills are the contraceptive of choice for many adolescents early in their sexual careers because using pills is independent of sexual intercourse. Such hormonal methods are safe and highly effective, but because they afford essentially no protection against sexually transmitted diseases including HIV, the additional use of condoms with nonoxynol-9, a spermicide with some STD protection, is recommended. Oral contraceptives are associated with a number of minor side effects including nausea, breast tenderness, occasional weight gain, and breakthrough bleeding, especially within the first 3 months of use. However, there is now evidence that the progesterones in the new combined formulations (see below) markedly decrease such side effects. There are also absolute and relative contraindications for use of hormonal contraception, which must be compared on an individual basis to the risk for pregnancy. Absolute contraindications include abnormal vaginal bleeding of unknown cause, estrogen-dependent tumor, liver disease, thromboembolic disease, and cerebrovascular disorders. Relative contraindications include metabolic diseases such as diabetes mellitus, current seizures, vascular headaches (migraine), and marked hypertension. An immature hypothalamic-pituitary-ovarian axis as exhibited by a lack of regular menses for more than 12 to 18 months postmenarche is a relative contraindication because the risks with pregnancy probably outweigh the theoretical risk of hormonal contraceptive impact on the developing axis. Diseases of other organ systems that may be considered as contraindications to hormonal therapy include sickle cell disease, depression, and hepatic, pancreatic, cardiovascular, renal, and neurologic diseases. In addition, increased cardiovascular complications have been shown in older women of reproductive age who smoke. Major compliance problems with medical regimens may make oral contraception less than ideal.

Recent advances have been made in contraception. New fixed-combination oral contraceptive pills employing three new progestins derived from L-norgestrel (gestodene, nogestimate, desogestrel) are now available. These preparations have weak antiestrogenic and weak androgenic effects, have a longer half-life (18 to 58 hours), produce less breakthrough bleeding and amenorrhea, and have a positive effect on acne and lipids. Such formulations are excellent choices for the adolescent patient. Depo-medroxyprogesterone acetate has now been improved for contraceptive use and is given in a 150-mg IM dose every 3 months. This intramuscular preparation has all the benefits of oral progestins and can be used safely by lactating mothers.

Another advance in contraception has been achieved with the development of the L-norgestrel (36 mg) contraceptive implant. Consisting of the subcutaneous implantation of six silicone rubber capsules usually placed under the skin of the inner surface of the upper arm, this form of contraceptive is ideal for the patient desiring long-term (up to 5 years) contraception but not sterilization. Both depo-medroxyprogesterone and the L-norgestrel implant are excellent alternative contraceptive methods for those adolescents who want long-term contraception not linked to coitus, have compliance problems, are unable to use oral contraceptives, or cannot use estrogen-containing preparations. Possible progesterone-related side effects associated with these progesterone-only products include amenorrhea, breakthrough bleeding, acne, and depression. As with oral contraceptives, these formulas do not protect against STDs, and the adolescent should be encouraged to use condoms in addition.

EMERGENCY CONTRACEPTION

Regimens for emergency contraception (postcoital contraception) have been known and well accepted in countries other than the United States for years. However, more recently there has been an effort to educate health professionals and young women (and young men) about its effectiveness and availability. Although not well studied, it is felt that the most commonly used medications (combined oral contraceptive pills) work in a number of ways including the prevention of ovulation and implantation. Formats have included using the fixed dosage first reported by Yuzpe of 100 μg of ethinyl estradiol and 1.0 mg of norgestrel divided into two doses 12 hours apart. Common side effects include significant nausea and vomiting and menstrual irregularities. Dosage regimens are outlined in Table 3-15. The Yuzpe method prevents approximately 74% of expected pregnancies, but this rate decreases to about 58% as the interval from unprotected sexual intercourse increases from 1 to 3 days. It is therefore imperative to educate those at risk to be evaluated and treated as soon as possible up to 72 hours after unprotected sexual intercourse. Other methods include using a progestin-only format, which has fewer side effects and has been shown to prevent 94% of expected pregnancies if used within 24 hours of sexual intercourse. However, this progestin-only format requires taking 40 pills (20 tablets to start and 20 tablets 12 hours later). Finally, mifepristone (RU-486) has been shown to prevent up to 100% of pregnancies when taken within 72 hours; has few side effects, which have been shown to be dose related; and does not decrease in effectiveness as the time interval from intercourse to treatment increases to 72 hours.

Evaluation of the perspective at-risk adolescent includes determination of risk (unprotected sexual intercourse at midcycle), performing a pregnancy test to eliminate the possibility of an existing pregnancy if necessary, and determining if there are any medical indications to prevent the use of a short course of high-dose estrogen (if choosing the most common formats). Although many

TABLE 3-15

COMMON REGIMENS FOR EMERGENCY CONTRACEPTION

I. COMBINED PILL	(100 μg ethinyl estradiol plus 0.5−1.0 mg norgestrel)
Fixed dosage	
Ovral®	2 tabs start, repeat in 12h
LoOvral®	4 tabs start, repeat in 12h
Preven®	2 tabs start, repeat in 12h
Nordette®	4 tabs start, repeat in 12h
Levlen®	
Levora®	
Alesse®	5 tabs start, repeat in 12h
Triphasic	
Tri-Levlen®	4 tabs start, repeat in 12h
Tri-Levora®	(yellow tabs only)
Triphasil®	
II. PROGESTIN-ONLY PILL	0.075 mg norgestrel (equals 0.0375 L-norgestrel)
Ovrette®	20 tabs start, repeat in 12h
III. PROGESTERONE ANTAGONIST	200 mg mifepristone (RU-486)

young women and their physicians are concerned about short-and long-term sequelae of taking high-dose hormones, no data support these concerns as emergency contraception has been shown to be effective and very safe. Although carefully studied to date in adolescents, it does not appear that the availability of emergency contraception discourages the use of more consistent and long-term contraception. Some clinicians give their more mature adolescents and young adult patients a prescription for, or a prepackaged packet of, emergency contraception to be used after a telephone consult with the clinician in order to minimize the time interval to treatment. Others prefer to have the adolescent evaluated in an urgent care setting before prescribing the emergency contraception.

MEDICAL ASSESSMENT AT THE CONTRACEPTIVE VISIT

A complete medical and sexual history and physical assessment, including a pelvic examination (see Sec. 3.4), are recommended as a part of the first contraceptive visit to evaluate specific needs and eliminate serious contraindications to contraceptive use, especially hormonal. Laboratory screening tests should include a urinalysis, serum triglycerides and cholesterol, and a Papanicolaou smear when possible. Pregnancy testing should be done when indicated. Screening for sexually transmitted disease, especially chlamydia and gonorrhea, should be done for both female and male teenagers (see Sec. 3.6.1). To ensure compliance with any method recommended, the first follow-up contraceptive visit should be scheduled approximately 1 month later. For girls using oral contraceptives, the follow-up schedule for the first year includes assessments at 1, 3, 6, and 12 months. For girls using IM progesterone, follow-up is done at each visit for medication (every 3 months). Implant patients should be followed as needed every 3 to 6 months. Weight and blood pressure should be recorded at each visit. A discussion of any side effects and difficulties in taking the medication and the need for continued contraception should be reviewed briefly with the patient at each visit. For the male adolescent, a brief review of need and type of contraceptive should be done at each well visit.

References

Common Reproductive Health Problems

Breast Masses (Female)

Diehl T, Kaplan DW: Breast masses in adolescent females. J Adolesc Health Care 6:353, 1985

Drukker BH, deMendonca WC: Fibrocystic change and fibrocystic disease of the breast. Obstet Gynecol Clin North Am 14:685, 1987

Frank JW, Mai V: Breast self-examination in young women: More harm than good? Lancet 2:654−657, 1985

Greydanus DE, Parks DS, Farrell EG: Breast disorders in children and adolescents. Pediatr Clin North Am 36:601, 1989

Minton JP, Foecking MK, Mathews RH, et al: Caffeine, cyclic nucleotide and breast disease. Surgery 86:105, 1979

Neinstein LS: Breast disease in adolescents and young women. Adolescent gynecology: Part 1. Common disorders. Pediatr Clin North Am 46(3): 607−629, 1999

Osuch JR: Benign lesions of the breast other than fibrocystic change. Obstet Gynecol Clin North Am 14:703, 1987

Rohan TE, Cook MG, McMichael AJ: Methylxanthines and benign epithelial disorders of the breast in women. Int J Epidemiol 18:626, 1989

Schairer C, Brinton LA, Hoover RN: Methylxanthines and benign breast disease. Am J Epidemiol 124:603, 1986

US Department of Health and Human Resources: Surveillance Epidemiology End Results, Incidence and Mortality Data 1973−1977. NCI Monograph 57, June 1981

Williams SM, Kaplan PA, Peterson JC: Mammography in women under age 30. Radiology 161:49, 1986

Gynecomastia

Mahoney PC: Adolescent gynecomastia: Differential diagnosis and management. Pediatr Clin North Am 37(6):1389−1404, 1990

Simmons PS: Diagnostic considerations in breast disorders of children and adolescents. Obstet Gynecol Clin North Am 19(1):91−102, 1992

Zachmann M, Eiholzer U, Muritano M, et al: Treatment of pubertal gynecomastia with testolactone. Acta Endocrinol 279(suppl):218, 1986

Scrotal Masses

Edelberg J, Surh Y: The acute serotum. Emerg Med Clin North Am 6:521−546, 1988

Kapphahn C, Schlossberger N: Male reproductive health: painful scrotal masses (part 1). Adolesc Health Update 4(3):1−8, 1992

Kapphahn C, Schlossberger N: Male reproductive health: painless scrotal masses (part 2). Adolesc Health Update 5(1):1−8, 1992

Muller G, Skakkebaek NE: The prenatal and postnatal development of the testis. In: deKretser DM, guest ed: The Testis. Balliere's Clin Endocrinol Metab 6(2):251−271, 1992

Peckham M: Testicular cancer. Acta Oncol 27:439−453, 1988

Sheldon CA: Undescended testis and testicular torsion. Surg Clin North Am 65(5):1303, 1985

Tumeh S, Benson C, Richie J: Acute diseases of the scrotum. Semin Ultrasound, CT, MR 12:115−130, 1991

Common Menstrual Problems

Coupey SM, Ahlstrom P: Common menstrual disorders. Pediatr Clin North Am 36:551−571, 1989

Davis S: Pregnancy in adolescents. Pediatr Clin North Am 36:665–680, 1989

Speroff L, Glass RH, Kase NG, eds: Menstrual disorders. In: Clinical Gynecologic Endocrinology and Infertility, 6th ed. Baltimore, Lippincott Williams & Wilkins, 1999, 557–574

Stephenson JN: Pregnancy testing and counseling. Pediatr Clin North Am 36:681–696, 1989

Pregnancy and Contraception

Ammerman S, Shafer MA, Snyder D: Ectopic pregnancy in adolescents. J Pediatr 117:677–686, 1990

Anon: Depo-medroxyprogesterone acetate: an overview of DMPA and its FDA approval. Contracept Rep 3:4–8, 1992

Buster JE, Pisarska MD: Medical management of ectopic pregnancy. Clin Obstet Gynecol 42:22–30, 1999

Carson SA, Buster JE: Ectopic pregnancy. N Engl J Med 329:1175–1181, 1993

Chow WH, Daling JR, Cates W, et al: Epidemiology of ectopic pregnancy. Epidemiol Rev 9:70–94, 1987

Darney PD: Hormonal implants: contraception for a new century. Obstet Gynecol 170:1536–43, 1994

Ectopic pregnancy—United States, 1988–1989. Morb Mortal Wkly Rep 41:591–594, 1992

Ectopic pregnancy. ACOG Tech Bull 150:1–7, 1990

Ellertson C, Shochet T, Blanchard K, Trussell J: Emergency contraception: a review of the programmatic and social science literature. Contraception, 61(3):145, 2000

Gaspard V: Metabolic effects of oral contraceptives. Am J Obstet Gynecol 157:1029, 1987

Gelletlie R, Nielson JB: Evaluation and comparison of commercially available pregnancy tests based on monoclonal antibodies to human choriogonadotropin. Clin Chem 32:2166–2170, 1986

Gold MA: Prescribing and managing oral contraceptive pills and emergency contraception for adolescents. Ped Clin N Am 1999; 46:695.

Hatcher RA, Trussel J, Stewart F, et al: Contraceptive Technology, 17th rev ed. New York, Ardent Media Inc, 1998

Ho PC: Emergency contraception: methods and efficacy. Curr Opin Obstet Gynecol 12(3):175, 2000

London RS: The new era in oral contraception: Pills containing gestogene, norgestimate, and desogestrel. Obstet Gynecol Survey 47(11):777–782, 1992

Mishell DM, Fisher HW, Haynes PJ, et al: Menorrhagia: A symposium. J Reprod Med 29:763–782, 1984

Owens PR: Prostaglandin synthetase inhibitors in the treatment of primary dysmenorrhea: Outcome trials reviewed. Am J Obstet Gynecol 148:96, 1984

Pisarska MD, Carson SA: Incidence and risk factors for ectopic pregnancy. Clin Obstet Gynecol 42:2–8, 1999

Rebar RW, Zeserson K: Characteristics of the new progestins in combination oral contraceptives. Contraception 44:1–10, 1991

Reindeollar RH, Novak M, Tho SPT, McDonough PG: Adult onset amenorrhea: A study of 262 patients. Am J Obstet Gynecol 155:531, 1986

Stevens-Simons C: Reproductive health care and contraceptives. Pediatr Rev 19:399–478, 1998

Taylor RN: Ectopic pregnancy and reproductive technology. JAMA 259:1862–1864, 1988

The Contraceptive Report: Health benefits of oral contraceptives. Emerg Contracept Options 8(2), May 1997

Trussel J, Kost K: Contraceptive failure in the United States: A critical review of the literature. Stud Family Plan 18:237–238, 1987

Trussell J, Rodriguez G, Ellertson C: Updated estimates of the effectiveness of the Yuzpe regimen of emergency contraception. Contraception 59:147, 1999

Washington AE, Gove S, Schachter R: Oral contraceptives, *Chlamydia trachomatis* infection and pelvic inflammatory disease. JAMA 253:2246, 1985

3.6   SEXUALLY TRANSMITTED INFECTIONS

Mary-Ann Shafer and Anna-Barbara Moscicki

Currently, more adolescents are engaging in sexual intercourse than 15 years ago: 50% have experienced their sexual debut by age 16 and 75% by 19 years of age. An increase in the prevalence of reported sexually transmitted infections (STIs) has accompanied a changing pattern of adolescent sexual activity.

The STDs are epidemic among teenagers, who represent 3 million STI cases reported annually in the United States. The STDs place our youth at risk for pelvic inflammatory disease and associated sequelae of ectopic pregnancy and infertility, genital cancers, and even death through complications of STIs, especially HIV infection. Therefore, pediatricians must be able to recognize symptomatic STIs; screen and treat STIs, both symptomatic and asymptomatic; and prevent STIs among youth.

PREVALENCE

Commonly reported prevalences of STIs among sexually active adolescent girls both with and without lower genital tract symptoms include *Chlamydia trachomatis* (10 to 25%), *Neisseria gonorrhoeae* (3 to 18%), syphilis (0 to 3%), *Trichomonas vaginalis* (8 to 16%), and herpes simplex virus (2 to 12%). Among adolescent boys with no symptoms of urethritis, isolation rates include *C. trachomatis* (9 to 11%) and *N. gonorrhoeae* (2 to 3%).

By use of molecular genetic techniques, human papillomavirus (HPV) DNA has been detected in 20 to 60% of female adolescents. The increasing rate of SIL among young women is an indicator of the impact of STIs on young women. The highest incidence of LSIL occurs in women aged 15 to 19 years.

Although adolescents currently represent fewer than 1% of reported cases of acquired immunodeficiency syndrome (AIDS) in the United States, the number of cases among ages 20 to 24 is tenfold greater. Because of the long latency period of the disease (2 to 7 years or more), it is probable that many young adults with AIDS acquired their HIV infections during adolescence. The HIV seropositivity data available from screening programs show a rate of <1/1000 for military recruits, 3.6/1000 for Job Corps applicants, and 50/1000 for runaway youth. The greatest increase in new AIDS cases is among heterosexuals, including adolescents.

AGE, GENDER, ETHNICITY

Gonorrhea rates, used as a measurable indicator of STD risk, continue to show that adolescents have the highest rate of reportable STIs relative to sexual activity. From individual studies and sentinel centers, it is obvious that adolescents have the highest rate of chlamydial infections, with females having the associated morbidities of pelvic inflammatory disease (PID) and ectopic pregnancy. Gender is an important factor in the epidemiology of STIs because both the rates of infection and sequelae are disproportionately higher among females compared to males. In 1997, among 15- to 19-year-olds, the female:male ratio for chlamydia was 7.7, for gonorrhea 2.0, and for primary and secondary syphilis 2.2. During the same year the ratios of gonorrhea for African-American, Native American, Hispanic and white youth were 25:3:2:1. The ratios for primary and secondary syphilis among these same groups were 40:10:4:1, and for chlamydia the ratios were 7:4:2:1.

Trends in rates of gonorrhea among youth show a decrease over the past 10 years. Between 1990 and 1997, the gonorrhea rate has decreased about 46% among youth. However, rates from 1994 to 1997 show little to no change among 15- to 19-year-old Native Americans and Hispanic males and small increases in Native American and Hispanic females. It is important to note that the relationships between the ethnicity and STIs including AIDS have been confounded by socioeconomic factors. In addition to age, gender, and ethnicity, a number of important biological and behavioral factors may help to explain these epidemic rates of STIs among adolescents.

CONTRACEPTIVES AND SEXUALLY TRANSMITTED DISEASES

Condoms have been shown consistently to prevent STDs, especially gonococcal and chlamydial infections, and assist in preventing HIV infection as well. Inadequate contraceptive use by adolescents is reflected in the high pregnancy and STD rates in this age group. Only one-third of female and one-half of male adolescents reported using condoms at last intercourse.

In addition to condoms, spermicides have also been shown to inhibit some STD agents. Nonoxynol-9, a major component of many spermicides, acts as a surfactant to destroy the STD agent's cell walls and has been shown to inhibit *N. gonorrhoeae, Treponema pallidum, T. vaginalis, Candida,* and herpes simplex virus I and II in studies in vitro. Nonoxynol-9 has also been shown to kill HIV. Although a combination of a barrier method of contraception (condoms, diaphragms) and a spermicide seems to be the most effective protection against STDs for adolescents, fewer than 10% of adolescents use spermicides and fewer than a third use condoms.

Oral contraceptives have been linked to some STD infections. For example, candidal infections have long been associated with oral contraceptive use. Controversy surrounds the role of oral contraceptives and the establishment of endocervical infection and development of PID with *N. gonorrhoeae* and *C. trachomatis.* It appears that oral contraceptive users have fewer gonococcal endocervical infections, and when gonococcal PID occurs, it is less severe. The impact of oral contraceptives on the establishment of chlamydial endocervical infections is less clear, but most authors show an increased risk for chlamydial infection among oral contraceptive users. Oral contraceptive users, however, appear to have less chlamydial PID.

CLINICAL ASPECTS OF SEXUALLY TRANSMITTED DISEASES

An overview of STDs by agents, pathogenesis, common clinical syndromes, diagnosis, and treatment is outlined in Table 3-16 for common bacterial, fungal, and viral infections.

3.6.1   Bacterial Infections

NEISSERIA GONORRHOEAE

Pathogenesis

Neisseria gonorrhoeae is a gram-negative bacterium that has the unique genetic ability to change the antigenic expression of its surface-exposed proteins. This ability has made the development of a gonococcal vaccine difficult. The pathogenesis of infection includes the presence of pili, which are hair-like appendages needed for attachment, and the lipooligosaccharide (LOS) gonococcal endotoxin, which damages host epithelial cells such as fallopian tube cells.

Clinical Syndromes

The most common manifestation of gonococcal disease among men is urethritis, which may be asymptomatic. After urethral inoculation with the organism during sexual activity, it is estimated that 2 to 4 days elapse before symptoms of dysuria and/or discharge appear. The discharge may be scant and mucoid or may present as a profuse purulent discharge. Untreated gonococcal urethritis in men typically resolves over 1 to 2 months but may progress in up to 10% of cases to acute epididymitis and urethral strictures. An outline of the evaluation of urethritis is presented in Fig. 3-6.

Although women have urethral infections, they are usually associated with endocervical infection. Most gonococcal infections in women affect the lower genital tract with a particular predilection for the columnar cells of the endocervix. Syndromes in both men and women are outlined in Table 3-16. In particular, disseminated gonococcal infection (DGI), a blood-borne infection manifested by skin lesions, tenosynovitis, and/or septic arthritis (culture-positive joint fluid in approximately 50% of cases only), occurs in 2 to 5% of infected individuals. However, it is more common in African-Americans than in other race/ethnicity groups. Pelvic inflammatory disease is another important complication of gonococcal infection and is discussed in Sec. 3.6.5.

Diagnosis and Treatment

Diagnostic tests are outlined in Table 3-16, evaluation of both urethritis and vaginitis is found in Figs. 3-6 and 3-7, and treatment regimens are summarized in Table 3-17. As stated by the Centers for Disease Control in the STD treatment guidelines (1993), treatment of gonococcal infections in the United States is based on the following: (1) the anatomic site of infection; (2) the antibiotic resistance [penicillinase-producing strains (PPNG), tetracycline-resistant strains (TRNG), and chromosomally mediated resistance to multiple antibiotics]; (3) high prevalence of concurrent chlamydial infections in patients with gonococcal infection; and (4) the side effects and costs of different treatment regimens. While treating for gonorrhea, screen for syphilis by serology. Treatment regimens that include ceftriaxone or a 7-day course of doxycycline (or erythromycin) may be effective against incubating syphilis, but few studies are available. Therefore, all patients with an STD should be screened for syphilis serologically.

Treatment for disseminated gonococcal infection (DGI) requires initial parenteral therapy and evaluation for possible meningitis or endocarditis. The recommended regimen is ceftriaxone, 1 g IM or IV q24h; an alternative regimen (allergy to β-lactams) is spectinomycin, 2 g IM q12h. Compliant patients may be discharged in 24 to 48 hours after symptom resolution or oral medication to complete a total 7-day course using ciprofloxacin, 500 mg BID PO (if not pregnant), or cefixime, 400 mg PO BID, or ofloxacin, 100 mg PO bid.

CHLAMYDIA TRACHOMATIS

Pathogenesis

The pathogenesis of *C. trachomatis* infections has not been clearly defined. Chlamydiae are obligate intracellular parasites, and disease

TABLE 3-16

COMMON SEXUALLY TRANSMITTED DISEASES IN ADOLESCENTS

NAME	PATHOGENESIS	COMMON SYNDROMES	DIAGNOSIS	TREATMENT[a]	COMMENTS
I. Bacterial					
Neisseria gonorrhoeae (Gonorrhea) Gram (−) diplococcus (Sec. 3.6.1)	Genetic ability to frequently change antigenic surface structures	*Uncomplicated* Urethritis Endocervicitis Pharyngitis Proctitis Conjunctivitis *Complicated* Disseminated gonococcal infection PID Epididymitis	*Male: Urethritis* Gram stain [Gram (−) intracellular diplococci] Culture *Female: Cervicitis* Endocervical culture Gram stain but ↓ sensitivity DNA probe and NAATs applied to genital and FCU specimens[d]	See Table 3-17[b]	Many asymptomatic infections in men and women Screen all gonorrhea patients for syphilis, chlamydia; R/O HIV
Chlamydia trachomatis (Chlamydia) (Sec. 3.6.1)	Obligate intracellular bacteria that cause cell damage directly at end of their growth cycle and indirectly by stimulation of inflammatory host immune response	*Uncomplicated* Endocervicitis Urethritis Proctitis Conjunctivitis *Complicated* PID Pharyngitis Epididymitis	*Male: Nongonococcal urethritis* (NGU) Negative gonococcal culture and/or Gram stain ≥ 4 PMNs/oil (mean of 5 hpf × 1000×) immersion and no GNID Urethral culture (+) Nonculture tests *Female: Endocervicitis* Mucopus and/or ≥ 10–30 PMNs/hpf on Gram stain (confirm with specific chlamydia test) DNA probe and NAATs applied to genital and FCU specimens	See Table 3–17[b]	Many asymptomatic infections in men and women; most common cause of urethritis in adolescent boys and cervicitis in adolescent girls
Treponema pallidum (Syphilis) (See Sec. 13.2.33)	Enters through small abrasions in mucosa during intercourse and stimulates a local immune response and spreads hematogenously (secondary)	*Primary:* chancre *Secondary:* generalized skin rash especially palms and soles *Early, late latent, and tertiary:* rare in adolescents	*Primary:* treponemes on dark-field microscopy *Secondary:* VDRL or RPR, confirmed by FTA-ABS or MHA-TP (Sec. 13.2.33)	Benzathine[b] Pen G: 2.4 × 10⁶ UI IM or, if penicillin allergy, Doxycycline 100 mg PO BID or Tetracycline 500 mg PO qid × 14 days	Screen with VDRL or RPR if contact history, at diagnosis of any STD, or in population with high syphilis rate; penicillin in pregnancy; screen for HIV.
II. Viral					
Herpes simplex virus (HSV) (Sec. 13.4.6) HSV type 1 HSV type 2	Enters host through mucosa or abraded epithelium Replicates in host cell nucleus Predilection for sensory autonomic nerve cells Latency, reactivation states Host immune response related to disease severity	Genital herpes Primary (systemic) Recurrent (local) Vulvovaginitis Cervicitis Proctitis Penile lesions Urethritis Oropharyngitis	1. Based on symptoms and signs at presentation 2. HSV culture with fluorescent antibody	1. Primary: acyclovir 200 mg PO 5 × day for 7–10 days or until resolved 2. Recurrent: see CDC Treatment Guidelines	Infection in clinical presentation in adolescents often primary disease

(continued)

Benzathine[b] Pen G: 2.4 × 10⁶

TABLE 3-16 Continued

NAME	PATHOGENESIS	COMMON SYNDROMES	DIAGNOSIS	TREATMENT[a]	COMMENTS
Human papillomavirus (HPV)	Requires direct access to basal epithelial cells, eg, transformation zone of the cervix and active cellular replication to sustain viral replication which result in the cytohistologic manifestations	*Condyloma acuminata* Visible genital skin wart *Subclinical HPV* Flat condylomas invisible to unaided eye that occur anywhere in anogenital tract	*Condyloma acuminata* Visible inspection of genital skin *Subclinical HPV* Pretreat area—3% acetic acid wash Colposcopic (magnify) examination: dense, white areas: HPV HPV DNA detection (hybridization techniques)	Based on type, location, extent *condyloma acuminata*: Podophyllin, liquid nitrogen TCA (85% trichloroacetic acid) Extensive/recalcitrant: topical 5-FU, interferon, laser Subclinical HPV (LGSIL/ HGSIL): Refer for TCA, 5-FU, cryotherapy, laser, LEEP	*Condyloma acuminata* Liquid nitrogen: pain on application Podophyllin: systemic toxicity, teratogenicity precludes use on mucosa and pregnancy TCA: Safe with mucosa and pregnancy; local sensitivity LGSIL/HGSIL: Refer all patients with visible warts for evaluation and treatment
III. Fungal/protozoal *Candida albicans*	Unclear mechanisms: Host factors Disease states Medications	Vulvovaginitis Balanitis	1. Symptoms of vulvovaginitis 2. Presence of pseudohyphae in KOH preparation or Gram stain (only 40% accurate) 3. Vaginal pH < 4.5 4. Culture prn	Clotrimazole,[b,c] two 100-mg vaginal tablets hs for 3 doses or 500-mg vaginal tablet once	Controversy over diagnosis of disease when *Candida* present and asymptomatic
Trichomonas vaginalis	Unclear mechanisms: Host factors Local environment Asymptomatic carrier	Vaginitis Cervicitis Urethritis	1. Symptoms of vulvovaginitis 2. Vaginal pH > 5.0 3. Trichomonads (motile) on NaCl wet mount, PAP smear, direct culture, or by direct monoclonal antibody technique	Metronidazole: 2.0 g PO once (nonpregnant)[b] or 500 mg BID for 7 days	Classic frothy yellow-green discharge found in only 12%, and "strawberry cervix" or punctate hemorrhages on exocervix seen in only 2%

[a] Screen and treat all partners and encourage use of condoms.
[b] STD treatment guidelines, Centers for Disease Control, 1993.
[c] Other comparable medications include butoconazole, miconazole, tioconazole, and terconazole; most creams are oil-based and may weaken latex condoms; over-the-counter preparations are available, but self- medication by the adolescent is not encouraged because of the risk of other STDs causing symptoms.
[d] NAATs = nucleic acid amplification tests, eg, ligase or polymerase chain reactions; FCU = first-catch urine (first 10–20 mL urine)
5-FU = 5-fluorouracil; GNID = gram-negative intracellular diplococci
LGSIL = low-grade squamous intraepithelial lesion
HGSIL = high-grade squamous intraepithelial lesion
LEEP == loop electrosurgical excision procedure

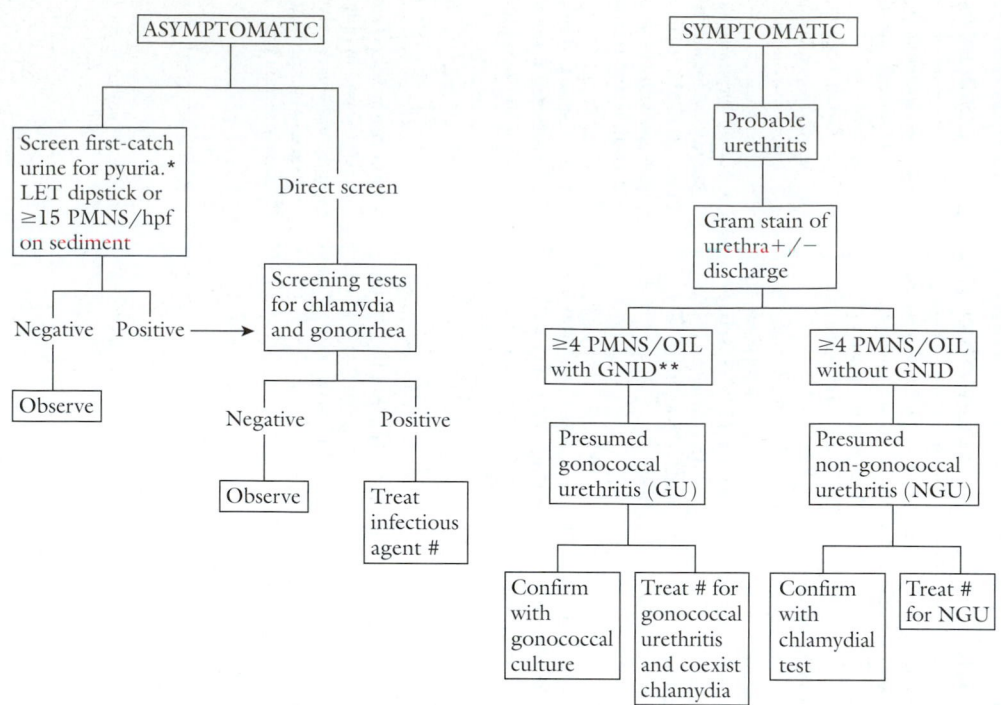

FIGURE 3-6 Assessment of urethritis in sexually active male adolescents. *First 15 mL of micturition of urine sample tested. (a) Spun-resuspended shows ≥10 polymorphonuclear leukocytes per high-power field, or (b) unspun urinary leukocyte esterase test (LET) for activity. **GNID = Gram-negative intracellular diplococci; # = do partner tracing to refer for evaluation and treatment; PMNS = polymorphonuclear leukocytes.

appears to result from both the destruction of cells during the growth cycle and the body's immune response to the infection producing inflammation.

Clinical Syndromes

Uncomplicated infections include asymptomatic and symptomatic urethritis in men and women. In men, 20 to 50% of those with gonococcal urethritis are also infected with *Chlamydia. Chlamydia* is responsible for 23 to 55% of nongonococcal urethritis in men, with higher rates among young boys. Endocervicitis is the most common clinical manifestation of infection in sexually active female adolescents. Pelvic inflammatory disease presents as the most serious complication of endocervical infection, including a subclinical form that lacks the typical symptoms, which may also lead to infertility. An overview of syndromes, diagnosis, and treatment is found in Tables 3-16 and 3-17.

C. trachomatis is the most common cause of nongonococcal urethritis (NGU) in men. Men with NGU may present with discharge and dysuria. The infection is identified through contact tracing from a chlamydial-positive partner or often by screening of symptomatic men. Among women, 50% or more of chlamydial lower genital infections are asymptomatic. An uncomplicated endocervicitis can be associated with the clinical signs consistent with mucopurulent cervicitis (MCP), which presents with a yellow endocervical discharge on a swab sample or by identification of increased polymorphonuclear cells on a Gram stain from the discharge (more than 10–30 per high-power field). Although it is asymptomatic in many young women, chlamydial cervicitis is sometimes accompanied by abnormal vaginal discharge and abnormal vaginal bleeding, especially after intercourse. *Chlamydia* has been identified in from 9 to 51% of MPC cases, and the gonococcus is

also responsible for some cases as well. However, MPC is not a sensitive indicator of infection because most women with either chlamydial or gonorrheal endocervical infection do not have MPC. Diagnosis by direct testing for *Chlamydia*, when possible, is encouraged (Table 3-16). *Candida albicans, Trichomonas vaginalis,* human papillomavirus, and herpes simplex virus can also produce urethritis in men and women as well as endocervicitis in women.

Diagnosis and Treatment

There are a number of situations such as NGU, PID, epididymitis, and confirmed gonococcal infection (5 to 30% of men and 25 to 50% of women with gonorrhea have concurrent chlamydia) that are associated frequently with chlamydia infections and necessitate immediate "presumptive" treatment to alleviate symptoms and to prevent complications and further transmission to partners. However, chlamydia testing and partner tracing and treatment should still be undertaken when possible. Testing for chlamydia is performed by using either the traditional "gold standard"—the cell culture—or the newer nonculture techniques. Although cell culture is being surpassed by nonculture techniques, the following conditions warrant the continued use of cell culture as the test of choice because nonculture methods have not been developed, have been inadequately tested, or yield poor performance profiles in these situations: urethral and rectal specimens in men and women and vaginal specimens in prepubertal girls.

Currently available tests for *Chlamydia* include the direct fluorescent antibody (DFA) test, the enzyme immunoassay (EIA) test, the DNA probe test, the rapid chlamydia test, and the leukocyte esterase dipstick test (LET). Except for the MicroTrak DFA (Syva) test and the Chlamydiazyme EIA (Abbott) test, evaluation by available tests is limited. Quality assurance is essential to the perfor-

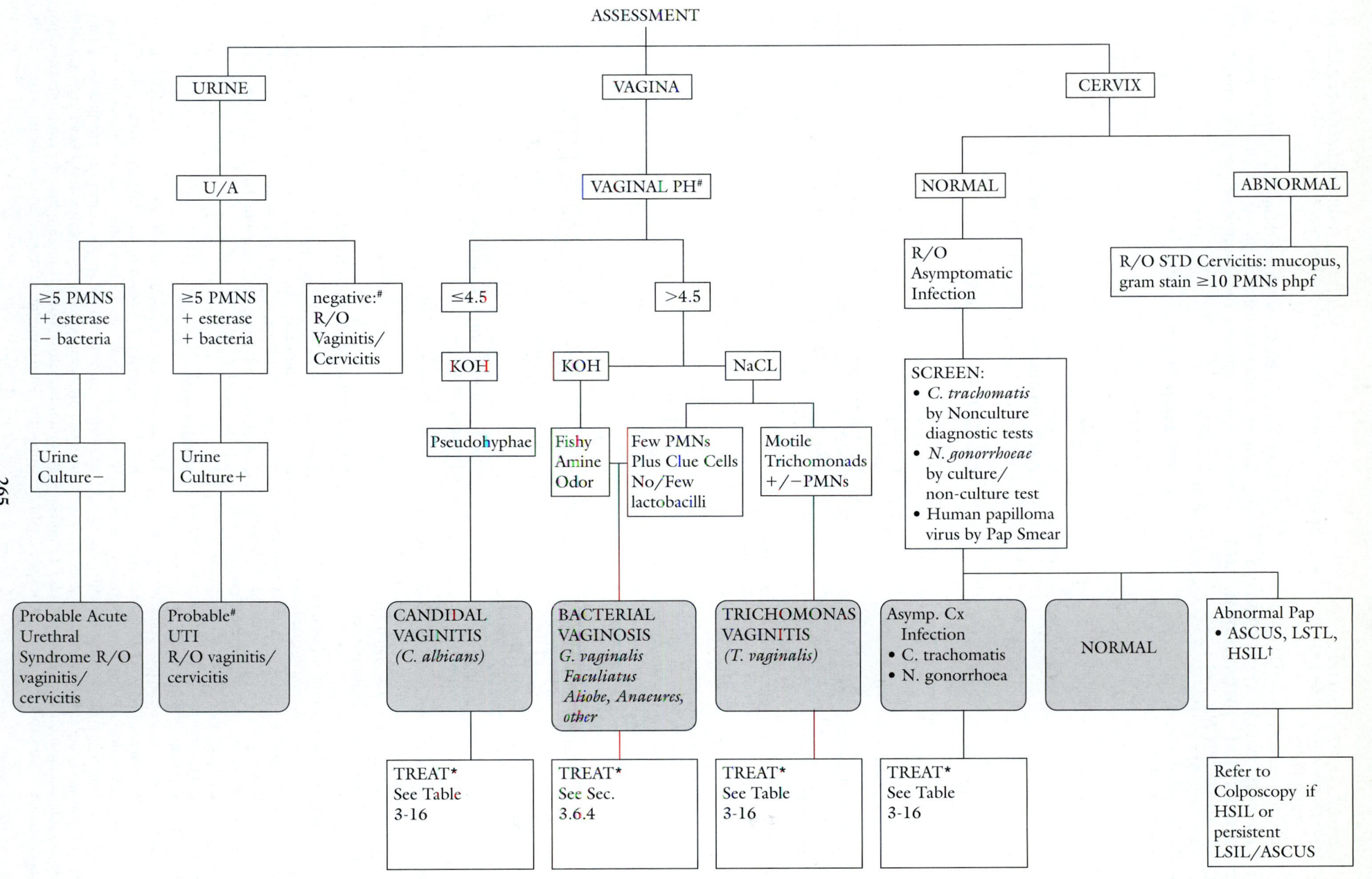

FIGURE 3-7 Assessment of lower genital tract infection in sexually active female adolescents. This should be done whether or not symptoms are present. #Vaginal discharge, pruritus, dysuria/frequency; *R/O pregnancy before treatment. PMNS = polymorphonuclear leukocytes. †Abnormal Pap smear with ASCUS or LSIL should be repeated in 3–4 months. If it persists, refer to colposcopy. ASCUS = atypical squamous cells of undetermined significance; HSIL = high-grade intraepithelial lesion; LSIL = low-grade intraepithelial lesion; R/O = rule out; UTI = urinary tract infection.

TABLE 3-17

TREATMENT OF UNCOMPLICATED GENITAL, ANAL, AND PHARYNGEAL[b] CHLAMYDIAL AND GONOCOCCAL INFECTIONS

For uncomplicated chlamydial infection:
   azithromycin 1 g orally × 1 dose[a]
                    or
   doxycycline 100 mg orally twice daily × 7 days
For uncomplicated gonococcal infection:
   cefixime 400 mg orally × 1 dose[a]
                    or
   ceftriaxone 125 mg IM × 1 dose[b]
                    or
   ciprofloxacin 500 mg orally × 1 dose[a–d]
                    or
   ofloxacin 400 mg orally × 1 dose[a,c,d]
                   plus
   (always treat for possible chlamydial coinfection)
   azithromycin 1 g orally × 1 dose[a]
                    or
   doxycycline 100 mg orally twice daily × 7 days
For pregnancy:
   erythromycin base 500 mg PO qid × 7 days;
                    or
   amoxicillin 500 mg PO qid × 7 days
For sexual partners:
   Contact, evaluate, and treat partners in the past 30 days for symptomatic (past 60 days for asymptomatic) infections for both chlamydial
   and gonococcal disease. Condoms should be used.
For follow-up:
   Although not currently recommended by CDC, 4–7 days after treatment test of cure can be considered when compliance is not assured
   or documentation of partner(s) treatment is not possible.

---

[a] It is now possible to treat both uncomplicated chlamydial and gonococcal infections with one-dose oral regimens. Cost factors must be evaluated locally. The effect of such regimens on incubating syphilis is not known. Although azithromycin and ofloxacin have been FDA-approved for those 16 years or older and 18 years or older, respectively, recent studies have shown them to be safe in younger adolescents as well.
[b] ≥ 90% effective against gonococcal pharyngitis.
[c] When STD identified, screen for syphilis by serology. Quinolones are not active against *T. pallidum*, are not contraindicated in pregnant/lactating women and in those ≤ 17 years (however, they have been used safely in adolescents).
[d] Pregnant women should not be treated with quinolones.

mance of any tests, especially the nonculture techniques, where false-positive results can lead to adverse psychosocial outcomes for the patient and partner. It is therefore essential for the clinician to know the performance capabilities of both the test and the laboratory being employed.

There had been increased interest in evaluation of the nonculture test on urine specimens. The *Chlamydia*-specific tests, such as the currently available EIA and DNA probe tests, show promise in their ability to detect *Chlamydia* in a urine specimen. More recently the new technologies—including the polymerase chain reaction (PCR) and the ligase chain reaction (LCR) with their capacity to amplify *Chlamydia* DNA in specimens—have also been applied to urine specimens with early success. Of interest to the primary-care clinician is the ability to screen asymptomatic adolescent boys with the nonspecific LET applied to the first-void urine specimen (first 10 to 15 mL voided into premarked container) for urethritis, which is most frequently caused by chlamydia or gonorrhea. Because the sensitivity of the LET in screening for chlamydia and gonorrhea is 46 to 100% (it is a nonspecific indicator of the presence of polymorphonuclear cells), it is necessary to follow up all positive LETs

with more specific gonorrhea and chlamydial tests (eg, EIAs, DFA). Data are insufficient to support the use of the LET to screen young women for chlamydia. The treatment protocols are outlined in Table 3-17.

TREPONEMA PALLIDUM

Treponema pallidum, the etiologic agent of syphilis, is a member of the order of Spirochaetales. The pathogenesis, common syndromes, diagnosis, and treatment are discussed in detail in Sec. 13.2.33.

3.6.2   Protozoan and Fungal Infections

CANDIDA ALBICANS

Among the 500 species of yeast that have been isolated from humans, 90% are pathogenic, and 50% cause genital infections. Approximately 90% of candidal species detected in vaginal secretions are *C. albicans*. Of the remaining 10% non-*albicans* species, *C. glabrata* (*Torulopsis*) is the next most common. Vulvocandidiasis (VVC) caused by the *albicans* and non-*albicans* species are identical with the non-*albicans* species more resistant to therapy. It is estimated that 75% of women will have one episode of VVC, with 40 to 45% having a recurrence, and about 5% will have retractable infection. Although sexual transmission of *C. albicans* occurs, the role of such transmission in promoting infection among sexually active women is unclear.

Pathogenesis

The pathogenic mechanism of *Candida* infection has yet to be defined. Colonization occurs mainly from perianal areas. Although the number of organisms is not related to production of disease, other factors are related to establishment of infection, including host factors, disease states (eg, diabetes mellitus, AIDS), medications, oral contraception, and degree of the organism's adherence to vaginal epithelia.

Clinical Syndromes, Diagnosis, and Treatment

These topics are reviewed in Table 3-16. Although it is nonspecific, the most common symptom related to infection is vulvovaginal itching with or without vaginal discharge.

TRICHOMONAS VAGINALIS

Trichomonads are flagellated protozoans with three species linked to disease in humans: *Trichomonas tenax* (mouth): *Pentatrichomonas hominis* (intestine), and *Trichomonas vaginalis* (genital organs of men and women). *T. vaginalis* has been shown to be sexually transmitted.

Pathogenesis

The pathogenesis of disease in humans is not completely understood. *T. vaginalis* is known to attach to epithelial cells. The response to infection varies from little or no reaction (carrier state) to an acute inflammatory response marked by the presence of numerous polymorphonuclear leukocytes. It is known that half of all asymptomatic carriers of *T. vaginalis* become symptomatic within 6 months. Development of disease appears to be related to the menstrual period, pubertal development, vaginal pH, environmental microbiological flora, and gender.

Clinical Syndromes

Syndromes associated with the organism include vaginitis and cervicitis in women and urethritis in both men and women. In women, genitourinary symptoms include vaginal discharge, dyspareunia, pruritus, lower abdominal pain, dysuria, and frequency. On examination, the vulva is often erythematous, and copious vaginal discharge may be present. On speculum examination, the vaginal walls appear granular in over half the cases. Although a discharge is common, the "classical" frothy yellow-green discharge occurs in only 12% and has been described in other causes of vaginitis. The "strawberry cervix" (punctate hemorrhages on the exocervix), which was erroneously considered pathognomonic for *T. vaginalis* cervicitis, occurs in only 2% of the infections. In men, the infection is usually self-limited, and most men are asymptomatic or present with features of nongonococcal urethritis (Table 3-16). Infrequently, epididymitis or proctitis may develop.

Diagnosis and Treatment

The diagnosis of *Trichomonas* vaginitis is made in the presence of vulvovaginal symptoms, a vaginal pH over 5.0, and identification of organisms on wet mount, Pap cytology, or direct culture. Detection of the organism depends on their number in the inoculum for both wet mount and culture and on the ability to maintain the specimen at body temperature and examine the wet mount immediately to preserve motility of the organism. The wet mount and Pap smear detect only about 60% of infections, with the Pap smear having the disadvantage of a 31% false-positive rate. Culture techniques (Diamond's media) and direct monoclonal antibody techniques detect 82 to 95% of infections. There is a commercially available culture technique (Trich In-Pouch). An overview of the diagnostic assessment is outlined in Figs. 3-6 and 3-7, and treatment is described in Table 3-16.

3.6.3   Viral Infections

Herpes simplex virus (HSV) is discussed in detail in Sec. 13.3.8 with a brief clinical description outlined in Table 3-16.

HUMAN PAPILLOMAVIRUS

Human papillomavirus (HPV) is a member of the Papovavirus family and is a closed, circular, double-stranded DNA virus. The viral genome is enclosed in an icosahedral capsule composed of several protein capsomeres and lacks the lipid-containing envelope common to many other viruses such as herpes simplex. Unlike other human STD virus infections such as herpes simplex, however, HPV growth in cell culture has been difficult because its replication is dependent on epithelial cell differentiation and maturation.

The common clinical presentation of HPV is the genital wart or external condyloma acuminatum. However, with the advent of DNA amplification techniques, it has become clear that HPV has extensive clinical expression ranging from latency to condyloma to invasive cancers, particularly of the anogenital tract. Subclassification of HPV into over 100 types has been based on differences in degree of DNA homology. Common skin warts are associated with types 2 and 4, whereas benign genital condyloma is usually associated with HPV type 6 or 11. In contrast, anogenital neoplasias are commonly associated with types 16, 18, 31, 33 or 35, 45, and 56.

Pathogenesis

The definitive mechanisms of HPV infection are unclear. The HPV appears to require direct access to basal epithelial cells to establish infection, and active cell division and differentiation are required for HPV replication. Vulnerable human sites where basal cells not only are physically accessible to viral inoculation but also are actively dividing include the active squamous metaplasia of the transformation zone of the female cervix and areas of wound healing in the genital area. In adolescents and young women, 70 to 90% of HPV infections are transient. On the other hand, persistent infection has been closely linked to the development of anogenital cancers. Recent information has linked several viral–host protein interactions with the loss of cell cycle control, a likely step in the development of these cancers. The natural progression from infection to cancer is not well understood. However, cofactors thought to play important roles include HSV, hormonal influences, cigarette smoking, and altered immunologic responses to infection or injury.

Clinical Syndromes

The HPV can cause multicentric disease including much of the anogenital area: the vaginal introitus, vulvar labia minora and majora, clitoris, perineum, anus, and cervix in women; and the penis, including the prepuce, frenulum, corona, glans, and shaft, with the anus and scrotum in men. The common genital warts, condyloma acuminatum, which are seen on the skin surfaces, present as polypoid masses with fissured and irregular surfaces. They are often multiple and polymorphic and commonly coalesce into large masses. When on mucosal surfaces, condyloma acuminatum appears as finger-like projections with central dilated capillary loops.

Subclinical infections are characteristically defined as lesions visualized with the aid of colposcopy and acetic acid. These include low-grade intraepithelial lesions (LSIL) and high-grade intraepithelial lesions (HSIL) and are typically identified by cytology screening. Typical appearances on colposcopy associated with LSIL, HSIL, and invasive cancers can assist in directing biopsy. Final diagnosis is dependent on histologic interpretation of the biopsy, not colposcopic appearance. Latent HPV DNA is also common in women, specifically young women. It is thought that this type of latency is transient in most. On the other hand, persistence of infection has been shown to be associated with a significant risk of HSIL and invasive cancer development.

Diagnosis and Treatment

Screening for HPV infections in adolescents is currently limited to visual inspection for external genital warts and cytology screening for LSIL, HSIL, and invasive cancers during the pelvic examination. Diagnosis of genital warts by visual inspection is considered adequate, and HPV testing plays little to no role in confirming the diagnosis unless the diagnosis is questioned. In this case, biopsy is the best confirmation. The differential diagnosis includes bowenoid papulosis, vulvar intraepithelial neoplasia, Bowen disease, condylomata lata, skin tags, nevocellular nevus, benign tumors, sebaceous glands, seborrheic keratosis, pearly penile papules, molluscum contagiosum, squamous cell carcinoma, vulva papillomatosis, and vestibular papillae. Treatment for genital warts includes primary ablative therapy including application of 85% trichloroacetic acid to the wart itself. Cryotherapy with liquid nitrogen is also quite effective. Treatments are usually applied weekly up to 4 to 6 weeks. If there is no improvement, therapy should be switched, or the diagnosis should be questioned. The current role of podophyllin resin in therapy is questioned because its potency is unpredictable, and it is contraindicated on mucosal surfaces and in pregnancy. Other methods include excisional and laser therapy. Self-applied therapies are also available and may be more cost-effective. Podofilox is applied directly to the warts twice daily for 3 consecutive days and repeated weekly up to 4 to 6 weeks. A recent novel therapy, imiquimod, which is a cytokine-inducing agent, appears to have equal efficacy as other therapies, and its advantage is the ability to self-apply treatment. Disadvantages to all therapies include irritation, inflammation, and ulceration from local applications.

Although cytology has known limitations in sensitivity, the primary screening tool for SIL and invasive cancers in adolescents remains cytology. Although HPV testing has recently been shown to help in SIL screening in older women, its role appears less specific in adolescents because of the high rates of HPV infections and LSIL and low rates of HSIL and invasive cancer in this age group. Currently, annual Pap smears are recommended in sexually active women. Pap smears in sexually inactive adolescents are not necessary.

Abnormalities on cytology, including a single HSIL, two LSIL, or two ASCUS on repeated cytologies, should prompt referral to colposcopy and biopsy. Confirmed HSIL by histology should be treated with either excisional therapy (LEEP) or cryotherapy. Lesions that are high into the endocervical canal may require conization. Confirmed LSIL may be observed with repeated Pap smears at 4- to 6-month intervals. Treatment is recommended for persistent LSIL at 18 months or if the lesion has progressed at any time to HSIL. Referral of partners to women with condyloma or SIL is controversial because most partners of women appear to have latent HPV infection. However, most agree that partners should be encouraged to have a genital examination by their physician for signs of infection. As with all STIs, examination should include tests for other co-sexually transmitted infections.

There are no treatments available or indicated for latent HPV infection.

HUMAN IMMUNODEFICIENCY VIRUS

Human immunodeficiency virus (HIV) is the newest viral STD to infect youth. An in-depth description of its clinical syndrome, AIDS, is beyond the scope of this section. For primary-care clinicians, the focus regarding HIV infection is prevention, and this is addressed in Sec. 3.6. See Sec. 13.4.12 for a detailed description of HIV infection.

3.6.4 Sexually Transmitted Disease Syndromes

A constellation of symptoms and signs is characteristic of specific sexually transmitted disease syndromes. Common lower genital tract syndromes in women include urethritis, vaginitis, endocervicitis, and bacterial vaginosis (Table 3-16 and Fig. 3-7). In men, urethritis is the most common STD syndrome (Table 3-16, and Fig. 3-6), but epididymitis also occurs. Proctitis occurs in both sexes.

BACTERIAL VAGINOSIS

Bacterial vaginosis (BV) results from the replacement of vaginal *Lactobacillus* spp. with a number of anaerobic bacteria in high con-

centrations including *Bacteroides* spp., *Mobiluncus* spp., and other bacteria such as *G. vaginalis* and *Mycoplasma hominis*. Although BV is responsible for a majority of cases of abnormal vaginal discharge (half the women who meet the clinical criteria for the diagnosis have no symptoms), it is not exclusively sexually transmitted. The diagnosis criteria and treatment are outlined in Table 3-16 and Fig. 3-7.

Treatment of nonpregnant women is linked only to relief of symptoms; male partners of infected women are asymptomatic, and treating men does not affect the woman's disease course. Metronidazole, 500 mg orally BID for 7 days, yields a 95% cure rate compared to the alternative regimen of 2 g orally in a single dose (84% cure rate). Although experience is limited, use of intravaginal clindamycin cream, 2%, one applicator at bedtime for 7 days and metronidazole gel, 0.75%, one applicator BID for 7 days appear efficacious. Because BV may be related to prematurity and postpartum endometritis, treatment of pregnant women is encouraged using intravaginal clindamycin.

PELVIC INFLAMMATORY DISEASE

Pelvic inflammatory disease (PID) represents the most important cause of chronic reproductive morbidity in young women, with over 1.25 million cases diagnosed annually in the United States. The term PID is used to described a sexually transmitted infection involving the uterus, ovaries, and peritoneal tissues as well as the fallopian tubes and leading to ectopic pregnancy and/or involuntary infertility. Risk factors that may predispose young women to develop acute PID include (1) *youth,* with sexually active female adolescents diagnosed three times more frequently than 25- to 29-year olds; (2) endocervical *STD infection,* especially *C. trachomatis* and *N. gonorrhoeae* (other vaginal flora, eg, anaerobes, *G. vaginalis, H. influenzae,* enteric gram-negative rods, *Streptococcus agalactiae, M. hominis,* and *U. urealyticum* have been implicated); (3) previous gonococcal salpingitis resulting in tubal damage, which may predispose to recurrent episodes of infection; (4) sexual behaviors, such as a number of sexual partners, that place women at increased risk for STD infection; (5) intrauterine devices (IUDs), which are associated with a two- to fourfold increase in PID and the presence of which encourages the development of a local endometritis; and (6) recent gynecologic interventions, eg, therapeutic abortion or endometrial biopsy. Although the relationship of oral contraceptives to acute PID has been controversial, most current research supports a protective role of oral contraceptives in the development of PID.

Pathogenesis

The proposed pathogenesis of PID involves ascending canalicular spread of the causative sexually transmitted agent(s) from the vaginocervical compartment during sexual intercourse. The organisms pass through the mechanical and immunologic barriers of the endocervix, along the endometrial surface to the tubal mucosa, and finally onto peritoneal surfaces by leakage from the tubal fimbria. Modes of transport are discussed above.

Diagnosis and Treatment

Symptoms and signs of acute PID include lower abdominal pain, vaginal discharge, cervical motion tenderness, and uterine and adnexal tenderness (Table 3-18). Only about 60% of cases are correctly diagnosed, based on verification by laparoscopy. The differential diagnosis to be considered in a young woman presenting with

TABLE 3-18

DIAGNOSTIC CRITERIA FOR PID

Major diagnostic criteria
Treat empirically for PID if all are present and no other causes are plausible:
  Lower abdominal tenderness
  Adnexal tenderness
  Cervical motion tenderness
Additional criteria
These criteria help in differential diagnosis and increase the specificity of the diagnosis:
  Oral temperature > 38.3°C
  Abnormal cervical or vaginal discharge
  Elevated erythrocyte sedimentation rate
  Laboratory-documented *N. gonorrhoeae* or *C. trachomatis* cervical infection
Definitive criteria (selected cases)
These criteria are based on findings consistent with PID delineated during additional testing when appropriate and available:
  Evidence of endometritis on biopsy
  Tuboovarian mass on transvaginal ultrasound or other imaging techniques
  Laparoscopic findings of PID

SOURCE: *Sexually transmitted diseases in adolescents: Prevention, diagnosis, and treatment in pediatric practice. Adolescent Health Update 6:1–7, 1994.*

acute lower abdominal pain, in addition to PID, includes acute appendicitis, acute cystitis, acute cholecystitis, acute pyelonephritis, ectopic pregnancy, endometriosis, hemorrhagic ovarian cyst, intrauterine pregnancy, mesenteric lymphadenitis, ovarian cyst with or without torsion, ovarian tumor, septic abortion, severe constipation, and trauma. Because laparoscopy is not warranted in most cases to define PID, reliance must be placed on an accurate sexual history and application of clinical criteria (Table 3-18).

Principles to remember in the clinical approach to PID include these: (1) rule out pregnancy; (2) use the standardized clinical criteria to guide, not dictate, the diagnosis; (3) err on the side of "overdiagnosis" of PID when in doubt to prevent sequelae, especially in view of the possibility of subclinical chlamydial infections; (4) treat with broad-spectrum antibiotics and begin the course immediately on diagnosis; and, finally, (5) follow up with clinical evaluations (within 24 to 48 hours) to confirm the original clinical diagnosis and reevaluate the treatment regimen. Treatment regimens are outlined in Table 3-19. Criteria for hospitalization include all adolescents; uncertain diagnosis; presence of a pelvic or tuboovarian abscess; pregnancy; severe illness, nausea, and vomiting; inability to take oral medications; failure of outpatient therapy within 48 hours; inability to arrange follow-up within 72 hours of starting antibiotics; and patient being HIV-positive. A major serious complication to acute PID is the development of a tuboovarian abscess. Although most abscesses can be managed medically, occasional surgical intervention is necessary when medications fail. Screening and treatment of the sexual partner is an important part of PID management, as with any STD.

EPIDIDYMITIS

Epididymitis is an inflammation of the epididymis caused by infection or trauma. The causative agent responsible for infection is a function of age and sexual behavior. In adolescents, *C. trachomatis* and *N. gonorrhoeae* are most common, responsible for approximately two-thirds of adolescent infection, but coliform organisms,

Pseudomonas, and gram-positive cocci must be considered in youth who have engaged in anal intercourse.

The patient will present with an acute onset of scrotal pain and swelling, often accompanied by urinary frequency, dysuria, and urethral discharge. Fever is a sign of systemic infection. The epididymis is swollen and tender. Early in the course of the infection, the epididymis is easily discernible from the testicle, but with progression, the testis becomes involved, producing epididymoorchitis, thereby making it difficult to differentiate the epididymis from a swollen and tender testicle. The cremasteric reflex may be present or absent.

Proper STD evaluation is similar to that outlined for urethritis (Fig. 3-6). Epididymitis is often difficult to differentiate from torsion of the spermatic cord. Radiologic techniques can be used to distinguish these two clinical entities (Fig. 3-6 and Table 3-13). Scrotal masses are discussed in Sec. 3.5.2.

If chlamydial or gonococcal epididymitis is suspected, treatment should include ceftriaxone, 125 mg IM, followed by a 10-day course of doxycycline, 100 mg BID (Table 3-17). For infection likely caused by enteric organisms or in those with allergies to cephalosporins or tetracyclines, suggested treatment includes ofloxacin, 300 mg PO BID for 10 days. All sexual partners should be contacted for evaluation and treatment. Additional therapy should include scrotal elevation and analgesics.

Epididymitis usually resolves without sequelae if treatment is administered promptly. However, there are some indications that oligo- or azoospermia may result, particularly if *C. trachomatis* was the etiologic agent. Other sequelae include atrophy, infarct, or abscess formation.

TABLE 3-19

TREATMENT REGIMENS FOR ACUTE PID[a]

Recommended inpatient regimens
  Parenteral regimen A
    Cefotetan[b] 2 g IV q12h, plus doxycycline, 100 mg IV q12h. Use IV for minimum of 48 hours after patient improves. After discharge, continue doxycycline 100 mg PO BID to complete 14-day course
                                  or
  Parenteral regimen B
    Clindamycin, 900 mg IV q8h, plus gentamicin 2 mg/kg IV or IM in one loading dose, followed by a maintenance dose of 1.5 mg/kg IV q8h in patients with normal renal function.
    Use IV for minimum of 48 hours after patient improves. After discharge, continue doxycycline 100 mg PO BID to complete 14 days total; or continue clindamycin 450 mg PO QID to complete 14-day course as an alternative.
Recommended outpatient regimens
  Ceftriaxone, 250 mg IM
                                  or
  Cefoxitin, 2 g IM, plus probenecid 1 g PO
                                  or
  Other third-generation cephalosporin (ceftizoxime or cefotaxime)
                                  plus
  Doxycycline, 100 mg PO BID for 14 days
Recommended to have a test of cure evaluation (7–10 days if use culture; 1 month if testing with NAATs)
Management of sex partners
  As in any STD, partners should be evaluated for other STDs and treated empirically for *N. gonorrhoeae* and *C. trachomatis* infection

[a] *CDC STD Treatment Guidelines, 1998.*
[b] Other cephalosporins such as ceftizoxime, cefotaxime, or ceftriaxone provide adequate gonococcal, other facultative gram-negative aerobic, and anaerobic coverage and may also be used in appropriate doses.
NAATs = nucleic acid amplification tests.

PROCTITIS

Proctitis is defined as an inflammation of the rectal mucosa, which is the tissue identified between the anal canal and the colon. Many infections involve the anus as well and are therefore considered "anorectal" infections. Although STD-related rectal infections are frequently associated with anal intercourse among homosexual men, they may also occur in women. Such infections in women are less well defined and, with gonorrhea, are often asymptomatic and associated with endocervical gonorrhea. The microbiological etiologic agents of anorectal infection among sexually active adolescents include *N. gonorrhoeae*, *C. trachomatis* (lymphogranuloma venereum, LGV, strains), HSV, *T. pallidum,* and food-borne enteric organisms. Sexually transmitted enteric organisms, such as *Giardia, Entamoeba, Campylobacter, Shigella,* and hepatitis A, can be associated with anal intercourse. HIV-infected individuals may also have severe herpes proctitis or be infected with organisms generally not sexually transmitted, including CMV, *Mycobacterium avium-intracellulare,* and others.

Whereas the anus is highly innervated, resulting in pain with inflammation, the rectum lacks such innervation; thus, proctitis that does not involve the anus is usually painless. Symptoms of anorectal disease include mucus or blood in the stools, loose stool, cramping, anal itching, pain with defecation leading to constipation, and tenesmus. On examination, the anus may appear inflamed and tender. Mucopurulent discharge with or without blood may be present. Anoscopy may reveal the presence of mucopurulent discharge and erythema of the mucosa with friability and ulceration. Diagnostic evaluation includes a careful sexual history to determine risk for anal intercourse; STDs; testing for STD-related urethritis in men (Fig. 3-6) and endocervicitis in women (Fig. 3-7); rectal cultures for *N. gonorrhoeae, C. trachomatis,* and HSV; appropriate stool and rectal specimens for enteric bacteria and parasites; and syphilis serology (Table 3-16). Treatment is outlined in Table 3-16 and depends on the etiologic agent responsible.

References

Sexually Transmitted Diseases

Berger RE, Alexander ER, Harnisch JP, et al: Etiology, manifestations and therapy of acute epididymitis: Prospective study of 50 cases. J Urol 121: 750–754, 1979

Bingham JS: Vulvo-vaginal candidosis—An overview. Acta Derm Venereol 121(suppl):39–46, 1986

Blake DR, Duggan A, Quinn T, Zenilman J, Joffe A. Evaluation of vaginal infections in adolescent women: can it be done without a speculum? Pediatrics 102:939–944, 1998

Broker TR, Botchan M: Papillomaviruses: Retrospectives and prospectives on cancer cells 4. Cold Springs Harbor Laboratory 17–36, 1986

Burgher SW: Acute scrotal pain. Emerg Med Clin North Am 16:781–809, 1998

Campion MJ: Clinical manifestations and natural history of genital human papillomavirus infection. Obstet Gynecol Clin North Am 14:363–388, 1987

Centers for Disease Control and Prevention: *Chlamydia trachomatis* genital infections—United States, 1995. Morb Mortal Wkly Rep 46:193–198, 1997

Centers for Disease Control and Prevention: 1998 Sexually transmitted disease treatment guidelines. Morb Mortal Wkly Rep 47:1–116, 1998

Chernesky MA: Nucleic acid tests for the diagnosis of sexually transmitted diseases. FEMS Immunol Microbiol 24(4):437–46, 1999

Corey L, Spear PG: Infections with herpes simplex viruses, part I. N Engl J Med 314:686–691, 1986

Corey L, Spear PG: Infections with herpes simplex viruses, part II. N Engl J Med 314:749–757, 1986

Division of STD Prevention: Sexually Transmitted Disease Surveillance, 1998. US Department of Health and Human Services, Public Health Service. Atlanta; Centers for Disease Control and Prevention, September 1999.

Fiumara NJ: Treatment of primary and secondary syphilis: Serologic response. JAMA 243:2500–2502, 1980

Holmes KK, Mardh PA, Sparling PF, et al, eds: Sexually Transmitted Diseases, 3rd ed. New York, McGraw-Hill Health Professions Division, 1999

Johnston JH: Acquired lesions of the penis, the scrotum and the testes. In: Williams DI, Johnston JH, eds: Pediatric Urology. London, Butterworth Scientific, 1982

Levi MH, Torres J, Piana C, et al: Comparison of the InPouch TV culture system and Diamond's modified medium for detection of *Trichomonas vaginalis.* J Clin Microbiol 35:3308–3310, 1997

Madico G, Quinn TC, Rompalo A, McKee KT Jr, Gaydos CA: Diagnosis of *Trichomonas vaginalis* infection by PCR using vaginal swab samples. J Clin Microbiol 36:3205–3210, 1998

Meisels A, Morin C: Human papillomavirus and cancer of the uterine cervix. Gynecol Oncol 12:S111–S123, 1981

Melekos MD, Asbach HW, Markou SA: Etiology of acute scrotum in 100 boys with regard to age distribution. J Urol 139:1023–1025, 1987

National Guidelines for the Management of Epididymo-orchitis. Clinical Effectiveness Group (Association of Genitourinary Medicine and the Medical Society for the Study of Venereal Diseases). Sex Transm Infect 75(Suppl 1):S51–S53, 1999

National Guidelines for the Management of *Trichomonas vaginalis.* Clinical Effectiveness Group (Association for Genitourinary Medicine and the Medical Society for the Study of Venereal Diseases). Sex Transm Infect 75(Suppl 1):S21–S23, 1999

Paavonen J, Eggert-Kruse W: *Chlamydia trachomatis:* impact on human reproduction. Human Reprod Update 5:433–447, 1999

Quinn TC: DNA amplification assays: a new standard for diagnosis of *Chlamydia trachomatis* infections. Ann Acad Med Singapore 24:627–633, 1995

Shafer MA, Blain B, Beck A, et al: *Chlamydia trachomatis:* Important relationships to race, contraceptive use, lower genital tract infection and Papanicolaou smears. J Pediatr 104:141–146, 1984

Shafer MA, Pantell R, Schachter J: Is the routine pelvic examination needed with the advent of urine-based screening for sexually transmitted diseases? Arch Pediatr Adolesc Med 153:119–125, 1999

Shafer MA, Prager V, Shalwitz J, et al: Prevalence of urethral *Chlamydia trachomatis* and *Neisseria gonorrhoeae* among asymptomatic sexually active adolescent males. J Infect Dis 156:223–224, 1987

Shafer MA, Sweet RL, Ohm-Smith MJ, et al: The microbiology of the lower genital tract of post-menarchal adolescent females. Differences by sexual activity, contraception, and presence of nonspecific vaginitis. J Pediatr 107:974–981, 1985

Sonda PL, Wang S: Evaluation of male external genital diseases in the emergency room setting. Emerg Med Clin North Am 6(3):473–486, 1988

Stamm WE: *Chlamydia trachomatis* infections: Progress and problems. J Infect Dis 179(Suppl 2):S380–383, 1999

Stamm WE, Koutsky LA, Benedette JK, et al: *Chlamydia trachomatis* urethral infections in men. Ann Intern Med 100:47–51, 1984

Stary A: Correct samples for diagnostic tests in sexually transmitted diseases: Which sample for which test? FEMS Immunol Med Microbiol 24(4): 455–459, 1999

Taylor-Robinson D, Renton A: Diagnostic tests that are worthwhile for patients with sexually transmitted bacterial infections in industrialized countries. Int J STD AIDS 10(1):1–4, 1999

Washington AE, Goves S, Schachter J, et al: Oral contraceptives, *Chlamydia trachomatis* infection and pelvic inflammatory disease. A word of caution about protection. JAMA 124:2246–2250, 1985

THE ACUTELY ILL INFANT AND CHILD

Julio Pérez Fontán and George Lister, Associate Editors

4.1 ASSESSMENT AND STABILIZATION OF THE ACUTELY ILL CHILD

The development of emergency medicine and critical care medicine as specialties within pediatrics is a consequence of the uniqueness of the knowledge and technical skills required to provide the care to the acutely ill infant and child. These relatively new specialties are, in part, defined by the setting where human and technical resources are concentrated to provide sophisticated care and, most importantly, by the common features of the disease processes that result in critical illness. Although unrealistic for every pediatrician to be knowledgeable in all the aspects of this care, it is essential that those who are involved in the medical management of children be able to recognize the signs of potentially life-threatening disease, to evaluate the severity of its manifestations, and to initiate the stabilization of infants or children who suffer these problems. Accordingly, this chapter provides an overview of the most common life-threatening problems that afflict infants and children. Rather than engaging in an exhaustive review of all the illnesses or injuries that qualify as life-threatening, we provide a framework for the rapid evaluation, initial management, and monitoring of the patient at risk for these clinical entities. And, we provide the pediatrician with information about some of the contemporary techniques that are used to provide life support in anticipation of recovery from critical illness.

4.1.1 Respiratory Distress and Respiratory Failure

Julio Pérez Fontán

The adaptation to air breathing at birth and the accelerated lung growth that follows during infancy require profound transformations in the structure and function of the respiratory system. The complexity and critical timing of these transformations increase the susceptibility of the immature respiratory system to the development of respiratory disease. Immaturity of the neural control of breathing, the small caliber of the airways, and a limited respiratory muscle reserve combine to render the infant, and especially the newborn, more vulnerable to congenital or acquired anomalies of the lungs and chest wall and to alterations in the function of other systems, especially the cardiovascular system. It is thus not surprising that, regardless of geographic location and socioeconomic state, the majority of patients admitted to a pediatric intensive care unit

develop respiratory dysfunction at some point in their course. Respiratory failure is acknowledged by the American Heart Association in its *Pediatric Advanced Life Support* textbook as the most common precipitant of cardiac arrest in childhood. Thus, it is essential that clinicians who care for children recognize the manifestations of respiratory disease and be familiar with the principles of its treatment.

REGULATION OF RESPIRATION

In healthy individuals, respiratory and circulatory functions are linked to tissue metabolic activity by a responsive regulatory system that translates biochemical and neural signals from the tissues into adjustments in cardiac output, vascular tone, and minute ventilation. The purpose of this system is to assure that all the cells in the organism receive a supply of O_2 commensurate with their metabolic needs without accumulating excessive amounts of CO_2. The system relies both on local circulatory reflexes, which alter the caliber of the supplying blood vessels in accordance with tissue metabolic activity, and on central circulatory and respiratory reflexes, which modify the pumping function of the heart and the intensity of the respiratory effort in response to changes in blood pressure (see Sec. 4.1.2) or respiratory gas composition in blood. An example is the chemoreceptor response, which adjusts neural activation of the respiratory muscles to optimize the P_{O_2} and P_{CO_2} of the arterial blood.

The chemoreceptor reflex plays a singularly important role in the genesis of the manifestations of respiratory disease (Fig. 4-1). Alterations in the P_{O_2}, P_{CO_2}, and pH of the blood are sensed by specialized chemoreceptor cells located in the carotid bodies (peripheral chemoreceptors, P_{O_2}) and reticular nuclei of the medulla oblongata (central chemoreceptors, P_{CO_2} and pH). These cells then relay the information to a medullary neuronal network, which regulates the activation of respiratory muscle motorneurons located at various levels of the spinal cord. The medullary regulatory network also receives inputs from mechanical and chemical sensors distributed throughout the lungs, airways, and chest wall. It is for this reason that the pattern of respiratory muscle use in any respiratory disease depends not only on the severity of the blood gas derangement but also on how the disease alters the mechanical function of the respiratory system. For instance, upper-airway obstruction (eg, croup; see Sec. 23.6) impairs inspiration more than expiration, thus it is characterized by a selective increase in the contraction force of inspiratory muscles such as the diaphragm or the scalene muscles. Intrathoracic obstruction (eg, asthma; see Sec. 23.7), in contrast, impairs expiration more than inspiration, and therefore it is accompanied by prominent use of the abdominal muscles to facilitate exhalation.

FIGURE 4-1 Chemoreceptor reflex and the signs of respiratory distress. Decreases in the partial tension of O_2 or increases in the partial tension of CO_2 are sensed by chemoreceptor cells in the carotid bodies and reticular formation of the medulla oblongata, respectively. The impulses produced by these cells are integrated in the medulla oblongata and transmitted to inspiratory and expiratory premotor neurons, which regulate directly the activity of diaphragmatic (inspiratory) and other respiratory muscle (inspiratory or expiratory) motor neurons in the spinal cord. Activation of this reflex causes an increase in respiratory neural output and results in the progressive activation of all muscles of respiration, including the upper-airway musculature. Nasal flaring, tachypnea, the recruitment of accessory inspiratory and expiratory muscles, and retractions are all manifestations of the increased neural output. Nasal flaring, increased vocal cord abduction during inspiration, and dilation of the pharyngeal passages may not be apparent to the observer. Alterations in the breathing frequency (usually tachypnea) or intercostal and subcostal retractions, however, are prominent in practically every child with acute respiratory disease.

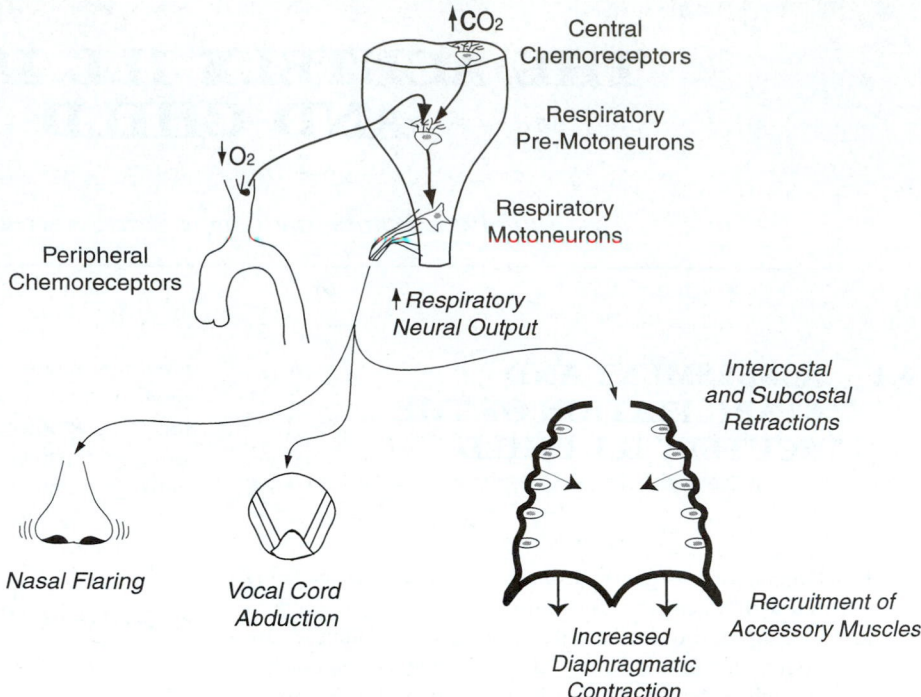

DEFINITION OF RESPIRATORY DISTRESS AND FAILURE

The phrase *respiratory distress* denotes an abnormal increase in the effort of the respiratory muscles, typically to overcome an impairment in the mechanical function of the lungs or the chest wall. The increased effort may only be noticeable to the patient, who perceives it as shortness of breath (*dyspnea*), or may also be apparent to an external observer as physical signs. Depending on the severity of the impairment (Table 4-1), these usually include a high breathing frequency (tachypnea), nasal flaring (from activation of the normally quiescent alae nasae muscles), retractions of the intercostal spaces (from the negative swings in pleural pressure generated by the diaphragmatic contractions), and recruitment of accessory muscles (muscles whose primary function is not respiratory, but which can contribute to pump air in and out of the lungs). The abdominal muscles (rectus abdominis, oblique muscles, and transversus abdominis) are the most frequently used among the latter. They take advantage of their insertions on the costal cartilages and ribs to stabilize the abdominal wall during inspiration and to accelerate lung emptying during expiration. The scaleni and sternocleidomastoids are also accessory muscles, but, in contrast to the abdominal muscles, they act only to augment rib cage volume through their distal insertions on the first and second rib and the sternal manubrium, respectively. Increases in the production of CO_2 (eg, fever or exercise) or in the concentration of hydrogen ions in the blood (metabolic acidosis) also augment neural output to the respiratory muscles, mimicking respiratory distress. However, a healthy respiratory system raises ventilation primarily by increasing tidal volume (hyperpnea). The presence of mechanical lung or chest wall dysfunction makes this strategy intolerable because it is too energy consuming, leaving tachypnea as the only alternative to raise ventilation. Thus, rapid and shallow breathing, particularly when combined with other physical findings such as

abnormal breath sounds, should always alert the clinician to the presence of an intrinsic respiratory anomaly.

Often, the increase in respiratory effort that defines respiratory distress is sufficient to prevent any substantial alteration in pulmonary gas exchange. On occasions, however, either the neural mechanisms that regulate ventilation fail or, more frequently, the compensatory effort of the respiratory muscles is insufficient to restore gas exchange to normality, and arterial hypoxemia (an abnormally low arterial P_{O_2}) and hypercapnia (an abnormally high P_{CO_2}) develop. This situation, known as *respiratory failure*, burdens the circulatory system, which must increase systemic blood flow to mitigate the reduction in arterial O_2 content as well as supply the increased needs of the respiratory muscles.

DIAGNOSIS OF RESPIRATORY DYSFUNCTION IN INFANTS AND CHILDREN

The emergency evaluation of any patient—child or adult—should always begin with an assessment of the adequacy and characteristics of the patient's respiratory effort. This is especially important in children who suffer from a known respiratory disturbance that has worsened or is not improving as expected. *In these circumstances, the presence of respiratory distress, as defined above, is a clear indication that the impairment affects the mechanical properties of the airways, lungs, or chest wall.* Rarely, patients with neuropathy or myopathy can develop signs of respiratory distress, manifested by dyspnea and activation of the respiratory muscles spared by the disease.

The finding of hypoxemia and hypercapnia (respiratory failure) without respiratory distress, on the other hand, alerts the clinician that either the neural control of breathing is disabled or, less frequently, that the respiratory muscles cannot respond to the increased output of the respiratory premotor neurons. This is partic-

TABLE 4-1
SEVERITY SCALE OF SIGNS OF RESPIRATORY DISTRESS

	MILD - MODERATE	SEVERE
Respiratory pattern	Normal or tachypnea	Tachypnea
Chest wall deformity	Subcostal retractions	Subcostal, intercostal, and suprasternal retractions; pectus excavatum
Breath sounds	Normal or decreased; adventitious sounds	Markedly decreased or inaudible
Consciousness and attention	Normal or anxious	Obtunded or apathetic
Breathing pattern	Regular	Irregular; head bobbing; expiratory pauses; alternation between muscle groups
Other signs		Nasal flaring; grunting

ularly evident when the patient has an abnormally low respiratory rate (bradypnea), shallow breathing movements, or no respiratory movements at all (apnea). The breathing control becomes disabled when the central nervous system, especially the brainstem, has suffered a direct injury (eg, cranial trauma, compression by an expanding cerebral tumor or hemorrhage) or is functionally impaired by hypoxia, acidosis, or depressants (eg, opioids or barbiturates). The respiratory muscles will fail to respond appropriately to an increased respiratory drive in patients with severe forms of neuromuscular dysfunction or after the administration of neuromuscular blockers.

RESPIRATORY DISTRESS: MECHANICAL DYSFUNCTION OF THE LUNGS AND CHEST WALL

We defined respiratory distress as a detectable increase in the effort of the respiratory muscles to compensate a mechanical impairment in the function of the airways, lungs, or chest wall. The increased effort is a reflex response directed at overcoming forces generated during breathing in the diseased lung or chest wall. These forces originate from two types of physical phenomena: one relates to lung inflation, the other relates to gas flow. Inflation-dependent forces arise from well-defined elements within the lungs or the chest wall, which oppose inflation and therefore produce retractive or recoil forces; thus, these forces are lung volume-dependent. The elastic fibers contained in the alveolar interstitium and in the airways and blood vessels of the lung are a good example. When stretched during inspiration, these fibers behave very much like a rubber band, accumulating energy in their molecular structures, which is then released as they recover their shape during expiration. The more the elastic fibers are stretched, the greater is their tendency to return to their original state or the greater is the overall recoil of the lung. The alveolar gas-liquid interface acts also as a recoil element, although its behavior is somewhat more complex. When a liquid like the water-based solution lining the alveoli contacts air, water molecules within the liquid phase experience a net push to leave the solution. This push translates into a net force, known as surface tension, that acts to reduce the volume of the alveolus. In the healthy lung, the tendency is relieved greatly by the presence of a lipid monolayer (alveolar surfactant), which separates the water and gas phases and makes the recoil generated from surface tension manageable. Even under these circumstances, and certainly when disease or immaturity interfere with surfactant function (see Sec. 2.16.1), surface phenomena contribute to overall lung recoil. Because lung inflation requires the active contraction of the inspiratory muscles (expiration is passive and therefore facilitated by recoil), the manifestations of the diseases in which lung or chest-wall

recoil is increased are always more prominent during inspiration than during expiration.

Flow-dependent forces are the result of brief molecular interactions between either the gas flowing through the airways and the airway walls or among tissue components as the lungs change volume. The forces generated by these interactions oppose both inflation and deflation. Just like the velocity of a vehicle determines the fuel consumption incurred in overcoming road and air drag, the magnitude of these forces (often grouped as *resistive forces*) depends primarily on the speed (or flow rate) at which the lungs inflate or deflate.

The clinical manifestations of respiratory distress usually contain important clues about whether the disease process involves predominantly an increase in lung recoil or resistive forces and about how the patient is tolerating this increase. These clues are often sufficient to establish a first distinction between two types of mechanical impairments: *restrictive* and *obstructive*.

Restrictive Impairments

Restrictive impairments are characterized by an abnormal increase in lung or chest-wall recoil, and therefore they interfere primarily with lung inflation. Examples include pulmonary edema, pneumonitis, interstitial lung disease, and chest-wall deformities that limit lung and chest-wall expansion (see Sec. 23.17). In some of these conditions, the presence of fluid (pulmonary edema or pneumonitis), inflammatory cells (pneumonitis), or scar tissue (lung fibrosis) in the interstitial spaces diminishes the ease with which the lung scaffolding can accommodate stretch. In others, water (advanced pulmonary edema) or exudate (pneumonia) in the alveolar spaces raises surface tension at the gas-liquid interface and reduces the space available for gas in the alveoli. Chest-wall deformities limit lung inflation by making the rib cage more rigid, often in an asymmetric fashion. Space-occupying lesions such as pneumothoraces, pleural effusions, and lung cystic anomalies are by definition restrictive, although frequently they distort neighboring airways, thereby creating simultaneous obstructive manifestations.

Restrictive impairments affect the relationship between lung volume changes and the effort that is required to produce them. Accordingly, their severity is best characterized by relating, graphically or mathematically, the volume change of the lungs to the force that the respiratory muscles must generate to overcome the recoil. Because force is a one-dimensional entity and the respiratory system has three dimensions, pressure is usually substituted for force. The graphical result of this substitution is the volume–pressure relationship of the respiratory system (Fig. 4-2). When plotted in a graphical format, the relationship is curvilinear, with two relatively flat portions, one at low lung volume and the other at high lung volume, where relatively large changes in pressure are needed to

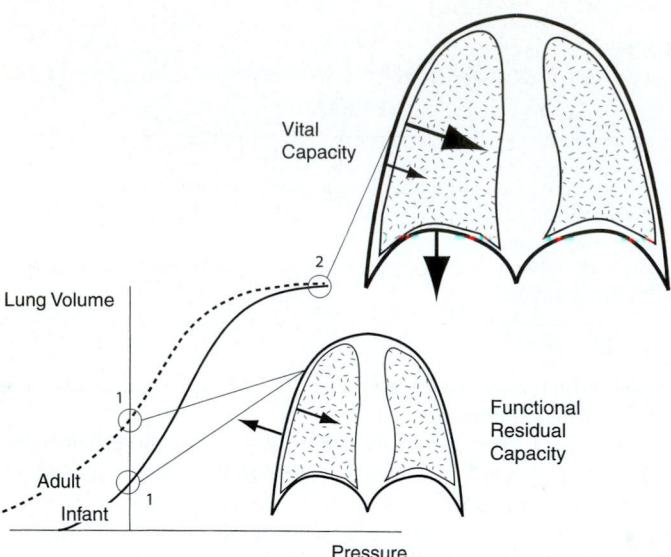

FIGURE 4-2 **Comparison of the combined static volume-pressure relationships of the lungs and chest wall in an infant and an adult. The relationships shown here are obtained by plotting lung volume (*ordinate*) against the pressure that the respiratory muscles must generate to maintain the lungs and chest wall at that particular volume (*abscissa*). These are determined by measuring lung volume and airway pressure while the lungs are held at a constant volume and the subject relaxes all respiratory muscles against a closed airway, or while the lungs are inflated passively in a stepwise manner. The interaction between the lungs and the chest wall is depicted at two points of interest indicated by *circles* in the volume-pressure relationships. The first point (labeled *1*) is the intersection with the ordinate, a volume that requires no muscle activity to be maintained. It is the relaxation volume of the respiratory system, which, under most circumstances, coincides with the functional residual capacity of the lungs. At this volume the outward elasticity of the chest wall equilibrates with the inward elasticity of the lungs (*arrows*). Because the immature chest wall has a much smaller tendency to recoil in the outward direction than does the mature chest wall, the relaxation volume of the infant's respiratory system is considerably lower than that of the adult. The second point of interest (labeled *2*) is the maximal volume that the lungs can reach during a voluntary inflation (*vital capacity*). At this volume, both lungs and chest wall generate inward-acting pressures, which are additive. At any point in the volume-pressure relationship between relaxation volume and vital capacity, the inward-acting forces of the lung predominate and the respiratory muscles must generate pressure accordingly (*down arrow*).**

produce small volume changes, and a steeper portion in the middle, where smaller pressure changes result in larger volume changes. Healthy individuals breathe in the range of lung volumes corresponding to the steep portion of the relationship. However, disease, or sometimes therapeutic interventions, can force the lungs toward one of the flat portions, increasing considerably the effort that the respiratory muscles must make to generate a given tidal volume. Mathematically, the volume–pressure relationship is often described by the *compliance* of the respiratory system, which is defined as the quotient of lung volume and pressure changes (also the slope of the volume–pressure relationship). A reduction in respiratory system compliance for any given lung volume is the fundamental characteristic of restrictive disease. It is important to realize, however, that because the slope of the volume–pressure relationship changes with lung volume, compliance can be decreased without

underlying abnormality of the lung or chest-wall tissue. A child with status asthmaticus, for example, may not have a primary restrictive disease of the lung in a strict sense, but will likely have a decreased lung compliance because of the combined presence in the lungs of overinflated and collapsed alveoli as a direct result of the airway obstruction.

Lung volume is influenced by the state of contraction of the respiratory muscles. When these muscles are completely relaxed, for example, at the end of an expiration, the lungs adopt a volume at which the recoils of chest wall (outward) and lungs (inward) neutralize each other (Fig. 4-2). Incomplete ossification of the rib cage causes the chest wall to be considerably more compliant in newborns and infants than in adults. This feature is a definite advantage during the birth process. Immediately after birth, however, a highly compliant chest wall leaves the inward-acting recoil of the lungs as the predominant factor in determining lung volume. As a result, when the respiratory muscles are fully relaxed, the lungs of the newborn or small infant tend to adopt a smaller volume relative to the lungs of older children or adults. The newborns of most species, including humans, confront this potential mechanical limitation by adopting a number of strategies to delay expiration, all in an effort to maintain the functional residual capacity of the lungs (the volume of gas contained in the lungs at the end of a normal expiration) above the relaxation volume of the respiratory system. They include partially closing the glottis during expiration, prolonging the activation of the diaphragm during part of the expiratory phase, and initiating the next inspiration before exhalation is complete. Neurologic dysfunction, anesthesia and sedation, and neuromuscular blockade render these strategies ineffective, making the newborn vulnerable to alveolar collapse and hypoxemia even in the absence of preexisting lung disease.

Manifestations of Restrictive Disease

The manifestations of restrictive respiratory disease can be attributed to the mechanical impairment itself, the ensuing increase in the respiratory drive, or the alterations of pulmonary gas exchange that develop if the impairment is not compensated.

From a mechanical point of view, restrictive diseases, independent of whether they affect primarily the lungs or the chest wall, always increase the inward recoil of the thorax as a whole. As a result, both tidal volume and functional residual capacity tend to decrease (Fig. 4-3). The consequences of this decrease can be appreciated during auscultation of the chest, which demonstrates diminished breath sounds, frequently accompanied by inspiratory and expiratory crackles or rales created by reopening of collapsed air spaces as the effort of the inspiratory muscles exceeds the critical opening pressure. To mitigate the decrease in lung volume, newborns and young infants often close their glottis before exhalation is complete. This may result in a characteristic grunting noise, which should be interpreted as a sign of unstable lung volume and an indication that oxygenation is endangered. Radiographically, restrictive disease is characterized by the small size of the lung fields and the general appearance of reduced aeration of the lungs. Alveolar collapse may occur in areas of the lung fields where an inefficient cough promotes mucus plugging or the effects of gravity neutralize the net forces that maintain alveoli open.

The increase in the respiratory drive is triggered by alterations in the blood gas tensions (chemoreceptor reflexes) or by disease-related changes in the tensile forces within the tissues of the lungs and chest wall (mechanoreceptor reflexes). The resultant increment

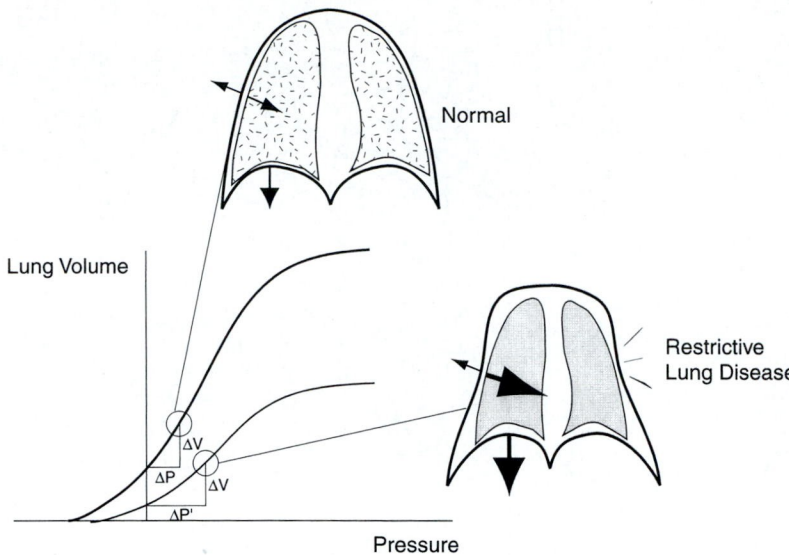

FIGURE 4-3   Effect of restrictive lung disease on the mechanical interaction of lung and chest wall. Restrictive disease flattens the volume-pressure relationship of the lungs. As a result, the decrease in pleural pressure needed to produce a given volume change in the lungs (ΔV) is larger than when the lungs are healthy ($\Delta P'$ versus ΔP). A more negative pleural pressure reduces the outward movement of the chest wall or causes it to move inward in weak areas such as the intercostal, subcostal, and suprasternal spaces, causing chest-wall retractions. This inward movement may be augmented at the level of the costal insertions of the diaphragm by the increased contraction force of the diaphragmatic muscle. Chest-wall retractions detract from lung ventilation and waste energy because they increase the displacement of the inspiratory muscles without increasing effective ventilation of the lungs.

in motor neural output to the respiratory muscles is aimed at increasing alveolar ventilation. In patients with restrictive disease, the increase is accomplished typically by adopting a pattern of rapid and shallow respirations. The increased respiratory frequency more than compensates for the reduced tidal volume of the shallow breaths. These, in turn, minimize the average force that the inspiratory muscles must generate over a given period of time (remember that elastic recoil increases proportionally to lung volume) and the energy cost of breathing. The finding of tachypnea as the leading sign of respiratory distress is often a reasonable indication that the disease is primarily restrictive. The only exception to this rule is in patients with severe respiratory dysfunction, for whom tachypnea may simply be a sign of respiratory muscle fatigue. Other manifestations of increased respiratory drive are less specific. Recruitment of accessory inspiratory muscles such as the scalene and sternocleidomastoid muscles, for example, can be detected in children with both restrictive disease and upper-airway obstruction, because in both instances the increased effort is mainly inspiratory. Conversely, recruitment of abdominal muscles during expiration is particularly prominent in patients with intrathoracic obstruction, but may also be found in patients with restrictive disease or upper-airway obstruction. In these situations, the contraction of the abdominal muscles helps stabilize the lower rib cage and increases respiratory frequency by accelerating expiration. Chest-wall retractions are a very common manifestation of respiratory distress in children, but their presence has little value in distinguishing the mechanism responsible for the respiratory distress. The retractions occur during inspiration, when the increased effort of the diaphragm and other inspiratory muscles to overcome lung recoil creates very negative pressures in the pleural space (Fig. 4-3). These pressures cause inward deformation of the cartilages and soft tissues of the chest wall, especially at the intercostal, subcostal, and suprasternal areas. The compliant chest wall of the newborn and infant undergoes considerably more deformation for the same degree of lung mechanical impairment than that of older children and adults. In premature and term newborn infants, entire sections of the cartilaginous rib cage can cave during inspiration, adding considerably to the work that the diaphragm has to perform to ventilate the lungs.

The abnormalities caused by restrictive disease on gas exchange depend both on the ability of the respiratory system to maintain alveolar ventilation and on the effectiveness of the local vascular and airway reflex mechanisms that preserve regional ventilation-perfusion ratios within the lungs. These are discussed in more detail later in this chapter.

Obstructive Impairments

Obstructive impairments are characterized by an increase in the flow-dependent forces generated through interactions among moving gas and tissue molecules during breathing. The largest portion of these forces originates from friction between air and the relatively narrow airway passages of the infant and child. A smaller proportion of flow-dependent forces originates from molecular interactions within the tissues of the lung and chest wall or in the gas-liquid interface. (These forces may increase in some forms of pulmonary disease, but their contribution to the overall mechanical dysfunction of the respiratory system is not well characterized.)

From a mechanical perspective, obstructive impairments have two distinguishing characteristics. First, any work that the respiratory muscles perform to overcome the obstruction is ultimately dissipated as heat (unlike restrictive disease, where the work done by elastic forces is stored during inspiration and used to facilitate expiration). Because energy that is transformed into heat leaves the system immediately, the relationship obtained by plotting the pressure generated by the respiratory muscles against the volume change of the lungs follows a different trajectory during inspiration and expiration (indicating that pressure diminishes even if volume is the same), a phenomenon known as *hysteresis* (Fig. 4-4). In addition, the magnitude of the energy losses incurred at the obstruction (and thus the pressure necessary to compensate these losses) depends on the velocity of the gas. Gas velocity, in turn, is determined by the gas flow rate and thus depends on the speed with which the lungs inflate and deflate.

Accordingly, the pressure that the respiratory muscles must generate to overcome obstruction increases as respiratory rate rises. The exact terms of the relationship between pressure and gas flow, however, are defined by the manner in which the gas molecules travel in the flow stream. During normal breathing, flow in most airways adopts a layered or laminar pattern, whereby the molecules in the most central layers travel faster than those in the outer layers, which are slowed down by the drag of the airway wall. Under such con-

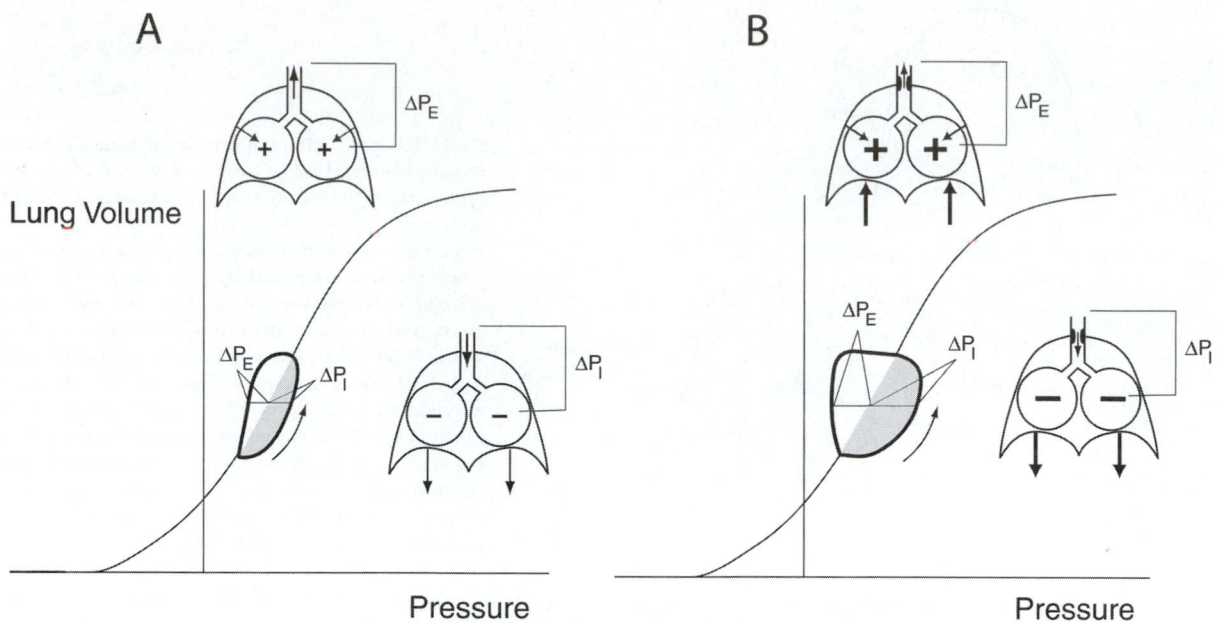

FIGURE 4-4 **Effect of airway obstruction on the volume-pressure relationships of the respiratory system. Whenever there is flow in the airways, friction and other energy-consuming processes create a pressure gradient in the direction in which the gas is moving. Alveolar pressure is therefore lower than atmospheric pressure during inspiration (negative sign) and higher during expiration (positive sign). The difference (ΔP_I during inspiration and ΔP_E during expiration) is determined by the magnitude of the frictional pressure losses and, when divided by the gas flow, yields the resistance of the airways. Because friction generates heat, which is carried away, the volume-pressure relationship follows a different trajectory during inspiration and expiration (direction shown by *arrow*), forming a loop (*hysteresis*). Airway obstruction (B) increases frictional pressure losses, widening the volume-pressure loop and forcing the respiratory muscles to increase the pressure difference between alveolar and atmospheric pressure (compare to normal on A).**

ditions, frictional pressure losses are proportional to the length of the airways and viscosity of the gas and inversely related to the fourth power of the airway's radius (Poiseuille's law). As flow velocity increases, or when irregularities develop in the airway wall, the laminar organization becomes disturbed and gas molecules start to move randomly, sometimes in directions opposite to the general progression of the flow. The resultant pattern, known as turbulent flow, dissipates more energy than laminar flow and therefore makes inefficient use of the effort of the respiratory muscles. Furthermore, because pressure losses during turbulence are caused by molecular collisions, the magnitude of these losses depends on gas density rather than on gas viscosity. This is one of the reasons why patients with obstructive airway disease may improve when breathing high concentrations of helium, which has a lower density than air or O_2 (even though its viscosity is slightly greater).

In normal airways, viscous friction predominates. The loss of energy dissipated as heat causes the pressure inside the airways to decline gradually in the direction of flow. For this reason, alveolar pressure is always lower (or more negative) than the pressure measured elsewhere in the airway tree during inspiration and higher (or less negative) during expiration. When there is an obstruction, the gradual decline in pressure turns into a sudden step. Gradual or sudden, the changes in the pressure inside the airways have important effects on the size of the airway lumen. Indeed, unlike rigid pipes, airways vary their caliber depending on the net balance of pressures acting on their inside and outside wall surfaces (*airway transmural pressure*). A positive transmural pressure (inside pressure greater than outside) increases airway caliber; a negative transmural pressure (outside pressure greater than inside pressure) de-

creases airway caliber and, depending on the rigidity of the airway wall, may cause the airway lumen to collapse altogether. If, for the time being, we ignore the factors that determine the outside pressure, an airway obstruction can reduce the pressure acting on the inside of the wall by two different mechanisms. First, as discussed earlier, increased friction and, when present, turbulence cause a step reduction in pressure downstream from the obstruction. In addition, to accommodate flow through an airway narrowing, the gas molecules must undergo acceleration, gaining in kinetic energy. Because of the principle of conservation of energy, the kinetic energy gain can only occur at the expense of the potential energy contained in flow stream. Because potential energy is stored in the forces applied laterally on the airway wall, the pressure of the gas against the wall decreases. (This is the basis for the Venturi effect, which makes it possible for airplanes to fly and for sailboats to tack against the wind.) The pressure reduction draws the wall of the airway into the flow, further worsening the obstruction. Independent of whether they are borne out by friction (related to viscosity) or by the shift from potential to kinetic energy (related to density), these effects of the obstruction on airway caliber diminish further the amount of flow that the obstructed airway can accommodate. An increase in contraction force of the respiratory muscles may compensate partially, forcing more flow through the obstruction. However, there is a limit at which the increase in driving pressure is offset by a further reduction in airway caliber caused either by the increase in pressure applied on the outside surface of the airway (*viscous flow limitation*) or by the decrease in the inside pressure as flow needs to be accelerated even more (*wave-speed flow limitation*). The maximum flow achievable under those circumstances depends on the location and severity of the obstruction and on the rigidity of the airway wall. *Flow limitation* is common in diseased airways and contributes substantially to the manifestations of airway obstruction.

Manifestations of Obstructive Disease

The manifestations of obstructive respiratory disease depend on the hierarchy of the obstructed airways and the severity of the obstruction. Obstructions of the larynx and trachea affect gas flow to both lungs and therefore represent a much greater threat for the patient's life than localized bronchial obstruction.

Mechanically, obstructive disease is characterized by local or generalized impairment in gas flow though the airways. Because gas flow determines the rate at which the lungs change volume, some delay in the time course of inspiration, expiration, or both is always detectable. The delay lengthens the total duration of each breath. Thus, tachypnea is a less prominent sign of respiratory distress (when not absent altogether) in patients with airway obstruction than in patients with restrictive disease.

Determining whether the impediment to gas flow is predominantly inspiratory or expiratory helps considerably in the differential diagnosis of airway obstruction. As a rule, obstructions of the extrathoracic airway (nose, pharynx, larynx, and cervical segment of the trachea) are exacerbated during inspiration; obstructions of the intrathoracic airway (thoracic segment of the trachea, bronchi, and bronchioles), in contrast, are exacerbated during expiration. These changes are an exaggeration of the normal fluctuations of the airway caliber during unobstructed breathing. They result from differences in how breathing affects the transmural pressure of the extra- and intrathoracic airways (Fig. 4-5).

The pressure acting on the inside surface of the extrathoracic airways is transmitted from the alveoli through the gas column. It is therefore slightly negative (subatmospheric) during inspiration, and slightly positive (above atmospheric) during expiration. The pressure acting on the outside surface of these airways, on the other hand, is similar to atmospheric pressure throughout the respiratory cycle. Consequently, extrathoracic airways are exposed to a negative (collapsing) transmural pressure during inspiration and to a positive (dilating) transmural pressure during expiration. Although small, the negative swings of the transmural pressure during inspiration are sufficient to collapse the lumen of the pharynx. The well-timed inspiratory contraction of the pharyngeal and laryngeal dilator muscles prevents this collapse, providing a protective mechanism that is absent in patients with brainstem dysfunction, who sometimes require tracheal intubation or tracheostomy to bypass the upper segment of the airway. When the extrathoracic airway is obstructed, increased friction and turbulence at the level of the obstruction force the respiratory muscles to augment their contraction force. Pleural and alveolar pressures become more negative during inspiration, and so does the pressure inside the airways downstream from the obstruction point. If the effort is sufficient, flow is restored to the levels needed to maintain alveolar ventilation. As a consequence, however, transmural pressure becomes substantially more negative during inspiration in the airway segment comprised between the obstruction point and the thoracic inlet. This, coupled with the Venturi effect created by the acceleration of the gas in the narrow segment, causes a reduction of the airway lumen, which further aggravates the obstruction and may create the conditions for flow limitation. Inward deformation of the chest wall is present and frequently severe during inspiration in patients with airway obstruction, as contraction of the diaphragm and recruitment of ac-

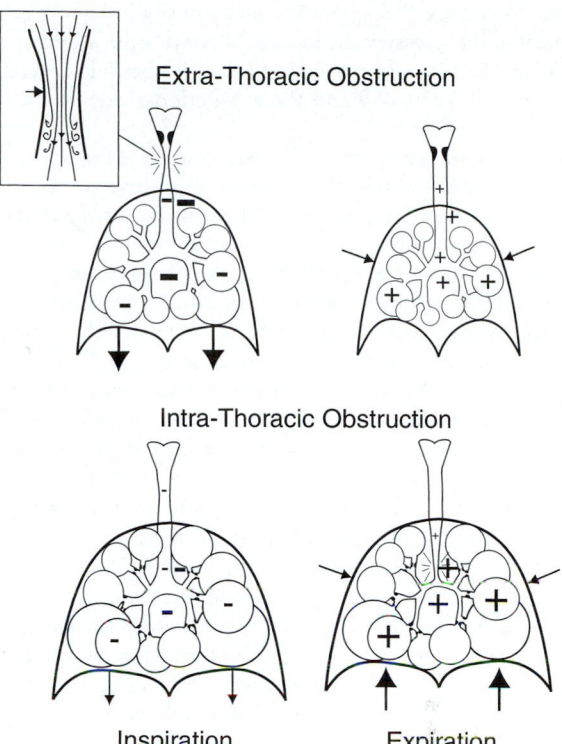

FIGURE 4-5 **Effects of extra- and intrathoracic airway obstruction on the caliber of the airways.** During inspiration, both forms of obstruction cause the inspiratory muscles to increase their effort to force air through the obstruction. As a result, pleural pressure and the pressure inside the airways decrease. When the obstruction is in the extrathoracic airways (*top left*), the decrease in the pressure inside the airway lumen (caused by combination of friction, turbulence, and the Venturi effect produced by the accelerated flow, *see inset*) causes a decrease in the airway caliber downstream from the obstruction point. When the obstruction is in the intrathoracic airways (*bottom left*), the decrease in pressure inside the airways is offset by a greater decrease in pleural pressure, which mitigates the effects of the obstruction of airway gas flow. During expiration, pressure in the airway lumen increases as a result of the passive recoil of the lungs and chest wall and, when activated, the contractile force of the expiratory muscles. When the obstruction is extrathoracic (*top right*), the increase in the pressure inside the airway dilates the airway lumen, improving the airflow. When the obstruction is intrathoracic (*bottom right*), however, pressure losses in the direction of flow (once again due to friction, turbulence, or acceleration) cause the pressure inside airways downstream from the obstruction to decrease below pleural pressure. As a result, the airway caliber decreases and the obstruction becomes exacerbated. Additional effort by the expiratory muscles to increase flow may worsen the obstruction by widening the gradient between pleural and intraluminal pressure.

cessory inspiratory muscles decrease pleural pressure well below atmospheric levels. Turbulence in the gas column and vibrations induced in the airway wall by the rushing gas create a high-pitch inspiratory noise known as *stridor*, which often can be heard without a stethoscope. The most prominent clinical feature of extrathoracic airway obstruction, however, is the prolongation of the inspiratory time. Expiration proceeds normally or may also be lengthened if the obstruction is severe enough to impede air exit despite the relative dilation of the airway lumen during expiration. Any circumstance that shortens the duration of inspiration compounds the negative effects of the obstruction because a shorter inspiration can only be accomplished by increasing gas velocity and by making the pressure inside the airways even more negative. Moreover, if viscous or wave-speed flow limitation is present, gas flow cannot be increased and the extra effort made by the subject is wasted.

The inside surface of the intrathoracic airways is also exposed to negative pressure during inspiration and positive pressure during expiration. The pressure acting on the outside surface of these airways, however, is similar to pleural pressure and therefore varies substantially during the breathing cycle. To understand how this variation affects airway transmural pressure, it is useful to keep in mind the two premises that define the relationship between the pressures in the pleural space and inside the airways. First, regardless of effort and breathing phase, pleural pressure must remain lower than alveolar pressure (the difference being the recoil pressure of the lungs). Second, the pressure inside the airways must be higher than alveolar pressure during inspiration and lower during expiration (otherwise flow cannot proceed). Based on these premises, the transmural pressure of the intrathoracic airways can only be positive during inspiration. During expiration, however, the pressure inside these airways decreases rapidly as friction steals energy from the flow stream and may, beyond a certain point, become lower than pleural pressure. Consequently, the transmural pressure of the intrathoracic airways can be positive or negative, depending on the location of an airway and the magnitude of the frictional losses, during expiration. When there is an obstruction in the intrathoracic airways, the decrease in the pressure applied to the inside surface is more than offset by the decrease in pleural pressure during inspiration, and the obstruction is partially relieved. However, during expiration, the steep decrease in the pressure inside the airways causes the transmural pressure to become negative and the caliber of the airways smaller somewhere between the obstruction point and the thoracic inlet. The decrease in caliber is dependent on the severity of the obstruction, the velocity of the flow (which draws the airway wall further into the flow stream), and the stiffness of the airway wall. Airways with abnormally soft cartilage or poor muscle tone are particularly vulnerable and may become obstructed during normal breathing (tracheobronchomalacia) or crying. Activation of the expiratory (abdominal) muscles may accelerate flow, but it also increases pleural pressure. Flow limitation (viscous or wave speed) develops eventually, and the muscle effort becomes wasted or counterproductive.

From a clinical point of view, the most distinguishing characteristic of intrathoracic airway obstruction is the prolongation of expiration. Usually, a high pitched noise or wheezing produced by high-frequency vibrations of the airway wall and gas column can be auscultated over the obstructed area or, if the obstruction is diffuse (eg, asthma), over the entire lung fields. Inspiration is less affected than expiration because the obstruction is partially relieved by the decrease in pleural pressure during this phase of the breathing cycle. However, severe intrathoracic airway obstruction also causes inspiratory difficulty, manifested as recruitment of accessory inspiratory muscles and inward chest-wall deformation. The preferential impairment of expiratory gas flow may not be compensated entirely by the prolonged expiratory phase. If so, the alveolar spaces serviced by the obstructed airways do not empty entirely before the next inspiration starts and the volume of the affected alveoli at end-expiration increases (a condition frequently referred to as *gas trapping*). The increase, however, is limited by the effects of distention on lung recoil, which dictate an equilibrium whereby the increased recoil limits tidal volume and accelerates exhalation enough to compensate for the low expiratory flow. The development of lung distention in patients with intrathoracic airway obstruction adds a restrictive component to the manifestations of their lung disease. This may be one of the reasons why children with asthma or other forms of bronchial obstruction have tachypnea as a prominent sign. The increase in lung volume is evident radiographically as decreased density denoting overinflation in the affected areas. When the disease is diffuse, the diaphragmatic curvature is reduced. Shortening of the phrenic fibers further diminishes the patient's ability to sustain ventilation. Complete bronchial obstruction also causes alveolar collapse due to reabsorption of the gas.

RESPIRATORY FAILURE

The main functions of the respiratory system are to replenish the venous blood's content of O_2 while removing its excess of CO_2. In general terms, respiratory failure is the inability to carry out this function in a manner commensurate with the needs of the organism. When considered in more specific terms, however, the definition is not as obvious. It is common, for example, to state that respiratory failure exists when the partial tensions of O_2 (PO_2) and CO_2 (PCO_2) in the arterial blood remain persistently outside the range found in normal humans (values of PO_2 <50 mm Hg or PCO_2 >45 mm Hg are often cited). However, this definition ignores the fact that breathing O_2-enriched gas can by itself restore the arterial PO_2 to the normal range, even though the gas-exchanging mechanism is faulty and may not sustain the needs of the individual while breathing air. Conversely, the same definition would categorize children with congenital cyanotic heart disease (who are hypoxemic) or with diuretic-induced metabolic alkalosis (who, as a compensatory mechanism, are hypercapnic) as suffering from respiratory failure, even though their respiratory system may be perfectly functional.

For these reasons, rather than detecting specific aberrations in blood gas content, the clinician's primary concern should focus on whether the respiratory system can support metabolic demands under all the circumstances that the patient is likely to encounter. Fever or exercise often unveil otherwise compensated anomalies of gas exchange by adding to the ventilatory load of the respiratory muscles or by increasing demand for pulmonary blood flow. Hypoxemia and hypercapnia interfere most noticeably with the function of the central nervous and cardiovascular systems. Agitation, somnolence, apathy, combativeness, or even stupor in an infant or child with respiratory distress or decreased respiratory effort should at least prompt the administration of O_2, even if blood gas analysis is unavailable. Increasing tachycardia, arterial hypertension, or, by way of progression, decreased perfusion, arterial hypotension, and bradycardia are worrisome signs in a patient with a respiratory derangement and, under most circumstances, constitute indications for the institution of ventilatory support.

Disruption of Gas Exchange: Hypoxemia and Hypercapnia

An understanding of the mechanisms that lead to blood gas aberrations in infants and children with respiratory failure is essential both to interpret clinical information and to plan treatment. Basic to such understanding is the notion that the interactions between the inspired gas and the blood in the lungs materialize into two simultaneous products: the expired gas and the arterial blood. Each of these products is a composite of the contributions of millions of alveolar-capillary units, weighted by the amount of oxygen or carbon dioxide in blood or gas from each unit. In every one of these units, and in the lung as a whole, the gas contents of the alveolar gas and the capillary blood are linked reciprocally by relatively simple laws, which establish a framework for the understanding of the gas-exchanging process and its abnormalities. Moreover, in alveolar-capillary units where there is an exchange of gas, it is generally assumed that the pressure of O_2 and CO_2 develop equilibrium between the blood and gas phase.

Because both O_2 and CO_2 are highly diffusible gases, diffusion impairments play little role in the genesis of hypoxemia or hypercarbia in children with respiratory disease. Accordingly, it is safe to assume that the PO_2 and PCO_2 of the blood exiting a given pulmonary capillary reflects the PO_2 and PCO_2 of the gas contained in the corresponding alveolus. The composition of the alveolar gas is determined by the rate at which gas that has undergone exchange with blood is replaced by fresh gas (ventilation) and by the relative rates of O_2 and CO_2 exchange across the alveolar-capillary membrane (O_2 uptake and CO_2 elimination). The relationship between alveolar PO_2, ventilation, and O_2 uptake is relatively complicated, among other reasons because O_2 is present in both the inspired and the expired gas. The relationship between PCO_2, ventilation, and CO_2 elimination, on the other hand, is relatively simple because the inspired gas does not contain CO_2. For the whole lung, the average alveolar PCO_2 is directly proportional to the amount of CO_2 produced by the body and inversely proportional to the volume of gas that participates in alveolar gas exchange per unit of time. The latter is known as *alveolar ventilation* (as opposed to *minute ventilation*, which is the total amount of gas that exits the lungs per unit of time or the product of tidal volume by breathing frequency).

Physiologists have taken advantage of the inverse relationship between alveolar PCO_2 and alveolar ventilation to compute the portion of the minute ventilation that does not participate in CO_2 exchange. This quantity, known as the *dead space* or *wasted ventilation*, provides a partial but useful view into the efficiency of the gas-exchanging process. By envisioning that each breath is a mixture of gas from dead space ($PCO_2 = 0$) and the alveolar space ($PCO_2 = PA_{CO_2}$), the ratio of the dead space ventilation to the tidal volume (V_T) can be calculated as:

$$V_D \,/\, V_T = (PA_{CO_2} - PE_{CO_2}) \,/\, PA_{CO_2}$$

where PE_{CO_2} is the PCO_2 of the mixed expired gas. Alveolar PCO_2 cannot be measured directly, but can be estimated using widely available monitoring tools. The end-tidal PCO_2, for instance, measures the PCO_2 of the gas exhaled at end-expiration on the assumption that it contains only alveolar gas. Along the same lines, the arterial PCO_2 is similar to the end-capillary PCO_2 and, barring any shunting of venous blood into the arterial circulation, it should be similar to the alveolar PCO_2 (in clinical practice the end-tidal PCO_2 is monitored as a surrogate of the arterial PCO_2; see (see Sec. 4.2.1). However, the end-tidal PCO_2 and the arterial PCO_2 may be quite different, especially in the presence of lung disease. The reason is that alveoli, which are relatively underperfused, have very low alveolar PCO_2 values; thus the gas that exits these alveoli lowers the end-tidal PCO_2 considerably. Alveoli that are relatively underventilated, in contrast, cannot have PCO_2 values greater than the mixed-venous blood (which is only a few mm Hg greater than the arterial PCO_2); thus, they are underrepresented in the end-tidal PCO_2. It follows that substituting the end-tidal or the arterial PCO_2 for the alveolar PCO_2 in the equation above yields two different values of the dead space. When the end-tidal PCO_2 is used, the result estimates the volume of gas contained in the conducting airways (fresh gas during inspiration and a mixture of fresh gas and

alveolar gas during expiration), away from the gas-exchanging regions of the lung (*anatomic* or *series dead space*). When the arterial PCO_2 is used, on the other hand, the resulting value (*physiological dead space*) is greater because it includes not only the anatomic dead space but also all the gas that enters the alveoli without undergoing CO_2 exchange (*alveolar* or *parallel dead space*). Dead-space calculations are impractical in clinical practice because they require cumbersome collection of the expiratory gas. The difference between arterial and end-tidal PCO_2, however, can be used as a simple bedside tool to assess disease or treatment-related changes in the distribution of perfusion in the lungs. Pulmonary emboli, for example, can be detected as a conspicuous decrease in the end-tidal PCO_2 relative to the arterial PCO_2 when the expired PCO_2 is monitored continuously (see Sec. 4.2.1). Similarly, redistribution of pulmonary blood away from overinflated areas of the lung during the application of positive end-expiratory pressure (PEEP) widens the difference between arterial and end-tidal PCO_2 in a fashion that can be used to adjust the therapy.

Another factor that contributes to the complex relationship between PO_2, ventilation, and oxygen uptake is that O_2 and CO_2 are often exchanged at an uneven rate; this creates a volume deficit that must be filled with O_2-containing fresh gas (typically O_2 consumption exceeds CO_2 production by 20%). Physiologists have circumvented these difficulties by recognizing that the reduction in PO_2 as gas equilibrates with blood in the alveolus is directly related to the increase in CO_2. The alveolar PO_2 can then be calculated by determining the PO_2 of the inspired gas and by subtracting the PO_2 decline produced by the CO_2-O_2 exchange between alveolus and pulmonary capillary. The resultant expression is the *alveolar gas equation*, in which the inequality of the CO_2-O_2 exchange is represented by the *respiratory exchange ratio* (R), or the result of dividing the CO_2 production by the O_2 consumption:

$$PA_{O_2} = FI_{O_2}\,(PB - PH_2O) - PA_{CO_2}\,[FI_{O_2} + (1 - FI_{O_2})/R]$$

where FI_{O_2} is the fractional concentration of O_2 in the inspired gas, PB is the atmospheric pressure, and PH_2O is the partial pressure of water vapor at body temperature. This formulation illustrates well the point that alveolar PO_2 and PCO_2 are linked to each other in such a way that, when one of them is specified, only one value can exist for the other in any particular alveolus. The alveolar gas equation can also be used to take a global view of the lung as if gas exchange were homogenous. Under such ideal circumstances, the alveolar PO_2 represents the highest PO_2 that could be expected in arterial blood. Thus, any difference between the calculated alveolar PO_2 and the actual arterial PO_2 (the *alveolar-arterial PO_2 difference*) is an important means for detecting and understanding aberrations in gas exchange.

When alveolar ventilation decreases globally (hypoventilation), alveolar PCO_2 and, by extent, arterial PCO_2 increase with the reduction in alveolar ventilation. As shown by the alveolar gas equation, alveolar and arterial PO_2 decline, and the decrease in arterial PO_2 is proportional to the increase in alveolar or arterial PCO_2 (the proportionality constant being R). Useful as the alveolar-arterial PO_2 difference is for detecting an abnormality in gas exchange, its magnitude changes considerably with the inspired O_2 concentration, which cannot always be controlled or known with precision. Thus, physiologists have developed an alternative strategy to quantify derangements in gas exchange. Just as dead space is an index of the efficiency (or rather the inefficiency) of CO_2 exchange in the lungs, *shunt* or *venous admixture* provides a similar quantitative index for the efficiency of O_2 exchange by dividing the pulmonary blood flow into two compartments. Shunt is composed of pulmonary capillary blood that undergoes ideal O_2 exchange with the alveolar gas, and the venous admixture is composed of venous blood that travels unaltered to the arterial side of the circulation. Venous admixture ($\dot{Q}s$) is usually expressed as a fraction of the systemic blood flow ($\dot{Q}t$), calculated by performing an O_2 mass balance across the pulmonary circulation:

$$\dot{Q}s/\dot{Q}t = (Cc'_{O_2} - Ca_{O_2}) / (Cc'_{O_2} - C\bar{v}_{O_2})$$

where Cc'_{O_2}, Ca_{O_2}, and $C\bar{v}_{O_2}$ are the O_2 contents (total volume of O_2 per 100 mL of blood) of the pulmonary capillary (estimated by the alveolar gas equation), the arterial blood (measured directly in a systemic artery), and mixed venous blood (measured directly in the pulmonary artery). Carrying further the comparison with the concept of dead space, pulmonary venous blood has two components. One consists of systemic venous blood that bypasses the alveoli and hence cannot take up O_2. The other arises from blood that undergoes perfect exchange of O_2 and CO_2 with alveolar gas, thereby attaining the blood gas composition predicted by the alveolar gas equation applied to the region of interest. The mixture of these two components determines the actual arterial blood PO_2.

For simplicity, the source of the blood that bypasses alveoli has conventionally been viewed as arising from several discrete pathways. First, *true anatomic shunt* follows anatomic communications between the venous and arterial side of the circulation. Some of these communications are found in normal individuals (eg, thebesian veins, which connect the coronary circulation to the left ventricle, or the bronchial vessels, which direct venous blood into the pulmonary veins). Others are the result of cardiac malformations or lung disease resulting in alveolar collapse or consolidation (ventilation-perfusion ratio of 0). Second, areas with a barrier to diffusion reduce the end-capillary PO_2 and thus contribute to venous admixture (which is not an important source of hypoxemia in infants or children). Finally, ventilation-perfusion inequality is the most common mechanism of venous admixture in patients with lung disease. The latter two conditions are also known as *virtual shunt* because the amount of shunt decreases with O_2 breathing (Table 4-2). In contrast, when an anatomic shunt exists, O_2 administration can only increase the oxygen content of the arterial blood by raising the volume of O_2 dissolved in the pulmonary capillary blood.

Ventilation-perfusion inequality is the most common mechanism of hypoxemia and hypercapnia both in children and adults with respiratory disease. Ventilation-perfusion differences are a natural consequence of the parallel organization of the bronchial and arterial networks of the lungs, which permits an infinite combination of ventilation-perfusion ratios to coexist in the same lung. Gravity causes a certain degree of ventilation-perfusion inequality

in normal lungs by directing a larger share of blood flow to dependent areas. Bronchial obstruction, consolidation or collapse of alveolar spaces, and abnormalities in pulmonary vascular function exaggerate this inequality greatly.

The cause of hypoxemia in ventilation-perfusion inequality lies primarily with the alveolar-capillary units that have a low ventilation-perfusion ratio (Fig. 4-6). Because renewal of the alveolar gas through ventilation cannot keep up with O_2 uptake by the blood, these units have a low alveolar PO_2, usually in a range where the O_2-hemoglobin dissociation curve is steep. As a result, the end-capillary blood is not fully loaded with O_2, and when mixed with blood from other units, it creates a substantial venous admixture. Units with high ventilation-perfusion ratios have a high alveolar PO_2. However, these units cannot compensate for the venous admixture caused by units with low ventilation-perfusion ratios because, at high PO_2 levels, the O_2-hemoglobin dissociation curve is flat and the blood cannot increase its O_2 content substantially.

Alveolar-capillary units with low ventilation-perfusion ratios cannot decrease their alveolar PCO_2 much below the mixed-venous level; thus, their ability to remove CO_2 from the blood is impaired. However, units with a high ventilation-perfusion ratio may lower their alveolar PCO_2 considerably. This establishes an efficient mechanism of compensation, which makes hypercapnia less prominent than hypoxemia, provided that the infant or child has sufficient respiratory muscle reserve to support the necessary increase in ventilation.

Clinical Manifestations

The majority of infants and children who develop respiratory failure suffer from some form of mechanical dysfunction of the lungs or chest wall. Respiratory distress is then the leading manifestation of the failure and the usual reason why medical attention is sought. Careful assessment of the incumbent physical signs usually provides helpful insight not only into the restrictive or obstructive character of the dysfunction but also into the exact nature of the disease that causes it (Fig. 4-7). Occasionally, however, an infant or child presents with respiratory failure caused by a primary or secondary dysfunction of the respiratory control or its neural connections. Under such circumstances, it is often the suspicion that the respiratory effort is insufficient to support the patient's ventilatory requirements that prompts the clinician to analyze pulmonary gas exchange and diagnose the presence of respiratory failure.

Increased Respiratory Effort and Mechanical Dysfunction

Severe respiratory disease inevitably interferes with both the mechanical and gas-exchanging functions of the respiratory system.

TABLE 4-2

RESPONSE OF ARTERIAL HYPOXEMIA TO O_2 BREATHING IN PULMONARY DISEASE

PHYSIOLOGIC ANOMALY	CALCULATED SHUNT FRACTION	ALVEOLAR-ARTERIAL PO_2 DIFFERENCE	EFFECT OF BREATHING 100% O_2
True or anatomic shunt	Increased	Increased	Calculated shunt is unchanged. Arterial PO_2 increases by addition of O_2 in ventilated areas (increase is small and depends on initial arterial PO_2).
Diffusion defects	Increased	Increased	Calculated shunt decreases. Arterial PO_2 increases.
Ventilation-perfusion inequality	Increased	Increased	Calculated shunt usually decreases. Arterial PO_2 increases.
Global hypoventilation	Unchanged	Unchanged	Calculated shunt is unchanged. Arterial PO_2 increases.

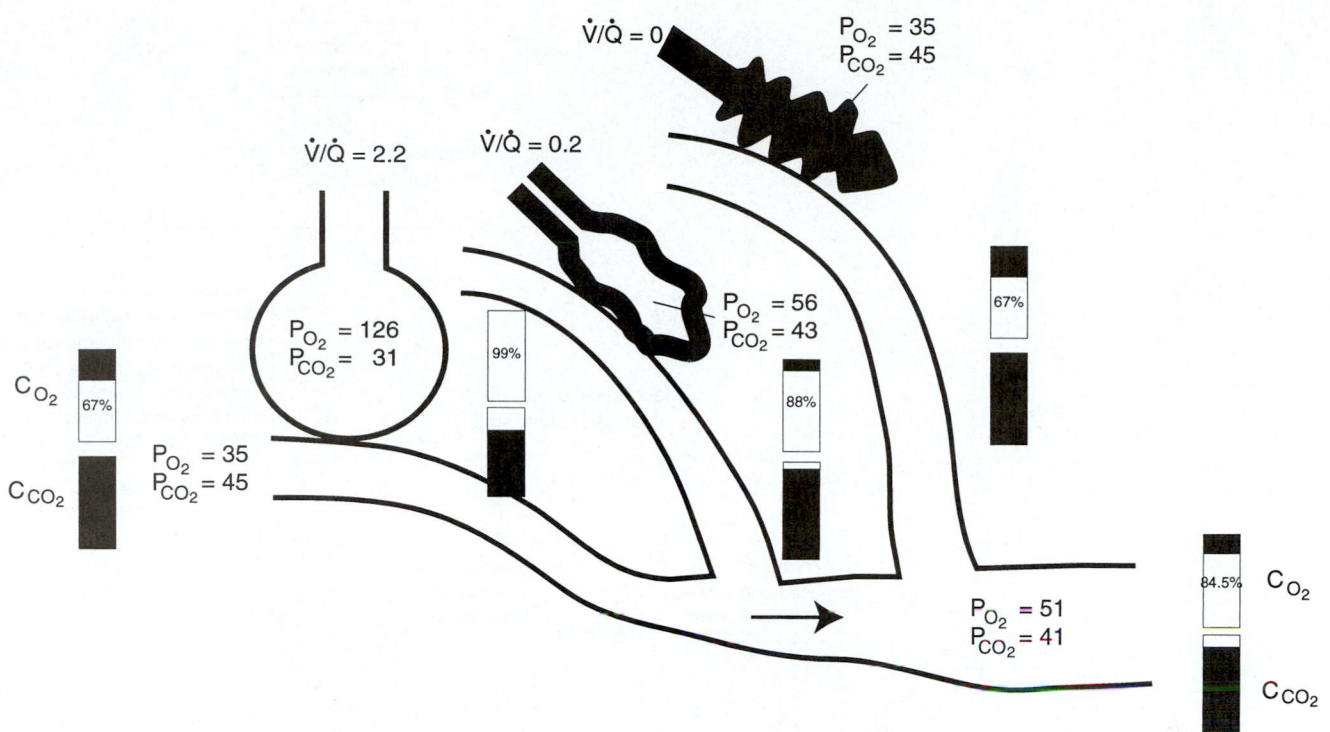

FIGURE 4-6   **Effect of ventilation-perfusion inequality on gas exchange. The diagram depicts three alveolar-capillary units, with ventilation/perfusion ratios ($\dot{V}/\dot{Q}$) of 2.2, 0.2, and 0. The alveolar P_{O_2} and P_{CO_2} of each unit were calculated for atmospheric air at sea level. The P_{O_2} and P_{CO_2} of the mixed-venous blood were assumed to be 35 and 45 mm Hg, respectively. The O_2 (C_{O_2}) and CO_2 (C_{CO_2}) contents of the mixed venous blood, the end-capillary blood for each unit, and the arterial blood were determined by assuming a hemoglobin concentration of 15 g/dL and that each unit contributed equally to the arterial outflow. The proportion of O_2-unsaturated hemoglobin (closed portion of the C_{O_2} box) in the arterial blood originates from the units with a reduced ventilation/perfusion ratio. Even if hypoxemia or hypercapnia induces a hyperventilatory response, units with a high ventilation-perfusion ratio cannot mitigate the hypoxemia because the shape of the hemoglobin dissociation curve prevents a substantial increase in the contribution of these units to the arterial O_2 content. Most of the CO_2 volume removed from the mixed-venous blood (open portion of the C_{CO_2} box) is eliminated in units with a high ventilation-perfusion ratio, a feature that frequently allows patients to maintain the arterial P_{CO_2} within normal range. However, severe ventilation-perfusion inequality may cause hypercapnia because the relationship between CO_2 content and P_{CO_2} is not perfectly linear and limits compensation by units with a high ventilation/perfusion ratio.**

Increased demands on the respiratory muscles combined with incipient arterial blood gas abnormalities trigger a compensatory response that is the essence of respiratory distress. Whether compensation is achieved or not depends on two conditions: the respiratory muscles must be able to perform and sustain the necessary work and the gas-exchange abnormalities must be correctable by an increase in ventilation. The situation in which the respiratory muscles are no longer capable of performing work commensurate with the ventilatory needs of the organism has been described as *respiratory muscle fatigue,* drawing an analogy with the behavior of skeletal muscle when subjected to excessive work. Recognizing its imminence is fundamental to preventing the development of life-threatening hypoxemia and hypercapnia, usually through the institution of mechanical ventilatory support.

The ability of the respiratory muscles to carry an increased mechanical load depends on the balance between the amount of energy that the muscles can transform into physical work and the magnitude of the work demands imposed by breathing. On one side of the balance, energy is provided to the respiratory muscles in the form of substrates (nutrients and O_2) carried by a well-regulated blood flow. Although the respiratory muscles, especially the diaphragm, can increase their blood supply severalfold, cardiovascular disease often imposes limitations to this ability by forcing the muscles to compete with other organs for their apportionment of the cardiac output. Respiratory failure may then result from respiratory workloads that would be tolerable, or even normal, under other circumstances. On the other side of the balance, the work demands of breathing are defined by the volume-pressure relationships of the respiratory system. Restrictive and obstructive impairments raise the pressure required to generate a certain minute ventilation. Moreover, by increasing physiological dead space, both forms of respiratory disease increase the minute ventilation needed to achieve a given alveolar ventilation, adding to the burden of the respiratory muscles.

Not all the energy processed by the respiratory muscles, however, is transformed into physical work. The result of dividing the pressure-volume work that the respiratory muscles do on the lungs and chest wall during a period of time by the energy that they

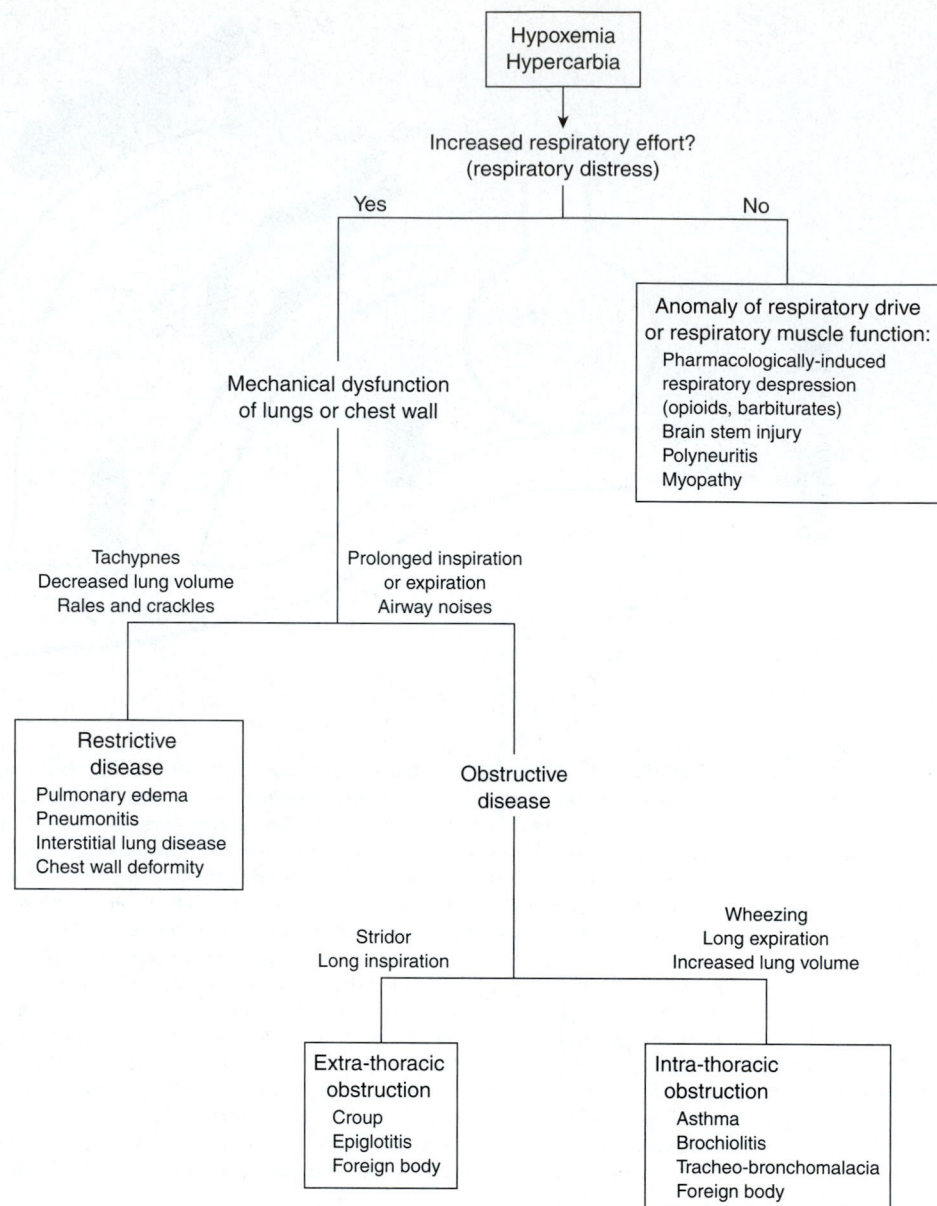

FIGURE 4-7   Diagnostic algorithm of hypoxemia and hypercarbia.

consume during the same period defines the *efficiency of the respiratory system*. The term is somewhat misleading because there are energy-consuming processes, such as the contraction of postural muscles that stabilize the chest wall, that do not change lung volume and therefore do not count as respiratory work. The best estimates suggest that respiratory efficiency does not exceed 15% in adults and is considerably lower in infants (values lower than 5% have been reported in premature newborns). Despite these limitations, the concept of efficiency is helpful to understand that the ability of the respiratory muscles to perform work is determined not only by the magnitude of the work itself but also by the factors that translate the work into energy cost. These factors include the respiratory pattern, the identity and state of conditioning of the respiratory muscles, and the configuration of the chest wall.

Breathing pattern is influenced by the nature and extent of the mechanical derangements produced by the disease. Although no plausible neural mechanism has been identified to date, the practical reality is that infants and children modify their tidal volume and

breathing frequency in a manner that minimizes energy expenditure. Thus, any conditions—external or internal—that interfere with a patient's ability to adopt an optimal pattern diminish by definition the efficiency of the respiratory system. Rapid breathing caused by agitation, for example, may precipitate respiratory muscle fatigue and failure in a child with croup or epiglottitis who is ill-advisedly separated from his or her mother to be examined in more detail. Similarly, bradypnea caused by central nervous system depression is a very disadvantageous breathing pattern in a child with pulmonary edema or other form of restrictive lung disease. Respiratory muscle fatigue appears to dictate respiratory pattern requirements of its own. Patients who are experiencing a decrease in the contraction force of their diaphragm often breathe rapidly and shallowly, regardless of whether their disease is predominantly restrictive or obstructive. It is also common for such patients to alternate the respiratory load between several muscle groups in a fashion that suggests that intermittent resting may make the effort more sustainable. Interestingly, some have proposed (but never demonstrated) that apnea and periodic breathing are indeed strategies to prevent respiratory fatigue in prematurely born and small infants whose diaphragm is burdened by excessive chest-wall distortion during inspiration.

Which specific muscles or muscles groups are activated in an effort to overcome a mechanical impairment has substantial bearing on breathing efficiency. The diaphragm is capable of increasing its work with only limited increases of its O_2 consumption and blood-flow requirements. Other accessory inspiratory and expiratory muscles are much less economic relative to the increase in ventilatory output that they generate, and as a consequence, their energy demands may quickly overburden the patient. This may be the case of the abdominal muscles, for which this disadvantage is often compounded by the presence of expiratory flow limitation, which renders their effort to increase expiratory flow even more wasteful. Poor nutrition, atrophy from lack of use (eg, in patients who have their ventilation fully supported for long periods of time), and myopathy all decrease the efficiency of the respiratory muscles by raising their energetic demands out of proportion with the work that they perform.

Limited ossification of the rib cage and the short axial dimension of the thorax makes the newborn and small infant's chest wall particularly prone to distortion. This may affect respiratory muscle efficiency by several mechanisms. First, all muscles achieve their maximal ratio of work-to-energy consumption at an optimal length. Overinflation of the lungs and abdominal distention flatten the diaphragmatic dome and reduce the effective length of the phrenic muscle fibers, degrading not only the maximal force that these fibers are able to develop but also the overall energetic efficiency of the muscle. In addition, developmental and disease-induced changes in the geometry of the chest influence the area of contact between the lateral surface of the diaphragm and the internal surface of the rib cage. This area, known as the *area of apposition* of diaphragm and the rib cage, facilitates lung inflation by translating the increase in intra-abdominal pressure produced by the diaphragmatic descent into an outward-directed force acting on the ribs. Because infants have a relatively wide lower chest, the costal insertions of the diaphragm are spread out, making their area of apposition small. Overinflation of the lungs and abdominal distention can further limit the lateral contact between diaphragm and rib cage, thereby wasting the work that the diaphragm does on the abdominal organs. Finally, inward distortion of the rib cage increases the shortening that the phrenic fibers must undergo in order to generate a certain volume change in the lungs. In the absence of distortion, the volume displaced by the diaphragmatic contraction is approximately the same as the volume increase of the lungs. When inward distortion occurs, however, the volume displaced by the diaphragm is divided between the volume increase of the lungs and the volume created by the inward movement of the rib cage (Fig. 4-8). Although strictly speaking the diaphragm performs real work to distort the rib cage, the energy used in the process is wasted in terms of ventilation. In this waste lies one of the major disadvantages that the immature child faces when developing lung disease: Chest wall distortion can multiply severalfold the work performed by the diaphragmatic muscle and may lead rapidly to respiratory muscle fatigue, even in the absence of a serious mechanical derangement of the lungs.

Decreased Ventilatory Effort and Hypoventilation

Abnormal decreases in the respiratory effort lead to *hypoventilation,* a condition in which the renewal of the alveolar gas is insufficient

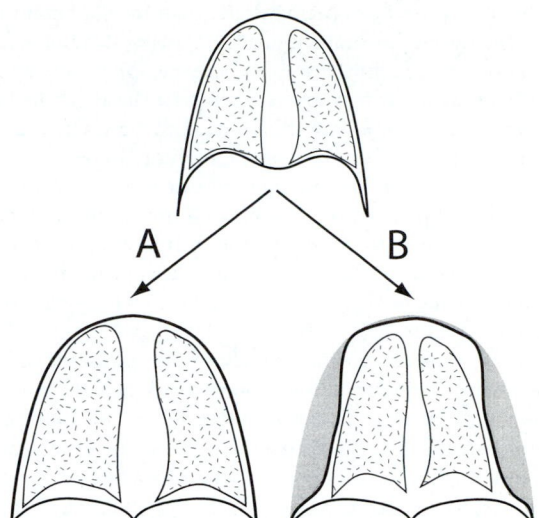

FIGURE 4-8   **Effect of rib cage distortion on lung volume change and diaphragmatic displacement. Inward distortion during inspiration is common in the newborn and small infant, particularly when pleural pressure is decreased to overcome lung disease. The diagram shows how the same inspiratory displacement of the diaphragm is applied entirely to inflate the lungs in the absence of distortion (A) and divided between the inward volume change of the rib cage (*shaded area*) and lung inflation when distortion exists (B).**

to maintain normal CO_2 and arterial O_2 tensions. The mechanisms underlying the blood-gas abnormalities that ensue are (a) the dependence of alveolar PCO_2 on alveolar ventilation and (b) the combined effects of the poor renewal of the alveolar gas and the continued uptake of O_2 by the pulmonary capillaries on the alveolar PO_2. Hypoventilation may be difficult to detect unless it occurs in a patient whose gas exchange is already being monitored or it is accompanied by other clinical findings such as upper-airway obstruction. Hypoxemia is present if the patient is breathing room air, but it is not always evident as cyanosis, especially in the presence of anemia or when the light conditions are unfavorable. Hypercapnia produces nonspecific clinical manifestations, somnolence usually being the most prominent.

The finding of a reduced respiratory effort, particularly when the patient is hypercapnic and hypoxemic, should raise immediate suspicion about the integrity of the central nervous system's function (see Fig. 4-7). Direct injuries to the brain, such as those caused by ischemia, an expanding intracranial mass, or infection, can lessen the brainstem's response to chemoreceptor stimulation. Metabolic toxins or exogenous pharmacologic agents may have similar consequences. Opioids, in particular, are effective inhibitors of the respiratory drive, a property that is often exploited to reduce spontaneous breathing and facilitate mechanical ventilation. Their advantages under such circumstances, however, often turn to disadvantage when it becomes appropriate to discontinue ventilatory support. Overdosing with opioids and benzodiazepines is a frequent cause of persistent respiratory failure in mechanically ventilated infants and children. Although it is not always easy to distinguish medication-induced hypoventilation from mechanical dysfunction and especially from muscle weakness, the clinician should be alerted to this possibility whenever a patient has a decreased arterial pH (acidemia) without signs of respiratory distress.

The respiratory control appears to be under more dominant inhibitory influences from supramedullary centers in newborn infants, especially if they are born prematurely, than in older children and adults. This developmental singularity explains why newborn infants may breathe shallowly or even become apneic in response to alveolar hypoxemia. It may also explain why these infants become apneic when their pulmonary stretch receptors are activated by excessive lung inflation (the basis of the Hering-Breuer reflex) or by stimuli that arise from the lung interstitium and airway walls in the presence of lung disease. An exaggerated inhibitory response to a combination of alveolar hypoxemia and mechanoreceptor stimulation is likely to be responsible for the frequency with which small infants have apnea as the first manifestation of lung diseases such as viral pneumonitis.

In rare circumstances, the anomaly of the respiratory control is isolated to the respiratory premotor network and the only manifestation of the disease is hypoventilation, usually during sleep, when supramedullary excitatory influences on the respiratory control are at a minimum (Ondine's curse). More frequently, the decrease in respiratory drive is part of a more extensive dysfunction of the central nervous system, involving supratentorial areas of the brain or other centers in the brainstem. Because the medullary neuronal networks that control the inspiratory muscles (eg, diaphragm) and the muscles that dilate the upper airway (eg, genioglossus or cricoarytenoid) are integrated functionally, hypoventilation is usually associated with upper-airway obstruction caused by decreased pharyngeal tone and glottic obstruction. This is manifested as snoring (stertor), stridor, and reduced air entry into the lungs during inspiration. The neuronal reflexes responsible for airway-protective mechanisms such as coughing and gagging are part of these networks, and they are also frequently impaired. In such case, accumulation of mucus and saliva in the upper airway and bronchi compounds the airway obstruction. Because the amplitude of the respiratory excursions and absolute lung volume are decreased, alveolar collapse becomes inevitable. Thus, it is not unusual to find alveolar densities in the chest radiograph of patients in whom the primary alteration is a reduction of the respiratory drive, a feature that may create confusion by leading the clinician toward a diagnosis of primary lung disease.

MANAGEMENT OF RESPIRATORY FAILURE

Mechanical ventilation, whether provided through an endotracheal tube or a mask, is often the only viable alternative to restore gas exchange and to unload the respiratory muscles when respiratory failure is imminent or already present. The physiological bases and practical applications of the various techniques of ventilatory support are discussed in Sec. 4.2.2.

Initial Management of the Child with Respiratory Distress and Failure

Patients with respiratory dysfunction are best served when even the initial treatment addresses the cause, or at least the mechanism, of the dysfunction. Pulmonary edema in a child with left ventricular failure, for example, is best treated with diuretics and, if appropriate, with inotropic medications. Bacterial pneumonia demands the use of antibiotics selected for the causal organism. Life-threatening upper-airway obstruction should be relieved by bypassing the obstructed airway segment with an endotracheal tube or other type of artificial airway. However, etiologic or mechanistic approaches require time and may not be possible if the cause of the disease is not apparent. Under such circumstances, the goal of the therapy is to guarantee the adequacy of gas exchange with minimal discomfort, pain, and complications for the patient. On occasion, this goal can be achieved by simple measures that increase the efficiency of the respiratory system, while avoiding interventions that may render it inefficient. For example, lifting the head of the bed in a patient with severe orthopnea may reduce upper-airway resistance and increase the initial length of the diaphragmatic fibers, improving the diaphragm's ability to handle its load enough so as to turn an unstable situation into a more stable one. Emptying a filled stomach may also improve the efficiency of the diaphragmatic contraction and increase lung volume at end-expiration. Avoiding actions that may frighten or upset a severely distressed child with croup or epiglottitis, on the other hand, allows the child to continue making use of an advantageous breathing pattern while preparations for safe intubation of the trachea are made.

Of all the alterations found in respiratory failure, hypoxemia is by far the most life-threatening. Every clinician must remember that the administration of O_2 to a child with respiratory distress is inherently safe and should not be delayed until the hypoxemia is corroborated by blood-gas analysis. The only notable exceptions are in patients for whom hyperoxia-induced pulmonary vasodilation may divert systemic blood flow to the pulmonary circulation through a large left-to-right shunt (eg, large ventricular septal defects, hypoplastic left-heart syndrome) or in newborns with ductal-dependent lesions whose ductus arteriosus may constrict in response to an increasing Po_2. Oxygen can be administered with a variety of devices. Nasal prongs are widely used at all ages because they are comfortable and usually well tolerated by infants and toddlers. Unfortunately, they provide only limited O_2-enrichment and humidification of the inspired gas and are not useful in patients who breathe through their mouth. Hoods can raise the concentrations of inspired O_2 to close to 100%, but they are cumbersome and threatening to small children. Masks and face tents are best tolerated by older patients. When equipped with a bag reservoir and a one-way exhalation valve (nonrebreathing masks), they approach the O_2 delivery efficiency of a hood.

References

Bryan AC, Wohl MEB: Respiratory mechanics in children. In: Macklem PT, Mead J, eds: Handbook of Physiology: The Respiratory System, Vol III, Part 2. Bethesda, MD, American Physiological Society, 1986: 179–191

Heldt GP, McIlroy MB: Distortion of chest wall and work of diaphragm in preterm infants. J Appl Physiol 62:164–169, 1981

Mead J: Respiration: pulmonary mechanics. Ann Rev Physiol 35:169–192, 1973

Pérez Fontán JJ: Mechanics of breathing. In: Gluckman PD, Heymann MA, eds: Pediatrics & Perinatology: The Scientific Basis. London, Arnold, 1996:845–855

Pérez Fontán JJ, Lister Q: Respiratory failure. In: Touloukian RJ, ed: Pediatric Trauma. St. Louis, Mosby, 1990:46–76

Roussos C, Campbell EJM: Respiratory muscle energetics. In: Macklem PT, Mead J, eds: Handbook of Physiology: The Respiratory System, Vol III, Part 2. Bethesda, MD, American Physiological Society, 1986:481–509

Weibel ER: The Pathway for Oxygen: Structure and Function of the Mammalian Respiratory System. Cambridge, MA, Harvard University Press, 1984

West JB: State of the art. Ventilation-perfusion relationships. Am Rev Resp Dis 116:919–943, 1977

West JB: Causes of carbon dioxide retention in lung disease. N Engl J Med 284:1232–1236, 1971

4.1.2   Poor Systemic Perfusion and Circulatory Shock

George Lister

Systemic perfusion can be reduced by a wide variety of processes and diseases that affect the infant and child. If there is not prompt recognition of the poor perfusion and appropriate intervention, there can be rapid progression to circulatory shock, a life-threatening state. While the regulatory mechanisms that control circulatory function are similar at all ages, some developmental features render the child vulnerable to circulatory dysfunction. For example, the high surface-to-mass ratio of the infant causes relatively high insensible water loss when there is fever, hypermetabolism, or a dry environment. The inability of the infant to have free access to fluids simultaneously limits the infant's capacity to respond and to restore any fluid-volume deficit (provoked by either loss of insensible water or enteric fluid with electrolytes). The young infant and certain other patients (eg, children with sickle cell disease) are susceptible to overwhelming infection, which as a consequence causes circulatory shock. And, the closure of the ductus arteriosus after birth can aggravate the obstruction to ventricular outflow with aortic stenosis or coarctation, thereby producing circulatory shock during this early postnatal period. It is the task of the clinician that confronts the child with poor perfusion to make a thorough, rigorous, and rapid assessment of the extent of the impairment and to determine the most likely mechanism(s) contributing to the circulatory disturbance as described in this section.

PATHOGENESIS

Reduced systemic perfusion provokes physical manifestations that are nonspecific, as well as physical manifestations that relate to the consequence or adaptation to the particular disturbance. Any of these types of signs may be responsible for signaling the need for medical attention. Nonspecific signs (eg, lassitude, hypotension, delayed capillary refill) provide information about severity of the dysfunction, but are not unique to a specific circulatory disturbance. Other, more specific signs (eg, crackles, gallop rhythm) relate to adaptation or result from the unique physiological alterations produced by the particular disturbance; these often provide valuable clues about the cause and mechanism of the derangement.

In considering both nonspecific and specific manifestations, it is useful to start by explaining some terms. Impaired perfusion here describes any state in which blood flow to the tissues is appreciably decreased. It encompasses a wide range of problems, from mild decreases in the circulating blood volume to cardiovascular collapse. *Shock* is the extreme form of impaired perfusion in which systemic blood flow is insufficient to sustain vital functions. An essential component of shock is that it is an unstable state; if left untreated, and possibly if treated, it causes progressive dysfunction of multiple organs and signs of severe tissue ischemia (eg, lactic acidemia). *Congestive circulatory failure* (see Sec. 22.4.4) is another form of impaired perfusion in which the compensatory mechanisms put forth by the cardiovascular system permit the maintenance of vital functions, but cause the patient to suffer complications of the adaptations (eg, peripheral and pulmonary edema, azotemia). Congestive circulatory failure also differs from shock because it is a more stable state.

The assessment of the child with impaired systemic blood flow is greatly facilitated by an understanding of how the normal mechanisms that maintain and regulate tissue perfusion can be altered by disease.

REGULATION OF TISSUE PERFUSION AND BLOOD PRESSURE

Blood flow and the supply of nutrients are normally in great excess of metabolic demands. Nearly 70% of the oxygen in arterial blood is returned to the right heart. This large reserve permits maintenance of metabolic balance even when there is a moderate decrease in cardiac output or increase in metabolic demands. However, when systemic blood flow is decreased relative to the tissues' needs, a variety of compensatory mechanisms are usually activated to redistribute the circulation and to maximize the extraction of oxygen and other nutrients from the blood. In the process, there are substantial changes in the perfusion and function of organs. As stated earlier, these changes provide important signs of an impaired circulation. The ability to acclimate to an imbalance between metabolic demands and tissue perfusion depends on the rapidity of onset of the disturbance and the presence of intact adaptive responses, some of which may be disturbed by the illness.

In general, blood flow is distributed to match the metabolic needs of an organ and blood pressure is tightly regulated so that organs such as the brain and heart remain well perfused when posture or activity change. Some organs, such as the skin and kidney, receive blood flow well in excess of their nutritive needs, because they perform specialized functions, for example, heat exchange and filtration, which necessitate high perfusion rates. When cardiac output is reduced, there are both local and systemic responses that sustain perfusion to metabolically active organs and that serve to maintain blood pressure (see Fig. 4-9). The redistribution of blood flow away from organs, such as the skin, gut, and kidneys, produces some characteristic changes in the physical examination that commonly help identify the child with a compromised circulation. To understand the nature of these changes it is worth briefly reviewing the mechanisms by which blood pressure and regional blood flow are regulated. Blood pressure provides the driving force to perfuse the organs and tissues. Because there is very little pressure drop within the large arteries, most organs receive blood at the same perfusion pressure. However, there are large intraorgan differences in the resistance to blood flow so that perfusion to individual organs varies widely despite the relative uniformity of perfusion pressure. Thus, blood flow to each organ is determined by both its perfusion pressure and its vascular resistance. Blood pressure is maintained by both neural and humoral influences, which serve to sustain perfusion pressure to organs throughout a wide range of cardiac output. For this reason, mean blood pressure is an insensitive measure of circulatory dysfunction and can be normal (or even increased) despite a marked reduction in cardiac output. This is well demonstrated by considering the relationship between pressure (P), flow (F), and resistance (R): $F \times R = P$. When flow, or cardiac output, is reduced, the host of neural and humoral responses that increase resistance sustain mean blood pressure near normal ($\downarrow F \times \uparrow R$ = near-normal P), although pulse pressure diminishes. Furthermore, processes such as sepsis, which interfere with vasoconstriction, can produce hypotension even though flow is not reduced.

When intravascular volume is reduced there is venous and arterial constriction (mediated by the sympathetic nervous system) and tachycardia (from disinhibition of the tonic vagal tone and increased circulating epinephrine). Whenever arterial blood pressure is reduced, there is a rapid (within seconds) reflex constriction of

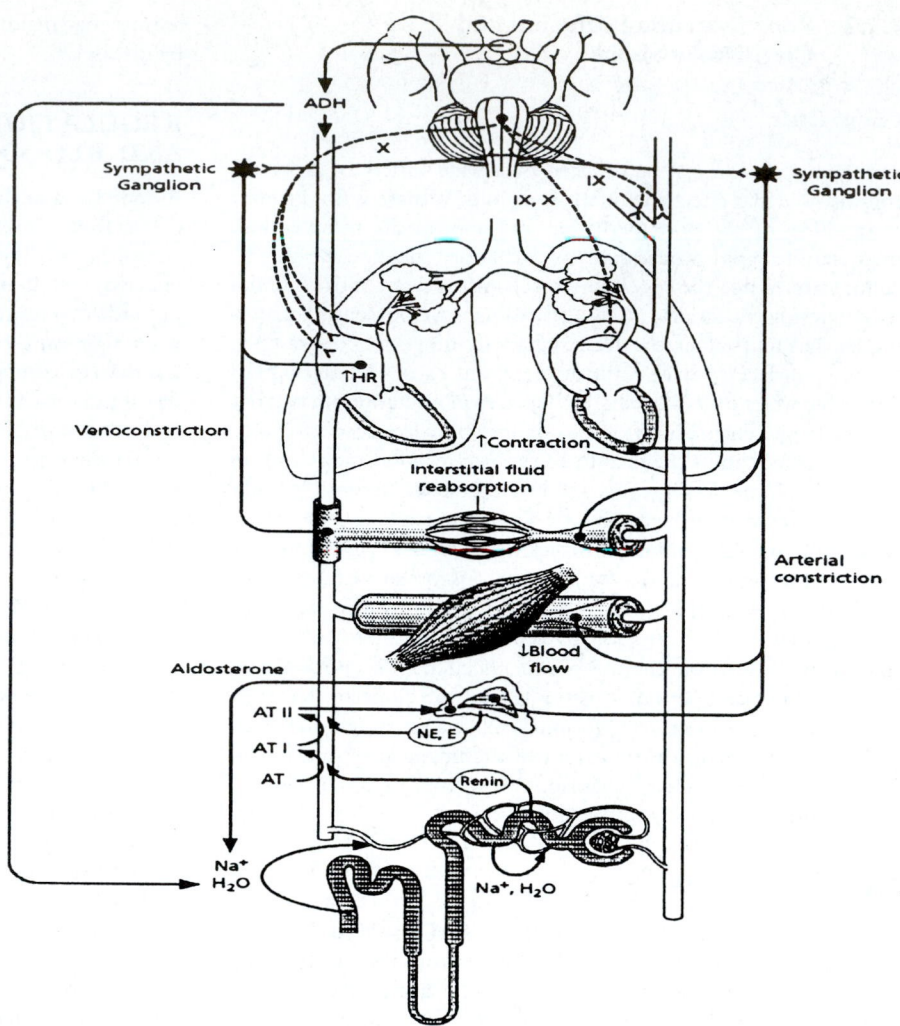

FIGURE 4-9 Diagram of neural and humoral responses to low cardiac output. The figure shows the important hormones and major afferent and efferent pathways that serve to restore perfusion when cardiac output is reduced. HR, heart rate; AT, angiotensin; NE, norepinephrine; E, epinephrine; ADH, antidiuretic hormone; roman numerals refer to respective cranial nerves. **SOURCE:** *Reproduced with permission from Lister G, Apkon M: Circulatory shock. In: Allen HD, Clark EB, Gutgesell HP, Driscoll DJ, eds: Moss and Adams Heart Disease in Infants, Children and Adolescents: Including the Fetus and Young Adult, 6th ed. Baltimore, MD, Lippincott Williams & Wilkins, 2000.*

most veins and arteries also mediated by the sympathetic nervous system. Intravascular volume is sensed by low-pressure stretch receptors located in the atria and pulmonary vessels, and arterial blood pressure is sensed by carotid sinus and aortic baroreceptors. The constrictive responses elicited by these receptors increase venous return, raise vascular resistance, and restore blood pressure. Although the venoconstriction can transiently increase venous return to the right heart, it also raises venous resistance, so it is necessary for other responses to raise the driving pressure for blood to return to the heart. Some of the increase in pressure is accomplished by *autotransfusion*, a process by which arteriolar constriction transiently lowers capillary hydrostatic pressure and promotes absorption of interstitial fluid into the capillaries.

In addition to the rapid responses to decreased blood pressure or volume, sympathetic stimulation of the adrenal gland causes the release of epinephrine and norepinephrine. These neural and humoral responses constrict renal afferent arterioles and stimulate renin release because of the decreased perfusion of the macula densa. Renin metabolizes angiotensinogen to angiotensin I, which is then hydrolyzed to angiotensin II by angiotensin-converting enzyme, an enzyme on the lumenal surface of endothelial cells. The angiotensin II stimulates release of aldosterone and antidiuretic hormone, and each of these hormones is a potent vasoconstrictor that raises blood pressure. Furthermore, antidiuretic hormone and aldosterone promote water and sodium reabsorption, respectively,

which helps restore intravascular volume. Thus, the humoral responses complement the neural reflexes and provide long-range regulation of the circulation.

REGULATION OF REGIONAL BLOOD FLOW

Even when arterial blood pressure decreases, some organs maintain blood flow by local vasodilation. In several organs (eg, brain, kidney, heart), a change in perfusion pressure causes the tone of the conducting vessels to change, such that blood flow stays constant (*autoregulation*). Autoregulation opposes the neural and humoral stimulation by the sympathoadrenal system and the release of vasoactive peptides that tend to cause vasoconstriction when cardiac output is decreased. How much a given organ responds to the vasodilatory or the vasoconstrictive influences depends on the inherent capacity to autoregulate, the α-adrenergic innervation (causing constriction), and the density and nature of the vascular receptors. Local metabolism also influences blood flow such that arteries perfusing active tissue (eg, working muscle) dilate and maintain blood flow even in the presence of neurohumoral stimulation. Therefore, when cardiac output is decreased, organs that are usually active metabolically or have little autonomic innervation (eg, brain or heart preserve their perfusion, whereas organs that have a low metabolic rate (eg, skin) or that have rich autonomic innervation (eg, kidney or gut) have intense vasoconstriction. These responses improve matching of blood flow to metabolism and, by increasing total vascular resistance, raise blood pressure.

When perfusion to an organ or tissue is reduced, local responses, including opening of previously closed capillaries and reduction in hemoglobin O_2 affinity can also serve to maximize the extraction of oxygen and other nutrients from arterial blood. The increased capillary density increases vascular surface area, reduces the diffusion distance, and increases the (transit) time for exchange. The reduced affinity because of the local decrease in pH permits more oxygen to be released from hemoglobin at any given venous PO_2. If oxidative metabolism cannot be sustained, the tissue produces excess H^+ and lactate, the metabolic rate declines, and the function of that tissue is reduced. Thus, when there is compromised perfusion to tissues, such as the skin, the cooler temperature (less perfusion with warm blood, less metabolism), prolonged capillary refill time (less perfusion), bluish or cyanotic discoloration (increased oxygen extraction and lower capillary and venous oxygen saturation), and diminished pulsation of the artery serving that tissue (vasoconstriction) all signal the impaired perfusion.

In addition to redistributing the limited blood flow, humoral responses serve to augment cardiac output by three mechanisms. Heart rate is increased (response to epinephrine and reduced vagal stimulation); sinus tachycardia is an expected adaptive response in any child with compromised perfusion unless there is also a problem in cardiac conduction or catecholamine response. Sinus tachycardia is also a sensitive barometer for the state of perfusion, because it is expected to decrease as perfusion improves. Contractility will also be enhanced by the catecholamine stimulation (norepinephrine and epinephrine), but the effectiveness of this adaptation depends on the capacity of the myocardium to respond and whether there is adequate cardiac filling. Finally, venous return will be increased by the venous and arterial constriction and by the mechanisms that promote fluid retention.

CAUSES OF INADEQUATE SYSTEMIC PERFUSION

Impaired perfusion arises when cardiac output to the tissues cannot keep pace with the demands for blood flow imposed by the body's metabolism. Because cardiac output is the product of stroke volume and heart rate, it depends directly on three factors: end-diastolic or filling volume, ejection fraction, and heart rate. If any of these was decreased, a decline in systemic blood flow would be expected, unless adaptive responses compensate. Alternatively, if metabolic demands were extraordinarily increased, perfusion might be insufficient, even if systemic blood flow were within the normal range. Mechanisms for low cardiac output are shown in Fig. 4-10, and examples of disturbances that decrease systemic perfusion are shown in Table 4-3.

Reduced cardiac filling occurs with intravascular volume depletion, increase in vascular capacity, or impedance to venous return. Whereas loss of intravascular volume from the body is apparent from history and measurement of body weight, loss within the body or increased vascular capacity can be subtle and only recognized by careful physical examination, especially when fluid has leaked into the interstitial space, bowel lumen, or peritoneum. Increased vascular (predominantly venous) capacity is a particularly difficult problem to detect because the blood volume remains in the vascular space and there is no sign of vascular congestion or weight loss. Finally, impedance to venous return dramatically reduces end-dia-

stolic volume of the heart but produces signs of increased systemic venous pressure (hepatic enlargement, jugular venous distention, fullness of the fontanel). Thus, the difference between collapsed veins and small cardiac silhouette with volume depletion or increased vascular capacity, and venous engorgement with increased impedance to venous return, is an important distinction in the physical examination.

Reduced ejection fraction results from poor contractile function or impedance (resistance) to outflow from the heart. With impaired contractile function, there is often a gallop rhythm and signs of systemic and pulmonary venous congestion. It is very important to recognize that the respiratory distress—including tachypnea, wheezing, air trapping, or alveolar collapse—from the congested and edematous lungs may mimic a primary pulmonary disease and obscure the diagnosis of cardiac dysfunction; a useful finding that implicates cardiac rather than respiratory disease is the presence of cardiomegaly. An increased afterload, the pressure against which the ventricle must pump during ejection, can also depress cardiac ejection, especially when the process is abrupt, for example, infants with aortic stenosis or coarctation in whom the ductus arteriosus closes or narrows. With an increased afterload there are also signs of systemic or pulmonary venous congestion, depending on which ventricle(s) is predominantly affected. However, circulatory shock can be the first obvious sign of the disturbance if the load on the heart rises abruptly before compensatory responses (eg, hypertrophy) can occur.

Although a slow heart rate is uncommon as a primary problem in children, it often occurs in response to asphyxia or when a patient is in extremis. Bradycardia can also aggravate other causes of poor perfusion because tachycardia is the expected adaptive response.

With any of these physiological disturbances, peripheral perfusion and cardiac output can be further disturbed by factors that increase the demands for blood flow, such as anemia, hypoxemia, fever, and excessive respiratory work. The importance of recognizing such factors is that they may sometimes be alleviated (eg, fever, anemia) and, in the process, significantly improve the balance between blood flow and metabolic demands.

ASSESSMENT

The first goal in assessment, which can usually be determined by careful physical examination, is to determine whether the child's perfusion is adequate to sustain vital functions or whether the circulatory disturbance is uncompensated. The physical findings of the child with poor perfusion reflect both the changes that occur primarily from the decrease in blood flow and those changes that occur in response to the adaptations. Superimposed on this picture may also be factors that relate to the underlying illness or injury that has disturbed the perfusion (Fig. 4-11). For example, the child with dehydration will have poor peripheral arterial pulses, cold and cyanotic extremities, and decreased capillary refill, whereas a child with sepsis might have warm extremities, edema, and easily felt peripheral pulses, even though there is acidosis and signs of organ dysfunction (see Sec. 13.1.7). With these general principles in mind, Table 4-4 gives an overview of the physical examination of the child with reduced systemic perfusion. These signs are sensitive to the degree of circulatory compromise, but are not specific for a particular cause of poor perfusion. And, as shown in Table 4-4, certain signs are particularly suggestive that the child may be in a state of uncompensated shock. Agitation, confusion or apathy, undetectable peripheral pulses, cold extremities, and hypotension

Reduced Cardiac Filling   **Impaired Ejection**

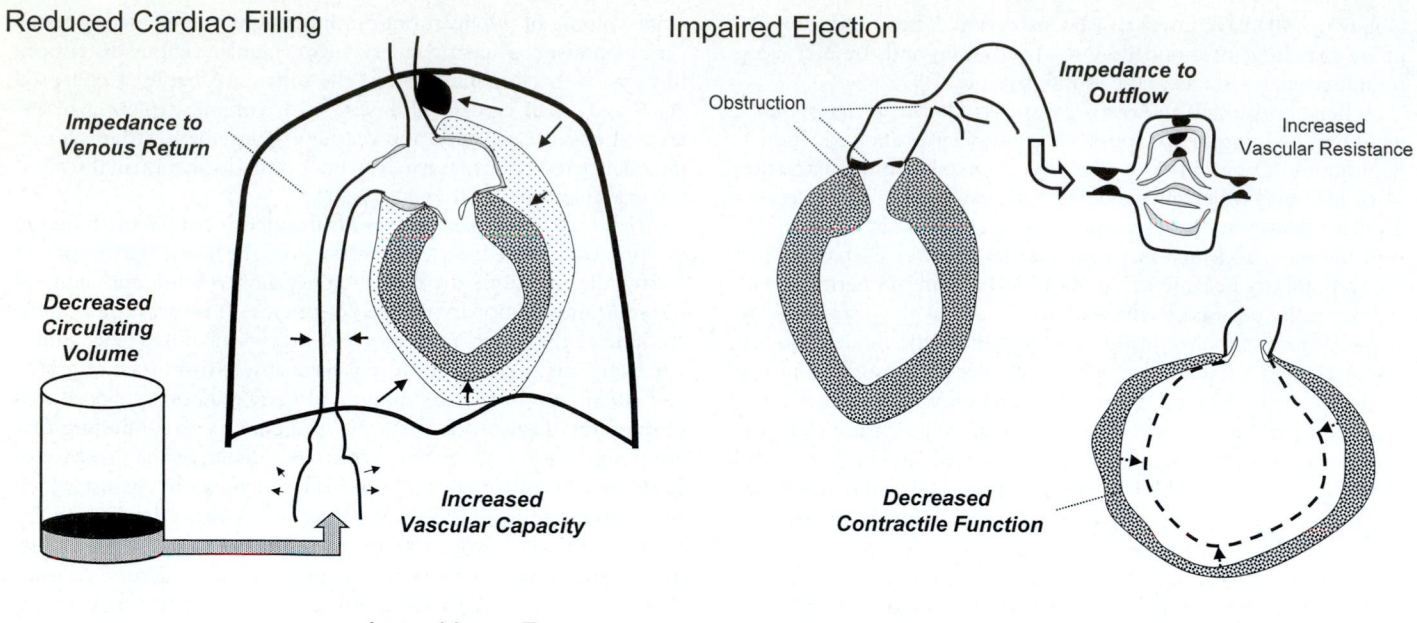

Low Heart Rate

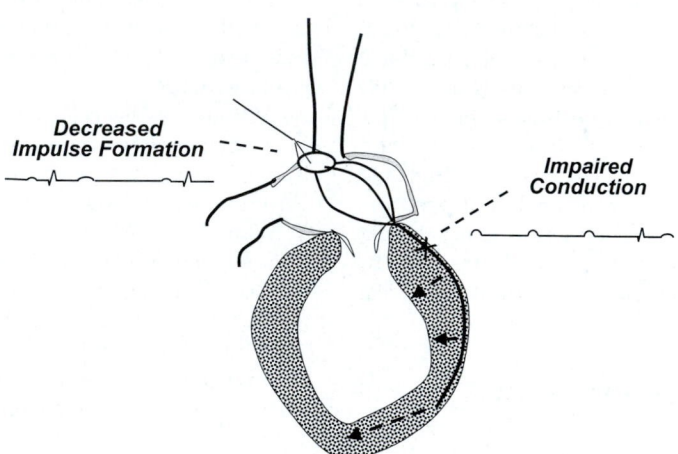

FIGURE 4-10   **General mechanisms for decreased cardiac output. A: Causes of reduced cardiac filling, which include decreased volume, increased capacity and impedance to venous return. Impedance to venous return is caused by a variety of processes within the thorax. The arrows in the thorax represent fluid, air, or masses that compress the vena cavae, and stippling in the pericardium represents air or fluid in that space. B: Causes of impaired ejection, which include impedance to outflow (obstruction, increased vascular resistance) and decreased contractile function, as shown by a dilated heart and decreased stroke volume. The stippled line shows a large end-systolic volume and arrows show that the stroke volume is decreased. C: Causes for low heart rate. The figure shows severe sinus bradycardia and third-degree atrioventricular block as examples.**

are findings that should prompt immediate attention and intervention.

In all patients with potentially impaired perfusion, vital signs should be measured and put in perspective with other physical findings. It is important to consider whether the findings are internally consistent or whether more information is needed. Both systolic and diastolic blood pressure should be measured because with peripheral vasoconstriction, systolic blood pressure can be normal but pulse pressure will be narrow. Blood pressure should be measured in an upper- (preferably right arm) and lower-body extremity in an infant because of the possibility of aortic coarctation. As discussed above, the neural and humoral responses preserve blood pressure over a wide range of cardiac output.

Certain signs are valuable because they yield insight into the nature or site of the specific disturbance. In particular, findings that locate disruption in cardiac function are useful. Pulmonary venous congestion and edema might be detected by tachypnea, crackles, wheezing, or grunting respiration. The tachypnea results from activation of stretch receptors in the lung with interstitial pulmonary edema. The wheezing, sometimes referred to as *cardiac asthma*, arises from congestion of the small airways and may be associated with gas trapping on radiography. Grunting, which may appear to represent a weak cry, is a response to reduced functional residual capacity of the lung. Interestingly, grunting can also be seen with low-perfusion states even when there is no primary or secondary pulmonary involvement. It is also worth noting that when the lungs

TABLE 4-3

CAUSES OF INADEQUATE SYSTEMIC PERFUSION

PHYSIOLOGICAL DISTURBANCE	MECHANISM	EXAMPLES
Reduced cardiac filling	Decreased circulating volume	Loss from body: hemorrhage, diarrhea, vomiting, heatstroke
		Loss within body: peritonitis, ileus, intracranial hemorrhage, sepsis
	Increased vascular capacity	Drug-induced venodilation, spinal trauma, sepsis, anaphylaxis
	Impedance to venous return	Tamponade, tension pneumothorax or pneumomediastinum, positive-pressure ventilation, tachyarrhythmia
Impaired ejection	Impedance to outflow	Aortic coarctation, aortic stenosis, increased pulmonary or systemic vascular resistance
	Decreased contractile function	Asphyxia, myocarditis, sepsis
Low heart rate	Disorder of impulse formation	Sick sinus syndrome, hypoxia
	Disorder of impulse conduction	Second- or third-degree atrioventricular block, tricyclic drugs
Increased demand for blood flow	Reduced arterial O_2 content	Hypoxemia, anemia
	Impaired nutrient utilization	Cyanide toxicity, sepsis
	Maldistribution of flow	Sepsis, arteriovenous fistula
	Increased metabolic rate	Fever, nonneutral thermal environment, excessive work of breathing, malignant hyperthermia

are congested, the response to the metabolic acidosis is tachypnea, whereas when the lungs are relatively normal, hyperpnea is expected.

Systemic venous congestion might be detected by hepatomegaly, jugular venous distention, or peripheral edema. (Peripheral edema without other signs of venous distention often indicates injured capillary endothelium, as is common in sepsis or other inflammatory processes.) In the presence of these congestive findings, the cardiothymic silhouette would usually be enlarged on the radiograph, although hyperinflated lungs, alveolar collapse, or pulmonary edema might obscure the detection of this enlargement. Murmurs help locate a site of turbulence, which suggests excess flow through an orifice or a narrowing of that orifice. A gallop rhythm suggests that the particular ventricle has diminished compliance. An active precordium is found when there is a large stroke volume; a quiet precordium might suggest a reduced stroke volume or a

cushion of fluid or air between the chest wall and the heart, as with tamponade. These findings could help the clinician establish a mechanism for the impaired circulation.

Some patients with apparently poor organ function but relatively brisk flow to the skin are often described as having distributive shock and may have signs of reduced extraction of oxygen by the tissues, which can be assessed from mixed venous blood (see Fig. 4-12). These patients often have signs and data consistent with inflammation (eg, fever, flushed skin, leukocytosis) and evidence that many somatic functions are impaired (eg, uremia). They also frequently have brisk capillary refill despite hypotension. Thus, they are an excellent example of a patient where a cursory examination might be misleading.

After it is established that perfusion is impaired, data should be sought to determine the primary factors interfering with perfusion

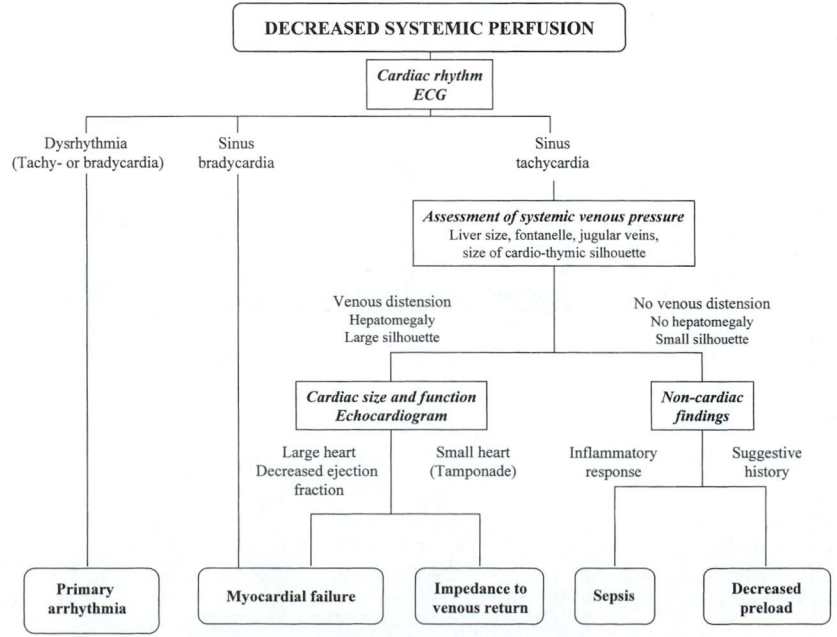

FIGURE 4-11 States of decreased perfusion: Differential diagnosis.

TABLE 4-4
SIGNS OF REDUCED SYSTEMIC PERFUSION

ORGAN SYSTEM	↓ PERFUSION	↓ ↓ PERFUSION (COMPENSATED)	↓ ↓ PERFUSION (UNCOMPENSATED)
Central nervous system	—	Restless, apathetic	Agitated-confused, stuporous
Respiration*	—	↑ Ventilation	↑ ↑ Ventilation
Metabolism	—	Compensated metabolic acidemia	Uncompensated metabolic acidemia
Gut	—	↓ Motility	Ileus
Kidney	↑ Specific gravity, ↓ volume	Oliguria	Oliguria-anuria
Skin	Delayed capillary refill	Cool extremities	Mottled, cyanotic, cold extremities
Cardiovascular system	↑ Heart rate	↑ ↑ Heart rate, weak peripheral pulses	↑ ↑ Heart rate, hypotension, central pulses only

↑, Slightly increased; ↑ ↑, greatly increased; ↓, slightly decreased; ↓ ↓, greatly decreased.
* The pattern of breathing depends on the mechanical state of the lung.

and a rational approach to reestablish adequate circulation. To determine the cause(s) of the poor perfusion, it is particularly useful to assess whether intravascular volume is expanded or depleted by examining the size of the liver and fullness of the anterior fontanel or of the jugular veins and, when possible, weighing the patient (see Fig. 4-11). Laboratory data are usually not needed to decide whether perfusion is adequate but are useful in determining how perfusion has been disturbed. An electrocardiogram (to determine whether there is the expected sinus tachycardia or any dysrhythmia), a radiograph of the chest (to determine whether the circulation is engorged or depleted and whether the heart is large or small), and a measure of acid/base status to determine the adequacy of metabolic compensation and whether asphyxia has contributed to myocardial dysfunction are generally of value. Measurement of hemoglobin concentration and/or hematocrit and

blood electrolyte, glucose (particularly in the infant or the child who has been ill for a while), creatinine, and urea nitrogen concentration are helpful to discern the etiology of the circulatory disturbance and to determine which fluid will be most appropriate after the initial treatment.

Certain monitoring should also be initiated to assist with the assessment and to judge the adequacy of the response to treatment. This should include frequent measurements of blood pressure, continuous display of the heart rate or ECG and arterial O_2 saturation, and measurement of urine output (consider inserting a bladder catheter). Ultrasound imaging and Doppler analysis are exceptionally valuable for evaluation and monitoring of myocardial contractile function and cardiac filling volume and for detection of pericardial effusion. However, these techniques require expertise that may not be available.

FIGURE 4-12 Diagram demonstrating the effect of different rates of organ perfusion: metabolism during conditions of normal cardiac output, low cardiac output, and low cardiac output with flow maldistribution. The percent of total cardiac output distributed to three organs with differing metabolic rates is shown. The venous O_2 saturation and PO_2 for any organ are influenced by the relationship of blood flow to metabolic rate for that organ, whereas the mixed systemic venous O_2 saturation and PO_2 are the volume-weighted means for all of the organs. As shown at the *top*, some organs (eg, the heart) extract a high fraction of the O_2 ("high" metabolism), whereas other organs (eg, the kidney) extract little O_2 ("low" metabolism). When cardiac output is decreased (*middle*) the blood flow and proportion of total cardiac output to organs with low or moderate metabolism decreases, thereby reducing the O_2 saturation and PO_2 of venous blood from those organs as O_2 extraction increases. Thus, there is more homogeneity of venous O_2 saturations and lower mixed venous O_2 saturation and PO_2. When there is not proper matching of flow to metabolism, as in the case of maldistribution of flow, arteriovenous shunting, or sepsis, mixed venous PO_2 and O_2 saturation are elevated despite the presence of poor organ perfusion. **SOURCE:** *Reproduced with permission from Lister G, Apkon M: Circulatory shock. In: Allen HD, Clark EB, Gutgesell HP, Driscoll DJ, eds: Moss and Adams Heart Disease in Infants, Children and Adolescents: Including the Fetus and Young Adult, 6th ed. Baltimore, MD, Lippincott Williams & Wilkins, 2000.*

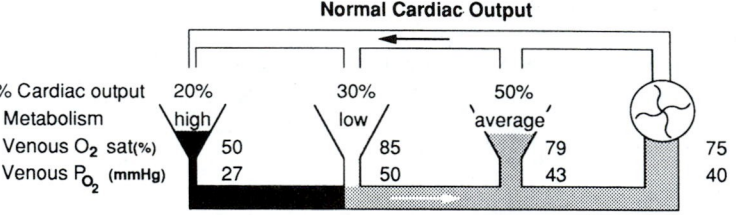

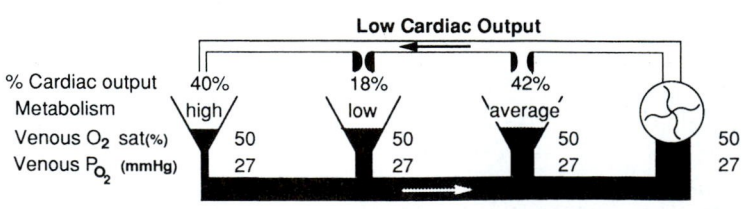

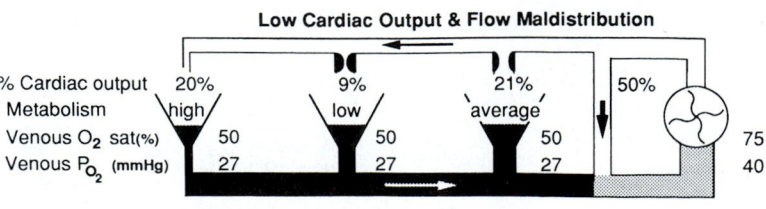

INITIAL STABILIZATION

When it is clear that the patient needs restoration of perfusion, vascular access must be established (see Sec. 4.2.4). The route of catheter placement is dictated by the urgency for care. It is often quite difficult to place a catheter percutaneously in a peripheral vein when the patient's circulating volume is decreased; alternative approaches may be needed even in the child who is not necessarily deteriorating, but who needs intravenous therapy. Techniques such as percutaneous cannulation (Seldinger technique) of a large central vein, venisection, or intraosseous cannulation are appropriate when the patient is in shock and there is no means for fluid and medication administration.

Supplemental oxygen should be provided (by face mask, nasal cannulae, or head box in the infant) to maximize oxygen delivery and to keep the lungs filled with oxygen, even if arterial oxygen saturation is normal. If, however, oxygen administration worsens the patient's perfusion, as can occur in the infant with critical left-heart obstruction in whom the ductus arteriosus constricts, then the supplemental oxygen (like any other drug which causes an adverse outcome) should be stopped immediately.

Improvement of Cardiac Output

In the course of the physical assessment, it should be determined which of the factors—heart rate, cardiac ejection, or cardiac filling—are impaired, so that therapy can commence. It is quite possible, depending on how far the underlying process has progressed, that circulatory function is impaired by more than one mechanism. For example, with sepsis, a child can have poor contractile function, diminished preload, and increased metabolic demands. However, in any child with poor perfusion, it is essential to start restoring circulatory function before there is further deterioration. If the circulation is not engorged, perfusion will usually be aided by rapid and repetitive infusion of crystalloid fluid in an isotonic mixture (eg, normal saline or Ringer's lactate) in aliquots of 5 to 10 mL/kg. After assessing serum glucose concentration, glucose should be given with the initial fluid whenever there is hypoglycemia. Although there is a long-standing and unresolved controversy about the merits of colloid versus crystalloid in resuscitation, crystalloid remains a practical initial therapy in recommended Pediatric Advanced Life Support courses. Following initial attempts at restoration of perfusion with crystalloid, subsequent choice of fluid should be based on the type of deficits and specific problems identified. For example, if there is anemia and circulating volume depletion, packed red blood cells are needed.

The quantity of fluid required for restoration of perfusion might be quite large when one considers that normal blood volume is 70 to 80 mL/kg. However, in states in which fluid volume has been lost over an extended period of time, the interstitial or cellular compartments may have also become depleted so that isotonic fluid distributes widely during the resuscitation. In addition, in states in which capillary integrity is damaged, fluid may readily extravasate from the plasma into the interstitium, even though the effective circulating plasma volume is inadequate. These phenomena are some of the reasons why colloid therapy is preferred by some clinicians.

If, during the course of fluid infusion, venous congestion develops before perfusion is normal, then it is very likely that there is impaired ejection of blood or impedance to filling of the heart. Inotropic support should be provided whenever there is direct evidence of depressed myocardial function (eg, venous congestion, cardiomegaly in the presence of a gallop rhythm) or when there is a progressive increase in venous engorgement without improvement in perfusion during fluid administration. Even with the risks of venous congestion, when myocardial function is depressed, it is appropriate to provide sufficient intravascular volume so that inotropic medications will be effective in increasing stroke volume (for any given ejection fraction, the stroke volume will increase when the filling of the heart is increased). The inotropic drugs that are most appropriate are given by intravenous route, they are rapidly metabolized, and the dose can be adjusted as conditions change. The most commonly used drugs (see Table 4-5) are the direct- and indirect-acting β agonists, including epinephrine, isoproterenol, dopamine, and dobutamine, and the phosphodiesterase (PDE) inhibitors milrinone and amrinone. Because these drugs also have important effects on the peripheral vasculature, it is worth considering whether some degree of vasoconstriction is needed to increase blood pressure (eg, dopamine, epinephrine) or whether vasodilation would be beneficial (eg, dobutamine, milrinone, amrinone, isoproterenol). Generally, the former group of drugs is most useful initially until it is clear whether blood pressure is sufficient to support perfusion. More sophisticated approaches to the support of

TABLE 4-5

INOTROPIC DRUGS IN COMMON USE FOR TREATMENT OF POOR SYSTEMIC PERFUSION

DRUG	RECEPTOR SITE OR ACTION	NET IN VIVO CARDIOVASCULAR EFFECTS	USUAL INITIAL DOSE
Norepinephrine	$\alpha_1, \alpha_2, \beta_1$	Vasoconstriction, inotropy	0.1 μg/kg/min
Epinephrine	$\alpha_1, \alpha_2, \beta_1, \beta_2$	Inotropy, vasoconstriction, tachycardia	0.05–0.1 μg/kg/min
Isoproterenol	β_1, β_2	Inotropy, vasodilation, tachycardia	0.05–0.1 μg/kg/min
Dopamine	α_1, β_1, D_1	Inotropy, vasoconstriction, renal vasodilation, +/−tachycardia	2–5 μg/kg min
Dobutamine	**$\alpha_1, \beta_1, \beta_2$	Inotropy, +/−vasodilation	2–5 μg/kg/min
Amrinone	PDE inhibitor	Inotropy, vasodilation	5–10 μg/kg/min [*following loading dose of 0.75 (older patients)– 4 (infants) mg/kg]
Milrinone	PDE inhibitor	Inotropy, vasodilation	0.3–0.6 μg/kg/min (*following loading dose of 0.5 mg/kg)

* Precise loading doses for amrinone and milrinone have not been established, and it is not clear that a loading dose is necessary.
** Sites of action are generally less important.
PDE, phosphodiesterase.

the circulation, such as left-ventricular assist devices balloon counterpulsation, are not widely available and are appropriate only in specialized settings (see Sec. 4.2.3).

If heart rate is not appropriately increased, there should be immediate concern that there is severe hypoxemia or asphyxia or that the myocardium is intrinsically injured. In this circumstance, oxygen should be given, cardiac rhythm should be checked closely, and consideration should be given to the use of an inotropic drug with chronotropic properties, such as isoproterenol, or use of a pacemaker if the rhythm is not sinus.

The response to therapy can be judged by repetitive physical examinations and measurements of vital signs. In particular, one should expect to find a decreasing heart rate, enhanced peripheral perfusion, and possibly increasing blood pressure or pulse pressure as the circulation is improved. If, on the other hand, signs of pulmonary congestion or edema (eg, tachypnea, crackles, wheezing, retractions) develop or worsen, or signs of systemic venous congestion (eg, enlarged liver or fontanel) develop without appropriate restoration of peripheral perfusion, it is necessary to consider more invasive monitoring and more extensive evaluation of cardiac function by echocardiography. Placement of a central venous catheter can be useful for measuring filling pressure of the right heart and for monitoring oxygen extraction. When there is reason to believe that the right and left ventricles have markedly different filling pressures or disparate function, a balloon flotation catheter can be passed into the pulmonary artery to measure wedge pressure and cardiac output and to assist in the evaluation of cardiac function and response to therapy.

Reduction in Demands and Adjuncts to Treatment

Special attention should be paid to factors that can reduce the demand for systemic blood flow. Anemia, hypoxemia, and fever should be corrected whenever possible. It is important to recognize, however, that fever may not abate until perfusion is restored because the vasoconstriction interferes with heat dissipation. This is in keeping with a common finding of an increased core temperature in the presence of cold extremities.

An important adjunct to therapy can be the use of positive-pressure ventilation in the patient with shock, even when there are no overt signs of respiratory distress. Supplanting the work of breathing can decrease overall metabolic rate and can divert blood flow from respiratory muscles to other vital tissues. Tracheal intubation and initiation of assisted ventilation is not without risk, so that it should be performed in a controlled environment with appropriate personnel. Moreover, positive-pressure ventilation can reduce venous return and decrease cardiac output. Therefore, it is important to be prepared to restore cardiac filling if this occurs.

There are some special considerations related to the neonate with left-heart obstruction, coarctation, aortic stenosis, or atresia that merit consideration because of the frequency with which these conditions occur and the potential for improvement with infusion of prostaglandin E_1 (see Sec. 22.4.4). These conditions commonly produce circulatory shock within the first week after birth; there will be little, if any, improvement in perfusion by using the conventional approaches described above, but prostaglandin, by opening a constricted ductus arteriosus, can provide a dramatic increase in perfusion until more definitive therapy is initiated.

After therapy for poor perfusion is started it is incumbent to search for an underlying etiology to treat (eg, antibiotics for sus-

pected sepsis), to consider additional strategies for improving circulatory function, and to plan a transfer to a facility equipped to provide extended monitoring and management.

References

Aubier M, Trippenbach T, Roussos C: Respiratory muscle fatigue during cardiogenic shock. J Appl Physiol 51:499–508, 1981

Carcillo JA, Davis AL, Zaritsky A: Role of early fluid resuscitation in pediatric septic shock. JAMA 266:1242–1245, 1991

Fahey J, Lister G: Response to low cardiac output: Developmental differences in metabolism during oxygen deficit and recovery in lambs. Pediatr Res 26:180–187, 1989

Jakschik BA, Marshall GR, Kourik JL, Needleman P: Profile of circulating vasoactive substances in hemorrhagic shock and their pharmacologic manipulation. J Clin Invest 54:842–852, 1974

Lister G, Apkon M: Circulatory shock. In: Allen HD, Clark EB, Gutgesell HP, Driscoll DJ, eds: Moss and Adams Heart Disease in Infants, Children and Adolescents: Including the Fetus and Young Adult, 6th ed. Baltimore, MD, Lippincott Williams & Wilkins, 2000, pp 1413–1431

Notterman DA: Pharmacology of the cardiovascular system In: Fuhrman BP, Zimmerman JJ, eds: Pediatric Critical Care, 2nd ed. St. Louis, MO, Mosby Year Book, 1998, pp 320–346

Parrillo JE, Burch C, Shelhamer JH, Parker MM, Natanson C, Schuette W: A circulating myocardial depressant substance in humans with septic shock. Septic shock patients with a reduced ejection fraction have a circulating factor that depresses in vitro myocardial cell performance. J Clin Invest 76:1539–1553, 1985

Sylvester J, Goldberg HSP: The role of the vasculature in the regulation of cardiac output. Clin Chest Med 4:111–126, 1983

Viires N, Sillye G, Aubier M, Rassidakis A, Roussos C: Regional blood flow distribution in dog during induced hypotension and low cardiac output. Spontaneous breathing versus artificial ventilation. J Clin Invest 72:935–947, 1983

4.1.3   Coma and Altered Consciousness

Susan T. Arnold

Acute alterations in the level of consciousness always indicate a serious medical problem, which must be comprehensively evaluated and closely monitored. They may arise from both primary processes within the central nervous system, or be caused by the secondary effects of other systemic disorders. In either case, if the disruption is severe enough, central control of respiratory or cardiovascular function can rapidly deteriorate, leading to a life-threatening situation. The differential diagnosis for altered consciousness or coma is broad, and imaging studies and laboratory tests alone may not identify an etiology. A careful history of the events leading up to the change in mental status and a full multisystem examination are essential and will help to guide the choice of diagnostic tests.

Normal consciousness requires both maintenance of arousal and the ability to respond to the environment with a full range of cognitive functions. Maintenance of arousal is mediated by a complex network of interactions within the brain, prominently involving the reticular activating system. This is a poorly delineated brainstem structure extending from the medulla to the rostral midbrain. It receives input from the cerebral cortex and all major sensory systems and projects to local structures within the brainstem, as well as, via ascending pathways, to the thalamus, hypothalamus, and cerebral cortex. Stimulation of the reticular activating system results in increased alertness, and destructive lesions produce unresponsiveness.

TABLE 4-6
GLASGOW COMA SCALE

Eye Opening	
Spontaneous	4
To speech	3
To pain	2
None	1
Verbal Response	
Oriented	5
Confused conversation	4
Inappropriate words	3
Incomprehensible sounds	2
None	1
Motor Response	
Obeys commands	6
Localizes pain	5
Withdraws	4
Abnormal flexion	3
Extensor response	2
None	1
Total Score	3–15

The cerebral hemispheres direct conscious response to environmental stimuli. In contrast to the brainstem, where even small lesions affecting the reticular activating system may produce coma, extensive bilateral injury of the cerebral cortex is necessary to cause severe impairment of consciousness. Diffuse cortical injury produces a global encephalopathy. Focal lesions rarely impair consciousness unless they cause compression or edema of the contralateral hemisphere, or when multiple, bilateral hemispheric lesions are present.

Altered consciousness usually begins with mild confusion or *lethargy*. More severe cases progress to *obtundation* where the patient is somnolent but arousable, then *stupor* where a patient responds only to vigorous stimuli and immediately becomes unresponsive when stimulation ceases. *Coma* refers to true unresponsiveness to external stimuli, although there may be reflexive, nonlocalizing motor responses to pain. Because terminology is used inconsistently among observers, and because a patient's exam may fluctuate, scoring systems such as the Glasgow Coma Scale (Table 4-6) are useful in documenting a patient's level of consciousness and changes over time. Although these scales provide

prognostic information when the etiology of altered consciousness is known, they do not assist in establishing a diagnosis and are not a substitute for a comprehensive history and examination.

INITIAL EVALUATION

The initial approach to the patient with altered consciousness, as with all critically ill patients, requires a systematic approach (Table 4-7) that pays first attention to the correction of life-threatening respiratory and cardiovascular dysfunctions (see Secs. 4.1.1 and 4.1.2). There is no value in diagnosing accurately the location of a cerebral hemorrhage if the patient dies in the CT scanner. Altered consciousness may result from or lead to further physiological derangements, which, if not recognized and treated, may cause extension of cerebral damage. Metabolic disorders, respiratory failure, cardiac rhythm disturbances, sepsis, and shock can all present with acute alteration of consciousness. Airway protection and ventilatory support are usually required in patients with significant respiratory abnormalities. Even if adequate respiratory effort is present, endotracheal intubation is usually required to prevent aspiration due to impairment of airway-protective reflexes. Circulatory disturbances may occur, especially in the setting of hypoxic-ischemic injury, and should be treated with intravenous fluid, vasoactive medications, and inotropic medications, if needed. Laboratory assessments of arterial blood gases, serum glucose and electrolyte concentrations, renal and liver function, a complete blood count, and comprehensive screening for drug toxicity should be a routine part of the initial evaluation of any patient with decreased responsiveness or coma of unknown cause. The primary focus of care should be to discover and treat conditions that may cause ongoing brain injury.

The initial physical evaluation should include a multisystem examination with special attention to focal or localizing neurologic signs. Signs of elevated intracranial pressure must be searched for specifically, and the condition should be treated aggressively if present. The Cushing response, including hypertension (the systolic pressure usually being more elevated than the diastolic pressure), bradycardia, and a significant impairment of consciousness, is an indication of acute intracranial hypertension and is frequently associated with an irregular breathing pattern. Papilledema is a hallmark of chronic intracranial hypertension but is not seen immediately, and its absence does not imply a normal intracranial pressure. Unilateral pupillary dilation and hemiparesis (ipsilateral or contra-

TABLE 4-7
INITIAL MANAGEMENT OF ACUTE ALTERATIONS OF CONSCIOUSNESS

STEPS IN MANAGEMENT

1. Respiratory or cardiovascular instability?	Yes → Stabilize respiratory/cardiac function.	No → Next Step
2. Signs of cerebral herniation syndromes?	Yes → Endotracheal intubation, mechanical ventilation, neurosurgical consultation.	No → Next Step
3. Survey for other life-threatening conditions. Obtain IV access, obtain blood for screening tests.		
4. Serum glucose low or results not immediately available?	Yes → Administer intravenous dextrose.	No → Next Step
5. Signs of opiate intoxication?	Yes → Administer intravenous naloxone.	No → Next Step
6. Obtain detailed general and neurologic examination and Glasgow Coma Scale.		
7. Impaired cough and gag reflexes?	Yes → Endotracheal intubation for airway protection.	No → Next Step
8. Obtain neuroimaging study.		
9. Evidence of increase intracranial pressure or mass effect?	Yes → Lumbar puncture is *contraindicated.*	No → Next Step
10. Perform lumbar puncture.		

lateral) may occur with transtentorial herniation of the temporal lobe. When diffuse cerebral edema occurs, or when the mass effect is in the posterior fossa, these findings may not be present. The management of increased intracranial pressure is discussed below.

After the patient's immediate stabilization needs are met, consideration can be given to further diagnostic testing. Neuroimaging is usually performed early in the course of evaluation. CT scans are rapid and readily available in most centers, but may not detect acute ischemic injury and are of limited value in assessing subtle cortical changes, brainstem lesions, and posterior fossa abnormalities. MRI is superior for these purposes, but the length of time required and the difficulty involved in monitoring an acutely ill patient during the test limit its use. Examination of the CSF assesses for infection, subarachnoid hemorrhage, and can also help the identification of some neoplastic and demyelinating disorders. *Because of the risk of herniation, however, lumbar puncture should never be performed in the unconscious patient until neuroimaging and examination have excluded the possibility of increased intracranial pressure.* An EEG can identify subclinical seizures, which, if present, will cause continued impairment of consciousness. It may also reveal patterns of prognostic significance and is occasionally of value in localizing a lesion not evident on imaging studies. It must be emphasized that, in most cases, none of these studies alone is sufficient to explain coma. Often, their results provide only part of the answer, and the findings must be interpreted in the individual clinical situation. For example, an ischemic stroke may result from a cardiac embolus, vasculitis, or infectious etiology. An intracranial hemorrhage could be due to a coagulopathy, arteriovenous malformation, or trauma. Careful history and a full physical examination are needed to complete the clinical picture and guide therapy.

GLOBAL ENCEPHALOPATHY

The clinical picture of diffuse encephalopathy is characterized by alteration in consciousness often associated with generalized seizures, but lacking focal or lateralizing signs. It can be the end result of a variety of different pathologic processes, which may occur alone or in combination with one another. Except for hypoxic-ischemic injury, alteration of consciousness usually begins gradually and brainstem function is typically preserved. Movement disorders, such as tremor, myoclonus, or asterixis, are characteristic of some of the syndromes described below. With more severe injury, symmetric motor findings occur, such as hyper- or hypotonia and hyperreflexia. Abnormal posturing and primitive reflexes such as the Babinski develop, reflecting widespread cortical dysfunction.

Toxic-Metabolic Encephalopathy

Toxic ingestions are not uncommon in children and should always be suspected in the setting of acute changes in mental status. In young children the ingestion is usually accidental. In adolescence, it is often intentional, although the individual may not be fully aware of the danger involved. Screening blood or urine for the presence of toxins may be diagnostic, but the tests take time, and no test will include all possible toxins. A careful history of all medications present in the home should be obtained, even if they are not believed to be accessible to the child. Physical examination may reveal findings characteristic for a specific ingestion (toxidromes, see Sec. 4.3.3). For example, pupillary constriction with hypercapnic hypoventilation is typical of opioid intoxication. Salicylate poisoning is manifest as hyperpnea with respiratory alkalosis and/or metabolic acidosis. Other common toxins such as alcohol (in

young children often due to ingestion of alcohol-containing household products), anticholinergic agents, and carbon monoxide poisoning also have characteristic physical and laboratory findings. Intoxication with iron supplements can present with coma at several points in its course and is the most frequent cause of pediatric fatality from accidental ingestion. Rapid identification of the toxic agent may allow use of specific antidotes or therapies. Regarding the latter, it is important to remember that, when there is a depressed level of consciousness, the airway should be protected if possible with a cuffed endotracheal tube before any attempt at gastrointestinal decontamination.

Encephalopathy can also result from endogenous toxins when normal homeostatic mechanisms are disrupted and allow excessive accumulation of metabolic products. In infants with inborn errors of metabolism, this can occur rapidly. In older children, the evolution is usually more gradual. The history may reveal evidence of a preexisting illness or of a genetic disorder causing unexplained infant mortality in the family, such as those affecting amino acid or urea metabolism. Examination may reveal characteristic findings such as the odors associated with diabetic ketoacidosis or maple syrup urine disease. Metabolic acidosis with a marked anion gap is prominent in amino and organic acidemias, diabetic ketoacidosis, and renal failure. In contrast, urea cycle defects cause hyperammonemia and coma without metabolic acidosis. Hepatic failure is often associated with hyperpnea and hypocapnia. Certain movement disorders are frequently seen with metabolic encephalopathies. Asterixis, although classically associated with hepatic failure, can occur early in the course of any metabolic brain disease. Multifocal myoclonus is more often seen in deeper states of unresponsiveness. Tremor occurs in hyperthyroidism and in association with the ingestion of many drugs. These bilateral, symmetric movement disorders almost never occur with focal cerebral lesions, unless they are associated with an underlying metabolic disorder. Imaging is usually normal, but the EEG may show patterns suggestive of metabolic encephalopathy.

Hypoglycemia

Hypoglycemia deserves special attention as a common and easily reversible etiology for metabolic encephalopathy. In the newborn, it may occur in the absence of other provoking factors. In older children, it presents more frequently as a complication of an underlying metabolic or endocrine disorder. It should also be suspected in situations in which glycogen stores in the liver are deficient (starvation, hepatic disease, very young infant), especially if there is another physical stress such as a concurrent infection. If untreated it can cause permanent brain injury. The administration of dextrose-containing intravenous solutions is advisable in virtually all cases of unexplained coma unless the serum glucose can be immediately and reliably determined to be normal. (If significant malnutrition is suspected, thiamine may be coadministered to prevent the rare complication of Wernicke encephalopathy.) Reversible focal neurologic signs are occasionally seen in association with hypoglycemia, but their presence should always prompt a search for an underlying focal cerebral lesion.

Infections of the Central Nervous System

The early signs of central nervous system infection may be difficult to recognize in children. Irritability is often attributed to fever, and in children under the age of 18 months, typical features of meningeal irritation, such as nuchal rigidity or the Kernig or Brudzinski signs, may be absent. The clinician must have a high suspicion of meningeal or cerebral infection in the child presenting with seizures or mental status changes, especially if accompanied by fever or leukocytosis. Bacterial meningitis usually presents initially as a global encephalopathy, without localizing signs. However, the leptomeningeal inflammation may progress to the development of subarachnoid infiltrates, which then extend into the perivascular spaces around small arteries and veins, causing focal vessel wall necrosis and thrombosis. This, in turn, can lead to localized cortical infarction and the development of focal features later in the course of the illness. A similar process occurring around the cranial nerve sheaths can result in cranial neuropathies, especially involving the third, fourth, and sixth cranial nerves, which have long intracranial segments. Obstructive or communicating hydrocephalus develops if the fibrinous exudate interferes with normal pathways of CSF flow or its reabsorption by the arachnoid granules. Diagnosis requires lumbar puncture to identify the responsible organism. When antibiotic treatment precedes CSF examination, latex agglutination testing of the CSF or urine may identify a bacterial organism. Management of bacterial meningitis requires the use of antibiotics with good CSF penetration. Inappropriate antidiuretic hormone (ADH) secretion occurs commonly, and fluid balance and serum electrolyte concentrations must be carefully monitored. If a pathologic bacterial organism cannot be identified, antibiotic coverage should include antiviral therapy for herpes encephalitis, which may have devastating consequences unless it is treated at an early stage. Focal seizures and an abnormal EEG, especially involving the temporal lobes, are commonly associated with herpes encephalitis, but may also be seen with other infections causing focal destructive lesions of the central nervous system.

With the exception of herpes encephalitis, other serious viral encephalitides are relatively uncommon but should be suspected in endemic areas, especially in the summer and fall months, when the incidence of arboviral encephalitis is higher. CSF studies typically show a lymphocytic pleocytosis, in contrast to the polymorphonuclear predominance of bacterial infections, but this pattern may not be evident early in the course of the disease. Cases of herpes and other viral encephalitides have been reported with normal CSF studies. Cat-scratch disease can present with precipitous onset of stupor or coma and a normal-appearing CSF. Antibody testing for *Bartonella henselae* is available, and antibiotic therapy is indicated. Central nervous system infections are discussed in detail in Chapter.

Seizures

Seizures are relatively common in children and frequently present with acute alterations in consciousness during or after the event. Most seizures are associated with a postictal period of drowsiness or obtundation that may last from minutes to hours. If the seizure is unwitnessed, the correct diagnosis may be overlooked. If a patient fails to show a gradually improving level of alertness following a seizure, the possibility of nonconvulsive status epilepticus (persistent seizure activity without motor movements) should be considered. This is particularly true following treatment for convulsive status epilepticus as continued depression of mental status may be wrongly attributed to medication. Nonconvulsive status epilepticus should also be considered in any patient with prolonged coma. This form of status epilepticus is often overlooked as a complication of diffuse or multifocal cerebral injury from other etiologies, especially when use of sedating medications or muscle relaxants masks signs of seizure activity. An EEG can establish the presence or absence

of status epilepticus, but may not be diagnostic if a seizure has already terminated. The evaluation and treatment of epilepsy is reviewed in greater detail in Chapter.

Hypoxic-Ischemic Encephalopathy

Hypoxia and ischemia trigger a complex cascade of events. These produce cerebral injury both directly as the result of an arrest of aerobic metabolism and accumulation of lactic acid, and via secondary injury from the generation of oxygen free radicals, accumulation of excitotoxins such as glutamate, and disturbance of intracellular calcium homeostasis. The secondary processes can lead to neuronal apoptosis (programmed cell death) occurring in an ongoing fashion for hours to days after the initial injury. Areas of the brain with higher density of amino acid receptors appear to be more vulnerable to hypoxic-ischemic insult, and these features, along with changes in cerebral metabolism and vasculature, contribute to the differing appearance of hypoxic-ischemic injury at different ages. After the neonatal period, the hippocampus, caudate nucleus, and cerebellar Purkinje cells are particularly at risk, as are the border zones between areas supplied by the major cerebral arteries, especially in the posterior parietal and occipital lobes. With less-severe injury, lesions are restricted to these areas; in that case, brainstem function is not impaired and residual deficits are few. In the most severe cases, however, the injury involves both the cerebrum and the brainstem, and coma is associated with loss of all cranial nerve function. The degree of injury is determined not only by the extent and duration of the hypoxic or ischemic event but also by features individual to the child, such as age, concurrent disease, and body temperature. In particular, hypothermia has a relatively protective effect, and the prognosis after prolonged hypoxia from cold water immersion may be better than with similar duration exposure under different conditions.

Hypoxic-ischemic injury is not always readily evident by history, and particularly with lesser degrees of injury, the diagnosis may be uncertain. Evidence of injury to other hypoxia-sensitive organs such as the heart, liver, or kidneys may provide clues to the diagnosis. Seizures are common, particularly early in the course of the disorder, and may be refractory to medical management. CT scans are usually unremarkable in the first 24 hours following ischemic injury. MRI demonstrates changes within a few hours. Diffusion-weighted MR in particular is abnormal very early after ischemic injury. EEG is helpful in identifying subclinical seizures and in predicting outcome. Severe suppression or a burst suppression pattern are indicative of a poor prognosis, unless associated with large doses of central nervous system depressant medication.

Trauma

Traumatic brain injuries may cause focal or diffuse cerebral lesions, often as a combination of several types of injury. When a localized insult is evident, concurrent signs of diffuse injury may be overlooked, although these have important implications for prognosis. The examiner must also be alert for evidence of cervical injury, and cervical spine radiographs should be obtained on every patient with known or suspected head trauma. The cause of injury is usually known, except in situations involving child abuse, where retinal hemorrhages or the evidence of fractures on a skeletal survey may suggest the diagnosis in the absence of visible external signs of injury. Trauma often produces cerebral edema and increased intracranial pressure, which must be carefully managed to prevent extension of the initial injury due to compression of adjacent structures. A deteriorating level of consciousness following an initial more lucid period should always raise the suspicion of intracranial bleeding and prompt an urgent evaluation for epidural or subdural hematoma, which requires emergent neurosurgical intervention.

FOCAL ENCEPHALOPATHY

In contrast to the diffuse processes described earlier, focal brain lesions have a wide variety of clinical presentations, depending on the structures involved (Table 4-8). A detailed neurologic examination is essential for correct localization and diagnosis of the pathologic process. Neuroimaging studies support the diagnosis, but are not a substitute for a careful examination. The most visible lesion on an image may not be the most clinically significant one; for example, brainstem lesions are difficult to see on some imaging studies, but, due to their proximity to vital structures, they may have more serious implications than cerebral hemisphere lesions of much larger size. Common etiologies for focal encephalopathy include hemorrhage, infarction, neoplasm, demyelination, and compression. Infectious and traumatic processes can cause focal or diffuse injury as discussed earlier.

Supratentorial lesions involving the cerebral hemispheres or basal ganglia are often associated with focal signs on examination. Headache and behavioral changes are common early in the course of an enlarging supratentorial mass lesion. Unilateral weakness, visual field deficits, hemineglect, and aphasia may occur, providing clues to localization. Seizures are frequent and typically have focal features. Consciousness is not usually impaired unless extensive bilateral lesions are present or a unilateral lesion causes compression of the contralateral hemisphere either by direct extension or by causing edema and shifting of adjacent structures, as occurs in the herniation syndromes described below.

The posterior fossa contains the brainstem and cerebellum, which are separated from the more rostral structures by an unyielding dural membrane, the tentorium cerebelli. Clinical findings from lesions in this space may include multiple cranial nerve palsies, ataxia, and abnormal pupillary responses. In contrast to supratentorial processes, where extensive bilateral injury is required to produce alteration of consciousness, relatively small infratentorial lesions can produce coma by injuring or compressing the brainstem reticular activating system. Lesions in the posterior fossa require particular vigilance, as even small amounts of edema in this confined area may lead to compression and infarction of brainstem respiratory and autonomic centers. More extensive swelling, as often occurs with cerebellar lesions, can produce herniation downward through the foramen magnum or upward through the tentorium. In either case, there is a high risk of developing hydrocephalus due to obstruction of CSF flow through the cerebral aqueduct and fourth ventricle, compounding the infratentorial process by causing compression and injury to supratentorial structures. Emergent surgical decompression of the posterior fossa may be indicated to halt this chain of events.

INTRACRANIAL HYPERTENSION

Intracranial hypertension can result from diffuse or focal cerebral processes as outlined above. In the newborn period, the open fontanel and cranial sutures provide a mechanism of adaptation to sudden increases in intracranial volume, as occurs, for example, after an intraventricular hemorrhage. (In these instances, a bulging fontanel and split sutures provide valuable signs of the increased pressure within.) Beyond this period, however, the cranial vault becomes a relatively fixed container for the brain parenchyma, CSF, and cerebral blood volume. An increase in one of these components raises the intracranial pressure. With slowly growing tumors or hydrocephalus, the remaining structures partially compensate the increase in pressure by decreasing or redistributing their volume. In children, the incompletely ossified cranial vault may also enlarge over time. The faster course of a more acute process such as hemorrhage or rapidly evolving edema does not allow for even such limited degrees of accommodation. The resulting increase in pressure initially causes headache, nausea, and somnolence, but can rapidly progress to stupor or coma. The neurologic examination reveals increasing obtundation often associated with ocular palsies (especially abducens palsy), and papilledema becomes evident over time. The classic Cushing response, with raised systolic blood pressure and bradycardia may not occur until late in the course, when medullary compression occurs. Severe intracranial hypertension leads to the cerebral herniation, which is a neurologic emergency. The patient should undergo tracheal intubation, and mechanical ventilation should be instituted. An emergent neurosurgical evaluation should be obtained, unless it is certain that no surgical intervention is possible. The nature of the pathologic process dictates the probable time course of intracranial hypertension and may help guide therapy. Cerebral hemorrhages cause acute, often catastrophic increases in intracranial pressure. Brain infarcts produce edema that usually reaches its maximum after 48 hours and then gradually improves. Abscesses and metastatic tumors are typically associated with extensive surrounding edema of longer duration.

As the intracranial pressure increases, it interferes with cerebral blood flow, causing further cerebral injury and edema. Cerebral perfusion pressure is defined as the difference between the mean arterial pressure and the intracranial pressure. Cerebral vessels have the ability to autoregulate, adjusting their caliber to maintain cerebral blood flow at a relatively constant level throughout a range of cerebral perfusion pressures. This mechanism cannot compensate for severe intracranial hypertension, however, or for significant systemic hypotension. Cerebral vessels are also responsive to changes in oxygen and carbon dioxide concentrations in the blood, increasing cerebral blood flow in response to metabolic demands. The medical management of intracranial hypertension, therefore, depends upon controlling those factors that can be externally modified in order to preserve cerebral perfusion pressure and vascular autoregulation and prevent extension of neuronal injury.

When intracranial hypertension is not severe, supportive therapies that maximize cerebral perfusion may be sufficient. Unless the

TABLE 4-8
LOCALIZING FINDINGS IN COMA

Probable lesion of the cerebral cortex
  Seizures
  Gaze preference
  Primitive reflexes (Babinski, snout, palmomental)
  Hemiplegia with ipsilateral facial weakness
  Decorticate posturing
  History of cortical deficit (aphasia, neglect, behavior change)
Probable lesion in the posterior fossa
  Multiple cranial nerve palsies
  Hemiplegia with contralateral or no facial weakness
  Pinpoint pupils (pontine lesion)
  Acute obstructive hydrocephalus
  Decerebrate posturing
  Irregular respirations
  History of ataxia

patient has arterial hypotension, the head should be elevated to facilitate venous drainage. Hypoxemia and hypercarbia cause cerebral vasodilation and should be avoided by using supplemental oxygen and, if necessary, mechanical ventilation. When endotracheal intubation is required, it should be performed by the most experienced person available, with appropriate sedation to prevent hypoxemia, hypoventilation, and coughing during laryngoscopy. Systemic hypotension should be avoided, and if arterial hypertension is present, it should be treated cautiously, weighing the risk of hypertensive complications against the risk of worsening neuronal injury from further decreasing the cerebral perfusion pressure. Seizures increase cerebral blood flow and should be treated aggressively. Agitation also increases intracranial pressure by increasing cerebral blood flow and impeding venous return. Attempts should be made to keep the patient calm, keeping in mind that sedative medications interfere with the assessment of a patient's level of consciousness. In the intubated patient, coughing or fighting against mechanical ventilation can produce dramatic increases in intracranial pressure, and sedation and muscle relaxation is usually necessary.

In the setting of more severe intracranial hypertension, specific measures are used to reduce the volume of the intracranial contents and to lower the pressure. When possible, these directly address the source of the disorder. Increased pressure due to intracranial hematoma or obstructive hydrocephalus, for example, represents a neurosurgical emergency, requiring surgical drainage or decompression. When direct surgical intervention is impossible or poses too great a risk of injury to adjacent structures, reduction of intracranial pressure is achieved indirectly, addressing those components that can most rapidly and effectively be modified. Mechanical hyperventilation lowers arterial PCO_2, causing cerebral vasoconstriction, which decreases the intracranial blood volume and produces an immediate reduction in the intracranial pressure. Unfortunately, the efficacy lessens with time, as bicarbonate levels in the CSF rise in response to hypocarbia. Osmotic diuretics such as mannitol or glycerol decrease the intracranial pressure by creating an osmotic gradient that shifts water from brain parenchyma to the intravascular space, thereby reducing brain volume. The decreased blood viscosity may also induce a reflex cerebral vasoconstriction, further lowering intracranial pressure. Unfortunately, hyperosmolarity increases the risk of complications such as hemolysis, rhabdomyolysis, or renal failure, and serum osmolarity should be monitored and kept below 315 mOsm/L. Osmotic diuretics do not act specifically on areas of edema; they are more effective in uninjured regions of the brain with an intact blood-brain barrier and may in some circumstances exacerbate focal edema. Steroid therapy has often been used to treat cerebral edema. It appears to be effective when the edema is caused by tumors or infectious processes, but has no role in traumatic or hypoxic-ischemic injury.

The effective treatment of intracranial hypertension requires the ability to assess the effect of therapy on intracranial pressure and to adjust treatment accordingly. When herniation is impeding, recovery of cranial nerve or brainstem function provides a clinical measure of efficacy. The clinical examination, however, is a limited source of information in these circumstances, especially if sedative medication or muscle relaxation is being used. Simultaneous monitoring of arterial and intracranial pressures permits a continuous assessment of cerebral perfusion pressure, as described above. Intracranial pressure can be measured by placing a fluid-filled catheter or transducer-tipped catheter into the subarachnoid space or brain parenchyma. Intracranial pressure monitoring is not indicated in all

clinical settings and should be used only when the risks are outweighed by the potential benefits. After cranial trauma, for example, edema from focal injury may jeopardize the viability of intact structures, and careful monitoring of the intracranial pressure may significantly improve outcome. In contrast, in diffuse brain injury, edema may be widespread, aggressive medical management already in place, and little to be gained by invasive measurement techniques. This is the case in hypoxic-ischemic encephalopathy, in which studies have shown no improvement in outcome with the use of intracranial pressure monitoring in children. Complications of intracranial pressure monitoring include infection and hemorrhage, as well as the possibility that inaccurate measurements caused by faulty calibration, displacement, or obstruction of the device may lead to inappropriate therapy. The devices are best employed by personnel familiar with their use and interpretation.

BRAIN HERNIATION SYNDROMES

Focal cerebral lesions, which undergo rapid expansion or are associated with massive edema, may displace surrounding brain tissue into an adjacent cranial compartment. In the process, surrounding blood vessels, cranial nerves, or adjacent brain parenchyma may be further injured. Unilateral edema, especially in the frontal lobe, may force the cingulate gyrus under the midline falx cerebri, compressing the ipsilateral anterior cerebral artery. Uncal herniation occurs when an expanding temporal or frontotemporal lesion forces the medial temporal lobe downward over the edge of the tentorium, compressing the third nerve, midbrain, and posterior cerebral artery. This produces the characteristic clinical sign of ipsilateral pupillary dilation, which is always associated with profound coma and often with the respiratory irregularities and the Cushing response (described earlier).

Central or transtentorial herniation is the result of caudal displacement of the diencephalon (thalamus and hypothalamus) through the tentorial notch, compressing the structures below. As the herniation progresses, injury extends from the diencephalon to the midbrain and lower portions of the brainstem, and a pattern of progressive loss of higher-level functioning may be evident. Diencephalic injury is characterized by preservation of conjugate oculocephalic responses. The pupils are small, but if carefully examined, still show constriction to light (unless the ipsilateral third nerve has been injured in concurrent uncal herniation). A Cheyne-Stokes respiratory pattern is often present, and noxious stimuli provoke nonpurposeful decorticate posturing with flexion of the arms and leg extension. As the midbrain and upper pons become involved, oculomotor movements become dysconjugate and may be difficult to elicit. The pupils are midposition and unresponsive to light. The respiratory pattern shifts to sustained tachypnea, and decerebrate posturing (with extension of all extremities) replaces decorticate posturing in response to stimulation. The development of these signs is associated with a grim prognosis. In most cases, medullary compression soon follows, announced by loss of oculovestibular responses, flaccid muscle tone, and slow, irregular breathing, which eventually progresses to apnea. In clinical situations, the progression from higher to lower stages of functioning is often less distinct, and findings are commonly asymmetric, but the ominous implications of the later stages are the same.

ASSESSMENT OF BRAIN DEATH

Brain death occurs when all cerebral functions are irreversibly absent. Accordingly, its diagnosis implies not only an evaluation of physical findings but also a judgment that brain function is not likely to recover. It is particularly the latter that puts an overpowering responsibility in the hands of the physician. To help the process and provide uniformity, several expert bodies have elaborated guidelines, which provide a very valuable framework for conducting the diagnostic procedures described below. The guidelines are by nature nonbinding and, especially those regarding the timing of various assessments, need to be complemented by careful consideration of the circumstances and mechanism of the neurologic injuries, the age of the patient, and the presence of other organ or system dysfunctions.

It is commonly accepted that the diagnosis of brain death requires at least two careful and detailed examinations by an experienced clinician, followed by formal documentation of apnea as described below. All central motor and autonomic responses to external stimuli must be absent, including reflexive decorticate or decerebrate posturing. Spinal motor reflexes may persist. Lack of brainstem function is documented by careful testing of individual cranial nerves. Vestibular and oculomotor functions are examined by testing the cold caloric responses. The head is elevated 30° and up to 120 mL of ice water are instilled over several minutes into a clear auditory canal. The respiratory control is assessed by performing an oxygenated apnea test. Although variations are often introduced, depending on the circumstances, it is common to start the test by ventilating the lungs with 100% oxygen for at least 10 minutes, documenting the presence of a normal arterial pH or P_{CO_2} (pH is generally the most relevant measurement because, in the presence of compensatory changes in bicarbonate concentration, an elevated P_{CO_2} may not be a stimulus for breathing). Mechanical ventilation is then discontinued or slowed. Hypoxemia may be prevented by continuous flow apneic oxygenation, allowing oxygen to flow through a catheter inserted into the trachea through the endotracheal tube (maximum care must be put into preventing the catheter from wedging itself into a bronchus to avoid lung injuries). The patient is observed for respiratory effort for 10 minutes while oxygen saturation is monitored. Persistent apnea despite a significant decrease in arterial pH (7.2 or less) or an increase in arterial rise in P_{CO_2} (60 mm Hg or more if the serum bicarbonate concentration is normal) confirms the absence of respiratory neural drive.

Clinical guidelines published in 1987 recommend using the EEG as a confirmatory test in children under 1 year of age. According to these guidelines, from age 7 days to 2 months, two examinations and EEGs should be performed with an interval of at least 48 hours. Between the ages of 2 months and 1 year, the examinations should be separated by 24 hours, and the interval may be decreased, and the second EEG eliminated, if radionuclide angiography shows no cerebral blood flow. After 1 year of age, laboratory testing is not required and the exams should be separated by 12 hours when an irreversible condition exists, or by 24 hours if the reversibility is difficult to assess, as in acute hypoxic-ischemic injury. No guidelines have been specified for the first week after birth. It should be noted that EEG is occasionally confounding if traces of cerebral activity are present on the test when all other signs are consistent with brain death. Laboratory testing in children over 1 year of age is most helpful when the ability to perform a clinical examination is impaired (for example by concurrent medication use), when there is a desire to reduce the observation interval between examinations, or when such testing is necessary to support the patient's family in coming to terms with the clinical situation.

References

Grigg MM, Kelly MA, Celesia GG, Ghobrial MW, Ross ER: Electroencephalographic activity after brain death. Arch Neurol 44:948–954, 1987

Le Roux PD, Jardine DS, Kanev PM, Loeser JD: Pediatric intracranial pressure monitoring in hypoxic and nonhypoxic brain injury. Childs Nerv Syst 7(1):34–39, 1991

Litovitz T, Manoguerra A: Comparison of pediatric poisoning hazards: an analysis of 3.8 million exposure incidents. A report from the American Association of Poison Control Centers. Pediatrics 89(6):999–1006, 1992

Plum F, Posner JB: The Diagnosis of Stupor and Coma, 3rd ed. Philadelphia, FA Davis, 1982

Task Force on Brain Death in Children. Guidelines for the determination of brain death in children. Pediatrics 1987, 80:298–300, 1987

Towne AR, Waterhouse EJ, Boggs JG, et al: Prevalence of nonconvulsive status epilepticus in comatose patients. Neurology 2000 54(2):340345, 2000

4.1.4   Pathophysiology of Systemic Inflammation

Brett P. Giroir

The distinction between infection and inflammation underlies our current paradigm for the diagnosis and treatment of severe childhood infections and their consequences. While *infection* denotes the presence of microorganisms in a normally sterile tissue or body fluid, *inflammation* is the host response to that infection, to an injury, or to any number of noninfectious stimuli. A distinction between infection and inflammation is evidenced by the presence of inflammatory responses in children without infections, as well as the persistence of severe inflammation in children after antibiotics have killed the pathogen. An example is severe meningococcemia, in which meningococci are rapidly killed by systemic antibiotics, yet fever, vasodilation, cardiac failure, disseminated intravascular coagulopathy, and organ failure persist and frequently progress for hours or even days.

Because advances in antibiotic potency have failed to substantially improve survival or the development of multiple organ failure, it has become obvious that treatment of infections with antimicrobials must be coupled with immunomodulation. However, because host responses have been optimized by evolution, any attempt at modulation of inflammation, particularly in the context of an ongoing infection in a developing immune system, requires a comprehensive understanding of the relationships between clinical signs and the underlying inflammatory cascades that they evidence.

SYSTEMIC INFLAMMATORY RESPONSE SYNDROME, SEPSIS, AND SEPTIC SHOCK

Whether caused by infectious or noninfectious stimuli, the *systemic inflammatory response syndrome (SIRS)* is diagnosed by the presence of hyper- or hypothermia, tachycardia, tachypnea, or alteration (increase or decrease) in the white blood cell count. The diagnosis of SIRS lacks specificity, as a large fraction of hospitalized patients and a majority of intensive care patients will fulfill SIRS diagnostic criteria. When SIRS is the result of an infection, the diagnosis of *sepsis* is made. However, *sepsis* does not require positive cultures, but can also be diagnosed by the presence of SIRS together with specific signs of infection such as purulent drainage, lobar infiltration, and extending purpura.

Severe sepsis denotes the presence of organ dysfunction or hypoperfusion abnormalities, such as lactic acidosis, oliguria, changes in mental status, or transient hypotension. In contrast to severe sepsis, the diagnosis of *septic shock* requires the persistence (>1 hour) of hypoperfusion or hypotension despite adequate fluid resuscitation.

The concepts of sepsis, severe sepsis, and septic shock describe an increasingly severe spectrum of systemic inflammatory responses that are associated with progressive mortality, morbidity, and risk of multiple organ failure. Recent clinical trials have also demonstrated that the diagnosis of severe sepsis and septic shock, irrespective of underlying pathogen or source of infection, can serve to indicate treatment with immunomodulatory-anticoagulant therapy that improves both survival and organ function. These novel data can be explained only if we understand that the systemic inflammatory response syndrome, in whatever form or severity, is the clinical manifestation of *innate immune system activation*.

SEPSIS AND INNATE IMMUNE ACTIVATION

Adaptive immunity is the biological process in which exquisitely specific immune effector mechanisms are generated in response to pathogen (or vaccine) exposure. Adaptive immunity requires days or weeks for development and often involves somatic gene rearrangements. Components of the adaptive immune system include immunoglobulins and specific T- and B-cell recognition molecules and their responses.

In contrast, *innate immunity* is a prepositioned defense, always vigilant, rapidly activated, encoded in the genome, and highly conserved throughout the evolution of plants, invertebrates, and mammals. Components of innate immunity are responsible for the *immediate recognition* of pathogens, their *localization* to prevent dissemination, and the initiation of pathogen *killing* mechanisms. These three functions are integrated, often self-perpetuating, and now known to be responsible for the clinical manifestations of SIRS and sepsis and their sequelae.

PATHOGEN RECOGNITION

The cells of the innate immune system (macrophages, neutrophils, NK cells, and dendritic cells) must accurately recognize pathogens and distinguish them from *self*. The innate immune system accomplishes this by identifying *pathogen-associated molecular patterns (PAMPs)*, which are primarily composed of lipids or carbohydrates essential to pathogen survival yet having no homologue in humans. The prototypical PAMP of gram-negative bacteria is LPS (lipopolysaccharide or endotoxin). The discovery of the LPS recognition system has revolutionized our understanding of innate immune recognition, and thereby our understanding of SIRS.

LPS, when present in tissues or the circulation, is first bound to LBP (LPS-binding protein) a 60-kDa acute-phase glycoprotein synthesized in the liver and present in the plasma. LBP facilitates transfer of LPS to a cell-surface complex consisting of the CD14 molecule and the recently discovered toll-like receptor 4 (TLR-4) molecule. The discovery of TLR-4 as the mammalian LPS receptor provided the key to understanding innate immune recognition. There are 10 TLRs thus far identified in humans. These receptors are strikingly homologous to receptors in plants and *Drosophila*, in which TLRs are essential for antipathogen responses. For example,

deficiency of the toll protein in *Drosophila* results in overwhelming *Aspergillus* infection and death from the fly equivalent of fungal sepsis. TLR-4 is responsible for recognition of endotoxin in mammals. Deficiency of TLR-4 results in complete protection from LPS challenge, yet complete lethality from challenge with even a few gram-negative organisms.

The functions of other TLRs have also been elucidated. TLR-2 recognizes essential components of gram-positive bacteria, such as peptidoglycans and lipoteichoic acids, and also recognizes cell wall components of yeast and mycobacteria. Another receptor in this family recognizes DNA sequences that are found in viruses, bacteria, parasites, and other potential pathogens ("CpG DNA"), but which are not found in mammals. The function of the other TLRs remains unknown, but they are likely to recognize other pathogens, or perhaps injury-associated molecular-pattern molecules.

SIGNALING

TLR recognition likely occurs in the phagosome following ingestion of pathogens by cells of the innate immune system. Binding of TLR-2 or TLR-4 to their pathogen substrates results in dimerization, recruitment of adapter proteins (MyD88 and TRAF6), and a critical serine threonine kinase named IL-1 receptor-associated kinase (IRAK). At least two signal transduction pathways are then activated: the IκB kinase pathway leading to NF-κB translocation, and the mitogen-activated protein kinase (MAP kinase) pathway activating the AP1 family of transcription factors.

PATHOGEN KILLING

Recognition of pathogens by TLRs signals for production of cytokines (TNF-α, IL-1, and chemokines) by macrophages and other sentinel cells. These cytokines, through up-regulation of adhesion molecules on phagocytic and endothelial cells, facilitate homing of neutrophils to the site of infection. Recognition of pathogen also primes neutrophil pathways for microbial killing. In addition to these "rapid response" cytokines, at least one additional cytokine (HMG-1) is induced many hours after initial pathogen identification and signaling; in early animal studies, HMG-1 mediates, at least in part, delayed mortality and multiple system organ failure following LPS challenge.

In addition to cytokine biosynthesis and secretion, the alternative complement pathway is activated by LPS and other PAMPs. Activated complement contributes to plasma microbicidal activity along with other antimicrobial proteins such as bactericidal/permeability-increasing protein (BPI), defensins, and lactoferrin.

LOCALIZATION OF INFECTION BY COAGULATION

Compelling data now indicate that the extrinsic pathway of coagulation is a central, critical component of the innate immune system. Endotoxin, peptidoglycan, and other PAMPs, via the induction of TNF-α and IL-1, stimulate the expression of tissue factor on monocytes and possibly on endothelial cells. The surface expression and release of tissue factor activates factor VII, which initiates the extrinsic coagulation cascade leading to activation of factor X to factor Xa, which, in the presence of factor Va, converts prothrombin to thrombin, resulting in the cleavage of fibrinogen to fibrin. The deposition of fibrin at the site of pathogen recognition can serve to localize microorganisms and thereby limit systemic dissemination. In addition, via several direct and indirect mechanisms, thrombin further activates NF-κB in monocytes and neutrophils, enhancing the production of cytokines within the vicinity of initial pathogen recognition.

REGULATORS OF INNATE IMMUNITY

SIRS is accompanied, to varying degrees, by a compensatory anti-inflammatory response which is at least as complex and integrated as its proinflammatory counterpart. Anti-inflammatory proteins such as IL-1 receptor antagonist (IL-1Ra), IL-10, and soluble TNF receptors mitigate inflammation and its propagation. Several hormones, including cortisol, epinephrine, α-melanocyte-stimulating hormone (α-MSH), and vasoactive intestinal peptide (VIP, from macrophages as well as the CNS) potently inhibit transcription and translation of cytokine genes.

Surprisingly, the innate immune system is also subject to direct neural control. This new paradigm of immune regulation was recently elucidated by the finding that afferent vagus nerve fibers instruct the brain that an innate immune response has been triggered. Subsequently, efferent vagus nerve fibers fire, release acetylcholine, and inhibit cytokine production by the liver and gut (the primary sources of TNF-α during sepsis). In experimental models, division of the vagus nerves leads to markedly increased systemic TNF levels following endotoxin challenge; whereas division of the vagus nerve followed by hyperstimulating efferent vagus fibers with a nerve stimulator not only decreases cytokine production but also preserves systemic arterial pressure and improves survival. Verification of this novel immunomodulatory neural network in humans is ongoing.

SIRS AND SEPSIS AS THE INNATE IMMUNE RESPONSE SYNDROME

The innate immune system of humans is ancient and strikingly homologous to that of lower animals, invertebrates, and even plants. It is clear, therefore, that human innate immunity developed in an evolutionary context of recognizing, containing, and killing a limited number of pathogens that breached a single tissue barrier. Innate immunity is highly successful in achieving this goal. The innate immune system is not evolved, however, to contend with overwhelming bacteremia, multiple trauma with massive transfusion, and other major insults of modern civilization. As such, Bruce Beutler (The Margaux Conference on Critical Illness, 2000) concluded that "septic shock reflects an unusual situation in which the microbial pathogens have achieved an intolerable burden, and caused coordinated activation of the innate immune receptors throughout the host."

As discussed previously, it is already proven that gram-positive and gram-negative bacteria, as well as yeast and mycobacteria, activate the innate immune system via TLRs. Because there is significant sharing of signal transduction pathways (including IRAK) among TLRs, the innate immune response is stereotyped, at least to a degree. This stereotyped response partially explains the clinical similarities of sepsis and SIRS caused by a wide range of microbial pathogens. Perhaps as important, TLR-4 has also been reported to be a specific receptor for heat-shock protein 60 (HSP 60), which may be induced by a variety of infectious and noninfectious stimuli, such as trauma, heat stress, and hypoxia. This finding suggests a potential molecular mechanism explaining how noninfectious insults can also cause SIRS that is clinically indistinguishable from SIRS caused by infection.

In the context of a disseminated and massive microbial load, TLR recognition and innate immune activation come with a phys-

iological price. High tissue and circulating levels of TNF-α and IL-1, both directly and indirectly, depress systolic and diastolic cardiac function, resulting in myocardial failure. The anaphylatoxins C3a and C5a, produced as a result of activation of complement, contribute directly to vasodilation and vascular permeability. In addition, activation of the contact system of coagulation results in the generation of kallikrein, which, in turn, releases the potently vasoactive bradykinin molecule from high-molecular-weight kininogen. TNF-α and IL-1 also cause transcription and translation of the inducible form of nitric oxide synthase (iNOS), resulting in markedly enhanced NO production. Although NO participates in microbial killing, particularly of intracellular pathogens, high levels of NO cause profound vasodilation and vasoplegia, as well as the uncoupling of cardiac β-adrenergic receptors from adenyl cyclase, thereby limiting the effects of β-receptor–dependent inotropes.

Transmigration of neutrophils, evolutionarily intended to occur only at an infected site, occurs diffusely into organs because of massive innate immune activation. Already primed via TLR-dependent mechanisms, neutrophils release free radicals and proteases, which are important for pathogen killing and also contribute to lung injury. High levels of NO react with released superoxides to form the highly reactive free radical peroxynitrite. Peroxynitrite has numerous deleterious effects, including lipid peroxidation of cell membranes, S-nitrosylation of proteins, and inhibition of heme-containing enzymes responsible for mitochondrial respiration. In addition, peroxynitrite induces strand breaks in DNA, with subsequent NAD$^+$ depletion secondary to continuous activation of poly-ADP ribose synthase.

High levels of TNF-α, IL-1, IL-6, and other cytokines up-regulate tissue factor diffusely on circulating monocytes, and possibly on endothelial cells, leading to disseminated intravascular coagulation (DIC). Removal of fibrin (fibrinolysis) is impeded by exaggerated release of plasminogen activator inhibitor -1 (PAI-1) from platelets and endothelial cells. Ongoing consumption of the coagulation regulators antithrombin, protein S, and protein C cause uninhibited coagulopathy. This dysregulation is worsened because thrombomodulin, which is absolutely required to activate protein C, is itself profoundly down-regulated on the endothelium via cytokine-dependent mechanisms.

The human sepsis phenotype is procoagulant and antifibrinolytic. As a result, disseminated microthromboses occur, further exacerbating endothelial injury and tissue ischemia. This self-perpetuating, and until recently, inevitable spiral of further capillary injury, inflammation, and coagulation resulted in vasomotor collapse, multiple organ dysfunction, and death.

THE SEARCH FOR NOVEL THERAPEUTICS

The conceptual framework for improving the outcome of SIRS, sepsis, and multiple organ failure can be found in the following equation, which was developed by Drs. Steve Opal, Patrick Scannon, and Brett Giroir for the Defense Sciences Research Council (2000).

$$\text{Probability of Death} = \frac{\text{\# organisms} \times \text{virulence} \times \text{route} \times \text{immune collateral damage}}{\text{host defenses}}$$

Currently, clinical practice is directed primarily at reducing the microbial load (# organisms) through prevention and the use of increasingly sophisticated antibacterial, antifungal, antiviral, and antiparasitic agents. Until now, immune collateral damage has generally been accepted as a nonmodifiable variable primarily determined by the patient's genetic predispositions. Instead, intensive care has focused only on the consequences of immune collateral damage, for example, organ failures, rather than the specific processes involved in the induction and propagation of the innate immune response itself. This focus on antimicrobials and organ support has been theoretically justified, because many interventions that limit immune collateral damage (in the numerator), directly and adversely affect host defenses (in the denominator). As a result, nonspecific immunosuppression, particularly in the context of inadequately treated infections, enhances mortality, instead of reducing it.

EFFECTIVELY TARGETING INNATE IMMUNITY

In the last 20 years, the failure of multiple clinical trials aimed at reducing the mortality of sepsis raised debate concerning the legitimacy of the current paradigm and its corollary hypotheses. Very large clinical trials conducted on septic adults, designed to block endotoxin, TNF-α, IL-1, platelet-activating factor (PAF), or nitric oxide, either showed no benefit or actually caused harm. Recent evidence, however, clearly demonstrates that the failure of these early trials stemmed primarily from inadequate study design and/or experimental agents, rather than from flaws in the infection-inflammation paradigm itself.

As a primary inducer of innate immunity, LPS (endotoxin) is an ideal therapeutic target in severe gram-negative sepsis, as well as in other conditions in which there is endotoxin translocation across the gut, such as burns, hemorrhage, and polytrauma. In children, severe meningococcemia is the prototype disease of massive innate immunity initially targeted for novel interventions. A large body of research has indicated that meningococcal septic shock, coagulopathy, multiple organ failure, and death result primarily from the shedding of endotoxin-containing blebs from the etiologic bacteria *Neisseria meningitidis*. This robust shedding of blebs, even prior to antibiotic administration, yields plasma endotoxin concentrations greater than those found in any other human infection.

The first large-scale randomized trial of immune modulation in meningococcemia was designed to mitigate endotoxin toxicity via administration of HA-1A, a monoclonal antibody that bound (but did not neutralize) endotoxin. Although this trial failed to demonstrate a statistically significant benefit, there was a strong trend toward survival advantage in the group treated with HA-1A. Unfortunately, HA-1A treatment was also associated with a trend toward enhanced morbidity in survivors.

More recently, pediatric investigators supplemented severe meningococcemia patients with an important component of their innate immune system, BPI. From earlier studies, BPI was known to be deficient in infants and relatively deficient in severely affected older children. Unlike HA-1A, BPI completely neutralizes endotoxin, in addition to binding it and facilitating its removal from the circulation. Moreover, BPI is itself a bactericidal agent that potently and rapidly kills both smooth and rough forms of gram-negative bacteria, including *Neisseria meningitidis*. Data from the Phase III randomized placebo-controlled trial (n=393 children) demonstrated that treatment with a recombinant N-terminal fragment of BPI ($rBPI_{21}$) reduced clinically significant morbidities (including severe amputations) and enhanced overall functional outcome. Although there was a numerical mortality advantage in the BPI-treated group, the study was underpowered to prove a survival advantage

with statistical confidence. The BPI trial data have been submitted to the FDA, and discussions regarding the fate of $rBPI_{21}$ therapy are ongoing.

Finally, the most important trial of innate immunomodulation targeted neither TLR ligands nor cytokines, but the coagulation-inflammation network. As previously indicated, a primary regulator of coagulation, fibrinolysis, and coagulation-induced inflammation is protein C. In both children and adults, acquired deficiencies in protein C (due to consumption in DIC) and deficits in protein C activation (due to thrombomodulin down-regulation) are directly correlated with morbidity and mortality in septic shock from all observed etiologies (gram-positive, gram-negative, fungal, and parasitic). The commonality of protein C deficiency is not surprising, because diverse pathogens all stimulate the extrinsic pathway of coagulation through cytokine enhancement of tissue factor expression.

In a 1690-patient randomized, placebo-controlled trial, administration of recombinant activated protein C (rhAPC) to adults with sepsis and organ failure resulted in a nearly 20% relative risk reduction in mortality ($P = .005$). Supplementation of rhAPC caused a prompt cessation of coagulopathy and also reduced inflammation as evidenced by a statistically significant reduction in IL-6. Preliminary data suggest that the dosing and safety profile of rhAPC is similar in children and adults, although the completion of a multicenter pediatric safety and pharmokinetics study is pending at the time of this publication.

CONCLUSIONS

With an improved understanding of the benefits and limitations of human innate immunity, it is likely that other therapies, in addition to rhAPC, will prove effective. These new therapies are likely to target multiple sites in the innate immune network and are likely to be immunomodulatory instead of immunosuppressive. The $rBPI_{21}$ and rhAPC trials also strongly suggest that the optimum drugs for modulating the innate immune system will be natural regulatory molecules evolved for that purpose. These natural regulators have only become inadequate given the challenge of modern disseminated infections and catastrophic injuries, in children provided the opportunity for survival by advanced pediatric transport, in pediatric emergency resuscitation, and in pediatric critical care.

References

Anderson KV: Toll signaling pathways in the innate immune response. Curr Opin Immunol 12:13–19, 2000

Bernard GR, Vincent J-L, Laterre P-F, et al: Efficacy and safety of recombinant human activated protein C for severe sepsis. N Engl J Med 334(10):699–709, 2001

Beutler B: Endotoxin, toll-like receptor 4, and the afferent limb of innate immunity. Curr Opin Microbiol 1:23–28, 2000

Esmon CT, Fukudome K, Mather T, et al: Inflammation, sepsis, and coagulation. Haematologica 84:254–259, 1999

Fijnvandraat K, Derkx B, Peters M, et al: Coagulation activation and tissue necrosis in meningococcal septic shock: severely reduced protein C levels predict a high mortality. Thromb Haemost 73:15–20, 1995

Hoffmann JA, Kafatos KC, Janeway CA, et al: Phylogenetic perspectives in innate immunity. Science 284:1313–1318, 1999

Janeway CA, Medzhitov R: Introduction: the role of innate immunity in the adaptive immune response. Semin Immunol 10:349–350, 1998

Levin M, Quint PA, Goldstein B, et al: Recombinant bactericidal/permeability-increasing protein (rBPI21) as adjunctive treatment for children with severe meningococcal sepsis: a randomised trial. Lancet 356:961–967, 2000

Nadel S, Newport MJ, Booy R, Levin M: Variation in the tumor necrosis factor-alpha gene promoter region may be associated with death from meningococcal disease. J Infect Dis 4:878–880, 1996

Rosenberg RD, Aird WC: Vascular-bed–specific hemostasis and hypercoagulable states. N Engl J Med 340:1555–1564, 1999

Wang H, Bloom O, Zhang M, et al: HMG-1 as a late mediator of endotoxin lethality in mice. Science 285:248–251, 1999

4.1.5   Assessment of the Child with Fever

David M. Jaffe

Fever is the most common symptom prompting sick child visits to the pediatric office and emergency department. By the age of 2 years, 65% of children in the United States will have visited a physician for fever. Under normal circumstances, body temperature is tightly regulated by the hypothalamus. Fever has been defined as a regulated rise in body temperature. As such, it is one of several acute-phase responses to infection, trauma, inflammation, and malignancy. Of these, infection is the most frequent. Fever can be distinguished from hyperthermia, in which the temperature rises above the thermoregulatory set point as a result of environmental heat. Hyperthermia is associated with a failure of hypothalamic thermal regulation caused by excessive heat, inadequate heat dissipation, or defects of hypothalamic regulation (see Sec. 4.3.7).

Normal core body temperature varies among individuals. In addition, there is diurnal temperature variation of as much as 1.3°C, the temperature being typically highest in the late afternoon (1700–1900 hours) and lowest in early morning (0200–0600 hours). Younger children also tend to have higher average body temperatures than do older children and adults. Measurement of temperature introduces additional sources of variability depending on the site and device used. Based on these considerations, any single temperature used to define fever threshold is arbitrary but nonetheless useful in clinical practice. The temperature most commonly used to define fever threshold in children is 38°C, rectal, although lower oral temperatures in adolescents and adults (37.2–37.8°C) may indicate a febrile response.

PATHOGENESIS OF FEVER

Fever is the result of a complex series of events initiated in the preoptic area of the anterior hypothalamus, which regulates core body temperature like a thermostat. Core body temperature is defined as the temperature of the blood that supplies the preoptic area of the hypothalamus. When the appropriate signal is received, the hypothalamic thermostat increases the set point for core body temperature. A number of autonomic, endocrine, and behavioral thermoregulatory responses follow, resulting in a rise of core body temperature by as much as 4°C. Blood flow is redirected from cutaneous to deep vascular beds, sweating decreases, and pulse rate and blood pressure increase. Heat is also generated by increased metabolic rate. Endocrine responses include decreased secretion of vasopressin and increased production of corticotropin-releasing hormone resulting in increased glucocorticoid levels. The liver produces acute-phase reactants. Behavioral responses include shivering, search for warmth, anorexia, and somnolence.

Pyrogens are substances that can cause fever. Exogenous pyrogens originate outside the body. Examples include bacteria, virus, fungi, and toxins. Exogenous pyrogens stimulate a variety of host cells, especially monocytes and macrophages, but also neutrophils, lymphocytes, endothelial cells, glial cells, and certain mesangial and mesenchymal cells to produce endogenous pyrogens. A variety of substances that originate within the host can also induce the production and release of endogenous pyrogens. These include antigen-antibody complexes, bile acids, complement components, and androgenic steroid metabolites.

Endogenous pyrogens are cytokines that, in addition to their other effects on the immune response, can induce fever. Interleukin-1 (IL-1), tumor necrosis factor (TNF)-α, interferon (IFN)-γ, and interleukin-6 (IL-6) are the most important and well studied of the cytokines. Other cytokines with pyrogenic properties include those that can bind to the common receptor gp 130: IL-6, interleukin-2 (IL-2), leukemic inhibitory factor, ciliary neurotropic factor, cardiotropin, and oncostatin M.

Endogenous pyrogens produced outside the central nervous system reach the brain from the systemic circulation, but do not cross the blood-brain barrier. Instead, they are thought to exert their effect in the organum vasculosum laminae terminalis (OLVT), a vascular network of fenestrated capillaries close to a cluster of neurons in the preoptic hypothalamus. Neurons in this region are accessible to circulating cytokines. It is not known whether systemic cytokines affect neurons in the OLVT directly. There is evidence, however, that arachidonic acid metabolites, primarily prostaglandin E_2 (PGE_2), are elaborated in the OLVT in response to circulating cytokines and function to mediate the febrile response in the hypothalamus. Because the response to injected cytokines occurs within minutes, it is likely that PGE_2 activates intrinsic neuronal pathways, which contact the neuron groups responsible for coordinating the autonomic, behavioral, and hormonal elements of the febrile response (Fig. 4-13).

Recent discoveries suggest that there may be alternatives to the "classic" mechanism of fever production. Vagal afferents in the liver can be activated by locally produced pyrogenic cytokines. Signal delivery occurs in the nucleus of the tractus solitarius, which is important in modulating metabolic responses and may also have neural connections with thermogenic area of the hypothalamus.

The precise limit of the febrile response is unknown, but core body temperature rarely rises above 41 to 42°C. This is the temperature range at which adverse physiological effects begin to occur. These include acid-base disturbances, arrhythmias, disseminated intravascular coagulation, thrombocytopenia, hemorrhage, and organ congestion.

The mechanism of control and limitation of the rise in body temperature characterizing the febrile response is largely unknown. However, it is likely composed of neuronal and hormonal elements. There are a number of substances that have been found to have cryogenic, or temperature-lowering, properties. Arginine vasopressin (AVP) was the first to be demonstrated. Subsequently, α-melanocyte-stimulating hormone (α-MSH), thyroliberin, gastric inhibitory polypeptide, neuropeptide Y, and bombesin were shown to have similar effects. Even TNF-α under some conditions lowers body temperature. There is also evidence that the release of pyrogenic cytokines down-regulates cytokine receptors, suggesting the existence of a self-regulatory negative feedback loop.

While there is no conclusive evidence that fever itself improves human survival and/or recovery from microbial infection, there are several arguments that support this hypothesis. Moderate increases in temperature enhance the immune response. Neutrophil function is enhanced by increasing both chemotactic responses and superoxide production. Fever increases interferon production and augments T-cell proliferation and B-cell antibody production. In animal experiments, fever improved survival rates, while suppression

Cytokines as Endogenous Pyrogens

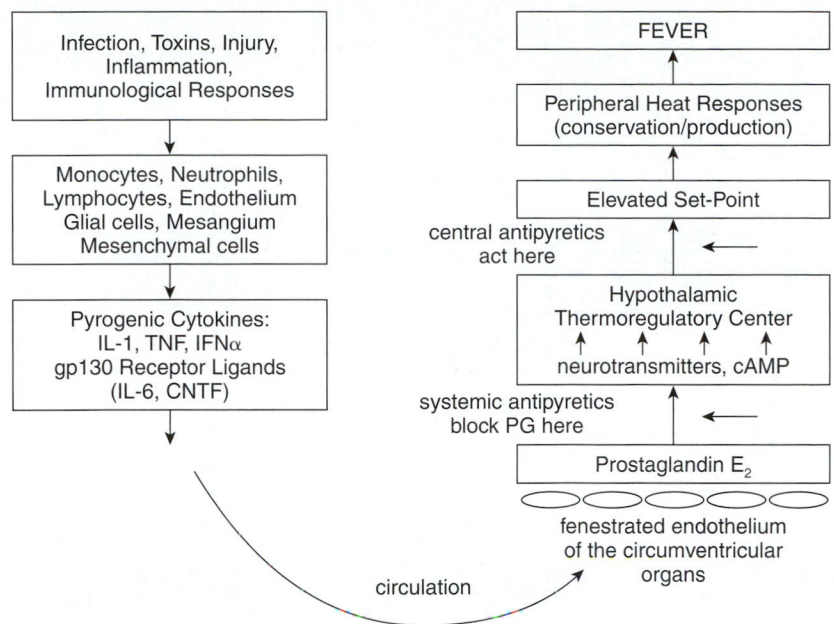

FIGURE 4-13 Schema for pathogenesis of fever. IL, interleukin; TNF, tumor necrosis factor; IFN, interferon; PG, prostaglandin; CNTF, ciliary neurotrophic factor. SOURCE: Reproduced with permission from: Dinarello CA: Cytokines as endogenous pyrogens. J Infect Dis 1999; 179 (Suppl 2):S294–304.

of fever increased mortality. Fever occurs in many animal types and at the expense of energy, which suggests that it has evolutionary survival value.

TREATMENT OF FEVER AND FEVER PHOBIA

Because fever is a sign of illness, the major medical task is to determine the specific cause of fever and to prescribe the most appropriate therapy. Nonetheless, it has become customary to prescribe additional treatment aimed at lowering core body temperature in children with fever.

Many parents and extended family members believe that fever is itself a disease and that it may cause permanent harm, including brain damage. Many common and reasonable pediatric practices inadvertently reinforce fever phobia. Among these are warnings to notify the physician about any fever in neonates and the aggressive search for bacterial infection frequently recommended in young children with fever. Protocols for investigation of occult bacteremia often specify a temperature threshold of 39.0 or 39.5°C, thereby ascribing significance to height of temperature. Physicians sometimes prescribe regimens of alternating acetaminophen and ibuprofen to prevent febrile seizures, although recent evidence suggests that aggressive antipyretic use does not alter the incidence of recurrent febrile seizures.

Permanent tissue damage is unlikely to occur at core temperatures associated with fever. However, fever causes or is associated with unpleasant experiences such as chills, anorexia, body ache, irritability, and mild dehydration. The main indication for treating fever is to reduce the associated discomfort. The well or happy-appearing child with fever requires diagnosis but does not necessarily require antipyretic therapy. The rare child with core temperature greater than 41.0°C should be treated with antipyretics to avoid reaching temperatures associated with tissue damage.

Acetaminophen and ibuprofen are antipyretic agents widely used to treat fever. Both agents decrease prostaglandin synthesis in the brain, thereby lowering the hypothalamic set point and reversing the metabolic, endocrine, and behavioral events that maintain

fever. Ibuprofen inhibits both central and peripheral prostaglandin synthesis and has both antipyretic and anti-inflammatory properties. Because acetaminophen does not provide effective blockade of prostaglandin synthesis in the peripheral tissues, it is not an effective anti-inflammatory agent. Aspirin was the first popular antipyretic, but its use as a standard pediatric antipyretic has been abandoned because of its association with Reye's syndrome. Recommended dosing of acetaminophen is 15 mg/kg as often as every 4 hours; the recommended dosing of ibuprofen is 10 mg/kg as often as every 6 hours.

APPROACH TO DIAGNOSIS AND MANAGEMENT

Routine skills of history taking and physical examination are essential in diagnosing the cause of fever. Special considerations apply to children with immune compromise, neonates, and children between the ages of 3 months and 3 years in whom no obvious focus of infection is found (Fig. 4-14).

In all cases, consideration should be given first to detection of life-threatening conditions such as meningitis, sepsis, severe pneumonia, acute cardiac infection, and acute appendicitis (Table 4-9). Children with life-threatening infections often appear "toxic" at the time of initial observation. No clinical skill is more important for the pediatric caretaker than the ability to recognize toxic-appearing children. Toxic appearance is characterized by listlessness, agitation, and/or failure to recognize the parents. There may be signs of respiratory distress or inadequate circulation such as cool extremities; weak, rapid pulse; or poor capillary refill. Color may be cyanotic, gray, or mottled. In this context, purpura is also an ominous skin sign.

Toxic appearance is a medical emergency. Rapid action may prevent septic shock and a cascade of events leading to multiple organ failure and death. After obtaining cultures of blood, urine, and cerebrospinal fluid, a broad-spectrum antibiotic should be administered parenterally. Cefotaxime or ceftriaxone at 50 mg/kg are effective against most agents causing sepsis. If penicillin-resistant *S. pneumoniae* is a concern, vancomycin (40 mg/kg/d) is added to the

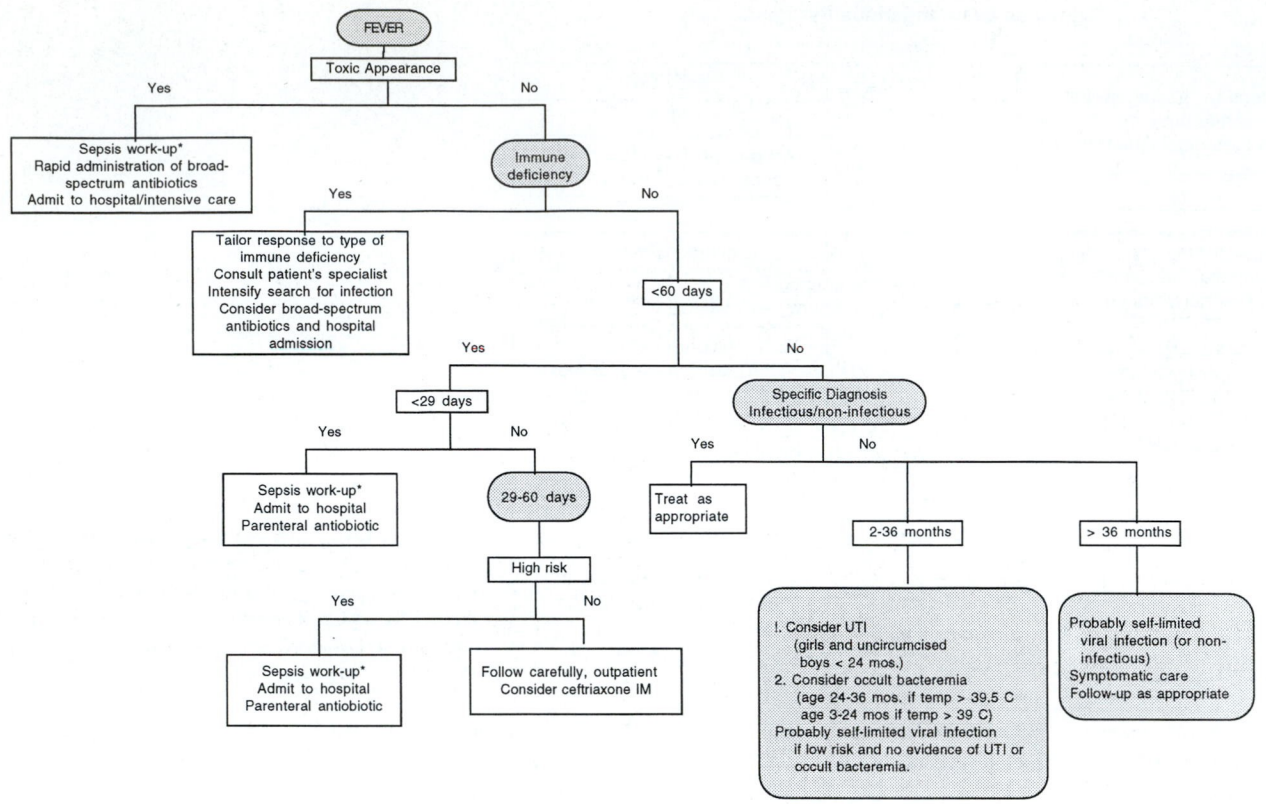

FIGURE 4-14   Algorithm for evaluation and management of febrile infant or child.

initial regimen. If disseminated herpes or herpes meningitis is suspected, acyclovir (30 mg/kg/d) should be given. Antibiotic administration should not be delayed significantly by prolonged attempts to obtain specimens for culture.

Febrile children with immune deficits also require special consideration. Profound neutropenia (absolute neutrophil count of less than 500 per cubic millimeter), actual or functional splenectomy, and advanced HIV disease are associated with significant risk of life-threatening infection. Degree and duration of neutropenia and the presence of breeches in host defenses modify the severity of risk. For example, neutropenia secondary to cytotoxic chemotherapy for cancer is often associated with mucosal ulceration. There may also be alterations in cellular immunity and hypogammaglobulinemia, which increase vulnerability to infection. In contrast, virally induced neutropenia carries a lower risk of significant bacterial infection. Patients who are functionally asplenic are especially vulnerable to life-threatening infections caused by encapsulated bacteria such as *S. pneumoniae, N. meningitidis,* and *H. influenzae.*

In the United States and Western Europe, the dominant organisms responsible for acute bacterial infections in immunocompromised hosts are gram-positive organisms, especially coagulase-negative staphylococci. *S. aureus* and enterococci are also important pathogens. Gram-negative organisms such as *Pseudomonas aeruginosa, E. coli,* and *Klebsiella* species still predominate in developing countries and can cause rapid development of life-threatening sepsis syndrome. Viral and fungal infections can also occur.

HIV-infected children with fever may develop recurrent, and sometimes severe, infections with a wide range of pathogens. The infections often have the same anatomic locations as seen in febrile children without HIV infection. Otitis, sinusitis, pneumonia, gastroenteritis, meningitis, urinary tract infection, and dermatitis are

all common. Most infections are also caused by organisms typically found at these locations. *S. pneumoniae* is a particularly important pathogen in respiratory, blood, and central nervous system infections. When CD4 counts are low, however, children become susceptible to opportunistic organisms as well. *Pneumocystis carinii* pneumonia is the most common opportunistic organism. Children with absolute neutrophil count less than 500 per cubic millimeter are highly susceptible to gram-negative bacterial infection and sepsis (see Sec. 13.4.12).

Treatment is guided by the type of immune deficiency, as well as by its severity and duration. For children with prolonged or severe neutropenia, empiric broad-spectrum antibiotic coverage is recommended, using ceftriaxone, cefotaxime, or combinations of antibiotics designed to combat the common gram-positive and gram-negative organisms. Outpatient regimens are becoming more popular for children at lower risk for overwhelming sepsis. After obtaining appropriate cultures, for example, children with sickle cell disease with fever are often managed with ceftriaxone as outpatients. Of course, if careful examination reveals a specific site of infection, more specific antimicrobial therapy can be given. It is often useful to consult with the specialists who provide longitudinal care for immunocompromised children with fever.

NEONATAL FEVER

Fever in the neonatal period (0–60 days) raises special concerns. During this period, neutrophils exhibit decreased chemotaxis, adherence, transendothelial migration, and bactericidal activity. Monocytes also have decreased chemotaxis, and secretion of interferon-γ is low. Germinal centers in the spleen and lymph node are underdeveloped until 4 to 8 weeks. Splenic T cells are predominantly suppressor, which prevents B cells from producing antibody.

TABLE 4-9
LIFE-THREATENING ACUTE FEBRILE ILLNESS

I. Infection
   A. Central nervous system
      1. Acute bacterial meningitis
      2. Encephalitis
   B. Upper Airway
      1. Retropharyngeal abscess
      2. Bacterial tracheitis
      3. Acute epiglottitis (rare)
      4. Laryngeal diphtheria (rare)
   C. Pulmonary
      1. Pneumonia (severe)
      2. Tuberculosis, miliary
   D. Cardiac
      1. Myocarditis
      2. Bacterial endocarditis
      3. Suppurative pericarditis
   E. Gastrointestinal
      1. Acute gastroenteritis (fluid/electrolyte losses)
      2. Appendicitis
      3. Peritonitis (other causes)
   F. Musculoskeletal
      1. Necrotizing myositis (gas gangrene)/fasciitis
   G. Systemic
      1. Meningococcemia
      2. Other bacterial sepsis
      3. Rickettsial disease (Rocky Mountain spotted fever, ehrlichiosis)
      4. Toxic shock syndrome
II. Collagen-Vascular
   A. Acute rheumatic fever
   B. Kawasaki disease
   C. Stevens-Johnson syndrome
III. Miscellaneous
   A. Acute poisoning, atropine, salicylate, amphetamine, cocaine
   B. Malignancy
   C. Thyrotoxicosis (rare in children)

SOURCE: *Adapted from Alper ER, Henretig FM: Fever. In: Fleisher GR, Ludwig S, eds: Textbook of Pediatric Emergency Medicine, 4th ed. Philadelphia, Lippincott Williams & Wilkins, 2000.*

There is reduced natural killing (NK) activity against herpes-virus-infected cells. IgG levels fall rapidly during the first 3 months, whereas IgM increases rapidly from birth to 25 days. Complement levels and opsonic activity are decreased.

The effect of these maturational deficiencies is that neonates tend to have more difficulty localizing infection and are particularly susceptible to infections by certain organisms. The incidence of sepsis in the first month is estimated at 1 to 8 per 1000 live births. Group B streptococci and gram-negative enteric organisms are the most prevalent, but *Listeria monocytogenes, H. influenzae, Enterococcus, S. aureus,* and herpes virus can also cause neonatal sepsis.

The comparatively limited neonatal behavioral repertoire also makes detection of serious infection more challenging than for other age groups. The manifestations of serious illness may be subtle and overlap those of benign or normal conditions. Changes in feeding habit, sleep and wake cycles, and stool pattern have been associated with neonatal sepsis. More obvious signs, such as seizures, respiratory distress, lethargy, or irritability, may also be present.

Although there has been significant controversy and variation in practice, there is general agreement that special precautions should

TABLE 4-10
PARENTERAL ANTIBIOTICS FOR NEONATAL FEVER

Ampicillin
   <1 wk, 100 mg/kg/d, divided b.i.d.
   >1 wk, 200 mg/kg/d, divided q.i.d.
Plus cefotaxime:
   <1 wk, 100 mg/kg/d, divided b.i.d.
   1–4 wk, 150 mg/kg/d, divided t.i.d.
Or plus gentamicin:
   <1 wk, 5.0 mg/kg/d, divided b.i.d.
   1–4 wk, 7.5 mg/kg/d, divided t.i.d.

SOURCE: *Adapted from Baker DM: Evaluation and management of infants with fever. Pediatr Clin North Am 46:1061, 1999.*

be taken when fever occurs in neonates. For infants younger than 1 month, cultures of blood, spinal fluid, and urine should be obtained. Chest radiograph and stool culture should also be obtained in the presence of symptoms referable to the respiratory and gastrointestinal systems, respectively. Parenteral antibiotics effective against the significant pathogens of neonates should be given (Table 4-10).

For neonates 29 to 60 days old, there remains controversy and practice variation. The vast majority of these febrile children are likely to have self-limited viral disease. Policies that prescribe hospitalization and intravenous antibiotics are costly and have documented complications. For these reasons, significant efforts have been directed at developing criteria to distinguish between febrile neonates at low versus high risk for serious bacterial infection. Two strategies have been developed and tested prospectively, one in Philadelphia and one in Boston. A third strategy, developed in Rochester, was designed to apply to all neonates, including those in the first month of life (Table 4-11). The Rochester criteria do not include CSF analysis, and the Boston criteria are slightly more specific and less sensitive than the Philadelphia criteria. There is evidence that neither the Rochester nor the Philadelphia criteria perform as well when applied to other populations, and the same is likely to be true for the Boston criteria. There is also preliminary evidence from a large, office-based clinical study that office pediatricians perform better than any of these guidelines when managing infants in their own practices.

It is reasonable to choose any of these published strategies for management of febrile neonates from 29 to 60 days. Many unnecessary hospitalizations can be avoided at relatively low risk. However, the prudent pediatrician will maintain close contact with the "low-risk" patient until the febrile episode is resolved.

DIAGNOSIS AND MANAGEMENT

After evaluating for toxic appearance and considering immune compromise and the special status of the newborn separately, the remaining patients require specific diagnosis whenever possible. Diagnosing fever requires meticulous gathering of data from the medical history and physical examination and knowledge of the common causes (see Table 4-9). Particular attention needs to be paid to the onset of symptoms, which often provides important diagnostic clues. Organ-specific symptoms such as cough, rhinorrhea, ear or abdominal pain, sore throat, vomiting, and/or diarrhea should be investigated. Otitis, pharyngitis, rhinitis, gastroenteritis, and pneumonia occur frequently and can be diagnosed without laboratory testing. Similarly, illnesses such as measles, chickenpox,

TABLE 4-11

NEONATAL FEVER: LOW-RISK CRITERIA FOR SERIOUS BACTERIAL ILLNESS

	ROCHESTER (0–3 MONTHS)	PHILADELPHIA (1–2 MONTHS)	BOSTON (1–3 MONTHS)
Hx	Term (>37 weeks) No antimicrobials Never hospitalized No unexplained hyperbilirubinemia No chronic or underlying illness Not hospitalized longer than mother	No immune deficiency syndrome	No antibiotics, immunizations past 48h
PE	Appears generally well No evidence of skin, bone, soft tissue, joint, or ear infection	Infant observation score ≤10 No sign of bacterial infection	Nontoxic—no clinical need for hospitalization No focal infection (ear, soft tissue, joint, bone)
Labs	WBC 5–15K Absolute band <1500 Spun urine <10 WBC/HPF Stool <5 WBC/HPF (if diarrhea)	WBC <15K Band/neutrophil ratio <0.2 Spun U/A <10 WBC/HPF, fever/no bacteria Stool <5 WBC/HPF if diarrhea CSF <8 WBC/HPF, negative Gram stain CXR—no discrete infiltrate	WBC <20K U/A <10 WBC/HPF or negative leukocyte esterase CXR—no infiltrate if obtained

Infants meeting these criteria are considered at low risk for serious bacterial infection. Authors of the Rochester and Philadelphia criteria recommend no antibiotic treatment for low-risk patients, whereas the Boston authors recommend parenteral ceftriaxone (50 mg/kg/d). In all cases, careful follow-up is recommended.
Hx = history; PE = physical examination; Labs = laboratory studies; WBC = white blood cells; U/A = urine analysis; HPF = high-power field; CSF = cerebral spinal fluid; CXR = chest radiograph.

hand-foot-mouth disease, erythema infectiosum, and scarlet fever can be diagnosed by the appearance of characteristic rashes. While the vast majority of children with fever have infections, noninfectious causes of fever, including vasculitis syndromes, neoplasms, poisonings, central nervous system disorders, and metabolic diseases, should also be considered. Miscellaneous conditions capable of causing fever are dehydration, hemolysis, hemorrhage into an enclosed space, familial Mediterranean fever, sarcoidosis, and inflammatory bowel disease.

Because noninfectious causes of fever are much less common than infectious causes in children, diagnosis can be challenging. There may be a history of ingestion of salicylate, cocaine, atropines, amphetamines, and antihistamines, or evidence of characteristic toxidromes (see Sec. 4.3.3). Vasculitis syndromes are often associated with arthritis and characteristic rash. Rheumatic fever and Kawasaki disease have clinical criteria established for diagnosis (see Sec. 22.4.12 and 12.6.2). For acute rheumatic fever, major diagnostic criteria include carditis, chorea, subcutaneous nodules, arthritis, and erythema marginatum. For Kawasaki disease, diagnostic criteria, in addition to prolonged fever, include conjunctivitis, oropharyngeal mucositis, cervical adenopathy, polymorphous rash, and extremity changes such as erythema, edema, or periungual desquamation.

Fever associated with childhood cancer often occurs in conjunction with signs and symptoms indicative of the specific neoplasm. For example, leukemia may be associated with pallor, splenomegaly, bone pain, or weight loss. Central nervous system tumors may be associated with headache or progressive neurologic deficits. The majority of children with chronic fever or fever of unknown origin will eventually be diagnosed with infections, and some chronic fevers will resolve without diagnosis. The remainder will have less common diagnosis in the noninfectious categories (Table 4-12).

Fever Without Focus

It is common to fail to find a specific focus of infection or to arrive at a specific diagnosis in relatively well-appearing febrile children. Most often, these children will have self-limited viral illnesses that can be managed expectantly with supportive measures. History of exposure to family or visitors with a similar febrile illness, or daycare attendance, supports this diagnosis, as does the appearance of nonspecific, diffuse macular or maculopapular rash. Two common occult bacterial infections occur in young children with fever without focus: urinary tract infection and occult bacteremia.

Urinary Tract Infection (see Sec. 21.6) The overall prevalence of urinary tract infection in febrile children younger than 2 years is estimated to be between 3 and 6%. The highest rates (16%) have been reported for white girls. The rates in circumcised boys is lower than 1% after 1 year of age, but may be as high as 8% in uncircumcised boys. Symptoms of urinary tract infection are nonspecific in children younger than 2 years, and fever is the most common symptom. It is difficult to distinguish cystitis from pyelonephritis clinically in this age group, and there is evidence to suggest that the renal parenchyma is often infected when fever, pyuria, and bacteriuria occur.

Girls and uncircumcised boys younger than 2 years and circumcised boys younger than 1 year with fever without focus, especially with temperatures greater than 39.0°C, should be evaluated for urinary tract infection. Evidence of pyuria and bacteriuria in a urine specimen collected by catheter or suprapubic puncture provides sufficient evidence to begin therapy presumptively. Urine culture should also be obtained. Oral antibiotics and outpatient care are generally sufficient; however, children who are unable to tolerate oral medications, who are toxic or particularly ill-appearing, who have known underlying urologic abnormalities, or in whom adherence to prescribed antibiotic regimen is in doubt should be treated

TABLE 4-12

FINAL DIAGNOSES IN 100 PATIENTS WITH FEVER OF UNKNOWN ORIGIN*

<6 YR (N = 52)		≥6 YR (N = 48)	
DIAGNOSIS	**NO. OF PATIENTS**	**DIAGNOSIS**	**NO. OF PATIENTS**
Infectious	34	Infectious	18
Viral syndrome	13	Viral syndrome	4
Urinary tract infection	3	Endocarditis	3
Bacterial meningitis	3	Infectious mononucleosis	2
Pneumonia	3	Streptococcosis	2
Tonsillitis	3	Osteomyelitis	1
Septicemia	2	Sinusitis	1
Sinusitis	2	Tonsillitis	1
Generalized herpes simplex	1	Tuberculosis	1
Malaria	1	Typhoid fever	1
Peritonsillar abscess	1	Urinary tract infection	1
Osteomyelitis	1	Pneumonia	1
Enteric fever	1		
Collagen-inflammatory	4	Collagen-inflammatory	16
Rheumatoid arthritis	3	Rheumatoid arthritis	7
Henoch-Schönlein purpura	1	Lupus erythematosus	3
		Regional enteritis	4
		Ulcerative colitis	1
		Vasculitis (undefined)	1
Malignancy	4	Malignancy	2
Leukemia	3	Lymphosarcoma	1
Reticulum cell sarcoma	1	Leukemia	1
Miscellaneous	7	Miscellaneous	3
Central nervous system fever	2	Beçhet syndrome	1
Agranulocytosis	1	Hepatitis, anicteric	1
Lamellar ichthyosis	1	Ruptured appendix	1
Milk allergy	1		
Aspiration pneumonia	1		
Agammaglobulinemia	1		
Undiagnosed	3	Undiagnosed	9

* From Pizzo PA, et al: *Pediatrics* 1975; 55:468–473.

in the hospital with parenteral antibiotics. Common urinary tract pathogens are *E. coli, Proteus, Klebsiella, Enterococcus, Enterobacter, Pseudomonas, Group B streptococci, Serratia,* and *Staphylococcus aureus.* Although resistance to popular antibiotics has increased, clinical response often occurs even with resistant organisms, because of high antibiotic concentrations that are achieved in the urine. Amoxicillin (30–50 mg/kg/d), cotrimoxazole (8–10 mg trimethoprim/kg/d), nitrofurantoin (5–7 mg/kg/d), cefixime (8 mg/kg/d), or cephalexin (20–50 mg/kg/d) are reasonable choices for initial oral antibiotic regimens for urinary tract infections. Specific antibiotic choice should be guided by knowledge of the pathogen involved in specific cases, as well as by local resistance patterns. Intravenous regimens include ampicillin, gentamicin, and ceftriaxone or cefotaxime.

Occult Bacteremia

Bacteremia can be detected in approximately 3% of children age 3 to 36 months, who have temperatures greater than or equal to 39°C. *Streptococcus pneumoniae* accounts for more than 90% of these infections, while *Neisseria meningitidis* and *Salmonella* cause the vast majority of the rest. The *Haemophilus influenzae B* conjugate vaccine has virtually eliminated this organism as a cause of occult bacteremia. Most children with occult bacteremia are clinically indistinguishable from febrile children with self-limited viral illness.

High- and low-risk groups can be established based on the absolute neutrophil (ANC) count. Children with ANCs greater than 10,000 per cubic millimeter have an 8% risk of bacteremia, whereas those with lower (but still normal) ANCs have a risk of less than 1%. Combinations of very high temperature (>41°C) and ANC may increase the risk to as much as 20%. Children with unsuspected meningococcemia tend to have elevated band counts (greater than 10% in 60% of cases).

While the majority of children with *S. pneumoniae* bacteremia recover spontaneously, approximately 3 to 5% develop meningitis, and another 5% develop other focal infections such as pneumonia, cellulitis, bone or joint infections, and persistent bacteremia. The data regarding the natural history of meningococcal and *Salmonella* bacteremia are limited. Retrospective data suggest that the meningitis rate may be as high as 40 to 50% in meningococcal bacteremia, with sepsis, extremity necrosis, and death occurring as additional untoward outcomes. Occult nontyphoidal *Salmonella* bacteremia is responsible for rare cases of sepsis, osteomyelitis, and persistent bacteremia, but tends otherwise to have benign outcomes.

Children with known meningococcal bacteremia, regardless of clinical appearance, require rapid investigation of cerebrospinal fluid; initiation of intravenous antibiotics, either penicillin or cefotaxime; and hospitalization. Children with *S. pneumoniae* and *Salmonella* bacteremia should be evaluated according to clinical appearance. Those who appear well and are afebrile will likely resolve successfully by completing a course of oral antibiotic therapy. Despite emerging antibiotic resistance among *S. pneumoniae* species, amoxicillin (40 mg/kg/d) should suffice in well-appearing children. Those with persistent fever or ill appearance should have blood and cerebrospinal fluids cultured and should receive parenteral antibiotics and inpatient care. Ceftriaxone (50 mg/kg/d) and cefotaxime (50 mg/kg/d) are most commonly used in this circumstance. Use of antibiotics for nontyphoidal *Salmonella* bacteremia is controversial because of evidence that they may prolong the carrier state and have inconsistent efficacy in eradicating the organism from the blood. Because serious invasive salmonellosis tends to occur in children younger than 3 months, documented *Salmonella* bacteremia in this age group warrants admission, "sepsis workup," and parenteral antibiotic therapy. Amoxicillin or chloramphenicol can be used. Similar management is indicated for children 3 months or older who are febrile or ill appearing. Those who appear well at the time of reevaluation may be managed as outpatients without antibiotics.

There is evidence that expectant treatment of children at risk for *S. pneumoniae* bacteremia either with oral amoxicillin or parenteral ceftriaxone reduces the rate of subsequent meningitis approximately 10-fold. In high-risk children with fever without focus (ie, ANC >10,000) this means reducing the meningitis rate from approximately 1 in 1000 to 1 in 10,000. Because many febrile children with self-limiting viral disease would also be treated unnecessarily, and because some consider the risk reduction to be insufficient to warrant the intervention, there has been significant controversy about selection of the most appropriate strategy for managing children at risk for occult bacteremia. There are strong advocates for a strategy of watchful waiting for all of these patients, symptomatic relief, and careful instructions about signs of worsening suggestive of sepsis or meningitis. Others have recommended a strategy that depends on the ANC (or WBC) combined with important age and temperature characteristics to select a subgroup of children at higher (approximately 8–10%) risk for occult bacteremia, and treat these children expectantly with antibiotics. This author uses the following strategy: for children between 24 and 36 months, treat with antibiotics if temperature is greater than or equal to 39.5°C and ANC is greater than 10,000 per cubic millimeter; for children between 3 and 24 months, treat with antibiotics if temperature is greater than or equal to 39.0°C and ANC is greater than 10,000 per cubic millimeter. The antibiotic with the best documented efficacy is ceftriaxone (50 mg/kg IM), but subsequent to the vaccine-related reduction in *H. influenzae* bacteremia, amoxicillin (40–60 mg/kg/d for 7–10 days) is an acceptable alternative. Blood culture should be obtained prior to initiating antibiotic therapy. Children not meeting these high-risk criteria may be followed with symptomatic care and home observation.

S. pneumoniae Vaccine   These considerations are likely to be significantly altered by the availability of conjugated *S. pneumoniae* vaccine. Clinical trials suggest that the vaccine is at least 90% effective in preventing invasive pneumococcal disease. While it is too early to predict whether serotypes not included in the vaccine will cause significant invasive disease in vaccinated children, it is likely that the rates of *S. pneumoniae* bacteremia and meningitis will diminish significantly in vaccinated populations. The rates of occult bacteremia as a result of all organisms will probably become low

enough that laboratory testing to determine high- and low-risk groups and expectant antibiotic therapy will no longer be cost-effective.

References

Alper ER, Henretig FM: Fever. In: Fleisher GR, Ludwig S, eds: Textbook of Pediatric Emergency Medicine, 4th ed. Philadelphia, Lippincott Williams & Wilkins, 2000, 257–266.

American Academy of Pediatrics, Committee on Quality Improvement, Subcommittee on Febrile Seizures: Practice parameter: long-term treatment of the child with simple febrile seizures. Pediatrics 102:1307–1309, 1999

American Academy of Pediatrics, Committee on Quality Improvement, Subcommittee on Urinary Tract Infection: Practice parameter: the diagnosis, treatment, and evaluation of the initial urinary tract infection in febrile infants and young children. Pediatrics 103:843–852, 1999

Baker MD: Evaluation and management of infants with fever. Pediatr Clin North Am 46:1061–1072, 1999

Baker MD, Bell LM, Avner JR: The efficacy of routine outpatient management without antibiotics of fever in selected infants. Pediatrics 103:627–631, 1999

Baraff LJ, Oslund SA, Schriger DL, Stephen ML: Probability of bacterial infections in febrile infants less than three months of age: a meta-analysis. Pediatr Infect Dis J 11:257–265, 1992

Baskin MN, O'Rourke EJ, Fleisher GR: Outpatient treatment of febrile infants 28 to 89 days of age with intramuscular administration of ceftriaxone. J Pediatr 120:22–27, 1992

Black S, Shinefield H, Fireman B, et al: Efficacy, safety and immunogenicity of heptavalent pneumococcal conjugate vaccine in children. Pediatr Infect Dis J 19:187–195, 2000

Cimpello LB, Goldman DL, Khine H: Fever pathophysiology. Clin Pediatr Emerg Med 1:84–93, 2000

Dinarello CA: Cytokines as endogenous pyrogens. J Infect Dis 179(Suppl 2):S294–S304, 1999

Jaffe DM: What's hot and what's not: the gold standard for thermometry in emergency medicine. Ann Emerg Med 25:97–99, 1995

Jaffe DM: Occult bacteremia in children. In: Aronoff SC, Hughes WT, Kohl S, Speck WT, Wald ER, eds: Advances in Pediatric Infectious Diseases. St. Louis, MO Mosby-Year Book, 1996, 237–260

Jaskiewicz JA, McCarthy CA, Richardson AC, et al: Febrile infants at low risk for serious bacterial infection—an appraisal of the Rochester criteria and implications for management. Pediatrics 94:390–396, 1994

Kluger MJ, Kozak W, Leon LR, Soszynski D, Conn CA: Fever and antipyresis. Prog Brain Res 115:465–475, 1998

Kuppermann N: Occult bacteremia in young febrile children. Pediatr Clin North Am 46:1073–1110, 1999

Mackowiak PA: Concepts of fever. Arch Intern Med 158:1870–1881, 1998

McCarthy CA: The febrile infant [commentary]. Pediatrics 94:391–399, 1994

Netea MG, Kullberg BJ, Van der Meer JWM: Do only circulating pyrogenic cytokines act as mediators in the febrile response? A hypothesis. Eur J Clin Invest 29:351–356, 1999

Pizzo PA: Fever in immunocompromised patients. N Engl J Med 341:893–900, 1999

Pizzo PA, Lovejoy FJ Jr, Smith DH: Prolonged fever in children: review of 100 cases. Pediatrics 55:468–473, 1975

Saper CB, Breder CD: The neurologic basis of fever. N Engl J Med 330:1880–1886, 1994

Shaw KN, Gorelick MH: Urinary tract infection in the pediatric patient. Pediatr Clin North Am 46:1111–1124, 1999

Toltzis P, Husson RN: Fever and AIDS. In: Kliegman RM, ed: Practical Strategies in Pediatric Diagnosis and Therapy. Philadelphia, WB Saunders, 1996, 904–918

van Stuijvenberg M, Derksen-Lubsen G, Steyerberg EW, Dik F, Habbema J, Moll HA: Randomized, controlled trial of ibuprofen syrup administered during febrile illnesses to prevent febrile seizure recurrences. Pediatrics 102:1200, 1998

4.2 SUPPORTIVE TECHNIQUES AND MANAGEMENT

4.2.1 Monitoring of Vital Function

George Lister

Many patients with serious illness or injury or life-threatening states require observation to detect changes in function or state. Although nothing supplants direct physical examination, electronic monitoring and surveillance provide (a) warning signals for physiological disturbances that permit staff to observe multiple patients simultaneously; (b) repetitive or continuous assessment that does not disturb the patient; and (c) means for detecting the effect of interventions. Current monitoring devices also frequently have the capacity to store data that can be reviewed subsequently for analysis. Because of the vital importance of circulatory and respiratory function, much of the monitoring in common use tracks activity of these systems, and such monitoring is the focus of this section.

RESPIRATORY RATE

Monitoring of respiratory rate provides valuable clues about disturbances in respiratory function. Processes that decrease respiratory system compliance often cause respiratory rate to increase; processes that depress ventilatory drive or produce fatigue cause respiratory rate to decrease. Such monitoring may be useful both in hospitalized patients and in those at home who are at risk for breathing disturbances. Respiratory rate is assessed by devices that monitor either a mechanical correlate of breathing, gas flow, or gas exchange. Each approach is described briefly below, and the techniques to derive data are contrasted in the Table 4-13.

The mechanical correlate of breathing most commonly used is a change in thoracic volume. Electrical impedance devices pass a small current between two electrodes placed on opposite sides of the chest. Increases in the gas volume of the chest with inspiration cause a small increase in impedance to current that can be detected by an electronic circuit. The periodicity in this variation in impedance permits determination of respiratory rate. This approach is simple, safe, readily applicable to patients of all sizes, and is, by far, the most common approach used for bedside monitoring in the hospital; it has also been employed widely for home monitoring. It is essential, however, to recognize important constraints inherent in this technique (see Table 4-13): the signal is *not* quantitatively related to a change in lung volume, movement unrelated to breathing can be mistaken for breathing, and impedance changes resulting from movement can completely obliterate the breathing signal. Another major limitation of the transthoracic impedance method is that there can be impedance changes associated with breathing movements even though there is no ventilation of the lungs. Thus, conditions of airway obstruction cannot be detected with this method.

Another approach to detect changes in thoracic volume relies on the electrical impedance changes in electrical conductors in elastic bands surrounding the thorax or abdomen. If the bands contain strain gauges, the impedance (or, more correctly, resistance) of the bands varies with circumference. If the bands contain wires in a sinusoidal pattern so that they do not reduce the compliance of the bands, the impedance (or, more correctly, inductance) varies with the transverse area of the chest subtended by the bands. By recording these changes in both thoracic and abdominal circumference or area, it is possible to derive information about respiratory rate and, in the case of inductance, tidal volume. This latter approach, known as *inductance plethysmography*, requires proper positioning of the bands, and it is subject to artifact; however; it has the potential to provide considerable information about mechanical function and mechanisms for breathing disturbances. It may also identify breathing movements when the airway is obstructed.

Other, somewhat less common means for monitoring breathing use a signal from expired gas to detect a change from one phase of respiration to the other. A thermistor placed by the nares detects a difference between the warmed gas breathed out during expiration from the cooler inspired air. Because the temperature signal has no quantitative relation to change in lung volume this technique can only be used to determine breathing rate. It is primarily used in a laboratory setting rather than for routine monitoring, because breathing through the mouth interferes with the ability to sense a breath and the equipment requires attention. Measurement of PCO_2 at the nares (*capnometry*) can also be used to sense a breath (see below) as well as to provide information about gas exchange.

GAS EXCHANGE

General Principles

The measurement of respiratory gases provides inference about both ventilatory and circulatory function, depending on which gas is considered and where it is sampled. A few general principles help elucidate this point. Because there is no appreciable CO_2 in inspired gas, the arterial PCO_2 is proportional to the rate of production (metabolic rate) and inversely proportional to the rate of excretion (ventilation). Furthermore, arterial PCO_2 changes rapidly with rapid alterations in ventilation.

Oxygen is taken up in the lungs and extracted by the tissues at about the same rate that carbon dioxide is produced by the tissues and excreted in the lungs (under normal conditions the ratio of CO_2 production to O_2 consumption ranges from 0.7–1). The arteriovenous content difference for either gas depends on the relationship between the metabolic rate for that gas and the blood flow rate (metabolic rate/blood flow = arteriovenous O_2 or CO_2 content difference). Thus, the difference between arterial and venous blood gas content increases when blood flow is reduced relative to metabolism. Because there is no net storage of O_2 or CO_2, the *fall* in O_2 content between arterial and mixed venous blood is roughly the same as the *rise* in CO_2 content from arterial to mixed venous blood (see Fig. 4-15). However, because the relationship between blood PCO_2 and content is generally more linear and much steeper than that between PO_2 and O_2 content, the arteriovenous PCO_2 difference is much smaller than the PO_2 difference under most conditions. The following section addresses means for estimating arterial and venous blood gas concentrations.

Carbon Dioxide

Arterial PCO_2 can be measured directly in small samples (<1 mL) of arterial blood using an electrode that measures the pH of a bicarbonate solution separated from the blood by a CO_2-permeable membrane. (Measurement of CO_2 content is more technically demanding and not practical for clinical medicine.) Because of the rapid response of arterial PCO_2 to changes in ventilation, anything

TABLE 4-13

COMMON TECHNIQUES FOR MONITORING RESPIRATORY FUNCTION IN CHILDREN

VARIABLE MONITORED	
SOURCE/SITE AND METHOD/MEASUREMENT	**COMMENTS AND PRECAUTIONS**

RESPIRATORY RATE	
Transthoracic impedance	Simple, easy to use; not quantitatively related to change in lung/chest wall volume; movement may appear like breath; obstructive apnea not detected; breath can be undetected
Inductance plethysmography	Provides estimate of relative tidal volume; signals apnea when tidal volume below arbitrary threshold; can aid in determining etiology of disordered breathing; false detection of breath, failure to detect breath
Nasal airflow thermistor	Simple; not quantitatively related to change in volume or flow; thermistor easily dislodged; mouth breathing can cause failure of breath detection

GAS EXCHANGE, INVASIVE	
Arterial Blood	Gold standard for evaluating ventilation and pulmonary gas exchange; sampling may disturb patient unless from indwelling catheter
Po_2	Usually need ≤ 0.2 mL; estimate HbO_2 saturation, which can be erroneous when HbCO, MetHb, or fetal Hb present
HbO_2	Usually need 0.1 mL; can also measure HbCO, MetHb, not sensitive to alterations in blood gas exchange when $>95\%$
Pco_2	Usually need ≤ 0.2 mL; $\geq$ arterial Pco_2 but generally within small range; disparity increased with poor perfusion
Peripheral Venous Blood	
Po_2	Not reliable estimate of arterial Po_2
Pco_2	Sensitive and reliable only when local perfusion is normal but usually exceeds arterial value by ≥ 6 mm Hg
Capillary Blood	
Po_2 or HbO_2	Unpredictably less than arterial value when local perfusion poor
Pco_2	Sensitive and reliable only when local perfusion is normal; usually exceeds arterial value slightly
Central Venous Blood	
Po_2 or HbO_2	Normally ~ 40 mm Hg and not reliable estimate of arterial Po_2; a very useful guide to cardiac output and decreases when cardiac output declines
Pco_2	Reliable estimate that usually exceeds arterial value by ≥ 6 mm Hg; venous-arterial difference will be increased by very low cardiac output

GAS EXCHANGE, NONINVASIVE	
Expired Gas, End-Tidal Pco_2	Provides estimate that is usually $\leq$ arterial Pco_2
Nasal gas	Water condensation and mucus can obstruct tubing; may entrain room air and dilute sample, yielding very low value
Tracheal gas	Intubated patient, in-line, or sidestream measurement from tracheal tube
Skin Surface (Transcutaneous)	Most useful in young infant; unpredictable estimate of arterial value when perfusion of skin is poor
Po_2	As above, variably $<$ arterial value; easily dislodged with movement
Pco_2	As above, variably $>$ arterial value; easily dislodged with movement
Arterial Pulse Oximetry	Estimate of arterial HbO_2; difficult to obtain when there is motion, very poor perfusion, or arrhythmia; error increases with severe hypoxemia; overestimate of HbO_2 when there is HbCO; reads close to 85% with high levels of MetHb
Sa_{O_2}	

that alters the ventilation (eg, discomfort, fright) can change the Pco_2 and the interpretation of findings. For these reasons, in critically ill patients, an indwelling catheter is sometimes used, or arterial Pco_2 is estimated by techniques that are less likely to disturb the child than arterial puncture. Owing to the narrow difference between arterial and venous Pco_2, a reasonable, but slightly high estimate of arterial Pco_2 can be obtained from freely flowing peripheral venous blood or from capillary blood where skin perfusion is adequate. Furthermore, when the skin is relatively thin, as in an infant, there is a small amount of diffusion of CO_2 through warmed superficial capillaries, which can be detected and measured noninvasively using an electrode attached to the skin surface (transcutaneous monitoring). Another noninvasive approach is derived from the fact that the Pco_2 of the gas in a hypothetical ideal alveolus

equilibrates with that in the adjacent pulmonary capillary blood (which eventually contributes to the systemic arterial blood). This alveolar gas can be sampled during exhalation to estimate arterial Pco_2, when some practical conditions are satisfied. The gas is analyzed by a capnometer, which monitors the inspiratory and expiratory Pco_2 and either provides a continuous recording or the value at end-expiration. The expiratory gas can be sampled through a small nasopharyngeal catheter using a withdrawal pump or, in an intubated patient, by withdrawing gas from the side of the tube (sidestream) or by having the sensor in series with the tracheal tube (in-stream). Typically, the Pco_2 of the gas is measured using an infrared sensor or, less commonly, by mass spectrometry. During inspiration the Pco_2 of gas in the nares or trachea decreases to 0. During expiration, the anatomic dead space, which has a Pco_2

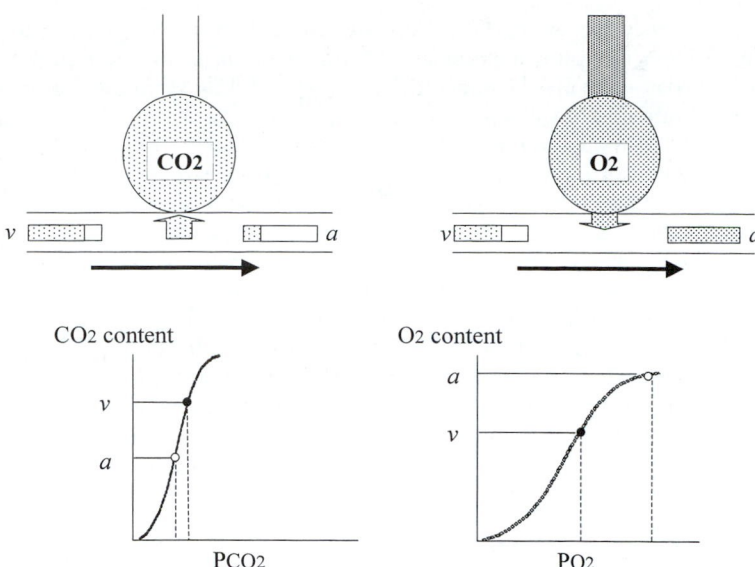

FIGURE 4-15 Unloading of CO_2 and loading of O_2 as blood passes through the lung. **Left:** As CO_2 (*stippled area*) is eliminated from venous (v) blood into the alveoli, the CO_2 content and blood PCO_2 decrease to arterial (a) levels as shown at the bottom. Note that this CO_2 content–PCO_2 relationship is steep, so that arterial and mixed venous PCO_2 are quite close under most circumstances. However, when flow slows, the arterial–mixed venous PCO_2 difference widens. **Right:** As O_2 (*stippled area*) is taken up from the alveoli and equilibrated with mixed venous (v) blood, the O_2 content and blood CO_2 increase to arterial (a) levels as shown at the bottom. Note that this O_2 content–PO_2 relationship is more gradual, so that arterial and mixed venous PO_2 differ considerably under most circumstances. Normally arteriovenous O_2 contents differ by 4–5 mL O_2/dL blood. When flow slows, the arterial–mixed venous PO_2 difference widens, and mixed venous PO_2 decreases, both of which provide evidence of a cardiac output that is low in proportion to metabolic demands.

equal to 0, is exhaled first, followed by gas from alveoli, which participate in gas exchange and contain CO_2. Under these circumstances expired CO_2, when viewed as a function of time, is 0 until the dead space is emptied; it then rises rapidly to near alveolar level, and then rises with a small slope to the end-expiratory value. Because areas of the lungs with different ventilation/perfusion ratios ($\dot{V}/\dot{Q}$) have alveolar PCO_2 values that differ, considerable information can actually be derived from the shape of the expiratory curve. Moreover, areas with low ventilation/perfusion ratios, which have higher PCO_2 values, generally, empty slowly. When there is relatively homogenous ventilation, the plateau (Fig. 4-16) is rela-

tively flat and the end-expiratory value is within 1 to 2 mm Hg of arterial PCO_2. However, when there is marked heterogeneity in the ventilation/perfusion ratios within the lung, a plateau may not be reached and the PCO_2 will rise throughout exhalation; under these conditions, end-tidal CO_2 could actually overestimate arterial PCO_2. More typically with parenchymal lung disease the end-tidal value will underestimate arterial PCO_2 by an unpredictable and variable amount for these conditions: areas of the lung with extraordinarily high ratios of alveolar ventilation to capillary perfusion have very low PCO_2 values, and the gas from these alveoli dilutes that from alveoli, with more normal ventilation/perfusion reducing the end-tidal PCO_2. Because the perfusion of these alveoli is low relative to the others, they contribute little to the arterial PCO_2, thereby generating an end-tidal–arterial CO_2 gradient. This is quite common in processes with airflow obstruction, such as asthma or bronchopulmonary dysplasia. The end-tidal PCO_2 may also be factitiously reduced if there is contamination of expired gas from air drawn into the system (in the patient whose trachea is not intubated or who has an air leak around the tracheal tube), which occurs particularly when the sample rate is high relative to alveolar ventilation. Capnometry may be particularly susceptible to underestimation of arterial PCO_2 in the small infant who breathes at such a high rate that a plateau is not achieved. Despite these important constraints, capnography is a valuable technique for monitoring gas exchange noninvasively, especially because of the risks and difficulties in maintaining an indwelling arterial catheter in many infants and children.

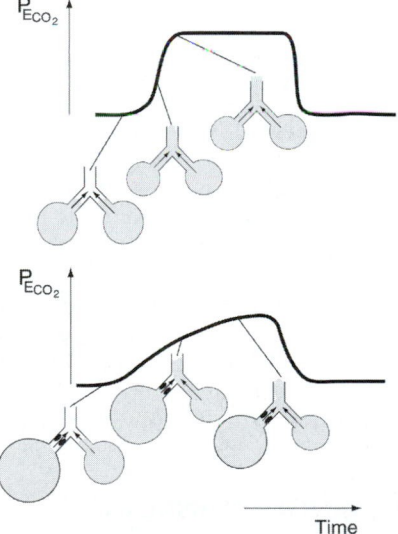

FIGURE 4-16 Expired PCO_2 (P_ECO_2) shown as a function of time. The shaded gas represents CO_2 as it goes from the alveoli to the bronchioles and to the trachea. The dark line shows the mixed expired PCO_2, which is derived from multiple alveoli as they empty. **Top:** Because the alveoli and conducting airways normally eliminate CO_2 at relatively similar rates, the P_ECO_2 is initially 0 as dead space gas is exhaled; it rises abruptly and then reaches a plateau (end-tidal P_ECO_2 or $P_{ET}CO_2$) close to the value for the arterial PCO_2. **Bottom:** When there is airflow obstruction or marked heterogeneity in the emptying of alveoli, the various rates of CO_2 elimination produce a gradually rising P_ECO_2, which underestimates arterial PCO_2.

Oxygen

Measurement of oxygen in arterial blood provides information about the adequacy of gas exchange in the lung and can be useful for quantifying the impairment in pulmonary function. Because arterial oxygenation can be decreased by an intracardiac right-to-left shunt, it is also useful for detecting certain cardiac defects. Oxygen can be measured from small volumes of blood using electrodes that detect PO_2. Hemoglobin O_2 saturation can also be measured in blood using an oximeter that compares the transmitted light at different wavelengths to determine the proportions of oxyhemoglobin, and, if needed, COHb and MetHb, relative to total hemoglobin. Machines that measure PO_2 may also provide a calculated value for HbO_2 that are based on the measured PO_2 and pH and on *assumptions* about the position and shape of the oxygen dissociation curve. The HbO_2 values obtained from the blood gases in this manner are only estimates and are not as valid as those obtained from a blood oximeter. It is important to remember the relation between PO_2, HbO_2 saturation, and O_2 content ([HbO_2 × Hb × 1.34 + PO_2 × 0.003] = O_2 content) and to remember that the relationship between HbO_2 and PO_2 is not linear.

Owing to the large arteriovenous difference, venous PO_2 is rarely useful for estimating arterial PO_2 except under unusual circumstances. O_2 can be measured in arterial blood from an indwelling catheter or by arterial puncture, with many of the same constraints raised for CO_2. When skin blood flow is adequate, capillary PO_2 will provide an estimate of arterial PO_2. Within the last 30 years the advent of noninvasive techniques has dramatically simplified the estimation and monitoring of arterial oxygenation. Unfortunately, the information provided can also be confusing because even healthy subjects have episodes when arterial oxygenation transiently decreases below what is perceived to be normal, and the implications of periods when arterial oxygenation decreases on potentially unhealthy infants, especially premature babies, is often unclear. As with CO_2, placement of an electrode on warmed skin allows detection of O_2 diffusing from the superficial capillaries, although the technique is only practical in the small infant.

Pulse oximetry has virtually replaced all monitoring of arterial blood oxygenation except that from an indwelling catheter. With pulse oximetry, a small band is placed on the skin, usually on a digit, and a light beam with two different wavelengths is periodically emitted from a light source on one side of the digit. The band also contains a light detector that is sensitive to both wavelengths and is located on the opposite side of the finger. The light detector picks up the light transmitted through the finger from the light source. The pulsating arterial blood in the tissue between the light source and detector absorbs some of the light, causing small variations in detected light intensity at the patient's pulse rate. These pulsations are analyzed by the instrument to determine the relative fraction of oxygenated to total hemoglobin. This ratio (HbO_2/total Hb) is often reported as %HbO_2. Because only two wavelengths are used, there can be interference caused by absorption by hemoglobin in other forms, and by a variety of other factors. Of particular importance, COHb causes falsely high readings, high concentrations of MetHb cause the pulse oximeter to read close to 85%, and external light can interfere with recognition of the pulsations. It is also useful to recognize that there are some variations among devices in the means for determining and calculating the Sa_{O_2}, such that some oximeters give falsely low values and others falsely high values when the true Sa_{O_2} is very low; these errors are not trivial. Pulse oximeters generally average the ratio of transmitted light intensity over several cardiac cycles to minimize the effects of interference with the signal from several sources. Some devices average the signal over a period of 3 minutes, while others use a shorter averaging time. Needless to say, the duration of the averaging period can affect the calculated Sa_{O_2} when there are transient changes in arterial blood oxygenation. Finally, the nature and degree of the error may not be well appreciated, because the clinician is usually not aware of the algorithm used by a particular instrument. Pulse oximeters also detect heart rate from the pulse. Some devices display a pulse waveform, but this should not be interpreted as a tracing of pulse pressure, because it is amplified and not calibrated to pressure. Although relatively insensitive to modest changes in circulation, the oximeter must be able to detect a pulse to determine arterial Sa_{O_2}, so states with poor peripheral perfusion can interfere with this technique and give a value unpredictably

lower than arterial Sa_{O_2}. Although normal arterial Sa_{O_2} is close to 95% in healthy children and adults, studies of infants have shown that there may be periodic decreases to <90% even in the absence of respiratory illness.

Although venous PO_2 is generally much lower than arterial PO_2 and not useful for gauging gas exchange, it is quite valuable for judging perfusion (see Fig. 4-15). By the relationship shown earlier, whenever flow decreases relative to metabolic rate, arteriovenous O_2 content difference increases. Therefore, in the subject with normal arterial oxygenation a decrease in cardiac output would be detected by a decline in mixed systemic venous PO_2, which is approximately 39 to 40 mm Hg (equivalent to a fractional HbO_2 of ~0.75) in the normal individual. Mixed venous blood can be measured in critically ill patients from a catheter placed in the pulmonary artery or in the superior vena cava or right atrium. The latter two sites are easier to access, but may not provide as well-mixed a sample as the pulmonary artery.

HEART RATE AND ECG

ECG can be monitored continuously from electrocardiographic electrodes generally placed on the chest, and a cardiotachometer determines heart rate from the frequency of the "QRS" signal. Although an invaluable tool for monitoring and for observing responses to therapy, there are important sources of error. The electrical signal may detect the T wave as well as the QRS and report a value that is twice normal. Failure to detect a signal can occur when the QRS amplitude changes, for example, with respiration, repositioning of the leads, or changes in posture. Finally, it is essential to recognize that the ECG recording used in patient monitoring is filtered to help reduce the amount of artifact and does not provide a complete view of cardiac forces. It is quite easy to misinterpret rhythm disturbances or even fail to detect them by observing the monitor or reading a single "rhythm strip." Whenever there is concern for an arrhythmia or the rate of the peripheral pulse does not concur with the monitor, a complete ECG should immediately be obtained.

There are two ways that a cardiac monitor determines heart rate from detected QRS complexes. An averaging cardiotachometer counts the number of QRS complexes that occur over a known period of time and then determines heart rate in much the same way a clinician does from palpating the peripheral pulse. The beat-to-beat cardiotachometer, on the other hand, measures the interval between each successive pair of R waves and determines the heart rate for each cardiac cycle. This latter method is essential for determining heart rate variability, but it can be distracting when the heart rate displayed by the monitor changes with each cardiac cycle. The averaging method is better for providing data to a digital display.

ARTERIAL BLOOD PRESSURE

Measurement of arterial pressure is essential for detecting abnormalities in the circulation and determining responses to therapy. It can be measured continuously in very sick patients by using an indwelling arterial catheter attached to an electronic manometer, or intermittently by a number of techniques. Determination of pressure using a sphygmomanometer in conjunction with a cuff that occupies about two-thirds of the length of the limb segment remains the standard approach. The cuff is inflated to a pressure well above that occluding the arterial systolic pulse and is gradually deflated while listening for Korotkoff sounds. The first sound corresponds to arterial systolic pressure, and the muffling of the second sound corresponds to the arterial diastolic pressure. The systolic pressure can also be determined by palpating the artery distal to the cuff and noting the pressure at which the pulse is first felt when the cuff is deflated. Alternatively, a Doppler device can be used to auscultate the arterial pulse when the cuff is deflated; this is particularly useful when the pulse is weak and difficult to feel consistently. A similar approach relies on detection of the return in the arterial waveform from a pulse oximeter at the systolic pressure when a blood pressure cuff is deflated. There are several devices that can automatically inflate a cuff and determine the Korotkoff sounds or other indications of arterial pulsations as the cuff is deflated. These instruments can be programmed to measure blood pressure at regular and very frequent intervals. Some of these devices tend to yield diastolic pressures lower than those obtained from auscultation or with an indwelling arterial catheter. It is important to recognize that there are some regional variations in blood pressure and that these can be accentuated in pathologic states. Normally, systolic pressure is higher and diastolic lower when comparing the legs to the arms. In states of poor cardiac output, systolic blood pressure from a large central artery is higher than values from peripheral vessels by a variable amount that depends on how impaired perfusion is. It is also important to realize that central systolic blood pressure may be sustained near normal levels even in the presence of shock, owing to severe vasoconstriction.

CENTRAL VENOUS PRESSURES

Central venous pressure is used as a proxy for central vascular volume. In general, as the volume in the vasculature increases, the central venous pressure rises. The pressure from a catheter in the right atrium or large central vein is used as a monitor of cardiac filling. Because systemic perfusion depends on left ventricular filling, there are conditions when measurement of right atrial pressure is insufficient. Specifically, when there is any site of obstruction between the chambers, dysfunction of one of the ventricles, or pulmonary vascular disease, the pressure in the right atrium may not reliably reflect that in the left atrium. For these reasons, a catheter may be placed in the pulmonary artery, which is then used to estimate left atrial pressure by measurement of the wedge or occlusion pressure (obtained by inflating a small balloon at the tip of the catheter that propels the catheter into a small distal vessel while occluding flow there). It is important to recognize that in certain circumstances venous and atrial pressures can be elevated because the atrium is compressed by air (pneumothorax), fluid (pericardial or pleural), or even inflated lungs, all of which will impede cardiac filling but create an erroneous impression that the atrium is filled. With these constraints in mind, central venous pressure can serve as a useful guide to effects of therapies or interventions on cardiac filling in patients where responses are not very predictable (eg, the child with congestive circulatory failure in whom positive end-expiratory pressure is administered) or in patients in whom there is a narrow margin of safety (eg, the child with elevated intracranial pressure and low cardiac output). Normal values for central venous pressure range from −3 to +3 mm Hg in the infant to 5 to 10 mm Hg in the child and young adult. These values, however, can be greatly affected by the use of positive-pressure breathing and are most useful to judge relative changes rather than to serve as absolute targets for therapy. Monitoring of pulmonary arterial or wedge pressures and sampling of mixed venous blood from the catheter also can provide very useful data regarding the mechanism for circulatory dysfunction or the response to therapy, especially in the patient in whom there is reason to believe that there is dysfunction

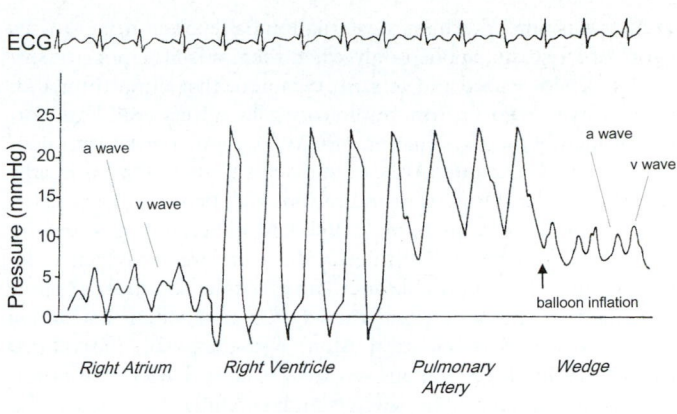

Catheter Position

FIGURE 4-17 **Representative recording of pressures as a balloon flotation catheter is inserted through a central vein into the right side of the heart into the pulmonary artery. The first recorded waveform is a right atrial tracing with characteristic *a* and *v* waves (note that the *a* wave is usually larger than the *v* wave in the right atrium and, conversely, in the left atrium or wedge, below). In the right ventricle, note that end-diastolic pressure is zero. In the pulmonary artery, a normal pressure waveform is recorded. (Note that the pressure in the pulmonary artery decreases during diastole as opposed to the increase in the diastolic pressure in the right ventricle; this difference in pressure contour helps distinguish catheter position during placement, because the actual values for systolic and diastolic pressures can be virtually identical.) The catheter is then advanced to the wedge position with the balloon inflated. The wedge pressure tracing shows *a* and *v* waves transmitted from the left atrium. The wedge tracing is not always this clear, but it should not be overly damped. The pressures shown here are in the range of normal.**

of either the left or right ventricle. Proper placement of a central venous or pulmonary arterial catheter is essential to reduce the risk of arrhythmias or untoward complications. The contour of the pressure tracing during placement of the catheter provides essential information to discern this position and is an invaluable aid in the process of catheter insertion (Fig. 4-17).

References

Matthay MA: Invasive hemodynamic monitoring in critically ill patients. Clin Chest Med 4:233–249, 1983

Ralston AC, Webb RK, Runciman WB: Potential errors in pulse oximetry: III. Effects of interference, dyes, dyshaemoglobins and other pigments. Anaesthesia 46:291–295, 1991

Tobin MJ: Respiratory monitoring in the intensive care unit. Am Rev Respir Dis 138:1625–1642, 1988

Severinghaus JW: History and recent developments in pulse oximetry. Scand J Clin Lab Invest 53(Suppl 214):105–111, 1993

Weese-Mayer DE, Corwin MJ, Peucker MR, et al: Comparison of apnea identified by respiratory inductance plethysmography with that detected by end-tidal CO_2 or thermistor. Am J Respir Crit Care Med 162:471–480, 2000

4.2.2 Life-Support Systems: Mechanical Ventilation

Julio Pérez Fontán

The past three decades have seen immense advances in the technologies used to replace the functions of failing organs or systems.

During this time, mechanical ventilation has evolved from the category of a last rite, applied only when there was little hope of survival, to a widely used and versatile technique that allows thousands of patients to recover from respiratory failure every year. Extracorporeal membrane oxygenation (ECMO), reintroduced into neonatal and pediatric intensive care medicine in the 1980s, is rapidly reaching similar status, as its indications and, perhaps more importantly, its limitations are better defined. More recently, external and implantable ventricular assist devices have undergone sufficient development to become viable alternatives for the continued support of patients with severe circulatory dysfunction, often as a bridge toward cardiac transplantation. Along with the possibilities offered by these technologies, intensive care specialists have the responsibility of using them wisely by selecting carefully the patients who can benefit, by providing patients and families with realistic assessments of their potential, and by evaluating carefully the results to define better indications and improve efficacy.

Perhaps because of the animistic significance assigned to the act of breathing life into a dying body, the ventilation of the lungs by artificial means has intrigued many in the history of medicine. Galen, Vesalius, and Paracelsus all employed primitive techniques of mechanical ventilation during their vivisection experiments with animals. Mouth-to-mouth breathing was used sporadically in the 18th century to resuscitate human drowning victims. Renewed interest after the industrial revolution led to the patent of several types of negative-pressure boxes conceived for the treatment of polio sufferers at the beginning of the 20th century. However, ventilatory support did not become a realistic option in the treatment of respiratory failure until the polio epidemics that swept through Europe in the 1940s. Cumbersome and inefficient, but for the first time successful, the iron lungs of this period soon gave way to new generations of positive-pressure ventilators in the 1960s and 1970s. Advances in pneumatic design coupled with improved understanding of the mechanical and gas exchange abnormalities found in patients with respiratory failure have improved considerably the versatility and, as a by-product, the complexity of ventilatory support. Today, any modern intensive care unit has at its disposal a wide array of ventilator models, many of them capable of ventilating effectively the lungs of adults as well as the lungs of premature infants. Although these devices certainly make the task easier, their application to the treatment of infants and children requires more than a passing knowledge of respiratory physiology and careful attention to monitoring the patient's responses.

PHYSIOLOGICAL PRINCIPLES

All commonly used methods of mechanical ventilation increase transthoracic pressure to force gas flow into the lungs during inspiration and allow the passive recoil of lungs and chest wall to force gas out of the lungs during expiration. The inspiratory increase in transthoracic pressure (the pressure difference between the alveoli and the external surface of the chest wall) is usually accomplished by generating positive pressure in the airway lumen, either through a cannula inserted in the trachea or through a mask applied around the mouth and nose *(positive-pressure ventilation)*. Rarely, transthoracic pressure is raised by lowering the pressure around the chest with an enclosing box *(negative-pressure ventilation)* while the trachea is cannulated to prevent closure of the pharynx and larynx out of synchrony with the ventilator's own cycle. The outward pull applied by the box on the chest wall reduces pleural and alveolar pressures relative to atmospheric pressure. Because inspi-

ratory gas is drawn directly from the atmosphere (or from O_2-enriched gas at atmospheric pressure), inspiratory gas is forced into the alveolar spaces. Contrary to common misconception, positive- and negative-pressure ventilation generate similar stresses and strains within the lungs for a given lung volume. Thus, it is unlikely that one method produces less lung injury than the other. By reducing rather than increasing pleural pressure relative to the atmosphere, negative-pressure ventilation may have a more beneficial effect on venous return to the heart than positive-pressure ventilation. This advantage, however, does not make up for the impracticalities of negative-pressure ventilators, which include bulkiness, poor access to the patients, and inefficiency when high levels of support are needed. For these reasons they are seldom used in modern intensive care units.

The choice of an appropriate ventilatory strategy involves careful consideration of both the characteristics of the patient's respiratory dysfunction and the capabilities of the ventilator. In general, the clinician must reconcile two fundamental and sometimes competing goals while designing such a strategy: (a) to maintain adequate gas exchange at the lowest possible inspired O_2 concentration and (b) to minimize the accumulative stretch of the lungs and airways.

Strategies to Improve Gas Exchange

The choice of optimal ventilatory pattern depends on the mechanical alterations produced by the disease in the lungs and airways, the homogeneous or heterogeneous distribution of these alterations, and the ability of the patient to contribute to the ventilatory effort. In practice, this choice materializes in a combination of several ventilatory settings, including ventilatory rate, tidal volume, inspiratory time, and inspiratory flow. These settings are organized into *modes of ventilation,* which are defined by the mechanisms that initiate, limit, and end (cycling) inspiration.

It is well established by both experimentation and clinical experience that no positive-pressure ventilator can duplicate the efficiency of the respiratory muscles. Even in individuals with healthy lungs, tidal volume, minute ventilation, and sometimes inspired O_2 concentration must be raised above physiological levels to compensate for the increase in dead space and venous admixture that follows the institution of ventilatory support. The mechanisms of such increased requirements include the excessive distention of the conducting airways, the effacement of the vertical ventilation/perfusion gradients within the lungs, and the limitations imposed to movement and posture by the need to keep the endotracheal tube safely in place.

Selection of Tidal Volume and Ventilatory Rate

The product of ventilatory rate by the tidal volume determines the contribution of the ventilator to the total minute ventilation, the remainder of it being supplied by the patient's spontaneous effort (if any). Tidal volume is usually preset by adjusting either the volume delivered into the ventilator's circuit *(volume-controlled ventilators)* or the pressure generated at the airway opening *(pressure-controlled ventilators)*. Some infant ventilators are time-cycled. When the safety pressure limit in these ventilators is set higher than the peak airway pressure, tidal volume is determined by the inspiratory flow circulating constantly through the circuit and the duration of the inspiratory time (when the airway pressure exceeds the safety pressure, the ventilator behaves as if it were in the pressure-controlled mode). Many ventilators combine options for volume-, pressure-, and sometimes time-cycled control of tidal volume.

When instituting ventilatory support in a volume-controlled mode, the tidal volume generated by the ventilator is always greater than the actual tidal volume delivered into the lungs. The difference usually results from leaks and compression of the gas in the ventilator tubing. Leaks may be apparent as a discrepancy between the inhaled and exhaled volume. Although their exact magnitude is difficult to estimate, they can be quite large with the uncuffed endotracheal tubes commonly used in infants and small children and often vary with the position of the head. Compression volume may not be as readily detected, but can be estimated easily based on the volume of the circuit and the airway pressures (0.001 mL/mL of circuit/cm H_2O of pressure is a reasonable presumption). It becomes larger at the expense of the actual tidal volume as the severity of the lung disease and the pressures needed to ventilate the lungs increase. Because of gas leaks and compression (not to mention frequent inaccuracies in volume measurement by the ventilator), the selection of an appropriate tidal volume should always be corroborated by the size of the chest wall excursions, independent of the information provided by the ventilator.

During pressure-controlled ventilation, tidal volume is determined by the magnitude and timing of the airway pressure increase during inspiration. In making these adjustments, it is important to remember that it is alveolar and not airway opening pressure that drives the change in lung volume. How airway and alveolar pressures relate to each other depends on the inspiratory flow and the combined resistance of the endotracheal tube and airways (Fig. 4-18). When inspiratory flow is constant (as is common during volume-controlled ventilation and always the case in infant constant-flow time-cycled ventilators), airway opening pressure is greater than alveolar pressure throughout inspiration. Thus, the peak inspiratory pressure at the airway opening underestimates the peak alveolar pressure by a magnitude proportional to the inspiratory flow and the resistance of the tube and airways. When a decelerating inspiratory flow is applied (as is common during pressure-controlled ventilation), airway opening and alveolar pressures equilibrate after gas flow ceases at the end of inspiration. Accordingly, peak airway opening and alveolar pressures are similar.

The choices of tidal volume and ventilatory rate are clearly interrelated. It is a good rule that their combination should mimic the patient's own ventilatory pattern. Small tidal volumes at a relatively high ventilatory rate may offer some advantage in infants and children with severe restrictive disease (see "Minimizing Lung Stretch" below). In contrast, larger tidal volumes and a slower ventilatory rate are appropriate in patients with airway obstruction. Especially when the obstruction is intrathoracic, enough time must be allowed for expiration to be completed. Otherwise, expiratory flow becomes interrupted by the subsequent inspiration, causing pressure in the alveoli to exceed that in the proximal airway (Fig. 4-19). The resultant increase in lung volume is difficult to detect. If uncorrected, it may flatten the combined volume-pressure relationship of the lungs and chest wall, decrease tidal volume, and interfere with venous return to the heart.

Positive End-Expiratory Pressure

When lung volume decreases as a result of disease (eg, surfactant deficiency, pulmonary edema), alveoli lose their mechanical stability and collapse easily. Under such conditions, the number and volume of the alveoli that remain open is very sensitive to the volume of the preceding inflations (a property that physiologists call *volume history-dependence*). This is why early ventilators were designed to provide periodic intermittent sighs or breaths larger than the prev-

alent tidal volume. Unfortunately, such practice resulted in a high rate of complications, especially air leaks. A more effective alternative was to support alveolar inflation by raising the functional residual capacity of the lungs (FRC) by increasing the airway pressure at the end of expiration. Ostensibly, the objectives of positive end-expiratory pressure (PEEP) are to recruit collapsed alveoli and to prevent the closure of those that are open. When these goals are achieved, the ventilation/perfusion profile of the lungs improves and venous admixture decreases (Fig. 4-20). As an added benefit, lung compliance and alveolar ventilation increase, improving the efficiency of mechanical ventilation while reducing the workload of the respiratory muscles in patients who also breathe spontaneously. However, when PEEP fails to recruit a predominance of collapsed or underventilated alveoli, well-ventilated alveoli become overdistended. Blood flow may then be forced through alveolar-capillary units with a low ventilation/perfusion ratio, overcoming their hypoxic vasoconstriction. As a result, venous admixture increases and lung compliance and alveolar ventilation decrease. The unpredictable nature of these changes emphasizes the importance of careful clinical assessment after introducing changes in ventilatory strategy.

Inspiratory Flow and the Distribution of Ventilation

The amplitude and time profile of the inspiratory flow influences greatly the distribution of tidal volume in the lungs, especially when lung disease has a heterogeneous distribution. When inspiratory time is shortened and the tidal volume is delivered at a high flow rate, gas tends to flow preferentially toward areas of the lung that have a low resistance or a low compliance (or a short *time constant* as the product of compliance by resistance is known). Consequently, areas served by obstructed airways receive a small proportion of the tidal volume, which in some situations may be an advantage, because these areas take longer to empty during expiration and are therefore prone to overdistention. Areas where the alveoli are prone to collapse because of pulmonary edema or surfactant deficiency, for example, receive a disproportionate apportionment of the tidal volume. In contrast, when inspiratory time is lengthened, there is more time for pressures to equilibrate across high-resistance airway segments, especially if flow ceases at the end of inspiration (see Fig. 4-18). Under such circumstances, tidal volume is distributed primarily to areas in which alveolar compliance is higher, regardless of whether the airways that serve these areas are obstructed or not. The resultant pattern of ventilation may be beneficial if the less-ventilated areas are also less perfused, but the preferential flow to areas with a long time constant renders the duration of the expiratory time critical to avoid gas trapping.

Mean Airway Pressure In patients with homogeneous restrictive disease, mean airway pressure (the integral of the pressure at the airway opening divided by the duration of the respiratory cycle) correlates well with arterial P_{O_2}. Although this observation cannot be safely extrapolated to situations in which the disease is nonhomogeneous or, much less, when it is obstructive, it has become common practice to characterize the level of ventilatory support based on the mean airway pressure value needed to achieve satisfactory arterial oxygenation. The value of mean airway pressure as a predictor of arterial P_{O_2} originates from the direct link that exists between this pressure and mean lung volume. Increases in tidal volume or peak inspiratory pressure, ventilatory rate, inspiratory time, inspiratory flow, and PEEP all have the effect of raising mean airway pressure and mean airway volume.

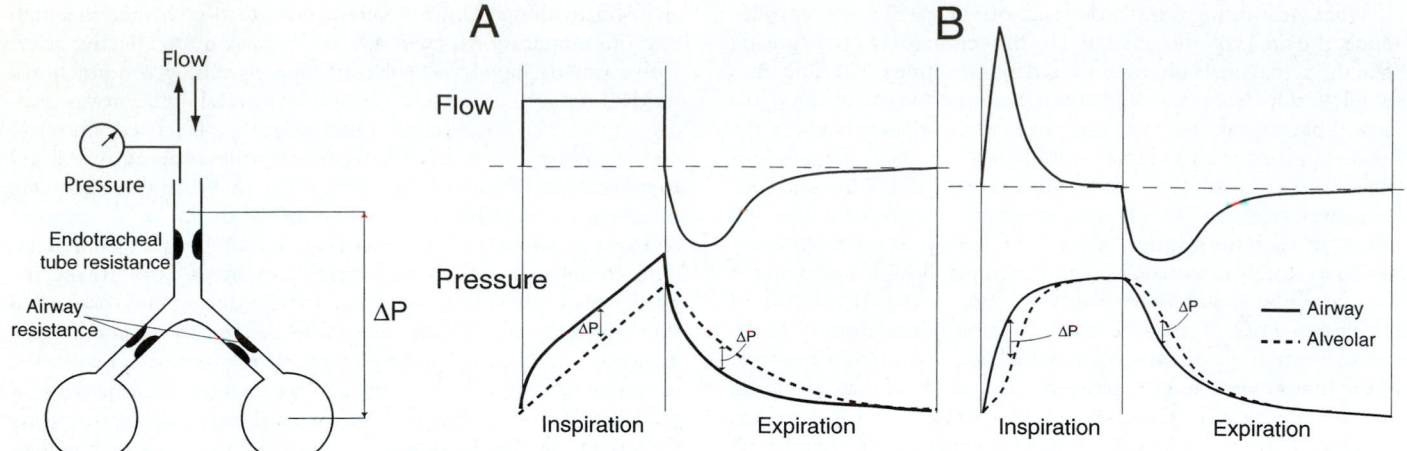

FIGURE 4-18   Relationship between airway and alveolar pressure during mechanical ventilation with constant (*A*) and decelerating (*B*) inspiratory flow. When flow is constant, the combined resistance of the endotracheal tube and airways (see diagram on the *left*) establish a constant pressure gradient between the airway opening and the alveoli (ΔP) during inspiration. Consequently, after the gradient is established, both airway opening and alveolar pressure form parallel ramps separated vertically by ΔP. Because the peak airway pressure is reached while gas is still flowing into the lungs, the peak pressure recorded by the ventilator underestimates peak alveolar pressure. When flow follows a decelerating course, ΔP is large at the beginning of inspiration when flow is high, but fades quickly and disappears when airway flow ceases at the end of inspiration. From that point on, airway opening and alveolar pressures are similar and lung volume is held constant until expiration starts. Both methods of ventilation generate the same peak alveolar pressure for a given tidal volume. However, the decelerating flow pattern does it with a lower peak airway opening pressure, a feature that sometimes is incorrectly claimed to offer advantages in terms of lung stretch. Constant inspiratory flow is typical of volume-controlled ventilation and time-cycled infant ventilators; decelerating flow is characteristic of pressure-controlled ventilation.

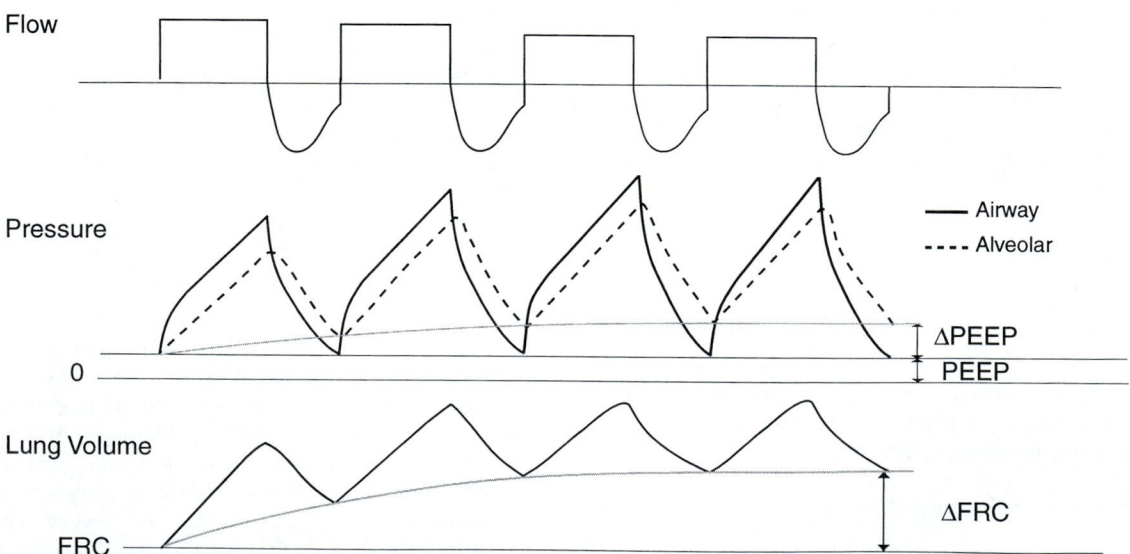

FIGURE 4-19   Increase in functional residual capacity (FRC) produced by shortening expiratory time during mechanical ventilation. When expiratory flow becomes interrupted by the following inspiration, alveolar pressure remains higher than the positive end-expiratory pressure (PEEP) measured at the airway opening. The difference (ΔPEEP), often referred to as *auto-PEEP* or *inadvertent PEEP,* increases lung volume at end-expiration relative to the previous breath. FRC continues to increase breath after breath until the increased recoil of the lungs equilibrates with ΔPEEP. The increased lung volume may only be apparent as an increased peak airway pressure.

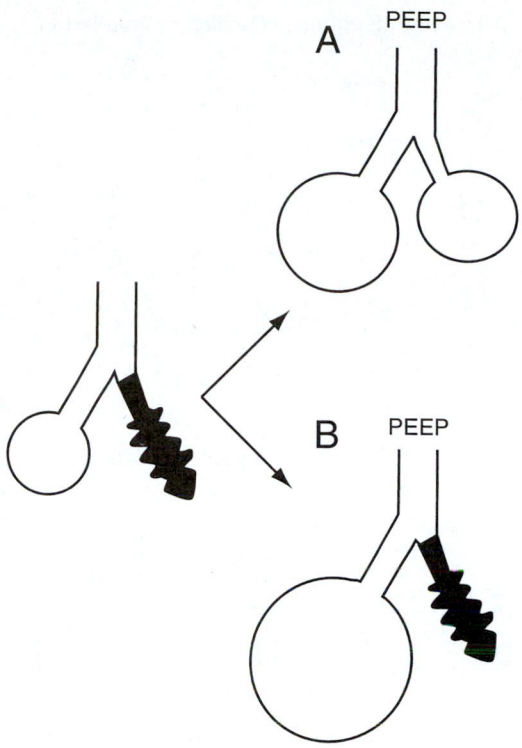

FIGURE 4-20   Representation of two potential effects of positive end-expiratory pressure (PEEP) on ventilated and nonventilated alveoli. A: PEEP may open collapsed alveoli, recruiting them into contributing to alveolar ventilation. Ventilated alveoli become further distended. B: PEEP may fail to open collapsed alveoli, limiting its effect to overdistending alveoli that are already open. Depending on whether A or B predominates, venous admixture may decrease or increase as PEEP is raised.

Administration of Supplemental O$_2$

Increasing the concentration of O$_2$ in the inspired gas is the most predictable and rapid method to increase arterial PO$_2$ in patients with increased venous admixture caused by ventilation/perfusion inequality, decreased ventilation, and diffusion abnormalities (see Table 4-2). Unfortunately, O$_2$ administration has no beneficial effect on the alterations that cause the hypoxemia. Moreover, the use of O$_2$ can compound the gas exchange derangements. The presence of high concentrations of O$_2$ in poorly ventilated alveolar-capillary units can cause reabsorption atelectasis as the O$_2$ in the alveolar gas is removed by pulmonary capillaries without being replaced by N$_2$. In the same areas, O$_2$ can abolish hypoxic vasoconstriction, increasing the contribution of these units to venous admixture. Oxygen is in itself highly toxic to the lung tissues, even though its continued administration up-regulates local antioxidant responses. Based on these considerations, it is reasonable, when ventilatory support is started, to increase inspired O$_2$ concentration as much as needed to correct hypoxemia. Thereafter, it is advisable to adopt other strategies, similar to the ones outlined above, that minimize the continued need for O$_2$.

Minimizing Lung Stretch

The idea that ventilation-induced lung injury is caused by excessive stretch of the lung tissues rather than by a direct effect of the pressures needed to ventilate the lungs has reached axiomatic category in the past few years. The intimate mechanisms that lead to the disruption of the interalveolar septa and small airways, and the inflammatory and fibroproliferative response that follows, are far from clear. It is reasonable to assume, however, that the interplay between lung volume and the modifications produced by disease in the elastic properties of the lung determines how much deformation and damage occurs. The absence of lung surfactant in the newborn's respiratory distress syndrome, for instance, reduces lung volume by promoting alveolar collapse. When positive pressure is applied to the airway in order to restore alveolar patency, the stresses generated within the lung tissues can become very high, even if the lung volume remains lower than it would be if the lungs were healthy. The reason is that the increased surface tension of the alveolar gas-liquid interface is transmitted through the alveolar septa to airways, blood vessels, and neighboring alveolar walls. The resultant stress in these tissue elements can disrupt their integrity, as well as stimulate the release of inflammatory cytokines and growth factors that alone can initiate a response of inflammation and repair.

Thus, reducing stress within the lungs is an important priority in planning ventilatory strategy. To do so, the clinician is often faced with a basic conflict between the need to preserve oxygenation and ventilation and the clear long-term advantage of reducing tidal volume, ventilatory rate, and PEEP to a minimum. The recognition of this conflict gave rise to ventilatory strategies that allow arterial PCO$_2$ to rise above its physiological values (*permissive hypercapnia*) and arterial PO$_2$ to decrease to the lowest levels compatible with tissue oxygenation, all the while keeping tidal volumes to a minimum. These strategies, which are not new to neonatologists and pediatricians, demonstrate promise in reducing the complications of ventilatory support in adults with acute respiratory failure.

MODES OF VENTILATION

As mechanical ventilators increase their complexity, the clinician faces new choices regarding the ventilatory rate and tidal volume that are most appropriate for a given patient, as well as determining the mechanism (pressure or flow) and interval in which the breaths are triggered, whether inspiratory flow is constant or decelerating, and the extent to which the patient's own breathing effort is complemented by the machine (Fig. 4-21). Many of the modes of

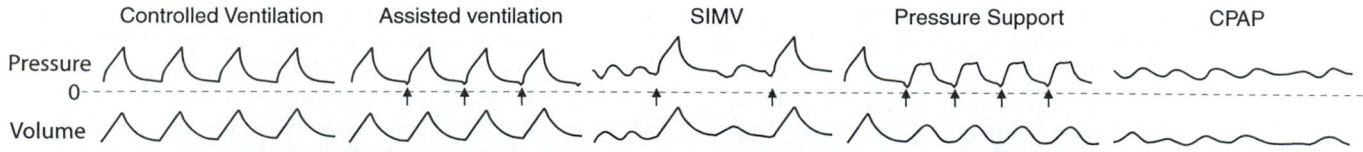

FIGURE 4-21   Diagrams of pressure and lung volume changes with several modes of ventilatory support. *Arrows* indicate triggered breaths. **SIMV = synchronized intermittent mechanical ventilation; CPAP = continuous positive airway pressure.**

mechanical ventilation defined by these options are designed to facilitate the patient's adaptation to the ventilator or the discontinuation of ventilatory support (a process often referred to as *weaning* from mechanical ventilation).

Controlled mechanical ventilation is a volume-targeted mode, in which all breaths are initiated and completed by the ventilator, without the possibility of triggering by the patient (Fig. 4-21). *Pressure-controlled ventilation* is a similar, but pressure-targeted, modality. It is frequently applied with inspiratory times that exceed the expiratory time *(pressure-controlled inverse-ratio ventilation)* as a means to increase mean airway pressure in patients with severe restrictive lung disease. Controlled ventilation and pressure-controlled ventilation usually require that the patient receive sedatives and, on occasion, neuromuscular blockers.

Assist-control ventilation allows the patient to trigger an unlimited number of ventilator breaths, with a back-up rate activated when the patient's own breathing rate decreases below a certain threshold. Rarely applied in children, this mode has the potential of resulting in lung hyperinflation when breaths are triggered too close to each other.

Intermittent mandatory ventilation (IMV) is a commonly used weaning mode in which ventilator breaths are delivered at a preestablished rate, allowing the patient to breathe freely from the ventilator circuit (from a constant flow or by opening a demand valve) in the interval between ventilator breaths. In most modern devices, the mandatory breaths can be triggered by the patient if the spontaneous breath falls within a certain window of time established by the ventilator's software *(synchronized IMV or SIMV)*.

Pressure support is also a weaning mode in which the early phase of the patient's inspiratory effort is complemented by the ventilator at a preestablished inspiratory pressure. The ventilator's contribution is triggered by the detection of the patient's breath (by a decrease in airway pressure or the initiation of inspiratory flow). The pressure is released when the inspiratory flow decreases below a preset level, signaling that the breath is completed and expiration may start. The advantages of pressure support are that it is initiated by the patient and allows the tidal volume to vary depending on the patient's respiratory drive. A potential disadvantage in children is that a large leak around an endotracheal tube may prevent the ventilator from initiating expiration in a timely manner. This will result in a prolonged inspiratory phase and patient discomfort. It is often combined with SIMV.

BiPAP is a mode named after a commercial ventilator that provides ventilatory support through a nasal mask. A pressure-controlling valve switches between inspiration and expiration by alternating two levels of positive airway pressure, expiratory positive airway pressure (EPAP) and inspiratory positive airway pressure (IPAP), depending on whether the patient's inspiratory flow exceeds a preset limit (EPAP to IPAP) or inspiratory flow decreases below a preset threshold or ceases altogether for a preset time (IPAP to EPAP).

Continuous positive airway pressure (CPAP) is a mode in which the patient is allowed to breathe spontaneously from a pressurized constant flow circuit or by activating a demand valve at a constant expiratory pressure. It is often applied to newborns and small infants through a facial or nasal mask, nasal prongs, or a pharyngeal cannula, thus avoiding endotracheal intubation. Care must be exercised when a demand valve system is used because the high resistance of the valve can impose an intolerable load on the diaphragm, especially in infants and small children.

High-Frequency Oscillatory Ventilation

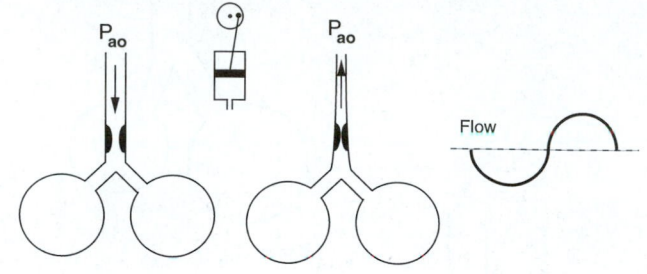

High-Frequency Jet Ventilation

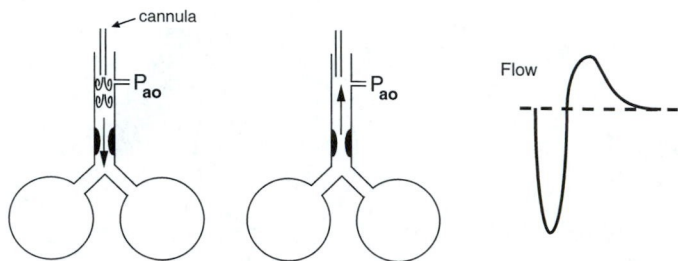

FIGURE 4-22   **Diagrams comparing the inspiratory and expiratory phase (as indicated by the *arrow direction*) and gas flow profile during high-frequency oscillation and jet ventilation. High-frequency oscillation uses a piston or a vibrating membrane to generate a quasi-sinusoidal flow in the airways. Expiration is facilitated by the vacuum action of the piston or membrane, resulting sometimes in airway collapse. Although modern oscillators minimize this problem by lengthening expiration, mean alveolar pressure may be underestimated by mean proximal airway pressure. High-frequency jet ventilation uses a cannula to deliver a burst or jet of inspiratory gas into the trachea. Additional gas is entrained from an indwelling endotracheal tube. Expiration is passive, a feature that poses a lower limit to the maximal frequency achievable by this method. PA_{O_2} = airway outflow pressure.**

High-Frequency Ventilation

The idea of ventilating the lungs at frequencies well above the physiological range began as a creative method to support gas exchange while suppressing spontaneous respirations in experimental animals. It soon became clear that ventilatory rates higher than 2 Hz (breath/second) and as high as 12 Hz provided adequate oxygenation and ventilation, with tidal volumes that appeared lower than the estimated dead space. This observation gave rise to extended speculation that alveolar ventilation during high-frequency ventilation involved singular mechanisms of gas transport. These mechanisms, according to the same speculation, made it possible to ventilate the lungs with airway pressures lower than those needed to produce the bulk movement of gas characteristic of spontaneous and conventional mechanical ventilation. Today's consensus is that gas exchange during high-frequency ventilation follows the same principles as during conventional mechanical ventilation. Any advantages of the former probably lie with the stability conferred to the alveoli by a higher end-expiratory volume.

Although high-frequency ventilation has been adopted by many as a routine form of ventilatory support in patients with severe lung disease, there is still little evidence of its superiority even in such situations. Comparisons with conventional modalities of ventilatory support are often hampered by lack of agreement regarding the physiological variables used to normalize the comparison. Airway pressures in particular are difficult to measure under the rapidly changing flow conditions created by high-frequency ventilators.

Two types of devices are used to provide high-frequency ventilation (Fig. 4-22) *High-frequency oscillators* generate a sinusoidal pressure waveform, which in modern ventilators is rectified to lengthen the expiratory phase and to minimize the gas trapping that was common in early prototypes. In addition to the ventilatory frequency, the operator can adjust the duration of the inspiratory time, the amplitude of the pressure oscillations, and the estimated mean airway pressure. Expiration is facilitated, a feature that may under some conditions limit expiratory flow. High-frequency jet ventilators use a cannula that is built into the wall of a special endotracheal tube or that is inserted directly into the airway lumen to deliver a rapid burst of inspiratory gas. Expiration is passive, a feature that limits the ventilatory frequencies achievable by this method to levels considerably lower than those used during high-frequency oscillatory ventilation.

SEDATION AND NEUROMUSCULAR BLOCKADE

Infants and children usually require sedation to alleviate the hardship and discomfort that are inevitable during ventilatory support, facilitate adaptation to the ventilator, and prevent movements that may result in dislodgement of the endotracheal tube when one is used. A combination of benzodiazepines and opioids is commonly used, taking advantage of the anxiolytic properties of the former and the analgesic and cough-suppressant effects of the latter. Both types of medications have the advantage of decreasing ventilatory drive when high levels of support are needed. This advantage turns into a disadvantage at the time of weaning, when the continued need for sedation must be balanced against the imperative that the patient sustains an appropriate ventilatory effort. Nondepolarizing neuromuscular blockers are given on rare occasions to suppress all respiratory muscular activity. The use of these medications should be reduced to a minimum because they increase the risks of hypoxemia and hypercarbia should the endotracheal tube become dislodged and prevent appropriate assessment of the patient's state of sedation and neurologic function.

References

Chang HK: Mechanisms of gas transport during ventilation by high-frequency oscillation. J Appl Physiol 56:553–563, 1984

Suter PM, Fairley HB, Isenberg MD: Optimum end-expiratory airway pressure in patients with acute pulmonary failure. N Engl J Med 292:284–289, 1975

Tobin MJ: Mechanical ventilation. N Engl J Med 330:1056–1061, 1994

Tobin MJ: Principles and Practices of Mechanical Ventilation. New York, McGraw-Hill, 1994

Truwit JD, Marini JJ: Evaluation of thoracic mechanics in the ventilated patient. Part 1: primary measurements. J Crit Care 3:133–150, 1988

Wagner PD: Summary: HFV and pulmonary physiology. Acta Anaesthesiol Scand 33(Suppl 90):172–175, 1989

4.2.3 Other Life-Support Systems

Fiona Howard Levy

EXTRACORPOREAL MEMBRANE OXYGENATION

The development of extracorporeal membrane oxygenation (ECMO) as an alternative to other forms of respiratory and cardiac support was a direct consequence of the success of the heart-lung machine during open-heart surgery. Advances in the immunologic tolerance of the materials used to build membrane oxygenators and in the reliability and efficiency of the blood pumps made it possible in the 1970s to begin expanding the benefits of cardiopulmonary bypass from the operating room to the intensive care unit. The initial interest in the application of ECMO to support adult patients with acute respiratory failure waned quickly, however, after initial controlled studies failed to demonstrate differences in outcome compared to conventional mechanical ventilation.

Despite early disappointment, the reversibility of some forms of neonatal lung disease continued to fuel interest in ECMO as an extraordinary, but feasible, form of respiratory support. As a result of the effort of committed pioneers, ECMO was soon recognized by many as a potentially salvaging therapy in some of these infants, triggering an explosion in the number of centers that offered the therapy in the United States. Based on encouraging results from early studies, often limited in their interpretation by the use of historic rather than concurrent controls, ECMO was applied in an increasing variety of situations, including to children with hypoxemic respiratory failure and, perhaps as a more natural extension of the origins of the therapy, to infants and children with cardiogenic shock after surgical correction of complex congenital heart lesions or cardiomyopathy. A collaborative group, the Extracorporeal Life Support Organization (ELSO), was formed, and a registry of patients receiving extracorporeal support was established. An analysis of ELSO's collective data shows current cumulative survival rates of 43 to 86%, depending on age and diagnosis. Newborns with acute respiratory failure continue to have the highest survival rate, while patients placed on ECMO to treat myocardial dysfunction have the lowest survival rate. The reversibility of lung and myocardial injury is the single most significant determinant of survival and therefore should be the most important consideration in establishing indications. In recent years, the introduction of new therapeutic options and generally improved care by more conventional means have resulted in a steady decline in the use of ECMO to support neonatal patients with acute respiratory failure.

ECMO is usually provided using two alternative circuit designs (Fig. 4-23). At least in the United States, *venoarterial ECMO* is used most frequently in pediatric patients, both for reasons of familiarity and because it can be used simultaneously to support gas exchange and cardiac output. In the typical arrangement, a portion of the patient's venous return is redirected via a cannula placed in the right atrium (usually through the internal jugular vein) to a venous reservoir in the ECMO circuit, where a rotary or centrifugal pump forces it sequentially through a membrane oxygenator and a countercurrent heat exchanger before returning it to the arterial circulation via another cannula positioned in the ascending aorta (usually through the carotid artery). In the oxygenator, blood flows in contact with a permeable membrane that separates it from a flow of oxygen and carbon dioxide. The composition and flow rate of

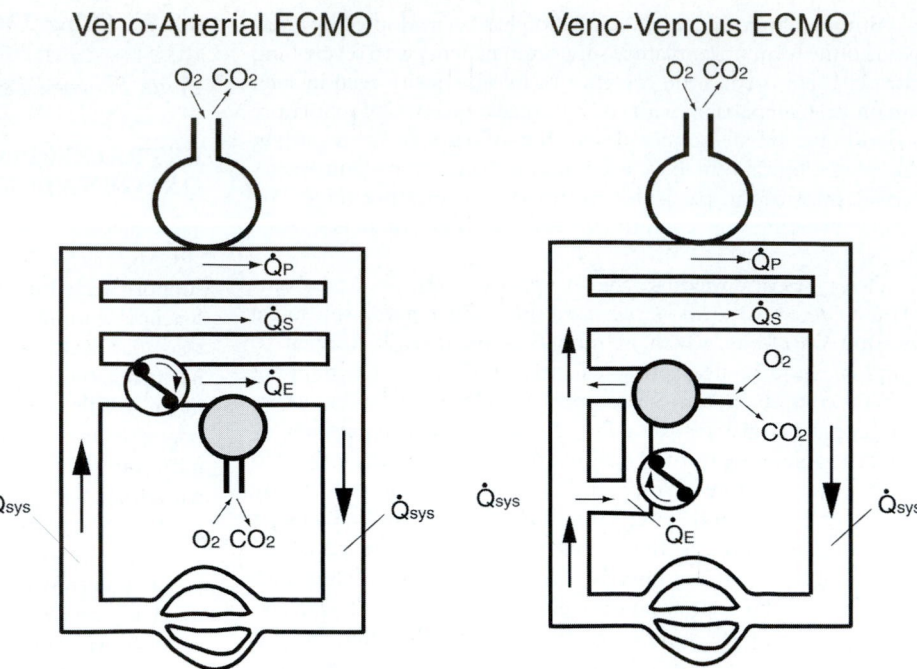

FIGURE 4-23 Diagram of blood flow during venoarterial *(left)* and venovenous *(right)* extracorporeal membrane oxygenation (ECMO). During venoarterial ECMO, a portion of the venous return to the heart ($\dot{Q}_E$) is diverted into the ECMO circuit, where it undergoes O_2 and CO_2 exchange in the membrane oxygenator and is then returned under pressure to the aorta where it mixes with blood from ventilated ($\dot{Q}_P$) and unventilated ($\dot{Q}_S$) areas of the lung. Systemic blood flow (Q_{SYS}) is the sum of $\dot{Q}_E$, $\dot{Q}_P$, and $\dot{Q}_S$. Arterial O_2 content reflects the flow-weighted sum of these three components. During venovenous ECMO, Q_E is diverted from the central venous circulation and then returned at a more proximal point in the same venous circulation. In this case, Q_P and Q_S have already undergone partial gas exchange in the membrane oxygenator.

the gas are adjusted to optimize the oxygen and carbon dioxide contents of the blood exiting the oxygenator.

The ECMO pump provides the driving force for the return of blood to the aorta. Because blood is removed from the right atrium by gravity, it is the flow of venous blood that limits ECMO flow. Lowering the venous reservoir relative to the right atrium increases the flow of blood into the circuit. The increase becomes limited, however, by the collapse of the right atrium or the systemic veins (Fig. 4-24). Increases in intrathoracic pressure (eg, PEEP), decreases in the circulating blood volume, or venous dilation reduce the maximal flow that can be achieved for a given right atrial pressure.

In *venovenous ECMO*, blood is removed and returned to the venous system. Consequently, this method supports only gas exchange and is not suitable for patients requiring cardiac support. Unlike venoarterial ECMO, systemic and pulmonary blood flow are the same. *Extracorporeal carbon dioxide removal* has been used successfully in adults with hypercapnic respiratory failure. It capitalizes on the extreme diffusibility of carbon dioxide across synthetic membranes to remove large volumes of this gas without the

need for a substantial extracorporeal diversion of venous blood. Extracorporeal carbon dioxide removal has no advantages in patients with refractory hypoxemia and is rarely applied in pediatrics patients.

VENTRICULAR ASSIST DEVICES

Infants and children with uni- or biventricular failure often have no intrinsic abnormalities in lung function, and therefore they might not benefit from the use of an external oxygenator and carbon dioxide exchanger. In recent years, the medical industry has produced a number of increasingly smaller ventricular assist devices that can be used to support the function of one or both ventricles. Many of these devices are now practical for use in small children and infants. Potential indications include cardiogenic shock after bypass surgery and cardiomyopathies. The availability of implantable devices has improved considerably the autonomy and quality of life of many pediatric heart transplantation candidates, often allowing them to be discharged from the hospital while they await their new organs.

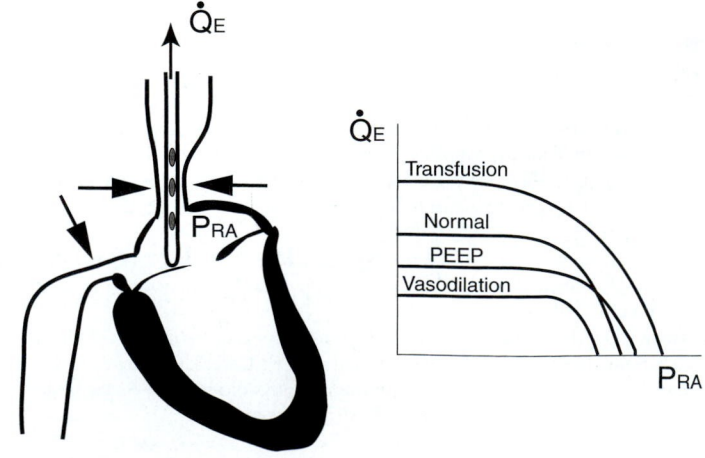

FIGURE 4-24 Representation of the factors that determine blood flow into the ECMO circuit. Gravitational force transmitted via the ECMO cannula lowers right atrial pressure (P_{RA}) relative to intrathoracic pressure. This decreases the transmural pressure and the lumen of the atrium and vena cavae, establishing a limitation for ECMO blood flow ($\dot{Q}_E$). The relationship between $\dot{Q}_E$ and P_{RA} is influenced by blood volume, intrathoracic pressure, and venous capacitance. Transfusion increases the maximal achievable flow, while application of positive end-expiratory pressure (PEEP) and vasodilation decrease it.

References

Bartlett, RH, Roloff DW, Custer JR, Younger JG, Hirschl RB: Extracorporeal life support: the University of Michigan experience. JAMA 283: 904–908, 2000

Delius RE, Bove EL, Meliones JN, et al: Use of extracorporeal life support in patients with congenital heart disease. Crit Care Med 20:1216–1222, 1992

Duncan BW, Hraska V, Jonas RA, et al: Mechanical circulatory support in children with cardiac disease. J Thorac Cardiovasc Surg 117:529–542, 1999

Gattinoni L, Pesenti A, Mascheroni D, et al: Low-frequency positive-pressure ventilation with extracorporeal CO_2 removal in severe acute respiratory failure. JAMA 256:881–886, 1988

Levy FH, O'Rourke PP, Crone RK: Extracorporeal membrane oxygenation. Anesth Analg 75:1053–1062, 1992

O'Rourke PP, Crone RK, Vacanti JP, et al: Extracorporeal membrane oxygenation and conventional medical therapy in neonates with persistent pulmonary hypertension of the newborn: a prospective randomized study. Pediatrics 84:975–963, 1989

4.2.4   Vascular Access

Andreas A. Theodorou and Robert A. Berg

Rapid establishment of vascular access is necessary for aggressive fluid resuscitation and administration of medications such as catecholamines, antibiotics, narcotics, and sedatives during emergencies. However, attaining vascular access during a life-threatening illness in a child is difficult and often consumes precious time. An organized approach to vascular access can minimize this potentially life-threatening delay in treatment. This section discusses the priorities in vascular access during emergent, urgent, and stable situations. Various techniques for achieving vascular access are reviewed, as well as the relative indications and potential complications.

PRIORITIES OF VASCULAR ACCESS

Time is of the essence in regard to attainment of vascular access for life-threatening emergencies such as cardiopulmonary arrest or decompensated shock. Of course, any preexisting intravenous catheter should be utilized in the initial resuscitation efforts, regardless of how small such a catheter might be. If there is no vascular access, especially in children <6 years old, intraosseous access should be attained as rapidly as possible. A practical approach is to pursue intraosseous and peripheral venous access simultaneously. However, time should not be wasted waiting for attempts at peripheral venous catheterization before attempting intraosseous access, because intraosseous access can be attained more rapidly and more reliably. Similarly, skilled clinicians may attempt placement of central venous catheters during life-threatening emergencies, but such attempts should not preclude simultaneous attempts at intraosseous access. After attaining intraosseous access for initial fluid resuscitation and infusion of emergency medications, peripheral or central venous catheterization is the next priority in order to assure a more reliable, long-lasting vascular access. Moreover, if needed, a central venous catheter can be placed in a more controlled manner.

For urgent situations, such as fluid resuscitation of a child with compensated shock/dehydration, the risk-benefit ratio shifts. Generally, it is most appropriate to initially insert a peripheral venous over-the-needle catheter. If multiple attempts are not successful, or if the child requires fluids or medications that are potentially problematic in a peripheral vein, central venous catheterization should be attempted by a qualified individual. Of course, if the child's clinical condition deteriorates prior to achievement of vascular access, priorities should be reassessed and it may be necessary to attain intraosseous access.

Relatively stable children may need vascular access for maintenance fluids or intravenous medications. Generally, peripheral venous cannulation with an over-the-needle catheter is adequate. If vascular access is necessary for more than 2 to 3 weeks, or if solutions to be infused are potentially dangerous when provided by peripheral vein, some form of central venous catheter may be necessary. However, central venous catheterization entails added risks, and its inherent risks and benefits deserve consideration (Table 4-14).

PERCUTANEOUS PERIPHERAL VEIN CANNULATION

Small-caliber plastic catheters have allowed for increasingly easy and reliable peripheral venous cannulation. Small over-the-needle catheters (22–24 gauge) are available to cannulate even the small veins of the hand, foot, or scalp of neonates and premature babies. Such peripheral venous catheters are generally all that are necessary for short-term delivery of intravenous fluids and/or intravenous medications.

The most common complication of peripheral venous cannulation is catheter displacement and infiltration of the tissues with the infusing fluid. Most intravenous solutions are isotonic or hypotonic and easily absorbed from the tissues. Infiltration with these solutions is generally treated by removal of the catheter and elevation of the limb. However, solutions that are very hypertonic (eg, those containing greater than 12.5% dextrose, 3% sodium chloride, or 8.4% sodium bicarbonate) or irritating substances, such as calcium or potassium salts, some antibiotics (eg, erythromycin), or medications with an extreme pH (eg, phenytoin), can cause substantial tissue injury and lead to sloughing of the skin. Importantly, extravasation of vasoconstricting agents such as dopamine, epinephrine, and norepinephrine can result in profound local vasoconstriction and subsequent significant tissue injury. Even without extravasation of the above noted medications and fluids, local vascular injury can result in aseptic thrombophlebitis. This aseptic thrombophlebitis may serve as a nidus for suppurative thrombophlebitis. The risks of aseptic and suppurative thrombophlebitis increase with the duration of the indwelling catheter.

Selection of catheter size and peripheral venous site are important issues. For a patient in shock, the widest and shortest catheter is optimal, because longer, narrower catheters result in more resistance to flow.

For the trauma victim, an uninjured limb, or at least a limb apparently free from major vascular trauma, is preferable. The greater saphenous vein, median cubital vein, and external jugular vein are three sites that are often used because they are relatively large and consistent in location. In older children, veins in the back of the hands and forearms are commonly used. Avoidance of the dominant hand or the hand with the finger or thumb that the infant prefers to suck allows for improved patient comfort and function, although such choices are not always available.

Before the vein is cannulated, the operator should wash his or her hands well and use universal precautions, including protecting the operator's hands with gloves. The extremities should be adequately immobilized, and the site should be cleansed with alcohol

TABLE 4-14
VASCULAR ACCESS TECHNIQUES

	INDICATIONS	BENEFITS	RISKS
Peripheral	Short-term infusion of fluids or medications	• Minimal training required • Minimal risk	• Local -Hematoma, infiltrations, infections • Systemic sepsis • Time-consuming (especially if vascular collapse)

Intraosseous	Emergent vascular access
	• Cardiac arrest
	• Decompensated shock
		Attained rapidly and reliably	• Adverse effects *rare*
			  -Osteomyelitis
			  -Compartment syndrome
			  -Fracture
			  -Soft-tissue necrosis

Central Venous—Acute	• Emergent vascular access
	• Hemodynamic monitoring
	• Infusion of:
	  -Irritating medications
	  -Vasoactive agents
		• More secure than peripheral
		• Safer for infusions of:
		  -Irritating medications
		  -Vasoactive agents
			• Pneumothorax
			• Chylothorax
			• Arrhythmia
			• Thrombosis
			• Embolus (air, catheter, wire)
			• Advanced skills necessary
			• Often time-consuming
			• Hemothroax
			• Hematoma
			• Malposition
			• Infection

Central Venous—Chronic (eg, Broviac, Hickman, peripherally inserted central catheter)	• Long-term parenteral (TPN) • Medications (antibiotics, chemotherapy, etc.)	Compared to central venous—acute • More secure • Lower infection risk • Lower thrombosis risk	Same as above (central venous—acute)

or iodine-containing solutions and allowed to dry. A tourniquet should be applied in order to engorge and distend the vein. The skin can be stretched taut with the operator's nondominant hand in order to immobilize the vein. The operator should puncture the skin at a 15 to 30° angle, 5 to 10 mm distal to the expected entrance site into the vein. The vein is subsequently punctured by the needle, with blood return into the catheter hub. When this blood return is noted, the catheter is advanced a few millimeters to ensure that the catheter tip, as well as the needle, is in the lumen of the vein. The catheter is then advanced over the needle into the vein, and the needle is removed. The tourniquet is released, and saline is flushed intravenously to ensure patency of the catheter and vein. After the needle is removed, it should generally not be reinserted while the catheter is in the subcutaneous space or in the vein, because this could lead to shearing the tip of the catheter and generate a small plastic embolus.

Adequate immobilization of the extremity is an important aspect of successful peripheral vein cannulation. Moreover, it is important to adequately secure and protect the catheter after successful cannulation. Attention to these details can minimize preventable failures.

INTRAOSSEOUS INFUSION

Although emergency intraosseous infusions were common in the 1940s and 1950s, the arrival of butterfly needles and plastic catheters, and widespread use of venisection led to virtual extinction of this technique for several decades. There has been a resurgence in

the use of intraosseous infusions since the early 1980s. Its increasing popularity is primarily because intraosseous infusions can be performed rapidly and reliably. Medical personnel can usually attain intraosseous access in less than 1 minute during emergencies. The bone marrow cavity is effectively a noncollapsible vascular space, even in the setting of shock or cardiac arrest. Therefore, intraosseous access is the initial vascular access site of choice in patients with life-threatening problems such as cardiopulmonary arrest or decompensated shock.

Almost any medication that can be administered into a central or peripheral vein can be safely infused into the bone marrow. Crystalloid solutions, colloid solutions, and blood products can be safely infused through the bone marrow, as can hypertonic solutions. In particular, all of the American Heart Association recommended medications for pediatric advanced life support can be safely and effectively administered via the intraosseous route, including catecholamine infusions. Pharmacokinetic variables, such as onset of action and plasma concentrations, are similar with intraosseous or peripheral venous administration in the settings of circulatory shock or cardiac arrest with CPR. Emergency medications should be followed by a saline flush to ensure rapid delivery into the circulation. In addition, the initial bone marrow aspirate is a reliable specimen for venous pH and PCO_2, blood typing and cross-matching, serum glucose, electrolytes, and blood cultures. The results of such studies may be less reliable after the administration of drugs through the intraosseous needle during CPR due to stasis in the bone marrow.

The greatest obstacle to successful intraosseous cannulation is psychological. For the inexperienced provider, the thought of forcing a needle into a child's bone seems cruel and inappropriate. The more experienced provider understands that time is crucial. The greatest obstacle for the experienced provider is overconfidence in his or her ability to provide rapid central venous catheterization or peripheral vein cutdown catheterization. Clearly, the less elegant intraosseous access technique is quicker and more reliable. Not surprisingly, even this relatively safe procedure can result in rare complications, including osteomyelitis, fractures, extravasation of toxic medications (eg, epinephrine, calcium), skin necrosis, and compartment syndrome. Compartment syndrome is easily avoided by monitoring the site for swelling and discontinuing the infusion if significant swelling occurs. Microvascular pulmonary fat and bone marrow emboli have been demonstrated, but do not appear to be clinically significant. The risk of such complications is acceptable in the dire circumstances of decompensated shock or cardiac arrest. Such risks, and the pain involved, may not be acceptable when the clinical indications are less stringent.

The most commonly utilized site for intraosseous access is the medial surface of the tibia, 1 to 3 cm below the tibial tuberosity. Alternative sites include the distal tibia above the medial malleolus, the distal femur, and the anterior superior iliac spine. There are various styles of intraosseous needles. They are all designed to go through the cortex, and they all have a stylet to avoid needle obstruction from core of bone during insertion. Aseptic technique and universal precautions should be followed if possible. The needle should be twisted into, rather than pushed through, the bone marrow. Evidence for successful entrance into the marrow includes (a) the lack of resistance (or a "give") after the needle passes through the cortex, (b) the ability of the needle to remain upright without support, (c) aspiration of the bone marrow into a syringe, and (d) free flow of the infusion without significant subcutaneous infiltration. Aspiration of bone marrow into the intraosseous needle is not always possible, especially in a very dehydrated patient. Infiltration of fluid into tissues around the bone is common when this route of infusion is used for a prolonged period of time, or if the fluid is infused under great pressure. Infiltration will manifest as an enlarging leg circumference, fluid leaking out from the skin insertion site, or resistance to the flow of the infusate.

CENTRAL VENOUS CATHETERIZATION

Central venous catheterization provides a more stable, reliable vascular access than does peripheral venous catheterization. In addition, central venous catheters permit hemodynamic monitoring and laboratory sampling of central venous blood. However, the convenience of central venous catheters must be balanced against the added risks.

Central venous cannulation obviates problems with irritating medications or vasoconstrictive medications, which are diluted during central venous administration. In addition, central venous catheterization is often indicated because of the difficulties in attaining peripheral venous access, particularly in the settings of circulatory shock, cardiac arrest with CPR, or the need for prolonged vascular access. Moreover, central venous catheterization allows for hemodynamic monitoring of the critically ill child. Specialized central venous catheters, including pulmonary artery catheters, may be used to monitor cardiac output, mixed venous oxygen saturation, pulmonary artery pressure, and pulmonary artery occlusion pressure, among many other important variables.

In the critical care setting, polyurethane central venous catheters are generally inserted percutaneously through a large central vein.

For chronic vascular access, silastic catheters are frequently placed. These catheters tend to be less thrombogenic and have lower infection rates. Examples include peripherally inserted central catheters (PICC), tunneled Broviac or Hickman catheters, and catheters that end in a port that is embedded in the subcutaneous tissue (Port-A-Cath). These catheters are most commonly inserted for provision of long-term chemotherapy, total parenteral nutrition, or antibiotics. The PICC catheters are placed peripherally (eg, brachial vein) and advanced into a thoracic vascular location. The Broviac and Hickman catheters are placed in a central vein and tunneled out through a distant exit site in the skin. The Hickman catheters have Dacron cuffs that are very fibrogenic. The resultant fibrous scar around the Dacron allows for the catheter to be more securely anchored and decreases the risk of ascending catheter infection from the skin. Finally, the catheters that end in a totally implanted vascular port do not exit the skin, and thereby further minimize the risk of infection ascending from the skin exit site. These totally implantable venous access devices are most useful when only intermittent infusions are necessary.

There are unavoidable risks associated with all central venous catheters. During attempts to cannulate the internal jugular or subclavian veins, inadvertent needle puncture of the lungs can result in pneumothorax. Perforation of a large vessel with resultant leak into the pleural space can lead to hemothorax, and mechanical damage to the thoracic duct or thrombosis of the left brachiocephalic vein downstream from the insertion of the thoracic duct can lead to chylothorax. In addition, injuries to nerves and arteries near the insertion site have been well-documented. When the catheter is open to the atmosphere and the patient creates negative intravascular pressure with a spontaneous breath, it is possible for air embolism to occur. This can be minimized by keeping the needle or catheter exit site in a dependent position (eg, Trendelenburg position during internal jugular or subclavian catheterization). The small radius of the catheter lumen of central venous catheters placed in infants increases the resistance to flow, minimizing the risk of air embolism. The Seldinger technique (see below), or guidewire technique, is convenient but increases the risk of vessel perforation by the guidewire and catheter malposition because of the potential for an unexpected course of a guidewire in the vascular system.

After initial insertion, central venous catheters can be a nidus for thrombosis and suppurative thrombophlebitis. The risks of each increase with time and are especially high among children who are hypercoagulable or have immune deficiencies. Critically ill children with central venous thrombosis associated with central venous catheters have a high incidence of hypercoagulable states. Detailed evaluation of their coagulation and thrombolytic systems should be considered. Newer catheter materials (polyurethane, silastic) and heparin bonding of the catheters are attempts to minimize the risks of thrombosis. Antibiotic bonding of the catheters has been used to decrease the risk of infection. The most important preventative measures for central venous catheter thrombosis and suppurative thrombophlebitis are (a) only place central venous catheters when indicated, and (b) remove the central venous catheter as soon as possible.

Local hemorrhage is common on removal of the central venous catheters. Applying direct pressure as the catheter is removed can minimize the size of the hematoma. Air embolism is a rare life-threatening complication associated with catheter removal. As during insertion, negative intrathoracic pressure with spontaneous respiration can result in negative intravascular pressure and entrapment of air into the vascular space. The major determinants of airflow are the difference in the atmospheric and vascular pressure and the size of the hole. Therefore, the risk is greater with a large, strong adolescent than a small baby; and, similarly, the risk is greater with a large-bore catheter than it is with a small-bore central venous catheter. The risk of air embolism can be minimized by placing the patient in the Trendelenburg position, removing the catheter at the end of deep inspiration, and immediately covering the exit site with petroleum jelly gauze.

The most common approaches to central venous catheterization in the critical care setting are via the internal jugular, external jugular, and femoral veins. The subclavian veins are also often used by experienced clinicians, although the risk of pneumothorax and hemothorax are higher than with the other techniques. The femoral vein is the safest approach for less-experienced providers. Prior to catheterization of the internal or external jugular or subclavian veins, the child should be placed in the Trendelenburg position to help engorge the veins and minimize risk of embolism. Conversely, if the femoral vein is used, a slight reverse Trendelenburg position will engorge the veins and improve the success rate. To minimize the risk of infection, the area is prepared with an iodine-containing solution and sterilely draped, and the health-care provider should use surgical gowns, caps, and masks after good hand washing. If a patient is conscious, local anesthesia with 1% lidocaine should be provided subcutaneously. A syringe and needle are used to locate the vein and aspirate blood. For femoral vein catheterization, the vein is located immediately medial to the artery, one to two finger's breadths below the inguinal ligament. The introducer needle is inserted into the vein at a 45° angle. When the blood is aspirated freely, the syringe is removed and the hub of the needle is covered with the thumb of the nondominant hand. A guidewire is then placed through the needle, and the needle is removed (Seldinger technique). A dilator is advanced over the wire in order to dilate the subcutaneous space and the entrance into the vein. The dilator is then removed, and the catheter is placed over the guidewire. After the catheter is introduced into the vein, the guidewire is removed, and blood is aspirated through the catheter to confirm intravascular placement. An electrocardiogram should be monitored during the procedure because the guidewire can trigger arrhythmias when advanced into the heart. Proper position of the catheter should be confirmed. The method of confirmation depends somewhat on the particular intended site for the catheter tip. Blood gas analysis can distinguish arterial from venous blood. Transduction of vascular pressure during the procedure is essential if the catheter is to be inserted into the pulmonary artery. The pressure contour is useful to ensure that a central venous catheter has not been inserted into the right ventricle, and it can distinguish accidental insertion of a catheter into a systemic artery (see Fig. 4-17 and Sec. 4.2.1). A radiograph can also be used to confirm position, but sometimes a single projection is insufficient to determine the precise distal site of the catheter (eg, distinguishing right atrium from right ventricle).

ANALGESIA AND SEDATION FOR PROCEDURES

An important, yet frequently neglected issue for any invasive procedure on a child is that of pain management and sedation. In the nonemergency situation, topical or local anesthetics should be used. The psychological milieu during the procedure should also be optimized. Music, toys, and interaction with family members can be important tools for improving comfort, thereby increasing the likelihood of cooperation and technical success. Moreover, minimizing discomfort during the procedure generally encourages better cooperation during the next potentially painful procedure for

that child. However, when sedation is provided, personnel qualified to handle sedation-induced respiratory failure or shock should be present.

References

American Heart Association: Emergency Cardiovascular Programs: Pediatric Advanced Life Support. Dallas, American Heart Association, 2001

Fiser D: Intraosseous infusion. N Engl J Med 322:1579–1581, 1990

Storvroff M, Teague WG: Intravenous access in infants and children. In: Caty MG, Irish MS, Glick PL, eds: The Pediatric Clinics of North America, Pediatric Surgery for the Primary Care Pediatrician. Part II. Philadelphia, WB Saunders, 1998:1373–1393

4.2.5   Management of Acute Neurologic Injury and Intracranial Hypertension

J. Michael Dean and Julio Pérez Fontán

STABILIZATION AND EMERGENCY MANAGEMENT

Although the search for neurologic abnormalities can easily monopolize attention in a comatose patient, the clinician must always adhere first to the emergency principles of assessing airway, breathing, and circulation. While appreciating the magnitude and implications of serious brain injury, the clinician's first priority is to ensure that respiratory and cardiovascular function are adequate. Then the clinician can assess the degree of neurologic injury in a rapid fashion to facilitate planning of further evaluations, such as neuroimaging, or surgical intervention. Finally, there must be vigilance for further neurologic deterioration and a preparedness to deal with possible cerebral edema and herniation.

Comatose children will frequently require ventilatory support, if only for protection of the airway and provision of supplemental oxygen. The potential for loss of a cough and gag reflex and aspiration of foreign materials into the airway may be unappreciated, especially if blood gases are adequate. Hypotension, hypoxemia, and hypercarbia can lead to worsening of an existing cerebral injury by extending a region of infarction or increasing intracranial pressure. Blood pressure must be high enough to maintain an appropriate cerebral perfusion pressure and coronary perfusion. A key to improved outcome of children with neurologic injury is excellent supportive care. The clinician must therefore be aggressive about instituting ventilatory and circulatory support early in the management of children with neurologic injury.

After addressing ventilation and circulation, it is important to assess neurologic function. Evidence of increased intracranial pressure and impending brain herniation should prompt immediate intervention. In a comatose patient, unequal pupils should be considered indicative of herniation (unless there is a clearly documented alternative explanation). Even if pupils are equal, a change in the motor exam from symmetric withdrawal to asymmetric posturing should also alert the clinician to possible impending herniation. Hypertension and bradycardia may occur (Cushing response), but these findings often are absent. Increased ventilation or hyperventilation, usually controlled via positive-pressure ventilation, is the most effective measure to reduce rapidly an increased intracranial pressure that is manifested by signs of brainstem compression. The titration point is usually the return of pupillary reactivity, but other detectable improvements in neurologic function may be considered an indication of temporary success (eg, restoration of withdrawal in response to pain). In these circumstances, the goal of hyperventilation is to allow time for the institution of other diagnostic and therapeutic measures, including administration of osmotic diuretics and, if appropriate, neurosurgical intervention.

Early assessment of neurologic injury helps the clinician to gauge the extent of intervention needed and allows physicians caring for the child afterward to determine the clinical course by comparing later exams to the initial evaluation. Furthermore, some of the therapies, such as anticonvulsants and muscle relaxants, used in the emergency room may obscure subsequent neurologic examinations, at least temporarily, making the baseline assessment critical. The Glasgow Coma Scale (see Table 4-6) is useful in the emergency setting because the information required for this score is quickly obtained and places no reliance on history. Scores less than 9 are suggestive of very severe injury. Patients with this degree of impairment usually require airway and ventilatory support and are potential candidates for intracranial pressure monitoring, as well as for invasive hemodynamic monitoring.

When coma or neurologic dysfunction is associated with trauma involving the head or other areas of the body, the essential question to answer is whether the cranial injury itself constitutes an acute threat to the patient's life. If the pupils are unequal or focal signs are present, a subdural or epidural hematoma may be strongly suspected and neurosurgical evaluation and intervention may proceed in the operating room while other injuries are managed. Even when trauma is believed to be restricted to the head, a search for occult systemic injury should be done. In all cases of head trauma, fractures of the cervical spine should be excluded with appropriate radiographic examinations. If, on the other hand, there is life-threatening abdominal or thoracic injury that requires operative intervention, its treatment must proceed without delay, while simultaneously making every effort to recognize and treat cerebral edema or herniation. Under these circumstances, initiation of intracranial pressure monitoring might be particularly useful because anesthetic agents will further impair consciousness and the physical examination will not reliably reflect the patient's neurologic injury.

When coma is not associated with known head trauma, the differential diagnosis is broad and the most important tool for the clinician is the physical examination. Signs of toxic, metabolic, neoplastic, and infectious processes should be assessed. The processes that present with acute focal or global encephalopathy are discussed in more detail in Sec. 4.1.3.

INCREASED INTRACRANIAL PRESSURE

Mechanisms

The location of the brain inside the cranial vault has important protective advantages. However, the rigidity of the bone enclosure also limits any changes in the volume of the intracranial contents, especially after the newborn and infant period, when fontanels and open sutures may still offer a partial mechanism of decompression. The expansion of any of the tissues and fluids contained within the skull carries with it an inevitable increase in intracranial pressure (Fig. 4-25), a condition known as intracranial hypertension.

Most forms of acute head injury increase the volume of the intracranial contents. Cerebral edema, hemorrhage, acute hydrocephalus, or rapidly growing tumors all result in intracranial hypertension. The relationship between the volume increase (although

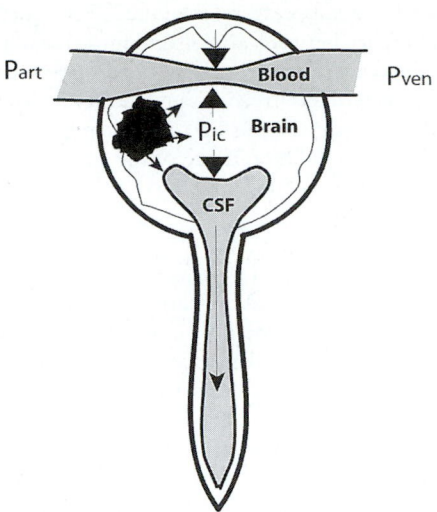

FIGURE 4-25 Mechanism and consequences of intracranial hypertension. The schema shows the contents of the cranial cavity, including the brain tissue, blood contained in the cerebral and meningeal vessels, and cerebrospinal fluid (CSF). A small increase in the volume of any of these three components (for instance as a result of cerebral edema, hemorrhage, or hydrocephalus) can be balanced by displacement of CSF into the spinal canal *(small arrow)*. This mechanism, however, offers only limited compensation. If the volume increase is larger (as shown by the dark image on the *left side*), intracranial pressure increases rapidly. When the pressure exceeds venous pressure (Pven), cerebral vessels become compressed and the perfusion pressure that determines cerebral blood flow (cerebral perfusion pressure) is the difference between the pressure in the arteries as they enter the cranial vault (Pa) and the intracranial pressure (Pic).

sanctioned by practice, the term "mass effect" is incorrect) and the rise in intracranial pressure is not linear. Small volumes can be accommodated either by stretch, if the cranial sutures are still open, or by displacement of CSF into the spinal canal (this is why in most forms of intracranial hypertension, with the notable exception of hydrocephalus, the ventricles appear small). To a lesser extent, the blood contained at any time in the cerebral vessels, especially the cerebral veins, diminishes. As the volume increase produced by the injury becomes larger, however, the pressure increases more rapidly, a circumstance that can be described as a volume-dependent decrease in the compliance of the cranium. Any additional volume causes a disproportionate elevation in intracranial pressure.

The most immediate and dangerous consequence of an increased intracranial pressure is a reduction in cerebral blood flow. Cerebral herniation (see Sec. 4.1.3) tends to be a later development. In most organs, blood flow is directly proportional to the difference between arterial and venous pressure (the perfusion pressure) and inversely proportional to the resistance of the organ's vascular bed. Some organs, such as the heart and the brain, regulate their vascular tone (and thus their vascular resistance) to maintain blood flow constant over a wide range of perfusion pressures appropriate for age (autoregulation) (see Sec. 4.1.2). Below or above this autoregulation range, blood flow changes in proportion to perfusion pressure. (Other organs, such as the intestine and the skin, have their flow regulated by neural and humoral inputs in response to a variety of physiological circumstances, sometimes without change in the blood pressure.) The presence of the cranial enclosure introduces a new variable for consideration. The outside surface of the cerebral blood vessels is exposed to intracranial pressure. If this pressure exceeds venous pressure, then the effective perfusion pressure is the difference between arterial and intracranial pressure, the venous pressure becoming irrelevant in defining blood flow (just as the height of a waterfall is irrelevant in determining the flow of the river). Intracranial hypertension can reduce cerebral perfusion pressure below the autoregulation range of the cerebral blood vessels, resulting in cerebral ischemia.

Monitoring

The monitoring of intracranial pressure is a useful clinical tool that should be applied in those instances in which the clinician suspects or anticipates the presence of intracranial hypertension based on the clinical signs (Table 4-15), and when access to the patient is obstructed, the physical examination is altered significantly by exogenous factors (necessary administration of medications) or where control of this hypertension is likely to improve the outcome. The most important purpose of monitoring intracranial pressure is to detect and then treat circumstances in which the cerebral perfusion pressure decreases enough to cause cerebral ischemia. Simultaneous monitoring of arterial pressure is thus advisable, making sure that the pressure-recording systems for both variables, arterial and intracranial pressure, have a common zero (the relevant arterial pressure is the one measured at the level of the cranium, but, because it is the difference that matters, both pressures could be measured in reference to the level of the heart). As an additional advantage, intracranial pressure monitoring also facilitates the detection of new pathologic events such as acute hydrocephalus or intracranial hemorrhages.

Intracranial pressure may be monitored by using catheters or by using transducer-tipped devices inserted into the cerebral ventricles, the epidural space, the subdural space, or the brain parenchyma itself. External monitors have been used to estimate intracranial pressure based on the tension of the anterior fontanel in infants, but their poor record of accuracy disqualifies them in most instances. The choice of monitoring location depends on the mechanisms of the disease and the age of the patient. Intraventricular catheters offer the advantage of allowing CSF drainage, which can have a substantial benefit in the control of intracranial hypertension. They are difficult to place, however, when the size of the ventricles is decreased, a circumstance that also limits their usefulness as a draining device. Subdural and epidural catheters are prone to obstruction, a disadvantage that has been eliminated by transducer-tipped catheters; these are routinely placed into the ventricles, subdural space, or the brain tissue, but cannot be used to drain fluid.

Regardless of the device chosen, the underlying assumption of intracranial pressure monitoring is that intracranial pressure is homogeneous. This assumption is not always valid because of the compartmentalization of the intracranial cavity by the reflections of the dura (the development of pressure differences is the reason for the herniation syndromes, see Sec. 4.1.3). Moreover, the monitoring device itself can cause tension within the tissue, which interferes with the measurements. Thus, it is imperative that a continuous recording of the intracranial pressure be displayed. A flattened or dampened waveform is often an indication of catheter or transducer dysfunction.

Aside from artifactual readings that may misguide treatment, the most common complication of intracranial pressure monitoring is infection. Intraventricular catheters carry the largest risk, which is compounded by the location of the infection (ventriculitis) and the difficulty of eradicating bacteria from the ventricular system. Risk of infections can be reduced by compulsive surgical technique and

TABLE 4-15
SIGNS OF INTRACRANIAL HYPERTENSION

Decreased consciousness
Papilledema
Headache
Sixth-nerve palsy
Unilateral pupillary dilation

by avoiding opening the monitoring system for fluid sampling. Hemorrhage may occur at the time of placement or thereafter. Whether caused by the catheter or preexisting, intraventricular hemorrhage increases the risk for occlusion of intraventricular catheters.

Treatment of Intracranial Hypertension

The treatment of intracranial hypertension has evolved considerably in the last 10 years as our understanding of both the mechanisms that cause and extend brain injury and the regulation of cerebral blood flow in health and disease states has progressed (Table 4-16). Some of this progress has involved the realization of the competing needs of injured and noninjured tissue. The focus has often become the prevention of injury extension to viable areas of the brain. The main aim of therapy, however, continues to be a reduction of the volume of the intracranial contents to avoid cerebral ischemia in viable areas and herniation. Whenever possible this approach should address the mechanism of disease. Tumors and abscesses should be resected as soon as it is safe. Extravascular accumulations of blood should be drained by craniotomy whenever possible.

A number of supportive measures are helpful in decreasing intracranial pressure or in mitigating its consequences. Some of these measures also affect the intracranial volume. For instance, administration of supplemental oxygen not only limits additional brain hypoxia, but it also corrects increases in cerebral blood flow initiated by hypoxemia (hyperoxia has no substantial effect on cerebral vascular tone, but hypoxemia can increase cerebral blood flow markedly). Similarly, mechanical ventilation not only stabilizes gas exchange but also facilitates manipulation of the arterial PCO_2 to influence cerebral vascular resistance and blood volume. Cardio-

TABLE 4-16
TREATMENT OF INTRACRANIAL HYPERTENSION

I. Supportive measures
      Supplemental oxygen
      Mechanical ventilation
      Vasoactive and inotropic medications
      Minimize agitation
      Control seizures
II. Interventions aimed at reducing cerebral blood volume
      Hyperventilation
      Elevation of head
      Sedation and control of seizures
      Cough suppression
      Hypothermia
III. Treatment of cerebral edema
      Osmotic and loop diuretics
IV. Direct interventions
      CSF shunt if hydrocephalus
      Drain hemorrhage
      Resect tumor and abscess
      Craniotomy for decompression

vascular support and treatment of hypotension with inotropic and vasoactive medications are fundamental in the preservation of cerebral perfusion pressure, although the loss of cerebral vascular autoregulation can cause the intracranial pressure to increase in response to these measures.

Hyperventilation to increase cerebral pH through decreases in cerebral PCO_2 is a still widely used and effective method of decreasing intracranial pressure rapidly by reducing cerebral blood volume. The caliber of cerebral vessels is highly sensitive to changes in cerebral (extracellular and CSF) pH and PCO_2 within the physiological range of these variables. Alkalemia and hypocapnia both increase vascular tone and decrease cerebral blood flow and volume. Unfortunately, vessels in healthy areas of the brain are more responsive to these changes than those in injured areas; thus, the potential exists for diversion of blood flow away from healthy areas causing ischemia and leading to further extension of the injury. For this reason, hyperventilation is no longer used as the mainstay of intracranial hypertension treatment, being generally reserved for control of acute crisis, especially in the presence of signs of herniation. As an additional disadvantage, continued hypocapnia results in compensatory reduction of bicarbonate in the extracellular compartment and CSF. As this reduces pH toward "normal," it blunts the effect of the therapy over time; furthermore, the lowered bicarbonate with near-normal pH creates a situation in which a reduction in ventilatory support (ie, increase in PCO_2) later in the course can cause a decrease in interstitial and CSF pH that may result in a recurrence of the intracranial hypertension.

Osmotic diuretics such as mannitol, glycerol, and urea have been used for a long time in the treatment of cerebral edema and intracranial hypertension. These molecules are small enough to be eliminated easily by glomerular filtration, but too large to penetrate the blood-brain barrier. Accordingly, where this barrier is intact, they act as an osmotic attractant for water, reducing the volume of the brain. A dose of 0.25 to 0.5 g/kg of mannitol is usually sufficient to produce a substantial reduction in intracranial pressure and can be repeated every few hours. However, the increases in serum osmolality limit the usefulness of the osmotic diuretics in the most severe cases of intracranial hypertension. Osmolalities greater than 320 mOsm/kg are associated with tissue and organ injury, including injury of the brain, and should not be exceeded. Loop and other diuretics increase plasma oncotic and osmotic pressure and therefore are also effective in reducing cerebral edema and intracranial pressure. They may be used after the full potential of the osmotic diuretics is exploited.

Other measures directed at reducing cerebral blood volume include the administration of sedatives and cough suppressants. Many sedating substances, including benzodiazepines and opioids, reduce cerebral metabolism and, because blood flow and metabolic activity are coupled, they also decrease blood flow and blood volume. In addition, eliminating agitation has the additional advantage of preventing acute increases in intrathoracic pressure, which can be transmitted via the blood column to the intracranial veins. Although venous pressure has no direct effect on cerebral blood flow when intracranial pressure is elevated, intracranial venous distention can cause marked increases in intracranial pressure. Cough suppressants such as opioids and local anesthetics such as lidocaine are often given before suctioning the endotracheal tube for similar reasons. However, these therapies become limited by progressive accumulation of the drugs.

Hypothermia was recently reintroduced into the treatment of intracranial hypertension. The principle is to reduce brain metabolism and, consequently, the need for blood supply, although the

reduction in temperature may have other salutary effects in brain preservation. It requires deep sedation and neuromuscular blockade to avoid shivering, which, similar to cough, can have negative effects on intracranial pressure.

Finally, craniotomy is applied in some centers as a measure of last resort in the control of refractory intracranial hypertension. It is performed by removing a section of the skull, which can be preserved for later replacement. The benefits of this measure have not been established conclusively.

References

Javaheri S, Corbett W, Wagner K, Adams JM: Quantitative cerebrospinal fluid acid-base balance in acute respiratory alkalosis. Am J Resp Crit Care Med 150:78–82, 1994

McManus ML, Churchwell KB, Strange K: Regulation of cell volume in health and disease. NEJM 333:1260–1266, 1995

Metz CM, Holzschuh M, Bein T, et al: Moderate hypothermia in patients with severe head injury: cerebral and extracerebral effects. J Neurosurg 85:533–541, 1996

Mitchell RA, Singer MM: Respiration and cerebrospinal pH in metabolic acidosis and alkalosis. J Appl Physiol 20:905–911, 1965

Polin RS, Shaffrey ME, Bogaev CA, et al: Decompressive bifrontal craniectomy in the treatment of severe refractory posttraumatic cerebral edema. Neurosurgery 41:84–94, 1997

4.2.6   Cardiopulmonary Arrest and Resuscitation

J. Michael Dean and George Lister

Cardiopulmonary arrest is unusual in infancy and childhood, but it is important for all pediatric clinicians to be knowledgeable about the fundamental steps in resuscitation and to be prepared to implement resuscitation on an immediate basis until assistance is available. In children, cardiopulmonary arrest is caused by primary cardiac failure (rare) or by cardiac arrest secondary to respiratory compromise (common). The prognosis of cardiopulmonary arrest is related to the underlying cause and the delay before cardiopulmonary resuscitation is undertaken. It is obvious that a patient who suffers cardiopulmonary arrest in a witnessed setting within a pediatric-equipped medical facility has a better chance of survival than the patient who suffers cardiopulmonary arrest in a setting that is less equipped for resuscitation. This is almost certainly a consequence of the speed with which effective resuscitation can be accomplished. On the other hand, children in the hospital who suffer cardiopulmonary arrest often have complicated medical or surgical problems and commonly do not survive to discharge.

The principles of resuscitation have been recognized (although not necessarily successfully enacted) for many centuries. Most early descriptions of resuscitation seem to focus on restoration of breathing (eg, the earliest attempts were directed at artificial respiration for drowning victims). However, a variety of devices and strategies used simultaneously augment respiration and circulation because chest compression also expels blood from the heart (eg, the rolling of a subject over a barrel to compress the chest as used first in the mid-1700s, or the encircling of the thorax with a long cloth that was pulled in opposite directions by two resuscitators). Despite understanding the principles, a consistent approach to resuscitation was not developed in the United States until well after World War II. Kouwenhoven first reported successful closed chest compression in 1960. Following this, the National Academy of Science recommended that the American Heart Association take responsibility for educating health care professionals in this new technique.

In 1978, the American Heart Association established a working group to develop just such an organized and uniform approach to resuscitation of the infant and child, following similar earlier efforts directed at resuscitation of the adult. There were at least two compelling reasons to develop distinct approaches for children: the difference in the common causes for cardiopulmonary arrest and a largely different set of health-care providers. This extraordinary effort culminated in the production of didactic materials and routinized guidelines, currently published by the American Heart Association in conjunction with the American Academy of Pediatrics and seven other international resuscitation councils, and the derivation of organized courses for both providers and teachers of Pediatric Advanced Life Support (PALS), Pediatric Basic Life Support (BLS), and Neonatal Resuscitation Programs. These courses provide detailed instruction in the techniques of cardiopulmonary resuscitation, recognition of signs of respiratory failure and circulatory insufficiency, and management of states that could proceed to cardiac or pulmonary arrest. Clinicians who provide care to infants and children should consider the courses as a valuable resource for themselves and for the other professionals with whom they work. This section does not replicate the didactic materials provided by these courses nor does it teach the technical skills, which require practical experience. Rather, this section familiarizes the clinician with the essential issues, highlights the need and nature of preparation, and discusses the considerations that arise following resuscitation, whether successful or unsuccessful.

ETIOLOGIES OF CARDIOPULMONARY ARREST

The most common causes in the postneonatal infancy period, when the majority of childhood cardiopulmonary arrests occur, are sudden infant death syndrome (SIDS) and respiratory failure. SIDS accounts for approximately 40% of all childhood cardiopulmonary arrests. Shock, metabolic disorders, and drug reactions or overdose might also lead to cardiopulmonary arrest, typically mediated by hemodynamic impairment and ischemia. Trauma deserves special emphasis as a cause of pediatric cardiopulmonary arrest (see Sec. 4.3.1). Injuries are the dominant problems encountered in prehospital pediatric emergency care and are the most common cause of death in children over 1 year of age. Events involving motor vehicle crashes (occupant, bicyclist, or pedestrian), fires, and falls comprise the primary mechanisms of injury. In some regions, drowning is frequent (see Sec. 4.3.4). Pediatric trauma is mainly blunt, although penetrating trauma is increasing in the urban areas. Fatal injury often includes trauma to the head, chest, and abdomen. Central nervous system injury usually is the determining factor in ultimate outcome from pediatric trauma. Identifying and managing the prearrest state in pediatric trauma are especially important because of high salvage rates for trauma victims treated within well-organized emergency medical service (EMS) systems.

Of all common causes, respiratory conditions—the most frequent etiologies for medical cardiopulmonary arrest throughout childhood—are especially important because they are usually treatable and reversible. Untreated respiratory insufficiency may lead to respiratory arrest and then to cardiopulmonary arrest. Survival from respiratory arrest alone, if identified prior to hemodynamic collapse and pulselessness, ranges from 44 to 97%. Respiratory failure may be caused by airway obstruction; restrictive lung disease, which can

cause fatigue; and depression of the respiratory drive. As noted earlier (see Sec. 4.1.1), when obstructive or restrictive lung disease becomes severe, there are signs of respiratory distress. When the patient's compensatory adaptations become disrupted, fatigue ensues, which eventually causes a respiratory arrest. The resultant hypoxemia and hypercarbia from insufficient ventilation can impair myocardial function (and function of other organs), ultimately resulting in cardiopulmonary arrest. Central nervous system depression, whether related to trauma, or to illness, or to the effects of drugs, can also cause apnea, followed by cardiopulmonary arrest. Shock (see Sec. 4.1.2), a state in which the circulation is insufficient to sustain vital function, has numerous causes in infants and children; all of these lead to inadequate coronary and cerebral blood flow and inadequate provision of oxygen and substrate to systemic tissues.

Primary cardiac failure with cardiopulmonary arrest is unusual in children, especially in the out-of-hospital setting, but can occur in children with cardiomyopathies, myocarditis, or congenital heart disease. Such events are often in-hospital events and may happen immediately after cardiac surgery, in children with dysrhythmias (eg, prolonged QT syndrome) or who are receiving various antiarrhythmic drugs, during cardiac catheterization and angiography, and after general anesthetics.

An important goal of medical care is to avoid a resuscitation by recognizing the signs of impending cardiac or respiratory insufficiency and reversing the process. However, when such an opportunity is not possible, an orderly resuscitation with expedient restoration of oxygen delivery to tissues may be possible. Whether the resuscitation occurs outside of a medical facility, in a clinician's office, or in the hospital, the initial management approach is the same.

RESUSCITATION

The sequence of resuscitation may be remembered as A-B-C-D-E, for airway, breathing, circulation, drug delivery, and electricity. There is a logic to this sequence, as oxygen cannot be delivered to the lungs unless the airway is patent, and oxygen cannot be circulated in the bloodstream unless oxygen arrives in the lungs via breathing. Drug therapy is entirely oriented toward improving the effectiveness of this circulation of oxygen. Finally, electrical countershock is indicated for treatment of specific cardiac arrhythmias such as ventricular fibrillation or supraventricular tachycardia.

Airway

The airway should be assessed and its patency must be assured. This may be accomplished by the head-tilt or chin-lift maneuver. The neck should not be hyperextended as this may occlude the trachea in an infant. In cases of cervical trauma, the chin-lift maneuver should be used. After the airway is clear, patients frequently begin breathing, and cardiopulmonary arrest may be averted.

Foreign-body aspiration is a frequent cause of airway obstruction, and if it is not possible to achieve a patent airway by positioning the chin and neck, the clinician should use back blows (in infants) or chest thrusts (in children) in an attempt to evacuate a possible foreign body from the airway (see Sec. 4.3.5). Magill forceps can be used to remove the object after it is within the oropharynx.

In most instances of cardiopulmonary arrest, the airway should be secured with endotracheal intubation to facilitate the remainder of the resuscitation sequence. However, ventilation should be instituted immediately after the airway is patent and should not be delayed while preparing for endotracheal intubation.

It is very important to recognize that fatigue commonly contributes to a respiratory arrest in infants and children. Thus, manual ventilation using a self-inflating bag-valve device applied to the face via a properly fitting mask can frequently be used to sustain adequate gas exchange, even for extended periods of time. Because intubation of the trachea requires specialized equipment and technical skills (as well as practice), it is not reasonable to expect most clinicians to be facile with this approach for airway support. In contrast, provision of ventilation with bag-valve and mask is a skill that can be easily learned and maintained by clinicians who care for ill children.

Breathing

After the airway is opened, the patient may begin spontaneous breathing. If this does not occur, it is necessary to provide assisted ventilation with a properly fitted bag and mask apparatus. The chest should be assessed to verify that ventilation is accomplished. If it is impossible to ventilate the child, the clinician should be concerned that the airway remains obstructed, perhaps due to a foreign body in the airway. Despite proper positioning of the head and neck, there are times when manual ventilation with bag-valve and mask is ineffective. In the patient who is comatose or who has stopped breathing, use of an oral airway is often sufficient to keep the tongue from obstructing the hypopharynx. In addition, suctioning of the hypopharynx may aid in clearing vomitus or mucus that interferes with manual ventilation.

If a bag and mask is not available, mouth-to-mouth, mouth-to-nose, or mouth-to-mouth and nose ventilation should be performed. Total-body substance precautions should be used to protect the clinician from disease transmission.

Circulation

After the airway is assessed and effective ventilation is started, check the pulse. If it is absent, then circulatory support with cardiopulmonary resuscitation must be started. It is important to note that provision of effective ventilation and oxygenation is the first priority. It is not helpful to check the pulse at the beginning of the resuscitation sequence and then to begin chest compressions—if there is an obstructed airway or lack of oxygen in the lungs, no amount of artificial circulation will deliver oxygen to the myocardium.

The mechanism by which external cardiac compression restores circulation has been the subject of much study over the past three decades. There are two predominant explanations for blood flow during cardiopulmonary resuscitation. First, the heart itself may be squeezed during compressions, ejecting blood in a manner similar to the normal circulation. Second, the entire intrathoracic cavity is clearly compressed during cardiopulmonary resuscitation, and a generalized rise in intrathoracic pressure can eject blood from the thorax. Both mechanisms have been demonstrated to occur in animal models, and a number of investigators have attempted to improve the efficiency of cardiac compressions by accentuating cardiac compression or intrathoracic pressure elevation. The most effective way to provide cardiac compression is by an open chest technique. The most effective way to increase intrathoracic pressure is to provide ventilations simultaneous to chest compressions.

In practice, it is likely that both mechanisms play a role in artificial circulation in children. However, simultaneous ventilation and compression is likely to impair effective ventilation. Because ventilatory problems are the most frequent etiologies for cardiac arrest in children, simultaneous compression and ventilation is not recommended in cardiopulmonary resuscitation of children.

Drugs

The most important drug used in cardiopulmonary resuscitation is epinephrine. Other drugs that are currently recommended for in-hospital resuscitation are shown in Table 4-17. The most frequently used drugs are epinephrine, atropine, lidocaine, and sodium bicarbonate.

Drug administration is important if cardiopulmonary resuscitation has proceeded as far as cardiac compressions, as the circulatory efficiency of cardiac compressions is poor unless vascular tone is maintained. Some drugs may be administered by endotracheal tube (epinephrine, atropine, lidocaine, naloxone), but vascular access is important for delivery of these and other drugs (sodium bicarbonate) as is provision of fluid resuscitation to treat underlying shock that may have precipated cardiac arrest in the older child. Vascular access may be technically difficult, but rapid access to the vascular compartment can be effectively obtained with an intraosseous bone marrow needle (see Sec. 4.2.4).

Epinephrine is used to cause vasoconstriction via its α-adrenergic agonist effect. Considerable laboratory evidence shows that cerebral and myocardial blood flow are increased during cardiac compressions by maintaining a high vascular tone. These experiments have led to clinical trials of very-high-dose epinephrine (compared with "standard"-dose epinephrine); these trials have generally not shown any superiority of high-dose epinephrine. It is obvious, however, that if standard-dose epinephrine and external compressions fail to restore spontaneous circulation (in the presence of effective ventilation and oxygenation), there is nothing to lose by administering a subsequent, higher dose.

When a spontaneous cardiac rhythm is present, but is too slow to support adequate circulation, atropine may be useful. Atropine was frequently used in the past, but recent recommendations have been to rely on epinephrine in this setting, because epinephrine has potent chronotropic agonist activity.

Lidocaine and other antiarrhythmic drugs will be used for specific cardiac rhythm disturbances. Lidocaine may be administered via endotracheal tube if vascular access has not been successfully obtained.

Cardiopulmonary arrest results in acidosis, and sodium bicarbonate has traditionally been used to treat this acidosis. Over the past several decades, however, much evidence has suggested that bicarbonate use should be restrained. The predominant cause of acidosis in cardiopulmonary arrest is carbon dioxide retention rather than lactic acidosis. Following restoration of ventilation and circulation, much of this respiratory acidosis will resolve without sodium bicarbonate administration. After spontaneous circulation is achieved, and fluids are administered to combat shock, sodium bicarbonate administration may be titrated according to arterial blood gas results.

Electricity

Electrical countershock may be necessary during cardiopulmonary resuscitation. While primary cardiac disease is not a common cause of cardiopulmonary arrest, arrhythmias may develop during resuscitation even in the absence of primary cardiac disease. Ventricular fibrillation, ventricular tachycardia, and supraventricular tachycardia are the most common treatable conditions in this circumstance and are treated with defibrillation or synchronized countershock.

TABLE 4-17

DRUGS USED IN PEDIATRIC ADVANCED LIFE SUPPORT

DRUG	DOSAGE (PEDIATRIC)	REMARKS
Adenosine	0.1–0.2 mg/kg	Rapid IV bolus
	Maximum single dose: 12 mg	
Atropine sulfate*	0.02 mg/kg	Minimum dose: 0.1 mg
		Maximum single dose: 0.5 mg in child, 1.0 mg in adolescent
Bretylium	5 mg/kg; may be increased to 10 mg/kg	Rapid IV
Calcium chloride 10%	20 mg/kg	Give slowly
Dobutamine hydrochloride	2–20 μg/kg per min	Titrate to desired effect
Dopamine hydrochloride	2–20 μg/kg per min	α-Adrenergic action dominates at $\geq$15–20 μg/kg per min
Epinephrine for bradycardia*	IV/IO: 0.01 mg/kg (1:10,000, 0.1 mL/kg)	
	ET: 0.1 mg/kg (1:1000, 0.1 mL/kg)	
Epinephrine for asystolic or pulse-less arrest*	First dose:	
	IV/IO: 0.01 mg/kg (1:10,000, 0.1 mL/kg)	
	ET: 0.1 mg/kg (1:1000, 0.1 mL/kg)	
	IV/IO doses as high as 0.2 mg/kg of 1:1000 may be effective.	
	Subsequent doses:	
	IV/IO/ET: 0.1 mg/kg (1:1000, 0.1 mL/kg)	
	Repeat every 3–5 min.	
	IV/IO doses as high as 0.2 mg/kg of 1:1000 may be effective.	
Epinephrine infusion	Initial at 0.1 μg/kg per min	Titrate to desired effect
	Higher infusion dose used if asystole present	(0.1–1.0 μg/kg per min)
Lidocaine*	1 mg/kg	
Lidocaine infusion	20–50 μg/kg per min	
Naloxone*	If $\leq$5 years old or $\leq$20 kg: 0.1 mg/kg	Titrate to desired effect
	If >5 years old or >20 kg: 2.0 mg	
Prostaglandin E$_1$	0.05–0.1 μg/kg per min	Monitor for apnea, hypotension, hypoglycemia
Sodium bicarbonate	1 mEq/kg per dose or 0.3 × kg × base deficit	Infuse slowly and only if ventilation is adequate

* For ET administration, dilute medication with normal saline to a volume of 3 to 5 mL and follow with several positive-pressure ventilations.
SOURCE: *Pediatric Advanced Life Support. American Heart Association Dallas, TX, 1997.*

If pediatric paddles are not available, adult paddles may be used by placing one anteriorly and the other posteriorly.

ORGANIZATION

Whether resuscitation is in or out of the hospital, it is essential to maintain organization, order, and coordination of activities so that there is proper attention to detail. It is valuable to keep all materials together and properly labeled. It is also useful to keep readily accessible and easily visible copies of written materials of doses or sizes of specific equipment because most individuals are not well enough versed to recall this information from memory. In any setting in which resuscitation is not a rare event, it is worth assigning specific roles and rehearsing these periodically as an educational tool. In settings in which such events are rare, it is also worth reviewing where resource materials (handbooks, drug lists, resuscitation cards) and equipment are kept and what resources are most available for care of emergencies and for subsequent management following successful resuscitation.

DECISIONS REGARDING TERMINATION OF RESUSCITATION

Customs regarding care of the seriously ill vary considerably among cultures, and the patients and families we serve have differing views of what constitutes life. Greek physicians believed that the heart was the seat of life and that the heartbeat was the feature that distinguished one who was alive. The ancient Hebrews viewed the breath as a defining feature of life. Others looked to the seat of the soul as the source of life. Accordingly, early physicians often disagreed on the definition of death. Even today there are varying views, and often ambiguous actions, despite the adoption of the Model Uniform Determination of Death Act. This act states that a person is legally dead when there is irreversible cessation of circulation and respiratory function *or* irreversible cessation of all functions of the entire brain including the brainstem. However, it is worth recognizing how frequently physicians state that a patient has brain death but later (sometimes hours or more) they declare and write in the chart that the patient "died" because of cessation of breathing or cardiac function. Such ambiguity is easily transmitted to families. Thus, clinicians who are involved in resuscitation should be prepared for the possibility that families may not share their perception of life and death. Furthermore, strong personal beliefs may be coupled with a lack of trust in prognosis provided by physicians who are not well known to the family. Thus, it may be confusing when to cease a resuscitation.

In the United States, it is generally expected that individuals first on the scene of a cardiopulmonary arrest will initiate resuscitative measures unless they are specifically aware of an advanced directive not to resuscitate. Decisions to cease resuscitation are much more complex and should, where possible, be made by an experienced clinician or by protocols written for emergency care providers. There is no compulsion to continue resuscitation if there is reason to believe that there will be no return of vital function, or if, based on knowledge of the patient, there is general belief that care is futile (see Sec. 7.8). However, knowledge of what represents futile care often varies with the level of experience of the clinician and with the viewpoint of the parents. Therefore, once a resuscitation has commenced, it is essential to attempt to contact the parents (or guardians) and the senior physician responsible for the care of that child. This physician is usually the most able judge of when a sufficient and reasonable effort has been made for restoration of function, and can convey this assessment to a family. Recognizing the value of input from the senior physician, nursing staff and parents, and from friends or members of the clergy who understand the parents' religious views, it is highly desirable to engage in discussions in advance of a resuscitation whenever this is possible (see Sec. 7.8). Such discussions help to provide direction to the caregivers and to reduce the risk of having management decisions at odds with family wishes.

With these thoughts in mind, there are some useful guidelines that help the individuals involved in the resuscitation. The following questions deserve primary consideration in establishing an endpoint:

1. Was the cardiopulmonary arrest witnessed?
2. What is the presenting rhythm?
3. Do extenuating factors exist, especially hypothermia, drug overdose, or electrolyte imbalance?
4. Did the child respond to critical advanced life-support interventions: endotracheal intubation, attempted defibrillation, or epinephrine?
5. What is the total cardiopulmonary arrest time?

An unwitnessed child in cardiopulmonary arrest with either asystole or slow, wide, pulseless electrical activity as the presenting rhythm is unlikely to respond to any therapy. If the child is warm and no extenuating factors are present, resuscitation should continue through intubation and reversal of hypoxia and respiratory acidosis. If hypothermia is suspected, efforts to revive the child are indicated until the heart is warm because hypothermia may confer a powerful protective effect on brain and organ survival. Documented survival from full cardiopulmonary arrest has occurred in a hypothermic child suffering more than 45 minutes of cardiopulmonary arrest time.

If the cardiopulmonary arrest rhythm is not asystole or bradycardia (VF, VT, SVT, or normal to fast, pulseless electrical activity), resuscitation should usually continue until either reperfusion or asystole is established. Multiple defibrillation attempts may be necessary. Protracted resuscitative efforts are often indicated for patients with intermittent periods of spontaneous circulation. However, mortality is likely in the child with no response and no extenuating factors.

Sometimes cardiovascular function returns, but the child has suffered overwhelming brain injury. As our technologies for resuscitation continue to evolve, this may become more common until better strategies for cerebral resuscitation are available. The child who dies warrants consideration for organ donation. Currently, there are "required request" laws that mandate documentation that families of potential organ donors were offered the option of donation and that the local procurement organization was notified. This discussion requires a sensitive approach to the bereaved family and can make caregivers feel quite uncomfortable. Other laws are being considered that will presume consent unless otherwise stated. Fortunately, trained professionals who are abreast of current options and laws that should be considered are often available for consultation and can assist with such delicate discussions.

TRANSPORT FOLLOWING RESUSCITATION

After resuscitation, it is likely that the patient will need to be transported to a facility where there can be intensive monitoring and additional interventions until stability is achieved or the inciting process abates. Such a resource is close by if the resuscitation is within a hospital, or there may be a need for transfer by land or air to another facility. Within the hospital, there are usually teams of individuals (including physicians, nurses, respiratory therapists, and possibly pharmacists) who are part of an organized resuscitation service; they are trained to provide safe intrahospital transport. The precise means for transport to another medical facility is more complex, varies from one community or region to the next, and depends on a number of factors, including distance, terrain, weather conditions, human resources and skills, possible modes of transport, and stability of the patient. It is valuable for each group of clinicians to be aware of the options for such transport, especially if critical care services are not within the community, and to have ready access by telephone to a regional resource and to skilled clinicians that can assist with consultation, triage, and transfer. While awaiting such transfer, it is important to have a plan to maintain the patient in as stable a condition as possible and to begin initiating treatment for the precipitating events (eg, sepsis, hypovolemia, meningitis, critical coarctation, etc.). During the process of obtaining additional history, a more thorough physical examination, or laboratory data to help with stabilization, cardiorespiratory function should be monitored as closely as possible (see Sec. 4.2.1). Consultants at regional facilities might also be able to provide cognitive assistance while waiting for the transport, so that that time can be used most effectively for initiating important management.

PROGNOSIS

For children, outcome from true cardiopulmonary arrest is dismal. Twelve pediatric cardiopulmonary arrest studies from 1983 to 1995 document an aggregate out-of-hospital survival of 11% (42/392 patients). In-hospital survival is higher, but not well documented. However, these data probably overstate true survival, because of inconsistencies and ambiguities in the inclusion criteria, definitions of cardiopulmonary arrest, and reporting of core data. Moreover, patient outcomes are often not further stratified by short- and long-term neurologic status, using quantifiable methods for assessing performance. Lastly, the denominator for all pediatric cardiopulmonary arrest studies is small, making it difficult to interpret objectively reported data, response to treatment, and survival characteristics.

When restoration of ventilation succeeds without need for external cardiac compressions, the prognosis is much better, presumably because intervention was carried out earlier in the course of events. Similarly, cardiopulmonary arrest in the hospital is more likely to be survived than cardiopulmonary arrest out of hospital. If the clinician is able to intervene earlier, the prognosis is better.

The cause of cardiac arrest in the hospital might be more treatable. For example, cardiac arrest may follow injection of dye at cardiac catheterization or may result from tension pneumothorax

TABLE 4-18

PERCENT OF OFFICES IN SUBURBAN AREA WITH AT LEAST MINIMAL OR OPTIMAL PREPARATION FOR OFFICE EMERGENCIES

TYPE OF EMERGENCY	PERCENT OF OFFICES SURVEYED			
	MINIMAL EQUIPMENT	OPTIMAL EQUIPMENT	MINIMAL TRAINING	OPTIMAL TRAINING
Status asthmaticus	73	4	73	4
Airway obstruction	61	2	24	2
Shock	29	8	29	6
Trauma	29	6	29	2
Status epilepticus	24	22	24	10
Endocrine	6	4	10	6
Cardiac arrest	6	0	6	0
Approximate initial cost (based on 1996)	$550	$6200		

SOURCE: *Adapted from Flores G. Weinstock DJ: The preparedness of pediatricians for emergencies in the office. What is broken, should we care, and how can we fix it? Arch Pediatr Adolesc Med 150(3):249–256, 1996.*

in the intensive care unit. These etiologies of cardiac arrest, while more rare than respiratory failure or shock, are more specifically treated. Hence, the likelihood of surviving cardiac arrest from these causes is greater. On the other hand, if a child is involved in a suffocation incident in the home, the cause of cardiac arrest is pro-

TABLE 4-19

SUGGESTED EMERGENCY EQUIPMENT FOR PHYSICIAN OFFICES (BASED ON RECOMMENDATIONS OF PEDIATRIC ADVANCED LIFE SUPPORT, 1997)

Airway Management
    Nasal cannulas: infant, child, and adult sizes 1–3
    Oral airways: 0–5
    Oxygen masks: infant, child, adult
    Oxygen source with flowmeter (to deliver >15 mL/min)
    Self-inflating bag-valve-mask resuscitators, including reservoir: infant, child, adult
    Suction catheters: Yankauer, 8F, 10F, 14F
    Suction: wall or machine
    Optional for intubation
      - Endotracheal tubes, uncuffed sizes 2.5–6.0 and cuffed 6.0–8.0
      - Laryngoscope handle with Miller or Wishipple blades: 0, 1, 2, 3
      - Laryngoscope batteries and bulbs
      - Magill forceps: pediatric and adult
      - Stylets: pediatric and adult sizes for endotracheal tubes
Fluid Management
    Intraosseous needles: 15 and 18 gauge
    Intravenous catheters: 14–24 gauge
    Isotonic fluids (normal saline or lactated Ringer solution)
    IV boards, tape, alcohol swabs, tourniquet
    Pediatric drip chambers and tubing
    Optional: central venous catheters—3F, 4F, 5F
Miscellaneous Equipment
    Blood pressure cuffs: infant, child, adult
    Cardiac arrest board
    Feeding tubes: 3F, 5F
    Foley urine catheters: 8F, 10F
    Nasogastric tubes: 10F, 14F
    Sphygmomanometer
Optional Equipment
    Noninvasive blood pressure monitor
    Portable ECG monitor/defibrillator
    Pulse oximeter

longed hypoxia. In addition, the location of cardiac arrest is in the home, away from skilled medical assistance. This delays effective cardiopulmonary resuscitation, lowering survival.

PREPARATION IN OFFICE

It is recognized that the types of emergencies that occur in offices have a different frequency distribution than those that occur in the hospital. Surveys of the level of training and availability of equipment and supplies to meet the most common emergencies also show that preparation may be inadequate and that preparation varies widely in settings with similar patient populations (see Table 4-18). The perceived rarity of emergencies, the lack of time of the clinician, and expense are most commonly cited as factors limiting such preparation. Accordingly, several authors have developed a list of suggested equipment for physician offices that may be tailored to the specific needs and population of the primary care provider (Table 4-19).

References

Anonymous: Guidelines for the determination of death. Report of the medical consultants on the diagnosis of death to the President's Commission for the Study of Ethical Problems in Medicine and Biomedical and Behavioral Research. JAMA 246(19):2184–2186, 1981

Chameides L, Hazinski MF: Pediatric Advanced Life Support. American Heart Association, Dallas, TX 1997

Denton R, Thomas AN: Cardiopulmonary resuscitation: a retrospective review. Anaesthesia 52:324–327, 1997

Fiser DH, Wrape V: Outcome of cardiopulmonary resuscitation in children. Pediatr Emerg Care 3(4):235–238, 1987

Flores G, Weinstock DJ: The preparedness of pediatricians for emergencies in the office. What is broken, should we care, and how can we fix it? Arch Pediatr Adolesc Med 150(3):249–256, 1996

Frand MN, Honig KL, Hageman JR: Neonatal cardiopulmonary resuscitation: the good news and the bad. Pediatr Clin North Am 45:587–598, 1998

Ginsberg HG, Goldsmith JP: Controversies in neonatal resuscitation. Clin Perinatol 25:1–15, 1998

Jarvis AS: Parental presence during resuscitation: attitudes of staff on a paediatric intensive care unit. Intensive Crit Care Nurs 14:p3–7, 1998

Kouwenhoven W, Jude JR, Knickerbocker GG: Closed chest cardiac massage. JAMA 173:1064–1067, 1960

Lewis JK, Minter MG, Eshelman SJ, Witte MK: Outcome of pediatric resuscitation. Ann Emerg Med 12:297, 1983

Omnibus Budget Reconciliation Act of 1986 (OBRA), Public Law 99-509, October 21, 1986

Otto CW: Airway management and ventilation during CPR. Acta Anaesthesiol Scand Suppl 111:52–54, 1997

Thel MC, O'Connor CM: Cardiopulmonary resuscitation: historical perspective to recent investigations. Am Heart J 137:39–48, 1999

Uniform Determination of Death Act. Uniform Laws annotated. (West Supp.) Title 12, 320–323, 1990

Weston CF, Wilson RJ, Jones SD: Predicting survival from out-of-hospital cardiac arrest: a multivariate analysis. Resuscitation 34:27–34, 1997

Young KD, Seidel JS: Pediatric cardiopulmonary resuscitation: a collective review. Ann Emerg Med 33:195–205, 1999

4.2.7 Perioperative Care

Deborah Schwengel

PREOPERATIVE CARE

The care of patients in the perioperative period has changed over recent years because surgical procedures are frequently performed without hospital admission, and when an admission is needed, stays are shorter. At the same time, procedures have gained in complexity and are often performed in a minimally invasive way, establishing the need for creative approaches for analgesia and sedation.

Same-day surgery provides significant medical, psychological, and economic benefits to children and their families, but also creates challenges for both pediatricians and anesthesiologists to deal effectively with common postoperative problems such as pain, nausea, and vomiting. Proper preoperative screening and evaluation is critical to success of both outpatient surgery and to care of complex inpatients; children are often sent to their pediatrician or family practitioner for this assessment. That same primary care provider might also be called on to address postoperative questions or problems. Thus, the pediatrician must have knowledge of appropriate perioperative evaluation and management.

The general goals of a preoperative visit are to estimate risk based on presenting problem, proposed surgical procedure, preexistent medical problems, family history, and physical examination; to obtain indication laboratory data; to adjust treatment for a preexisting condition; to begin psychological preparation and preoperative instruction; and to communicate concerns to the surgeon or anesthesiologist.

THE PREOPERATIVE HISTORY

The preoperative evaluation involves an assessment of the child's baseline health and a discussion with the child and family about what to expect in the perioperative period. Based on the preoperative visit, the patient can be prepared for an outpatient or an inpatient procedure, and psychological preparation can begin in the pediatrician's office.

Healthy children or those with well-controlled chronic illnesses are usually reasonable candidates for outpatient surgery. Most surgeries will proceed uneventfully, but there are times that it is appropriate to delay a procedure because a chronic condition is not as well controlled as possible or because an acute illness creates unnecessary risk for an elective procedure. Some very healthy children do not require a preoperative evaluation if they have no significant medical history and if the surgical procedure is simple enough to assume that the postoperative course will be uncomplicated. However, if the patient has a chronic medical condition or will be having complex surgery, a preoperative examination should be sought, and preoperative testing or medication might be required to make the patient fit enough for the proposed surgery.

When a primary care provider is requested to perform a preoperative assessment, several components of the evaluation are of special importance. Essential components are responses to previous anesthetics; family history of anesthetic problems; examination of the airway; history of breathing problems; assessment of circulation; and estimation of bleeding risk. It is of paramount importance that chronic disorders are as well controlled as possible prior to undergoing anesthesia.

An easy way to include the pertinent components of the preoperative history and physical examination is to follow a systems approach and to use a checklist (Fig. 4-26). Most departments of anesthesiology will share their preoperative evaluation form with regional doctors' offices.

EXAMINATION

Each body system should be examined in enough detail to reveal possible perioperative problems. The patient's weight, body habitus, and vital signs are of first importance. Both cachectic and obese patients have increased perioperative risk. Evidence of neurologic deficits, increased work-of-breathing, abnormal heart sounds, impaired systemic perfusion, and abdominal organomegaly or masses should be specifically noted. New abnormalities should initiate further workup. The extent of the patient's exercise endurance should be evaluated if there are abnormalities of the cardiopulmonary systems.

An appropriate airway exam includes measurements of oral excursion and thyromental distance, evaluation of dentition, assessment of neck flexion and extension, and the Mallampati examination. The Mallampati examination is an account of the pharyngeal structures visible through an open mouth and is related to the ease with which the vocal cords can be viewed with laryngoscope (Fig. 4-27). Patients are graded as easy or grade 1 if the uvula is visible; as grade 2 if the uvula is not visible but the soft palate and the faucial pillars are seen; as difficult or grade 3 if only the soft palate is visible; and as most difficult or grade 4 if only the hard palate is visible. It is less important to remember the exact Mallampati class than to fully describe which of the pharyngeal structures are visible on the preoperative examination. This examination requires a cooperative patient who can sit up and protrude the tongue without vocalizing, and not all children are able to comply. When examining young children or infants, look for features suggestive of a normal airway: a mouth that opens widely, a chin that is normally prominent (and not micrognathic), and a neck that moves easily.

LABORATORY TESTING OR IMAGING

Both the patient's medical condition and the proposed surgical procedure help to determine whether preoperative laboratory, imaging, or other diagnostic investigations are necessary (see Table 4-20). Healthy patients having minimally invasive surgery do not need laboratory testing before surgery because the data do not alter perioperative outcomes. Moreover, preoperative chest radiographs, urinalyses, and electrocardiography add unnecessary expense to the preoperative evaluation and are of uncertain value. The use of preoperative complete blood count is also questionable except when significant blood loss at surgery is anticipated; the amount of blood loss in most minor surgeries is usually negligible, and the incidence of undetected anemia in children having elective surgery is as low as 0.29%. Sickle cell screening is prudent in any African-American

Preanesthesia Assessment

Patient: **Date:**
Procedure: **Diagnosis:**
Medications/Dose: **Allergies:**
Last Oral Intake:

Previous Anesthetic Experience: **Fears/Concerns Expressed:**

History (mark Y or N)	
Neonatal History	**Anesthesia Issues**
Prematurity	Difficult Airway
Congenital Abnormalities	Snoring/Stridor/Croup
Apnea	Family History
Other	Malignant Hyperthermia
Cardiovascular	**Pulmonary**
CHD	Asthma
Hypertension	BPD
Arrhythmia	Other
SBE Prophylaxis	
	Neurologic
Renal	Seizure
Renal Failure	Elevated ICP
Other	Neuromuscular Disorder
	Other
Endocrine	
Diabetes	**Hematologic**
Other	Sickle Cell
	Coagulopathy
Gastrointestinal/Hepatic	Previous Transfusion
GE Reflux	Accept Transfusion
Hepatitis	
Other	

Explanation of Abnormalities:

Physical Examination				Laboratory Data
Age	Gender			
Wt	Ht			
BP	HR	R	T	
Other				
Mallampati: I II III IV				**ASA Status:** P1 P2 P3 P4 P5 P6

FIGURE 4-26   Elements of a preanesthesia assessment.

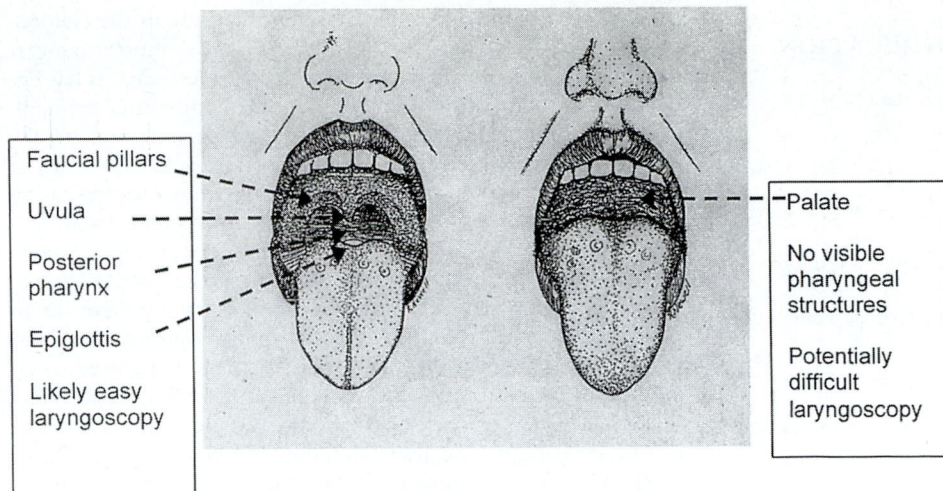

Faucial pillars

Uvula

Posterior pharynx

Epiglottis

Likely easy laryngoscopy

Palate

No visible pharyngeal structures

Potentially difficult laryngoscopy

FIGURE 4-27 The Mallampati examination of the airway. Figure on the *left* shows visible faucial pillars, the soft palate, and the uvula (grade 1). No pharyngeal structures are visible on the *right* (grade 4).

infant that has not already been screened for sickle cell anemia. Preoperative pregnancy tests should be obtained for a teenager or young adult female patient because anesthetics increase the risk of abortion and teratogenicity, and because pregnancy increases the woman's risk of pulmonary aspiration. The primary caregiver is the ideal person to broach the subject of possible pregnancy and to obtain the test. Patients with chronic medical conditions or known laboratory abnormalities or those patients who are taking medications with the potential to alter laboratory values should have preoperative laboratory testing relative to their area of risk. Thus, two factors determine the value of laboratory testing in apparently healthy patients: risks related to an undetected condition (eg, sickle cell trait, pregnancy) and risks related to the surgery (eg, anticipated bleeding).

Sleep studies prior to adenotonsillectomy in patients with suspected obstructive sleep apnea (OSA) are controversial. Patients with moderate to severe OSA need to be admitted postoperatively. Some insurance companies require a sleep study to qualify for a postoperative inpatient stay. Several studies have evaluated patient risk of postoperative respiratory difficulty following adenotonsillectomy, and they suggest postoperative monitoring except in mild OSA.

MANAGEMENT OF MEDICATIONS

Whether a medication is continued through the perioperative period or suspended is a matter to be decided for each patient. Most patients will tolerate the effects of anesthesia better if their chronic medical problem is well controlled. However, if a drug is known to have specific interactions with anesthetic agents or sympathomimetic agents, or if it will potentially cause an increase in intraoperative or postoperative bleeding, then it might be prudent to stop the drug preoperatively. Nonessential medications, especially diet and herbal drugs, that might have unknown interactions with anesthetic drugs should be stopped before surgery. Some patients need to have medications added to prepare them for surgery and anesthesia. Diabetics usually need adjustment of their insulin on the morning of surgery because of the preoperative fasting. The proposed duration of fasting and intraoperative management of the blood sugar determines the insulin regimen. Patients for tonsillectomy should usually have aspirin or nonsteroidal anti-inflammatory drugs (NSAIDs) withheld for several days preoperatively to reduce the risk of bleeding. Patients taking Coumadin might need to discontinue it and receive temporary treatment with a heparin until several hours before surgery, depending on their risk of thrombosis preoperatively. Patients taking mood-altering drugs might be at risk of altered reactions (eg, MAO inhibitors) with indirect-acting sympathomimetic drugs such as ephedrine. MAO inhibitors should be stopped 2 weeks prior to surgery. However, if a patient's risk of suicide is too high without the MAO inhibitor, the drug should be continued and the anesthesiologist consulted to establish a plan preoperatively.

ANESTHETIC RISK ASSESSMENT

To prepare patients and their families emotionally for a planned surgery an initial determination of risk is necessary. The risk of an-

TABLE 4-20
GUIDELINES FOR PREOPERATIVE LABORATORY TESTING

PATIENT CONDITION	SEVERITY OF SURGERY	SUGGESTED TESTS
Healthy	Minor	None
Healthy	Major	CBC, T&C, PT/PTT
Sick or potentially sick	Minor	Applicable to known disorder; ie, electrolytes if renal failure or on diuretics or digitalis, liver enzymes and PT/PTT if liver disease, CBC if anemic, anticonvulsant levels if on anticonvulsants, theophylline level if on theophylline, etc.
Sick	Major	CBC, T&C, PT/PTT, electrolytes, plus anything applicable to known disorders
Neonate	Minor or major	CBC, T&C, glucose + electrolytes, bilirubin
African-American	Minor or major	Sickle cell screen if never done
Menstruating female	Minor or major	Pregnancy test

CBC, complete blood count; T&C, type and crossmatch; PT/PTT, prothrombin time/partial thromboplastin time.

TABLE 4-21

THE ASA PHYSICAL STATUS CLASSIFICATION SYSTEM

P1	A normal healthy patient
P2	A patient with mild systemic disease
P3	A patient with severe systemic disease
P4	A patient with severe systemic disease that is a constant threat to life
P5	A moribund patient who is not expected to survive without the operation
P6	A declared brain-dead patient whose organs are being removed for donor purposes

esthesia and surgery depends on the health of the child coupled with the degree of difficulty of the surgery. Nevertheless, the risk of death under anesthesia is very small even in children undergoing complex surgery. Between 1978 and 1982, mortality for children less than age 15 years was 1 in 40,000 in France. An American study reported a mortality rate of 0.9 in 10,000 anesthetics during the period 1969 to 1983. The rate of complications is highest in the youngest patients; cardiac arrest was usually due to complications of airway management including laryngospasm, difficult intubation, or aspiration of gastric contents. Infants less than 1 month of age have the greatest risk of cardiac arrest and perioperative death because they are often sicker and are more likely to be having major or emergent surgery.

A system of stratifying patients according to their preoperative physical condition is used by anesthesiologists to describe the patient's baseline and may be used to define relative risk (Table 4-21). The main problem of this classification system is that it does not account for the risk of the surgery itself or for the existence of multiple diseases.

PSYCHOLOGICAL PREPARATION

Frequently the normal stress of an impending surgery is increased by parental anxieties, exposure to an unfamiliar environment, needle-phobia, waiting, fasting, fear of separation from the parent, and previous stressful experiences in the hospital or doctor's office. In contrast to inpatient procedures, outpatient surgery may cause fewer disruptions in sleep patterns, less developmental regression, fewer behavioral problems, and less nocturnal enuresis. Behavioral benefits have been demonstrated in children who were given an interactive book to prepare for surgery. A sensitive, honest, and factual conversation might be very useful in preparing the child and the parent, who has fears and anxieties that are commonly transmitted to the child. The content of the conversation with the child should be geared to the child's developmental level and psychological state. Children between 2 and 6 years of age are five times more likely to have preoperative anxiety reactions than are older children, whose reactions probably relate to the child's lack of familiarity with the place and the plan and to fears of separation from the child's parents. School-aged children may have fears of mutilation or torture, and in many age groups, needles are a major focus of anxiety. Consequently, eliminating unnecessary preoperative blood testing, if possible, might help to decrease fears. The pediatrician will be able to allay fears and put a positive spin on the events to come, but will not have control over the quality of the relationship between the child and the hospital personnel or the style of the anesthetic induction. In one study, mothers were the best predictors of behavioral distress in their children, and a history of previous

surgery was also predictive of the level of anxiety in the children studied. The study also showed that anxiety was most intense at the time of induction of inhalational (mask) anesthesia. It has become quite common for anesthesiologists to administer premedications that help to promote anxiolysis and amnesia prior to the induction of anesthesia. Also, many institutions have policies of allowing parents to accompany their children into the operating room. Some anesthesiologists maintain that parental presence decreases or eliminates the need for premedication; however, no two situations are alike in terms of parental anxiety and patient preparation. Common sense dictates evaluation of each patient on an individual basis and administration of premedications when indicated, especially when the child's parents suggest the need to do so. The medications available allow enough flexibility and safety that the clinician can offer preoperative sedation or anxiolysis to almost any patient. The available routes of administration offer an acceptable choice to most children. One of the drugs commonly used by anesthesiologists is midazolam because it provides reliable anxiolysis, some sedation, and amnesia in many patients to whom it is given.

Parents and patients should be told that there are several options for inducing anesthesia, including inhalational and IV induction techniques. It might be possible for the patient to choose how the patient wants to go to sleep, but in some situations, the patient's state of health might dictate the route of induction. Consequently, it is best not to promise a style of induction but simply to state that the anesthesiologist will probably be able to offer several choices on the day of surgery.

FASTING REQUIREMENTS FOR THE PREOPERATIVE PATIENT

Pulmonary aspiration of gastric contents is a dreaded complication of anesthesia. For many years, 8 hours was considered the standard fasting time, but this recommendation has been revised to take into account the fact that patient age and the composition of food or drink influence the speed of gastric emptying. The relationship between gastric emptying and fasting times is not uniformly predictable; however, ingestion of clear liquids up to 2 to 4 hours preoperatively decreases gastric volume in comparison with fasting for 8 hours (Table 4-22). More liberal intake of clear liquids might additionally increase gastric pH. Consequently, there is now fairly uniform agreement that clear liquids can be given up to 2 hours preoperatively in infants and up to 4 hours preoperatively in older children and adults. The duration of withholding breast milk and infant formulas is more controversial. Foods with particulate natures are likely to cause more pulmonary injury than clear liquids,

TABLE 4-22

FASTING GUIDELINES FOR THE HEALTHY PREOPERATIVE PATIENT

TYPE OF FOOD	AGE OF PATIENT	FASTING GUIDELINE
Clear liquids (last drink not more than 8 oz)	Infant to adult	2–4 hours
Breast milk	Infant	4 hours
Nonhuman milk	Infant	6 hours
Solids	All ages	8 hours

Note: These guidelines may not represent the opinions of every anesthesiologist, nor will they be appropriate for every patient.

and fat-containing foods slow gastric emptying. Nevertheless, most studies show that gastric emptying is faster following human breast milk meals than cow's milk formula; most recommendations for fasting therefore grant a shorter fasting interval for patients receiving breast milk than for those fed infant formulas. Fasting for solid foods is typically for 8 hours, although some anesthesiologists believe that a light carbohydrate such as toast or crackers can be given 6 hours prior to the induction of anesthesia. There is insufficient evidence to establish an absolute safe fasting time for the intake of nonhuman milk or solid foods. It is important to emphasize that some patients (eg, those with symptomatic gastroesophageal reflux; dysphagia; esophageal dysmotility; delayed gastric emptying as in diabetes mellitus; pregnancy; chronic renal failure) might require stricter fasting rules than the healthy patient.

ACUTE AND CHRONIC MEDICAL PROBLEMS

Allergy

A history of drug or food allergy should be elicited. Frequently, patients are wrongly labeled as having drug allergies when they have had a history of acute drug side effects, for example, "red-man's syndrome" is common when vancomycin is given too quickly.

Food allergies can be important clues to latex allergy. Patients who are allergic to latex are often intolerant of tropical foods including bananas, kiwi, avocado, and chestnuts. Patients with latex allergy also often have a history of atopy, and the parents might be able to relate stories of hives or swelling after contact with rubber balloons or other natural rubber products. The incidence of latex allergy in the general population is about 8%, but it is much higher in patients sensitized to latex; for example, in patients with spina bifida, the rate ranges from 34 to 64.5%. Factors that influence the risk of becoming allergic to latex include spina bifida; bladder exstrophy; multiple ventriculoperitoneal shunts; multiple operations; history of atopy; and multiple exposure to latex in infancy. The role of preoperative pharmacologic preparation, including desensitization, corticosteroids, or antihistamines, is not well established, even in patients with histories of anaphylaxis. Such preparation has been reported in isolated cases, but because pretreatment has never been shown to prevent IgE-mediated allergic reactions and because pretreatment might mask early signs of anaphylaxis, its use is generally not recommended. The role for preoperative allergy testing is also controversial. Whether the patient is tested and found allergic or not, the best strategy for treating the patient at risk is latex avoidance. Because latex is ubiquitous both within and outside the hospital, vigilance is required to avoid exposing the sensitized patient. Patients with spina bifida, bladder exstrophy, or a history of multiple surgical procedures should be considered at risk for latex allergy and should be treated in a latex-safe environment in the operating room, the doctor's office, and at home. Extremely allergic patients and health-care workers have had anaphylactic reactions simply while in a room where removal of latex gloves have caused aerosolization of latex particles. Powdered latex gloves lead to the highest aerosolized antigen levels in operating rooms. More information can be obtained online at *ww.cdc.gov/niosh/latexalt.html.*

Inherited Reactions to Anesthetics

Patients must be questioned about their response to prior anesthetics. Perioperative difficulties usually relate to nausea and vomiting. It is not unusual for families to have histories of elderly family members having intraoperative problems, but such problems are usually related to preexisting cardiac or pulmonary diseases and usually do not raise the risk of the pediatric relative. Occasionally, a family history of anesthetic problems will reveal a serious risk related to malignant hyperthermia, muscular dystrophy, or pseudocholinesterase deficiency.

Malignant hyperthermia is a rare clinical syndrome triggered by anesthetic medications and neuromuscular blocker. Its hallmark is uncontrolled skeletal muscle activity. Susceptible individuals can have life-threatening reactions resulting in mortality as high as 70% before the availability of dantrolene. With the advent of newer anesthetic drugs, nontriggering agents can be chosen and the at-risk patient safely anesthetized, but the patient must first be identified as malignant hyperthermia susceptible. Dantrolene is used to rescue patients once an episode is suspected. Initially malignant hyperthermia was thought to be autosomal dominant, a pattern most commonly observed in this disorder. However, it is more genetically complex than once thought, and several genetic loci are linked to this disorder. Anyone with a positive family history (unless proven negative by muscle biopsy or genetic testing), personal history, or an associated neuromuscular disorder is at risk, although there is considerable uncertainty about which neuromuscular disorders place the patient at risk. Central core disease, the King-Denborough syndrome, and Duchenne muscular dystrophy patients are considered high-risk individuals. Other myopathic disorders place the patient at high risk of anesthetic complications in general and at the risk of hyperkalemic cardiac arrest if succinylcholine is used, but there is usually not an increased risk of malignant hyperthermia.

Pseudocholinesterase deficiency is an autosomal recessive disorder that can result in prolonged neuromuscular blockade from succinylcholine or mivacurium. These drugs usually have a brief duration of action because they are normally rapidly hydrolyzed by pseudocholinesterase. When pseudocholinesterase is genetically abnormal, the duration of paralysis can exceed 6 hours. When not known preoperatively, this problem is not life-threatening, but it will require an unanticipated period of postoperative mechanical ventilation after succinylcholine or mivacurium administration.

Birth History and Congenital Abnormalities

Many premature infants or former premature infants need to have surgical procedures in the first year of life, and a history of their neonatal course and assessment of their current state of health should be obtained. If the patient had a prolonged course of mechanical ventilation in the neonatal intensive care unit, a history of subglottic stenosis should be sought or investigated. Concerning signs include stridor, recurrent episodes of "croup," and dyspnea with feedings (diaphoresis, tachypnea, head bobbing and retracting). Patients with signs of airway obstruction should be evaluated by an otolaryngologist prior to the planned surgical date.

A significant problem faced by the premature or former premature infant is postoperative apnea. This problem has been well documented, but there is uncertainty about how long a former premature infant is at risk for apnea after anesthesia, and interpretation of studies is difficult because of differences in the definition of apnea, small sample sizes, differences in anesthetic techniques, and differences in surgical procedures. Apnea has been described in a few infants as old as 55 to 60 postconceptional weeks, but infants younger than 46 postconception weeks have the greatest risk. Although term infants have a much lower incidence of postoperative apnea, the risk is not zero. Unfortunately, pneumocardiograms fail to predict which infants will have postoperative apnea. In premature infants younger than 42 postconception weeks, prolonged postoperative apneic episodes occurred in 62% of those studied. Some of the apnea episodes are not easily resolved and mechanical ventilation is required, although caffeine has decreased risk of postoperative apnea in formerly premature infants. Spinal or other regional anesthetics have been suggested as superior alternatives to general anesthesia in order to reduce the risk of postoperative apnea, but spinal anesthesia techniques do not eliminate the risk. Most pediatric anesthesiologists admit all high-risk patients for overnight monitoring after anesthesia regardless of the anesthetic technique used. Whenever possible, elective surgery should be postponed until the former premature infant is older than 50 weeks postconception.

Patients with trisomy 21 have a high risk of perioperative problems related to hypotonia, large tongues, and risk of obstructive sleep apnea, and congenital heart disease. They also have a 10 to 20% incidence of cervical spine instability. Flexion and extension neck films have been used to predict atlantooccipital instability; however, cervical spine films are considered by some to be unreliable identifiers of symptomatic atlantoaxial subluxation, and many patients are too young to perform flexion and extension films. Once recommended by the American Academy of Pediatrics (AAP) to determine sports participation, the value of routine cervical spine films is now considered uncertain. In the preoperative patient with trisomy 21, screening x-rays should be done on symptomatic patients or those about to undergo surgical procedures in which the neck will be extended or rotated, such as adenotonsillectomy or suspension microlaryngoscopy. Structural heart disease occurs in 40 to 50% of patients with trisomy 21. If a screening echocardiogram was not done in the neonatal period, one should be done preoperatively.

Cardiovascular System

Cardiac disorders should always be investigated because many anesthetic agents have negative inotropic effects, decrease systemic vascular resistance, or cause dysrhythmias. A history of exercise intolerance, respiratory difficulty, diaphoresis, and cyanosis during feeding, or failure to thrive can be an indication of significant cardiac disease. History of or presence of abnormal heart rate or rhythm, syncope, myocarditis, cardiomyopathy, significant anthracycline exposure especially with irradiation of the chest, or previous cardiac surgery should be evaluated by a pediatric cardiologist. Cardiac murmurs in healthy preschool or school-aged children usually do not need to be investigated unless an aspect of the history and physical examination suggests a cardiac defect (see Sec. 22.2.1). Finally, patients at risk of subacute bacterial endocarditis should be identified to receive prophylactic antibiotics (see Sec. 13.1.10 for guidelines).

Respiratory System

The respiratory system plays a fundamental role in the delivery and recovery from anesthesia. All general anesthetic agents alter airway reflexes, the drive to breathe, lung volumes, airway tone, and mucociliary clearance. Patients with chronic lung disease or neuromuscular disorders should be expected to have a transient decrease in respiratory function. Parents should be warned that the patient with chronic lung disease having major surgery might be intubated and mechanically ventilated in the postoperative period. Asthma is the most common chronic illness of childhood, with an estimated prevalence of 8.6 to 12.7%, and many children with asthma need to be anesthetized. Preoperative pulmonary function testing is not

necessary in the known asthmatic unless used to optimize the drug regimen in the patient with severe disease. When not properly prepared for surgery, the asthmatic patient can develop bronchospasm upon tracheal intubation. Fortunately, well-prepared asthmatic patients usually have uncomplicated intraoperative courses. It is recommended that all preoperative treatments be continued through the morning of surgery. Many anesthesiologists will administer a nebulized β-agonist before inducing anesthesia in asthmatic patients who do not routinely use β-agonists. Although there is no consensus, use of oral steroids, 1 mg/kg/d of methylprednisolone for 3 days preoperatively, is a practical means for reducing risk of airflow obstruction during surgery. This practice does not appear to have an increased risk of adrenocortical crisis, impaired wound healing, or postoperative infections in adults. Asthmatic children with exacerbations of their asthma or with upper respiratory tract infections (URIs) should have elective surgical procedures delayed for 3 to 6 weeks.

Infants with bronchopulmonary dysplasia (BPD) should have their pulmonary status fully optimized by continuing usual medications and by possibly increasing or adding β-agonists and corticosteroids, as in the asthmatic patient. Parents of these children should be prepared for an inpatient stay and perhaps a period of postoperative intubation and mechanical ventilation.

Children commonly present for surgery with a concurrent URI. Most children under age 2 average 5 to 10 URIs per year and might not have a healthy period in which to schedule a surgical procedure. Children who attend daycare or who have a chronic illness might have an even greater likelihood of having a current or recent URI. There are variable points of view about the risk of airway and pulmonary complications in children with current or recent URIs. Some studies show a greater risk of laryngospasm, bronchospasm, intraoperative or postoperative desaturation, or unspecified airway obstructive complications, whereas other studies fail to demonstrate any increased risk in children with URIs undergoing myringotomy. In most of the available studies, problems encountered under anesthesia were deemed easily managed and therefore did not pose significant threats to the patients, despite the many theoretical concerns. The question then is which patients should have their procedure canceled in the face of a URI (Table 4-23). Many pediatric anesthesiologists agree that procedures on the febrile or ill-appearing child should be canceled. In addition, anyone with wheezing, crackles, or other abnormal chest sounds suggestive of a chest infection should have their procedure canceled. It may also be prudent to cancel if the patient has purulent nasal drainage. It is reasonable for major surgeries, especially those involving the cardiopulmonary systems, to apply a lower threshold for cancelation. However, surgeries treating recurrent infections of the upper airway, such as adenotonsillectomies and myringotomies, may never proceed if the same stringent criteria are applied because the child always appears to be ill. If the abnormal findings are part of the patient's baseline disorder, such as purulent nasal drainage or abnormal chest sounds in the patient with cystic fibrosis, the procedure should probably proceed. In conclusion, each patient situation must be evaluated individually, and prudence would suggest a discussion with the anesthesiologist if it were not clear whether the procedure should proceed as planned.

Children with mild OSA uncomplicated by comorbid conditions have improved airway function postoperatively and do not need intensive monitoring and can possibly have an outpatient procedure. Postoperative admission is recommended for children under 3 years of age because of a high risk of airway obstruction. Some

TABLE 4-23

PREOPERATIVE DECISION-MAKING FOR THE CHILD WITH AN UPPER AIRWAY INFECTION

PATIENT	CLINICAL MANIFESTATIONS	SURGERY	DECISION
Normal	Simple - Afebrile - Feels well - No abnormal chest sounds	Minor - Brief and minimally invasive	Likely to proceed with or without endotracheal intubation
		Major - Intracavitary, long duration, significant blood loss expected	Lower threshold for cancelation if prone or postoperative endotracheal intubation a risk
		Emergent	Proceed
Normal	Complicated - Febrile - Purulent rhinorrhea - Abnormal chest sounds - Symptoms of croup	Minor - Brief and minimally invasive	Likely cancelation, especially if endotracheal intubation required
		Major - Intracavitary, long duration, significant blood loss expected	Cancel
		Emergent	Proceed, but expect problems
Chronic illness	Simple - Afebrile - Feels well - No abnormal chest sounds	Minor - Brief and minimally invasive	Lower threshold for cancelation, especially if intubation required. If patient has asthma, cancel unless preoperative steroids have been given
		Major - Intracavitary, long duration, significant blood loss expected	Cancel
		Emergent	Delay if possible to improve baseline with medications; expect problems if procedure must go on
Chronic illness	Complicated - Febrile - Purulent rhinorrhea - Abnormal chest sounds - Croup	Minor - Brief and minimally invasive	Cancel
		Major - Intracavitary, long duration, significant blood loss expected	Cancel
		Emergent	Delay if possible to improve baseline with medications; expect problems if procedure must be performed

children with very severe OSA will have pulmonary hypertension and cor pulmonale as a result of long-standing hypoxemia and hypercarbia. High-risk children should have a preoperative hematocrit and HCO_3^- measured, and those suspected to have secondary cardiac disease should be evaluated to determine the significance. Snoring and difficulty breathing are clinical hallmarks of OSA in children; unlike adults, daytime somnolence is not present in the majority of these patients. Polysomnography can be helpful for differentiating obstructive from central apneas and identifying severity of disease.

Endocrine System

Diabetes mellitus can be managed in a number of different ways, and it is valuable to consult with the anesthesiologist to determine the patient's fasting time. When possible, the operation should be planned to start early in the day to avoid a prolonged fast. Diabetic patients are often given only a portion of their usual insulin dose in the morning, with plans to monitor blood glucose levels intraoperatively and given insulin accordingly, either intermittently or

as a continuous infusion. A common regimen is to give half of the usual morning NPH insulin and no regular insulin.

Adrenal insufficiency requires the administration of stress steroid doses that can be administered in the operating room. Contrary to common belief, chronic glucocorticoid treatment is not an absolute indication for stress dosing preoperatively. Recent information suggests that the dosing of stress steroids should be graded according to the duration of steroid use, daily dose, and magnitude of the proposed surgical stress. This means that patients having minor surgery coupled with a history of low-dose glucocorticoid requirements probably only need a single preoperative steroid dose or none at all. Daily steroid users requiring major surgery should receive true stress doses perioperatively. Patients with Addison disease or congenital adrenal hyperplasia need complete stress steroid replacement beginning preoperatively and extending 2 to 3 days into the postoperative period.

Patients with diabetes insipidus should receive their usual doses of DDAVP. They should also be given clear fluids by mouth (up to 2–4 hours preoperatively; see fasting guidelines in Table 4-22) to help ensure an adequate intravascular volume.

Renal and Hepatic Systems

For patients on dialysis it is important to ensure that serum electrolytes are near normal and that intravascular volume is not significantly reduced or expanded. For patients with liver disease, hepatocellular enzymes and prothrombin time should be assessed preoperatively, and possibly postoperatively, because anesthetics and many surgical procedures reduce hepatic blood flow, and liver function can worsen.

Gastrointestinal System

Patients with a history of hiatal hernia or gastroesophageal reflux are at increased risk for aspiration of gastric contents during induction of anesthesia. Accordingly, the preoperative fasting period should be observed particularly carefully in these patients, continuing the use of antireflux and antacid medications if any are being used. The anesthesiologist must be made aware of the existence of easy reflux not only to adapt the induction technique (avoiding the use of mask ventilation or of medications that may result in vomiting before tracheal cannulation) but also because chronic aspiration may cause airway and lung parenchymal abnormalities relevant to the care of the patient during and after the surgery.

Hematologic System

A history of a coagulopathy such as easy bruising should be elicited. Drugs that cause platelet dysfunction should be withheld for 5 to 10 days before surgery with a risk of intraoperative or postoperative bleeding. It is helpful to acknowledge previous blood transfusions and a history of transfusion reactions. A discussion of the likelihood of transfusion is mandatory for major procedures. The risks of transfusion (see Sec. 19.11) should be discussed with the parents if they are anxious, even though these details will be covered in the discussion with the anesthesiologist. It is increasingly common for parents to request direct donation of blood before surgery. Although it is a good practice to honor this request when possible, direct donation procedures often require extra time and expense. Autologous donation is possible for some teenagers preparing for major surgery, but many weeks of preparation are required, especially if more than one unit is needed. The child will need iron therapy and time to replace the lost red cells.

Patients with sickle cell anemia are at high risk of perioperative complications. Hypovolemia, hypothermia, hypotension, hypoxemia or regional hypoxia, and acidosis may precipitate sickling crises. In addition, many older patients with sickle cell disease have baseline organ dysfunction manifested as baseline hypoxemia, heart failure, neurologic deficits, decreased glomerular filtration rate, or tubular dysfunction, and sometimes hepatocellular failure. It has long been felt that any patient with sickle cell disease, unless having the most minor surgery, should receive some preoperative transfusion, but recent studies with transfusion that raised hemoglobins to 10 g/dL were as successful in preventing perioperative complications as the more aggressive regimens that reduced the percentage of hemoglobin S to less than 30%. The extent of preexisting disease and the severity of proposed surgery should be factored into the plan for preparing the patient. The authors of recent studies that demonstrate silent cerebral infarcts and psychometric abnormalities in children with sickle cell disease advocate baseline therapeutic intervention, including a hematocrit of more than 27%.

Central Nervous System

Disorders of the central nervous system can result in abnormalities of respiration, poor pharyngeal muscle tone, or an inability to maintain or protect the airway. Seizures should be controlled and recent anticonvulsant levels obtained. Patients with neuromuscular disorders should be at their best possible baseline state. If they are prone to atelectasis or to recurrent pulmonary infections, pulmonary toilet should be maximized preoperatively and antibiotics used if indicated. Significantly weak patients usually require postoperative mechanical ventilation and need aggressive pulmonary toilet. These patients should have their procedures delayed if an intercurrent infection develops in the days preoperatively. Any patient with changes in mental status should be urgently evaluated.

POSTOPERATIVE MANAGEMENT

Postoperative nausea and vomiting are common problems in pediatric patients, and those having strabismus, ear surgery, herniorrhaphy, or orchiopexy are at particular risk. Opioids can induce nausea or vomiting, but pain also delays gastric emptying and can lead to vomiting. Vomiting can be severe and persist after discharge from the surgical area, although hospital admissions are rarely necessary. Postoperative vomiting usually does not persist beyond the first postoperative day, and therefore dehydration is uncommon. However, persistent vomiting may preclude oral pain medications from being effective. In the early postoperative period, nonsedating antiemetics, the serotonin antagonists (such as ondansetron), are favored as the first-line of treatment. Although expensive, these medications have no substantial side effects. Droperidol is an effective antiemetic and antinausea drug, but it is very sedating and produces marked dysphoria in some patients. Phenothiazines are sometimes effective when the serotonin antagonists have failed to control nausea and vomiting, but they are sedating and can cause extrapyramidal reactions. The glucocorticoids also have antiemetic effects and seem to be most effective when used in combination with a serotonin antagonist. When treating a postoperative patient with nausea and vomiting, it is important to reassure the patient and family that the problem usually resolves within 24 hours. Pharmacologic treatment is used in conjunction with dietary instructions; patients should limit intake of solids and should ingest electrolyte-containing clear liquids. If pain management is problematic, rectal antiemetics and analgesics can be considered. Patients having persistent vomiting might need a change in pain or other drug regimens; codeine is a common cause of vomiting. Frequent or prolonged postoperative vomiting requires additional investigation and treatment.

Emergence delirium is a short-term alteration that occurs sometimes during the recovery from anesthesia. Behavioral problems are quite common after surgery, although most common after overnight hospitalization. Patients may be sleepier than normal but should be easily arousable. Any concern about a decline in mental status is not explainable by an outpatient anesthetic and therefore needs to be evaluated like any other decline in mental status.

References

Hackmann T, Steward DJ, Sheps SB: Anemia in pediatric day-surgery patients: prevalence and detection. Anesthesiology 75:27, 1991

Keenan RL, Boyan CP: Cardiac arrest due to anesthesia: a study of incidence and causes. JAMA 253:2373, 1985

Kinney TR, Sleeper LA, Wang WC, et al: Silent cerebral infarcts in sickle cell anemia: a risk factor analysis. The Cooperative Study of Sickle Cell Disease. Pediatrics 103:640–645, 1999

Kurth CD, Spitzer AR, Broennie AM, Downes JJ: Postoperative apnea in preterm infants. Anesthesiology 66:483–488, 1987

Mallampati SR, Gatt SP, Gugino LD, et al: A clinical sign to predict difficult tracheal intubation: a prospective study. Can Anaesth Soc J 32:429–434, 1985

Niggemann B, Buck D, Michael T, Wahn U: Latex provocation tests in patients with spina bifida: who is at risk of becoming symptomatic? J Allergy Clin Immunol 102:665–670, 1998

O'Connor ME, Drasner K: Preoperative laboratory testing of children undergoing elective surgery. Anesth Analg 70:176–180, 1990

Tait AR, Knight PR: Intraoperative respiratory complications in patients with upper respiratory tract infections. Can J Anaesth 34:300–303, 1987

Tiret L, Nivoche Y, Natton F, et al: Complications related to anaesthesia in infants and children: a prospective survey of 40,240 anaesthetics. Br J Anaesth 61:263, 1988

Vichinsky EP, Haberkern CM, Neumayr L, et al: A comparison of conservative and aggressive transfusion regimens in the perioperative management of sickle cell disease. The Preoperative Transfusion in Sickle Cell Disease Study Group. N Engl J Med 333:206–219, 1995

Welborn LG, DeSoto H, Nannallah RS, et al: The use of caffeine in the control of post-anesthetic apnea in former premature infants. Anesthesiology 68:796–798, 1988

4.2.8   Pain Management

Deborah Schwengel

Increased attention is being paid to the recognition and control of pain in children, especially infants. In addition to the moral imperative to treat pain, the stress response to pain may itself be detrimental to patient outcomes. It is safe to provide potent analgesics to even the youngest pediatric patient when proper safeguards are used. Patient- (or parent) controlled analgesia (PCA) and indwelling epidural catheters with local anesthetic infusions are now commonplace and should be considered the current standard of care for acute management of either severe medical or surgical pain. Most patients with acute pain have relief with one drug or a combination of drugs when administration is timely and doses are appropriate. Management of chronic pain is more complex and may require a multifaceted approach that includes PCA, epidural infusions, nerve blocks, and adjuvant drugs. Adjuvant drugs, such as anticonvulsants, antidepressants, and neuroleptic drugs, are useful for neuropathic pain and chronic pain syndromes and pain associated with depression. Alternative therapies such as acupuncture, hypnosis, and massage have been successful in reducing pain, usually in conjunction with pharmacologic therapies.

Part of the problem of treating pain in infants, young children, or nonverbal older patients is accurate assessment of what they are feeling. Assessment tools can be useful but must be used in conjunction with vital signs, facial expression, patient activity, and knowledge of the pain-inducing event and expected time-course of recovery. A number of scales have been developed to help caregivers compare the changes in the state of an infant or child during the course of care. The scales do not define how much pain a patient has; rather, they provide one convenient means to determine whether it changes with time or intervention. The cues and methods of assessment account for difference in age and types of response. Examples of some of the most common tools are as follows: Neonatal Infant Pain Scale for 0 to 1 month; Objective Pain Scale for 1 month to 3 years or for children who cannot help with self-rating; Faces scales (eg, Oucher or Wong-Baker) for >3 to 4 years old, in which the child provides the rating by comparing self to a facial expression; or a numeric scale for school-age children to young adults, in which the patient rates pain on a 1 to 10 scale.

Parents are likely to be the most accurate assessors of their child's pain; their opinions must be solicited. Parents might also be able to provide nonmedicinal comfort measures that either eliminate or decrease the need for analgesics. In addition, an overlay of fatigue, fears, or other psychosocial problems might lower the pain threshold or patient coping mechanisms. Consequently, judicious doses of anxiolytics or sleep-agents might decrease the need for analgesics.

Considering the source of pain and nature of injury, choose a drug that offers a potency commensurate with the degree of pain and a route of administration appropriate to the urgency of treatment or the ability of the patient to take medications by mouth. Pain management can be considered in a step-wise fashion of escalating potency and invasiveness (Fig. 4-28).

PAIN MANAGEMENT

Nonopioid Analgesics

The nonopioid analgesics (Table 4-24), often considered mild analgesics, may provide relief to intense pain. The nonsteroidal anti-inflammatory drugs (NSAIDs) inhibit the formation of eicosanoids from arachidonic acid. The eicosanoids are mediators of fever, inflammation, and pain (especially headache and dysmenorrhea). The original NSAIDs are nonselective inhibitors of the enzyme cyclooxygenase (COX). There are two identified COX isoenzymes: COX-1 and COX-2. COX-1 catalyzes synthesis of prostaglandins that help to regulate normal cellular activity. Inhibition of COX-1 results in GI irritation, inhibition of platelet aggregation, and renal injury. COX-2 catalyzes synthesis of prostaglandins at sites of inflammation. The new, selective COX-2-inhibitors show promise in reducing inflammation and providing analgesia while not producing the GI, platelet, and renal side effects seen with the nonselective NSAIDs. Consequently, the NSAIDs are very useful in treating pain associated with inflammation or pain directly associated with the production of prostaglandins and can be more effective than opioids in dealing with these types of pain. The side effects of these drugs include impairment of platelet aggregation and gastrointestinal irritation that can lead to ulceration and bleeding. Another side effect is impairment of osteoblastic or osteoclastic activity resulting in poor bone repair and remodeling. Aspirin can cause hypersensitivity reactions and bronchoconstriction; NSAIDs are less likely but also capable of causing bronchoconstriction in susceptible individuals.

Opioid Analgesics

There are numerous opioid agonists or agonist-antagonists in clinical use. All of the opioid drugs act at receptors in the central nervous system (Table 4-25). The opioid receptors Mu, Kappa, Delta, and Sigma produce different effects and bond selectively to different drugs. It is the pattern of receptor activation that characterizes the clinical effects produced by the various opioid drugs. The respiratory depressive effects of the opioid drugs are well known. These drugs can also cause cardiovascular depression, gastrointestinal, genitourinary, and endocrine side effects. Ideally, the opioid drugs should be titrated to effect and patients should be monitored for proper effect and signs of adverse reactions. The adverse effects depend on the drug, dose, route of administration, interaction with other drugs, and condition of the patient. A variety of conditions are commonly associated with increased risk of apnea, airway obstruction, or hypotension following administration of sedatives or opioids; these include early infancy (<42 postconception weeks in term infants or <60 weeks in preterm infants), history of apnea or

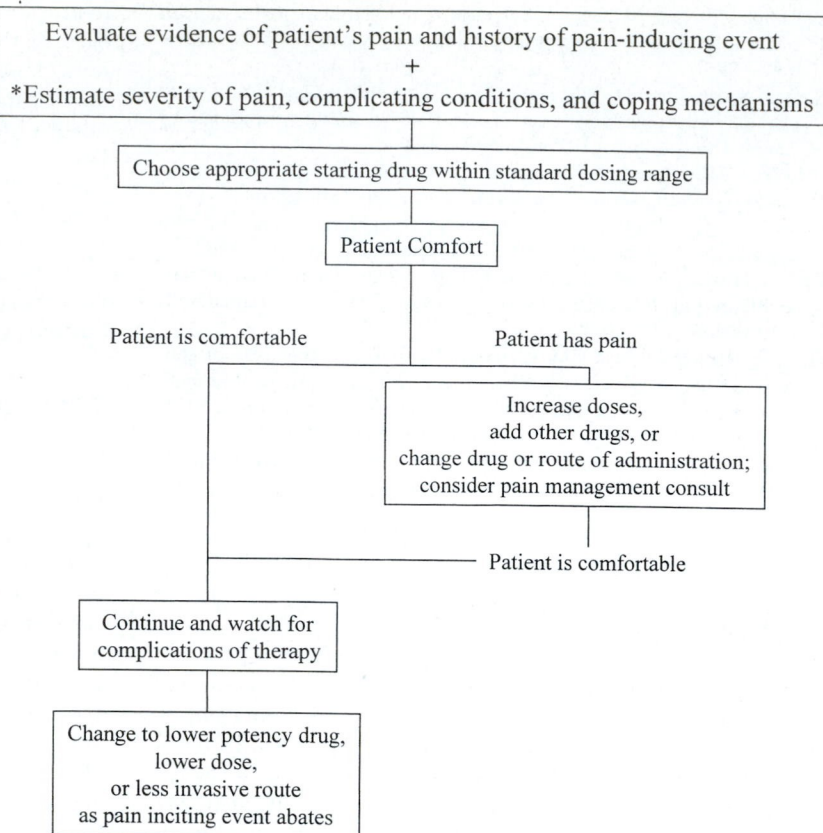

FIGURE 4-28 Algorithm for management of pain. *Possibly use one of scales for comparison of change after intervention.

airway obstruction, cardiovascular dysfunction, coma, neuromuscular disease, renal disease, or liver disease.

Pure Agonists

The pure agonists (Table 4-26) are primarily Mu agonists. At equianalgesic doses, they are all effective analgesics and they all potentially produce physical dependence, respiratory depression, bradycardia, sedation, nausea and vomiting, pruritus, urinary retention, and constipation. The side effects of the opioids can be quite bothersome, but there is often a treatment for these (Table 4-27).

Agonist-Antagonists

These drugs were originally synthesized in an effort to develop analgesics without abuse potential. Their effects depend on their CNS receptor activity (see Table 4-28). Whether a drug acts as an agonist or antagonist at a particular receptor is sometimes dose-dependent. Both the pure antagonists and the agonist-antagonists can produce withdrawal symptoms in susceptible patients.

Regional and Local Anesthetic Therapies

Local anesthetics are the only pharmacologic agents that can provide anesthesia or analgesia to a specified part of the body without producing systemic effects such as sedation. They have toxicity, however, and safe dosing is determined by the drug, its concentration, and the route used. Topical anesthetics or local infiltration of local anesthetics (field block) are applicable in many situations of injury or simple procedures such as repair of laceration, circumcision, venipuncture, and lumbar puncture. EMLA (eutectic mixture of local anesthetics) cream is an emulsion of lidocaine and prilocaine that can be used to anesthetize skin for superficial procedures.

It is very effective if applied to the treatment area at least 60 to 90 minutes prior to the procedure. Its drawback is that it causes vasoconstriction and may make venipuncture more difficult, although painless. Even without pain, children will still often cry due to fear of needles and a dislike of tourniquet placement. Care must be used when treating neonates because of risk of methemoglobinemia induced by the prilocaine component of the cream. Nevertheless, a single application is usually safe and effective in full-term newborns undergoing circumcision. Other combinations of local anesthetics can be used for laceration repair. TAC (tetracaine, adrenaline, cocaine) is an effective drug but difficult to use because the addition of cocaine makes it a controlled substance. In addition, cocaine can easily cause toxicity if applied to mucus membranes or very vascular areas. The epinephrine content makes its use contraindicated in tissues supplied by end-arteries (digits, nose, penis, pinna). It is also contraindicated in patients taking MAO inhibitors. An effective alternative to TAC is LET (lidocaine, epinephrine, tetracaine). It is designed for laceration repair but is also contraindicated for digits, nose, penis, and pinna because of its epinephrine content. LET can be mixed as a liquid or gel and is applied with a cotton-tip applicator or cotton ball. One to 3 mL is held in place for 20 to 30 minutes.

Injection of local anesthetics is quite painful but can be made significantly more comfortable by injecting slowly, using a small (27 or 30 gauge) needle, and by buffering the drug to raise the pH. Lidocaine is buffered by mixing 1 mL (1 mEq) sodium bicarbonate with 9 mL of 1% lidocaine. The buffering volumes of sodium bicarbonate used for other local anesthetics can be determined by mixing just until the combination begins to precipitate in the syringe.

Both topical application and local field block have risk of systemic toxicity, especially if an open wound, highly vascular area, or a mucous membrane is being anesthetized. Systemic local anes-

TABLE 4-24
NONOPIOID ANALGESICS

DRUG	DOSE	TYPE OF PAIN	COMMENTS
Acetaminophen	10–15 mg/kg q4–6h PO or PR Max total dose 75 mg/kg/d or 4 g/d adult dose	Mild	Toxicity: hepatic failure, dose related No anti-inflammatory effect
Aspirin	10–15 mg/kg q4–6h PO or PR Max total dose 4 g/d	Mild arthritis; rheumatoid disorders	Toxicity: acid-base, hepatitis Gastric irritation Reye syndrome risk Platelet inhibition Hypersensitivity
Choline magnesium trisalicylate	7.5–15 mg/kg q6h PO	Mild bone pain	Some gastric irritation (less than aspirin or NSAIDs) Reye syndrome risk No platelet inhibition
Diclofenac	1–1.5 mg/kg q12h PO	Powerful anti-inflammatory; bone, joint pain	Gastric irritation Elevated hepatic transaminases CNS effects
Ibuprofen	4–10 mg/kg q6h PO Max dose 40 mg/kg/d or 2400 mg/d	Stronger than acetaminophen; dysmenorrhea; rheumatoid disorders	Gastric irritation Platelet inhibition
Indomethacin	0.5 mg/kg q6h PO or 0.5–1 mg/kg q6h PR Max dose 4 mg/kg/d or 200 mg/d	Ankylosing spondylitis	Platelet inhibition Hepatitis Renal insufficiency CNS effects Promotes closure of ductus arteriosus in neonates
Ketorolac	0.5 mg/kg q6h IV/IM Max dose 120 mg/d Adults: 10 mg q6h PO or max dose 40 mg/d Do not exceed 5 days of therapy	Very potent, bone pain	Gastric irritation Platelet inhibition Nephritis Only parenteral NSAID
Naproxen	5 mg/kg q8–12h Max dose 1.5 g/d	Dysmenorrhea	Gastric irritation common Thrombocytopenia CNS effects
Tolmetin	5–7 mg/kg q6–8h Max dose 30 mg/kg/d or 2 g/d		Gastric irritation common CNS effects Hypersensitivity
Cyclooxygenase-2 inhibitors (Celecoxib, Melicoxam, Nimesulide, Vioxx)	Limited pediatric dosing information	Have been studied for arthritis and dental extractions	No significant GI side effects No reductions in platelet aggregation Unclear effect on bone repair and remodeling activity

thetic toxicity occurs immediately in the event of direct intravenous injection or is delayed in the event of intravenous diffusion of a large depot of drug. The signs of local anesthetic toxicity need to be distinguished from those of an allergic reaction. Mild toxicity causes tinnitus, headache, visual disturbances, and anxiety. Moderate toxicity causes agitation and hypotension; severe toxicity causes coma, seizures, respiratory arrest, ventricular arrhythmias, and cardiovascular collapse.

In addition to stopping the local anesthetic, the treatment of toxicity is supportive and, when resuscitation is needed, follows

TABLE 4-25
OPIOID RECEPTORS AND THEIR CLINICAL EFFECTS

RECEPTOR	CNS LOCATION	CLINICAL EFFECTS
Mu	Brain: cortex, thalamus, periaqueductal gray matter Spinal cord: substantia gelatinosa	Mu_1: cortical-level analgesia, physical dependence Mu_2: respiratory depression, decreased gastrointestinal motility, bradycardia
Kappa	Brain: hypothalamus, periaqueductal gray matter, claustrum Spinal cord: substantia gelatinosa	Spinal analgesia, sedation, inhibition of antidiuretic hormone release
Delta	Brain: pontine nucleus, amygdala, olfactory bulbs, deep cortex	Analgesia, euphoria, physical dependence
Sigma	Unknown	Dysphoria, hallucinations

TABLE 4-26

OPIOIDS AND THEIR DOSING

DRUG/CNS RECEPTOR ACTIVITY	DOSE & INDICATIONS	COMMENTS
Alfentanil Mu agonist	Anesthesia: 10–150 µg/kg IV	Short duration of action (20–30 minutes) Apnea, bradycardia common
Codeine Mu agonist	Analgesia: 1 mg/kg PO q4h	Often poorly tolerated because of nausea and vomiting Converted to morphine in the liver (10% of dose) Use with caution in renal failure
Fentanyl Mu agonist	Analgesia: • IV dosing 0.5–1 µg/kg titrated to 5 µg/kg single dose 1–3 µg/kg/h infusion • Transmucosal Fentanyl lollipop (Oralet®) PO 10–15 µg/kg • Transdermal Patch 25–100 µg/h, not for acute pain management • Epidural management by anesthesiologist Anesthesia: higher IV doses	Short duration of action (<60 minutes) Apnea, bradycardia common Chest wall rigidity possible with high dose and/or bolus doses (usually >5 µg/kg) Multiple administration routes 100X more potent than morphine
Hydromorphone Mu agonist	Analgesia: • IV/IM 0.02 mg/kg q4–6h • PO 0.03–0.08 mg/kg q 4–6 h • PR Adult dose 3 mg • Epidural management by anesthesiologist Anesthesia: higher IV doses	5–7X more potent than morphine Carries all the risks of other opioids Sometimes produces less sedation, pruritus, or nausea than morphine Variable oral absorption
Meperidine Mu agonist	Analgesia: 1–2 mg/kg IV/IM q3–4h	Greater euphoric effects than morphine Causes tachycardia Causes some histamine release Normeperidine, a toxic metabolite with 15–20-hour half-life, causes seizures Contraindicated in patients taking MAO-inhibitors, and not recommended when increased ICP or cardiac arrhythmias Use caution in patients taking any CNS-acting agents Can be effective in stopping shivering Preparation contains bisulfite Use caution in renal insufficiency
Methadone Mu agonist	0.1 mg/kg q4–6h max dose 10 mg/dose	Multiple dosing results in prolonged duration of action
Morphine Mu agonist Weak Sigma agonist	Analgesia: • IV/IM 0.05–0.1 mg/kg q2–4h • PO 0.2–0.5 mg/kg q4h • Epidural management by anesthesiologist Anesthesia: higher IV doses	Induces histamine release Poor GI absorption Seizures reported in newborns Pruritus and urinary retention are common
Oxycodone Mu agonist	Analgesia 0.1 mg/kg q4–6h max dose 10 mg/dose	Produces less nausea than codeine May contain bisulfite
Remifentanil Mu agonist	Anesthesia 0.5-µg/kg bolus followed by infusion	Ultrashort acting, half-life 3–5 minutes Eliminated by plasma cholinesterase Significant risk of chest wall rigidity and apnea 100X more potent than morphine

(continued)

TABLE 4-26 Continued

DRUG/CNS RECEPTOR ACTIVITY	DOSE & INDICATIONS	COMMENTS
Sufentanil Mu agonist	Anesthesia 0.1 μg/kg, starting dose	High incidence of chest wall rigidity, apnea and nausea 1000X more potent than morphine

Tramadol
  Mu agonist and nonopioid re-
  ceptor activity
	Analgesia 50–100 mg, adult dose (FDA approved for
	  adults)
		Synthetic analogue of codeine
		Low side-effect profile
		Use for weak to moderate pain

TABLE 4-27

TREATMENT OF OPIOID-INDUCED SIDE EFFECTS

- Respiratory depression:
  1. Support the airway, provide oxygen and manual breaths as necessary
  2. Stop opioid
  3. Naloxone administration as described in Table 4-28
- Excessive sedation:
  1. Reduce dose
  2. Add amphetamine as a morning dose
- Nausea and vomiting:
  1. Administer ondansetron OR
  2. Diphenhydramine OR
  3. Metoclopramide OR
  4. Droperidol
- Pruritus:
  1. Administer diphenhydramine OR
  2. Agonist-antagonist such as butorphanol OR
  3. Naloxone infusion
- Constipation:
  1. Administer one or a combination of laxatives
  2. Lubricant
  3. Stimulant
  4. Surfactant
  5. Bulk-producing agent

usual guidelines (see Sec. 4.2.6). Multifocal premature ventricular contractions with sustained cardiac output and blood pressure can be treated with magnesium, phenytoin, or bretylium. Seizures should be treated with benzodiazepines or sodium thiopental.

Regional nerve blocks (eg, digital block) and neuraxial applications of local anesthetics (eg, epidural or subarachnoid blocks) are techniques useful for anesthetizing specific areas that have the potential for providing anesthesia without compromising airway function or responsiveness of the patients. These techniques, however, require specialized training to administer.

SEDATION AND SLEEP MANAGEMENT

New procedures, sicker patients, and more humane approaches to the care of children require that physicians who prescribe or administer sedatives be well prepared to deal with the challenges of inadequate sedation, pain management, drug side effects or overdose, and monitoring of vital functions (see Fig. 4-29). It is incumbent on the person ordering or administering sedating drugs to assess the patient's airway patency and to consider the risks of sedation. One should also consider whether a patient requires care by an anesthesiologist. High-risk patients are the same as those who are susceptible to apnea, airway obstruction, or hypotension with opioid administration. In addition to the patient conditions listed, procedures placing patients in awkward positions (eg, knee to chest), those limiting access and visibility, and those requiring immobility are situations in which the patency of the airway is a concern. It is generally accepted that nonanesthesiologists can provide a level of sedation in which spontaneous breathing and airway-protective reflexes are maintained. An appropriate level of sedation is one that allows the child to respond appropriately to verbal or tactile stimulation; a deeper level of sedation does not assure maintenance of the airway. The situations of applicability are usually for

TABLE 4-28

THE OPIOID ANTAGONISTS AND AGONIST-ANTAGONISTS

DRUG	DOSE	CNS RECEPTOR ACTIVITY	COMMENTS
Butorphanol	Analgesia, sedation, treatment of pruritus 10–20 μg/kg IV/IM q6h 50 μg/kg PO q6h	Mu antagonist Kappa, Sigma agonist	Very sedating
Nalbuphine	Analgesia, sedation, treatment of pruritus 0.1 mg/kg IV/IM 0.5 mg/kg PO	Mu antagonist Kappa weak agonist	
Naltrexone	Treatment of addiction following detoxification Adult dose: 50 mg PO q24h	Pure antagonist	2–10× more potent than naloxone

Naloxone	Respiratory arrest:
	0.1 mg/kg/dose, can repeat
	Nonarrest situation:
	Titrate dose to desired effect, starting with doses
	  of 0.5 μg/kg
	Pruritus:
	0.5 μg/kg/hr by IV infusion and increase dose
	  if necessary
		Pure antagonist	1. Prompt reversal of respiratory depression resulting from Mu-receptor agonists
			2. Use with caution in patients with cardiac disease
			3. Expect development withdrawal symptoms in susceptible patients

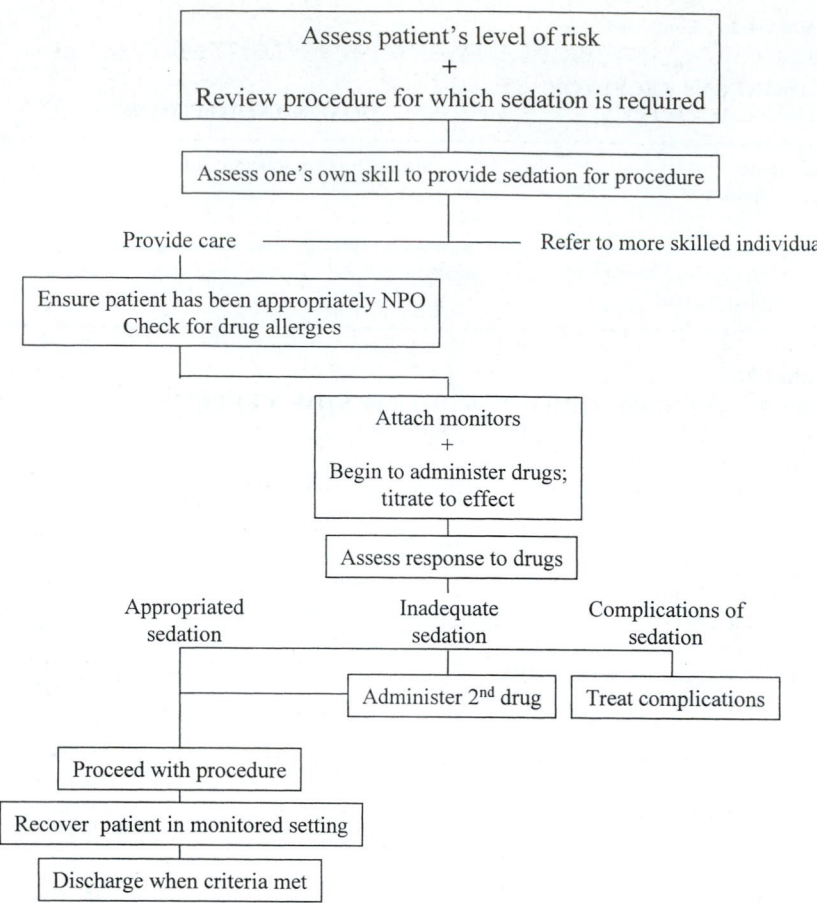

FIGURE 4-29 Algorithm for management of sedation.

short-duration, noninvasive procedures or painful procedures where sedation plus analgesia is provided. For this level of sedation, the American Academy of Pediatrics, the American Society of Anesthesiologists, and other professional medical and dental organizations have published sedation policy guidelines, which include recommendations for patient preparation, equipment setup, monitoring requirements, essential personnel, and recovery [see, eg, Guidelines for Monitoring and Management of Pediatric Patients During and After Sedation for Diagnostic and Therapeutic Procedures (RE9252) *http://www.aap.org/policy/04789.html*]. Guidelines for fasting are similar to those for general anesthesia (see Table 4-22). The practitioner providing sedation must devise both sedation and rescue strategies. This is most important in remote areas of the hospital and procedure rooms (such as imaging suites) where

access to the patient may be challenging. Trouble can be averted by proper monitoring and oxygen administration. Essential monitors include ECG, blood pressure, and continuous pulse oximetry; temperature and capnography monitoring are recommended. Essential equipment includes suction, oxygen, positive-pressure ventilation equipment (bag and mask), equipment for endotracheal intubation (endotracheal tubes, laryngoscope and blades, stylets), and a nearby resuscitation cart. The minimal qualifications for personnel include basic life-support training, training in the use of controlled substances, airway management, monitoring the unconscious patient, and use of resuscitation equipment.

Once the procedure is completed, the child must be taken to a monitored recovery area where an appropriate discharge time is based on the child's return to a safe level of consciousness. The following criteria are useful in judging when it is safe to discharge the child: (a) Cardiovascular function and airway patency is satisfactory and stable; (b) the patient is easily arousable, and protective reflexes are intact; (c) the patient can talk (if age-appropriate); (d) the patient can sit up unaided (if age-appropriate); (e) for a very young or handicapped child, incapable of the usually expected responses, the presedation level of responsiveness or a level as close as possible to the normal level for that child should be achieved; and (f) the state of hydration is adequate.

There are three general situations for which sedation is often required for children: (a) painful procedures, (b) frightening but nonpainful procedures; and (c) sleep management in the ICU or other hospital locations. It must be stated that painful procedures cannot be managed under "conscious sedation" alone. Analgesics or anesthetics must be given in addition to sedatives; ideally, a local

TABLE 4-29

SEDATION GOALS AND SUGGESTED CLASSES OF DRUGS

MEDICATION GOALS	DRUG OPTIONS
Amnesia	Anticholinergics (scopolamine), benzodiazepines
Analgesia, anesthesia	Opioids (see Tables 4-25 and 4-26), local anesthetics
Anxiolysis	Benzodiazepines
Sleep	Antihistamines, barbiturates, benzodiazepines, butyrophenones, chloral hydrate, phenothiazines

TABLE 4-30

SPECIFIC SEDATIVE DRUGS, DOSING, AND SIDE EFFECTS

CLASS OF DRUGS	DRUG/DOSING	BENEFITS	SIDE EFFECTS
Anticholinergics	Scopolamine 0.01–0.02 mg/kg IM/IV	Amnesia, drowsiness, sleep, antiemetic, antisialagogue	Delirium: coadministration of morphine minimizes delirium Disorientation Blurry vision Contraindicated in glaucoma and urinary obstruction
Antihistamines	• Diphenhydramine 0.5–1 mg/kg q4–6h PO, IV, IM; max dose 50 mg • Hydroxyzine 0.5–1 mg/kg q4–6h PO or IM (cannot be given IV); max dose 100 mg	Antiemetic, antipruritic, tranquilization and sleep, treatment of extrapyramidal reactions	Paradoxical excitement, occasionally
Barbiturates	Pentobarbital 0.5–1 mg/kg IV, titrated to max dose of 6 mg/kg or 200 mg; 2–6 mg/kg IM/PO/PR, max dose 6 mg/kg or 200 mg	Sedation, sleep, anticonvulsant, treatment of opioid withdrawal	Respiratory depression, airway obstruction Coma Paradoxical excitement Residual sedation Acute intermittent porphyria attack
Benzodiazepines	• Diazepam 0.1–0.2 mg/kg IV or 0.2–0.3 mg/kg PO/PR; cannot be given IM • Lorazepam 0.03–0.05 mg/kg IV or 0.05–0.2 mg/kg PO/PR • Midazolam 0.05–0.15 mg/kg IV or 0.5–1mg/kg PO/PR	Anxiolysis, sedation, amnesia, anticonvulsant, relieve muscle spasms	Respiratory depression, airway obstruction Hypotension Paradoxical excitement Phlebitis
Butyrophenones	Droperidol 0.03–0.75 mg/kg IV/IM; max dose 1.25 mg	Sedative, antiemetic, inhibits shivering	Hypotension Decreased seizure threshold Extrapyramidal reactions Dysphoria
Chloral hydrate	25–100 mg/kg PO/PR; max dose 1 g/dose, 2 g/d	Sedation, sleep	Unreliability or ineffective sedation Respiratory depression and airway obstruction especially in young infants placed in car seats Gastrointestinal effects: vomiting, diarrhea Residual sedation or paradoxical excitement Dermatologic effects Acute intermittent porphyria attacks Hyperbilirubinemia, acidosis, prolonged half-life in newborns
Phenothiazines	• Chlorpromazine 0.5–1 mg/kg q6–8h IV/IM, PO, PR; max dose 40 mg/d <5 yr old, 75 mg/d 5–12 yr old • Promethazine 0.5–1 mg/kg q6–8h IV, IM, PO, PR; max dose 50 mg/dose	Tranquilizer, anxiolytic, antiemetic, antipruritic	Extrapyramidal reactions more common in children with varicella, measles, and dehydration Neuroleptic malignant syndrome Hypotension Decreased seizure threshold

anesthetic or an opioid, plus a sedative, would be given. Physicians skilled in giving sedatives consider "conscious sedation" a myth. Many infants or young children who truly retain airway-protective reflexes (the definition of conscious sedation) are uncomfortable, and those who sleep through a procedure often were given deep sedation or general anesthesia. General anesthesia is required for some procedures or for some patients with special needs. Table 4-29 lists suggested drug classes to achieve amnesia, anxiolysis, an-

algesia or anesthesia, or sleep. *Any of the drugs in any class can cause respiratory depression when used in high dose; when used in combination with other sedating drugs, opioids, or alcohol; or when given to patients at high risk for respiratory complications.* Specific drugs, their effects, and dosing are listed in Table 4-30.

A common question from pediatricians and radiologists is how to provide safe sedation for a healthy, young child needing computed tomography (CT). There are at least two strategies to deal with this issue. Fortunately, CT scans are very brief and nonpainful, but they do require a motionless patient. The first strategy utilizes a parent, nurse, play therapist, or another person who can accompany the patient into the scanning area to provide coaching, reassurance, and physical contact for the 5 minutes required to complete the scan. The second strategy utilizes sedative drugs solely or in combination with the first strategy. Rational drug choices to provide sleep and a still patient include barbiturates, chloral hydrate, or benzodiazepines. (See Table 4-30 for dosing guidelines.)

References

Ho ML, Chang JK, Chuang LY, Hsu HK, Wang GJ: Effects of nonsteroidal anti-inflammatory drugs and prostaglandins on osteoblastic functions. Biochem Pharmacol 58:983–990, 1999

Mandell BF: COX 2-selective NSAIDs: biology, promises, and concerns. Cleve Clin J Med 66:285–292, 1999

Taddio A, Stevens B, Craig K, et al: Efficacy and safety of lidocaine-prilocaine cream for pain during circumcision. N Engl J Med 336:1197–1201, 1997

Wong DL: Whaley and Wong's Essentials of Pediatric Nursing, 5th ed. St. Louis, Mosby-Year Book, 1997

4.3   INJURIES AND UNTOWARD EVENTS

4.3.1   Major Trauma in Children

M. Douglas Baker

Each year in the United States, nearly 1 of every 3 children younger than 16 years of age sustain injuries serious enough to require medical attention—60,000 children are injured each day, and 22 million children are injured each year. Injuries in childhood are so common that 40 to 45% of all child and adolescent visits to emergency departments are injury-related. Although the number has declined over the past decade, motor vehicle crashes remain the most common cause of death in children in the United States. Alarmingly, during the same period of time, the incidence of homicide increased tremendously. Homicide is the second leading cause of death in children younger than 4 years of age, and the most common cause of death for all African-American children. Data from the National Center for Health statistics linked infant birth-death certificate data sets indicate that the leading causes of death in infants less than 1 year of age are homicide, suffocation, motor vehicle crashes, and inhalation of food or other objects. While falls are a very common cause of injury for children of all ages, they infrequently result in death. Most childhood trauma involves blunt mechanisms of injury. Although they are less common, penetrating injuries are increasing in childhood and adolescence, especially in large urban areas of the United States.

FEATURES UNIQUE TO PEDIATRIC TRAUMA PATIENTS

Several unique characteristics of children significantly affect the assessment and management of childhood trauma and distinguish it from its adult counterpart. The obvious size discrepancy between children and adults is one such important feature. When there is impact with a moving object, the mechanical energy applied to the smaller body mass of a child results in a greater force applied per unit body. When transmitted to a body with less fat and close proximity of multiple organs, that energy frequently causes multiple organ injuries. More than two-thirds of children with significant chest injury have other organ system injuries.

Another factor that contributes to the occurrence of multiple organ injuries in children is their skeletal structure. Because children's skeletons are incompletely calcified and contain multiple active growth centers, they are more pliable. As a result, internal organ damage is often noted without overlying bony fracture. For instance, significant thoracic trauma will infrequently result in rib fractures, but frequently result in pulmonary contusion. The occurrence of rib fractures in a young child suggests the transfer of a massive amount of energy and the possibility of multiple, serious organ injuries.

The young child's head constitutes a relatively high proportion of the total body mass (19%) when compared to an adolescent or an adult (9%). The combination of immature coordination skills and relatively large head atop a proportionately smaller frame contributes to the frequency of serious head injuries in infants. In fact, head injuries are the leading cause of trauma-related deaths in children. This is one reason why injury-prevention strategies for children often include efforts to increase utilization of effective head-protection gear.

Infants and young children have open fontanels and mobile cranial sutures. Therefore, they may develop an expanding intracranial mass before there are signs of compression of vital structures. Thus, the infant who has stable vital signs but who has a bulging fontanel following trauma should be managed as having a severe injury.

The examination of a child with a possible spinal injury must consider some developmental singularities of the human spine. The cervical spine of the child differs from that of the adult because the interspinous ligaments and joint capsules are more flexible, the vertebral bodies are wedged anteriorly and tend to slide forward with flexion, and the facet joints are flat. Because the child's head is relatively large compared to the neck, during injury, the force applied to the neck is relatively greater than it is in the adult and the fulcrum for injury is more cephalad. Nevertheless, only 5% of all spinal cord injuries occur in the pediatric age-group.

The anatomic differences of the child's cervical spine account for several unique radiographic findings. Approximately 40% of children younger than 7 years of age demonstrate pseudosubluxation, anterior displacement of C2 on C3. Pseudosubluxation is also noted in 20% of children up to 16 years of age. This finding is seen less commonly at C3 to C4. Pseudosubluxation is made more pronounced by flexion of the cervical spine and is minimized by placing the child's neck in the neutral position. An increased distance between the dens and the anterior arch of C1 also occurs in about 20% of young children. Gaps exceeding the upper limit of normal for adults are frequently seen.

Children sustain spinal cord injury without radiographic abnormality (SCIWORA) more commonly than adults; this injury is detected by MRI and often is diagnosed well after the initial assessment. Approximately two-thirds of children with spinal cord injuries have normal cervical spine radiographs. Thus, normal radiographs do not exclude significant spinal cord injury in children with suggestive historical or physical findings.

The ratio of body surface area to body volume is greatest in young infants and decreases as the child achieves adult size. The relative amount of body fat is also considerably less in young children. Accordingly, thermal energy loss is a significant concern in children. Hypothermia can occur quickly and can complicate resuscitation efforts. The smaller amount of internal fat also provides less protective cushion for internal organs and contributes to the high rate of organ injury following blunt trauma.

As mentioned previously, the child's skeleton differs from that of the adult. It is less calcified and more flexible. As a result, trauma to extremities can cause incomplete greenstick or buckle (torus) fractures. Actively growing children have open growth plates that are far weaker than the tendons or ligaments that insert near them. Injuries to the physes (Salter-Harris fractures) are common, often difficult to demonstrate radiographically, and can significantly alter future growth of the injured bone.

A further consideration is the effect that any injury might have on subsequent childhood growth and development. In children, even minor injuries can cause prolonged neurologic, psychological, or other organ-system disabilities. Up to 60% of children who sustain severe multisystem trauma have residual personality changes 1 year after hospital discharge. Half of all seriously injured children manifest cognitive and physical handicaps, or social or learning disabilities. Trauma can affect immediate survival, as well as the subsequent quality of life.

MANAGEMENT

For the severely injured child, resuscitation should follow the same prioritized general format used for those with nontrauma-related illnesses. In all instances, universal precautions should be used. Trauma management is often categorized into three phases: the primary survey, the secondary survey, and the definitive care phase (Fig. 4-30). There are some special considerations that add to the management priorities for severely injured children. However, as is the case for all resuscitations, the provision of adequate oxygenation and ventilation is of paramount importance.

Primary Survey

The management of the injured child begins with the primary survey and includes attention to the adequacy of the airway, breathing, and circulation (the ABCs). These are the "automatic" life-saving measures required by all children during resuscitation.

Monitoring of the injured child should commence at the time management is initiated and should continue throughout the evaluation and resuscitation. At the very least, continuous monitoring of heart rate, respiration, and oxygen saturation, and intermittent monitoring of blood pressure are essential (see Sec. 4.2.1). Physical examination, history, and response to interventions should dictate needs for additional monitoring.

Because the possibility exists for a spinal injury that has severe consequences in the unexamined child, care must be taken to fully protect the cervical spine until such injury has adequately been excluded. In the uncooperative or unresponsive child, in the young child who is unable to supply reliable or meaningful responses to questions, or in the child with painful distracting injuries, significant spinal injuries cannot be excluded by physical examination alone. For those children and for any children with neck pain on active movement of the neck, tenderness on palpation of the cervical vertebrae, detectable cervical spine deformity, or neurologic abnormality referable to the neck, immobilization and protection of the cervical spine should be provided until spinal injuries have been definitively ruled out (see "Secondary Survey" later in this section).

Cervical spine immobilization can be effectively accomplished in a number of ways. While most prehospital care providers and

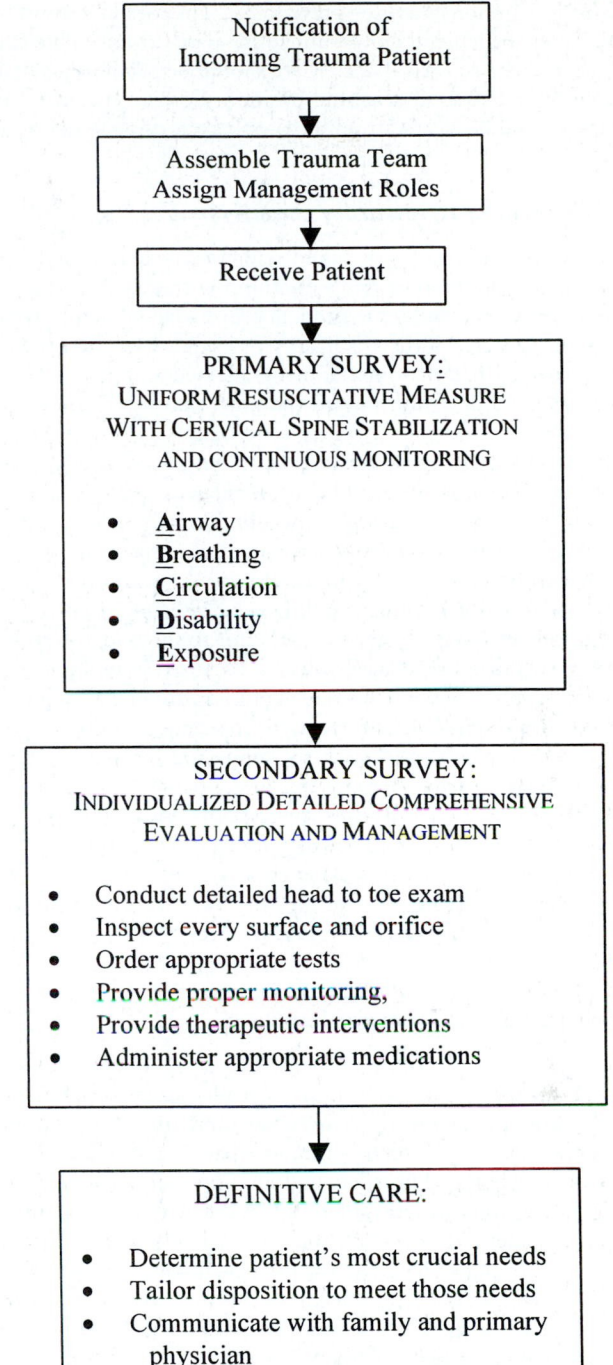

FIGURE 4-30 **Organization of the evaluation and management of a child with trauma.**

emergency medicine physicians use rigid collars for this purpose, simple criss-cross taping of the skin of the forehead to a spine immobilization board is also effective. Alternatively, placing one's fingers bilaterally on the mastoid and mandible to fix the position of the head and to impede both lateral movement and flexion-extension can provide manual stabilization.

Before, during, and after cervical spine immobilization, attention should be focused on adequacy of respiration. Inadequate oxygenation and ventilation is the most common cause of cardiac arrest in children. Secondary injury to the brain resulting from hypoxemia is common and often preventable. The person responsible for airway management should utilize standard advanced life-support techniques (see Sec. 4.2.6). Care should be taken to maintain the spine and airway in a neutral position. Foreign materials and vomitus should be cleared from the oropharynx using large-caliber suction.

Treatment of Respiratory Impairment

Some injuries can restrict the child's ability to expand the lungs. Accumulation of blood or free air within the thorax should be diagnosed promptly and evacuated appropriately. Pneumothorax should be suspected if there is history or evidence of chest trauma and diminished breath sounds on the affected side. In some instances, tracheal deviation toward the side opposite the injury can also be felt.

Once detected, a pneumothorax that compromises circulation or oxygenation should be promptly evacuated. This can first be achieved by aspiration through a needle or small catheter placed through the chest wall at the second intercostal space in the midclavicular line. Subsequently, more effective evacuation of either free air or blood can be accomplished by inserting a chest tube through the fifth intercostal space, anterior to the midaxillary line.

When two or more adjacent ribs are fractured in multiple locations, flail chest can occur. In this condition, the negative pleural pressure with inspiration causes inward movement of the flail segment, which limits expansion of the lungs and reduces the functional residual capacity. Because this interferes with gas exchange and requires excess energy to breathe, positive-pressure ventilation may be the only means to provide adequate tidal volume. Penetrating injuries can result in sucking chest wounds that also impede the development of negative pressure and interfere with breathing. These can be quickly remedied by placing an occlusive dressing over the open wound.

Treatment of Abnormal Perfusion

While airway and breathing problems are being addressed, circulatory status should be assessed, and vascular access should be attained. Although it is preferable to secure more than one large-bore intravenous line in the multiple trauma patient, resuscitation can be adequately initiated in most children using one site of access. If peripheral intravenous access is not achievable within a few minutes, an alternate method of access should be attempted. That method should be determined based on the individual skills of those present and the urgency of the child's needs. Central venous access, intraosseous infusion, or surgical exposure of a peripheral or central (femoral) vein are viable options (see Sec. 4.2.4).

After vascular access is established, the need for fluid resuscitation should be determined (see Sec. 4.1.2). Quick assessment of four organ systems (cardiac, renal, central nervous system, and skin) can help in that determination. Tachycardia is often the first sign of hypovolemia, while hypotension is a late finding. In fact, 25% of a child's blood volume can be lost before low blood pressure is manifest. Decreased urinary output or less quantitative findings, such as weak pulses, cool or clammy skin, or confusion may suggest the need for large amounts of additional fluids. Delayed capillary refill is also suggestive of poor tissue perfusion that occurs following substantial blood loss. Care must be taken, however, to weigh limiting factors such as the temperature of ambient air, which can significantly alter results. Laboratory studies might not be useful when evaluating vascular status. The child's hematocrit will not reflect blood loss until sufficient time has elapsed for the plasma volume to equilibrate.

Fluid resuscitation should be initiated with the administration of 20 mL/kg of either lactated Ringer solution or normal saline. If needed, additional boluses may be given. If the child requires more than three or four such boluses of fluid to support the circulation, it can be assumed that there is undetected bleeding and 10 mL/kg of packed red blood cells should be infused. Whenever possible infused blood should be type-specific. In more urgent situations, O-negative blood can be used.

Some patients may not improve with the volume resuscitation because of continued hemorrhage, and they require rapid detection of the site of bleeding and hemostasis, often with surgical intervention. Occasionally, a patient may even worsen with continued fluid administration, because of progressive venous engorgement. Accordingly, continued assessment for liver size, venous congestion, or central venous pressure are essential; when this suggests high venous pressure and poor response to fluid infusion, it may be an indication of cardiac and pericardial involvement, previously undetected tension pneumothoraces or hemothorax, or, more rarely, venous obstruction.

Following the ABCs is an assessment of neurologic disability. At this point, the assessment is brief and consists of checking pupillary size and response and obtaining a rapid neurologic evaluation by determining whether the patient is alert; responsive to vocal stimuli; responsive to painful stimuli; or unresponsive. This rapid assessment forms the basis of the AVPU system, an acronym that derives from the neurologic responses (Table 4-31). Another approach to assessment comes from the elements in the modified Glasgow Coma Scale (see Table 4-6). If not yet accomplished, the child's body must be inspected in its totality to complete the primary survey. Compression should be applied to sites of active bleeding.

Secondary Survey

After completion of the primary survey, and after life-saving measures have been initiated, the secondary survey can be performed. During this phase of management, the physician conducts a comprehensive head-to-toe examination of the child. Different from the primary survey, in which all children receive the same standardized assessment, during the secondary survey, diagnostic testing and therapeutic intervention are individualized for each patient. Every part of the body should be palpated, and every orifice inspected. The chest and abdomen should be auscultated, and the patient "log-rolled" to enable examination of the back and rectum. All findings should be comprehensively documented in the medical record.

Like the primary survey, the secondary survey should proceed in a logical, regimented order, beginning with the head, neck, and central nervous system. In infants, the condition of the fontanel (open, closed, depressed, flat, bulging) should be noted. All children should be inspected for signs of skull fracture, including hemotympanum, raccoon eyes, Battle sign (ecchymosis near the tip

TABLE 4-31

RAPID NEUROLOGIC EVALUATION

A: Alert
V: Responsive to vocal stimuli
P: Responsive to painful stimuli
U: Unresponsive

of the mastoid process from basilar skull fracture), or persistent clear fluid drainage from either the nostrils or external auditory canals, which might indicate leakage of cerebrospinal fluid. Signs of intracranial injury, history of loss of consciousness or persistent depressed consciousness merit further evaluation by CT scan. In addition, a patient with a low Glasgow Coma Scale score (eg, ≤8) might warrant intracranial monitoring.

Determination that there is no significant injury to the cervical spine by physical examination, that is, "clinical clearance," is an issue that has generated many spirited debates and will likely continue to do so. Nonetheless, this can be accomplished in selected patients. To qualify for clinical clearance, the child must be awake and fully cooperative, able to understand and respond to instruction, and have no injuries that are painful enough to distract attention. Under those circumstances, the child should first be instructed to not move the head or neck unless asked to do so. After that condition is acknowledged, with the patient's head manually immobilized, the cervical restraint (collar, tape, etc.) can be removed. Keeping the head and neck immobilized, both should be visually inspected for injury and deformity. The cervical spine should then be palpated from the base of the skull to T1. The patient should be asked to indicate the location of any pain generated during palpation. If any deformity, swelling, or bone pain on palpation is noted, the cervical spine should be again immobilized, and diagnostic imaging of the spine, preferably by CT, obtained. If there is no evidence of deformity, swelling, or bone pain on palpation, the child should be asked to actively rotate his or her neck from side to side, and to then flex and extend it. If these movements likewise generate no bone pain, clinical clearance has been achieved, and diagnostic imaging can be avoided. However, if any bone pain results from these maneuvers, spinal immobilization should be reinstituted, pending diagnostic imaging.

It is particularly difficult to determine the need for cervical spine immobilization in infants and preschool-age children. Those children often arrive in the emergency department alert, upset, unrestrained, and uncooperative. Many (or most) display full, active, head and neck movement and resist attempts to restrict that movement. In the absence of visible signs of head or neck injury, many physicians choose to observe, rather than to restrain forcefully and obtain radiographic images.

Comprehensive examinations of the chest, abdomen, genitalia, and extremities complete the secondary survey. During each of these remaining portions, care should be taken to auscultate, palpate, and probe appropriately. Diagnostic tests and therapeutic interventions should be ordered only as needed for each patient. Open wounds should be covered, injured bones splinted, and analgesics and other appropriate medications (eg, vaccines, antibiotics) administered.

Omissions or oversights commonly involve the abdomen or back. In a frightened or anxious child, or a child who has sustained significant head injury, the abdominal examination can be particularly difficult. If an adequate examination cannot be obtained, diagnostic imaging should be considered. In children who require CT imaging of their head, subsequent CT imaging of the abdomen might be in order. Diagnostic peritoneal lavage has been generally replaced by CT imaging. However, diagnostic peritoneal lavage (DPL) might be a useful diagnostic adjunct for the child who is hemodynamically unstable, or who would otherwise be at risk if placed in the CT scanning device away from immediate medical support. For such children, ultrasound might also be a useful alternative diagnostic tool. The mere presence of intraperitoneal blood on CT, DPL, or ultrasound does not mandate operative intervention. It has been well-demonstrated that bleeding from an injured spleen, liver, or kidney generally is self-limiting. However, rupture of a hollow viscus requires early operative intervention.

The secondary survey is not complete until the patient's back is inspected. To avoid the aggravation of possible spinal injury, each patient should be carefully log-rolled. This requires a coordinated effort by several personnel. Care must be taken to sustain in-line cervical, thoracic, and lumbosacral spinal immobilization during this maneuver. Once rolled, the back should be visually examined and palpated, and a rectal examination performed. If, for any reason it is unsafe to log-roll the patient, palpation should carefully be attempted by slipping a gloved hand between the patient's back and the stretcher.

Factors that contribute to increased morbidity and mortality in trauma patients include uncorrected hypoxemia and acidosis, uncorrected shock, inadequate stabilization of spinal or other bony or ligamentous injuries, and unrecognized internal or external blood loss. In general, any significant delay in timely recognition and management of major injuries is potentially life-threatening. To achieve optimal results, one must use a comprehensive, standardized approach for all patients, and must efficiently enlist the aid of other specialists according to the specific needs of each patient.

Definitive Care

The third phase of management of acute trauma is that of definitive care. At this point, decisions regarding disposition of the patient from the acute care setting and future care are made. Many management issues should be reviewed at this time, including the need for medications (eg, antibiotics, immunizations, analgesics, sedatives), additional diagnostic studies (eg, MRI, selective vascular studies) or monitoring (eg, intravascular, intracranial), or consultations to special services. Prior to engaging in any such intervention, one must substantiate the need by evaluating the specific risks and benefits of each for the patient. Patients requiring transfer should be directed to trauma referral centers that provide the best level of care for their most serious injuries. Patients should never be transported from facility to facility unless they are judged to be stable enough to endure the move. Urgency must be balanced by safety. Transport must always be performed by appropriately trained and equipped medical personnel. A comprehensive exchange of information regarding the patient should take place between the referring and receiving physicians prior to the transfer of any patient. Patients should be accompanied by a complete written account of the events that transpired at the referring center and (whenever possible) by copies of results of diagnostic imaging and other tests or evaluations.

References

American College of Surgeons Committee on Trauma. Pediatric trauma. In: Advanced Trauma Life Support Program for Doctors. 6th ed. Chicago, IL: American College of Surgeons; 1997, pp 353–375

Schwartz GR, Wright SW, Fein JA, Sugarman JS, Pasternack J, Salhanick S: Pediatric cervical spine injury sustained from low heights. Ann Emerg Med, 30:249–252, 1997

Young GM, Eichelberger MR: Evaluation, stabilization, and initial management after multiple trauma. In: Fuhrman BP, Zimmerman JJ, eds: Pediatric Critical Care, 2nd ed. Mosby Year Book, St. Louis, MO, 1998, pp 1212–1220

4.3.2 Apparent Life-Threatening Events

Michael J. Corwin

The assessment and management of infants who are described as having had a frightening, perhaps life-threatening, event is a challenging problem for clinicians. The fear that the infant may experience additional episodes, perhaps a fatal one, heightens the anxiety level of both families and medical professionals.

DEFINITION

An apparent life-threatening event (ALTE) was defined in 1986 at a National Institutes of Health (NIH) Consensus Development Conference on Infantile Apnea and Home Monitoring as an "episode that is frightening to the observer and that is characterized by some combination of apnea (central or occasionally obstructive), color change (usually cyanotic or pallid but occasionally erythematous or plethoric), marked change in muscle tone (usually limpness), choking, or gagging." In addition, it was recommended that previously used terminology such as "aborted crib death" or "near-miss sudden infant death syndrome (SIDS)" be abandoned to avoid implication of a causal association between this type of spell and SIDS.

ALTE episodes were described in the Consensus Development Conference statement as a "chief complaint that describes a general clinical syndrome." This general clinical syndrome may be secondary to a specific diagnosis or may remain idiopathic despite a thorough evaluation. The definition of an ALTE appears straightforward; however, in practice, the decision regarding whether or not an infant experienced an ALTE can be extraordinarily difficult for clinicians. Although 15 years have passed since the adoption of the ALTE definition, the published literature regarding the epidemiology, clinical course, and prognosis of ALTE remains limited, and there is no evidence that these events arise from any single mechanism. Nor is there evidence that the manifestations represent a consistent pattern. Factors that contribute to the difficulty in studying infants who experience ALTE episodes include:

- Marked heterogeneity of clinical presentation
- Lack of symptoms during initial assessment by medical professionals
- Parents or other caretakers who have been very frightened and have difficulty accurately describing symptoms
- Possibility that some symptoms are fabricated or inflicted

INCIDENCE

Data regarding incidence of ALTEs are limited. In a large national study of SIDS and control infants born in the late 1970s, 3% of parents of control infants with a birthweight ≥2500 g and 6% of parents of low birth weight infants reported that their infant experienced at least one postnatal episode in which the infant "turned blue or stopped breathing." Parents of infants who died of SIDS reported having observed similar episodes in 6% and 11% of infants with a birth weight ≥2500 g and <2500 g, respectively. Most likely, however, few of these episodes would have met the definition of an ALTE.

Some perspective on the occurrence of idiopathic ALTE can be obtained from the Collaborative Home Infant Monitoring Evaluation (CHIME study), which was conducted at five medical centers (located in Cleveland, Toledo, Chicago, Los Angeles, and Honolulu) during the mid-1990s. This study included a systematic review of infants who presented with diagnoses consistent with ALTE and found that a typical urban medical center hospital provides care for about one case of possible ALTE each week and that approximately 20% of such cases will be considered an idiopathic ALTE.

CLINICAL PRESENTATION

Infants Who Are Asymptomatic at the Time of Presentation

Most commonly infants are no longer experiencing respiratory or circulatory dysfunction by the time they are first seen by medical professionals. Even in cases where an emergency medical team has been called, the signs commonly have resolved by the time emergency medical technicians arrive. In some cases, during a routine well-child visit, a parent may describe an event that was witnessed days or weeks in the past.

Among the most difficult tasks for the clinician is to identify the signs that the infant actually experienced. The ability of the caretakers to provide an accurate history is diminished by the fact that they may have been frightened to the point of panic. The situation may be further confounded by circumstances such as a dark room, clothes, or covers obscuring the view of the infant, or inexperience evaluating infant behavior.

The first step is to try to establish whether the symptoms were indeed life-threatening or, as is often the case, are consistent with normal behavior or common minor symptoms. To this end, it is important to ascertain the following:

1. Characteristics of the event
   - Was the infant making breathing efforts? If so, was there anything observed that might suggest obstruction of the airway? This information helps to identify episodes of airway obstruction and, on further questioning, determine if there is an obvious explanation (eg, foreign body, airway secretions, food), or if further evaluation may be necessary.
   - What was the longest period that the infant was not making breathing efforts? Infants normally have irregular breathing patterns. It is not unusual for parents to express a concern because they noticed a 10- to 15-second pause in breathing. Such pauses are not unusual and should not be a cause for concern unless accompanied by other symptoms.
   - Were there changes in the infant's color? Reports of the baby turning blue (ie, cyanosis) are consistent with a genuine ALTE. However, it is important to distinguish perioral cyanosis from generalized cyanosis. Infants described as having turned red or who appear pale are unlikely to have experienced a genuine ALTE.
   - Was the infant asleep or awake? If the child is awake and alert, obstruction is more likely to be the cause.
   - Was the infant crying or making other noises during the episode? Color changes associated with vigorous crying (ie, turning red or blue in the face) may scare parents but are generally not life-threatening events.
   - Were there changes in the infant's muscle tone or abnormal body movements? Genuine ALTE events frequently are associated with changes in muscle tone. Loss of tone is most common. However, normal infants who are sleeping may also appear hypotonic. Alternatively, families may describe body movements consistent with seizure activity.
   - Was the episode associated with feeding or emesis? This association may suggest gastroesophageal reflux, problems

with feeding technique, swallowing dyscoordination, or possible airway obstruction.

- How long did the symptoms persist and what intervention was provided? Symptoms that resolve within 30 to 60 seconds, especially if no or minimal intervention was provided, should generally not be considered life-threatening. In cases in which substantial intervention is provided, it is important to consider that a frightened caretaker may have provided more intervention than required.

2. Current health status of the infant, including acute illnesses (eg, respiratory infections), chronic health problems (eg, neurologic problems, presence of gastroesophageal reflux, congenital abnormalities), and medications
3. Previous history of life-threatening events
4. Other previous medical problems including perinatal and neonatal problems (eg, prematurity, chronic lung disease, birth asphyxia)
5. History of life-threatening events or SIDS in other family members
6. Family history of inborn errors of metabolism

Ultimately, a judgment must be made regarding whether or not to categorize the infant as having experienced an ALTE. At one extreme is the judgment that the event was not severe enough to be considered a significant clinical problem (ie, it was not genuinely life-threatening) or perhaps was clearly misinterpreted normal behavior. Alternatively, the nature of the described symptoms may be such that it is clear that the event was a genuinely life-threatening episode. In practice, however, in the absence of persistent symptoms or sequelae, it is difficult to be confident that a life-threatening event actually occurred.

Infants Who Are Symptomatic at the Time of Presentation

In a relatively small proportion of infants who are evaluated as having experienced a possible ALTE, the infant is symptomatic when first seen by medical professionals. In addition to the assessment described above for asymptomatic infants, the opportunity to observe the nature and severity of persistent symptoms permits a greater degree of confidence when determining whether the episode was indeed life-threatening. In some instances, the life-threatening nature of the event is clear. These include episodes where the initial medical responders may need to initiate or continue resuscitative efforts, as well as those where the infant may be stable but still has symptoms such as respiratory distress, cyanosis, or loss of muscle tone. In other cases, the symptoms may be less clearly indicative of a life-threatening event but may point toward an underlying illness that could contribute to such an event (such as a seizure).

EVALUATION

In cases in which an infant has indeed experienced a genuine ALTE, a careful investigation should be undertaken to try to identify a cause. Recognizing that most of the signs potentially relate to disturbed breathing, the initial focus in an evaluation is often directed at respiratory function unless there are other cues in the history. Some of the most common potential causes of an ALTE include: disturbed respiratory control or mechanical function (respiratory infection, especially respiratory syncytial virus; seizures; CNS tumor; gastroesophageal reflux; drug-induced respiratory depression; poisoning; postanesthetic depression; upper airway obstruction);

arrhythmias; inborn error of metabolism; child abuse (Munchausen by proxy). Based on the results of the history and physical examination, one should identify those conditions that require further investigation. Table 4-32 lists the tests commonly used in the evaluation of these infants. The most common diagnoses identified include infections, gastroesophageal reflux, and seizures. The relative proportion of each diagnosis may vary widely depending on the manner in which the ALTE criteria are applied or the referral pattern for a particular locale. For example, a given center might not use the ALTE designation in cases of suspected gastroesophageal reflux, or might receive few referrals of such cases. In addition, among infants who were born prematurely, while no specific etiology may be identified, ALTE episodes may be attributable to persistent apnea of prematurity. In some cases, it may be possible to document features that suggest an immature respiratory control based on physiological recordings; however, no prognostic value of these recordings has been demonstrated.

PROGNOSIS

Data are quite limited regarding the prognosis for infants who experience an ALTE. In rare cases, the ALTE itself results in persistent residual organ damage or neurodevelopmental impairment. Usually, however, infants have no obvious residual problems following the ALTE. Among infants in whom a cause for the ALTE is identified, the prognosis is determined by the particular diagnosis and by the ability to successfully provide treatment. In those cases in which ALTE is associated with prematurity, no further episodes are usually observed beyond the 43 to 44 weeks postconception age. Although premature infants have a higher rate of sudden unexpected death than do term infants, the occurrence of apnea has not been shown to add to this risk.

Among infants with idiopathic ALTE, there is no convincing evidence that these infants are at increased risk for neurodevelopmental problems. The rate of recurrent ALTE episodes or subsequent death is not well studied but appears to be less than 5%. One difficulty in understanding the prognosis of recurrent ALTE is the difficulty in disentangling child abuse from other causes. Although, the proportion of ALTE cases that may be attributable to child abuse is unknown, such cases have been well documented. Factors that increase the suspicion of child abuse include recurrent ALTE requiring CPR, history of SIDS or ALTE in siblings, and episodes that occur only in the presence of a single caretaker. Infants who have ALTE features suggestive of child abuse are at particularly high risk of recurrent episodes or death.

TABLE 4-32

DIAGNOSTIC TESTING FOR INFANTS WITH ALTE

Initial assessment appropriate in most infants requiring evaluation
- Complete blood count with differential (evidence of infection)
- Serum electrolytes (evidence of CO_2 retention or bicarbonate loss, hyponatremia)
- Cardiorespiratory monitoring (evidence of dysrhythmia or irregular breathing)

Tests occasionally indicated based on other findings
- Neurologic testing (EEG, brain imaging)
- Cardiac evaluation (ECG, echocardiogram)
- Evaluation for gastroesophageal reflux (pH monitoring)
- Polysomnography (simultaneous recordings of multiple physiological signals, usually for at least 8 hours, with channels selected based on nature of symptoms)

ALTE, apparent life-threatening events.

MANAGEMENT

A general strategy for management of infants who have experienced a possible ALTE is provided in Fig. 4-31. In the majority of cases, a careful history and physical will suggest that the event was either misinterpreted normal behavior or was relatively trivial (eg, minor choking episodes). In these cases, families need reassurance with a clear explanation of why no further intervention is needed and, if appropriate, need advice regarding childcare practices that will decrease the likelihood of recurrence (eg, proper feeding technique to reduce choking). Although, there is often reluctance on the part of both families and clinicians to accept simple reassurance and counseling, there is no evidence that these episodes are associated with increased risk of morbidity or mortality. In this setting, undertaking an extensive work-up that may be both intrusive and expensive has little justification and may heighten, rather than reduce, anxiety.

Alternatively, when findings are suggestive that the event was truly life-threatening, further evaluation, generally in the hospital, is warranted and will dictate subsequent management strategies.

Infants in Whom a Cause for the ALTE Is Identified

If a specific cause for the ALTE is identified, then a treatment plan can be developed related to that specific entity. In general, to the extent such therapy is successful, home cardiorespiratory monitoring for recurrent ALTE is not warranted. However, if there is a concern that treatment will not be entirely successful, especially if presenting symptoms were severe, short-term cardiorespiratory monitoring may be useful. In these cases, a home monitor may be prescribed if clinicians feel that early caretaker intervention for events might be beneficial (ie, monitor use as part of a therapeutic approach) or a home monitor with memory may be prescribed to document the frequency of events, to distinguish true events from false alarms, and to document the nature of physiological changes associated with events (ie, monitor use as a diagnostic strategy). On the other hand, the use of a home monitor as a diagnostic or therapeutic tool has considerable limitations owing to constraints in current technology. Transthoracic impedance is used to detect respiratory effort, and there is a high risk of failing to detect obstructive apnea or having an alarm despite the presence of a breath (see Sec. 4.2.1).

Infants in Whom No Cause for the ALTE Is Identified

The 1986 NIH Consensus Development Conference Statement, recommended that home cardiorespiratory monitoring or an alternative therapy is indicated for infants who have experienced one or more ALTEs requiring cardiopulmonary resuscitation or vigorous stimulation. This recommendation was based on limited data available at that time suggesting the possibility of a high risk for death among these infants. Recent data from the CHIME study suggest that, at least among term infants, the risk of recurrent severe cardiorespiratory events or death may not be sufficiently high to justify a recommendation for home monitoring. Given the heterogeneous nature of this population, a selective approach seems more reasonable. Circumstances that would push one toward the use of a home monitor include persistent symptoms, neurologic impairment, a high level of family anxiety, an infant who was born prematurely, or a history that raises suspicion of child abuse.

Infants Who Experience Multiple ALTEs

Infants who experience multiple events that meet criteria to be considered an ALTE are at very high risk for substantial morbidity including death. In such cases, it is critical to identify the underlying cause, so that appropriate intervention can be initiated. The most common causes of recurrent ALTE include infections, seizures, gastroesophageal reflux, and child abuse. Of these, the most difficult and the most important to diagnose is child abuse. However, an appropriate index of suspicion and a careful look for features consistent with abuse (described earlier) can be life-saving. In cases of multiple ALTE, where a specific diagnosis cannot be identified, use of a home monitor with memory may be of value in determining whether the events described are in fact genuine and, if they are genuine, to define physiological changes that occur during the event.

CONCLUSION

Management of the infant who has experienced a possible ALTE is a challenge for clinicians that elicits great anxiety and frustration. Despite the absence of means for establishing an accurate prognosis based on clinical presentation or results of testing, decisions must be made regarding need for hospitalization, scope of testing, and need for home cardiorespiratory monitoring. Given the lack of proven efficacy for intrusive and expensive management strategies, families and clinicians should be reassured that the vast majority of infants with a possible ALTE appear well within minutes and will have no subsequent significant problems. Hospitalization and intensive evaluation should be reserved for the relatively small number of infants who have had clearly life-threatening events with persistent symptoms placing them at higher risk for recurrent events.

References

Brooks JG: Apparent life-threatening events and apnea of infancy. Clin Perinatol 19:809–838, 1992

Consensus Statement: National Institutes of Health consensus development conference on infantile apnea and home monitoring, Sept 29 to Oct 1, 1996. Pediatrics 79:292–299, 1987

Cote A, Hum C, Brouillette RT, Themens M: Frequency and timing of recurrent events in infants using home cardiorespiratory monitors. J Pediatr 312:783–789, 1998

Southall DP, Plunkett MC, Banks MW, Falkov AF, Samuels MP: Covert video recordings of life-threatening child abuse: lessons for child protection. Pediatrics 100:735–760, 1997

4.3.3   Toxic Ingestions and Exposures

Milton Tenenbein

Accidental poisoning has always been a concern for those caring for children. In the United States during the 1940s, accidental poisoning was estimated to cause 500 deaths per year in children under the age of 6 years. This unacceptable mortality has been addressed by several approaches, including the development of poison control centers and a sophisticated poison management database; governmental regulation; development of safer medications and child-resistant closures for medication and consumer product containers; education and anticipatory guidance; and a growing understanding of the environmental and pharmacologic foundations of toxicol-

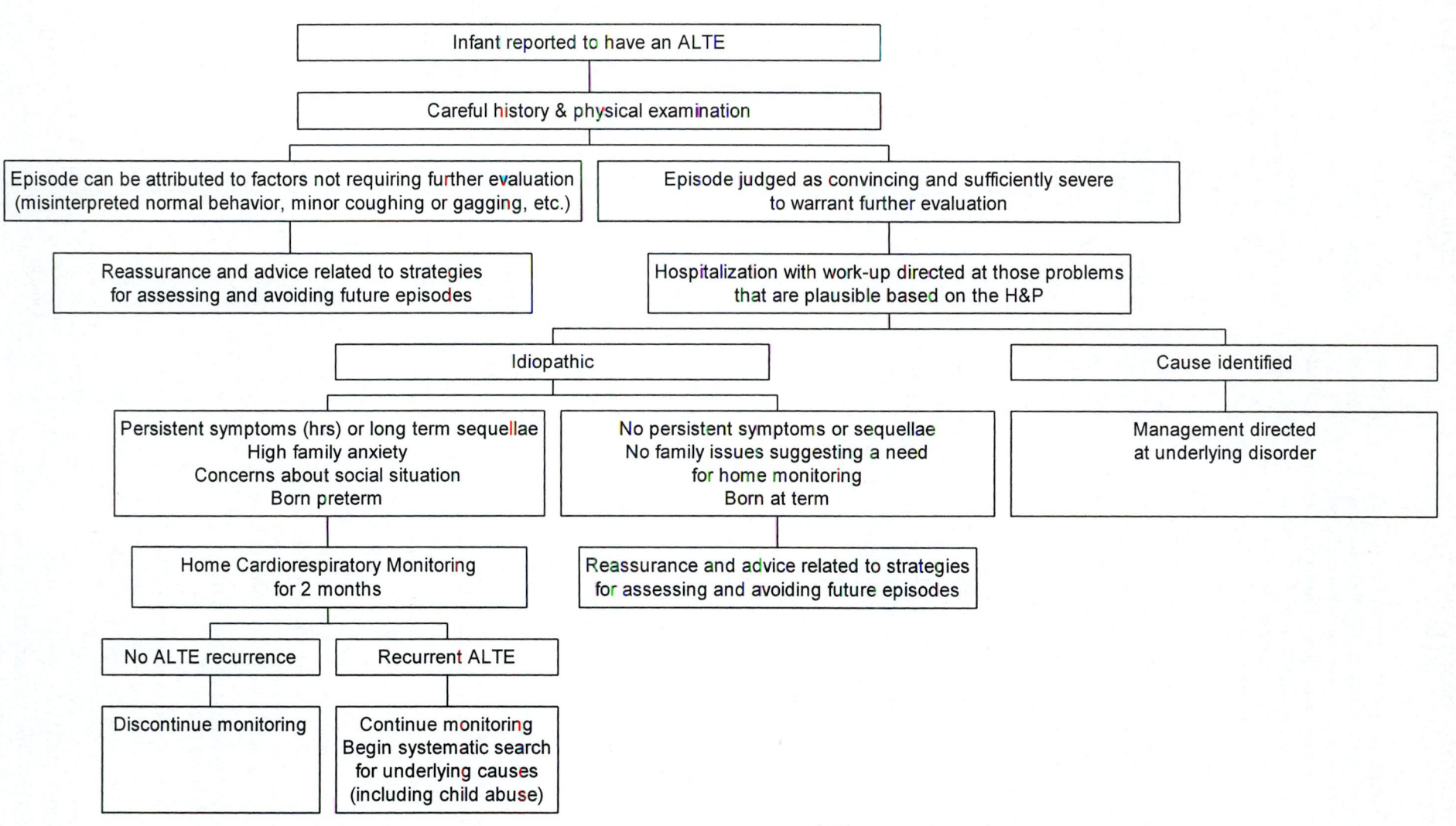

FIGURE 4-31 Algorithm for management of an infant reported to have an apparent life-threatening event (ALTE).

ogy. When viewed from the perspective of mortality rates, the results have been extraordinary. During the 1990s, fewer than 25 children per year under the age of 6 years died of acute poisoning.

However, poisoning remains an important pediatric concern. There are greater than one million telephone calls to American poison control centers each year, and the presentation of a child to an emergency department because of poisoning is a common event.

POISON PREVENTION

As for all injuries, the goal is to prevent the poisoning from occurring, and there have been great strides toward that end. However, there will always be the need for active preventive strategies, with the most important being parental education. The best way to deliver this is through anticipatory guidance during well-child visits. Although advocated by some, poison education as a "teachable moment" during a child's presentation to the emergency department because of poisoning is not uniformly well received. Brochures and other materials for poison prevention can be obtained from local poison control centers or national pediatric societies.

EPIDEMIOLOGY

There are two common scenarios for poisoning related to the age of the child. In the first scenario, a toddler or a preschooler who, as a function of the child's curiosity, may sample a substance in the child's immediate environment. The little taste of a single substance makes significant morbidity or mortality unlikely. The American Association of Poison Control Centers consistently reports that greater than 98% of ingestions in this age group are trivial; most are asymptomatic, and the remainder result in minor symptoms and signs. Commonly sampled objects include medications, consumer products, and plants. The most common ingestions reflect product prevalence and are acetaminophen, cleaning substances, cosmetics, and personal care products. The most common fatal poisoning is iron. As with other injuries in this age group, there is a male preponderance.

In the second scenario, an adolescent is poisoned as a result of a suicide attempt or of recreational ingestion. Although the majority of cases involve a single substance, the ingestion of multiple agents is common. Typically, large amounts are ingested, often making the consequences more serious than in accidental ingestions. Acetaminophen is the most commonly ingested medication in this circumstance, and cyclic antidepressants are the medications that result in most fatalities. Most clinically important poisonings are a consequence of ingestion. However, not all intoxications involve the alimentary tract. Other routes of exposure include ocular, dermal, injection, and inhalation. Ocular and dermal exposures rarely result in systemic toxicity. Injection is usually the consequence of adolescent recreational substance use. Inhalation typically originates from an environmental exposure, which is more common at the work place and less likely to occur in children.

PRINCIPLES OF MANAGEMENT OF THE POISONED PATIENT

There are five steps in the management of the poisoned patient: patient evaluation; resuscitation and stabilization; decontamination; enhancing elimination; and, when appropriate, administration of an antidote.

Patient Evaluation

A complete evaluation (a history, a physical examination, and clinical investigations) follows after assuring the stability of the patient.

In the unstable patient, resuscitative measures must proceed simultaneously with the evaluation.

History

Exposure to a presumed toxic substance is usually the chief complaint. Ingestion, followed by ocular and dermatologic exposures are most common in children, whereas injection and inhalation exposures are uncommon. Ingestion of a potentially toxic substance should be suspected in any seriously ill child or adolescent with altered mental status of unknown etiology, whenever there is apparent willful withholding of history, and in cases of potential child abuse. What and how much was ingested, and how much time has passed since the ingestion are important to derive from the history. The answers to these questions help define the need for and the extent of treatment required. Many substances are nontoxic (Table 4-33), and the ingestion of one of these requires no intervention other than appropriate counseling on poison prevention.

It is usually difficult to assess the dose of ingested medication or toxin with any degree of certainty: the young child has ingested something when not being directly supervised, while the adolescent may withhold information. When a container is available, it is safe to assume that the ingested dose included the number of dosage forms remaining from the original number in the container. There are two practical tips regarding the young child: (a) One dosage form independently ingested by a young child usually will not pro-

TABLE 4-33
COMMON NONTOXIC INGESTIONS

Household Products	Cosmetics
Artificial sweeteners	Baby products
Ballpoint pen ink	Body conditioners
Bath oil	Cologne
Candles	Deodorants
Crayons	Eye makeup
Dehumidifying packets	Hand lotions and cream
(silica gel or charcoal)	Hydrogen peroxide
Deodorizers	(household, 3%)
Fertilizers	Lanolin
Fish bowl additives	Lipstick
Household bleach	Perfume
Shaving cream	Suntan lotion
Shoe polish	Toilet water
Thermometers (mercury)	Miscellaneous
Water colors	Abrasives
Soaps and Detergents	Chalk
Bar soap	Cigarettes
Bath products	Clay
Bubble bath	Felt-tip pens
Fabric softener	Glues and paste
Hand and dishwashing soap	Greases
Laundry detergent	Lubricating oil
Shampoo	Magic markers
Pharmaceuticals	Matches
Antacids	Motor oil
Antibiotics	Paint
Contraceptives	Paraffin
Corticosteroids	Pencil lead
Diuretics	Play-Doh
Laxatives	Silly Putty
Mineral oil	
Topical preparations	
Vitamins (without iron)	
Zinc oxide	

duce clinically important toxicity, except when oral hypoglycemic agents, clonidine, or a large, single dose of morphine is consumed. (b) Young children rarely develop clinically important toxicity from the ingestion of a liquid from a small aperture (soda bottle size). This is because they lack the skill to allow air to enter as the fluid leaves. The usual amount ingested is only a few milliliters with the rest being either on the child or on the floor. Only highly caustic or corrosive liquids can produce significant toxicity at these small doses.

The time since ingestion is important and frequently given insufficient consideration. In general, if 4 hours have passed without significant clinical effect, it is unlikely that one will occur, except when acetaminophen, enteric-coated, or other delayed-release drugs have been ingested. The importance of this is underscored by the fact that the average time for an adolescent to present for care after an overdose is 3 to 4 hours.

Physical Examination

Assuming a stable or a stabilized patient, a complete physical examination is then performed to ascertain whether there are signs attributable to the poison in question or to other mechanisms (other unsuspected substances or trauma). Table 4-34 describes clinical findings commonly observed in poisonings, which may help focus attention on important signs.

Much has been written about toxidromes, which are sets of symptoms and signs produced by various poisons. Many toxidromes are based on dysfunction of the autonomic nervous system caused by sympathomimetic, sympatholytic, anticholinergic, or cholinergic effects of a drug. Toxidromes represent an attempt to diagnose a specific poisoning in an ill patient when little or no history is provided. Unfortunately, there is often so much overlap amongst toxidromes that they are of little practical bedside application. However, there are three important toxidromes that must be recognized because these are present in life-threatening poisonings, which require urgent diagnosis and intervention. These are the opioid, cyclic antidepressant, and cholinergic toxidromes.

The opioid toxidrome consists of decreased level of consciousness, respiratory depression, and miosis. The cyclic antidepressant toxidrome consists of decreased level of consciousness, wide QRS interval, dysrhythmias, and seizures. The cholinergic toxidrome, consequent to organophosphate or carbamate insecticide poisoning, consists of bronchospasm, bronchorrhea, salivation, lacrimation, and diaphoresis.

Detection of a Toxin

Oxygen saturation, ECG, CBC, serum electrolytes and osmolality, blood gases, and abdominal x-rays are often useful in the initial evaluation of the potentially poisoned child. When the specific toxin is known, then a quantitative serum drug concentration is most useful, and many laboratories have capacity to measure common toxins within a short time (preferably within 1 hour). A drug screen is a battery of tests performed upon a biological specimen for the purpose of identifying the presence of a drug. Urine is the preferred specimen because it is easier to work with and most common toxic drugs are found in higher concentrations in urine than in blood. However, as demonstrated in several studies, drug screens obtained on an emergency basis have negligible impact upon patient management and outcome. Even if the drug found in the urine is quantified, there is no relationship between this value and clinical effect, because the screen can not differentiate between therapeutic dosing and an overdose. Because a drug screen cannot

possibly identify all drugs, false-negatives can occur. However, there are situations (for forensic or mental health) where a drug screen may have potential value. For these situations, specimens can be obtained and analyzed later.

TABLE 4-34

COMMON SIGNS OBSERVED IN VARIOUS POISONINGS

Tachycardia
  Amphetamines
  Anticholinergics
  β-Adrenergics
  Caffeine
  Cocaine
  Cyclic antidepressants
  Theophylline
Hypertension
  Amphetamines
  Cocaine
  Ephedrine
  Phencyclidine
  Phenylpropanolamine
  Pseudoephedrine
Ventricular Dysrhythmias
  Amphetamines
  β-Adrenergics
  Caffeine
  Chloral hydrate
  Cocaine
  Cyclic antidepressants
  Digoxin
  Quinidine
  Theophylline
Miosis
  Carbamate insecticides
  Cholinergics
  Clonidine
  Opioids
  Organophosphate insecticides
  Phencyclidine
Hyperthermia
  Amphetamines
  Anticholinergics
  Antipsychotics
  Cocaine
  Cyclic antidepressants
  MAO inhibitors
  Phencyclidine
  Salicylates
Convulsions
  Amphetamines
  Anticholinergics
  Antihistamines
  Caffeine
  Camphor
  Cholinergics
  Cocaine
  Cyclic antidepressants
  Isoniazid
  Lindane
  Organophosphates and carbamates
  Phencyclidine
  Phenothiazines
  Strychnine
  Theophylline

Bradycardia
  β-Blockers
  Calcium channel blockers
  Clonidine
  Cyclic antidepressants
  Digoxin
  Opioids
  Sedative hypnotics
Hypotension
  β-Blockers
  Calcium channel blockers
  Cyanide
  Cyclic antidepressants
  Clonidine
  Opioids
  Phenothiazines
Wide QRS Interval
  Cyclic antidepressants
  Encainide
  Flecainide
  Potassium
  Propranolol
  Quinidine
  (Other type Ia antiarrhythmics)
Midriasis
  Amphetamines
  Anticholinergics
  Antihistamines
  Cocaine
  LSD
  MAO inhibitors
Hypothermia
  Alcohol
  Clonidine
  Opioids
  Sedative hypnotics
Coma
  Alcohol
  Benzodiazepines
  Clonidine
  Cyclic antidepressants
  Opioids
  Phenothiazines
  Sedative hypnotics

Some toxins can be detected because they produce small molecules that are not normally measured in serum. The anion gap, which detects the presence of unmeasured anions, is estimated by subtracting the sum of the prevalent serum anions, chloride and bicarbonate, from the serum sodium: $Na^+ - (Cl^- + HCO_3^-)$. The normal value is 12 ± 4 mEq/L, and this is often increased with ingestions. Therefore, the mnemonic MUDPILES has been used to remember common causes for an increased gap, many of which relate to toxins: methanol; uremia; diabetic ketoacidosis; paraldehyde and phenformin; iron and isoniazid; lactic acidosis; ethylene glycol; and salicylates and solvent (toluene).

The osmol gap, which detects unmeasured osmotically active molecules, is estimated by subtracting the calculated osmolality from the measured serum osmolality. The former is derived from one of the following formulae:

$$2Na \ (mEq/L) + Glucose \ (mg/dL)/18 + BUN \ (mg/dL)/2.8$$

or

$$2Na + Glucose + BUN \ (for \ SI \ Units)$$

The normal value is 5 ± 10 mOsm/kg, and when this is increased, an unmeasured osmotically active molecule is presumed to be present. Important toxins that commonly produce an increased anion gap include ethanol, isopropanol, methanol, and ethylene glycol. The osmolar gap is often recommended as a screening test for the presence of methanol or ethylene glycol. However, this is not a particularly sensitive test because 64 mg/dL of methanol or 120 mg/dL of ethylene glycol, both highly toxic levels, only increase serum by 20 mOsm/kg. Therefore, if either of these is the poison of concern, specific quantification should be obtained along with an osmolar gap to ensure against a false-negative.

The abdominal x-ray is a very important procedure for the patient who has ingested iron. It validates the ingestion and directs gastrointestinal decontamination. Historically, abdominal x-rays were recommended for several ingestions including chloral hydrate, heavy metals, iron, phenytoin, and slow-release tablets. These recommendations were based on in vitro data without clinical validation. Therefore, the abdominal x-ray should be limited to suspected iron and heavy metal ingestions.

Resuscitation and Stabilization

Attention to the patency of the airway, adequacy of the breathing effort, and efficiency of the circulation is paramount. Initial treatment of problems involving any of these areas should follow the same general guidelines applied to other life-threatening illness or injury. Appropriate monitoring should include measurement of arterial oxygen saturation and recording of heart rate and ECG. Intravenous access should be obtained promptly, especially if circulatory dysfunction is present. A decreased respiratory effort or an obstructed airway are usually indications for tracheal intubation and institution of mechanical ventilation, unless there is strong suspicion that the toxic agent is an opioid, in which case administration of an opioid antagonist may restore airway and ventilatory functions.

Decontamination

The goal of decontamination is to prevent the absorption of an ingested poison from the gastrointestinal tract into the bloodstream or to remove a potentially damaging substance from the eye or the skin. The use of decontamination has been the subject of five position statements by the American Academy of Clinical Toxicology and the European Association of Poison Centres and Clinical Toxicologists. These statements suggest an approach different from the traditional use of either syrup of ipecac–induced emesis or orogastric lavage, followed by a slurry of activated charcoal combined with a cathartic. The American Academy's recommendations for most ingestions include only the use of activated charcoal (with no cathartic, gastric lavage, or ipecac). In selected situations, whole-bowel irrigation should be considered.

Another important aspect of gastric decontamination is its decreasing likelihood of benefit as time since ingestion increases. Traditional recommendations were to perform these interventions up to 4 to 6 hours after ingestion. Current practice is to limit gastric decontamination to the period of 1 to 2 hours after ingestion.

Activated charcoal acts as an adsorbent. Many organic and inorganic molecules bind to it in the intestine, preventing them from being absorbed, but it is not useful for adsorbing iron, lithium, cyanide, alcohols, and strong acids and bases, for example, hydrochloric acid and sodium hydroxide. Although charcoal can bind to ethanol and methanol, the amounts of charcoal required to produce benefit generally exceeds the patient's tolerance. Even though the more charcoal given, the greater the amount of toxin bound, the dose of charcoal is based on the maximum amount that the patient can tolerate. For toddlers and preschoolers a slurry of 25 g of aqueous-activated charcoal (not in sorbitol) can generally be given; for adolescents 50 to 100 g can generally be given. Young children who will not drink charcoal must be given it by nasogastric tube. The complication of charcoal is from aspiration so it is important to reduce the risks for this. Whole-bowel irrigation is an intervention intended to prevent the absorption of ingested poisons from the gastrointestinal tract into the bloodstream. Whole-bowel irrigation is the rapid administration of polyethylene glycol electrolyte lavage solution (proprietary solutions used as colonoscopy or bowel surgery preparations) by nasogastric tube. It flushes potentially toxic substances out of the gut. Administration rates are 500 mL/h for toddlers and 1.5 to 2.0 L/h for adolescents. The endpoint is a clear rectal effluent, which may take many hours. The indications for this procedure are the ingestion of substances not absorbed by charcoal, such as iron and lithium, and the ingestion of modified-release pharmaceuticals. These can persist in the small intestine for many hours, and whole-bowel irrigation is the only decontamination strategy with the potential to be effective beyond the pylorus.

For ocular and dermal exposures, copious irrigation with tap water may decontaminate the area and prevent or ameliorate injury caused by ongoing contact from the substance.

Decontamination in the Home

Tap-water irrigation should be begun immediately after ocular or dermal exposure. For several decades, keeping ipecac in the home was a prominent aspect of poison prevention education in the United States. However, many poison control centers have reconsidered the recommendation of home ipecac use. Chief issues are the efficacy of this intervention and that it delays and hampers charcoal administration. Activated charcoal therapy in the home, promoted by some manufacturers of this product, has problems, including the inability to administer appropriate doses effectively.

Enhancing Elimination

The goal of elimination enhancement is to hasten the excretion of toxins from the blood at a rate greater than endogenous clearance. Interventions purported to achieve that end include forced diuresis, urinary alkalization or acidification, multiple-dose charcoal therapy, hemodialysis, and hemoperfusion. Forced diuresis and urinary acidification are either ineffective or fraught with adverse effects and are not recommended.

Multiple-Dose Charcoal Therapy

Although multiple doses (every 1–4 hours) of activated charcoal can be given to hasten the excretion of some drugs (eg, phenobarbital, theophylline) from the blood, this intervention is not beneficial to poisoned patients. Unfortunately, multiple-dose charcoal therapy is indiscriminately used for many poisonings, much like hemodialysis a generation ago. The position statement of the American Academy of Clinical Toxicology and the European Association of Poison Centres and Clinical Toxicology on multiple-dose charcoal recommends that it should only be considered for phenobarbital, theophylline, phenytoin, carbamazepine, and dapsone poisonings. Dosing varies from 10 to 25 g every 1 to 4 hours. Complications include charcoal aspiration and bowel obstruction, and the risks often outweigh the purported benefits.

Urinary Alkalization

This intervention is aimed at increasing the clearance of toxins that are weak acids. The increase in urinary pH raises the ionization ratio of the toxin, rendering it less soluble in the membrane lipids and thus less likely to be reabsorbed into the bloodstream. The goal of this intervention is to trap weak acids in the renal tubular fluid. The most commonly used alkalinizing agent is sodium bicarbonate, which is administered at doses of 1 to 2 mEq/kg intravenously and continued as an infusion adjusted to produce a urinary pH of 7.0 to 8.0. This method of enhanced clearance has been proposed for salicylate and phenobarbital poisonings. Increasing the urinary pH by one unit enhances salicylate excretion 20-fold, but urinary alkalinization is typically difficult to achieve in salicylate poisoning. In fact, the administration of sodium bicarbonate may produce a state of paradoxic aciduria (alkaline plasma and acid urine), because the potassium depletion, which is virtually always present, is aggravated by the alkaline infusion.

Hemodialysis

Hemodialysis can correct fluid, electrolyte, and acid-base imbalances and can hasten the removal of toxic substances from the blood. It is effective for toxins that have small volumes of distribution (less than 1.0 L/kg) and that have low protein binding, and should be considered for methanol, ethylene glycol, salicylate, and lithium poisonings.

Hemoperfusion

Hemoperfusion is similar to hemodialysis except for the substitution of the dialysis membrane by a cartridge containing an adsorbent material (typically charcoal). Unlike dialysis, however, this is accomplished without the need for the toxin to undergo ultrafiltration and thus the method is more suitable to larger molecules. In the past, its chief indication was for theophylline poisoning. Because this is rarely seen, this procedure is used infrequently.

Antidotes

An antidote is an agent that prevents the development of, or that reverses the symptoms and signs of, poisoning. An ideal antidote has no other drug action beyond reversing the poisoning. Antidotes may be true competitive antagonists, physiological antagonists, or dispositional antidotes. A competitive antagonist directly competes with the poison for receptor sites. Physiological antagonists alter the physiological effect produced by the poison, for example, atropine and physostigmine for anticholinergic and cholinergic poisonings, respectively. Most antidotes are dispositional antidotes, which decreases the poison's action by altering its absorption, metabolism, disposition, or excretion, eg, N-acetylcysteine for acetaminophen poisoning.

Serious poisonings may require large and unpredictable antidote doses. For most antidotes, dosing is limited by the potential for adverse effects. However, there are some antidotes for which this is not the case and their dosing is by titration. Examples include naloxone for opiate poisoning, atropine for organophosphorus insecticide poisoning, and pyridoxine for isoniazid poisoning.

Table 4-35 provides a list of poisons and their antidotes. Indications and doses are discussed in sections that follow. Flumazenil, the benzodiazepine antagonist, deserves special comment because it is generally not recommended for poisonings from this group of drugs. Benzodiazepine ingestion is not a particularly hazardous poisoning. Virtually all patients do well with a brief period of supportive care. Flumazenil is a hazard for patients who are thought to have benzodiazepine poisoning when, in fact, their altered mental status is caused by a neuroleptic or cyclic antidepressant, either alone or in combination with the suspected benzodiazepine. Many neuroleptics and cyclic antidepressants lower the seizure threshold, and the blockade of GABA-inhibitory receptors by the administration of flumazenil has provoked seizures that can be difficult to

TABLE 4-35

ANTIDOTES OR TREATMENTS USEFUL FOR COMMON POISONINGS

POISON	ANTIDOTE
Acetaminophen	N-Acetylcysteine
Benzodiazepines	Flumazenil[1]
β-Blockers	Glucagon
Calcium channel blockers	Glucagon
Carbamate insecticides	Atropine
Carbon monoxide	Oxygen
Cyanide	Cyanide antidote kit
Cyclic antidepressants	Sodium bicarbonate
Digoxin	Antidigoxin Fab antibody fragments
Ethylene glycol	Fomepizole or ethanol[2]
Heavy metals	Chelators
Isoniazid	Pyridoxine
Iron	Deferoxamine
Jimson weed	Physostigmine
Methanol	Fomepizole or ethanol[2]
Methemoglobinemia	Methylene blue
Opioids	Naloxone
Organophosphate insecticides	Atropine + pralidoxime
Sulfonylureas	Diazoxide or octreotide
Warfarin	Vitamin K

[1]Flumazenil is generally not recommended for benzodiazepine poisoning.
[2]Fomepizole is favored over ethanol.

treat. It is important to remember that specific antidotes are available for a very small number of poisonings and that the cardinal principle of management of the poisoned patient is meticulous supportive care. Moreover, it can be dangerous to try to determine the toxin by testing the response to specific antidotes.

SPECIFIC TOXINS

Acetaminophen

Acetaminophen is the most common drug overdose of all ages, an obvious function of its widespread use as an analgesic and antipyretic. It is available in many forms including concentrated drops (80 mg/mL), children's suspensions and elixirs (160 mg/5 mL), children's tablets (80 and 160 mg), adult solid dosage (500 mg), and as a modified-release product (325 mg conventional-release and 325 mg delayed-release). It is also marketed in several combinations with drugs including codeine, antihistamines, decongestants, antitussives, and muscle relaxants.

Toxicology

The chief target organ of acetaminophen poisoning is the liver, with the kidneys being involved in about 10 to 20% of those patients with hepatotoxicity. Rarely, nephrotoxicity may occur without significant hepatic involvement. The metabolism of this drug helps explain the pathogenesis of liver injury and the basis of the antidote. After therapeutic dosing, most of this drug is glucuronidated or sulfated in the liver and then excreted in the urine. A small amount is oxidized in the liver by the cytochrome P_{450} system. An intermediary metabolite of this oxidative transformation, N-acetyl-p-benzoquinonenemine (NAPQI), is highly reactive with cell proteins and produces hepatotoxicity. To a lesser extent, a similar process takes place in the kidneys. The amount of NAPQI generated after therapeutic dosing is easily conjugated by glutathione, as part of the scavenging mechanisms that dispose of the oxidants generated during normal metabolic activity. Organ damage does not occur until reserve glutathione is consumed to a level of 30% of normal. The antidote, N-acetylcysteine, replenishes glutathione.

The dose required to produce significant hepatotoxicity in adults is 7.5 to 10.0 g. The commonly stated hepatotoxic dose for children is 150 mg/kg. However, this is an extrapolation of adult data because there are few reports of toxicity from a single overdose of acetaminophen in children under the age of 6 years. Recently, amounts as high as 200 to 250 mg/kg have been suggested as doses of concern for young children. Children are well known to be less sensitive to acetaminophen overdose than adults if the dose is normalized for weight. Although the reason proposed is that acetaminophen undergoes greater levels of sulfation in prepubertal children, the total amount metabolized through sulfation and glucuronidation is quite similar. Rather, the reason for the relative resistance in young children seems to be that they clear drugs more efficiently than adults because on a gram per kilogram basis, their livers and kidneys are larger than in adults. Hepatotoxicity in young children has been reported in association with subacute overdosing. This occurs when children receive multiple marginally supratherapeutic doses over several hours to a few days, or therapeutic doses at too frequent intervals. In many instances liver transplantation has been required.

Clinical Presentation and Management

During the first few hours after the ingestion of a toxic dose the patient will be either asymptomatic or have mild gastrointestinal symptoms, including anorexia, nausea, vomiting, and abdominal pain. If the patient has abnormal vital signs or altered mental status, another poison, either alone or in addition to acetaminophen, must be considered. Hepatotoxicity manifests at 24 to 48 hours after acetaminophen ingestion with right upper-quadrant pain and tenderness and laboratory evidence of hepatic dysfunction, including elevated transaminase values and prolonged prothrombin time. Those patients destined to develop nephrotoxicity often have detectable elevations in serum creatinine concentrations at this time. Clinical and laboratory evidence of liver dysfunction peaks at 72 to 96 hours, after which spontaneous resolution is common and the prognosis for recovery is very good. A minority of patients develop irreversible hepatotoxicity, typically between days 3 and 5.

Treatment of acetaminophen must be based on a careful assessment of risk and includes gastric decontamination and administration of the specific antidote N-acetylcysteine (Fig. 4-32). Patients with irreversible hepatotoxicity need to be considered for liver transplantation. Patients are at risk if greater than 150 mg/kg or 7.5 g of acetaminophen have been ingested. If less than 1 to 2 hours have elapsed since the ingestion, activated charcoal in water should be administered at doses of 25 g to a child less than 6 years old, 25–50 g to a 6- to 12-year-old, and 50 to 100 g to a teenager (or about 1 g/kg). After this precautionary measure is taken, it is appropriate to assess drug absorption by determining the serum acetaminophen concentration. N-acetylcysteine is indicated if the serum concentration is above the treatment line on the nomogram (Fig. 4-33) or if the serum acetaminophen concentration will not be known within 8 hours of drug ingestion. The nomogram has two lines, the lower "possible hepatotoxicity" and the upper "probable toxicity." In the United States, the usual recommendation is to initiate therapy if the value is above the lower line, but others recommend antidote administration when the serum concentration is above the upper line. It is important to initiate N-acetylcysteine therapy within 8 hours of drug ingestion because its efficacy diminishes thereafter. If subsequent acetaminophen concentration falls below the treatment line, the antidote can be discontinued.

There are three potential dosing protocols for N-acetylcysteine (Table 4-36). The oral route is the only one with FDA approval. The 20-hour intravenous protocol is favored in most countries other than the United States, while the 48-hour protocol has support from published studies in the United States. Recently, some clinicians have recommended discontinuing the oral protocol as soon as acetaminophen is undetectable in the blood.

The disadvantages of the oral protocol are that it takes longer (3 days vs. 20 hours), it is often poorly tolerated because of vomiting, and the concern regarding the potential for decreased bioavailability because of previous administration of activated charcoal. The disadvantage of the intravenous protocol is that it induces histamine release and hence the risk for an anaphylactic reaction. This is typically mild, manifesting as flushing and urticaria, and its risk is minimized by giving the loading dose over 1 hour rather than over 15 minutes.

There are data that support the use of intravenous N-acetylcysteine beyond 24 hours in patients with acetaminophen-induced hepatic failure. Its use for this indication has been associated with a less severe clinical course and a decreased likelihood for liver transplantation. There are several speculations for its mechanism of action.

Assuming that any mental health issues requiring attention have been addressed, indications for discharge are a nontoxic ingestion or the completion of antidote therapy. All patients receiving a

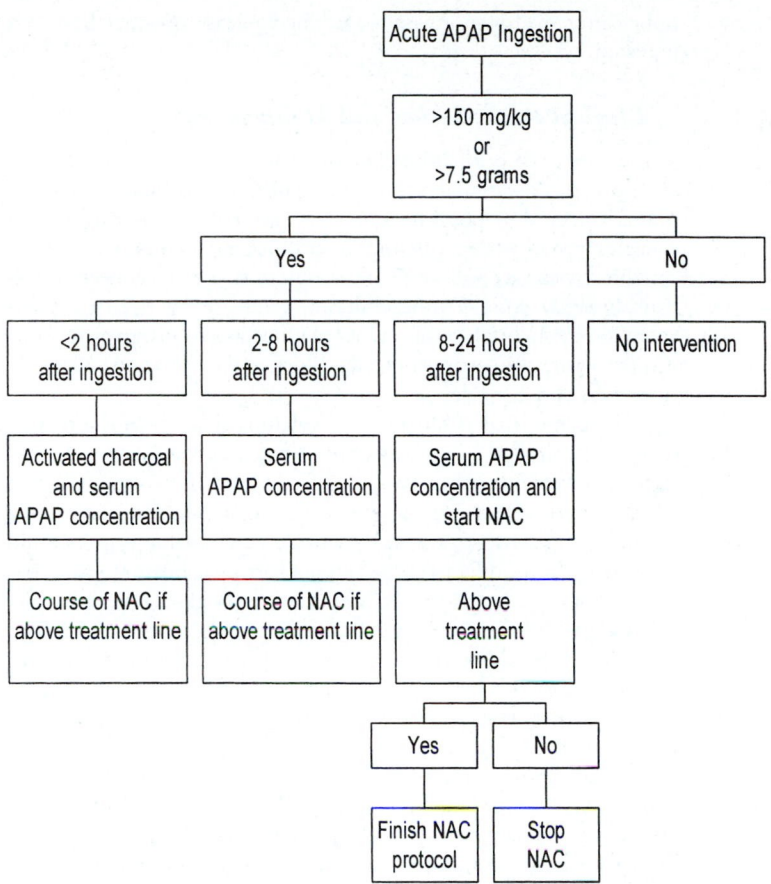

FIGURE 4-32 Algorithm for management of acetaminophen ingestion. APAP = acetaminophen; NAC = N-acetylcysteine.

course of *N*-acetylcysteine should have laboratory assessment of liver and kidney function following treatment.

Anticoagulants

Most anticoagulant exposures involve young children who sample a rodenticide that had been left out to exterminate mice or rats. Because rodents are relatively resistant to the original warfarin rodenticides, these rodenticides were replaced by the more potent second-generation superwarfarins. The superwarfarins comprise two classes: 4-hydroxycoumarin (brodifacoum, bromadiolone and difenacoum) and indandione (diaphacinone and chlorphacinone), both of which are marketed in very low concentrations as pellets, treated seeds, or oatmeal. Typically, the rodent requires multiple exposures for extermination. Children can also ingest pharmaceutical warfarin, but this is much less likely because of the low penetrance of this agent in their environment.

Toxicology

The warfarins work by inhibiting vitamin K, a cofactor in the synthesis of clotting factors II, VII, IX, and X, which prolongs prothrombin time. The toxic effect of warfarin poisoning is hemorrhage, but this is not expected from a single ingestion of a superwarfarin rodenticide by a young child. Massive ingestion with suicidal intent or chronic ingestions are required to produce poisoning. The superwarfarins are 100 times more potent and have a duration of action at least 3 times greater than that of warfarin.

Clinical Presentation and Management

Ingestion is most commonly by a small child who has tasted a rodenticide that was left out to exterminate mice or rats. In this sit-

uation, no interventions or evaluation are indicated. In contrast, if the child has ingested a potentially toxic dose of pharmaceutical warfarin, measurement of prothrombin time and gastric decontamination should be considered. Most significant cases of warfarin poisoning present as bruising or bleeding with laboratory confirmation of coagulopathy but no history of ingestion. In these cases children are victims of child abuse by poisoning or have surreptitiously and chronically ingested the superwarfarin rodenticide. The differential diagnosis of an unknown coagulopathy is very broad and reviewed elsewhere. Superwarfarin poisoning is confirmed by specific assay of the blood, which requires the services of a reference laboratory. Coagulopathy from superwarfarin poisoning is typically severe and can persist for months. It is often refractory to large parenteral doses of vitamin K, with the only effective treatment being repeated fresh-frozen plasma transfusions.

β-Blockers and Calcium Channel Blockers

Although β-blockers and calcium channel blockers (see Tables 4-37 and 4-38) are two distinct classes of drugs, they are considered together because of their similar effects. The management of poisoning from these two drug classes has several aspects in common. Their chief uses are to treat hypertension, angina pectoris, and cardiac dysrhythmias, and overdose is not infrequent. Poisonings are difficult to treat and have significant morbidity and mortality.

Toxicology

β-Blockers competitively inhibit the binding of norepinephrine and epinephrine by β-adrenergic receptors. There are several $β_1$-selective agents, but in overdose, selectivity may be lost. Several β-blockers have membrane-stabilizing effects that manifest after overdose.

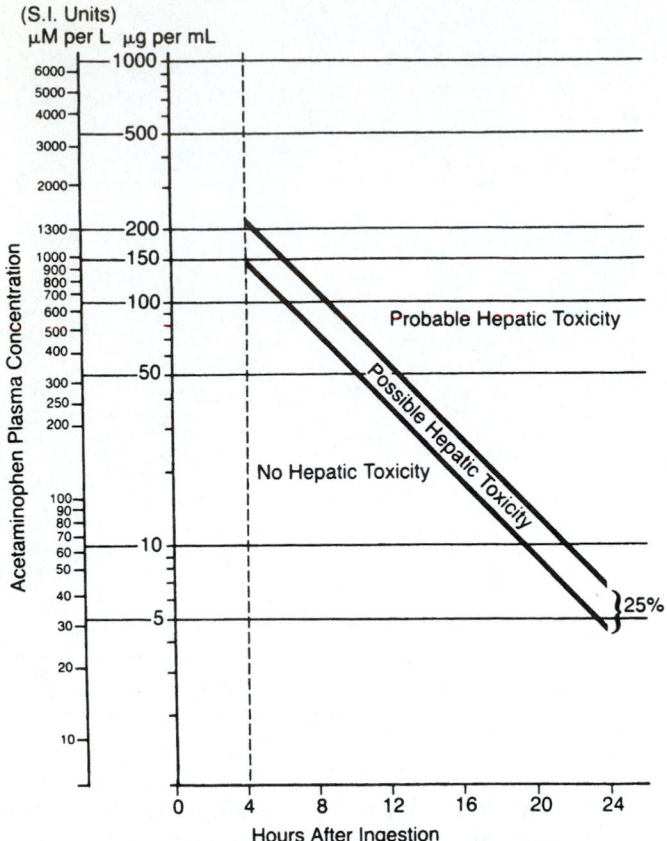

FIGURE 4-33 **Nomogram for predicting hepatotoxicity after a single acute overdose of acetaminophen; preferred time to obtain serum concentration is approximately 4 hours after ingestion. The lower line (25% below upper line) is used in the United States to determine need for antidotal therapy (see text).**

This results in reduced membrane permeability to the fast influx of sodium ions. Membrane stabilization is a significant contributor to the adverse cardiac and central nervous system effects seen in β-blocker overdose. These include bradycardia, hypotension, coma, and seizures. Calcium channel blockers inhibit calcium entry into cells, which causes decreased inotropy and chronotropy and decreased vascular smooth muscle tone. Calcium channel blockers are well absorbed after ingestion, and signs are expected within 1 to 2

TABLE 4-36

N-ACETYLCYSTEINE PROTOCOLS FOR THE TREATMENT OF ACETAMINOPHEN POISONING

20-hour intravenous
  150 mg/kg over 15 minutes*
  50 mg/kg over 4 hours
  100 mg/kg over 16 hours
72-hour oral
  140 mg/kg loading dose
  70 mg/kg given every 4 hours (17 doses)
48-hour intravenous
  140 mg/kg loading dose
  70 mg/kg given every 4 hours (12 doses)

* Giving the loading dose over 1 hour rather than over 15 minutes minimizes the likelihood of adverse effects from histamine release.

hours after overdose unless a sustained-release product has been ingested.

Clinical Presentation and Management

The hallmark of both β-blocker and calcium channel blocker poisoning is cardiovascular depression manifested as bradycardia, hypotension, and hypoperfusion. The cerebral hypoperfusion can cause altered mental status, and the β-blockers, such as propranolol, can directly cause coma and convulsions or decreased consciousness from hypoglycemia. Young children are at greater risk than teenagers for the hypoglycemia. ECG manifestations progress from sinus bradycardia to atrioventricular block and on to ventricular dysrhythmias and asystole.

Management of β-blocker and calcium channel blocker overdose is very similar. Patients with moderate to severe symptoms and signs require close observation in a facility where treatment can be administered. If less than 2 hours have elapsed since ingestion of a potentially toxic dose, a dose of activated charcoal in water should be given. If a modified-release dosage form has been ingested between 2 and 12 hours before presentation, begin whole-bowel irrigation at 500 mL/h for a child less than 6 years old and 1.5 to 2.0 L/h for the older child or teenager. Gastrointestinal decontamination should not be employed in patients manifesting significant signs of toxicity because it is too late to provide clinically important benefit. Rather, supportive care is most effective at this time. Atropine can be tried for bradycardia, but it frequently fails. Intuitively, β-agonists and calcium are logical interventions for these two respective poisonings, but both frequently fail, even at very large dosages, when the antagonistic effect of the toxin precludes their effect completely. The most effective pharmacologic intervention is glucagon, which increases intracellular cyclic adenosine monophosphate independent of stimulation of β-adrenergic receptors. Because of its short duration of action, it must be given as a bolus dose followed by a constant infusion. The doses are 0.5 to 1.0 mg followed by 1 to 5 mg/h in adult-sized patients and 50 to 150 μg/kg followed by 10 to 50 μg/kg/h, not to exceed the adult dose, in smaller children. Unfortunately, many hospital pharmacies do not maintain sufficient stock of glucagon to support this therapy. If pharmacologic interventions are unsuccessful, consider transcutaneous or transvenous cardiac pacing. Other interventions for very severe poisoning include intra-aortic balloon pump or cardiopulmonary bypass.

Blood sugar should be frequently monitored in β-blocker poisoning and hypoglycemia treated with intravenous dextrose. Mon-

TABLE 4-37

β-BLOCKERS IN COMMON USE

DRUG	β_1-SELECTIVE	MEMBRANE STABILIZATION
Acebutolol	Yes	Yes
Atenolol	Yes	No
Labetalol	No	No
Metoprolol	Yes	No
Nadolol	No	No
Oxyprenolol	No	Yes
Pindolol	No	Yes
Propranolol	No	Yes
Sotalol	No	No
Timolol	No	No

TABLE 4-38

CALCIUM CHANNEL BLOCKERS AND THEIR CARDIOVASCULAR ACTIONS

CLASS AND DRUG	RESTING HEART RATE	AV NODE CONDUCTION	BLOOD PRESSURE	SYSTEMIC VASCULAR RESISTANCE	CARDIAC CONTRACTILITY
Phenylalkylamine (verapamil)	−	− − −	−	−	− −
Benzothiazepine (diltiazem)	−	− −	−	− −	−
Dihydropyridine (nifedipine, amlodipine, nicardipine, nimodipine, felodipine, isradipine)	± or +	±	− −	− − −	±
Diarylaminopropylamine (bepridil)	−	− −	−	−	±

itoring or measurement of serum concentrations of β-blockers or calcium channel blockers does not contribute to management, and extracorporeal drug removal is potentially useful only for atenolol and sotalol.

Patients who manifest no symptoms and signs and have a normal cardiac rhythm at 4 hours after ingestion can be discharged. If a modified-release dosage form has been ingested, longer observation (~18 hours), including a period without supportive care, is warranted prior to discharge.

Carbon Monoxide Poisoning

Carbon monoxide (CO) is generated from the combustion of carbon-containing material. It is the most common cause of poisoning death, usually resulting from home fires or from exposure to incomplete combustion of carbon fuels. Most victims die before arrival to the hospital from smoke inhalation. Other sources of CO include heating and cooking fuels such as wood, coal, kerosene, methane, propane, automobile exhaust, and methylene chloride, which is metabolized to CO and is found in many paint strippers and in some spray paints.

Toxicology

The pathogenesis of CO toxicity is a direct result of its high affinity for heme-containing molecules. In the case of hemoglobin, CO's affinity is 240 times greater than that of oxygen. CO binding to hemoglobin has two consequences. The most obvious is the displacement of oxygen molecules from their binding sites, which reduces the oxygen content of the arterial blood and oxygen delivery to tissues. In addition, the combination of CO with hemoglobin to form carboxyhemoglobin produces an increase in the affinity of the hemoglobin molecule for the oxygen molecules that are bound to it, reducing the release of oxygen into the tissues. CO also binds to myoglobin and intracellular cytochrome oxidase, causing additional impairment of oxidative metabolism.

The half-life of carboxyhemoglobin in patients breathing room air is approximately 4 hours. Because CO and O_2 compete for hemoglobin binding, increasing arterial P_{O_2} by breathing 100% oxygen at 1.0 and 2.5 atmospheres will decrease half-life to approximately 60 minutes and 20 minutes, respectively.

Clinical Presentation and Management

Any victim of a house fire or any subject found unconscious inside a running automobile should be considered as suffering from CO poisoning until proven otherwise. However, most CO exposures are inadvertent, and the symptoms and signs are nonspecific, making this diagnosis a distinctive challenge. Symptoms and signs include headache, nausea, vomiting, lightheadedness, general malaise, dyspnea, confusion, and syncope. More serious exposures may present with seizures, coma, or dysrhythmias. Because exposure is often unknown and because the symptoms and signs are nonspecific, mild cases are often undiagnosed. Mistaken diagnoses include flu-like illness, tension or migraine headache, gastroenteritis, food poisoning, and depression. The sign of cherry-red coloration of skin and mucous membranes is inconsistently found.

The diagnosis is confirmed by measurement of the percentage of carboxyhemoglobin present in the blood. The normal range is 0 to 5% in nonsmokers. It can approach 10% in heavy smokers. There is a reasonably consistent relationship between percentage of carboxyhemoglobin and symptoms and signs (Table 4-39). The presence of carboxyhemoglobin reduces arterial blood hemoglobin oxygen saturation. However, arterial P_{O_2} is normal because dissolved O_2 in blood is unaffected by carboxyhemoglobin, and the HbO_2 saturation *calculated* from the P_{O_2} is reported as normal. Furthermore, the oxygen saturation measured by routine pulse oximetry is falsely normal because the device does not detect carboxyhemoglobin (see Sec. 4.2.1). However, oxygen saturation measured from a blood sample with a device that is sensitive to carboxyhemoglobin, such as a co-oximeter, will detect the arterial hypoxemia. Because of the potential for confusion in how the hemoglobin oxygen saturation is determined, the laboratory should be specifically alerted to the concern for detection of carboxyhemoglobin.

The treatment for CO poisoning is aimed at reducing the amount of CO bound to heme proteins by administering 100% oxygen to increase the partial pressure of oxygen in the blood and tissues, until the carboxyhemoglobin decreases to the normal range.

TABLE 4-39

SIGNS AND SYMPTOMS OF CARBON MONOXIDE POISONING

PERCENT CARBOXYHEMOGLOBIN	SYMPTOMS AND SIGNS
0–10	None
10–20	Headache
20–40	Increasing headache, nausea, vomiting, dyspnea, fatigue, lightheadedness, impaired judgment
40–60	Tachypnea, tachycardia, confusion, syncope, seizure, coma
60–70	Hypotension, dysrhythmias, coma, death
>70	Rapidly fatal

Hyperbaric oxygen administration takes this strategy one step further, creating in the process a meaningful increase in the blood and tissue PO_2. However, outcome data showing benefit are lacking. Unless a hyperbaric facility is readily available it seems inappropriate to transfer the patient to another center if the transfer time is longer than the CO elimination time while breathing 100% oxygen. If the patient is unstable, the potential risk of transport must be factored into the risk-benefit analysis. Proponents of hyperbaric oxygen therapy for CO-poisoned patients list the following as indications for this intervention: coma, a history of loss of consciousness, cardiovascular dysfunction, pulmonary edema, acidosis, and a carboxyhemoglobin of 30 to 40%.

Caustic or Corrosive Ingestion

Caustic and *corrosive* are terms that are used interchangeably for the ingestion of strong alkalis or acids. The most commonly ingested alkali is sodium hydroxide, while the most commonly ingested acids are hydrochloric, phosphoric, and sulfuric acids. Caustic ingestions are chiefly seen in children less than 4 years of age, and rarely in suicidal adolescents. They are found in various consumer products such as drain cleaners, oven cleaners, rust removers, toilet bowl cleaners, and tile cleaners. Fortunately, the incidence of serious caustic injury is infrequent compared to that of a generation ago. The reason for this is the requirement for child-resistant closures for most consumer products containing strong alkalis or acids.

Toxicology

Serious injury is associated with agents whose pH is >12 or <2. Acids denature protein resulting in coagulation necrosis, while alkalis saponify fats and dissolve protein resulting in liquefaction necrosis.

Clinical Presentation and Management

The chief symptom is pain, which may be oral, thoracic, or abdominal depending on the site of caustic injury. Young children may manifest pain by crying, drooling, refusing to swallow, and vomiting. Stridor or hoarseness usually indicates laryngeal injury. Rarely, hematemesis or melena may occur. Examination may find evidence of dermatologic or ocular burns. The presence of oral or pharyngeal burns does not predict the presence of esophageal or gastric injury. Conversely, the absence of oral or pharyngeal burns does not preclude distal injury, particularly if a liquid alkali or acid has been ingested. Full-thickness esophageal or gastric injury cause perforation or subsequent fistula formation.

Initial management should focus on the support of vital functions, when these are threatened. Airway injury might necessitate endotracheal intubation or, in rare cases, performance of an emergency tracheostomy. Esophageal perforation and mediastinitis should also be considered as a severe initial complication. Pain control with opioids and avoidance of fluid or solid ingestion are the principles of management. Gastric decontamination with activated charcoal or gastric lavage is contraindicated. However, some clinicians advocate the administration of small volumes to dilute any remaining alkali or acid. This view is opposed by those who think that it is unlikely that any ingested caustic would still be present by the time of emergency department presentation.

Patients with alkali or acid caustic injury will require endoscopic evaluation and they may need surgical intervention. Asymptomatic patients can be monitored for the development of symptoms. A 12-hour symptom-free period usually indicates that no intervention will be needed. Prophylactic antibiotics are not indicated, and there is no evidence for benefit of corticosteroid therapy to prevent alkali-induced esophageal stricture.

Clonidine

Clonidine is a centrally acting antihypertensive agent that is also used to treat attention-deficit hyperactivity disorder, Tourette syndrome, and withdrawal from various types of recreational substance abuse. It is available as 0.1-, 0.2-, and 0.3-mg tablets, in combination with chlorthalidone or as a transdermal patch.

Toxicology

Clonidine is an α-agonist with primary α_2-adrenergic activity. Stimulation of the presynaptic α_2-adrenergic receptors in the medulla oblongata results in decreased sympathetic outflow from the central nervous system. This results in a reduction of heart rate and cardiac output. Clonidine also has weak peripheral α_1-adrenergic activity, which manifests as arterial vasoconstriction. The central α_2 predominates over the peripheral α_1; hence its use as an antihypertensive agent. In addition, clonidine is thought to stimulate the secretion of endogenous opioids within the central nervous system, which explains the opioid-like effects often observed in clonidine poisoning.

Young children are especially sensitive to clonidine. Toxicity has been reported in infants after the ingestion of a single tablet. In teenagers, significant toxicity occurs only after the ingestion of 1.0 to 2.0 mg. Clonidine patches represent a notable hazard for young children who can develop significant toxicity even after the ingestion of a used patch.

Clinical Presentation and Management

Onset of toxicity occurs within 1 hour of ingestion for the majority of patients and within 2 hours for most others. Activated charcoal should be given if the patient is seen within 2 hours of ingestion and has not yet developed significant symptoms and signs. Symptoms and signs include decreased level of consciousness, miosis, respiratory depression, hypothermia, bradycardia, and hypotension. Paradoxically, a transient episode of hypertension may occur early in the course because of clonidine's α_1-agonist effect.

The mainstay of treatment is support of vital functions. Endotracheal intubation may be required for respiratory support and fluid infusion for hypotension. Although there are several reports of reversal of the depressed level of consciousness, respiratory depression, and miosis after naloxone administration, the response to this antidote is inconsistent. Tolazoline, an α-adrenergic antagonist, was touted as a potential antidote; however, experience with it is inconclusive. On balance, it is probably best to limit pharmacologic interventions. The duration of toxicity usually subsides within 24 hours. Measurement of serum concentrations and extracorporeal removal are not indicated.

Cyclic Antidepressants

Cyclic antidepressants produce significant morbidity and mortality. Fortunately, their use has declined because of the introduction of selective serotonin reuptake inhibitors for the treatment of depression. Databases of the American Association of Poison Control Centers show that the number of cyclic antidepressant ingestions decreased by 38% and the proportion of deaths decreased by 45% from 1988 to 1998, a finding attributable to the introduction of less-toxic antidepressants. Still, in 1998, tricyclic agents were implicated in 12.6% of all poison-related deaths. Commonly prescribed agents are the tricyclics imipramine, amitriptyline, doxepin, and nortriptyline, and the tetracyclics maprotiline and mianserin.

Toxicology

When ingested at toxic doses, cyclic antidepressants are especially hazardous because their effects are centered primarily on the cardiovascular and central nervous systems. The pharmacologic effects of cyclic antidepressants include inhibition of norepinephrine uptake by synaptic terminals, muscarinic cholinergic inhibition, and α_1-adrenergic blockade. These effects are manifest in both the central and autonomic nervous system as variable combinations of signs and symptoms, the final make of which depends on the specific drug, the dose, and the age of the subject. Central nervous system toxicity causes euphoria and irritability, followed in severe cases by myoclonus and seizures, leading finally to a state of unresponsiveness associated with depression of breathing and airway-protective reflexes. Autonomic system toxicity is often dominated by findings of muscarinic inhibition, including midriasis, dry skin and mucosae, ileus, urinary retention, and tachycardia. Tricyclic antidepressants have specific effects on the heart muscle, delaying conduction through the His-Purkinje system, depressing muscle fiber contractility, and inducing a quinidine-like effect (thus prolongation of the QRS and QT intervals), which render the heart susceptible to ventricular dysrhythmias. Absorption is rapid after overdose, with symptoms and signs occurring within 2 hours of ingestion. Most of the deaths occur within several hours of the overdose. Cholinergic blockade may cause unexpected delays in toxicity by prolonging gastric emptying.

Clinical Presentation and Management

The clinical presentation may vary substantially, often progressing in severity within minutes. Early cardiovascular effects include tachycardia and hypertension. These are related to the anticholinergic and norepinephrine uptake-blocking actions. The hypertension is usually mild and transient, and soon gives way to hypotension because the blockade of reuptake rapidly results in norepinephrine depletion (hypotension also relates to α_1 blockade). Decreased cardiac output due to myocardial depression or dysrhythmias can also contribute to the hypotension. Serious ventricular dysrhythmias, such as ventricular tachycardia and torsades de pointes (a form of ventricular tachycardia), may supervene the more common supraventricular tachycardia. Central nervous system manifestations include a depressed level of consciousness, agitation, delirium, coma, seizures, myoclonus, and hyperthermia. Seizures may be a direct consequence of the cyclic antidepressant or may be due to decreased cerebral perfusion when cardiac output is decreased. Some of the more common anticholinergic effects include absent bowel sounds, ileus, and urinary retention. There are no consistent pupillary findings in cyclic antidepressant-poisoned patients. Although overdose of most drugs in this group can lead to any of the above problems, amoxapine and maprotiline infrequently produce significant cardiac toxicity.

Management of cyclic antidepressant poisoning is mainly supportive. Intravenous access and cardiac monitoring should be immediately established. Endotracheal intubation is indicated if central nervous system depression is present. Hypotension should be treated with rapid crystalloid infusion and, if this fails, pharmacologic support. Norepinephrine is often recommended because of its predominant vasoconstrictive effects with minimal β_1 activity, which limits its tendency to cause ventricular arrhythmias; phenylephrine, a pure α-agonist has similar benefits. No specific interventions are indicated for hypertension because it is typically transient and usually followed by a fall in the blood pressure. A QRS duration of >100 msec is associated with seizures, while a duration of >160 msec is associated with ventricular dysrhythmias. Values less than these do not rule out the possibility of these adverse events. Treatment of dysrhythmias can be quite challenging. Supraventricular tachycardia generally requires no intervention. Sodium bicarbonate, 1.0 mEq/kg to a maximum of 100 mEq, with alkalinization of the plasma to a pH of 7.45 to 7.55 should be considered for all patients with a QRS duration >100 msec or with ventricular dysrhythmias. Seizures typically occur within the first few hours of overdose, are brief, and typically subside before anticonvulsants can be given. The agent of choice is diazepam or lorazepam, although phenytoin has also been proposed because of its antiarrhythmic properties. Activated charcoal in water, 25 g for a young child and 50 g for a teenager, should be given to all patients who have ingested a potentially toxic dose of a cyclic antidepressant within 2 hours and who have no or minor symptoms and signs. It is unlikely that symptomatic patients will derive clinically important benefit from any type of gastrointestinal decontamination procedure and there is a greater risk for adverse effects from these interventions in this population. Measurement of serum concentrations of these drugs and extracorporeal elimination procedures play no role in the management of this poisoning.

Patients who develop no symptoms or signs of cyclic antidepressant toxicity (normal cardiac rhythm and level of consciousness) can be discharged at 4 hours after ingestion. Patients with tachycardia and lethargy require monitoring until they have had a 6-hour symptom-free period. Those patients with ventricular dysrhythmias, hypotension, seizures, or coma require a critical care setting.

Digoxin and Cardiac Glycosides

In addition to pharmaceutical digoxin and digitoxin, cardiac glycosides are present in potentially toxic amounts in common plants such as oleander, yellow oleander, lily of the valley, and foxglove. Poisoning in children from digoxin and digitoxin is, fortunately, uncommon. Most cardiac glycoside poisonings are seen in the elderly as a consequence of adverse drug reactions or chronic toxicity.

Toxicology

Cardiac glycosides inhibit the sodium-potassium-adenosine-triphosphatase pump, increasing sodium and calcium influx and potassium efflux from cells. In myocardial cells, this results in a positive inotropic effect, increased excitability and automaticity, and decreased conduction velocity. Digoxin also augments vagal tone, resulting in a negative chronotropic effect.

Digoxin and digitoxin are relatively well absorbed after ingestion. The distribution phase is very long, lasting many hours, during which time there is no correlation between serum and tissue concentrations. This accounts for the lack of relationship between the serum digoxin concentration and toxicity after acute overdose. Values 10-fold greater than the therapeutic serum concentration can be seen in asymptomatic patients during the first few hours after acute overdose, sometimes without development of toxicity. Similar concentrations in a patient with subacute or chronic toxicity would be fatal. Previously well young children can tolerate acute digoxin ingestions of 2.0 mg and adolescents can tolerate ingestions of 5.0 mg without toxicity.

Clinical Presentation and Management

Hyperkalemia is the typical serum electrolyte abnormality of acute digoxin overdose because of the inhibition of the sodium-potassium-adenosine-triphosphatase pump. It is both an indicator of toxicity and of prognosis after acute ingestion.

There are cardiac and noncardiac symptoms and signs of acute digoxin overdose. The noncardiac symptoms and signs include gastrointestinal manifestations such as anorexia, nausea, vomiting, and abdominal pain; neurologic manifestations such as confusion, drowsiness, headache, and hallucinations; and visual manifestations such as transient amblyopia, photophobia, blurred vision, scotomata, and aberrations of color vision.

Cardiac glycoside toxicity has been included for a long time in the differential diagnosis of virtually every dysrhythmia. There is, however, a typical sequence for the rhythm abnormalities seen after ingestion of a toxic dose. Bradycardia due to delayed conduction through the AV node as a result of vagal stimulation is an early manifestation, characterized electrocardiographically by PR prolongation. Sinoatrial arrest and second- and third-degree blocks are not infrequent, often followed by ectopic rhythms such as premature atrial and ventricular beats, junctional tachycardia, and ventricular tachycardia resulting from increased automaticity. The treatment of symptomatic patients includes airway support and circulation as required. Intravenous access and cardiac monitoring should be instituted immediately and serum electrolytes measured. The early sinus bradycardia, or AV blocks, often respond to atropine. However, life-threatening ventricular dysrhythmias, a serum potassium greater than 5.0 mEq/L, or bradycardia unresponsive to atropine mandate the use of the antidote, digoxin-specific Fab antibody fragments. This is administered intravenously. There are dosing guidelines based on serum digoxin concentrations; however, these are irrational because in acute overdose there is not a steady-state relationship between the plasma and tissue concentrations. Other dosing guidelines are based on the history of the amount ingested, which is notoriously imprecise. Therefore, this author recommends an empiric dose of 10 vials (38 mg immune Fab/vial) intravenously for both children and adults. This is given over 30 minutes, and if a clinical response does not occur within 30 to 60 minutes after completion of the infusion, another 10 vials can be given. The serum potassium often falls precipitously after dysrhythmia reversal by this antidote, and potassium supplementation is frequently required.

If the patient is asymptomatic upon presentation, if greater than 2.0 mg has been ingested by a young child or greater than 5.0 mg has been ingested by an adolescent, and if less than 2 hours have elapsed since ingestion, then activated charcoal in water is indicated. Gastric lavage and induction of emesis should be particularly avoided in digoxin overdose because of concern for cardiac dysrhythmias due to vagal stimulation. All patients with dysrhythmias require a critical care setting for monitoring and management.

Patients with chronic toxicity usually respond to smaller doses of Fab antibody fragments. One vial in an infant and four to six vials in an adolescent are empiric doses that can be repeated if there is no clinical response.

Measurement of the serum digoxin concentration contributes little, if anything, to the management of the acute overdose; however, it is crucial for the diagnosis of chronic toxicity. After admin-

istration of Fab antidigoxin antibody fragments, the serum digoxin concentration dramatically increases because both free and bound digoxin are measured by routine laboratory methods. Therefore, this test is of no use in this situation. Extracorporeal removal is not useful in this poisoning.

Patients who remain asymptomatic with normal cardiac rate and rhythm for 6 hours after ingestion may be discharged. Symptomatic patients require a 12-hour asymptomatic period with normal cardiac rate and rhythm before discharge can be considered.

Hydrocarbons

Hydrocarbon is a generic term for organic compounds that contain only hydrogen and carbon; most are products of the distillation of petroleum, but some are derived from plant (eg, turpentine and pine oil) and animal sources. Hydrocarbons are divided into aliphatic (straight chain) and aromatic (central benzene ring) groups, either of which can be halogenated. Hydrocarbon-containing consumer products are found in every home. Common examples include cleaning agents, polishes, fuels, lubricants, and automotive products. Kerosene was a common and serious problem within this group; however, its prevalence as a toxic agent has diminished as a consequence of the decline of its use as a fuel for heating and illumination. Serious hydrocarbon ingestion has become a sporadic and uncommon event. An important reason for this is the legislated requirement for child-resistant closures for most hydrocarbon consumer products.

Toxicology

Most hydrocarbons are poorly absorbed after ingestion and lack systemic toxicity. The chief concern is that some of them have the potential for producing aspiration pneumonitis. This risk is a function of their low viscosity, which allows them to circumvent closure of the laryngeal opening by the epiglottis and the vocal cords as an airway-protective mechanism. Hydrocarbons with low viscosity values (measured in Saybolt universal seconds), such as kerosene, gasoline, lighter fluid, turpentine, mineral seal oil (a common constituent of furniture polish), and mineral spirits, have the highest risk for aspiration. In contrast, more viscous hydrocarbons, such as petroleum, lubricating oil, and paraffin, represent a lower risk. Mineral oil has different grades of viscosity, ranging from low in baby oil to the relatively viscous mineral oil used as a laxative. The former is associated with the risk of aspiration pneumonitis, whereas the latter is not. A good rule in establishing a preliminary assessment of risk after an ingestion is that hydrocarbons that have textures similar to polishes have a high risk for aspiration pneumonitis, whereas those that feel like lubricating oils are of negligible risk. Although not as important, another physical characteristic of hydrocarbons that contributes to the determination of the risk of aspiration pneumonitis is surface tension. A low surface-tension chemical has the ability to creep or spread along a surface. A third characteristic of hydrocarbons is volatility, the ability to vaporize: the more volatile the agent, the greater the likelihood for adverse central nervous system effects. Volatile hydrocarbons are inhaled by older children and adolescents as a common type of recreational substance abuse.

Aspiration pneumonitis is a consequence of direct contact of a hydrocarbon within the lower respiratory tract. These chemicals interfere with surfactant and directly irritate respiratory epithelium. The results are alveolar collapse, bronchospasm, direct damage to the airway epithelium and endothelium, and interstitial pneumonitis resulting in ventilation perfusion mismatch and hypoxemia and hypercapnia. Some hydrocarbons have inherent systemic toxicity.

The most important of these are the highly halogenated species, of which carbon tetrachloride is the most toxic. The ingestion of a small volume of this chemical can cause fatal hepatotoxicity. Camphor is of concern because of its ability to cause seizures. Other hydrocarbons commonly discussed within the group having systemic toxicity are really mixtures containing more-toxic substances such as heavy metals and pesticides; the hydrocarbon is present as a solvent. The management of these situations should be directed at treating the effects of the more-toxic agent, with the issue of the concomitant hydrocarbon being a secondary consideration.

Clinical Presentation and Management

Choking, gagging, and coughing occur virtually immediately on exposure. There may be oral pain if an irritating hydrocarbon has been ingested. Vomiting is common, and this may increase the risk of aspiration, but it is not necessary for aspiration. In most children, the initial symptoms resolve without the development of aspiration pneumonitis. Signs of significant exposure are continued cough, tachypnea, increased respiratory effort, rib cage retractions, grunting, wheezes, and rales on chest auscultation. An altered level of consciousness is usually a consequence of respiratory failure; however, some hydrocarbons, such as camphor and aromatics, may produce this directly. Fever and leukocytosis are common early signs of the acute inflammatory response. Chest x-ray findings are heterogeneous and may include perihilar, basal, or lobar densities. These findings occur within a few hours and can be found in asymptomatic patients. Occasionally, pneumatoceles develop after several days and may take weeks to resolve.

Initial management involves attention to vital functions with focus upon support of respiration. Use of supplemental oxygen is guided by oxygen saturation and presence of respiratory distress. Measurement of blood gases and the chest x-ray guide further management. Tracheal intubation and mechanical ventilation may be required for the management of respiratory failure. Admission to an intensive care unit is recommended for patients with early symptoms and signs of lower respiratory involvement because further deterioration of the respiratory function can be rapid. Prophylactic antibiotics and corticosteroids were used in the past, but are no longer favored by most authors.

Most children that have ingested a hydrocarbon will have no signs or symptoms at the time of seeking medical attention. There has been greater controversy regarding gastrointestinal decontamination for this ingestion than for most other ingestions. Charcoal is thought to have poor adsorptive capacity for most hydrocarbons and it may promote vomiting. Therefore, its use is generally discouraged. Some authorities continue to recommend ipecac-induced emesis or orogastric lavage for those few agents with systemic toxicity. This is probably not a good idea for those hydrocarbons that produce neurotoxicity directly, such as camphor and aromatics, because the onset of symptoms and signs is very rapid, thus risking altered mental status or seizures during these interventions, which increases the risk for aspiration. It is prudent to consider gastric emptying for extremely hazardous hydrocarbons such as carbon tetrachloride, if this can be done within 1 to 2 hours of ingestion. Analysis of blood or urine specimens for hydrocarbons and extracorporeal removal play no role in the management of hydrocarbon ingestion.

Symptoms and signs of aspiration pneumonia are apparent within 4 to 6 hours of ingestion, making observation beyond this period for the asymptomatic patient unnecessary. The course of aspiration pneumonia varies with severity and ranges from several days to a few weeks.

Iron

Iron overdose is a serious health threat in children. Iron compounds are available as preparations intended for children and for adults, either alone or combined with vitamins and other mineral nutritional supplements. Overdose of products intended for children rarely lead to clinically significant toxicity because of the relatively small doses of iron that they contain. However, the overdose of iron-containing products intended for adults can lead to serious and potentially fatal toxicity.

Toxicology

Iron is a potent promoter of free-radical production resulting in tissue damage from lipid peroxidation. The superoxide anion in the presence of ferric ion will produce the hydroxyl radical (via the Fenton reaction), which causes the lipid peroxidation and tissue inflammation and injury. Target organs are those with high metabolic activity or exposure to high concentrations of this metal. These include the stomach, small intestine, liver, and heart. The upper gastrointestinal tract is exposed to the highest concentration of iron after ingestion. The result is necrosis of the stomach and proximal small intestine. First-pass hepatic extraction of absorbed iron is relatively high, resulting in potentially fatal hepatic injury, which is apparent in the periportal region of the liver.

Clinical Presentation and Management

Five clinical stages of iron poisoning that follow from the pathogenesis of the iron toxicity have been identified. The earliest signs (Stage I with onset ~2–6 hours after ingestion) result from the direct effects of iron on the stomach and intestine. These include abdominal pain, nausea, vomiting, diarrhea, hematemesis, and hematochezia. The gastrointestinal blood loss can be life-threatening, often starting as early as 30 minutes after ingestion and usually resolving within 6 to 12 hours. If there are no gastrointestinal symptoms or signs within the first 6 hours after iron ingestion, it is unlikely that the patient will suffer substantial complications. An exception is the ingestion of enteric-coated iron where the onset of toxicity can be delayed for several hours. As toxicity progresses (Stage II, ~6–12 hours after ingestion), the patient may appear improved, but have early signs of hypoperfusion and a modest metabolic acidosis. Later (Stage III, 6–24 hours after ingestion), shock and metabolic acidosis account for the majority of iron-poisoning deaths. The shock is multifactorial. The early onset is caused by gastrointestinal blood loss, but usually there is distributive shock thought to be due to the direct vasodilatory effects of iron on the peripheral vasculature. Shock persisting at 48 hours or longer may be cardiogenic as a result of the direct effects of iron on the myocardium. The acidosis of iron poisoning can be very severe. It is caused by hypoperfusion as well as by the hydration of nonprotein-bound ferric ions in the plasma. The next (Stage IV, onset ~12–36 hours after ingestion) consequences result primarily from hepatotoxicity, which is dose-dependent. It is the second most common cause of death in iron poisoning. Finally (Stage V, ~2–4 weeks after ingestion), there can be intestinal obstruction caused by a subacute inflammatory reaction after gut injury. The most common site is at the pylorus; however, it can occur anywhere in the small bowel if an enteric-coated iron preparation was ingested.

The risk for toxicity is a function of the amount of elemental iron ingested. It is important to differentiate isolated gastrointestinal adverse effects of iron overdose from systemic iron poisoning. Elemental iron doses of 20 to 40 mg/kg will routinely cause nausea, vomiting, diarrhea, and abdominal pain, but are unlikely to result in systemic toxicity. A dose of 40 mg/kg is a dose of concern with the potential to produce systemic toxicity. The peak serum iron concentration, which occurs at 2 to 4 hours after iron ingestion, helps to define the severity and prognosis of iron poisoning. Peak values of 350 to 500, 500 to 1000, and >1000 μg/dL are mild, moderate, and severe iron poisonings, respectively.

Management of critically ill patients requires support of vital functions. For iron poisoning, the most critical problem is support of circulation. The usual reason for shock at the outset is gastrointestinal fluid and blood loss. Therefore, bolus crystalloid infusions and blood transfusion are frequently needed. Very high hyperferremia is associated with a coagulopathy unrelated to hepatic dysfunction, which may require fresh-frozen plasma if hemorrhage is uncontrolled. The patients are profoundly acidemic, typically out of proportion to their hypoperfusion, and require prodigious doses of sodium bicarbonate. Altered mental status is a function of the hypoperfusion, not a direct result of the iron poisoning.

The management of the stable patient begins with an estimation of the amount of iron ingested. If it is certain that <40 mg/kg of elemental iron was ingested, then no intervention is indicated. However, abdominal symptoms, such as nausea, vomiting, diarrhea, and pain, are expected if 20 to 40 mg was ingested. If it is estimated that >40 mg/kg was ingested, an abdominal x-ray should be obtained immediately. If the x-ray does not demonstrate iron in the gut, and if the patient is asymptomatic, no interventions are needed. Patients with opacities attributable to the presence of iron require gastrointestinal decontamination. Charcoal does not adsorb iron well. The gut decontamination procedure of choice is whole-bowel irrigation with polyethylene glycol electrolyte lavage solution by nasogastric tube. The dose is 500 mL/h for children <6 years old and 1.5 to 2.0 L/h for older children. The endpoint is a clear rectal effluent.

One or two serum iron concentrations (at least 1 hour apart) should be obtained between 2 and 4 hours after ingestion from patients who ingested >40 mg/kg of elemental iron and from patients who have symptoms or multiple opacities in their abdominal x-ray. Blood gases should also be obtained from these patients because acidosis is a sensitive indicator for iron poisoning. Patients with serum iron concentrations >500 μg/dL should be admitted to hospital, and continuation of the treatment in an intensive care unit is justified if the serum iron is >1000 μg/dL. Early establishment of vascular access and invasive physiological monitoring should be considered in these patients because of the high risk of circulatory shock. Serial monitoring of hepatic and renal function and coagulation is advisable. Serum transaminase values greater than 2000 to 3000 U/L have a grave prognosis, and liver transplantation should be considered early.

Deferoxamine is a specific chelator of iron. Indications for deferoxamine are a serum iron concentration >500 μg/dL, acidemia, or evidence of systemic toxicity. It should be given by intravenous infusion at 15 mg/kg/h for a minimum of 8 hours preceded by intravenous administration of crystalloid to minimize the risk of acute renal failure. Infusions longer than 24 hours may cause pulmonary toxicity. Serum iron studies are not a reliable guide to therapy during deferoxamine infusions. Acidosis can be used as a criterion for continuing the deferoxamine infusions. Many patients will have a rusty-orange-colored urine during deferoxamine infusion if they are hyperferremic. However, this is neither a reliable positive nor negative criterion for deferoxamine therapy.

A follow-up visit at 2 to 4 weeks after discharge from hospital should be considered to assess for possible gut obstruction in those patients who experienced significant iron poisoning. Patients with abdominal pain persisting for longer than a week after iron ingestion are especially at risk for this sequela.

LEAD
Howard A. Pearson and David J. Schonfeld

Lead poisoning, a problem that affects nearly one million children nationwide, is widely considered to be the most common environmental health issue of American children. Its management has evoked considerable controversy among health care professionals. Almost all significant lead poisoning in the United States is a consequence of house paints that contain lead pigment. The major source of lead exposure is ingestion of lead-containing paint chips or lead-contaminated dust or dirt, by the hand-to-mouth activity of young children residing in homes that were constructed before 1980. Although lead-based paint was banned in 1978 for residential use, lead is still present in maritime paints and paints used on bridges and large external industrial structures. Pica has long been implicated in cases of lead poisoning, but the eating of paint chips is not necessary to result in lead poisoning. More commonly, children ingest dust and soil contaminated with paint flakes or chalks, which are disturbed during home renovation or maintenance and renovation activities. Lead paint on interior and exterior window components is often a cause because it is abraded into dust by repetitive opening and closing of the window. Lead-contaminated dust, ingested because of normal repetitive hand-to-mouth activity, is the major source of increased body lead burden in American children. Gasoline containing tetraethyl lead used to prevent engine "knocking" that was extensively used until the early 1980s, contributed to an increased concentration of lead in the soil. Less commonly, and particularly in certain ethnic groups, lead poisoning may result from use of folk remedies, cosmetics, and ceramic cooking utensils. Lead poisoning has also been caused by drinking water contaminated from solder in home plumbing. Inhalation of lead-containing air may occur in children living in the vicinity of lead smelting and automobile battery plants and from clothing brought into the home by family members working in lead-related industries. However, despite these many possible sources of lead exposure, the major source of lead poisoning in American children is the ingestion of lead-containing chips and dust by children living in homes built prior to 1980. It has been estimated that as as many as three-quarters of dwellings built prior to 1980 have lead-containing paint on their interior surfaces. These housing units are prevalent in inner-city neighborhoods and are often substandard and poorly maintained. Although lead poisoning is disproportionately a disease of poor, inner-city minority children, and most initiatives to prevent and detect lead poisoning are based on this premise, it must be remembered that it can occasionally occur in other contexts and venues.

TOXICOLOGY Lead is an obligate toxin that serves no physiologic function. Ingested material containing lead is solubilized by gastric hydrochloric acid and then absorbed, primarily in the upper gastrointestinal tract. About 10% of ingested lead is absorbed by adults, but as much as 50% may be absorbed by children. This may be increased further by concomitant iron and other trace metal deficiencies, malnutrition, and increased fat in the diet. When taken into the body, lead is distributed to the skeleton, soft tissues, and blood. About 70 to 90% of body lead is deposited in the bones and teeth, and about 5% is present in the red blood cells and the RBC precursors in the bone marrow. Lead is very slowly excreted from the body, primarily in the urine, and its biological half-life has been estimated to be more than 15 years.

The toxic effects of lead are primarily related to its binding to sulfhydryl ligands, leading to inhibition of a large number of enzymes. Lead toxicity is a function of the level of lead in the blood and tissues as well as the duration of exposure. In the RBC precursors, lead interferes with several steps in the heme synthetic pathway, which leads to an increased level of the heme precursors, free erythrocyte protoporphyrin (FEP), and zinc protoporphyrin (ZPP) in the mature RBC and is evident by blood ZPP levels $> 35 \ \mu g/$ dL in whole blood. At higher levels, lead reduces iron utilization resulting in anemia. In the central nervous system, particularly in the immature, developing brain, even moderate elevations of lead cause neurobehavioral abnormalities and decreases of I.Q, which appear to be permanent. Lead can cause neuronal demyelinization, decreased numbers of neurons, decreased neuronal growth, and interferes with neuronal transmission. Sensorineural hearing loss has been described that may result in significant delays in the acquisition of language and difficulty in auditory processing in children poisoned with lead in the first 2 years of life. At very high levels, lead can cause encephalopathy and cerebral edema resulting in death or severe neurologic damage in survivors. Peripheral neuropathy and nephropathy that occur in adults are unusual in children.

LABORATORY CRITERIA FOR LEAD POISONING AND SCREENING The magnitude of body lead is indicated by the level of lead in blood, and laboratory assessment is based primarily upon blood levels determined by atomic absorption analysis and by measurement of ZPP by photofluorometry. Elevations in ZPP do not occur immediately after acute ingestion of lead, but the level of ZPP provides an assessment of the chronicity of exposure. However, increased levels of ZPP do not usually occur until the blood lead level is $> 40 \ \mu g/dL$, so it is insensitive to moderate degrees of poisoning. Blood lead concentrations can be measured in capillary blood, but abnormal findings should be confirmed using venous blood because finger-stick capillary blood can be contaminated by trace amounts of lead-containing dust on the skin.

Over the past four decades, the Centers for Disease Control and Prevention (CDC) have issued a series of guidelines concerning blood levels that should be considered toxic. In the 1960s, a blood lead level $\geq 60 \ \mu g/dL$ was the definition of lead poisoning. In response to accumulating evidence of toxicity at lower levels, the guideline was decreased to 30 $\mu g/dL$ in 1975 and 25 $\mu g/dL$ in 1985. CDC guidelines issued in 1991 acknowledged that there were deleterious effects associated with lower blood lead levels and established the threshold for lead poisoning prevention activities at $\leq 10 \ \mu g/dL$ and recommended a "multitiered" approach based upon blood lead levels (see Table 4-40). The CDC also recommended universal screening of children between 6 months and 6 years of age. This approach was endorsed by the Committee on Environmental Health of the American Academy of Pediatrics in 1993. Minimal blood lead screening is therefore recommended at both 12 and 24 months. Because blood lead levels usually peak at about 18 to 24 months of age, a single blood lead level at 12 months of age is not sufficient. If either of these levels are $>10 \ \mu g/$ dL, follow-up with additional testing is indicated. Additional blood lead screening is indicated for any child up to 6 years of age with

TABLE 4-40

BLOOD LEAD CONCENTRATION AND SUGGESTED MANAGEMENT*

Class I: $< 10 \ \mu g/dL$.
Children with this degree of exposure are not considered to have lead poisoning.

Class IIA: $10-14 \ \mu g/dL$.
A large number of children with levels in this range in a particular neighborhood indicate the need for community-wide activities. Individual children in this class should be retested every 3 to 4 months until level is below 10 on two consecutive measurements, or below 15 on three consecutive measurements, then retested in 1 year.

Class IIB: $15-19 \ \mu g/dL$.
Parents should receive education on preventing further exposure and nutritional counseling.
Children should be retested at least every 3 to 4 months. If elevation continues at this level, environmental inspection and intervention are indicated.

Class III: $20-44 \ \mu g/dL$.
Full medical evaluation is indicated, not necessarily including drug treatment. Environmental sources of lead should be identified and eliminated.

Class IV: $45-69 \ \mu g/dL$.
Requires both medical and environmental interventions, including chelation therapy.

Class V: $> 70 \ \mu g/dL$.
Represents a medical emergency requiring immediate hospitalization and chelation, as well as environmental management.

---

* Based on CDC recommendations, 1991.

suspected increased risk of exposure and for children with developmental delays, particularly if they exhibit pica. The need for universal screening has been questioned, resulting in recent recommendations to consider "targeted" blood lead screening when adequate data are available to confirm a very low prevalence in a specific geographic area. If targeted screening is to be performed, a regular assessment of possible increased risk factors should be done (Table 4-41). Any child who has increased risk factors should have a blood lead level checked. Health-care providers may choose to utilize a risk assessment questionnaire to assess possible increased exposure as well as for anticipatory guidance.

CLINICAL PRESENTATION AND TREATMENT Clinical symptoms do not usually occur unless the blood lead level exceeds 50 $\mu g/$ dL, and symptoms may not be present in children with levels even higher. Symptoms that may be associated with lead poisoning are

TABLE 4-41

GUIDELINES FOR INCREASED RISK ASSIGNMENT

1. Children 9 months to 6 years of age who live in or are frequent visitors in older dilapidated housing or who live in neighborhoods with known high prevalence of lead poisoning.
2. Children 9 months to 6 years of age who are siblings, housemates, visitors, or playmates of children with known lead toxicities.
3. Children of any age living in older housing where renovation is ongoing.
4. Children 9 months to 6 years of age who live near lead smelteries or automobile battery plants or whose parents or other household members participate in a lead-related occupation or hobby.
5. Children with pica or neurodevelopmental retardation.

relatively nonspecific and include gastrointestinal complaints such as anorexia, constipation, abdominal pain, and vomiting. Signs and symptoms suggestive of central nervous system involvement include irritability, lethargy, changes in sleep pattern, and alterations in behavior and coordination. Seizures, hypertension, coma, and signs of increased cranial pressure are indicative of lead encephalopathy, which is usually associated with blood levels >70 μg/dL.

The most important interventions are to remove the child from further exposure and to initiate a course of therapy, which is determined by the blood lead level. As indicated on Table 4-40, children with a blood level <10 μg/dL are not considered to be lead poisoned. Chelation treatment of children with levels between 10 and 44 μg/dL is somewhat controversial. A recent study indicated that chelation therapy for children with blood lead levels between 25 and 45 μg/dL did not have a beneficial effect on chronic neuropsychological abnormalities. However, medical evaluation, repeated testing, nutritional intervention to increase iron and calcium intake and decrease fat consumption, to treat iron deficiency anemia and investigation of the source of lead exposure are indicated.

Children with blood levels of 45 to 69 μg/dL should receive chelation therapy. A Health Department inspection should be conducted to ascertain that the home is safe. Until this is possible, the child should be hospitalized or relocated to a known lead-free environment. If home therapy is being considered, a Health Department inspection should be done prior to starting treatment. Since oral chelating agents can increase lead absorption from the intestine, an abdominal x-ray should be done to look for radiopaque particles in the gastrointestinal tract (Fig. 4-34). If these are present, an oral cathartic (magnesium citrate or polyethylene glycol solution, Golytely) should be given to cleanse the bowel.

If there is no history or clinical findings suggestive of symptomatic lead poisoning, chelation therapy with oral 2,3-dimercaptosuccinic acid (DMSA, succimer, Chemet) should be considered. Baseline laboratory studies (CBC, liver function tests) should be obtained prior to starting chelation therapy. The dose of succimer is 350 mg/m^2 (10 mg/kg) three times a day for 5 days and then twice a day for an additional 14 days to complete a 19-day course of therapy. The most frequent side effects are nausea, loss of appetite, and diarrhea, but these are usually not severe enough to require stopping treatment. Mild and transient elevations of serum transaminase levels occur in 5 to 10% of patients. Granulocytopenia (absolute neutrophil count <1200/mm^3) rarely occurs but should be monitored by periodic blood counts. Blood lead levels decrease with succimer therapy, but then frequently rebound sometimes to pretreatment levels. Multiple courses of succimer therapy may be necessary until the blood level is consistently below 45 μg/dL. An alternative to oral chelation therapy, is a 5 day course of CaNa$_2$EDTA, given as a continuous 24-hour infusion in a dose of 1000 mg/m^2/day. Because the major toxicity of this drug is renal, adequate hydration should be given to keep the urinary specific gravity <1.020. Blood urea nitrogen and creatinine levels and urinalyses should be done at baseline and at 3 and 5 days of therapy.

Children with a blood lead level of ≥70 μg/dL, or any child with symptoms suggestive of central nervous system involvement, should be immediately hospitalized for emergency therapy with intravenous CaNa$_2$EDTA combined with intramuscular dimercaprol (BAL). Prior to beginning therapy, allergy to peanuts must be ascertained because BAL is suspended in peanut oil. BAL may also produce hemolysis in glucose-6-phosphatase–deficient individuals, and G6PD levels should be measured before starting therapy. Iron therapy should not be given during intramuscular or intravenous

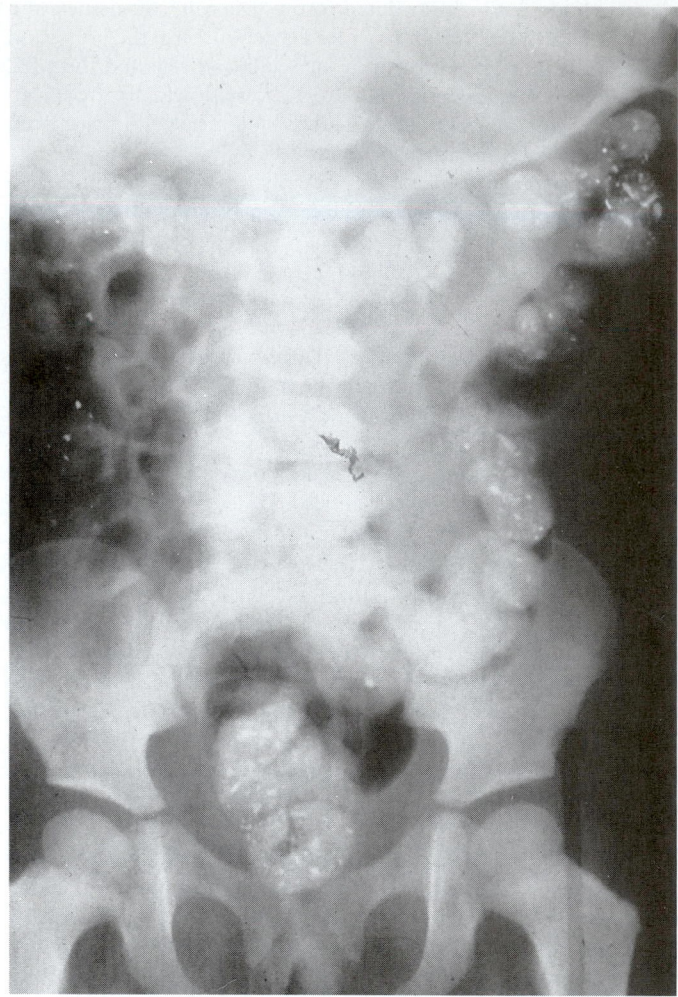

FIGURE 4-34   Abdominal roentgenogram of a child with lead poisoning secondary to ingestion of lead-containing paint chips. The radiopaque paint chips containing lead are evident throughout the intestinal tract.

therapy. An abdominal x-ray should be obtained to determine whether there is particulate radiopaque material in the intestine.

Chelation is begun with intramuscular BAL at a dose of 75 mg/m^2 every 6 hours. BAL crosses the blood-brain barrier, while CaNa$_2$EDTA chelates only from the intravascular space and may aggravate symptoms or precipitate encephalopathy in patients with very high levels if used alone. Four hours after the first dose of BAL, if urinary output is adequate, a continuous 24-hour infusion of intravenous CaNa$_2$EDTA should be started and continued for 5 days. Both drugs are usually continued for 5 days; however, if the child was asymptomatic prior to treatment and if the blood level is <50 μg/dL 2 hours after the fourth dose, discontinuation of BAL can be considered.

If there are signs of acute lead encephalopathy, the child should be admitted to an intensive care unit or comparable facility. Only maintenance fluid should be given. BAL should be started, followed by CaNa$_2$EDTA infusion as above. CaNa$_2$EDTA should be given intramuscularly at a dose of 250 mg/m^2 every 8 hours to minimize fluid intake. Both drugs should be continued for 5 days. It is important to note that lumbar puncture is contraindicated in children who have signs of encephalopathy.

Children with large body burdens of lead may require multiple courses of chelation therapy. Children requiring inpatient chelation therapy should not be discharged until lead hazards in their homes have been eliminated or alternative lead-free housing has been ensured.

References

Centers for Disease Control: Preventing lead poisoning in young children. A statement by the Centers for Disease Control. Atlanta: Centers for Disease Control, October, 1991

Chisolm JJ Jr: The road to primary prevention of lead toxicity in children. Pediatrics 107:581–583, 2001

Committee on Environmental Health American Academy of Pediatrics: Lead poisoning—from screening to primary prevention. Pediatrics 92:176–181, 1993

Rogan WJ, Dietrich KW, Ware JH, Dockery DW et al, for the Treatment of Lead Exposed Children Trial Group: The effect of chelation therapy on neuropsychological development inn children exposed to lead. New Eng J Med 344:1421–1426, 2001

Rosen JF, Mushak P: Primary prevention of childhood lead poisoning—the only solution. (Editorial). New Eng J Med 344:1470–1471, 2001

Schonfeld DJ, Needham D: Lead: a practical perspective. Contemp Pediatrics 11:64–96, 1994

Methanol and Ethylene Glycol

Toxicology

Like acetaminophen, methanol and ethylene glycol produce toxicity because their metabolites are injurious. Both alcohols are metabolized sequentially by alcohol and aldehyde dehydrogenases. The toxic metabolites are formic acid for methanol and glycolic and oxalic acid for ethylene glycol. Metabolic acidosis is a prominent feature of both of these poisonings, and because the metabolites are cellular poisons, virtually any organ can be damaged. Particular targets are the retina in methanol poisoning and the kidney in ethylene glycol poisoning, which can cause blindness and renal failure, respectively.

The fatal dose of both alcohols can be as low as 5 to 10 mL in a toddler. Both are rapidly absorbed after ingestion, with peak plasma concentrations occurring within 1 to 2 hours. However, the rates at which they are metabolized into their toxic metabolites are decidedly different. The half-life for methanol is 14 to 20 hours, whereas that of ethylene glycol is 2 to 4 hours. This difference has implications for the managements of these two poisonings.

Clinical Presentation and Management

Methanol is a component of many consumer products, including windshield-washing fluids, fuels, solvents, and various paint products, while the most common source for ethylene glycol is antifreeze. Most methanol and ethylene glycol ingestions occur in young children. The exception is the rare instance of an adolescent who ingests methanol in the mistaken belief that it is a beverage alcohol. Young children are typically brought to medical attention very soon after ingestion and before they become symptomatic. The most likely symptom is vomiting. Methanol is not particularly inebriating; however, ethylene glycol is inebriating. Poisoned patients presenting later in their course will be tachypneic because of their acidosis. Depending on the severity of the poisoning, there may be hypoperfusion and a decreased level of consciousness. For those

TABLE 4-42

FOMEPIZOLE VERSUS ETHANOL AS ANTIDOTES FOR METHANOL AND ETHYLENE GLYCOL POISONINGS

	FOMEPIZOLE	ETHANOL
Inebriation	No	Yes
Hypoglycemia	No	Yes
Dosing	12 hourly	Constant infusion
Serum concentrations	Reliable	Fluctuate
Monitoring of serum concentrations	No	Yes
Dosing calculations	Simple	Complex
Requirement for ICU setting	No	Yes
Need for hemodialysis (ethylene glycol)	No (nonsevere cases)	Yes
Cost	High	Low

presenting late and with symptoms, the history of ingestion is often unknown. Diagnosis of these patients can be challenging, with the most important clue being the presence of an anion gap metabolic acidosis.

Management of the young child presenting with a history of ingestion depends on the serum methanol or ethylene glycol concentration. The osmol gap can be calculated, but because these molecules are large and have an important effect when blood levels are low, the osmolality is an insensitive means to detect toxic ingestions. For example, a toxic dose of methanol is in the range of 120 mg/kg, and 1 mg of methanol only increases the serum osmolality 0.34 mOsm/kg H_2O; a toxic dose of ethylene glycol is also 120 mg/kg, but 1 mg of ethylene glycol increases the serum osmolality 0.20 mOsm/kg H_2O. The anion gap may also not be increased much early in the intoxication.

The treatment of methanol and ethylene glycol poisonings includes blocking of alcohol dehydrogenase (preventing formation of the toxic metabolites) and extracorporeal removal of the alcohol in conjunction with supportive therapy. There are two options for the blockade of alcohol dehydrogenase: ethanol and fomepizole. Fomepizole has been approved for the treatment of ethylene glycol poisoning, and at the time of the writing of this section, its approval for methanol poisoning is under consideration. Curiously, ethanol, the traditional antidote, has not been approved for either. Although there is limited pediatric experience with fomepizole, it has many advantages (Table 4-42). Because of the shorter half-life of ethylene glycol, a loading dose of fomepizole should be administered while waiting for the results of the serum concentration. This is unnecessary after methanol ingestion if the patient is asymptomatic. If the methanol or ethylene glycol serum concentrations cannot be measured immediately, a loading dose of fomepizole should be given and a strategy for obtaining blood levels developed (access to a laboratory or transfer of the patient). Metabolic acidosis is treated with sodium bicarbonate. Hemodialysis is recommended for patients with methanol poisoning. When the methanol concentration level is >50 mg/dL, there is metabolic acidosis, or neurologic or visual impairment, because the elimination can be prolonged. Hemodialysis is also indicated in ethylene glycol poisoning if either profound acidosis or renal failure is present.

Methemoglobinemia

Methemoglobinemia is further discussed in Sec. 19.5.3.

Toxicology

Methemoglobinemia is not a poisoning, but it can be a consequence of poisoning from several drugs and chemicals (see Table 19-7). Methemoglobin (MetHb) is produced by the oxidation of the ferrous iron in hemoglobin to ferric iron. MetHb is normally found in the blood with its proportion being <2% of circulating hemoglobin. MetHb cannot transport oxygen, and its presence shifts the oxyhemoglobin dissociation curve to the left, potentially impeding oxygen unloading.

MetHb is measured in a blood sample using an oximeter designed to distinguish Met from CO from oxyhemoglobin. It is important to remember that MetHb cannot be estimated from a hemoglobin oxygen saturation derived from arterial PO_2 because the calculated oxygen saturation is erroneous in the presence of MetHb. Equally as important, pulse oximetry provides an erroneous estimate of arterial hemoglobin oxygen saturation when there is more than 5 to 15% MetHb; the pulse oximeter under these conditions usually reads ~85% saturation, independent of the actual MetHb or hemoglobin oxygen saturation (see Sec. 4.2.1).

Clinical Presentation and Management

MetHb is dark brown, and when it is present in concentrations >1.5 g/dL the blood appears chocolate brown. Cyanosis occurs when greater than 5.0 g/dL of reduced hemoglobin is present. Symptoms and signs are a function of the proportion of MetHb present (Table 4-43).

Methemoglobinemia should be suspected in any cyanotic patient without a history of cardiac or respiratory disease. Failure to improve with oxygen therapy is an additional clue. Another presentation is the unexpected pulse oximetry finding of an oxygen saturation of 85 to 90% in an otherwise well child. In both situations, methemoglobinemia must be confirmed by measurement in blood (see above). A bedside screening test is to compare the color of a few drops of the patient's blood with a control on a piece of filter paper. If the blood appears more brown, then a significant amount of MetHb is likely. (Details of treatment are discussed in Sec. 19.5.3.)

Opioids

Opioid is a generic term that includes all drugs with morphine-like action (Section 4.2.8 discusses opioid therapeutic use). There are natural (eg, morphine, codeine), semisynthetic (eg, heroin, hydrocodone, hydromorphine, oxycodone, and oxymorphone), and synthetic opioids (eg, fentanyl, perperidine, methadone). They are used in clinical medicine for analgesia and cough suppression and for the treatment of diarrhea. Poisonings in the pediatric age group include unintentional ingestions in the young and suicidal gestures or substance abuse mishaps in adolescents.

Toxicology

Opioids mediate their actions by binding to various specific receptors in the central nervous system and elsewhere (see Table 4-25). They are well absorbed after oral dosing, but some of them, morphine in particular, have decreased bioavailability by this route because of significant first-pass metabolism. Other potential routes of absorption include intravenous, intramuscular, rectal, nasal, buccal, respiratory, and transdermal (fentanyl patches). The pharmacokinetics are drug-specific. Those with particularly long half-lives, such as methadone and levorphanol, are of particular concern in overdose situations because of possible relapse after antidote therapy.

Clinical Presentation and Management

Serious poisonings present with the classic triad of coma, respiratory depression, and miosis. Respiratory depression causes decreased tidal volume, but in severe intoxication, the bradypnea is prominent. Attention should be focused on support of ventilation with a bag-valve-mask device and supplemental oxygen. Endotracheal intubation is usually not required because of the rapid response to the opioid antidote naloxone, which is best given intravenously at a dose of 0.1 mg/kg, up to 2.0 mg. A response is expected within 5 minutes, and if not seen, this dose should be repeated every 5 minutes. If there is no response after three cycles, consider another etiology for the patient's condition. If the intravenous route is unavailable, naloxone can be administered by the endotracheal, intramuscular, or intralingual routes. Naloxone has an extremely wide therapeutic index except in patients with opioid addiction. In such patients, rapid and full reversal would likely precipitate a withdrawal syndrome, and it should be given more cautiously. Repeat doses of 0.1 and 0.4 mg should be given, titrated against the patient's clinical condition with the endpoint being satisfactory ventilation. Naloxone should also be given with considerable caution in patients with cardiovascular instability and at much lower doses (0.001 mg/kg), because of its potential to produce hypertension.

Activated charcoal should be given to alert patients presenting within 1 to 2 hours after ingestion of a potentially toxic dose. Give 25 g to a child less than 6 years of age and 50 g to an older child. Observation for 4 hours after the time of ingestion suffices if the patient remains asymptomatic. All patients treated with naloxone should be observed for relapse, even if apparently well, for 8 to 12 hours after the last dose because the half-life of many opioids is longer than that of naloxone. Some patients require continuous naloxone infusions, particularly if they have ingested a very large dose or a long-acting opioid such as methadone or levorphanol. The usual indications for infusion therapy are relapse after naloxone therapy or the requirement of a particularly large dose of naloxone for initial reversal.

Serum concentration determinations and extracorporeal removal play no role in the management of opioid poisonings.

Oral Hypoglycemic Agents

Oral hypoglycemic agents are used for the treatment of noninsulin-dependent diabetes mellitus. These agents are either sulfonylureas or biguanides. The sulfonylureas include acetohexamide, chlorpropamide, glipizide, glyburide, and tolbutamide, while metformin is

TABLE 4-43

SYMPTOMS AND SIGNS OF METHEMOGLOBINEMIA IN PATIENTS WITHOUT ANEMIA

% METHEMOGLOBIN	SYMPTOMS AND SIGNS
0–15%	Cyanosis
20–40%	Headache, dyspnea, tachypnea, tachycardia
40–50%	Confusion, lethargy, metabolic acidosis
>50%	Coma, seizures, dysrhythmias
>70%	Lethal

the only available biguanide. Because these drugs are widely prescribed, poisonings are frequent.

Toxicology

Sulfonylureas stimulate insulin secretion from the pancreas and may decrease insulin clearance by the liver. Biguanides enhance the cellular effects of insulin and reduce neoglucogenesis, thereby decreasing glucose levels usually without causing hypoglycemia. Young children are especially sensitive to sulfonylureas. There is the potential for hypoglycemia after the ingestion of a single adult therapeutic dose. Large overdoses can result in a profound, sustained, and difficult to treat hypoglycemia. The hypoglycemia of metformin overdose is mild and easily managed. However, the condition of concern is biguanide-induced lactic acidosis, which has significant morbidity and mortality.

Clinical Presentation and Management

The principal feature of sulfonylurea overdose is profound hypoglycemia. These patients present with coma and seizures. Lack of response to 50% dextrose in water in the presence of hypoglycemia virtually confirms the diagnosis. The pharmacologic agents normally used to increase blood sugar—glucagon and corticosteroids—are usually ineffective because they aggravate the hyperinsulinemia. The agent of choice is an inhibitor of insulin secretion, either diazoxide or octreotide. There is more experience with diazoxide; a dose of 3 to 5 mg/kg intravenously is appropriate. Hypotension has not been described at this dose, but remains a concern. Relapse of hypoglycemia may result in the need for repeat bolus dosing or constant infusion. Octreotide is an attractive therapeutic alternative because it has no substantial side effects. However, there are insufficient data for sound pediatric dosing recommendations. Octreotide can be given subcutaneously or intravenously with a starting dose of 25 to 50 μg. Relapse of hypoglycemia may result in the need for repeat dosing.

The principal feature of severe metformin overdose is lactic acidosis. Vital functions require support as indicated with particular attention to intravascular volume expansion. Hypoglycemia, if present, is easily managed. The administration of intravenous bicarbonate in lactic acidosis is controversial, and there are data suggesting that it may be ineffective and potentially harmful. If used at all, the goal should be to correct the pH, for example, to a value of 7.2.

For asymptomatic patients who have ingested a sulfonylurea within the past 1 to 2 hours, a dose of charcoal in water is indicated (25 g to a child less than 6 years old and 50 g to an older child). Blood glucose should be monitored frequently, allowing free access to glucose-containing fluids. Parenteral dextrose is not indicated in euglycemic patients because it prolongs the observation period, which makes ascertaining whether the patient is dependent on exogenous sugar difficult. Hypoglycemia is treated with increasing concentrations of hypertonic dextrose solutions as needed, but if unsuccessful, prompt diazoxide or octreotide therapy should be considered.

Because of chlorpropramide's long half-life, there is concern for late-occurring hypoglycemia. However, for this to occur, there must have been hypoglycemia early in the course. Therefore, observation periods of 24 hours of euglycemia are unnecessary. For the asymptomatic patient who has ingested a sulfonylurea or a biguanide, a 4- to 6-hour observation period from the time of inges-

TABLE 4-44

SELECTED ORGANOPHOSPHATE AND CARBAMATE INSECTICIDES

	HIGH TOXICITY	LOW TOXICITY
Organophosphate	Parathion	Malathion
	Phosdrin	Diazinon
	Tetraethyl pyrophosphate	Dichlorvos
Carbamate	Aldicarb	Carbaryl
	Carbofuran	Propoxur

tion suffices. If the blood sugar and blood gases remain normal, then discharge is appropriate.

Organophosphate and Carbamate Insecticides

Organophosphate and carbamate insecticides are widely available consumer products. The most prevalent ones are low-concentration aerosol products marketed for use in the home and are often referred to as "over-the-counter bug bombs." Insecticides for garden and agricultural uses have a higher potential for toxicity because they are intrinsically more toxic and more concentrated. Table 4-44 lists some examples of high- and low-toxicity products.

Toxicology

The organophosphate and carbamate insecticides inhibit the enzyme acetylcholinesterase by binding to it. Organophosphates form a stable bond and thus produce irreversible inhibition; carbamates form bonds that undergo spontaneous hydrolysis, causing reversible acetylcholinesterase inhibition. Acetylcholinesterase breaks down acetylcholine, the neurotransmitter for parasympathetic and sympathetic ganglia, postganglionic parasympathetic nerves, and neuromuscular junctions. Acetylcholinesterase inhibition results in an excess of acetylcholine and continued stimulation of muscarinic, nicotinic, and central nervous system receptors.

Although cholinesterase-inhibiting insecticide poisoning produces dysfunction in many body systems (Table 4-45), it is the effects upon the respiratory system that are most critical. Death is usually due to respiratory failure, which is a consequence of bronchospasm, bronchorrhea, respiratory muscle weakness, and central respiratory depression. Many of these insecticides are dissolved in a

TABLE 4-45

EFFECTS OF ORGANOPHOSPHATES AND CARBAMATES

Muscarinic	
Lungs	Bronchorrhea; bronchospasm
Cardiovascular	Decreased heart rate; decreased blood pressure
Apocrine glands	Salivation; lacrimation; diaphoresis
Gastrointestinal	Cramps; vomiting; diarrhea; tenesmus
Nicotinic	
Cardiovascular	Increased heart rate, increased blood pressure
Skeletal muscle	Fasciculations; twitching; cramps; weakness; paralysis
Central Nervous System	Altered consciousness; seizures; respiratory depression; Cheyne-Stokes respirations; anxiety; restlessness; ataxia; dysarthria; tremor

hydrocarbon carrier, making hydrocarbon aspiration pneumonitis yet another potential factor in the pathogenesis of respiratory failure.

These insecticides can be absorbed after ingestion or inhalation or percutaneously. Onset of action can be delayed for several hours because some, such as parathion, require metabolism to an active agent. Duration of toxicity is shorter for carbamates because their bond with acetylcholinesterase undergoes spontaneous hydrolysis.

Clinical Presentation and Management

Being a heterogeneous group of substances, toxicity varies among substances. The most common exposure is to an "over-the-counter bug bomb," which, because of its low concentration of active ingredient, is unlikely to produce clinically important toxicity.

The principal feature of severe cholinesterase-inhibiting insecticide is acute respiratory distress. Symptoms and signs include dyspnea, increased respiratory muscle effort, decreased air entry, rales, rhonchi, wheezes, and cyanosis. Apocrine gland hypersecretion manifests as salivation, lacrimation, and diaphoresis. Pupils are usually constricted. Typically, the nicotinic effect (tachycardia) predominates over the muscarinic effect (bradycardia). Central nervous system effects include coma and seizures. Peripheral muscular weakness and paralysis may be present, but usually are not appreciated because they are overshadowed by the severity of respiratory involvement. However, skeletal muscle fasciculations may be apparent. Milder poisonings may be very difficult to diagnose in patients presenting without a history of exposure because of the many possible presentations. One helpful clue is a garlic-like odor that is typical of these insecticides.

Treatment is focused upon the respiratory system. Oxygen should be administered. Frequent suctioning is usually necessary, and intubation and mechanical ventilation are frequently required. Atropine, often in very-high doses, can dry the copious respiratory secretions related to muscarinic effects of the insecticides. Atropine competes with acetylcholine at muscarinic and central nervous system receptors, but has no effect at nicotinic receptors. Administer a trial dose of 0.05 mg/kg up to 1 to 2 mg intravenously, and an absence of signs and symptoms of atropinization confirms the diagnosis of organophosphate or carbamate poisoning. Repeat doses will be necessary, with the amount and the frequency being dependent on the patient's response. Severely poisoned patients may require a constant infusion. Pralidoxime reverses the organophosphate acetylcholine bond at the nicotinic receptor and is indicated for poisoning with insecticide when there is muscle weakness. It is not necessary for carbamate poisoning because of the rapid spontaneous hydrolysis of the carbamate acetylcholinesterase complex. It must be given within the first 24 to 48 hours for it to be effective. The dose is 25 to 50 mg/kg to a maximum of 1 to 2 g intravenously and may be repeated every 6 hours to treat skeletal muscle weakness and fasciculations. Improvement of these adverse effects usually occurs within 15 to 60 minutes after pralidoxime administration.

Consider a dose of activated charcoal in water for asymptomatic patients presenting within 1 to 2 hours with a history of a significant organophosphate or carbamate ingestion. Dermal exposures require aggressive washing with soap and water.

Plasma cholinesterase activity can be measured and will be depressed; however, this rarely contributes to the management of the patient.

Plants

Approximately 5 to 10% of all telephone calls to poison control centers are a consequence of plant ingestion. A large proportion involves children less than 3 years of age. These children lack the interest and the ability (no molars) to consume significant amounts of plant material. Most plant ingestions are trivial, with fatalities being extremely rare.

Toxicology

Tables 4-46 and 4-47 are lists of nontoxic and toxic plants. If any adverse effect may result from the ingestion of a plant, that plant is included in the toxic list. Many of these adverse events are best described as nuisances rather than as causes of significant morbidity. Examples include dermatitis, mild gastrointestinal upset, and oropharyngeal irritation. For most toxic plants, amounts larger than can readily be consumed by a young child are required to produce clinically important toxicity.

TABLE 4-46
NONPOISONOUS PLANTS

African daisy	Geranium (dermatitis)
African palm	Gloxinia
African violet	Grape ivy
Airplane plant	Hawthorn
Aluminum plant	Hibiscus
Aralia, false	Honeysuckle
Araucaria	Hoya
Arbutus	Impatiens
Asparagus fern (dermatitis)	Jade Plant
Aspidistra (cast-iron plant)	Kalanchoe
Aster	Lily (Day, Easter, or Tiger)
Baby's tears	Lipstick plant
Bachelor buttons	Lysima Croton (house variety)
Bamboo	Magnolia
Begonia	Marigold
Bird's-nest fern	Monkey plant
Blood leaf plant	Mother-in-law tongue
Boston fern	Mountain ash
Bougainvillea	Norfolk Island pine
California poppy	Orchid
Camelia	Oregon grape
Christmas cactus	Peperomia
Chrysanthemum (dermatitis)	Petunia
Coleus species	Piggy-back plant
Corn plant	Prayer plant
Cotoneaster	Primrose (dermatitis)
Crap apples	Purple passion
Creeping Charlie	Pyracantha
Creeping Jennie, Moneywort Rose	Rubber plant
Dahlia	Salal
Daisies	Sansevieria
Dandelion	Schefflera
Dogwood	Sensitive plant
Donkey tail	Swedish ivy
Easter Lily	Tulip (bulb dermatitis)
Echeveria	Umbrella tree
Eucalyptus (caution)	Violets
Eugenia	Wandering Jew
Ficus (dermatitis)	Wax plant
Fuchsia	Yucca
Gardenia	Zebra plant

TABLE 4-47
POISONOUS PLANTS

PLANT CATEGORY	EXAMPLES	TOXICITY
Gastrointestinal irritants	Daffodil (*Narcissus pseudonarcissus*) Holly (*Ilex* sp.) Pokeweed (*Phytolacca americana*) Mistletoe (*Phoradendron serotinum*)	Gastroenteritis is usually mild and self-limited, but may be severe with significant fluid and electrolyte losses.
Dermatitis	Poison ivy (*Toxicodendron radicans*) Poison sumac (*T. vemix*) Poison oak (*T. quercifolium*)	Resins or other components may induce dermatitis.
Oxalates Insoluble	Dumbcane (*Dieffenbachia sp.*) Philodendron (*Philodendron sp.*) Elephant's ear (*Colocasia sp.*)	Insoluble oxalate crystals may cause intense pain and local swelling on contact with skin or mucous membranes.
Soluble	Boston ivy (*Parthenocissus tricuspidata*) Rhubarb (*Rheum rhabarbum*)	Soluble oxalate salts may cause kidney damage by precipitating as calcium oxalate.
Alkaloids Atropine	Jimsonweed (*Datura stramonium*) Angel's trumpet (*D. suaveolans*) Potato (*Solanum tuberosum*) Tomato (*S. lycopersicum*) Eggplant (*S. melonoena*)	Anticholinergic syndrome; mydriasis, flushed skin, tachycardia, delirium, hallucinations, xerostomia, urinary retention. Nausea, vomiting, diarrhea; rarely CNS depression.
Cyanogenic glycosides	Apricot pits (*Prunus armeniaca*) Bitter almonds (*P. dulcis* var. *amara*) Peach pits (*P. persica*) Black cherry pits (*P. serotina*) Apple seeds (*Malus sylvestris*) Pear seeds (*Pyrus communis*)	Pulverized or thoroughly chewed seeds may release glycosides, which are then hydrolyzed to cyanide by stomach acid. Serious poisonings require large quantities and are rare.
Cardiac glycosides	Foxglove (*Digitalis purpurea*) Oleander (*Nerium oleander*) Lily of the valley (*Convallaria majalis*)	A few foxglove or oleander leaves may cause vomiting, cardiac arrhythmias, and hyperkalemia. Poisoning from lily of the valley is rare. The glycosides may cross-react as digoxin on serum assays and respond to treatment with digoxin Fab antibodies.
Toxalbumins	Rosary pea (*Abrus precatorious*) Castor bean (*Ricinus communis*)	Severe gastroenteritis is common and dehydration may occur. Liver and kidney toxicity may occur.
Convulsants	Strychnine (*Strychnos nux vomica*) Jessamine (*Gelsemium sempervirens*) Water hemlock (*Cicuta sp.*)	Strychnine and jessamine produce tetanus-like muscular contractions. Water hemlock causes gastroenteritis followed by generalized convulsions.
Nicotine-like compounds	Tobacco (*Nicotiana tabacum*) Indian tobacco (*Lobelia inflata*) Poison hemlock (*Conium maculatum*)	Toxicity includes salivation, muscle weakness, diaphoresis, tachycardia, hypotension. Pupils may be small. Coma and paralysis may occur in severe poisonings.
Hepatotoxins	Comfrey (*Senecio, Symphytum*) Heliatropium Crotalaria	Hepatotoxic pyrrolizidine alkaloids produce hepatitis with features of hepatic vein thrombosis. May be found in some herbal teas.

Clinical Presentation and Management

Plants containing calcium oxalate comprise one of the most common groups ingested by young children. This chemical is very irritating to the oropharynx with the potential to produce pain and swelling. Airway obstruction is a theoretic concern; however, this has never been documented. Common examples of this group include the dieffenbachia (dumb cane), philodendron, elephant ear, and caladium.

The poinsettia, a frequent Christmas-time plant ingestion, at one time was considered hazardous; however, the worst outcome is mild gastrointestinal symptoms.

Salicylates

Salicylate poisoning in children is uncommon because of the progressive replacement of aspirin as an analgesic-antipyretic with acetaminophen and modern nonsteroidal anti-inflammatory agents. Salicylates have a relatively narrow therapeutic index, and the treatment of aspirin poisoning is very challenging. The case fatality rate

is an order of magnitude higher for salicylate poisoning than for acetaminophen poisoning.

Toxicology

Aspirin's metabolism is an important factor contributing to its narrow therapeutic index. After routine dosing, it is metabolized in the liver and its breakdown products are excreted in the urine. However, hepatic metabolism is easily saturated, and this occurs in the upper portion of the therapeutic serum-concentration range. In this situation, there is increasing reliance on the less-efficient renal excretion of parent salicylate, resulting in a disproportionate increase in the elimination half-life with larger total-body burdens of salicylate.

Salicylates initially stimulate the respiratory center of the medulla, which causes the early finding of hyperventilation. Compensation for the resultant respiratory alkalosis occurs from renal excretion of HCO_3^-, restoring pH toward (but not reaching) normal. At higher doses, salicylates also uncouple oxidative phosphorylation; block metabolism of pyruvic, lactic, and acetoacetic acids; inhibit amino acid metabolism; stimulate gluconeogenesis, glycolysis, and lipid metabolism; and depress respiratory drive. The metabolic disturbances cause a marked increase in metabolic rate (CO_2 production), sweating, and flushed skin. Furthermore, the serum HCO_3^- will be very low from the previous loss during hyperventilation, or from the metabolic acidosis with the deranged intermediary metabolism. Respiratory acidosis can further compound the metabolic disturbance, producing severe acidosis. This is the basis for the myriad of toxic effects, with the major ones being acid-base imbalances, fluid and electrolyte abnormalities, and central nervous system toxicity. Aspirin also produces platelet dysfunction and in overdose can lead to decreased production of various coagulation factors. However, hemorrhagic complications are rare in salicylate-poisoned patients.

The combination of acid-base disturbances depends on the amount ingested and metabolized. Accordingly, the combined respiratory and metabolic acidosis is common in infants and toddlers, whereas teenagers often have a respiratory alkalosis and metabolic acidosis. There may also be problems regulating serum glucose, causing either hyperglycemia or hypoglycemia.

Fluid and electrolyte abnormalities are always present in the aspirin-poisoned patient. Water loss is a consequence of vomiting, hyperventilation, hyperthermia, diaphoresis, and the diuresis associated with obligatory excretion of Na^+, K^+, and HCO_3^- as a response to the respiratory alkalosis.

Central nervous system abnormalities are prognostically very important because they are associated with significant mortality. Acidemia is an important contributor because its presence promotes the ingress of salicylate into the brain. With the uncoupling of oxidative phosphorylation, the brain is reliant on glycolysis as its energy source. There may be intracellular decreased glucose concentrations despite normoglycemia. Central nervous system toxicity is clinically manifested as agitation, confusion, altered mental status, seizures and coma, and cerebral edema.

Clinical Presentation and Management

Vomiting is a common early manifestation of aspirin poisoning, as is tinnitus and tachypnea. As the poisoning progresses there may be fever and evidence of dehydration and, in young children particularly, central nervous system toxicity manifested by irritability, agitation, and altered mental status. Laboratory findings include respiratory alkalosis followed by metabolic acidosis, leukocytosis, and hyperglycemia (which may be followed by hypoglycemia). The potassium concentration is usually normal, but it often precipitously decreases later in the course. More severe cases will have hypokalemia, hyponatremia, elevated BUN and creatinine, and a frank metabolic acidosis, which may contribute to the development of seizures, coma, and cardiac dysrhythmias.

Treatment of moderate to severe salicylate poisoning focuses on support of vital functions, the most pressing being the fluid-electrolyte and acid-base disturbances. Hypoperfusion requires fluid administration with supplemental potassium as soon as urine flow is assured. Bladder catheterization is required to monitor urine output. There is an increased demand for glucose in the central nervous system, and it should be supplemented even if the patient is normoglycemic. Acidemia should be treated with sodium bicarbonate to reduce the ingress of aspirin into the central nervous system. An additional reason for bicarbonate administration is derived from the fact that an increase of urine pH by 1.0 increases aspirin excretion

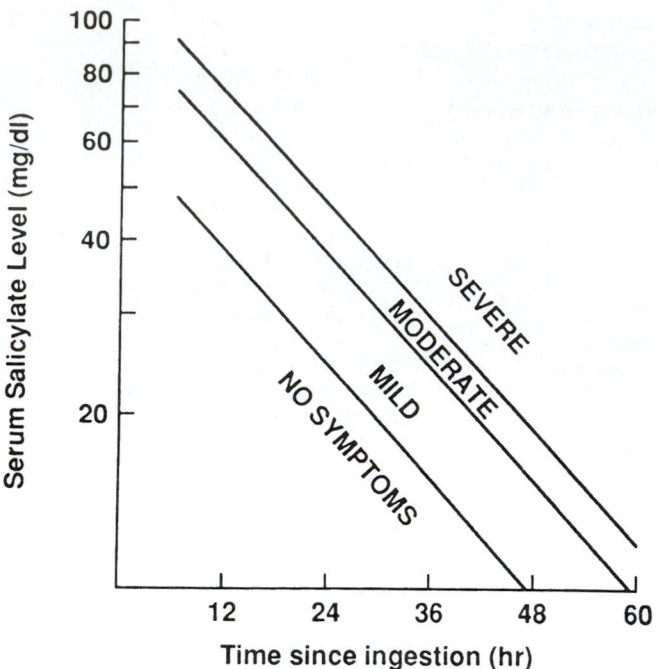

FIGURE 4-35 Salicylate nomogram.

20-fold. Raising the urine pH to the desired levels can be difficult, however, because potassium depletion causes a paradoxic aciduria (alkaline plasma with acid urine). Serum salicylate concentrations help define the severity of the aspirin poisoning using the Done nomogram (Fig. 4-35). This nomogram is only applicable to young children who have ingested a single, acute overdose of a nonenteric-coated aspirin product. Values in the severe range require intensive care and hemodialysis. Hemodialysis may be indicated for severe fluid electrolyte, acid-base disturbances, or acute renal failure.

For the patient presenting within 1 to 2 hours who has ingested greater than 150 mg/kg of aspirin, give 25 g of charcoal in water to a child and 50 to 100 g to a teenager (about 1 g/kg). A blood specimen should be drawn for plotting on the Done nomogram. Although the initial data point on this nomogram is at 6 hours after ingestion, earlier specimens, for example at 2 to 3 hours, can be helpful if they demonstrate no salicylate, which is a frequent finding when the ingestion is uncertain. Multiple-dose activated charcoal therapy was recommended in the past, but was subsequently shown to be of no benefit.

Patients can be discharged if their serum salicylate concentrations are in the mild or nontoxic portions of the nomogram.

SUBSTANCE ABUSE

Substance abuse is a common problem among adolescents, making the presentation to hospital for adverse effects from this practice a frequent experience. Occasionally, a young child may present after unwittingly ingesting a street drug and the diagnosis may be challenging if the caretaker is not forthcoming with the history. Child abuse by poisoning should always be considered whenever a young child presents with poisoning from substances of abuse. In most instances, the acute adverse effects from drugs of abuse are managed with supportive care. However, counseling and treatment of the underlying issues related to substance abuse is extremely difficult, often requiring referral to specialized agencies or services.

Alcohol

Ethanol is a central nervous system depressant. It is the most common substance of abuse, and the presentation of frankly inebriated adolescents for medical care is a frequent occurrence. The diagnosis is rarely challenging, even if the history is not forthcoming, because of alcohol's characteristic odor. Ethanol is a CNS depressant. However, by depressing some inhibitory control mechanisms, it can initially produce stimulation and excitement, although aggressive or abusive behavior can also result. Initially, processes such as memory, concentration, and insight are depressed. With further intoxication, there is general impairment of all nervous system functions, eventually producing general anesthesia. All incapacitated, apparently inebriated patients require careful assessment to exclude comorbidities. Occasionally, CNS toxicity may be severe enough to produce respiratory failure, hypotension, and death. Management is largely supportive to maintain cardiorespiratory function, and assisted ventilation may be needed in the most serverely intoxicated patients. Ethanol intoxication commonly coexists with ingestion of other psychotropic drugs, so it is important to consider these as confounding factors in the management of patients when the history is unclear.

Young children may unwittingly ingest ethanol-containing substances. A particularly hazardous consumer product is mouthwash. Ethanol-poisoned infants and toddlers are particularly at risk for hypoglycemia, making the monitoring of blood sugar very important in this age group.

Amphetamines and Related Drugs; Cocaine

These drugs may be either illicit or pharmaceuticals. Legitimate uses include the treatment of attention-deficit hyperactivity disorder, narcolepsy, and refractory obesity. Examples include amphetamine, dextroamphetamine, methamphetamine, and methylphenidate. Caffeine, ephedrine, and phenylpropanolamine are frequently sold as if they were amphetamines. Methylenedioxymethamphetamine, commonly known as MDMA or ecstasy, is a hallucinogenic amphetamine. It is discussed with the hallucinogens. Depending on the specific agents, these drugs may be ingested, injected, snorted, or smoked, with onset of action being route-dependent.

Amphetamines stimulate the release of catecholamines, while cocaine blocks the presynaptic reuptake of these neurotransmitters. Thus, these agents are sympathomimetics. Effects occur both within the central nervous system and peripherally. These include changes of mood, excitation, tachycardia, and hypertension. Hypertension is the most serious of these and can be life-threatening. Dysrhythmias may occur. Central nervous system manifestations include anxiety, agitation, confusion, psychosis, and seizures. Hyperthermia is seen in patients with moderate to severe toxicity.

Treatment should be directed at lowering the blood pressure if hypertension is present, because of the risk of a cerebral vascular accident. Nifedipine or nitroprusside should be considered if systolic or diastolic blood pressures are greater than 170 or 110, respectively. Agitation may be controlled by reduction of external stimulation; however, a benzodiazepine may be required. Sedation has the advantage of decreasing heat production. Severe hyperthermia requires external cooling measures. Seizures are treated with diazepam or lorazepam.

Hallucinogens

The hallucinogens include marijuana, LSD, phencyclidine (also known as PCP or angel dust), and MDMA. They produce sensory misperceptions, disordered thought processes, and mood changes. Marijuana is typically smoked and is the most frequently used hallucinogen, yet it is a very uncommon reason for presentation for medical care. LSD use waxes and wanes. It is colorless, odorless, and tasteless, and is ingested as a tablet, capsule, or powder or impregnated in sugar cubes or pieces of blotter paper. Phencyclidine is usually ingested but may be smoked, while MDMA is taken orally.

Hallucinogen use does not result in frequent presentation for medical care. Occasionally, there may be excessive persistent or unpleasant reactions, or ingestion may have been accidental rather than intended. These are the usual reasons for seeking medical help. Possible effects range from mild alterations of mental status to agitation, acute panic, and anxiety reactions or an acute toxic psychosis. In most cases, a short period of observation and limitation of stimulation is all that is needed. Occasionally, sedation with a benzodiazepine may be required. However, PCP and MDMA can produce life-threatening toxicity.

Marijuana is an infrequent reason for presentation for medical care, but occasionally a toddler finds a hidden supply and ingests it. In addition to the above symptoms, young children may develop central nervous system depression. LSD use is more likely to result in acute toxic psychosis. PCP intoxication can be striking, including agitation, belligerence, coma, and seizures. Physical findings include nystagmus, ataxia, hypertension, increased muscle tone, hyperreflexia, twitching, tremors, diaphoresis, and hyperthermia.

Methylenedioxymethamphetamine is frequently associated with prolonged dancing parties known as raves. The hallucinogenic-induced symptoms and signs described above can be seen with this drug, and stimulant effects of amphetamines on the CNS and cardiovascular systems are usually manifest with an overdose. Because of decreased fluid intake and increased physical activity, patients ingesting amphetamines are at risk for hyperthermia, dehydration, electrolyte disturbances, and seizures. Treatment is dictated by the particular adverse effects and is supportive.

Heroin (see Opioids)

Inhalant Abuse

Inhalant abuse is the deliberate inhalation of a volatile organic compound for recreational purposes. It is also known as glue sniffing, sniffing, huffing, and volatile substance abuse. It is a common type of pediatric substance abuse with approximately one in five children experimenting with inhalants. The active chemicals are aliphatic and aromatic hydrocarbons, aliphatic nitrites, esters, and ketones. These are available in countless consumer products. Inhalants are depressants related to anesthetic gases. In fact, anesthetic gases can be abused in this fashion. The physiological effects of inhalants are those of the early stages of anesthesia including stimulation, disinhibition, and impulsive behavior. Speech becomes slurred and the gait becomes staggered. Euphoria, frequently with hallucinations, is followed by drowsiness and sleep, particularly after repeated cycles of inhalation. Coma is unusual, because as the user becomes drowsy, exposure to the inhalant is terminated.

It is rare for a child to receive care for acute toxicity unless the child is brought in by the police. The most feared adverse event of sniffing is sudden death, which is caused by a ventricular dysrhythmia. If this develops in an acute care setting, standard advance cardiac life-support protocols should be followed with no proscription against the use of epinephrine.

Some chemicals commonly abused are associated with significant sequelae after chronic use. Examples include white-matter degeneration, dementia, and cerebellar encephalopathy of chronic toluene abuse, and the peripheral neuropathy of chronic *n*-hexane abuse.

References

Poison Prevention

American Academy of Clinical Toxicology, European Association of Poisons Centres and Clinical Toxicologists: Position statement: ipecac syrup. J Toxicol Clin Toxicol 35:699–709, 1997

American Academy of Clinical Toxicology, European Association of Poisons Centres and Clinical Toxicologists: Position statement: gastric lavage. J Toxicol Clin Toxicol 35:711–719, 1997

American Academy of Clinical Toxicology, European Association of Poisons Centres and Clinical Toxicologists: Position statement: single-dose activated charcoal. J Toxicol Clin Toxicol 35:721–741, 1997

American Academy of Clinical Toxicology, European Association of Poisons Centres and Clinical Toxicologists: Position statement: cathartics. J Toxicol Clin Toxicol 35:743–752, 1997

American Academy of Clinical Toxicology, European Association of Poisons Centres and Clinical Toxicologists: Position statement: whole-bowel irrigation. J Toxicol Clin Toxicol 35:753–762, 1997

Acetaminophen

Prescott LF, Illingworth RN, Critchley JAJH, Stewart NJ, Addam RD, Proudfoot AT: Intravenous *N*-acetylcysteine: the treatment of choice for paracetamol poisoning. Brit Med J 2:1097–1100, 1979

Smilkstein MJ, Bronstein AC, Linden C, Augenstein WL, Kulig KK, Rumack BH: Acetaminophen overdose: 48-hour intravenous *N*-acetylcysteine treatment protocol. Annals of Emergency Medicine 20(10): 1058–1063, 1991

Smilkstein MJ, Knapp GL, Kulig KK, Rumack BH: Efficacy of oral *N*-acetylcysteine in the treatment of acetaminophen overdose. N Engl J Med 319:1557–1562, 1988

Anticoagulants

Mullins ME, Brands CL, Daya MR: Unintentional pediatric superwarfarin exposures: Do we really need a prothrombin time? Pediatrics 105:402–404, 2000

Watts RG, Castleberry RP, Sadowski JA: Accidental poisoning with a superwarfarin compound (bradifacoum) in a child. Pediatrics 86:883–887, 1990

B-Blockers and Calcium Channel Blockers

Critchely JA, Ungar A: The management of acute poisoning due to beta-adrenoceptor antagonists. Med Toxicol Adverse Drug Exp 4:32–45, 1989

Pearigen PD, Benowitz NL: Poisoning due to calcium antagonists. Experience with verapamil, diltiazem and nifedipine. Drug Saf 6:408–430, 1991

Carbon Monoxide Poisoning

Baker MD, Henretig FM, Ludwig S: Carboxyhemoglobin levels in children with non-specific flu-like symptoms. J Pediatr 113:501–504, 1988

Sheinkestel CD, Bailey M, Myles PS, et al: Hyperbaric or normobaric oxygen for CO poisoning: a randomised controlled clinical trial. Med J Aust 170:1203–1210, 1999

Caustic or Corrosive Ingestion

Anderson KD, Rouse TM, Randolph JG: A controlled trial of corticosteroids in children with corrosive injury of the esophagus. N Engl J Med 323:637–640, 1990

Crain EF, Gershel JC: Symptoms as predictors of esophageal injury. Am J Dis Child 138:863–865, 1984

Clonidine

Caravati EM, Bennet DL: Clonidine transdermal patch poisoning. Ann Emerg Med 17:175–176, 1988

Wiley JF, Wiley CC, Torrey SB, Henretig FM: Clonidine poisoning in young children. J Pediatr 116:654–658, 1990

Cyclic Antidepressants

James LP, Kearns GL: Cyclic antidepressant toxicity in children and adolescents. J Clin Pharmacol 35:343–350, 1995

Walsh DM: Cyclic antidepressant overdose in children: a proposed treatment protocol. Pediatr Emerg Care 2:28–35, 1986

Digoxin and Cardiac Glycosides

Antman EM, Wenger TL, Butler VP Jr, Haber E, Smith TW: Treatment of 150 cases of life-threatening digitalis intoxication with digoxin-specific Fab antibody fragments. Final report of a multicentre study. Circulation 81:1744–1752, 1990

Woolf AD, Wenger TL, Smith TW, Lovejoy FH Jr: Results of multicenter studies of digoxin-specific antibody fragments in managing digitalis intoxication in the pediatric population. Am J Emerg Med 9(Suppl 1): 16–20, 1991

Hydrocarbons

Anas N, Namasonthi V, Ginsburg CM: Criteria for hospitalizing children who have ingested products containing hydrocarbons. JAMA 246:840–843, 1981

Eade NR, Taussig LM, Marks MI: Hydrocarbon pneumonitis. Pediatrics 54:351, 1974

Iron

Banner W Jr, Tong TG: Iron poisoning. Pediatr Clin North Am 33:393–409, 1986

Tenenbein M: Whole-bowel irrigation in iron poisoning. J Pediatr 111: 142–145, 1987

Methanol and Ethylene Glycol

Brent J, McMartin K, Phillips S, et al: Fomepizole for the treatment of ethylene glycol poisoning. Methylpyrazole for toxic alcohols study group. N Engl J Med 340:832–838, 1999

Jacobsen D, McMartin KE: Antidotes for methanol and ethylene glycol poisoning. J Toxicol Clin Toxicol 35:127–143, 1997

Methemoglobinemia

Curry S: Methemoglobinemia. Ann Emerg Med 11:214–221, 1982

Ralston AC, Webb RK, Runciman WB: Potential errors in pulse oximetry: III effects of interferences, dyes, dyshaemoglobinemias and other pigments. Anesthesia 46:291–295, 1991

Opioids

Aronow R, Paul SD, Woolley PV: Childhood poisoning. An unfortunate consequence of methadone availability. JAMA 219:321–324, 1972

Tenenbein M: Continuous naloxone infusion for opiate poisoning in infancy. J Pediatr 105:645–648, 1984

Oral Hypoglycemic Agents

Krentz AJ, Boyle PJ, Justice KM, Wright AD, Schade DS: Successful treatment of severe refractory sulfonylurea-induced hypoglycemia with octreotide. Diabetes Care 16:184–186, 1993

Palatnick W, Meatherall RC, Tenenbein M: Clinical spectrum of sulfonylurea overdose and experience with diazoxide therapy. Arch Intern Med 151:1859–1862, 1991

Organophosphate and Carbamate Insecticides

Sofer S, Tal A, Shalak E: Carbamate and organophosphate poisoning in early childhood. Pediatr Emerg Care 5:222–225, 1989

Zwiener RJ, Ginsburg CM: Organophosphate and carbamate poisoning in infants and children. Pediatrics 81:121–126, 1988

Plants

Kunkel DB, Spoerke DG: Evaluating exposures to plants. Emerg Med Clin North Am 2:133–144, 1984

Mrvos R, Dean BS, Krenzelok EPK: Philodendron/dieffenbachia ingestions: are they a problem? J Toxicol Clin Toxicol 29:485–491, 1991

Salicylates

Snodgrass WR: Salicylate toxicity. Pediatr Clin North Am 33:381–391, 1986

Yip L, Dart RC, Gabow PA: Concepts and controversies in salicylate toxicity. Emerg Med Clin North Am 12:351–364, 1994

Substance Abuse

Kulberg A: Substance abuse: clinical identification and management. Pediatr Clin North Am 33:325–361, 1986

McGuigan MA: Toxicology of drug abuse. Emerg Med Clin North Am 2: 87–101, 1984

4.3.4   Drowning and Near-Drowning in Children and Adolescents

Linda Quan

EPIDEMIOLOGY

Drowning is defined as death following submersion injury and near-drowning is survival from submersion injury. Drowning is a leading cause of unintentional death in children worldwide. It is the second leading cause of nonintentional injury death in children less than 10 years old, and the third leading cause of injury death in adolescents in the United States and in most countries where injury death has been evaluated. Drowning rates are highest in the western United States, and it is the leading cause of pediatric injury-related death in Alaska and California. Drowning rates in children have steadily decreased over the past two decades, though less so among infants. Interestingly, in the state of Washington a decrease in drownings was not related to improvements in medical care, but was associated with decreased alcohol use.

The availability of statistics regarding near-drowning are more limited, but those available also show a strong influence of age. The ratio of hospitalization for near-drowning to drowning deaths is 1.5 in children less than 15 years old and 0.5 for older adolescents in the state of Washington. This age-related ratio reflects the high lethality of submersion injury in adolescents and may explain why pediatric medical literature has concentrated on drowning and near-drowning in preschoolers. Preschoolers are less likely to die at the scene and are more likely to reach hospitalization than are adolescents; the adolescent submersion-victim is far less likely to enter the prehospital or hospital system for medical care because the adolescent may be inebriated or alone. These ratios also reflect the lethality of submersion injury: nearly 50% of all pediatric submersion-victims die, making it one of the most lethal injuries studied.

Submersion injury is a set of complex, multifaceted events that vary with the victim's age, socioeconomic status, and proximity to bodies of water. Drowning, however, can occur in inches of water. In inner cities, large buckets as well as bathtubs represent the major risk for infants and toddlers; in wealthy populations in warm climates, the home swimming pool is the site of submersion injury for 90% of victims <5 years of age. Even in coastal settings, freshwater such as lakes, rivers, and canals are the most likely sites for submersion injury for older children and adolescents.

Risk factors for drowning relate to gender, age, race, and season. As in all other injuries, males predominate after age 1 year, and they account for 85% of drownings. The male to female ratio of 3:1 among young children increases to 6:1 among older adolescents. In all states or countries reporting drownings, the incidence of drowning and near-drowning is highest in children <5 years old and next highest incidence rate is in 15- to 24-year-olds. The activity that leads to the submersion also tends to vary with age. Examples include the infant who has been left unattended or with a young sibling in a bathtub; the unsupervised preschooler who falls into the pool or a lake who is unable to swim; or the eager adolescent who goes to an unsupervised, remote, open-water setting who is unable to swim as well as his or her friends or who had a boating mishap. Most drownings and near-drownings occur during the summer months when water-related activity is highest.

Other risk factors for drowning are epilepsy, alcohol use, and intentional trauma. Drowning represents the highest risk for unintentional death in patients with seizure disorders. Epilepsy increases the risk 13-fold for both near-drowning and drowning. The bathtub is the most common lethal setting for these patients because victims are usually unattended and not found in a timely manner.

Alcohol consumption increases the risk for drowning 4- to 31-fold. Reported alcohol use is extraordinarily prevalent among males while boating. This is reflected in the finding of positive blood-alcohol levels in 10 to 50% of adolescent drownings, especially those involving males, use of boats or motor vehicles, or suicide. Not only may alcohol increase the likelihood of the submersion occurring, its effects may limit the victim's ability to reach safety.

Intentional injury should always be considered and evaluated when there is submersion. Bathtub submersions in children, especially, require evaluation because they are the most commonly recognized setting for intentional submersion in patients admitted to tertiary pediatric centers. An inconsistent history, or a history incompatible with the victim's developmental abilities, is the key to recognition of child abuse in drowning or near-drowning (see Sec. 5.6.9). In older children, suicide, in addition to abuse and homicide, should be considered a potential cause of the submersion injury.

Water conditions play a role in adolescent drownings and near-drownings. Hypothermia is frequently unrecognized as a risk factor for submersion injury. Adolescents are often unaware that their endurance and swimming ability decrease markedly while immersed in cold water.

PATHOPHYSIOLOGY

The sequence of events triggered by submersion in animals includes efforts to surface and breathe, followed by laryngospasm and swallowing of water, and finally loss of consciousness and cardiac arrest. A critical distinction between young human drowning victims and the animals used in the experiments leading to these observations is that the former may only struggle minimally. Many parents have unfortunately relied on the notion that submersion is a noisy event; this has misled them to think that aural supervision is an adequate substitution for visual supervision.

The major consequence of the submersion is global hypoxia. While aspiration of water or gastric contents and hypothermia may add to the injury, hypoxia-induced cell death in multiple organs is the main injury. Each organ system's response to hypoxic injury follows a relatively predictable timetable. Central nervous system and myocardium manifest the most acute responses. Unresponsiveness and apnea may develop in 1 to 3 minutes; ventricular dysrhythmias and asystole may develop within 3 to 4 minutes.

The diving reflex is postulated to provide cerebral protection by producing bradycardia while preserving blood flow to the brain and heart. It occurs in some sea mammals submerged in cold water, but its importance in humans is questionable and difficult to demonstrate.

It may be hours after a severe submersion event that signs of organ-system death become manifest. The brain is the organ that generally exhibits the greatest sensitivity to both hypoxic injury and to the additional ischemic injury that ensues in the event of cardiac arrest. Neuronal death by necrosis or apoptosis are the final results of these injuries. Their clinical manifestations include the development of cerebral edema, which may be evident in imaging studies within 6 to 8 hours after the event. As in other forms of hypoxic-ischemic encephalopathy, the clinical course of the severe injuries is often indolent and characterized by slow progression toward brain death or vegetative states. Myocardial pump failure or multisystem organ failure is a less common cause of death.

Pulmonary injury from submersion causes less morbidity and is far more treatable than the cerebral injury. Aspiration may have several mechanisms of causing hypoxia. In 10% or less of victims, fluid is not found in the lungs, suggesting that entry of water into the pharynx provokes reflex closure of the glottis, which is maintained until the subject is unconscious or even apneic. When this protective mechanism becomes inoperative, aspirated water fill completely some alveoli, diluting in others the concentration of surfactant, which then leads to alveolar collapse. Even in the cases in which water is aspirated into the alveolar spaces, the volume tends to be small. Furthermore, aspirated water is usually absorbed rapidly. The swallowing of large amounts of water may set up the patient for aspiration of stomach contents, a more threatening condition. Nonbacterial pneumonitis is common and may explain the fever encountered on the first day of hospitalization. Acute respiratory distress syndrome (ARDS) develops in only 5 to 10% of hospitalized submersion victims, most of whom suffer concomitant posthypoxic cardiac or central nervous system injury.

Acute renal tubular necrosis and acute cortical necrosis may occur after severe hypoxic or ischemic events. Vascular endothelial damage is manifested by disseminated intravascular coagulopathy. Damage to the gastrointestinal tract may be manifest by bloody diarrhea with mucosal sloughing. Multisystem organ damage usually indicates irreversible injury.

Hypothermia can be an additional injury or could be somewhat protective of the brain and other organs if it develops prior to onset of hypoxia. However, for the majority of submersion victims, hypothermia (core temperature <35°C) represents the second major injury incurred, rather than a protective phenomenon. The effects of severe hypothermia include hypotension from reduced myocardial contractility and loss of vascular and other muscular tone. Below 29°C, bradycardia, ventricular fibrillation, or asystole occur. Coma, apnea, and dilated pupils ensue as a result of brainstem depression. The condition mimics death.

CLINICAL FINDINGS

The clinical state of submersion victims is determined by the severity of the hypoxic insult, which, in turn, is usually related to the duration of submersion. Victims are best approached by deriving a rapid assessment of their cardiopulmonary and neurologic function (most importantly the level of consciousness) and by determining whether there are other potentially life-threatening injuries consequent to the event (eg, head or neck trauma).

Alert Patients

Many children may be cyanotic or apneic upon rescue, but may respond readily to a few rescue breaths or stimulation to breathe and resume spontaneous breathing with good respiratory control. They quickly regain consciousness at the scene. After that, the majority are alert or mildly confused on arrival at the hospital. They may demonstrate mild to moderate metabolic acidosis that resolves without treatment. Some children develop mild respiratory distress within hours of the submersion. A smaller subset of alert patients develop full-blown pulmonary edema heralded by frothy pink sputum in transport to the hospital. Respiratory distress and oxygen requirement often resolve with treatment within 5 to 8 hours, and almost always resolve in the alert patient within 24 hours.

Comatose Patients

Victims who remain unresponsive following initial life-resuscitative interventions to stimulate or support breathing and correct hypoxia have suffered severe injury. This is reflected by cardiopulmonary arrest, severe metabolic acidosis, and signs of brainstem injury; they often have concomitant hypothermia. Following cardiac resuscitation, some patients develop myocardial pump failure, and dysfunction of multiple organs is commonly seen in these patients.

THERAPEUTIC APPROACHES

The goal is to minimize the risk of additional hypoxia and treatable complications of the submersion. Almost 90% of pediatric submersion victims survive if submerged less than 5 minutes; almost 90% die with longer submersions.

Scene Care

As soon as water rescue is safely accomplished, hypoxemia must be treated with oxygen. Ventilation should be supported mechanically if needed. For the alert child, oxygen is usually enough. Wet clothing should be removed, and the child transported to an emergency facility with ongoing observation for signs of developing respiratory distress. For the unresponsive child, rescuers should provide basic life-support interventions, including mouth-to-mouth or bag-and-mask mechanical ventilation, if available. If the child is pulseless, cardiopulmonary resuscitation should be started and the child's trachea intubated if advanced life support is available. Vascular access and administration of normal saline or lactated Ringer solution is indicated for medication administration. Treatment of submersion victims should follow the usual algorithms for both basic and advanced life support. Cervical spine immobilization should be provided if the submersion involved diving, surfing, a motor vehicle accident, attempted homicide, or other injuries that put the victim at risk for multisystem trauma. At this time, treatment for hypothermia in the field is restricted to removal of wet clothing.

Emergency Department Care

Monitoring of the responsive child should include noninvasive oxygen saturation (there is little need for assessment of arterial blood gas tensions) and vital signs. The child who appears well can be observed for several hours. Children who improve within 5 to 6 hours and who appear well can be discharged home if the social setting permits.

The child with respiratory distress merits assessment by blood gas analysis, chest radiograph, and continuous oxygen-saturation monitoring, while providing supplemental oxygen. If there are signs of severe or progressive respiratory distress, the breathing should be supported or assisted (see Sec. 4.1.1). Blood alcohol should be measured in adolescents. A social worker assessment should be conducted when child abuse or neglect is suspected, especially in young children whose submersion involved the bathtub.

The unresponsive child in the emergency department should be placed on cardiorespiratory monitoring, and an intravenous infusion of isotonic fluid should be given; the stomach should be decompressed and emptied with an orogastric or nasogastric tube (use the former if there is any concern about head trauma). Arterial blood gas tensions and pH, blood glucose, complete blood count, electrolytes, and chest radiograph should be obtained. Endotracheal intubation is indicated if the patient is cyanotic, has inadequate cardiac or respiratory function, or remains unresponsive. Wheezing may be improved with inhaled bronchodilators, but may

reflect persistently low lung volume or cardiac congestion. As in any child with shock, fluid resuscitation should commence and there should be consideration for use of inotropic support based on the response to volume expansion (see Sec. 4.1.2). Hypoglycemia may be present and should be treated with 0.5 to 1.0 mL/kg of 50% dextrose or 2 to 4 mL/kg of 10% dextrose IV. Hyperglycemia, a glucose >300 mg/dL, is associated with a poor outcome but does not require treatment. Unresponsive patients should be admitted or transported to a pediatric intensive care unit.

Hypothermia should be assessed using a rectal thermometer capable of detecting low temperatures. Rewarming efforts are based on the patient's temperature with a goal of restoring the core temperature to 32 to 34°C. For temperatures >32°C, external rewarming with lights and warm blankets may suffice to stop shivering. For temperatures <32°C, active internal rewarming measures, including warmed isotonic intravenous fluids (40–43°C), are needed. For severe hypothermia, <30°C, more internal rewarming measures, including gastric, bladder, peritoneal, or thoracic lavage with warm fluids, may be necessary; if there is asystole with severe hypothermia, cardiopulmonary bypass may be more effective.

Hospital Care

Hospital care focuses on cardiorespiratory support. Supplemental oxygen may be needed only for a brief time in the majority of alert children. Continuous positive airway pressure (CPAP) may be used in alert patients who are significantly hypoxemic and who do not improve with oxygen alone. Frequent reassessment is needed to identify developing respiratory distress. The intubated and ventilated patient requires more extensive monitoring and often needs adjustments in ventilation to sustain adequate gas exchange (see Sec. 4.2.2). Diuretics are given for pulmonary edema (indications may vary), and sodium bicarbonate can be used for severe, uncompensated metabolic acidosis. Antibiotics and corticosteroids are not routinely recommended.

There are no unique factors to consider in managing or monitoring depressed circulatory function (see Sec. 4.1.2). In the patients who are presumed to be euvolemic and who have adequate circulatory function, fluids and free water are often mildly restricted to limit the severity of cerebral edema.

Neurologic function should be monitored frequently by physical examination in the patient with a depression level of consciousness. In the comatose patient, interventions should focus on preventing or limiting increases in intracranial pressure (see Secs. 4.1.3 and 4.2.5). Generalized seizures are treated with conventional medications, but may be quite refractory to anticonvulsants. Cerebral resuscitation measures, such as corticosteroids, generalized hypothermia, barbiturate coma, hyperventilation, and intracranial pressure monitoring have failed to improve the outcome of drowning and are not used.

Finally, owing to the likelihood of global organ dysfunction in the comatose patient, renal, metabolic, hematologic, and gastrointestinal systems need evaluation and support.

PROGNOSIS

The published statistics for overall mortality rate is 40 to 60% for near-drowning in children and adolescents, although it varies by age group. The outcome from submersion injury is bimodal. Most survivors are neurologically intact; less than 10% of all pediatric submersion victims survive with severe neurologic sequelae, spastic quadriplegia with no self-help skills, or persistent vegetative state. However, 50% of submersion patients admitted to pediatric intensive care unit represent this small group of children with devastating neurologic handicap.

Outcome is determined by duration of submersion. Multiple studies document that submersions of 5 minutes or less generally result in normal survival, while submersions greater than 5 minutes are associated with death or survival with severe neurologic sequelae. From 1975–1995 in King County, Washington, there were no survivors of non-icy-water submersions greater than 25 minutes.

Survival following prolonged (>25 minutes) icy-water (<5°C) submersions has been described, although the data remains anecdotal, and predictors for icy-water submersions do not exist. In contrast, submersion in cold but not icy water is not protective; hypothermia is not a favorable prognostic factor. Contrary to common wisdom, age is not a protective factor either; there is no evidence that young children tolerate submersion better. Instead, the survival advantage of preschoolers relates to their greater likelihood of supervision for rescue, submersion in bodies of water, such as pools, where rescue is easy when compared to rescues in lakes and rivers, and thus shorter submersion durations.

The most reliable predictors for outcome relate to the patient's ability to recover immediately from the episode. These are the patient's mental status (cerebral cortex), pupillary responses (brainstem), glucose, and resuscitation interval (duration of cardiopulmonary resuscitation needed). The patient who is alert in the field or who develops spontaneous, purposeful movements within 24 hours of admission should survive intact. Conversely, the patient who remains unresponsive and lacks normal brainstem function at 24 hours will die or sustain severe neurologic sequelae. For example, in western Washington from 1980–1991, 75% of comatose patients died from 1980–1991.

Similarly, the longer the need for cardiopulmonary resuscitation, the worse the prognosis. From 1985–1989, overall survival following cardiopulmonary resuscitation of pediatric submersion patients in Seattle and King County Emergency Medical Systems was 21%, with one-third of survivors having good neurologic outcomes. Based on data from 1974–1989, 87% of patients who had cardiac arrest developed spontaneous return of circulation and a measurable blood pressure within 10 minutes of cardiopulmonary resuscitation and survived. However, following 25 minutes of continuous cardiopulmonary resuscitation, there were no survivors. Thus, after 25 minutes of resuscitation, the futility of continued efforts make it reasonable to consider discontinuing the resuscitation.

The occurrence of hyperglycemia (glucose >300 mg/dL) in the postischemic brain predicts a bad outcome. It is unclear, however, whether hyperglycemia is a cause of neuronal injury or a marker for massive catecholamine response to a major injury.

PREVENTION

The societal costs of the mortality and morbidity of drowning and near-drowning are significant. In California and Washington state, the average hospital charge for submersion injury and for submersion injury leading to death is $13,000 (1995 dollars), and for injury leading to severe neurologic sequelae it is $61,000, with estimated subsequent annual medical costs of $100,000. Long-term effects on families have not been measured but are probably sizeable, as parental divorce and depression are common aftermaths of pediatric drowning deaths. Prevention is a more effective means of controlling this scourge.

Efforts have focused on preventing preschool children's drowning in swimming pools. Most communities require only three-sided fencing of swimming pools, which permit the child access to the pool from the house. Where local ordinances have required four-sided fencing of pools with self-closing gates and latches, drowning rates decreased by 50%. Federal legislation is needed to protect children in all communities. In addition, pool owners should be required to learn CPR as only 44% of pool-owner households in the 1980s include someone who knew CPR.

Less attention has been focused on adolescent submersion in open water. Adolescents are the group with the next largest drowning incidence. Personal flotation devices, commonly called life vests, remain the most reliable technologic prevention intervention for boating-related drownings for all age groups. However, in 1998, only 33 states required children to wear life vests while boating, defining children as ages 6 to 12 years old. And, in 1995, only 63% of 5- to 14-year-olds and 13% of those over 14 years old wore life vests while boating in Washington state. Swimming lessons, swimming pool covers, and alarms are not effective interventions. Further efforts are needed to identify and prove effective interventions.

References

Alderson P, Fleminger S, Klassen T, et al: Drowning. Injuries Group (formerly Brain and Spinal Cord Injury Module of the Cochrane Database of Systemic Reviews). Available in The Cochrane Library [database on disk and CDROM]. The Cochrane Collaboration; Issue 1: Oxford: Update Software, 1998 (updated quarterly)

Bratton SL, Jardine DS, Morray JP: Serial neurologic examinations after near drowning and outcome. Arch Pediatr Adolesc Med 148:167–170, 1994

Brenner RA, Smith GS, Overpeck MD: Divergent trends in childhood drowning rates, 1971 through 1988. JAMA 271:1606–1608, 1994

Diekema DS, Quan L, Holt VL: Epilepsy as a risk factor for submersion injury in children. Pediatrics 91:612–616, 1993

Gillenwater J, Quan L, Feldman K: Inflicted submersion in childhood. Arch Pediatr Adolesc Med 150:298–303, 1996

Graf WD, Cummings P, Quan L, Brutocao D: Predicting outcome in pediatric submersion victims. Ann Emerg Med 26:312–319, 1995

Howland J, Hingson R, Heeren T, Mangione T: Alcohol use and aquatic activities—United States, 1991. Morb Mortal Wkly Rep 42:675–682, 1993

Kyriacou DN, Arcinue EL, Peek C, Kraus JF: Effect of immediate resuscitation on children with submersion injury. Pediatrics 94:137–142, 1994

Noonan L, Howrey R, Ginsburg CM: Freshwater submersion injuries in children: a retrospective review of seventy-five hospitalized patients. Pediatrics 98:368–371, 1996

Quan L, Gore EJ, Wentz K, Allen J, Novack AH: Ten-year study of pediatric drownings and near-drownings in King County, Washington: lessons in injury prevention. Pediatrics 83:1035–1040, 1989

Quan L, Kinder D: Pediatric submersions: prehospital predictors of outcome [see comments]. Pediatrics 90:909–913, 1992

Smith G, Brenner R: The changing risks of drowning for adolescents in the United States and effective control strategies. Adolesc Med 6:2, 1995

Suominen PK, Korpela RE, Silfvast TGO, Olkkola KT: Does water temperature affect outcome of nearly drowned children. Resuscitation 35:111–115, 1997

Wintemute GJ: Childhood drowning and near-drowning in the United States. Am J Dis of Child 144:663–669, 1990

4.3.5   Foreign-Body Aspiration

M. Douglas Baker

Foreign-body aspiration (FBA) is the cause of death for more than 300 children each year in the United States; nonfatal FBA occurs in thousands more. Although children of all ages are at risk, most (75–90%) documented aspirations of foreign bodies by children involve preschoolers. The approximate distribution by age is: <1 year = 10 to 15%; 1 to 2 years = 40 to 50%; 2 to 3 years = 15 to 25%; and >3 years = 15 to 20%. Two factors contribute significantly to the high incidence in infants. During their orally focused phase of development, these children are likely to place anything that will fit into their mouths. Because they have not yet developed molar teeth, they are unable to chew certain edibles finely enough to swallow them. Reportedly, boys aspirate foreign bodies more often (2:1) than girls. Large case series indicate that nuts and peanuts account for approximately half of all foreign-body aspirations by children. Other foods or organic materials are involved in an additional 25% of cases. Toys and other small objects of a variety of compositions make up the remaining number. One report of 103 asphyxiation deaths of young children by food identified hot dogs (17%) as the single most common aspirated food, followed by candy, peanuts, nuts, and grapes.

PATHOGENESIS

The pathophysiology of upper-airway obstruction by foreign-body aspiration is as follows: With the foreign body in the posterior pharynx, discomfort and irritation causes the child to cough or cry. The initial phase of this response is a vigorous inspiration that causes foreign-body impaction within the airway. In that confined space, the foreign body increases resistance to inspiratory and expiratory flow. Because it can create a "valve-like" effect, the foreign body can cause more airflow obstruction during expiration than inspiration and can produce generalized or asymmetric gas trapping (one of the signs of foreign-body impaction in a bronchus). Surface sensory receptors of the respiratory tract will become adapted to prolonged pressure caused by a foreign body lodged in its site. Coughing will not recur until other sensory receptors are stimulated either by movement of the foreign body or by secretions. Thus, a latent period free of symptoms may occur and last from hours to months or longer.

CLINICAL PRESENTATION

Aspiration of a foreign body can cause a variety of respiratory signs, although cough is the most common (Table 4-48). The manifestations are determined by many factors, including the size, shape, composition, and location of the aspirated material, as well as the

TABLE 4-48
SIGNS AND SYMPTOMS ASSOCIATED WITH IMPACTED FOREIGN BODIES

	BRONCHIAL (n = 163)	LARYNGOTRACHEAL (n = 35)
Cough	95%	66%
Decreased air entry	62%	20%
Wheezing	60%	26%
Dyspnea	59%	74%
Fever	36%	3%
Cyanosis	34%	40%
Rales	32%	26%
Stridor	13%	63%
Hoarseness	1%	11%
Other	9%	3%
Asymptomatic	1%	—

TABLE 4-49
LOCATION OF IMPACTED FOREIGN BODIES

Right main bronchus	30–40%
Left main bronchus	30–35%
Right lobar bronchus	5–15%
Left lobar bronchus	5–15%
Trachea	5–15%
Larynx	1–5%

time elapsed since the aspiration. The acute event is marked by a sudden onset of choking or coughing and is often followed by wheezing, dyspnea, and stridor. Symptoms and signs are somewhat different, depending on whether the aspirated foreign body has lodged in a bronchus (most common) or in the larynx or trachea (Table 4-49). Unilaterally decreased air entry (on auscultation), wheezing, and fever are more commonly observed with bronchial foreign bodies, while stridor and hoarseness are more often associated with laryngotracheal foreign bodies.

The diagnosis of foreign-body aspiration is sometimes delayed. As many as 15 to 20% of cases of foreign-body aspiration are diagnosed more than 1 month after aspiration. A similar proportion of children with subsequently retrieved airway foreign bodies have been reported to be completely free of clinical symptoms and radiologic signs when first examined by a physician. The classic history of sudden onset of choking, coughing, dyspnea, and stridor should signal the need to rule out any possibility of foreign-body aspiration. A similar suspicion should be raised by the presence of otherwise unexplained chronic cough, wheezing, or recurrent pneumonia.

Although the majority of aspirated foreign bodies are radiolucent, the radiograph is a useful tool because of the secondary effects on the lungs produced by the aspiration (Table 4-50). The most commonly demonstrated abnormality on chest radiograph is obstructive asymmetric hyperinflation, which is present in up to 65% of children with bronchial foreign bodies. Evidence of pneumonia, atelectasis, radiopaque foreign body, or pneumothorax are less commonly seen. Overall, 10 to 25% of children with subsequently documented airway foreign bodies (up to 60% of those in a laryngotracheal location) will demonstrate no abnormality on plain chest radiographs. For that reason, some have suggested the use of other diagnostic techniques, such as fluoroscopy, as supplemental tools.

MANAGEMENT

The management of foreign-body aspiration (Fig. 4-36) varies according to presentation of the disorder and age of the patient. If the child presents with acute signs and symptoms of upper-airway obstruction due to foreign-body aspiration and can cough, breathe, or speak, the child should be encouraged to utilize his or her cough to dislodge the foreign body. However, if the child is observed to have either complete obstruction or partial obstruction with either

TABLE 4-50
RADIOGRAPHIC FINDINGS ASSOCIATED WITH IMPACTED FOREIGN BODIES

Obstructive emphysema	50–65%
Normal	10–25%
Atelectasis	5–15%
Pneumonia	1–15%
Radiopaque foreign body	5–10%

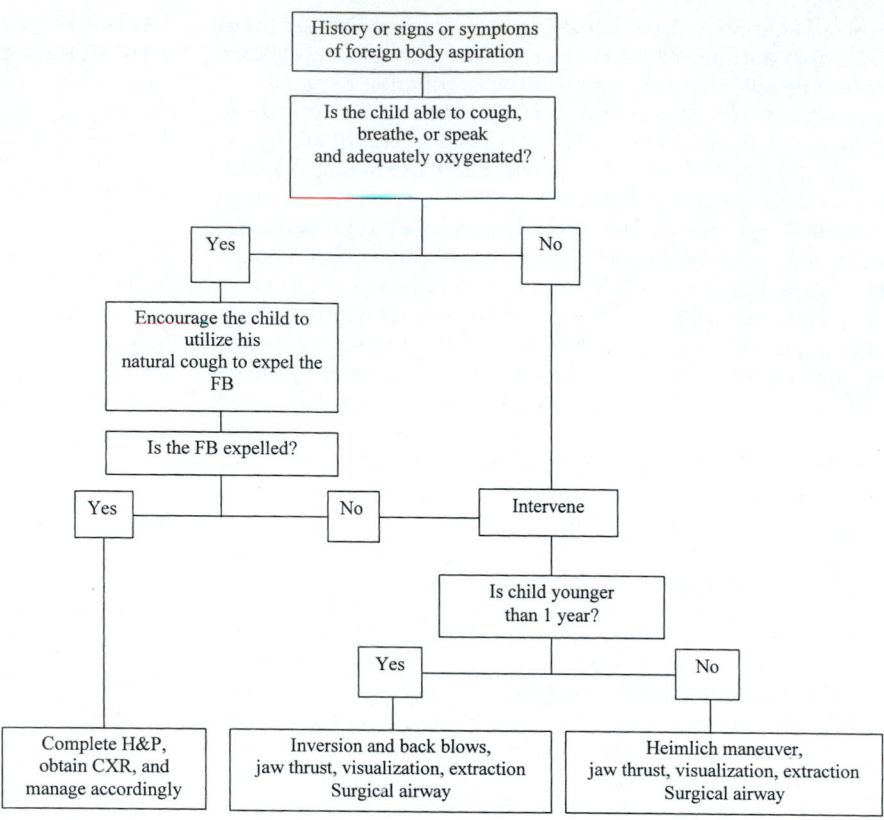

FIGURE 4-36   Suggested management of foreign body aspiration.

cyanosis or poor air exchange, or if the child's cough is ineffective in expelling the foreign body, then the rescuer should intervene. Based on current recommendations, the most appropriate intervention for infants younger than 1 year consists of inversion (face down) followed by five forceful back blows. For children older than 1 year, the Heimlich maneuver (subdiaphragmatic abdominal thrusts) should be the first mode of intervention.

Blind finger-sweeps are to be avoided in infants and children because the foreign body could be pushed back into the airway, causing further obstruction. In the young child who is unable to control his or her actions, this maneuver also puts the rescuer at risk for digit injury.

When initial interventions fail, a jaw thrust should be performed, with the hope of partially relieving the obstruction. If the foreign body can be visualized, it should be manually removed, using Magill or other large forceps. In the unconscious, nonbreathing child, a tongue-jaw lift can be performed by grasping both the tongue and lower jaw between the thumb and finger and lifting. If other methods of reestablishment of adequate air exchange fail, a surgical airway distal to the suspected site of obstruction should be established.

For children who present with signs and symptoms suggestive of bronchial foreign-body aspiration beyond the oropharynx, endoscopy should be performed by those experienced with the procedure. Unless the foreign body has been present for an unusually prolonged period of time or there is other evidence of accompanying infection, antibiotics need not be administered to these patients.

A final word of caution: There are many instances when the history suggests that a child has aspirated or ingested a foreign object and subsequently expelled it, resulting in a normal physical examination. Although it is tempting to omit the radiograph from the evaluation of such an asymptomatic child, that temptation should be resisted. Even the asymptomatic child might harbor a retained foreign body. Numerous medical and legal case reports suggest that it is prudent to carefully rule out the silent presence of such a foreign body. To minimize subsequent complications, airway foreign bodies must be promptly detected and removed.

References

Black RE, Johnson DG, Matlak ME: Bronchoscopic removal of aspirated foreign bodies in children. J Pediatr Surg 29:682–684, 1994

Blazer S, Naveh Y, Friedman A: Foreign body in the airway, a review of 200 cases. Am J Dis Child 134:68–71, 1980

Metrangolo S, Monetti C, Menoghini L, et al: Eight years' experience with foreign body aspiration in children: what is really important for a timely diagnosis? J Pediatr Surg 34:1229–1231, 1999

4.3.6   Burn Injuries

Robert P. Foglia

Trauma accounts for almost 50% of all deaths in children between 1 month of age and 14 years of age. Burn injuries are the third most common cause of death due to trauma in children in the United States, accounting for 2500 deaths and over 10,000 cases of severe, permanent disability annually. Many of these injuries are preventable. Approximately 55 to 60% of the admissions for treatment of burns at St. Louis Children's Hospital are in children under 2 years of age. The majority of burns to younger children, particularly those under 3 years of age, are caused by hot liquids, and by fire to older children and adults. Burns occur most commonly in the kitchen and bathroom. The outcome for the burned patient is related to the magnitude of the injury and is influenced substantially by the quality of the care provided. The initial resuscitation has a fundamental role in this care, particularly in the case of large-body-surface area burns.

The skin serves a number of functions including acting as a barrier against infection and injury, preventing fluid loss, regulating of body temperature, and facilitating sensory contact with the environment. Its attributes help to define a person's uniqueness and recognition from other individuals. Burns can be categorized as the result of thermal, electrical, chemical, or radiation causes. The vast majority of burns in children have a thermal mechanism. A number of factors, such as body surface area to body mass ratio and thickness of the skin, account for differences in response to a burn injury between infants and children and adults. The child has a larger body surface area to body mass ratio. For example a 1-year-old weighing 10 kg has one-seventh the body mass of an adult and one-third of the adult's body surface area. Accordingly, the child has larger evaporative fluid loss and greater difficulty maintaining temperature regulation for a similar body surface area burn. The child's skin is less thick than the adult's, and thus can burn more deeply after the same duration of contact with a heat source.

The severity of tissue damage is related to several factors: (a) temperature of the heat source responsible for the burn; (b) duration of exposure; (c) area of the body burned; and (d) age of the patient. Grease, casseroles, and other hot liquids that tend to stick to the skin will have a longer exposure time and have the potential to cause a deeper burn than a hot liquid of the same temperature that remains in contact with the skin for a shorter length of time. Burns to the palms of the hand and soles of the feet tend to be less deep than similar burns to other parts of the body because of the relative thickness of the epidermis in those areas. Likewise, while a shoulder burn may require a skin grafting because of the depth of burn, a facial burn after a similar exposure may heal spontaneously because the rich blood supply of the face limits the injury by dissipating heat more rapidly from the area.

DETERMINATION OF SURFACE AND DEPTH OF A BURN

The accurate determination of the surface area burned is an essential part of burn-wound management. In adults, the rule of nines is a simple and accurate way of doing it. Each upper extremity represents 9% of the body surface area; each lower extremity represents 18% of the body surface area; and the anterior and posterior trunk represent 18% of the body surface area each. The head and neck encompass 9% and the external genitalia represent the remaining 1% of the body surface area. Unfortunately, the rule is not applicable to children. For instance, the head and neck of a child younger than 1 year of age accounts for as much as 21% of the body surface area. Tables like the modified Lund-Browder body surface area chart shown in Fig. 4-37 divide the body in sectors known to represent a certain proportion of the body surface area. By drawing the burn on the corresponding sector, it is easy to estimate the percent of the body surface area involved in the burn. Except in "stocking-glove"-type burns that extend from the tip of an extremity to the trunk, it is often necessary to approximate the magnitude of involvement of a body part. Especially in the case of irregular burns, it is useful to know that the palm of a child represents approximately 1% of the body surface area.

Burn depth is categorized as either partial or full thickness. *Partial-thickness burns* involve the epidermis and portions of the dermis. They correspond to the older nomenclature's first-degree burns, which are exemplified by the sunburn, and second-degree

burns, which are characterized by a red or mottled appearance, blisters, edema, and a weeping, moist surface. Because of involvement of the dermal nerve endings, they are both painful to the touch and sensitive to cold air. Partial-thickness burns are subclassified as superficial or deep partial-thickness burns. Superficial partial-thickness burns tend to heal spontaneously over 7 to 14 days after the injury. Deep partial-thickness burns may heal spontaneously, but over a longer period of time, and may require tangential excision and skin grafting. *Full-thickness* or third-degree burns involve all skin layers. Their color can be variable. The tissue appears usually dry and inelastic, and the area is insensitive. Full-thickness burns will not heal spontaneously. As a norm, they require excision and skin grafting. Small full-thickness burns may heal by wound contracture. In some burns, the central portion is full thickness and the peripheral portion is partial thickness.

TREATMENT OF BURNS

Immediate Treatment

The first measure of immediate burn care in the field is to make sure that there is no ongoing injury. If there is any clothing or object that may still be a significant source of heat, it should be immediately removed from the patient. Jewelry should be removed from the area and the burn should be wrapped with a clean, dry cloth. Cold liquids should not be applied to burns larger than 1 or 2% of the body-surface area because the cold can result in diminished local perfusion, which may worsen the injury. The patient should be made as comfortable as possible, and rapid transport should be arranged to a hospital.

Admission and Fluid Resuscitation

Criteria for hospital admission include: (a) partial-thickness burn of greater than 5% body surface area; (b) full-thickness burn of greater than 1% body surface area; (c) inhalation injury; (d) chemical burn; (e) electrical burn; (f) circumferential burn of an extremity or trunk; and (g) burns involving the hands, face, feet, or perineum. Intravenous access should be obtained in any patient with greater than a 10% body surface area burn, and fluid resuscitation should be initiated. The often-stated guideline is to achieve a urine output of 1 mL/kg/h in young children and 30 to 50 mL/h in adolescents. A Foley catheter should be inserted to monitor urinary output. If there is a perineal burn, bladder catheterization should be performed before edema formation makes this difficult.

Airway and Lung Injuries

Any patient with a potential for a smoke-inhalation injury requires a rapid physical examination with special attention to the integrity of the airway and to gas exchange. Carbonaceous material in the oropharynx, nasopharynx, or sputum should be noted. Pharyngeal burns, stridor, significant bronchorrhea, dyspnea, or a decreased arterial oxygen saturation are indications of airway or lung injuries. Supplemental oxygen should be started if it was not started during transport. If there is a concern about airway patency, the trachea should be intubated. Arterial blood gas and carboxyhemoglobin levels should be determined.

Three important complications are associated with smoke-inhalation injuries: carbon monoxide poisoning, a thermal injury to the upper respiratory tract, and chemical injury by combustion products to the lower respiratory tract. Carbon monoxide intoxication is discussed in detail in Sec. 4.3.3. It should be suspected in

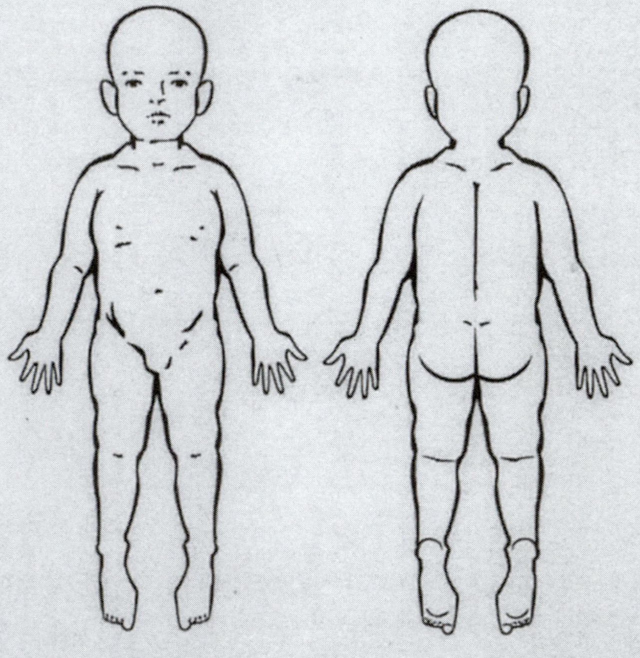

Area	Age-Years					%	%	%
	0-1	1-4	5-9	10-15	Adult	2°	3°	Total
Head	19	17	13	10	7			
Neck	2	2	2	2	2			
Ant. Trunk	13	13	13	13	13			
Post. Trunk	13	13	13	13	13			
R. Buttock	2-1/2	2-1/2	2-1/2	2-1/2	2-1/2			
L. Buttock	2-1/2	2-1/2	2-1/2	2-1/2	2-1/2			
Genitalia	1	1	1	1	1			
R. U. Arm	4	4	4	4	4			
L. U. Arm	4	4	4	4	4			
R. L. Arm	3	3	3	3	3			
L. L. Arm	3	3	3	3	3			
R. Hand	2-1/2	2-1/2	2-1/2	2-1/2	2-1/2			
L. Hand	2-1/2	2-1/2	2-1/2	2-1/2	2-1/2			
R. Thigh	5-1/2	6-1/2	8-1/2	8-1/2	9-1/2			
L. Thigh	5-1/2	6-1/2	8-1/2	8-1/2	9-1/2			
R. Leg	5	5	5-1/2	6	7			
L. Leg	5	5	5-1/2	6	7			
R. Foot	3-1/2	3-1/2	3-1/2	3-1/2	3-1/2			
L. Foot	3-1/2	3-1/2	3-1/2	3-1/2	3-1/2			
				Total BSA Burn				

Modified from Lund and Browder

• Hand Method for non-uniform burns—palm of child's hand approximates 1 percent of child's total BSA burn.

FIGURE 4-37   The Lund-Browder body surface area chart.

any patient who was exposed to combustion products, especially if the exposure occurred in a closed environment and if the patient has an altered state of consciousness or signs of poor oxygen delivery to the tissues, such as a metabolic acidosis.

Thermal burns can affect the pharynx, the nasopharynx, and the upper airway, causing edema and mucosal sloughing. Direct thermal injuries are rare below the glottis, although steam may carry sufficient heat to cause burns in the trachea and bronchi. Inhalational injuries in the subglottic respiratory tract are almost invariably due to chemical damage to the lower respiratory tract, including the bronchi, terminal bronchioles, and alveoli. Their severity varies from bronchial irritation causing cough, increased mucus production, and bronchospasm to more serious alveolar-capillary disruption resulting in respiratory failure (adult respiratory distress syndrome). In patients with burns greater than 25 to 30% of their body surface area, pulmonary edema is a common complication, independent of smoke inhalation. Its mechanism involves fluid overload, hypoalbuminemia, and systemic inflammation initiated by the burn. Infection of the respiratory tract is common and carries a high morbidity and mortality. Respiratory failure resulting from any of the mechanisms discussed above occurs in more than half of the children who die as a result of their burns.

Fluid Resuscitation

Fluid resuscitation within the first 24 hours can be done with crystalloid alone, crystalloid and colloid, or hypertonic saline. Each regimen has its rationale and proponents. We favor a crystalloid resuscitation based on an initial intravenous infusion of 4 mL of Ringer lactate solution by kilogram of body weight by percent unit of body surface area burned, in addition to the patient's calculated maintenance fluids. Half of the fluid is given in the first 8 hours of the resuscitation and the remaining half in hours 9 through 24. In the course of the treatment, the volume of Ringer lactate infusion is adjusted to maintain urine output at 1 mL/kg/h. In this manner, the patient's homeostatic mechanisms are used to guide the therapy and to avoid over- and underhydration. Edema, although unavoidable, can cause complications of its own. A partial-thickness burn of the back may progress to a full-thickness burn because of dependent edema. In patients with myoglobinuria or hemoglobinuria, a larger urine output is desirable and consideration should be given to the administration of sodium bicarbonate to raise urine pH.

A number of metabolic disturbances can occur with fluid resuscitation. Metabolic acidosis is most often due to inadequate perfusion and is best treated by increasing fluid volume. Hyperkalemia can be seen in patients with electrical burns and is the consequence of red blood cell breakdown. Moderate hyponatremia is common after fluid resuscitation with Ringer lactate. If the patient is symptomatic, the judicious use of hypertonic saline may be indicated.

Circumferential Burns

Circumferential burns deserve specific attention because they have a high potential to cause additional vascular or respiratory derangements. In the case of an extremity injury, burned skin and subcutaneous tissue constrict the extremity, limiting venous outflow. Continued arterial inflow causes edema in the distal portion of the extremity, eventually occluding the arterial vessels. Arterial inflow is prevented. Cyanosis, paresthesia, weakness, or a decreased or absent pulse are indications for escharotomy involving both sides of the finger, hand, or arm. For circumferential burns to the chest, a limited tidal volume or chest rise and laboratory evidence of gas exchange abnormalities should prompt similar action. The escharotomy can be done at the bedside because these burns are full thickness in nature and are anesthetized.

Burn-Wound Management

It is often difficult to assess the depth of burn in a child shortly after the child has been injured. The initial treatment consists of debridement of the wound injury and application of a topical antibiotic, usually silver sulfadiazine (Silvadene). Daily wound care follows, including submersion in a whirlpool and wound debridement of the burn eschar. The likelihood of spontaneous reepithelialization and the formation of capillary buds in the burn area is assessed on these opportunities, followed by the application of more silver sulfadiazine, assessment of the mobility by a physical therapist, and wrapping. Sedation is often used in these treatments to facilitate aggressive wound debridement and to obviate the anxiety associated with repetitive care. The use of split-thickness skin grafting is carried out in full-thickness and deep partial-thickness burns. We feel that an early decision to do grafting has the advantage of a lower risk of infection, shorter hospitalization, and improved outcome.

Ancillary Considerations

Burn patients have perhaps the largest caloric needs of any single group of pediatric patients. In a child who has suffered a large body surface area burn, the caloric needs may be 50% greater than the calculated basal needs for body weight or surface area. Many of these patients will not take a sufficient amount of calories orally. In addition, because of the need for daily burn-wound debridement and procedural sedation, the patient may not ingest nutrients for a number of hours before or after the debridement procedure. The use of enteral feeding via a nasogastric tube is an excellent method for supplying the appropriate caloric needs and carries a much lower risk of morbidity when compared to intravenous nutrition. Enteral feedings can be started as soon as 24 hours after the burn.

The type of bacterial flora that colonizes burn injuries changes with time. In the first week, gram-positive organisms predominate. By week 2, gram-negative organisms increase in frequency and number. By week 3, infections due to fungal organisms and antibiotic-resistant organisms are often found. There has been no proven benefit of using prophylactic antibiotic therapy in burn patients. In contrast, the use of topical antimicrobials is well documented to be efficacious in their management. Silver sulfadiazine is the topical agent used most frequently throughout the United States because it affords good gram-positive and gram-negative coverage and because it is relatively easy to apply. A disadvantage to its use is the development of leukopenia in a small number of patients. It is often unclear whether this leukopenia is the result of using the silver sulfadiazine or the result of infection. Sulfamylon is an alternative agent that has the advantage of better penetration of the burn eschar. It is of particular benefit in ear burns, where the cartilage may be involved. Its disadvantages are that it acts as a carbonic anhydrase inhibitor and that it may be painful when applied. Acticoat is a new antimicrobial product that is also silver-based. Purportedly it reduces the number of dressing changes needed.

A major principle in burn care is to obtain coverage of the burn wound. This can be achieved by spontaneous reepithelialization or by graft coverage. The vast majority of superficial partial-thickness burns heal well spontaneously and do not require skin grafting for a satisfactory cosmetic result. Tangential excision of the burn eschar and split-thickness skin grafts are indicated in children with full-thickness burns and partial-thickness burns. Tangential excision removes the dead burn tissue to the point that capillary bleeding is identified. This recipient bed is then covered with a meshed graft (1.5:1, 3:1, or 6:1) of approximately 14/1000-inch thickness. The meshing allows for expansion of the skin graft, an important consideration in the patient with an extensive burn. The cosmetic result, however, declines as more widely meshed grafts are used.

A major research interest for decades in the field of burn injury has been in the area of biological dressings. Ideally, the patient's own skin would and should be used. However, in large-surface-area burns, there is often not enough skin that can be used. The use of cultured epidermal autografts began in 1985. This technique consists of taking a portion of skin from a patient and growing that tissue in culture. Large sheets of autograft can be harvested and applied to a recipient bed on the patient. However, the tissue is very fragile and the cost of producing the cultured autografts is high. Another technique is to place a thinner (6–7/1000-inch) split-thickness skin graft on a donor dermal base. This allows for earlier reharvesting of a graft from the same donor site of the burn patient. In patients where there is a clear need for wound coverage but not enough tissue available for skin grafting, cadaveric homograft or porcine xenograft can be used as a temporary biological dressing. These types of grafts would typically be recognized as foreign tissue by an immunocompetent recipient and rejected in 4 to 5 days. In patients with significant burns, there often is a degree of immune dysfunction and these grafts may last for up to 10 to 14 days. Biological dressings decrease the risk of infection on the same principle as do grafts. They also decrease fluid loss and discomfort with dressing changes, while allowing spontaneous epithelialization of the native skin. Thus, they can be used in patients where (a) there is not enough native skin to cover a burn and a cover is needed until sufficient skin is available for grafting, (b) there is a burn-wound infection and a split-thickness skin graft is likely to become infected, and (c) there is a reasonable likelihood that the wound will epithelialize spontaneously and thus will not require a skin graft, but prompt coverage is desirable.

Nonbiological Dressing Coverage

An ideal dressing for burn wounds should have adherence, flexibility, permeability, transparency, lack of antigenicity, sterility, ease of application, a long shelf-life, and low cost. Materials such as Opsite or Tegaderm have many of these characteristics. Additionally, we have found that the use of Biobrane, consisting of an ultrathin semipermeable silicone membrane, mechanically bonded to a flexible knitted nylon fabric and coated with hydrophilic collagen peptides, offers good wound coverage and allows water-vapor transport.

References

Blot S, Hoste E, Colardyn F: Acute respiratory failure that complicates the resuscitation of pediatric patients with scald injuries. J Burn Care Rehabil 21:289–290, 2000

Burke JF: Current concepts in pediatric burn care: artificial skin—its place in the system of pediatric burn care. Eur J Pediatr Surg 2:205–206, 1992

Carvajal HF: Fluid resuscitation of pediatric burn victims: a critical appraisal. Pediatr Nephrol 8:357–366, 1994

Ebach DR, Foglia RP, Jones MB, et al: Experience with procedural sedation in a pediatric burn center. J Pediatr Surg 34:955–958, 1999

Engelhardt VJ, Clark SM: Early enteral feeding of a severely burned pediatric patient. J Burn Care Rehabil 15:293–297, 1994

Haith LR, Patton ML, Goldman WT: Cultured epidermal autograft and the treatment of the massive burn injury. J Burn Care Rehabil 13:142–146, 1992

Herndon DN, Rutan RL, Rutan TC: Management of the pediatric patient with burns. J Burn Care Rehabil 14:3–8, 1993

Sheridan RL, Hinson MI, Liang MH, et al: Long-term outcome of children surviving massive burns. JAMA 283:69–73, 2000

Sheridan RL, Remensnyder JP, Schnitzer JJ, et al: Current expectations for survival in pediatric burns. Arch Pediatr Adolesc Med 154:245–249, 2000

4.3.7 Heat-Stress-Induced Illness

Michael Apkon

Hyperthermia is a state in which body core temperature rises as a result of heat generation and absorption exceeding heat loss. Given that body temperature reflects the balance between heat gain and heat loss, hyperthermia is found most frequently under conditions such as exercise, in which heat production is increased, or in subjects, such as infants, who lack the ability to increase their heat loss in response to environmental heat. Thus, individuals who engage in athletic activities and infants are at particular risk for heat-related illness. Heat stress has been recognized as a cause of illness for more than 2000 years. It is responsible for perceptible increases in the death rates for populations of people exposed to high environmental temperatures during hot times of the year, and increases morbidity related to other diseases. Heatstroke, the most serious form of heat-related injury, is the second most common cause of athletics-related death after head injury.

PHYSIOLOGY OF TEMPERATURE REGULATION

It is important to differentiate fever, where the body temperature set-point is elevated as a result of the influence of pyrogenic cytokines, from hyperthermia, where temperature is elevated above normal because the heat-dissipating homeostatic mechanisms activated at temperatures above the set-point are overwhelmed. In febrile patients, homeostatic mechanisms, including vasoconstriction and shivering, are activated to raise body temperature, whereas in hyperthermic patients, homeostatic mechanisms are attempting to lower body temperature.

Metabolic activity leads to heat production. If no heat were lost to the environment, resting heat production would raise body temperature by ~1°C/h. This increase would be even greater during exercise, when heat production may rise as much as fourfold. Heat may also be absorbed from the environment by radiation from the sun or the ground, or by convection when the air temperature exceeds body temperature.

Heat production and absorption are balanced by heat loss via four mechanisms. Conduction carries heat between a body and a contacting surface along a temperature gradient. This is the primary mechanism of cooling during ice or water immersion. Convection transfers heat from the body surface to or from a gas or fluid circulating around the body. With conduction, heat transfer stops when the contacting surface temperature reaches body temperature, whereas with convection, circulation of fresh gas or fluid around the body preserves the temperature gradient between the body and the circulating gas or fluid, thus increasing the efficiency of heat transfer. Radiation transfers heat from a warmer to a colder body via electromagnetic waves. Evaporation removes heat by using it to promote a phase transition from liquid to a gas. Of these four mechanisms, radiation is the principal mechanism of heat elimination in temperate environments. Heat loss by convection and radiation are increased by cutaneous vasodilation, a neurally mediated response to hyperthermia. As either heat production or environmental temperature increase, evaporation of sweat becomes the principal mechanism for heat elimination. It is important to recognize that sweating is the only mechanism for heat loss at environmental temperatures above body temperature, because for heat to be lost by conduction, convection, or irradiation, body temperature must be warmer than the gas, fluid, or objects to which heat is dissipated. In fact, conduction, convection, and irradiation lead to heat gain when environmental temperatures exceed body temperature. Under these conditions, the adaptation to heat stress relies on both a greater rate of sweating at a lower degree of exercise and a lower electrolyte content of sweat. Sweating (or evaporation) is a very effective mechanism of temperature control, provided that the environment's humidity is low enough to permit evaporation. This does not occur when the air becomes saturated with water vapor at humidity levels of 90 to 95% and is reduced at humidity levels greater than 75%. In addition, sweating, which occurs at the rate of 1 L/h/m^2 of body surface area, can cause a substantial water and electrolyte loss. This may contribute to the clinical manifestations found in a child exposed to excessive heat.

CAUSES OF HYPERTHERMIA

Under most circumstances, hyperthermia in children is the result of decreased heat elimination, either because the subject has a limited ability to vasodilate (dehydration, shock, autonomic dysfunction, medications that impair thermal control) or sweat (dehydration, ectodermic dysplasia, medications that inhibit sweating), or because the normal mechanisms of heat dissipation are precluded by the circumstances of the environment (high ambient temperature, lack of convective flow, high humidity). Occasionally, however, hyperthermia occurs when the amount of heat generated by the body overwhelms the normal mechanisms of heat dissipation (strenuous exercise, thyrotoxicosis, malignant hyperthermia of anesthesia). Even then, however, the increase in temperature is limited unless the ambient conditions are also unfavorable.

CLASSIFICATION OF HEAT-RELATED ILLNESSES

Heat-related illnesses are a spectrum of disorders varying in the severity of their manifestations from heat cramps, heat syncope, and heat exhaustion, to the life-threatening condition usually described as heatstroke. Heat cramps are thought to be caused by electrolyte disturbances resulting from thirst-driven replacement of large sweat losses with hypotonic fluid. They affect large muscle groups and are more common after exercise. Heat syncope occurs as a result of decreased cerebral blood flow secondary to vasodilation-induced peripheral blood pooling, dehydration, and gravitational redistribution of blood in upright individuals.

Heat exhaustion and heatstroke refer to the more severe forms of heat-related illness and represent a continuum with poorly defined boundaries. With both conditions, illness is in part a consequence of homeostatic attempts at temperature regulation. With heatstroke, those homeostatic mechanisms become overwhelmed and temperature rises above normal. Heat exhaustion, the most common form of heat-related illness, is characterized by intravas-

cular volume depletion under conditions of heat stress and encompasses a poorly defined array of nonspecific symptoms. Signs and symptoms of heat exhaustion include weakness, malaise, headache, dizziness, orthostatic or nonorthostatic hypotension, dehydration, tachycardia, nausea, and vomiting. Typically, mental function is preserved, sweating persists and may be profuse, and body temperature is normal or mildly elevated.

In heatstroke, body temperature is elevated (rectal temperature >40°C), there are deficits in mental function (ranging from disorientation to coma), and there is a history of heat exposure. Classically, there is cessation of sweating, although some individuals may continue to sweat, even profusely. Heatstroke may be characterized as exertional or nonexertional. Individuals succumbing to exertional heatstroke tend to be young, healthy individuals engaged in vigorous activity. The impact of heat stress on these individuals may be exacerbated by limited access to water. Even when there is free access to water, heat-stressed individuals frequently voluntarily replace only a fraction (approximately two-thirds) of the fluids that they lose. Nonexertional heatstroke develops more slowly in individuals without the capacity to regulate their environment or to replace ongoing losses of fluid. Infants and individuals with chronic disease are, therefore, at highest risk.

EFFECTS OF ELEVATED BODY TEMPERATURE

Hyperthermia has negative effects on both cellular and organ functions. At a cellular level, it raises metabolic activity, increasing heat production as well as the demand for oxygen delivery. At an organ or system level, the characteristic response of the organism to a heat stress is cutaneous vasodilation. This results in a shift in the blood volume from the central venous circulation to the skin and a decrease in systemic vascular resistance. These effects are partially compensated for by splanchnic vasoconstriction. Cardiac output initially rises to compensate for both the increased metabolic activity and the vasodilation. The rise in cardiac output results from an increase in heart rate and myocardial contractility, as well as from the reduction in afterload. Redistribution of blood volume from the central veins and reduction in intravascular volume by dehydration limit this rise in cardiac output. When intravascular volume depletion and redistribution become severe, cardiac output will fall. When temperature elevation is more severe, cardiac output may be reduced further because of myocardial injury and conduction disturbances. Cardiovascular collapse may ensue when the circulatory disturbances become sufficiently severe that homeostatic processes defending against circulatory shock (ie, peripheral vasoconstriction) compete with those defending against hyperthermia (ie, cutaneous vasodilation).

Even before cardiovascular collapse occurs, when cardiac output and oxygen delivery are insufficient to meet the demands of an accelerated metabolic rate, cell function may be disrupted by depletion of their energy stores. Some authors suggest that there is a critical maximal temperature above which cellular injury is likely to occur. However, it is perhaps more accurate to consider injury to represent the integrated effect of the extent and duration of hyperthermia.

All organ systems may be affected by severe hyperthermia. Alterations in mental function are universal in heatstroke and range from delirium, convulsions, and opisthotonus to coma. Cerebellar injury leading to ataxia is common, and its manifestation may be delayed and progressive. Despite cooling, the liver may be particularly sensitive to the effects of hyperthermia because of its high

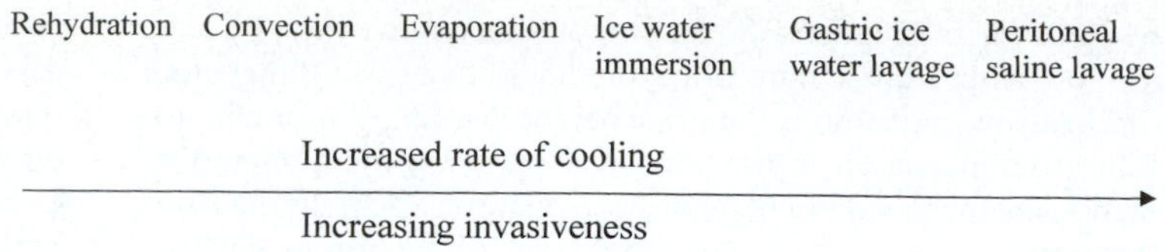

Rehydration   Convection   Evaporation   Ice water   Gastric ice   Peritoneal
                                          immersion   water lavage   saline lavage

Increased rate of cooling

FIGURE 4-38   Methods of cooling of child with heat-stress-induced illness.

Increasing invasiveness

metabolic rate, which leads to a normal temperature above body core temperature. A consumptive coagulopathy and edema are both common, indicating activation of systemic inflammation of a magnitude sufficient to cause an endothelial injury. Muscle injury may be manifest as rhabdomyolysis. The myoglobinuria that results from muscle injury may precipitate acute renal failure and acute tubular necrosis. Diminished cardiac output, hypotension, and direct heat injury may also cause or contribute to renal failure. Impaired respiration usually results from pulmonary edema that may develop as a result of myocardial failure (ie, cardiogenic pulmonary edema) or as a result of increased pulmonary capillary permeability. Hyperventilation is common, leading to development of a respiratory alkalosis that may be manifest as tetany from the reduction of ionized calcium concentrations that accompanies alkalosis.

Although many of the consequences of hyperthermia may be ascribed to the direct effects of temperature elevation, it is likely that some effects are secondary to the generation of inflammatory cytokines, particularly interleukin-1 (IL-1). In animals, immunization against bacterial endotoxin before heat stress markedly reduces heat-induced elevations in interleukin levels and mortality. Moreover, treatment of animal subjects with an IL-1 receptor antagonist at the time of heat exposure reduces the cardiovascular dysfunction caused by hyperthermia. It is not known to what extent cytokines play a role in human heat-related disease.

TREATMENT OF HYPERTHERMIA

Therapy for heat-related illness is aimed at supporting cardiorespiratory function, repleting intravascular volume, and reducing temperature. For milder forms of heat injury, reducing the level of physical activity, transport to a cooler environment, and oral rehydration are typically sufficient. When heat cramps are present, salt as well as water may be replaced using a 0.1 to 0.2% salt solution ($\sim\frac{1}{4}$ tsp table salt per 8 oz water).

Heatstroke is a medical emergency and temperature reduction is a central priority. Cooling is the mainstay of first aid and can be initiated by removing clothing and drenching with cool water. Cooling should continue during and following transport to a hospital, but should be terminated when the core temperature is less than 38.5 to 39°C to prevent hypothermia. A number of methods are effective at reducing body temperature (Fig. 4-38). Ice-water immersion produces the greatest rate of temperature decrease ($\sim$0.15–0.2°C/min) using noninvasive means. Some authors suggest that this method is inadequate because it is possible that cutaneous vasoconstriction limits heat dissipation or that shivering leads to heat production. Paradoxical increases in rectal temperature with ice-water immersion have not been observed. Shivering, if it occurs, may be well controlled using diazepam. Other noninvasive therapies are less effective than ice-water immersion but include spraying the patient with atomized water spray combined with fanning to increase convection. Core cooling may also be accomplished by ice-water gastric lavage, cold saline peritoneal or pleural lavage, or by cardiopulmonary bypass. Antipyretics are not indicated in the management of heatstroke. Acetaminophen may

potentiate hepatic injury, and other nonsteroidal anti-inflammatory drugs may potentiate renal injury and coagulopathy.

PROGNOSIS AND OUTCOME

Prognosis following the milder forms of heat-related illness is generally excellent after appropriate cooling and rehydration. In contrast, heatstroke is a life-threatening disease with morbidity and mortality being largely determined by the degree of injury to the nervous system, the liver, and the kidneys. With appropriate supportive care, mortality is less than 10%. Renal failure occurs in as many as 5% of patients with nonexertional heatstroke and in as many as 25% with exertional heatstroke. Long-term sequelae of heatstroke are well recognized. Specific injuries to the cerebellum and basal ganglia have been described. Such injuries may not be evident at the time of hospital discharge and may develop over days or weeks later. Radiographic abnormalities, including generalized cerebellar atrophy, may be absent on presentation, appear up to several weeks after presentation, and progress for up to 1 year following heatstroke.

PREVENTION

Heatstroke is a preventable disease caused by circumstances largely under human control. Prevention requires an awareness of risk factors as well as appropriate behavioral responses to heat stress. Anticipatory guidance should focus on education of parents, young athletes, and coaches about the need for both rest between exertions and appropriate hydration when exercising in warm environments. Athletic events should be planned with environmental conditions and the need for ready access to water in mind. Parents of young children should also be aware of the dangers of heat exposure in automobiles and that window openings need to be substantial before internal temperatures remain close to ambient air temperatures. Temperatures inside closed automobiles may rapidly rise to as high as 70°C. Finally, parents, coaches, and childcare supervisors need to be aware of the signs of heat-related illness to allow detection prior to the full manifestation of heatstroke.

References

Chiu WT, Kao TY, Lin MT: Increased survival in experimental rat heatstroke by continuous perfusion of interleukin-1 receptor antagonist. Neurosci Res 24:159–163, 1996

Harker J, Gibson P: Heat-stroke: a review of rapid cooling techniques. Intens Crit Care Nursing 11:198–202, 1995

Hubbard RW: Heatstroke pathophysiology: the energy depletion model. Med Sci Sports Exerc 22:19–28, 1990

King K, Negus K, Vance JC: Heat stress in motor vehicles: a problem in infancy. Pediatrics 68:579–582, 1981

Mehta AC, Baker RN: Persistent neurological deficits in heat stroke. Neurology 20:336–340, 1970

Noakes TD: Fluid and electrolyte disturbances in heat illness. Int J Sports Med 19(Suppl 2):S146–149, 1998

Squire DL: Heat illness. Fluid and electrolyte issues for pediatric and adolescent athletes. Pediatr Clin North Am 37:1085–1109, 1990

4.3.8 Poisonous Bites and Stings

Dee Hodge, III

This section addresses the clinical diagnosis and management of injuries that result from bites and stings. Although a large proportion of the morbidity and mortality from these injuries occurs in the pediatric age group, there are few studies on specific treatments for children. An overall assessment should include vital signs; location and size of fang or sting marks; pain; swelling; color of surrounding skin; and any systemic symptoms. General care should include relief of pain and itching; tetanus prophylaxis; antibiotics if needed; and emotional support. Animals must be identified as venomous or not. In evaluating any potential venomous bite or sting, the physician must distinguish between the asymptomatic and the symptomatic bite or sting. Clinical observation may be the only means of distinguishing between the two.

AQUATIC STINGS

A large number of venomous marine animals cause mild, debilitating, or even fatal envenomization. These are seen most frequently in tropical or temperate waters of North America and the Indo-Pacific region. Because of the marked increase in recreational water sports, especially diving, exposure to marine-animal envenomization has become more frequent.

Phylum Coelenterata (Cnidaria)

Members of this group are divided into three large classes: the Hydrozoa (hydras, Portuguese man-of-war), Scyphozoa (true jellyfish), and Anthozoa (soft corals, stone corals, anemones). All of these animals are present in temperate, subtropical, and tropical environments. All members of the phylum have specialized organelles called *nematocysts* (ie, *cnidae*) that are used for entrapping and poisoning prey. Envenomation or dermatitis results from encounters with representatives of this phylum. When the tentacles touch a victim, the nematocysts fire, releasing toxin on or through barbed threads. The firing of the nematocysts is not fully understood; the process may be protein- or cation-mediated. The severity of envenomation is related to the species (toxicity of venom), number of nematocysts discharged, general condition of the victim, and prior sensitization of the victim. Mild to severe local and/or systemic reactions may ensue. Stings from sessile species are, in general, not as severe as stings from free-floating forms. Paralysis and central nervous system (CNS) effects appear to be related primarily to toxic proteins and peptides. Burning pain and urticaria are secondary to the presence of serotonin, histamine, and histamine-releasing agents in the venom.

The hydrozoans include the feathered hydroid (*Pennaria tiarella*) and the Portuguese man-of-war (*Physalia physalis*). The mild sting of the feathered hydroid occurs with handling and may be treated with local care. The Portuguese man-of-war is commonly considered a jellyfish, but in reality, it is a hydrozoan colony. The tentacles hang from the float and may reach a length of more than 75 feet. Each tentacle contains about 750,000 nematocysts. Because of the length and transparency of the tentacles in the water, swimmers are often stung without seeing the animal. Nematocysts may discharge even when the animal is dead and on the beach. The toxin injected is one of the most powerful marine toxins. Local effects are immediate and include intense pain and irritation. The affected area usually has the appearance of deeply erythematous, vesicular, whip-like striations crisscrossing over one another and delineating the pattern of the tentacles on the skin. The lesions may become necrotic, ulcerate before healing, and leave long-lasting, pigmented striae. Systemic reactions include headache, myalgias, fever, abdominal rigidity, arthralgias, nausea and vomiting, pallor, respiratory distress, hemolysis, renal failure, and coma. Death may occur if the area stung is extensive in relation to the size of the victim.

Of the scyphozoans (true jellyfish), the common purple jellyfish (*Pelagia noctiluca*) and the sea nettle (*Chrysaora guinguecinda*) are only mildly toxic. Local skin irritation is the major clinical manifestation. Lion's mane (*Cyanea capillata*) is highly toxic. Lion's mane is found along both North American coasts. Contact with its tentacles produces severe burning. Prolonged exposure causes muscle cramps and respiratory failure.

Treatment of hydrozoan and scyphozoan stings is based on the same general principles: relief of pain, stopping further envenomation, alleviating effects of venom, and controlling shock. The most important step is to remove any adherent tentacles. As long as the tentacle adheres to the skin, the nematocysts continue to discharge. The unexploded nematocysts can be inactivated by topical application of vinegar (3% acetic acid), slurry of baking soda, or meat tenderizer (papain) for 30 minutes. The area should then be washed with normal saline. Fresh water should not be used because it causes nematocysts to discharge. Any adherent tentacles should be removed with instruments or gloved hands and the wound area should be immobilized. Removal of nematocysts may be difficult. Some physicians recommend applying aerosol shaving cream and then shaving off the nematocysts with a safety razor. General supportive measures for local and systemic reactions include oral antihistamines, oral corticosteroids, and oral narcotics for pain. Anaphylaxis may require administration of epinephrine and cardiac and respiratory support. Muscle spasms have been treated with calcium gluconate or a benzodiazepam given intravenously. There is no antivenin available for *Physalia* or the other scyphozoans. A specific antivenin is available for stings by the highly venomous and sometimes fatal box jellyfish *Chironex fleckeri* of Australia. It is effective and, if used promptly, can be life-saving. Local dermatitis should be treated with a topical corticosteroid cream.

The anemones and corals (class Anthozoa) found within United States tidal zones are mildly toxic at worst. Sea anemone stings usually occur in shallow water. Almost instantaneously, they produce severe burning, which is followed by intense itching. An area of central pallor frequently appears, surrounded by erythema and petechial hemorrhage. The envenomed area can become edematous and, in severe envenomation, may become ecchymotic and hemorrhagic. The lesion may ulcerate and heal after eschar formation. Milder envenomizations usually resolve uneventfully within several days. In the United States, fire corals (*Millepora spp.*) are among the most common cause of mild coelenterate stings. Contact with these sessile creatures result in immediate, intense burning or stinging sensation. Severe pruritus and urticaria that may last for several days follow the pain. Wheals reach maximum size 30 to 60 minutes after contact. Untreated, the wheals flatten over 14 to 24 hours and resolve over 3 to 7 days. The wheals may leave an area of hyperpigmentation, which gradually fades after several months. Hours after contact, a delayed reaction can appear, presenting as papules or hemorrhagic vesicles. At times, an erythema nodosum−like reaction can recur repeatedly over several months.

The stinging ability of stony corals is not well defined but is considered to be of minor significance. Coral cuts, however, can result in serious injury because they combine laceration of tissue, nematocyst venom, persistence of foreign debris in the wound, and secondary bacterial infection. The presentation typically includes a stinging sensation followed by wheal formation and itching. If the wound is untreated, then an ulcer with an erythematous base may form within a few days. Cellulitis, lymphangitis, fever, and malaise commonly occur. Treatment consists of cleaning the wound and irrigation with copious amounts of saline. Foreign particles must be removed, and debridement may be necessary. Seawater provides an excellent inoculum for wound infections. Organisms include *Vibrio* species, *Erysipelothrix rhusiopathiae,* and *Mycobacterium marinum.* Wounds should be left open. Broad-spectrum antibiotic therapy, particularly tetracycline, has been advocated for children older than 8 years of age. For children less than 8 years of age, cephalexin or trimethoprim-sulfamethoxazole should be used.

Seabather's eruption is a pruritic, usually benign, dermatitis that is caused by planula larvae of the phylum Coelenterata (Cnidaria). Typically, these larvae possess more than 200 nematocysts. Off the northeast coast of the United States, the planula larva of the sea anemone *Edwardsiella lineata,* and off the coast of Florida, the planula larva of the jellyfish *Linuche unguiculata,* have been identified as the probable cause. Onset typically occurs 4 to 24 hours after exposure. The eruption consists of erythematous maculopapules, or wheals with pruritus. Some people have reported a prickling sensation or develop urticarial lesions immediately, while others may be asymptomatic for 3 to 4 days. The duration of symptoms varies from several days to weeks. Children may have high fevers, which may lead to extensive medical studies for meningitis, sepsis, or fever of unknown origin. Treatment is symptomatic with antihistamines or corticosteroids.

PHYLUM ECHINODERMATA

This phylum includes starfish, sea urchins, and sea cucumbers. Of the three classes, the Echinoidea—sea urchins—account for the greatest threat to children. Only 1 to 2% of the known species are poisonous. Of the poisonous species, either hollow venom-filled spines or jaw-like organelles called *pedicellariae* inject venom. The most severe envenomations occur from those species in which the venom is injected by the pedicellariae. Most commonly, the long-spined urchins (eg, Diadema) cause injuries. Most of the spines are solid and do not possess venom (as do some of the tropical urchins), but the spines, composed of calcium carbonate, are dangerous when stepped on or handled. The spines easily pierce the skin and lodge deep in the flesh. The spines can penetrate wet suits and sneakers, and may break off in the wound. Penetration is accompanied by intense pain followed by redness, swelling, and aching. Complications include tattooing of the skin, secondary infection, and granuloma formation.

Treatment consists of immersion of the punctured extremity in hot water (40–45°C). All spines should be removed as completely as possible. If spines break off in the wound, debridement should be performed with local anesthetic. Analgesics may be needed for pain. Systemic antistaphylococcal antibiotics should be used if infection develops.

Phylum Chordata

Stingrays

Stingrays are the single most important group of venomous fishes, accounting for an estimated 750 envenomations per year in North America. Stingrays are bottom feeders that have a habit of burying themselves in sand or mud. Envenomations usually occur when an unsuspecting swimmer steps on the back of the animal, causing it to hurl its barbed tail upward into the victim as a reflex defense response. Most injuries are confined to the lower extremities, although wounds to the chest and abdomen have been reported. The venom is delivered by a serrated, retropointed, dentinal caudal spine located on the dorsum of the tail. The spine is encased in an integumentary sheath that contains specialized secretory cells. When the barb strikes the victim, it penetrates the skin, rupturing the integumentary sheath over the spine and causing the venom to pass along the ventrolateral grooves of the barb into the wound. The venom is a heat-labile toxin that has been shown to contain at least 15 fractions, including serotonin, 5-nucleotidase, and phosphodiesterase. The toxin produces severe local pain, depresses medullary respiratory centers, and interferes with the cardiac conduction system.

Wounds vary in length and are a combination of puncture and laceration. The sting is followed immediately by pain, which spreads from the site of injury and usually reaches its greatest intensity within 90 minutes. Pain and edema are most often localized to the area of injury. The wound often has a jagged edge that bleeds profusely, and the wound edges may be discolored. Discoloration may extend several centimeters from the wound within hours after injury and may subsequently necrose if untreated. Syncope, weakness, nausea, and anxiety are common complaints. Generalized symptoms include vomiting, diarrhea, sweating, and muscle fasciculations of the affected extremity. Generalized cramps, paresthesias, hypotension, arrhythmias, and death may occur.

Treatment at the scene includes wound irrigation with cold salt water. Irrigation can help remove much of the venom. Bleeding should be controlled with direct pressure and shock treated. At the site of definitive care, an attempt should be made to remove any remnants of the integumentary sheath, if it can be seen in the wound. The extremity should be placed in hot water (40–45°C) for 30 to 90 minutes. This inactivates the venom and relieves pain. After soaking, the wound should be reexplored. Further debridement can be accomplished and the wound can be loosely closed. Additional pain relief may be achieved with narcotic analgesia. Tetanus prophylaxis should be given as needed.

Scorpaenidae

The family Scorpaenidae includes the zebrafish, the scorpionfish, the stonefish, and the sculpin. Scorpaenidae are generally found in shallow water, around reefs, kelp beds, or coral. All members of the family are nonmigratory and slow swimming, and are often buried in sand. The venom apparatus consists of a number of dorsal, anal, and pelvic spines covered by integumentary sheaths containing venom glands that lie within anterolateral grooves. The venoms are unstable, heat-labile compounds. Envenomation usually occurs when the fish are handled during fishing excursions.

Signs and symptoms vary among the species in degree only. Severe pain at the site of the wound is the primary clinical sign. The wound and surrounding area becomes ischemic and then cyanotic. Paresthesia and paralysis of the extremity may occur. Other signs and symptoms include nausea, vomiting, hypotension, tachypnea progressing to apnea, and myocardial ischemia.

Treatment involves irrigating the wound with sterile saline. The injured extremity is then immersed in hot water (40–45°C) for 30 to 60 minutes or until the pain is completely relieved. In addition, narcotic analgesics may be required. The patient should be monitored carefully for cardiotoxic effects and respiratory depression. The only antivenin available is for the stonefish of Australia.

Catfish

The catfish is a popular food and sport fish found throughout the United States. The venom apparatus consists of a number of spines located in the dorsal and pectoral fins. The integumentary sheaths covering the spines contain venom glands. The venoms are unstable, heat-labile compounds. Envenomation usually occurs when the fish are handled during fishing excursions. Combinations of injuries are seen: wounds secondary to puncture and laceration, foreign body reaction, and the effects of venom.

The spines inflict a puncture wound or laceration. The spines may become imbedded in the flesh of the victim, causing soft tissue swelling and possibly a cellulitis and foreign-body reaction. The venom produces a local inflammatory response: local intense pain, edema, local hemorrhage, and tissue necrosis. To treat, first irrigate the wound with sterile saline, then immerse the injured extremity in hot water (40–45°C) for 30 to 60 minutes or until pain is relieved. Narcotic analgesia may be required. The wound should be explored to locate and remove any retained spines. Systemic antibiotics to cover gram-negative organisms are recommended. Wounds may be closed using a delayed primary closure.

TERRESTRIAL BITES AND STINGS

Phylum Arthropoda

The arthropods make up the largest phylum in the animal kingdom. All arthropods have an exoskeleton with jointed appendages. The phylum is divided into two subphyla: the Chelicerata—including spiders, scorpions, ticks, and mites—and the Mandibulata, which includes insects.

Spiders

More than 100,000 species of spiders (class Arachnida) are known to exist. All are carnivorous and have fangs and venom that they use to immobilize and kill their prey. The risk of serious bites is small, because in most species, the fangs are too short and fragile to penetrate human skin, and the venom is mild. Contrary to common belief, most spiders are harmless and shy. However, two species in the United States are capable of producing more severe reactions.

Loxoscelism (Bite of the Brown Recluse Spider) Two species of *Loxosceles* have caused envenomation in the Western Hemisphere. *Loxosceles reclusa* is found primarily in the southern and midwestern states (Arkansas, Missouri, and Texas). *L. laeta* is found in South and Central America. These small spiders (1–1.5 cm in length) are characterized by a brown violin-shaped mark on the dorsum of the cephalothorax. They establish nests indoors, especially in closets and basements, and when disturbed, the spider bites. The venom is cytotoxic and contains a factor similar to hyaluronidase.

Initially, the bite appears innocuous, but the site can become painful within hours of the bite. Because the bite is often unnoticed at first, there is sometimes a delay in seeking medical attention. The spectrum of reaction ranges from minor local reaction to severe necrosis. The local reaction is characterized by mild to moderate pain, generally 2 to 8 hours after the bite. At the site of the bite, erythema develops with a central blister or pustule. A bulla may develop, and concentric areas of ischemia and erythema may appear. During the ensuing 24 to 48 hours, the lesion becomes cyanotic and ulcerates. The necrotic ulcer slowly expands and can reach 10 to 20 cm in diameter during the subsequent weeks to months. The local reaction varies with the amount of venom injected. Scar formation is rare if there is no clinical evidence of necrosis within 72 hours of the bite. Systemic reaction is most commonly seen in small children. Symptoms are noted 24 to 48 hours after the bite and include fever, chills, malaise, weakness, nausea, vomiting, joint pain, morbilliform eruption with petechiae, intravascular hemolysis, hematuria, and renal failure.

Unless the spider is brought for identification, definitive diagnosis cannot be made. There is no specific serologic, biochemical, or histologic test to diagnose envenomation. Several other spiders found in the United States are also known to cause necrotic lesions. Serious complications are rare, and the vast majority of victims will heal with supportive care. If large areas of necrosis have become demarcated, surgical excision and skin grafting may be required, but grafting is usually not needed. Administration of steroids or heparin does not seem to alter the extent of necrosis. The use of dapsone should be limited to adults with proven brown recluse bites because of methemoglobinemia. Antivenin is not commercially available. For systemic manifestations, vigorous supportive care is needed. Laboratory monitoring is needed for evidence of hemolysis and renal failure.

Latrodectism (Bite of the Black Widow Spider) The *Latrodectus mactans* (black widow spider) is the leading cause of death from spider bites in the United States. The female is shiny black with a brilliant-red hourglass marking on the abdomen. A similar marking may also be present on the male. The average width of the abdomen is 6 mm, and the overall length (with legs extended) is 40 mm. The male is not a threat because it is only one-quarter the size of the female and its fangs are unable to penetrate human skin. The webs are usually found in out-of-the-way places such as vacant rodent burrows, hollow stumps, or dark corners of barns, privies, and garages. The female is not aggressive unless guarding her egg sac or provoked. The venom, a complex protein that includes a neurotoxin, stimulates myoneural junctions, nerves, and nerve endings.

The bite of the female black widow spider resembles a pinprick, sometimes accompanied by slight swelling. Immediately after the attack, lymphatic absorption of the toxin begins, and the patient experiences local sharp, throbbing pain that increases in intensity for several hours, by which time vascular spread has occurred. One to 8 hours after the bite, cramping pain is felt in the abdomen, flanks, thighs, and chest. Nausea and vomiting are often reported in children. Respiratory distress is not unusual. Chills, urinary retention, and priapism have been reported. There is an overall 4 to 5% mortality rate, with death resulting from cardiovascular collapse.

Symptoms generally are more severe in children and the elderly. A child who presents with severe pain and muscle rigidity after a spider bite should be considered a potential *Latrodectus* bite victim. In children who weigh less than 40 kg, treatment with *Latrodectus* antivenin (Lyovac; Merck, Sharp & Dohme) should be administered as soon as a bite is confirmed. The usual dose is 2.5 mL (one vial) in 50 mL of saline administered by slow IV injection after skin testing for sensitivity to horse serum. For children who weigh more than 40 kg, it is not as urgent to give antivenin treatment, but indications for its use include patients under 16 years old, respiratory difficulty, or marked hypertension. Antivenin is usually effective within 30 minutes and may be repeated within 2 hours if necessary. Serum sickness is a possible side effect but is uncommon. Muscle relaxants such as diazepam have been advocated, but they are variably effective and the effects are short-lived. Analgesia may be achieved with morphine or meperidine.

Tarantulas and Other Spiders   Tarantulas, although fearsome in size and appearance, do not bite unless provoked. The venom is mild, and envenomation is not a problem. The wolf spider *(Lycosa spp.)* and the jumping spider *(Phidippus spp.)* also have been implicated in bites. Like the tarantula, they have a mild venom that causes only local reactions. Bites from all three of these spiders should be treated with local wound care.

Scorpions

There are many scorpion species that accidentally sting humans. Only a limited number are dangerous to man. In Mexico, for example, where scorpions have been responsible for 82% of 24,627 deaths from poisonous animals over a 10-year period, more than 80% of these fatalities have occurred in children under 5 years of age, and 94% in children under 10 years. In the southwest United States, *Centruroides sculpturatus (C. exilicauda)* is the lethal inhabitant. The animal has two pinching claws anteriorly and a tail or pseudoabdomen that ends in a telson. The telson houses a pair of poison glands and a stinger. The animals are nocturnal. During the day they may crawl into sleeping bags and unoccupied clothing.

The scorpion's venom consists of a local cytotoxin and a neurotoxic component that also has hemolytic properties. The general neurotoxicity is excitatory, affecting the autonomic and skeletal neuromuscular system. Following a sting there is an immediate sharp pain. Common symptoms include restlessness, hyperactivity, roving eye movements, and respiratory distress. Other associated signs may include convulsions, drooling, wheezing, hyperthermia, cyanosis, and respiratory failure. Pulmonary and gastrointestinal hemorrhage may occur. Death occurs because of respiratory paralysis, pulmonary edema, or intractable hypotension and shock. A history of a sting may not be elicited, making the diagnosis difficult. There is no laboratory test for confirmation of envenomation.

Treatment should be initiated as soon as possible. General supportive care is critical. Cryotherapy of the site of sting has been advocated to reduce swelling and local induration. Specific anti-scorpion serum generally is available in those areas where these dangerous animals exist. Its administration is the single most important treatment for severe envenomization. Antivenin should be considered after general supportive care has been instituted if the following symptoms persist: tachycardia, hyperthermia, severe hypertension, and agitation. In the United States, the available antivenin is not approved by the Federal Drug Administration (FDA) and is only available through the Antivenin Production Laboratory at Arizona State University in Tempe, Arizona. Sedative-anticonvulsant, in particular phenobarbital, has been used to treat persistent hyperactivity, convulsions, and agitation. A recent study shows the benefit of continuous IV midazolam in severe envenomation. Calcium gluconate has been given IV to reduce muscular contractions and associated pain, but its benefit is unproven. Corticosteroids and antihistamines have no proven benefit.

Ticks

Both tick bites and tick-borne diseases have become more frequent, especially along the east coast of the United States. Ticks are blood-sucking ectoparasites in all of their stages, and they can be recognized easily by the organization of their mouthparts and body. They

are subdivided into two major groups: (a) the argasids, or soft ticks; and (b) the ixodids, or hard ticks.

Ticks are widespread in nature and may transmit numerous infectious diseases including spirochetes, viruses, rickettsiae, bacteria, and protozoa. In addition they cause mechanical injury at the bite wound. Occasionally, they may release toxic substances of their own, as in the case of the tick-induced paralysis. Ticks attach to their host by their highly specialized mouthparts, and they may engorge themselves with blood for days or weeks before dropping off. During this period, they may become so enlarged that they resemble a pedunculated wart or fibroma. The North American deer tick *Ixodes scapularis* is minute and may go unnoticed. After a tick bite and detachment, a granuloma may form at the bite wound. This generally resolves during the subsequent few months.

Tick paralysis most often is reported in children, in whom almost all fatalities occur. Approximately 20 species of ticks, in the genera *Dermacentro, Amblyomma, Rhipicephalus, Ixodes, Ornithodoros, Haemaphysalis,* and *Argas,* have been implicated. In North America, tick paralysis in humans is usually associated with species of *Dermacentor* and *Amblyomma.* Symptoms may begin with motor weakness and progress as an ascending, flaccid, motor paralysis, which often is mistaken for Guillain-Barré syndrome or poliomyelitis. Sensory involvement is uncommon. Symptoms of paralysis may become evident 4 to 7 days after the blood-sucking starts, although cases as soon as 1 day have been reported. The ascending paralysis may progress in a matter of hours to bulbar signs with facial and lingual paralysis. Patients may die of respiratory failure or aspiration pneumonia. Laboratory data, including cerebrospinal fluid are usually normal, but lymphocytic pleocytosis has been reported. It is believed that the gravid female tick secretes in her saliva a neurotoxin that blocks the release of acetylcholine at neuromuscular junctions. If not too far advanced, removing the tick is associated with prompt, and often dramatic, reversal of the symptoms. Patients usually are afebrile. A tick will be found after careful examination. It is important to search the scalp, axilla, and pubic regions to locate the ticks.

Ticks normally should be removed manually by gentle traction using blunt forceps or tweezers. The tick should be grasped as close to the skin surface as possible and pulled upward with a steady, even pressure. A twisting or jerking motion may cause the mouthparts to break off. The entire tick, including the mouthparts, must be removed. If the mouthparts are left behind, they usually cause a severe granulomatous lesion that may not heal for months. Squeezing or crushing the body of the tick may facilitate inoculation of infective agents into the host. Ticks can be controlled with benzene hexachloride sprays. Dogs should wear tick collars that are changed every 30 to 60 days. Clothing can be impregnated with tick repellents such as dimethylphthalate, diethyltoluamide, or indalone. Dogs should be inspected every day to prevent infesting the home.

Centipedes

Centipedes (class Myrapoda) are worm-like arthropods possessing many repetitive body segments, each of which has one pair of segmented legs. Immediately below the mouth are modified legs of the first body segment (ie, the maxillipeds), which are powerful poison claws that are used to attack and kill prey. Although centipedes are greatly feared for their appearance, they rarely bite. However, bites can be extremely painful. The toxin causes only local reaction. The pain usually diminishes rapidly and may require nothing more than a cold compress and local wound care. Injection of local anesthetic at the wound site is used for extreme pain. More generalized reactions, such as nausea, vomiting, and dizziness, occur infrequently. General supportive care is warranted in these cases. A single death in a 7-year-old child has been reported.

Insects

The stings of bees, hornets, yellow jackets, wasps, and fire ants introduces a venom that in nonsensitized individuals causes immediate pain, induration, and redness lasting several hours or longer. Serious allergic reactions, including death, may occur, especially in those who are previously sensitized. Hymenoptera are responsible for 50% of human deaths from venomous bites and stings. While higher in adults than in children, only approximately 8% develop an allergic reaction following a repeat sting. It is not clear whether subsequent experiences are associated with progressively more severe reactions. Stings may cause a profound systemic reaction such as nausea, vomiting, hypotension, loss of consciousness, and death. However, in most cases, individuals who have had local reactions continue that pattern with each sting. Systemic reactions occur more frequently in individuals who have had multiple stings.

The venoms of the bee, hornet, yellow jacket, and wasp contain protein antigens that can elicit an immunoglobulin (IgE antibody) response in those persons who are stung. In addition, venoms contain various biogenic amines, phospholipase, phosphatase, and hyaluronidase. The barbed stinger of the bee remains in the victim's skin. The wasp, in contrast, may sting many times. The allergic reactions may be grouped by severity. Group I reactions consist of a local response at the site of bite or sting. Group II reactions include generalized pruritus and urticaria (mild systemic reactions). Group III reactions include wheezing, angioneurotic edema, nausea, and vomiting (severe systemic reactions). Group IV reactions include laryngoedema, hypotension, and shock (life-threatening systemic reactions).

The barbed honeybee stinger with venom sac is avulsed and often remains in the victim's skin. It must be removed if seen. A recent study showed that the method of removal is irrelevant; however, delays in removal are likely to increase the dose of venom received. Treatment is based on the severity of the allergic reaction. Group I reactions need only cold compresses at the site of sting; group II reactions are treated with diphenhydramine orally for several days; group III reactions are treated with subcutaneous injection of epinephrine 1:1000 (0.01 mL/kg, 0.3 mL max). It may be necessary to repeat epinephrine twice at 10-minute intervals to arrest the symptoms, followed by oral diphenhydramine. H_2-blockers such as ranitidine or cimetidine may provide additional benefit. The patient should be admitted for observation for 24 hours. Group IV reactions may require intubation if upper-airway obstruction is present. Wheezing refractory to epinephrine should be treated with aminophylline. Hypotension should be treated with a fluid bolus of saline or lactated Ringer solution. IV epinephrine may be indicated if hypotension fails to respond to subcutaneous epinephrine and fluid bolus. In addition, intravenous steroids should be given for 4 days.

Children who have had a group III or IV reaction need to be followed by an allergist for hyposensitization. Because immunotherapy may reduce the risk of anaphylaxis to approximately 3%, many advocate that venom-sensitized patients be immunized against the appropriate venoms. Allergic individuals who have not had immunotherapy should be advised to carry an anaphylaxis emergency treatment. Parents should receive information regarding the avoidance of situations and behaviors that would attract stinging insects.

Ant stings frequently occur in the southern United States and are caused by various species of fire ants of the genus *Solenopsis*. Multiple stings and mass attacks can cause severe reaction. Harvester ants (ie, *Pogonomyronex*) attack humans readily and cause a painful sting. The venom differs from the venom of other Hymenoptera in that it is an alkaloid with a direct toxic effect on mast cell membranes. There is no cross-reactivity with other members of the order. Severe and fatal reactions have been reported in farm animals; fortunately, these are rare in humans. The fire ant bites with well-developed jaws and then uses its head as a pivot to inflict multiple stings. Immediately after a sting, an erythematous wheal appears, which vesiculates after a few hours. A pustule forms within 24 hours; in several days to a week this ruptures, encrusts, and finally forms a small fibrous nodule or scar. Pain can persist for 3 to 10 days. Systemic reactions can occur, especially if there are multiple stings. Treatment is symptomatic. Local care, such as ice applied to the reactive area, and frequent cleansing of the lesions to prevent secondary infection is all that is usually required. Systemic therapy does not appear to prevent pustule formation. Antihistamines are useful for pruritus. Systemic reactions are rare and should be treated similarly to other Hymenoptera reactions.

Phylum Chordata

Venomous Snakebites

Although only 15% of the 120 snake species found in the United States are venomous, an estimated 8000 persons are bitten annually by poisonous snakes. Predictably, the pediatric population, especially males age 5 to 19 years, accounts for a disproportionately large number of these victims. The highest incidence occurs in the Southeast and Southwest between April and October. If treated properly and early, these injuries have a remarkably low mortality and morbidity. Only 10 to 15 deaths are reported per year, but the morbidity in limb dysfunction and other complications, though unknown, is undoubtedly higher.

The poisonous snakes indigenous to the United States are members of the Crotalidae (pit viper) or Elapidae families. The Crotalidae contain three genera: *Crotalus,* or large rattlesnake, with about 30 species including the Eastern and Western diamondback, timber, prairie, and pacific rattlesnakes; *Sistrurus,* or ground rattlers, which include the massasauga and the pygmy rattlesnake; and *Agkistrodon,* or moccasins, which include the cottonmouth and copperhead. The pit vipers have several characteristic features that distinguish them from nonvenomous snakes: (a) the pit from which their name originates contains heat-sensitive organs that assist in the localization of prey and are located on each side of the head between the eye and nostril; (b) their pupils are elliptical and vertically oriented in contrast to the round pupil of harmless snakes; (c) they have two 5- to 20-mm-long curved fangs or hollow maxillary teeth that are folded posteriorly against the palate and advance forward when the pit viper strikes; in larger snakes, they may be spaced as wide as 3 cm; (d) a relatively more triangular head than that of most nonvenomous snakes; and (e) a single-row scute, or scales, on the ventral portion caudad to the anal plate as opposed to the double-row seen in nonpoisonous snakes. Physicians who might treat snakebite victims should become familiar with the particular species in their areas.

The family Elapidae, which includes cobras and mambas, is represented by two species of coral snake, the eastern (*Micrurus ful-*

vius) and the Arizona (*Micruroides euryxanthus*). *M. fulvius* is responsible for the majority of human envenomation and is found in most of the southeastern states. *M. euryxanthus* is indigenous only to Arizona and New Mexico. The relatively passive coral snake is responsible for only 10 to 15 snakebite cases per year in the United States. Coral snakes are 2 to 3 feet long and do not share the pit viper's distinctive physical characteristics (ie, it has round pupils, a blunt head, ventral caudal scuta, and lacks pits). Unlike nonpoisonous snakes, the coral snake does have two small maxillary fangs. A small amount of highly toxic venom is produced. The snout of the coral snake is always black and is followed by brightly colored transverse bands of yellow, red, and black.

Venoms

Snake venoms are an evolutionary adaptation for obtaining food. As such, venoms are complex mixtures of potent enzymes, primarily proteinases and low-molecular-weight peptides that possess toxic properties. Certain components are intended to immobilize prey, while other components are digestive enzymes that penetrate throughout the prey's tissues. Crotalid venom is often a combination of necrotizing, hemotoxic, neurotoxic, nephrotoxic, and/or cardiotoxic substances. Elapid venom contains neurotoxic and cardiotoxic components. The neurotoxins make up a large fraction of the venom of the Mojave rattlesnake. These toxins are related to phospholipase A and bind the nicotinic acetylcholine receptors, thus preventing the depolarizing action of acetylcholine. Proteolytic enzymes aided by hyaluronidase cause much of the local tissue destruction. Many of the venoms induce increased endothelial permeability and venous pooling, decreasing intravascular volume. Transient hemoconcentration may be present as a result of plasma extravasation. Respiratory failure may occur because of pulmonary edema or hypovolemic shock. Hemotoxic effects include hemolysis and fibrinogen proteolysis. Thrombocytopenia is frequently present. Elapid snake venoms may cause considerable necrosis in addition to exhibiting neurotoxicity.

The venom enzymes typically found in crotalid and viperid venoms are esterases with procoagulant and bradykinin-releasing activity. They cause intravascular clotting either by a thrombin-like action (pit vipers) or by activation of factor X (eg, Russell viper). The thrombin-like activity of many North American pit viper venoms differ, however, from that of thrombin in that other clotting factors are not usually activated and the resulting microclots are friable, unstable, and readily lysed by the activation of the plasminogen-plasmin system. This results in defibrination and a clinical picture resembling disseminated intravascular coagulation in which the defibrinating agent is presumed to be thrombin. Snake venom procoagulants, however, do not usually cause platelet aggregation, nor do they activate and destroy factors V and VIII. Inhibition by heparin is incomplete or does not occur. The defibrination produced is readily corrected by antivenin.

Pit Viper

Signs and Symptoms The effects of a snakebite depend on the characteristics of both victim and snake. The victim's size and state of health influence how the toxins are tolerated; the characteristics of the wound inflicted by the bite and its location affect venom absorption. Fang penetration of a vessel or subfascial compartment ensures a more rapid absorption and serious systemic effects. Likewise, a bite on the head, neck, or trunk (3% of snakebites) hastens systemic absorption. Approximately one-third of snakebites involve

the upper extremity and cause a higher long-term functional morbidity than do lower-extremity wounds.

The snake's size, the amount of venom injected, and the potency of the particular species' venom also influence the bite's outcome. Venom secretion is under voluntary muscular control. Thus, any condition that facilitates it (eg, long, healthy fangs or full stores of venom) adds to the toxicity of the bite.

Local pain after a crotalid envenomation is typically intense. A sensation of burning occurs almost immediately (within 5 to 10 minutes). The pain increases as edema develops and is dependent on the size of the venom inocula. Victims of a significant rattlesnake bite often complain within minutes of perioral numbness and paresthesias extending to the scalp and periphery. These paresthesias may be accompanied by a metallic taste in the mouth. Nausea, vomiting, weakness, chills, sweating, and syncope are also frequent. A copperhead or pygmy rattlesnake envenomation usually produces less-local symptoms, and systemic consequences are often minimal, unless the victim is a small child, there are multiple bites, or a larger than average snake is involved. The effects of the water moccasin's envenomation are more variable. Severe pain and swelling are absent after Mojave rattler bites, although, as in other crotalid bites, the patient may complain of paresthesia in the affected extremity. Within several hours, neuromuscular symptoms, such as diplopia, swallowing difficulty, lethargy, nausea, and progressive weakness, develop.

The wound should be inspected for fang punctures, and if two are present, the distance between them should be noted. In general, less than 8 mm interfang distance suggests a small snake; 8 to 12 mm suggests a medium-sized snake; and greater than 12 mm suggests a larger snake. Fang wounds by small snakes such as the pygmy rattler may be extremely subtle. There may be bloody serosanguineous fluid dripping from the fang punctures. Depending on the time to presentation, the fang marks may be hidden within hemorrhagic blebs and edema. Occasionally, only one puncture or two simple scratches are present. In these wounds, there is still the potential for envenomation. However, 10 to 20% of known rattlesnake strikes do *not* inject venom. Other etiologies for puncture wounds also must be kept in mind—notably rodent bites or thorn wounds. Nonpoisonous snakes sometimes leave an imprint of their two rows of teeth, but the wounds should lack fang puncture marks.

Progressive swelling usually develops over the next 8 hours and may continue to some degree for an additional 24 hours, depending on the size of the inoculum. In a severe diamondback rattlesnake bite, an entire extremity may be swollen within 1 hour. The swelling looks impressive and the skin may feel tense and look shiny. Subfascial compartmental pressures are generally not increased, and compartment syndromes requiring fasciotomy are rare. Bluish discoloration of the bitten part is common, and ecchymoses, blebs, and blisters may develop. Local ecchymoses and vesicles usually appear within the first few hours, and, commonly, by 24 hours hemorrhagic blebs are present. Lymph node enlargement or lymphadenitis also may become apparent. Without appropriate therapy, these local manifestations progress to necrosis and may extend throughout the bitten extremity. However, local necrosis may occur even in optimally treated patients.

Other systemic signs are dependent on the species and the amount of venom injected. Tachycardia and decreased capillary perfusion may be seen. In severe cases, hypotension and shock develop. Increased respiratory effort may result from metabolic acidosis or from developing pulmonary edema. Respiratory failure has been described. Oliguria may be secondary to shock or renal failure. Hemoglobinuria and hematuria are the result of the bleeding diathesis, which can develop (hemoglobinuria cannot be the result of the bleeding problem alone). Neurologic signs include fasciculation, weakness, paralysis, and convulsions.

Treatment

Therapy for poisonous snake bites remains controversial because they are uncommon, few physicians have extensive experience with treatment, and controlled studies are infeasible. In spite of this, certain tenets of management are not in question. As in all medical emergencies, the airway, breathing, and circulation of the patient must be assessed and guaranteed before attending to the snakebite. The first priority of prehospital care of the snakebite victim is rapid transport to a medical facility. Time is of the essence, and all activities in the field must be tempered by this fact.

Prehospital Care

It is important to approach the patient with reassurance and to place the patient at rest. The affected extremity should be stripped of any jewelry or clothing and immobilized in a position of function below the level of the heart. Tight tourniquets are not recommended. However, a *constriction band* that obstructs lymph and venous flow can be valuable when a transport longer than 30 to 60 minutes is anticipated. The band should be at least 2 cm wide, made of non-stretchable material, and placed 5 to 10 cm proximal to the wound. Only the lymphatics and superficial veins need to be occluded, and good distal arterial pulses should be preserved (band loose enough to admit a finger). Observation for adequate perfusion is necessary because of progressive edema; the constriction band should be shifted to remain proximal to the swelling. The band must be applied initially within 1 hour of a pit viper bite.

Incision and suction cannot be routinely recommended. Studies show that Sawyer's Extractor, which provides approximately 1 atmosphere of negative pressure, is effective in extracting venom from the bite site provided it is started within 5 minutes of the snake's strike. (Note that constriction bands and incision and suction are not recommended in coral snake envenomation.)

In the rare situation in which skilled personnel and supplies are at the scene and a long transport is expected, it is reasonable to allow one or two attempts at IV access. Many also suggest capturing or killing the snake for later verification; however, an inexperienced person should not risk the bite of an agitated snake. If the snake arrives in the emergency department or office, treat it with respect—"dead" snakes have been known to bite, and decapitated snakes can bite reflexively for up to 1 hour.

In the past, the use of ice to cool the bitten part was advocated. However, cryotherapy should *never* be used in snakebite. Cryotherapy causes more damage because frostbite is easily produced in a limb with circulation already impaired by the action of the venom. Cooling does not slow the action of the venom. Recently, the use of electric shock therapy has received a great deal of publicity in the lay press. The use of high-voltage, low-current shocks in experimental studies have failed to demonstrate any beneficial effects and should not be used.

Emergency Department Care

The keys to management of snakebite in the emergency department are: (a) establish a baseline of physical findings and physiologic parameters; (b) grade the level of envenomation; (c) administer an-

tivenin if indicated; and (d) provide other supportive and therapeutic measures.

Establish a Baseline A brief history should be obtained and an initial physical examination including vital signs, an inspection of the bite site for fang and/or tooth marks, and evaluation of current neurologic status should be done. Next, the circumference of the injured extremity at the leading point of edema and 10 cm (4 inches) proximal to this level should be measured every 30 minutes for 6 hours and then at least once every 4 hours for a total of 24 hours. If the history and physical examination on arrival in the emergency department are consistent with a venomous snakebite, immediate laboratory evaluation and IV access are indicated. Aggressive supportive medical care must be available if signs of major system dysfunction are present. Any prehospital care (eg, extremity immobilization) should be rechecked. If an occluding tourniquet is present, it should be removed after placing a more proximal constriction band, being prepared to respond to a systemic release of venom.

Therapy is based on the clinician's overall grading of venom toxicity. Local and systemic manifestations, as well as laboratory findings, weigh heavily in this judgment. A complete blood count, coagulation studies, platelet count, urinalysis, and blood cross-matching should be obtained on all patients with suspected venomous snakebite. In moderate or severe poisoning, serum electrolytes, BUN, creatinine, fibrinogen, and arterial blood gases are indicated because of the findings described below. The laboratory studies may need to be repeated every 6 hours to ensure that no significant changes occur. The clinical pattern may change dramatically as the venom's effects unfold. Frequent reassessment is crucial.

Grade Severity of Envenomation The Scientific Review subcommittee of the American Association of Poison Control Centers has suggested a grading system. The grading system only applies to pit viper bites.

No envenomation—Little or no pain and no swelling after 4 hours.

Mild envenomation—Local findings include pain, tenderness, and swelling within 10 cm of the bite. There may be a slight bluish discoloration around the site of the bite. There are no systemic symptoms and no laboratory abnormalities.

Moderate envenomation—Local findings include those seen in mild envenomation with progressive swelling. There may be a bluish discoloration of the entire limb. Systemic symptoms include nausea, vomiting, weakness, perioral and scalp paresthesias, and fasciculation. Laboratory abnormalities include thrombocytopenia, hypofibrinogenemia, and hemoconcentration.

Severe envenomation—Local findings include rapidly progressing pain and swelling. There is development of vesicles/bullae and ecchymoses. Systemic symptoms include those seen in moderate envenomation plus hypotension, shock, bleeding diathesis, and respiratory distress. Laboratory abnormalities include thrombocytopenia, hypofibrinogenemia, anemia, and metabolic acidosis.

Antivenin One antivenin (antivenin Crotalidae polyvalent: Wyeth Laboratories) is effective for rattlesnake, water moccasin, and copperhead envenomations. For maximal venom binding, the antivenin should be given within 4 hours of the snake strike. The benefits of crotalid antivenin administration after 12 hours is questionable, and use is not indicated after 24 hours. An exception may be continued coagulopathy. The initial recommended dosage varies with the severity of the envenomation. Dosages in the higher range are used when snake or human variables associated with higher morbidity/mortality are present. Antivenin is highly antigenic horse serum, therefore, skin testing is mandatory. The standard skin test involves an intradermal injection of 0.02 mL of 1:10 dilution of reconstituted antivenin. If the history suggests a likely reaction, a more diluted (1:100 or greater) preparation should be used. A saline control in the opposite extremity is useful for judging a positive-reaction wheal, which is usually seen within 15 minutes. Resuscitation equipment, including airways and oxygen, IV epinephrine (1:10,000), antihistamines, and steroids must be kept in close proximity. If the skin test is negative, the reconstituted antivenin is diluted 1:4 with normal saline. Start to infuse the antivenin by IV slowly (1–2 mL/h). If no signs or symptoms of an allergic reaction occur, increase the rate of infusion so that the total volume is completed over 2 to 4 hours. Extremity edema and vital signs should be measured every 15 minutes for evidence of progression and venom toxicity. The initial dose of antivenin should be repeated every 2 to 4 hours until the progression of the swelling has stopped. Fluid overload is a potential complication in small children. The number of antivenin vials initially anticipated is a rough estimate; more or less antivenin may be required as the clinical reassessments dictate (as many as 75 vials have been used in a child). As a general rule, start with 5 vials for mild envenomation, 10 vials for moderate envenomation, and 15 vials for severe envenomation.

In the event of a pronounced hypersensitivity reaction, further antivenin is contraindicated unless the severity of the bite is judged to be life-threatening. If mild allergic manifestations develop, stop the infusion and give intravenous diphenhydramine. After the allergic symptoms have resolved, wait a minimum of 5 minutes, and then restart the infusion at a slower rate. If symptoms recur, stop the antivenin again; further therapy at this point is controversial. Some physicians recommend an epinephrine infusion titrated to minimize any allergic phenomena when the antivenin is restarted. Intravenous steroids are also recommended. An alternative desensitization method for allergic reactions is described in the product insert, but requires at least 3 hours to achieve; thus, it is impractical in severe envenomation. If life-threatening anaphylaxis occurs, diphenhydramine and steroids are given immediately IV, and other supportive measures are instituted as needed.

Other Supportive Care Wound care includes irrigation, cleansing, a loose dressing, and tetanus prophylaxis if the patient is judged to lack immunity. The affected extremity should be maintained just below the level of the heart and in a position of function. Cotton padding between swollen digits is useful. As in any animal wound, secondary infection is a risk. Broad-spectrum prophylactic antibiotics may be indicated. Analgesics for pain should be given. Surgical excision of the wound, routine fasciotomy, and application of ice are contraindicated. Fasciotomy should be reserved for the very rare case of a true compartment syndrome. Necrosis is usually the result of the proteolytic enzymes or inappropriate therapy and is not caused by compartmental pressure. Superficial debridement may be required at 3 to 6 days. Physical therapy is beneficial during the healing phase.

The major goal of supportive care is correction of the intravascular volume depletion that results from increased venous capacitance, interstitial edema, and hemorrhagic losses. Moderate or severe envenomation requires placement of two IV catheters for separate but simultaneous antivenin therapy and volume replacement. Shock usually develops between 6 and 24 hours after the snakebite but may present within the first hour in severe envenomation. Signs of hypovolemia deserve aggressive therapy (see Sec. 4.1.2). Central vascular monitoring and accurate urine output measurements are desirable for optimal therapy. Normal saline or lactated Ringer solution (20 mL/kg over 1 hour), followed by fresh whole-blood or other blood components, frequently corrects the hypovolemia. Vasopressors are usually needed only transiently in the most severe cases. A bleeding diathesis is best managed with fresh whole-blood, or blood-component therapy, in addition to antivenin. With life-threatening bleeding, platelets and cryoprecipitate should be considered. Abnormal clotting parameters, including fibrinogen and platelet and blood counts, should be reevaluated every 4 to 6 hours. Respiratory support also is frequently required when shock has developed. Renal failure is another potential problem in this setting.

Serum sickness syndrome may develop approximately 4 days to 3 weeks after antivenin treatment. Serum sickness is almost assured with doses greater than seven vials of antivenin. Rashes, arthralgias, edema, malaise, lymphadenopathy, fever, and/or gastrointestinal symptoms evolve over several days. High-dose prednisone (2 mg/kg/d, maximum 80 mg) given until symptoms abate (and then a tapering schedule) has been used with success in most cases. In mild cases, diphenhydramine has been given alone.

Coral Snake

Signs and Symptoms Symptoms seen after coral snake bite differ from those seen after the bite of pit vipers. The signs and symptoms reflect the neurotoxic nature of the venom. The bite may have one or two punctures, at most 7 to 8 mm apart, as well as other small teeth marks, as opposed to the one or two fang marks of pit viper bites. There is usually only mild pain and little, if any, swelling. Local necrosis does not occur. Systemic symptoms are delayed and occur over several hours. Initial symptoms include generalized malaise and nausea, vomiting, and paresthesias in the bitten part. Fasciculations and weakness develop insidiously. The patient may complain of diplopia and may have difficulty talking or swallowing. Physical examination reveals bulbar dysfunction and generalized weakness. Paralysis of skeletal muscles follows, beginning with the limb girdles and progressing distally. Respiratory failure may ensue. Paralysis persists for 3 to 4 days followed by recovery, although minor effects may linger for several weeks.

Treatment All patients bitten by the eastern coral snake, even if asymptomatic, should receive antivenin for *Micrurus fulvius* (Wyeth). This is an equine serum and requires preliminary skin testing (see package insert). The initial recommended dosage is five vials by IV; additional five vials may be given as needed for signs of venom toxicity. There is no antivenin available for the Arizona coral snake (*Micruroides euryxanthus*). If itching, hives, or other evidence of hypersensitivity to horse serum develops, the infusion should be stopped and the patient given diphenydramine. The infusion may be restarted at a lower rate with careful monitoring. Additional supportive care measures as outlined in the management of pit viper bites should be followed.

Exotic Snakes

The clinician confronted with an exotic snakebite or a clinician inexperienced in snakebites should consult a local medical herpetologist, poison control center, or the Oklahoma Poison Control Center (1-405-271-5454), which indexes the availability of unusual antivenins. Report all illegally possessed reptiles to the police or to the appropriate fish and game agency.

References

Auerbach PS: Marine envenomation. N Engl J Med 325:486–493, 1991

Baden HP, Burnett JW: Injuries from sea urchins. South Med J 70:459–460, 1977

Berg RA, Tarantino MD: Envenomation by the scorpion *Centruroides exilicauda* (*C. sculpturatus*): severe and unusual manifestations. Pediatrics 87:930–933, 1991

Bitseff EL, Garoni WJ, Hardison CD, Thompson JM: The management of stingray injuries of the extremities. South Med J 63:417–418, 1970

Clark RF, Wethern-Kestner S, Vance MV, Gerkin R: Clinical presentation and treatment of black widow spider envenomation: a review of 163 cases. Ann Emerg Med 21:782–787, 1992

Cruz NS, Alvarez RG: Rattlesnake bite complications in 19 children. Pediatr Emerg Care 10:30–33, 1994

Freudenthal AR, Joseph PR: Sunbathers' eruption. N Engl J Med 329:542–544, 1993

Gibly R, Williams M, Walter FG, McNally J, et al: Continuous IV midazolam infusion for *Centruroides exilicauda* scorpion envenomation. Ann Emerg Med 34:620–625, 1999

Gold BS, Wingert WA: Snake venom poisoning in the U.S.: a review of therapeutic practice. South Med J 87:579–589, 1994

Haller JS, Fabara JH: Tick paralysis. Am J Dis Child 124:915–917, 1972

Kizer KW, McKinney HE, Auerbach PS: Scorpaenidae envenomation: a five-year poison center experience. JAMA 253:807–810, 1985

Jerrard DA: ED management of insects stings. Am J Emerg Med 14:429–433, 1996

Lawrence WT, Giannopoulos A, Hansen A: Pit viper bites: rational management in locales in which copperheads and cottonmouths predominate. Ann Plast Surg 36:276–285, 1996

McGoldrick J, Marx JA: Marine envenomations: Part 1. Vertebrates. J Emerg Med 9:497–502, 1991

McGoldrick J, Marx JA: Marine envenomations: Part 2. Invertebrates. J Emerg Med 10:71–77, 1992

Needham G: Evaluation of five popular methods for tick removal. Pediatrics 75:997–1002, 1985

Visscher PK, Veller RS, Camazine S: Removing bee stings. Lancet 348:301–302, 1996

Wright SW, Wrenn KD, Murray L, Segar D: Clinical presentation and outcome of brown recluse spider bite. Ann Emerg Med 30:28–32, 1997

Zeman MG: Catfish stings: report of three cases. Ann Emerg Med 18:211–213, 1989

DEVELOPMENTAL-BEHAVIORAL PEDIATRICS

W. Thomas Boyce and Jack P. Shonkoff, Associate Editors

INTRODUCTION

Jack P. Shonkoff

The scope and organization of this chapter demonstrates the continuing maturation of the knowledge base underlying the developmental and behavioral content of pediatric medicine. As in sophisticated clinical practice, the material presented here moves beyond the traditional reliance on memorized developmental milestones and packaged behavioral recommendations, and it reflects a rich conceptual perspective on a broad range of pediatric concerns.

The chapter begins with an overview of seven fundamental concepts in child development that inform enlightened clinical problem-solving and effective patient care. Drawn from a diverse array of disciplines, including psychology, neurobiology, epidemiology, psychiatry, and sociology, these concepts provide a strong foundation for a sophisticated approach to the assessment, diagnosis, and management of the full spectrum of developmental and behavioral issues arising within the context of comprehensive child health care.

The remaining five sections of the chapter address a broad, multidimensional clinical agenda. The first section examines special challenges inherent in the task of developmental and behavioral diagnosis, often focusing less on the identification of categorical entities and more on an understanding of the elusive continuum of normal variation, transient dysfunction, and frank disability. The second section addresses common functional concerns related to everyday behavioral regulation. The third section provides an overview of the clinical spectrum of developmental and behavioral variability that straddles the range from normality to dysfunction. The fourth section addresses major psychopathologic disorders that affect children and adolescents. The fifth section explores a representative set of psychosocial issues that affect contemporary family and community life, thereby presenting challenges to the practicing pediatrician that extend the boundaries of traditional medical care.

The essence of developmental-behavioral pediatrics is reflected in its integrative nature. Its underlying knowledge base draws on the conceptual and empiric contributions of a broad range of biological and social sciences. Perhaps the most important integrative feature, however, is the extent to which contemporary developmental-behavioral pediatrics provides intellectual and clinical unity for what previously were viewed as separate domains labeled "developmental," "behavioral," and "psychosocial." Under the old model, developmental pediatrics focused on the assessment and management of children with significant neurologically based disabilities such as cerebral palsy, mental retardation, spina bifida, and autism. Behavioral pediatrics dealt with the evaluation and management of common functional challenges such as difficulties related to discipline, sleep, and aggression in otherwise normally de-

veloping children. Psychosocial pediatrics referred to the influences of sociopolitical and cultural factors such as poverty, adolescent pregnancy, and changes in family structure, or both child development and behavior.

In recent years, as our knowledge of human development has grown, the interacting influences of biology and environment have become better appreciated. Consequently, continuing distinctions among developmental, behavioral, and psychosocial pediatrics are conceptually unwarranted and clinically misleading. Children with neurologically based developmental disabilities often have problems in behavioral regulation that demand clinical intervention. Similarly, many of the common behavioral concerns brought to a pediatrician's attention originate in underlying constitutional differences or biological dysfunctions. Finally, whether our concerns are focused on developmental competence or behavioral style, all aspects of human performance unfold within a broad social context and are determined, in part, by the characteristics of that context.

5.1 FUNDAMENTAL CONCEPTS OF CHILD DEVELOPMENT

5.1.1 Homeostasis and Adaptation

W. Thomas Boyce

No single construct has been more central in the development of the biological sciences than homeostasis. Although the term *homeostasis* was coined in the 20th century, its conceptual origin can be traced to the notion of a stable, relatively unchanging internal environment, which was first described by Bernard in the 19th century. Bernard recognized the fragility of life, surrounded as it is by a constantly threatening, aversive, and often pathogenic environment, and he argued that viability in the face of external challenge depends on an organism's capacity for protecting its internal milieu. In this context, homeostasis is a dynamic, self-regulating process that ensures constancy and permanence in the internal physiological state through complex, multilevel feedback systems that respond to a deviation in one direction with a countering adjustment in the opposite direction. Thus, the fundamental goal of a homeostatic system is to maintain an inerrant "set point" that assures stable and continuous biological functioning. The regulation of body temperature, cortisol suppression of adrenocorticotropic hormone (ACTH) secretion, and glycogenolysis during periods of hypoglycemia are all examples of feedback loops that protect the continuity and equilibrium of an organism's interior.

Whereas homeostasis governs regulatory strategies within the tissue, cell, or subcellular structures, the closely related concept of adaptation refers to the behavioral and biological activities that promote the survival of individuals or groups. In Darwin's evolutionary theory, adaptation involves the selective preservation and reproduction of organisms that are able to adjust to external threats. Beyond evolution, however, adaptation has been used to describe complex social and individual developmental processes that respond to specific environmental challenges. For example, daytime continence emerges in a 3-year-old child within a context of growing parental expectations for toilet training; a preschooler clings to a tattered but revered blanket (a so-called transitional object) to calm his or her uncertainties and fears about attending a new child-care center; and a 12-year-old girl exhaustively discusses her first menstrual period with friends as a means to cope with the complications and challenges of sexual maturation. At all stages of development, the capacity to weather, absorb, and find meaning in the vicissitudes of life is one of the defining characteristics of humankind.

Many novel life experiences are normative and accessible to a range of homeostatic and adaptive strategies. However, children also encounter circumstances that strain their adaptive capacities and may present acute or chronic stressors that exceed their ability to cope. Indeed, psychosocial stress has been defined as environmental demands or threats that overtax an individual's ability to adapt. When such conditions are encountered, a variety of biological and behavioral responses are evoked; if sufficiently intense or prolonged, such responses can lead to the development of a diagnosable disorder.

Recent studies in humans suggest that three interactive systems are involved in the neurobiological response to stress: (a) the corticotropin-releasing hormone (CRH) system, (b) the locus ceruleus-norepinephrine (LC-NE) system, and (c) the limbic system. The CRH system stimulates the release of ACTH and β-endorphin by cells of the anterior pituitary gland, which, in turn, triggers secretion of adrenal glucocorticoids, thereby altering blood pressure, glucose metabolism, and behavior. Norepinephrine-producing neurons from the LC-NE system activate the sympathetic arm of the autonomic nervous system, which raises blood pressure and heart rate and promotes vigilance. The limbic system, which includes the hippocampus, amygdala, and other neural structures, plays an important role in the retrieval of memories and the emotional appraisal of environmental stressors.

These three highly interrelated response systems mediate successful biological adaptation to stressors, as well as the pathogenesis of stress-related physical and mental health disorders. In some cases, such disorders constitute a failure of homeostatic and adaptive processes; in other cases, they reflect the capacity of dysfunctional, exaggerated adaptive processes to *cause* disease. Recently, associations between emotionally stressful experiences and adverse health outcomes have become increasingly well substantiated in both adults and children. Although debate continues about whether stressors cause specific pathologic conditions or simply alter host susceptibility, little doubt remains that both chronic adversities and acute stressful events elevate the risk of physical and mental disorders.

Both clinical experience and epidemiologic observation suggest that not all children are equally vulnerable to psychosocial stressors. In fact, homeostatic and adaptive capacities appear to be distributed very *un*evenly within populations. Some children succumb to minimally stressful events, while others seem to be able to sustain normal functioning and good health through even the most adverse and emotionally trying circumstances. Observations of children with unusual levels of resilience or vulnerability to environmental challenges raise questions about the universality of stress-illness

linkages and underscore the importance of individual differences in children's behavioral and biological responses to the social world.

A common occurrence in pediatric practice is a parent's expression of elation or dismay on discovering how different in personality and behavior a second child is from the first. In families with several children, one may be highly susceptible to broken bones, falls from heights, unusual rashes, or a seemingly endless series of ear infections or colds. One child may be thoroughly outgoing, while another is timid and withdrawn. A daughter may be an outstanding athlete, while a son has not even a passing interest in sports. Physicians certainly are aware of the range from quiet calm to noisy fearfulness that accompanies the intrusion of a physical examination or the discomfort of an immunization.

Each of these experiences is a reminder that one of the more celebrated and universal characteristics of childhood is its marked diversity. A central task of pediatric medicine is to discover, honor, and respond to this diversity in a manner that supports parents in their efforts to nurture the individual talents of their children.

While observations regarding differences in personal style extend back to ancient Greek civilization, the systematic study of temperamental differences began with the New York Longitudinal Study of Chess and Thomas. Although researchers differ in the extent to which they view temperament as a stable, inherent characteristic, all agree that the concept itself describes a set of individual predispositions that underlie and modulate the expression of activity, emotionality, and sociability. In Chess and Thomas' original work, clusters of behavioral styles were constructed to identify "easy," "difficult," and "slow to warm-up" children. Further study has suggested that temperament has both behavioral and psychobiological aspects. Behavioral differences generally are arrayed along dimensions such as activity level, adaptability, intensity, and mood; psychobiological differences include the physiological responses to stress that reflect internal reactivity to environmental events.

Developmental researchers now have a greater understanding of the significant associations between the behavioral and psychobiological facets of temperament. For example, three components of autonomic nervous system reactivity—threshold (ie, the stimulus intensity required to elicit a response), dampening (ie, return to baseline following a stimulus), and reactivation (ie, rearousal with repeated stimulation)—may be biological analogues of the original behavioral descriptions that defined distinct temperament clusters. Thus, the child with an "easy" temperament might have a high threshold and strong capacity for dampening, whereas a "difficult" child might have a low threshold and capacity for dampening but be strongly predisposed to reactivation.

The origins of differences in behavioral and psychobiological "style" are not completely known, but they appear to be determined by both genetic endowment and environmental experience. For example, individual differences in shyness are derived from constitutional factors as well as personal experience. In a similar fashion, irritability is an interactive product of both molecular and social influences ranging from genetically encoded monoamine levels in the central nervous system to the prevalence of stressors and supports in the social environment.

An appreciation of individual temperament differences is important in the practice of pediatrics, not only because of their impact on development and behavior but also because of their potential link to both mental and physical health. For example, preschool children with extreme shyness may be at heightened risk for anxiety disorders during middle childhood or for panic disorder and agoraphobia (ie, fear of being in large, open spaces) as adults. Reactive individuals displaying the type A behavior pattern have higher rates of cardiovascular disease injuries and minor respiratory illnesses, and children with exaggerated cardiovascular or immunologic responses to stressors appear to have an elevated incidence of injuries and respiratory infections during periods of naturally occurring stressors such as a residential move or parental divorce.

While the mechanisms underlying these associations are unknown, available data suggest that certain subsets of children may have an impaired ability to self-regulate their behavior, physiological functions, and subjective experiences of somatic pain. One possible explanation for impaired self-regulation is that children who display certain behavioral and psychobiological phenotypes (eg, shyness and its associated predisposition to autonomic arousal) have an underlying hypersensitivity to external stimuli and a relative inability to monitor and constrain their behavioral and physiological responses.

A capacity for recognizing and controlling the emotional "coloring" of environmental events is a critical early developmental achievement. Infants' interactions with caregivers, principally with their mothers, appear to guide and shape the unfolding of affective experience and expression during the first months of life. Later, as maturation proceeds, the regulation of emotional experience becomes less dependent on caregivers and more accessible to a child's emerging self-control. In future years, individual differences in the capacity for such self-regulation may emerge as an important determinant of mental and physical well-being. In what may have been a moment of prescience 250 years ago, Sydenham wrote that the cause of "nervous disorders" may lie in "the temperament of the body . . . given us by nature."

5.1.2   Attachment and Individuation

Jack P. Shonkoff

Unlike almost all other species, humans experience a prolonged period of helplessness and total dependence early in life. In fact, it is striking that the species demonstrating the greatest capacity to control its environment is so incapable of meeting even its most basic survival needs on its own during infancy. Consequently, the relationship between an infant and his or her primary caregiver(s) is a fundamental requirement for healthy human development.

The initial bond and growing attachment that characterize an infant–caregiver relationship are grounded firmly in biology. As described by Bowlby, newborns and their parents are genetically programmed to form strong attachments to each other. Young infants respond preferentially to the image of a human face and to the higher pitched sound of a mother's voice. In turn, caregivers are naturally captivated by the magnetism of a baby's smile and the urgency of his or her cry. These core attachment behaviors have been documented in a variety of family configurations and across a broad range of cultures.

The defining characteristics of healthy, growth-promoting, early human relationships are embodied in the social concepts of reciprocity and contingency. Thus, when young children and their caregivers are "tuned in" to each other, their interactions are adaptive. During the early years of an infant's life, much of the responsibility for promoting a harmonious relationship rests on the caregiver's ability to read the baby's cues and to respond appropriately. When a caregiver's responses are contingent, predictable, and attuned to the infant's feelings, the young child experiences an early sense of security, personal efficacy, and positive self-worth. This leads to what Erikson labeled "basic trust," or the phenomenon through which outer predictability leads to a sense of inner cer-

tainty. For most parents, getting to know their babies and learning to read their signals is a highly rewarding experience that evolves naturally without the need for professional assistance. However, challenges to this relationship-building process may originate in either partner; from the infant who is relatively unresponsive or "difficult to read" as a result of prematurity, neurologic impairment, chronic illness, or extreme temperamental style; or from the caregiver whose capacity to nurture is compromised by inexperience, psychological disturbance, or severe external stressors such as poverty or social isolation.

Establishment of a secure attachment with one or a small number of key caregivers provides a firm foundation for healthy cognitive, social, and emotional development. Essential to this process is the need for a secure and trusted base from which the developing child can venture forth to explore the larger environment and to develop a differentiated identity as an autonomous, yet socially connected, individual. Thus, the average 1-year-old child seeks maternal closeness, the 15- to 18-month-old child begins to stray cautiously from the parental orbit (with frequent returns for "refueling"), and the healthy 2-year-old child is off and running (and rarely looks back!). As the process of separation and individuation unfolds, the adaptive child navigates a delicate balance between the maintenance of strong interpersonal bonds and the mastery of both physical and psychological independence.

During the first 6 months of life, most infants respond positively to anyone; during the second 6 months, they seek preferential closeness with their primary caregivers and begin to show signs of stranger anxiety when confronted by unfamiliar persons. Throughout the second year, children and caregivers negotiate a gradual disengagement from their intense, highly personalized attachment relationship. Whereas the younger infant assumed that "mother is always there," the emerging toddler becomes acutely aware of his or her own separateness and demonstrates varying degrees of "separation anxiety" behaviors that mark this important phase of development. For many children, a transitional object, such as a special blanket or stuffed animal, serves a vital symbolic function to facilitate the mastery of this fundamental separation challenge. By the end of the third year, most children are able to tolerate the temporary absence of their primary caregivers and accept the company of unfamiliar adults with minimal difficulty.

Extensive research has demonstrated the far-reaching benefits of strong, early attachments and the adaptive resolution of necessary and inevitable separations. During infancy, children with secure attachments engage in richer exploratory behavior, demonstrate more sophisticated problem-solving skills, and exhibit more positive affect. During the preschool years, secure attachments are associated with better peer relationships, higher self-esteem, and a greater capacity for empathy. The ability to form increasingly mature and stable relationships into adulthood is presumed to be influenced by one's early attachment experiences. Ongoing tensions between the development of personal autonomy and the nurturance of meaningful social relationships represent a fundamental life challenge.

5.1.3   Mastery and Achievement

Jack P. Shonkoff

The concept of individual competence and the intrinsic drive to master one's environment are basic features of human development throughout the life cycle. This begins in early infancy with the inductive process, through which babies learn about the nature of the physical and social world by their own experiences and actions. For elderly people, the inherent drive for mastery persists with attempts to maintain a sense of autonomy, dignity, and self-sufficiency despite the inevitable dependence that accompanies physiological decline.

To a certain extent, differences in the level and quality of performance among individuals are manifestations of differences in biological endowment. However, human abilities do not develop independent of the context in which people live. Thus, individual competencies in children are shaped by the degree to which the early caregiving environment and ongoing life experiences provide both opportunities to learn and the support needed to take advantage of such opportunities. The talented athlete who combines natural grace with a commitment to long hours of practice and the musical prodigy whose parents arrange for piano lessons in the preschool years are examples of this dynamic interplay between biology and the environment. Long-standing battles over the extent to which human competence is influenced by nature (ie, genetics/constitution, as underscored in the maturational model popularized by Gesell) *or* by nurture (ie, experience/environment, as emphasized in the learning theory developed by Watson and Skinner) reflect exercises in futility. The question is not *which* is important but *how* each contributes to ultimate outcomes.

The traditional approach to studying and assessing children's abilities has been to focus on a core set of performance domains. Although these domains are interdependent and the boundaries among them can be somewhat arbitrary, it is helpful to review each independently.

In the physical realm, increasingly refined *motor control* develops in a cephalocaudal and proximal-to-distal pattern. Influenced by both neuromaturation and practice, the development of discrete motor skills continues from early infancy through adult life. In the gross motor area, children begin by establishing head control and the ability to roll over, progressing to maintaining a sitting position and walking independently. They then progress through the mastery of increasingly complex skills such as riding a bicycle, participating in competitive sports, and, in rare circumstances, pursuing a successful career as a professional dancer or gymnast. In the fine-motor area, children begin by reaching for objects and establishing a fine pincer grasp. They then move on to more complex tasks such as cutting with scissors and writing legibly and, in some instances, may achieve ultimate success during adulthood in the arts of calligraphy or microsurgery.

The development of *cognitive competence* reflects a range of intellectual capacities that distinguish humans from all other living creatures. From earliest infancy, children are programmed biologically to learn about the world through their own actions and the ongoing construction of their own internal mental representations. Much learning depends on the extent to which a child's environment provides appropriate opportunities and supports, but much of the energy fueling the development of cognitive competencies arises from the child's own initiative.

In the early years, the thinking of young children is characterized as "egocentric" (ie, they are unable to view the world from any but their own perspective). Thus, a great deal of cognitive maturity is embedded in the process of gradual "decentration," whereby children develop a growing appreciation of how the world is perceived and understood by others.

Based on the seminal work of Piaget, cognition can be viewed as progressing through four discrete stages. The first stage, termed *sensorimotor,* extends from birth to approximately 18 months of age. During this period, the child's knowledge of the world is grounded in his or her motor activities and sensory experiences. Coinciding with the emergence of a sense of one's existence as a separate human being, children learn that objects exist even when they are no longer visible (ie, "object permanence"), and they develop an appreciation for the relation between actions and consequences (ie, "causality"). The second stage of cognitive development, termed *preoperational,* generally extends from 18 months to 7 years of age. The hallmark of this period is development of the capacity for representational thinking, symbolic functioning, and the emergence of fantasy in language as well as in play. The "magical thinking" of the preschool years results in delightful explanations of natural phenomena (eg, "rain comes from God crying") as well as the risk of viewing illness as a punishment for misbehavior. The third cognitive stage, termed *concrete operational,* typically extends from ages 7 to 11 years. During this period, children are capable of logical mental manipulations, and their thinking reflects an ability to appreciate several dimensions of an issue at the same time. For example, as demonstrated in Piaget's classic experiments, the school-aged child can understand that a short, fat cup can hold as much water as a tall, thin glass. Finally, beginning in early adolescence or later, the cognitive stage of *formal operations* is reached; during this period, individuals engage in abstract reasoning, which gives them the power to manipulate ideas rather than remain restricted to the concrete world. For the reflective adolescent and young adult, this provides a framework for passionate discussions about morality, values, and philosophic principles.

Closely related to the realm of cognition is the development of a symbol-based system of communication known as *language.* Comparable to the emergence of their knowledge about the physical world, children develop communicative competence because they have the innate ability to "discover" the rules that underlie language function and not simply to imitate what they have heard. Although we generally take for granted these abilities to interpret what we hear and to speak, it is important to appreciate how remarkable it is that young children are able to process the verbalizations of people around them and to produce unique word combinations that they have never before heard.

The study and assessment of communication distinguishes between *speech,* which refers to the physical act of talking, and *language,* which refers to the underlying symbol system. During the first 12 months of life, infants progress from cooing (ie, vowel sounds) to babbling (ie, consonant sounds) in conjunction with a growing appreciation of the social context of communication, which is characterized by selective attention to conversation, turn taking, and interpretation of a repertoire of nonverbal signals. By the end of their first year, most children have mastered virtually all sounds of their native language and have produced their first true words. During their second year, expressive language progresses competence in syntax (ie, rules of grammar). By 3 years of age, most children are able to communicate their thoughts through coherent narratives, and by age 5 years, the structure of their language begins to approximate that of adults.

Beyond the domains of physical and cognitive/linguistic skills, expanding competence in the realms of *emotional development* and *social relationships* represents another critical maturational agenda. From the basic reciprocal interactions that characterize the early infant–caregiver bond through the intense process of separation-individuation and the development of core family ties, peer relationships, and mature adult intimacies, humans are essentially feeling and social creatures. Thus, as children develop a growing sense of themselves as separate individuals, they develop the capacity to look both inward and outward.

The identification and understanding of affect, capacity for empathy, emerging sense of morality, ability to form meaningful relationships, and growth of both self-concept and social perspective are some of the central dimensions of social-emotional development that show continued growth from early childhood through the later adult years. Attempts to understand the underlying processes in this domain of personal competence have generated some of the richest theoretic contributions to our understanding of human maturation. In the classic Freudian formulation, social and emotional well-being depend on the successful resolution of intense conflicts between the child's innate pleasure-seeking drives and the limits placed on the satisfaction of those urges by parental control and cultural mores. Following Freud's seminal theories, Mahler and her colleagues viewed the early process of separation and individuation as the essential means through which young children achieve "psychological birth" and a beginning sense of their own individual identity. Erikson developed an elaborated life span conceptualization of psychological identity extending from the fundamental establishment of a basic sense of trust in early infancy through the sequential challenges of increasing autonomy, skill, and a sense of personal efficacy, intimate relationships, and generativity. As in all other areas of development, success in the emotional and social domains depends on both intrinsic constitutional abilities (eg, temperamental style, sensitivity to social cues) and the influence of supportive relationships (both within and outside of the core family unit).

In summary, human competence manifests in a wide range of domains involving physical prowess, mental problem-solving and abstract reasoning, emotional regulation, and social sensitivity. The range of abilities in the general population is broad, and the relative value assigned to differential achievement varies among families and across cultures. In a highly competitive society, the natural human drive toward mastery is exaggerated by intense social and economic pressures. In contrast, a culture characterized by nonhierarchic egalitarian values offers broader acceptance and support of a wider range of ability. The transmission of these values, through both the family unit and the wider culture, is likely to have a major influence on the evolution of individual self-concept as well as on how people view each other.

5.1.4 Continuities and Discontinuities in Developmental Trajectories

Jack P. Shonkoff

The extent to which human development is a continuous or a segmented process is the focus of much debate. Proponents of a discontinuous model point to the dramatic qualitative changes that are apparent when one takes a long-term view over the course of the full childhood period. Thus, 15-year-old children do not simply know *more* than 7-year-old children (or 7-year-old children more than 2-year-old children); they also know things in a *different* way. On the other hand, qualitative changes occur gradually, not by great leaps, which suggests an essentially continuous process.

Many of the greatest contributions to our knowledge of child development have been conceptualized within the context of stage models; for example, Piaget's work on cognition and Freud's stages of psychosexual development discontinuities (Table 5-1). Despite

TABLE 5-1
PERSPECTIVES ON HUMAN BEHAVIOR

AGE	FREUD	ERIKSON	PIAGET	LANGUAGE	MOTOR	PSYCHOPATHOLOGY
Birth to 18 months	Oral	Basic trust vs mistrust	Sensorimotor	Body actions; crying; naming; pointing	Reflex sitting, reaching, grasping, walking	Autism; anaclitic depression; colic; disorders of attachment; feeding, sleep problems
18 months to 3 years	Anal	Autonomy vs shame, doubt	Symbolic (preoperational)	Sentences; telegraph jargon	Climbing, running	Separation; negativism; fearfulness; constipation; shyness; withdrawal
3 to 6 years	Oedipal	Initiative vs guilt	Intuition (preoperational)	Connective words; can be understood	Coordination; tricycle; jumping	Enuresis; encopresis; anxiety; aggression; phobias; nightmares
6 to 11 years	Latency	Industry vs inferiority	Concrete operational	Subordinate sentences; reading/writing; reasoning	Increased skills; sports, recreational games	School phobias; obsessive reactions; conversion reactions; depressive equivalents
12 to 17 years	Adolescence (genital)	Identity vs role confusion	Formal operational	Reason abstract; using language; abstract manipulation	Refinement of skills	Delinquency; promiscuity; schizophrenia; anorexia nervosa; suicide
17 to 30 years	Young adulthood	Intimacy vs isolation	Formal operational	Same	Same	Schizophrenia; borderline personality; adjustment disorders; development of intimate difficulties with relationships
30 to 60 years	Adulthood	Generativity vs stagnation	Formal operational	Same	Same	Depression; self-doubts; career development issues; family, social network; neuroses
>60 years	Old age	Ego integration vs despair	Formal operational	Same	Loss of function?	Involutional depression; anxiety, anger, dependency

SOURCE: *Modified from Dixon SD, Stein MT: Encounters with Children: Pediatric Behavior and Development. 2nd ed. Chicago: Year Book, 1992.*

the salience of stage-related theories of development, however, the day-to-day reality of individual human function is certainly not marked by dramatic qualitative shifts. A reconciliation of these seemingly contradictory positions can be found in the concept of a *developmental transition,* which refers to the transformation from one discrete stage to the next. One way to understand developmental transitions is to think of them as times of structural reorganization (ie, periods of psychological disequilibrium reflecting elements of both the stage being completed and the stage yet to begin). Intense negativism in a toddler who is attempting to reconcile strong feelings of attachment to his mother with the natural drive for autonomy is one example. The need to balance core family ties with adolescent rebellious impulses to achieve a healthy adult identity is another example.

One important consequence of the qualitative change that characterizes human development is the relative instability of individual differences in competence. This is to say that except in cases of severe disability, the rank ordering of individuals within specific developmental domains often shows dramatic variability over time. Part of the variance in performance relates to the ongoing influences of differential life experiences. However, beyond the role of environmental impact is the inherent nature of stage-related, qualitative developmental discontinuities. For example, the "brightest" 15-month-old child will not necessarily be the "smartest" 10-year-old child, because block stacking and the rapid completion of formboards reflect different skills from those needed to excel in verbal and quantitative reasoning.

A related phenomenon is the concept of "critical periods" of development. Derived from the discipline of ethnology, it is postulated that certain developmental accomplishments must be mastered within a particular time frame, after which the "window of opportunity" is lost irrevocably and permanent dysfunction becomes inevitable. Although critical periods have been demonstrated for a number of behaviors in a variety of species (eg, imprinting in geese), these have not been documented for any specific aspect of competence in humans. Alternatively, the concept of "sensitive periods" has been suggested to indicate that although their later emergence is not impossible, certain developmental achievements are best mastered during particular periods in the life cycle. The establishment of basic trust in early infancy and the development of language by the end of the preschool period are two examples of competencies that have been postulated to be difficult to achieve beyond their sensitive periods.

Perhaps the construct that best captures the complex issue of developmental continuity-discontinuity is the concept of epigenesis. Derived from the science of embryology, the epigenetic model depicts a dynamic process in which a highly differentiated organism evolves from a completely structureless germ cell through the complex, reciprocal impacts of environment and protoplasm. Thus, like the dramatic changes that characterize the marked transformation from zygote to embryo to fetus to neonate, human development and behavior unfold through a highly interactive process marked by progressive differentiation, individual continuity, and dramatic qualitative change.

5.1.5 Environmental Supports and Adversities

Jack P. Shonkoff

An important advance in our knowledge of human development over the past few decades has been a growing appreciation of the contextual nature of complex developmental processes. Stated simply, despite its strong biological underpinnings, the development of children is highly influenced by the multiple environments in which they live, a phenomenon described by Bronfenbrenner as the ecology of human development. In different circumstances, the environment can be viewed as either supportive or detrimental. Most frequently, different aspects of the same environment can serve as sources of both protection and risk.

The most proximal aspect of a child's care-giving environment is the family unit, and at its core is the special intimacy characterizing the daily interactions that take place between an infant and his or her primary caregiver(s). These dyadic relationships are themselves embedded within a dynamic family system that can be highly variable in structure and in the way it affects the development of its members. As children grow older, they are influenced by a wider variety of overlapping relationships that make up the larger family unit. These may include ties to parents, siblings, grandparents, and other members of the extended family. Within these relationships, differences in personal investment, overt or covert rivalries, and temperamental matches or mismatches all contribute to the considerable diversity of family experiences shaping the personalities of children as they grow up.

In addition to variations in their membership and structure, other important differences in family characteristics can have significant impacts on the development of children. Families may be cohesive, fragmented, or enmeshed. They may be flexible and highly adaptable, or rigid and incapable of adjusting to change. Attitudes toward child-rearing may be strict and authoritarian or permissive and nonhierarchic. Standards for individual performance and behavior may be high or low. Approaches to discipline and punishment may be harsh or forgiving. Interactions may foster intense competition or convey a strong egalitarian message.

All children who live in the same household experience both a shared and a unique environment. To the extent that a distinctive ambiance characterizes the family unit, the environment is shared. However, the fact that individual family members influence and experience each other in different ways means that each child occupies a relatively unique environmental niche.

Above and beyond the powerful impacts of their family, children also are influenced by the communities in which they grow up. Similar to the family, a community can be an important source of protection or vulnerability, depending on its material and spiritual resources. For example, a local neighborhood may provide high-quality, easily accessible, and affordable child care, or it may have a fragmented and poor-quality infrastructure for working families. Available recreational facilities may include safe and attractive parks and playgrounds or dangerous and foreboding abandoned buildings and empty lots. A school system may be well supported and rich in creativity and nurturance, or it may be poor in resources and diminished in morale. A community may embody a sense of pride and joint ownership in its shared way of life, or it may be depleted in spirit and devoid of any sense of meaningful interconnection.

Finally, families and communities are themselves embedded, like nested cubes, in a broader culture that reflects a particular set of values and traditions. Cultural characteristics that are likely to influence the development of children include religious rituals, attitudes toward gender roles, traditional approaches to discipline, and the extent to which ethnic discrimination and racism influence social, economic, and political institutions. For minority groups and newly immigrated families, conflicts with the majority culture present significant challenges to personal development, which may result in both positive and negative outcomes.

5.1.6   Constitution and Context

W. Thomas Boyce

The ultimate mystery of human development is the complex process through which threads of genetic endowment and contextual experience are woven together to form the fabric of a maturing individual. Indeed, all developing persons are products of nature, nurture, and what Sameroff described as their complex transactions.

A vast array of phenotypic characteristics is encoded in the genome of each individual. Such characteristics define an array of physical parameters such as facial features, hair and eye color, and potential for linear growth. Experienced pediatricians are well attuned to the atypical phenotypic features of children with chromosomal anomalies (eg, trisomies, deletions, nondysjunctions) and the metabolic consequences of specific gene mutations (eg, sickle cell anemia, phenylketonuria). Typically less well-known or understood, however, are the genetic influences on psychological development, including those involved in the regulation of intelligence, temperament, and personality.

Heritable psychological characteristics are polygenic in origin (ie, the products of multiple interacting genes). For example, genetic analyses suggest that polygenic influences account for approximately one-half of the variance in IQ scores. Other research raises the possibility that both subtle differences in personality style and the manifestations of character disorders may be determined, in part, by genetically determined levels of neurotransmitters (eg, dopamine, norepinephrine, serotonin) in selected regions of an individual brain. Although the emerging science of behavioral genetics is beginning to elucidate the magnitude of such influences, it cannot identify the specific genes that are responsible for a given behavioral trait or developmental dysfunction. In this regard, research focused on efforts to locate and clone the genes responsible for various psychological disorders offers a promising new frontier.

As observations of the genetic influence on behavior and development have grown, evidence for the power of environmental effects also has been increasing. In fact, nongenetic impacts on behavior appear to be at least as important as genetic factors, because genetic variation rarely accounts for more than one-half of the variability in behavioral traits. Because children in the same family share *both* genomic and environmental influences on their development, disentangling the effects of each is a challenging task. Furthermore, the techniques of selective breeding and experimental exposure to different environments are restricted to studies of laboratory animals, so human behavioral genetics must rely on the less definitive findings of family, adoption, and twin studies. For example, pairs of monozygotic (ie, identical) and dizygotic (ie, fraternal) twins raised in the same family can be examined to ascertain the degree to which genetic relatedness results in similarities of behavior or psychopathology. Conversely, environmental effects can be assessed by studying differences in outcomes among monozygotic twins who were separated during infancy and raised in different families; to whatever extent variations in outcome are not attributable to environmental causes, the remaining variance generally can be assigned to the genome.

Research on schizophrenia, for example, shows a concordance rate of 30% among monozygotic twins, a figure that is 30 times higher than the 1% base rate of the disorder in the general population. While this finding suggests a strong genetic contribution to schizophrenia, the 30% concordance rate is far from the rate of 100% that would be expected if the disorder were purely inherited. Thus, data on schizophrenia suggest that nongenetic factors also play a strong, complementary role in its pathogenesis. Adoption studies of individuals with bipolar and unipolar depression have shown both genetic and environmental influences as well, as have studies of autism, anorexia nervosa, attention-deficit hyperactivity disorder, and delinquent behavior. In some conditions, genetic potentialities are triggered or revealed only in specific environmental contexts. For example, phenylketonuria in human infants results in mental retardation only in the presence of dietary phenylalanine; heterozygotes for sickle hemoglobin are resistant to malaria, which conveys a selective advantage that probably augments the prevalence of the gene in certain parts of the world. In each of these examples, expression of a genotype depends on the child's exposure to specific environmental triggers.

Another example of the complexity of gene–environment interaction involves the traditional assumption that two children raised in the same family experience the same child-rearing environment. This conventional wisdom has been challenged by recent observations that siblings growing up under the same roof often experience quite different "families" and that these *unshared* aspects of the family environment can have important effects on behavioral and developmental outcomes. Indeed, it now appears that the most powerful environmental influences on behavior and psychopathology are those that derive from these unshared family experiences. Such differences in experience probably occur through a variety of mechanisms. A parent in an unsatisfying marriage, for example, may single out one child for maltreatment. Alternatively, children may have a different experience because of the unique perspective each brings to the family system and because of the differential responses each child elicits from all other family members.

While context cannot change the structure or sequence of the genome, certain experiences appear to have direct regulatory effects on the translation and transcription of genetic material. For example, environmental stressors play a much stronger etiologic role in the development of a first major episode of clinical depression than they do in subsequent episodes of the same disorder. One way of accounting for this observation is the possibility that repeated neuronal transmission in certain central nervous system (CNS) structures sets in motion intracellular processes, known as *kindling,* that may alter gene transcription. Such alterations in gene expression may leave behind memory traces, at the level of neuronal function, that produce a sustained increase in the risk of subsequent depressive episodes.

Waddington proposed a visual metaphor for the complex developmental transactions that unfold between genes and environment. He suggested that development is like a ball rolling downhill through a landscape of valleys and ridges. The further the ball rolls, the deeper the valleys and the steeper the walls of the ridges, thus making diversion into different paths less likely as the process proceeds. Developmental trajectories that are deeply ingrained, with little potential for environmental influence (eg, limb morphology, development of gender, independent ambulation) are referred to as *canalized* characteristics. Other pathways, such as those that direct a child into normal or disturbed trajectories of emotional development, have less-steep walls and remain susceptible to the effects of life experiences. Thus, the likelihood that a child will enter a path of abnormal emotional development is a product of both genetic "momentum" and environmental constraints derived from the influences of family, siblings, teachers, and friends.

The importance of the continuing debate about the origins of variability in human development and behavior lies in the increasing prevalence of psychosocial pathologies in contemporary societies. In far too many circumstances, children and their families are surrounded by a grim harvest of increasingly maladaptive development, the seeds of which can be found among problems such as poverty, racism, mental illness, substance abuse, and other risk-taking behaviors. It is hoped that an understanding of the underlying science of developmental-behavioral pediatrics will contribute to the search for preventive interventions and effective management techniques that will provide truly comprehensive care for all children and their families.

References

Brazelton TB: Touch Points: Your Child's Emotional and Behavioral Development. Reading, MA, Addison-Wesley, 1992

Bronfenbrenner U: The Ecology of Human Development. Cambridge, MA, Harvard University Press, 1979

Cole M, Cole SR: The Development of Children, 2nd ed. New York, Scientific American Books, 1993

Dixon SD, Stein MT: Encounters With Children: Pediatric Behavior and Development, 2nd ed. Chicago, Year Book, 1992

Dubos RJ: Man Adapting. New Haven, CT, Yale University Press, 1965

Erikson EH: Childhood and Society, 2nd ed. New York, Norton, 1963

Fraiberg S: The Magic Years. New York, Charles Scribner's Sons, 1959

Ginsberg H, Upper S: Piaget's Theory of Intellectual Development. Englewood Cliffs, NJ, Prentice Hall, 1979

Konner MJ: The Tangled Wing: Biological Constraints on the Human Spirit. New York, Henry Holt, 1990

Leach P: Your Baby and Child, 2nd ed. New York, Knopf, 1989

Mahler MS, Pine F, Bergman A: The Psychological Birth of the Human Infant: Symbiosis and Individuation. New York, Basic Books, 2000

Thomas A, Chess S: Temperament and Development. New York, Brunner/Mazel, 1977

Zelazo PR, Barr RG, eds: Challenges to Developmental Paradigms: Implications for Theory, Assessment and Treatment. Hillsdale, NJ, Lawrence Erlbaum Associates, 1989

5.2   BRAIN DEVELOPMENT AND BEHAVIOR

Charles A. Nelson

Over the past two decades, we have witnessed impressive growth in our understanding of how the brain develops and, in particular, a growing appreciation of the phenomenal changes in both the circuitry and neurochemistry of the brain that occur during prenatal and early development. In the sections that follow, each major phase of brain development is summarized, followed by a discussion of critical or sensitive periods and of the general role of experience in influencing brain development.

5.2.1   Phases of Brain Development

The brain develops over a prolonged period of time; the most rapid period of development occurs prenatally and during the first few postnatal years. This includes neurulation (formation of the neural tube), cell migration and proliferation, and, finally, cell differenti-

ation. However, important aspects of brain development, such as myelination and synaptogenesis, continue for many years thereafter.

NEURULATION

Between the second and third week of gestation, the dorsal region of the ectodermal layer of the embryo begins to thicken and form a pear-shaped plate. As cell proliferation continues, this plate becomes a groove and then a tube. Toward the end of the third week of gestation, the anterior end of the neural tube forms a set of swollen enlargements that give rise to three primary vesicles: the *forebrain* (which will become the cerebral hemispheres), the *midbrain* (which will contain important pathways to and from the forebrain), and the *hindbrain* (which will consist of the brainstem and cerebellum). The remainder of the neural tube gives rise to the spinal cord, peripheral nerves, and certain endocrine glands in the body. The neural tube completes its closure by the end of the third prenatal week.

This phase of development may be compromised, leading to a class of disorders referred to as *neural tube defects*. For example, anencephaly is a disorder in which the entire cortex fails to develop due to an opening in the most rostral portion of the neural tube. A less devastating (although still handicapping) condition is spina bifida, in which there is an opening further down along the spinal cord, generally leading to motor disabilities.

NEUROGENESIS

After the neural tube has closed, a new phase of brain development commences. Within the neural tube, the innermost cells divide rapidly and repeatedly, giving rise first to the cells that primarily become neurons, and later to precursors of both neurons and the supportive tissue components called *glia* (which will include elements such as astrocytes, oligodendrocytes, etc.). In most areas of the brain, the process of *neurogenesis* is completed by the third trimester of pregnancy, except for the cells that line the olfactory bulb, which turn over on a near-weekly basis for the entire life span. Recently, exciting discoveries of postnatal neurogenesis were observed among the cells that make up the dentate gyrus, a region of the hippocampus, and in portions of the frontal and parietal cortex. It is not clear what functional role these new cells play.

CELL MIGRATION

As cells are formed anew, a complementary process of migration commences. Specifically, the wall of the recently closed neural tube consists of a single layer of *epithelial* cells. These cells are connected to each other, and they rapidly proliferate and the layer thickens. The neuroblasts that line the neural tube attach themselves to a specialized type of glial cell, the *radial glia fiber*, and essentially climb along this fiber until the cell has reached its target destination. Once this has occurred, a process that takes 10-20 hours, the neuroblast essentially detaches itself from the glial fiber and begins the process of differentiation.

The initial formation of the *cortical plate* occurs by migration of cells to the deepest layer (VI) of the cortex, and subsequent migrations follow in what is called an *inside-out* pattern. In this manner, young (postmitotic) neurons leave their zone of origin and typically migrate past older cells to reach their final position. As a result, the earliest formed cells come to inhabit the deepest cortical layer (VI), whereas progressively later-formed cells will occupy positions at progressively more superficial layers. An exception to this is in the cerebellum, where granule cells are formed in the external germinative layer and move in an *internal* direction.

The cells trapped between the ectodermal wall and the neural tube are *neural crest cells*. This zone of cells will extend effectively from the forebrain downwards along an axis. The cells on each side of this axis migrate to the dorsolateral side of the neural tube and eventually give rise to the *sensory ganglia* (or dorsal root ganglia) of the spinal and cranial nerves (V, VII, IX, and X).

After cell migration is complete, usually by the sixth prenatal month, neurons must begin the arduous process of differentiating (making *processes*, or axons and dendrites) and then making connections.

SYNAPTOGENESIS

After neurons have differentiated, their axons begin to reach out to neighboring cells. Here they typically form the synaptic connections through which they can communicate with the target cell, with another neuron, or with a nonneuronal cell such as a muscle. In most parts of the nervous system, the stability and strength of these synapses are determined to some degree by the activity (neural firing) of these connections.

Not surprisingly, the formation of synapses to some degree follows the form-followed-by-function rule in which those regions of the brain that are the first to develop functioning synapses become functional first, and those that develop synapses later function last. In addition, in all areas of the cortex, there is an initial overproduction of synapses that far exceeds adult numbers, followed by a pruning back or retraction of synapses. For example, the peak of overproduction in the visual cortex occurs between 3 and 4 postnatal months, with maximum density reached at 4 months. Synaptogenesis in Heschl's gyrus, the primary auditory cortex, follows a similar timetable and is 80% complete by 3 months of age. In contrast, overproduction in the middle frontal gyrus is not achieved until nearly 1 year of age. Despite the similarity across areas, the retraction of synapses differs greatly in these three areas. Thus, adult levels of synapses in the visual and auditory cortices are obtained between the second and sixth postnatal year, whereas adult levels of synapses in the middle frontal gyrus are not reached until middle to late adolescence.

Collectively, synapse elimination in the human brain appears to occur late in gestation and early in the postnatal period, during a time when the nervous system is highly sensitive to environmental influences. Indeed, it has been suggested that the main purpose of this overproduction followed by retraction is to "capture" synapses on a systemwide basis. In so doing, there is both selective confirmation and elimination that is based on experience.

MYELINATION

Like synapse development, the development of myelin is a protracted developmental process that extends well into the postnatal period. Myelin is produced by a specialized glia element called *oligodendroglia*. Myelin essentially insulates the cell and increases conduction velocity. The formation of myelin is a genetically defined process that is preceded by the proliferation and differentiation of glial cells proximate to the pathways to be myelinated, and is most prominent during the period of rapid brain growth. Although this process is genetically determined, it can be influenced during the postnatal period by environmental factors such as diet.

As a rule, motor roots myelinate first, followed by sensory roots, followed by primary somesthetic, visual, and auditory cortices. Next to myelinate (during the first postnatal months) are the secondary association areas that surround the primary sensory or motor cortices. Myelination of the classic association areas that are involved with higher cortical functions, most notably in the frontal cortices, extends well into the postnatal period and possibly into adolescence.

5.2.2   Role of Experience in Brain Development

Although most aspects of prenatal brain development are not dependent on experience (with the exception of obvious deleterious experiences, such as exposure to poor nutritional environments and teratogens), the same cannot be said of postnatal development. Indeed, many elements of postnatal development depend critically on experience. For example, although the initial formation of ocular dominance columns in the visual cortex occurs independent of experience, full elaboration and differentiation of these columns depends heavily on experience; thus, untreated strabismus inalterably leads to abnormal visual development. Furthermore, several aspects of language development depend on experience. For example, the infant's ability to discriminate speech sounds from the infant's native language depends considerably on hearing the sounds of that language. Thus, before 6-12 months of age, infants from around the world are quite adroit at discriminating the sounds of most of the world's languages. However, after this age infants behave more like adults and discriminate best the sounds of their native language. Moreover, we know that infants begin to profit from hearing their mother's voice weeks before they are born (assuming a term pregnancy) because they can recognize this voice within hours of being delivered. Finally, it is currently believed that an infant or toddler's vocabulary can vary as a function of the words heard in the child's home.

Outside of sensory development, little is known about the specific role of experience, and the timing of such experiences, in influencing brain development. Based on studies of deprivation, such as in children who are neglected or abused, we suspect that a very broad sensitive period may exist for the formation of initial human attachments. For example, children reared in Romanian orphanages and adopted into homes in Canada, Britain, or the United States typically have better developmental outcomes if they were adopted before 6-12 months of life. Here it is assumed that the myriad of deprivations that occurred in those first months derailed the infant from a normal trajectory and that the longer this deprivation continued, the worse the outcome and/or the harder it is to bring the infant back onto a normal trajectory.

Moving beyond basic abilities such as seeing, hearing, and forming attachments, we know that there is considerable plasticity in both the cognitive and motor domains. With regard to the cognitive domain, we know that learning and memory are possible throughout the life span; we also know that in the rat these experiences can be powerfully influenced by how the rats are housed. Thus, rats living in so-called complex environments (those with lots of toys and other rats) perform better on maze tasks and have more synapses per unit area in the areas of the brain that underlie memory and visual function than do rats housed in single cages (the typical laboratory rat environment). With regard to motor skills, we know that the area of the somatosensory cortex that represents the fingers of the left hand in trained right-handed musicians is larger than both their right hand and the left hand of nonmusicians. Similarly, we know that motor training following an ischemic stroke can recruit neighboring areas of the motor cortex that lead to recovery of motor ability. Finally, with regard to language, there are reports that children with language-learning impairments who receive intensive training in speech perception can show remarkable and seemingly long-lasting improvements in their language ability.

Overall, the most *rapid* period of brain development occurs shortly after conception through the first few postnatal years. However, the establishment of the extensive network of interconnections that underlies behavioral change occurs for many years thereafter. More importantly, many forms of plasticity occur throughout the life span. Thus, the prevailing urgency to provide specific and enriching experiences to infants and toddlers during their first 3 years of life (such as listening to classical music) is largely unwarranted based solely on neuroscience evidence.

References

Black JE, Jones TA, Nelson CA, Greenough WT: Neuronal plasticity and the developing brain. In: Noshpitz JD, Alessi N, Harrison S, eds: Handbook of Child and Adolescent Psychiatry. Vol. 6. Basic Psychiatric Science and Treatment. New York, John Wiley, 1998:31–53

Kolb B, Forgie M, Gibb R, Gorny G, Rowntree S: Age, experience, and the changing brain. Neurosci Biobehav Rev 22:143–159, 1998

Nelson CA: The neurobiological bases of early intervention. In: Shonkoff JP, Meisels SJ, eds: Handbook of Early Childhood Intervention, 2nd ed. New York, Cambridge University Press, 2000

Nelson CA, Bloom FE: Child development and neuroscience. Child Dev 68:970, 1997

Nelson CA, Bosquet M: Neurobiology of fetal and infant development: implications for infant mental health. In: Zeanah CH, ed: Handbook of Infant Mental Health, 2nd ed. New York, Guilford Press, 2000

Tallal P, Miller SL, Bedi G, et al: Language comprehension in language-learning-impaired children improved with acoustically modified speech. Science 271:81–84, 1976

5.3   THE DILEMMA OF DEVELOPMENTAL AND BEHAVIORAL DIAGNOSIS

W. Thomas Boyce

Formulating a diagnosis in developmental and behavioral pediatrics is a thorny clinical dilemma. However, it is unique neither to development and behavior, nor to pediatric medicine, nor to medicine itself. Rather, diagnosis of a distinct clinical "abnormality" is simply the medical version of a larger scientific problem—the choice between categoric and continuous descriptions of natural phenomena. A central issue in 20th century physics, for example, was crafting a plausible reconciliation between the view of light as a particle and the view of light as a wave. Consequently, the principle of complementarity states that light is both photon and wave and both a discrete categoric unit with measurable mass and a continuous waveform lacking discontinuities.

Developmentalists and pediatricians also struggle with how certain symptoms or clinical problems might fit within taxonomies of disease. Within this context, all clinicians are familiar with both continuous and categoric descriptions of biological parameters. The concentration of hemoglobin, for example, varies along a continuous spectrum, with a theoretically large range of values. Pediatricians measure linear growth as a continuously distributed range of heights, and auditory acuity is assessed along an unbroken con-

tinuum of sound levels. On the other hand, clinicians also are accustomed to categoric discriminations between normal and abnormal conditions. Conventional standards such as the Jones criteria for rheumatic fever place discrete limits on the clinical circumstances in which some diagnoses can be made. Similarly, cutoff points along a continuum of possible results, such as a 1:32 positive VDRL titer for syphilis or 10 mm of induration on a tuberculin skin test, are assigned for distinguishing disease from nondisease. Thus, while clinicians are familiar with the interpretation of data along continuous distributions, medical diagnosis is often focused on the location of symptoms and signs in a set of discrete, non-overlapping clinical profiles.

In the mental health domain, past approaches to diagnosis also have emphasized matching clinical presentations to categoric disorders. In the 18th century, a variety of mental health conditions, including hypochondria, hysteria, "spleen," and "the vapors," were collapsed into the single, largely undifferentiated diagnosis of "nervous disorders." In the 19th and in much of the 20th centuries, such disorders were regarded as illegitimate medical conditions (ie, highly prevalent but disconcertingly unassociated with a "lesion" toward which interventions could be directed). In recent decades, the American Psychiatric Association produced its *Diagnostic and Statistical Manual of Mental Disorders,* now in its fourth edition (*DSM-IV*), to disaggregate mental disorders into an explicit nosology of discrete clinical entities. This categoric approach to psychiatric diagnosis has both fostered and been advanced by recent growth in neurobiological knowledge, which has brought psychological medicine close to the identification of psychopathological changes at the neuronal and molecular level.

Despite the successes of the *DSM-IV,* there are important ways in which the spectrum of developmental behavioral and psychiatric disorders defies categorization. From a clinical perspective, developmental and behavioral difficulties often appear as multidimensional clusters of problems rather than as discrete, unitary entities. Attention-deficit hyperactivity disorder, for example, has high rates of comorbidity with other "categories" of behavioral concern such as depression, anxiety, and tic disorders; affective disorders are often accompanied by symptoms that fulfill the diagnostic criteria for an anxiety disorder. While diagnostic taxonomies draw clean lines among the various disorders, reality is more often a clinical "soup" comprising symptoms from several categories of mental impairments.

Even more challenging than comorbidity is the task of deciding where normal variation ends and diagnosable pathology begins (ie, differentiating noncases from cases). While diagnostic "gold standards" are often available in other areas of medicine (eg, the results of two concurrent throat cultures in assessing the accuracy of a rapid streptococcal antigen screen), external validators often are unavailable in developmental-behavioral pediatrics, where firm pathologic signs are less prevalent. Consequently, developmental-behavioral diagnosis begins in a difficult position by virtue of its frequent inability to confirm the presence or absence of pathology.

If a gold standard criterion *were* available for a given developmental diagnosis, patients with and without the diagnosis would show the distributions displayed in Fig. 5-1 on a typical diagnostic test. When a threshold value or "positivity criterion" is chosen along a range of test results, the decision almost always results in the misclassification of some individuals to both the normal and disordered groups. Some children with the disorder will score sufficiently low to be categorized as normal, and some normal children will score so high that they are misclassified as disordered. Thus, placement of the threshold value along the spectrum of test scores

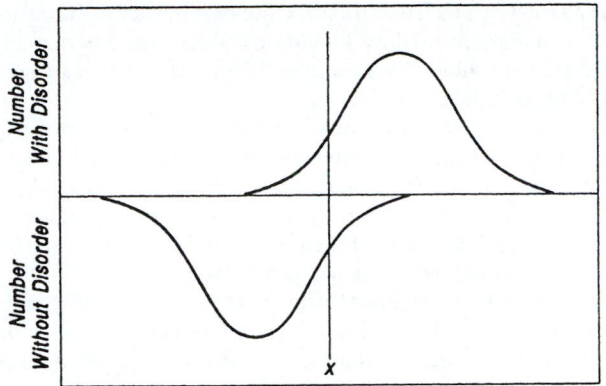

Any cutoff (here shown at point x) will result in some false results.

FIGURE 5-1   Results of a typical diagnostic test plotted separately for subjects with and without disorders. SOURCE: *From Zarins DA, Earls F: Diagnostic decision making in psychiatry. Am J Psychiatry 150: 197–206; 1993.*

determines the relative prevalences of false-negative and false-positive results. The balance of these false results and their comparative importance is a function of the clinical or research question being asked.

A deeper question is how well a given diagnostic approach conforms to the underlying reality of developmental and behavioral difficulties encountered by children. Thus, it is important to assess the clinical *utility* of categoric and dimensional views of diagnosis and to ask which approach more accurately reflects the real character of developmental psychopathology. For example, assigning a diagnosis of colic to infants who occupy the extreme end of a normative crying distribution may be a misuse of the conventional distinction between normal and abnormal. Rather, crying behavior in early infancy may be better evaluated according to its functional significance in the life of the child and family.

Examples of categoric versus dimensional views of developmental-behavioral disorders are plentiful. Whether autism and Asperger syndrome are distinctive disorders with different etiologies or simply two different locations on an "autism spectrum" remains unanswered. While many regard Asperger syndrome as a variant of autism, the IQ profiles of patients with this syndrome are quite distinct from those of children with classic autism. Similarly, there is conflicting evidence regarding the categoric or continuous nature of reading disabilities or dyslexia. Neurobiological studies suggest that children with such disabilities have a distinctive abnormality in the early components of visually evoked cortical electroencephalographic potentials, indicating a slowing in transmission along CNS visual pathways. On the other hand, the discrepancy between observed and predicted reading achievement shows a normal distribution, suggesting that dyslexia is simply the tail of a continuously distributed skill.

Although this chapter cannot resolve these ongoing clinical dilemmas, the chapter's structure takes a clear position. Underlying the following discussions is an assumption that developmental-behavioral diagnosis is most accurate and useful when conceptualized as the location of a child along the spectrum of functioning. It is acknowledged that *qualitative* differences among children may be important, but continuous, dimensional views most often provide clinicians with useful diagnostic approaches to developmental-behavioral problems. To this end, this section is organized largely into clinical continua representing the spectrum from normal variation to developmental-behavioral disorder.

References

Barr RG: Normality, a clinically useless concept: the case of infant crying and colic. J Dev Behav Pediatr 14:264–270, 1993

Hare E: The history of "nervous disorders" from 1600 to 1840, and a comparison with modern views. Br J Psychiatry 159:37–45, 1991

Kagan J, Snidman N: Temperamental factors in human development. Am Psychol 46:856–862, 1991

Zarin DA, Earls F: Diagnostic decision-making in psychiatry. Am J Psychiatry 150:197–206, 1993

5.4   STANDARDIZED ASSESSMENT INSTRUMENTS: THEIR BENEFITS AND THEIR LIMITATIONS

Melvin D. Levine

Many justifications are given for the use of standardized assessment instruments in the practice of developmental-behavioral pediatrics. Such tools are presumed to minimize observer subjectivity, thereby facilitating reliable diagnosis.

STANDARDIZATION

Instruments are considered "standardized" if they have undergone tests of their reliability and validity and appropriate normative data have been gathered and analyzed. Reliability testing establishes that the findings will be stable and unlikely to change soon after the test's first administration (ie, test-retest reliability) and that the test will be consistent across users (ie, interobserver reliability) and scorers (ie, inter-rater reliability). Validation establishes that the instrument measures what it purports to measure. A tool may be validated against another, previously validated instrument, or it may be validated by studying its associations with current function (ie, concurrent validity) or future outcomes (ie, predictive validity).

Good diagnostic instruments are based on strong conceptual models as well as scientific evidence that the constructs being measured correspond to important definable domains. For example, a test of a child's attention strength should conform to what is known in the literature regarding the parameters of normal and deficient attention.

APPLICATIONS

A well-standardized instrument can find many specific applications in a pediatric setting. These functions commonly include:

- The establishment of a specific diagnosis to facilitate the formulation and implementation of an intervention plan;
- The determination of the severity and, possibly, the prognosis of a condition;
- The measurement (on a continuum) of functional strengths and weaknesses compared with other individuals (as on intelligence, developmental, or achievement testing);
- The derivation of a label or diagnostic category needed to establish eligibility and/or reimbursement for services; and

• The clarification of problematic patterns of behavior and/or development to prevent the negative effects of their misinterpretation (eg, accusing a child with language problems of not really trying in school).

To be well-suited to the practice of pediatrics, instruments must be practical to administer and interpret within the constraints of the clinical setting. Not all of these instruments need to be administered by a pediatrician; in many clinical settings, diagnostic tools are used mainly by other members of a multidisciplinary assessment team, who must receive adequate training and practice in their use to prevent misinterpretation. Nevertheless, pediatricians need to be familiar with the applications and limitations of these instruments themselves.

Commonly used standardized measures and their indications, are summarized in Table 5-2. These types of standardized instruments can be applied in pediatrics, namely tests, interviews, and questionnaires. In the following sections, the benefits and limitations of these formats are considered.

STANDARDIZED TESTS

BENEFITS Tests permit the direct sampling and observation of abilities and/or behaviors in children. As such, they can help a clinician derive a profile or description of a child's strengths, deficits, and preferred styles. Results may help to explain a wide range of phenomena such as poor school performance, difficulty concentrating, or diminished athletic ability. Some measures, such as the Brazelton Neonatal Behavioral Assessment Scale, help to account for difficult behaviors or problems that parents may have nurturing or relating to a young child. Projective tests (eg, interpretations of inkblots, provocative images, children's drawings) are used as indirect measures of personality as well as indicators of personal preoccupations, self-concept, family problems, and fears.

TABLE 5-2

COMMON STANDARDIZED MEASURES AND THEIR INDICATIONS

STANDARDIZED MEASURE	INDICATIONS
Intelligence testing	When there is a need to assess overall cognitive ability and/or seek evidence for strengths and weaknesses in specific domains (eg, memory)
Language testing	When delayed receptive and/or expressive language function is suspected because of observed delay or academic problems
Neuropyschological or neurodevelopmental testing	When there is a need to examine specific areas of cognitive and/or developmental function (eg, motor skills, visual spatial abilities)
Projective testing	When a child shows behavioral or affective problems, and there is a need to understand problematic perceptions or conflicts
Achievement testing	When a student is suspected of having academic delays, and there is a need to specify which skills are strong and which are weak
Behavioral questionnaire	When a child exhibits symptoms of emotional distress, and there is a need to document and/or categorize the symptoms
Standardized interview	When a child or youth has problems and there is a need to tap his or her self-perceptions and insights into the difficulties

LIMITATIONS Clinicians who make use of standardized tests need to be keenly aware of their limitations. When any instrument is viewed as an infallible "gold standard" it can become hazardous to the child and family.

Measures of ability are especially imperfect and controversial. Included in this category are intelligence tests, neurodevelopmental examinations, neuropsychological assessment procedures, achievement tests, and more focused tests such as scales of language or motor development. Some of the principal limitations of such tests are discussed in the following paragraphs.

Standardized tests may not always measure exclusively what they purport to measure. For example, a child may perform poorly on a language test because the child has an attention deficit disorder. Thus, although the scored results may indicate weak receptive language skills, the child was simply "tuning in and tuning out" during the examination. In fact, whenever a child performs poorly on a full assessment, or a section, or individual item on a test, there can be multiple reasons for the poor performance. Rigid or glib interpretations that "go by the book" can delude diagnosticians.

The measure may not evaluate all relevant domains. An overall score on an IQ test may be low because the test failed to measure the child's areas of intellectual strength. This is particularly important in view of the growing interest in the existence of "multiple intelligences." Thus, traditional tests of intelligence may only tap a narrow band of cognitive competencies, thereby underrating, and potentially undervaluing, certain kinds of minds. Even within developmental domains, a test may fail to tap critical dimensions of function. For example, the verbal subtests of the Wechsler Intelligence Scale for Children (WISC-III) do not assess several vital components of language (eg, phonologic awareness, verbal fluency, discourse comprehension). Consequently, a child with serious language problems may look verbally intact on the verbal subtests of an intelligence test.

The use of tests for service eligibility determinations can be especially misleading. Often a student must reveal an arbitrary discrepancy between his IQ and achievement scores to obtain special help in school. Another child may be denied services because a standardized achievement test fails to detect the child's problem with writing, organization, or the use of memory during reading because the instrument simply does not measure those (and many other) critical academic parameters. It is also possible that a child's IQ score may fail to reflect specific cognitive deficits, or that one or two subtest results may significantly lower the overall score, making it appear as if the child has low academic "potential."

Test norms may be biased. Many assessment procedures run the risk of discriminating against certain cultural groups. This is especially true for examinations that demand considerable linguistic proficiency. Ideally, clinicians should have access to local norms that are calibrated specifically for the population they serve.

Tests that generate diagnostic labels may drastically oversimplify a child's status and service needs. For example, if a test allegedly shows that a child has attention-deficit hyperactivity disorder, the result may distract the clinician from diligently examining the child for learning disorders or depression, both of which may be crucial elements in the overall clinical picture.

Some children simply are better test-takers than are other children. Artifacts introduced by the testing situation may prevent certain individuals from revealing their authentic profiles. The unfamiliar examination setting, situational anxiety, timed conditions, skill of the examiner, and quality of the rapport established with the child all can make it difficult to distinguish between transient states and stable traits. Some children have problems with particular test formats. For example, there are individuals whose cognitive styles render them unable to excel on multiple-choice tests; other formats are more likely to elicit their strengths.

Tests designed to elucidate emotional problems are especially susceptible to misinterpretation or overinterpretation. Clinicians must be aware that many projective tests have not been validated rigorously in the pediatric age group. Therefore, their interpretation must be considered highly subjective and exceptionally vulnerable to observer biases of various kinds.

STANDARDIZED QUESTIONNAIRES

BENEFITS   Standardized questionnaires have become a mainstay in developmental-behavioral pediatrics. They are used to diagnose a multitude of conditions, including attention deficits, depression, and the full gamut of behavior problems. Questionnaires also are employed to characterize specific behavioral qualities such as temperament, self-esteem, and social skills. These instruments may be completed by parents or teachers, or by the children themselves.

Questionnaires can greatly facilitate the practice of pediatrics. They save time, enabling the efficient gathering and integration of a substantial amount of information, and they permit systematic comparison of same-age children. They help to identify variations in the perceptions of a child by different observers (eg, parent and teacher). They also enable clinicians to detect clusters of traits and suggest behavioral or personality patterns that conform to certain established diagnoses (eg, bipolar illness) that may have treatment and/or prognostic implications.

LIMITATIONS   Like standardized tests, questionnaires have substantial limitations, including those discussed below.

The reading and observational skills of the person completing the questionnaire are likely to affect that which is recorded. Some individuals are more skilled questionnaire responders than are other individuals.

Halo effects often distort the results. For example, a parent who feels angry with a child may check off nearly every undesirable trait, and a child completing a questionnaire might practice denial, seeking to represent himself or herself as a behavioral paragon.

Political or economic agendas may contaminate the findings. Thus, a school that is either unwilling or unable to offer appropriate services may underrate a child's learning problems on a questionnaire. Alternatively, a parent may want a child to be given a particular diagnosis and might skew the responses either intentionally or unconsciously to obtain that diagnosis. Such distortion might occur, for example, in custody cases or when specific services are sought.

The assumption that the number of traits a child demonstrates can determine whether he or she has a particular condition may well be questionable. Many questionnaires depend heavily on this dubious premise. For example, if a child sets fires but has relatively few other abnormal symptoms, the child's overall score on a behavioral questionnaire could result in an erroneous assessment as mentally healthy.

Concerns over confidentiality may prevail. Parents, teachers, or children may not feel comfortable revealing highly personal information on a document that could be disseminated.

INTERVIEWING

An old but valid medical adage goes, "If you want to know what's wrong with the patient, ask him." All too often clinicians miss an opportunity by not having systematic ways of interviewing families

and children to define and refine diagnosis. A well-conducted interview also can go a long way toward establishing a level of rapport and trust that is unlikely to result from the application of a questionnaire or test. Standardized interviews can yield useful clues regarding affect, learning styles, and social experience, among other parameters. One such interview, the STRANDS, is used to uncover specific breakdowns and strengths in learning among high school students. In this age group, when asked appropriate questions in a systematic fashion, students are able to pinpoint where their learning breakdowns are occurring. Clinicians should seek interview formats that are as well-designed and validated as standardized tests and questionnaires.

OVERALL SAFEGUARDS

Standardized developmental-behavior assessment instruments will continue to play an important role in pediatrics. They can be used most effectively if all findings are subjected to cross-validation. That is, there ought to be a prerequisite for multiple data sources before any definitive assessment result or diagnosis is confirmed. This process is facilitated best when a pediatrician serves on a multidisciplinary team within which somewhat overlapping observations are made. For example, to evaluate a child's affect, evidence could be harvested from a parent questionnaire, an interview with the child, and direct observations made during testing, as well as from a report from the school. In this way, the process of assessment becomes a search for recurring themes from multiple sources.

Rigid decisions based on overall test scores must be avoided. Many newer forms of assessment are made flexible and often more revealing than traditional measures. So-called dynamic assessment procedures encourage clinicians to change the nature of the tasks to determine what it takes for a child to succeed. Semistandard interview techniques enable children and parents to elaborate on responses in a way that is not possible on questionnaires. Such flexible testing in skilled hands can enrich our appreciation of a child's highly individualized needs.

No single test, task, or observational look should ever be considered as the ultimate explicator of a developmental or behavioral problem. Moreover, clinicians need to be aware of the multiple possible interpretations of any single finding or score. Evaluation processes should evolve longitudinally as one follows the progress of a child or family over time. Standardized assessment is most likely to be helpful when there are multiple data points and when clinicians can retain an open mind, infuse their own informal observations, minimize their personal or professional biases, and recognize that standardized instruments must never replace rigorous clinical reasoning, eclectic argument, and informed judgment.

References

Brazelton TB: Neonatal behavioral assessment scale. Clin Dev Med, No. 50 London, Spastics Society, 1973

Carey WB, Levine MD: Comprehensive diagnostic formulation. In: Levine MD, Carey WB, Crocker A, eds: Developmental-Behavioral Pediatrics, 3rd ed. Philadelphia, Saunders, 1998

Gardner H: Frames of Mind. New York, Basic Books, 1983

Knoff H: The Assessment of Child and Adolescent Personality. New York, Guilford Press, 1986

Levine MD: Developmental Variation and Learning Disorders 2nd ed. Cambridge, MA, Educators Publishing Service, 1998

Weinberg RA: Intelligence and IQ: landmark issues and great debates. Am Psychol 44:98, 1989

5.5 COMMON FUNCTIONAL CONCERNS

5.5.1 Crying and Colic

Ronald G. Barr

DEFINITIONS AND EPIDEMIOLOGY

Colic syndrome refers to a cluster of behaviors that are presumed (but not yet demonstrated) to represent a distinct condition. There are three characteristic dimensions.

First, crying usually clusters in the late afternoon or evening, peaks in the second month, and resolves by 3 to 4 months of age. Second, there are associated motor behaviors (eg, legs over abdomen, clenched fists), an atypical facial expression (eg, pain facies), gastrointestinal symptoms (eg, distention, gas, regurgitation), and lack of response to soothing (including lack of quieting with feeding). Third, the prolonged crying bouts are "paroxysmal," beginning and ending without warning, and unrelated to events in the environment. Colic is variably defined, but the most widely known is Wessel's "rule of threes": crying more than 3 hours per day for more than 3 days per week for more than 3 weeks. Such quantitative definitions capture neither the quality nor the overlap with normal crying. They are helpful, but not sufficient, for clinical evaluation.

To reflect the range of crying complaints, it is more helpful to consider a spectrum of behavioral clusters for which a clear etiology may be demonstrable only for "organic" cases. Based on controlled studies, this spectrum could include:

Organic, with clear evidence for disease;
Wessel's crying (a), a group with excessive crying that meets Wessel's criteria who *also* have physical signs of hypertonia (eg, arched back, clenched fists, hypertonic arms/legs), crying bouts perceived as particularly intense, high pitched, or pain-like behavioral signs of distress;
Wessel's crying (b), a group that meets Wessel's criteria for quantity with a typical diurnal rhythm, unsoothable bouts, and occasional pain facies and qualitatively different cries, but who are otherwise normal;
Non-Wessel's crying, a group whose crying does not meet quantitative criteria for excessive crying but who may have qualitatively different (eg, sick-sounding) cries; and
Normal concern, in which the crying pattern is typical, and the complaint results wholly from lack of information about typical crying characteristics at this age.

Estimated incidence varies by site (primary or referral), but all complaints together could include 40-50% of infants. Wessel's and Wessel's-"plus" crying together account for approximately one-third of all complaints. Organic causes are demonstrated in 5% or less of all complaints.

ETIOLOGY AND PATHOGENESIS

Infant behavior is organized as a set of discontinuous and distinct modes or behavioral "states." States have the features of:

Being self-organizing; that is, the characteristic behavioral clusters (eg, vocalizations, respirations, facial and motor activity) are constrained to occur together because of the organizational relationships between the components;
Being stable over time (minutes rather than seconds); and
Having qualitatively distinct reactions to stimuli depending on behavioral state (ie, the responses are state-specific and nonlinear).

In transitions between states, the organism is less well organized and less stable. In Wolff's classification of infant behavior, crying and awake activity represent behavioral states, and fussing represents a transition. Thus, intermittent crying vocalizations can become incorporated into a state of the organism that is prolonged, self-sustaining, and resistant to soothing, which is consistent with a "discontinuous" colic bout in other healthy infants. This may explain why a soothing maneuver that is otherwise successful for unsustained whimpering or fussiness can fail if initiated during the crying state.

Both internal and external stimuli (ie, physiological or behavioral) can act alone or together to enhance the stability of states, or transitions to a different state. Consequently, "etiologies" are not restricted to pathologic organic or behavioral interactions. Cry/colic syndromes are equally likely in well infants in optimal caregiving contexts. Thus, it is more accurate to consider *determinants* of prolonged crying states rather than specific etiologies. Recognized probable determinants of crying include maturation, nutrients, gut hormones and transmitters, and caregiving behaviors, as well as diseases and pathophysiological processes. In addition, there are a number of "myths" about factors inaccurately assumed to be relevant to colic.

Maturation

Rapid growth and differentiation of the central nervous system (CNS) are reflected in the reorganization of crying, waking, and sleeping behavioral states in the first 3 months after birth. Noncry wakefulness is increasingly stable, less disrupted by internal and external stimuli, and more responsive to psychologically significant stimuli such as human voice and face. For crying, these maturational changes are reflected in longer, but usually not more frequent, crying bouts.

Nutrients

Nutrients can both exacerbate and reduce crying. More than 20 potentially antigenic cow's milk proteins may be passed through formula or breast milk, may stimulate gastrointestinal hypersensitivity reactions, and may contribute to increased crying. However, results of controlled diet trials are mixed; positive results are more likely in small, highly select samples of Wessel's-plus infants who manifest additional gastrointestinal symptoms. Incomplete carbohydrate (especially lactose) absorption contributes to gas symptoms but not to crying. Nutrients can also reduce crying by a number of mechanisms. Sucrose taste recruits central opioid-mediated distress reduction systems, but this is less effective in infants with colic. Nutrient effects may be mediated by cholecystokinin-mediated motility changes and by ingestion of exogenous opioids.

Gut Hormones and Transmitters

Variability in gut hormone and transmitter release due to individual differences, maturational stage, feeding pattern, or pathologic insult could contribute to prolonged crying by inducing motility changes.

Caregiving Behaviors

Behaviors such as carrying, frequent feeding, use of a pacifier, car rides, and close mother–infant proximity—all involving postural change, repetition, constancy, and/or rhythmicity—tend to maintain a noncrying state. However, behavioral modifications have mixed results when used as treatment modalities in infants with well-established colic. They tend to modify crying during the time they are used, but do not "cure" colic.

Diseases and Pathophysiology

Almost any disease or illness, from minor to severe, provokes acute crying in infants. However, only a few infants have presented with nonfebrile, nonacute colic-like syndrome before 4 months of age (see Definition earlier). Although rare, there is good evidence that cow's milk protein intolerance, isolated fructose intolerance, maternal fluoxetine hydrochloride (Prozac) via breastmilk, infantile migraine, and anomalous left coronary artery can present with a colic-like syndrome. Evidence for reflux esophagitis is moderate to weak. Of particular concern are those syndromes that may have no other symptoms or visible signs, such as infant abuse.

ETIOLOGIC "MYTHS"

There are no differences in crying or colic incidence in breast versus formula-fed infants, or in first- versus later-born infants. Changing from breast to formula feeding does not reduce crying or colic. By observing "sham" diaper changes, Wolff showed that wet diapers were not a cause of infant crying. There is no evidence that crying, especially colic, is caused by responsive parenting. Nor is there evidence that being attentive to crying spoils the infant or causes colic. However, parental caregiving should be "responsive" rather than "intrusive."

CLINICAL MANIFESTATIONS

Crying is the first and most salient communicative behavior of infancy. Paradoxically, crying functions to ensure adaptively "positive" consequences of adequate nutrition, protection, and prosocial mother–infant interaction, as well as potentially "negative" consequences of discontinuing breast-feeding, complaints of excessive crying, maternal depression and erosion of confidence, and, in extreme instances, child abuse and death. Human infants cry more in the first 3 months of life than during any other time in their lives, and this crying has four robust characteristics. First, there is an *early peak pattern* (increasing during the first 2 months and decreasing thereafter) and clustering during the evening hours. The early peak is demonstrable in most caretaking contexts, including age-corrected preterm infants, and is probably a behavioral universal of infancy. Second, the peak results primarily from changes in bout *length* of intermittent crying ("fussing"), while bout *frequency* remains constant. Duration but not frequency varies with the caretaking context and is modifiable by caretaking practice. Third, individual differences in crying quantity are substantial. However, crying is *variable* from day to day, and even week to week, for any one infant despite consistency in caretaking practice. Finally, with the exception of crying following pain stimuli or periods without a feed, early crying is *paroxysmal*, variously referring to its recurrent, unpredictable, precipitous, unexplained, and apparently spontaneous occurrence.

In the clinical setting, *colic* refers to crying problems that are presented as *complaints* and to a *syndrome* in which crying is the cardinal symptom. Regardless of etiology, colic complaints are always dyadic, that is, a product of both infant behavior and parental tolerance. Thus, prolonged crying with a tolerant parent will not present as colic, while mild crying with a less-tolerant parent will. Notable predispositions to lower parental tolerance are:

- Expectations of a happy infant and the reality of a crying one;
- Lack of explanation for the peak and paroxysmal character of crying;
- Social pressure from spouses, parents, and friends;
- The postpartum tendency toward maternal emotional lability and depression; and
- Fatigue accompanying sleep disruption.

Presentation of a complaint is associated both with prolonged crying and parental anxiety. While first- and later-born infants cry the same amount, crying first-born infants are more often taken to health-care facilities. With the possible exception of clinically depressed parents, however, there is little justification for attributing increased crying to parental distress or personality. Furthermore, even anxious parents are remarkably accurate in reporting quantity and quality of crying.

ASSESSMENT AND DIAGNOSIS

The presentation of a crying complaint must be taken seriously regardless of the quantity of crying. There are always two problems: namely, the infant's behavior and the parent's tolerance for it. Crying has negative consequences for the infant if caregiver frustration exceeds the caregiver's tolerance. The crying may indicate none to severe organic, behavioral, or psychological illness in the infant. Neglect of the complaint could lead to severe consequences such as abuse or even death.

There are three important tasks for the clinician presented with a crying complaint: (a) detecting organic disease; (b) managing the crying and the caregiver's concern; and (c) providing appropriate follow-up. Figure 5-2 presents an algorithm incorporating important decision points in regard to these tasks. Acute presentation and/or febrile infants require an investigation for organic disease. Nonfebrile infants with persistent crying who are older than 4 months do not have colic syndrome. If they do not have organic disease, they may have persistent mother–infant distress syndrome (seen in high-risk infants in high-risk families where normal "intuitive" parenting has broken down), be temperamentally "difficult" infants, or meet criteria for dysregulated infants with generalized problems with crying, feeding, and sleeping.

If infants do present with colic-like syndrome, there are four clues that are more common, although not diagnostic, in infants with organic etiologies:

- A cry described as "high-pitched" from an infant who regularly arches his or her back (even during fussing bouts) and whose crying does not manifest a diurnal pattern (more in the afternoon and evening);
- Crying is not the only symptom or sign following a complete history and physical;
- A late onset of crying (ie, it begins in the third month), especially following a switch from breast to formula feeding (suggesting cow's milk protein intolerance);
- Unusual and excessive crying persisting beyond 4 months (suggesting an organic cause).

Infants that do not have organic clues but who meet Wessel's-plus criteria (less than 10%) are candidates for a *therapeutic diet*

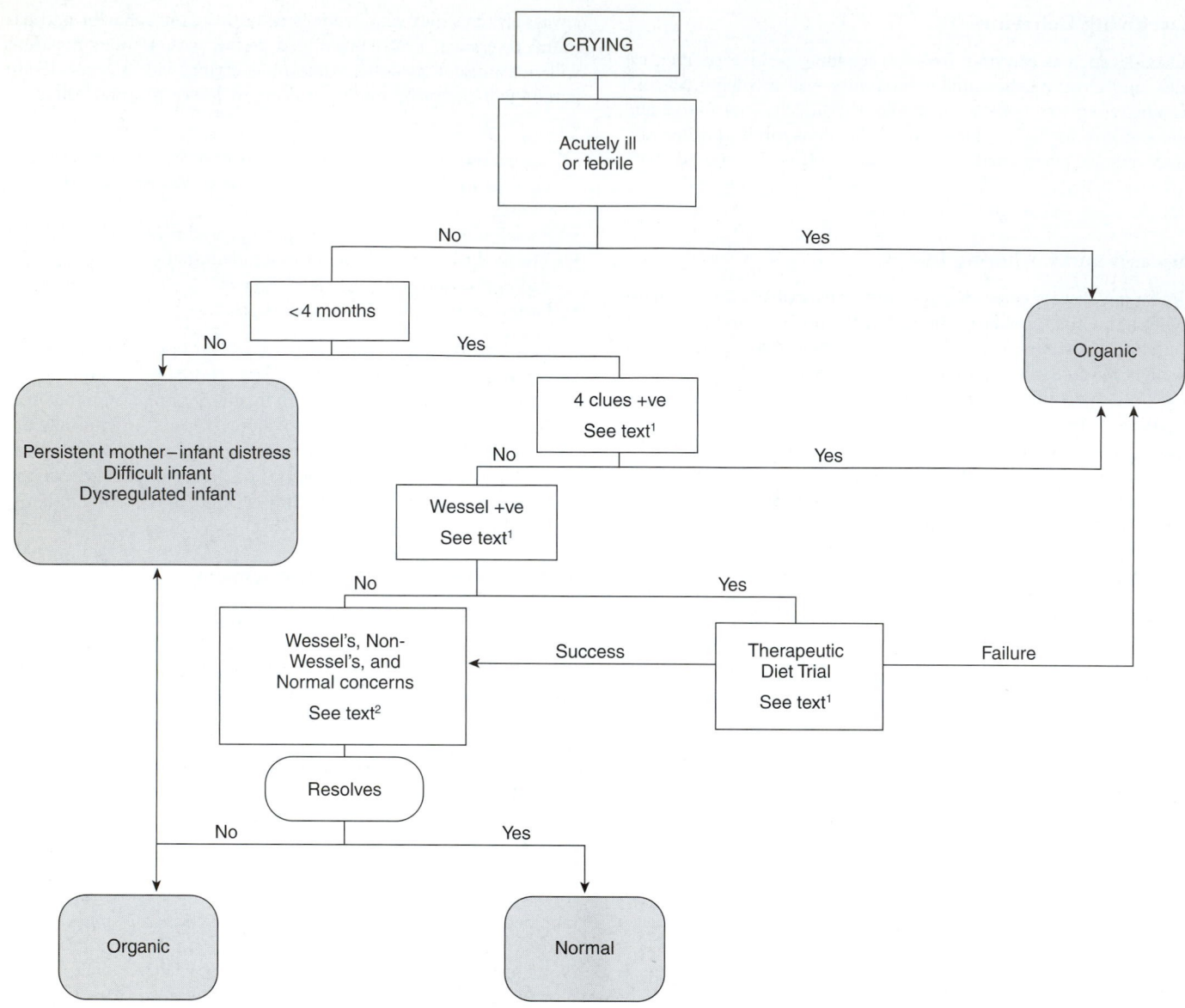

FIGURE 5-2   Algorithm showing an assessment of crying in infants. 1. See "Assessment and Diagnosis" 2. See "Definitions and Epidemiology."

trial (formula change to protein hydrolysate, or elimination of cow's milk from mother's diet). There is no indication to switch from breast-feeding to formula. This practice increases maternal perception of the "vulnerability" of the infant. If a diet trial fails, an organic workup is indicated. Prior to 3 months of age, success will probably be only partial. Even if successful, these infants should be followed until crying resolves completely.

For the remainder, it is less important to diagnose colic than to assess its functional significance for the infant and the parents. This can be facilitated by standard assessments for organic etiologies, sensitive interviewing, and by assessment on more than one occasion. All caregivers should be asked whether

- The frustration is too great;
- They are no longer attracted to their infant because of the crying; and
- They have depressive symptoms.

Diary recording of the infant's behavior (including crying and fussing), feeding, and weight by the parents is helpful for both parents and clinicians. A diurnal rhythm and weight gain make disease less likely.

MANAGEMENT

Based on current knowledge, management includes providing information, focusing parental anxiety, modifying the caretaking style, providing preventive advice, and making environmental modifications. If caregiver tolerance is strained, more intense monitoring or referral to specialized services is indicated.

PROVIDING INFORMATION

Information should be provided to parents about the typical pattern of crying, lack of responsivity to soothing, and the excellent outcome.

FOCUSING PARENTAL ANXIETY

This is accomplished by ruling out disease processes, involving parents in data gathering (eg, maintaining a diary), and removing the guilt of "bad parenting."

MODIFYING CARETAKING STYLE

The caretaking style should move the parent toward behaviors that encourage a state of alert wakefulness rather than crying. These include carrying or rocking the baby, responding promptly to signals from the infant, decreasing feeding intervals, and using a pacifier. The more frequently these measures are provided, the more likely they are to be effective.

PREVENTIVE ADVICE

All parents should be instructed never to shake the infant when frustrated. Instead, parents should be given someone supportive to call as an alternative.

ENVIRONMENTAL MODIFICATIONS

These capitalize on the responsiveness of infants to constant, rhythmic stimulation. The best modification is increased time and contact with the infant. Alternatives include music, car or stroller rides, and devices that produce a rhythmic motion. The practice of using washer or dryer vibrations requires secure placement of the infant seat to prevent injury to the infant from falling off the appliance.

Short and predictable periods of *respite* for the primary caretaker are essential.

The only medication demonstrated to be effective is dicyclomine hydrochloride. However, colic has been removed as an indication for its use because respiratory distress and apnea have been reported with its use.

NATURAL HISTORY AND PROGNOSIS

In most infants, the condition resolves by 3 months of age, but in about 30% of infants it persists to 4 months of age. If it does not resolve, organic causes should be reconsidered. To date, there is no evidence of growth, developmental, health, or temperament sequelae in infants with colic. However, parental *perception* of their infants as "difficult" or of themselves as less effective or symptomatically depressed caregivers is increased. Unresolved crying is more likely in families who are themselves at risk and who have an infant with colic (a "double hit"). In the absence of infant or parental illness, the outcome, including mother–infant interaction, is excellent.

References

Barr RG: In: Walker WA, Durie PR, Hamilton JR, Walker-Smith JA, Watkins JB, eds: Pediatric Gastrointestinal Disease: Pathophysiology, Diagnosis, and Management, 2nd ed. St. Louis, Mosby, 1996

Barr RG: Excessive crying. In: Sameroff AJ, Lewis M, Miller SM, eds: Handbook of Developmental Psychopathology. New York, Plenum Press, 2000

Barr RG: The early crying paradox: a modest proposal. Hum Nature 1: 355–389, 1990

Barr RG, Rotman A, Yaremko J, Leduc D, Francoeur TE: The crying of infants with colic: a controlled empirical description. Pediatrics 90:14–21, 1992

Forsyth BW, McCarthy PL, Leventhal JM: Problems of early infancy, formula changes, and mothers' beliefs about their infants. J Pediatr 106: 1012–1017, 1985

Gormally SM, Barr RG: Of clinical pies and clinical clues: proposal for a clinical approach to complaints of early crying and colic. Ambulatory Child Health 3(2):137–153, 1997

St James-Roberts I, Halil T: Infant crying patterns in the first year; normal community and clinical findings. J Child Psychol Psychiatry 32:951–968, 1991

Singer JI, Rosenberg NM: A fatal case of colic. Pediatr Emerg Care 8:171–172, 1992

Wessel MA, Cobb JC, Jackson EB, Harris GS, Detwiler AC: Paroxysmal fussing in infancy, sometimes called "colic." Pediatrics 14:421–434, 1954

Wolff PH: The Development of Behavioral States and the Expression of Emotions in Early Infancy: New Proposals for Investigation. Chicago, University of Chicago Press, 1987

5.5.2   Sleeping

Deborah Madansky

Sleep is a complex human behavior. It is determined by the changing neurophysiological patterns of the growing child and shaped by the interpersonal, social, and cultural practices of the child's family. Sleep problems are the most commonly reported behavioral concerns in early childhood, and they are a source of fatigue, frustration, and concern for parents. Understanding and managing a particular sleep difficulty requires knowledge of normal sleep patterns during childhood as well as a thorough review of parental behaviors and expectations.

DEFINITIONS AND EPIDEMIOLOGY

Childhood sleep problems most commonly present as symptoms that fall into two broad categories: (a) disruptive behaviors interrupting nighttime sleep (ie, "night waking"), and (b) difficulties with or resistance to going to sleep (ie, "bedtime struggles").

Night Waking

Nighttime has generally been defined as the period extending from 1 hour after bedtime until the start of the next day or, more narrowly, as midnight to 5 a.m. Waking refers to physiological arousals or partial arousals that occur during this sleep period. Although these episodes can be detected almost universally in children by an EEG or a videotape, clinically significant night waking is that which is reported as problematic by parents.

Night waking is commonly experienced during the first 3 years of life. Its prevalence varies from 10 to 44% in children during the first year, 20 to 40% during the second year, and 14 to 33% between second and fourth years of age. Night waking at later ages has not been well studied.

Bedtime Struggles

Reluctance or resistance to going to sleep is a common feature of childhood. Several studies have defined a bedtime struggle in children under 4 years as taking more than 1 hour to fall asleep, accompanied by active protest, more than 3 nights a week. This problem does not generally arise until the latter half of the first year, and it has been reported in 20 to 62% of children less than 4 years of age, with a greater prevalence in children who also are night wakers.

ETIOLOGY AND PATHOGENESIS

Night Waking

Normal Developmental Pattern

During the first few months of life, sleep periods lengthen and cluster at night, so that by 3 months of age, 70% of children "settle" or sleep from midnight to 5 a.m. without parental intervention. By 6 months of age, 83% do so, and 90% have done so by 1 year. Between 6 and 12 months of age, 50% of those who have settled previously will begin crying again during wakeful periods, a phenomenon that is probably related to separation anxiety generated by the newly developed cognitive attainments of recall memory and object permanence. Persistent, disruptive night waking develops when children have not learned to handle their normal arousals [which typically occur at the end of the sleep cycle, including a period of rapid eye movement (REM) and non-REM sleep] quietly and by themselves. Many factors contribute to this need for persistent parental intervention at night.

Sleep Onset Associations

Children who are held, rocked, sung to, or otherwise lulled to sleep by parents at bedtime have learned to associate sleep onset with some parental intervention. Being unused to and unable to soothe themselves after later awakenings, such children protest and require parental intervention for sleep reinduction.

Nocturnal Feeding

After 6 months of age, eating or drinking at night is a learned habit rather than a physiological need. Continued night feeding may contribute to night waking because it represents a positive reinforcement and stimulation to the gastrointestinal, hormonal, and urinary systems.

Positive Reinforcements

Child-waking behavior that is rewarded by parental attention at night, such as removing the child from the crib or the bed and engaging the child in play, television viewing, or parental activities, is likely to persist as long as the positive reinforcement continues.

Temperamental Characteristics

A child's innate behavioral style is associated with night waking. "Difficult" children (those described as highly active, poorly adaptable, intense, and negative) seem to have fewer self-soothing behaviors and therefore greater reliance on their parents for nighttime comforting. Those with a low sensory threshold seem to wake more often.

Medical Factors

Adverse perinatal events correlate with increased night waking. However, this finding has been difficult to interpret because of inconsistent definitions among studies and no clear differentiation between the possible direct neurologic influences of the perinatal events and their indirect influence on subsequent parental behavior and expectations. Furthermore, both acute and chronic medical problems may interrupt nighttime sleep because of intruding symptoms or untoward effects of medication.

Psychosocial Factors

Traumatized children often sleep poorly because of increased physiological arousal and distress over disturbing dreams. A variety of family stressors are associated with night waking in children, including financial difficulties, changes in employment, family injury or illness, marital discord, and maternal depression. These factors seem to contribute indirectly to wakeful behavior, as preoccupied parents often have ineffective child-management skills and their children may not get their emotional needs met during the day, thus increasing the pressure for attention at night.

Cosleeping

At least occasional sleeping in the parental bed is reported in 35 to 55% of children under 4 years of age. In most studies, parents of frequent cosleepers report more night waking. Cultural and ethnic differences must be considered, however, as the prevalence of cosleeping is higher among African-American and Latino families.

Parasomnias

Events reported by parents as night waking may be caused by childhood parasomnias. These are defined as specific events happening during sleep or that are induced or exacerbated by sleep.

A *nigthmare* is a disturbing dream that occurs during REM sleep. It is usually followed by an awakening, during which the child exhibits distress about the dream content. The peak age of onset is 3 to 5 years, and the prevalence ranges between 25 and 50% of children in this age group. Occasional nightmares occur in most individuals throughout the life span, but recurrent nightmares and their subsequent night waking often indicate significant distress in a child's daytime life.

A *night terror* (ie, *pavor nocturnus*) is often described as a wakeful episode or a nightmare, but it actually represents a distinct non-REM parasomnia. It is a partial arousal, resulting from a rapid transition from stage 4 non-REM sleep to near arousal. The EEG during these episodes shows a mixture of light sleep, deep sleep, and wakefulness. Because of the electrophysiological basis of night terrors, most occur during the first third of the night. The child appears to be awake but is unresponsive; later the child is amnesiac for the episode. Night terrors are more common in males and are reported in 1 to 6% of all children. Onset is usually in the preschool years; in about one-third of the cases, the phenomenon persists until adolescence. A family history of partial arousals is common. Although not stemming primarily from physical or emotional causes, night terrors have been reported to occur more often at times of emotional turmoil or physical exhaustion.

Somnambulism (Sleepwalking)

Another clinical phenomenon in which the child may appear to be awake at night is *sleepwalking* (ie, *somnambulism*). This event, however, represents a non-REM parasomnia occurring during stage 4 non-REM sleep. The most common age of onset is 4 to 8 years, with approximately 15% of children affected before puberty.

Sleeptalking (ie, *somniloquy*) may occur during any stage of sleep, including a dream or partial arousal. Parents often are aroused or alarmed by their child's verbalizations during the night and initially may mistake the phenomenon for an arousal. This phenomenon is not well studied and is probably more common than its reported prevalence of 7 to 8%. Sleeptalking is most common in 4- to 5-year-old children but is present throughout the life span.

Bedtime Struggles

Several factors contribute to difficulty in falling asleep at bedtime.

Developmental Factors

Healthy young children are engaged in a continuous love affair with life and are reluctant to relax and withdraw from the events of the day. In infants and toddlers, difficulties with separation from caregivers are common; in toddlers and preschoolers, oppositionality (borne of a desire for autonomy) is virtually universal. These control struggles may persist in older children. Age-related nighttime fears also may contribute to a reluctance to sleep.

Scheduling Factors

Most children get a fixed amount of sleep within a 24-hour period, and a regular routine enables the child's sleep circadian rhythm to develop. Some children, however, are not sleepy at a prescribed bedtime because of schedule problems or because of a delayed sleep phase. A late afternoon nap might preclude a desired early bedtime. Too many naps may shorten the nighttime sleep period, and avoiding naps altogether might result in a child who is irritable and oppositional at bedtime. Children with a delayed sleep phase (ie, "owls") struggle at an earlier bedtime, but they fall asleep easily at a later bedtime and sleep well into the morning if left undisturbed.

Parental Handling Factors

The most common cause of bedtime struggles is the absence of clear and consistent limits set by parents regarding acceptable bedtime behavior. This may take the form of lack of bedtime routine, which allows the child to fall asleep when and where he or she wishes; responding to every demand by the child; having the parent lie down with the child; or any other request that continues to engage parental attention. Bedtime struggles are also commonly reported among families who cosleep frequently with their children.

CLINICAL MANIFESTATIONS

The typical manifestations of problematic night waking in childhood are crying, whining, verbally protesting, or requesting parental presence and attention during the night. The child who is able may get out of the crib or bed. In most cases, the child appears alert and is responsive to parental attempts at calming and consoling. In children manifesting parasomnias as the etiology of nighttime disruptions, however, this may not be the case. A child awakening from a nightmare will be alert and able to describe a disturbing dream. However, a child experiencing a night terror may scream, cry, thrash in bed, sit up, and stare glassily ahead, but he or she is not actually awake. Under such circumstances, the child is very difficult to arouse or engage; the child does not acknowledge parental presence or remember the episode in the morning. Similarly, sleepwalkers typically sit up, get out of bed, and move about in a distant, confused, and clumsy state while being difficult or impossible to arouse to full awareness. Persistent efforts to "wake up" the sleepwalker may lead to agitation.

Bedtime struggles usually manifest as crying, whining, oppositionality, leaving the bedroom, or a variety of verbal requests for food, drink, trips to the bathroom, "one more story," or any other attempt to engage parental attention.

ASSESSMENT AND DIAGNOSIS

The key to assessment and diagnosis of childhood sleep problems is a careful history. This history should include information about the child's schedule (including the bedtime hour; time of sleep onset; time of night wakings; time of morning awakening; and the usual timing of daytime snacks, meals, and naps); the child's behaviors at bedtime and during the night; the exact timing and nature of parental behaviors and interventions; the child's medical history; a description of the child's temperament; a family psychosocial history, including significant stressors; the family history of sleep problems; and the nature of any other concurrent concerns. A complete physical examination also should be performed to screen for medical problems and to assess the child's neurologic and developmental status.

Although the history and physical examination are usually sufficient to understand the factors contributing to a child's sleep problem, additional diagnostic aids—such as sleep charts, questionnaires, and audio, video, or nighttime recordings of the child's behavior and parental interventions—also may be effective. The gold standard for the diagnosis of physiologically based problems is polysomnography, which includes the simultaneous recording of an EEG, electromyogram, electro-oculogram, heart rate, respiratory rate, and behavior in a sleep laboratory setting.

MANAGEMENT AND TREATMENT

The prevention and treatment of sleep problems in childhood often can be handled within the context of routine health-maintenance visits. Most commonly, effective management involves changing parental interventions rather than prescribing medication.

Appropriate sleep management involves establishing a regular daily routine in which the expectation for total sleep decreases as the child ages. Infants should be placed in a crib that is located separate from the parents' bedroom, if possible, and put to sleep when drowsy but still awake. Nighttime interventions should be minimal, and middle-of-the-night feedings should be discontinued as soon as feasible, usually by 4 to 6 months of age.

In toddlers and preschoolers, a pleasant, calming bedtime routine should be instituted. Typically, this might involve bathing, changing clothes, having a snack, brushing teeth, toileting, reading books, or playing with quiet toys or games. A night light may help to allay fears of the dark. The routine might end with a positive statement such as, "go to sleep now; sweet dreams," or "see you in the morning." Further bids for parental attention should be handled in a neutral but firm fashion. School-aged children need less assistance to meet their physical needs but often enjoy parental contact at the end of the day. Adolescents generally prefer to arrange their own bedtime activities.

Bedtime struggles in sleepy children are usually solved by firm handling and a definite time for "lights out." When children know that nothing else will happen no matter what they do, they usually give in to their fatigue and fall asleep. Children who are not sleepy should have their schedules adjusted gradually, by 15 minutes per day, eliminating unnecessary naps or shifting naps to the early afternoon and moving the bedtime and wake-up time until the desired schedule has been achieved.

Night waking in infants may be handled successfully by discontinuing maladaptive sleep-onset associations, night feeding, parental physical contact, and other positive reinforcements. Such waking may be handled by systematically ignoring it (which may result in excessive crying, but often is successful within a week) or by a gradual withdrawal of parental attention, with verbal reassurance given every so often on a consistent or gradually decreasing basis. The parent may also elect to provide bedside reassurance for three nights by placing a cot in the child's room and providing only verbal reassurance during nighttime awakenings.

A child who wakes after a nightmare should be reassured that the dream is over and he or she is safe in bed. The child also may be helped by talking about the dream the next day. It is helpful for parents to be aware of violent themes in movies, television shows, or the news, because the nightmare may replay these vicarious experiences. Frequent nightmares also may be a symptom of more serious distress that deserves an initial psychosocial assessment by the pediatrician, with referral to a mental health practitioner for further assessment and treatment if necessary.

The parents of a child experiencing a night terror should be reassured of the benign nature of the event. Effective management requires simple observation, because efforts to promote full wakefulness only prolong the event. When night terrors are recurrent and frequent, several nights of anticipatory awakening before the usual time of the event have been reported to eliminate the phenomenon. For the sleepwalking child, the environment should be made safe and the child merely observed or gently led back to bed. It has been reported that awakening the child for several nights before the usual time of sleepwalking will eliminate future episodes. Sleeptalking requires no intervention.

NATURAL HISTORY AND PROGNOSIS

Between 6 months and 4 years of age, problematic night waking and bedtime struggles are reported to persist for up to several years if no intervention is provided. By school age, children typically are not put to bed, are given a certain leeway about how and when they fall asleep, and generally can handle night wakings without parental intervention. The spontaneous resolution of night terrors can be expected, although a subsequent history of sleepwalking is common. Sleepwalking usually resolves spontaneously by adolescence. The relation between early childhood sleep problems and adult sleep difficulties has not been well studied.

References

Adair RH, Bauchner H: Sleep problems in childhood. Curr Probl Pediatr 23:147–170, 1993

American Sleep Disorders Association: International classification of Sleep Disorders: Diagnostic and Coding Manual. Lawrence, KS, Alan Press, 1990

Cuthbertson J, Schevill S: Helping Your Child Sleep Through the Night. New York, Doubleday, 1984

Dahl RE: The development and disorders of sleep. Adv Pediatr 45:73–91, 1998

Ferber R: Solve Your Child's Sleep Problems. New York, Simon & Schuster, 1985

Lozoff B, Askew AW, Wolf AW: Cosleeping and early childhood sleep problems: effects of ethnicity and socioeconomic status. J Dev Behav Pediatr 17:9–15, 1996

Madansky D, Edelbrock C: Cosleeping in a community sample of 2- and 3-year-old children. Pediatrics 86:197–203, 1990

5.5.3   Eating

Barbara J. Howard

Eating is a basic requirement for human survival. Parents may consciously or unconsciously equate their ability to feed their child with their own success as parents, and their child's willingness to eat with the child's love for them. The emotional issues associated with feeding can produce a variety of problems, ranging from daily irritation with messes to life-threatening malnutrition. The forms of potential interactional problems change as the child and the parent negotiate the shift in balance between the child's early need for dependence and the child's later quest for independence. Constitutional reasons for feeding problems, while much less common and often subtle, also must be considered.

EARLY INFANT FEEDING PROBLEMS—BIRTH TO 6 MONTHS

Suckling begins at 34 weeks of gestation but coordination of suckling and breathing does not emerge until 36 weeks. Neonates who are slow to make the adjustment to oral feedings, especially those born prematurely, may have an inadequate suck that keeps them from taking in enough calories to grow. Such infants often require transient tube feedings. Immaturity of gastrointestinal motility patterns also may result in excessive spitting and erratic feeding schedules. Careful attention to feeding cues, setting a regular schedule for erratic feeders, and gradual advancement of feeding times and volumes all will help during the few months that such problems of homeostasis may take to resolve.

Temperamentally irregular, poorly adaptable, overly sensitive infants often have erratic feeding cues that are difficult to recognize. However, even infants whose cues are easily recognizable can be challenging to feed if caregivers cannot adjust to their individual style. Parents may not respond to their infant's feeding signals because of anxiety; depression; other serious mental illness; substance use; a sense that the baby is vulnerable or that weight gain is critical; concern about their own adequacy or willingness to nurture; pressure from others; psychosocial stresses; or an intense desire to succeed. The frustration and concern that often develop can seriously complicate feedings, interfere with breast milk let down, and result in negative feelings toward the infant.

After obtaining a careful history of feeding and temperamental patterns, and preferably after observing a feeding interaction, the pediatrician can help parents to understand their infant's style, recognize feeding cues, wait for the baby's initiatives, respect pauses and satiety cues, and find nonnutritive ways of consoling the baby between feedings. Generally, the most important part of the management is eliciting the parents' expectations of the child and of themselves as caregivers (which often are based on how they themselves were parented), identifying the psychosocial stresses the parents are experiencing, and assuring that the parents have adequate supports. Most interactional feeding problems can be resolved in days to weeks, depending on the depth of the underlying psychological difficulties. When disregarded, the problems often continue for years and may evolve into other interactional problems. Because 30% of child abuse cases occur to infants under 6 months of age, parenting frustrations during this period should not be considered trivial.

Excessive spitting up occurs in 15% of normally developing infants. This can result from gastroesophageal reflux (GER), overfeeding, temperamental sensitivity, or tension in the feeding interaction. A modest amount of reflux of stomach contents through an insufficient lower esophageal sphincter is normal during the first year of life. However, if sufficient nutrition is lost or an aversion to feeding develops, the child can fail to gain, or even lose, weight. Tense or sensitive infants may have higher gastric motility, or simply become aversive in the feeding situation, because of the associated negative emotions. If spitting is persistent but growth and the parent–child relationship are good, and the child is not being overfed, the parents can be reassured. Even spitting because of true GER resolves in 60 to 80% of children between 9 and 18 months of age. When feedings are given to ease crying and overfeeding occurs, oral intake should be reduced, and alternative consoling methods such as swaddling, pacifiers, or carrying should be taught. If there is significant tension during feedings, this should be explored in depth and counseling provided. Excessive spitting, when accompanied by gagging, choking, aspiration, apnea, or poor weight gain, usually indicates GER, which can be treated with thickened feeds, pharmacologic interventions, prone positioning, and attention to associated complications (see Sec. 17.10.4).

Rumination, or apparently pleasurable, habitual regurgitation and reswallowing of the stomach contents, may occur with or without GER as a result of increases in intraabdominal pressure. The fingers or fist are often inserted into the mouth to initiate a gag. This behavior also may be a symptom of esophagitis. Psychogenic rumination is a symptom of inadequate nurturing in infancy, with an average age at onset of 5 months. Self-stimulatory rumination presents at any age but almost exclusively in children with severe or profound mental retardation. However, the latter also can be perpetuated by the secondary gain of the attention it attracts, especially if nurturing is inadequate. Five times as many males as females develop either kind of rumination.

Clinically significant rumination is rare, making up less than 1% of admissions to children's hospitals. However, the complications of malnutrition, electrolyte imbalance, and aspiration account for a 15% mortality rate. Persistent rumination requires an evaluation for GER, developmental assessment, and investigation of all the child's caregiving environments. Most symptoms of psychogenic rumination resolve in 1 week if the caregivers hold the infant for 15 minutes before, during, and after feedings, although problems related to parenting dysfunction may require months of treatment. Rumination in children with mental retardation may require behavioral feedback such as "time out," which generally improves the problem in 2 to 4 weeks.

Around 4 months of age, infants become more visually attentive and socially interactive, and they often turn away from the breast or bottle. Some parents interpret these exploratory moments as a personal rejection and either terminate feedings inappropriately or begin to wean the child prematurely, unless techniques for avoiding distractions are suggested. Midline play skills also emerge around 4 months, making it possible for infants to hold their own bottles. Although some parents take this as an opportunity to leave the baby alone with feedings, bottle propping is more common in neglectful or disturbed parent–child relationships. Supine self-feeding can result in otitis media, milk-bottle caries, chronic bronchitis, and occasionally, aspiration and death.

INFANT AND TODDLER FEEDING— 6 MONTHS TO 3 YEARS

By 6 months of age, infant desires begin to be expressed more clearly, yet some parents are unprepared to accept their child's strong preferences regarding texture and flavor. If parents push unwanted foods, they may promote feeding aversion. However, if a variety of textures are not introduced during this sensitive developmental period, difficulty in accepting solids may result later. When infants begin to show an interest in feeding themselves, starting around 6 months, parents may resist to avoid the mess, because they feel unready for their infant to "grow up," or because they are overly controlling. In turn, some infants react by refusing to eat,

even to the point of failing to gain weight. One strategy is to offer the infant finger foods and avoid spoon-feeding entirely. Advising the parents to feed the child over newspapers, with a bath to follow, can make the messiness more tolerable. Beyond providing concrete suggestions, parental concerns must be explored so that they do not interfere with the child's opportunities for self-feeding.

EATING PROBLEMS IN PRESCHOOL AND SCHOOL-AGED CHILDREN

Twenty-four percent of 2-year-old children, 19% of 3-year-old children, and 18% of 4-year-old children are reported to have problems with feeding, especially regarding "pickiness" related to taste, texture, and food combinations. Even during the first year of life, children will select a balanced diet over a period of weeks if offered only nutritionally valuable foods, but they will prefer sweet or sweet-fat combinations if they are available. Thus, to assure adequate nutrition for picky eaters, it is essential to limit foods with little nutritional value.

Intake generally tends to improve when a variety of foods are offered. The most powerful influences on a child's food preferences are cultural traditions, modeling by family members (especially siblings), and the emotions expressed around food. It takes more than 10 to 15 tasting exposures to increase the likelihood that a child will eat a previously rejected food. Using food as a reward heightens its desirability, but bribing a child to eat a certain food actually increases an aversion to it. Severe constipation also can produce poor appetite. The best strategy to improve eating includes establishing regular mealtime routines, ensuring a pleasant eating atmosphere, providing models of eating a variety of nutritious foods, facilitating multiple exposures to new foods, offering small servings, reducing between-meal calories (to enhance appetite), and avoiding pressure related to either the type or volume of intake.

Mealtime misbehaviors, such as getting up and down from the table, playing with food, and fighting with siblings, primarily occur when parents have not established control over the child's behavior in general. An effective management technique to prevent these types of problems is to serve the child in a highchair, or at the table, and to terminate the meal calmly when playing with food exceeds eating or there is significant misbehavior, regardless of how much the child has consumed. One hour later, the child may be offered either the same food or a healthy snack. This "second chance" to eat makes it more likely that all involved adults will be consistent in setting mealtime limits, because they need not feel as if they are depriving the child of food.

Older children often are picky because of the control it provides them, even to the point of refusing known favorite foods. This can be a sign that meals are being hurried, that the parents are overly concerned about the details of the diet, or that the child is oppositional overall. Advise parents that their job is to offer nutritious foods and to leave eating to the child as long as the child is capable of self-feeding. Children generally should be given limited choices, with at least one acceptable food or form of preparation. If all are rejected, no other food should be served at that meal. Other behavioral problems related to control should be explored and managed as well.

Beginning in preschool, some children demonstrate excessively emotional reactions to eating that manifest by food refusal, begging, or gorging as a response to overregulating, underregulating, or rejecting parenting. Such parent–child relationship problems must be addressed through family or individual counseling. In general, focal reactions to food can be separated from larger interpersonal dynamics quite quickly, and successful interventions can be provided. One simple management strategy is based on ensuring that the child has continuous access to a variety of nutritious finger foods kept on a low tray. If the parents are anxious, the amounts of these foods that are consumed by the child may be recorded, but there should be absolutely no comments about food made in the child's presence. The child should be brought to the table for meals and served a small portion, but not required to stay and eat. Begging can be dealt with by pointing to the tray. Gorging, which is common initially, should be ignored. It usually takes 4 to 7 days after the parents are capable of implementing this plan for the child to feel comfortable about the availability of food, for the social aspects of the meal to become more important than the struggles, and for the child to stop begging, gorging, or refusing food.

Food "phobias," which are defined as anxious avoidance of certain foods or textures, are almost universal in small degrees. Resistance usually develops following an episode of choking or nausea after eating, or in association with a traumatic incident. Chewing and swallowing also can take on symbolic psychological meaning, usually because of conflict over aggressive or sexual feelings or experiences. When simple avoidance is inconvenient, desensitization is the treatment of choice. Traumatic, symbolic, or intransigent cases may require psychotherapy. Resistance to certain textures of food also may be a sign of oral motor dysfunction, hyperactive gag reflex, pervasive developmental disorder, or tactile defensiveness. The refusal of certain categories of food, especially high-calorie types, may be associated with anorexia nervosa or bulimia.

Oral motor dysfunction may manifest by inadequate sucking or chewing; excessive or prolonged drooling; uncoordinated swallow; regurgitation; aspiration; hoarseness; nasal voice; posturing of the head or neck during feeding; and/or gagging or choking. Such difficulties can be associated with cerebral palsy, orofacial anomalies (including submucous cleft palate), and neuromuscular disease. Suprabulbar palsies may be subtle. Fully one-third of children with developmental disabilities affecting motor function have some feeding problem; the prevalence rises to 80% of children with severe or profound mental retardation. In the latter case, feeding can take 2 to 12 times longer than it would for children without special needs, and 15 to 20% of these children will have inadequate caloric intake. In such cases, symptoms are usually present from birth, but they also may appear at later ages. Treatment for oral motor dysfunction must be individualized and may include oral desensitization; swallowing training; provision of altered food textures; special positioning; pharmacotherapy and/or fundoplication for GER; and partial or total gavage or gastrostomy feedings. Prolonged reliance on normal feeding may result in difficulty weaning the child from the tube. Prognosis varies, but these problems often are difficult to resolve completely.

ASSESSMENT

A thorough history (including specific details about feeding, general child behavior, caregiver–child interaction, and family functioning) and the careful measurement of growth parameters are all that are required for assessing most eating concerns. Evidence of failure to thrive, or symptoms of oral motor dysfunction, GER, or rumination, indicate the need for a more complete evaluation. This should include a detailed feeding history focused on methods; positioning; duration (abnormal, >30 minutes); transitions to solid foods of different consistencies (including the child's reactions); timing of the emergence and management of self-feeding skills; and signs of oral motor dysfunction. The physical examination should focus on growth parameters; skinfold thickness; signs of cardiac or renal abnormalities; features of genetic syndromes; and evidence of orofacial anomalies (including bifid uvula and nasal septum suggestive of a submucous cleft). Any signs of chronic illness should be investigated further. The neurologic examination should focus on developmental skills, muscle tone, and primitive reflexes (especially the feeding reflexes of rooting, sucking, gag, and biting). A nutritional assessment, including a complete dietary record, should also be obtained. Therefore, a nutritionist or dietitian who is familiar with pediatric feeding problems is a key team member in the management of children with significant dysfunction. Direct observation of feeding with several types of provocative foods is needed, including an assessment of feeding position; pacing; parental sensitivity to cues; signs of tension or anxiety; child responses and signals; child self-feeding skills; and parental response to cooperative or oppositional child behaviors. This is best done by a team that includes either an occupational therapist or a speech pathologist with expertise with feeding problems who will address abnormal feeding behaviors such as tongue thrust; bite reflexes; aversive movements; choking; gagging; drooling; regurgitation; or rumination. Assessment scales are available to standardize or quantitate these observations.

When organic dysphagia is suspected, video fluoroscopy (ie, videotaping a fluoroscopic study of the swallowing of barium-treated foods) is essential for both diagnosis and treatment planning. This can confirm the presence of oral motor incoordination, aspiration, anatomic abnormalities, and responses to different food consistencies. Pharyngeal manometry is needed only if specific esophageal motor disorders are suspected. Overnight pH monitoring and a technetium-labeled milk scan can diagnose GER; the latter also determines transit time, gastric emptying, and aspiration. If these assessments are considered, a feeding team consultation is also indicated.

References

Hammer LD: The development of eating behavior in childhood. Pediatr Clin North Am 39:379–394, 1992

Howard BJ: Common issues in feeding. In: Levine MD, Carey WB, Crocker AC, eds: Developmental-Behavioral Pediatrics, 2nd ed. Philadelphia, Saunders, 1992

Kenny DJ, Koheil RM, Greenberg J, et al: Development of a multidisciplinary feeding profile for children who are dependent feeders. Dysphagia 4:16–28, 1989

Mayes SD, Humphrey FJ II, Handford HA, Mitchell JF: Rumination disorder: Differential diagnosis. J Am Acad Child Adolesc Psychiatry 27:300–302, 1988

Satter E: The feeding relationship: Problems and interventions. J Pediatr 117:S181–S189, 1990

Tuchman DN: Cough, choke, sputter: The evaluation of the child with dysfunctional swallowing. Dysphagia 3:111–116, 1989

Whitehead WE, Schuster MM: Behavioral approaches to the treatment of gastrointestinal motility disorders. Med Clin North Am 65:1397–1411, 1981

5.5.4 Pain

Kathy Ann Merritt

Pain is a ubiquitous phenomenon that observes no boundaries of age. Although pediatric health professionals frequently see children suffering pain, few efforts were made to understand pain phenomena in pediatric populations before the 1980s. Pain was rarely indexed in pediatric textbooks, and when it was discussed, the focus was on pain characteristics of specific disease states, not on pain as a distinct entity deserving dedicated evaluation and intervention. Past management of children with postoperative and procedural pain included physical restraint, separation from parents, and only rarely adequate pharmacologic intervention. Patients with nonspecific, recurrent pain syndromes were often managed with both over- and underindulgence by parents and the medical profession.

For years, a misconception existed regarding children's ability to perceive pain. Neurologic immaturity and incomplete myelinization were believed to protect young children from pain. This unfortunate myth was discredited by data demonstrating that the pain pathways and the cortical and subcortical centers necessary for pain perception are well developed by late in gestation. Additionally, neurochemical responses occur to normally pain-inducing stimuli, and these responses are attenuated by anesthesia. For humanitarian reasons, all pediatric patients must be protected from painful experiences. Religious and societal attitudes that defend pain as punishment, character building, or a sign of weak character are being effectively challenged by those who care for children in pain. It is no longer acceptable to perform a bone marrow aspiration, burn debridement, circumcision, lumbar puncture, or surgery without adequate attention to pain control.

As defined by the International Association for the Study of Pain (IASP), pain is "an unpleasant sensory and emotional experience associated with actual or potential damage, or described in terms of such damage." As such, it is a relevant variable throughout this general pediatric textbook. Within the IASP, a special interest group is dedicated to advancing the understanding, prevention, and treatment of pain in children. Empiric data continue to accumulate despite the subjective nature of pain, absence of gold standards for identifying and quantifying pain, and ethical constraints that limit the study of pain in children. Many improvements in the current "standard of care" reflect the findings of such data.

To guide the recognition, assessment, and management of pediatric pain, several authors have attempted to categorize pain experiences. Four generally accepted categories include:

1. Pain associated with a disease state (eg, arthritis, sickle cell disease);
2. Pain associated with an observable physical injury or trauma (eg, burns, fractures);
3. Pain not associated with a well-defined or specific disease state or physical injury (eg, tension headaches, recurrent abdominal pain); and
4. Pain associated with medical and dental procedures (eg, circumcisions, injections).

These categories are not mutually exclusive or exhaustive. For example, a child with cancer may have both chronic, intermittent pain associated with tumor infiltrating the periosteum and anticipatory, acute pain associated with a venipuncture. Common to each category, however, is the fact that pain, although unpleasant, serves to protect against continued noxious stimulation by alerting the sufferer and those charged with her or his protection to the importance of removing the source of discomfort. For the child with sickle cell disease, a painful crisis may herald an infection that, left untreated, may lead to significant morbidity or mortality. Pain felt when touching a hot skillet or during a medical procedure will prompt a child to withdraw to avoid further tissue damage. Complaints of recurrent abdominal pain may alert the physician to emotional concerns that are interfering with school performance and thus allow for timely intervention.

FACTORS THAT MODIFY CHILDREN'S PAIN PERCEPTIONS

Children can perceive pain without obvious injury, and they can sustain injury without experiencing pain. The pain perceived and/or expressed in response to noxious stimuli varies both among children and within the same child at different times depending on multiple factors, including age; cognitive development; gender; previous learning experiences; temperament; cultural and family factors; and situational factors.

Age

The anatomic and functional components required to perceive painful stimuli are present in the newborn. Pain-associated increases in heart rate, respiratory rate, cortisol, and palmar sweating, along with decreases in transcutaneous oxygen, are reliably observed in preterm and full-term neonates undergoing circumcision, heel stick, intubation, and endotracheal tube suctioning. Clearly, children's interpretation and expression of pain experiences evolve over time. Learning, previous experiences, and more sophisticated communication skills all contribute to differences in pain experiences, expressions, and behaviors. There is, however, no evidence to suggest that specific age-related changes in children's sensitivity to pain are responsible for the observed differences. In fact, it is likely that the differences reflect developmental experimental variability that is independent of age.

Cognition

Cognitive functioning is an important modulator of children's perception of pain. Children's ability to communicate and understand issues related to etiology, diagnosis, and treatment changes over time. Developmental transitions in pain reactivity correspond to three major Piagetian stages: (a) preoperational; (b) concrete operational; and (c) early formal operational. With maturity, shifts in thinking occur; concrete perceptions become more abstract, sophisticated, and psychologically oriented; subjective, egocentric thinking becomes more objective; and the prelogical child becomes increasingly logical. With these shifts, children's definitions of pain evolve. Initially, pain is described in very concrete terms as "a thing," "something," or "it," and it is defined by a location in the body or by unpleasant physical properties. With time, the definition includes feeling or sensation, but without a specific location. Ultimately, pain can be described by a child in physiological, psychological, or psychophysiological terms.

In the minds of young children, an association between pain and transgression is supported by the findings of several studies on children's understanding of illness causality. When pain is experienced as an imagined "punishment for wrongdoing," children should be reassured with age-appropriate explanations of the etiology and plans for pain management. Specific reassurances should be gauged by the patient's level of cognitive functioning. For example, caution should be used when using references to time or discussing distant benefits of painful procedures. A healthy 2-year-old child will not be comforted when told "this shot will just hurt for a minute," because the child's concept of time is still ill defined. Similarly, a 5-year-old child will not be comforted when told "this shot will keep you from getting sick with measles." A teenager, however, is capable of understanding that discomfort from immunization is brief, minor, and necessary to protect against a preventable disease. Finally, with the stress of acute and chronic illness, children may regress, and chronologic age may not be the most appropriate indicator of their cognitive developmental level.

Gender

While there is evidence of both infants and older children that males are more tolerant of pain, it remains unclear whether observed gender differences result from genetic dissimilarities, gender-specific child-rearing practices, or societal biases in measurement.

Previous Pain Experience

Children's understanding of the sensory qualities, emotional impact, and coping strategies associated with pain are influenced by their previous experiences. There is evidence that inadequate analgesia during a child's initial experience with a medical procedure may be a more important factor driving subsequent reactions than the number of exposures to a specific procedure. Whether or not a child is likely to remember an upcoming painful procedure, efforts should be made to minimize negative associations with the first and subsequent procedures because of the potential impact on similar, subsequent events.

Temperament

Interest is growing in learning more about the association between temperament and children's responses to pain. Temperament is one way to describe characteristic behavioral styles; it is assumed to be biologically determined and reasonably stable. Adaptability (ie, ease or difficulty with which reactions to situations can be modified in a desirable way), rhythmicity (ie, predictability or unpredictability in the timing of biological functions), and approach-withdrawal (ie, nature of initial responses to a new stimulus) are three temperamental dimensions that correlate with pain-related distress behavior.

Cultural and Family Factors

The role of the family and the culture of origin on a child's experience with pain is not limited to genetic factors. Although certain pain-associated diseases are genetically determined (eg, sickle cell disease, cystic fibrosis) or influenced (eg, irritable bowel), pain responses in other clinical settings are shaped by family members' responses to their own pain and to the child's pain. Children learn from people they admire, and realistic parental reassurance teaches effective coping strategies. In some cultures, specific pain experiences may be perceived as essential, and thereby may enhance coping. When pain tolerance is viewed as a virtue, the child may be hesitant to complain, and therefore less likely to receive appropriate pain relief. Children who believe they have some control often tolerate pain more easily than those forced into a state of helplessness. Hence, children should be given control when appropriate, by using language such as, "Please hold this Band-Aid. When the lumbar puncture is over and there is no more 'hurt,' I'll take the Band-Aid and put it on your back."

Situational Factors

Psychological and contextual factors that are unique to each clinical situation exert broad influences on specific painful experiences. For example, adult behaviors have an impact on children's responses to pain. Medical staff demonstrate their respect for children and encourage coping by including them in discussions, listening responsively, and offering control when appropriate. Distress in children undergoing procedures is exacerbated by anxious parents, criticism of the child by adults, and apologies. Other influences that modify a child's experience of pain include the child's understanding of why the pain is occurring, expectation of relief, and available coping strategies.

ASSESSMENT AND MEASUREMENT

When referring to pain, the terms *assessment* and *measurement* are sometimes used interchangeably. Strictly speaking, assessment reflects a more global appraisal of the pain experience, and measurement involves quantifying specific aspects of that experience. Currently available techniques for assessing and measuring pain include behavioral measures (both verbal and nonverbal), psychological measures (eg, galvanic skin response, salivary cortisol, transcutaneous oxygen saturation, cardiovascular responses), subjective judgments of the experience (eg, by parent, physician, or nurse), and self-report (eg, drawings, interviews, visual analogue scales).

Given differences in children and the crudity of available techniques to measure pain reactions, it is not surprising that the relation between measures of pain intensity and pain perception is not linear. Judgments of pain that compare findings between behavior, self-report, and physiological indicators show that factors contributing to one outcome measure may be different and independent from those contributing to another. Furthermore, the function of specific pain behaviors can vary among different children. For example, crying may serve as an emotional release, an adaptive coping strategy, or a means of achieving secondary gains.

RECURRENT PAIN SYNDROMES

Pain that is not associated with a specific disease state or identifiable physical injury can be very debilitating. Headache pain, abdominal pain, limb pain, and chest pain are four of the common recurrent pain syndromes reported in childhood. Each has the potential to be frightening, frustrating, and costly. Involving the patient and parent in the diagnostic evaluation by requesting a symptom diary (a description of pain, time of onset, duration, associated environmental events and symptoms, mitigating interventions) often facilitates diagnosis and medical management.

Headache

Epidemiology

Headaches are the most common recurrent pain in childhood. There are three general categories: (a) migraine; (b) tension; and (c) organic. Estimates of headache prevalence (ie, number of children with headache complaints at a given point in time) and incidence (ie, number of children who develop chronic headaches each year) vary dramatically. The majority of estimates reflect data from retrospective chart reviews and questionnaires completed by parents after their child's diagnosis. There is, however, general agreement that tension headaches are more common than migraines, that the average age of headache onset is approximately 7 years, and that headache prevalence is higher among girls and older children.

Clinical Manifestations

Migraine headaches, which are caused by vascular disturbances, must meet certain criteria. They must occur 5 or more times, last 2 to 72 hours, and have no identified etiology. Two of the following characteristics must be present: unilateral pain, pulsating/throbbing pain, moderate or severe intensity, and/or increasing severity with activity. In addition, the patient must report either associated nausea, photophobia, or phonophobia. Although usually spontaneous, migraines can be precipitated by psychological stress and other events.

Tension headaches, which are caused by muscular contraction, tend to become more severe later in the day. A pressing, dull, persistent tightness, often described as a band of pain, is characteristic.

Organic headaches are associated with structural pathology and metabolic or infectious disease. The severity and frequency generally increase, mild pain medications fail to relieve the discomfort over time, and the physical examination, history, and laboratory or imaging results will reveal the etiology. Additionally, headaches caused by tumor are frequently present on awakening in the morning.

Abdominal Pain

Epidemiology

Recurrent abdominal pain (RAP) is a common problem. It is reported that more than one-third of children complain of abdominal pain lasting 2 weeks or longer. Prevalence studies report the peak incidence among children between 7 and 10 years of age, more complaints in girls (12 to 19%) than boys (9 to 12%), and a higher incidence of abdominal pain and other somatic complaints in families of children with RAP than in families of nonaffected children.

Clinical Manifestations

RAP occurs in children 3 years and older. RAP is defined as pain that has occurred at least 3 times in 3 or more months. It is described as dull, crampy, or sharp pain in the periumbilical area. Although it interferes with daily living, there are periods of complete resolution, and, importantly, growth and development are normal. The traditional, simple "organic versus psychogenic" distinction fails to emphasize the multidimensional factors that place a child at risk for RAP. Evaluation and management of RAP is facilitated when attention is directed to identifying a somatic predisposition such as autonomic instability or gut motility. Similarly, environmental stress (eg, academic, athletic, social, familial), a model (eg, a vocal relative with ulcers), specific temperament characteristics, and learned response patterns (eg, secondary gain associated with abdominal pain) can exacerbate complaints. Organic etiologies that may present with abdominal pain include constipation, cholelithiasis, inflammatory bowel disease, lactase deficiency, pregnancy, and urinary tract infection. An organic etiology is reportedly responsible for only 5% of children diagnosed with RAP.

Limb Pain

Epidemiology

Recurrent limb pain, otherwise known as "growing pains," is the most common musculoskeletal problem of children, with prevalence estimates ranging between 5 and 15% of school-aged children. Consistent findings across surveys include a peak incidence

between 8 and 12 years of age and a gender difference, with girls being affected 1 to 2 times more often than boys.

Clinical Manifestations

Growing pains are benign limb pains (not due to growing) that are typically bilateral and characterized by deep, aching pain in the muscles of the legs. The pain varies in frequency, duration, and intensity. Most complaints are reported late in the day and resolve by morning. The pain does not involve joints, and it has no associated inflammation.

As with other recurrent pain syndromes, the diagnosis of growing pains requires thorough consideration and evaluation of the differential diagnoses. Conditions with organic etiologies include:

1. Trauma (eg, stress fracture, myositis ossificans);
2. Orthopedic problems (eg, chondromalacia patellae, Osgood-Schlatter disease);
3. Collagen vascular disorders (eg, juvenile rheumatoid arthritis, fibromyalgia);
4. Infections (eg, viral, bacterial, vaccine injection);
5. Neoplasms (eg, leukemia); and
6. Miscellaneous (eg, endocrine, storage diseases).

Psychosomatic conditions include school phobia, reflex neurovascular dystrophy, and hysteria-conversion reactions.

Chest Pain

Epidemiology

Chest pain in pediatric patients is least likely to be cardiac in origin and rarely a symptom of a life-threatening condition. One large, urban pediatric emergency room reported chest pain as the chief complaint for 6 in 1000 visits, and it is the second most common reason for referral to pediatric cardiologists. The differential is exhaustive, although the etiology is most often idiopathic. In patients older than 13 years, the cause is more likely psychogenic. Females and males are equally represented. The average age of presentation of 13 years is older than for other common pain syndromes.

Clinical Manifestations

In the pediatric patient, specific complaints of chest pain generally reflect the benign, although often chronic, course. Nevertheless, the evaluation must include a thorough history, physical examination, and if indicated, laboratory evaluation if one is to diagnose the rare, life-threatening event and allow for a timely intervention. Once a life-threatening disease is excluded, the diagnosis and management plan necessary for healing can continue.

Cardiac etiologies can be grouped as anatomic lesions, acquired lesions, and arrhythmias. Findings on history include fatigue, decreased exercise tolerance, irregular heart rate/rhythm, crushing chest pain, and shortness of breath. A review of systems directed toward cardiac, gastrointestinal, musculoskeletal, psychiatric, and pulmonary disease can be used to refine the physical examination. On physical examination abnormalities of the cardiovascular system (a pathologic murmur, gallop, rub, distant heart sound), the abdomen (hepatomegaly), and/or the endocrine system (thyromegaly) can direct the laboratory investigation. A 12-lead ECG, chest x-ray, echocardiogram, and blood values of specific interest can guide treatment strategies when necessary.

ASSESSMENT, MANAGEMENT, AND TREATMENT OF RECURRENT PAIN SYNDROMES

Several general principles to guide the assessment, diagnosis, and management of recurrent pain syndromes should be noted. First, children and parents may find it helpful to acknowledge that the complaint reflects real pain and requires a specific treatment plan. Second, scheduling adequate time for the evaluation increases the likelihood that the diagnosis can be based on positive evidence; in other words, avoid approaching the diagnosis by "ruling out" organic etiologies. An interactive history and physical examination can blur the conventional distinction between diagnosis and treatment by facilitating an alliance between the child, parent, and physician. A heightened awareness of the dynamics of the pain syndrome is facilitated, and an interpretation of the findings and implementation of management strategies is underway from the beginning. Third, search for positive evidence that explains the pain by interviewing the child and parent separately. This enhances the opportunity for inquiry about known constitutional predispositions to specific pain and other variables with an impact on pain experiences such as (a) family, school, and personal routines; (b) temperament and coping skills; and (c) critical events in the child's environment. Explore specific diagnoses that frighten the child or parent. Find out why they chose to seek medical attention when they did. If the pain is interfering with school attendance, facilitating the child's immediate return to school is of paramount importance, because social isolation can exacerbate the perception of pain. Consider adding adjuncts to the history, such as a quantitative estimation scale for a description of pain, a drawing of the pain and symptoms, and/or a pain diary (eg, time of onset, duration, severity, activities, diet, relief). This information can be used in the initial assessment; at follow-up visits, the information will provide comparison data against which to evaluate and quantify improvement. Fourth, clinicians and patients benefit when requests for the laboratory and imaging procedures are based on historical and clinical data. Avoid the shotgun approach of ordering laboratory and imaging procedures regardless of specific questions generated from the unique features of the patient under evaluation. Fifth, after reviewing all data, consider a referral or a consultation. The usefulness of a referral will vary depending on the patient, complaint, and experience of the referring physician and consultant. Sixth, present the working diagnosis and management plan to the family in a timely fashion. Include a description of the pain and reassure the child and family that the problem is common and not likely to be life-threatening. A discussion of specific diagnoses that the child and/or parent feared is critical. Include an explanation of management strategies and arrangements for ongoing follow-up.

Treatment options for the patient with recurrent pain must reflect the type and severity of pain as well as the situational, emotional, familial, and behavioral factors that trigger and exacerbate the pain. In general, it is advisable for patients to avoid known precipitating events and emotional or environmental factors that exacerbate pain syndromes. Behavioral, dietary, and pharmacologic therapy as well as reassurance are interventions associated with symptom reduction.

PAIN MANAGEMENT

Managing pain responses in children is challenging and involves attention to multiple factors. The goal is to facilitate adaptive coping.

Nonpharmacologic Interventions

Nonpharmacologic interventions with demonstrated efficacy in reducing procedural pain in pediatric patients include behavioral, cognitive, and physical strategies.

Behavioral Strategies

Behavioral interventions, including biofeedback, desensitization, exercise, and play therapy, reduce pain via a combination of mechanisms. Biofeedback teaches the child with pain to distinguish between relaxed and tense body states. Electrical and thermoregulatory activities of the body are translated into visual or auditory signals that the child can use to direct self-induced relaxation strategies. Biofeedback is particularly useful when pain is temporarily associated with stress or tension (ie, headaches, abdominal pain, preprocedural anxiety). Desensitization requires systematic pairing of an anxiety-arousing event with a response that is incompatible with anxiety. By coupling coping strategies that increase relaxation, control, and understanding of the treatment with gradual exposure to the noxious stimulus, the child learns to reduce his or her anxiety and to cope with the painful experience.

Exercises, such as jumping rope, swimming, and walking, are also recommended for patients with chronic and recurrent pain. By normalizing and routinizing daily activities, the focus on pain is redirected to age-appropriate recreation. Anxiety decreases, and depression accompanying the pain is reduced through serotonin production and β-endorphin release associated with exercise. Play therapy reduces emotional and physical pain by providing distraction, relaxation, and stress reduction. Trained therapist (ie, child-life workers) offer books, clay, games, paint, puppets, and toys to evaluate children's understanding of illness and pain, to assess and model coping strategies, and to facilitate children's efforts to gain mastery over their fears.

Children experiencing pain are almost unanimous in their desire to have a parent present. Separating children from parents intensifies feelings of vulnerability and likely exacerbates pain, yet to some pediatric professionals, parental presence remains a controversial issue. Consequently, preparing parents and actively supporting their presence during painful procedures is an underused technique in pediatric settings. Parents are a valuable source of information regarding the coping strategies likely to help their child during painful experiences. With guidance and appropriate support, most parents are eager to accept instruction on how they can facilitate coping. For example, a parent may be told, "You can help your child by sitting in this chair, holding her hand, and singing her favorite tune. We will assume responsibility for helping her hold still during this blood draw." Educating, empowering, and supporting parents facilitates positive involvement during their child's painful procedures. Additionally, when they are present, parents can gain comfort from seeing staff members doing everything possible to provide optimal care. Excluding a parent simply for the convenience of the professional staff is unacceptable.

Cognitive Interventions

Cognitive interventions, including distraction and hypnosis, actively reduce pain by focusing the child's attention away from a noxious stimulus and toward nonthreatening, pleasant experiences. Both strategies are readily available, inexpensive, and highly valuable.

Common distraction techniques that can be used with children include bubble blowing, coughing or whistling, hand-holding, visual or auditory involvement with intriguing toys, and singing.

When using hypnosis, the clinician enters the child's world. After helping the child achieve a relaxed physical state, the power of fantasy and imagination is used to focus attention and to create an altered state of consciousness. Unpleasant experiences can be modified through suggestions for altering sensations. Suggested hypnotic techniques for infants include rocking, singing, and playing peek-a-boo. Preschoolers respond to pretend situations such as blowing candles at a birthday party (ie, deep breathing), storytelling, puppets, bubble blowing, and singing. School-age children can use favorite-place imagery (eg, riding on a roller coaster, lying on the beach), stories with superheroes and superheroines, drawing, and metaphors to refocus. With increasing maturity, progressive relaxation, create-a-story, and computer activities are beneficial. To use hypnosis requires training and experience. Workshop information is available through various pediatric and hypnosis societies.

Physical Interventions

Physical interventions include anesthetic blocks, topical anesthetics, and multiple physical therapies. These strategies reduce pain by blocking peripheral or central nerve pathways. Anesthetic nerve blocks with lidocaine and bupivacaine temporarily interrupt transmission of nociceptive stimuli and can provide pain relief during circumcision, dental procedures, and minor orthopedic procedures. Topical anesthetics, such as lidocaine and, more recently, EMLA (eutectic mixture of local anesthetics) cream, are available to numb the skin surface for venipuncture, immunization, and minor surgical procedures. Physical therapies modify pain sensations by stimulating a region with pressure (eg, massage), heat, cold, or weak electrical currents (eg, transcutaneous electrical nerve stimulation).

Pharmacologic Interventions

Pharmacologic interventions are critical for certain children and certain situations. "Analgesic" refers to drugs that decrease pain without a loss of consciousness.

Orally Administered Analgesia

In pediatrics, nonnarcotic analgesics that are used to manage fever, inflammation, and mild levels of pain include acetaminophen, aspirin, and other nonsteroidal anti-inflammatory drugs. Narcotic analgesics required for relief of moderate to severe pain include morphine, codeine, and synthetic/semisynthetic agents (eg, meperidine, oxycodone). Combinations of aspirin or acetaminophen with codeine are available and provide anti-inflammatory properties, as well as pain relief.

Local Anesthesia

Local anesthetics are agents that reversibly block conduction of neural impulses along nerve pathways. An appropriate agent must be physically deposited by injection of topical application. Fibers carrying stimuli from pain receptors have relatively smaller diameters and less myelin than larger, heavily myelinated fibers carrying pressure and touch sensation, and they are blocked first and by lesser amounts of anesthesia. To minimize discomfort accompanying injection, sodium bicarbonate can be added in a 1:10 ratio to buffer an acidic pH of the anesthetic, the anesthetic can be warmed to 37 degrees Celsius, and a slow rate of injection through a 30-gauge needle can begin as soon as the needle enters the skin.

The two major classes of local anesthetic agents are esters (procaine, chloroprocaine, tetracaine, and cocaine) and amides (lidocaine, mepivacaine, bupivacaine). To block nerve conduction, a minimum concentration (influenced by fiber diameter, degree of myelination, anesthetic pH, tissue calcium concentration, and rate of nerve stimulation) of the desired agent is required. The quality and duration of action of a block can be enhanced by the addition of a vasoconstrictor. Epinephrine delays absorption of the agent, thereby prolonging its action. By decreasing the need for a concentrated solution, the potential for toxicity is reduced. And, finally, by causing local vasospasm, bleeding is reduced. For this reason, epinephrine should not be used in tissue supplied by an end artery, such as digits, the ear pinna, nasal alae, or the penis because of the risk of tissue ischemia or necrosis.

Topical anesthetics are understandably popular in pediatrics and should be considered when appropriate. One must review onset of action, presence of epinephrine, site requiring analgesia (open or closed wound and location), potential toxicity, and known allergies to determine the best preparation of those preparations currently available (TAC—tetracaine, adrenaline, cocaine; LET—lidocaine, epinephrine, tetracaine; EMLA, lidocaine and prilocaine).

Patient-Controlled Analgesia

Another approach to managing children's pain is patient-controlled analgesia (PCA), which allows the child to press a button and self-administer a small dose of analgesic drug via an intravenous catheter and a programmable pump device. The therapeutic benefits of PCA for managing pain have been demonstrated in children with postoperative pain. PCA eliminates insufficient dosing of pain medication that is associated with staff reluctance to administer drugs resulting from fears of addiction and side effects. Children's preference to endure pain to avoid a feared intramuscular injection is obviated. Finally, pain and anxiety are diminished by providing the patient with control. When compared to more conventional routes and p.r.n. scheduling, patients prefer PCA and use less analgesia postoperatively.

In summary, pediatric pain was ignored until recently by many in the medical profession. Fortunately, major efforts continue to learn more about the biological, psychological, and social underpinnings of pediatric pain, and to integrate new knowledge into clinical pediatric settings. As expertise in understanding, preventing, assessing, and managing pediatric pain increases, the goal must be to place the welfare of the child above all other considerations, including the convenience of the physician and the hospital rules.

References

Anand KJ, Hickey PR: Pain and its effects in the human neonate and fetus. N Engl J Med 317:1321–1329, 1987

Boyce WT, Barr RG, Zeltzer LK: Collection of papers from the William T. Grant Foundation Research Consortium on the Developmental Psychobiology of Stress. Pediatrics 90:483–513, 1992

Bush JP, Harkins SW, eds: Children in Pain, Clinical and Research Issues from a Developmental Perspective. New York, Springer-Verlag, 1991

Coleman WL: Recurrent pain and Munchausen syndrome by proxy. In: Levine MD, Carey WB, Crocker AC, eds: Developmental-Behavioral Pediatrics. Philadelphia, Saunders, 339–349, 1992

Dahlquist LM, Gil KM, Armstrong D, Delawyer DD, Greene P, Wuori D: Preparing children for medical examinations: The importance of previous medical experience. Health Psychol 5:249–259, 1986

Emslander HC: Local and topical anesthesia for pediatric wound repair: A review of selected aspects. Pediatr Emerg Care 14:123–130, 1998

Frothingham TE: Chronic pain. In: O'Quinn A, ed: Management of Chronic Disorders of Childhood. Boston, Hall, 164–178, 1985

Kocis KC: Chest pain in pediatrics. Pediatr Clin North Am 46:189–203, 1999

McGrath PA: Pain in Children: Nature, Assessment, and Treatment. New York, Guilford Press, 1990

Olness K: Hypnosis and Hypnotherapy with Children, 2nd ed. Philadelphia, Grune & Stratton, 1988

Ross DM, Ross SA: Childhood Pain: Current Issues, Research, and Management. Baltimore, Urban & Schwarzenberg, 1988

Schechter HL, ed: Acute pain in children. Pediatr Clin North Am 36:781–1052, 1989

Schechter NL, Bernstein BA, Beck A, Hart L, Scherzer L: Individual differences in children's response to pain: Role of temperament and parental characteristics. Pediatrics 87:171–177, 1991

5.5.5   Adaptation to Illness

David J. Schonfeld and Ellen C. Perrin

Children frequently experience minor illnesses; during their first year alone, children experience an average of 5 to 7 respiratory or gastrointestinal illnesses. Many children also have a long-term illness that may be associated with restrictions in daily activities, physical disabilities, and repetitive, often painful, treatments and hospitalizations. Estimates of the prevalence of chronic illness range from 15 to 20% of children, with estimates even higher if less serious conditions are included. Approximately 2% of children from birth to 21 years of age have a chronic condition that is severe enough to significantly alter their daily lives.

Illnesses and their treatment are predictably upsetting experiences for children and their families. They represent potential stressors that can *interfere* with normal development, but they also provide an opportunity for mastery, which can enhance self-esteem and *promote* development. It is important to appreciate how children of various ages typically interpret and react to physical illness and its treatment to identify ways of minimizing the negative impact of such experiences and of maximizing their positive potential. This section reviews the developmental process by which children come to understand physical illness and its treatment; children's reactions to acute and chronic illness; the normative reactions of children to the treatment process, including medical procedures and hospitalization; and guidelines for assisting children to understand and cope with illness and treatment.

CHILDREN'S UNDERSTANDING OF PHYSICAL ILLNESS AND ITS TREATMENT

Children develop an increasingly sophisticated understanding of physical illness and its treatment as the result of both biological maturation and the accumulation of relevant experiences. Developmental theorists (such as Piaget) describe important qualitative differences in the basic ways that children at different developmental stages see, interpret, and come to understand various phenomena, including physical illness and its treatment. Effective support and assistance at the time of illness is predicated on an appreciation of this developmental process.

Very young children often rely on magical thinking and phenomenistic explanations and may attribute the cause of illness to *immanent justice,* the belief that good is naturally rewarded and misdeeds are punished. Such beliefs lead to a child's adopting explanations for illness etiology based on personal guilt or the attribution of guilt to others. Immanent justice explanations are used more persistently in situations in which the child has had less personal experience and for which more adequate explanations have not been provided.

As young children develop a more accurate understanding about the causes of illness, the concept of contagion appears in their explanations of illness cause and transmission. Initially, such explanations are often overextended to include even noninfectious conditions. By about 9 or 10 years of age, children believe that germs must be internalized to cause illness, but usually are not able to elaborate on the process or mechanism by which illness results. By 12 or 13 years of age, children begin to appreciate the complicated interactions between host and agent in disease causation and recovery from illness. It is often not until at least adolescence that children can associate apparently unrelated symptoms (eg, sore throat and a rash) or different stages of an illness and appreciate that they belong to a single disease process. During adolescence, children develop a better understanding of physiology, enabling them to appreciate the rationale underlying many common treatments, such as the use of insulin in diabetes or bronchodilators for asthma.

Young children may fail to accurately report symptoms of physical illness because they can only describe the processes of bodily functioning or illness causality without understanding the processes. They may not understand the relationship of symptoms to a disease process (eg, that dizziness or headache might be symptoms of hypoglycemia). Magical thinking and egocentrism may lead children to conclude that they can deal with symptoms on their own, without reporting them to adults. In addition, immanent justice beliefs may encourage the withholding of information out of shame or fear of punishment. In frustration, parents, and even health-care providers, may unwittingly reinforce maladaptive views of treatment as a form of punishment by "threatening" the child with worsening health or invasive procedures (eg, "If you don't take your asthma medicine, your wheezing will get worse and you'll have to go to the hospital and get a shot."). While such strategies might yield short-term compliance with treatment regimens, they fail to help a child reach a better understanding of underlying health concepts or the rationale for a treatment. These issues are particularly relevant for children with a chronic medical condition, who are often asked to identify and report subtle symptoms (eg, shortness of breath) that may result in unpleasant or painful treatments.

Less is known about how children come to understand the cause of psychological conditions. Children younger than 10 or 11 years of age appear to attribute the causes of psychological symptoms to genetic and perinatal difficulties, while older children more often impute social and intrafamilial difficulties.

CHILDREN'S REACTIONS TO ACUTE ILLNESS

Many factors, such as those listed in Table 5-3, may influence children's reactions to acute illness and its treatment. Influencing factors include those that are intrinsic to the child or related to the nature of the family support as well as specific characteristics of the illness and the treatment process. The child's understanding of the illness and its treatment becomes increasingly more important for children after 4 years of age. Systematic preparation of the child with specific information and developmentally appropriate explanations facilitates the psychological and physiological adjustment of children to illness, difficult procedures, and hospitalization. Preparation also enhances a child's ability to cooperate with treatment, and assists parents by decreasing their anxiety and improving their satisfaction with the treatment process.

TABLE 5-3

FACTORS AFFECTING THE IMPACT OF ILLNESS AND ITS TREATMENT

Child-Dependent Factors
  Child's age and developmental capabilities
  Temperament, personality, coping style, locus of control
  Genetic predisposition (eg, pain threshold)
  Past experiences with illness and hospitalization
  Prior preparation regarding procedures and hospitalization
Characteristics of Family
  Perceived meaning of illness for family
  Degree of support among family members
  Nature of preexisting parent–child relationship
  Practical resources to deal with problems (eg, financial resources)
Characteristics of Illness and Its Treatment
  Perceived meaning of illness for child
  Nature of illness, injury, or treatment
    Stability and predictability of course; prognosis
    Visibility of disability; limitations on cognitive abilities; functional
      impairments
  Amount of pain/discomfort associated with illness and treatment
  Requirement for procedures/surgery
  Length and frequency of hospitalization

The experience of minor acute illness provides children with some opportunities for constructive learning, which may help them in coping with their own or other family members' illnesses in the future. They learn, for example, that acute illnesses are generally transient and time-limited, that simple remedies may help to relieve the symptoms, and that their bodies are equipped with remarkable restorative mechanisms. For both parents and children the symptoms provide a salient "laboratory" from which to observe and learn about the processes of bodily functioning and dysfunction.

Both during and following a serious illness, a broad range of behavioral sequelae can be anticipated. Many of these effects represent behavioral regression (eg, thumb sucking, enuresis, sleep and feeding problems) or emotional and social regression (eg, increased dependency, decreased ability to share). Some regression during illness is appropriate, allowing the child to accept care and nurturance and to adjust to the stressors at hand. Severe regression (eg, biting in a 5-year-old child, incontinence in a child who has been toilet trained for several years), on the other hand, can be especially uncomfortable to the child as well as the family, and it may necessitate intervention. Children may also manifest a broad range of internalizing behaviors (eg, aggressive behavior, acting out). It should be noted as well that serious illness and hospitalization may act as stressors that exacerbate preexisting emotional or family problems, which may then become evident and accessible to intervention.

CHRONIC ILLNESS AND CHILD DEVELOPMENT

Chronic illness and physical disabilities may pose different challenges to children and their families, depending on the developmental stage of the child as outlined in Table 5-4. The presence of a chronic illness during infancy, along with the attendant physical discomfort and disruption in routines, may compromise the consistency and dependability of an infant's environment, as well as undermine development of basic trust. An illness may also pose a serious challenge to the parents' emerging sense of competence and confidence in their new roles as parents. During later developmental stages, the necessity for parental involvement in the management

of a child's illness may interfere with toddlers' or older children's need for increasing independence and undermine their sense of self-control and autonomy. School-age children and adolescents may be concerned as well that restrictions, medication requirements, and visible disabilities associated with their condition could identify them as different from their peers (and thereby label them as "imperfect") and interfere with peer acceptance. Limitations imposed by the chronic condition may conflict with the need for increasing independence during adolescence, and it may compromise peer relationships and the emergence of a secure physical and sexual identity. Many of the factors affecting the impact of illness and its treatment that can be found in Table 5-3 apply to chronic illness as well.

While most children and their families find ways to adapt successfully to the extra demands of a chronic physical condition, children with a chronic condition have about twice the risk of experiencing some difficulty with emotional, social, or school functioning as compared with healthy peers. Children with chronic conditions

---

TABLE 5-4

CHALLENGES FOR CHILDREN WITH A CHRONIC HEALTH CONDITION AT DIFFERENT DEVELOPMENTAL STAGES

Infants and Toddlers
  Developmental Task
    Development of trust and security
  Challenges
    Chronic discomfort or pain
    Hospitalizations and painful procedures
    Altered eating/feeding experiences
    Restriction of movement
    Parental grief
Preschoolers
  Developmental Task
    Development of autonomy
  Challenges
    Need for adult supervision
    Repeated separations
    Medication requirements
    Dietary and mobility restrictions
    Impaired limit-setting by parents
    Limitations on peer interactions
School-Age Children
  Developmental Task
    Development of sense of mastery
  Challenges
    Requirements for adult monitoring
    Restrictions on independence
    Dependence on medical care
    Medication and dietary requirements
    Activity restrictions
    School absence
    Differences from peers
Adolescents
  Developmental Task
    Development of personal identity separate from family
  Challenges
    Requirements of medical supervision
    Enforced dependency
    Altered body image and visible deformity
    Decreased growth
    Medication and dietary requirements
    Vocational limitations
    Challenges to sexuality

are most likely to show evidence of low self-esteem, anxiety, depression, and social withdrawal. While the prevalence and types of adjustment problems may depend in part on the unique characteristics of specific conditions, most difficulties that children and their families encounter result from challenges common to a broad range of chronic illnesses.

CHILDREN'S REACTIONS TO HOSPITALIZATION

Approximately 5% of children in the United States are hospitalized each year. It is often difficult to separate the stress of hospitalization from that of the illness itself and its treatment. In fact, the impact may be synergistic and not simply additive. Hospitalization is almost universally stressful because of various factors related to the stress of separation, disruptions in routines, unfamiliarity with the people and surroundings, and fear and pain related to the illness and its treatment. Separation from parents and other significant family members is a particularly painful issue for children between 6 months and 4 years of age because of their physical, social, and cognitive immaturity and close, dependent relationship with their parents. It is important to minimize hospitalizations by using home-based treatment or day-surgery units and to restrict the use of invasive or painful procedures to situations in which alternatives are unavailable. Optimal control for any pain associated with the illness or its treatment should be a primary goal of pediatric medicine. By setting up a scenario in which the child can master an anticipated stressor (eg, allowing the child to administer injections to a doll), therapeutic play can be used to allow the child to turn helpless, passive feelings into a sense of active mastery. Additional principles to consider in reducing the stress associated with illness and hospitalization are found in Table 5-5.

TABLE 5-5

TECHNIQUES TO MINIMIZE THE STRESSES ASSOCIATED WITH ILLNESS AND HOSPITALIZATION

Prior preparation
General education for children before illness through media, schools, and during well-child pediatric visits
Prehospitalization tours, videos, educational material (eg, coloring books)
At the time of illness
Involve child and family members, including siblings, in discussions regarding the illness and its treatment
Support self-care and optimize child's sense of control and mastery by involving child in treatment decisions; offer choices when possible
Optimize pain control, including for procedures, and minimize functional limitations of illness
Maintain normal home and family routines
Maintain age-appropriate expectations of behavior, including chores, homework, and so on
Promote continued peer group involvement
Adapt family and school requirements as necessary
During hospitalization
Minimize length and number of hospital stays
Encourage and facilitate rooming-in and visiting of family members and friends
Child-life programs (recreation and therapeutic play); inpatient school programs
Provide continuity of care; minimize number of physicians, nurses, and students involved in care
Provide family-centered care

THE ROLE OF PREVENTIVE HEALTH EDUCATION

Health education should begin when children are well. Children should be taught more than to "just say no" to bad health decisions, and they must be helped to understand the rationale behind positive choices. Not only do children need to develop refusal skills with which to avoid risky behaviors but they also need to learn informed and responsible health decision-making skills in a context of gradually increasing personal responsibility. Health-care providers should use routine health-care visits as opportunities to advance not only parents' but also children's understanding of illness and its treatment. Unfortunately, while children bring many relevant questions about their health to these visits, pediatricians typically spend little time in direct discussion with the child; most of these questions go unaddressed. Brief educational interventions for children, parents, and physicians have been shown to enhance physician–child communication during well-child visits and to support the child in assuming a more active role. Health education in other settings (eg, school) is also effective in conveying factual information and in advancing a child's level of conceptual sophistication about illness processes.

References

Bauman LJ, Drotar D, Leventhal JM, Perrin EC, Pless IB: A review of psychosocial interventions for children with chronic health conditions. Pediatrics 100:244–251, 1997

Goslin ER: Hospitalization as a life crisis for the preschool child: A critical review. J Commun Health 3:321–346, 1978

Lavigne JV, Faier-Routman J: Psychological adjustment to pediatric physical disorders: A meta-analytic review. J Pediatr Psychol 17:133–157, 1992

Newacheck PW, Taylor WR: Childhood chronic illness: Prevalence, severity, and impact. Am J Public Health 82:364–371, 1992

Perrin EC: Hospitalization, surgery, and medical procedures. In: Levine MD, Carey WB, Crocker AC, eds: Developmental-Behavioral Pediatrics, 3rd ed. Philadelphia, Saunders, 1999:324–329

Perrin EC, Gerrity PS: Development of children with a chronic illness. Pediatr Clin North Am 31:19–31, 1984

Schonfeld DJ: The child's cognitive understanding of illness. In: Lewis M, ed: Child and Adolescent Psychiatry: A Comprehensive Textbook, 2nd ed. Baltimore, Williams & Wilkins, 1996:943–947

Schonfeld DJ, Johnson SR, Perrin EC, O'Hare LL, Cicchetti DV: Understanding of acquired immunodeficiency syndrome by elementary school children—A developmental survey. Pediatrics 92:389–395, 1993

Wallander JL, Varni JW, Babani L, Banis HT, Wilcox KT: Family resources as resistance factors for psychological maladjustment in chronically ill and handicapped children. J Pediatr Psychol 14:157–173, 1989

5.6 THE CONTINUUM FROM DEVELOPMENTAL VARIATION TO DISORDER

5.6.1 Hyperactivity: Overactivity to Attention-Deficit Disorder

Paul H. Dworkin

Few clinical concerns in pediatric care are as complex and controversial as questions about attention and activity. The very existence of a discrete disorder characterized by short attention span, impulsivity, and overactivity, termed *attention-deficit hyperactivity disorder,* is the subject of intense debate. Nonetheless, a group of children who have difficulty directing their attention and activity, and who consequently experience low educational achievement and a higher frequency of social and emotional problems, undeniably exists.

DEFINITIONS AND EPIDEMIOLOGY

The range for presentations of children with problems of attention and activity is extremely broad. The challenge for the clinician is to differentiate those behavioral traits that reflect normal developmental variations and temperamental characteristics from those that interfere with children's learning and behavior.

Behaviors Related to Normal Developmental Stages

A high level of activity and short attention span are normal developmental characteristics of infants and toddlers. During the preschool years, most children continue to have short attention spans and are unwilling to focus on tasks for more than a brief moment. Significant impulse control generally is not achieved until around 4 years of age. Despite the normality of such stage-related behaviors during the preschool years, they still may elicit parental concern and anxiety.

Variations in Temperament

Activity level, distractibility, persistence, and attention span are core manifestations of a child's temperament or behavioral style, and they vary widely in their expressions. The extent to which such traits contribute to school-related problems depends on their "goodness of fit" with the child's classroom environment (ie, the demands and expectations of teachers and the content of the curriculum). For example, children with a high activity level, high distractibility, and low persistence are noted to have "low task-orientation" in the classroom. A tendency toward inattention may be potentiated in the "difficult" child who is slowly adaptable to change, while such inattentiveness may be minimized in the "easy" child who adapts readily to new situations in the classroom.

Situational Inattention

So-called situational inattention may result when a young child is faced with developmentally inappropriate expectations in a highly academically oriented preschool setting, or when a school-age child is confronted with unrealistic curriculum demands. Such children do not display pervasive problems with attention and behave appropriately for their age under most circumstances.

Inattention Secondary to Various Conditions and Disorders

A child with a subtle language or learning disorder or mild cognitive impairment might be inattentive in the classroom because of difficulties in processing information or understanding directions and expectations. Symptoms of anxiety include decreased attention span and increased motor activity. Inattention and overactivity are often associated with primary neurologic disorders such as epilepsy, the sequelae of CNS infections or severe traumatic brain injuries, and with sensory impairment, lead poisoning, iron deficiency anemia, congenital infections, hyperthyroidism, and Sydenham chorea. Similar symptoms may appear as side effects of certain medications such as phenobarbital, antihistamines, and possibly theophylline, or they may be associated with social stressors such as domestic violence, child abuse or neglect, and loss of a family member.

Psychiatric Comorbidity

Children with attention deficits often fit the diagnostic criteria for oppositional defiant disorder, conduct disorder, autism/pervasive developmental disorder, and anxiety or affective disorders (eg, depression). Most children with learning disorders also demonstrate impaired attention, and up to 25% of children with specific learning disabilities also meet criteria for a diagnosis of attention-deficit hyperactivity disorder. Attention deficits are found among most children with Tourette syndrome.

Attention-Deficit Hyperactivity Disorder

A cluster of problems with attention, concentration, impulsivity, and overactivity emerging during early childhood and present under a variety of circumstances characterizes a behavioral syndrome termed *attention-deficit hyperactivity disorder (ADHD).* According to the American Academy of Pediatrics, the "disorders known as the attention-deficit hyperactivity disorders are chronic neurological conditions resulting from a persisting dysfunction within the central nervous system and are not related to gender, level of intelligence, or cultural environment." Examples of the behaviors that comprise the diagnostic criteria for ADHD, as published in the *DSM-IV,* are listed in Table 5-6.

Conservative estimates suggest that 2 to 4% of school-age children fulfill the diagnostic criteria for ADHD, with a male preponderance of about 3:1. However, cross-cultural differences in the ratings of hyperactive and disruptive behaviors have been found. For example, in Great Britain, the diagnosis of ADHD is applied sparingly for those children who demonstrate severe overactivity and inattentiveness in nearly all situations, and the diagnosis of "conduct disorder" is preferred for the majority of children with less-severe attentional problems.

TABLE 5-6

EXAMPLES OF INATTENTIVE, HYPERACTIVE, AND IMPULSIVE BEHAVIORS INCLUDED WITHIN THE CRITERIA FOR DIAGNOSIS OF ATTENTION-DEFICIT HYPERACTIVITY DISORDER

Inattentive Behaviors
  Is easily distracted by extraneous stimuli
  Makes careless mistakes in schoolwork or other activities
  Has difficulty sustaining attention in tasks or play activities
  Does not seem to listen to what is being said to him or her
  Fails to finish schoolwork, chores, or other duties
  Loses things necessary for tasks or activities
  Has difficulty organizing tasks and activities
  Forgetful in daily activities
Hyperactive/Impulsive Behaviors
  Runs about or climbs excessively in situations where it is inappropriate
  Fidgets with hands or feet or squirms in seat
  Has difficulty awaiting turn in games or group situations
  Blurts out answers to questions

SOURCE: *Based on the Diagnostic and Statistical Manual of Mental Disorders, 4th ed. Washington, DC: American Psychiatric Association, 1994.*

ETIOLOGY AND PATHOGENESIS

For most children with ADHD no etiology is identified. Longitudinal studies have failed to support the concept that neurologic damage during the pre- or perinatal period is a major cause of attention deficits. Although the demonstration of "soft neurologic signs" among some children with ADHD is cited to suggest delayed maturation of the CNS, such findings also are observed among normal children, as well as among those children with other behavior disorders. Evidence from family studies supports the role of genetic factors for at least a subgroup of children with ADHD; the increased prevalence of alcoholism, sociopathy, and hysteria among parents of children with ADHD suggests potential contributions from both the environment and genetics. Some data suggest a relationship between ADHD and dysfunction of the catecholamine neurotransmitters dopamine and norepinephrine, but further study is needed to substantiate this association. Furthermore, although neuroanatomic and neurophysiological variations have been reported in studies of individuals with ADHD (using such techniques as magnetic resonance imaging; single-photon emission tomography to quantify regional blood flow; positron-emission tomography scanning to examine rates of regional cerebral glucose metabolism; and EEG power spectral analysis to examine CNS arousal levels), their clinical significance remains speculative.

Prenatal and childhood exposures to a variety of toxins have also been associated with attention deficits. In addition, problems of activity and attention secondary to fetal alcohol exposure and lead poisoning are well documented. The effects of artificial food additives, sugar, and naturally occurring salicylates are controversial, and controlled studies generally have failed to substantiate such claims.

A recent theory proposes that the clinical manifestations of ADHD reflect an underlying problem with inhibitory control and difficulties with goal-directed persistence, rather than a deficit in attention per se. Barkley reframes ADHD as a "behavioral inhibition disorder" in which symptoms are primarily genetically mediated and psychosocial factors are unimportant. A fundamental deficit in time perception and poor linking of past actions to future planning contribute to a "temporal (time) neglect syndrome." The validity of this theory remains speculative.

Attention deficits do not have a single, specific cause. Rather, they represent the consequence of multidimensional "transactions" among intrinsic characteristics of the child and environmental factors, which is consistent with the biopsychosocial model. The documentation of such "polycausality" awaits multivariate investigations in which genetic, neurologic, and environmental variables are all studied.

CLINICAL MANIFESTATIONS

Children with attention deficits typically display some or all of the following symptoms.

Inattentiveness and Easy Distractibility. The child has significant difficulty selecting an appropriate stimulus and focusing on necessary tasks within a classroom, particularly when such tasks are protracted and tedious. Easy distractibility results in overfocusing on inappropriate stimuli and activities.

Impulsivity. Such children act quickly and without considering the consequences of their actions. Lack of planfulness is evident as careless errors are made and written work is messy.

Motor Restlessness and Hyperactivity. Early history frequently describes a child who wore a hole in the crib mattress, never walked but ran, and climbed over the crib bars despite extra precautions.

Manifestations in the school-aged child may include excessive fidgeting, squirming, and restlessness. Whether the presence or absence of hyperactive and impulsive behaviors distinguishes a specific subgroup of children with ADHD is uncertain.

Difficulties with Planning and Organizing Tasks. Children may display difficulties with several so-called executive functions that regulate learning and adaptation. These may include problems with planning, organizing, or performing tasks in the correct order; appropriately beginning and ending activities; or shifting from one task to another.

Emotional Lability. Socially undesirable behaviors such as temper outbursts, fighting, and overexcitement may result from an inability to perform expected tasks and a low frustration tolerance.

All of these behavioral characteristics can lead to educational, social, and emotional consequences. Children with attention deficits generally have an increased need for special education services, their impulsivity and emotional lability contribute to poor peer relationships, and lowered self-esteem is a common outcome.

ASSESSMENT AND DIAGNOSIS

Children who demonstrate significant problems with inattention, impulsivity, and overactivity require a comprehensive assessment that considers the myriad factors that might contribute to such behaviors. Communication with school personnel is essential to obtain critical information about classroom functioning.

History

Detailed information regarding the child's behavior at school and at home should be sought, particularly regarding the frequency, severity, and context of problems with attention, impulsivity, and overactivity. The presence of associated behaviors such as emotional lability and poor organizational skills should also be ascertained. Other important aspects of school functioning include the child's academic achievement, results of past psychoeducational testing, and any special school services provided.

The perinatal history should be reviewed for problems associated with attention deficits such as maternal alcohol or drug intake during pregnancy. Early childhood health problems of special relevance include recurrent or persistent otitis media, lead poisoning, iron deficiency anemia, and frequent injuries because of overactivity. Family and social history may identify contributing genetic or environmental factors.

Physical Examination

Physical examination assumes a limited but important role in the evaluation of children with attention deficits. General observation may indicate moodiness, sadness, or anxiety. Tics may suggest Tourette syndrome. Direct observations of attention span and activity level must be interpreted cautiously, because a child's behavior in the office may be remarkably different from that in the classroom or at home. Phenotypic features may suggest specific syndromes known to be associated with attention deficits (eg, fetal alcohol effects), but the significance of so-called minor congenital anomalies is uncertain. Some studies have suggested an increased number of atypical features such as "electric" hair, epicanthal folds, low-set ears, high-arched palate, clinodactyly, and an increased gap between the first and second toes among children with ADHD. However, most children with ADHD show no such signs. The physical examination must include vision and hearing screening because sensory deficits can result in inattentiveness and overactivity.

The role of an "extended" neurologic examination is controversial. Increased incidence of "soft" neurologic signs has been noted among some boys, but not among girls, with attention deficits. Examples include dystonic posturing of the upper extremities with heelwalking, marked "mirror" movements of the opposite hand in conjunction with rapid opposition of the thumb and forefinger, and "overflow" tongue movement when the child is occupied with writing his name.

Laboratory Studies

Laboratory studies are of limited value. Lead screening should be considered for all children and is definitely indicated for those at risk by virtue of past history, living environment, pica, or parental occupational exposure. Screening for iron deficiency anemia should be performed for children who are at risk because of nutritional history or socioeconomic status. The prevalence of thyroid abnormalities reportedly is higher in children with ADHD than in the normal population, so thyroid function studies may be performed. There is no role for routine neuroanatomic studies (eg, computer tomography or magnetic resonance imaging) or neurophysiological studies (eg, EEG, neurometrics, brain electrical activity mapping) in children with attention deficits.

Rating Scales

In view of the importance of sampling behavior in multiple settings (ie, school and home) and the impracticality of direct observations outside the office, teacher and parent questionnaires are useful as supplements to a complete history. A variety of questionnaires are available. So-called "diagnostic" scales, such as the SNAP (Swanson, Nolan, and Pelham) Rating Scale and DuPaul's ADHD Rating Scale, focus specifically on ADHD. Others, such as Achenbach and Edelbrock's Child Behavior Checklist, focus on a broad range of behaviors in addition to attention deficits. Conners' Parent and Teacher Rating Scales often are used to monitor the effectiveness of drug treatment. Such scales can be helpful in confirming suspicions of ADHD based on history.

Performance Tests and Direct Measures of Motor Activity

A variety of tests have been developed to measure a child's ability to sustain attention. Vigilance tests (eg, Children's Checking Task) assess a child's capacity to maintain concentration over time while performing a monotonous task. Impulsivity may be measured with instruments such as the Matching Familiar Figures Test. Computerized devices (eg, the Gordon Diagnostic System) include a delay task that requires the child to inhibit responses to earn points, a vigilance task such as the Continuous Performance Task, and a distractibility task such as the Continuous Performance Task with added visual distractors. The clinical applicability of such performance tests remains to be proven, however, and they should not serve as the sole basis for a diagnosis of attention deficits. Measurements of actual motor activity with devices such as a wrist or leg actometer or a movement-recording seat cushion are not appropriate for clinical assessment.

Psychoeducational Evaluation

No individual psychological test or battery of tests should be used to make a specific diagnosis of ADHD. Nevertheless, psychological testing may be an important component of evaluation, especially when learning problems exist. An IQ test provides an opportunity for behavioral observation under standardized conditions, and it may suggest an attention problem that is secondary to deficits in cognition, auditory or visual processing, or memory. Tests of academic achievement document the impact of attention deficits on classroom performance and may suggest the possibility of learning disabilities.

MANAGEMENT AND TREATMENT

The treatment of children with attention deficits must be individualized, must address both intrinsic characteristics of the child and relevant environmental factors, and must coordinate a variety of interventions within multiple settings (ie, school, home, and community).

Behavior Management

Behavioral modification methods that have been used with varying success include (a) positive reinforcement, with use of praise or tangible rewards such as tokens; (b) punishment strategies such as time-out or social isolation, verbal reprimand, and nonverbal gestures; and (c) extinction techniques such as the systematic ignoring of undesirable behaviors. Close communication between teachers and parents is essential to ensure consistency between school and home management. A well-structured, highly organized classroom in which instructions are brief and consistent, and responses to the child are clear, is desirable. Examples of additional classroom strategies include preferential seating in an area with few distractions, use of checklists and desk diaries, and modification of the classroom routine to enable the child to change activities and move about periodically.

Special Education

Special education services and tutoring should address academic delays and specific learning disabilities when present. The educational program should be designed to create opportunities for the child to experience success and enhanced self-esteem.

Drug Treatment

Stimulant medications have a beneficial effect on the behavior of 60 to 80% children with ADHD. Studies demonstrate a variety of short-term effects, including enhanced attention span and concentration; decreased task-irrelevant behavior and impulsivity; reduced activity level; shortened response latency on measures of reaction time; and enhanced performance on vigilance and discrimination tasks. Despite such well-documented, favorable behavioral impacts, stimulant drugs do not appear to influence academic performance directly. Improved handwriting and mathematics performance are often noted, but the gains most likely are secondary to enhanced attention span and concentration rather than from the direct acquisition of new skills or knowledge. Stimulant medication does not appear to substantially influence long-term academic or occupational outcomes. Thus, drugs should not be used in isolation but rather as one component of a multimodal treatment approach.

The most commonly used stimulant medications in the treatment of ADHD include methylphenidate, dextroamphetamine, and the closely related Adderall, mixed salts of a single-entity amphetamine product. Although their precise mechanisms of action are not known, these drugs affect the function of multiple CNS neurotransmitters. They increase the release and inhibit the reuptake of dopamine and norepinephrine from neurons in the CNS, and their beneficial effects are similar. The stimulant drugs generally are well tolerated and safe. Adverse effects typically are transient and may include sleep disturbances, decreased appetite, irritability, and abdominal pain. More significant concerns include the potential for growth suppression and exacerbation of a tic disorder. Pemoline, another form of stimulant medication, is no longer recommended for routine use due to problems with hepatic toxicity.

A variety of medications have been proposed as alternatives to stimulants. Tricyclic antidepressants, primarily desipramine and imipramine, may be considered when stimulant drugs are ineffective or produce unacceptable side effects. Clonidine, an α_2-noradrenergic agonist, may be helpful when children also display aggressive or "hyperaroused" behaviors. Studies have yet to demonstrate the efficacy of monoamine oxidase inhibitors, fluoxetine, or major tranquilizers.

Adjunctive Therapies

Psychotherapy can be beneficial in addressing low self-esteem, depression, and anxiety. Family therapy may be helpful in addressing conflicts in relationships. Parent training programs in behavior management and support groups such as CHADD (Children with Attention Deficit Disorders) can offer concrete assistance. Cognitive-behavioral training has been suggested to help students self-monitor, achieve self-control, and develop problem-solving strategies, whereas social skills training teaches children how to listen and participate in group situations, give and receive praise, and cope with frustration.

A variety of nonconventional treatments also have been proposed for children with attention deficits. Therapies that are alleged to have a biochemical basis include orthomolecular medicine (eg, megavitamins, mineral therapy), dietary manipulation (eg, exclusion of sugar and food additives), and treatment of presumed hypoglycemia. Neurophysiologically based interventions include patterning, optometric training, sensory integration therapy, and α-wave conditioning. None of these approaches has been supported by controlled studies.

NATURAL HISTORY AND PROGNOSIS

Although the symptom of hyperactivity typically diminishes over time, problems secondary to inattentiveness and impulsivity persist in about 50 to 70% of adolescents and young adults with a prior diagnosis of ADHD. Adolescents are at particular risk for low self-esteem, problems with peer relationships, and antisocial or high-risk behaviors. Longitudinal studies suggest that the majority of individuals with ADHD fare reasonably well in adulthood, are employed, and are not more prone to severe psychopathology or antisocial behavior. However, persistence of some difficulties with social adjustment are suggested by a greater number of moves, more car accidents, completion of fewer years of education, and a higher risk of alcohol and drug abuse when compared with control subjects not having a history of attention problems.

Favorable prognostic factors for individuals with ADHD include higher levels of intelligence and socioeconomic status. Poor long-term outcomes are associated with early aggression and conduct problems, parental psychopathology, poor academic achievement, emotional instability, and poor social relations. Studies have yet to prove that specific treatment approaches influence prognosis. The most promising results to date have been reported for multimodality therapies, which combine behavioral management, appropriate use of medication, and psychotherapy. Important studies of specific therapies are now being conducted that will guide clinical practice.

References

Barkley RA: Attention-deficit/hyperactivity disorder, self-regulation, and time: toward a more comprehensive theory. J Dev Behav Pediatr 18: 271–279, 1997

Brown FR, Voight RG, Elksnin N: AD/HD. A neurodevelopmental perspective. Contemp Pediatr 13:25–44, 1996

Culbert TP, Banez GA, Reiff MI: Children who have attentional disorders: interventions. Pediatr Rev 15:5–14, 1994

Kelly DP, Aylward GP: Attention deficits in school-aged children and adolescents. Current issues and practice. Pediatr Clin North Am 39:487–512, 1992

Mannuzza S, Klein RG, Bessler A, Malloy P, LaPadula M: Adult outcome of hyperactive boys. Educational achievement, occupational rank, and psychiatric status. Arch Gen Psychiatry 50:565–576, 1993

Reiff MI, Banez GA, Culbert TP: Children who have attentional disorders: diagnosis and evaluation. Pediatr Rev 14:455–464, 1993

5.6.2 Learning Problems: Differences in Learning Styles to School Failure

J. Lane Tanner

Experiences with both mastery and failure powerfully shape the process of human development. In most industrialized countries, a child's emerging sense of competence is influenced in a fundamental way by the child's accomplishments in school. Within the context of overall health supervision, the pediatrician can play an important role both in helping families to understand variations in learning styles and in identifying children at risk for developmentally disabling school failure.

DEFINITIONS AND EPIDEMIOLOGY

Success in school draws on a broad range of developmental abilities. Developmental variation with respect to learning and school performance is determined by the maturity and efficiency of such neurodevelopmental modalities as cognition, speech and language, memory, social functioning, motor and sensory capabilities, and attention.

Differences in Learning Styles

These differences are the manifestations of complex profiles of distinct, although interdependent, biologically based abilities. The concept of "learning styles" emphasizes the different approaches to academic and other learning tasks that children naturally use according to their available strengths and areas of relative weakness. Each child possesses a unique profile of such strengths and weaknesses.

Success in school also depends on factors that are extrinsic to the specific learning profile of the child. Schools themselves exert powerful pressures and expectations, which may or may not match an individual child's strengths and weaknesses. The physical and emotional health of the child as well as the stability and supportive qualities of the family all determine the degree to which the child can mobilize his or her intrinsic abilities for learning. Cultural and linguistic heterogeneities also affect an increasing proportion of children in American classrooms. Thus, assessments of children experiencing school failure must address the contexts, conditions, and supports for learning as well as the individual qualities of the learner.

Learning Disabilities

Historically, these disabilities have been understood as deriving from specific neurodevelopmental weaknesses or dysfunctions, which, in turn, prevent expectable learning in one or more academic areas. It has been a defining principle that such deficiencies are unexpected given the overall intellectual functioning of the child. Learning disabilities thus are not simply the result of global delays in learning capacities, of major sensory impairments such as vision or hearing handicaps, or a consequence of major social or emotional stressors. Approximately 5% of public school children in the United States receive special education services for learning disabilities; prevalence estimates for the actual need for such services are two to three times that number.

ETIOLOGY AND PATHOGENESIS

The dramatic variations that are observable in the learning styles of normal children can be readily understood if one considers the evolutionary pressures that formed our species. Certain "wired-in" skills, adaptations, or forms of intelligence may have carried crucial survival benefits in our formative stages, yet be unused or counterproductive in today's schools.

Some support for this link between past evolutionary pressures and current learning variability is found in the seemingly greater vulnerability to insult, and greater variation of expression, of the more recently evolved brain systems (eg, the language centers of the left hemisphere; the attentional and executive functions associated with the prefrontal cortex). Today, language-based learning disorders and attentional problems comprise the great majority of referred learning problems.

At the same time, our social systems have moved toward strikingly increased levels of organizational complexity. It must be remembered, for example, that the expectation for universal literacy is historically quite new. In this sense, we are applying an evolutionarily old brain to the tasks of a new world, and inherent variations of learning profiles are to be expected.

Differences in learning style as well as learning disabilities may be described according to specific neurodevelopmental modalities. Table 5-7 presents a scheme of such modalities and examples of learning functions within each. These categories reflect specialized brain systems that are distinct yet interconnected to varying degrees.

Learning differences also may be organized according to (a) input (ie, sensory input for visual, auditory, and tactile information); (b) processing (ie, making meaning out of incoming stimuli, accessing memory, referencing and bridging content across modalities); and (c) output (ie, planning and executing vocal, written, and motor expressions). Hence, a child with hearing or vision impairments has special needs that are mainly limited to problems with input. A child with moderately severe cerebral palsy, however, may have very significant impairments of speech and motor output yet basically intact input and processing capacities. A third child might have dramatic difficulties in entering rote information into memory storage, which is a specific processing weakness.

As noted, certain modalities are more liable to learning dysfunctions. For example, the majority of classically defined learning disorders have their basis in language-processing problems. *Developmental dyslexia,* which is the failure to acquire reading skills along the usual time course, most often results from a core difficulty in reliably recalling and linking specific speech sound units (ie, phonemes) with their representative letters, and vice versa. This most common of identified learning disabilities is largely an inherited and

TABLE 5-7

NEURODEVELOPMENTAL MODALITIES THAT DETERMINE THE LEARNING PROFILE

MODALITY	EXAMPLES OF RELATED LEARNING FUNCTIONS
Motor/sensory	Fine-motor manipulations (eg, pencil use, scissors, daily living tasks)
	Sensory (eg, tactile and positional sense)
	Gross motor (eg, postural, athletic)
Language	Spoken language, receptive and expressive
	Written language (eg, reading, spelling, writing)
	Social (pragmatic or interactive) language
Visual/spatial	Visual discrimination and pattern recognition (eg, identification of written symbols)
	Spatial analysis (eg, for math, handwriting, art, organization or written products)
Memory	Short-term vs long-term memory
	Memory for verbal vs memory for visual material
	Long-term memory for meanings and facts vs for events and experiences
Integration	Efficiency of integration between modalities [eg, visual-motor coordination, sound (auditory)-to-letter (visual) association]
Executive functions	Directing and maintaining attention; organizational and planning skills; self-monitoring
Higher cognitive skills	Reasoning and problem-solving; capacity to use general concepts, contextual meanings and stored knowledge
Social cognition	Emotion perception; development of social reciprocity (eg, turn-taking, awareness of another's needs or state of mind)

familial disorder and is frequently associated with other kinds of difficulties in the development of language and speech. Recent prevalence data show dyslexia to be a disorder with varying degrees of severity that affects boys and girls in roughly equal proportion. Treatment includes the explicit teaching of phonemes and their associated letters. With proper teaching, most such children become successful readers. However, for those with more severe forms of dyslexia, reading is likely to remain effortful and nonautomatic throughout their lives. By being alert to the child who presents with early language delays and/or a family history of reading problems, pediatric clinicians can play a vital role in the early identification and appropriate teaching of children at greatest risk for dyslexia.

In addition to learning disorders connected to the language centers of the brain, a cluster of *"nonverbal" learning disabilities* has received considerable attention. In children with normal language abilities, there is an association with disorders of spatial perception, handwriting, and mathematical understanding. These so-called right hemisphere disorders have in common underlying deficits of spatial cognition and analysis. Children with such difficulties have trouble understanding the whole picture, or gestalt, of visually presented tasks (ie, they "miss the forest for the trees"). They are said to have problems with *simultaneous* as opposed to *sequential* cognitive processing. Deficits in social judgment and understanding also seem to be frequent in this group and may be the main presenting problem.

Executive functions, including attentional, organizational, planning, and self-monitoring/modulation capacities, are necessary, although not sufficient, requirements for success across all other learning functions. Confusion thus may arise in determining whether a learning disorder is the consequence or the cause of observed deficits in attention, organization, and impulse control. For example, a child with a significant disorder in auditory sequential memory may be referred for attention-deficit disorder yet be struggling principally with the understanding of oral directions and information (see Sec. 5.6.1).

In addition to the expectable variations in neurodevelopment, etiologies for learning disorders may include inherited disabilities, neurologic insults, predisposing disorders of health or development, socioemotional preoccupations, and/or mismatches between child characteristics and school expectations. (See Table 5-8 for examples.)

CLINICAL MANIFESTATIONS

Learning problems emerge only as external expectations require performance in the area(s) of the child's vulnerability or weakness. This timetable of challenges might be seen as having four qualitatively distinct periods:

1. School readiness;
2. Acquisition of basic skills;
3. Self-organization of tasks and processing of greater volumes of information; and
4. Uses of higher cognitive skills and abstract thinking.

For the child of kindergarten age, *school readiness* requires an ability to "settle," that is, to inhibit motor impulses to allow attention and focus on demand. Basic language and communicative abilities are necessary, as are the sensory capacities to discriminate auditory and visual differences in spoken sounds and letter shapes, respectively. Fine-motor competency must be sufficient for pencil use. Success is enhanced with a fund of basic language and numerical concepts, and social demands require that the child be able to take turns and express his or her own needs verbally. Pediatricians are confronted with children who adapt poorly to their first year or two of school because of specific weaknesses in any of the previously mentioned areas or because of global immaturities. The latter is especially common with children who are chronologically young at the start of school, and it is more often true of boys than of girls.

The period from first through fourth or fifth grade is heavily focused on the *acquisition of basic skills* in reading, writing, spelling, and arithmetic. The child at this stage is absorbing a tremendous amount of rote knowledge with respect to the symbol systems of letters, words, and numbers, and the rules by which they are combined. Children are asked to use a broad array of facilities in concert. Delays in language understanding and usage put early learners at particular risk of failure. Memory is heavily relied on in all its forms (eg, active working memory, recent recall, long-term information storage and retrieval). Motor output for writing may be an exceedingly frustrating, rate-limiting step for children with fine-motor delays. By the end of elementary school, these basic learning skills should be rendered nearly automatic and require a minimum of effortful concentration.

Toward the end of elementary school and throughout middle school, the child is faced with a new set of challenges, namely, *self-organization of tasks and the processing of greater volumes of information*. Task requirements now emphasize an increased volume of received information, both written and spoken, and increased demand for written products. At the same time, the child is expected, both at home and at school, to be substantially more self-reliant and responsible. Thus, the special capacities that are newly tested during this time are those that assist in (a) planning, organizing,

TABLE 5-8

THE PEDIATRICIAN'S ROLE IN THE COMPREHENSIVE EVALUATION OF A CHILD WITH SCHOOL FAILURE[a]

Ascertaining concern
  Routine developmental screening
  Review of school information
    Initial: parent's report regarding grades, school behavior, and social relations
    Follow-up: teacher/school reports such as teacher questionnaire, telephone contact, achievement scores, past school-based assessments
Directed pediatric evaluation
  History with special emphasis on the following etiologic categories:
    Heritable: family history of learning/neurodevelopmental disorders, such as dyslexia; speech and language disorders; genetic syndromes such as fragile X, Turner, Klinefelter, or phenylketonuria
    Neurologic dysfunction: fetal alcohol syndrome and other toxic intrauterine exposures; neonatal asphyxia; complications of prematurity; major head trauma; seizure disorder; lead poisoning; central nervous system irradiation
    Predisposing disorders of health and development: speech and language delay; sensory organ deficits, including recurrent otitis media with hearing impairment; chronic illness affecting general health and development such as anemia, malnutrition
    External stress/socioemotional preoccupation: parental divorce, conflict, or depression; family turmoil or violence; death or illness of a family member
    Child–school mismatch: immature child/academically advanced school; differences in home and school environments about social and behavioral expectations; misunderstood temperamental differences
  Physical examination
    General examination: rule out chronic medical conditions; check growth and head circumference; appraise for genetic syndrome phenotype
    Hearing and vision screening
    Neurologic examination: standard and extended
  Laboratory assessment: where indicated screen for anemia, lead toxicity, metabolic disorders, fragile X syndrome
  Options for more in-depth pediatric assessments
    Child interview
    Neurodevelopmental and educational screening
    Family interview
Referral for academic evaluation
  Psychological, educational, and speech and language evaluations
Collaboration and advocacy
  With multidisciplinary assessment team and/or school "Individualized Educational Plan" team
Ongoing monitoring as needed

---

[a] A child's failure to progress in school usually has biological, psychological, and social roots as well as significant psychosocial consequences. Evaluations and interventions therefore require multidisciplinary collaborations. This table displays the elements, in sequence, of a comprehensive evaluation which begins in the pediatrician's office.

monitoring, and efficiently performing tasks and activities (ie, "executive functions"); and (b) processing larger volumes of information, reading, homework, and written work. For those children who continue at this stage to struggle with some aspects of their basic skills, managing this increased volume will clearly be compromised. For those who have had prior success in early rote learning, difficulties at this level are often experienced as baffling and demoralizing.

By the end of middle school and throughout high school, academic skills are increasingly used as a means of information gathering and understanding and less as an end in themselves. Literature, mathematics, and the social and natural sciences all rely on basic skills acquired earlier, but also introduce *higher cognitive skills and abstract thinking.* Issues of individual interest, future orientation, and directed motivation increasingly apply.

ASSESSMENT AND DIAGNOSIS

For pediatric clinicians, the principal goal of assessment is the identification of children who are at risk for learning disorders and school failure. The definitive diagnostic description of the child's functioning in most cases will be the task of the educational specialist, psychologist, and speech and language specialist. The medical provider's particular responsibilities and roles are listed in Table 5-8.

Screening for school problems begins with simply asking about the school experience. The child's grades, the child's general level of enjoyment of school, reports of classroom behaviors and peer interactions, school attendance records, and class-administered achievement test scores all are global measures that help the clinician decide whether to expand the inquiry. In-the-office screening tasks provide direct observations to assist in determining the direction for further assessment and referral. Contact with the teacher via phone or questionnaire is invaluable in clarifying the nature of the concerns. The clinician must be alert to the array of predisposing factors to learning disorders, such as those listed on Table 5-8, and be prepared to intensify the screening process in such cases.

Office screening procedures may include grade-normed reading, spelling, and mathematics samples, which take little time to administer yet provide vivid examples of the elementary school child's academic difficulties. Asking a younger child to write the alphabet (while the clinician is occupied taking the history with the parent) gives an easily acquired view of the child's developing memory and visual-motor capabilities. Asking a child to draw a person is an excellent screening measure of the child's cognitive, visual-spatial, and fine-motor sophistication. The content of the drawing, as well as the child's comments about it (elicited simply by asking, "Tell me about your drawing"), frequently reveal pressing psychosocial concerns.

Other tools also have been devised to help the clinician screen for strengths or weaknesses within particular modalities (eg, language, visual-spatial perception, memory). Some of these screening tools have been developed specifically for the pediatric context.

The neurologic assessment comprises both a standard neurologic examination and an extended neurodevelopmental assessment. The developmental examination is intended to demonstrate the child's neurologic maturity and the qualitative efficiency of motor, sensory, and position-sense functions. Gross-motor examples might be stressed-gait tasks such as tiptoe walking, sustained hopping, and skipping. Fine-motor examples include rapid alternating movements of the fingers, hand, or forearm, with the examiner testing for speed and ease of movement as well as freedom from mirror movements (ie, synkinesia) of the opposite hand. An example of the sensory examination might include the accurate detection of two fingers touched simultaneously. In addition to allowing the direct observation of samples of these specific motor and sensory functions, the extended neurologic examination also provides supportive evidence for determining whether a child's CNS difficulties are diffuse across many modalities or specific to one or two.

American pediatric clinicians should be aware of the provisions of the Individuals with Disabilities Education Act (IDEA). This national legislation guarantees a free appropriate public education for eligible children and youth with disabilities and mandates educational services appropriate to their needs in the least restrictive educational environment. Recent revisions in IDEA also require assessment and early intervention programs for children from infancy to school-age who are at risk for significant developmental and learning disabilities. The school-based evaluative process results in an Individualized Educational Plan (IEP) that guides special education placements and teaching objectives. Pediatricians play an important role in informing parents of their option to pursue an IEP.

In addition, many pediatricians work closely with particular consultants of other disciplines, especially educational specialists, psychologists, and speech and language specialists. Through this professional team approach, the pediatrician may extend his or her role to that of case manager or consultant for ongoing learning evaluations.

MANAGEMENT AND TREATMENT

Whether speaking of differing learning styles or major learning disorders, the philosophy of management and treatment is the same, that is, the individual child's unique learning profile must be appreciated, and teaching must aim to challenge the child in ways to which the child can successfully respond. Where weaknesses are significantly disabling, teachers and parents must help the child to compensate for them, as much as possible, by capitalizing on the available strengths and skills.

Educational therapy and special education programs vary greatly. They may involve in-class adaptations, part-time resource assistance programs within and outside the classroom, full-day self-contained classrooms, free-standing schools for children with more significant learning problems, or out-of-school private remediation. Services also may include speech and language therapy, physical/occupational therapy, or mobility training. The child's educational progress, as measured on yearly academic achievement tests, as well as the child's enjoyment of school become central evaluative measures of the success of the educational program.

In addition, appropriate treatment may include psychological therapy for children whose emotional needs stand in the way of learning. For those who also have significant neurodevelopmentally based learning disorders, choosing a psychotherapist who is versed in disorders of child development is essential. Consultation and/or therapy with the family is often a critical component of this work. For cases in which social cognition and understanding are significant weaknesses, training programs in social skills are more widely available as well.

Finally, the pediatrician may be asked to institute medication for attention deficit and other behavioral problems. The details of this decision and treatment are covered in Sec. 5.6.1.

NATURAL HISTORY AND PROGNOSIS

The natural history of learning differences and disorders depends on their nature and severity. With most neurodevelopmentally based disorders of learning, it is common for early weaknesses to persist, regardless of intervention, to varying degrees into adulthood. Whether such weaknesses become disabling in the long run depends on (a) the child's ability to compensate and cope through his or her unaffected strengths; (b) appropriate teaching and accommodations in school programs; (c) the development over time of self-valued and socially respected competencies; and (d) the degree to which the child comes to understand the disability as a real but limited part of the self and not a feature that devalues the whole. The pediatrician is uniquely positioned to encourage the school and parents to understand and be responsive to the whole child.

References

Dworkin PH: School failure. Pediatr Rev 10:301–312, 1989

Levine MD: Developmental Variation and Learning Disorders. Cambridge, MA, Educators Publishing Service, 1987

Montgomery TR: The pediatric neurodevelopmental assessment of school-age children. In: Capute AJ, Accardo PJ, eds: Developmental Disabilities in Infancy and Childhood. Baltimore, P.H. Brookes, 1991, p. 151–164

Pennington BF: Diagnosing Learning Disorders: A Neuropsychological Framework. New York, Guilford, 1991

Shaywitz SE: Current concepts: dyslexia. N Engl J Med 338:307–312, 1998

Wender E, ed: School Dysfunction in Children and Youth: The Role of the Primary Health Provider for Children who Struggle in School. Report of the 24th Ross Roundtable on Critical Approaches to Common Pediatric Problems. Columbus, OH, Ross Laboratories, 1993

Whitmore K, Hart H, Willems G, eds: A neurodevelopmental approach to specific learning disorders. In: Clinics in Developmental Medicine #145. London, Cambridge University Press, 1999

5.6.3   Developmental Delays: Maturational Lags to Mental Retardation

Yvette Yachmirk

DEFINITIONS AND EPIDEMIOLOGY

Development is a multidimensional process that influences performance in all spheres of life. Consequently, impairments in development may affect one or several domains of ability, and they can have an impact on both intellectual and adaptive function across the life span. The boundaries between "normal" and "delayed" developmental progress are often indistinct, particularly during a child's first and toddler years.

A diagnosis of mental retardation has crucial clinical, educational, and social implications for the child and the child's family. In 1992, the American Association on Mental Retardation (AAMR) revised its official definition and system of classification to reflect the shift from a view of mental retardation as an intrinsic individual trait to an emphasis on the interaction between a person with limited intellectual functioning and his or her environment. Consequently, the new definition of mental retardation is:

> Significantly subaverage functioning (defined as an IQ score of below 70 to 75) existing concurrently with related limitations in two more of the following applicable adaptive skill areas: communication, self-care, home-living, social skills, community use, self-direction, health and safety, functional academics, leisure, and work.

The definition has evolved from a conceptual model that emphasizes the *adoptive functioning* of individuals with limited *capabilities* within the *context* of specific sociocultural *environments*. Thus, impaired intellectual functioning is a necessary, but not sufficient, criterion for determining a diagnosis of mental retardation. This model provides a useful framework for understanding influences on developmental progress in children with mental retardation, as well as in those with less-significant maturational lags. It emphasizes the

importance of attitudes and expectations within the family, and in the broader community, when determining the adaptation of individuals to specific impairments.

Because the long-term intellectual and adaptive function of very young children is difficult to predict, both infants and toddlers who acquire skills more slowly than their chronologic peers are often diagnosed as having a "developmental delay." Frequently, this slower timetable for the attainment of specific developmental skills represents a normal maturational variation, and many infants with such "delays" eventually "catch up." Furthermore, because the sensory motor skills (eg, block stacking) that indicate mastery during infancy are different from the cognitive and adaptive competencies essential for later functioning, their delayed acquisition does not necessarily predict later impairment. Thus, the traditional diagnostic tools that are available for assessing development in infants do not identify stable intellectual deficits that erupt in children with severe developmental disabilities. In most cases, a diagnosis of mental retardation can be made only after multiple longitudinal observations that document persistent lags in the acquisition rate of developmental skill.

Traditionally, the severity of mental retardation has been determined solely on the basis of an individual's performance (IQ score) on a standardized intelligence test. In the past, this taxonomy resulted in the classification of a disability as borderline (IQ 68 to 83), mild (IQ 52 to 67), moderate (IQ 36 to 51), severe (IQ 20 to 35), or profound (IQ below 20). In contrast, the newly revised AAMR classification system deemphasizes IQ scores and characterizes individuals with mental retardation by the degree of support they need to function in their usual environments. This approach recognizes the individual's unique profile of strengths and weaknesses, as well as specific demands of different settings. Four levels of support are defined:

1. Intermittent: does not require constant support but may need support on a short-term basis for special occurrences
2. Limited
3. Extensive: needs daily support in some aspects of living, such as with handling finances, or may need time-limited support for employment training
4. Pervasive: requires constant, high-intensity support for all aspects of life

Over the years, inconsistencies in definition and classification schemes have made epidemiologic data about developmental delays and mental retardation highly imprecise. Estimates of prevalence based on standard psychometric tests given *in the past* indicate that just under 3% of the general population have "significantly subaverage intellectual functioning" (ie, have test scores that fall more than 2 standard deviations below the norm). However, in 1993, data from the United States Department of Education indicated the prevalence of mental retardation among school-age children (6–17 year) is 1.14%. Recent estimates suggest that approximately 90% of people with mental retardation function within the mild range of impairment. The prevalence of mild mental retardation is highest among children from poor families, whereas individuals with more severe disabilities are represented equally in all income groups. Approximately 5% of the population with mental retardation is severely or profoundly affected.

The epidemiology of mental retardation is further obscured by the focus on functional adaptation within varying environmental contexts. Research consistently indicates that mental retardation is most prevalent among school-age children, with lower numbers in both the preschool and postschool periods. In the early years, this reflects a tendency by clinicians to recognize only the more severely impaired children. Because many individuals who are classified as mentally retarded within the context of form education adapt more readily to the postschool environment, they lose their label in late adolescence.

ETIOLOGY AND PATHOGENESIS

Historically, many theorists in the field of child development have advocated a "defect" or "difference" approach to intellectual impairments, arguing that all individuals with mental retardation approach cognitive tasks in a biologically based, qualitatively direct manner. More recently, the model was replaced by one that distinguishes between individuals with and individuals without a clearly delineated organic cause for their retardation. According to this latter approach, most individuals with mental retardation represent the lower end of normal developmental continuum, while the subset with identifiable organic insults remains qualitatively distinct. Although attempts are still made to distinguish between "origin" and "cultural–familial" etiologies of retardation, current developmental thinking emphasizes the interdependence of both biological and environmental factors as determinants of individual competence. Consequently, a "transitional" approach to the pathogenesis of both transient maturational lags and persistent developmental disabilities recognizes that the ultimate intellectual and adaptive functioning of all individuals is determined by the integrity and the maturational status of their CNS as well as the impacts of their life experiences.

As medical technology continues to become more sophisticated, previously unrecognized insults to the developing brain are being identified as etiologic factors for a variety of cognitive disabilities. Specific impairments in CNS development are attributable to a heterogenous group of factors, including chromosomal abnormalities, *recognizable syndrome,* structural or metabolic abnormalities of the brain, and CNS insults resulting from infections, toxins, malnutrition, anoxia, or trauma. In a parallel fashion, a range of adverse environmental experiences correlate with impaired intellectual functioning including family disorganization, parental psychopathology, parental substance abuse, and severely dysfunctional parent–child interactions. Despite our growing understanding of the pathogenesis of developmental impairments, a specific etiology *can be identified in only 40–60% of all patients undergoing evaluation,* and it generally is difficult to unravel the complex interacting factors that produce individual variability within diagnostic groups.

CLINICAL MANIFESTATIONS

Clinical signs of developmental delay and mental retardation are as diverse as their etiologies and individual expressions. Children with discrete congenital disorders or syndromes associated with impaired intellectual development, such as Down syndrome, trisomy 13, trisomy 18, Williams syndrome, or fetal alcohol syndrome, can be identified early in infancy by characteristic clusters of phenotypic features.

The majority of children who are eventually diagnosed with mental retardation, however, appear to be "normal" and are identified only when they fail to meet age-appropriate developmental expectations. Children with the most severe impairments are most likely to be identified relatively early in the first year of life; when they lag in the acquisition of sensory motor skills. On the other hand, moderate degrees of disability often do not become apparent until the emergence of the Piagetian preoperational stage of development in the second year, when the first behavioral manifes-

tations of symbolic thought (ie, representational play and language) are expected to appear. In contrast, children with mild impairments generally are identified only after they enter school, when they demonstrate difficulties with academic tasks that require more abstract thinking. Aspects of normal development are presented in Sec. 1.2.1 and Table 1-9. A brief outline of developmental expectations during the preschool years is shown in Table 5-9.

ASSESSMENT AND DIAGNOSIS

Early identification of children with developmental impairments is best achieved within the pediatric primary-care setting by clinicians who ask appropriate, targeted questions and who make sensitive, informed observations. Attention to concerns raised by parents and other caregivers (eg, childcare providers, teachers) in conjunction with the judicious use of office surveillance and screening techniques can facilitate the timely identification of children who deserve a more formal developmental assessment.

The diagnostic evaluation of a child with suspected developmental impairments should include a comprehensive medical, social, and family history that identifies both risk and protective factors within the child and the environment. A careful physical examination including a detailed neuromotor assessment must be performed. An approach to the diagnostic evaluation is shown in Tables 1-10 and 1-11. Laboratory studies, when appropriate, can provide insight into the etiology and expected course of the disorder. Table 5-10 lists indications for relevant laboratory assessments, particularly as related to specific signs and symptoms. Although a comprehensive medical evaluation of the child with developmental delay is an essential component of the diagnostic workup, it is usually inconclusive.

Ultimately, the diagnosis of mental retardation is made by demonstrating "significantly subaverage intellectual functioning," in conjunction with "related limitations in . . . adaptive skill areas." Impaired intellectual functioning can be confirmed by the administration of a standardized psychometric instrument (eg, the Bayley Scales of Infant Development, McCarthy Scales of Children's Abilities, Stanford Binet Intelligence Scale, or the Wechsler Intelligence Scales for Children) by an appropriately trained professional. Limitations in adaptive functioning can be confirmed by the administration of a behavioral instrument such as the Vireland Adaptive Behavior Scales or the AAMR Adaptive Behavior Scale.

MANAGEMENT AND TREATMENT

The pediatrician's role in the management of developmental delay or mental retardation is to assist family members with their adaptation to the initial diagnosis as well as facilitate their acquisition of appropriate services. A major challenge for the clinician is to recognize the unique needs of each child and family and to develop an individual approach for each situation.

The initial sharing of diagnostic information with family members is among the most intellectually and emotionally challenging responsibilities that a clinician will face. If handled sensitively and skillfully, this process can be rewarding to the physician and supportive for the family, and it can provide the foundation for ongoing parent–professional collaboration. All available information should be shared as soon as the physician suspects a problem exists, even if the information is incomplete and reflects some uncertainty. The skilled clinician will identify areas of relative competency and the potential areas for growth, and will invite affective responses from family members. It is essential that the clinician answer all questions openly and honestly, as well as ensure that family mem-

TABLE 5-9

DEVELOPMENTAL EXPECTATIONS

AGE	MOBILITY/DEXTERITY	COMMUNICATION	PLAY/PROBLEM SOLVING
By 6 months	Rolls over Reaches for objects	Reciprocal vocalizations	Mouths and shakes objects Watches dropped objects
By 12 months	Crawls Pulls to stand Cruises Pincer grasp Finger feeds	Babbling Word-like vocalizations Response to verbal requests	Nonspecific manipulation (eg, banging, shaking, mouthing) Nonspecific exploration (eg, fingering, turning, examining) Searches for hidden object Simple means–ends action
By 18 months	Walks well Feeds self with spoon	Uses intelligible single words to express needs Recognizes named objects	Functional use of objects on own body (eg, brushing hair) Container play (eg, filling/dumping) Finds object after multiple visible displacements
By 24 months	Walks up and down stairs Feeds self with fork and spoon Removes clothes	Uses more than 50 words and 2-word phrases Follows 2-step commands Understands some prepositions 50% intelligibility	Groups toys in meaningful way Representational play (eg, feeds doll) Finds object after multiple invisible displacements
By 30 months	Jumps with both feet	Identifies actions in pictures and objects by use Uses pronouns, adjectives, and adverbs 75% intelligibility	Sequenced representational play (eg, child stirs spoon in cup, feeds doll, puts doll to sleep) Discovers causal mechanisms without seeing them work
By 36 months	Stands on one foot briefly Pedals tricycle Dresses with supervision	Uses sentences of 3 or more words Uses negatives and plurals Knows own full name Recognizes colors	Fantasy play Interactive peer play

bers reach a well-informed and balanced understanding of the child's disability. Finally, the physician should work with the family to formulate specific plans for appropriate therapeutic, educational, and/or supportive services.

The role of the physician varies with the needs of individual children and families. All children must have a regular source of primary care to provide routine immunizations, to monitor health and growth, and to care for minor illness. Subspecialty medical services are indicated selectively for the children with specific conditions that occur with greater frequency among individuals having developmental disabilities, such as seizure disorders, orthopedic problems, and vision and hearing deficits. Genetic counseling also must be provided whenever the diagnosis is of a heritable disorder.

An evolving societal commitment to the needs of families and children with developmental impairments culminated in the 1986 enactment of the Education for All Handicapped Children Amendments (reauthorized in 1991 as the Individuals with Disabilities Education Act). This legislation meant to ensure individualized special education and related services in the least-restrictive environment for all children with disabilities from 3 to 22 years of age. In addition, the Amendments established a discretionary program for eventual full implementation in each participating state of a "comprehensive, coordinated, multidisciplinary, interagency program of early intervention services for all handicapped infants and their families." Although implementation of these laws varies across communities and states, educational services for children with developmental disabilities are becoming established as a right. The standard approach to young children with developmental disabilities has evolved from almost universal placement in residential institutions to coordinated efforts to develop community-based services both for children and their families.

The two cardinal features of all treatment approaches for children with developmental disabilities are that they are individual and

family focused. The optimal therapeutic and educational plan for each individual child must be developed through the collaborative efforts of professionals and family members. Early intervention programs for infants and toddlers emphasize the central role of the parents, and they are designed to support the family's ability to

TABLE 5-10

LABORATORY STUDIES RECOMMENDED FOR THE CHILD WITH DEVELOPMENTAL DELAY AND SPECIFIC SIGNS AND SYMPTOMS

SIGN OR SYMPTOM	LABORATORY STUDIES
Neurologic regression Sensory abnormalities Unexplained new or progressive neurologic finding Failure to thrive accompanied by neurologic findings	Urine for organic acids Serum amino acid lactate, pyruvate, and long-chain fatty acid concentrations (peroxisomal disorders)
Cranial abnormalities (eg, microcephaly)	Viral titers for congenital infection Urine for cytomegalovirus Cranial computed tomography or magnetic resonance imaging
Gross-motor delay with associated hypotonia, weakness, and hyporeflexia	Serum creatine phosphokinase Aldolase concentrations Electromyography Nerve conduction velocity
Congenital malformations Many atypical physical features	Chromosomal karyotype
Family history of unexplained mental retardation	Chromosomal analysis for fragile X syndrome
Language delay	Audiologic evaluation

nurture the child's development. As children move into the school system, professionals must be prepared to work closely with families in the development of individualized educational programs. The long-term goals of both health care and educational professionals are to facilitate positive self-esteem, social competence, and adaptive living skills so as to promote the optimal development of each individual.

NATURAL HISTORY AND PROGNOSIS

The natural history of developmental delays and mental retardation varies with the level of severity, presence of associated disabilities, quality of the caregiving environment, and caliber of therapeutic and educational services that are provided. The revised AAMR classification system is based on the assumption that most people with mental retardation will improve their functioning with effective supports, enabling them to live more productive, independent, and integrated lives. With the exception of a small group of children having progressive neurologic disorders that are characterized by a deterioration in functioning over time, individuals with mental retardation continue to develop new skills throughout a lifetime.

References

Curry CJ, Stevenson RE, Aughton D, et al: Evaluation of mental retardation; recommendations of a consensus conference. Am J Med Genet 72: 468–477, 1997

Drew CJ, Logan DR, Hadman MI: Mental retardation: A Life-Cycle Approach, 5th ed. Columbus, OH, Merrill, 1992

Hodapp RM, Burack JA, Zigler E, eds: Issues in the Developmental Approach to Mental Retardation. Cambridge, Cambridge University Press, 1990

Jons KL: Smith's Recognizable Patterns of Human Malformation, 4th ed. Philadelphia, Saunders, 1988

King BH, Stake MW, Shoh B, Davanzo P, Dylers E: Mental retardation: a review of the past 10 years. Parts I and II. J Am Acad Child Adolesc Psychiatry 36:12, 1997

Meisels SJ: Handbook of Early Childhood Intervention. New York, Cambridge University Press, 2000

Mental Retardation: Definition, Classification, and Systems of Supports, 9th ed. Washington, DC, American Association on Mental Retardation, 1992

Richardson SA, Koler H, Schonkoff JP: Twenty-Two Years: Causes and Consequences of Mental Retardation. Cambridge, MA, Harvard University Press, 1996

Smith R, ed: Children with Mental Retardation. A Parent's Guide. Rockville, MD, Woodbine House, 1993

5.6.4   Language Delay: Late Talking to Communication Disorder

Jack P. Shonkoff

Except for the first independent step, no milestone of early child development is awaited with greater anticipation than a baby's first word. This momentous achievement represents an important marker along an extraordinary continuum that extends from the earliest differentiated cries to the most sophisticated conversation. Development of competence in language unfolds through a complex, highly interactive process that is influenced by both neuromaturation and human relationships. It is not simply an imitative function in which children learn to repeat what they hear; it is a creative process through which children master a rule-based, symbolic system that ultimately enables them to articulate unique thoughts. In most cases, language abilities emerge in an apparently effortless manner. The assessment and management of delayed or atypical development in this area, however, can present a formidable challenge.

DEFINITIONS AND EPIDEMIOLOGY

The study of language development focuses on five essential dimensions: (a) phonology (ie, the sound system); (b) semantics (ie, the meaning attached to words); (c) morphology (ie, the rules of word formation such as adding "-ed" for past tense); (d) syntax (ie, the rules of sentence formation); and (e) pragmatics (ie, the social uses of language for communication). Development of communicative competence consists of both receptive and expressive components. Receptive abilities refer to what a child understands; expressive communication refers to what the child can produce. Generally, receptive skills are inferred from behavioral observation. Expressive abilities are observed directly and evolve from the early cooing (ie, vowels), babbling (ie, consonants), and gestures (eg, pointing) of infants through the verbalizations (ie, recognizable words) of toddlers and the elaborate conversations of preschoolers. The difference between the concept of *language,* which refers to an underlying symbol system, and the act of *speech,* which refers to the physical act of talking, is an important clinical distinction. For example, a problem in expressive language, which primarily involves difficulty in symbolic formulation may or may not be accompanied by a speech problem, which may be manifested by an impairment of articulation (eg, a lisp) or a dysfluency (eg, stuttering), each of which requires a different treatment approach. Dysfluencies are hesitations, interruptions, or disruptions in speech that typically appear during the period of advancing from two-word utterances to more complex sentence production.

The development of communicative competence is characterized by substantial variability. The boundaries between normal variation and transient maturational delays are difficult to determine, so accurate data on the prevalence of "late talking" are unavailable. It has been estimated that between 5 and 10% of children have a significant language disorder, and that 4% go through a period of stuttering that lasts for 6 months or more. Thus, the average pediatrician is likely to see at least one or two young children each day with a problem in language development that is worthy of investigation.

ETIOLOGY AND PATHOGENESIS

In view of the complex and highly interactive process through which language competence is achieved, it is not surprising that the cause of a delayed or atypical pattern is rarely simple and discrete. Thus, it is more fruitful to abandon the search for a *single* etiology and focus on understanding the relative contributions of *multiple* causal factors. Furthermore, a speech or language delay may result from dysfunction at any of several levels, including *sensation* (ie, auditory or visual acuity), *perception* (ie, the ability to differentiate speech sounds), *comprehension* and *processing* (ie, higher cortical function), and *production* (ie, the formulation of linguistic concepts and the mechanical production of intelligible speech sounds). Specific language delays may result from a focal impairment in one domain, or reflect problems throughout this complex input-output system.

The extent to which the etiology of late talking is intrinsic or extrinsic is an important question for the clinician. Most commonly, the pathogenesis is interactive, and the controversy surrounding the role of recurrent otitis media as a cause of language delay or disorder provides a useful illustration. It is hypothesized that fluctuating conductive hearing losses associated with middle-ear fluid produce distortions in auditory input that can be particularly disabling in the period of rapid language development during the first 2 years of life. More specifically, it has been suggested that these distortions interfere with the development of receptive language and lead to subsequent expressive difficulties. Support for this hypothesis comes from several retrospective studies that documented higher rates of otitis media in the early pediatric histories of school-age children with language-based learning disabilities. However, most children with recurrent otitis media have normal language development, and many children with significant learning disabilities have no history of significant middle-ear disease. Thus, without more definitive data, it seems logical to assume that children with preexisting constitutional problems in the area of language development may be more susceptible to the adverse effects of the fluctuating conductive hearing losses, whereas children without underlying vulnerabilities can be expected to progress in a satisfactory manner in spite of transient hearing impairment.

The relative role of the caregiving environment in the development of language can be viewed in a similar manner. Young children are exposed to a wide variety of language experiences. Some grow up in homes with a great deal of interactive conversation among family members and where reading books to young children is commonplace. Others are raised in environments characterized by the extremes of minimal verbal interaction or noncontingent, auditory overload. However, some children exhibit language delays despite a highly facilitating environment; others have limited exposure to good language models yet develop strong communicative skills. Thus, children living in suboptimal environments who develop language problems are likely to have intrinsic vulnerabilities, whereas many youngsters who develop normal language skills might have exhibited difficulties had they been reared under less-favorable circumstances.

The etiology and pathogenesis of language delays or disabilities is multifactorial and often obscure. There is a widespread agreement, however, that late talking is not caused by either "laziness" or tongue tie, and there are no consistent data to support a role for birth order. Furthermore, although children who are raised in bilingual environments may make early syntactic errors (related to word order) as they begin to speak in short sentences, delayed talking indicates a probable underlying language problem rather than a consequence of exposure to more than one language. Finally, the normal rate of early language development in twins often is slower than that of single children, with eventual "catch up" not achieved until the end of the preschool period.

CLINICAL MANIFESTATIONS

In view of the considerable variation in the rate of normal language development and given the high prevalence of transient maturational delays, the determination of true "late talking" is a major clinical challenge. Communication involves more than word production, so it is important to look for signs of potential difficulties beginning in early infancy. Moreover, language must be viewed as one domain among several areas of development and behavior. For example, a paucity of early vocalizations (ie, cooing, babbling) and later verbalization (ie, producing recognizable words) may reflect a specific problem in language, a more global cognitive impairment, or a temperamental variation in a quiet, yet normally developing child. Because it is common for young children to be relatively

silent in unfamiliar places, even if they are chatterboxes at home, the extent to which reliable observations can be recorded in the office setting may be limited; therefore, a parental report is most important. During the late toddler and early preschool years, significant language delays often present as behavior problems. Fueled largely by frustration, such children may display excessive impatience, tantrums, and aggression. Children with normal receptive language, especially bright youngsters, are particularly vulnerable to this frustration. Normal dysfluency is most common between 18 and 36 months of age but can persist up to age 5 years. It is characterized by intermittent repetitions of sounds, syllables, and words, especially at the beginning of sentences. Stuttering is manifested by a higher frequency and longer duration of such repetitions, often accompanied by eye blinking and other signs of tension. Based on the importance of using a flexible approach in determining the range of normal expectations, Tables 5-11 and 5-12 provide guidelines for assessing normal progress in both receptive and expressive language performance.

ASSESSMENT AND DIAGNOSIS

Pediatric assessment of language development in young children is based on a careful history and on opportunistic observation in the clinical setting. Information from parents or other caregivers is best obtained through open-ended questions. In the receptive domain, one simply asks, "What do you think (the child) understands?" Because the parents of a typical toddler often report that the child

TABLE 5-11
RECEPTIVE LANGUAGE DEVELOPMENT

6 months
 Own name
12 months
 Names of family members
 Names of familiar objects
 Simple phrases (eg, "all gone," "bye-bye," "peek-a-boo")
 Simple requests (eg, "give me the ___")
15 months
 Names of family members and familiar objects
 Body parts
 Simple phrases (eg, "no more")
 Simple instructions without gestural cues (eg, "go get your ___")
18 months
 Names of people, objects, and pictures
 Body parts
 Simple instructions without gestural cues (eg, "give the ___ to Mommy")
24 months
 Names of people, objects, and pictures
 Body parts (at least seven)
 Simple instructions without gestural cues (eg, "put the ___ on the table")
3 years
 Names of almost all common objects
 Physical relations (eg, "on," "in," "under")
 Concept of "two"
 Gender differences
 Two- or three-step instructions (eg, "put the ___ on the chair, and put the ___ under the table")
4 years
 Identification of colors
 Concepts of "same" and "different"
 Three-step instructions

TABLE 5-12

EXPRESSIVE LANGUAGE DEVELOPMENT

6 months
  Vocalizations (eg, screeching, babbling)
  Differential cries
12 months
  Gestures (eg, pointing, head shaking)
  Words (eg, "mama," "dada")
15 months
  Gestures
  Words (other than "mama" or "dada")
18 months
  Gestures
  Words (15 to 20)
  Phrases (2 to 3 words)
  Intelligibility to family members
24 months
  Gestures
  Words (rapidly expanding vocabulary)
  Phrases (2 to 3 words)
  Fluency (eg, stuttering)
  Intelligibility to strangers (25%)
3 years
  Words (regular plurals, pronouns, prepositions)
  Complete sentences (3 to 4 words)
  Short paragraphs
  Fluency
  Intelligibility to strangers (75%)
4 years
  Words (past tense)
  Complete sentences (4 to 5 words)
  Short paragraphs
  Ability to describe a recent experience/tell a story
  Fluency
  Intelligibility to strangers (almost 100%)

TABLE 5-13

"RED FLAGS" IN SPEECH AND LANGUAGE DEVELOPMENT

Referral by 12 to 15 months
  Child is not babbling or using a variety of consonant and vowel sounds
Referral between 18 and 24 months
  Child uses only a few single words spontaneously and no significant increase in vocabulary is noted
Referral by 2 years
  Child listens but does not appear to understand simple directions unless accompanied by pointing or demonstration
  Child indicates wants by pointing or using descriptive sounds rather than specific words
  Child is not producing two-syllable words and/or combining words
Referral between 2.0 and 2.5 years
  Child attempts to say words but cannot be understood most of the time
  Child seems to consistently omit the beginning and/or final consonants or reduces the number of syllables in a word
  Child is not using two- to three-word sentences
  Child does not appear to understand or remember two-step directions
  Child does not pronounce the following sounds clearly: m, p, b, w, n, h
Referral by 3 years
  Child has difficulty repeating a four- to five-word sentence related to an activity in which he or she is involved
Referral by 3.5 years
  Child frequently uses indefinite words like "that," "those," or "there" instead of naming specific objects, persons, or places
  Child omits words in sentences, or uses incorrect adjectives, verb endings, or pronouns
  Child does not pronounce the following sounds clearly: d, t, g, k, f
Referral by 4 years
  Child has difficulty telling a simple story or explaining an event that has just happened
Referral by 5 years
  Child does not pronounce the following sounds clearly: v, l, j, ch, sh
Referral by 6 years
  Child does not pronounce the following sounds clearly: z, s, r, th, st

understands "everything," it may be necessary to ask for specific examples. In the expressive domain, it is useful to inquire, "How does (the child) communicate what he/she wants?" This provides a baseline impression of how easy or difficult it is for the child to make his or her needs known. After the initial parental responses to these open-ended inquiries are recorded, one can follow up with specific probes using the landmarks presented in Tables 5-11 and 5-12 as guidelines. Once a descriptive database has been obtained, it is necessary to determine whether the child's abilities fall within the range of normative expectations. "Red flags" indicating a threshold for seeking a more thorough evaluation and possible intervention are provided in Table 5-13.

The differential diagnosis of late talking is summarized in Table 5-14. Any child with a significant delay in language development must have a formal hearing assessment by an audiologist who is trained to evaluate young children. Hearing screening in a pediatric office setting is not sufficient in such cases, and such screening is particularly vulnerable to missing a mild, high-frequency, sensorineural hearing loss that can result in a substantial language problem. Because few children with mild mental retardation exhibit early motor delays, late talking is the most common early manifestation of a global intellectual impairment, which must be ruled out by a comprehensive developmental assessment. Children with a pervasive developmental disorder or autism are recognizable by their stereotypic mannerisms and significant impairments in social interaction. Children with oral-motor dysfunction secondary to dysarthria (eg, cerebral palsy) or dyspraxia (eg, motor planning

problem) may have a history of feeding difficulties, excessive drooling, or other evidence of oral-motor incoordination. Both maturational delays and specific language disorders are found more frequently in association with a positive family history. Finally, although an "impoverished language environment" may be an important contributory factor in the delayed onset of talking, a careful clinical evaluation is needed to identify constitutional problems in the child that may make the child more vulnerable to the effects of an adverse environment. Most children with expressive language delays have normal receptive abilities, and the differential diagnosis generally is clear after a complete history, physical examination, hearing evaluation, and developmental assessment have been completed. An EEG should be considered for children with significant

TABLE 5-14

DIFFERENTIAL DIAGNOSIS OF LATE TALKING

Hearing impairment
Mental retardation
Specific language disorder
Pervasive developmental disorder/autism
Oral-motor dysfunction (dysarthria, dyspraxia)
Maturational delay
"Impoverished language environment"

receptive language abilities, which occasionally are related to subclinical seizure activity in the temporal lobes. In the absence of any suspicion of a specific health condition, no additional laboratory tests are indicated.

MANAGEMENT

Although children with significant language disorders benefit from specialized early intervention services, management of late talking begins in the pediatric primary-care setting. Once it is determined that the child has normal hearing and that the child's problems fall within the domain of a simple maturational delay or specific language disorder, early treatment focuses on assuring that the caregiving environment is oriented toward language facilitation. A supportive health-care provider can provide valuable guidelines to parents in this regard.

Throughout the infant and toddler period, children are provided with labels for objects and words to describe their everyday experiences *in context.* Any attempt by a child to imitate a sound should be followed by verbal praise. The imitation of verbal intonation patterns or the first sounds of a word can be reinforced over time as the child's responses come closer to matching the adult model. This process is known as *shaping* a response. In general, children are reinforced more effectively when an adult imitates what they say, rather than when they are pressured to produce a specific sound or word.

Whenever a child does produce a meaningful sound or specific word, it is important to provide a response that will facilitate more sophisticated language development. This process, termed *modeling* or *extension,* is illustrated by the following examples:

- If the child says a word but does not articulate the first or last sound clearly, it is helpful to repeat the word, emphasizing that sound; and
- If the child says a single word clearly, the listener should respond by expanding the word to a two-word utterance (eg, child sees a dog and says "doggie"; parent responds "Hi, doggie").

Finally, a number of behaviors that are important to encourage generally emerge between 18 and 24 months. These behaviors include:

- Exclamatory expressions such as "oh-oh" and "no-no";
- Combining verbal expressions with pointing or gesturing to obtain objects (provides an opportunity for shaping and modeling);
- Jabbering during play (can be reinforced by comments such as "nice talking");
- Echoing the last word spoken (adult reinforcement is likely to stimulate continued talking);
- Imitating environmental sounds (eg, animals, motors, and so on);
- Attempting to sing along (using familiar tunes such as "Happy Birthday" and nursery rhymes); and
- Vocalizing wishes and needs during familiar routines such as mealtime (provides an opportunity to praise *any* attempt at vocalizing and to give the child the words that he or she needs through modeling).

In general, children will not respond to confrontation or pressure to speak. Reinforcement, encouragement, shaping, and modeling are the keys to language facilitation.

Children less than 2 years of age with significant language delays should be referred to an early intervention program. After 3 years of age, the specialized services of a speech and language pathologist are essential; between 2 and 3 years of age, the relative indications for generic developmental services versus specialized therapeutic intervention must be determined on an individual basis. Normal dysfluencies and mild stuttering are best treated by providing reassurance and support for the parents. Persistent or severe stuttering indicates the need for consultation with a speech and language pathologist.

NATURAL HISTORY AND PROGNOSIS

Long-term data on "late talkers" are extremely limited. A large percentage of children with isolated expressive language delays eventually "catch up" and exhibit no significant developmental sequelae. A significant subgroup, however, have continued problems in language performance and ultimately are at greater risk for language-based learning difficulties during the school-age years. Some children with an early language delay may experience an "illusory recovery period" during the preschool years but subsequently have difficulty in learning to read during the early elementary grades because of problems with phonetic awareness (ie, difficulty recognizing individual parts of words such as sounds or syllables). Most stuttering is resolved by late childhood, leaving 1% of the population with long-term problems into the adult years. Unfortunately, there are limited data to assist in formulating specific prognoses for individual children.

Youngsters with problems in receptive as well as expressive language are at much greater risk. Children who live in high-risk environments have a more guarded prognosis. Although there are no hard data to assess the impact of age of intervention on long-term outcomes, the relative benefits of earlier treatment for children with more significant disorders has received widespread endorsement. This is particularly important for children who develop significant behavior problems secondary to their communication difficulties and for whom long-term problems in social development are a major concern.

References

Coplan J: Evaluation of the child with delayed speech or language. Pediatr Ann 14:203–208, 1985

Paul R: Late bloomers: language development and delay in toddlers. In: Butler KG, ed: Topics in Language Disorders, Vol 11, Number 4. Gaithersburg, MD, Aspen Publishers, 1991

Prizant BM, Wetherby AM: Assessing the communication of infants and toddlers: integrating a socioemotional perspective. Zero to Three 11: 1–12, 1990

Resnick TJ, Allen DA, Rapin I: Disorders of language development: diagnosis and intervention. Pediatr Rev 6:85–92, 1984

Rice ML: Children's language acquisition. Am Psychologist 44:149–156, 1989

Richardson S: The child with "delayed speech." Contemp Pediatr 9:55–74, 1992

5.6.5   Difficult Behavior: Temper Tantrums to Conduct Disorders

Martin T. Stein

All children and adolescents display some disruptive behaviors while growing up. These behaviors come to clinical attention when a parent, teacher, clinician, or other adult experiences the behavior as troublesome or unsettling. It is often the adult's perceptions of the behavior, their tolerance, emotional response, and social expectations that determines whether a child's behavior comes to the attention of a pediatrician. Disruptive behaviors become a part of a pediatric encounter under three circumstances: (a) when the behavior is overwhelming to parents or teachers and is interfering with social interactions; (b) when a pediatrician systematically surveys family function and childhood behavior as part of a periodic health supervision visit; or (c) when a disruptive behavior occurs during an office visit.

Disruptive behaviors in children include temper tantrums, angry outbursts that may be physical or verbal, hitting, biting, pushing, as well as more serious antisocial behaviors such as stealing, setting fires, truancy from school, destruction of property, animal cruelty, and physical confrontations with other people. A common clinical pitfall when confronted with a disruptive behavior is for the clinician to respond with a well-intentioned suggestion or intervention, without exploring the nature of the behavior in the context of the child's developmental stage, the environmental factors that may trigger the behavior, or the parental response to the episodes. Each of these elements is critical to answer the following questions:

Is the behavior a normative phenomenon at this particular stage of development?

- Infants are characteristically more irritable in late afternoon and early evening.
- Strangers may initiate a fear response in some infants at the end of the first year of life and during the second year.
- All toddlers experience temper tantrums during moments of frustration when their journey toward psychologic autonomy is threatened.
- Separation experiences from parents are commonly associated with emotional outbursts, crying, and sleep disturbances at this age.

These examples reflect the importance of the developmental tasks of attachment during the first year of life and autonomy in the second year. Exploring disruptive behaviors at this time of life in the context of the continuum from attachment and trust to autonomy and independence provides a clinical framework for insight as well as guidance.

What characteristics of the child's family, peer, and school environments contribute to or modify the behavior? The social context in which behaviors unfold may trigger, exacerbate, or ameliorate those behaviors. Emotional responses in younger children may be modified by verbal and nonverbal responses of parents and other caretakers. School-aged children and adolescents are influenced by peers and teachers. The media, neighborhood, and the expectations generated from school are additional potent environmental influences on the behavior of children.

How have the parents (and other providers of childcare) responded to the disruptions? Parental responses to disruptive behaviors in their children span a broad continuum, from active intervention to withdrawal. Each response reflects parental temperament, understanding of developmental expectations, family stress in economic and psychological, domains, and, perhaps most significantly, their own experiences growing up and memories of parent–child encounters. An exploration of these factors often yields insights into the interventions and responses that parents have experienced as they attempt to alter disruptive behaviors. In addition, the information provides a basis for the clinician to tailor pediatric guidance to the needs of a particular family and child.

DEFINITIONS AND EPIDEMIOLOGY

The spectrum of disruptive behaviors in childhood is broad and, to a large extent, depends on developmental stage. *Episodic crying* of less than 3 cumulative hours each day occurs in all infants in the first 3 months after birth. Approximately 15% of young infants experience longer periods of fussiness at this stage. These "colicky" babies are typically calmer as they enter the fourth month. *Temper tantrums* are reported by parents in as many as 80% of 2- to 4-year-old children. Tantrums occur at least once each day in about 20% of 2-year-old children and 10% of 4-year-old children. Moderate to severe tantrums are reported in 5% of 3-year-old children.

Some infants and children hold their breath during a temper tantrum. *Breath-holding* usually occurs at the initiation of a tantrum when the emotion (eg, fear, anger, frustration) is triggered by an environmental event. At least one breath-holding spell occurs in 5% of children. Family pedigree analysis of children with severe breath-holding spells suggests an autosomal dominant trait with reduced penetrance. A positive family history for breath-holding or fainting is common. These behaviors usually appear in the second year of life and may continue until 5 years of age; they also may occur in some infants after 6 months of age. Two physiological types have been described: (a) a cyanotic form in which the face turns blue until breathing resumes, and (b) a pallid type in which the face is pale secondary to vasovagal syncope. In both forms, the child ceases breathing following a period of intense crying. Syncope occasionally develops at the moment the child begins to cry; this may be seen with the pallid spells and be associated with a rigid, arching posture. Breathlessness is brief and followed by spontaneous respiration and normal behavior. A minority of these children will have symmetric tonic-clonic movements before awakening. Although benign, breath-holding spells are dramatic and frightening to many parents; those with a family history of breath-holding spells may be less concerned as a result of awareness of their benign nature. They do not cause irreversible hypoxic brain injury or epilepsy, and subsequent cognitive development and behavior are normal. There is emerging evidence that iron therapy is effective in reducing the frequency of recurrent breath-holding spells in children with and without biochemical evidence of iron deficiency. The mechanism for this response is unknown.

ETIOLOGY AND PATHOGENESIS

The etiology of socially disruptive behaviors is multifactorial and can be framed in the context of developmental expectations and temperament patterns of the child and other family members; expectations and responses of caretakers to disruptive behaviors; family patterns including interpersonal relationships, socioeconomic class, and educational levels; and biological predisposition for specific patterns of psychological dysfunction.

Development and Temperament

Frustration, anger, and aggressive outbursts are experienced during all stages of the life cycle, with a predictable decline in frequency and intensity through time. Age-specific developmental tasks account for some of these behaviors. For example, the toddler's struggle for emotional independence as he or she separates from an infantile attachment to parents frequently manifests with tantrums or nightmares; these behaviors reflect the child's struggle with the "push-pull" process of emotional separation and individuation. In a similar fashion, adolescent defiance directed to parents, verbal and physical outbursts of anger, and isolated acts of social defiance may reflect the requisite quest for autonomy as he or she strives for independence from family and searches for a personal identity.

Behaviors that are beyond the borders of the expected developmental range may result from individual temperament styles. Temperament refers to stable biological–psychological traits that focus on an individual's reactive style and are under some degree of genetic control. Even in the absence of social, economic, or other environmental stressors, a child's temperament may be a significant contributor to a particular behavior. Irritable and colicky infants, excessively clinging 1-year-old children, easily frustrated and tantrum-prone toddlers, and physically intrusive preschoolers represent particular specific temperament-regulated patterns of behavior that manifest at various developmental stages.

Temperament may play an even larger role in the etiology of a disruptive behavior when the temperament of an infant, child, or adolescent is not in harmony with that of an adult authority (eg, parents, other caretakers, teachers). Coping strategies in response to developmentally appropriate disruptive behaviors require parental composure, reflection, and recognition of the need for a cooling-off period, which may not be a natural response for some temperamentally highly reactive parents. In addition, an inhibited 2- or 3-year-old child may be at risk for development of a disruptive behavior only when a poor temperament fit between child and parent exists or when a family is disorganized and troubled.

Expectations and Responses

The behavioral expectations of adult caretakers and teachers may mediate the intensity, frequency, and outcome of disruptive behaviors in children. It is clinically useful to view childhood behaviors as transactional phenomena. A behavior does not stand alone. Its quality and quantity is influenced by other persons in the immediate environment (eg, peers, parents, teachers). In fact, a behavioral dialogue can be seen as an emotional conversation between two individuals, each influencing the other by verbal and nonverbal responses.

In this transactional model, the expectations of parents and teachers will modify the behavior of a child. When a school-age child repeatedly refuses to clean his or her room, parental expectations of personal responsibilities for tidiness and the youngster's desire to please the parent will interact and guide the next response. The parent may make a reasoned request, an angry demand, or physically punish the child; a reward system or series of punishments may follow. The adult response to a disruptive behavior is mediated by both the adult's expectations and the effect that the behavior evokes in the adult.

Family Patterns

The quality of early attachment experiences influences subsequent behavior, especially in response to frustration. The emotional security and nutritional adequacy that are required for healthy infant–maternal attachment during the first year yields a sense of trust in oneself and others as the infant enters the second year. The development and maintenance of psychological attachment to a parent or other family member over time provides the emotional foundation to manage and make sense out of the many moments of ambiguity and uncertainty that become prominent after the child's first birthday. Children who experience family disruptions, serious physical or emotional illness in a parent, family violence that is directed toward the child or parent, or major economic hardship are at risk for disruptive behaviors. Social, economic, or psychological stressors within the family may be a primary cause of the behavior

or act as secondary triggers for a child or family where a biological predisposition exists.

Families also act as systems in which each component member depends on other members. A disruptive behavior pattern in a child may reflect a more generic pathology in the social or psychological makeup of the family system. At times, a family may appear to be functionally and socially intact, while a child's externalizing behavior presents as the problem. Drug or alcohol abuse in a parent, marital disharmony, and chronic sexual abuse are examples of family dynamics that may influence disruptive behavior in children.

Biological Factors

Several different lines of research strengthen the argument that genetic endowment plays a role in the etiology of disruptive behaviors. Perhaps the strongest evidence is the continuity of temperament in some groups of infants. For example, vigilant, alert babies who experience relatively smooth state transitions tend to be less irritable infants and more uninhibited toddlers and school-age children. Their risk for oppositional behavior and conduct disorder is considerably less than that in irritable infants who develop inhibited toddler temperaments.

Injury to the CNS correlates with disruptive social behaviors in particular situations. Temporal lobe epilepsy is an example of a focal abnormality that may be associated with episodic disruptive behaviors. CNS tumors and encephalitis may be associated, or even present, with behavioral outbursts and mood lability.

Chromosome disorders (eg, XYY and 5p-deletion), progressive encephalopathies (eg, Rett syndrome), inborn errors of metabolism (eg, Lesch-Nyhan syndrome and Wilson disease), and toxic encephalopathy (eg, lead, mercury, alcohol, cocaine, methamphetamine, hallucinogen poisoning) are examples of biological disorders that are associated with severe manifestations of disruptive behaviors. Although the precise anatomic and neurochemical abnormality remains uncertain, it does appear that function in the amygdala portion of the limbic system may be altered in these disorders.

A genetic component for aggressive and antisocial behavior has been demonstrated in studies that show a concordance for criminality among monozygotic twins. In addition, children of male and female criminals who are raised in adoptive homes demonstrate more antisocial behaviors than adopted children of noncriminal parents do.

CLINICAL MANIFESTATIONS

Symptoms of disruptive behaviors are specific to each developmental stage. The pattern of expressed behavior will reflect a child's verbal, motor, and affective developmental capacities. Boundaries for behavior set by adults will also determine the characteristics of the behavior. The challenge for clinicians is to separate those behaviors that are normal developmental variations from those that represent an emotional disorder or are symptoms of a specific disease process. Prognosis and intervention strategies will be guided by this distinction. When distinguishing developmental variation from a disorder, specific clinical patterns of disruptive behavior are often less important than an assessment of duration, intensity, and effect on family function, school performance, and socialization skills.

Oppositional Defiant Disorder

Frequent temper tantrums occur in some children with an intensity, frequency, and duration that disrupts the family, school, or neighborhood. These children often experience frequent loss of temper in response to apparently minimal frustrations. They may express a pattern of behavior that is argumentative, negativistic, and hostile. Lability of mood, limited tolerance to frustrating events, and low esteem may be associated with the disruptive behavior in these children. A formal diagnostic category, *oppositional defiant disorder*, has been used to describe these children in whom a specified pattern of behavior lasting at least 6 months can be documented (Table 5-15). Importantly, these behaviors occur in normal children at the school-aged and adolescent stages of development. When these behaviors present frequently and with a greater-than-expected intensity, an oppositional defiant disorder should be considered.

Conduct Disorder

Disruptive behaviors that are repetitive, persistent (ie, at least 6 months), and violate the rights of other people or their property suggest a behavior pattern consistent with a *conduct disorder* (Table 5-16). Children who have a conduct disorder do not respond with guilt or remorse when confronted with their misconduct. These quarrelsome school-aged and adolescent children are typically seen by pediatricians after recurrent episodes of stealing, lying, fighting, setting fires, perpetration of sexual abuse, or drug abuse.

Two distinct groups of children and adolescents with a conduct disorder have been identified. The *undersocialized* form demonstrates an impairment in interpersonal relationships that manifests as unpopularity, lack of any close friendships, and generalized social isolation. These children may lack empathy for peers and are hostile and argumentative toward adults. This form of aggressive and undersocialized behavior is pervasive, typically occurring at school, at home, and in the community. Those children with the *socialized* pattern of conduct disorder participate in antisocial behaviors (eg, criminal acts, school truancy) in the context of a peer group. Interpersonal attachments are strong and binding, but relationships with adults are inconsistent and characterized by confrontation with authority.

TABLE 5-15
DIAGNOSTIC CRITERIA FOR OPPOSITIONAL DEFIANT DISORDER

A. A pattern of negativistic, hostile, and defiant behavior lasting at least 6 months, during which four (or more) of the following are present:
   (1) Often loses temper
   (2) Often argues with adults
   (3) Often actively defies or refuses to comply with adults' requests or rules
   (4) Often deliberately annoys people
   (5) Often blames others for his or her mistakes or misbehavior
   (6) Is often touchy or easily annoyed by others
   (7) Is often angry and resentful
   (8) Is often spiteful or vindictive
   Note: Consider a criterion met only if the behavior occurs more frequently than is typically observed in individuals of comparable age and developmental level.
B. The disturbance in behavior causes clinically significant impairment in social, academic, or occupational functioning
C. The behaviors do not occur exclusively during the course of a Psychotic or Mood Disorder.
D. Criteria are not met for Conduct Disorder, and if the individual is age 18 years or older, criteria are not met for Antisocial Personality Disorder.

SOURCE: *Reprinted with permission from the Diagnostic and Statistical Manual of Mental Disorders, Fourth Edition. Copyright 1994 American Psychiatric Association.*

TABLE 5-16
DIAGNOSTIC CRITERIA FOR CONDUCT DISORDER

A. A repetitive and persistent pattern of behavior in which the basic rights of others or major age-appropriate societal norms or rules are violated, as manifested by the presence of three (or more) of the following criteria in the past 12 months, with at least one criterion present in the past 6 months:
   Aggression to people and animals
   (1) Often bullies, threatens, or intimidates others
   (2) Often initiates physical fights
   (3) Has used a weapon that can cause serious physical harm to others (eg, a bat, brick, broken bottle, knife, gun)
   (4) Has been physically cruel to people
   (5) Has been physically cruel to animals
   (6) Has stolen while confronting a victim (eg, mugging, purse snatching, extortion, armed robbery)
   (7) Has forced someone into sexual activity
   Destruction of property
   (8) Has deliberately engaged in fire setting with the intention of causing serious damage
   (9) Has deliberately destroyed others property (other than by fire setting)
   Deceitfulness or theft
   (10) Has broken into someone else's house, building, or car
   (11) Often lies to obtain goods or favors or to avoid obligations (ie, "cons" others)
   (12) Has stolen items of nontrivial value without confronting a victim (eg, shoplifting, but without breaking and entering; forgery)
   Serious violations of rules
   (13) Often stays out at night despite parental prohibitions, beginning before age 13 years
   (14) Has run away from home overnight at least twice while living in parental or parental surrogate home (or once without returning for a lengthy period)
   (15) Is often truant from school, beginning before age 13 years
B. The disturbance in behavior causes clinically significant impairment in social, academic, or occupational functioning.
C. If the individual is age 18 years or older, criteria are not met for Antisocial Personality Disorder.
Specify type based on age at onset:
   Childhood-Onset Type: onset of at least one criterion characteristic of Conduct Disorder prior to age 10 years
   Adolescent-Onset Type: absence of any criteria characteristic of Conduct Disorder prior to age 10 years
Specify severity:
   Mild: few if any conduct problems in excess of those required to make the diagnosis and conduct problems cause only minor harm to others
   Moderate: number of conduct problems and effect on others intermediate between "mild" and "severe"
   Severe: many conduct problems in excess of those required to make the diagnosis or conduct problems cause considerable harm to others

SOURCE: *Reprinted with permission from the Diagnostic and Statistical Manual of Mental Disorders, Fourth Edition. Copyright 1994 American Psychiatric Association.*

ASSESSMENT AND DIAGNOSIS

The diagnostic assessment process has four major goals:

- To describe the child's or adolescent's behavior in detail, with attention to triggering events and environmental setting;
- To define psychological, economic, and social stressors within the family or community that may affect the behavior;
- To delineate the content and style of parental responses to the behavior; and

- To explore the strengths that exist within the child as well as the family and the community environment that may be protective factors or, alternatively, that may be recruited as a treatment.

As in most areas of diagnostic decision-making, it is important to prevent premature diagnostic impressions. A behavioral diagnosis does not need to be daunting in a pediatric practice when the requisite data are obtained with care and in some detail. A comprehensive, developmentally based personal and family history will assure the primary-care pediatrician that important data are included. Pediatricians who follow children longitudinally for developmental surveillance and comprehensive health supervision will have the advantage of previous knowledge about the child's development and the family's level of functioning and will thus be positioned to assess disruptive behavior at an early stage.

A request should be made to the parent or school for past psychoeducational evaluations, disciplinary reports, and report cards. A brief narrative from the teacher, specifically discussing classroom and playground behaviors, learning style and output, and perceived strengths, will be helpful. During an initial interview, observation of the child's and parent's affective state and the parent–child interactions should be recorded in the medical record. Assessment of independent and interactive play in a pediatric office is possible when toys are available. Some pediatricians find it useful to supplement the initial interview with a brief behavioral screening test. A pediatric assessment for a behavioral problem is not complete without an examination by a physician.

Parents can be interviewed alone and with the child, and adolescents should be given an opportunity to tell their story without the presence of a parent. When possible, a family interview, including parents and siblings, will yield important information about interpersonal dynamics. Focused questions such as the following will delineate important details about the behaviors and contributing factors:

- Describe your child's tantrum (or troubling behavior) as you experience it.
- Do you know what brings on these behaviors?
- In what settings does the behavior occur (eg, home, school, with peers, in public places)?
- What is your response to the behavior? Your spouse's response? Other children's response?
- Have you tried other responses in the past? Describe them.
- Who manages most disruptive behaviors in your home?
- Describe some of your child's strengths. When does your child make you happy or proud?
- Does your child have friends? A best friend? What activities do they participate in together?
- Can you recall how tantrums and other difficult child behaviors were managed during your childhood? Tell me about those experiences.

While asking these questions, the clinician is also beginning the treatment process. Questions should be asked empathically and without conveying a hurried atmosphere. Recognition of helpful parent interventions will go far in the development of a therapeutic alliance.

Inquire about anger outbursts, physical or verbal violence, and specific encounters with a mental health professional by other members of the immediate and extended family. A family history of related problems such as dropping out of school, truancy, job dissatisfaction or chronic unemployment, and alcohol or drug abuse

may be helpful in formulating a diagnosis. Some pediatricians may resist exploring the family dynamics in areas of marital discord, sexual dissatisfaction, and childhood experiences of parents. However, this information informs and expands the diagnostic process, especially during an evaluation for disruptive childhood behaviors.

Inquire about social forces that may influence childhood behaviors. Does violence permeate the neighborhood? Are guns available in the home? How much television does the child watch each day? What kind of programs does he or she watch? Are violent shows or those with overt sexual messages monitored? Do the parents discuss violent themes or socially controversial topics on television with the child? This line of questioning is also appropriate for movie-watching behavior.

The final step in the diagnostic formulation is to decide which behaviors are developmentally appropriate, which reflect a moderate variation from a predictable norm, and which patterns of behavior represent one of the disruptive behavior disorders. This formulation may not be apparent after the initial interview; at other times, the pattern of behavior may not fit into a single category. The assessment process for disruptive behaviors may not require a specific pediatric diagnosis, but rather the development of insight about the place on the continuum from normal variation to psychopathology at which this child's and family's behavior fits. Further diagnostic "tuning" may occur at future office visits or in association with a referring mental health professional.

MANAGEMENT AND TREATMENT

The approach to management of disruptive childhood behaviors depends on the intensity, frequency, and number of settings in which the behavior occurs, as well as the pediatrician's willingness to spend a modest amount of time with the family. When confronting a pattern of repetitive disruptive behaviors, the process of clinical evaluation begins the treatment process. For most parents, a setting to explore the troublesome behavior with a pediatric clinician is therapeutic in itself. An empathic clinician listens carefully and actively while asking focused questions about the child's temperament; social interactions with peers, parents, siblings, and teachers; and the responses of parents and other caretakers. A clear demonstration of respect for different parenting styles encourages a therapeutic bond between parent and clinician. This bond can be used to explore family values with regard to child-rearing and specific responses to disruptive behavior. Focused questions such as the following directed to the parent may clarify the nature of discipline:

- What are you trying to teach?
- Why is it important to you?
- How are you trying to teach it?
- What is your child learning?

In some situations, a parent may be reassured about the range of normal developmental expectations, with the clinician emphasizing that an isolated disruptive behavior may in fact reflect an adaptive response and a strength in overall development. The clinician may point out that the toddler or adolescent is expressing his or her autonomy and quest for emotional independence in a healthy, affirmative way. In other cases, an assessment will suggest that the behaviors are outside the expected developmental range and require intervention. Pediatricians can manage most children with toddler tantrums, episodic breath-holding spells, and mild forms of oppositional defiant disorders. School-age children and adolescents with a conduct disorder generally require long-term behavioral and psychotherapeutic intervention programs. Referral to a mental health specialist is usually necessary in these cases.

A common pitfall in the management of disruptive behaviors is to limit the intervention to a plan for behavior modification. While a therapeutically powerful and useful treatment to be sure, a management plan that is limited to behavioral techniques risks inattention to other important diagnostic concerns such as parental depression, school refusal or truancy, disorders of attention, learning disabilities, and child or spousal abuse. These problems frequently coexist with disruptive behaviors. Assessment and management of these associated disorders may be as important or even more significant than the disruptive behavior with regard to prognosis and outcome.

TABLE 5-17

APPROACHES FOR PARENTS TO DISRUPTIVE BEHAVIORS

Anticipating Disruptive Behaviors. Suggest that parents list situations in which places where disruptive behaviors are more likely to occur. Suggest strategies for avoiding or altering those difficult moments. For example, shop with children when they are rested and bring along a distraction (toys, dolls, or books); use appropriate videos or *Sesame Street* when preparing dinner. Parents can restructure their physical environment at home in order to limit recurring and frustrating moments. They can also anticipate a disruptive behavior by preparing the child for a predictable transition (eg, "Five more minutes to play before bedtime.")

Parent–Child Communication Skills. Teach parents to use clear and unequivocal directions. "It's time to go to bed." versus "Would you like to go to bed?" Educate parents of toddlers that receptive language matures before expressive language. They can use words that are beyond the young child's speech capacity to communicate ideas, feelings, and expectations.

Active Listening. Some parents benefit by examples that demonstrate this technique. "You seem real angry now!" or "You're really upset with your sister!" These brief verbal reflections of the child's emotional state are to be followed by a moment of silence which allows children to reflect on the experience of hearing their parents express their emotional feelings. A new level of parent–child communication may follow.

Distracting a Child. When a disruptive behavior is in an early stage, it is often useful to distract the child to another activity. Offering a toy or book or even taking the child to another room may defuse a difficult moment. Intuitive parents know this technique; others require direction and examples.

Time-Out. This form of discipline may be useful as a response to more severe disruptive behaviors, including tantrums. Placing the child in his/her room for a brief period (1 minute for each year of age with a maximum of 5 minutes) or an older child in a chair in the corner of a room may be helpful. The parent should explain the reason for a time-out. A time-out should be followed by a "time-in" period when the child is welcomed back into the social group. A hug and a few kind words demonstrates genuine affection. This experience provides the child with an opportunity to regulate an out-of-control emotional response, to reconstitute his/her affective state, and, simultaneously, it provides a focused response for parents. Time alone should never be excessive.

Behavioral Reinforcement. All children require parental reinforcement when appropriate and healthy behaviors occur. Children with disruptive behaviors need a heavier dose! Self-esteem and conscience formation are enhanced when parents praise a child for a positive behavior or action. Parents can be taught to recognize and respond to positive behaviors with frequent words and facial expressions of praise. Negative and disruptive behaviors that are not excessive or intrusive should be ignored. Attention to negative behavior encourages those behaviors when the child experiences them as the primary access to a parent's attention.

One of the most challenging and frequent inquiries for pediatricians in the area of behavioral pediatrics is discipline. Knowing that the Latin verb *disciplinare* is the root of the English word *discipline* is illuminating to many parents when they learn that it means *to teach* or *to instruct*. A parent's ability to discipline and to teach is central to raising emotionally healthy children who can learn societal rules; live, play, and eventually work with others; develop a positive sense of self; and discern right from wrong (ie, the development of a conscience). Modeling positive behaviors by means of language and actions remains the most effective disciplinarian tool for parents. Punishments for unwanted and disruptive behaviors should be consistent (from time to time and among family members), logical, and reasonably immediate. Loss of privileges (eg, television, meals with the family, a sleepover with a friend) usually gives a strong message that the disruptive behavior will not be tolerated.

Physical punishment in the form of spanking is a common practice in American families. Its use appears to be the result of historical tradition with biblical and puritanical roots. The initial rapid suppression of a disruptive behavior after physical punishment is attractive to many parents. Many well-meaning and effective parents frequently use physical punishment to teach acceptable behavior; in some cultures and ethnic groups, physical punishment toward children is more acceptable than in others.

The argument against physical punishment focuses on two issues. First, there are other effective methods for managing disruptive behaviors that teach children self-regulation, provide alternatives to uncontrolled anger, and assist in the attainment of self-esteem (Table 5-17). Second, physical punishment models an adult method of conflict resolution that children should not be taught to use. It is a form of behavior modification that cannot be internalized in the child's quest for learning to regulate feelings and conflicts. In fact, it may be experienced as a form of resolving unpleasant situations that is counterproductive to their emerging sense of self-worth. Child-oriented advocacy that focuses on anticipatory guidance, behavior modification, improved parent–child communication skills, and effective limit-setting is more appropriate for pediatric counseling.

References

American Academy of Pediatrics, Committee on Psychosocial Aspects of Child and Family Health: Policy statement on guidance for effective discipline. Pediatrics 101:723, 1998

American Academy of Pediatrics: The short- and long-term consequences of corporal punishment. Part 2. Pediatrics 98:803, 1996

Clark L: The Time-Out Solution. Chicago, Contemporary Books, 1989

Daoud AS, Batieha A, Al-Sheyyab M, et al: Effectiveness of iron therapy on breath-holding spells. J Pediatr 130:547–550, 1997

Dimario FJ JR: Breath-holding spells in childhood. Am J Dis Child 146:125–131, 1992

Dixon SD, Stein MT: Encounters with Children: Pediatric Behavior and Development, 2nd ed. St. Louis, MO, Mosby-Year Book, 1992

Faber A, Mazlish E: How to Talk so Kids Will Listen and Listen so Kids Will Talk. New York, Avon, 1980

Gordon T: P.E.T. Parent Effectiveness Training: The Tested New Way to Raise Responsible Children. New York, New American Library, 1975

Gottlieb SE, Friedman SB: Conduct disorders in children and adolescents. Pediatr Rev 12:218–223, 1991

Howard BJ: Discipline in early childhood. Pediatr Clin North Am 38:1351–1369, 1991

Lombroso CT, Lerman P: Breathholding spells (cyanotic and pallid infantile syncope). Pediatrics 39:563–581, 1967

Smith EE, Van Tassel E: Problems of discipline in early childhood. Pediatr Clin North Am 29:167–176, 1982

Vaughan VC, Litt IF: Child and Adolescent Development: Clinical Implications. Philadelphia, Saunders, 1990

Wolraich ML: The Classification of Child and Adolescent Mental Diagnosis in Primary Care (DSM-PC). Elk Grove Village, IL, American Academy of Pediatrics, 1996

5.6.6   Separation Difficulties: Clinging Behaviors to School Refusal

Constance Helen Keefer

Most children will display shyness with strangers, fear of new places, clinginess with mother, or reluctance to go to school at some time in their early years of life, depending on their stage of development, temperament, and circumstance. These behaviors reflect normal development of attachment, autonomy, and self-esteem, and the range of individual differences in temperament. Certain children persist in these reactions, however, in a way that interferes with their social development and that indicates problems in socioemotional development or the family situation. Even when not reflecting pathology in the child or the family, certain extreme variations in behavioral styles stress parents and require special pediatric guidance and support.

Pediatricians learn of these kinds of behavioral deviations through screening questions ("How is she adjusting to school?" and "How has he taken to the new baby sitter?"), through direct observations of the separations and stresses that occur in health supervision and sick visits, and through parents' spontaneous descriptions of these behaviors as problems. When such problems are presented, the pediatrician has an important role in locating the behavior along a spectrum from developmentally normal to serious disorder. Within this spectrum of shy and clingy behaviors, six clusters, or syndromes, can be identified: (a) expected for age and stage of development; (b) expected given the situation or circumstances; (c) temperamental style that is either extreme or perceived by a parent as problematic; (d) insecure attachment; (e) school refusal; and (f) separation anxiety disorder (SAD).

DEFINITION AND EPIDEMIOLOGY

Developmentally predictable clingy behavior around strangers becomes noticeable some time after 6 months of age, when all infants begin to show a preference for their mothers, especially when stressed, and a wariness with strangers or new situations. These behaviors intensify between 9 and 18 months, and wane by 2.5–3 years. Even after age 3, children experience some discomfort with the unfamiliar, but are able to deal with it internally or verbally so that no behavioral symptoms are manifest.

Acute situational factors, such as concurrent stressors (fatigue or illness) and recent losses (father's travel for work, death of a grandparent, a friend moving away), may be associated with symptoms throughout childhood.

Children vary in their styles of behaving along a number of dimensions of activity, reactivity, and emotionality. These are referred to as *temperamental characteristics* and are presumed to reflect constitutional traits that are relatively persistent, in some cases over many years, but are also shaped by interactions with caregivers. In short, temperament refers to the "how" of behavior, as opposed to the "what" or the "how well." The nine dimensions (Table 5-18)

TABLE 5-18
DIMENSIONS OF TEMPERAMENT

Activity level
The motor component present in a child's functioning and the diurnal proportion of active and inactive periods.

Rhythmicity[a]
The degree of predictability in time of any function (eg, sleep, hunger, elimination)

Approach-withdrawal
The nature of the child's initial responses to new or altered stimulus (eg, new food, toy, or person)

Adaptability[a]
The nature of a child's responses to new or altered situations regarding the ease with which they are modified in a desired direction (irrespective of the initial response)

Intensity of reaction
The energy level or vigor of a child's response independent of its direction (either negative or positive)

Threshold of responsiveness
The intensity level of stimulation that is necessary to evoke a discernible response

Quality of mood
The amount of pleased, joyful, and friendly behavior versus the amount of displeased, crying, and unfriendly behavior

Distractibility
The ease with which a child can be diverted from an ongoing activity by extraneous peripheral stimuli

Attention span/persistence
The length of time that a particular activity is pursued by a child and the continuation of an activity by a child in the face of obstacles to the maintenance of activity

---

[a] Scored on behaviors occurring over days or weeks.
SOURCE: *Adapted from Chess S, Thomas A: Dynamics of Individual behavioral development. In: Levine MD, Carey WB, Crocker AC, eds: Developmental-Behavioral Pediatrics. Philadelphia, WB Saunders, 1992.*

from Chess and Thomas are the most commonly used categorizations for assessment of temperament by parent questionnaire. Most of these dimensions can be identified in brief encounters with the child and match meaningfully the experience of many parents.

Using the Chess and Thomas categories, 65% of children can be classified into one of three constellations: the "difficult child" (10%), the "slow-to-warm-up child" (15%), and the "easy child" (40%). The temperament dimensions that define each cluster are shown in Table 5-19. Because these are not true syndromes but variations along a continuum of behavioral tendencies, and because 35% of children do not fall into any of the three constellations, the pediatrician should be prepared to explore all nine dimensions in order to explain extreme behavior in the child. For example, while the cluster of low adaptability and negative, but low-intensity, responses to new stimuli identifies the classic "slow-to-warm-up" child, clusters of other temperament dimensions might also contribute to a child's caution or anxiety in novel situations. A child who is highly persistent, poorly distractible, and tends to a negative affect does not fit one of the three temperamental types, but may appear to be shy by not noticing a new stimulus or by reacting negatively to the approach of visitors. In addition, the possibility of the problem being one of parental perception should be considered, because many studies show that certain children who are perceived by their parents as temperamentally difficult are not described that way when either the parents or the professionals use objective behavioral ratings rather than global characteristic ratings.

The *development of attachment* to caregivers, and the subsequent development of comfortable autonomy from them, are fun-

TABLE 5-19
CLUSTERS OF TEMPERAMENT DIMENSIONS

CLUSTERS	DIMENSIONS
Easy	Rhythmicity: Highly regular
	Approach-withdrawal (to novelty): Approaches
	Adaptability (to change): Highly adaptive
	Intensity of reaction: Mildly or moderately intense
	Mood: Positive
Difficult	Rhythmicity: Highly irregular
	Approach-withdrawal (to novelty): Withdraws
	Adaptability (to change): Nonadaptive or slowly adaptive
	Intensity of reaction: Extremely intense
	Mood: Negative
Slow-to-warm-up	Approach-withdrawal (to novelty): Withdraws
	Adaptability (to change): Slowly adaptive
	Intensity of reaction: Mildly intense
	Mood: Variable

damental tasks of the early years of life. In studies of attachment, Ainsworth and colleagues discovered four relatively inclusive and robust patterns of reaction to separation. The defining characteristics of the four patterns are the child's response to separation from the mother and her subsequent return and to the presence of a stranger during the mother's absence.

The most common response pattern is that of the securely attached child, who protests the mother's leaving, but can be consoled and distracted to attend to the toys in the room. This child seeks contact with the mother in the reunion, but once consoled, the child's attention can turn to play. The next most common is the insecure/avoidant child who barely notices the mother's leaving and return, and who actively moves away from the mother's attempts at contact upon reunion. The third pattern is the insecure/ambivalent child, who suffers the greatest distress in the mother's absence and seeks contact on the mother's return, but who can neither be consoled by her nor turned away from her, maintaining a period of clingy fussiness. The fourth is the disorganized child, who shows both avoidant and ambivalent behaviors.

As measured by this laboratory assessment in low-risk U.S. samples, 63% are secure, 18% avoidant, 9% ambivalent, and 10% disorganized. These attachment behaviors do vary across cultures, however, probably because of parental child-rearing behaviors and socioemotional goals that inform those parental practices.

The average child's stability within a given category is quite high between 12 and 18 months, although stability is less for high-risk populations, and in the face of environmental stress, secure infants tend to move into an insecure category. Attachment behavior has been studied principally in small samples or clinical populations, such as abusive families or depressed mothers, and the distribution of the four types in large, primary-care populations has not been adequately tested. The four behavioral types have been replicated by many investigators, however, and show high correlation with in-home observation.

School refusal is defined by at least 2 weeks of persistent school absences, 2 to 3 days per week, based on a preference to be at home and with the knowledge of the parents. The absence is usually due to discomfort at the thought of being in school and is often associated with somatic complaints. This definition excludes truancy, in which the child does not want to be at home or at school, and the parents are generally unaware of the school absence. Psycho-

biological signs of anxiety, phobia, and behavioral inhibition may be found in some children with school-avoidance behavior.

Thirty percent of 11-year-olds and 75% of grade school children would be absent from school if given the choice, but school refusal itself occurs in 3 of 1000 of a general population of school children, 10 of 1000 of high school children, and 5 of 100 of disturbed children. It is most frequent in the early teen years and more common among boys than girls; no effect of socioeconomic status, race, or IQ is seen. School refusal is the number three cause of school absence, falling after acute illness and truancy but before the child being "required at home for service to the family." *Separation anxiety disorder (SAD)* may be diagnosed when the refusal persists beyond 4 weeks, is associated with fears of harm to parents or excessive anxiety about separation from the parent even for sleep, or causes disturbance in other social functions.

ETIOLOGY AND PATHOGENESIS

The child's normal developmental preference for the mother and wariness of strangers are due to a psychobiological process of attachment that serves to keep the infant physically close to those who would feed and protect. Such nurturance and protection allows development of social and emotional interactions that will ultimately shape the child into an acceptable member of society. Developmental changes, such as walking, that thrust children into new situations can challenge their sense of security, leading to increased demand for proximity to the parent. Object permanence appears as a cognitive change at 9 months of age, enabling the child to remember, and call for, an absent parent.

Even as the young child achieves secure attachment to parents, the child will remain vulnerable to situational changes causing separation anxiety disorder. Abrupt or prolonged separations or stressful family dynamics can overwhelm the child's regulation of affect. More serious problems, such as maternal depression and anxiety disorders; marital discord, especially when one parent seeks closer contact with the child; father absence; or an abusive environment can lead to anxiety over separation, even into middle childhood.

The etiologic mechanisms involved in the extremes of temperament and the clustering of temperament traits remain unknown. These traits are presumed to reflect constitutional patterns of CNS reactivity that are relatively persistent, in some cases over many years, but are also shaped by interactions with caregivers. The "shy child syndrome" (negative mood and tendency to withdraw from novelty or change) is associated with a significantly lower threshold for arousal of the sympathetic nervous system. Children with less iris pigmentation are overrepresented in this syndrome, as are infants born to women who experience extended day length. Twin studies reveal the effects of both genetics and gender on separation anxiety, but most have been retrospective studies.

The etiology of insecure attachment behavior is not known. Interactions with attachment figures are presumed to lead to the development of an "internal working model" of the attachment figure, the primary relationship, and the self as worthy and intact. This elemental model of relationship with other human beings prepares the child for building and maintaining other significant relationships. When the attachment figure is withdrawn, overly involved, or abusive, the internal working model will be distorted, and the child's behavior will be extreme, as seen in the avoidant, ambivalent, and disorganized child. In addition, mothers of nonsecurely attached children are far more likely to have a history of an abusive or withdrawn mother themselves, possibly suggesting transgenerational transmission of environmental influences on behavior.

School refusal is a disorder of social function that stems from psychological disorders, from disorders of the primary relationships, or from temperamental or environmental factors. A pathologic tie to the parent is often a key element; that is, a child responds to a mother who is unavailable or angry or depressed by wanting to protect or cling to her. The child is believed to be projecting on to others his or her own prohibited aggressive impulses toward the mother. Left aware only of the danger to the mother, the child is then overwhelmed by the need to defend her and cannot tolerate a separation. Finding anxiety or panic disorders in families of children who avoid school indicates both genetic and environmental etiologic mechanisms.

CLINICAL MANIFESTATIONS

Clinical manifestations are often shared within this spectrum of normal behaviors and disorders; the child is (or is described to be) extremely intense in rejecting contact with new people or unfamiliar situations and in favoring one or a few caregivers. At times even familiar adults are rejected in the consoling role. This is particularly problematic when those familiar adults are as important as father, grandmother, or babysitter.

Distinguishing features among the five clusters are not always present, but the following tend to be found. Behavior that reflects *normal development or reaction to the environment* is usually temporary and resolves spontaneously. Growing familiarity with one person can be transferred to another by the child playing or being cared for in the presence of both; time, and eventually reasoning, can break down the resistance. Normative separation behavior is also often situation specific, which is generally not the case with temperamental complaints.

Children who withdraw from new people or situations because of *extreme temperament* are usually difficult across situations and beyond single stages of development. Their difficulty with novelty will extend to foods, sights, and sounds, as well as to places and people. Such temperamental styles often lead to problems in functional areas such as sleep and limit setting.

Insecure attachment manifests itself primarily in situations involving threatened loss of mother or the presence of the unfamiliar. The problem behaviors persist beyond the mother's return or the stranger's absence. The parade of children through well-child office visits serves as a lively demonstration of these variations in attachment behaviors.

Typically in school refusal children resist going to school for no reason other than a sense of fear about being away from home and a desire to be near the parent. These children can be tearful at the thought of school or at the time of the actual, enforced separation at the school door. They are often very resistant with their parents even though they tend to appear compliant in the pediatrician's office. Some have somatic complaints, most typically abdominal pain, diarrhea, anxiety, anorexia, or pallor in younger children, and dizziness or palpitations in older children, while others have obvious impairments in social relations. Those with somatic complaints may say that they like school but cannot go because of the symptom. Psychological symptoms more often reflect depression than anxiety.

Most children are actually relieved of their anxiety and their symptoms once in school. Some children remain miserable, on the other hand, and these children may have true anxiety disorder or phobia, and may be beset by distracting and depressive worries about the safety of a parent. Some continue to have somatic complaints that get them out of the classroom and into the nurse's office.

ASSESSMENT

No single diagnostic tool is available, but the most helpful diagnostic approach is to examine the behavior in detail and to look beyond the symptom to other areas of the child's and family's life. In this type of work, in fact, the assessment becomes the first therapeutic step, blurring the distinction between diagnosis and intervention. As the parents' description of the child and the child's behavior are juxtaposed to their reflections on other areas of family function, they often discover connections hitherto unrecognized. The problem becomes a story to be worked on, not an undifferentiated experience.

The clinical presentation within this spectrum of behavior problems could include a 9-month-old who purportedly cries all day at the new babysitter's home; a 2-year-old who has defeated the pediatrician in examining his heart for the past three well-child visits and fights his mother even as she gives him the hugging that he demands; an 8-year-old who has been refusing to go to school for the past 2 weeks. In each case, the fundamental assessment tool is the ability to make specific behavioral observations and elicit objective behavioral descriptions, while searching for the larger story within which the behaviors are being interpreted. For example, discovering that the mother of the fearful 2-year-old believes she must prevent an out-of-control 16-year-old by her responses now enables you to free her from the constraints of that future story and to help her understand the current behaviors in the more benign story of a young child who is overwhelmed by his or her own sense of being out-of-control.

Guiding the elicitation, observation, and interpretation of these descriptions is a set of step-wise assessments. First, with regard to the child:

- Where is this child developmentally, especially in cognitive, attachment, and motor skills? (These are the areas of development that change a child's relation to herself and her caregivers.)
- Has a recent developmental spurt occurred? (These can disrupt the child's sense of self, as well as violate his mother's expectations.)
- How is the child characterized on the nine temperamental dimensions as assessed by direct observation or, in more problematic cases, by a parent questionnaire? Questionnaires are designed for parents to rate either: (a) many discrete behaviors which are then clustered to give relative scores on temperamental dimensions or (b) the nine dimensions directly.

In general, eliciting careful observations of actual behaviors (as opposed to judgments or global ratings) provides the pediatrician with the most reliable data from which to distinguish temperamental style from behaviors that are more reactive or from parental perceptions. The clinician's own observations of the child should be checked against those of the parent, and feedback should be elicited on whether what the clinician is seeing is what the parents are experiencing. Often this level of assessment will clarify whether it is a normal developmental, situational, or temperamental problem.

When the parents cannot accept that the behavior is normal or cannot be helped by suggestions for adaptation to a temperamental style or a particular stage, then the exploration should go further. Parents should be asked to describe the child's typical day or a recent day, especially in terms of transitions, separations, and reunions, and how they are handled by adult caregivers. Clinicians should listen carefully for impressions, judgments, and assumptions, as distinct from actual observations, in the answers to these questions. The responsivity and affect of parents and caregivers should be carefully evaluated. The clinical focus should be widened to include questions about what is happening in the family, with an ear to recent losses or changes. Changes in parental work, health, and mood should be explicitly elicited, because their connection to the child's symptom and behavior are often not apparent to the parent. A child's behavior is a barometer for family tensions and changes. Evidence of abuse or neglect at home and in the school setting should be actively solicited. Eventually, even the parents' own histories with their parents should be discussed, along with any history of depression, anxiety, panic, or phobic disorders in the family.

Especially in the assessment of school refusal, interviewing the child alone may be helpful, perhaps during the physical examination. The child's relations with teachers and other students should be explored along with the child's attitudes toward the academic and extracurricular work and the child's perspective on events in the home. A detailed physical exam is important in order to give the family and the child the message that the complaints are being taken seriously and to reinforce their acceptance of a conclusion that the child is physically normal and healthy despite the symptoms. In addition, children who are avoiding school may have associated physical problems.

After the history and physical exam, a large battery of screening tests should be avoided, because it is far more likely to lead to false-positive results, which will only prolong the uncertain phase in which the child is missing school and the parents are confused. Specific findings should be followed by specific laboratory assessments; for example, eliciting a history of soiling and finding palpable stool on abdominal exam should be followed by an x-ray of the abdomen and an encopresis workup; a CBC and differential blood count might be indicated if the child is truly pale. Follow-up of results should be done swiftly, and the results and their implications should be made clear to the child, the parents, and the school. The pediatrician's willingness to consider these symptoms seriously and to clarify their status quickly is an important part of the assessment and therapeutic process. The pediatrician should remain involved in the management even after medical problems are ruled out.

MANAGEMENT AND TREATMENT

The following principles apply to the management of separation difficulties at all ages.

1. Reshape the story. Through the assessment process, a presumptive working model, or story of the child and the child's environment can be reconstructed as a way of generating not only explanations, which are themselves often therapeutic, but also management suggestions for helping the child adapt to the new environment. Accepting that the parents' perceptions (of themselves and their child) are a major factor linking temperament in infancy to behavior problems in childhood, pediatricians can play an important preventive mental health role by helping parents (a) to become aware of their perceptions and the sources of those perceptions; (b) to separate those perceptions from the actual child; and (c) to reconstruct their images closer to the reality. The concept of a story, with its ele-

ments of characters, plot, and moral, is often helpful as a heuristic device in this restructuring.

2. Bring nonjudgmental terms—judgmental of neither the child nor the parents—to the description and explanation. Temperament terms such as "slow approach-withdrawal" are much less judgmental than "bad" or "stubborn." A constitutional or developmental explanation is also much less judgmental of parents. Break the global impression of "bad" behavior into its components; these are more manageable than the whole constellation.

3. Both the child's behavior and the parents' reactions should be the focus of intervention. Changes in the environment should be attempted simultaneously or at least alternatingly with adjustments in the child's behavior.

4. Advice is best received after the problem is clearly understood. Advice given during the course of developing an understanding of the problem can be helpful, but should be given tentatively with the understanding that it might change as the problem becomes redefined. Advice can be part of the diagnostic process, as the response to the advice may help clarify the nature and the source of the problem. Management should not end with the giving of the advice, however, but should include support of the parents in dealing with the actual or feared responses to the recommended changes in their child-rearing practices.

5. The specific content of advice must be related to the context and not just to the behavior itself. For example, parents who are overly protective need permission to leave the child to cry and recover alone, or to set a limit despite some tears. Such parents need to be shown that the distress is not harmful and that the child's experience of distress and recovery from it are important developmental steps, which may allow for more effective coping with fearful situations in the future.

Other parents, in response to the same clingy behavior, need encouragement to accept the behavior and to not respond with punishment. These more rigid and withholding parents often need help in lowering their expectations of the child's abilities and in allowing greater control by the child. Many clingy children are just asking, with their behavior, the important question, "Will you be there for me?" The parent who holds off the child who is clinging for this reason may be unknowingly reinforcing the behavior. When the parent is open and available to the child's demands for contact, the result can often be paradoxical—the child actually becomes less clingy. Testing the meaning of the behavior for the child in this way is an example of how thoughtful advice can be used as a diagnostic probe.

6. Empathetic information-gathering and collaborative problem-solving are most appropriate in working with parents in the pediatric office. Many child behaviors and family dynamics can be transformed through parental reflection and careful advice regarding child-rearing practices. Some pediatricians can do this level of counseling; a physician who cannot do this level of counseling should refer these families either to a developmental-behavioral pediatrician or to a psychologist or psychiatrist. Certainly, when the child's behavior is extreme or intractable, referral to mental health services for children and families is indicated. Psychosocial treatments can be effective, especially when the therapy is directed to the entire family. Pharmacotherapy with tricyclics (imipramine, with behavior therapy) has been effective with separation anxiety and school

refusal. Benzodiazepines (chlordiazepoxide, with psychotherapy, clonazepam, alprazolam) have had favorable effects on separation anxiety, school phobia, and SAD.

7. For school refusal, the primary intervention should be to insist that the child attend school despite any associated symptoms. This should be instituted even before a diagnostic workup is complete, as the exploration of family and school dynamics may take several sessions. Only a potentially abusive situation in the school should prevent the consistent return of the child to the school setting. The child who is allowed to miss more school only becomes further behind academically, thereby generating even greater fearfulness of an eventual return. Persistent, recurrent, or severe refusal, or the discovery of significant family psychopathology, are definite indications for mental health referral, which should, in general, have a family focus. The pediatrician's continued involvement and availability throughout the management is essential. The child, the parents, and the school officials need reassurance that the condition does not warrant absence from the classroom, and reexamination of the child or review of the symptoms may be necessary to support that reassurance. The child and parents benefit from seeing that medical and school personnel are in agreement about the importance of the child remaining in the classroom despite symptoms, and that agreement comes about mainly through direct contact and shared decision-making.

NATURAL HISTORY AND PROGNOSIS

Some difficult temperamental styles persist throughout childhood and even into adulthood, but more often they are transformed or lost. Even when not problematic in the home, they may become problematic in school, where the demands are different and the environment is often less forgiving. When persistent, and when identified as troublesome by parents, difficult temperament is likely to be associated with later behavior problems. The mechanisms of that evolution are not clear, but the association is robust. However, management of behavior problems in young children always presents an opportunity for prevention of more serious problems at a later stage.

Children who are insecurely attached are also more likely to have difficulty with separation and other behavior problems throughout childhood and possibly to have difficulty in adult relations. Eventually they may interact with their own children in ways that encourage insecure attachment behavior. This makes it even more important that pediatricians be alert to these behavior problems in early childhood and that pediatricians be prepared to intervene.

In school refusal, the prognosis is good for most children, especially when the onset is acute in young children who return to school early in the course of the problem. Adolescents and children with underlying psychopathology have a more guarded prognosis, with some studies showing as many as one-third developing serious problems with schooling or anxiety disorders in adulthood.

References

Bernstein GA, Hektner JM, Borchardt CM, McMillan MH: Treatment of school refusal: one-year follow-up. J Am Acad Child Adolesc Psychiatry 40:206, 2001

Carey WB: Temperament issues in the school-aged child. Pediatr Clin N Amer 39:569–584, 1992

Elliott JG: School refusal: issues of conceptualization, assessment, and treatment. J Child Psychol Psychiatry 40:1001, 1999

King NJ, Bernstein GA: School refusal in children and adolescents: a review of the past 10 years. J Am Acad Child Adolesc Psychiatry 40:197, 2001

5.6.7   Fears: Worries to Anxiety

John M. Jemerin

FEARFULNESS IN NORMAL PSYCHOLOGICAL FUNCTIONING

Definition

Fear and anxiety are essential to normal psychological organization and central to abnormal mental states. Mechanisms for withdrawal in response to danger are crucial to survival in most animal species. *Fear* refers to the emotional uneasiness associated with an objective, external threat. *Anxiety* and *worry*, on the other hand, are used to describe apprehension accompanying the anticipation of future or imagined danger. Fearfulness and worry can be accompanied by a wide range of physical and behavioral manifestations, including (a) subjective sensations such as tension, nervousness, preoccupation, and restlessness; (b) physiological reactions such as tachycardia, increased respiratory rate, increased blood pressure, flushing, pallor, increased sweating, diarrhea, nausea, abdominal pain, headache, chest pain, lightheadedness, urinary frequency, increased muscle tone, and tremulousness; (c) behavioral signs such as agitation, hypervigilance, insomnia, nightmares, exaggerated startle, clinginess, shyness, social withdrawal, cautiousness, reckless behavior, and irritability; and (d) cognitive changes such as distractibility, impulsivity, and memory impairment.

Fears and Worries in Normal Development

Fears and worries arise in a predictable developmental sequence from infancy through adolescence. In early infancy, fear is expressed through general distress signs such as startle reactions and crying. By several months of age, infants begin to display gaze aversion or sobering in response to fear-evoking stimuli. Mobile infants actively avoid threatening situations or seek contact with the primary caregiver. In all cultures studied, infants between 6 and 15 months of age begin to show fear responses when encountering unfamiliar people. In Western societies, "stranger anxiety" typically begins in the last quarter of the first year. In the preschool and older child, fearfulness or worry may be expressed indirectly through behaviors such as bed-wetting, temper tantrums, or somatic complaints such as stomach aches. While preschool children's worries are often of imaginary or formless threats such as monsters or "the dark," school-age children's worries focus more on realistic concerns such as bodily injury or natural hazards. During later school-age and adolescence, school achievement and social relations become the chief sources of worry. Older children report fewer fears, and girls tend to report more fears than boys.

Theoretical Perspectives on Fearfulness

The *ethnological* perspective postulates that the human infant is genetically programmed to fear stimuli and events that threaten survival. In early infancy, when the organism is highly dependent and its behavioral repertoire most limited, the presence of programmed distress responses serves a protective function by signaling the caregiver. As the infant begins to move away from caretakers, fearfulness of strangers serves a protective function by reducing the likelihood of predation or abduction by unrelated adults. *Learning theory* views fear as resulting from "classical conditioning," the coupling of physiological reactions to previously neutral stimuli through associative learning. In a well-known experiment, human fear acquisition by classical conditioning was demonstrated in a normal 11-month-old by pairing exposure to a rabbit with a loud noise. *Psychodynamic* conceptualizations call attention to the fact that fear arises not only in response to external threats, but also in response to internal thoughts or desires that threaten to lead the individual into situations of danger.

Biological Correlates of Fear

Fear is accompanied by activation of the "fight or flight" response, a general neuroendocrine response to stress that integrates arousal of the sympathetic-adrenomedullary system and the hypothalamic-pituitary-adrenocortical axis. Sympathetic arousal underlies many of the physiological correlates of fearfulness, including tachycardia; increased blood pressure; shifting of blood to skeletal muscles and away from visceral organs; glycogen breakdown; and increased alertness. Empathetic activation by itself, however, is neither necessary nor sufficient to produce the subjective sensation of fear. Rather, neuronanatomic studies implicate the limbic system, or visceral brain, in the regulation of emotions in general, and in fearfulness in particular. At the molecular level, inhibitory, gamma-aminobutyric acid receptors, widely distributed throughout the brain, are thought to be important in anxiety regulation. There is also evidence of a general inhibitory function for serotonin, and it is possible that higher levels of central serotonin may be related to the inhibition of behavior seen in anxiety.

CONTINUA OF FEARFULNESS IN CHILDHOOD

Fearfulness and worries in childhood can be conceptualized as falling along a number of continua ranging from a normal developmental variation at one end to an anxiety disorder at the other. Between the extremes lie fearful manifestations that are troublesome to the child or family, but lacking the severity, persistence, or associated features of the corresponding psychiatric disorder.

Definitions and Clinical Manifestations

The Specific Fear Continuum

Circumscribed fears are an expectable developmental phenomenon. At the normative end of the specific fear continuum are single, transient fears limited to a single period of development. A second level of fearfulness is represented by multiple specific fears at one developmental stage. Transient fears are common in nonclinical populations; however, specific fears that persist across developmental stages probably occur in no more than 20% of children who report fears. Persistent fears may engender some limitation of functioning or subjective distress, although they are not necessarily seriously disabling. At the pathologic end of the specific fear continuum are persistent, excessive, or unreasonable fears of specific objects or situations that are associated with clinically significant impairment of a child's social, educational, or occupational functioning. In the current psychiatric nomenclature, the *Diagnostic*

and Statistical Manual: Fourth Edition, or *DSM-IV,* such fears are referred to as *simple phobias.*

The Worry Continuum

As with fears of specific objects or situations, transient worries about imagined, past, or future events are a normal developmental phenomenon. Such worries normally do not persist, cause undue distress, or interfere with optimal functioning. At a second level of the worry continuum are isolated worries that cause some degree of distress or interference with functioning. For example, a school-age child's avoidance of sports because of concern about competence is problem-level worry. With progression across the continuum, worries become (a) more persistent, (b) more excessive in relation to the actual demands or impact of the anticipated (or past) event, and (c) less under the worrier's control. Children who have multiple, persistent, and excessive worries that cause marked subjective distress or significant difficulty in their relationships, schoolwork, or other activities are given the diagnosis generalized anxiety disorder (GAD). Children and adolescents with GAD may worry about performance in school, sports, and relationships and about natural catastrophes or other threats to safety. Such children tend to be perfectionistic and overly oriented toward approval. In addition, they often express somatic symptoms such as restlessness, fatigue, sleep disturbance, and head- or stomachaches.

The Inhibition Continuum

Transient episodes of social anxiety are common in early childhood. They are generally limited to specific situations and do not interfere with developmental goals. A minority of children exhibit a stable pattern of withdrawal in response to unfamiliar situations and tend to remain on the sidelines during peer group activities. Prospective study of such behaviorally inhibited toddlers through the early school-age years has shown that most remain unusually shy. Marked shyness in early childhood is associated with negative mood, worries and fears, and behavior problems. Furthermore, children with inhibited responsiveness to novel or challenging situations demonstrate increased arousal of limbic and central noradrenergic pathways when compared to sociable, outgoing children.

Shyness in itself is a normal developmental variation. At the extreme, however, shyness may compromise social development as a result of excessive sensitivity to criticism and difficulties with self-assertion. When fear of one or more social or performance situations is sufficiently severe and persistent to interfere significantly with the child's functioning in school or relationships, or to cause marked distress, a diagnosis of social phobia may be warranted. Children with social phobia have normal relationships with family members and other familiar people, but experience marked anxiety in interactions with unfamiliar peers and adults. Social phobia tends to have a later onset than simple phobia, generally after puberty, and is highly associated with depression.

The Responses to Stress Continuum

Throughout development, environmental stress is associated with transient alterations in behavior. All of these manifestations are expectable responses to events that disrupt a child's relationships or usual activities and normally last no more than several weeks. Occasionally, anxiety symptoms will persist for a number of months following a relatively common childhood stressor and may cause mild to moderate distress or impaired functioning. *DSM-IV* refers to anxious responses to stressful events lasting no more than 6 months as adjustment disorders with anxious mood.

Individuals who are exposed to extreme, unusual stressors often experience states of intense fear, helplessness, and horror. In children, such experiences may be accompanied by disorganized or agitated behavior. After extremely traumatic events, some individuals develop a constellation of persistent behavioral and emotional changes in three areas: (a) persistent reexperiencing of the traumatic event; (b) avoidance of stimuli associated with the trauma or a reduction in general responsiveness ("emotional numbing"); and (c) increased arousal. Children may develop such symptoms following events involving threatened death or serious injury, after witnessing the death or serious injury of another person, or in relation to acute or chronic sexual abuse. When children have symptoms in all three areas lasting at least 1 month accompanied by significant distress or impairment of functioning, the term *posttraumatic stress disorder* (PTSD) is applied. As compared to adults, children with PTSD are more likely to reexperience the traumatic event through repetitive play rather than intrusive memories. Emotional numbing in children may be indicated by diminished interest in usual activities, and increased arousal may take the form of physical symptoms such as stomachaches or headaches. Children with PTSD often have a foreshortened sense of the future with diminished expectations for career or marriage.

The Acute Fear to Panic Continuum

As noted, fear is normally accompanied by subjective uneasiness and physiological arousal. Individuals vary in the extent to which they are susceptible to activation of a fear response. At one end of this continuum are individuals who are relatively resistant to experiencing acute fear at a subjective or physical level. At the pathologic end of this continuum, some individuals experience discrete episodes of extreme physiological arousal called panic attacks. Panic attacks typically have rapid onset; last minutes to hours; and consist of terror, a fear of dying, going crazy, or losing control, and somatic symptoms such as palpitations, tremulousness, nausea or abdominal distress, paresthesias, hot flushes or chills, and chest pain. Panic attacks can occur in a variety of anxiety disorders in response to the feared object or situation. In panic disorder, panic attacks occur spontaneously and unexpectedly in the absence of a situational trigger. Panic disorder often presents in late adolescence and occurs rarely in prepubertal children.

Epidemiology

Recent epidemiologic research has found that child anxiety disorders in the aggregate represent the most prevalent psychiatric conditions of childhood and adolescence. Depending on the age group studied and the method of case identification used, prevalence estimates have varied from about 9% to 21%. Childhood anxiety disorders usually do not occur in isolation. All have a high degree of comorbidity with other anxiety disorders and depression, and a less-strong but significant association with attention deficit and behavior disorders.

Relatively little information is available about the epidemiology of individual childhood anxiety disorders. Prevalence estimates of simple phobias range between 2 and 9%, and they are thought to be more common in girls. Because of recent changes in the classification of childhood anxiety disorders, no information is available on the epidemiology of GAD in children, but 1-year prevalence rates in adult populations are about 3%. Reliable prevalence data

on social phobia are not available; however, social phobia is diagnosed more frequently in boys. Panic disorder has a 1-year prevalence of between 1 and 2% in the general population. Although accurate estimates for children are unavailable, the incidence of childhood PTSD is thought to be rising as more children become witnesses or victims of violence.

Etiology and Pathogenesis

There is growing evidence that anxiety disorders aggregate within families. Both genetic and environmental factors appear to contribute. A genetic contribution to the etiology of fearfulness and anxiety disorders is supported by research on children adopted at birth showing that shyness in 2-year-old children is related to shyness in the biological mother. Furthermore, twin studies indicate that genetic factors contribute to the etiology of panic disorder. The finding of neurologic soft signs in children of adults with anxiety disorders also suggests a biological contribution to the transmission of anxiety disorders within families.

Environmental pressures within the family system are also central to the ontogeny of childhood fearfulness. Fearful parents model risk avoidance for their children and are less likely to encourage children to take on challenging tasks. Children of adults with anxiety disorders may thus be at double risk; they may be genetically predisposed to develop anxiety disorders, as well as exposed to a family environment that unwittingly supports fearfulness and avoidance.

Anxious children demonstrate a cognitive processing bias that may contribute to the pathogenesis of anxiety disorders. Both clinically referred and nonreferred anxious children demonstrate selective attention toward threatening information. The presence of such an attentional bias may help to explain how children progress along the fear continua from points within the normal range to points representing significant anxiety problems or disorders.

Assessment and Diagnosis

Normal Fearfulness, Problem, and Disorder

Because fears and worries are normative phenomena throughout childhood, the clinician is faced with the problem of differentiating normal developmental fears from fearfulness that is beyond the range of normal developmental variation and problematic for the child or family. Further assessment is warranted if: (1) the distress associated with a child's fear is prolonged and persists despite comforting by the parent; (2) fears or worries limit the activities of the child or family; (3) children experience fears that are not appropriate to their stage of development; or (4) children suffer from multiple, diverse, or persistent fears.

If initial inquiry indicates the presence of clinically significant fearfulness or worry, a full history and examination is needed to define the symptom more precisely and to establish its context. As it may not be possible to obtain all of the information needed in the course of a routine pediatric visit, it is often helpful to have the family return at a later time to complete the assessment. Some practitioners schedule longer appointments to evaluate psychosocial problems at the end of regular office days when they are not pressured by waiting patients.

History

Children and parents often will not bring up concerns about fearfulness spontaneously. Hence, clinicians should be alert to common manifestations of child and adolescent anxiety disorders, including school avoidance or refusal, a decline in school performance, decreased participation in usual pastimes, social withdrawal, and physical symptoms not explained by somatic illness. If a complaint about fearfulness is elicited, further history is needed. Both the child and the parents should be interviewed, and adequate symptoms definition may also require information from the child's school or other relevant sources.

If the clinician suspects fearfulness or anxiety outside the range of normal developmental variation, the *present history* should be defined by establishing (a) whether the fear (or worry) is associated with a specific stimulus versus diffuse or anticipatory; (b) how the symptoms, or avoidance resulting from the symptom, restricts or interferes with the activities of the child or family; (c) other psychological symptoms; and (d) factors within the family that reinforce or maintain the symptom.

Other components of the history include (a) *developmental history,* with attention to temperamental characteristics; (b) *medical history,* including physical illnesses and medications that may produce anxiety or anxiety-like symptoms; (c) *school history,* emphasizing absences, academic and athletic functioning, and social skills and behavior; (d) *social history,* including age-appropriateness of peer relationships, and major past stressors such as separation, illness or death of family members, history of physical or sexual abuse, and exposure to violence; and (e) *family history,* including anxiety or other major psychiatric disorders in family members, family history of medical disorders associated with anxiety-like symptoms, and the parents' level of stress and success in coping with stress.

Examination

The clinician should make note of behavioral signs of anxiety such as tremulousness, motor restlessness, worried facial expression, or unusual timidity. Signs of anxiety that may be noted on physical examination include tachycardia, hyperventilation, heightened motor tension, and sweating. A full physical examination is needed to evaluate the presence of medical and neurologic conditions that may present with anxiety-like symptoms.

Differential Diagnosis

The differential diagnosis of anxiety symptoms includes:

(a) *Normal anxiety:* In contrast to normal developmental anxiety or transient anxiety following stressful events, symptomatic anxiety is likely to be experienced as beyond the child's control, pervasive or multiply focused, highly distressing, or associated with restricted functioning.

(b) *Medical disorders:* Medical conditions that can produce anxiety-like symptoms include hypoglycemia; pheochromocytoma; hyper- and hypothyroidism; hypercortisolism; growth hormone deficiency; acute bronchospasm; cardiac arrhythmias; and seizure disorders. Medical syndromes less commonly associated with anxiety-like symptoms are migraine; brain tumors of the third ventricle or diencephalon; collagen-vascular diseases; pulmonary embolus; and chronic obstructive pulmonary disease. Mitral valve prolapse can produce panic-like symptoms including palpitations, chest pain, and lightheadedness.

(c) *Drugs:* In general, anxiety-like symptoms are produced by central nervous system stimulants and by withdrawal from CNS depressants. Prescribed medications include beta-agonists; stimulating psychotropic medications such as methyl-phenidate, dextroamphetamine, and fluoxetine; and withdrawal from sedating anticonvulsants such as phenobarbital and benzodiazepines. Drugs of abuse that cause anxiety symptoms include amphetamines, cocaine, and other stimulants, and withdrawal from depressants such as alcohol, barbiturates, and other sedatives. Heavy use of caffeine can also mimic anxiety.

(d) *Other psychiatric disorders:* Anxiety can be associated with virtually every psychiatric disorder. To be classified as an anxiety disorder, anxiety must be the central feature of the disturbance. If anxiety occurs in the context of a severe disturbance of thought form or content, incoherence, perceptual features such as hallucinations, or pervasive developmental disturbance, a psychotic disorder such as *schizophrenia* or a *pervasive developmental disorder* should be diagnosed. The motor restlessness and difficulty concentrating seen in children with *attention deficit hyperactive disorder* (ADHD) may confer a "nervous" appearance suggestive of an anxiety disorder. On interview, however, the child with ADHD alone will not reveal prominent worries or fearfulness. In contrast to ADHD, agitation and attentional difficulties occurring in the context of an anxiety disorder typically wax and wane with the child's level of subjective worry, and the marked impulsivity associated with ADHD is less characteristic of children with anxiety disorders. When pervasive overactivity, impulsivity, and distractibility are present in addition to marked fearfulness or worry causing significant distress or limitation of functioning, the clinician should diagnose both ADHD and an anxiety disorder.

Anxiety symptoms are often seen in children with *depressive disorders.* In the child with a depressive disorder alone, if anxiety symptoms are present as a secondary feature, they typically begin after the depressed mood and are not the most prominent feature of the disturbance at any point. Conversely, the restriction of activities associated with severe anxiety disorders may lead to a depressed mood; however, the depressive symptoms follow the anxiety symptoms temporarily, and depressive features such as guilt or feelings of unworthiness are not present. If a child meets the full criteria for both a depressive and an anxiety disorder, both disorders should be diagnosed.

Management and Treatment

Successful management of problems related to fearfulness depends upon accurate assessment. The pediatrician provides a valuable intervention solely by recognizing the presence of a concern in parent or child and correctly locating it on the continuum from normal developmental fearfulness to problem-level anxiety and anxiety disorder. This step in itself can be reassuring to parents and leads to other interventions that can prevent the development of future problems.

Parental concerns about normal developmental fearfulness as well as many anxiety problems can be managed effectively by the general pediatrician. More severe problems or full anxiety disorders will usually require referral to a mental health specialist. If assessment indicates that fearfulness is a response to ongoing circumstances that are realistically threatening, intervention should focus on altering the child's environment. For example, a child who is being tormented by older children at school may appropriately fear going to school, and a child living with an abusive parent may have generalized worry. Changing the child's environment may require the assistance of other professionals, such as school personnel or social workers.

Pediatricians and other primary health-care providers can intervene at a number of levels in the management of childhood fearfulness, including education and anticipatory guidance, advice about parenting, use of psychopharmacologic agents, monitoring symptoms over time, and referral.

Education and Anticipatory Guidance

Parents may express great concern about fears or worries that, on assessment, are found to be developmentally appropriate. In such cases, education about fearfulness in the course of normal development may be quite helpful. When expressions of worry have emerged following a stressful or frightening but not catastrophic event, parents should be reassured that such increases in fearfulness are common and usually temporary. Parents of shy, behaviorally inhibited children may benefit from an explanation of temperament emphasizing that healthy children differ in their characteristic manner of reacting to new people and things and that one style is not inherently better or worse than another. The pediatrician should explain that although shy children may initially withdraw in novel contexts, in time they will often warm up and engage fully with a new person or situation.

Parenting Advice: Normal Fearfulness

Parents should be helped to respond to normal childhood fears and worries in a manner that is tolerant and emphatic, but at the same time not encouraging of fearfulness or avoidance. For example, a 4-year-old who is worried that a robber will come in through the window might wake during the night and enter the parents' bedroom. The pediatrician might advise the parent to spend a few minutes showing the child that all the windows are locked, and then redirect the child to the child's own bed. Parents should be counseled to take children's worries seriously, but not to confirm worries by accommodating rules or expectations more than is necessary. Parents of shy children should be guided to accept the child's reticence noncritically. By using encouragement and praise, parents may be able to ensure that even extremely shy children obtain a sufficiently rich range of experience to build social confidence and a positive self-image.

Parenting Advice: Problem-Level Fearfulness

When a child exhibits problem-level fearfulness in the context of a reasonably safe and well-organized environment, pediatric management via parent counseling may be possible if the onset of symptoms is relatively recent and the impairment of functioning relatively mild. Parents may perceive the child's avoidant behavior as stubborn or intentionally "contrary." A first step in enlisting parents' collaboration is helping them to understand the connection between the child's fears and the resistant behavior. As in the management of normal developmental fearfulness, it is important that parents talk with children about their fears and that they listen and respond noncritically. When fears have begun to limit functioning, however, it is imperative that parents take an active role in assisting children to broaden their range of activities. Parents most express to children both in words and actions that fear is a normal and understandable response to challenging tasks, but that it is necessary to pursue activities despite the presence of fear. The pediatri-

cian should also explain that praise of desirable behaviors is a powerful tool in shaping children's behavior.

Pharmacologic Agents

Pharmacologic agents can be of help in the short-term management of acute situational anxiety. The pediatrician should consider use of medications for relief of agitation or insomnia following a major life event, such as bereavement, and for severe anxiety in association with painful or frightening medical procedures. Benzodiazepines may effectively reduce acute anxiety in children and are well tolerated. The major side effects are sedation and decreased mental acuity, and behavioral disinhibition has also been reported. Because of their capacity to induce tolerance and a withdrawal syndrome including seizures, treatment with benzodiazepines should be of short duration and the medication should be tapered gradually. Antihistamines such as hydroxyzine and diphenhydramine are widely used in the management of acute anxiety in children. They are extremely well tolerated by children and have the advantage of not inducing dependence. The major side effect is sedation. Antidepressant medications are also effective agents for reducing anxiety. In particular, the group of of antidepressants known as serotonin selective reuptake inhibitors are being used increasingly in the management of childhood anxiety disorders.

Follow-Up

Concerns about fearfulness should be carefully monitored over time to verify that symptoms diminish rather than increase in severity. In the management of problem-level fearfulness, the pediatrician should schedule return visits on a monthly or more frequent basis to monitor treatment and to track improvement. In some families, parental anxiety or marital difficulties will prevent parents from being able to function as cotherapists in the management of a child's anxiety problem. If symptoms persist or increase, referral to a mental health specialist is warranted.

Referral

When needed, referral should be thought of as an intervention requiring skillful handling; its success may well determine the child's chances for recovery. A separate time should be scheduled to effect the referral, as a rushed recommendation given at the end of a regular office visit is likely not to be followed. The diagnosis and reason for referral should be explained. It is important that the clinician direct comments to the child as well as the parents, and that each family member be given an opportunity to ask questions and express concerns.

The status of the referral must be checked at subsequent pediatric visits, the obstacles to obtaining treatment discussed, and a new referral made if necessary. Once the referral has been accomplished, the pediatrician should communicate with the mental health provider and continue to follow the course of the problem and treatment. Children who have concurrent physical illness or who are likely to require psychopharmacologic intervention are best referred to a developmental-behavioral pediatrician or to a child and adolescent psychiatrist. Psychologists and psychiatric social workers also treat children with emotional difficulties.

Most mental health professionals employ a multimodal approach combining a range of psychotherapeutic methods, collateral work with parents, consultation with school personnel and the primary care pediatrician, and, in some cases, medication. Psychopharmacologic agents should be used as an adjunct to other treatment components as they do not by themselves alleviate the psychological and environmental factors underlying the disorder. Psychotherapeutic modalities that are clinically useful in anxiety disorders include:

- *Behavior therapy,* which is a set of techniques based on learning theory that work by altering the contingencies associated with specific behaviors. Behavioral approaches involve working with parents, schools, and children to pair positive feelings with desired behaviors, and to eliminate rewards for undesirable behaviors. Because behavior therapy is concerned with manifest behavior rather than the feeling states underlying behavior, it is most appropriate as a sole treatment in situations where the problem is relatively circumscribed and not associated with broader family or personality difficulties.

- *Dynamic psychotherapy,* which is derived from psychoanalytic theory, is a therapy that integrates support, practical guidance, and active work with parents with exploration of the meaning of the child's anxiety symptoms in relation to current developmental crises. Dynamic psychotherapy uses the child's relationship with the therapist to introduce more adaptive ways of responding to internal and external pressures. Because of its focus on the larger context of the child's developing personality, dynamic psychotherapy is often the treatment of choice for anxiety problems that are associated with more widespread difficulties in self-esteem or social functioning.

- *Cognitive-behavioral therapy,* which is a derivative of behavior therapy that works to alter the negative and self-defeating thoughts that often accompany states of fearfulness or anxiety.

- *Family therapy,* which is a treatment modality that explores the meaning of symptoms in relation to family functioning. Family therapy works directly on the relationship and role patterns within the family.

Most psychotherapies require weekly visits during the active phase of treatment, in addition to regular meetings with parents. Relatively circumscribed problems, such as simple phobias, may resolve in 8 to 12 sessions. Despite increasingly limited insurance coverage for mental health treatment, however, clinical experience shows that children with more severe anxiety disorders usually require treatment for a minimum of 6 to 12 months to achieve lasting clinical improvement.

Natural History and Prognosis

Few longitudinal studies of treated or untreated children are available; however, the outcome of childhood anxiety disorders appears to be extremely variable. There is evidence that children who present later and with more symptoms have worse outcomes. Uncomplicated simple phobias in children eventually remit with or without treatment; when they persist, they are likely to be associated with other psychopathology. Social phobia, on the other hand, frequently has a chronic course that may be complicated by secondary depression, substance abuse, and dropping out of school. Significant morbidity has also been described in children with PTSD at 3-year follow-up. Moreover, recent evidence indicates that the effects of severe trauma experienced in childhood often persist into young adulthood and that chronic PTSD is associated with other anxiety disorders and depression. Children with anxiety disorders and comorbid depression have more psychological problems and worse outcomes as young adults than do children with anxiety

disorders alone. Although the evidence is preliminary, current findings indicate that some anxiety disorders in children and adolescents have a chronic course and that their prognosis is improved by treatment. Early identification by primary health-care providers has the potential to enhance developmental outcomes and to reduce long-term morbidity in children who have fear-related difficulties.

References

American Academy of Child and Adolescent Psychiatry: Practice parameters for the assessment and treatment of anxiety disorders. J Am Acad Child Adolesc Psychiatry 32:1089–1098, 1993

Craske MG: Fear and anxiety in children and adolescents. Bull Menninger Clin 61(2 Suppl A):4–36, 1997

Kovacs M, Devlin B: Internalizing disorders of childhood. J Child Psychol Psychiatry 37:47, 1998

Last CG, Hansen C, Franco N: Anxious children in adulthood; a prospective study of adjustment. J Am Acad Child Adolesc Psychiatry 36:645–652, 1997

Pollock RA, Rosenbaum JF, Marrs A, et al: Anxiety disorders of childhood: implications for adult psychopathology. Psychiatr Clin North Am 18:745–766, 1995

Stevenson-Hinde J, Shouldice A: 4.5 to 7 years; fearful behavior, fears, and worries. J Child Psychol Psychiatry 36:102, 1995

VanAmeringen M, Mancini C, Oakman JM: The relationship of behavioral inhibition and shyness to anxiety disorder. J Nerv Ment Dis 186:425–431, 1998

5.6.8 Compulsive Behaviors: Habits to Tics

Tina Gabby

Parents often express concern about the repetitive behaviors their young infant or toddler displays during tantruming, bedtime, or boredom. Head banging, body rocking and rolling, and hair pulling are all normal behaviors that are frequently misinterpreted and, consequently, distressing to parents. Because some repetitive behaviors occur more often in children with severe neurologic or emotional problems, such behaviors may be interpreted as signs of significant neurologic impairment. Even thumbsucking, when it persists into school age, may create concern.

Repetitive, stereotypic movements are evident during fetal development. Sonographic observations of the fetus sucking his or her thumb in midgestation and the presence of sucking blisters on the lips of neonates confirm the early, prenatal nature of these behaviors. The inherent electrical activity of the brain is rhythmic, and rhythmicity is characteristic of many bodily functions that are controlled at the level of the brainstem (eg, breathing). In certain children, this intrinsic rhythmicity may not be inhibited at birth; as a result, rhythmic behaviors may emerge during childhood. Accordingly, although the etiology of the rhythmic, repetitive habits of early childhood remains obscure, these behaviors may be attributed to variability in the normal patterns of neuronal regulation.

Evidence of stereotypic behaviors seen in individuals who suffer cortical damage and the increased frequency of rhythmic habit patterns in children with severe mental disabilities together imply a cortical locus to these behaviors. The observation of rhythmic movement disorders in cases of human amphetamine overdose, and following intracerebral injection of dopamine and amphetamines in animal studies, supports the conjecture that neurotransmitters play a central etiologic role.

Learning theorists contend that rhythmic movements begin as normal behaviors that are reinforced over time. To the extent that infants find these activities pleasurable or tension-relieving, such behaviors would tend to be repeated. Others postulate that an organism requires an optimal amount of stimulation, and when a threshold amount of stimulation is not experienced, rhythmic behaviors emerge. These behaviors may serve to alleviate monotony in a child's environment, as evidenced by the frequent rocking observed in blind children or institutionalized children with mental retardation. Self-stimulatory, repetitive behaviors are common in children with depression or autism and in those children with pervasive developmental disorder, all entities that may be characterized to some degree by social isolation.

As children age, motor stereotypies are seen less often during times of boredom or sleep and more often when concentrating. Given the prevalence of many of these conditions, it is likely that they serve an important function for the developing child. Nervous habits have been observed more frequently during structured times of the day and with negative mood states. Most people assume that rhythmic behaviors are multifactorial in nature and that it is important for parents and professionals to consider the functions of the behavior.

HABITS AND REPETITIVE BEHAVIORS

Stereotypies of Infancy

Body Rocking

Body rocking occurs in 6 to 19% of young children, with a mean age of onset of 6 months. In either the sitting or the crawling position, a child rocks forward and backward, gently or violently. Vigorous rockers have been known to move their cribs across the room and may cause damage as the crib repeatedly strikes the wall. Frequently occurring when the child is tired or near the child's bedtime, this behavior usually continues for 15 to 30 minutes. Body rocking usually ceases by 2 to 3 years of age and rarely persists into later childhood and adolescence.

Head Rolling and Nodding

Although occasionally described in very young infants, head rolling occurs in 6 to 10% of normal infants between 7 and 9 months of age. A supine child will roll his or her head from side to side, the resultant friction often creating a large patch of hair loss on the back of the head. Head nodding, with similar ages of onset, occurs when the sitting child vigorously nods his or her head or shakes it from side to side. Most head rolling occurs when the child is alone, tired, or listening to music. The duration of head rolling is usually less than 30 minutes, and the behavior generally disappears by 2 years of age.

Head Banging

Head banging, which occurs in 5 to 15% of normal children, concerns parents because of the apparent potential for injury. Head banging typically begins at 8 to 9 months of age and ceases by 4 years. This stereotypy is more frequent in males (male:female, 3:1) and most often occurs at bedtime or during awakening from sleep. Episodes of head banging may last from less than 15 minutes to 3 or 4 hours. Familial patterns reveal that head banging may be seen in 20% of siblings. It also often is associated with other rhythmic movements, most commonly thumbsucking.

Children may bang their heads in various positions. Poised on their hands and knees, some may rock forward and strike their heads on the front of the crib or wall. Sitting children often head bang to the rear, with their occiput striking a carseat or crib. Still other children, while lying prone, repeatedly drop their head onto a mattress or pillow, often creating significant frontal bruising or callus formation.

Given that EEG and neurologic follow-up studies of children with this habit have revealed no abnormalities, parents should be reassured that their child does not have a significant neurodevelopmental problem. An explanation of the behavior as pleasurable and a tension release often is comforting to the worried parent; parents should appreciate the potential for secondary gain and reinforcement of the behavior if parental anxiety is extreme. Attempts to decrease head banging with the introduction of daytime, purposeful rhythmic movements (eg, rocking horses, swings, metronomes) have had variable results. Parents should be instructed to pad the areas of contact to minimize bruising and callus formation, especially for vigorous head bangers. Children with autism or mental retardation, who may physically injure themselves while head banging, may need medication to diminish the frequency and intensity of self-injurious behaviors; phenothiazines and haloperidol are the drugs of choice. Protective helmets also may be necessary.

Oral Habits

Thumbsucking

Nonnutritive sucking emerges by the 28th week of gestation in the human fetus, and it is considered normal until approximately 5 years of age. Although the neonate who discovers his or her thumb probably does so accidentally, the child typically finds thumbsucking pleasurable, and the behavior is reinforced. Thumbsucking occurs in 13 to 31% of North American children less than 4 years of age, with an equal distribution between boys and girls. Because thumbsucking is thought to be a learned behavior, it is not surprising that studies of Eskimo children, who are swaddled and carried on their mother's back for up to 3 years, reveal no evidence of this behavior. Although more breast-fed infants suck their thumbs than bottle-fed infants (34 vs. 17%), the mean duration of thumbsucking is less for the breast-fed infant (21 vs. 51 months). Thumbsucking peaks between 18 and 21 months of age, and most children spontaneously drop the habit by 4 years. Persistent thumbsucking into adolescence occurs more frequently in girls and may signal underlying insecurities or other psychological problems.

Like other repetitive behaviors in early childhood, thumbsucking often occurs at times of fatigue or anxiety. Illness may exacerbate the behavior, and during times of family stress, thumbsucking may return, along with other regressive behaviors. A thumbsucking child may have associated behaviors such as hair twisting and pulling or manipulating a favorite object (eg, a blanket or stuffed animal).

A child who thumbsucks beyond 4 years of age should be referred for dental evaluation. The potential for dental problems is significant during the period of 4 to 14 years, when major dentofacial development occurs. Displacement of the upper front teeth can be problematic; deciduous baby teeth form the pathway for the permanent teeth to follow. If the upper teeth are displaced forward and the lower incisors pushed back, the permanent teeth may emerge at abnormal angles. Self-correction by pressures from the lips and tongue will occur if the habit ceases before permanent teeth are in place. Abnormal swallowing and speech defects also may be seen in children who thumb- or fingersuck. Specific consonants, especially the *t* and *d* sounds, require an effective seal with the tip of the tongue behind the incisors. If their teeth have been displaced, children may talk with a significant lisp. Chronic inflammation of the thumb and paronychia may occur as well.

Before 4 years of age, parents should be reassured that thumb-sucking is a normal part of early childhood behavior and likely to resolve spontaneously. Parents' attempts to dissuade a child from this habit may only reinforce it. Insecurity, unhappiness, and resentment may result from parent's constant reprimands. Ignoring the habit is often helpful, and positive feedback during times when the child is not sucking should be promoted. Encouraging the child to become an active participant in the management of his or her own habit is crucial. Elimination of the favored object associated with thumbsucking may decrease thumbsucking behaviors. Hypnotherapy has been described as a treatment modality with great potential for this and other habit disorders in childhood, and while punitive measures have little effectiveness, aversive training with bitter-tasting nail polishes may be successful. If a thumbsucking child appears to be withdrawn or depressed, a more thorough psychosocial evaluation may be needed. Dental appliances may be indicated in the older child to correct malocclusion and to discourage sucking; these appliances generally consist of a plate fitted with a palatal bar or rake that prevents the comfortable insertion of the thumb.

Nail-Biting

Habitual nail-biting, or onychophagia, is a common, disturbing habit of both children and adults. Onychophagia includes biting of the nail itself, the surrounding cuticles, and soft tissues, and it often may cause significant inflammation (ie, onychia), bleeding, and infection (ie, paronychia). Although dental malocclusion has not been associated with nail-biting, severe onychophagia may play a role in tooth root resorption because of the persistent, downward pressure applied to the top of the tooth.

Nail-biting occurs most frequently between the ages of 10 and 18 years, but it may begin as early as age 4. Approximately 50% of children at one time or another display this habit, and prevalence figures decline with increasing age. By 18 years of age, 23% of people continue to bite their nails. Although there are no significant gender differences between 5 and 10 years of age, nail-biting is more common in males after this age. This habit is seen in 10% of men over 30 years of age. There also may be a familial tendency for nail-biting, because an increased frequency is found in the parents of an index case and studies of monozygotic twins show concordance rates twice that of dizygotic twins.

Nail-biting rarely requires treatment other than when bleeding or infection occur. As with thumbsucking, aversive reinforcement techniques have not proven to be consistently helpful. Behavioral techniques, including positive reinforcement, relaxation training, and habit reversal procedures (eg, patients engage in a hand grasp whenever they feel the urge to nail-bite) are superior to the negative techniques of punishment, scolding, and bitter nail polishes. Children should be taught good nail-grooming habits and should be praised for the times they do not engage in nail biting.

Bruxism

Bruxism is clenching or grinding of the teeth, which produces a high-pitched, audible sound. The habit is typically nocturnal and occurs during REM (rapid eye movement) sleep. Bruxism may cause tenderness in the muscles of mastication, temporomandibular joint pain, tension headaches, facial pain, and neck stiffness. The etiology of bruxism remains obscure, but most authorities suspect a relationship between bruxism and psychological stress, anxiety, or tension. Organic conditions associated with bruxism include middle-ear effusion, allergic rhinitis, anal pruritus or pinworms, chronic abdominal disorders, and neurologic conditions such as meningitis or cerebral palsy.

Because it occurs during sleep, the epidemiology of bruxism is difficult to ascertain. While incidence figures vary widely, parents acknowledge this habit in 15% of children between the ages of 3 and 17 years. Bruxism is more common in boys, and familial patterns are common.

Teeth and supporting structures may be permanently damaged, and children may complain of pain with mastication. Splints and bite guards serve to protect the teeth and also may cure bruxism. Alternative behavioral modalities, including hypnotherapy, acupressure, physical therapy, and psychotherapy, are beneficial for certain individuals.

Trichotillomania

Trichotillomania, which is the recurrent failure to resist impulses to pull out one's own hair, is an uncommon, troubling disorder. Hair is typically pulled from the scalp, creating patchy bald spots, but hair also may be pulled from the eyebrow, lashes, and pubic areas. Hair loss is characterized by short, broken strands of hair adjacent to normal length hair in affected areas. Children may perform this activity openly or secretly. Hair may be chewed and swallowed (ie, trichophagy), and massive accumulations of hair may form in the stomach (ie, trichobezoar), often causing abdominal discomfort and occasionally requiring surgical removal. Trichotillomania is described in the *DSM-IV* as a disorder of impulse control and currently is thought to fall along the spectrum of obsessive compulsive disorders.

Although incidence figures are unavailable in adults, there appears to be a female predominance. Trichotillomania may be separated into two categories. Early-onset trichotillomania presents before age 5 years; a second group typically presents in later childhood, during adolescence, or in young adulthood. Early-onset trichotillomania presents at a mean age of 4 years, usually with a long history of hair pulling. These children typically pull hair during periods of tension or boredom or at bedtime. The clinical course is episodic, with frequent periods of relapse and remission. Episodes may be associated at times with thumbsucking or hair twirling. Typically, late-onset trichotillomania presents around the start of puberty. Associated psychopathology, including depression, anxiety disorders, bipolar disorders, substance abuse, and personality disorders, is common in the late-onset form.

The patchy alopecia noted in trichotillomania should be differentiated from alopecia areata, tinea capitis, hair loss associated with cytotoxic drug use, and traumatic and traction alopecia. Because iron deficiency anemia has been associated with trichotillomania and trichophagia, screening for anemia should be considered.

The benign, self-limited trichotillomania that is occasionally seen in young infants and children usually responds to simple behavioral management techniques, including positive reinforcement with "time-outs" and "time-ins." The later-onset form is chronic, more difficult to treat, and may signal underlying psychopathology. Cognitive-behavioral strategies have been used for treatment, but no controlled studies support their efficacy. Comorbid psychiatric diagnoses may have an impact on treatment outcomes. Preliminary data appear promising in studies of antidepressants and serotonin reuptake-inhibiting drugs as adjuncts to behavioral management.

TIC DISORDERS

Tics are sudden, spasmodic, repetitive movements or utterances that are involuntary and purposeless. Muscle groups of the eyes, mouth, face, and neck are most frequently involved. Extreme tic behaviors may include obscene gestures (ie, copropraxia), self-injury, or phonic tics, which range from simple throat clearing to repetitive obscene vocalizations (ie, coprolalia). Although tics usually cease during sleep and may be temporarily suppressed, they often become worse with emotional stress.

Estimates indicate that 10% of the population experience a tic that persists for 1 month or longer. The estimated incidence of tic behaviors during childhood ranges from 1 to 13%. Tic behaviors are most common in school-aged children and males, with a male: female preponderance of 2:1. The prevalence of tic disorders is estimated at 1 to 2%. The *DSM-IV* classifies tic disorders of childhood as being either transient, chronic, Tourette syndrome, or "tic disorder not otherwise specified." The latter category includes the atypical patterns of tic behaviors that do not fall into other categories.

Transient Tic Disorder

With an onset of before 18 years of age, the transient tic disorder persists for at least 4 weeks but no longer than 12 consecutive months. Tics typically occur many times a day, nearly every day. Symptoms may wax and wane in severity over time. Eye blinking or facial tics are most common, although vocal tics also may occur. Boys display this tic disorder more commonly than girls, and presentation typically occurs between 3 and 10 years of age. Although rarely incapacitating, the tic may be a source of social embarrassment and withdrawal in the school-age child.

Chronic Motor or Vocal Tic Disorder

Chronic tics may be of varying intensity and frequency, but they often are more severe than the transient tic disorder. This rare disorder presents before age 18 and may include either vocal or motor tics (ie, involuntary, sudden, rapid, recurrent, nonrhythmic, stereotyped motor movements or vocalizations), but not both. The tics occur many times a day, nearly every day, or intermittently throughout a period of over 1 year. This condition may continue into adulthood in a residual state in which tic symptoms are seen only during times of stress or fatigue. This diagnosis excludes those patients who display tic behaviors because of substance abuse, a general medical condition (eg, Huntington's chorea, postviral encephalitis), or Tourette syndrome.

Tourette Syndrome

The most severe of the tic disorders, the Gilles de la Tourette syndrome, typically begins in early childhood with simple motor tics such as eye blinking or facial twitching. Tic character varies as the syndrome evolves; more complex motor tics involving touching, squatting, and twirling while walking may appear later. Simple vocal tics, which appear 1 to 2 years after the onset of motor tics, may give way to more complex phonic tics, including grunts, barks, sniffs, coughs, echolalia, or coprolalia. There may be associated symptoms of mental coprolalia (ie, sudden and intrusive obscene thoughts), obsessions, and compulsions. Attention-deficit hyper-

activity disorder (ADHD) and obsessive compulsive disorder are frequent comorbid diagnoses. Following the introduction of stimulant medication in children with ADHD, tic disorders, including Tourette syndrome, may be unmasked and should be an indication to stop the drug.

This disorder is at least three times more common in males, and the estimated prevalence rate is 0.5 per 1000 children. The median age of onset is 7 years, with the majority presenting before age 14. Tic disorders tend to improve in late adolescence and early adulthood, showing a diminished frequency of both motor and vocal tics. The etiology of this and other tic disorders remains obscure; hypotheses regarding the involvement of various neurotransmitters is supported by the knowledge that dopaminergic blockers modify tic behavior. Tourette syndrome is common among first-degree relatives, and there is a 50% concordance rate in monozygotic twins. Recent evidence suggests an autosomal dominant pattern of inheritance, although a genetic locus has not been identified. Because obsessive compulsive disorder also is more common in first-degree relatives of patients with Tourette syndrome, these diseases may represent varying expressions of the same underlying disorder.

Treatment

Because self-esteem, family functioning, social adaptation, and school performance may be affected, the approach to the child with a tic disorder should be comprehensive. Children with transient tic disorders should be followed clinically, because this is a diagnosis of exclusion. Parental reassurance is warranted, because many tic disorders improve or resolve spontaneously. Dietary and behavioral treatments, including relaxation therapy and hypnotherapy, have not yet provided consistent positive effects in the treatment of Tourette syndrome. Although many medications have been used for Tourette syndrome, it is a relatively selective dopamine-receptor antagonist, haloperidol, that relieves symptoms in 80% of patients. Because side effects are common with haloperidol, low doses of clonidine, which diminishes central noradrenergic and serotonergic activity, have also been used. Additionally, psychotherapy may be a useful adjunct in some individuals.

References

American Psychiatric Association: Diagnostic and Statistical Manual of Mental Disorders, 4th ed. Washington, DC, American Psychiatric Association, 1994

Cohen DJ, Riddle MA, Leckman JF: Pharmacotherapy of Tourette's syndrome and associated disorders. Psychiatr Clin North Am 15:109, 1992

Foster LG: Nervous habits and stereotyped behaviors in preschool children. J Am Acad Child Adolesc Psychiatry 37:711, 1998

Gardner GG: Hypnotherapy in the management of childhood habit disorders. J Pediatr 92:838, 1978

Hoder EL, Cohen DJ: Repetitive behavioral patterns of childhood. In: Levine MD, Carey WB, Crocker AC, eds: Developmental-Behavioral Pediatrics, 2nd ed. Philadelphia, Saunders, 1992:407

Leckman JF, Cohen DJ: Tic disorders. In: Lewis M, ed: Child and Adolescent Psychiatry: A Comprehensive Textbook. Baltimore, Williams & Wilkins, 1991:613

Mitchell R, Etches P: Rhythmic habit patterns (stereotypies). Dev Med Child Neurol 19:545, 1977

Peterson JE, Schneider PE: Oral habits: a behavioral approach. Pediatr Clin North Am 38:1289, 1991

Sallustro F, Atwell CW: Body rocking, head banging, and head rolling in normal children. J Pediatr 93:704, 1978

Shevlov SP: Thumbsucking. Pediatr Rev 16:73, 1995
Swedo SE, Leonard HL: Trichotillomania: an obsessive compulsive spectrum disorder? Psychiatr Clin North Am 15:777, 1992

5.6.9   Child Maltreatment: Neglect to Abuse

John M. Leventhal

The spectrum of parental feelings and behaviors toward children can extend from those that are positive and nurturing to those that are negative, harmful, and culturally unacceptable. At the negative extreme are behaviors that result in child maltreatment including physical abuse, neglect, or sexual abuse. Although such negative behaviors are often viewed as deviant and separate from normal parenting, in fact, many "normal" parents have feelings and behaviors that may extend to those considered to be maltreatment. Thus, a parent's anger at the child and use of physical punishment may border on physical abuse, ignoring the child and providing inadequate nurturance or supervision may border on neglect, and close bodily contact and sensual feelings toward the child may border on sexual abuse.

DEFINITIONS AND EPIDEMIOLOGY

Maltreatment of children includes physical abuse, neglect, sexual abuse, and emotional maltreatment. Physical abuse is defined as an act of commission toward the child by a parent or other caregiver that results in harm or intended harm to the child. It can include bruises from a beating, broken bones, or even death. Neglect is defined as an act of omission, such as failure to provide adequate nutrition, shelter, clothing, or supervision; abandonment; or failure to ensure that the child receives adequate health care or education. Physical abuse and neglect must be distinguished from unintentional or "accidental" injuries, and health neglect must be distinguished from less serious lapses in attending to a child's medical care, such as poor adherence to medical recommendations or missing a few appointments for health care.

Sexual abuse is defined as the involvement of children or adolescents in sexual activities that they do not fully understand, to which they cannot give informed consent because of their developmental understanding, and that break societal or family taboos. It includes behaviors such as sexual intercourse, genital fondling, and exposing children to pornography.

Emotional maltreatment, which is the most difficult form of maltreatment to define, includes repeated verbal denigration, belittling, or scapegoating so that the child develops a sense of worthlessness and low self-esteem. Because emotional maltreatment often coexists with other forms of maltreatment, it is difficult to identify and enumerate as a separate type, and thus is substantially underreported.

Although abuse of children and infanticide have occurred over the centuries, pediatric recognition of and concern about the *battered child syndrome* did not begin formally until the 1960s. By the mid-1960s, each state had passed laws requiring the reporting of suspected maltreatment to the state's child protection agency, and since 1976, there have been annual tabulations of these states' reports. The results of the 1997 survey identified almost 3.2 million reports of maltreatment in children less than 18 years of age and about 1200 deaths due to abuse or neglect. The types of maltreatment reported were neglect (52%), abuse (26%), sexual abuse (7%), emotional abuse (4%), and other (11%). Reports were approximately equal for males and females, except for sexual abuse in which 75% of the victims were female. Approximately 40% of reported children were younger than 6 years of age, and 30% were older than 10. Of the reported cases, 34% were substantiated, meaning that the protective service agency found enough evidence to believe that maltreatment occurred. An unsubstantiated report, however, does not necessarily mean that maltreatment did not occur; rather, it means that there was insufficient evidence to meet the state's definition of maltreatment. Because states have different requirements for reporting, use different criteria to decide whether a report is a substantiated case of maltreatment, and use different approaches to classification and to counting multiple reports on the same child, it is difficult to compare rates from one state to another.

Since yearly national statistics were first collected in 1976, reports of maltreatment have increased annually. One explanation for this increase is that changes in society have made it more difficult for parents to care for their children; an alternative explanation, however, is that professionals caring for children have broadened their definition of maltreatment and both parents and professionals have become more aware of the problem and more likely to recognize less serious forms of maltreatment.

Reports of sexual abuse peaked in the early 1990s (more than 400,000 reports, representing about 13% of all reports). Since then, the number of reports has decreased substantially, so that in 1997 there were approximately 225,000 reports (representing only 7% of all reports). It is unclear how much of this recent decrease is due to prevention programs that teach young children about sexual abuse, changes in reporting criteria, a decrease in the backlog of cases detected in the 1980s, or a true change in the occurrence of the phenomenon.

Although reported cases of maltreatment come from all social classes, abuse and neglect are reported more commonly in families who are poor and less educated. Other factors associated with reports of physical abuse or neglect are young maternal age, single-parent households, ethnic minority status, and parental alcohol or drug abuse. Most maltreatment occurs in the child's home. Males inflict physical abuse more often than females. Perpetrators of sexual abuse are almost all males, and about 20% of them are juveniles. The child who has been sexually abused often knows the perpetrator, who may be the father, stepfather, another male relative, or a family friend. The small proportion of sexually abused children who do not know the perpetrator are usually older children or adolescents who are victims of forceful sexual assault or rape.

Reported cases of maltreatment are those that are recognized by clinicians and therefore may substantially underestimate the true rate of maltreatment that occurs in society. Two additional epidemiologic approaches have been used to determine the true prevalence of the problem. First, parents have been interviewed to determine their behaviors, particularly those that are violent, toward their children. For example, a random telephone survey conducted in 1985, found that 11% of parents had reported one of the following severely violent behaviors toward their child in the previous year: kicking, biting, punching, beating up, or threatening with or using a gun or a knife. A second approach has surveyed adults about how they were treated as children, particularly to determine the prevalence of childhood sexual abuse. Although the rates of reported past sexual abuse vary based on the population sampled, the type and number of questions asked of adults, and the operational definitions used, reasonable estimates are that 20% of adult women and 5 to 10% of adult men in North America report being sexually abused before age 18.

ETIOLOGY AND PATHOGENESIS

The causes of maltreatment are complex and tend to vary with the type of maltreatment, as well as with factors in the social setting, family, parents, and child.

Physical abuse typically occurs when a parent loses control and injures a child. Perhaps most important in understanding this behavior are the parent's attitudes and feelings toward the child. An abusive parent often has very negative views of the child, which may be fixed so that the abuser cannot recognize any of the child's positive qualities. These negative feelings may be long-standing and have their origin in the fact that the child was unwanted, or they may be related to the parent's unconscious view of the child, in which the parent comes to hate the part of him or her that is represented in the child. Such negative feelings often lead to constant denigration of the child so that the child experiences emotional abuse as well.

Nonabusive parents also may have negative feelings toward their child, such as upset or anger, which are episodic and associated with the child misbehaving. Although such parents may inflict physical punishment, they usually do not lose control and, on balance, have more positive feelings and attitudes toward their child.

Factors that have been associated with the occurrence of abuse are listed in Table 5-20. The presence of any single factor, or even several factors, may make it more difficult for a parent to provide appropriate nurturance to the child, but does not necessarily mean that abuse will occur. For example, although there is a strong association between a history of abuse as a child and abusing one's own child (the so-called "intergenerational transmission of abuse"), the majority of parents who were abused as children do not abuse their own children.

Although abusive parental behaviors often are directed toward a specific child in the family, in some families more than one child is affected. In families where abuse occurs, an acute stressful event may upset a parent and lead to abusive behaviors toward a child. Sometimes these triggers are normal childhood behaviors, such as crying, spilling a glass of milk, or wetting oneself.

Neglecting parents fail to provide the basic care necessary to ensure the child's growth, development, or safety. Although children may be injured from a single episode of neglect, neglect is usually a chronic problem. For many neglecting parents, negative feelings toward the child result in inadequate nurturing. For others, although there may be significant positive feelings toward their child, the parents lack the basic skills, interest, or energy to provide adequate care. For example, a parent with mental retardation may lack the basic skills necessary to provide appropriate food or stimulation to a child, while a depressed mother may lack the energy and vigilance to supervise the child adequately. Table 5-20 highlights some of the risk factors associated with neglect. An important factor to consider is parental drug or alcohol abuse, which can have profound negative influences on parents' abilities to care for their children. For example, over the past two decades, the epidemic of crack cocaine has resulted in a marked increase in the incidence of neglect.

The sexual abuse of children is more difficult for most clinicians to understand than is the occurrence of physical abuse or neglect. The two prerequisites for this form of maltreatment include sexual arousal to children and the willingness to act upon this arousal. Factors that may contribute to this willingness include alcohol or drug abuse, poor impulse control, and a belief that the sexual behaviors are acceptable and not harmful to the child. The past history of the perpetrator (eg, having been sexually abused during childhood), the particular vulnerability of the child (eg, a developmental delay), and a circumstance that enables the perpetrator to have increased contact with the child (eg, a mother who is hospitalized) all contribute to the likelihood that sexual abuse may occur.

CLINICAL MANIFESTATIONS

Like other forms of family violence, the maltreatment of children often occurs in the privacy of a home and is seldom witnessed by another person. Because the child is often too young or too frightened to explain what happened and the correct history often is not known or not provided by the parents, clinicians should be aware of suspicious histories and recognize the typical behaviors and physical findings of maltreated children. Although three types of maltreatment (physical abuse, neglect, and sexual abuse) are described separately, a child may suffer from more than one type.

Physical Abuse

Five types of histories should raise the suspicion of abuse: (a) a child with a serious injury, such as a fracture, but no history of preceding trauma (eg, "I noted that his arm was limp."); (b) a history that is inconsistent with the severity, mechanism, or timing of the injury; (c) a delay in seeking medical care for a significant injury; (d) a history that changes during the course of the evaluation; and (e) a history of recurrent injuries, especially those that are poorly explained.

Children who have been abused display a variety of behaviors. They may be excessively fussy, frightened, or depressed due to recurrent pain, maltreatment, and the impact of living in a threatening and unpredictable environment. Older children may demonstrate role reversal in their interactions with their parents: instead of the parent caring for the child's needs, the children learn to be particularly sensitive to the parents' needs and, in part, to avoid being hurt, may provide care for the parents. Such children may attempt to be well-behaved around adults in order to avoid offending them and being punished. Some children who have been abused repeatedly do not cry during medical procedures, such as blood drawing, because crying at home may have resulted in additional punishment.

TABLE 5-20

FACTORS ASSOCIATED WITH ABUSE OR NEGLECT

Social Setting:	Poverty
	High level of violence
	Unemployment
Family:	Family violence
	Isolated family
	Single parent
	Inadequate supports
	Many children under 5 years of age
Parent:	Maltreated as child
	Serious psychiatric illness
	Mental retardation
	Substance abuse
	Mother less than 19 years old at child's birth
	Unrealistic expectations of child
Child:	Unwanted
	Disabled
	Twin

The spectrum of physical abuse extends from a single episode, such as a slap on the face, to recurrent and more serious injuries. Children who sustain injuries from abuse that are mistakenly diagnosed as unintentional injuries are at substantial risk of being more seriously hurt or even of dying from abuse.

Soft tissue injuries are the most common clinical manifestation of physical abuse. These include hand marks from slapping, bruises from punches, linear and curved marks from belts, cords, or switches, and bite marks. In evaluating injuries to the skin, it is important to consider the child's developmental level. For example, 1-year-olds who are learning to walk often fall forward and bruise their face, and it is not uncommon for preschool children to bruise their shins. Studies of bruises in young children have demonstrated that it is unusual to see bruises in children who are not cruising. "Black eyes," and bruises around the ears, in the genital region, or on the posterior surface of the body are highly suspicious of abuse at any age. Bruises result from bleeding into the skin or subcutaneous tissues. Fresh bruises are usually tender and swollen, with maximum swelling in 1 or 2 days. Bruises change color from deep purple/red to green to yellow/brown. The rate of these changes depends on the depth of the bruise, the amount of bleeding, and the location of the injury.

Burns are another common type of abusive injury. These can include scald burns from hot liquids or burns from hot objects, such as irons, stoves, or cigarettes. Although burns that are due to abuse are often difficult to distinguish from unintentional injuries or those due to neglect, the location and pattern can be helpful. Children who have been immersed in hot water may have bilateral burns of the upper or lower extremities or burns of the buttock or back. These inflicted burns often have a sharp demarcation between the injured and noninjured skin. A child who has been held in hot water in a tub may have a spared area of buttocks, as a result of the area having been pressed against the tub. In contrast, nonabusive scalds tend to be asymmetric from one extremity to the other, have less sharply demarcated borders, and reveal splash marks that indicate the child tried to avoid the injury. Other commonly occurring unintentional scald burns occur when young children spill containers of hot liquid on themselves.

Cigarette burns are another type of suspicious injury. An isolated, unintentional cigarette burn, which tends to be superficial, can occur when a young child comes in contact with a cigarette held by an adult. In contrast, inflicted cigarette burns tend to be deeper, are located on areas for which accidental contact would be unlikely, and may be multiple.

Head injuries are the most common cause of death due to child abuse. In children less than 1 year of age, shaking of the infant is the most common mechanism of injury and can result in intracranial bleeding due to repeated accelerations and decelerations of the brain that produce shearing of the bridging veins (resulting in subdural or subarachnoid hemorrhages) and retinal hemorrhages, which often can be extensive, involve different layers of the retina, and extend to the periphery. Other cerebral injuries can include diffuse axonal injury, cerebral edema, and intracerebal hemorrhages.

Biomechanical studies have suggested that shaking alone may not cause sufficient accelerations of the brain to cause the observed injuries; in addition, some so-called "shaken babies" have some evidence of injuries due to impact, such as skull fractures and intracerebral bleeding. Such injuries are the result of the infant's head striking the crib, bed, floor, or other hard surface. Because it is often difficult to be certain whether intracranial bleeding is due to shaking and/or impact, the term *shaken baby* has been replaced with *shaken baby/impact syndrome.*

Children with abusive head injuries may present with seizures, signs of increased intracranial pressure, coma, or apnea and cardiac arrest. Often, there are other signs of child abuse, such as bruises or healing fractures. Rib fractures are seen commonly with shaken baby/impact syndrome; these fractures occur when the infant is held around the thorax, and the abuser squeezes the chest and shakes the infant. Because rib fractures are usually not visible on chest radiographs until callus formation has begun to occur 10 to 14 days after an injury, the presence of an acute head injury and healing rib fractures indicates that the child has been injured on at least two occasions.

In head injuries due to abuse, there usually is no clear history of severe head trauma to direct the clinician toward the right diagnosis. In contrast, when children sustain serious unintentional intracranial injuries, such as those due to major falls or automobile accidents, there is a clear history to explain the injury, and retinal hemorrhages occur much less commonly. Most minor falls from heights of less than 36 inches do not result in serious head injuries, although skull fractures or epidural bleeding can occur. Similarly, subdural hematomas are not expected after such minor falls, but small ones have been noted on rare occasions.

Fractures of bones are another common type of abusive injury in young children. In a series of 215 children less than 3 years of age with fractures, 24% were believed to be due to abuse. Fractures of the skull were the most common, followed by fractures of the extremities. Although skull fractures that are depressed, branching, or diastatic have been associated with physical abuse, the most common type of skull fracture found as a result of abuse (as well as with unintentional injuries) is a linear fracture of the parietal bone. Fractures of the humerus (especially midshaft or proximal) and fractures of the femur (especially in children less than 1 year of age) should be considered suspicious of abuse. In contrast, a 2- or 3-year-old child may have a supracondylar fracture of the humerus from a fall on an elbow, or a spiral fracture of the femur or tibia from falling and twisting. Whether the fracture is spiral or transverse is not by itself diagnostic for abuse. Two types of fractures that are considered more specific for abuse are metaphyseal, or "bucket handle," fractures and rib fractures, particularly those that are posterior and adjacent to the spine. Several studies have indicated that rib fractures are unlikely to occur during cardiopulmonary resuscitation in young children.

Other types of injuries that should raise the suspicion of abuse are intentional poisonings and abdominal injuries (including lacerations of the liver, spleen, or intestines). Children with abdominal injuries are at particular risk of hypovolemic shock and even death, when the internal injury is unrecognized and the history of blunt trauma is not provided by the caregiver.

An additional type of abuse that is often difficult to recognize is Munchausen syndrome by proxy (MSBP) in which a parent (usually the mother) fabricates symptoms of an illness in the child resulting in an extensive medical evaluation, or causes the child to be ill by poisoning or some other means (eg, injecting contaminated fluid into an intravenous line). MSBP has a high fatality rate because the recognition of this condition often occurs too late.

Studies of MSBP have focused on two other conditions—ALTE (apparent life-threatening event) and multiple SIDS in families—that can be caused by abusive behaviors, such as suffocation or strangulation. In a British study of 39 children (age range of 2 to

44 months) who were referred because of suspicion of an induced illness, 36 presented with ALTE. In the 39 families, 12 previous children had died suddenly and were labeled as deaths due to SIDS. Covert video recordings in the hospital revealed abuse in 33 cases, and there was documentation of suffocation in 30 of these children. In 11 of the cases of suffocation, the children had bleeding from the nose and/or mouth.

In a related development, the infants who were identified by Steinschneider in a 1972 article, in which prolonged apnea was described as the cause of multiple SIDS in a family, were determined to be victims of abuse by suffocation. When more than one infant in a family dies unexpectedly and is labeled SIDS, child abuse and other causes, such as metabolic ones, need to be considered.

Neglect

Neglected children are recognizable by the chronic failure of their parents to provide adequate physical care or ensure appropriate medical care or education, or when the child is brought for medical attention because of an injury or ingestion. Worrisome histories include evidence of inadequate provision for the child's basic needs, inadequate supervision, or a delay in seeking medical care.

In infants and young children, a common manifestation of neglect is poor growth and developmental delay due to decreased nutritional intake and understimulation. Such children, who are labeled as having nonorganic failure-to-thrive, often are recognized first because of poor weight gain or because they fall off the growth curve. Initially, the child's length and head circumference may be relatively spared, but if the nutritional deprivation continues, these parameters also are affected. The general pattern of growth for decreased nutritional intake, regardless of the cause, is for weight to be most affected, and head circumference least affected; this pattern can be ascertained by plotting each of the growth parameters on the 50th percentile curve and determining the child's age at the respective points (eg, the child's "weight age"). In many children whose failure-to-thrive is due to neglect, there also is a developmental delay, particularly affecting the child's language and social interactions. Such children may appear listless, have a flat affect, and demonstrate indiscriminate attachment behaviors.

Older children who are neglected often appear as emotionally needy. They may be depressed or adult-like in their behaviors, as a result of having to learn to care for themselves.

Acute problems, such as ingestions, burns, or injuries from falls are common presentations in neglected children and should be distinguished from abuse or unintentional injuries.

Sexual Abuse

Children who have been sexually abused generally come to the attention of clinicians because the child has told an adult about an uncomfortable experience (eg, "My uncle touches me down there, and I don't like it."), the parent becomes concerned about the child's behaviors (eg, sexualized acting out) or symptoms (eg, vaginal discharge), or a genital or anal abnormality is noted on physical examination.

Although the child's statement is one of the clearest indications that the child has been sexually abused, a very young child may have difficulty explaining what happened, and an older child may retract a relatively clear statement after the child begins to understand how upsetting the disclosure is to the family. In certain circumstances, such as disputes about custody or visitation, it may be particularly difficult to determine the truthfulness of the child's statements because of the complexities of the relationships in the family.

Children who have been sexually abused demonstrate a variety of behaviors and symptoms. Many are nonspecific and are seen in response to other childhood stresses as well, such as poor school performance, generalized anxiety, encopresis, or suicidal gestures. Others are more suggestive such as excessive masturbation, sexualized behaviors, vaginal discharge or bleeding, or rectal bleeding. Even a symptom such as vaginal discharge, however, has a low likelihood of being due to sexual abuse. In several studies of premenarcheal girls with the complaint of vaginal discharge, the most frequent diagnosis was poor hygiene, and sexual abuse was found in less than 5% of cases.

Although all children suspected of being sexually abused should have a complete physical examination, only 15 to 20% of such exams will reveal a genital or anal finding suspicious of sexual abuse. A normal exam, however, does not rule out sexual abuse, as there may have been no injury to the genital area, or if there was an injury, it might have healed without leaving any signs. Even in cases in which there has been a conviction of the perpetrator, it is unusual for the victims to have an abnormal physical finding. In a series of 236 children where the perpetrators were convicted, 23% of genital exams of girls and 7% of anal exams of all the children were considered abnormal or suspicious.

There has been considerable research in the last several years to define normal and abnormal genital and anal anatomy in prepubertal children. Acute abrasions, lacerations, or hematomas of the female genitals are particularly worrisome for a recent episode of sexual abuse. Findings considered suspicious of past abuse include U- or V-shaped clefts (notches) in the posterior rim of the hymen or attenuation or decreased hymenal tissue posteriorly. These findings should persist when the child is examined in the prone, knee-chest position. Scarring, such as of the posterior fourchette, also is indicative of previous trauma. Although an enlarged horizontal diameter of the hymenal opening has been considered suspicious of sexual abuse in a prepubertal girl, the size of the hymenal opening varies with different examination techniques and with the child's state of relaxation. The finding of an enlarged hymenal opening, therefore, should not by itself be used to make a diagnosis of sexual abuse. Abnormalities of the male genitals due to sexual abuse are unusual. Anal findings, such as acute fissures or thickened ruggae also can be seen in sexually abused children.

Children who have been sexually abused may acquire a sexually transmitted disease, and adolescents are at risk of becoming pregnant. The most common infections are gonorrhea, chlamydia, and human papillomavirus. Also, there have been several reports of HIV infection that were transmitted by sexual abuse.

ASSESSMENT AND DIAGNOSIS

When evaluating a child for suspected maltreatment, the clinician must decide whether an alternative explanation such as an unintentional injury, a medical problem, or an acceptable parental behavior can help explain the child's problem. The evaluation should include a complete history, careful physical examination, appropriate laboratory tests, and full documentation of the findings. In many settings, these tasks are divided among professionals, so that a physician might obtain a medical history and conduct the examination while a social worker obtains a psychosocial history. When available, community-based or hospital-based child-protection teams can guide clinicians in their assessments and offer specialized evaluations or treatment services.

A careful history concerning the events leading to the child's condition, the child's health status and development, and the family's strengths and weaknesses can help determine what happened to the child and the important contributory factors (Table 5-21). Data should be collected from the parents, the professionals who know the child and family, and from the child directly.

It is not uncommon for caregivers who were not actually present when the child was injured to report about the events causing the injury as if they were present. Careful questioning can help distinguish eyewitness accounts from secondhand information. It is important to note inconsistencies in reports (either from different caregivers or over time from the same caregiver) about how an injury occurred or how an injury/behavior evolved. Sometimes, however, inconsistencies may reflect different styles of history-taking or variable documentation, rather than inconsistencies because of intentionally confusing and misleading information. When maltreatment is being considered, supportive interviews of the parents alone and together may result in an admission of an abusive episode, a chronic pattern of neglect, or failure to nurture the child adequately.

When failure-to-thrive due to neglect is suspected, a careful feeding history should be obtained to estimate the child's caloric intake and to determine how the formula (or food) is prepared, what is offered to the child and how the child responds, whether there have been feeding problems in the past, and what the parental concerns and fears are. Information also should be obtained about the child's developmental milestones, temperament, affect, and the child's interactions with parents and others.

When sexual abuse is suspected, the parents must be asked explicitly about what the child said, as well as about the child's symptoms, such as vaginal discharge or bleeding, rectal bleeding, constipation, encopresis, sexualized behaviors, or unusual or recurrent fears. Important data about the family include whether the parents are separated or divorced, what kind of visitation schedule exists, and whether there is a dispute about custody or visitation. De-

TABLE 5-21

HISTORY TO EVALUATE SUSPECTED MALTREATMENT

A. Event(s) "causing" injury:
  What happened to child
  Who was present
  How the child responded
  How the adults responded
  Who cares for the child
B. Child:
  Previous injuries or concerns
  Past medical history, including immunizations and missed appointments
  Developmental history
  Parents' descriptions of child
  Parents' feelings toward child
C. Family:
  Care of other children
  Parents' own nurturing
  Parents' physical and mental health
  Family violence
  Substance abuse
  Resources and supports
  Recent stresses

pending upon their age, children should be interviewed directly about what may have happened to them. This interview or series of interviews should be done with the child alone if possible, and the interviewer should be skilled at such assessments and careful to avoid leading questions. To help young children describe what may have happened to them, interviewers have used stimulus props, such as anatomic drawings or anatomically correct dolls. Although controversy exists about whether these dolls are overly suggestive, research indicates that few nonsexually abused children respond in sexual ways with the dolls and that the dolls help children provide more details about what happened to them.

The physical examination should focus on the child's growth, development, affect, and interactions with parents and health professionals, as well as on the state of hygiene, signs of new and old injuries, and signs of sexual abuse. The examination of children suspected of having been sexually abused should include a careful inspection of the genitals and anus. The clinician should remain alert to signs that might point to an alternative diagnosis. In premenarcheal girls, the genital exam is best performed in the supine position; when abnormalities of the hymen are noted, the child also should be examined in the prone, knee-chest position to determine whether the abnormality persists. To visualize the hymen, the examiner can use two maneuvers: labial separation—separating the labia majora and pulling down at an angle of 45°—and labial traction—gently pinching the labia majora and pulling out and toward the examiner. Girls with suspicious findings should be examined by an expert examiner who uses a video- or photocolposcope, which provides magnification and the ability to document the findings.

In some cases, more extensive diagnostic studies are indicated. For children with serious head injuries, an ophthalmologic examination should be performed to determine whether retinal hemorrhages are present. A child's course can be followed clinically and with CT scans as necessary; an MR scan can be helpful in dating the age of an intracranial injury. Where there is a suspicion of abuse or neglect in a child less than 3 years of age, a skeletal survey (radiographs of all the bones) can reveal unsuspected recent or old fractures, as well as provide information about an underlying medical problem, such as osteogenesis imperfecta. Because rib fractures are difficult to detect on plain films until callus formation occurs 10 to 14 days after the acute injury, a bone scan can help to detect acute rib fractures. The rate of detection of unsuspected fractures depends upon the sample investigated; in one study of children less than 36 months of age with fractures, 31% of skeletal surveys were positive.

Initial laboratory tests in abused or neglected children should include a complete blood count, lead level (in children younger than 6 years of age), and urinalysis. In children with bruises or bleeding, a platelet count, prothrombin time, and partial thromboplastin time are appropriate screens. When suspected clinically, more detailed tests for bleeding disorders should be ordered. A recent study of abused children suggested that liver transaminase might be a helpful screen for occult liver injury.

In children with failure-to-thrive, laboratory tests may include a sedimentation rate, blood urea nitrogen, creatinine, and electrolytes. Additional tests to search for an underlying disease should be directed by concerns noted in the history or abnormalities noted on the physical examination.

When a child is evaluated within 72 hours of an episode of suspected sexual abuse, the clinician should gather appropriate forensic information, such as swabs to detect semen. Tests for sexually transmitted diseases, including gonorrhea, chlamydia, syphilis, hepatitis

B, and HIV infection, should be obtained in children when the abuse might have resulted in transmission of such a disease. In adolescents, a pregnancy test may be necessary.

Detailed documentation of the data collected, with direct quotations of the parents' or child's statements, and a clear description of the child's injuries, both in writing and with sketches is important. Many states have a specific form for recording information from an examination to determine whether sexual abuse has occurred. Photographs of the child's injuries, labeled with the date and the child's name and record number, can be very helpful.

Differential Diagnosis

The most common distinction that must be made in a case of suspected maltreatment is between frank abuse or willful neglect and an unintentional injury or inadequate nurturance. In addition, a variety of alternative explanations should be considered in the differential diagnosis. Bruises must be distinguished from birthmarks (eg, Mongolian spots), coagulation abnormalities (eg, idiopathic thrombocytopenic purpura), dermatitis (eg, phytodermatitis), or the result of folk medicine practices (eg, coin rubbing). Burns due to maltreatment can be confused with skin diseases that develop bullae, unintentional scalds, or unusual burns, such as seat belt buckle burns; cigarette burns may be confused with impetigo. When evaluating a young child with a fracture, the clinician must consider the possibility of an underlying disease such as osteogenesis imperfecta, rickets, or congenital syphilis. In such cases, there usually are other clinical signs or radiographic features to help make the correct diagnosis.

When evaluating concerns of sexual abuse, the clinician should consider the possibility of a false allegation in the differential diagnosis. In young children, particular attention should be paid to the use of open-ended or forced-choice questions, and to avoiding the overinterpretation of vague statements, such as, "He touched me." Also, clinicians should consider the possibility of a false allegation if the child has a serious mental health problem; if the child is caught in a bitter dispute, such as a custody battle, between parents; or if the child's statements about what happened have important inconsistencies, are vague and lack details, or seem rare in nature.

In cases of suspected sexual abuse, the examiner will have to identify abnormalities that are secondary to trauma due to sexual abuse from normal variations of anatomy. Physical conditions also can be mistaken for sexual abuse. Two common examples are streptococcal infection, which can cause marked redness of the vagina and perianal region, and lichen sclerosis, which can cause thinning of the skin and subepidermal hemorrhages of the vulva and perianal area. Straddle injuries, which usually have a clear history of a fall and are associated with external injuries of the female genitalia, also must be distinguished from sexual abuse. A foreign body, such as toilet paper in the vagina, can present with foul smelling, serosanguineous fluid and can be confused with sexual abuse.

Children with failure-to-thrive due to neglect must be distinguished from children who are not growing well because of an underlying disease (eg, cystic fibrosis or a congenital infection) or whose poor nutritional intake is due to an interactional problem between the primary caregiver (usually the mother) and the child. For example, if an infant is fussy and spitting during feeding, a vulnerable mother may not enjoy feeding her child, lose patience, and thus provide inadequate calories. A proposed developmental framework for considering these interactional problems and the development of feeding disturbances includes three distinct stages. In the first, which occurs from birth to 2 months, the developmental task of an infant is the regulation of state. Disorders of homeostasis (eg, poor sucking) may result in poor intake. If the parent fails to recognize the infant's cues, then underfeeding may occur with resultant failure-to-thrive. In the second stage, from 3 to 6 months, disorders of attachment may result in feeding problems; a parent who is depressed and apathetic may have a quiet and poorly interactive infant who feeds poorly and thus fails to thrive. In the third stage, from 7 to 36 months, disorders of separation and individuation may lead to feeding problems. For example, a struggle can occur between the child's wish to feed him- or herself and the parent's desire to ensure that the child receives adequate nutrition. If the struggle results in the child's regular refusal of food, poor growth will result. Because this type of feeding pattern may develop over several months, interventions that are aimed at rapid changes in feeding, such as short-term hospitalization, are unlikely to be successful.

MANAGEMENT AND TREATMENT

There are six important steps in the management of suspected child maltreatment. First, there must be appropriate communication with the family about the child's condition and the physician's concerns. The physician must communicate clearly that there are questions about how the child got hurt and worry that the child may have been abused. The family should be informed that the physician is a mandated reporter who must notify the state's child protection agency about "suspected" maltreatment and not just cases of confirmed abuse.

The second step is appropriate medical care for the child; third is ensuring the child's safety. Although some abused and neglected children are admitted to the hospital for protection and further evaluation, it is not uncommon for children who are not seriously injured to be placed by the child protection agency in foster care or with relatives. Fourth, the physician must assess the child's medical, developmental, emotional, and educational needs so that appropriate services can be provided. Fifth, the parents' and family's needs also must be evaluated so that adequate parenting can be ensured. And sixth, siblings should be assessed carefully to determine whether they have been maltreated.

These steps, which usually are carried out over time by professionals from several disciplines, including primary care clinicians, experts in child abuse and forensic pediatrics, child-protection service workers, police, and mental health clinicians, help determine the kinds of interventions needed. Services for the child might include ensuring appropriate medical care, participation in an early intervention program or a crisis nursery, or mental health counseling for an older child. For families, services might include concrete assistance (eg, ensuring adequate housing or transportation for the child's medical care), treatment programs for the parents own problems (eg, drug treatment, mental health counseling, or counseling about domestic violence), or treatment programs that focus on parenting (eg, Parents' Anonymous or parent–child programs).

If the suspected maltreatment is substantiated, the child-protection agency can help the family obtain the necessary services and monitor the child's safety. Unfortunately, most state protective service agencies are understaffed due to budgetary constraints and often have difficulty providing the necessary supervision of families whom they are mandated to serve. Pediatricians can help monitor families by providing follow-up care that focuses on the child's needs. This includes re-reporting the child to protective services if new injuries occur or if the child continues to be at substantial risk of maltreatment.

Maltreated children whose safety cannot be ensured in the home usually are placed in foster care or with relatives. Surveys of these children have noted a high rate of unrecognized medical, nutritional, developmental, educational, and emotional problems. To help with the recognition and management of these problems, foster care clinics were developed to provide multidisciplinary evaluations and recommendations for services. These types of programs have been successful at identifying problems and ensuring that the child is linked to appropriate services.

An alternative approach to out-of-home placements for children who are in imminent danger of continued maltreatment is to involve the family in an intensive family preservation service. This approach provides intensive, home-based services (while the child remains with the family) for 2 to 4 months by a paraprofessional who is often teamed with a social worker. The purpose of this intensive involvement is to mobilize the family at a time of crisis, to help reorganize the family to focus on the child's needs, and to connect the family to longer-term community services. Despite the philosophical appeal of such intensive services and a federal commitment of almost one billion dollars for family preservation from 1994 to 1998, evaluations have not provided clear evidence that such programs result in reduced rates of placements in foster care compared to standard care, nor are there sufficient data to indicate whether the children are functioning better because of these interventions.

Although most efforts concerning maltreated children have focused on recognition and treatment, there has been increasing interest in attempting to prevent maltreatment. Home-based outreach programs, which begin prenatally or shortly after birth and continue during the first 1 to 2 years of the child's life, have shown promising results in reducing the occurrence of abuse or neglect. Additional studies are needed to determine the intensity and duration of services needed, and whether high-risk families, such as those in which the mother uses cocaine, can be helped.

Most attempts to prevent sexual abuse have targeted young children who are the potential victims. For example, school-based programs have been developed to help children recognize good and bad touches and to learn how to respond to unwanted advances by telling an appropriate adult. Children as young as first graders are able to learn and retain these concepts, at least over a short period of time. Evaluations, however, have not been able to provide systematic data about whether such programs have resulted in the prevention or earlier recognition of sexual abuse.

NATURAL HISTORY AND PROGNOSIS

Maltreatment can have long-lasting and devastating effects on the development of children, adolescents, and adults. Although a child can be physically harmed from maltreatment, and brain injuries can have serious, long-term consequences, it is likely that the major consequences of maltreatment are related to its emotional impact. Moreover, there are many other factors that can affect the development of a maltreated child such as malnutrition, placement in multiple foster homes, or exposure to family violence. Thus, the link between child maltreatment and subsequent outcomes is not straightforward. Studies of abused and neglected children indicate that they have a higher rate of delayed intellectual development, poor school performance, and low self-esteem compared to nonmaltreated children. There also is an increased occurrence of emotional difficulties, including depression, suicide attempts, and self-

mutilation. Children who were maltreated are likely to have difficulty in forming trusting relationships with adults and in viewing adults as helpful people in their lives. Children who were neglected may be indiscriminate in seeking adult relationships.

There is clear evidence that children who have been maltreated have substantial problems with social interactions with peers. Children who were physically abused, in particular, have been noted to be physically aggressive and antisocial. Both abused and neglected children are at an increased risk of juvenile delinquency, substance abuse, and self-destructive behaviors during adolescence.

Adults who have been abused or neglected as children often have difficulty forming intimate relationships and often choose partners with similar problems. Parents who were abused as children are at increased risk of abusing their own children (the "intergenerational transmission of abuse"), but the link between experiencing childhood abuse and abusing one's own child is not a simple linear association. Although some investigators have estimated that 30% of abused parents will abuse their own children, more research is needed to define this risk more clearly.

Sexual abuse also has a major adverse impact on development. Children who have been victims of sexual abuse may develop low self-esteem and feelings of guilt and shame and may learn to use sexual behaviors inappropriately in their interactions with peers and adults. Teenage girls and adult women are at increased risk of promiscuity, have difficulties forming intimate relationships, and may be revictimized. They also are at increased risk of having mental health problems, such as depression, suicide, eating disorders, multiple personality disorders, and posttraumatic stress disorder. Males who were sexually abused as children are at increased risk of having mental health problems, abusing substances, or becoming perpetrators.

There are little data about the long-term effects of specific treatments of maltreated children. The expectation is that early recognition and appropriate treatment for the child and family will minimize adverse outcomes. The presence of a supportive adult who is able to respond to the emotional needs of the child seems to minimize the short-term psychological effects of maltreatment, but less is known about long-term sequelae.

References

Adams JA, Harper K, Knudson S, Revilla J: Examination findings in legally confirmed child sexual abuse: it's normal to be normal. Pediatrics 94:310–317, 1994

American Academy of Pediatrics, Committee on Child Abuse and Neglect: Guidelines for the evaluation of sexual abuse of children: subject review. Pediatrics 103:186–191, 1999

Atabaki S, Paradise JE: The medical evaluation of the sexually abused child: lessons from a decade of research. Pediatrics 1204(suppl):178–186, 1999

Behrman RE, ed: Sexual abuse of children. Future Child 4(2), 1994

Belsky J: The determinants of parenting: a process model. Child Dev 55:83–96, 1985

Berenson AB, Hegar AH, Hayes JM, Bailey RK, Emans SJ: Appearance of the hymen in prepubertal girls. Pediatrics 9:387–394, 1992

Chatoor I, Schaefer S, Dickson L: Non-organic failure to thrive: a developmental perspective. Pediatr Ann 13:829–842, 1984

Duhaime AC, Christian CW, Rorke LB, Zimmerman RA: Nonaccidental head injury in infants—the "shaken baby syndrome." N Engl J Med 333:1822–1829, 1998

Faller KC: Understanding Child Sexual Maltreatment. Newbury Park, Sage, 1993

Heger A, Emans SJ, ed: Evaluation of the Sexually Abused Child: A Medical Textbook and Photographic Atlas. New York, Oxford University Press, 1992

Helfer RE: The neglect of our children. Pediatr Clin North Am 37:923–942, 1990

Helfer ME, Kempe RS, Krugman RD, eds: The Battered Child Syndrome. 5th ed. Chicago, University of Chicago Press, 1997

Henegan AM, Horwitz SM, Leventhal JM: Evaluating intensive family preservation programs: a methodologic review. Pediatrics 97:535–542, 1996

Hobbs CJ: Skull fracture and the diagnosis of child abuse. Arch Dis Child 5:246–252, 1984

Holmes WC, Slap GB: Sexual abuse of boys: definition, prevalence, correlates, sequelae, and management. JAMA 280:1855–1862, 1998

Kempe CH, Silverman FN, Steele B, Droegemuller W, Silver HR: The battered child syndrome. JAMA 18:17–24, 1962

Kerns DL, guest ed: Establishing a medical research agenda for child sexual abuse. Child Abuse Negl 22:453–660, 1999

Kleinman PK, ed: Diagnostic Imaging of Child Abuse. 2nd ed. St Louis, Mosby, 1998

Leventhal JM: Twenty years later: we do know how to prevent child abuse and neglect. Child Abuse Negl 20:647–653, 1996

Leventhal JM, Thomas SA, Rosenfield NS, Markowitz RI: Fractures in young children: distinguishing child abuse from unintentional injuries. Am J Dis Child 147:87–92, 1993

McCann J, Kerns DL: The Anatomy of Child and Adolescent Sexual Abuse: A CD-ROM Atlas/Reference. St Louis, Intercorp, 1999

McCann J, Wells R, Simon M, Voris J: Genital findings in prepubertal girls selected for nonabuse. A descriptive study. Pediatrics 86:428–439, 1990

Meadow R: Munchausen syndrome by proxy—the hinterland of child abuse. Lancet ii:343–345, 1977

National Research Council: Understanding Child Abuse and Neglect. Washington, DC, National Academy of Sciences, 1993

Nelson KE, Landsman MJ: Alternative Models of Family Preservation: Family-Based Services in Context. Springfield, Charles C. Thomas, 1992

Olds DL, Eckenrode J, Henderson CR, et al: Long-term effects of home visitation on maternal life course and child abuse and neglect: fifteen-year follow-up of a randomized trial. JAMA 278:637–643, 1997

Olds DL, Henderson CR, Kitzman H: Does prenatal and infancy nurse home visitation have enduring effects on qualities of parental caregiving and child health at 25 to 50 months of life? Pediatrics 93:89–98, 1994

Reece RM, ed: Child Abuse: Medical Diagnosis and Management. Philadelphia, Lea & Febiger, 1994

Southall DP, Plunkett MCB, Banks MW, Falkow AF, Samuels MP: Covert video recordings of life-threatening child abuse: lessons for child protection. Pediatrics 100:735–760, 1997

Stier DM, Leventhal JM, Berg AT, Johnson L, Mezger J: Are children born to young mothers at increased risk of child maltreatment? Pediatrics 91:642–648, 1993

Sugar NF, Taylor JA, Feldman KW, and the Puget Sound Pediatric Research Network: Bruises in infants and toddlers: Those who don't cruise rarely bruise. Arch Pediatr Adolesc Med 153:399–403, 1999

5.6.10   Gender and Sexuality: Normal Development to Problems and Concerns

Suzanne D. Dixon

A child's identity as a boy or a girl is a component of the child's own individuality, emerging in predictable stages through interactions between biology and culture, family and peers. A clearer sense of self as a person with a sexual dimension grows from infancy through adolescence and into adulthood through normative developmental change.

NORMAL DEVELOPMENT

Infancy

The genetic sex of a child influences more than in utero genital formation. Cognitive processes such as visual-spatial perceptual abilities, verbal abilities, level of activity, and the degree of assertiveness are examples of areas of differential gender-specific neurobehavioral development that influence a child's responsiveness to postnatal experiences. Also, less-rigid cerebral lateralization is evident in girls. The family's image of the child as a boy or girl begins prior to birth through speculation or with ultrasound or chromosomal evidence. Most parents do obtain this information if it's available, perhaps accelerating parental attachment to the fetus. At birth, if not before, the confirmation of the child's gender immediately begins to influence parent-child interaction: the way the infant is handled, talked to, ascribed emotions and intentionality by parents and others, all vary by the infant's gender. Once announced, this attribute of the child is extremely difficult to alter in the parents' mind; delivery room announcements in all cases must be very accurate. The infant thus has a gender-specific life experience as well as constitution from the start.

Healthy sexuality begins in infancy with the pleasurable bodily sensations of touching and holding. Self-exploration of the infant's genitals occurs in the second half of the first year of life, although this has been observed in utero. Erections in boys may now be purposely induced by the infant. Similar behavior is seen in infant girls, usually a little later. This usually involves rhythmically rubbing against objects.

Toddlerhood/Preschool

Children have increased interest in the genitals themselves at 16 to 19 months, followed several months later by naming of the genitals if labels are provided. Genital exploration continues through toddler and preschool years, peaking at about 4 years, and becomes increasingly private through parental responses to this behavior and the child's growing awareness that it is unacceptable public behavior.

Gender identity, the concept of oneself as a boy or a girl emerges in the second year (see Table 5-22). Children younger than 2 years can reliably identify themselves as the appropriate sex and will be able to correctly classify others and associate particular traits with gender. Hair and clothing attributes appear to be more salient than the genitals in making these early assignments. Men and women are also correctly classified at this age, but the continuity between youth and maturity (gender constancy, eg, girl to woman) still remains a fuzzy connection until 4 to 5 years of age. Children younger than this believe they can change into or grow up into the opposite sex. Fantasy and dress-up switches, boasts of "sex changes" are evidence of developmental work in this area. By age 4 to 5, children know they will always be a boy/a girl and will grow up to be the same-sex adult—they have achieved gender stability, another aspect of self-concept.

Children's ideas of sex-appropriate activities, toys, and clothing are solidified in preschool. This is the public expression of the internal construct of gender identity that includes the behaviors and attitudes considered appropriate for males and females. These ideas are often more stereotyped than adults' ideas. This rigidity of what is gender appropriate peaks at about 5 to 6 years and is stronger in boys than in girls. No gender-specific toy preferences are seen by age 1; by age 2 there are substantial differences, and by age 5 these preferences are very clear. Boys and girls learn what is regarded as

TABLE 5-22
TERMS IN THE DEVELOPMENT OF THE SEXUAL SELF

TERM	CONCEPT/BELIEF	APPROXIMATE AGE OF ACQUISITION	VARIATION
Gender recognition	That person is a man. That voice belongs to a lady.	10 to 18 months	Tracks with cognitive abilities
Gender identity	I am a boy/I am a girl. (The internal or private belief.)	18 to 30 months	Fixed very early in life
Gender understanding			Varies with cognitive development
Stability	I will always be a boy. I was a baby boy, and I will grow to be a man.	3 to 4 years	
Constancy	Even if I dress up like a girl, I am still really a boy underneath.	4 to 5 years	
	Julie is still a girl even if she puts on her brother's clothes. Later: I'm still a boy, because I have a penis.	4 to 6 years	
Gender role definition (the public expression of gender identity)	Boys always play football. Ladies work in offices. Boys push in line. Girls talk too much.	2 years up; play differential from 4 years onward	Varies by age, culture, social circumstances, and temperament. More narrow in boys. Most rigid in preschoolers.
Sexual orientation	I feel attracted to girls. I think about sex with boys.	8 to 11 years (may be present much earlier) 11 years and older	May be uncertain, indeterminate, particularly among young teens. "Coming out" means recognizing and being open with a same-sex orientation.

"appropriate" behaviors, even at this early age. Children in family systems with a strict gender stereotype (an organized set of beliefs about gender characteristics) adapt same-gender toys and dress slightly earlier and more restrictively, but these are only short-term differences. These gender-specific activities come from the cognitive processes within the child, the inherent drive to classify people, things, and activities, influenced by broad societal forces. Play activities, toys, and styles of physical and verbal interaction become very distinctly "boy" and "girl" during this time, no matter how flexibly these lines are drawn by a family. Boys are stricter than girls in this process and will remain so. Attempts at androgynous play environments may encourage children to explore a wider range of play activities but do not appear to alter gender-specific play or playmate preferences over the long-term. Recent social changes have not altered societal gender stereotypes as much as might be expected.

Children increasingly segregate themselves into same gender groups if given free choice of playmates, and in these, they play in a gender-specific ways. Boys interact in groups with more physical bumping, pushing, and shoving, engage in one-upmanship in games and stories, and play hierarchical team games. Girls interact verbally, seek to be included and inclusive, have "best friends," play in small groups, and attempt to influence through verbal suggestions and demands. They work to be noncompetitive and cooperative, but subtly coercive in the exercise of control. Although individual children will vary in these dimensions of play, these basic patterns appear broadly in all cultural groups and settings.

Genital anatomic differences have focused interest by 4- to 5-year-olds and are now important in one's perception of gender of self and others. Few children, particularly girls, are given accurate names for their genitals in order to find out more about this part of themselves. The avoidance of genital naming in the home is often echoed in the pediatric office. This avoidance of discussion conveys a sense of forbiddenness that shuts off questions and concerns. It may also mean that the adults are unprepared to deal with sexual issues in a straightforward way. Clinicians can be models for more accurate, forthright naming and explaining this part of a child to him- or herself.

Seductive behavior toward opposite-sex parents or toward other adults is typical at this age, partly because of the exploration of what is the appropriate gender role. Teaching restraint and providing an emotionally safe environment allows for healthy resolution and healthy emotional expression.

School Age

Grade-school children are very rigid in their view of sex-appropriate attire, behavior, talk, and associations. They tend to be very modest, easily embarrassed, and avoid overt sexual events. Their concrete thinking and underlying sexual tension appear to be the origins of this strict delineation. They will flee from cross-gender interaction but remain curious. Sexual concerns bubble to the surface occasionally as manifest by such behaviors as cross-sex teasing and chasing or severe embarrassment at the sight of kissing or other sexual behavior by others. Grade-school children are very anxious about being seen nude, even by parents, and certainly by health providers. "Bad" words and jokes about elimination or implied sexual function are regarded as extremely funny; public hugs and kisses by parents are agony (while private ones are still much needed). A child at this age has learned to be circumspect regarding sexual matters, the child's own and that of others, but still needs healthy affection expressed from family.

Adolescence

The work of adolescence requires the development of a self-concept that includes sexual dimensions. In young adolescents, this process begins with increased interest in sexual matters and initiates a process of consolidation of sexual orientation, or the specific focus of sexual attraction toward one or both genders. Remote targets of these sexual attractions such as teachers, coaches, music idols, and sports figures offer safe ways to imagine oneself sexually and are typical of the late grade school, early teen years. Crushes lessen with age in intensity as real sexual encounters become a possibility. Opposite-sex pairings in early or mid-adolescence are often regarded as means to acquire status or prestige, or to try out a sexual role, posturing primarily for same-sex friends. Labeling oneself as "going with" someone may precede dating by years. Adults may worry about this impersonal, commodity-like approach, but it is fairly typical of the junior high student. Youngsters at this age still are usually found in same-sex groups whose opinions and attitudes are paramount. Group activities with the opposite sex are usually safer, offering group support.

Young adolescents may have concerns regarding their own sexual orientation at this time. Almost 25% of 12-year-olds are unsure of their sexual orientation. Limited homosexual attractions, fantasies, or encounters increases in masturbation and transient interest in some type of pornographic materials are not unusual at this age as a result of these processes. In one study, 11% of males and 6% of females have had at least one homosexual experience, although the numbers were lower (2.8%, and 0.9%, respectively) in another study. Some youngsters may become anxious or guilty afterwards. Assurance by the clinician of the common occurrence of such events and the fact that these do not, in themselves, define future sexual orientation may be helpful. Conversely, by bringing up homosexuality as an issue, the clinician offers the opening to discuss this issue further if indicated.

Some youngsters begin to experience sexual intercourse at this age, although this is not the norm. About one-quarter of 14-year-olds have been sexually active; the average age of initiation of intercourse for boys is about 15; for girls, it is about 16. The psychological backdrop for early sexual intercourse is almost always egocentric or as a means to obtaining something that is perceived as missing, such as enhanced self-esteem, affection, peer approval, status, freedom from abuse, or sexual reassurance. Entering into sexual relationships at this time in psychological development may inhibit one's further maturation as an independent sexual person who is capable of sustained intimacy in long-term relationships. Difficulties down the line have been associated with the factors that track with this early imitation of intercourse. Psychological and physical risks accompany this early initiation of intercourse.

Many adolescents of high school age develop sexual friendships or intimate relationships with others varying in intensity and duration. Dating may be initiated or accelerated by the acquisition of a driver's license. By their 18th birthday, 75% of boys and 50% of adolescent girls will be sexually active, although 18% will finish high school as virgins. Most healthy adolescents have only one relationship at a time (termed *serial monogamy*), are not promiscuous, and have an emotional relationship to their dating partner. The healthcare provider should be comfortable in addressing the issues surrounding initiation of sexual intimacy, both physical and psychological. Counsel regarding delays in the initiation of intercourse and responsible actions (eg, birth control, sexually transmitted disease protection) at this stage in development is effective but may be hampered by the youngster's sense of invulnerability (ie, "It can't happen to me."). Peer counseling may have enhanced effectiveness in these areas.

PARENTAL CONCERNS

Masturbation

Self-stimulation of the genitals is nearly universal from infancy to adulthood, reported by more than 90% of males and more than 50% of females. It occurs at all ages, with peak occurrence at about 4 years and in adolescence. Masturbation may masquerade as abdominal pain, motor tics, epilepsy, dystonia, or other unusual behavioral patterns in young children. It may be triggered by vulvovaginitis, tight clothing, or urethral irritation. Counsel about keeping this behavior private should be provided to all children. In families with religious prohibition, simple teaching and redirecting behavior should be provided. Dramatically negative reactions or punishments set the stage for feelings of shame in one's sexual self and for the need to hide sexual issues from parents. Punishment may even solidify, rather than eliminate, this behavior.

Compulsive, excessive, or intense masturbation that interrupts other activities, involves objects, or is persistently public is not normative at any age, and usually signals a disturbance in some aspects of the child's emotional life. Some children masturbate when tense, when feeling rejected, or when bored. The behavior may be a symptom of some disturbance in the interpersonal sphere, usually a perceived or real lack of affection or an experience of sexual exploitation or exposure to explicit sexual material or events. The origins of this behavior need to be identified before any management plan is developed. Treatments designed around providing additional, nongenital tactile input such as rocking or holding, along with addressing the underlying interactional issues, are successful in changing this behavioral pattern. Punishment does not work and may only reinforce the pattern of turning to oneself for comfort. Masturbation *with objects* is very unusual in childhood and should raise questions of atypical sexual experiences.

Masturbation increases during adolescence, with about half or more of boys less than 13 years old and about one-third of girls self-reporting masturbation with regularity. These numbers increase with age and with a higher male frequency. In spite of changed societal attitudes, many adolescents may have feelings of guilt and worry. Parents with conservative beliefs or religious prohibitions may be distressed. The pediatric position should be that there is no scientific evidence that masturbation causes any physical or mental difficulties at any age and that it is a very common behavior. No particular concern needs to be addressed unless the behavior is compulsive, serves to isolate the child from healthy interpersonal relationships, signals a lack of such relationships, or is a source of conflict between a youngster and his or her parents. If conflicts exist, the pediatric care provider should help those families resolve the issues involved.

Sexual Exploration

During the first 3 years of life, sexual exploration includes the curious handling of one's own and others' genitalia, and curiosity about anatomic sexual differences and behaviors such as kissing and stroking of others. Touching of another child's genitals, observing toileting and bathing, showing one's own genitals to others, flirtatious behavior, and nude parading are very common, ranging from 10 to 60% in one large series of normal young children. Exhibitionistic and voyeuristic behaviors are very common in the 3 to 6 year age range but are remarkably unusual by grade school and require further explanation if present beyond age 6. An overly sexualized experience, lack of impulse control, and cognitive delays are all possibilities in explaining this unusual pattern.

The boundaries of acceptable behaviors vary widely among both parents and professionals. However, certain activities that are both uncommon and judged by most professionals to be very worrisome cluster around "adult" sexual behaviors and those behaviors accompanied by aggression. Behaviors that are not usually seen in this culture are frank imitation of sexual intercourse, requests to engage in intercourse, doll play that includes oral, anal, or vaginal penetration, or putting one's mouth on another's genitals. Children with such behavior have often witnessed multiple sexual acts—distinctly atypical in this culture—or they themselves have been involved with adult sexual behavior (ie, sexual abuse). This situation needs to be explored further to identify its origins. Typical children do not imitate sexual intercourse from movies or television exposure alone, although they may pick up models for provocative, seductive behavior. School-age children, particularly, filter sexual behavior seen in the media, to either push it out of consciousness or inhibit their own modeling of it. Differences in families regarding openness of discussion of sexual issues, family nudity, and attitudes toward sexual issues generally create differences in the clinical presentation of problems. The frequency of (recognized) common sexual behaviors is greater in families with more liberal attitudes than in families who describe themselves as conservative. Specific questions and open-ended queries from the clinician may identify parental concerns not brought up spontaneously.

Children with other behavioral problems (eg, conduct disorder, attention deficit hyperactivity disorder) are also more likely to act out in sexual ways. Children with poor impulse control and patterns of externalizing behavioral problems, particularly boys, are more likely to present with concerns that have a sexual aspect. These children should not be labeled "sexually deviant." The clinician will do well to place the sexualized behaviors in a broader explanatory context and provide referrals for the management of the troublesome behavioral profile overall.

Children with retarded development generally have the sexual exploration patterns appropriate for their developmental age rather than physical age. Genital touching, seductive behavior, or "sexualized behavior" may be a disturbing complaint in the older grade-school child with a toddler's cognitive level. This "acting out" should be placed in its proper developmental context. Simple behavior modification techniques can be used to help these youngsters learn appropriate behaviors, times, and places.

Adolescents who repeatedly engage in exhibitionistic behavior need a mental health referral. Although this behavior may be based on the need for assurance of one's sexual self, more commonly it is a sign of underlying aggression directed toward the viewer or others who might be angered by it (ie, parents or teachers). Exhibitionism, in general, should decrease with age across the school-age population as children learn socially acceptable patterns of sexual expression and become both more private and circumspect. Those who will be consistent exhibitionists have a typical onset of this behavior as problematic at 15 years of age. This often comes out of feelings of needing reassurance of one's sexuality while keeping the targets distant. There is a complex origin in most situations that requires specialized referral. A resurgence in overt or inappropriate sexualized behaviors should signal a need for assessing the child and environment and identifying etiology. Children who have been sexually abused are reported to have more sexual behavior problems as well as other psychosocial concerns. This etiology

should be one of several considered in evaluating the basis for these sexual concerns.

Sexual Assault

Violent sexual activity directed at others, such as forced genital touching, genital injury, sexually explicit demands, or sexual activity with animals, finds its origins in uncontrolled aggression and early poor attachments, not in uncontrolled sexual arousal, although these may have become linked over time. Children who assault others sexually have histories of isolation, lack of empathy, loneliness, and sexualized coping behaviors to handle stress. These children need referral to a mental health professional. They themselves may have been sexually victimized, raised in a nonnormative sexual environment, been prompted by peers or adults to act out in this way, or have a large store of anger and lack of a trusting relationship. These are major behavioral issues that need professional intervention.

"Dirty Pictures"

Children aged 3.5 to 5 years often include genitals in their drawings. After 4 years of age, clothing and hair become more gender specific, with drawings by boys and girls becoming distinct. It is distinctly unusual for older grade-school children to include genitals in human figure drawing or to have sexually ambiguous figures in their drawings. Like the privatization of their behavior generally, their drawings demonstrate restraint. Particularly if persistent and combined with aggressive themes, these unusual drawings should trigger further investigation by clinicians, including the possibility of sexual abuse. The presence of genitals is *not* diagnostic for child abuse; it is a sign of an atypical developmental course in a grade-school child, requiring more assessment to define its meaning.

Many children, particularly older grade-school children and young teens, may show an interest in pornographic material. Exposure through the Internet is an increasing possibility for many children and adolescents. There is no evidence that one or two episodes are unusual or are, in themselves, inciting of further sexual activity. However, the exploitative nature of many of these materials should be identified to all young people through an open discussion with parents, clinicians, or counselors. Further investigation is warranted if such interest becomes continual over months, becomes compulsive or dominant in interests, occurs in the context of an isolated youngster with atypical social relationships, or is combined with aggressive actions or plans. Atypical sexual development, depression, or major psychiatric disturbance may be present. However, one or a few such events should not be regarded as unduly alarming in a child who is functioning well in other domains of his life. It does require parental involvement that clinicians may need to encourage.

Exposure to sexually explicit movies and videos does harm through a similar display of violent or exploitative sexual interactions. The separation of genuine affection, commitment, and consequences from sexual activity is the wrong message for teens. Parents need to stay involved with their child's viewing choices in all media, with opportunities for open discussion of context in line with family values. Television, movies, magazines, the Internet, and music are all forums for teens/parents discussion of limits and acceptable content. Sexual interest is developmentally based; acceptable norms should be family-based.

Cross-Dressing

It is entirely normal for children under age 5 to dress up in the outer clothes of the opposite sex as they work on the psychological tasks of gender role and gender understanding during this time (see above). These costumes are usually part of an elaborate fantasy that is shared with interested audiences (eg, playmates, parents) and one that regularly shifts and changes. If secretive, this behavior is abnormal in the school-age child or adolescent, and requires further evaluation by the health-care provider. Undergarments of a parent may be treasured as a comfort item by a young toddler, but hoarding or wearing these clothing items by the preschooler or beyond is very atypical and, with increasing age, carries a sexual dimension with it. Older children and adolescents who experience sexual pleasure with cross-dressing (transvestitism), often with undergarments, do so covertly and with deep shame and stress. Heterosexual orientation is the likely outcome for these youngsters, although some may have the emergence of a homosexual orientation. Behavior modification techniques can be used to change this activity, provided the youngster is motivated and there is an absence of other psychological problems.

Older children and youth who dress exclusively or flamboyantly in the outer garments of the opposite sex raise consideration of gender identity disorder (see below) or effeminate homosexuality in boys. This clinical complaint should not be dismissed without further evaluation. Cross-dressing of any etiology should not be punished. It is healthy in the young child and needs further investigation in the older child.

Sissy Boys and Tomboy Girls

Issues of childhood sexuality may present clinically with a parental concern: a boy who is more effeminate in behavior, dress, or interests than is seen as appropriate, or, less commonly, a girl who is described as being "too interested" in boys' things—a tomboy. Nearly 6% of boys and 12% of girls in a sample of typical children sometimes or frequently behave like the opposite sex and have such labels. A smaller number of children actually said they wish to be of the opposite sex. Although temperamental mismatch between the youngster and family is the most common explanation for these concerns as they emerge in clinical settings, disorders of gender identity, atypical sexual orientation, or other sexual issues must be considered with this presenting complaint. The spectrum runs from normal variation in behavior, to problematic behavior, to a behavior disorder as laid out in the *DSM-IV* (Table 5-23).

Children with gender-identity disorder (GID) truly and persistently believe they are the opposite of their genetic sex. They are distressed with every aspect of their gender from genitals to clothes, activities to friends. Little girls with GID consistently assert such things as they will grow a penis or refuse to urinate sitting down. A boy may say his penis will disappear or that he will grow up to be a woman. Although transient fantasy for change or dissatisfaction of ones' sexual self is common in all children, children with GID have a deep, persistent abhorrence and denial of their genetic sex.

This is a rare disorder, occurring in perhaps 1 in 25,000 males and 1 in 125,000 females, the numbers being estimates. All ethnic and income groups are represented. GID usually presents clinically between 2.5 and 5 years in boys, a little later in girls. Boys are significantly overrepresented in clinical samples, thought to be due to the poor tolerance of feminized behavior in boys in Western culture. The disorder does not go away in older children, who may

hide their ideas, wishes, and concerns so that the problem may appear to lessen with time.

There is no clear etiology, although constitutional factors in the child are increasingly implicated. There is no evidence that parental behavior causes this disorder, although there is a higher-than-expected level of parental psychopathology, particularly depression, in such families. However, high family stress levels are usually present at the time of clinical presentation. Other psychopathologies are more common in youngsters with GID, including anger and depression. These are unhappy youngsters.

Play activities and peer choices may give clues to this disorder. Fantasy and play for boys with GID show a preference for feminine roles, activities, and playmates. Traditional male activities are avoided. These boys are often described as shy and anxious, particularly with separations. In one study, nearly two-thirds of the re-

TABLE 5-23

DIAGNOSTIC CRITERIA FOR IDENTITY DISORDER OF CHILDHOOD

A. A strong persistent cross-gender identification (not merely a desire for any perceived cultural advantages of being the other sex).

   In children, the disturbance is manifested by four (or more) of the following:
   1. Repeatedly stated desire to be, or insistence that he or she is, the other sex.
   2. In boys, preference for cross-dressing or simulating female attire; in girls, insistence on wearing only stereotypical masculine clothing.
   3. Strong and persistent preferences for cross-sex roles in make-believe play or persistent fantasies of being the other sex.
   4. Intense desire to participate in the stereotypical games and pastimes of the other sex.
   5. Strong preference for playmates of the other sex.

   In adolescents and adults, the disturbance is manifested by symptoms such as a stated desire to be the other sex, frequent passing as the other sex, desire to live or be treated as the other sex, or the conviction that he or she has the typical feelings and reactions of the other sex.

B. Persistent discomfort with his or her sex or sense of inappropriateness in the gender role of that sex.

   In children, the disturbance is manifested by any of the following:
   In boys, assertion that his penis or testes are disgusting or will disappear, assertion that it would be better not to have a penis, or aversion toward rough-and-tumble play and rejection of male stereotypical toys, games, and activities.
   In girls, rejection of urinating in a sitting position, assertion that she has or will grow a penis, assertion that she does not want to grow breasts or menstruate, or marked aversion toward normative feminine clothing.

   In adolescents and adults, the disturbance is manifested by symptoms such as preoccupation with getting rid of primary and secondary sex characteristics (eg, request for hormones, surgery, or other procedures to physically alter sexual characteristics to simulate the other sex) or belief that he or she was born the wrong sex.

C. The disturbance is not concurrent with physical intersex condition.

D. The disturbance causes clinically significant distress or impairment in social, occupational, or other important areas of functioning.

SOURCE: *From American Psychiatric Association: Diagnostic and Statistical Manual of Mental Disorders, Fourth Edition. Washington, DC, American Psychiatric Association, 1994.*

ferred group met criteria for separation anxiety disorder. Heightened and atypical perceptual sensibilities also have been described in taste, touch, and hearing. Drawings and other projective techniques demonstrate feminine patterns. Girls with GID have the mirror-image profile with activities, playmates, and fantasy that are more typically male.

Most effeminate boys do not have GID. Although their style, mannerisms, and interest are not conventionally male, they neither hate their gender nor wish to be a girl. This factor distinguishes the variation and problem-level concern from the real disorder. Similarly, most tomboys do not have GID. Although these girls may be athletic, competitive, and like the more active life of boys, they see themselves as girls and do not have an aversion to their sex. These distinctions are important as the prognosis and management for the youngster with true GID is substantially different than for the youngsters who have untraditional gender roles but solid same-sex gender identity.

The *DSM-IV* (see Table 5-23) gives criteria to distinguish profiles that are really just temperamental variations or are at the problem level from those of true GID. Core gender identity is at the base of these distinctions. The variation profile, a temperamental dimension, needs reassurance; the problem profile needs some intervention, perhaps in primary care. GID needs specialized help and referral over both the short- and long-term.

There is no convincing evidence that youngsters with true GID will change in gender identity with therapy. Experienced therapists can address secondary adjustment problems, depression, separation anxiety, family stress, and the high degree of concomitant psychopathology. Redirection and support of gender-appropriate play and interests may minimize stigma. About three-quarters of youngsters with GID will have a homosexual, bisexual, or indeterminate sexual orientation as adults; most homosexual adults do not have GID. Those with the strongest cross-gender behavior were more likely to evolve into transsexualism. For those adolescents with GID who continue to cross-dress, considerable gender dysphoria persists with many secondary problems.

Some adolescents and adults with clear heterosexual orientation and typical gender identity continue to cross-dress. This transvestitism provides erotic arousal. The issues, evolution, and secondary concerns here are substantially different than those with GID or transsexual individuals.

The pediatric clinician should take very seriously the youngster who doesn't like himself or herself, even if the child is very young. This applies to the abhorrence or denial of one's sexual self. Parental concerns regarding effeminate boys and tomboy girls should lead to additional history about patterns, persistence, pervasiveness, observation for play, interests, and peers, and, in some cases, specialized referral.

Gay and Lesbian Parents

It is estimated that 6 to 14 million children have a homosexual parent, so every child health-care provider will encounter families with this issue. The data to date all suggest that there is no deleterious effect on the children raised with a homosexual parent on social functioning, psychological well being, or peer and adult interactions. Children of homosexual parents have no increased behavioral or developmental risk in any area, including gender identity, gender role acquisition, and sexual orientation. Children raised in these widely varying circumstances may experience changing parental partners, the economic struggles of a single-parent home in some cases, and alienation from the extended families, stressors that

also are present in the homes of heterosexual parents. Two "parents," no matter the gender, improve developmental outcome over single-parent families. For example, children raised by a lesbian mother do better if the mother has a stable partner rather than in a single-adult household or one with changing partners. The sexual orientation of their parents per se does not appear to have any additional influence on several aspects of development. Families with low levels of stress and conflict, and with strong, positive emotional ties, expectedly have well-adjusted children, irrespective of the sexual orientation of the parents.

The health-care provider should support these atypical families' care of their children with a generic evaluation of the family's ability to meet the child's physical and psychological needs. These include the need to be valued as an individual, including one's sexual identity, the involvement in healthy, supportive community, role models of both sexes and consistency in love and affection.

Homosexuality

Homosexuality is a persistent pattern of same-sex arousal accompanied by a weak or absent heterosexual arousal. One's sexual orientation is toward members of the same gender. For the vast majority, one's gender identity is in concordance with one's own biological sex. All societies have identified homosexuality in some members, although the incidence, acceptance, and roles vary widely. Biological factors, including genetic influences on the prenatal development of the central nervous system via sex steroids, are gaining prominence in etiologic formulations. Some differences in CNS structures, family, and twin studies add to the evidence regarding biological origins.

Prevalence reports suggest that between 1 and 8% of men and 1 and 4% of women say they have a homosexual orientation, although methodology in studies makes it difficult to determine. Many adolescents are unsure of their sexual orientation and may engage in interactions and fantasies that do not indicate long-term sexual problems. Homosexual attractions, fantasies, and some activities are reported more often in adolescents than in adults; only about one-third of these will describe themselves as homosexual or bisexual. Homosexual orientation does not appear to be a matter of volition, although sexual behaviors and life-style are matters of choice.

Many individuals become aware of their homosexuality during adolescence and struggle with "coming out," telling the world of their sexual orientation. Internal psychological struggles and external conflicts make this an extremely vulnerable group for behavioral problems. Academic issues, truancy, and peer difficulties, even physical attacks; parental rejection; and homelessness; running away; and substance abuse occur singly or in combination in the majority of this group. Adolescents in this group may beat themselves up, engaging in self-destructive behavior, acceptance of discrimination, and severe self-doubt. From 25 to 40% of homeless youth are homosexual. Many (20–42% by one study) contemplate or attempt suicide. These youngsters account for about 30% of all teen suicides. Gay teens (males) are more at risk than lesbian (female) youth. Eating disorders, particularly among gay men, and poor body image are prominent in this group. The clinician should consider struggles with sexual orientation as possible etiology for behavioral problems including suicide attempts among youth. An open, nonjudgmental environment in the clinical setting may assist the youth in accepting him- or herself and dealing with these issues. Formal therapeutic intervention may help young people to clarify their sexual orientation or to deal with secondary struggles. Therapy directed toward changing a homosexual orientation is contraindicated; it has not been successful and it may instill lowered self-esteem and guilt. Appropriate care for this group of youngsters, like those with a heterosexual orientation, includes counsel regarding safe and responsible sexual behavior, the avoidance of sexual exploitation and of promiscuity. Acceptance of oneself, responsible actions, and developing a strong life plan in line with one's strengths are the focus of care.

Disorders of Sexual Differentiation: Psychological Issues

The biological influences on sexual differentiation, including psychosocial processes, are highlighted in situations in which the biology is altered very early in life. For example, youngsters with congenital adrenal hyperplasia (CAH) develop a gender identity based on the sex of rearing, with this more solid in children with early gender assignment and unambivalent child rearing by parents (see Sec. 24.4.8). Gender roles and behavior, however, may be influenced by this early alteration in hormonal environments. Early exposure to androgenizing hormones results in more masculine play preferences, patterns, and playmates with emotional and cognitive processes skewed in the masculine direction for this group. Girls with congenital adrenal hyperplasia raised as girls, although most commonly oriented toward males, have a high rate of homosexual, bisexual, and ambivalent orientations. Conversely, prenatal exposure to nonandrogenizing progesterones results in girls who generally have a more "feminized" behavior, although the differences in similarly exposed boys are less clear.

Girls with Turner syndrome (XO) consistently develop an unequivocal female gender identity, engage in typically feminine interests and activities, and have a heterosexual sexual orientation. Cognitive difficulties in spatial processing, issues of short stature, and confronting infertility are issues facing this group. Youngsters with androgen insensitivity syndrome are genotypically male but are phenotypically female. They develop very traditional female behavioral patterns and maintain a strong female gender identity even if some masculinization occurs at puberty, as occurs in a small subpopulation. The behavioral profiles of individuals are dominated by developmental delays. Sexual development shows no systematic irregularities in these cases. In fact, the vast majority of patients with any type of gender ambiguity are heterosexual based on the sex of rearing. The only exception may be those with 5-alpha-reductase deficiency. Born as genetic males, their genitalia appear female at birth. At puberty, virilization occurs. In at least some of these individuals, there is an apparent switch to a masculine identity at this time.

These observations suggest that there is considerable genetic and prenatal influence on the development of our sexual selves. This body of information is increasing. However, the social, family, and personal environments of rearing also have considerable influence on how these differences evolve.

References

Alan Guttmacher Institute: Sex and America's Teenagers. New York, Alan Guttmacher Institute, 1994

American Academy of Pediatrics: The Classification of Child and Adolescent Mental Disorders in Primary Care (DSM-PC). Elk Grove Village, IL AAP, 1996

Bradley SJ, Zucker KL: Gender identity disorder: a review of the past 10 years. J Am Acad Child Adolesc Psychiatr 36(7):872–880, 1997

Chan RW, Raboy B, Patterson CJ: Psychosocial adjustment among children conceived via donor insemination by lesbian and heterosexual mothers. Child Devel 69(2):443–457, 1998

Friedrich WN, Grambsch P, Broughton D, Kuiper J, Beilke RL: Normative sexual behavior in children. Pediatrics 88:456–464, 1991

Gold MA, Perrin EC, Futterman D, Friedman SB: Children of gay or lesbian parents. Pediatr Rev 15:354–358, 1994

Golombok S, Fivush R: Gender Development. Cambridge, Cambridge University Press, 1994

Heiman MI, Leiblum S, Cohen Esquilin S, Menendez Palletto L: A comparative survey of beliefs about "normal" childhood sexual behaviors. Child Abuse Negl 22(4):289–304, 1998

Leung AKC, Robson WLM: Childhood masturbation. Clin Pediatr (April): 238–241, 1993

Marcus IM, Francis JJ, eds: Masturbation: From Infancy to Senescence. New York: International Universities Press, 1975

McCauley E: Disorders of sexual differentiation and development. Curr Iss Pediatr Adoles Endocrinol 37(6):1405–1420, 1990

Money J, Ehrhardt AA: Man and Woman, Boy and Girl: The Differentiation and Dimorphism of Gender Identity from Conception to Maturity. Baltimore, MD, Johns Hopkins University Press, 1972

Patterson CJ: Children of lesbian and gay parents. Child Devel 63:1025–1042, 1992

Remafedi G: Adolescent homosexuality: psychosocial and medical implications. Pediatrics 79:331–337, 1987

Ryan GD, Lane SL, eds: Juvenile Sexual Offending: Causes, Consequences and Correction. Lexington, MA: Lexington Books, 1991

Stronski Huwiler SM, Remafedi G: Adolescent homosexuality. Adv Pediatr 45:107–144, 1998

Tasker F, Golombok S: Adults raised as children in lesbian families. Am J Orthopsychiatry 65(2):203–215, 1995

Weinraub M, Clemens LP, Sockloff A, Ethridge T, Gracely E, Myers B: The development of sex role stereotypes in the third year: relationships to gender labeling, gender identity, sex-typed toy preferences, and family characteristics. Child Devel 55:1493–1503, 1984

Zucker KJ, Bradley SJ, Lowry Sullivan CB, Kuksis M, Berkenfeld-Adams A, Mitchell JN: A gender identity interview for children. J Pers Assess 61(3):443–456, 1993

Zucker KJ, Green R: Psychosexual disorders in children and adolescents. J Child Psychol Psychiatry 33:107–151, 1992

5.6.11 Weight Gain: Overeating to Obesity

Thomas N. Robinson and William H. Dietz

DEFINITION AND EPIDEMIOLOGY

Obesity results from an interaction of genetic, environmental, developmental, and behavioral processes, and reflects a broad continuum from normal variation to a pathologic condition. This is clearly demonstrated by the limited usefulness of available definitions. During childhood and adolescence, obesity is most commonly defined as weight greater than 120% of the median weight for height, or a triceps skinfold thickness or body mass index (ie, weight/height^2) greater than the 85th or 95th percentile for children of the same age and sex. However, these standards are limited by the representativeness of the samples from which they are derived. Until recently, available reference samples generally have not reflected sufficient racial, cultural, or socioeconomic diversity. The newly revised growth standards from the National Center for Health Statistics now include nationally representative samples of whites, African-Americans, and Mexican Americans, but not large numbers of children or adolescents from other racial and/or ethnic groups. Nevertheless, the greatest limitation of threshold definitions of obesity is lack of evidence for their clinical validity. Although recent data suggest that more than half of children who meet traditional definitions of obesity show evidence of associated physiological morbidities, few data confirm that children and adolescents who are "above" one or more of the previously mentioned definitions, are much worse off from a clinical standpoint than those who fall just below the cutoff points. Instead, body fatness is related to morbidity in a continuous, up-sloping, curvilinear manner, without the thresholds suggested by the common cutoff definitions.

For epidemiologic purposes, conventional definitions may provide useful information on trends in the population and differences among various groups. Data from the most recent national surveys demonstrated that the prevalence of obesity among children and adolescents has more than doubled from the 1970s to the early 1990s. The increases appear to have occurred across all ethnic groups, although the highest rates are among Mexican American boys and girls and African-American adolescent girls. More detailed analysis of the trends in being overweight has demonstrated the worrisome finding that most of the increase has occurred in the upper extremes of the distribution, resulting in larger numbers of extremely overweight children and adolescents, those who are most likely to suffer from obesity-associated morbidities.

By far, the strongest risk factor for obesity in children and adolescents is having an obese parent. Whether it is the mother or the father makes little difference; as expected, having two obese parents is a greater risk factor than having only one obese parent. Parent weight status also strongly influences the likelihood of a child becoming an obese adult. In one retrospective cohort study, for example, 3- to 5-year-olds were 3 times more likely to be overweight in their twenties if they had one overweight parent and about 15 times more likely if both parents were overweight. As children age, the child's weight becomes a better predictor of adult obesity than parent weight. In the same study, overweight 10- to 14-year-olds were about 20 times more likely to be overweight in their twenties than their normal-weight peers, while having at least one overweight parent at age 10 to 14 years doubled the risk of obesity in young adulthood.

ETIOLOGY AND PATHOGENESIS

Obesity results from an energy imbalance. Experimental evidence shows that obesity develops when energy intake exceeds energy expenditure, and weight is lost when energy expenditure exceeds energy intake. Nevertheless, controversies remain over the specific mechanisms that lead to this imbalance. Obese children do not appear to have lower metabolic rates or lower energy expenditures than nonobese children. Obese children do tend to underestimate their food intake and overestimate their physical activity compared to nonobese children, although data are inconsistent on whether obese children actually consume more calories (ie, eat more) than their nonobese peers. However, methods used to measure energy intake and expenditure have limited accuracy. Extremely small energy discrepancies can lead to large changes in body weight over time. For example, one extra 12-ounce can of regular soda per day is the caloric equivalent of about 15 pounds of excess weight gain over the course of a year.

The genetic contribution to obesity is receiving increased attention. Some data have even been interpreted to suggest that heredity explains nearly all obesity. However, a careful look at the evidence suggests that the role of genes in the etiology of obesity is more complex. Many candidate obesity genes have been identified in rodents. However, most linkage studies have yet to offer strong evidence of a role in human obesity, and the human mutations that have been identified to date are unlikely responsible for the most common forms of obesity. Although body fatness is correlated in families, the strength of these correlations is much greater in the normal weight range than among the obese. This and other methodologic factors may account for exaggerated estimates of the genetic contribution to obesity in twin studies. Some of the most informative evidence comes from experimental energy balance manipulations among adult twin pairs. These studies confirm a significant hereditary component to changes in body composition. However, even in controlled experimental settings, heredity accounts for a maximum of only about 25% of the variation in weight (and fat) gain and loss. As a result, 75% or more is left to be explained by nongenetic influences. Heredity appears to play its primary role in the susceptibility to obesity, but environmental and behavioral influences determine how genetic susceptibility is expressed.

The timing of weight gain also may play a role in the onset and persistence of obesity. At least three critical periods occur during childhood when the onset of obesity is more likely to persist into adulthood. These include the prenatal period, the period of normal adiposity rebound (ie, about 5 to 7 years of age), and the early adolescent years associated with puberty. All three periods are characterized by normal changes in the growth and distribution of adipose tissue. Overnutrition (ie, more calorie consumption than calorie expenditure) during any of these periods may entrain an obese physiology. Thus, preventive interventions may be more successful if they specifically target these periods.

CLINICAL MANIFESTATIONS

In addition to advanced height, growth, and sexual maturation, obesity in childhood and adolescence is associated with a number of other clinical manifestations (Table 5-24). These problems are more common at the upper extremes of obesity, and most are

TABLE 5-24

CLINICAL MANIFESTATIONS OF OBESITY IN CHILDREN AND ADOLESCENTS

Cardiovascular
  Hypertension
  Hypercholesterolemia
  ↑ Triglycerides
  ↑ Low-density lipoproteins (LDL)
  ↑ Very-low-density lipoproteins (VLDL)
  ↓ High-density lipoproteins (HDL)
Pulmonary
  Obstructive sleep apnea
  Primary alveolar hypoventilation
Endocrine
  Hyperinsulinemia and insulin resistance
  Early menarche
  ↑ Estradiol and estrone
  Oligospermia
Musculoskeletal
  Slipped capital femoral epiphysis
  Blount disease
Gastrointestinal
  Cholelithiasis
  Hepatic steatosis
Neurologic
  Pseudotumor cerebri
Dermatologic
  Acanthosis nigricans
Immunologic
  Impaired cell-mediated immunity

found in a minority of obese children and adolescents. The more common obesity-associated problems (ie, dyslipidemias, hyperinsulinemia), however, are found in more than half of overweight children and adolescents. In addition, the results of several longitudinal studies suggest that overweight children and adolescents may have increased risks of morbidity and mortality in adulthood regardless of their adult weight status. The greatest risks are associated with persistence of obesity into adulthood or adult-onset obesity. Among obese adults, the clinical manifestations become more prevalent and serious. In addition to the problems noted in Table 5-24, obese adults are at increased risk of overall mortality and death from cardiovascular diseases, cancer, diabetes, and digestive diseases. They also are more likely to suffer from osteoarthritis and have complications of pregnancy. Recent studies suggest that the economic costs of obesity in the United States approach $100 billion per year.

While the physical complications of obesity pose significant problems to a minority of overweight children and adolescents, the psychological and social consequences may be much more common. In several studies during the 1960s, diverse samples of children and adults associated negative stereotypes with representations of obese children and ranked them as less likable than representations of children with physical disabilities. Obesity has been associated with lower college acceptance rates, lower desirability to employers, prospective attainment of lower social class, and increased risk for body dissatisfaction and binge eating and purging behaviors among adolescent girls. However, some studies have shown that children's actual rating of liking and disliking are unrelated to the weight status of their peers, and obese children do not score consistently lower than normal-weight peers on formal assessments of social and emotional functioning. Similarly, although low self-esteem and more depressive symptoms have been documented in some clinical samples of obese children, this has not been the case in population-based, nonclinical samples.

ASSESSMENT AND DIAGNOSIS

The goal of the initial clinical evaluation should be:

- To assess the extent of overweightness;
- To identify existing associated morbidity;
- To assess the level of associated risk;
- To identify important family or environmental factors;
- To rule out the rare endocrinologic and genetic disorders that an associated with obesity; and
- To design a treatment plan.

An approach to assessing obesity in children is shown in Fig. 5-3. Rare congenital and endocrinologic disorders that may be associated with obesity include Alström syndrome; Carpenter syndrome; Cohen syndrome; Cushing syndrome; growth hormone deficiency; hyperinsulinemia (eg, pancreatic tumor, pancreatic beta-cell hypersecretion, hypothalamic lesion); hypothyroidism; Laurence-Moon (Bardet-Biedl) syndrome; polycystic ovary (Stein-Leventhal) syndrome; Prader-Willi syndrome; pseudohypoparathyroidism; and Turner syndrome. With the exception of hyperinsulinemia, all of these disorders generally are associated with short stature; delayed growth and sexual maturation; developmental delay or mental retardation; and other distinct functional, morphologic, or physiological abnormalities. In contrast, "primary" obesity generally is associated with advanced height, growth, and sexual maturation. Thus, genetic and endocrinologic disorders with as-

sociated obesity, which account for less than 1% of obesity among children and adolescents, usually can be ruled out based on a careful history and physical examination.

Initial assessment of an overweight child should include a history of linear growth as well as weight, age at onset of obesity, pubertal history (if applicable), and detailed diet and physical activity histories. An informal diet and activity history, reviewing the intake of total and saturated fat and calorically dense foods on a typical day, also may be sufficient. A careful review should seek symptoms associated with the congenital and endocrinologic "causes" and complications listed in Table 5-24 such as headaches; visual changes; menstrual history (if applicable); polydipsia; polyuria; nocturia; lower extremity pain; daytime somnolence; snoring; or abdominal discomfort, as well as an assessment of depressive symptoms and disordered eating attitudes and behaviors. A family history should include questions about obesity, diabetes, hypertension, hyperlipidemias, cerebrovascular disease, coronary heart disease, and gallbladder disease. The parents' and child's opinions regarding the cause, as well as impact of the problem, should be explored in detail, with particular attention paid to lack of consensus among parents and children, impact on other family members, assignments of blame, denial, and expectations for weight loss.

A full physical examination is indicated, with emphasis on findings associated with obesity and symptoms identified by the history (eg, if headaches are present, a funduscopic and neurologic exam should be performed), as well as dysmorphic features; acanthosis nigricans; hirsutism; violaceous striae; abdominal tenderness; undescended testes; limited hip range of motion; and lower leg bowing. If height is greater than or equal to the 50th percentile for age and the history and physical examination are not suggestive, endocrinologic and congenital causes can essentially be ruled out. Every patient should have blood pressure measured.

A fasting insulin and lipid profile are recommended to detect the more common obesity-associated morbidities and to monitor during treatment. Otherwise, laboratory assessments are rarely useful unless they are specifically indicated based on findings from the history and/or examination. Thyroid function tests or a bone age may be helpful only to reassure children or parents who are convinced of the "glandular" nature of the obesity, but these are not necessary for a child with normal linear growth. If daytime somnolence or snoring are reported, further workup may include pulmonary function tests, arterial blood gases, sleep study, and otolaryngology evaluation. Complaints of lower extremity pain or bowing should be evaluated with appropriate radiologic studies and an orthopedic evaluation. Right-upper-quadrant abdominal discomfort and/or suggestive findings on physical examination should be followed up with ultrasound evaluation for cholelithiasis.

Body mass index (BMI), which is defined as weight in kilograms divided by the square of the height in meters (kg/m^2), is recommended as the primary method for assessing obesity in children and adolescents. Recent national standards by age and sex are now available along with the height and weight growth charts from the National Center for Health Statistics. The 95th percentile has been recommended as the most appropriate cut-off for the clinical definition of obesity. The 95th percentile identifies children who are at a substantial risk for obesity-associated morbidities and likely to become obese adults. Children with a BMI between the 85th and the 95th percentile are defined as overweight, and should also be evaluated thoroughly for obesity-associated complications. In the U.S. population, the 85th and 95th percentiles in children also correspond to adult BMI's of 25 and 30, respectively, the accepted

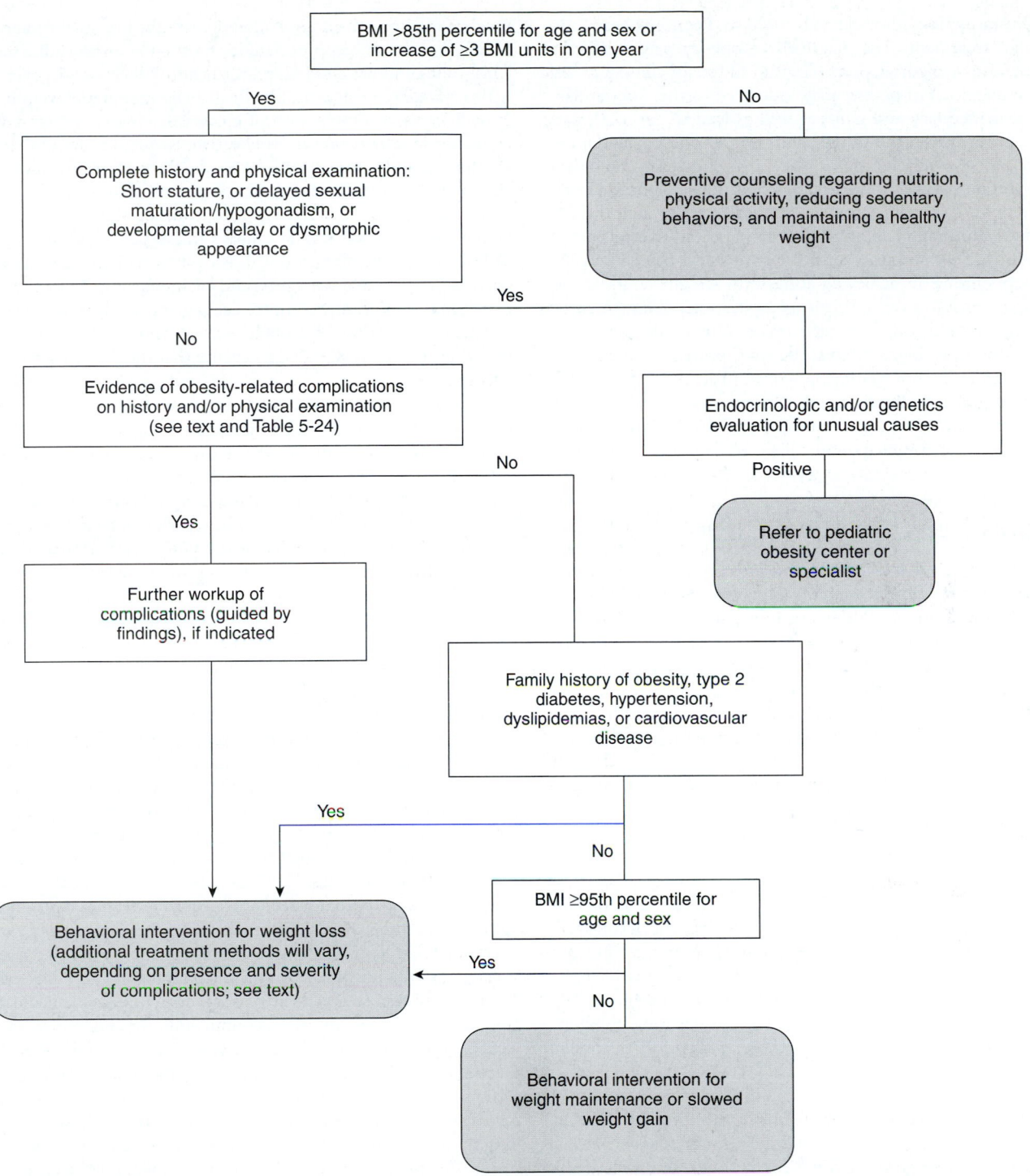

*Children under the age of 7 years requiring weight loss should be evaluated and treated under the supervision of a pediatric obesity center or specialist.

FIGURE 5-3   Algorithm for the evaluation and management of obesity in children ≥ 7 years of age* (see text for details).

definitions of adult overweightness and obesity. Clinicians who are practiced at using skinfold calipers may also wish to measure a triceps skinfold thickness. The triceps skinfold thickness and BMI are about equally predictive of associated morbidity. The BMI tracks better into later adolescence and adulthood, however, and is easier and more reliable because it depends only on accurate measures of

height and weight. Children and adolescents with increased frame size and well-developed musculature may be overweight for height without being overfat. Skinfolds are most helpful in distinguishing the overfat from the overmuscled child. However, reliable skinfold thickness measurement is difficult and therefore less appropriate for the general clinical setting.

Weight status alone should not be used to diagnose obesity and recommend treatment. The diagnosis of obesity may itself have significant adverse medical, psychological, and social consequences. A medical diagnosis of obesity may induce or further substantiate feelings of inadequacy and guilt, as well as lead to "special treatment" by parents. On the other hand, not all obese children experience adverse psychological or social consequences, and only a minority sustain significant medical complications. Clinical samples tend to differ considerably from nonclinical samples, and there is evidence for ethnic and cultural variations in perceived ideal weight and body shape. In addition, available treatments have been relatively disappointing in achieving long-term weight control, and treatments themselves can result in complications. Consequently, the clinician should judge the appropriateness of diagnosis and treatment on a case-by-case basis, focusing primarily on children and adolescents demonstrating physical (Table 5-24) or psychosocial complications, those at highest risk of developing obesity-related morbidity, and those patients and families who are most highly motivated and most likely to be successful in treatment.

MANAGEMENT AND TREATMENT

Some treatments involving children and adolescents have produced substantial short-term improvements in percent overweight, blood pressure, and lipid profiles. However, longer-term effects of treatment generally have been disappointing. The most successful interventions have been family based and behaviorally oriented. Such treatments include parents in the treatment process, usually as a target of treatment along with the child; a diet program that promotes adherence and provides sufficient nutrition for growth; modification of the child's food environment at home and in school; a physical activity program emphasizing life-style activities instead of a specific exercise regimen; specific strategies to reduce sedentary time; behavior modification techniques, including self-monitoring of diet and activity behaviors; identification of potential barriers and problem-solving; cognitive restructuring techniques to help the child cope with difficult situations, stressful times, and dietary lapses; parental skills training and role modeling; and a contracting and reward system emphasizing positive reinforcement for both proximal and distal goals. State-of-the-art programs incorporating these elements in research settings have produced 10-year success in up to about one-third of participating children. These are much better results than those from adult treatment programs.

Perhaps the most important factor in weight control treatment is the readiness of the child and the family. Although the clinician participates in treatment, the family has the primary role. A clinician can provide the requisite knowledge and methods, but until a family is ready to change, the necessary changes will not occur. Therefore, when there is a lack of agreement between parent and child, or between two parents, it is appropriate to defer treatment until a consensus is reached. In some cases, participation of a family therapist may facilitate treatment. Although family therapy–based interventions for obesity have yet to be proven effective, a child's weight problem is often a focus of family conflict within treatment-seeking families. Consequently, changes made as part of a treatment program may substantially alter family dynamics.

In children without complications of obesity that require immediate weight reduction, the initial goal of treatment should be to maintain weight or to slow the rate of gain. Once weight maintenance is achieved, progression to a weight loss goal of about 1 pound per month is appropriate for most children and adolescents. This strategy allows children to "grow into" their weight over time without risking adverse health effects from more rapid weight loss. In such cases, a combination of increased activity levels and moderate calorie restriction can be effective. Reductions in total dietary fat content and calorically dense foods, through substitutions and eliminations alone, can produce a sufficient caloric deficit without changing the general pattern of food consumption for the child or family. Diets that are low in calories and fats and high in complex carbohydrates and fiber are not associated with complications in older children and adolescents, and such diets lead to loss of body fat without significantly compromising growth in height. However, frequent monitoring of growth and intermittent assessment by a nutritionist is recommended to ensure that the diet is nutritionally adequate.

Sedentary behavior, and television viewing in particular, has received much attention as an etiologic factor for obesity. Recent experimental studies suggest that reducing television viewing, and videotape and video game use, may be an effective strategy for primary prevention of obesity and for weight control among obese children. When obese children are heavy television viewers, reduced viewing time may result in increased activity levels, decreased eating in front of the TV, and decreased exposure to high-fat, high-calorie food advertising.

Children with more severe obesity or significant associated complications (eg, pickwickian syndrome, imminent slipped capital femoral epiphysis, noninsulin-dependent diabetes mellitus, pseudotumor cerebri) demand more restrictive dietary interventions because of the immediacy of their problems. For these patients, very-low-calorie diets, also known as protein-modified fasts, may be indicated. The goal of the protein-modified fast is to maximize loss of fat while minimizing loss of protein. These diets generally provide from 800 to 1000 Kcal/d of energy and from 2.0 to 2.5 g of protein per kg ideal body weight per day. Such patients require vitamin and mineral supplements, particularly potassium and calcium, and sufficient fluids. These diets tend to produce mean weight losses of approximately 3.0 kg during the first week and 1.0 kg per week thereafter, with broad variation. They should not be recommended for patients with renal, hepatic, or cardiac disease. Inadequately supervised, commercially available, very-low-calorie diets have been associated with cardiac arrhythmias, cardiac arrests, and death, and they are not recommended for children or adolescents. Even when properly supervised, very-low-calorie diets have been associated with hair loss, thinning of the skin, cold intolerance, orthostatic hypotension, and arrhythmias. Patients treated with such diets require close, frequent follow-up by physicians thoroughly trained in clinical nutrition and experienced in the use of these therapies. Therefore, most clinicians will refer such patients to a specialized childhood obesity treatment program.

Current pharmacologic therapies should be reserved for use in children or adolescents who have failed behavioral and nutritional treatments and who are participating in monitored clinical trials. The results of pharmacologic treatment studies in obese adults suggest that weight gain generally returns after medication use is discontinued. This suggests that pharmacologic treatments may eventually need to be used for long-term treatment. As a result, long-term safety and efficacy should be established before they are routinely used in children and adolescents. Similarly, surgical treatments, gastroplasty and gastric bypass, are occasionally being used in the adolescent age group as an extension of their use in adults, although clinical trials are needed to assess the safety and efficacy of these approaches in adolescents.

NATURAL HISTORY AND PROGNOSIS

Long-term effects of weight control treatments have been somewhat disappointing. After an initial rapid weight loss, most subjects gradually regain their original excess fat. The best results suggest that average weight losses of 5 to 10% in relative weight may be maintained at up to 10 years after treatment, which leaves the majority of patients obese. These results are further limited by the recognition that subjects and families who volunteer for treatment studies may not represent the average obese patient or family. Population-based natural history studies have found that less than 50% of obese preadolescents but about 75% of obese adolescents go on to be obese adults. In addition, not all obese children and adolescents suffer from obesity-associated physical morbidities.

A number of factors associated with increased risk of adiposity or morbidity in adulthood have been identified. Because of a combination of genetic, environmental, and behavioral influences, obesity clusters strongly in families, and the presence of obese parents or siblings is a strong risk factor. Similarly, a family history of potential comorbidities such as hypertension, diabetes, or coronary heart disease may be helpful in predicting greater risk for an individual child. Tracking studies demonstrate that both the absolute severity of obesity and the age of the child are predictors of future obesity; the more overweight and the older the overweight child, the more likely that the child will be an obese adult. Several researchers have also noted an association between adult adiposity and timing of the normal second rise in body fat, usually occurring around 6 years of age. An early "adiposity rebound," assessed by plotting serial BMI or triceps skinfold thickness measures, and usually defined as younger than 5.5 years of age, is a better predictor of adult obesity than childhood weight status alone. Finally, a relative predominance of truncal or abdominal fat, as indicated by an increased ratio of waist circumference to hip circumference, has been associated with increased obesity-associated morbidity among adolescents. However, the clinical utility of this measure among prepubertal children is questionable. The presence or absence of these factors may help the clinician to decide on the appropriate intensity of intervention to recommend.

References

Barlow SE, Dietz WH: Obesity evaluation and treatment: expert committee recommendations. Pediatrics 102(3):e29, 1998 (http://www.pediatrics.org/cgi/content/full/102/3/e29)

Dietz WH: Health consequences of obesity in youth: childhood predictors of adult disease. Pediatrics 101:518–525, 1998

Dietz WH: Critical periods in childhood for the development of obesity. Am J Clin Nutr 59:955–959, 1994

Epstein LH: New developments in childhood obesity. In: Stunkard AJ, Wadden TA, eds: Obesity: Theory and Therapy, 2nd ed. New York, Raven, 1993:301–312

Epstein LH, Valoski A, Wing RR, McCurley J: Ten-year outcomes of behavioral, family-based treatment for childhood obesity. Health Psychol 13:373–383, 1994

Robinson TN: Defining obesity in children and adolescents: clinical approaches. Crit Rev Food Sci Nutr 33:313–320, 1993

Robinson TN: Behavioural treatment of childhood and adolescent obesity. Int J Obesity 23(Suppl 2)S52–S57, 1999

Troiano RP, Flegal KM: Overweight children and adolescents: description, epidemiology, and demographics. Pediatrics 101:497–504, 1998

Wadden TA, Stunkard AJ: Social and psychological consequences of obesity. Ann Intern Med 103:1062–1067, 1985

5.6.12   Coordination Problems: Clumsiness to Major Motor Disorders

Janice Prontnicki and Lawrence Taft

The normal development of both fine and gross motor coordination involves interplay among multiple components of the neuromuscular system. The positional feedback loop enters the dorsal horn cells to give position sense, the cortex determines the adjustments needed for the desired movement, and a message is sent down through the pyramidal tracts to the spinal cord, out the anterior horn cells, and through the peripheral nerves and neuromuscular junction to the muscle. Any complex movement such as walking or riding a bicycle requires such continuous feedback and fine-tuning adjustments. The more well-developed the system, the more smoothly these movements are executed. A problem in any portion of the loop, be it neurosensory, neurostimulatory, or located in a peripheral nerve or muscle, will have an adverse impact on motor performance.

The age at which common motor milestones are achieved can vary greatly. For example, while 25% of children are able to walk by 11 months of age, 10% of normal children have not yet done so by 15 months of age. Similarly, the ability to scribble with a crayon will be present in approximately 50% of infants by 13 months of age but not yet developed in 10% by 17 months of age. There is a certain point, however, beyond which motor development may be considered to be delayed or pathologic.

Parental reporting or actual observation of attained developmental milestones offers the examiner insight into motor maturation. If a delay is suspected, a formal neurologic examination is necessary. Such an examination includes the classic deep-tendon reflexes and also determines the presence or absence of both primitive and postural reflexes (Table 5-25). Primitive reflexes (eg, Moro, asymptomatic tonic neck) are brainstem-mediated movement patterns that are normally present from birth or shortly thereafter, and many have their origins in fetal life. As these primitive

TABLE 5-25

SELECTED PRIMITIVE AND POSTURAL REFLEXES: AVERAGE AGE OF EMERGENCE AND INTEGRATION

REFLEX	EMERGES	INTEGRATED
Sucking	28 wks' gestation	4 mo
Moro	30 wks' gestation	5 mo
ATNR	26 wks' gestation	9 mo
Galant	30 wks' gestation	6 mo
Stepping	Birth	2 mo
Landau	3 mo	15 mo
Protective extension:		
Forward	6 mo	Persists
Sideways	7 mo	Persists
Backward	9 mo	Persists
Tilting reaction (standing)	12 mo	Persists

ATNR = Asymmetric tonic neck reflex

reflexes come under more voluntary control, they gradually fade during the latter part of the first year, but may persist in children with abnormalities of motor development. Concurrently, the more functional postural reflexes (eg, protective extension responses) are integrated as cortical control of volitional motor movements emerges.

The classic neurologic examination also evaluates the child's muscle tone (ie, resistance of the muscles or joints to passive movement when the child is at rest). Tone can be increased (hypertonia) or decreased (hypotonia). Abnormalities in this area affect posture and may inhibit normal movements.

Much information can also be obtained by careful observation of the quality of a child's movements. For example, the school-aged child may be able to draw a human figure with the expected number of parts for age, but the child may hold the crayon with a clumsy, tight-fisted grasp, like that of a younger child. Another example is the 6-year-old child who can balance on each foot for more than 5 seconds but requires an extraordinary amount of concentration, and who demonstrates motor overflow such as tongue protrusion while the arms are held in exaggerated or dystonic posture. In each of these examples, there may be no "hard" neurologic findings (eg, changes in tone, strength, or reflexes), and both children may have reached all of their developmental milestones on schedule. Such findings are considered to be subtle indicators of neuromaturational delays (ie, "soft signs").

DEFINITION AND EPIDEMIOLOGY

A centrally based motor deficit implies a lesion affecting the cortical motor tracts rather than the peripheral nerves or muscles. In such circumstances, muscle atrophy is rare or appears later as a secondary response to decreased use. Involuntary movements such as ataxia, athetosis, dystonia, or chorea may be present. The hallmark of a static encephalopathy is the absence of regression (or loss of skills) despite slow development. Children with static encephalopathic motor impairments range in their degree of functional involvement from mild clumsiness to an inability to sit and/or walk (Sec. 25.5).

Clumsy child is a phrase that has been in use for approximately 25 years. It describes a child whose fine and/or gross motor skills are qualitatively like those of a younger child. Movements may be described as slow, disorganized, or careless. The frequency of such a coordination disorder is estimated at 6 to 7% of school-aged children. Another term in use is *developmental coordination disorder* (DCD). In the *Diagnostic and Statistical Manual, 4th Edition* (*DSM-IV*), this is defined as "performance in daily activities that require motor coordination substantially below that expected given the person's chronological age and measured intelligence, . . . clumsiness." Furthermore, these coordination difficulties must interfere with the child's academic achievement or activities of daily living and not be the result of a general medical condition or pervasive developmental disorder.

Cerebral palsy is a disorder of movement and/or posture caused by a static encephalopathy. It is found in children whose disability is more clinically obvious than that of the clumsy child. By definition, cerebral palsy is a nonprogressive, central disorder. The incidence of cerebral palsy is estimated to be from 1 to 2 cases per 1000 live births. This includes children with all subtypes and a variety of degrees of cerebral palsy.

ETIOLOGY AND PATHOGENESIS

The etiology of clumsiness has not been clearly delineated. A majority of cases are believed secondary to heredity, subtle brain injury,

or a combination of the two. The poor coordination is believed to represent a mild type of cerebral dysfunction related to dyspraxia, sensory feedback deficits, or sensory-motor integration difficulties.

Dyspraxia is a condition in which voluntary movements are performed in an irregular or inconsistent manner despite normal sensorimotor pathways. It is characterized by difficulty in motor planning and learning complex motor tasks because of premotor cortical dysfunction.

Clumsiness also may result from a sensory feedback deficiency. An example is the 12-year-old child who cannot do rapid alternating finger movements (ie, touching the thumb to each other finger in succession) without holding the hand in front of his or her face. Normally, children at this age can execute such movements without visual input simply based on proprioception (ie, knowing where their fingers are in space).

Cerebral palsy results from a brain injury or malformation, which may have occurred prenatally, perinatally, or during early childhood before brain maturation was complete. Prenatal causes include maternal infections, toxic exposures, chromosomal abnormalities, or hypoxic-ischemic encephalopathy secondary to placental insufficiency. Children with congenital abnormalities of the brain and who experience an adverse fetal environment appear to be especially susceptible to hypoxic-ischemic insults to the brain during labor. Premature infants are especially susceptible to hemorrhage into the area of the pyramidal tract fibers controlling the lower extremities. After birth, meningoencephalitis, head trauma, toxic exposure, and cardiac arrest are factors that can result in cerebral palsy. In many cases, however, there is no clear etiology. While the risk of cerebral palsy increases with younger gestational age, most affected children were born at full term.

CLINICAL MANIFESTATIONS

Because the "clumsy child syndrome" represents a subtle motor problem, the diagnosis often is not made earlier than school age, if at all. Frequently, the child is first aware of his or her own motor difficulties. Such children tend to shy away from competitive sports and avoid physical competition with peers. This behavior may be a source of concern for the parents, who then bring it to the attention of the pediatrician. Often, preschool teachers will comment on difficulties the child is having in coloring within the lines, learning to use scissors, or buttoning. Such difficulties are often detected on a kindergarten readiness screen. In more subtle cases, clumsiness may not be detected until the child enters the older grades and concerns emerge about handwriting.

The importance of relatively minor motor impairments is not insignificant. Such children frequently sustain blows to self-esteem because of their poor athletic skills. For both boys and girls in the younger grades, physical abilities on and off the playground are especially important. For teenage boys, organized sports seem to be a rite of passage, and one from which the clumsy child is often excluded. This exclusion can be especially handicapping for children who also have a learning difficulty. In such cases, excelling at sports could have been one means of achieving the respect from peers that is not being obtained within the classroom.

The identification of clumsiness also may be important in signaling the need for further developmental investigation. For example, clumsiness has been considered one of the "soft" neurologic findings that are seen with increased frequency in children who have other cerebral dysfunctions such as learning disabilities or attention-deficit hyperactivity disorder (ADHD). Indeed the association of a DCD with learning problems and ADHD is considered so frequent that the Scandinavian literature has introduced the terminology DAMP (Deficits in Attention, Motor Control, and Perception). Boys are more often affected with DAMP than girls. There is considerable overlap between ADHD and DCD, with about half of each diagnostic group also meeting criteria for the other diagnosis. The sooner such difficulties are detected, the sooner specific therapies and educational interventions can be instituted.

Another difficulty associated with clumsiness relates to family dynamics. In some cases, parents resent their children's slow and inconsistent abilities, and they may criticize these children for taking so long to finish tasks such as tying their shoes. When parents tire of waiting and dress the child themselves, this can lead to overdependence, foster immature behavior, and limit the child's opportunities to practice and eventually master the tasks in question.

The signs of cerebral palsy result from a lack of inhibition from the brain to the lower CNS. Because of this diminished inhibition, there is a persistence of primitive (ie, brainstem) reflexes beyond the normal duration. In affected infants, exaggerated extensor posturing secondary to an abnormal tonic labyrinthine reflex frequently is perceived by the parent as "stiffness" or "resistance" to snuggling. This misperception can lead to difficulties in parent–child interaction.

As the cerebral hemispheres also are responsible for the coordination of more complex motor tasks, infants suffering from cerebral palsy may have problems with sucking and swallowing as well as overflow drooling, which makes the feeding process less pleasant for both the parent and child. Other motor skills also are delayed, and frequently abnormal, in their achievement. For example, infants with hemiplegia crawl asymmetrically. Children with diplegia crawl by using their arms in a reciprocal manner while pulling their lower body behind. If or when the child with cerebral palsy learns to walk, increased tone (ie, tightness) of the involved muscles frequently results in an abnormal pattern characterized by toe walking, a crouched gait, "scissoring," and exaggerated use of the upper extremities for balance.

ASSESSMENT AND DIAGNOSIS

To make the diagnosis of clumsy child, parent reports and teacher observations are essential. Developmental milestones usually are achieved within the normal time frame, although often at a later end. The classic neurologic examination is normal except for occasional mild hypotonia. In the examining room, the diagnosis generally is supported by functional testing (ie, the child is observed while performing age-appropriate motor activities and the skillfulness of the movements compared with the fluency expected for that age). Watching a school-age child write or dress provides a good indication of fine-motor abilities. Regarding gross motor skills, the clumsy child will skip and run in an uncoordinated, inconsistent manner. In younger children, articulation difficulties, persistent drooling, and feeding problems signal oral-motor dyspraxia.

In children with cerebral palsy, motor developmental milestones are usually delayed. The classic neurologic examination reveals abnormalities of tone and reflexes, and a functional assessment reveals the extent of impairment.

Cerebral palsy is frequently classified by the predominant neurologic sign. The most common type, spastic cerebral palsy, is characterized by increased muscle tone with exaggerated deep tendon reflexes. Other, less common types include choreoathetoid, ataxic, dystonic, hypotonic, and mixed forms (see Sec. 25.5). An approach to assessment of the child with impaired motor skills is shown in Fig. 5-4.

MANAGEMENT AND TREATMENT

After the diagnosis of clumsy child is made, the first step in treatment is to explain the coordination to the child and family—a process known as *demystification*. The child needs to know that this is not an uncommon condition so that the child does not feel very different from peers. On the other hand, the problem cannot be minimized, because the child is likely to be painfully aware of the difference between him- or herself and others. Clumsy children can be told that with time and maturity, their coordination will improve. However, they should not be told that they will catch up completely; clumsy children frequently grow up to be clumsy adults.

Clumsy children should be encouraged to participate in any activity, including sports, that they enjoy, no matter how good (or poor) they are at it. However, there are certain sports in which the clumsy child appears to be less handicapped than others, including swimming, soccer, karate, and horseback riding. In all cases, it is important that children not be pushed beyond their abilities, which only leads to more frustration and to loss of self-esteem. Furthermore, parents must understand that while it may be necessary to assist their child more, they should not limit the child's opportunities to practice these tasks. For example, although Velcro may be best for the early morning rush to school, a child who has difficulty tying shoelaces should be allowed to practice tying shoelaces when there are no time constraints. The teacher also should be made aware of the child's difficulties. Interventions such as allowing a student to hand in typed or taped reports rather than handwritten papers will lead to rewards for creative talent rather than criticism for poor penmanship.

For the more affected clumsy child, occupational therapy (using sensory integration and/or sensory motor techniques) may be helpful. Speech and language therapy may improve the child's oral-motor abilities, and adaptive physical education, which is more individualized and less competitive than the typical gym class, may be appropriate. However, enrollment in any such programs must be weighed carefully, because children often feel stigmatized by such special treatment.

The comprehensive care of a child with cerebral palsy requires an interdisciplinary team of physicians, nurses, and therapists. For the child who is identified before 3 years of age, such services should be provided through an early intervention program. For older children, therapies are provided through the local school system.

Traditionally, physical therapy concentrates on the gross motor areas of development and seeks to improve posture, tone, and functional ability, whereas occupational therapy involves a task-oriented, sensory-motor integrational approach to fine-motor difficulties. In the context of a comprehensive intervention program, therapists educate the family about cerebral palsy and its complications as well as help the family learn how to care for the child's special needs. For example, a therapist can encourage a family to facilitate their baby's development in ways that are appropriate for the child's functional level, and the parents can be taught ways to handle the baby, particularly around the time of feeding, to make this a more pleasurable experience for all concerned. By pointing out their child's advances and positive attributes, parents can be helped to develop an optimistic yet realistic attitude toward the future.

Orthopedic interventions, including bracing, serial casting, and surgical tendon releases or transfers, may be helpful for later potential complications such as contractures or muscle atrophy. For selected cases, medications, nerve blocks, selective dorsal rhizotomy

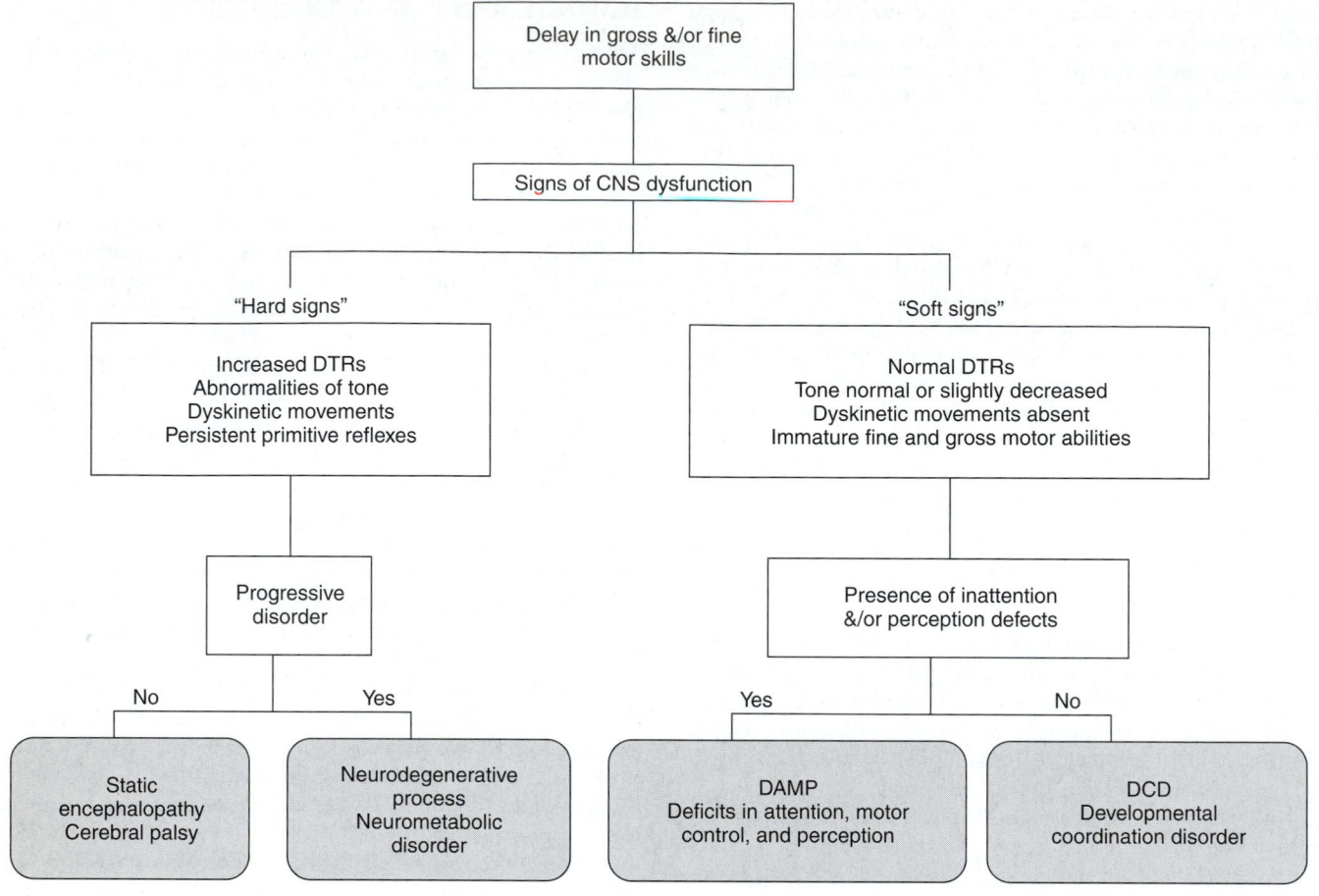

FIGURE 5-4   Algorithm showing assessment of a child with delayed development of motor skills (clumsy child). DTRs - deep tendon reflexes.

and intrathecal baclofen pump may be used to decrease the degree of spasticity.

NATURAL HISTORY AND PROGNOSIS

It is generally believed that the degree of clumsiness lessens with maturity. This may be the result of several factors. First, repetition and practice of a given motor activity itself leads to improved performance. Second, for most adults, there is less emphasis on physical prowess than there was during childhood. Also, adults can modify their environment to avoid those areas in which they do not do well.

Studies have demonstrated that many clumsy children have significant motor difficulties as teenagers. Clumsy children can grow up to be clumsy adults. Adaptive individuals choose careers emphasizing their strengths rather than their weaknesses. It is only in school that we expect children to excel simultaneously in sports, academics, and social interactions; we do not necessarily expect a world-renowned scientist to be artistic or athletically inclined.

If a clumsy child has associated learning disabilities or ADHD, these, too, can have an adverse impact on the child's wellness. The most damaging effects on long-term outcome are actually secondary. That is, the child with lowered self-esteem becomes socially withdrawn because of the child's clumsiness and other people's reaction to it; consequently, the child suffers the most from this "in-

visible handicap." Such secondary effects may linger long after any trace of clumsiness has resolved.

Despite the static nature of the underlying lesion of cerebral palsy, its symptoms and signs can change throughout the life span. For example, low muscle tone may evolve to high muscle tone or frank spasticity. In contrast, at the mildest end of the spectrum are well-documented cases of children with all the classic findings of cerebral palsy in the first years of life but who later showed no such findings on neurologic examination and were said to have "outgrown" their cerebral palsy.

Although motor impairment is the hallmark of cerebral palsy, coexisting neurologic morbidity is not uncommon. Approximately one-half of the individuals with cerebral palsy are also mentally retarded; the remainder frequently have learning difficulties and attention problems.

Those children who previously were noted to have outgrown their cerebral palsy (in terms of the classic motor findings) are more at risk than the general population for low intelligence, epilepsy, articulation problems, and behavioral difficulties. Even affected children with normal cognitive abilities may have limited opportunities for normal childhood experiences because of physical restrictions. In addition, physical disabilities place considerable stress on the family system which, in turn, may lead to increased risk of family breakup, financial difficulties, and child overprotection, all of which can further hinder a child's developmental progress. Thus, intervention must seek to maintain both the child's self-esteem and the family's integrity, neither of which should be overshadowed by the medical or surgical needs of the condition itself.

References

American Psychiatric Association: Diagnostic and Statistical Manual of Mental Disorders, 4th ed (DSM-IV). Washington, DC, American Psychiatric Association, 1994

Gubbay SS: The Clumsy Child; A Study of Developmental Apraxia and Agnosia. London/Philadelphia, Saunders, 1975

Kabesjo B, Gillberg C: Attention deficits and clumsiness in Swedish 7-year-old children. Dev Med Child Neurol 40(12):796–804, 1998

Kuban KC, Leviton A: Cerebral palsy. N Engl J Med 330:188–195, 1994

Losse A, Henderson SE, Elliman D, et al: Clumsiness in children—do they grow out of it? A ten-year follow-up study. Dev Med Child Neurol 33: 55–68, 1991

Nelson KB, Ellenberg JH: Children who "outgrew" cerebral palsy. Pediatrics 69:529–536, 1982

Taft LT, Barowsky EI: Clumsy child. Pediatr Rev 10:247–253, 1989

Wallace HM, Biehl RF, Taft LT, Ogelsby AC, eds: Handicapped Children and Youth: A Comprehensive Community and Clinical Approach. New York, Human Sciences Press, 1987

5.6.13   Hearing Problems: Impairment to Deafness

Desmond P. Kelly

Hearing is a critical element of language and social development. The newborn infant shows a preference for the mother's voice over that of other females, and by 2 to 3 months of age, infants are able to detect and discriminate most speech sounds and recognize prosodic elements of their native language. While expressive language largely does not emerge until the second year, critical exposure to spoken language has occurred long before then. Unfortunately, hearing impairment, especially in its milder forms, too often remains undetected during these critical developmental stages. Although the median age at diagnosis of children in the United States with severe congenital hearing loss has decreased from 2.5 years to 1.5 years, this is still too late for too many children. Infants and young children also are especially vulnerable to the detrimental effects of milder degrees of hearing loss such as that associated with chronic otitis media and middle-ear effusion. Thus, health professionals working with young children should be attuned to the protean manifestations and far-reaching consequences of hearing impairment.

DEFINITIONS AND EPIDEMIOLOGY

The term *hearing impairment* encompasses a broad range of disability, as outlined in Table 5-26. Hearing loss in children can vary by type, cause, age of onset, degree, and audiometric configuration. Sound is quantified in terms of loudness or amplitude (measured in decibels [dB]) and pitch or frequency (measured in hertz [Hz]). Vowel sounds are generally of lower frequency, while consonants are higher pitched. Hearing loss is conventionally reported and categorized as an average across frequencies. *Deafness* denotes a profound hearing loss of greater than 90 dB, resulting in an inability to distinguish elements of spoken language. While the threshold

TABLE 5-26
THE HEARING SPECTRUM

INTENSITY LOUDNESS (dB)	FAMILIAR SOUNDS	DEGREES OF HEARING LOSS	FUNCTIONAL IMPAIRMENT
0	Water dripping	Normal	None
15			
20	Clock ticking	Slight	May miss some consonants
25			
30	Whisper	Mild	Mild speech problems
			Only hears louder voice sounds
40	Conversational	Moderate	Hears speech as a whisper
50	speech		
55	Baby crying	Moderate to	Understands loud
60		severe	speech at 3–5 feet
70			
80	Loud shout	Severe	Hears shout as a
90	Telephone		whisper
100	Lawn mower	Profound	Not able to discriminate speech
110	Plane		
120	Discomfort		sounds

Frequency Pitch (Hz)	250	500	1000	2000	4000	8000
Sound	Vowels	a,e,i,o,u	p,h,g,ch	Consonants	f,s,th	Whistle

An appreciation of the loudness of familiar sounds assists in understanding of the functional impairment associated with different degrees of hearing loss.

for mild hearing loss has been defined as 25 dB, losses of 15 dB or greater in children can influence speech perception.

Conductive hearing loss follows disruption of the mechanical components that are required for the transduction of sound wave energy into hydraulic waves in the inner ear. This pathway includes the external ear canal, tympanic membrane, and the middle-ear ossicles connecting to the oval window. Accumulated fluid in the middle ear is the most common cause of conductive hearing loss. The affected child can hear loud speech, but distortions can inhibit early language discrimination. Conductive hearing loss is limited to 50 dB, because sounds louder than this are conducted directly via bone to the cochlea. *Sensorineural* hearing loss denotes dysfunction of the sensory epithelium, the cochlea, or the neural connections to the auditory cortex via the eighth cranial nerve and central pathways. Severe or profound hearing loss is always sensorineural, and higher frequency sounds usually are most affected. Not infrequently, there is a combination of these types, termed a *mixed* hearing loss. Hearing impairment also can occur at the cortical level, with difficulty related to auditory perception and processing.

While significant hearing loss reflects bilateral involvement, unilateral sensorineural hearing loss has been associated with behavioral difficulties and academic problems.

Congenital hearing loss is present at birth and can be either *hereditary* or *acquired* (eg, secondary to congenital infection). Postnatal hearing loss is usually acquired, although some forms of hereditary deafness have delayed onset and are associated with progressive impairment (see Sec. 15.1.4).

Severe to profound hearing loss is relatively rare, affecting 1 to 2 per 1000 children at birth in developed countries and probably twice that number in developing nations. A further 2 to 3 per 1000 children subsequently acquire severe loss. Up to 67% of young children experience some degree of intermittent conductive hearing loss secondary to otitis media.

ETIOLOGY AND PATHOGENESIS

The causes of the various types of hearing impairment are summarized in Table 5-27. Deafness is inherited in 50% of cases, either as an isolated trait or as part of a recognizable syndrome. Approximately 80% of genetic deafness is inherited as an autosomal recessive trait, 18% is autosomal dominant, and 2% is X-linked recessive. The spectrum of acquired causes is broad. The incidence of congenital rubella, previously one of the most common causes of congenital deafness, has declined because of childhood immunizations, and the same is true for measles and mumps. However, other infections, such as congenital cytomegalovirus and toxoplasmosis, remain significant factors. Infants who have been treated in neonatal intensive care units are at particularly increased risk for hearing loss. Bacterial meningitis has been a relatively common cause of sensorineural hearing loss, with this sequela in up to 10% of cases. The introduction of *Haemophilus influenzae* type B immunization and early steroid therapy have decreased its impact. Prolonged exposure to loud noise, either environmental or recreational (eg, audio headphones), can damage cochlear hair cells and result in a predominantly high-frequency hearing loss.

CLINICAL MANIFESTATIONS

Obvious manifestations of hearing loss include the failure of an infant to startle at loud noises or turn to localize a sound. Toddlers might not respond to requests or instructions. In most cases, however, hearing impairment is subtle and can evade detection quite easily. Infants with even a profound hearing loss will begin to vocalize before 6 months of age, with delays in further language development only later becoming apparent. Dysfunctional behavioral patterns and/or impaired social interactions secondary to hearing problems might be ascribed incorrectly to disorders such as autism, oppositional behavior, or mental retardation.

ASSESSMENT AND DIAGNOSIS

An approach to assessment and management of the child with suspected hearing impairment is shown in Fig. 5-5. The key to an optimal outcome for the child with a hearing impairment is early diagnosis and intervention. Use of a "high-risk register" was previously promoted to identify those children at most significant risk for hearing loss. The key neonatal variables identified by the Joint Committee on Infant Hearing were: family history of sensorineural hearing loss; congenital infection associated with hearing loss; presence of craniofacial anomalies; birth weight under 1500 g; neonatal jaundice requiring exchange transfusion; ototoxic medications; bacterial meningitis; evidence of severely depressed physiological status at birth (eg, Apgar score of 3 or less at 5 minutes); and

TABLE 5-27

SOME CAUSES OF HEARING LOSS

CATEGORY			CONDUCTIVE	SENSORINEURAL
Hereditary	Autosomal	Dominant	Mandibulofacial dysostosis (Treacher Collins)	Clinically undifferentiated deafness Syndromes: Waardenburg (pigmentary anomalies) Alport (nephritis)
		Recessive	(Rare) Cryptophthalmos syndrome Paget disease	Clinically undifferentiated deafness Syndromes: Usher (retinitis pigmentosa) Pendred (goiter) Jervell and Lange-Nielsen (abnormal ECG)
	X-linked		Otopalatodigital syndrome	Hunter syndrome Deafness with pigmentary anomalies
Acquired	Cogenital		(Rare)	Maternal Infection: Rubella Cytomegalovirus Toxoplasmosis Syphilis Maternal diabetes
	Postnatal		Otitis media: acute chronic Tympanic membrane disruption Ossicular dislocation Cholesteatoma	Ototoxins Acoustic injury Tumor
Malformation deformation conditions			Goldenhar syndrome Hemifacial microsomia	Klippell-Feil syndrome (Wildervanck)

Conductive loss follows damage to structures extending from the external ear to the oval window. Sensorineural hearing loss involves the cochlea or neural connections to the auditory cortex (see Sec. 15.1.1). Causes of hearing variation can be classified by timing and locus of effect and whether they are hereditary or acquired.

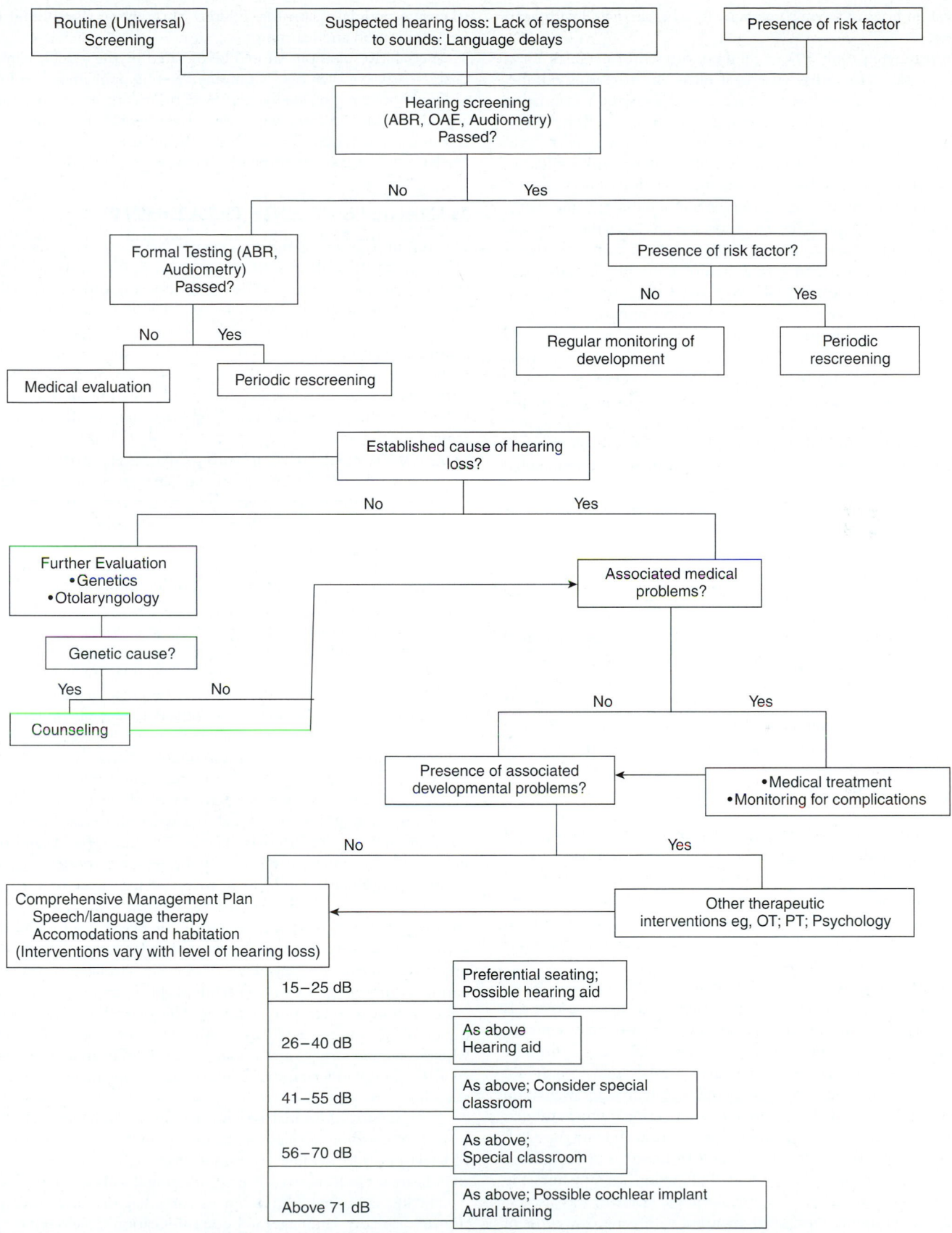

FIGURE 5-5 Effective management of the child with hearing loss hinges on early and accurate diagnosis and intervention plus attention to potential associated medical and developmental problems. ABR = auditory brain response; OT = occupational therapy; PT = physical therapy.

physical findings of a syndrome known to be associated with hearing loss.

Unfortunately, only 50% of children with sensorineural deafness manifest one of these risk criteria at birth. An increasing number of states in the United States have passed legislation mandating universal newborn hearing screening programs. The Joint Commission on Infant Hearing and The American Academy of Pediatrics have set a goal of identification of all infants with significant congenital hearing loss by 3 months and initiation of necessary intervention by 6 months. Improvements in technology and methodology have decreased the false-positive rate of screening tests. However, there is still a need to be vigilant for hearing loss that is of delayed onset or progressive in nature. Current methodologies for physiological screening include evoked otoacoustic emissions (EOAE) and automated auditory brainstem response (ABR) testing. Otoacoustic emissions are a form of energy produced by active movements of the outer hair cells of the cochlea during the normal hearing process. EOAE testing entails the introduction of clicks through a probe in the external ear canal, with measurement of the emissions from the inner ear by a microphone. This technique is relatively simple and highly sensitive, but it is less specific than auditory brainstem-evoked response testing, which is recommended as a second-stage test for babies failing EOAE screening.

In children with recurrent or persistent otitis media, the level of hearing loss should be documented and monitored closely. Perfunctory assessments of hearing in a clinical setting can be misleading. Response to a bell, hand clap, or other loud sound does not rule out milder levels of hearing loss or discriminate a loss at specific frequencies.

Hearing can be assessed accurately in children at any age. By 6 months, audiometry is possible using conditioned responses to speech or tones from speakers in a soundproof booth. For younger infants and for those children who either cannot or will not cooperate, auditory brainstem-evoked response testing is accurate and reliable and can detect unilateral loss. A click is introduced at the external canal, and transmission of the evoked potential through the brainstem pathways to the auditory cortex is recorded by means of scalp electrodes.

Tympanometry entails measurement of acoustic energy passed through the middle-ear system (ie, admittance) or reflected back (ie, impedance). Mobility of the tympanic membrane and middle-ear pressure can be gauged. The presence of the acoustic reflex (ie, contraction of the stapedius muscle in response to sounds of greater than 70 dB) confirms the presence of hearing but is not an acceptably sensitive measure.

When hearing loss has been identified, further medical assessment is necessary. In children with sensorineural hearing loss, it is essential to rule out any associated conductive component that could be treated relatively easily but that may be exaggerating the degree of loss. Thus, a detailed general physical examination should include pneumatic otoscopy. Comprehensive neurologic evaluation is important to look for associated disabilities, including vestibular dysfunction. Unexplained fainting spells in a deaf child might signal a cardiac conduction defect (eg, long QT interval) of Jervell and Lange-Nielsen syndrome. Thyroid dysfunction accompanies the Pendred syndrome. Careful ophthalmologic evaluation is also essential. For example, retinitis pigmentosa with progressive loss of vision indicates a probable diagnosis of Usher syndrome, and chorioretinitis is a further complication of some of the congenital infections. Finally, routine evaluation for refractive errors is essential to ensure optimal vision for children who rely on visual input for communication and learning.

Special investigations should be dictated by the specific clinical characteristics of each case. Computed tomography imaging of the temporal bone region can be helpful in ruling out structural anomalies that could have implications for treatment. It is important to recognize that certain forms of hearing loss can be progressive, so the level of hearing loss should be reevaluated routinely.

MANAGEMENT AND TREATMENT

Hearing impairment demands a comprehensive management approach. This incorporates attention to medical treatment, educational interventions, use of assistive devices, and support as well as advocacy. The initial evaluation and treatment of a child with hearing loss is often best performed by a team of professionals representing pediatrics, otolaryngology, audiology, speech and language pathology, and aural habilitation. Other specialty areas, such as genetics, neurology, psychology, and social work, might also be involved, depending on the special circumstances of the child and family.

Antibiotic therapy of acute otitis media has eliminated the suppurative complications that were previously seen. Persistent middle-ear effusions warrant careful monitoring. Any child with a middle-ear effusion persisting for longer than 2 months should have a formal hearing evaluation. It has been suggested that significant hearing loss for more than 3 months in a child under 2 years of age is an indication for surgical intervention with insertion of middle-ear ventilation tubes (see Sec. 15.1.9).

In cases of established hearing loss, the child should be fitted with a hearing aid as soon as possible. A variety of formats are available, ranging from the traditional, body-worn receiver to behind-the-ear aids and units that are self-contained in a mold within the pinna and external canal. Hearing aids generally amplify all sounds, which results in some distortion. Technologic advances have produced devices that amplify sounds differentially in the frequency spectra most affected. Bone-conduction devices are used for children with malformations of the external canal. A newer form of hearing augmentation for children with profound loss is the cochlear implant. This consists of an external microphone and amplifier with an induction coil set in the temporal bone and connected to a multichannel electrode that is passed through the round window into the scala tympani of the cochlea. Cochlear implants are being performed with increased frequency in young children with profound sensorineural hearing loss who have received negligible benefit from hearing aids. Longitudinal studies have revealed continued improvements in speech perception and expressive language as long as 4 years postimplant. This procedure is now being performed in children as young as 18 to 24 months of age. Children who receive any form of amplification device need auditory training to help them understand the meaning of the newly amplified sounds.

A number of additional assistive devices are available, including telecommunication devices for the deaf (TDD), closed captioning of television, and adapted warning devices such as flickering lights to indicate fire, adverse weather, or a ringing doorbell or telephone.

The key to successful outcome is early diagnosis and intervention to promote language and communication development. In cases of profound hearing loss, the child, parents, and other immediate caregivers should receive professional assistance in establishing a functional system of communication as soon as possible.

Opinions differ among those involved in the education of deaf children regarding the most appropriate communication and instructional techniques. Options include sign language (ie, manual communication) or lip reading and use of speech (ie, oral communication). Educational interventions should be tailored to the individual needs of each child. Options range from the use of interpreters in a regular classroom, to special programs in a regular school, to enrollment in a school for the deaf. Children with hearing impairment must have the opportunity for full participation in academic and social activities. The optimal school setting to achieve this goal depends on the individual characteristics of the child and the educational system in that geographic region.

The primary-care physician is a vital source of information and support for the families of children with severe hearing impairment. A number of specialists often are involved, and parents might receive conflicting advice regarding both medical and educational interventions that are deemed necessary for their child. The stress of adjusting to the diagnosis, coupled with the need to learn new forms of communication and to initiate interventions, affirms the need for care, coordination, and advocacy.

NATURAL HISTORY AND PROGNOSIS

The long-term sequelae of milder forms of hearing loss associated with otitis media are not defined clearly. While the fluid collections associated with acute infections are time-limited, a significant proportion of children develop serous effusions (eg, otitis media with effusion) that can be prolonged, with accompanying conductive losses during important periods of early language development. The conclusions of the many studies that have addressed developmental outcomes for children having otitis media with effusion are conflicting, with some studies suggesting an increased risk for language disabilities (particularly related to phonologic awareness), and other studies indicating an association with later attention problems.

Children with severe or profound hearing loss generally have normal nonverbal intelligence, but they do not achieve levels of academic functioning congruent with their hearing peers. Consequently, there is concern in the field of deaf education that expectations for deaf students are unnecessarily low.

There are many determinants of outcome in addition to the more obvious factors such as degree of hearing loss. Children who have had the opportunity to acquire and assimilate a language structure before losing their hearing are better able to communicate orally than those with deafness of prelingual onset (ie, less than 2 years of age). Deaf children born into families with other deaf members benefit from earlier adaptations and efforts to promote communication. Associated disabilities have been reported in up to 30% of children with deafness, especially those with acquired causes such as congenital infections or extreme prematurity. Problems can include visual impairment, neuromotor difficulties, seizure disorders, and learning disabilities. Although attentional problems do not appear to be more prevalent in deaf children as a whole, certain subgroups (eg, those with acquired deafness) appear to be at increased risk.

New technologies, including the Internet, continue to broaden the opportunities for individuals with hearing impairment to participate more fully socially, in school, and in the workplace. The Americans with Disabilities Act adds legal safeguards and provisions. Gallaudet University and the National Technical Institute for the Deaf are highly respected institutions of higher learning for the deaf, and many colleges and universities now incorporate services for those with hearing impairment.

References

American Academy of Pediatrics Task Force on Newborn and Infant Hearing: Newborn and infant hearing loss: detection and intervention. Pediatrics 103(2):527–530, 1999

Brookhouser PE, Beauchaine KL, Osberger MJ: Management of the child with sensorineural hearing loss. Pediatr Clin North Am 46(1):121–141, 1999

Davidson J, Hyde ML, Alberti PW: Epidemiologic patterns in childhood hearing loss: a review. Int J Pediatr Otorhinolaryngol 17:239–266, 1989

Kelly DP, Kelly BJ, Jones ML, Moulton NJ, et al: Attention deficits in children and adolescents with hearing loss: a survey. Am J Dis Child 147:737, 1993

Lotke M: The sounds of silence: the hearing-impaired child. Contemp Peds 12(10):104–114, 1995

Marschark M: Psychological Development of Deaf Children. New York, Oxford University Press, 1993

Meadow KP: Deafness and Child Development. Berkeley, University of California Press, 1980

Northern JL, Downs MP: Hearing in Children, 4th ed. Baltimore, Williams & Wilkins, 1991

Rapin I: Hearing disorders. Pediatr Rev 14:43–49, 1993

Roberts JE, Wallace IF: Language and otitis media. In: Roberts JE, Wallace IF, Henderson FH, eds: Otitis Media in Young Children. Baltimore, Paul H. Brookes, 1997:133.

Roizen NJ: Etiology of hearing loss in children. Pediatr Clin North Am 46(1):49–61, 1999

Van Naarden K, DeCoufle P, Caldwell K: Prevalence and characteristics of children with serious hearing impairment in metropolitan Atlanta, 1991–1993. Pediatrics 103(3):570–575, 1999

5.6.14   Vision Problems: Impairment to Blindness

Deborah Orel-Bixler

BACKGROUND

In the United States, vision disorders are the fourth most common disability of children and the leading cause of handicapping conditions in childhood. The most prevalent vision disorders include amblyopia (2–3%), strabismus (3–4%), significant refractive error (15–30%), color vision deficits (4–5%), and ocular disease (<1%). The prevalence for significant refractive error includes hyperopia (20%), myopia (4%), anisometropia (1%), astigmatism (10%), and color vision deficits (8–10% males; 0.5% females). Although the prevalence of ocular disease is less than 1%, it has public health significance due to the association of ocular disease with visual impairment, blindness, morbidity, and mortality.

VISION IMPAIRMENT TO BLINDNESS: DEFINITIONS

The World Health Organization (WHO) lists five categories of visual impairment (Table 5-28).

The terms *partially sighted, low vision, legally blind,* and *totally blind* are used in the educational context to describe students with visual impairments. These terms are defined as follows:

TABLE 5-28

WHO CATEGORIES OF VISUAL IMPAIRMENT

CATEGORY	TERMINOLOGY	VISION, BETTER EYE, BEST CORRECTED
1	Visually impaired	<6/18 to 6/60 (<20/30 to 20/200)
2	Severely impaired	<6/60 to 3/60 (<20/200 to 20/400)
3	Blind	<3/60 to 1/60 (<20/400 to 20/2400)
4	Blind	<1/60 to LP (<20/2400 to light perception)
5	Blind	NLP (no light perception)

- *Partially sighted* indicates some type of visual problem has resulted in the need for special education. People are partially sighted if their visual acuity is better than 20/200 but worse than 20/70 in the better eye with refractive correction.
- *Low vision* generally refers to a severe visual impairment, not necessarily limited to distance vision. Low vision applies to all individuals with sight who are unable to read the newspaper at a normal viewing distance, even with the aid of eyeglasses or contact lenses. People with low vision use a combination of vision and other senses to learn, although they may require adaptations in lighting or the size of print and sometimes Braille.
- *Legally blind* indicates that a person has less than 20/200 vision in the better eye or a very limited field of vision (20 degrees at its widest point).
- *Totally blind* students cannot visually detect light with either eye and learn via Braille or other nonvisual media.

Different classifications have been used to describe the causes of blindness and severe visual impairment in children. The classification based on anatomy is determined by the part of the eye or visual system that has been damaged and includes the categories cornea, lens, retina, optic nerve, glaucoma, and other. The classification based on time of insult includes the categories prenatal (including hereditary factors and intrauterine insults), perinatal, and postnatal factors.

Data on the number and demographic characteristics of blind and visually impaired persons are difficult to obtain for a variety of reasons. The lack of consensus on the definition of blindness and visual impairment confounds the difficulty in data collection. Comparison of data is difficult due to varying definitions or classifications of visual impairment and varying age ranges. There is no central registry for persons with disabilities in the United States. Children with limited vision are usually not reported to any data collection agency until they reach school age.

EPIDEMIOLOGY OF AMBLYOPIA

A total of 6 million Americans experience loss of vision due to amblyopia, with an additional 75,000 3-year-olds developing amblyopia each year. Amblyopia is responsible for loss of vision in more people younger than 45 years than all other ocular disease and trauma combined. The National Plan of the National Eye Institute concluded that if the risk factors for the development of amblyopia are detected in infancy or early childhood, amblyopia,

in principle at least, is completely preventable. Using a 2% prevalence of amblyopia in children and including only today's preschool population, it has been estimated amblyopia will cause 20 million people years of preventable vision loss.

EPIDEMIOLOGY OF VISION IMPAIRMENT AND BLINDNESS

By recent estimates, 3.8% of worldwide blindness involves children younger than 15 years. By the WHO criteria, there are 1.5 million children worldwide who are blind: 1.0 million in Asia, 0.3 million in Africa, 0.1 million in Latin America, and 0.1 million in the rest of the world.

There are marked geographic differences in causes of vision loss in children across the world. In the United States and industrialized nations, the cause of childhood blindness is due to perinatal (24%) and hereditary factors (18%). This is compared with hereditary factors (66%) in the Middle East and Sri Lanka, and childhood factors (47%) in Africa, which include corneal opacification caused by measles, vitamin A deficiency, and traditional eye medicine complex. Retinal disease causes most pediatric blindness in the United States and industrialized nations, compared with cataract in Latin America and the Middle East and corneal opacities in Asia and Africa. The regional differences in the causes of pediatric blindness are also based on socioeconomic factors. It has been estimated that, in developing countries, 30 to 72% of blindness is avoidable, 9 to 58% is preventable, and 14 to 31% is treatable.

Available data from 2553 students at 26 of the 126 US schools for the blind suggest that the leading causes of blindness are cortical visual impairment (19%), retinopathy of prematurity (13%), and optic nerve hypoplasia (7%). There has been a significant increase in cortical visual impairment (CVI) and retinopathy of prematurity (ROP) in the past 10 years. Other causes of blindness include (in decreasing order of prevalence, ranging from 5% to 2% of the total) albinism; optic atrophy; cataract and cataract/cataract surgery complications; retinitis pigmentosa; microophthalmia/anophthalmia; aniridia; and glaucoma. Other conditions, which each had a prevalence of about 1%, include Leber's congenital amaurosis; cone-rod dystrophy; coloboma of the retina/optic nerve; retinal detachment; trauma; diabetes; and the TORCH infections. Ocular trauma is the most common cause of acquired blindness in children in the United States. Eye injuries occur two to four times as often in boys as in girls. The most frequent cause of eye injury is accidental or intentional trauma by another child; sports-related injuries are the second most frequent cause.

There is a need for more complete and more uniform data on blindness and visual impairment based on the WHO reporting format. The current estimate for the rate at which visual impairments occur in individuals under the age of 18 is 12.2 per 1000; severe visual impairments (legally or totally blind) occur at a rate of 0.06 per 1000.

Of the nearly 1 in every 1000 US children who have low vision or who are legally blind, nearly two-thirds also have one or more other developmental disabilities including mental retardation, cerebral palsy, hearing impairment, or epilepsy. Infants with cerebral palsy, Down syndrome, and other genetic conditions associated with mental retardation have a higher prevalence of refractive errors, strabismus, cortical visual impairments, and other ocular problems than do those children without disabilities (see Table 5-29). Children with more severe disabling conditions have more severe vision problems.

TABLE 5-29

RELATIVE OCCURRENCE OF OCULAR PROBLEMS IN CHILDREN (1950 TO 1992)

	REFRACTIVE ERROR %	STRABISMUS %	OTHER %
Normal	15 to 30	2 to 4	<1
Cerebral palsy	21 to 76	15 to 60	1 to 25
Mental retardation	52	16 to 40	21
Down syndrome	42 to 73	23 to 44	33
Fragile X syndrome	59	30 to 50	13
Deafness	29	13	9

SOURCE: *From Wesson MD and Maino DM: Oculovisual findings in children with Down syndrome, cerebral palsy, and mental retardation without specific etiology. In: Maino D, ed: Diagnosis and Management of Special Populations. St. Louis, MO, Mosby-Year Book, 1995.*

Normal Visual Development

The visual system of infants is relatively mature at birth and undergoes rapid development in the early postnatal years. Formation of eye begins at 22 days of fetal life and develops from an outpouching of the developing brain. By 6 weeks postconception, the ocular structures and differentiation of the brain are fairly well developed. Teratogenic factors (drug abuse, infection, medications) occurring in the first trimester of pregnancy often result in ocular defects.

The eye is one of the most fully developed organs at birth. The eye of the newborn is two-thirds of the adult size. It undergoes its most rapid growth during the first year of life and finally reaches the adult length and size by adolescence. At birth, the anterior structures of the eye (cornea, lens, iris) are more developed than the posterior structures (retina). Within the retina, the photoreceptors consisting of rods (responsible for night vision) and cones (responsible for day vision, detail vision, color vision) are all present at birth but are immature in size and spacing. The inner layers of the retina differentiate further after birth in particular, the fovea (central area of the retina specialized for acute vision) is very immature and the peripheral retina develops sooner. The optic nerve is relatively full size at birth, and myelination of this visual pathway is not complete until age 2 years. The lateral geniculate nucleus has the full complement of neurons present at birth, but they enlarge and establish more connections to other neurons with age. The visual cortex of the brain has all the neurons of one's lifetime present at birth, but these migrate to superficial layers of the brain and increase in their neural connections.

The anatomic and physiological developments of the visual system are accompanied by a rapid improvement in visual capabilities. Most aspects of vision function reach adult levels during the first year of life. Visual fixation by the newborn is evident at birth and accurate fixation is achieved by 6 to 9 weeks. The newborn's eye movements change from saccadic, fixational movements to smooth pursuit eye movements by 2 to 3 months of age. Optokinetic nystagmus (OKN) and the vestibular ocular reflex (VOR) are involuntary eye movements important for providing stability of visual images on the eye when objects in the world move (OKN) or the infant moves (VOR). OKN is present at birth but immature until 3 months of age. The newborn is unable to suppress the VOR (reflexive eye movements induced by spinning) until 2 months of age. Accommodation, the ability to focus the intraocular lens of the eye for near viewing, is present at birth but inaccurate until 2

to 3 months of age. Fortunately, the small pupils of the neonate permit a relatively large depth of focus (range over which visual objects remain clear without focusing effort). The average refractive error of newborns is hyperopic (farsighted) due to the strong optics of the eye and short axial length, with an incidence of astigmatism from 15 to 30%. The prevalence of hyperopia and astigmatism decrease with age. The refractive error in the majority of infants disappears by 9 to 12 months.

Visual capabilities improve rapidly during the first year of life and have been quantified with preferential looking (PL) and visual-evoked potential (VEP) techniques. Contrast sensitivity, the ability to detect brightness differences or subtle shades of gray, for large objects is adult-like by 10 weeks of age. Infants have measurable color discrimination as early as 2 weeks of age, and color vision improves over the first 3 months of life. Visual acuity, the ability to discern fine details, reaches adult levels by 6 to 8 months of age as measured with VEP, and 3 years of age as measured behaviorally with PL. Stereopsis, the ability to discern fine depth or 3D vision, has a rapid onset at 3 months of age and reaches near adult levels in most infants by 6 months of age.

Health-care professionals recognize the need to identify ocular conditions that might interfere with the development of normal vision such as ocular disease (cataracts and corneal opacities), strabismus, and significant refractive errors (anisometropia, astigmatism, and high ametropias). Early detection of vision problems allows intervention at a time when the problems are highly amenable to treatment.

Anomalous Visual Development

Normal eye movements do not develop in visually impaired infants. Abnormal eye movements are often the first symptom of significant vision impairment. Sensory nystagmus occurs with bilateral disruption of central vision if the visual defect is congenital or acquired during the first 2 years of life. The onset of congenital nystagmus usually occurs between 8 and 12 weeks of age. Acquired nystagmus appears about 1 month after the vision loss. If central vision can be restored, the nystagmus may disappear. With longer delays in visual rehabilitation, the nystagmus becomes irreversible. The presence of roving eye movements in infants indicates severely reduced vision, usually worse than 20/200. The differential diagnosis for an infant with visual impairment, nystagmus, and nonobvious ocular findings includes Leber's congenital amaurosis; albinism; nystagmus; congenital stationary night blindness; achromatopsia; and optic nerve atrophy and/or hypoplasia. Blind infants are unable to suppress the VOR. Infants with infantile esotropia and amblyopia retain an asymmetric optokinetic nystagmus. Tracking and following an object with eye movements may be irregular and accommodation may be insufficient or lacking in an infant with visual impairment.

While neonates show rudimentary binocular alignment of the eyes, 88% show brief periods of misalignment up to 6 months of age; orthotropia is the rule, however, 97% by 6 months. Normal development of binocular fusion and disparity detection by 3 months of age lays the foundation for the development of stereopsis (fine depth perception). A lack of stereopsis may indicate the presence of strabismus, anisometropia, and/or amblyopia. Sensory strabismus is a deviation of one eye secondary to a severe reduction or loss of vision caused by an abnormality in that eye. Any strabismus, constant or intermittent, past 4 months of age should be referred for evaluation by a pediatric ophthalmologist or optometrist.

The mean refractive error of newborns is hyperopia in full-term and myopia in premature infants. The refractive error in the majority of infants disappears by 9 to 12 months. Visual impairment and blindness interfere with the emmetropization process, and high refractive errors are often associated with structural or functional abnormalities of the eye and visual system. Greater than +3.50D of hyperopia at 6 to 8 months of age, when left untreated, led to a 13-fold increase in having amblyopia by the age of 4 years.

IMPACT OF ABNORMAL VISION ON GENERAL CHILD DEVELOPMENT

Vision is the most important sense for general development and education. Much of early learning is through imitation, primarily visual imitation. The infant with visual impairment has limited access to this mode of learning. Visual impairment and blindness affect all areas of development. The most important areas are communication; bonding; level of wakefulness; motor development; spatial concepts; balance; object permanence; picture perception; incident learning; language development; and social interaction. Blindness has a profound impact on motor development and achievement of developmental milestones. Indirect influences including the characteristics of the visual impairment, lack of visual stimulation, inability to make use of imitative learning, and environmental factors can have an impact on the motor developmental process.

In the first few months of life, the motor development of infants with visual impairment is not markedly different from that of fully sighted infants. Postural milestones such as independent sitting and standing can be achieved within expectations for sighted infants. Sighted babies raise their heads and look about by 12 weeks; blind babies are unhappy in this position and prefer to be on their backs, which may delay motor control of head and trunk. There are qualitative differences in motor development. It has been reported that an infant who is blind sits motionless and that the infant's self-initiated mobility is delayed. Even blind infants "look" at their hands by bringing them to their face by 16 weeks, but reaching out is delayed beyond the norm of age 3 to 4 months. Early visual tracking motivates the infant to reach and grasp, whereas lack of vision deprives the infant of this critical motivation and leads to delay in acquisition of physical skills in using the body, hand coordination, and development of fine muscles. The ability to grasp an object (6 months) may be delayed until 1 year. By age 7 months, sighted infants localize with their eyes a part of the body that has been "touched," whereas infants who are blind may take up to 2 years to do so. In general, infants who are blind are slow to localize sounds by reaching out to touch them; instead, they tend to remain motionless in response to sounds. Both sighted and visually impaired infants start to babble at the same age, but lack of visual input slows progress, as words are less meaningful without the corresponding visual symbols.

Infants who are visually impaired and have additional disabilities are an extremely diverse group. They have great variation in the etiology of the vision loss, the range of vision loss, the types of other disabilities, and in severity of other disabilities. Given the heterogeneity of the population, it is not surprising to find little research on the effects of visual impairment, and infants with additional disabilities have more significant developmental delays than do infants who are only visually impaired. In infants with additional disabilities, selected developmental milestones are attained later than they are attained in infants with visual impairment and no other disabilities. When an infant is visually impaired and has additional disabilities, the infant has to develop specific ways to assess sensory information and to interact with the environment. Learning how to obtain and interpret information and becoming motivated to explore surroundings and to undertake activities are essential for development in many areas such as cognitive and linguistic abilities.

CLINICAL MANIFESTATIONS

Signs and Symptoms of Prevalent Vision Problems in Infancy and Childhood

Amblyopia is a loss of visual acuity that is not due to ocular pathology and is not correctable with glasses or contact lenses. Amblyopia may result from the abnormal visual experience in early childhood induced by significant refractive errors (anisometropia, astigmatism, high bilateral ametropia, or blur), strabismus, or visual deprivation from media opacities (cataract or corneal opacity). The monocular vision loss in amblyopia often goes unnoticed because a child with reduced visual acuity may not be able to express difficulties with his or her vision nor convey the loss of depth perception.

Strabismus is a misalignment of the eyes in which one or the other eye is turned in (esotropia), out (extopropia), up (hypertropia), or down (hypotropia), some or all of the time (intermittent or constant). The most common forms of strabismus in children include infantile and accommodative estropia. Amblyopia occurs frequently with esotropia (see Sec. 26.13.1).

Significant Refractive Error

Modest, symmetric refractive error in the youngest age groups do not generally require refractive correction and do not lead to vision loss. The manifestations of refractive error are shown in Table 5-30. High refractive errors, particularly when unequal between eyes, can lead to both temporary and more permanent (and difficult to treat) loss of vision (ie, amblyopia). Anisometropia (unequal refractive error between eyes) is the leading cause of amblyopia with studies indicating that up to 60% of all amblyopia is due to anisometropia. A child with hypermetropic anisometropia is more likely to become amblyopic than a child with myopic anisometropia. Hyperopia is also a risk factor for esotropia, which has an additional role in causation of amblyopia. High uncorrected hyperopia also has been linked to reading difficulties. High refractive errors are more often associated with both structural and functional abnor-

TABLE 5-30

SIGNS AND SYMPTOMS OF UNCORRECTED REFRACTIVE ERROR IN YOUNG CHILDREN

Difficulty with depth perception
Eye–hand and coordination difficulties
Confuses likeness and minor differences
Frequently rubs eyes
Blinks excessively
Complains of double vision
Cannot maintain fixation on a task
Frequently closes or covers one eye
Lack of interest in outdoor activities
Lack of interest in near tasks
Positions self close to television or books
Squints
Displays no signs or symptoms

SOURCE: *Adapted from Ciner E. In: Moore BD, ed: Eye Care for Infants and Young Children. Woburn Butterworth-Heinemann, 1997.*

malities of the eye and visual system. Children with low vision tend to have a greater amount of astigmatism than do children with normal vision.

Color-Vision Deficits

Identification of color-vision deficiency before school age is important because a large part of the early educational process involves the use of color identification and discrimination. Hue discrimination (red-green) is probably present at birth with an ability to match colors by 2 years of age. Abnormal color vision includes X-linked inheritance protan and deutan (red-green) deficits, which occur in 8 to 10% of males and in less than 0.5% of females, and other rare deficits, which affect up to 0.007% of both males and females. Changes in color-vision capabilities may be an early indicator of retinal or optic nerve disorders.

Color-vision deficits have negative impacts on learning, particularly with color-coded educational materials, and impose restrictions on career choice because many service occupations (military, police, and fire) require normal color vision.

Ocular disease encompasses a wide range of disorders in isolation or associated with other systemic conditions. There are several ocular anomalies that result in poor vision and lead to visual inattention in infants, including:

1. Opacities of the ocular media including bilateral cataracts or corneal opacities associated with congenital glaucoma;
2. Disorders of the retina including achromatopsia; Leber's congenital amaurosis; albinism; congenital stationary night blindness; retinal degeneration associated with rare syndromes and metabolic disorders; retinopathy of prematurity; vitreous hemorrhage; and macular lesions;
3. Optic nerve disorders including optic nerve hypoplasia and optic nerve atrophy; and
4. Disorders of the brain including cortical visual impairment secondary to a significant perinatal problem such as hypoxic-ischemic encephalopathy.

All of these conditions can be diagnosed with a vision examination, but not all of these conditions present with obvious signs to the parents other than visual inattention. The signs during infancy that a parent may recognize and that may indicate a serious vision-threatening problem are listed in Table 5-31. These signs should prompt a visit to the infant's pediatrician and eye-care professional.

The specific behaviors of an infant that suggest poor vision may include staring at lights, nystagmus, eye poking, failure to smile, or disinterest in the visual environment. The apparent visual difficulty may be present only under specific conditions such as dim or bright illumination. The infant may become upset when a night light is turned off or when he or she is taken out of bright sunlight. If the infant has older siblings, the parents can compare the younger child's development to the older child's achievement of visual milestones. Often, the open-ended question, "How well does your baby see?" prompts the parents to recall these specific behaviors of concern.

Prevalent Ocular Conditions Causing Visual Impairment in the United States

Cortical visual impairment (CVI) is a loss of vision secondary to damage to the geniculostriate pathways (visual cortex and optic radiations). It is characterized by reduced vision, absence of optokinetic nystagmus (OKN) with normal ocular examination find-

TABLE 5-31

SIGNS DURING INFANCY THAT MAY INDICATE A SERIOUS VISION-THREATENING PROBLEM

Lack of eye contact by 3 months
Lack of visual fixation or following by 3 months
Lack of accurate reaching for objects by 6 months
Persistent lack of the eyes moving in concert or the sustained crossing of one eye after about 4 months
Frequent horizontal or vertical jerky eye movements (nystagmus)
Lack of a clear black pupil (haziness of the cornea, a whitish appearance inside the pupil, or a significant asymmetry in the usual "red eye" appearance in a flash photograph)
Persistent tearing when the infant is not crying
Significant sensitivity to bright light (photophobia)
Persistent redness of the normally white conjunctiva
Drooping of an eyelid sufficient to obscure the pupil
Any asymmetry of pupil size
Any obvious abnormalities of the shape or structure of the eyes (keyhole pupil)

SOURCE: *Adapted from Tamplin SW: Visual impairment in infants and young children. Inf Young Children 8:18, 1995*

ings, and intact pupillary light responses. CVI results from hypoxic insults, meningitis, encephalitis, metabolic disturbances, head trauma, or hydrocephalus. The recovery of vision is often protracted and only partial, although, in some cases, recovery may be complete and rapid. For this reason cortical visual impairment, not cortical blindness, is the appropriate terminology. The most common cause of CVI is generalized cerebral hypoxia at the striate, parietal, and premotor regions, as well as vascular lesions of the striate cortex. Most children with CVI have associated neurologic abnormalities, including seizures, cerebral palsy, hemiparesis, and hypotonia. Associated eye problems include strabismus, optic nerve atrophy, ocular motor apraxia, nystagmus, and retinal disease.

Retinopathy of prematurity (ROP) was first reported in 1942 as a condition confined to premature infants and as a disorder of the immature retinal vasculature. ROP became the leading cause of blindness in the United States and parts of Europe during the 1940s and 1950s. Restriction of oxygen use in premature neonates has dramatically decreased the incidence of ROP. The incidence and severity of ROP increase with the level of immaturity (birth weight and gestational age). Severe ROP occurs mainly in infants with <1250 g birth weight and <30 weeks gestational age. Associated eye problems include vision impairment, strabismus, and refractive error with a tendency toward myopia, astigmatism, and anisometropia (see Sec. 26.11).

Optic nerve hypoplasia (ONH) is a nonspecific manifestation of damage to the visual system that was sustained at any time before its full development. ONH has been associated with maternal diabetes, alcohol abuse, use of antiepileptic medications, young age (age 20 years or under), and maternal exposure to a toxic substance. There is a wide variation in the appearance of hypoplastic optic discs, and their effect on vision is also widely variable. Bilateral severe ONH presents as blindness in early infancy with roving eye movements and sluggish pupil reactions. Lesser degrees of ONH may cause minor visual defects or sensory strabismus. ONH may be associated with a variety of endocrine disorders such as hypothyroidism, growth hormone deficiency, or neonatal hypoglycemia. Children with ONH in the first 4 years of life should be considered for neuroimaging to confirm or exclude associated cerebral malformations and other deficits.

Retinoblastoma is the most common malignant ocular tumor of childhood, but it is quite rare at 1 in 20,000 live births. Close to 50% of retinoblastomas are heritable. This ocular tumor arises from primitive retinal cells, with the majority of cases in children less than 4 years of age. Untreated, the tumor is almost uniformly fatal; with treatment the survival rate is greater than 90%. The presenting symptoms and signs for retinoblastoma include leukokoria (white pupil) 56%, strabismus 20%, glaucoma 7%, and poor vision 5%; about 3% of retinoblastomas are asymptomatic but noted on routine examination.

ASSESSMENT AND DIAGNOSIS

Most parents in the United States rely on the child's primary medical provider to detect eye or vision problems that need diagnostic evaluation. It is important to detect these problems early in order to provide proper intervention. Those conditions that are noncorrectable through medical or optical means must be understood, so that appropriate vision rehabilitation and educational programs can be implemented.

The priority for early visual assessment is to detect:

1. Ocular pathologies that may have life- or sight-threatening potential or that may require medical/surgical intervention. These include tumors (retinoblastoma and rhabdomyosarcoma); neurologic diseases; cranial nerve palsies; papilledema (raised intracranial pressure due to brain tumor, brain hemorrhage, or infections); and infections (toxoplasmosis, toxocariasis).
2. Visual impairment that cannot be treated but of which early detection is desirable for management and early intervention strategies.
3. Threats to binocular vision development, which includes amblyopia, strabismus, and significant refractive errors.

Vision problems of infants and children are detectable with a comprehensive vision examination. The current recommendations of both the American Academy of Optometry and the American Academy of Ophthalmology include complete eye examinations to be given to all infants at 8 months of age, followed by examination at age 2.5 to 3 years. The basic components of a vision examination include a review of the infant's medical and family history; evaluation of the alignment and binocularity of the eyes; determination of refractive error; quantification of visual capabilities including visual acuity, color vision, contrast sensitivity, depth perception, and visual fields; and assessment of the health of the eyes. The clinical examination includes discussion of findings with parents, recommendations for treatment and follow-up, and referral of the infant for early intervention service or other diagnostic tests, such as electroretiongram (ERG) to assess the health of the eyes or neuroimaging to assess the health of the central nervous system.

It is estimated that only 14% of children younger than age 6 years receive vision examinations. Vision examinations are not available to all children in the United States. Screening is an established public health strategy for the detection of people with or at risk of developing significant health problems, and is used when the signs and symptoms of those problems are not obvious. Vision screening is advocated to detect the presence or absence of general categories of vision problems and is a cost-effective way to identify unexamined children in need of further vision care. The ideal screening programs are those that use simple, noninvasive, and inexpensive tests. Guidelines for vision screening programs, including specific tests to be used, have been issued by several organizations for preschool and school-age children; however, no comparable guidelines exist for infants.

To detect ocular abnormalities and visual impairment the following combinations of screenings and clinical examinations are recommended: (a) examination of newborn; (b) screening of low-birth-weight infants for retinopathy of prematurity; (c) examination of infants and high-risk groups; (d) preschool vision screenings; and (e) school vision screenings. Any questions concerning vision should be referred to a pediatric ophthalmologist or optometrist who can provide further evaluation.

Examination of the Newborn

Examination of the eyes and adnexa of all newborn babies shortly after birth should be performed by a pediatrician or neonatologist using a direct ophthalmoscope to examine the external eye, pupillary reflexes, and the red reflex to detect obvious structural abnormalities such as microophthalmus, cataract, iris colobomas, and buphthalmos. Pupillary responses to direct illumination are present at birth in full-term infants and premature infants at the conceptual age of 30 weeks. Consensual pupillary responses are present at birth. Newborns should be able to fixate and follow a human face or high-contrast target for 30 to 60 degrees horizontally. Alignment of the eyes should be attained by 6 to 12 weeks. Any constant strabismus beyond 6 weeks should be referred. The prognosis for congenital cataract is poor unless it is detected and treated by 6 weeks of age. With early treatment, good visual acuity outcome is possible provided there are no associated ocular anomalies and there is good management of the aphakia with optical correction.

Screening of Low-Birth-Weight Infants for Retinopathy of Prematurity

Infants at risk for ROP are those born at less than 32 weeks gestation and those weighing less than 1500 g at birth. A dilated fundus examination by an ophthalmologist is recommended at 5 to 7 weeks after birth and repeated every 1 to 2 weeks until the infant has reached 36 weeks gestational age; or until there are signs of regression; or until the temporal retinal periphery is completely vascularized. Cryotherapy favorably influences the anatomic and functional outcome of stage 3+ ROP.

Examination of Infants and High-Risk Groups

Clinical vision examinations are recommended for infants at 8 months of age for high-risk groups. High-risk groups include infants and children with multiple disabilities; a difficult pre-, peri-, or postnatal course; a prenatal exposure to cigarettes, alcohol, or drugs; and a premature birth/or low birth weight. Examinations are recommended for all children born to families with genetic disease (ie, retinoblastoma, familial cataract, aniridia). Children with certain systemic diseases, when there is a high risk of eye disease, should be examined on a regular basis.

Infants and children in early services may also receive a functional vision assessment. This assessment supplements the clinical exam and is done by a low-vision specialist or a teacher of the visually impaired. A functional vision assessment is a systemic way of observing and assessing an infant's ability to use vision for certain tasks under different conditions and in both familiar and unfamiliar settings. It builds on the findings of the clinical eye examination to describe how the infant's responses vary with motivation, levels of alertness, and environmental conditions such as the time of day, lighting, and contrast conditions. It highlights the infant's areas of strength and needs in using vision as the basis for identifying priorities for learning.

Preschool Screenings

In countries with good primary health-care clinics, children with major structural abnormalities, strabismus, and/or severe visual impairment will already have been identified by 2 to 3 years of age. Identification of children with unilateral or bilateral visual impairment because of refractive errors, amblyopia, or less obvious structural abnormalities (retinal lesions, optic nerve disease, or media opacities) is problematic.

Table 5-32 lists the ages, vision disorders, and associated methods for detecting vision problems in preschoolers as recommended by six nationally recognized organizations or programs. The guidelines show a general agreement toward screening preschool children at 3 years of age and some agreement toward the targeted vision disorders (amblyopia and strabismus). One national group lists refractive error and color-vision deficits as targeted vision disorders. There is less agreement on the screening tests or methods recommended for use. Some guidelines fail to provide the referral criteria for determining the pass or fail status, and none specify the personnel eligible to screen the vision of preschool children.

In 1998, a Preschool Children's Vision Screening task force was convened to evaluate the "state of the art" of vision screening for preschool children (36 to 59 months old). This panel of experts was assembled at the request of the Maternal and Child Health Bureau in the Health Resources and Services Administration and the National Eye Institute of the National Institutes of Health. The task force concluded that there is an urgent need for large-scale, generalized studies aimed at answering basic questions about the reliability and validity of commonly used screening methods, as well as new technologies. Two components of vision screening were recommended for preschoolers: monocular distance visual acuity and stereopsis. Recommendations for the distance (3 m) visual acuity test include the HOTV, LEA, or tumbling E symbols arranged in lines on a chart. Single optotype testing was not acceptable due to the underreferral for amblyopia. Achievement of a visual acuity of 20/40 in 36- to 47-month-olds and 20/30 from 48- to 59-month-olds constituted a pass on the screening. The Random Dot E stereotest at 40 cm (630 arc sec) was also recommended for vision screening because both good ocular alignment and visual acuity is a prerequisite for stereopsis.

School Vision Screenings

Most industrialized countries have school vision-screening programs for 5- to 6-year-olds that serve adequately as a safety net to identify children with visual or refractive problems, particularly myopia.

Although a vision-screening program is worthwhile, it is a screening, not a complete vision examination of children. Cases are bound to be missed by the very nature of the vision disorders being screened, the training of the screeners, and the tests employed. Factors in screening programs such as who does the screening, the availability of local resources for the cases detected, and what tests are used, all have a significant bearing on making the vision-screening program cost-effective.

TABLE 5-32
GUIDELINES CURRENTLY RECOMMENDED FOR PRESCHOOL VISION-SCREENING PROGRAMS

PRESCHOOL VISION-SCREENING GUIDELINES			
ORGANIZATION	**AGE (Y)**	**VISION ANOMALIES**	**METHOD**
Am. Acad. of Pediatrics Am. Acad. of Ophthalmology Am. Assoc. of Pediatric Ophthalmology & Strabismus	3–5	Reduced visual acuity Ocular misalignment	Snellen letters/numbers Tumbling E HOTV Allen figures Lea symbols Unilateral cover test (3 m) Random E stereotest
American Optometric Association	2–6	Amblyopia High refractive error Ocular misalignment Color-vision deficiencies	Monocular visual acuity Patient history plus lens test Bruckner test Monocular visual acuity Bruckner/Hirschberg/CT Ishihara plates or equivalent

Prevent Blindness America	3–4	Eye health
		Reduced visual acuity
		
		Other (unspecified)
			Observation/questions
			Lea chart (at 3 m)
			Tumbling E
			HOTV
			Optional tests include cover
			    test, corneal reflex, stereop-
			    sis, plus lens test

Head Start Program	3	Reduced visual acuity Strabismus	Tumbling E (at 3 m) Cover test Hirschberg test

SOURCE: *From Ciner EB, Schmidt PP, Orel-Bixler D, et al: Vision screening of preschool children: Evaluating the past, looking toward the future. Optom Vis Sci 75:571, 1998.*

MANAGEMENT AND TREATMENT

Early identification of infants and children with ocular abnormalities and visual impairment is important. Early management of treatable conditions (cataract, glaucoma, retinopathy of prematurity, infantile esotropia) favorably influences the visual outcome. Appropriate early intervention can prevent or minimize the psychomotor developmental delay, which often accompanies visual loss of early onset.

The prevalence, negative associations, and intervention strategies for vision disorders of the preschool child are summarized in Table 5-33.

Early identification of visual impairment is important. The earlier the identification of causative factors of visual impairment, the better the prognosis for any therapeutic interventions. The infant's visual system is still developing, and reversal of amblyogenic factors may prevent the occurrence of visual deficits before they become embedded. Parents can provide toys and visual stimulation to match the infant's visual abilities and participate actively in enabling their infant's optimal visual development.

It is generally recognized that there are developmental periods for amblyopia. In the critical period from birth to 6 months, amblyopia requires aggressive treatment, otherwise the infant runs the risk of remaining legally blind. In the sensitive period from 6 months to 8 years, amblyopia requires aggressive treatment, otherwise the outcome is visual impairment. Some clinicians note that this also represents the upper age limit for the development of amblyopia.

Does amblyopia treatment make a difference in the life of a patient? Both adults and children with amblyopia have a 6 to 16 times greater risk, respectively, of losing their fellow eye to trauma than does the general population. There is strong consensus among clinicians that both screening for and treatment of amblyopia are worthwhile. The number of children requiring screening is considerable. Furthermore, the treatment process for anisometropia and strabismus does not appear to cause long-lasting psychological harm to children or their families.

Strabismus usually develops in infancy or early childhood. Esotropia is three times as frequent as exotropia, and infantile esotropia is the most common form of strabismus, accounting for 28 to 48% of all individuals with esotropia. The prognosis for accommodative esotropia is good provided the child is given glasses before the strabismus becomes constant. Single binocular vision with bifixation can be permanently lost after 2 to 3 months of nonuse. It is important that the evaluation not be delayed after onset of strabismus even if the deviation initially presents as intermittent.

Left untreated, strabismus commonly results in amblyopia and impaired binocularity, or both. Strabismus may result in delayed developmental milestones within the first 2 years of life, and may have a negative impact on the parent–child relationship and the child's psychological development. Strabismus that is cosmetically displeasing can have adverse effects on a person's self-image, interpersonal relationships, schooling, work, and sports activities.

Because normal vision from birth is necessary for proper eye development, failure to treat amblyopia and strabismus before school age may later result in irreversible visual deficits, permanent amblyopia, loss of depth perception and binocularity, cosmetic defects, and educational and occupational restrictions.

The diagnosis, management, and treatment of vision disorders is the primary responsibility of eye-care professionals (pediatric ophthalmologists). Promotion of adaptive behavior is the pediatrician's responsibility.

Severe visual impairment frequently places an infant at a disadvantage beginning at birth. Lack of early eye contact can retard the bonding that is necessary between mother and infant. Some parents react negatively to lack of eye contact, thereby setting up a cycle of reinforcement that may retard the development of an adequate and meaningful relationship between parent and child. The relationship with siblings is affected because the visually impaired child requires more of a parent's attention and the child does not meet expectations of being a companion.

Opportunities to satisfy the basic need for movement and activity must be provided from earliest infancy, otherwise the child will gain his or her satisfaction from seemingly aimless physical activities or stereotypic behaviors, which are sometimes referred to as blindisms. The most common behaviors include eye pressing, eye poking, body rocking, head swaying, and head banging. Most of these behaviors have been observed in other disabled children. They are characterized as being repetitive and not directed toward the attainment of any specific goal. Eye poking is a social problem because it causes negative feelings even in caregivers and may lead to

TABLE 5-33
PREVALENT CHILDHOOD VISION DISORDERS

VISION DISORDER	PREVALENCE	NEGATIVE ASSOCIATION	INTERVENTION STRATEGIES
Amblyopia	2–3%	Visual impairment	Patching
		Loss of stereopsis	Spectacles
		Occupational limitations	Vision therapy
Strabismus	3–4%	Amblyopia, cosmesis	Spectacles, prism
		Binocular dysfunction	Surgery
		Occupational limitations	Vision therapy
Refractive errors	15–30%	Amblyopia, loss of stereopsis	Spectacles
		Binocular dysfunction	Contact lenses
		Decreased reading abilities	
Ocular Disease	<1%	Visual impairment	Low-vision devices
		Illness/loss of life	Medical/surgical
			Rehabilitation services
Color-vision deficits	4–5%	Loss of learning potential	Education
		Occupational limitations	

SOURCE: *Adapted from Ciner EB, Schmidt PP, Orel-Bixler D, et al: Vision screening of preschool children: Evaluating the past, looking toward the future. Optom Vis Sci 75:571, 1998.*

further vision loss due to retinal detachments. Eye pressing leads to atrophy of orbital rim bone and fat tissue, and the eyes become sunken in appearance.

Intervention must begin in early infancy with providing substitutes for visual tracking. For the blind child, knowledge of the object world comes primarily through tactile channels, and only secondarily through auditory channels. Thus, to make use of sound as a motivation for reaching and grasping, the child must first have attached a meaning to that sound, and second be interested in the object with the sound. The hands, mouth, feet (all parts of the body) should be used to explore and learn about the object world. Activities that require the use of fine hand coordination, manipulation blocks, and beads are essential if the child is to be successful in those school tasks that require that skill such as Braille reading and writing. Children who lose their vision after age 5 years may have greater difficulty becoming tactile rather than visual learners; may evidence accompanying difficulty becoming tactile rather than visual learners; and may evidence accompanying emotional reactions to their loss of vision. Teachers and parents must be sensitive to potential educational and emotional effects that the time of onset might have on development and behavior.

Intervention during the early school years should include activities that continue to develop fine hand coordination and the ability to move about in the environment with freedom and ease, as well as direct teaching of the skills that are usually acquired through imitative learning. Early work in these areas will facilitate the later work of the orientation and mobility instructor in developing the child's social skills.

Children with vision impairment often need services such as special education programs to assist in their development. In the 1995–96 school year, costs for these programs for visually impaired children exceeded $145 million. Computers and low-vision optical and video aids enable many partially sighted, low vision, and blind children to participate in regular class activities. Educational materials are available through large-print books, books on tape, and Braille books.

Students with visual impairments may need additional help with special equipment and modifications in the regular curriculum to emphasize listening skills, communication, orientation and mobility, vocation/career options, and daily living skills. Students with low vision or who are legally blind may need help using their residual vision more efficiently and may need help working with special aids and materials. Students who have visual impairment combined with other types of disabilities have a greater need for an interdisciplinary approach and may require greater emphasis on self-care and daily living skills.

Schools for the blind concentrate teaching resources on dealing with issues such as maximum use of remaining vision, special technology providing education means (closed circuit televisions), and practical vocational counseling. These schools also make an effort to allow contact with sighted peers and to encourage incorporation of the blind child into the sighted society.

It is estimated that 50% of all cases of childhood blindness are avoidable through the provision of preventative services at the community level, specialized surgical services in pediatric ophthalmology units, and provision of low-vision devices and services to those children with established visual loss.

SUMMARY

The first 3 years of life are the most critical years in every child's development. Recognition of their significance has resulted in fed-

eral legislation that mandates early intervention services for infants who have disabilities and for their families. The primary purpose of early intervention services is to support families in enhancing their infants' development and to ensure optimal outcomes for these children. When infants are diagnosed with visual impairments and additional disabilities, early intervention services are even more critical in promoting optimal developmental outcomes for them. The term *early intervention* refers to the comprehensive system of multidisciplinary services from the fields of education, medicine, mental health, and social welfare that are provided to infants who have disabilities and to their families.

Habilitation of visually impaired infants and children is mostly the domain of pediatrics and special education. Pediatric ophthalmologists and optometrists have an important role in the team. They provide information as to the role of optical factors; accommodation; problems related to corrective lenses; structural changes in the eyes and binocularity; and can measure visual function and provide guidance for the team. Together, they should interpret clinical findings and give a report that answers questions related to the role of vision in each developmental area: communication, motor functions, spatial concepts, exploration, and incidental learning. Visually impaired infants are cases of developmental emergency. The need for habilitation does not decrease with age; it only changes in content to fit the needs of the child at each different stage of development.

The effective pediatrician listens to what parents say, provides information about the child's condition, assures the availability of appropriate services and resources, and assists parents in advocating for their child's needs by coordinating the diagnostic and educational process.

References

American Foundation for the Blind: Internet http://www.afb.org/services.asp

Chen D: Essential Elements in Early Intervention: Visual Impairment and Multiple Disabilities. New York, American Foundation for the Blind Press, 1999

Ciner EB, Schmidt PP, Orel-Bixler D, et al: Vision screening of preschool children; evaluating the past, looking toward the future. Optom Vis Sci 75:571–584, 1998

Ferrel KA: Infancy and early childhood. In: Scholl GT, ed: Foundations of Education for Blind and Visually Handicapped Children and Youth. New York, American Foundation for the Blind Press, 1986:119–144

Foster A, Gilbert C: Epidemiology of visual impairment in children. In: Taylor D, ed: Pediatric Ophthalmology. Osney Mead, Oxford, Blackwell Science, 1997:3–12

Fraiberg S: Insights from the Blind Comparative Studies of Blind and Sighted Infants. New York, Basic Books, 1977

Good WV, Jan JE, De Sa L, Barkovich J, Groenveld M, Hoyt CS: Cortical visual impairment in children. Surv Ophthalmol 38:351–364, 1994

Huo R, Burden SK, Hoyt CS, Good WV: Chronic cortical visual impairment in children: etiology, prognosis, and associated neurological deficits. Br J Ophthalmol 83(6):670–675, 1999

Hyvarinen L, Lindstedt E, eds: Early visual development—normal and abnormal. Acta Ophthalmol (Copenh) (Suppl. 157):1–122, 1983

Isenberg SJ: The Eye in Infancy. St. Louis, MO, Mosby Year Book, 1994

Jan JE, Freeman RD, Scott EP, eds: Visual Impairment in Children and Adolescents. New York, Grune and Stratton, 1997

Maino D, ed: Diagnosis and Management of Special Populations. St. Louis, MO, Mosby-Year Book, 1995

Moore BD: The epidemiology of ocular disorders in young children. In: Moore B, ed: Eye Care of the Infant and Young Child. Newton, MA, Butterworth-Heinemann, 1997:21–27

Orel-Bixler D: Clinical vision assessments for infants. In: Chen D, ed: Essential Elements in Early Intervention: Visual Impairment and Multiple Disabilities. New York, American Foundation for the Blind Press, 1999: 105–156

Steinkuller PG, Du L, Gilbert C, Foster A, Collins ML, Coats DK: Childhood blindness. J Am Acad Pediatr Ophthalmol Strabismus 3(1):26–32, 1999

Vision screening in the preschool child. Proceedings of a conference held in Bethesda, Maryland, September 10–11, 1998. Copies available at no charge from: National Maternal and Child Health Clearinghouse 8201 Greensboro Drive, Suite 600 McLean, VA 22102.

Templin SW: Visual impairment in infants and young children. Infants Young Child 8(1):18–51, 1995

Warren DH: Blindness and Children. An Individual Differences Approach. New York, Cambridge University Press, 1994

World Health Organization: Manual of the International Statistical Classification of Disease, Injuries, and Causes of Death, vol. 1. Geneva, WHO, 1977

5.7   MAJOR PSYCHOPATHOLOGIC DISORDERS

5.7.1   Autistic Disorder and Other Pervasive Developmental Disorders

Glen R. Elliott

In the mid-1940s, Kanner described a group of children with a distinctive combination of dysfunctions that include poor or absent communication, marked impairment in social interactions, and an array of odd behaviors. The notable inability of these children to develop social relationships with people, whether adults or peers, led Kanner to suggest the term *infantile autism.* Subsequent studies clarified key clinical aspects of autism, and childhood disorders with similar features are clustered under the broader term *pervasive developmental disorders* (PDDs). The current definition of autistic disorder (AD), as set forth in *DSM-IV,* still incorporates the major elements of Kanner's initial description.

DESCRIPTION AND EPIDEMIOLOGY

DSM-IV defines PDDs as a cluster of syndromes that share marked abnormalities in the development of both social and communicative skills (Table 5-34). Mental retardation is a common comorbid condition with most of these disorders, but specific delays in social skills and communication must be worse than expected for the mental age of the child and can occur even in individuals with normal or superior intelligence.

AD is by far the most common and best studied of the PDDs. In *DSM-IV,* the diagnosis is made based on 12 criteria divided

TABLE 5-34
PERVASIVE DEVELOPMENTAL DISORDERS

Autistic disorder
Rett disorder
Childhood disintegrative disorder
Asperger disorder
Pervasive developmental disorder not otherwise specified

equally within 3 broad domains of impairment: (a) social interaction; (b) verbal and nonverbal communication; and (c) behaviors and activities. For most children with AD, problems begin quite early, often from birth; in fact, *DSM-IV* requires that a delay must have occurred before 3 years of age in the development of social interaction, use of language for social purposes, or imaginative and symbolic play. In addition, the patient must meet at least two criteria that relate to problems in social interaction and at least one criterion in each of the other two domains, and qualify for at least six criteria across all three domains.

Children with Rett syndrome may have many of the same signs and symptoms as children with AD. Early development, up to at least 5 months of age, typically appears to be normal. After 5 months of age, however, head growth decelerates, hand skills are lost, stereotyped handwringing movements appear, gait and trunk movements become poorly coordinated, and language development becomes severely impaired. This disorder has been described almost exclusively in females (see Sec. 25.6.3).

Childhood disintegrative disorder is a relatively old syndrome that has been resurrected in the past decade. It is notable mainly for seemingly normal development through the first 2 years, with the appearance by at least age 10 of marked loss of at least two of the following: (a) language; (b) social skills and adaptive behavior; (c) bowel or bladder control; (d) play; or (e) motor skills. The result is a clinical picture much like AD.

Asperger syndrome is the most recent addition to the PDDs. It shares with AD a severe and pervasive impairment in social interaction, as well as restricted, repetitive, and stereotyped behaviors. However, these problems occur without any general delays in language skills and in cognitive development. Problems with physical coordination are common but are not part of the diagnostic criteria.

Finally, pervasive developmental disorder not otherwise specified describes children with problems in reciprocal interaction and communication who do not meet the criteria of other PDD diagnoses.

Epidemiologic data on the PDDs is improving and has been a major source of concern during the late 1990s because of some evidence suggesting that the prevalence of these disorders may be on the rise. AD remains by far the most commonly diagnosed of the PDDs, although Asperger syndrome is diagnosed with increasing frequency. The best available evidence suggests a prevalence rate for all PDDs of 5 to 7 per 10,000 people, with studies done during the 1990s showing consistently higher rates than did earlier studies. Except for Rett syndrome, the PDDs are much more common in males; the male to female ratio for AD is about 4:1. There does not appear to be notable shifts in either prevalence or gender ratios across ethnicity or geographic settings.

ETIOLOGY

Despite considerable investigative effort over the past 50 years, the cause(s) of AD and other PDDs remains unknown. An early focus on parenting styles or other early experiential factors has largely given way to a search for biological causes. Convincing evidence exists to suggest a genetic contribution to at least some cases of AD and Asperger syndrome, especially among individuals with spared cognitive function. Monozygotic twins have a high concordance for AD, and other siblings also have a slightly increased risk. Furthermore, the PDDs all share the following risk-augmenting factors: (a) pre- and perinatal birth complications; (b) prenatal infections with certain viruses, especially rubella and cytomegalovirus;

and (c) abnormalities on computed tomography or magnetic resonance imaging. However, no specific defects in brain structure have emerged, as yet, nor have neuropathologic studies identified consistent patterns on autopsy. One uniform unexplained finding is that about one-third of individuals with AD have relatively high concentrations of platelet serotonin, as is true also for a similar proportion of individuals with mental retardation who do not have AD. For neither group is there a hypothesis linking the finding to the disorder, and mental retardation is not the common factor. Hypotheses that some AD might result either from problems with intestinal absorption or as an adverse reaction of immunizations during the first few years of life are of great interest to the general public but have yet to receive substantive research support.

ASSESSMENT, DIAGNOSIS, AND EVALUATION

Diagnosing AD or other PDDs has two elements: (a) ruling out other possible causes of the presenting problems and (b) identifying disorders that are known to increase the risk of having AD. Table 5-35 lists diagnoses that are often confused with PDDs because of similar signs and symptoms.

For younger children, the most common cause of diagnostic confusion is mental retardation. All criteria for AD and other PDDs are based on the child's estimated mental age. For example, regardless of the chronologic age, a child with a mental age of 2 years or less is not apt to be able to display consistent peer friendships. One important distinction between AD and expressive language disorders is the relative absence in AD of communicative intent or drive. Children with AD often display a remarkable lack of interest in using even the language that is available to them. Concerns about possible hearing problems is a common presenting complaint for children below age 3 years who subsequently prove to have AD or another PDD; indeed, children with PDD do have a high incidence of unsuspected ear infections and may merit closer clinical monitoring for such infections, because they often fail to show typical signs and symptoms. However, successful treatment of ear infections seldom results in a marked or sustained increase of verbal productions and comprehension in children with AD. Children with selective mutism typically have had normal language that disappears with an external stressor; their social interactions are generally normal.

In older children, the major diagnostic dilemma is correctly identifying Asperger syndrome and AD in individuals with average

TABLE 5-35
KEY DIFFERENTIAL DIAGNOSES FOR PERVASIVE DEVELOPMENTAL DISORDERS

Infants and Toddlers
  Mental retardation, especially fragile X syndrome
  Expressive and receptive language disorders
  Deafness
  Selective mutism
Latency Age—Children and Adolescents
  Anxiety disorders
  Attention-deficit hyperactivity disorder
  Nonverbal learning disability
  Obsessive compulsive disorder
  Tourette syndrome
  Schizophrenia
  Schizoid personality disorder

or superior cognitive function. For example, children with ADHD may have poor nonverbal skills and may fail to develop appropriate peer friendships, but they do not have the bizarre or unusual preoccupations or the consistent inability to engage socially and emotionally that characterizes Asperger syndrome or AD. Children with Tourette syndrome or obsessive compulsive disorder may have odd behaviors, but their ability to interact with others is unimpaired. Schizoid personality disorder produces less-severe impairment in socialization and is not accompanied with the bizarre behaviors or preoccupations typical of Asperger syndrome and AD. Schizophrenia requires the presence of hallucinations or delusions, as well as marked impairments in reality testing. Although its prodromal phase may include social isolation, schizophrenia does not impair language development or early socialization skills, nor do the PDDs produce a clear disturbance in reality testing.

AD and related disorders remain purely clinical diagnoses; no specific laboratory tests yet exist to aid in making the diagnosis. However, there are a variety of associated disorders for which testing may be useful. For example, encephalitis, phenylketonuria, tuberous sclerosis, maternal rubella, and fragile X syndrome are all reported to increase the risk of AD. Evaluation of a child with possible AD should include a detailed family history; developmental and behavioral history; physical and neurologic examination; and formal testing of cognitive and functional abilities. Depending on the findings, additional testing may be indicated, including urine and blood samples for genetic screening and chromosomal examination, as well as audiologic testing. EEG, magnetic resonance imaging, or computed tomography are appropriate only if the clinical picture is suggestive of seizures, which may be present by adolescence in up to one-third of children with AD.

MANAGEMENT AND TREATMENT

Home and school are the primary sites for managing children with AD and other PDDs. Especially for children under 5 years of age, the major focus should be to foster and enhance effective communication and establish good behavioral control.

Communication approaches must be tailored to the child's mental age and existing abilities. Children with AD differ from those with other forms of language disabilities in several important ways. First, they are much less likely to learn passively; teaching usually requires one-on-one interaction with heavy use of primary rewards, such as food, as motivators. Second, they may have a low communicative drive, resorting to efforts to communicate only when forced to do so. Third, they do not generalize readily; new principles must be taught in small increments, with much repetition. Many teachers use a "total communication" approach that includes a range of techniques such as symbols, sign, and spoken language; they then capitalize on whatever avenues of communication seem to work for a particular child.

Behavior modification programs can be exceedingly helpful with these children, and parents need to become expert in applying such principles to their child. Parent self-help books can be enormously valuable, as can targeted consultations with behavior experts. The major principles are: (a) identify a manageable problem; (b) find a reward that works for that child, usually food in the case of young children; and (c) try to modify the behavior both consistently and repeatedly. Parents are likely to be particularly frustrated around issues of punishment for bad behavior, toilet training, and inappropriate behaviors in public. These, and many more problems, can respond to good behavioral programs. A behavior program called

Discrete Trial Learning, developed by Ivar Lovaas, sometimes seems to help improve the long-term prognosis of individuals with AD. It probably needs to be applied before age 3 years, and seems most apt to be of help with children who have normal cognitive functioning who are especially resistant to direction from adults.

Existing medications do not alter the course of PDDs, although many families try a variety of nonprescription medications, with or without their doctor's blessing. Traditional preparations to which parents resort include vitamin B_6 plus magnesium and dimethylglycine. In the late 1990s, Secretin was added to that list. In general, such interventions seem to carry minimal risk, but efforts to show benefit in well-designed studies have been uniformly unimpressive.

From one-third to one-half of individuals with AD may need medication for a behavior that is dangerous to themselves or others or that interferes with their ability to function (Table 5-36). For prepubertal children, the most common problems that lead to medication use are excessive physical activity and poor attention. A diagnosis of AD formally precludes a diagnosis of ADHD, and it is important to determine whether a child is "inattentive" because of mental age or lack of motivation. Even so, a small subgroup of children with AD may have symptoms of inattention and hyperactivity that respond well to stimulants. For most, low doses of a high-potency antipsychotic agent seem to be more effective in reducing overall activity levels, disruptive stereotypes, and poor attention. Such drugs also can produce mild benefits in social relatedness and school functioning. For unclear reasons, many children with AD are highly sensitive to the side effects of such drugs, leading to the general dictum, "start low and go slow."

Especially as children enter adolescence, intermittent assaultive behavior may become more of a problem, either because of the onset of puberty or simply because of their greater size. Again, antipsychotics are the conventional treatment of first choice, although anticonvulsants and lithium also are used at times. No systematic studies exist to help clinicians choose among these options for a particular patient. Compelling evidence does exist that children and adolescents with PDD can have concurrent symptoms of anxiety, depression, obsessions, or compulsions; when such comorbid conditions occur, they seem to respond well to pharmacologic interventions typically used for those disorders.

NATURAL HISTORY AND PROGNOSIS

Developmental studies of children with AD have all been retrospective. Typically, parents report that they first developed concerns about their child's development relatively early, often from birth and almost always by 18 to 24 months of age. As many as one-third of children with AD reportedly have normal language from 12 to 18 months, which language then fails to progress or even disappears completely. A large proportion of children with AD receive an initial diagnosis of "developmental delay," which may not be refined until 4 to 5 years of age or even later. However, most children with AD and other PDDs can be diagnosed unambiguously much earlier than that, and the studies of the benefits of early intervention, especially in enhancing communication skills, underscores the importance of early, careful assessments when language and social development clearly are not progressing smoothly.

All of the PDDs carry a poor prognosis. Except for Asperger syndrome, all are associated with a high incidence of mental retardation, usually in the mild to severe range. Rett syndrome appears to be a degenerative neurologic process, although the majority of individuals with this diagnosis live into adulthood; childhood disintegrative disorder also has many of the features of a degenerative process. At most, 1 to 2% of individuals with AD go on to be "normal" as adults; the rest will have marked impairments that typically cause them to function at roughly one level of mental retardation worse than their formal testing would suggest. Thus, a child with AD and mild mental retardation usually functions more like someone with moderate mental retardation. Overall, at least two-thirds of children with PDD will require high levels of supervision and structural support throughout their lives.

At present, not enough is known about the causes of AD and other PDDs to comment meaningfully on their prevention. It is important to inform parents with one AD child that they have a somewhat higher risk of having a second AD child, although the actual risk of most couples probably is relatively slight. Possibly more important are the associated genetic disorders such as fragile X, for which good screening tests are available. More promising are efforts of secondary prevention to minimize unnecessary disability through the early diagnosis of AD, thus enabling parents to obtain appropriate placements for their child during the key educational years of 3 to 6. Early diagnosis may ensure that such children have the best possible opportunity to learn to communicate and develop appropriate behavioral control, two key factors in determining their ability to function later in life.

TABLE 5-36

COMMON BEHAVIORS IN CHILDREN WITH PERVASIVE DEVELOPMENTAL DISORDERS THAT MEDICATIONS MAY ALLEVIATE

DISORDER	MEDICATION
Uncontrollable motor activity, including perseverations	Antipsychotics (eg, risperidone, olanzapine, haloperidol, or thioridazine)
Severe, ongoing self-abuse	Anticonvulsants (eg, carbamazepine, valproic acid, gabapentin)
Persistent assaultiveness	Lithium
Mental-age inappropriate hyperactivity and inattention	Stimulants (eg, methylphenidate, amphetamine)
	Alpha-adrenergic agonists (eg, clonidine, guanfacine)
	Tricyclic antidepressants (eg, imipramine)
Markedly disturbed sleep with sleep refusal, frequent awakenings, or early awakenings	Trazodone, mirtazapine, tricyclic antidepressants (especially imipramine or clomipramine)
Persistent, severe anxiety	Buspirone, tricyclic antidepressants
Repetitive, obsessive, or compulsive behaviors	Selective serotonin reuptake inhibitors (eg, citalopram, clomipramine, fluoxetine, fluvoxamine, paroxetine, sertraline)
Seizures	Anticonvulsants (eg, carbamazepine, gabapentin, valproic acid)

References

American Psychiatric Association: Diagnostic and Statistical Manual of Mental Disorders, 4th ed. Washington, DC, Author, 1994

Ellaway C, Christodoulou J: Rett syndrome; clinical update and review of recent genetic advances. J Paediatr Child Health 35:419, 1999

Fombonnie E: The epidemiology of autism: a review. Psychol Med 29:769, 1999

Kanner L: Autistic disturbances of affective contact. J Nerv Child 2:217, 1943

Malhotra S, Gupta N: Childhood disintegrative disorder. J Autism Devel Disord 29:491, 1999

Siegel B: The World of the Autistic Child: Understanding and Treating Autistic Spectrum Disorders. New York, Oxford University Press, 1996

Smith T, Eikeseth S, Klevstrand M, Lovaas OI: Intensive behavioral treatment for preschoolers with severe mental retardation and pervasive developmental disorder. Am J Ment Retard 102:238, 1997

Trottier G, Srivastava L, Walker CD: Etiology of infantile autism; a review of recent advances in genetic and neurobiological research. J Psychiatry Neurosci 24:103, 1999

Tsai LY: Psychopharmacology in autism. Psychosom Med 61:651, 1999

Volkmar FR, ed: Autism and Pervasive Developmental Disorders. New York, Cambridge University Press, 1998

5.7.2   Affective Disorders and Suicide

Ronald E. Dahl and David Brent

Some experiences of sadness or depressed mood arise during the course of most children's lives. However, there has been increasing recognition that some children and adolescents suffer from serious and pervasive disorders of mood regulation and that these disorders are associated with significant morbidity (ie, impairment in psychosocial function) and mortality (ie, suicide). Consequently, the critical clinical task is to differentiate the serious disorders from the larger spectrum of children and adolescents with some symptoms of sadness or grief. Because our understanding of the pathophysiology of emotional dysregulation is just emerging, diagnosis of major depressive disorders can be clinically challenging and relies entirely on clinical history and mental status. There currently are no reliable tests to assist or to confirm a diagnosis. Judgments must be based on the best available data from clinical studies, epidemiologic research, and careful observations of longitudinal course.

DEFINITION AND EPIDEMIOLOGY

Currently, depressive illnesses are classified into three broad categories:

1. *Major Depressive Disorder:* Requires at least 2 weeks of sad, bored, or irritable mood at least 50% of the time as well as an additional four depressive symptoms. Table 5-37 lists the symptoms of major depressive disorders. In contrast, adjustment disorder with depressed mood is a milder and relatively brief disturbance following a serious life stressor.

2. *Dysthymic Disorder:* A more chronic disorder of depressed and irritable mood with at least three other symptoms that have been present for at least 1 year without evidence of specific major depressive episodes.

3. *Bipolar Affective Illness or Cyclothymic Disorder:* Involves periods of depressed mood with alternating periods of mania or hypomania (eg, significant elevation of mood, increased energy, decreased need for sleep, pressured speech, associated symptomatology).

Major affective illnesses are relatively uncommon before puberty. Estimates of the point prevalence of major depression are approximately 1.5 to 2.5% in prepubertal children, increasing to 4

TABLE 5-37

MAJOR DEPRESSIVE DISORDER

Major Symptoms:
  Depressed mood (in children and adolescents, can be irritable mood)
  Diminished interest
Additional Symptoms May Include:
  Significant weight loss or weight gain
  Decrease or increase in appetite
  Insomnia or hypersomnia
  Psychomotor agitation or retardation
  Fatigue or loss of energy
  Feelings of worthlessness
  Excessive or inappropriate guilt
  Diminished ability to think or concentrate
  Recurrent thoughts of death

to 5% during adolescence. Bipolar affective illness is estimated at a point prevalence of 0.2 to 0.4% among prepubertal children, increasing to approximately 1% among adolescents. Depressive illnesses do not show gender differences in children; however, at puberty, there is a significant increase in major depression among females, resulting in a female-to-male ratio of 2:1 during adolescence, a gender difference that endures throughout the adult life span. Bipolar disorders are equally common in males and females across the life cycle.

ETIOLOGY AND PATHOGENESIS

Most etiologic models of early onset depression focus on the interactions between individual vulnerabilities and adverse life events. The central question is: Why do some children grow up amidst chronic adverse conditions with no signs of significant mood disturbances, while others develop severe affective illnesses following relatively mild difficulties? Although many types of emotional trauma have been associated with the early onset of depressive disorders (eg, physical and sexual abuse, loss of a parent, loss of a sibling or close friend), the single most important risk factor associated with development of an early depressive illness is having at least one depressed parent. Increased risk for early onset depression is associated with greater familial loading for depression, early age at onset of depression in the parent, family history of either bipolar affective illness or recurrent unipolar depression, and major affective illness present in three generations. The best evidence suggests that parental depression contributes to illness in their children through both genetic and shared environmental sources of transmissions, including disruption of the parental role, decreased family support, and increased parent–child discord. Parent–child discord has been shown to be significantly worse in families of depressed children when compared with those of nondepressed control children. Studies also provide evidence that is consistent with a genetic component to affective illness. Physiological changes associated with early onset depression include abnormalities of growth hormone regulation and abnormalities in CNS serotonergic function. Some of these abnormalities have been found in nondepressed children who have very high rates of affective illnesses on both sides of the family, suggesting that these changes may represent a vulnerability trait for major depressive disorder. Other psychobiological changes seen in adult depression, including EEG sleep and cortisol abnormalities, appear to be relatively infrequent in young depressed subjects.

Child and adolescent depression also have been associated with the use of medications including antihypertensive agents, glucocorticoids, and phenobarbital. Similarly, depression has been associated with certain chronic illnesses including epilepsy, inflammatory bowel disease, and juvenile onset diabetes.

CLINICAL MANIFESTATIONS

Typically, depressed children show periods of disturbed mood that are often accompanied by somatic complaints; decreased school performance; apathy and loss of interest; social withdrawal; increased irritability; and sleep and appetite changes. They may sometimes demonstrate suicidal ideation or behavior. Among adolescents, depressive illnesses frequently are associated with tobacco, alcohol, or substance use; promiscuous sexual behavior; and risk-taking behavior. Depression often may follow severe stressors such as physical or sexual assault and bereavement, particularly if the child or adolescent has a personal or family history of depression. A family history increases the risk of depressive disorders at least threefold. *Depressed mood in children and adolescents can present as sadness, irritability, or boredom.* Depressed children also are likely to have somatic complaints and may present with psychotic features related to their mood disorder (ie, delusions of worthlessness, hopelessness, sin, or guilt; self-deprecatory or auditory hallucinations; paranoid ideation). Anxiety symptoms and behavioral problems also are more frequent among children with major depression. Evidence from one longitudinal study suggests that anxiety disorders often *antedate* depressive symptomatology, whereas conduct symptoms generally follow an affective illness.

An episode of mania indicates a bipolar affective disorder and is usually characterized by euphoria or grandiosity (ie, an unrealistic sense of being grand, powerful, or famous). It can be associated with anger and irritability as well. Mania can be differentiated from attention-deficit hyperactivity disorder (ADHD) insofar as mania is much more likely to be associated with increased energy, increased sexuality, euphoria, and grandiosity. Clinically, it can be quite difficult to detect mania or hypomania in younger children; however, in severe forms, the children and adolescents with mania can display bizarre behaviors such as leaping from a building with the belief that one can fly. More typically, young adolescents during manic episodes show periods of prolonged excitation, euphoria, rapid speech, grandiosity, sensation seeking, and promiscuous sexual behavior. When children and adolescents with bipolar disorder are depressed, they often present as anergic (ie, low energy and slow), hypersomnic, and psychotic.

ASSESSMENT AND DIAGNOSIS

Any persistent disturbance of mood that is associated with functional impairment (ie, deterioration of school or social function) should raise the suspicion of a major depressive disorder. Both the child and parents are likely to contribute important information to be used in the diagnosis of depression. The child is a more accurate reporter for symptoms of internal state, including depressed mood, guilt, worthlessness, and suicidal thoughts; the parents most often note externally validated symptoms such as irritability, decline in school performance, and withdrawal from social and other pleasurable activities. Affective illness in children often is associated with moods not only described as sad but also with other pervasive negative moods such as "grouchy, mad, or bored."

The primary goals of clinical assessment are to determine (a) the presence of symptoms of mood disorder, (b) the extent that these symptoms are interfering with school or social functions, and (c) the potential for suicidal risk. Definitive diagnosis of child and adolescent depression usually is best achieved by structured or semi-

structured diagnostic interviews. The two most extensively examined instruments are the Schedule for Affective Disorders in Schizophrenia for School-Aged Children (K-SADS) and the Diagnostic Interview Schedule for Children (DISC). Structured interviews typically include information from both the child and the parent, with specific rules for combining information from the two sources. Rigorous criteria for making the diagnosis are established, including reliability and validity data for these instruments. Self-report screens for depressive disorder include the Children's Depression Inventory (CDI) for 8- to 13-year-olds, and the Beck Depression Inventory for older adolescents.

MANAGEMENT AND TREATMENT

The most common mood problems among children and adolescents typically represent depressive symptoms that are associated with an adjustment disorder revolving around specific stressors, family discord, school failure, or difficulty with peers. Often, such difficulties will respond to a few sessions of supportive counseling, with the pediatrician and adolescent working together to focus on problem identification and strategies to manage specific problems and stressors. If family discord appears to be prominent, problem-solving interventions should involve the entire family.

Children and adolescents with a severe mood disorder are probably best managed by a child psychiatrist with clinical expertise in this area. Psychiatric intervention typically includes three components: (a) psychoeducation, (b) psychotherapy, and (c) pharmacotherapy. Family psychoeducation is designed to improve compliance, to reduce tensions of living with an affectively ill patient, and to sensitize the family to recognizing early signs for recurrence of the disorder. In addition, the assessment of suicide risk and, when indicated, the achievement of a "no-suicide contract" with the patient and family are critical aspects of family psychoeducation. Psychotherapy should be aimed at ameliorating interpersonal and social deficits that are associated with depressive symptoms. Clinical trials have demonstrated the efficacy of cognitive-behavior therapy (CBT) and interpersonal therapy (IPT) for child and adolescent depression. In CBT, treatment focuses on correcting maladaptive and negative thinking patterns that predispose to and reinforce depression, whereas IPT focuses on improving interpersonal interactions that may be related to depressive experiences. Between 25 and 40% of children will fail to respond to psychotherapy and may require pharmacotherapy. Pharmacotherapy with selective serotonin reuptake inhibitors (SSRIs) is increasingly becoming the first-line treatment for early onset depression. Clinical trials have established the efficacy of SSRIs relative to both placebo and to tricyclic antidepressants, which do *not* appear to be efficacious for early onset depression and should not be used as first-line agents. Treatment should be continued for at least 6 months to minimize the probability of relapse. Bipolar disorder requires prophylaxis with a mood-stabilizing agent, either lithium or an anticonvulsant such as valproic acid or carbamazepine.

Most patients who are affectively ill can be managed outside the hospital. Inpatient psychiatric referrals should be considered for those who are psychotic, acutely suicidal, manic, abusing substances, or refractory to outpatient treatment.

NATURAL HISTORY AND PROGNOSIS

Naturalistic studies indicate that when untreated, major depressive disorders in children and adolescents typically last from 7 to 12 months. Longitudinal studies reveal that most children with serious major depressive disorders in childhood and adolescence go on to have recurrent episodes of depression, with persistent social impairment between episodes. The risk of both suicide attempts and completed suicides is markedly increased in early onset depression.

Suicide and Suicidal Behavior

Among adolescents from 15 to 19 years of age, the rate of suicide in 1997 was 9.5 per 100,000 in the United States. This rate is 3.5 times higher than the 2.7 per 100,000 cases in 1950, but it is not significantly elevated over the rate of 8.5 per 100,000 in 1980. In addition to completed suicides, suicidal behavior has also become increasingly common. Data from 1990 indicate that 4% of high school students made a suicidal attempt within the previous 12 months, and 8% made some suicidal attempt during their lifetime. Only a fraction of adolescent suicide attempts ever come to medical attention. Although suicide attempts appear to be twice as frequent among female adolescents, completed suicide rates are four times higher among 15- to 19-year-old males when compared to females in this age range. Completed suicide is relatively rare among prepubertal children. Suicidal ideation is commonly associated with major depressive disorders in children, and the risk for suicide among depressed children should not be taken lightly. Approximately 50% of completed suicides occur following previous suicidal threats or attempts. Precipitants for suicidal behavior are frequent interpersonal conflict, interpersonal loss, physical or sexual abuse, and legal or disciplinary problems. The most common method of suicide among adolescents in the United States is firearms, followed by hanging, jumping, carbon monoxide, and self-poisoning. By contrast, suicide attempters (ie, those not completing suicide) most frequently use self-poisoning, followed by cutting their wrists.

Identification of Youth at Risk for Suicide

Studies have established that the following factors place adolescents at risk for suicide:

- Psychiatric difficulties, including depression, substance abuse, conduct problems, psychosis, or past suicidal threats or attempts;
- Poor social adjustment, including school failure, legal problems, and social isolation with severe interpersonal conflicts;
- Severe family or environmental discord;
- Family history of psychiatric disorder or suicide;
- Significant interpersonal loss, abuse, or neglect; and
- The availability of firearms in the home.

There is also growing evidence that a homosexual or bisexual orientation is a risk factor for suicidal behavior in males.

Any child who is suspected of being at risk should be directly questioned concerning suicidal ideation, moving from nonspecific to more specific questions if the answers are positive. Examples of this line of questioning include: Have you ever thought that life was not worth living? Have you ever wished that you were dead? Have you ever thought about trying to hurt yourself? Do you intend to hurt yourself? Do you have a plan to hurt yourself? Have you ever attempted suicide? Pediatricians should avoid promises of confidentiality that would be necessary to break to protect and properly treat the child or adolescent. The patient's parents must be given some feedback about the assessment, because parental involvement is usually a critical factor in compliance and treatment. On discovering that a patient is suicidal, it is critical to obtain a "no suicide agreement" in which the patient promises to refrain from hurting him- or herself and to notify the physician or another designated, responsible adult if the child feels suicidal again. It also is

critical to ensure that potential means of suicide, particularly firearms, are removed from the home. No method of storing firearms should be regarded as safe.

When a child has actually attempted suicide, the child should not be discharged directly from the emergency room, regardless of the medical condition. At least a short-term admission (eg, 48-hour hospitalization in a medical hospital) to evaluate the patient and the family is recommended. In the most severe cases of highly suicidal and psychiatrically disturbed patients, direct admission to a psychiatric facility may be warranted.

References

Birmaher B, Ryan ND, Williamson DE, et al: Childhood and adolescent depression: a review of the past ten years, Part I. J Am Acad Child Adolesc Psychiatry 35(11):1427–1439, 1996

Birmaher B, Ryan ND, Williamson DE, et al: Childhood and adolescent depression: A review of the past ten years, Part II. J Am Acad Child Adolesc Psychiatry 35:1575–1583, 1996

Brent DA, Poling K, McKain B, Baugher M: A psychoeducational program for families of affectively ill children and adolescents. J Am Acad Child Adolesc Psychiatry 32:770–774, 1993

Brent DA, Ryan ND, Dahl RE, Birmaher B: Early onset affective illness. In: Bloom FE, Kupfer DJ, eds: Psychopharmacology: The Fourth Generation of Progress, vol 140. New York, Raven, 1995:1631–1642

Dahl RE, Ryan N: The psychobiology of adolescent depression. In: Cicchietti D, Toth SL, eds: Rochester Symposium on Developmental Psychopathology, Volume VII: Adolescence: Opportunities and Challenges. Rochester, NY, University of Rochester Press, 1996:197–232

Kaufman J, Birmaher B, Brent D, et al: Schedule for affective disorders and schizophrenia for school-age children: present and lifetime version (K-SADS-PL). Initial reliability and validity data. J Acad Child Adolesc Psychiatry 36:980–988, 1997

5.7.3   Obsessive-Compulsive Disorder

Lewis W. Sprunger

Normal children across the age spectrum have fears, worries, and superstitions. They engage in repetitive and ritualistic activities. The recently toilet-trained 2-year-old may become very rigid about cleanliness as this developmental step is consolidated. A 5-year-old may repeatedly request one more bedtime story or glass of water in order to allay fears for which there are no words. Grade-school-age children remind each other to hold their breath when passing a cemetery. Adolescents may spend inordinate amounts of time in front of the mirror until every hair is in place. Such thoughts and behaviors are most often age-appropriate, and they often appear to be propelling an ongoing, forward, developmental thrust. When rituals and superstitions lose their age appropriateness, when they develop abnormal content (such as excessive washing or hoarding), or when they begin to impede socialization, the possibility of childhood obsessive-compulsive disorder (OCD) should be considered.

DEFINITION AND EPIDEMIOLOGY

The American Psychiatric Association's *Diagnostic and Statistical Manual of Mental Disorders, 4th Edition (DSM-IV)*, provides diagnostic criteria for OCD based on two fundamental definitions. *Obsessions* are persistent, recurrent, senseless ideas, images, or impulses that are intrusive and not voluntarily produced. An example is a teenager's repeated, unwelcome thoughts of murdering a younger sibling. *Compulsions* are repetitive, seemingly purposeful behaviors that are performed either in response to an obsession (often in an attempt to neutralize it), according to certain rules, or in a stereotyped fashion. Compulsive behaviors are done with a sense of subjective urgency or necessity, and are not experienced as particularly pleasurable. They are aimed at preventing or reducing distress or are designed to prevent some dreaded event or situation. An example is a child who showers excessively in an attempt to cope with an obsessive fear of contracting AIDS.

The *DSM-IV* diagnostic criteria for OCD apply to children and adolescents, as well as to adults. Either obsessions or compulsions or both must be present. The person with obsessions attempts to suppress, ignore, or neutralize them, and recognizes that they are the product of his or her own mind, although this last feature does not always apply to children. If a second psychiatric disorder is present, the content of the obsessions is unrelated to that second disorder. For example, the food obsessions of a person with anorexia nervosa would not meet criteria for a diagnosis of OCD. Compulsions are also generally experienced by the child as unwelcome, excessive, and unreasonable. Important to the definition of the disorder are three features: (a) the obsessions or compulsions cause marked distress; (b) they consume more than an hour per day; and (c) they significantly interfere with the patient's normal life routines, social activities, or relationships with others.

The incidence of OCD in children and adolescents has been difficult to determine due to methodologic difficulties and a general lack of population-based studies. Children with OCD are often secretive about their symptoms. Case definition can also be difficult, because some subjects who appear to meet diagnostic criteria do not claim significant functional compromise. The Isle of Wight study, which surveyed 10- and 11-year-olds, found mixed obsessional/anxiety disorders in 0.3% of the children surveyed. The most thorough US study to date found weighted point and lifetime prevalences of 0.8% and 1.9%, respectively, in a large population of adolescents.

ETIOLOGY AND PATHOGENESIS

Numerous findings over the past two decades have led to increasing focus on OCD as a neurobiological disorder. Dysfunction of the frontal lobe-limbic-basal ganglia system has been proposed, based on CNS imaging studies and on the association of obsessive-compulsive symptoms with neurologic disorders such as Sydenham chorea. The successful treatment of OCD with the selective serotonin reuptake inhibitors (SSRIs) has led to numerous investigations of the role of serotonin and its effects on CNS receptor systems. Genetic investigations have shown an increased incidence of OCD in the first-degree relatives of child and adolescent probands. The content of the presenting obsessions and/or the nature of the specific presenting compulsions of patients and their parents are typically dissimilar, arguing against straightforward social or cultural transmission. Genetic bases for OCD are also suggested by its familial links with Tourette syndrome (TS). Many patients with TS have clinically significant obsessive-compulsive features, and many of those with OCD have significant tics.

Findings that patients with Sydenham chorea often have clinically significant obsessions and compulsions raise the possibility that at least some persons with a sudden onset or recurrence of OCD may be experiencing a nonsuppurative sequela of a group A beta-hemolytic streptococcal (GABHS) infection, or even the after-effects of other acute infectious illnesses. Recent work has used the acronym PANDAS (pediatric autoimmune neuropsychiatric disor-

ders associated with streptococcal infections) to describe a subgroup of patients identified by: (1) the presence of OCD and/or a tic disorder; (2) prepubertal symptom onset; (3) episodic course of symptom severity; (4) association with GABHS infection; and (5) association with neurologic abnormalities. These criteria point to an underlying hypothesis that autoimmune phenomena, primarily directed at the basal ganglia, are responsible for the symptoms.

Attention to neurobiological etiologies has resulted in less focus on the "functional" aspects of OCD and the psychodynamic theories that traditionally view the overt symptoms as maladaptive defenses against internal guilt, conflict, or anxiety. While these theories have not been subjected to rigorous, systematic research, they do raise important questions about the specific content of obsessions or compulsions, which are largely ignored by many investigators.

CLINICAL MANIFESTATIONS

Patients with a wide variety of clinical histories and symptoms can meet *DSM-IV* criteria for OCD. Clinical samples generally show a preponderance of boys, who tend to have an earlier age of onset than girls, although sex differences may disappear by adolescence. A large NIMH study of severely ill children and adolescents revealed several children whose symptoms had begun prior to age 7 years. Significant symptoms can exist for years before children (or their families) come to professional attention.

The most frequently reported ritual in childhood OCD involves cleaning or washing (handwashing, showering, tooth-brushing). Other common compulsions include repetitive behaviors (going in and out of doors, restating, rereading), checking (doors, windows, locks), counting (performing behaviors a specified number of times), and ordering or arranging objects. Rituals are often disguised or incorporated into innocuous-appearing activities.

The most common obsessions reported by children involve dirt and germs. Others include preoccupation with something terrible happening, the feeling that something has not been done correctly, concern about symmetry and order, and worry about forbidden sexual or aggressive impulses and thoughts.

ASSESSMENT AND DIAGNOSIS

Parents (and, in turn, pediatricians) may become concerned over behaviors that are less obvious than those described above. These can include inordinate amounts of time spent doing unproductive homework; excessive erasing; increasing and unreasonable amounts of laundry; rigidity about cleanliness; rapidly disappearing soap; chronically chapped hands; hoarding objects or supplies; exaggerated needs for reassurance; and ongoing fears of self or others being harmed. The pediatrician's ability to elicit such symptoms and address them directly can be a relief to parents, because it is not infrequent that families become reluctantly, but intimately, involved in the child's system of obsessions or compulsions and share their child's embarrassment, secrecy, and fear. The message that OCD is a known condition that can be treated is helpful and a source of comfort and hope.

The differential diagnosis is broad and sometimes confusing, because OCD has been shown to co-occur with several other conditions. TS can involve complex tics that may be difficult to distinguish from compulsive rituals (which are usually preceded by a specific thought). Obsessive rumination on gloomy thoughts or ideas is a common feature of major depression, but it is usually seen by the depressed patient as making sense, whereas the patient with true obsessions generally views such thoughts as alien. Anxiety disorders in childhood also involve worries and fears, but they are not viewed as senseless and are unaccompanied by rituals. Severe OCD frequently includes phobic features, but these do not disappear when the feared object or situation is removed. Eating disorders, while involving many obsessions and compulsions, are excluded, by *DSM-IV* definition, from OCD.

Because of the associations between OCD and TS, the possibility of an obsessive-compulsive spectrum of disorders has been raised. Such a spectrum might include conditions such as trichotillomania (pathologic hair-pulling) and onychophagia (habitual nail-biting), which share with OCD not only the repetitive behaviors, but also the patient's subjective urge and sense of obligation to perform the action.

Two additional issues arise in relation to the diagnosis of OCD. First, nearly all children experience age-related and transient superstitions and rituals during their development. These enhance socialization and help the child to attain mastery and control. The opposite applies to the rituals associated with OCD. For example, 10-year-old boys may collect and elaborately store and catalog baseball cards. For most, this activity is enjoyable and provides a means of social interchange with friends, even though the parents may despair of the time, energy, and intensity involved. In contrast, a boy who obtains no pleasure from his collection and determinedly stores his cards in plastic sleeves to protect himself from the germs his friends' fingers may have left would be thought of as having a compulsion aimed at keeping him safe from an obsessive fear. Second, many children and adolescents develop personality styles characterized by neatness, orderliness, rigidity, and perfectionism. These traits may increase during periods of personal or familial distress. In the extreme, these individuals may meet *DSM-IV* criteria for obsessive-compulsive personality disorder (OCPD). This disorder describes an enduring set of character traits in which there is a pervasive and cross-situational pattern of preoccupation with orderliness, perfectionism, and mental and interpersonal control, at the expense of flexibility, openness, and efficiency. OCPD does not include the presence of either obsessions or compulsions, making OCD and OCPD clearly distinguishable disorders. Most studies have not found evidence for an increased incidence of past or present OCPD in persons with OCD, indicating that the two disorders do not occur on a continuum.

Currently, diagnosis of OCD is accomplished on the basis of clinical history, which may be augmented by the use of structured inventories or questionnaires. There are no pathognomonic physical or laboratory findings.

MANAGEMENT AND TREATMENT

While most current authorities do not recommend psychodynamically oriented psychotherapy as the primary treatment approach for OCD, nearly all believe that the expressive and supportive psychotherapies have an important treatment role to play. The majority of patients can profit from attention to issues of self-esteem, interpersonal relationships, and the challenges of living with a long-term illness. Families also need attention because there are often boundary and relationship issues directly related to the havoc that OCD can wreak within the family setting. Both individual and family therapies can form a solid base on which other therapeutic modalities can be more successfully used.

Behavioral therapies are widely recommended for patients with OCD across the age spectrum, but are probably underused in children and adolescents. They depend on interest, commitment, and an ability to sacrifice short-term comfort in the interest of long-

term gain by the child and the family. The most commonly used method involves deliberate exposure of the patient to a feared or provocative stimulus (such as dirt), while simultaneously preventing the usual response (washing) for increasing lengths of time. Positive responses in motivated patients who have mild to moderate OCD are usually seen within the first 2 weeks. Behavior therapy typically needs to be an ongoing process because the disorder is chronic.

Pharmacologic treatment of OCD has been revolutionized in the past decade with the introduction of the SSRIs. Used originally in adults, they have rapidly become a prominent and important treatment for children and adolescents. Fluoxetine in doses ranging from 20 to 60 mg/d is effective. Its side effects, though generally more tolerable, can include agitation, increased anxiety, insomnia, and loss of appetite. Sertraline, fluvoxamine, and paroxetine can also be used. Clomipramine (CMI), a tricyclic antidepressant, is effective in doses ranging from 3 to 5 mg/kg/d. Recommendations for maximum daily dose vary from 150 to 250 mg, with doses in this range requiring electrocardiogram and liver function monitoring. Like other tricyclic antidepressants, CMI often has troubling anticholinergic side effects that limit its usefulness. While CMI also functions well as an antidepressant, its non-SSRI chemical relatives, such as desipramine, have not been found useful in OCD. When OCD is associated with other conditions, such as movement disorders or depression, pharmacologic approaches may be varied to include additional drugs.

NATURAL HISTORY AND PROGNOSIS

Follow-up studies of children and adolescents with OCD have shown that at least half are still symptomatic as adults. This is consistent with the finding that many adults with OCD can retrospectively pinpoint the onset of their symptoms to their childhood or adolescence. One study of a community-wide sample of adolescents found that approximately half were still affected 2 years later. Studies of patient samples indicate that OCD in childhood can be expected to run a waxing and waning course. Some patients' symptoms disappear; many have periods of seeming remission followed by relapse. Nearly all patients whose OCD is chronic experience changes in their symptom constellations as time passes. Why this disorder disappears in approximately half its affected individuals remains a mystery.

The increased clinical and research attention paid to this disorder, coupled with the encouraging behavioral and pharmacologic treatments currently available, bring hope for more effective approaches to managing this chronic illness and perhaps for finding cures.

References

American Academy of Child and Adolescent Psychiatry: Practice parameters for the assessment and treatment of children and adolescents with obsessive-compulsive disorder. J Am Acad Child Adolesc Psychiatry 37(Suppl. 10):275, 1998

American Psychiatric Association: Diagnostic and Statistical Manual of Mental Disorders, 4th ed. (DSM-IV). Washington, DC, 1994

Lenane MC, Swedo SE, Leonard H, et al: Psychiatric disorders in first-degree relatives of children and adolescents with obsessive compulsive disorder. J Am Acad Child Adolesc Psychiatry 29(3):407, 1990

Leonard HL, Goldberger EL, Rapoport JL, et al: Childhood rituals: normal development or obsessive-compulsive symptoms? J Am Acad Child Adolesc Psychiatry 29(1):17, 1990

Leonard HL, Swedo SE, Lenane MC, et al: A 2- to 7-year follow-up study of 54 obsessive-compulsive children and adolescents. Arch Gen Psychiatry 50:429, 1993

Rettew DC, Swedo SE, Leonard HL, et al: Obsessions and compulsions across time in 79 children and adolescents with obsessive-compulsive disorder. J Am Acad Child Adolesc Psychiatry 31(6):1050, 1992

Swedo SE, Leonard HL, Garvey M, et al: Pediatric autoimmune neuropsychiatric disorders associated with streptococcal infections: clinical descriptions of the first fifty cases. Am J Psychiatry 155(2):264, 1998

Swedo SE, Rapoport JL, Leonard H, et al: Obsessive-compulsive disorder in children and adolescents: clinical phenomenology of 70 consecutive cases. Arch Gen Psychiatry 46:335, 1989

Towbin KE, Riddle MA: Obsessive-compulsive disorder. In: Lewis M, ed: Child and Adolescent Psychiatry: A Comprehensive Textbook, 2nd ed. Baltimore, Williams & Wilkins, 1996:684

5.7.4   Munchausen by Proxy Syndrome

W. Peter Metz

DEFINITION AND EPIDEMIOLOGY

Munchausen by proxy syndrome (MBPS) (also named factitious disorder by proxy) describes a disturbance in the patient–child relationship in which a caregiver, almost always the mother, deliberately fabricates a history of illness in her child and/or harms the child to create illness. This form of child maltreatment is quite distinct from the more commonly occurring physical, sexual, or emotional abuse and neglect. However, MBPS was only recently recognized as a significant problem. The name for this disorder is derived from the adult disorder, Munchausen syndrome, which is characterized by self-induced or fabricated illness to gain medical attention.

To date, MBPS has been the subject of over 300 publications, which constitute a growing body of mostly anecdotal data that confirm its protean manifestations and that children of any age may be at risk. However, little systematic or longitudinal information regarding this syndrome is available. Its incidence and prevalence are unknown, but the disorder probably is not rare. One prospective study from the UK found an annual incidence of MBPS in the range of 0.5 per 100,000 for children aged under 16 years and 2.8 per 100,000 for children aged under 1 year. In 42% of diagnosed families with more than one child, a sibling had previously suffered some form of abuse. Children in a family usually are victimized serially rather than simultaneously.

ETIOLOGY AND PATHOGENESIS

Determining the etiology of this form of child abuse must account for the fact that 95% of reported MBPS cases involve mothers and that this syndrome centers on the mother's need to form an intense, ambivalent connection with pediatric-care providers. The past history of mothers with MBPS generally does not reveal the overt, gross abuse or neglect that is so commonly noted in the early lives of parents who commit other forms of child abuse. Rather, these mothers frequently grew up in families in which, in a more subtle but nevertheless profound way, the mother felt unloved and unwanted as a child. Having been deprived of enough love in childhood, the mother with MBPS experiences enormous gratification in the close relationship she achieves with her child's medical-care provider at the same time that she conveys enormous covert hostility toward this authority figure through deception and betrayal of trust.

Because mothers with MBPS usually are very convincing in their presentation as devoted, concerned, and knowledgeable parents, they typically are perceived as conscientious parents by pediatric-care providers. Such acceptance and close connection, particularly when the child is hospitalized, powerfully reinforces the mother's illness-producing behavior.

Munchausen by proxy syndrome has been described as a type of disorder in which mothers engage in compulsive behavior to avoid overwhelming anxiety and with the aim of revenge. Because such persons feel a sense of elation when brazenly defying moral authority, they often appear to be remarkably calm at exactly the moment when their child is most ill. The compulsive behavior of a mother with MBPS does not result from psychotic thinking. However, like the compulsive starvation of a patient with anorexia nervosa, it can be relentless and driven by great urgency.

Consistent with the view of MBPS as a type of perversion, the child serves a dehumanized function for the mother as a fetish. This fetish, whether an object (ie, the child) or a fantasy (ie, the conviction that the child must be ill), enhances feelings of power and wards off fear. Mothers with MBPS are aided in their sometimes gruesome acts of harm to their children precisely because the child is dehumanized.

CLINICAL MANIFESTATIONS

Over 100 different presenting signs and symptoms have been described in victimized children, including psychiatric symptoms. The most common signs and symptoms are seizures, vomiting, diarrhea, fever, and apnea. Children at any age may be at risk, although this syndrome has been recognized most commonly in infants and preschool-age children, whose younger age does not require active participation on their part. When older children are involved, there generally is some degree of collusion between the child and other family members. Family and social characteristics often include a distant or absent father and a socially isolated mother who appears to be extremely devoted to her child and usually knowledgeable about the child's illness. The mother may have a background in health care and, in a significant proportion of cases, have a history of Munchausen syndrome in herself. Children of mothers with MBPS are high-volume users of pediatric health-care, although this use may not appear to be excessive to the pediatric-care provider. Some "red flags," which suggest the possibility of MBPS, are listed in Table 5-38.

ASSESSMENT AND DIAGNOSIS

Munchausen by proxy syndrome should be included in the differential diagnosis of any child with recurrent serious illness for which a satisfactory explanation cannot be found. The atypicality of the child's medical problems may manifest in the constellation of symptoms, an unusual course, and/or a failure to respond to usual treatments. Independent verification of symptoms reported by the mother is critically important, and this may be the most direct means to clarify a diagnosis of MBPS in cases in which the mother limits herself to fabricating symptoms rather than active induction of physical signs. Diagnosis of MBPS in parents of children who have objective signs of physical illness may be confirmed by documentation that signs of illness resolve when the child is separated from the abusing parent, although such separation may be difficult to effect. Gaining independent verification of other parts of the history provided by the mother also can be helpful, including allegations of previous illness in the child and/or mother or other

TABLE 5-38

"RED FLAGS" FOR THE DETECTION OF MUNCHAUSEN BY PROXY SYNDROME[a]

Recurrent serious illness for which a satisfactory explanation cannot be found.

Failure of an illness to respond to usual therapeutic interventions.

Symptoms reported by the mother which can not be verified by an independent observer.

Determination that the mother has fabricated any aspects of the child's or family's history.

History of unexplained illness or death in siblings of a currently ill child.

A mother who appears inappropriately calm or euphoric when her child is most acutely ill in the hospital.

A history of Munchausen syndrome in the mother.

A mother who goes out of her way to ingratiate herself to hospital staff and care providers when her child is hospitalized.

[a] While none of these findings are diagnostic, the presence of one or more should alert the pediatric care provider to the possibility of Munchausen by proxy syndrome in the differential diagnosis.

dramatic and unusual aspects of the family history. Confirmation that the mother has fabricated other aspects of the history is an important warning sign in alerting one to the possibility of MBPS. While it is observed less commonly, a history of unexplained sibling illness or death is also an important warning sign.

The diagnosis of MBPS needs to be established by a treatment team that includes all involved health-care professionals, especially mental health professionals who are familiar with this disorder. A team approach often is achieved most speedily and effectively in the hospital.

Careful surveillance of the suspected parent and child in the hospital setting is critical and must include controls so that the parent does not have unmonitored access to the medical record, including nursing notes, and does not bring in food or give the child medications. It is important to retain all samples (eg, vomit, urine, stools, or blood) that may be useful for analysis. Careful documentation of all suspicious findings is necessary for subsequent legal action once the diagnosis is made.

The potential for harm in a misdiagnosis of MBPS is significant and not dissimilar to the family trauma that is precipitated by incorrect assertions of physical or sexual abuse. Although there are few reported cases of misdiagnosis of MBPS, health-care providers must be cautious of being overzealous about asserting this disorder, particularly in a child with genuine chronic illness. It is sometimes difficult to distinguish mothers with MBPS from anxious mothers who perceive their children as vulnerable.

MANAGEMENT AND TREATMENT

When compelling evidence of MBPS is obtained, the state's child protective agency must be notified. Such notification is best given before confronting the parent so that the protective services social worker can be educated, if necessary, about MBPS, and arrangements made for emergency placement of the child (and possibly other children in the family). Confrontation of the family regarding the diagnosis should occur in the hospital, and care should be taken to ensure that a court order can be obtained, if needed, to prevent the parent from fleeing with the child. When presenting the diagnosis, it is important to include the spouse and/or other family members in the confrontation and to ensure the availability of immediate psychiatric help for the mother, who may become suicidal.

The more problematic, and probably more common, management challenge regarding MBPS is associated with situations in which the harm that is done to the child is limited to excessive medical visits, diagnostic tests, and prescription of medications. Entertainment of the diagnosis may be based on a history of persistent assertions of symptoms by the mother, such as seizures or vomiting, that no one else has witnessed. In these circumstances, the best strategy may be careful follow-up of the child while avoiding intrusive medical or surgical interventions that lack clear indications based on more than just the mother's history. Concurrently, efforts must be made to engage the mother and her spouse or other family members in psychotherapy. If the mother refuses to be seen by a mental health professional, consultation from someone knowledgeable about MBPS regarding the possibility of the diagnosis should be obtained. The primary-care provider also is in a key position to alert subspecialists who may be engaged in care of the child to the possibility of MBPS and to attempt to monitor "doctor shopping" by the mother.

When MBPS is suspected but not confirmed, the primary-care provider has the difficult but important task of remaining vigilant about the possibility of child abuse, while maintaining a supportive, positive relationship with the parents. Consultation with a colleague or mental health professional may be helpful in managing conflicting feelings of betrayal and ongoing trust of the parent suspected of MBPS. Maintaining a viable treatment relationship with the parent is crucial in limiting the harm, especially iatrogenic harm, that may be done to the child in cases of unconfirmed MBPS.

NATURAL HISTORY AND PROGNOSIS

Little is known about the natural history or prognosis of this disorder. Reported mortality rates for MBPS of 9 to 10% are probably high because of underdiagnosis of less-severe cases. One long-term (ie, 1 to 14 years) follow-up study found "unacceptable outcomes" in 50% of the victims and 65% of their siblings. However, these involved less-severe cases in which the children were returned to their parents, suggesting that the long-term sequelae of this disorder may be frequent and severe. There is some evidence that older children who were subjected to MBPS may go on to develop adult Munchausen syndrome, although it is not known how frequently this occurs.

The natural history of MBPS appears to range from the extreme of murder (usually unintentional) in severe cases in which the compulsive behavior pursues a relentless course, to intermittent or isolated episodes of MBPS at times of particular stress and isolation for the parent who is less compulsively caught up in the disorder. Additional prospective follow-up studies are needed to help clarify questions of natural history, prognosis, and the effect of treatment for this underdiagnosed and serious form of child abuse.

References

Asher R: Munchausen's syndrome. Lancet ii:339–341, 1951

McClure RJ, David PM, Meadow SR, Sibert JR: Epidemiology of Munchausen syndrome by proxy, non-accidental poisoning, and non-accidental suffocation. Arch Dis Child 75:57–61, 1996

McGuire TL, Feldman KW: Psychologic morbidity of children subjected to Munchausen syndrome by proxy. Pediatrics 83:289–292, 1989

Meadow R: Suffocation, recurrent apnea, and sudden infant death. J Pediatr 117:351–357, 1990

Neale B, Bools C, Meadow R: Problems in the assessment and management of Munchausen syndrome by proxy abuse. Child Society 5:324–333, 1991

Rosenberg DA: Web of deceit: a literature review of Munchausen syndrome by proxy. Child Abuse Negl 11:547–563, 1987

Schreier HA, Libow JA: Hurting for Love: Munchausen by Proxy Syndrome. New York, Guilford Press, 1993

Schreier HA: Factitious presentation of psychiatric disorders. When is it Munchausen by proxy? Child Psychol Psychiatry Rev 2:108–115, 1997

Sovid AK, Keith DV, Cunningham AS: Munchausen syndrome by proxy. Clin Pediatr 37(8):497–503, 1998

5.7.5 Childhood Schizophrenia

Fred R. Volkmar

Historically, the definition of schizophrenia in childhood has been controversial, reflecting changing views of "psychosis" in children. Available evidence suggests a basic similarity in presentation in children and adults; accordingly the condition is defined as for adults on the basis of characteristic psychotic symptoms (hallucinations, delusions, and other symptoms of thought disorder) accompanied by deficits in adaptive functioning for at least 6 months. Some aspects of the disorder may present slightly differently in children; for example, delusions may be less complex and systematized.

For many years there was considerable confusion about the relationship of autism to schizophrenia. However, present data suggest that autism is *not* a form of schizophrenia. Indeed, the concept of psychosis, as applied to children, is problematic in multiple respects, because it is clear that children experience marked shifts in their understanding of reality over the course of development. Changes in the definition of the disorder also complicate interpretation of the research literature. Most recent studies suggest that, in childhood, schizophrenia is probably less common than autism (ie, with fewer than 2 cases per 10,000). In contrast to autism, no marked male predominance is noted. Consistent with research using adult samples, there is evidence suggesting that schizophrenia in children may be more frequent in families of lower socioeconomic status and that the condition has a genetic component.

ETIOLOGY AND PATHOGENESIS

Various lines of evidence suggest the importance of neurobiological factors in pathogenesis. Neuropsychological studies reveal deficits in attentional capacities and the processing of information; there may be cortical gray matter volume over time. Family studies (eg, of adopted children) suggest that rates of schizophrenia are substantially elevated among children whose parents have schizophrenia. Earlier research tended to emphasize the possible contribution of psychological factors in the pathogenesis, but data supporting this notion are limited. However, there is evidence that stressful life experiences may be important in precipitating psychotic episodes in children. As is true for adults with schizophrenic illness, exposure to certain pharmacologic agents (eg, stimulants) may produce a schizophrenic-like psychosis.

CLINICAL MANIFESTATIONS

Although studies of *adults* who develop schizophrenia suggest some childhood precursors of the condition, the applicability of this research to childhood schizophrenia is limited. The available data do suggest that children who develop schizophrenia may demonstrate various premorbid features, such as problems with attention, inhibition, withdrawal, and sensitivity.

This condition rarely is manifest before age 5 years. Three patterns of onset are noted: (a) acute; (b) insidious with gradual deterioration; and (c) insidious onset with an acute exacerbation of disturbance. Males are more likely to have an earlier onset of the disorder. Although differing in certain respects from the thought disturbance observed in adults with schizophrenia, children with this condition exhibit similar problems with hallucinations, delusions, and thought process.

Hallucinations are the most frequently reported symptom. Auditory hallucinations with persecutory content (eg, voices commenting about the child) are most common, whereas somatic and visual hallucinations are less frequent. Hallucinations and delusions are typically less detailed or less complex in younger children. A formal thought disorder is difficult to assess, although rating instruments are available.

ASSESSMENT AND DIAGNOSIS

The diagnosis of schizophrenia is least complicated in older children and adolescents. It should be made after very careful evaluation with due consideration of other factors, such as substance abuse and seizure disorder. Schizophrenia of childhood onset should be differentiated from the mood disturbances seen in psychotic depression or mania. On occasion, children with obsessive-compulsive disorder may exhibit ideas that are difficult to distinguish from delusions; however, an affected child usually is cognizant of the irrational nature of such ideas. Hallucinations occasionally occur as an isolated symptom, and a diagnosis of childhood schizophrenia should not be made in such cases. In some circumstances, the diagnosis is confirmed only as the course becomes more clear. In clinical practice, it is often the case that delays in diagnosis reflect both the technical difficulties inherent in making the diagnosis in children, as well as a reluctance to seriously consider it. It is also the case that some children exhibit psychotic conditions that are poorly differentiated and do not simply correspond to current diagnostic categories.

The assessment of the child with possible schizophrenia should include a detailed and comprehensive history, psychological and/or communicative examinations, psychiatric examination, physical examination, and neurologic consultation or toxicologic screen if indicated. The presence of other developmental or psychiatric disorders should be noted. Psychological testing may be helpful diagnostically and for designing an intervention program. Several assessment instruments have been developed explicitly for the evaluation of psychosis or thought disorder in childhood, such as the Kiddie Formal Thought Disorder Rating Scale. Given the low frequency and severity of this condition, the expertise of an experienced child and adolescent psychiatrist should be obtained.

MANAGEMENT AND TREATMENT

The management of the child with schizophrenia should build on specific patterns of strength and weakness, with recognition of the stage of the illness (ie, the presence of active psychotic symptoms). Usually an intensive, multimodal treatment program is indicated, which includes medications, individual psychotherapy, educational intervention, and family support. Inpatient treatment may be appropriate, particularly during the active psychotic phase and in cases in which the diagnosis is unclear.

Available data suggest that, as with adults, major tranquilizers may diminish certain "positive" symptoms, such as hallucinations and delusions. The newer "atypical" neuroleptics have some advantages for treatment. Family interventions should be focused on supporting the child's ongoing development and adaptation; any associated problems in development or learning also should be addressed.

NATURAL HISTORY AND PROGNOSIS

Changes in the definition of childhood schizophrenia complicate the interpretation of previous research on its natural history. However, if the condition is defined strictly, it appears that the outcome is generally poor. In a minority of cases, a remission is observed; in most cases, problems persist over time. Early onset (before age 10 years) is a negative prognostic sign. As with adult schizophrenia, "negative" symptoms in childhood schizophrenia (eg, anhedonia) are probably less responsive to pharmacologic intervention. Relatively positive outcome is related to acute onset, older age at onset, better premorbid adjustment, and well-differentiated symptoms.

References

Caplan R, Guthrie D, Fish B, Tanguay P, David-Lando G: The Kiddie Formal Thought Disorder Rating Scale: clinical assessment, reliability, and validity. J Am Acad Child Adolesc Psychiatry 28:408–416, 1989

McClellan J, Werry J: Practice parameters for the assessment and treatment of children and adolescents with schizophrenia. J Am Acad Child Adolesc Psychiatry 36:177S–193S, 1997

Rapoport JL, Giedd JN, Blumenthal J, et al: Progressive cortical change during adolescence in childhood-onset schizophrenia. A longitudinal magnetic resonance imaging study. Arch Gen Psychiatry 56:649–654, 1999

Sourander A: Risperidone for treatment of childhood schizophrenia [letter]. Am J Psychiatry 154:1476, 1997

Volkmar FR: Childhood schizophrenia. In: Louis M, ed: Child and Adolescent Psychiatry: A Comprehensive Textbook, 2nd ed. Baltimore, MD, Williams & Wilkins, 1996

Volkmar FR, Becker DF, King RA, et al: Psychotic processes. In: Cicchetti D, Cohen D, eds: Handbook of Developmental Psychopathology. New York, John Wiley, 1994:512–534

5.8   PSYCHOSOCIAL ISSUES IN CONTEMPORARY FAMILY AND COMMUNITY LIFE

5.8.1   Changing Concepts of the Family

Laurie J. Bauman and Ruth E.K. Stein

AN INTRODUCTION TO FAMILIES

Pediatricians provide care for children who live in a variety of family forms. Children may live with two working parents, unmarried parents, grandparents or another nonparental caregiver, in single-parent families where the mother may have divorced or never married, or with gay parents, in foster homes, or in blended families. The *traditional nuclear family,* consisting of a mother and father who are married to each other and living with their biological children,

is becoming less common. Although it was the norm three decades ago, only 50% of American households today include a married couple, and only 50% of those have children. Only one-third of preschoolers are raised in a two-parent home with a working father and a full-time homemaker mother. Given the diversity of family forms, it is important to identify the central ideas in the definition of *family.*

The notion of family is universal in all cultures and societies, but the definition is changing, confused, and often vague. At a broad conceptual level, the family is a system of social relationships that are shaped by expectations and values and based on distinctions of age and sex. Each member occupies a particular position or status that governs behavior toward other family members. On a more practical level, the US Bureau of the Census defines a family as two or more persons who live together and are related by blood, marriage, or adoption.

Characteristics of Families

Given the difficulty in defining family, it may be useful to conceptualize the characteristics and functions of family units. First, many families share biology, including temperament, personality, talent, and disease vulnerability. Second, families typically have a power hierarchy that is determined in part by age, generation, culture, personality characteristics, and gender. Third, families tend to have their own *culture,* which includes a family-specific set of values, goals, and expectations. Although they are unique to each family, these *microcultures* reflect the larger societal and ethnic cultures. Fourth, every family has an *invisible boundary* that defines who is a member and who is not.

Another set of family characteristics are developmental and arise from a family's common history and future. Family history may extend back for generations, and it usually reflects both ethnic and religious beliefs. A family's future course usually follows a pattern of successive developmental phases that depend in part on both *biology* and *social norms.* The *phase of expansion* includes the initial union and continues until the youngest child becomes an adult. This period spans fertility and the physical and emotional maturation of children. The *phase of dispersion* occurs when the first child achieves adulthood and leaves home. The *phase of independence* begins when all the children have left and the parents are alone. The *phase of replacement* covers the period of retirement to death.

Societal Functions of the Family

Historically, the family as a social institution has served a number of functions. Its primary purpose was the care, rearing, and socialization of children. Families retain the major role in child-rearing and in regulating sexual relationships. Marriage was the social institution that was used to legitimize sexual union; however, over time, sexual liaisons outside of marriage have become more common and accepted. An important function of the family was to regulate reproduction, but childbirth has occurred with increasing frequency outside of the marital tie. In 1950, only 4% of children were born out of wedlock; now a majority of first births are to unmarried mothers. The family also meets the subsistence needs of its members, but a recent survey found that 30% of US families had no member who worked. Another role of the family was to provide love and emotional intimacy. This is more characteristic of Western than of Eastern societies, but American notions include the expectation that partners will provide affection and emotional support.

TYPES OF FAMILIES

There are many ways to classify types of families, but family types are most often described by their structure. In its simplest form, a family consists of the husband, wife, and nonadult children, and it is called the *nuclear,* conjugal, elementary, immediate, or simple family. This family structure consists of two generations. In industrial societies, nuclear families tend to live in a separate household that often is far removed from relatives.

In *extended* families, several generations live together, and grandparents often have some responsibility for child-rearing. As a result of parent incapacity, abandonment, or death, 1.4 million children in the US live in families headed by a grandparent. In such configurations, the children may have experienced the loss of a parent and may have had to move, leaving behind home, friends, and school. Sometimes, custody is a matter of legal question or family controversy. Although many children develop loving, caring relationships with new caregivers, some relationships between children and custodians are ambivalent or antagonistic, and on occasion, custodians may be antagonistic to the biological parent(s). If a parent has died, all may be grieving. Recently, parental death from AIDS has generated a host of AIDS orphans, who, it is estimated, number more than 125,000 children in the United States alone. Little is known about custodial arrangements of many of these vulnerable children. Regardless of the reason for the transfer of custody, many grandparents find it difficult to parent again.

Single-parent families are increasingly common. More than 25% of all children under 18 years of age and more than 50% of all black children in the United States live in single-parent families. It is projected that 70% of children who were born in 1980 will live for a time with a single parent. Single-parent families also include never-married mothers, some of whom choose to parent alone, and parents who are divorced, some of whom share the custody of their children.

Single parents face special challenges. Most importantly, they tend to have far fewer economic resources and a much lower standard of living. Divorced parents and their children find the first year to be very painful, but research suggests that children who have a supportive, understanding, and affectionate parent tend to do well. Although these fathers often are uninvolved with their children, many children remain emotionally connected to both parents, even when contact with the noncustodial parent is limited. Eighty percent of divorced women work outside the home, and adequate sources of child care are difficult to find. Older siblings may be given significant responsibility, and some may experience school and peer problems. Despite the many problems that single parents confront, there is strong evidence that most single families raise healthy, secure children. Resources facilitating a positive outcome include parental organizational skills, adequate support networks, and closer proximity to extended family.

Blended families are found with increasing frequency. Seventy-five percent of divorced people remarry, usually within 3 years. Remarriage often eases the financial problems of single parenthood, but complex new family relationships result. For example, there may be significant friction between the child and the stepparent as they struggle for the biological parent's attention and negotiate new roles. These relationships may be more complicated when both of the child's biological parents are involved with new partners. In addition, new siblings may be introduced from the stepparent's family or as a product of the parent's new relationship. It may be difficult for the child to maintain these multiple new relationships and live by the rules and standards of the child's different families, especially if the families have different cultural values.

Many children live with *unmarried parents* who have made a commitment to stay together. In some instances, one parent lives with children who are not his or her own but who are from the partner's previous relationship. Although this arrangement may be a transitional step toward planned marriage, this cannot be assumed. The lack of permanence can be difficult for all family members; there may be conflict between partners about where the relationship is going. The instability of the relationship may draw attention away from the children, but if the parental figure and the child have a strong bond, this family form can work well.

Homosexual families are often overlooked as a family form. Sometimes, parents realize after having children that they are gay. Divorce may result, and the child may live with or visit a homosexual parent. Both the resulting family separation and need for the child to adjust to a new adult in the home may be stressful. Furthermore, the child may be taunted by peers or experience rejection from the larger community or other parent. To avoid the many possible problems, some parents choose secrecy. In other instances, a homosexual couple form a primary relationship and actively choose to parent a child. The small body of research on the children of homosexual parents documents that children can be nurtured effectively in this family form.

Few adolescents are prepared for the demands of *teenaged* parenthood. Married teenagers with children are more likely than married teenagers without children to have marital problems, to have additional children at an accelerated pace, and to leave school earlier. Inherent in children parenting children is the tension between the developmental needs of the adolescent and those of the child. Some teenagers set up an independent household, either as a single parent or with the infant's father. However, most adolescent parents live at home with their parents, which creates an extended family system. There may be conflict between the adolescent and her mother over caregiving responsibilities for the infant and the adolescent's own independence and autonomy.

EFFECTS OF SOCIAL TRENDS ON FAMILIES

Several social changes in the United States are affecting families of many structures. One that affects an increasing number of families is the *deinstitutionalization* of elderly, disabled, and mentally ill persons. Mothers of young and adolescent children may confront the additional demands of caring for an ill or elderly parent, spouse, or child. Social, economic, and psychological supports for these women are often inadequate, and this may have an adverse impact on child-rearing and the responsibilities of older children in the family unit.

Another societal evolution that will continue to affect families is *changing gender roles*. More married mothers are in the workforce, and more men are sharing or taking primary responsibility for child-rearing.

Recent economic trends have meant that many families need two incomes. In two-thirds of nuclear households with children, both parents work. *Families with two working parents* tend to be smaller, younger, have a higher level of education, and have a higher income; 25% of two-paycheck families are two-career families. Child-rearing in families with two working parents can be stressful, and it requires effective and flexible external sources of child care. When both parents work, there may be special concerns; these families are likely to have latchkey children who are left alone after school until the parents come home from work. It is especially important for health professionals to provide anticipatory guidance to caretakers concerning when this is developmentally appropriate as well as guidelines for accident prevention.

CLINICAL IMPLICATIONS OF THE CHANGING FAMILY

The variability of family forms and the different values and norms that they reflect pose challenges to physicians. Families often behave in ways that are counter to the health-care providers' own beliefs or to traditional health advice. Doctors, nurse practitioners, or social workers may find their own values and standards differ from those of the patients. At times, these differences may create problems in communication or inappropriate attempts to enforce family conformity.

The clinician must be aware of the potential for family differences and recognize them during interactions with a wide range of different families. There are many ways that family structure and values influence child development and behavior. The degree to which understanding of the family affects a clinician's practice depends on the nature of the encounter and the type of information and interaction that are required to meet the needs of the child and to care for the child's condition.

Health-Care Maintenance Visit

The clinician who is aware of variations in family structure can be sensitive to these differences. At a very basic level, this sensitivity is reflected in the way that the initial registration data and history are obtained. For example, many conventional registration forms ask for information on the child's mother and father, but they do not entertain the possibility or allow the inclusion of alternate family structures such as foster, blended, extended, or gay and lesbian families. Inquiring about caregivers, guardians, and their relationship to the child, as well as asking the person who brings in the child for care to identify the primary adults in the child's family structure, allows the accompanying adult to define that structure without prejudgment or defensiveness. It also is helpful to know how the child refers to these individuals. Information can be obtained on each of the named family members and on his or her relationship to the child. The range of information should include each member's health and mental status, because it affects the child's health and emotional well being, and the role and responsibility of other family members for the child's care. When the biological parents differ from the caregivers, it is important to obtain information about their health as well as to determine their relationship to the child.

Because family structure may not be stable over the course of childhood, the clinician should inquire periodically about changes in caregiving, living arrangements, and responsibility for the child. Inquiries that are made without assumptions of family type are perceived as supportive by those whose family configuration is not traditional and allows them to feel welcome in the practice. Such questions ease communication and create an atmosphere that reflects concern and interest in the child as well as family. However, it also is important to remember that knowing about family issues does not necessarily require the clinician to do anything about them.

Child development and the internal adjustment of family pressures occur in the context of two worlds: the world defined by the family's own norms, and the larger social world in which the family must function. Learning to navigate these two worlds is part of normal child development. As children mature, they become aware of the ways in which their own family differs from others. Differences in family composition, socioeconomic circumstances, health status, physical appearance, behavior, religion, or education are often sources of distress or embarrassment, especially during latency and early adolescence, and the child may go through a phase of discomfort with the child's own family members. The clinician who is sensitive to these feelings may be able to help the child be more comfortable with stresses generated by the awareness of differences between the two worlds.

Acute Intercurrent Illness

Issues of family organization and management are often relevant in the care of children with acute intercurrent illness. When a child is on a short course of antibiotics, for example, it may be desirable to know whether the person who brings in the child for health care also can depend on other caregivers to adhere to the medication schedule, and whether the babysitter or daycare provider will cooperate. It also may be important to obtain history about the onset of symptoms from the person who was actually with the child when the problem first presented. When there are marked differences in health beliefs, other family frictions, or conflicting agendas such as in custody disputes, cooperation may be impaired and the acute care of the child jeopardized. The clinician may need to address such issues if they interfere with the delivery of effective pediatric care.

Management of Chronic Conditions

Issues that relate to the care of children with acute illness become accentuated in the face of serious ongoing health conditions. These conditions are inherently long-lasting and often interfere with daily functioning or require special attention and care. Such conditions pose significant burdens for all families, and they require building a therapeutic alliance between health-care professionals and the family members, including the affected child. Unless all members of the family unit are known to the pediatrician, and unless all family members understand the implications of the condition and its care, there is substantial opportunity for miscommunication and misunderstanding that can impede the development and implementation of an appropriate care plan.

It is essential that the pediatrician speak with all the primary caregivers in the family at the time of the initial diagnosis of a chronic health condition as well as at periodic reassessments or when there are major decisions to make. When the daily life of a child with a chronic condition involves a great deal of direct personal care, communication among all caregivers is critical, especially when they do not overlap in their time of child care. Changes in symptoms or adjustments of medications must be communicated carefully and compulsively. This can be especially difficult around times of stress, such as during an episode of major illness involving another family member, or when there are changes in the family structure, such as separation or divorce. In such instances, the pediatrician can play an important role in helping the family members to focus on the child's needs and in identifying potential supports to help stabilize the situation.

RESPECTING DIVERSITY

Although family forms vary from society to society, across social classes, and by place of residence, certain norms of family behavior are so rooted in fundamental social values that they are legally enforceable. These usually involve the physical and moral safety of children, as well as the care that parents are expected to provide. In contrast, minor violations are handled informally by neighbors, family members, and health-care providers. Within legal limits, a great variation of behavior is observed. Idiosyncratic or eccentric families that provide consistent and nurturing environments rarely produce serious disturbance in their children's personalities or adjustment.

The majority of children who are reared in any given family type will grow and thrive. During the course of normal child development, the stability of caregiving arrangements and provision of supportive and affectionate nurturance for the child are central issues, and the availability of multiple adults who are related to the child may offer some advantage to the child's emotional development. The clinician who has a trusting and respectful longitudinal relationship with a child and family can play a critical role in helping them through a wide range of adaptive challenges.

References

Bond LA, Wagner BM: Families in Transition: Primary Prevention Programs that Work. Newbury Park, CA, Sage, 1988

Burden D: Single parents and work settings: the impact of multiple job and home life responsibilities. Fam Relat 35:37, 1987

Copons S: Children in Family Contexts. New York, Guilford, 1989

Fiese BH, Sameroff AJ: Family context in pediatric psychology: a transactional perspective. In: Roberts MC, Wallander JL, ed: Family Issues in Pediatric Psychology. Hillsdale, NJ, Lawrence Erlbaum Associates, 1992:239–260

McCubbin HI, Figley C, eds: Stress and Family Coping with Normative Transitions. New York, Brunner/Mazel, 1983

Roberts MC, Wallander JL: Family issues in pediatric psychology: an overview. In: Roberts MC, Wallander JL, eds: Family Issues in Pediatric Psychology. Hillsdale, NJ, Lawrence Erlbaum Associates, 1992:1–24

Tanner L, ed: Children, Families and Stress. 25th Ross Roundtable. Columbus, OH, Ross Laboratories, 1994

Turk DC, Kerns RD: Health, Illness, and Families: A Life Span Perspective. New York, Wiley, 1985

Wallerstein JS: Second Chances: Men, Women and Children a Decade after Divorce. New York, Ticknor & Fields, 1989

5.8.2 Nonparental Child Care

Abbey D. Alkon

Nonparental child-care arrangements for children under age 6 years increased over the last 20 years as the demographics of our society changed. In 1997, 25% of children lived in single-parent households, 32% of births were to single women, and 65% of married mothers with children under age 6 years were in the labor force. Women work out of the home primarily for economic reasons, but also for intellectual stimulation, a sense of accomplishment and self-worth, and a source of social networks.

TYPES OF NONPARENTAL CHILD-CARE ARRANGEMENTS

Parents seek nonparental child care that is affordable, conveniently located, dependable, and of high quality. The three most common types of nonparental child-care arrangements are in-home care, family child care, and center care. From 1965 to 1993, child-care arrangements changed from primarily in-home care to center care. In-home care decreased from 77% to 53%, and child-care center enrollment increased from 6% to 30%, respectively. Family child care has remained stable at 17%.

In-home care, individual care provided by a relative or nonrelative in the child's or provider's home, is most common for children under 2 years of age. In-home care is not regulated in most states, and the majority of providers do not have specialized training. In-home care is also the most expensive type of child care, if provided by a nonrelative. *Family child care,* small groups of children from different families cared for in a caretaker's home, is the most prevalent child-care arrangement for children under 5 years of age. Family child care is usually located in the child's neighborhood and has flexible hours. Children who receive state or federally subsidized care are most likely to be in family child care (56%). Unfortunately, family child care is not adequately regulated, and thus the quality varies tremendously across sites. *Child-care centers,* group care in licensed facilities by staff meeting regulatory standards, have structured hours of operation and are usually more expensive than family child-care homes. Because they are licensed by the state, requirements for staff-to-child ratios, group size, space, health and safety conditions, and staff training vary greatly across the country. Centers are known to employ trained staff and provide adequate space, equipment, toys, and organized activities as required by licensure, which varies for each state.

CHILD CARE QUALITY

High-quality child care, whether in family child-care home or center settings, provides healthy and safe environments that are appropriate to the child's background, age, and stage of development. Unfortunately, many of our children in the United States are not receiving high-quality child care. Several recent national studies rated the overall quality of child care in the United States as mediocre. In a study of 401 child-care centers in 4 states, 86% of the centers provided only medium- or poor-quality services. A full 40% of the infants and toddler centers were judged low quality, had poor general health practices, and had inadequate interaction with caregivers. Infants in families at either extreme of socioeconomic levels—poverty or affluence—received higher-quality infant child care than infants in near-poverty. Family child care did not fare better. In an observational study of 225 children in family child-care homes or relative care, 35% of the homes were rated as inadequate in quality. Children from low-income homes were in lower-quality care than the children from higher-income homes.

Higher-quality centers have low child:staff ratios, small group size, teachers with early childhood education, low teacher turnover, higher teacher wages, and more experienced administrators than lower-quality centers. Because there are no federal standards for child care, the responsibility for maintaining quality lies with the individual states or child-care sites. In response to the need for higher standards in child care, the National Association for the Education of Young Children (NAEYC) and the National Association for Family Child Care (NAFCC) began voluntary programs for accreditation of child-care centers and family child-care homes. Quality criteria were established by these professional associations to improve the quality of care and education for children in out-of-home care settings. The American Academy of Pediatrics and the American Public Health Association also developed standards for health and safety in out-of-home programs. The National Center for the Early Childhood Work Force showed that centers with high quality were more likely to have nonprofit status, to pay higher wages to teaching staff, to retain skilled teachers, and to achieve NAEYC accreditation than were lower-quality centers.

EFFECTS OF NONPARENTAL CHILD CARE

The effects of nonparental child care on young children have been controversial for many years. The effect of child care on children's development depends on a number of interrelated factors, including characteristics of the family, child, and care setting. Some of these factors are the stability of nonparental care arrangements and the length of time in nonparental care.

For children from low-income families, studies show strong positive effects of high-quality child care on children's growth and development, academic achievements, and success in adult life. A long-term evaluation of the Perry Preschool Program showed that low-income children enrolled in half-day child-care centers from 3 to 5 years of age were more likely as adults to complete high school, to stay married, to maintain employment, and to have lower delinquency rates, when compared to children who did not participate in their program. Another longitudinal study, the Carolina Abecedarian Project, provided child care for infants through age 5 and found that participating children had higher cognitive test scores from the toddler years to age 21, and higher reading and math scores from primary school to young adulthood. In addition, as adults the intervention children completed more years of education, were older when their first child was born, and achieved higher maternal employment status than families that did not participate in the Project.

The newest longitudinal and comprehensive child-care study, the NICHD Study of Early Child Care, enrolled 1364 infants from 10 sites in 1991 to study the effect of child care on children's development. The recent study findings show that family characteristics and the quality of the mother's relationship with the child were stronger predictors of children's development than were child-care factors. Infants' attachment to their mothers at 15 months of age was not generally affected by length of time in child care. Family and home characteristics (eg, income, maternal education, maternal sensitivity, maternal depression), rather than child-care experiences, predicted the quality of the mother–child interaction and children's behavior at age 3 years. Children who spent time in group care with three or more children had fewer behavior problems and were more cooperative in child care than children who were not in group care.

EFFECTS OF CHILD-CARE QUALITY

A number of studies have found significant social and cognitive benefits from high-quality child care. Children's cognitive and social development are positively related to the quality of the child-care experience. Children in better child-care centers display more advanced language and premath skills, have better relationships with their teachers, and have more advanced prosocial skills than do children in lower-quality care. Children who attended higher-quality child care were more sociable, self-confident, and had more positive peer relationships than children in lower-quality centers. The positive effects of better quality child care on children's cognitive and socioemotional outcomes were found for both boys and girls, for children from different ethnic backgrounds, and for children whose mothers had different levels of education.

A follow-up study of preschool children who attended child-care centers in the Cost, Quality & Outcomes Study when they were in second grade, showed that children who attended high-quality centers had better math skills and fewer problem behaviors through second grade than did children who went to lower-quality centers. Children with closer teacher–child relationships in child care had better classroom skills, particularly thinking/attention skills, and fewer problem behaviors in second grade.

ROLE OF THE CHILD-HEALTH PROFESSIONAL

Primary Care

Child-health professionals can promote successful child-care experiences for young children by discussing family needs and plans for nonparental child-care arrangements during the prenatal *and* postnatal periods. It can be stressful finding an affordable, conveniently located, high-quality child-care program that also meets an individual child's emotional needs and fits the child's temperament. There are numerous national and local organizations that provide information about child-care availability, licensure requirements, and indicators of high-quality child care (Table 5-39). For example, the National Association of Child Care Resource and Referral Agencies (NACCRRA) lists local agencies that help families find child care, and the National Association for the Education of Young Children (NAEYC) provides information about quality in child care. Health and safety information is provided by the American Academy of Pediatrics (AAP) and the US Department of Health and Human Services' Child Care Bureau.

Health Consultants

Growth in the number of children in nonparental child care presents both challenges and unique opportunities for child-health professionals. At the community level, there are new roles for primary-care providers to become child-health consultants for family child-care homes and child-care centers. Because children attending group-care settings are at elevated risks for infectious disease and injuries, there is a growing need for health professionals to advise local child-care programs about health and safety standards. Health professionals can also work with child-care providers to identify children with developmental, health, social, and/or behavioral problems. Primary-care providers can help parents and staff to develop appropriate care plans for children with special needs.

There have been several recent national campaigns to promote the health and safety of children in nonparental care settings. In 1995, the Child Care Bureau and the Maternal and Child Health Bureau initiated the Healthy Child Care America Campaign, which outlined ten steps communities could take to promote healthy and safe child care. In 1999, The National Training Institute for Child Care Health Consultants at the University of North Carolina, Chapel Hill, developed a curriculum for training health professionals as child-care health consultants that is being disseminated at the state level. The Institute's purpose is to prepare health-care consultant trainers who will, in turn, train health-care consultants to work with their local child-care programs to improve the health and safety of young children in group settings.

Advocacy

To improve the quality of child care for all children, child-health professionals should lobby for federal and state standards that lower child-staff ratios, increase teacher educational requirements, limit group size, and improve health and safety standards. Additional

TABLE 5-39

CHILD-CARE HEALTH CONSULTANT RESOURCES: NATIONAL ORGANIZATIONS AND PUBLICATIONS

ORGANIZATION	SERVICES PROVIDED AND PUBLICATION(S)	WEBSITE ADDRESS http://
American Academy of Pediatrics (AAP) Committee on Early Childhood, Adoption, and Dependent Care (CECADC) Elk Grove Village, IL 800-433-9016	Pediatricians involved in child-care health collaborate on projects, policies, etc. *Health in Day Care: A Manual for Health Professionals,* 2000 (in press); *Healthy Child Care America Campaign—Blueprint for Action,* and AAP newsletter.	www.aap.org
Child Care Law Center San Francisco, CA 415-495-5498	Quarterly newsletter, *Legal Update.* Resource about legal issues related to Americans for Disabilities Act and child care.	www.childcarelaw.org
Early Childhood Education Linkage System (ECELS) Rosemont, PA	Pennsylvania's AAP chapter created the ECELS program and provides information, guidelines, manual, checklists for health consultants. Resource library, training materials, and workshops available.	www.paaap.org/ecels/
National Association of Child Care Resource and Referral Agencies (NACCRRA) Washington, DC 202-393-5501	Publishes directory of local resource and referral agencies, checklist for choosing quality child care.	www.naccrra.net
National Association for Family Child Care Des Moines, IA 515-282-8192	Provides technical assistance for family child-care organizations, biannual conferences, quarterly newsletter. Accreditation provided for family child care.	www.nafcc.org
National Association for the Education of Young Children (NAEYC) Washington, DC 800-424-2460	Publishes books and established accreditation process for centers. *Healthy Young Children: A Manual for Programs* (1995) Kendrick, Kaufmann, Messenger, eds. *Model Child Care Health Policies* (1993) Pennsylvania AAP Chapter.	www.naeyc.org
National Association of Pediatric Nurse Associates and Practitioners (NAPNAP) Cherry Hill, NJ 609-667-1773	Professional organization of Pediatric Nurse Practitioners (PNP) involved in child-care health. *Child Care Special Interest Group News:* published 4 times/year	www.napnap.org
National Child Care Information Center Vienna, VA 800-616-2242	Maintains central database for child-care-related information. Bimonthly newsletter, *Child Care Bulletin.*	nccic.org
National Resource Center for Health and Safety in Child Care University of Colorado, Health Sciences Center; School of Nursing Denver, CO 800-598-KIDS	Links to child-care Web sites (eg, organizations, conferences, child-care training, research study results), lists states' child-care regulations, and APHA and AAP's *National Health and Safety Performance Standards.*	nrc.uchsc.edu
The National Training Institute for Child Care Health Consultants Department of Maternal and Child Health, University of N. Carolina Chapel Hill, NC 919-966-5976	Developed and implemented a standardized national training program for Child Care Health Consultants.	cdlhc.sph.unc.edu/courses/childcare/
Child Care Bureau, US Department of Health and Human Services, Administration on Children, Youth, & Families (ACYF), Washington, DC 202-690-5641	Information on child care and development block grants; links to other ACYF sites and child-care sites; *Healthy Child Care America—Blueprint for Action,* compiled by the National Center for Education in Maternal and Child Health (US Govt. Printing Office; 1996–719-428).	www.acf.dhhs.gov/programs/ccb

federal and state issues are the lack of accessible, affordable, high-quality child care, especially for the low-middle-income families and families living in rural and migrant agricultural communities. Other issues that affect child care are parents' need for flexible work schedules, income tax credits for child care, and support for the Parental Leave Act.

High-quality nonparental child care is important for all children's social, emotional, and cognitive development. The nation should increase its investment in young children by supporting better salaries and educational opportunities for child-care teachers and improved standards for family child-care homes and child-care centers. Both government agencies and businesses should increase their financial support of our children by subsidizing the cost of good

quality child care for low-income families, and those investments should be tied to incentives for care providers to increase quality. Primary-care providers can get involved locally, regionally, or nationally to ensure that all young children who have parents working in the labor force have access to affordable, high-quality nonparental care.

References

American Public Health Association and American Academy of Pediatrics: Caring for Our Children; National Health and Safety Performance Standards: Guidelines for Out-of-Home Child Care Programs. Washington, DC, American Public Health Association, 1992

Clarke-Stewart K: Predicting child development from child care forms and features: the Chicago Study. In: Phillips DA, ed: Quality in Child Care: What Does Research Tell Us? Washington, DC, NAEYC, 1993

Cost Quality and Outcomes Study Team: Cost, Quality, and Child Outcomes in Child Care Centers, Public Report, 2nd ed: Denver, CO, University of Colorado, 1995

Galinsky E, Howes C, Kontos S, Shinn M: The Study of Children in Family Child Care and Relative Care. New York, Families and Work Institute, 1994

Helburn S, Howes C: Child care cost and quality. Fut Child 6:62–82, 1996

Hofferth S, Brayfield A, et al: National Child Care Survey, 1990. Washington, DC, The Urban Institute, 1991

NICHD Early Child Care Research Network: Child care and mother–child interaction in the first 3 years of life. Dev Psychol 35:1399, 1999

Schweinhart L, Weikart D: Young Children Grow Up: The Effects of the Perry Preschool Program on Youths Through Age 15. Ypsilanti, MI, High/Scope Educational Research Foundation, 1980

Whitebrook M, Howes C, et al: The National Child Care Staffing Study— Who Cares? Child Care Teachers and the Quality of Care in America. Washington, DC, Center for the Child Care Work Force, 1990

Whitebrook M, Sakai L, et al: NAEYC Accreditation as a Strategy for Improving Child Care Quality. Washington, DC, National Center for the Early Childhood Work Force, 1997

Zigler E, Lang M: Child Care Choices: Balancing the Needs of Children, Families, and Society. New York, The Free Press, 1991

5.8.3 Vulnerable Child Syndrome

Michael Thomasgard

DEFINITIONS AND EPIDEMIOLOGY

Green and Solnit introduced the term *vulnerable child syndrome* based on their observations of 25 children who had recovered from potentially fatal medical conditions (eg, congenital heart disease, seizures, apnea). The parents of these children shared the common experience of having been told by their child's physician, or of personally concluding, that their child would likely die. Following the child's full recovery, these children were considered by their parents, for reasons that were not founded in reality, to be at continued risk for serious illness or premature death. The syndrome includes a distinct cluster of characteristics, including parental difficulty in setting limits, that often result in impulsive child behavior, persistent overconcern about the child's health with excessive use of medical services, indulgent parental behaviors toward the child that are often demonstrated through infantilization, and difficulties with separation. Data on the prevalence of this behavioral syndrome are unavailable.

ETIOLOGY AND PATHOGENESIS

The defining feature of the vulnerable child syndrome is a parental perception of heightened child vulnerability to illness or injury, secondary to a threatened separation or loss of the child. Several markers have been postulated that lead to a parent's unconscious perception of excessive child vulnerability:

- History of a previous serious illness from which the parent did not believe the child would recover;
- The child representing for the parent an important figure from the past who died prematurely;
- Stresses occurring around the time of the child's conception (eg, death of a significant individual in the parent's life, series of

devaluing experiences, knowledge of close friends or relatives who had children with impairments);
- Health events that are associated with past pregnancies or the child's perinatal period (eg, history of stillbirth, abortion, infertility, prematurity, feeding problems, jaundice); and
- The mother's fear of her own dying during childbirth.

How perceptions of child vulnerability become reinforced in a parent's mind often can be traced to the period of recovery from illness, at a time when the parent was still anticipating the child's death. Subsequently, the child may sense the parent's lingering fear and anxiety and engage in behaviors designed to test parental limit setting.

CLINICAL MANIFESTATIONS

A broad spectrum of parental reactions to illness or other developmental stresses exists for all families, including those whose children have chronic medical conditions. Even highly adaptive parents may experience a transient sense of anxious guilt concerning subsequent illnesses their child may have. Parents who retain the perception of their child being uniquely vulnerable often face the fear of losing the child, albeit unconsciously, with every minor illness that follows. In such circumstances, the normal parenting tasks of facilitating the child's increasing independence and setting appropriate limits are thwarted. Consequently, successive illnesses or developmental transitions call forth an unconscious resurgence of previous fears related to potential loss and separation from the child, rather than providing an opportunity to promote growth for both the parent and child. The parent does not experience any meaningful resolution of his or her fear of loss; instead only negative child outcomes are imagined for the future.

Variants of the vulnerable child syndrome have been described in association with parental reactions to false-positive test results and what has been termed *nondisease*. For example, a false-positive screening for a metabolic disorder such as phenylketonuria or hypothyroidism has led some parents to continue believing that their child will be mentally retarded despite subsequent negative tests and reassurances from their physician. Similar concerns have been documented in children with innocent heart murmurs whose activities were restricted by their parents over fear of sudden cardiac death. The common denominator for true life-threatening conditions and benign events that provoke excessive parental concern generally relates more to parental variables (eg, anxiety, compulsive behavior, past unresolved ambivalent relationships involving loss or separation) than to the child's intrinsic health.

ASSESSMENT AND TREATMENT

Diagnosis and management of the vulnerable child syndrome are closely linked. The clinician must address both the parent's concerns about the child and the child's pattern of health, behavior, and development. Thus, the child must be viewed in the context of the parent–child relationship and its historical unfolding. This contextual approach is particularly important when managing a parent whose anxious appearance and concern about the child's health seem to be disproportionate to the child's biological status and life circumstances.

The care of families who manifest such difficulties begins with a thorough history and physical examination. The clinician must be sensitive to the fact that parents often are not aware of the connection between past health events, their unconscious perceptions, and their current behaviors and interactions with the child. Statements such as "You seem very worried about your child's health" and "What is it about this illness that concerns you the most?" can help the story to emerge in a nondefensive manner. Follow-up inquiries such as "Was your child ever seriously ill?", "How sick was your child at that time?", and "Were you afraid that your child might die?" often uncover previously unspoken concerns. The clinician must tolerate the parent's anxiety and suspend premature judgment about the child's condition. Attempts to minimize the parent's concerns or to confront the parent's feelings abruptly are generally counterproductive. Meeting with the child's other parent or caregiver provides an opportunity to explore how the responsibilities of parenting and feelings of anxiety are shared.

The prevention of an enduring parental sense of child vulnerability can be accomplished by not overstating the dangers of a serious illness at the initial diagnosis, having continued conversations with parents during the acute phase of the illness and the recovery period, and helping parents to regain their sense of competence in caring for their child as the child improves. A follow-up meeting with parents after the acute phase of a serious disease can help them to gain closure on the episode in a constructive and reassuring manner.

NATURAL HISTORY AND PROGNOSIS

Reported outcomes range from complete resolution of both the grieving process and the child's illness, with normal subsequent psychosocial development, to significant parent–child difficulties focused on separation and autonomy (eg, sleeping, eating, dressing, feeding, discipline, temper tantrums). Perceived child vulnerability is frequently followed by permissive parenting behaviors manifested by difficulties with limit setting or, less frequently, as overprotective parenting manifested by highly controlling parental behaviors toward the child. Behavioral outcomes have included school underachievement and increased child internalizing (eg, somatic, anxiety) and/or externalizing (aggressive, impulsive) symptoms.

In the case of permissive parenting, both parental anxiety and unresolved feelings of guilt or grief continue to resurface as the child develops more independence. The dilemma for the parent is reflected in the challenge of setting age-appropriate limits without risking separation from the child, which may represent the psychological equivalent of the child's death. At times of stress, guilt may be overtaken by anger, and the parent may suddenly become punitive toward the child, with a shift from overly indulgent to overly controlling and demeaning interactions. The clinical challenge is to understand the parent's anxiety regarding limit setting and to help the parent develop more consistent and effective behavior-management strategies.

It may be challenging and time-consuming to address parents' anxieties about their children in a busy office practice. However, the alternative often results in a repeated cycle of excessive medical encounters to address both perceived child vulnerability and parental anxiety.

References

Bergman AB, Stamm SJ: The morbidity of cardiac nondisease in schoolchildren. N Engl J Med 276:1008–1013, 1967

Boyce WT: The vulnerable child: new evidence, new approaches. Adv Pediatr 39:1–33, 1992

Forsyth BWC, Canny PF: Perceptions of vulnerability 3 1/2 years after problems of feeding and crying behavior in early infancy. Pediatrics 88:757–763, 1991

Forsyth BWC, McCue Horwitz S, Leventhal JM, Burger J, Leaf PJ: The child vulnerability scale: an instrument to measure parental perceptions of child vulnerability. J Pediatr Psychol 21:89–101, 1996

Green M: Vulnerable child syndrome and its variants. Pediatr Rev 8:75–80, 1986

Green M, Solnit AJ: Reactions to the threatened loss of a child: a vulnerable child syndrome. Pediatrics 34:58–66, 1964

Kemper KJ, Forsyth BW, McCarthy PL: Persistent perceptions of vulnerability following neonatal jaundice. Am J Dis Child 144:238–241, 1990

Levy J: Vulnerable children: parents' perspectives and the use of medical care. Pediatrics 65:956–963, 1980

Perrin EC, West PD, Culley BS: Is my child normal yet? Correlates of vulnerability. Pediatrics 83:355–363, 1989

Thomasgard M: Parental perceptions of child vulnerability, overprotection, and parental psychological characteristics. Child Psychiatry Hum Dev 28:223–240, 1998

Thomasgard M, Metz WP: The two-year stability of parental perceptions of child vulnerability and parental overprotection. J Dev Behav Pediatr 17:222–228, 1996

Thomasgard M, Metz WP: Parent–child relationship disorders: what do the child vulnerability scale and the parent protection scale measure? Clin Pediatr 38:347–356, 1999

5.8.4   Major Family Transitions: Birth of a Sibling and Bereavement

Lauren Heim Goldstein

The lives of children often are filled with an inexhaustible series of joys and sadness, triumphs and defeats, and times of stability and change, as are the lives of their parents. The vicissitudes in children's lives comprise not only severe, unexpected events that test their ability to cope but also a long succession of predictable and normative events that issue milder, more frequent challenges to a child's adaptive capability. Indeed, it has been argued that one of the principal forces driving cognitive and emotional development is the *challenge to adapt* that is inherent in adversity and hardship. From a developmental perspective, it is often the crises in human experience, and an individual's efforts to move through and past these crises, that invoke a capacity for growth, regeneration, and mastery. Ironically, the very difficulties that distress and dispirit a child often prompt the setting of new trajectories and guide the child's emergence into new and richer developmental landscapes.

Transitions often are stressors by virtue of their capacity to confront children with novelty and change, disrupt homeostatic family processes and alter the character of relationships, aggravate previously existing difficulties, and close or open opportunities for change. For example, it is known that even an eagerly anticipated transition such as a 5-year-old child's entry into kindergarten is capable of evoking psychobiological and behavioral changes characteristic of a classical stress response. Gross motor skills that are acquired near the end of the first year of life allow independent, self-guided mobility, but fundamentally change the nature of a toddler's relationships to his or her parents. An 11-year-old child who has struggled with feelings of self-deprecation may be depressed on entering the disorienting world of middle school. An adolescent's graduation from high school signals not only new possibilities for autonomy and growth but also the end of the adolescent's tenure as a child in the family home. It is at the cusp of these major transitions that children experience both the irrepressible elation of new possibilities and a troubling, unsettled sense of their "world" being forever changed.

Two of the most challenging adaptive transitions in childhood are a younger sibling's birth and the death of a parent or loved one. The birth of a younger brother or sister is a memorable turning point in which the family is transformed by the advent of a new life and new relationships. No family is unchanged after gaining a new member. The death of a loved one, however, especially the death of a parent or a much-loved grandparent, marks the *end* of a relationship and the beginning of a long, often painful struggle to understand and accommodate its ending.

Although births and deaths seem to have antithetical effects on children's lives, both events share deep commonalities. While the birth of a sibling is usually and logically viewed as a joyful gain to the family, it also heralds important, inevitable *losses* in the child's experience of his or her parents and family. It is those losses attending a birth that often are emotionally the most salient for an older brother or sister. Similarly, while the death of a parent or grandparent is most importantly and profoundly experienced as a loss, there are often ways in which a child may *gain* through that death new insights into the meaning of personal relationships, new appreciation for the presence of family, and new capacities for pondering the deeper questions of life.

The psychological meanings of these family transitions thus comprise for children both the losses and gains that regularly accompany births and deaths of family members. The pediatrician's ability to assist children and families through such troubling events requires knowledge of the developmental and behavioral sequelae of major transitions, a capacity for eliciting and responding to emotional information, and an understanding of the adaptive strategies useful to children in coping with stressful life events. In the midst of these transitions, it is crucial to assess the resources available to the child, the developmental skills required to master the transition, and the family's appraisals of the event or transition. The developmental, family, and community contexts in which children experience these events will largely shape a child's psychological experiences and understanding of the events. The distinctive features of these two transitions (ie, the birth of a sibling and the death of a loved one) are first addressed individually, then followed by a general discussion of the pediatric management of childhood transitions.

BIRTH OF A SIBLING

Pediatricians often help parents to understand the misgivings that a first child may feel at the birth of a younger brother or sister by drawing a simple analogy to the parent's own experience. How would you feel, the parent (eg, the mother) is asked, if your husband came home one evening with another, younger woman and said, "I want you to meet Julie. You know how much I have always loved you, but now I also love Julie, and she will be living with us from now on." Parents usually understand, with vivid recognition, the conflicted and seemingly unacceptable feelings that a child may experience in confronting the arrival of a younger sibling. Especially for a first child, but even for the second, third, or fourth in a large family, a newborn brother or sister brings an end to life as they have known it, along with new complexities, parental demands and expectations, and constraints on behavior and activity. Suddenly, the parental lap that was once the older child's throne is occupied by a smaller, and more demanding, infant. Maternal attention to the older sibling decreases significantly; more controlling, punitive parenting styles are often implemented; and short-term changes in the security of the mother–child attachment relationship often occur. There is evidence that during this time period fathers can usefully provide the older sibling with more attention, thereby compensating for the mother's preoccupation with the new infant.

Along with the older sibling's adjustment to an infant's presence, parents themselves also must face and adjust to difficult and emotionally draining changes. Night wakings, periods of infant fussiness, new financial obligations, and the infant's unique set of personal needs all place new and taxing demands on parents. Family patterns and routines are likely to be disrupted, and care for older children is often transferred, at least temporarily, to other family members or extrafamilial caretakers. Within such a context, there is little wonder that an older child may feel displaced, unsettled, or abandoned.

Responses to the Birth of a Sibling

Some degree of felt or expressed hostility toward the new baby is an almost universal occurrence for the older child. Parents should be told that while the infant must be protected from active, physical aggression, the older sibling's feelings should be acknowledged, named, and addressed with understanding and care. Older children's emotional and behavioral responses to a birth will depend importantly on aspects of both temperament and development. Parents therefore must be attentive to the characteristic signs of distress of both their own child and of most children at their child's particular developmental stage. While some may exhibit developmental regression such as a return to thumb-sucking or loss of toilet training, others may show sadness or withdrawal, and still others may develop aggressive behavior problems at home or in child care, or problems with peer relationships. Boys are more likely to show increases in peer conflict following the birth of a sibling, and girls more frequently experience an increase in anxious-depressive behaviors. A 4-year-old child may revert to wetting the bed at night; a highly independent 3-year-old child with months or years of child-care experience suddenly may develop difficulties with separation from parents on arrival at the child-care center. Older children may either distance themselves from parents and family or immerse themselves in the activities surrounding the care and feeding of the infant. The increase in problem behaviors, although common during this transition, is short-lived and should decrease within approximately 1 year after the birth of the new sibling.

Recommendations for Pediatricians

Given these age-dependent differences in response, some parents seek pediatric advice regarding the spacing of children and the optimal age for an older child at the birth of a new baby. While evidence in this regard is sparse, it appears that a birth interval of at least 2 years is associated with better verbal skills and academic achievement in the older child, which is an observation most likely related to early developmental acceleration with individual parental attention. When the spacing of children is less than 18 months, there may be a tendency toward treating both the older child and the infant in a similar manner, leading to an infantalization of the older sibling. While too narrow an interval between children logically might be discouraged, parents should be told that there is no single best time to have a second, third, or fourth child.

Other aspects of pediatric counsel that may be useful to parents during this transition include:

During pregnancy:

- Encourage parents to be open with older children about the pregnancy and expected birth. Allowing children to share in the anticipation of a new birth assists them in finding ways to cope and adapt to the prospect of a younger sibling.
- Allow the older child to participate in the care of the baby. During pregnancy, the older child should be invited to come to obstetric appointments, listen to the fetus' heart beat or watch it on an ultrasound image, and feel the baby move. After delivery, the older child can be involved by holding, feeding, and comforting the newborn under parental supervision.
- Changes in the configuration of the older child's bed or bedroom should be carried out well in advance of the delivery. Efforts should be made to cast such changes in a positive light. Switching the older child to a regular bed, for example, should be accompanied by statements of pride in the child's growth and in the child's new ability to sleep in a real bed, "just like a big person." If possible, some decision-making discretion should be given to the older child, for example, allowing the child to help with decisions about where in the bedroom the baby's crib will be placed.
- Local librarians or children's booksellers can assist parents in choosing books on the birth of a younger sibling from the broad children's literature on difficult family transitions. Especially when a parent is available to read and discuss the book, this may offer the older child a valuable chance to "rehearse" the arrival of the baby and begin thinking and talking about all it will mean.
- Encourage parents to foster their child's positive peer relationships by having play dates when possible. Children's early friendships provide opportunities to learn social skills, to learn to tolerate frustration, and to resolve conflicts. These skills enable children to interact with siblings in positive ways.

Following the birth of the new sibling:

- A father's increased involvement and attention, perhaps more than any other intervention, can provide the comfort and reassurance that older children often need at this time. Encourage fathers to use the postnatal period as an opportunity not only to meet and get to know a new son or daughter but to spend more intensive and extended time with the older children as well. A father's genuine attentiveness to the older child's needs will do much to assuage the complicated and difficult feelings that often emerge at this time. If no father is present in the family, having another relative (eg, grandparent, aunt, or uncle) or a close friend spend additional one-on-one time with the older child is beneficial.
- Parents can encourage the older child to express his or her emotions and reactions to the birth of the baby. Role play, fantasy play, and drawing may help children cope with their new emotions during this time. Parents can help the older child to understand the advantages and benefits of becoming a big sister or brother by emphasizing the behaviors and privileges of which the newborn is incapable.

BEREAVEMENT

While the death of a parent or loved one is universally recognized as a profoundly painful family transition, bereavement also is an intensely personal process with great individual variability in its meaning, complexity, and degree of difficulty. Death is experienced and interpreted within the family's social, cultural, ethnic, and religious contexts. A child's understanding of death and responses to the mourning process depend on the child's cognitive and emotional development, the child's family background, and the amount and quality of support the child receives. Death is understood by children of different ages in different ways. Four central ideas that emerge with the maturation of death concepts during the middle childhood years have been identified:

1. Irreversibility (ie, an understanding of death as permanent and irrevocable);
2. Finality (ie, an understanding of the cessation of all life processes);
3. Inevitability (ie, death's inescapability for all living beings); and
4. Causality (ie, the development of a rational understanding of the causes of death)

Developmental Understanding of Death

Although losing a loved one during a child's preschool years may result in a precocious understanding of death, children younger than 5 years of age generally have rudimentary and cognitively incomplete interpretations of death and the process of dying. Under 5 years of age, a child's normatively egocentric view of the causes for events may result in feelings of guilt or persistent, unspoken concerns that something the child did was implicated in the parent's death. Early experiences with the death of pets or other creatures may enable a child to explore the meaning of dying in a context with less traumatic emotional implications. Until approximately 6 or 7 years of age, children are typically not able to understand the finality and irreversibility of death. During the period between 5 and 10 years, cognitive and emotional development results in a gradual acquisition of the four basic death concepts, and by the second decade of life, adolescents generally have arrived at a fully mature cognitive understanding of death.

Behavioral and Emotional Responses to Death

Behavioral and emotional responses to the loss of a parent or loved one at any age often are severe and deeply troubling. Young children may harbor strong feelings of anger toward either the deceased or the surviving parent. Many preschool children at first may seem to sustain little visible reaction to their loss, returning almost too soon or too readily to the normal activities of daily life. However, sleep disturbances, separation anxiety, and/or aggressive behaviors are common problems seen in reaction to loss in this age group. Other children may show regressive behaviors, social withdrawal, or expressions of inconsolable sadness and despair over their loss. This wide range of behaviors may be the child's way of indirectly asking for help. School-age children may appear to deny that a death occurred and try to act "grown up"; in this age group, many children find it important not to stand out as different among their peer group and thus may hide their feelings of pain and grief. Ultimately, a child's ability to overcome bereavement and move back onto a path of healthy psychological and emotional development will depend on a number of interacting factors, including the security of the child's relationships with both parents, opportunity for open grieving, and continuing presence of nurturing, supportive adults in the child's social environment.

Tasks of Bereavement

A child must accomplish a series of tasks to accommodate to loss and to move on with his or her life and relationships in a healthy, functional manner. The early tasks include understanding the death in an age-appropriate way and being protected. A child must be given an accurate, prompt, age-appropriate explanation of how, when, and why the person died. Next, the child needs to feel safe and protected following the loss of a loved one. Questions such as, "Who will take care of me now?" and "Who will take me to school?" are common as children try to figure out what the new roles will be.

The next series of tasks involve accepting the loss emotionally, reevaluating the relationship with the deceased, and bearing the emotional pain. Because the painful feelings accompanying the loss of a parent or close loved one can be unbearable and overwhelming, a child often experiences the pain in small, more manageable doses over a longer period of time. Thus, the mourning process for children is often more prolonged than for adults. This may help to explain why a bereaved child may be deeply involved in play and normal childhood activities at one point in time only to appear extremely distressed later the same day.

Finally, a child needs to invest in new relationships and to return to developmental tasks. A child may avoid forming new relationships after the loss of a parent or loved one because the child does not want to risk losing anyone else. Because children may take a long time to work through the mourning process, it may take them longer than it takes adults to be able to accept new people in their lives such as a stepparent. After the loss of a parent or loved one, the child eventually must return to age-appropriate developmental tasks. Although the tasks of development have not changed, the family context has changed, and the child's identity may have changed as well.

Risk Factors

Risk factors for a poor psychiatric outcome in the short- or long-term include: (a) bereavement of a child less than 5 years of age or in early adolescence; (b) death of the mother for girls younger than 11 years and death of the father for boys in adolescence; (c) a child with prior psychological difficulties or a conflictive prior relationship with the parent who died; (d) a surviving parent who becomes emotionally dependent on the child; (e) a family or community context characterized by instability and lack of support; and (f) a death that was unexpected and/or violent in nature, as in suicide or homicide.

Recommendations for Pediatricians

Surviving parents who are confronted with the psychological management of their grieving children may bring a broad range of questions regarding appropriate responses to a child's bereavement to the pediatric clinician. Should children be allowed to attend funerals and memorial services? How much should I, as a parent, hide my own grief in the service of my child's emotional well-being? How much should children be told during a terminal illness? What else could I be doing to help?

Some recommendations for physicians helping families cope with parental loss are:

- Parents should be told that efforts to "protect" children from the emotional pain of a family's grieving most often are ineffective and, at times, even counterproductive. Parents should be advised to provide their children with honest and direct answers to questions about a dying parent and be reassured that children generally request only the information they are ready to hear. Children should be given accurate, age-appropriate explanations of the death.

- Children should be included according to their individual needs and interests in all formal events and informal stages of the mourning process and be allowed to either attend or avoid a funeral according to their own individual preferences.

- Within the family, open expression of feelings regarding the loss should be encouraged by the surviving parent's own visible willingness to share his or her emotions. Children should be encouraged to express their feelings verbally or through play and drawing.

- Parents should recognize the phenomenon of anniversary grieving (ie, the tendency for feelings of abandonment and sadness to recur on the yearly anniversary of the death) even when the date itself is not consciously remembered or recognized.

- Children need to feel safe and secure during a time of intense loss. Adults should assure the child that the child will be taken care of and loved. Support, reassurance, and affection should be continuously available. Adults who have developed a long-standing basis of mutual trust and love are most able to help a child cope with the loss of a parent. It is important to have a substitute father or mother figure to which the child can turn.

- Bereavement support groups for children may serve an important function. Support groups provide children with the opportunity to meet others their age who have also experienced similar losses. Bereavement support groups provide children with a safe place in which feelings can be shared.

- Children who have lost a parent are likely to be more sensitive in subsequent years to various kinds of natural disasters and sad events that occur in their community or in the world. Because one terrible, unexpected event happened in their lives, they may fear that a tragedy may be more likely for the surviving parent or for other loved ones. The surviving parent and other close relatives should be aware of this possible response and be sensitive to the child's perspective.

GENERAL PRINCIPLES IN MANAGING FAMILY TRANSITIONS

Children's responses to these major family transitions are determined by a combination of their chronologic and developmental ages, temperaments and personalities, past experiences with transitions and adversities, and the preparation, support, and encouragement they receive from parents and others. While parental interventions must be carefully shaped to fit the needs of individual children, a number of approaches can help children regardless of their individual dispositions and circumstances.

Often, one of the more damaging or discomforting aspects of a major transition is the disarray that it can cause in the day-to-day life of a family. Children depend on families to provide daily predictability and "sameness," which offer a child a sense of permanence and stability within a rapidly changing and challenging world. Contemporary children are regularly confronted with a dizzying profusion of novelty and change. Families provide an antidote to this disarray, offering a stable point of reference and a reassuring place to which a child can return. During stressful transitions, parents should continue, to whatever degree is possible, the *routines* and *rituals* that children count on to provide this sense of predictability. Bedtime rituals, family meals, and simple chores all are examples of routines that offer stable, reliable structures during periods of upheaval and adversity. It is the "changelessness" of these routines of family life that can balance the disorienting change that is inherent in many transitions.

Another characteristic of major transitions is their tendency to be accompanied by a great proliferation of stressful life events. Indeed, a major finding of stress research is that over an individual life span, stressful events tend to occur in clusters within relatively brief periods of time. It is not so much individual events that are responsible for stress-related declines in physical or mental health; rather, it is the combined effects of many small stressors sustained over a few short weeks or months. Parents can assist children during family transitions by *slowing the pace of change*. For example, if a move to a new home is contemplated following the birth of another child, parents may want to delay the move for several months, allowing older children to adapt first to the presence of the new child.

Often unacknowledged in the counseling that pediatricians do with parents is the extraordinary effect of a parent simply *spending time* with children. A great cultural myth has arisen in Western societies during the waning years of the 20th century: that pre-planned, high-intensity "quality time" between parents and children is an adequate or even optimal approach to the provision of parental attention and guidance. Quality time is a social illusion in need of active debunking by pediatric clinicians. Throughout the developing years, and especially during stressful family transitions, children need the gift of *regular* and *abundant parental time*. Moments of real "connection" between parents and children most often happen when they are least expected and when adequate provision has been made for large segments of time together. While much of this family time will be allotted to mundane events and interactions, it is during these unexceptional moments that parents' encouragement, support, and nurturing are most likely to occur. The best thing that a parent can spend on their children is time.

Parents should also be taught that *fantasy* and *play* are important means of coping with stressful transitions, particularly in young children. Children naturally use play as a self-therapeutic tool for managing and processing aspects of their lives that are troubling or upsetting. For example, it has been noted that among children living in war-torn areas of world, those who engage in "war play" remain psychologically more intact than children who avoid such play. Providing children with an opportunity to play and fantasize about births, deaths, and other significant transitions may constitute an important means of assistance in their emotional recovery from them.

Parents can be encouraged to share with their children the adaptive "tricks" and strategies that were acquired over the years of the parents' own lives. Such strategies may include dividing the transition task into smaller and more manageable segments, intentionally "stopping" the thoughts that are upsetting or saddening, or using exercise and games to reduce stress during periods of difficult change. Parents often are rich repositories of such accumulated wisdom, and they can be usefully encouraged to assist their children by sharing adaptive experiences and techniques.

Pediatricians and other child-health clinicians have the uncommon privilege of assisting families and children during the most critical and unsettling periods of their collective lives. A legitimate and important pediatric role thus is the provision of insight, encouragement, support, and care during the inevitable moments of painful and difficult family transition.

References

Baydar N, Hyle P, Brooks-Gunn J: A longitudinal study of the effects of the birth of a sibling during preschool and early grade school years. J Marriage Fam 59:957–965, 1997

Bowlby J: Attachment and Loss. Vol 3: Loss. New York, Basic Books, 1980

Boyce WT, Goldstein LH: Critical life events: sibling births, separations, and deaths in the family. In: Levine MD, Carey WB, Crocker AC, eds: Developmental-Behavioral Pediatrics, 3rd ed. Philadelphia, Saunders, 1999:141–148

Corr CA, Corr DM: Handbook of Childhood Death and Bereavement. New York, Springer, 1996

Kramer L, Gottman JM: Becoming a sibling: "with a little help from my friends." Dev Psychol 28:685–699, 1992

Kreppner K: Changes in dyadic relationships within a family after the arrival of a second child. In: Hinde RA, Hinde JS, eds: Relationships within Families: Mutual Influences. New York, Oxford University Press, 1988:143–167

Lewis M, Lewis DO, Schonfeld DJ: Dying and death in childhood and adolescence. In: Lewis M, ed: Child and Adolescent Psychiatry: A Comprehensive Textbook. Baltimore, Williams & Wilkins, 1991:1051–1059

Stewart RB: The Second Child: Family Transition and Adjustment. Newbury Park, CA, Sage, 1990

Teti DM, Sakin JW, Kucera E, Corns KM, Eiden RD: And baby makes four: predictors of attachment security among preschool-age firstborns during the transition to siblinghood. Child Dev 67:579–596, 1996

Yamamoto K, Davis OL, Dylak S, Whittaker J, Marsh C, Van Der Westhuizen PC: Across six nations: stressful events in the lives of children. Child Psychiatry Hum Dev 26:139–150, 1996

5.8.5   Foster Care and Adoption

Brad D. Berman

Raising a child outside the child's biological family of origin, as in foster care or adoption, presents a unique set of psychosocial challenges involving interplay between transition and adaptation. The child must contend with separation and possible reunification with the birth-parent; adjustments to one or more families; and changes in physical environment, social support, and care providers. The foster or adoptive parents are challenged with helping the child integrate into a new family, taking into account the child's previous experiences, and facing the possibility of further transitions in the future. The child's and family's success in adapting to these changes in care are influenced by a complex interaction between innate, individual capabilities and external resources. Nowhere is the traditional role of the pediatric provider more important in providing continuity of care, family guidance, and support for the physical, neurodevelopmental, and emotional needs of the child and family.

EPIDEMIOLOGY AND DEFINITIONS

Foster Care

It is estimated that there are almost 500,000 children in foster care at any given time in the United States. The number of these children undergoing more than one foster home placement has risen to nearly 50%, of which half have had three or more placements. The average length of stay in a foster placement has decreased to around 2 years. Of children entering foster care, it is currently estimated that one-third of the children are younger than age 5 years and one-third are adolescents. There is an approximately equal distribution of males and females. Minority representation and children living in poverty or economically disadvantaged circumstances is high.

Children enter foster care for a variety of reasons, including the negative impact of acute and chronic family stressors, abandonment, parental inability to care for a child, homelessness, parental substance abuse, and, increasingly, child neglect and/or physical and sexual abuse. Foster care is intended to be a temporary legal arrangement in which the child is protected and nurtured while supportive services are provided to the biological parent(s) to achieve family reunification. Risk factors for a child entering foster care are family poverty and homelessness, parental substance use, neglect, and exposure to physical and/or sexual abuse.

Foster placement is coordinated through the courts and the foster care agency, whose role (as delineated by the Child Welfare League of America) is to establish and maintain suitable substitute care; to work toward establishing a safe and permanent home for the child while maintaining biological family connections; to help children receive appropriate and necessary services; and to assist children in adjusting to the temporary care arrangement. A number of children are now being placed in *kinship foster care* with a family relative. Ironically, there may be less supervision in this type of care, with less services available for children and less economic support to the kinship foster parent. Approximately 75% of children are placed in foster care by court order. Roughly half of these children will be reunited with their biological families, often within the first 6 months, with an estimated 5 to 16% remaining in long-term foster care, 14% being adopted, and 9% being emancipated at age 16. Emancipation is legally declared in court if the child is self-supporting and not living at home. It is estimated that 25% of children in foster care will remain in the foster care system for 2 or more years and that more than 25% will experience at least three separate foster placements.

Adoption

Despite the lack of a comprehensive national adoption data system, it is estimated that 1 million children live with adoptive parents and that 2 to 4% of US families have an adopted child. The core participants in this process [ie, the child, birth parent(s), and adoptive parent(s)] are called the *adoption triad*. Adoption arrangements vary extensively, including *informal* adoption, often with a relative, in which legal approval for adoptive care is not obtained.

The typology of adoption has expanded from the traditional *closed* adoption, in which there is little ongoing communication between the birth parent(s) and adoptive parent(s), to include *open* adoption in which there is a greater sharing of information. In an open adoption, the birth parent(s) usually meet the adoptive parent(s) and agree on future communication and contacts between them and the child. Increasingly, children are being adopted through *transracial* adoptions, both domestic and international, and *special needs* adoption (ie, children with physical neurodevelopmental or emotional disorders). The trend toward *international* adoption has also steadily increased with approximately 13,000 children having been adopted from foreign countries in 1997. Currently, the largest representation is from China, Korea, Russia, and Central America. The majority of children adopted internationally are below age 4 years, often below age 1, and female.

Most adoptions are coordinated through public or private agencies, although about 31% are either independently or privately arranged. The majority of children placed for adoption are under 2 years of age and generally from premarital births. Adoptions may fail following placement approximately 10% of the time; risk factors for failure include advancing age of the child, two or more prior placements, and greater length of time spent in foster care.

BIOPSYCHOSOCIAL ISSUES IN FOSTER CARE

Health care for children who are in foster care is often compromised by insufficient access, poor programmatic planning, inadequate communication and funding, and improper parental care before the foster placement. Foster parents often are provided scant information on preplacement health issues or on services already provided if a child has changed foster homes. Medical care is often inconsistent, leading to inadequate immunizations and limited screening for lead exposure, iron deficiency and anemia, vision, and hearing. Such children are at risk for poor nutrition, and short stature has been reported to be twice as prevalent in these children as it is among the general population. Up to one-third of children in foster care are estimated to have significant dental decay and malocclusion.

Chronic health problems also abound, estimated to affect between 40 and 75% of children in foster care. Congenital infections; neurodevelopmental consequences of in utero drug, tobacco, and alcohol exposure; HIV infection; and hepatitis B assume increasing prominence as sources of morbidity within this group. Common illnesses are more frequent, including recurrent upper respiratory infections, otitis media, and asthma. Higher rates are reported for congenital anomalies and for cardiovascular, gastrointestinal, dermatologic, ophthalmologic, and musculoskeletal problems. Inconsistent record-keeping and tracking may lead to inadequate treatment and follow-up for acute and chronic medical conditions.

Neuromaturational lags, mild to moderate developmental delays, and speech or language disorders are frequent. As a group, children in foster care often function in the low-average range of cognitive abilities, and they are overrepresented in grade retention, school failure, and need for special education services. There is a significant need in this population for both inpatient and outpatient mental health services. Common diagnostic comorbidities include attention-deficit hyperactivity disorder (ADHD), oppositional defiant disorders, conduct disorders, and anxiety disorders. However, some children show improvement in school attendance and academic growth when they are placed in a supportive foster home environment.

The life-course trajectory for children in foster care is disrupted by virtue of cumulative experiences with adversity and change; one estimate is that more than 50% of children experience mental health problems. These children may be confused about parent–child roles and display such behaviors as insecurity in their attachment to the foster parent and "parentalization" or precocious competence. Maladaptive behaviors include hoarding food and hyperphagia, stealing, encopresis, enuresis, aggression, and sexual acting out. These children have been removed from their homes, parents, and siblings, which leads to reactions ranging from acute grief to depression and apathy. The child may become confused, adding to a sense of abandonment, rejection, and a damaged self-esteem. Frequent fears, possibly resulting from worries about continuing abuse or future moves to yet another home, are common. Some children may repeat disruptive behaviors in their new foster home to "recreate" familiar relationships, unfortunately reinforcing their notion of a neglectful or abusive world. This often leads to profound confusion and frustration for the foster parent.

An additional challenge that foster children often experience is the transition into and following visitations with their natural parent(s). The consistency and quality of visitation is the predictor of family reunification. For some, this is a welcome opportunity to reunite with their parent(s) before ultimately returning home; for others, it may be an uncomfortable reminder of prior neglect or inappropriate care. It is not unusual for a child in foster care to regress behaviorally or act out for a brief time after a visit with their parent(s).

BIOPSYCHOSOCIAL ISSUES IN ADOPTION

Each member of the adoption triad must adjust to the transition of the child moving from the care of one family to the care of another. The birth mother may experience a sense of loss and unresolved grief long after the adoption process ends.

The adopted child must blend life experiences and feelings toward the adoptive family with the reality of a birth mother who resides outside the family. Confusion over identity, fantasies about the birth-parent and her reasons for relinquishing the child, and feelings of rejection all may arise and influence the child's sense of belonging and self-esteem. An open and accepting family attitude toward adoption has been shown to be predictive of a child's positive adjustment to these psychological issues. Discussing adoption with children should begin at about 5 to 7 years of age, when the child can begin to understand cognitively the difference between an adoptive and a birth-parent. From 8 to 11 years, questions regarding their permanence within the adoptive family may arise, possibly mixed with fantasies of being reclaimed by a birth-parent. During early to midadolescence, the child struggles to consolidate different notions of self with beginning interest about information on the birth family and heritable traits. By mid- to late adolescence, there is a clearer understanding of the emotional and legal permanence of the adoption. At this time, adopted children also may begin to seek contact with their birth mother or other members of the birth family.

The challenge to adoptive parents consists of raising the child within their own family while helping them to understand their "dual identity." Meeting this challenge requires sharing important information with the adopted child in a careful, understandable, and age-appropriate manner.

An open adoption may facilitate resolution of these dilemmas by providing an opportunity for the birth and adoptive parents to meet before and after the birth and to develop continuing (although different) relationships with the child. Currently, the adoptive family usually determines the extent of the birth-parent's relationship with the child and adoptive family once the adoption is finalized. This "openness" can provide a conduit of accessible information that allows the child to learn more about him- or herself and provides an opportunity for both sets of parents to share in the child's life without unnecessary fantasies or fears.

Adopted children show somewhat higher rates of neurodevelopmental and psychological morbidity, especially early in childhood. Adopted children are overrepresented among those with learning disabilities, with an estimated prevalence of school problems three to four times national norms. Adopted children represent 5% of children seen in outpatient mental health settings and 10 to 15% of children in inpatient mental health facilities. Externalizing behaviors such as oppositional-defiant and conduct disorders, aggression, and ADHD occur more frequently, as do personality disorders. However, most adopted individuals perceive their experiences positively and mature as healthy, normal children with successes and failures similar to their nonadopted peers.

Children adopted internationally represent a unique group. The prospective adopted parent(s) must go through the effort and expense of working with an agency specializing in international adop-

tion, fulfilling the legal requirements of both the United States and the child's country of origin, and of traveling to that country to receive the child, commonly with only scant or inaccurate information about the child, the child's family history, and the child's health. Often neglected with poor nutrition and inadequate health care, these children present a distinct challenge for their adoptive parents. The challenges range from acute and chronic medical problems and inadequate immunizations to developmental delays, speech and language disorders, and disrupted emotional development/behavior. These children need to adjust not only to their new parent(s), but they need to cope with the transition to a strange country, home, and language. The supportive role of the pediatrician is never more apparent than in this circumstance (Table 5-40).

HEALTH-CARE PROVIDER'S ROLE

The pediatrician occupies an ideal position to assist in the foster or adoptive child's adaptation to a new family by (a) providing thorough health supervision, (b) assisting families in the coordination of services and providing professional advocacy, and (c) serving as a counselor to the child and family (Table 5-41).

The health professional also is in a unique position to achieve a global view of the child's strengths and needs within the context of the family, thus helping to facilitate planning for individual or family interventions when necessary. Such a role requires a working familiarity with local educational, social, and mental health resources for children.

Physicians may find themselves in the role of counseling the adoptive or foster family, the child, and the biological parent(s). Feelings of guilt, confusion, and frustration require an empathic ear. An understanding, "neutral" health professional can be a valuable resource for children as questions of self-identity arise in the

---

TABLE 5-40

SUPPORTIVE ROLE OF THE PEDIATRICIAN IN THE PREADOPTION VISIT

Preview information on child, eg, medical records, videotape
Advise on supplies to take to pick up child, eg, medicines, formula
Plan for evaluation of the child upon return
Refer family to support group for international adoption
Anticipatory guidance for new parents
Medical evaluation

Immediate (1st week)
    Evaluate/treat acute illnesses
    Measure baseline growth

Comprehensive Examination (4–6 weeks)
    Complete PE: look for congenital anomalies, chronic conditions, nutritional disorders
    Screen: vision, hearing, dental
    Update immunizations
    Recheck newborn screening if <3 months old
    Screening medical tests to include: CBC, Pb, Fe (look for hemoglobinopathies), U/A, TB (PPD), O + P for parasitic infections, Hep B, HIV, syphilis, malaria (if appropriate)
    Developmental evaluation: gross and fine motor, communication skills, initial behavior/coping responses
    Anticipatory guidance—refer to support groups, literature

Periodic Surveillance
Well-child care, update immunizations
Monitor growth, nutrition
Check for late signs of infections
Close developmental surveillance
Counsel or refer for developmental/behavioral problems

TABLE 5-41

TASK OF THE PEDIATRICIAN IN ASSISTING ADAPTATION OF A CHILD TO A NEW FAMILY

Child enters foster care
Health-care supervision
  Screen for: growth, infectious diseases, eg, TB, HIV, Hep B
  Pb, Fe, anemia
  Vision, hearing, dental screen
  Chronic medical, congenital disorders
  Update immunizations
  Generate portable medical record; "medical passport"
Neurodevelopmental supervision
  Screen/refer for: speech/language delays, developmental delays, school
    difficulties, cognitive impairment/learning disabilities, ADHD
Mental health supervision
  Screen/refer for: behavioral disruptions, anxiety, depression
Examination for ongoing signs of abuse; physical, sexual
Supportive role to foster parent

ADHD = attention-deficit hyperactivity disorder

middle-school years. Clinicians also may serve as a sounding board to prospective parents about decisions regarding foster or adoptive care. Families often need guidance regarding normal child development and behavior and sometimes ask for assistance when innate or adaptive behaviors become dysfunctional. At times, appropriate referral to a mental health professional will be necessary. The pediatric health-care provider thus occupies a central role in monitoring the well-being of the child and family and of supporting their adaptation to the sequence of transitions experienced in foster care and adoption.

References

Adoptive Families of America: Guide to Adoption, St. Paul, MN, Author, 1999

Barnett E, Miller L: International adoption: the pediatrician's role. Contemp Pediatr 13:29, 1996

Behrman R, ed: The Future of Children: Adoption. Los Altos, Center for the Future of Children, David and Lucille Packard Foundation, 1993

Brodzinsky D, Singer L, Braff A: Children's understanding of adoption. Child Dev 55:869, 1984

Child Welfare League of America: Standards for Health Care Services for Children in Out-of-Home Care. Washington, DC, Author, 1998

Committee on Early Childhood, Adoption, and Dependent Care: Health Care of Children in Foster Care. Pediatrics 93:335, 1994

Quarles C, Brodie J: Primary care of international adoptees: Am Fam Physician. 58:2025, 1998

Rosenfeld AA, Pilowsky DJ, Fine P, et al: Foster care: an update. J Am Acad Child Adolesc Psychiatry 36:448, 1997

Sherry SN: Helping families adapt to adoption. Contemp Pediatr Nov:96, 1986

Simms M: Foster children and the foster care system. Curr Probl Pediatr 21:197, 1991

Szilagyi M: The pediatrician and the child in foster care. Pediatr Rev 19:39, 1998

5.8.6   Family Discord, Divorce, and Remarriage

Michael Jellinek

Few events in an individual's life are as dramatic and meaningful as a divorce. For a child and family, divorce is a disintegration of expectations, hopes, the family unit, and, if the child must move from his or her community or school, much of what is familiar. The divorce is a legal landmark that often reflects years of tension, coldness, confusing emotions, anger, and loss. After the divorce, the child faces an ongoing effort at each developmental level to understand the past, to maintain parental attachments, to feel secure in his or her emerging identity, and to invest in relationships (eg, peers, teachers, stepparents) with trust and intimacy. Divorces that end discord or abuse may be a welcome relief, yet still require an understanding of the emotional damage sustained throughout the divorce process.

Pediatricians often miss the opportunity to provide guidance during this critical process. Although more than 1 million divorces each year involve 1 million children, many pediatricians are not routinely aware of family discord, divorces, or remarriages among parents. Without such awareness, pediatricians cannot provide anticipatory guidance for children in typical divorces, or mental health referral and long-term follow-up in virulent divorces characterized by ongoing discord.

RECOGNITION

Because of divorce, out-of-wedlock birth, or parental death, approximately 60% of children in the United States live with a single parent at some time in their lives. Based on this high prevalence, if pediatricians could ask only three mental health screening questions during an annual physical, they should be: (a) Is there any ongoing discord in the marriage? (b) Do you (the parent) feel that the child needs mental health services? and (c) Is either parent, especially the mother, depressed?

EXPECTED PSYCHOLOGICAL REACTIONS

Parents may ask whether it is better to stay married "for the sake of the children" than to "put them through a divorce." The tensions in discordant marriages may result in verbal or physical confrontations, compound other psychological problems such as depression or substance use, and create a bitter emotional tone in the home. Children who live with chronic family discord, tension, and unhappiness become vigilant as to how their parents are feeling and assume responsibility for causing or trying to relieve tension and unhappiness. Many children wonder what they are supposed to do to help. Over time, these children often harbor intense anger at their parents and grow up suspicious of, yet longing for, intimacy. Thus, as young adults they may feel unable to tolerate intimacy, or they may begin marriages dominated by the ghosts of their parents' discord.

For parents, divorce represents a loss of both initial marital hopes and the family unit. Dashed hopes, selfish behavior, scorn, substance use, or infidelity may fuel one spouse's intense anger and disappointment about the other. As a consequence of this rage, some parents cannot distinguish the needs of the child from their total commitment to hurt their spouse. Pediatricians face a dilemma because sometimes the request by one parent to protect the child from the other is appropriate (eg, abuse, neglect, substance use), while at other times it is part of one parent's anger or legal strategy to rationalize his or her fury. During the divorce, and often for a year or more thereafter, a substantial percentage of mothers may suffer clinical depression, while some men continue to be dominated by ongoing anger or to distance themselves from the parenting role by limiting visits to their children.

For the child, divorce is a loss that is reexperienced at various times throughout childhood and adolescence. Some children recall feelings of loss when seeing well-functioning two-parent families, and during events such as birthdays, holidays, graduation, or a college visit. Up to a half of school-aged children manifest some symptoms in the first year after their parents' divorce. Approximately 10%, largely those exposed to ongoing discord, experience sustained emotional difficulties and dysfunction through adolescence and young adulthood, and commonly require mental health services.

Infants and toddlers are heavily influenced by their caregivers; thus, these children suffer when their caregiving parent (most commonly their mother) is preoccupied, overwhelmed, or clinically depressed. Children under 3 years of age require special consideration in terms of visitation, because they have less tolerance for long absences, especially if one parent is the predominant caregiver. Given the language and cognitive limitations of the early years, as well as the many life events that add cumulative variance over time, it is difficult to determine the specific long-term consequences of divorce into adulthood.

Children 4 and 5 years of age have access to more sophisticated language, but they also have important cognitive limitations that influence their ability to grasp the implications of a divorce. These children have a rich fantasy life, and their cognitive stage results in their taking responsibility for most of what happens, including parental discord. Thus, many children in this age group feel guilty about having caused the divorce, which is a feeling reinforced by any overheard arguments that mentioned their name.

School-aged children can begin to understand more realistically and in concrete terms the issues causing and related to the divorce. These children often feel caught in loyalty conflicts, wishing their parents would reunite, and wondering about whether the parents would have divorced if they (ie, the children) had been "better." School-age children often are moody and preoccupied, and boys are commonly more aggressive, especially toward their mother. The sources of this increased aggression may be the propensity for boys to be more aggressive, a sense of security and permission derived from the mother being the custodial parent, and the son possibly eliciting some of the mother's unresolved anger toward her husband.

Older children and adolescents are vulnerable to psychosomatic disorders, which may be an emotional solution to avoiding angry feelings directed at the parents or reflecting their helplessness during the divorce. A secondary result of both psychosomatic symptoms and oppositional behavior might be to gain the attention of both parents, sometimes jointly, as during medical visits when worry about a potential illness temporarily replaces parental tensions.

Although adolescents have the cognitive capacity to understand the divorce process, they are at a particularly vulnerable point, having had so many years of both positive and ill effects from the marriage. In addition, adolescents are in the process of developing their own sense of mature autonomy, identity, and capacity for intimacy, which only increases their need for a stable base and sense of trust. Divorce calls into question the adolescent's basic assumptions about the meaning of both trust and intimacy. Faced with the rapid, real loss of what was their "home," adolescents may flee into young adult behavior (eg, premature autonomy or sexuality), feel depressed (and resort to self-medication with substances), or give up their own developmental path to take care of other family members. For some, a sense of intimacy may be hard to achieve in their own later relationships, and psychotherapy may be needed during young adulthood.

COMMON ISSUES

Beyond the loss of daily parental contact, divorce has a major impact on the child's life outside the home. Many activities become complicated by visitation schedules, lack of money, or parental discord. Everyday experiences, such as going over to a friend's house, sleepovers, team sports, and music lessons, now must be double-checked and approved by two often busy and less than cooperative households. In addition to scheduling problems, the costs of summer camp or school tuition suddenly may be beyond the family's means, or may provoke tense negotiations through lawyers or the courts. If the family's home is a major asset, it may have to be sold, with the consequence that the child will have to change communities, thereby threatening the stability of school, friends, and recreational activities.

A physician may be used by one parent against the other to substantiate charges of poor parenting while in a custody or financial struggle. Thus, pediatricians should be wary of requests for letters or recommendations unless the issues are clear-cut, valid, and known firsthand. If the pediatrician has a better preexisting relationship with one parent than the other, it is essential to offer the less-familiar parent an opportunity to be heard. Whenever possible, medical instructions and reports should be given to both parents. If the child has a serious acute or chronic disease, routine scheduling of meetings with both parents should be a high priority.

In the heat of a divorce, many parents may not be able to meet their child's basic needs, may be irritable or more violent, and may be depressed or blur boundaries so as to be unable to differentiate their child's needs from their own. In such cases, the child is at greater risk for abuse and neglect, unintentional injuries, and psychological damage, especially if the child is being used to meet one or both parents' own agenda.

Visitation and custody arrangements are particularly complex. They should depend on the child's age, temperament, and personality. Often there is a tension between the clarity and flexibility of being raised in a single-parent household (especially for younger children) in the exclusive custody of the mother versus efforts at coparenting, which are inherently more cumbersome but often more effective in supporting the father's ongoing involvement. In recent years, the courts and legislative statutes have shifted away from automatically favoring mothers to a more neutral stance, especially for school-age children and adolescents, which encourages parents to negotiate the details of joint physical and legal custody. Joint physical custody implies a close to equal time-sharing arrangement; legal custody relates to shared authority in decision-making, which is relevant to such issues as obtaining consent for medical care. If joint physical or legal custody is used only to expedite contentious cases, implementation of such orders often is an ongoing basis for discord. Under such circumstances, every hour, activity, vacation, and option in the child's life is a potential vehicle to express anger and initiate another round of poor faith negotiations. In a positive context, joint custody offers an opportunity for both parents to remain highly involved in their child's daily life. However, such arrangements require cooperative, flexible parents who are able to focus on the child's needs and who are willing to live in reasonable proximity of each other for many years.

MANAGEMENT

An approach to management of a family with discord is shown in Fig. 5-6. Pediatricians should ask about the quality of the parents' marriage or relationship on an annual basis. Larger group practices

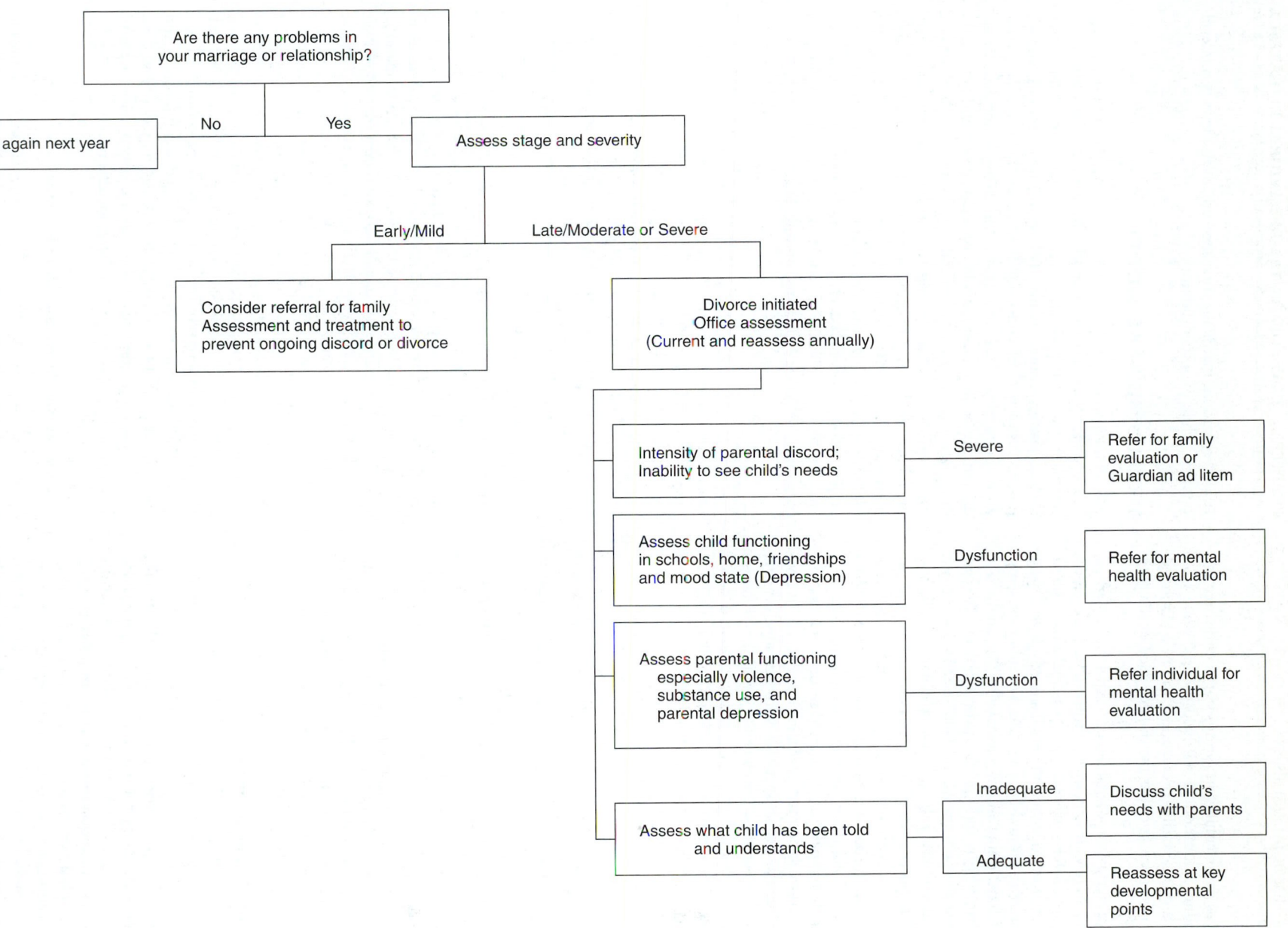

FIGURE 5-6 Approach to assessment and management of a family with discord.

are likely to have so many families in various stages of divorce that facilitating or leading education or self-help groups, alone or in conjunction with a mental health professional, can be a highly valued clinical service to prevent either the divorce itself or the harm of ongoing discord.

Any evidence of significant marital discord, separation, or intention to divorce should initiate a multiyear protocol that assesses the child's acute reaction, level of parental interpersonal anger, the capacity of the parents to understand the child's needs distinct from their own feelings of anger and loss, and the screening for symptoms of impaired functioning in any member of the family. The best time to initiate help is early in the divorce process. Recommending a mediator and focusing on the child's needs from an early point can be critical in limiting the extent to which intrafamily hostility can seriously damage a child's sense of trust and self-esteem. Pediatric guidance and review should span from initial attempts at preventing the divorce throughout adolescence until young adulthood. If advice or referral does not seem to be able to break a contentious gridlock, the pediatrician should recommend that the parents consider a court-appointed guardian ad litem, who is generally a lawyer or mental health specialist with investigatory and arbitration authority to serve on behalf of the child's best interest. In the face of significant ongoing hostility and argument, or when a child demonstrates substantially impaired functioning, a mental health evaluation should be initiated, preferably with the support of both parents.

References

Jellinek MS: Sounding board. The present status of child psychiatry in pediatrics. N Engl J Med 306:1227–1230, 1982

Jellinek MS, Nurcombe B: Two wrongs don't make a right. Managed care, mental health, and the marketplace. JAMA 270:1737–1739, 1993

Maccoby EE, Mnookin RH: Dividing the Child: Social and Legal Dilemmas of Custody. Cambridge, MA, Harvard University Press, 1992

Norton A, Glick PC: One-parent families: a social and economic profile. Fam Relat 35:9–17, 1986

Stolberg AL, Ellwood M, Draper DA: The pediatrician's role in children's adjustment to divorce. J Pediatr 114:187–193, 1989

Wallerstein JS, Blakeslee S: Second Chances: Men, Women, and Children a Decade after Divorce. New York, Ticknor & Fields, 1989

Wallerstein JS, Kelly JB: Surviving the Breakup: How Children and Parents Cope with Divorce. New York, Basic Books, 1980

5.8.7   Parental Substance Abuse

Barry S. Zuckerman

In the early 1960s, the significant effects of thalidomide brought attention to the possible dangers of drug use during pregnancy. Structural damage, like that of the limbs in children affected by thalidomide or like the alteration of the facial features of children with severe fetal alcohol syndrome, are severe but rare consequences of prenatal substance exposure. Intrauterine growth retardation and neonatal neurobehavioral dysfunction are more common consequences of prenatal exposure to drugs, especially psychoactive substances. However, the threshold of effect on behavior may be lower than that of effects on in utero growth; a specific amount of drug exposure during pregnancy might result in neurobehavioral dysfunction yet not impair growth. Findings from studies of developmental outcome in children exposed prenatally to drugs are inconsistent as well. For example, of two longitudinal

studies regarding marijuana, one showed adverse effects on development, while the other did not.

DEVELOPMENTAL MODEL

The development of a child affected by prenatal exposure to drugs is best understood through a multifactorial model consisting of interrelated pre- and postnatal factors. Postnatal health problems, such as lead exposure, anemia, failure to thrive, injuries, and exposure to violence, affect development adversely and are more common among drug-exposed infants. Caretaking is impaired by addiction. An addicted mother's life is organized around getting the drug, not around taking care of children. Mothers may not respond to their infant's needs. During the toddler and preschool years, discipline may be inconsistent, and promises are made and then forgotten. Even threats to remove a child may not alter an addicted mother's drug use, because addiction involves continued drug use despite adverse consequences. While not all substance-using parents are addicted, those with addiction are at high risk for poor parenting, including child abuse and neglect.

Cocaine

Cocaine blocks the presynaptic reuptake of dopamine, norepinephrine, and epinephrine, resulting in an exaggerated signal at the postsynaptic membrane, which leads to decreased uterine blood flow, constriction of umbilical arteries, euphoria, and decreased appetite. Cocaine is highly water and fat soluble, and it has been found in the brain in concentrations four times higher than the peak plasma concentration.

Newborn Outcome

Maternal cocaine use has been associated with decreased newborn length, weight, and head circumference for gestational age, even when confounding variables are controlled. Rare but serious congenital abnormalities, including urogenital anomalies, distal limb deformities, gastroschisis, cardiac lesions, and CNS malformations, have been noted. However, there is no consistent pattern of malformations associated with prenatal cocaine exposure or definitive scientific evidence that cocaine causes such anomalies.

Neonatal neurobehavioral abnormalities following cocaine exposure have been reported in some studies. No differences are noted in Neonatal Abstinence Scale scores between cocaine-exposed and comparison groups, however. Results of studies using the Brazelton Neonatal Behavioral Assessment Scale (BNBAS), which provides a more sensitive assessment of newborn behavior, do show adverse effects, including increased tremulousness and startle, decreased motor function, and decreased habituation. Even so, even among studies that show adverse effects, most areas of function measured by the BNBAS are not affected.

Long-Term Developmental Outcome

In one longitudinal study, cocaine nonopiate-exposed infants achieved scores on assessments of global development similar to unexposed infants at 2 to 3 years of age. However, prenatal drug exposure, which was defined as use of alcohol, cigarettes, or marijuana with or without cocaine, was associated with lower IQ scores at 3 years of age. In another longitudinal study, infants exposed to cocaine and PCP showed deficits in unstructured play at 18 months and high rates of insecure, disorganized attachment.

Opiates

Opiates include morphine, codeine, heroin, and meperidine hydrochloride. These substances bind at specific sites in the CNS.

Newborn Outcome

Prenatal exposure to narcotics does not appear to result in an increased rate of congenital malformation. The primary effects on the fetus are intrauterine growth retardation and abstinence syndrome that includes significant neurobehavioral dysfunction. When the supply of drugs is terminated following delivery, the newborn develops withdrawal symptoms consisting of irritability, tremulousness, sweating, stuffy nose, difficulty in feeding, diarrhea, and vomiting.

A narcotic abstinence-syndrome scoring system is used for quantifying the severity of withdrawal symptoms to determine when pharmacotherapy is indicated and guide therapy once it is begun. Approximately 60 to 75% of infants will exhibit sufficiently severe withdrawal symptoms that pharmacotherapy is indicated. The remainder can be treated with swaddling, pacifiers, and decreased environmental stimuli. The most common pharmacologic treatment for narcotic abstinence syndrome is a narcotic [paregoric or denatured tincture of opium (DTO) and/or phenobarbital]. Paregoric or DTO are the drugs of choice for infants of women using narcotics alone. Once a maintenance dose has been established for either drug, the dose is decreased by approximately 10% per day so that the mean duration of therapy ranges between 2 and 3 weeks.

Long-Term Developmental Outcome

There is no convincing evidence that exposure to narcotics in utero causes a significant delay in global development between ages 2 and 5 years. However, in preliminary studies of later school performance, many heroin-exposed children require special education classes or repeat one or more grades, and their teachers report high rates of impulsivity and inattention. The relative contributions of prenatal narcotic exposure and adverse social experiences require further study.

Marijuana

The principal psychoactive chemical in marijuana is Δ^9 tetrahydrocannabinol (THC). THC is stored in the fatty tissues, has a half-life in humans of 7 days, and may take up to 30 days to be excreted completely in the feces and urine.

Newborn Outcome

Some, but not all, studies show that prenatal marijuana is associated with a small decrement (ie, 70 g) in birth weight when confounding variables are controlled. Prenatal marijuana exposure is associated with increased tremors, alterations in acoustic cry characteristics, and alterations in sleep EEG. When present, these effects are small. Their implications are unknown.

Long-Term Developmental Outcome

Few studies have evaluated the developmental and behavioral functioning of children who are exposed prenatally to marijuana. In one study, no effect of prenatal marijuana use on developmental scores was noted at 12 or at 24 months. While prenatal marijuana use does not appear to be associated with decreased global developmental scores, it has been associated with lower scores on memory and verbal ability at 4 years of age, and with small impairments of specific functions (eg, sustained attention, visual perceptual functioning, visual memory, language comprehension) at 5 and 6 years of age. Firm conclusions about the long-term impact of prenatal marijuana exposure on developmental functioning are difficult to make at this time.

Alcohol

Alcohol is quickly absorbed from the gastrointestinal tract by passive diffusion. Because it is water soluble, it is distributed rapidly throughout the body, and it crosses the placenta.

Newborn Outcome

Fetal alcohol syndrome is a specific pattern of malformation. It is discussed in detail in Sec. 10.3.8. Fetal alcohol syndrome has been described only among women who are alcoholic. Approximately 2 to 10% of alcoholic women will have a child with this syndrome.

Heavy maternal drinking that does not lead to full fetal alcohol syndrome may result in children with fetal alcohol effects or alcohol-related birth defects. These children generally show characteristics from one or two of the categories that define fetal alcohol syndrome. Whether there is a threshold or linear relationship between prenatal alcohol consumption and adverse newborn outcomes is controversial. In some studies, two drinks or fewer per day do not appear to have an adverse effect on birth weight if the mother is well nourished and healthy. Some studies show that neurobehavioral dysfunction, such as poorer habituation and poor arousal, is related to alcohol consumption.

Long-Term Developmental Outcome

Children with fetal alcohol syndrome may have a variety of developmental problems, including developmental delay in early childhood, mental retardation, attention-deficit hyperactivity disorder (ADHD), selective learning disabilities, motor incoordination, and conduct disorders in older childhood and adolescence. Some longitudinal studies of children exposed to alcohol prenatally but without fetal alcohol syndrome show an adverse affect on development at age 3 years and older. In the longest follow-up study to date, prenatal alcohol exposure, especially binge drinking, was shown to adversely effect children's attentional abilities and gross and fine motor skills at 7 years.

Tobacco

Nicotine, which is the most pharmacologically active of the more than 2000 compounds in cigarette smoke, is known to cross the placenta. The effects of nicotine on the fetus are thought to be primarily indirect, through maternal vasoconstriction and reduced oxygen availability.

Newborn Outcome

Cigarette smoking during pregnancy increases perinatal mortality, especially through spontaneous abortions, and reduces fetal growth by approximately 200 g. Some, but not all, studies assessing neurobehavioral functioning by the BNBAS show an association between maternal cigarette smoking and transient adverse effects on newborn behavior.

Long-Term Developmental Outcome

Most, but not all, long-term follow-up studies show lowered cognitive scores associated with prenatal maternal smoking. In some studies, positive findings disappear when confounding social and environmental factors are controlled; if positive findings occur, the differences between the exposed and nonexposed groups are small. Recent studies show that independent of prenatal exposure, passive smoking is associated with behavior problems.

Clinical Implications

Because maternal drug and alcohol abuse are part of a life-style that frequently involves more than one drug and other associated risk factors such as parenting dysfunction, children of parents who abuse drugs are at high risk for developmental and behavioral problems. The primary care clinician should ensure that basic needs of the family for food, housing, health care, and safety are met; that nondrug-using adults are available and supportive; and that the health and development of the child is promoted and monitored. The primary care pediatrician should discuss with parents in a non-judgmental manner their drug and alcohol use, refer them to drug treatment services if needed, and support their recovery.

References

Frank DA, Bresnahan K, Zuckerman BS: Maternal cocaine use: impact on child health and development. Adv Pediatr 40:65−99, 1993

Sonderegger TB, ed: Perinatal Substance Abuse: Research Findings and Clinical Implications. Baltimore, MD, Johns Hopkins University Press, 1992

Zagon IS, Slotkin TA, eds: Maternal Substance Abuse and the Developing Nervous System. San Diego, CA, Academic Press, 1992

Zuckerman B, Bresnahan K: Developmental and behavioral consequences of prenatal drug and alcohol exposure. Pediatr Clin North Am 38:1387−1406, 1991

5.8.8   Family and Community Violence

Joy D. Osofsky

Violence and children-witnessing of violence have been characterized as a public health epidemic in the United States. Violence among youth (ie, ages 11 to 17 years), including murder, rape, robbery, and aggravated assault, has increased 25% in the last decade. Yet, the grim statistics do not adequately denote the extent to which violence has infiltrated the lives of all of our young people. Homicide ranks as the second leading cause of death among males between 15 and 24 years of age, and even more striking it has become the third leading cause of death among elementary school children. Gun violence is the second leading cause of death for children ages 10 to 19 years. A recent survey at a public hospital-based pediatric clinic in a major US city found that 1 of every 10 children under the age of 6 years reported having witnessed a shooting or stabbing.

It is important to understand the meaning that an experience of violence may have for a child. The meaning will be influenced by the nature of the threat and the damage; the child's relationship with the victim or perpetrator; the severity and duration of the violence; and its proximity to the child. Different types of violence have different effects on children and families. While it is possible to differentiate community from family violence, as we learn more about the perpetrators and victims, it has become clear that at least half of the violence reported in the United States involves people who know each other.

Recent data on approximately 300 children between 6 and 12 years of age indicate that school-age children are victims and witnesses of significant amounts of violence. In one moderate-sized city, 51% of the fifth graders had been direct victims of violence, and 91% had personally witnessed some type of violence. Children's reports of distress syndromes indicated a significant relation to violence exposure. Very early in their lives, many children must learn to deal with loss and cope with grieving for family members and friends who have been killed. Parents often feel helpless and hopeless as they try to help their children deal with such trauma.

Parallels have been drawn between children growing up in US inner cities and those living in war zones. In many urban areas, children, many of whom have behavior control problems, commonly tell pediatric health-care providers that they hear gunshots outside their homes, witness shootings on playgrounds and in their neighborhoods, and have a family member or relative who has been a victim or a perpetrator of violence. The majority of elementary-school-age children attending inner-city schools report having witnessed shootings or stabbings, often of a family member or close friend. In addition to their exposure to community violence, at least 33 million children witness domestic violence each year, which ranges from attacks by hitting and slapping to fatal assaults with guns and/or knives.

Recent studies of television and movies indicate that children of all ages also are exposed to a great deal of media-based videos, which exposure has a demonstrable effect on the development of aggressive behavior as well as on attitudes toward violence. There is little doubt that the adverse effects are most significant among children who are at greatest risk, including those who are exposed to domestic and community violence and who receive less supervision and parental monitoring of such exposure. However, the substantial outbreak of suburban and rural school violence in the past year indicates that children from all parts of the country, urban and rural, have been influenced by the glorification of violence in our society.

EFFECTS OF EXPOSURE TO VIOLENCE ON THE CHILD

Developmental Model

The impact of exposure of children to violence depends on many factors, including the age of the child, characteristics of the neighborhood (eg, degree of community resources), amount and quality of support from key caregivers and other significant adults, child's experience of previous abuse, child's proximity to the violent event, and the child's level of familiarity with the victim or the perpetrator. The capacity of children to perceive and remember a violent experience affects the presence and pattern of symptoms, as well as the circumstances under which they are likely to occur. Exposure to violence also may affect the way that children think about themselves and the world around them, particularly regarding the extent to which they view relationships as trustworthy and dependable.

Reactions to violence exposure vary depending on the child's age and developmental level. During the first 3 years of life, children show increased irritability and sleep disturbances as well as fears of being alone. Exposure to trauma interferes with their normal development of trust and the later emergence of autonomy through exploration. Regression is common in developmental achievements such as toileting and language. For preschool children, cognitive confusion is common, with decreased verbalization and more precocious use of trauma-related expressions in play and language.

Sleep disturbances, night terrors, and other manifestations of increased anxiety are common as well. School-age children also experience increases in anxiety and sleep disturbances. They may have difficulty paying attention and experience intrusive thoughts. For preschoolers, as well as school-age children, there is often a decrease in mastery motivation, including lack of pleasure in exploring the physical environment. For adolescents, learning problems are common, with difficulties in concentration, school decline, and failure. Resulting secondary problems with self-esteem often lead to increased risk of aggressive acting-out behavior, substance abuse, and secondary psychiatric morbidity. Any evaluation of the effects of violence exposure on children must consider that parents or caregivers may also be numbed, frightened, depressed, and often unable to be available emotionally to their children. When children at any age cannot depend on the trust and security that comes from caregivers who are emotionally available, they may withdraw and show disorganized behaviors.

Short-Term Symptoms

Overall, most children demonstrate the same patterns of behavior and physiological reactivity and symptoms following trauma as do adults. Many show increased anxiety at bedtime or difficulty going to sleep, exaggerated startle reactions, persistent hyperviolence, difficulty in regulation (including either increased aggression and/or social withdrawal), and new fears (including fear of being alone). Posttrauma psychopathology may include posttraumatic stress disorder symptoms (including reexperiencing, avoidance, emotional numbing, and hyperviolence), phobic and overanxious disorder, depression, substance abuse, and dissociative sleep, or somatization disorders.

Infants and toddlers have fewer ways to express their feelings than do older children who are able to use words, play, or drawings to communicate their experience. Many kinds of stress, including exposure to violence, can contribute to sleep and eating difficulties, withdrawal, nightmares, and night terrors in children of all ages. School-aged boys are more likely to show aggressive responses and girls are more likely to withdraw. Violence exposure may contribute significantly to the development of secondary symptoms and problematic behaviors. Symptom clusters that are associated with posttraumatic stress in children include reexperiencing the traumatic event (ie, nightmares or play that includes reexperiencing the trauma), avoiding people or situations that remind the child of the fearful event, numbing of responsiveness (ie, emotionally subdued, socially withdrawn, constricted in play), and increased or decreased arousal (ie, hypervigilance, exaggerated startle responses, night terrors, increased aggression, withdrawal).

Long-Term Sequelae

Less is known about children's later adaptation and the long-term sequelae of exposure to violence. Children who have been mistreated or exposed to the homicide of someone familiar to them have more difficulty with later school adjustment relationships, and with interpersonal relationships in general. Long-term outcomes are likely to be related to the child's gender, age at experience, comprehension of danger, developmental status, and functioning before the exposure to violence, and to the availability of support after the event. The nature of the available support following violence exposure likely is crucial for facilitating adaptation. The child should be able to experience some sense of safety in his or her environment. Also, the parents' ability to deal with their own trauma and/or grief is important to their children's progress so that the child can express anxieties, fears, and concerns with people the child trusts.

MANAGEMENT

Acute Case

Concurrent with the problems that children who have been exposed to violence face directly, pediatricians are increasingly confronted with the concerns of parents and/or other caregivers who often have difficulty coping with their own fears, living in a situation neither they nor the physician can change.

Developmental and behavioral issues should be kept in mind. Problems that may arise include regressions in communication ability; loss of previously established bladder and bowel control; sleep disturbances; excessive clinging and fear of separating from the primary caregiver; learning difficulties; and generally more difficult patterns of behaviors. Parents may bring these concerns to the attention of the pediatrician, and it is important to be aware that violence exposure may be playing an important etiologic role in these problems.

Referral for Specialized Treatment

An important decision regarding the treatment of children exposed to violence relates to which referral to a mental health professional is indicated. Many children who are exposed to violence do not receive the help that they need. Parents may want to avoid dealing with the experience themselves and may not realize that the child has been traumatized. Many parents, teachers, community workers, and health-care professionals are not sure how to deal with the problem and may prefer to avoid it entirely. Health-care professionals besieged by overflowing clinics and managed-care demands may not be able to take the time to carefully evaluate the extent of the child's exposure to violence, or the impact on the child and the parent, or to determine what is the most advantageous course of treatment. Many children who grow up with chronic violence in their homes and/or neighborhoods exhibit patterns or symptoms of behaviors that generally are difficult for their parents or caregivers to manage. Any child who has been exposed to a significant level of violence and is symptomatic should be referred to a mental health specialist, preferably one who has had experience treating children exposed to violence.

Presentation and Advocacy

Violence in the United States has grown to epidemic proportions. Effective pediatric advocacy can best be focused in three main areas: (a) a family centered approach to the prevention of violence and treatment of its aftermath; (b) a national campaign to change attitudes toward violence and tolerance to violent behavior; and (c) informed public policy at all levels of government that is designed to reduce violence and to prevent violence.

References

Drell M, Siegel C, Gansbauer T: Post-traumatic stress disorders. In: Zenah CH Jr, ed: Handbook of Infant Mental Health. New York, Guilford Press, 1998

Fingerhut LA, Kleinman JC: International and interstate comparisons of homicide among young males. JAMA 263:3292–3295, 1990

Giabarino J, Dubrow N, Kostehy K, Pardo C: Children in Danger: Coping With the Consequences of Community Violence. San Francisco, Jossey-Bass, 1992

Groves BM, Zuckerman B, Manans S, Cohen DJ: Silent victims. Children who witness violence. JAMA 269:262–264, 1993

Osofsky JD. Children in a Violent Society. New York, Guilford Press, 1997

Osofsky JD, Ferichel ES: Caring for Infants and Toddlers in Violent Environments. Hurt, Healing and Hope. Arlington, VA, National Center for Clinical Infant Programs Publications, 1994

Osofsky JD, Wevers S, Hann DM, Fick AC: Chronic community violence, what is happening to our children? Psychiatry 56:36–45, 1998

Prothrow-Stuih D: Deadly Consequences. New York, Harper Collins, 1991

Teri L: Too Scared to Cry: Psychic Trauma in Childhood. New York, Harper & Row, 1990

5.8.9   Poverty, Homelessness, and Social Disorganization

Teresa M. Kohlenberg and Barry S. Zuckerman

POVERTY AND CHILD DEVELOPMENT

Children who live in poor families face pervasive challenges to their health and development. These challenges result in increased rates of illness, developmental delay, behavioral problems, school failure, and social dysfunction. Family dysfunction and environmental deterioration combine to amplify the impact of biological vulnerabilities on the child. However, as with other threats to health and development, poverty's effects can be offset by individual, family, and community buffering factors that offer both protection and support.

THE EPIDEMIOLOGY OF POVERTY

In the 1990s, one-fifth of all US children lived below the poverty line, while one-third spent at least 1 year of their childhood in poverty. Contrary to stereotypes, almost two-thirds of poor children have parents who work, and over one-half of poor children live in the suburbs or rural areas. There are enormous racial disparities: a greater proportion of African-American and Latino children live in poverty (ie, one-half of all African-American children and one-third of all Hispanic children live in poverty), but there are more poor white than poor African-American or Latino children.

THE DIMENSIONS OF POVERTY

The concept of "poverty" encompasses not only insufficient income but also the range of conditions that families who are poor encounter. Poverty's impact varies, depending on whether it is normative within a given society; urban or rural; brief, intermittent, or chronic; relative; or at a level that compromises physical survival. For example, abject material poverty (ie, lack of food, clothing, shelter, and health care) may be common for families in the developing world; relative material poverty (ie, lack of access to goods and services that most members of the society can afford) is more widespread in the United States. Income inequality is now thought to be a more sensitive indicator of health problems than mean income. This may be mediated through social marginalization, the end product of the experience of social inequalities such as poor schools, poor health services, and poor homes. Some US families may have members who are disabled by mental illness, alcoholism, or other chronic conditions, and local economic stagnation or racism may limit their access to educational opportunities and better jobs, leading to multigenerational poverty.

Families in such variable settings experience different social environments and have different expectations for themselves and their children. For example, families who fall under the poverty level for shorter periods because of transient unemployment may have more economic and psychological reserves with which to endure its effects than families who have been in poverty for several generations. Families living in urban poverty have increased exposure to lead, household allergens, and airborne pollutants, while rural families typically have less access to the array of helping agencies that are available in cities.

RISK AND PROTECTIVE FACTORS IN POVERTY

Many of the biomedical risks of poverty affect the CNS directly and are linked to behavioral and developmental problems. Factors that affect poor women of childbearing age also affect pregnancy outcomes (ie, undertreated vaginal infections are associated with preterm delivery; poor nutritional status is associated with multiple perinatal risks) as well as child health outcomes not limited to the prenatal period. The consequences of some of these risk factors for children are summarized in Table 5-42. For example, a child who is born prematurely and has iron deficiency anemia and lead poisoning is at high risk for early language delay, later learning problems, and school failure. Such a child is less likely to succeed in school or at work unless these factors are recognized, and treatment, early intervention, and support are provided.

Poverty also presents psychosocial challenges to child development. While these stressors may be conferred by poverty, the same kinds of protective factors and coping strategies found among more affluent families can serve as buffers that enable poor families and children to surmount such challenges. Poor families who successfully overcome these stressors often do so by developing strong and flexible networks among extended family and friends, as well as among community resources such as churches and neighborhood

TABLE 5-42

THE IMPACT OF BIOMEDICAL FACTORS ASSOCIATED WITH POVERTY

PREGNANCY RISK FACTOR	EFFECTS ON CHILD
Maternal malnutrition	Preterm delivery, low birth weight, neural tube defects
Undertreated sexually transmitted diseases	Preterm delivery, congenital infections
Stress-related hypertension	Low birth weight, stunting
Cigarette use	Increased respiratory problems and otitis media
Substance use (self-medication)	Withdrawal syndromes, low birth weight, impaired brain development

POSTNATAL RISK FACTOR	EFFECTS ON CHILD
Child malnutrition (protein/calorie, micronutrients such as iron)	Decreased growth and maturation; decreased energy for exploration and learning; decreased emotional expression inhibits interaction and relationships
Lead exposure/toxicity	Apathy; irritability; anemia; attention deficit; coordination problems; learning disabilities

associations. The ability to form such relationships (social capital) is critical to the survival of families in poverty.

THE IMPACT OF CHRONIC POVERTY

Prolonged poverty fosters a number of coping styles that are maladaptive in other settings. For example, children who are raised in poorer families may be socialized for early independence and toughness, traits that are adaptive to their neighborhood, if not for school. Furthermore, living amid a culture of much higher material expectations, chronically poor families in an affluent society endure a sense of persistent helplessness and hopelessness, which can grow into depression and rage that are as devastating as the lack of access to goods or services.

Families living in poverty can develop the kinds of coping strengths that are often seen in intact preindustrial cultures. These include individual resilience, resourcefulness, and endurance; flexible extended family networks that provide child care and a sense of belonging, and help with practical needs in times of crisis; and churches and other religious institutions that further extend the family network.

THE EFFECTS OF POVERTY ON CHILDREN AND FAMILIES

Poverty has direct effects on children (eg, from exposures to lead or street violence), as well as indirect effects through its impact on the parents and other adults. Indeed, parental well-being is the critical mediator for the impact of poverty on the child. Responsive caregivers provide the context for later behavioral and cognitive competence, through daily interactions that establish trust, safety, a sense of cause and effect, and the ability to express curiosity.

The high, persistent levels of stress that are associated with poverty undermine parents' physical and mental health, leading to high rates of stress-related medical conditions (such as hypertension and asthma) and psychological problems (such as depression, anxiety, troubled relationships, and substance abuse). Joblessness is linked to domestic violence and child abuse, particularly by fathers. In addition, many institutions that are meant to serve poor families (eg, welfare and public housing agencies) impose further stress through demeaning and time-consuming hurdles. This stress can powerfully affect parenting.

Recent research has begun to delineate the physiological processes linking sensitive and nurturant caregiving with optimal infant brain development. For example, research has shown that children who have formed more secure attachments with their mothers are more protected from the effects of stress on cortisol release. Excessive and poorly modulated cortisol release in response to stress is associated with neuronal damage, particularly in the hippocampus. Injury to the hippocampus is, in turn, associated with problems in memory, learning, and emotional regulation. Atrophy of the hippocampus has been shown in adults with posttraumatic stress disorder due to childhood abuse. Thus, factors that affect parental well-being can be seen as modulators of structural brain effects in children which increase their risk for learning and psychological problems.

HOUSING: A CASE IN POINT

Stable, safe housing is necessary for children's health and development. It has been estimated that 100,000 children in the United States are homeless every night and that many more sleep on couches and floors in the homes of relatives or friends. In addition to homelessness, marginal housing has negative biomedical and psychosocial effects, including injuries, lead poisoning, asthma, stunted growth, developmental delays, and early onset of mental health problems.

Homeless children cannot count on a quiet place to sleep or a safe place to play and learn. They do not have the support of regular routines, and their parents are often stressed and preoccupied by the struggle to survive. They may spend their days on the streets and their nights in cars or doorways, or they may live in homeless shelters. Such shelters often are noisy and dangerous, leaving children tired and hypervigilant when and if they reach school.

THE ROLE OF HEALTH-CARE PROVIDERS FOR POOR CHILDREN

Although adequate health care can buffer children from some of the adverse consequences of poverty, broad-based policies that provide for basic needs (eg, food, shelter, income support) are needed to attenuate other negative impacts. As we come to understand the powerful role of interactions during infancy, we see that support for parents' ability to nurture their children is as critical as enhancing early childhood and school-based programs. Health-care providers have three important roles to play for poor children and their families: (a) screening and identification; (b) the provision of supportive relationships; and (c) advocacy.

Advocacy

Health-care providers can and should function as advocates for children and families whether they need food, medication, early intervention services, family counseling, or household lead abatement. Disenfranchised families facing multiple crises generally cannot convince agencies or governments of the wisdom or cost-effectiveness of the services they need. Health-care providers can be particularly effective voices for such families and their children, whether through individual advocacy or through policy-related research.

References

Children's Defense Fund (US): The State of America's Children, 1992. Washington, DC, 1992

Duncan G, Brooks-Gunn J: Consequences of Growing Up Poor. New York: Russell Sage, 1997

Garbarino J: The meaning of poverty to children. In: Korbin JE, ed: The Impact of Poverty on Children. American Behavioral Scientist. Vol 35, No 3. Beverly Hills, Sage Publications, 1992

Gelles RJ: Poverty and violence towards children. In: Korbin JE, ed. The Impact of Poverty on Children. American Behavioral Scientist Vol 35, No. 3. Beverly Hills, Sage Publications, 1992

Huston AC, McLoyd VC, Coll CG: Children and poverty: issues in contemporary research. Child Dev 65(2 Spec No):275–282, 1994

McEwen BS: Protective and damaging effects of stress mediators. N Engl J Med 338:171–179, 1998

McLoyd VC: The impact of economic hardship on black families and children: psychological distress, parenting, and socioemotional development. Child Dev 61:311–346, 1990

Parker S, Greer S, Zuckerman B: Double jeopardy: the impact of poverty on early child development. Pediatr Clin North Am 35:1227–1240, 1988

CHILDHOOD DISABILITY AND REHABILITATION

Linda J. Michaud, Associate Editor

6.1 INTRODUCTION

A century ago, infectious disease was the principal threat to health in the young. With immunization practices and the antibiotics available as we begin the 21st century, chronic diseases and injuries have replaced acute illnesses as the major causes of mortality and morbidity for children in the United States. Chronic illness and significant injury in childhood usually result in impairment, defined by the World Health Organization (WHO) as any loss or abnormality of psychological, physical, or anatomic structure or function. Congenital or acquired impairment may have an impact on the child's age-appropriate activity, affecting mobility, self-care, communication, cognition, and/or psychological and social function. Disability is the limitation in activity, in the manner or within the range considered normal, caused by impairment. Handicap exists when an impairment or disability limits or prevents participation in a role that is normal for age and gender, within the social and cultural milieu. Goals of management of pediatric chronic disease and disability include minimizing the impairment and maximizing activity and participation in age-appropriate life roles (school, play, work). The approach to care is often interdisciplinary and should be coordinated, comprehensive, and family-centered.

Specific impairments are discussed elsewhere in this text. In this section, the focus is on the common issues of limitations in activity and restrictions in participation that cross impairments of varied organ systems. Principles and interventions discussed are applicable to a heterogeneous population of children with congenital or acquired conditions. The major objective in disability management is to facilitate independent function in the particular areas of functioning, referred to as domains, that are affected. Function is promoted in mobility, self-care, communication, cognition, and/or psychosocial domains. In each area, efforts are initially directed toward assisting the child to accomplish skills independently, when possible. This is accomplished through treatment strategies that enhance the functional capacity either of the affected system, when skills can be restored or developed, or through compensatory strategies using systems unaffected by the pathologic condition. Secondary disability should be prevented to the extent possible. When necessary, prescription of equipment or modifications to the physical or social environment may provide the child with greater independence. Psychological and educational techniques may also enhance patient performance. Prescriptions for therapy programs, adaptive equipment, orthoses, and prostheses should be age-appropriate and include consideration of the child's ongoing growth and development.

6.1.1 The Epidemiology of Pediatric Disability

Sarah L. Winter

An estimated 31% of children are affected by chronic conditions, according to data collected in the 1988 National Health Interview Survey. Severe disabilities are much less prevalent, affecting approximately 1 to 5% of children, but have a greater impact on the daily lives of children and their families. A broad spectrum of disorders with a low prevalence cause pediatric impairment resulting in significant disability. The types of pediatric chronic illness and disability have changed dramatically over the past several decades as medical therapies have evolved. Infectious diseases, such as polio, tuberculosis, and rheumatic fever, previously accounted for a large percentage of childhood disability. Children with disabilities secondary to these infectious diseases were hospitalized for long periods of time in convalescent facilities, away from their families and schools. Children with birth defects such as spina bifida or congenital heart disease often did not survive. Children experiencing severe head trauma or spinal cord injury frequently did not survive their initial injuries. Now polio, rheumatic fever, and tuberculosis and their secondary conditions are rare. With improved medical and surgical technology, many children with spina bifida and congenital heart defects have a normal life expectancy. With improvements in emergency medical care and intensive care, children with severe neurotrauma have increased survival, often with sequelae. Children with cerebral palsy, multiple congenital anomalies, and neurosensory impairments are living longer and healthier lives.

Collecting and reporting population-based data are the ideal methods to follow epidemiologic trends. Although there is a long history of monitoring selected disabilities in some European countries, few sources of population-based studies exist to examine trends in childhood disability in the United States. Recent prevalence data for the most common causes of childhood disability are presented in Table 6-1.

These numbers are relatively small compared to the higher prevalence of chronic illnesses such as eczema, allergies, repeated ear infections, and asthma, but severe disabilities have significantly more impact on the daily lives of the child and family. In the National Health Interview Survey of 1988, children with severe chronic conditions spent an average of 10 days in bed and missed 11 days of school annually. These children had an average of 16 physician contacts annually and accounted for 33% of all hospital days resulting from chronic conditions.

The National Health Interview Survey data suggest that among children with mild to severe disability caused by chronic conditions,

TABLE 6-1

PREVALENCE OF MAJOR CHILDHOOD DISABILITIES

DISABILITY	PREVALENCE: NO. OF CASES/1000
Mental retardation[a]	12.0
Cerebral palsy[a]	2.3
Arthritis[b]	1.4
Hearing impairment[a]	1.1
Vision impairment[a]	0.7
Spina bifida[c]	0.6
Severe traumatic brain injury[d]	0.6
Spinal cord injury[e]	0.1

[a] Metropolitan Atlanta Developmental Disabilities Surveillance Program, CDC, number of cases/1000 live births.

[b] Southwestern Sweden; point prevalence of active cases.

[c] Metropolitan Atlanta Congenital Defects Program, CDC, number of cases/1000 live births.

[d] Southwestern Sweden; incidence of functional impairment following TBI.

[e] United States; individuals 24 years of age or younger; number of cases/1000 population; Vogel LC, DeVivo MJ.

21% had two or more chronic conditions. Among children with cerebral palsy, 75% had one or more other disabilities. As would be expected, children with multiple chronic physical conditions have a higher prevalence of developmental delay, learning disabilities, and emotional and behavioral disorders.

Racial and gender distributions vary with the etiology of the disability. Overall, there is little difference noted in prevalence for race and gender for cerebral palsy, severe to profound mental retardation, or vision and hearing impairment. Boys over 9 years of age are four times more likely to experience spinal cord injury. In younger children there are no racial trends for spinal cord injury. However, in adolescents, there is a higher prevalence of African-Americans experiencing spinal cord injury than is proportionate to their representation in the general population. Boys experience twice the incidence of traumatic brain injury. Girls are almost twice as likely to have chronic active arthritic conditions.

Many pediatric disabilities are complicated by a host of secondary conditions that exacerbate existing dysfunction or create new dysfunction. Examples of secondary conditions include skin breakdown secondary to the insensate skin in persons with spinal cord injuries or spina bifida and depression in individuals with restricted activities as a result of immobility. The identification and prevention of secondary conditions or disabilities has recently emerged as a new focus for epidemiologic study.

6.1.2 Outcome Measures for Children with Disabilities

Jilda Vargus-Adams

Establishing the impact of a disability on the daily life of a child is challenging. Functional outcome measures provide information regarding the ability to accomplish day-to-day tasks in a typical fashion. Understanding the true function of a child requires consideration of each dimension included in the WHO framework of disability described above. Good functional outcome measurement should identify functional status in a meaningful manner, which

requires information at the levels of impairment, limitation in activity, and restriction in participation.

Numerous instruments have been developed to measure function and development in children. Because function varies with age in children, there is overlap of functional and developmental measures. Examples of these follow.

The Vineland Adaptive Behavior Scales (VABS) were developed largely for use by child psychologists. The VABS are applicable to all ages of children and include domains of communication, daily living skills, socialization, and motor skills. In typical usage, the VABS are administered in 30 to 60 minutes. This instrument describes function well in children and adolescents with developmental disabilities but may prove less informative for children with severe motor or cognitive impairments. Traditionally, the VABS have not been employed in the pediatric rehabilitation setting.

The Battelle Developmental Inventory (BDI) has been used primarily in the realm of early childhood education. The BDI is recommended for use in children 0 to 8 years of age. Content areas include personal-social, adaptive, motor, communicative, and cognitive functioning. The various forms of testing include a screening battery and typically take 30 to 45 minutes to administer. The BDI is standardized, valid, and reliable and provides a good description of development in young children.

The Child Health Questionnaire (CHQ) was developed as a measure of health outcomes in children. The CHQ is intended not to specifically measure functional outcomes but rather to provide information on the overall health of children. Fourteen concepts are addressed with this instrument, including physical functioning, role/social function in terms of emotion, behavior, and physical limitation, bodily pain, general behavior, mental health, self-esteem, general health perceptions, change in health, parental impact in terms of emotion and time, and family activities and cohesion. The CHQ is intended for children over the age of 5 years. Like the BDI and VABS, the CHQ is not an ideal outcome measure specifically for rehabilitation outcomes but provides data that relate to quality of life as well as parent and child perceptions and evaluations of health status.

The Pediatric Evaluation of Disability Inventory (PEDI) is designed for use in pediatric rehabilitation settings and is intended for children ages 6 months to 7 years. The PEDI is administered in several forms and includes domains of self-care, mobility, and social function. Within each domain, functional skill level or capacity, caregiver assistance, and modifications are recorded. Administration of the PEDI takes 45 to 60 minutes. The PEDI has been demonstrated to be valid.

The Functional Independence Measure for Children (WeeFIM) was also developed for use in the pediatric rehabilitation setting. The WeeFIM is modeled after the Functional Independence Measure (FIM), an instrument used widely in tracking functional gains in adult rehabilitation patients. The WeeFIM measures the amount of assistance required for children in the six domains of self-care, sphincter control, mobility, locomotion, communication, and social-cognitive function. The WeeFIM is intended for children 6 months to 8 years of age but may be used in children with developmental disorders up to 12 years of age or with a mental age of less than 7 years. The WeeFIM can be administered in 15 to 45 minutes. The WeeFIM is valid, reliable, and demonstrates good interrater agreement.

The VABS and BDI focus on a developmental hierarchy and patterns of skill acquisition that are well described in typical children or in those with developmental delay. Frequently, children with disabilities do not follow typical patterns of functional gains, as their specific impairments may present variable limitations in accomplishing the tasks of daily life. Children with disabilities may have the skills or abilities to perform some activities but may not actually accomplish them because of a lack of time, appropriate aids, or a supportive environment. In addition, children with disabilities may perform like their typical peers in some domains of function and demonstrate significant limitations in other domains. For these reasons, instruments that attempt to place children with disabilities on a developmental continuum may not provide the most meaningful analysis of function. Adult outcome criteria are generally not applicable to children because children with disabilities remain "works in progress" in that they continue to grow and develop. The expected or desired level of functioning for a child may change dramatically over time. Functional gains are anticipated as children with disabilities recover from injury or undertake rehabilitation programs while ongoing skill acquisition and altered functioning because of childhood growth and development are also expected.

The PEDI and WeeFIM are instruments that provide functional data related to the specific outcomes of children with congenital or acquired disability. These data can be used to track function over time or to analyze the efficacy of therapeutic interventions on the basic tasks of daily life (often called self-care or activities of daily living), including grooming, feeding, and bathing, as well as issues of mobility, transfers, and cognitive and social function. The instruments discussed above represent only a sampling of the currently available tools, and new measures are being developed. The use of standardized, objective instruments is important for evaluating the efficacy of various interventions and to assure that the care of children with disabilities improves over time. Pediatric rehabilitation and related fields will need to employ functional outcome measures in the future as a way to justify resource allocation and policy decisions for a growing population of children with chronic illness and disability.

6.1.3 The Medical Home

Roberta E. Bauer

As health care has become more complex, services exist in multiple settings from multiple specialized professionals. A medical home is an approach to providing continuous and comprehensive primary pediatric care from infancy through young adulthood, securing optimal services from the community's and region's resources to meet a child's needs. Healthy children may obtain immunizations, nutritional advice, and anticipatory guidance safely from multiple health care providers, still securing appropriate and high-quality care. When chronic health care conditions exist, coordination of care is not a luxury but is essential to effective care. Active management of cost-effective and appropriate anticipatory guidance, of utilization of outpatient and inpatient services, and of coordination of information exchange and subspecialty treatment provision is required to meet the needs of children with special health care needs. The concept of a medical home requires a compassionate managing physician to know the family's and child's needs, the community's resources for educational, recreational, and mental health support services, and the history of a child's and family's strengths and resiliencies in meeting the challenges of both the medical complications of illness and negotiating the health care system.

The American Academy of Pediatrics recommends that every child should have a medical home addressing seven elements defin-

ing quality of care. Care should be *accessible* to the family, both geographically and economically. Medical decision makers should recognize the family's role as the ultimate support and center of ongoing care provision. Physicians should provide unbiased and complete information to parents allowing *family-centered* planning, decision making, and treatment. Care provision is *continuous* from infancy to adolescence and available through transitions from home to school and to adult service sites. The physician provides centralized information and records to *coordinate comprehensive care* for primary, preventive, and tertiary health care among educational, supportive, and community-based services. Beyond state-of-the-art care, the physician demonstrates respect and concern for the well-being of the child. The physician–family partnership is valued and respected with *compassionate* and *culturally competent* care. By working together in a medical home, physicians and parents work to identify and access all the medical and nonmedical services needed to help children with chronic illness and disability maximize their health and developmental and functional potential.

References

DeLisa JA, Currie DM, Martin GM: Rehabilitation medicine: past, present, and future. In: DeLisa JA, Gans BM, eds: Rehabilitation Medicine: Principles and Practice, 3rd ed. Philadelphia, Lippincott-Raven, 1998:3–32

Hays RM, Michaud LJ: Principles of pediatric rehabilitation. In: Hays RM, Kraft GH, Stolov WC, eds: Chronic Disease and Disability: A Contemporary Rehabilitation Approach to Medical Practice. New York, Demos Publications, 1994:215–229

ICIDH-2: International Classification of Impairments, Activities, and Participation. A Manual of Dimensions of Disablement and Functioning. Beta-1 draft for field trials. Geneva, World Health Organization, 1997

Epidemiology

Emanuelson I, v Wendt L: Epidemiology of traumatic brain injury in children and adolescents in south-western Sweden. Acta Paediatr 86:730–735, 1997

Gare BA, Fasth A: Epidemiology of juvenile chronic arthritis in southwestern Sweden: A 5-year prospective population study. Pediatrics 90:950–958, 1992

Hays RM, Michaud LJ: Principles of pediatric rehabilitation. In: Hays RM, Kraft GH, Stolov WC, eds: Chronic Disease and Disability: A Contemporary Rehabilitation Approach to Medical Practice. New York, Demos Publications, 1994:215–229

Murphy CC, Yeargin-Allsopp M, Decoufle P, Drews CD: Prevalence of cerebral palsy among ten-year-old children in metropolitan Atlanta, 1985 through 1987. J Pediatr 123:S13–S19, 1993

Newacheck PW, Stoddard JJ: Prevalence and impact of multiple childhood chronic illnesses. J Pediatr 124:40–48, 1994

Newacheck PW, Taylor WR: Childhood chronic illness: prevalence, severity, and impact. Am J Public Health 82:364–371, 1992

Vogel LC, DeVivo MJ: Etiology and demographics. In: Betz RR, Mulcahey MJ, eds: The Child with a Spinal Cord Injury. Rosemont, IL, American Academy of Orthopaedic Surgeons, 1996:3–12

Yeargin-Allsopp M, Murphy CC, Oakley GP, Sikes RK, and the Metropolitan Atlanta Developmental Disabilities Study Staff: A multiple-source method for studying the prevalence of developmental disabilities in children: the Metropolitan Atlanta Developmental Disabilities Study. Pediatrics 89:624–630, 1992

Yen IH, Khoury MJ, Erickson JD, James LM, Waters GD, Berry RJ: The changing epidemiology of neural tube defects: United States, 1968–1989. Am J Dis Child 146:857–861, 1992

Outcome Measurement

Braun SL, Msall ME, McCabe M, Granger CV: Guide for the Use of the Functional Independence Measure for Children (Wee-FIM) of the Uniform Data Set for Medical Rehabilitation, version 4.0. Buffalo, NY, Center for Functional Assessment Research, State University of New York at Buffalo, 1994

Haley SM, Coster WJ, Ludlow LH: Pediatric functional outcome measures. Phys Med Rehabil Clin North Am 2:689–723, 1991

Haley SM, Coster WJ, Ludlow LH, et al: Pediatric Evaluation of Disability Inventory (PEDI), Version 1: Development, Standardization and Administration Manual. Boston, New England Medical Center, PEDI Research Group, 1992

ICIDH-2: International Classification of Impairments, Activities, and Participation. A Manual of Dimensions of Disablement and Functioning. Beta-1 draft for field trials. Geneva, World Health Organization, 1997

Landgraf JM, Abetz L, Ware JE: The CHQ User's Manual. Boston, The Health Institute, New England Medical Center, 1996

Newborg J, Strock J, Wnek L: Battelle Developmental Inventory. Allen, TX, DLM Teaching Resources, 1984

Sparrow SS, Ballo DA, Cicchetti DV: Vineland Adaptive Behavior Scales. Circle Pines, MN, American Guidance Service, 1984

Medical Home

Ad HOC Task Force on Definition of the Medical Home, American Academy of Pediatrics: The medical home. Pediatrics 90:774, 1992

6.2   SPECIFIC ISSUES IN CHILDHOOD DISABILITY

6.2.1   Care of the Child with a Tracheostomy

Virginia Simson Nelson and Elizabeth A. Grady

Children with varied disabling conditions may require long-term tracheostomy. The most common abnormalities are airway disorders such as subglottic stenosis or vocal cord paralysis, where the tracheostomy bypasses an obstructed upper airway, severe oral-pharyngeal problems with aspiration, where the tracheostomy allows access for airway suctioning, and neuromuscular disorders, where the tracheostomy allows mechanical ventilation. Before electively placing a tracheostomy, a team should discuss the indications and expected use of the tracheostomy. This team should include the surgeon (usually otolaryngologist), primary pediatrician, speech-language pathologist, nurse, respiratory therapist, and managing physician. The type of tracheostomy tube should be decided on the basis of airway anatomy, patient comfort, the child's size, and the ability to communicate orally. Ideally, the smallest tube that provides an adequate airway and optimizes vocalization should be used. It is not always necessary to upsize the tracheostomy tube as the child grows. Occasionally, a custom tube may need to be designed to meet the needs of the child. See Table 6-2 for the advantages and disadvantages of various types of tracheostomy tubes.

Patient and family education is a critical part of successful tracheostomy tube placement in patients to be discharged home with a tracheostomy tube. Education should begin before elective placement or on the day of surgery in emergency situations. The anat-

TABLE 6-2

ADVANTAGES AND DISADVANTAGES OF VARIOUS TRACHEOSTOMY TUBES

TUBE TYPE	ADVANTAGES	DISADVANTAGES
Uncuffed	Lowest incidence of tracheal damage Easy insertion Allows vocalization	Air leak Fixed diameter
Low pressure air cuff (LPA)	Offers option to seal air leak Variable diameter depending on volume of air in cuff Vocalization with cuff down	More difficult to insert Potential for tracheal damage if pressure too great
Fenestrated	Vocalization possible with cuff inflated	Formation of granulation tissue
Bivona Tight to Shaft™ Aire-Cuff®	Easier insertion than LPA Vocalization with cuff down	High tracheal wall pressure with cuff inflated Cuff is permeable, making it difficult to keep cuff inflated
Bivona Fome-Cuff®	Lowest tracheal wall pressure of cuffed tubes	Difficult to insert Cuff self-inflates, so cannot be used in deflated position for long Poor vocalization
Metal	Reusable	Needs adapter to use with Ambu bag More expensive than standard plastic tubes

omy and physiology of the airway, purpose of the tracheostomy, assessment of the child, suctioning, use of the manual resuscitation bag, stoma care, tracheostomy tube tie changes, tracheostomy tube changes, emergency procedures, and cardiopulmonary resuscitation (CPR) via tracheostomy should all be reviewed. The use of a "go bag" should be discussed, and before discharge the family should be given assistance in preparation of an appropriate bag that contains a suction machine and suction catheters, extra tracheostomy tubes of the same size and one size smaller, tracheostomy tube ties, nonsterile gloves, small containers of saline to use with suctioning, an extra artificial nose, speaking valve, or tracheostomy tube cap, and inhaled medications. Caregivers and teachers should be fully trained in suctioning, bagging, tracheostomy tube changes, use of inhaled medications, and CPR via tracheostomy. Use of metered dose inhalers and nebulizers and secretion clearance techniques should be taught as needed. The clinical nurse specialist and/or respiratory therapist should provide the teaching with reinforcement regarding its importance by the physician.

HOME MANAGEMENT OF THE CHILD WITH A TRACHEOSTOMY

Management of a tracheostomy tube in a child at home is different from management in the hospital. A tracheostomy is not sterile, and none of the procedures associated with it are sterile. Nonsterile gloves may be used to protect the caregiver, but many families choose not to use gloves. Suction catheters may be reused, if desired, without an increased risk of pneumonia. Reuse of a plastic tracheostomy tube is not recommended because degradation of the plastic material after prolonged use may cause separation of the tube from the connector. The tube should be changed as needed, but at least once a month. Tracheostomy tubes with inner cannulas should be considered for patients with copious secretions, allowing for frequent changing of the inner cannula without changing the tracheostomy tube. Smaller or cuffed tubes may need to be changed more frequently. Prolonged intervals between changes may cause difficulty in tube removal.

Tracheostomy tube changes with the same size tube are not medical procedures but routine care. The physician should perform the first tracheostomy tube change and subsequent changes when the type or size of the tube is changed. Tracheostomy tube ties should be changed daily or as needed and should not be too tight. A general guideline is that the tie should be loose enough to allow the placement of one or two adult fingers between the neck and the tie. Gauze ("trach pants") may be placed under the tracheostomy tube to catch secretions, but this is not always necessary. An antifungal cream may be used as needed around the tracheostomy site. With prospective management, children with tracheostomies may participate in school and community activities. Their tracheostomies should be covered with an artificial nose, speaking valve, tracheostomy tube mask, or cap to prevent dry air from directly entering the trachea. They should always take their "go bag" with them. If the child rides a school bus, a trained aide should accompany him or her. The managing physician should provide the patient with a data sheet that contains necessary medical information related to the tracheostomy and physician contact information.

6.2.2 Nutritional Management of Children with Disability

Ann E. Weidenbenner

Specific aspects of formula selection and nutritional management are discussed in Sec. 17.3 and 17.6. Selection of supplemental feeding devices is reviewed below in Sec. 6.2.3 and in Sec. 17.6. Children with chronic illness or disabilities frequently have additional nutrition needs related to their underlying disorder. As many as 40% of children with special health care needs experience nutrition-related problems. Nutrition screenings completed in four states among children with disabilities between the ages of 1 and 3 years revealed that 20% were below the fifth percentile weight for height, 30% had feeding difficulties, and 25% were on chronic medications. A total of 46% of these children had more than one nutrition risk factor, and 25% had more than three nutrition risk factors.

A study of children with special health care needs in Washington state found major nutrition and feeding problems among 30% of children with special health care needs, ages 11 days to 17 years. These problems included altered growth, inappropriate or inadequate nutrient intake, delayed or impaired feeding skills, need for specialized feedings, and oral motor feeding problems. Following nutrition or feeding team intervention, positive outcomes for these children included appropriate growth in the children who had slow growth or failure to thrive; improved dietary intake and adequacy in all of the children who had inappropriate or inadequate intake; decreased illness and hospitalization; improved feeding skills; improved feeding behavior; decreased constipation; and developmental feeding progress. The greatest improvements were in growth and dietary intake, which addressed the frequent initial problems of poor growth and inadequate diet. The estimated medical cost savings achieved by providing nutritional or feeding team services ranged from $180 to $5000 per year depending on the patient's diagnosis, with the overall cost saving far exceeding the costs of the nutritional consultation and intervention.

Children with special needs require ongoing and periodic nutrition assessments followed by appropriate intervention and ongoing follow-up and coordination of care. Many of the feeding and nutrition problems are complex and require expertise of the multidisciplinary team (see Sec. 17.8).

Cooperation among community-based physicians, dietitians, and tertiary center facilities provides the most effective continuity of care. Both community and tertiary center dieticians can be enlisted for the cooperative, ongoing care of children with chronic illness and disability. A system is most successful when all health, education, and social agencies, as well as family members, are able to collaborate in making decisions that will benefit the child.

6.2.3 Enteral Feeding Management in Childhood Disability

Deborah Mason

As discussed above, children with disabilities benefit from adequate nutrition to promote growth and expedite healing of injuries. The oral feeding route is not always appropriate. Atypical development of or disruption in oral feeding abilities frequently occurs in chronic illness and disability and may be temporary or long-term. The decision to replace or supplement oral feeding with alternative methods is based on an assessment of the child's impairment, oral motor skills, and acceptance of the family. Alternative feeding routes are selected according to the age and size of the child, gastrointestinal tract function, the anticipated period needed for enteral feedings, risk for aspiration, and the need for abdominal surgery. In all cases the risks and benefits of selected approaches must be carefully balanced, as discussed in Sec. 17.6.1.

If a child is unable or unwilling to eat by mouth, and the anticipated period needed for supplemental feedings is less than 4 to 6 weeks, a nasogastric or nasojejunal tube may be inserted through the nose into the stomach or intestinal tract. Nasogastric tubes are generally placed in children who are at low risk for aspiration and have normal gastric emptying. Nasojejunal tubes may be useful in children who are at high risk of aspiration or have impaired gastric emptying. Advantages of these types of tubes are that they avoid surgery, are easy to use, and are inexpensive. Disadvantages of these types of tubes are that they are visible on the face, aversive to place, and easily dislodged. Nasally placed tubes also increase the risk for sinusitis and otitis media. The presence of a nasally placed tube in the posterior pharynx may also cause discomfort for the child and may interfere with the assessment of a child's oral motor functioning and the ability to resume oral feeding. For those tubes placed into the small intestinal tract, placement requires radiographic guidance. Repeated placement increases radiation exposure of the child and is an inconvenience for the family.

If the need for enteral feedings is anticipated to be over 6 weeks, placement of a gastrostomy or jejunostomy tube should be considered. For long-term enteral feeding, the gastrostomy tube is more common. When the gastrocutaneous fistula is well healed (usually 3 months) a skin-level device may be placed. This is generally recommended, as it increases the mobility of a child for therapies, promoting motor development, and is cosmetically more pleasing.

For a child who is bedridden, skin-level devices may not provide an advantage.

Before tube feedings are initiated, proper placement of the tube must be confirmed. A feeding tube's position is checked when the tube is placed, before feedings, every 4 to 8 hours during continuous feedings, or at any time tube position is questioned.

Even though a child may require enteral feedings, families should be instructed to keep mealtimes as normal as possible. Young children should be held during feedings to promote normal development and bonding. Older children should be fed at the same time as other family members to promote normal family relationships.

Understanding the child's nutritional needs and absorption process is critical in selection and administration of enteral feedings. Nasogastric and gastrostomy feedings are given either by bolus or continuous feeding methods. Bolus feedings are given at intervals and only when the feeding tube is in the stomach. Continuous feedings are given over a longer period of time and are required when the feeding tube is in the small intestine because of the limited tolerance of the small intestine for bolus feedings. Jejunostomy tubes are frequently placed in a newly injured child because of concerns about a decreased level of responsiveness, reflux, and aspiration. An important goal for a child undergoing rehabilitation after acquired injury is to return to the most normal feeding regimen as soon as possible. Therefore, it is often helpful to convert the child from continuous feedings to intermittent bolus feedings as soon as the child demonstrates that these types of feedings can be tolerated without undue risk of aspiration.

When the decision has been made to initiate enteral feedings, routine monitoring is necessary. Feedings must be adjusted to meet changing requirements related to the child's growth and activity level as well as those related to potential ongoing recovery of neurologic function in children with recently acquired injury. Families should be instructed to follow up regularly with the child's interdisciplinary rehabilitation team, which should include a clinical dietician.

In caring for a child with a feeding tube, special attention must be given to the tube, surrounding skin, and stoma site. Specific issues regarding care of feeding tubes and complications of feeding tubes are summarized in Table 17-17. The skin should be washed with mild soap and water and allowed to air dry once or twice daily. Surgically placed tubes should be rotated in a full circle during cleaning to prevent the tube from adhering to the tract and to evaluate for proper fit. When nasogastric tubes are changed, the tube should be alternated between nares to avoid consistent irritation of a single naris. All tubes should be properly secured to prevent excessive pulling on the tube. This prevents increased irritation on the nares or stoma site, with decreased potential of dilating the stoma. In addition, the length of the tube should be inspected to make sure that tube position has not changed.

The decision to discontinue enteral feedings is made after the child has demonstrated the ability to take all of his or her feedings, liquids, and medications by mouth. If a child has been fed through a nasally placed tube, trial periods of withholding the tube feedings may easily be accomplished. If a child has a surgically placed tube, the decision for removal must be carefully considered. Generally, the minimum criterion for removal of a surgically placed tube is no use of the tube for 3 to 6 months with documented maintenance or gain in weight. Depending on the underlying medical condition, if the child is at an acceptable weight but has minimal nutritional reserves or is expected to be at risk for additional physiological stressors and/or medical or surgical interventions, it may be advisable for the child to demonstrate that he or she can meet all nutritional requirements for a longer period, such as through an illness.

6.2.4   Management of the Child with a Neurogenic Bladder

Stephanie R. Ried

Neurogenic bladder dysfunction is characterized by impairment of the lower urinary tract's ability to function as a coordinated system for urinary collection, storage, and excretion. In the pediatric population, impairment may result from a variety of congenital or acquired etiologies. The most common cause is myelomeningocele, although neurogenic bladder disorder may result from any congenital condition affecting the spine and involving neural elements. The child with cerebral palsy whose cognitive capacity is adequate for toilet training, but who experiences persistent incontinence, may have central nervous system involvement at the level of the brainstem or spinal cord, resulting in a neurogenic bladder. In end-stage Duchenne muscular dystrophy, bladder dysfunction may occur secondary to degenerative changes in the bladder resulting in poor contractility. With pelvic, retroperitoneal or spinal involvement with a neoplasm, such as in association with neurofibromatosis, bladder function may be impaired as a result of obstruction, direct nerve involvement, or spinal cord compression.

Inflammatory processes involving the spinal cord or brainstem, as seen in transverse myelitis and meningitis, are among the acquired conditions that can cause neurogenic bladder dysfunction. Traumatic spinal cord injury invariably results in some degree of bladder dysfunction. Infarcts of the spinal cord secondary to arteriovenous malformation or any process that interrupts the blood supply to the anterior spinal artery may also result in impaired bladder function.

PATHOPHYSIOLOGY

Normal micturition is a complex of finely integrated neuromuscular events involving somatic, parasympathetic, and sympathetic pathways with final coordination of these events occurring in the rostral pons of the brainstem. The micturition cycle may be divided into two major phases, a filling phase (storage) and an emptying phase (voiding). The external urinary sphincter and striated muscles in the pelvic floor are innervated primarily by sacral roots S2 through S4 via the pudendal nerve. Primary innervation of the bladder's detrusor muscle is parasympathetic, via the pelvic nerve, and also arises from S2 through S4. Sympathetic innervation of the lower urinary tract comes from T10 to L2 via the hypogastric nerve and has both α- and β-adrenergic activity. α-Adrenoreceptors mediate closure of the smooth muscle of the internal sphincter in addition to blocking neuronal transmission between pre- and postganglionic parasympathetic nerve. β-Adrenoreceptors mediate relaxation of the body of the bladder wall to increase bladder compliance during the filling phase. In voluntary voiding, micturition is accomplished by complete relaxation of the striated muscle of the external sphincter and pelvic floor, which is the initial event in activation of the "micturition reflex." The urethra and bladder neck gradually open, the detrusor contracts, and urine flow begins. These complex coordinated events are integrated in the pontine micturition center.

Lesions at the level of the pons may impair the coordinated functioning of the lower urinary tract. As with spinal cord injury, manifestations are usually upper motor neuron in nature, with involuntary detrusor contractions, failure of the external sphincter to relax during detrusor contractions, and subsequent development of bladder wall thickening, trabeculations, and decreased compliance and storage capacity because of detrusor hyperactivity. Lower motor neuron dysfunction resulting from anterior horn cell and/or peripheral nerve damage causes detrusor areflexia, poor bladder emptying and normal or decreased sphincter pressure, with a long-term risk of developing low bladder compliance. It is critical to recognize that many patients, particularly those with multiple injuries, incomplete spinal cord injury, nontraumatic spinal cord injury, and myelomeningocele, can have a mixed pattern of upper and lower motor neuron involvement that cannot be predicted from the neurologic history. Additionally, there is a significant incidence of neurogenic bladder dysfunction in otherwise apparently neurologically intact individuals, particularly those with thoracolumbar spinal injuries. Thorough urologic evaluation is, therefore, required when there is clinical suspicion of abnormality. Incontinence following central nervous system lesions above the level of the pons is usually a result of disinhibition rather than lower urinary tract dysfunction.

EVALUATION AND MANAGEMENT

Accurate diagnosis depends on careful evaluation of the child's history, physical examination, laboratory and imaging studies, and urodynamic assessment. Lower urinary tract dysfunction is generally related to bladder-filling and storage problems, bladder-emptying problems, or a combination of both. Bladder symptoms may be irritative or obstructive in nature. Urinalysis and urine culture should be done to rule out infection, which is the most remediable cause of urinary symptoms. Further diagnostic evaluation should include renal and bladder ultrasound to assess anatomy. Urodynamic evaluation includes simultaneous recordings of detrusor and sphincter activity and is invaluable in the diagnosis of desynchronization of detrusor and sphincter function in detrusor–external sphincter dyssynergia. The synchronous addition of cystourography in video urodynamics adds a functional dimension, with the use of fluoroscopy. It is considered the "gold standard" for evaluation of voiding abnormalities. When this is not available, the voiding cystourethrogram provides data on bladder capacity, postvoid residual volumes, and vesicoureteral reflux and is an appropriate complement to the pressure-flow urodynamic study.

The primary goal in managing neurogenic bladder dysfunction is adequate storage at low intravesical pressures, thus avoiding deleterious changes to the upper urinary tract. Treatment is based on the functional impairment demonstrated. The cornerstone for management of the neurogenic bladder is clean intermittent catheterization. This is often supplemented with pharmacotherapy. Inadequate storage capacity may be addressed by lowering detrusor tone and decreasing uninhibited detrusor contractions with an anticholinergic medication, such as oral or intravesical oxybutynin. α-Adrenergic agents such as ephedrine sulfate or imipramine can be used to address internal sphincter dysfunction. The frequency of catheterization should be adjusted to limit overdistension of the bladder. In general, bladder capacity can be estimated by the formula *age in years* + 2 = *volume in ounces* until 14 years of age, when normal bladder volume approximates that of an adult, about 500 ml. It is critical that detrusor–external sphincter dyssynergia

be addressed early, to limit the risk of transmitting excessive intravesical pressures to the upper urologic tracts with resultant renal damage. When medical management with intermittent catheterization and anticholinergic medication fails to maintain intravesical pressure within an acceptable range, surgical interventions such as vesicostomy, bladder augmentation, or diversion procedures may be considered. Antibiotic treatment is not recommended for asymptomatic bacteriuria in the absence of vesicoureteral reflux because this bacteriuria is not associated with renal scarring. Antibiotic prophylaxis for urinary tract infections is of uncertain value and invariably results in emergence of drug-resistant organisms.

PROGNOSIS

Before the advent of appropriate bladder-emptying regimens, urologic complications were the main cause of death in children with myelomeningocele and spinal cord injuries. With appropriate management, mortality from renal failure is uncommon. Favorable prognosis depends on compliance with an appropriate bladder management program and lifelong annual urologic surveillance with renal ultrasounds and/or urodynamic studies as indicated. Multiple studies have documented that in children with myelomeningocele, early intervention, beginning in the newborn period, with clean intermittent catheterization improves compliance with the procedure and acceptance of this method of bladder emptying as a regular part of daily life. This results in significantly decreased risk of irreversible bladder dysfunction and need for bladder augmentation as these children mature.

6.2.5   Bowel Management in Children with Disabilities

Janice L. Cockrell

Defecation difficulties are common in children with disabilities. Factors contributing to incontinence and/or difficulty with evacuation include neurologic dysfunction, prolonged recumbent positioning or lack of ambulation, inappropriate toileting position, inadequate fluid intake, diets low in fiber, and medication side effects. Recommendations for bowel management can be generalized within a diagnosis; for example, an upper motor neuron bowel needs to be managed differently than a lower motor neuron bowel. At the same time, it is most important to individualize the program to the habits and preferences of the child and his or her family. It is also important to assure that other causes of constipation are excluded before assuming that the problem is solely a result of the disability. The overall approach to the management of constipation is discussed in Sec. 17.7.6.

The establishment of a bowel management program begins with a thorough history, which, in addition to the medical diagnosis, should include current medications, fluid intake including fluid types as well as volumes, stool timing and consistency, and frequency of stool incontinence. The physical examination should focus on observation (abdominal/rectal area, looking for masses, asymmetry and skin breakdown), palpation (looking for size and consistency of any abdominal masses), auscultation for bowel sounds, sensory exam (sacral dermatomes), evaluation of anal reflexes (anal wink, bulbocavernosus), and finally a digital rectal examination to evaluate sphincter tone and the ability to voluntarily contract the sphincter and to assess the presence and consistency of stool in the rectal vault.

The bowel program itself will consist of several elements. Even in individuals reportedly having daily bowel movement, there may be a large amount of stool present, often extending as far as the ascending colon. A "clean-out" is often the most effective way to initiate a bowel program. This may consist of Fleets, saline, or tap water enemas, which could be repeated once or twice on the first day of the program or, in the case of persons with patulent sphincters, an oral agent such as magnesium citrate or mineral oil. Caution should be exercised in the use of oral agents (especially mineral oil) in patients at risk for potential aspiration. In severe cases of impaction, initial clean-out may require inpatient admission with nasogastric administration of balanced electrolyte–polyethylene glycol solutions, pulsed irrigation evacuation, and/or manual disimpaction under anesthesia.

Following the initial clean-out and disimpaction, the oral maintenance (or enteral) aspects of the program should be addressed with bulk-producing agents (such as Miller bran or psyllium), stool softeners (such as milk of magnesia or docusate), and adequate fluid intake. The importance of bulking agents such as fiber and psyllium in the bowel management of children with spinal disorders cannot be underestimated. Stimulation of defecation using glycerin suppositories or digital stimulation are additional elements that prove useful in bowel programs, particularly for persons with upper motor neuron findings. In spinal cord injury, this may be required on a daily basis and has no adverse effects. If bowel stimulants are necessary, bisacodyl suppositories can be employed for the first few weeks of the bowel program until a regular schedule is established, but the associated crampy pain may lead to a negative psychological association with rectal manipulation, making the child resist any further management attempts with suppositories or digital stimulation.

Scheduling the bowel program is one of the most important aspects of treatment. The family must have a clear understanding of the gastrocolic reflex and appreciate the importance of a regular time for a bowel movement in order to successfully manage their program. It is helpful to assist the family in identifying a time of day that could consistently be utilized for a bowel program. In some cases right after dinner is practical, but in other cases right after breakfast is more convenient. Morning timing also prevents soiling during school attendance. An appropriate upright positioning system, such as a commode with armrests and positioning straps, may also be useful.

Newer techniques for neurogenic bowel management, which may be particularly helpful for patients with flaccid sphincters who often smear during the day even on an appropriate bowel program, include the catheter enema and cecostomy with daily lavage. Some recent work using anterior sacral root stimulator implants has shown potential to improve bowel and bladder control in adults with upper motor neuron dysfunction causing incontinence. Trials in the pediatric population are likely in the near future.

6.2.6 Management of the Child with Spasticity

Douglas G. Kinnett and Mary A. McMahon

Spasticity is a velocity-dependent increase in muscle tone that is associated with upper motor neuron lesions. Resistance to passive range of motion (ROM) increases with higher speed of movement.

For example, an examiner extending an elbow from a position of flexion can demonstrate spasticity if, with more rapid extension, more resistance is felt. The presence of hyperactive muscle stretch reflexes, the spreading of the reflex response beyond the muscle stimulated, and clonus can all be associated with spasticity.

Conditions in which spasticity may be seen in childhood include cerebral palsy, traumatic brain injury, spinal cord injury, and other developmental anomalies and acquired lesions of the central nervous system, such as infections and vascular accidents. Children present a unique challenge in spasticity management because of the early onset of spasticity in combination with significant future linear growth. Different rates of growth in bone and muscle length can lead to joint deformities and the development of permanent muscle contractures. Spasticity should be detected early so that appropriate treatment can be initiated before the onset of secondary complications.

The treatment of spasticity in children begins with the identification of spasticity that interferes with function, positioning, care, or comfort. Pediatric centers that see children with the above conditions often have a team that can provide a comprehensive evaluation and treatment plan for spasticity. These interdisciplinary teams may include physiatrists, orthopedic surgeons, neurosurgeons, developmental pediatricians, neurologists, therapists, and nurses who are knowledgeable about the many options available for spasticity management.

The initial intervention in many cases is with the therapist. Physical and occupational therapists can provide thorough evaluations and ongoing treatment for children with spasticity. Documentation of baseline spasticity, ROM, and motor skills by the therapist can be helpful in monitoring progress following interventions. Education of families in home exercise, including stretching and strengthening, programs is done with periodic reevaluations for further modifications. Bracing (described in Sec. 6.3.4) can be done across a joint to maintain muscle length and bony alignment for the promotion of functional activities or to prevent contracture in the child with spasticity.

Many times therapy alone is not sufficient to prevent secondary complications related to spasticity in a child. Pharmacologic management can be used for generalized spasticity adjunctively with therapy interventions. There are three antispasticity medications that are currently commonly used in children with spasticity: dantrolene sodium, baclofen, and tizanidine. These can be used alone or in combination, as each has a different mechanism and site of action. These medications are taken orally to reduce spasticity and allow easier ROM and greater ease and comfort with positioning. The advantage of oral antispasticity medications is ease of use with widespread effects, but each has potential negative side effects, including sedation. Maximal doses may not be enough to sufficiently reduce severe spasticity.

When a few spastic muscles cause problems in function for a child, a focal approach is indicated. Nerve blocks and soft tissue releases lend themselves well to management of focal spasticity. Botulinum toxin and phenol can be used to block the nerve impulse to individual muscle groups, resulting in temporary relaxation. Repeat nerve blocks can be done, which is especially helpful in the growing child. Soft tissue releases provide a more permanent surgical approach to obtain needed ROM and may be necessary if a fixed contracture has occurred across a joint. Multiple releases can be done at the same time if there is involvement of several joints.

Children who have severe generalized spasticity are at significant risk for developing musculoskeletal deformities that can result in decreasing functional abilities and the development of chronic pain.

For these children more invasive procedures should be considered. *Selective dorsal rhizotomy* is a neurosurgical procedure that can dramatically reduce spasticity, in lower extremities more than upper extremities. This procedure involves severing a portion of the sensory nerve roots in the lumbar and upper sacral levels of the spinal cord. An *intrathecal baclofen infusion pump* is another method of significantly reducing spasticity. This involves implantation of a pump in the abdominal wall with a catheter under the skin; the catheter extends from the pump through a lumbar foramen superiorly along the spinal cord up to the thoracic level. Spinal dorsal rhizotomy is a more permanent approach to relieving spasticity, whereas intrathecal baclofen is a more readily adjustable, reversible approach that requires more intensive follow-up and maintenance care. The treatment of spasticity in a single child can involve one or many of the approaches mentioned above, depending on the age of the child, degree of spasticity, presence of fixed contractures, and amount of underlying voluntary strength.

6.2.7 Immunizations for Children with Chronic Conditions

Mary Allen Staat

Routine immunizations are important for all children, and this component of well-child care is equally important in children with chronic illness and disability. Certain chronic conditions may increase susceptibility to and complications from infections with some of the vaccine-preventable diseases. Specific conditions may also contraindicate selected routine immunizations. In addition, those who live in residential institutions may benefit from other immunizations such as pneumococcal and influenza vaccine. Table 6-3 lists recommendations for both routine and special immunizations for children with chronic conditions. Further information regarding these immunizations is provided in Sec. 1.00.

6.2.8 Dental Care for Children with Disabilities

William A. Greenhill

Children with chronic illness and disability are at greater risk than the general pediatric population for dental decay. Because of abnormal oral-motor reflexes, it may be very difficult for some caregivers to adequately provide good oral hygiene. Swallowing difficulties can lead to retention of food particles in the mouth, which can promote further dental problems. Children with chronic conditions often take many medications, which can have detrimental influences on the oral environment. For instance, phenytoin promotes gingival hyperplasia. Other medications promote tooth decay with their high sugar content: some liquid medications contain 30 to 50% sucrose. Abnormal positioning of the lips, tongue, or cheeks contributes to malocclusion, which can be associated with such problems as an anterior open bite, crowding, or poor tooth position. Bruxism, a habitual grinding of the teeth, is also a common finding, as well as lip and cheek biting. Poor dental health leads to needless pain, loss of appetite, and infection. Adequate prevention is an important first step in managing special care patients.

Because children with special health care needs are at high risk for dental decay, they should be seen for regular dental check-ups,

TABLE 6-3

SPECIAL ISSUES IN IMMUNIZATIONS FOR CHILDREN WITH CHRONIC CONDITIONS

IMMUNIZATION	RECOMMENDATIONS
Routine immunizations	
Diphtheria/tetanus/ pertussis vaccine	Defer in children with specific or yet undefined neurologic conditions until condition is diagnosed and found to be nonprogressive
Hemophilus influenzae type b vaccine	Recommended for asplenic children who have not received this vaccine as an infant
Inactivated polio vaccine	Recommended for all children
Hepatitis B vaccine	Recommended for all children
Measles/mumps/rubella vaccine	Contraindicated in immunocompromised children except for HIV-infected children who are not severely immunocompromised; contraindicated in children requiring steroids
Varicella vaccine	Contraindicated in immunocompromised children; contraindicated in children requiring steroids
Special immunizations	
Pneumococcal vaccine	Recommended for those at risk for disease or complications (chronic pulmonary disease, cardiac disease, liver disease, diabetes mellitus, asplenia, or cerebrospinal fluid leaks)
Meningococcal vaccine	Recommended for those with functional or anatomic asplenia
Influenza vaccine	Recommended for those with chronic pulmonary (including asthma) or cardiovascular disorders, chronic metabolic diseases, renal dysfunction, hemoglobinopathies, immunosuppressive conditions, or for those on long-term aspirin therapy or who live in chronic care facilities
Hepatitis A vaccine	Recommended for children with clotting factor disorders, chronic liver disease, or those awaiting or who have received liver transplants

at least every 6 months. Children and their families should be instructed in proper hygiene. Adaptations to toothbrushes can be made to improve the child's ability to grip the toothbrush. Electric toothbrushes may also be helpful. For those patients who cannot adequately brush, caregivers should be instructed in providing proper hygiene. Using several tongue blades taped together can serve as an excellent prop to hold the mouth open, improving access for the caregiver. At the completion of brushing and flossing with a floss holder, the child can be offered water through a straw or a plastic squeeze bottle. The water can be swallowed, but if the child elects it can be spit or trickled into a washbasin. Another important preventive consideration is whether the patient is receiving adequate amounts of fluoride, both dietary and topical. Strict use of bottled water by the caregiver may not provide adequate fluoride. Also, there are water filters that remove most of the fluoride from the water. These products can negatively impact the child's preventive dental care. For those children using chronic medications with high sugar content, sugar-free medications can be requested from the pharmacist. For children with bruxism, an acrylic appliance such as a lip bumper may occasionally be needed to help prevent self-injury.

Routine oral health care may require innovative approaches because of physical limitations. For example, positioning the child with limited trunk strength or control or excessive muscle tone may present challenges. Many children with disabilities have wheelchairs with special features, such as tilt-in-space or recline mechanisms, that give them adequate support for better head and trunk control. It may be better to treat these children in their own wheelchairs. This will provide better support, facilitating head and oral-motor control and thus improving access for the child's dental examination. Some patients may be able to adequately maintain good muscular control sitting in the dental chair. Beanbags or pillows may further support the child with physical disabilities. Generally, dental examinations should be kept as short as possible. The use of a stainless steel mirror and mouth prop will help protect both the patient and the examiner. If restorative treatment becomes necessary, this often needs to be done with the use of a general anesthetic.

The dental community, in collaboration with other health professionals, must develop unique treatment strategies aimed at the specific needs of children with a variety of medical conditions associated with disability. A team approach to managing these children will ensure that adequate dental care is an important part of their overall well-child care. Pediatric dentists usually have had special training on proper management of children with disability and can recommend appropriate plans for prevention and intervention.

6.2.9 Complementary and Alternative Therapy in Children with Chronic Conditions

Bonnie J. Patterson

The use of complementary and alternative medicine (CAM) has increased significantly in the past decade. Fifty to 70% of children with chronic disorders use some type of alternative or complementary therapy. Alternative therapies are health care interventions offered in place of conventional therapies, whereas complementary medicine refers to care provided in conjunction with traditional medical practices. The term integrative medicine is now being used in many areas instead of alternative or complementary.

The CAM therapies can be divided into four distinct groups. Biochemical interventions include herbal preparations and nutritional supplements. Many of the medicines we use today were derived from plants and therefore were "herbal" in origin. Medications are more highly purified forms of the active ingredients. The purity and quality control of herbal preparations can vary. Some have had contaminants, such as lead and mercury. Nutritional supplements are frequently given to children with chronic conditions and often include megadoses of vitamins and minerals as well as other supplements such as amino acids and digestive enzymes. Although most vitamins and minerals are safe, some can cause serious side effects when given in high doses. Vitamin A overdose can affect the liver and brain, vitamin C can cause diarrhea, and chronic use of zinc can lower copper levels in the body.

The three other groups of CAM therapies include life-style, biomechanical, and bioenergetic interventions. Life-style interventions include dietary modifications and exercise, which are increasingly becoming part of traditional medical management. Massage and craniosacral manipulation are examples of biomechanical interventions. Massage is an ancient healing technique, which many parents use informally when they burp their child or rub the child's back.

Massage techniques can contribute to relaxation and well-being. Acupuncture is a good example of a bioenergetic therapy. There is evidence to support its expanding use within conventional medicine, which is currently occurring. Other examples of bioenergetic therapies that are more controversial would include therapeutic touch and homeopathy. Table 6-4 lists CAM therapies commonly used in children with chronic illness and disability.

Parents of children with chronic disorders often find that CAM therapies give them a sense of hope, in contrast to traditional medicine. Parents of children with chronic conditions are frequently given conflicting information and recommendations related to traditional interventions. In the case of children with developmental disorders such as autism, chromosomal disorders, and ADHD, the treatments offered are most often educational and behavioral rather than medical. The need to be actively involved in their child's care and to have a feeling of control often leads parents to investigate CAM therapies. Some parents express the fear they may miss the opportunity to "cure" or help their child if they do not explore the options for therapies that are recommended on the Internet or by friends.

The primary care physician has an important role in working with families as they try to explore the ever-increasing array of CAM therapies that may be recommended for their child. It is in the best interest of the child that the parents and the physician have an open and honest relationship so that the parents will feel comfortable in telling the physician what therapies they are considering or already using. Information regarding CAM therapies should be discussed at the time the initial management plan is developed. If the physician is not involved, only the advocates of the therapy will provide information to the family, and this may be limited and biased. If the parents feel the health care professional is not supportive or will ridicule their use of these types of interventions, they may keep their use hidden, and this could result in harm to the child. This could be particularly true with the use of certain herbal remedies, which could interact negatively with the child's regular medications, or with the use of spinal manipulation in a child at risk for atlantoaxial instability. It is important for the health care professional to be educated regarding the various types of CAM therapies so that they can support their use and/or discuss realistic concerns regarding dangerous interventions and be able to identify "red flags" such as high cost or unsubstantiated claims of cure or of benefit for every child with the disorder.

TABLE 6-4

COMMON COMPLEMENTARY AND ALTERNATIVE THERAPIES USED IN CHILDREN WITH DISABILITY

Nutritional supplements
Hypoallergenic diets
Herbs
Facilitated communication
Auditory integration
Craniosacral manipulation
Music therapy
Massage/brushing
Melatonin
Sicca cell therapy
Intravenous immunoglobulin
Secretin
Patterning

Research in the field of alternative therapy is the key to future widespread acceptance and use of these interventions within conventional medicine. The US Congress created the National Center for Complementary and Alternative Medicine (NCCAM) in 1998. The mission of this program is to support research to determine the safety and efficacy of CAM therapies, provide information, and support training programs. The Complementary and Alternative Medicine Citation Index comprises over 180,000 bibliographic records describing much of the research in this area over the last 35 years. The Web site for NCAAM is http://nccam.nih.gov. The US Food and Drug Administration monitors adverse effects of conventional and nonconventional medical and food additive products (www.fda.gov/medwatch/).

References

Tracheostomy Care

Bahng SC, Van Hala S, Nelson VS, et al: Parental report of pediatric tracheostomy care. Arch Phys Med Rehabil 79:1367–1369, 1998

Ramsey AM, Grady EA: Long-term airway management for the ventilator-assisted child. In: Driver LE, Nelson VS, Warschausky SA, eds: The Ventilator-Assisted Child: A Practical Resource Guide. San Antonio, Communication Skill Builders, 1997

Ramsey AM, MacPherson C: Growing and Thriving with a Tracheostomy. Ann Arbor, University of Michigan Medical Center, 1994

Nutritional Care

Baer MT, Blyer EM, Cloud HH, McCammon SP: Providing early nutrition intervention services: preparation of dietitians, nutritionists, and other team members. Infants Young Children 3(4):56–66, 1991

Center on Hunger, Poverty and Nutrition Policy: The Link Between Nutrition and Cognitive Development in Children. Medford, MA, Tufts University School of Nutrition, 1994

Lucas B, Nardella M, Feucht S: Cost considerations: the benefits of nutrition services for a case series of children with special health care needs in Washington State. Developmental Issues 17(4):1–4, 1999

Position of The American Dietetic Association: Nutrition services for children with special health needs. J Am Diet Assoc 95:809–812, 1995

Enteral Feeding

Gibbons K, Cyr N, Christensen M, Helms R: Techniques for Pediatric Enteral and Parenteral Nutrition. Silver Spring, MD, ASEN, 1998:1–10

Krach LE, Kriel RL: Traumatic brain injury. In: Molnar GE, Alexander MA, eds: Pediatric Rehabilitation, 3rd ed. Philadelphia, Hanley & Belfus, 1999:254

Neurogenic Bladder

Bauer S: Neurogenic bladder dysfunction. Pediatr Clin North Am 34:1121–1124, 1987

Blaivas J, Chancellor M: Atlas of Urodynamics. New York, Williams & Wilkins, 1996

Churchill B, Gilmour R, Williot P: Urodynamics. Pediatr Clin North Am 34:1133–1157, 1987

Kaefer M, Pabby A, Kelly M, Darbey M, Bauer S: Improved bladder function after prophylactic treatment of the high-risk neurogenic bladder in newborns with myelomeningocele. J Urol 162:1068–1071, 1999

Wu I, Baskin L, Kogan B: Neurogenic bladder dysfunction due to myelomeningocele: neonatal versus childhood treatment. J Urol 175:2295–2297, 1997

Bowel Management

Cardenas DD, Mayo ME, King JC: Urinary tract and bowel management in the rehabilitation setting. In: Braddom RL, ed: Physical Medicine and Rehabilitation. Philadelphia, WB Saunders, 1996:569–579

Creasey G: Restoration of bladder, bowel and sexual function. Top Spinal Cord Injury Rehabil 5:21–32, 1999

Liptak GS, Reveli GM: Management of bowel dysfunction in children with spinal cord disease or injury by means of the enema continence catheter. J Pediatr 120:190–194, 1992

Spasticity

Armstrong RW, Steinbok P, Cochrane DD, Kube SD, Fife SE, Farrell K: Intrathecally administered baclofen for treatment of children with spasticity of cerebral origin. J Neurosurg 87:409–414, 1997

Glenn MB, Whyte J: The Practical Management of Spasticity in Children and Adults. Philadelphia, Lea & Febiger, 1990

Koman LA, Mooney JF 3rd, Smith BP: Neuromuscular blockade in the management of cerebral palsy. J Child Neurol 11(Suppl 1):S23–28, 1996

Nishida T, Thatcher SW, Marty GR: Selective posterior rhizotomy for children with cerebral palsy: a 7-year experience. Childs Nerv Syst 11:374–380, 1995

Parziale JR, Akelman E, Herz DA: Spasticity: pathophysiology and management. Orthopedics 16:801–811, 1993

Immunizations

American Academy of Pediatrics, Pickering LK, ed: 2000 Red Book: Report of the Committee on Infectious Diseases, 25th ed. Elk Grove Village, IL, American Academy of Pediatrics, 2000

Centers for Disease Control and Prevention: Control and prevention of meningococcal disease and control and prevention of serogroup C meningococcal disease: evaluation and management of suspected outbreaks: recommendations of the Advisory Committee on Immunization Practices (ACIP). MMWR 46(no. RR-5):1–21, 1997

Centers for Disease Control and Prevention: Measles, mumps, and rubella-vaccine use and strategies for elimination of measles, rubella, and congenital rubella syndrome and control of mumps: recommendations of the Advisory Committee on Immunization Practices (ACIP). MMWR 47(no. RR-8):1–57, 1998

Centers for Disease Control and Prevention: Prevention and control of influenza: recommendations of the Advisory Committee on Immunization Practices (ACIP). MMWR 48(no. RR-4):1–28, 1999

Centers for Disease Control and Prevention: Prevention and hepatitis A through active or passive immunization: recommendations of the Advisory Committee on Immunization Practices (ACIP). MMWR 45(no. RR-15):1–30, 1996

Centers for Disease Control and Prevention: Update: vaccine side effects, adverse reactions, contraindications, and precautions: recommendations of the Advisory Committee on Immunization Practices (ACIP). MMWR 45(no. RR-12):1–35, 1996

Dental Care

Children with Disabilities. New Brunswick, NJ, Johnson & Johnson Consumer Products, 1989

Grundy MC, Shaw L, Hamilton DV: An illustrated Guide to Dental Care for the Medically Compromised Patient. Aylesbury, England, Wolfe Publishing, 1993

National Oral Health Information Clearinghouse: http://www.aerie.com/nohicweb/special.html

Nowak AJ: Helping Persons with Disabilities Clean Their Teeth. Chicago, The National Easter Seal Society, 1977; rev 1985

Alternative and Complementary Therapy

Acupuncture. NIH Consensus Statement 15(5):1–34, 1997

Eisenberg DM, Kessler RC, Foster C, Norlock FE, Calkins DR, Delbanco TL: Unconventional medicine in the United States: prevalence, costs, and patterns of use. N Engl J Med 328:246–252, 1993

Kemper K: The Holistic Pediatrician. New York, Harper Collins, 1996:3–15

Nickel RE: Controversial therapies for young children with developmental disabilities. Infants Young Children 8(4):29–40, 1996

Spigelblatt L, Laine-Ammara G, Pless IB, Guyver A: The use of alternative medicine by children. Pediatrics 94:811–814, 1994

6.3   THERAPY SERVICES AND ANTICIPATORY GUIDANCE FOR THE CHILD WITH DISABILITY

6.3.1   Physical Therapy and Occupational Therapy

Lisa A. Kurtz

Because of their central role in coordinating care for children with disabilities, physicians need to clearly understand the roles and functions of other professional consultants, including physical and occupational therapists. Physical therapy (PT) addresses problems associated with neuromuscular dysfunction and gross motor delay as they influence the child's ability to be mobile within the environment. Occupational therapy (OT) addresses problems with neuromuscular dysfunction, sensory perception, psychosocial competence, and fine motor delay as they influence the child's ability to participate in self-care, play, and school activities, which are the primary *occupations* of childhood. Especially with younger children, play is the medium of choice for achieving therapeutic objectives. Many other interventions, including exercises, splinting or casting, use of adapted equipment, environmental modifications, and developmental intervention, are used to help children with disabilities achieve the highest possible level of functional independence. In practice, there is often considerable overlap in the methods and techniques used by the two disciplines, especially with very young children. Table 6-5 provides an overview of how physical and occupational therapists approach common rehabilitation objectives from different perspectives.

Children with a variety of chronic and disabling conditions may benefit from physical and/or occupational therapy. In general, children should be referred for physical therapy evaluation when there is a delay in gross motor development or concern about the child's quality of movement. Children should be referred for occupational therapy evaluation when there is reason to suspect impairment in the performance of age-appropriate daily tasks or routines, including self-care, play, social interaction, or in the execution of school-related activities that have a perceptual-motor component. Depending on state regulatory guidelines for practice and insurance requirements, written referral from a physician may be required before treatment may begin. Referral should include a complete diagnosis, information about relevant precautions (eg, allergies, weight-bearing status, exercise tolerance), and the reason for refer-

TABLE 6-5

COMPARISON OF OCCUPATIONAL (OT) AND PHYSICAL (PT) THERAPY

REHABILITATION GOAL	TYPICAL OT EMPHASIS	TYPICAL PT EMPHASIS
Maintain or increase strength and mobility	Upper body	Lower body
Teach functional skills for daily living	Dressing, eating, toileting, personal hygiene, household chores	Ambulation, transfers, other mobility demands
Promote developmental progression of skills	Fine motor, adaptive, personal-social domains	Gross motor domain
Promote environmental accessibility	1. Organizing work/play areas for efficiency 2. Modifying the environment to facilitate attention and information processing	1. Reducing architectural barriers for mobility (eg, ramps/lifts) 2. Providing adapted car seats or other devices for safe transportation
Provide assistive technology	Adapted toys, school materials, computers, self-care aids, environmental controls	Wheelchairs, ambulation aids, transfer equipment

SOURCE: *Batshaw ML, ed: Children with Disabilities, 4th ed, Baltimore: Paul H Brookes 1997:710.*

ral. In addition, copies of previous evaluations help the therapist avoid repeating unnecessary interviews pertaining to the child's medical background or developmental history.

Treatment approaches may include *exercises* that are routinely used to strengthen weak muscles, increase range of motion (ROM), improve endurance for activity, or promote cardiovascular fitness. Passive exercises and slow static stretching exercises are helpful in lengthening muscle-tendon units that have been shortened through disuse or spasticity. Active exercises, graded from movement in a gravity-eliminated plane to movement against strong resistance, are used for strengthening. Exercise is often embedded within play to ensure the child's cooperation. For example, squeezing and molding clay of gradually increasing density encourages the child to strengthen the finger flexors.

Therapeutic positioning and handling is used to attempt to control abnormal tone and patterns of movement. This approach is used extensively with children with cerebral palsy or other neurologic impairment and is often referred to as *neurodevelopmental therapy*. Individualized handling techniques are selected according to the child's specific problems with muscle tone and motor control as well as his or her cognitive abilities and motivation to engage in tasks. Parents and other relevant caregivers are taught to incorporate these handling procedures into the child's daily routine so that he or she has frequent opportunities for sensorimotor experiences that more closely approximate those of a typically developing child. This approach also incorporates the use of positioning equipment, such as adapted chairs, sidelyers, or prone standing boards. These may be used to support improved skeletal alignment, to compensate for abnormal postures, to promote the proximal stability needed for controlled upper extremity movements, or to prepare the child for more independent mobility.

Physical and occupational therapists also may recommend and/or fabricate a variety of *orthotic devices* (see Sec. 6.3.4) and assistive technology (see Sec. 6.3.3) for children. For rehabilitation efforts to be effective, they must become integrated into the child's typical daily routine, involving much practice and repetition. For this reason, *parent education* is an integral part of therapy. Because parental involvement with therapy programs offered in school settings is variable, it is sometimes advisable to provide supplemental therapy for purposes of parent education.

6.3.2 Speech Pathology for the Child with Disability

Ann W. Kummer

Communication is a fundamental human skill that has a direct effect on the way that an individual is able to learn and function in society. In fact, verbal and written communication is essential for social interactions and many activities of daily living. Children with developmental delay or other disabling conditions often have difficulty with receptive and/or expressive communication skills for a variety of reasons.

Speech-language pathologists are professionals who are educated in the study of human communication, including normal development and communication disorders. Speech-language pathologists are also trained to recognize neurologic and upper aerodigestive disorders that affect speech and swallowing. Therefore, children with suspected communication disorders or difficulty with feeding or swallowing can benefit from the services provided by a speech-language pathologist.

By evaluating the speech, language, cognitive-communication, and swallowing skills of children with disabilities, the speech-language pathologist can determine specific deficits, the severity of the disorder (often based on age level norms), and possible etiologic and contributing factors. This information forms the basis of a treatment plan for the child. The recommendations may include formal therapy or parent training and consultation with periodic rechecks.

Therapeutic intervention usually involves a variety of strategies that consider not only the child's specific deficits but also the child's strengths and abilities. Depending on the type of disorder, therapy may include exercises to improve oral-motor skills, exercises to develop appropriate articulation placement, or activities to develop functional language skills. Some children lack the basic prerequisites for verbal communication for a variety of causes (ie, tracheostomy, significant hearing loss, neuromuscular disorder, etc.). For those children, augmentative or alternative communication systems are developed (see Sec. 6.3.3). Regardless of the type of therapy, parent involvement is a key component of the treatment process. Therefore, parents are encouraged to observe the therapy sessions whenever possible and are given instructions for working with the child at home.

Physicians should refer patients to a speech-language pathologist whenever there is a suspicion of a communication or feeding/swallowing disorder. See Table 6-6 for some referral guidelines. Children are appropriate for referral as early as the first few months of life if they exhibit feeding problems or do not begin to coo and babble appropriately. In addition, "high-risk" infants, such as those

TABLE 6-6

INDICATIONS FOR REFERRAL FOR SPEECH PATHOLOGY SERVICES

Articulation
- The infant is very quiet and doesn't coo by 4 or 5 months of age
- The child doesn't babble using consonant sounds (particularly b, m, d, and n) by 8 or 9 months of age
- The child uses mostly vowel sounds and gestures for communication after 18 months
- The speech is usually unintelligible at the age of 3
- The child frequently omits consonants in words at the age of 3
- The speech is difficult to understand at the age of 4
- At the age of 6, the child is still unable to produce many sounds
- The child is omitting, substituting, or distorting any sounds after the age of 7
- The child is embarrassed or disturbed by his or her speech at any age

Language
- The child shows poor attention to the speech of others
- The child has difficulty understanding the speech of others or following directions
- The child's vocabulary is limited, or the child often uses inappropriate words
- The child uses short, "telegraphic" phrases and sentences
- Sentence construction is often faulty

Voice
- The voice is hoarse, harsh, breathy, or of poor quality
- The voice is always too loud or too soft
- The pitch is inappropriate for the child's age or sex
- Pitch breaks occur frequently
- The voice is hyponasal or hypernasal

Fluency
- The parents have expressed a concern about stuttering
- The child has an abnormal number of repetitions, hesitations, prolongations, blocks, or disruptions in the natural flow of speech
- The child exhibits tension during speech
- The child avoids speaking situations because of a fear of stuttering
- The child considers him- or herself to be a stutterer

Feeding or swallowing
- The child doesn't suck normally
- The child has difficulty sucking or drinking from a cup
- The child has difficulty taking foods from a spoon or has difficulty chewing foods
- The child avoids certain types of foods or certain food textures
- The child gags, chokes, or coughs with feeding

with a traumatic birth history or hearing loss, are appropriate for referral so that the infant's development can be monitored and the parents can be counseled regarding methods of stimulation. It is important to note that early intervention is critical for the best long-term prognosis. Intervention is best started during the preschool years because this is the time when the brain is particularly receptive to speech and language learning. Early intervention is also important because habit strength becomes a factor as the child gets older. Finally, early intervention can help to avoid the social, emotional, and learning problems that can result from the inability to communicate adequately.

6.3.3 Assistive Technology

Jill Jump, Margaret Bouwkamp, and Claire Morress

Assistive technology enables children with disabilities to become more active participants in the world around them. The assistive technology devices available are as diverse as the needs and characteristics of the children who use them (Table 6-7). Children with a variety of acquired, congenital, or developmental disabilities may benefit from assistive technology.

The *Technology-Related Assistance for Individuals with Disabilities Act of 1988* (Tech Act) defines assistive technology devices as "any item, piece of equipment, or product system . . . that is used to increase, maintain, or improve functional capabilities of children with disabilities" [20 USC Chapter 33, Section 1401 (25)]. Assistive technology devices improve a child's ability to play, learn, compete, and interact with peers, family, and friends. This legislation mandates and provides a model for assistive technology services as any service that directly assists a child with a disability in the selection, acquisition, or use of an assistive technology (AT) device [20 USC Chapter 33, Section 1401 (26)], so that services covered by this law include evaluation; acquisition; customizing, adapting, and repairing devices; coordinating and using other therapies, interventions, or services with AT devices; and training or technical assistance for the child, family, professionals, employers, and others. Assistive technology is not only a desirable addition to instruction and the learning process, it is now mandated by federal law to be incorporated into educational programs for children with disabilities, when appropriate. The need for AT should be an integral part of a comprehensive assessment for students with disabilities in all areas related to their disabilities, as appropriate for each student, and must be considered by the Individual Educational Plan (IEP) team.

It is important to understand that not all technologies are appropriate for all children. Each child has his or her own unique set of strengths, weaknesses, interests, and experiences. The purpose of an assessment is to determine which AT, if any, is appropriate to assist an individual child in achieving a specific goal (such as mobility, communication). A feature match approach should be used that considers the device characteristics and the individual child's abilities, functional limitations, specific objectives, and preferences. The equipment recommended should conform to ergonomic design principles, ie, maximize function, comfort, and safety and minimize injury to the user. Multiple strategies should be considered, including low-tech and high-tech solutions. Device trials are an essential part of the assessment process. Trials can reduce costly mistakes and abandonment of technology. Funding of assistive technology has historically been a barrier to acquiring systems. Despite recent legislation and funding mandates, access to equipment is not always readily achieved. Key elements in obtaining funding include extensive knowledge of funding sources and appropriate documentation for justification.

Early identification of technical support and personnel to provide services in each of the child's daily environments is important. Thorough training of the child, family, and all support people in the setup, maintenance, use, and programming of the device is vital for successful outcomes. The child will often require additional therapeutic support such as occupational, physical, and speech ther-

TABLE 6-7

EXAMPLES OF ASSISTIVE TECHNOLOGY DEVICES

AREA OF ASSISTIVE TECHNOLOGY	DEFINITION	EXAMPLES OF EQUIPMENT	
		LOW TECH	HIGH TECH
Aids of daily living	Adapted or modified tools, objects, and utensils for performing self-care activities	Reachers, adapted feeding utensils, bath seats	Electric feeder, page turner, switch toys
Augmentative/alternative communication	Devices or systems designed to support, enhance, or augment the communication of individuals who are not independent communicators	Manual picture boards, eye-gaze letter boards	Electronic voice-output communication devices, voice amplifiers, electrolarynx
Auditory aids	Amplification devices to provide increased clarity and volume or visual feedback to individuals with hearing loss	Visual alerts, amplified phones	Hearing aids, FM listening system, TTY
Visual aids	Devices or tools to provide access to visual materials through alternative means, including magnification, hearing, or touch	Large-print books, magnifying glass, cane	TV projected magnifiers (CCTV), talking organizers, screen readers, Braille keyboards
Computer utilization	Devices that replace the traditional keyboard and mouse to provide text entry and cursor control or software that compensates for impaired physical or cognitive abilities	Keyguards, enlarged key labels, ergonomic wrist pad	Alternative keyboards, voice recognition software, head pointing, switch scanning, touch screens
Seating and positioning	Adapted positioning components, devices, or seating systems that enable an individual with impaired posture, equilibrium, or muscle function to assume appropriate positions or postures	Prone and supine standers, floor sitters, prone wedges	Wheelchair seating systems
Wheelchairs and mobility	Devices that assist or replace ambulation	Walkers, gait trainers, adapted tricycles, wheeled standers	Power wheelchairs, ultralight and sport wheelchairs
Prosthetics and orthotics	A device that is added to part of an individual's body to support, position, immobilize, restore function, assist weak muscles, modify tone, or substitute for the loss of a body part	Splints, braces, mobile arm support	Myoelectric hand
Environmental control and access	A system or single device that allows access or control of the environment and/or objects in the environment	Universal design door handles, ramps	Computer controlled house, remote appliance control

TTY = teletypewriter; CCTV = closed-circuit television.

apies in an outpatient setting for specific skill development and to increase independent use of the device. Typical skills that require intervention include communication, literacy and spelling, and mobility concepts and motor skills for physical access of the device. Ongoing follow-up and evaluation should be provided to ensure that the technology is upgraded as necessary and that the child's needs continue to be met as indicated by developmental and physical changes.

Specific developmental issues that can be addressed with assistive technology include play, mobility, communication, and learning. Children learn about their world through independent manipulation of real objects during play. Children who are unable to participate in play can experience deficits in language, cognitive, and social skills. If a child is unable to select and interact with toys on his or her own, her or she may assume the role of a passive observer to the play of siblings and peers. Assistive technology can provide a means for children with disabilities to engage in vigorous interactive play. A battery toy adapted with a large button switch can help develop the concept of cause and effect. A child using a communication device can role-play with peers during pretend play. Familiar turn-taking games, such as Checkers and Connect Four, become accessible to all children when played on a computer.

Independent mobility is usually acquired in the first 2 years of life. Restricted mobility in early childhood has long-lasting adverse developmental effects that include decreased curiosity and decreased self-initiated behaviors. Independent mobility enables a child to engage in self-initiated, self-directed exploration, resulting in control of and interaction with the environment. Assistive devices that offer functional, effective, and self-directed mobility should be considered for children with a disability after the age of 1 year. This includes consideration of ambulation aids, wheeled devices, and powered devices. Mobility should not require so much time and effort that it restricts the child's natural ability to explore and interact with the environment. Propulsion speed, effort, and physical endurance should be among the factors considered in recommending manual or power mobility.

Powered mobility devices for young children have often been considered a "last-resort" intervention. Professionals are often reluctant to prescribe power mobility because of concerns about the effect on motivation for further development of independent physical/ambulation skills and fears that the child will injure him- or herself or peers. However, it is now evident that power mobility has a positive effect on skill development, including head and postural control, self-initiated exploration, social interaction, and communication. The early prescription and provision of mobility devices can be instrumental in enhancing the cognitive, emotional, and social development of young children with disabilities.

Children learn to control their world through communication. Children with disabilities should be afforded the same early communication opportunities as their peers. An augmentative or alternative communication (AAC) system should combine all of the modalities available to the child, including vocalizations, word approximations, gestures, signs, eye gaze, manual communication boards, and voice-output communication devices. The use of a voice-output communication device does not discourage the development of oral language. On the contrary, an increase in vocalization and word approximations may occur after the use of a voice-output device. Voice-output devices can range from a single switch with a recorded phrase to a computer system with complicated vocabulary/language systems and a range of access methods. A number of key factors should be considered in selecting a communication system for a child. These include the vocabulary and language abilities of the device and child, physical abilities and access, cognitive abilities, literacy skills, communication environments and partners, the individual child's preferences, and future potential for expansion. Successful use of a communication system requires a team approach during all phases of assessment and intervention.

6.3.4   Orthoses

Teresa L. Massagli

Orthoses (also called braces or splints) are external devices applied to the body that may be used to restrict motion, enhance function, or provide support. They can be used to immobilize painful joints, correct or prevent contractures, aid or substitute for weak muscles, and stabilize joints for weight bearing.

SPINAL ORTHOSES

Cervical orthoses are used with stretching and strengthening exercises in infants with congenital muscular torticollis. A foam collar can be modified to obstruct the head tilt but trimmed on the other side to permit movement in other directions. A plastic tubular orthosis can also be adapted for the infant. A loop of plastic tubing is flattened into an oval, placed behind the neck, and held together in front with a clip. On the side of the head tilt, two plastic struts are inserted to block tilting. The struts can be lengthened as the range of motion improves. With either the foam or the tubular orthosis, the neck is not immobilized. The infant is able to move actively in other directions away from the head tilt, thereby maintaining strength.

The *Milwaukee brace* is used in idiopathic scoliosis if sensation and the ability to make corrective movements away from the support pads are intact. The *thoracolumbosacral orthosis* (TLSO) is used more commonly for the conservative treatment of neuromuscular scoliosis. There are many styles, including back-opening, front-opening, or bivalved TLSOs. The anterior portion should extend from just below the clavicles to the anterior superior iliac spine without pinching the thighs when the child is seated on a firm surface. There should be no pressure in the axillae. Posteriorly, the TLSO should extend from at least the spine of the scapula to about 2 cm above the table surface. In some neuromuscular disorders, although bracing rarely prevents surgery, it may delay it until the child has achieved sufficient growth to undergo spine fusion. In Duchenne muscular dystrophy, bracing to slow the progression of scoliosis is not indicated, as declining pulmonary function over the period of the delay may increase surgical complications.

UPPER EXTREMITY ORTHOSES

Upper extremity orthoses may be used to treat or prevent contractures caused by weakness, spasticity, arthritis, arthrogryposis, or burns. Loss of range of motion (ROM) at the shoulder as a result of burns is often managed with an airplane splint. This orthosis is fabricated to hold the arm in abduction and flexion and can be worn during the day and/or at night. In upper motor neuron disorders such as cerebral palsy and stroke, shoulder ROM is usually well maintained using manual stretching alone. In the first few weeks after a stroke, the shoulder may be at risk for subluxation. The arm can be supported with a sling during ambulation and with an arm rest or tray while seated.

Elbow, wrist, and finger flexion contractures that develop over weeks to months (eg, after traumatic brain injury or stroke) are often best initially treated by serial application of casts to stretch the muscles. Serial casting can be combined with botulinum toxin injections or phenol motor point blocks to hasten correction. It can be followed with orthosis provision to maintain the gain in ROM. The most common contractures with chronic upper extremity spasticity are of the fingers and wrists. Orthoses worn during the day or night can help prevent loss of ROM and may allow some relaxation of spastic muscles to permit voluntary movement. Wrist orthoses can be applied to either the dorsal or volar surface. A resting splint for the spastic hand should place the wrist in about 30° of extension, the metacarpophalangeal joints in about 45° of flexion, the fingers in extension, and the thumb in abduction and extension. A neoprene hand splint may be used to hold the thumb in abduction and opposition when the child has spasticity of the thumb adductors.

In the most common form of arthrogryposis, amyoplasia, the child has extension contractures of the elbow, flexion contractures at the wrist, and reduced movement at the interphalangeal joints. Serial splinting and manual stretching can be very effective in the first few years of life in increasing passive range of motion in elbow flexion, wrist extension, and finger flexion. Hand splints may need to be adjusted every few weeks.

Children with tetraplegia from spinal cord injury may use orthoses to enhance function. Mobile arm supports can be mounted on a wheelchair. The forearm is supported with a trough. With a minimum amount of shoulder and elbow flexion strength, the child can bring the hand to his or her mouth. If the child has elbow flexion but no wrist or hand movement, a ratchet splint can be applied to the wrist, with the thumb supported in a position of opposition to the index and middle fingers. When the wrist is ratcheted into extension, the fingertips will oppose due to tenodesis of the finger flexors. If the child has active wrist extension, the same concept is used without the ratchet. A universal cuff around the hand can be fit with utensils to allow self-feeding and with a range of other adaptive aids to assist with other age-appropriate activities of daily living and writing.

LOWER EXTREMITY ORTHOSES

The *supramalleolar orthosis* is a plastic orthosis that encompasses the malleoli and extends around the foot. It can control hindfoot varus/valgus instability and forefoot abduction or adduction. It does not control dynamic equinus. The child must be able to clear the toes in swing. It is often used in children with sacral myelomeningocele. *Ankle-foot orthoses* (AFOs) extend from below the fibular head to the sole of the foot. In nonambulatory children AFOs can be used to prevent contractures. During the gait cycle, an AFO can provide medial-lateral stability to the ankle in stance, toe pick-up in swing, and aid in pushoff. If the child does not have active dorsiflexion or plantarflexion, a solid ankle with no movement is used. The AFO can be made with a hinged ankle or constructed with thinner plastic to allow bending into dorsiflexion (dynamic AFO: DAFO). The sole of the AFO should extend to the metatarsal heads, allowing a toe break during pushoff. If control of the toes is needed, the end of the sole plate should be of thinner plastic to allow the toe break. Without a toe break, knee hyperextension can occur. DAFOs can be fabricated with "tone-reducing"

foot plates. These are custom contoured and built up under the toes, the lateral and medial arches, and the transverse metatarsal arch. They are recessed under the metatarsal and calcaneal pad areas. They are believed to decrease spasticity by stretch of the triceps surae and toe flexors and to protect the foot from tactile-induced reflexes. In a comparative study, both the solid AFO and DAFO improved stride length in children with cerebral palsy and reduced plantar flexion at foot contact and in midstance, but there were no advantages of one over the other except that DAFOs are lighter in weight and may be more cosmetically attractive.

Knee-ankle-foot orthoses (KAFOs) can provide all the functions at the ankle of an AFO and also compensate for an unstable knee. Children with neuromuscular disease, paraplegia, myelomeningocele, or polio who lack antigravity strength in the knee extensors use them. At higher levels of paralysis, the *reciprocating gait orthosis* (RGO) can be used. The RGO couples hip flexion with reciprocal extension of the contralateral hip. The RGO is most effective if the child has some active hip flexion; otherwise, it requires the child to initiate gait by extending the trunk over the weight-bearing leg to initiate a step with the other foot. Crutches or a walker must be used. Although the RGO is designed to produce an alternating gait pattern, most children ambulate more quickly using a swing-through pattern.

Community ambulation is most likely for the child who requires no more than one KAFO to walk; at a minimum, one leg has at least antigravity strength in hip flexion and knee extension, and no significant contracture or uncontrolled spasticity is present. Ambulation with bilateral KAFOs or RGOs requires 5 to 10 times the energy of normal ambulation. To avoid anaerobic metabolism, the child must walk more slowly. In contrast, wheelchair mobility approximates the energy expenditure of ambulation and may provide the child with greater mobility, especially outside of the home for community distances.

6.3.5   Prostheses

Linda J. Michaud

Prostheses are devices that substitute for absent body parts. Upper or lower extremity prostheses may be indicated for children with congenital limb deficiencies or acquired amputations. Normal developmental milestones guide prescription of a prosthetic device and its components.

UPPER EXTREMITY PROSTHESES

The initial prosthesis for the child with an upper extremity deficiency is provided at about 6 months of age, when he or she is able to sit and is making attempts at lateral propping. Some clinicians favor earlier fitting, at about 3 to 4 months of age, as the infant is bringing hands to mouth and before development of two-handed activities, for incorporation into body image. Late initial fit, especially after 2 years of age, is associated with a high rate of prosthetic rejection, related to lack of incorporation of the prosthesis into the body image and development of compensatory techniques. The initial upper extremity prosthesis for an infant is a passive device that allows holding large objects and weight bearing and also provides sensory feedback. Cable activation of a prehensile terminal device is not done until 18 to 24 months of age, when the child is able to learn to operate the device. If the level of deficiency is above the elbow, the elbow joint is activated at about 3 years of age. Early fitting with myoelectric systems is controversial. Until there is development of lighter, smaller components and systems, there is unlikely to be consensus that these systems are appropriate for children younger than 2 years of age. Hybrid systems consist of combinations of electric and body-powered control and are options for older children, especially if they have bilateral or proximal deficiencies.

LOWER EXTREMITY PROSTHESES

The initial prosthesis for the child with a lower limb deficiency is provided at about 9 months of age, when the child starts to pull to stand. Fitting earlier may interfere with development of earlier gross motor skills, such as crawling. If the level of deficiency is above the knee, a knee joint is either not provided or is locked and not activated until about 3 years of age, when the child is developmentally able to reciprocally climb stairs.

Growth raises challenges in pediatric prosthetic management. Replacement for growth is typically required annually until 5 years of age, every 2 years between ages 5 and 12 years of age, and then every 3 to 4 years until adulthood. Prosthetic adjustments may be required three or four times per year. Many strategies have been developed to accomodate growth. These include substituting thinner for thicker socks, starting with five plies at initial fitting and gradually reducing to a single ply; using double or triple wall sockets, and peeling out the inner layers; using flexible thermoplastic inner sockets that can be heated and stretched or replaced; and using components that can be lengthened or switched easily, such as to a larger foot. Materials appropriate for use in children's prostheses should be durable, comfortable, cosmetic, and age-appropriately simple in construction and requirements for operation. Weight should approximate that of the replaced limb.

Not all children with congenital limb deficiencies or amputations will benefit from the provision of a prosthesis. There are high rates of rejection of prostheses at the extremes of residual limb length. Children with very distal amputations are usually more functional using the residual hand or foot than a prosthesis. The use of prostheses for proximal lower extremity amputations may result in excessively high energy requirements. Prostheses for some proximal upper extremity deficiencies may be cumbersome and offer only minimal functional advantage. Children born with one intact upper extremity generally become completely independent in activities of daily living without a prosthesis. Children born with absence of both upper extremities can be expected to be independent in most activities of daily living using their feet. Parental acceptance is a major factor in long-term prosthetic acceptance by the child. Education should be provided for the family regarding application, removal, and care for the prosthesis and also for recognition of signs of growth that require prosthetic modification.

The child amputee generally can and should be as active as his or her able-bodied peers. Specialized components for both upper and lower limb prostheses can be used to enhance the child's participation in a variety of sports and recreational activities, such as interchangeable sports-specific terminal devices for holding rackets, ski poles, or baseball gloves, and lower limbs designed exclusively for swimming. Children with limb deficiencies and amputations typically require little formal therapy for training in use of prosthetic devices, especially for the lower extremity. If a prosthesis fits well and improves the child's function, it will usually be accepted.

6.3.6   Recreational Therapy

Lisa Jo Hicks

Play is a vital component of the life of a child and adolescent. When a child or adolescent experiences a traumatic injury or disability, the child's activities of daily living and ability to play are affected, which may have an impact on subsequent normal development. Treatment and medical procedures may cause significant anxiety that delay recovery or adjustment. An allied health discipline that assists children who have experienced a traumatic injury or disability is recreational therapy or therapeutic recreation.

The role of recreational therapy in a pediatric setting is to provide functional activities to achieve treatment goals identified through an individual assessment and to provide opportunities for normal development through play. Recreational therapists use various interventions as a form of active treatment to improve the cognitive, emotional, physical, and social functioning of individuals who are impaired or disabled as a result of trauma or disease. Qualified and competent professionals use the following four-step process to deliver recreational therapy services: (1) complete an assessment based on specific information obtained from an interview, observation, and/or evaluation tool(s), (2) formulate a plan to identify specific therapeutic goals, objectives, and interventions that will address specific needs of the individual being served, (3) implement the plan developed, and (4) evaluate the progress an individual makes toward meeting the therapeutic goals. Recreational therapy is not always about playing, nor is playing always therapeutic. Children may play for the simple outcome of fun. Recreational therapists may use play to facilitate certain outcomes. All interventions are designed to maximize independent skills and improve opportunities for a productive and meaningful life style.

An important factor in development or recovery is for the individual child or adolescent to take some control over his or her own environment. Recreational therapists are creative professionals who focus on assisting individuals to make choices and exercise some control. When a child becomes disabled, treatment modalities may include the following: sensory stimulation, animal-facilitated therapy, horticulture therapy, developmental play skills, social interaction skills, adaptive play skills, cognitive retraining, reality orientation, behavior management, expressive therapy, coping skills, aquatic therapy, self-esteem exercises, leisure education, sibling intervention, family training, community resources, and community reintegration. A Certified Therapeutic Recreation Specialist (CTRS) provides interventions in individual or group therapy sessions. Some recreational therapists cotreat with other interdisciplinary team members such as physical, occupational, or speech therapists and psychologists.

6.3.7   Education and Employment of Youth with Disabilities

J. Erin Riehle and Susan Rutkowski

Making a successful entry into the adult community and work life is particularly challenging for a child with a disability. The pediatrician can play a pivotal role in increasing the likelihood of a successful school-to-work transition by imparting knowledge regarding the development of a work personality, transition to work, vocational rehabilitation services, and available community resources.

DEVELOPMENT OF A WORK PERSONALITY

There are numerous theories about how a person develops a work personality. Despite the diversity of opinions, there is general agreement that for people with disabilities the process needs to begin at diagnosis and should mirror developmental milestones for typical peers. Development of a successful work personality can be fostered through simple discussion and modeling of events that are common for most youth.

Children with disabilities need to perceive themselves as valuable, contributing members of their families and society. They need to have a meaningful role in the family and the same expectations as their siblings. Even though it may be more difficult for children with disabilities to perform chores, they need to be held responsible for increasingly more difficult tasks. The performance of these chores has been found to be one of the most critical determinants of future successful employment. The physician can guide the development of high expectations for success by encouraging the individual to explore, take risks, understand failure, and develop a sense of accomplishment. By setting the expectation that the child with a disability can be a productive member of society, the pediatrician guides the family in the establishment of a vision that sees employment and productivity as a realistic outcome.

The physician should expect that the individual with a disability *will* work. Like any other child, children with disabilities need to be asked at an early age about future career plans. Questions should continue to focus on more complex job issues such as work environment, areas of interest, work strengths and weaknesses, and training and education opportunities. The disability should not drive the career decision; rather, the career decision should be based on interest, skills, and ability and accomplished through training, adaptations, and accomodations.

The development of social competencies and work habits is critical to the child's successful entry to the world of work. Physician and family expectations, appropriate educational goals, and meaningful community activities all contribute to this important skill acquisition. Most people lose jobs because of behavior rather than lack of skills or knowledge. For all individuals, including those with disabilities, there are certain work prerequisites that must be nurtured and developed. These include:

- Appropriate social skills
- Ability to work with others
- Attendance and punctuality
- Proper grooming and hygiene
- Basic activities of daily living
- Ability to take direction
- Basic communication skills

Adolescents can gain appropriate social and work skills in two major ways: work experiences and participation in school and community activities. Both promote the development of social competencies and work habits and assist with carrying out the long-term vision of successful employment.

TRANSITION TO WORK

The IDEA (Individuals with Disabilities Education Act) Reauthorization Act of 1997 (formerly Public Law 94-142) provides a comprehensive plan (Individualized Educational Plan: IEP) of services to be "wrapped around" each child. Children can be served under

this law until they are 22 years old if they have a disability in any of the following 13 categories:

- Multihandicaps (MH)
- Hearing impaired (HI)
- Speech handicaps (SH)
- Severe behavior handicaps (SBH)
- Severe learning disabilities (SLD)
- Deaf blind (DB)
- Visually impaired (VI)
- Orthopedic handicaps (OH)
- Developmental handicaps (DH)
- Pervasive developmental disabilities (PDD)
- Autism
- Traumatic brain injury (TBI)
- Other health impairments (OHI)

Many children with significant health impairments who do not fit into the above categories may qualify for services under the Other Health Impairment label. If a condition such as cystic fibrosis or sickle cell disease significantly interferes with the learning process, the child can qualify for special education services under this label. Because of chronic medical conditions, many youth are at risk and would be better served by having their educational and vocational services coordinated under a comprehensive plan, but the stigmatization that may result from being identified as having a disability causes many families to reject services. The physician can assist the family in discussing the pros and cons of sacrificing labels for services.

The IEP includes many other areas, such as behavior, assessment, and transition. The law mandates the development of transition goals by age 14, but these activities can and should start much younger. Children who have other disabling conditions but don't fit into the 13 categories of IDEA may qualify for educational adaptations under section 504 of the Rehabilitation Act. A "504 plan" may not be as comprehensive as an IEP but often makes it possible for a student to be successful in the school environment. To qualify, a student must have a disability that significantly interferes with his or her ability to learn. The 504 plan is designed to make accommodations and adaptations to the educational environment, whereas the IEP is a special education "service plan."

In both cases, a team of people designs the plan with representation from families, schools, vocational rehabilitation, and service agencies. This plan lays the cornerstones for vocational training and employment. Traditionally, health care professionals have not been a part of the team. Physician participation in the development of these plans can greatly influence the outcome.

The length of formal education has been shown to be a greater predictor of successful work outcome than IQ. For this reason, it is important that families and schools take advantage of all the educational and vocational opportunities available. "Deferred graduation" is one method that encourages students with disabilities to participate in high school graduation ceremonies with their peers, receive a blank diploma, and continue in the educational process in additional high school training programs or vocational school. Students with disabilities who participate in a vocational training program are nine times more likely to become employed than those who graduate from a special education program. It is also known that students who participate in vocational education programs at an older age (20–22 vs 17–18) and who receive transition services have better vocational outcomes.

Most states have a continuum of vocational education options designed to meet the needs of students with a variety of cognitive and physical challenges. "Hands-on" learning and integrated academics, the cornerstones of vocational education, are successful elements for youth with disabilities. Vocational education programs include all types of students, with and without disabilities.

Work experiences and other career development activities need to be an integral part of any school program, especially vocational education. Physicians should encourage youth to work as early as possible. Students may have several jobs before they finish high school; most typical teenagers do! It is one of the most meaningful ways for them to practice appropriate employability and social skills in a real work environment.

Every state has a vocational rehabilitation agency. The mission of this agency is to work with people who have disabilities to reach their vocational goals. Vocational rehabilitation counselors can begin working with students in their last several years of high school. They provide valuable input and resources toward fulfilling the child's vocational vision. These agencies offer services such as vocational assessment, job coaching, and work-related adaptations and accommodations.

The Ticket to Work and Work Incentives Improvement Act of 1999 afford individuals with disabilities increased opportunities to obtain the services and supports needed to secure and maintain meaningful employment. Implementation may be expected to greatly reduce restrictions to participation in the workplace in the future for youth with disabilities.

6.3.8   Psychosocial Adjustment to Disability

Juliet M. Coscia and Shari L. Wade

A child's psychosocial adjustment to chronic disability is a matter of concern to parents, pediatricians, mental health professionals, and teachers. The majority of children are resilient in the face of chronic physical and cognitive disabilities, but a proportion of these children are at increased risk for overall maladjustment, internalizing (eg, anxiety) and externalizing (eg, oppositional) symptoms and problems with self-esteem, as compared to their healthy peers.

The risk of psychosocial dysfunction may vary across impairment groups. Whether the condition is congenital or acquired may differentially impact a child's self-concept. For example, the child with a traumatic brain injury often must adapt to significant changes in his or her thinking and learning skills and other functional limitations, typically after a period of normal functioning in these areas. In contrast, a child with a disability that is present from birth does not face acute loss and significant changes in functioning. Children with chronic neurologic conditions (eg, cerebral palsy, spina bifida, traumatic brain injury) are at increased risk for emotional and behavioral problems in comparison to physically healthy peers and to children with nonneurologic chronic conditions. Included in this group at risk for psychosocial maladjustment are children with sensory disabilities. One factor hypothesized to account for the increased risk in children with neurologic, including sensory, impairments is difficulty developing age-appropriate social competence and peer relations. Finally, children with visible physical impairments (ie, burns, physical deformities) are potentially more vulnerable to social difficulties and low self-esteem related to social rejection and avoidance by peers.

Potential protective factors that are associated with adjustment in children with disabilities include cognitive appraisal of stress, social support, and physical appearance. Positive psychosocial adaptation among children with limb deficiencies appears to be related to having an intact social support network and fewer concerns about physical appearance. Other potential protective factors relate to the family. Children with disabilities have more favorable psychosocial outcomes when they are in more cohesive, supportive families that are low in conflict. Lower levels of maternal distress are also related to better child adjustment. Socioeconomic status, sex, and age of the child are not reliably related to psychological adjustment.

Psychosocial interventions typically utilize education, cognitive-behavioral approaches (eg, relaxation and social skills training) and biofeedback procedures to reduce the stress associated with chronic disabilities. Interventions that target the family as well have the potential to yield better outcomes, given the critical role of family in the adjustment of the child. Although most children adapt successfully, adjustment changes may occur over time in conjunction with critical events (eg, diagnosis), changes in the course of illness (eg, exacerbations or lapses in symptoms), developmental changes (eg, emerging autonomy in adolescence), and changing family structure and dynamics (eg, divorce, death, birth of a sibling).

6.3.9   Transition to Adulthood

Kevin P. Murphy

Life expectancy of adults in the United States is increasing with time, including that for individuals with chronic illness and disability. More than 90% of children with chronic illness and/or disability now survive into adulthood. Growing older with a chronic condition of childhood onset is associated with unique challenges. A teenager or young adult with cerebral palsy or other congenital or acquired condition associated with childhood disability often finds that adult health-care providers know little about their condition or the secondary conditions that may occur with increased frequency with aging. The pediatric provider knows little about secondary and acquired conditions associated with aging and is not trained or experienced with differential diagnoses and treatment plans for this population of adults. The result is often that neither adult nor pediatric health-care providers feel comfortable in providing holistic care for the adult with a chronic condition of childhood onset. Thus, the young adult with childhood-onset disability is challenged in finding health-care provision during adulthood.

In the 1980s, Bax and colleagues reviewed the health needs of 104 young adults with physical disabilities living in the United Kingdom. On the basis of a medical examination and personal interview, the state of health of all subjects was judged to be poor. In the group of individuals with cerebral palsy, 60% were poorly nourished, 71% had lower extremity contractures, and bowel and bladder problems were found in 56% and 53%, respectively. A total of 60% had speech and other communication difficulties. Murphy and colleagues studied 101 adults with cerebral palsy between the ages of 19 and 74 years. A total of 76% had multiple musculoskeletal problems, including 63% under the age of 50 years. These authors suggested that abnormal biomechanical forces and immobility had led to excessive physical stress and strain, overuse syndromes, and possibly early joint degeneration. A number of patients had urinary complaints because of difficulties with toilet accessibility and neurologic involvement of the bladder. General health-care seemed satisfactory for acute illnesses, but there was lack of preventive health-care. Treatment for the musculoskeletal problems and access to technology, seating systems, and adaptive devices had not generally been provided. Formal transition clinic teams have been widely recommended for young adults with chronic conditions, including by the American Academy of Pediatrics.

Transition from a pediatric to adult health-care delivery system requires a change in paradigm. Pediatric health-care is typically child and family centered. Adult health-care models are focused on mature patients who are often self-reliant, assertive, and well-informed decision makers, with family members assuming more of a peripheral role. Interdisciplinary team health-care is generally more available in pediatrics but is not the rule in adult health-care. All of these differences create a challenging transitional process for the young adult and family working to facilitate autonomy, independence, and community living.

Providers of transition services must recognize that transition is a process and not an event. The transition process should begin at the day of diagnosis and continue into young adulthood. The adolescent and family should both be involved in the decision process, preparing to renegotiate their roles as they enter the adult health-care model. Coordination of services and providers is essential. Medical and surgical specialists are needed within the adult health-care system to address problems that may not be within the realm of expertise of pediatric subspecialists. Physical, occupational, and speech therapists and sports and recreational specialists are vital for many adults with disabilities to optimize their quality of life. Vocational issues are paramount, as addressed in Sec. 6.3.7. Prior work experience, effective communication (including augmentative communication devices when necessary), mobility (including power wheelchairs), ergonomically correct workstations, and high self-esteem are key. The transition team thus should include access to social services, vocational specialists, the local center for independent living, home care staff, and counselors. Sexuality and other psychosocial issues should be addressed. Teens with disabilities have a 68% higher poverty rate and 37% higher incidence of being raised in a single-parent household. Lower academic achievement is common, with an elevated high school dropout rate. Sexual abuse is four times that of able-bodied peers, with a higher rate of teen pregnancy. Lack of sexual knowledge and skills is prevalent, complicated by learning difficulties, poor social skills, low self-esteem, and lack of formal education. People with disability are often seen by society as asexual when such is not the case. Discussions regarding sexuality and disability are often avoided, as parents and health-care providers find themselves uncomfortable in dealing with the topic. Meeting potential partners is a common frustration for single able-bodied adults, but the challenges are often much greater for those with disabilities. An increase in adult and family support groups with organized social and recreational gatherings across the life span will, we hope, lessen some of these problems.

As parents age, concerns arise as to who will care for their child with a disability when they are no longer able. Life care planning is essential, coinciding with all transitional endeavors. Each plan must be individualized in adults with childhood-onset conditions.

Life-span care should provide a broader perspective on how best to care for the individual and family at all ages. Currently, preexisting medical conditions may limit or even preclude insurance eligibility for many individuals with chronic conditions with onset in childhood. Life insurance may be difficult to find or afford for the adult with childhood-onset disability, who may be married and raising a family. Estate planning can be complicated by false assumptions that an adult with physical disability is not cognitively able to manage his or her financial affairs. Societal expectations and attitudes toward children with disabilities must continue to evolve as

well, to facilitate their transition to independent adulthood, whenever possible.

6.3.10 Family Adaptation

Shari L. Wade and Juliet M. Coscia

A child with significant physical or cognitive disabilities poses an array of potentially significant stresses for families, with implications for parents, siblings, and marital and family relationships. These stresses include increased caregiving demands, the financial burden of medical treatments, the reactions of family and friends, the loss of the anticipated healthy child, and worries for the future. However, despite these stresses, there is considerable variability in family adaptation and outcome, and many, if not most, families cope successfully with the demands of raising a child with a disability.

Mothers or primary caregivers are at greatest risk for a variety of adverse consequences, including increased parenting stress and higher levels of psychological symptoms, when compared to caregivers of typically developing children. Primary caregivers may also have smaller social networks and fewer opportunities for work and leisure outside of the home. Social support networks limited to health-care professionals and extended family may contribute to a sense of role restriction and an impoverished quality of life. Although less well documented, fathers may also experience less parenting satisfaction and a decrease in friendships outside the home.

The presence of a disabled child has the potential to affect the marital relationship in both positive and negative ways. Many couples report increased closeness and marital satisfaction derived from facing new parenting challenges together. However, for a subset, differences in coping styles and the division of parenting responsibilities may result in mounting dissatisfaction and disengagement. Mothers may assume a disproportionate degree of responsibility for the child's care, and fathers may become increasingly uninvolved and withdrawn. Other family roles may shift, with older female siblings being given increased responsibilities for caregiving tasks while younger, unimpaired siblings may be required to function independently at an earlier age. Although some children appear to benefit from this increased responsibility, others may feel unfairly burdened and isolated from peers who don't share those demands.

Given the wide variability in family outcomes, it is important to identify risk and protective factors that are associated with successful versus unsuccessful family adaptation, thereby enabling physicians to identify families at increased risk. Within the domains of disease and disability parameters, the extent of neurologic or behavioral involvement appears to be a much more important predictor of caregiver distress than the specific type of disability or the extent of physical disability. For example, caregivers of children with traumatic brain injury report higher levels of injury-related burden and psychological distress than caregivers of children with physical disabilities and no neurologic involvement. Whether the disability is congenital or acquired (ie, traumatic brain injury) may also influence family adaptation because acquired disabilities require grieving the loss of the normal child who is alive yet permanently altered.

Because of the importance of the family to the development and adjustment of the child with disabilities, it is critical for health-care providers to facilitate family adaptation. Families with many preexisting stresses and few supports should be linked to supportive services at the time of diagnosis, including counseling when appropriate. Support groups focused on a specific condition can provide a useful forum to address questions and connect with other families encountering similar challenges. Most caregivers require encouragement and support to continue social and leisure activities outside the home because of the perceived need to dedicate themselves to remediating the child's disability. However, families of children requiring nearly constant supervision and care may particularly benefit from respite services that would enable them to engage in activities outside the home on a regular or episodic basis.

The family's need for support and anticipatory guidance is likely to change with the child's age and the developmental stage of the family. Developmental transitions such as adolescence or early adulthood may pose challenges for previously well-functioning families. Because many families adapt successfully to having a child with a disability, parental stress and depression or marital conflict should be viewed as an indication of problems rather than as normative.

6.3.11 Ethical Issues in Chronic Illness and Disability in Childhood

Rita Ayangar

The ethical conflicts encountered in pediatric chronic care and rehabilitation typically involve issues such as therapeutic goal setting, patient–provider team relationships, and quality of life rather than the dramatic life-death issues seen in acute care settings. In chronic care, the emphasis is not on cure but on developing, adapting, and learning to live despite disease or disability. Successful rehabilitation restores wholeness and integrity to the person and develops or preserves a meaningful life and self-identity through an educative process. Children with chronic illness and disability often require treatment in a variety of settings (acute care, rehabilitation facilities, home, and community) and over a long period of time. Resource allocation therefore becomes a frequent source of conflict in rehabilitation medicine.

SETTING REHABILITATION GOALS

Patients and families are expected to assume responsibility for their actions and decisions and work with the rehabilitation professionals to establish their rehabilitation goals. However, these patients and families generally have high levels of stress related to their recent losses and feel frightened, insecure, or vulnerable from anxiety, fatigue, or depression. The responsibility of setting goals for rehabilitation may impose an undue additional stress. A moral conflict is raised regarding whether it is right to expect the patient and family to set goals in the early stages of rehabilitation, when they are so vulnerable. Who then should set the goals: the patients or the providers? The health-care provider faces a strong temptation to assume an "I know better" paternalistic attitude and establish goals for the patient.

Patients and families may best know their life styles, habits, and the amount of energy and resources they wish to expend on therapy. Parents and other family members may continue in their caregiving capacity with a greater burden of care, and the disability may necessitate major changes in life style. Caregivers may be more objective than the child in assessing needs. On the other hand, they may themselves have impairments (depression, alcoholism, back pain) that can compromise their ability to assist the child with disability. There may be tensions between the principles of autonomy and beneficence. Rehabilitation professionals may be very uncomfortable letting a child with spastic cerebral palsy and his family do things their way, especially if time, money, and effort will be wasted or a needlessly poor health outcome may result (eg, letting the child feed orally to meet nutritional needs when the swallowing studies demonstrate severe aspiration). The process of goal setting is also influenced by health-care reimbursers, who may have limits on the duration of treatment, total expenditures, or use of specialists or special types of treatments.

PATIENT–PROVIDER RELATIONSHIPS

There are many ethical implications of professionals working as a team to care for patients. How does a team member balance loyalty and responsibility to the team while maintaining confidentiality and moral obligation to the patient when a 16-year-old girl with a brain tumor shares in confidence that she is "doing drugs"? How do teams avoid coercion or condescending treatment of patients and families? How should medical care be balanced with other priorities of rehabilitation, such as addressing the psychological, social, educational, and vocational needs necessary for successful integration into society?

Several models of relationships between patient and provider exist. The traditional Hippocratic method is one of medical paternalism. The contractual model provides patients and families the right to make choices about the type and extent of care they receive, and they may, for example, reject care that is known to be beneficial. Caplan and Jennings suggest a third "fiduciary" model of relationship that respects the need for time to allow the patient and family to adjust to the reality of severe disability. According to this model, the practitioner may start with a paternalistic approach, and the relationship will evolve to a balanced, interactive relationship where "choices" and "decisions" and the "patient's good" are mutually discovered over time.

QUALITY-OF-LIFE DECISIONS

Rehabilitation seeks a better balance between longevity and quality of life (QOL), adding not just years to life but life to years. QOL is often measured based on factors relevant to able-bodied individuals. Physicians and others in society may misapply their own personal perspective to justify withholding or implementing treatments, eg, life-sustaining therapeutic interventions for the ventilator-dependent adolescent with advanced neuromuscular disease. Instead, decisions should be made by examining the life satisfaction of patients and families of competent individuals who have already chosen these options. The great majority of severely disabled ventilator-assisted individuals with neuromuscular disease or spinal cord injury are satisfied with their lives, despite inability to achieve many of the "usual" goals linked with QOL in the physically able population, deriving satisfaction from social relationships, school, and reorganization of goals enhanced by the use of assistive technological aids. With improved medical management, the life expectancy of a child with high cervical spinal cord injury is increased well into adulthood. Quality of life may be addressed with rehabilitation, which should include planning for adulthood, with vocational training, and with independent living with personal assistance services. Considerations related to QOL appear to be playing an increasing role in the allocation of societal resources.

References

Physical and Occupational Therapy

American Academy of Pediatrics, Committee on Children with Disabilities: The role of the pediatrician in prescribing therapy services for children with motor disabilities. Pediatrics 98:308–310, 1996

Campbell SK, ed: Physical Therapy for Children. Philadelphia, WB Saunders, 1994

Case-Smith J, Allen AS, Pratt PN: Occupational Therapy for Children, 3rd ed. St Louis, Mosby-Yearbook, 1996

Kurtz LA, Harryman SE: Rehabilitation interventions: physical therapy and occupational therapy. In: Batshaw ML, ed: Children with Disabilities, 4th ed. Baltimore, Paul H Brookes, 1997:709–725

Solomon R: Pediatricians and early intervention: everything you need to know but are too busy to ask. Infants Young Children 7(3):38–51, 1995

Speech Pathology

Capute AJ, Accardo PJ: Linguistic and auditory milestones during the first two years of life. Clin Pediatr 17:847–853, 1978

Capute AJ, Shapiro BK, Palmer FB: Marking the milestones of language development. Contemp Pediatr 4:24–41, 1987

Coplan J: Normal speech and language development: an overview. Pediatr Rev 16:91–100, 1995

Glascoe FP: Can clinical judgment detect children with speech-language problems? Pediatrics 87:317–322, 1991

Kummer AW: Normal speech and language development. In: Baker RC, ed: Handbook of Pediatric Care. Boston, Little, Brown, 1995

Kummer AW: Assessment of speech and language disorders. In: Cotton RT, Myer CM III, eds: Practical Pediatric Otolaryngology. Philadelphia, Lippincott-Raven, 1999

Olswang LB: Developmental speech and language disorders. ASHA 35:42–44, 1993

Ruben RJ: Communication disorders in children: a challenge for health care. Prev Med 22:585–588, 1993

Assistive Technology

AbleData Web Site on Assistive Technology: www.abledata.com

Cook AA, Hussy SM: Assistive Technologies: Principles and Practice. St. Louis, Mosby Year Book, 1995

Glennen SL, Decoste DC: Handbook of Augmentative and Alternative Communication. London, Singular Publishing Group, 1997

Gray DB, Quatrano LA, Lieberman ML: Designing and Using Assistive Technology: The Human Perspective. Baltimore, Paul H Brookes, 1998

Judge SL, Parette HP: Assistive Technology for Young Children with Disabilities. Cambridge, MA, Brookline Books, 1998

Orthoses

Carlson WE, Vaughan CL, Damiano DL, Abel MF: Orthotic management of gait in spastic diplegia. Am J Phys Med Rehabil 76:219–225, 1997

Jacques C, Karmel-Ross K: The use of splinting in conservative and postoperative treatment of congenital muscular torticollis. In: Karmel-Ross K, ed: Torticollis: Differential Diagnosis, Assessment and Treatment, Surgical Management and Bracing. Binghamton, Haworth Press, 1997: 81–90

Luna-Reyes OB, Reyes TM, So FY, Matti BMS, Lardizabal AA: Energy cost of ambulation in healthy and disabled Filipino children. Arch Phys Med Rehabil 69:946–949, 1988

Merritt JL: Knee-ankle-foot orthotics: Long leg braces and their practical applications. Phys Med Rehabil State Art Rev 1:67–82, 1987

Radtka SA, Skinner SR, Dixon DM, Johanson ME: A comparison of gait with solid, dynamic, and no ankle-foot orthoses in children with cerebral palsy. Phys Ther 77:395–409, 1997

Prostheses

Cummings DR: Pediatric prosthetics: current trends and future possibilities. Phys Med Rehabil Clin North Am 11:653–679, 2000

Herring JA, Birch JG, eds: The Child with a Limb Deficiency. Rosemont, IL, American Academy of Orthopaedic Surgeons, 1998

Jain S: Rehabilitation in limb deficiency. 2. The pediatric amputee. Arch Phys Med Rehabil 77:S9–13, 1996

Recreational Therapy

Austin D: Therapeutic Recreation Processes and Techniques, 3rd ed. Champaigne, IL, Sagamore Publishing, 1997

Austin D, Crawford M: Therapeutic Recreation: An Introduction, 2nd ed. Needham Heights, MA, Allyn and Bacon, 1996

Education and Employment

Coughran L, Daniels JL: Early vocational intervention for the severely handicapped. J Rehabil 49:37–41, 1983

Fraser RT: Career development and school-to-work transition for adolescents with traumatic brain injury. In: Ylvisaker M, ed: Traumatic Brain Injury Rehabilitation: Children and Adolescents, 2nd ed. Boston, Butterworth-Heinemann, 1998:417–427

National Institute of Disability and Rehabilitation Research: School to Work Transitions for Youth with Disabilities: Report from Consensus Validation Conference. Arlington, VA, National Institute of Disability and Rehabilitation Research, 1994

White PH: Success on the road to adulthood: issues and hurdles for adolescents with disabilities. Rheum Dis Clin North Am 23:697–707, 1997

Psychosocial Adjustment to Disability

Lavigne JV, Faier-Routman J: Psychological adjustment to pediatric physical disorders: a meta-analytic review. J Pediatr Psychol 17:133–157, 1992

Lavigne JV, Faier-Routman J: Correlates of adjustment to pediatric physical disorders: a meta-analytic review and comparison with existing models. J Dev Behav Pediatr 14:117–123, 1993

Wallander JL, Thompson RJ: Psychosocial adjustment of children with chronic physical conditions. In: Roberts M, ed: Handbook of Pediatric Psychology. New York, Guilford Press, 1995:124–141

Transition to Adulthood

American Academy of Pediatrics Committee on Children with Disabilities and Committee on Adolescents: Transition of care provided for adolescents with special health care needs. Pediatrics 98:1203–1206, 1996

Bax MCO, Smyth DPL, Thomas AP: Health care of physically handicapped young adults. Br Med J 296:1153–1155, 1988

Bronheim S, Fiel S, Schidlow D, Magrab P, Boczar K, Dillon C: Crossings: A Manual for Transition of Chronically Ill Youth to Adult Health Care. Washington, DC, Georgetown University Child Development Center, 1996

Murphy KP, Molnar GE, Lankasky K: Medical and functional status of adults with cerebral palsy. Dev Med Child Neurol 37:1075–1084, 1995

Rosen D: Between two worlds: bridging the cultures of child health and adult medicine. J Adolesc Health 17:10–16, 1995

Sharpland C: Sexuality Issues for Youth with Disabilities and Chronic Health Conditions. An Occasional Policy Brief of the Institute for Child Health Policy. Gainesville, FL, Institute for Child Health Policy, 1999

White PH: Success on the road to adulthood: issues and hurdles for adolescents with disabilities. Rheum Dis Clin North Am 23:697–707, 1997

Family Adaptation

Breslau N, Staruch KS, Mortimer EA: Psychological distress in mothers of disabled children. Am J Dis Child 136:682–686, 1982

Kazak A, Marvin RS: Differences, difficulties and adaptation: stress and social networks in families with a handicapped child. Family Relations 33: 67–77, 1984

Taylor HG, Yeates KO, Wade SL, Drotar D, Klein S, Stancin T: Influences on first-year recovery from traumatic brain injury in children. Neuropsychology 13:76–89, 1999

Wade SL, Taylor HG, Drotar D, Stancin T, Yeates KO: Family burden and adaptation during the initial year after traumatic brain injury in children. Pediatrics 102:110–116, 1998

Wallander JL, Varni JW, Babani L, DeHaan CB, Wilcox KT, Banis HT: The social environment and the adaptation of mothers of physically handicapped children. J Pediatr Psychol 14:371–387, 1989

Wallander JL, Venters TL: Perceived role restriction and adjustment of mothers of children with chronic physical disability. J Pediatr Psychol 20:619–632, 1995

Ethics

Bach JR, Barnett V: Ethical considerations in the management of individuals with severe neuromuscular disorders. Am J Phys Med Rehabil 73: 134–140, 1994

Haas J: Ethical considerations of goal setting for patient care in rehabilitative medicine. Am J Phys Med Rehabil 72:228–232, 1993

Jennings B, Callahan D, Caplan AL: Ethical challenges of chronic illness. Hastings Center Rep 18(Suppl):1–16, 1988

Matthews DJ, Meier RH, Bartholme W: Ethical issues encountered in pediatric rehabilitation. Pediatrician 17:108–114, 1990

Meier RH, Purtillo RB: Ethical issues and the patient–provider relationship. Am J Phys Med Rehabil 73:365–366, 1994

COMPLEX DECISIONS IN PEDIATRICS LAW, ETHICS, AND CARE NEAR THE END OF LIFE

Angela R. Holder and Bernard Lo, Associate Editors

7.1 LAW, ETHICS, AND CLINICAL JUDGMENT

As citizens, physicians have an obligation to obey the law. On such issues as confidentiality of medical records and informed consent by minors, laws and regulations give clear guidance. However, on many other issues, the law provides only general guidance, gives great discretion to physicians to implement their professional responsibilities, or is largely silent.

In many situations, physicians will need to follow their professional ethics, which may impose obligations beyond legal requirements. From a legal perspective, pediatricians need only obtain the authorization of the parent or guardian of a child. However, professional ethics requires pediatricians to provide pediatric patients information about their condition and care in ways that are developmentally appropriate and also to try to obtain the assent of children for care. Furthermore, ethical standards require pediatricians to act with compassion and integrity.

In many cases, sound clinical judgment and good communication allow pediatricians to resolve ethical issues within the framework set by professional ethics and legal requirements. For instance, adolescents may ask pediatricians not to tell their parents that they are seeking care for substance abuse or psychiatric illness. Although the law in most states allows adolescents to obtain such care without parental authorization, the pediatrician has an ethical obligation to act in the patient's best interests. Usually it is in the adolescent's best interests to have a parent involved in such care. The pediatrician can help the adolescent understand that parental involvement is usually beneficial in these situations and that parents are likely to learn of their situation in any case. Often the physician can help the adolescent decide how to discuss his or her problems with a parent or another adult relative and help the parents play a constructive role in their child's care. In any case, the physician must also be careful not to make agreements that constrain appropriate clinical care.

7.2 THE PEDIATRICIAN, THE PARENTS, AND THE CHILD

The pediatrician's patient is the child, and the pediatrician's main ethical obligations are to the child. The pediatrician should be guided primarily by the child's best interests. Pediatricians also should treat children with respect, compassion, and honesty. To the extent it is developmentally appropriate, doctors should provide children with information about their condition and care, obtain their assent or consent, offer them realistic choices regarding their care, and respect their privacy.

Because children are dependent, parents or guardians play a crucial role in children's health care. Parents have responsibility for children and are given considerable latitude in raising them. Furthermore, it is in the child's best interest to grow up within a closely knit family. Therefore, within broad limits set by society, parents are given great discretion to inculcate values in children and to choose how to rear them. For example, children must attend school, but parents may decide whether to send their children to public school, private school, religious-based school, or home schooling. Within a family, what is best for the family as a whole or for other members of the family must be balanced against what is best for an individual child. Parents cannot be expected to devote all their energy and resources to one child, to the exclusion of the needs of other children or themselves. Similarly, parental authority and discretion extend to health care decisions.

Children depend on their parents to seek medical attention and to follow dietary, lifestyle, and pharmaceutic regimens. In the vast majority of cases, the interests of children and the actions of parents coincide. However, when the parent's decisions and actions seriously compromise the well-being of the child, the physician's role is to promote the best interests of the child. Advocacy by pediatricians is essential because children cannot represent themselves. Usually it is better for pediatricians to try to work with the parents in providing health care, making recommendations, and arranging in-home assistance as needed. The alternatives of imposing treatment over the parent's objections or taking the child away from the family often are unsatisfactory.

Parents are given discretion to make decisions within parameters set by law and sound clinical practice. Thus, parents have the authority to accept or decline treatment such as elective surgery or medications for mild or self-limited conditions. Even in serious conditions, such as the care of infants with extreme prematurity or severe birth defects, parents are not obligated to accept all possible medical interventions. Physicians and society have set limits at the extremes of care: parents may not demand futile treatments, and parents may not forego short-term interventions that are highly likely to correct medical problems, such as transfusions for severe anemia, antibiotics for life-threatening infection, or surgery for tracheoesophageal fistula. However, between these extremes, the parent's informed preferences and values should guide medical care. In extreme situations, physicians may need to oppose the parents, for example, asking the courts to order transfusions or antibiotics over parental objections or reporting child abuse or neglect to appropriate officials.

In some situations, laws and regulations that would compel parental behaviors are not enforced because the child would be harmed by conflict between the parents and the medical or health care system. For instance, some parents object to immunizing their children because of religious objections to medical interventions, fears of side effects, or distrust of the medical system. Although immunizations generally are required for entrance into school, many states allow for exemptions based on parental religious beliefs or other objections. Furthermore, requirements for immunizations may not be enforced, provided that the number of children not immunized is sufficiently small that the risk of an epidemic is slight. For the child, the benefits of enforcing the parent's legal responsibilities do not seem worth the risk of alienating the parents. However, if an epidemic does break out, the risk to unimmunized children increases, and public health officials rapidly enforce requirements for immunization.

As children develop, they gain the capacity to make informed decisions about their care. Physicians can foster and respect such maturation by providing information to adolescents in terms they can understand, helping them deliberate about decisions, and respecting their informed preferences. With adolescents, the law and the standard of practice have set additional limits on parental authority. Adolescents commonly engage in behavior of which parents disapprove, such as sexual intercourse or drug use. Parents may want the pediatrician to inform them of such adolescent behaviors so that they can respond in their parental role. However, many adolescents are unwilling to be candid with physicians about these activities if parents will be told. Because sexually transmitted diseases, pregnancy, and substance abuse are major health problems for adolescents, society has determined that adolescents should be allowed to seek medical care for these conditions without their parent's consent. Furthermore, adolescents' requests for confidentiality should be respected if possible.

7.3 INFORMED CONSENT: WHO DECIDES?

7.3.1 Informed Consent and the Preadolescent Child

Giving an "informed consent" to medical treatment means that the person agreeing to treatment for him or herself (or for another) understands the nature of the proposed treatment, why it is necessary, the risks and benefits of the therapy proposed, and what alternatives might be available. In urgent as well as nonurgent cases a patient has the right to know what will happen if nothing is done.

In virtually all cases, parental consent is required to treat a young child. The exception to the rule of parental consent is that emergency treatment may be provided if the parent is not available, and the courts have construed "emergency" in this context very broadly. The situation may be one in which care should be provided quickly. It certainly does not have to be a situation in which the child might die or be disabled if treatment is not provided. For example, if a child in day care falls off a sliding board, cuts her head, and is taken to the Emergency Department, someone should try to find her parents, but if they are not immediately available, the child's cut should be sutured. To make the child wait in pain, fear, and misery until a parent is located to give permission is not only

unnecessary but bad pediatric practice. If the child needs surgery or a risky treatment, if possible, it is well to wait until the parent is contacted, but setting a simple fracture or suturing a cut may certainly be done before the parent can be found.

A noncustodian may not bring a child to a physician for a nonurgent problem and have the child treated without parental consent. A teacher, for example, cannot expect a pediatrician to treat a child if she brings him for a diagnosis of attention deficit disorder and asks the physician to write a prescription for methylphenidate (Ritalin) without discussing the situation with the child's parent.

Children are much more likely to be cooperative if they are told what will happen and if they are allowed to make some choices, so even with young children, an explanation of what is going to happen—the shot will sting for just a minute—and being allowed to decide if the red bandaid or the blue bandaid will be applied thereafter is probably good pediatric practice. Under no circumstances, however, would this be considered "consent," any more than "No, I don't want the shot" would be acceptable as an informed refusal from a 4-year-old who needs an immunization. If a sick child needs medication (or, for that matter, surgery), although sensible health care providers will make every effort to engage the child in conversation about why it is necessary, why it tastes nasty, and why it will make him better, the child has no right to refuse. It would be perfectly legal, for example, for an 8-year-old, to be taken to surgery for an appendectomy over his most vigorous protests, and in fact would be very bad medical care if his refusal is accepted and he dies of peritonitis.

An older child may be allowed to choose among alternatives if they genuinely exist. To the extent that the child seems to understand what is wrong with him or her, why the problem needs to be treated, and what the options are should be explained. The child's developmental stage is the controlling factor in this analysis, but it is clear that a preadolescent child has no right to consent to or to refuse medical care.

7.3.2 Informed Consent and the Adolescent Patient

Almost always adolescents and their parents agree on medical care, the physician finds the choices reasonable, and treatment proceeds. This is not, however, always the case. On occasion, both parent and child want some therapy provided that the physician thinks is wrong or unwise. Suppose, for example, a 14-year-old with leukemia and his parents wish the physician to treat him with laetrile or one of the other "alternative" medicines? The physician not only does not have to do so, but in an urgent case, if the child and family refuse conventional therapies in addition to insisting on some course of treatment the physician thinks may be harmful, there is always the option of obtaining a court order to treat the young patient. Other interventions may not be inherently harmful, but the physician believes that they are unwise. For example, a teenager and her parents may agree on cosmetic plastic surgery for an imagined defect. (She thinks her nose is ugly and her parents agree, when, in truth, her nose is not at all abnormally large.) Although there is certainly no objection to rhinoplasty in appropriate cases, if, in this instance, the plastic surgeon believes that the real problem is psychosocial, she certainly does not have to do a procedure just because the patient wants it.

The adolescent patient and his or her parent may also disagree about therapy. When the issue is not life-threatening, counseling would appear to be in order, but it should be remembered that unless the therapy is clearly necessary, parents are not obliged to pay for elective treatment to which they object. If the teenager in the example above wants a rhinoplasty, and her parents think she is being ridiculous and that there is nothing wrong with her nose, although she may be sufficiently mature to consent on her own, her parents certainly would not have to pay the surgeon's bill. On the other hand, if therapy is clearly needed, and there is serious disagreement between the patient and the parents, the decision should be made in the best interests of the patient, not the parents. If, for example, a teenager who is a Jehovah's Witness decides that she wants blood transfusions for treatment of her leukemia and the parents object on religious grounds, the patient's interests should prevail. The medical team, however, should consider the effects on the family unit of such a conflict and attempt to provide support and conflict resolution as necessary—in this case, for example, the parents might refuse to allow the "sinful" patient to come home after discharge from the hospital.

If the parents want the therapy and the adolescent patient does not, a court order might be required before a mature minor can be treated against his or her will. In most cases, however, negotiation will resolve the issue. If a teenager wants to stop chemotherapy because her baldness is causing her great distress, purchase of a wig may be more to the point than protracted discussion of the limits of her autonomy or legal action to force her to accept it. In these cases of family disagreement, there are usually underlying family conflicts, often about control of the adolescent, that are presented as conflicts about specific issues of therapy. Attention to the real problems may resolve the therapeutic conflicts. In any case, however, strapping an adolescent down and administering therapy to which the patient vehemently objects is extremely unwise because cooperation of the patient is usually essential to the treatment.

The parameters of the child's right to consent or to refuse to participate in clinical research is a subject of such complexity that it cannot be covered adequately in this chapter. The reader is referred to the references at the end of the text.

7.3.3 Informed Consent and Adolescents Who Do Not Wish to Involve Their Parents

Many states, by statute, fix an age at which a minor may consent on his or her own to medical treatment. If such a statute applies, and the minor declines to involve his or her parents, and counseling by the physician does not change the patient's mind, in most cases the patient may consent to treatment as an adult would do. Even in states where there are no such statutes, courts recognize the "mature minor" rule. This grants adolescents who are as capable as an adult of understanding the proposed treatment and its risks and benefits the right to consent. Most of these situations involve outpatient care because most hospitals are more interested in who will pay the bill than they are in the patient's right to autonomy. Thus, they will not admit a nonemergency patient unless the parents agree to have their insurance available or are otherwise willing to assume responsibility for payment. Also, there may be no problem at all with treating a 14-year-old for acne at the adolescent clinic without parental involvement, but no oncologist would be willing to treat the same teenager for leukemia without parental knowledge. So the limits of adolescent decision making reflect not only the age and maturity of the patient but the nature of the condition for which treatment is necessary.

Emancipated minors are those who are not under the care and control of their parents. By definition, the adolescent is not dependent on them for support and is usually not living with them. Married minors, by definition, are emancipated, and in most states a minor mother, even if she lives with her parents, is considered emancipated for purposes of making medical decisions for herself and her baby. Runaways are usually considered, by default, emancipated because if an adolescent needs treatment and refuses to disclose how to find his or her parents, treatment must be given. Where an adolescent meets the criteria for emancipation, parents do not have to be included in the decision-making process and are not liable for any of the emancipated minor's expenses, medical and otherwise.

7.4 REFUSAL OF TREATMENT: WHO DECIDES?

7.4.1 Handicapped Newborns

Until a few years ago, parents and physicians together often decided that a child born with non-life-threatening but severe handicaps would be "allowed to die" even when treatment, such as surgery, would have cured some of the baby's problems and would have routinely been done except for the handicap. During the Reagan years, the "Baby Doe" rules attempted to require treatment of virtually all children born alive, even when the prognosis was dire and the outcome at best one of insentient existence. Few noticed at the time that physicians already had the legal authority to obtain court orders for treatment of children whose parents were refusing to permit therapy. Failure to obtain reasonable medical treatment for a child, by definition, constitutes child neglect, and courts will virtually always order treatment to be given if a hospital or physician asks for such an order.

The legal impact of the "Baby Doe" rules was, therefore, minimal. They did, however, create great anxiety among pediatricians, and that anxiety has probably resulted in insistence on treatments for some handicapped babies whose physicians actually believed the treatments unwise. As a result of the public discussion on this issue, however, many hospitals established pediatric ethics committees to advise parents and physicians in case of conflicts and to provide a forum where disputes may be aired and perhaps resolved.

7.4.2 Young Children and Parental Refusal of Treatment

WHERE THE PROGNOSIS IS GOOD

If a child has an injury or illness and medical care can produce a cure or at least a recovery with minimal disability, the courts almost always override parental refusal of treatment. For example, if a child is hit by a car and requires surgery but parents refuse on grounds that blood transfusions are necessary and their religion forbids the use of blood products, a court order, if sought, will always be granted for treatment. A court order, however, in practical terms requires physical custody of the child during the treatment period. Parents who object to chemotherapy for a child with an excellent chance of recovery from cancer may, during the period when the child is ordered to come for outpatient care, simply remove the child from the jurisdiction and perhaps from the country if their objections are sufficiently heartfelt. Thus, for practical purposes, court-ordered treatment is useful only if the intervention is predicted to be effective and can be completed while the child is hospitalized. Long-term therapies, such as chemotherapies, in these circumstances may require asking the court to place the child in a foster home; thus, the trauma to child and parents should always be balanced against the predicted success of the treatment.

WHERE THE PROGNOSIS IS NOT GOOD

Parents may wish to refuse treatment when the child's prognosis, under the best of circumstances, is not good; the side effects are substantial; and they feel that they would like the child to live as comfortably as possible for whatever time remains. Hospice care, appropriate and usually available for adults in this circumstance, is unfortunately less readily available for young children, but that goal may be the best possible outcome for the situation. There is no legal duty whatever on a physician to insist on treatment that will delay death in a terminal illness, regardless of the age of the patient.

If the reason the parents (or the child) wish to refuse treatment is their understanding of the suffering the child must endure, the conflict may often be resolved by careful explanation of the pain relief and palliative care available even as therapy continues in hopes of a remission or possible cure.

If the physician insists on obtaining a court order for treatment, it is probable that one will be issued, but in recent years courts are increasingly likely to side with the parents' decision in a case of this nature. In case of a profound disagreement between physician and family in these cases, the most humane course of action may be to assist the parents in finding a physician who shares their perspective and who is willing to assume the responsibility for care of the child.

7.4.3 Adolescents and Refusal of Treatment

Adolescents can and do object to treatment that their parents wish them to have. Short of forcibly medicating a patient or physically restraining him or her, it is often best just to negotiate what the adolescent finds acceptable because the alternatives, whatever the legal issues involved, are so difficult. "No" may be many things other than a death wish, and the physician should spend enough time with the young person to find out what the real agenda is. A teenager who refuses chemotherapy may be making a statement that she wants a normal social life for a while; if possible, the regimen might be changed to allow her more freedom to go about her life for a bit, without taking her refusal at face value as a permanent statement of intent. Younger children as well as adolescents often benefit when they are allowed to participate in and control some aspects of treatment decisions, even when they have no right to refuse to have the treatment. The child's or adolescent's feelings of helplessness in the face of serious illness or an injury should be understood and respected, and that respect may lessen the likelihood of outright refusal.

If the treatment is an unpleasant one for a condition for which the adolescent will recover eventually anyway, the adolescent has a fair amount of latitude in the legal right to refuse. The right of refusal is virtually absolute in a situation where the treatment is entirely elective. If a parent brought a teenager to a plastic surgeon for cosmetic surgery and the teenager did not wish to have it, that should end the matter. The same rule would apply if a parent presents a pregnant adolescent for an abortion and the girl wishes to have her baby. If, however, the adolescent may die if treatment is not provided, it is most unlikely that a court would accept the patient's decision as final.

When treatment violates an adolescent's religious beliefs (such as a blood transfusion for a Jehovah's Witness) and the parents agree with the patient, extreme care is necessary to find out if the patient is being intimidated or coerced by his or her family before deciding that the adolescent has a "right to die." Before a 16-year-old Jehovah's Witness is allowed to die when blood would save him, at the very least the physician and other members of the health care team should discuss the situation with the patient *outside* the presence of the parents and assure him that if he wants to receive blood, the health care team will administer it where his parents will not find out unless he chooses to tell them. Even if the patient is mature enough to make the decision, parental coercion must be totally eliminated before the choice is accepted. Most courts will not, if asked, allow a minor to make a decision to refuse life-saving therapy, but there are a few cases, all involving religious beliefs about blood transfusions, in which judges have found that teenagers who are 15 and up and who demonstrate an understanding of the situation and are not being coerced by their parents may make these decisions. In other courts, on identical facts, life-saving treatment has been ordered for adolescents within weeks of their 18th birthdays and adulthood.

Where the prognosis is poor, however, the courts seem to be awarding increasingly respect to an adolescent's right to refuse treatment and to "die in peace."

7.5 EMERGENCY TREATMENT

In an emergency, treatment should be given to the child on the basis of implied consent if delaying care in order to seek parental authorization would jeopardize the health of the child. Thus, if a child suffers trauma and has a possible fracture, appropriate emergency treatment should be initiated while a parent or responsible adult is being contacted. The ethical rationale is that if asked, almost all parents would want such emergency treatment to be provided rather than delayed in order to contact them. The exception is that treatment should not be provided if there has been a previous decision to forego it, as in the case of withholding resuscitation in terminal illness. After the emergency situation is stabilized and there is time for deliberation, parents need to authorize continued treatment.

7.6 CONFIDENTIALITY

In pediatrics, especially with adolescent patients, a promise of confidentiality may be the only means to obtain honest information with which to diagnose and treat the patient's problem. Although some parents sincerely believe that they have the right to know absolutely everything about their child's life, failing to respect the child's confidences, regardless of parental views on the matter, may yield an inability to discover serious medical or behavioral problems. As a rule of thumb, the right to expect confidentiality from one's physician increases with maturity, and thus, if a young person has the right to consent to or to refuse treatment, that treatment can be given confidentially.

7.6.1   Confidentiality and the Younger Child

The right of confidentiality of younger children is severely limited. In most cases, however, it does not occur to very young children that their parents do not already know everything about them. The concept of confidentiality requires a certain level of maturity. A parent is usually present at the interaction between the physician and the child in any case, and thus, the issue rarely if ever arises.

7.6.2   Adolescents and Disclosures to Parents

All states have statutes providing that treatment for venereal diseases, drug abuse, and alcohol problems may be provided without parental involvement. It became obvious as early as the 1960s that teenagers with these problems would not go for help if they thought their parents would find out. State legislators concluded that it was better to provide confidential treatment than for the epidemic of STDs to spread or for teenagers with drug and alcohol problems to be involved with illegal activities for want of help.

In some states, these statutes specifically forbid billing the parent for the child's care without the consent of the patient. In almost all situations if the parent's insurer is billed for the care, the parent will find out, so if treatment is to be given confidentially (for any reason), the physician can look only to the adolescent for payment.

Contraception provided by a clinic or other entity receiving federal funding under Title X of the Public Health Act (the Family Planning program) must be provided confidentially to adolescents. There have been attempts, all held unconstitutional, to require either parental consent or postprescription parental notification, but courts have held that in this area the adolescent has the same rights to privacy as an adult.

State laws vary on parental involvement with abortion decisions. Thirty-eight states require either parental consent or a court determination that the girl is sufficiently mature to make the decision on her own. (If the judge concludes that she is too immature to decide whether to have an abortion, the judge is, by definition, concluding that she is sufficiently mature to be a mother, of course.) If there is no such requirement in the state, the assumption is that the minor may consent to abortion just as she could consent to other medical procedures as a mature minor.

When a young teenager (for example, a girl under 15) asks for a pregnancy test, or when it is found that she is pregnant, independent of confidentiality issues, the physician should investigate whether she is the victim of some form of sexual abuse or coercion or whether her situation is the result of a relatively age-appropriate relationship. It may well be the case that a child abuse report is required; thus, confidentiality as to the parent may be beside the point.

When a teenager demands confidentiality before revealing a problem or consenting to treatment, the pediatrician should realize that there may be family problems. If the pediatrician is the teenager's regular physician, attempts to help the patient work out the relationship with his or her parents may be more valuable than viewing the question as one of confidentiality on a specific issue. On the other hand, although "my mother would kill me if she knew I was pregnant" is usually hyperbole, it should not be assumed to be such unless the physician knows the family well and has confidence that such is not the case. In the absence of information about the family, the physician should be most unwilling to override a teenager's plea for confidentiality.

Of course, a developmentally disabled adolescent cannot make decisions about care at the same level of autonomy allowed for the usual adolescent, and thus, the corresponding right to confidential care is diminished.

Even when confidentiality is respected, there are some instances in which parents should be notified. For example, if a child is threatening to harm him- or herself or someone else, whatever promises of confidentiality have been made are less important than making sure the parents can keep the child safe. Furthermore, if the risk is sufficiently high to consider having the child committed to a mental hospital, it would be impossible to do so without parental knowledge.

7.6.3   Disclosures to Others

REPORTS TO AUTHORITIES

All states mandate reporting of child abuse, and thus confidentiality must give way to legal mandates. If a 15 year-old girl is pregnant and her 16-year-old boyfriend is the father of the fetus, confidentiality is probably required. On the other hand, if the physician discovers that the pregnancy is the result of a coerced relationship with the mother's live-in companion, that would be reportable as child abuse. The mother would thus be informed of the situation. Infectious diseases are usually reportable to state authorities as well, even if the adolescent patient has the right of confidentiality as to his or her parents.

REPORTS TO SCHOOLS

Health information sent to a school nurse or to a school-based clinic is not necessarily confidential. It may well be accessible by the principal and, from there, to the faculty. Thus, the physician should be aware that informing a school nurse about a patient's medical condition is not the same thing as sharing medical information with another physician in private practice or with the adolescent clinic at the local hospital. This lack of confidentiality and potential invasion of privacy, coupled with the concern that children with HIV may be unfairly treated or abused in school, cause many physicians simply to refuse to notify the school when their patient is HIV+. Rather, the physicians hope that teachers understand that universal precautions are necessary in dealing with all children. In any case, the parent of a young child, and the adolescent and his or her parent, should know exactly what information is being sent to the school and in most cases decline to allow it to be disclosed.

REPORTS TO OTHERS

Other relatives without responsibilities for the child have no more right to know about the child's medical problems than the next door neighbor does. At the least, no such information should ever be disclosed without the knowledge and consent of the parent and the adolescent child.

7.7   TERMINAL ILLNESS

Serious illness such as extreme prematurity, cancer, or HIV infection may worsen despite the best pediatric care. As prognosis worsens, the side effects of treatment may become more burdensome, relative to the limited benefits. Pediatricians need to take the lead in discussing with parents and children (if they are able) what course of care is in the child's best interests. To start, pediatricians should ask the parents and child what their understanding of the current situation and prognosis is and what their concerns, fears, and hopes are regarding their illness. Such questions are essential because the pediatrician needs to ascertain that the parents and child understand the medical situation. If the parents or child is unrealistic, the pediatrician can gently correct their misunderstandings. Next, the pediatrician needs to develop a plan of care that is mutually acceptable. If the parents and child appreciate that the illness is progressing despite treatment, the pediatrician should focus attention on positive goals for care. What would be important for the child to do in whatever time is left? Is it to spend time at home rather than in the hospital? Is it to have relatives visit? Is it to be free of physical suffering?

Relief of pain and other symptoms is essential in the management of terminal illness. As prognosis dims, palliation of symptoms may become the paramount goal of care. Sometimes parents or children need to be reassured that use of narcotics to relieve pain in terminal illness is morally appropriate, and concerns about addiction need to be addressed. Pediatricians should not hesitate to use high doses of narcotics and sedatives if lower doses have not successfully alleviated symptoms in terminally ill patients. Even if high doses of narcotics and sedatives may hasten death, they are ethically and legally appropriate if lower doses have failed to relieve distressing symptoms. Use of high doses of narcotics and sedatives to relieve distressing symptoms can be distinguished from active euthanasia. According to the doctrine of double effect, the pediatricians' intent is important. If the intention is to relieve pain, the possibility of hastening death is acceptable as a potential but unintended consequence of using high doses of medication. Two other aspects of the doctrine of double effect are important. The child's death must not be the intended means to relieve suffering. Furthermore, the risk of the undesired effect must be proportional to the benefit. This requirement of proportionality is satisfied if lower doses have failed to palliate the patient's suffering and the child's death is not the means by which the goal of relieving suffering is accomplished.

Many parents and children will choose to limit medical interventions, as described in Section 7.4. Pediatricians need to make plans to implement these decisions. Often a DNR order is the first topic discussed. When a child is found to be in cardiopulmonary arrest, CPR needs to be administered immediately to have any chance at success. Therefore, CPR is attempted unless a DNR order has been written. Pediatricians caring for children with terminal or chronic illness need to raise the issue of DNR orders with parents and mature minors. DNR orders direct nurses, paramedics, and physicians not to attempt CPR in case of cardiopulmonary arrest. DNR orders are appropriate if the parents or an informed, competent adolescent refuses CPR or if the child would not survive the hospitalization even if CPR were attempted.

In the hospital, the attending pediatrician needs to write a formal DNR order in the medical record as well as a progress note explaining the decision. If the child will be at home, appropriate forms need to be completed so that if paramedics are called because of distressing symptoms, they can provide palliation without initiating CPR. Oral DNR orders are unacceptable because misunderstanding is likely and because nurses are placed in legal jeopardy if they do not initiate a code. "Slow" or shadow codes, in which CPR is perfunctorily administered in a manner known to be ineffective, are unethical because they deceive families into believing that maximal care is being provided.

The pediatrician will also need to discuss what other medical interventions may be withheld or provided. Everyone needs to understand that DNR does not mean withdrawal of all care or abandonment of the patient. Although a DNR order means only that CPR will be withheld, the same considerations that lead to a DNR order may also lead to limitations of other medical interventions. Such specific issues as intravenous lines, antibiotics for infection, and intensive care may need to be discussed. Many pediatricians and parents have an intuitive sense that "extraordinary" interventions should be withheld but "ordinary" measures continued. These terms, however, are ambiguous and confusing. Extraordinary measures are often considered to be high technology, invasive, or unusual. However, it is misleading to regard technologies as being intrinsically categorized as extraordinary or ordinary; the appropriateness of an intervention depends on the patient's condition and the desired goals of care. Thus, mechanical ventilation may be "extraordinary" for a patient with leukemia who has developed pneumonia after failing chemotherapy, but it would be considered ordinary care for a healthy child undergoing appendectomy. Hence, it is better to focus discussions on the goals of care and the benefits and burdens of interventions in the context of the child's prognosis.

Some interventions have symbolic significance. Many parents and health care workers regard tube feedings as "ordinary" care that should always be provided. To them, withholding artificial feeding would be like withholding nursing, formula, or food from a child, which would cause distress from hunger and thirst. Also, feeding a child is a basic responsibility for parents. Such deeply held feelings need to be acknowledged. However, pediatricians need to point out that in the terminal stages of illness, patients often stop taking oral food and fluids. Although caregivers should continue to offer sips of fluid and favorite foods, most patients do not experience hunger and thirst in the final days. Furthermore, good oral care and administration of analgesics if needed prevent symptoms of dry mouth and thirst. In addition, placing a feeding tube or intravenous line involves discomfort and invasiveness without proportionate benefits. The caring often associated with feeding can be provided directly, by cuddling an infant or holding an older child's hand.

Organizational arrangements for palliative care may be crucial. Often arrangements need to be made for visiting nurses or home hospice care. Hospice can provide in-home services, education for parents, rapid access to a skilled nurse, and attention to psychosocial and spiritual issues.

7.8   FUTILE CARE

A physician is under no legal or ethical obligation to provide treatment requested by parents that will offer little or no benefit to the child, and the parents should be told that the requested intervention is not an available option. This may be particularly likely to occur if a child has a disease for which the prognosis is extremely poor and the parent has discovered some "alternative" therapy, such as shark cartilage as a treatment for cancer, but the rule equally applies to ill-advised "conventional" therapies. Before discussions of "futility" commence, however, the physician should remember that the family of a dying child might have an entirely different definition of the term than the physician's. Simply having a child who is not dead may not seem "futile" to many parents; if that view cannot be respected by the physicians involved, the discussions about future care are themselves likely to be futile. This is never "business as usual" for a family.

Futility is a controversial concept that has several different interpretations. In its strict sense, futility refers to interventions that have no pathophysiological rationale, have already failed in the patient, or will not achieve the goals of care. In these situations, physicians have no ethical obligation to provide such interventions, and parents are not entitled to demand such interventions. In some cases, physicians use the term "futile" in a looser sense when they believe that the probability of success is unacceptably low, that the parents' goals for care are not worth pursuing, that the child's quality of life is unacceptable, or that the costs of the intervention do not justify a very small likelihood of benefit. Terming such care futile requires value judgments, not simply scientific expertise. In this looser sense, futility does not justify unilateral decisions by physicians to withhold interventions despite the objections of parents. However, it is appropriate for physicians to recommend to parents that such interventions be limited and to try to persuade them.

References

Blustein J, Levine C, Dubler N, eds: The Adolescent Alone: Decision Making in Health Care in the United States. New York, Cambridge University Press, 1999

Grodin MA, Glantz LH, eds: Children as Research Subjects: Science, Ethics, and Law. New York, Oxford University Press, 1994

Holder AR: Legal Issues in Pediatrics and Adolescent Medicine, 2nd ed. New Haven, Yale University Press, 1987

Koocher GP, Keith-Spiegel PC: Children, Ethics and the Law. Lincoln, University of Nebraska Press, 1990

Koren G, ed: Textbook of Ethics in Pediatric Research. Malabar, FL, Krieger Publishing Co, 1993

Melton GB, Koocher Gerald P, Saks MJ, eds: Children's Competence to Consent. New York, Plenum Press, (1977) 1983

Morrisey JM, Hofmann AD, Thrope JC: Consent and Confidentiality in the Health Care of Children and Adolescents: A Legal Guide. New York, The Free Press, 1986

Stanley B, Sieber JE, eds: Social Research on Children and Adolescents. Newbury Park, CA, Sage Publications, 1992

7.9   CARING FOR CHILDREN DYING FROM CHRONIC DISEASE

Arthur R. Ablin

The doctor, being himself a mortal man, should be diligent and tender in relieving his suffering patients, inasmuch as he himself must one day be like a sufferer.
Thomas Sydenham 1624–1689

The care and treatment of a child with chronic illness from which he or she is not expected to recover and is expected to die from sometime in childhood is one of the most difficult challenges we face as physicians and caregivers. Children who are dying deserve no less care than is given to those who are expected to live. This chapter is about the special aspects of giving that care to the approximately 10,000 children with chronic and incurable disease in the United States who are expected to die sometime in their childhood. It is also about the concept that comfort care, which requires at least the same or perhaps more planning, preparation, and forethought than we routinely give to children not expected to die, *is* treatment. Further, the suggestions herein are based on the indisputable fact that the death rate is one per person, and that includes the caregiver. What is good for our young patients is good for *our* children, and what is good for the parents of our young patients is good for *us*. We should treat our patients with the same care and compassion that we would wish our children and ourselves to receive.

The problems faced by children who will die in childhood from chronic disease are somewhat different from those of infants in the neonatal nursery or victims of accidents or acute illness in the emergency room or intensive care unit. Those equally devastating tragedies have some important differences that are valuable to recognize: (1) the caregivers have not had as much time to develop bonds of trust with the patient (possibly not at all) and family; (2) there may be few options for the patient to exert autonomy or control over the management; and (3) the family and patient may have had no time to prepare for the shock of the circumstances. However, the overwhelming grief requires many of the same sensitivities brought forth in discussions when there is time to prepare for a child's death. Furthermore, despite the relatively brief initial encounter with the physician, there is a need for continued contact to provide closure on personal issues and to address unresolved questions, many of which cannot even be thought of, let alone asked, at the time of the tragedy. Accordingly, it is an important obligation of caregivers to be available to the family long after the death of a child from an acute illness or accident and valuable for these caregivers to consider many of the same issues raised in the sections to follow.

It is my position that it is possible to teach a bright recent high school graduate how to successfully treat a newly diagnosed child with acute lymphoblastic leukemia. However, it is impossible to teach that high school graduate how to care for a child with an incurable disease who is expected to die and his or her family. The skills required are vastly different. In the imminently dying, the physician's own judgment, sensitivity, and communication skills in large part replace the drug, the scalpel, and the x-ray beam. Palliative care with the intent to prolong life and palliative care when death appears to be imminent place enormous responsibilities on the physician and his or her immediate helpers. Those burdens are great, but rewards from fulfilling the responsibilities the burdens bring can far outweigh them. No areas of medicine cause more sadness or emotional turmoil to the professional caregiver than caring for dying children, and likewise, none has the potential for bringing greater personal satisfaction or reward. It is my hope that this section will aid physicians and other caregivers to achieve those benefits.

CHRONIC ILLNESSES FROM WHICH CHILDREN DIE AND SOME OF THEIR SYMPTOMS

CANCER Cancer is the chronic disease that accounts for the greatest number of deaths during childhood. Although there have been remarkable improvements in survival since the 1970s, about 2200 children between 1 and 19 years of age die each year in the United States. Childhood cancers, most commonly acute leukemias, brain tumors, embryonal tumors, and soft tissue and bone sarcomas, are generally more rapidly growing and aggressive than adult carcinomas. Once the disease becomes resistant to therapy, the course to death is shorter and more fulminant than that observed in adults. Pain control is the major concern for symptom control for many. Anemia and thrombopenia secondary to bone marrow failure may cause asthenia and bleeding. Dyspnea secondary to pulmonary metastasis or pneumothorax, although not uncommon in children, generally is not a cause for the severe breathlessness seen in adults. Children with brain tumors have the multiple distressing symptoms of ataxia, diplopia and/or blindness, endocrinopathies, paralysis, headache, and vomiting, depending on the location of the tumor.

NEURODEGENERATIVE AND METABOLIC DISEASES These are individually rare diseases, but taken together they constitute a fair portion of children with chronic disease who may be expected to die before adulthood. This distressed group of children have disorders of lipid, amino acid, carbohydrate, or lysosomal enzyme metabolism that result in disease such as Nieman-Pick, Tay-Sachs, Krabbe disease, metachromatic leukodystrophy, Hurler syndrome, and Morquio syndrome. These sometimes intellectually impaired and severely physically ill children often have problems with mobility, vision, speech, incontinence, breathing, and convulsions. Symptom control is a major problem from birth to death.

CYSTIC FIBROSIS Cough, pulmonary infection, breathlessness, hemoptysis, and esophageal varices are very troublesome symptoms that increase in intensity as these children grow older and sicker. With improved care these children are now dying later and later in life, some even living long enough to have children of their own, bringing new social and ethical issues to their care. When near death, often in their 20s and 30s, these young adults are keen participants in the decision making concerning their care. The demands on the communication skills of the professional caregiver are great.

DISORDERS OF MUSCLE Death occurs after just a few years of life in children with spinal muscular atrophy and later in muscular dystrophy, the most common form of which is Duchenne muscular dystrophy. Inability to handle secretions, to swallow, or to cough, together with progressive respiratory failure necessitating assisted ventilation, are among the most distressing symptoms with disease progression in patients who remain mentally intact and intellectually alert. Loss of mobility and contractures add to the patient's struggles and increase the already taxed requirements for constant, demanding around-the-clock care.

CARDIAC DISEASES Congenital anomalies, acquired cardiomyopathies, or cardiac failure associated with cystic fibrosis or muscular dystrophy are the most common etiologic entities associated with cardiac death in children. Death may be unexpected and swift secondary to an arrhythmia or less surprising, as in the hospital postoperatively. Long-standing symptoms of fatigue, dyspnea, and edema become severe as death approaches.

HEPATIC FAILURE Congenital bile duct obstruction, chronic hepatitis resulting in jaundice, failure to survive, pruritus, variceal bleeding, ascites, hepatorenal syndromes, and encephalopathies are some of the symptoms that must be dealt with. Many children in the United States have organ transplantations and die secondary to transplant failure. As a result, most deaths occur in the hospital following attempts to correct the problems.

RENAL FAILURE Death from real failure may be rapid when secondary to electrolyte imbalance or may be over a period of months and years following failure of one or more transplants. Uremia, acidosis, and anemia may require chronic dialysis and result in fatigue, nausea, edema, fluid overload, and dyspnea.

DEFINITIONS

Palliative care with intent to prolong life: All treatments and care that occur when it has been agreed by consensus between patient or family and the caregivers that cure is no longer possible, but an attempt to prolong life will be the goal for treatment, as long as the quality of that life is considered equal to or greater than the emotional and physical costs of the treatment.

Palliative care for the imminently dying child: All care and treatments whose goals are to provide comfort when it is agreed by patients, families, and caregivers that the quality of life is so poor that prolonging life is not of value to the patient. Only interventions that bring comfort are considered treatments, and other interventions are avoided. If taking a temperature does not add to comfort, it is not done.

Treatment versus intervention: Physicians are prone to call what they do or cause to be done with the expectation of cure or relief "treatments." It is also the expectation of our patients that they will derive some benefit from these treatments. When the results of procedures or medications are unknown, we must refrain from referring to them as treatments, lest we introduce our understandable but misleading bias and unwisely influence our patients to accept them. In the desperation that occurs in patients, families, and caregivers when disease is no longer curable, there is the temptation to call "interventions" with unknown but hoped-for effects "treatment." We must call them what they are: "drugs or procedures with unknown but hoped-for effects." Honesty is imperative, especially in the care of incurable patients, if we are to retain their confidence and trust.

Hope and hopelessness: Approaching death is absolutely not a hopeless situation if it occurs with the closeness of those loved and is accompanied by genuine concern, honesty, openness, and expression of mutual grief and caring. Is this not our own "hope" when we reflect on our own inevitable death? We should not confuse an ill-placed hope for immortality with the reasonable expectation of hope for compassionate support during dying.

My own definition of hopelessness includes care lacking in expertise, abandonment, and insensitivity in times of great distress, whereas hope is expertise, attentiveness, and compassion at those same times. Hopelessness, is a toothache attended by an incompetent dentist who pulls the wrong tooth, followed by reaction from a family that is uncaring and unconcerned in a spiritually empty individual.

ABOUT COMMUNICATING BAD NEWS

ESTABLISHING A MODEL FOR COMMUNICATION The very first meeting at the original diagnosis of a chronic disease and every one after that set the stage for communication among the physician, patient, and family. The caregivers must provide a model for sensitivity, openness, honesty, and excellent listening skills. It may be expected that the model the physician establishes at the beginning of a relationship will define roles for the patient and family during the subsequent course of the illness. If a good dialogue is established at the beginning of a long-term relationship, the difficult discussions around end-of-life issues may be significantly eased.

PHYSICAL ARRANGEMENTS The key meeting with patients and families, where goals are set and important treatment decisions are made, should be well thought out beforehand and carefully planned. The physical aspects of the meeting are of utmost importance: a quiet, uncrowded room with all persons seated at the same level, and thought given to the body language expressed by each person's position. The physician should not sit behind a desk. Sufficient time needs to be set aside for adequate discussion and for questions to be answered. Care must be taken that all who are closely involved are present, and introductions must be made. Tape-recording the meeting allows patients to hear again, at less stressful times, the information shared. These are life-and-death issues and must be respected as such.

SEEKING INFORMATION The purpose of the meeting must be agreed on and clearly stated, and the discussion directed to achieve that purpose. The intent to receive as well as to give information should be mentioned. If it is not known, it is wise to start out by inquiring about the patient's and family's understanding of the present status of the illness. Much information may thereby be obtained that influences the content of the subsequent discussion. Remember that most patients and families want to be heard, so one must be a skilled listener. Do not feel compelled to fill in silences, which may be used by the patient or family for thinking. Inquire into the family's cultural and religious beliefs and indicate a respect for them. Make every effort to include the child patient at the appropriate cognitive level. Acknowledge awareness of the emotional strain this discussion puts on the patient and/or family. When the patient or a family member describes particularly difficult situations, indicate a willingness to understand and show compassion. "That must have been very difficult for you!" or "How terrible!" The intent to receive as well as to give information should be made clear.

SHARING INFORMATION After this initial interchange, the physician should disclose the medical information known to him or her in lay terms at an appropriate level for each family. The tremendous emotional strain for patients and families must be recognized, and communication must be clearly presented. Because retention is poor, important parts of the discussion should be repeated over and over both at the meeting and probably in the future. The physician

can recommend an appropriate goal for treatment for consideration by the family. Treatments compatible with the goal should be discussed. Care must be taken to give as much information as is desired and understood. The advantages and disadvantages of each treatment recommended should be included. Allow time for questions and gather from them the family's reaction to the recommendations. Consider alternative recommendations. When possible offer choices and seek family and patient opinions about which would be their preference and why. It is acceptable to give reassurance about the competency of the physician and institution to handle the situation if such is the case, or to express a willingness to arrange a second opinion if the family or patient chooses.

REACTIONS Anticipate that a flood of emotions may arise during the discussion: anger, hostility, frustration, grief, denial, guilt, or depression. Avoid being judgmental, acknowledge the behavior, and express empathy and a willingness to understand. Remember that when things go bad, most of the time people understand they may not be fixable but want their feelings acknowledged and respected.

AGREEING ON A PLAN Keep in mind the purpose of the meeting and adopt a goal for treatment and then a treatment plan to achieve that goal. All players must be in accord. The physician may have a recommendation in goal setting and may so state it but recognize that he or she is an advisor: the final decision lies with the patient and family. Success is achieved when all accept a plan. This is the time to summarize the discussion and agree on a method for accomplishing the plan.

TALKING WITH CHILDREN ABOUT DEATH

ADULT'S UNDERSTANDING OF DEATH It has been my experience that seriously ill children older than 2 to 3 years of age have an understanding of the seriousness of their illness and its potential fatal complications. However, it is important to recognize that the adult meaning of death is not usually achieved until approximately 7 to 8 years of age, and until then the consequence of a fatal illness is interpreted according to the cognitive development achieved at that time. We adults understand the permanent separation that occurs with death as well as its irrevocable condition. There is no calling back, no recovery, and no continuation. Further, we understand that death is logically caused by the cessation of all body functions and not by grievous spells, misdeeds, or witches. Death brings with it, as understood by adults, insensitivity and immobility. There is total absence of sensory input, no feeling, no coldness, pain, or hunger. We know all living creatures are destined to die, the concept of universality. There is no immortality, and mothers, fathers, sisters, and even we are not exceptions.

CHILDREN'S UNDERSTANDING OF DEATH Jean Piaget, a Swiss psychologist in the early 1900s, recognized that it takes time to acquire these associations, and children do so in an orderly fashion influenced by many factors in the cultural and family environment as well as the child's own psychological and cognitive makeup. Before 2 years of age all interactions with the outside world are sensory and motor, and there is probably no intellectual concept of death. Starting in early childhood, at 2 years and up to 7, orientation is self-centered, and the outside world is considered only from the child's personal and subjective point of view. It is a world in which reality exists primarily as it is manufactured from within and is not limited by logic. Imaginary and magical things are important determinants of occurrences. The concept of all things dying is not yet developed, and dead things should be able to eat and feel and breathe. Parents can be immortal, and dying animals should be able to return. With further development, from 7 to 11 years, thinking is less and less egocentric and, although more realistic, object orientated. Abstractions are still difficult. Reasoning is based on direct observation, and concepts of death are present. Their concerns of death are of separation and less concerned with afterlife and its abstractions. After age 12, full intellectual capacities develop, and with them the ability to deal in abstractions. The adult concepts of death are fully developed. Honesty, full disclosure, and directness are needed in dealing with adolescents.

TALKING WITH CHILDREN ABOUT THEIR OWN DEATH Given these benchmarks of child cognitive development, the following suggestions are offered for discussing their own impending death with children with incurable disease. Under 2 years of age no discussion of death is going to be understood, and, therefore, none needs to made. Symptom relief, comfort care, holding, and hugging are the requirements as death approaches. For the 2 to 7-year-old, death is seen as temporary, like sleep, and reversible and, perhaps, a result of magical actions originating within the child. It is necessary for this group to attempt to correct misperceptions about the cause of their grave illness and to correct feelings of guilt and self-blame. Separation and abandonment are major concerns and need to be addressed by the availability of the parents and stabilization of nursing care. Children starting about 7 begin to know that animals and people do not die because of a magical spell they or others cast but perceive reality and causation. They need to know the details of their care and to be reassured that pain and suffering will be treated and how. Truthfulness is paramount, and a description of details that adults might take for granted is necessary, as, for example, in death there is no pain or hunger or coldness. An adolescent's concerns about his or her changed physical appearance, hair loss, and weakness need to be acknowledged, and they must be given opportunity to express their anger.

Children deserve the same rights and privileges as adults: compassion, honesty, and respect. If it is felt wise and compassionate to discuss issues about death with seriously ill adults in order to allow them to share their concerns and fears, then it is equally wise to bring up such matters with children at a level compatible with their cognitive development. The physician should involve appropriate nurses, psychologists, art therapists, child study workers, and social workers, some of whom may bring valuable insights and expertise to the discussion. All questions about possible death are to be answered honestly and directly, as this presents the ideal opportunity to explore the subject. What has worked for me is a simple statement that it must be so very difficult to be so ill, and then ask: What is the hardest thing about it? Other open-ended questions that generate conversation are: How do you think your treatment is going? What do you think will happen to you? Do you think you will be able to go back to school? Do you want to keep taking your medicines? What do you think would happen if you stopped your medicines? It must always be remembered that people of all ages in great stress, and especially children, don't expect those stresses to be fixed, they just want acknowledgment that the listener has some appreciation of how great those stresses really are. Great good comes from just listening and shaking one's head. It is seldom that a seriously ill child asks, "Am I going to die?" If they do, it is almost certainly because they know they are, and they are probing if it is safe to talk about it. False, overly reassuring answers are only evasive and certain to stop meaningful conversation. Answers like "I'm worried for you because the last medications, as you know, did not work. It's possible but I am not sure. What do you think?" Also if the conditions are such "I think it's the transfusions and oxygen or antibiotics that are keeping you alive. If we stopped them, you would die. You probably knew that, didn't you? That opens another opportunity for discussion like -"I'm not sure what happens to people when they die. What do you think?" Since none of us know, it is best to help others find their answers rather than provide one for them.

Some children have questions but are hesitant or unable to express them. Also, they may be willing to talk at certain times or with certain individuals but not at others. Appropriate nurses, psychologists, art therapists, child life workers, and social workers have valuable *expertise and availability and should freely be called on to assist.*

HOW WILL I DIE? Children over 5 to 7, like adults, worry not only if they will die but also how they will. "What is it going to be like?" Both children and adults seldom ask even if very concerned for fear of going into territory too difficult for the caregiver or because of the risk of breaking a mutual pretense that such a problem doesn't exist and, therefore, is best avoided. Imagination can run rampant and be much worse than the truth. Inaccuracies can be corrected, and horror stories dispelled. Fortunately, most children die a relatively peaceful death. Depending on the diagnosis, they can usually be reassured their death will be peaceful with pain controlled and with their parents and loved ones present. This is an opportunity to give reassurance for continuity of care, pain control, and intensification of supportive and comfort care. The risks for producing apprehension are great, but when such discussions are entered with great sensitivity, caution, and judgment, the opportunity to bring relief is greater.

LAST GOOD-BYES Like adults, children need time for their last good-byes and to put their affairs in order. To whom they would give their favorite baseball cards or dolls, stamp collections, or varsity sweaters is as important to children as putting financial affairs and saying goodbye to spouses and friends is to adults. Verbalization is difficult for some children, and here again, art therapy, puppet play, and music are alternatives to talking. Child life workers are especially trained in such techniques and should be called on. Care providers must understand that it is necessary to set aside time for these discussions, which are every bit as important as anything else in the therapeutic armamentarium.

SPECIAL PROBLEMS OF ADOLESCENTS

Just as adolescents have a full adult understanding of the implications of incurable disease and impending premature death, they are aware of the joys and satisfactions that are so unfairly being denied to them. They realize that they are in the spring of their lives and should be thrilled with anticipation of the future rather than facing the bleakness and emptiness of death. This should be a time of discovery, growth, seemingly limitless energy, and strength and invincibility. Instead they are aware their lives are being cut short, and they are being robbed of the opportunity to see their expectations achieved. At a time they are most sensitive about their physical appearance their body shames them to themselves and, in their perception, to their peers. When they so vividly anticipate independence, want privacy, and seek out social relationships with their schoolmates, they become dependent on parents and physicians, lose in the most intimate way their privacy, and are separated from peers. Understandable reactions to the condition thrust on them through no fault of their own are denial, anger, depression, and withdrawal. Who can blame them? How do we help them?

HELPING WITHOUT FIXING

It is appropriate here, to retell the story of the broken bicycle. Johnny, a boy of 9, is sent by an awaiting family on a 5-minute errand to pick up milk for dinner. He returns after 20 minutes to an impatient household. After being severely chastised for taking so long he is asked for an explanation. "Just outside the door on the way home," he explains, "my friend, Billy, was crying because his bicycle was broken. I stopped to help him." The father questions, "What do you mean you helped him? You're only 9; you don't know how to fix a bicycle!" Johnny answers almost incredulously: "Why, I helped him cry."

Similarly we caregivers must realize not everything has to be or can be fixed in order to be helped. Children will die. The depths of the despair of our patients, children, adolescents, and also adults sometimes cannot be fixed but almost certainly can be helped by acknowledgment, empathy, and compassion. The power of these tools is too often underestimated by physicians and, therefore, not chosen for use when they may be the most effective forms of treatment.

DIFFICULTIES FACED BY SIBLINGS AND GRANDPARENTS

SIBLINGS Depending on their age, brothers and sisters of chronically ill children face a set of problems unique to them. If they are in the 2- to 10-year-old range, there may be feelings of guilt that they might have caused their sibs incurable illness. They may have concerns that they may become ill like their sib or perhaps even wish that they had the same illness so that they would receive similar lavish attention. Falling school performance, resentment, enuresis, and acting-out behavior have all been described. Including them in family decision making, giving them meaningful responsibilities in the family, providing honest reassurance about the chances of two in the family acquiring the same disease, and relieving guilt if it is determined that the sib feels instrumental in causing the illness are all helpful measures. Parents should be advised of the special problems of sibs and encouraged to anticipate them during the entire course of the patient's illness.

GRANDPARENTS Grandparents, often among the most serious of the unforgotten emotionally injured, deserve special consideration in the care of children with incurable and terminal disease. They are in double jeopardy, having both a grieving child and a dying grandchild. In addition, they are a step removed from making decisions about care and thus have heightened feelings of helplessness and frustration. Caregivers, after receiving patient and/or parental permission, should include them when possible in information sharing and take time to listen to their concerns. A special consultation with them is always appreciated and may make them feel less helpless and, therefore, less critical.

GOAL SETTING AND DECISION MAKING

WHEN CURE IS NO LONGER POSSIBLE When cure is no longer a possibility, decisions must be made about future care. Palliation with a goal to prolong life and palliative care with the goal to achieve maximum comfort but not to prolong life are the treatment options available. Health care professionals, patients, and family members must all be involved as these difficult decision-making processes evolve. Until the goals of care are established and accepted by all parties, the necessary treatment decisions are made in a vacuum and proceed in no apparent direction. Too often consensus-derived goals are not established before an intervention course is started. Confusion, disagreement, anger, and frustration within the family and among caregivers often are the result because goals are different among all members.

WHY ACCEPTANCE OF THIS GOAL IS SO DIFFICULT

THE PATIENT AND FAMILY Acceptance of the reality that cure is no longer possible is required to permit decision making about treatment once disease, in fact, becomes incurable. Many reasons, however, stand in the way of both patients and families accepting this condition. Hope for cure must be cast aside, and the reality of impending death must be faced. This is an extremely difficult admission in a society in which children are not supposed to die and the concept of childhood death is unacceptable. Guilt, most often unjustified, is an ever-present emotion. "What if I had gotten my child to the doctor sooner?" or other "what ifs" are on almost every parent's mind. Denial, the ability to not recognize facts because of their unacceptability, itself becomes unacceptable once incurability is recognized. To even discuss incurability is so emotionally painful and almost intolerable for all parties, it is frequently avoided. This barrier to communication has been termed "mutual pretense" in which only safe topics are discussed as all parties pretend nothing is wrong. Conversations are terminated or the topic is changed when there is danger of crying or breaking down. As a result, the necessary decision making about the goals of subsequent treatment is left undone.

THE HEALTH PROVIDER Coupled with this are the pain and bias of the health provider who finds confrontation with death issues difficult both for him or herself and the patients and families as well as extremely time consuming. A sense of failure may exist because the previous attempt for cure has been unsuccessful. There exists a perceived need to protect patients and families, and an attempt is often made to do so by avoiding full disclosure, to be overly reassuring and optimistic. It is also time saving to avoid very troubling, emotion-laden discussions.

THE UNCERTAINTY OF DEATH It is not always possible for the physician to know with absolute certainty that cure is no longer possible. Rare reported survivals and experimental therapies might offer a modicum of chance for cure. This complicates the already difficult problems faced by the patient and family and explains even more why such decisions are made too late in the dying process, sometimes hours before death. Futile attempts at cure can result in terrible hardship and are to be avoided. Acceptance of the incurability of disease is hard enough when honest and open discussion is possible but nearly impossible when it is not.

PALLIATIVE CARE WITH LIFE-PROLONGING GOAL Once the goal for cure must be abandoned, what options for treatment are available? Children with incurable disease may still have months or even years of good quality of life. Life-prolonging treatments that are not so arduous that they eliminate or minimize the quality of life are acceptable. Antibiotics, chemotherapy, radiation therapy, diagnostic testing, and surgery are compatible with the goal of life-prolonging measures as long as they do not destroy the good quality of remaining life. Caregivers must frequently reassess the patient's quality of life together with the physical and emotional burdens of the treatment that may be prolonging it. As the disease become more resistant to intervention and unresponsive, it is inevitable that even palliation with prolongation of life will no longer be an available goal or one in which the burdens exceed the benefits. It is important that this recognition is not delayed by the continuing use of burdensome interventions that deny the dying child the good quality of life that still may be available to him or her. The physician should be assisted when possible by the patient and certainly the family in this important decision-making process. Physicians and other health providers should not be doing this alone.

COMFORT CARE Most difficult of all decision-making discussions are those about the necessity to giving up both cure and life-prolonging palliative goals and the adoption of comfort care as the goal for treatment. It is here that the patient, family, and physician must be convinced that comfort care *is* treatment and that a time has arrived when death is the therapeutic option of choice. There is no such entity as "no treatment." Comfort care is treatment and not abandonment or lessening of treatment or care but is, in fact, intensification. No one should say or murmur or even think that there is "no treatment" when the end of life approaches. It is not a giving up but an acceptance of reality and a wise and compassionate change in direction with great intensity. This is an often-missed therapeutic window that has the opportunity to prolong living and shorten dying. If, sooner rather than later, the physical and psychosocial burdens associated with fruitlessly attempting to prolong life are removed, the benefits of being alive, overshadowed by the burdens of intervention, can become realized. When this is understood by all, it is possible to make a decision for this optimal treatment. Treatment at this stage is intensive, demanding, time consuming, and highly personal for both the patient and the physician. There must be no slacking back of treatment when comfort care is the goal.

DO NOT RESUSCITATE ORDER

When comfort is chosen as the goal for treatment of the imminently dying child, invasive and heroic measures to prolong life are not consistent with that goal. An important part of that decision-making discussion should be the wisdom of instituting or not a "Do Not Resuscitate" order. Unless specifically contravened, at the time of cardiac or pulmonary collapse, resuscitation must be attempted, unfortunately, sometimes with grave results. The physician, after discussion with the patient, if reasonable, and family, must document in the chart their willingness to not have a resuscitation attempt started. This discussion and with whom must be documented in the progress notes, and a specific "Do Not Resuscitate" order written in the order sheet. A carefully considered and unhurried discussion should occur during the period of transition from the goal of palliative therapy with prolongation of life to the goal of

comfort care when there is no imminent threat of death and adequate time to consider it. It should be viewed by the patient and family as another step for them, assisted by the physician, to secure control of the dying process and of its treatment. When accord is properly obtained, there should be the realization that nothing beneficial is being withheld, but the treatment for comfort is obtained.

HOME, HOSPITAL, OR HOSPICE DEATH?

ABSENCE OF EMERGENCIES When the goal for treatment becomes comfort care rather than the prolongation of life, events that, up to that time, were considered emergencies because they were threatening to life are no longer such. They can be cared for equally well in the hospital, a free-standing hospice, or in the home. Fevers require neither blood cultures nor antibiotics; bleeding does not have to be halted, and convulsions can be treated with expectation to stop or, when prolonged, with medications that can be made available in the home. In the United States, care of the child expected to die imminently generally occurs in the hospital or home and much less commonly in a freestanding hospice. Where death occurs depends in large part on the wishes, psychosocial status, and special circumstances of the family including the child. The physical characteristics of the home must also be considered. Acceptance of a "no emergency" philosophy allows the home to be the place of choice for many families.

HOME For end-of-life care to be at home, the family must be able and willing to accept the not to be underestimated taxing responsibility that comes with this decision. The child must want to be at home. Basic physical needs must be available, such as telephone, transportation, and a space for the sick child that offers some degree of quiet and privacy. The physician for the child and home health care services should be available to provide medical, nursing, and pharmacy assistance. Respite facilities provided by the community or extended family and friends should be available to the family to provide the intermittent relief they will desperately need. In case the family becomes overwhelmed, the opportunity of readmission to the hospital must be available.

The benefits of dying at home are many. If one asks what is missed most by families and chronically sick children in this situation, it is the opportunity to be normal; nothing special, "just normal." Few can appreciate more the beauty and tranquility of being "just normal." Children are more comfortable in their own home environment and have a sense of normality. A family living at home instead of existing around a hospital, even with a dying child, can carry on some aspects of their normal activities, eg, eating together, continuing at school or work part time, being close to friends. Parents, siblings, and other family members have the opportunity to participate first hand in the care of the child and reap the benefits that come with fulfilling a need and taking responsibility. Great satisfaction comes with taking charge and having a sense of control. There is an opportunity for family interaction and communication, permitting a strengthening of relationships that is very much treasured after the child's death. Local health professionals also are able to participate in care and enjoy the satisfactions that would not be possible were death to occur in the tertiary hospital.

HOSPITAL But home death is not for all families or children. There may be cultural or ethnic contraindications that must be respected. Other families do not have the physical space, the emotional stability, or the support to handle the difficult task. The location of the home may make the opportunity for in-home supportive services difficult or impossible. Some children and families develop great security with the hospital and staff and are more comfortable there. Each child and family, with their attendant special circumstances, require individual considerations. Family decisions must be supported and care taken not to be critical of families who refuse the chance to have a home death for their child.

HOSPICE Although free-standing and in-home hospice services are increasingly available for adults, few such services are available in the United States for children. Free-standing children's hospices that provide either total care or temporary respite care for children who are near the ends of their lives and their families are more available in Europe and Canada. They provide a service and ambiance intermediate to the institutional atmosphere of the hospital and the informality and familiarity of home and provide a niche of care that is of great benefit. Many primarily adult hospices will provide in-home services to families of dying children. Their services are invaluable and should be sought.

RESPONSIBILITIES OF THE PHYSICIAN AT THE TIME OF A HOSPITAL DEATH

PRONOUNCEMENT A task required of almost every physician, sometime in his or her career, is the pronouncement of death. When the death is that of a child, the task is particularly onerous. On reflection, it is not the determination of death that is so difficult, but rather the interaction with the family that occurs immediately thereafter. I would like to share my thoughts with the reader of how a not unexpected death in the hospital can be handled. What follows is my own style and represents only one way and certainly leaves room for many other styles.

It must be remembered the reason the physician is called for the pronouncement of death of a child is to remove any doubt that death has occurred. The pronouncement, therefore, should include the word death or died rather than a euphemism, which may evade the issue. "I'm sorry to share with you that Johnny has died" or "I'm sorry to say Johnny has died" is a suitable example of compassionate definitive statement.

TOUCHING After such tragic news, no matter how long death had been expected, an emotional dam is broken, and there is no way or need to stop it. For a time, words become meaningless, and nothing needs to be said or done other than standing next to or touching the parent's shoulder or hand. One should not underestimate the helping quality of touch at such a time, perhaps because it connects people and is an expression of empathy. Respectful silence and touching acknowledge compassion for the moment in a way as good as or better than any other.

SIBLINGS If other family members are not in the room but elsewhere in the hospital, particularly if there are siblings, they should be sent for. Siblings over 2 to 3 years are best with the family at this point rather than separated and "protected." If possible, they should be met outside the room to prepare them for what follows. In announcing the death to others not in the room at the time of pronouncement, one should address the youngest in the group. Children under 3 should not be ignored but be addressed directly and told that their sib has just died. "Your brother Tommy has just

died. Your Mom is in the room, and I want to tell you about Tommy and how you can help your Mom and Dad." It will be helpful to tell them that their dead brother or sister will look as they always had but that they will not be able to hear, respond, move, or feel anything. When touched, their body may feel cold. They should be told that the death was not their fault. Parents will, of course, understand what is said to the child, but the language has to be geared to the understanding of the youngest family member.

PRIVACY Once the family is together, an offer should be made to give them time and privacy as a family to be with the dead child. If accepted, one should return at intervals to visually check when the family has had enough time. This is generally indicated by their drawing back from the bed and not touching the deceased and having some conversation among themselves.

REASSURANCE Among the first comments on reentry could be to reassure the family that they have done all that it was possible for them to do and shown great love and devotion for the deceased. This addresses an overriding concern that they will most likely have and helps to partially relieve the inevitable guilt that parents almost always feel. As the caregiver physician, wouldn't you like someone to say the same to you at that time? Our families or our colleagues often do this for us.

VENTILATION AND ACKNOWLEDGEMENT Allow the family members to vent their frustration, anger, or disappointment by, perhaps, bringing up some outstanding characteristic of the dead child and waiting for a response. "I don't think I ever heard him omit saying thank you when we brought something to him." Another observation that may stimulate ventilatory remarks from the family is "What is so exceptionally difficult about a child's death is that it is not just the child who dies but everything he or she might have been. He was a whiz with Legos, wasn't he?" Most families will seize this opportunity to emote. The physician's willingness to open such a discussion indicates empathy and compassion, which is exactly what people in great crisis need to know; ie, their pain is recognized and acknowledged. They know that he death cannot be undone or fixed. The most help comes with the recognition that others are aware of their pain. One needs to listen and almost only nod.

CHECKLIST At the time of a child's death, caregivers should avoid asking the already burdened family what they would like done but rather offer suggestions they may accept or decline. A checklist should be kept in mind and could be as follows: "I will call the doctor who referred you here. I am certain he or she will want to know," or "There are probably others who will want to know. We can call whomever you would like." This will serve as a reminder to the family that others may need to be informed. "We have a chaplaincy program in the hospital and a chaplain or rabbi would be pleased to come if you would like. I can call them." "Where are you staying? We can call them and let them know what happened." "Can we help you gather your things together." "Will you need something for sleep tonight? I can order it for you." "If you are going home today, driving may be a problem for you. We can call someone you know to pick you up." "If you have arranged for a funeral home, we will take care of calling them. You do not have to decide on any details of a service at this time." If the family has not made a choice of mortuary services, the "If you do not know of a funeral home, we can call the doctor who referred you here, and he or she may be able to help us with some names."

AUTOPSY An autopsy should be requested on every child who dies in the hospital. It is the best way to insure that errors in diagnosis and treatment have not occurred and that unsuspected pathology has not been overlooked. There is something to be learned from each death and each autopsy. It is the obligation of the attending physician to request permission for the postmortem examination of every child who dies in the hospital. This request must be approached sensitively while respecting the ethnic and religious customs of the family, yet recognizing a need to obtain permission. In circumstances when most answers are believed known before death, then any reluctance of the family may be accepted. On the other hand, when important questions for the family or physicians can be answered only by the autopsy, a cautious, sensitive, and considerate request for permission is acceptable.

One reasonable way to approach the subject is as follows: "It is our belief that a postmortem examination (autopsy) will clarify the cause of death, answer any questions that we or you may have had about treatments, or even learn about anything that was unsuspected. We ask your permission." Some families will have a reluctance to grant permission, and it is acceptable to determine why. It is often possible that the examination can be modified to accommodate those concerns by omitting a part of the procedure and still obtain necessary and important information. When it is of exceptional importance to answer clinical questions and the family is still reluctant, one can limit the examination to just an abdominal incision through which a significant portion of the routine exam can be completed. Even an appendectomy-sized incision offers many opportunities to obtain tissues. When families are reluctant to do even that, it should be remembered that a postmortem examination limited to needle biopsies can reveal answers to clinical conditions, and this opportunity can be offered to the family. Families should be informed of the preliminary results of the exam within a day or two by phone. When the final histologic examination is completed, many families would welcome the opportunity to return for a discussion of the findings and to review the entire course of the illness. This is a therapeutic visit of considerable value in the bereavement process.

BEREAVEMENT

EXPRESSING CONCERN Bereavement is the emotional state that individuals in families of a dead child are in for a period after the death. Anticipatory grief is the emotional state contemplating bereavement. Not uncommonly, all family members of a dying child minimize or deny their own emotional reactions, feeling either that it is selfish to be concerned about themselves while a child is dying or that they must not dilute the care to the child. Encouraging them to express those concerns, however, may ease some of their own tensions and even allow more open communication with the dying child. Expression of anticipatory grief may ease the travail of the bereavement after death.

EMPTINESS Death of a child causes an emptiness and sense of missing in the family that must be dealt with in the bereavement period. Recognized patterns of behavior are attempting to forgive and forget, to put the death behind them as if it were God's will or nature at work. Another is filling the missing space by increasing work and preoccupation as if replacing the emptiness produced by the death with something more acceptable. The most effective form of bereavement is keeping a connection with the deceased by continuing to talk about him or her and acknowledging his or her absence while seeing the value of continuing on with life and family matters.

PROGNOSTIC DETERMINANTS One of the most emotionally traumatic of all events is for a parent to lose a child. Guilt, despair, depression, grief, anger, frustration, and disappointment are the normal components of the initial bereavement period. In spite of the gravity of those reactions, when they are accompanied by an ability to communicate about them to other family members and friends, the outlook is good. Likewise, parents who are able to look out at life continuing about them, are willing to participate, and who retain flexibility in actions and thought can be reassured that their grief, though overwhelming at times, is proper and within the normal limits. Focus and chat groups are helpful in allowing expression of feelings to an empathetic audience while dispelling the idea that they are alone in their despair. They can be reassured, however, of the normality of their reaction and that psychiatric referral is unnecessary.

Those in need of additional help are those who become uncommunicative, withdrawn, and choose to stay apart from society in semiisolation. They may become frozen in the time of the death of the child and have diminished sense of the world, which continues to go on about them. Frequent and continued communication with the pediatric team and psychiatric referral are indicated.

DURATION The length of the bereavement period is highly variable from family to family and among individuals within that family, and no definite time period for normal bereavement can be stated. Years after the death of a child or sibling, there may be short periods of intense grief brought about by a birth date that recalls the deceased child to mind. In this fashion bereavement may never end. However, when the bereaved are able to reenter into social and economic activities, to view current activities as relevant to their lives, and to look to the future in anticipation of better things, the bereavement period can be considered to be reasonably resolved. Being able to talk in a cheerful way about the deceased child, remembering both the good and mischievous parts of his or her life, are healthy signs of that resolution.

HELPING THE BEREAVED FAMILY The key to helping the family of a recently deceased child is continued involvement and contact, with as many members as possible realizing that each is affected in his or her own way. The assistance of all members of the health care team is invaluable during this time. All must realize is that what the bereaved need most is reassurance, if true, that their feelings of grief are normal and expected and that time and the work of grief will help to dull the pain. Further, the most important role the health professional can serve is in acknowledging to the bereaved the appropriateness of their grief. No one expects that the deceased can be recalled, but if the grief of the bereaved can be understood and validated by the health care worker, that is of enormous benefit and is all that can be expected. Encourage talk about the deceased child, both the good and the bad qualities, because this promotes reality and resolution. Participation in focus groups or sometimes even computer chat rooms may allow outlets for emotion or give insight into an individual's difficulties.

SIBLINGS' BEREAVEMENT Siblings, perhaps as much as parents, have a sense of emptiness, especially if they are close in age to the deceased child and have been close companions in play or at school. Their behavioral reaction to the death may be wide ranging, from loneliness to anger or attention seeking. They may even become more fearful of falling ill themselves and facing death.

Siblings need reassurance about their own role in their sibling's death. The level of reassurance is age- and development-related. Children less than 8 or 9 years of age may not have a good understanding of the causes of death, leading them to think that they or their wishes might have caused the death. This could result in guilt, self-incrimination, and fear of reprisal and to subsequent behavioral dysfunction. Siblings should be routinely followed after the child's death for evidence of related disabilities. Referral to counseling or psychiatric help should be made for those sibs with worsening school performance, erratic behavior, or withdrawal.

GRANDPARENTS' BEREAVEMENT Besides parents, grandparents may be hard hit in the postdeath period, mourning the loss of a grandchild at the same time as witnessing the grief of their own child. They may be hesitant to seek help, feeling that others in the family are in greater need and not wishing to distract from the needs of others. They may be behind the scene and less noticeable to the treating team. It is well to inquire about their welfare.

CARE OF MEDICAL PROFESSIONALS

Medical caregivers, not at all unlike the patients and families they treat, are subject to the great emotional pain that accompanies the care of a chronically ill child who ultimately dies. The repeated exposure to such tragedy makes even more difficult the burdens attendant with caregiving. With repeated death can come frustration, a prolonged sense of failure, helplessness, sadness, and even depression. With so much suffering around them in their patients and families, it is not difficult to think that there is reluctance of the professionals to admit to or discuss their own difficulties. Almost unbelievably, there is no one on the treatment team part of whose purpose is to care for the professional caregivers. Where then do the professionals find help?

SOURCES OF SUPPORT FROM WITHIN One source of support must come from within and from the realization of the great satisfaction that comes with providing care at the end of life. There is the opportunity to be of great help to those experiencing one of life's greatest tragedies. An immensely personal and close direct relationship exists between physician and patient. If one is able to reach out to help, he or she will certainly find a hand appreciatively grasping for it from a truly needy individual. There are few greater satisfactions in medicine, and from these the caregiver can find the strength to continue, often with even greater enthusiasm. With the realization and appreciation of these rewards, the caregiver can avoid the noxious effects leading to burnout and depression. Prevention is a much better therapeutic modality than treatment.

COLLEAGUES Important sources of support include other members of the treatment team. Open communications about the dilemmas of care, difficult families, the futility of treatments, the social injustices, and the apparent inhumanity of our God are fair game in periodic team support meetings. It is important that team members, like our patients, have this opportunity to express their frustrations and to release their own burdens. A well-functioning treatment team is of great help to one another.

SYMPTOM MANAGEMENT

Most symptoms faced by dying children are treated in much the same fashion as in the acute or chronically ill. The significant differences when they occur are in the matter of intensity and the realization that the goal is as complete relief and comfort as possible. Some side effects such as sedation, perhaps intolerable in the nondying child, may be acceptable in the dying. It is also to be realized that ordinarily one treats symptoms by eliminating their cause. In the imminently dying that is usually not possible. The symptom generally must be eliminated pharmacologically, and often sedation or obtundation is the most effective approach. A few remarks follow about the special problems encountered in the treatment of symptoms of dying children. The reader is also referred to longer and more detailed discussion than space allows here in the list of references.

PAIN Patients under our care have the right to pain control and we physicians have the obligation to do all in our power to relieve the pain while avoiding the morbidity that may be associated with the treatment.

BENEFICENCE, NONMALEFICENCE, AND THE DOUBLE EFFECT Beneficence, the quality of causing benefit, must be balanced by nonmaleficence, the quality that requires no harm be done. Nowhere more than in the management of sedation and pain control in the imminently dying is the balance between beneficence and nonmaleficence more sharply defined. The achievement of adequate pain control may require doses of opiates that lead to oversedation, hypoxia, and subsequent death and therefore may do harm. Inadequate pain control fails to control symptoms and produces no benefit. This may create a moral and ethical dilemma in the care of the dying child with severe pain. The principle of the "double effect" addresses the dilemma by looking into intent. If the intent is to relieve pain, beneficence, possible untoward and unintended consequences, even death, are acceptable. The physician's intent in providing pain-relieving medications, however, should not be to cause or hasten death, which would not be consistent with the principle of nonmaleficence, that no harm be done.

THE PAIN LADDER The ladder approach promoted by the World Health Organization selects progressively stronger analgesic drugs based on the severity of the pain. It provides an excellent guideline and is of proven effectiveness. One moves up a ladder from simple acetaminophen-like drugs to codeine to opiates, not abandoning previous drugs but adding to them and increasing doses in a stepwise fashion. Children, like adults, experiencing chronic pain may become tolerant of opioids and require increasing doses. Standard doses commonly become inadequate, and the prescriber must become aware that the *correct* dose is the amount required to control the symptoms. That is the test. The route of administration when repeated doses and continuous effect are necessary is important. Oral, sublingual, transdermal, and intravenous routes through a central catheter with patient-controlled devices each have specific places. Intramuscular and rectal routes are so traumatic to children that they are almost always unacceptable.

EMOTIONAL PAIN In addition to nociceptive pain, the caregiver must be aware of the overwhelming emotional pain that can occur with dying. Pain should be considered multifactorial, including not only the physical reasons but also the contributions coming from the familial, psychosocial, and ethnic milieu. For many, the emotional pain is equal to or greater than the pain from identifiable physical causes. Both pharmacologic and nonpharmacologic approaches are necessary. Benzodiazapenes such as diazepam, lorazepam, and midazolam may be needed to relieve accompanying agitation. Consideration of the use of antidepressants such as amitriptyline or imipramine, neuroleptics such as chlorpromazine or haloperidol, and stimulants such as dextroamphetamine or methylphenidate should be part of the pharmacologic armamentarium.

In some circumstances such as cord or root compression, neurosurgical and anesthetic approaches to pain relief may be necessary, such as epidural anesthesia or cordotomy.

Nonpharmacologic approaches are important additions and should be included relatively early in the planning of care. Cognitive treatments such as psychotherapy, hypnosis, and imagery are tailored to both caregiver and patient. Physiotherapy and massage, biofeedback, behavior modification, and relaxation therapy may all be useful. Pain control is a multidisciplinary endeavor and must be recognized as such in the treatment of the dying child.

NUTRITION AND HYDRATION For the dying child who can no longer be fed by mouth, feeding by nasogastric or nasoduodenal tube or gastrostomy and intravenous hydration raise ethical and cultural problems requiring individual solutions. A part of the answer to provide alternative feeding and hydration routes is to be found when a clear concept of the goals of treatment has been mutually adopted by the patient, family, and physician. If palliative care with the intention of prolonging life is the goal of treatment because the quality of life is acceptable, one must ask if the tube feeding, gastrostomy, or intravenous line so destroys the quality of life that goals must change. Then one can reasonably question the use of such invasive measures. Thirst in the imminently dying is not a bothersome symptom, and any mentioned discomfort is usually relieved with mouth swabs. There is no moral or ethical requirement demanding alternative feeding routes. The wishes of the family and their ethnic and religious orientation should strongly influence decision making.

SEIZURES For some children with neurodegenerative disorders or brain tumor, seizures may be a part of their routine care. Seizures, on the other hand, may not be a problem for many children, but all parents caring for an imminently dying child at home should be prepared for this possibility. Families need be reassured that seizures that prove to be short may need nothing more than observation. In the case of prolonged seizures, when an intravenous line is not available, parents should be instructed in the use of either rectal diazepam or lorazepam diluted in saline at specific doses for individual patients. It may never need to be used but brings confidence and reassurance to parents participating in a home care program that they have a program for action in case this trying situation develops. Anticipatory discussion should include any conditions in which convulsion might cause consideration of rehospitalization, so hasty decision making might be avoided.

BREATHLESSNESS Anxiety is the major symptom to be controlled when oxygen does not relieve symptoms associated with breathlessness. Opioids in doses necessary to relieve anxiety with no top dose recognized, coupled with the benzodiazepines, diazepam or lorazepam, are the important drugs to manage this troublesome symptom. If secretions are troublesome, then atropine or glyco-

pyrrolate may offer additional support by their anticholinergic effectiveness.

SLEEP DISTURBANCES Sleeplessness may be associated with pain, side effects of medications, or anxiety. It may be extremely troublesome for patients and their families. A wide variety of agents should be considered, such as hydroxyzine, chloral hydrate, barbiturates, and benzodiazepines. For depression amitripyline may be considered. Nonpharmacologic considerations are guided imagery, music therapy, and relaxation tapes.

ETHICAL CONSIDERATIONS

Children who have chronic illness have surprising insight into their disease based on their personal experience with the symptoms they have, the effects of the medications they have taken, and the procedures they have endured. If they are cognitively mature enough to be able to understand the significance of their own morbidity and death, then they should be accorded the autonomy that allows them the right of participation in decision making. This requires disclosure of diagnosis, treatment options, and prognosis. They deserve to be treated with honesty, openness, and respect for their rights. They should give assent to planned procedures and medical treatments before they are performed. It is important that the rights of parents are not placed above those of the child.

SPIRITUAL MATTERS

There is need in the care of the dying to address matters other than the physical. Older children and parents almost all express a need that transcends the material and addresses concepts that go beyond oneself: questions like "For what purpose do we live?" and "What are my correct values?" and "What exists beyond myself?"

A formal system with established rules and customs may be considered a religion. Although not all individuals may embrace a religion, almost everyone has a spiritual identification. As death approaches, this sense of spirituality increases. Our patients welcome the opportunity to discuss these highly personal values with those they respect and with whom they feel safe. All members of the health care professional team, and not only the chaplain, are such individuals. Attending to the spiritual matters of the mind and soul of our patients as well as to their physical ailments is not beyond the borders of what physicians are allowed, and may have some responsibility, to do.

References

Ablin AR, ed: Supportive Care of Children with Cancer, 2nd ed. Baltimore, Johns Hopkins University Press, 1997

Baile WF, Kudelka AP, Beale EA, et al: Communication skills training in oncology. Cancer 86:867–897, 1999

Doyle D, Hanks WC, MacDonald N: Oxford Textbook of Palliative Medicine. Oxford, Oxford University Press, 1998

Martinson IM: Improving care of dying children. West J Med 163:258–262, 1995

Mcgrath PA: Pain in Children: Nature, Assessment and Treatment. New York, Guilford Publications, 1990

Wolfe J, Grier HE, Klar N, et al: Symptoms and suffering at the end of life in children with cancer. N Engl J Med 342:326–333, 2000

CONTEMPORARY DIAGNOSTIC TECHNIQUES

Norman Siegel, Associate Editor

CONTEMPORARY APPROACH TO PATIENT EVALUATION AND DIAGNOSIS

With increasing frequency, it is possible to establish a specific diagnosis for children who have complex and sometimes obscure disorders. A systematic approach and in-depth understanding of childhood diseases requires the use of a variety of modalities from imaging studies to molecular genetics. Moreover, implementing evidence-based practice requires an ability to understand, assess, and interpret both clinical studies and diagnostic tests. Four major aspects of a contemporary approach to the evaluation of patients and establishing a diagnosis are reviewed from the perspective of the information that can be gained and the application of that knowledge to the care of patients. Specific tests and/or diagnostic criteria as related to a defined disorder are provided in other chapters, which discuss those specific disease states. Molecular genetics provides the backbone for our understanding of a number of disorders and represents a technology that will advance our understanding of both susceptibility to and the pathogenesis of many child health-related problems. An understanding of the systematic approach to children with serious biochemical problems related to inborn errors provides a context from which less complicated problems can be approached and ensures that these rare cases of inborn errors are not missed inadvertently. Imaging studies continue to represent the backbone of diagnosis for a variety of disorders. With the increasing use of noninvasive techniques that provide even greater sensitivity for defining anatomic structure and, possibly in the future, physiological function, it is important to know the advantages and weaknesses of different modalities. Interpretation of the medical literature is key to sustaining diagnostic skills at a high level, but concomitantly requires an interpretation of published materials and the evaluation of diagnostic tests so that appropriate new advances can be incorporated into practice. To this end, the sections that follow provide the basics that enable the embodiment of new knowledge to contemporary practice.

8.1 MOLECULAR DIAGNOSTICS IN CHILDHOOD DISORDERS

Rachel Sparks and Jeffrey R. Gruen

8.1.1 Introduction

Genetic principles and technologies have evolved beyond the domain of the laboratory and have taken hold in the field of pediatric medicine, primarily through the diagnosis of childhood disorders. These diagnostic capabilities are due largely to advances in genetic technology over the last 10 years and the rapid increase in the identification and characterization of the estimated 100,000 genes that are encoded by the DNA contained in each human cell. The discovery and functional characterization of these 100,000 genes have been the ultimate goals of the Human Genome Project, an ambitious multinational initiative to sequence the human genome, the 3×10^9 (3 billion) base pairs of DNA in each human cell. Applied technologies will determine the genetic components of common diseases such as diabetes and cancer, and molecular diagnostics will enable preventative measures and novel treatments of infectious and nongenetic disorders. Understanding the theory and application of these technologies to serve patients is the purpose of this section as well as a glimpse of applications currently under development and the potential impact on medicine over the next several years.

8.1.2 DNA: the Basic Blueprint of All Cells

Each nucleated cell in the human body contains all 3×10^9 DNA base pairs of the human genome wrapped around special protein cores called *histones* and organized into chromosomes. The DNA in our cells is a long chain composed of individual links; each link is one of four deoxynucleotide bases: deoxyadenylate (A), deoxythymidylate (T), deoxyguanylate (G), and deoxycytidylate (C). In most cases, a single strand of a DNA chain anneals (binds) to its complementary strand because the A bases bind to the T bases and the C bases bind to the G bases. This complementary binding between As and Ts and Cs and Gs is the basis of high-fidelity DNA replication in all cells. It also provides an opportunity to manipulate DNA using synthetic short chains of deoxynucleotides called *oligonucleotides* (oligos). Oligos bind (or anneal) to the DNA sequence with a high degree of specificity. Depending on the conditions of the annealing reaction (ie, salt concentration, temperature, and reactant concentrations), the oligo will not anneal if one or more of the deoxynucleotide bases do not perfectly complement the DNA sequence of the opposite strand.

Just as nucleotide bases are the links of short oligonucleotide chains, they are also the building blocks of genes, the basic unit of the human genome. Each functional gene encodes the amino acid sequence of one or more proteins along with specific regulatory instructions which are encoded in the promoter region of the gene. The promoter dictates in which cells the protein is to be expressed, when expression is to occur, and the level of expression. Proteins are the functional molecules of the cell. Among their many diverse and specialized functions, proteins make up receptors, enzymes, and structural components of cellular organization. But it is the gene that determines the amino acid sequence and contains the regulatory instructions for the protein. To generate a protein, the

DNA sequence of a gene is first copied into an RNA version in a process called *transcription* that takes place in the nucleus (Fig. 8-1). RNA and DNA are chemically similar and differ only at a single position in the ribose ring of both compounds; the hydroxyl group (OH) in RNA is replaced by hydrogen in DNA. The RNA version of the gene is called messenger RNA, or mRNA. The mRNA migrates from the nucleus to the cytoplasm where it is then "read" by ribosomes that assemble an amino acid chain reflecting the nucleotide bases specified by the mRNA sequence. This process of protein synthesis that occurs in the cytoplasm is called *translation*.

Errors in the sequence of the deoxynucleotide bases that encode a gene, commonly called *mutations,* are transcribed into mRNA and read by the ribosomes. DNA mutations are reflected in the amino acid sequence of the corresponding protein. These mutations can generate proteins with altered or no activity, prevent the protein from being synthesized at all, or alter the normal regulation of expression (as a result of mutations in the promoter). If a mutation ultimately results in abnormal cellular function, then disease can result. For example, in Duchenne muscular dystrophy, the dystrophin protein is either not made or is inactive due to a mutation in the dystrophin gene DNA sequence. Accurate and timely mutation discovery therefore requires a robust and efficient method of determining gene sequence.

8.1.3   DNA Diagnostic Testing: the Polymerase Chain Reaction: An Enabling Technology

For a long time, generating quantities of DNA large enough for sequencing presented a significant technological barrier. To faithfully replicate many identical copies of a segment of DNA, the segment had to be "glued" (enzymatically inserted or "ligated") into a larger biologically engineered DNA circle called a *vector*. The vector contained information for DNA replication and for conferring antibiotic resistance. Bacteria were coaxed to take up the large circle of DNA (vector plus insert) and replicate many copies. Antibiotic mixed into the growth media provided selective pressure so that only those bacteria that acquired the vector would survive and grow. Following sufficient growth, the vector and insert were separated from the larger host bacterial DNA. This process was called *DNA cloning* because the bacterial hosts took up and replicated the vector/insert constructs so that all the construct copies were genetically identical. While the accuracy of the replication was high, extraction of the vector/insert was a labor-intensive process and not cost-effective for investigating many samples.

The polymerase chain reaction (PCR) represented a major revolution in the amplification and isolation of specific segments of DNA (Fig. 8-2). The technique was invented by Kary Mullis who had been working with oligonucleotides and their application to the process of DNA sequencing. He proposed to synthesize an oligonucleotide with a sequence complementary to a specific stretch of DNA. He would then use a special enzyme called a *polymerase,* which adds another deoxynucleotide to the end of the oligonucleotide. The newly added deoxynucleotide would not be random, but would be complementary to the opposing base on the long strand of DNA to which the oligonucleotide was annealed. Mullis contemplated what would happen if he applied his technique to both strands of double-stranded DNA at the same time. He would design two oligonucleotides, one for each strand, and as the new deoxynucleotides were added to the end of the oligonucleo-

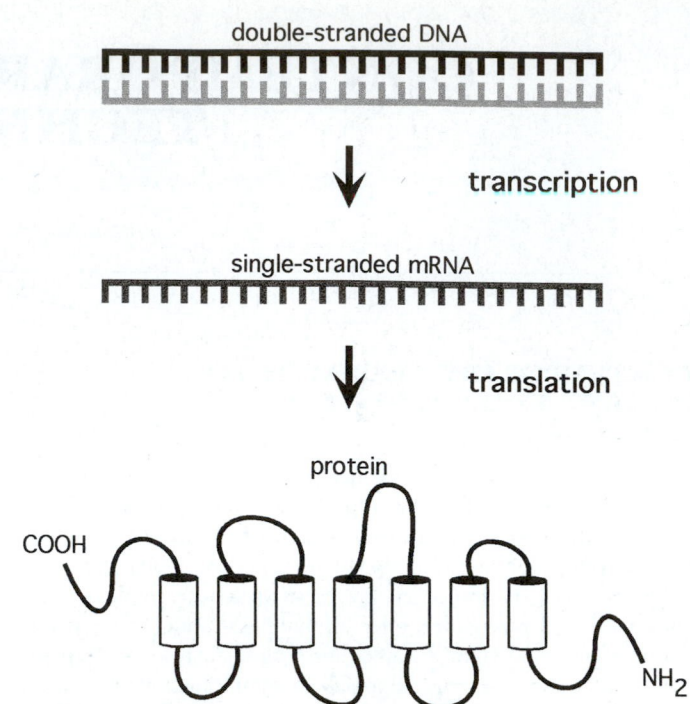

FIGURE 8-1   DNA *transcription* to mRNA occurs in the nucleus. mRNA molecules then migrate to the cytoplasm where they associate with ribosomes and serve as templates that order the amino acids within the polypeptide chains of proteins. This process is called *translation* because the nucleotide sequence of genes is translated into the amino acid sequence of proteins.

tides, the distance between them would shorten by two bases. Mullis realized that many polymerases do not add a single deoxynucleotide to the end of an oligonucleotide, but add many nucleotides, each complementary to the base in the opposite DNA strand to which the now-growing oligonucleotide anneals. Mullis' epiphany is the foundation of what is now the most widely used technique in molecular genetics, the polymerase chain reaction, for which he was awarded the Nobel Prize for Medicine in 1993. The beauty of PCR resides in its simultaneous power and simplicity. PCR can be used to amplify DNA from samples for many diagnostic purposes including (a) detection of sequences or genes of an infectious agent such as bacteria, parasites, or viruses; (b) identification of sequence differences in genomic DNA responsible for genetic disease or predisposing to disease; and (c) identification of sequences that identify a family relationship.

A powerful application of PCR has been in the area of infectious diseases in which rapid, sensitive, and accurate tests have accelerated diagnosis and initiation of specific therapies. For example, conventional methods for diagnosing *Mycobacterium tuberculosis* can require up to 6 weeks, but diagnosis can be made within a few hours using PCR. The diagnostic sample, perhaps sputum or blood, contains DNA from both the human host and the mycobacterium. The DNA of both organisms are biochemically identical and differ only in their unique sequence of nucleotide bases that encode the genes specific for each organism. For the PCR diagnostic assay (Fig. 8-2), oligonucleotides are chosen based on the mycobacterium genomic sequence and will not find a suitable complementary sequence in the human genome to which to anneal. The sample collected from the patient, the oligonucleotides (also known as *primers* because they prime the polymerase reaction), free deoxy-

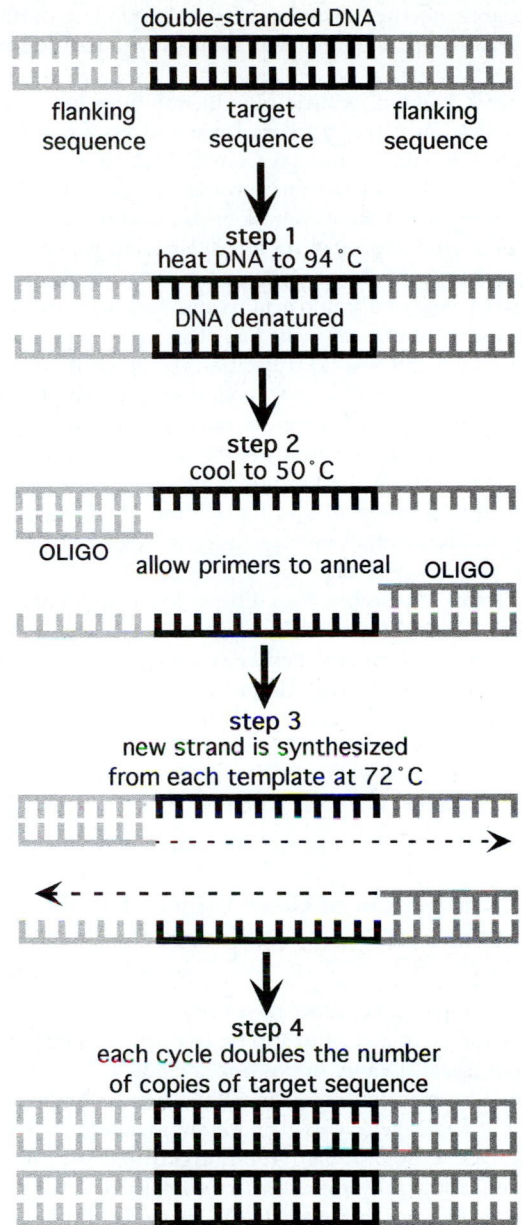

FIGURE 8-2 **The double strands of the DNA helix (the template) are separated, or denatured, by heating to 94°C. After the two strands are separated, the temperature of the reaction is lowered to allow the oligonucleotides (or "primers") to anneal to the template. The temperature is then raised to the temperature optimum for the activity of the thermostable polymerase, usually 68 to 72°C. The polymerase adds free deoxynucleotides to the end of the primer and the length of the primer extends. After a specific length of DNA is amplified the reaction mixture is again heated to separate the strands of DNA and the procedure is repeated. As each cycle is repeated, the number of copies of the target sequence grows exponentially.**

nucleotides, and a special thermostable polymerase (*Taq*) are mixed in the same tube. The tube containing the reaction mixture is heated so as to separate, or denature, the double-stranded DNA in the patient sample. The oligonucleotide primers can only anneal to single-stranded DNA; hence the two strands must be heated to separate them.

After the two strands are separated, the temperature of the reaction is lowered to allow the primers to anneal to the DNA. Find-

ing the correct temperature for primer annealing is critical. If the temperature is too high, the primers will not anneal to the DNA, but if the temperature is too low, the primers can anneal to imperfect matches. At the optimal temperature, the primers will only anneal to the DNA sequences that are perfectly complementary to their own. After the primers are annealed, the temperature is raised to the optimum temperature for the activity of the thermostable polymerase, which adds the free deoxynucleotides to the end of the primers and the length of the primers extends (see Fig. 8-2). The number of deoxynucleotides that the polymerase adds is dependent on the amount of time that the reaction remains at optimal temperature (generally 1 to 2 minutes), and on how quickly the polymerase can add new deoxynucleotides. After a specific length of DNA is amplified, the reaction mixture is again heated to separate the strands of DNA and the procedure is repeated. The number of DNA copies doubles with each successive cycle of denaturation, annealing, and extension. Twenty cycles yield 1 million-fold amplification (10^6), and 40 cycles yield 10^{12}-fold amplification. In practical terms, this means that starting with 25 ng of total genomic DNA, any 1000 base pair-amplified segment (representing approximately 0.00003% of the total DNA) would typically yield 10 to 500 ng, or more than a 1 million-fold amplification. This enormous increase in the amount of specific DNA that can be amplified from a few nanograms of the total genome demonstrates the robust nature of PCR, a quality due largely to the hearty nature of the DNA template. Unlike proteins that are typically unstable with short half-lives, DNA can remain intact and in good condition for a relatively long time depending on the conditions in which it is stored. For this reason, PCR has a significant advantage over other diagnostic techniques that rely on less stable targets.

Many different biological substances have been used as DNA templates for PCR, including blood, stool, mummified remains, and a single hair. PCR is so sensitive that DNA from even the smallest entities can be used as a template. Using only a single sperm, the entire sperm genome can be amplified using a mixture of random oligonucleotide primers that are 15 bases long. In addition, the mRNA transcript of a gene can be used as a template for a unique type of PCR reaction called *reverse transcriptase PCR (RT-PCR)*. In this reaction, the mRNA is primed with a single DNA primer and a special polymerase called *reverse transcriptase* is added. Reverse transcriptase generates a DNA copy of an RNA template. After generating a DNA copy with reverse transcriptase, a standard PCR reaction using two primers and *Taq* polymerase further amplifies the newly synthesized DNA sequence. Among its many applications, RT-PCR is used to detect HIV, an RNA virus, in patients with viral loads as low as 20 copies per mL. This technology enables diagnosis in the period between initial infection and the detection of anti-HIV antibodies, in addition to enabling determination of HIV viral loads and measuring the effectiveness of antiretroviral therapy even when standard techniques can no longer detect the virus.

In clinical diagnosis, PCR is used many fields, but it has been most successful in the areas of infectious disease diagnosis and the identification of genetic disorders. In addition to positively identifying organisms such as HIV, *Mycobacterium tuberculosis*, rabies, and human papillomavirus, PCR can also distinguish between different strains of each organism. This permits the tracking of infectious outbreaks and surveillance for resistance as organisms evolve in response to environmental pressures and antimicrobial therapies. Perhaps better known is the application of PCR to the diagnosis of genetic disorders such as cystic fibrosis, fragile X syndrome, and myotonic dystrophy (Table 8-1). While this use of PCR is still com-

TABLE 8-1

EXAMPLES OF HEREDITARY DISORDERS DIAGNOSED BY PCR

DISORDER	INCIDENCE	GENE	MUTATION DETECTION RATE
Monogenic			
Cystic fibrosis	1:4000	*CFTR*	98%
Duchenne muscular dystrophy	1:4000	*DMD*	About 90%
Fragile X syndrome	1:4000	*FMR*	100%
Huntington disease	1:5000–1:10,000	*HD*	100%
Hemophilia A	1:10,000	*F8C*	About 90%
Phenylketonuria	1:10,000	*PAH*	99%
Polycystic kidney disease	1:1500	*PKD1* *PKD2*	About 15%
Inherited cancers			
Breast-ovarian cancer	1:4000	*BRCA1* (80%) *BRCA2* (20%)	50–65% 35%
Li-Fraumeni syndrome		*p53*	50%
Ataxia-telangiectasia		*ATM*	70%
Familial polyposis coli	1:4000	*APC*	87%
Hereditary nonpolyposis coli	1:2000	*MLH1* (30%) *MSH2* (60%) *MSH6*	33% 12%
Cardiovascular disorders			
Familial hypercholesterolemia	1:500	*LDLR*	60%
Hyperlipidemia		*APOE*	10%

mon and the number of disorders to which it can be applied is increasing, PCR has also entered the domain of preimplantation genetic diagnosis and prenatal genetic diagnosis for which there are a number of detectable mutations.

With the exception of germ cells (sperm and egg cells), each nucleated cell of the body is diploid, meaning that it contains two copies of the entire human genome—one complete haploid copy inherited from each parent. Therefore, any diploid cell can be interrogated for inherited mutations that would affect proteins unrelated to the specific function of that cell. For example, the DNA in a circulating white blood cell can be evaluated for particular mutations affecting only the retina or Kupffer cells. Also, placental cells of the chorionic villi comprising the fetal side of the placenta can be analyzed for inherited mutations as early as the tenth week of gestation, enabling very early prenatal diagnosis. Pleuripotential cells of the preimplanted embryo can be studied as early as the 6- to 10-cell stage. All applications of PCR-based molecular diagnoses are restricted to only those genes and mutations that are previously known to segregate within a particular family or population. Because primers must be highly specific in order to amplify a defined nucleotide sequence, each test (and often each mutation) requires its own primer design. Thus, careful consideration and discussion must precede the ordering of DNA diagnostic tests because there are no global mutation screens that identify all possible mutations

for all possible inherited disorders. Misunderstanding of this concept can lead to disappointment in families who have undergone testing.

In general, DNA diagnostic tests identify four types of DNA mutations that alter the transcriptional process from DNA to mRNA, the translational process from mRNA to protein, or the amino acid sequence of the final protein product encoded by a particular gene. All of these alterations can lead to gain or loss of function of a specific protein on a cellular level, which results in pathologic changes at the tissue or organ level: (a) missense mutations that change one amino acid to another; (b) nucleotide deletions or insertions that cause the loss of an amino acid or alter the translation of the mRNA; (c) truncation (or nonsense) mutations that introduce a premature stop codon thereby shortening the translated protein; and (d) trinucleotide expansions. In addition, the location of a mutation within a gene sequence can alter protein function. Mutations in the promoter region can change the expression pattern of a particular protein without changing the amino acid sequence itself, either up-regulating or down-regulating protein expression in key cells.

Trinucleotide expansions are a distinct form of mutation with a strong clinical correlation and have been found exclusively in inherited neurologic disorders such as Huntington disease and myotonic dystrophy (see Chaps. 10 and 25). In these disorders the severity of the symptoms increases over successive generations, a clinical phenomenon called *anticipation*. This effect is due to a large expansion of a trinucleotide codon (typically increasing in number each generation) that interferes with normal protein processing or function.

8.1.4   Identification of Gene Targets: Family Studies

Identifying a gene that encodes for a certain protein or one that is responsible for a human disease can be accomplished by functional cloning, positional cloning, or positional-candidate cloning.

As would be expected, it was initially easiest to study disorders caused by a single gene and that follow mendelian inheritance within families. From 1955 to 1988, approximately 100 disease genes were identified by *functional cloning*, such as the gene for globin that is responsible for sickle-cell anemia and the adenosine deaminase gene that is mutated in some children with severe combined immunodeficiency. Genes identified through functional cloning are located based on information about the basic biochemical defect of the disorder with no information about the chromosomal location of the gene responsible for the disease. In the case of sickle cell, a defective globin protein causes the red blood cell to deform under certain conditions. Because the underlying biochemical mechanism responsible for most diseases is unknown, this method of gene identification has limited potential.

Between 1988 and 1998, a gene-identification approach called *positional cloning* was used to identify genes responsible for diseases that were transmitted from generation to generation in families. The process of positional cloning does not require knowledge of the putative function of the gene. In this approach, unrelated individuals are not expected to share a high degree of DNA similarity, but related individuals tend to have small areas of identical DNA. Using extended pedigrees of families who carry the disease, segments of identical DNA in affected family members are identified and assumed to contain the disease gene; unaffected family members are assumed not to carry the identical stretch of DNA. After the identical regions are identified, the sequence in affected individuals is compared to that in unaffected individuals. Any differences in sequence common in affected individuals but not seen in the unaffected population might be a mutation responsible for the disease. By using this technique to identify shared DNA sequences in family members with hereditary diseases, many disease genes have been isolated, including the genes for Duchenne muscular dystrophy, retinoblastoma, and the breast cancer genes BRCA1 and BRCA2.

As more genes are identified and their functions elucidated, gene identification has shifted from positional cloning to *positional-candidate* strategies that still use pedigrees to locate the region where the responsible gene is located. The stretches of DNA shared by pedigrees of people with a given disease (yielding positional data, or the chromosomal location of a gene) and the genes in that region are identified. Genes potentially responsible for the disease are selected (the genes are considered candidates for the disease and are hence referred to as "candidate genes"). The candidate gene sequences of the patients are compared with those of unaffected individuals in order to identify possible mutations. Any difference in the sequence of a gene between people with the disease and those unaffected suggests that particular gene could be responsible for the disease. For example, Marfan syndrome was mapped to a region on chromosome 15 by positional cloning and the fibrillin gene was located in the identified region. This gene was a very attractive candidate gene and mutations in the fibrillin gene were quickly identified in Marfan patients (see Chap. 10).

8.1.5   Mutations and Polymorphisms

Mutations and polymorphisms are both differences in DNA sequence, but the distinction between the two is not always clear. In general, mutations are sequence differences that alter protein function, while polymorphisms do not alter protein function. These alterations in the DNA sequence may be inherited (transmitted through male and female germ cells) or acquired (perhaps due to ionization damage of DNA by the UV component of sunlight). For example, a tumor-suppressor gene might acquire nucleotide changes that would causes the protein made by the gene to be inactive. The effect would be unbridled cell division and malignant transformation. Because the function of the protein is altered by the nucleotide change of the gene, this is an example of a mutation. In contrast, many sequence differences within the coding region of genes do not alter the amino acid sequence of the protein because an amino acid can be specified by more than one three-nucleotide codon, termed *degeneracy*. For example, the genetic codes for the amino acid leucine are CTT, CTC, CTA, and CTG. Because the third position of the codon can vary, a nucleotide change in this position will not result in a different amino acid. These DNA sequence variations that do not change the protein sequence are considered polymorphisms.

Distributed throughout the human genome, approximately once every 100 base pairs, are minor differences in the DNA sequence, called *polymorphisms,* that are of no consequence to protein formation or function. These single-nucleotide polymorphisms, or SNPs, occur mostly in the expanses of sequence of DNA between genes (intergenic DNA) that actually make up 95% of the human genome and are also present in the coding regions of many genes. These tiny differences can be used as "markers" of the genome, akin to road signs that tell their specific subchromosomal localization. Because SNPs are so numerous, an effort is underway to build a dense genetic map with a panel of SNP markers distributed throughout all 22 autosomes and 2 sex chromosomes. SNPs are important because it is assumed that there are a finite number of variations in the human genome that contribute to genetic susceptibility for common diseases. Because these single-base-pair changes can distinguish individuals genetically, SNP can be used as markers in the human genome for both single-gene disorders and for disorders caused by multiple genes that are difficult to characterize. Using SNPs as location markers, genes associated with disease will be identified with a much higher precision.

8.1.6   Future Directions

To date, most disease genes have been identified through (a) biochemical information about the nature of the disease; (b) abnormalities in a karyotype, such as deletions, translocations, or rearrangements, that suggest a subchromosomal location; or (c) analysis of hereditary patterns within families (classical genetic linkage analysis). However, as more genes are located and more genetic markers (such as SNPs) are defined, disease genes will be located and genetic disorders that lack a strong hereditary pattern or for which large pedigrees of families do not exist will be studied. One such mapping approach, called *genetic association,* compares unrelated cases with a narrowly defined condition or illness to unaffected controls that are closely matched for ethnicity, race, sex, and age. For example, comparing individuals with and without cardiovascular disease might reveal a higher frequency of some common markers (SNPs) in the affected individuals and suggests that a gene in the region linked to the SNPs might contribute to the clinical condition. Association is an extraordinarily powerful technique. When used in conjunction with family mapping, association has successfully localized disease genes to within 60,000 base pairs.

While the underlying genetics of an individual can be very useful in determining predisposition to a certain illness, comparing differences in gene expression in tissues or organs is an alternative strategy for identifying genetic abnormalities. New techniques termed *expression profiling* determine the levels of expression of hundreds or thousands of genes in a given tissue. In this technique, the coding sequences of tens of thousands of genes are spotted onto a single glass slide or silicon surface (microchip) to which DNA naturally binds. Fluorescent-labeled RNA from the tissue to be queried is applied to the chip, and the levels of expression of the genes in the tissue can be determined by measuring the relative fluorescence from each spot where the RNA has annealed to the immobilized gene sequences. This technique can indicate suppressed and induced pathways by comparing normal and disease states, and can also increase the understanding of complex genotype-phenotype correlations. In addition, expression profiling has the potential to become a very powerful diagnostic tool. Diseases may be characterized by a gene expression pattern typified in certain tissues; ie, a gene "signature" can potentially be used in differential diagnosis and to evaluate the potential for disease progression. In addition, the genetic signature of a particular disorder will be useful in deciding the most effective course of treatment.

The Human Genome Project and related technologies will enable the interrogation of an individual's genome with increased sensitivity and specificity. Through the analysis of a given set of genes, it may be possible to determine those diseases to which one is strongly predisposed and the appropriate preventative measures could be taken. This best-case situation will have to be balanced by the propensity for discrimination against those with a certain genetic "fingerprint," despite the fact that the individual remains clinically unaffected. As with any increase in information, these "problems of knowledge" must be resolved and ever-anticipated as new, powerful technologies continue to provide us with more information about our genetic fabric.

References

Mullis KB: The unusual origin of the polymerase chain reaction. Sci Am 262(4):56, 1990.

Risch N, Merikangas K: The future of genetic studies of complex human diseases. Science 273(5281):1516, 1996.

Van Ommem GJB, Bakker E, den Dunnen JT: The human genome project and the future of diagnostics, treatment and prevention. Lancet 354: S15, 1999.

Zhang L, Cui X, Schmitt K, Hubert R, Navidi W, Arnheim N: Whole genomic amplification from a single cell: implications for genetic analysis. Proc Natl Acad Sci U S A 89:5847, 1992.

Initial Sequencing and Analysis of Human Genome. Nature 6822(Feb): 860, 2001

8.2　BIOCHEMICAL DIAGNOSIS OF INBORN ERRORS OF METABOLISM

Piero Rinaldo and Dietrich Matern

8.2.1　Biochemical Genetics

Approximately 10% of diseases among hospitalized children have been ascribed to mendelian traits inherited as single-gene defects. Approximately 1000 inborn errors of metabolism (IEM) have been identified primarily through the detection of endogenous metabolites in biological fluids and tissues. Because of the stereotypical clinical presentation of many IEM, a major role of the biochemical genetics laboratory is to analyze complex metabolite profiles to reach a rapid, but preliminary, diagnosis that must always be confirmed by enzymatic and/or molecular studies. Accordingly, a major function of biochemical genetics is a screening process that can be divided as follows: (a) at-risk screening (prenatal diagnosis); (b) newborn screening (testing of presymptomatic patients); (c) high-risk screening (testing of symptomatic patients); and (d) postmortem screening (metabolic autopsy).

8.2.2　At-risk Screening: Prenatal Diagnosis of IEM

Despite constant progress in medical treatment, several IEM result in severe morbidity and inevitable mortality in early life. Most IEM are autosomal recessive disorders and have a recurrence risk of 25% in subsequent pregnancies. Thus, at-risk screening for prenatal diagnosis usually involves the prior diagnosis in an index case. Figure 8-3 shows an algorithm of sequential steps to be taken in determining indications, prerequisites, and methods necessary to perform a prenatal diagnosis of an IEM. Genetic counseling of a couple seeking a prenatal diagnosis is essential to identify risk factors, provide a risk/benefit assessment, and to consider the possible impact of medical, religious, and social issues. Risk factors identifiable prior to conception include parental consanguinity, ethnic origin, and a positive family history. Risk assessment includes the possibility of pregnancy loss as a consequence of the sampling procedure (0.5–1% by chorionic villus sampling, 0.5% by amniocentesis) and the potential fallacy of "experimental" procedures or test results such as the occurence of either false-negative or false-positive results. Benefit assessment is not limited to the option of terminating an affected fetus; it is also for gaining the foreknowledge of the fetus's status and to plan immediate implementation of postnatal treatment and preventive measures.

A precise understanding of the biochemical phenotype and genotype of the IEM in the index case of the family under consideration is mandatory; indeed, the performance of a prenatal diagnosis under less defined circumstances is prone to mistakes and should be strictly avoided. Similarly, the validity of undertaking a prenatal diagnosis when the biological parents are not the same as the index case is questionable because the recurrence risk in most cases is greater than 1 in 500. Other prerequisites include evidence that the IEM is expressed in accessible fetal tissue(s) and fluids, and reliance on laboratories with sufficient experience in performing the analysis and interpreting the results. Confirmation of results by a second and independent method, and approval of testing costs, which may be substantial, is also needed.

Methods used for prenatal diagnosis of IEM have different requirements in terms of timing, sample collection, and options for independent confirmation. Chorionic villus sampling (CVS) either by transcervical (<10 weeks of gestational age) or transabdominal (>10 weeks) procedure has the advantages of being performed earlier in the pregnancy and allowing direct enzymatic analysis that can be verified later in cultured cells. Disadvantages of CVS include a higher risk of fetal loss, the possibility of inconclusive results requiring follow-up by amniocentesis, and the risk of artifactual results, which has made this approach very unreliable in specific disorders (for example, methylmalonic acidemia). Amniocentesis is performed later in pregnancy (16–19 weeks) but is a safer procedure and, more importantly, provides both amniocytes and amniotic fluid that can be used for independent and complementary diagnostic methods. Direct assay of amniocytes, however, is not possible, and it may take 2 to 3 weeks to grow a sufficient amount of cells in culture. The possibility of contamination with cells of maternal origin needs to be prevented and actively monitored. For these reasons, the combination of enzyme assay in cultured cells and the direct metabolite analysis in the cell-free supernatant of the amniotic fluid offers the preferred approach to the prenatal diagnosis of IEM, in which separate tests based on independent methods are performed to reach a consensus diagnosis. When this is not technically feasible, at least two separate laboratories should perform the same test independently to minimize the risk of incorrect results. Direct analysis of metabolites in amniotic fluid is based on positive identification of target metabolite(s) by mass spectrometry in combination with other techniques (stable isotope dilution, selected ion monitoring) to provide the degree of specificity and sensitivity needed to confidently detect and quantitate very low concentrations of the diagnostic metabolites. The major advantages of direct metabolite analysis in amniotic fluid are the independence from tissue expression and the rapid availability of a result (usually within 24 hours), which also allows a prompt verification of equivocal results by another laboratory. In addition to a written interpretation, a report should include: (a) quantitative results matched against a statistically validated range of normal controls; (b) evidence of quality control (results of duplicate analysis, simultaneous negative and positive controls); and (c) a summary of the labora-

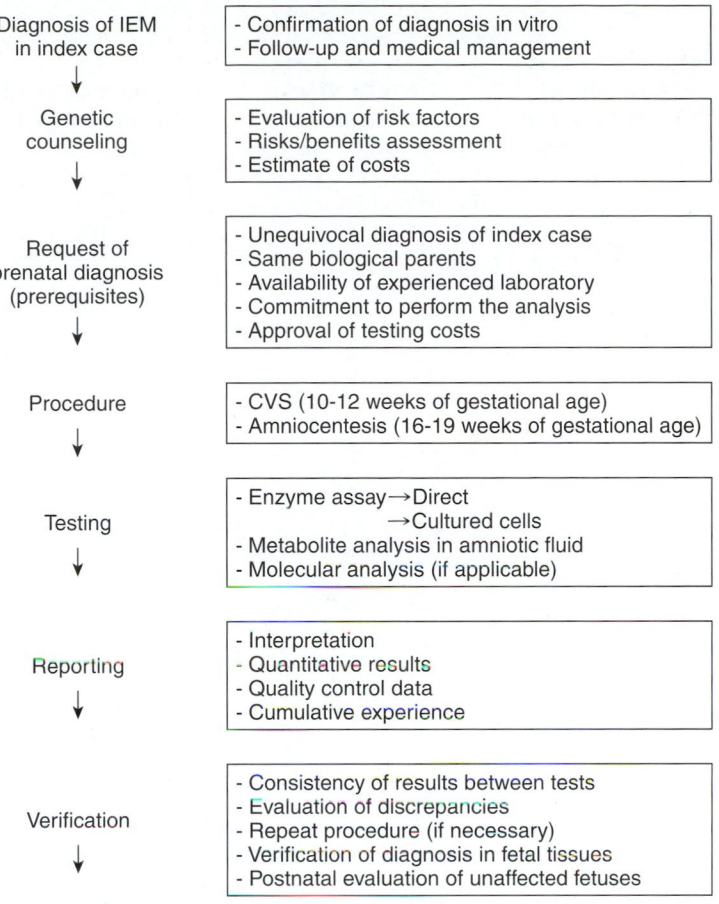

AT-RISK SCREENING: PRENATAL DIAGNOSIS

Diagnosis of IEM in index case
- Confirmation of diagnosis in vitro
- Follow-up and medical management

Genetic counseling
- Evaluation of risk factors
- Risks/benefits assessment
- Estimate of costs

Request of prenatal diagnosis (prerequisites)
- Unequivocal diagnosis of index case
- Same biological parents
- Availability of experienced laboratory
- Commitment to perform the analysis
- Approval of testing costs

Procedure
- CVS (10-12 weeks of gestational age)
- Amniocentesis (16-19 weeks of gestational age)

Testing
- Enzyme assay→Direct
           →Cultured cells
- Metabolite analysis in amniotic fluid
- Molecular analysis (if applicable)

Reporting
- Interpretation
- Quantitative results
- Quality control data
- Cumulative experience

Verification
- Consistency of results between tests
- Evaluation of discrepancies
- Repeat procedure (if necessary)
- Verification of diagnosis in fetal tissues
- Postnatal evaluation of unaffected fetuses

FIGURE 8-3   **At-risk screening: Algorithm for the prenatal diagnosis of IEM. Abbreviations:** *CVS* = **chorionic villus sampling;** *IEM* = **inborn errors of metabolism.**

tory's overall experience (number of cases tested, results obtained in affected and unaffected fetuses, respectively) with the prenatal diagnosis of that particular disorder.

Parents must be counseled that a preliminary diagnosis of an affected fetus by metabolite analysis (typically available within 24 hours from the time of amniocentesis) should not be the basis for termination of a presumably affected fetus. Instead, parents should defer the decision until results of enzyme assays in cultured cells become available, usually in 2 to 3 weeks. Although it is a rare occurrence, discordant results are occasionally obtained, and a correct diagnosis may require a repeat amniocentesis. Finally, the prenatal diagnoses that the fetus is unaffected should be followed up by routine biochemical testing of the newborn.

8.2.3   Newborn Screening: Presymptomatic Diagnosis of IEM

Newborn screening was initiated in 1962 for the identification of infants affected with phenylketonuria (PKU), but soon was expanded to include other genetic and nongenetic conditions (eg, infectious disorders such as toxoplasmosis and HIV). However, the number of disorders that are screened is not uniform in all regions, and only PKU and congenital hypothyroidism are included in all screening programs in the United States. The goal of newborn screening is to detect diagnostic markers of the selected disorders in blood samples collected from presymptomatic newborns. A population-wide screening is justified based on the documented pre-

vention of morbidity by early diagnosis, availability of a suitable screening method amenable to large-scale testing, and resources to provide treatment, follow-up care, and genetic counseling. In addition, the disease should be frequent enough to allow for a positive cost-benefit ratio. The current methods used to identify genetic diseases are not always reliable in identifying patients during their first day of life, which is important because of increasingly early discharge of well babies from the hospital. Currently, blood spots are collected on filter paper prior to discharge of the newborn to home but not later than 7 days of age. If infants are discharged in the first 24 hours of life, a second sample should be collected before 14 days of age to minimize the occurrence of false-negative results.

More than 30 years after the initial implementation of testing for phenylketonuria, newborn screening programs are undergoing substantial revisions in terms of objectives (eg, selection of disorders to be screened) and the methods used for screening. The driving force behind these changes is the introduction of tandem mass spectrometry (MS/MS).

Analyses of amino acids, acylcarnitines, and a rapidly expanding number of other metabolites are now routinely performed by MS/MS to evaluate patients suspected of having IEM. MS/MS is currently being incorporated in newborn screening laboratories worldwide because the detection of several IEM can be accomplished in a single dried blood spot in a timely and cost-efficient manner (Table 8-2). Among them, medium-chain acyl-CoA dehydrogenase (MCAD) deficiency and glutaric acidemia type I clearly meet the requirements for newborn screening on the basis

TABLE 8-2
NEWBORN SCREENING

GENETIC DISORDER	ESTIMATED INCIDENCE	PREVENTION OF MORBIDITY BY EARLY DIAGNOSIS	CONVENTIONAL SCREENING PROGRAM[1]	DETECTABLE BY MS/MS ANALYSIS
Classic phenylketonuria (PKU)	1:10,000	+++	Yes	Yes
Other hyperphenylalaninemias	1:20,000	+	Yes	Yes
Homocystinuria	1:150,000	+++	Yes	Yes
Maple syrup urine disease (MSUD)	1:180,000	+++	Yes	Yes
Biotinidase deficiency	1:100,000	+++	Yes	Yes
Hemoglobinopathies	1:2,000	+++	Yes	Yes
Congenital adrenal hyperplasia	1:12,000	+++	Yes	Possible
Congenital hypothyroidism	1:4,000	+++	Yes	No
Galactosemias	1:50,000	+++	Yes	No
Cystic fibrosis	1:2,000	+	Yes	No
MCAD deficiency	1:17,000	+++	No	No
Glutaric acidemia type I	1:30,000	+++	No	No
Tyrosinemias	1:100,000	+++	No	No
CPS deficiency	1:80,000	+	No	Possible
OTC deficiency	1:80,000	+	No	Possible
Citrullinemia	1:80,000	+	No	Yes
Argininosuccinic aciduria	1:80,000	+	No	Yes
Arginase deficiency	1:100,000	+	No	Possible
HHH syndrome	Unknown	+	No	Possible
Nonketotic hyperglycinemia	1:250,000	−	No	Yes
Propionic acidemias	1:50,000	+	No	Yes
Methylmalonic acidemias	1:50,000	+	No	Yes
Isovaleric acidemia	1:50,000	+	No	Yes
Methylcrotonyl-CoA carboxylase deficiency	Unknown	+	No	Yes
HMG-CoA lyase deficiency	Unknown	+	No	Yes
Glutaric acidemia type II, severe form	1:100,000	−	No	Yes
Glutaric acidemia type II, mild form	1:100,000	+	No	Yes
Carnitine uptake defect	Unknown	+++	No	Possible
Translocase deficiency	Unknown	+	No	Yes
CPT II deficiency	Unknown	+	No	Yes
VLCAD deficiency	1:50,000	+	No	Yes
TFP/LCHAD deficiency	1:40,000	+	No	Yes
SCAD deficiency	Unknown	+	No	Yes

Genetic disorders currently included in newborn screening programs and metabolic disorders detectable by MS/MS analysis of blood spots. Symbols and abbreviations: *CPS,* carbamylphosphate synthetase; *CPT,* carnitine palmitoyltransferase; *HHH,* hyperornithinemia-hyperammonemia-homocitrullinuria; *HMG-CoA,* 3-hydroxy-3-methylglutaryl-coenzyme A; *LCHAD,* long-chain 3-hydroxyacyl-CoA dehydrogenase; *MCAD,* medium-chain acyl-CoA dehydrogenase; *OTC,* ornithine transcarbamylase; *SCAD,* short-chain acyl-CoA dehydrogenase; *TFP,* trifunctional protein; *VLCAD,* very-long-chain acyl-CoA dehydrogenase.
[1]With the exception of PKU and congenital hypothyroidism, testing for individual disorders is not offered by all screening programs; +++, effective treatment is available; +, treatment is available but the prognosis is guarded in most patients;−, disorders that will be detected by MS/MS but are currently considered untreatable.

of their incidence, difficulty to detect before the onset of symptoms, and an outcome that could be substantially improved by early treatment (see Chap. 9).

8.2.4 High-Risk Screening: Symptomatic Diagnosis of IEM

High-risk screening refers to the laboratory evaluation of patients who present with signs and symptoms suggestive of an underlying IEM, often under circumstances of a life-threatening situation. Testing for metabolic disorders has gradually shifted from highly specialized and esoteric activity to an integral component of the evaluation of pediatric patients with signs or symptoms suggesting an IEM. The great expansion of the metabolite and enzyme activities that can be assayed in human body fluids and tissues for diagnostic purposes requires increased awareness to avoid diagnostic oversights and to enhance early recognition.

Inborn errors of amino acid, organic acid, carbohydrate, and fatty acid metabolism share a natural history of presenting with life-threatening episodes of acute metabolic decompensation. Morbidity and mortality are high, justifying the need for at-risk and newborn screening as preventive measures. When the diagnosis of IEM is suspected, the analysis shown in Table 8-3 represents a first step in the evaluation process and should be followed by specialized investigations chosen based on the initial results. Although blood gases, serum electrolytes, and glucose are routinely part of the evaluation of any acutely ill pediatric patient, analysis of plasma for ammonia, lactate, and pyruvate is infrequently obtained at admission. In urine the qualitative determination of ketonuria and evaluation of the serum anion gap are particularly important in the early stage of evaluation of an acutely ill patient with a possible IEM. The pattern of changes of this sequence of the tests should allow a differential diagnosis, and the selection of appropriate specialized investigations (Table 8-3).

TABLE 8-3

HIGH-RISK SCREENING FOR SUSPECTED INBORN ERRORS OF METABOLISM

| | ORGANIC ACIDURIAS | PRIMARY LACTIC ACIDEMIAS— DEFECTS OF: | | | | FAO DISORDERS | UREA CYCLE DEFECTS | AMINO ACID DEFECTS | |
		PYRUVATE OXIDATION	GLUCONEO- GENESIS	PYRUVATE CARBOXYLASE	RESPIRATORY CHAIN			MSUD	NKHG
Metabolic acidosis	+++	+++	+++	+++	+++	+	−	+	−
Ketoaciduria	+++	−	+	++	++	−	−	+	−
Hyperammonemia	+	+	+	+++	+	+	+++	−	−
Hypoglycemia	+	−	+++	+	+	+++	−	−	−
Lactic acidemia	+	+++	+++	+++	+++	+	−	−	−
L/P Ratio		N	↑↑	↑↑	↑↑↑				
Number of IEM	>50	7	3	3	>100	22	8[1]	4	1
Specialized investigations[2]	OA (U) AA (P) AC (P) CAR (P)	AA (P) OA (U)	AA (P) OA (U)	AA (P) OA (U)	AA (P) AA (U) OA (U)	AC (P) CAR (P) FFA (P) OA (U) AG (U)	AA (P) AA (U) Orotic (U)	AA (P) OA (U)	AA (P) AA (CSF)

Diagnostic orientation by routine and specialized laboratory investigations in IEM presenting with life-threatening episodes of metabolic decompensation. Symbols and abbreviations: *FAO*, fatty acid oxidation; *IEM*, inborn errors of metabolism; *MSUD*, maple syrup urine disease; *NKHG*, nonketotic hyperglycinemia; +, possibly present; +++, typically present with high diagnostic significance;−, not typically present; *N*, normal (controls: 10–20); ↑↑, higher than normal; ↑↑↑, much higher than normal. Codes for specialized investigations: *AA*, amino acids; *AC*, acylcarnitines; *AG*, acylglycines; *CAR*, carnitine (total and free); *FFA*, free fatty acids: *OA*, organic acids. Letters between parenthesis indicate the preferred specimen:*CSF*, cerobrospinal fluid; *P*, plasma; *U*, urine; L/P Ratio, Lactate/Pyruvate Ratio.

[1]Number includes transport defects of dibasic amino acids which also present with hyperammonemia.

[2]The diagnostic specificity of these analyses may vary considerably under acute asymptomatic conditions.

SOURCE: Modified from Rinaldo P: Laboratory diagnosis of inborn errors of metabolism In: Suchy FJ, ed: Liver Disease in Children. St. Louis, Mosby, 1994.

Quantitative profiling of amino acids, carnitine, acylcarnitines, and free fatty acids in plasma, and urine organic acids and acylglycines are the methods of choice to reach a biochemical diagnosis in a vast majority of metabolic disorders. These tests are highly specialized and difficult to interpret, and the results must be integrated with clinical findings. Other relevant factors include the residual activity of the defective enzyme in vivo, the dietary load of precursors, and the degree of and response to medical management at the time of sample collection. For these reasons, an interpretative report of any of these tests should include: (a) an overview of positive and negative results (eg, ketotic vs nonketotic dicarboxylic aciduria, methylmalonic aciduria with or without homocystinuria); (b) quantitative determination in comparison to age-matched reference values; (c) a list of possible diagnoses with correlation to available clinical information; (d) criteria of differential diagnosis; (e) recommendations for additional biochemical testing and in vitro confirmatory studies (enzyme assay, molecular analysis); (f) name and mean(s) to contact investigators able to provide such studies; and (g) a phone number to reach the biochemical geneticist who wrote the report in case the referring physician has additional questions.

8.2.5   Postmortem Screening: the Metabolic Autopsy

In most cases, IEM present with life-threatening episodes of metabolic decompensation that occur early in life. In view of the high mortality rate that is a common feature of these disorders, it is not surprising that sudden infant death syndrome (SIDS) has been sporadically associated with inborn errors of amino acid, organic acid, and energy metabolism. These anecdotal reports represent instances of a delayed diagnosis possibly combined with atypical or mild clinical phenotypes. On the other hand, the number of patients who have been found to be affected with fatty acid oxidation (FAO) disorders (either postmortem or after the diagnosis of an affected sibling) has soared in the last few years. Based on these observations, it is possible that FAO disorders might be responsible for up to 5% of children who die suddenly and unexpectedly in the period from birth to 5 years of age, particularly with evidence of acute infection. The postmortem diagnosis of FAO disorders is important for genetic counseling and for the evaluation of siblings who may be at risk for significant, yet often preventable, morbidity and mortality (see Chap. 9).

Figure 8-4 summarizes a diagnostic protocol that enables the detection of multiple disorders based on the evaluation of independent diagnostic criteria. If permission to perform an autopsy is not granted, an immediate effort should be made to retrieve available specimens; if death occurred in a nursery or hospital setting, the laboratory should be immediately contacted and asked to hold any unused portions of blood and urine specimens previously collected for routine tests. If available, these specimens should be analyzed for carnitine, acylcarnitine, and free fatty acid in plasma and organic acid and acylglycine profiles in urine. If death occurs at home, retrieval of any unused portion of the blood spots collected for new-

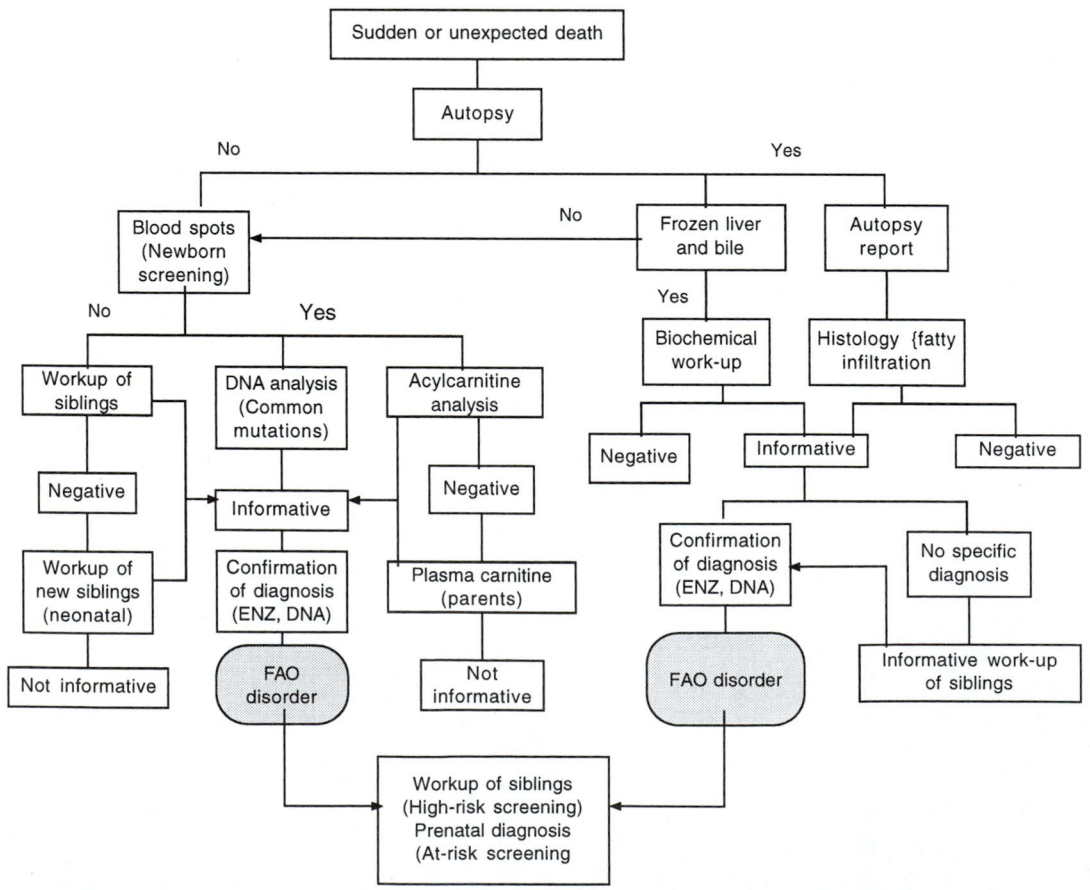

FIGURE 8-4   A protocol for the biochemical diagnosis of fatty acid oxidation disorders. Abbreviations: *DNA* = molecular analysis; *ENZ* = enzymatic assay; *FAO* = fatty acid oxidation. Reproduced with permission from Rinaldo et al: Inherited metabolic disorders in neonate. Semin Perinatol 23:204, 1999.

born screening might be arranged with the state laboratory. Blood spots should be sent for acylcarnitine analysis by electrospray MS/MS to allow screening for multiple conditions and to avoid missing patients carrying less common mutations. If the acylcarnitine profile is not informative, testing of parental plasma carnitine levels is indicated to detect heterozygosity for carnitine uptake defects. As a last resort, a biochemical screening of all siblings should be considered. Although this approach needs to consider the potentially concealed biochemical phenotype of several FAO disorders, it has been very effective, particularly in the case of medium-chain acyl-CoA dehydrogenase (MCAD) deficiency.

If permission to perform an autopsy is granted, analysis of fatty acids, glucose, and carnitine and histology for steatosis can be performed on a frozen samples of liver obtained up to 72 hours after death. This set of analyses is complemented by acylcarnitine profiling of bile, in which levels of carnitine and its easters are considerably higher than in plasma. The reliance on multiple independent diagnostic criteria minimizes the risk of false-negative results.

Because it is unrealistic to recommend routine screening in all cases of sudden or unexpected death, pathologists, pediatricians, and geneticists should select cases with risk factors for the presence of a possible FAO disorder, which include the finding of fatty infiltration of the liver and other organs, a family history of sudden death, Reye syndrome, or myopathy, and especially a history of lethargy, vomiting, and/or fasting (decreased caloric intake) prior to death. Ideally, a frozen specimen of liver and bile should be preserved in all cases. IEM typically exacerbate during even minor infections when higher energy requirements and decreased caloric intake are common. Therefore, postmortem screening for FAO disorders should not be excluded in infants who die suddenly and unexpectedly with an infection, particularly if associated with any degree of fatty infiltration of the liver.

References

Blau N, Duran M, Blaskovics M: Physician's Guide to the Laboratory Diagnosis of Metabolic Diseases. London, Chapman & Hall, 1996.

Boles RG, Buck EA, Blitzer MG, et al: Retrospective biochemical screening of fatty acid oxidation disorders in postmortem liver of 418 cases of sudden unexpected death in the first year of life. J Pediatr 132:924, 1998.

D'Alton ME, Gross I: Inherited metabolic disorders in the neonate. Semin Perinatol 23:99, 1999.

Millington DS, Chace DH, Hillman SL, Kodo N, Terada N: Diagnosis of metabolic disease. In: Matsuo T, Caprioli RM, Gross ML, Seyama Y, eds: Biological Mass Spectrometry: Present and Future. New York, Wiley, 1994.

8.3   BASICS OF DIAGNOSTIC IMAGING

Wendy Zolotor Stiles, Brian D. Davison, and Johan G. Blickman

8.3.1   Introduction

To be of most help to a clinician, a radiologist must be a consultant, not only on imaging matters, but also on a clinical level. The radiologist should be thoroughly acquainted with the patient's clinical situation before undertaking a study. Moreover, both patients and parents should be aware of special preparation for selected studies (Table 8-4).

On the other hand, the imager should be considered part of the health-care delivery team and used to judge the necessity of an imaging study in relationship to radiation exposure, as well as the cost of a study, both financial and emotional. The primary-care physician and the radiologist should be versed in the manner in which pediatric disease processes and their diagnoses, treatments, and follow-up can be best assessed with different imaging modalities allowing for efficiency in diagnostic imaging and a less traumatic experience for the patient.

TABLE 8-4

PATIENT PREPARATION BEFORE SELECTED IMAGING

PROCEDURE	NPO	BOWEL PREPARATION NEEDED	SEDATION NEEDED (USUAL AGE GROUP)	OTHER NOTES
UGI	<2 yo: 3–4 h >2 yo: after MN	n/a		
Barium enema	4 h	No[+]		No solids on day of examination.
IVP	4 h	Yes, if patient >2 yo		No solids on day of examination.
CT	Infant: 4 h Child: after MN	n/a	4 mo–4 yo	Abdominal CT: use oral and IV contrast.[++]
MRI	4 h	n/a	<6 yo	
Nuclear imaging	2 h (8 h for gastric emptying)	n/a	1–4 yo	Liver/spleen scan should be performed before contrast studies. Renal scan: oral fluids to tolerance about 2 h preprocedure (ensure adequate hydration).
US	<4 yo: 4 h >4 yo: 8 h	n/a		

MN = midnight; n/a = not applicable. [+]Bowel preparation is not necessary in the children, and is contraindicated in suspected Hirschsprung disease. [++]Oral contrast not necessary in trauma situation. IV contrast contraindicated if renal stones are suspected. UGI = upper gastrointestinal, IVP = intravenous pyelogram, CT = computed tomography, MRI = magnetic resonance imaging, US = ultrasound.

8.3.2   Radiation Exposure

The amount of radiation to which the patient is exposed is a major concern for patients, parents, and practitioners alike. The quantity of exposure decreases as the distance of the object (patient) increases from the radiation source and varies with the type of source (ie, the intensity of the x-ray beam). In medical imaging, a more accurate measure of the ionizing radiation dose received by the patient can be made through determining the radiation level actually absorbed by the patient rather than simply exposure during an imaging procedure. The human body absorbs 90% of the radiation to which it is exposed, making the quantification of this small but definite health risk important. The rem (Roentgen Equivalent Man) is the most frequently used unit expressing the risk of biological damage caused by deposition of radiation dose in tissues and is dependent on the energy of the particles being deposited. The dose to which a patient is exposed varies with the diagnostic procedure (Table 8-5).

Although the effects of an atomic radiation event have been well described, radiation hazard is not nearly as easily defined in the doses used in diagnostic imaging. The gonads and bone marrow are most at risk, as is a developing fetus in the first trimester, but the exact amount at which the potential gene damage occurs is not known. The amounts of radiation exposure that state and federal guidelines allow are much lower than what has been potentially linked to human mutational effect. A typical diagnostic examination exposes the gonads to radiation ranging from 0 to 60 mrad, well under the projected significant gonadal dose.

Quantifying this information can best be done by putting radiation exposure factors in context. The radiation a person is exposed to every day comes from many sources; exposure to ionizing radiation for diagnostic studies is one of the smallest sources. Natural background (ie, from the soil, sun, etc.) radiation is estimated to be about 95 mrad/year, but varies with geographical location and skin pigmentation. As a rule of thumb, one chest x-ray is roughly equivalent to radiation exposure during a transcontinental airplane flight, one pack of cigarettes, or the exposure to radon of a person living in the northeastern United States in the winter. The acute lethal dose of radiation has been found to be 5000 rad. Thus, to accumulate enough radiation exposure to ensure death, a person

would have to undergo 2500 CT examinations consecutively! For comparison, the goal of radiation therapy is the eventual death of a target tissue using high-dose radiation (6000 rad).

8.3.3   Conventional Radiographs

During radiograph studies, anatomic position is extremely important. Nomenclature is based on which anatomic surface the x-ray beam passes through first. The difference between an anterior-posterior view (AP) and a posterior-anterior view (PA) is that in an AP view the beam passes from anterior to posterior, while the opposite is true for a PA. Most AP radiographs are carried out at the bedside, portably; a PA view is usually performed in the imaging suite. Contrary to adult images, this difference in technique does not affect magnification significantly in infants and young children.

THE CHEST

To evaluate a chest radiograph correctly, the reader should be aware of the type of view (AP, PA), appropriate exposure (such as easy identification of the thoracic bodies through the cardiothymic silhouette), alignment (symmetry of the clavicles and ribs), age of the child (both gestational and temporal), and clinical history. If there is a question of asymmetry of the lungs, fluoroscopy is preferred over inspiration/expiration films.

THE AIRWAY

Evaluation of the size, shape, position, and density of the trachea, pharynx, retropharynx, nasopharynx, epiglottis, tonsils and adenoids, and the bony skeleton can be achieved with AP and lateral imaging of the neck. Stridor is one of the most common indications, while other reasons for imaging the neck include snoring, hoarseness, abnormal cry, neck mass, suspected foreign body, epistaxis, trauma, and caustic ingestion.

The lateral film is most efficacious in shedding light on conditions such as: (a) encroachment of the adenoidal tissue on the nasopharyngeal airway; (b) retropharyngeal swelling/abscess (air in the retropharyngeal space); (c) degree of hypopharyngeal airway distention as a measure for airway encroachment (croup); and (d) identification of a radiopaque foreign body. The AP radiograph is best for evaluation of tracheal position. Normally, the trachea is slightly deviated to the right by the aortic arch (deviation to the left is always abnormal) and a normal thymus will not affect the position of the trachea.

ABDOMEN/PELVIS

Plain radiographs of the abdomen have traditionally been and should continue to be the initial examination in the workup of abdominal and pelvic symptoms. A supine *and* upright radiograph should be routine, except if encopresis is the clinical condition.

The most useful way to look at an abdominal radiograph is to imagine the anatomic structures individually in the area where they should be located. Then, "trace" them and identify potential abnormalities. Often, a soft tissue mass can be "seen" after consciously "tracing" the liver, spleen, stomach, and transverse colon.

Abnormal air patterns can also be distinctive. In the neonate, duodenal atresia may result in a characteristic plain film appearance, the *double-bubble* appearance. An *hourglass-* or *caterpillar-shaped* dilated stomach may suggest pyloric stenosis in the 4- to 8-week-old infant or midgut volvulus in a newborn, while in the 6- to 20-

TABLE 8-5

DOSE EQUIVALENTS (MREM) RELATED TO SELECTED DIAGNOSTIC PROCEDURE

PROCEDURE	EQUIVALENT DOSE (MREM)	MEAN GONADAL DOSE MALE (M), FEMALE (F) (MREM)
Chest x-ray	1–10	M: 1, F: 1
Skull or sinus series	10–22	M: 1, F: 1
Cranial CT	100–400	n/a
Barium enema (2× UGI)	300–800	M: 175, F: 903
Nuclear medicine study	200–1000	n/a

n/a = data not available.
NOTE: rem = roentgen equivalent man, absorbed dose, measure of risk of biological damage, dependent on energy of particles deposited; GU = nuclear scan 30 mrem to bladder wall 2–5 mrem for male.

month-old child with abdominal symptoms the density of a soft tissue mass created by an intussusceptum suggests intussusception. As the colon is an absorptive organ, air-fluid levels in the colon are always abnormal and this finding may indicate the presence of gastroenteritis (diarrhea) or a localized ileus due to neighboring inflammatory change. Tentative diagnoses may be made when abnormal collections of air are present in the scrotum or inferior to the inguinal ligament (an inguinal hernia), within the bladder (anorectal malformations, fistulae), or in the bowel wall (necrotizing enterocolitis (NEC)).

The characteristic feature of NEC is pneumatosis intestinalis, which is air within the subserosal or submucosal layers of the bowel wall. It may be a harbinger of perforation, yet the clinical course may wax and wane, or even resolve. If perforation occurs, free air may be seen between the liver and the abdominal wall on a left decubitus abdominal radiograph or resulting in the "football sign," on a supine film.

Adynamic ileus may display a characteristic pattern of increased intraluminal air without the usual stepladder configuration of obstruction. Erect or decubitus films may, however, demonstrate air-fluid levels because of the lack of peristalsis. The etiology is varied and includes patients who are postsurgery, septic, having electrolyte disturbances, dehydrated, or on morphine-like or anticholinergic drugs.

A paucity of colonic air, the stepladder pattern of air-fluid levels in distended loops of bowel, or a mass may all be findings in dynamic ileus. Usually this form of bowel obstruction has an anatomic cause. The differential diagnosis includes appendiceal inflammation, intussusception, inguinal hernia, adhesions, and malrotation.

While conventional radiography can be used for assessment of ascites with "central" location (floating) of air-filled bowel loops, ultrasound and CT are more sensitive and specific.

Finally, the normal appearance of air throughout the bowel can be important. Newborns should have air in the stomach at birth; if no gastric air is seen by 1 hour of life, esophageal obstruction should be considered. Similarly, air should pass through the small bowel by 12 hours and to the rectum within 24 hours after delivery.

SKELETAL

Conventional radiography is the traditional way to examine the bony skeleton, is excellent at revealing detail, and is less costly than more modern technology. Therefore, it remains the initial study in the evaluation of skeletal disease, in some cases rivaling pathology in diagnostic accuracy (bone tumors) (see Chap. 20). Adequate imaging includes at least two perpendicular or orthogonal planes (ie, AP and lateral). Comparison views are only obtained if a suspected abnormality is noted, and a possible normal variant must be differentiated.

CENTRAL NERVOUS SYSTEM

A skull series should include frontal views and horizontal-beam lateral views. The orbits, facial bones, and paranasal sinuses are evaluated with upright AP (Caldwell) and (angled) Waters views, as well as lateral projections. Conventional radiographs of the skull and sinuses are not used routinely but occasionally provide a starting point in evaluating trauma, infection, or craniofacial anomalies.

Conventional radiographs of the spine are the initial study in any child with suspected dysraphism, scoliosis, torticollis, or neurologic symptoms, or with clinical signs relating to the spine.

8.3.4   Contrast Studies/Fluoroscopy

TYPES OF CONTRAST AGENTS

Barium is an inert, inexpensive contrast agent that provides excellent mucosal coating. In the event of barium spilling from the gastrointestinal tract, it may cause granuloma formation. In general, the use of barium as a contrast agent is contraindicated with suspected bowel perforation or high-grade obstruction. Aspirated barium in a nonneurologically impaired patient is usually coughed up rapidly. Otherwise, chest physical therapy is employed.

Water-soluble agents are manufactured in three types: high-, iso-, and low osmolar varieties. In contrast to barium, these agents only fill the bowel lumen rather than coating the mucosa, decreasing their efficacy in evaluating mucosal lesions.

Hyperosmolar agents should not be used routinely in the upper or lower gastrointestinal tract as they may cause massive fluid shifts. With proper dilution, however, these agents can be made near isotonic and used in suspected perforation or to evaluate anatomic integrity, such as in NEC or bowel anastomoses after surgery. Also, these agents can be used as a therapeutic enema in conditions such as meconium ileus or plug by facilitating an increase in fluid in the bowel lumen to effect evacuation. Caution should be exercised when a patient is at risk for pulmonary aspiration, as the high osmolar agents often cause pulmonary edema or death when aspirated secondary to the release of histamine or histamine-like substances in the lung.

Advantages of the newer nonionic contrast agents are that dilution does not occur in the gastrointestinal tract and that the effect on the lungs with aspiration is minor when compared to osmolar agents. On the other hand, their cost is somewhat prohibitive.

Air is an alternative contrast agent and is especially advantageous in cases such as suspected esophageal atresia, in which a small amount of air could outline the atretic pouch, while liquid contrast media would carry a high risk for aspiration. Reduction of intussusception can be accomplished using air insufflation. If perforation occurs (rarely), extravasation of air does not result in any harm; unfortunately, the perforation rate is somewhat higher for air reduction than for barium reduction (2.5 vs 0.5%) of intussusception.

Double contrast makes use of both air and barium to better visualize the mucosa of the bowel. It is sometimes used in cases of suspected inflammatory bowel disease or to evaluate for the presence of polyps, but it is rarely used in the pediatric population.

UPPER GASTROINTESTINAL (UGI) STUDY

Anatomically, the UGI study evaluates the contour and mucosal lining of the naso-, oro-, and hypopharynx; esophagus; gastroesophageal (GE) junction; stomach; and duodenum, as well as localizing the ligament of Treitz (the duodenojejunal junction). Identifying the ligament of Treitz constitutes proof that normal rotation of the gastrointestinal tract has occurred in utero. Functionally, the UGI study provides visualization of the swallowing mechanism from the oral cavity to the stomach, in addition to peristalsis throughout the UGI tract. Anomalies in function, such as the presence of nasopharyngeal reflux or achalasia can be readily documented. Vomiting, abdominal pain, and GI bleeding are common indications for a UGI study.

Vomiting often is a sentinel sign of mechanical or functional obstruction of the GI tract. The abnormalities that can be detected with a UGI study encompass duodenal atresia, malrotation or midgut volvulus, and hypertrophic pyloric stenosis (HPS). Duodenal atresia might be identified on plain film and HPS may be detected by other noninvasive means, such as palpation or ultrasound. In an infant with bilious vomiting, the possibly fatal condition of midgut volvulus should be considered and a classic *corkscrew* appearance of the second and third portions of the duodenum is seen on UGI study when the small bowel is malpositioned in this condition.

Another common indication for UGI study is abdominal pain, including dysphagia and dyspepsia. In achalasia, the classic *bird's beak* appearance of the lower esophagus and associated disordered peristalsis will be identified on a supine radiograph with contrast. Gastroesophageal reflux (GER) cannot be fully evaluated by a UGI in the pediatric population without other studies. While a UGI study helps to rule out GER, the pH probe is the gold standard for diagnosis. In infants less than 9 to 12 months of age, the lower gastroesophageal junction sphincter is still maturing and GER may be detected but represent normal maturation. Therefore, imaging for GER in this age group is not fruitful.

A third common indication for a radiographic UGI evaluation is bleeding. In the neonate, NEC and infectious colitis are likely, while in the infant, a stress ulcer, Meckel diverticulum, and intussusception top the list of potential dignoses. The older child is more likely to have polyps or inflammatory bowel disease (IBD). In IBD, the UGI study may reveal involvement of the terminal ileum, fistulas, "cobblestoning," or a mass.

SMALL BOWEL FOLLOW-THROUGH

This extension of a UGI study enables the assessment of transit time and mucosal fold pattern—which may be helpful in evaluating patients with diarrhea/malabsorption, IBD, or unexplained gastrointestinal bleeding, chronic/recurrent abdominal pain, and vomiting.

BARIUM ENEMA (BE)

Barium enemas are used in the anatomic evaluation of suspected large bowel obstructions such as neonatal small left colon, meconium plug syndrome, ileal atresia, or Hirschprung disease. Localization of the colon to rule out malrotation has a low specificity, as the cecum in infants often is "floppy," a reflection of the intrauterine rotational process not being quite complete.

In intussusception, barium enema is used as both a diagnostic and therapeutic modality: identification of the intussusceptum and then possibly reduction. Postevacuation films should be obtained after intussusception reduction and after all single-contrast enema examinations to evaluate mucosal detail and rule out a lead-point lesion.

In Hirschsprung disease, the barium enema is 70% specific for definitive diagnosis by identifying a transition zone—a caliber change from a distended proximal portion to a more narrowed (aganglionic) distal bowel or rectum.

A contrast enema should not be performed if toxic megacolon is suspected or identified on conventional radiograph or if the patient has pseudomembranous colitis, peritonitis, or free intraperitoneal air.

Prominent lymphoid follicles found throughout the entire gastrointestinal tract are normal findings in children.

VOIDING CYSTOURETHROGRAM (VCUG)

The VCUG is used to evaluate for vesicoureteral reflux (VUR) and bladder function, as well as to depict bladder and urethral anatomy. Labial adhesions represent a relative contraindication to VCUG because imaging cannot be performed until these adhesions are released.

VCUG is most commonly performed on young children with a documented urinary tract infection (UTI) or for evaluation of a significantly dilated renal collecting system (for specific indication see Chap. 21). Other indications for performing VCUG include voiding dysfunction and delineation of anatomy and function of the bladder in patients with anorectal malformations, myelodysplasia, and prune-belly (Eagle-Barrett) syndrome.

The performance of a VCUG necessitates placing a 5- or 8-French pediatric feeding tube into the bladder with the use of a topical anesthetic. Psychological preparation for the child and parents is mandatory.

EXCRETORY UROGRAPHY (INTRAVENOUS PYELOGRAM OR IVP)

The IVP enables visualization of the entire urinary tract by an intravenously administered nonionic contrast agent excreted by the kidneys. An IVP can demonstrate anatomy (size, shape, and position) and can semiquantitatively evaluate renal function. Except for posturologic surgery, an IVP is rarely performed.

Abnormal ultrasound examination of the upper urinary tracts (shrunken/scarred kidney or hydronephrosis), suspicion of an obstructing urinary tract calculus, incontinence (in girls), and suspected neurogenic dysfunction of the bladder constitute the major indications for this examination.

Dehydration and shock are absolute contraindications to performing an IVP, whereas previous allergic reaction to contrast agents or shellfish is only a relative contraindication. In neonates, an IVP is limited because of the intrinsically low GFR.

8.3.5 Ultrasound (US)

The principle of ultrasound involves the use of high-frequency sound waves to detect the interface of two tissues with different densities. Energy is reflected based on the density of the tissue and converted into two-dimensional images. When sound waves encounter a moving object, the reflected frequency is changed and can be detected. This shift in frequency is proportional to the velocity of the moving object and can be used to evaluate blood flow to organs and tissues. Termed *Doppler imaging,* this technique facilitates identification of vessel patency and flow.

The advantages of ultrasound are numerous: (a) noninvasive; (b) superb imaging quality because of a paucity of fat in children; (c) easy and quick to perform; (d) portable; (e) minimal patient preparation; (f) no ionizing radiation; (g) no known risks; (h) seldom necessary to use sedation; and (i) inexpensive when compared to computed tomography or magnetic resonance imaging.

Disadvantages of ultrasound include the impossibility of imaging air-containing structures or bone, limited image quality in the obese patient, and dependency on the operator's skill.

ABDOMEN/PELVIS

Ultrasound is the screening modality of choice in the pediatric patient with suspected intra-abdominal pathology. In the diagnosis of appendicitis, the accuracy of ultrasound is 93% with sensitivity and specificity of 95% in the pediatric population. Ultrasound can also rule out other causes of right lower quadrant pain, such as ovarian cyst, ectopic pregnancy, IBD, or endometriosis. In hypertrophic pyloric stenosis (HPS) a "bull's-eye" or "donut" representing the hypertrophied pyloric muscle can be identified as well as elongation of the pyloric channel greater than 14 mm. When visualized on ultrasound, intussusception has been described as a "donut" or "pseudo-kidney."

The diagnosis of acute cholecystitis or cholelithiasis is often made by ultrasound. Ultrasound has a 95% accuracy in the diagnosis of "sludge," hyperconcentrated bile that presents as echogenic densities that change position with gravity, and thickening or irregularity of the gallbladder wall. Biliary duct dilation may also be seen. A hypoechoic halo may surround the gallbladder in the case of acute cholecystitis.

Ultrasound can reliably assess liver texture and anatomy, while splenic anomalies may be difficult to assess because of the spleen's limited accessibility. Splenomegaly is suggested if the tip of the spleen reaches below the lower pole of the kidney.

Ultrasound is 95% accurate in detecting pancreatic abnormalities if gastric air does not obstruct the ultrasound waves. The normal pancreatic duct may be visualized up to 3 mm. Cystic fibrosis manifests as an echogenic pancreas with occasional cysts.

GENITOURINARY

Ultrasound can delineate renal and retrovesical anatomy. The most common cause of a neonatal abdominal mass is hydronephrosis, which is best evaluated with ultrasound. In addition, hydronephrosis discovered in the prenatal period should be followed by reevaluation after birth. It is the screening modality of choice in infants and neonates with urosepsis, and in children at high risk for renal anomalies, tumors, and genital tract anomalies (see Chap. 21). Renal US provides good evaluation of renal size and growth of the kidneys for which standardized growth charts are available. In addition, assessment of bladder anomalies and bladder wall thickening can be achieved.

Ultrasound accuracy is high in the diagnosis of painful scrotal masses, such as acute and chronic torsion, epididymoorchitis, hydrocele, and tumor. Absent intratesticular flow in a prepubertal boy suggests torsion while normal or increased flows suggest epididymitis (see Sec. 21.16).

SKELETAL

Ultrasound is the gold standard in the screening evaluation of developmental dysplasia of the hip (formerly called congenital dislocation) in a dynamic fashion, as well as in the follow-up after repositioning. Evaluating the child's hip for toxic synovitis or an elbow for a joint effusion, possibly a supercondylar fracture, is another use for skeletal ultrasound.

CENTRAL NERVOUS SYSTEM

Ultrasound through the anterior fontanelle is noninvasive and provides rapid real-time and multiplanar imaging of the brain anatomy in the fetus and the preterm or term infant. It provides screening for intracranial hemorrhage, congenital malformations (Dandy-Walker, agenesis of the corpus callosum), ventricular size, atrophy, and large extracerebral fluid collections and cysts. Color-flow Doppler can be used in the evaluation of intracranial blood flow for the determination of brain death and to evaluate a patient with suspected galenic or other vascular malformation. In the screening of spinal dysraphism, ultrasound delineates the conus medullaris, which normally terminates above the L2 level. A tethered cord with a thickened filum and tethering masses such as lipomas can be reliably identified by ultrasound.

8.3.6   Computed Tomography (CT)

The principles of CT involve variable attenuation (absorption) of an x-ray beam as it passes through tissue based on the tissue's density, providing the computer with information to generate cross-sectional images. The technological advantage of CT is that CT can distinguish a difference in tissue attenuation of 0.1%, unlike conventional radiographs that record differences in attenuation of about 10%, preventing detailed characterization of various soft-tissue densities.

Conventional tomography evolved into incremental conventional CT and then into helical or spiral CT. Prior to spiral CT, the data were acquired with the patient on a table that was kept in a fixed position. In general, with spiral CT, the table and the gantry containing the x-ray generator and detectors are in continuous motion. The technological advance of spiral CT benefits patients by halving the scan time, thus leading to a proportional decrease in the exposure to radiation and to a near 45% reduction in the use of sedation. In addition, spiral CT provides volume acquisition of data, allowing after-the-fact reconstruction of any portion of the scanned volume (decreasing rescans), as well as production of three-dimensional images.

Noncontrast CT studies are useful for detecting calcium or hemorrhage (ie, renal stone or intracranial hemorrhage). For abdominal and pelvic CT, oral contrast helps distinguish normal bowel and prevents misinterpretation of unopacified bowel as being abnormal. Administration of oral contrast is contraindicated when a patient lacks a gag reflex or might require general anesthesia. Nonionic IV contrast is almost universally used and has reduced the incidence of contrast reactions by 90% but is contraindicated in suspected intracranial hemorrhage because leakage across the blood-brain barrier may cause focal cerebral edema and seizures. In children, the lack of abdominal fat limits delineation of retroperitoneal structures. In some cases, sedation may be required to limit motion artifacts.

CHEST

Indications for chest CT include further definition of anatomy, if it is not clear on conventional radiographs. Specifically, CT defines airway obstruction (foreign bodies), mediastinal pathology, and pulmonary metastatic disease, as well as subpleural, tracheal, chest wall, and major bronchial lesions.

ABDOMEN/PELVIS

CT is superior to ultrasound or plain radiographs in assessing solid abdominal masses and staging tumors, in delineating retroperitoneal anatomy, and in guiding drainage-catheter placement. For hemodynamically stable pediatric trauma patients, CT is the gold standard for evaluating the abdomen. Helical CT has a high sensitivity and specificity for vascular lesions (hemangiomas) of the liver and the evaluation of possible appendicitis or flank pain.

SKELETAL

CT is the appropriate imaging choice for delineating the extent of a bony lesion, as in stress or comminuted fractures, in addition to defining metastatic and primary bone lesions. CT also provides improved visualization of the bony skeleton through cast material and complex osseous structures, as well as pre- and postoperative imaging that uses three-dimensional reconstruction capability.

CENTRAL NERVOUS SYSTEM

For CNS studies, CT is the mainstay in imaging trauma victims and in evaluation of synostosis.

8.3.7 Magnetic Resonance Imaging (MRI)

MRI is based on the fact that a nucleus with an odd number of protons or neutrons has inherent spin, allowing it to behave as a magnet. Usually nuclei are randomly oriented, resulting in no net magnetization. In the presence of a static magnetic field, nuclei orient their axes parallel to the magnetic field. For example, hydrogen, having one proton, has inherent spin and will align with an applied magnetic field, resulting in a net magnetization occurring in the direction of the static field when the proton is in the ground state.

The spin on these nuclei is tilted; therefore, the spin actually appears more like wobbling. The wobbling nuclei-magnets have a characteristic frequency, known as the resonance frequency. If a radiofrequency signal is applied at this characteristic resonance frequency, the nuclei become excited and orient such that magnetization occurs in the transverse plane to the applied magnet, as opposed to the nuclei-magnets in the ground state, which arrange parallel to the applied magnet. This net magnetization in the transverse plane generates a radiofrequency signal that is detected by the receiving coil of the MRI system. As the excited nuclei return to ground state, loss of MRI signal intensity results. Thus, MRI takes advantage of the ability to induce and monitor the resonance of the magnetic moment of nuclei in magnetic fields

The interplay of the relaxation times (T1 and T2) and the concentration of hydrogen ions in tissue determine the intensity of signals that are converted to images. Each tissue has a characteristic T1 and T2 relaxation time as well as hydrogen ion concentration, whereby specific characteristics can be detected. Fat appears white because of its high concentration of hydrogen on T1 images and short T1 and long T2 relaxation times, whereas muscle is gray because of a high hydrogen concentration and intermediate T1 and T2 relaxation times. Air is black because of its extremely low concentration of hydrogen, and cortical bone is black because of its lack of mobile protons in addition to long T1 and short T2 relaxation times. Flowing blood is black on spin-echo images because of the flow of protons away from the area before the signal can be received.

Contrast-enhanced MRI employs gadolinium to perturb the local magnetic field, which allows the extent of perfusion of an organ or lesion to be delineated in much the same manner that IV contrast enhances CT imaging studies.

MRI produces images of superb diagnostic quality with the added ability to obtain data in almost any anatomic plane without employing ionizing radiation. There is excellent tissue and vessel contrast resolution even without the administration of gadolinium, resulting in high sensitivity, as well as specificity of diagnosis.

The disadvantages include the need for sedation to prevent movement artifact in most patients less than 6 years old, possible claustrophobia, and higher cost. Also, motion artifacts are more likely with MRI than with spiral CT because increased scan time. Currently available oral contrast agents do not opacify small bowel distal to the ligament of Treitz.

CHEST

MRI coupled to the electrocardiogram (gated MRI) and MR angiography (MRA) are becoming more widely used in the evaluation of mediastinal vasculature and for characterization of the vascular supply of bronchopulmonary foregut malformations. Anatomic and functional imaging of congenital heart disease, anomalies of the great vessels, and vascular lesions of the lung are frequently indicated. Even lung parenchymal imaging with hyperpolar gases shows promise, further evidence that the capability to connect structural and functional imaging is rapidly improving.

ABDOMEN

Peristalsis is a limiting factor for optimal intraperitoneal MR imaging. MRI is used primarily for retroperitoneal oncologic studies.

CENTRAL NERVOUS SYSTEM

In most instances, MRI is the modality of choice for evaluating intracranial anatomy, the extent of CNS development and myelination, the degree of blood-brain barrier breakdown (with the addition of gadolinium), and vascular integrity (with MRA). MRI T2-weighted imaging may be useful in the assessment of bacterial infections, if meningeal enhancement occurs. For vascular occlusive conditions, MRI has greater sensitivity and specificity than ultrasound or CT.

While ultrasound or CT detects the majority of intracranial masses, MRI defines the extent of lesions, particularly treatment-related responses of tumors. For the evaluation of tumor seeding, gadolinium enhancement is necessary. MRI is diagnostic for extradural extension of metastatic disease, such as neuroblastoma.

Unexplained hydrocephalus or seizures, as well as neuroendocrine disorders, are best approached by MRI, as are neurocutaneous syndromes, migrational anomalies, neurodegenerative diseases, encephalitis, cerebritis, abcesses, and orbital inflammation.

MRI of the spine offers improved depiction of developmental malformations (tethered cords), myelination disorders, neoplasm, infection, and trauma.

Head and neck masses, such as hemangiomas and their arterial and venous flow, lymphangiomas, branchial cleft anomalies, and nodal enlargement are best evaluated by sequential ultrasound and MRI.

SKELETAL

MRI can directly image the bone marrow, joints (osteonecrosis or Legg-Calvé-Perthes of the hips), cartilaginous structures, and soft tissues in the search for infection or tumor. Also, the extent of tumor and degree of vascular compromise are best depicted by this modality.

For example, osteosarcoma can be detected on plain x-ray by "sunburst" periosteal new-bone formation, while MRI defines bone marrow and soft tissue involvement before and after therapy (see Sec. 20.9). By outlining the extent of a chondrosarcoma on

MRI, the surgeon can more confidently map the area for wide excision of tumor. MRI delineates leukemia/lymphoma (or metastatic neuroblastoma) from fatty marrow (see Chap. 20).

8.3.8 Radionuclide/Nuclear Imaging

Radionuclide imaging provides functional data because studies reflect selective uptake or transit of radiopharmaceuticals in various organs. Radiopharmaceuticals may be used individually, such as 131-iodine (^{131}I), or bound to an organ-specific molecule, such as 99m technetium-DTPA (^{99m}Tc-DTPA). These studies are limited by poor anatomic resolution, yet the functional data acquired through dynamic (flow) or static (accumulation) methods may be useful in diagnosing disease processes that would alter tissue function before changing anatomic structure.

CHEST

Evaluation for pulmonary embolism employs a V/Q scan, which uses a radioactive gas such as xenon (^{133}Xe) or aerosolized radioactive particles for the ventilation study and intravenous radioactive macroaggregated albumin (^{131}I-MAA) particles for the perfusion study.

Cardiac structure and function can be assessed through multiple-gated acquisition (MUGA) of data in which a series of images representing an average cardiac cycle can be retrieved by using ^{99m}Tc-albumin.

Imaging cardiac shunts involves the injection of a radionuclide (^{99m}Tc-pertechnetate) through the jugular vein with digital acquisition of 0.5-second frames documenting transit through the heart and lungs. The pulmonary-to-systemic flow ratio is generated and provides precise quantification of left-to-right shunts. For identification of right-to-left shunts, the method uses the radionuclide ^{99m}Tc-MAA. The difference in the distribution of activity between the systemic circulation and lungs is a measure of the size of the shunt.

For staging of neoplastic lesions, 67-gallium citrate (^{67}Ga-citrate) is used most often. Imaging to localize inflammation (an abscess) can employ 111-indium (^{111}In) white blood cells (WBCs) or ^{67}Ga-citrate taking advantage of its avidity for white cells.

ABDOMEN

If GER is suspected clinically but not detected by other imaging techniques, then nuclear imaging may be helpful. The "milk scan" involves the mixture of ^{99m}Tc-sulfur colloid with the patient's normal meal (milk or formula, in the case of infants) and delivery into the stomach by way of bottle, nasogastric tube, or orogastric tube. GER is defined as spikes of increased activity above background on a time-activity curve. The frequency and magnitude of reflux can also be determined.

When the etiology for symptoms such as nausea, vomiting, distention, and weight loss is not revealed with other studies, a gastric-emptying ^{99m}Tc-sulfur colloid (mixed with solid) or ^{111}In-DTPA (in a liquid) nuclear scan is warranted. The amount of activity remaining in the stomach after the radionuclide meal is serially measured in order to determine the rate of emptying.

GI bleeding can be evaluated using ^{99m}Tc red blood cells (RBCs). In the case of ectopic gastric mucosa located in a Meckel diverticulum, such mucosa will selectively concentrate ^{99m}Tc-pertechnetate with an accuracy of 90 to 98%. This procedure should be performed before endoscopy or barium studies due to the possibility of localization of radionuclide to iatrogenically created areas of irritation. Barium may also mask the localization of the radionuclide.

Liver and spleen scans using ^{99m}Tc-sulfur colloid or ^{99m}Tc-albumin colloid are indicated in the (a) evaluation of functional liver disease, such as cirrhosis and hepatitis, (b) detection of hepatic lesions for biopsy, and (c) investigation of hepatomegaly, jaundice, ascites, and liver enzyme abnormalities. Static images are obtained at different time intervals. This examination has a high sensitivity, but poor specificity. The minimum detectable lesion is 1.5 cm in diameter. A unique distinguishing feature of hepatic hemangioma is that this lesion retains labeled RBCs for at least 2 hours.

A biliary scan using ^{99m}Tc-diSIDA can be useful to differentiate between neonatal hepatitis and biliary atresia. Images are obtained at various intervals up to 24 hours or until radioactivity is demonstrated in the gastrointestinal tract.

GENITOURINARY

Agents filtered by the glomerulus or secreted by the tubules are employed to assess renal function. Renal parenchyma is investigated with agents that are retained for prolonged periods of time.

The agent ^{99m}Tc-DTPA is freely filtered and neither reabsorbed nor secreted by the tubules of the kidney and evaluates renal function (GFR), prerenal blood flow, and postrenal collecting system integrity. Also, it can identify obstruction at the level of the ureteropelvic junction or ureterovesical junction, in addition to roughly estimating renal size and shape. When there is delayed excretion of the radiopharmaceutical from the collecting system, a diuretic (eg, furosemide) may be administered to further evaluate the functional significance of the obstruction.

In the past, tubular agents such as methenamine (Hippuran) evaluated renal plasma flow, but a more versatile agent, ^{99m}Tc-MAG3, is used today. It is freely filtered with near total tubular secretion and no tubular reabsorption, and provides better image quality at a lower absorbed radiation dose. Renal function curves can then be constructed from the digitally acquired information, determining the percent differential renal function.

In renal cortical scintigraphy, agents such as ^{99m}Tc-DMSA and ^{99m}Tc-glucoheptonate are utilized. These radionuclides can evaluate renal morphology, assess degree of scarring, and identify local inflammatory processes. Parenchymal transit time of the radionuclide may help to differentiate between etiologies of hydronephrosis.

Radionuclide cystography with ^{99m}Tc-pertechnetate can be used to evaluate for VUR. Although the sensitivity for VUR detection is higher, and the radiation dose is but 5% of a VCUG, the specificity for identification of lower urinary tract anatomic abnormalities is significantly lower than with VCUG (see Sec. 21.6).

SKELETAL

A three-phase bone scan involves dynamic acquisition of the area of interest immediately after injection of ^{99m}Tc-methylene diphosphonate, as well as extracellular (blood pool) imaging acquired within the first few minutes of injection, and delayed static images acquired at 2 to 3 hours postinjection of the radionuclide. This sequence reveals areas with increased blood flow, making it sensitive for pathology such as bone tumors, trauma, and avascular necrosis, as well as the diagnosis, staging, and assessment of response to therapy.

Furthermore, a bone scan is the most sensitive and specific test for differentiating septic arthritis, cellulitis, and osteomyelitis when conventional studies may appear normal. ^{33}Ga-citrate can then be used to further differentiate cellulites from osteomyelitis (see Chap. 13).

CENTRAL NERVOUS SYSTEM

Single-photon emission CT (SPECT) uses ^{99m}Tc bound to either an agent that can or cannot penetrate the blood-brain barrier and a gamma-camera to generate computer images. SPECT is useful in the evaluation of patients with epilepsy, differentiation of tumor progression, and determination of blood flow during seizures.

The extent of a tumor can be pinpointed better with SPECT imaging than with CT or MRI. SPECT can distinguish between tumor and gliosis (radiation necrosis) in patients with a change in neurologic status postradiation therapy. SPECT is also useful in the determination of brain death (see Chap. 25).

References

Blickman JG: Pediatric Radiology: The Requisites, 2nd ed. St. Louis, Mosby, 1999.

Katz DS, Math KR, Groskin SA: Radiology Secrets. Philadelphia, Hanley and Belfus, 1998.

Swischuk LE: Imaging of the Newborn, Infant and Young Child, 4th ed. Baltimore, Williams & Wilkins, 1998.

8.4   THE INTERPRETATION OF CLINICAL STUDIES AND DIAGNOSTIC TESTS

John M. Leventhal

Caring for patients is both an art and a science. The art depends in part on the clinical and personal experiences of the physician, the physician's relationship with the patient and family, and the physician's knowledge of the patient's wishes and desires. In contrast, the science depends upon what is known about the disease—including its pathophysiology, clinical characteristics, epidemiology, prognosis, and treatment. Most of the chapters in this book review what is known about the science of childhood diseases. This chapter takes a step back from the specific diseases and focuses on basic epidemiological principles for the interpretation of studies and diagnostic tests. These principles should be particularly helpful when relating the medical literature to specific patients' conditions. The topics covered are: (a) basic research designs and levels of evidence; (b) evaluation of diagnostic tests; and (c) reading the medical literature.

8.4.1   Research Designs and Levels of Evidence

When reviewing a clinical study there are at least four questions to be asked:

1. Who is being studied and are the results relevant to one's own patients?
2. What kind of study design is used and what effect should that have on interpreting the findings of the study?
3. Are the conclusions of the study valid?
4. How will the results affect one's practice?

WHO IS BEING STUDIED

To determine who is being studied and whether the results are generalizable to other populations and, in particular, one's own patients, it is necessary to examine the characteristics of the study population and the criteria for inclusion and exclusion. For some research questions, the similarity of the population being studied and one's own patients is less critical than for other questions. For example, the results of a study on the rate of urinary tract infections in uncircumcised males who are identified at birth at a large urban hospital and followed to 2 years of age should be generalizable to almost all practice settings. In contrast, the results of a study of child abuse in children born to adolescent mothers may not be relevant to all settings. If the study only includes children of impoverished adolescents who are followed in an inner city clinic, these results may not be generalizable to children of adolescents from rural or suburban communities, and clearly are not generalizable to children of all mothers.

STUDY DESIGNS

Three types of designs are reviewed: (a) experimental designs in which an intervention or maneuver is applied to one group in an attempt to change the rate of the occurrence of an outcome; (b) observational studies, in which the authors examine the relationship (or association) between an exposure and an outcome; and (c) descriptive studies. Experimental studies, or randomized controlled trials, with an intervention group and a control group, are considered the most powerful of the research designs and are used frequently to test new medications and interventions. Despite the importance of such studies in answering specific types of questions, many research questions cannot be answered using a randomized controlled study design. Such questions include: Does exposure to low levels of lead affect developmental outcomes? Are former premature infants more likely to have school problems when compared to former full-term infants? Which young children with fever are most likely to have bacteremia?

Experimental Studies

Randomized controlled trials (RCTs) are the gold standard when considering the validity of a study. They have the advantage of an experimental paradigm in which the intervention is imposed by the investigator and the process of randomization provides two groups of patients with equal susceptibility to the occurrence of the outcome. In such a study, the clinical population is identified and often narrowed to minimize the heterogeneity of the group. Patients are then assigned to the intervention or control group based on the randomization process. If the sample size is reasonably large, then the various characteristics of the patients that will influence the likelihood that the outcome will or will not occur will be evenly distributed by the randomization into the two groups. It is important to ensure that the patients in the intervention group actually receive the intervention. For example, if an oral medication is taken, a research nurse might watch the patient take the medication, pills might be counted, or a blood or urine level of the medication checked periodically. The control group should be free of the intervention. At a specific interval after the assignment of the patients to the two groups, the outcome is ascertained. To minimize bias, this determination should be done in an equivalent fashion for both groups. The best way to accomplish this is to have the investigators who are determining whether the outcome has occurred "blinded" to the patient's group assignment.

In an RCT, the rate of the occurrence of the outcome in each group can be calculated; this rate represents the incidence of the outcome. The incidence in each group can be compared by calculating the risk ratio (dividing the incidence in the treatment group by the incidence in the control group) and determining the 95% confidence interval. If the rate of the outcome in the intervention group is statistically different from the rate in the control group, and if the groups are equivalent in the important variables other than the intervention, then one can conclude that the difference is due to the intervention

While the major strength of an RCT is the experimental design, there also are four important limitations. The first relates to generalizability because often many patients are excluded from such studies. If there are too many restrictions and exclusions, the population studied might not be comparable to those in one's practice. For example, in a study of a new antimicrobial to treat otitis media, patients with other illnesses (eg, asthma or other chronic conditions) or with recent treatment for otitis media might be excluded from the RCT, and thus the study would provide no data about the effectiveness of the medication in these excluded patients. Second, RCTs usually only provide information about whether the intervention is helpful in a group of patients, not whether it will be helpful to a specific patient sitting in the physician's office. The results of RCTs are unlikely to provide information about which patients will benefit from the treatment and under what conditions. Third, RCTs are expensive to conduct and often require large sample sizes. Finally, RCTs can answer only a limited range of scientific and clinical questions because of either ethical constraints or because of the clinical questions being posed.

Observational Studies

In observational studies, the intervention is not imposed by the investigator; rather, the investigator identifies a risk factor or exposure variable and examines its association with an outcome. This type of design can be used to examine the association between child sexual abuse and adult depression, respiratory syncytial virus (RSV) during infancy and the subsequent occurrence of asthma, or the presence of coronary aneurysms in Kawasaki disease and the later occurrence of death. Studies can be designed prospectively in which subjects are followed forward over time, retrospectively in which data are collected about past events, or using a combination of the two approaches. For observational studies, the three research designs are the cohort study in which sampling is done based on the exposure or risk factor; the case-control study in which sampling is based on the outcome; and cross-sectional studies in which information about the exposure and outcome is obtained at the same time by interview or questionnaire.

Cohort Studies

In cohort studies, two groups are identified based on the exposure or risk factor. One group has been exposed to the factor (eg, prematurity) and the other group has not (full-term infants). The two groups are then followed over time, and the outcome (low IQ) is determined. In a cohort design, the analysis is similar to an RCT; the incidence of the outcome in each group and the risk ratio are calculated. If the outcome occurs more commonly in the group with the factor and the two groups are comparable on variables that affect the occurrence of the outcome, then this factor is considered a risk factor for the outcome. The individuals with and without the risk factor might be prospectively identified by the investigators and followed forward in time. Alternatively, a cohort can be identified

in the past and divided into the two groups based on the exposure. The outcome also can be identified in the past, so the entire study is done retrospectively.

Because patients are not allocated to the two groups by randomization, the research design is a less powerful one than an RCT. The validity of the results depends on the methodologic rigor of the study. Bias can occur because of at least three methodologic problems: (a) failure to ensure the comparability of the two groups at baseline; (b) an inadequately defined risk factor; or (c) unequal ascertainment of the outcome in the two groups.

Comparability of the Two Groups In an RCT, the two groups should only differ by one variable: the presence or absence of the imposed intervention. In a cohort study, however, the risk factor is not randomly assigned and the two groups will likely differ on other variables at baseline. If, for instance, one of these other variables occurs more commonly in the group with the risk factor and that same variable affects the likelihood of the outcome occurring, then it would be false to conclude that the difference in the rates of the outcomes in the two groups is due to the presence or absence of the risk factor being studied. Failure to adjust or control in the analysis for this other variable, termed a *confounder,* would lead to a biased result. Because of the importance of baseline differences in the two groups, a table describing these baseline characteristics is a critical feature in assessing a cohort study.

The issue of the failure to control for potential confounders, which leads to biased results, is important. For example, studies that examine early experiences (eg, in utero exposure to drugs, breast feeding vs bottle feeding, frequent episodes of otitis media, or the occurrence of child maltreatment) and later developmental outcomes (eg, intelligence, language development, school performance, or attachment) may have a major limitation if potential confounders (either those that are measured, such as socioeconomic status, or those that might not be measured, such as parental stimulation of the child) are not assessed.

Investigators commonly use two different strategies in an attempt to minimize bias and control for confounders. One strategy is "matching," which occurs in the selection of the comparison group (ie, the group without the risk factor). In this strategy, after the group with the risk factor (index group) has been identified, a comparison group without the risk factor is chosen by selecting subjects who are identical to the index group on predefined variables such as age, socioeconomic status, ethnicity, and so on. Such matching ensures comparability of the index and comparison groups for these potential confounders. The other strategy is controlling in the analysis for baseline differences in potential confounding variables and reporting the unadjusted and adjusted results, the latter having been adjusted for the potential confounders.

Clear Definition of the Risk Factor In an RCT, the intervention is imposed by the investigators. In a cohort study, the groups are defined by the presence or absence of the risk factor, so it is important for this factor to be clearly defined and for adequate information to be obtained to ensure its absence in the comparison group.

Equal Ascertainment of the Outcome The duration of follow-up and the approach to determining whether the outcome has occurred should be comparable in both groups of a cohort study. It is important that the investigators describe the rate of follow-up in each group and whether the rates are comparable. Because the group with the risk factor may be followed more carefully or intensely than the comparison group, the rate of the outcome might be falsely elevated in this group because of detection bias. "Blinding" of the investigators also helps to ensure comparable ascertainment and to minimize detection bias.

Case-Control Studies

In case-control studies, sampling is based on the presence or absence of the outcome: cases are subjects identified with the outcome (low IQ) being investigated, and controls are those without the outcome (normal IQ). The investigator then looks backward in time to determine the presence of the exposure or risk factor (prematurity) in each group. The rate or prevalence of the risk factor in each group can be compared and is termed an *odds ratio*. If the prevalence of the exposure is significantly higher in the cases than in the controls, then that exposure is considered a risk factor for the outcome that was used to define the cases. It is important to note that in this research design, the frequency or incidence of the outcome cannot be determined since it was used to define the cases being selected for study.

In case-control studies, the directionality of the data collection depends on the research question. In a retrospective study, cases might be selected from a cancer registry and controls from similar neighborhoods to examine the exposure to in utero radiation. For a prospective study, cases may be identified by active surveillance for an outcome such as varicella; controls might be chosen from the same pediatric practice and the exposure might be whether the varicella vaccine was received.

Case-control studies are usually considered the least scientifically valid of the research designs and the most subject to bias. Critical aspects of the design include (a) how the cases and controls are selected and (b) how the exposure or risk factor is ascertained.

Selection of Cases and Controls Cases should be representative of children with the outcome, as opposed to the most severe or obvious cases. It is important that the investigators ensure that the control group does not have the disease or outcome. Often controls are chosen from the general population. If the outcome is relatively rare, it would be unlikely for the controls to have the outcome; on the other hand, if the outcome of interest is relatively common, it would be important for the investigators to explicitly delineate how it has been determined that the selected controls are actually free of the disease.

A second critical methodologic issue in the selection of the two groups is their comparability. Cases and controls should be chosen from populations that have the equivalent potential of being exposed to the risk factor. For example, in a study of the association of child abuse and adolescent pregnancy, if the cases of abuse are from an urban, underserved area where the rate of adolescent pregnancy is high, then the controls should be chosen from a similar population. If on the other hand, controls are chosen from a suburban population with a very low rate of teen pregnancy, then cases and controls will not be comparable. Comparability can be ensured by matching controls to cases on important sociodemographic variables or choosing controls from a similar population such as a pediatric practice or geographic location. If the groups of cases and controls are large enough, important differences between the groups can be adjusted in the analyses. An alternative strategy is to select cases and controls from a diagnostic registry; for example, cases might be children with a positive lumbar puncture for bacterial meningitis and the controls those children with a negative culture. The risk factor might be the height of the child's fever.

Ascertainment of the Risk Factor To minimize bias in the ascertainment of the risk factor, information about the presence of the risk factor needs to be obtained in an identical manner in both groups. Detection or recall bias can occur if one group, usually the case group, has an added incentive to remember differently than the control group. For example, mothers of children with mental retardation may recall more difficulties with pregnancy, labor, or delivery than mothers of normal children. In such a study, it might be important to determine whether such differences are due to differences in the recall of the events versus true differences in the occurrences of certain risk factors related to pregnancy or delivery.

In ascertaining the risk factor, the investigators should ensure that the risk factor preceded the occurrence of the outcome. For example, in a case-control study to determine whether RSV infection is a risk factor for the subsequent development of asthma, it would be important for the investigators to ensure that in the cases of children with asthma, the RSV infection actually occurred before the occurrence of asthmatic symptoms.

Despite these limitations, this research design has several advantages. First, the necessary sample size is much smaller than that of a cohort study; second, the study can be conducted over a shorter period of time because the investigators do not have to wait for several years for the outcome to occur; and third, such studies are often much less expensive than longitudinal studies. This methodology can be particularly useful when investigating relatively rare events, such as specific childhood cancers, new diseases, such as fibromyalgia or Reye syndrome, or outbreaks of illnesses, such as hemolytc uremic syndrome.

Cross-Sectional Studies

A common approach to data collection is to obtain information about the risk factor and outcome at the same time. The investigator can then analyze the data using either a cohort or case-control approach. For example, a questionnaire might be used to survey high school seniors about sexual abuse (the risk factor) and suicidal ideations or gestures (the outcomes). In the analysis, the investigators could divide the adolescents by the presence or absence of sexual abuse and determine the rates of suicidal ideations or gestures. Alternatively, these same data could be analyzed as a case-control study. Clearly, it is important in such a study to be sure that the risk factor preceded the outcome.

Descriptive Studies

Single case reports or case series may describe a new disease, interesting features of a patient or group of patients, or the natural history of a disease. Although such descriptions usually do not involve research hypotheses or comparison groups, these descriptive studies can be very helpful: for instance, the descriptions of the battered child syndrome, specific clinical findings associated with a metabolic disease, or a genetic abnormality.

Level of Evidence

The validity of a study refers to whether the results are true or accurate. This validity depends upon the methodologic rigor of the study design. In a well-designed study, bias, which can lead to a systematic error in measurement, is minimized; thus the results are likely to be valid. In general, experimental studies are least likely and observational studies are most likely to be subject to bias. With appropriate rigor and evaluation, bias can be minimized and valid conclusions obtained.

Whether the results change one's practice depends on several factors. First, are the results clinically, as well as statistically, significant? With large samples, statistical significance can occur, but the clinical difference between the groups might be small and less meaningful to patient care. In an RCT, the clinical significance of the results might be more clearly presented by reporting on the number needed to be treated. For example, if one needs to treat 100 patients to cure 1 child, the clinician can decide whether this treatment option is clinically wise. Second, have the results been replicated in other studies? In other words, there should be evidence that the findings are reproducible. Third, have others endorsed the results? Finally, can the intervention or new approach to diagnosis be implemented in practice or are substantive changes necessary to achieve the reported outcome.

8.4.2   Evaluation of Diagnostic Tests

Many clinical studies compare the accuracy of a medical test, such as a screening or diagnostic test, to an outcome, such as a disease state. For example, a screening test might be compared to a diagnostic or more detailed and expensive test (eg, capillary lead to venous lead or the Denver Developmental Screening Test to the Bayley Scales of Infant Intelligence), or a test might be compared to a disease state (eg, in a febrile 6-week-old, the WBC to bacteremia or in a child with abdominal pain, a spiral CT scan to appendicitis). Studies evaluating such screening or diagnostic tests are designed with two groups: those with the outcome or disease and those without. To determine the accuracy of a test, the investigator compares the results of the test in the two groups, as shown in Table 8-6. The sensitivity of a test is defined as the capability of a test to detect the disease or outcome when the disease is actually present $(a/(a+c))$. When the test is negative, but the disease is present, a false-negative has occurred and the false-negative rate is represented as $1-$sensitivity. Specificity is defined as the capability of a test to detect the absence of a disease when the disease is not present $(d/(b+d))$. If the test is positive, but the disease is not present, one has a false-positive and the false-positive rate is represented as $1-$specificity.

Two other important characteristics of a test provide information about the likelihood of the occurrence of the disease when the test is positive or negative. The positive predictive value is defined as the ratio of subjects with a positive test and disease (a) to all subjects with a positive test $(a+b)$: $(a/(a+b))$. The negative predictive value is defined as the proportion of subjects with a negative test who do not have the disease (d) to all subjects with a negative test $(c+d)$: $(d/(c+d))$. These predictive values are of particular relevance for the clinician who wants to know what the likelihood of the occurrence of the disease is, given the result of a test.

If the test being examined were perfect in distinguishing between diseased and nondiseased subjects, the sensitivity, specificity, and predictive values would be 100%. Because most tests have errors, clinicians are faced with the challenge of interpreting imperfect tests. A highly sensitive test would detect most of the cases of the disease, regardless of the specificity (eg, an ANA test for patients with suspected SLE). Such a test would be a good screening test, but additional tests might be necessary to confirm who has the disease (eg, an anti-ds DNA test to specifically diagnose SLE). Table 8-7 compares a test with high sensitivity (Table 8-7a) to a test with high specificity (Table 8-7b) with a highly sensitive test (sensitivity is 99%, and the specificity 50%). A negative test means that the disease can be "ruled out" because the false-negative rate is a very low 0.2% (1/501). A positive result in this setting is less helpful because the positive predictive value is only 16.5% (99/599). With a test that is highly specific (Table 8-7b), the sensitivity is 90% and specificity is 99.5%; it is very rare for subjects without the disease to have a positive test. In this situation, the positive predictive value is 94.7% (90/95). Thus, tests with high specificity are useful in "ruling in" a specific diagnosis.

The frequency or prevalence of a disease in a population affects the predictive values of a test and thus the interpretation of the results. In Table 8-7, the prevalence of disease is represented by $(a+c)/(a+b,+c+d)$. The importance of prevalence is shown in Table 8-8. The prevalence of the disease is high (20%) in Table 8-8a and low (5%) in Table 8-8b. The sensitivity and specificity of the test are 95% in both Table 8-8a and b. When the prevalence is high the positive predictive value is 82.6%. Accordingly, if the clinician treats all patients with positive tests, the majority will have the disease. In contrast, when the prevalence of the disease is low (Table 8-8b), the positive predictive value is 50%, so only half the patients with a positive test will actually have the disease. When the prevalence is low, the clinician might decide that (a) the treatment

TABLE 8-6
CHARACTERISTICS OF A TEST

TEST RESULT	DISEASE		
	PRESENT	ABSENT	
Positive	a	b	a+b
Negative	c	d	c+d
	a+c	b+d	a+b+c+d

Sensitivity = a/(a + c)
Specificity = d/(b+d)
Positive predictive value = a/(a+b)
Negative predictive value = d/(c+d)

TABLE 8-7
EXAMPLES OF TESTS WITH HIGH SENSITIVITY OR HIGH SPECIFICITY

a. Test with High Sensitivity

TEST RESULT	DISEASE		TOTAL
	PRESENT	ABSENT	
Positive	99	500	599
Negative	1	500	501
Total	100	1000	1100

Sensitivity = 99/100 = 0.99
Specificity = 500/1000 = 0.50

b. Test with High Specificity

TEST RESULT	DISEASE		TOTAL
	PRESENT	ABSENT	
Positive	90	5	95
Negative	10	995	1005
Total	100	1000	1100

Sensitivity = 90/100 = 0.90
Specificity = 995/1000 = 0.995

TABLE 8-8

EFFECTS OF DIFFERENT PREVALENCES ON POSITIVE PREDICTIVE VALUE

a. High Prevalence (20%) of the Disease

| | DISEASE | | |
TEST RESULT	PRESENT	ABSENT	TOTAL
Positive	1,900	400	2,300
Negative	100	7,600	7,700
Total	2,000	8,000	10,100

Positive predictive value = 1,900/2,300 = 0.826

b. Low Prevalence (5%) of the Disease

| | DISEASE | | |
TEST RESULT	PRESENT	ABSENT	TOTAL
Positive	475	475	950
Negative	25	9,025	9,050
Total	500	9,500	10,100

Positive predictive value = 475/950 = 0.50

is relatively benign so it is tolerable to treat many patients without the disease, (b) the test is not useful in the population and a different test must be chosen, or (c) a second confirmatory test is necessary when the initial test result is positive.

In some studies of diagnostic testing, the investigators aim to determine the best demarcation or cutoff for a test that does not have a discrete positive or negative result. An example of such a test might be a continuous variable such as the WBC or height of fever in predicting bacteremia or serious illness. The investigators can determine the best demarcation for the WBC by developing a Receiver Operating Characteristic (ROC) curve. To develop this curve, the investigators choose a series of demarcations for the WBC (eg, 12,500, 15,000, 17,500, 20,000) and plot the sensitivity versus 1–specificity for each WBC value. The demarcation that maximizes sensitivity and minimizes 1–specificity can then be chosen from the curve that is developed. An alternative demarcation might be chosen if the goal is to maximize sensitivity regardless of 1–specificity.

8.4.3   Reading the Medical Literature

With the availability of computerized searches and access to the medical literature (both abstracts and full texts), reading of the literature has become both easier because of almost instantaneous access and more challenging because of the need to synthesize large quantities of information. In general, two different approaches to medical information are used "keeping up" and reading about a specific patient or problem.

Current journals are read for a variety of reasons—keeping abreast of current knowledge, learning about controversies, finding relevant information about a recent patient, or even recognizing an article by a colleague. Although individualized approaches to scanning the current literature are developed, a helpful approach in deciding what to read might focus on these questions:

1. Is the topic of interest?
2. Are the patients in the study similar to one's practice?

3. Is this the optimal research design to answer the question?
4. Are there important biases that affect the validity of the results?
5. What are the results?
6. Are the findings clinically meaningful?
7. Is there an editorial to place the results in context?
8. When are there side effects of the intervention?
9. What are the costs of changing practice (or implementing the intervention)?
10. Is there enough information to change practice?

A second approach to reading is to focus on a specific clinical problem or question related to patient care and to read the relevant literature. Although this scientific approach to answer questions has been used for some time, recent attention to evidence-based medicine has emphasized critical examination and synthesis of relevant articles that use methodologically sound research designs.

When reading about a problem, several types of articles are available, from those that use different research designs to those that attempt to summarize or synthesize current knowledge. Over the last several years, there has been increasing attention on efforts to summarize the extant literature on a specific topic or question. Four general approaches have been used: (a) generalized clinical reviews, which summarize what is known and which provide advice about diagnosis and management; (b) meta-analyses; (c) methodologic reviews; and (d) practice guidelines. Because the first approach is well known, only the other three approaches are described.

In a *meta-analysis,* investigators attempt to provide a summary estimate of the effectiveness of an intervention from multiple individual studies. For example, a meta-analysis could summarize the effects of all the randomized trials of antimicrobial agents compared to placebos in the treatment of otitis media. The summary value, because of the increased sample size due to the inclusion of patients from many studies, will have a narrower confidence interval than the results of a single study. Meta-analyses also have been used to summarize the results of observational studies, for example, the effects of the exposure to low levels of lead on intelligence.

When evaluating a meta-analysis, there are several challenges to be considered. First, have the investigators identified all relevant studies, and are all the relevant data published? For example, studies that show no effect are less likely to be published than studies showing an effect. Second, are the target populations, interventions, and outcomes in the various studies comparable enough to be included in the meta-analysis? For example, if the dose of the medication used in one RCT is markedly higher than the dose used in other trials, should the RCT with this higher dose be included? Third, in a meta-analysis, poorly and well designed studies are often combined. If there are more poorly designed studies that show a large effect, but the few well-designed studies show no effect, combining these studies would produce a biased meta-analysis. An effort to produce, update, and collate meta-analyses on all interventions is called the Cochrane collaboration. Methodologists and clinicians volunteer to provide systematic reviews of interventions, and these reviews are available through publication and/or on the Internet.

A somewhat different approach to summarizing studies is taken in a *methodologic review*. In such a review, the investigators systematically analyze the critical methodologic strengths and weaknesses of the relevant studies, and attempt to identify those studies that are less likely to be flawed. The conclusions of those studies are then summarized in an effort to provide the best answer to the question posed by the studies. This approach to summarizing studies can be particularly helpful when reviewing clinical issues that cannot be studied with an experimental intervention.

An additional approach to reviewing studies and to linking the finding to a clinical problem is the development of clinical practice guidelines. Such guidelines often are published by an authoritative organization after an extensive review of the relevant literature. The American Academy of Pediatrics, for example, has published many guidelines on topics such as hyperbilirubinemia of the newborn, febrile seizures, and minor head trauma. These guidelines attempt to guide practice, to help clinicians make decisions that are based on evidence from the literature, and to indicate where there is inadequate evidence to provide clear guidelines. This third point should help to stimulate relevant clinical research so that important gaps in knowledge can be filled.

References

Bailar JC: The promise and problems of meta-analysis. N Engl J Med 337: 559, 1997.

Evidence-Based Medicine Working Group: Evidence-based medicine: a new approach to teaching the practice of medicine. JAMA 268:2420, 1992.

Horwitz RI: The dark side of evidence-based medicine. Cleve Clin J Med 63:320, 1996.

Jekel JF, Elmore JG, Katz DL: Epidemiology, Biostatistics, and Peventive Medicine. Philadelphia, WB Saunders, 1996.

Lau J, Ioannidis JPA, Schmid CH: Summing up evidence: one answer is not always enough. Lancet 351:123, 1998.

Oxman AD, Cook DJ, Guyatt GH: Users' guide to the medical literature. VI. How to use an overview. JAMA 272:1367, 1994.

METABOLIC DISORDERS

Roderick R. McInnes and Joe T. R. Clarke

9.1 A CLINICAL APPROACH TO INBORN ERRORS OF METABOLISM

Joe T. R. Clarke, Pranash K. Chakraborthy, and Roderick R. McInnes

9.1.1 General Principles

HOW TO USE THIS CHAPTER

This introductory section on inborn errors of metabolism provides a clinically oriented guide to the use of the other sections of the chapter. It is organized according to the clinical presentation or the most prominent clinical feature of various inherited metabolic diseases, with more detail about the specific defects provided in subsequent sections that are organized biochemically or by organ system. The two parts of the chapter are, therefore, complementary. This overview addresses a problem confronted by pediatricians: when to consider that the problems presented by a patient might be the result of an inborn error of metabolism, and what to do next to approach a specific diagnosis (see Sec. 8.2). The introductory section meets the need for a broad clinical framework to facilitate the recognition and preliminary investigation of inborn errors of metabolism. The later sections provide more detail about the pathophysiology, diagnosis, and management of various specific metabolic diseases. The biochemical organization of these later sections facilitates the discussion of pathophysiology and a rational approach to the diagnosis and management of specific diseases.

WHAT ARE INBORN ERRORS OF METABOLISM?

The expression *inborn error of metabolism* was coined almost a century ago by Sir Archibald Garrod, who used it to describe four rare, relatively benign, hereditary metabolic curiosities—albinism, alkaptonuria, cystinuria, and benign pentosuria—explainable by point defects in metabolism inherited in a mendelian fashion as autosomal recessive traits. The concept has since expanded to include more than 400 conditions involving deficiencies of specific enzymes or transport proteins causing diseases affecting virtually every system of the body. Although most of these disorders are inherited as autosomal recessive conditions, a significant minority are transmitted as X-linked recessive disorders and a few as dominant diseases. Mutations in the mitochondrial genome, which is inherited matrilineally, make up a rapidly growing subgroup of inborn errors of metabolism; these disorders exhibit some unique genetic and clinical characteristics (see Sec. 9.7.3).

HOW DO INBORN ERRORS OF METABOLISM CAUSE DISEASE?

The key to understanding how inborn errors of metabolism cause disease is to understand the primary and remote metabolic consequences of defects in specific metabolic processes. This knowledge also facilitates a logical approach to the diagnosis of these disorders through analytical biochemical and physiological investigations (see Sec. 8.2).

The primary consequences of point defects in metabolism are shown in Fig. 9-1. The pathophysiology of most metabolic defects, for example in the conversion of compound B to C, arises from the accumulation of B, the deficiency of C, or from some combination of the two. The accumulation of B may also inhibit other reactions such as the conversion of E to F. Occasionally, normally minor metabolites, such as D, accumulate and contribute to the pathogenesis. The accumulation of G_{M2}-ganglioside in the brains of children with Tay-Sachs disease, caused by deficiency of β-hexosaminidase A, is a good example of a condition in which substrate accumulation is important in the pathogenesis of the disease. Defects in hormone biosynthesis and some of the inherited defects of amino acid metabolism exemplify diseases that result from deficiency of a product. Secondary or more remote metabolic consequences of inborn errors of metabolism may be particularly important in the production of disease, such as the lactic acidosis and hypoglycemia that are prominent features of hereditary fructose intolerance. Awareness of the possibility of metabolically remote effects of inborn errors of metabolism is important in the interpretation of diagnostic laboratory information. For example, hyperglycinemia is a prominent feature of some of the organic acidurias, such as propionic aciduria. However, the primary defect in

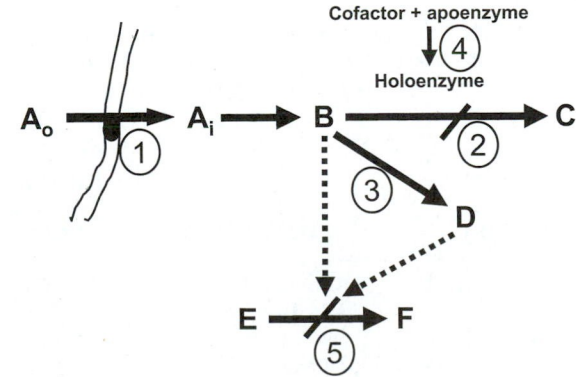

FIGURE 9-1 The metabolic consequences of inborn errors of metabolism. 1, Transporter-mediated movement of A from one compartment to another; 2, defect in the conversion of B to C; 3, increased conversion of B to D resulting from accumulation of B; 4, defect in the reaction or interaction between an apoenzyme and a cofactor required for enzyme activity; and 5, secondary inhibition of the conversion of E to F by excess B or D.

the disease, deficiency of propionyl-CoA carboxylase, does not involve glycine, and accumulation of glycine does not appear to play a significant role in the pathogenesis of the disease.

HOW ARE INBORN ERRORS OF METABOLISM INHERITED?

Autosomal Recessive Inheritance

The majority of known inborn errors of metabolism are transmitted as autosomal recessive conditions. The overall frequency of heterozygous carriers of any specific autosomal recessive mutations in most populations is relatively low, and the majority of inborn errors are rare, with an incidence of less than 1 in 15,000 births. However, the incidence of disease in various subgroups within the general population may be much higher as a result of assortative mating, the tendency for individuals to marry within their own ethnic or cultural groups. Certain inborn errors of metabolism are so common in some ethnic groups or genetically isolated populations that the diseases are often identified with the group. Some examples of inborn errors of metabolism occurring at a particularly high frequency in specific groups are shown in Table 9-1.

The most extreme example of this phenomenon is marriage within the family, and as Garrod himself noticed, the incidence of consanguinity is much higher among the parents of children with rare inborn errors of metabolism than in the general population.

Specific mutant alleles often reach high frequencies in genetically isolated populations. For example, two mutant *HEXA* alleles account for almost 95% of all mutations causing Tay-Sachs disease in Ashkenazi Jews; in non-Jews, the same mutations account for less than a third of the mutant alleles found in Tay-Sachs disease carriers. This concentration of specific mutant alleles can be used to advantage in the diagnosis of disease, as well as in carrier detection, among members of the group in question. In contrast, in members of the general population, specific mutation analysis is less useful for diagnosis and is generally of little value for carrier detection.

X-Linked Recessive Inheritance

Some important inborn errors of metabolism, such as X-linked adrenoleukodystrophy, are transmitted as X-linked recessive traits.

TABLE 9-1

SOME EXAMPLES OF INBORN ERRORS OF METABOLISM OCCURRING IN HIGH FREQUENCY AMONG SPECIFIC ETHNIC GROUPS

DISEASE	ETHNIC GROUP	ESTIMATED INCIDENCE (PER 100,000 BIRTHS)
Gaucher disease, type 1	Ashkenazi Jews	100
Tay-Sachs disease	Ashkenazi Jews	33
Gaucher disease, type 3	Swedish (Norrbottnia)	uncertain
Congenital adrenal hyperplasia	Yupik Eskimos	200
Hepatorenal tyrosinemia	French-Canadians	54
Porphyria variegata*	South African whites	300
Maple syrup urine disease	Pennsylvania Mennonites	568

* Actually transmitted as an autosomal dominant condition with highly variable expressivity.

The incidence of these disorders is not affected by inbreeding, and they tend not to be concentrated within specific ethnic groups. On the other hand, because the inheritance of only one mutant gene is sufficient to cause disease, there is more often a family history of these diseases than is the case for autosomal recessive conditions. Affected individuals are usually male, although females can also be affected as a result of the random inactivation of one X-chromosome in every cell, a process known as *lyonization* (see Chapter 10). As many as a third of boys with X-linked recessive inborn errors, without a family history of the condition, are found to have the disease as a result of a new germline mutation occurring either in them or in their mothers. Finally, because of the much greater contribution of new mutations to the occurrence of X-linked recessive inborn errors, disease-causing mutations tend to be much more variable than the mutations causing autosomal recessive conditions. Each family tends to have its own mutation, which are known as *private* mutations. This characteristic severely limits the usefulness of specific mutation analysis for the diagnosis and carrier detection of X-linked recessive inborn errors of metabolism.

Autosomal Dominant Inheritance

Few inborn errors of metabolism are inherited as autosomal dominant conditions. In general, autosomal dominant diseases more often involve structural or receptor proteins, rather than catalytic proteins. For example, a common autosomal dominant disorder, familial hypercholesterolemia, is most often caused by mutations in the low-density lipoprotein receptor. One autosomal dominant disease due to an enzyme defect is acute intermittent porphyria caused by mutations in porphobilinogen deaminase.

Mitochondrial Inheritance

A family history of matrilineal disease transmission, with males and females equally affected, but with no instance of transmission from an affected male to his offspring, is typical of the inheritance of mutations of the mitochondrial genome. A high proportion of disease caused by mitochondrial mutations in children is the result of new mutations, and the family history is often unremarkable. On the other hand, the manifestation of disease resulting from mitochondrial mutations is strongly influenced by heteroplasmy, a phenomenon in which the likelihood and severity of disease and the tissues affected depends on the proportion of mutant mitochondria in each cell. In these cases, the family history may be complex, with several members of the family, all related matrilineally, being affected with conditions that appear superficially to be quite different, but which are all caused by the same mitochondrial mutation. Taking a family history is much more demanding than it is in the case with simple autosomal recessive conditions—one must inquire about *all* disease in blood relatives, not just the specific disease presenting in the index case.

WHAT CLINICAL CLUES SHOULD MAKE ONE SUSPECT THE POSSIBILITY OF AN INBORN ERROR OF METABOLISM

By their very nature, inborn errors of metabolism may present with symptoms referable to virtually any system or combination of systems in the body. The large number of inborn errors known to affect children, their comparative rarity, the general paucity of pathognomonic physical findings, and the need to "think metabolically," make this a daunting group of disorders to diagnose and manage. The situation is further complicated by the experience that inborn errors often mimic more common, acquired conditions, such as infections, intoxications, or nutritional disorders (see Sec. 8.2). Although inborn errors may present in many different ways, a large proportion present in one of five ways (Table 9-2).

9.1.2 Neurologic Syndrome

Many inborn errors of metabolism present with neurologic symptoms. Delineation of the extent of the pathology often provides important clues to the underlying nature of the condition. Evidence that more than one component of the nervous system is involved with the disease, or evidence of nonneural involvement, is not only suggestive of an inborn error of metabolism but helps to guide specific metabolic investigation. Among the inborn errors of metabolism, there are five particularly common neurologic presentations: acute encephalopathy; chronic encephalopathy; movement disorder; myopathy; and psychiatric or behavioral disturbance (see Chapter 25).

ACUTE ENCEPHALOPATHY

Acute metabolic encephalopathy is a common presentation of metabolic disease that often presents as deterioration of consciousness, often with seizures. Although inborn errors of metabolism causing acute encephalopathy can present at any age, neonates and young infants are the most commonly affected. Characteristics suggesting that the illness is the result of an inherited metabolic disease are: (a) it often occurs with little warning, without an adequate explanation, in a previously healthy child; (b) it may initially present as a behavioral disturbance; (c) it often progresses rapidly; and (d) it is usually not associated with focal neurologic deficits. A summary of the most common inborn errors presenting as acute encephalopathy is shown, along with helpful laboratory studies, in Fig. 9-2. Most of the inborn errors presenting as acute encephalopathy are "small-molecule" diseases involving defects in the metabolism of water-soluble metabolites, such as glucose, ammonium, amino acids, and organic acids. An important exception is acute encephalopathy caused by mitochondrial electron transport defects. However, the plasma lactate concentration is almost invariably elevated

TABLE 9-2
COMMON GENETIC METABOLIC "SYNDROMES"

Neurologic syndrome
    Acute encephalopathy
    Chronic encephalopathy
    Movement disorder
    Myopathy
    Psychiatric or behavioral disturbance
Metabolic acidosis
    Renal tubular dysfunction
    Accumulation of fixed anion
Hepatic syndrome
    Jaundice
    Hepatomegaly
    Hypoglycemia
    Hepatocellular dysfunction
Cardiac syndrome
    Coronary disease
    Cardiomyopathy
"Storage" syndrome and dysmorphism

in these cases, providing an important clue to the nature of the underlying problem. The investigation of possible inborn errors of metabolism should not be delayed—appropriate treatment is often lifesaving.

Clinical Presentations

Metabolic diseases resulting in acute encephalopathy classically present in the newborn period, but may not manifest until later in life. Infants with a small-molecule disease associated with acute encephalopathy are usually born following an unremarkable pregnancy and are healthy at birth. Following parturition, the maternal metabolism is no longer able to supplement the metabolism of the fetus. Also, the transition to extrauterine life involves an initial catabolic period and adaptation to a new, nonplacental, source of nutrition. Over the first days to weeks, during which an affected baby usually remains well, a diffusible substrate or metabolite begins to accumulate to toxic levels in the brain due to the metabolic defect. Alternatively, an essential product becomes deficient. The baby begins to experience feeding problems, lethargy, irritability, and vomiting. If the illness is not recognized and appropriate therapy not initiated, the encephalopathy progresses with a decreasing level of consciousness and seizures; if there is acidosis and/or hyperammonemia, tachypnea may also be present. This presentation could very well be a description of a baby who is developing a significant infection or who has been asphyxiated. Alternative etiologies for the syndrome of acute encephalopathy in infants include accidental or nonaccidental trauma, intoxications, malignancies, or congenital malformations (eg, cardiac). Given the nonspecific nature of the syndrome of acute encephalopathy, the most difficult step in the diagnosis of an inborn error of metabolism as the cause is considering the possibility that one exists.

Inborn errors presenting later in life with acute encephalopathy can be more challenging to recognize than the classic neonatal presentation. Older patients with small-molecule disease may present with ataxia, disorientation, or frank psychosis, as well as loss of consciousness. Children who present later in life often have a higher residual enzyme activity than do those who present in the newborn period, and are able to maintain homeostasis until challenged by a catabolic stress (see below). An example is the intermittent variant of maple syrup urine disease (MSUD), in which the child is biochemically normal except when challenged by the catabolism of intercurrent illness, at which time ataxia and decreased consciousness develops because of an accumulation of the branched-chain α-ketoacids. A later presentation in an X-linked disorder may reflect the phenomenon of X-inactivation (see above). For example, ornithine transcarbamoylase deficiency may cause acute encephalopathy in a female carrier of the disease after she has given birth—a time of massive maternal catabolism.

Acute Metabolic Encephalopathy After the Initial Presentation

A common feature of the inborn errors being considered in this section is that their metabolic consequences are more pronounced during a period of catabolic stress. During these periods, there is increased breakdown of endogenous proteins and fats which results in increased delivery of metabolites to the blocked pathway causing an accumulation of a toxic metabolite. This accumulation leads to an acute deterioration of the clinical status, a *metabolic crisis*. As mentioned above, the first catabolic stress that a baby undergoes is during the transition to extrauterine life. Infants who escape a newborn presentation (often because they have slightly more residual

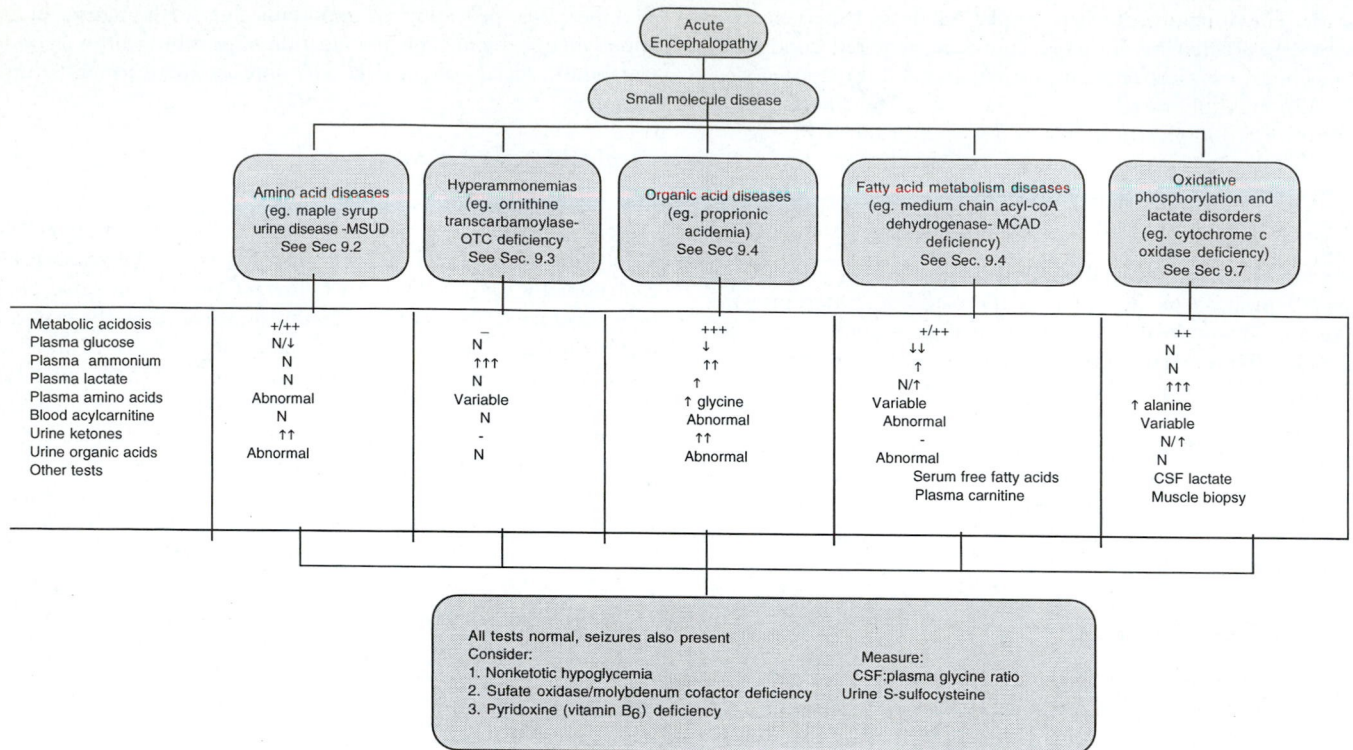

FIGURE 9-2 **Inborn errors of metabolism commonly presenting as acute encephalopathy, and the laboratory studies that are required to identify and differentiate between them. + Mild, ++ moderate, +++ severe; ↑ mildly increased, ↑↑ moderately increased, ↑↑↑ markedly increased; ↓ decreased, ↓↓ moderately decreased; N, normal; AbN, abnormal; CSF, cerebrospinal fluid.**

enzyme activity, with a less severe metabolic block) may present after the postnatal period when they are exposed to other stresses including infections, starvation, trauma, surgery, and parturition. A similar phenomenon occurs with increased exposure to exogenous nutrients that can enter the blocked pathway. For example, a protein load resulting from a change in diet from breast milk to formula, or from a gastrointestinal bleed, can lead to hyperammonemia in a patient with a urea cycle defect (see Sec. 9.3). Most of the encephalopathic metabolic crises that periodically affect even well-treated patients with inborn errors are precipitated by catabolic stress. Therefore, a cornerstone of the long-term management of these disorders is the avoidance and early recognition of impending catabolic situations and stresses. The parents of older patients often recognize subtle signs (such as changes in behavior) of impending metabolic decompensation early enough to prevent progression of the episode to acute encephalopathy.

Approach to Laboratory Investigation

The initial approach to inborn errors of metabolism causing acute encephalopathy follows the same principles as for an acute illness of any other etiology. Whenever faced with an acute encephalopathy in an infant or child, it is useful to consider three questions: (a) How sick is the child? (b) Is any immediate intervention required to stabilize the child? (c) What is the underlying etiology of the child's medical problems? That is, what is the diagnosis? A failure to institute therapy (see below) while trying to pinpoint a diagnosis can lead to severe neurologic damage, or even to death.

A number of simple, readily available laboratory investigations should be undertaken to explore the possibility of an inborn error of metabolism and to delineate the initial differential diagnosis in a

child with acute encephalopathy. These investigations are summarized in Fig. 9-2. Blood gases and electrolytes should be obtained to identify acidosis, or an increase in the anion gap, as well as the respiratory alkalosis often associated with hyperammonemia syndromes. Plasma and urine amino acids should be quantified. Hypoglycemia can be a feature of the underlying disease, and may also contribute to the encephalopathy. An elevated plasma ammonium concentration is the primary indication of urea cycle diseases and is also seen as a secondary metabolic abnormality in organic acidurias and fatty acid oxidation diseases. In errors of oxidative phosphorylation and pyruvate metabolism, plasma lactate concentration is often elevated. Plasma lactate can also be secondarily elevated in organic acidurias and in fatty acid metabolism defects. The presence or absence of urinary ketones can also be helpful in the initial assessment. Ketosis is expected to occur when a child is in a catabolic state, but can be pronounced in some errors of amino acid and organic acid metabolism. Conversely, an inability to produce ketones is a hallmark of fatty acid oxidation defects, because ketone bodies are the final products of fatty acid catabolism. Although it may take some time to obtain a result from an assay for urine organic acids, it is critical to obtain a urine sample for this test prior to, or as soon as possible after, instituting acute therapy. Organic acid abnormalities may not be detectable after the catabolic state is corrected, and failure to obtain a urine sample during the acute illness can delay the diagnosis of organic acid and fatty acid oxidation diseases (see Sec. 8.1).

Approach to Therapy

The acute therapy of acute encephalopathy due to any of the likely inborn errors of metabolism involves measures to decrease the production of offending metabolites and to increase their excretion. Treatment should include:

1. Ensuring adequate cardiorespiratory function to allow delivery of oxygen and nutrients and to enable removal of any accumulating metabolites. Adequate hydration is essential to maintain good urine output because many of the offending diffusible metabolites are freely filtered at the glomerulus.

2. Reversing the catabolic state and reducing exposure to the offending nutrients. A useful initial fluid protocol to achieve these first two therapeutic objectives is 10% dextrose in 0.45% saline, with 20 mEq/L of potassium (if patient is voiding), run intravenously at 150% of maintenance fluid requirements. This regimen provides approximately 9 to 10 mg/kg/min of glucose to neonates and infants. Fluid restriction may be necessary if cerebral edema is present (see Sec. 21.4).

3. Correction of the metabolic acidosis by sodium bicarbonate administration if the serum bicarbonate level is less than 15 mEq/L. Beware of overcorrection: stop once the bicarbonate level has reached 15 mEq/L. Also, beware of iatrogenic hypernatremia, although this may be unavoidable (see Sec. 21.4).

4. After these measures have been instituted, and even before a precise biochemical diagnosis has been made, begin hemodialysis or hemofiltration to remove the offending small molecule as quickly as possible if the patient is comatose or semicomatose.

5. Provide specific therapy appropriate to the disease; for example:
   a. Nutritional modification, such as appropriate caloric supplements free of the offending precursor nutrients (eg, leucine, isoleucine, and valine in MSUD [see Sec. 9.2]).
   b. Cofactor administration, which will sometimes improve the function of a genetically defective enzyme (eg, vitamin B_{12} in some cases of methylmalonic aciduria, because methylmalonic acid is a cofactor for methylmalonyl-CoA mutase [see Sec. 9.4]).
   c. Metabolic manipulation, such as the administration of sodium benzoate in hyperammonemias (see Sec. 9.3), to divert a toxic substrate to a benign excretable form.

CHRONIC ENCEPHALOPATHY

The psychomotor retardation or developmental delay caused by inborn errors of metabolism tends to be global. In addition, it is usually progressive, is often associated with severe irritability (infants) or behavior problems (older children), and is usually associated with other objective evidence of neurologic dysfunction. One approach to the problem is shown in Fig. 9-3. Some inborn errors of metabolism may present as cerebral palsy, with generalized spasticity and developmental delay. For example, a history of a period of apparent normalcy, the absence of a history of perinatal insult, and evidence that the cerebral palsy is becoming more severe are typical of children with arginase deficiency. It is also a common presenting feature in children with glutaric aciduria type I or Lesch-Nyhan disease.

While the inborn errors of metabolism that result in acute encephalopathy are usually small-molecule diseases, Fig. 9-3 reveals a wider metabolic etiology of chronic encephalopathy. These etiologies can be divided into two broad groups: small-molecule diseases and diseases of organelles. The small-molecule diseases that cause chronic encephalopathy are of two types: the less-severe variants of enzyme deficiencies that are also associated with acute encephalopathy (see above), and a distinct group of conditions, exemplified by phenylketonuria (PKU), that lead to chronic encephalopathy.

The organelle diseases include the lysosomal storage diseases, diseases of mitochondrial energy metabolism, and peroxisomal disorders.

Chronic Encephalopathy Due to Small-Molecule Diseases

Patients with mild forms of many small-molecule diseases may present with static or relatively nonprogressive developmental delay or mental retardation. Such patients have escaped the extreme accumulations of metabolites noted in the more severely affected infants, generally because they tend to have more residual enzyme activity. The investigations outlined in Fig. 9-3 for disorders of amino acid, organic acid, and ammonium metabolism should be performed in these patients. For example, with the intermediate variant of maple syrup urine disease, the amino and ketoacid concentrations are chronically increased to levels that damage the brain but do not alter consciousness (except with a catabolic stress). Patients with less-severe forms of organic acidopathies may never accumulate enough of the abnormal organic acid to become overtly acidotic. In those with mild urea cycle defects (for example, some carrier females with ornithine transcarbamoylase deficiency), blood ammonia levels may only be increased postprandially (2–3 hours after finishing a protein-containing meal). Key small-molecule diseases that can result in chronic encephalopathy are PKU and homocystinuria (see Sec. 9.2).

Chronic Encephalopathy Due to Organelle Diseases

The diseases of organelles that must be considered in patients with slowly deteriorating or static neurologic dysfunction are those that impair the ability of mitochondria to produce energy, lysosomal storage diseases, and peroxisomal disorders. As indicated above, diseases of oxidative phosphorylation (mitochondrial energy metabolism) often present with acute encephalopathy, in addition to being responsible for much chronic neurologic disease. They must be considered in any patient with chronic encephalopathy, particularly if there is evidence of muscle weakness, by measuring serum lactate and pyruvate concentrations. Depending on the disease, patients with this group of chronic encephalopathies may have intellectual handicap, dementia, or motor deficits (see Sec 9.7). The lysosomal and peroxisomal diseases, in contrast, are usually associated only with chronic progressive neurologic abnormalities.

Lysosomal storage diseases are caused either by enzyme defects that impair the degradation of macromolecules in lysosomes or by disruptions in the efflux of molecules from the lysosome to the cytoplasm. Cell death results from the consequent intralysosomal "storage" of the undigested macromolecule, or from the accumulation of a nontransportable substrate. Macromolecules are integral structural components of cells. The major function of the lysosome is to degrade such molecules, including glycosaminoglycans, glycoproteins, gangliosides, and glycolipids (the latter two collectively known as sphingolipids) into their small-molecule components, which can then be recycled in metabolism and biosynthesis. In contrast to diseases that disturb the metabolism of small diffusible molecules, the pathology of the lysosomal diseases is restricted to tissues in which the macromolecule is normally degraded. Examples of lysosomal storage diseases include the mucopolysaccharidoses, the oligosaccharidoses, and the gangliosidoses. These conditions are all recessive, and are either autosomal or X-linked in their inheritance (see Secs. 9.8 and 9.9).

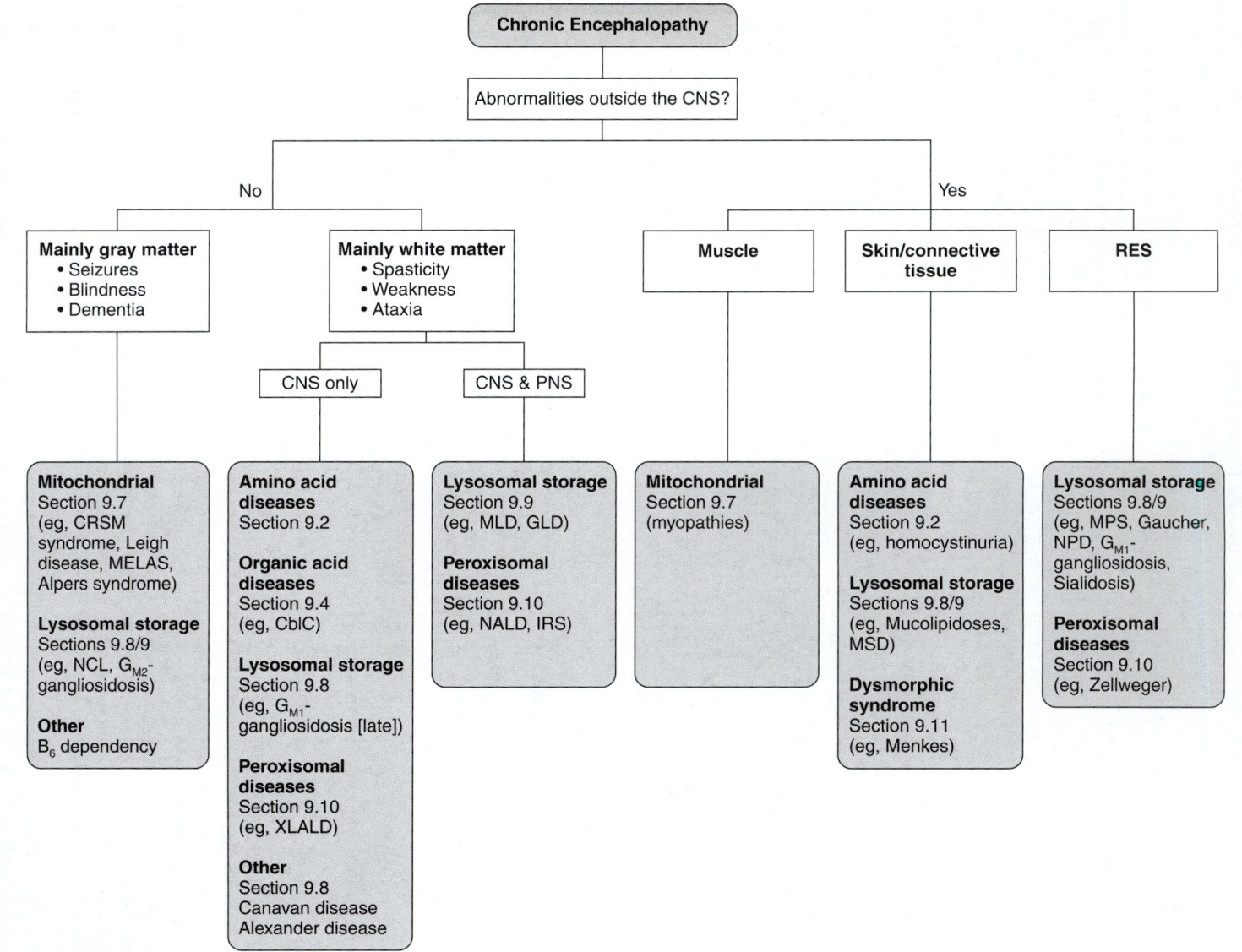

FIGURE 9-3 An approach to the identification of inborn errors of metabolism causing chronic encephalopathy. CNS = central nervous system; PNS = peripheral nervous system; CRSM = cherry-red spot myoclonus; MELAS = mitochondrial encephalomyopathy, lactic acidosis, and stroke-like episodes syndrome; NCL = neuronal ceroid lipofuscinosis; CblC = cobolamin C disease; XLALD = X-linked adrenoleukodystrophy; MLD = metachromatic leukodystrophy; GLD = Krabbe globoid cell leukodystrophy; NALD = neonatal adrenoleukodystrophy; IRS = infantile Refsum syndrome; MSD = multiple sulfatase deficiency; RES = reticuloendothelial system; MPS = mucopolysaccharide storage disorder; NPD = Niemann-Pick disease.

TABLE 9-3

SOME INBORN ERRORS OF METABOLISM IN WHICH MOVEMENT DISORDERS ARE PROMINENT

DISORDERS	EXAMPLES
Progressive ataxia	
Sphingolipidoses and other lysosomal disorders	Late-onset G_{M2}-gangliosidosis
	Late-onset metachromatic leukodystrophy
	Late-onset Krabbe globoid cell leukodystrophy
	Late-onset galactosialidosis
	Niemann-Pick disease, type C
	Infantile neuronal ceroid lipofuscinosis
Organic acidopathies	L-2-Hydroxyglutaric aciduria
Aminoacidopathies	Hartnup disease
Disorders of neutral lipid metabolism	Abetalipoproteinemia
	Refsum disease
	Cerebrotendinous xanthomatosis
Mitochondrial disorders	Ataxia may be a prominent feature of many different mitochondrial ETC defects
Intermittent ataxia	
Aminoacidopathies	Mild or intermittent MSUD
Organic acidopathies	Methylmalonic aciduria
	Propionic aciduria
	Isovaleric aciduria and others
Urea cycle enzyme defects	Mild variants of OTC deficiency, CPS deficiency, argininosuccinic aciduria, citrullinemia
Mitochondrial disorders	Mild pyruvate dehydrogenase deficiency (boys)
	Various mitochondrial ETC defects
Dystonia/choreoathetosis	
Organic acidopathies	Glutaric aciduria, type I
	4-Hydroxybutyric aciduria
Disorders of purine metabolism	Lesch-Nyhan disease
Disorders of glycolysis	Triose phosphate isomerase deficiency
Disorders of trace element metabolism	Wilson disease
Disorders of neurotransmitter metabolism	Segawa syndrome
Parkinsonism	
Disorders of trace element metabolism	Wilson disease

ETC, electron transport chain; MSUD, maple syrup urine disease; OTC, ornithine transcarbamoylase; CPS, carbonyl phosphate synthetase.

Peroxisomes participate in a number of unique anabolic processes, including bile acid and plasmalogen (other phospholipids found in almost all membranes, most notably myelin) biosynthesis, and catabolic processes including the oxidation of very-long-chain fatty acids (VLCFA), phytanic acid, and pipecolic acid. More than 20 peroxisomal disorders have been identified, and they can be divided into (a) peroxisomal biogenesis defects in which peroxisomes are absent, abnormal, or lacking multiple enzyme activities, and (b) single-enzyme defects. The cardinal feature of most peroxisomal diseases is severe, progressive central nervous system dysfunction, usually evident in infancy. Other features that should raise suspicion of these diseases in early life are facial dysmorphism, hepatomegaly and liver dysfunction, hypotonia, renal cysts, and various

ocular abnormalities. In older patients, the phenotype is more variable, and may include, in addition to the above findings, diverse manifestations of neurodegeneration, including ataxia and other signs of white matter disease. Unfortunately, these diseases are almost uniformly untreatable. They are all autosomal recessive in their inheritance, except for X-linked adrenoleukodystrophy. (See Sec. 9.10. and Chapter 25.)

MOVEMENT DISORDER

An extrapyramidal movement disorder may be the most prominent neurologic problem in children with certain inborn errors of metabolism. However, it is almost always associated with signs referable to other parts of the nervous system, and many patients with these movement disorders also exhibit significant nonneurologic signs. Intermittent or episodic ataxia—generally in periods of catabolic stress—is a common finding in children with variant forms of aminoacidopathies, such as mild maple syrup urine disease, or organic acidopathies, such as mild methylmalonic aciduria. Ataxia is also the most prominent finding in many children with "channelopathies," hereditary defects in ion channels required for the maintenance of membrane potentials and controlled depolarization.

Dystonia and choreoathetosis are prominent features of glutaric aciduria, type 1, and Lesch-Nyhan disease. Parkinsonism, dystonia, and cerebellar dysfunction are common presenting features of Wilson disease. Table 9-3 summarizes various types of movement disorder and associated inborn errors of metabolism.

MYOPATHY

Marked generalized muscle weakness or exercise intolerance with cramps and myoglobinuria are prominent features of inherited metabolic diseases affecting muscle energy metabolism. Unlike congenital nonmetabolic myopathies, the muscle weakness caused

TABLE 9-4

INBORN ERRORS OF METABOLISM IN WHICH MYOPATHY IS PARTICULARLY PROMINENT

Fatty acid oxidation defects
Systemic carnitine deficiency
Carnitine palmityltransferase II deficiency
Long-chain acyl-CoA dehydrogenase deficiency
Long-chain 3-hydroxyacyl-CoA dehydrogenase deficiency or trifunctional protein deficiency
Short-chain acyl-CoA dehydrogenase deficiency
Short-chain hydroxyacyl-CoA dehydrogenase deficiency
Defects of carbohydrate metabolism
Pompe disease (acid maltase deficiency)
Myophosphorylase deficiency (McArdle disease)
Glycogen storage disease, type III
Glycogen storage disease, type VIII
Phosphofructokinase deficiency
Phosphoglycerate kinase deficiency
Lactate dehydrogenase deficiency
Myoadenylate deaminase deficiency
Mitochondrial electron transport chain defects
Kearns-Sayre syndrome (KSS)
Myoclonic epilepsy and ragged-red fiber disease (MERRF)
Mitochondrial encephalomyopathy, lactic acidosis, and stroke-like episodes (MELAS)

TABLE 9-5

SOME COMMON FEATURES OF DEFECTS IN THE MITOCHONDRIAL ELECTRON TRANSPORT CHAIN

Present in most mitochondrial conditions
Lactic acidosis
Failure to thrive
Muscle weakness and hypotonia
Psychomotor retardation
Seizures
Present in many mitochondrial conditions
Ophthalmoplegia
Retinitis pigmentosa
Cardiomyopathy, usually hypertrophic
Cerebellar ataxia
Sensorineural hearing impairment
Diabetes mellitus
Stroke
Renal tubular dysfunction
Episodic apnea and tachypnea
Cardiac arrhythmias

TABLE 9-6

SOME INBORN ERRORS OF METABOLISM IN WHICH PSYCHIATRIC OR BEHAVIOR ABNORMALITIES ARE PROMINENT

Sanfilippo disease (MPS III)
Hunter disease (MPS II)
X-linked adrenoleukodystrophy
Late-onset metachromatic leukodystrophy
Late-onset G_{M2}-gangliosidosis
Porphyria
Wilson disease
Lesch-Nyhan disease
Urea cycle enzyme defects, especially HHH syndrome
Cerebrotendinous xanthomatosis
Homocystinuria due to MTHF reductase deficiency

MPS, mucopolysaccharide storage disorder; HHH, hyperammonemia, hyperornithi-nemia, homocitrullinemia; MTHF, methylenetetrahydrofolate.

by inborn errors of energy metabolism is usually progressive or intermittent. The defect may involve fatty acid oxidation, carbohydrate metabolism, or the mitochondrial electron transport chain (Table 9-4).

In some cases, such as myophosphorylase deficiency and carnitine palmityltransferase (CPT) II deficiency, the association of the

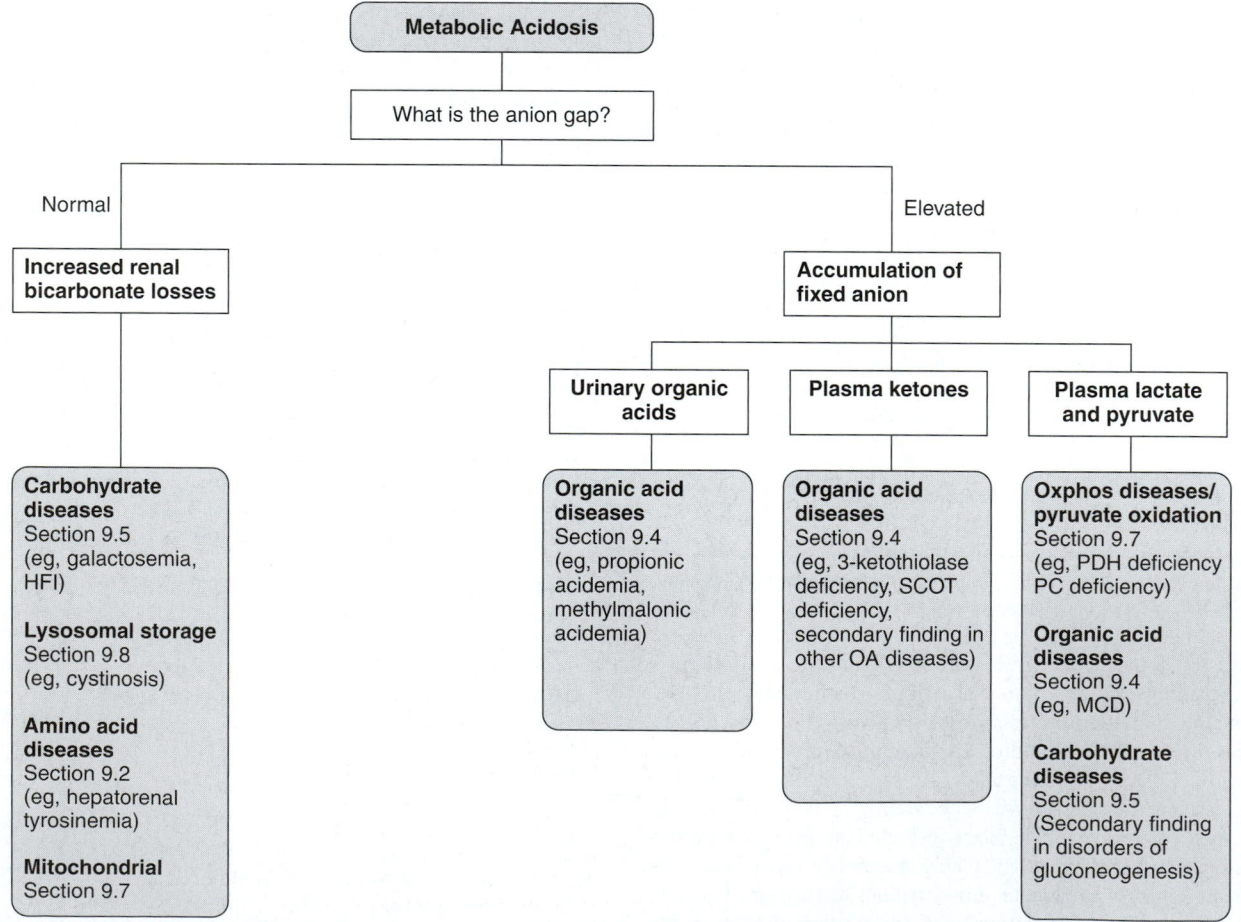

FIGURE 9-4   An approach to the diagnosis of inborn errors of metabolism associated with metabolic acidosis. HFI = hereditary fructose intolerance; SCOT = succinyl-CoA:3-oxoacid CoA transferase; Oxphos = oxidative phosphorylation; PDH = pyruvate dehydrogenase; PC = pyruvate carboxylase; MCD = multiple carboxylase deficiency.

weakness, muscle cramps, and pigmenturia with rigorous or prolonged exercise is typical of the disorders. In others, like the mitochondrial electron transport chain defects, the myopathy is associated with prominent evidence of chronic, multisystem involvement (Table 9-5).

PSYCHIATRIC OR BEHAVIOR DISTURBANCE

Psychiatric disorders or severe behavior disturbance may be the first or only clinical manifestation of a wide range of inborn errors of metabolism (Table 9-6). The late-onset defects of ureagenesis are particularly prominent causes of psychiatric disturbance or intermittent changes in behavior. These psychiatric problems tend to be severe and particularly resistant to conventional psychotropic medication, and this feature is sometimes the only clue to the underlying nature of the disease.

9.1.3   Metabolic Acidosis

Metabolic acidosis resulting from inborn errors of metabolism may develop as a result of accumulation of fixed anion or loss of bicarbonate, which is usually due to renal tubular dysfunction. The two are relatively easy to distinguish. In metabolic acidosis resulting from accumulation of fixed anion, the plasma chloride concentration is generally normal and the anion gap, a reflection of the concentration of unmeasured anions, is increased. In patients with metabolic acidosis caused by loss of bicarbonate, the plasma chloride level is elevated and the anion gap (the difference between the plasma sodium and the sum of the chloride and bicarbonate) is generally normal (ie, 10–15 mmol/L).

ACCUMULATION OF FIXED ANION

Metabolic acidosis caused by accumulation of organic anions due to a defect of organic acid catabolism is usually persistent and often severe, particularly during stress-induced metabolic decompensation (see Sec. 21.4). It is commonly associated with a history of feeding difficulties and chronic failure to thrive. Secondary hypoglycemia and hyperammonemia, along with the metabolic acidosis, often precipitate acute encephalopathy with vomiting, lethargy, ataxia, and stupor. The sweat and urine may have a peculiar odor. An approach to the diagnosis of inborn errors presenting with metabolic acidosis is shown in Fig. 9-4. In addition to these genetic defects, ketoacidosis and lactic acidosis are common metabolic responses to a wide variety of physiologic and pathologic conditions, including simple starvation (producing ketoacidosis) and sepsis or shock (producing lactic acidosis). Ketone bodies and lactic acid also frequently accumulate secondary to primary disorders of organic acid metabolism or gluconeogenesis (see Secs. 9.4 and 9.5, respectively).

LOSS OF BICARBONATE

Proximal renal tubular dysfunction, with bicarbonate wasting, is a major feature of only a small handful of inborn errors of metabolism—usually it is traceable in children to some acquired condition, such as infection, poisoning, or nutritional vitamin D deficiency. In cystinosis, the persistence and severity of the renal tubular defect typically causes severe growth retardation and rickets, the most prominent clinical features of the early stages of the disease. In other inborn errors of metabolism, such as galactosemia, evidence

TABLE 9-7

INBORN ERRORS OF METABOLISM ASSOCIATED WITH RENAL TUBULAR DYSFUNCTION

Cystinosis
Galactosemia
Hepatorenal tyrosinemia
Hereditary fructose intolerance
Mitochondrial cytopathies
Glycogen storage disease, type I
Wilson disease
Vitamin D dependency
Osteopetrosis with renal tubular acidosis
Lowe syndrome

of renal tubular dysfunction is associated with other more obvious clinical problems (Table 9-7). (See Sec. 21.11.)

9.1.4   Hepatic Syndrome

An outline of inherited metabolic disorders commonly presenting as "hepatic syndromes" is shown in Table 9-8, and some of the conditions are described in detail in Chapter 18. The breakdown in Table 9-8 is somewhat contrived because there is considerable overlap in the clinical presentations of the various inborn errors that affect the liver. The hepatomegaly in glycogen storage disease, type

TABLE 9-8

SOME INBORN ERRORS PRESENTING AS "HEPATIC SYNDROME"

Hepatomegaly
   Glycogen storage diseases
   Lysosomal storage diseases
Jaundice
   Defects of bilirubin metabolism
   Congenital nonspherocytic hemolytic anemia
   Wilson disease
Hypoglycemia
   Glycogen storage disease, especially type I
   Defects in gluconeogenesis
   Fatty acid oxidation defects
   Galactosemia (in the newborn)
   Hereditary fructose intolerance
Hepatocellular dysfunction
   Early infancy
     Galactosemia
     Hepatorenal tyrosinemia
     Fatty acid oxidation defects
     α_1-Antitrypsin deficiency
     Glycogen storage disease, type IV
     Wolman disease
     Mitochondrial DNA depletion syndrome
   Early childhood
     Glycogen storage disease, type III
     Gaucher disease, type 3
     Niemann-Pick disease, type C
     CPT I deficiency
   Adolescence or later
     Wilson disease
     Cholesterol ester storage disease
     Niemann-Pick disease, type B

CPT, carnitine palmitoyltransferase.

I, is usually massive, but most infants with the disease probably come to attention more often as a result of hypoglycemia. With the other glycogen storage diseases, such as type III, the enlargement of the liver is usually not as severe as in type I, but hypoglycemia is less common as a presenting problem. The hepatomegaly in children with lysosomal storage diseases, such as Gaucher disease and Niemann-Pick disease, type B, is usually associated with significant splenomegaly. However, the spleen may be only minimally enlarged in children with cholesterol ester storage disease (lysosomal acid lipase deficiency). Hepatomegaly is present in virtually all the metabolic conditions presenting as severe liver failure. However, the prominence of hepatocellular dysfunction, such as coagulopathy, ascites and anasarca, hypoglycemia, and elevated transaminases, sets this group apart from the others in which live function is usually not severely affected.

9.1.5   Hypoglycemia

Hypoglycemia is common in many inborn errors of metabolism (Fig. 9-5). In some, such as the inborn errors of gluconeogenesis, it is the result of primary defects of glucose homeostasis; in most, it is a secondary metabolic phenomenon. The disorders discussed are those in which diagnostic studies aimed specifically at the identification of primary disorders of carbohydrate or fatty acid metabolism are likely to be helpful.

9.1.6   Cardiac Syndrome

Cardiac involvement is an important feature of many inborn errors of metabolism. The valvular disease in patients with mucopolysaccharidoses is, for example, a significant cause of morbidity and mortality. However, the noncardiac manifestations of these disorders are generally obvious and provide the basis for clinical diagnosis. By contrast, in some inborn errors, the clinical features of the metabolic defect are dominated by cardiac or vascular abnormalities.

Vascular disease, including premature coronary artery disease and stroke, is a prominent clinical characteristic of familial hypercholesterolemia (see Sec. 9.14). Vascular disease is also a clinically significant complication of homocystinuria (see Sec. 9.2) and Fabry disease, a lysosomal storage disease (see Sec. 9.9).

Cardiomyopathy is a particularly prominent feature of a wide range of inborn errors (Table 9-9), especially those involving defects in myocardial energy metabolism. The type of defects in energy metabolism that cause skeletal myopathy also often involve the

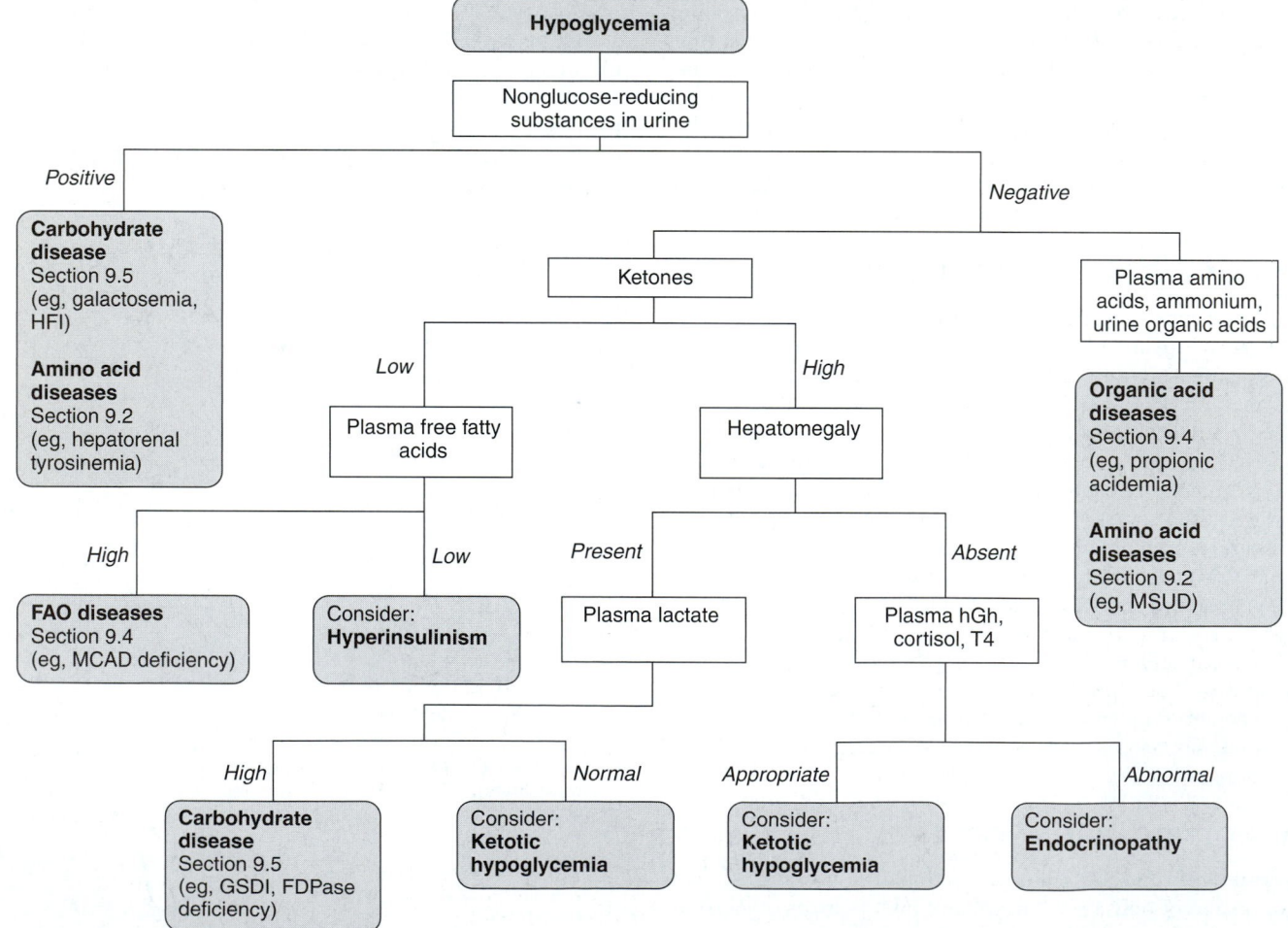

FIGURE 9-5   **An approach to the diagnosis of inborn errors of metabolism associated with severe hypoglycemia. HFI = hereditary fructose intolerance; FAO = fatty acid oxidation defect; MCAD = medium-chain acyl-CoA dehydrogenase; GSD I = glycogen storage disease, type I; FDPase = fructose 1,6-diphosphatase; hGH = growth hormone; T4 = thyroxine; MSUD = maple syrup urine disease.**

TABLE 9-9

INBORN ERRORS OF METABOLISM IN WHICH CARDIOMYOPATHY IS PROMINENT

Disorders of glycogen metabolism
  Pompe disease (GSD II)
  Glycogen storage disease, type III
  Phosphorylase β kinase deficiency
  Glycogen storage disease, type IV
Fatty acid oxidation defects
  Systemic carnitine deficiency
  LCAD deficiency
  LCHAD deficiency
  Carnitine-acylcarnitine translocase deficiency
Organic acidopathies
  Propionic aciduria
  Methylmalonic aciduria
  HMG-CoA lyase deficiency
  β-Ketothiolase deficiency
  Glutaric aciduria, type II
Lysosomal storage diseases
  Fabry disease
  Hurler disease (MPS IH)
  Hunter disease (MPS II)
  Maroteaux-Lamy disease (MPS VI)
  G_{M1}-gangliosidosis
  Gaucher disease
Mitochondrial cardiomyopathies
  Kearns-Sayre syndrome
  Lethal infantile cardiomyopathy
  Hypertrophic cardiomyopathy and myopathy
  Barth syndrome
Aminoacidopathies
  Hepatorenal tyrosinemia

GSD, glycogen storage disease; MPS mucopolysaccharide storage disease; LCAD, long-chain acyl-CoA dehydrogenase deficiency; LCHAD, long-chain 3-hydroxyacyl-CoA; HMG-CoA, 3-hydroxy-3-methylglutaryl-CoA.

myocardium, including many of the disorders of glycogen metabolism, the fatty acid oxidation defects, and defects in the mitochondrial electron transport chain. Myocardial involvement may dominate the clinical presentation. Usually, however, the presence of noncardiac problems, such as skeletal myopathy, hepatomegaly, and skin lesions, or a history of episodic hypoglycemia, metabolic acidosis or hyperammonemia, or particular physical findings, provide clues to the underlying nature of the cardiac disease.

9.1.7   Storage Syndrome and Conditions with Dysmorphic Physical Findings

A diagnostically challenging group of inborn errors of metabolism is that associated with somatic dysmorphism. These disorders present a challenge because (a) they are rare; (b) they often involve the metabolism of large, water-insoluble metabolites that are technically difficult to isolate and analyze; (c) the defect is often in a relatively inaccessible subcellular organelle (eg, peroxisomes, mitochondria, lysosomes); (d) the techniques required to demonstrate the presence of the specific biochemical abnormality are difficult to master; (e) the basic defect often impairs the *synthesis* of some compound so that substrate accumulation does not occur and therefore cannot help in making a diagnosis; and (f) there are few screening tests that are useful for ruling out entire classes of disorders, such as amino acid analysis for aminoacidopathies.

Although the dysmorphism (see Chapter 10) associated with inborn errors may be severe, with some prominent exceptions, it generally involves disturbances of shape (distortions), rather than fusion or cellular migration defects (disruptions) or abnormalities of number, such as polydactyly (true malformations). The dysmorphism tends to become more pronounced with age, and histologic and ultrastructural abnormalities obtained by tissue biopsy are often prominent. Table 9-10 summarizes the inborn errors associated with significant dysmorphism (see Sec. 9.11).

9.1.8   How Does Laboratory Investigation Help?

The definitive diagnosis of inborn errors of metabolism is based on a wide range of biochemical studies, most of which are not readily available in community hospitals or in routine diagnostic laboratories (see Sec. 8.2). In recent years, biochemical testing has been supplemented by molecular genetic studies. Although molecular testing has undeniably enhanced the investigation of these disorders, the first line of investigation is invariably biochemical or metabolic in nature. The biochemical phenotype is central to the identification of the primary metabolic defect (see Sec

TABLE 9-10

INBORN ERRORS OF METABOLISM IN WHICH DYSMORPHISM IS PROMINENT

Lysosomal disorders
  Mucopolysaccharide storage diseases
    Hurler disease, Hunter disease, Morquio disease, and others
  Multiple sulfatase deficiency Glycoproteinoses
    Infantile G_{M1}-gangliosidosis
    Infantile sialidosis
    Galactosialidosis
    Fucosidosis
    α-Mannosidosis
    β-Mannosidosis
    Aspartylglucosaminuria
    I-cell disease
  Sphingolipidoses
    Farber lipogranulomatosis
Mitochondrial disorders
  PDH deficiency
  Glutaric aciduria, type II
  3-Hydroxyisobutyric aciduria
  Mitochondrial ETC defects
Peroxisomal disorders
  Zellweger syndrome
  Rhizomelic chondrodysplasia punctata
  Neonatal adrenoleukodystrophy
  Infantile Refsum disease
Biosynthetic defects
  Mevalonic aciduria
  SLO syndrome
  CDG syndrome
  Albinism
  Primary defects in hormone biosynthesis
  Homocystinuria
  Menkes disease
Receptor defects
  Familial hypercholesterolemia
  Pseudohypoparathyroidism

SLO, Smith-Lemli-Opitz; CDG, carbohydrate-deficient glycoprotein; ETC, electron transport chain.

TABLE 9-11

SOME CLINICAL DIFFERENCES BETWEEN SMALL-MOLECULE DISEASES AND ORGANELLE DISEASES

CLINICAL FEATURE	ORGANELLE DISEASE	SMALL-MOLECULE DISEASE
Onset	Gradual	Often sudden, especially with stress
Course	Slowly progressive	Characterized by relapses and remissions
Physical findings	Often typical and helpful	Nonspecific
Histopathology	Often reveals typical changes	Generally nonspecific
Response to supportive therapy	Poor, incomplete	Often brisk
Some examples	Most lysosomal storage diseases; most peroxisomal disorders; many mitochondrial ETC defects[1]	Many of the aminoacidopathies[2]; most organic acidopathies

[1]Some mitochondrial disorders, such as Leigh subacute necrotizing encephalomyopathy, may pursue a salutatory course, with episodes of sudden deterioration, followed by improvement.

[2]There are some important exceptions, such as phenylketonuria, homocystinuria, and hyperargininemia, that do not have the typical small-molecule disease presentation described. ETC, electron transport chain.

8.2). The pattern and extent of tissue involvement in inborn errors of metabolism often provides important clues to the underlying nature of the condition. Imaging studies, electrophysiological testing (eg, nerve conduction velocities, brainstem auditory-evoked responses, EEG, EMG), and histopathologic, histochemical, and ultrastructural studies on tissue obtained by biopsy are all useful. Analysis of various metabolic intermediates, such as amino acids, organic acids, lactate, free fatty acids, in plasma, urine, and CSF may also provide critical leads to the diagnosis.

At this stage of investigation, it is often helpful to consider whether the condition is more likely to be an inborn error of small-molecule metabolism, such as an aminoacidopathy or organic acidopathy, or an organelle disease. Table 9-11 shows some general characteristics of each, although there is considerable overlap. The distinction is useful because the investigation of each group differs, especially with respect to the analysis of metabolic intermediates. In small-molecule diseases, analysis of water-soluble metabolites, such as amino acids and organic acids, is helpful. It is also technically easier than analysis of the high-molecular-weight, often water-insoluble metabolites that accumulate in organelle diseases, such as the lysosomal storage diseases. With amino acid and organic acid defects, a single laboratory test often covers a wide range of diseases and has some of the characteristics of metabolic screening. This is less common in organelle diseases, in which secondary accumulation of other high-molecular-weight compounds is common and diagnostically confusing. The diagnostic value of the analysis of metabolic intermediates is greatly enhanced in children with small-molecule diseases by provocative physiological testing such as carefully monitored prolonged fasting. This type of investigation is inherently dangerous, however, and it should only be undertaken under carefully monitored circumstances in a hospital.

Ultimately, identification of the biochemical phenotype in children with inborn errors of metabolism requires specific analysis of the activity of the mutant gene product, the catalytic protein, such as the enzyme or transporter involved. This is particularly true of the organelle diseases in which clinical overlap often creates diagnostic confusion. For example, Gaucher disease, type 1, is easily confused clinically with Niemann-Pick disease, type B; confident differentiation requires measurement of the relevant lysosomal enzyme activities in an appropriate tissue, such as leukocytes or cultured skin fibroblasts.

The highest level of definition of an inborn error of metabolism is, as with all genetic diseases, demonstration of disease-causing mutations in the relevant genes (see Sec. 8.1). Because genetic and allelic heterogeneity is often enormous, however, mutation analysis

is only rarely useful as a first line of investigation. However, mutation analysis does provide powerful confirmation of defects identified on the basis of biochemical data, such as enzyme deficiencies or particular typical patterns of intermediate metabolite concentrations in plasma, urine, or CSF. After a mutation is identified as responsible for disease within a family, testing for the molecular defect provides a relatively simple and reliable method for carrier detection and prenatal diagnosis (see Sec. 8.2).

References

Clarke JTR: A Clinical Guide to Inherited Metabolic Diseases. Cambridge, Cambridge University Press, 1996

Fernandes J, Saudubray J-M, van den Berghe G (eds): Inborn Metabolic Diseases: Diagnosis and Treatment, 3rd ed. Heidelberg, Springer-Verlag, 2000

Hommes FA (ed): Techniques in Diagnostic Human Biochemical Genetics. New York, Wiley-Liss, 1991

Pourmand R (ed): Metabolic myopathies. Neurol Clin 18:1, 2000

Scriver CR, Beaudet AL, Sly WS, Valle D (eds): The Metabolic and Molecular Bases of Inherited Disease, 8th ed. New York, McGraw-Hill, 2001

Thompson MW, McInnes RR, Willard HF (eds): Thompson and Thompson Genetics in Medicine, 5th ed. Philadelphia, Saunders, 1991

9.2 DISORDERS OF AMINO ACID METABOLISM

Markus Grompe

The disorders of amino acid metabolism provide a significant challenge for diagnosis and management. Defects in amino acid catabolism represent the largest group, but abnormalities also exist in amino acid biosynthesis and transport. The clinical manifestations vary widely and involve many different organ systems (Table 9-12). Therefore, this group of single-gene deficiencies must be considered in the differential diagnosis of many disease states. Systemic manifestations are common because of the presence of high levels of circulating small-molecule metabolites, and many of these abnormalities cause mental retardation. Importantly, most disorders of amino acid metabolism can be diagnosed by quantitative analysis of plasma amino acids. The examination of urine organic acids is often the single most valuable diagnostic test.

9.2.1　Phenylalanine-Tyrosine Group

PHENYLKETONURIA

Phenylketonuria (PKU) is an autosomal recessive disorder of metabolism in which phenylalanine cannot be converted to tyrosine. Blood phenylalanine levels are elevated and phenylpyruvic acid is excreted in the urine (Fig. 9-6). Since the advent of newborn screening programs, it has become evident that there are other varieties of hyperphenylalaninemias in addition to classic PKU.

Clinical Findings

In classic PKU, the most important clinical characteristic is mental retardation. Most untreated patients have severe retardation with intelligence quotients under 30 because persistently elevated phenylalanine levels are toxic to the central nervous system. The damage exerted by phenylalanine begins to become irreversible by 8 weeks after birth, making early screening and treatment important. Phenylketonuric infants appear normal at birth, but early symptoms occur in more than 50% of these infants. Vomiting, irritability, an eczematoid rash, or a peculiar odor may also be present in the early months. The characteristic smell has been described as mousy, wolf-like, or musty, and has been correlated with excretion of phenylacetic acid in the urine. General physical development is usually normal. Over 90% are fair-haired, fair-skinned, and blue-eyed, but dark skin, dark hair, or dark irises do not exclude the diagnosis. Peripheral neurologic findings are usually not prominent, but one-third of phenylketonic infants have minimal signs, such as hyperactive deep-tendon reflexes or hypertonicity. Seizures occur in about one-fourth of patients, predominantly in those most severely retarded. Electroencephalographic abnormalities have been described in approximately 80% of patients, and CT or MRI scan may reveal cortical atrophy.

Clinical manifestations may also occur in patients who were treated early in life but who subsequently discontinued therapy. Behavioral problems, including restlessness, aggression, and sleep disturbances, are common.

Maternal PKU

High phenylalanine levels are exquisitely toxic to the developing fetal brain, and thus the fetuses of mothers with PKU can be severely affected even though they do not have PKU themselves. Affected children have microcephaly at birth and suffer severe, irreversible mental retardation. This outcome can be prevented if the maternal phenylalanine levels are kept below 6 mg/dL from the time of conception.

Biochemical Findings

Phenylalanine is normally converted to tyrosine by hepatic phenylalanine hydroxylase (PAH), which is undetectable in classic PKU. In the absence of PAH, tyrosine becomes an essential amino acid, and alternate pathways are used to metabolize phenylalanine. In PKU, phenylalanine and these alternate metabolic products (including phenylpyruvic and phenylacetic acids) accumulate in body fluids. These compounds are not abnormal metabolites, but normal metabolites in abnormal amounts (see Sec. 9.1 and Fig. 9-1). Plasma phenylalanine concentrations range from 6 to 80 mg/dL in patients with PKU, in contrast to normal values of about 1 mg/dL. Patients with classic PKU virtually always have concentrations over 20 mg/dL throughout infancy. There is a fairly linear relationship between blood levels of phenylalanine and urinary excretion of phenylpyruvic acid.

Genetics

PKU occurs in 1 per 10,000 to 20,000 persons. It is an autosomal recessive disease occurring around the world with a carrier frequency in most populations of ~1 to 2%. The gene for phenylalanine hydroxylase has been cloned and mapped to chromosome 12q24.1. More than 240 mutations have been defined, but no single mutation accounts for a majority of patients. Carrier detection and prenatal diagnosis are possible with molecular genetic methods.

Diagnosis and Screening

PKU should be diagnosed in the neonatal period. This is initiated through the routine screening of all infants after a few days of life and after the initiation of feeding (see Sec. 8.2).

After identifying patients from positive screening tests, the first step in diagnosis is quantitative analysis of the concentrations of phenylalanine and tyrosine in the blood. Most infants identified in the screening programs simply have delayed maturation of amino-acid-metabolizing enzymes and very high tyrosine concentrations; they can be excluded and followed expectantly. The patient with classic PKU generally has a very rapid rise in serum concentration of phenylalanine on a normal diet to levels well over 30 mg/dL, and the concentration of tyrosine is low. About 1 to 2% of patients with hyperphenylalaninemia do not have defects in PAH, but in synthesis or recycling of biopterin. Every patient must be tested for this group of disorders.

Therapy

All clinical manifestations of classic PKU can be completely prevented by restriction of dietary intake of phenylalanine. This provides strong support for the concept that the clinical disease is an intoxication produced by the abnormal chemical milieu. Commercial preparations make long-term treatment economically feasible and palatable. Dietary therapy readily lowers levels of phenylalanine in the blood; concomitantly, phenylpyruvic acid and its metabolic products disappear. Extensive experience indicates clearly that early diagnosis and consistent treatment will prevent the development of mental retardation.

The treatment of infants with a low-phenylalanine diet is challenging and requires specialized expertise. The general approach is to reduce total protein intake and supplement essential amino acids as necessary for growth and development. This requires the use of special phenylalanine-free formulas. The phenylalanine tolerance must be individually established in each patient. Newly diagnosed babies are generally started on a diet containing ~40 mg/kg/d of phenylalanine. The blood levels are tightly monitored (every 2 days), and the diet is adjusted to establish phenylalanine levels of 2 to 6 mg/dL. If parental cooperation is good, this can be done in an outpatient setting, and hospitalization is not necessary. Breast milk is relatively low in phenylalanine content and breast-feeding can be continued, but usually in conjunction with a phenylalanine-free supplement. Frequent (at least biweekly) monitoring of blood phenylalanine levels is recommended throughout childhood.

All infants, including those with PKU, require a certain amount of phenylalanine; the minimal requirements are similar to those of normal infants. Patients with PKU often vomit or refuse feedings, and infections may complicate the metabolic state. If restriction of phenylalanine is too severe, tissue breakdown may occur and levels

TABLE 9-12

DISORDERS OF AMINO ACID METABOLISM

DISORDER	ENZYME DEFECT	MANIFESTATIONS
Phenylalanine and tyrosine		
Phenylketonuria	Phenylalanine hydroxylase	Mental retardation, fair complexion, hyperphenylalaninemia, positive $FeCl_3$ test
Biopterin deficiency (malignant PKU)	Dihydropteridine reductase Tetrahydrobiopetrin synthesis	Progressive neurologic deterioration even with well-controlled blood phenylalanine; hypotonia, seizures
Tyrosinemia type 1 (hepatorenal)	Fumarylacetoacetate hydrolase	Liver failure, renal Fanconi syndrome, urinary succinylacetone
Tyrosinemia type 2 (oculocutaneous)	Tyrosine aminotransferase	Corneal ulcers, keratoses on palms and soles
Tyrosinemia type 3	4-hydroxy-phenylpyruvate dioxygenase	Mental retardation
Alkaptonuria	Homogentisic acid dioxygenase	Dark urine, adult onset of ochronosis and arthritis
Infantile parkinsonism	Tyrosine hydroxylase GTP cyclohydrolase I	Dystonia, rigidity, dopa responsive
Branched-chain amino acids		
Maple syrup urine disease	Branched-chain ketoacid decarboxylase	Hypotonia, coma, urinary odor, death
Propionic acidemia	Propionyl CoA carboxylase	Hypotonia, vomiting, ketosis, acidosis, hypoglycemia, hyperammonemia, coma, death
Methylmalonic acidemia	Methylmalonyl-CoA mutase Cobolamin pathway	As in propionic acidemia Psychomotor retardation, hypotonia, seizures, thrombosis, homocystinuria, death
3-Ketothiolase deficiency	3-Ketothiolase	As in propionic acidemia, but milder, mental retardation
Isovaleric acidemia	Isovaleryl-CoA dehydrogenase	As in propionic acidemia, sweaty sock odor, mental retardation, death
3-Hydroxy-3-methylglutaric aciduria	3-Hydroxy-3-methylglutaryl-CoA lyase	Hypoketotic hypoglycemia, coma, acidosis, death
Beta-methylcrotonylglycinuria	3-Methylcrotonyl-CoA carboxylase	Milder than propionic acidemia, Reye syndrome-like, recurrent ketosis, hypoglycemia, seizures
3-Methylglutaconic aciduria	3-Methylglutaconyl-CoA hydratase	Psychomotor retardation
Mevalonic aciduria	Mevalonate kinase	Failure to thrive, psychomotor retardation, hypotonia, ataxia, dysmorphic features
Multiple carboxylase deficiency	Holocarboxylase synthase; biotinidase	Failure to thrive, alopecia, eczema-like skin rash, hypotonia, ataxia, psychomotor retardation
Lysine, hydroxylysine, and tryptophan		
Glutaric aciduria type I	Glutaryl-CoA dehydrogenase	CNS degeneration, macrocephaly, spasticity, involuntary movements
2-Ketoadipic acidemia	2-Ketoadipic acid dehydrogenase	Probably normal variant
Hyperlysinemia	α-Aminoadipic semialdehyde synthase	Probably normal variant
Glutaric aciduria type II	ETF; ETF dehydrogenase	Variable presentation, neonatal acidosis, hypoglycemia, sweaty sock odor, death or dysmorphic facies; macrocephaly, renal cysts
Sulfur-containing amino acids		
Homocystinuria	Cystathione β-synthetase	Psychomotor retardation, Marfanoid habitus, lens dislocation, thrombosis, high methionine levels
	Methylenetetrahydrofolate reductase; methionine synthase	Psychomotor retardation, thrombosis, normal or low methionine levels
	Cobalamin pathway	Psychomotor retardation, hypotonia, seizures, thrombosis, death, low methionine levels, methylmalonic acidemia
Cystathioninuria	Cystathionase	Probably normal variant
Sulfite oxidase deficiency	Sulfite oxidase Molybdenum cofactor	Seizures, hypotonia, psychomotor retardation, lens dislocation
Pyroglutamic aciduria	Glutathione synthetase	Psychomotor retardation, hemolysis, acidosis
γ-Glutamylcysteine synthetase deficiency	γ-Glutamylcysteine synthetase	Hemolytic anemia, spinocerebellar degeneration
Glutathionuria	γ-Glutamyltranspeptidase	Mental retardation
Glycine and Proline		
Nonketotic hyperglycinemia	Glycine cleavage system	Seizures, hypotonia, death
Sarcosinemia	Sarcosine dehydrogenase	Probably normal variant
Hyperoxaluria type 1	Alanine:glyoxylate aminotransferase	Nephrocalcinosis, oxalate stones, renal failure, systemic oxalosis

(continued)

TABLE 9-12   Continued

DISORDER	ENZYME DEFECT	MANIFESTATIONS
Hyperoxaluria type 2	D-Glycerate/glyoxylate reductase	Nephrocalcinosis, oxalate stones, renal failure
Guanidinoacetate methyltransferase deficiency	Guanidinoacetate methyltransferase	Hypotonia, progressive extrapyramidal movement disorder, seizures, low creatine level
Hyperprolinemia	Proline oxidase 1-pyrroline-5-carboxylate dehydrogenase	Probably normal variant
Hydroxyprolinemia	4-Hydroxy-1-proline oxidase	Probably normal variant
Miscellaneous		
Carnosinemia	Carnosinase	Probably normal variant
γ-Hydroxybutyric aciduria	Succinic semialdehyde dehydrogenase	Mild psychomotor retardation, hypotonia, seizures
GABA transaminase deficiency	γ-Aminobutyrate aminotransferase	Progressive psychomotor retardation, hypotonia
Pyridoxine dependency with seizures	Glutamate decarboxylase	Neonatal seizures
Histidinemia	Histidine ammonia-lyase	Probably normal variant
Urocanase deficiency	Urocanase	Progressive psychomotor retardation, seizures

of phenylalanine increase; hypoglycemic convulsions may occur, and death has been reported.

There is general agreement that classic PKU must be treated; opinion on the other hyperphenylalaninemias, however, is divergent. Many centers believe that any patient with blood phenylalanine levels over 8 mg/dL or who excretes phenylalanine metabolites in the urine should be treated. The necessity for treatment should be evaluated repeatedly by dietary challenge; treatment may be discontinued if it can be established that a patient is of the benign variant type.

It was common to discontinue the dietary restriction of phenylalanine after a few years of age, but several studies show that this leads to IQ loss and behavioral disturbances. Therefore, many metabolic centers now keep classic PKU patients on the diet lifelong, including adulthood. It also has been documented that many adult PKU patients who were not treated in childhood, and who are retarded, nonetheless benefit from a low-phenylalanine diet in terms of psychiatric manifestations of the disease.

HYPERPHENYLALANINEMIA

Widespread screening of populations has led to the recognition that not all patients with hyperphenylalaninemia have classic PKU. It is now recognized that a variety of mutations in the hydroxylase gene lead to different clinically phenotypic variants with varying enzyme activity, level of phenylalanine, and tolerance to dietary phenylalanine.

Whereas most infants with classic PKU cannot tolerate more than 75 mg/kg/d of phenylalanine, a patient with hyperphenylalaninemia will have a rise in serum phenylalanine levels to less than

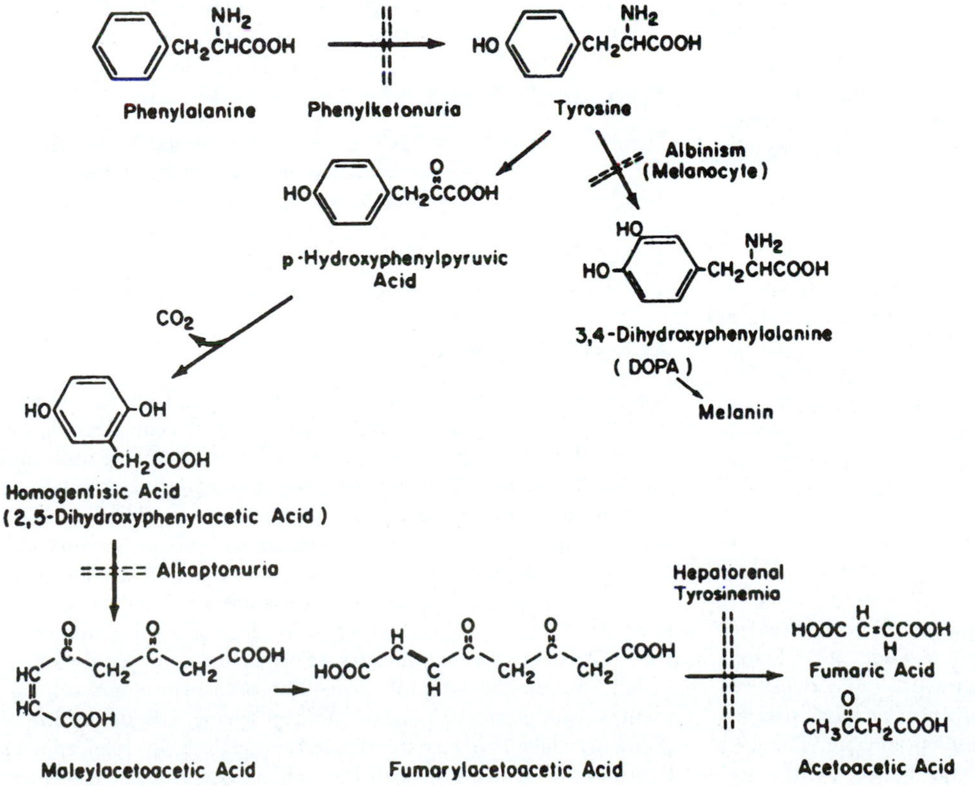

FIGURE 9-6   Metabolism of phenylalanine and tyrosine. Sites of metabolic blocks in alkaptonuria, albinism, phenylketonuria, and hepatorenal tyrosinemia are indicated.

20 mg/dL when challenged with 180 mg/kg/d of phenylalanine for 72 hours.

DEFECTS IN SYNTHESIS OR RECYCLING OF BIOPTERIN

A group of patients with hyperphenylalaninemia have neurologic symptoms that are progressive in spite of dietary treatment that maintained normal phenylalanine levels (malignant PKU). These patients have defects in the synthesis of tetrahydrobiopterin, the cofactor for phenylalanine hydroxylase, or the enzymes that regenerate tetrahydrobiopterin from dihydrobiopterin. Each of these defects results in deficient conversion of phenylalanine to tyrosine, even though the phenylalanine hydroxylase apoenzyme itself is normal. Tetrahydrobiopterin is also the cofactor for the hydroxylation of tryptophan and tyrosine, and its deficiency interferes with the synthesis of serotonin, dihydroxyphenylalanine (dopa), and norepinephrine. Severe neurologic disease may occur with only mild hyperphenylalaninemia, suggesting that tetrahydrobiopterin levels may be relatively more adequate for phenylalanine hydroxylation than for that of tryptophan or tyrosine. Affected patients have had marked hypotonia, as well as spasticity and dystonic posturing. Some have seizures, myoclonus, and EEG abnormalities. Drooling is common. The delay in psychomotor development is usually profound. Defective biosynthesis of tetrahydrobiopterin can be diagnosed by assay of the pattern of excretion in the urine, as well as by quantitative assay of tetrahydrobiopterin in the plasma, especially after a phenylalanine load. Testing should be done routinely in all patients with hyperphenylalaninemia, because early treatment is vital. The diagnosis of specific enzyme deficiency can be confirmed by assay in cultured fibroblasts.

The treatment for this group of patients consists of phenylalanine restriction and the administration of biogenic amine precursors, such as 5-hydroxytryptophan and dopa, which do not require hydroxylation. Carbidopa is a necessary adjunct to prevent decarboxylation of these precursors before they reach the central nervous system. Tetrahydrobiopterin is used in patients with synthesis defects, but by itself, it is insufficient. To optimize the drug dosages, monitoring of neurotransmitter levels in cerebrospinal fluid is indicated. Unfortunately, however, even early and aggressive therapy does not prevent progressive neurologic deterioration and eventual death in some patients.

TYROSINEMIA

The tyrosinemias are a group of disorders in which elevated quantities of tyrosine are found in body fluids. The most common form is transient tyrosinemia of the newborn resulting from delayed maturation of tyrosine-metabolizing enzymes. It is particularly common in premature infants. Tyrosinemia also occurs in scurvy and many forms of liver disease. In addition, there are several genetic deficiencies of enzymes involved in tyrosine catabolism, all of which are autosomal recessive diseases.

Hepatorenal Tyrosinemia (Hereditary Tyrosinemia Type 1)

This disease is caused by deficiency of fumarylacetoacetate hydrolase, the last enzyme in tyrosine catabolism (see Fig. 9-6). Symptoms may begin early in infancy with an acute rapid course to demise, or they may progress more chronically. Most patients present with failure to thrive and hepatosplenomegaly. The liver disease is progressive, causing cirrhosis, and icterus, ascites, and

hemorrhage often ensue. Patients display renal tubular acidosis of the Fanconi type, and typical radiographic changes of rickets are often present. Mental retardation is not a feature. Surviving patients have a high risk for developing hepatocarcinoma (see Chapter 18).

Biochemical alterations include elevated plasma concentrations of tyrosine and methionine and the excretion of tyrosyl compounds in the urine. The presence of succinylacetone in urine is diagnostic. Highly elevated concentrations of α-fetoprotein are seen, even before the elevation in tyrosine. Hypoglycemia may occur, and coagulation defects are common.

The liver failure and renal Fanconi syndrome of hepatorenal tyrosinemia can be effectively treated with a new drug, 2(2-nitro-4-trifluoromethylbenzoyl)-1,3-cyclohexane dione (NTBC), which blocks tyrosine metabolism by inhibiting the second step (see Fig. 9-6), thus preventing the accumulation of toxic metabolites. NTBC raises blood tyrosine levels and thus needs to be combined with a diet low in phenylalanine and tyrosine. The prognosis of patients with this disease has vastly improved with this new therapy.

The gene for fumarylacetoacetate hydrolase has been cloned and can be used for prenatal diagnosis and carrier detection. Hepatorenal tyrosinemia is common in the Canadian province of Quebec, where a single founder mutation is responsible for most cases.

Oculocutaneous Tyrosinemia (Tyrosinemia Type 2)

Tyrosine aminotransferase, the first step of tyrosine degradation, is deficient in oculocutaneous tyrosinemia. The characteristic features of this disease are corneal ulcers or dendritic keratitis early in life and erythematous papular or keratotic lesions on the palms and soles. About 50% of patients display mental retardation. Tyrosine itself is not hepatotoxic, and the liver and kidney are not affected in this disorder. Plasma concentrations of tyrosine are higher than in other forms of tyrosinemia, and the urine contains large amounts tyrosine metabolites. The lesions on the palms and soles and in the eyes relate directly to the accumulation of tyrosine. Both respond rapidly to treatment with diets low in tyrosine.

Tyrosinemia Type 3

The second step in tyrosine catabolism is catalyzed by 4-hydroxyphenylpyruvate dioxygenase. Several patients lacking this enzyme have been identified, and all suffer from mild psychomotor retardation, but no other organ systems are involved. Plasma tyrosine levels are elevated, but usually not to levels that cause corneal ulcers or hyperkeratosis. Treatment consists of a low-tyrosine diet.

ALKAPTONURIA

Alkaptonuria results from defective activity of the enzyme homogentisic acid dioxygenase, the third enzyme in tyrosine degradation (see Fig. 9-6). However, blood tyrosine levels are not elevated, and the disorder is characterized by the excretion of dark-colored urine. Fresh urine appears normal, but on standing and particularly after alkalinization, oxidation of homogentisic acid proceeds, and a dark brown or black pigment appears. This should permit the condition to be recognized early in life, but the diagnosis is usually first made in adult life during routine urinalysis or during investigation of arthritis. Persons with alkaptonuria are usually asymptomatic in childhood. After the third decade, deposition of brownish or bluish pigment is seen, particularly in the ears and sclerae. The deposition of pigment, which may be extensive in fibrous tissues, is referred to as ochronosis. Ochronotic arthritis, which occurs later, produces symptoms resembling rheumatoid arthritis or osteoarthritis, with limitation of motion; complete ankylosis is common.

Garrod's suggestion that the disorder results from absence in the liver of the enzyme that catalyzes the oxidation of homogentisic acid (see Fig. 9-6) gave rise to the one-gene, one-enzyme hypothesis and the field of biochemical genetics.

INFANTILE PARKINSONISM

An autosomally recessive inherited isolated deficiency of tyrosine hydroxylase causes severe parkinsonism in infancy. A less-severe form of the disease is termed *Segawa syndrome* or *dopa-responsive dystonia*. Dystonic posture or movement of one limb appears insidiously between ages 1 and 9 years. Intelligence is normal. This disorder can also be autosomal dominant. In these families, the mutated gene is GTP cyclohydrolase I, which is involved in the biosynthesis of tetrahydrobiopterin. The diagnosis can be made by finding abnormally low levels of homovanillic acid in cerebrospinal fluid. All forms of the disease respond to treatment with L-dopa.

9.2.2   Branched-Chain Amino Acid Group

Defects in the degradation of the branched-chain amino acids valine, leucine, and isoleucine result in the accumulation of organic acid intermediates. High levels of these compounds are toxic, particularly to the central nervous system. These diseases are most readily detected by analysis of urine organic acids, and in many cases, there is a characteristic odor. There are many different enzymes involved in this pathway, and autosomal recessive inheritance has been described for many. An elevation in the branched-chain amino acids is often seen in maple syrup urine disease. The remainder of the enzyme defects in this catabolic pathway result in elevated levels of the intermediate organic acids, but normal concentrations of valine, leucine, and isoleucine (see Sect. 9.4.)

MAPLE SYRUP URINE DISEASE

In maple syrup urine disease (branched-chain ketoaciduria), major cerebral symptoms appear early in the newborn period, and the urine has an odor reminiscent of maple syrup. The branched-chain amino acids—leucine, isoleucine, and valine—are present in high concentration in the blood and urine, and the ketoacid analogues are found in the urine.

Clinical Findings

Infants with maple syrup urine disease appear well at birth. In the typical patient, symptoms begin after 3 to 5 days and progress rapidly to death within 2 to 4 weeks. Early manifestations include feeding difficulty, irregular respirations, or progressive loss of the Moro reflex. Severe hypoglycemia may occur. Characteristically these patients develop convulsions, opisthotonos, and generalized muscular rigidity with or without intermittent flaccidity. Death usually occurs after decerebrate rigidity develops. Cortical atrophy may be seen on CT or MRI scan, and the myelin is usually hypodense. This is consistent with the defective myelinization that has been observed at autopsy. The feature that distinguishes any form of branched-chain ketoaciduria from other cerebral degenerative diseases of infancy is the characteristic maple syrup, or caramel, odor of the urine, skin, or hair. The odor may become evident 1 or 2 days after birth and may persist, but varies in intensity and may not be detected in some specimens.

Milder forms of the disease occur that are known as intermittent branched-chain aminoaciduria; they represent variant mutations in the same enzyme complex as in classic maple syrup urine disease. Ataxia and repeated episodes of lethargy progressing to coma occur without mental retardation; these episodes may be precipitated by infection or anesthesia.

Biochemical Findings and Genetics

Increased quantities of leucine, isoleucine, and valine are found in the plasma and urine. The presence of an abnormal amino acid, alloisoleucine, is diagnostic for MSUD. The catabolism of branched-chain amino acids is initiated by a transamination reaction to generate the respective ketoacids which then undergo decarboxylation to coenzyme A (CoA) derivatives. The defect in MSUD is in this oxidative decarboxylation of the ketoacids, which is catalyzed by a mitochondrial multienzyme complex similar to pyruvate dehydrogenase and to α-ketoglutarate dehydrogenase. For this reason, autosomal recessive mutations in four different genes can cause MSUD. Patients have been identified with defects in the $E_1\alpha$, $E_1\beta$, E_2, and E_3 subunits of the complex. The E_3 subunit is shared by all three complexes, and patients with defects in this gene have simultaneous deficiency of branched-chain ketoacid dehydrogenase, pyruvate dehydrogenase, and α-ketoglutarate dehydrogenase. MSUD is rare in most populations with an incidence of ~1/150,000.

Therapy

Experience has now been accumulated with prolonged use of special diets in which the intakes of leucine, isoleucine, and valine are closely controlled. Concentrations of the branched-chain amino acids in plasma can be maintained within normal limits. This therapy is difficult. Many patients have had permanent brain damage before treatment is started, but experience with siblings of previous patients, in whom very early diagnosis is possible, and with patients detected by neonatal screening programs, indicates that a normal IQ may be achieved. Commercial products are available that are useful in management. Intravenous solutions of amino acids that exclude the branched-chain amino acids take advantage of protein synthesis to reduce concentrations of leucine and the other amino acids and reverse coma in acute episodes of metabolic imbalance. Rare patients have a thiamine-responsive form of MSUD, and therefore this vitamin should be tried in all patients.

KETOTIC HYPERGLYCINEMIAS

Secondary elevation of plasma glycine is found in some defects of branched-chain amino acid metabolism, particularly in propionic acidemia, methylmalonic acidemia, and 3-ketothiolase deficiencies. Because these conditions are also associated with ketoacidosis, they are grouped as the ketotic hyperglycinemias and contrasted with nonketotic hyperglycinemia, a primary defect in the glycine cleavage system. Urine organic acids should be analyzed in any patient with elevated plasma glycine concentration.

9.2.3   Lysine, Hydroxylysine, and Tryptophan Group

Only one clinical disorder, glutaric aciduria type I, is caused by an enzyme defect in the catabolic pathway of lysine, hydroxylysine, and tryptophan. A second form of glutaric aciduria, designated glutaric aciduria type II, is characterized by severe illness in the neonatal period; it has been uniformly fatal. Organic acid analysis in type I reveals glutaric aciduria and glutaric acidemia. In type II, there are, in addition, accumulations of a wide variety of organic acids, including adipic and ethylmalonic acids. In type I, there is a specific defect in glutaryl-CoA dehydrogenase, whereas in type II, there is a general deficiency in the activity of many acyl-CoA dehydrogenases (see Sec. 9.4.).

HYPERLYSINEMIA

Deficiency of the bifunctional protein α-aminoadipic semialdehyde synthase causes familial hyperlysinemia. The clinical significance of this enzyme deficiency is controversial. Psychomotor retardation has been reported in many, but not all, affected individuals.

2-KETOADIPIC ACIDEMIA

Individuals who lack 2-ketoadipic acid dehydrogenase excrete large amounts of 2-ketoadipic acid and 2-hydroxy adipic acid in their urine. Although there are some reports of neurologic disease in this condition, other patients have been clinically normal.

9.2.4   Sulfur-Containing Amino Acid Group

HOMOCYSTINURIA (CYSTATHIONE β-SYNTHETASE DEFICIENCY)

Homocystinuria (elevated urinary levels of homocystine) is a hallmark of several disorders in the metabolism of sulfur-containing amino acids. The term is sometimes used to specifically indicate the classic form of the disease which is caused by defective activity of the enzyme cystathionine β-synthetase (CBS). However, several other enzyme defects can also cause elevated homocysteine, including defects of B_{12} metabolism. Thus, homocystinuria is not a single disease, but a heterogeneous group of disorders. Plasma methionine, cystine, and B_{12} levels, as well as urine organic acids, should be measured in all patients with homocystinuria.

Deficiency of CBS, which is inherited in an autosomal recessive manner, is the most common cause of homocystinuria.

Clinical Findings

The classic presentation of cystathionine β-synthetase deficiency includes marfanoid habitus, developmental delay, lens dislocation, and predisposition for blood clotting. Presentation is usually in the first decade with the exception of embolism, which occurs later. Homocystinuria is one of the few disorders of amino acid metabolism in which clinical manifestations tend to be progressive in adulthood, because many clinical manifestations result from thrombotic complications. Classic tests of clotting function are normal, but elevated homocystine levels cause increased platelet adhesiveness. The most characteristic feature of this disorder is subluxation of the ocular lens. Mental retardation is common, although not always present. Most patients have osteoporosis and skeletal abnormalities similar to those seen in Marfan syndrome. In homocystinuria, however, the joints tend to be limited in mobility rather than hypermobile. There is also lenticular subluxation in both conditions; however, in Marfan syndrome the lens is usually displaced upwards, whereas in homocystinuria it is displaced downwards and medially (see Chapter 10).

Biochemical Findings and Genetics

The normal biosynthesis of the sulfur amino acid cysteine involves the demethylation of methionine to homocysteine, followed by its reaction with serine to form cystathionine. This latter step is catalyzed by the pyridoxine-requiring enzyme cystathione β-synthetase. Homocystine is derived from the condensation of homocysteine to form the disulfide homocystine and is not normally detected in the usual assays of amino acids in body fluids. In CBS deficiency, elevated homocystine levels can be detected in both urine and blood. Levels of methionine are usually also elevated, and levels of cystine are reduced. Because homocystine is unstable, testing should be done only on fresh urine. Homocystine binds to plasma proteins, and it is therefore important to rapidly remove protein during the processing of blood specimens. Urine can be screened by adding nitroprusside following treatment with cyanide. Because homocystinuria can be caused by several genetic defects, it is important to specifically confirm the diagnosis of CBS deficiency by measuring the enzyme in liver, cultured skin fibroblasts, or lymphoblasts. Importantly, CBS is a pyridoxine-dependent enzyme, and in many patients some activity can be restored by pharmacologic doses of pyridoxine.

CBS deficiency is autosomal recessive, and the gene has been cloned and mapped to chromosome 21q. Many disease-causing mutations have been described, and DNA-based diagnosis can be used for prenatal detection of the condition.

Therapy

All patients should be treated with large doses (100–500 mg/d) of pyridoxine to determine their degree of responsiveness. If the homocystine levels normalize, no additional therapy may be needed. Those who do not respond may be treated with a diet low in methionine and supplemented with L-cystine. In addition, the compound betaine may be used to aid in the conversion of homocysteine to methionine. Medications aimed at reducing platelet adhesiveness can be prescribed, but do not abolish all thromboembolic events.

OTHER CAUSES OF HOMOCYSTINURIA

Homocystinuria may result from defects other than CBS. Two of these defects—methylenetetrahydrofolate reductase deficiency and methionine synthase deficiency—are associated with low, rather than high, plasma methionine levels. The deficient enzymes are involved in the recycling of homocysteine to methionine. Clinically, both disorders lack the eye and skeletal involvement of CBS deficiency, but display the same clotting propensity. The specific enzyme diagnosis can be made on cultured skin fibroblasts. Treatment is similar to CBS deficiency, but no pyridoxine is given and methionine is supplemented rather than restricted in the diet. Folate administration may also be beneficial.

As mentioned earlier, homocystinuria and methylmalonic aciduria occur jointly in disorders of vitamin B_{12} transport or metabolism because MetCbl is required for recycling of homocystine to methionine. These conditions are often associated with neurologic deterioration and have a poor prognosis. For this reason, it is important that every patient with homocystinuria have a urine organic acid analysis. If a vitamin B_{12} defect is found, B_{12} injections are used in addition to the usual treatments for homocystinuria.

CYSTATHIONINURIA

Cystathioninuria, an inborn error of amino acid metabolism in which there is a deficiency of the activity of cystathionase, was first reported in two adults with mental deficiency. Subsequently, however, cystathioninuria has been found in a number of individuals with no clinical signs and is currently considered a benign variant.

SULFITE OXIDASE AND MOLYBDENUM COFACTOR DEFICIENCY

The terminal step in the oxidative degradation of cysteine and methionine, the conversion of sulfite to sulfate, is catalyzed by the molybdenum-containing enzyme sulfite oxidase. Severe neurologic disease is associated with deficiency in this system.

Clinical Findings

Most patients present with neonatal neurologic disease including severe hypotonia, seizures, and myoclonic spasms. Symptoms are progressive and usually lead to early death. Patients with milder forms of the disease have progressive cerebral palsy and choreiform movements. Infantile hemiplegia has been reported, and lens dislocation is a frequent finding even in neonates.

Biochemical Findings and Genetics

Sulfite oxidase deficiency can be caused by a defect in the gene for this protein or by defects in the synthesis of the molybdenum cofactor required for its function. In all cases, the disease is autosomal recessive in inheritance. Sulfite oxidase functions in the oxidative degradation of the sulfur-containing amino acids cysteine and methionine. Deficiency results in increased amounts of sulfite, thiosulfate, and S-sulfocysteine in the urine. These compounds are not readily detected during routine metabolic studies, and the diagnosis needs to be suspected to initiate appropriate testing. The elevated urinary sulfite levels can be detected using commercial strip tests normally utilized for wine making. Mutations in two genes (MOCS1 and 2) can cause molybdenum cofactor deficiency, resulting in absent aldehyde oxidase and xanthine dehydrogenase, in addition to sulfite oxidase. Very low uric acid levels in blood and urine are a clue to this condition. In molybdenum cofactor deficiency, the urinary excretion of hypoxanthine and xanthine is highly elevated. The genes for all three proteins have been cloned and prenatal diagnosis can be performed.

Therapy

Currently, no effective therapy is available.

DISORDERS OF THE γ-GLUTAMYL CYCLE

The synthesis and recycling of the sulfur-containing tripeptide glutathione involves a series of six enzymatic reactions termed the *γ-glutamyl cycle*. Deficiencies in several of these enzymes are associated with disease (see Table 9-12).

Pyroglutamic Aciduria

Pyroglutamic aciduria, or 5-oxoprolinuria, is caused by autosomal recessive deficiency of glutathione synthetase. Pyroglutamic acid is 2-pyrrolidone-5-carboxylic acid, a cyclized condensation product of glutamic acid or glutamine. It can be readily detected by urine organic acid analysis.

Clinically, the disease is characterized by neurologic symptoms that include spasticity, ataxia, and mental retardation. Patients can experience episodes of acidosis and hemolysis. Glutathione deficiency is considered the likely underlying cause of the disease, and

therapeutic attempts are aimed at increasing cellular glutathione concentrations and antioxidant activity. Unfortunately, this intervention does not completely eliminate neurologic problems. Drugs such as acetaminophen, which require glutathione for detoxification, should be avoided.

9.2.5 Glycine, Oxalate, and Proline Group

NONKETOTIC HYPERGLYCINEMIA

Nonketotic hyperglycinemia (NKH) is an inborn error of metabolism in which large amounts of glycine are found in body fluids, without detectable accumulation of organic acids.

Clinical Findings

Nonketotic hyperglycinemia usually presents with intractable seizures in the neonatal period. Hypotonia, lethargy, hyperreflexia, hiccoughing, and myoclonic jerks are frequent. Many patients require assisted ventilation, and death is a common outcome. The EEG is abnormal and displays a typical burst-suppression pattern. Most patients who survive have severe mental retardation. Patients with later-onset forms have been described but are rare.

Biochemical Findings and Genetics

In NKH, elevated glycine levels are found in all body fluids including blood, urine, and CSF. In contrast to ketotic hyperglycinemia described above, plasma ketone levels are not elevated and no abnormal organic acids are found in the urine. Glycine levels are most elevated in the central nervous system. The ratio of the CSF concentration of glycine to that of the plasma is substantially higher in patients with nonketotic hyperglycinemia than in hyperglycinemic patients with organic acidemia.

The basic defect is in the glycine cleavage system, which catalyzes the conversion of glycine to CO_2 and hydroxymethyltetrahydrofolic acid. The enzyme is multimeric with four distinct protein components designated P, H, T, and L. All forms of NKH are autosomal recessive in inheritance. The genes for all four proteins have been cloned and mapped. Mutations in the P and T genes have been found, with the P protein being most commonly affected. A single mutation is responsible for most cases in Finland. Prenatal diagnosis can be performed by biochemical analysis of chorionic villus sample biopsies.

Therapy

Recently, there has been modest success in the treatment of NKH, particularly in late-onset cases. Large doses of sodium benzoate may reduce CSF concentrations of glycine and decrease seizures. Glycine is a neurotransmitter, and anticonvulsants that block the N-methyl-D-aspartate (NMDA) receptor may be beneficial. Dextromethorphan has been used and resulted in some improved outcome.

SARCOSINEMIA

Sarcosine is the N-methyl derivative of glycine. It is formed from dimethylglycine, which may be a product of betaine or choline. Sarcosine is not normally present in blood or urine in detectable amounts, although sarcosinuria may occur after the ingestion of lobster and some other foods. Sarcosine dehydrogenase deficiency causes sarcosinemia and has been found in individuals with short stature and mental retardation, but a causal relationship has not been established.

HYPEROXALURIA (OXALOSIS)

Clinical Findings

Primary hyperoxaluria is a metabolic disorder in which large amounts of oxalate are excreted in the urine, leading to calcium oxalate lithiasis and nephrocalcinosis (see Sec. 21.12). Two distinct types are known, with type 1 generally being more severe than type 2. When extrarenal deposits of calcium oxalate ensue, the condition is known as oxalosis. Renal failure is common, and first symptoms appear before 5 years of age.

Biochemical Findings and Genetics

Primary hyperoxaluria type 1 is caused by deficiency of the liver enzyme alanine:glyoxylate aminotransferase and type 2 by deficiency of D-glycerate/glyoxylate reductase. Both types are characterized by hyperoxaluria, but in type 1 there is additional excretion of glycolic acid. In type 2, the urine contains high amounts of L-glycerate.

Oxalic acid is a dicarboxylic acid that forms a calcium salt of very low solubility. Oxalate in the urine is clearly of endogenous origin, and glycine is a precursor. Patients with hyperoxaluria may excrete 30 times as much oxalate as normal.

Both types of hyperoxaluria are autosomal recessive. The genes have been cloned, and disease-causing mutations have been identified. Prenatal diagnosis is available.

Therapy

Dietary and pharmacologic treatment are ineffective. However, several patients have been successfully treated with combined hepatorenal transplantation. Renal transplantation alone has been unsuccessful because systematically generated oxalate is deposited in the transplanted kidney.

GUANIDINOACETATE METHYLTRANSFERASE DEFICIENCY

This autosomal recessive disease affects the biosynthesis of creatine from glycine via the intermediate metabolite guanidinoacetate. The deficient enzyme is guanidinoacetate methyltransferase (GAMT). Clinically, the disease has a neurologic presentation with hypotonia, progressive movement disorder, and seizures. Creatine levels are very low. Importantly, treatment with creatine monohydrate has been reported to reverse neurologic symptoms. The gene for GAMT is located on chromosome 19p, and disease-causing mutations have been found.

HYPERPROLINEMIA AND HYDROXYPROLINEMIA

Hyperprolinemia and hydroxyprolinemia are inborn errors of metabolism of the amino acids that are now generally accepted as metabolic markers unassociated with clinical disease. Three distinct metabolic defects have been identified: proline oxidase is deficient in type I hyperprolinemia; 1-pyrroline-5-carboxylate dehydrogenase is deficient in type II hyperprolinemia; and hydroxyproline oxidase is deficient in hydroxyprolinemia.

9.2.6   Miscellaneous Disorders

CARNOSINEMIA

A number of patients with carnosinemia have been reported. Most have had abnormalities of the central nervous system, but further experience has revealed a number of completely normal people who have the same defect. Therefore, this metabolic curiosity probably does not cause human disease.

γ-HYDROXYBUTYRIC ACIDURIA

Succinic semialdehyde dehydrogenase (SSAD) deficiency is a disorder in the catabolism of GABA (γ-aminobutyric acid), a neurotransmitter. GABA is transaminated to form succinic semialdehyde, which is then reduced by SSAD to succinate. In the presence of a block at this step, succinic semialdehyde is reduced to γ-hydroxybutyric acid which accumulates in the urine, serum, and CSF. Patients with this disease have severe ataxia and hypotonia, convulsions, and mild psychomotor retardation. γ-Hydroxybutyric aciduria is an interesting model disorder of metabolism because the basic defect leads to the accumulation of a compound of known neuropharmacologic activity. γ-Hydroxybutyric acid was originally developed by the pharmaceutical industry as an analogue of GABA that could readily cross the blood-brain barrier and be used as an intravenous anesthetic. It had to be abandoned for clinical use because it produced convulsions and coma.

The gene for SSAD has been cloned and many disease-causing mutations have been found. Prenatal diagnosis is available by enzymatic analysis of cultured amniocytes. Treatment is supportive and employs standard anticonvulsant drugs.

GABA-TRANSAMINASE DEFICIENCY

GABA transaminase deficiency has been reported in patients with progressive neurologic deterioration, leukodystrophy, and hypotonia resulting in eventual death. CSF levels of GABA and homocarnosine were markedly elevated.

PYRIDOXINE DEPENDENCY

The biosynthesis of GABA occurs via decarboxylation of glutamate in a pyridoxine-dependent reaction. Several patients with neonatal seizures and deficiency of this enzyme in tissue extracts have been described. The seizures respond well to pharmacologic doses of pyridoxine, providing the rationale for vitamin B_6 administration in neonates with convulsions (see Sec. 25.10).

HISTIDINEMIA AND UROCANASE DEFICIENCY

Histidinemia is a disorder of intermediary metabolism in which large amounts of histidine are found in blood and urine. The condition must be included in the differential diagnosis of PKU because it produces a positive ferric test in the urine. Although there may be no clinical manifestations, more than half of these patients have speech retardation; mental and growth retardation also may occur. Relatively fair hair and blue eyes are common.

Histidine is normally converted by histidase to urocanic acid, which is further metabolized to form iminoglutamic acid and, ultimately, glutamic acid. In histidinemia, histidine levels are increased in plasma, urine, and CSF. Many patients also have hyperalaninemia. Deficiency of histidase (histidine ammonia-lyase) has been demonstrated by direct assay of the enzyme in skin. Recent prospective studies have shown conclusively that histidinemia does not cause disease.

Rare case reports have associated autosomal recessive deficiency of urocanase, the next enzyme in histidine metabolism, with severe mental retardation and neurologic deterioration.

References

Phenylketonuria

Eisensmith RC, Woo SL: Population genetics of phenylketonuria. Acta Paediatr Suppl 407:19–26, 1994

Hanley WB, Clarke JT, Schoonheyt W: Maternal phenylketonuria (PKU)—a review. Clin Biochem 20(3):149–156, 1987

Scriver CR, Waters PJ: Monogenic traits are not simple: lessons from phenylketonuria. Trends Genet 15(7):267–272, 1999

Smith I, Lobascher ME, Stevenson JE, et al: Effect of stopping low-phenylalanine diet on intellectual progress of children with phenylketonuria. Br Med J 2(6139): 723–726, 1978

Biopterin Defects

Hyland K, Arnold LA, Trugman JM: Defects of biopterin metabolism and biogenic amine biosynthesis: clinical diagnostic, and therapeutic aspects. Adv Neurol 78:301–308, 1998

Tyrosinemia

al-Hemidan AI, al-Hazzaa SA: Richner-Hanhart syndrome (tyrosinemia type II). Case report and literature review. Ophthalmic Genet 16(1): 21–26, 1995

Holme E, Lindstedt S: Diagnosis and management of tyrosinemia type I. Curr Opin Pediatr 7(6):726–732, 1995

Kvittingen EA: Hereditary tyrosinemia type I—an overview. Scand J Clin Lab Invest Suppl 184:27–34, 1986

Ney D, Bay C, Schneider JA, et al: Dietary management of oculocutaneous tyrosinemia in an 11-year-old child. Am J Dis Child 137(10):995–1000, 1983

Alkaptonuria

Brenton DP, Krywawych S: Alkaptonuria. Clin Rheum Dis 12(3):755–769, 1986

Garrod AE: The incidence of alkaptonuria: a study in chemical individuality. Lancet 2:1616, 1902

La Du BN, Zannoni VA, Laster BC, et al: The nature of the defect in tyrosine metabolism in alcaptonuria. J Biol Chem 230:251, 1958

Infantile Parkinsonism

Gorke W, Bartholome K: Biochemical and neurophysiological investigations in two forms of Segawa's disease. Neuropediatrics 21(1):3–8, 1990

Maple Syrup Urine Disease

Chuang DT: Maple syrup urine disease: it has come a long way. J Pediatr 132(3 Pt 2):S17–23, 1998

Clow CL, Reade TM, Scriver CR: Outcome of early and long-term management of classical maple syrup urine disease. Pediatrics 68(6):856–862, 1981

Peinemann F, Danner DJ: Maple syrup urine disease 1954 to 1993. J Inherit Metab Dis 17(1):3–15, 1994

Hyperlysinemia

Dancis J, Hutzler J, Cox RP: Familial hyperlysinemia: enzyme studies, diagnostic methods, comments on terminology. Am J Hum Genet 31(3): 290–299, 1979

Homocystinuria

Barber GW, Spaeth GL: The successful treatment of homocystinuria with pyridoxine. J Pediatr 75(3):463–478, 1969

De Franchis R, Sperandeo MP, Sebastio G, et al: Clinical aspects of cystathionine beta-synthase deficiency: how wide is the spectrum? The Italian Collaborative Study Group on Homocystinuria. Eur J Pediatr 157(Suppl 2):S67–70, 1998

Dillon MJ, England JM, Gompertz D, et al: Mental retardation, megaloblastic anaemia, methylmalonic aciduria and abnormal homocysteine metabolism due to an error in vitamin B_{12} metabolism. Clin Sci Mol Med 47(1):43–61, 1974

Harpey JP, Rosenblatt DS, Cooper BA, et al: Homocystinuria caused by 5,10-methylenetetrahydrofolate reductase deficiency: a case in an infant responding to methionine, folinic acid, pyridoxine, and vitamin B_{12} therapy. J Pediatr 98(2):275–278, 1981

Kraus JP, Janosik M, Kozich V, et al: Cystathionine beta-synthase mutations in homocystinuria. Hum Mutat 13(5):362–375, 1999

Sulfite Oxidase Deficiency

Aukett A, Bennett MJ, Hojking GP: Molybdenum co-factor deficiency: an easily missed inborn error of metabolism. Dev Med Child Neurol 30(4): 531–535, 1988

Kisker C, Schindelin H, Pacheco A, et al: Molecular basis of sulfite oxidase deficiency from the structure of sulfite oxidase. Cell 91(7):973–983, 1997

Pyroglutamic Aciduria

Wellner VP, Sekura R, Meister A, et al: Glutathione synthetase deficiency, an inborn error of metabolism involving the gamma-glutamyl cycle in patients with 5-oxoprolinuria (pyroglutamic aciduria). Proc Natl Acad Sci 71(6):2505–2509, 1974

Nonketotic Hyperglycinemia

Deutsch SI, Rosse RB, Mastropolo J: Current status of NMDA antagonist interventions in the treatment of nonketotic hyperglycinemia. Clin Neuropharmacol 21(2):71–79, 1998

Hamosh A, McDonald JW, Valle R, et al: Dextromethorphan and high-dose benzoate therapy for nonketotic hyperglycinemia in an infant [see comments]. J Pediatr 121(1):131–135, 1992

Hayasaka K, Tada K, Kikuchi G, et al: Nonketotic hyperglycinemia: two patients with primary defects of P-protein and T-protein, respectively, in the glycine cleavage system. Pediatr Res 17(12):967–970, 1983

Sarcosinemia

Gerritsen T, Waisman HA: Hypersarcosinemia: an inborn error of metabolism. N Engl J Med 275(2):66–69, 1966

Levy HL, Coulombe JT, Benjamin R: Massachusetts Metabolic Disorders Screening Program: III. Sarcosinemia. Pediatrics 74(4):509–513, 1984

Hyperoxaluria

Cochat P: Primary hyperoxaluria type 1 [clinical conference]. Kidney Int 55(6):2533–2547, 1990

Kemper MJ, Conrad S, Muller-Wiefel DE: Primary hyperoxaluria type 2. Eur J Pediatr 156(7):509–512, 1997

Tarn AC, von Schnakenburg C, Rumsby G: Primary hyperoxaluria type 1: diagnostic relevance of mutations and polymorphisms in the alanine: glyoxylate aminotransferase gene (AGXT). J Inherit Metab Dis 20(5): 689–696, 1997

Guanidinoacetate Methyltransferase Deficiency

Schulze A, Hess T, Wevers R, et al: Creatine deficiency syndrome caused by guanidinoacetate methyltransferase deficiency: diagnostic tools for a new inborn error of metabolism [see comments]. J Pediatr 131(4):626–631, 1997

γ-Hydroxybutyric Aciduria

Gibson KM, Hoffmann GF, Hodson AK, et al: 4-Hydroxybutyric acid and the clinical phenotype of succinic semialdehyde dehydrogenase deficiency, an inborn error of GABA metabolism. Neuropediatrics 29(1): 14–22, 1998

Histidinemia

Lam WK, Cleary MA, Wraight JE, et al: Histidinaemia: a benign metabolic disorder. Arch Dis Child 74(4):343–346, 1996

Urocanase Deficiency

Kalafatic Z, Lipovac K, Jezerinac Z, et al: A liver urocanase deficiency. Metabolism 29(11):1013–1019, 1980

9.3   INHERITED UREA CYCLE AND RELATED DISORDERS

Mendel Tuchman and Mark L. Batshaw

Urea cycle disorders are caused by specific defects in genes encoding enzymes or membrane transporters involved in ureagenesis (Fig. 9-7). Their overall prevalence is about 1:30,000 births. These diseases, summarized in Table 9-13, should be distinguished from other inborn errors of metabolism with secondary hyperammonemia, including fatty acid oxidation disorders, organic acidurias, and nonketotic hyperglycinemia; congenital disorders must also be differentiated from the acquired hyperammonemia seen in liver disease of various causes and following chemotherapy and organ transplantation. Finally, there is a rare and severe condition termed *transient hyperammonemia* of the neonate, found predominantly in premature infants, the etiology of which remains obscure.

9.3.1 Biochemical Basis of the Congenital Hyperammonemias

The congenital hyperammonemias include: (a) Urea cycle enzyme defects in carbamoyl phosphate synthetase I (CPS); ornithine transcarbamylase (OTC); argininosuccinate synthetase (AS) (a disorder known as citrullinemia); argininosuccinate lyase (AL) (a disorder called argininosuccinic aciduria); arginase (ARG) (also called argininemia); and N-acetylglutamate synthetase (NAGS); and (b) membrane transport defects of dibasic amino acids: hyperdibasic aminoaciduria, also called lysinuric protein intolerance (LPI), and hyperornithinemia, hyperammonemia, homocitrullinuria (HHH syndrome). Awareness of these disorders is important, because failure to recognize hyperammonemia often leads to brain damage or death, and because these are genetically inherited disorders that frequently affect more than one family member.

Ammonia exerts its toxicity almost exclusively on the brain. The exact mechanism is unclear, although interference with energy or neurotransmitter metabolism has been implicated. Brain edema rapidly develops during hyperammonemic coma, and swelling of astrocytes has been observed on postmortem analysis. Plasma ammonia levels as low as 100 to 200 μmol/L are usually associated with clinical symptoms of lethargy, confusion, and vomiting, while higher levels usually result in coma.

The complete urea cycle resides exclusively in periportal hepatocytes and is an essential biochemical pathway for waste nitrogen excretion. A cascade of enzymatic transformations converts the toxic ammonia molecule to nontoxic water-soluble urea, which contains two amino groups (one deriving from free ammonia and the other from aspartate) and is eliminated in the urine (Fig. 9-7). Ammonia is also taken up by "scavengers" (eg, glutamate, pyruvate, and aspartate) and is used in the synthesis of nitrogen-containing compounds (eg, glycine and pyrimidines, including orotic acid). A functional block of the urea cycle results either from an enzyme deficiency (CPS, OTC, NAGS, AS, AL, and ARG) or depletion of an amino acid that is essential to the normal function of the cycle resulting from a transport defect (HHH syndrome and LPI). A recently identified, separate mitochondrial transporter, the function of which is unknown, causes citrullinemia type II and is seen in Japanese adults.

Except for OTC deficiency, which is transmitted as a partially dominant X-linked trait, all other known urea cycle disorders are autosomal recessive traits. The gene associated with the enzyme deficiency has been identified in each of these disorders except NAGS, and deleterious mutations have been found in the respective genes of affected patients. Thus, DNA analysis for mutation detection is possible for each, enhancing both prenatal and postnatal diagnosis as well as carrier detection in affected families. The degree of the deleterious effect of the mutation on the respective protein's function tends to correlate with the severity of the clinical course. However, the milder the mutation, the more heterogeneous the resulting clinical picture. Unfortunately, newborn mass screening is not currently available for the early diagnosis of these disorders.

9.3.2 Clinical Presentation

Generally, the more proximal the enzyme defect, the more severe and resistant to treatment is the hyperammonemia; that is, CPS and OTC deficiencies are the most severe. However, as noted above, there is considerable heterogeneity in the severity of hyperammo-

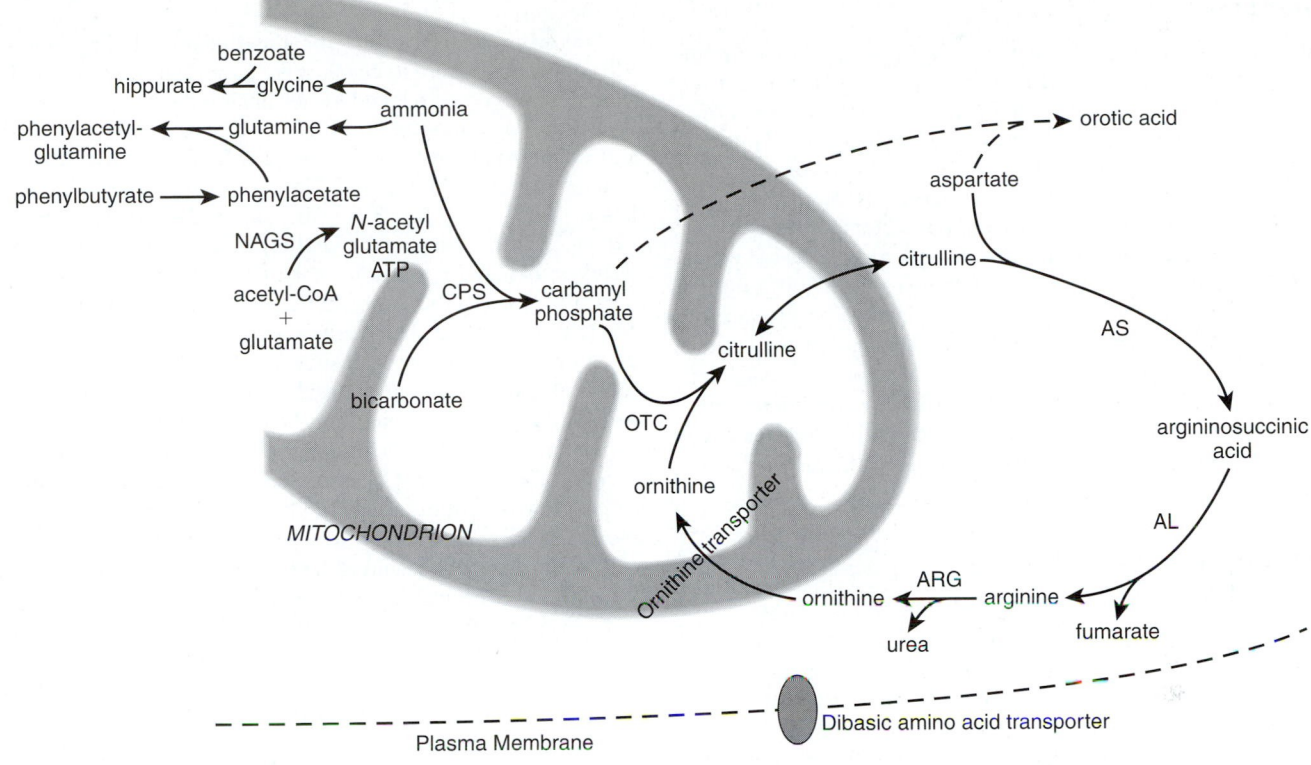

FIGURE 9-7   The complete urea cycle pathway that resides in the liver is illustrated. Also shown are the alternative pathways used to eliminate nitrogen in patients with urea cycle defects. CPS = carbamoylphosphate synthetase; OTC = ornithine transcarbamoylase; AS = argininosuccinate synthetase; AL = argininosuccinate lyase; ARG = arginase; NAGS = *N*-acetylglutamate synthase.

nemia and the age of initial presentation, based not only on the position of the block within the urea cycle but also on the degree of enzyme deficiency. The most severe cases have absent enzyme activity and present with hyperammonemic coma in the first week of life, while patients with the milder forms have some residual enzyme activity and their clinical presentation occurs later in life

(from infancy to adulthood) with recurrent episodes of hyperammonemia. Approximately 15% of OTC-deficient heterozygotes develop symptoms of hyperammonemia sometime in their lives, presumably as a result of skewed lyonization. Conversely, occasional asymptomatic adults have been found to harbor the same genetic defect causing symptoms in a family relative.

TABLE 9-13

THE INBORN ERRORS OF UREAGENESIS

DISORDER	GENETICS	ENZYME DEFECT	MANIFESTATIONS
Enzyme Defects			
Carbamoyl phosphate synthetase deficiency	autosomal recessive	carbamoyl phosphate synthetase	encephalopathy
NAGS deficiency	autosomal recessive	*N*-acetylglutamate synthetase	encephalopathy
Ornithine transcarbamoylase deficiency	X-linked recessive	ornithine transcarbamoylase	encephalopathy
Citrullinemia	autosomal recessive	argininosuccinate synthetase	encephalopathy
Argininosuccinic aciduria	autosomal recessive	argininosuccinate lyase	trichorrhexis nodosa
Argininemia	autosomal recessive	arginase	progressive spastic diplegia or quadriplegia, tremor, ataxia, and choreoathetosis
Transporter Defects			
Lysinuric protein intolerance (LPI)	autosomal recessive	amino acid transporter gene SLC7A7 (positive amino acid transporter)	pulmonary alveolar proteinosis, glomerulonephritis and osteoporosis, immune deficiency
HHH syndrome	autosomal recessive	mitochondrial ornithine transporter ORNT1	progressive spastic diplegia or quadriplegia, retinal depigmentation, and chorioretinal thinning

NAGS = *N*-acetylglutamate synthetase; HHH = hyperornithinemia, hyperammonemia, homocitrullinuria.

NEONATAL-ONSET UREA CYCLE DISORDERS

Infants with complete enzyme deficiencies are usually born at term with normal Apgar scores because the maternal circulation detoxifies the accumulating ammonia. Between 1 and 5 days of age, however, they become lethargic and hypotonic, feed poorly, vomit frequently, and may hyperventilate. The diagnosis of sepsis is frequently considered. These patients progressively develop tremor, stupor, seizures, apnea, coma, increased intracranial pressure, and death if the hyperammonemia is not diagnosed and treated effectively. Plasma ammonia levels may be higher than 1000 μmol/L (normal <35). Other clinical findings may include hepatomegaly, mild serum liver enzyme elevations, and a coagulopathy. Initial blood gas measurement typically shows a respiratory alkalosis, which can be quite important since in most cases the clinical presentation would suggest an acidemia. Pulmonary bleeding has been reported as a terminal event, but more frequently the cause of death is vascular compromise of the CNS.

LATE-ONSET UREA CYCLE DISORDERS

In patients with partial enzyme deficiencies, the first recognized clinical episode may be delayed for months or years; the hyperammonemia is less severe, and the symptoms more subtle. The clinical abnormalities vary somewhat with the specific disorder. In most urea cycle disorders, the hyperammonemic episodes are marked by loss of appetite, cyclical vomiting, lethargy, and behavioral abnormalities. Sleep disorders, delusions, hallucinations, and psychosis have also been reported. An encephalopathic (slow wave) EEG pattern may be observed during hyperammonemia, and nonspecific brain atrophy may be present subsequently on MRI (see Sec. 25.4).

ASSOCIATED CLINICAL ABNORMALITIES

In addition to the symptoms of hyperammonemia, a number of hyperammonemic disorders have other, more specific clinical abnormalities. In argininemia, there is a progressive spastic diplegia or quadriplegia that has also been observed in HHH syndrome. Tremor, ataxia, and choreoathetosis have been reported in argininemia as well, whereas retinal depigmentation and chorioretinal thinning have been observed in HHH syndrome. Interstitial pneumonia due to pulmonary alveolar proteinosis is seen in LPI, as is glomerulonephritis and osteoporosis; there may be an underlying immune deficiency in this disorder as well. Trichorrhexis nodosa, a node-like appearance of fragile hair, is pathognomonic for argininosuccinic aciduria.

9.3.3 Differential Diagnosis

The diagnosis of congenital hyperammonemia should be entertained upon finding an elevated plasma ammonia level in association with only mild or no liver dysfunction, and in the absence of ketoacidosis. A precipitating catabolic event such as an infection, traumatic injury, ingestion of large amounts of protein, or other yet unknown metabolic stresses can precipitate hyperammonemia in these patients. Valproate or haloperidol administration has unmasked undiagnosed urea cycle defects in some patients, while

other patients have erroneously been diagnosed as having Reye syndrome.

Following an algorithm for the differential diagnosis (Fig. 9-8), the first measure to be taken is a plasma ammonia level. Blood should be placed on ice and ideally analyzed within 30 minutes of collection. Most hospitals now have automated analyzers that measure ammonia and require less than 1 mL of blood with an analysis time of less than 30 minutes. Normal plasma ammonia levels are less than 35 μmol/L (63 μg/dL). In symptomatic hyperammonemia, levels are usually above 100 μmol/L. Other routine laboratory tests may be useful in making the diagnosis. A low blood urea nitrogen (BUN) concentration and respiratory alkalosis in a severely ill child are characteristic of urea cycle disorders. On the other hand, a metabolic acidosis or ketoacidosis is more commonly seen in hyperammonemia caused by an organic acidemia or congenital lactic acidosis. These can be further discriminated by measuring urinary organic acids for the former and plasma lactate/pyruvate for the latter. Organic acidemias and fatty acid oxidation defects can be distinguished by measuring acylcarnitine esters in blood.

Quantitative plasma and urinary amino acids are most helpful in establishing a specific diagnosis of a defect in urea synthesis (Fig. 9-8). Concentrations of glutamine, alanine, and asparagine, serving as storage forms of waste nitrogen, are increased. Plasma arginine concentration is decreased in all urea cycle disorders, except in argininemia in which it is increased 10- to 20-fold. Plasma citrulline levels help discriminate between the proximal and distal urea cycle defects because citrulline is the product of OTC and CPS activity and a substrate for the distal enzymes. As a result, no citrulline, or only a trace, is detected in plasma in neonatal-onset CPS and OTC deficiencies; concentrations are low to low-normal in late-onset disease, but are markedly elevated in blood and urine in citrullinemia and argininosuccinic aciduria. To distinguish CPS from OTC deficiency, urinary orotic acid is measured; concentrations are significantly elevated in OTC deficiency, and normal or low in CPS deficiency. In addition to OTC deficiency, urinary orotic acid excretion can be increased in argininemia, citrullinemia, HHH syndrome, and LPI. Patients with citrullinemia have up to a 100-fold elevation in plasma citrulline levels, while those with argininosuccinic aciduria show a more moderate increase in citrulline of about 10-fold, associated with the presence of normally absent argininosuccinic acid. The argininosuccinate chromatographic peak may coelute with leucine or isoleucine, resulting in an apparent increase in one of these amino acids, but its anhydrides eluting later in the run should allow the correct identification of argininosuccinate. In HHH syndrome, plasma ornithine and urine homocitrulline levels are elevated, whereas in LPI, urinary lysine, arginine, and ornithine levels are elevated.

Citrullinemia, argininosuccinic aciduria, and argininemia, as well as LPI and HHH syndrome, can be diagnosed on the basis of the amino acid pattern. NAGS deficiency requires enzymatic diagnosis on hepatic tissue. In OTC deficiency, 75% of patients have an identifiable mutation by DNA studies, and mutation analysis can be done for the other disorders as well. A definitive diagnosis of CPS or OTC deficiency depends on enzyme determination on a liver biopsy specimen.

9.3.4 Treatment Approaches

Treatment approaches rely on a combination of dietary nitrogen restriction, replacement of deficient amino acids, and stimulation

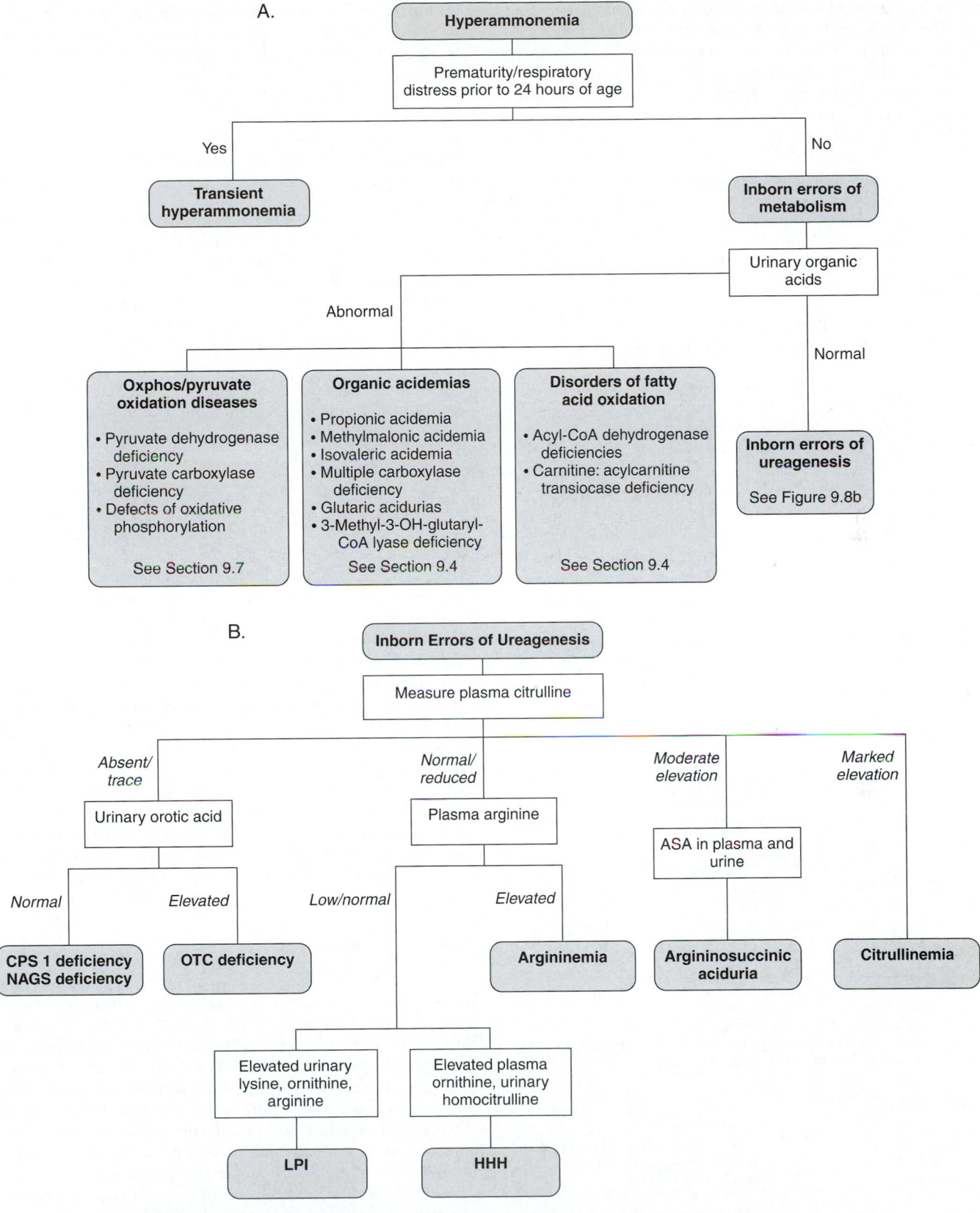

FIGURE 9-8 A, Algorithm for the differential diagnosis of congenital hyperammonemia. B, Algorithm for the differential diagnosis of the inborn errors of ureagenesis. ASA = argininosuccinic acid; LPI = lysinuric protein intolerance; HHH = hyperornithinemia, hyperammonemia, and homocitrullinuria syndrome.

of alternate pathways for waste nitrogen excretion. The protein-restricted diet is often supplemented with essential amino acids. Arginine is deficient in all disorders except argininemia, and it must be replaced. Hair fragility and rash are associated with arginine deficiency, which can develop if arginine replacement is inadequate. Alternate pathway therapy (Fig. 9-7) entails the use of sodium benzoate, which is conjugated in the liver with glycine to form hippuric acid, and sodium-phenylacetate (or its precursor sodium-phenylbutyrate), which is conjugated in the liver with glutamine to form phenylacetylglutamine. Both hippurate and phenylacetylglutamine are readily eliminated in the urine, thereby providing an alternate pathway for waste nitrogen excretion. In addition, arginine stimulates waste nitrogen excretion in citrullinemia and argininosuccinic aciduria.

TREATMENT OF ACUTE HYPERAMMONEMIA IN NEWBORNS

Acute hyperammonemia represents a medical emergency. Studies have shown that hyperammonemic coma lasting longer than 72 hours invariably leads to brain damage and mental retardation. Plasma ammonia levels above 200 μmol/L in the newborn, when associated with coma, should trigger the use of hemodialysis if at all possible, or hemofiltration or peritoneal dialysis if hemodialysis is not available. Protein intake is discontinued until ammonia levels come under control, and intravenous glucose and lipids are administered to decrease catabolism (Fig. 9-9). In addition, alternative pathways are exploited to eliminate nitrogen by the intravenous administration of sodium-benzoate and sodium-phenylacetate. Arginine hydrochloride 10% solution is given to prevent arginine deficiency and, in the case of citrullinemia and argininosuccinic aciduria, to prime the urea cycle to incorporate nitrogen into citrulline and argininosuccinic acid, which are excreted in the urine. Steri-

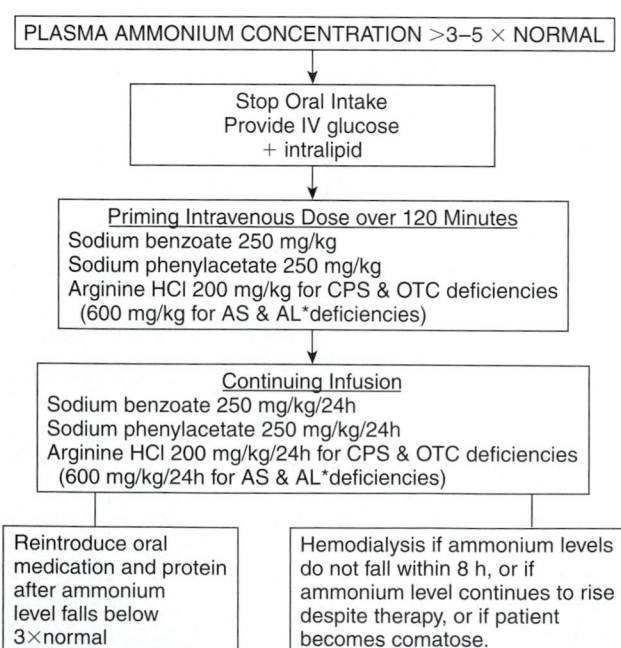

FIGURE 9-9 **Protocol for treatment of hyperammonemia episodes in patients with urea cycle disorders. CPS = carbamoylphosphate synthetase; OTC = ornithine transcarbamoylase; AS = argininosuccinate synthetase; AL = argininosuccinate lyase. *Treatment of AL deficiency usually requires only arginine without benzoate or phenylacetate.**

lization of the gut may also be useful in reducing ammonia absorption. Treatment of increased intracranial pressure is also very important. The comatose child should be placed on a ventilator with mild hyperventilation and drugs should be administered to reduce intracranial pressure.

TREATMENT OF ACUTE HYPERAMMONEMIA IN OLDER CHILDREN

In children with partial (late-onset) defects, and in those children with neonatal-onset disease who are on alternate pathway therapy, intercurrent hyperammonemic episodes may be initially treated in a more conservative manner than in the newborn period (Table 9-14). If plasma ammonia levels are less than 200 μmol/L and the child is not in coma, intravenous treatment with benzoate, phenylacetate, and L-arginine can be tried initially. However, if the plasma ammonia level does not fall within hours and/or the clinical condition worsens, dialysis should be started. To ameliorate catabolism, glucose and lipids should also be given.

LONG-TERM THERAPY

Chronic management (Table 9-14) includes a high-caloric, protein-restricted diet, with or without replacement of some dietary protein by an essential amino acid mixture. Minerals, vitamins, and trace elements are supplemented because modified diets are often deficient in some essential nutrients. L-Citrulline or L-arginine (free base) is supplemented depending on the disorder. Citrulline contains one less nitrogen atom than arginine, making it a useful substitute in treatment of CPS, OTC, and NAGS deficiencies, and LPI. Alternative pathway therapy with oral phenylbutyrate (Buphenyl) or with benzoate and phenylacetate (Ucephan) can be employed to eliminate nitrogen in all these disorders. A deficiency of aspartic acid may occur in argininosuccinic aciduria, thus, supplementation of a precursor such as citrate has been used. In NAGS deficiency, N-carbamylglutamate has been used to replace the deficient product, N-acetylglutamate, which activates CPS. In HHH syndrome, L-ornithine or L-citrulline supplements have been effective. For the most severe cases, which are not amenable to the above therapy, liver transplantation has been used with relative success. Gene therapy may eventually replace liver transplantation as the curative procedure in the future.

9.3.5   Outcome

Prior to the development of alternate pathway therapy, virtually all children with neonatal-onset disease died rapidly. Approximately half of affected neonates still succumb to hyperammonemic coma. However, long-term survival has improved, with about half of the infants who survive neonatal hyperammonemic coma living 5 years or more. Survival is obviously better in partial defects, but these children still remain at risk for intercurrent life-threatening hyperammonemic crises. Although mortality has improved, morbidity remains high. There is a significant risk for multiple developmental disabilities, including mental retardation, cerebral palsy, and seizure disorders in children with a neonatal-onset disorder. Children with partial defects and those who have been treated prospectively from birth because of a previously affected sibling have a better outcome, although there is a high incidence of more subtle cognitive deficits, including learning disabilities and attention deficit hyperactivity disorder.

TABLE 9-14

LONG-TERM TREATMENT OF UREA CYCLE DISORDERS (g/kg/d, UNLESS OTHERWISE SPECIFIED)

DISORDER	PROTEIN INTAKE[1]	CITRULLINE	ARGININE FREE BASE	SODIUM PHENYLBUTYRATE[2]
Neonatal-onset CPS or OTC deficiency	1.4–1.9	0.17 or 3.8 g/M²/d	—	0.45–0.60 if <20 kg; 9.9–13.0 g/M²/d in larger patients
Late-onset OTC or CPS deficiency	1.2–1.4	0.17 or 3.8 g/M²/d		0.45–0.60 if <20 kg; 9.9–13.0 g/M²/d in larger patients
Citrullinemia	1.2–1.9	—	0.40–0.70 or 8.8–15.4 g/M²/d	0.45–0.60 if <20 kg; 9.9–13.0 g/M²/d in larger patients
Argininosuccinic aciduria	1.2–1.9	—	0.40–0.70 or 8.8–15.4 g/M²/d	Usually not required
Argininemia	0.5–1.4	—	—	0.45–0.60 if <20 kg; 9.9–13.0 g/M²/d in larger patients
NAGS deficiency[3]	1.2–1.9	0.17 or 3.8g/M²/d	0.17 or 3.8 g/M²/d	0.45–0.60 if <20 kg; 9.9–13.0 g/M²/d in larger patients
LPI[4]	1.0–1.5	0.17 or 3.8g/M²/d	0.17 or 3.8 g/M²/d	0.45–0.60 if <20 kg; 9.9–13.0 g/M²/d in larger patients
HHH[5]	1.0–1.5	0.17 or 3.8g/M²/d		0.45–0.60 if <20 kg; 9.9–13.0 g/M²/d in larger patients

[1]Caloric requirement may be completed using a protein-free formula. In general, the minimum daily protein intake for growth was used: for 1–4 mo, 1.6–1.9 g/kg/d; for 4–12 mo, 1.7 g/kg/d; for 1–3 yr, 1.4 g/kg/d. Daily protein intake may include an essential amino acid formula.
[2]If intolerant of phenylbutyrate, Ucephan (Na-benzoate + Na-phenylacetate) can be given orally at a dose of 0.25–0.5 g/kg/d each.
[3]N-Carbamoylglutamate may also be given at a dose of 0.32–0.65 g/kg/d.
[4]Ornithine or lysine can also be given at a dose of 0.1–0.25 g/kg/d.
[5]Ornithine 0.18 g/kg/d can be substituted for citrulline.
CPS = carbamoylphosphate synthetase deficiency; HHH = hyperornithinemia, hyperammonemia, homocitrullinuria; LPI = lysinuric protein intolerance; OTC = ornithine transcarbamoylase deficiency.

References

Batshaw ML: Carbamyl phosphate synthetase I deficiency. Arginase deficiency. Argininosuccinic acidemia. Citrullinemia. N-Acetylglutamate synthetase deficiency. Ornithine transcarbamylase deficiency. In: Gilman S, Goldstein GW, Waxman SG, eds: Neurobase. La Jolla, CA, CD-ROM, 1998

Batshaw ML: Inborn errors of urea synthesis: a review. Ann Neurol 35:133, 1994

Batshaw ML, Brusilow SW: Treatment of hyperammonemic coma caused by inborn errors or urea synthesis. Pediatrics 97:893–900, 1980

Brusilow SW, Horwich AL: Urea cycle enzymes. In: Scriver CR, Beaudet AL, Sly WS, Valle D, eds: The Metabolic and Molecular Basis of Inherited Disease, 7th ed. New York, McGraw-Hill, 1995, 1187–1232

Cederbaum SD: Treatment of urea cycle disorders. Int Pediatr 7:61, 1992

Maestri NE, Hauser ER, Bartholomew D, Brusilow SW: Prospective treatment of urea cycle disorders. J Pediatr 119:923–928, 1991

Tuchman M: Inherited hyperammonemia. In: Blau N, Duran M, Blaskovics ME, eds: Physician's Guide to the Laboratory Diagnosis of Metabolic Diseases. London, Chapman & Hall Medical, pp 209–222, 1996

Tuchman M: The clinical biochemical and molecular spectrum of ornithine transcarbamylase deficiency. J Lab Clin Med 120:836–850, 1992

9.4 ORGANIC ACIDEMIAS AND DISORDERS OF FATTY ACID OXIDATION

Stephen Irwin Goodman

9.4.1 Organic Acidemias

Organic acidemia, that is, the accumulation of one or more non-amino organic acids in the blood, occurs both in physiological states, such as ketosis, and in a number of acquired and inherited disorders. These organic acids are intermediate metabolites of the catabolism of amino acids, fatty acids, and carbohydrates. The organic acidurias described in the first part of this section arise mainly from defects in amino acid catabolism and are summarized in Table 9-12. The latter part of this section describes those disorders caused by defects in fatty acid metabolism. Organic acidemias arising from carbohydrate metabolism generally involve the primary or secondary elevations of pyruvic and lactic acids and are described in Secs. 9.5 and 9.7.

Except for lactic acid, most organic acids are effectively cleared from the bloodstream by the kidney, and organic acidemias are thus much more easily detected when the characteristic organic acids are sought in urine. Any changes in amino acid levels that occur in these conditions, such as the hyperglycinemia of propionic and methylmalonic acidemias, are not diagnostic, and diagnosis of these conditions depends on methods to separate and identify organic acids (see Sec. 8.2).

ISOVALERIC ACIDEMIA

Isovaleric acidemia was the first condition to be recognized as an organic acidemia when the "odor of sweaty feet" of an infant with episodic encephalopathy was shown to be caused by isovaleric acid. The disorder is the result of a defect in isovaleryl-CoA dehydrogenase, a FAD-containing enzyme that converts isovaleryl-CoA, an intermediate in leucine oxidation, to 3-methylcrotonyl-CoA, and is inherited as an autosomal recessive trait.

Clinical Features

Isovaleric acidemia may present in the newborn period with encephalopathy, metabolic acidosis, and the characteristic odor of sweaty feet, but more often presents in infancy or childhood with episodes of encephalopathy, hepatomegaly, and odor, brought on by infections or protein intake. Severe hyperammonemia is rare. If untreated, the condition is often fatal, and mental retardation is common.

Diagnosis

Metabolites characteristic of the condition include isovalerylglycine and 3-hydroxyisovaleric acid; isovaleric acid itself is not detected by most analytic methods. Most of the isovaleryl-CoA that accumulates behind the metabolic block is excreted normally as nontoxic isovalerylglycine, but the amounts that accumulate during infection or after protein loading exceed the capacity of the liver to esterify it, and it then appears as isovaleric and 3-hydroxyisovaleric acids. Acylcarnitine analysis will identify accumulation of isovalerylcarnitine.

The enzyme defect can be demonstrated in many tissues, including leukocytes and cultured fibroblasts, and prenatal diagnosis of an affected fetus can be made by demonstrating enzyme deficiency in cultured amniocytes or chorionic villus cells. Isovalerylglycine is also increased in the amniotic fluid surrounding an affected fetus, but is difficult to detect by standard methods. The gene encoding isovaleryl-CoA dehydrogenase has been cloned and localized to chromosome 15 (15q12-15), and several disease-causing mutations have been identified. Prenatal diagnosis can be established on this basis if the mutations in the family are already known.

Treatment

Acute episodes of acidosis may require treatment with intravenous glucose and bicarbonate or lactate. Long-term treatment is by restricting leucine intake to amounts necessary for normal growth and development and by providing exogenous glycine to increase excretion of isovaleryl-CoA as isovalerylglycine. The use of carnitine to increase excretion of the carbon skeleton as isovalerylcarnitine is less-well established.

ISOLATED 3-METHYLCROTONYL-CoA CARBOXYLASE DEFICIENCY

3-Methylcrotonyl-CoA carboxylase (MCC) is a biotin-containing enzyme that converts 3-methylcrotonyl-CoA to 3-methylglutaconyl-CoA, and enzyme deficiency can exist alone or as part of multiple carboxylase deficiency. Isolated MCC deficiency is inherited as an autosomal recessive trait.

Clinical Features

Most patients present between the ages of 1 and 3 years with an infection-induced episode of vomiting, hypoglycemia, hepatomegaly (due to fatty infiltration), hyperammonemic encephalopathy, and hypotonia. Earlier and later presentations have been described, as have several enzyme-deficient asymptomatic siblings of affected patients. Serum carnitine levels may be very low, probably as a consequence of 3-hydroxyisovalerylcarnitine excretion.

Diagnosis

Urine organic acid analysis shows increased excretion of 3-methylcrotonylglycine and 3-hydroxyisovaleric acid, and tandem mass spectrometry (MS-MS) shows increased 3-hydroxyisovalerylcarnitine. MCC deficiency can be demonstrated in several tissues, including leukocytes and cultured fibroblasts, and prenatal diagnosis can probably be established by enzyme assay in cultured amniocytes

or chorionic villus cells, or by demonstrating increased 3-methylcrotonylglycine in amniotic fluid.

Treatment

Acute episodes should be treated with fluids, glucose, and electrolytes, and long-term treatment relies on modest protein (or leucine) restriction and oral carnitine to correct carnitine deficiency. Biotin is almost always tried, but does not reduce the organic acid excretion. Acute episodes may be fatal, but providing that irreversible brain damage does not occur at this time, the ultimate prognosis is quite good.

3-HYDROXY-3-METHYLGLUTARIC ACIDURIA

3-Hydroxy-3-methylglutaric acidemia is due to deficiency of 3-hydroxy-3-methylglutaryl-CoA lyase, which hydrolyzes its substrate, an intermediate in leucine oxidation and ketone-body synthesis, to acetyl-CoA and acetoacetic acid. The defect limits ketone-body biosynthesis during hypoglycemia, and is characterized by fasting-induced hypoketotic hypoglycemia. The disorder is inherited as an autosomal recessive trait.

Clinical Findings

The condition can present in the newborn with severe hypoglycemia, metabolic acidosis, and hyperammonemia, or as episodes of hypoglycemia, hepatomegaly, and encephalopathy that follow intercurrent infection. The latter form of the disease is often mistaken for Reye syndrome. If not promptly treated, cerebral atrophy, neurologic signs, and mental retardation may follow.

Diagnosis

Urine organic acid analysis shows increased 3-hydroxy-3-methylglutaric, 3-methylglutaconic, and 3-methylglutaric acids, and MS-MS shows increased 3-hydroxy-3-methylglutarylcarnitine. The absence of ketonuria during acute illness is characteristic. Liver function tests may be abnormal at times of acute illness. The enzyme defect can be demonstrated in many tissues, including fibroblasts and peripheral leukocytes, and fetal disease can be diagnosed by enzyme assay on cultured amniocytes or chorionic villus samples, or by demonstrating the characteristic organic acids in amniotic fluid.

Treatment

Acute management requires intravenous fluids, electrolytes, and glucose, and long-term management is directed to avoiding fasting and the resulting hypoglycemia. The possible life-threatening consequences of fasting make it imperative that parents bring the child to hospital as soon as possible when oral intake is compromised.

MITOCHONDRIAL ACETOACETYL-CoA THIOLASE DEFICIENCY

Mitochondrial acetoacetyl-CoA thiolase removes acetyl-CoA from acetoacetyl-CoA and 2-methylacetoacetyl-CoA, which is an intermediate in isoleucine oxidation. Enzyme deficiency is inherited as an autosomal recessive trait.

Clinical Features

Like propionic acidemia the disease can present in the newborn period with hyperammonemia, metabolic acidosis, and severe ketosis, or later in infancy or childhood with fasting- or protein-induced episodes of vomiting, hepatomegaly, ketoacidosis, and encephalopathy.

Diagnosis

The urine organic acids characteristic of mitochondrial acetoacetyl-CoA thiolase deficiency are 2-methyl-3-hydroxybutyric acid, 2-methylacetoacetic acid, and tiglylglycine, but large amounts of normal ketone bodies (ie, 3-hydroxybutyric and acetoacetic acids) may obscure them during acute illnesses. The diagnostic metabolites may be detectable only when the patient is symptom-free or after an oral load of L-isoleucine (100 mg/kg). Glycine concentration is often elevated in blood and urine.

While usually not necessary to establish the diagnosis, the enzyme defect can be demonstrated in fibroblasts and leukocytes, and probably in amniocytes for prenatal diagnosis. The gene encoding the enzyme has been cloned and localized to chromosome 11 (11q22.3-23.1), and a few disease-causing mutations have been identified.

Treatment

Acute episodes should be treated with intravenous glucose and sodium bicarbonate. Long-term treatment with a low-protein diet, coupled with the avoidance of fasting, decreases the frequency and severity of acute episodes and permits normal growth and development if irreversible neurologic damage has not already occurred.

PROPIONIC ACIDEMIA

Propionic acidemia was first described, albeit unknowingly, when ketotic hyperglycinemia was reported in 1960 as a syndrome of mental retardation and episodic ketoacidosis, neutropenia, thrombocytopenia, osteoporosis, and hyperglycinemia induced by protein intake or infection. The discovery that the condition could be caused by propionic acidemia (or methylmalonic acidemia or mitochondrial acetoacetyl-CoA thiolase deficiency) was made only when methods to examine and identify organic acids became available.

The disorder is due to a defect in propionyl-CoA carboxylase (PCC), a biotin-containing enzyme that converts propionyl-CoA,

an intermediate in the oxidation of isoleucine, threonine, valine, and methionine, to D-methylmalonyl-CoA (Fig. 9-10), and is inherited as an autosomal recessive trait.

Clinical Findings

Like many other organic acidemias, propionic acidemia can present in the neonate as severe and life-threatening ketoacidosis, hyperammonemic, encephalopathy, and bone marrow suppression. An equally common more chronic course presents later in infancy with episodes of vomiting, ketoacidosis brought on by infections, failure to thrive, and osteoporosis severe enough to cause pathologic fractures. Acute striatal damage may occur, usually but not always during an episode of ketoacidosis. Developmental delay is occasionally present, and is probably caused more by newborn hyperammonemia or recurrent illness in infancy than by the disease itself.

Diagnosis

Urine organic acid analysis shows large amounts of 3-hydroxypropionic and methylcitric acids, often with propionylglycine, tiglylglycine, and abnormal ketone bodies such as 3-hydroxy- and 3-keto-n-valeric acids. Acylcarnitine analysis by MS-MS shows increased propionylcarnitine, and glycine levels in blood and urine are often elevated.

The defect in PCC can be demonstrated in many tissues, including leukocytes and cultured fibroblasts, and prenatal diagnosis of an affected fetus can be made by demonstrating enzyme deficiency in cultured amniocytes or chorionic villus cells, or by demonstrating an elevation of methylcitric acid concentration in amniotic fluid.

PCC is an octamer of four α and four β subunits. The genes encoding the α and β subunits have been cloned and localized to chromosomes 13 and 3, respectively. Several disease-causing mutations have been identified so that, when the mutations in a proband are known, prenatal diagnosis can also be made on this basis.

Treatment

Dietary restriction of protein or propiogenic amino acids to amounts necessary to support normal growth and development

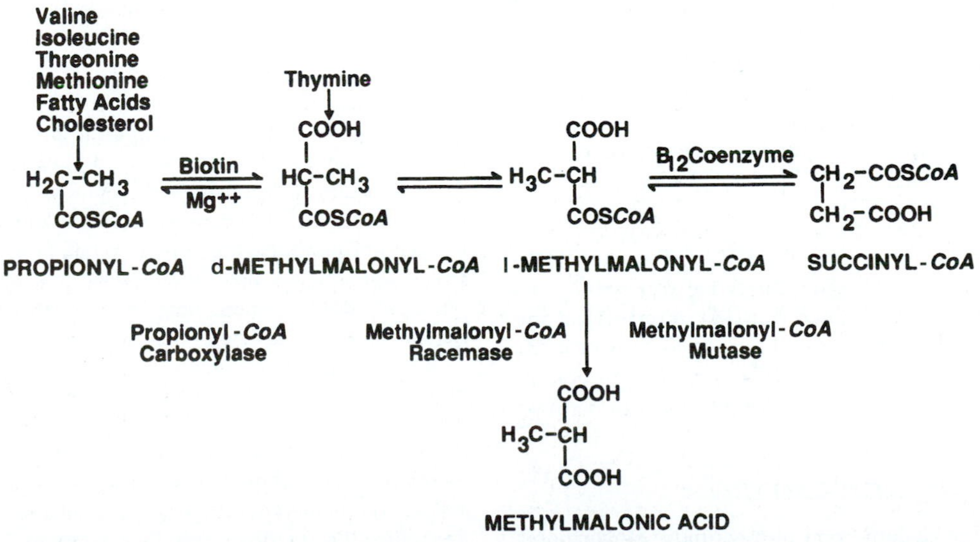

FIGURE 9-10 Metabolism of propionic acid. Sites of the defect in propionic acidemia and methylmalonic acidemia are in propionyl-CoA carboxylase and methylmalonyl-CoA mutase.

is indicated; this usually amounts to protein intake of less than 1 g/kg/d. Treatment with carnitine is useful in secondary carnitine deficiency and may increase excretion of propionyl-CoA as propionylcarnitine. Attacks of ketoacidosis that complicate infections should be treated with fluid and electrolytes. Biotin is usually tried, but is rarely effective. Therapy often reduces the frequency and severity of attacks of ketoacidosis, and some patients treated in this manner do well and have normal intelligence; most, however, die in early childhood.

MULTIPLE CARBOXYLASE DEFICIENCY

Multiple carboxylase deficiency is caused by defects in incorporating biotin into the carboxylases that act on propionyl-CoA, 3-methylcrotonyl-CoA, acetyl-CoA, and pyruvate. It can be the result of deficiency of holocarboxylase synthetase, which attaches biotin to the apocarboxylases, or of biotinidase, which makes biotin available for the synthetase reaction by releasing it from the peptide form (biocytin) in which most of it exists in nature. Both conditions produce a triad of alopecia, skin rash, and encephalopathy, and are inherited as autosomal recessive traits.

Clinical Findings

Holocarboxylase synthase deficiency usually causes earlier and more severe disease than biotinidase deficiency, with life-threatening ketoacidosis, alopecia, and a red, scaly, total-body eruption. Coma, apnea, and death often follow unless therapy is instituted. Biotinidase deficiency usually presents later in infancy with periorificial dermatitis resembling acrodermatitis enteropathica, patchy alopecia, and neurologic abnormalities such as ataxia, neurosensory defects, developmental delay, and convulsions. In both conditions the rash may be complicated by superinfection with monilia. The defect in neonatal disease is usually in holocarboxylase synthetase and in most later-onset patients in biotinidase, but there is extensive overlap and accurate diagnosis can only be made by enzyme assay.

Diagnosis

Urine organic acid analysis shows increased 3-methylcrotonylglycine and 3-hydroxyisovaleric acid, often with methylcitric, 3-hydroxypropionic, and lactic acids. Acylcarnitine analysis by MS-MS shows propionyl- and 3-hydroxyisovalerylcarnitine. Holocarboxylase synthetase deficiency can be demonstrated in fibroblasts or leukocytes; biotinidase activity can be assayed even in serum. Enzyme assay in amniocytes and/or demonstration of abnormal organic acids in amniotic fluid can be used for prenatal diagnosis of holocarboxylase synthetase deficiency.

Treatment

Patients with multiple carboxylase deficiency are very sensitive to free biotin, and doses of 5 to 20 mg/d usually reverse all of the disease manifestations. Because it can cause permanent neurologic sequelae and because it is so easily and effectively treated, biotinidase deficiency is often screened for in the newborn period (see Sec. 8.2).

METHYLMALONIC ACIDEMIAS

Accumulation of methylmalonic acid in inherited methylmalonic acidemias is due to deficiency of methylmalonyl-CoA mutase, an adenosyl-B_{12}–requiring enzyme that converts L-methylmalonyl-CoA to succinyl-CoA (see Fig. 9-10). In some patients, mutase deficiency is caused by a defect in the mutase gene, but in other patients, it is caused by a defect in the biosynthesis of adenosyl-B_{12} from vitamin B_{12}. If the defect in the biosynthetic pathway also blocks the synthesis of methyl-B_{12}, which is required (by N^5-methyltetrahydrofolate:homocysteine methyltransferase) for the remethylation of homocysteine to methionine, homocystinuria is also present.

Cells from patients with these conditions cannot incorporate radiolabel from [^{14}C] propionic acid into protein. As many enzymes in the pathway of B_{12} coenzyme biosynthesis are not known, patients with defects in the pathway are classified by determining if their cellular defect can be corrected by cells from other patients. Cells that do not correct each other have the same defect and are said to belong to the same complementation group. Cells from patients with defects in adenosyl- and methyl-B_{12} biosynthesis form the cb1C, cb1D, and cb1F complementation groups, and those from patients with a defect only in adenosyl-B_{12} biosynthesis form the cblA and cblB groups. All forms of methylmalonic acidemia are inherited as autosomal recessive traits.

Clinical Findings

As in propionic acidemia, patients with methylmalonic acidemia due to mutase deficiency can present with life-threatening hyperammonemia, ketoacidosis, and thrombocytopenia in the first weeks or months of life, or later with the more chronic course of ketotic hyperglycinemia, with vomiting, intermittent attacks of life-threatening ketoacidosis, and failure to thrive. As a rule, patients with defects in adenosyl-B_{12} biosynthesis have somewhat milder disease. Acute striatal damage may occur, often but not always during an episode of ketoacidosis, and late-developing interstitial nephritis is common.

Patients with both homocystinuria and methylmalonic aciduria are quite different, and usually present during the first months of life with failure to thrive; macrocytic anemia; megaloblastosis; nonspecific neurologic manifestation such as hypotonia; and, unexpectedly, hemolytic-uremic syndrome. Thromboembolism and episodes of ketoacidosis are rare.

Diagnosis

Organic acid analysis shows increased urine methylmalonic acid and, especially in patients with defects in methylmalonyl-CoA mutase, tiglylglycine, 3-hydroxypropionic and methylcitric acids, and the same abnormal ketone bodies found in propionic acidemia. Analysis of acylcarnitines by MS-MS shows propionylcarnitine, and glycine levels are often elevated in blood and urine. Blood concentrations of vitamin B_{12} are normal. When homocystinuria is present, amino acid analysis also shows low methionine and high cystathionine; in addition, methylmalonic acid excretion is usually lower than in mutase deficiency.

The defect in methylmalonyl-CoA mutase can be demonstrated in many tissues, including leukocytes and cultured fibroblasts. Prenatal diagnosis can be established by enzyme assay on cultured amniocytes or chorionic villus cells, or by demonstrating increased methylmalonic and methylcitric acids in amniotic fluid. If it is necessary, complementation analysis is available in a few centers. The gene encoding methylmalonyl-CoA mutase has been cloned and localized to chromosome 6 (6p.12-21.1). Several disease-causing mutations have been identified, and prenatal diagnosis can also be made on this basis when the mutations in the family are known.

Treatment

Like that of propionic acidemia, treatment of mutase-deficient methylmalonic acidemia relies on restricting dietary protein (or propiogenic amino acids) to amounts necessary to support normal growth and development. Carnitine is useful to treat secondary carnitine deficiency, and attacks of ketoacidosis should be treated with fluid and electrolytes. Some patients treated in this way do well, but most die in early childhood. Liver transplantation may be curative, and successful outcome after combined liver-kidney transplantation in a patient with chronic renal failure has been reported. Large doses of vitamin B_{12} lower methylmalonic acid excretion only in patients with defects of adenosyl-B_{12} biosynthesis.

Patients with methylmalonic aciduria and homocystinuria are treated with betaine, another methyl donor for the conversion of homocysteine to methionine, and intramuscular vitamin B_{12}. These measures reduce excretion of methylmalonic acid and homocystine, but often without appreciable clinical response. Many patients succumb because of hemolytic-uremic syndrome or cardiorespiratory arrest during childhood, but long-term survival, often with neurologic sequellae, is not unknown.

GLUTARIC ACIDEMIA (TYPE I)

Glutaric acidemia is the result of a defect in glutaryl-CoA dehydrogenase, a FAD-containing enzyme that converts glutaryl-CoA, an intermediate in the oxidation of lysine, tryptophan, and hydroxylysine, to crotonyl-CoA, and is inherited as an autosomal recessive trait.

Clinical Features

Most patients with glutaric acidemia are born with macrocephaly, and develop normally until they suddenly develop hypotonia and dystonia during or after an intercurrent infection; this usually occurs during the first 2 to 3 years of life. CT-MRI scans show frontal and cortical atrophy from birth and, after the onset of dystonia, degeneration of the caudate nucleus and putamen. Some patients gradually develop signs of striatal degeneration during the first years of life, and others, probably less than 5% of patients, remain asymptomatic. Metabolic acidosis, the usual indication for organic acid screening, is rare.

Diagnosis

Urine organic acid analysis shows increased excretion of glutaric and 3-hydroxyglutaric acids, and acylcarnitine analysis by MS-MS shows increased glutarylcarnitine. Some patients do not have prominent organic aciduria, and some patients show it only when ill. Most patients have low serum-carnitine levels by the time they are diagnosed.

The enzyme defect can be demonstrated in many tissues, including leukocytes and cultured fibroblasts, and prenatal diagnosis of an affected fetus can be made by demonstrating enzyme deficiency in cultured amniocytes or chorionic villus cells, or by demonstrating increased glutaric acid concentrations in amniotic fluid. The gene encoding glutaryl-CoA dehydrogenase has been cloned and localized to chromosome 19 (19p.13.2), and many disease-causing mutations have been identified. Prenatal diagnosis can also

be made on this basis when mutations in a particular family are known.

Treatment

Treatment of symptomatic patients with a diet low in lysine and tryptophan, or drugs such as depakene and lioresal, is of limited benefit. However, treatment with diet and L-carnitine before the onset of symptoms prevents striatal degeneration in about 80% of patients, especially if catabolism accompanying infection is treated with intravenous fluids and glucose, and, if necessary, insulin. The responsiveness of asymptomatic patients to such treatment has been used to argue for newborn screening for this disease.

MEVALONIC ACIDEMIA

Mevalonic acidemia is due to deficiency of mevalonate kinase, an enzyme involved in the biosynthesis of cholesterol and nonsterol isoprenes from 3-hydroxy-3-methylglutaryl-CoA.

Clinical Features

The most severely affected patients have profound developmental delay, distinctive facial dysmorphism, cataracts, and hepatosplenomegaly, and die in infancy. Less severely affected patients have milder retardation, hypotonia, myopathy, and ataxia. All patients have recurrent episodes of fever, lymphadenopathy, arthralgia, subcutaneous edema, and rash. Neuroimaging shows progressive cerebellar atrophy developing after infancy. Metabolic acidosis is not present. No effective treatment is available.

Diagnosis

Urine organic acid screening shows elevated levels of mevalonic acid lactone, and measurement of mevalonic acid in blood and urine can be done by stable isotope dilution gas chromatography-mass spectrometry (GC-MS). Mevalonic kinase deficiency can be demonstrated in fibroblasts and lymphoblasts, and prenatal diagnosis of an affected fetus can be made by demonstrating enzyme deficiency in cultured amniocytes or chorionic villus cells, or by demonstrating increased mevalonic acid levels in amniotic fluid.

D- AND L-2-HYDROXYGLUTARIC ACIDEMIAS

2-Hydroxyglutaric acid can exist as D- or L- isomers, and disorders are known in which large amounts of one or the other are found in blood and urine. The metabolic pathways in which D- and L-2-hydroxyglutaric acid occur, and thus the enzyme defects that cause the conditions, are not known. Both disorders are inherited as autosomal recessive traits.

Clinical Manifestations

L-2-Hydroxyglutaric acidemia typically presents in childhood or adult life with developmental delay and signs of cerebellar dysfunction such as ataxia and intention tremor. MRI scans show changes in subcortical white matter, cerebellar atrophy and signal changes in the putamen and dentate nuclei. D-2-Hydroxyglutaric acidemia usually presents with hypotonia, apnea, seizures, and developmental delay during the first few months of life, but symptoms in some patients are milder and appear later. The most consistent MRI finding is enlargement of the lateral ventricles, especially in the occipital region. There is no treatment.

Diagnosis

Organic acid analysis shows increased amounts of 2-hydroxyglutaric acid, but does not usually distinguish between the D- and L-isomers. Definitive diagnosis requires separation on a chiral column or use of special derivation procedures that will permit separation even on the standard columns. Prenatal diagnosis of both conditions is possible and is based on measuring 2-hydroxyglutaric acid in amniotic fluid.

9.4.2 Disorders of Fatty Acid Oxidation

Fatty acid oxidation in mitochondria provides the main source of energy for heart and skeletal muscle and, by generating acetyl-CoA for ketone-body production, also provides energy for other tissues when the supply of glucose is limited. Fatty acids must first be conjugated to carnitine, transported across the mitochondrial membrane, and released in the matrix as an acyl CoA before they can be catabolized in the β-oxidation spiral (Fig. 9-11). Disorders that limit β-oxidation, by reducing carnitine uptake by cells, by entry of fatty acids into mitochondria, or by blocking β-oxidation itself, limit energy production by heart and skeletal muscle at rest

and lessen the ability of other tissues, including brain, to cope with a low-glucose milieu.

Most patients with such disorders present before the age of 2 years, about 25% of them in the first week of life. Presentation in neonates may be with cardiac arrhythmias and/or sudden death, occasionally with facial dysmorphism and malformations, including renal cystic dysplasia. Symptoms in infancy and early childhood may relate to the liver, or to cardiac or skeletal muscle, and thus include fasting- or stress-related hypoketotic hypoglycemia or Reye-like syndrome; conduction abnormalities; arrhythmias or dilated or hypertrophic cardiomyopathy; and muscle weakness or fasting- and/or exercise-induced rhabdomyolysis.

Diagnosis may be difficult even when the presentation is characteristic. Probably the most important single diagnostic test is analysis of acylcarnitine esters in serum or plasma by MS-MS, which identifies characteristic esters in many disorders, even when patients are symptom-free (see Sec. 8.2). Other tests that may be useful include analysis of urine organic acids and free and total carnitine in serum and urine, loading tests with medium- and long-chain fats, and enzyme assays in leukocytes or fibroblasts.

Treatment of acute encephalopathy associated with hypoketotic hypoglycemia is by intravenous 10% glucose and L-carnitine. Long-

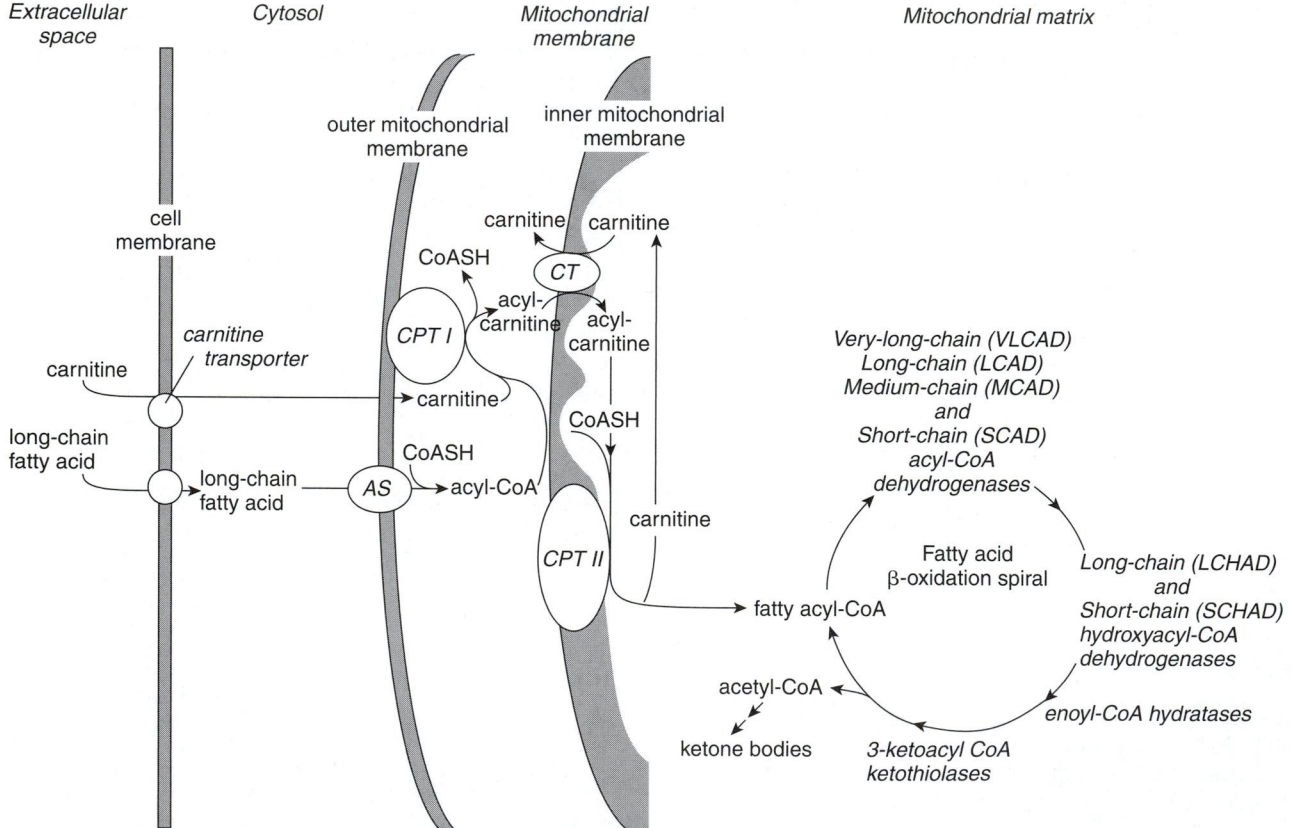

FIGURE 9-11 Transport and metabolism of fatty acids. To cross the mitochondrial membrane, long-chain fatty acids must be ligated to carnitine by carnitine palmitoyltransferase I (CPTI) and transferred by a translocase (CT). Carnitine palmitoyltransferase II (CPTII) releases the acyl group from carnitine into the mitochondrial matrix. Medium- and short-chain fatty acids can freely enter the mitochondria, and do not require the carnitine system. Fatty acids are oxidized in a cycle that removes one acetyl-CoA moiety per turn. Dehydrogenases specific to very-long-, long-, medium-, and short-chain fatty acids catalyze the first reaction. As described in the text, defects have been found in many of the transporters and enzymes shown. Ketone bodies are formed in the liver from acetyl-CoA moieties. All defects of fatty acid oxidation are inherited as autosomal recessive diseases. AS = acyl-CoA synthetase; CT = carnitine-acylcarnitine translocase.

term therapy involves replenishing carnitine stores with L-carnitine and preventing hypoglycemia. This may be accomplished by providing a snack before bedtime, but continuous intragastric feeding may be required. Except for MCAD deficiency and the disorders that respond dramatically to carnitine (eg, carnitine uptake defect), the long-term prognosis for most of these conditions is guarded, with sudden death often occurring due to a conduction defect or an arrhythmia.

CARNITINE UPTAKE DEFECT (PRIMARY CARNITINE DEFICIENCY)

This disorder is the result of a defect in the sodium-dependant high-affinity carnitine transporter in the plasma membrane, which ultimately limits β-oxidation by reducing entry of acyl-CoA esters into mitochondria (see Fig. 9-11). The defects in the kidney and gut cause very-low levels of free carnitine in serum, and the disorder responds dramatically to L-carnitine. It is inherited as an autosomal recessive trait. (See also Chapter 22.)

Clinical Features

The condition may present in early infancy or in late childhood, usually with dilated cardiomyopathy or recurrent episodes of encephalopathy and hypoketotic hypoglycemia. Skeletal muscle involvement may be apparent as hypotonia or proximal limb weakness. Conduction defects and arrhythmias are rare. Sudden death is common, with autopsy showing fat in the heart, liver, renal tubules, and skeletal muscle.

Diagnosis

Diagnosis is based on finding extremely low levels of carnitine in serum and tissues; serum carnitine may be 1 μmol/L or undetectable (normal = 30–70). Organic acid and acylcarnitine analysis are usually normal. Carnitine transport is deficient in fibroblasts, and fetal diagnosis is possible based on the same assay on amniocytes. The gene encoding the carnitine transporter has been cloned and localized to chromosome 5 (5q31), and several disease-causing mutations have been described.

Treatment

The response to L-carnitine supplementation is dramatic and life-saving; 100 to 200 mg/kg/d can be given intravenously in emergency situations, and then administered orally.

DEFECTS OF FATTY ACID ENTRY INTO MITOCHONDRIA

Short- and medium-chain fatty acids can enter mitochondrial directly, but CoA esters of fatty acids longer than C_{12} are transported into mitochondria by carnitine palmitoyltransferases (CPT) I and II, and by carnitine-acylcarnitine translocase (see Fig. 9-11). CPT I in the outer mitochondrial membrane first transfers the acyl moiety from CoA to carnitine, and the translocase then moves the acylcarnitine ester across the inner membrane in exchange for free carnitine. CPT II on the inside of the inner membrane then reconstitutes the CoA esters, which enter the β-oxidation spiral. Defects of CPT I, CPT II, and translocase are inherited as autosomal recessive traits.

Clinical Findings

CPT I deficiency usually presents in infancy with episodes of fasting-induced hypoketotic hypoglycemia. There are two distinct phenotypes of CPT II deficiency. The more common muscular form presents with exercise-induced muscle pain and rhabdomyolysis in adult life; only the rare hepatocardiomuscular form occurs in infants and children. Those that present as neonates die in 1 to 2 weeks with hepatomegaly, cardiomyopathy, and encephalopathy, and often have renal cystic dysplasia. Those presenting later usually have hypoketotic hypoglycemia, cardiomyopathy, and muscle disease, and are at risk for sudden death due to conduction defects or arrhythmias.

Translocase deficiency usually presents as life-threatening disease in the newborn period with hyperammonemia, conduction defects, and arrhythmias, and evidence of skeletal muscle involvement, with high creatine phosphokinase. The ultimate prognosis of this condition is good if the child survives the neonatal period.

Diagnosis

The serum acylcarnitine profile is usually normal in CPT I deficiency, but may show elevated C_{16} esters in CPT II and translocase deficiency. There are no changes in amino acids (eg, high or low citrulline) to indicate a urea cycle defect as the cause of the hyperammonemia in translocase deficiency, and urine organic acids are normal or show only mild dicarboxylic aciduria. Free carnitine concentration in serum is 2 to 3 times normal in CPT I deficiency, and very low in CPT II and translocase deficiency.

All three enzymes can be assayed in fibroblasts and leukocytes, and while prenatal diagnosis by enzyme assay on amniocytes should be possible in all of these disorders, it has been accomplished only in CPT II and translocase deficiency. In some instances, prenatal diagnosis of CPT II can also be made by demonstrating enlarged echogenic kidneys by ultrasonography. Disease-causing mutations have been identified in all of the genes.

Treatment

Acute episodes of hypoketotic hypoglycemia should be treated with intravenous glucose-containing fluids, and treatment of hyperammonemia may require dialysis (see Fig. 9-9). Preventing fasting is simple in CPT I deficiency, but continuous intragastic feeding may be necessary in CPT II and translocase deficiency. Carnitine should be given when serum carnitine level is low.

DEFECTS OF β-OXIDATION

Once in the mitochondrial matrix, acyl-CoA esters enter the β-oxidation spiral, in which a series of four reactions successively remove two-carbon fragments of acetyl-CoA. FAD-containing acyl-CoA dehydrogenases oxidize the acyl-CoA to 2,3-enoyl-CoA, which becomes hydrated to a 3-hydroxyacyl-CoA by hydratases. Oxidation to a 3-ketoacyl-CoA by NAD-requiring hydroxyacyl-CoA dehydrogenases and removal of acetyl-CoA by 3-ketothiolases follow, and the acyl-CoA, which is now two carbons shorter, reenters the spiral.

All these reactions are catalyzed by enzymes with distinct (and often overlapping) chain-length specificities. For example, different FAD-containing acyl-CoA dehydrogenases act on very-long-chain (C_{12-24}), long-chain (C_{6-20}), medium-chain (C_{4-14}), and short-chain (C_{4-6}) acyl-CoAs, and similar specificities exist for the hydratases, hydroxyacyl-CoA dehydrogenases, and thiolases.

Inherited disorders in almost all these enzymes have been described. As a rule, defects in long-chain-specific enzymes block β-oxidation more completely and cause the most severe clinical disease. Most of these conditions are rare, but very-long-chain acyl-

CoA dehydrogenase (VLCAD) deficiency, medium-chain acyl-CoA dehydrogenase (MCAD) deficiency, and long-chain hydroxyacyl-CoA dehydrogenase (LCHAD) deficiency are relatively common, and therefore important. All three are inherited as autosomal recessive traits.

VERY-LONG-CHAIN ACYL-CoA DEHYDROGENASE (VLCAD) DEFICIENCY

Clinical Findings

VLCAD deficiency can present in the newborn period with arrhythmias and sudden death, or with hepatic, cardiac, or muscle presentations later in infancy or childhood. The hepatic presentation is characterized by fasting-induced hypoketotic hypoglycemia, encephalopathy, and mild hepatomegaly, often with mild acidosis, hyperammonemia, and elevated liver transaminases. Some patients present with arrhythmias or dilated or hypertrophic cardiomyopathy in infancy or childhood, and a few patients present with exercise-induced muscle pain, rhabdomyolysis, elevated creatine kinase levels, and myoglobinuria. Most VLCAD- deficient patients present early with severe cardiomyopathy, and their outcome is poor.

Diagnosis

Analysis of serum acylcarnitines by MS-MS usually shows elevations of saturated and unsaturated C_{14-18} esters, even between episodes. Urine organic acid analysis during acute illness often shows increased C_6 (adipic), C_8 (suberic), and C_{10} (sebacic) dicarboxylic acids but, because very similar changes are seen in resolving ketosis and after ingesting medium-chain triglycerides, will not raise suspicion of disease unless C_{12} and C_{14} dicarboxylic acids are also present. Serum concentration of free carnitine is usually low.

VLCAD deficiency can be demonstrated in fibroblasts or leukocytes, and enzyme assay in cultured amniocytes can be used for prenatal diagnosis. The gene encoding the enzyme has been cloned and localized to 17p13. Several disease-causing mutations have been described, and those that affect enzyme function the most cause the most severe and early presenting clinical disease.

Treatment

Management involves avoiding fasting, maintaining high-carbohydrate intake, and treating episodes of acute disease with glucose-containing intravenous fluids. Continuous intragastric feeding may be necessary. Oral carnitine may also be useful. Medium-chain triglycerides, whose oxidation does not involve VLCAD, can be administered to provide calories, but should not be used until the diagnosis of VLCAD deficiency is certain.

MEDIUM-CHAIN ACYL-CoA DEHYDROGENASE (MCAD) DEFICIENCY

Clinical Findings

MCAD deficiency usually presents during the first 2 years of life with episodes of fasting-induced vomiting, lethargy progressing to coma and seizures, hypoketotic hypoglycemia, and hepatomegaly, often with mild hyperammonemia. Misdiagnosis as Reye syndrome or, because the initial episode is fatal in about 25% of patients, sudden infant death syndrome is common. Levels of uric acid, liver transaminases, and creatine kinase are often elevated during the

acute episode, and liver biopsy shows microvesicular steatosis. Autopsy shows fatty infiltration of the liver, renal tubules, and heart and skeletal muscle. A few enzyme-deficient individuals do not develop symptoms.

Diagnosis

Analysis of serum acylcarnitines by MS-MS shows elevations of C_8, $C_{8:1}$, and $C_{10:1}$ esters, even between episodes. Urine organic acids during acute illness often show increased C_6 (adipic), C_8 (suberic), and C_{10} (sebacic) dicarboxylic acids, together with hexanoylglycine, suberylglycine, and phenylpropionylglycine. The dicarboxylic aciduria also occurs during resolving physiological ketosis and after ingestion of medium-chain triglycerides, and will not be perceived as abnormal unless the glycine esters, or unsaturated and/or longer-chain dicarboxylic acids, are also present. Free-carnitine level in serum is usually low.

The enzyme defect can be demonstrated in several tissues, including fibroblasts and leukocytes, but molecular diagnosis is often easier. The gene encoding MCAD has been localized to 1p31. Several disease-causing mutations have been identified but the K304E mutation, which changes the lysine residue at position 304 of the mature enzyme to glutamic acid, accounts for 90 percent of mutant alleles found in whites. Ninety-nine percent of affected whites have at least one copy of this mutation (81% are homozygous, and 18% are heterozygous), and analysis for this one mutation will confirm the diagnosis in many patients.

Treatment

Acute episodes should be treated with intravenous glucose and bicarbonate. Long-term treatment consists of avoiding fasting, usually by providing carbohydrate snacks at bedtime. Oral carnitine (100 mg/kg/d) is useful, both to replenish depleted stores and to augment excretion of toxic intermediates as carnitine esters. Developmental delay, behavioral problems, and other chronic CNS problems are not uncommon outcomes of the initial episode, but if such damage did not occur, prognosis is quite good. Newborn screening for MCAD deficiency has been advocated, and is based on the responsiveness to treatment and the frequency of death and other sequelae following the initial episode (see Sec. 8.2).

LONG-CHAIN 3-HYDROXYACYL-CoA DEHYDROGENASE (LCHAD) DEFICIENCY

NAD-dependent 3-hydroxyacyl-CoA dehydrogenases catalyze oxidation of 3-hydroxyacyl-CoA esters to their 3-keto analogues. LCHAD, the long-chain-specific enzyme, acts on acyl groups longer than C_8 and exists in mitochondria as part of a protein with three activities. This mitochondrial trifunctional protein (MTP) is an $\alpha_4\beta_4$ octamer, with the α subunit carrying LCHAD and long-chain enoyl-CoA hydratase, and the β subunit carrying long-chain β-ketothiolase. LCHAD deficiency can exist alone or with deficiency of the other two enzymes.

Clinical Findings

Patients with isolated LCHAD deficiency often present in infancy with fasting-induced hypoketotic hypoglycemia; however, patients may also present with neonatal cardiomyopathy or, much later, with exercise-induced rhabdomyolysis. History often reveals a pregnancy complicated by acute fatty liver or HELLP (*h*emolysis, *e*levated *l*iver enzymes, and *l*ow *p*latelets). Unlike most other fatty acid oxidation disorders, severe and progressive cholestatic liver disease is common, and many patients develop retinopathy with hypopigmentation or focal pigmentary aggregations. Most patients die in early childhood. The presentation of patients with MTP deficiency is similar to that of isolated LCHAD deficiency, but it is usually earlier and more severe.

Diagnosis

Acylcarnitine analysis by MS-MS is usually diagnostic and shows elevated saturated and unsaturated C_{16} and C_{18} hydroxyacylcarnitines. Organic acid analysis often shows elevated C_{6-14} 3-hydroxydicarboxylic acids, but the same abnormalities are seen in patients with respiratory-chain defects and glycogenoses and are not specific. The enzyme defect can be demonstrated in fibroblasts and leukocytes and, for prenatal diagnosis, in amniocytes. The gene encoding the α subunit has been cloned and localized to 2p24.1-23.3. The E510Q mutation, which changes the glutamic acid residue at position 510 to glutamine, accounts for nearly 90% of mutant alleles in Europeans.

Treatment

Therapy is much the same as that of VLCAD and MCAD deficiency. As in VLCAD deficiency, it may be necessary to completely eliminate fasting by continuous intragastric feeding, and medium-chain triglycerides may be used to provide calories. Carnitine is probably useful to replenish depleted stores. Oral supplements of docosahexaenoic acid, a polyunsaturated C_{20} acid, may be useful in reversing retinopathy.

GLUTARIC ACIDEMIA TYPE II

Electrons from acyl-CoA dehydrogenases involved in fatty acid and amino acid oxidation (eg, isovaleryl-CoA dehydrogenase and glutaryl-CoA dehydrogenase) are transferred from the FAD coenzymes into the respiratory chain via electron transfer flavoprotein (ETF) and ETF:ubiquinone oxidoreductase (ETF:QO). The electrons first move into the flavin of ETF, and then through flavin and iron-sulfur clusters of ETF:QO to coenzyme Q in the inner mitochondrial membrane. Defects in ETF and ETF:QO cause glutaric acidemia type II (GA2), and are transmitted as autosomal recessive traits.

Clinical Findings

Glutaric aciduria type II may present in the neonatal period with severe hypoglycemia, metabolic acidosis, hyperammonemia, and the odor of sweaty feet typical of isovaleric acidemia, often with cardiomyopathy, facial dysmorphism, and severe renal cystic dysplasia. Most such patients die within the first days or weeks of life, often of conduction defects or arrhythmias. Fatty infiltration of the liver, renal tubules, and heart and skeletal muscle are consistent findings at autopsy. Milder disease, sometimes called ethylmalonic adipic aciduria, may present with episodic hypoketotic hypoglycemia and hepatomegaly in childhood, or simply as hypoglycemia in adult life.

Diagnosis

Acylcarnitine analysis by MS-MS shows glutarylcarnitine, isovalerylcarnitine, and straight-chain esters of chain length C_4, C_8, C_{10}, $C_{10:1}$, and C_{12}. Urine organic acids show increased ethylmalonic, glutaric, 2-hydroxyglutaric, and 3-hydroxyisovaleric acids, together with C_6, C_8, and C_{10} dicarboxylic acids and isovalerylglycine. Serum carnitine concentration is usually low. Elevated serum sarcosine on amino acid analysis is common in patients with mild disease.

Enzyme assays on fibroblasts show that some patients with GA2 are deficient in ETF and that other patients are deficient in ETF:QO. The genes encoding ETF:QO and the α and β subunits of ETF have been cloned and mapped to 4q32>ter, 15q23-25, and 19q13.3, respectively, and disease-causing mutations in all three genes have been identified in different patients.

Treatment

Patients with complete defects die during the first weeks of life, usually of conduction defects or arrhythmias; but those with incomplete defects can survive well into adult life. As in other fatty acid oxidation disorders, treatment relies on the avoidance of fasting, sometimes with continuous intragastric feeding, and carnitine to replenish lost stores. Medium-chain triglycerides cannot be oxidized in this condition because all of the acyl-CoA dehydrogenases are deficient.

References

Isovaleric Acidemia

Mehta KC, Zsolway K, Osterhaut KC, et al: Lessons from the late diagnosis of isovaleric acidemia in a five-year-old boy. J Pediatr 129:309, 1996

Tanaka K, Budd MA, Efron ML, Isselbacher KJ: Isovaleric acidemia: a new genetic defect of leucine metabolism. Proc Natl Acad Sci U S A 56:236, 1966

Isolated 3-Methylcrotonyl-CoA Carboxylase Deficiency

Elpeleg O, Havkin S, Barash V, et al: Familial hypotonia of childhood caused by isolated 3-methylcrotonyl-coenzyme A carboxylase deficiency. J Pediatr 121:407, 1992.

Gibson KM, Bennett MJ, Naylor EW, Morton DH: 3-Methylcrotonyl-coenzyme A carboxylase deficiency in Amish/Mennonite adults identified by detection of increased acylcarnitines in blood spots of their children. J Pediatr 132:519, 1998

Lehnert W, Niederhoff H, Suormala T, Baumgartner ER: Isolated biotin-resistant 3-methylcrotonyl-CoA carboxylase deficiency: long-term outcome in a case with neonatal onset. Eur J Pediatr 155:568, 1996

3-Hydroxy-3-Methylglutaryl-CoA Lyase Deficiency

Bakker HD, Wanders RJA, Schutgens RBH, et al: 3-Hydroxy-3-methylglutaryl-CoA lyase deficiency: absence of clinical symptoms due to a self-imposed dietary fat and protein restriction. J Inherit Metab Dis 16:1061, 1993

Mitochondrial Acetoacetyl-CoA Thiolase Deficiency

Robinson BH, Sherwood WG, Taylor J, et al: Acetoacetyl CoA thiolase deficiency: a cause of severe ketoacidosis in infancy simulating salicylism. J Pediatr 95:228, 1979

Propionic Acidemia

Hommes FA, Kuipers JRG, Elema JD, et al: Propionic acidemia, a new inborn error of metabolism. Pediatr Res 2:519, 1968

North KN, Korson MS, Gopal YR, et al: Neonatal-onset propionic acide-mia: neurologic and developmental profiles, and implications for man-agement. J Pediatr 126:916, 1995

Multiple Carboxylase Deficiency

Haagerup A, Andersen JB, Blichfeldt S, Christensen MF: Biotinidase defi-ciency: two cases of very early presentation. Dev Med Child Neurol 39: 832, 1997

Touma E, Suormala T, Baumgartner ER, et al: Holocarboxylase synthetase deficiency: report of a case with onset in late infancy. J Inherit Metab Dis 22:115, 1999

Wolf B, Pomponio RJ, Norrgard KJ, et al: Delayed-onset profound biotin-idase deficiency. J Pediatr 132:362, 1998

Methylmalonic Acidemias

Enns GM, Barkovich AJ, Rosenblatt DS, et al: Progressive neurological deterioration and MRI changes in *cblC* methylmalonic acidemia treated with hydroxycobalamin. J Inherit Metab Dis 22:599, 1999

Shih VE, Axel SM, Tewksbury JC, et al: Defective lysosomal release of vitamin B_{12} (cblF): a hereditary cobalamin metabolic disorder associated with sudden death. Am J Med Genet 33:555, 1989

Stokke O, Eldjarn L, Norum KR, et al: Methylmalonic aciduria: a new inborn error of metabolism which may cause fatal acidosis in the neo-natal period. Scand J Clin Lab Invest 20:313, 1967

Van't hoff WG, Dixon M, Taylor J, et al: Combined kidney-liver transplan-tation in methylmalonic acidemia. J Pediatr 132:1043, 1998

Glutaric Acidemia (Type I)

Brismar J, Ozand PT: CT and MR of the brain in glutaric acidemia type I: a review of 59 published cases and a report of 5 new patients. Am J Neuroradiol 16:675, 1995

Hoffmann GF, Zschocke J: Glutaric aciduria type I: from clinical, biochem-ical and molecular diversity to successful therapy. J Inherit Metab Dis 22:381, 1999

Mevalonic Acidemia

Hoffmann GF, Charpentier C, Mayatepek E, et al: Clinical and biochemical phenotype in 11 patients with mevalonic aciduria. Pediatrics 91:915, 1993

D- and L-2-Hydroxyglutaric Acidemias

Barth PG, Hoffmann GF, Jaeken J, et al: L-2-Hydroxyglutaric acidemia: a novel inherited metabolic disease. Ann Neurol 32:66, 1992

Van der Knapp MS, Jakobs C, Hoffmann GF, et al: D-2-Hydroxyglutaric aciduria: further clinical delineation. J Inherit Metab Dis 22:404, 1999

Disorders of Fatty Acid Oxidation General

Brivet A, Boutron A, Slama A, et al: Defects in activation and transport of fatty acids. J Inherit Metab Dis 22:428, 1999

Saudubray JM, Martin D, de Lonlay P, et al: Recognition and management of fatty acid oxidation defects: a series of 107 patients. J Inherit Metab Dis 22:488, 1999

Vianey-Saban C, Guffon N, Delolne F, et al: Diagnosis of inborn errors of metabolism by acylcarnitine profiling in blood using tandem mass spec-trometry. J Inherit Metab Dis 20:411, 1997

Wanders RJA, Vreken P, den Boer MEJ, et al: Disorders of mitochondrial fatty acyl-CoA β-oxidation. J Inherit Metab Dis 22:442, 1999

Carnitine Uptake Defect

Rinaldo P, Stanley CA, Hsu BYL, et al: Sudden neonatal death in carnitine transporter deficiency. J Pediatr 131:304, 1997

Defects of Fatty Acid Entry into Mitochondria

Chalmers RA, Stanley CA, English N, Wigglesworth JS: Mitochondrial car-nitine-acylcarnitine translocase deficiency presenting as sudden neonatal death. J Pediatr 131:220, 1997

Haworth JC, Demaugre F, Booth FA, et al: Atypical features of the hepatic form of carnitine palmitoyltransferase deficiency in a Hutterite family. J Pediatr 121:553, 1992

North KN, Hoppel CL, de Girolami U, et al: Lethal neonatal deficiency of carnitine palmitoyltransferase II associated with dysgenesis of the brain and kidneys. J Pediatr 127:414, 1995

Defects of β-Oxidation

Andresen BS, Olpin S, Poorthuis BJHM, et al: Clear correlation of genotype with disease phenotype in very-long-chain acyl-CoA dehydrogenase de-ficiency. Am J Hum Genet 64:479, 1999

Iafolla AK, Thompson RJ, Roe CR: Medium-chain acyl-coenzyme A de-hydrogenase deficiency: clinical course in 120 affected children. J Pediatr 124:409, 1994

Isaacs JD, Sims HF, Powell CK, et al: Maternal acute fatty liver of pregnancy associated with fetal trifunctional protein deficiency: molecular charac-terization of a novel maternal mutant allele. Pediatr Res 40:393, 1996

Kjaergaard S, Graem N, Larsen T, Skovby F: Recurrent fetal polycystic kidneys associated with glutaric aciduria type II. APMIS 106:1188, 1998

Loehr JP, Goodman SI, Frerman FE: Glutaric acidemia type II: heteroge-neity of clinical and biochemical phenotypes. Pediatr Res 27:311, 1990

Przyrembel H, Wendel U, Becker K, et al: Glutaric aciduria type II: report on a previously undescribed metabolic disorder. Clin Chim Acta 66:227, 1976

Smelt AHM, Poorthuis BJHM, Onkenhout W, et al: Very-long-chain acyl-coenzyme A dehydrogenase deficiency with adult onset. Ann Neurol 43:540, 1998

Tyni T, Palotie A, Vinikka L, et al: Long-chain 3-hydroxyacyl-coenzyme A dehydrogenase deficiency with the G1528C mutation: clinical presen-tation of thirteen patients. J Pediatr 130:67, 1997

9.5 DISORDERS OF CARBOHYDRATE METABOLISM

Yuan-Tsong Chen

Carbohydrate synthesis and degradation play a vital role in cellular function by providing the energy required for most metabolic pro-cesses. The carbohydrates to be discussed include three monosac-charides—glucose, galactose, and fructose—and a polysaccha-ride—glycogen. The relevant biochemical pathways of these carbohydrates are shown in Fig. 9-12.

Glucose is the principal substrate of energy metabolism in hu-mans. Metabolism of glucose generates ATP via glycolysis (con-version of glucose or glycogen to pyruvate) or mitochondria oxi-dative phosphorylation (conversion of pyruvate to carbon dioxide and water), or both. A continuous source of glucose from dietary intake, gluconeogenesis (glucose made de novo), and degradation of glycogen maintains normal blood glucose levels. Sources of glu-

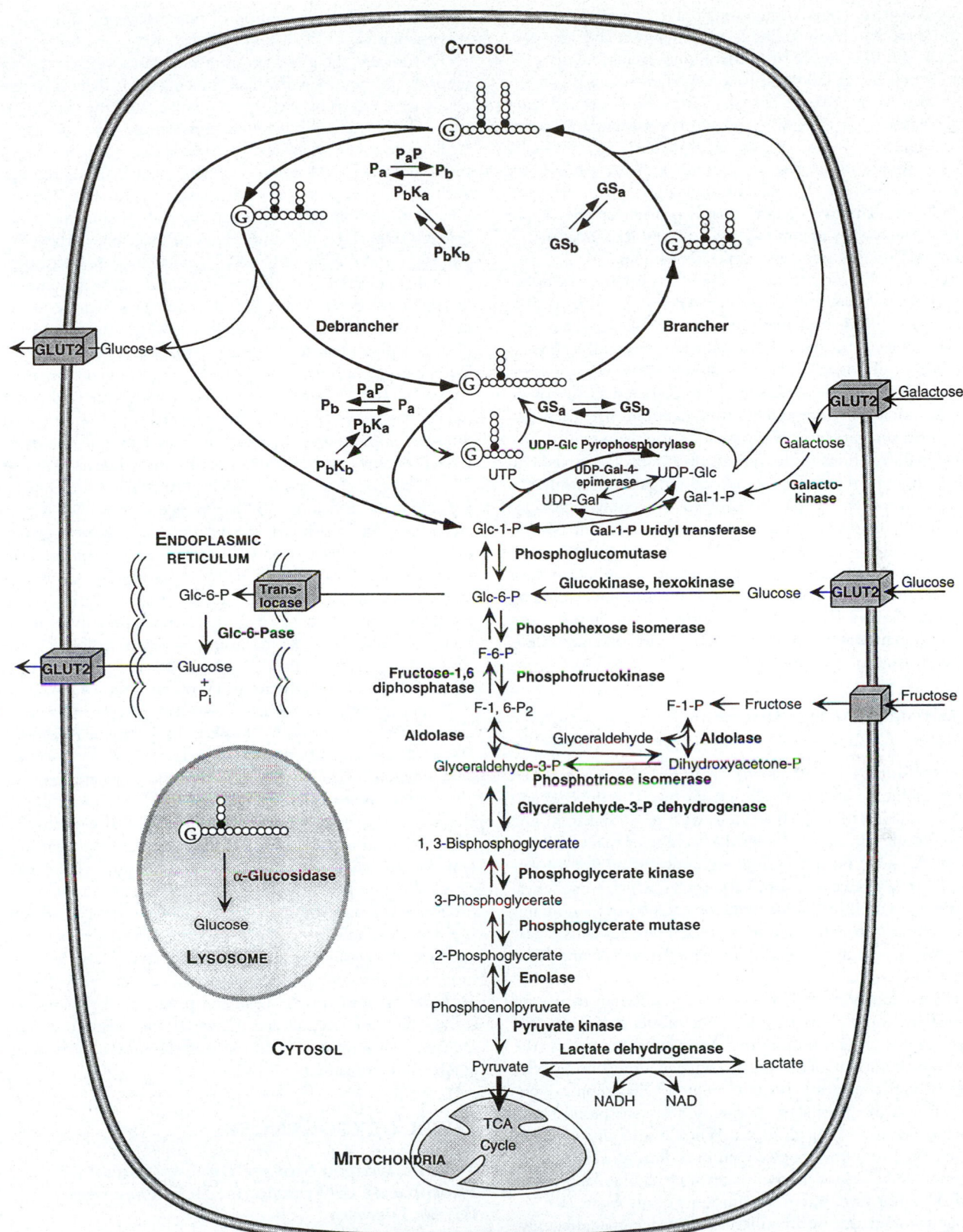

FIGURE 9-12   Metabolic pathways related to glycogen storage diseases and to galactose and fructose disorders. Nonstandard abbreviations are as follows: GSa = active glycogen synthase; GSb = inactive glycogen synthase; Pa = active phosphorylase; Pb = inactive phosphorylase; PaP = phosphorylase *a* phosphatase; PbKa = active phosphorylase *b* kinase; PbKb = inactive phosphorylase *b* kinase; G = glycogenin, the primer protein for glycogen synthesis. *Modified from AR Beaudet: Glycogen storage diseases. In: Isselbacher KJ, et al, eds: Harrison's Principles of Internal Medicine, 13th ed. New York, McGraw-Hill, 1994.*

cose in our diet are obtained by ingesting polysaccharides, primarily starch, and disaccharides including lactose, maltose, and sucrose.

Galactose and fructose are two other monosaccharides that provide fuel for cellular metabolism; however, their role is much less significant than is the role of glucose. Galactose is derived from lactose (galactose + glucose) which is found in milk and milk products. If necessary, galactose can be incorporated into glycogen, becoming a source of glucose. Galactose is also an important component for certain glycolipids, glycoproteins, and glycosaminoglycans. The two dietary sources of fructose are sucrose (fructose + glucose), a commonly used sweetener, and fructose itself which is found in fruits, vegetables, and honey.

This section is devoted to the inherited disorders of carbohydrate metabolism caused by defects in enzymes or transport proteins involved in glycogen metabolism, gluconeogenesis, and glycolysis. The defects in glycogen metabolism typically cause an accumulation of glycogen in the tissues, hence the name *glycogen storage disease (GSD)*. The defects in gluconeogenesis or glycolytic pathway, including galactose and fructose metabolism, do not usually result in an accumulation of glycogen in the tissues.

Clinical manifestations of the various disorders of carbohydrate metabolism differ markedly. The symptoms range from harmless to lethal. Unlike disorders of lipid metabolism, mucopolysaccharidosis, or other storage diseases, dietary therapy has been effective in many of the carbohydrate disorders. Almost all the genes responsible for the inherited defects of carbohydrate metabolism have been cloned and mutations identified. Advances in understanding the molecular basis of the disease are being used to improve the diagnosis and management of the disorders, and some are candidates for early trials of gene therapy.

9.5.1   Glycogen Storage Disease

Glycogen, the storage form of glucose in animal cells, is composed of glucose residues joined in straight chains by $\alpha 1-4$ linkages and branched at intervals of 4 to 10 residues with $\alpha 1-6$ linkages. The tree-like molecule can have a molecular weight of many millions and may aggregate to form structures recognizable by electron microscopy. In muscle, glycogen forms β particles, which are spherical and contain up to 60,000 glucose residues. Each β particle contains a covalently linked protein called *glycogenin*. Liver contains β particles and rosettes of glycogen called α particles, which appear to be aggregated β particles.

The primary function of glycogen varies in different tissues. In skeletal muscle, stored glycogen is a source of fuel that is used for short-term, high-energy consumption during muscle activity; in the brain, the small amount of stored glycogen is used during brief periods of hypoglycemia or hypoxia as an emergency supply of energy. In contrast, the liver takes up glucose from the bloodstream after a meal and stores it as glycogen. When blood glucose levels start to fall, the liver converts glycogen back into glucose and releases it into the blood for use by tissues such as brain and erythrocytes that cannot store significant amounts of glycogen.

Glycogen storage disease are inherited disorders that affect glycogen metabolism. Disorders in virtually every enzyme involved in the synthesis or degradation of glycogen and its regulation cause some type of glycogen storage disease (see Fig. 9-12) in which glycogen is abnormal in quantity, quality, or both. Excluded from this section are those conditions in which tissue glycogen accumulation is secondary, such as overtreatment of diabetes mellitus

with insulin or administration of pharmacologic amounts of glucocorticoids.

Historically, the glycogen storage diseases were categorized numerically in the order in which the enzymatic defects were identified. Classification by the organs involved and the clinical manifestations is the system followed in this section.

Because liver and muscle have abundant glycogen, they are the most commonly and seriously affected tissues. The glycogen storage diseases that principally affect the liver (see Fig. 9-12) include glucose-6-phosphatase deficiency (type I); debranching enzyme deficiency (type III); branching enzyme deficiency (type IV); liver phosphorylase deficiency (type VI); phosphorylase kinase deficiency (type IX); glycogen synthetase deficiency (type 0); and glucose transporter-2 defect (type XI). Because carbohydrate metabolism in the liver affects plasma glucose levels, the disorders of hepatic glycogen degradation and glucose release typically cause fasting hypoglycemia and hepatomegaly. Some glycogen storage diseases (types III and IV) are also associated with liver cirrhosis. Other organs besides liver may also be involved, for example, renal dysfunction in glycogen storage disease type I, and myopathy in types III and IV, and some rare forms of phosphorylase kinase deficiency.

The role of glycogen in muscle is to provide substrates for the generation of sufficient ATP for muscle contraction. The muscle glycogen storage diseases can be divided into two groups (see Fig. 9-12). The first group is characterized by progressive skeletal myopathy and/or cardiomyopathy and is represented by a lysosomal enzyme deficiency (acid α-glucosidase, type II). The second group is a muscle-energy disorder characterized by muscle pain, exercise intolerance, myoglobinuria, and susceptibility to fatigue. This group includes type V (McArdle disease), a muscle phosphorylase deficiency, and deficiencies of phosphofructokinase (type VII), phosphoglycerate kinase, phosphoglycerate mutase, lactate dehydrogenase, fructose 1,6-bisphosphate aldolase A, and pyruvate kinase. Some of these enzyme deficiencies are associated with a compensated hemolysis, suggesting a more generalized defect in glucose metabolism. The overall frequency of all forms of glycogen storage disease is approximately 1 in 20,000 live births. Most of them are inherited as autosomal recessive traits, but phosphoglycerate kinase deficiency and one form of phosphorylase kinase deficiency are X-linked disorders. The most common childhood disorders are glucose-6-phosphatase deficiency (type I), lysosomal acid α-glucosidase deficiency (type II), debrancher deficiency (type III), and liver phosphorylase kinase deficiency (type IX). The most common adult disorder is myophosphorylase deficiency (type V, or McArdle disease). In the past, the prognosis for many glycogen storage diseases was guarded. However, early diagnosis and better management have improved the survival rates, and many affected children are now adults.

LIVER GLYCOGENOSES

Type I Glycogen Storage Disease (Glucose-6-Phosphatase or Translocase Deficiency, von Gierke Disease)

Type I glycogen storage disease is due to a defect in glucose-6-phosphatase in liver, kidney, and intestinal mucosa. It can be divided into two subtypes: type Ia, in which the glucose-6-phosphatase enzyme is defective, and type Ib, which is caused by a defect in the translocase that transports glucose-6-phosphate across the microsomal membrane. The defects in both type Ia and Ib lead to inadequate conversion in liver of glucose-6-phosphate to glucose and thus make affected individuals susceptible to fasting hypoglycemia.

Clinical and Laboratory Findings

Patients with type I disease may develop hypoglycemia and lactic acidosis during the neonatal period, but more commonly present at 3 to 4 months of age with hepatomegaly and/or hypoglycemia. These children often have doll-like faces with fat cheeks, relatively thin extremities, short stature, and a protuberant abdomen that is the result of massive hepatomegaly; the kidneys are enlarged, and the spleen and heart are of normal size.

The hallmarks of the disease are hypoglycemia, lactic acid acidosis, hyperuricemia, and hyperlipidemia. Hypoglycemia and lactic acidosis can develop after a short fast. Hyperuricemia is present in young children, but gout rarely develops before puberty. Despite hepatomegaly, liver enzymes are usually normal or near normal. Intermittent diarrhea may occur (the mechanism is not known). Easy bruising and epistaxis are associated with a prolonged bleeding time as a result of impaired platelet aggregation/adhesion.

Hypertriglyceridemia may cause the plasma to appear "milky," and cholesterol and phospholipid concentrations are also elevated. The lipid abnormality resembles type IV hyperlipidemia and is characterized by increased levels of very-low-density lipoprotein (VLDL); low-density lipoprotein (LDL); increased levels of apolipoproteins B, C, and E; and normal or reduced levels of apolipoproteins A and D. The hepatocytes are distended by glycogen and fat with large and prominent lipid vacuoles. There is little associated fibrosis.

All these findings apply to both type Ia and Ib glycogen storage diseases, but type Ib has the additional feature of recurrent bacterial infections due to neutropenia and impaired neutrophil function (see Chapter 19). Oral and intestinal mucosa ulcerations are common, and inflammatory bowel disease may occur.

Long-Term Complications

Although type I glycogen storage disease mainly affects the liver, multiple organ systems are also involved. Gout usually becomes symptomatic around puberty as a result of the long-term hyperuricemia. Puberty is often delayed, but fertility appears to be normal. Hypertriglyceridemia causes an increased risk of pancreatitis, but premature atherosclerosis has not been documented. Impaired platelet aggregation may reduce the risk of atherosclerosis.

By the second or third decade, most patients with type I glycogen storage disease develop hepatic adenomas that can hemorrhage and, rarely, become malignant. Other complications include pulmonary hypertension and osteoporosis.

Renal disease is a late complication, and almost all patients above age 20 have proteinuria. Many have hypertension, kidney stones, nephrocalcinosis, and altered creatinine clearance. Glomerular hyperfiltration, increased renal plasma flow, and microalbuminuria can occur before the onset of gross proteinuria. In young patients, hyperfiltration and hyperperfusion may be the only signs of renal abnormalities. With advanced renal disease, focal segmental glomerulosclerosis and interstitial fibrosis are evident on biopsy. In some patients, renal function deteriorates and progresses to failure, requiring dialysis or transplantation. Other abnormalities in renal function include amyloidosis, Fanconi-like syndrome, and distal renal tubular acidification defect. The increases in renal perfusion and maternal blood volume that normally occur in pregnancy can ex-

acerbate renal problems. In addition, hypoglycemia may also become more difficult to control.

Diagnosis

The diagnosis of type I disease can be suspected based on clinical presentation and abnormal plasma lactate and lipid values. In addition, administration of glucagon or epinephrine causes little or no rise in blood glucose, but increases lactate levels significantly. Prior to cloning of glucose-6-phosphatase and glucose-6-phosphate translocase genes, a definitive diagnosis required a liver biopsy to demonstrate a deficiency. Gene-based mutation analysis now provides a noninvasive way of diagnosis for the majority of type Ia and Ib patients.

Treatment

Treatment is designed to maintain normal blood glucose levels and is achieved by continuous nasogastric infusion of glucose or oral administration of uncooked cornstarch. Nasogastric drip feeding in early infancy may consist of an elemental enteral formula or may contain only glucose to maintain normoglycemia during the night; frequent feedings with a high-carbohydrate content are given during the day.

Uncooked cornstarch acts as a slow-release form of glucose and can be given at a dose of 1.6 g/kg of body weight every 4 hours for infants under the age of 2 years. As the child grows older, the cornstarch regimen can be changed to every 6 hours, and it can be given by mouth as a liquid (1:2, weight:volume) at a dose of 1.75 to 2.5 g/kg of body weight. Because fructose and galactose cannot be converted to free glucose, their dietary intake should be restricted, and dietary supplements of multivitamins and calcium are required. Allopurinol is given to lower the levels of uric acid. In patients with type Ib glycogen storage disease, granulocyte and granulocyte-macrophage colony-stimulating factors have been used successfully to correct the neutropenia, to decrease the severity of bacterial infection, and to improve the chronic inflammatory bowel disease.

Prior to surgery, the bleeding status should be evaluated, and good metabolic control should be established. Prolonged bleeding time can be corrected by the administration of a constant intravenous glucose infusion for 24 to 48 hours prior to surgery. Vasopressin can be given during surgery to reduce bleeding complications, and normal glucose levels should be maintained throughout surgery.

Prognosis

In the past, many patients with type I glycogen storage disease died, and the prognosis was guarded for those who survived. The long-term complications occur mostly in adults whose disease was not adequately treated during childhood. Early diagnosis and initiation of effective treatment have improved the outcome, but it is not known if all long-term complications can be avoided through good metabolic control.

Genetics

Type I glycogen storage disease is an autosomal recessive disorder. Both type Ia and Ib diseases have been reported in many ethnic groups, but type Ia is rarely seen in blacks. The structural gene for glucose-6-phosphatase is located on chromosome 17q21; three common mutations (R83C, 130X, Q347X) are responsible for 70%

of the known disease alleles. The structural gene for glucose-6-phosphate translocase is located on chromosome 11q23; two mutations, G339C and 1211delCT, appear to be prevalent in white patients, while W118R appears to be most common in Japanese patients. Carrier detection and prenatal diagnosis are possible with the use of molecular techniques.

Type III Glycogen Storage Disease (Debrancher Deficiency, Limit Dextrinosis)

Type III glycogen storage disease is caused by a deficiency of glycogen debranching enzyme. Debranching enzyme and phosphorylase are responsible for complete degradation of glycogen; when debranching enzyme is defective, glycogen breakdown is incomplete, and an abnormal glycogen that has short outer chains and that resembles limit dextrin accumulates.

Clinical and Laboratory Findings

Deficiency of glycogen-debranching enzyme causes hepatomegaly, hypoglycemia, short stature, variable skeletal myopathy, and cardiomyopathy. The disorder usually involves both liver and muscle and is termed *type IIIa glycogen storage disease*. However, in about 15% of patients, the disease appears to involve only the liver and is classified as *type IIIb*.

During infancy and childhood, the disease may be almost indistinguishable from type I disease because hepatomegaly, hypoglycemia, hyperlipidemia, and growth retardation are common features of both. Splenomegaly may be present, but kidneys are not enlarged in type III. Remarkably, hepatomegaly and hepatic symptoms in most type III patients improve with age and usually disappear after puberty. However, progressive liver cirrhosis with failure may occur, which seems especially common in Japanese patients.

In patients with muscle involvement (type IIIa), muscle weakness is usually minimal during childhood but can become severe during the third or fourth decade of life, as evidenced by slowly progressive weakness and muscle wasting. Electromyographic (EMG) changes are consistent with a widespread myopathy, and nerve conduction may be abnormal. Ventricular hypertrophy is frequent, but overt cardiac dysfunction is rare. Hepatic symptoms may be so mild that the diagnosis is not made until adulthood, when neuromuscular disease becomes manifest. Polycystic ovary appears to be a common finding in female patients; fertility, however, does not seem to be affected.

Hypoglycemia, hyperlipidemia, and elevated liver transaminases occur in childhood. In contrast to type I disease, fasting ketosis is prominent, and blood lactate and uric acid concentrations are usually normal. The administration of glucagon 2 hours after a carbohydrate meal causes a normal rise of blood glucose levels, but after an overnight fast, glucagon may provoke no change in blood glucose. Serum creatine kinase levels can sometimes be used to identify patients with muscle involvement, but normal levels do not rule out muscle enzyme deficiency.

The histology of the liver is characterized by a universal distention of hepatocytes by glycogen and by the presence of fibrous septa. The fibrosis and the paucity of fat distinguish type III from type I glycogenosis. The fibrosis can range from minimal periportal fibrosis to micronodular cirrhosis.

Diagnosis

In glycogen storage disease type IIIa, deficient debranching enzyme activity can be demonstrated in liver, skeletal muscle, and

heart. In contrast, type IIIb patients have debranching enzyme deficiency in the liver, but not in muscle. In the past, definitive assignment of subtype required enzyme assays in both liver and muscle. DNA-based analyses now provide a noninvasive way of subtyping in the majority of patients.

Treatment

Dietary management of type III disease is less demanding than in type I. If hypoglycemia is present, frequent high-carbohydrate meals with cornstarch supplements or nocturnal gastric drip feedings are usually effective. A high-protein diet during the daytime plus overnight protein enteral infusion may be tried in patients with myopathy, but it is not established whether such a regimen is effective. Patients do not need to restrict dietary intake of fructose and galactose, as do those with type I disease.

Prognosis

Liver symptoms improve with age and usually disappear after puberty. Cirrhosis of the liver may occur later in life. In type IIIa disease, muscle weakness and atrophy worsen during adulthood.

Genetics

The type III glycogenoses are inherited as autosomal recessive traits. The disease has been reported in many different ethnic groups, and the frequency is relatively high in non-Ashkenazi Jews of North African descent. The gene for debranching enzyme is located on chromosome 1p21. At least 20 different mutations that cause type III disease have been identified. Two mutations (17delAG and Q6X), both located in exon 3 at amino acid codon 6, are exclusively found in the subtype IIIb. Carrier detection and prenatal diagnosis are possible using DNA-based linkage or mutation analysis.

Type IV Glycogen Storage Disease (Branching Enzyme Deficiency, Amylopectinosis, or Andersen Disease)

Deficiency of branching enzyme activity results in accumulation of an abnormal glycogen with poor solubility. The disease is referred to as *type IV glycogen storage disease*, or *amylopectinosis*, because the abnormal glycogen has fewer branch points, more (1–4) linked glucose units, and longer outer chains, resulting in a structure resembling amylopectin.

Clinical and Laboratory Findings

This disorder is clinically variable. The most common form is characterized by progressive cirrhosis of the liver and is manifest in the first 18 months of life as hepatosplenomegaly and failure to thrive. The cirrhosis progresses to cause portal hypertension, ascites, esophageal varices, and liver failure that leads to death by age 5 years. Less frequently, patients survive without progression of liver disease.

Tissue deposition of amylopectin-like materials can be demonstrated in liver, heart, muscle, skin, intestine, brain, spinal cord, and peripheral nerve. The histologic findings in the liver are characterized by both micronodular cirrhosis and faintly stained basophilic inclusions in the hepatocytes. The inclusions consist of coarsely clumped, stored material that is periodic acid–Schiff-positive and partially resistant to diastase digestion. Electron microscopy shows, in addition to the conventional glycogen particles, an accumulation of fibrillar aggregations typical of amylopectin. Definitive diagnosis requires demonstration that branching enzyme activity is deficient in liver, muscle, cultured skin fibroblasts, or leukocytes.

A neuromuscular form of type IV glycogen storage disease has also been reported. These patients may (a) present at birth with severe hypotonia, muscle atrophy, and neuronal involvement, and die during the neonatal period; (b) present in late childhood with myopathy or cardiomyopathy; or (c) present as adults with diffuse central and peripheral nervous system dysfunction accompanied by accumulation of polyglucosan bodies in the nervous system (adult polyglucosan body disease). Definitive diagnosis of the adult disease requires assay of branching enzyme in leukocytes or nerve biopsy, as the deficiency is limited to those tissues.

Treatment

There is no specific treatment for type IV glycogen storage disease. For progressive hepatic failure, liver transplantation has been performed, but caution should be taken in selecting patients for liver transplantation as a nonprogressive hepatic form of the disease exists and extrahepatic manifestation of the disease may occur after transplantation (see Sec. 18.14).

Genetics

Type IV glycogen storage disease is a rare autosomal recessive disease. Prenatal diagnosis is available by using cultured amniocytes or chorionic villi to measure the level of enzymatic activity. The glycogen-branching enzyme gene is located on chromosome 3p12. Both hepatic and neuromuscular forms of the disease are caused by the mutation in the same branching enzyme gene; its characterization in individual patients may be useful in predicting the clinical course.

Type VI Glycogen Storage Disease (Liver Phosphorylase Deficiency, or Hers Disease)

The number of patients with enzymatically documented liver phosphorylase deficiency is small. It appears that patients with liver phosphorylase deficiency have a benign course. These patients present with hepatomegaly and growth retardation early in childhood. Hypoglycemia, hyperlipidemia, and ketosis are usually mild if present. Lactic acid and uric acid concentrations are normal. The heart and skeletal muscles are not involved. The hepatomegaly and growth retardation improve with age and usually disappear around puberty. Treatment is symptomatic. A high carbohydrate diet and frequent feeding are effective in preventing hypoglycemia, but most patients require no specific treatment. The liver phosphorylase gene is located on chromosome 14q21. A splicing-site mutation in intron 13 was identified in a large Mennonite kindred, and four other mutations were found in patients with different ethnic background.

Type IX Glycogen Storage Disease (Liver Phosphorylase Kinase Deficiency)

Defects of phosphorylase kinase cause a heterogeneous group of glycogenoses. The heterogeneity is the result of the complexity of the phosphorylase kinase gene, which consists of four subunits (α, β, γ, δ), each encoded by different genes on different chromosomes (X chromosomes as well as autosomes) and differentially expressed in different tissues. Based on the gene/subunit involved, tissues that are primarily affected, and the mode of inheritance, the phosphorylase kinase deficiency can be divided into several subtypes.

Clinical and Laboratory Findings

X-Linked Liver Phosphorylase Kinase Deficiency. X-linked liver phosphorylase kinase deficiency is one of the most common liver glycogenoses. Phosphorylase kinase activity may also be deficient in erythrocytes and leukocytes, but it is normal in muscle. Typically, a child between the ages of 1 and 5 years presents with growth retardation and hepatomegaly. Levels of cholesterol, triglycerides, and liver enzymes are mildly elevated. Ketosis may occur after fasting. Lactate and uric acid levels are normal. Hypoglycemia is mild, if present. The rise in blood glucose concentration following the administration of glucagon is normal. Hepatomegaly and abnormal blood chemistries gradually return to normal with age. Most adults achieve a normal final height and are practically asymptomatic, despite a persistent phosphorylase kinase deficiency.

Liver histology shows glycogen-distended hepatocytes. The accumulated glycogen (α particles, rosette form) has a frayed or burst appearance and is less compact than in type I or type III disease. Fibrous septae and low-grade inflammatory changes may be present.

The structural gene for the liver isoform of the phosphorylase kinase α subunit is located on chromosome Xp22, and mutations of this gene have been found in the disorder. Subtle mutations tend to retain the phosphorylase kinase activity in the blood cells, while nonsense mutations cause the enzyme deficiency in both liver and blood cells.

Autosomal Liver and Muscle Phosphorylase Kinase Deficiency. An autosomal recessive form of liver and muscle phosphorylase kinase deficiency has been reported in several patients. As in the X-linked form of the disorder, hepatomegaly and growth retardation are the predominant symptoms in early childhood. Some patients also exhibit muscle hypotonia and have reduced activity of phosphorylase kinase in muscle. This form of the phosphorylase kinase deficiency is caused by mutations in the β subunit of the gene located on chromosome 16q12-13.

Autosomal Liver Phosphorylase Kinase Deficiency. In contrast to the benign course of X-linked phosphorylase kinase deficiency, patients with autosomal recessive form of liver phosphorylase kinase deficiency have more severe phenotypes and often develop cirrhosis of the liver. This form of the phosphorylase kinase deficiency is due to mutations in the testis/liver isoform of the γ subunit of the gene located on chromosome 16p.

Muscle-Specific Phosphorylase Kinase Deficiency. Muscle-specific phosphorylase kinase deficiency causes cramps and myoglobinuria on exercise or progressive muscle weakness and atrophy. The activity of the enzyme is decreased in muscle but (when determined) normal in liver and blood cells. There is no hepatomegaly or cardiomegaly. The disorder could be due to mutation in the muscle isoform of the α subunit located on X chromosome.

Cardiac-Specific Phosphorylase Kinase Deficiency. Several sporadic cases with cardiac-specific phosphorylase kinase deficiency have been reported. All died during infancy from cardiac failure due to massive glycogen deposition in the myocardium. The molecular basis has not been defined.

Diagnosis

Definitive diagnosis of phosphorylase kinase deficiency requires demonstration of the enzymatic defect in affected tissues. Although phosphorylase kinase can be measured in leukocytes and erythrocytes, the enzyme has many tissue-specific isozymes, and the diagnosis can be missed without studies of the liver, muscle, or heart.

Treatment

The treatment for liver phosphorylase or phosphorylase kinase deficiency is based on symptoms. A high-carbohydrate diet and frequent feedings are effective in preventing hypoglycemia, but most patients require no specific treatment. Prognosis is usually good; adult patients have normal stature and minimal hepatomegaly. There is no treatment for the fatal form of isolated cardiac phosphorylase kinase deficiency.

Type 0 Glycogen Storage Disease (Glycogen Synthase Deficiency)

Strictly speaking, this is not a type of glycogen storage disease, as the deficiency of the enzyme leads to decreased glycogen stores. The patients present in early infancy with early-morning drowsiness and fatigue, and sometimes convulsions associated with hypoglycemia and hyperketonemia. There is no hepatomegaly or hyperlipidemia. Prolonged hyperglycemia and elevation of lactate with normal insulin levels after administration of glucose suggest a possible diagnosis of glycogen synthase deficiency. Definitive diagnosis requires a liver biopsy to measure the enzyme activity. Treatment is symptomatic and involves frequent feedings rich in protein and nighttime supplement with uncooked cornstarch to alleviate hypoglycemia. Prognosis seems good as patients survive to adulthood with resolution of hypoglycemia except during pregnancy. The liver glycogen synthase gene is located on chromosome 12p12.2. Mutations in this gene that cause glycogen synthase deficiency have been identified.

Type XI Glycogen Storage Disease (Hepatic Glycogenosis with Renal Fanconi Syndrome, Fanconi-Bickel Syndrome)

This rare autosomal recessive disease is caused by defects in the facilitative glucose transporter 2 (GLUT2), which transports glucose in and out of hepatocytes, pancreatic cells, and the basolateral membranes of intestinal and renal epithelial cells. The disease is characterized by proximal renal tubular dysfunction, impaired glucose and galactose utilization, and accumulation of glycogen in liver and kidney.

Clinical and Laboratory Findings

The affected child presents in the first year of life with failure to thrive, rickets, and a protuberant abdomen caused by hepato- and renomegaly. Laboratory findings include glucosuria, phosphaturia, generalized aminoaciduria, bicarbonate wasting, hypophosphatemia, increased serum alkaline phosphatase levels, and radiologic findings of rickets. Mild fasting hypoglycemia and hyperlipidemia may be present. Liver transaminases, plasma lactate, and uric acid concentrations are usually normal. Oral galactose or glucose tolerance tests show intolerance to these sugars, which could be explained by the functional loss of GLUT2 preventing liver uptake.

Tissue biopsies show marked accumulation of glycogen in hepatocytes and proximal renal tubular cells, presumably due to the altered glucose transport out of these organs.

Treatment

There is no specific therapy. Growth retardation persists through adulthood. Symptomatic replacement of water, electrolytes, and vitamin D; restriction of galactose intake; and a diabetes mellitus-like diet, presented in frequent and small meals with cornstarch supplement and an adequate caloric intake may improve growth.

Genetics

The low prevalence of Fanconi-Bickel syndrome (less than 100 cases reported worldwide) is underlined by the fact that consanguinity of the parents was found in 72% of reported families and in 70% of the cases with a detectable GLUT2 mutation. The gene for GLUT2 is located on chromosome 3q26, and most mutations detected so far predicted a premature termination of translation.

MUSCLE GLYCOGENOSES

The muscle glycogenoses can be separated into two categories: muscle energy impairment or myopathy of skeletal muscle with or without cardiac muscle involvement. The disorders that fall into the first category are (a) type V GSD (muscle phosphorylase deficiency), (b) type VII GSD (muscle phosphofructokinase deficiency), and (c) five other rare glycogenoses resulting from defects in terminal glycolysis. The inborn error resulting in the phenotype of skeletal and/or cardiac myopathy is type II GSD (Pompe disease). This glycogenosis is distinct from all others in that the enzyme that is deficient is not involved in the cytosolic metabolic pathways used to release glucose from glycogen. Rather, the deficient acid maltase enzyme is a lysosomal glycogenolytic enzyme.

Type V Glycogen Storage Disease (Muscle Phosphorylase Deficiency, or McArdle Disease)

Deficiency of muscle phosphorylase is the prototype muscle-energy disorder. Deficiency of this enzyme in muscle limits ATP generation by glycogenolysis and results in glycogen accumulation.

Clinical and Laboratory Findings

Symptoms usually develop first in adulthood and are characterized by exercise intolerance with muscle cramps. Two types of activity tend to cause symptoms: (a) brief exercise of great intensity, such as sprinting or carrying heavy loads, and (b) less intense but sustained activity, such as climbing stairs or walking uphill. Moderate exercise, such as walking on level ground, can be performed by most patients for long periods. Many patients experience a characteristic "second wind" phenomenon; if they rest briefly at the first appearance of muscle pain, they can resume exercise with more ease. About half report burgundy-colored urine after exercise, the consequence of myoglobinuria secondary to the rhabdomyolysis. Intense myoglobinuria after vigorous exercise may cause renal failure (see Sec. 21.4). Although most patients are diagnosed in the second or third decade, many report weakness and lack of endurance since childhood. In rare cases, EMG findings may suggest an inflammatory myopathy, and the diagnosis can be confused with polymyositis.

The level of serum creatine kinase is usually elevated at rest and increases more after exercise. Exercise also increases the levels of blood ammonia, inosine, hypoxanthine, and uric acid. The latter abnormalities are attributed to accelerated recycling of muscle purine nucleotides in the face of insufficient ATP production.

Clinical heterogeneity is not common, but late-onset disease with no symptoms as late as the eighth decade and an early-onset, fatal form with hypotonia, generalized muscle weakness, and progressive respiratory insufficiency have been reported.

Diagnosis

Lack of an increase in blood lactate levels and exaggerated blood ammonia elevations after an ischemic exercise test are indicative of muscle glycogenosis and suggest a defect in the conversion of glycogen or glucose to lactate. The abnormal exercise response, however, is not limited to type V disease and can occur with other defects in glycogenolysis or glycolysis, such as deficiencies of muscle phosphofructokinase or debranching enzyme (when the test is done after fasting). Definitive diagnosis is made by enzymatic assay in muscle tissue or by mutation analysis of the myophosphorylase gene.

Treatment

In general, avoidance of strenuous exercise can prevent the major attack of the rhabdomyolysis. Aerobic training, or oral administration of glucose or fructose, can augment exercise tolerance. A high-protein diet may increase exercise endurance in some patients. Longevity does not appear to be affected.

Genetics

Type V glycogen storage disease is an autosomal recessive disorder that does not appear to have ethnic predilection. The gene for muscle phosphorylase is located on chromosome 11q13. The most common mutation in North American patients is a nonsense mutation that changes an arginine to a stop at codon 49 (R49X), and the most common mutation in Japanese patients is deletion of a single codon (F708). This allows DNA-based diagnosis and carrier detection in these two populations.

Type VII Glycogen Storage Disease (Muscle Phosphofructokinase Deficiency, or Tarui Disease)

Type VII disease is caused by a deficiency of muscle phosphofructokinase, which catalyzes the conversion of fructose-6-phosphate to fructose-1, 6-diphosphate and is a key regulatory enzyme of glycolysis.

Phosphofructokinase is composed of three isozyme subunits (M, muscle; L, liver; and P, platelet), which are encoded by different genes and are differentially expressed in tissues. Skeletal muscle contains only M subunit isozymes, and red blood cells contain a hybrid of L and M forms. Type VII disease is due to defective M isoenzyme, which causes complete enzyme deficiency in muscle and partial deficiency in red blood cells.

Clinical and Laboratory Findings

The features are similar to those in type V disease, namely, early onset of fatigue and pain with exercise. Vigorous exercise causes severe muscle cramps and myoglobinuria. However, several features of type VII disease are distinctive: (a) Exercise intolerance is usually evident in childhood, is more severe than in type V disease, and may be associated with nausea and vomiting. (b) A compensated hemolysis occurs as evidenced by an increased level of serum bili-

rubin and reticulocyte count. (c) Hyperuricemia is common and becomes more marked after exercise. (d) An abnormal glycogen-resembling amylopectin is present in muscle fibers; it is periodic acid–Schiff-positive and resistant to diastase digestion. (e) Exercise intolerance is particularly acute following meals rich in carbohydrate because glucose cannot be utilized in muscle and because the ingested glucose inhibits lipolysis, thereby depriving muscle of fatty acid and ketone substrates. In contrast, patients with type V disease can metabolize glucose derived from either liver glycogenolysis or exogenous glucose. Indeed, glucose infusion improves exercise tolerance in type V patients.

Two rare type VII variants have been reported. One presents in infancy with hypotonia and limb weakness, and a rapidly progressive myopathy leads to death by age 4. The other presents in adults and is characterized by a slowly progressive, fixed muscle weakness rather than by cramps and myoglobinuria.

Diagnosis

The M isoenzyme defect must be demonstrated in muscle, red blood cells, or cultured skin fibroblasts by biochemical or histochemical techniques.

Treatment

There is no specific treatment. Avoidance of strenuous exercise prevents acute attacks of muscle cramps and myoglobinuria.

Genetics

Type VII glycogen storage disease is inherited as an autosomal recessive trait. The disease appears to be rare, and most reported patients are either Japanese or Ashkenazi Jews. The gene for the M isoenzyme is located on chromosome 12q13.3. In Ashkenazi Jews, 95% of mutant alleles are either a splicing defect or a nucleotide deletion.

Other Muscle Glycogenoses with Muscle-Energy Impairment

Five additional enzyme defects produce muscle glycogenoses, namely, deficiencies in phosphoglycerate kinase, phosphoglycerate mutase, lactate dehydrogenase, fructose 1,6-bisphosphate aldolase A, and pyruvate kinase. All five enzymes affect terminal glycolysis, and deficiency causes muscle-energy impairment similar to that in type V and VII disease. The failure of blood lactate to increase in response to exercise can be used to separate muscle glycogenoses from disorders of lipid metabolism, such as carnitine palmitoyl transferase II deficiency and very-long-chain acyl-coenzyme A dehydrogenase deficiency, which also cause muscle cramps and myoglobinuria. Muscle glycogen levels may be normal in the disorders affecting terminal glycolysis, and definitive diagnosis is made by assaying the enzymatic activity in muscle.

Glycogen Storage Disease Type II (Acid α-1,4-Glucosidase Deficiency, or Pompe Disease)

Glycogen storage disease type II is caused by a deficiency of lysosomal acid α-1,4-glucosidase (acid maltase), an enzyme responsible for the degradation of glycogen in lysosomal vacuoles. This disease is characterized by accumulation of glycogen in lysosomes as opposed to its accumulation in cytoplasm in the other glycogenoses.

Clinical and Laboratory Findings

The disorder encompasses a range of phenotypes, each including myopathy but differing in age of onset, organ involvement, and clinical severity. The most severe is the infantile-onset disease with cardiomegaly, hypotonia, and death prior to 1 year of age. Infants appear normal at birth but soon develop generalized muscle weakness with feeding difficulties, macroglossia, hepatomegaly, and congestive heart failure due to a hypertrophic cardiomyopathy. Electrocardiographic findings include high-voltage QRS complexes and a shortened PR interval. Death usually occurs from cardiorespiratory failure.

The juvenile or late-childhood form is characterized by skeletal muscle manifestations, usually without cardiac involvement, and a slowly progressive course. The juvenile form typically presents as delayed motor milestones (if age of onset is early enough) and difficulty in walking, and is followed by swallowing difficulties, proximal muscle weakness, and respiratory muscle involvement; it can cause death before the end of the second decade.

An adult form of type II disease presents as a slowly progressive myopathy without cardiac involvement and has its onset between the second and seventh decades. The clinical picture is dominated by slowly progressive proximal muscle weakness with truncal involvement and greater involvement of the lower than the upper limbs. Pelvic girdle, paraspinal muscle, and diaphragm are the most seriously affected. The initial symptoms may be respiratory insufficiency manifested by somnolence, morning headache, orthopnea, and exertional dyspnea.

Laboratory findings include elevated levels of serum creatine kinase, aspartate transaminase, and lactate dehydrogenase, particularly in infants. Muscle biopsy shows the presence of vacuoles that stain positively for glycogen, and muscle acid phosphatase is increased, presumably from a compensatory increase of lysosomal enzymes. Electron microscopy reveals the glycogen accumulation. EMG reveals myopathic features with irritability of muscle fibers and pseudomyotonic discharges. Serum creatine kinase concentration is not always elevated in adults, and, depending on the muscle biopsied or tested, muscle histology or EMG may not be abnormal. It is prudent to examine affected muscle.

Diagnosis

Diagnosis can be established by demonstration of absence or reduced levels of acid-glucosidase activity in muscle or cultured skin fibroblasts. Deficiency is usually more severe in the infantile form than in the juvenile and adult disorders.

Treatment

No effective treatment for the infantile form is currently available. Enzyme replacement is a promising therapy for this fatal lysosomal storage disease, and clinical trials are ongoing to test its safety and efficacy. A high-protein diet may be useful for the juvenile and adult forms. Nocturnal ventilatory support can improve the patient's quality of life.

Genetics

Pompe disease is an autosomal recessive disorder and does not appear to have an ethnic predilection. The gene for acid-glucosidase is on chromosome 17q25. A splice-site mutation (IVS1-13TG) is commonly seen in patients with adult-onset disease. Prenatal diagnosis using amniocytes or chorionic villi is available.

9.5.2 Disorders in Galactose Metabolism

GALACTOSE 1-PHOSPHATE URIDYL TRANSFERASE DEFICIENCY GALACTOSEMIA

"Classic" galactosemia is a serious disease with early onset of symptoms; the incidence is 1 in 60,000. The newborn infant normally receives up to 20% of caloric intake as lactose, which consists of glucose and galactose. Without the transferase the infant is unable to metabolize galactose 1-phosphate (see Fig. 9-12), the accumulation of which results in injury to parenchymal cells of the kidney, liver, and brain.

Clinical and Laboratory Findings

The diagnosis of uridyl transferase deficiency should be considered in newborn infants or older infants or children with any of these clinical manifestations: jaundice; hepatomegaly; vomiting; hypoglycemia; convulsions; lethargy; irritability; feeding difficulties; poor weight gain; aminoaciduria; cataracts; vitreous hemorrhage; hepatic cirrhosis; ascites; splenomegaly; or mental retardation. Patients with galactosemia are at increased risk for *E. coli* neonatal sepsis; the onset of sepsis often precedes the diagnosis of galactosemia. When the diagnosis is not made at birth, damage to the liver (cirrhosis) and brain (mental retardation) becomes increasingly severe and irreversible.

Diagnosis

The preliminary diagnosis of galactosemia is made by demonstrating a reducing substance in urine specimens collected while the patient is receiving human or cow's milk or another formula containing lactose. The reducing substance found in urine by Clinitest can be identified by chromatography or by an enzymatic test specific for galactose. Definitive diagnosis requires the demonstration of a deficient activity of galactose 1-phosphate uridyl transferase in erythrocytes or other tissues, which also exhibit increased concentrations of galactose 1-phosphate.

Treatment

Because of widespread newborn screening for galactosemia, patients are being identified early and treated early (see Sec. 8.2). Elimination of galactose from diet reverses growth failure and renal and hepatic dysfunctions. Cataracts regress, and most patients have no impairment of eyesight. Early diagnosis and treatment have improved the prognosis of galactosemia; on long-term follow-up, however, patients still manifest ovarian failure with primary or secondary amenorrhea, developmental delay, and learning disabilities, which increase in severity with age. In addition, most will manifest speech disorders, while a smaller number demonstrate poor growth and impaired motor function and balance (with or without overt ataxia). The relative control of galactose 1-phosphate levels does not always correlate with long-term outcome, leading to the belief that other factors, such as UDP-galactose deficiency (a donor for galactolipids and proteins), may be responsible.

Genetics

Transferase deficiency galactosemia is inherited as an autosomal recessive trait. There are several enzymatic variants of galactosemia. Duarte variant is the most common and has a carrier frequency of

12% in the general population. Individuals with Duarte variant homozygote have diminished red cell enzyme activity (50% of normal), but usually no clinical manifestations. Individuals with Duarte galactosemia (D/G) compound heterozygosity have 25% of the enzyme activity and galactose 1-phosphate levels are often elevated. These children are usually asymptomatic, but most physicians restrict lactose intake if the erythrocyte galactose 1-phosphate levels are elevated. Some African-American patients have milder symptoms despite absence of measurable transferase activity in erythrocytes; these patients retain 10% enzyme activity in liver and intestinal mucosa, while most white patients have no detectable activity in any of these tissues. The gene for galactose 1-phosphate uridyl transferase is located on chromosome 9p13. In African-Americans, 48% of alleles are represented by the S135L mutation; a mutation may be responsible for the milder disease. In the white population, 70% of alleles are represented by the Q188R missense mutation. Carrier testing and prenatal diagnosis can be carried out by direct enzyme analysis of amniocytes or chorionic villi. Also, testing can be DNA-based.

GALACTOKINASE DEFICIENCY

In contrast to the multiple systems that are affected in transferase-deficiency galactosemia, cataract is usually the sole manifestation of galactokinase deficiency. The affected infant is otherwise asymptomatic. These patients have an increased concentration of blood galactose levels with normal transferase activity and an absence of galactokinase activity in erythrocytes. Treatment is dietary restriction of galactose intake. The gene coding for galactokinase is located on chromosome 17q24. Mutations leading to galactokinase deficiency have been identified.

URIDINE DIPHOSPHATE GALACTOSE 4-EPIMERASE (UDP GAL 4-EPIMERASE) DEFICIENCY

The abnormally accumulated metabolites are very much like those seen in transferase deficiency; however, there is also an increase in cellular UDP-galactose. There are two distinct forms of epimerase deficiency. A benign form was discovered incidentally through a neonatal screening program. Affected persons in this case are healthy and without problems; the enzyme deficiency is limited to leukocytes and erythrocytes, without deranged metabolism in other tissues. No treatment is required. The second form of epimerase deficiency is severe, with clinical manifestations resemble transferase deficiency, and the additional symptoms of hypotonia and nerve deafness. The enzyme deficiency is generalized, and clinical symptoms respond to restriction of dietary galactose. Although this form of galactosemia is rare, it must be considered in a symptomatic patient who has normal transferase activity. The gene for epimerase is located on chromosome 1p35-36; mutations responsible for both forms of the epimerase deficiency have been identified.

9.5.3 Disorders in Fructose Metabolism

DEFICIENCY OF FRUCTOKINASE (BENIGN FRUCTOSURIA)

This condition is not associated with any clinical manifestations. It is an accidental finding usually made through the detection of fructose as the reducing substance in the urine. No treatment is necessary.

DEFICIENCY OF FRUCTOSE 1,6-BISPHOSPHATE ALDOLASE (ALDOLASE B, OR HEREDITARY FRUCTOSE INTOLERANCE)

This severe disease of infants, appearing with the ingestion of fructose-containing food, is caused by deficiency of fructose 1,6-bisphosphate aldolase B activity in the liver, kidney, and intestine. The enzyme catalyzes the hydrolysis of fructose 1-phosphate and fructose 1,6-bisphosphate into the 3-carbon sugars, dihydroxyacetone phosphate, glyceraldehyde 3-phosphate, and glyceraldehyde (see Fig. 9-12). Deficiency of this enzyme activity causes a rapid accumulation of fructose 1-phosphate and initiates severe toxic symptoms when exposed to fructose.

Clinical and Laboratory Findings

Patients with fructose intolerance are perfectly healthy and asymptomatic until fructose or sucrose (table sugar) is ingested (usually from fruit, fruit juice, or sweetened cereal). Clinical manifestations may resemble those of galactosemia and include jaundice, hepatomegaly, vomiting, lethargy, irritability, and convulsions. Laboratory findings include prolonged clotting time, hypoalbuminemia, elevation of bilirubin and liver transaminase levels, and proximal tubular dysfunction. If the disease is not diagnosed and intake of the noxious sugar persists, hypoglycemic episodes recur, and liver and kidney failure progress, eventually leading to death.

Diagnosis

Suspicion of the enzyme deficiency is fostered by the presence of a reducing substance in the urine during an attack. The diagnosis is supported by an intravenous fructose tolerance test that will cause a rapid fall, first of serum phosphate, then of blood glucose, and a subsequent rise of uric acid and magnesium concentrations. Oral-tolerance testing should not be done as patients may become acutely ill. Definitive diagnosis is made by assay of fructose 1,6-bisphosphate aldolase B activity in the liver.

Treatment

Treatment consists of the complete elimination of all sources of sucrose, fructose, and sorbitol from the diet. With treatment, liver and kidney dysfunction improve and catch-up growth is common. Intellectual development is usually unimpaired. As the patient matures, symptoms become milder even after fructose ingestion, and the long-term prognosis is good. Owing to dietary avoidance of sucrose, affected patients have few dental caries.

Genetics

The true incidence of hereditary fructose intolerance is not known but may be as high as 1 in 23,000. The gene for aldolase B is on chromosome 9q22.3. Several mutations causing hereditary fructose intolerance have been identified. A single missense mutation, a G to C transversion in exon 5, which results in the normal alanine at position 149 being replaced by a proline, is the most common mutation identified in northern Europeans. This mutation plus two other point mutations account for approximately 80 to 85% of hereditary fructose intolerance in Europe and the United States. Diagnosis of hereditary fructose intolerance can thus be made by screening of these mutations in the majority of patients. Prenatal diagnosis should be possible from both amniocentesis and chorionic villi, utilizing DNA mutational or linkage analysis.

9.5.4   Disorders of Gluconeogenesis

FRUCTOSE 1,6-DIPHOSPHATASE DEFICIENCY

Fructose 1,6-diphosphatase deficiency is a defect in gluconeogenesis. The disease is characterized by life-threatening episodes of acidosis, hypoglycemia, hyperventilation, convulsions, and coma. These episodes are triggered by a decrease in oral food intake during febrile illness or gastroenteritis. Laboratory findings include low blood glucose, high lactate and uric acid concentrations, and metabolic acidosis. In contrast to hereditary fructose intolerance, there is usually no aversion to sweets, and renal tubular and liver functions are normal. Treatment of acute attacks consists of correction of hypoglycemia and acidosis by IV infusion, and the response is usually rapid. Later, avoidance of fasting and elimination of fructose and sucrose from the diet prevent further episodes. For long-term prevention of hypoglycemia, a slowly released carbohydrate such as cornstarch is useful. Patients who survive childhood seem to develop normally.

Diagnosis

The diagnosis is established by demonstrating an enzyme deficiency in either the liver or an intestinal biopsy specimen. The enzyme defect may sometimes be demonstrated in leukocytes. The gene coding for fructose 1,6-diphosphatase is located on chromosome 9q22. In patients with known mutations, carrier detection and prenatal diagnosis are possible using the DNA-based test.

PHOSPHOENOLPYRUVATE CARBOXYKINASE (PEPCK) DEFICIENCY

PEPCK is a key enzyme in gluconeogenesis. It catalyzes the conversion of oxaloacetate to phosphoenolpyruvate. PEPCK deficiency has been described both as a mitochondrial and as a cytosolic enzyme deficiency. The disease has been reported rarely. The clinical features are heterogeneous, with hypoglycemia, lactic acidemia, hepatomegaly, hypotonia, developmental delay, and failure to thrive as the major manifestations. Hepatic and renal dysfunction may be present. The diagnosis is based on the reduced activity of PEPCK in liver, fibroblasts, or lymphocytes. Fibroblasts and lymphocytes are not suitable for diagnosing the cytosolic form of PEPCK deficiency because these tissues possess only mitochondrial PEPCK.

9.5.5   Disorder of Pentose Metabolism

Pentosuria is observed in normal individuals if the dietary pentose intake is increased, as with the excessive ingestion of fruit containing pentose. Under these circumstances there may be urinary excretion of xylose and arabinose up to 200 mg/24 h. Ribosuria (D-ribose) has been demonstrated in some patients with muscular dystrophy. The only condition in which excretion of pentose is marked is essential pentosuria.

ESSENTIAL BENIGN PENTOSURIA

This benign condition is characterized by a reducing substance in the urine of an otherwise healthy individual. Care should be taken not to mistake the reducing substance for glucose. The pentose in the urine reacts with Clinitest but not with glucose oxidase test papers.

L-Xylulose dehydrogenase converts L-xylulose (which can arise from D-glucuronate) to xylitol. Xylitol is converted to D-xylulose, which becomes D-xylulose-5-phosphate and enters the pentose phosphate shunt. Deficiency of this enzyme leads to increased concentration of L-xylulose in blood and urine. This rare defect is most common in Jews. No therapy is required.

References

Ali M, Rellos P, Cox TM: Hereditary fructose intolerance. J Med Genet 35:353–65, 1998

Bao Y, Kishnani P, Wu JY, et al: Hepatic and neuromuscular forms of glycogen storage disease type IV caused by mutation in the same glycogen branching enzyme gene. J Clin Invest 97:941, 1996

Chen Y-T, Burchell A: Glycogen storage diseases. In: Scriver CR, Beaudet AL, Sly WS, Valle D, eds: The Metabolic and Molecular Bases of Inherited Disease, 8th ed. New York, McGraw-Hill, 2001, pp 1521–1552

Chen Y-T, Cornblath M, Sidbury JB: Cornstarch therapy in type I glycogen storage disease. N Engl J Med 310:171, 1984

Daude N, Gallaher TK, Zeschnigk M, et al: Molecular cloning, characterization, and mapping of a full-length cDNA encoding human UDP-galactose 4-epimerase. Biochem Mol Med 56:1, 1995

DiMauro S, Bruno C: Glycogen storage disease of muscle. Curr Opin Neurol 11:477–84, 1998

Elpeleg ON: The molecular background of glycogen metabolism disorders. J Pediatr Endocrinol Metab 12:363–379, 1999

el-Schahawi M, Tsujino S, Shanske S, et al: Diagnosis of McArdle's disease by molecular genetic analysis of blood. Neurology 47:579, 1996

Fernandez J, Chen Y-T: The glycogen storage disease. In: Inborn Metabolic Disease: Diagnosis and Treatment, 2nd ed. Saudubray JM, Van Den Berghe G, eds: New York, Springer-Verlag, 1995: p 71–87

Gerin I, Veiga-da-Cunha M, Achouri Y, et al: Sequence of a putative glucose 6-phosphate translocase, mutated in glycogen storage disease type lb. FEBS Lett 419:235–238, 1997

Gitzelmann R, Steinmann B, Van Den Berghe G: Disorders of fructose metabolism. In: Scriver CR, Beaudet AL, Sly WS, Valle D, eds: The Metabolic and Molecular Bases of Inherited Disease, 8th ed. New York, McGraw-Hill, 2001: pp 1489–1520

Hendricks J, Dams E, Coucke P, et al: X-linked liver glycogenosis type II (XLG II) is caused by mutations in PHKA2, the gene encoding the liver alpha subunit of phosphorylase kinase. Hum Mol Genet 5:649, 1996

Hirschhorn R: Glycogen storage disease type II: acid α-glucosidase (acid maltase deficiency). In: Scriver CR, Beaudet AL, Sly WS, Valle D, eds: The Metabolic and Molecular Bases of Inherited Disease, 8th ed. New York, McGraw-Hill, 2001: pp 3389–3420

James CL, Rellos P, Ali M, et al: Neonatal screening for hereditary fructose intolerance: frequency of the most common mutant aldolase B allele (A149) in the British population. J Med Genet 33:837, 1996

Kikuchi T, Yang HW, Pennybacker M, et al: Clinical and metabolic correction of Pompe disease by enzyme therapy in acid maltase deficient quail. J Clin Invest 101:827–833, 1998

Kroos MA, Van der Kraan M, Van Diggelen OP, et al: Glycogen storage disease type II: frequency of three common mutant alleles and their associated clinical phenotypes studied in 121 patients. J Med Genet 32:836, 1995

Lai K, Langley SD, Singh RH, et al: A prevalent mutation for galactosemia among black Americans. J Pediatr 128:89, 1996

Lei K-J, Shelly LL, Pan C-J, Sidbury JB, et al: Mutations in the glucose 6-phosphatase gene that cause glycogen storage disease type Ia. Science 262:580, 1993

Maichele AJ, Burwinkel B, Maire I, et al: Mutations in the testis/liver isoform of the phosphorylase kinase γ subunit (PHKG2) cause autosomal liver glycogenosis in the gsd rat and in humans. Nat Genet 14:337, 1996

Ratner-Kaufman F, Reichardt JKV, Ng WG, et al: Correlation of cognitive, neurologic, and ovarian outcome with the Q188R mutation of the galactose-1-phosphate uridyltransferase gene. J Pediatr 125:225, 1994

Santer R, Schneppenheim R, Dombrowski A, et al: Mutations in *GLUT2*, the gene for the liver-type glucose transporter, in patients with Fanconi-Bickel syndrome. Nat Genet 17:324–326, 1997

Schweitzer S, Shin Y, Jakobs C, et al: Long-term outcome in 134 patients with galactosaemia. Eur J Pediatr 152:36, 1993

Segal S, Berry GT: Disorders of galactose metabolism. In: Scriver CR, Beaudet AL, Sly WS, Valle D, eds: The Metabolic and Molecular Bases of Inherited Disease, 8th ed. New York, McGraw-Hill, 2001: pp 1553–1588

Shen J-J, Bao Y, Liu H-M, et al: Mutations in exon 3 of the glycogen debranching enzyme gene are associated with glycogen storage disease type III that is differentially expressed in liver and muscle. J Clin Invest 98:352, 1996

Stambolian D, Ai Y, Sidjanin D, Nesburn K, et al: Cloning of the galactokinase cDNA and identification of mutations in two families with cataracts. Nat Genet 10:307, 1995

Tolan DR, Brooks CC: Molecular analysis of common aldolase B alleles for hereditary fructose intolerance in North Americans. Biochem Med Metab Biol 48:19, 1996

Van den Berg IET, Van Beurden EACM, Malingre HEM, et al: X-linked liver phosphorylase kinase deficiency is associated with mutations in the human liver phosphorylase kinase α subunit. Hum Mol Genet 3:1983, 1994

Veiga-da-Cunha M, Gerin I, Chen YT, et al: A gene on chromosome 11q23 coding for a putative glucose 6-phosphate translocase is mutated in glycogen storage disease type Ib and type Ic. Am J Hum Genet 63(4):976–983, 1998

Walter JH, Collins JE, Leonard JV, et al: Recommendations for the management of galactosemia. UK Galactosemia Steering Group. Arch Dis Child 80:93–96, 1999

Wolfsdorf JI, Crigler JF Jr: Effect of continuous glucose therapy begun in infancy on the long-term clinical course of patients with type I glycogen storage disease. J Pediatr Gastroenterol Nutr 29:136–148, 1999

9.6   METABOLIC LIVER DISEASE

Metabolic disorders affecting the liver are discussed in Chapter 18.

9.7   OXIDATIVE PHOSPHORYLATION DISEASES AND DISORDERS OF PYRUVATE OXIDATION

John M. Shoffner

The phenotypic spectrum of diseases of oxidative phosphorylation (OXPHOS) and disorders of pyruvate metabolism is very broad. For over three decades, the neuromuscular manifestations of OXPHOS diseases played an important role in formulating the criteria used by clinicians to diagnose the disease. Diagnosis depended on the recognition of characteristic phenotypes, the identification of histologic and ultrastructural abnormalities in skeletal muscle mitochondria, and the identification of abnormalities in OXPHOS

enzyme activities. Although the mitochondial DNA (mtDNA) encodes only 13 polypeptide subunits of the OXPHOS enzymes, there are more than 70 nuclear-encoded subunits and a much larger number of factors necessary for the assembly and maintenance of a functional respiratory chain. This degree of complexity makes the diagnosis of OXPHOS diseases a challenging process. Disorders of pyruvate metabolism are less commonly encountered than OXPHOS diseases. The clinical overlap between these two classes of disorders of cellular energetics is large, requiring a complex synthesis of clinical, biochemical, pathologic, and genetic information.

9.7.1   Biochemistry

Mitochondria are cytoplasmic structures of about 0.1 to 0.5 μm in diameter with an inner and outer membrane separated by an intermembrane space. The outer membrane is permeable to most small molecules and ions, and it contains a variety of proteins such as monoamine oxidase, long-chain acyl-CoA synthetase, carnitine palmitoyl transferase 1 (CPT1), and mitochondrial protein import proteins. The inner mitochondrial membrane is impermeable to most metabolites. It has a convoluted structure with multiple folds called *cristae*. The inner membrane has a high content of protein and cardiolipin. It contains the enzymes of oxidative phosphorylation, as well as multiple classes of translocases. The space surrounded by the inner mitochondrial membrane, called the *mitochondrial matrix*, contains an array of enzymes including those for the Krebs cycle (tricarboxylic acid cycle); the pyruvate dehydrogenase complex (PDC); β-oxidation of fatty acids; urea cycle; ketone metabolism; amino acid metabolism; heme metabolism; nucleotide metabolism; and the peptidases plus chaperonins necessary for mitochondrial protein import and OXPHOS enzyme assembly and maintenance. The matrix also contains mitochondrial DNA.

Pyruvate is the product of glycolysis, an extramitochondrial process (Fig. 9-12). After it is formed in the cytosol, pyruvate has a variety of possible metabolic fates, depending on cellular energetics requirements (see Fig. 9-13). When anaerobic metabolism predominates, pyruvate can be reduced to lactate by lactate dehydrogenase or transaminated to alanine by alanine aminotransferase. In the fasting state, pyruvate is used to maintain blood glucose by conversion to phosphoenolpyruvate by the hepatic enzymes

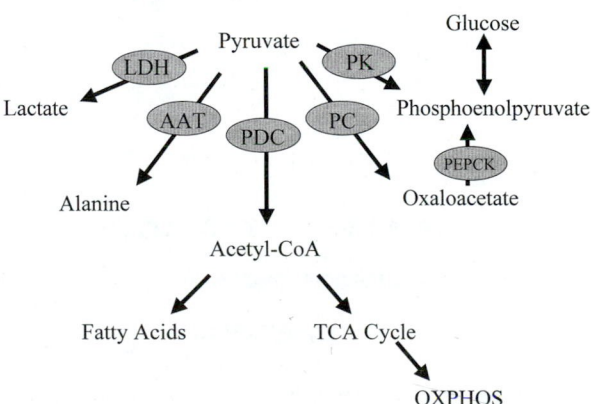

FIGURE 9-13   Metabolic alternatives for pyruvate. Depending on metabolic demands, pyruvate can be converted to lactate, alanine, acetyl CoA, oxaloacetate, or phosphoenolpyruvate. LDH = lactate dehydrogenase; AAT = alanine aminotransferase; PDC = pyruvate dehydrogenase complex; PC = pyruvate carboxylase; PK = pyruvate kinase; PEPCK = phosphoenolpyruvate carboxykinase.

pyruvate carboxylase and phosphoenolpyruvate carboxykinase. During aerobic metabolism, pyruvate is used by the PDC, the citric acid cycle, and OXPHOS to maintain adequate production of cellular ATP.

The PDC is responsible for converting pyruvate to acetyl-CoA, which can then enter the citric acid cycle (Fig. 9-14). The PDC consists of three enzymes: pyruvate dehydrogenase (two E1α and two E1β subunits), dihydrolipoamide acetyltransferase (E2 monomer), and dihydrolipoamide dehydrogenase (E3 homodimer). The E3 component is also found in two other multienzyme complexes: α-ketoacid dehydrogenase and branched-chain α-ketoacid dehydrogenase. Two regulatory components are also part of PDC and alter pyruvate metabolism by inactivation of PDC through dephosphorylation (E1-specific kinase) or by activation of PDC through phosphorylation (phospho-E1 phosphatase). A lipoyl-containing component designated protein X is an integral part of PDC, but its precise function is unclear. Product inhibition of PDC activity by NADH and acetyl-CoA are also important regulatory mechanisms.

OXPHOS uses about 95% of the oxygen delivered to tissues, producing most of the ATP that is required by cells. The expression of the genes involved in the OXPHOS pathway and the assembly of the five OXPHOS enzyme complexes (Complex I to Complex V) into the inner mitochondrial membrane is a highly ordered and coordinated process that depends on gene expression from the mitochondrial DNA, as well as from the nuclear DNA. The mtDNA is a 16,569-nucleotide pair, double-stranded, circular molecule that codes for 2 ribosomal RNAs (rRNA), 22 transfer RNAs (tRNA), and 13 polypeptides that are integral components of the enzyme complexes that constitute the mitochondrial respiratory chain. A much larger number of proteins (perhaps hundreds) are estimated

to be necessary for proper OXPHOS function and are encoded by nuclear DNA genes. OXPHOS enzymes are located in the mitochondrial inner membrane. As shown in Fig. 9-14, the OXPHOS enzymes are designated as Complex I (NADH:ubiquinone oxidoreductase, EC 1.6.5.3), Complex II (succinate:ubiquinone oxidoreductase, EC 1.3.5.1), Complex III (ubiquinol:ferrocytochrome c oxidoreductase, EC 1.10.2.2), Complex IV (ferrocytochrome c: oxygen oxidoreductase or cytochrome c oxidase, EC 1.9.3.1), and Complex V (ATP synthase, EC 3.6.1.34). Complex I transfers electrons to ubiquinone (coenzyme Q_{10}) through a long series of redox groups that include flavin mononucleotide (FMN) and six iron-sulfur clusters. This large and fragile enzyme is composed of approximately 43 subunits—7 encoded by mtDNA and 36 encoded by nuclear DNA. Complex II performs a key step in the citric acid cycle in which succinate is dehydrogenated to fumarate and the electrons are donated to ubiquinone in the mitochondrial inner membrane. It is localized to the matrix side of the mitochondrial inner membrane and is the only OXPHOS enzyme in which all subunits are coded by nuclear DNA. Complex III catalyzes electron transfer between two mobile electron carriers, ubiquinol and cytochrome c, and also translocates protons across the mitochondrial inner membrane. This enzyme is composed of 11 polypeptides, only 1 of which is encoded by mtDNA. Complex IV, or cytochrome c oxidase, is the terminal enzyme complex of the electron transport chain. It collects electrons transferred from reduced cytochrome c and donates them to oxygen, which is then reduced to water. In conjunction with this process, protons are pumped across the mitochondrial inner membrane into the intermembrane space. Mammalian Complex IV is composed of 13 polypeptide subunits, 3 of which are encoded by mtDNA. Complex V uses the electrochemical gradient created by Complexes I, III, and IV as a source of energy for synthesizing ATP from ADP + P_i. This enzyme is composed of two parts, the F_1 segment, which catalyzes ATP synthesis, and the F_0 segment which translocates protons into the mitochondrial matrix. It is composed of 12 to 13 subunits, 2 encoded by mtDNA (ATPase 6 and 8 genes) and 11 to 12 subunits encoded by nuclear DNA. The synthesis of ATP by Complex V is functionally coupled to electron transport through Complexes I, III, IV, and the reduction of oxygen. In coupled mitochondria, electron transport and oxygen consumption increase when ADP is available, and decline to a minimum constant level when ADP is limiting.

The transmission of mtDNA in mammals is, as far as is known, strictly maternal (see Chapter 10). Thus, in humans, transmission of mtDNA mutations is expected to occur exclusively along maternal lineages. When a pathogenic mtDNA mutation is present, the consequences of maternal transmission are influenced by whether the mtDNA is homoplasmic (all mtDNAs share the same sequence) or heteroplasmic (different sequence variants coexist). As the majority of pathogenic mutations are heteroplasmic it is important to understand the transmission genetics of mtDNA sequence variants. Although oocytes contain about 100,000 copies of mtDNA, rapid shifts in the proportion of mutant mtDNAs have been observed between generations. This is the result of a genetic bottleneck for mtDNA in early oogenesis. The practical consequence of this phenomenon is that the risk of having affected offspring is not trivial at any degree of heteroplasmy.

When heteroplasmy exists in somatic cells, the normal and mutant mtDNAs segregate randomly during cytokinesis to the daughter cells. The rate of replicative segregation is faster than expected because the replication of mtDNA is not tied to the cell cycle. Thus mtDNA templates can replicate more than once or not at all during the cell cycle. After the mutant mtDNAs reach a critical level, the

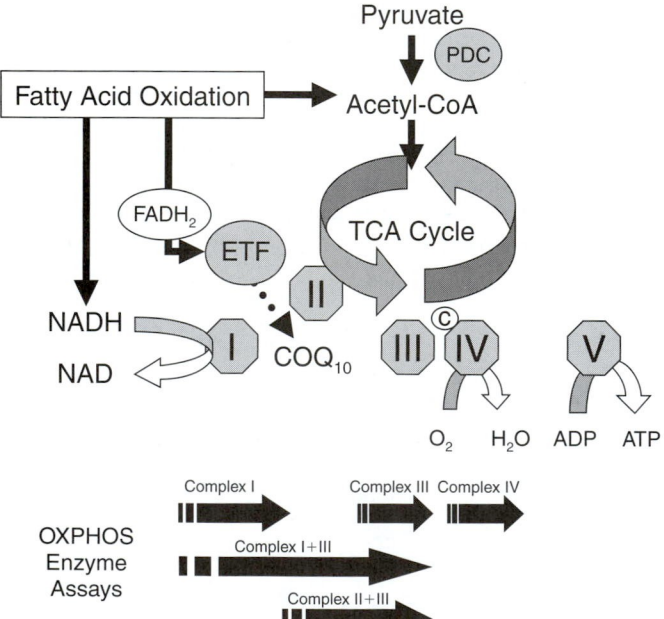

FIGURE 9-14   Pyruvate metabolism, oxidative phosphorylation, tricarboxylic acid cycle, and fatty acid oxidation. Due to the close interrelationship among these pathways, primary abnormalities in OXPHOS or pyruvate metabolism may cause a variety of metabolic abnormalities. Common enzyme assays used to assess OXPHOS are listed. Arrows indicate the flow of electrons through the enzyme assays (Complex I, Complex I+III, Complex II+III, Complex III, and Complex IV).

cellular phenotype changes rapidly from normal to abnormal. The relationship between genotype and phenotype is more complex for pathogenic mtDNA mutations that are homoplasmic. Disease expression appears to be influenced by poorly understood genetic and environmental interactions.

9.7.2 Algorithm for Patient Diagnosis

OXPHOS defects can result from mutations in any of the mitochondrial genes or in any of the nuclear OXPHOS genes. Because the genes for OXPHOS are located in two distinct genomes, the inheritance of OXPHOS diseases can be either maternal, mendelian (autosomal dominant, autosomal recessive, X-linked), or sporadic. Pyruvate metabolism disorders demonstrate X-linked or autosomal recessive inheritance patterns as well as sporadic mutations. In most patients considered to have sporadic mutations, germ cell line mosaicism is difficult to exclude. The basic elements of the algorithm are (a) phenotype recognition, (b) metabolic testing, (c) assessment for skeletal muscle pathology, (d) enzymology, and (e) genetic testing (Fig. 9-15).

PHENOTYPE RECOGNITION

Because of the large number of phenotypes that are described, phenotype recognition can be difficult. Tables 9-15 and 9-16 outline major classes of phenotype-genotype associations in patients with OXPHOS diseases and pyruvate metabolism disorders.

METABOLIC TESTING

In general, a urine sample is best for assessment of organic acids and blood is best for assessment of amino acids. A 24-hour urine collection is useful because it can provide an integrated evaluation of organic and amino acids as well as insight into the function of proximal renal tubules, which are highly OXPHOS-dependent. Although this is easily accomplished in adults, a 24-hour urine collection is difficult in pediatric patients, thus, spot urine collection may be used. Analysis of organic and amino acids in venous blood can be complicated by technical factors such as duration of tourniquet application, activity such as recent seizures or vigorous crying and struggling that occurs in some children during venipuncture, and delays in sample processing. In addition, lactate and pyruvate quantitation in blood and in cerebrospinal fluid (CSF) is more accurate when assessed by enzymatic techniques rather than by chromatographic techniques due to alterations of the lactate and pyruvate levels that can be introduced by the preparation process. In rare patients, the metabolic abnormalities are evident only in CSF.

Abnormalities in oxidative phosphorylation can produce identifiable defects in related metabolic pathways such as glycolysis, py-

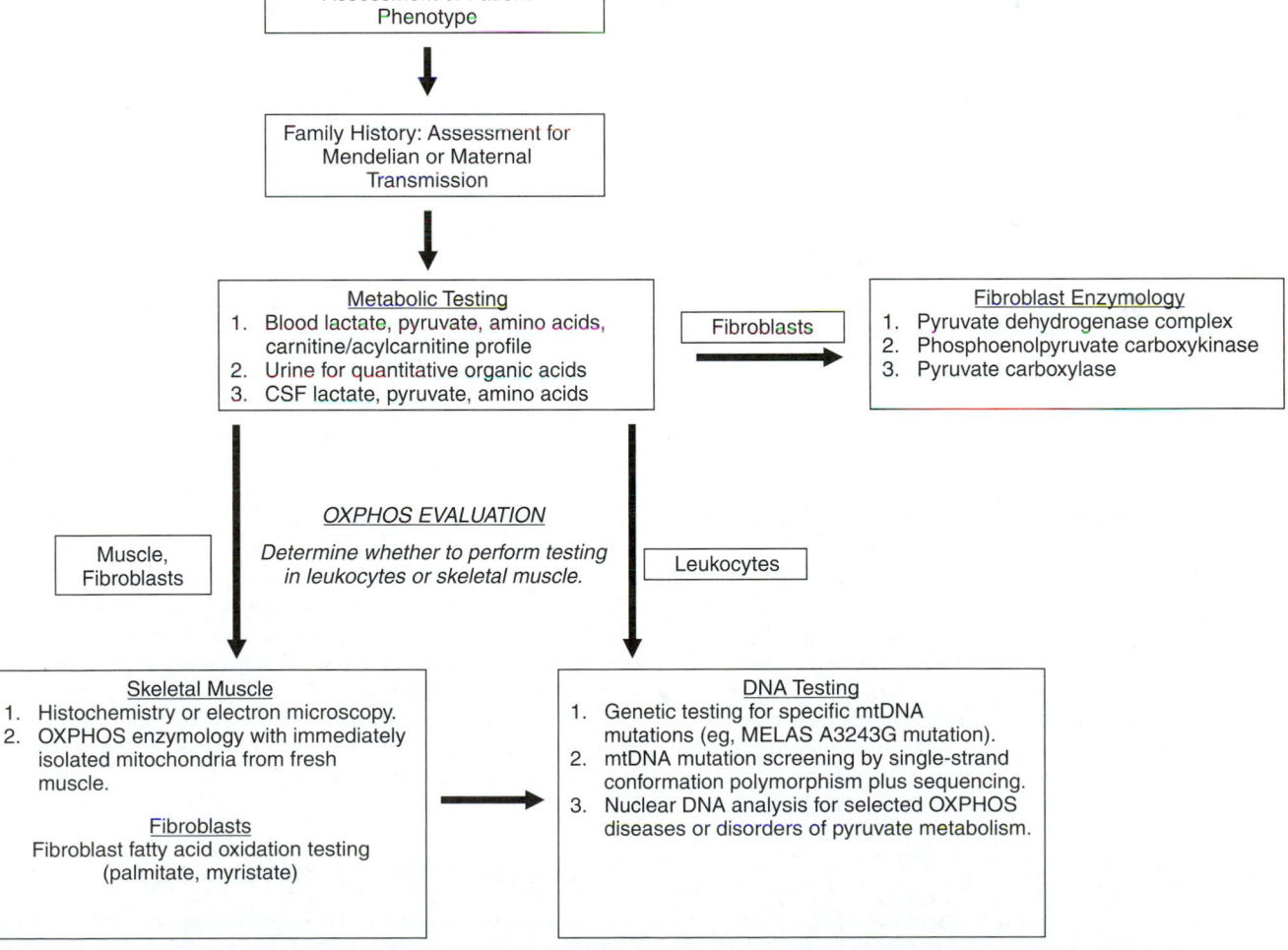

FIGURE 9-15 Diagnostic algorithm for assessment of oxidative phosphorylation diseases and disorders of pyruvate metabolism.

TABLE 9-15

THE MOST COMMON OXPHOS DISEASES CAUSED BY mtDNA GENE MUTATIONS

DISEASE	MANIFESTATIONS	GENETIC DIAGNOSIS
Kearns-Sayre syndrome and chronic progressive external ophthalmoplegias	**Common manifestations** CPEO or KSS; ragged-red fiber myopathy; cardiomyopathy; cardiac conduction defects; sensorineural hearing loss; pigmentary retinopathy; gastrointestinal motility dysfunction; seizures; diabetes mellitus; peripheral neuropathy; ataxia; lactic acidemia; short stature; gastrointestinal dysmotility; failure to thrive **Uncommon manifestations and reported associations** Hypoparathyroidism; MELAS; pernicious anemia; Pearson syndrome; choroideremia-like fundus; anhydrosis; oculocerebrorenal syndrome (Lowe syndrome); de Toni-Fanconi syndrome; Bartter syndrome; Leigh disease; hypogonadotropic hypogonadism; adrenal insufficiency; cataracts; leukodystrophy; glomuerulosclerosis and renal failure; Wolfram syndrome	mtDNA Southern blot and/or long-range PCR for single (clonal) mtDNA deletions/duplications. Most cases are sporadic. Rare cases are maternally transmitted.
Mitochondrial encephalomyopathy, lactic acidosis, and stroke-like episodes (MELAS)	**Common manifestations** Stroke; migraine headaches; retinitis pigmentosa; optic atrophy; sensorineural deafness; ragged-red fiber myopathy; diabetes mellitus; cardiomyopathy and conduction blocks; ophthalmoplegia; seizures; mental retardation; gastrointestinal dysmotility; failure to thrive; ataxia; lactic acidemia **Uncommon manifestations and reported associations** Renal failure; cataracts; supranuclear ophthalmoplegia; Leigh disease; myoclonic epilepsy; hypothalamic hypogonadism; pancreas exocrine dysfunction; diabetic embryopathy; VACTERL (vertebral, anal, cardiovascular, tracheoesophageal, renal, limb defects); demyelinating polyneuropathy; cerebral calcifications	mtDNA point mutation analysis for the tRNA$^{Leucine(UUR)}$ A3243G and tRNA$^{Leucine(UUR)}$ A3271C mutations
Myoclonic epilepsy and ragged-red fiber myopathy (MERRF)	**Common manifestations** Myoclonic epilepsy; generalized seizures; deafness; ataxia; ragged-red fiber myopathy; lactic acidemia; optic atrophy; dementia; mental retardation **Uncommon manifestations and reported associations** Leigh disease; dystonia; multiple symmetric lipomatosis; ophthalmoplegia; MELAS; atypical Charcot-Marie-Tooth presentation; retinitis pigmentosa	mtDNA point mutation analysis for the tRNA^{Lysine} A8344G and tRNA^{Lysine} T8356G mutations
Neurogenic muscle atrophy and retinitis pigmentosa (NARP) and Leigh disease	**Common manifestations** Neuropathy; ataxia; developmental delay; mental retardation; Leigh disease; retinitis pigmentosa; lactic acidemia	mtDNA point mutation analysis for the ATP6 T8993G and ATP6 T8993C mutations

ruvate metabolism, the tricarboxylic acid cycle, protein catabolism, and fatty acid oxidation. Traditional explanations of the effects of OXPHOS defects on lactate levels hold that the OXPHOS defects alter the cellular redox potential (increased NADH/NAD$^+$ ratio). Accumulation of NADH inhibits the pyruvate dehydrogenase complex, which leads to a decrease in pyruvate oxidation. The increase in pyruvate shifts the lactate dehydrogenase equilibrium in favor of lactate formation (see Fig. 9-12). Although the quantitation of organic acids and amino acids in blood, urine, and cerebrospinal fluid can provide useful diagnostic information, normal values for metabolic tests are common in patients with OXPHOS diseases and do not exclude the diagnosis. Metabolic acidosis, as well as elevations of lactate, pyruvate, lactate/pyruvate ratio (>20), alanine, tricarboxylic acid cycle intermediates, dicarboxylic acids, and/or a generalized aminoaciduria, can be important diagnostic clues to the presence of an OXPHOS disease. Other metabolites that may also be increased are tiglylglycine, ethylmalonic acid, 3-methylglutaconic acid, 2-ethylhydracrylic acid, 2-methylsuccinate, butyrylgly-

cine, isovaleryl glycine, and ammonia. Excretion of carnitine esters may be associated with reduced blood and tissue carnitine levels.

Similar abnormalities may be observed in patients with disorders of pyruvate metabolism. Urine organic acid analysis can demonstrate increases in lactate, pyruvate, β-hydroxybutyrate, α-hydroxyvalerate, and α-ketoglutarate. A normal lactate/pyruvate ratio is often used by clinicians to distinguish patients with OXPHOS defects from patients with pyruvate metabolism disorders. As more has been learned about these disorders, it is clear that lactate/pyruvate ratios are not very sensitive for discriminating these disorders.

SKELETAL MUSCLE PATHOLOGY

Most patients who are suspected of having an OXPHOS disease require a muscle biopsy. The primary goals of the muscle biopsy are (a) to assess the muscle for other diseases; (b) to isolate mitochondria for biochemical testing; (c) to isolate DNA for testing;

TABLE 9-16

OXPHOS DISEASES CAUSED BY NUCLEAR GENE MUTATIONS

DISEASE	MANIFESTATIONS	GENETIC DIAGNOSIS
Autosomal dominant progressive ophthalmoplegia and Kearns-Sayre syndrome	**Common manifestations** CPEO or KSS; ragged-red fiber myopathy; cardiomyopathy; sensorineural hearing loss; pigmentary retinopathy; gastrointestinal motility dysfunction; diabetes mellitus; peripheral neuropathy; ataxia; lactic acidemia; elevated CSF protein **Uncommon manifestations and reported associations** Hypogonadism; multiple symmetric lipomatosis; myoclonic epilepsy; Leigh disease; rhabdomyolysis; hyperthermia; Brachmann-de Lange syndrome; subacute-onset flaccid tetraplegia; alcohol intolerance; periodic paralysis; parkinsonism; leukoencephalopathy; male infertility; polymyalgia rheumatica; multiple sclerosis variant; chronic fatigue syndrome	mtDNA Southern blot and/or long-range PCR for multiple mtDNA deletions; although deletions are apparent in the mtDNA, the identity of the nuclear gene lesion is unknown
Autosomal recessive CPEO	**Common manifestations** Similar manifestations as the autosomal dominant patients; rare cause for CPEO **Uncommon manifestations:** Wolfram syndrome; Pearson syndrome	Same
Autosomal recessive myoneurogastrointestinal encephalopathy	**Common manifestations** CPEO; dementia; progressive leukodystrophy; ragged-red fiber myopathy; peripheral neuropathy; prominent gastrointestinal mobility abnormalities; lactic acidemia; elevated CSF protein	mtDNA Southern blot; long-range PCR for multiple mtDNA deletions; mutation analysis of the thymidine phosphorylase gene
Autosomal recessive mtDNA depletion diseases	**Common manifestations** Ragged-red fiber myopathy; hepatopathy; liver failure; hypoketotic hypoglycemia; lactic acidemia; fatal infantile encephalomyopathy; psychomotor delay; Leigh disease **Uncommon manifestations and reported associations** Alpers disease; nephropathy; cataracts; spinal muscular atrophy	mtDNA Southern blot to detect mtDNA depletion; quantitative PCR and in situ hybridization of muscle mtDNA may be helpful in some cases
Leigh disease (autosomal recessive)	**Common manifestations** Bilateral basal ganglia lesions (increased signal with T_2-weighted MRI images); optic atrophy; ophthalmoplegia; nystagmus; respiratory failure; ataxia; hypotonia; spasticity; developmental delay or regression; myopathy; abrupt deterioration with viral or bacterial infections; variable degrees of lactic acidemia; Complex I and Complex IV defects **Uncommon manifestations and reported associations** Hepatopathy; cardiomyopathy; Alexander disease	OXPHOS enzymology is central to the diagnosis due to the molecular heterogeneity. OXPHOS genes: succinate dehydrogenase (flavoprotein subunit); Complex I (NDUFS4 subunit); Complex I (NDUSF8 subunit); Complex I (NDUFV1 subunit); SURF1. Pyruvate metabolism genes: pyruvate dehydrogenase
Friedreich ataxia (autosomal recessive)	**Common manifestations** Ataxia; nystagmus; vibratory and proprioceptive sensation loss; corticospinal tract dysfunction; cardiomyopathy; diabetes mellitus **Uncommon manifestations and reported associations** Psychiatric syndromes, mental retardation	Genetic testing for trinucleotide repeat (GAA) expansion in the frataxin gene(first intron)
Autosomal recessive spastic paraplegia with ragged-red fibers	**Common manifestations** Weakness; spasticity; decreased vibratory sensation **Uncommon manifestations and reported associations** Dysphagia; scoliosis; optic nerve atrophy	Muscle biopsy demonstrating ragged-red fibers; genetic testing of the paraplegin gene
Barth syndrome (X-linked)	**Common manifestations** Congenital dilated cardiomyopathy; endocardial fibroelastosis; mitochondrial myopathy; growth retardation; decreased free and muscle carnitine level; increased urinary 3-methylglutaconic acid and 2-ethylhydracrylic acid; variable OXPHOS defects **Uncommon manifestations and reported associations** Mental retardation	Cardiac biopsy or muscle demonstrating abnormal mitochondria; OXPHOS biochemistry; genetic testing of the tafazzin gene (G4.5)

CPEO = chronic progressive external ophthalmoplegias; CSF = cerebral spinal fluid; KSS = Kearns-Sayre syndrome.

(d) to look for pathologic changes in the muscle such as fibrosis and inflammation that would produce secondary abnormalities in the muscle biochemistry; and (e) to search for histochemical and ultrastructural changes that support the presence of an OXPHOS disease.

There are only a few histochemical changes that are predictive of the presence of an OXPHOS disease: (a) ragged-red fibers; (b) abnormal succinate dehydrogenase reactions; and (c) cytochrome c oxidase–deficient fibers. Ragged-red fibers are characterized by large proliferations of subsarcolemmal mitochondria and replacement of some of the contractile elements with intermyofibrillar accumulations of mitochondria. They appear red as detected by Gomori-trichrome staining, and have a moth-eaten appearance due to the loss of some of the contracile elements. The percentage of ragged-red fibers shows large interindividual variability, ranging from approximately 2% to 70% of the total fibers. Ragged-red fibers also have mild accumulations of glycogen and neutral lipid. Pathologic alterations are segmental and do not extend the length of the myofiber, thus emphasizing the heterogeneous nature of the skeletal muscle manifestations. The abnormal myofiber segments can have sharp boundaries as in Kearns-Sayre and chronic progressive external ophthalmoplegia syndromes or be somewhat diffuse. Ragged-red fibers usually show increased reactivity for succinate dehydrogenase (which is a more sensitive indicator of mitochondrial proliferation than the Gomori-trichrome stain) and a decreased activity for cytochrome c oxidase (COX) reaction (COX-negative or COX-deficient fibers). Frequently, the number of COX-negative or COX-deficient fibers are larger than the number of ragged-red fibers, suggesting that the biochemical abnormality is a prerequisite for the morphologic abnormality. These changes are observed in a wide variety of oxidative phosphorylation diseases, including mtDNA depletion, mtDNA deletions, and mitochondrial transfer RNA mutations. The mitochondrial transfer RNA A3243G mutation in the tRNA$^{Leucine(UUR)}$ gene is an important exception to this pattern of histopathology. This mutation is the most common cause for mitochondrial encephalomyopathy, lactic acidosis, and stroke-like episodes (MELAS). In many patients, the ragged-red fibers may be COX deficient or show a positive COX reaction. In addition, the blood vessels characteristically show an increased succinate dehydrogenase reaction. COX-deficient fibers, increased succinate dehydrogenase reaction, and ragged-red fibers may be observed in a variety of conditions, including normal aging; zidovudine myopathy; myotonic dystrophy; limb-girdle dystrophy; inclusion body myositis; inflammatory myopathies; and nemaline myopathy.

Electron microscopy of muscle from most patients with OXPHOS diseases will show only nonspecific changes. Mitochondria may be pleomorphic and show variable degrees of intramyofibrillar and subsarcolemmal accumulation. However, in some patients, the ultrastructural analysis of the muscle can be important and may reveal structurally abnormal mitochondria with paracrystalline inclusions, which are intermembranous condensations of mitochondrial creatine kinase and possibly other mitochondrial proteins. When this ultrastructural abnormality is found in conjunction with ragged-red fibers, increases in succinate dehydrogenase reactivity, and cytochrome c oxidase–deficient fibers, the presence of a mtDNA mutation that impairs mitochondrial protein synthesis, such as a mtDNA deletion, mtDNA depletion, or a mitochondrial transfer RNA point mutation, is highly likely. This can be important in focusing the genetic testing.

Unfortunately, most patients with OXPHOS diseases do not show any of the above characteristic muscle changes. The muscle

pathology may show neurogenic changes; internal nuclei; fiber splitting; myofiber hypertrophy or hypotrophy involving either type I or type II fibers; accumulations of lipid; or mild increases in glycogen. In some individuals, the muscle histology may even be normal. Patients with OXPHOS defects (mtDNA or nuclear DNA) do not usually display dystrophic changes in muscle such as increased connective tissue or significant myonecrosis. This observation can be important in distinguishing patients with OXPHOS diseases from other classes of neuromuscular diseases (see Chapters 10 and 25).

The muscle pathology from patients with pyruvate metabolism disorders is nonspecific. Although the biochemical defect is expressed in muscle, the histology is normal or may show nondiagnostic changes such as accumulation of neutral lipid or evidence of mild denervation.

ENZYMOLOGY

The presence of an OXPHOS disease or of a pyruvate metabolism disorder can be confirmed by enzymology. To perform accurate assessments of this OXPHOS, immediate isolation of mitochondria from fresh muscle biopsies is helpful. This approach avoids artifacts in OXPHOS enzyme analysis that are associated with freezing the biopsy prior to mitochondrial isolation. Although it is now possible to achieve a precise diagnosis of certain OXPHOS diseases by DNA analysis alone, particularly when the syndrome is clinically evident, OXPHOS enzymology is necessary for diagnosis of the majority of cases. To determine the specific activities of OXPHOS enzymes, Complex I, Complex III, and Complex IV assays are used to assess electron flow across single OXPHOS complexes and the Complex I+III and Complex II+III assays assess the movement of electrons between complexes (see Fig. 9-14). The specificity of these assays is demonstrated by using respiratory inhibitors.

Due to the complexities associated with the measurement of respiratory chain enzyme activities, corroborative data can be sought by testing for abnormalities in skin fibroblast β-oxidation. β-Oxidation of substrates such as palmitate ($C_{16:0}$) and myristate ($C_{14:0}$) is often reduced in patients with OXPHOS defects. In our experience, β-oxidation defects (reduced palmitate and myristate oxidation rates) were observed in about 24% of fibroblast cultures from patients who had skeletal muscle OXPHOS defects, most commonly Complex I defects. OXPHOS defects, particularly those involving Complex I, reduce the oxidation of palmitate and myristate to levels that are approximately 40 to 60% of the control mean. This contrasts with diseases, such as carnitine palmitoyl transferase deficiency and medium-chain acyl-CoA dehydrogenase deficiency, which reduce the oxidation of these fatty acids to <10% and <20% of the control means, respectively (see Sec. 9.4). Assessment of long-chain fatty acid oxidation by the trifunctional protein is normal in patients who harbor OXPHOS defects.

The enzymologic analysis of pyruvate metabolism disorders can be complex. In most patients who have pyruvate dehydrogenase complex (PDC) defects, or defects in other enzymes of pyruvate metabolism, the enzymologic defect is present in essentially all tissues. However, due to lability of some of the enzymes, the analysis of enzyme activity in cultured fibroblasts is the best approach for diagnosis. In a few cases of PDC deficiency, the defect was not evident in cultured fibroblasts, possibly due to tissue-specific disease expression. For this reason, muscle is frozen in liquid nitrogen at the time of biopsy and stored at −80°C. If the fibroblast enzymology is normal and a PDC defect is still suspected, the muscle can be used for further investigations. Immunoblot analysis of PDC also may be useful in characterizing the defect, particularly in patients who have defects of the E1 enzyme.

GENETIC TESTING

At the time of muscle biopsy, a small portion of the biopsy is frozen in liquid nitrogen for DNA isolation. The integrated clinical-genetic, metabolic, and biochemical-genetic protocol increases the probability of reaching the correct biochemical and genetic diagnosis that is necessary for accurate genetic counseling and effective patient management. Although a large number of mtDNA mutations are known, most are private or semiprivate mutations (ie, occurring in relatively few families). If one of the known mtDNA mutations is not found in a proband, then it can be useful to exclude a mtDNA mutation. This can be done with a comprehensive analysis of mtDNA by single-strand conformation polymorphism (SSCP) and DNA sequencing. This is a highly accurate approach to mutation detection. Similar approaches can be used for genetic assessment of pyruvate metabolism disorders.

9.7.3   Mitochondrial DNA Mutations: Frequently Encountered Oxphos Diseases (see Table 9-15)

Three classes of pathogenic mtDNA mutations exist: (a) mtDNA rearrangements in which mtDNA genes are deleted or duplicated; (b) mtDNA point mutations in tRNA or ribosomal RNA genes resulting in defects in mitochondrial protein synthesis; and (c) missense mutations that change an amino acid, thus altering a critical function of an OXPHOS polypeptide.

KEARNS-SAYRE AND CHRONIC PROGRESSIVE EXTERNAL OPHTHALMOPLEGIA (CPEO) SYNDROMES

Ptosis, ophthalmoplegia, and a ragged-red fiber myopathy represent a clinical triad that is highly predictive for the presence of a mtDNA mutation. Patients with these manifestations can be classified into one of three groups according to their age of onset and the severity of their clinical symptoms. The most severe variant is the Kearns-Sayre syndrome, which is characterized by infantile, childhood, or adolescent onset of disease manifestations and significant multisystem involvement that can include cardiac abnormalities (cardiomyopathies and cardiac conduction defects), diabetes mellitus, cerebellar ataxia, deafness, and evidence of multifocal neurodegeneration. Some patients present in infancy with an atypical variant called Pearson syndrome; they manifest anemia, leukopenia, and thrombocytopenia, requiring frequent transfusions (see Chapter 19). Exocrine pancreatic dysfunction is an important manifestation of this disease. Patients with Pearson syndrome may have severe systemic manifestations or may be oligosymptomatic. However, if patients survive infancy and early childhood, Kearns-Sayre syndrome develops.

CPEO-plus refers to a disorder of intermediate severity that has an adolescent or adult onset and variable involvement of tissues other than the eyelids and eye muscles. The mildest variant is isolated CPEO in which clinical signs and symptoms worsen with age. Individuals who are initially classified as isolated CPEO can progress to CPEO-plus, and patients with Kearns-Sayre syndrome often develop more severe multisystem involvement.

The most common cause of Kearns-Sayre and CPEO syndromes is a rearrangement of mtDNA. The mtDNA deletion mutation has the simplest structure, consisting of a mtDNA molecule that is missing contiguous tRNA and protein-coding genes, thus yielding a mtDNA molecule that is smaller than the normal 16.6-kb mtDNA. The structurally more complex mtDNA duplication mutation produces a mtDNA molecule that is larger than the normal mtDNA and contains two tandemly arranged mtDNA molecules consisting of a full-length 16.6-kb mtDNA coupled to a mtDNA deletion. Leukocytes and platelets containing mtDNA rearrangements tend to be lost from the circulation. By contrast there is evidence for an accumulation of mtDNA deletions in skeletal muscle. Assessment for mtDNA deletions in blood samples is probably the most common mistake made when requesting mtDNA genetic testing. Skeletal muscle is nearly always necessary for detection of large-scale mtDNA rearrangements.

Approximately 80% of patients with Kearns-Sayre syndrome, 70% with CPEO-plus, and 40% with CPEO harbor mtDNA rearrangements. In most patients with mtDNA rearrangements, the mutation was not inherited, but appears to be a spontaneous event that occurred during oogenesis or very early embryogenesis. Due to replicative segregation of mutant and wild-type mtDNAs, the identification of maternal inheritance of a mtDNA rearrangement by clinical criteria can be difficult and often requires analysis of skeletal muscle mtDNA from maternal lineage relatives of the proband. The mtDNA duplication mutation has the greatest probability of being maternally transmitted. Point mutations in mitochondrial tRNA genes, which are usually maternally inherited, are also an important cause for Kearns-Sayre and CPEO syndromes. Characterization of the mtDNA mutation in a patient with either Kearns-Sayre or CPEO syndrome is important for genetic counseling of the patient and family members.

MYOCLONIC EPILEPSY AND RAGGED-RED FIBER DISEASE (MERRF)

MERRF can begin at any age, ranging from late childhood to adulthood. The clinical features that are most predictive are epilepsy (myoclonic epilepsy, generalized seizures, or focal seizures), cerebellar ataxia, and a ragged-red fiber myopathy. Other manifestations include dementia, corticospinal tract degeneration, peripheral neuropathy, optic atrophy, deafness, proximal renal tubule dysfunction, cardiomyopathy, and lactic acidemia plus hyperalaninemia. Myoclonic jerks occur at rest and increase in frequency and amplitude with movement. The myoclonus in MERRF patients is best categorized as cortical reflex myoclonus and can be associated with epileptiform discharges and photic sensitivity with large-amplitude occipital waveforms on EEG, as well as giant cortical somatosensory-evoked repsonses. As many as 80 to 90% of the MERRF cases are caused by an A-to-G mutation that alters a conserved nucleotide in the tRNA^{Lysine} at position 8344 of the mtDNA.

MITOCHONDRIAL ENCEPHALOMYOPATHY, LACTIC ACIDOSIS, AND STROKE-LIKE EPISODES (MELAS)

Disease manifestations in patients with MELAS can appear at essentially any age. Patients are generally younger than 45 years of age and are characterized as "stroke in the young." They present with a large or small vessel stroke that can be associated with a migraine headache and/or seizures. Delineating this presentation from the long list of other causes of stroke in the young can be difficult and is assisted by recognizing myopathy, ataxia, cardiomyopathy, diabetes mellitus (see Sec. 25.8). Biochemical and genetic studies are essential in establishing the diagnosis. Cerebellar ataxia is often observed in patients with MELAS and may precede the development of stroke by many years. However, careful patient evaluation usually reveals manifestations in other organs, thus distinguishing these patients from other classes of cerebellar ataxia (see Sec. 25.15).

An A-to-G mutation in the tRNA$^{Leucine(UUR)}$ gene (A3243G) accounts for approximately 80% of MELAS cases. A mutation at position 8356 of the tRNA^{Lysine} gene was associated with features of both MERRF and MELAS. As many as 1% of randomly selected patients with adult-onset diabetes mellitus may harbor the A3243G mutation. OXPHOS diseases are important considerations in the differential diagnosis of patients with diabetes mellitus and stroke. The A3243G mutation is an important cause of Kearns-Sayre and CPEO syndromes and should be considered in the differential diagnosis of these disorders. The identification of this mutation is important in these patients because it is maternally inherited and is associated with a greater risk of stroke than the mtDNA rearrangements.

LEIGH SYNDROME AND CEREBELLAR ATAXIA AND PIGMENTARY RETINOPATHY SYNDROMES

Leigh syndrome or subacute necrotizing encephalopathy is suspected when cranial nerve abnormalities, respiratory dysfunction, and ataxia are observed in conjunction with bilateral hyperintense signals on T2-weighted MRI images in the basal ganglia, cerebellum, or brainstem. The age of onset for disease manifestations is usually during infancy or early childhood. Two mtDNA mutations, T8993G or T8993C in the ATPase 6 gene are important causes for Leigh disease. The T8993G mutation is the most frequently encountered of the two mutations; it changes an evolutionarily conserved leucine to an arginine in the proton channel of the ATPase 6 polypeptide, impairing ATP synthesis and was originally identified in patients with retinitis pigmentosa plus cerebellar ataxia syndromes.

The T8993G mutation acts in a recessive manner. Patients generally have no manifestations when the levels of the T8993G mutation in tissues is less than approximately 60 to 70% of the total mtDNA. Patients that harbor between approximately 70 and 90% mutant mtDNAs in their tissues have highly variable disease manifestations. The neurologic features are discussed in Chapter 25. Additional manifestations that can be observed are hypertrophic cardiomyopathy, sensory and motor neuropathies, muscle weakness, and elevated lactate or alanine levels in blood or urine. Approximately 7 to 20% of patients with Leigh disease harbor the T8993G mutation.

MITOCHONDRIAL DNA DEPLETION DISEASES

Mitochondrial DNA depletion diseases are an important group of disorders affecting infants and neonates in which a quantitative reduction in mtDNA copy number exists within various tissues. Patients have variable combinations of mitochondrial myopathy with cytochrome c oxidase–negative fibers, hypotonia, hepatopathy, progressive external ophthalmoplegia, and severe lactic acidosis. The diagnosis is made using quantitative Southern blot analysis

which demonstrates that the copy number of the mtDNA is greatly reduced in affected tissues. Interestingly, the unaffected tissues of some patients may show normal levels of mtDNA. Prenatal diagnosis of mtDNA depletion diseases is difficult. Only about 5% of amniocytes express depletion. The disorder appears to be usually transmitted in an autosomal recessive fashion.

9.7.4   Nuclear DNA Mutations and Oxphos Disease (See Table 9-16)

KEARNS-SAYRE AND CHRONIC PROGRESSIVE EXTERNAL OPHTHALMOPLEGIA (CPEO) SYNDROMES

Kearns-Sayre and chronic progressive external ophthalmoplegia syndromes can be transmitted in an autosomal dominant or recessive fashion. The mtDNA analysis of affected individuals in these families revealed that each harbors an array of deleted mtDNAs. Clinical manifestations include ophthalmoplegia, proximal muscle weakness, sensorineural hearing loss and abnormal vestibular responses, tremor, ataxia, and sensorimotor neuropathy. Although multiple mtDNA deletions accumulate in various tissues of some patients, clinical manifestations within the same pedigree are often highly variable, ranging from individuals with severe manifestations to individuals who are asymptomatic. In one family with this disorder, the male proband exhibited the manifestations of Kearns-Sayre syndrome and Leigh disease. Elevations in blood lactate, a ragged-red fiber myopathy, and OXPHOS defects primarily affecting Complexes I and IV occur. The biochemical abnormalities are typical of mutations which cause defects in mitochondrial protein synthesis. The mtDNA deletions are best detected in skeletal muscle biopsies. These mutations are generally absent in populations of rapidly dividing cells such as cultured fibroblasts, peripheral blood cells, cultured myoblasts, myotubes, or in vitro innervated muscle cells. Autosomal dominant forms of the disease map to chromosome 10q23.3-24.3 and chromosome 3p14.1-21.2.

MYONEUROGASTROINTESTINAL DISORDER AND ENCEPHALOPATHY (MNGIE)

MNGIE is an autosomal recessive disorder characterized by a progressive external ophthalmoplegia, dementia with a progressive leukodystrophy, mitochondrial myopathy, peripheral neuropathy, and prominent involvement of the gastrointestinal tract. The gastrointestinal manifestations are heralded by diarrhea, malabsorption, and weight loss with normal pancreatic function. Radiologic investigations may show marked thickening of the small intestines which reflects the pathologic findings of extensive mural thickening and fibrosis of the submucosa and subserosa. Lactate levels may be elevated along with other tricarboxylic acid cyle intermediates. This disorder is linked to chromosome 22q13.32-qter. Recent investigations demonstrated that it is caused by loss-of-function mutations in the thymidine phosphorylase gene. Thymidine phosphorylase converts thymidine to 2-deoxy-D-ribose-1-phosphate and may function to regulate thymidine availability for DNA synthesis. Thymidine phosphorylase is widely expressed in human tissues. Interestingly, this enzyme is apparently not expressed in skeletal muscle, even though disease manifestations are identifiable in this tissue.

LEIGH SYNDROME

Leigh syndrome can be caused by defects in aerobic energy metabolism including pyruvate dehydrogenase; however, OXPHOS defects (Complexes I and IV) are the most commonly identified biochemical abnormality in this group of patients. All nuclear OXPHOS gene mutations reported are transmitted in an autosomal recessive fashion.

Four mutations in nuclear-encoded respiratory chain subunits have been identified in Leigh syndrome patients. One is in the gene coding for the flavoprotein subunit of Complex II. The other three mutation groups involve Complex I subunits. One is a mutation in the 18-kDa (AQDQ) Complex I subunit which maps to chromosome 5, the second in the NDUSF9 (TYKY) subunit, and the third in the 51-kDa subunit (NDUFV1). The Complex I mutation in the 18-kDa subunit showed normal organic and amino acids, skeletal muscle light microscopy, and electron microscopy. The Complex I defect was present in both skeletal muscle and in fibroblasts. This patient provides genetic confirmation for the common observation that Complex I defects generally do not produce detectable metabolic abnormalities. Additional phenotypic heterogeneity was observed with the 51-kDa subunit mutations.

Although Complex IV defects are frequently observed, mutations affecting the nuclear encoded subunits of Complex IV were not found in Leigh syndrome patients. Alternatively, three complementation groups appear to encompass the majority of these patients. In one complementation group, mutations in a highly evolutionarily conserved gene, the SURF1 gene (chromosome 9q34) were found to be the cause of systemic cytochrome c oxidase (Complex IV) deficiency in these patients, all of whom had Leigh syndrome with early-onset hypotonia, ataxia, brainstem abnormalities, regression, and the characteristic bilateral basal ganglia lesions. The SURF1 gene appears to be essential for Complex IV assembly. Mutations in the SURF1 gene are heterogeneous, consisting of small deletions and insertions, nonsense mutations, and donor splice-site mutants, and most patients are compound heterozygotes. All reported mutations are loss-of-function mutations and predict a truncated protein product.

A group of Leigh syndrome patients, referred to as the Saguenay Lac-Saint-Jean type, shows Complex IV deficiency. Although phenotypically similar to the patients harboring mutations in the SURF1 gene, this recessively transmitted disorder maps to chromosome 2. Whereas the Complex IV defect in the group with SURF1 mutations is systemic, the Saguenay Lac-Saint-Jean group has 50% activity in muscle, fibroblasts, and amniocytes; less than 10% activity in brain and liver; and normal activity in kidney and heart.

HEREDITARY SPASTIC PARAPLEGIA WITH RAGGED-RED FIBER MYOPATHY

An autosomal recessive form of spastic paraparesis was identified at chromosome 16q24.3. Patients experience progressive weakness, spasticity, mild decreases in vibratory sensation as their major manifestations, and have ragged-red, COX-deficient fibers in their skeletal muscle. Dysphagia, scoliosis, and optic nerve atrophy have also occurred. This unique form of hereditary spastic paraplegia is caused by mutations in the gene called "paraplegin" that is localized to the mitochondria. Paraplegin has a high degree of homology with a subclass of ATPases belonging to the AAA family. These ATPases are metalloproteases with both proteolytic and chaperonin

functions, suggesting that paraplegin plays a role in the assembly and maintenance of the respiratory chain enzyme complexes.

FRIEDREICH ATAXIA

Friedreich ataxia was recently discovered to be a mitochondrial disease. Clinical manifestations are systemic and include hypoactive or absent deep-tendon reflexes, ataxia, corticospinal tract dysfunction, impaired vibratory and proprioceptive function, hypertrophic cardiomyopathy, and diabetes mellitus. This autosomal recessive disorder was mapped to chromosome 9q13. This disease is caused by a GAA trinucleotide repeat expansion in the first intron of the frataxin gene. Frataxin is a mitochondrial protein that is involved in iron homeostasis. Frataxin gene mutations result in impaired activity of the iron-sulfur–containing enzymes within the mitochondria: Complex I, Complex II, Complex III, and aconitase (see Sec. 25.15.)

9.7.5   Disorders of Pyruvate Metabolism

PYRUVATE DEHYDROGENASE COMPLEX DEFECTS

PDC defects are important causes of primary lactic acidosis and progressive neurologic disease of infancy and childhood. Most cases are caused by a defect in the E1α subunit of pyruvate dehydrogenase which is located on the X-chromosome at p22.1-22.2. Rare cases are encountered with defects in the dihydrolipoamide acetyltransferase (E2), dihydrolipoamide dehydrogenase (E3), phospho-E1 phosphatase, or protein X. Clinical features are not predictive of the precise biochemical defect.

The patient phenotypes are heterogeneous. Neonates with PDC defects may present with severe acidosis caused by progressive lactate and pyruvate accumulation, hypotonia, microcephaly, partial or total agenesis of the corpus callosum, and dysmorphic features similar to those seen in fetal alcohol syndrome (see Chapter 10).

The acidosis is refractory to treatment, but thiamine pyrophosphate and dichloroacetate are often administered. If these infants survive this initial phase, they have severe neurologic impairment and typically die by about 3 years of age. Some children present later during the first year of life with Leigh disease. The clinical manifestations can be indistinguishable from forms caused by OXPHOS defects.

Milder variants can present during infancy or childhood with episodic cerebellar ataxia which may occur spontaneously, be precipitated by carbohydrate intake, or occur in conjunction with mild infections. Lactic acidosis is usually not found during testing of these patients.

PYRUVATE CARBOXYLASE DEFICIENCY

As discussed above, pyruvate carboxylase is important in regulating gluconeogenesis, allowing pyruvate to be converted through a series of enzymatic steps to glucose during fasting. Due to difficulties in measuring the activity of this enzyme in tissues such as liver and kidney where it is most active, it is preferred to measure it in fibroblasts. Three major clinical presentations are described. One group of patients had symptoms that included psychomotor retardation; lactic acidemia; elevated blood alanine and proline concentrations; elevated urine α-ketoglutarate; and sometimes proximal renal tubular acidosis. A second group of patients had lactic acidosis and elevated blood alanine, proline, citrulline, lysine, and ammonia levels. Both groups are recognized either at birth or during the first few months of life and are rapidly fatal. A rare group is characterized by intermittent lactic acidosis, elevated blood alanine, lysine, and proline and urinary α-ketoglutarate concentrations. One patient had normal development at 7 years of age.

PHOSPHOENOLPYRUVATE CARBOXYKINASE (PEPCK) DEFICIENCY

A defect in this enzyme is rare and the diagnosis is difficult. PEPCK exists as two isoforms, one within the mitochondria and one localized to the cytosol. Deficiencies are the result of defects in either isoform. Measurement of the enzyme activity in cultured fibroblasts is the diagnostic method of choice. Clinical manifestations include failure to thrive; hypoglycemia; hepatomegaly because of fat accumulation; hypotonia; episodes of idiopathic hyperpyrexia; and muscle weakness.

9.7.6   Treatment

The treatment of patients with OXPHOS diseases or disorders of pyruvate metabolism is frustrating for the patients, their families, and the clinicians. At best, therapies are palliative. Metabolic therapies for OXPHOS diseases aim to increase mitochondrial ATP production and thus arrest the progression of the clinical manifestations; those that may have a positive therapeutic effect include coenzyme Q_{10}, phylloquinone, menadione, succinate, ascorbate, nicotinamide, dichloroacetate, L-carnitine, and riboflavin. However, assessment of the efficacy of treatment has been difficult because of the clinical and genetic heterogeneity of these disorders.

Specific supplements do not appear to be helpful in patients with pyruvate carboxylase or PEPCK defects. Patients with PDH defects have been treated with thiamine, low-carbohydrate or ketogenic diets, and L-carnitine. In most patients with disorders of pyruvate metabolism, proper diagnosis permits establishment of reasonable management plans. Advances in genetic testing allow families to obtain information that can be important for future pregnancies and for providing genetic counseling to other family members.

References

General

Shoffner JM, Wallace DC: Oxidative phosphorylation diseases. In: Scriver CR, Beaudet AL, Sly WS, Valle D, eds. The Metabolic and Molecular Bases of Inherited Disease. New York, McGraw-Hill, 2001:2367

Diagnosis

Mita S, Tokunaga M, Kumamoto T, Uchino M, Nonaka I, Ando M: Mitochondrial DNA mutation and muscle pathology in mitochondrial myopathy, encephalopathy, lactic acidosis, and stroke-like episodes. Muscle Nerve 3:S113, 1995

Yamamoto M, Koga Y, Ohtaki E, Nonaka I: Focal cytochrome c oxidase deficiency in various neuromuscular diseases. J Neurol Sci 91:207, 1989

Zheng XX, Shoffner JM, Voljavec AS, Wallace DC: Evaluation of procedures for assaying oxidative phosphorylation enzyme activities in mito-

chondrial myopathy muscle biopsies. Biochim Biophys Acta 1019:1, 1990

(mtDNA) Kearns-Sayre and Chronic Progressive External Ophthalmoplegia (CPEO) Syndromes

Holt IJ, Harding AE, Cooper JM, et al: Mitochondrial myopathies: clinical and biochemical features of 30 patients with major deletions of muscle mitochondrial DNA. Ann Neurol 26:699, 1989

Moraes CT, DiMauro S, Zeviani M, et al: Mitochondrial DNA deletions in progressive external ophthalmoplegia and Kearns-Sayre syndrome. N Engl J Med 320:1293, 1989

Rowland LP: Progressive external ophthalmoplegia and ocular myopathies. In: Rowland LP, DiMauro S, eds: Handbook of Clinical Neurology. New York, Elsevier Science Publishers BV, 1992

(Nuclear DNA) Kearns-Sayre and Chronic Progressive External Ophthalmoplegia (CPEO) Syndromes

Kaukonen JA, Amati P, Suomalainen A, et al: An autosomal locus predisposing to multiple deletions of mtDNA on chromosome 3p. Am J Hum Genet 58:763, 1996

Servidei S, Zeviani M, Manfredi G, et al: Dominantly inherited mitochondrial myopathy with multiple deletions of mitochondrial DNA: clinical, morphologic, and biochemical studies. Neurology 41:1053, 1991

Suomalainen A, Kaukonen J, Amati P, et al: An autosomal dominant locus predisposing to deletions of mitochondrial DNA. Nat Genet 9:146, 1995

Myoclonic Epilepsy and Ragged-Red Fiber Disease

Shoffner JM, Lott MT, Lezza AM, Seibel P, Ballinger SW, Wallace DC: Myoclonic epilepsy and ragged-red fiber disease (MERRF) is associated with a mitochondrial DNA tRNA (Lys) mutation. Cell 61:931, 1990

Zeviani M, Muntoni F, Savarese N, et al: A MERRF/MELAS overlap syndrome associated with a new point mutation in the mitochondrial DNA tRNA(Lys) gene [published erratum appears in Eur J Hum Genet 1(2): 124, 1993]. Eur J Hum Genet 1:80, 1993

Mitochondrial Encephalomyopathy, Lactic Acidosis, and Stroke-Like Episodes (MELAS)

Koo B, Becker LE, Chuang S, et al: Mitochondrial encephalomyopathy, lactic acidosis, stroke-like episodes (MELAS): clinical, radiological, pathological, and genetic observations. Ann Neurol 34:25, 1993

Van den Ouweland JMW, Lemkes HHPJ, Trembath RC, et al: Maternally inherited diabetes and deafness is a distinct subtype of diabetes and associates with a single point mutation in the mitochondrial tRNA-Leu(UUR) gene. Diabetes 43:746, 1994

(mtDNA) Leigh Syndrome and Cerebellar Ataxia Plus Pigmentary Retinopathy Syndromes

Rahman S, Blok RB, Dahl HH, et al: Leigh syndrome: clinical features and biochemical and DNA abnormalities. Ann Neurol 39:343, 1996

Santorelli FM, Shanske S, Jain KD, Tick D, Schon EA, Dimauro S: A T to C mutation at nt 8993 of mitochondrial DNA in a child with Leigh syndrome. Neurology 44:972, 1994

Shoffner JM, Fernhoff PM, Krawiecki NS, et al: Subacute necrotizing encephalopathy: oxidative phosphorylation defects. Neurology 42:2168, 1992

(Nuclear DNA) Leigh Syndrome

Loeffen J, Smeitink J, Triepels R, et al: The first nuclear-encoded complex I mutation in a patient with Leigh syndrome. Am J Hum Genet 63: 1598, 1998

Schuelke M, Smeitink J, Mariman E, et al: Mutant NDUFV1 subunit of mitochondrial complex I causes leukodystrophy and myoclonic epilepsy. Nat Genet 21:260, 1999

Tiranti V, Hoertnagel K, Carrozzo R, et al: Mutations of SURF-1 in Leigh disease associated with cytochrome c oxidase deficiency. Am J Hum Genet 63:1609, 1998

van den Heuvel L, Ruitenbeek W, Smeets R, et al: Demonstration of a new pathogenic mutation in human complex I deficiency: a 5-bp duplication in the nuclear gene encoding the 18-kD (AQDQ) subunit. Am J Hum Genet 62:262, 1998

Zhu Z, Yao J, Johns T, et al: SURF1, encoding a factor involved in the biogenesis of cytochrome c oxidase. Nat Genet 20:337, 1998

mtDNA Depletion Diseases

Moraes CT, Shanske S, Tritschler HJ, et al: mtDNA depletion with variable tissue expression: a novel genetic abnormality in mitochondrial diseases. Am J Hum Genet 48:492, 1991

Telerman-Toppet N, Biarent D, Bouton JM, et al: Fatal cytochrome c oxidase-deficient myopathy of infancy associated with mtDNA depletion. Differential involvement of skeletal muscle and cultured fibroblasts. J Inherit Metab Dis 15:323, 1992

Tritschler HJ, Andreetta F, Moraes CT, et al: Mitochondrial myopathy of childhood associated with depletion of mitochondrial DNA. Neurology 42:209, 1992

Myoneurogastrointestinal Disorder and Encephalopathy (MNGIE)

Blake D, Lombes A, Minetti C: MNGIE syndrome: report of 2 new patients. Neurology 40(Suppl 1):294, 1990

Nishino I, Spinazzola A, Hirano M: Thymidine phosphorylase gene mutations in MNGIE, a human mitochondrial disorder. Science 283:689, 1999

Simon LT, Horoupian DS, Dorfman LJ, et al: Polyneuropathy, ophthalmoplegia, leukoencephalopathy, and intestinal pseudo-obstruction: POLIP syndrome. Ann Neurol 28:349, 1990

Hereditary Spastic Paraplegia with Ragged-Red Fiber Myopathy

Casari G, De Fusco M, Ciarmatori S, et al: Spastic paraplegia and OXPHOS impairment caused by mutations in paraplegin, a nuclear encoded mitochondrial metalloprotease. Cell 93:973, 1998

Friedreich Ataxia

Campuzano V, Montermini L, Molto MD, et al: Friedreich's ataxia: autosomal recessive disease caused by an intronic GAA triplet repeat expansion. Science 271:1423, 1996

Rotig A, de Lonlay P, Chretien D, et al: Aconitase and mitochondrial iron-sulphur protein deficiency in Friedreich ataxia. Nat Genet 17:215, 1997

Pyruvate Dehydrogenase Complex Defects and Pyruvate Carboxylase Deficiency

Kretzchmar HA, DeArmond SJ, Koch TK, et al: Pyruvate dehydrogenase complex deficiency as a cause of subacute necrotizing encephalopathy (Leigh's disease). Pediatrics 79:370, 1987

Robinson BH: Lactic acidemia (disorders of pyruvate carboxylase, pyruvate dehydrogenase). In: Scriver CR, Beaudet AL, Sly WS, Valle D, eds: The Metabolic and Molecular Bases of Inherited Disease. New York, McGraw-Hill, 2001

Van Coster RN, Fernhoff PM, DeVivo DC: Pyruvate carboxylase deficiency: a benign variant with normal development. Pediatr Res 30:1, 1991

9.8
MUCOPOLYSACCHARIDOSES, GLYCOPROTEINOSES, AND MUCOLIPIDOSES

J. Edmond Wraith

9.8.1 Mucopolysaccharidosis

The mucopolysaccharidoses (MPS) are a family of disorders that are caused by inherited defects in the catabolism of sulphated components of connective tissue known as glycosaminoglycans (GAGs). In affected patients, one or more of three specific polymers—dermatan sulfate (DS), heparan sulfate (HS), and keratan sulfate (KS)—accumulate within the cells, interfering with normal function and are, in addition, excreted to excess in the urine.

The enzymes associated with GAG catabolism are all lysosomal hydrolases, and patients with an MPS disorder usually have less than 1% residual enzyme activity. Heterozygote detection based on enzyme activity alone is inaccurate and now, fortunately, no longer necessary, as the genes encoding the enzymes involved in GAG catabolism have been identified and sequenced. Phenotypic variability (heterogeneity) is very much a feature of MPS disease, and within each specific enzyme deficiency there is a very wide spectrum of clinical effects. Although the disorders are most often known by their eponymous titles (eg, Hurler syndrome), this has led to an oversimplification in the classification of the subtypes, which should be borne in mind when interpreting the data in Table 9-17.

CLINICAL PRESENTATION

MPS disorders, like all lysosomal storage diseases, are progressive conditions. Affected infants are usually normal at birth and the disease only comes to light as the phenotype evolves with time. Infants with an MPS-like phenotype present at birth are most likely to have mucolipidosis type II (I-cell disease) or G_{M1}-gangliosidosis.

The MPS disorders tend to present in one of three ways:

- As a dysmorphic syndrome; eg, MPS IH, MPS II, MPS VI
- With learning difficulties, behavioral disturbance, and dementia; eg, MPS III
- As a severe bone dysplasia; eg, MPS IV

The diagnosis is based on clinical suspicion, supported by appropriate clinical and radiologic examinations followed by urinary examination for GAG excretion and then by specific enzyme assay, usually on white blood cells. Urinary *screening* tests for MPS disorders may be inaccurate and false-negative results, especially in MPS III and IV, are well recognized. Furthermore, patients with mucolipidosis or glycoproteinases do not have excessive excretion of GAG. Therefore a negative screening test should not dissuade the clinician from vigorously pursuing a diagnosis in a clinically suspicious case. Although algorithms aimed at helping the diag-

TABLE 9-17

BIOCHEMICAL AND GENETIC CHARACTERISTICS OF THE MUCOPOLYSACCHARIDOSES AND RELATED DISORDERS

DISEASE	ENZYME DEFICIENCY	STORAGE MATERIAL	SCREENING TEST	DIAGNOSTIC TEST	CHROMOSOME LOCATION	GENE MUTATION	PRENATAL DIAGNOSIS
Mucopolysaccharidoses							
MPS I (Hurler, Scheie, Hurler/Scheie)	α-Iduronidase	DS, HS	Urine GAGs	WBC enzyme assay	4p16.3	W402X, Q70X, plus many others	CVB[1]
MPS II (Hunter)	Iduronate 2-sulfatase	DS, HS	Urine GAGs	Plasma enzyme assay	Xq27-28	No common mutations	CVB[2]
MPS III (Sanfilippo)							
MPS IIIA	Heparan N-sulfatase	HS	Urine GAGs	WBC enzyme assay	17q25.3	R245H, R74C, plus many others	CVB
MPS IIIB	N-acetylglucosaminidase	HS	Urine GAGs	Plasma enzyme assay	17q21.1	No common mutations	CVB
MPS IIIC	Acetyl-CoA:glucosamine N-acetyltransferase	HS	Urine GAGs	WBC enzyme assay	Uncertain	Unknown	CVB
MPS IIID	N-acetylglucosamine-6-sulfatase	HS	Urine GAGs	WBC enzyme assay	12q14	Very few patients studied	CVB
MPS IV (Morquio)							
MPS IVA	Galactose-6-sulfatase	KS	Urine GAGs	WBC enzyme assay	16q24	I113F (Britain and Ireland)	CVB
MPS IVB	β-Galactosidase	KS	Urine GAGs	WBC enzyme assay	3p21-pter	No common mutations	CVB
MPS VI (Maroteaux-Lamy)	Galactosamine-4-sulfatase	DS	Urine GAGs	WBC enzyme assay	5q13-q14	No common mutations	CVB[3]
MPS VII (Sly)	β-Glucuronidase	HS, DS	Urine GAGs	WBC enzyme assay	7q21.1-q22	Very few patients studied	CVB
MPS IX	Hyaluronidase	HA	None	Cultured cells enzyme assay	3p21.3	One patient	Unknown
Mucolipidoses							
ML I (Sialidosis I)	α-Neuraminidase	SA	Urine sialic acid	Cultured cells enzyme assay	10pter-q23	Unknown	Cultured cells
ML II and III	Transferase[4]	Many compounds	Urine oligosaccharides	Plasma enzyme assay[5]	Unknown	Unknown	Cultured cells or AF
ML IV	Unknown	Unknown	None	Ultrastructure	19p13.2-13.3	Unknown	Ultrastructure of CVB

(continued)

TABLE 9-17 Continued

DISEASE	ENZYME DEFICIENCY	STORAGE MATERIAL	SCREENING TEST	DIAGNOSTIC TEST	CHROMOSOME LOCATION	GENE MUTATION	PRENATAL DIAGNOSIS
Glycoproteinoses and other disorders							
Mannosidoses							
α-Mannosidosis	α-Mannosidase	Mannosyl-oligos	Urine oligosaccharides	WBC enzyme assay	19p13.2-q12	R750W (20%)	CVB
β-Mannosidosis	β-Mannosidase	Mannosyl-oligos	Urine oligosaccharides	WBC enzyme assay	4q21-25	One patient studied	CVB
Fucosidosis	α-Fucosidase	Fucosyl-oligos	Urine oligosaccharides	WBC enzyme assay	1p34.1-36.1	Q422X plus many others	CVB
Schindler disease	α-N-Acetylgalactos-aminidase	Oligos and Oligopeptides	Urine oligosaccharides	WBC enzyme assay	22q13.1-13.2	Very few patients	CVB
Aspartylglucosaminuria	Aspartylglucosaminidase	Aspartylglucosamine	Urine oligosaccharides	WBC enzyme assay	4q23-q27	C163S, R161Q (Finland)	CVB
G_{M1}-gangliosidosis	β-Galactosidase	Galactosyl-oligos and G_{M1}-ganglioside	Urine oligosaccharides	WBC enzyme assay	3cen-p21	No common mutations	CVB
Galactosialidosis	Combined α-neuraminidase + β-galactosidase	Sialyloligos	Urine oligosaccharides	WBC and cultured cells enzyme assay	20q13.1	Very few patients studied	Cultured AF cells
Mucosulfatidosis (Austin disease)	Multiple sulfatases	Various	Urine oligosaccharides	Plasma and WBC enzyme assays	Unknown	Unknown	CVB
Salla disease	Sialic acid transporter	Sialic acid	Urine oligosaccharides	Urine sialic acid	6q14-15	Unknown	CVB[6]

DS, dermatan sulfate; HS, heparan sulfate; KS, keratan sulfate; HA, hyaluronic acid; SA, sialic acid; GAGs, glycosamoinoglycans; Oligos, oligosaccharides; CVB, chorion villus brops.

[1]Low activity in CVB: danger of contamination with maternal decidual.

[2]Always do fetal sexing as some unaffected female fetuses will have very low enzyme results.

[3]Difficult because of X-reactivity from other sulfatases.

[4]UDP-N-Acetylglucosamine:lysosomal enzyme N-acetylglucosaminyl-l-phosphotransferase.

[5]Deficiency on many enzymes in leukocytes, elevated values of some in plasma.

[6]Sialic acid concentration measured rather than an enzyme assay.

nostic process have been developed, in clinical practice their use is limited by the extreme heterogeneity in this group of disorders.

If urinary GAG analysis by electrophoresis is negative, one needs to consider other diagnostic possibilities. Urine oligosaccharide and sialic acid analysis should be undertaken to exclude oligosaccharidoses and other glycoproteinoses. White cell and plasma lysosomal enzyme studies should be performed to confirm abnormalities and to exclude galactosialidosis. Radiographs should be reviewed to confirm the presence of dysostosis multiplex (Fig. 9-16 A, B, & C), and abnormal lysosomal storage should be confirmed by electron microscopy of a skin biopsy. If all of these investigations are normal, it is important to remember that some nonlysosomal disturbances can mimic storage disease (eg, Coffin-Lowry syndrome, Williams syndrome, and geleophysic dysplasia).

All MPS disorders are multisystem diseases, and effective management is dependent on a multidisciplinary approach involving many different clinical specialities, as well as access to expert support services. The pediatrician has a major role in orchestrating the various members of the therapeutic team. Anesthesia is particularly difficult in these patients, and surgery should only be performed in centers in which there is access to anesthetists who are used to dealing with difficult pediatric airways and who have access to pediatric intensive care.

Many patients survive through adolescence and into adult life, and careful planning of the transition between pediatric and adult services is necessary.

There is a tendency to classify the individual MPS disorders into "mild" and "severe" subtypes, based on either survival or on the presence or absence of CNS disease. This is a gross oversimplification; it is preferable to consider the disorders a clinical spectrum. Although many conditions are compatible with prolonged survival, for the majority of patients, these are not benign conditions.

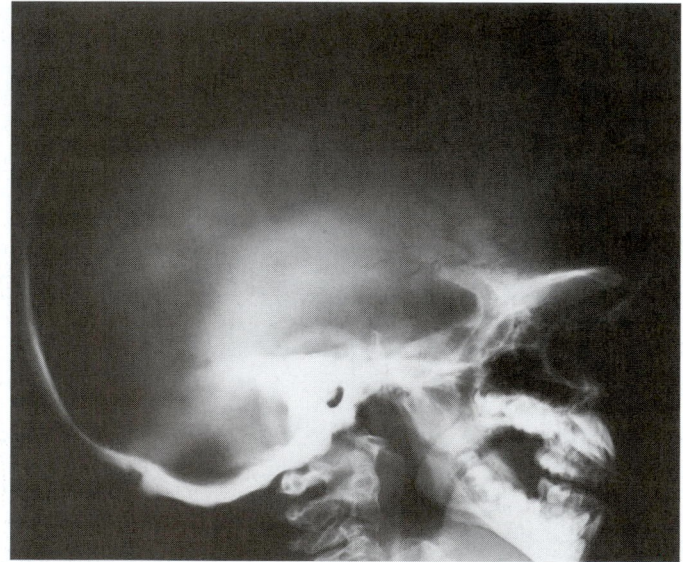
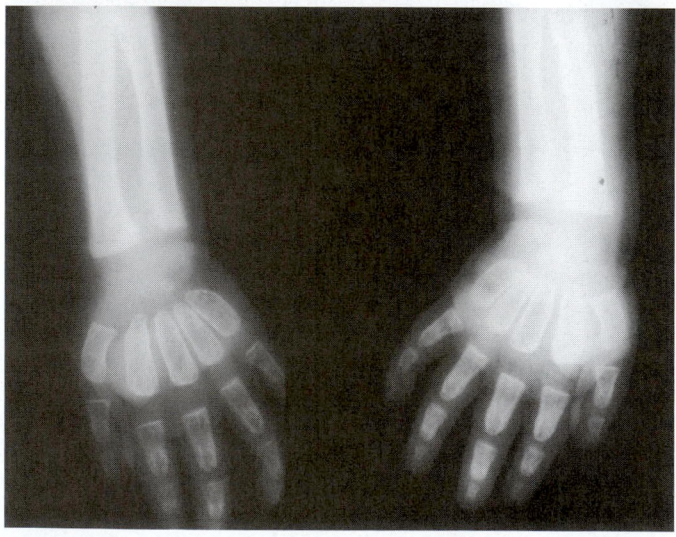
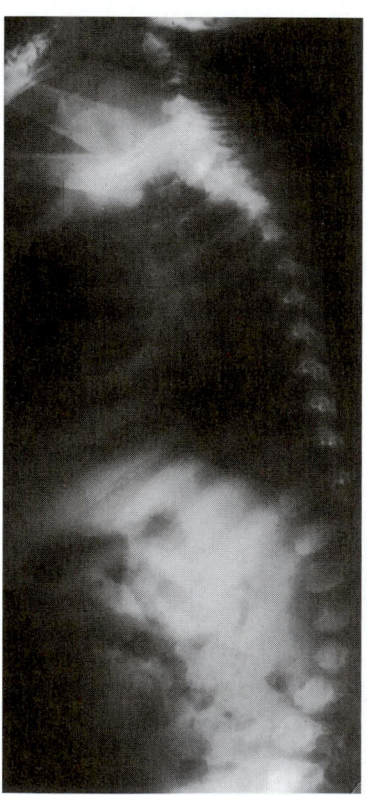

FIGURE 9-16 **Radiographic findings in MPS disorders. A, Lateral radiograph of the skull of patient with MPS IH showing massive enlargement of the sella turcica. B, Radiograph of the hand in MPS showing pointing of the metacarpals. C, Lateral radiograph of the spine in MPS IV showing universal platyspondylisis (*left*) and MPS IH showing hypoplastic lumbar vertebrae and gibbus anomaly (*right*).**

Mucopolysaccharidosis Type I
(α-L-Iduronidase Deficiency; MPS IH: Hurler Syndrome; MPS IH/S: Hurler/Scheie Syndrome; MPS IS: Scheie Syndrome)

Patients with MPS IH (Hurler syndrome) are usually diagnosed toward the end of the first year of life when the facial phenotype becomes obvious (Fig. 9-17). Many will have presented with inguinal and umbilical hernias and recurrent respiratory infections before the diagnosis is established. Parents often notice the lower thoracic–upper lumbar gibbus, but are usually reassured that the abnormality is only postural and not of importance. A number of patients will have a large head circumference, and communicating hydrocephalus will develop in up to 40% of patients. The early clinical picture is dominated by the upper respiratory tract obstruction secondary to the mid-face hypoplasia and the large tongue. Obstructive sleep apnea is usual, and all affected children require expert ear, nose, and throat surgery. Although growth for the first 12 to 18 months of life is normal, the effects of the skeletal dysplasia eventually lead to severe growth restriction. In addition all patients have a dysplastic odontoid process and are at risk of sudden and severe spinal cord damage secondary to atlantoaxial subluxation. Hepatosplenomegaly and progressive cardiac disease develops, and corneal deposition of GAG becomes clinically apparent as corneal clouding during the second year of life in most patients. Although learning difficulties are a feature of all patients with the severe forms of iduronidase deficiency, developmental progress can be surprisingly good over the first 2 or 3 years and often contrasts greatly with the affected child's physical appearance. Deafness is usually present and must be diagnosed early and treated appropriately.

Prognosis depends upon the severity of cardiac involvement. This can range from a very severe cardiomyopathy causing death in the early months of life to progressive valve involvement (usually mitral and aortic) with relatively good left ventricular function and survival up to the end of the first decade and occasionally beyond. Coronary artery disease can be severe and episodes of cardiac ischemia and infarction can occur. Although corneal clouding can be significant, severe visual loss is usually due to retinal or postretinal involvement. Sudden blindness can occur due to compression of the optic nerve within the optic sheath.

At the other end of the clinical spectrum are those patients diagnosed in late childhood or early adult-life, usually because of their orthopedic or ophthalmologic problems. In MPS IS (Scheie syndrome), intellectual development is normal and the disorder is compatible with a normal life span. Some patients require cardiac valve surgery, but the clinical picture tends to be dominated by the bone and joint involvement. Carpal tunnel syndrome is an almost universal finding in this type of MPS disorder. In some patients, corneal haze limits vision to such a degree that corneal transplan-

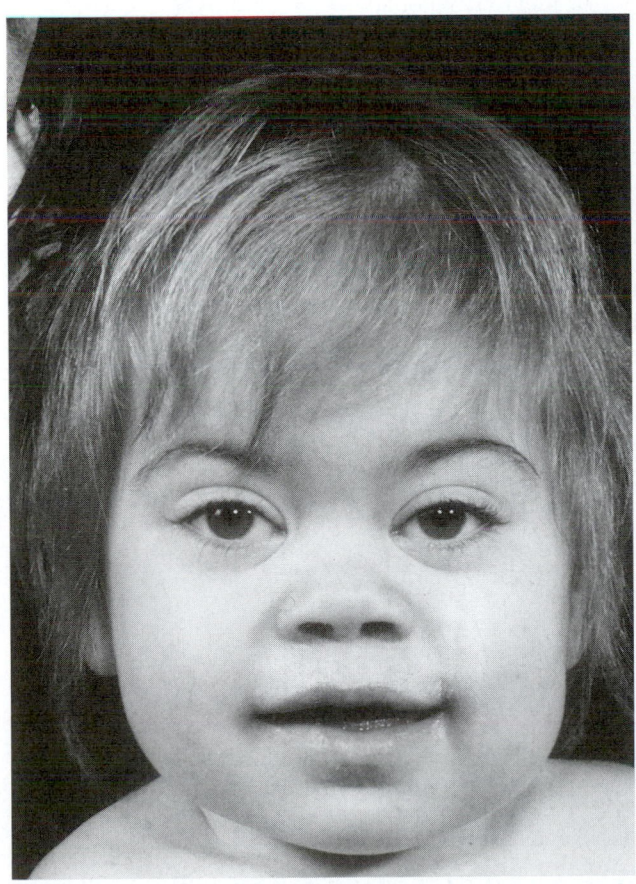 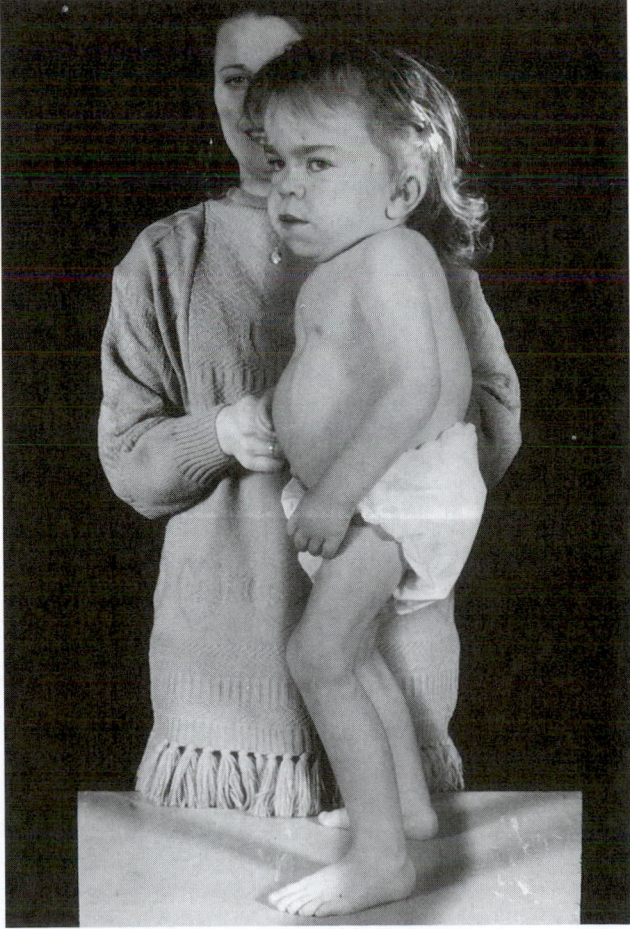

FIGURE 9-17   Clinical features of Hurler disease. A, At diagnosis age 14 months and B, at age 2 years 6 months.

tation is necessary. Most patients tolerate this procedure well and the transplanted cornea remains clear. Before embarking on this surgery, however, a careful assessment of retinal function is necessary to ensure that the visual loss is not secondary to retinopathy, which also occurs in MPS IS.

Between these two extremes is a continuous clinical spectrum that is often labeled MPS IH/S (Hurler/Scheie syndrome) (Fig. 9-18). These patients may develop late-onset neurologic deterioration, but most of the active clinical problems relate to the progressive joint stiffness and to degenerative bone disease that commonly occurs. Spondylolisthesis of L5/S1 is very common and requires surgical repair. Progressive visual loss due to a combination of corneal clouding and retinal disease is usual, and many patients will develop progressive cardiac disease. Frequent chest infections, limited chest expansion, and upper respiratory obstruction are common. In addition many patients have a relative micrognathia and are unable to open their mouths widely. Sleep apnea can be troublesome, and routine pulse oximetry overnight during sleep should be performed annually. Some patients require continuous positive airway pressure (CPAP) via a nasal mask. In patients who cannot tolerate the tight-fitting mask or the noise of the machine, tracheostomy remains the only alternative. In general, this is poorly tolerated in MPS disorders; in addition, it is often associated with an increase in airway secretions that requires frequent suction.

The gene coding for α-L-iduronidase is on chromosome 4p16.3 and consists of 14 exons. Many different mutations have been described, especially in the more severe forms of MPS I. W402X and Q70X, two nonsense mutations, are relatively common in Europe, although their incidence varies from country to country.

Mucopolysaccharidosis Type II (Iduronate-2-Sulfatase Deficiency; MPS II: Hunter Syndrome)

The clinical features in MPS II are even more heterogeneous than in MPS I. At the severe end of the clinical spectrum, the disorder is very similar to MPS IH, but generally milder, allowing for survival up to mid-teen years. At the other end of the spectrum, survival into adult life with reproduction is possible. There are two important differences from MPS I: first, the disorder is inherited as an X-linked recessive condition (it is the only X-linked MPS disorder—all the rest are recessives), and second, corneal clouding does not occur to any significant degree in the vast majority of patients.

In severely affected patients, the diagnosis is usually established around the second birthday because of a combination of learning difficulties, middle-ear disease, a history of hernia repairs, and a coarse facial appearance. Many patients have troublesome diarrhea and most develop joint stiffness and organomegaly. A nodular rash around the scapulae and on the extensor surfaces is said to be pathognomonic of the disorder, but is actually rare in childhood. The learning difficulties are different from those in MPS IH, as most patients with MPS II make more developmental progress than the typical MPS IH patient. The behavioral phenotype is also different, with challenging behavior, attention deficit disorder, and seizures being much more common in MPS II as compared to MPS IH. Cardiomyopathy (apart from asymmetric septal hypertrophy) is rare in MPS II, but progressive valve lesions can occur, although these rarely lead to symptoms.

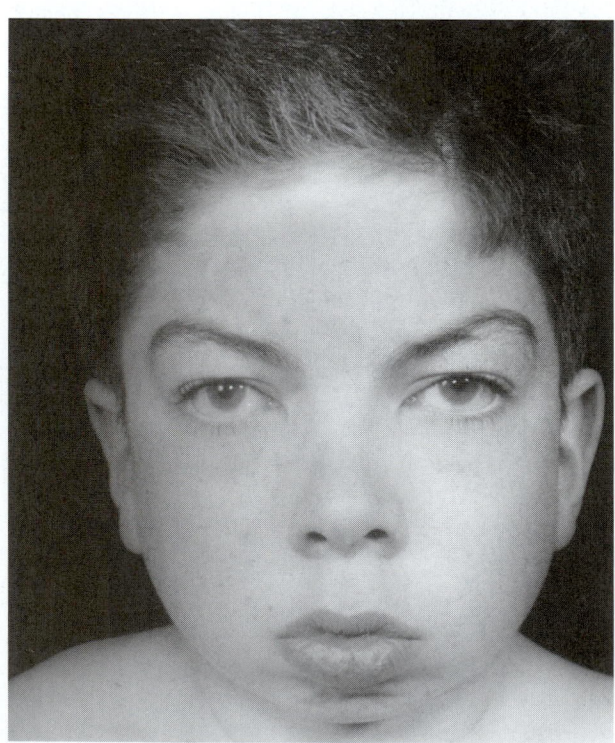 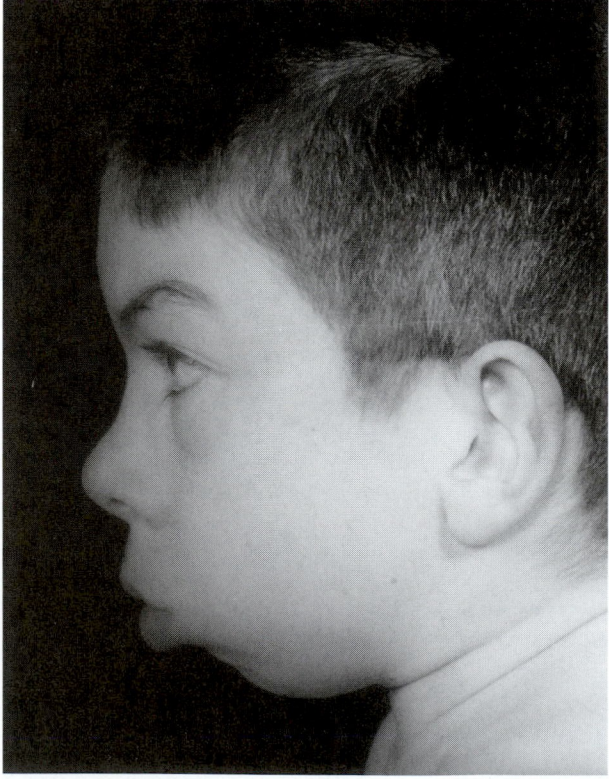

FIGURE 9-18 Facial appearance in MPS IH/S (Hurler-Scheie syndrome). Note the relative underdevelopment of the lower jaw. This appearance is similar to that seen in juvenile chronic arthritis and greatly increases the anesthetic risk in these patients.

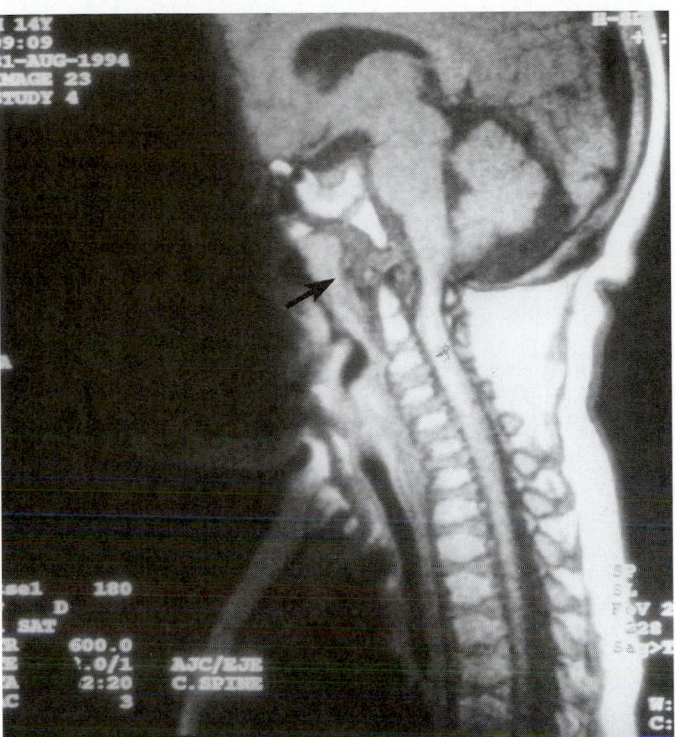

FIGURE 9-19   MRI of the craniocervical junction in a patient with a less severe form of MPS II. Abundant soft tissue at the tip of the odontoid peg has caused posterior displacement of the spinal cord and subsequent compression.

In patients with less-severe forms of MPS II, cervical cord compression due to hyperplasia of the dura and ligamentum flavum can lead to a progressive cervical myelopathy (Fig. 9-19). This usually presents with decreasing exercise tolerance that can be mistaken for a progression of the joint stiffness unless a careful neurologic examination is performed. From the age of 10 years, these patients should be routinely evaluated by magnetic resonance imaging (MRI) of the craniocervical junction, and posterior decompression should be performed in all patients with cervical compromise. Fortunately, atlantoaxial instability is not a feature of MPS II as the odontoid is usually well developed.

Despite often gross abnormality on cerebral imaging, intellectual development is normal in this form of MPS II, but the severe somatic features present in some intellectually normal men lead to considerable psychosocial problems, which require sensitive and careful handling.

Most adults with MPS II develop upper respiratory obstruction and sleep apnea. Many benefit from the use of nasal CPAP devices, although the nasal masks often have to be shaped individually because of the abnormal facial anatomy.

Although MPS II is an X-linked disorder, an occasional affected female patient has been described. This can occur as a result of chromosomal translocation or nonrandom X-inactivation.

The MPS II gene is large and located at Xq27-28. In affected boys, a whole range of molecular pathologies have been described, including insertions, deletions, point mutations, and splice-junction mutations. There are no common mutations, and it is often difficult to predict severity from the molecular lesion. In some patients, no abnormalities are detected despite sequencing of the whole coding region, and it is assumed that other regulatory elements must be involved in the disease.

Mucopolysaccharidosis Type III (Heparan N-Sulfatase Deficiency; Sanfilippo Syndrome: MPS IIIA, α-N-Acetylglucosaminidase Deficiency; Sanfilippo Syndrome: MPS IIIB, Acetyl-CoA:α-Glucosamine N-Acetyltransferase Deficiency; Sanfilippo Syndrome: MPS IIIC, N-Acetylglucosamine-6-Sulfatase Deficiency; Sanfilippo Syndrome: MPS IIID)

This MPS disorder is a clinically similar, but biochemically heterogeneous, group of four recognized conditions all associated with an inability to catabolize heparan sulfate. MPS IIIA is the most common MPS disorder in the UK, accounting for 80% of all MPS III patients. The remaining patients are mainly MPS IIIB; types IIIC and IIID are rare. The hallmark of MPS III is severe central nervous system (CNS) involvement in the presence of a mild somatic phenotype. As a consequence of this combination the diagnosis is usually established much later in life (4–5 years) when compared to other MPS disorders, and the condition is less heterogeneous than MPS I or II. In a typically affected patient, a triphasic illness can be recognized. The first phase, often before diagnosis, consists of developmental delay alone. There is often a history of recurrent upper respiratory infections and most patients have troublesome diarrhea. Sleep disturbance can present early in life, and in its extreme form produces a reversal of the normal sleep/wake cycle. Gradually the characteristic behavioral phenotype evolves as the second phase of the illness starts, usually in late infancy. This comprises severe challenging behavior with severe hyperactivity and often aggression. In addition, there is a complete lack of acknowledgement of danger and the children are a risk to themselves and others, and need constant attention. Temper tantrums are frequent and normal family life for many families becomes impossible. It is during this phase that the diagnosis is established in the majority of patients. As the disease advances developmental milestones are lost and increasing spasticity leads to progressive loss of motor skills. Precocious pubertal development is a well-recognized association. The third and final stage of the illness usually begins in early teenage years and is characterized by further loss of skills leading to swallowing dysfunction; eventually the disorder culminates in a vegetative existence in mid-late teens. Death usually occurs around the second decade. Seizures are common in the later stages in some patients, and can be difficult to control, while other patients develop a severe movement disorder resistant to treatment. Mood disturbance with prolonged crying can be extremely distressing for the parents of affected children.

Somatic features are usually mild except in some patients from the Asian subcontinent who can develop severe cardiac involvement (usually mitral valve disease).

The disorder is probably underdiagnosed at the less severe end of the clinical spectrum as these patients may have only mild learning difficulties until the age of 20 to 30 years.

Mutation analysis has been performed extensively in MPS IIIA and IIIB. The MPS IIIA gene is located on chromosome 17q25.3 and consists of eight exons. Considerable genetic heterogeneity has been demonstrated and a wide range of mutations described; R245H and R74C have a combined frequency of over 50% in some European populations.

The MPS IIIB gene is situated on chromosome 17q21.1 and consists of six exons. An even greater degree of genetic heterogeneity is seen in this disorder, and there are no common mutations.

Mucopolysaccharidosis Type IV (Galactose-6-Sulfatase Deficiency; Morquio Syndrome: MPS IVA, β-Galactosidase Deficiency; Morquio Syndrome: MPS IVB)

Patients with MPS IV have a severe skeletal dysplasia and, unlike the other MPS conditions, are not dysmorphic. In addition, CNS involvement does not occur and the clinical course is dominated by the severe bone disease and resulting extreme short stature. The diagnosis can be established in the newborn period, but more commonly is made toward the end of the first year of life when the sternal protrusion, which occurs as a result of the short trunk, becomes obvious. The radiologic abnormalities are different from the classic dysostosis multiplex seen in MPS I, II, VI, and VII, and are characterized by vertebral platyspondylisis as well as other features of a generalized spondyloepiphyseal dysplasia (see Fig. 9-16C).

Most severely affected adults are under 105 cm in height and have a typical clinical phenotype of fixed hip flexion, genu valgum and pes planus with mid-thoracic gibbus, sternal protrusion, and a very short neck. The greatest immediate danger to these patients is the inevitable odontoid dysplasia that is present in all severely affected patients (Fig. 9-20). Without treatment 60% of MPS IV patients suffer an irreversible neurologic deficit by age 6 years. Chronic cervical myelopathy presents with an insidious loss of motor function and evolves into a slowly progressive tetraparesis unless the instability in the cervical region is detected and corrected. Flexion/extension radiographic views of the cervical spine are helpful in identifying those patients likely to benefit from early spinal fusion. MRI scanning of the cervical region will demonstrate the degree of cervical involvement and should be performed routinely at regular intervals following diagnosis. The timing of cervical fusion remains contentious, but most groups are moving toward prophylactic fusion in those patients with atlantoaxial subluxation demonstrated radiologically. The situation requires continual vigilance as instability may develop further down the vertebral column.

Very little else can be done for the bone deformities present in this condition. Corrective surgery for the genu valgum often only produces a temporary cosmetic improvement and does not greatly improve mobility. Most adults with the severe form of this disease prefer to use a motorized wheelchair.

Although this disorder is commonly reported to be associated with "ligamentous laxity," this is not the case. The ligaments and tendons are generally stiffer than normal (similar to other MPS disorders), but the skeleton is poorly ossified. The excess movement present at the wrist is due to the cartilaginous nature of the carpal bones, as readily demonstrated by hand x-rays.

Dental decay is common, secondary to enamel hypoplasia, and the teeth are generally pointed and wide-spaced.

A number of patients will develop aortic insufficiency or mild corneal haze as adults, but these rarely need treatment. The biggest problem for older patients is the restrictive respiratory disease that often leads to respiratory failure in adult life and is the most common cause of death.

At the less-severe end of the spectrum, the odontoid is not dysplastic and the patients are not at risk from cervical myelopathy. Growth may be normal or marginally affected, and the usual complaints relate to hip involvement that may require corrective surgery.

The MPS IVA gene is located on chromosome 16q24, and extensive allelic heterogeneity has been demonstrated on mutation analysis. In British/Irish patients, the I113F mutation is relatively common (20%) and produces a severe form of the disease when homoallelic.

Mucopolysaccharidosis Type VI (Galactosamine-4-Sulfatase Deficiency; Maroteaux-Lamy Syndrome: MPS VI)

MPS VI is an uncommon disorder and, like other MPS conditions, displays considerable heterogeneity. In the typical or severe form of the disease, the clinical phenotype is similar to MPS IH, but the intellect is preserved. All patients, even those at the less-severe end of the clinical spectrum, are at risk from cervical myelopathy secondary to dural and ligamentous hyperplasia. Atlantoaxial subluxation is variable, and it is often not possible to predict whether cervical fusion will be necessary in addition to decompression in patients with cervical cord disease until the time of operation.

Upper respiratory obstruction, middle-ear disease, corneal clouding, and progressive joint stiffness all occur. Cardiac involvement is universal and can be severe, including a neonatal presentation with endocardial fibroelastosis. With age, in severely affected patients, diffuse airway narrowing can lead to cor pulmonale (see Chapter 22).

The MPS VI gene is located on chromosome 5q13-q14 and no common mutations have been detected.

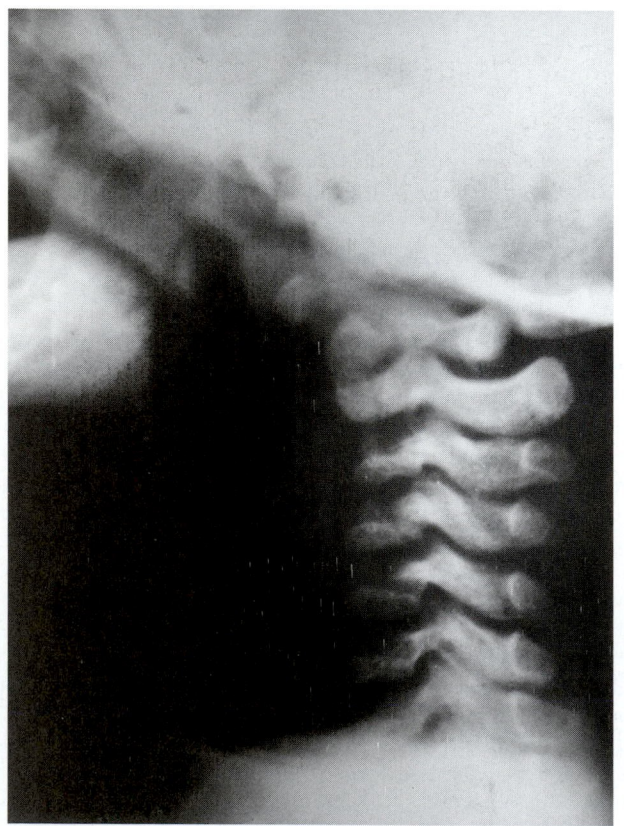

FIGURE 9-20   **Lateral x-ray of the cervical spine in the neutral position from a patient with MPS IV. Anterior subluxation of C1 on C2 and a dysplastic odontoid.**

Mucopolysaccharidosis Type VII (β-Glucuronidase Deficiency; Sly Disease: MPS VII)

MPS VII is a rare disorder and its importance is largely due to the research work that has been carried out on the murine model of the disease. This work has provided important information about therapeutic options in MPS disorders in general, including response to bone marrow transplantation, enzyme replacement therapy, and gene augmentation. Affected patients are few in number, as one of the main modes of presentation is with hydrops fetalis. Patients that survive to delivery often have a severe Hurler phenotype, although, like other MPS disorders, there is considerable heterogeneity.

The MPS VII gene is located on chromosome 7q21.1-q22 and consists of 12 exons. The relative rarity of MPS VII has rendered mutation analysis to be of academic interest only.

Mucopolysaccharidosis Type IX (Hyaluronidase Deficiency; MPS IX)

A 14-year-old girl with mild short stature and multiple periarticular soft-tissue masses has been described. There was no other visceral or CNS involvement, although synovial histology revealed abundant lysosomal storage. The patient was subsequently shown to have a mutation in the HYAL1 gene on chromosome 3p21.3 which results in a deficiency of hyaluronidase and accumulation of hyaluronic acid (hyaluronan, HA), a large GAG abundant in the extracellular matrix. The disorder has been tentatively labeled MPS IX.

MANAGEMENT OF MPS

Definitive/curative treatment for MPS disorders is still not possible despite a number of recent advances. Even in the most severely affected patients, however, careful attention to palliative therapies can have a beneficial effect on quality of life, and all patients should be under regular pediatric review.

Palliative Therapy

Palliative therapies in severe MPS I, II, and VI include treatment of hydrocephalus, middle-ear disease, and regular analgesia for joint pain and stiffness. More aggressive therapies, such as surgical correction of the gibbus abnormality or cardiac surgery, are not indicated in MPS I and II in view of the limited life expectancy. Appropriate education, speech therapy, physiotherapy, and occupational therapy should be offered, and parents should be given help with regard to appropriate financial support, aids, and adaptations (see Chapter 10).

In patients with less-severe forms of these disorders a more aggressive approach is justified. These patients may require neurosurgical interventions to prevent cervical cord disease, and many require regular ENT and orthopedic assessments. Cardiac status requires monitoring, and in patients with MPS I and VI, ophthalmologic follow-up is essential.

Patients with MPS III provide a very different clinical challenge. The behavioral problems and sleep disturbance require attention, although both are resistant to treatment. It is preferable to try and improve the child's sleep pattern first as the parents are more able to deal with the challenging behavior if fully rested. Chronic exhaustion due to sleep deprivation magnifies the clinical problems and creates an unsuitable therapeutic environment within the home. Hypnotic medication can be successful, but is usually only of transient benefit. The use of melatonin has been encouraging with a positive response obtained in at least 75% of those treated.

Respite care on a regular basis is essential to allow the parents time for themselves and for normal siblings. The challenging behavior responds poorly to a psychological or behavioral approach, and the children are effectively "untrainable." The use of a major tranquilizer is often necessary to modify aggressive or destructive behavior, and the hyperactivity generally responds poorly to amphetamine derivatives. Environmental modification within the home is an essential part of management.

Seizures usually respond well to a normal anticonvulsant regimen, although there are exceptions.

When swallowing dysfunction starts to produce coughing, often with drinks before solids, a formal assessment from a speech and language pathologist should be performed. This usually involves performing a special radiologic study of the swallowing process—videofluoroscopy. If the child is at risk from aspiration, nonoral feeding should be instituted; most parents prefer a surgically placed gastrostomy tube rather than a nasogastric tube for this purpose.

In MPS IV, attention should be focused on the cervical cord and the prevention of irreversible neurologic disease. In older patients, management of the respiratory failure is difficult as the patients do not respond to nasal CPAP. It is important to ensure that the patients receive influenza vaccine and that any respiratory infection is treated with the utmost seriousness. Efforts to improve sitting posture and breathing exercises may be helpful for patient morale but probably achieve very little clinically.

"CURATIVE" TREATMENT

Bone marrow transplantation (BMT) has been used as a crude form of "gene therapy" in patients with MPS since 1981 (see Sec. 20.4). Initially, many different types of MPS disease were treated, but it is now accepted that the therapy is of no benefit in MPS III and IV and there remains considerable doubt about its efficacy in severe MPS II.

In carefully selected patients with MPS IH and VI, there is no doubt that BMT will alter the natural history of the disease, although the indications for treatment in both disorders differ. In MPS IH, the prime objective is to avoid the intellectual deterioration and, consequently, BMT has to be performed at an early age (<18 months). In MPS VI, the aim of treatment is to prevent the cardiorespiratory decline that is responsible for early death.

Following a successful BMT, urinary GAG excretion quickly increases and then falls to the normal range after 3 to 6 months. Organomegaly resolves and there is incomplete clearing of the cornea. Cardiomyopathy, if present, is also successfully treated. In MPS IH, developmental progress is maintained in the majority of patients who receive BMT earlier than 18 months of age and the final DQ (developmental quotient) is usually identical to the DQ at the time of BMT. In both MPS IH and MPS VI, the skeletal disease is very resistant to correction. Although remodeling of the facial bones can change the coarse facial appearance and the long bones grow better, the vertebral bodies are not significantly improved and marked spinal deformity can result over time. Almost all patients with MPS IH who have had a successful BMT require complex corrective spinal surgery. Despite this, the majority of successfully transplanted patients have a good quality of life, and this therapy can no longer be regarded as experimental. For many patients it offers them their only chance of long-term survival.

Enzyme replacement therapy is intuitively attractive as a treatment, and the relevant enzymes can now be manufactured in large quantities by molecular means. Clinical trials in MPS IH, H/S, and S are currently underway. Gene augmentation (gene therapy) has also been attempted in patients with MPS IH, and a number of other studies have been performed on various animal models of MPS. Like the majority of other attempts at this form of treatment, none has produced any therapeutic benefit.

9.8.2 Mucolipidoses

The terminology used for this group of conditions is confusing, and mucolipidoses (ML) I and IV are very different conditions from ML II and III, which are allelic. The conditions are considered together for simplicity, but it is important to note that the enzyme basis, stored material, and clinical disturbance is very different despite common use of the term mucolipidosis.

CLINICAL PRESENTATION

Mucolipidosis Type I (Neuraminidase Deficiency; Sialidosis I, Cherry-Red Spot Myoclonus Syndrome, ML I)

This is a very heterogeneous disorder ranging in presentation from hydrops fetalis to a more chronic disorder (juvenile sialidosis) presenting with myoclonus and ataxia associated with a macular cherry-red spot. Dementia occurs very late, if at all, in this variant, and prolonged survival is usual. The most common mode of presentation is between these two extremes (childhood sialidosis), which produces a mild Hurler-like phenotype as well as mild dysostosis multiplex and a cherry-red spot. Death usually occurs in late teenage years (see Chapter 25).

Mucolipidosis Types II and III (UDP-*N*-Acetylglucosamine:Lysosomal Enzyme *N*-Acetylglucosaminyl-L-Phosphotransferase Deficiency; I-Cell Disease: ML II; Pseudo-Hurler Polydystrophy: ML III)

ML II and ML III represent two ends of the same disease spectrum. The basic biochemical defect involves an abnormality in the post-translational modification of lysosomal enzymes in which a targeting sequence (mannose-6-phosphate) fails to be added to the maturing enzyme. As a consequence lysosomal enzymes are not routed to the lysosome but are lost to the extracellular spaces where they are inactive. As a result, a variety of substrates accumulate within the lysosomes interfering with normal cellular function.

ML II produces very severe clinical and radiologic abnormalities and can present in the newborn period with a Hurler phenotype, as well as with a severe dysostosis that may be associated with intrauterine or neonatal fractures. Periosteal new bone formation is often very prominent. Hyperplastic gums soon after birth are an important clue to diagnosis (Fig. 9-21). Affected patients often make little developmental progress and are often extremely difficult to feed; some succumb early to cardiomyopathy. In contrast to other storage disorders, the head circumference in ML II is usually small and premature sutural synostosis can occur. Death usually occurs in infancy due to cardiac failure or infection.

ML III, on the other hand, can be a very mild disorder with survival into the fifth and sixth decades of life. Mild developmental problems are usual, although not present in all patients. The disorder produces severe orthopedic problems secondary to the progressive joint stiffness. The underlying dysostosis differs from that seen in MPS and characteristically affects the ball-and-socket joints most severely. Affected patients are unable to raise their arms above

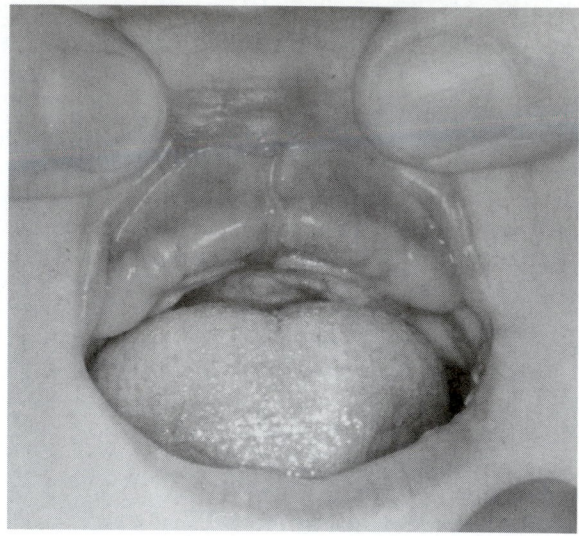

FIGURE 9-21   Hyperplastic gums in ML II.

their heads, and progressive hip dysplasia (Fig. 9-22) often leads to severe problems with mobility by early adult life. Most patients have carpal tunnel syndrome, and cardiac valve lesions (usually aortic incompetence) can develop later in life.

Mucolipidosis Type IV (Basic Biochemical Defect Unknown)

ML IV is a very rare disorder that is most commonly seen in children of Ashkenazi-Jewish extraction. Although the basic biochemical defect remains unknown, the ML IV gene maps to chromosome 19p13.2-13.3 by linkage analysis. Affected children present in the first year of life with corneal opacity and developmental delay and generally have a nonprogressive disorder. There is no organomegaly or dysostosis, and diagnosis depends on clinical suspicion and electron microscopy of skin fibroblasts.

MANAGEMENT OF MUCOLIPIDOSES

Unfortunately, there is no effective curative treatment for any of the mucolipidoses and palliative care is all that can be offered.

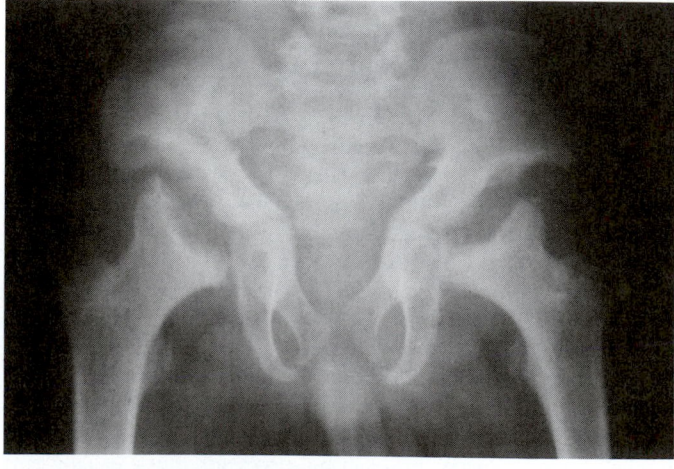

FIGURE 9-22   Radiograph of the hips in ML III showing almost complete loss of the femoral heads.

9.8.3 Glycoproteinoses and Other Related Disorders

CLINICAL PRESENTATION

Mannosidoses (α-Mannosidase Deficiency, α-Mannosidosis; β-Mannosidase Deficiency, β-Mannosidosis)

The term *mannosidosis* usually refers to α-mannosidosis, which is the most common of the mannosidoses. In this heterogeneous disorder, presentation can be severe in the first months of life with a Hurler-like disorder, or much later with a more prolonged clinical course with survival into middle age. Immunologic abnormalities are noted in most patients. Severe middle ear and respiratory infections are common, and immune deficiency caused by inadequate antibody production and decreased white-cell killing has been demonstrated in affected patients.

β-Mannosidosis was known to exist in goats long before it was identified in humans. The clinical phenotype is not well characterized, as there have been very few reported cases in humans. The first patients described with an isolated deficiency of β-mannosidase were adults who presented with angiokeratoma and mild learning difficulties; a severe presentation with infantile epileptic encephalopathy has also been reported.

Fucosidosis (α-Fucosidase Deficiency)

Fucosidosis is a rare disorder that produces symptoms and signs similar to mannosidosis, although the neurodegeneration has a tendency to be more aggressive in progression. In addition, the dysostosis and somatic abnormalities tend to be less obvious than in mannosidosis. Angiokeratoma can be extensive in some older patients with less-severe forms of the disease (sometimes called fucosidosis type II).

Schindler Disease (α-N-Acetylgalactosaminidase Deficiency)

Although only a few patients with this disorder have been reported, a wide clinical spectrum has been described. The condition was first described in infants with severe neurologic involvement, including myoclonus, spasticity, and rapidly progressive dementia. Histologic studies suggested a form of neuroaxonal dystrophy. Subsequent patients have been described with a very mild disorder consisting of angiokeratoma, but no overt neurologic disease.

Aspartylglucosaminuria (Aspartylglucosaminidase Deficiency)

Although this disorder occurs in all ethnic groups, it is relatively more common in the Finnish population. The disorder usually presents in infancy or early childhood with speech delay, middle-ear disease, and behavioral disturbance that can mimic Sanfilippo syndrome. With time, however, the somatic features become more obvious with facial coarsening and dysostosis multiplex, and by teenage years these features are usually well developed. Survival well into adult life is usual.

G_{M1}-Gangliosidosis (Isolated β-Galactosidase Deficiency)

β-Galactosidase activity is required for the catabolism of G_{M1}-ganglioside, galactose-containing glycoproteins, and keratan sulfate.

Different mutations in the β-galactosidase gene appear to affect activity toward these substrates differently, resulting in a tremendous variability in clinical effect in β-galactosidase-deficient patients. The most severely affected patients present in the newborn period with generalized gangliosidosis. In this rapidly progressive disorder, a Hurler phenotype can be noted at or soon after birth. Most severely affected infants make little or no developmental progress and die in infancy from progressive neurodegeneration. Later onset variants known as late-infantile, juvenile, and adult G_{M1}-gangliosidosis have been described. Finally, as described above, several patients with a phenotype indistinguishable from that of MPS IVA (Morquio syndrome) have been described. Here, the β-galactosidase mutation seems predominantly to affect keratan sulfate catabolism.

Galactosialidosis (Sialidosis Type II, Combined Neuraminidase and β-Galactosidase Deficiency)

Galactosialidosis is a heterogeneous disorder that manifests in utero with hydrops fetalis or later in infancy (infantile), childhood (juvenile), or adult life. The basic biochemical defect is in protective protein/cathepsin A (PPCA), which, when defective, leads to an intralysosomal proteolysis of β-galactosidase and neuraminidase. The majority of reported patients present with mild clinical features and the majority are of Japanese ancestry. The clinical features are similar to the cherry-red spot myoclonus syndrome, although the skeletal disease is usually more obvious. Mental retardation is usually mild and the disorder is only slowly progressive.

Mucosulfatidosis (Multiple Sulfatase Deficiency, Austin Syndrome)

Mucosulfatidosis results from a deficiency of *all* sulfatases, both lysosomal and microsomal. The multiple enzyme deficiency results from a deficiency of an enzyme that converts a specific cysteine thiol residue to an aldehyde. Biochemical testing reveals accumulation of GAGs, sulfatides, and gangliosides in the brains of affected children. Cerebral white-matter histology and biochemistry reveals features similar to those in metachromatic leukodystrophy. Clinically affected patients are ichthyotic due to a deficiency in steroid sulfatase and have profound neurologic handicap. Mild dysmorphism is usually present along with radiologic evidence of dysostosis multiplex, and death usually occurs in childhood.

Salla Disease [Sialic Acid Transporter Defect, Infantile Sialic Acid Storage Disease (ISSD)]

ISSD and Salla disease (so-called because it is seen in the Salla area of Finland) are variants of the same basic defect: a deficiency in the transport of free sialic acid across the lysosomal membrane. Along with excessive intracellular accumulation of sialic acid is excessive urinary excretion that is readily detected by urinary oligosaccharide analysis.

In ISSD, a dramatic neonatal presentation can occur with hydrops fetalis, hypopigmentation, recurrent severe infection, and failure to thrive. Dysostosis multiplex, vacuolated lymphocytes, and cardiac disease are usual, and the facial features often coarse. Most affected patients die in the first year of life. Salla disease is a less-severe presentation of the same disease. Most patients of Finnish origin present in the first year or two of life with learning difficulties, but progression is slower and patients survive well into adult life.

MANAGEMENT OF GLYCOPROTEINOSES AND RELATED DISORDERS

For the majority of disorders treatment is palliative only. BMT has been performed in α-mannosidosis, fucosidosis, and aspartylglucosaminuria, and although the numbers treated remain small, BMT may prove to be a useful therapy in carefully selected patients.

9.8.4 Genetic Counseling, Prenatal Diagnosis

All of the conditions discussed in this chapter are genetic (see Table 9-17) and diagnosis within a family should be followed by referral for appropriate counseling. In some conditions, for example, the X-linked disorder MPS II (Hunter syndrome), carrier detection may be a priority within the family. Prenatal diagnosis is possible for all the disorders. In some conditions, this can be done by direct enzyme assay on uncultured chorion villus material, providing a speedy result at an early stage in pregnancy (10–12 weeks). In other disorders, cultured cells or analysis of amniotic fluid may be more relevant. Because of the clinical overlap between these disorders, it is imperative that an accurate biochemical diagnosis be established in the index case before embarking on prenatal testing and that the various possibilities be discussed with the metabolic laboratory *before* samples are collected (see Sec. 8.2).

Because these disorders are relatively rare, the management should be centralized within the regional metabolic or genetics unit.

9.8.5 Other Disorders Presenting with Progressive Chronic Encephalopathy

The neuronal ceroid lipofuscinoses, Canavan disease, and Alexander disease all cause a syndrome of progressive neurodegeneration (see Sec. 25.17).

NEURONAL CEROID LIPOFUSCINOSES

The neuronal ceroid lipofuscinoses (NCLs) are a group of eight autosomal recessive lysosomal storage diseases characterized by the classic triad of blindness, seizures, and dementia, with a combined incidence of about 1:12,500. The light microscopic finding of a light-brown fluorescent storage material (ceroid lipofuscin) in subcellular vacuoles is shared amongst all of the NCLs; it is for this reason, and because of their clinical similarities, that they have been grouped together.

CANAVAN DISEASE

Canavan disease is an autosomal recessive disorder causing a chronic, progressive encephalopathy in infancy. It is characterized by early macrocephaly, initial hypotonia, and global developmental delay. Head control is often very poor. As the disease progresses, hypertonia and seizures develop. Episodic vomiting and sweating, as well as hyperthermia, are frequent. Optic atrophy and visual loss are common findings. Death usually ensues in the few years of life (see Sec. 25.17).

ALEXANDER DISEASE

This autosomal recessive disease is phenotypically very similar to Canavan disease. Macrocephaly develops early in infancy and may be associated with hydrocephalus. Spasticity, dementia, ataxia, and seizures ensue. Vision is spared. Death usually occurs within months to a few years of the onset of symptoms. The genetic etiology has not yet been characterized (see Sec. 25.17).

References

Amir N, Zlotogora J, Bach G: Mucolipidosis type IV: clinical spectrum and natural history. Pediatrics 79:953–959, 1987

Bartz H-J, Wiesner L, Wappler F: Anaesthetic management of patients with mucopolysaccharidosis IV presenting for major orthopaedic surgery. Acta Anaesthesiol Scand 43:679–683, 1999

Cleary MA, Wraith JE: Management of mucopolysaccharidosis type III. Arch Dis Child 69:403–406, 1993

Cleary MA, Wraith JE: The presenting features of mucopolysaccharidosis type IH (Hurler syndrome). Acta Paediatr 84:337–339, 1995

Fischer TA, Lehr H-A, Nixdorff U, Meyer J: Combined aortic and mitral stenosis in mucopolysaccharidosis type I-S (Ullrich-Scheie syndrome). Heart 81:97–99, 1999

Keulemans JL, Rueser AJ, Kroos MA, et al: Human alpha-N-acetylgalactosaminidase (alpha-NAGA) deficiency: new mutations and the paradox between genotype and phenotype. J Med Genet 33:458–464, 1996

Krivit W, Peters C, Shapiro EG: Bone marrow transplantation as effective treatment of central nervous system disease in globoid cell leukodystrophy, metachromatic leukodystrophy, adrenoleukodystrophy, mannosidosis, fucosidosis, aspartylglucosaminuria, Hurler, Maroteaux-Lamy, and Sly syndromes, and Gaucher disease type III. Curr Opin Neurol 12:167–176, 1999

Lemyre E, Russo P, Melancon SB, Gagne R, Potier M, Lambert M: Clinical spectrum of infantile free sialic acid storage disease. Am J Med Genet 82:385–391, 1999

Natowicz MR, Short MP, Wang Y, et al: Clinical and biochemical manifestations of hyaluronidase deficiency. N Engl J Med 335:1029–1033, 1996

Okamura-Oho Y, Zhang S, Callahan JW: The biochemistry and clinical features of galactosialidosis. Biochim Biophys Acta 1225:244–255, 1994

Patel MS, Callahan JW, Zhang S, et al: Early infantile galactosialidosis: prenatal presentation and postnatal follow-up. Am J Med Genet 85:38–47, 1999

Peters C, Shapiro EG, Anderson J, et al: Hurler syndrome: II. Outcome of HLA-genotypically identical sibling and HLA-haploidentical related donor bone marrow transplantation in fifty-four children. Blood 91:2601–2608, 1998

Ransford AO, Crockard HA, Stevens JM, Modaghegh S: Occipito-atlanto-axial fusion in Morquio-Brailsford syndrome. J Bone Joint Surg Br 78B:307–313, 1996

Schindler D, Bishop DF, Wolfe DE, et al: Neuroaxonal dystrophy due to lysosomal α-N-acetylgalactosaminidase deficiency. N Engl J Med 320:1735–1740, 1989

Tomatsu S, Fukuda S, Cooper A, et al: Mucopolysaccharidosis IVA: identification of a common missense mutation I113F in the N-acetylgalactosamine-6-sulfate sulfatase gene. Am J Hum Genet 57:556–563, 1995

Triggs-Raine B, Salo TJ, Zhang H, Wicklow BA, Natowicz MR: Mutations in HYAL1, a member of a tandemly distributed multigene family encoding disparate hyaluronidase activities, cause a newly described lysosomal disorder, mucopolysaccharidosis IX. Proc Natl Acad Sci U S A 96:6296–6300, 1999

Vafiadaki E, Cooper A, Heptinstall LE, Hatton CE, Thornley M, Wraith JE: Mutation analysis in 57 unrelated patients with MPS II (Hunter's disease). Arch Dis Child 79:237–241, 1998

Vellodi A, Young EP, Cooper A, et al: Bone marrow transplantation for mucopolysaccharidosis type I: experience of two British centers. Arch Dis Child 76:92–99, 1997

Walker RWM, Dorowski M, Morris P, Wraith JE: Anaesthesia and mucopolysaccharidoses. Anaesthesia 49:1078–1084, 1994

Willems PJ, Seo HC, Couke P, Tonlorenzi R, O'Brien JS: Spectrum of mutations in fucosidosis. Eur J Hum Genet 7:60–67, 1999

Wraith JE: The mucopolysaccharidoses: a clinical review and guide to management. Arch Dis Child 72:263–267, 1995

9.9   SPHINGOLIPIDOSES

Joe T. R. Clarke

Inborn errors of sphingolipid metabolism are a clinically heterogeneous group of disorders characterized by inherited point defects in the breakdown of complex lipids resulting in the accumulation of compounds containing a large, lipophilic core, called *ceramide,* and either a hydrophilic oligosaccharide (glycosphingolipids) or phosphorylcholine (sphingomyelin). Ceramide is composed of a long-chain fatty alcohol containing an amine group in amide linkage with a long-chain fatty acid.

The glycosphingolipids are classified into three groups, which differ metabolically and in the structure of the oligosaccharides (Fig. 9-23). The *globo* series of glycosphingolipids is characterized by an oligosaccharide containing galactose(α1-4)galactose(β1-4)glucose. The name of the series is derived from the neutral glycosphingolipid, globoside, the principal glycosphingolipid of red cell membranes. Globoside and ceramide trihexoside also occur in relatively high concentration in kidney. The *ganglio* series of glycosphingolipids is characterized by an oligosaccharide containing N-acetylgalactosamine(β1-4)galactose(β1-4)glucose. This series includes the gangliosides, which are distinguished by the presence in the molecule of one or more molecules of N-acetylneuraminic acid (one of a series of nine-carbon monosaccharides called *sialic acid*). Gangliosides containing up to three sialic acid residues are particularly enriched in gray matter of the brain, where they are localized primarily in synaptic terminals. The *galacto* series of glycosphingolipids includes galactocerebroside and galactocerebroside-O-3-sulfate (also called *sulfatide*).

9.9.1   Tissue Distribution and Function

Glycosphingolipids and sphingomyelin are ubiquitously distributed, predominantly as components of membranes, throughout the body. They are concentrated primarily in plasma membranes, including specialized plasma membrane derivatives, such as myelin. The concentrations of sphingolipids in all tissues are very low, when compared with other lipid constituents of plasma membranes, except in the brain. The concentration of higher-molecular-weight gangliosides, such as G_{M1}-ganglioside and di- and trisialogangliosides, is 10 to 15 times higher in cerebral gray matter than in any other tissue. Similarly, the concentrations of galactocerebroside and sulfatide are 100 to 1000 times higher in cerebral white matter than in any other tissue. Not surprisingly, in inherited defects in ganglioside metabolism, such as Tay-Sachs disease, neurologic involvement, particularly affecting gray matter function, is prominent. In contrast, inherited disorders of the catabolism of glycosphingolipids of the galacto series, such as metachromatic leukodystrophy and Krabbe globoid cell leukodystrophy, are characterized by clinical signs of cerebral white matter involvement; that is, leukodystrophy. The concentrations of neutral glycosphingolipids of the globo series are particularly high in leukocytes, erythrocytes, and macrophages. Hepatosplenomegaly is a prominent clinical feature of defects in the catabolism of this class of glycosphingolipids, such as Gaucher disease. Kidney is particularly rich in galNAc(β1-3)gal(α1-4)gal(β1-4)glc(β1-1')ceramide (globoside) and gal(α1-4)gal(β1-4)glc(β1-1')ceramide (ceramide trihexoside). Renal disease is a par-

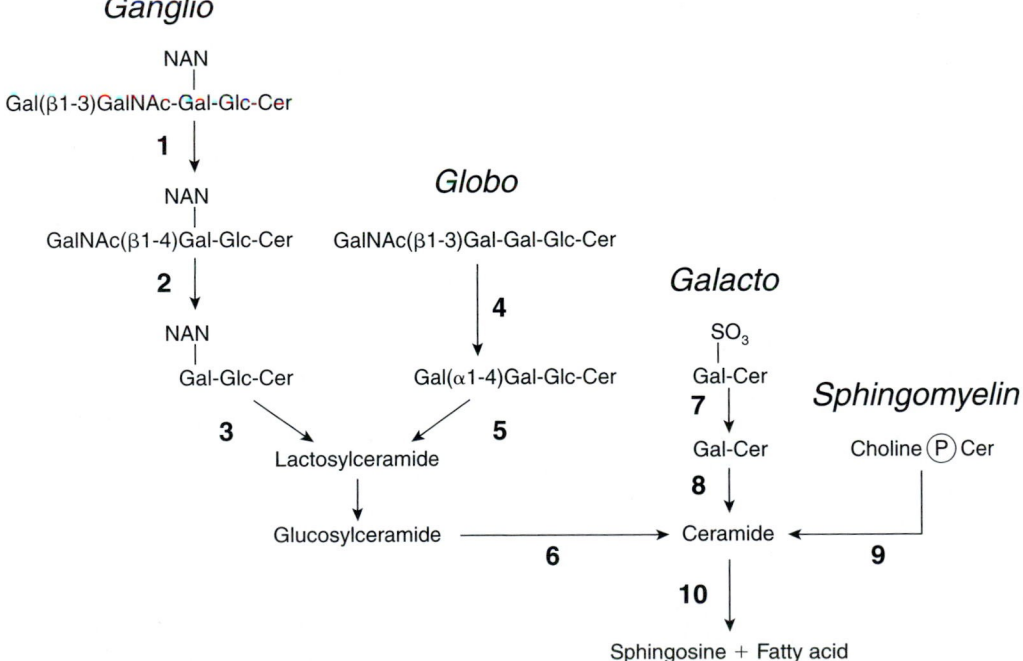

FIGURE 9-23   **Summary of the structure and catabolism of sphingolipids. 1, β-Galactosidase; 2, β-hexosaminidase A + G_{M2}-activator protein; 3, α-neuraminidase (sialidase) + saposin B; 4, β-hexosaminidase A; 5, α-galactosidase + saposin B; 6, glucocerebrosidase + saposin C; 7, arylsulfatase A; 8, galactocerebrosidase; 9, acid sphingomyelinase; 10, acid ceramidase + saposin D and C.**

ticularly prominent clinical feature of Fabry disease. The tissue distribution of sphingomyelin mirrors that of glucocerebroside, except in brain, where sphingomyelin is a major constituent of myelin and glucocerebroside concentrations are very low. The similarity of Gaucher disease and Niemann-Pick disease clinical phenotypes is explainable in part by the similarities in the tissue distributions of the sphingolipid substrates of the enzymes involved.

Sphingolipids appear to function in two general capacities. In some membrane systems, their role is primarily structural. Galactocerebroside, sulfatide, and sphingomyelin are important constituents of myelin, in which they are critically important to the ordered structure of the membrane. Glucocerebroside appears to be important to the structural integrity of the skin. In other membranes, they play a more functional role, as receptors (eg, blood group antigens) or as important intermediaries in signal transduction. Considerable evidence has been accumulated to indicate that ceramide and sphingomyelin turnover play important roles in the regulation of cell proliferation and apoptosis. The functional significance of higher-molecular-weight glycosphingolipids is still unclear. The concentration of higher gangliosides in neurons and synaptic nerve-endings suggests that they are important in neurotransmission.

9.9.2   Metabolism

The normal lysosomal degradation of glycosphingolipids occurs by the sequential hydrolysis of single monosaccharides from the nonreducing end of the oligosaccharide, ultimately yielding ceramide, which is then hydrolyzed to produce sphingosine and a free fatty acid. Sphingomyelin is catabolized by enzymic cleavage of the lipid into ceramide and phosphorylcholine. The sequence of reactions is summarized in Fig. 9-23. Each step in the hydrolytic catabolism of the sphingolipids is catalyzed by one of a series of enzymes having several properties in common. They are all glycoproteins, which are localized intracellularly in lysosomes. They all have complex, waterinsoluble, lipid substrates, and they are all hydrolases; that is, they cleave covalent bonds by the addition of a molecule of water to the substrate. They all have acidic pH optima, and they are all relatively robust, stable to long-term storage in frozen tissues. Some of the enzymes require the presence of a separate, noncatalytic polypeptide activator protein for activity toward their natural substrates.

All of the glycosphingolipid hydrolases exhibit relaxed substrate specificity. Although they are, for the most part, highly specific for the structure of the monosaccharide and the anomeric configuration of the glycosidic bond being cleaved, the structure of the aglycone, that is, the noncarbohydrate part of the molecule, is relatively unimportant. For the purposes of making the diagnosis of disease caused by deficiency of one of the glycosphingolipid hydrolases, this is an important property. Instead of having to use the natural substrate to measure enzyme activity, one may use synthetic, chemical substrates that change color or fluoresce when the glycosidic bond is broken.

The natural substrates of the lysosomal sphingolipid hydrolases are insoluble in water, and measurement of enzyme activity in vitro requires the addition of a detergent to solubilize the substrate. The catabolism of the glycosphingolipids in vivo requires the presence of naturally occurring protein cofactors called *sphingolipid activator proteins.* Four activator proteins, called *saposins,* are products of the proteolytic cleavage of prosaposin, a common precursor, coded by a gene located on chromosome 10. A fifth activator protein, G_{M2}-activator protein, is encoded by a separate gene, located on chro-

mosome 5. Mutations involving prosaposin or G_{M2}-activator protein cause diseases clinically indistinguishable from those caused by deficiency of the specific enzymes. Deficiencies of saposin or G_{M2}-activator do not affect the activities of sphingolipid hydrolase activities measured with the use of synthetic substrates. Disease variants caused by defects in prosaposin or G_{M2}-activator protein are rare and diagnostically challenging (see Sec. 9.9.5).

Another diagnostic challenge traceable to the substrate specificities of lysosomal sphingolipid hydrolases is the phenomenon of pseudodeficiency. Some nucleotide sequence changes result in the production of enzyme proteins that are catalytically active toward the natural substrates in vivo, but are inactive toward synthetic substrates in vitro. This is a relatively common phenomenon affecting β-hexosaminidase A and arylsulfatase A. For example, among non-Jews, up to 40% of individuals who test as carriers of Tay-Sachs disease by enzyme assay are actually carriers of one of three pseudodeficiency alleles. Homozygosity for pseudodeficiency alleles is not associated with disease. Arylsulfatase A pseudodeficiency is a particularly common polymorphism affecting as much as 10% of the normal population and is not associated with disease. The possibility of pseudodeficiency is important to keep in mind when the diagnosis of metachromatic leukodystrophy is undertaken for the purposes of presymptomatic treatment by bone marrow transplantation.

9.9.3   Clinical Features (Table 9-18)

NEONATAL ONSET

Nonimmune Fetal Hydrops

Infants with very severe variants of various lysosomal storage disorders, including the sphingolipidoses (especially Gaucher disease, Niemann-Pick disease, and G_{M1}-gangliosidosis), may present before birth or in the newborn period with nonimmune fetal hydrops. Severe ascites and generalized anasarca, associated with respiratory distress and disseminated intravascular thrombosis, often progress rapidly to death in the first few days of life. Radiographs may show subtle skeletal changes typical of severe variants of the same diseases presenting later in infancy. Rarely, affected infants may survive, with clearing of the edema and ascites, to present later in infancy with classic variants of the diseases. The diagnosis of a specific lysosomal disorder generally requires analysis of enzyme activities in cultured skin fibroblasts or tissues obtained at autopsy.

Neonatal Gaucher Disease (Type 4)

Infants with very severe Gaucher disease (type 4) present in the newborn period with thick, shiny, collodion skin; multiple congenital anomalies; hepatosplenomegaly; marked paucity of spontaneous movement; hypertonicity and hyperreflexia; neck retraction; and poor suck. In some cases, nonimmune hydrops is severe. Survival is generally measured in days or weeks.

EARLY INFANCY (1 TO 6 MONTHS)

Gaucher Disease, Type 2

Type 2 (acute neuronopathic) Gaucher disease is a rare, panethnic disease caused by deficiency of lysosomal glucocerebrosidase. It is characterized by accumulation of glucocerebroside in macrophages of the reticuloendothelial system and the brain. Glucocerebroside

TABLE 9-18

CLINICAL, BIOCHEMICAL, AND GENETIC CHARACTERISTICS OF THE SPHINGOLIPIDOSES

	DISORDER	ENZYME DEFECT	GENE	GENE LOCUS	CLINICAL FEATURES
Onset in early infancy (1–6 months of age)	Gaucher disease, type 2	Glucocerebrosidase	GBA	1q21	Early and severe neurologic involvement, marked hepatosplenomegaly, panethnic
	Gaucher disease with normal glucocerebrosidase	Saposin C	PSAP	10q22.1	Early and severe neurologic involvement, marked hepatosplenomegaly, extremely rare
	Globoid cell leukodystrophy	Galactocerebrosidase	GALC	14q31	Early onset, rapidly progressive, severe neurodegeneration, seizures
	Niemann-Pick disease, type A	Acid sphingomyelinase	SMPD1	11p15.4-p15.1	Rapidly progressive neurodegenerative disease, hepatosplenomegaly, failure to thrive, ±cherry-red spot, higher incidence in Ashkenazi Jews
	Farber lipogranulomatosis	Ceramidase	ASAH	8p22-p21.3	Painful subcutaneous nodules, chronic pulmonary disease, hepatosplenomegaly, neurodegeneration
Onset between 6 months and 2 years of age	G_{M1}-gangliosidosis	β-Galactosidase	GLB1	3p21.33	Early neurodegeneration, hepatosplenomegaly, dysostosis multiplex
	Metachromatic leukodystrophy (late-infantile form)	Arylsulfatase A	ARSA	22q13.31-qter	Early motor problems, ataxia, peripheral neuropathy, progressive cerebral deterioration
	Metachromatic leukodystrophy with normal arylsulfatase A	Saposin B	PSAP	10q22.1	Clinically indistinguishable from late-infantile MLD
	Multiple sulfatase deficiency	Multiple lysosomal and non-lysosomal sulfatases	MSD	?	Clinically resembles combination of MLD and mild MPS disorder with ichthyosis
	Tay-Sachs disease (classic TSD)	β-Hexosaminidase A	HEXA	15q23-q24	Early onset, rapidly progressive neurodegenerative disease, macrocephaly, hyperacusis, seizures, blindness, cherry-red spot, higher incidence in Ashkenazi Jews
	Sandhoff disease	β-Hexosaminidase A and B	HEXB	5q13	Early onset, rapidly progressive neurodegenerative disease, macrocephaly, hyperacusis, seizures, blindness, cherry-red spot
	Tay-Sachs disease (AB variant)	G_{M2}-activator protein	GM2A	15q31.3-q33.1	Early onset, rapidly progressive neurodegenerative disease, macrocephaly, hyperacusis, seizures, blindness, cherry-red spot
	Gaucher disease, type 3	Glucocerebrosidase	GBA	1q21	Slowly progressive neurologic involvement, variable hepatosplenomegaly, panethnic
	Niemann-Pick disease, type C	Intracellular cholesterol trafficking defect	NPC1	18q11-q12	Progressive neurodegeneration, hepatosplenomegaly, failure to thrive, dystonia, ataxia, dysarthria, vertical supranuclear gaze palsy
Onset between 2 and 18 years of age	Gaucher disease, type 1	Glucocerebrosidase	GBA	1q21	Hepatosplenomegaly, "bone crises," no neurologic involvement, common in Ashkenazi Jews
	Metachromatic leukodystrophy (juvenile form)	Arylsulfatase A	ARSA	22q13.31-qter	Progressive intellectual deterioration, ataxia, dysarthria, dystonia
	Late-onset G_{M2}-gangliosidosis	β-Hexosaminidase A or both A and B	HEXA or HEXB	15q23-q24 or 5q13	Progressive ataxia, incoordination, dysarthria, progressive psychomotor regression, spasticity, seizures, no cherry-red spot, progressive dementia, acute schizophrenia
	Niemann-Pick disease, type B	Acid sphingomyelinase	SMPD1	11p15.4-p15.1	Hepatosplenomegaly, sea-blue histiocytes in marrow, ±cirrhosis, ±bone lesions
	Niemann-Pick disease, type D (Nova Scotia variant)	Intracellular cholesterol trafficking defect	NPC1	18q11-q12	Progressive neurodegeneration, ±hepatosplenomegaly, dystonia, ataxia, dysarthria, vertical supranuclear gaze palsy
	Fabry disease	α-Galactosidase	GLA	Xq22	Burning pain in hands and feet, acroparesthesias, angiokeratomata, proteinuria, progressive renal disease

is derived from the catabolism of both the ganglio and globo series glycosphingolipids. The lipid accumulating in the brain is derived predominantly from the breakdown of gangliosides. In other tissues, it is derived primarily from neutral glycosphingolipids of the globo series (see Fig. 9-23).

Infants with the disease generally appear normal for the first several weeks of life. However, by 2 to 4 months of age, developmental progress slows. Over the next few weeks, the baby experiences feeding difficulties, resulting in failure to thrive. The abdomen becomes protuberant, and the infant often develops strabismus, obvious difficulty swallowing, and opisthotonic posturing. Examination of the abdomen reveals massive hepatosplenomegaly, with the spleen often extending into the left lower quadrant of the abdomen. Both organs are firm, but smooth, and nontender. In a few infants, funduscopic examination may reveal the presence of a macular cherry-red spot.

Hematologic studies show evidence of hypersplenism, with anemia, leukopenia, and marked thrombocytopenia. Liver function tests are usually normal or only mildly abnormal. The plasma tartarate-resistant acid phosphatase is generally increased as a nonspecific, though characteristic, feature of the disease. Bone marrow aspiration shows the presence of typical Gaucher storage cells. These are large, mononucleated histiocytes, with cytoplasm distended with basophilic material resembling wrinkled tissue paper by light microscopy. Similar storage cells occur throughout the reticuloendothelial system, including liver and spleen. Electron microscopic examination of liver tissue obtained by biopsy shows that the storage cells contain masses of twisted, filamentous inclusions. Unlike patients with later-onset variants of the disease, infants with neonatal-onset or with acute neuronopathic Gaucher disease show little or no radiographic evidence of skeletal involvement. Along with the characteristic clinical findings, the presence of Gaucher cells in bone marrow is virtually diagnostic of the disease. However, the diagnosis is confirmed by the demonstration of deficiency of β-glucosidase in peripheral blood leukocytes, cultured skin fibroblasts, or tissues obtained by biopsy or at autopsy.

Treatment of the disease is primarily supportive. Enzyme replacement therapy, which is dramatically effective in the management of nonneuronopathic variants of Gaucher disease, is of little value in the treatment of type 2 disease. Bone marrow transplantation is also ineffective. Infants with type 2 Gaucher disease generally succumb to severe inanition and pneumonia before age 2 years.

Krabbe Globoid Cell Leukodystrophy

This is a very rare, panethnic, rapidly progressive, neurodegenerative disease caused by deficiency of lysosomal galactocerebrosidase, resulting in accumulation of galactocerebroside, derived from myelin, in the brain and peripheral nerves. The absolute concentration of galactocerebroside in brain in globoid cell leukodystrophy has been found to be unexpectedly low. However, histopathologic studies show marked demyelination and the presence of giant multinucleated cells, called *globoid cells,* in perivascular spaces, and the ratio of galactocerebroside to sulfatide, a marker of myelination, is abnormally high. The extensive demyelination, which is such a characteristic feature of this disease, appears to be the result of accumulation of psychosine (galactosylsphingosine), normally present in only trace amounts (for detailed discussion see Sec. 25.17).

Niemann-Pick Disease, Type A

Niemann-Pick disease, type A, is a rare, degenerative neurovisceral disease caused by deficiency of lysosomal acid sphingomyelinase, resulting in accumulation of sphingomyelin in a wide range of tissues, particularly in elements of the reticuloendothelial system. It is much more common among Ashkenazi Jews than in other populations (for detailed discussion see Sec. 25.17).

G$_{M1}$-Gangliosidosis

G$_{M1}$-gangliosidosis, caused by deficiency of lysosomal β-galactosidase, is characterized by accumulation of G$_{M1}$-ganglioside in brain and other tissues. However, the principal cause of pathology is accumulation of β-galactoside-terminated oligosaccharides derived from glycoprotein catabolism. The disorder is discussed in Sec. 25.17.

Farber Lipogranulomatosis

Farber lipogranulomatosis is a rare autosomal recessive multisystem disorder resembling a generalized inflammatory disease. It is caused by deficiency of lysosomal ceramidase. Accumulation of ceramide causes granulomatous reactions in the lungs and subcutaneous and submucosal connective tissues throughout the body. Ceramide accumulation is also found in neurone of the CNS.

Clinically, the disease is characterized by a hoarse cry; painful, swollen joints; palpable subcutaneous nodules over the joints; and respiratory problems. Dysphagia, recurrent vomiting, pulmonary consolidation, and fever also occur. In some affected infants, hepatomegaly may be prominent and associated with significant hepatocellular dysfunction. Death from progressive neurologic deterioration, inanition, and chronic pulmonary disease usually occurs within several months of the onset of the disease. The diagnosis is established by demonstrating deficiency of acid ceramidase activity in cultured skin fibroblasts. Treatment is supportive.

LATE INFANCY AND EARLY CHILDHOOD (6 MONTHS TO 2 YEARS)

Gaucher Disease, Type 3

Like other variants of the disease, subacute neuronopathic (type 3) Gaucher disease is caused by a deficiency of lysosomal glucocerebrosidase. Originally considered to be limited largely to natives of the northern Swedish provinces of Norrbotten and Västerbotten, this variant is now recognized to be panethnic and much more common than was formerly thought. It is clinically highly heterogeneous. Generally, patients with the disease fall into one of two clinical groups, which have been designated type 3a, with prominent neurologic abnormalities and relatively mild visceral involvement, and type 3b, in which the visceral disease is severe and aggressive.

Patients with type 3a disease typically present in early-to-middle childhood with myoclonus, dementia, and ataxia. An apparently constant feature of the condition is the early development of an isolated, horizontal, supranuclear gaze palsy characterized by slowing of horizontal sacchadic eye movements, often with blinking and superimposed upward looping of the eyes and head thrusting. Smooth-pursuit eye movements are also generally abnormal, although they may be normal. Treatment-resistant generalized tonic-clonic seizures and spasticity develop later. Ultimately, the disease ends with death in the second or third decade of life. The spleen and liver are usually enlarged, but typically do not cause the problems seen in patients with type 3b or severe type 1 disease. Skeletal lesions, similar to those seen in patients with type 1 disease, occur in most patients.

Patients with type 3b Gaucher disease may appear to have particularly severe type 1 disease. However, they are generally much younger, averaging 2 to 3 years of age, and the degree of hepatosplenomegaly is greater and more rapidly progressive than in children with nonneuronopathic disease. Evidence of hepatocellular dysfunction is particularly prominent, with failure to thrive, ascites, peripheral edema, easy bruising, and nosebleeds. Portal hypertension, bleeding from esophageal varices, and other evidence of cirrhosis may be prominent. Infiltration of the lungs with storage cells causes restrictive pulmonary disease. The progression of visceral disease may be so rapid that death occurs, from hepatic or respiratory failure, before involvement of the nervous system is appreciated. The most common, and sometimes the only, sign of neurologic involvement is oculomotor apraxia. In addition, affected children often show some developmental or intellectual impairment, although this may be mild and the significance is often obscured by the severity of their visceral disease. Bone marrow aspirates invariably show the presence of typical Gaucher storage cells. The diagnosis is confirmed by measurement of β-glucosidase in leukocytes or cultured skin fibroblasts. Treatment by bone marrow transplantation or by enzyme replacement invariably produces improvement in the organomegaly and hematologic abnormalities of the disease. Further studies are necessary to determine the impact of these treatments on the inexorably progressive neurologic deterioration.

Niemann-Pick Disease, Type C

Niemann-Pick disease, type C, is relatively common compared with the other sphingolipidoses involving the central nervous system; it affects 250 to 500 children each year in the United States. It is the only lysosomal disorder under discussion here that is not caused by a defect in a specific lysosomal enzyme. Although the details of the pathophysiology have not yet been fully elucidated, the primary defect appears to be in the intracellular trafficking of cholesterol esters. The disease is characterized by intralysosomal accumulation of cholesterol, predominantly in tissues of the reticuloendothelial system. Neurologic deterioration is a prominent feature of the disease, but the mechanism of the neurologic abnormalities is still unknown. This condition is discussed in Sec. 25.17.

Late-Infantile Metachromatic Leukodystrophy

Late-infantile metachromatic leukodystrophy is an uncommon, rapidly progressive neurodegenerative disease caused by deficiency of arylsulfatase A resulting in accumulation of sulfatide in cerebral and cerebellar white matter and peripheral nerve. The disease usually presents in the second year of life with ataxia, hypotonia, and muscle weakness. Deep tendon reflexes are depressed. Generally, within a few months, muscle tone increases, progressing to generalized spasticity and, ultimately, to decerebrate posturing. Developmental regression is initially slow, but becomes more prominent as the disease progresses. Ophthalmoscopic examination may show the presence of grayish discoloration of the macula, resembling the cherry-red spot of Tay-Sachs disease. Seizures are a common, but invariably late, manifestation of the disease.

Nerve conduction velocities are slow, and CSF protein concentrations are elevated. CT studies show progressive attenuation and loss of periventricular white matter, followed by marked loss of myelin throughout the central nervous system and the corticospinal tracts of the cord. Ultrasound examination of the abdomen shows nonfunctioning of the gallbladder, with thickening of the mucosa and stones, a curiosity characteristic of this disorder (see Sec. 25.17).

Tay-Sachs Disease

This disorder, which predominantly affects the nervous system, is discussed in Sec. 25.17.

Sandhoff Disease

Sandhoff disease is a very rare, progressive, neurodegenerative condition caused by total β-hexosaminidase deficiency. The most prominent pathologic and clinical changes in this disease are the same as are seen in Tay-Sachs disease. In most cases, Sandhoff disease is clinically virtually indistinguishable from Tay-Sachs disease. In some patients, however, mild-to-moderate enlargement of the liver and spleen occur, and radiographs may show subtle evidence of dysostosis multiplex. (For detailed discussion see Sec. 25.17.)

Multiple Sulfatase Deficiency

This is a rare condition caused by a defect in the posttranslational processing of a number of lysosomal and nonlysosomal sulfatases, including arylsulfatases A, B, and C, iduronate-2-sulfate sulfatase N-acetylgalactosamine-6-sulfate sulfatase, and N-acetylglucosamine-6-sulfate sulfatase (see Sec. 9.8).

LATE CHILDHOOD AND ADOLESCENCE (2 TO 18 YEARS)

Gaucher Disease, Type 1

Nonneuronopathic (type 1) Gaucher disease is the most common lysosomal storage disease. Among Ashkenazi Jews, in whom it is particularly common, the disease may affect 1 of every 500 individuals. Like the other variants of Gaucher disease, it is caused by deficiency of lysosomal glucocerebrosidase. Although visceral manifestations of the disease may be severe, there is no primary involvement of the central nervous system.

The disease often comes to medical attention as a result of the incidental discovery of painless splenomegaly. The spleen may be very large, extending into the left lower quadrant of the abdomen. It is generally smooth, mobile, and nontender. The liver is also usually enlarged, but only rarely as enlarged as the spleen. It is usually smooth, firm, and nontender. Cirrhosis is rare. Enlargement of the liver and spleen often produces abdominal protuberance. Decreased exercise tolerance and fatigability are common complaints in patients with Gaucher disease. Enlargement of the spleen and liver is occasionally accompanied by episodes of acute abdominal pain caused by splenic or hepatic infarction.

Patients may also come to attention as a result of a history of excessive bleeding. The hemorrhagic complications of the disease are primarily the result of thrombocytopenia caused by hypersplenism. The bleeding is sometimes severe. Mild bleeding problems, not related to decreased platelets, are common in children with moderate disease. Young children with Gaucher disease may present with "growing pains," aching pain in the lower extremities, resulting from skeletal infiltration with storage cells. The pain is typically worse at night, sometimes waking the child from sleep. Children with the disease may develop fractures, including crush fractures of vertebrae, with avascular necrosis of the hips resembling Legg-Calvé-Perthes disease, or as a result of bone crises clinically difficult to distinguish from pyogenic osteomyelitis. Children with severe type 1 Gaucher disease often show growth retardation.

On physical examination, children with Gaucher disease often have a sallow complexion, out of proportion to any anemia, and sometimes associated with increased pigmentation of the skin. The skeletal manifestations of Gaucher disease are clinically variable, depending on the degree of secondary bone and joint destruction. Children with type 1 Gaucher disease often look remarkably healthy for the degree of splenomegaly.

The bone marrow contains typical Gaucher storage cells. As is the case with other variants of the disease, the diagnosis is confirmed by demonstrating marked deficiency of β-glucosidase in leukocytes or cultured skin fibroblasts. The three clinical variants of Gaucher disease are indistinguishable by routine enzyme assays. Mutation analysis is somewhat more helpful in predicting the course of the disease in individual patients.

Mild normocytic normochromic anemia is a typical feature of Gaucher disease. Iron stores in the bone marrow are characteristically increased, and treatment of anemia with iron supplements is generally inappropriate. Bleeding resulting from thrombocytopenia caused by hypersplenism may require aggressive intervention. The response to splenectomy is generally rapid and complete. Because of the risks associated with total splenectomy, some have resorted to partial removal of the organ, but the response is unpredictable and usually of limited duration (see Chapter 19). Treatment of painful bone crises often requires intravenous administration of narcotic analgesics.

Enzyme replacement therapy has dramatically changed the management of Gaucher disease (see Sec. 9.9.6).

LATE-ONSET METACHROMATIC LEUKODYSTROPHY

Children with late-onset metachromatic leukodystrophy generally present at 4 to 10 years of age, often with a history of deteriorating school performance. It is often associated with personality changes, including obsessiveness, emotional lability, and social withdrawal, as well as ataxia and dysarthria. Progression of the disease is usually slow, and seizures, though common, generally occur later in the course of the disease. Survival into the late teens or later is common. Treatment is supportive (see Sec. 25.17).

LATE-ONSET G$_{M2}$-GANGLIOSIDOSIS

This variant of G$_{M2}$-gangliosidosis is characterized by the onset at age 2 to 10 years of progressive ataxia, incoordination, dysarthria, progressive psychomotor regression, spasticity, seizures, and blindness with retinal pigmentary changes, but no cherry-red spot. The disease may be dominated by progressive dystonia, choreoathetosis, ataxia, muscle wasting, and dementia, or by dysarthria, ataxia, and other cerebellar signs, spasticity, muscle wasting, and pes cavus deformity, with relative preservation of intelligence. It may also present in adolescence as acute schizophrenia, paranoia, or recurrent psychotic depression. Treatment is supportive.

Niemann-Pick Disease, Type B

Niemann-Pick disease, type B, is caused by incomplete deficiency of acid sphingomyelinase. It is more common among Ashkenazi

Jews than in other populations. Clinically, it is virtually indistinguishable from Gaucher disease, type 1. It presents most often in middle or late childhood as asymptomatic splenomegaly. The liver and spleen increase in size with time. Hematologic complications and skeletal involvement are generally less severe than in Gaucher disease; however, the risk of cirrhosis is higher. Bone marrow aspirates show the presence of foamy storage histiocytes, identical to those seen in Niemann-Pick disease, type A. However, the marrow often also contains sea-blue histiocytes. Treatment is supportive. Severe disease responds to bone marrow transplantation.

Fabry Disease

The only sphingolipidoses transmitted as an X-linked recessive disorder, Fabry disease is also one of the most protean. Affected boys generally present around the time of puberty with complaints of pain, usually in the hands and feet. The pain is usually episodic, severe, and of a particularly unpleasant, burning, quality. Painful crises are often precipitated by extremes of environmental temperature, especially heat by physical exertion or by physical debilitation. Pain in the joints may be clinically indistinguishable from acute pauciarticular arthritis. Abdominal pain may resemble an acute abdomen. The response to conventional analgesics is generally incomplete. Decreased or absence of sweating is typical of the disease. The explanation for the pain is often not recognized, causing significant psychological problems for the boys and their families.

By the mid-to-late teens, affected boys gradually develop increasing numbers of tiny, red-to-black, papular lesions, called *angiokeratomata*, in the umbilicus and on the skin of the buttocks, scrotum, penis, and buccal mucosa. The lesions are not associated with inflammatory changes, itching, or secondary skin changes, although they often bleed when traumatized. Slit-lamp examination of the eyes shows the presence of characteristic corneal opacities, which are subtle and never interfere with vision. Proteinuria, progressive renal impairment, premature coronary artery disease, and stroke occur later in life. Heterozygous girls may experience painful crises similar to those occurring in affected boys. Corneal lesions are common. However, angiokeratomata are rare, even in severely symptomatic girls. The neurologic manifestations are discussed in detail in Sec. 25.17.

The disease is caused by deficiency of lysosomal α-galactosidase, which causes accumulation of ceramide trihexoside in the walls of small arteries throughout the body, in the glomerulus and renal tubular epithelium, and in dorsal root ganglia and small, unmyelinated nerve fibers. The diagnosis is confirmed by demonstration of deficiency of the enzyme in plasma, leukocytes, or cultured skin fibroblasts. Painful crises respond to treatment with carbamazepine and are preventable by long-term treatment with gabapentin. In some patients, gastrointestinal signs of autonomic dysfunction may be prominent. These often respond to treatment with metaclopramide. The pain associated with the disease appears to respond to intravenous infusions of purified α-galactosidase. The role of enzyme replacement in the long-term management of the disease is still under investigation.

9.9.4 Genetics

Some important clinical features and the genes involved in the various sphingolipidoses are summarized in Table 9-18. All but one of the sphingolipidoses are transmitted as autosomal recessive conditions; Fabry disease is inherited as an X-linked recessive disorder.

The genes encoding the sphingolipid hydrolases are relatively un-complicated, "housekeeping" genes, expressed in all tissues.

Some generalizations are possible regarding genotype-phenotype correlations among the sphingolipidoses. For example, sequence changes resulting in complete absence of functional gene product, such as the common *HEXA* mutations causing Tay-Sachs disease, invariably cause severe disease. On the other hand, changes producing amino acid substitutions may cause almost any disease phenotype, depending on the stability of the mutant protein and the relationship of the sequence change to the active site of the enzyme. For example, patients with Gaucher disease who carry the common Asn370Ser mutation always have type 1 disease. By contrast, patients with the Leu444Pro mutation are at high risk for neuronopathic disease (type 2 or 3), especially if they are homozygous for the mutation. However, within these groups of patients, the clinical variability between individual patients with identical genotypes, even within families, may be enormous.

9.9.5   Diagnosis

The extent of visceral and neurologic involvement in the sphingolipidoses is helpful in guiding diagnostic laboratory investigation (Fig. 9-24). There is no established screening test for the sphingolipidoses. However, recent studies on the potential role of measurements of plasma levels of lysosome-associated membrane proteins (LAMP) for early detection of infants affected with these diseases are promising. Diagnosis requires a high index of suspicion, based on the history and findings on physical examination, and systematic consideration of the various etiologic possibilities. The diagnosis of a particular condition may be strongly suspected on the basis of clinical and morphologic studies, such as examination of bone marrow aspirates or other types of tissue biopsy. Ultimately, definitive diagnosis requires the demonstration of marked deficiency of specific sphingolipid hydrolases or identification, by molecular genetic techniques, of specific mutations known to cause a particular disease.

DEMONSTRATION OF STORAGE

MORPHOLOGIC STUDIES   Histopathologic studies on bone marrow aspirates or on tissue obtained by biopsy generally show evidence of accumulation of complex lipid. Although the nature of the lipid and localization in lysosomes may be determined by histochemical and ultrastructural studies on appropriately prepared tissue samples, the changes are generally not specific enough, except in the case of Gaucher disease, to make the diagnosis of a specific sphingolipidosis. The demonstration of metachromatic granules in peripheral nerve biopsies is typical of metachromatic leukodystrophy. The positive filipin staining of cultured fibroblasts is a characteristic finding in Niemann-Pick disease, type C.

CHEMICAL ANALYSES   Chemical analysis of tissues is rarely practical or necessary for the diagnosis of the sphingolipidoses. However, glycosphingolipid analysis of urinary sediment is often helpful for confirmation of the diagnosis of metachromatic leukodystrophy when clinical signs may be minimal and the possibility of arylsulfatase A pseudodeficiency needs to be considered. Glycosphingolipid analysis of urinary sediment is also helpful for carrier detection of Fabry disease.

DEMONSTRATION OF ENZYME DEFICIENCY

The demonstration of profound deficiency of lysosomal enzyme activity in an appropriate tissue, especially cultured skin fibroblasts, is the gold standard for the laboratory diagnosis of the sphingolipidoses. In most cases, enzyme assay using synthetic substrates is adequate for the establishment of a specific diagnosis. However, problems arise when disease is caused by deficiency of sphingolipid activator protein (saposin) or G_{M2}-activator protein, and enzyme activity measured with the use of synthetic substrates is normal. The diagnosis of activator deficiency requires analysis of enzyme activity using the natural substrates or analysis of the activator itself.

Visceral Involvement ↓	None	CNS[1] only	CNS + PNS[2]	PNS only
		Neurologic Involvement		
None		Tay-Sachs disease Sandhoff disease	Late-onset G_{M2}-gangliosidosis MLD[3] GCLD[4]	Fabry disease (early)
Enlarged liver and spleen	Gaucher disease, type 1 NPD[5], type B	Gaucher disease, type 2 Gaucher disease, type 3 NPD, types A or C		
Cardiac, renal, vascular, or pulmonary	Fabry disease	NPD, type A Farber lipogranulomatosis		Fabry disease
Skin lesions	Fabry disease	Farber lipogranulomatosis		Fabry disease

[1]Central nervous system; [2]peripheral nervous system; [3]metachromatic leukodystrophy; [4]Krabbe globoid cell leukodystrophy; [5]Niemann-Pick disease

FIGURE 9-24   **Summary of the extent of visceral and neurologic involvement in the sphingolipidoses.**

MUTATION ANALYSIS

Mutation analysis is useful for diagnosis of the various sphingo-lipidoses when the mutant alleles responsible for the disease in a particular family are known. In some populations, the most cases are caused by a small number of specific mutant alleles, and specific mutation analysis is useful for primary diagnosis. The best-studied examples are sphingolipidoses occurring with particularly high frequency among Ashkenazi Jews.

CARRIER DETECTION

Carrier detection by measurement of lysosomal enzyme levels in peripheral blood leukocytes is possible for most of the sphingoli-pidoses. For some, the identification of carriers on the basis of enzyme activities in plasma or leukocytes is relatively simple and reliable. Tay-Sachs carrier detection represents a special case: the measurement of HexA and HexB by differential heat-inactivation is reliable, but the measurement of the enzymes is cumbersome and fastidious. Nonetheless, the procedure has become routine in many specialized laboratories around the world and is used for large-scale carrier detection among high-risk populations, such as Ashkenazi Jews. Wide acceptance of Tay-Sachs carrier detection, coupled with prenatal diagnosis and selective termination of pregnancy, has led to a marked decrease in the incidence of the disease.

Selected carrier testing of relatives of infants affected with any of the sphingolipidoses, except Niemann-Pick disease, type C, is possible by enzyme assay, although it is technically difficult and unreliable in some cases. Screening by mutation analysis is easier and more reliable, when the mutant allele segregating in the family is known. Screening for carriers of Gaucher disease or of Niemann-Pick disease, type A, is offered by some centers to individuals without a family history of disease, but who are from high-risk populations. These centers rely more on specific mutation analysis than on enzyme assay, taking advantage of the observation that a small number of mutant alleles account for the majority of disease in the population.

Carrier detection among asymptomatic women is often possible by measurement of leukocyte α-galactosidase activities. However, in 15% or more of carriers, enzyme activity is in the normal range. Carriers generally have subtle corneal opacities, visible only by slit-lamp examination, and they excrete increased amounts of ceramide trihexoside in their urine.

PRENATAL DIAGNOSIS

Midtrimester prenatal diagnosis, by chorionic villus sampling or by amniocentesis, is possible for all the sphingolipidoses. Except in the case of Niemann-Pick disease, type C, diagnosis is generally based on enzyme assay of appropriate cells, although mutation analysis is also used. Misdiagnosis of normalcy is a potential problem with chorionic villus analysis, especially if the cells are expanded by culturing the sample. Only laboratories with specialized experience and expertise in lysosomal diseases usually do these procedures (see Sec. 8.2).

9.9.6   Treatment

SUPPORTIVE

General

Caring for children with progressive neurovisceral storage diseases is emotionally and physically demanding. Any approach to sup-portive care should take the needs of the entire family, especially those of healthy siblings, into account. The presence of extended family members or close friends is particularly important to help take over some of the care of the child to avoid parental exhaustion.

Nutritional Issues

Most young children with severe neurodegenerative disorders have difficulty feeding, and most are associated with severe inanition as the disease progresses. Nutritional supplements administered by mouth are of only limited value as swallowing becomes increasingly impaired. At some stage, most physicians and parents consider the initiation of feeding by nasogastric tube or gastrostomy. The decision is often a difficult one. Some argue that tube feeding is technically cumbersome and merely prolongs the life of the terminally ill child. They cite evidence that starvation in these severely neurologically impaired children is not associated with the discomfort experienced by neurologically intact individuals. Others point out that tube feeding decreases the time required for feeding, decreasing the tension associated with feeding and increasing the opportunity for other emotionally more rewarding interactions, including attention to healthy siblings. The presence of a nasogastric tube or gastrostomy also facilitates the administration of drugs and fluids, especially during intercurrent illnesses. What is best for one family is often quite different from what is best for another.

Respiratory Care

Patients with neurodegenerative sphingolipidoses are at high risk for aspiration, even when feeding is entirely by nasogastric tube or gastrostomy. Immobility and depressed gag and cough reflexes increase the risk of aspiration pneumonia. Frequent changes in posture, postural drainage, gentle chest physiotherapy, and oropharyngeal suctioning improve the quality of life of these patients.

Pain

With the important exception of Fabry disease, pain is not a common or prominent feature of the sphingolipidoses. In the case of Fabry disease, however, the pain is not only particularly severe, but it is also extraordinarily unpleasant in quality. Arising from glyco-lipid accumulation in dorsal root ganglia and small nonmyelinated nerves, it is neuritic in character, often causing a chronic, unremitting burning sensation, especially in the hands and feet. It may also occur as episodes of indescribably unpleasant acroparesthesias, with lightning-like radiation along the extremities. The pain is characteristically exacerbated by exposure to extremes in temperature, especially heat. Relief by administration of conventional analgesics is usually incomplete. However, many patients benefit from treatment with phenytoin, carbamazepine, or gabapentin. Patients with late-onset G_{M2}-gangliosidosis may also experience similar, neuritic pain, although rarely as severe as in Fabry disease.

Seizures

Seizures are a common and prominent feature of many of the sphingolipid storage diseases involving the central nervous system. They are often complex partial seizures, which may be frequent and difficult to control with conventional anticonvulsants. In some cases, such as Tay-Sachs disease, a compromise needs to be made between complete seizure control, which is very difficult to achieve, and unacceptable drowsiness or other side effects. In some diseases, such as Gaucher disease, type 2, and Niemann-Pick disease, type

C, myoclonic seizures are particularly common and difficult to control.

BONE MARROW TRANSPLANTATION

Bone marrow transplantation is effective in the treatment of sphingolipidoses in which the disease primarily affects elements of the reticuloendothelial system (see Sec. 20.4). Diseases such as Gaucher disease, type 1, and Niemann-Pick disease, type B, respond well to this treatment. It may also delay the progression of neurologic deterioration in children with late-infantile metachromatic leukodystrophy and in late-onset Krabbe globoid cell leukodystrophy. Experience with bone marrow transplantation is still too limited to determine its role in the long-term management of these disorders.

ENZYME REPLACEMENT THERAPY

The demonstration that the tissue uptake of infused glucocerebrosidase was manipulable by modification of the oligosaccharide of the enzyme after purification revolutionized this approach to therapy. Biweekly infusions of glucocerebrosidase, purified from human placenta or produced by recombinant Chinese hamster ovary cells, is safe and invariably effective in reversing the hematologic and early skeletal complications of Gaucher disease, irrespective of the type. The effect on neurologic disease, in types 2 and 3, is only modest.

Treatment requires regular intravenous infusions of enzyme, which often requires the installation of some device to facilitate venous access, particularly in young children. The greatest obstacle to treatment is the cost. The success of enzyme replacement therapy in Gaucher disease has prompted studies of the possibility that other sphingolipid storage diseases might also respond to this approach to treatment. Studies are currently in progress to evaluate the effectiveness of the treatment of Niemann-Pick disease by infusions of acid sphingomyelinase and of Fabry disease by infusions of α-galactosidase.

INHIBITORS OF GLYCOSPHINGOLIPID SYNTHESIS

Experiments are currently being performed in humans to evaluate the effectiveness of controlling glycosphingolipid accumulation in some disorders, such as Gaucher disease and Fabry disease, by administration of inhibitors of the synthesis of glucosylceramide, the precursor of all the glycosphingolipids of the globo and ganglio series. This approach to treatment is not expected to be effective in patients with no residual enzyme activity, such as in classic Tay-Sachs disease. It is more promising for the treatment of sphingolipidoses such as Gaucher disease, type 1, in which significant enzyme activity is preserved.

GENE TRANSFER THERAPY

Most researchers agree that supplementation of the mutant genome with one or more copies of the wild-type gene responsible for the disease is the ultimate way to cure the sphingolipidoses. The feasibility of treatment by retrovirus-mediated gene transfer treatment has been demonstrated for many lysosomal storage diseases by in vitro studies with cultured cells. In some cases, especially in Gaucher disease, the results of studies in mice have been promising. However, experiments in patients with the disease have, so far, been disappointing.

References

Baldinger S, Pierpont ME, Wenger DA: Pseudodeficiency of arylsulfatase A: a counselling dilemma. Clin Genet 31:70–76, 1987

Balicki D, Beutler E: Gaucher disease. Medicine (Baltimore) 74(6):305–323, 1995.

Barth ML, Ward C, Harris A, Saad A, Fensom A: Frequency of arylsulphatase A pseudodeficiency-associated mutations in a healthy population. J Med Genet 31:667–671, 1994

Barton NW, Brady RO, Dambrosia JM, et al: Replacement therapy for inherited enzyme deficiency—macrophage-targeted glucocerebrosidase for Gaucher disease. N Engl J Med 324:1464–1470, 1991

Berger J, Löschl B, Bernheimer H, et al: Occurrence, distribution, and phenotype of arylsulfatase A mutations in patients with metachromatic leukodystrophy. Am J Med Genet 69:335–340, 1997

Brady RO: Sphingolipidoses. Annu Rev Biochem 47:687–713, 1978

Desnick RJ, Ioannou YA, Eng CM: Alpha-galactosidase A deficiency: Fabry disease. In: Scriver CR, Beaudet AL, Sly WS, Valle D, eds: The Metabolic and Molecular Bases of Inherited Disease, 8th ed. New York, McGraw-Hill, 2001 p. 3733–3774

Eng CM, Desnick RJ: Molecular basis of Fabry disease: mutations and polymorphisms in the human alpha-galactosidase A gene. Hum Mutat 3:103–111, 1994

Fink JK, Filling-Katz MR, Sokol J, et al: Clinical spectrum of Niemann-Pick disease type C. Neurology 39:1040–1049, 1989

Grabowski GA, Leslie N, Wenstrup R: Enzyme therapy for Gaucher disease: the first 5 years. Blood Rev 12:115–133, 1998

Hakomori S: Glycosphingolipids in cellular interaction, differentiation, and oncogenesis. Annu Rev Biochem 50:733–764, 1981

Hua CT, Hopwood JJ, Carlsson SR, Harris RJ, Meikel PJ: Evaluation of the lysosome-associated membrane protein LAMP-2 as a marker for lysosomal storage disorders. Clin Chem 44:2094–2102, 1998

Johnson WG: The clinical spectrum of hexosaminidase deficiency disease. Neurology 31:1453–1456, 1981

Kaback M, Lim-Steele J, Dabholkar D, Brown D, Levy N, Zeiger K: Tay-Sachs disease—carrier screening, prenatal diagnosis, and the molecular era: an international perspective, 1970 to 1993. JAMA 270:2307–2315, 1993

Karlsson KAG: On the character and functions of sphingolipids. Acta Biochim Pol 45:429–438, 1998

Kobayashi T, Goto I, Yamanaka T, Suzuki Y, Nakano T, Suzuki K: Infantile and fetal globoid cell leukodystrophy: analysis of galactosylceramide and galactosylsphingosine. Ann Neurol 24:517–522, 1988

Kolodny EH: Niemann-Pick disease. Curr Opin Hematol 7:48–52, 2000

Kolodny EH, Raghavan S, Krivit W: Late-onset Krabbe disease (globoid cell leukodystrophy): clinical and biochemical features of 15 cases. Dev Neurosci 13:232–239, 1991

Levade T, Moser HW, Fensom AH, Harzer K, Moser AB, Salvayre R: Neurodegenerative course in ceramidase deficiency (Farber disease) correlates with the residual lysosomal ceramide turnover in cultured living patient cells. J Neurol Sci 134:108–114, 1995

Luberto C, Hannun YA: Sphingolipid metabolism in the regulation of bioactive molecules. Lipids 34 (Suppl):S5–S11, 1999

Mahuran DJ: The biochemistry of HEXA and HEXB gene mutations causing G_{M2}-gangliosidosis. Biochim Biophys Acta 1096:87–94, 1991

Mahuran DJ, Triggs RB, Feigenbaum AJ, Gravel RA: The molecular basis of Tay-Sachs disease: mutation identification and diagnosis. Clin Biochem 23:409–415, 1990

Meikle PJ, Hopwood JJ, Clague AE, Carey WF: Prevalence of lysosomal storage disorders. JAMA 28:249–254, 1999

Natowicz MR, Prence EM, Chaturvedi P, Newburg DS: Urine sulfatides and the diagnosis of metachromatic leukodystrophy. Clin Chem 42:232–238, 1996

O'Brien JS, Kishimoto Y: Saposin proteins: structure, function, and role in human lysosomal storage disorders. FASEB J 5:301–308, 1991

Pastores GM, Einhorn TA: Skeletal complications of Gaucher disease: pathophysiology, evaluation, and treatment. Semin Hematol 32 (Suppl 1): 20–27, 1995

Pentchev PG, Brady RO, Blanchette-Mackie EJ, et al: The Niemann-Pick C lesion and its relationship to the intracellular distribution and utilization of LDL cholesterol. Biochim Biophys Acta 1225:235–243, 1994

Ricketts MH, Goldman D, Long JC, Manowitz P: Arylsulfatase A pseudodeficiency-associated mutations: population studies and identification of a novel haplotype. Am J Med Genet 67:387–392, 1996

Salvetti A, Heard JM, Danos O: Gene therapy of lysosomal storage disorders. Br Med Bull 51:106–122, 1995

Schiffmann R: Niemann-Pick disease type C—from bench to bedside. JAMA 276:561–564, 1996

Schuette CG, Doering T, Kolter T, Sandhoff K: The glycosphingolipidoses—from disease to basic principles of metabolism. Biol Chem 380: 759–766, 1999

Shamburek RD, Pentchev PG, Zech LA, et al: Intracellular trafficking of the free cholesterol derived from LDL cholesterol ester is defective in vivo in Niemann-Pick C disease: insights on normal metabolism of HDL and LDL gained from the NP-C mutation. J Lipid Res 38:2422–2435, 1997

Sidransky E, Sherer DM, Ginns E: Gaucher disease in the neonate: A distinct Gaucher phenotype is analogous to a mouse model created by targeted disruption of the glucocerebrosidase gene. Pediatr Res 32:494–498, 1992

Stoffel W: Sphingolipids. Annu Rev Biochem 40:57–82, 1971

Vanier MT, Suzuki K: Recent advances in elucidating Niemann-Pick C disease. Brain Pathol 8:163–174, 1998

Zhao HG, Li HH, Bach G, Schmidtchen A, Neufeld EF: The molecular basis of Sanfilippo syndrome type B. Proc Natl Acad Sci USA 93:6101–6105, 1996

Zimran A, Kay A, Gelbart T, et al: Gaucher disease. Clinical, laboratory, radiologic, and genetic features of 53 patients. Medicine (Baltimore) 71:337–353, 1992

9.10 PEROXISOMAL DISORDERS

David Valle and Gerald V. Raymond and Stephen J. Gould

9.10.1 Peroxisome Biology and Metabolism

Peroxisomes are single membrane-bound organelles present in all cells except for erythrocytes. In human cells, peroxisomes are spherical in shape and range in number from a few hundred to a few thousand per cell. They contain a dense proteinaceous matrix composed of 50 or more enzymes that participate in a variety of metabolic processes. Prominent among these is a set of enzymes catalyzing β-oxidation of fatty acids that are analogous to, but distinct from, those catalyzing mitochondrial β-oxidation (see Fig. 9-11) and are encoded by different genes. The β-oxidation systems of peroxisomes and mitochondria have distinct but overlapping substrate specificities, with the peroxisomal system oxidizing very-long (C20-C26)- and long (C12-C18)-chain fatty acids, and the mitochondrial system oxidizing long (C12-C18)-, medium (C12-C6)-, and short (C6-C4)-chain fatty acids. An additional difference is that the flavin adenine dinucleotide (FAD)-linked acyl-CoA oxidase, which catalyzes the first step in the peroxisomal β-oxidation spiral, is reoxidized by molecular oxygen to produce H_2O_2 while the analogous enzymes in mitochondria transfer their electrons to the respiratory chain via electron transport flavoprotein

(ETF) and ETF-dehydrogenase. The H_2O_2 produced in the first step of the peroxisome β-oxidation spiral and by other peroxisomal oxidases is efficiently eliminated by catalase, another peroxisomal matrix enzyme. Additional metabolic processes that involve peroxisomal matrix enzymes include glyoxylate transamination, lysine degradation, α-oxidation of phytanic acid and other β-methyl-branched fatty acids, and synthesis of cholesterol, bile acids, and ether lipids such as plasmalogen.

9.10.2 Genetic Disorders of Peroxisomes: Overview

Peroxisomal disorders can be divided into two classes: first, the peroxisomal biogenesis disorders (PBD) characterized by deficiency of multiple peroxisomal functions; and, second, the single-function disorders in which only one peroxisomal function is deficient. The PBD are a genetically heterogeneous set of disorders comprising at least 12 complementation groups as determined by somatic cell hybridization studies. All are inherited as autosomal recessive traits and have an aggregate frequency of about 1 in 50,000. Zellweger syndrome (ZS) and rhizomelic chondrodysplasia punctata (RCDP) are the paradigms for the PBD clinical phenotypes. At the cellular level, most PBD complementation groups demonstrate aberrant cytosolic localization of matrix proteins, relatively empty peroxisomes, and no defect in the import of peroxisomal membrane proteins or in the synthesis of peroxisomal membranes. By contrast, a few PBD complementation groups have no detectable peroxisomal membranes.

The single-function peroxisome disorders include at least 11 different disorders inherited either as autosomal or X-linked recessive traits, nearly all of which are uncommon, with frequencies of less than 1 in 50,000. The clinical exemplar for this class of peroxisomal disorders is X-linked adrenal leukodystrophy (X-ALD), a neurologic disorder with abnormal accumulation of very-long-chain fatty acids (VLCFA) and an incidence in males of about 1 in 20,000. At the cellular level, peroxisomes in the single-function disorders appear normal and have normal import of matrix proteins.

9.10.3 Peroxisome Biogenesis Disorders (PBD)

CLINICAL PHENOTYPES

The clinical consequences of the PBD can be organized into two broad phenotypic spectra. The largest of these, the Zellweger spectrum, accounts for about 80% of PBD patients and includes at least three phenotypes originally thought to represent discrete disorders, but which are now recognized as segments of a continuous spectrum. From the most to the least severe, these are Zellweger syndrome (ZS), neonatal adrenoleukodystrophy (NALD), and infantile Refsum disease (IRD). The second PBD phenotypic spectrum, accounting for about 20% of PBD patients, is RCDP. The phenotype of most RCDP patients is severe and relatively uniform, but milder variants have been described.

Zellweger Spectrum

Zellweger syndrome, a metabolic disorder with dysmorphic features (see Chapter 10 and Table 10-10), represents the severe end of the Zellweger spectrum. These infants have a characteristic facial appearance with a high forehead, epicanthal folds, a small nose with

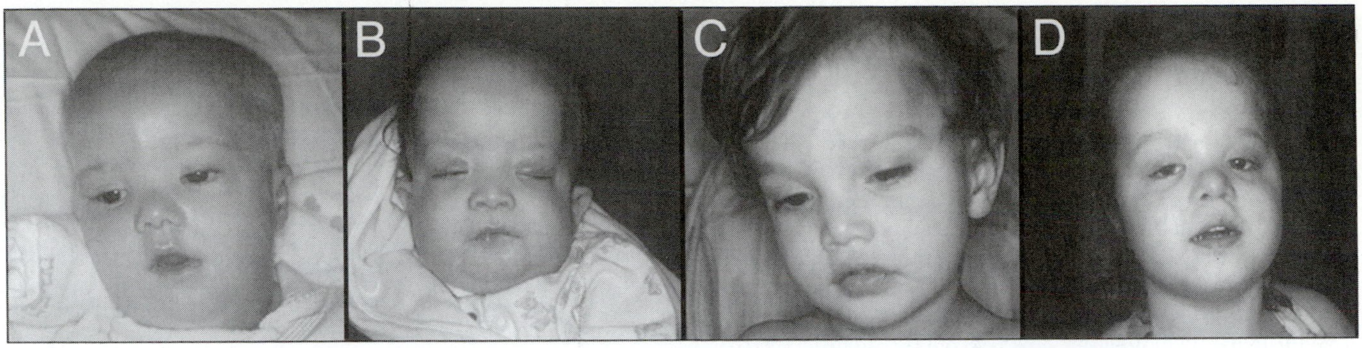

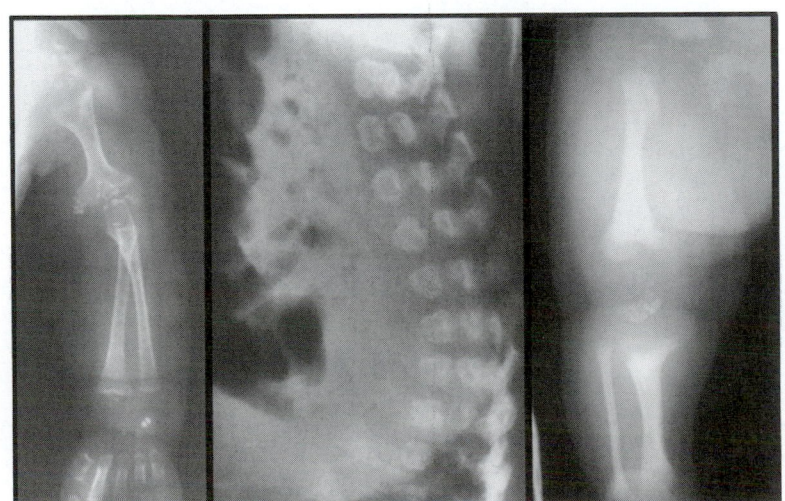

FIGURE 9-25 Facial appearances of PBD patients in the Zellweger spectrum. (A) Four-month-old infant with Zellweger syndrome; (B) three-month-old infant with Zellweger syndrome; (C) two-year-old child with neonatal adrenoleukodystrophy (NALD); (D) four-year-old child with infantile Refsum disease (IRD).

a broad nasal bridge, anteverted nares, and micrognathia (Fig. 9-25 A, B). The anterior fontanelle is large. Cataracts and a pigmentary retinopathy are common. There is profound hypotonia, feeding problems, and growth failure. Most have neonatal seizures relatively resistant to medical management. Liver function is abnormal with conjugated hyperbilirubinemia. Radiologic examination reveals punctate calcifications ("calcific stippling") in the patella and epiphyses of the long bones. Multiple small renal cysts are common but may not detected by ultrasound examination. Infants with ZS rarely live to be 1 year of age.

Neonatal adrenoleukodystrophy is similar to, but less severe than, ZS. Dysmorphic facial features are less severe or may even be absent (Fig. 9-25C). Hypotonia and seizures are common. Because of their flat facial features and hypotonia, NALD patients are sometimes thought to have Down syndrome. Survival ranges from several months to several years. The older patients have profound mental retardation often accompanied by sensorineural hearing loss and retinopathy.

Infantile Refsum disease patients have mild dysmorphic features and hypotonia (Fig. 9-25D). As they get older virtually all IRD patients develop sensorineural hearing loss and pigmentary retinopathy. They usually learn to walk but have severe mental retardation. Patients with IRD may live into the second decade of their life or beyond.

Milder variants of the Zellweger spectrum with normal development and appearance may present in adult life with sensorineural hearing loss and pigmentary retinopathy.

Rhizomelic Chondrodysplasia Punctata Spectrum

Patients with classic RCDP (see Chapter 10 and Table 10-10) present at birth with severe skeletal involvement that distinguishes them from those in the Zellweger spectrum (Fig. 9-26). There is rhizomelia (shortening of the proximal limbs) and limited range of movement of the large joints of the extremities. Radiologic examination shows extensive calcific stippling involving the epiphyses of long bones, most prominent in the knees, elbows, hips, and shoulders (Fig. 9-26). Additionally, coronal clefts of the vertebral bodies are apparent on lateral spine films. RCDP patients also have a flat face with frontal bossing. Cataracts are common and an ichthyotic skin rash may develop after birth. Severe psychomotor retardation is present, and most die before 2 years of age. In addition to this classic RCDP phenotype, mildly affected patients with little or no rhizomelia have been described, some with mild intellectual defects as their only manifestation. Classic RCDP is caused by mutations in *PEX7*, the gene encoding the receptor for PTS2 proteins. A few patients with the classic RCDP phenotype (<10% of the total number of patients) have single-function defect in PTS2-targeted peroxisomal matrix enzymes necessary for normal synthesis of plasmalogen.

FIGURE 9-26 Radiographs of an infant with rhizomelia chondrodysplasia punctata (RCDP). (A) Forearm showing extreme rhizomelia and punctate calcifications; (B) lateral spine showing coronal clefts of the vertebral bodies; (C) lower extremity.

BASIC DEFECTS

Over the last decade, research involving model organisms and genetic studies of PBD patients has identified a set of genes and their protein products, termed *PEX* genes and *peroxins,* respectively, that are necessary for peroxisome assembly. Most of these are involved in the targeting and uptake of matrix proteins into the organelle.

Peroxisome matrix proteins are synthesized on free cytosolic ribosomes and directed to the organelle by targeting sequences of two types (Fig. 9-27). Peroxisome-targeting signal 1 (PTS1) is utilized by more than 90% of the matrix proteins. PTS2, located 5 to 10 residues from the N-terminus, is utilized by a few peroxisomal matrix proteins, including one involved in β-oxidation (peroxisomal thiolase 1), one involved in α-oxidation, and one involved in plasmalogen synthesis. The PTS1 or PTS2 motifs are bound by specific cytosolic receptors encoded by *PEX5* and *PEX7,* respectively. Docking of the receptor and its bound cargo on the peroxisome membrane is mediated by binding to specific peroxisomal membrane proteins (*PEX13, PEX14, PEX17*). With the action of additional peroxisomal membrane proteins (*PEX2, PEX8, PEX10, PEX12*), the newly synthesized matrix proteins are translocated into the organelle and the receptors are recycled to the cytosol. The recycling process appears to be facilitated by the action of *PEX1, PEX6, PEX22,* and *PEX4.* Genetic defects in this subset of *PEX* genes are responsible for eight PBD complementation groups that are characterized by mislocalization of matrix proteins to the cytosol.

The mechanism and signals involved in targeting peroxisomal membrane proteins to the organelle are less well understood. A few *PEX* genes encoding proteins that function in this process have been identified (*PEX3, PEX16, PEX19*). Not surprisingly, genetic defects in this subset of peroxins are responsible for the three PBD complementation groups that lack detectable peroxisomes.

LABORATORY DIAGNOSIS OF PBD

The most frequently utilized diagnostic laboratory tests for the PBD detect abnormalities of peroxisomal metabolic processes in-
cluding VLCFA β-oxidation, phytanic acid α-oxidation, and plasmalogen synthesis. VLCFA are elevated about 10-fold in ZS, about 5-fold in NALD, and about 3-fold in IRD. Similarly, plasma phytanic acid concentration is increased 10 to 100-fold in Zellweger spectrum patients who are old enough to be ingesting dietary precursors of this compound. Red cell plasmalogens are reduced by 10-fold or more. Other laboratory abnormalities in Zellweger spectrum patients include increased urinary excretion of medium- and long-chain dicarboxylic acids and pipecolic acid, and reduced levels of plasma bile acids.

In RCDP, plasma VLCFA levels are normal, possibly because peroxisomal thiolase 2 (sterol carrier protein X) substitutes for the lack of the PTS2-targeted peroxisomal thiolase 1. RBC plasmalogens are reduced in RCDP to an extent similar to that in Zellweger spectrum patients. In RCDP patients ingesting foods containing phytanic acid precursors, the levels of phytanic acid in plasma are usually higher than in Zellweger spectrum patients.

Confirmation of diagnoses made on the basis of clinical phenotype and the above metabolite assays should be confirmed by studies of peroxisomal β-oxidation and plasmalogen synthesis in cultured skin fibroblasts. These are available at reference labs (see *www.genetests.org* or *www.peroxisome.org*) and can be supplemented by immunohistochemical studies localizing PTS1- and PTS2-targeted matrix proteins and peroxisomal membrane proteins. Complementation analysis is a useful preliminary test for molecular studies to identify the responsible *PEX* gene but has little prognostic value because patients representing different segments of the Zellweger spectrum have been identified in most complementation groups. Recent progress in identification of the *PEX* genes provides the opportunity for molecular diagnosis of nearly all PBD patients.

TREATMENT OF PBD

The pathophysiology of the PBD is complex and often begins in utero. For these reasons, treatment of these disorders is only supportive. Feeding difficulties are frequent, and placement of a gastrostomy tube is often indicated to improve nutrition and facilitate

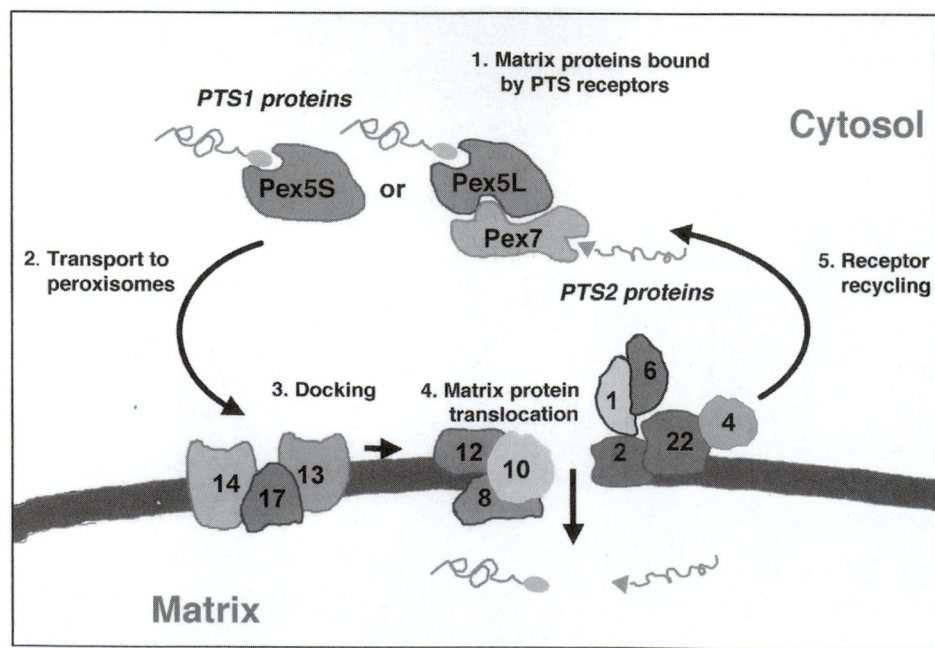

FIGURE 9-27   Model of import of peroxisomal matrix proteins. Matrix proteins targeted by either a PTS1 or a PTS2 signal bind their respective receptors (PEX5, PEX7) in the cytosol. PEX5 has two isoforms, a long (PEX5L) and a short (PEX5S); the former interacts with PEX7. The PEX proteins or peroxins involved in docking of the receptors, translocation of the matrix protein into the organelle, and recycling of the receptors are indicated by the numbered structures at the peroxisome membrane. See the reference by Collins et al for the data supporting the order of action of the various peroxins in this dynamic system.

care. Anticonvulsant medications are indicated to control seizures. In older individuals, plasma phytanic acid should be followed and dietary phytanic acid and its precursors (phytol) limited. The consequences of the severe skeletal involvement should be carefully assessed in RCDP patients. Moderate cervical spine stenosis in a patient with RCDP was recently recognized.

COUNSELING ISSUES

Age at demise is often listed as one of the criteria used to categorize phenotypic severity in the Zellweger spectrum. At the time of diagnosis, however, the phenotypic features of ZS, NALD, and IRD overlap; thus, in most cases, it is unwise to make precise survival predictions.

All known PBD are inherited as autosomal recessive traits with a 25% recurrence risk for each subsequent pregnancy to couples identified because they have had one PBD infant. Prenatal diagnosis is possible by biochemical methods and is provided by several reference labs (see Web sites above). If the molecular basis of the index case is known, similar studies can be used for prenatal diagnosis in subsequent pregnancies.

9.10.4   Single-Function Defects

In contrast to the PBD, peroxisomes in this class of disorders have a normal structure and function except for an isolated deficiency or abnormality of a particular peroxisomal protein. At least 11 well-defined disorders meet this criterion and they can be grouped according to the disrupted peroxisomal function (Table 9-19).

X-LINKED ADRENOLEUKODYSTROPHY

This highly variable X-linked neurodegenerative disorder is caused by mutations in *ALD,* the gene encoding ALDP, an ATP-binding cassette (ABC) transporter located in the peroxisomal membrane.

Clinical Phenotype

There are multiple phenotypic presentations for males with X-ALD. The most severe, the childhood cerebral form, is a rapidly progressive, inflammatory, central demyelinating disease that begins between ages 3 and 10. About 35% of X-ALD males manifest this phenotype with progressive behavioral, cognitive, and neurologic abnormalities leading to total disability within 3 years, and eventually to death. Nearly all of these patients have adrenal insufficiency. The T2-weighted MRI shows symmetric areas of increased signal in the parieto-occipital region.

A second, distinct phenotype, known as adrenomyeloneuropathy (AMN), begins in the third to fourth decade and is characterized by a distal axonopathy, mainly involving the spinal cord. AMN patients manifest a slowly progressive gait disturbance and progressive urinary sphincter dysfunction. About two-thirds of AMN patients have adrenal insufficiency and about 40% eventually develop cerebral involvement.

Other phenotypic presentations include adults with adrenal involvement only, but many of these men eventually develop AMN symptoms (see Sec. 25.17 for detailed description of neurologic manifestations).

TABLE 9-19

SUMMARY OF DISORDERS WITH ABNORMAL FUNCTION OF A SINGLE PEROXISOMAL PROTEIN

PEROXISOMAL FUNCTION	N	DISORDER	OMIM #	PHENOTYPE(S)	DEFECTIVE PROTEIN	BIOCHEMICAL ABNORMALITIES
Fatty acid β-oxidation	1	X-ALD	300100	Progressive neurodegeneration of variable severity	ALDP	↑ VLCFA
	2	Acyl-CoA oxidase deficiency	264470	Zellweger spectrum	Acyl-CoA oxidase	↑ VLCFA
	3	D-Bifunctional protein deficiency	261515	Zellweger spectrum	D-Bifunctional protein	↑ VLCFA
	4	Thiolase deficiency	261510	Zellweger spectrum	Peroxisomal thiolase 1	↑ VLCFA
	5	Racemase deficiency	604489	Combined peripheral motor and sensory neuropathy	Peroxisomal α-methyl-acyl-CoA racemase	↑ Pristanic acid ↑ DHCA ↑ THCA
Fatty acid α-oxidation	6	Refsum disease	266500	Combined peripheral motor and sensory neuropathy with retinal degeneration	Phytanoyl-CoA hydroxylase	↑ Phytanic acid
Etherphospholipid	7	RCDP, type 2	222765	Rhizomelia with mental retardation and cataracts	DHAPAT deficiency	↓ Plasmalogens ↑ Phytanic acid
	8	RCDP, type 3	600121	Rhizomelia with mental retardation and cataracts	Alkyl-DHAP synthase deficiency	↓ Plasmalogens ↑ Phytanic acid
Isoprenoid biosynthesis	9	Mevalonic aciduria	251170	Retardation, FTT episodic fevers	Mevalonate kinase	↑ Urine mevalonic acid
		hyper IgD/periodic fever	260920	Abdominal pain, episodic fevers		
Hydrogen peroxide degradation	10	Acatalasemia	115500	Oral ulcers	Catalase	
Glyoxylate detoxification	11	Hyperoxaluria type 1	259900	Progressive nephrocalcinosis	Alanine:glyoxylate aminotransferase	Hyperoxaluria; hyperglycolic aciduria

ALDP = adrenoleukodystrophy protein; FTT = failure to thrive; OMIM, online mendelian inheritance in man; RCDP, rhizomelic chondrodysplasia; VLCFA, very-long-chain fatty acids; X-ALD, X-linked adrenoleukocystrophy.

Basic Defect

There is no correlation between the nature of the *ALD* mutation and phenotypic severity. In fact, multiple affected members in a single family, all with the same mutant *ALD* allele, may manifest the extremes of phenotypic expression; individuals with the childhood cerebral form occur in the same family as individuals with AMN or adrenal insufficiency only.

ALDP, the protein product of *ALD,* is a peroxisomal membrane transporter. The functional transporter is either a homodimer of two ALDP subunits or a heterodimer of ALDP with one of three other related ABC transporters found in the peroxisome membrane. The ligands for these transporters are not known with certainty but are likely to be long-chain fats, fatty acyl-CoAs, or other hydrophobic substances.

Laboratory Diagnosis of X-ALD

Regardless of their phenotype, X-ALD patients have a marked elevation of plasma VLCFA levels, particularly $C_{26:0}$. In cultured skin fibroblasts, β-oxidation of VLCFA is impaired. These observations suggest that ALDP function is required for entry of these fats into peroxisomes where they are degraded by peroxisomal β-oxidation.

Prenatal diagnosis is possible by measurement of VLCFA in amniotic fluid and by molecular analysis of ALD.

Treatment

The highly variable phenotypic manifestations of X-ALD makes evaluation of any therapy difficult. Reduction of plasma VLCFA by dietary measures does not seem to prevent the development of symptoms. Although more work needs to be done in this area, current evidence indicates that in boys manifesting the early stages of the childhood cerebral phenotype, bone marrow transplantation may be highly efficacious in blocking progression of the disease.

Counseling

X-ALD is inherited as an X-linked recessive trait. The combination of plasma VLCFA determination and molecular analysis can identify all X-ALD hemizygotes and heterozygotes. Reliable prenatal diagnosis of affected individuals can be utilized to prevent transmission of the disease. The inability to predict phenotypic severity complicates this process.

DISORDERS OF PEROXISOMAL FATTY ACID β-OXIDATION

Three inherited disorders have been identified: (a) straight-chain acyl-CoA oxidase deficiency; (b) D-bifunctional protein deficiency; and (c) peroxisome thiolase 1 deficiency. Interestingly, the phenotype of inherited deficiency of any of the three enzymes in the β-oxidation spiral is indistinguishable from that of PBD patients at the severe end of the Zellweger spectrum (ZS and NALD). Eight acyl-CoA oxidase-deficient patients, more than 40 D-bifunctional–deficient patients, and 1 peroxisomal thiolase 1–deficient patient have been identified.

The clinical phenotype of patients with deficiency of one of these three enzyme-catalyzing steps in the peroxisomal β-oxidation spiral resembles that of PBD patients in the Zellweger spectrum. This observation suggests that disruption of peroxisomal β-oxidation plays a major role in the pathophysiology of the PBD.

Diagnosis of these patients depends on evidence for disruption of peroxisomal β-oxidation (increased VLCFA, pristanic acid, and bile acid precursors) without evidence for lack of other peroxisomal functions (plasmalogen synthesis) or of problems in peroxisomal assembly. All of these disorders are inherited as autosomal recessive traits and prenatal diagnosis is available.

DEFICIENCY OF α-METHYLACYL-CoA RACEMASE

This peroxisomal racemase catalyzes a step in the oxidation of long-branch-chain fatty acids and bile acids upstream of their entry into the β-oxidation spiral. A recent report describes two unrelated adults presenting with a combined peripheral sensory and motor neuropathy plus features suggesting either Refsum disease or X-ALD. Both, however, had essentially normal levels of VLCFA and phytanic acid, excluding both diagnoses, but very high levels of pristanic acid, suggesting a defect in pristanic acid oxidation upstream of the β-oxidation spiral. Subsequent studies in fibroblasts clearly showed deficiency of the racemase, which was confirmed at the molecular level.

REFSUM DISEASE

This abnormality in the peroxisomal α-oxidation of phytanic acid typically presents in the second decade, although about a third of patients experience their first symptoms before age 10 years. Virtually all patients develop retinitis pigmentosa with night blindness as an initial symptom. The electroretinogram is extinguished and the visual field gradually constricts. Progressive combined sensory and motor neuropathy affecting mainly the lower extremities are later symptoms, as is cerebellar dysfunction. Other less-uniform symptoms include early-onset anosmia, cardiomyopathy, mild epiphyseal dysplasia, and ichthyotic skin rash.

The primary defect is deficiency of phytanoyl-CoA hydroxylase caused by mutations in the *PAHX* gene. Plasma phytanic acid levels are markedly elevated (100–1000-fold). Cerebrospinal fluid protein is elevated without a pleocytosis. The enzymatic defect can be demonstrated in cultured skin fibroblasts.

Refsum disease is an autosomal recessive disorder, and prenatal diagnosis by biochemical and/or molecular methods is possible.

The sole sources of phytanic acid are dietary phytanic acid and its precursor, phytol. Meat, ruminant fat, dairy products, and fish are rich sources of phytanic acid. Diets restricted in these substances produce a gradual but dramatic decline in plasma and tissue phytanic acid. This can be hastened by plasmapheresis. Patients who maintain their phytanic acid at near-normal levels often improve clinically. For these reasons, dietary treatment should be instituted as soon as possible and maintained for life.

References

Collins CS, Kalish JE, Morrell JC, Gould SJ: The peroxisome biogenesis factors Pex4p, Pex22p, Pex1p, and Pex6p act in the terminal steps of peroxisomal matrix protein import. Mol Cell Biol 20:7516, 2000.

Ferdinandusse S, Denis S, Clayton PT, et al: Mutations in the gene encoding peroxisomal alpha-methylacyl-CoA racemase cause adult-onset sensory motor neuropathy. Nat Genet 24:188, 2000

Gould SJ, Raymond GV, Valle D: The peroxisome biogenesis disorders. In: Scriver CR, Beaudet AL, Sly WS, Valle D, eds: The Metabolic and Molecular Bases of Inherited Disease, 8th ed. New York, McGraw-Hill, 2001

Gould SJ, Valle D: Peroxisome biogenesis disorders: genetics and cell biology. Trends in Genetics 16(8):340, 2000

Moser HW, Smith KD, Watkins PA, Power JM, Moser AB: X-linked adrenoleukodystrophy. In: Scriver CR, Beaudet AL, Sly WS, Valle D, eds: The Metabolic and Molecular Bases of Inherited Disease, 8th ed. New York, McGraw-Hill, 2001

Poll-The BT, Saudubray J-M: Peroxisomal disorders. In: Fernandes J, Saudubray J-M, van den Berghe G, eds: Inborn Metabolic Diseases. Berlin, Springer-Verlag, 2000

Sacksteder KA, Gould SJ: The genetics of peroxisome biogenesis. Annu Rev Genet 34:623, 2000.

Shapiro E, Krivit W, Lochman L, et al: Long-term effect of bone marrow transplantation for childhood-onset cerebral X-linked adrenoleukodystrophy. Lancet 356:713, 2000

Wanders RJ, Barth PG, Heymans HSA: Single peroxisomal enzyme deficiencies. In: Scriver CR, Beaudet AL, Sly WS, Valle D, eds: The Metabolic and Molecular Bases of Inherited Disease, 8th ed. New York, McGraw-Hill, 2001

Wanders RJ, Jakobs C, Skjeldal OH: Refsum disease. In: Scriver CR, Beaudet AL, Sly WS, Valle D, eds: The Metabolic and Molecular Bases of Inherited Disease, 8th ed. New York, McGraw-Hill, 2001

9.11 INHERITED METABOLIC DISEASES WITH DYSMORPHIC FEATURES

Heidi L. Peters and Stephen G. Kahler

9.11.1 Introduction

There are a number of inborn errors of metabolism with recognized distinctive dysmorphic features (Tables 9-20 and 10-10). The individual inborn errors involving lysosomes and peroxisomes have well-described facial dysmorphism and structural malformations/deformations (see Sec. 9.8 and Sec. 9.10). The dysmorphic features associated with lysosomal disorders occur largely as a result of impaired turnover of structural macromolecules within cells and extracellular matrix. As a result of ongoing storage there is progressive deformation of shape and growth. The lysosomal storage disorders present with various combinations of progressive facial coarsening, developmental delay and regression, hepatosplenomegaly, and progressive skeletal changes of dysostosis multiplex, contractures, and short stature.

The dysmorphic features and malformations associated with peroxisomal disorders, when they occur, are usually present at birth. They are typically characterized by various combinations of craniofacial abnormalities; retinitis pigmentosa and cataracts; profound hypotonia; structural brain malformations; skeletal changes of chondrodysplasia punctata; hepatocellular dysfunction; and developmental delay.

Abnormalities in cell energy production may also result in structural malformations such as those recognized with respiratory chain disorders. Such infants frequently have pre- and postnatal growth retardation, microcephaly, structural brain malformations (especially agenesis of the corpus callosum), and a constellation of facial features consisting of long eyelashes, hirsutism, high forehead, flat philtrum, low-set ears, and full, slightly droopy cheeks (see Sec. 9.4).

The rare disorders of valine metabolism, methacrylic aciduria and 3-hydroxyisobutyric aciduria, may also cause dysmorphism and malformations.

Homocystinuria, principally due to cystathionine β-synthase deficiency, results in abnormal collagen cross-linking and consequently affects tissue structure and growth. Affected individuals often have a Marfanoid body habitus, pectus excavatum/carinatum, ectopia lentis, kyphoscoliosis, and varying severity of intellectual impairment (see Sec. 9.2).

Maternal phenylketonuria (PKU) syndrome is an example of a teratogenic affect of metabolites. This syndrome occurs when a fetus is exposed to high levels of phenylalanine during pregnancy in women with inadequately treated or unrecognized PKU (see Sec. 9.2).

Subtle dysmorphic features in organic and aminoacidurias, which present with the classic acute or chronic metabolic decompensation, especially droopy, full cheeks, are usually not diagnostic in themselves. However, many of these patients appear similar. An inborn error of metabolism should be considered in the differential diagnosis of nonspecific dysmorphic features, especially if associated with acute or chronic decompensation or neurologic impairment, and appropriate investigations performed (see Chapter 10).

9.11.2 Metabolic Diseases

MENKES DISEASE

Menkes disease is a rare X-linked recessive disorder caused by mutations in the Menkes (*MNK*) gene resulting in abnormal intracellular copper utilization. Copper is taken up into the cell normally but cannot be transported to the site of synthesis of a number of copper-dependent enzymes. The deficient function of these enzymes explains the characteristic features of this condition. These cuproenzymes include lysyl oxidase, which is important for collagen and elastin cross-linkage; dopamine-β-hydroxylase; cytochrome oxidase; tyrosinase; superoxide dismutase; and ceruloplasmin.

Affected individuals classically present in the neonatal period, often following a premature delivery, with temperature instability, hypothermia, and hypoglycemia. The characteristic facial appearance includes pudgy cheeks and sagging jowls and lips. The hair and eyebrows are hypopigmented, sparse, stubby, and broken. Microscopic examination of the hair shows pili torti, hence the alternate name "kinky hair disease." By 2 to 3 months, progressive neurodegeneration becomes apparent with loss of milestones and the development of ataxia and seizures. Abnormalities in collagen formation result in bladder diverticuli, tortuous vessels, hypermobile joints, and osteoporosis. Radiologic examination demonstrates wormian bones, metaphyseal spurs, and osteoporosis, which may result in fractures. Abnormalities in dopamine β-hydroxylase may result in blood pressure instability and hypotension. Chronic diarrhea is an additional complication.

The natural history is of progressive neurologic deterioration with survival rare beyond 2 to 3 years of age (see Sec. 25.17). Treatment with copper histidinate injections can modify the course of the disease if commenced prior to the onset of neurologic symptoms. This may necessitate premature delivery and commencement of treatment immediately. Later treatment has not improved the long-term prognosis.

Individuals with a milder form of Menkes disease have been described. The occipital horn syndrome (previously known as Ehlers-Danlos syndrome, type IX) is a mild allelic form of classic Menkes disease. This syndrome has the connective tissue features of Menkes syndrome without the neurodegeneration, although mild mental retardation may occur.

TABLE 9-20

DISEASES ASSOCIATED WITH SPECIFIC DYSMORPHIC FEATURES

Abnormal skin
- Holocarboxylase deficiency: rash
- Albinism: depigmented
- Alkaptonuria: pigmented
- Untreated PKU: rash
- Oculocutaneous tyrosinemia: hyperkeratosis
- Menkes: depigmented, loose skin
- Mucopolysaccharidoses (MPS): thickened skin, nodular skin lesions (Hunter)
- Hypercholesterolemia: xanthoma
- Mevalonic aciduria: morbilliform rash
- Lipoprotein lipase deficiency: eruptive xanthoma
- Fabry, G_{M1}, fucosidosis, galactosidosis: angiokeratoma
- Ethylmalonic aciduria: acrocyanosis, petechiae
- CDG: lipodystrophy, fat pads

Abnormal head size
- Glutaric aciduria type I: macrocephaly
- D-2-Hydroxyglutaric aciduria: macrocephaly
- L-2-Hydroxyglutaric aciduria: macrocephaly
- Succinic semialdehyde dehydrogenase deficiency: macrocephaly
- Glutaric aciduria type II: macrocephaly
- MPS: macrocephaly
- Canavan disease: macrocephaly
- Tay-Sachs disease: macrocephaly
- Propionic aciduria: microcephaly
- Phenylketonuria: microcephaly
- Hyperargininemia: microcephaly
- HMG-CoA lyase deficiency: microcephaly
- Menkes disease: microcephaly
- CDG syndromes: microcephaly

Abnormal hair
- Alopecia: holocarboxylase/biotin deficiency, argininosuccinic aciduria, 3-methylglutaconic aciduria, lysinuric protein intolerance
- Albinism
- Phenylketonuria

- Menkes disease
- Hirsute: MPS, mucolipidosis, etc.

Abnormal mouth
- Enlarged tongue: Pompe disease
- Thick gums/tongue: MPS, mucolipidosis, G_{M1}-gangliosidosis

Hypoplastic/inverted nipples
- Propionic aciduria
- CDG syndrome

Stature
- Homocystinuria: tall
- Glycogen storage diseases: short
- Cystinosis: short
- MPS: short
- Mucolipidosis: short
- G_{M1}-gangliosidosis: short
- Fucosidosis: short
- Mevalonic aciduria (failure to thrive): short

Abnormality of eyes
- Albinism: depigmentation
- Alkaptonuria: pigmented
- Homocystinuria: ectopia lentis, retinal detachment
- Oculocutaneous tyrosinemia: corneal ulcers, photophobia, blisters
- Galactosemia: cataracts
- Zellweger syndrome: cataracts, retinitis pigmentosa
- Cystinosis: corneal deposits, photophobia, abnormal cornea
- Wilson disease: Kayser-Fleischer rings
- MPS: corneal clouding
- Mevalonic aciduria: cataracts, uveitis, retinitis
- Lipoprotein lipase deficiency: lipemia retinalis
- Fabry disease: corneal lenticular opacities
- G_{M1}-gangliosidosis, Tay-Sachs disease, Sandhoff disease, G_{M2}-gangliosidosis, Niemann-Pick disease, galactosialidosis: cherry-red spot
- Fucosidosis, mannosidosis: cataracts, corneal clouding
- Canavan disease: optic atrophy

Estimates of the incidence of Menkes disease range from 1 in 50,000 to 1 in 250,000 births. Diagnosis is established on the basis of a classic clinical phenotype and history suggestive of X-linked inheritance. Serum copper and ceruloplasmin levels are low when measured after the first week after birth. Copper accumulation and kinetic studies performed on cultured fibroblasts may also give additional supportive evidence. Copper measurement in intestinal biopsies is high, while levels in liver are low.

Prenatal testing, by measurement of copper in chorionic villi or copper studies on amniotic fluid cells, will detect affected males. DNA-based diagnosis is now possible, with large deletions and smaller mutations within the *MNK* gene described. To date there does not appear to be a common mutation.

Female carriers may have the subtle clinical features of patchy skin hypopigmentation and microscopically abnormal hair. Fibroblast copper studies may also be helpful in detecting carriers. However-normal results do not exclude carrier status; molecular testing is the preferred method of carrier detection.

CARBOHYDRATE-DEFICIENT GLYCOPROTEIN SYNDROMES

The carbohydrate-deficient glycoprotein syndromes (CDGS), now called *congenital disorders of glycosylation,* are a complex group of disorders characterized by hypoglycosylation of multiple serum and cellular glycoproteins. Because of the numerous proteins affected, these disorders all result in multisystemic abnormalities, including specific dysmorphic features.

Glycoproteins are proteins with *N*- or *O*-linked oligosaccharide trees. Most proteins are glycosylated. Defects that affect the pathway for *N*-glycosylation result in CDG. In this pathway, an oligosaccharide tree is formed on a lipid dolichol pyrophosphate backbone on the endoplasmic reticulum membrane. After the oligosaccharide tree is formed, it is transferred to a peptide chain where it may undergo further modification. Defects may occur in one of the many enzymes required for this process or in the availability of sugar substrates. To date, at least six subtypes of CDGS have been identified and it is likely that there are more. Current classification is into two main groups: CDG-I (with subtypes a, b, c, d, and e) and CDG-II, based on specific patterns detected on transferrin isoelectric focusing and clinical phenotype. The CDG-I syndromes are due to defects in the assembly and transfer of the oligosaccharide tree, whereas CDG-II is the result of abnormalities in the trimming of the protein-bound oligosaccharides.

A majority of patients have CDG-Ia, which is inherited in an autosomal recessive manner. The incidence is estimated to be 1 in 80,000. Four clinical stages are recognized. The first stage is referred to as the infantile alarming multisystem stage. In the neonatal period, there may be failure to thrive; mild facial dysmorphism (high bridge of nose, large ears, and prominent jaw); abnormal subcutaneous adipose tissue with anomalous fat pads over buttocks, the inguinal/pubic region, and axillae; areas of lipoatrophy; and inverted nipples. Hypothyroidism (due to deficiency of thyroid-binding globulin) may be detected on newborn screening. Neurologic involvement is prominent with strabismus, roving-eye movements, hypotonia, psychomotor retardation, ataxia, and hyporeflexia. Olivopontocerebellar hypoplasia is frequently present.

Infants may also develop pericardial effusions, cardiomyopathy, severe infections, nephrotic syndrome, or hepatic failure. Carnitine deficiency may be detected. These complications are associated with a high mortality.

In the childhood ataxia-mental retardation stage, neurologic signs of ataxia and static mental retardation dominate. During this stage, stroke-like episodes may occur, related to intercurrent infections. Pigmentary retinal degeneration may also develop. These features may stabilize; then, the teenage leg atrophy stage follows. During this phase, there are symptoms of lower-limb neuropathy with weakness and leg atrophy, joint contractures, and development of kyphoscoliosis. The fourth stage is called adult hypogonadic. Adults are usually moderately to severely intellectually impaired and frequently wheelchair-bound. Failure of puberty usually occurs in females.

Isoelectric focusing of transferrin is used routinely in the diagnosis. Several bands are normally seen, predominantly those indicating 4 and 5 sialic acid residues. Deficiency of the negatively charged terminal sialic acid of transferrin results in an increase in asialo- and disialo-transferrin instead of the usual penta- and tetra-sialo-transferrin. This altered charge can be detected on isoelectric focusing (and quantitated by densitometry). Many other glycoproteins in the blood, such as antithrombin III, thyroid-binding globulin (TBG), ferritin, α_1-antitrypsin, α_1-antichymotrypsin, α_1-acid glycoprotein, ceruloplasmin, and complement C1, C3a, and C4a may show similar defects and have functional impairment.

Most patients with CDG-Ia have deficient activity of phosphomannomutase (PMM). This enzyme converts mannose-6-phosphate to mannose-1-phosphate, which, in turn, is converted to GDP-mannose, the donor of mannose for oligosaccharide side chains. PMM activity can be measured in cultured fibroblasts.

Two phosphomannomutase genes have been identified: *PMM1* and *PMM2*. All cases of PMM deficiency so far are caused by mutations within *PMM2*.

Approximately 20% of patients with CDG-I do not have a detectable deficiency of the PMM enzyme, suggesting that there are other subtypes. CDG-Ib, due to phosphomannose isomerase deficiency, is dominated by gastrointestinal symptoms: protein-losing enteropathy and hepatic fibrosis, in addition to coagulopathy and hypoglycemia. Affected individuals have normal psychomotor development and normal facial features. CDG-Ic (previously type V) has been described in at least one patient who had a defect in a glucosyltransferase; mutations in *hAlg6* gene have been identified in such patients. Clinical and laboratory features were similar to PMM deficiency.

CDG-Id and CDG-Ie (previously type IV) are clinically similar. A number of patients have been described with severe psychomotor delay, epilepsy, hypotonia, and microcephaly. Dysmorphic features include hypertelorism, Gothic palate, small hands with dysplastic nails, knee contractures, and failure to thrive. The classic features of CDG-Ia are absent. Reduced activity of a dolichol phosphate mannose synthase has been identified as the cause for CDG-Ie and

defects in the gene *Dpm1* described. The defect in CDG-Id is in the gene *hAlg3*, which encodes a mannosyltransferase.

CDG-IIa is rare. Mental retardation (more severe than in CDG-I) and dysmorphic features occur, but there is no neuropathy or cerebellar pathology. There is a deficiency of the enzyme *N*-acetylglucosaminyltransferase II.

All forms of CDG syndrome are inherited in an autosomal recessive manner. Therapy directed at symptoms can be somewhat helpful. Treatment with oral mannose is being studied for types Ia, Ib, and Ie, with initial data indicating success in treating type Ib at least.

SMITH-LEMLI-OPITZ SYNDROME

Smith-Lemli-Opitz (SLO) or RSH syndrome is an autosomal recessive multiple malformation syndrome caused by a defect in cholesterol biosynthesis. Cholesterol plays an important role in embryogenesis, which is reflected in the range of abnormalities detected in this disorder. The spectrum of clinical phenotypes ranges from isolated 2/3 toe syndactyly to severely malformed fetuses that die in utero. A previous classification of type I (milder) and type II (lethal in infancy) was used before the biochemical defect was found.

In the most typical form, the characteristic facies consists of microcephaly; anteverted nostrils; broad nasal tip; ptosis; hypertelorism; low-set ears; narrow bifrontal diameter; cleft palate; and micrognathia. Postaxial polydactyly, short, low-set thumbs, overlapping fingers, and partial 2/3 toe syndactyly may be present. Genital abnormalities ranging from mild hypospadias to ambiguous genitalia can be found in males. Pre- and postnatal growth retardation frequently occur. Various lung, cardiac, hepatic, renal, and cerebral malformations have been described. Intellectual impairment may be severe.

The fundamental biochemical defect is deficient activity of 7-dehydrocholesterol reductase, which catalyzes the conversion of 7-dehydrocholesterol to cholesterol. Affected individuals typically have elevated serum levels of 7-dehydrocholesterol, and normal to low levels of cholesterol. Serum cholesterol levels, or cholesterol as a fraction of total sterols, inversely correlate with clinical severity, whereas levels of 7-dehydrocholesterol do not correlate with clinical symptoms. The incidence of this disorder is thought to be in the order of 1 in 20,000 to 1 in 40,000 births. Mutations in the *DHCR 7* gene have been identified. Affected fetuses may be detected prenatally by maternal serum screening (unconjugated estriol levels are low), and increased nuchal translucency has also been described. In a previously identified family, prenatal diagnosis by enzyme assay or DNA analysis may be available.

Treatment with dietary cholesterol and bile-acid supplements has been tried with varying success. Therapy corrects the serum cholesterol level and may ameliorate some of the growth and behavioral/developmental abnormalities. Further long-term studies are required. The discovery of a defect in cholesterol biosynthesis as the cause for SLO prompted a search for other defects within this pathway that may also result in malformation syndromes. Desmosterolosis and X-linked dominant Conradi-Hünermann-Happle syndrome were subsequently identified. It is unclear whether the malformations associated with these disorders result from cholesterol deficiency or from a toxic effect of sterol precursors.

DESMOSTEROLOSIS

Desmosterolosis is the result of a defect in 3β-hydroxysterol $S\Delta^{24}$-reductase, with the accumulation of desmosterol. The malformations include macrocephaly; cleft palate; hypoplastic nasal bridge; thick alveolar ridges; gingival nodules; rhizomesomelic limb shortness; structural cardiac defect; generalized osteosclerosis; and ambiguous genitalia. Some of the facial features may suggest a lysosomal storage disorder.

X-LINKED DOMINANT CONRADI-HÜNERMANN-HAPPLE SYNDROME

The Conradi-Hünermann-Happle syndrome is an X-linked dominant disorder characterized by chondrodysplasia punctata. Affected individuals typically have rhizomesomelic short stature with asymmetric limb shortening. The skin is often ichthyotic with areas of follicular atrophoderma and there may be patchy alopecia. The hair is otherwise coarse and lusterless. Facial features described include flat facies, hypoplasia of the malar eminences, and cataracts. Defects in an intermediate step of cholesterol metabolism at 3β-hydroxy-steroid-Δ^8, Δ^7-isomerase have been found, and mutations detected in a number of patients.

MEVALONIC ACIDURIA

Mevalonic aciduria is caused by a defect in mevalonate kinase, an early step in the pathway of cholesterol and nonsterol isoprenoid biosynthesis. A characteristic facial dysmorphism consists of dolichocephaly, frontal bossing, low set and posterior rotated ears, long eyelashes, down-slanting palpebral fissures, blue sclera, and cataracts (see Sec. 9.4.1).

References

Bankier A: Menkes disease. J Med Genet 32:213–215, 1995

Braverman N, Lin P, Moebius FF, et al: Mutations in the gene encoding 3β-hydroxysteroid-Δ^8, Δ^7-isomerase cause X-linked dominant Conradi-Hünermann syndrome. Nat Genet 22:291–294, 1999

Clayton PT, Thompson E: Dysmorphic syndromes with demonstrable biochemical abnormalities. J Med Gen 25:463–472, 1988

Cunniff C, Kratz LE, Moser A, Natowicz MR, Kelley R: Clinical and biochemical spectrum of patients with RSH/Smith-Lemli-Opitz syndrome and abnormal cholesterol metabolism. Am J Med Genet 68:263–269, 1997

Fernandes J, Saudubray J-M, van den Berghe G, eds: Inborn Metabolic Diseases: Diagnosis and Treatment, 3rd ed. Heidelberg, Springer-Verlag, 2000

Fitzpatrick DR, Keeling JW, Evans MJ, et al: Clinical phenotype of desmosterolosis. Am J Med Genet 75:145–152, 1998

Hoffmann GF, Charpentier C, Mayatepek E, et al: Clinical and biochemical phenotype in 11 patients with mevalonic aciduria. Pediatrics 91:915–921, 1993

Houten SM, Kuis W, Duran M, et al: Mutations in MVK, encoding mevalonate kinase hyperimmunoglobulinaemia D and periodic fever syndrome. Nat Genet 22:175–177, 1999

Jaeken J, Matthijs G, Earone R, Carchon H: Carbohydrate deficient glycoprotein (CDG) syndrome type I. J Med Genet 34:73–76, 1997

Jaeken J, Stibler H, Hagberg E: The carbohydrate-deficient glycoprotein syndrome. A new inherited multisystemic disease with severe nervous system involvement. Acta Paediatr Scand Suppl 375:1–71, 1991

Kahler SG: Menkes disease. Adv Pediatr 41:263–304, 1994

Kelley R: RSH/Smith-Lemli-Opitz syndrome: mutations and metabolic morphogenesis [invited editorial]. Am J Hum Genet 63:322–326, 1998

Kelley RI, Wilcox WG, Smith M, Kratz LE, Moser A, Rimoin DS: Abnormal sterol metabolism in patients with Conradi-Hünermann-Happle syndrome and sporadic lethal chondrodysplasia punctata. Am J Med Genet 83:213–219, 1999

Niehues R, Hasilik M, Alton G, et al: Carbohydrate-deficient glycoprotein syndrome type lb. Phosphomannose isomerase deficiency and mannose therapy. J Clin Invest 101:1414–1420, 1998

Orlean P: Congenital disorders of glycosylation caused by defects in mannose addition during N-linked oligosaccharide assembly. J Clin Invest 105:131–132, 2000

Scriver CR, Beaudet AL, Sly WS, Valle D, eds: The Metabolic and Molecular Bases of Inherited Disease, 8th ed. New York, McGraw-Hill, 2001

9.12   THE INBORN ERRORS OF HEME BIOSYNTHESIS: THE PORPHYRIAS

Robert Desnick

The porphyrias are a group of inherited and acquired disorders resulting from the deficient activity of specific enzymes in the heme biosynthetic pathway. These disorders are classified as either hepatic or erythropoietic depending on the primary site of overproduction and accumulation of the porphyrin precursor(s) or porphyrin(s) (Table 9-21). Although some have overlapping features, manifestations of the hepatic porphyrias are neurologic, including abdominal pain, neuropathy, and mental disturbances, whereas the erythropoietic porphyrias characteristically cause cutaneous photosensitivity. The reason for neurologic involvement in the hepatic porphyrias, which does not usually occur before puberty, is poorly understood. Cutaneous sensitivity to sunlight may occur in infancy because of the excitation of excess porphyrins in the skin by long-wave ultraviolet light, which leads to cell damage, scarring, and deformation. Steroid hormones, drugs, and nutrition influence the production of porphyrin precursors and porphyrins, thereby precipitating or increasing the severity of some porphyrias. Thus, the porphyrias are actually ecogenic disorders in which environmental, physiological, and genetic factors interact to cause disease.

Many symptoms of the porphyrias are nonspecific, and diagnosis is often delayed. Laboratory testing can confirm or exclude the diagnosis of a porphyria. Table 9-21 summarizes the major metabolites that accumulate in each porphyria. Urinary 5-aminolevulinic acid (ALA) and porphobilinogen (PBG) are easily quantitated by chemical methods, and the urinary porphyrin isomers can be separated and quantitated by high-performance liquid chromatography. The diagnostic profile of accumulated precursors and/or porphyrins in each disorder can also be defined by extraction and thin-layer chromatography of fecal porphyrins. However, a definite diagnosis requires demonstration of the specific enzyme or gene defect. The isolation and characterization of the genes, encoding all eight heme biosynthetic enzymes have permitted the identification of the molecular lesions that cause each porphyria. Such molecular analyses make it possible to provide precise heterozygote identification and prenatal diagnosis in families with known mutations or with informative polymorphisms.

9.12.1   Heme Biosynthesis

The first and last three enzymes in the heme biosynthetic pathway are located in the mitochondrion, whereas the other four are in the cytosol (see Fig. 9-28). The first enzyme, 5-aminolevulinate synthase (ALA-synthase), catalyzes the condensation of glycine, activated by pyridoxal phosphate and succinyl coenzyme A, to form ALA. In the liver, this rate-limiting enzyme can be induced by a

TABLE 9-21

CLINICAL, METABOLIC, AND GENETIC CHARACTERISTICS OF THE HUMAN PORPHYRIAS

TYPE/PORPHYRIA	DEFICIENT ENZYME	INHERITANCE	PHOTO-SENSITIVITY	NEURO-VISCERAL SYMPTOMS	INCREASED ERYTHROCTYE PORPHYRINS	PORPHYRIN EXCRETION	
						URINE	STOOL
Hepatic Porphyrias							
ALA-dehydratase deficiency (ADP)	ALA-dehydratase	AR	—	+	PROTO	ALA, COPRO III	—
Acute intermittent porphyria (AIP)	HMB-synthase	AD	—	+	—	ALA, PBG	—
Porphyria cutanea tarda (PCT)	URO-decarboxylase	AD	+++	—	—	URO I, 7-carboxylate porphyrin	ISOCOPRO
Hepatoerythropoietic porphyria	URO-decarboxylase	AR	+++	+/−			
Hereditary coproporphyria (HCP)	COPRO-oxidase	AD	+	+	—	ALA, PBG, COPRO III	COPRO III
Variegate porphyria (VP)	PROTO-oxidase	AD	+	+	—	ALA, PBG COPRO III	PROTO IX, 5-carboxylate porphyrin
Erythropoietic Porphyrias							
X-linked sideroblastic anemia (XLSA)	ALA-synthase	XLR	—	—	—	—	—
Congenital erythropoietic porphyria (CEP)	URO-synthase	AR	+++	—	URO I	URO I	COPRO I URO I
Erythropoietic protoporphyria (EPP)	Ferrochelatase	AD	+	—	PROTO IX	—	PROTO IX

AR, autosomal recessive; AD, autosomal dominant, XLR, X-linked recessive; ALA, 5-aminolevulinic acid; PBG, porphobilinogen; COPRO I, coproporphyrin I; COPRO III, coproporphyrin III; ISOCOPRO, isocoproporphyrin; URO I, uroporphyrin I; URO III, uroporphyrin III, PROTO, protoporphyrin IX.

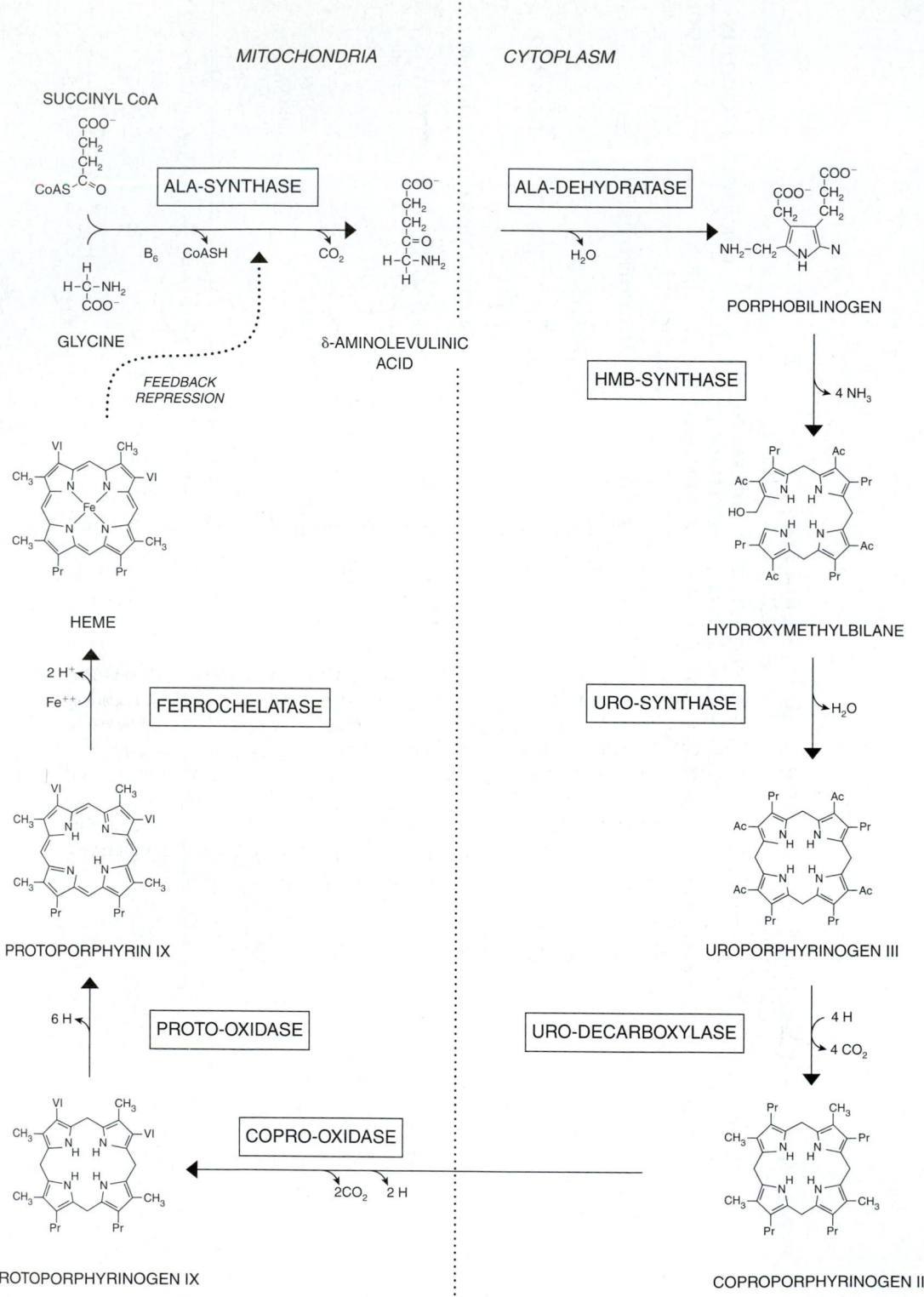

FIGURE 9-28   The human heme biosynthetic pathway.

variety of drugs, steroids, and other chemicals. Distinct erythroid-specific and housekeeping forms of ALA-synthase are encoded by separate genes. Defects in the X-linked erythroid cause X-linked sideroblastic anemia (see Chapter 19).

The second enzyme, 5-aminolevulinate dehydratase (ALA-dehydratase), catalyzes the condensation of two molecules of ALA to

form PBG. Four molecules of PBG condense to form the tetrapyr-role uroporphyrinogen III by a two-step process catalyzed by hydroxymethylbilane (HMB)-synthase (also known as PBG-deaminase or uroporphyrinogen I synthase) and uroporphyrinogen III (URO) synthase. HMB-synthase catalyzes the head-to-tail condensation of four PBG molecules by a series of deaminations to form the linear tetrapyrrole hydroxymethylbilane. URO-synthase catalyzes the rearrangement and rapid cyclization of HMB to form the asymmetric, physiological, octacarboxylate porphyrinogen uroporphyrinogen III isomer.

The fifth enzyme in the pathway, uroporphyrinogen decarboxylase (URO-decarboxylase), catalyzes the sequential removal of the four carboxyl groups from the acetic acid side chains of uroporphyrinogen III to form coproporphyrinogen III, a tetracarboxylate porphyrinogen. This compound then enters the mitochondrion, where coproporphyrinogen (COPRO)-oxidase, the sixth enzyme, catalyzes the decarboxylation of two of the four propionic acid groups to form the two vinyl groups of protoporphyrinogen IX, a dicarboxylate porphyrinogen. Next, protoporphyrinogen (PROTO)-oxidase oxidizes protoporphyrinogen IX to protoporphyrin IX by the removal of six hydrogen atoms. The product of the reaction is a porphyrin (oxidized form), in contrast to the preceding tetrapyrrole intermediates, which are porphyrinogens (reduced forms). Finally, ferrous iron is inserted into protoporphyrin IX to form heme, a reaction catalyzed by the eighth enzyme in the pathway, ferrochelatase (also known as heme synthetase or protoheme ferrolyase).

Each of the heme biosynthetic enzymes is encoded by a separate gene. Full-length human cDNAs for each of the enzymes, including those for both forms of ALA-synthase, have been isolated and sequenced, and the chromosomal locations of the genes have been identified (Table 9-22).

9.12.2   Regulation of Heme Biosynthesis

About 85% of the heme produced in the body is synthesized in erythroid cells to provide heme for hemoglobin, and most of the remainder is produced in the liver where the biosynthetic pathway is under negative feedback control. "Free" heme in the liver regulates the synthesis and mitochondrial translocation of the housekeeping form of ALA-synthase. Heme represses the synthesis of the ALA-synthase mRNA and interferes with the transport of the enzyme from the cytosol into mitochondria. ALA-synthase is inducible by many of the same chemicals that induce the cytochrome P450 enzymes in the endoplasmic reticulum of the liver. Because most of the heme in the liver is used for the synthesis of cytochrome P450 enzymes, hepatic ALA-synthase and the cytochrome P450 enzymes are regulated in a coordinated fashion.

Different regulatory mechanisms control production of heme for hemoglobin. The erythroid-specific ALA-synthase encoded on the X-chromosome is expressed at higher levels than the hepatic enzyme, and an erythroid-specific control mechanism regulates iron transport into erythroid cells. During erythroid differentiation, the activities of the heme biosynthetic enzymes are increased.

9.12.3   The Hepatic Porphyrias

The acute hepatic porphyrias are characterized by the rapid onset of neurologic manifestations. During the acute attack, individuals have markedly elevated plasma and urinary concentrations of the porphyrin precursors ALA and PBG, which originate in the liver.

ALA-DEHYDRATASE–DEFICIENT PORPHYRIA

This disease is a rare autosomal recessive trait that has been described in only a few patients. Onset and severity of the disease are variable, presumably depending on the amount of residual ALA-dehydratase activity. Treatment and prevention of the neurologic complications are the same as for other acute porphyrias.

Clinical Features

The clinical presentation is variable. The first reported cases were in two unrelated German men who had clinical onset during adolescence of abdominal pain and neuropathy, resembling acute intermittent porphyria (AIP). A Swedish infant presented with failure to thrive and required transfusions and parenteral nutrition. Presumably, the earlier age of onset and more severe manifestations reflect a more severe enzyme deficiency. A Belgian man developed an acute motor polyneuropathy and polycythemia at age 63. Re-

TABLE 9-22

THE HUMAN HEME BIOSYNTHESIS GENES*

GENE	CHROMOSOME LOCATION	cDNA/Protein	GENOMIC ORGANIZATION LENGTH/#EXONS
ALA-synthase			
Housekeeping	3p21.1	2199 bp/640 aa	17 kb/11 exons
Erythroid-specific	Xp11.21	1937 bp/587 aa	22 kb/11 exons
ALA-dehydratase	9q34		
Housekeeping		1149 bp/330 aa	15.9 kb/exons 1A, 2–12
Erythroid-specific		1154 bp/330 aa	15.9 kb/exons 1B, 2–12
HMB-synthase	11q23.3		
Housekeeping		1086 bp/361 aa	11 kb/exons 1, 3–15
Erythroid-specific		1035 bp/344 aa	11 kb/exons 2–15
URO-synthase	10q25.2→q26.3		
Housekeeping		1296 bp/265 aa	34 kb/exons 1, 2B–10
Erythroid-specific		1216 bp/265 aa	34 kb/exons 2A, 2B–10
URO-decarboxylase	1p34	1104 bp/367 aa	3 kb/10 exons
COPRO-oxidase	3q12	1062 bp/354 aa	14 kb/7 exons
PROTO-oxidase	1q23	1431 bp/477 aa	5.5 kb/13 exons
Ferrochelatase	18q21.3	1269 bp/423 aa	45 kb/11 exons

* cDNA base pairs (bp), number of encoded amino acids (aa), genomic length in kilobases (kb), and number of exons are indicated.

cently, a Japanese woman was described who had her first acute attack and the syndrome of inappropriate secretion of antidiuretic hormone at age 69.

Diagnosis

Patients have increased urinary levels of ALA and coproporphyrin. ALA-dehydratase activity in erythrocytes is <5% of normal. Because either lead or succinylacetone (which accumulates in hereditary tyrosinemia and is structurally similar to ALA) can inhibit ALA-dehydratase, increase urinary excretion of ALA, and cause manifestations that resemble those of the acute porphyrias, lead intoxication (see Sec. 4.3) and hereditary tyrosinemia (fumarylacetoacetase deficiency; see Sec. 9.2) should be considered in the differential diagnosis of ALA-dehydratase–deficient porphyria. Immunologic studies in the reported cases demonstrated the presence of nonfunctional enzyme proteins that cross-reacted with anti-ALA–dehydratase antibodies. DNA analysis revealed different missense mutations that resulted in the amino acid substitutions G133R and V275M in the infantile-onset patient, and R240W and A274T in a juvenile-onset patient.

Heterozygotes are clinically asymptomatic and do not excrete increased levels of ALA, but they can be detected by demonstration of intermediate levels of erythrocyte ALA-dehydratase activity or by demonstrating a specific mutation in the ALA-dehydratase gene. Prenatal diagnosis of this disorder is possible by determination of the ALA-dehydratase activity in cultured chorionic villi or amniocytes.

Treatment

Treatment is similar to that of AIP.

ACUTE INTERMITTENT PORPHYRIA

This hepatic porphyria is an autosomal dominant condition resulting from the half-normal level of HMB-synthase (also termed PBG-deaminase) activity. The disease is widespread but is especially common in Scandinavia and perhaps Great Britain. The enzyme deficiency can be demonstrated in most heterozygous individuals, but clinical expression is highly variable. Activation of the disease is related to ecogenic factors, such as drugs, diet, and steroid hormones, which can precipitate the manifestations. Attacks can be prevented by avoiding known precipitating factors.

Clinical Features

Most heterozygotes remain clinically asymptomatic (latent) unless exposed to factors that increase the production of porphyrins. Endogenous and exogenous gonadal steroids, porphyrinogenic drugs, alcohol ingestion, and low-calorie diets, usually instituted for weight loss, are common precipitating factors. Table 9-23 lists the major drugs that are harmful in AIP [and also in hereditary coproporphyria (HCP) and variegate porphyria (VP)] and some drugs and anesthetic agents known to be safe. More extensive lists of drugs considered harmful or safe are available (*www.enterprise.net/apf/index.html*), but information is incomplete for many drugs. Attacks also can be provoked by infections and by surgery.

Because the neurovisceral symptoms rarely occur before puberty and are often nonspecific, a high index of suspicion is required to make the diagnosis. The disease can be disabling but is rarely fatal. Abdominal pain, the most common symptom, is usually steady and poorly localized, but may be cramping. Ileus, abdominal distention,

TABLE 9-23

CATEGORIES OF UNSAFE AND SAFE DRUGS IN AIP, HCP, AND VP

UNSAFE	SAFE
Barbiturates	Narcotic analgesics
Sulfonamide antibiotics	Aspirin
Meprobamate	Acetaminophen
Glutethimide	Phenothiazines
Methyprylon	Penicillin and derivatives
Ethchlorvynol	Streptomycin
Mephenytoin	Glucocorticoids
Succinimides	Bromides
Carbamazepine	Insulin
Valproic acid	Atropine
Pyrazolones	
Griseofulvin	
Ergots	
Synthetic estrogens and progestogens	
Danazol	
Alcohol	

AIP, acute intermittent porphyria; HCP, hereditary coproporphyria; VP, variegate porphyria.

and decreased bowel sounds are common. However, increased bowel sounds and diarrhea may occur. Abdominal tenderness, fever, and leukocytosis are usually absent or mild because the symptoms are neurologic rather than inflammatory. Nausea; vomiting; constipation; tachycardia; hypertension; mental symptoms; pain in the limbs, head, neck, or chest; muscle weakness; sensory loss; dysuria; and urinary retention are characteristic. Tachycardia, hypertension, restlessness, tremors, and excess sweating are due to sympathetic overactivity.

The peripheral neuropathy is the result of axonal degeneration (rather than demyelination) and affects primarily motor neurons. Significant neuropathy does not occur with all acute attacks; abdominal symptoms are usually more prominent. Motor neuropathy affects the proximal muscles initially, more often in the shoulders and arms. The course and degree of involvement are variable. Deep-tendon reflexes may be normal or hyperactive, but are usually decreased or absent with advanced neuropathy. Motor weakness can be asymmetric and focal and may involve cranial nerves. Sensory changes such as paresthesias and loss of sensation are less prominent. Progressive muscle weakness can lead to respiratory and bulbar paralysis and death when diagnosis and treatment are delayed. Sudden death may result from sympathetic overactivity and cardiac arrhythmia.

Mental symptoms such as anxiety, insomnia, depression, disorientation, hallucinations, and paranoia can occur in acute attacks. Seizures can be caused by neurologic effects or by hyponatremia. Treatment of seizures is difficult because virtually all antiseizure drugs (except bromides) may exacerbate AIP (clonazepam may be safer than phenytoin or barbiturates). Hyponatremia results from hypothalamic involvement and inappropriate secretion of antidiuretic hormone, or from electrolyte depletion due to vomiting, diarrhea, poor intake, or excess renal sodium loss. Persistent hypertension and impaired renal function may occur. When an attack resolves, abdominal pain may disappear within hours, and paresis begins to improve within days, and may continue to improve over several years.

Diagnosis

ALA and PBG levels are increased in plasma and urine during acute attacks. The excretion of these compounds generally decreases with clinical improvement, particularly after hematin infusions. A normal urinary PBG level effectively excludes AIP as a cause for current symptoms. Fecal porphyrins are usually normal or minimally increased in AIP, in contrast to HCP and VP. Most asymptomatic ("latent") heterozygotes with HMB-synthase deficiency have normal urinary excretion of ALA and PBG. Therefore, measurement of HMB-synthase in erythrocytes may be useful to confirm the diagnosis and to screen asymptomatic family members.

The enzyme deficiency is detectable in erythrocytes from most AIP heterozygotes (*classic AIP*). Note that the activity is higher in young erythrocytes and may increase into the normal range in AIP when erythropoiesis is increased due to a concurrent condition. However, patients with the rare erythroid form of AIP (*erythroid* or *variant AIP*) have normal enzyme levels in erythrocytes and deficient activity in nonerythroid tissues. The erythroid and housekeeping forms of HMB-synthase are encoded by a single gene, which has two promoters. One promotes transcription of a messenger RNA for the housekeeping form found in all tissues, and the other promotes formation of the erythroid-specific transcript only in erythroid cells. Several deletions and over 150 different point mutations in the coding region of the gene have been found in unrelated AIP families. These mutations alter the kinetic properties and/or stability of the mutant enzymes or create premature termination codons. Mutations that cause erythroid AIP variants with half-normal enzyme in nonerythroid tissues, but normal activity in erythrocytes, include point mutations in the initiation methionine codon (that prevent translation) or in the 5′ donor splice site of intron 1 (that cause abnormal splicing of the HMB-synthase transcript).

Heterozygotes can be identified by restriction fragment length polymorphism (RFLP) studies in informative families using various polymorphic sites in the HMB-synthase gene. Efforts are now under way to identify the specific mutations in the HMB-synthase gene in all AIP families; this information will make it possible to identify all heterozygotes in affected families and to advise them to avoid the factors known to cause acute attacks. The prenatal diagnosis of a fetus at risk can be made with cultured amniotic cells or chorionic villi.

Treatment

During acute attacks, narcotic analgesics may be required for abdominal pain, and phenothiazines are useful for nausea, vomiting, anxiety, and restlessness. Chloral hydrate can be given for insomnia, and benzodiazepines in low doses are probably safe if a minor tranquilizer is required. Although intravenous glucose (at least 300 g/d) can be effective in acute attacks of porphyria, a more complete parenteral nutritional regimen may be beneficial if oral feeding is not possible for a prolonged period. However, intravenous heme is more effective than glucose in reducing porphyrin precursor excretion and probably leads to a more rapid recovery. The response to heme therapy is reduced if therapy is delayed. Therefore, 3 to 4 mg of heme, in the form of hematin, heme albumin, or heme arginate, may be infused daily for 4 days beginning as soon as possible after onset of an attack. Heme arginate and heme albumin are chemically stable and are less likely than hematin to produce phlebitis or an anticoagulant effect. The rate of recovery from an acute attack depends on the degree of neuronal damage and may be rapid (1 to 2 days) with prompt therapy. Recovery from severe motor neuropathy may continue for months or years. Identification and avoidance of inciting factors can hasten recovery from an attack and prevent future attacks. Multiple inciting factors may contribute to a symptomatic episode. Frequent clear-cut cyclical attacks occur in some women and can be prevented with a luteinizing hormone-releasing hormone analogue (this indication is not approved by the US Food and Drug Administration).

PORPHYRIA CUTANEA TARDA

Porphyria cutanea tarda (PCT), the most common of the porphyrias, can be sporadic (type I) or familial (types II and III), and also can develop after exposure to halogenated aromatic hydrocarbons. Hepatic URO-decarboxylase is deficient in all types of PCT. In type I PCT, URO-decarboxylase activity is normal in erythrocytes. In type II PCT, an autosomal dominant trait, the enzyme is deficient in erythrocytes and other tissues. In type III PCT, which clusters in families, deficiency of the enzyme activity is limited to the liver. Deficient hepatic URO-decarboxylase and a porphyrin pattern resembling PCT can be produced by exposure of normal individuals to a number of halogenated aromatic hydrocarbons. Hepatoerythropoietic porphyria (HEP) is an autosomal recessive form of porphyria that results from the marked systematic deficiency of URO-decarboxylase activity.

Clinical Features

Cutaneous photosensitivity is the major clinical feature. Neurologic manifestations are not observed. Fluid-filled vesicles and bullae develop on sun-exposed areas such as the face, the dorsa of the hands and feet, the forearms, and the legs. The skin in these areas is friable, and minor trauma may lead to the formation of bullae. The appearance of small white plaques, termed *milia*, may precede or follow vesicle formation. Bullae and denuded skin heal slowly and are subject to infection. Other features include hypertrichosis and hyperpigmentation, especially of the face, and thickening, scarring, and calcification resembling the cutaneous changes of systemic sclerosis.

A number of factors contribute to the development of hepatic URO-decarboxylase deficiency, including excess alcohol, iron, and estrogens. Recently, the importance of excess hepatic iron as a precipitating factor was documented by finding that the incidence of the common hemochromatosis-causing mutations, *HFE* C282Y and H63D, were increased in types I and II PCT patients. PCT also can be induced by various chemicals; an epidemic of PCT occurred in eastern Turkey in the 1950s, from the consumption of wheat contaminated with the fungicide hexachlorobenzene. Hexachlorobenzene produces a disorder similar to PCT and induces hepatic URO-decarboxylase deficiency in animals. PCT in humans has occurred after exposure to other chemicals, including di- and trichlorophenols and 2,3,7,8-tetrachlorodibenzo-(*p*)-dioxin (TCDD, dioxin). Patients with PCT characteristically have liver damage and are at risk for hepatocellular carcinoma (see Sec. 18.10). These carcinomas do not produce porphyrins.

Hepatoerythropoietic porphyria (HEP) resembles congenital erythropoietic porphyria (CEP) and usually presents with blistering skin lesions, hypertrichosis, scarring, and red urine in infancy or childhood.

Diagnosis

Porphyrin levels are increased in the liver, plasma, urine, and stool. The urinary ALA level may be slightly increased, but the PBG level is normal. Urinary porphyrins consist mostly of uroporphyrin and 7-carboxylate porphyrin, with lesser amounts of coproporphyrin and 5- and 6-carboxylate porphyrins. Plasma porphyrins also are increased in a pattern that resembles that in urine. Isocoproporphyrins are increased in feces, and sometimes also in plasma and urine. The finding of increased isocoproporphyrins is diagnostic for a deficiency of hepatic URO-decarboxylase.

Type II PCT and HEP can be diagnosed by finding decreased URO-decarboxylase activity in erythrocytes. URO-decarboxylase activity in liver, erythrocytes, and cultured skin fibroblasts in type II PCT is approximately 50% of normal in affected individuals and in family members with latent disease. In HEP, the URO-decarboxylase activity is markedly deficient, with typical levels of 3 to 10% of normal. Several point mutations have been identified in the coding region of the URO-decarboxylase gene from unrelated type II PCT and HEP patients. Excess hepatic iron contributes to development of sporadic and familial forms of PCT. As noted above, the coinheritance of *HFE* mutations causing hemochromatosis is a PCT precipitating factor. In the familial forms (types II and III), iron inhibits the residual normal enzyme, so that enzymatic activity in liver is less than 50% of normal. In type I PCT, the decreased hepatic URO-decarboxylase activity is not accompanied by a decreased amount of enzyme protein, suggesting that the enzyme is present in an inactive form, and hepatic URO-decarboxylase activity gradually increases after a remission is induced by phlebotomy.

Treatment

Alcohol, estrogens, iron supplements, and, if possible, any drugs that may exacerbate the disease, should be discontinued, but this step does not always lead to improvement. A complete response can almost always be achieved by repeated phlebotomy to reduce hepatic iron. A unit (450 mL) of blood can be removed every 1 to 2 weeks. Because iron overload is not marked in most cases, remission may occur after only five or six phlebotomies. Hemoglobin levels or hematocrits and serum ferritin should be followed closely to prevent development of iron deficiency and anemia. After remission, continued phlebotomy may not be needed even if ferritin levels return to normal. Relapses are treated by additional phlebotomy.

PCT also can be treated with chloroquine or hydroxychloroquine, both of which complex with the excess porphyrins and promote their excretion. Small doses (eg, 125 mg chloroquine phosphate twice weekly) should be given, because standard doses can induce transient, sometimes marked, increases in photosensitivity and hepatocellular damage. Hepatic imaging can diagnose or exclude complicating hepatocellular carcinoma. Treatment of PCT in patients with end-stage renal disease is facilitated by administration of erythropoietin.

HEREDITARY COPROPORPHYRIA

Hereditary coproporphyria (HCP) is an autosomal dominant form of hepatic porphyria that results from half-normal levels of COPRO-oxidase activity. Photosensitivity may occur. A few cases of homozygous dominant HCP have been reported.

Clinical Features

HCP is influenced by the same factors that cause attacks in AIP. The disease is latent before puberty, and symptoms are more common in women. Neurovisceral symptoms and other manifestations are virtually identical to those of AIP. Photosensitivity may resemble that in PCT and VP. Cutaneous lesions may begin in childhood in the rare homozygous dominant cases.

Diagnosis

Coproporphyrin concentrations are markedly increased in the urine and feces when the disease is symptomatic, and sometimes when there are no symptoms. Urinary ALA and PBG levels are increased during acute attacks but may return to normal when symptoms resolve. Although the diagnosis can be confirmed by measuring COPRO-oxidase activity, these assays are not widely available and require cells other than erythrocytes.

Treatment

Neurologic symptoms are treated as in AIP. Phlebotomy and chloroquine are ineffective when cutaneous lesions are present.

VARIEGATE PORPHYRIA

VP, a hepatic porphyria that results from the deficient activity of PROTO-oxidase, is inherited as an autosomal dominant trait, and can present with neurologic symptoms, photosensitivity, or both.

Clinical Features

Neurovisceral signs and symptoms develop after puberty and are similar to those of AIP or HCP. Attacks are provoked by the same drugs, steroids, and nutritional factors that are detrimental in AIP. Skin manifestations are more common than in HCP, but usually occur apart from the neurovisceral symptoms. Because the skin lesions in VP, HCP, and PCT are not distinguishable by clinical examination or biopsy, these conditions must be diagnosed by assay of porphyrins and porphyrin precursors in blood, urine, and feces.

VP is particularly common in South Africa, where 3 in 1000 whites have the disorder. Most are descendants of a couple who emigrated from Holland to South Africa in 1688. Homozygous dominant VP is associated with photosensitivity, neurologic symptoms, and developmental disturbances, including growth retardation in infancy or childhood; all cases had increased erythrocyte levels of zinc protoporphyrin, a characteristic finding in all homozygous porphyrias so far described.

Dual porphyria, the simultaneous occurrence of VP and type II PCT, has been documented in several kindreds. *Chester porphyria* was described in a large British family in which individuals had acute porphyric attacks and deficiency of both PROTO-oxidase and HMB-synthase. Photosensitivity was not observed. It is unclear whether Chester porphyria is a variant of VP or AIP.

Diagnosis

When VP is symptomatic, levels of fecal protoporphyrin and coproporphyrin and of urinary coproporphyrin are increased. Urinary ALA and PBG levels are increased during acute attacks. Plasma levels of porphyrins are increased, particularly when there are cutaneous lesions. VP can be distinguished rapidly from all other porphyrias by examining the fluorescence emission spectrum of porphyrins in plasma at neutral pH. This test is particularly useful for differentiating VP from PCT.

Assays of PROTO-oxidase activity in cultured fibroblasts or lymphocytes are not widely available. Some latent cases of VP can be diagnosed by measurement of fecal porphyrins in relatives of VP patients.

Treatment

Acute attacks are treated with hematin as in AIP. Other than avoiding sun exposure, there are few effective measures for treating the skin lesions. β-Carotene, phlebotomy, and chloroquine are not helpful.

9.12.4 The Erythropoietic Porphyrias

In the erythropoietic porphyrias, porphyrins from bone marrow erythrocytes and plasma are deposited in the skin and lead to cutaneous photosensitivity.

X-LINKED SIDEROBLASTIC ANEMIA

X-linked sideroblastic anemia (XLSA) results from the deficient activity of the erythroid form of ALA-synthase and is associated with ineffective erythropoiesis, weakness, and pallor.

Clinical Features

Typically, males with XLSA develop refractory hemolytic anemia, pallor, and weakness during infancy. They have secondary hypersplenism, become iron overloaded, and can develop hemosiderosis. The severity depends on the level of residual erythroid ALA-synthase activity and on the responsiveness of the specific mutation to pyridoxal 5-phosphate supplementation. Peripheral blood smears reveal a hypochromic, microcytic anemia with striking anisocytosis, poikilocytosis, and polychromasia; the leukocytes and platelets appear normal. Hemoglobin content is reduced, and the mean corpuscular volume and mean corpuscular hemoglobin concentration are decreased. Recently, patients with milder later-onset disease have been reported.

Diagnosis

Bone marrow examination reveals a hypercellular marrow with a left shift and megaloblastic erythropoiesis with an abnormal maturation. A variety of Prussian blue–staining sideroblasts are observed. Levels of urinary porphyrin precursors and of both urinary and fecal porphyrins are normal. The level of erythroid ALA-synthase is decreased in bone marrow, but this enzyme is difficult to measure in the presence of the normal ALA-synthase housekeeping isozyme. Definitive diagnosis requires the demonstration of mutations in the erythroid ALA-synthase gene.

Treatment

The severe anemia may respond to pyridoxine supplementation. This cofactor is essential for ALA-synthase activity, and mutations in the pyridoxine-binding site of the enzyme have been found in several responsive patients. Cofactor supplementation may make it possible to eliminate or reduce the frequency of transfusion. Unresponsive patients may be transfusion-dependent and require chelation therapy.

CONGENITAL ERYTHROPOIETIC PORPHYRIA

Congenital erythropoietic porphyria (CEP) is an autosomal recessive disorder, also known as *Gunther disease*, that is the result of markedly deficient activity of URO-synthase and is associated with hemolytic anemia and cutaneous lesions. CEP is characterized by accumulation of uroporphyrin I and coproporphyrin I isomers.

Clinical Features

Severe cutaneous photosensitivity begins in early infancy. The skin over sun-exposed areas is friable, and bullae and vesicles are prone to rupture and infection. Skin thickening, focal hypo- and hyperpigmentation, and hypertrichosis of the face and extremities are characteristic. Secondary infection of the cutaneous lesions can lead to disfiguring of the face and hands. Porphyrins are deposited in teeth and bones. As a result, the teeth are reddish brown and fluoresce on exposure to long-wave ultraviolet light. Hemolysis is probably due to the marked increase in erythrocyte porphyrins and leads to splenomegaly. Adults with a milder form of the disease have been described.

Diagnosis

Uroporphyrin and coproporphyrin (mostly type I isomers) accumulate in the bone marrow, erythrocytes, plasma, urine, and feces. The diagnosis should be confirmed by demonstration of markedly deficient URO-synthase activity. The disease can be detected in utero by measuring porphyrins in amniotic fluid and URO-synthase activity in cultured amniotic cells or chorionic villi. Molecular analyses of the mutant alleles from over 20 unrelated patients have revealed the presence of gene rearrangements, an mRNA processing defect, and several point mutations that cause amino acid substitutions.

Treatment

The transfusion of sufficient blood to suppress erythropoiesis is effective but results in iron overload. Splenectomy may reduce hemolysis and decrease transfusion requirements. Protection from sunlight and from minor skin trauma is important. β-Carotene may be of some value. Complicating bacterial infections should be treated promptly. Recently, bone marrow transplantation has proven effective in several transfusion-dependent children, providing the rationale for stem-cell gene therapy.

ERYTHROPOIETIC PROTOPORPHYRIA

Erythropoietic protoporphyria (EPP) is caused by the partial deficiency of ferrochelatase and is inherited as an autosomal dominant trait. Protoporphyrin accumulates in erythroid cells and plasma, and is excreted in bile and feces. EPP is the most common erythropoietic porphyria and, after PCT, the second most common porphyria.

Clinical Features

Skin photosensitivity usually begins in childhood. The skin manifestations differ from those of other porphyrias. Vesicular lesions are uncommon. Redness, swelling, burning, and itching can develop within minutes of sun exposure and resemble angioedema. Symptoms may seem out of proportion to the visible skin lesions. Sparse vesicles and bullae occur in 10% of cases. Chronic skin changes may include lichenification, leathery pseudovesicles, labial grooving, and nail changes. Severe scarring is rare, as are pigment changes, friability, and hirsutism.

The primary source of excess protoporphyrin is the bone marrow reticulocyte. Erythrocyte protoporphyrin is free (not complexed with zinc) and is mostly bound to hemoglobin. In plasma, protoporphyrin is bound to albumin. Hemolysis and anemia are usually absent or mild.

Liver function is usually normal, but in some patients accumulation of protoporphyrin causes chronic liver disease that can progress to liver failure and death. The hepatic complications are often preceded by increasing levels of erythrocyte and plasma protoporphyrin, and probably result, in part, from protoporphyrin accumulation in the liver. Protoporphyrin is insoluble; it forms crystalline structures in liver cells, and can decrease hepatic bile flow. Gallstones composed at least in part of protoporphyrin occur in some patients.

Some obligate heterozygotes are asymptomatic and have little or no increase in erythrocyte protoporphyrin. Thus, there is phenotypic variation in this disease.

Diagnosis

Protoporphyrin levels are increased in bone marrow, circulating erythrocytes, plasma, bile, and feces. Urinary levels of porphyrin and porphyrin precursors are normal. Ferrochelatase activity in cultured lymphocytes or fibroblasts is decreased.

Treatment

Oral β-carotene improves tolerance to sunlight in many patients. The dosage may need to be adjusted to maintain serum carotene levels in the recommended range of 10 to 15 μmol/L (600–800 μg/dL). Mild skin discoloration due to carotenemia is the only significant side effect. The beneficial effects of β-carotene may involve quenching of singlet oxygen or free radicals. Unfortunately, this drug is less effective in other forms of porphyria associated with photosensitivity.

Treatment of hepatic complications is difficult. However, cholestyramine and other porphyrin absorbents, such as activated charcoal, may interrupt the enterohepatic circulation of protoporphyrin and promote its fecal excretion, leading to some improvement. Splenectomy may be helpful when the disease is accompanied by hemolysis and significant splenomegaly or secondary hypersplenism. Caloric restriction and drugs or hormones that may induce the heme pathway or impair hepatic excretory function should be avoided. Iron deficiency should be prevented or treated. Transfusions or intravenous heme therapy may suppress erythroid and hepatic protoporphyrin production and are sometimes beneficial. Liver transplantation has been carried out in some patients with severe liver complications.

References

Anderson K, Sassa S, Bishop D, Desnick R: Disorders of heme biosynthesis; X-linked sideroblastic anemia and the porphyrias. In: Scriver CR, Beaudet AL, Sly WS, Valle D, eds. The Metabolic and Molecular Bases of Inherited Disease, 8th ed. New York, McGraw-Hill, 2001, 2961–3062

Anderson KE, Spitz IM, Bardin CW, Kappas A: A GnRH analogue prevents cyclical attacks of porphyria. Arch Intern Med 150:1469, 1990

Astrin KH, Desnick RJ: Molecular basis of acute intermittent porphyria. Hum Mutat 4:243, 1994

Bonkovsky HL, Poh-Fitzpatrick M, Pimstone N, et al: Porphyria cutanea tarda, hepatitis C and HFE gene mutations in North America. Hepatology 27:1661, 1998

Cotter PD, May A, Fitzsimons EJ, et al: Late-onset X-linked sideroblastic anemia. Missense mutations in the erythroid delta-aminolevulinate synthase (ALAS2) gene in two pyridoxine-responsive patients initially diagnosed with acquired refractory anemia and ringed sideroblasts. J Clin Invest 96:2090, 1995

Cotter PD, May A, Li L, Al-Sabah AL, Fitzsimons EJ, Cazzola M, Bishop DF: Four new mutations in the erythroid-specific 5-aminolevulinate synthase (ALAS2) gene causing X-linked sideroblastic anemia: increased

pyridoxine responsiveness after removal of iron overload by phlebotomy and coinheritance of hereditary hemochromatosis. Blood 93:1757, 1995

De Siervi A, Rossetti MV, Parera VE, Astrin KH, del C batlle AM, Desnick RJ: Identification and characterization of hydroxymethylbilane synthase mutations causing acute intermittent porphyria: evidence for an ancestral founder of the common G111R mutation. Am J Med Genet 86:366, 1999

Desnick RJ, Anderson KE: Heme biosynthesis and its disorders: porphyrias and sideroblastic anemias. In: Hoffman R, Benz EJ, Jhattil SJ et al: Hematology: Basic Principles and Practices, 2d ed. New York, Churchill Livingstone, 1995, pp 523–545

Desnick RJ, Glass IA, Xu W, Solic C, Astrin KH: Molecular genetics of congenital erythropoietic porphyria. Semin Liver Dis 18:77, 1998

Lindberg RL, Martini R, Baungartner M, et al: Motor neuropathy in porphobilinogen deaminase-deficient mice imitates the peripheral neuropathy of human acute porphyria. J Clin Invest 103:1127, 1999

May A, Bishop DF: The molecular biology and pyridoxine responsiveness of X-linked sideroblastic anaemia. Haematologica 83:56, 1998

Mendez M, Sorkin L, Rosetti MV, et al: Familial porphyria cutanea tarda: characterization of seven novel uroporphyrinogen decarboxylase mutations and frequency of common hemochromatosis alleles. Am J Hum Genet 63:1363, 1998

Moore MR, Kenneth EL, Rimington C, Goldberg A: Disorders of Porphyrin Metabolism. New York, Plenum, 1987

Mustajoki P, Nordmann Y: Early administration of heme arginate for acute porphyric attacks. Ann Intern Med 153:2004, 1993

Plewinska M, Thurnell S, Holmberg L, Wetmur JG, Desnick RJ: δ-Aminolevulinate dehydratase deficient porphyria: identification of the molecular lesions in a severely affected homozygote. Am J Hum Genet 49:167, 1991

Tezcan I, Xu W, Gurgey A, et al: Congenital erythropoietic porphyria successfully treated by allogeneic bone marrow transplantation. Blood 92:4053, 1998

Xu W, Warner CA, Desnick RJ: Congenital erythropoietic porphyria: identification and expression of 10 mutations in the uroporphyrinogen III synthase gene. J Clin Invest 95:905, 1995

9.13   INHERITED PURINE AND PYRIMIDINE DISORDERS

Mendel Tuchman and Mark L. Batshaw

Purine and pyrimidines exist in living organisms as free bases, ribonucleosides (attached to ribose or deoxyribose sugars) and ribonucleotides (base-sugar-phosphate) that are the building blocks of DNA and RNA, or as conjugates with other sugars such as galactose and glucose or other compounds. Because of their diverse biological role, disorders of purine and pyrimidine metabolism involve many different functions and systems, including the central nervous system, hematologic system, muscle, and kidney. Inborn errors of purine and pyrimidine metabolism have been described that affect the de novo synthesis, "salvage," and degradation pathways of purine and pyrimidine metabolism, each producing markedly different clinical syndromes. This section deals with these pathways, excluding those disorders causing immune deficiencies and hematologic disorders, which are addressed in Chapters 11 and 19.

The metabolic pathway of purine metabolism is illustrated in Fig. 9-29. Purine ribonucleotides are synthesized to form ATP and GTP that serve as substrates for DNA and RNA synthesis. Phosphorylated ribonucleotides are partially degraded to nucleosides and their bases and can be "salvaged" to reform phosphorylated nucleotides again. In addition, purines consumed in the diet are

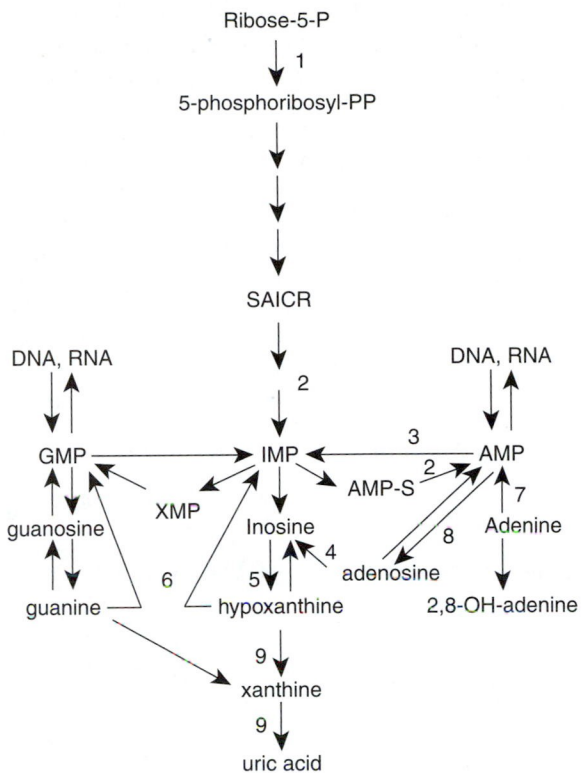

FIGURE 9-29 Purine metabolism. 1, Phosphoribosylpyrophos-phate synthetase; 2, adenylosuccinate lyase; 3, adenylate deaminase; 4, adenosine deaminase; 5, purine-nucleoside phosphorylase; 6, hypoxanthine guanine phosphoribosyltransferase; 7, adenine phosphoribosyltransferase; 8, purine 5-nucleotidase; 9, xanthine oxidase. AMP, adenosine monophosphate; AMP-S, adenylsuccinate; IMP, inosine monophosphate; GMP, guanosine monophosphate; P, phosphate; SAICR, succinyl aminoimidazole carboxamide ribotide; XMP, xanthine monophosphate.

available to form ribonucleotides via the salvage pathway. The catabolic end product is uric acid, a compound that cannot be further metabolized and that is excreted in the urine. Thus, there are two pathways leading to purine ribonucleotide synthesis: the de novo pathway and the salvage pathway. The synthesis of purines is regulated as feedback inhibition by the purine nucleotides of the initial synthesis steps, especially by the formation of phosphoribosylpyrophosphate (PPRP).

9.13.1 Disorders of De Novo Purine Synthesis

PHOSPHORIBOSYLPYROPHOSPHATE SYNTHETASE OVERACTIVITY

This disorder, which accounts for a small proportion of patients with gout, is inherited as an X-linked recessive trait. It results from superactivity of the enzyme PPRP synthetase, one of the initial steps in purine synthesis (see Fig. 9-29). A defect in this enzyme leads to resistance to feedback from the purine nucleotides and to overproduction of purines. In turn, this leads to enhanced degradation of purines and overproduction of uric acid, resulting in gout and urolithiasis in early adulthood. There is, however, a more severe phenotype that presents in males during early childhood with gout, neurodevelopmental impairment, and sensorineural deafness. Gout

and deafness can also develop in a subgroup of heterozygous females, presumably as a result of skewed lyonization.

A late juvenile–adult-onset variety of this disorder is restricted to males who show gout and/or uric acid urolithiasis but no neurologic signs. Two genes (*PRPS 1* and *PRPS 2*) that code for isoforms of the enzyme have been identified on the X-chromosome, one on the long arm and the other on the short arm. For diagnostic purposes, elevated activity of the enzyme can be found in red blood cells, lymphocytes, and cultured skin fibroblasts. Therapy is designed at reducing the production of uric acid by using allopurinol, avoidance of dehydration, and alkalinization of the urine.

ADENYLOSUCCINASE DEFICIENCY

This enzyme in the de novo pyrimidine pathway was found to be deficient in certain children with severe mental retardation, autistic behavior, and seizures. These children have elevated levels of succinylaminoimidazole carboxamide riboside and succinyladenosine in their CSF and urine, both usually undetectable in body fluids. Liver and cultured skin fibroblast activity of adenylosuccinase is markedly reduced. The disorder is transmitted as an autosomal recessive trait. The responsible gene has been cloned and sequenced, and disease-causing mutations have been identified. Adenine replacement and allopurinol have been tried with little success.

ADENYLATE DEAMINASE DEFICIENCY

This enzyme deficiency occurs in 1 to 2% of the population manifesting in some individuals as muscle weakness and cramping following vigorous exercise. It is usually diagnosed in adulthood, but may be a common cause of benign hypotonia in infancy. The disorder is transmitted as an autosomal recessive trait, but most affected homozygotes are asymptomatic. For detailed description see Sec. 25.17.

9.13.2 Disorders of Purine Salvage Pathway

ADENINE PHOSPHORIBOSYLTRANSFERASE (APRT) DEFICIENCY

APRT deficiency is inherited as an autosomal recessive trait caused by an inability of cells to salvage the purine base adenine (see Fig. 9-29). The accumulated adenine is oxidized by the enzyme xanthine oxidase to 2,8-dihydroxyadenine, but cannot be further metabolized. Dihydroxyadenine is very insoluble in water, leading to precipitation and formation of crystals and stones within the urinary tract. The dihydroxyadenine stones are reddish-brown when wet, and gray when dry. They are soft, friable, and radiolucent, and may be mistaken for uric acid stones. Clinical symptoms, which may become apparent at any age, including the neonatal period, include renal colic, hematuria, urinary tract infections, and dysuria. However, the clinical spectrum is wide and the disease severity is variable; some homozygous individuals are asymptomatic. Elevated urinary levels of 2,8-dihydroxyadenine, 8-hydroxyadenine, and adenine are diagnostic of this condition. The pathologic changes in the kidney are similar to those seen in uric acid nephropathy.

APRT activity can be measured in erythrocytes, lymphocytes, and cultured skin fibroblasts. Based on enzyme studies in red blood cells, the disorder has been classified into type I and type II. Patients with type I have no detectable enzymatic activity, while those with type II (found only in Japan) have reduced but not absent activity. The APRT gene has been cloned and sequenced, and several disease-causing mutations have been detected.

Treatment includes dietary purine restriction and a high fluid intake. Allopurinol has been used to prevent oxidation of adenine and formation of stones. Use of alkaline substances should be avoided as it may favor precipitation of purine bases. Renal transplantation has been used successfully for end-stage renal disease.

HYPOXANTHINE GUANINE PHOSPHORIBOSYLTRANSFERASE (HGPRT) DEFICIENCY

This X-linked recessive disorder, known as *Lesch-Nyhan disease,* is caused by a deficiency of HGPRT (see Fig. 9-29). This enzyme salvages the purine bases hypoxanthine and guanine and converts them to nucleotides. The two main clinical consequences of this enzyme deficiency are (a) a severe neurologic disorder of self-mutilation, mental retardation, and dyskinetic cerebral palsy, and (b) hyperuricemia resulting in uric acid stones and in gout.

Affected male infants appear normal at birth and develop clinical signs by 3 to 6 months of age with irritability, spasticity, recurrent emesis, and failure to thrive. In early childhood extrapyramidal signs become evident, including choreoathetosis and dystonia, which interfere with attempts at ambulation. The most singular manifestation of this disease is self-injury that usually develops between 2 and 3 years of age. Affected children tend to bite their lips and fingers, often causing severe loss of tissue. There seems to be a compulsive quality to the self-injury. When physically restrained to prevent self-mutilation, they appear to be less agitated and more content. Although some degree of mental retardation is usually present, cognitive skills are often underestimated because of the motor deficits and self-injurious behavior. The pathophysiology of the neurologic manifestations is unclear, although a developmental deficit in dopaminergic cells has been observed in patients and in an animal model of self-injury.

Other abnormalities associated with this disorder are renal stones, resulting from a 200-fold increase in uric acid production, macrocytosis, and megaloblastosis. Heterozygous females are usually healthy, although hyperuricemia and gout have been described in some.

HGPRT deficiency can be documented in red blood cells and cultured skin fibroblasts. Severely affected patients have a complete deficiency. Partial deficiencies confer a less-severe phenotype, with hyperuricemia and gout and few neurologic symptoms. Interestingly, heterozygous females show normal HGPRT activity in their cells rather than the expected 50% activity, suggesting a negative selection of cells with deficient HGPRT activity. As a result, enzyme determination cannot be used for carrier testing. The gene encoding HGPRT is located on the long arm of the X-chromosome; it has been cloned and sequenced. Many different mutations have been identified in affected families. DNA analysis can be used for carrier testing and prenatal diagnosis. Therapy for the gout includes allopurinol and alkalinization of the urine. There is no effective therapy for the neurologic deficits.

HEREDITARY XANTHINURIA

Xanthine oxidase deficiency, an autosomal recessive disorder, blocks the conversion of hypoxanthine and xanthine to uric acid, resulting in their accumulation (see Fig. 9-29). About half of the homozygotes are clinically asymptomatic, having only biochemical evidence of low serum-uric-acid levels and increased urinary xanthine excretion. Symptomatic individuals develop renal stones and subsequent urinary tract complications that can lead to chronic renal failure. Xanthine stones are brownish-yellow and, like all other purine stones, are radiolucent. Xanthine oxidase deficiency can be documented in liver and intestinal tissues. No specific therapy is available, but patients do benefit from increased fluid intake and a diet low in purines.

Because xanthine oxidase requires molybdenum as a cofactor, disorders that interfere with molybdenum cofactor metabolism cause a secondary deficiency of xanthine oxidase. Such is the case of inherited molybdenum cofactor deficiency, a severe neurologic disorder. It should be noted that although xanthine metabolism is affected in this disorder, it is not the main clinical problem.

9.13.3 Disorders of De Novo Pyrimidine Synthesis

HEREDITARY OROTIC ACIDURIA

This rare autosomal recessive disorder is caused by a deficiency of both orotate phosphoribosyltransferase and orotidine 5'-monophosphate decarboxylase. These two reactions are catalyzed by a single bifunctional enzyme encoded by a single gene called *uridine monophosphate synthetase.* The consequence of this deficiency is the inability to synthesize pyrimidine nucleotides, resulting in megaloblastic anemia and excretion of large amounts of orotic acid. Some patients additionally have psychomotor retardation, growth retardation, and cellular immunodeficiency (humoral immunity is normal). The urine is saturated with orotic acid, which may precipitate to form crystals causing an obstructive uropathy. The enzymatic defect can be documented in liver, erythrocytes, lymphoblasts, and cultured skin fibroblasts. Treatment with the pyrimidines uridine, uridylic acid, or cytidilic acid is effective in reversing the megaloblastic anemia and in reducing orotic acid formation by restoring the feedback inhibition for the pathway.

9.13.4 Disorders of Pyrimidine Degradation

HEREDITARY PYRIMIDINEMIA

This autosomal recessive disorder is caused by a deficiency of dihydropyrimidine dehydrogenase (DPD) or, less commonly, dihydropyrimidine amidohydrolase, the subsequent enzyme in the pyrimidine degradation pathway. The clinical presentation is variable, ranging from normal health to mental retardation. The deficiency predisposes even asymptomatic individuals to enhanced toxicity to fluorouracil (5-FU), because the pyrimidine bases uracil and thymine, as well as their fluorinated analogues, are degraded by these enzymes. The diagnosis of DPD deficiency is suggested by finding elevated levels of uracil and thymine (as well as 5-hydroxymethyluracil) in urine, blood, or cerebrospinal fluid. DPD activity can be measured in white blood cells and cultured skin fibroblasts. The DPD gene has been cloned and sequenced, and DNA analysis can be used in diagnosis and carrier testing.

Defects in the next pyrimidine degradation enzyme, dihydropyrimidine amidohydrolase, should be suspected when both pyrimidine bases and their dihydro derivatives are present in high concentrations. Because of the variable clinical presentation of patients with pyrimidine base degradation defects (except for enhanced

5-FU toxicity), the exact relationships between the clinical findings and the enzymatic defects remain to be defined.

References

General

Gresser U: Molecular Genetics Biochemistry and Clinical Aspects of Inherited Disorders of Purine and Pyrimidine Metabolism. Berlin, Springer-Verlag, 1993

Scriver R, Beaudet AL, Sly WS, Valle D, eds: Purine and pyrimidines. In: The Molecular and Metabolic Bases of Inherited Disease 7th ed. New York, McGraw-Hill, 1995

Simmonds HA: Purine and pyrimidine disorders. In: Holton JB, ed: The Inherited Metabolic Diseases. Edinburgh, Churchill Livingstone, 1994

Simmonds HA: Diagnosis and treatment of inborn errors of purine and pyrimidine metabolism: an overview. Adv Exp Med Biol 370:73–76, 1994

Simmonds HA: Purine and pyrimidine disorders. In: Blau N, Duran M, Blaskovics ME, eds: Physician's Guide to the Laboratory Diagnosis of Metabolic Diseases. London, Chapman & Hall Medical, 1996

9.14 DISORDERS OF LIPID AND LIPOPROTEIN METABOLISM

Peter O. Kwiterovich, Jr.

This section presents a theoretical and practical approach to disorders of plasma lipid and lipoprotein metabolism in infants, children, and adolescents. Three groups of disorders are discussed: the hyperlipoproteinemias, those associated with normal lipid levels, and the hypolipoproteinemias. Although the biochemical and genetic bases for these disorders differ considerably, the clinical complications generally include premature atherosclerosis and deposition of lipid in various tissues. Children with profound hypertriglyceridemia are at high risk of pancreatitis.

9.14.1 Plasma Lipid and Metabolism

LIPOPROTEIN CLASSIFICATION AND PROPERTIES

Plasma lipoproteins are usually spherical particles consisting of a core that contains hydrophobic lipids, mostly triglyceride and cholesteryl ester, surrounded by a surface coating consisting of proteins (apolipoproteins), phospholipids, and free (unesterified) cholesterol. The plasma lipoproteins have been classified by their density and electrophoretic mobility into four major groups: chylomicrons, very-low-density (pre-β) lipoproteins (VLDL), low-density (β) lipoproteins (LDL), and high-density (α) lipoproteins (HDL) (Table 9-24). After electrophoresis, chylomicrons remain at the origin, and VLDL, LDL, and HDL migrate in the same positions as pre-β-, β-, and α globulins, respectively. The hydrated density of the lipoproteins is related to their chemical composition and the relative content of lipid and apolipoprotein. Chylomicrons are 99% lipid, most of it being triglyceride (Table 9-24). After plasma has stood overnight, these large particles (80–500 nm) will rise to the top, where they appear as a creamy layer. VLDL are about 90% lipid, the majority of it being triglyceride, with lesser amounts of cholesterol. When present in plasma in increased amounts, VLDL are large enough (30–80 nm) to impart a cloudy or turbid appearance to plasma. LDL are the major carriers of cholesterol in plasma, and about 50% of their weight is cholesteryl ester and cholesterol. LDL are a heterogeneous group of particles whose hydrated densities range from 1.019 to 1.063 g/mL. HDL (1.063–1.21 g/mL) comprise about equal amounts of apoprotein and lipid, principally phospholipids and cholesterol.

APOLIPOPROTEINS

Plasma lipoprotein classes are associated with a number of apolipoproteins (Table 9-25). Nomenclature for the apolipoproteins follows an alphabetical scheme. The characteristics of the 10 major apolipoproteins are summarized in Table 9-25. The nucleotide sequences of cDNA for these apolipoproteins have been determined.

TABLE 9-24

CLASSIFICATION AND PROPERTIES OF THE MAJOR HUMAN PLASMA LIPOPROTEINS

	CHYLOMICRONS	VERY-LOW-DENSITY (PRE-β) LIPOPROTEIN	LOW-DENSITY (β) LIPOPROTEIN	HIGH-DENSITY (α) LIPOPROTEINS
Hydrated density ranges (g/mL)	<0.95	0.95–1.006	1.019–1.063	1.063–1.21
Electrophoretic migration	Origin	Pre-β	β	α
Average composition (%)				
Cholesterol*	3	22	50	20
Triglyceride	90	55	5	5
Phospholipid	6	15	25	25
Protein	1	8	20	50
Major apoproteins	ApoB-48 ApoC-I, II, III ApoA-I, II, IV, ApoE	ApoB-100 ApoC-I, II, III ApoE	ApoB-100	ApoA-I, II ApoC-I, II, III ApoE
Origin	Intestine	Liver, intestine	Metabolic product of VLDL catabolism	Liver, intestine
Function	Transport dietary triglycerides	Transport hepatic triglycerides	Provide cholesterol to cells	Reverse cholesterol transport

* Includes the mass of cholesteryl ester and unesterified cholesterol.

TABLE 9-25

CLASSIFICATION AND PROPERTIES OF MAJOR HUMAN PLASMA APOLIPOPROTEINS

APOLIPOPROTEIN	MOLECULAR WEIGHT	CHROMOSOMAL LOCATION	FUNCTION
ApoA-I	29,016	11	Cofactor LCAT
ApoA-II	17,414	1	Inhibit HL and VLDL hydrolysis
ApoA-IV	44,465	11	Activates LCAT
ApoB-100	512,723	2	Secretion of triglyceride from liver; binding ligand to LDL receptor
ApoB-48	240,800	2	Secretion of triglyceride from intestine
ApoC-I	6630	19	Inhibits apoE
ApoC-II	8900	19	Cofactor LPL
ApoC-III 0–2	8800	11	Inhibits ApoC-II activation of LPL
ApoD	19,000	3	Reverse cholesterol transport
ApoE	34,145	19	Facilitates uptake of chylomicron remnant and IDL

LCAT, lecithin cholesteryl acyltransferase; HL, hepatic lipase; LPL, lipoprotein lipase; VLDL, very-low-density lipoprotein; IDL, intermediate-density lipoprotein; LDL, low-density lipoprotein.

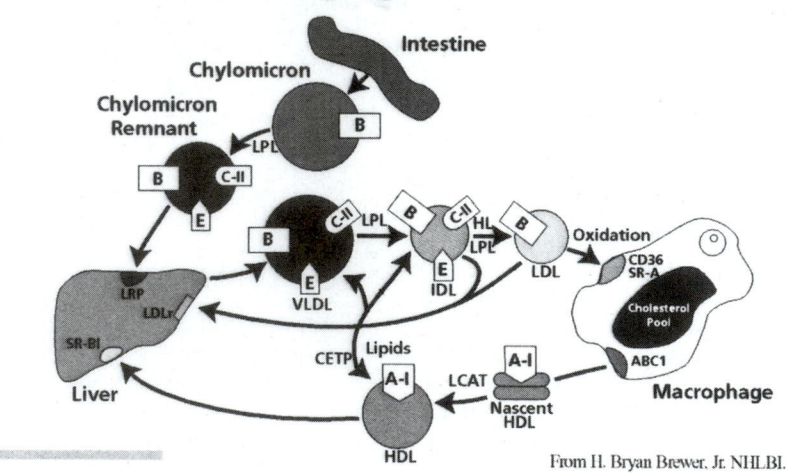

From H. Bryan Brewer, Jr. NHLBI.

FIGURE 9-30   Overview of lipoprotein metabolism. Three major pathways of plasma lipoprotein metabolism are shown: 1) transport of dietary (exogenous) fat; 2) transport of hepatic (endogenous) fat (middle); 3) reverse cholesterol transport (bottom). Dietary fat is secreted from intestinal cells on chylomicrons, a process that requires apoB (apoB-48). The triglycerides in the core of chylomicrons are hydrolyzed by lipoprotein lipase (LPL), with apoC-II as a cofactor, producing a smaller chylomicron remnant. This remnant is removed primarily by a chylomicron remnant receptor on the liver, called LRP, or the low-density lipoprotein-like receptor protein. Triglyceride-rich VLDL is synthesized and secreted from the liver, a process that requires apoB (apoB-100). In plasma, the triglyceride in the core of VLDL is broken down by lipoprotein lipase (LPL) and apoC-II, its cofactor, producing smaller VLDL remnants that end with IDL, the final remnant particle. Some of the IDL particles are removed though the interaction of apoE with the LDL receptor on the surface of the liver, or the TG in IDL can be hydrolyzed further by hepatic lipase (HL) to produce LDL. LDL is normally removed by the interaction of apoB-100 with the LDL receptor (LDLr). If LDL is oxidized, it can enter the macrophage through the scavenger receptors, CD36 and SR-A. A "cigar-shaped" nascent HDL produced in the liver and intestine contains very little cholesterol, and is mostly comprised of phospholipid and apoA-1. Nascent HDL interacts with the ABC1 transporter on the surface of extrahepatic cells and removes cellular cholesterol. Through its cofactor apoA-1, LCAT (lecithin-cholesterol acyl transferase) esterifies the cholesterol in nascent HDL in plasma, resulting in mature, spherical HDL, enriched in core cholesteryl ester (CE). The cholesteryl esters in spherical HDL can be (1) delivered directly to the liver where they are selectively taken up by the HDL (SRB-1) receptor, or (2) transferred by CETP (cholesterol ester transfer protein) from HDL to the apoB-containing lipoproteins, i.e., VLDL, IDL, and LDL; the cholesteryl esters in IDL and LDL are internalized into the liver by the LDLr.

ORIGIN AND FATE OF PLASMA LIPIDS AND LIPOPROTEINS

The transport of plasma lipids by lipoproteins may be divided into exogenous (dietary) and endogenous systems (Fig. 9-30).

EXOGENOUS LIPID TRANSPORT

Most dietary lipid is in the form of neutral fat or triglyceride (75–150 g/d). The amount of cholesterol in the diet usually varies from 300 to 600 mg/d. In the small intestine, triglyceride and cholesteryl esters are emulsified by bile acids and hydrolyzed by pancreatic lipases. Triglyceride is broken down into fatty acids and 2-monoglycerides; cholesteryl ester is hydrolyzed into fatty acids and unesterified cholesterol. These components are then absorbed, primarily in the ileum. In intestinal cells, the monoglyceride is reesterified into triglyceride, which is packaged into chylomicrons, together with dietary cholesterol and apolipoproteins apoA-I, apoA-II, apoA-IV, and apoB-48. The chylomicrons are secreted into the thoracic duct from which they enter the peripheral circulation where they acquire apoC-II and apoE from HDL. Chylomicrons are too large to cross the endothelial barrier, and apoC-II, a cofactor for lipoprotein lipase (LPL), facilitates the hydrolysis of triglyceride near the endothelial lining of blood vessels. The fatty acids that are released are taken up by muscle cells for energy utilization, or by adipose cells for reesterification into triglyceride. As a result, a chylomicron remnant is produced that is enriched in cholesteryl ester and apoE. This remnant is rapidly taken up by the liver by a process that involves an initial sequestration of remnant particles on hepatic cell surface proteoglycans, followed by receptor-mediated endocytosis of remnants by the chylomicron remnant receptor (LRP) or by the low-density lipoprotein receptor (LDLr) on the surface of hepatic parenchymal cells (Fig. 9-30). The initial binding to proteoglycans may be facilitated by LPL, which possesses both lipid and heparin binding domains. The uptake of dietary cholesterol by this process regulates the synthesis of endogenous cholesterol by inhibiting the rate-limiting enzyme of cholesterol synthesis, hydroxymethylglutaryl (HMG)-CoA reductase. Exogenous cholesterol is secreted into bile, converted to bile acids, or used for lipoprotein synthesis. There is now evidence that dietary saturated fat and cholesterol suppress the production of LDLr in liver.

ENDOGENOUS LIPID TRANSPORT

In the fasting state, most triglyceride in plasma is carried by VLDL. Triglyceride is synthesized in the liver and packaged into VLDL with other lipids and apolipoproteins (Table 9-24), primarily apoB-100 and apoE, and secreted into plasma. VLDL triglyceride is subsequently hydrolyzed by LPL to produce remnant intermediate-density lipoproteins (IDL; d, 1.006–1.019 g/mL). In this process, some surface lipid is transferred to HDL (Fig. 9-30). Compared with VLDL, IDL are relatively enriched in cholesteryl ester and depleted in triglyceride. Some IDL are taken up directly by the liver, but others are hydrolyzed by hepatic lipase (HL) to produce LDL, the final end product of VLDL metabolism (Fig. 9-30).

The apoB-100 component of the cholesteryl ester-rich LDL is recognized and bound by a high-affinity LDL receptor either in the liver or in extrahepatic cells (Fig. 9-30). The bound LDL are internalized by absorptive endocytosis. In lysosomes, apoprotein B-100 is broken down into amino acids, cholesteryl esters hydrolyzed, and cholesterol released. Excess cholesterol is reesterified by acylcholesterol acyltransferase (ACAT). The preferred substrate for ACAT is oleic acid. Excess saturated fatty acids decrease ACAT activity. As unesterified cholesterol increases, it inhibits the proteolysis and release of a transcription factor, sterol regulatory element binding protein (SREBP) from the nuclear membrane, preventing the entry of SREBP into the nucleus. SREBP is unavailable to upregulate the genes for HMG-CoA reductase and the LDLr. Conversely, a decrease in hepatic cholesterol causes an enhanced proteolysis and release of SREBP into the nucleus, where it interacts with the sterol regulatory element on the HMG-CoA reductase and LDLr genes and increases their transcription.

Some plasma LDL enter scavenger cells by a low-affinity, LDL-receptor-independent mechanism through interaction with scavenger receptors, CD36 and SRA (Fig. 9-30). Entry of LDL through this mechanism is not subject to the feedback inhibition by LDL-derived cholesterol on LDLr synthesis. Conditions that favor an increased uptake of LDL through the scavenger pathway promote the production of foam cells and the associated atherosclerosis and xanthomas.

The other major class of plasma lipoproteins, HDL, are synthesized as nascent particles primarily in the liver, but also in intestine. After entering plasma, HDL participate in two important reactions. In the process of lipolysis, apoA-I is transferred from chylomicrons to HDL, and apoC-II and apoE on HDL are transferred to the triglyceride-rich lipoproteins. ApoA-I is a cofactor for the enzyme lecithin cholesterol acyltransferase (LCAT) (Tables 9-24 and 9-25). Unesterified cholesterol is removed from peripheral cells through the ATP-binding casette protein (ATP1) and esterified through the action of LCAT and apoA-I (Fig. 9-30). These cholesteryl esters are then transferred from HDL to IDL by the cholesteryl ester transfer protein (CETP). Such cholesteryl ester in IDL can then be taken up by the liver, or can end up in LDL. Cholesteryl ester may also be delivered directly to the liver through an HDL receptor (SRB1). These reactions reflect a process called *reverse cholesterol transport*, and may explain the protective effect that HDL and apoA-I have against the development of atherosclerosis. Conversely, factors that impede this process appear to promote atherosclerosis.

PLASMA LIPID AND LIPOPROTEIN LEVELS

The plasma lipid and lipoprotein levels result from the above complex metabolic processes that are under the control of a number of genetic and environmental (eg, dietary) influences. Consequently, the concentrations of plasma cholesterol, triglycerides, and lipoproteins in children are distributed over a wide range of values (Tables 9-26 and 9-27). After the age of 2 years, the mean and the extreme percentiles remain relatively constant up to the age of 19 years. However, a relatively small, temporary decrement occurs in the total and LDL cholesterol levels during adolescence, while the triglyceride levels increase and remain so. After adolescence, males have an average HDL cholesterol level that is 5 to 10 mg/dL lower than females.

Plasma Lipid and Lipoprotein Levels in Infancy and Early Childhood

Human plasma cholesterol levels are lowest during intrauterine life. At birth, the mean (1 SD) plasma levels (mg/dL) are: total cholesterol 74 (11); LDL cholesterol 31 (6); HDL cholesterol 37 (8); and triglyceride 37 (15). The plasma total and LDL cholesterol levels increase rapidly in the first weeks of life. The kind and source

TABLE 9-26

NORMAL PLASMA LIPID CONCENTRATIONS (PERCENTILE) IN THE FIRST TWO DECADES OF LIFE*

AGE (YEARS)	NO.	CHOLESTEROL (mg/dL)			TRIGLYCERIDE (mg/dL)		
		5TH	MEAN	95TH	5TH	MEAN	95TH
0–4							
Males	238	114	155	203	29	56	99
Females	186	112	156	200	34	64	112
5–9							
Males	1253	121	160	203	30	56	101
Females	1118	126	164	205	32	60	105
10–14							
Males	2278	119	158	202	32	66	125
Females	2087	124	160	201	37	75	131
15–19							
Males	1980	113	150	197	37	78	148
Females	2079	120	158	203	39	75	132

* Data are from the Lipid Research Clinic Book (1979). Lipids were determined on plasma from 11,219 fasting, white subjects (5749 males; 5470 females) who were studied in seven North American Lipid Research Clinics, using common protocols and laboratory methods.

of the milk in the infant's diet can markedly influence the cholesterol levels. Measurement of plasma lipid and lipoprotein levels is not recommended before 2 years of age.

Abnormal Plasma Lipid and Lipoprotein Levels in Infancy, Childhood, and Adolescence

A given level of plasma lipid or lipoprotein is not diagnostic of a disorder of lipid or lipoprotein metabolism. The age- and sex-adjusted 5th and 95th percentile values for plasma cholesterol and triglyceride (Table 9-26) have been used to arbitrarily define a subset of patients in the pediatric age group. Hyper- or hypolipidemia is often accompanied by hyper- or hypolipoproteinemia; that is, by increased (or decreased) levels of one or more of the major lipoprotein classes (Table 9-27).

9.14.2 Hyperlipidemia and Hyperlipoproteinemia

SCREENING

Whom to Screen

Considerable epidemiologic, pathologic, metabolic, and genetic data indicate that the early lesions of atherosclerosis begin in youth. A variety of lipid (high LDL and VLDL, low HDL) and nonlipid (high blood pressure, obesity, cigarette smoking) risk factors are associated with the development of such lesions. However, most attention has been given to the role of plasma cholesterol and its major carrier, LDL, in the atherosclerotic process. The National Cholesterol Education Program (NCEP) Expert Panel on Blood

TABLE 9-27

NORMAL PLASMA LIPOPROTEIN CONCENTRATIONS (PERCENTILE) IN THE FIRST TWO DECADES OF LIFE*

AGE (YEARS)	HDL CHOLESTEROL (mg/dL)				LDL CHOLESTEROL (mg/dL)			
	NO.	5TH	MEAN	95TH	NO.	5TH	MEAN	95TH
5–9								
Males	145	38	56	75	132	63	93	129
Females	127	36	53	73	114	68	100	140
10–14								
Males	298	37	55	74	288	64	97	133
Females	248	37	52	70	245	68	97	136
15–19								
Males	300	30	46	63	298	62	94	130
Females	297	35	52	74	295	59	96	137

* Data are from the Lipid Clinic Data Book (1979). Lipoproteins were determined on plasma from 1415 fasting, white subjects (743 males; 672 females) who were studied in seven North American Lipid Research Clinics, using common protocols and laboratory methods.

TABLE 9-28

CHARACTERISTICS OF STEP ONE AND STEP TWO DIETS FOR CHILDREN AND ADOLESCENTS WITH DYSLIPIDEMIAS

	RECOMMENDED INTAKE	
NUTRIENT	**STEP ONE DIET**	**STEP TWO DIET**
Total fat, % of calories	Average of no more than 30	Same
Saturated fatty acids, %	<10	<7
Polyunsaturated fatty acids, %	Up to 10	Same
Monounsaturated fatty acids, %	Remaining total fat calories	Same
Cholesterol, mg/dL	<300	<200
Carbohydrates, % of calories	About 55	Same
Proteins, % of calories	About 15–20	Same
Calories	To promote normal growth and development and to reach or maintain desirable body-weight	Same

From the National Cholesterol Education Program Report of the Expert Panel on Blood Cholesterol in Children and Adolescents.

Cholesterol Levels in Children and Adolescents recommends two complementary strategies to lower plasma total and LDL cholesterol levels. First, a population approach is advocated in which all healthy American children older than 2 years follow a Step One diet moderately reduced in total fat, saturated fat, and cholesterol (Table 9-28). The second strategy is an individualized approach aimed at detecting those children and adolescents who are more likely to develop premature coronary artery disease (CAD) because of a family history of early CAD, a dyslipidemia, or because of the aggregation of two or more other risk factors. Such children need a more detailed clinical evaluation a more structured, and often a more stringent, diet (Step Two, Table 9-28); and, in some cases, drug treatment.

The individual approach for screening includes four recommendations:

1. Obtain a lipoprotein profile in children and adolescents whose parents and grandparents at age 55 years or younger had coronary arteriography and were found to have coronary atherosclerosis (often leading to coronary artery bypass surgery and balloon angioplasty).
2. Perform a lipoprotein profile in children and adolescents whose parents, grandparents, or aunts and uncles, at age 55 years or younger, had a previously documented myocardial infarction, angina pectoris, peripheral vascular disease, cerebral vascular disease, or sudden cardiac death.
3. Screen for hypercholesterolemia in offspring of a parent who has high blood cholesterol (>240 mg/dL).
4. When the parental or grandparental history is unobtainable, children and adolescents who have two or more risk factors may be screened at the physician's discretion. These risk factors include a positive family history of premature coronary artery disease (before 55 years of age), high blood pressure, cigarette smoking, low HDL cholesterol levels, obesity (>30% overweight), physical inactivity, and diabetes mellitus.

When and How to Sample

A child can be screened any time after the age of 2 years. The blood sample is obtained after a 12-hour overnight fast (fasting is not required for the measurement of total cholesterol alone). A venipuncture is preferred, because lipid determinations on capillary plasma from a finger stick are not as dependable.

What to Measure

The simplest and least-expensive screening tool is a total cholesterol level. The optimal diagnostic assessment includes measurement of total cholesterol, total triglyceride, and HDL cholesterol following an overnight fast of 12 hours. This allows LDL cholesterol to be estimated by the formula:

$$\text{LDL cholesterol} = \text{Total cholesterol} - \left[\text{HDL cholesterol} + \frac{\text{Total triglyceride}}{5}\right]$$

The concentration of cholesterol on VLDL in this formula is estimated by dividing the total triglyceride by 5. This formula is valid provided the patient is fasting, the triglyceride is below 400 mg/dL, and type III hyperlipoproteinemia is not present.

Interpretation

The laboratory should provide accurate and reproducible lipid and lipoprotein results (less than 5% coefficients of variability). Cutpoints recommended as guidelines for interpreting plasma levels of total and LDL cholesterol in children and adolescents are summarized in Table 9-29. The high total and LDL cholesterol levels approximate the 95th percentiles (Tables 9-26 and 9-27). Youths screened on the basis of the above recommendations may also have a low HDL cholesterol level alone (<35 mg/dL, approximately 5th percentile, Table 9-27), an elevated triglyceride level alone (>95th percentiles, age and sex specific, Table 9-26), or a combi-

TABLE 9-29

CUTPOINTS FOR PLASMA TOTAL AND LDL CHOLESTEROL LEVELS IN CHILDREN AND ADOLESCENTS FROM HIGH-RISK FAMILIES

CATEGORY	TOTAL CHOLESTEROL mg/dL	LDL CHOLESTEROL mg/dL
High	≥200	≥130
Borderline high	170–199	110–129
Acceptable	<170	<100

From National Cholesterol Education Program Expert Panel on Blood Cholesterol Levels in Children and Adolescents.

nation of a high LDL cholesterol and triglyceride levels, with or without a low HDL cholesterol level.

Occasionally, a child will have turbid plasma, indicative of a triglyceride level above 250 mg/dL and a more marked endogenous hypertriglyceridemia. Rarely, the plasma may be lactescent, indicating the presence of chylomicrons, which can be visualized as a thick creamy layer at the top of plasma which has stood at 4°C overnight. The presence of chylomicrons reflects an exogenous hypertriglyceridemia (Fig. 9-30).

Evaluation

The approach recommended by the NCEP Pediatric Panel is summarized in Fig. 9-31. The average LDL cholesterol level is derived from two lipoprotein profiles obtained at least 3 weeks apart. Those children with an average LDL cholesterol level ≥130 mg/dL return for more detailed clinical and family assessment (Fig. 9-31). Those familial dyslipoproteinemias generally characterized by elevated LDL cholesterol levels will be discussed first. Some children from high-risk families may have low HDL cholesterol level or elevated triglyceride level without a high LDL cholesterol level.

PRIMARY VERSUS SECONDARY DYSLIPOPROTEINEMIA

Before considering a dyslipoproteinemia to be primary, secondary causes must be excluded (Table 9-30).

9.14.3   Metabolic Disorders with Hyperlipoproteinemia

FAMILIAL DISORDERS OF LDL METABOLISM

Familial Hypercholesterolemia

Familial hypercholesterolemia (FH) is the most commonly recognized and best understood disorder of lipoprotein metabolism in childhood.

Studies in cultured fibroblasts from FH-homozygous patients by Goldstein and Brown formed the basis for the elucidation of the LDLr pathway (see Fig. 9-30) and for the demonstration that FH was caused by any one of more than 150 genetic mutations at the locus that specified the LDLr protein. These mutations include insertions, deletions, and missense and nonsense mutations, which can affect the normal synthesis, transport, LDL-binding ability, and clustering (in coated pits) of the LDLr. FH is an autosomal dominant inherited condition that has a gene-dosage effect. FH heterozygotes have plasma concentrations of total and LDL cholesterol elevated about two- to three-fold above normal; FH homozygotes have levels that are elevated five- to six-fold above normal. Subjects with FH have large, rather than small, dense LDL particles. The HDL cholesterol level is often below average in FH patients. FH is completely expressed at birth and early in childhood. Estimates of the frequency of FH heterozygotes range between 1 in 200 and 1 in 500.

Typical plasma lipid and lipoprotein levels for FH heterozygotes are found in Table 9-31. The heterozygous FH child is clinically asymptomatic in the first decade; 10 to 15% of heterozygotes develop tendon xanthomas during the second decade, most commonly in the Achilles tendon and extensor tendons of the hands. Achilles tendinitis and tenosynovitis may be the initial clinical man-

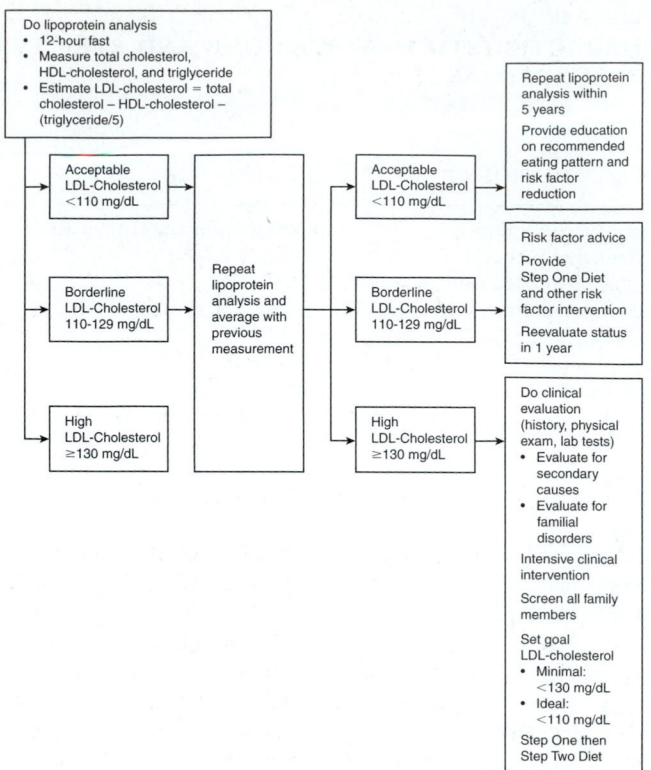

FIGURE 9-31   A diagnostic algorithm and recommendation for the clinical evaluation of children with high LDL cholesterol levels. From the report of the Expert Panel on Blood Cholesterol Levels in Children and Adolescents. National Cholesterol Education Program, 1992.

ifestations of FH in the teenage patient. Rarely, a FH heterozygote will develop angina pectoris in the late teenage years. However, many FH heterozygotes already manifest endothelial cell dysfunction.

TABLE 9-30

CAUSES OF SECONDARY HYPERLIPIDEMIA AND HYPERLIPOPROTEINEMIA IN CHILDREN AND YOUNG ADULTS

Exogenous	Renal
Alcohol	Chronic renal failure
Contraceptives	Hemolytic-uremic syndrome
Prednisone	Nephrotic syndrome
Anabolic steroids	Hepatic
13-*cis*-Retinoic acid	Benign recurrent intrahepatic
Endocrine and metabolic	cholestasis
Acute intermittent porphyria	Congenital biliary atresia
Diabetes mellitus	Acute and transient
Hypopituitarism	Burns
Hypothyroidism	Hepatitis
Lipodystrophy	Others
Pregnancy	Anorexia nervosa
Storage disease	Idiopathic hypercalcemia
Cystine storage disease	Klinefelter syndrome
Gaucher disease	Progeria (Hutchinson-Gilford
Glycogen storage disease	syndrome)
Juvenile Tay-Sachs disease	Systemic lupus erythematosus
Niemann-Pick disease	Werner syndrome
Tay-Sachs disease	

TABLE 9-31

PLASMA LIPID, LIPOPROTEIN, AND apoB LEVELS IN PEDIATRIC PROBANDS WITH FH, FCHL, AND HYPERapoB*

			PLASMA CONCENTRATION (mg/dL)				
LIPID DISORDER	AGE	TOTAL CHOLESTEROL	TRIGLYCERIDES	HDL CHOLESTEROL	LDL CHOLESTEROL	apoB	LDL-C/apoB RATIO
FH (n=20)	8.0 ± 4.7	323 ± 44	86 ± 36	44 ± 8	262 ± 45	219 ± 42	1.22 ± 0.22
FCHL (n=65)	9.3 ± 4.7	220 ± 51	120 ± 91	45 ± 11	140 ± 46	153 ± 39	0.98 ± 0.19
HyperapoB (n=11)	7.8 ± 4.6	200 ± 20	91 ± 35	52 ± 7	130 ± 16	138 ± 21	0.95 ± 0.10
Control Children (n=110)	8.7 ± 1.8	182 ± 30	70 ± 39	51 ± 10	79 ± 27	85 ± 20	1.15 ± 0.20

* Values represent the mean ± one standard deviation; FH, familial hypercholesterolemia; FCHL, familial combined hyperlipidemia. Data are from Cortner, Coates, and Gallagher, 1990.

Homozygous FH children have cholesterol levels of 600 to 1000 mg/dL. Planar xanthomas, flat orange-colored skin lesions, may be present at birth and usually occur by 5 years. Planar xanthomas are located on buttocks, on extensor surfaces, between the fingers, and in the popliteal fossa. Tendon and tuberous xanthomas develop between the ages of 5 and 15 years. Angina pectoris and myocardial infarction are ordinarily delayed to the second decade, but they have occurred as early as 6 years of age. The generalized atherosclerosis affects the aortic valve as well as the aorta and coronary vessels, resulting in aortic stenosis. Many patients with homozygous FH are genetic compounds; that is, they have two different mutant alleles at the LDLr locus.

Phenocopies of Familial Hypercholesterolemia

Many instances of primary (and usually moderate) hypercholesterolemia will not indicate FH. The presence of notably elevated LDL cholesterol levels (with normal triglyceride levels) in about half the first-degree relatives, or of tendon xanthomas in a parent, helps to confirm the diagnosis of FH heterozygosity in a given infant or child. The combination of planar xanthomas and profound hypercholesterolemia is clinically diagnostic of homozygous FH, but the status of LDLr activity should be determined in such a child. Most other disorders associated with cutaneous lipid deposition have other clinically salient findings. Examples include biliary cirrhosis, congenital biliary atresia, myelomas, and Wolman disease. The diagnosis of sitosterolemia should be considered in a child who has tendon xanthomas in the first decade but only moderate hypercholesterolemia.

Familial Defective apoB-100

In 1 of 20 families, the presence of high LDL cholesterol levels and xanthomas is related to a mutation in the ligand, apoB (Arg3500Glu; Arg3531Cys; and Arg3500Trp). The mutant apoB in this disorder, familial defective apoB-100, is not bound normally by the LDLr, often leading to elevated LDL cholesterol levels. However, most patients with familial defective apoB-100 do not have tendon xanthomas, and the LDL cholesterol level in children or adults with this disorder may be normal or moderately or markedly elevated. This defect appears to account for only a small portion (perhaps 1–2%) of premature CAD. For the purpose of treatment, it is not necessary to distinguish FH from familial defective apoB-100.

Monogenic Hypercholesterolemia with Normal LDL Receptor and apoB Genes

In some families, the hypercholesterolemia does not segregate with either the LDLr gene or the apoB gene. Tendon xanthomas and premature CAD can be present. A locus in a 9-cM interval at 1p34.1-p32 has been found. As well, a small subset of patients with the phenotype of homozygous FH have a normal LDLr gene, but fail to internalize LDL, perhaps because of a defect in some component of endocytosis through clathrin-coated pits.

DISORDERS OF INCREASED LDL PRODUCTION

Familial Combined Hyperlipidemia

In certain children and adolescents from high-risk families who have elevated LDL cholesterol levels, the LDLr activity is normal, and the increased number of LDL particles results from the overproduction of VLDL particles and apoB in the liver (Fig. 9-30). One disorder due to such increased LDL production is familial combined hyperlipidemia (FCHL); representative values from children with FCHL are summarized in Table 9-31. FCHL is believed to result from the influence of a major gene. Affected patients may have elevated LDL cholesterol alone (type IIa), elevated LDL cholesterol and triglyceride (type IIb), or normal LDL cholesterol with elevated triglyceride (type IV). In adults, this pleiotropic presentation is often accompanied by premature coronary artery disease. Xanthomas are not present in FCHL, but corneal arcus may be. FCHL is not completely expressed until after 20 years of age. However, FCHL has an estimated prevalence of 1:100. Children with FCHL also manifest endothelial dysfunction, and young affected adults show decreased coronary flow reserve.

Hyperapobetalipoproteinemia

Hyperapobetalipoproteinemia (hyperapoB) is a lipoprotein phenotype characterized by an elevated LDL apoB level with a normal LDL cholesterol level; the triglyceride level can be normal or elevated. Representative values in children with hyperapoB are found in Table 9-31. HyperapoB also results from the overproduction of VLDL, and leads to an increased number of small, dense LDL particles, as reflected by a low ratio of LDL cholesterol to apoB (Table 9-31). HyperapoB and FCHL are metabolically and, in some families, genetically related. Other syndromes also appear related to FCHL and hyperapoB; namely, LDL subclass pattern B, familial dyslipidemic hypertension, and syndrome X. Children with hyperapoB may be overweight and hyperinsulinemic, and have higher blood pressure levels but lower HDL cholesterol levels. In the Bogalusa Heart Study, syndrome X was characterized by linking a metabolic entity (hyperinsulinemia/insulin resistance, dyslipidemia, and obesity) to a hemodynamic factor (hypertension) through shared correlation with hyperinsulinemia/insulin resistance. The clustering of these clinical features was independent of sex and age in both black and white youth.

Candidate Genes for Small, Dense LDL Syndromes In addition to enhanced VLDL production in these syndromes, delayed clearance of postprandial triglyceride-rich lipoproteins, namely, chylomicrons and chylomicron remnants, may also occur (Fig. 9-30). A number of genes have been linked to FCHL and to other small, dense LDL syndromes. These are believed to be "modifying genes" and include LCAT, manganese superoxide dismutase, apoAI-CIII-AIV gene cluster; LDLr; and CETP. The fundamental defect has proven to be elusive; in Finnish families, FCHL was linked to a locus on 1q21-q23, and a mouse model of FCHL, Hyplip1, was linked to a chromosome region syntenic to human 1q21-q23. To date, the fundamental defect(s) remain to be precisely elucidated.

FAMILIAL METABOLIC DISORDERS OF TRIGLYCERIDE-RICH LIPOPROTEINS

Metabolic disorders involving the triglyceride-rich lipoproteins—chylomicrons, VLDL, and their remnants—are heterogeneous. Hypertriglyceridemia may result from increased synthesis or decreased catabolism of one or more of these lipoprotein classes, or from a combination of enhanced synthesis and suppressed catabolism.

Endogenous Hypertriglyceridemia

Familial Hypertriglyceridemia

In some children, the plasma total and LDL cholesterol levels will clearly be normal and the VLDL cholesterol and triglyceride levels elevated (type IV lipoprotein pattern). A genotypic diagnosis requires study of the parents and other siblings to distinguish familial hypertriglyceridemia (FHT) from FCHL. In those families in which the type IV phenotype "breeds true," the genotypic designation of FHT is appropriate. In adults with FHT, glucose intolerance, obesity, hyperuricemia, and peripheral vascular disease are often found. The disorder is probably inherited as an autosomal dominant trait with reduced penetrance; the phenotype is expressed in only 1 in 5 children under the age of 20 years born to an affected parent.

In FHT, the HDL cholesterol level is often low; the LDL cholesterol and LDL apoB levels are quite normal, in contrast to FCHL, in which they are borderline high or elevated. The VLDL particles in FHT tend to be triglyceride enriched, and in liver, VLDL triglyceride, but not apoB, is being overproduced. There is some controversy about whether CAD is increased in FHT; as a general rule, if a family has premature CAD and FHT, then the dyslipoproteinemia in affected family members is potentially atherogenic until proven otherwise.

Exogenous Hypertriglyceridemia

The lipolytic activity in plasma is measured after the intravenous injection of heparin (60 U/kg) that releases the membrane-bound lipases into the bloodstream [postheparin lipolytic activity (PHLA)]. LPL, hepatic lipase (HL), and phospholipases are released. There are two inherited disorders in which LPL activity is absent or markedly deficient.

Defective or Missing LPL

When the enzyme LPL is defective or missing, massive increases in chylomicrons with marked hypertriglyceridemia (as high as 10,000 mg/dL) occur. The marked chylomicronemia, indicating inability to clear dietary fat, is manifested by a thick, creamy layer over a clear infranate in a tube of plasma left to stand overnight at 4°C. Hypercholesterolemia is usually present, but the ratio of triglyceride to cholesterol is at least 5 and is usually 10. VLDL cholesterol is normal, but HDL and LDL cholesterol levels are low. LPL activity is absent from the plasma and adipose tissue of patients with this disease (also called type I hyperlipoproteinemia). The half-life of chylomicrons is prolonged to 100 minutes (normal, 17 minutes). The cofactor for LPL, apoC-II, is present in normal concentrations. The disorder ordinarily presents before the age of 10 years. Abdominal pain is the usual initial symptom, presenting as colic in the first year of life or as an acute abdominal condition later in childhood. Other clinical features may include eruptive xanthomas, hepatosplenomegaly, and lipemia retinalis. The disorder is rare; it is the result of a homozygous state for a mutant allele. Parents of affected children may have normal lipid levels, or appear to have FCHL (see above). The absence of atherosclerosis in type I suggests that chylomicrons, unlike chylomicron remnants, are not atherogenic.

To date, more than 80 mutations in the LPL gene have been reported. The human LPL gene is approximately 30 kb in length and consists of 10 exons interrupted by 9 introns. Missense mutations typically predominate in the LPL gene, with a preferential location in exons 3, 4, and 5, and have been described in the catalytic triad, Asp_{156}, His_{241}, and Ser_{132}.

Deficiency of Apolipoprotein C-II

If a deficiency of apolipoprotein C-II (the cofactor for LPL) is present, hypertriglyceridemia can range from 800 to almost 10,000 mg/dL; the lipoprotein pattern may be type I or the elevated chylomicrons may be accompanied by elevated VLDL (type V). The total cholesterol concentrations can also be normal or increased (151–980 mg/dL). The LDL and HDL cholesterol levels are below the fifth percentile of normal persons. PHLA activity is absent or very low. ApoC-II is present in only trace amounts. However, addition of apoC-II to plasma of these patients in vitro, or by blood or plasma transfusion in vivo, restored normal PHLA activity. The disorder is rare and inherited as an autosomal recessive trait. The problem usually presents in adulthood with pancreatitis, although one homozygote developed pancreatitis at the age of 6 years. Abnormalities of the apoC-II gene are caused by either small deletions or by splice-site mutations.

Endogenous and Exogenous Hypertriglyceridemia

Type V Hyperlipoproteinemia

Patients with a type V lipoprotein phenotype have marked hypertriglyceridemia caused by increased amounts of both chylomicrons and VLDL. Common clinical findings include pancreatitis, eruptive xanthomas, lipemia retinalis, and abnormal glucose tolerance with hyperinsulinism. The atherosclerosis associated with some of the other familial hyperlipidemias is not as prevalent in type V, although some patients have premature peripheral vascular or coronary artery disease. The increased VLDL in type V hyperlipoproteinemia may be the result of increased synthesis or decreased clearance of VLDL, or a combination of both. Although this phenotype is usually expressed only in young adulthood, several preadolescent children with type V hyperlipoproteinemia have been described. Affected relatives may have type V or, more commonly, type IV lipoprotein phenotypes. A pattern of autosomal dominant inheritance has been found in several large collections of kindreds whose probands had type V phenotypes.

Dysbetalipoproteinemia (Type III Hyperlipoproteinemia)

Patients with dysbetalipoproteinemia present with elevations in both cholesterol and triglyceride levels, often above 300 mg/dL. Dysbetalipoproteinemia, or type III hyperlipoproteinemia, is conventionally defined by a plasma VLDL that is cholesterol-enriched and has β, rather than pre-β electrophoretic mobility. Ultracentrifugation of plasma, without density (d) adjustment (d <1.006 g/mL), is required to make the diagnosis. The ratio of VLDL cholesterol to plasma total triglyceride is usually greater than 0.3 (normal, 0.15–0.25). Such "beta" VLDL reflects the accumulation of cholesterol-enriched remnants of both hepatic VLDL and intestinal chylomicrons. The levels of LDL cholesterol and HDL cholesterol are usually low.

The recessive defect involves a polymorphic genetic locus that specifies the structure of apoE. ApoE binds to receptors on the surface of liver cells, promoting the hepatic uptake of remnant lipoproteins. Human apoE exists as three major isoforms (E_2, E_3, and E_4), each of which is specified by an independent allele at the locus

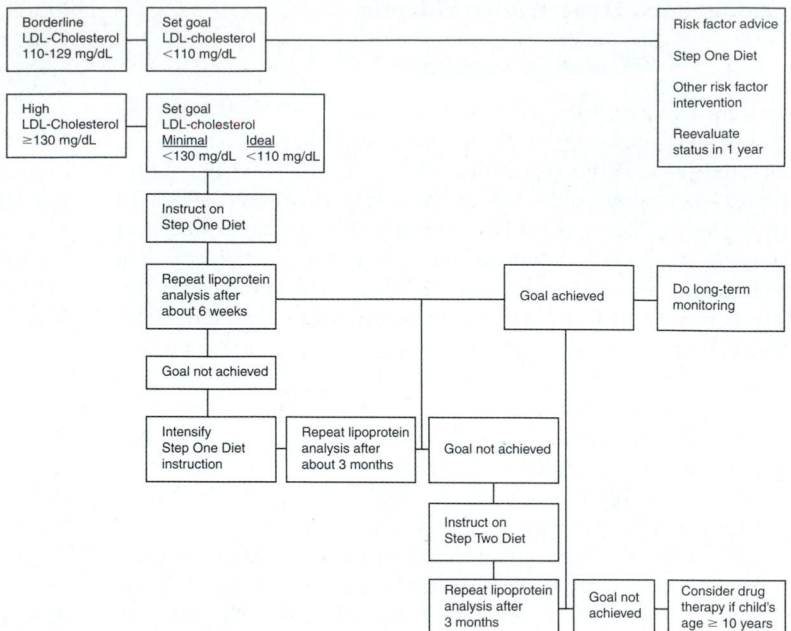

FIGURE 9-32   A treatment algorithm for dietary management of children with high LDL cholesterol levels. From the report of the Expert Panel on Blood Cholesterol Levels in Children and Adolescents. National Cholesterol Education Program, 1992.

for the apoE gene. The most common allele is $apoE_3$ and the rarest allele is $apoE_2$. The most frequent variant of $apoE_2$ has a cysteine substituted for arginine at residue 158. One in 100 persons is homozygous for the $apoE_2$ allele. Most patients with dysbetalipoproteinemia are $apoE_2$ homozygotes; because the prevalence of the disorder is only 1:10,000, other modifying factors, such as an overproduction of VLDL in liver (seen in FCHL), or hormonal and environmental conditions (such as hypothyroidism, low-estrogen state, obesity, or diabetes) are necessary for full-blown clinical expression. This recessive form of dysbetalipoproteinemia has a delayed penetrance.

The dominant form of dysbetalipoproteinemia is a consequence of one of several rare variants of apoE that usually involve the substitution of neutral or acidic amino acids for basic ones in residues 136 to 150—the region of apoE that interacts directly with the LDLr. Examples include Arg142Cys; Arg145Cys; Lys146Gln or Glu. The dominant form can be expressed in childhood and does not require the presence of modifying factors.

The clinical features of the disease are often delayed until adulthood. Affected patients often develop xanthomas, particularly yellowish deposits in the creases of the palms of the hands (xanthoma striata palmaris) and the tuberous and tuberoeruptive xanthomas over the elbows, knees, and buttocks. Tendon xanthomas are much less frequent. Premature atherosclerosis of the coronary, carotid, abdominal, and femoral arteries is prevalent. Hyperuricemia and glucose intolerance occur in up to half the patients with this syndrome.

FAMILIAL METABOLIC DISORDERS OF HDL METABOLISM

Hypoalphalipoproteinemia

In many children from families with premature coronary artery disease, the low HDL cholesterol level is not the primary abnormality; instead, it accompanies the pleiotropic presentation of an LDL or triglyceride-rich lipoprotein disorder. Some children have a primary genetic defect in HDL metabolism as the etiology for their low HDL cholesterol level (also called *hypoalphalipoproteinemia*). These disorders are under the hypolipidemias.

Hyperalphalipoproteinemia

In distinct contrast to hypoalphalipoproteinemia, some children have very high HDL cholesterol levels (>95th percentile), termed *hyperalphalipoproteinemia*. The total cholesterol level may actually be elevated as a result of the high HDL cholesterol level; the LDL cholesterol level is usually quite normal and the triglyceride level is normal or low. Hyperalphalipoproteinemia is associated with longevity and a decreased risk of coronary artery disease.

Defects in Hepatic Lipase and Cholesterol Ester Transfer Protein

Several kindreds with hyperlipidemia have been described with defects in HL or in CETP. Both are associated with hypercholesterolemia and hypertriglyceridemia, but the HDL cholesterol levels are normal or markedly increased. Few data are available on the expression of these disorders in children.

TREATMENT OF METABOLIC DISORDERS OF HYPERLIPOPROTEINEMIA

Dietary Treatment of Hyperlipidemia

The first form of therapy for children with metabolic disorders of hyperlipoproteinemia is a diet containing decreased amounts of total fat, saturated fat, and cholesterol. The intake of complex carbohydrates is increased while that of simple sugars is decreased. No decrease in total protein is recommended. The NCEP Expert Panel on Blood Cholesterol Level in Children and Adolescents recommended two steps of dietary therapy (Table 9-28) for children over 2 years of age.

Children Less Than 2 Years of Age

Dietary therapy is not recommended for those less than 2 years of age. Occasionally, an infant or toddler with homozygous or heterozygous FH may require a modified-fat diet. A commercially available formula (lower in cholesterol than human or cow's milk) can be used. The selection of appropriate preparations of baby and junior foods and kinds and amounts of solid foods is encouraged.

Reduction to or Maintenance of Ideal Body Weight

Calories sufficient for growth are needed and the percent nutrient intake (Table 9-28) varies depending on the total daily caloric intake (eg, 1200–2300 cal/d). However, children with these disorders, particularly those involving hypertriglyceridemia, are often either obese (weight for height >120%) or overweight for height. Reduction to a weight appropriate for height (ideal body weight) is an important part of the dietary management for hyperlipidemic children, and can be best achieved by keeping the weight constant while the height is increasing. Exercise is an important part of this approach. These measures often decrease the plasma levels of total cholesterol, LDL cholesterol, VLDL cholesterol, and triglyceride, but increase HDL cholesterol.

Severe Exogenous Hypertriglyceridemia

A child with profound hypertriglyceridemia requires an even more stringent restriction in fat to 10 to 15 g/d. It is important to maintain intake of linoleic acid as 1% of the calories. With severe hyperchylomicronemia, medium-chain triglycerides (MCT), which are absorbed directly through the portal vein, can be added to the diet as 15% of calories to increase compliance. Infants with type I may take a formula high in MCT. A subset of LPL-deficient children with unique, possibly posttranscriptional genetic defects, respond to therapy with MCT oil or omega-3 fatty acids by normalizing the fasting triglyceride levels; a therapeutic trial with MCT oil should be considered in all children presenting with the familial chylomicronemia syndrome. A dramatic response to antioxidant therapy has been reported in a small number of patients with LPL deficiency who had failed dietary measures and had frequent severe episodes of pancreatitis.

Response to Dietary Treatment and Follow-Up

The NCEP Expert Panel on Blood Cholesterol Levels in Children and Adolescents developed an algorithm for dietary treatment and follow-up of children with LDL disorders (Fig. 9-32). After 6 to 12 months of treatment with diet, drug therapy can be considered in those 10 years of age or older whose LDL cholesterol levels are still too high. Children with metabolic disorders of triglyceride-rich lipoproteins can be treated with diet alone and do not need lipid-lowering drugs.

Potential Side Effects of Diet

The Step One and Step Two diets (Table 9-28) appear to be safe, provided that sufficient calories are given. The diets are not restricted in animal protein and must include sufficient iron, zinc, and calcium. Available data indicate that even a balanced vegetarian diet can support normal growth and development. The Dietary Intervention Study in Children (DISC) demonstrated that the more stringent Step Two diet was safe and efficacious in adolescents with moderately elevated LDL levels. The use of weight-reduction diets in obese children can temporarily alter the growth curve.

Drug Therapy

The LDL cholesterol level will decrease, on average, about 10 to 15% with dietary treatment. In some patients, particularly those

with heterozygous FH, dietary therapy alone is insufficient. The NCEP panel recommendations for the initiation of drug treatment are summarized in Table 9-32. These recommendations are made for children older than 10 years, but exceptions to these guidelines may be made based upon clinical judgment.

The NCEP only recommended the use of bile acid sequestrants (cholestyramine, or Questran; and colestipol, or Colestid). These drugs have been used over long periods, clinically appear free of adverse effects, and can effectively lower LDL cholesterol levels. These anion-exchange resins bind bile acids and prevent their resorption through the enterohepatic circulation. Hepatic cholesterol is converted to bile acids at an accelerated rate. The pool of liver cholesterol is perturbed, including increased LDLr activity on the surface of hepatocytes. Total and LDL cholesterol can be lowered in most heterozygous children treated with bile sequestrants. The dosage of cholestyramine required to lower LDL cholesterol into the normal range is directly proportional to the postdietary LDL cholesterol levels and is not related to the body weight of the children. The dose can be effectively and conveniently given twice daily. The drug is more effective when combined with dietary treatment.

Agents other than cholestyramine are not recommended for routine use in children. Nicotinic acid is usually reserved for use in a specialty lipid clinic. The inhibitors of the rate-limiting enzyme of cholesterol biosynthesis hydroxymethylglutaryl (HMG) CoA reductase are not approved by the FDA for use in individuals younger than 18 years of age. A randomized, placebo-controlled trial, found that lovastatin, in a dose of 20 or 40 mg/day, lowered LDL-C an average of 26% in male adolescent FH heterozygotes without any adverse effect on growth, development, or hepatic enzymes. The degree of response to statins may be related to the nature of the LDL receptor mutation. In 63 children and adolescents with heterozygous FH, simvastatin, 20 mg/day, reduced LDL cholesterol in patients with the W66G mutation 31%, whereas in the deletion >15 kb and C646y mutation groups, it was 33% and 42%, respectively.

In FH homozygotes, studies at the National Institutes of Health found that with diet alone, plasma total cholesterol level fell an average of 11.5%. After the addition of cholestyramine, in a dose of 16 to 48 g/d (0.62–1.52 g/kg/d), the plasma total cholesterol level decreased an average of 31.6% (range, 4–52%). Nicotinic acid, in divided doses of 55 to 87 mg/kg/d, was added to diet and cholestyramine therapy in 6 of the 10 FH homozygotes who were treated as inpatients. In five of these six FH homozygotes, an additional average fall of 33% (range, 19–49%) was observed; one homozygote did not respond at all to either cholestyramine or the

TABLE 9-32

GUIDELINES FOR THE USE OF DRUG THERAPY IN CHILDREN 10 YEARS OR OLDER WITH PRIMARY LDL CHOLESTEROL ELEVATION

RISK FACTORS FOR CAD	POSTDIETARY LDL CHOLESTEROL LEVEL
None	>190 mg/dL
(1) Positive family history for premature CAD, or (2) Two or more other CAD risk factors	>160 mg/dL

SOURCE: *From the National Cholesterol Education Program Report of the Expert Panel on Blood Cholesterol Levels in Children and Adolescents.*

combination of the resin with nicotinic acid. In South Africa, treatment of 15 FH homozygotes with either simvastatin or atorvastatin prevented the progression of carotid intima-media thickening. Statins may decrease VLDL production independent of their effect on inducing LDL receptors, leading to decreased LDL production. The statins may also improve endothelial function and increase nitric oxide production. Although intensive dietary and drug therapy can be effective in the FH homozygote, additional measures such as plasma exchange are often necessary.

Side Effects of Drug Therapy

The side effects of bile acid sequestrants are less prominent in children than in adults. The most prominent side effect is transient gastric fullness. About one in five children develops constipation, but this is not usually persistent. Steatorrhea occurs in adults who receive cholestyramine. Restricting fat intake to 30% of calories (see Table 9-28) can minimize such steatorrhea. While bile acid sequestrants might theoretically decrease the absorption of fat-soluble vitamins, a number of studies in children have reported that the plasma levels of vitamins A and E remain within the normal range. No consistent changes have been observed in either calcium or phosphate metabolism in children treated with bile acid sequestrants. An anion exchange resin can interfere with the absorption of negatively charged molecules such as folate. Some decrease in serum folate levels usually occurs in FH heterozygotes treated with the resin, but this has not been associated with anemia. After treatment with cholestyramine, a few children develop transient mild increases in serum aspartate transaminase.

Serum concentrations of fat-soluble vitamins (A, D, E) and erythrocyte folate, liver function tests, and a complete blood count should be monitored annually in children receiving bile sequestrants. A daily supplement of multivitamins containing both iron and folic acid should also be given.

Treatment with statins is not usually associated with clinical side effects. Tests of liver function should be followed routinely and symptoms of myositis monitored. Erythromycin, systemic antifungal agents, and cyclosporin should not be used when children are on statins.

9.14.4   Metabolic Disorders of Lipid and Lipoprotein Metabolism Associated with Normal Lipid Levels

These disorders are associated with the deposition of lipid and premature atherosclerosis in the absence of marked hyperlipidemia.

SITOSTEROLEMIA

Sitosterolemia is a rare, inherited disorder that invariably presents with tendon and tuberous xanthomas before the age of 10 years, and atherosclerosis of the coronary arteries and aortic valve (producing aortic stenosis) can occur as early as the second decade of life. In sitosterolemia, plasma levels of total plant sterols are elevated (range, 13–37 mg/dL) and constitute 7 to 16% of the total plasma sterols. Sitosterol is the plant sterol that is predominantly elevated (range, 8–27 mg/dL), whereas the levels of campesterol and stigmasterol are much lower. In normal individuals, the plasma concentration of sitosterol is very low (range, 0.3–1.7 mg/dL) and represents less than 1% of the total plasma sterol. In addition to being elevated in plasma, the plant sterols are found along with

cholesterol in xanthomas, atherosclerotic lesions, erythrocytes, and adipose tissues. In sitosterolemia, there is greatly increased (5–10 times greater) intestinal absorption of dietary plant sterols that are only minimally absorbed in normal individuals. Patients with phytosterolemia also have a reduced clearance of sitosterol and cholesterol from plasma. Thus, two factors—increased absorption coupled with reduced removal—apparently lead to the enhanced tissue deposits of plant sterols and cholesterol in this disease. The plasma cholesterol levels are often normal in sitosterolemia, although they can be moderately elevated. Sitosterolemia is inherited as an autosomal recessive trait. The basic defect is not known, although the disorder has been linked to an area on 2p21.

CEREBROTENDINOUS XANTHOMATOSIS

Cerebrotendinous xanthomatosis (CTX) is a rare inherited disorder characterized by progressive neurologic findings such as dementia, cerebellar ataxia and spinal cord paresis, cataracts, tendon xanthomas, and premature atherosclerosis. Intelligence is often subnormal. The initial stage may begin in childhood; it is characterized by dementia. The onset of symptoms is often insidious and unpredictable. In the second and third decades of life, cataracts and tendon xanthomas (particularly of the Achilles tendon) are common. The major chemical finding is significant elevation of cholestanol, the α-saturated derivative of cholesterol. The plasma cholesterol and triglyceride levels are often normal, but are occasionally elevated. CTX is inherited as an autosomal recessive trait. The underlying biochemical defect involves a deficiency of hepatic mitochondrial 26-hydroxylase, causing a block in bile acid synthesis and resulting in a marked deficiency of cholic acid and chenodeoxycholic acid and the excretion of bile acid precursors such as bile alcohol glucuronides (see also Sec. 18.4).

ELEVATED LEVELS OF LP(a) LIPOPROTEIN

Lp(a) lipoprotein is a very large lipoprotein (M_r 3×10^6) found in the density range 1.050 to 1.080 g/mL. Its lipid composition is similar to LDL, but Lp(a) contains two proteins, apoB-100 and a large glycoprotein called apo(a). Apo(a) is attached to apoB-100 through a disulfide bond. Apo(a) is very similar to plasminogen and has many homologous kringle four regions. The variation in the number of kringle four regions in apo(a) is under genetic control, and there is an inverse relation between the size of apo(a) and the levels of Lp(a). Lp(a) is measured by immunochemical methods. High levels of Lp(a) appear inherited and are often strongly associated with premature cardiovascular disease in some families.

TREATMENT OF SYNDROMES OF LIPOPROTEIN METABOLISM INVOLVING NORMAL LIPID LEVELS

Patients with sitosterolemia require great care in their dietary management. Because these patients have enhanced intestinal absorption of plant sterols, dietary enrichment of polyunsaturated fats of vegetable origin cannot be recommended; vegetable oils and margarines are prohibited. Thus, fats of both animal and plant origin must be decreased. The plasma concentrations of all sterols in sitosterolemia can be decreased about 50% by treatment with cholestyramine. Treatment with the statins is not recommended.

Treatment of CTX also requires certain precautions based on the tenet that the disease results from a block in bile acid synthesis. As a result of reduced synthesis, the enterohepatic circulation of cholic acid and chenodeoxycholic acid is low. Treatment with chenodeoxycholic acid expands the deficient bile acid pool, and results in a marked decrease in plasma cholestanol levels. In some patients, neurologic findings are reversed. In contrast, cholestyramine aggravates the bile acid synthetic defect in CTX and produces a fourfold rise in plasma cholestanol levels, so that treatment of CTX with cholestyramine is contraindicated.

Lp(a) levels do not respond to a low-fat diet or to most lipid-lowering drugs. Niacin (nicotinic acid) may be effective.

9.14.5 Metabolic Disorders with Hypolipoproteinemia

DEFICIENCIES IN ApoB-CONTAINING LIPOPROTEINS

Abetalipoproteinemia

Abetalipoproteinemia (Bassen-Kornzweig syndrome) is a rare autosomal recessive disorder whose clinical expression in childhood includes fat malabsorption, severe hypolipidemia, retinitis pigmentosa, cerebellar ataxia, and acanthocytosis (Table 9-33). Three of the four major plasma lipoprotein classes (chylomicrons, VLDL, and LDL) are absent from the plasma. The concentrations of both plasma cholesterol and triglyceride are low (Table 9-34). Both apoB-48 and apoB-100 are absent in plasma.

The disorder presents soon after an uncomplicated neonatal period with abdominal distention, steatorrhea, and decreased rate of growth. The misdiagnosis of celiac disease is often made. Neurologic signs such as clumsiness, ataxia, and decreased muscular strength usually begin before the age of 10 years. Muscular weakness may also be associated with ocular symptoms such as nystagmus and strabismus. Decreased visual acuity and scotomata accompany the development of atypical retinitis pigmentosa. The diagnosis is based on the demonstration of large intracellular fat particles in biopsy specimens of the jejunum, on the failure to form chylomicrons following a meal, and on the absence of apoprotein B in plasma as determined by immunochemical techniques.

The pathophysiology of abetalipoproteinemia is important because the clinical findings result from defects in absorption and transport of ligands, especially the fat-soluble vitamins A, D, E, and K. The digestion of dietary triglyceride and the uptake of FFA and monoglyceride proceed normally. The mucosal cells fail to make chylomicrons, presumably because apoB-48 is not available. The jejunal cells become fat laden, and most of the dietary fat is excreted in the stools. Most patients with abetalipoproteinemia do not have a clinical deficiency in vitamin D, because vitamin D does not depend upon lipoproteins for absorption or transport. Deficits in vitamins A and K do occur, because these vitamins are absorbed from the intestine and transported to the liver via the chylomicron pathway (Fig. 9-30). However, after vitamins A and K reach the liver, they are not secreted on VLDL, but have their own independent transport systems. In contrast, vitamin E requires the chylomicrons to reach the liver, after which it is secreted on VLDL and subsequently ends up in LDL (Fig. 9-30). The significant impairment in the delivery of vitamin E to peripheral tissue appears to be the most clinically important vitamin deficiency in patients with abetalipo-

proteinemia, and most of the major symptoms, particularly of the retina and nervous system, appear to be the result of vitamin E deficiency.

Abetalipoproteinemia is not caused by a defect in the apoB gene. The defect in the synthesis and secretion of apoB is secondary to the absence of a microsomal triglyceride transfer protein (MTP) from liver and intestine, which mediates the intracellular transport of membrane-associated lipids and their transfer to apoB. MTP is a heterodimer composed of both the ubiquitous multifunctional protein disulfide isomerase and a unique 97-kDa subunit. Mutations that lead to the absence of the functional 97-kDa subunit cause abetalipoproteinemia. At least 13 mutant 97-kDa–subunit alleles have been described.

Hypobetalipoproteinemia

Hypobetalipoproteinemia is characterized by very low levels of LDL, usually defined as the lower fifth percentile of a normal distribution. The concentration of plasma cholesterol is low; VLDL cholesterol and plasma triglyceride levels are low or normal (see Table 9-34). Occasionally, hypobetalipoproteinemia is secondary to anemia, dysproteinemias, hyperthyroidism, intestinal lymphangiectasia with malabsorption, myocardial infarction, severe infections, and trauma. Familial hypobetalipoproteinemia has been detected at birth, but children or adults with primary hypobetalipoproteinemia have few clinical symptoms (see Table 9-33). Neurologic signs and symptoms of a spinocerebellar degeneration similar to those of Friedreich ataxia have been found in several affected members. The concentrations of fat-soluble vitamins in plasma are low to normal. Like familial hyperalphalipoproteinemia, hypobetalipoproteinemia may confer a decreased risk for coronary artery disease and concomitant increase in life span. The disorder is inherited as an autosomal dominant. At least 25 mutations in the *APOB* gene causing hypobetalipoproteinemia have been described. Almost all of the mutations are either nonsense mutations or frameshift mutations resulting from the deletion of 1 to 5 bp that create a premature stop codon. A truncated apoB is usually found in the plasma.

Homozygous Hypobetalipoproteinemia

The clinical presentation of children with this disorder depends on whether they are homozygous for null alleles in the *APOB* gene (ie, make no detectable apoB) or homozygous (or compound heterozygotes) for other alleles, and whether their lipoproteins contain small amounts of apoB or a truncated apoB. Null-allele homozygotes are similar phenotypically to those with abetalipoproteinemia and may have fat malabsorption, neurologic disease, and hematologic abnormalities as their prominent clinical presentation (Table 9-33). However, the parents of these children are heterozygous for hypobetalipoproteinemia. Patients with homozygous hypobetalipoproteinemia may develop less-marked ocular and neuromuscular manifestations, and at a later age, than those with abetaliporoteinemia. The concentrations of fat-soluble vitamins are low. In those homozygotes whose plasma contains small amounts of apoB, the total and LDL cholesterol values are as low as those with the null alleles, but the triglyceride levels, in distinct contrast, are normal (Table 9-34).

Chylomicron Retention Disease

A syndrome known as chylomicron retention disease, or Andersen disease, is characterized by a selective inability to secrete apoB from

TABLE 9-33

CLINICAL FINDINGS IN HYPOLIPOPROTEINEMIA CAUSED BY DEFICIENCIES IN ApoB-CONTAINING LIPOPROTEINS

FAMILIAL DISORDER	NEUROLOGIC	GASTROINTESTINAL	HEMATOLOGIC	OPHTHALMOLOGIC	CARDIOLOGIC	BIOPSY FINDINGS	OTHER FINDINGS
Abetalipoproteinemia	Cerebellar ataxia	Severe fat malabsorption	Acanthocytes	Atypical retinitis pigmentosa	Arrhythmias	Gross intracellular fat in jejunal cells	Myopathy (occasionally) depleted adipose mass
Heterozygous hypo-betalipoproteinemia	Usually absent[a]	Minimal fat malabsorption	Acanthocytes (occasionally)	Usually absent[b]	None	None	—
Homozygous hypo-betalipoproteinemia[c]	Ataxia	Severe fat malabsorption	Acanthocytes	Atypical retinitis pigmentosa	—	Gross intracellular fat in jejunal cells	—
Homozygous hypo-betalipoproteinemia[d]	Usually absent	Minimal to mild fat malabsorption	Mild acanthocytes	Usually absent	None	None	—

[a] Spinocerebellar degeneration and peripheral neuropathy have been described in some patients.
[b] Atypical retinitis pigmentosa has been reported in some patients.
[c] Homozygotes for "null alleles" in apoB gene.
[d] Usually compound heterozygotes for truncated apoB.

TABLE 9-34

LABORATORY FINDINGS IN HYPOLIPOPROTEINEMIA DUE TO DEFICIENCIES IN ApoB-CONTAINING LIPOPROTEINS

	PLASMA LIPIDS		PLASMA LIPOPROTEINS				
FAMILIAL DISORDER	CHOLESTEROL (mg/dL)	TRIGLYCERIDES (mg/dL)	CHYLOMICRONS	VLDL	LDL	HDL	LCAT ACTIVITY
Abetalipoproteinemia	Low (35–70)	Very low (1–10)	Absent	Absent	Absent	Low apoC-III$_{0,1}$; both absent	Decreased
Heterozygous hypobetalipopro-teinemia	Low (55–146)	Low or normal (20–146)	Low	Low	Low (10–50% of normal)	Normal	—
Homozygous hypobetalipopro-teinemia[a]	Low	Very low	Absent	Absent	Absent	Low	—
Homozygous hypobetalipopro-teinemia[b]	Low (25–75)	Normal	Low	Low	Very low (0–21)	Low to high (20–77)	—

[a] Homozygotes for "null alleles" in apoB gene.
[b] Usually compound heterozygotes for truncated apoB.

the intestinal cells, leading to fat malabsorption and neurologic disease. The basic defect is not known, but appears distinct from that of abetalipoproteinemia and hypobetalipoproteinemia.

HYPOLIPOPROTEINEMIAS CAUSED BY DEFICIENCIES IN HDL

Hypoalphalipoproteinemia

Hypoalphalipoproteinemia is defined as a low level of HDL cholesterol (<5th percentile, age and sex specific) in the presence of normal lipid levels. Patients with this syndrome have a significantly increased prevalence of coronary artery disease but do not manifest the clinical findings typical of other forms of HDL deficiency (Table 9-35). Low HDL cholesterol levels of this degree are most often secondary to disorders of triglyceride metabolism (see above). Consequently, hypoalphalipoproteinemia, although more prevalent than the rare recessive disorders, including deficiencies in HDL, is relatively uncommon. In some families, hypoalphalipoproteinemia behaves as an autosomal dominant trait, but the basic defect is unknown.

Apoprotein A-I Variants

A number of apoA-I variants, such as apoA-I Milano (see Tables 9-35 and 9-36) have been described. These apoA-I variants were detected by isoelectric focusing of apoA-I, and each has a specific amino acid substitution. For example, apoA-I Milano results from a mutation in the apoA-I gene at codon 173, changing arginine to cysteine. Heterozygous carriers for autosomal codominant traits often have low levels of HDL cholesterol (see Table 9-36), but are usually asymptomatic in regard to premature coronary artery disease. The mutant apoA-I variant can be catabolized more rapidly in plasma than normal apoA-I.

Tangier Disease

Tangier disease (see Tables 9-35 and 9-36) is a rare metabolic disorder in which plasma HDL is both abnormal and present in severely reduced concentrations. Tangier homozygotes have plasma apoA-I levels below 3% of normal. Immunochemically detectable apoA-I is synthesized by intestinal cells, but is rapidly catabolized in plasma.

The HDL in Tangier disease (termed HDL_T) are markedly abnormal; a chylomicron-like lipoprotein particle is present in the density range of HDL on a normal high-fat diet. These abnormal lipoproteins are rich in cholesteryl esters and are likely the lipoproteins that are sequestered by the reticuloendothelial cells in Tangier disease. These large, flattened, lucent particles, 100 nm in diameter, disappear with a low-fat diet. These observations suggest that HDL is necessary for normal metabolism of chylomicrons.

The compositions and amounts of the other lipoproteins are also abnormal (see Table 9-35). The level of total plasma cholesterol is decreased, with normal or elevated concentrations of plasma triglyceride. The lipoprotein abnormalities are accompanied by a striking deposition of cholesteryl ester in different tissues. The major clinical manifestations reflect the lipid storage and include enlarged orange-yellow tonsils, splenomegaly, and a relapsing peripheral neuropathy (see Table 9-35). Mild hepatomegaly, lymphadenopathy, and corneal infiltration (in adulthood) may also occur. Foam cells can be demonstrated on biopsy of the skin, bone marrow, peripheral nerves, or rectum. The disorder can be detected in children, but the age of detection has varied from 3 to 48 years.

The *APOA*-I gene is normal in Tangier disease. The basic defect resides in a double-dose of mutations in the ATP-binding cassette (ABC1) transport protein. The ABC1 protein normally mediates the efflux of cellular cholesterol onto the nascent plasma HDL particle for transport to the liver (see Fig. 9-30). The mutation in the original family from Tangier Island in the Chesapeake Bay is caused by deletion of nucleotides 3283 and 3284 in exon 22, resulting in a frameshift mutation and a premature stop codon at 3375.

Lecithin-Cholesterol Acyltransferase Deficiency and Fish-Eye Disease

LCAT esterifies cholesterol through association with HDL (α-LCAT) or, to a lesser extent, with VLDL/LDL (β-LCAT). In classic LCAT deficiency, both α-LCAT and β-LCAT activities are absent, resulting in a markedly reduced plasma cholesterol esterification rate, a low plasma cholesteryl ester content, and an abnormal lipoprotein profile with very low HDL (Table 9-36). Clinical findings include glomerulosclerosis, normochromic anemia, corneal opacities (that can be detected in childhood), and premature peripheral atherosclerosis (Table 9-35). Specific defects in the LCAT gene, including stop codons and amino acid substitutions, have been elucidated in several kindreds with classic LCAT deficiency.

Fish-eye disease is a phenotypically distinct syndrome of LCAT deficiency in which most, but not all, patients appear to have a selective defect in α-LCAT activity, which is accompanied by dense corneal opacities; HDL cholesterol is low, but premature atherosclerosis is not present (Tables 9-35 and 9-36). Several molecular defects have been described in the LCAT gene of patients with fish-eye disease, but an interesting mutation (LCAT[300-del]) has led to the postulate that the heterogeneity in the phenotypic syndromes of LCAT deficiency may be related to the residual amounts of total plasma LCAT activity.

Other Syndromes Associated with Deficiencies of HDL

Two such syndromes are distinguished here, based on clinical and laboratory findings (see Tables 9-35 and 9-36). In patients with apoA-I and apoC-III deficiency, there is corneal clouding, premature coronary artery disease, very-low HDL levels, and defective HDL production, because these homozygotes are unable to synthesize apoA-I. Examples of mutations include a rearrangement at the apolipoprotein gene locus that inactivates both apoA-I and apoC-III; the deletion of the entire locus, producing a deficiency in apoA-I, apo-III, and apoA-IV; and a small insertion in the *apoA-I* gene. Heterozygotes with one mutant allele have HDL levels that are about 50% of normal. HDL deficiency with planar xanthomas, although clinically similar to apoA-I and apoC-III deficiency (see Table 9-35), is distinguished from the latter by the elevated levels of apoC-III (see Table 9-36).

TREATMENT

Patients with abetalipoproteinemia, and those who are null-allele homozygotes for hypobetalipoproteinemia (Table 9-33) require similar treatment approaches. Steatorrhea can be controlled by reducing the intake of fat to 5 to 20 g/d. This measure alone can result in marked clinical improvement and growth acceleration. In addition, the diet should be supplemented with linoleic acid (eg, 5 g corn oil or safflower oil/d). MCT as a caloric substitute for long-chain fatty acids may produce hepatic fibrosis, and thus MCT

TABLE 9-35

CLINICAL FINDINGS IN HYPOLIPOPROTEINEMIA DUE TO DEFICIENCIES IN HDL

FAMILIAL DISORDERS*	NEUROLOGIC	GASTROINTESTINAL	HEMATOLOGIC	OPHTHALMOLOGIC	CARDIOLOGIC	BIOPSY FINDINGS	OTHER FINDINGS
Tangier disease	Relapsing peripheral neuropathy	Moderate splenomegaly, mild hepatomegaly	Normal; stomatocytosis	Corneal infiltration (adults)	CAD	Foam cells in bone marrow, skin, small nerves, and rectum	Enlarged orange tonsils
LCAT deficiency	Usually absent (occasionally peripheral neuropathy; sensorineural hearing loss)	Normal	Normochromic anemia; platelet environment disorder	Diffuse corneal opacities (childhood); normal visual acuity; corneal arcus	Premature atherosclerosis (peripheral)	Foam cells in bone marrow and renal glomeruli; sea-blue histiocytes in spleen and bone marrow	Proteinuria with late renal insufficiency; genetic linkage with haptoglobin
Fish-eye disease	Normal	Normal	Normal	Dense corneal opacities; reduced visual acuity	Atherosclerosis at old age	Not performed	
Apolipoprotein A-I and C-III deficiency	Normal	Normal	Normal	Corneal clouding; normal visual acuity	Premature CAD	Lipid-laden histiocytes in skin	Planar and tendon xanthomas
HDL deficiency with planar xanthomas	Normal	Hepatomegaly	Normal	Corneal opacity	Premature CAD	Foam cells in skin and rectal tumors	Planar xanthomas; xanthelasma

* Clinical findings in hypoalphalipoproteinemia confined to premature coronary artery disease (CAD); patients with apoprotein A-I variants are clinically normal.

709

TABLE 9-36

LABORATORY FINDINGS IN HYPOLIPOPROTEINEMIA DUE TO DEFICIENCIES IN HDL

FAMILIAL DISORDER	PLASMA LIPIDS CHOLESTEROL (mg/dL)	TRIGLYCERIDE (mg/dL)	PLASMA LIPOPROTEINS VLDL	LDL	HDL	LCAT ACTIVITY
Hypoalphalipopro-teinemia	Normal	Normal	Normal	Normal	Low (<5th percentile)	Normal
Apoprotein A-I variants ApoA-I Milano	Normal (184–231)	Elevated (181–319)	Normal	Normal or elevated; increased triglyceride content	Low (<1st percentile); enlarged particles; ApoA-I-cysteine variant	Normal
Tangier disease	Low (38–112)	Normal or high (116–332)	Beta mobility on electrophoresis; ApoC apoproteins low	Low (<10th percentile); increased triglyceride content	Barely detectable amounts of mutant HDL	Decreased (half-normal)
LCAT deficiency	Low, normal, or high (42–565)	Normal or high (105–900)	Beta mobility on electrophoresis	Low amounts of abnormal, large LDL	Low amounts of abnormal HDL	Markedly decreased (0–10% of normal)
Fish-eye disease	Normal	Elevated	Elevated	Normal level but increased triglyceride content; large particles	Low (<5th percentile)	Partial decrease
Apolipoprotein A-I and C-III deficiency	Normal	Normal	Reduced; ApoC-III apoprotein absent	—	Trace amounts	Decreased (half normal)
HDL deficiency with planar xanthomas	Normal	Normal or high	Elevated; broad beta band on electrophoresis; ApoC-III apoprotein increased	Normal level (increased triglyceride and ApoA-II content)	Trace amounts	Normal

should be used with caution, if at all. Fat-soluble vitamins should be added to the diet. Rickets can be prevented by normal quantities of vitamin D, but 200 to 400 IU/kg/d of vitamin A may be required to raise the level of vitamin A in plasma to normal. Enough vitamin K (5–10 mg/d) should be given to maintain a normal prothrombin time. Most importantly, massive doses (150–200 mg/kg/d) of vitamin E must be given. Neurologic and retinal complications may be prevented, or ameliorated, through oral supplementation with vitamin E. Adipose tissue rather than plasma may be used to assess the delivery of vitamin E.

In Tangier disease, a low-fat diet diminishes the abnormal lipoprotein species that are believed to be remnants of abnormal chylomicron metabolism. The large LDL species found in LCAT deficiency is also thought to be a remnant of abnormal chylomicron metabolism. Its disappearance on a low-fat diet may have a beneficial effect, because large LDL may be involved in the pathogenesis of renal disease. Patients with other syndromes associated with deficiencies of HDL and premature atherosclerosis are also treated with a diet modified in total fat, saturated fat, and cholesterol (see Table 9-28).

References

Plasma Lipids, Lipoproteins, and Apolipoproteins

American Academy of Pediatrics, National Cholesterol Education Program: Report of the Expert Panel on Blood Cholesterol Levels in Children and Adolescents. Pediatrics 89:515–584, 1992

Bachorik PS, Lovejoy K, Carroll MD, Johnson CL: Apolipoprotein B and AI distributions in the United States, 1988–1991: results of the National Health and Nutrition Examination Survey III (NHANES III). Clin Chem 43(12):2364–2376, 1997

Berenson GS, Srinivasan SR, Bao W, et al: The Bogalusa heart study. Association between multiple cardiovascular risk factors and atherosclerosis. N Engl J Med 338:1650–1656, 1998

Hussain MM, Strickland DK, Bakillah A: The mammalian low-density lipoprotein receptor family. Annu Rev Nutr 19:141–172, 1999

Disorders of LDL Metabolism

Cortner JA, Coates PM, Gallagher PR: Prevalence and expression of familial combined hyperlipidemia in childhood. J Pediatr 116:514–519, 1990

Couture P, Brun LD, Szots F, et al: Association of specific LDL receptor gene mutations with differential plasma lipoprotein response to simvastatin in young French Canadians with heterozygous familial hypercholesterolemia. Arterioscler Thromb Vasc Biol 18:1007–1012, 1998

DISC Collaborative Research Group: The efficacy and safety of lowering dietary intake of total fat, saturated fat, and cholesterol in children with elevated LDL-cholesterol: The Dietary Intervention Study in Children (DISC). JAMA 273:1429–1435, 1995

Haddad L, Day IN, Hunt S, et al: Evidence for a third genetic locus causing familial hypercholesterolemia J Lipid Res 40:1113–1122, 1999

Kawaguchi A, Miyatake K, Yutani C, et al: Characteristic cardiovascular manifestation in homozygous and heterozygous familial hypercholesterolemia. Am Heart J 137:410–418, 1999

Mietus-Snyder M, Malloy MJ: Endothelial dysfunction occurs in children with two genetic hyperlipidemias: improvement with antioxidant vitamin therapy. J Pediatr 133:35–40, 1998

Pitkanen OP, Nuutila P, Raitakari OT, et al: Coronary flow reserve in young men with familial combined hyperlipidemia. Circulation 99:1678–1684, 1999

Raal FJ, Pilcher GJ, Veller MG, et al: Efficacy of vitamin E compared with either simvastatin or atorvastatin in preventing the progression of atherosclerosis in homozygous familial hypercholesterolemia. Am J Cardiol 84:1344–1346, 1999

Stein AE, Illingsworth DR, Kwiterovich PO Jr, et al: Efficacy and safety of lovastatin in adolescent males with heterozygous familial hypercholesterolemia. A controlled trial. JAMA 281:137–144, 1999

Tybjaerg-Hansen A, Steffensen R, Meinertz H, et al: Association of mutations in the apolipoprotein B gene with hypercholesterolemia and the risk of ischemic heart disease. N Engl J Med 338:1577–1584, 1998

Disorders of Triglyceride Metabolism

Heaney AP, Sharer N, Rameh B, et al: Prevention of recurrent pancreatitis in familial lipoprotein lipase deficiency with high-dose antioxidant therapy. J Clin Endocrinol Metab 84:1203–1205, 1999

Mahley RW, Rall SC Jr: Type III hyperlipoproteinemia (dysbetalipoproteinemia): the role of apolipoprotein E in normal and abnormal lipoprotein metabolism. In: Scriver CR, Beaudet AL, Sly WS, Valle D, eds: The Metabolic Basis of Inherited Disease, 7th ed. New York, McGraw-Hill, 1995, p1953–1980

Polonsky SM, Bellet PS, Sprecher DL: Primary hyperlipidemia in a pediatric population: classification and effect of dietary treatment. Pediatrics 91:92–96, 1993

Rouis M, Dugi KA, Previato L, et al: Therapeutic response to medium-chain triglycerides and omega-3 fatty acids in a patient with the familial chylomicronemia syndrome. Arterioscler Thromb Vasc Biol 17:1400–1406, 1997

Metabolic Disorders with Normolipidemia

Bjorkhem I, Boberg KM: Inborn errors in bile acid biosynthesis and storage of sterols other than cholesterol. In: Scriver CR, Beaudet AL, Sly WS, Valle D, eds: The Metabolic Basis of Inherited Disease, 7th ed. New York, McGraw-Hill, 1995, p.2073–2102

Srinivasan SR, Dahlen GH, Jarpa RA, et al: Racial (black-white) differences in serum lipoprotein (a) distribution and its relation to parental myocardial infarction in children. Bogalusa Heart Study. Circulation 84:160–167, 1991

Hypolipoproteinemia

Klein HG, Lohse P, Duverger N, et al: Two different allelic mutations in the lecithin:cholesterol acyltransferase (LCAT) gene resulting in classic LCAT deficiency: LCAT (tyr^{83}/ra stop) and LCAT (tyr^{156}/ra asn). J Lipid Res 34:49–56, 1993

Klein HG, Santamarina-Fojo S, Duverger N, et al: Fish-eye syndrome: a molecular defect in the lecithin-cholesterol acyltransferase (LCAT) gene associated with normal alpha-LCAT-specific activity. Implications for classification and prognosis. J Clin Invest 92:479–485, 1993

Linton MF, Farese RV Jr, Young SG: Familial hypobetalipoproteinemia. J Lipid Res 34:521–541, 1993

Pessah M, Benlian P, Beucler I, et al: Anderson's disease: genetic exclusion of the apolipoprotein-B gene in two families. J Clin Invest 87:367–370, 1991.

Rader DJ, Brewer HB Jr: Abetalipoproteinemia. New insights into lipoprotein assembly and vitamin E metabolism from a rare genetic disease. JAMA 270:865–869, 1993

Remaley AT, Rust S, Rosier M, et al: Human ATP-binding cassette transporter 1 (ABC1): genomic organization and identification of the genetic defect in the original Tangier disease kindred. Proc Natl Acad Sci USA 96(22):12685–12690, 1999

Wang J, Hegele RJ: Microsomal triglyceride transfer protein (MTP) gene mutations in Canadian subjects with abetalipoproteinemia. Hum Mutat 15(3):294–295, 2000

CLINICAL GENETICS AND DYSMORPHOLOGY

John C. Carey and Michael J. Bamshad

10.1 THE GENETIC APPROACH TO DISORDERS OF CHILDREN

Michael J. Bamshad and Lynn B. Jorde

Genetic disorders and birth defects are sometimes perceived as being so uncommon that the general pediatrician will seldom encounter them. However, each day more than 400 babies with birth defects are born in the United States, and one of every five infant deaths is caused by these disorders. Virtually every medical condition, except for some cases of trauma, has a genetic component. Rapid advances in our knowledge of the structure and function of the human genome and an emerging understanding of the effects of various genetic changes (ie, mutations) on human disease are also rapidly transforming the practice of medicine (see Chap. 8).

Comprehensive databases of factual information about the identification of new disease genes, genotype-phenotype correlation, and the availability of genetic testing are becoming increasingly available online and in published review articles. Thus each of the following sections seeks to emphasize important fundamental concepts while providing paradigmatic examples.

Traditionally, various human conditions (eg, skin color, intelligence) and disorders (eg, phenylketonuria, achondroplasia) have been divided into those that are *genetic* versus those that are *nongenetic*, the latter usually referring to disorders "determined" by the environment (eg, infectious diseases, teratogens). However, this dichotomy separating gene and environment is largely artificial, and the distinction between the two has become increasingly blurred over the last decade. Disorders caused by mutations in a single gene (eg, cystic fibrosis, sickle-cell disease) can be heavily influenced by the environment, and diseases caused by the environment (eg, AIDS secondary to infection with HIV-1) can be substantially modified by the presence of certain polymorphisms. In other words, most diseases can be considered genetic and environmental, and some diseases are more strongly influenced by genes, whereas others are more strongly influenced by the environment.

Whether defined narrowly or broadly, genetic disorders and birth defects contribute substantially to morbidity and mortality in pediatric patients. For example, the percentage of deaths attributable to genetic disease in hospitals in the United Kingdom has risen from 16.5% in 1914 to 50% in 1976. Birth defects are also the leading cause of death in infancy (>20%) in the United States, and cardiovascular malformations are the leading cause of premature mortality from congenital anomalies. This reflects a better understanding of the etiology of pediatric diseases as well as the substantial reduction in infectious disease and perinatal mortality during the twentieth century. Recent population-based studies suggest that birth defects and genetic disorders account for about 10% of hospitalizations and about 30% of all hospitalization charges. Approximately 7% of pediatric admissions are for single-gene and chromosomal disorders, and another 15 to 20% for congenital malformations of different types. Moreover, the deaths of about 35% of children who die in a children's hospital are caused by a genetic condition and/or birth defect. Recent advances in therapeutics have substantially prolonged the survival of children with birth defects and/or genetic diseases, challenging practitioners to care for older children and young adults with genetic disorders.

CLASSIFICATION OF GENETIC DISORDERS

Classifications of genetic disorders depend, in part, on the delineation of a phenotypic trait (eg, mental retardation, craniosynostosis) and the judgment of whether this trait varies substantially from a "normal" trait. Whether a trait should be considered normal or abnormal (eg, a midline abdominal aorta, short digits) is not always clear, and the decision may depend, in part, on findings in other family members. Genetic disorders can be broadly classified into several major groups: chromosome disorders, single-gene disorders, multifactorial disorders, and disorders with nontraditional mechanisms of expression and inheritance.

Chromosome disorders result from abnormalities of chromosome number (ie, aneuploidy) and/or structure. These abnormalities include duplications, deletions, rearrangements, extra chromosomes (trisomy), and missing chromosomes (monosomy). Most chromosome disorders arise de novo and are not transmissible. However, some chromosome disorders are heritable because they are carried by an unaffected parent in a state that does not cause disease (eg, balanced rearrangements) but can be transmitted to an offspring to produce a state that does cause disease (unbalanced rearrangement). Most conceptions with chromosome abnormalities are spontaneously terminated early in gestation, and chromosome abnormalities are the leading known cause of pregnancy loss. Most individuals with chromosome disorders have major and/or minor malformations, variable degrees of mental retardation, and/or growth deficiency.

Disorders in which single genes have been altered are called *monogenic conditions*. Single-gene disorders can be transmitted from parent to offspring in autosomal-dominant or autosomal-recessive patterns and thus are sometimes known as *mendelian* conditions. Single-gene disorders can also be produced by new mutations in a single individual that are appearing for the first time in a family; the mutation has arisen de novo in the affected family member. Copies of genes that have different sequences are referred to as *alleles*. A gene's location on a chromosome is termed a *locus*. The four modes of inheritance of single-gene disorders are autosomal-recessive, in which both copies of a gene at a single locus on an autosome (nonsex chromosome) are altered; autosomal-dominant, in which only one allele of a gene at a single locus on an autosome is altered; X-linked recessive, in which one allele of a gene at a locus on the X chromosome is altered in affected males and both alleles of a gene at a locus on the X chromosome are altered in affected females; and X-linked dominant, in which one allele of a gene at a locus on the X chromosome is altered in affected males and females. Y-linked inheritance is uncommon for genetic disorders.

Substantial progress has been made toward identifying the genes that cause single-gene disorders. However, these conditions represent only a small fraction of the total burden of genetic disease. Most birth defects are not caused by alterations of a single gene or chromosome, and many common pediatric disorders are influenced by different combinations of alleles at various loci. Traits in which variation is caused by the effects of many different genes are called *polygenic*. If the variation of a polygenic trait is also affected by nongenetic factors (eg, environmental variables), the terms *multifactorial* or *complex* are often used to describe the trait. In contrast to single-gene disorders, multifactorial traits are not transmitted in mendelian patterns. The identification of the genetic and environmental determinants of multifactorial traits is a major objective of future genetic research.

Some genetic disorders do not segregate in the patterns expected of single-gene conditions or multifactorial traits and are transmitted from parent to offspring in nontraditional patterns of inheritance. Disorders exhibiting nontraditional patterns of inheritance include those caused by mutations in the mitochondrial genome, uniparental disomy (two alleles from the same locus inherited from one parent instead of both parents), and gene duplication. The expression of some conditions is influenced substantially by whether the altered allele is transmitted to a child by the mother or father, a so-called parent-of-origin effect. Some genetic conditions exhibit a nontraditional pattern of inheritance as a consequence of this parent-of-origin effect and are relatively uncommon.

KEY PRINCIPLES IN HUMAN GENETICS

The terms *congenital, hereditary,* and *familial* are not synonymous. Conditions that are present at birth are referred to as *congenital* conditions, whether genetic conditions or not. For example, infection with cytomegalovirus, clubfeet caused by oligohydramnios, and trisomy 21 are all congenital conditions. However, only trisomy 21 is clearly a genetic condition, and none of these conditions are usually hereditary.

The term *hereditary* defines conditions that can be transmitted from parent to offspring. All hereditary conditions are genetic conditions, but not all genetic conditions are hereditary (eg, trisomy 21). Conditions that appear to cluster within families are frequently called *familial* conditions and may include nongenetic conditions (eg, rotaviral or streptococcal infections) as well as genetic conditions. Nevertheless, although all hereditary conditions can be familial, not all genetic conditions are familial (eg, trisomy 21). Distinguishing which term most appropriately defines a condition facilitates diagnosis, management, and counseling of families about the risk of recurrence of a condition.

The probability that an individual who possesses a disease-related genotype (an individual's allelic constitution at a single locus is called a *genotype*) exhibits the disease phenotype is called *penetrance*. When this probability is less than 1, the disease is said to

exhibit *reduced* (or *incomplete*) penetrance. Penetrance levels are usually estimated by examining a large number of families and determining what proportion of the obligate carriers (ie, those individuals who have an affected parent and an affected child and thus must be carriers of the altered gene) or obligate homozygotes (in the case of autosomal-recessive disorders) develop the disease phenotype. Retinoblastoma is a good example of a genetic condition in which reduced penetrance is observed. Family studies have demonstrated that about 10% of obligate carriers of a mutation in the retinoblastoma susceptibility gene do not develop a retinoblastoma. The penetrance of the condition is thus about 90%.

Individuals with the same genetic condition or even the same genotype can have substantially different phenotypes. This is called *variable expressivity*. For example, within the same kindred, one sibling with neurofibromatosis type 1 (NF1) may have café-au-lait spots, axillary freckling, and sphenoid wing dysplasia, and another sibling with NF1 has café-au-lait spots, a plexiform neurofibroma, and pseudarthrosis of the tibia. Although each sibling has the same genotype, the expression of the NF1 phenotype is different between them.

Variable expressivity may be explained by the influence of other genes (ie, modifying genes), environmental factors (eg, earlier palliative intervention), or random variation. Variable expressivity among families is sometimes related to the presence of different genotypes. The causation of a disease phenotype by a variety of different genotypes at the same locus is called *allelic heterogeneity*. A potentially powerful strategy to provide affected individuals with better anticipatory guidance is to estimate the correlation between genotypes and specific phenotypic characteristics (genotype-phenotype correlation studies). The compilation of findings from many individuals with a genetic condition defines the phenotypic spectrum of a disorder. Although not every affected individual will have the same findings, variable expressivity is often confused with reduced penetrance. The absence of a disease phenotype in an obligate carrier (ie, reduced penetrance) is not considered variable expression of the condition.

Genes that have more than one discernible effect on the phenotype are said to be *pleiotropic*. A good example of a gene that has pleiotropic effects is the *cystic fibrosis transmembrane regulator* (*CFTR*). *CFTR* encodes a protein that forms cyclic-AMP–regulated chloride ion channels that span the cell membrane of specialized epithelial cells such as those that line the lungs and bowel. Mutations in *CFTR* result in abnormalities of the lungs, pancreas, and sweat glands. Other examples of genetic conditions that result from mutations in genes with pleiotropic effects include Marfan syndrome (characterized by ocular, cardiovascular, and skeletal defects) and osteogenesis imperfecta, in which the bones, teeth, and sclerae are affected. Thus pleiotropy can be caused by genes whose products play similar roles in different tissues and organs. Pleiotropy can also be caused by genes whose protein products play varied roles in different developmental programs. For example, individuals with campomelic dysplasia have a skeletal dysplasia that is sometimes accompanied by sex reversal. Campomelic dysplasia is caused by mutations in a gene called *SRY-related HMG-BOX 9* (*SOX9*), which plays an important regulatory role in skeletal development and sexual differentiation.

Some genetic conditions seem to display an earlier age of onset and/or more severe expression in the more recent generations of a pedigree, called *anticipation*. Some investigators had proposed that anticipation was an artifact of better observation and diagnostic tools available to the contemporary clinician: a disorder previously diagnosed at age 60 might now be diagnosed at age 40. Within the last 10 years, it has been demonstrated that for some disorders, anticipation has a biological basis. One of the best examples of anticipation comes from studies of myotonic dystrophy (DM), the most common muscular dystrophy that affects adults. Myotonic dystrophy is characterized by progressive deterioration of skeletal muscle, cardiomyopathy, testicular atrophy, and cataracts and is caused by mutations in a gene on chromosome 19 that encodes a protein kinase. Analysis of this gene has demonstrated that myotonic dystrophy is caused by the expansion of a CTG repeat in the 3′ untranslated region of the gene (ie, a region transcribed into mRNA but not translated into protein). Unaffected individuals have 5 to 30 copies of the repeat, mildly affected individuals may have 50 to 100 copies of the repeat, and severely affected individuals may have 100 to more than several thousand repeats. The number of repeats is positively correlated with the severity of the disease. Furthermore, the number of repeats often increases with succeeding generations, which have more severe disease compared to preceding generations.

MONOGENIC CONDITIONS: SINGLE-GENE DISORDERS

Autosomal-Dominant Disorders

For autosomal-dominant conditions, the presence of only one copy of an altered allele at a locus is sufficient to produce a disease phenotype. Genetic disorders that are inherited in an autosomal-dominant pattern are the most common single-gene disorders described in humans. Individually, however, each autosomal-dominant disorder is relatively uncommon. Thus, most affected offspring are produced from the mating of an affected parent and an unaffected parent or may suffer from a de novo mutation. A parent affected with an autosomal-dominant disorder can transmit either the normal or altered allele to his or her offspring. Each of these events has a probability of .5. Thus, on average, half of the children will be heterozygous for the altered allele and express the disease, and half will be homozygous for a normal allele. Matings between individuals affected by the same autosomal-dominant disorder are rare.

An idealized pedigree for autosomal-dominant inheritance (Fig. 10-1) illustrates several important characteristics: First, the two sexes exhibit the trait in approximately equal proportions, and males and females are equally likely to transmit the trait. Second, no generation is skipped. Every individual with the trait has an affected parent. Third, father-to-son transmission is observed. Although father-to-son transmission is not required to establish autosomal-dominant inheritance, its presence excludes some other modes of inheritance (eg, X-linked and mitochondrial). Last, an affected individual transmits the trait to half of her or his offspring, on average.

De novo mutations are an important cause of autosomal-dominant conditions. For autosomal-dominant conditions that are lethal in prereproductive age (eg, thanatophoric dysplasia), de novo mutations are the most common cause of the disorder. For some autosomal-dominant conditions (eg, achondroplasia, Marfan syndrome) the age of the father and the likelihood of transmitting a new mutation to his offspring are positively correlated. Sometimes, clearly unaffected parents have more than one child affected with an autosomal-dominant disorder. Recent studies have demonstrated that one of the parents in such families has two or more different cell lines in his or her germ cells (cells that produce sperm or eggs)—with at least one cell line containing an altered allele.

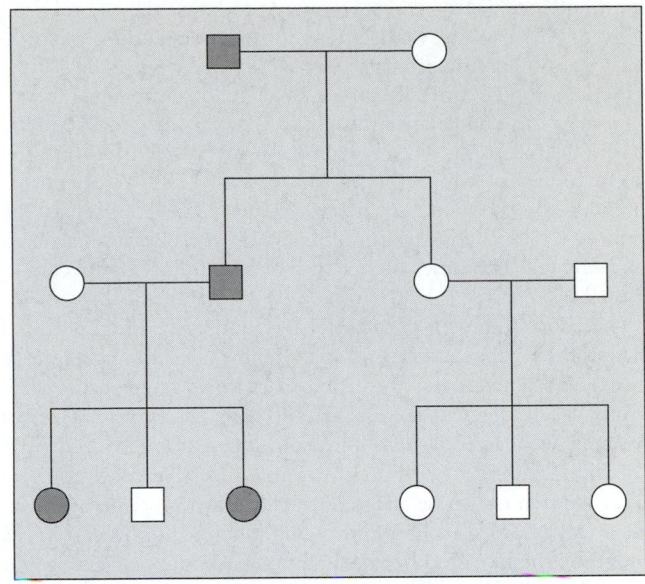

FIGURE 10-1   A pedigree illustrating an autosomal-dominant disorder. Affected individuals are represented by shading. Note the male-to-male transmission and that no generation is skipped.

This phenomenon is called *germ-line mosaicism*. Germ-line mosaicism appears to be much more common for some disorders (eg, osteogenesis imperfecta) and is another cause of autosomal-dominant conditions that are lethal in prereproductive age. Two or more cell lines can also be found in the somatic cells of an individual (somatic mosaicism). Individuals with somatic mosaicism may have all the same characteristics found in affected individuals, exhibit abnormalities limited to only tissues containing the mutant cell line, or appear unaffected.

Autosomal-Recessive Disorders

For autosomal-recessive conditions, the presence of two copies of an altered allele at a locus is required to produce a disease phenotype. Genetic disorders that are inherited in an autosomal-recessive pattern are less common than autosomal-dominant disorders in most populations. However, heterozygous carriers for recessive conditions are much more common than affected homozygotes. Thus the parents of individuals affected with autosomal-recessive conditions are usually heterozygous carriers. For example, the prevalence of cystic fibrosis is approximately 1 in 2500 in northern European populations. The Hardy-Weinberg law states that population frequencies of genotypes can be predicted on the basis of gene frequencies in a randomly mating population (random mating is also referred to as *panmixia*). Suppose that at a two-allele locus the frequency p of an allele A is 0.70. Then 70% of the sperm and egg cells in a population have this allele. Because the sum of allele frequencies at a locus must equal 1, the frequency q of the allele a is equal to $1 - p = q$ or $1.0 - 0.7 = 0.3$. Under panmixia the probability that a sperm carrying allele A unites with an egg carrying allele A is $p \times p = p^2$ or $0.7 \times 0.7 = 0.49$ (multiplication rule). This is the probability of producing an offspring with the AA genotype. The probability of producing an offspring with the aa genotype is $q \times q = q^2$ or $0.3 \times 0.3 = 0.09$.

Heterozygotes can be produced two different ways. A sperm carrying allele A can unite with an egg carrying allele a, or a sperm carrying allele a can unite with an egg carrying allele A. Thus, the frequency with which this occurs is equal to the product of the gene frequencies, $p \times q$. Since we want to know the overall probability of either event, we use the addition rule, adding the probabilities to obtain a heterozygote frequency of $pq + pq = 2pq$. Overall the genotype frequencies of a two-allele locus are equal to $p^2 + 2pq + q^2 = 1$. This relationship indicates that the gene frequency (q) for alleles causing CF is equal to $q^{1/2}$ or $(1/2500)^{1/2}$ or $1/50$. The frequency of normal alleles, p, is $(2499/2500)^{1/2}$ or approximately 1. The frequency of heterozygotes ($2pq$) is equal to $2(1)(1/50) = 1/25$. Thus, the frequency of heterozygous carriers is approximately 100 times higher than the frequency of affected individuals.

The probabilities of two carriers producing children with two normal alleles (homozygous normal), a normal allele and a disease-causing allele (heterozygous carriers), or two disease-causing alleles (homozygous affected) are .25, .5, and .25, respectively. Thus, on average, one-quarter of the children produced by heterozygous carriers will be affected with an autosomal-recessive condition. If a child is known not to be affected, the likelihood that he or she is a carrier is 2 of 3, ie, likelihood of being a heterozygous carrier (.5) divided by the likelihood of being a heterozygous carrier (.5) plus the likelihood of being homozygous normal (.25).

An idealized pedigree for autosomal-recessive inheritance (Fig. 10-2) illustrates several important characteristics: First, autosomal-recessive disorders are usually observed in one or more siblings but are not usually found in other generations. Second, similar to autosomal-dominant conditions, males and females are affected in equal proportions, and males and females are equally likely to transmit the disease-causing mutation. Third, on average about 25% of the offspring of two heterozygous carriers will be affected. Last, consanguinity is observed more often in pedigrees of autosomal-recessive disorders compared to autosomal-dominant conditions. *Consanguinity* refers to the mating of related individuals, who are more likely to share the identical disease-causing alleles of a locus because of descent from a common ancestor.

X-Linked Disorders

Genes that are located on the X or Y chromosome are known as sex-linked genes. The Y chromosome has relatively few genes and is the smallest of the human chromosomes, about 70 megabases (Mb). One important gene on the Y chromosome is called the *sex-determining region Y (SRY)* gene. Mutations of *SRY* can result in

individuals with normal external female genitalia and gonadal dysgenesis (ie, abnormal formation of the gonads). However, this is an uncommon cause of abnormalities of sexual differentiation in humans.

In contrast to the Y chromosome, the X chromosome is almost twice as large (about 160 Mb) and contains thousands of genes that play a variety of roles during development and adult life. A number of well-known pediatric genetic conditions are caused by alterations of X-linked genes, including hemophilia A, Duchenne and Becker muscular dystrophy, red-green color blindness, ocular albinism with neurosensory hearing loss, anhidrotic ectodermal dysplasia, and ornithine transcarbamoylase deficiency. In addition, genes causing more than 60 phenotypes associated with mental retardation (eg, fragile X syndrome) have been mapped to the X chromosome, although genes have been cloned for only a handful of these conditions.

Females have two copies and males one copy of the X chromosome. Yet the quality of product encoded by most X-linked genes does not differ between males and females. The equalization of X-linked gene products is called *dosage compensation* and is produced by the inactivation of one of the X chromosomes early in female embryonic development. This inactivation process is random, so the maternally and paternally derived X chromosomes will each be inactive in about half of the embryo's cells. Once an X chromosome is inactivated, the same X chromosome remains inactivated in all descendants of the cell. Thus, all normal females have at least two populations of cells (somatic mosaicism), one containing a paternally derived active X chromosome and the other containing a maternally derived active X chromosome, which becomes clearly evident if the maternally and paternally derived X chromosomes produce different products. For example, the retinas of women who are carriers for X-linked ocular albinism demonstrate alternating patches of pigmented and nonpigmented cells corresponding respectively to cells in which the disease-bearing X chromosome (nonpigmented) or the normal X chromosome (pigmented) has been inactivated.

Inactivation of the X chromosome takes place approximately 2 weeks after fertilization, begins in a region of the X chromosome called the *inactivation center,* and subsequently spreads along the chromosome. The X inactivation center contains at least one gene required for inactivation, *XIST. XIST* is transcribed only from the

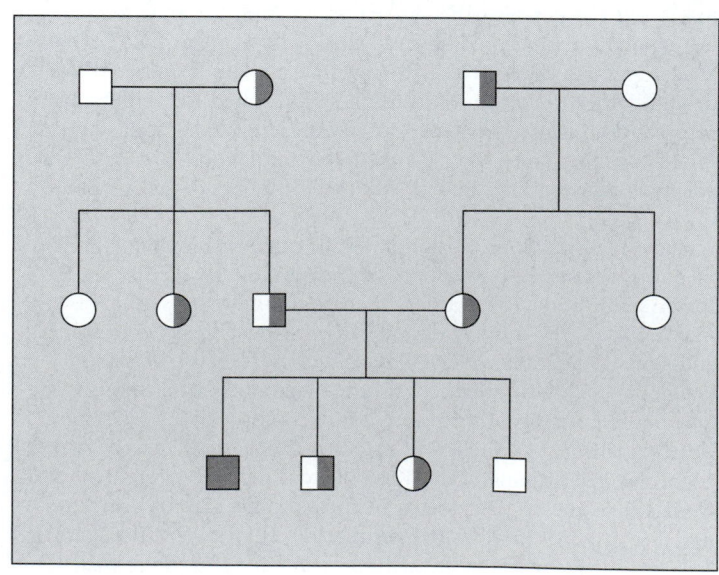

FIGURE 10-2   A pedigree illustrating the inheritance pattern of an autosomal recessive disorder. Affected individuals are represented by shading and heterozygotes by partial shading.

inactive X chromosome, but its mRNA never leaves the nucleus and is not translated into protein. The mRNA product of *XIST* appears to coat the portions of the X chromosome that are subsequently inactivated. Maintenance of inactivation appears to depend on methylation of CG dinucleotide repeats that are commonly found in the 5′ (upstream) regions of genes. Inactivation of the X chromosome is incomplete, and genes in several regions continue to be transcribed from the inactivated X chromosome. Some of these genes have transcribed homologues on the Y chromosome, and thus dosage compensation is maintained by their activation on both X chromosomes in females.

The inheritance patterns of X-linked conditions differ substantially from the inheritance patterns of autosomal disorders. Females can be homozygous for a disease allele at a given locus, heterozygous for a disease allele and a normal allele, or homozygous for a normal allele at a locus. Males have only one X chromosome and are considered hemizygous (*hemi* is half) for an allele at a locus on the X chromosome. If a male inherits the altered allele for a recessive disorder, he will be affected with the condition because the Y chromosome does not carry a normal allele that might compensate for the effects of the disease gene. In contrast, X-linked dominant disorders can cause the disease condition in either males or females because the presence of only one copy of an altered allele is sufficient for disease expression.

For X-linked recessive disorders, the frequency of the disease condition in males is equal to the gene frequency q. This is because all males with the altered gene have the disease condition. Because females need two copies of the altered allele to manifest the condition, the frequency of the disease condition is q^2. For example, hemophilia A has a prevalence of approximately 1/10,000 males ($q = 0.0001$). Thus, affected females will be observed in q^2 ($q^2 = 0.00000001$) or 1/100,000,000 individuals. Consequently, X-linked recessive disorders are likely to be found much more frequently in males than females.

A pedigree (Fig. 10-3) illustrates some of the important characteristics of an X-linked recessive trait. First, only females are able transmit the disorder to their sons; in other words, there is no male-to-male transmission for X-linked recessive conditions. Second, sibships containing only carrier females (unaffected) appear as "skipped generations." In these generations, carrier females appear unaffected, and the X chromosome transmitted to males by their mother contains a normal allele. An affected father transmits the disease allele to all his daughters, who in turn transmit it to half of their sons on average.

At least three mechanisms account for some female carriers of X-linked recessive disorders manifesting some of or all the characteristics of the condition. First, because inactivation of the X chromosome is a random process within each cell, sometimes a much higher proportion of X chromosomes bearing a normal allele is inactivated than X chromosomes carrying a disease allele. These affected carrier females are known as *manifesting heterozygotes*. For many disorders, manifesting heterozygotes have a milder form of the condition compared to affected males. For example, approximately 5% of women carrying an allele for hemophilia A have factor VIII levels low enough to exhibit a mild form of the disease. Second, some women have only a single X chromosome (ie, Turner syndrome, see below) and subsequently will manifest X-linked recessive conditions for which they would have otherwise been carriers. Last, chromosomal aberrations such as deletions or rearrangements involving the X chromosome and an autosome can also result in affected females. X chromosome rearrangements involving the mutation-containing X chromosome cause disease in females because the normal X chromosome will be preferentially inactivated to avoid inactivating the autosome attached to the other X chromosome. These events are relatively rare.

NONTRADITIONAL MECHANISMS OF DISEASE

Some single-gene conditions are caused by mechanisms that are transmitted in patterns that are distinct from those of autosomal and sex-linked conditions. Many of these conditions are relatively uncommon. Nevertheless, these nontraditional mechanisms of disease often explain cases that are otherwise inconsistent with the current state of knowledge of genetic disorders. For example, the expression of most traits is independent of the parent of origin of the causative allele. Recently, however, it has become apparent that this is not always true. The most striking example to date is caused

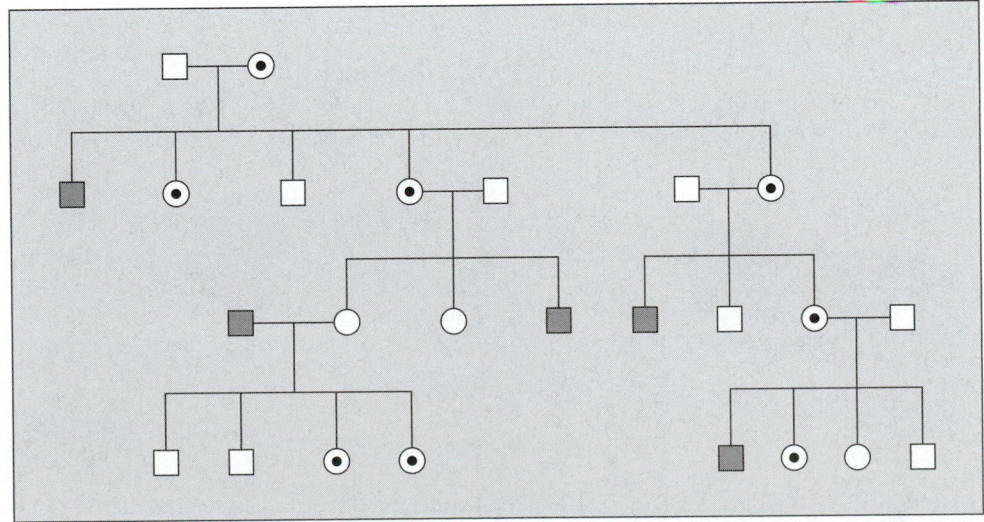

FIGURE 10-3   A pedigree showing the inheritance of an X-linked recessive condition. Solid symbols represent affected individuals, and dotted symbols represent heterozygous carriers. Only females can transmit the disorder to their sons. Fathers transmit trait to all daughters.

by a deletion of 2 to 4 Mb of chromosome 15. When this deletion is inherited from the father, the offspring is born with Prader-Willi syndrome: severe neonatal hypotonia, obesity, small hands and feet, and an unusual behavioral profile including mental retardation (Fig. 10-4). In contrast, when the deletion is inherited from the mother, the offspring manifests Angelman syndrome, appearing normal at birth but subsequently developing seizures, mental retardation, ataxia, and a characteristic posture.

Within the 2-4 Mb region of chromosome 15 that is deleted in patients with either Prader-Willi or Angelman syndrome lie several genes that are transcriptionally active on one of the chromosomes inherited from the mother or father but not both (ie, they are active on only one chromosome). If these genes are deleted, the result is a complete loss of the encoded product and a disease condition. If all of the paternally active genes are lost, the offspring has Prader-Willi syndrome (Fig. 10-5). Angelman results from the deletion of a maternally active gene called *ubiquitin-protein ligase E3A (UBE3A)* that is involved in the degradation of proteins within the brain (Fig. 10-5). The differential activation of genes contingent on whether they are maternally or paternally transmitted is called *genomic imprinting.*

Approximately 70% of cases of Angelman or Prader-Willi syndrome are caused by chromosome deletions. However, several additional mechanisms may also cause these disorders. One of these is the inheritance of both copies of a chromosome, in part or the whole chromosome, from only one parent, called *uniparental disomy.* Thus, if both copies of the maternal chromosome 15 are inherited, the resulting offspring lacks the paternally active genes and develops Prader-Willi syndrome. Conversely, uniparental disomy of paternal chromosome 15 causes Angelman syndrome. Uniparental disomy also has been found to be responsible for some cases of Beckwith-Wiedemann syndrome. Uniparental disomy has been re-

ported for most human chromosomes, although the overall clinical significance of this finding is unclear.

Other cases that have been difficult to explain until recently include the expression of autosomal-recessive conditions (eg, cystic fibrosis) in the offspring of matings between a carrier parent (ie, heterozygous for a disease allele and a normal allele) and an unaffected parent homozygous for two normal alleles. Using molecular markers that can identify specifically each of the four parental chromosomes, it was found that both copies of the chromosome bearing a disease allele were identical and inherited from the heterozygous parent (uniparental isodisomy). The proportion of genetic conditions caused by this type of abnormality is unknown but likely to be low.

The majority of genetic conditions are caused by abnormalities of the nuclear genome. Nevertheless, a growing number of conditions are caused by defects of the only genetic material existing outside of the nucleus, that of the mitochondria. In contrast to the nuclear genome, which is *diploid* (two copies of each gene), the mitochondrial genome contains only one copy of each gene and is thus *haploid.* Because of the unique properties of mitochondria, these disorders exhibit a characteristic pattern of inheritance and wide phenotypic variability. Each of the 100 to 100,000 mitochondria within a cell contains at least several copies of a 16,569-bp genome in the mitochondrial matrix, and each mtDNA molecule is identical. The state in which all copies of mtDNA are identical is called *homoplasmy.* The mtDNA molecule encodes 13 polypeptides that are components of the oxidative phosphorylation (OXPHOS) system (another approximately 90 components are encoded by the nuclear genome), 2 ribosomal RNAs, and 22 transfer RNAs. Replication and transcription of mtDNA take place within the mitochondria and are facilitated by nuclear-encoded proteins. In humans, mitochondria in the midpiece of the sperm may enter

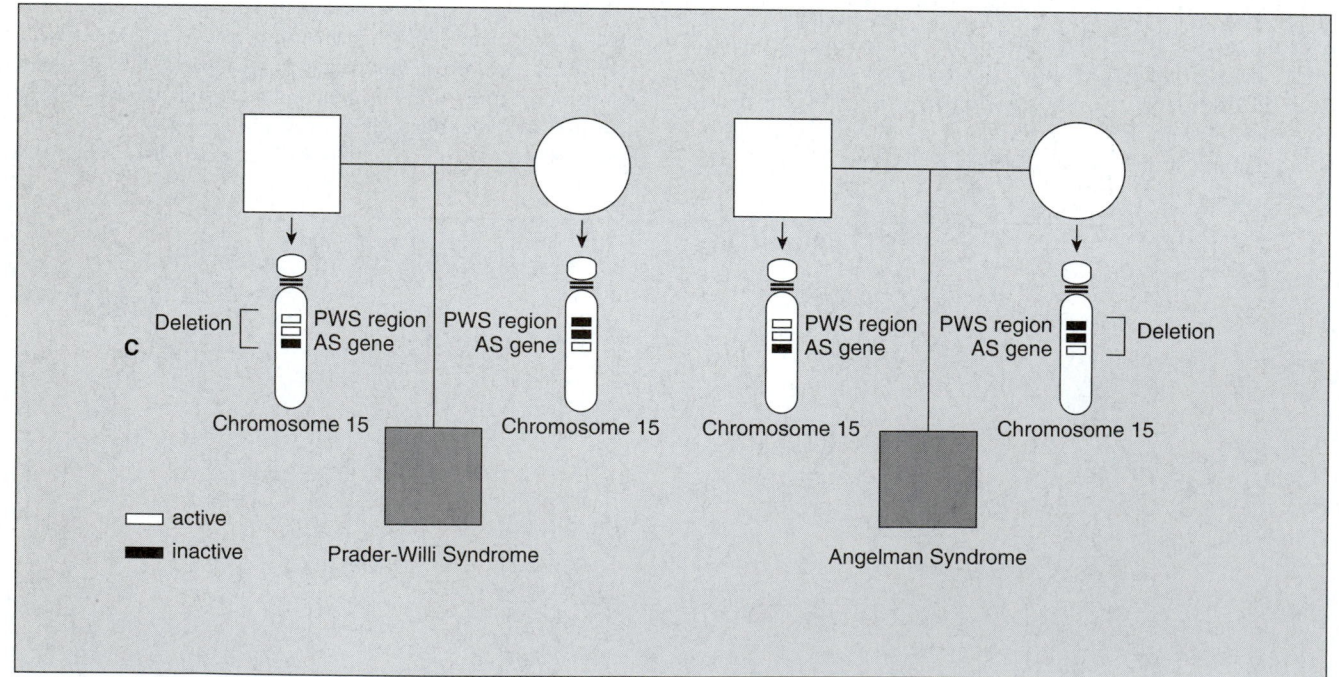

FIGURE 10-4 Pedigrees illustrate the inheritance pattern of the chromosome 15 deletion and the activation status of genes in the critical region. Inheritance of the deletion from the father produces Prader-Willi syndrome, and inheritance of the deletion from the mother produces Angelman syndrome. *(Modified from Jorde LB, Carey JC, Bamshad MJ, White RL: Medical Genetics. St. Louis, Mosby, 2000.)*

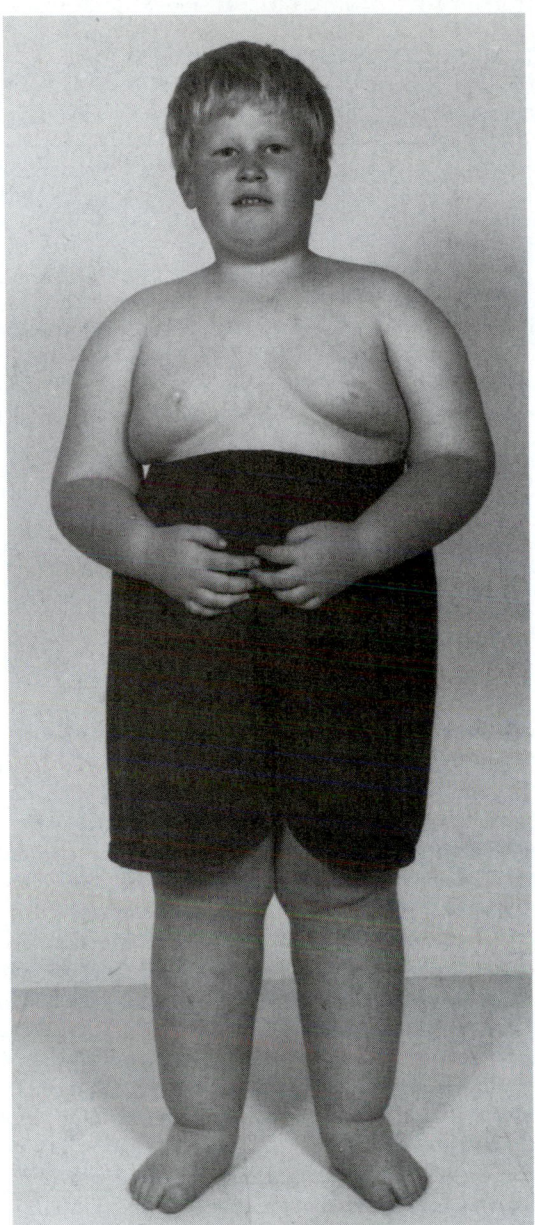 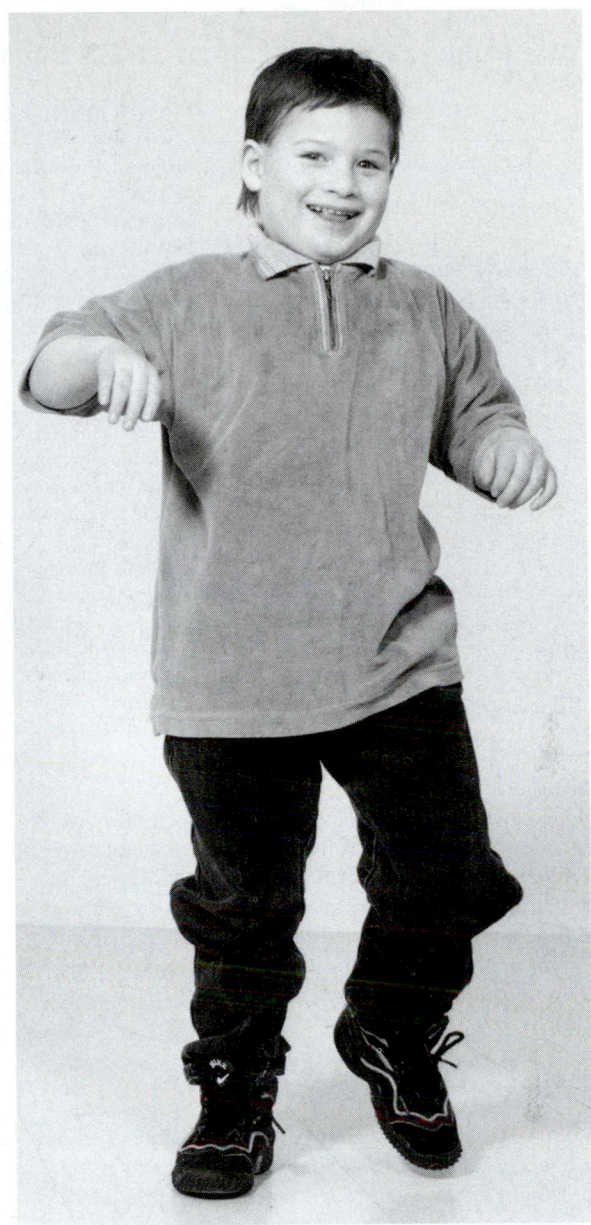

FIGURE 10-5   Illustration of the effect of imprinting on chromosome 15. A. Inheritance of the deletion from the father produces Prader-Willi syndrome (truncal obesity, small hands and feet, developmental delay). B. Inheritance of the deletion from the mother produces Angelman syndrome (seizures, developmental delay, characteristic gait). *(From Jorde LB, Carey JC, Bamshad MJ, White RL: Medical Genetics. St. Louis, Mosby, 2000.)*

the egg, but the mtDNA from the sperm rarely, if ever, persists in the embryo. Thus all the mitochondria of the offspring are descendants of those located within the cytoplasm of the egg. Consequently, the inheritance of mtDNA is exclusively maternal.

Because there is more than one copy of mtDNA within each mitochondrion, a new mutation in an mtDNA molecule will result in the emergence of two different mtDNA populations within a mitochondrion. The state of having two or more different populations of mtDNA molecules is called *heteroplasmy*. As cells divide and the mitochondria proliferate, the proportion of mutant mtDNA molecules within a cell and the proportion of cells in a tissue or organ containing mitochondria with mutant mtDNA molecules will change. Mutant mtDNA diminish the efficiency of OXPHOS metabolism and cause cells to die and tissues and organs to

deteriorate prematurely. A threshold of mutant mtDNA molecules within a mitochondrion (typically 85%) must be exceeded before a biochemical defect disrupts the normal function of the OXPHOS system. Thus, the larger the proportion of mutant mtDNA molecules within a cell or tissue, the higher the likelihood of expressing a disease phenotype or the greater the severity of disease.

Mitochondrial disorders are commonly classified according to the type of mutation that causes them or their clinical presentation (Table 10-1). In general, mutations in the mtDNA molecule are either rearrangements (ie, deletions and duplications) or point mutations (ie, missense or nonsense mutations). Many mtDNA disorders present with nonspecific neurologic findings such as coma, seizures, and ataxia. In the neonatal period, mitochondrial disorders commonly present with metabolic encephalopathy, cardiac or

TABLE 10-1

GENETIC DISORDERS CAUSED BY MUTATIONS IN THE MITOCHONDRIAL GENOME

DISORDER	MAJOR MANIFESTATIONS	ONSET	MUTATION TYPE
Myoclonic epilepsy and red ragged fibers (MERRF)	Progressive myoclonic epilepsy Myopathy Slowly progressive dementia Hearing loss	Late childhood to adult	Point mutations in tRNA^{Lys}
Mitochondrial encephalopathy, stroke-like episodes, and lactic acidosis (MELAS)	Progressive myopathy Stroke-like episodes	Toddlers to teenagers	Point mutations in t-RNA^{Leu}
Leber hereditary optic neuropathy (LHON)	Progressive loss of visual acuity	Teenagers to young adults	Missense mutations in *ND1, ND4, ND6, COI, CYTB*
Leigh disease	Basal ganglia defects Hypotonia, myopathy Optic atrophy, ophthalmoplegia	Infants to toddlers	Point mutations in ATP6
Kearns-Sayre syndrome (KSS)	Ophthalmoplegia Retinitis pigmentosa Myopathy Cardiac conduction defects	Before 20 years old	Predominantly deletions
Chronic progressive external ophthalmoplegia (CPEO)	Same as Kearns-Sayre syndrome	After 20 years old	Predominantly deletions
Pearson syndrome	Anemia, neutropenia Pancreatic dysfunction Myopathy	Infants	Deletions

ND = complex 1 subunit; ATP6 = ATPase 6 subunit a; COI = cytochrome oxidase subunit 1; CYTB = cytochrome oxidase subunit b

hepatic failure, and/or lactic acidemia. Although uncommon, mitochondrial disorders account for a substantial percentage of cerebrovascular accidents in children. Most mitochondrial disorders are uncommon, but mtDNA mutations also contribute to common disorders such as deafness and diabetes mellitus. Mitochondrial mutations have also been implicated in the process of aging. However, whether these mutations are a cause or a consequence of the aging process is unclear.

MECHANISMS OF MUTATION

The identification and characterization of a disease gene are the first steps in understanding the molecular pathogenesis of a condition. Further insight is often gained by understanding the mechanism by which mutations disturb the function of a cell. Most mutations result in either a gain of function or loss of function of the encoded product.

A disease allele occasionally results in a protein product with a novel function compared to the normal product. More commonly a disease allele causes the overexpression of its product or expression of its product at an inappropriate time or place. These types of mutations are known as gain-of-function mutations and commonly result in conditions transmitted in a dominant pattern. Huntington disease, a late-onset condition characterized by progressive neurologic deterioration, is caused by a gain-of-function mutation.

Some gain-of-function mutations extend the normal function of a gene. For example, mutations in fibroblast growth factor 3, *FGFR3*, result in the uncontrolled activation of the receptor leading to enhanced inhibition of the growth of long bones (eg, the femur). Depending on the location of the mutation, this produces hypochondroplasia, achondroplasia, or thanatophoric dysplasia.

Some mutations result in the loss of 50% of the encoded product, and 50% of the product remains available (encoded by the normal allele). Often, but not exclusively, these loss-of-function mutations are observed in recessive conditions (eg, galactosemia,

Hurler syndrome). Since carriers for most recessive disorders are asymptomatic, the availability of 50% of the encoded product is often enough to prevent disease. In circumstances in which 50% of the encoded product is not sufficient to prevent disease (*haploinsufficiency*), a loss-of-function mutation can also result in dominant disorders. For example, a deletion of the gene encoding the extracellular matrix protein, elastin, results in diminished incorporation of elastin into the wall of large arteries, producing supravalvular aortic stenosis.

Another type of loss-of-function mutation results when the encoded product is not only nonfunctional, but also interferes with the activity of the normal product and is known as *dominant negative mutation*. This type of mutation is usually observed in genes that encode proteins that are components of multimeric (containing two or more protein subunits) proteins. For example, mutations in one of the collagen genes (*COL1A1*) can impair the binding of collagen subunits into a normal trimeric complex, resulting in osteogenesis imperfecta.

Over the last decade a novel type of mutation produced by an expansion of a repeated nucleotide motif has been found to cause a variety of genetic conditions. Most commonly, these disorders are associated with an expansion of a trinucleotide repeat (eg, CAG, CTG). These repeats can be located within a gene or in the 5′ or 3′ untranslated portions of a gene. One of the most notable of the genetic conditions caused by an expansion of a trinucleotide repeat is fragile X syndrome, the most common cause of inherited mental retardation in males.

Fragile X syndrome is an X-linked dominant condition with 80% penetrance in males and 30% penetrance in females. It is caused by the expansion of a CGG repeat in the 5′ untranslated region of a gene called *FMR1*. In unaffected men, there are typically 6 to 50 CGG repeats. Males who carry the disease allele but do not have fragile X syndrome are called *transmitting males*. An intermediate number of repeats (ie, 50-230), or *premutation*, is found in transmitting males and their female offspring. When these female offspring transmit the gene to their offspring, the premutation expands to a full mutation ranging up to several thousand repeats. Men with full mutations have no *FMR1* mRNA in their cells, indicating that transcription of *FMR1* has been silenced. Furthermore, premutations tend to become larger in successive generations, and larger premutations are more prone to expansion to a full mutation. These expansions do not occur when a male transmits the premutation. This explains why males with a premutation cannot transmit the disease to their daughters and why grandsons and great-grandsons of normal transmitting males are more likely to be affected with fragile X syndrome.

Expansions of trinucleotide repeats are also associated with various progressive neurodegenerative disorders, including some of the spinocerebellar ataxias, Huntington disease, and myotonic dystrophy. As discussed previously, some of these trinucleotide repeat expansions are also associated with anticipation. More recently, the expansion of a 12-bp repeat from 2 or 3 repeats to approximately 60 repeats has been discovered to cause autosomal-recessive myoclonic epilepsy.

POPULATION VARIATION, CONSANGUINITY, AND INBREEDING

The prevalence of many genetic disorders varies extensively among human populations. For example, the prevalence of cystic fibrosis varies from 1/313 in the Hutterites of Alberta, Canada, to 1/90,000 in Asians, a difference of nearly 300-fold. Although mutation is ultimately the source of all variation in the genome, different mutation rates among populations are not a sufficient explanation for wide variation in prevalence rates of genetic conditions. Varied prevalence rates are the imprints left by evolutionary forces other than mutation (ie, natural selection, genetic drift, gene flow) on disease-related variation in human populations. Explaining these patterns of disease-related genetic variation facilitates understanding the etiology and pathogenesis of genetic conditions. However, estimating disease-related genetic variation depends on understanding the distribution of total genetic variation. Over the last decade a variety of new molecular and statistical tools for estimating genetic variation have been applied widely to human populations to further explain the genetic basis of various medical conditions and traits and have provided new insights about how evolutionary forces have shaped disease-related genetic variation in contemporary populations.

Genetic drift refers to the random fluctuations in gene frequencies that occur from generation to generation as the result of sampling a limited number of gametes. As the size of the population decreases, the degree of fluctuation increases. Genes that are rare in large populations may be common in small populations or vice versa. Genetic drift can be caused by a substantial reduction in the size of a population (a *population bottleneck*) or the separation of a subset of a larger population (*founder effect*). For example, according to well-maintained historical records, the Old Order Amish in Lancaster County, Pennsylvania, were established by approximately 50 couples. Nearly half of all the reported cases of Ellis-van Creveld (EVC) syndrome (an autosomal-recessive skeletal dysplasia characterized by short stature, polydactyly, and cardiac defects) have been identified in the Amish population. The gene for EVC syndrome was recently identified, although its function remains unknown. The relatively small founding population of the Amish and their custom of marrying only within their relatively isolated community (*endogamy*) have resulted in a very high carrier frequency of the disease-causing alleles of EVC.

Natural selection alters the frequency of a trait (*disease condition*) contingent on the relative fitness of a phenotype in a given environmental context. Phenotypes with a high fitness are positively selected, and phenotypes with a low fitness are negatively selected. Traditionally, fitness has been estimated by the number of descendants produced by those who possess a given genotype or phenotype. For example, individuals who die without descendants have a fitness of zero, whereas individuals with varying numbers of offspring have higher fitness values. Diseases maintained in a population by natural selection illustrate the relationship among genes, phenotypes, and the environment. *CC chemokine receptor 5 (CCR5)* is one of the cell surface receptors used by HIV-1 to enter certain T cells and macrophages. Individuals homozygous for a 32-bp deletion in *CCR5* are relatively resistant to infection with HIV-1. However, this polymorphism appears to have arisen relatively recently, and it has achieved a high frequency only in white populations, which has led to the hypothesis that this polymorphism was positively selected in Europeans, although the selective force that is responsible remains to be identified.

Consanguinity is defined as the mating of related individuals. Although consanguinity is relatively rare in Western populations, it is common in many populations of the world. Consanguinity increases the chances that a mating couple will both carry the same disease allele. Thus, consanguineous matings are more likely to produce offspring affected with autosomal-recessive disorders.

Many studies have shown that mortality rates among the offspring of first-cousin marriages are substantially higher than in the general population. Furthermore, the prevalence of genetic disease is approximately twice as high among the offspring of first-cousin marriages. There are few data about the mating of first-degree relatives (ie, incestuous matings), although the prevalence of mental retardation, short stature, and major congenital anomalies is clearly higher.

References

Collins FS: Shattuck Lecture-Medical and Societal Consequences of the Human Genome Project. N Engl J Med 341:28–37, 1999

OMIM: Online Mendelian Inheritance of Man: http://www.ncbi.nlm.nih.gov/omim/, 2000

Scriver CR, Beaudet AL, Sly WS, Valle D, eds: The Metabolic and Molecular Bases of Inherited Disease. New York, McGraw-Hill, 1995

Scriver CR, Waters PJ: Monogenic traits are not simple: lessons from phenylketonuria. Trends Genet 15:267–272, 1999.

Sinden RR: Trinucleotide repeats: biological implications of the DNA structures associated with disease-causing triplet repeats. Am J Hum Genet 64:346–353, 1999

Wallace DC: Mitochondrial diseases in man and mouse. Science 283:1482–1488, 1999

Zielenski J: Genotype and phenotype in cystic fibrosis. Respiration 67:117–133, 2000

10.1.1   Multifactorial Inheritance

Lynn B. Jorde

Although the genetics of most single-gene disorders is now relatively well understood, these disorders account for a relatively small proportion of the total disease burden in the pediatric population compared with diseases that are thought to arise from the interaction of multiple genetic and environmental factors: neural tube defects, congenital heart defects, isolated cleft lip/palate, and clubfoot. Many multifactorial disorders are present at birth and are thus considered to be congenital malformations, but others, such as infantile autism and type 1 diabetes, typically present later in childhood. This section will review basic concepts relating to the genetics of multifactorial disorders, with emphasis on diseases that occur in the pediatric population.

THE MULTIFACTORIAL MODEL

Many quantitative traits, such as height, blood pressure, and IQ, exhibit a normal distribution in human populations, which is the consequence of multiple genetic and environmental influences on the phenotype (hence the designation *multifactorial*). Most of the diseases to be considered in this chapter, however, are either present or absent in the individual. There is an underlying distribution for these disorders, which follows the familiar bell-shaped curve. If an individual has enough liability factors to exceed a threshold, then that person is affected with the disorder (Fig. 10-6).

In some cases, the threshold may be higher in one sex than in the other. Pyloric stenosis is a classic example of a multifactorial disease that appears to follow such a sex-specific threshold model. This birth defect, in which a narrowing of the pylorus produces constipation, chronic vomiting, weight loss, and electrolyte imbalance, affects approximately 1 in 1000 females and approximately 1 in 200 males, which indicates that the liability threshold is higher for females than for males. Accordingly, affected females should possess more liability factors than should affected males. Having more risk factors, affected females will be more likely to produce affected offspring. This prediction is borne out in Table 10-2, which shows that the recurrence risk is considerably higher for the offspring of affected females than for the offspring of affected males.

A similar pattern is seen in infantile autism, where the male-to-female ratio is approximately 4:1. The threshold is thought to be higher for females than males in this multifactorial disorder, and one large study showed that the recurrence risk for siblings of affected females is twice as high as the risk for siblings of affected males (7.0 versus 3.5%).

RECURRENCE RISKS FOR MULTIFACTORIAL DISEASES

Recurrence risks for single-gene diseases are known with considerable certainty (50% for an autosomal-dominant disease and 25% for an autosomal-recessive disease, although incomplete penetrance

TABLE 10-2

RECURRENCE RISKS FOR OFFSPRING OF INDIVIDUALS AFFECTED WITH PYLORIC STENOSIS

Affected parent	Male	Female
Affected sons	5.5%	19.4%
Affected daughters	2.4	7.3

SOURCE: From Kidd KK, Spence MA: Genetic analyses of pyloric stenosis suggesting a specific maternal effect. J Med Genet 13:290–294, 1976

may decrease these figures). In contrast, the number of genetic and environmental factors (not to mention their identity) is unknown for nearly all multifactorial disorders. For these diseases, empirical recurrence risks (ie, risks based on direct observation) are estimated by identifying a population of affected individuals and then tabulating the proportion of their relatives who are affected by the same disease. Suppose, for example, that 1000 siblings of individuals affected with a neural tube defect have been identified. If 30 of these siblings are also affected with a neural tube defect, the empirical recurrence risk is 3%.

Empirical recurrence risks can vary from one population to another because of interpopulation variation in risk factors or can vary temporally, as risk factors change. Thus, empirical risk factors, strictly speaking, are population-specific.

Patterns of recurrence risks for multifactorial disorders differ in several important ways from the patterns observed for single-gene disorders:

1. The recurrence risk increases as the number of affected individuals in the family increases. The sibling recurrence risk for a ventricular septal defect, for example, has been estimated to be 3% if one sibling is affected. If two siblings are affected in the same family, then the recurrence risk increases to 10%. Recurrence risks for single-gene disorders, in contrast, remain the same regardless of the number of affected individuals in the family. As increasing numbers of individuals affected with a multifactorial disorder are observed in a family, the risk itself does not actually change but it becomes apparent that the family lies higher on the liability distribution (ie, they have more genetic and/or environmental risk factors), resulting in a higher risk for each sibling.

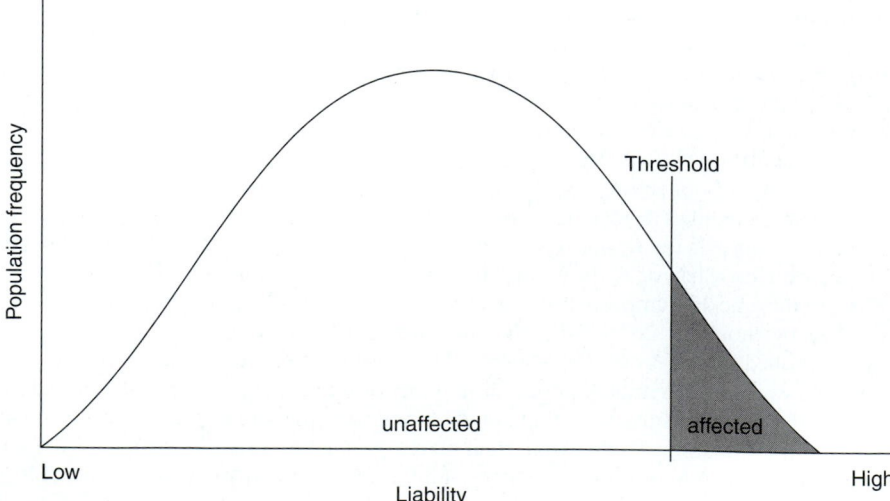

FIGURE 10-6 The liability distribution for a multifactorial disease. An individual must exceed a threshold on this distribution to be affected with the disease.

TABLE 10-3

PREVALENCE RATES AND RECURRENCE RISKS FOR SEVERAL MULTIFACTORIAL DISEASES

		RISK		
DISEASE	GENERAL POPULATION	FIRST-DEGREE RELATIVE	SECOND-DEGREE RELATIVE	THIRD-DEGREE RELATIVE
Cleft lip/palate	0.1%	4.0%	0.7%	0.3%
Clubfoot	0.1	2.5	0.5	0.2
Developmental dysplasia of hip	0.2	5.0	0.6	0.4
Infantile autism	0.04	4.5	0.1	0.05

2. The recurrence risk is higher if the affected individual (the *proband*) is a member of the less commonly affected sex. As in the pyloric stenosis and autism examples cited above, an affected individual who is a member of the less commonly affected sex is thought to lie higher on the liability distribution. Thus, relatives of this individual have a higher recurrence risk.

3. The recurrence risk tends to increase if the proband has a more severe expression of the disease. More severe expression of the disease is thought to be correlated with a greater number of liability factors in the family and should produce a higher risk for relatives of the proband. For example, the recurrence risk for relatives of an individual with bilateral cleft lip/palate is higher than that for relatives of an individual with a unilateral cleft.

4. The recurrence risk decreases rapidly as the degree of relationship decreases between the proband and his or her relatives. For single-gene disorders, the recurrence risk decreases by one-half for each successive degree of relationship (eg, for an autosomal-dominant disease, the recurrence risk is 50% for siblings, 25% for uncle-niece or grandparent-grandchild relationships, 12.5% for first cousins, and so on). The more rapid decrease seen for multifactorial disorders (see Table 10-3) reflects the fact that many genetic and environmental factors must typically combine to cause the trait, and these are unlikely to be present in less closely related family members.

5. The recurrence risk is correlated with the prevalence of the disease in a population. In single-gene disorders, the recurrence risk is largely independent of prevalence. But for multifactorial disorders, empirical studies have shown that if the population prevalence is p, the sibling risk is approximately $\sqrt{p}$. The data shown in Table 10-3 indicate that, for many multifactorial diseases, this relationship holds quite well. However, the relationship is only approximate, and some diseases, such as infantile autism, deviate from it (here, the population prevalence is approximately 1 in 2500 but the sibling recurrence risk is approximately 4%).

TWIN STUDIES: GAUGING THE RELATIVE INFLUENCE OF GENETICS AND ENVIRONMENT

The relative influences of "nature" and "nurture" in human traits have long been a subject of debate. A common method for assessing the relative influence of genetics and environment involves the study of twins, which occur with a frequency of approximately 1 in 100 births in whites (the prevalence is slightly lower in Asians and slightly higher in Africans). Sir Francis Galton, a cousin of Sir Charles Darwin, realized that monozygotic (or identical) twins could be compared with dizygotic (or fraternal twins) to shed light on the nature-nurture question. Monozygotic (MZ) twins, which

arise from the early cleavage of the embryo into two virtually identical embryos, share 100% of their genes. Dizygotic (DZ) twins, which are caused by the fertilization of two egg cells by two different sperm cells, are genetically the same as siblings, sharing 50% of their genes. Galton reasoned that a trait strongly influenced by genes should show greater similarity in MZ twins than in DZ twins. For quantitative traits such as height or blood pressure, this similarity is typically measured as an intraclass correlation coefficient, which varies from -1.0 to 1.0. An intraclass correlation of 1.0 indicates a perfect positive association for a trait in all twin pairs, and a correlation of -1.0 indicates a perfect negative association. A correlation coefficient of 0 indicates that there is no association. For present/absent traits, such as neural tube defect, a concordance rate is estimated (ie, if one twin has the trait, how often does the other twin have it?). For traits in which the prevalence varies according to gender, MZ twins are compared with like-sexed DZ twins.

As shown in Table 10-4, traits that are thought to be strongly influenced by genes (such as autism) show substantial differences in similarity in MZ versus DZ twins. Traits unlikely to have a large genetic component, such as measles infection, show little difference in similarity. Concordance rates and correlation coefficients can be used to estimate the *heritability* of a trait, which is defined as the proportion of variation of a trait that is caused by genetic factors. A common measure of heritability is given by $(C_{MZ} - C_{DZ})/(1 - C_{DZ})$, where C_{MZ} is the concordance rate (or correlation coefficient) for a trait in MZ twins and C_{DZ} is the rate in DZ twins. As the difference between the rates increases, heritability goes to 1.0. If there is no difference in the rates, the heritability is 0.

Although twin studies have been used widely to provide initial estimates of the relative influence of genes on a trait, a number of biases and difficulties confound such studies. Foremost among these is the assumption that the environments of MZ and DZ twins are equally similar. MZ twins are in fact often treated more similarly than are DZ twins, resulting in an environmental bias that tends to increase the MZ concordance rate. This environmental bias has

TABLE 10-4

MZ AND DZ TWIN CONCORDANCE RATES FOR SELECTED PEDIATRIC DISEASES

DISEASE	MZ CONCORDANCE	DZ CONCORDANCE
Autism	60%	0%
Cleft lip/palate	38%	8%
Clubfoot	32%	3%
Spina bifida	72%	33%
Measles	95%	87%

MZ = monozygotic twins; DZ = dizygotic twins.

been observed in studies of the heritability of blood pressure, in which heritability estimates based on twin studies are substantially higher than are estimates based on other types of relatives (eg, parents and offspring).

A factor that may work in the opposite direction is the fact that somatic mutations may occur after embryonic cleavage, resulting in MZ twins that are less than 100% genetically identical (clearly, if such a mutation occurs shortly after cleavage, the difference is likely to be greater). Still another factor that can influence the similarity of MZ twins is the uterine environment itself (ie, whether there are separate amnions and chorions, a shared chorion, or shared amnion and shared chorion).

MZ twins who were reared apart are still genetically identical but do not share common environments. Because of the rarity of this situation, few conditions have been studied. However, psychological inventories indicate a remarkable degree of behavioral resemblance in MZ twins reared in separate environments. Repeated analyses in many different populations have revealed enough consistency to support the use of twin studies to gain an initial impression of the role of genes in disease etiology. Twin studies, of course, do not pinpoint specific genes. Other techniques, such as linkage analysis and positional cloning, must be used to accomplish this goal.

COMMON APPROACHES FOR FINDING GENES UNDERLYING MULTIFACTORIAL DISEASES

Because of the complexity of multifactorial disorders, the identification of individual genes presents a difficult challenge but, several approaches for overcoming this challenge have been developed.

Identification of Highly Heritable Subsets

For some multifactorial disorders, subsets of families in which the disease follows mendelian transmission patterns have been identified: autosomal-dominant breast cancer (*BRCA1* or *BRCA2* mutations) and autosomal-dominant colorectal cancer (*APC* mutations and mutations in any of the several DNA repair genes that give rise to hereditary nonpolyposis colorectal cancer). Frequently, mendelian subsets of multifactorial diseases are expressed relatively early in life and may have especially severe expression.

In pediatric patients, maturity-onset diabetes in the young (MODY) is often inherited in autosomal-dominant fashion, which provides a useful subset of diabetes cases in which specific causative genes have been identified. About 50% of MODY cases are caused by mutations in the gene that encodes glucokinase, a rate-limiting enzyme involved in the conversion of glucose to glucose-6-phosphate. Mutations in four other genes are known to cause MODY, and the protein products of these genes are all transcription factors involved in insulin regulation or pancreatic development (hepatocyte nuclear factor 1-α, hepatic nuclear factor 1-β, hepatocyte nuclear factor 4-α, and insulin promoter factor 1). The identification of these specific genes and their protein products may lead to a better understanding of the pathophysiology of more common types of diabetes.

Hirschsprung disease (aganglionic megacolon) provides a second example of a childhood disease in which subsets of cases follow a mendelian transmission pattern. In approximately 10 to 20% of Hirschsprung patients, aganglionosis extends beyond the sigmoid colon, and the inheritance pattern is more likely to approximate that of a single-gene disorder. In some families exhibiting autosomal-dominant transmission (with reduced penetrance), loss-of-

function mutations in the *RET* proto-oncogene have been shown to cause the disease. Mutations in the endothelin B receptor gene have been seen in families in which Hirschsprung disease manifests a recessive mode of inheritance.

Linkage Analysis

Recurrence risks for multifactorial diseases usually decrease rapidly with more remote degrees of relationship (Table 10-3). Thus, it is difficult to assemble large, extended pedigrees with multiple affected individuals. An alternative is to study only closely related pairs of relatives (most commonly, pairs of sibs both affected with the disorder). To localize genes underlying the trait of interest, DNA polymorphisms located throughout the genome are assayed in each pair of sibs, (see Molecular Diagnostics, in Chap. 8). If a gene underlying the trait lies close to one of the polymorphisms (ie, the polymorphism and the disease gene are linked), then the affected sib pairs will share a higher proportion of alleles of the polymorphism than would be expected under standard mendelian inheritance. If there is no linkage between a polymorphism and a disease-causing gene, then 25% of sibs will share no alleles of the polymorphism, 50% will share one allele, and 25% will share both alleles. As seen in Table 10-5, a significant proportion of sib pairs share more alleles than would be expected if there were no linkage between type 1 diabetes and polymorphisms in the class I MHC region. This result provides support for a role of MHC genes in the causation of type 1 diabetes. In a typical sib-pair linkage analysis, approximately 400 DNA polymorphisms dispersed uniformly throughout the genome are tested (ie, about one polymorphism in every 10 million base pairs of DNA).

Quantitative Trait Locus Analysis

The goal of quantitative trait locus (QTL) analysis is to uncover genes that underlie quantitative variation in multifactorial traits. Experimental models in which breeding experiments can be undertaken to create animals with extreme values of a trait (eg, high blood pressure or low glucose tolerance) are usually employed. Such animals are more likely to be homozygous for genes responsible for the trait in question. A series of crosses are then performed (see Fig. 10-7) to produce animals that are optimized for linkage analysis. Linkage "maps" of DNA polymorphisms are available for experimental animals such as mice and rats, and these are used to identify the QTL. Because rodents and humans share a high degree of similarity in their DNA sequences homology, the location of a QTL in the animal model will give an important clue to its location in the human genome. A specific gene that is identified (cloned) in the animal model can be used to probe for the same gene in the human.

This approach (and many variations of it) has been applied to many human diseases, including type 1 diabetes. More than a dozen QTLs have been identified in the non-obese diabetic mouse and

TABLE 10-5

MHC CLASS I ALLELE SHARING IN SIBS AFFECTED WITH TYPE I DIABETES

	NUMBER OF ALLELES SHARED		
	0	1	2
Expected	25%	50%	25%
Observed	5%	41%	54%

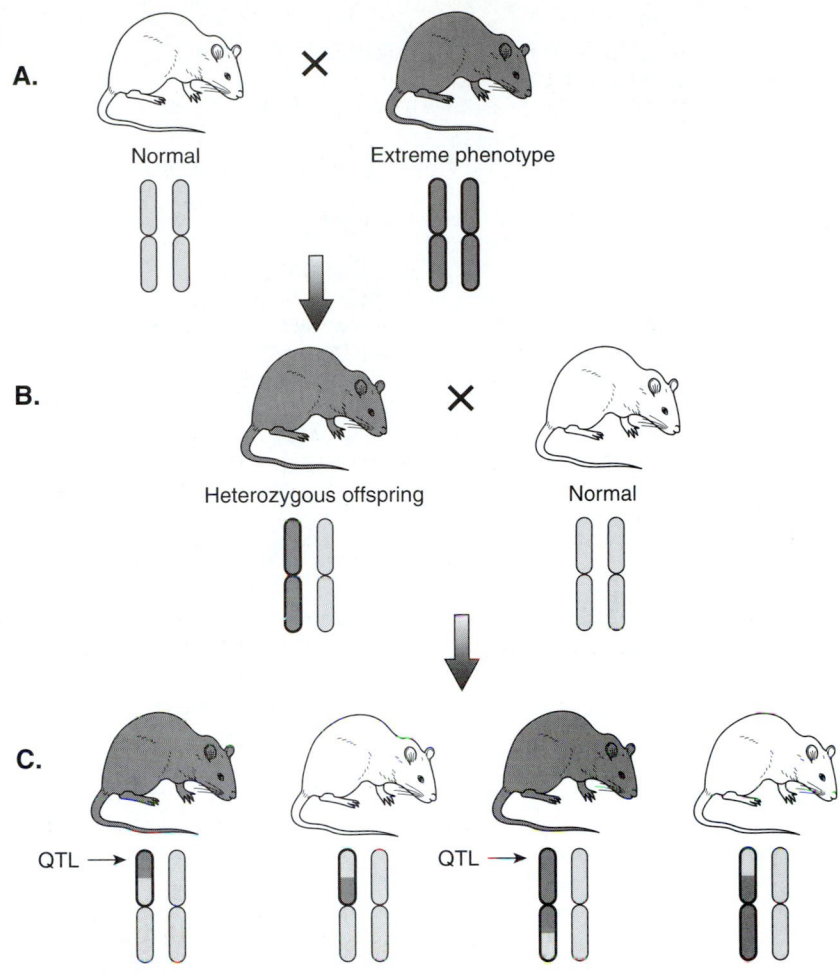

FIGURE 10-7 **A summary of the use of an animal model to isolate quantitative trait loci (QTLs). A. Animals with extreme values of a quantitative trait (eg, high blood pressure) are crossed with normal animals. The offspring of these animals are expected to have one chromosome that carries a gene encoding the extreme trait value, whereas the other chromosome should have the normal version of the gene (i.e., they are heterozygotes). B. The heterozygous animals are crossed with normal animals (a backcross) to produce individuals in the next generation in which recombinations have occurred between the chromosomes carrying the normal and extreme value genes. C. These recombinant chromosomes are highly useful in linkage analysis, which is then used to localize the QTL to a specific chromosome region. Molecular techniques are then used to isolate the QTL itself. Because of the extensive homology between humans and experimental animals such as mice and rats, the animal version of the gene can be used to probe the human genome for the human version of the QTL.**

provide important clues for diabetes pathogenesis in humans. The mouse QTLs do not necessarily correspond directly to human QTLs, in part because of differences in the penetrance and expression of diseases in humans and mice and because the patterns of interaction of gene products are likely to differ substantially between the two species. Nonetheless, this approach can offer important insights into the genes underlying susceptibility to multifactorial disorders.

Association Analysis

Association studies seek to demonstrate a causal relationship between a gene and a disease by showing that a specific allele is seen significantly more often in affected individuals than in unaffected controls. Whereas linkage analysis attempts to find the chromosomal location of a gene by using family data, association studies typically use population data: a set of cases and a set of controls.

An example of an association analysis is illustrated by neural tube defects (NTDs), which cluster strongly in families. Preconceptional dietary supplementation with folic acid has been demonstrated to prevent approximately 70% of NTDs. However, some women who receive dietary supplementation still produce children with NTDs, and most women who have a dietary deficiency do not produce offspring with NTDs. Thus, it is reasonable to suspect that other factors, including genes that influence the metabolism of folate, could affect this association, and genes that encode protein products involved in folate metabolism are "candidate genes" for association with NTDs. In fact, several studies have demonstrated

associations between polymorphisms in the methylene tetrahydrofolate reductase (MTHFR) gene in mothers and the probability of producing a child with a NTD. In addition, some studies indicate that the same polymorphism occurring in the fetus may be a predisposing factor for an NTD. This enzyme, and others involved in folate metabolism, may well be responsible in part for susceptibility to NTDs in the general population.

Although association studies are very common, a number of potential difficulties occur including stratification effects in the case and control samples: An apparent association may be caused by an extraneous factor that happens to differ in the two samples and has nothing to do with the causative factor in question. This limitation can be overcome by careful matching of cases and controls or by adopting a prospective study design (see in Chap. 8, Interpretation of Clinical Studies). Evidence for a true association is strengthened considerably by replication of an association result in multiple populations.

References

Botto LD, Moore CA, Khoury MJ, Erickson JD: Neural-tube defects. N Engl J Med 341:1509–1519, 1999

Thomsom G, Esposito MS: The genetics of complex diseases. Trends Cell Biol 9:M17–20, 1999

Todd JA: From genome to aetiology in a multifactorial disease, type 1 diabetes. BioEssays 21:164–174, 1999

10.1.2   Principles of Care for Children with Genetic Disorders

Claire O. Leonard

The contribution of genetic variation to health and disease has become increasingly clear as a result of our burgeoning understanding of the human genome. Genetics can no longer be considered as only the identification of rare syndromes and inborn errors of metabolism. Many genetic conditions can be treated effectively. Others require chronic, ongoing management, often of a multidisciplinary nature. Prevention of many diseases that can manifest later in life requires appreciation of genetic predisposition during childhood. No physician can hope to recognize and personally manage all genetic disorders, many of which are quite rare and/or have rapidly changing treatment options. Rather, the suspicion that a disorder is genetic, willingness to coordinate care, and advocacy for the child and family are critically important. Circumstances that may suggest a genetic disorder are outlined in Table 10-6. Single-organ diseases or birth defects (eg, cataracts, Hirshsprung disease, ichthyosis) may also be genetic. Once a genetic condition is suspected, diagnostic evaluation should be undertaken. In the majority of situations, the diagnosis is based on clinical criteria only, although the American College of Medical Genetics has developed protocols for evaluation of some common clinical situations such as the child with mental retardation. Confirmatory laboratory studies usually require a focused differential diagnosis. No set of screening tests can be recommended, and obtaining a karyotype often obscures a search for the actual genetic basis of a disorder. Several internet resources allow matching of signs and symptoms with a list of syndromes or genetic conditions (POSSUM, London Dysmorphology Database). Collaboration with a clinical geneticist will allow access to specialized tests to confirm a suspected diagnosis and provide an overview of expectations for the family and genetic counseling if desired.

Whether the parents are first told of the diagnosis (termed an *informing session*) by a consultant or the primary care physician should be decided on an individual basis. These informing sessions are critically important and guidelines to help facilitate interactions are given in Table 10-7. A process similiar to that described for counseling the family of a newborn with Down syndrome (see Sec. 10.2) can be adapted for most abnormalities.

Development of long-term care plans facilitates coordination and delivery of care to children with genetic conditions. Health maintenance guidelines for specific disorders address common complications, anticipate concerns, and focus on preventive care. Such guidelines have been developed by a variety of groups including disease-specific support groups and the Committee on Genetics

TABLE 10-6

SITUATIONS WITH HIGH PROBABILITY OF GENETIC DISEASE

1. Family history of genetic disorder or chronic disease
2. Prenatally diagnosed fetal anomalies
3. Positive newborn metabolic screening test
4. Multiple congenital anomalies
5. Neurodevelopmental disorders
6. Perinatal or neonatal death
7. Acute life-threatening event
8. Disorders of growth
9. Multisystem disorders

TABLE 10-7

SUGGESTIONS FOR THE INFORMING INTERVIEW

- Inform both parents together.
- Inform in private and with sufficient time to answer questions and concerns.
- Avoid distractions such as siblings, pagers, and hospital technology (monitors, ventilators).
- Avoid unnecessary delays in imparting the diagnosis.
- Have adequate information to answer common questions.
- Focus on the child not on the disease (use child's name, hold child, make positive statements about the child).
- Use understandable language, avoiding medical terminology (have a medical interpreter when needed rather than a friend or family member).
- Allow parents time to process information and feel natural emotions rather than moving too rapidly to discussions of management plans.
- Provide written information about the conditions, resources, and a follow-up plan.

of the American Academy of Pediatrics. A compilation covering many conditions is available (see reference). Many disorders require referral to a variety of subspecialists for management. For more common conditions, multidisciplinary teams, which consist of professionals who can address the medical, psychological, genetic counseling, social, nutritional, functional, and educational needs of the child during a single appointment may exist at children's hospitals, academic medical centers, and health departments. The primary care physician should receive prompt feedback from the team, interpret reports for the family, and assist the family in accessing appropriate care and support services. The family should know who will be responsible for acute illnesses and for specific aspects of a child's care to avoid confusion and delays in obtaining timely care and appropriate interventions. To facilitate communications and consistency of care, families of children with special health care needs should be provided a document specifying diagnosis, treatment information, potential acute complications, plans for emergency management, and source for consultation especially for children with metabolic disease where prompt recognition of a rare condition and appropriate treatment may limit morbidity and be lifesaving (see Chap. 9).

In the case of progressive conditions where death is likely during childhood, the primary care physician is often the most appropriate person to provide support for the family, including advice concerning post mortem diagnosis, if appropriate (see Sec. 8.2 and Chap. 7).

Obtaining up-to-date information on a specific genetic condition may be a challenge, and online resources are quite helpful. Mendelian Inheritance in Man (OMIM; *www.ncbi.nlm.nih.gov/ omim/*) is a catalogue of known single-gene disorders that provides general information and current references. Gene Clinics (*www.geneclinics.org/index/html*) provides clinical summaries for various types of genetic condition. Support groups for specific disorders also frequently have web pages or other online resources as well as printed materials for both parents and professionals. The Alliance of Genetic Support Groups (*www.geneticalliance.org*) is designed to connect a practitioner to a specific group. As defined by the American Society of Human Genetics,

Genetic counseling is a communication process that deals with human problems associated with the occurrence, or the risk of occurrence, of a genetic disorder in a family. This process involves an attempt by one or more appropriately trained persons to help the individual or family to (1) comprehend the medical facts, including the diagnosis, probable course of the disorder, and the available management; (2) appreciate the way heredity contributes to the disorder, and the risk of recurrence in specified relative; (3) understand the alternatives for dealing with the risk of recurrence; (4) choosing the course of action which seems to them appropriate in view of their risk, their family goals, and their ethical and religious standard, and to act in accordance with that decision; and (5) to make the best possible adjustment to the disorder in an affected family member and/or to the risk of recurrence of that disorder.

This definition includes much more than recurrence risk and reproductive counseling and requires ongoing attention over many years during the reproductive period of the family and the lifetime of the affected individual. The pediatrician should be the primary source of support for families and make referrals to subspecialists, including genetic counselors and obstetricians, specializing in high-risk pregnancies, when indicated. Areas where families frequently need assistance are summarized in Table 10-8. Effective assistance in these areas requires knowledge of both local and national organizations and services. The internet and parent support groups can be especially helpful for many families.

Reference

Wilson GN, Cooley WC: Preventive Management of Children with Congenital Anomalies and Syndromes. Cambridge University Press, 2000

10.1.3   Human Cytogenetics

Zhong Chen and John C. Carey

The field of clinical cytogenetics and the description of syndromes caused by gross chromosomal abnormalities laid the foundation for defining and delineating malformation syndromes. This was also,

TABLE 10-8

SUPPORT NEEDS OF SOME FAMILIES WITH GENETIC DISEASE

1. Adjustment to the diagnosis and its implications
2. Financial resources for coping with medical and other expenses
3. Assistance with health-care payors (documentation, education, advocacy, legislative efforts)
4. In-home nursing services, medical devices, equipment
5. Special educational services and therapies
6. Assistance with sibling adjustment
7. Behavioral counseling and psychotherapy
8. Antidiscrimination efforts
9. Emotional support, marriage counseling
10. Planning for long-term care or independent living
11. Transition to the adult health-care system
12. Bereavement counseling
13. Assurance that research is ongoing, relevant to their needs, and available to them in a timely fashion

in part, the foundation of the field of dysmorphology. This section provides the principles of cytogenetics.

Cytogenetics is the microscopic examination of chromosomes arrested during the metaphase stage of cell division. In the early 1960s chromosome analysis was limited to counting chromosomes and assigning them to seven groups, A through G, based upon their size and the location of the centromere (the ordered display of chromosomes is called a *karyotype*). Thus, cytogenetic abnormalities were detectable in only a few syndromes at that time. For example, three copies of a G group chromosome could be identified in individuals with Down syndrome. In 1970, banding techniques were introduced in which chemical or enzyme treatments produce characteristic light and dark patterns, called *bands*, along the arms of the chromosomes. Each of the 46 chromosomes could be identified individually. Comparisons of bands between homologs, or members of a pair of chromosomes, allowed identification of some rearrangements, including translocations, deletions, and duplications. The extra G chromosome in Down syndrome was subsequently identified as chromosome number 21.

As new cell culture techniques were developed, longer chromosomes in prophase or early metaphase with more band resolution were obtained, allowing for *high-resolution analysis*. Subtle chromosome abnormalities were observed using these techniques, which facilitated the characterization of syndromes associated with chromosome deletions, such as Prader-Willi and Miller-Dieker. Specialized media and manipulation of cultured cells with chemicals such as bromodeoxyuridine (BrdU) permitted the identification of even more chromosome abnormalities. Analyses for the exchange of material between chromatids (sister chromatid exchange studies) were developed to diagnose chromosome breakage syndromes, and DNA replication studies allowed the identification of the inactive X chromosome by differential staining.

Most recently, molecular techniques have expanded the repertoire of tools available for diagnosing genetic conditions (see Chap. 8). Molecular cytogenetic methods capitalize on the accuracy and detail of molecular studies, combined with the well-established techniques of cytogenetics, to gain a deeper understanding of chromosome structure. DNA probes for specific loci or genes on the chromosomes are used in fluorescence in situ hybridization (FISH). This method helps confirm structural chromosome changes and offers the capability of evaluating the chromosome complement in interphase or nondividing cells.

CYTOGENETIC ANALYSIS

Cytogenetic studies are more in demand today than ever before, and many different tissue types are amenable to study. Most commonly, lymphocytes from peripheral blood (1 to 5 mL of sterile whole blood anticoagulated with sodium heparin) are examined. Amniotic fluid and chorionic villus sampling are obtained for prenatal chromosome analysis for indications such as advanced maternal age, previous pregnancies with chromosome abnormalities, parental carrier of a chromosome anomaly, and abnormal maternal serum screen results. Skin or tissue samples (2- to 3-mm punch biopsies) from a fetus may also be useful in evaluating miscarriages and families with multiple spontaneous fetal loss. Bone marrow or solid tumor biopsies are examined as an aid in the diagnosis and prognosis of leukemias and cancers (see Chap. 20). Sterile collection and rapid transport of all specimens at room temperature is also critical, since living, growing cells are required for chromosome analysis.

A typical karyotype is performed by growing cells in culture, arresting each dividing cell, treating the cells to make them swell, and fixing the chromosomes and nuclei from nondividing cells. Subsequently the chromosomes of dividing cells are spread across the surface of the slide. The chromosomes are stained and are examined by light microscopy. In general, 20 metaphase spreads are analyzed before a result is rendered. Routine karyotyping techniques yield a chromosome complement with 400 to 600 bands, and high-resolution techniques can extend this to 850 bands or more. Review of a karyotype in conjunction with clinical information is essential for making an accurate diagnosis (Fig. 10-8).

NOMENCLATURE

Normally, each human has 46 chromosomes that are distributed in 23 pairs, 22 pairs of autosomes and 1 pair of sex chromosomes (XX in females and XY in males). Thus each individual has two copies of each chromosome (ie, *diploid*). A normal chromosome constitution is termed the *euploid* state, whereas an abnormal chromosome complement is called *aneuploidy*. The autosomes are divided into seven groups labeled *A* through *G* and pairs 1 to 22, with the numbers assigned in descending order of length, size, and centromere position of each chromosome pair, although chromosome 21 is actually smaller than chromosome 22. The position of the centromere varies among chromosomes and is classified into three categories: Metacentric chromosomes have centromeres in the middle, submetacentric chromosomes display centromeres closer to one end, and acrocentric chromosomes have centromeres at the end of the chromosome (Fig. 10-8). For example, the chromosomes of the D (13 to 15) and G (21 and 22) groups are referred to as *acrocentric*.

The centromere (*cen*) divides a chromosome into a short (*p*) arm and a long (*q*) arm (Fig. 10-9). Each arm ends in a terminus (*ter*). Thus the end of the short arm is called *qter*. The arm of each chromosome is divided into regions, regions are divided into bands, and bands into subbands. When a karyotype is reported, the total number of chromosomes is presented first, followed by the sex chromosomes' constitution, and then any numerical and structural anomalies are indicated to the level of the subbands. The International System for Human Cytogenetic Nomenclature (ISCN) 1995 provides additional information. Definitions of some common cytogenetic terms and abbreviations are given in Table 10-9. Some examples of normal and abnormal karyotype reports:

46,XY	A normal male
46,XX	A normal female
47,XX,+13	A female with an extra chromosome 13 (trisomy 13)
47,XXY	A male with two X chromosomes and one Y chromosome (Klinefelter syndrome)
46,XX,del(4)(p16)	A female with a terminal deletion and a breakpoint at band 4p16
45,XX,(15;21)(q10;q10)	A female with a robertsonian translocation involving chromosomes 15 and 21
46,XX,(15;21)(q10;q10),t21	A female with an unbalanced robertsonian translocation between chromosomes 15 and 21, resulting in trisomy 21
46,XY,t(9;22)(q34;q11)	A male karyotype with a balanced reciprocal translocation between chromosomes q and 22, with breakpoints at bands 9q34 and 22q11, generating the Philadelphia chromosome rearrangement
47,XY,+21/46,XY	A male with mosaicism for trisomy 21

CLASSIFICATION OF CHROMOSOME ABNORMALITIES

Abnormalities of chromosomes may be classified as numerical or structural, with numerical changes being the most common. The term *numerical abnormality* refers to gain or loss of chromosomes, which is always associated with physical or mental maldevelopment or both. *Trisomy* and *monosomy* refer to the presence of an extra autosome and the absence of an autosome, respectively. *Mosaicism* refers to the presence of two or more distinct cell populations within an individual.

Structural rearrangements result from chromosome breakage, followed by reconstitution in an abnormal configuration. Structural rearrangements are defined as either *balanced* or *unbalanced*, depending on whether all the normal complement of genetic information is still present. The most common type of structural rearrangement, a balanced translocation, is present in about 1 in 500 newborns and usually has no phenotypic effect, although an increased risk of having children with an unbalanced rearrangement occurs.

Reciprocal translocations refer to the exchange of segments between nonhomologous chromosomes (e.g., between chromosomes 9 and 22). *Robertsonian translocations* involve the fusion of two acrocentric chromosomes in which the short arms of each chromosome are lost in these rearrangements. These short arms contain redundant copies of ribosomal RNA genes, and thus their loss is of no clinical significance. Nevertheless, unbalanced robertsonian translocations result in partial trisomy for the long arms of acrocentric chromosomes.

Translocations between chromosomes 14 and 21, 21 and 22, and two 21 chromosomes are the most common robertsonian translocations and can result in the birth of a child with trisomy 21. In other unbalanced rearrangements, the phenotype is also likely to be abnormal because of a deficiency (resulting from partial monosomy) or excess (resulting from partial trisomy) of chromsomal material or a combination of both. When a chromosome undergoes two breaks and the broken ends of the chromosome reunite, a chromosome that looks like a ring is formed.

A marker chromosome is a structurally abnormal chromosome whose chromosome of origin cannot be identified. Cytogeneticists find marker chromosomes difficult to characterize specifically because the marker is usually so small that the banding pattern is ambiguous. Advanced molecular cytogenetic techniques sometimes allow identification of marker chromosomes. Small marker chromosomes are often composed of little more than heterochromatin from the centromere. However, larger marker chromosomes can create a significant imbalance of genetic material (eg, the marker chromosome derived from chromosome 22 observed in patients with "cat-eye" syndrome).

Chromosome abnormalities may occur spontaneously or they can be inherited. In general, numerical alterations and many bal-

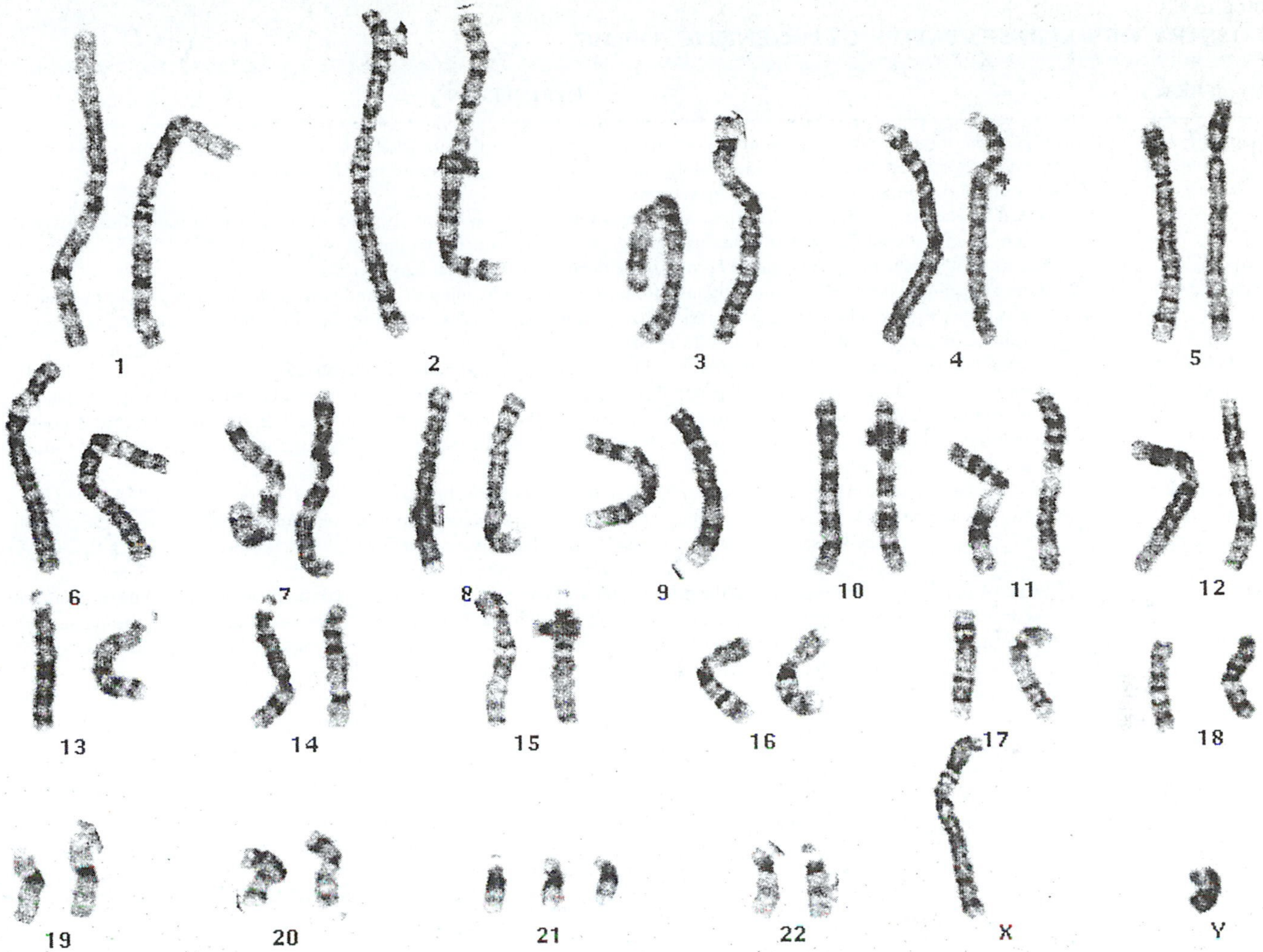

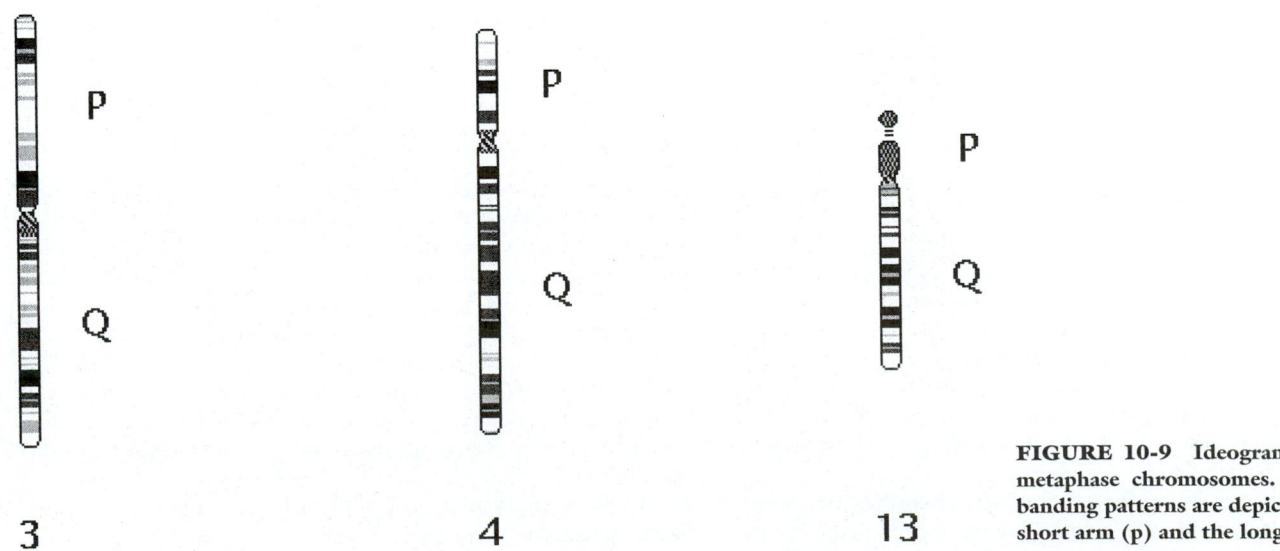

FIGURE 10-8   The karyotype of a male with three copies of chromosome 21 or trisomy 21. Note the arrangement of the chromosomes from largest to smallest.

FIGURE 10-9   Ideograms of human metaphase chromosomes. The specific banding patterns are depicted. Note the short arm (p) and the long arm (q).

TABLE 10-9

GLOSSARY OF REPRESENTATIVE CYTOGENETIC TERMS

TERM	DEFINITION
Aneuploidy	Deviation of the chromosome number from that characteristic for the species. In the human, a chromosome complement that is not an exact multiple of the haploid number (n) (23 chromosomes), eg, 46 chromosomes.
Autosome	Any chromosome other than the sex chromosomes.
Banding	The illumination of various intrachromosomal bands and/or regions of varying intensity by procedures of differential staining. The most commonly used procedures are Q-, G-, C-, R- and T-banding.
Breakpoint	Location of a break in a chromatid or chromosome denoted by the exact band involved.
Diploidy ($2n$)	State of having two full sets of homologous chromosomes (ie, containing the number of chromosomes present in somatic and primary germ cells). Each species has a characteristic number ($2n$), with the haploid number (n) being present in the gamete (sperm or ovum). In humans, $2n = 46$.
Hypodiploid	Containing fewer than the diploid number of chromosomes; in the human, fewer than 46.
Interphase	Portion of the cell cycle when the cell is not in mitosis. Interphase includes the G1, S, and G2 phases. During interphase, the chromosomes are active in RNA synthesis. At a certain, rather fixed, time before the cell next divides, the chromosomes replicate and thus double the amount of chromosomal material in the nucleus. The time at which they are doing this is known as the S (synthesis) *period*.
Interstitial deletion	Loss of chromosomal material not involving the terminal ends of the chromosome.
Karyotype	Systematic arrangement of the chromosomes into various groups according to size, centromere location, and other morphologic features. In the human, the karyotype consists of 22 pairs of autosomes and 2 sex chromosomes (XX in females, XY in males).
Metaphase	Phase of cellular division characterized by disappearance of the nuclear membrane and the nucleoli and arrangement of the chromosomes in one plane at the equator of the cells. This arrangement is called the *metaphase plate*. In this phase, the chromosomes are maximally condensed, most easily seen, and least genetically active and become attached to the spindle at the region along their length called the *centromere* through the kinetochore.
Modal chromosome number	Predominant number in cells with a wide range of chromosome numbers.
Monosomy	Absence of one member of a homologous pair of chromosomes.
p	Arm of chromosome above the centromere, generally a short arm of a chromosome.
Pseudodiploidy	In humans, the state of having 46 chromosomes but with an abnormal karyotype.
q	Arm of chromosome below the centromere, generally a long arm of a chromosome.
t	Translocation, the details of which are usually shown by two sets of parentheses, the first presenting the chromosomes involved and the second the bands affected by the breakpoints.
Trisomy	Presence of an extra (third) autosome in addition to a normal homologous pair. Also, presence of an extra sex chromosome.

anced and unbalanced translocations, deletions, partial duplications, and ring chromosomes arise de novo. When parents carry a balanced translocation, their offspring have an increased risk of inheriting an unbalanced chromosome constitution depending on how meiotic segregation takes place. The segregation of a balanced translocation from generation to generation can produce a family having unbalanced abnormal individuals in a pattern unlike the usual patterns of monogenic disorders. Thus, observing a nonmendelian segregation pattern of individuals affected with mental retardation, growth retardation, and/or major or minor congenital anomalies within a family should suggest that a chromosomal rearrangement might be the cause.

MOLECULAR CYTOGENETICS

In the 1980s the techniques of molecular biology were applied to cytogenetic preparations. This hybrid field is called *molecular cytogenetics* and is transforming the way chromosomal abnormalities in humans are studied. For example, the diagnostic confirmation of microdeletion syndromes has been advanced, the ability to determine the origin of supernumerary marker chromosomes and de novo derivative chromosomes is markedly improved, and the ability to predict phenotypes associated with these types of chromosome abnormalities is increasing.

With molecular cytogenetic techniques, chromosomal abnormalities in nondividing cells including those in fixed tissue can be detected. Some constitutional chromosome abnormalities and conditions associated with chromosomal mosaicism can be studied without growing cells in culture or in cells that are not amenable to growth in culture. Accordingly, chromosome studies can be performed more quickly and stored tissues can be investigated. Moreover, questions about chromosome organization and the tissue distribution of chromosome abnormalities can be addressed in ways that were not possible a few years ago.

Plate 27 illustrates one of the most popular molecular cytogenetic methods used today, fluorescence in situ hybridization (FISH). A piece of DNA called a *probe* is used to detect the presence or absence of a specific chromosomal segment. Three different types of probes are typically used in clinical FISH studies:

1. *Satellite repeat-sequence probes* target the centromeres of specific chromosomes and are useful in determining the number of chromosomes in cases of possible trisomies or sex chromosome aneuploidies. Indeed, these probes can be used to more rapidly diagnose trisomy 18 in newborns. Centromere probes can be used with interphase cells if metaphase cells are not available. In cancer studies, numeric changes such as trisomy 8 and 9, monosomy 7 in myeloid disorders, and trisomy 4, 10, and 21 in acute lymphocytic leukemia can be detected. The proportion of XX and XY cells following an opposite-sex allogeneic bone marrow transplant can also be monitored.

2. *Whole chromosome paint probes* cover an entire chromosome. Chromosome paints are especially helpful for identifying the chromosome of origin of marker chromosomes and translocated material.

3. *Unique sequence probes* target a specific locus (or gene) on a chromosome. Certain acquired translocations such as the t(9;22) in CML, the t(15;17) in AML-M3, and the t(12;21) in childhood ALL can be detected in interphase cells with dual-color unique sequence probes. In addition, this approach is also being used in the diagnosis of chromosome microdeletion syndromes such as the DiGeorge/velocardiofacial [(del(22)(q11.2)] and Prader-Willi and Angelman syndromes [(del(15)(q11-q13)].

Another new molecular cytogenetic technique, called *comparative genomic hybridization* (CGH), has been recently developed for detecting chromosomal imbalances in tumor genomes and some constitutional conditions. CGH is based on two-color FISH. Equal amounts of differentially labeled tumor DNA and normal DNA are mixed and hybridized under specific conditions to normal metaphase spreads. This allows CGH, in a single experiment, to identify gains and/or losses of genetic material and map the location of these changes on metaphase chromosomes. DNA extracted from either fresh or frozen tissues, cell lines, and formalin-fixed, paraffin-embedded samples is suitable for CGH. CGH becomes particularly advantageous when structural analysis of chromosomal changes in cancers is severely limited by quality of the karyotype. CGH has been an effective screening method for describing and establishing a phenotype-genotype correlation in solid tumor progression and other genetic conditions.

An additional new technique called *multicolor spectral karyotyping* (SKY) helps identify unknown chromosomal material in marker chromosomes (see Plate 28). This technique combines Fourier spectroscopy, charge-coupled device (CCD) imaging, and optical microscopy to measure chromosome-specific spectra after FISH with differentially labeled painting probes. Currently, work is underway to generate a multicolor banding pattern (bar code) of the human chromosome complement by using chromosome arm- and band-specific painting probes to identify intrachromosomal anomalies. Therefore, SKY may be a very promising approach to the rapid and automatic karyotyping of complex chromosome rearrangements in neoplastic cells and constitutional chromosome disorders.

Microdissection of individual chromosomes to obtain specific segments of DNA can be used to generate whole chromosome paint probes and band- or region-specific probes. This technique is particularly useful for identifying the origin of chromosomes or chromosomal regions that cannot be identified definitively by standard cytogenetic methods. The strategy of combining the production of probes from microdissected chromosomal DNA and subsequent FISH analysis has been called *micro-FISH analysis*.

References

Gersen SL, Keagle MB: The Principles of Clinical Cytogenetics. Totowa, NJ, Humana Press, 1999:1–31
Mitelman F, ed: ISCN: An International System for Human Cytogenetic Nomenclature. Basel, S. Karger, 1995

10.2   CHROMOSOME DISORDERS

John C. Carey

Chromosome disorders and their associated syndromes can be classified into abnormalities of chromosome number and defects of chromosome structure as well as divided into conditions involving autosomes and those involving sex chromosomes. Three autosomal trisomy syndromes involving chromosomes 21, 18, and 13 and the now well-recognized 22q11 deletion syndrome are the most common disorders involving the autosomes.

Abnormalities of chromosome structure involve duplication or deficiency of a chromosome region or a combination of both. The common deletion syndromes involving terminal monosomy of chromosomes 4p, 5p, 18p, and 18q were described in the 1960s. However, the introduction of banding techniques led to the recognition and delineation of many other partial monosomy and partial trisomy syndromes. Whereas many of the phenotypic defects and syndromes caused by chromosome abnormalities have been catalogued, most of these disorders are typified by a pattern of multiple anomalies and developmental disability. In this section the most common trisomy conditions will be presented; selected deletion syndromes and other aneuploid conditions will also be reviewed.

Chromosome abnormalities occur in about 1 in 150 live born infants, are responsible for a substantial proportion of genetic diseases, are a major contributor to fetal loss, and are a significant cause of congenital malformations and mental retardation. About 10% of all newborns with a congenital malformation and approximately 15 to 20% of persons with moderate to severe mental retardation have a chromosomal abnormality. Trisomy 21, the most common of the trisomy syndromes, accounts for nearly one-third of the infants born with a chromosome abnormality, and about 1 in 300 newborns will have an abnormality of one of the sex chromosomes. All the other autosomal disorders of number and structure combined have an overall frequency of less than 1/1000. Of note, balanced rearrangements such as translocations and inversions occur in about 1 in 500 individuals.

Each chromosome syndrome has its own natural history, list of component manifestations, and intrinsic variability. Most disorders of autosomes are associated with alterations of growth and development such as developmental disabilities, prenatal growth deficiency, short stature, and microcephaly. In addition, congenital heart defects are observed with increased frequency in all the well-established chromosome syndromes. Although the separate features of each chromosome syndrome are relatively nonspecific, the total constellation of phenotypic findings in each of the syndromes is distinctive enough to permit clinical recognition. In particular, this is true of the common autosomal trisomy syndromes and well-established deletion syndromes. Moreover, it is usually the minor anomalies of structure and the alterations of facial morphogenesis that provide the clinical clues that alert the clinician to the possibility of a chromosomal syndrome. Furthermore, a remarkable consistency of the facial gestalt of children with a well-established syndrome at similar ages occurs and is clearly evident by examining photographs of different children with Down syndrome.

The phenotypes of chromosome disorders of structure vary considerably because of differences in the size of chromosome duplication or deficiency and the involvement of nonhomolgous chromosomes. The clinical indications for performing cytogenetic analysis have become well established in the last two decades. Certainly all persons suspected of having a recognizable chromosome syndrome such as Down syndrome, Turner syndrome, or trisomy 18 need a karyotype. In addition, infants and children with unrecognizable patterns of multiple major or minor anomalies should have a karyotype to define the potential etiology of the condition. In recent years, most geneticists have recommended a cytogenetic analysis in all children and adults with idiopathic mental retardation, regardless of whether the individual is dysmorphic. Although this recommendation is somewhat controversial, discovery of a chromosome abnormality, even an uncommon one, will assist the clinician and the family in understanding the condition and organizing medical management.

Other indications for performing a cytogenetic analysis in the pediatric setting are situations in which certain individual findings bring to mind specific conditions. Examples include stillborns with no recognizable reason for fetal death, proportionate short stature in a female (a feature of Turner syndrome), adolescent males with small testes or significant gynecomastia (features of Klinefelter syndrome), infants with hypotonia (Prader-Willi syndrome), and newborns with ambiguous genitalia. Cytogenetic analysis of parents whose children have structural chromosome abnormalities, such as deletions and duplications, is also indicated. Karyotyping is usually not indicated in an infant or child with a single malformation (eg, a neural tube defect or cleft lip) or in the parents of children with a recognized trisomy syndrome (eg, trisomy 21).

COMMON TRISOMY SYNDROMES

The most common autosomal chromosome syndromes are trisomy 21, 18, and 13. The 22q11 deletion syndrome is probably as common as trisomy 18. Complete trisomy of other chromosomes such as 7, 8, 9, and 22 has been described in live born infants, although most individuals with these conditions are mosaic for the trisomic cell line. The catalogs of chromosome disorders listed at the end of the chapter provide further information on these less common chromosome syndromes.

Trisomy 21 (Down syndrome)

Down syndrome is caused by trisomy 21 and is the most common autosomal chromosome abnormality in humans. The condition occurs in about 1 in 800 infants and is the most common multiple congenital anomaly/mental retardation syndrome. The use of the term *mongolism* is no longer appropriate, because this designation is considered pejorative and stigmatizing. The etiology of Down syndrome is related to trisomy of the distal part of the long arm of chromosome 21. Over 90% of individuals with Down syndrome will have three copies of the entire chromosome 21, while less than 10% will have trisomy of only part of the long arm of chromosome 21. The latter is usually caused by unbalanced robertsonian translocation (see Sec. 10.1.3).

The phenotypic pattern of Down syndrome is characteristic and consistent enough to permit recognition of an affected neonate. Most of the facial and limb features of individuals with Down syndrome are not morphologically abnormal, but the specific constellation of manifestations is distinctive. The well-known list of phenotypic variations and minor anomalies is described in many sources and will not be summarized here. The brachycephaly, small ears (less than 3.2 cm in longest length in the newborn), upslanted palpebral fissures, flat midface, full cheeks, and distinctive shape of the mouth when crying are very consistent and together evoke a distinctive gestalt in a child of virtually any age. Small ears and hypotonia are observed in over 90% of newborns with Down syndrome. Although epicanthal folds and a single transverse crease (the so-called simian line) are commonly sought when considering the syndrome, these features are not only nonspecific but also occur in only about 50% of persons with Down syndrome. Short, broad fingers (brachydactyly), absent to very small nipple buds, and a central placement of the posterior hair whorl are more specific to Down syndrome than many other well-known findings. Systems for scor-

ing the clinical findings of children in whom the diagnosis of Down syndrome is being entertained have been developed but are rarely needed because of the ease of recognizing most infants with the syndrome (see Fig. 10-10).

Congenital heart malformations occur in about 40% of children with Down syndrome. About one-third of these malformations fall within the spectrum of an atrioventricular (AV) canal defect and about one-third are ventricular septal defects. Atrial septal defects of the secundum type and tetralogy of Fallot also occur, although they are less frequent. Since a heart murmur is frequently not present in a child with an AV canal defect, clinical examination alone is not enough to exclude the presence of a heart malformation in children with Down syndrome. Referral for an echocardiogram is now considered part of routine health supervision of infants with Down syndrome. If the diagnosis of a shunt lesion is missed in infancy, the early development of pulmonary hypertension characteristically seen in infants with Down syndrome could preclude some surgical options.

Obstructive gastrointestinal lesions including duodenal atresia and Hirschsprung "disease" occur in about 5% of infants with Down syndrome. However, no investigative studies are recommended unless an infant is symptomatic. Congenital cataracts occur in only about 5% of newborns as well, but other ocular problems (eg, strabismus, refractive errors) are common, warranting careful eye examinations in infancy. Other congenital malformations are uncommon in Down syndrome.

Individuals with Down syndrome, whether or not a heart defect is present, have an increased mortality rate compared to other children. The higher childhood mortality may, in part, be caused by

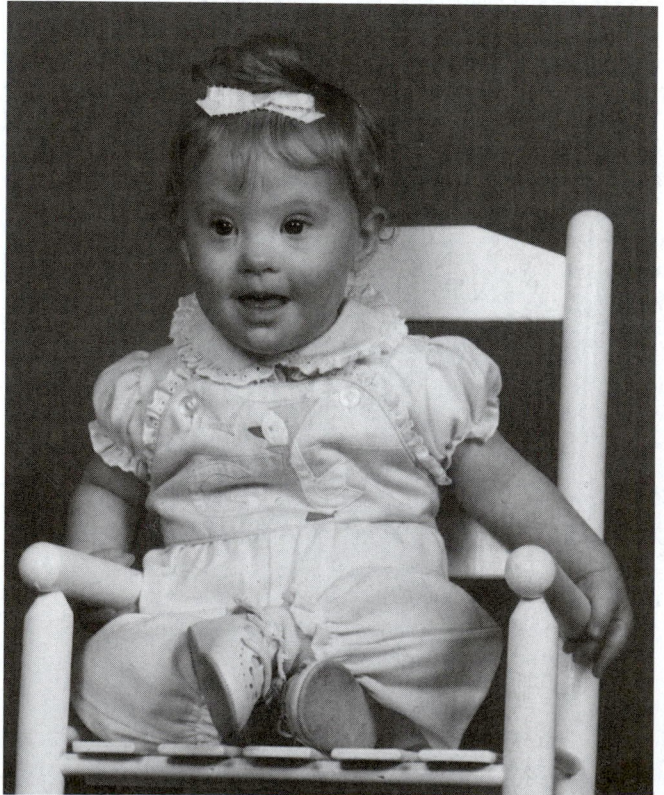

FIGURE 10-10   An infant with Down syndrome illustrating typical features of this disorder including upslanting palpebral fissures, epicanthic folds, and a flat facial profile. (*From Jorde LB, Carey JC, Bamshad MJ, White RL: Medical Genetics, St. Louis, Mosby, 2000.*)

an increased occurrence of infections, especially pneumonia. Abnormalities that affect the respiratory system, including gastroesophageal reflux, primary pulmonary hypertension, and obstructive sleep apnea, are often the basis for symptoms that occur in infancy including cyanosis, respiratory distress, apnea, and growth deficiency. Although a detailed evaluation of an infant with Down syndrome who has these symptoms is appropriate, a perspective on increased mortality needs to be communicated to families during the newborn period. For example, about 90% of children without heart defects will live into adolescence and early adulthood.

The degree of developmental disability in children with Down syndrome is quite variable, but children learn to walk and develop communication skills. The development of most children progresses steadily, albeit at a slower pace than usual. There is no evidence that function regresses during childhood or adolescence. Early intervention accelerates attainment of development skills in the preschool years, but the long-term effect of these programs on ultimate intellectual functioning is unknown. Nevertheless, referral to early intervention programs is recommended, because these programs help the family in areas other than acquisition of developmental skills by providing emotional support, information regarding the educational system, and feedback regarding a child's individual developmental strengths and weaknesses.

Older persons with Down syndrome have an increased risk for a variety of medical problems including atlantoaxial subluxation, cataracts, diabetes mellitus, hypo- and hyperthyroidism, leukemia, and seizures. Most of these problems occur infrequently, but the pediatrician should maintain a high level of suspicion. In the fourth decade of life, some adults with Down syndrome develop increasing cognitive dysfunction including a memory disorder. For this reason, baseline psychometric testing in the twenties is indicated in all young adults with Down syndrome.

Guidelines for health supervision and anticipatory guidance in infants, children, and adolescents with Down syndrome are available. The American Academy of Pediatrics (AAP) has published guidelines that are used commonly, and specific recommendations include cardiac evaluation with echocardiogram before 6 months of age; audiologic evaluation including tympanogram by 6 months of age; newborn screening for hypothyroidism and periodic T4 and TSH throughout childhood and into adulthood; ophthalmologic evaluation at 4 years of age; and routine immunizations.

Various alternative therapies have been proposed in the treatment and management of infants and children with Down syndrome and information on risks and benefits of these therapies should be discussed with parents.

Genetic Basis of Trisomy 21

Cytogenetic studies are recommended for all infants who have a clinical phenotype consistent with Down syndrome to rule out the few chromosome syndromes that could mimic Down syndrome (XXXY, partial 10q trisomy), especially in infancy, and to determine if the infant has three complete copies of chromosome 21 or a translocation involving chromosome 21. This latter finding is important because the recurrence risk for parents varies dependent on the type of chromosome abnormality found in the affected child.

If a child with trisomy 21 is found to have three complete copies of chromosome 21, the risk that a mother under the age of 35 will have a second affected child with trisomy 21 is about 1 to 2%. Compared to the background risk of having a child with trisomy 21 (1/800 or 0.125%), this is an 8- to 16-fold increase for women who have had one child with trisomy 21. If a woman is over the

age of 35, the recurrence risk is thought to be similar to the age-specific risk. Further cytogenetic testing of the parents is not indicated.

If a child with trisomy 21 is found to have an unbalanced translocation resulting in partial trisomy 21, cytogenetic analysis should be performed on the parents. If one of the parents carries a balanced translocation involving chromosome 21, the risk of recurrence will depend on the type of translocation and which parent is the carrier. Fathers carrying a balanced robertsonian translocation have a 1 to 2% recurrence risk, whereas mothers who carry it have a 10 to 15% recurrence risk. Families of children with Down syndrome caused by a translocation should be referred for genetic counseling. Prenatal testing of future pregnancies can be offered to the families of any child with trisomy 21.

The etiology and pathogenesis of trisomy 21 are unknown. The extra copy of chromosome 21 is thought to result from altered segregation of the chromosomes during meiosis, a phenomenon called *nondisjunction*, which may explain why the only factor that is consistent throughout all studies is that the prevalence of Down syndrome increases with advancing maternal age. No environmental factors have been implicated as causes for trisomy 21.

Counseling the Family of a Newborn with Down Syndrome

The pediatric practitioner often has the responsibility of informing the parents that their newborn baby has Down syndrome. The approach to this situation is complex because every family differs in their expectations and preconceived notions about developmental disability and about the meaning of children within their family. The principles around these informing sessions and guidelines for effective and empathetic communications are outlined in Table 10-7.

Several retrospective studies on parents' reactions to the birth of a child with Down syndrome indicate that families prefer to know the diagnosis as soon as possible. If the diagnosis is not in question and the infant does not have an associated life-threatening malformation, suggestions for planned counseling include the following: Arrange a private meeting with both parents together; avoid initiating the discussion while on an open postpartum ward or with other parents in the room; sit down with the family as opposed to standing; refer to the infant by first name if known; plan to meet the parents daily for the first few days of the infant's life and set up a structure for these interviews; use the initial interview to present the diagnosis and the concept of a syndrome; be realistic but hopeful about the information; mention that all children with trisomy 21 have developmental disability but that it varies in degree; have current and accurate information on natural history, the developmental disability, and health supervision available; and avoid presenting details about the genetic basis of trisomy 21 at the initial interview. Information on issues such as the recurrence risk and feasibility of prenatal diagnosis is usually not appropriate to present at the first meeting unless parents specifically ask for it. This additional information can be presented at follow-up visits.

Let the second interview attempt to assess the parents' feelings and their state of mind. Create an opportunity to discuss their various reactions, listen to their personal concerns, and recognize individual feelings of each parent. When the results of the chromosome analysis are available, discuss any further implications and confirmation of the diagnosis. When the infant is being discharged, use the physical exam to emphasize the many normal aspects of the child as well as manifestations of the syndrome.

During the first few days after the diagnosis has been made, recall that parents are not only grieving the loss of an expected normal child but also going through the natural process of bonding to a newborn baby. After the first few interviews, the parents should be acquainted with community resources and can be referred to the appropriate agency or infant programs that deal with children with developmental difficulties. Many parents express particular interest during this time in meeting other parents who have a child with Down syndrome and to have accurate and current reading material. The internet offers hundreds of contact points regarding Down syndrome. The web pages for two of the large support groups, Down Syndrome Congress and Down Syndrome Society, are excellent resources. Referral to a local support group or parent-to-parent contact is always appropriate in these situations and has become a component of routine care.

Each family will proceed through this adjustment process at a different rate. Feelings of denial, anger, guilt, and sadness mixed with natural tendencies to bond to their newborn baby will affect the family's understanding and perhaps even the reception of technical information. Over the last two decades, a clear trend toward presenting information in a hopeful and optimistic manner has been the approach rather than overemphasizing disabilities and problems. Eliminating the inappropriate and misleading stigma that has surrounded the diagnosis of Down syndrome for decades goes a long way toward improving parental adjustment in this setting.

Trisomy 18 (Edwards Syndrome)

The distinct pattern of malformation known as *Edwards syndrome* caused by trisomy 18 is the third most common autosomal disorder and occurs in about 1 in 6000 live-born infants. Trisomy 18 is also a common and important recognizable chromosomal cause of stillbirth, and among live-born cases, females comprise four times the number of cases as males. Similar to trisomy 21, trisomy 18 occurs with increased frequency as a woman ages. Infants with trisomy 18 have a recognized pattern of multiple congenital anomalies and an increased neonatal and infant mortality rate. The constellation of findings is as recognizable to the experienced clinician as Down syndrome (Fig. 10-11).

The pattern of abnormalities observed in infants with trisomy 18 consists of prenatal growth deficiency of length and weight, a distinctive face characterized by a high forehead and small facial structure and mouth, short sternum, and a characteristic set of hand findings consisting of overlapping fingers and hypoplastic nails (Fig. 10-11). Ninety percent of children with trisomy 18 have structural heart malformations, usually consisting of a ventricular septal defect with a polyvalvular dysplasia; some children will have more serious malformations such as hypoplastic left heart or a double outlet right ventricle.

Neonatal and infant mortality are increased; 50% of children with trisomy 18 syndrome die in the first week of life, and about 90% have died by 1 year of age. The cause of most infant deaths is probably central apnea. The common heart malformations observed in infants with trisomy 18 are rarely the sole cause of death but may contribute to early death of some children. Individuals who survive into later infancy and childhood consistently have a significant developmental disability. The degree of disability is marked enough that children with trisomy 18 do not usually walk unsupported or develop expressive language. However, all children progress slowly in attaining milestones, recognize their families, and demonstrate skills that are usually age-appropriate for a 6- to 12-month-old child. Some older children develop skills such as feeding themselves and understanding cause and effect comparable to the developmental age of a 2-year-old. The plight of families who have an infant with trisomy 18 is obviously overwhelming. Decisions around management during newborn and early infancy are complex, and practitioners who care for families of children with trisomy 18 have both the challenge and the opportunity to support the parents in a memorable and significant manner (see Chap. 7).

Ninety-five percent of infants with Edwards syndrome have three copies of the entire chromosome 18. The remaining 5% have either mosaicism or partial trisomy of most of the long arm of 18. The chance for recurrence in future pregnancies is about 1% in families where the mother is less than 35 years old, and it is most likely the age-specific risk for the older mothers. As in Down syndrome and all other chromosome syndromes, parents should be referred to a parents' support group. The Support Organization for Trisomy 18, 13, and Related Disorders (SOFT), *http://www.trisomy.org*, is a valuable resource for families of children with trisomy 18 and 13 and other chromosome syndromes that involve similar medical difficulties.

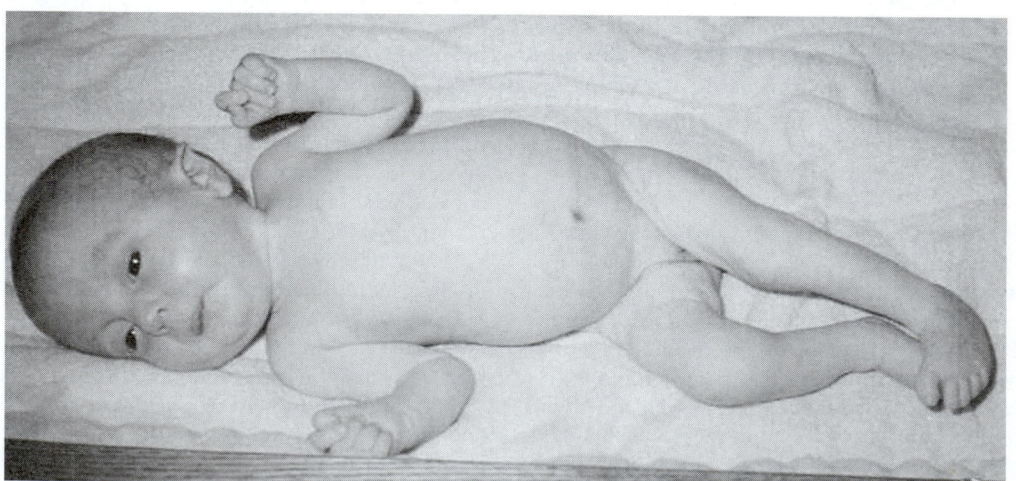

FIGURE 10-11   A newborn girl with trisomy 18 (Edwards syndrome). Note a short sternum, overlapping fingers with clenched fists, and a left-sided clubfoot. *(From Jorde LB, Carey JC, Bamshad MJ, White RL: Medical Genetics. St. Louis, Mosby, 2000.)*

Trisomy 13 (Patau Syndrome)

Trisomy 13, also referred to as *Patau syndrome,* is the fourth most common autosomal disorder in humans and has a prevalence of about 1/10,000 to 1/15,000 live births. The pattern of malformations observed in children with trisomy 13 is the combination of an orofacial cleft, microphthalmia, and posterior polydactyly of the limbs (Fig. 10-12A). The entire spectrum of the facial characteristics associated with holoprosencephaly, ranging from cyclopia to premaxillary agenesis, can be seen in infants with trisomy 13. Similar to trisomies 18 and 21, congenital heart malformations are common in infants with trisomy 13 and occur in about 80% of affected infants. The prognosis for both survival and development is similar to that of children with trisomy 18. However, for infants with trisomy 13, the presence of holoprosencephaly is probably the single most important finding that predicts survival. To this end, it should be noted that most children with trisomy 13 who survive early infancy usually do not have holoprosencephaly (Fig. 10-12B).

Approximately 80% of children with trisomy 13 have three complete copies of chromosome 13, and most of the remaining cases have three copies of the long arm of chromosome 13 caused by an unbalanced robertsonian translocation. Only a few percent of children with trisomy 13 are mosaic. The recurrence risk for trisomy 13 is similar to that for trisomy 18.

Common Deletion Syndromes

The first deletion or partial trisomy described in humans was 18p in 1963. Deletions of the distal portions of chromosomes 4p, 5p, and 18q have well-characterized patterns of malformation. Chromosome catalogs and the database of Schinzel provide further details. Unlike the classical autosomal trisomy syndromes, the phenotypic spectrum of these and other partial monosomy and trisomy conditions varies substantially, contingent on the size of the extra or missing chromosomal segments and whether one or more chromosomes are involved. However, determination of natural history of these conditions is often complex because of the selection bias of case reports that tend to report findings in infants and young children.

Wolf-Hirschhorn syndrome (WHS) was first described in the early 1960s and is related to partial loss of material from the distal short arm of chromosome 4. The frequency is estimated to be about 1/50,000 births with a female predominance. Early case reports suggested that about one-third of these children died in infancy, but there are now many adolescents and adults with WHS.

The phenotype of WHS is quite characteristic and consists of pre- and postnatal growth deficiency, microcephaly, a characteristic appearance of the nose, hypertension, a short philtrum, and hypotonia. Congenital heart malformations are observed in about one-half of cases. Problems in infancy consist primarily of severe feeding difficulties and a marked increased incidence of seizures, which occur in almost 90% of children with WHS. The severity of the seizures seems to diminish after the first few years of life, and they cease by the age of 10 years. The developmental disability of children with WHS is significant, but there are a number of older children who are able to walk unsupported and gain toilet control. A few children speak in phrases or sentences. Children with WHS should be monitored for visual and hearing problems when young and scoliosis as older children and adolescents. Similar to the autosomal trisomies, guidelines for routine supervision have been proposed, and there exists a support group for families of children with WHS.

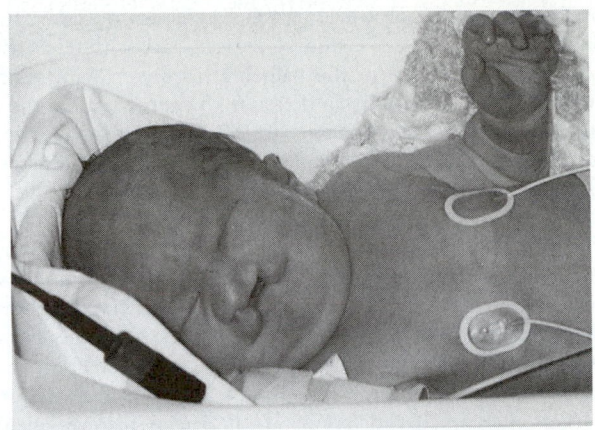

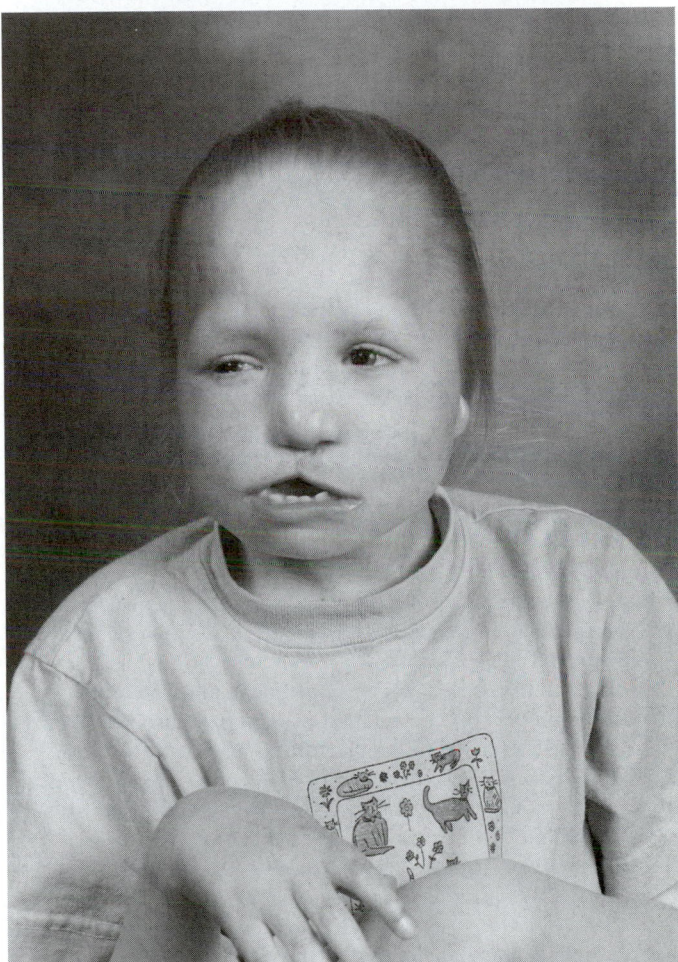

FIGURE 10-12   A. Newborn showing the features of trisomy 13 (Patau syndrome). Note the bilateral cleft lip and broad nasal bridge and posterior polydactyly of the left hand. (*From Jorde LB, Carey JC, Bamshad MJ, White RL: Medical Genetics. St. Louis, Mosby, 2000.*) B. An older child with trisomy 13. Note the repaired cleft lip.

Cri-du-chat syndrome is caused by a deletion of the short arm of chromosome 5p and is one of the most well-known chromosome disorders because of the famous and distinctive cry. Other than the cry, which is said to resemble the sound of a cat and is caused by an anatomic alteration of the larynx, none of the phenotypic abnormalities is specific. However, the facial characteristics are quite similar in early childhood, including a round face with telecanthus and mild down-slanting of the palpebral fissures. Major malformations are less common in 5p deletion syndrome than in the autosomal trisomes, although about 30% of children will have a heart defect. The degree of developmental disability is also significant, but similar to WHS, the original case reports probably reflected only the most severely affected children.

The 18q deletion syndrome, sometimes referred to as *De Grouchy syndrome,* is characterized by variable microcephaly and developmental disabilities. Growth deficiency is also observed, although it is less frequent than in the other autosomal syndromes. The severity of abnormalities appears to be related to the size of the monosomic region (ie, a larger deletion is associated with more problems than is a smaller deletion). Craniofacial features include deep-set eyes and a notable mid-facial hypoplasia, producing a facial gestalt that is characteristic. The fingers are thin, and there are often prominent dimples at the elbow and shoulder joints. Major malformations are less common than in the autosomal trisomy syndromes, but narrowed or atretic ear canals are a hallmark of the condition, and the presence of this finding in a child with multiple minor anomalies should raise the suspicion of 18q deletion syndrome.

Microdeletion Syndromes

The microdeletion syndromes are exemplified by the 11p monosomy syndrome, which is characterized by aniridia and Wilms tumors, previously known as the *WAGR syndrome,* which is owed to haploinsufficiency of two identified genes, *PAX6* and *Wilms tumor 1 (WT1).* The notion that these disorders may be caused by deficiency of contiguous genes in the deleted chromosome region led to the widely described concept of *contiguous gene syndromes.* This particular term is used less often now because it became clear that almost all deletion syndromes fall to some extent under this umbrella.

One of the most exciting discoveries surrounding microdeletion syndromes was the recognition in the late 1980s that a deletion of chromosome 15q11 caused two separate conditions, Prader-Willi syndrome and the Angelman syndrome, depending on whether the deleted region was on the paternal or maternal chromosome, respectively (Fig. 10-4). These observations eventually led to an increased understanding of the concept of genomic imprinting. Both conditions are currently diagnosed in the clinical setting using FISH techniques to identify the deleted region (see plate 27) or DNA methylation studies that can discriminate between the genes inherited from mother and father. Table 10-10 includes the other microdeletion syndromes (i.e., 22q11 deletion syndrome, trichorhinophalangeal syndrome, and Williams syndrome).

One microdeletion syndrome that warrants expanded discussion is the 22q11 deletion syndrome, which is a fascinating account of how technological advances helped explain seemingly disparate but previously recognized entities. The 22q11 deletion syndrome has been referred to by many different eponyms and labels, and this has led to considerable confusion. In the past, the 22q11 deletion syndrome was referred to as the *DiGeorge syndrome; Sprintzen syndrome; velocardiofacial syndrome;* or *cleft palate, absent thymus, congenital heart disease* (CATCH 22). All these labels have some merits but also considerable disadvantages. Thus, this condition is most properly referred to as the *22q11 deletion syndrome.*

Estimates of frequency of 22q11 deletion syndrome suggest that it occurs in about 1 of every 4000 to 5000 infants. Indeed, the 22q11 deletion syndrome is responsible for a substantial percentage of newborns with conotruncal heart malformations (eg, about 30% of infants with truncus arteriosus have a 22q11 deletion). However, a deletion of chromosome 22q11 produces an extremely variable syndrome.

The 22q11 deletion syndrome phenotype consistently includes a characteristic craniofacial appearance (Fig. 10-13), but this finding is particularly subtle in the newborn. By 6 to 12 months the facial features are usually recognizable, although they are not distinctive. The majority of patients have some T-cell dysfunction and are occasionally labeled as having the *DiGeorge syndrome.* However, this T-cell dysfunction is not a specific etiologic entity but an anomaly of pharyngeal development that is observed in many different conditions, although the most common cause is 22q11 deletion syndrome. Cleft palate or, more commonly, velopharyngeal insufficiency is observed in the majority of patients with 22q11 deletion syndrome. Learning disabilities are common in older children, but mental retardation is uncommon and not to be expected. A national support and foundation offer a number of valuable resources for the families of children with 22q11 deletion syndrome (*www.ggc.org/ucfsup.html*).

The microdeletion of chromosome 22q11 is sometimes visible on a routine karyotype. However, the diagnosis is confirmed most commonly using FISH (see Plate 27) to detect the absence of genes in the region deleted in most patients. Because of the heart defects observed in children with 22q11 deletion syndrome, all children with a conotruncal heart defect should be tested for the 22q11 deletion.

Other Aneusomy Syndromes

Other important chromosome syndromes include those caused by deletions of 9p and 13q. More than a hundred cases of each of these conditions have been reported and thus their clinical characteristics are well described. The 13q deletion syndrome is of particular importance, because children with deletions involving the q14 band are predisposed to the development of a retinoblastoma.

The most common partial trisomy syndromes involve trisomy of the 4p, 5p, and 9p. Patients with these less common aneusomy syndromes present with multiple congenital anomalies or developmental delay. As in the case of all aneusomy syndromes, the phenotypes of children affected with these conditions are relatively well delineated (see Table 10-10). In all cases of partial monosomy or trisomy, parental karyotypes should be performed to look for associated structural rearrangements that may predispose to a partial monosomy or trisomy. Consequently, the recurrence risk in these situations depends on parental karyotype.

It is beyond the scope of this chapter to describe the many uncommon chromosome syndromes associated with partial deletion or duplication of a chromosome. Clinical phenotypes have been associated with partial monosomy or trisomy of some portion of the long and short arms of every chromosome. The phenotypes associated with these chromosomal abnormalities are highly variable and hard to define because of the varying types of chromosome duplications and deficiencies. For example, several different phenotypes have been associated with deletions of different parts of the long arm of chromosome 1.

Sex Chromosome Abnormalities

About 1 in 500 live-born infants has an abnormality of the X or Y chromosomes. Three conditions—47,XXY (Klinefelter syndrome), 47,XYY, and 47,XXX—comprise over 80% of this group of disor-

TABLE 10-10

MULTIPLE CONGENITAL ANOMALY SYNDROMES

DISORDER	MAJOR MANIFESTATIONS	LABORATORY/X-RAY	INHERITANCE (OMIM #)	GENE LOCUS/ GENE PRODUCT
Chromosome Instability Syndromes				
Ataxia-telangiectasia (see Chap. 20)	Growth deficiency; CNS deterioration; ataxia; telangiectasia; frequent infections; malignancies	Immunodeficiency (deficient T cell, low IgA), increased frequency of some breaks; ↑ AFP, chromosome 11q22	AR (208900)	11q22/ATM peptide
Xeroderma pigmentosum	Extreme photosensitivity; skin atrophy; pigmentary changes; malignancies	Defective DNA repair in UV light; UV-induced sister chromatid exchange; several subtypes mapped to different chromosomes	AR (278700) multiple complement groups: A, C, D, E, F, G	9q22/XPA peptide
Bloom syndrome (see Chap. 20)	Prenatal growth deficiency; microcephaly; malar hypoplasia; facial telangiectasia; malignancies	Increased chromosome breaks and sister chromatid exchanges; chromosome 15q26.1	AR (210900)	15q26/DNA helicose
Fanconi anemia	(See syndromes of limb defects with hematologic abnormalities, below)			
Craniofacial syndromes				
Goldenhar (oculoauricularvertebral dysplasia spectrum/OAV)	See syndromes associated with branchial arch derivative anomalies (Table 10-11)			
Treacher Collins syndrome (mandibulofacial dysostosis)	See syndromes associated with branchial arch derivative anomalies (Table 10-11)			
Velocardiofacial syndrome	See syndromes associated with cleft lip and/or palate (Table 10-11)			
Van der Woude syndrome	See syndromes associated with cleft lip and/or palate (Table 10-11)			
Nager syndrome	See syndromes associated with branchial arch derivative anomalies (Table 10-11)			
Kabuki syndrome (Niiakawn-Kuroki)	See syndromes associated with cleft lip and/or palate (Table 10-11)			
Stickler syndrome	See syndromes associated with cleft lip and/or palate (Table 10-11)			
Oral-facial-digital syndrome type I	See syndromes associated with cleft lip and/or palate (Table 10-11)			
Coffin-Lowry syndrome	Coarse features; mental retardation, vertebral defects; tufted distal phalanges; scoliosis	Skeletal findings on x-ray	X-linked (303600)	Xp22/RSK2/kinase
Oto-palato-digital syndrome type I	Short stature; thick skull; hypertelorism; microstomia; hypodontia; cleft palate; small trunk; short and broad distal phalanges, nails, and metacarpals	Skeletal findings on x-ray	XR (311300)	Xq28/–
Alagille syndrome	Long, thin face; biliary and cardiac anomalies; Axenfeld eye anomaly	Cardiac abnormalities on echocardiogram	AD (118450)	20p12/JAGGEI
Waardenburg syndrome I	See syndromes associated with hypertelorism or frontonasal malformation (Table 10-11)			
Syndromes characterized by overgrowth				
Prader-Willi syndrome (Fig. 10-5) (see also Angelman syndrome)	Hypotonia; obesity; narrow bifrontal skull; almond-shaped eyes; hypoplastic genitalia; small hands and feet; mental retardation; polyphagia	Deletion of paternal chromosome 15q11 or maternal uniparental disomy 15q11; methylation studies	Sporadic (few inherited chromosomally) (176270)	15q11-13/–
Sotos syndrome	Large for gestational age; macrocephaly; prominent forehead; down-slanting eyes; hypertelorism; mental retardation	Advanced bone age	Sporadic (117550)	—
Weaver syndrome	Large for gestational age; macrosomia; camptodactyly; distinctive face	Advanced bone age	Sporadic (277590)	—
Beckwith-Wiedemann syndrome	Macrosomia; macroglossia; omphalocele; ear fissures; facial hemangioma; mental retardation	Polycythemia, hypoglycemia, duplication of paternal chromosome 11p on DNA studies	Sporadic, AD (130650)	11p15/–

(continued)

TABLE 10-10   Continued

DISORDER	MAJOR MANIFESTATIONS	LABORATORY/X-RAY	INHERITANCE (OMIM #)	GENE LOCUS/ GENE PRODUCT
Bardet-Biedl syndrome	Obesity, retinitis pigmentosa, syndactyly; polydactyly; hypoplastic genitalia; mental retardation; diabetes mellitus; renal disease	Serum glucose, urinalysis, renal findings	AR (209900, 605231)	Multiple loci/*MKK* gene
Proteus syndrome	Large hands or feet; hemihypertrophy; nevi; subcutaneous tumors; accelerated growth	Pelvic lipomas on abdominal ultrasound	Sporadic (176920)	—
Limb deficiency syndromes				
Femoral hypoplasia—distinctive face syndrome	Short nose; hypoplastic alae nasi; long philtrum; Robin cleft micrognathia; hypoplastic femurs and fibulae	Skeletal findings: vertebral defects short/absent femurs	Sporadic, occurs in infants of diabetic mothers (134780)	—
Ectrodactyly-ectodermal dysplasia-clefting (EEC) syndrome	Split hand/foot malformation; ectodermal dysplasia; cleft lip/palate	Renal defects on ultrasound	AD (604292)	3q27/p63
Hypoglossia-hypodactylia syndrome	Small to absent tongue; short to absent digits	—	Sporadic (10330)	—
Möbius syndrome	Cranial nerve defects; hypoplastic tongue or digits, limb deficiency, Poland anomaly	—	Sporadic (157900)	—
Holt-Oram syndrome	Variable upper limb deficiency; triphalangeal thumb, congenital heart defect, especially atrial septal defect	Cardiac abnormalities on ECG, echocardiogram	AD (142900)	12q24/TBX5
Syndromes of limb defects with hematologic abnormalities (see Chap. 19)				
Fanconi anemia syndrome	Pancytopenia; hypoplastic thumb and radius; hyperpigmentation; abnormal facies	Bone marrow hypoplasia; increased chromosome breakage; skeletal x-ray	AR (227650) Multiple complement groups	16p/A-FANC
Diamond-Blackfan syndrome (Aase syndrome)	Triphalangeal thumb; radial hypoplasia; hypoplastic anemia; congenital heart defect	Bone marrow	AD (105650)	19q13/ribosomal protein S19
Thrombocytopenia-absent radius (TAR) syndrome	Thrombocytopenia; absent radii; normal thumbs	Platelet count; bone marrow	AR (274000)	—
Arthrogryposes (multiple congenital contractures)				
Amyoplasia	Multiple contractures with shoulders in internal rotation, elbows in extension, wrists in plantar flexion, feet in equinovarus; facial hemangiomas	—	Sporadic (108110)	—
Freeman-Sheldon syndrome (whistling face syndrome)	Distal arthrogryposis; restricted mouth movement; ptosis and facial hypoplasia, scoliosis	—	AD (193700)	11p15/-
Congenital contractural arachnodactyly (Beal syndrome)	Arthrogryposis; arachnodactyly; kyphoscoliosis; abnormal helix of ear	—	AD (121050)	5q23/fibrillin-2
Pena-Shokier "syndrome" (fetal akinesia sequence)	Generalized arthrogryposis; hypertelorism; malformed ears; micrognathia; pulmonary hypoplasia; usually lethal	—	AR (208150)	—
Cerebro-oculo-facio-skeletal syndrome	Finger, knee, elbow contractures; microcephaly; blepharophimosis, serious CNS abnormalities, microphthalmia	—	AR (208150)	—
Multiple pterygium syndromes	Multiple joint webs; arthrogryposis; several types with variety of additional anomalies, some lethal	Skeletal finding on x-ray in cervical fusion	AR, AD, sporadic (253290) heterogeneous	—
Popliteal web syndrome	Popliteal webs, lip pits; cleft lip/palate; genital hypoplasia; nail dysplasia	—	AD (119500)	1q/32/-
Distal arthrogryposis Type IA	Camptodactyly, foot deformities	—	AD (108120)	9p2-9q2

(continued)

TABLE 10-10   Continued

DISORDER	MAJOR MANIFESTATIONS	LABORATORY/X-RAY	INHERITANCE (OMIM #)	GENE LOCUS/ GENE PRODUCT
Syndromes with severe neurologic abnormalities				
Meckel-Gruber syndrome	Encephalocele; polycystic kidney, polydactyly; lethal	—	AR (249000)	17q22/-
Miller-Dieker syndrome	Lissencephaly; microcephaly; micrognathia; anteverted nares	CT scan; MR imaging; deletion chromosome 17p13 by FISH	del 17p (146510)	17p/LIS1
Hall-Pallister syndrome	Hypothalamic hamartoblastoma; polydactyly; imperforate anus	CT scan; MRI; cranial ultrasonography; chromosome 3/7 translocation	Sporadic, AD (146510)	7p/GLI3
Angelman syndrome (see also Prader-Willi syndrome and Fig. 10-5)	Microcephaly; prognathism; ataxia; seizures; paroxysmal laughter; mental retardation	Deletion of maternal chromosome 15q11 or paternal uniparental disomy	Sporadic (few inherited) (105830)	15q11-13/ubiquitin-protein ligase
Warburg (HARD ± E) syndrome	Hydrocephalus; agyria; retinal dysplasia; encephalocele	CT scan; MR imaging, ophthalmology muscle evaluation	AR (236670)	—
Metabolic syndromes with congenital anomalies (see Chap. 9, 24)				
Congenital hypothyroidism	Large fontanelle; macroglossia, umbilical hernia	Hyperbilirubinemia; delayed bone age; decreased plasma T_4; increased plasma TSH	Sporadic, inherited forms uncommon	—
Menkes syndrome	Progressive neurologic deficit; sparse and broken hair; pili torti; skeletal changes	Decreased serum cooper and ceruloplasmin; skeletal x-ray	X (309400)	Xq13/ATPase copper transport protein
Zellweger syndrome	Hypotonia; flat occiput; extranuchal skin; epicanthal folds; camptodactyly; hepatomegaly; cerebral defects; retinal lesions; renal cortical cysts	Peroxisome defect; increased very long chain fatty acids; stippled bones; increased phytanic and pipecolic acids	AR (214100)	Locus heterogeneity/ peroxin gene
Glutaric acidemia type II	Hepatomegaly, facial dysmorphism, renal cysts, GU anomalies, acrid color	Nonketotic hypoglycemia; metabolic acidosis; hyperammonemia; organic aciduria	AR (231680)	15q23/electron transfer flavoprotein
Neonatal adrenoleukodystrophy	Seizures, demyelination, adrenal hypoplasia, retinitis pigmentosa, deafness, hepatomegaly	Peroxisome defect; increased phytanic, pipecolic, and very long chain fatty acids	AR (600414)	12p13/peroxisome receptor 1
Rhizomelic chondrodysplasia punctata	Short limbs, nasal hypoplasia, cataracts, ichthyosis	Peroxisome defect, increased phytanic, pipecolic acid; decreased plasmalogens; stippled bones; vertebral body clefts	AR (215100)	PEX7
Smith-Lemli-Opitz syndrome	Short stature; microcephaly; ptosis; epicanthal folds; anteverted nares; broad alveolar ridges; syndactyly toes 2–3; cryptorchidism; hypospadias; mental retardation	Cholesterol metabolism: elevated 7 dehydrocholesterol deficiency of delta-7 reductase	AR (270400)	11q12/delta-7-reductase
Associations				
VATER	Vertebral defects, anal atresia, tracheoesophageal fistula, radial dysplasia, renal dysplasia, congenital heart defect	Vertebral defects on x-rays; renal abnormalities on ultrasound	Sporadic (192359)	—
CHARGE	Coloboma, congenital heart defect, choanal atresia, growth and mental retardation; genitourinary anomalies (genital hypoplasia); characteristic ear anomaly	—	Sporadic (214800)	—
Other important syndromes				
MURCS	Müllerian duct aplasia, renal aplasia, cervicothoracic somite dysplasia	Cervical vertebral defects on x-ray	Sporadic (none)	—

(continued)

TABLE 10-10   Continued

DISORDER	MAJOR MANIFESTATIONS	LABORATORY/X-RAY	INHERITANCE (OMIM #)	GENE LOCUS/ GENE PRODUCT
Robinow syndrome	Mild shortness of stature; macrocephaly; hypertelorism; short and anteverted nose; short forearms and digits; hemivertebrae; hypoplastic genitalia	Skeletal findings on x-ray	AD, AR (180700, 268310)	—
Aarskog syndrome	Mild shortness of stature; hypertelorism, ptosis; anteverted nares; short fingers with webbing; clinodactyly; inguinal hernia; shawl scrotum	—	XD (305600)	Xp11/FGD1 protein
Trichorhinophalangeal syndrome I (TRPI)	Bulbous nose; hypoplastic nares; long philtrum; large ears; hypotrichosis; short metacarpals and metatarsals; cone-shaped epiphyses	Skeletal survey	AD (190350)	8q24/-
Langer-Giedion syndrome (TRPII)	Bulbous nose; thickened alae nasi with upward "tenting" long philtrum; hypodontia; cone-shaped epiphyses; exostoses; mental retardation	Skeletal survey, deletion 8q24	Sporadic; familial translocations (150230)	8q24/-
Opitz syndrome (BBB syndrome) (Opitz-Frias)	Hypertelorism; telecanthus; high and broad nasal bridge; cleft lip/palate; hypospadias; laryngo-tracheo-esophageal cleft	—	XD/AD (3000000)	Xp/MID1
Noonan syndrome	Short stature; congenital heart defect; pectus excavatum, webbed neck; hypertelorism; lymphedema; bleeding diathesis; possible mental retardation	Cardiac evaluation; bleeding studies	AD (163950)	12q.../...
Williams syndrome	Growth delay; mental retardation; stellate iris; hypoplastic nails; epicanthal folds; periorbital fullness; anteverted nares; supravalvular aortic stenosis	Microdeletion of chromosome 7q11	Sporadic (194050) deletion 7q	7q11/elastin
Rubinstein-Taybi syndrome	Short stature; mental retardation; antimongoloid slant of eyes; beaked nose; hypoplastic maxilla; broad thumbs and toes; congenital heart defect	Microdeletion of chromosome 16p13.3	Sporadic (180849)	16p13/CREB binding protein
McCune-Albright syndrome	Multiple bony fibrous dysplasia; café-au-lait spots; sexual precocity	Skeletal x-ray; G protein mutation mosaicism	Sporadic	20q13/G protein
Short stature syndromes				
De Lange syndrome	Prenatal growth retardation; microcephaly; hirsutism; synophrys; anteverted nares; downturned mouth; limb reduction defects; congenital heart defects; mental retardation	—	Sporadic (122470)	—
Dubowitz syndrome	Prenatal growth delay; telecanthus; ptosis; blepharophimosis; short palpebral fissures; eczema, hypotrichosis; behavioral problems	—	AR (223370)	—
Russell-Silver syndrome	Prenatal growth retardation; asymmetric, triangular facies; café-au-lait spots; hypoglycemia	Renal findings on ultrasound	Usually sporadic (180860)	—
Seckel syndrome	Pre- and postnatal growth retardation; microcephaly; characteristic nose; mental retardation	—	AR (210600)	—
Hallermann-Streiff syndrome	Proportionately small, hypoplastic mandible; microphthalmia; cataracts, hypoplastic nose; neonatal teeth; hypotrichosis	—	Sporadic (234100)	—

OMIM = Online Mendelian Inheritance of Man: <*http://www.ncbi.nlm.nih.gov/omim/*>, 1999

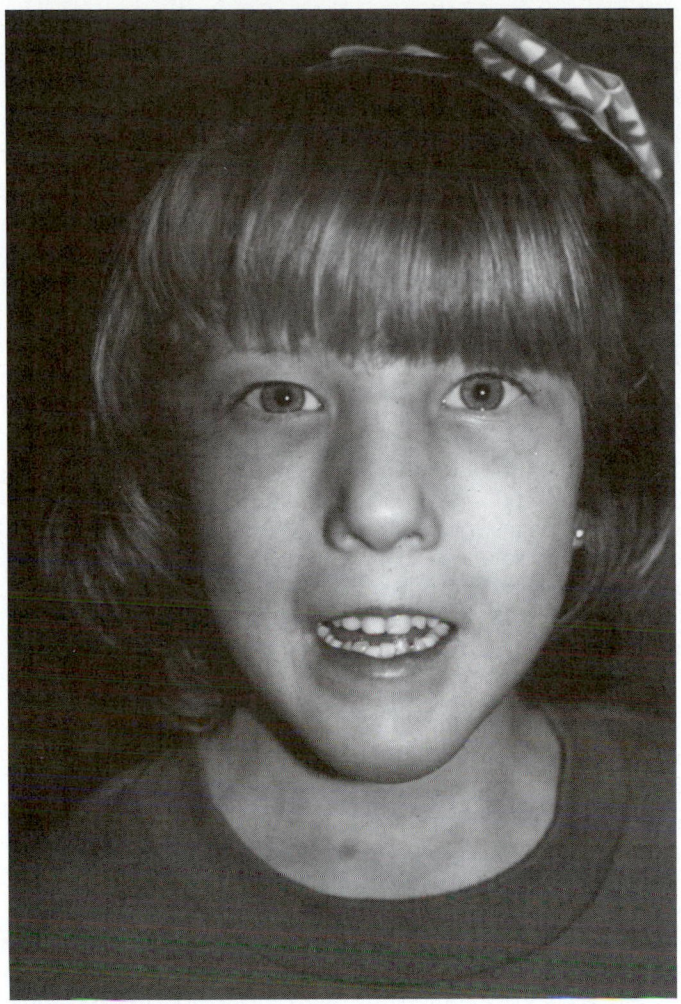

FIGURE 10-13 A 6-year-old girl with the 22q11 deletion syndrome illustrating the distinctive tall nasal root and bridge with a bulbous nasal tip and a small mouth.

ders. The phenotypic characteristics of these conditions are more subtle typically than those caused by abnormalities of the autosomes. Therefore, the diagnosis is not entertained unless there is a high index of suspicion. The phenotypes of children with Turner syndrome, 49,XXXXY, and 49,XXXXX are more distinct. Klinefelter syndrome is discussed in Chap. 24.

Turner syndrome was described in 1938 by Henry Turner in females with proportionate short stature, a lack of secondary sexual characteristics, and gonadal dysgenesis leading to infertility. Many patients with Turner syndrome also have congenital heart defects, most commonly obstructive lesions of the left side of the heart (bicuspid aortic valve in 50% and coarctation of the aorta in 15 to 20%). These abnormalities are the cause of the most significant medical problems in girls with Turner syndrome. However, affected individuals also have a characteristic physical appearance consisting of a triangular shaped face, posteriorly rotated ears, a broad neck, and lymphedema of the hands and feet at birth.

The prevalence of Turner syndrome is low compared to other sex chromosome abnormalities, with about 1/2500 to 1/5000 live-born females having the condition. If no heart abnormalities are present, the primary medical impact of the syndrome is the short stature and the associated infertility and lack of secondary sexual development. In many cases of newborn females with Turner syn-

drome, the phenotype is easily recognizable and diagnosed on clinical features alone. However, the range of abnormalities observed in children with Turner syndrome is much wider than many of the chromosome syndromes. Clues such as dorsal lymphedema, the presence of a left-sided obstructive cardiac lesion, or a webbed neck suggest ordering a katyotype. Guidelines for the routine medical care and health supervision of girls with Turner syndrome have been developed by the American Academy of Pediatrics. Various support groups for families have been established (*www.turner-syndrome-us.org/*).

About half of all females with the Turner syndrome phenotype will have the 45,X chromosome constitution. The remaining cases will have either 45X/46XX mosaicism or some degree of monosomy of the X short arm. There is a long listing of various karyotypic findings associated with the Turner syndrome phenotype.

In addition to the clinical settings mentioned above, the 45X karyotype will also be seen in the evaluation of fetal loss; over 90% of all conceptions with 45X die before birth. The characteristic fetal loss occurs in second trimester with massive hydrops and a nuchal bleb (cystic hygroma). The hydrops and nuchal bleb are related to a malformation of lymph channel development that is probably also responsible for the web neck in live-born females with Turner syndrome.

Other than the common autosomy-trisomy syndromes and the Turner syndrome, knowledge of the natural history of most human chromosome disorders is generally lacking. There are no multicenter studies that describe the occurrence of manifestations over time, and there is little information on children beyond infancy and early childhood.

Chromosomal Instability Syndromes

A number of autosomal-recessive conditions exhibit an increased occurrence of chromosome breaks under specific laboratory conditions. These disorders are termed *chromosome instability syndromes* and include ataxia-telangiectasia, Bloom syndrome, Fanconi anemia, and xeroderma pigmentosum (Table 10-10). Among patients with Fanconi anemia, the frequency of breaks can be increased further when the chromosomes are exposed to certain alkylating agents. Patients with Bloom syndrome have a high incidence of somatic cell sister chromatid exchange. All these syndromes are associated with a significant risk for cancer (Chap. 20).

Substantial progress has been made in understanding the etiology of these conditions. All the chromosome instability syndromes are thought to be the result of faulty DNA replication or repair, although only in the last decade have the genes responsible for these conditions been identified.

References

Baty BJ, Blackburn BL, Carey JC: Natural history of trisomy 18 and trisomy 13: I. Growth, physical assessment, medical histories, survival, and recurrence risk. Am J Med Genet 49:175–188, 1994

Baty BJ, Jorde LB, Blackburn BL, Carey JC: Natural history of trisomy 18 and trisomy 13: II. Psychomotor development. Am J Med Genet 49:189–194, 1994

DeGrouchy J, Turleau C: Clinical Atlas of Human Chromosomes. New York, Wiley, 1984

Jones KL: Smith's Recognizable Patterns of Human Malformation, 4th ed. Philadelphia, Saunders, 1988

Lindsay EA, Greenberg F, Shaffer LG, Shapira SK, Scamber PJ, Baldini A: Submicroscopic deletions at 22q11.2: variability of the clinical picture and delineation of a commonly deleted region. Am J Med Genet 56: 191–197, 1995

Schinzel A: Catalogue of Unbalanced Chromosome Aberrations in Man. 2nd ed., Hawthorne, NY, Walter De Gruyter, 2001

10.3   BIRTH DEFECTS, MALFORMATIONS, AND SYNDROMES

John C. Carey and Michael J. Bamshad

Birth defects are relatively common—about 2% of newborns will have a medically significant malformation recognized during the first day of life. However, approximately one-half of all defects that are present at birth are not diagnosed until later in infancy. Defects that may not be apparent at birth include abnormalities of the central nervous system, cardiovascular system, and sensory systems (eg, hearing, vision) among others. Collectively, it appears that 4% of infants have a medically significant structural anomaly diagnosed by 12 months of age.

Birth defects can be isolated abnormalities or be features of one of the thousands of known genetic syndromes. For example, approximately 75% of children with congenital heart disease have isolated defects, whereas additional birth defects are found in the remaining 25%. The etiology of most birth defects is unknown, although it is estimated that a substantial proportion are caused by mutations in genes that control normal development. Birth defects that arise from an intrinsically abnormal developmental process are called *malformations*. Birth defects can also result from an alteration of the form, shape, or position of a normally formed body part by mechanical forces and are termed a *deformation*. For example, oligohydramnios can result in abnormal mechanical constraints on the joint mobility of a fetus leading to the formation of contractures (eg, clubfoot). Birth defects may also be caused by external interference with an originally normal developmental process, known as a *disruption*. For example, strands of amniotic tissue that become tightly wound around a digit can result in truncation of the digit. An abnormal organization of cells into tissues (eg, a hemangioma) is also sometimes considered a type of birth defect. Of note, malformations and dysplasias are primary disturbances of embryogenesis and histogenesis, respectively. Deformations and disruptions are secondary to a primary extrinsic force.

The presence of a birth defect often evokes an aura of mystery or implies a difference in personhood. Furthermore, terms such as *elfin-like face* and *harelip* implicitly reinforce these differences. Yet families who experience the birth of a newborn with a birth defect wrestle with the same questions about cause, responsibility, and outcome as any other family of a child with a serious pediatric disease. Approaching the diagnosis and management of an infant or a child with a birth defect can also be overwhelming in that thousands of different conditions are associated with birth defects, and strategies to diagnose and treat these conditions change rapidly. Despite these challenges, a logical and systematic approach to the evaluation of children with birth defects and the collection of phenotypic data are important for both diagnostic and therapeutic reasons.

The recognition of a well-characterized disorder, even if the etiology is unknown, provides: (1) information on the pattern of inheritance and recurrence risk, (2) the framework and options for the management of future pregnancies, and (3) information that can be used to make general predictions about future manifesta-

tions and outcomes, including guidelines for routine care and suggestions for educational interventions, especially when a specific behavioral profile has been associated with a condition (eg, Williams syndrome). A specific diagnosis also eliminates the motivation to perform unnecessary testing and enables the use of appropriate screening tools for anticipated problems. For many families, explaining the diagnosis, natural history, and strategy for health care maintenance and anticipatory guidance helps with coping with the uncertainty that typically surrounds genetic disorders.

CLASSIFICATION OF BIRTH DEFECTS

Because our knowledge of the pathogenetic basis of birth defects is limited, all classification schemes of birth defects and malformations are somewhat arbitrary. Most medical textbooks classify birth defects according to the organ system or body part that is affected (eg, cardiovascular system, limbs). Such classifications can help develop intervention strategies (eg, for surgical palliation) and identification of the general causes of these defects. However, the utility of anatomical classifications becomes limited once specific information on the etiology, natural history, and recurrence is required.

Birth defects can also be classified depending on whether they occur as isolated findings or as a component of multiple congenital anomalies. This particular distinction is probably the most valuable in the evaluation of any infant and child with a birth defect. Compared to children with isolated birth defects, children with multiple birth defects have greater morbidity and mortality and are more likely to have a chromosomal abnormality and/or syndrome diagnosis. Birth defects can also be classified by etiologic categories such as chromosome, single gene, multifactorial, and teratogenic.

Categorization of defects by the developmental process that is perturbed is useful for generating hypotheses about causative pathogenetic mechanisms, although many birth defects can result from the perturbation of more than one pathway, making it difficult to identify the primary disturbance. Although no specific classification is appropriate for all cases, birth defects will be presented according to the developmental process that is disturbed to facilitate understanding of pathogenesis and provide a background for understanding future observations. Accordingly, a brief review of the genetic controls of development, and the cardinal processes that, when disturbed, cause birth defects is provided.

10.3.1   Basic Concepts of Development

Michael J. Bamshad

Development is the process by which a fertilized ovum becomes a mature organism capable of reproduction. Thus, a single fertilized egg divides and grows to form different cell types, tissues, and organs, all of which are arranged in a species-specific body plan (ie, the arrangement and patterning of body segments). Many of the instructions necessary for normal development are encoded by genes that are identical in each cell of an organism. The mechanisms by which identical genetic constitutions create a complex adult organism comprised of many different cells and tissues and the determinants of the fate of each cell, that is, what governs a cell, for example, to become a heart cell or a brain cell, are critical processes. Understanding the pathogenesis of human malformation and genetic syndromes is rooted in developmental biological principles.

Evolution of species requires that development of individual organisms be replicated with high fidelity. Otherwise, it might be difficult to recognize that a group of organisms share similar properties that define a species. In sexually reproducing species, the necessary tools and instructions for building an organism that closely resembles its parents are located in the fertilized ovum (zygote). Most of this information is transmitted from parent to offspring via genes that encode signaling molecules and their receptors, DNA transcription factors, components of the extracellular matrix, enzymes, transport systems, and many other proteins. Each of these genetic mediators is expressed in combinations of spatially and temporally overlapping patterns that are used repeatedly to control different developmental processes. Mutations in the genes mediating development are a common cause of human birth defects.

Interactions between neighboring cells are often controlled by proteins that can diffuse across small distances to induce a response and are termed *paracrine factors* because they are secreted into the space surrounding a cell, unlike hormones that are secreted into the bloodstream. Major paracrine-signaling molecules include the: (1) fibroblast growth factor (FGF) family; (2) hedgehog family; (3) wingless (Wnt) family; and (4) transforming growth factor β (TGF-β) family. Mutations in genes encoding these molecules may lead to abnormal communication between cells.

Many different mechanisms regulate the expression of a gene (see Sec. 8.1). Genes encoding proteins that function to activate or repress other genes are called *transcription factors*. Transcription factors commonly do not activate/repress only a single target, but regulate the transcription of many genes that, in turn, regulate other genes in a cascading effect.

Extracellular matrix proteins (EMPs) are secreted macromolecules that serve as scaffolding for all tissues and organs. These molecules include collagens, fibrillins, proteoglycans, and large glycoproteins such as fibronectin, laminin, and tenascin. EMPs are not simply passive structural elements. To facilitate cell migration, EMPs must transiently adhere to a cell's surface, which is accomplished by two families of receptors, integrins and glycosyltransferases. Integrins integrate the extracellular matrix and the cytoskeleton, allowing them to function in tandem.

PATTERN DETERMINATION

The process by which ordered spatial arrangements of differentiated cells create tissues and organs is called *pattern formation*. The general pattern of the animal body plan is laid down during embryogenesis, which leads to the formation of semiautonomous regions of the embryo in which the process of pattern formation is repeated to form organs and appendages. Such regional specification takes place in several steps: (1) definition of the cells of a region, (2) establishment of signaling centers that provide positional information, and (3) differentiation of cells within a region in response to additional cues.

For pattern formation to occur, cells and tissues communicate with each other through many different signaling pathways. These pathways are used repeatedly and integrated with one another to control specific cell fates. For example, patterning of the vertebrate neural tube, somites, and limbs, as well as the way the left is distinguished from right, employs the secreted protein, sonic hedgehog (Shh). In mouse, lack of Shh activity produces a loss of ventral midline development within the central nervous system. In humans, point mutations in *SHH*, the human homologue of *Shh*, cause abnormal midline brain development (eg, holoprosencephaly), severe mental retardation, and early death. However, not all affected individuals have holoprosencephaly; some have only minor birth defects such as a single upper central incisor. Interestingly, attachment of Shh to the lipophilic moiety, cholesterol, appears to be necessary for the proper spatial patterning of hedgehog signaling, which may partly explain how certain human teratogens that inhibit cholesterol biosynthesis as well as disorders of cholesterol metabolism (eg, Smith-Lemli-Opitz syndrome) cause midline brain defects.

Gastrulation

Gastrulation is the process whereby the cells of the blastula are given new positions and neighbors. In the human embryo, gastrulation occurs between days 14 and 28 of gestation. In this process, the embryonic bilaminar disk is transformed into a trilaminar embryo composed of three germ layers: outer ectoderm, inner endoderm, and the interstitial mesoderm. The formation of these layers is a prerequisite for organogenesis. The major structural feature of mammalian gastrulation is the primitive streak, which appears as a thickening of epiblast extending along the anterior to posterior axis.

Neurulation and Ectoderm

Once a trilaminar embryo is formed, the dorsal mesoderm and the overlying ectoderm interact to form the hollow neural tube. This event is called *neurulation* and is mediated by a process called *induction*, which occurs when the cells of one embryonic region influence the organization and differentiation of cells in a second embryonic region. Induction of the neural tube and transformation of the flanking mesoderm into an amphibian embryo with clear anterior/posterior and dorsal/ventral axes is controlled by a group of cells known as the Spemann-Mangold organizer.

Neurulation is a critical event in development that initiates organogenesis and divides the ectoderm into three different cell populations: (1) the neural tube, which will eventually form the brain and spinal cord, (2) the epidermis of the skin, and (3) the neural crest cells. In humans, neural tube closure begins at five separate sites that correspond to the locations of common neural tube defects such as anencephaly (absence of the brain), occipital encephalocele, and lumbar myelomeningocele. Neural crest cells migrate from the neuroepithelium along defined routes to tissues where differentiation into a variety of cell types such as sensory neurons, melanocytes, neurons of the small bowel, and smooth muscle occurs.

Mesoderm and Endoderm

The formation of a layer of mesoderm between the endoderm and ectoderm is one of the major events in gastrulation. Mesoderm can be divided into five components: the notochord; dorsal, intermediate, lateral, mesoderms; and head mesenchyme. The notochord is a transient structure that induces the formation of the neural tube and body axis. Dorsal (paraxial) mesoderm is observed on either side of the notochord and differentiates into sclerotomes, myotomes, and dermatomes that form the axial skeleton, appendicular skeleton and skeletal muscles, and connective tissue of the skin, respectively. Intermediate mesoderm forms the kidneys and genitourinary system. Lateral plate mesoderm differentiates into heart, connective tissue of viscera, and the connective tissue elements of the amnion and chorion. Finally, the muscles of the eyes and head arise from head mesenchyme.

The primary function of embryonic endoderm is to form the linings of the digestive tract and the respiratory tree. Outgrowths of the intestinal tract form the pancreas, gallbladder, and liver. A bifurcation of the respiratory tree produces the left and right lungs. The endoderm also produces the pharyngeal pouches that, in conjunction with cells derived from the neural crest, give rise to endodermal-lined structures such as the middle ear, thymus, parathyroids, and thyroids.

Axis Specification

Animal body plans have evolved into a wide variety of symmetries. Specification and formation of the axes are critical events in development that determine the orientation of the body plan. The proteins mediating these processes are rapidly being discovered. Many of these mediators have additional roles in patterning of the body plan and tissues.

Formation of the Anterior/Posterior Axis

The anterior/posterior axis of a developing mammalian embryo is defined by the primitive streak. At the anterior end of the primitive streak is a structure called the *node*, which is homologous to the Hensen node in birds and contains many of the same proteins found in the amphibian organizer. Patterning of the anterior/posterior axis is controlled by the HOX genes that encode transcription factors containing a DNA-binding domain of about 60 amino acids called the *homeodomain*. In *Drosophila* these genes compose the homeotic gene complex (HOM-C), which has two classes of genes, Antennapedia and Bithorax.

HOX genes are expressed along the dorsal axis from the anterior boundary of the hindbrain to the tail. Within each cluster, 3′ HOX genes are expressed earlier than 5′ HOX genes, termed *temporal collinearity*. Furthermore, the boundaries of expression of 3′ HOX genes extend more anteriorly than those of 5′ HOX genes, referred to as *spatial collinearity*. Thus, *Hoxa-1* expression occurs earlier and more anteriorly than the expression of *Hoxa-2*. These overlapping domains of HOX gene expression produce combinatorial codes that specify the positional commitment of cells and tissues. Collectively these codes identify various regions along the anterior/posterior axis of the trunk and limbs.

Formation of the Dorsal/Ventral Axis

Dorsal/ventral patterning of the vertebrate depends on the interaction between dorsalizing and ventralizing signals, which are mediated, in part, by molecules that act in a concentration-dependent fashion. Molecules that can promote multiple positive responses from a field of undifferentiated cells as a function of concentration are called a *morphogens*. The function of morphogens can be attenuated or inhibited by antagonists, which bind and inactivate them.

FORMATION OF ORGANS AND APPENDAGES

Subsequent to vertebrate axis determination and gastrulation is the formation of organs and limbs, called *organogenesis*. Many of the proteins used for patterning and growth of organs and limbs are the same molecules used earlier in blastogenesis. However, additional genes that were transcriptionally silent now become active and encode proteins that may act as switches for organ formation or receptors for recognizing patterning information or participate in the expected function of terminally differentiated cells. To date, most of the developmental genes known to cause human birth defects have prominent roles in this period of development. Mutations in genes that disrupt earlier developmental events may be lethal.

Craniofacial Development

Development of the craniofacial region is directly related to the formation of the underlying central nervous system. In mammalian embryos, neural crest cells from the forebrain and midbrain become the nasal processes, palate, and mesenchyme of the first pharyngeal pouch. This mesenchyme forms the maxilla, mandible, incus, and malleus. The neural crest cells of the anterior hindbrain migrate and differentiate to become the mesenchyme of the second pharyngeal pouch and the stapes and facial cartilage. Cervical neural crest cells produce the mesenchyme of the third, fourth, and sixth pharyngeal arches (in humans the sixth pharyngeal arch degenerates), which become the muscles and bones of the neck. The bones of the skull develop directly from mesenchyme produced by neural crest cells via a process called *intramembranous ossification*. Complete fusion of these bones usually does not occur until adulthood. Premature fusion (synostosis) of the skull bones (craniosynostosis) causes the head to be misshapen and can impair brain growth (see Sec. 10.3.4).

Development of the Limb

The developing tetrapod limb is one of the best understood classical models of morphogenesis. Many of the signaling pathways and transcriptional control elements that coordinate limb development in model organisms such as *Drosophila* and chick appear to be conserved in mammals, including humans.

The vertebrate limb is composed of elements derived from lateral plate mesoderm (bone, cartilage, and tendons) and somitic mesoderm (muscle, nerve, and vasculature). The signal that initiates induction of forelimbs and hindlimbs appears to arise in the intermediate mesoderm. Once initiated, proximal/distal growth of the limb bud is dependent on a region of ectoderm called the *apical ectodermal ridge* (AER), which extends from anterior to posterior along the dorsal/ventral boundary of the limb bud.

Mediation of proximal/distal growth by the AER is controlled, in part, by fibroblast growth factors (FGF2, FGF4, and FGF8) that stimulate proliferation of an underlying population of mesodermal cells in the so-called progress zone (PZ). However, maintenance of the AER depends on a signal from a region in the posterior mesoderm of the limb bud known as the *zone of polarizing activity* (ZPA). The signaling molecule of the ZPA is sonic hedgehog (Shh), which is also responsible for dorsal/ventral patterning of the central nervous system and establishment of the embryonic left/right axis. The ZPA also specifies positional information along the anterior/posterior of the limb bud.

Defects of the anterior and posterior elements of the upper limb occur in the Holt-Oram syndrome (HOS) and ulnar-mammary syndrome (UMS), respectively. HOS is caused by mutations in the gene *TBX5*, whereas UMS is caused by mutations in the tightly linked gene *TBX3*. *TBX3* and *TBX5* are members of a highly conserved family of DNA transcription factors containing a DNA-binding domain called a *T-box*.

Organ Formation

Many processes must be coordinated simultaneously to construct a specific arrangement of cells and tissues that manifests the properties of an organ. Similar to limb development, formation of parenchymal organs is notable for the reciprocal induction of the epithelium on the mesenchyme and vice versa. This interaction is mediated by secreted signaling molecules that bind to receptors, transduce the signal through various interconnected pathways, and stimulate or repress DNA transcription. Use of the same elaborate networks to form different organs allows for genomic economy while maintaining developmental flexibility.

Once a specialized cell within an organ is terminally differentiated, various proteins turn on its molecular machinery so that it may perform its fated function. Often development of the organ and function of the differentiated cell are interrelated. Epithelial-mesenchymal interactions are prominent in the development of cutaneous structures (eg, hair, sweat glands, breasts), parenchymal organs (eg, liver, pancreas), lungs, thyroid, kidneys, and teeth. These interactions are dynamic such that expression patterns in the epithelia and mesenchyme change over time.

One of the largest organs in the body is the skeleton. In contrast to the development of cranial bones by intramembranous ossification, most skeletal bone formation takes place using a cartilaginous template called *endochondral ossification*. However, both intramembranous and endochondral ossification are regulated by bone-forming cells called *osteoblasts*. The differentiation of osteoblasts is regulated by an osteoblast-specific transcription factor called *Cfba1*. Targeted disruption of *Cfba1* results in mice with a complete lack of ossification of the skeleton. Heterozygous mice have widened cranial sutures, shortened digits, and abnormalities of the shoulder girdle. Similar defects are found in individuals with cleidocranial dysplasia, which is caused by mutations in *CFBA1*, the human homologue of *Cfba1*.

References

Epstein CJ: The new dysmorphology: application of insights from basic developmental biology to the understanding of human birth defects. Proc Natl Acad Sci U S A 92:8566–8573, 1995

Gilbert SF: Developmental Biology. Sunderland, Sinauer Press, 1999

10.3.2 Approach to the Child with Birth Defects

John C. Carey and Michael J. Bamshad

In the mid-1960s, David W. Smith coined the term *dysmorphology* to describe the field of medicine devoted to the study of abnormal human development. His intent was to propose a term that both replaced teratology (whose literal meaning and reference to monsters was pejorative) and captured the essence of the discipline. The ability to recognize and interpret minor and major anomalies is an important skill that is required for evaluating a child with a birth defect.

A *syndrome* is a pattern of birth defects that are etiologically related and regularly recur in different individuals (eg, Down syndrome). In other areas of medicine, the word *syndrome* often refers to a specific set of symptoms that are not necessarily etiologically related (eg, nephrotic syndrome).

A *sequence* is a primary defect with a secondary cascade of structural changes. Birth defects that represent a sequence are usually localized to a single body area. Whereas a sequence can often be misinterpreted as a group of malformations, more critical inspection reveals a single malformation and a subsequent disruption or deformation. For example, the Pierre Robin sequence is caused by a primary abnormality in mandibular development that produces disruption of palatal closure and secondary obstruction of the airway by the tongue. A sequence can occur in isolation or be a component of an underlying syndrome diagnosis. For example, about 20% of children with Pierre Robin sequence have a disorder of connective tissue called *Stickler syndrome* (characterized by joint hyperextensibility and myopia).

An *association* is two or more primary defects that occur in the same individuals more often than is expected by chance: Defining a group of defects as an association suggests that the anomalies are etiologically related to each other, yet the nature and mechanism of that relationship remains unclear. For example, children with defects of the vertebrae, anus, trachea and esophagus, radius, and kidneys (renal) are often labeled with the acronym *VATER association*. Associations tend to be etiologically heterogenous more often than syndromes, and fewer characteristics of an association are observed in each affected child.

CLINICAL PRACTICE

The approach to a child with birth defects is multifaceted and includes the collection of phenotypic data, determination of the immediate and long-term issues of care, and the provision of the family with psychological support (Fig. 10-14).

Phenotypic data that should be collected include detailed obstetrical, medical, and family histories, a comprehensive physical examination, and ancillary laboratory, physiological, or imaging studies. The gestational and birth history needs to include exposures to over-the-counter and prescription medications as well as illicit drugs, frequency and vigor of fetal movements, intrauterine positioning, quantity and quality of amniotic fluid, maternal medical history, and the results of all prenatal testing. Documentation of at least a three-generation pedigree is also recommended. The pedigree should include information about the occurrence of sudden deaths, unexpected deaths, or early deaths (ie, deaths at less than 55 years of age); individuals with developmental disabilities, unusual behavioral profiles, and/or mental retardation; individuals with birth defects; degree of relatedness of parents (ie, level of consanguinity); and the ethnic background of the family. Examination of photographs of the parents taken when they were children, of siblings, and of extended family members is especially useful when attempting to determine whether a particular physical characteristic is a diagnostic clue, part of the phenotypic background of the family, or both (ie, when a parent or relative is unknowingly affected as well).

Differentiating between "normal" and "abnormal" physical findings represents the cornerstone of phenotype analysis. Many of the physical findings that are considered abnormal and clues to syndromes are found on the head and/or limbs.

For the cranium and face, the various relationships among the many individual components (hair, ears, forehead, nose, eyes, midface, philtral folds, lips, mouth, jaw, neck, and ears) should form a gestalt (ie, a subjective impression of the overall pattern of relationships). Does a particular feature (eg, a hemangioma or region of marked asymmetric growth) make the face look different from what might be anticipated? Are there several features that when juxtaposed with one another make a face look particularly distinguishable? If a physical feature differs from what one considers "normal," consider the mechanism that might have produced this impression. For example, if the ear of an infant appears set too low on the side of the head, is it because the ear is small, posteriorly rotated, or that the superior helix is overfolded? Each of these possibilities can produce the illusion that an ear is set too low. Alternatively, an ear with a normal size and structure but placed at the angle of the mandible indicates that the ear is genuinely set too low.

Each physical feature of the face (or hands or chest, etc.) can be classified as to whether the variation is a minor anomaly or mild malformation. Minor anomalies include both qualitative character-

Approach to management of the child with congenital anomalies

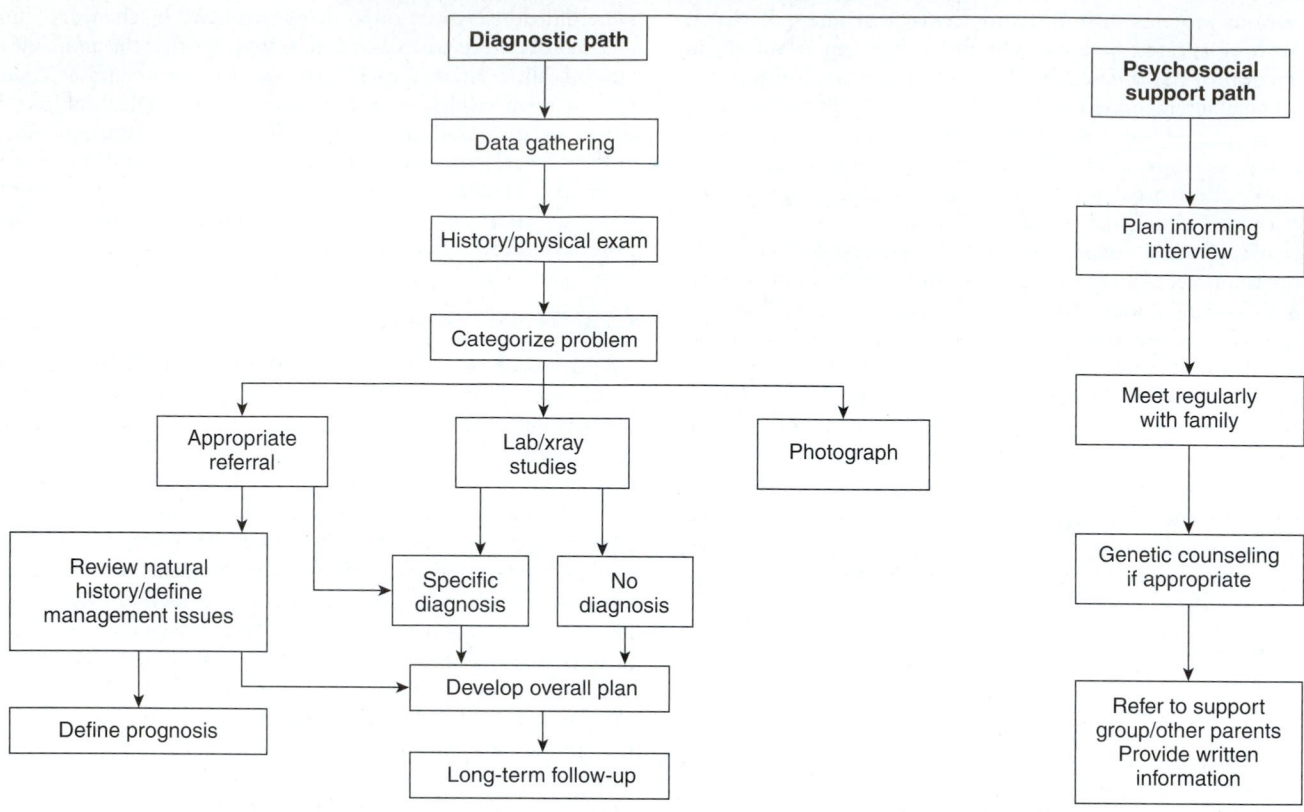

FIGURE 10-14 **The approach to the management of the child with congenital anomalies. Note the diagnostic pathway and the psychosocial path are in parallel. The step involving the categorization of the problem may lead to one of the other diagnostic algorithms.**

istics (eg, size of the nasal tip) that can be challenging to judge as normal versus abnormal as well as features that lend themselves to rapid quantitative measurement (eg, distance between the inner canthal folds). Measurement of many of the quantitative features can be compared to normative data collected from selected groups of individuals considered normal. Each physical characteristic must be considered in the context of the general morphology of the family, their ethnic group, and their continent of origin. Many of the physical findings that are used to distinguish among persons of Asian or African descent are quantitative traits that may differ substantially between groups, alone or in combination. For example, short palpebral fissures are a consistent finding in children with fetal alcohol syndrome. However, wide variation exists in the length of the palpebral fissures among individuals of European, Asian, and/or American-Indian ancestry, which makes the interpretation of the importance of short palpebral fissures challenging. Minor malformations are structural changes of a mild degree that have no intrinsic medical significance (unlike major malformations). Examples include auricular tags and posterior polydactyly.

The measurement of a body part or the relationships between parts is an important component of accurate diagnosis. For example, the length of the ear can be a valuable clue when evaluating a child for fragile X syndrome (characterized by a long ear) or trisomy 21 (characterized by a short ear). Apparently wide-spaced eyes can relate to the presence of epicanthal folds, telecanthus (soft-tissue displacement of the inner canthi), short palpebral fissures, or true ocular hypertelorism. Distinction among these possibilities requires astute observation, knowledge of normal facial structure relation-

ships/proportions, and measurements of the inner canthal/interpupillary and outer canthal distances. These distinctions are crucial, because different syndromes are characterized by different abnormalities of eye placement.

Examination of the limbs should be conducted similarly, and the general relationships among the parts of the hand (eg, length of digits, spacing between digits) should be assessed and subsequently each part should be examined individually. The thumb is a particularly complex body part that requires skill in differentiating between normal variations and abnormal findings. Alterations of the thumb include low-set thumbs (usually hypoplastic with an underdeveloped thenar eminence), tapered thumbs, bifid thumbs, and triphalangeal thumbs (three phalanges instead of two). Examination of the flexion creases on the digits including the thumbs is also a valuable observation because these creases develop between 8 and 10 weeks of embryogenesis, and perturbations of the flexion creases (eg, hypoplasia, absence) reflect an abnormality of fetal movement in the first trimester of gestation. For example, children with multiple congenital contractures caused by a reduced quantity of amniotic fluid in the third trimester may have normal flexion creases, whereas an infant with amyoplasia (a form of arthrogryposis) may have complete absence of the flexion creases.

The recognition of minor and major anomalies helps to determine whether a child may have a multiple congenital anomaly syndrome and, if so, how to proceed toward confirmation of a specific diagnosis. Comparing physical findings in members of a child's extended family may indicate that a child who *apparently* has multiple anomalies simply has an abnormal appearance related to combined

Diagnostic Process

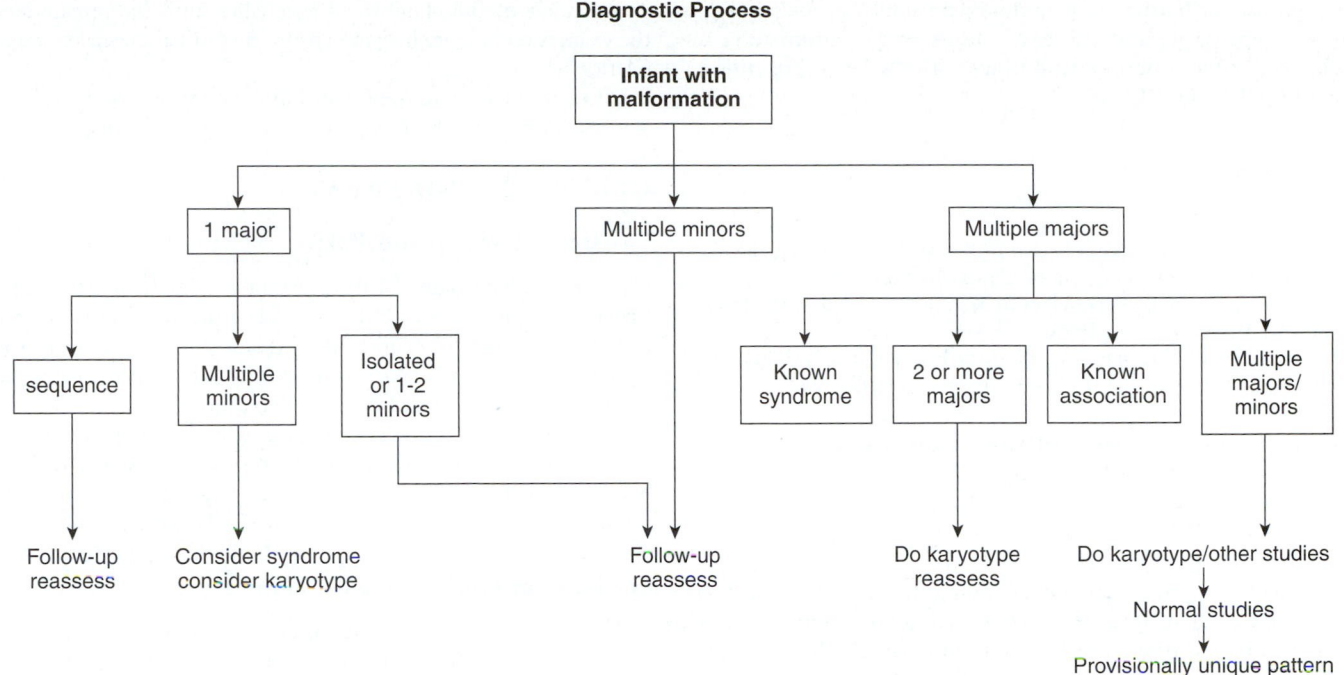

FIGURE 10-15   The diagnostic process for evaluating an infant with malformations, single or multiple. A karyotype is indicated in the child with multiple major anomalies or the child with a single major anomaly and multiple minor anomalies.

effects of the parents' unusual but normal physical characteristics. This underscores the point that overinterpretation of multiple minor anomalies in a child is troublesome. Although 10% of newborns have two or more minor anomalies, the overwhelming majority of these otherwise normal appearing infants do not have a specific syndrome and are unlikely to experience further physical and/or developmental problems.

Minor anomalies often provide useful clues as to whether a more severe defect of a body part or organ may be present. Many purported associations have been overstated in the past and probably have little significance (eg, the purported association of accessory nipples and renal defects). However, some minor anomalies are clearly markers for more important underlying defects. For example, the presence of a deep sacral dimple, commonly with an overlying patch of hair or a hemangioma, should prompt further investigation for spinal dysraphism. Pits in the skin or tags of skin near the external ear should bring to mind specific syndrome diagnoses (eg, branchial-otorenal syndrome) and are associated with an increased risk of hearing loss.

The most pivotal step in the diagnostic algorithm of a child with multiple congenital anomalies is categorizing the pattern of findings into a unifying etiologic mechanism (whether or not characteristic of a known syndrome) (Figs. 10-14 and 10-15). Concluding that a child's phenotypic findings probably fit a recognizable pattern in contrast to representing an isolated defect is critical (Fig. 10-15). A child with an isolated finding (eg, isolated cleft lip) may require no further diagnostic evaluation. In contrast, a child with a pattern of phenotypic findings consistent with a unifying etiologic mechanism may need substantially more testing to reach a diagnosis. For example, a karyotype is virtually always indicated in children with a recognizable but undiagnosed pattern of congenital defects. A skeletal survey may help resolve the diagnosis in a child

with a limb abnormality or who is suspected of having a skeletal dysplasia.

Most children who are being evaluated for multiple congenital anomalies do not need to be tested for an inborn error of metabolism (see Chaps. 8 and 9). For example, children who have disorders of amino acid metabolism do not present typically with birth defects. However, some conditions with inborn errors of metabolism do present with malformations and/or dysplasias (see Sec. 9.1.7 and Table 9-10). To complicate matters further, some very well-known multiple congenital anomaly syndromes have turned out to be caused by defects of metabolism. For example, Smith-Lemli-Opitz (SLO) syndrome, characterized by multiple malformations and variable cognitive abnormalities, has recently been shown to be a defect of cholesterol biosynthesis caused by mutations in the gene 7-dehydrocholesterol reductase.

If trisomy 21 is excluded, at least 50% of the remaining newborns with multiple congenital anomalies will not have a specific diagnosis. Because of improvements in our understanding of the breadth and evolution of phenotypes as well as advances in diagnostic testing, periodic reevaluation of this group of children will occasionally lead to identification of a diagnosis. Nevertheless, children without a specific diagnosis are frequently labeled with a provisionally unique pattern of anomalies, and their care should be determined via a prudent but flexible strategy of empirical management. Predictions about the outcome of a specific defect should be shared with the family. Genetic counseling about the recurrence risk can be based on empirical estimates. Depending on the organ system involved, an appropriate specialist may facilitate the management of a child with multiple congenital anomalies. Providing adequate psychosocial support for a family is crucial while they are both adapting to the reality that they have child with a birth defect, a child that may have special needs, and realizing that they may be at a high risk for having another child with similar problems (Fig. 10-14). Appropriate and effective delivery of this information is important, and long-term relationships with the family are critical (see Tables 10-7 and 10-8).

References

Hall JG, Froster-Iskenius UG, Allanson JE: Handbook of Normal Physical Measurements. New York, Oxford University Press, 1989

McKusick VM. Mendelian Inheritance In Man, 12th ed., Baltimore, Johns Hopkins University Press, 1998

POSSUM/OSSUM Database c/o Murdoch Institute, Royal Columbian Hospital, Flemington Rd., Parkville, Victoria, Australia 3052

10.3.3 Syndromes of Multiple Congenital Anomalies/Dysplasia

John C. Carey

Rather than memorize the essential findings for all or even most of the multiple congenital anomaly syndromes, it is far more useful to develop a strategy for syndrome recognition that is both logical and practical, yet flexible enough to generalize among genetic conditions. Part of this strategy requires availability of information about genetic disorders that is accurate, succinct, and complete. Many specific textbooks and online databases provide this information (see references for Sec. 10.3.2), and these resources increasingly are becoming available to the families of children with genetic conditions. Consequently, parents are frequently very knowledgeable about a diagnosis before their health care provider has had the opportunity to discuss it with them. Nevertheless, many of the concepts that are required to fully understand the implications of a diagnosis are difficult to grasp. Consequently, primary care physicians must be able to explain the principles of human genetics to the families of children with varied conditions.

It is beyond the scope of this section to provide a comprehensive description of the hundreds of relatively common genetic conditions or thousands of rare genetic disorders. Thus, Table 10-10 summarizes some of the multiple congenital anomaly/dysplasia syndromes.

10.3.4 Craniofacial Disorders

Michael L. Cunningham

Malformations of the face and skull represent a large portion of structural malformations in humans and can have significant morbidity, often requiring surgical management in the first few months of life. Many children with craniofacial disorders are managed in multidisciplinary teams including pediatricians, geneticists, plastic and reconstructive surgeons, maxillofacial surgeons, orthodontists, otolaryngologists, audiologists, speech pathologists, neurosurgeons, social workers, nutritionists, and nurse specialists. This section describes the major types of craniofacial malformations, their classification, and suggested management (Table 10-11).

All children born with structural malformations of the face and/or skull require a careful physical examination, because many have associated multisystem involvement (20%). The obvious malformations of craniofacial structures can be so dramatic that the examiner overlooks other less obvious associated anomalies that deserve attention and may help to establish a diagnosis. Leaving the

examination of the craniofacial anomalies until the remainder of the exam is completed helps to ensure that other anomalies are not overlooked.

There is a national support group for persons with craniofacial abnormalities, Let's Face It (www.faceit.org/letsfaceit).

CLEFT LIP AND PALATE

Isolated Cleft Lip and Palate

Cleft lip and/or palate (CLP) represent one of the most common structural malformations in humans. The incidence of CLP varies depending on race (1/250 births in some native American tribes, 1/350 in Asian-Americans, 1/700 in white Americans, and 1/3000 in black Americans). However, more recent studies indicate that these may be overestimations. Cleft lip and palate in combination is the most common form of orofacial clefting with isolated cleft lip and isolated cleft palate having the following relative frequencies: 1:1.2:2.5 (CL:CP:CLP) (Fig. 10-16).

Heredity of Cleft Lip and Palate

Although most cases of CLP represent sporadic (stochastic) events, recurrence in families with isolated CLP is well documented. CLP represents a multifactorial disorder that can have a hereditary component. If the first-born child of a couple has CLP, the risk of the next child having CLP is 3 to 4%. This risk is increased (1) with the birth of additional children with orofacial clefts and (2) if a parent has a cleft and is considered to have a "hereditary predisposition" of CLP (see Sec. 10.1.2). Presently, there is no way to discern sporadic from hereditary forms of isolated CLP, and thus statistically based risk estimates are currently used for genetic counseling. Recently, periconceptual folate supplementation has been suggested to reduce the risk of CLP in these "at risk" families, and some centers have implemented this recommendation.

Although the majority of cases of CLP represent isolated cases, over 290 known syndromes are associated with CLP. Relatively common syndromic forms of orofacial clefting include: Stickler syndrome, 22q11 deletion (velocardiofacial) syndrome, Van der Woude syndrome, and ectodermal dysplasia ectrodactyly and clefting (EEC) syndrome (Table 10-11). Isolated cleft palate, rather than cleft lip and/or palate, is more frequently associated with syndromic forms.

Airway Management

The specifics of management of children with orofacial clefting are center-specific. The first issue to be addressed with any child born with orofacial clefting is airway management. Although children with isolated cleft palate are more prone to airway difficulties, children with CLP can also have airway obstruction, particularly those with Robin sequence: association of micrognathia (small mandible) with isolated clefting of the secondary palate. Although the pathogenesis of Robin sequence has not been proved, it is thought that micrognathia leads to cleft palate in the sixth to seventh weeks of gestation because of superior displacement of the tongue into the nasopharynx preventing fusion of the palatal shelves. The combination of micrognathia and a palatal cleft often results in glossoptosis (pathologic position of the tongue leading to airway obstruction), which requires urgent care ranging from prone positioning to emergent tracheostomy. Some centers use other surgical and nonsurgical means of treatment for more severe obstruction (eg, nasopharyngeal intubation). The American Academy of Pediatrics

TABLE 10-11

MALFORMATIONS AND SYNDROMES INVOLVING CRANIOFACIAL STRUCTURES

SYNDROME NAME	CLINICAL PHENOTYPE	INHERITANCE	OMIM#	GENE	LOCUS
Syndromes associated with cleft lip and/or palate					
Velocardiofacial syndrome	Pierre Robin sequence, cleft palate, small open mouth, myopathic facies, retrognathia, prominent nose with squared-off nasal tip, hypoplastic nasal alae, learning disability, behavioral/psychiatric disorders, short stature, slender tapering digits (overlapping features with DiGeorge syndrome)	AD	192430	Microdeletion of chromosomal region containing multiple genes	22q11.2
Robin sequence	Micrognathia, cleft palate, glossoptosis, airway obstruction, feeding difficulties	Sporadic, associated with several syndromes with recessive and X-linked forms suggested	261800		
Stickler syndrome, type I; type II	Cleft palate, micrognathia, glossoptosis, severe myopia, risk of retinal detachment, midfacial hypoplasia, hearing impairment, arthropathy, pectus, short fourth, fifth metacarpals	AD	180300; 184840	Collagen, type XI, alpha-2 chain (COL11A2)	6p21.3
Van der Woude syndrome	Cleft lip and/or palate, lower lip pits/cysts, ankyloglossia	AD	119300		1q32
Smith-Lemli-Opitz syndrome (see Chap. 9)	Cleft palate, micrognathia, short nose, ptosis, high square forehead, microcephaly, hypospadias, cryptorchidism, VSD, TOF, hypotonia, mental retardation, postaxial polydactyly, 2-3 syndactyly of feet, defect in cholesterol biosynthesis	AR	270400	delta-7-reductase (DHCR7)	11q12-11q13
Ectrodactyly ectodermal dysplasia and clefting syndrome (EEC1; EEC2)	Cleft lip and/or palate, split-hand/split-foot, ectodermal dysplasia (sparse hair, dysplastic nails, hypohydrosis, anodontia), GU anomalies	AD	129900; p63 602077		3q27; 7q11.2-q21.3
Ankyloblepharon ectodermal dysplasia and clefting syndrome (AEC)	Cleft lip and palate, intraoral alveolar bands, maxillary hypoplasia, filiform eyelid fusion (ankyloblepharon), ectodermal dysplasia (sparse hair, dysplastic nails, hypohydrosis, anodontia)	AD	106260	p63	3q27
Kabuki syndrome (Niiakawn-Kuroki)	Cleft palate, arched eyebrow with sparse lateral hair, long palpebral fissures, eversion of lateral third of lower eyelid, brachydactyly, short fifth metacarpal, congenital heart defects, postnatal growth deficiency/dwarfism, mental retardation	Sporadic ?AD	147920		
Oral-facial-digital syndrome	Paramedian cleft of upper lip, asymmetric cleft palate, accessory oral frena, lobulate tongue with hamartomas, broad nasal root, small nostrils, syndactyly, brachydactyly, postaxial polydactyly, polycystic renal disease, agenesis of the corpus callosum, X-linked dominant lethal in males	X-linked	311200		Xp22.3-p22.2
Pallister-Hall syndrome	Cleft palate, flat nasal bridge, short nose, multiple buccal frenula, microglossia, micrognathia, malformed ears, hypothalamic hamartoblastoma, hypopituitarism, postaxial polydactyly with short arms, imperforate anus, GU anomalies, IUGR	AD	146510	GLI-Kruppel family member 3 oncogene (GL13)	7p13
Early amnion rupture sequence	Cleft lip and palate, oblique facial clefts, focal areas of scalp aplasia, constriction bands with terminal limb amputations and syndactylies, occasional anencephaly, encephalocele, and ectopia cordis	Sporadic	217100		
Syndromes associated with branchial arch derivative anomalies					
Hemifacial microsomia (craniofacial microsomia, oculo-auriculo-vertebral spectrum)	Unilateral or bilateral microtia/anotia/atresia, preauricular tags, conductive hearing loss, microphthalmia, mandibular hypoplasia, maxillary hypoplasia, macrostomia, vertebral anomalies (hemivertebra and fusions), structural renal malformations/agenesis	Sporadic	164210		

(continued)

TABLE 10-11 Continued

SYNDROME NAME	CLINICAL PHENOTYPE	INHERITANCE	OMIM#	GENE	LOCUS
Goldenhar syndrome	Unilateral or bilateral microtia/anotia/atresia, preauricular tags, facial tags, conductive hearing loss, epibulbar lipodermoids, microphthalmia, mandibular hypoplasia, maxillary hypoplasia, macrostomia, cervical vertebral anomalies (hemivertebra and fusions), congenital heart disease	Sporadic, ?AD	164210		
Branchiootorenal syndrome (BOR syndrome)	Branchial cleft fistulas, preauricular pits, cochlear and stapes malformation, mixed sensory and conductive hearing loss, renal dysplasia/aplasia	AD	113650	Eyes absent-1 gene (EYA1)	8q13.3
Treacher Collins mandibulo-facial dysostosis	Cleft palate, malar hypoplasia, micrognathia with prominent antigonial notch, down-slanting palpebral fissures, lower eyelid coloboma (missing medial lower lid lashes), microtia/atresia, conductive hearing loss	AD	154500	Treacle (TCOF1)	5q32-q33.1
Nager syndrome (preaxial acrofacial dysostosis)	Cleft palate, malar hypoplasia, down-slanting palpebral fissures, lower eyelid coloboma (missing medial lower lid lashes), mandibular hypoplasia, microtia/atresia, conductive hearing loss, radial ray hypoplasia, hypoplastic/absent thumbs, paternal age effect (dominant and recessive inheritance suggested)	AD/AR	154400		9q32
Miller syndrome (postaxial acrofacial dysostosis)	Cleft palate (occasional cleft lip), malar hypoplasia, down-slanting palpebral fissures, lower eyelid coloboma (missing medial lower lid lashes), mandibular hypoplasia, microtia/atresia, conductive hearing loss, postaxial limb deficiency, absent fifth digital rays, short forearms, gastric and midgut volvulus	AR	263750		
Syndromes associated with craniosynostosis					
Crouzon syndrome	Craniosynostosis (coronal>lambdoid>sagittal), proptosis, hypertelorism, strabismus, maxillary hypoplasia	AD	123500	Fibroblast growth factor receptor-2 (FGFR2)	10q26
Saethre-Chotzen syndrome	Coronal craniosynostosis (unilateral or bilateral), acrocephaly, brachycephaly, hypertelorism, strabismus, maxillary hypoplasia, ptosis, small ears, cutaneous 2-3 syndactyly of hands (variable)	AD	101400	Twist (TWIST)	7p21
Muenke syndrome	Unilateral coronal>bicoronal craniosynostosis, occasionally with limb anomalies similar to Jackson-Weiss syndrome (OMIM#123150), also known as *nonsyndromic craniosynostosis:* overlap with the Saethre-Chotzen (OMIM#101400) phenotype has been suggested	AD	602849	Fibroblast growth factor receptor-3 (FGFR3)	4p16.7
Apert syndrome	Craniosynostosis (coronal>lambdoid>sagittal), brachycephaly, acrocephaly, hypertelorism, proptosis, strabismus, maxillary hypoplasia, narrow palate (cathedral ceiling palate), invariable syndactyly (cutaneous and boney), "single nails"	AD	101200	Fibroblast growth factor receptor-2 (FGFR2)	10q26
Pfeiffer syndrome	Craniosynostosis (coronal>sagittal>lambdoid), acrocephaly, hypertelorism, proptosis, maxillary hypoplasia, broad first digits with radial deviation	AD	101600	Fibroblast growth factor receptor-1, 2 (FGFR1, FGFR2)	8p11.2-p11.1; 10q26
Jackson-Weiss syndrome	Craniosynostosis (usually coronal), midfacial hypoplasia, enlarged great toes, 2-3 syndactyly, tarsonavicular and calcaneonavicular fusions in the feet, widely variable expression (eg, foot anomalies without synostosis)	AD	123150	Fibroblast growth factor receptor-2 (FGFR2)	10q26
Crouzon syndrome with acanthosis nigricans	Coronal craniosynostosis with craniofacial appearance of Crouzon syndrome (OMIM#123500) associated with acanthosis nigricans	AD	134934.001	Fibroblast growth factor receptor-3 (FGFR3)	4p16.6
Craniosynostosis, type 2 (Boston-type craniosynostosis)	Coronal craniosynostosis, forehead retrusion, frontal bossing, turribrachycephaly, occasional Kleeblattschaedel deformity (cloverleaf skull), short first metatarsals	AD	123101	Msh homeobox homolog 2 (MSX2)	5q34-q35
Carpenter syndrome (acrocephalopolysyndactyly type II)	Craniosynostosis (coronal>lambdoid>sagittal), hypertelorism, proptosis, acrocephaly, preaxial polysyndactyly, mental retardation, only well described recessive craniosynostosis syndrome	AR	201000		

(continued)

TABLE 10-11   Continued

SYNDROME NAME	CLINICAL PHENOTYPE	INHERITANCE	OMIM#	GENE	LOCUS
Kleeblattschadel (cloverleaf skull deformity)	Cloverleaf skull (trilobar) coronal, lambdoid, sagittal, and metopic craniosynostosis, proptosis to exophthalmos, hydrocephalus, presumed dominant—all cases to date sporadic, can be seen as part of thanatophoric dysplasia (OMIM#187600) and most forms of syndromic craniosynostosis, a descriptive term for head shape in these cases of severe craniosynostosis	AD	148800		
Antley-Bixler syndrome	Coronal and lambdoid craniosynostosis, brachycephaly, proptosis, choanal stenosis/atresia, maxillary hypoplasia, humeroradial synostosis, camptodactyly, multiple contractures	AR	207410		
Syndromes associated with calvarial size/shape anomalies					
Holoprosencephaly 3 (HPE3)	Microcephaly, ocular hypotelorism to cyclopia, single central incisor, proboscis, midface hypoplasia, brain anomalies range from holoprosencephalon to a structurally normal brain, mental retardation to lethality	AD	142945	Sonic hedgehog	7q36, several other loci identified for this phenotype
Cleidocranial dysostosis	Brachycephaly, frontal and parietal bossing, wormian bones, persistent open anterior fontanelle, maxillary hypoplasia, delayed eruption of deciduous and permanent teeth, supernumerary and fused teeth, hypoplastic to absent clavicles, brachydactyly, joint laxity	AD	119600	Core-binding factor, runt domain, α subunit 1 (CBFA1)	6p21
Neurofibromatosis, type I	Macrocephaly, neurofibroma, plexiform neurofibroma (occasionally intraorbital), dysplasia of the sphenoid bone, hypertelorism, other malignancies, learning disabilities to mental retardation	AD	162200	Neurofibromatosis, type 1 gene (NF1)	17q11.2
Basal cell nevus syndrome (Gorlin syndrome)	Macrocephaly, broad facies, frontal and biparietal bossing, hypertelorism, mandibular prognathism, odontogenic keratocysts of jaws, cleft lip and palate, brachydactyly, rib anomalies, calcification of falx cerebri, mental retardation, paternal age effect	AD	109400	Patched (PTC)	9q22.3-q31
Syndromes associated with hypertelorism or frontonasal malformation					
Aarskog syndrome	Hypertelorism, widow's peak, ptosis, down-slanting palpebral fissures, strabismus, maxillary hypoplasia, broad nasal bridge with anteverted nostrils, occasional cleft lip and/or palate, floppy ears, brachydactyly, clinodactyly, joint laxity, shawl scrotum, cryptorchidism, moderate short stature, females mildly affected	X-linked	100050	Faciogenital dysplasia 1 (FGD1)	Xp11
Waardenburg syndrome (type I, type IIA)	Partial albinism, white forelock, premature greying, heterochromia iridis, wide nasal bridge, short philtrum, cleft lip and/or palate, occasional cochlear deafness, spina bifida, lumbosacral myelomenigocele, occasional Hirschsprung disease, dystopia canthorum and absent vagina specific to type I	AD	193500; 193510	Paired box homeotic gene-3 (PAX3); microphthalmia-associated transcription factor (MITF)	2q35; 3p14.1-p12.3
Craniofrontonasal dysplasia	Coronal synostosis (unilateral>bilateral), frontonasal dysplasia with marked hypertelorism, broad to bifid nose, brachycephaly, broad great toe, syndactyly, hypermobile shoulders with pseudoarthrosis of clavicle, female preponderance (more severe in females), males may have shawl scrotum	X-linked	304110		Xp22
Craniometaphyseal dysplasia	Craniofacial hyperostosis (leonine facies), hypertelorism, wide nasal bridge, cranial nerve compression (facial palsy, deafness, anosmia), characteristic diaphyseal sclerosis and metaphyseal dysplasia of long bone	AD/AR	123000		5p15.2-p14.1
Acrocallosal syndrome	Macrocephaly, prominent forehead and occiput, hypertelorism, absent corpus callosum, hypospadias and cryptorchidism, postaxial polydactyly and hallux duplication, hypotonia and severe mental retardation	AR	200990		12p13.3-p11.2

(continued)

751

TABLE 10-11 Continued

SYNDROME NAME	CLINICAL PHENOTYPE	INHERITANCE	OMIM#	GENE	LOCUS
Greig cephalopolysyndactyly syndrome	Macrocephaly without synostosis, high forehead and bregma, frontal bossing, hypertelorism, bifid great toe and thumb, polysyndactyly, advanced bone age	AD	175700	GLI-Kruppel family member 3 oncogene (GLI3)	7p13
Binder syndrome	Maxillonasal dysplasia, maxiallary hypoplasia, short nose with flat nasal bridge and absent anterior nasal spine, convex upper lip	AD	155050		
Reiger syndrome, type 1	Hypertelorism, telecanthus, iris dysplasia, microcornea, corneal opacity, maxillary hypoplasia, broad nasal root, prognathism, protruding lower lip, short philtrum, microdontia, hypodontia, cone-shaped teeth, hypospadias, anal stenosis	AD	180500	RIEG1	4q25-q26
Other craniofacial syndromes					
Sturge-Weber syndrome	Hemangiomata in the distribution of the trigeminal nerve can involve the choroid of the eye and the meninges, glaucoma, seizures (those with seizures often have learning disability), no clear evidence for mendelian inheritance	Sporadic	185300		
Beckwith-Wiedemann syndrome	Coarse facial features, macroglossia (often with secondary maxillary and mandibular deformity), ear lobe creases, posterior auricular pits, midface hypoplasia, omphalocele, generalized overgrowth or hemihypertrophy, visceromegaly, Wilms tumor (and other malignancies), cryptorchidism, cardiomyopathy	AD, imprinting at 11p15.5	130650	Cyclin-dependent kinase inhibitor IC (CDKN1C)	11p15.5
Cornelia de Lange	Microbrachycephaly, micrognathia, low hairline, synophrys, arched eyebrows, long eyelashes, thin upper lip, low-set ears, spade-like hands, 2-3 syndactyly of toes (more severe limb anomalies common), failure to thrive, prenatal growth deficiency, short stature	Sporadic, dominant forms suggested	122470		
Romberg syndrome (progressive hemifacial atrophy, Parry-Romberg syndrome)	Slowly progressive hemifacial atrophy, normal at birth, atrophy of facial soft tissue and bone, always unilateral with well-demarcated median border, malocclusion, hemiatrophy of tongue, enophthalmos on affected side, hyperpigmentation and vitiligo, can be associated with trigeminal neuralgia, migrane-like headaches, and contralateral Jacksonian epilepsy	AD	141300		
Freeman-Sheldon syndrome	Whistling facies (with small mouth and vertical skin folds on chin), hypertelorism, "sunken" eyes, small nose, adducted thumbs, ulnar deviation of hands, camptodactyly, clubfoot	AD	193700		
Trichorhinophalangeal syndrome (type I)	Micrognathia, "pear-shaped" nose, short stature, brachydactyly with short metacarpals, normal intelligence	AD	190350		8q24.12

752

Note: Not all phenotypic features listed will necessarily be present in every case. If considering one of these diagnoses, it is suggested to review one or more of the following references:
OMIM: Online Mendelian Inheritance of Man: <http://www.ncbi.nlm.nih.gov/omim/>, 1999; Gorlin RG, Cohen MM, Levin LS: Syndromes of the Head and Neck, 3rd ed. New York, Oxford University Press, 1990; Jones, KL: Smith's Recognizable Forms of Human Malformation, 5th ed. Philadelphia, Saunders, 1996; National Institute of Dental and Craniofacial Research: Listing of craniofacial-oral-dental diseases and disorders: <http://www.nidr.nih.gov/cranio/home.html>, 1998.

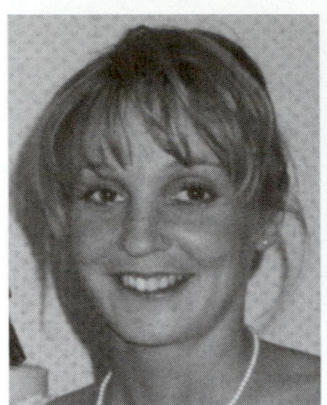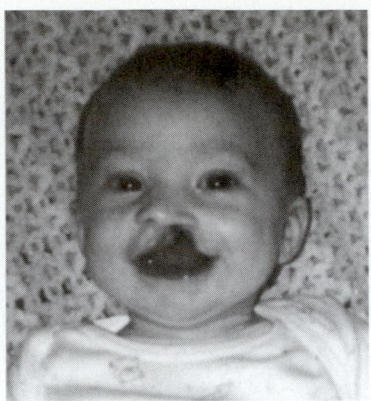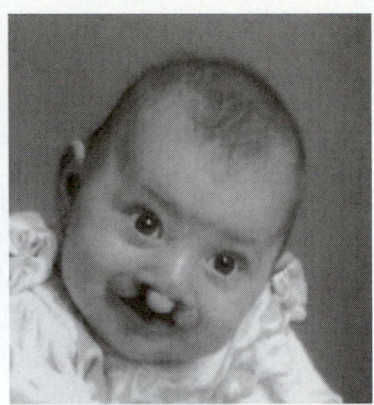

FIGURE 10-16 Variable expression of cleft lip and palate in two children born to different unaffected fathers. Their mother shows no manifestation of orofacial clefting.

supports prone positioning of infants with orofacial clefting (and other craniofacial malformations) to alleviate minor airway obstruction.

Feeding

Children with cleft palates usually cannot solely breast-feed because an intact palate is necessary to generate the negative pressure required for suckling. For this reason, a number of specialized feeding techniques (eg, squeeze bottles) have been devised. Any child with nonsyndromic cleft palate should be expected to have normal weight gain. A general rule of thumb is that the child should take approximately 2.5 ounces/pound per day to have good growth. Adequate weight gain is imperative in these children, who will require surgical interventions in the first year of life. Infants with cleft palate often have minor swallowing difficulties and/or gastroesophageal reflux (particularly syndromic forms such as 22q11 deletion syndrome).

Surgery

The timing and nature of surgical management for children with orofacial clefting differs from center to center. In general, closure of the lip occurs within the first 5 months of life, and the palate is repaired by age 12 months. The timing of palatal closure by 1 year of age is suggested to optimize speech and language development, but early palate closure (under 6 months) may impede normal midfacial development. Special attention needs to be given to the child with isolated cleft palate associated with respiratory difficulties (particularly in cases of Robin sequence with evidence of glossoptosis) because closure of the palate can exacerbate airway compromise. In addition to the obvious need for surgical management of the orofacial clefting, children with cleft palate (including submucous cleft palate) have an increased risk of persistent middle ear effusions (MEE) and/or chronic recurrent otitis media (OM). In these children, who are predisposed to language difficulties caused by their clefts, hearing must be optimized. The predisposition for MEE and OM is due to abnormal function of the distal eustachian tube. Most children with overt cleft palate require the placement of tympanostomy tubes in the first year of life. Additional surgeries that may be necessary in this population include bone grafting of the alveolar cleft when present, pharyngeal surgeries for improvement of speech, and midfacial advancement in cases of midfacial hypoplasia.

HEMIFACIAL MICROSOMIA (CRANIOFACIAL MICROSOMIA, OCULOAURICULOVERTEBRAL DYSPLASIA)

The association of external ear anomalies (microtia, anotia, canal atresia, and/or preauricular tags) with maxillary and mandibular hypoplasia is the second most common craniofacial malformation in humans. This condition is known as *hemifacial microsomia* (HFM) (also known as *craniofacial microsomia, oculoauriculovertebral dysplasia, lateral face dysplasia,* or *first and second branchial arch syndrome*) and can present with a wide degree of severity. HFM can present as an isolated malformation of craniofacial structures or as a component of a multiple malformation complex (eg, Goldenhar syndrome, VATER). Since approximately 30% of cases of HFM are bilateral, some clinicians prefer the term *craniofacial microsomia* for this disorder.

ISOLATED HEMIFACIAL MICROSOMIA

At birth, the most critical issues surround airway and feeding difficulties. Severe cases of HFM have airway obstruction caused by the combination of mandibular and maxillary hypoplasia. The management of upper airway obstruction can range from prone or side-lying positioning, to early mandibular surgery, to tracheostomy. Severe mandibular and/or maxillary deficiency can negatively impact oral feeding in the first months of life. Temporary nasogastric and, in some cases, gastrostomy feeding may be necessary.

In the first year of life, children with HFM should have renal ultrasonography to rule out clinically significant renal malformations (10 to 15% estimated to have some renal anomaly). In addition, between 25 to 30% of children with "isolated" HFM have cervical vertebral anomalies. As the structural malformations of the spine rarely have functional significance until later childhood, spine films can be delayed for the first few years to allow more complete ossification and improve the quality of the study. Any child over age 5 years with HFM participating in activities that put the cervical spine in jeopardy should have full c-spine (including flexion/extension views to rule out cervical instability) and thoracic/lumbar radiographs prior to participation. All children with unilateral or bilateral HFM should have formal audiologic evaluation (brainstem auditory evoked response, or other accepted means). Even in apparently unilateral cases, an increased incidence of bilateral hearing loss occurs and is most commonly conductive (owing to the mal-

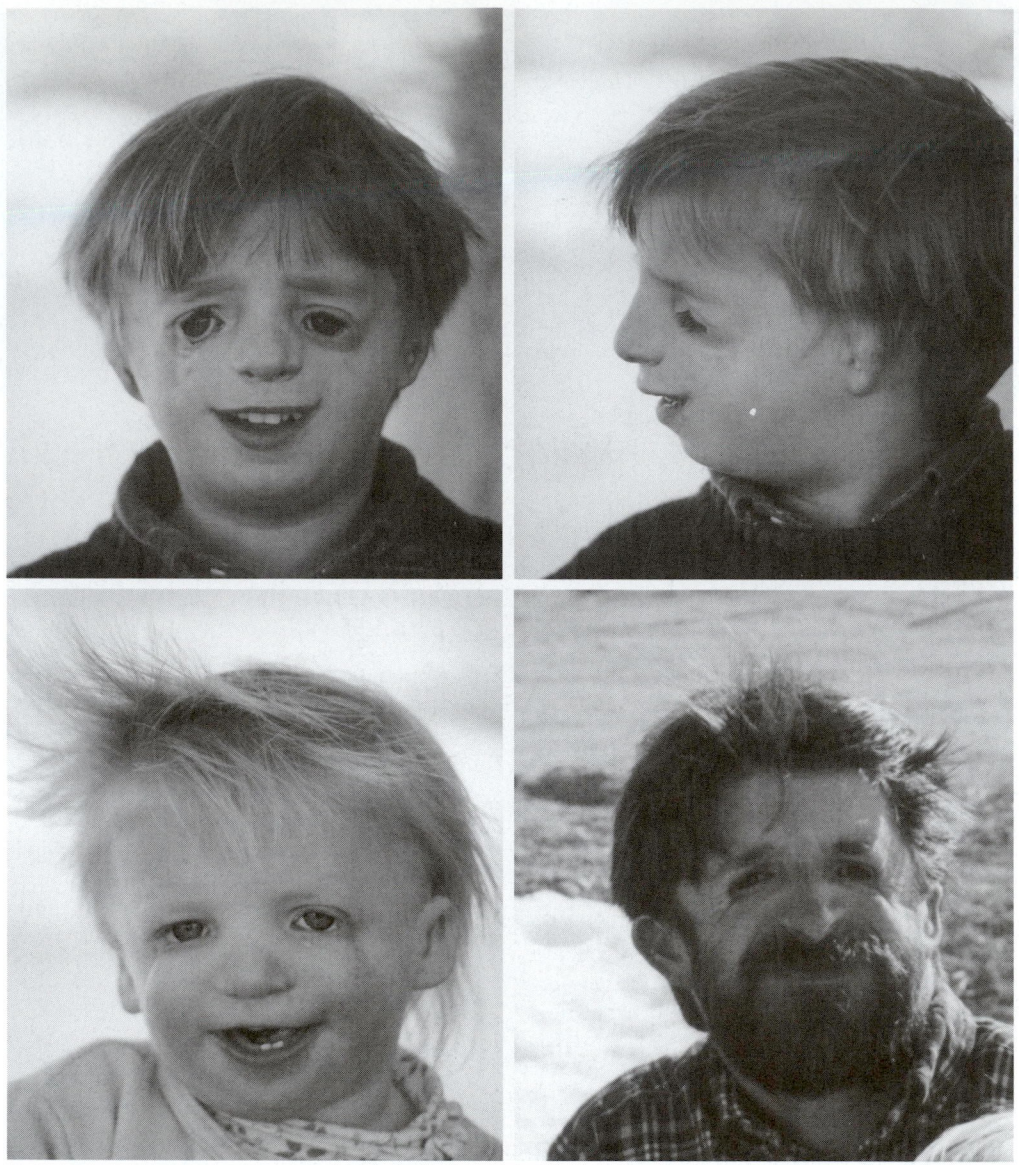

FIGURE 10-17 Two siblings top panels and lower left panel with variable manifestations of autosomal dominant Treacher Collins Syndrome. Their father, lower right panel was the first individual in his family known to have Treacher Collins Syndrome. Both children were born with cleft palate while their father has an intact palate.

formation of the middle ear ossicles), but a mixed sensory and conductive loss can be present (particularly in syndromic forms, BOR; see Table 10-11).

Beyond the issues present in the first months of life, the major issues for children with HFM are related to (1) hearing, (2) functional reconstruction of the maxilla and mandible, (3) orthodontic issues, and (4) external ear reconstruction.

GOLDENHAR SYNDROME

Goldenhar syndrome is the association of HFM, epibulbar lipodermoids (fibro-fatty masses on the globe of the eye, usually lateral and/or inferior), vertebral defects (fusions and/or hemivertebrae of the cervical-lumbar vertebrae), cardiac malformations (from VSD to outflow tract malformations), and structural kidney malformations. Many experts feel that Goldenhar may represent the more severe end of a clinical spectrum of isolated HFM. In fact,

up to 15% of children born with "isolated" HFM can present with cervical vertebral anomalies and/or structural kidney defects.

BOR SYNDROME

Branchio-oto-renal dysplasia (BOR syndrome) is an autosomal-dominant condition that shares many features with HFM. Although patients with BOR syndrome rarely have severe maxillary or mandibular deficiency, the syndrome is characterized by the presence of external ear malformations ("lop" ear), preauricular pits and occasional tags, branchial cleft fistulae of the neck (sometimes extending into the pharynx), mixed sensory and conductive hearing loss associated with cochlear and ossicular chain malformations, renal dysplasia/aplasia, and occasional pulmonary hypoplasia. Recently, a mutation of *EYA1* has been identified as the cause of some cases of BOR syndrome (Table 10-11).

TREACHER COLLINS SYNDROME (MANDIBULOFACIAL DYSOSTOSIS TYPE I)

Treacher Collins syndrome is an autosomal-dominant craniofacial malformation syndrome that shares some phenotypic features with HFM and is caused by a mutation in the *TREACLE* gene, although significant phenotypic variability between or within affected families occurs. The disorder is characterized by mandibular and maxillary hypoplasia, zygomatic arch clefts, and variable microtia/anotia/atreasia. The hypoplastic mandible usually has a characteristic exaggeration of the antigonial notch. Facial features are notable for downward sloping palpebral fissures (owing to lateral orbital clefts), and colobomata of the lower eyelids (Fig. 10-17). Cleft palate occurs in a minority of patients. Cognition is usually normal; other malformations (eg, cardiac) are rare, although conductive hearing loss is frequently associated. The clinical issues of Treacher Collins syndrome are very similar to those of bilateral HFM (respiratory, feeding, mandibular/maxillary surgery, external ear reconstruction). Two more rare forms of mandibulofacial dysostosis include Nager and Miller syndromes (see Table 10-11).

CRANIOSYNOSTOSIS

Craniosynostosis is the pathologic condition of premature fusion of calvarial sutures. The overall incidence of sporadic craniosynostosis is 1 in 1700 to 2500 live births, and the incidence of the hereditary forms is approximately 1 in 25,000. The most common form of single suture fusion is sagittal synostosis (followed by coronal, metopic, and lambdoid, with isolated lambdoid fusion representing only 2 to 3% of all forms of synostosis). Sagittal synostosis is much more common in males (M:F is 5:1). In humans, premature suture fusion results in abnormalities in calvarial shape owing to restriction of growth in the region of a fused suture. In general, the limitation in expansion along the fused suture leads to excessive growth perpendicular to the suture. Thus, a careful examination can usually predict the form of synostosis. In the case of sagittal synostosis, excessive anterior and posterior growth of the skull leads to long narrow head shape with frontal and occipital prominence (scaphocephaly). The head shape changes in cases of craniosynostosis can be associated with (1) increased intracranial pressure that may result in permanent brain injury and (2) alteration of craniofacial growth leading to midfacial hypoplasia, abnormalities in dental alignment, and orbital deformation. Cases with severe midfacial hypoplasia often have significant airway obstruction and may require tracheostomy. The combination of craniosynostosis and associated facial malformations leads to significant morbidity but rarely mortality.

Patients with craniosynostosis require one or more major reconstructive surgeries to correct the functional deficits associated with their malformations. Syndromic forms often have more midfacial involvement and require additional corrective surgeries. The timing of surgical corrections varies with the treating center and the severity of the malformation. In addition to the craniofacial manifestations of craniosynostosis, some hereditary forms (Apert, Saethre Chotzen, and Pfeiffer) have associated limb anomalies (syndactylies and synostoses) frequently requiring surgical intervention for restoration of function (Table 10-11).

The genetics of craniosynostosis is complex. All the major forms of hereditary craniosynostosis are inherited in an autosomal-dominant pattern. Each form demonstrates a high degree of phenotypic variability and in some instances incomplete penetrance (particularly Muenke and Crouzon syndromes) (Fig. 10-18). Mutations of the fibroblast growth factor receptor (FGFR) family occur in many syndromic forms; however, mutations in the *TWIST* and *MSX2* genes have also been found (Table 10-11). Some clinical molecular laboratories are currently offering mutational testing for these syndromic forms of synostosis. In general, the family of a child who presents with more than one fused suture should be counseled that a hereditary form of synostosis should be considered. Single-suture fusion in the absence of other phenotypic features of syndromic synostosis (eg, ptosis, midfacial hypoplasia, limb anomalies, proptosis) is thought to represent epigenetic events perhaps related to in utero positioning. One must be very careful during assessment of the family history because of numerous examples of "isolated" sagittal and/or coronal synostosis recurring in families.

The surgical management of craniosynostosis has three main purposes: (1) to increase intracranial volume to reduce the risk of intracranial hypertension, (2) to reduce secondary events related to calvarial suture fusion (facial asymmetry and/or maxillary/mandibular malalignment), and (3) to return the calvarial contour to a more acceptable shape (these conditions lead to progressive deformation of the craniofacial skeleton if left untreated).

POSITIONAL FLATTENING OF CALVARIA (PLAGIOCEPHALY)

Positional plagiocephaly is a postnatal oblique flattening of the skull caused by position preference of the infant. Often associated with torticollis, persistent positioning leads most commonly to flattening of the occipitoparietal area that can be of sufficient severity that secondary changes, including ipsilateral frontal prominence and anterior displacement of the ipsilateral ear, occur. The natural history of positional plagiocephaly is as follows: (1) normal head contour at birth (unless abnormal in utero positioning is present), (2) occipital flattening noted by 1 to 2 months of age (infant usually demonstrating a sleep position preference and/or torticollis at this time), (3) increasing severity until 4 to 5 months, (4) improvement in head contour between 4 to 7 months, and (5) static head deformation after 7 months. The final head shape can be improved by reducing back lying while awake and increasing side-lying position during sleep. Some investigators have suggested that the incidence of this postnatal deformation has increased with the supine sleep position recommended to reduce the incidence of SIDS. The most dramatic aspect of the deformation is the occipital skull flattening often leading to the misdiagnosis of unilateral lambdoid synostosis. Positional plagiocephaly can be distinguished from lambdoid synostosis by physical examination (Table 10-12) and skull radiography (sclerosis of lambdoid suture can be seen on plain films or, preferably, CT scan). Positional plagiocephaly can be left untreated if mild; however, a number of "orthotic" devices (eg, helmets) are available for more severe cases.

OCULAR HYPERTELORISM AND FRONTONASAL DYSPLASIA

The term *frontonasal dysplasia* (FND) refers to a constellation of findings ranging from hypertelorism (widely spaced eyes) to complex malformations of nasal, midfacial, and premaxillary structures. The most accurate means of quantitating eye position include measurement of interpupillary distance and/or interorbital distance on skull radiography. Standards for ocular measurements are available (see references for Sec. 10.3.2). Orbital spacing varies between races (eg, blacks have a greater interpupillary distance than whites). In addition, other facial features (lateral displacement of the inner canthi, short palpebral fissures, low nasal bridge, and exotropia) can

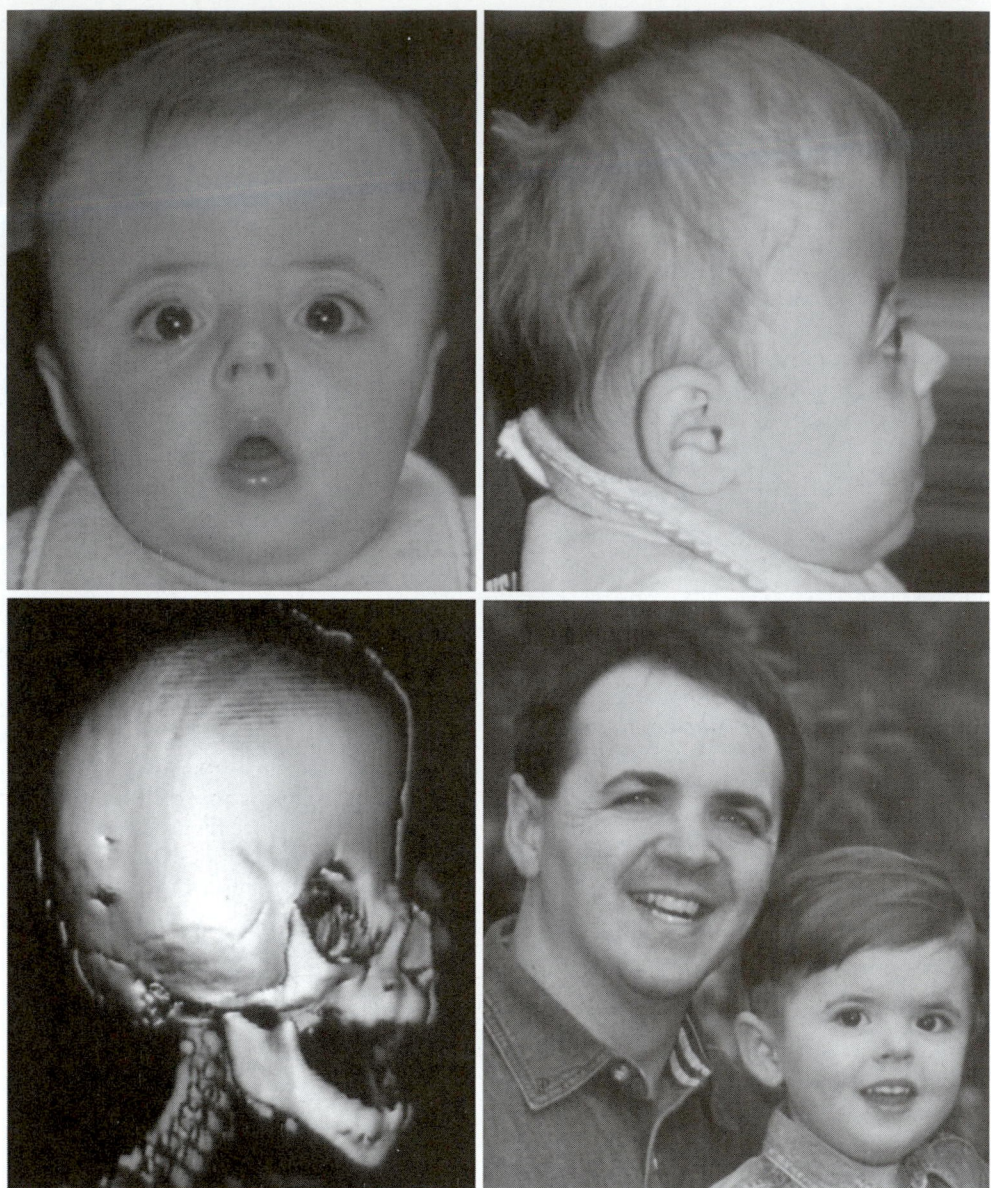

FIGURE 10-18   Clinical phenotype in a case of bilateral coronal craniosynostosis (top panels) subsequently found to be caused by a FGFR3 mutation Pro(250)Arg. Three dimensional CT scan demonstrating obliteration of the coronal sutures (bottom left panel). Mutational analysis of his parents determined that his father also had the FGFR3 mutation but resulted in minimal phenotypic manifestations (bottom right shown with proband after reconstructive surgery).

give the false impression of hypertelorism. As with most malformations, hypertelorism and FND can be an isolated finding or a part of a multiple malformation syndrome. Some syndromic examples of frontonasal dysplasia include: Opitz and Aarskog syndromes, the oral-facial-digital syndromes, craniofrontonasal dysplasia, and Waardenburg syndrome, among others (Table 10-11). Overall, 200 syndromes are associated with anomalies of frontonasal development.

The management issues for children with FND vary greatly depending on severity and the presence of associated or syndromic findings. Severe hypertelorism can affect the development of binocularity, and thus all children with FND should be evaluated by a qualified ophthalmologist. FND can be associated with central nervous system anomalies including frontonasal encephaloceles, tera-

tomas/lipomas of the ventral forebrain, agenesis/hypoplasia of the corpus callosum and/or septum pellucidum. Several other less common CNS anomalies can also be seen. In the case of frontonasal encephalocele, the anterior skull base is incompletely formed allowing for ventral displacement of the forebrain into the nasopharynx. Since frontonasal encephalocele occurs in mild cases, nasogastric or nasal suction tubes are not used when FND is present (unless necessary for emergent resuscitation efforts). Even more common than mild FND are congenital nasal dermal sinus tracts that are epithelial-lined and usually extend onto the midline of the nose (from base to tip) or even in the philtral groove. These malformations are thought to represent minor anomalies in embryonic facial growth and are of clinical significance in that they may extend through the cribriform plate (often through the crista galli), representing

TABLE 10-12

CLINICAL DIFFERENTIATION OF POSITIONAL PLAGIOCEPHALY AND LAMBDOID SYNOSTOSIS

PHYSICAL FINDING	POSITIONAL PLAGIOCEPHALY	LAMBDOID SYNOSTOSIS
Ear position (affected side)	Anterior displacement	Posterior and inferior displacement
Ipsilateral frontal prominence	Present (progressive to 7 months)	Absent
Contralateral occipito-parietal prominence	Absent	Present/progressive
Lambdoid ridge and submastoid prominence (affected side)	Absent	Present
Progressive after 7 months	No	Yes

a conduit for CNS infection. Any midline anomaly of nasal development requires high-resolution CT scan to rule out such anomalies.

References

Clarren SK, Anderson B, Wolfe LS: Feeding infants with cleft lip, cleft palate, and cleft lip and palate. Cleft Palate J 24:244, 1987

National Institute of Dental and Craniofacial Research: Listing of craniofacial-oral-dental diseases and disorders: *http://www.nidr.nih.gov/cranio/home.html*, 1998

Tolarova MM, Cervenka J: Classification and birth prevalence of orofacial clefts. Am J Med Genet 75(2):126–37, 1998

10.3.5 Constitutional Disorders of Bone

John C. Carey and Michael J. Bamshad

Skeletal dysplasias are generalized disorders of bone structure that can produce short stature, osseous deformity, and functional disabilities. More than 230 different skeletal dysplasias have been described by the International Working Group on Constitutional Diseases of Bone; collectively these dysplasias represent approximately half of all constitutional disorders of bone. The overall frequency of the skeletal dysplasias is about 1 in 4000 births, making this class of disorders as common as neurofibromatosis type 1 or Turner syndrome, much better known conditions. In contrast, disorders of bone structure that cause deformities and functional abnormalities of individual bones, either alone or in combination, are called *dysostoses*. Dysostoses and skeletal dysplasias comprise the constitutional disorders of bone and cause substantial morbidity in children and adults, yet many affected individuals lead relatively "normal" lives, albeit with some special challenges. This section describes the classification, distinguishing characteristics, and management of selected disorders of bone.

Conventionally, the skeletal dysplasias are often grouped according to the anatomic location of the bones that are most severely affected and the histologic abnormalities that are commonly observed. For example, skeletal dysplasias that affect the spine and the epiphyses are called *spondyloepiphyseal dysplasias*. However, the criteria used to categorize disorders into this classification are incon-

sistently applied to many skeletal dysplasias (eg, achondroplasia), and this diminishes its heuristic value. The classification schemes used to organize dysostoses are quite varied. No single system has become widely adopted, and, accordingly, the clinical presentation and varied expressions of the dysostoses tend to be difficult to remember accurately. Moreover, some disorders of bone share characteristics of both the skeletal dysplasias and the dysostoses.

The strategy of classifying malformations according to the developmental pathway that is disrupted can be applied to the skeletal dysplasias and dysostoses. The logic of the classification is to separate development of the skeleton into three primary phases: patterning, morphogenesis (ie, condensation, differentiation, and histogenesis), and growth. Dysostoses are typically produced by disturbances of skeletal patterning in a myriad of ways that have historically been categorized by the specific bone (eg, radial defects, fibular-femur complex) or anatomic location affected (eg, truncation defects, posterior polydactyly). Disturbances of bone growth lead to generalized disorders of bone as exemplified by most skeletal dysplasias (eg, achondroplasia). Skeletal disorders characterized by defects of the formation of individual bones have been more difficult to categorize. In these disorders, the patterning of the skeletal elements is normal and the growth of most skeletal elements is unaffected, but the morphogenesis of particular bones is disturbed. Thus, these conditions exhibit features of both skeletal dysplasias and dysostoses. For example, most of the bones in children with campomelic dysplasia exhibit normal patterning and growth. However, the long bones (femur, tibia) of children with campomelic dysplasia are bowed because histogenesis of these bones has been perturbed. Recent studies suggest that expression of the gene encoding type II collagen (*COL2A1*) is directly regulated by SOX9 protein and that abnormal regulation of *COL2A1* during chondrogenesis is a cause of the skeletal abnormalities associated with campomelic dysplasia.

Historically, the term *dwarf* has been used to refer to persons with bone dysplasias and disproportionate short stature. Because of the pejorative nature of this label and because it evokes thoughts of a different class of personhood, the term has been dropped from usage. The preferred terminology is to refer to a condition by its medical designation (eg, diastrophic dysplasia).

GENERAL APPROACH

The child with a bone dysplasia will present in primarily three ways: (1) as a newborn with short limbs (or trunk) in respiratory distress requiring ventilation, (2) as a newborn or older infant with disproportionate short stature, or (3) as a child with one of the various osseous manifestations associated with the bone dysplasias. An infant in the first group typically has one of the lethal chondrodystrophies (eg, thanatophoric dysplasia) and needs ventilatory support because of pulmonary hypoplasia or another respiratory feature of these conditions. A child with either the second or third presentation likely has one of the various disorders listed in Table 10-13. The systematic approach to the patient with any of the three presentations has been developed by Hall and other authorities in the field (Fig. 10-19).

The first step is the gathering of the history and physical examination with recognition of the decreased length or height. The pregnancy history may reveal that an abnormality was detected by ultrasonography (eg, short limbs or polyhydramnios), since prenatal diagnosis of a fetus with a presumed skeletal dysplasia is becoming more commonplace. As always, a detailed family history is

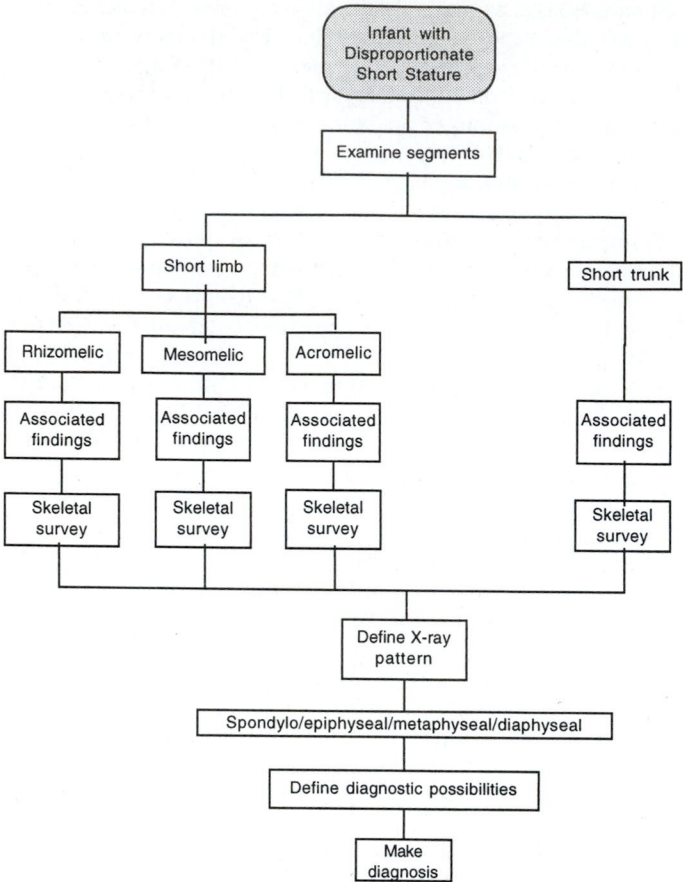

FIGURE 10-19   The diagnostic approach to the child with dispro-portionate short stature.

important and may reveal relatives with short stature or consanguinity.

The physical examination should include accurate measurements of length/height, weight, OFC, the arm span, and the upper/lower body ratio. The latter two measurements will define disproportion of the limbs to the trunk. The arm span is usually within 4 cm of the length/height at any age. If arm span is less than 5 cm of length, short limbs are suggested; if more than 5 cm of length, a short trunk is likely. The upper to lower ratio is taken by measuring the distance from the pubis to the heel (lower segment) and substracting this from the length/height to obtain the upper segment. The ratio of the upper to the lower (U/L) is 1.6 to 0.93 from the newborn to the adolescent. Children with an elevated U/L ratio (eg, greater than 1.8 in a newborn) have a short-limbed form of disproportionate short stature while those with a lowered ratio have a short-trunk form. Often the disproportion can be visualized just by simply looking at the infant or child; the upper limbs usually come to about one-third of the length of the thigh when held down by the side. When the fingertips of the hand are at or above the iliac crest, clinical disproportion is present.

The second step in the diagnostic process involves determining which segment of a limb or trunk is the shortest. Usually in any short-limb (or short-trunk) form of short stature there is a decrease in total length. However, one portion is often more shortened than the others, and this can be a clue to a diagnosis. If the upper portion of the limb (ie, the humerus or the femur) is the shorter part (as is the case in achondroplasia), this is referred to as *rhizomelic short-*

ening. If the middle segment of the limb (ie, forearm and lower leg) is the relatively shorter part, then this is called *mesomelic shortening.* Shortening of the distal part of the limb (ie, hands and feet) is called *acromelic shortening.* If the trunk is the predominant area of shortening (as in Morquio syndrome), then either the neck, thorax, or the entire spine will be short.

The next major step involves documenting all the nonskeletal physical features. Associated clinical findings, either malformations (eg, cleft palate, polydactyly) or important secondary findings (eg, dimples, bowing, contractures), are very helpful in leading to the diagnosis and will facilitate considering specific diagnostic paths. An important associated clinical finding is the presence or absence of serious respiratory difficulties at birth, the hallmark of the so-called lethal chondrodystrophies.

The fourth step in the process is a systematic categorization of the radiographic findings by area of involvement. A complete skeletal survey should include radiographs of the skull, long bones, AP pelvis, and spine and will be necessary in the evaluation of the child with a potential skeletal dysplasia. All the disorders shown in Table 10-13 are characterized by a specific pattern of skeletal abnormalities that are apparent on these radiographs. Most of the bone dysplasias have predictable and nonrandom adverse effects on the epiphyses, metaphyses, and the diaphyses, and spinal involvement varies with each condition. The architecture of the pelvic contour or the vertebral bodies is often distinctive enough to lead to a specific diagnosis (eg, thanatophoric dysplasia). Thus in this way each skeletal dysplasia can be categorized as predominantly involving the epiphyses, metaphyses, or diaphyses and/or the spine (spondylo-). For example, if one utilizes this approach radiologically, the bone findings could be classified as showing a spondyloepiphyseal dysplasia (Kniest dysplasia) or a spondylometaphyseal dysplasia (achondroplasia) and so on.

The final step in the evaluation, if necessary, is to confirm the clinical diagnosis using laboratory tests or histologic findings. For example, assay of skin fibroblasts for defects of type I collagen is sometimes necessary in the diagnosis of osteogenesis imperfecta. Some disorders show abnormalities of calcium and phosphorous (eg, hypophosphatemic rickets) or alkaline phosphatase (eg, hypophosphatasia) (see Sec. 24.11). In a lethal chondrodystrophy (eg, thanatophoric dysplasia type I) biopsy of the growth plate at postmortem examination may be helpful in confirming a clinical diagnosis.

Once a specific diagnosis is made, a plan for health supervision and management can be organized based upon the natural history of the condition. All the skeletal dysplasias, with rare exception (eg, warfarin embryopathy), are single-gene disorders, and with the exception of the few X-linked conditions, are inherited in an autosomal-dominant and/or recessive pattern. The risk of germ-line mosaicism is important for some conditions that are apparently new mutations (eg, osteogenesis imperfecta and campomelic dysplasia). The prenatal diagnosis of chondrodystrophies is also complicated because of changes in the technology and availability of genetic testing.

The psychological aspects of coping with the impact of a bone dysplasia are particularly unique. There are different implications for families in which average-sized parents have a child with a dysplasia or in which parents with achondroplasia (ie, heterozygotes) have a baby homozygous for the mutation causing achondroplasia, which is lethal. There are also different challenges for children with different conditions. In conditions such as achondroplasia or spondyloepiphyseal dysplasia congenita, where short stature is a prominent and consistent feature, a child has to cope with the stigma of short stature, a physical appearance of disproportion, the consequences of orthopedic and neurosurgical complications, and day-to-day challenges that medical professionals rarely encounter, such as clothing and bathroom needs and practical changes around the house. The Little People of America is an outstanding resource for families and children (*www.lpaonline.org*). Most individuals with these conditions deal with them effectively and adapt their lives to these challenges. Sensitivity to the many issues surrounding the emotional and psychological impact is obviously important, and a genuine acceptance of the differences in persons with skeletal dysplasias is also crucial to developing a relationship of caring.

Table 10-13 lists selected skeletal dysplasias, their clinical and radiographic features, and the molecular defect (when known); the conditions are grouped by gene product and function (if known). In addition achondroplasia and osteogenesis imperfecta are discussed in detail. Over 30 different skeletal dysplasias that include significant respiratory insufficiency that usually results in neonatal death have been described. A neonate with disproportionate short stature who has respiratory distress may have a lethal skeletal dysplasia.

SKELETAL DYSPLASIAS CAUSED BY MUTATIONS IN TRANSMEMBRANE RECEPTORS

The prototypic conditions that involve transmembrane receptors are the achondroplasia group and result from mutations in a gene encoding a receptor (fibroblast growth factor receptor 3, FGFR3) that negatively regulates the growth of cartilage. Thus, mutations in FGFR3 activate this receptor, and as a consequence growth is significantly inhibited. The phenotypic overlap between some of the conditions in this group had been observed for decades, and thus investigators were not surprised when different mutations of the same gene were discovered to cause achondroplasia, thanatophoric dysplasia, and hypochondroplasia (Table 10-13).

ACHONDROPLASIA

Achondroplasia is the best-known skeletal dysplasia in humans, occurs in about 1 in 20,000 newborns, and is usually recognized at birth. The syndrome pattern consists of disproportionate short stature with rhizomelic shortening, macrocephaly, and characteristic craniofacial findings including a flat nasal bridge, a prominent forehead, and midfacial hypoplasia (Fig. 10-20A). The hands are short, and the fingers are broad with digits 3 and 4 splayed more distally than proximally, giving the hand a "trident" appearance. The overall length is often in the low-average range at birth but by 2 to 3 months of age, the length is below the fifth percentile. A lumbar gibbus occurs in infancy but usually resolves. Children with achondroplasia usually do not have malformations such as cleft palate or polydactyly that are observed in other newborn skeletal dysplasias.

The diagnosis of achondroplasia is confirmed by the abnormalities found on the AP pelvis film that includes the upper femurs, which are quite characteristic (Fig 10-20B). The iliac bones are short and round, and the acetabulum is flattened. The shape of the ilia is similar to that found in other conditions, but the head of the femur exhibits a particularly distinctive contour. The other long bones have mildly flared metaphyses; the lumbar vertebrae have short pedicles and posterior scalloping. In general the findings are consistent with a spondylometaphyseal dysplasia.

Individuals with achondroplasia are at risk for a number of problems and complications, including a predisposition to serous otitis media, delay in motor milestones in infancy, bowing of the legs

(usually the tibia) presenting after ambulation has started, and orthodontic problems related to the maxillary hypoplasia. Growth curves are available for follow-up of the child with achondroplasia. Length and OFC can be monitored on well-child visits. Average adult height in males with achondroplasia ranges between 118 and 145 cm, and the range in females is between 112 and 136 cm. Limb-lengthening procedures have been performed on some adolescents with achondroplasia and resulted in an increase of several centimeters in height. However, this approach is controversial, and studies of long-term outcome are needed to help determine the risk/benefit ratio of this procedure. The most important manifestation of achondroplasia is related to the stenosis of the foramen magnum and spine. The former presents in infancy, whereas the latter occurs in later years, usually adulthood. Compression of the upper cord at the foramen magnum presents with a myriad of symptoms including apnea (both obstructive and central), quadriparesis, growth delays, and hydrocephalus. Any signs of compression or of hydrocephalus warrant referral to a neurosurgeon and/or neurologist. Some experts have suggested screening for compression using routine sonograms, but the American Academy of Pediatrics guidelines suggest measuring the size and shape of the fontanelle and monthly monitoring of the OFC. Standards of the size of the foramen magnum, as measured by computed tomography or magnetic resonance imaging, in children with achondroplasia are available and can be used to help decide if there is compression at the cervicomedullary junction.

Achondroplasia is an autosomal-dominant disorder with most children having a de novo mutation of *FGFR3*. Most patients with achondroplasia have an identical missense mutation that results in a substitution of codon 380 of FGFR3; this missense mutation causes a glycine residue to be replaced by an arginine. Patients with hypochondroplasia or thanatophoric dysplasia have different missense mutations in *FGFR3*.

THANATOPHORIC DYSPLASIAS

Two relatively distinct skeletal dysplasias also involving mutations of *FGFR3* are thanatophoric dysplasia I and II, which have similar clinical characteristics but different molecular defects. Both are lethal chondrodystrophies with only a few recorded survivors beyond the neonatal period. Death is usually caused by either compression at the cervicomedullary region by the foramen magnum or pulmonary hypoplasia. The presentation is always in the newborn with many cases now being diagnosed prenatally by ultrasound because of polyhydramnios or the detection of the short limbs.

As in achondroplasia there is true macrocephaly; the limbs are very short with obvious disproportion. There is a notable increase in folds of skin of the limbs and striking shortness and broadness of the digits. The radiographic findings are diagnostic with marked platyspondyly, flared metaphyses of long bones, and short iliac bones. In type I thanatophoric dysplasia the femurs are bowed, but in type II they are straight. Furthermore, the cranium of infants with type II thanatophoric dysplasia often shows the cloverleaf skull malformation.

Type I is caused by mutations in two regions of the extracellular domain of the FGFR3 while type II patients have mutations of codon 650, which is in the intracellular portion of the receptor protein. Both conditions are caused by de novo mutations of *FGFR3,* and thus parents are at very low recurrence risk. DNA testing for FGFR3 mutations is available both for prenatal diagnosis or confirmatory testing of an infant.

TABLE 10-13
SKELETAL DYSPLASIAS

CATEGORY OF DISORDER	MAJOR MANIFESTATIONS	LABORATORY/X-RAY	INHERITANCE (OMIM #)	GENE LOCUS/ GENE PRODUCT
Disorders of transmembrane receptors				
Achondroplasia (see text and Fig. 10-20A)				
Thanatophoric dysplasia type I*	Macrocephaly, rhizomelic shortening	Marked platyspondyly, short ilia, bowed femur with broad metaphyses	AD (187600)	4p16/FGFR3
Thanatophoric dysplasia type II*	Macrocepaly, cloverleaf skull anomaly	Platyspondyly, straight femur	AD (187610)	4p16/FGFR3
Hypochondroplasia	Mild rhizomelic shortening, macrocephaly	Short pedicles of vertebra; short/ broad ilia	AD (146000)	4p16/FGFR3
Disorders of cartilage matrix proteins and collagen				
Osteogenesis imperfecta (see text)				
Kriest dysphasia	Flat nose, midfacial hypoplasia, short stature, prominent joints	Broad metaphyses of femur; coronal clefts of spine	AD (156556)	12q13/type II collagen
Achondrogenesis type II*	Flat nose, very short limbs, hydrops	Short tubular bones, deficit/absent ossification of vertebrae	AD (200610)	12q13/type II collagen
Spondyloepiphyseal dysplasia congenita	Myopia, hearing loss, eventually short trunk	Flat vertebrae, odontoid hypoplasia, scoliosis	AD (183900)	12q13/type II collagen
Hypochondrogenesis*	Flat nose, very short limbs	Relatively normal long bones; vertebral hypoplasia	AD (120140)	12q13/type II collagen
Schmid metaphyseal dysplasia	Mild disproportinate short stature; tibial bowing	Metaphyseal broadening	AD (156500)	6q21/type X collagen
Pseudoachondroplasia	Long trunk, short limbs, leg joints	Platyspondyly, tongue-like projections anteriorly, epiphyseal dysplasia	AD (177170)	19p12/COMP
Multiple epiphyseal dysplasia	Mildly short limbs	Multiple epiphyseal changes, normal spine	AD (600969) (locus heterogeneity)	19p12/COMP
Disorders of transmembrane sulfate transporter				
Diastrophic dysplasia	Cleft palate, laryngeal abnormalities, transient swellings of ears	Short long bones, scoliosis, broad metaphyses	AR (222600)	5q32/sulfate transporter
Atelosteogenesis type II*	Flat nose, very short limbs, +/− cleft palate	Short humeri; fibular hypoplasia	AR (256050)	5q32/sulfate transporter
Achondrogenesis type I*	Flat nose, very short limbs, hydrops	Short tubular bones, poor ossification of vertebrae	AR (600972)	5q32/sulfate transporter
Disorders of DNA transcription factors				
Campomelic dysplasia*	Macrocephaly, flat nose, cleft palate, clubfeet, dimples over tibia	Short bowed femur and tibia; narrowed ilia; hypoplastic scapulae	AD (114290)	17q24/SOX9
Disorders of bone density				
Hypophosphatasia, congenital form*	Soft skull, short limbs	Very short underossified long bones with spikes; low alkaline phosphatase	AR (241500)	1p36/alkaline phosphatase
Disorders of unknown pathway				
Ellis-van Creveld syndrome	Sparse hair, natal teeth, postaxial polydactyly, long/thin chest; genu valgus	Short/broad ilia	AR (225500)	4p/
Jeune dysplasia	Relatively normal face	Short ribs, short/broad ilia	AR (208500)	—
Short rib/polydactyly type I*	Flat nose, postaxial polydactyly	Metaphyseal spurs; short/horizontal ribs, small ilia	AR (263530)	—
Short rib/polydactyly type II*	Flat nose; postaxial polydactyly	Short/horizontal ribs; oval-shaped tibiae	AR (263520)	—
Spondylometaphyseal dysplasia	Short trunk, tibial bowing	Platyspondyly, broad metaphyses	AD (120140)	—

* Lethal in neonatal period.
OMIM: Online Mendelian Inheritance of Man: <*http://www.ncbi.nlm.nih.gov/omim/*>, 1999.

DISORDERS OF STRUCTURAL PROTEINS OF CARTILAGE

Several different skeletal dysplasias are caused by mutations of genes encoding proteins involved in the extracellular matrix of cartilage (Table 10-13). Functional disturbances of a variety of proteins, including types II, IX, X, and XI collagen and the noncollagenous cartilage oligomeric protein (COMP), have been described.

A principal collagen of bone is type I collagen, a triple helical molecule consisting of two α-1 and one α-2 proteins. Mutations in

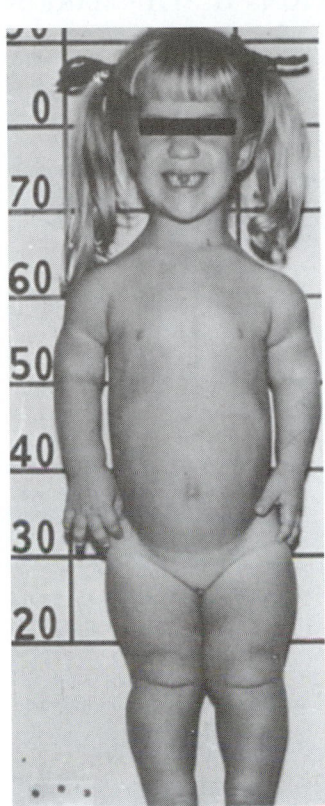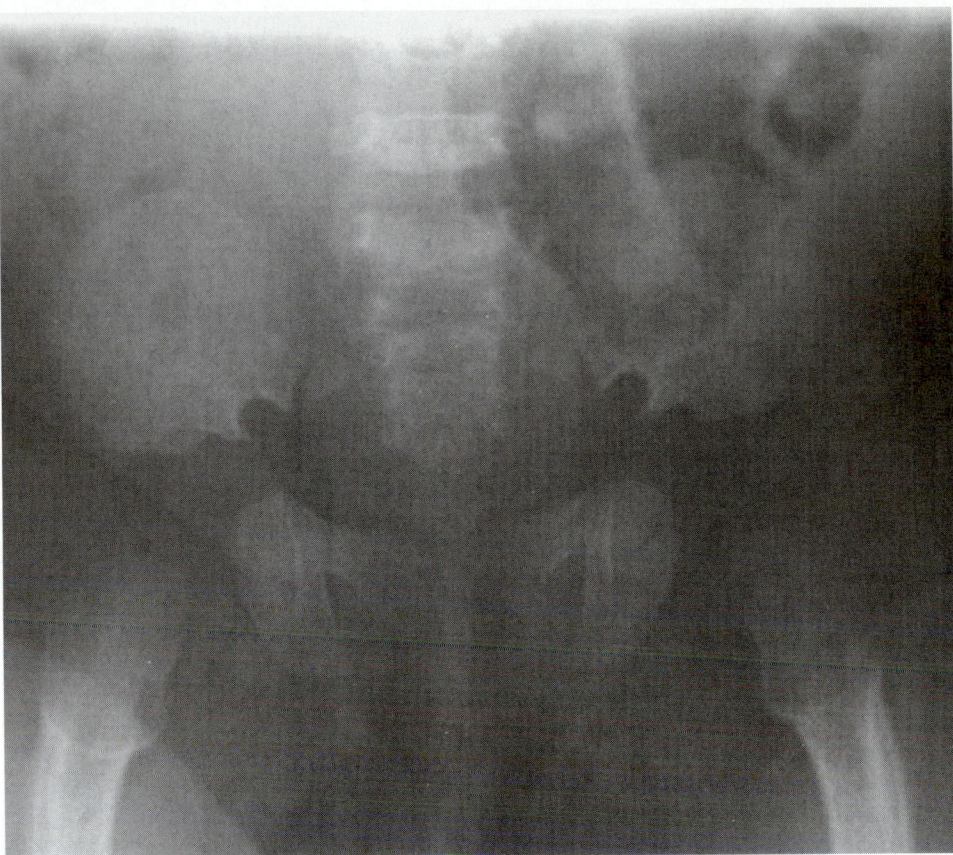

FIGURE 10-20   A. A child with achondroplasia. Note the rhizomelic shortening. B. Radiograph of the pelvis in a child with achondroplasia. Note the squared-off iliac wings, flat and irregular acetabular roofs, thick femoral necks, and ice-cream-scoop-shaped femoral heads.

the genes encoding these two proteins (*COL1A1* and *COL1A2*) cause the most common forms of osteogenesis imperfecta (OI), a group of skeletal dysplasias involving abnormalities of bone density.

OSTEOGENESIS IMPERFECTA

Osteogenesis imperfecta represents a heterogeneous group of bone dysplasias that are characterized by osseous fragility, short stature, and a wide range of other skeletal findings that vary with the type of OI. The classification of Sillence is most commonly used and another dozen disorders of bone density and osseous fragility can be placed in this category. However, aside from OI types I to IV, all these entities are very rare.

OI type I is well-known skeletal condition that is sometimes referred to as *brittle bone disease*, and this autosomal-dominant disorder consists of the variable presence of blue sclerae, delay in fontanelle closure, joint laxity, short stature, and multiple fractures. The prevalence is about 1 in 30,000 births, with the majority of cases being familial and a minority representing de novo mutations. Fractures are uncommon at birth. The sclerae are deep blue, often the hue of a robin's egg, and do not resolve with time as usually occurs in children as a normal variant. Primary or secondary deformities of long bones are uncommon, and the prognosis for normal function is excellent. Fractures from minimal trauma occurring throughout childhood are the rule, but by middle to late adolescence fracture frequency diminishes markedly. Sometimes, child abuse is incorrectly suspected, and can be challenging to resolve because the abnormalities observed in some children with type I OI can be subtle. Radiographs show mild osteopenia of the long

bones and wormian bones (bones within sutures). Some families exhibit the dental manifestation of dentinogenesis imperfecta. Scoliosis and hearing impairment from a conductive loss occur in the second or third decade. Biochemical analysis will often show a decrease in the synthesis of type I collagen, and inactivating mutations of either gene can occur.

OI type II is a serious condition usually resulting in newborn death caused by respiratory insufficiency and is the second most common lethal skeletal dysplasia behind the thanatophoric dysplasias. The skull is markedly soft on palpation, and the limbs are short and bowed even beyond the occurrence of fractures. The radiographic contour on the long bones is particularly characteristic with a crumpled appearance, and the ribs are beaded because of callus formation. Studies of *COL1A1* demonstrate that point mutations that disrupt helical assembly lead to abnormal collagen formation. Almost all cases are related to de novo mutation of a *COL1A1*. Because germ-line mosaicism has been documented in a number of families, recurrence risk for parents of a sporadic case is usually given as 6%, which is probably an overestimate of the actual risk because of ascertainment bias.

OI type III usually presents in the newborn infant with multiple fractures. This type of OI was formerly called (along with type II) *OI congenita* and is sometimes referred to as the *progressively deforming type* because there is severe osseous fragility leading to bowing and deformity. Indeed, short stature is significant. Many patients with type III OI are not able to ambulate owing to an inability to bear weight. The sclerae are usually blue at birth but lighten with age. Comprehensive rehabilitation emphasizing physical supports and bracing is suggested, and referral to a team or an OI clinic (several are located at Shriners' hospitals in North America) is always indicated for children with type III OI. Decisions regarding timing and appropriateness of surgery are complex and require input from experienced orthopedists. Most of the neurologic findings that have been described in patients with OI, including hydrocephalus and basilar skull invagination, occur in this type of OI. Newer therapies that are used in osteoporosis, such as bi-phosphonates, are being tried in type III OI with some efficacy and improvement. Most cases are caused by point mutations of *COL1A1,* similar to what is observed in type II and IV OI.

Type IV OI is characterized by marked variability with most cases having a milder phenotype like type I OI. Typically, there are only mild changes of the sclerae, which often become lighter with time. Delay in closure of the fontanelles is common, and fractures are often present at birth. The hallmark of type IV OI is the presence of tibial bowing, which is usually not seen in the other mild type of OI, type I. Dentinogenesis imperfecta is observed in some families. Most patients have point mutations or exon deletions affecting *COL1A2.*

The Osteogensis Imperfecta Foundation *(www.med.virginia. edu/medicine/admin/grants/osteo.html)* is an excellent resource for parents of newly diagnosed infants. Their written material helps parents learn how to handle their baby, since it is quite natural for parents to be hesitant to care for their child because of the osseous fragility. A checklist for routine care has been developed for follow-up of children with OI (as well as many other syndromes and skeletal dysplasias) by Wilson and Cooley.

References

Academy of Pediatrics Committee on Genetics: Health supervision for children with achondroplasia. Pediatrics 95:443–451, 1995

Hall BD: Approach to skeletal dysplasias. Pediatr Clin North Am 39:279–305, 1992

International Working Group on Constitutional Diseases of Bone International: Nomenclature of the osteochondrodysplasias. Am J Med Genet 79:376–382, 1997

Taybi H, Lachman RS: Radiology of Syndromes, Metabolic Disorders & Skeletal Dysplasias. Chicago, Year Book, 1996

Wilson GN, Cooley WC: Preventive Management of Children with Congenital Anomalies and Syndromes. Cambridge, Cambridge University Press, 2000

10.3.6   Connective Tissue Dysplasias

Maurice Godfrey

Like the skeletal dysplasias, primary disorders of connective tissue comprise a heterogeneous group of genetic conditions. Because of their importance in pediatric patients, this section focuses on Marfan syndrome and the Ehlers-Danlos syndromes.

MARFAN SYNDROME

Marfan syndrome is a serious heritable disorder of connective tissue with manifestations in many organs, including the eyes, heart, aorta, skeleton, skin, lung, and dura (Table 10-14). The disorder is transmitted in an autosomal-dominant pattern with virtually complete penetrance but variable expression. Without diligent clinical monitoring and treatment, life span may be significantly reduced. The major morbidity and mortality associated with the Mar-

TABLE 10-14

CLINICAL MANIFESTATIONS OF THE MARFAN SYNDROME

MAJOR CRITERIA	MINOR CRITERIA
Skeletal system	
Pectus carinatum	Moderate pectus excavatum
Pectus excavatum needing surgery	Joint hypermobility
Reduced U/L segment ratio or arm-span-to-height ratio	High arched palate
Wrist and thumb signs	
Scoliosis >20%	
Reduced extension at elbows (<170%)	
Pes planus	
Protrusio acetabuli	
Ocular system	
Ectopia lentis	Abnormally flat cornea
	Increased axial length of globe
	Hypoplastic iris or ciliary muscle
Cardiovascular system	
Dilation of the ascending aorta	Mitral valve prolapse
Dissection of the ascending aorta	Dilation of main pulmonary artery, without obvious cause, below age 40 years
Pulmonary system	
None	Spontaneous pneumothorax
	Apical blebs
Skin and integument	
None	Striae atrophicae
	Recurrent or incisional hernias
Dura	
Lumbosacral dural ectasia	None

fan syndrome is related to cardiovascular complications. The incidence of the Marfan syndrome has been estimated to be as high as 1 in 5000 individuals and is without gender or ethnic predilection.

Clinical Presentation

Ocular System

The hallmark manifestation of Marfan syndrome is ectopia lentis, or subluxation of the ocular lens, usually bilateral, which is found in 50 to 80% of patients and is often present at or soon after birth. Typically, the lens is displaced upward but the attached zonular fibers remain intact. Some patients can voluntarily replace the lens by head movement, and because the zonular fibers are intact, accommodation may occur. Iridodonesis, or tremor of the iris, indicates the presence of ectopia lentis. Slit-lamp examination as part of a complete ophthalmologic evaluation will directly demonstrate subluxation. Abnormally flat cornea, as measured by keratometry; increased axial length of the globe, as measured by ultrasound; and hypoplastic iris or ciliary muscle are all considered minor criteria for ocular involvement in the Marfan syndrome. Recent studies suggest the possibility of early development of cataracts and open-angle glaucoma.

Cardiovascular System

Progressive dilation of the aortic root and ascending aorta involving at least the sinuses of Valsalva and dissection of the ascending aorta are the major cardiovascular manifestations in the Marfan syndrome and may lead to rupture or aortic valvular incompetence with re-gurgitation. Echocardiography is the diagnostic procedure of choice for monitoring progression of aortic disease in children and adults with the Marfan syndrome. Uncommonly, dilation of the descending or abdominal aorta, or other major arteries, may occur, as well as dilation of the aortic annulus and may result in progressive aortic valvular incompetence with regurgitation manifested as heart failure. Mitral valve prolapse, a minor diagnostic criterion, can be demonstrated by echocardiography in about 80% of patients and may be associated with mitral regurgitation. Aortic regurgitation is both more common and hemodynamically more significant than mitral regurgitation.

Skeletal System

The skeletal manifestations that are characteristic of Marfan syndrome are common in the population, and, consequently, a constellation of several skeletal features must be present to meet diagnostic specificity. Typically, the affected individual is excessively tall for age and has disproportionately long and thin extremities (dolichostenomelia) (Fig. 10-21). Some patients have an apparent muscular hypoplasia, producing a gaunt and emaciated appearance. The palate may be narrow and high-arched, with dental crowding. Abnormality of the anterior chest (both pectus excavatum and carinatum) is common and often asymmetric. Scoliosis or kyphoscoliosis may develop, particularly during the adolescent growth spurt. The hands are narrow and the fingers long and thin (arachnodactyly or "spider fingers"). Joint hypermobility at major and minor joints is manifest by features such as genu recurvatum and flat feet (pes planus). Protrusio acetabuli, determined by radiography, is another skeletal finding useful for clinical diagnosis.

Skeletal disproportion is usually demonstrated in several ways. Arm span exceeds height, and the U/L ratio typically is greater than 2 standard deviations below the mean for race and age. Both these features reflect the relative increase in limb length as compared to trunk length. Metacarpal overgrowth (and joint hypermobility) may be demonstrated by the *thumb sign,* extension of the thumb past the ulnar border of the hand when apposed to the palm, and by the *wrist sign,* overlapping of the thumb and fifth finger when these fingers encircle the wrist.

Other Clinical Features

Spontaneous pneumothorax owing to rupture of pulmonary blebs, usually apical, may occur with or without thoracic deformity. Inguinal, femoral, or other hernias may be present and tend to recur following surgical repair. Striae distensae (striae atrophicae) of the skin are often present over buttocks, thighs, and shoulders. Dural ectasia may be an important diagnostic indicator in many patients. In fact, lumbosacral dural ectasia, determined by computed tomography or magnetic resonance imaging, is a major clinical criterion for diagnosis of the Marfan syndrome. Dural ectasia is usually asymptomatic and is thought to be less common in children.

Diagnosis

The clinical variability of Marfan syndrome makes unequivocal diagnosis difficult in mildly affected individuals and necessitates careful physical examination with anthropomorphic measurements, competent ophthalmologic and echocardiographic evaluations, and family studies. The accepted criteria for clinical diagnosis depend upon the presence or absence of an unequivocally affected first-degree relative. If there are no affected first-degree relatives, then

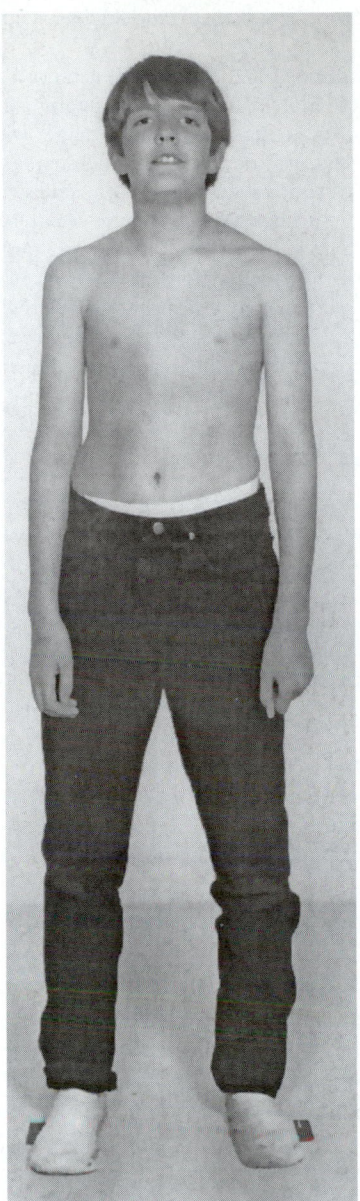

FIGURE 10-21   A young man with Marfan syndrome. Note his tall stature, narrow face, long limbs, and long fingers.

diagnosis requires the presence of major criteria in at least two different organ systems and involvement of a third (Table 10-14). In the presence of documented family history of the Marfan syndrome, the presence of one major criterion and involvement of a second organ system are sufficient for diagnosis.

Since the molecular etiology of the Marfan syndrome is known, genetic studies can contribute to clinical diagnosis. For example, the presence of a mutation in the gene encoding fibrillin-1, *FBN1,* known to cause the Marfan syndrome, or the presence of an *FBN1* haplotype, inherited by descent, and associated with unequivocal Marfan syndrome, is major diagnostic criterion. Both have been used for presymptomatic and prenatal diagnosis. In all instances, absence of homocystine in the urine in the absence of pyridoxine supplementation is necessary to rule out homocystinuria, a disorder that may share many features of Marfan syndrome. Other conditions often considered in differential diagnosis include familial or isolated mitral valve prolapse syndrome, familial or isolated annuloaortic ectasia (Erdheim disease), and Stickler syndrome (see Table 10-11).

Although definitive diagnosis will be achieved by adherence to specified criteria in most patients, there remains a group of patients with multiple features suggestive but not diagnostic of Marfan syndrome; such patients present a clinical dilemma. On the one hand, overenthusiastic diagnosis may provoke needless psychologic distress and may commit patient and family to extended and possibly lifelong intensive follow-up and drug therapy. On the other hand, nondiagnosis of the Marfan syndrome may place the patient at increased risk for unmanaged and potentially lethal complications. Molecular diagnosis should be strongly considered in such patients. Diagnosis of Marfan syndrome creates the obligation to carefully evaluate the patient's first-degree relatives for this disease.

Pathology and Etiology

The most extensive pathologic studies are those of the cardiovascular system, and the most common histologic manifestation is the so-called cystic medial necrosis, with degeneration of the elastic fibers, irregular hypertrophy of smooth muscle, and focal cystic areas filled with metachromatically staining materials. Valvular changes include thinned and stretched aortic valve cusps, endocarditis of the mitral valve, dilated mitral valve annulus, floppy mitral leaflets, and ruptured and elongated mitral chordae tendineae. Premature dilation of the sinuses of Valsalva is also seen and is a key feature for diagnosis. The glycoprotein fibrillin has been implicated in the etiology of Marfan syndrome. Molecular studies have now documented numerous mutations in the *FBN1* gene; most mutations have been unique and thus observed in only one patient or family.

Management

The major goal is the prevention of complications of the disease and anticipation of the need for definitive surgical intervention. Morbidity and mortality are governed primarily by cardiovascular complications, and secondarily by musculoskeletal (eg, kyphoscoliosis, pectus deformities) complications and response to treatment.

Cardiovascular

The most important tool in the management of the cardiovascular complications in the Marfan syndrome is routine, annual or semiannual monitoring by echocardiography. More frequent echocardiographic monitoring may become necessary as aortic dilation or valvular insufficiency progresses. Because progressive aortic dilation typically (but not invariably) precedes dissection, prevention or delay of dilation and surgery prior to dissection or rupture is a central goal. When the aortic diameter reaches 50 to 55 mm (in an adult), surgical intervention must be considered, and a decision for surgery is based on considerations of the rate of aortic dilation, presence of aortic or mitral regurgitation, pulmonary function, age, and, possibly, previous experience with other affected family members. The use of β-adrenergic blockade has become ubiquitous in Marfan patients in an attempt to delay aortic dilation. Some evidence suggests, however, that this treatment is more efficacious in children than adults. Dosage must be tailored for each patient and treatment closely monitored, especially at the beginning. The use of calcium-channel inhibitors is an alternative therapeutic approach. Strenuous physical activity (heavy lifting, isometric exercise) and competitive athletics are contraindicated, but aerobic, noncompetitive exercise is important to overall fitness. Normal play for young children gen-

erally needs no restriction. People with the Marfan syndrome are at increased risk for bacterial endocarditis, and prophylactic antibiotics are recommended prior to dental or genitourinary procedures.

Ocular

Annual ophthalmologic evaluations should be obtained beginning in childhood. Patients should be carefully instructed to seek immediate help for onset of visual symptoms, and failure to detect visual problems may result in amblyopia. Dislocated lenses cause few problems in most people, but if the lens interferes with vision, the use of eyeglasses or contact lenses helps to achieve satisfactory vision with correction of refraction. Removal of a subluxated lens is rarely necessary. The eyes need to be protected from injury (sports involving blows to the head, eg, boxing, football), because people with the Marfan syndrome are at increased risk for retinal detachment.

Skeletal

Annual evaluation is critical for the well-being of the patient. Deformity of the spine or anterior chest can be disfiguring and/or may compromise respiratory and/or cardiovascular function. Either reason may require surgery. Bracing may be effective in stabilizing the spine and to avoid surgery. Chest wall deformities, if surgically repaired too early, may recur and intervention in midadolescence or later is recommended unless respiratory or cardiovascular function is reduced. Induction of puberty by exogenous hormonal administration may limit the degree of curvature and deformity caused by scoliosis or kyphoscoliosis and reduce final adult height, which may be advantageous for those individuals, especially girls, whose projected final height exceeds 6 feet. Experience has been favorable and not associated with undue side effects. Joint laxity may delay walking, but stability increases as the child grows and should minimize associated problems. Other orthopedic or surgical complications such as joint instability or various hernias are repaired for the usual indications.

Other

Psychological problems can emerge as a result of a diagnosis of the Marfan syndrome. Although most people cope well, the lifelong stigma and exclusion from sports, especially for boys, may require psychological counseling as part of complete management. Because of the narrow palate, tooth crowding may occur and good dental care, with orthodontic intervention, is required.

Pregnancy imposes increased risk for accelerated aortic dilation in women with Marfan syndrome. Women with moderate to severe cardiovascular involvement are at greatest risk, whereas women with minimal involvement generally tolerate pregnancy well. Genetic counseling regarding recurrence risks should be performed at an appropriate age. Prenatal diagnosis has been done by chorionic villus sampling and genetic linkage analysis.

EHLERS-DANLOS SYNDROMES

The Ehlers-Danlos syndromes (EDS) are a heterogeneous group of connective tissue disorders that share, as fundamental features, alterations of the integrity of the supporting structures of the body. The cardinal manifestations of EDS are hyperextensible ("stretchy") skin, hypermobile joints, easy bruisability, and dystrophic scarring. Concomitant generalized or localized fragility of various connective tissues leads to a variety of additional features in some EDS variants. These manifestations, together with the pattern of inheritance, serve as the basis for the diagnosis and subclassification into several varieties or subtypes. Although the exact prevalence of EDS is unknown, they are believed to be the most common heritable disorders of connective tissue. The spectrum of severity ranges from mild manifestations (thus frequently undiagnosed) to severe debilitation. Certain varieties of EDS are associated with an ominous prognosis.

EDS result from abnormalities of the connective tissues, and the clinical and genetic heterogeneity reflect in part an underlying molecular and biochemical heterogeneity. Recently, a simplified classification of EDS into six major types has been proposed and will be used for describing clinical ascertainment, management, and molecular etiology of each type (Table 10-15).

All known molecular etiologies involve the biogenesis of the collagens, the major structural fibrous proteins of the body. Many varieties of collagens are known, each of which has a specific and unique distribution in the body, implying a specific functional role. Collagen biogenesis is complex and involves extensive modification of the proteins by different enzymes following synthesis and prior to assembly into biologically useful structural units (eg, fibrils, bundles). Thus, collagen defects might involve either a decrease or absence of a specific variety of collagen or structural abnormalities leading to defective assembly of collagen structural units.

Clinical Features

Skin

The skin in EDS is characteristic in texture and consistency but may vary in apparent thickness: Soft, doughy, and velvety to the touch, like the feel of wet chamois or of a fine sponge. Redundant skin over the hands and feet, is common, sometimes occurring over the stomach as well. When pulled, skin is hyperextensible, or "stretchy" (Fig. 10-22) but returns immediately to a normal configuration when released. Cutaneous hyperextensibility is virtually diagnostic of EDS, but this feature is minimal in several varieties. Hyperextensibility should be tested at a site not subject to mechanical forces or scarring (eg, volar surface of the forearm). Much subcutaneous fat in young children makes skin hyperextensibility difficult to assess.

Cutaneous fragility or dermatorrhexis, manifested by splitting of the skin after insignificant trauma, may be a prominent feature. Typically, these wounds occur over the shins, knees, elbows, forehead, and chin, or other areas prone to trauma and tend to bleed little and often present a gaping "fish-mouth" appearance owing to retraction of the adjacent skin. Sutures may pull out of this fragile skin, leading to dehiscence of the wound. The cellular phase of wound healing proceeds normally, but acquisition of tensile strength is delayed. Characteristic so-called cigarette-paper or papyraceous scarring may occur; these scars appear thin, atrophic, shiny, and broad, and are often hyperpigmented and corrugated by fine wrinkles.

Easy bruisability is a major feature, may vary in severity, and may be the initial symptom in young children (child abuse must be considered in the differential diagnosis). Bruising may be generalized or restricted to trauma-prone areas such as the shins. Bleeding from the gums after brushing or dental extractions is also fairly common. Tests for coagulopathy are normal with the exception of a positive test for capillary fragility.

Other skin manifestations of EDS include the so-called molluscoid pseudotumors found typically at pressure points such as the

heel, elbows, and knees; irregular firm subcutaneous masses resulting from fibrosis or calcification of hematomas; and small fat-containing cysts called *spherules*, which resemble phleboliths but may be easily distinguished by their subcutaneous location. Many EDS patients have highly wrinkled palms or soles manifested as adventitious palmar creases.

Joint Manifestations

Joint hypermobility is a cardinal feature of EDS but, as with the cutaneous manifestations, varies with the specific type of syndrome. Typically, joint hypermobility involves both large and small joints; with marked hypermobility, dislocations may be present at birth or occur later. The knees and elbows can be extended past 180° and the fingers extended past 90° from the palmar plane. Often the thumb can be apposed to the radius in flexion, extension, or both (Fig. 10-23). In some patients, feats of remarkable contortion, such as touching the elbows behind the back and placing the head between the knees while bending backward, may be performed easily. Joint mobility decreases with advancing age. Joint effusions may be relatively frequent. Hemarthrosis may occur, especially in vascular EDS. Ligamentous laxity is usually associated with joint hypermobility. Congenital clubfoot, apparently the result of ligamentous laxity and joint hypermobility coupled with intrauterine compression, is not uncommon. On occasions, marked apparent hypotonia with poor motor activity and muscular underdevelopment simulate neuromuscular disease in the newborn infant.

Varieties of Ehlers-Danlos Syndromes

Table 10-15 outlines the six types of EDS, previous designation, diagnostic criteria, mode of inheritance, and molecular defect. Forms of previously classified EDS that do not fit in any of the major types will be noted at the end of this section.

The *classical type* (previously *type I gravis* and *type II mitis*) comprises the bulk of cases of EDS and is characterized by a wide range of severity of skin manifestations including skin hyperextensibility, dystrophic scarring, and marked bruising. The skin may also be smooth and velvety. Other skin lesions include molluscoid pseudotumors, associated with scars at pressure points, and subcutaneous bodies that may be calcified and radiographically detected. Tissue fragility may present surgical difficulties, and hernias may result postoperatively.

Joint hypermobility is also an important diagnostic criterion. Complications of hypermobile joints include sprains and recurrent dislocations often in the shoulder, patella, or temporomandibular joints. Joint hypermobility together with muscle hypotonia may result in delayed gross motor development.

Electron microscopy findings in skin demonstrate large collagen fibrils, many of which are irregular in cross-section. Recently, classical type of EDS was found to be caused by abnormalities of type V collagen. Type V collagen is a heterotrimer composed of the products of two genes, *COL5A1* and *COL5A2*. Mutations have been identified in both genes. Genetic linkage studies can be used for prenatal or postnatal diagnosis in informative families. However, a few families have been excluded using these studies. Thus, the possibility that other genes may also cause EDS remains.

The *hypermobility type* (previously *type III hypermobile*) is the only major type of EDS in which the molecular basis remains unknown and is characterized by severe, generalized joint hypermobility with or without dislocations, hemarthroses, and precocious arthritis. Recurrent and frequent dislocations of the shoulders, patella, and temporomandibular joints are common. Skin manifesta-

TABLE 10-15

CHARACTERISTICS OF MAJOR VARIANTS OF EHLERS-DANLOS SYNDROME

NEW DESIGNATION	PREVIOUS DESIGNATION	DIAGNOSTIC CRITERIA—MAJOR	DIAGNOSTIC CRITERIA—MINOR	INHERITANCE	MOLECULAR DEFECTS
Classical type	Type I (gravis) Type II (mitis)	Skin hyperextensibility Tissue fragility Atrophic scars Joint hypermobility	Smooth velvety skin Easy bruising Molluscoid pseudotumors Subcutaneous spheroids Muscle hypotonia Delayed gross motor development	AD	Type V collagen
Hypermobility type	Type III (hypermobile)	Joint hypermobility Skin hyperextensibility and/or smooth velvety skin	Joint dislocations Chronic joint/limb pain	AD	Unknown
Vascular type	Type IV (ecchymotic)	Thin, translucent skin Arterial/intestinal/uterine fragility or rupture Extensive bruising Characteristic facial appearance	Hypermobility of small joints Acrogeria Tendon and muscle rupture Talipes equinovarus Early-onset varicose veins Gingival recession	AD	Type III collagen
Kyphoscoliosis type	Type VI (ocular-scoliotic)	Generalized joint laxity Severe muscle hypotonia at birth Progressive scoliosis from birth Scleral fragility	Tissue fragility Easy bruising Arterial rupture Marfanoid habitus	AR	Lysyl hydroxylase deficiency
Arthrochalasia type	Types VIIA and VIIB (arthrochalasis multiplex congenita)	Severe joint hypermobility; recurrent subluxations Congenital bilateral hip dislocation	Skin hyperextensibility Tissue fragility Easy bruising Muscle hypotonia Kyphoscoliosis	AD	Type I collagen
Dermatosparaxis type	Type VIIC (human dermatosparaxis)	Severe skin fragility Sagging redundant skin	Soft, doughy skin texture Easy bruising Large hernias	AR	Procollagen I N-proteinase deficiency

AD = autosomal dominant; AR = autosomal recessive

796

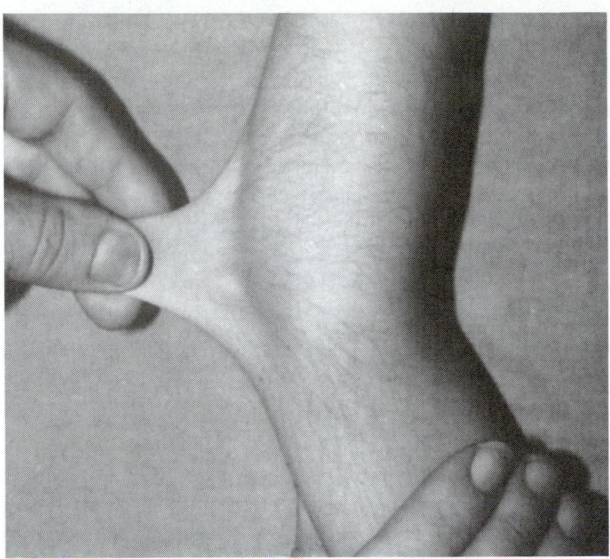

FIGURE 10-22   Cutaneous hyperelasticity at the elbow in a 6-year-old boy with Ehlers-Danlos type I.

tions (hyperextensibility and smooth and velvety) are mild but present, serving to distinguish this disorder from familial articular hypermobility syndrome. Musculoskeletal pain occurs early and becomes chronic. Inheritance is autosomal dominant.

The *vascular type* (previously *type IV arterial/ecchymotic*) exhibits considerable clinical heterogencity, ranging from nearly normal to extensive, wide ecchymoses. The major manifestations of the vascular type of EDS include thin, often semitransparent skin; arterial, intestinal, and/or uterine fragility or rupture; extensive bruising; and a characteristic face. Minor diagnostic features include joint hypermobility limited to digits; acrogeria; talipes equinovarus; early-onset varicose veins; arteriovenous and carotid-cavernous sinus fistula; pneumothorax; gingival recession; and family history that may include sudden death in a close relative.

A prominent venous network over the anterior trunk can be frequently seen through the thin, translucent skin. Bruisability ranges from mild to severe, and some patients may never be free of extensive ecchymoses resulting from inapparent trauma (child abuse must be considered in the differential diagnosis). Large varicose veins may be present. Vasular EDS carry a serious prognosis because of a liability to catastrophic bleeding from defects in major arteries, which may occur without antecedent dilation or dissection and often without apparent trauma. Major bleeding ensues, and operative attempts at vascular repair are almost uniformly unsuccessful because the vessel walls are friable; conservative treatment, whenever possible, is recommended. Aneurysmal dilation and dissection of major vessels may occur. The prognosis for successful repair in patients is at present unclear. Because of the vascular fragility in these patients, angiographic studies are hazardous and should be attempted only for adequate cause and with caution to avoid perforation or dissection of vessels. Arterial rupture generally occurs in the third and fourth decades but may present earlier.

Although less common than arterial rupture, spontaneous rupture of the bowel (primarily large bowel) may recur repeatedly, possibly after intramural bleeding. Transient intestinal obstruction without perforation may also occur. The patient with vascular type EDS who presents with abdominal pain often poses a considerable diagnostic and treatment problem because obstruction, perforation, and arterial bleeding must all be considered, as well as other pathologies. Patients with constipation should be treated with dietary fiber and laxatives, because the use of enemas has caused fatal intestinal perforation in patients, including adolescents. Obstetrical complications have also been reported.

The characteristic facial appearance consisting of thin, pinched nose, thin lips, hollow cheeks, and prominent eyes is due to a decrease in adipose tissue. However, these characteristics are not readily apparent in children, making diagnosis without family history difficult.

The biochemical and molecular basis for this autosomal-dominant form of EDS has been identified as the absence, diminution, or structural abnormality of type III collagen. Numerous mutations

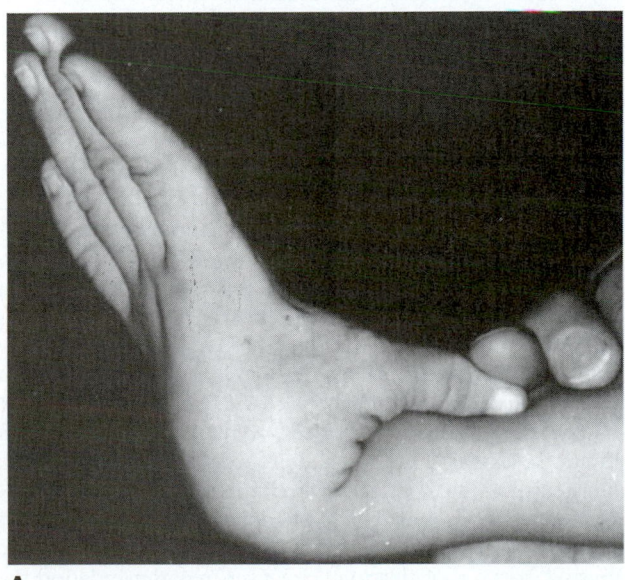

A

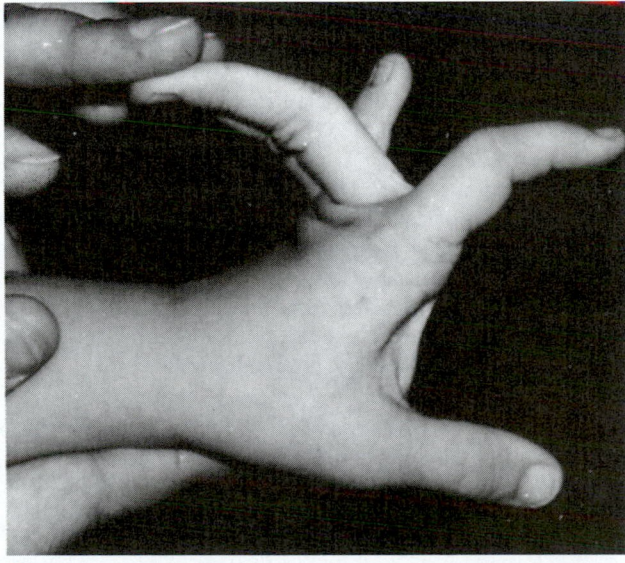

B

FIGURE 10-23   Joint hypermobility in a 5-year-old boy with Ehlers-Danlos syndrome, type III, benign hypermobile type.

in the *COL3A1* have now been identified. Type III collagen is found principally in tissues of those organs that normally undergo physiological distention, such as blood vessels and hollow viscera. Although prenatal diagnosis is possible in families, there is an inherent risk in obtaining tissue because of its fragility. If vascular EDS are suspected, a skin biopsy should be taken for protein and genetic analysis.

The *kyphoscoliosis type* (previously *type VI ocular-scoliotic*) is an autosomal-recessive form of EDS caused by a deficiency of a collagen-modifying enzyme, lysyl hydroxylase. Carriers have about one-half normal levels of enzymatic activity. The major diagnostic criteria consist of joint laxity, severe muscle hypotonia and scoliosis at birth, and scleral fragility. Minor criteria include tissue fragility, easy bruising, arterial rupture, marfanoid habitus, microcornea, and osteopenia (detectable radiographically). Serious ocular problems are not as frequent as previously believed. The severe muscular hypotonia leads to delayed gross motor development, and kyphoscoliosis is progressive. The severity of this phenotype often results in loss of ambulation in the second and third decades of life. Differential diagnosis includes the neonatal form of the Marfan syndrome. A diagnosis of kyphoscoliosis type of EDS should be considered in a "floppy infant."

Individuals who are either homozygous or compound heterozygotes for mutations in the gene encoding lysyl hydroxylase (PLOD) have been identified. Lysyl hydroxylase normally converts certain lysine residues in collagen to hydroxylysine. Measurement of total urinary hydroxylysyl pyridinoline and lysyl pyridinoline has a high degree of sensitivity and specificity. Dermal lysyl hydroxylase activity and *PLOD* mutation analysis can also be performed but are not generally available. A rarer and less severe form with normal lysyl hydroxylase activity has also been reported.

The *arthrochalasia type* (previously *types VIIA and VIIB arthrochalasis multiplex congenita*) is an autosomal-dominant condition. Typically, infants are born with bilateral hip dislocations and exhibit extreme ligamentous laxity with dramatic hyperextension at the knees and elsewhere. Recurrent joint subluxations are common. Minor diagnostic manifestations are muscular hypotonia, easy bruising, tissue fragility with atrophic scars, kyphoscoliosis, skin hyperextensibility, and mild osteopenia. These factors contribute to breech presentation and delayed gross motor development. The differential diagnosis should include Larsen syndrome.

The defect is caused by the skipping of exon 6 in either the 1 or 2 chains of type I collagen. Type I collagen is the most abundant collagen in skin and bones. Exon 6 encodes the cleavage site for the procollagen I N-terminal peptidase. The absence of the cleavage site causes the persistence of the N-propeptide and the secretion of longer than normal molecules. Biochemical analysis of skin fibroblast collagen may be used for laboratory diagnosis. Electron microscopy has shown irregular and loosely organized collagen fibrils.

The *dermatosparaxis type* (previously *type VIIC human dermatosparaxis*) is an autosomal-recessive form of EDS that is caused by a deficiency of the procollagen I N-terminal peptidase. The major diagnostic criteria are severe skin fragility and sagging, redundant skin. Minor manifestations include soft, doughy skin, easy bruising, premature rupture of fetal membranes, and large umbilical or inguinal hernias. Although skin fragility and bruising are prominent, wound healing is normal, and scars are not atrophic. Redundant skin produces a facial appearance similar to children with cutis laxa.

This type of EDS is the recently identified human counterpart of the long-known ovine and bovine disease dermatosparaxis. Electron microscopy of skin has demonstrated ribbon-like collagen fibrils and hieroglyphic shapes such as those seen in dermatosparactic

animals. Biochemical confirmation of type I collagen abnormalities is the same as that for the arthrochalasia type. Determination of N-proteinase activity and identification of genetic mutations are not generally available. Individuals either homozygous or compound heterozygotes for mutations have been identified.

Other forms of EDS have appeared in the literature, yet it is unclear whether they are separate entities. Type V, which is X-linked, has only been described in one family. Type VIII is similar to the classical type but presents with periodontal disease, is rare, and may not be a distinct entity. Finally, type X has also been described in one family with many of the cardinal features of EDS, autosomal-recessive inheritance, and abnormal platelet aggregation owing to a fibronectin defect.

Diagnosis of Ehlers-Danlos Syndromes

Most types of EDS are usually readily diagnosed by observation of soft, doughy, hyperelastic skin, joint hypermobility, and easy bruisability. Vascular EDS, by contrast, may be difficult to recognize owing to subtlety of cutaneous features and limited joint findings; easy bruisability, thin skin, and a prominent venous pattern over the anterior trunk may be the major clinical findings. Misdiagnoses typically occur because hyperelasticity of skin is missed and may result in inappropriate investigation (eg, extensive hematologic workup for easy bruising) or inappropriate diagnosis (eg, child abuse). The current revised classification of EDS was designed to refine more specifically the diagnostic criteria for each type of EDS. Because of the prognostic implications, biochemical or molecular confirmation of the vascular and kyphoscoliosis types should be obtained; the latter disease may also be ameliorated by therapy.

Treatment

Complications caused by tissue fragility and biomechanical incompetence may cause considerable morbidity. The major goals are preventive therapy and careful surgical repair of serious complications. Use of shin guards, high-topped boots, and knee pads and limiting physical contact activities have substantially decreased skin splitting, excessive bruising, and dystrophic scarring over the lower extremities. Prolonged wound fixation by stay sutures and taping may prevent dystrophic scarring and dehiscence, and these measures should be continued for about twice as long as usual. Surgical repair of hernias, diverticulae, prolapses, and the like should be accomplished with due consideration of the underlying tissue fragility and delayed recovery of tensile strength; the use of simple precautions to prevent postoperative disruption will almost always be successful.

Scarring and easy bruisability are sometimes a cosmetic problem, and vitamin or other hematinic therapy is of no value. Prolonged bleeding after surgery has been observed in some instances and should be considered prior to intervention. Patients with vascular EDS may be at risk for hemorrhage, and surgery is usually high risk.

The enzyme deficient in kyphoscoliosis type, lysyl hydroxylase, requires ascorbic acid as one cofactor. In selected patients, vitamin C supplementation has increased enzymatic activity. Recurrent dislocations, chronic effusions, and progressive kyphoscoliosis may require surgical repair (usually with limited success).

Recent evidence has begun to suggest that individuals with classical and perhaps hypermobility types of EDS are at risk for progressive aortic root dilation. However, recommendation that patients with these forms of EDS undergo routine echocardiography, similar to that for individuals with the Marfan syndrome, is, for now, premature.

References

Burrows NP: The molecular genetics of the Ehlers-Danlos syndrome. Clin Exper Dermatol 24:99–106, 1999

Depaepe A, Devereux RB, Dietz HC, et al: Revised diagnostic criteria for the Marfan syndrome. Am J Med Genet 62:417–426, 1996

Rossi Foulkes R, Roman MJ, Rosen SE, et al: Phenotypic features and impact of beta blocker or calcium antagonist therapy on aortic lumen size in the Marfan syndrome. Am J Cardiol 83:1364–1368, 1999

10.3.7   Neurocutaneous Disorders

David H. Viskochil

Neurofibromatosis types 1 and 2 (NF1 and NF2), tuberous sclerosis complex (TSC1 and TSC2), and von Hipple Lindau disease (VHL) are neurocutaneous disorders that are loosely classified as *phakomatoses* (Chap. 25). Additional neurocutaneous conditions are discussed in Sec. 25.18.

The phakomatoses are generally autosomal-dominant conditions that show a consistent pattern of abnormal growth of various tissue, and each affected individual has unique and unpredictable manifestations. The variability of clinical expression of cutaneous manifestations and tumors distinguishes these disorders from other genetic conditions and has multiple causes, including modifier loci, somatic mutation, and simple stoichiometry in cells with haploin-sufficiency of the respective neurocutaneous gene. Somatic mutation leading to inactivation of the normal neurocutaneous gene allele, termed *second hits,* in individuals who have a constitutional mutation is a common theme and suggests that genes causing neurocutaneous disorders fit the paradigm of "tumor suppressors." Characterization of these genes has led to the identification of biochemical pathways involved in intracellular growth-signaling, information that will lead to the development of novel therapeutic regimens strategically targeted to the regulation of growth of benign tumors associated with these conditions.

NEUROFIBROMATOSIS 1

Clinical Aspects

Neurofibromatosis type 1 is the most common neurocutaneous disorder, affecting about 1 in 3000 people worldwide. The hallmark features of NF1, café-au-lait spots and benign cutaneous neurofibromas, typically arise before the ages 5 and 15, respectively. Approximately two-thirds of individuals with NF1 have only these neurocutaneous manifestations, whereas the remaining one-third display myriad medical complications that are unpredictable, both in timing and severity.

Even though NF1 has been recognized as von Recklinghausen disease by the medical community since the nineteenth century, both its variability and age dependence of clinical manifestations made it essential to establish a well-accepted set of clinical criteria (Table 10-16). The presence of at least two of seven criteria establishes the diagnosis. The typical clinical manifestations allow the diagnosis to be established in children by age 10 years. By virtue of full penetrance in the adult population, NF1 is more straightforward to diagnose in familial cases because it requires only one physical manifestation in addition to an affected first-degree relative. In sporadic cases, NF1-related associations that are not part of the diagnostic criteria sometimes appear prior to the development of a second diagnostic sign.

TABLE 10-16

DIAGNOSTIC CRITERIA FOR NF1 (NEUROFIBROMATOSIS 1)

- Six or more cafe-au-lait macules of over 5 mm in greatest diameter in prepubertal individuals and over 15 mm in greatest diameter in post-pubertal individuals
- Two or more neurofibromas of any type or one plexiform neurofibroma
- Freckling in the axillary or inguinal regions
- Optic glioma
- Two or more Lisch nodules (iris hamartomas)
- A distinctive osseous lesion such as sphenoid dysplasia or thinning of the long bone cortex with or without pseudarthrosis
- A first-degree relative (parent, sibling, or offspring) with NF1 by the above criteria

Stumpf DA: Neurofibromatosis: NIH Consensus Statement. 6(12):1-19, 1987; Gutmann DH, et al: The diagnostic evaluation and multidisciplinary management of neurofibromatosis 1 and neurofibromatosis 2. JAMA, 278:51–57, 1997.

The typical pattern of clinical presentation in NF1 is age-dependent. Usually, multiple café-au-lait spots (CLS) are identified in the first 2 years of life (Fig. 14-13). The observation of greater than five CLS that are greater than 0.5 cm in diameter in toddlers is a classical presentation, but a number of other conditions include multiple CLS (ie, McCune-Albright syndrome), although other signs and symptoms generally enable exclusion of other diagnoses fairly easily.

Intertriginous freckling, which usually involves the axillae and groin areas, occurs in approximately three-quarters of individuals with NF1 who present with multiple CLS and this sign develops by late childhood (Fig 14-13). Lisch nodules can be identified by slit-lamp exam in over 75% of preadolescents.

Neurofibromas are benign peripheral nerve sheath tumors that are a collection of Schwann-like cells, fibroblasts, and extracellular matrix. Cutaneous neurofibromas tend to appear at the time of puberty and progress in number. Dermal neurofibromas can be difficult to detect at their outset and are often most easily palpated along the flanks and lower abdomen as slight depressions rather than bumps. Plexiform neurofibromas, however, are thought to be congenital malformations that tend to present before adolescence. Actively growing plexiform neurofibromas in infancy require a significant amount of medical attention, as these tumors are diffuse, and may extensively entwine internal organs. Only the larger plexiform neurofibromas have a propensity to undergo malignant transformation, and this is rare in the pediatric population.

Optic pathway tumors affect approximately 15% of individuals with NF1, and only half of these are symptomatic. Symptomatic tumors tend to arise in the toddler and early childhood years, and optic pathway tumors rarely develop after puberty.

The skeletal features of NF1 are also age-dependent. Sphenoid wing dysplasia, long-bone bowing with pseudarthrosis, and dysplastic scoliosis all tend to present in infancy or early childhood. The pathophysiology of the various skeletal features is not understood, and it challenges the paradigm of NF1 being a disorder of neural crest origin. Some of the skeletal manifestations are clearly of primary mesodermal origin rather than a secondary reaction to either altered blood supply or the presence of an associated tumor. Both dysplastic scoliosis and pseudarthrosis of long bones are primary defects that require significant orthopedic management and do not usually arise in the context of either plexiform or paraspinal neurofibromas. Like cutaneous neurofibromas, paraspinal neurofibromas tend to arise in later childhood and adolescence. In general, these tumors are asymptomatic unless they compress either nerve roots or adjacent spine.

Individuals with NF1 are prone to a number of medical complications that are quite varied, although it is rare that any one individual has more than one major complication. Approximately 40 to 50% have speech impediments and learning problems, which are not specific to NF1. Early recognition and treatment within the educational environment can effectively deal with NF1-related learning problems, which is one reason to provide a provisional diagnosis of NF1 in sporadic cases who only have multiple café-au-lait spots. Short stature, macrocephaly, hypertension, constipation, and chronic headaches are other NF1-related features. Dysplastic scoliosis, deep plexiform neurofibromas, low-grade astrocytomas of the CNS, spinal neurofibromas, malignant peripheral nerve sheath tumors, pheochromocytomas, rhabdomyosarcomas, and myelogenous leukemia are a few of the more serious medical complications associated with NF1.

Molecular Aspects

The NF1 gene spans approximately 335 kb of genomic DNA and is ubiquitously expressed, although the highest level of expression is in the central nervous system. *NF1* acts as a tumor suppressor by diminishing signaling through MAPK pathway.

The high sporadic incidence of NF1 suggests that the gene is highly mutable, and it has been calculated that 1 in 10,000 gametes harbor an inactivating *NF1* mutation. This propensity for mutation has yet to be adequately explained. The high germ-line mutation rate likely carries over to somatic mutation, which would support the "tumor suppressor" model for NF1 and provide an explanation for the variable and progressive nature of some clinical features. Random acquisition of somatic inactivation of the normal *NF1* allele (the second hit) in tissue showing abnormal growth could explain the age-related clinical presentation of many NF1 features, ie, neurofibromas, optic nerve pathways tumors, and dysplastic scoliosis. Leukemia cells, cutaneous neurofibromas, malignant peripheral nerve sheath tumors, and pheochromocytomas have all demonstrated either loss of heterozygosity or homozygous inactivation of *NF1*.

Management

Approximately half of the individuals with NF1 seen in North America and Europe are sporadic cases. Even though there is a high sporadic incidence, once it is established within a pedigree NF1 behaves like any other autosomal-dominant condition whereby there is a 50% risk for occurrence in each child conceived by an affected parent. However, unlike many other autosomal-dominant conditions, the lack of a genotype-phenotype correlation means that affected family members who have the same *NF1* mutation usually have different manifestations. To date, the only evidence for a genotype-phenotype correlation lies with the patients who have large whole-gene deletion and seem to share a phenotype marked by an unusually large number of neurofibromas that present at an earlier age, distinctive facial features differing from family background, and decreased level of intellectual functioning. Most medical complications of NF1 are managed surgically; however, there is clearly a role for "watchful waiting" in this condition.

The clinical recognition of NF1 signifies a need for periodic ophthalmologic evaluations that may not otherwise be performed. Anticipatory guidance counseling encompasses features that are not included in the diagnostic criteria (Table 10-17) but represents age-related concerns of NF1.

TABLE 10-17
ANTICIPATORY GUIDANCE IN NF1

Newborn–2 years
  Café-au-lait spots for diagnosis
  Long bone bowing
  Plexiform neurofibromas
  Optic pathway tumor
  Developmental delay
2–10 years
  Optic pathway tumors
  Plexiform neurofibromas
  Scoliosis
  Hypertension
  Freckling patterns
  Learning problems
10–20 years
  Onset of dermal neurofibromas
  Learning problems
  Self-esteem
  Scoliosis
  Plexiform neurofibromas
  Reproductive decisions
  Hypertension
Adult years
  Offspring
  Progression of dermal and plexiform neurofibromas
  Malignant peripheral nerve sheath tumors
  Hypertension

TUBEROUS SCLEROSIS COMPLEX

Clinical Aspects

Tuberous sclerosis is an autosomal-dominant condition that may affect as many as 1 in 5700 to 1 in 10,000 people, worldwide. Tuberous sclerosis complex (TSC) clinically manifests in many ways as evidenced in the diagnostic criteria outlined in Table 10-18. The hallmark cutaneous features include ash-leaf hypopigmented macules, shagreen patches, facial angiomas and forehead plaques, and ungual and gingival fibromas (Plate 7). The multisystem involvement of TSC is much broader than the other neurocutaneous disorders. Unlike the other common phakomatoses conditions, TSC carries a higher risk for mental retardation, especially when associated with seizures in the first year of life. A difficult diagnostic and counseling issue in TSC is the incomplete penetrance of this condition. Unlike NF1, where affected adults can be readily identified, mild cases of TSC have often been diagnosed only when an affected first-degree relative with TSC has prompted an imaging workup that identifies an asymptomatic manifestation (see Table 10-19). The broad variability of clinical expression within individuals and families with multiple affected members is similar to NF1.

The typical clinical presentation for TSC is much less predictable than for NF1. Recognition of TSC by physical examination in older children and adults is straightforward. However, the diagnosis is often complicated both by the age dependency of many features and by incomplete cutaneous manifestations of TSC. Identification of hamartomatous involvement of various organs in TSC is necessary for both diagnosis and anticipatory guidance. Prenatal cardiac rhabdomyomas identified by fetal ultrasonography may be the earliest sign of TSC and typically regress over an individual's lifetime. The prevalence of these tumors in TSC in infancy is over 50%, which makes echocardiography one of the more reliable diagnostic screening tests in that age group. Cardiac rhabdomyomas are not

TABLE 10-18
DIAGNOSTIC CRITERIA FOR TUBEROUS SCLEROSIS COMPLEX (TSC)

PRIMARY FEATURES	SECONDARY FEATURES	TERTIARY FEATURES
Facial angiomas	Affected first-degree relative	Hypomelanotic macules
Multiple ungual fibromas	Cardiac rhabdomyoma (histologic or radio-graphic confirmation)	Confetti skin lesions
Cortical tuber (histologically confirmed)		Renal cysts (radiographic evidence)
Subependymal nodule or giant cell astrocytoma (histologically confirmed)	Retinal hamartoma other than astrocytoma or achromatic patch	Randomly distributed enamel pits in deciduous and/or permanent teeth
Multiple calcified subependymal nodules pro-truding into the ventricle (radiographic evidence)	Cerebral tuber (radiographic confirmation)	Hamartomatous rectal polyps (histologic confirmation)
	Noncalcified subependymal nodules (radiographic confirmation)	Bone cysts (radiographic confirmation)
Multiple retinal astrocytomas	Shagreen patch	Pulmonary lymphangiomyomatosis (radiographic confirmation)
	Forehead plaque	
	Pulmonary lymphangiomyomatosis (histologic confirmation)	Cerebral white-matter migration tracts or gingival fibromas
	Renal angiomyolipoma (histologic or radiographic confirmation)	Hamartomas of other organs (histologic confirmation)
	Renal cysts (histologic confirmation)	Infantile spasms

DIAGNOSTIC DEFINITION OF TSC

1. Presence of either one primary feature and two secondary features *or* one secondary feature plus two tertiary features—*definite* TSC
2. Presence of either one secondary plus one tertiary feature *or* three tertiary features—*probable* TSC
3. Presence of either one secondary feature *or* two tertiary features—*suspected* TSC

SOURCE: Hyman MN, Whitemore VN, NIH Consensus Conference: Tuberous Sclerosis Complex. Arch Neurol 57: 662–665, 2000.

predictive of other TSC-related features and usually do not cause severe morbidity.

Infantile spasms are considered a tertiary feature of TSC, and approximately 50% of all infants with this type of seizure activity have TSC. The onset of seizures before 1 year of age predicts more significant mental impairment and greater numbers of cortical tubers on brain imaging studies. Regardless of seizure status, both cortical tubers and subependymal nodules become evident by brain imaging in early childhood.

Hypopigmented spots of ash-leaf character can be seen in all ages, even newborns, and, unlike the café-au-lait macules, enhancement with a Wood's lamp may be useful in the diagnostic clinical examination. The hypopigmented skin findings of TSC are not specific; however, the manifestation of clustered spots in a confetti-like

TABLE 10-19
TSC MANAGEMENT

		SURVEILLANCE INITIAL SCREEN OF		
	SUSPECTED CASE	KNOWN CASE WITH NO SYMPTOMS	KNOWN CASE WITH SYMPTOMS	FIRST-DEGREE RELATIVE AT TIME OF DIAGNOSIS OF AFFECTED INDIVIDUAL
Funduscopic examination	R	NR	R	R
Brain MR/head CT imaging	R	R[a]	R	R[b]
Brain EEG	NR[c]	NR	R[d]	NR
Cardiac ECG and ECHO	R	NR	R[e]	NR[f]
Renal MR, CT, or ultrasound imaging	R	R[g]	R[e]	R[h]
Dermatologic screening	R	NR	R[d]	R
Neurodevelopmental testing	R	R[i]	R[d]	NR
Pulmonary CT	NR	NR[j]	R[d]	NR

R = indicates screening recommended; NR = screening not recommended; MR = magnetic resonance, EEG = electroencephalogram; ECG = electrocardiogram; ECHO = echocardiogram; and CT = computed tomography.
[a] Every 1 to 3 years.
[b] With negative physical examination results, CT screen is recommended.
[c] Unless seizures are suspected, generally not useful for diagnosis.
[d] As clinically indicated.
[e] Every 6 months to 1 year until involution or size stabilization occurs.
[f] Probably less frequently than in children.
[g] Every 3 years until adolescence.
[h] Ultrasound is generally recommended because of cost, although local imaging expertise may vary.
[i] Recommended for children at the time of beginning first grade.
[j] Baseline screen at age 18.

presentation, in addition to the typical ash-leaf spots, may be the only physical features in the childhood years. Fibrous plaques involving the cranium can also occur in infancy, but other cutaneous features such as adenoma sebaceum and multiple ungual fibromas (primary criteria), and the shagreen patch (secondary criteria), typically present later in life, even after adolescence.

Of the renal manifestations, cysts usually are common in childhood and may be confused with polycystic kidney disease, whereas angiomyolipomas typically arise in middle age and have been found in approximately two-thirds of individuals with TSC who have had an autopsy. Retinal astrocytomas, pitted enamel hypoplasia, and rectal polyps are found in over one-half of TSC patients. All these findings can arise in childhood and should be considered in the diagnostic workup. Finally, pulmonary lymphangioleiomyomatosis, a rare complication of TSC, typically develops in females in the third or fourth decade. The age dependence of the various manifestations of TSC is an important concept that must be considered in the management of pediatric cases of TSC.

Molecular Aspects

Linkage studies have demonstrated that TSC is a genetically heterogeneous condition, mapping to either chromosome 9 (band 9q34.3) or chromosome 16 (band 16p13.3). The *TSC1* gene has been isolated, and the gene product, hamartin, is unique with no known function, although it interacts with the ezrin-radixin-moesin family of binding proteins. Complexes between hamartin and ERM-family proteins are proposed to act through a small GTP-binding protein, rho, to mediate a signal transduction pathway, which regulates cell adhesion properties.

The *TSC2* gene has also been cloned and partially characterized. *TSC2* encompasses approximately 43 kb of genomic DNA, and its 5.5-kb transcript encodes a novel 190- to 200-kDa protein designated tuberin. A small domain at the carboxyl end of tuberin bears homology to the catalytic domain of the GTPase activating protein called *rap1GAP*, which suggests that tuberin could down-regulate Rap1a-activated mitogenic signaling in specific cell types. Genetic analysis of the *TSC1* and *TSC2* locus supports a role as a loosely defined tumor suppressor.

Management Issues

TSC is so broad that individuals who may be only mildly affected are at risk of having offspring who may be severely affected. Likewise, the diagnosis of TSC could modify diagnostic evaluations for developmental delay and circumvent unneeded studies.

Like other neurocutaneous disorders, the clinical care of TSC patients is devoted to control of symptoms. Medical management of seizures and cardiac arrhythmias associated with cardiac rhabdomyomas is an important issue to consider. A recommendation of vigabatrin as the drug of first choice to treat TSC infantile spasms has been proposed by an NIH consensus conference. Implementation of surveillance protocols for renal and pulmonary tumors is also important to identify those rare cases early in tumor progression.

NEUROFIBROMATOSIS 2

Clinical Manifestations

Neurofibromatosis 2 (NF2) is an autosomal-dominant condition whose hallmark is the presence of bilateral vestibular schwannomas, previously called *acoustic neuromas*. The incidence of this condition is estimated at about 1 in 33,000 to 1 in 40,000. Even though NF2

is a neurocutaneous condition with variable clinical expressivity, there is almost complete penetrance by 60 years of age. Diagnostic criteria have been established as shown in Table 10-20. Even though the mean age of onset of symptoms is in the third decade, clinical presentation in childhood is not rare.

The presenting symptoms of NF2 are usually related to the vestibular schwannomas: hearing loss, tinnitus, imbalance, and facial weakness. Vestibular schwannomas are found in approximately 95% of individuals with NF2 and are bilateral in 90%. Other CNS tumors occur in approximately one-half of individuals with NF2 and include intracranial meningiomas, spinal schwannomas, cranial nerve schwannomas (the fifth cranial nerve being most common), and ependymomas. Presenile lens opacities or cataracts occur in 50 to 75% of individuals with NF2 and serve as an early clinical sign of the disorder that can be used as a screening modality in the pediatric population. Cutaneous manifestations of NF2 include CLS and skin tumors. Usually there are fewer than 5 CLS. The dermal tumors are either characteristic plaque-like lesions or subcutaneous nodules that are pathologically diagnosed as schwannomas. There are two major clinical forms of NF2. The Gardner subtype is milder with later onset of symptoms and few intracranial or spinal tumors, whereas the Wishart subtype is earlier in onset, more rapid in progression of hearing loss, and has an increased occurrence of intracranial and spinal tumors.

Mapping of NF1 to chromosome 17 and NF2 to chromosome 22 underscores the clinical impression that these two conditions are distinct entities, especially because NF2 does not have neurofibromas.

Molecular Aspects

NF2 genetically maps to the long arm of chromosome 22, and its gene encodes a 595-amino-acid cytoplasmic protein that shares homology with a family of cytoskeletal-associated proteins (ezrin, ra-

TABLE 10-20

DIAGNOSTIC CRITERIA FOR NF2 (NEUROFIBROMATOSIS 2)

- Bilateral vestibular schwannomas, either proven histologically or seen by MR imaging with gadolinium enhancement.
- A parent, sibling, or child with NF2 and either a unilateral vestibular schwannoma *or* two or more of the following:
  Schwannoma
  Posterior subcapsular lenticular opacities
  Cerebral calcification
- Unilateral vestibular schwannoma *and* two or more of the following:
  Meningioma
  Glioma
  Schwannoma
  Posterior subcapsular lenticular opacities
  Cerebral calcification
- Multiple meningiomas (two or more) *and* one or more of the following:

  Glioma
  Schwannoma
  Posterior subcapsular lenticular opacities
  Cerebral calcification

SOURCE: Evans DG, Huson SM, Donnai D, Neary W, Blair V, Newton V, Strachan T, Harris R: A genetic study of type 2 neurofibromatosis in the United Kingdom. II. Guidelines for genetic counselling. J Med Genet 29(12):847-852, 1992; adapted from Huson SM, Rosser EM: The phakomatoses. In: Rimon DL, Connor JM, Pyeritz RE, eds: Emery and Rimoin's Principles and Practice of Medical Genetics, 3rd ed. New York, Churchill-Livingstone, 1997, 2269-2302

dixin, and moesin). This ERM family of proteins mediates communication between the extracellular milieu and the intracellular cytoskeleton. The *NF2* gene product, called either *merlin* or *schwannomin,* is unusual because as a structural protein it has tumor suppressor properties. Inactivating mutations correspond to the more severe Gardner phenotype, whereas the milder Wiscott phenotype corresponds to missense and splice-site mutations. Somatic mutation also plays a significant role in the pathology of this condition. Loss of the normal allele in NF2-related tumors has been demonstrated, which supports the hypothesis that *NF2* is a bona-fide tumor suppressor gene.

Management

Individuals suspected of having NF2 should undergo a comprehensive initial investigation to identify CNS tumors, skin manifestations, and eye findings. Neurosurgical management provides many options, and referral to a center experienced in NF2-related tumors, both adult and pediatric, is warranted. Audiologic evaluations and early facilitation of communication skills in individuals who are at risk for either progressive deafness or acute hearing loss secondary to surgical intervention is important. Genetic linkage studies are warranted in established families. In informative families, linkage analysis could identify those individuals who carry a mutated *NF2* gene. Those who have not inherited the chromosome 22 harboring the mutated gene do not need to undergo routine and costly screening tests.

Hearing screens, ophthalmologic evaluations, and radiologic screening in presymptomatic individuals is an important component of NF2 management. Such screening could detect a significant number of presymptomatic adolescents. At-risk screening for vestibular schwannomas is recommended in late childhood with annual sensitive hearing evaluations, including brainstem evoked response testing. MR screening to detect vestibular schwannomas when the tumors are small enough to be surgically removed with preservation of hearing is recommended. A normal MR imaging in late adolescence reduces the likelihood that an at-risk individual has NF2 by 50%, and a normal scan at 30 years of age makes it unlikely that such an at-risk individual has NF2.

VON HIPPEL-LINDAU SYNDROME

Clinical Aspects

Von Hippel-Lindau disease (VHL) is an autosomal-dominant condition characterized by a predisposition to develop tumors in the eyes, central nervous system, kidneys, pancreas, and adrenal gland. Most manifestations of VHL initially present in early adulthood, except for the cardinal features, retinal angioma and cerebellar hemangioblastoma, which can present in the first decade and teenage years, respectively. The well-established diagnostic criteria for the diagnosis of von Hippel-Lindau syndrome are outlined in Table 10-21. The prevalence has been estimated to be about 1 in 40,000 to 50,000 people. Like other neurocutaneous conditions, VHL demonstrates marked variability of clinical expression and relatively high penetrance in the adult population. Imaging studies are helpful to identify asymptomatic individuals who have characteristic malformations and tumors.

The cerebellar hamangioblastoma associated with VHL differs from sporadic forms of this tumor, presents earlier in life, and consists of multiple tumors. Symptoms are similar to any posterior fossa tumor, but the majority of VHL-related tumors are cystic rather than solid. Angiomas of the eye occur in approximately half of pa-

TABLE 10-21

DIAGNOSTIC CRITERIA AND SCREENING PROTOCOL FOR VON HIPPEL-LINDAU SYNDROME

Diagnostic criteria:
More than one hemangioblastoma of the central nervous system or retina, or an isolated hemangioblastoma in association with a pheochromocytoma, renal carcinoma, or pancreatic involvement
A first-degree relative with von Hippel-Lindau syndrome and any one manifestation
Screening for affected individuals:
Annual physical examination and urine testing
Annual ophthalmology evaluations
Brain MR scan every 3 years to age 50 and every 5 years thereafter
Annual abdominal MR scan
Annual 24-h urine collection for vanillylmandelic acid
Screening for at-risk relatives:
Annual physical examination and urine testing after age of 5 years
Annual ophthalmology evaluations from age 5 until age 60
Brain MR scan every 3 years from age 15 to 40 years and every 5 years thereafter
Annual abdominal MR from age 20 to age 60
Annual 24-h urine collection for vanillylmandelic acid

SOURCE: Maddock IR, Moran A, Maher ER, Teare MD, Norman A, Payne SJ, Whitehouse R, Dodd C, Lavin M, Hartley N, Super M, Evans DG: A genetic register for von Hippel-Lindau disease. J Med Genet 33(2):120–127, 1996

tients with VHL, and about one-third are bilateral. Without screening, these retinal tumors are usually detected in the second and third decades of life. Hemorrhage, retinal detachment, and visual loss can all occur if not recognized early and treated. At-risk family members are routinely screened for these manifestations as shown in Table 10-21. Other CNS lesions and visceral tumors of VHL present later in life. Renal cell carcinoma usually presents in the fourth decade of life and occurs in approximately 25 to 40% of patients with VHL. A genotype-phenotype correlation with respect to pheochromocytoma in families with VHL occurs, and those families with pheochromocytoma appear less likely to develop renal carcinoma.

Molecular Aspects

VHL genetically maps to chromosome 3p25, and the disease-causing gene is composed of three exons that encode a protein of 213 amino acids. The gene is ubiquitously expressed, and the unique VHL protein (pVHL) is present both in the nucleus and cytoplasm of cells; pVHL plays a role in regulating expression of hypoxia-response genes. The most characterized function of pVHL is its role in transcription elongation. Thus, inactivation of pVHL by mutation of the gene leads to unregulated elongation of transcription of oncogenes and results in tumor growth.

Germ-line mutations can be detected in approximately 75% of families with VHL. The apparent genotype-phenotype correlation with respect to pheochromocytoma may arise as a consequence of missense mutations, whereas "inactivating" mutations are not associated with pheochromocytoma. The identification of second hits in the *VHL* gene in tumor tissue from individuals with VHL demonstrates that it is a classical tumor suppressor (see Sec. 20.2).

Management

The variability of age of onset of the various tumors makes diagnosis and screening for VHL somewhat ineffective. More than 60% of patients do not have the hallmark features of VHL. Thus, more than other neurocutaneous disorders, characterization of the *VHL* gene allows for effective and appropriate presymptomatic screening by DNA analysis to determine affected status of at-risk family members. The clinical screening protocols for VHL are more extensive than in the other neurocutaneous disorders; therefore clarification of the at-risk status by DNA analysis has a major impact on the diagnostic imaging performed in this condition.

References

Friedman JM, Gutmann DH, MacCollin M, Riccardi VM: Neurofibromatosis: Phenotype, Natural History, and Pathogenesis, 3rd ed. Baltimore, Johns Hopkins, 1999

Hyman MH, Whittemore VH: National Institutes of Health Consensus Conference: Tuberous sclerosis complex. Arch Neurol 57:662–665, 2000

10.3.8   Environmental Causes of Birth Defects

Lynne P. Martinez, Julia Robertson, and Marsha Leen-Mitchell

The very definition of a teratogen—any agent, external to the fetal genome, that induces structural or functional alterations during prenatal development—suggests that the clinicians' first encounter may be well after the (prenatal) exposure has occurred. Knowledge of the principles of teratology can direct diagnostic and treatment approaches to a child with dysfunction or dysmorphology of unknown etiology and can be instrumental in guiding initial evaluations well as physician-patient-parent interactions.

TYPES OF PRENATAL EXPOSURES

MEDICATIONS Few pregnancies progress to term without the use of at least one medication, whether prescription or nonprescription drugs, herbal remedies, or nutritional supplements. If vitamins and minerals are excluded, an average of three to four medications are used during the course of a pregnancy, with analgesics being the most commonly reported. Other common categories include cough and cold products, antacids, antihistamines, antiemetics, barbiturates or sedatives, and antibiotics.

CHEMICALS Given the growing number of chemical agents being developed or sold for both home and industrial environments, pregnant women are increasingly vulnerable to chemical exposures. Although many such compounds do not appear to be teratogenic to humans, limited human data exist to develop risk assessment. In most cases, however, symptoms of maternal poisoning are present when teratogenic chemical exposure occurs.

INFECTIONS Infections of primary concern during pregnancy include "childhood" diseases such as varicella and some sexually transmitted diseases such as HIV. When the mother only is exposed to the disease, the fetus is not at risk; fetal effect occurs only when the pregnant woman acquires the active infection.

CHRONIC MATERNAL CONDITIONS Chronic medical conditions such as insulin-dependent diabetes mellitus or systemic lupus can be teratogenic. In most cases, risk to the fetus increases with the severity of maternal disease and inadequate treatment, emphasizing the necessity of rigorous medical oversight.

OTHER PHYSICAL AGENTS High doses of ionizing radiation used for therapeutic indications can induce fetal anomalies. Diagnostic radiation (less than 5 rads directly to the uterus) has not been found teratogenic. Chorionic villus sampling is a procedure that carries some risk for the fetus.

FACTORS USED TO DETERMINE TERATOGENIC RISK

In weighing the possibility that a specific teratogen is responsible for a child's disease or defect, one of the most important factors to be considered is *background risk*. Any pregnancy carries an approximate 4% risk that the fetus will be affected with a major, life-affecting defect. While this level of risk can be increased by maternal teratogenic exposure, it cannot be decreased. A common misconception is that a majority of birth defects are a result of teratogenic exposure. However, teratogens cause only about 5% of the clinically significant congenital structural defects in humans.

Principles of teratology—timing (within the gestational period) of the exposure, dose of the agent, and duration of the exposure—are critical to an accurate determination of teratogen involvement.

TIMING OF EXPOSURE The time frame at which an exposure occurs during the pregnancy is, arguably, the most important factor to consider when determining teratogenicity. Contemporary understanding of embryology and embryopathy guides this principle. For example, teratogenic exposure between days 15 and 28 after fertilization can be the cause of a neural tube defect, because during this time neural tube closure occurs in the embryo. Parallels can be drawn between teratogenic exposure and development of virtually any other major organ or system. Thus, knowing that the mother was exposed during a critical time for induction of the child's anomaly is vital when evaluating a child for possible teratogenic effects.

DOSE OF THE AGENT The dosage or measure of exposure to a teratogen appears to have a direct association with effect on the fetus. Fortunately, threshold levels have been estimated for most known human teratogens. For example, the dosages of methotrexate required for therapeutic treatment of rheumatoid arthritis and psoriasis are considerably below those that could induce fetal defects.

DURATION OF EXPOSURE Since functional as well as structural development of the fetus can be affected by some teratogens, the duration of an exposure can have a significant impact. For example, smoking more than 10 cigarettes each day can affect the growth of the fetus if the smoking continues beyond the twentieth week of gestation. Alcohol can affect functional brain development, and thus heavy consumption of alcohol that continues beyond 24 weeks in the pregnancy is associated with developmental and learning disorders.

EPIDEMIOLOGIC PRINCIPLES

Knowledge of some of the primary tenets of epidemiologic investigation can be instrumental in assessing possible teratogenic etiologies of a patient's condition (see Chap. 8).

CONFOUNDING VARIABLES Confirmation of a specific drug, chemical, infection, or other exposure as cause for a child's outcome can be complicated by the fact that multiple exposures often take place concurrently in the same pregnancy. As an example, early investigations into caffeine led researchers to hypothesize that its consumption during pregnancy resulted in low birth weight infants. Only later was it discovered that heavy coffee drinkers are also more likely to be heavy tobacco users; smoking was thus the confounding variable in lower birth weight.

SPECIES SPECIFICITY Studies of pregnancy outcomes in animals are not predictive of human outcomes, since teratogenic agents tend to demonstrate species-specific effects. Genetic variability among species produces differences in drug absorption, distribution, and metabolism. Extrapolating from animal data to humans is problematic, because pharmacokinetic profiles vary depending on the drug and species. For example, the limb agenesis observed in children with thalidomide exposure is not seen in the usual animal studies. Other differences may be credited to animals' ability to carry multiple fetuses and variations in placental development and function. Thus, whereas animal models are useful in detecting the mechanisms by which known teratogens exert their influence, such studies are not beneficial in determining which agents are teratogenic in humans.

CLINICAL CONSISTENCY Most of the identified human teratogens show patterns of abnormalities presenting as syndromes rather than isolated or nonspecific single defects. Although statistically rare, these events have been the hallmark by which teratogens have been "discovered." Two examples can illustrate this point.

Within three years of release of isotretinoin, a vitamin A congener, three cases of isotretinoin embryopathy characterized by isolated anotia, microtia, and conotruncal heart defects were reported. All three infants had a combination of these anomalies that is rarely seen, heightening the statistical probability that there was a teratogenic agent involved. Based on just three reports, isotretinoin was suspected as a human teratogen, which was established by epidemiologic and clinical investigations.

Case reports of malformations among children exposed to Bendectin (a combination of doxylamine, disydomine, and pyridoxine) in utero were reported, but no pattern of defects could be detected, and epidemiologic analyses found the rate of malformations in patients exposed to the drug was no higher than the background risk of malformations, which demonstrated the lack of teratogenicity of the product. Therefore, the degree of certainty of cause depends on the rarity of the exposure and the distinctiveness of the outcome.

SELECTED ESTABLISHED HUMAN TERATOGENS

The proven human teratogens are relatively few in number, and Table 10-22 outlines a comprehensive list of well-established human teratogens.

Drugs

Carbamazepine Carbamazepine (Tegretol) carries a less than 1% risk for a neural tube defect (spina bifida) when exposure occurs between 15 and 29 days after conception. Although other fetal effects (growth retardation and possible developmental delay) have been attributed to carbamazepine, subsequent studies have failed to support an association. The level of risk caused by fetal exposure to carbamazepine is as yet unknown.

Methotrexate/Aminopterin Methotrexate can have a teratogenic effect when taken between weeks 6 and 9 of gestation at doses higher than 10 mg per week. Craniosynostosis (premature ossification of the skull and sutures), underossified skull, craniofacial abnormalities (wide-spaced eyes, broad nose, small chin, and flattened facies), and limb defects (absent toes, webbed fingers, or shortened limbs) have been reported. The level of fetal risk after exposure to methotrexate is not known.

Based on cases in which aminopterin was used as an abortifacient in high doses (12 mg or more per week), there is an increased risk for spontaneous abortion, low birth weight, craniofacial abnormalities, limb abnormalities, craniosynostosis (premature ossification of the skull and sutures), and possibly neural tube defects (spina bifida or anencephaly). The level of risk for birth defects associated with aminopterin use in the first trimester of pregnancy is unknown.

Thalidomide Thalidomide was one of the first drugs identified as a human teratogen. When exposure to the drug occurs during days 34 to 50 of gestation, there is a risk of at least 20% for limb reduction defects (missing arms and/or legs) and ear malformations, including deafness. Because of its effectiveness in treating some peripheral neuropathies associated with Hansen disease (leprosy), thalidomide was approved for marketing in the United States in the summer of 1998. The drug's parent company has established an extensive physician and pharmacy registration process along with a detailed patient consent procedure in an effort to avoid additional cases of thalidomide embryopathy in children.

Maternal Disorders

Alcoholism Heavy consumption of alcohol during pregnancy as a putative cause of poor infant outcome has been considered for more than 100 years. To establish a diagnosis of fetal alcohol syndrome (FAS), findings in at least three categories, in addition to a history of maternal ethanol exposure, must be present: (1) two facial characteristics (Fig. 10-24) including shortened palpebral fissures, epicanthic folds, hypoplastic nasal root, short, upturned nose, hypoplastic or absent philtrum, thin upper lip, and/or hypoplastic mid-face; (2) one abnormality of pre- and/or postnatal growth deficiency such as microcephaly, weight less than tenth percentile, or length/height less than tenth percentile; and (3) one cognitive abnormality including developmental or learning problems. The highest risk of affected infants of chronic alcoholic women who continue drinking throughout pregnancy has been placed at 10 to 15%, although some of the larger studies of pregnant alcoholics place the risk as low as 2%.

Unfortunately, the facial characteristics, growth deficiencies, and developmental or learning problems used to diagnose FAS are not specific, making the diagnosis in a particular child problematic. In fact, a FAS diagnosis should not be attempted until the child is at least 1 year of age and, because the face grows and changes, preferably not until the child is 4 to 8 years old. Additionally, prenatal ethanol exposure may manifest as developmental and/or learning difficulties in children of alcoholic mothers who drank heavily during the latter parts of pregnancy, with none of the facial signs of FAS present.

Ethnic variability is another critical consideration when determining whether a child has a "short, upturned nose" or "hypoplastic mid-face." Norms for length of a nose or palpebral fissures and other features are only now being established for ethnic groups not descended from Northern Europeans. So-called norms, then,

TABLE 10-22
KNOWN HUMAN TERATOGENS

TERATOGEN	POTENTIAL DEFECTS	CRITICAL PERIOD	PERCENT AFFECTED
Medications/metals			
ACE Inhibitors	Renal dysgenesis	Second to third trimester	Not established
	Oligohydramnios		
	Skull ossification defects		
Alcoholism	Fetal alcohol syndromes:	<12 weeks	10–15
	Craniofacial features		
	CNS abnormalities		
	Heart defects		
	Low birth weight	>24 weeks	Not established
	Developmental delay		
Aminopterin >12mg/week	Spontaneous miscarriage	<14 weeks	Not established
	Craniofacial anomalies	First trimester	Not established
	Limb defects		
	Craniosynostosis		
	Neural tube defects		
	Low birth weight	>20 weeks	Not established
Androgens/norprogesterones	Masculinization of external female genitalia	>10 weeks	0.3
Carbamazepine	Spina bifida	<30 days pc	1
Carbimazole/methimazole	Hypothyroidism		Not established
	Goiter, scalp defects		
Cigarette smoking			
>20/day	Miscarriage	<20 weeks	Not established
>10/day	Low birth weight	>20 weeks	Not established
Cocaine	Abruptio placentae	Second to third trimester	Not established
	Intracranial hemorrhage	Third trimester	Not established
	Premature labor/delivery		
Diethylstilbestrol	Uterine abnormalities	<12 weeks	Not established
	Vaginal adenosis		
	Vaginal adenocarcinoma		
	Cervical ridges		
	Male infertility		
Etretinate	See isotretinoin		
Isotretinoin	Fetal death	>15 days pc	45–50
	Hydrocephalus		
	CNS defects		
	Microtia/anotia		
	Small or missing thymus		
	Conotruncal heart defects		
	Micrognathia		
Lithium	Ebstein anomaly	<8 weeks	<1
Methotrexate	Craniosynostosis	6 to 9 weeks pc	Not established
>10 mg/week	Underossified skull		
	Craniofacial anomalies		
	Limb defects		
Penicillamine	Cutis laxa		Not established
Phenytoin	Craniofacial anomalies	First trimester	10–30
	Hypoplastic phalanges/nails		
	Vitamin K deficiency with resultant hemorrhage		
		Second to third trimester	Not established
Solvents, abuse (entire pregnancy)	SGA		Not established
	Developmental delay		
Streptomycin	Hearing loss	Third trimester	Not established
Tetracycline	Stained teeth and bone	≥20 weeks	Not established
Thalidomide	Limb reduction defects	38 to 50 post-LMP days	15–25
	Ear anomalies		
Thiouracil	Spontaneous miscarriage	First trimester	Not established
	Stillbirth	>20 weeks	Not established
	Goiter		Not established
Trimethadione	Developmental delay	First trimester	Not established
	V-shaped eyebrows		
	Low-set ears		
	Irregular teeth		

(continued)

TABLE 10-22   Continued

TERATOGEN	POTENTIAL DEFECTS	CRITICAL PERIOD	PERCENT AFFECTED
Valproic acid	Spina bifida	<30 days pc	1–2
	Craniofacial appearance	First trimester	Not established
	Preaxial defects		
Warfarin	Nasal hypoplasia	6 to 9 weeks	Not established
	Stippled epiphyses		
	CNS defects secondary to cerebral hemorrhage	>12 weeks	Not established
Methylmercury	Cerebral atrophy	Not established	Not established
	"Spasticity" seizures		
	Mental retardation		
Lead	Pregnancy loss	Not established	Not established
Polychlorbiphenyls (PCBs)	Low birth weight		
	Skin discoloration	Not established	Not established
Maternal infections			
Rubella	Deafness	Up to 8 weeks	85
	Cataracts	9–12 weeks	52
	Heart defects	12–20 weeks	16
	Mental retardation		
Cytomegalovirus	Low birth weight	<27 weeks	5
	Mental retardation		
	Microcephaly		
	Hearing loss		
Toxoplasmosis	Hydrocephalus	10–24 weeks	Not established
	Blindness		
	Mental retardation		
Varicella	Skin scarring	Up to 20 weeks	1
	Limb reduction defects		
	Chorioretinitis		
	Mental retardation		
Parvovirus	Miscarriage	10 to 25 weeks	7–10
	Fetal hydrops		
	Fetal death		
Syphilis	Abnormal teeth and bones	>5 months	Not established
(untreated)	Mental retardation		
	Proteinuria		
Venezuelan equine encephalitis	CNS abnormalities	Not established	Not established
	Stillbirth		
Genital herpes type II (primary)	Miscarriage	<20 weeks	Not established
Active genital herpes	Vertical transmission at term delivery	Not established	Not established
Maternal states			
Diabetes mellitus	Heart defects	First trimester	6–10
	Caudal deficiency sequence		
	Femoral hypoplasia		
	Renal vein thrombosis	>11 weeks	Not established
Hypo-/hyperthyroidism	Goiter		
	Mental retardation		
	Growth retardation		
Phenylketonuria (PKU)	Fetal death	Entire pregnancy	Not established
(untreated)	Microcephaly		
	Mental retardation		
	Craniofacial features		
	Heart defects		
Hypertension	Miscarriage	<20 weeks	Not established
	IUGR	>20 weeks	
	Placental insufficiency		
	Placental abruptio/previa		
Seizure disorder	Oral clefts	First trimester	6–8
(treated)	Heart malformations		
Hyperthermia	Neural tube defects	14–30 days pc	1
Systemic lupus erythematosus	SAB	<20 weeks	Not established
(SLE)	Stillbirth	>20 weeks	
	Prematurity		
	Congenital heart block		

pc = postconception.

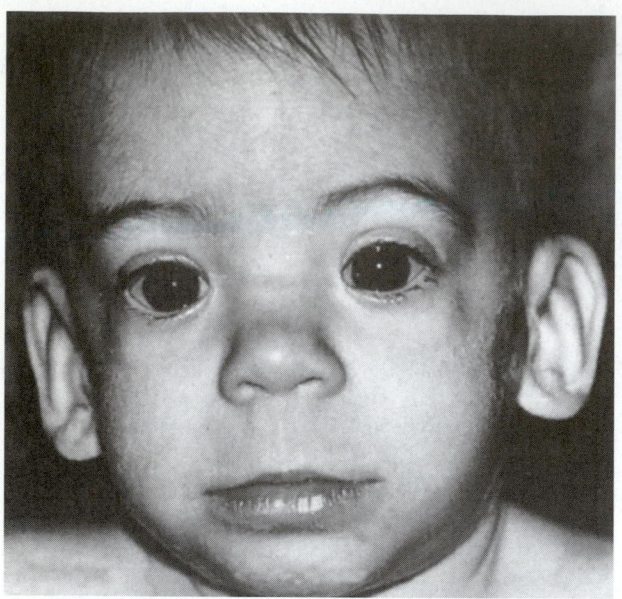

FIGURE 10-24   A 1-year-old infant with fetal alcohol syndrome. Note the facial features including a low nasal root, short palpebral fissures, and flat philtral folds.

when applied to native Americans, Latinos, blacks, or those of other ethnicity can lead to erroneous results. Studies have demonstrated that children of economically disadvantaged, nonwhite women are more likely to be evaluated for substance abuse than are their counterparts, leading to the possibility of overdiagnosis of FAS in certain populations.

The benefits and drawbacks of early FAS diagnosis remain controversial. Many argue that early identification of FAS can lead to interventions that will improve the child's life. Others note that the diagnosis of FAS can result in labeling of the child, limiting achievement expectations.

Diabetes Mellitus   Maternal diabetes mellitus is the most common human teratogenic state. Mothers with insulin-dependent diabetes have a 2 to 3 times increased risk for having a child with a congenital defect. The pattern of defects observed in children is not random and includes sacral agenesis, laterality defects (i.e., situs abnormalities), and holoprosencephaly. Improved control of glucose levels prior to conception decreases the risk substantially and underscores the importance of preconceptional counseling.

Human Parvovirus B19/Fifth Disease   Fatal congestive heart failure (hydrops) can occur in 10% of fetuses whose mothers contract this infection during pregnancy. Between 10 and 24 weeks of gestation is the most vulnerable exposure time, with the gestational period after 12 weeks and before 22 weeks comprising the greatest risk. There have been no reported congenital anomalies related to maternal parvovirus infection (see Chap. 13).

Varicella   When a pregnant woman contracts chickenpox during the first trimester, the risk of fetal effects is approximately 1%. If the infection occurs prior to or during limb bud formation, limb reduction defects can result. Other effects of varicella include chorioretinitis, scarring of the skin with muscle atrophy, and a possibility of developmental delay, which is less well established than the eye, skin, and limb effects (see Chap. 13).

Chemicals

Methylmercury   Methylmercury is an organic compound that can accumulate in animals (eg, fish) that are subsequently consumed by humans, and when a pregnant woman develops symptoms of methylmercury poisoning, there is a concern for fetal development at any stage of the pregnancy. The fetal effects of methylmercury poisoning can include cerebral atrophy, seizures, and developmental delay.

Solvents   Studies of solvent exposure in an occupational setting have shown pregnancy loss when mothers experience long-term high doses that create symptoms of toxicity (lightheadedness and headaches). In the absence of these signs of toxicity, no adverse fetal effects have been reported. Some pregnant women abuse solvents, and the fetal effects are discussed in the following section.

Substance Abuse

With the exception of alcohol and possibly cocaine and solvents, no substance of abuse has been conclusively associated with an increased risk of birth defects. However, reversible toxicity and/or withdrawal symptoms may occur in newborns whose mothers abuse certain drugs throughout the pregnancy or in large dosages near the time of delivery. Substance abuse throughout pregnancy has been associated with an increased risk for intrauterine growth retardation, prematurity, and low birth weight regardless of the particular substance abused (see Chap. 2). Also, with needle use, an increased risk for transmission of pathogens such as human immunodeficiency virus (HIV) or hepatitis B can cause adverse health effects for both the mother and infant (see Chap. 13).

Cigarette Smoking   Investigative evidence associates a greater risk of low birth weight commensurate with the number of cigarettes smoked during pregnancy. Also evidence suggests that heavy maternal smoking (more than 10 cigarettes/day) is associated with an increased risk for miscarriage, premature delivery, and stillbirth.

Cocaine   With cocaine use during pregnancy, an increased risk for abruptio placentae, which can result in a miscarriage, stillbirth, or premature delivery, occurs. Used near delivery, cocaine can also be associated with an increased risk for intracranial hemorrhage. Infants whose mothers use cocaine continuously throughout pregnancy or in large amounts near the time of delivery may be at an increased risk for irritability, tremulousness, and muscle rigidity, which usually develop several days after birth, resolve quickly, and seem to have no long-term effects on the infant or child (see Chap. 2).

Solvent Abuse   Case reports suggest an association between maternal solvent abuse and pregnancy loss, intrauterine growth retardation, prematurity, microcephaly, and development delay. However, the magnitude of risk remains unknown.

Most infants exposed to drugs in utero will not have physical signs of problems, but there are concerns that fetal drug exposure can lead to behavioral problems later in childhood. To date, no conclusive studies have been able to confirm this link, but it is presumed that at least a portion of these infants are at risk for learning and behavioral problems. Socioeconomic elements that can accompany maternal substance abuse (ie, inadequate parenting skills, poverty, lack of education) may ultimately prove to have as significant an impact on the long-term outcomes for these children as the physiological consequences (see Chap. 1).

COUNSELING PATIENTS ABOUT TERATOGENS

Counseling Parents

Most pregnancies in the United States are not planned, and a majority of women will have been exposed to some type of teratogen during their pregnancy. When a child is born with an anomaly, families are therefore likely to focus on a putative teratogen as the cause and frequently turn to their physicians for advice and counsel.

Preconceptional Counseling

Drug exposures early in pregnancy may result in a higher potential for teratogenicity, because this is the critical period of tissue differentiation and organ system development. Because many women are not yet aware that they are pregnant for much of this critical period, preconceptional counseling is critical for women during their reproductive years. Because more than 50% of pregnancies in the United States are not planned, this counseling should not be limited to only those anticipating a pregnancy.

Women who require routine management of medical conditions must be counseled carefully about potential pregnancies. Often, correction or improvement of the condition before conception can improve maternal health during pregnancy and result in a more positive fetal outcome. For example, strict periconceptional control of conditions such as diabetes mellitus and phenylketonuria is known to improve pregnancy outcomes. Ironically, many women are so concerned that their medications may pose a risk to the fetus that they stop taking drugs, which actually has an adverse effect on the fetus.

Counseling women regarding preconceptional use of multivitamins containing folic acid, which may reduce the risk of neural tube defects, is also important. The Centers for Disease Control and Prevention recommend that all women of childbearing years take either a multivitamin with folic acid or a folic acid supplement (0.4 mg) every day.

Counseling Pregnant Patients

The basic approach to counseling a patient about the risk of medication exposure during pregnancy usually includes the 3 to 4% background risk of congenital malformations and the risk-versus-benefit issues of medication use. If medication exposure has already occurred, counselors recommend notification of the pediatrician. One of the most important goals of patient counseling is to avoid unnecessarily alarming the patient. The Organization of Teratology Information Services (OTIS) provides referrals to local Teratology Information Services, which are comprehensive and multidisciplinary resources for medical consultation on prenatal exposures. For a referral to a local service, call 1-888-285-3410. A list of services is available on line at *www.ucsd.edu/otis.*

PATERNAL EXPOSURES

Although information is available regarding maternal exposures during pregnancy, limited information exists surrounding outcomes from paternal exposures. There is concern that environmental exposures could affect the egg or sperm cells. However, studies of such mutagenic exposures do not reveal an increased risk of birth defects; damage of the germ cells appears only to affect the fertility of those cells. Semen studies of men exposed to known teratogens did not suggested an increased risk of malformations. In addition, concentration of the agent in semen does not appear to have sys-

temic effects in women and therefore does not affect the pregnancy except when an infection is transmitted to the mother through the semen.

References

Briggs GG, Freeman R-K, Sumner J: Yaffe Drugs in Pregnancy and Lactation, 5th ed. Baltimore, Williams & Wilkins, 1998

Institute of Medicine Fetal Alcohol Syndrome: Diagnosis, Epidemiology, Prevention and Treatment. Washington DC, National Academy Press, 1996

Shepard TH: Catalog of Teratogenic Agents, 9th ed. Baltimore, Johns Hopkins, 1998

10.4   GENETIC ASPECTS OF DEVELOPMENTAL DISABILITIES

John C. Carey

Developmental and sensory disabilities are an important contributor to morbidity and to chronic illness in childhood. Establishing a diagnosis and etiology helps with the prediction of recurrence risks in genetic counseling, knowledge of the natural history of a condition, and the implementation of appropriate guidelines for health supervision and anticipatory guidance. The practical approaches to the diagnosis are also similar to the principles outlined for evaluation of congenital malformations (see Sec. 10.3.2, Fig. 10-14): The first question is whether the child's problem is an isolated one or a component of a broader syndromic pattern. The diagnosis of a syndrome is helpful in elucidating the etiology and prognosis whereas isolated findings are descriptive categories and obviously heterogeneous in etiology.

In addition, the principles used in the recognition of minor anomalies and subtle phenotypic variations, as well as the data-gathering process, are similar to what has been discussed in the section on congenital defects. Developmental delay/mental retardation, hearing loss, and microcephaly will be used to illustrate concepts because of their high frequency in the pediatric setting. The approach to the child who has autism or the autism spectrum disorder is quite similar to the child with developmental delay/mental retardation (see Sec. 5.7). The approach to the individual with a visual disability or so-called blindness is also very similar to the thought process surrounding the child with hearing loss (see Chap. 26). Referral for genetic consultation and counseling is appropriate for children in which there is no specific diagnosis present and where parents are asking questions regarding recurrence risk.

10.4.1   Approach to the Child with Developmental Disabilities/Mental Retardation

Agatino Battaglia

Medically, mental retardation (MR) is understood as a highly variable, heterogeneous manifestation of central nervous system dysfunction. According to the DSMIV (1995), the diagnostic criteria are: (1) onset before age 18 years, (2) an IQ of approximately 70 or below, and (3) concurrent deficits or impairments in two or more of the following areas: communications, self-care, home living, social and interpersonal skills, use of community resources, self-direction, functional academics, health and safety, and work and leisure.

MR is grouped into four degrees of severity by measure of tested IQ. *Mild* MR is defined as "educable"; patients possess an IQ level from 50 to approximately 70. *Moderate* MR is considered a "trainable" severity level and is seen in individuals with IQs of 35 to 55. In *severe* MR, the IQ level is 20 to 40, and profound MR is most frequently defined by an IQ level below 20 to 25. It has been estimated that about 85% of individuals with MR function within the mild range, whereas about 10% function within the moderate range, and only 5% are severely to profoundly impaired. Recently, the American Association on Mental Retardation proposed that a different system, one that utilizes the intensity of the support needed by the individual, would better express the functional limitations of the individual and thus hold more practical use. Intensity of intervention is quantified as intermittent, limited, extensive, or pervasive. However, grouping by degrees of severity is still useful from the clinical point of view.

Mental retardation may become evident during infancy or early childhood as developmental delay (DD), which is a common clinical problem in pediatrics and is estimated to occur in approximately 2 to 10% of the population (see Chap. 5). However, recent data from the United States Department of Education indicate that the prevalence of MR among schoolage children (6-17 years) is 1.14%. The different rates of prevalence of MR depend on definitions used, methods of ascertainment, and population studied. The individual's cultural and socioeconomic environments should also be taken into consideration when testing procedures are applied. Importantly, the prevalence of mild retardation varies inversely with socioeconomic status, whereas moderate to severe disability does not.

ETIOLOGY

Etiologic factors may be biological or socioenvironmental; in some cases, there may be combination of the two. The biological factors can be prenatal, perinatal, or postnatal. The prenatal factors can be further subdivided into preconceptual, embryonic, and fetal factors. Preconceptual factors include single-gene abnormalities such as neurocutaneous disorders, malformation syndromes, inborn errors of metabolism, and chromosome aberrations such as trisomy syndromes and polygenic familial syndromes. In the embryonic phase, chromosome abnormalities, infections (eg, TORCH), exposure to teratogens such as alcohol, placental dysfunction, and central nervous system malformations are considered factors that can result in MR. Fetal factors include infections, teratogens, maternal phenylketonuria, placental dysfunction, and intrauterine malnutrition. Prematurity, hypoxia/ischemia, hypoglycemia, hypomagnesemia, hyperbilirubinemia, and infections are perinatal conditions that can cause MR. Postnatal influences include infections, asphyxia, trauma, metabolic disorders, poisoning, and malnutrition.

McLaren and Bryson reviewed more than a dozen studies and found causes of mental retardation could be divided into the following categories and associated prevalence: chromosomal, 30%; CNS malformations, 10 to 15%; multiple congenital anomaly (MCA) syndromes, 4 to 5%; metabolic, 3 to 5%; acquired causes, 15 to 20%; and unknown, 25 to 38%. A genetic etiology was present in almost 50% of the cases.

Battaglia and colleagues conducted a retrospective analysis of the diagnostic yield of 120 patients with developmental delay or mental retardation referred to a university-based institute of child

neuropsychiatry. Diagnostic studies, which included up-to-date MRI techniques and video-electroencephalogram (EEG) polygraphy, yielded a causal diagnosis in 41.6% and a pathogenetic diagnosis in 39.2% of the patients. Etiology remained unknown in 19.1% of the 120 patients. Causal categories included chromosomal abnormalities in 14 patients, fragile X syndromes in 4 patients, known MCA/MR syndromes in 19 patients, fetal environmental syndromes in 1 patient, neurometabolic disorders in 3 patients, neurocutaneous disorders in 3 patients, hypoxic/ischemic encephalopathy in 3 patients, other encephalopathy in 1 patient, and congenital bilateral perisylvian syndromes in 2 patients. Notably, this study marks the first time that appropriately different forms of CNS malformations were defined, resulting in a better etiologic yield.

In summary, although the impact of specific factors on prevalence varies among the cited studies, all the reports classify causes of MR into five major categories: MCA syndromes, CNS malformations, metabolic disorders, acquired conditions, and so-called pure or nonspecific (idiopathic) mental retardation.

In about 20 to 55% of individuals seen in clinical settings, no clear etiology of MR can be determined, despite extensive efforts. However, recent developments in diagnostic testing, such as cytogenetic and molecular genetic techniques, neuroimaging, metabolic screenings, and detailed EEG studies, make it likely that the estimated percentage of idiopathic MR cases will decrease in the future. A better diagnostic yield will be obtained as an increasing number of patients originally diagnosed with developmental delay or MR are actually found to have an MCA/MR syndrome.

CLINICAL FEATURES

The overwhelming majority of children with MR are identified when age-appropriate expectations are not met. In fact, the cardinal symptom of MR is represented by delayed achievement of developmental milestones (see Chap. 5). Delay may be restricted to specific areas of development, as is often the case of the child with moderate to mild retardation. For example, a toddler or schoolage child may present with normal motor development but with delayed speech and language abilities.

The diagnosis of MR does not imply a constant state. Early stimulation, social interaction, caregiving, and access to and provision of special education services have a significant impact on functioning of children with MR. The development of cognitive abilities requires not only the integrity and maturation of the nervous system but also an adequate motivation and a harmonic, well-balanced personality organization. Some early personality changes noted in the first months of life, if not properly addressed, may lead to a progressive lowering of cognitive abilities. In early autistic conditions, evolution toward mental retardation can often be seen in an even more profound way. The quality of early reciprocal social interaction, particularly with the mother, is of the utmost importance for the adequate stimulation of cognitive abilities and for giving the child the interest and motivation to use them. Thus, the natural history of mental retardation is greatly variable and dependent on differences in etiology and associated disability as well as access to adequate educational and therapeutic experiences. However, children who lose developmental milestones previously attained have a progressive neurologic disorder and represent an important subgroup (see Chap. 25).

DIAGNOSIS

When mental retardation is identified in a child, there is a shared sense of urgency to determine the causative factor. Given the potential impact of an MR diagnosis, and the hundreds of conditions known to cause mental retardation, any number of investigations may be initiated to establish a diagnosis. A rising consensus, however, suggests an alternative to such a comprehensive diagnostic approach. *Rational evaluation* is an approach that promises to provide significant benefits to the patient, family, and practitioner.

Traditionally, the primary care physician weighs a variety of factors when deciding which screening tests to perform on a specific patient. The seriousness of the condition being evaluated, the acceptability (including risk, safety, yield, sensitivity, and specificity) of the test, and how important it is to make a diagnosis are usually considered before the tests proceed. Rational evaluation is an expansion and extension of this approach specific to MR (Fig. 10-25). Rational evaluation is based on two premises: (1) Making a diagnosis is important and (2) clinical signs, as well as family needs, will drive the evaluation. Making a diagnosis is essential to the individual and the family, who want to know not only why and how MR occurred in their child but also if it will happen again. A specific diagnosis also helps with genetic counseling; planning medical management and early diagnosis may help avoid costly and invasive tests.

Despite recent advances and continued intensive efforts directed at understanding the causes of MR, there remains a lack of uniformity concerning evaluation of patients. In 1995, the American College of Medical Genetics published a consensus report that suggested that three-generation pedigrees, complete history and physical examination, serial evaluations of the patient, selected chromosome or DNA testing, neuroimaging in the presence of neurologic symptoms, and metabolic testing were among the essential elements of the rational MR evaluation.

The importance of a thorough clinical history cannot be overestimated. Prenatal, birth, and family history should be noted. A careful, head-to-toe physical examination includes a neuromotor assessment and a meticulous search for skin changes. Documentation of abnormal findings, as well as measurements where indicated, is critical. Photographs and video can prove very useful. Videotap-

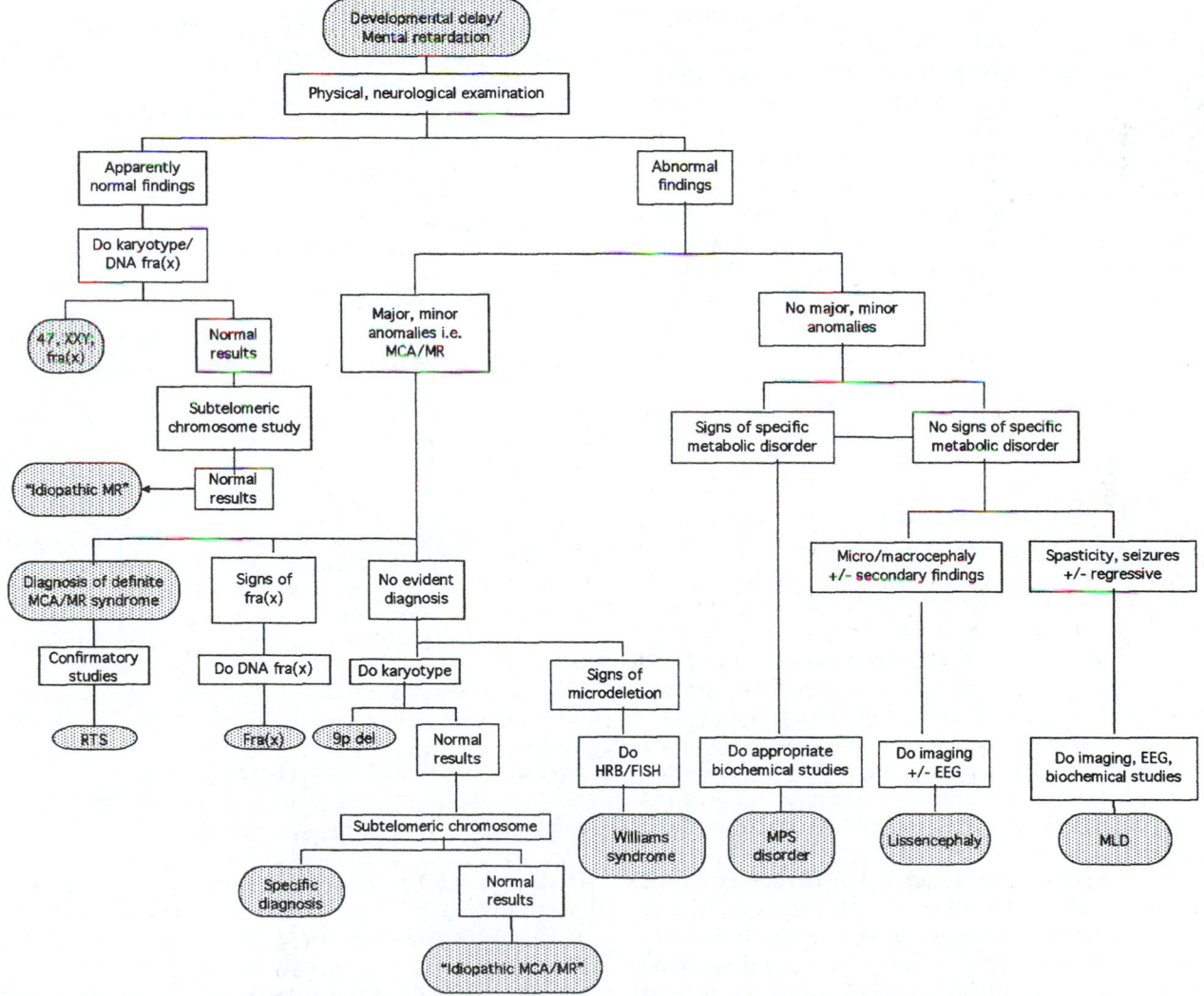

FIGURE 10-25   **The approach to defining the etiology of developmental delay or mental retardation. The initial step is to decide if there are anomalies or abnormal neurologic findings. Examples of diagnoses are given at the end of some pathways. (RTS) = Rubenstein-Taybi syndrome; MPS = mucopolysaccharide disorder; MLD = metachromatic leukodystrophy; MR = mental retardation; MCA = multiple congenital anomalies. Other similar diagnoses should be established using this approach.**

ing is an invaluable tool because it can document behavioral characteristics, gait, posture, and any movement disorders.

The information gleaned from the physical exam alone can help in determining a diagnosis in a number of cases or in postulating a provisional diagnosis for appropriate testing. For example, a patient presenting with DD, severe MR, absent speech, epileptic seizures, microbrachycephaly, ataxia, and jerky arm movements is very likely to have Angleman syndrome. The priority testing, then, would be molecular cytogenetics evaluation for Angleman syndrome and EEG for the exact definition of the seizures and movement disorder. Test results would thus guide the therapy modality; the first choice in this case would most likely be drug treatment. In another case, a floppy infant with no progress in motor functions, little or no reaction to environmental stimuli, minor anomalies, and epileptic seizures should undergo a metabolic workup, searching for a paroxysomal disorder (Zellweger syndrome); EEG and brain MRI would be the second-line investigation. A schoolage patient presenting with cognitive disturbances, behavior problems, and loss of vision is very likely to have X-linked adrenoleukodystrophy (paroxysomal disorder). In this case, confirmation of an excess of very long chain fatty acids (VLCFA) in tissues and body fluids should be made as well as a brain MRI. A child with "coarse facies," failure to thrive in spite of adequate food intake, liver and spleen enlargement, deafness, mental dysfunction, behavioral problems, poor motor performance, eye abnormalities, epilepsy, and myoclonus is very likely to have a storage disorder; appropriate biochemical studies should be the first step toward the diagnosis.

When to order cytogenetic studies can be an ongoing quandary. Opitz has suggested that reduced family resemblance may be one of the most sensitive indicators for the presence of chromosomal abnormalities. Minor anomalies observed in the infant or child but not seen in relatives may signal the necessity of cytogenetic evaluation (see Sec. 10.1.3). Conversely, it is worth noting that a number of MR patients thought to be nonsyndromal on physical examination were later found to demonstrate aneuploidy or fragile X.

Interestingly, there is no known association between chromosome abnormalities and the level of MR. Although chromosome studies are performed less often on individuals with mild MR, individuals with moderate MR show no greater positive rate of chromosomal abnormalities than do those with profound MR.

Little is reported in the literature on the value of the EEG in MR patients, but a recent study by Battaglia and colleagues found that the diagnostic yield of EEG investigations was relatively high (8.3%). An EEG (waking and sleeping) polygraphy, together with an accurate clinical history of epileptic seizures, could allow the clinician to narrow the diagnosis as a definite epileptic syndrome. Other specific clinical presentations could justify an EEG exam, such as significant language impairment (Landau-Kleffner syndrome), Angleman syndrome, Inv dup(15) syndrome, and Wolf-Hirschhorn syndrome.

It has been reported that neuroimaging can detect cerebral anomalies in 9 to 60% of individuals with MR. Many of these abnormalities are descriptive findings (agenesis or hypoplasia of the corpus callosum, ventricular enlargement) and have yet to add significantly to our knowledge of the causes of MR. However, when coupled with ongoing improvement in our knowledge surrounding the diverse brain malformation syndromes and sequences, the use of neuroimaging can undoubtedly complement the diagnostic process of the individual with MR.

In several syndromes and conditions, (Prader-Willi, Angelman, Williams, velocardiofacial, fragile X), the recognizable physical and behavioral phenotype evolves over time; observation of these changes through systematic clinical follow-up can guide confirmation of a diagnosis (increasing the number of diagnoses by 5-20%), selection of a differential diagnosis, or elimination of a diagnosis. Serial clinical evaluations represent an important approach to the patient with MR with the potential to eventually lead to a definite diagnosis or even the characterization of a novel syndrome.

TREATMENT AND MANAGEMENT

As with diagnosis, the first charge in the treatment and management of patients with MR is to recognize the individuality of each patient's condition, environment, and prognosis. A few disorders associated with MR, such as phenylketonuria and hypothyroidism, can be treated. Smith-Lemli-Opitz syndrome is an example of a condition that can improve with treatment. There remain a large number of conditions where little can be done in terms of treatment. Yet each patient has the inherent right to receive not just the ordinary care given to any child but also the extraordinary care necessary to the patient's well-being, as prescribed by his or her singular situation.

Early intervention is key to a productive treatment plan. MR patients receive a thorough "functional evaluation," accomplished by an appropriate professional at the earliest possible juncture. Whenever possible, enrollment in a habilitation program, personalized to the individual's function level, should occur. School placement at the appropriate time is considered mandatory. Vocational training, particularly when the child's overall level of function allows for progression toward independent or semi-independent adult living, should be introduced in secondary school.

Beyond health surveillance and treatment, listening to the family's primary concerns and addressing such concerns whenever possible is helpful. Referral to parent support groups or arrangement of a meeting with other parents of individuals with the same condition may be quite beneficial.

References

Battaglia A, Bianchini E, Carey JC: Diagnostic yield of the comprehensive assessment of developmental delay/mental retardation in an institute of child neuropsychiatry. Am J Med Genet 82: 60–66, 1999

Curry CJ, Stevenson RE, Aughton D, et al, American College of Medical Genetics: Evaluation of mental retardation: recommendations of a consensus conference. Am J Med Genet 72: 468–477, 1997

Majnemer A, Shevell MI: Diagnostic yield of the neurologic assessment of the developmentally delayed child. J Pediatr 127:193–199, 1995

10.4.2 The Child with Hearing Loss

Nathaniel H. Robin and Linda Bone Jeng

Deafness and hearing impairment represent one of the most common disabilities involving the sensory organs, affecting 1 in every 15 Americans. This means over 28 million Americans have some degree of hearing impairment, including more than 8 million schoolage children. Approximately 70% of pediatric hearing impairment is genetically determined, most commonly as an autosomal-recessive trait. However, hearing impairment is incredibly heterogeneous, with dozens of different genes involved.

Prelingual hearing impairment is that which occurs prior to the acquisition of speech or prior to 3 years of age, has an overall incidence of 1.2 to 5.7 per 1000 live births, and is a source of delays in language development and academic achievement, despite advances in hearing aid technology, education techniques, and a greater availability of intervention and habilitation services. The average deaf student graduates high school with language and academic achievement levels of a hearing fourth-grade student. With newborn screening for hearing loss becoming routine in many states, the diagnosis of an infant with hearing loss will become an increasingly common dilemma.

CLASSIFICATION OF THE HEARING IMPAIRMENT

Hearing impairment is classified by type (sensorineural, conductive, or mixed), severity (mild, profound), frequency range primarily affected, age of onset (prelingual, adult onset), and presence or absence of associated anomalies (syndromic, nonsyndromic). (See Fig. 10-26.) Approximately 70% of prelingual deafness/hearing impairment (D/HI) is isolated, or nonsyndromic. A genetic etiology is found in 60% of nonsyndromic D/HI; 85% of these cases are autosomal recessive (AR). Therefore, the majority of the cases with nonsyndromic D/HI are unexpected, as 90 to 95% of these children are born to normal hearing parents who have no family history of D/HI.

THE GENETICS OF NONSYNDROMIC DEAFNESS/HEARING IMPAIRMENT: UNPRECEDENTED HETEROGENEITY

Although over a dozen genes have been identified, more than 60 genetic loci have been defined that contain genes with important roles in hearing. Five of these genes have AR inheritance: *GJB2 (Cx26)* at the DFNB1 locus at 1p33-p35, *myosin VIIa* at the DFNB2 locus, *myosin 15* at the DFNB3 locus, *PDG* at the DFNB17 locus, and *α-tectorin* at the DFNB21 locus.

Mutations in *GJB2*, the *connexin 26 (Cx26)* gene, are known to cause over 50% of AR, D/HI and 30% of singlet cases (those with-

out a family history of D/HI). The difference between these two groups reflects unrecognized acquired causes of nonsyndromic hearing impairment, mostly undiagnosed cases of congenital cytomegalovirus (CMV) infection. In Americans, the carrier frequency for *Cx26* mutations is approximately 1/40 (2.5%) but varies according to racial background. *Cx26* is a member of the connexin family of gap junction proteins, which facilitate the transfer of small molecules and ions between neighboring cells, creating the almost instantaneous propagation of an action potential. Cx26 is expressed in many tissues, including many components of the auditory system, including the stria vascularis, spiral limbus, basement membrane, and spiral prominence of the cochlea. Studies have suggested that Cx26 is important in maintaining the high potassium concentration in the scala media and that Cx26 mutations alter the functional properties of the gap junction, which may cause potassium levels to remain elevated in hair cells.

COGNITIVE AND EDUCATIONAL PERFORMANCE IN CHILDREN WITH D/HI

Early identification of children with profound hearing loss has been shown to positively affect the long-term outcomes. A logical intervention for deaf children requires defining each child's specific educational needs relative to cognitive ability. Recent studies suggest that a hard-of-hearing person's intellectual capacity or ability to learn is not affected by D/HI.

Cognitive variability in D/HI may be explained by the etiology of deafness. There is an obvious difference between someone with a genetic disorder such as Zellweger syndrome, which has sensorineural D/HI and multiple other congenital anomalies, compared to individuals with isolated D/HI. What is not clear is if some of the variability in cognitive capacity among individuals with isolated D/HI may relate to the different etiologies of the D/HI.

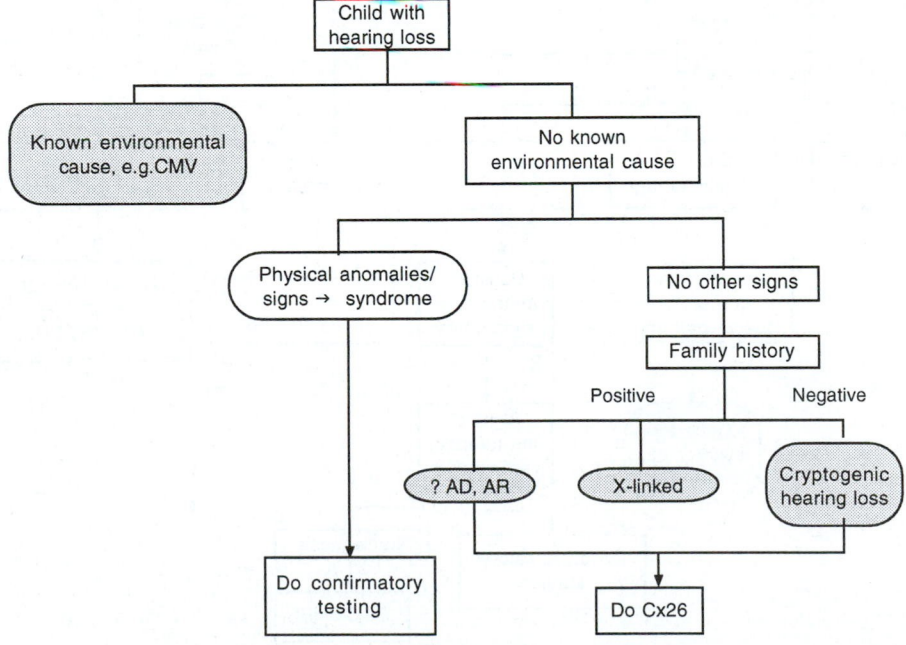

FIGURE 10-26   **The diagnostic approach to the child with hearing loss.**

The results of the studies that looked at the cognitive mechanisms of D/HI individuals have indicated underlying processing differences among deaf children. For example, intelligence testing results have shown that some deaf children are stronger in word knowledge and language development but weaker in abstract visual problem-solving ability when compared to other deaf children. These differences are not as apparent when the test results are compared to the norms of children with normal hearing. Previously, these findings have been explained as relating to the underlying differences in the children's learning strategies but may reflect the distinct genetic etiologies for the D/HI.

Comparing hard-of-hearing and deaf children's abilities with those of their normal hearing peers does not indicate the deaf child's intellectual capacity or ability to learn. The cognitive differences among deaf children may be attributable to the underlying cause of the hearing loss or deafness. For example, D/HI children with a Cx26 gene mutation can be habilitated with a cochlear implant and read at normal to above normal levels for hearing children, whereas other genetic causes of D/HI may have more generalized adverse effects on the central nervous system and therefore cognition.

References

Deaf World Web (2000) web page at HYPERLINK
   http://dww.deafworldweb.org/
National Institute on Deafness and Other Communication Disorders (1998) web page at *http://www.nih.gov/nidcd/genetic.htm*
Willems PJ: Genetic cause of hearing loss. NEJM 342:1101–1109, 2000.

10.4.3 Microcephaly

Agatino Battaglia and John C. Carey

Etymologically, microcephaly means a small head, but the term *micrencephaly* would be more appropriate to designate a small brain. A high correlation between the growth of the two structures exists. Tables of head circumference in fetuses and from birth to adulthood have been well established. Most investigators have defined *microcephaly* as an occipitol frontal circumference (OFC) of less than 3 standard deviations (SD) below the mean for age and sex. However, a surprising amount of controversy exists about whether 3 SD or 2 SD below the mean for age and sex is actually abnormal. For sure, the broader definition of 2 SD below the mean includes some persons with a normal brain who have a small head. Study of the head size of healthy schoolage children will detect a few persons with head measurements of less than −2 SD, because the definition is based on a normal distribution. In this group, however, persons with measurements of less than −3 SD are extremely unusual, and therefore an OFC of that size usually indicates a pathologic abnormality of brain growth. Small head size that is proportionate to chest size and length in infants and height in older children suggests proportionate small body size. However, in a child who is physically or neurologically abnormal, proportionate smallness should not be assumed. In addition, an individual whose height and OFC are both 3 SD below the mean usually has a generalized abnormality of growth affecting both the brain and linear growth rate and should be evaluated for a broad pattern of malformation (see Sec. 24.2). Because small head size can be a familial trait or a normal familial developmental pattern, the OFC of the

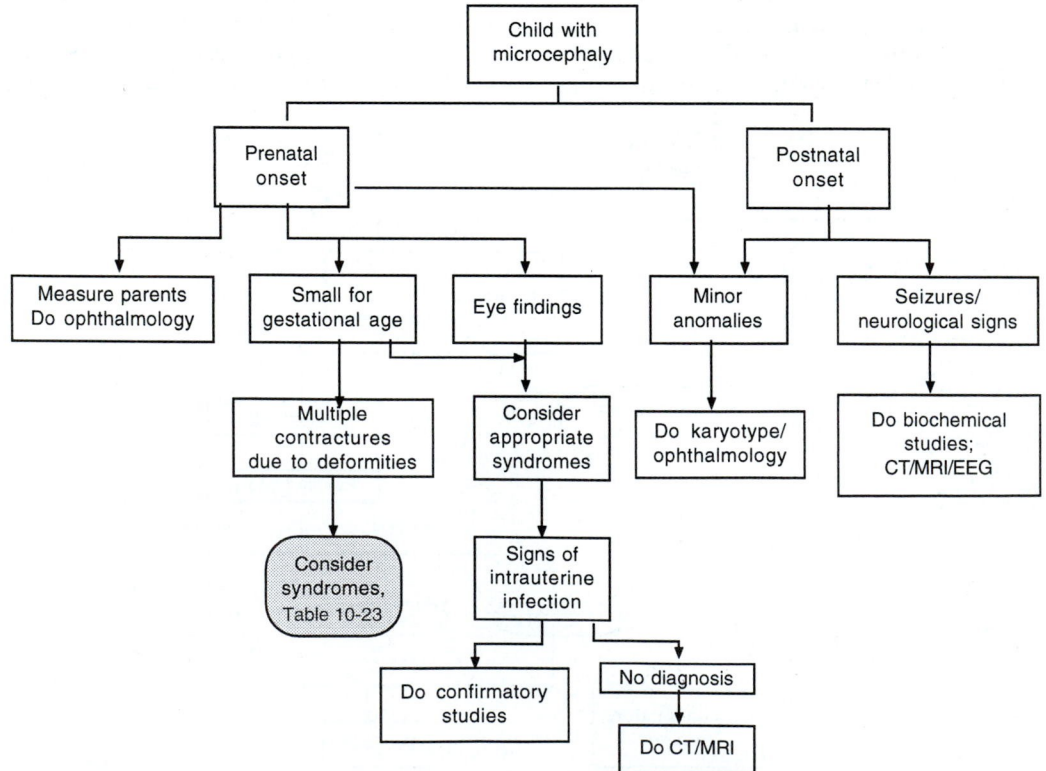

FIGURE 10-27 **The diagnostic approach to the child with microcephaly. CT = computed tomography; MRI = magnetic resonance imaging.**

parents and siblings should be recorded and compared with the head measurement of the proband.

Microcephaly is a descriptive term that does not refer to a particular etiology and covers a wide range of heterogeneous cases caused by multiple mechanisms. Most malformed brains are small. However, microcephaly is a relatively common finding in a large number of constitutional and acquired conditions. Many of the common autosomal chromosome syndromes have prenatal microcephaly as one feature of their recognizable pattern, and most have postnatal microcephaly as a finding (see Sec. 10.1). Interruption of neuronal production or secondary destruction and/or faulty migration, caused by intrinsic or extrinsic factors, may cause microcephaly.

By classical definition primary microcephaly is present by the seventh month of intrauterine life, and secondary microcephaly occurs after the seventh month of gestation. However, a child with disproportionately small head at birth is termed to have *primary microcephaly,* and a child with normal birth OFC, whose head circumference falls below normal centiles after birth, has *secondary microcephaly.*

Some authors prefer to classify microcephaly as *isolated* or *pure/nonsyndromic,* and *associated* or *syndromic.* Isolated or pure/nonsyndromic microcephaly was described in the 1950s in adults with mental retardation and called *microcephalia vera.* The only constant feature reported is severe microcephaly (OFC 3-6 SD below the mean), whereas morphologic anomalies vary from case to case. The classic pattern (poorly differentiated cortex with no horizontal lamination, severe depletion of neurons in layers II and III, polymicrogyria, and clusters of heterotopic neurons in the white matter) is inconsistent. Parodoxically, individuals with microcephalia vera do not show gross neurologic signs but only hypekinetic behavior and disturbances of fine motor coordination. The inheritance of microcephalia vera is most often autosomal recessive, whereas autosomal-dominant and X-linked transmission have also been recorded. Associated or syndromic microcephaly may be part of a distinct pattern of malformation (genetic, acquired, or of unknown origin).

Figure 10-27 presents a diagnostic approach to the child with microcephaly. The initial step in evaluating a child with microcephaly is to obtain the newborn head size and as many measurements on the OFC chart as possible. Prenatal microcephaly (abnormal OFC present at birth) implies an intrauterine onset of the abnormality of brain growth and has a different set of causes than does microcephaly with postnatal onset. The head measurement is then compared with linear growth and weight to determine whether the head size is disproportionately small for the body or if the subject has an overall pattern of growth deficiency. The head size can also be compared with chest size in infancy, since these two measurements are similar during the initial months after birth. Proportionate head circumference, chest size, and length in an otherwise normal individual with mild microcephaly would imply overall small size and not an abnormality of brain growth.

TABLE 10-23

RECOGNIZABLE CAUSES AND SYNDROMES OF MICROCEPHALY

PRENATAL ONSET	POSTNATAL ONSET
Frontal bone recession	**Primary abnormality in brain growth**
Holoprosencephaly/aprosencephaly	Chromosomal syndromes (eg, Down syndrome)
Trisomy 13	Malformations syndromes
Meckel-Gruber syndrome	Rubinstein-Taybi syndrome
Toxoplasmosis	Williams syndrome
Generalized microcephaly	Septo-optic dysplasia
Primary abnormality in brain growth	Angelman syndrome
Chromosomal syndromes, many	Aicardi syndrome
Malformation syndrome	Fanconi syndrome
De Lange syndrome	X-linked microcephaly syndromes—Renpenning syndrome
Smith-Lemli-Opitz syndrome	Structural brain malformations with postnatal onset of microcephaly
Dubowitz syndrome	**Secondary abnormality in brain growth**
Syndromes with primordial short stature	Acquired insult to brain (e.g., postanoxic encephalopathy)
Seckel syndrome	Metabolic insult associated with slowing of brain growth (PKU, Krabbe disease)
Microcephaly, osteodysplasia	Intrauterine viral syndrome
Heritable syndromes of microcephaly	Hypopituitarism, normal intelligence
Joint contractures and other abnormalities	**Microcephaly that is normal variant with normal intelligence**
Cerebro-oculo-facial-skeletal syndrome	Autosomal-dominant trait
Neu-Laxova syndrome	Part of overall pattern of generalized small body size
Bowen-Conradi syndrome	
Heritable syndromes of microcephaly and choreoretinal abnormalities (eg, falciform folds)	
Autosomal-recessive microcephaly	
Structural brain malformations (eg, lissencephaly)	
Secondary abnormality in brain growth	
Radiation exposure of greater than 0.2 Gy	
Chemical teratogenic syndromes (eg, alcohol)	
Intrauterine viral syndromes, rubella, CMV, toxoplasmosis	
Offspring of mother who has PKU	
Death of monozygotic twin in utero affecting surviving twin's brain development	

A complete pre- and perinatal history together with an extensive family pedigree (three-generation), including consanguinity, and measurements of parents' head sizes are an essential second step. Physical examination, including a careful search for dysmorphic features or structural defects, should follow to determine whether the child may have a malformation syndrome. Signs of prenatal abnormalities, such as frontal bone recession or absence of flexion creases on the fingers, are especially important. A thorough neurologic examination should be performed to ascertain the presence of any abnormal finding, such as alteration of tone and reflexes, and presence of abnormal movements, posture, gait, and behavior. The presence of seizures should be carefully documented. In the presence of the aforementioned findings and features, the small head almost certainly indicates an abnormal brain. A complete ophthalmologic evaluation with pupillary dilation is mandatory in all children with an abnormal head size, because the detection of chorioretinitis, optic nerve hypoplasia, optic atrophy, cataracts, retinal folds, or macular abnormalities may lead to a specific diagnosis or suggest a pathologic process.

Historical and physical/neurologic findings determine laboratory evaluation of the child with microcephaly (Fig. 10-27). If the child is dysmorphic or has multiple malformations and does not fit a recognizable syndrome, a karyotype should be performed; in case of normal results, other possible pathways are illustrated in the algorithm. If the child does fit a recognizable syndrome (eg, Smith-Lemli-Opitz), then the most appropriate tests to define that syndrome should be undertaken. If the child shows no major/minor anomalies but has a history of seizures, an accurate waking/sleep electroencephalogram (possibly with video-polygraphy) and neuroimaging should be carried out. Neuroimaging is also recommended in the child with pre- or postnatal microcephaly, with no specific diagnosis, in search of possible intracranial calcifications or structural defects. A metabolic screening is performed whenever signs of metabolic disorders are present. Appropriate microbiologic cultures and titers are suggested in the infant with signs of intrauterine infection syndromes or with no obvious diagnosis. Table 10-23 outlines the recognizable causes and common syndromes of microcephaly.

Without a specific diagnosis to explain the alteration or abnormality in brain growth, ultimate mental development cannot be predicted accurately. If the infant has an OFC of less than 3 SD below the mean and has abnormal neurologic signs, however, the probability of developmental retardation is high. With milder degree of decreased head size and no specific diagnosis, one must be cautious in predicting cognitive ability.

Genetic counseling regarding the risk of recurrence in a situation of undiagnosed sporadic microcephaly is not clear-cut. A child with severe nonsyndromic microcephaly whose parents are not consanguineous and who is the only affected person in the family may represent sporadic microcephaly caused by an autosomal or X-linked gene, or the child may have abnormal head size because of an unrecognized environmental cause. Without a specific physical or biochemical marker, these possibilities cannot be separated. Therefore, empirical recurrence risk figures must be used in this situation. Various investigators have arrived at different figures for the recurrence risk of microcephaly, ranging from 6 to 20%. The studies have differed in their methods of ascertainment of microcephaly and in the homogeneity of the ethnic groups. A risk range in unclassifiable, nonsyndromic cases of 5 to 10% seems to be a reasonable estimate.

Reference

Opitz JM, Holt MC: Microcephaly: general considerations and aids to nosology. J Craniofac Dev Biol 10:175–204, 1990

ALLERGY AND IMMUNOLOGY

Jonathan D. Gitlin

11.1 INTRODUCTION TO IMMUNOLOGY

The pioneering work of Harvard chemist E. J. Cohn preparing albumin for the battlefields of the Second World War initiated the era of plasma protein research. The era also witnessed the widespread introduction of antibiotics into clinical practice, and with the advent of these new therapeutic agents, individuals with recurrent infections began to be recognized. Armed with the new methods for the separation and analysis of plasma proteins, pediatricians soon reported the remarkable occurrence of children with recurrent infections and a complete absence of γ-globulins. The field of immunodeficiency was born. In the relatively short period of time since the initial description of these patients, a myriad of inherited diseases of the immune system have been described. The cellular and molecular bases of most of these disorders have now been elucidated.

Our current understanding of the human immune system is largely derived from the lessons learned from these patients. We now recognize the immune system as an aggregate of lymphoid and phagocytic cells as well as circulating antibody and complement proteins that work in a coherent fashion to defend the host against infectious agents. Knowledge of the specific host factors involved in any individual child's response to infection has become increasingly important as awareness of the environmental and genetic factors underlying susceptibility to infection has grown. Understanding the clinical and molecular aspects of the immunologic deficiency diseases of childhood provides the pediatrician with a solid foundation for evaluating the normal immune system in the developing child. These immunologic first principles provide the scientific rationale for childhood immunization and establish the framework for evaluation of any child suspected of having undue susceptibility to infection.

11.2 DEVELOPMENT OF THE IMMUNE SYSTEM

Calvin B. Williams

The development of the highly specific yet anticipatory human immune system begins with fetal hematopoiesis and continues throughout life. Although many nonspecific barrier mechanisms such as the skin and ciliated, mucus-covered membranes play a protective role, it is the development of specialized lymphoid cells and of specific immune responses that ultimately protects us from a universe of potential pathogens. These specialized cells include T, B, natural killer (NK), and antigen-presenting cells (APCs). Each

cell type expresses a unique collection of cell surface molecules, the composition of which changes during development and during an immune response. These surface molecules have been classified by the World Health Organization as "cluster of differentiation" antigens (CD), and the list includes coreceptors, adhesion molecules, and cytokine receptors (Table 11-1). The antigen-specific receptors found on B and T cells are not included in this general classification scheme, as each unique cell or clone possesses a distinct receptor.

Through combinatorial joining of gene segments and other mechanisms of diversity associated with DNA rearrangement, it is estimated that there are 10^{11} different B-cell antigen receptors and 10^{16} different T-cell antigen receptors. It stands to reason that with so many different receptors, some of them could potentially bind self-proteins and thereby direct the immune response toward self-tissues rather than infectious agents. Thus, the central task of the developing immune system is one of "education." The functional immune system must eliminate those cells with self-reactive receptors from the repertoire, thereby avoiding autoimmunity, while maintaining those cells capable of recognizing foreign proteins. Tolerance, or lack of reactivity to self-antigens, is an essential feature of the immune system.

The first progenitor cells of the immune system are found in the yolk sac at approximately 3 weeks of gestational age. These pluripotential hematopoietic stem cells (Fig. 11-1) seed the liver at 5 weeks, and hematopoiesis begins at 6 weeks of gestation. By the eighth week, stem cells have migrated to the primary lymphoid organs, the bone marrow, and the thymus. These organs serve as the site for the development of T cells (thymus) or B cells (bone marrow). Mature T and B cells first migrate to secondary lymphoid tissue, the lymph nodes, mucous-membrane-associated lymphoid tissue, and spleen, at 10 to 12 weeks of gestational age. It is in the secondary lymphoid tissues that most mature lymphocytes reside and where immune responses are generated. Responses to bloodborne antigens occur in the spleen, which is connected to the systemic circulation. Lymphocytes in lymph nodes respond to antigens delivered from the skin via the lymphatics. The tonsils, Peyer's patches, and lamina propria of the gut contain lymphocytes that respond to antigens entering through mucosal surfaces.

11.2.1 Thymus and T-Cell Development

The thymus itself is formed from the third brachial cleft and the third/fourth brachial pouch, which may contribute both endoderm and ectoderm. Embryonic tissue from these locations moves caudally to fuse in the midline, forming the two thymic lobes. Each lobe contains three regions with distinct structure and function: the cortex, the corticomedullary junction, and the medulla. The thymic cortex is composed of specialized epithelial cells that express class I and class II molecules of the major histocompatability complex (MHC) and mediate the early stages of maturation including positive selection. Multipotent $CD1a^-$, $CD5^-$, $CD34^+$, and $CD38^{low}$

TABLE 11-1

CLUSTER OF DIFFERENTIATION (CD) CLASSIFICATION AND FUNCTION OF SELECTED MOLECULES

CD NUMBER	DISTRIBUTION	FUNCTION
CD1	B, Mφ, DC, T	"Nonclassical" MHC molecule; presents glycolipids
CD2	T, NK	Binds CD58 (LFA-3); costimulation
CD3	T	Associated with TCR; signal transduction
CD4	T	Binds HLA class II; coreceptor
CD5	T, B	Binds CD72; increased adhesion and proliferation
CD7	T, NK	Modulates T and NK activation
CD8	T, NK	Binds HLA class II; coreceptor
CD11a	T, B, NK	CD11a/CD18 (LFA-1) binds ICAM 1–3; adhesion
CD11b	T*, M, G, Mφ, NK	CD11b/CD18 (Mac-1) receptor for iC3b and ICAM 1–3
CD11c	M, G, Mφ, NK	CD11c/CD18 receptor for ICAM 1, iC3b; adhesion
CD16	NK, M, G	Receptor for IgG Fc (FcγRIII); ADCC, activation
CD18	T, B, NK, M, G, Mφ	CD11$_{a,b,c}$/CD18 as above; adhesion
CD19	B	Forms complex with CD21, Leu-13; regulates signaling
CD20	B	Calcium channel; mediates activation
CD21	B	C3d/EBV receptor, associates with CD19 as above
CD23	B	Low-affinity Fc IgE receptor
CD25	T*, B*	α-Chain, low-affinity IL-2 receptor
CD28	T	Binds CD80 (B7-1) and CD86 (B7-2); costimulation
CD32	B, M, G, P	Receptor for Fc IgG (FcγRII)
CD34	SC, precursors	Adhesion
CD40	B	Activation and differentiation
CD40L	T*	Ligand for CD40
CD45	All leukocytes	Many isoforms, phosphatase in signal transduction
CD56	NK	Mediates homophilic adhesion (NCAM)
CD80	B*, Mφ, DC	Binds CD28 and CD152 on T cells; costimulation
CD86	B*, M, DC	Binds CD28 and CD152 on T cells; costimulation
CD95	Many cells	Fas, binds CD95L; programmed cell death (apoptosis)
CD95L	T*, NK, M, N	Mediates Fas+ targeted cell lysis
CD122	T*, B*, NK, M	β-Chain, with CD25 forms intermediate affinity IL-2R
CD132	T*, B*	γ-Chain, with CD25, CD122 forms high-affinity IL-2R
CD152	T*	CTLA-4, binds CD80, CD86 on APCs; negative signal

Key: T = T cell; T* = activated T cell; M = monocyte; DC = dendritic cell; B = B cell; B* = activated B cell; G = granulocyte; SC = stem cell; NK = natural killer cell; Mφ = macrophage; N = neutrophil; P = platelet.

stem cells enter the thymus at the corticomedullary junction and migrate into the cortex. These stem cells are slightly different from those found in fetal bone marrow in that they express high levels

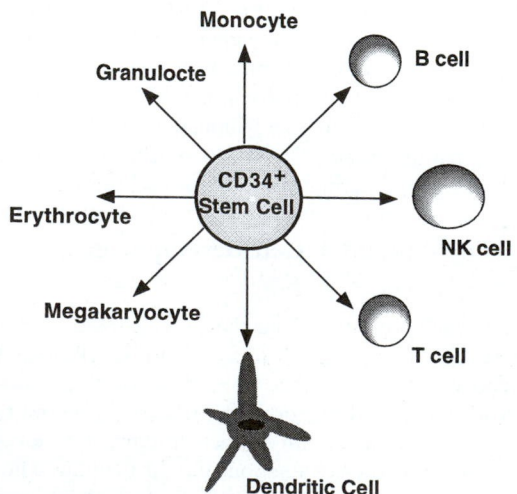

FIGURE 11-1 **CD34+ stem cells give rise to all cells in the hematopoietic lineage. This section focuses on the development of T, B, NK, and dendritic cells.**

of CD45RA and CD7. This implies that the stem cell progeny entering the thymus have undergone some differentiation since leaving the sites of hematopoiesis. Current data suggest that they may develop into dendritic cells (DCs), NK cells, or T cells, as indicated in Fig. 11-2.

Maturation of T cells continues in the thymic cortex through a series of developmental stages as cells migrate back through the cortex toward the corticomedullary junction. Expression of low levels of CD4 combined with rearrangement of T-cell receptor (TCR) δ genes marks the commitment to the T-cell lineage. Next, developing human thymocytes express low levels of CD8. This is followed by rearrangement at the TCR β locus, leading to expression of a pre-TCR on the cell surface. The pre-TCR mediates survival and proliferation, and serves as a developmental checkpoint. Cells that fail to express the pre-TCR die by apoptosis. This process is called β selection. Ultimately, the pre-T α chain is replaced by the TCR α chain, generating an antigen-specific TCR. These intermediate- to late-stage progenitors express low levels of the $\alpha\beta$ TCR and both CD4 and CD8. A parallel line of development occurs for $\gamma\delta$T cells.

Small double-positive (DP) cells (CD4+, CD8+, TCR^{low}) account for about 75% of all thymocytes. Maturation beyond this stage depends on the interaction between the unique TCR on each DP thymocyte and the self-peptide/MHC complexes expressed on the surface of thymic epithelial cells. Evidence supports the notion

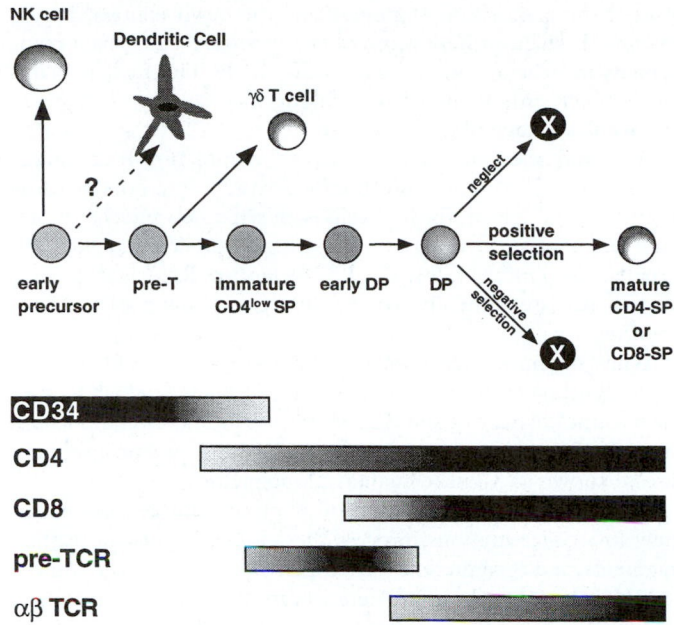

FIGURE 11-2   The stages of T-cell development that occur within the thymus. *Horizontal bar graphs* indicate the cell surface expression of four important T-cell receptors/coreceptors in relation to the stem cell marker CD34. The *gray scale* approximates the level and timing of expression, with *black* indicating a higher level. SP = single positive; DP = double positive.

that the strength and timing of these interactions determine cell fate. If the interaction between TCR and peptide/MHC complex is "weak," then the cells die by neglect, having failed to receive a positive signal. If the interaction is too "strong," then the cells die by activation-induced cell death (negative selection). This later process is the primary mechanism by which self-reactive T cells are eliminated from the repertoire. Last, if the interaction is "appropriate," then those thymocytes receive a positive signal and mature to become either CD4 or CD8 single-positive (SP) cells.

Both positive and negative selection begin at the DP stage in the thymic cortex, but the latter occurs most efficiently when thymocytes encounter professional APCs such as the thymic dendritic cells at the corticomedullary junction. Thymocytes in the medulla bear mature phenotypes. They express either CD4 or CD8 and a single TCR heterodimer associated with the polypeptide chains of the CD3 complex ($\gamma,\delta,\epsilon,\zeta$). CD4$^+$ cells recognize foreign antigen in association with HLA class II proteins, whereas those expressing CD8 are restricted to HLA class I molecules. The migration of the first naive, mature T cells from the thymic medulla to lymph node and spleen begins at 11 to 12 weeks of embryonic development and continues for many years thereafter. By 12 weeks, T cells can proliferate when stimulated by lectins such as PHA and ConA, and by 15 to 20 weeks the first antigen-specific responses are detected. Considerable maturation of the immune response continues throughout the first year of life, a factor limiting the immunogenicity of some vaccinations. Although the traditional view has been that thymic function declines rapidly after puberty, recent evidence indicates that some level of functional thymopoiesis continues well into adulthood.

Peripheral T-cell expansion and the development of memory T cells are the final components of T-cell development. These events have a profound effect on the repertoire and the precursor frequency of antigen-specific T cells. When the T cell's antigen-spe-

cific receptor is engaged by a specific peptide bound to an MHC molecule expressed on the surface of an antigen-presenting cell (APC), an "immunologic synapse" involving intracellular signal transduction and reorganization of signaling molecules in the membrane is initiated. The genes that are activated include cytokines, cytokine receptors, and transcription factors.

Activation of naive T cells requires a second signal other than that provided through the TCR. The best-characterized costimulatory molecule on the surface of naive T cells is CD28. CD28 binds to B7-1 and B7-2 on the surface of APCs and increases intracellular tyrosine phosphorylation.

On activation, naive T cells secrete interleukin 2 (IL-2), the most effective T-cell growth factor. Over a period of days those T cells that are CD4$^+$ will differentiate into either TH1 or TH2 effectors. TH1 cells secrete IL-2, interferon γ (IFN-γ), lymphotoxin (LT), and tumor necrosis factor β (TNF-β). These cytokines act synergistically to lyse virally infected cells and activate macrophages and granulocytes. Interferon γ also acts to enhance the differentiation toward TH1 cells and inhibit the development of TH2 cells. In contrast, TH2 cells secrete IL-4, IL-5, IL-10, and IL-13. IL-4 is the factor that induces immunoglobulin heavy chain class switching to the IgE isotype and uncommitted T cells to differentiate toward the TH2 phenotype. IL-5 is an eosinophil growth factor. Thus, TH2 cells enhance the allergic response by a number of mechanisms.

Most T cells generated by a primary immune response undergo apoptotic cell death. However, a small number of cells, proportional to the initial antigenic load and clonal burst size, survive by unknown mechanisms and differentiate into memory cells. In general, memory cells allow for a more rapid, more potent, and more enduring secondary response that is the basis for vaccine-induced immunity. The memory phenotype is not seen early in life but increases with age.

11.2.2 NK-Cell Development

"Natural killer" or NK cells are a subset of lymphocytes distinguished by their morphology, function, and expression of distinct surface molecules. Mature NK cells are larger than T or B cells and have a more granular cytoplasm. They selectively identify and kill virally infected cells and tumor cells but lack either the TCR or BCR. NK cells use cytotoxic mechanisms similar to cytotoxic T lymphocytes to lyse target cells. Following contact with a target cell, organelles are oriented toward the target by a calcium-dependent mechanism. This is followed by a release of granules containing granzyme A, perforin, and TGF-β. Perforin alone is sufficient for cell lysis. The NK cells are identified by their expression of CD16 (FcγRIII) and CD56 (NCAM-1) on the cell surface and comprise 10 to 15% of circulating lymphocytes. Mature NK cells can be found in the spleen, lungs, and liver. During the first trimester of pregnancy they are also found in the placental decidua.

NK cells first make their appearance in fetal liver as early as 6 weeks of gestation. However, committed CD34$^+$, CD56$^-$ NK progenitors have been identified in the fetal thymus, bone marrow, and liver, although the thymus is clearly not required for NK-cell development.

NK-cell development does not require gene segment rearrangements to generate a unique receptor. Instead, NK cells use an array of stimulatory and inhibitory receptors to trigger their cytolytic functions. A cluster of genes preferentially expressed in human NK cells has been identified on chromosome 12 (designated the NK complex or NKC). A cluster of inhibitory receptors was recently described on chromosome 19.

11.2.3   B-Cell Development

B cells are the progenitors of antibody-secreting plasma cells, which provide the main form of protection against some pathogens. B-cell development begins at the same gestational age as T-cell development, follows a similar time course, and utilizes similar developmental strategies. Like developing thymocytes, B-cell progenitors must be positively selected. Those with self-reactive receptors may be clonally eliminated in the bone marrow or reformed by generating new antigen receptors that are not self-reactive.

B-cell development begins before 7 weeks of gestational age in the fetal liver. By 8 to 10 weeks, CD34+ hematopoietic stem cells migrate to the bone marrow and begin a complex program of antigen-independent differentiation. This program can be divided into three distinct stages, as shown in Fig. 11-3. The first progenitors committed to the B-cell lineage are called early pro-B cells. These cells express CD34 and terminal deoxynucleotidyltransferase (TdT). Immunoglobulin gene rearrangement has not yet occurred in these progenitors. Intermediate pro-B cells express CD34, TdT, and B220, a receptor tyrosine phosphatase. Intermediate pro-B cells also express intracellular Igα and Igβ, two proteins that serve as the signal transduction apparatus in the BCR (analogous to CD3 proteins in T cells). Late pro-B cells have lost TdT expression but complete H chain rearrangement by rearranging V_H to $D_H J_H$ segments. They express surrogate light chains (ΨL) encoded by the *14.1* and $V_{\text{pre-B}}$ genes, both of which are invariant and expressed in the absence of DNA rearrangement.

The first developmental checkpoint occurs at the late pro-B to pre-B transition. If the rearranged H chain is functional, cytoplasmic expression of a μH chain can be detected, and the cells are now called *large pre-B cells*. Large pre-B cells mature to become small pre-B cells, which are TdT. Light chain rearrangement takes

place at this stage of development, and the newly expressed polymorphic L chain protein replaces the surrogate light chain components to generate an antigen-specific BCR. The BCR contains the complete mIgM molecule, marking the transition to the *immature B-cell* stage of development.

A second selection event occurs at the immature B-cell stage, when 10 to 20% of immature B cells derived in the bone marrow migrate to the spleen; those B cells with self-reactive receptors are eliminated. Those that survive the selection processes rapidly differentiate into mIgM+, mIgD+, B220+ *mature B cells,* which enter the follicular areas, thereby joining the recirculating pool of B lymphocytes.

When mature B cells contact antigen through the BCR, associated signaling events involve the Src-family kinases, which activate the tyrosine kinases Syk and Btk. Mutations in Btk result in a failure of pre-BCR signaling, compromised B-cell development, and in the disease known as X-linked agammaglobulinemia.

Antigen-specific B cells can capture protein antigens at vanishingly low concentrations, process the antigen into small peptide fragments, and then present the antigen to TH cells in the context of MHC class II molecules. Bacterial capsular polysaccharides also activate B cells but do so in the absence of T cells and lymphokines by extensive cross-linking of the BCR. On activation, the B cell becomes responsive to the effects of lymphokines. IL-4 and IL-10 have been shown to be important B-cell growth factors and to induce isotype switching.

Plasma cells are terminally differentiated B cells that secrete antigen-specific immunoglobulins, or antibodies. Antibodies are composed of two identical light chains and two identical heavy chains. Each heavy chain is covalently attached to a light chain, and the two heavy chains are joined together by extensive noncovalent interactions and by disulfide bonds to form the intact molecule. There are two light chain isotypes or classes (designated κ or λ) and five heavy chain isotypes (designated μ, γ, α, δ, and ε). Thus, IgM antibodies contain μH chains, IgG antibodies, γH chains, and so forth. Two heavy chain isotypes can be further divided into subclasses based on antigenic differences. These include four subclasses of IgG (IgG1, IgG2, IgG3, and IgG4) and two subclasses of IgA (IgA1 and IgA2).

The different isotypes and subclasses have different distributions and functions. IgM, the first immunoglobulin to be generated in a primary immune response, is secreted as a pentamer and is found in the secretory Ig at mucosal surfaces and in breast milk. Secreted IgD is present at very low concentrations in human serum, and its function is not known. Membrane IgD is found on the surface of most peripheral B cells, where it functions with IgM as an antigen-specific receptor. IgG is the most prevalent immunoglobulin in human serum, making up 75 to 85% of the total Ig. IgG is divided into four subclasses, which are both structurally and functionally different. The subclasses are named numerically in order of their serum concentration: IgG1 (8 mg/mL), IgG2 (4 mg/mL), IgG3 (0.8 mg/mL), and IgG4 (0.4 mg/mL). The structural differences are located primarily in the hinge region, where different numbers of amino acids and different numbers of interchain disulfide bonds create molecules with a variable ability to bind complement (C1q) and lyse cells. The affinity of each subclass for C1q is IgG3 > IgG1 > IgG2. IgG4 is unable to bind C1q and trigger the classical complement cascade. IgM antibodies also fix complement.

Binding of IgG molecules to the three classes of Fcγ receptors expressed on overlapping sets of macrophages, granulocytes, lymphocytes, NK cells, neutrophils, and eosinophils mediates such functions as antibody-dependent cellular cytotoxicity and transfer

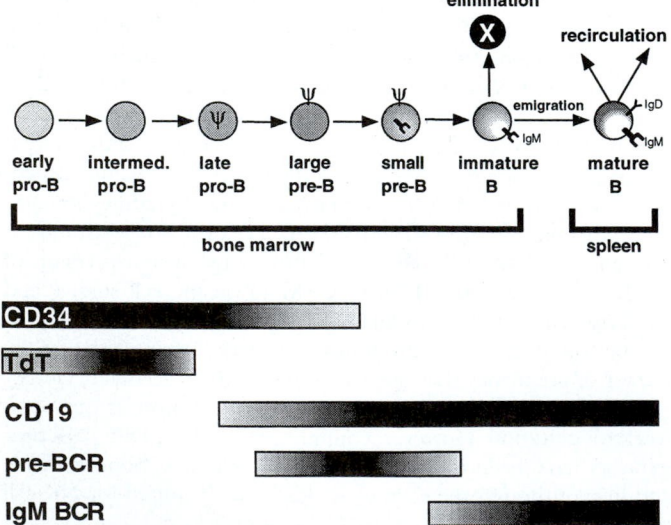

FIGURE 11-3 **The stages of B-cell development in the bone marrow and spleen. Expression of the intracellular enzyme TdT, the cell surface marker CD19, and the BCRs is shown. The *gray scale* estimates the timing and level of expression, with *black* indicating a higher level. BCR = B-cell receptor.**

of IgG from mother to fetus. IgA makes up 10 to 15% of serum Ig and contains two subclasses, IgA1 and IgA2. The two subclasses differ by the addition of 13 amino acids to the hinge region of IgA1. IgA1 is the dominant subclass in human serum, where it is found in monomeric form. Both IgA1 and IgA2 are secreted in saliva, breast milk, tears, and bronchial secretions. Secreted forms of IgA are dimers consisting of two IgA monomers, a joining (J) chain, and a secretory component (SC). IgE is the least prevalent Ig in human serum. IgE plays a role in defending against parasites and mediates allergic reactions.

Under normal circumstances, the first plasma cells can be found in fetal lymphoid tissue at about 20 weeks of gestation, and only in small numbers thereafter. Thus, the IgG found in fetal serum is predominantly of maternal origin. Transplacental transfer of IgG begins between 8 and 12 weeks of gestation, although levels remain below 100 mg/dL until 20 weeks. By 30 weeks, the fetal serum IgG concentration is about half of the maternal concentration, and it ultimately exceeds the maternal concentration by about 10% at term. Thus, 50% of IgG transfer takes place in the last 10 weeks of gestation. Very low levels of IgM and a few nanograms/mL IgA and IgE can be found in cord serum at term. These immunoglobulins are of fetal origin because they do not cross the placenta. After birth, as a consequence of increased antigen exposure, neonatal Ig synthesis increases as the passively acquired IgG levels fall. An IgG nadir of about 400 mg/dL is reached by 3 to 4 months of age. Synthesis of all immunoglobulins continues to increase, reaching adult levels at 1 year for IgM, 5 to 6 years for IgG, and adolescence for IgA.

11.2.4   Antigen-Presenting Cells

Although B cells are capable of recognizing epitopes on intact proteins, T cells require that the protein be processed and that the epitopes to be recognized be presented in the context of molecules of the major histocompatability complex. Specialized cells termed antigen-presenting cells have evolved for this purpose and include B cells themselves, macrophages, and dendritic cells (DCs).

Foremost among these is the dendritic cell, which both initiates and modulates the immune response. DCs are efficient APCs because they take up particles and antigen by phagocytosis, sample the extracellular fluid by macropinocytosis, and display an array of specialized receptors that enable them to recognize IgG, IgE, or mannose residues on the surface of pathogens.

Internalized antigen is targeted to specialized late-endosomal compartments, which degrade proteins to peptides. In a viral infection, endogenously synthesized viral proteins are also degraded, and peptides from them are presented in the context of MHC class I.

After contact with antigen, DCs begin a maturation process that drives them from peripheral tissues to the lymph nodes and spleen. In lymphoid organs, DCs complete this maturation process, resulting in the release of chemokines to attract T and B cells. Clearly, DCs play a central role in initiating and controlling immune responses.

References

English KB, Wilson CB: The neonatal immune system. In: Rich RR, ed-in chief; Fleisher TA, Schwartz BD, Shearer WT, Strober W, eds: Clinical Immunology: Principles and Practice, vol I. St Louis, Mosby-Year Book, 1996:779–788

Gans HA, Arvin AM, Galinus J, Logan L, DeHovitz R, Maldonado Y: Deficiency of the humoral immune response to measles vaccine in infants immunized at age six months. JAMA 280:527–532, 1998

Pillai S: The chosen few: positive selection and the generation of naive B lymphocytes. Immunity 10:493–502, 1999

Spits H, Blom B, Jaleco A, et al: Early stages in the development of human T, natural killer and thymic dendritic cells. Immunol Rev 165:75–86, 1998

11.3   UNDUE SUSCEPTIBILITY TO INFECTION

Talal A. Chatila

11.3.1   Clinical Presentations

Each year a large number of children are evaluated by their primary care physicians for recurrent infections, an especially common event in early childhood. The overwhelming majority of such cases are benign, and an extrinsic cause of recurrent infection is identified. Examples of extrinsic causes include heightened exposure to pathogens in a daycare setting, carriage of a pathogenic organism such as *Staphylococcus aureus* in the context of recurrent infection with this organism, or recurrent upper respiratory tract infections in the context of parental smoking. However, concern about an intrinsic pathologic underpinning is heightened on the basis of frequency of infections, their severity, and the nature of the offending organism. The coexistence of multisystem disease, autoimmunity, or lymphoreticular malignancy should also prompt evaluation for immunodeficiency. A family history of recurrent infections raises the index of suspicion.

One helpful clue to the presence of a host abnormality is a high frequency of infections. Examples include two or more systemic bacterial infections at any time (such as sepsis, deep-seated abcesses, or meningitis), three or more bacterial infections (eg, draining otitis media), or six to eight or more upper respiratory tract infections in 1 year. The last finding should be modified by the fact that many children, especially toddlers, suffer from recurrent upper respiratory tract infection from repeat exposure to respiratory (usually viral) pathogens, especially during the first year of daycare attendance.

Recurrent infections with a particular organism also point to abnormalities of the host. A case in point is meningococcemia, in which a second episode of this disease raises the prevalence of a terminal complement pathway abnormality in afflicted individuals from ≤1% to 30 to 40%. Other examples include *Staphylococcus aureus* infections in children with chronic granulomatous disease (CGD) or leukocyte adhesion deficiency (LAD).

The severity of the recurrent infection is reflective of the seriousness of the underlying disorder. The compromised child may fail to recover completely between infections. Failure to thrive, weight loss, and growth retardation are grave manifestations of immunodeficiency and call for immediate investigation. The need for surgical intervention provides yet another measure of the severity of the underlying infection. Such interventions may include myringotomy tube placement for chronic otitis media, sinus surgery for chronic sinusitis, lobectomy for chronic right middle lobe pneumonia, and drainage of superficial and deep abcesses.

The availability of effective antibiotic therapy may modulate the presentation, but in general the clinical picture may slowly but progressively worsen over a protracted period of time.

The nature of sites affected by the recurrent infections also provides valuable clues to the problem at hand. Humoral immunodeficiency, cystic fibrosis, and immotile cilia syndrome result in recurrent severe sinopulmonary infections including chronic sinusitis, pneumonia, and bronchiectasis. Humoral immunodeficiency may also result in chronic diarrhea as a consequence of infestations with pathogens such as *Giardia lamblia*. Recurrent infections affecting one particular site (eg, one specific lung lobe or one ear) may point to underlying anatomic abnormalities.

Recurrent upper respiratory infections in the absence of other organ system involvement may point to allergic disorders or to mild atypical forms of cystic fibrosis. Supporting evidence may come from a family history of allergic diseases including asthma and atopic dermatitis and findings on physical exam of allergic attributes such as allergic shiners, clear nasal discharge eczema, or wheezing. Diagnosis can be established by appropriate testing including allergen skin testing, serum IgE, and sweat test for cystic fibrosis.

The identity of the offending organism is particularly relevant to the investigation and often provides insight to the underlying diagnosis. Patients with defects in humoral immunity are susceptible to pyogenic organisms, including *Haemophilus influenzae, Streptococcus pneumoniae,* and *Staphylococcus aureus.* They suffer from recurrent sinopulomary infections, abcesses, cellulitis, and meningitis. Because complement proteins and phagocytes collaborate with antibodies in clearing these infections, deficiencies or abnormalities affecting complement proteins or phagocytes should be considered in evaluating recurrent bacterial infections. Patients with asplenia, whether acquired in the course of sickle-cell disease or more rarely congenital, may present with sepsis with encapsulated organisms.

Restricted sets of pyogenic pathogens also characterize other diseases. Patients with cystic fibrosis are particularly susceptible to respiratory infections with *Pseudomonas aeruginosa, Burkholderia* sp., and *Staphylococcus aureus.* Those with chronic granulomatous disease suffer from recurrent infections with catalase-positive organisms including *Staphylococcus aureus, Chromobacterium violaceum, Pseudomonas cepacia, Serratia marcescens, Candida,* and *Aspergillus* species.

Defects in cellular immunity predispose to recurrent, often disseminated viral infections, especially with herpes viruses. Patients with cellular immune defects may also suffer from atypical mycobacterial infections, mucocutaneous candidiasis, and *Pneumocystis carinii* pneumonia. Patients afflicted with the more serious cellular immune defects also suffer from ineffective antibody production because of lack of T-cell helper function. Infections attributable to defective cellular and humoral compartments herald combined immunodeficiency that may be congenital, such as in primary immunodeficiencies, or acquired, such as in the acquired immunodeficiency syndrome.

Of particular interest is the association of specific immune defects to susceptibility to a particular pathogen, which may constitute sufficient grounds for careful search for immunodeficiency or other abnormalities. Examples include susceptibility to neisserial infections in deficiency of terminal components of the complement cascade, *Pneumocystis carinii* pneumonia in patients with CD40 ligand deficiency, and atypical mycobacterial infections in patients with defects involving the IL-12–interferon-γ system including IL-12, IL-12 receptor, and interferon-γ receptor mutations. Another example includes enteroviral infections (echo, coxsackie, and polio viruses) in patients with X-linked agammaglobulinemia. A sometime tragic presentation of immunocompromised hosts involves morbid or disseminated infections with live viral or bacterial vaccine pathogens including polio, measles, mumps, or rubella viruses, varicella, or bacillus Calmette-Guérin (BCG) mycobacterium.

11.3.2   Investigation of the Child with Recurrent Infections

A carefully gathered medical history is the indispensable starting point and should focus on characteristics of infections, growth and development, and family history of infections, allergies, or other medical conditions. A history of severe or fatal infections in maternal uncles suggests an X-linked immunodeficiency disorder such as chronic granulomatous disease or severe combined immunodeficiency (SCID) in boys under investigation for undue susceptibility to infection, whereas a history of easy bruising in a boy with recurrent infections is suggestive of another X-linked disorder, the Wiskott-Aldrich syndrome. A history of delayed separation of the cord in the context of recurrent pyogenic infections may point to leukocyte adhesion deficiency or to neutropenia, conditions that result in too few neutrophils being present at the cord stump site to effect cord separation.

The physical exam can provide significant clues. Evidence of failure to thrive, the presence of allergic stigmata including allergic shiners, eczema, or respiratory wheezing, or the presence of thrush may be helpful. The absence of appreciable tonsilar tissue or the lack of an adenoid shadow on lateral neck views may point to failure of B-cell development. Characteristic facial features and cardiac murmurs may result from the DiGeorge syndrome, and dwarfism may point to immunodeficiency related to cartilage-hair hypoplasia. Ataxia with oculocutaneous telangiectasias may point to a diagnosis of ataxia-telangiectasia.

Documentation of infections by microbiological techniques (cultures, serologies, or DNA testing) or radiographic studies (sinus/chest x-rays, etc) is essential to confirm a history of recurrent infections and provides clues to pathogenesis (including anatomic abnormalities) and therapy. A comprehensive evaluation is outlined in Table 11-2.

Additional tests can be performed in cases in which suspicion for an underlying abnormality is high. Recurrent infections with catalase-positive organisms in conjunction with adenitis, osteomyelitis, hepatosplenic abscesses, and other deep-seated infections can point to the presence of CGD. Persistent thrush or the isolation of unusual organisms from sinopulmonary sites, including CMV and *Pneumocystis carinii*, should prompt evaluation of cellular immune status. The blood levels of specific complement components can be measured in case of an association with autoimmunity. A high index of suspicion for cystic fibrosis in the face of a normal sweat test may prompt DNA genotyping for unusual mutations in the cystic fibrosis transporter gene, whereas unrelenting sinus and lung infections may eventuate in biopsy for ciliary abnormalities.

11.3.3   Management of Recurrent Infections

The choice of therapy for patients with recurrent infections obviously depends on the underlying disorder. Patients whose recurrent infections have such causes as allergy or exposure to tobacco smoke can be helped by avoiding the trigger. For immunodeficiency, therapy is usually determined by the type and severity of the immune defect. Antibiotic prophylaxis may be successfully utilized in a num-

TABLE 11-2

INVESTIGATION OF THE CHILD WITH UNDUE SUSCEPTIBILITY TO INFECTION

General tests
  Complete blood count with differential
  Erythrocyte sedimentation rate
  Platelet count
  Examination of peripheral smear for Howell-Jolly bodies
  Sweat test
  Allergen skin testing
  HIV serology (as appropriate)
Tests for B-cell disorders
  Immunoglobulin levels
  Isohemagglutinins
  Antibody titers to common childhood vaccines
  Peripheral blood B-cell phenotyping by flow cytometry
Tests for T-cell disorders
  Intradermal delayed hypersensitivity skin testing
  Proliferation to antigens and mitogens
  Peripheral blood T-cell phenotyping by flow cytometry
Tests for phagocytic cell disorders
  Respiratory burst assay
  Peripheral blood neutrophil phenotyping by flow cytometry
Tests for complement protein disorders
  CH50 for the classical complement pathway
  CH50 for the alternative complement pathway, to include measurements of factors B and D
  Assay for other individual complement proteins if either of the above tests is abnormal

---

ber of disorders including transient hypogammaglobulinemia of infancy, drug-induced immunosuppression, phagocytic cell dysfunction, and AIDS. In particular, the AIDS epidemic has resulted in widespread use of antibiotics and other chemotherapeutic agents for prophylaxis against specific infections including trimethoprim-sulfamethoxazole prophylaxis for *Pneumocystis carinii* pneumonia and macrolides for atypical mycobacteria. Patients with complement component deficiency may benefit from penicillin prophylaxis for recurrent infections with pneumococci or *Neisseria*. Similarly, penicillin prophylaxis is beneficial in patients with sickle-cell disease or other causes of asplenia. Immunoglobulin replacement therapy is the definitive therapy for hypo- and agammaglobulinemia. To maintain preinfusion serum IgG concentrations at protective levels (>800 mg/dL), therapy is administered intravenously once every 3 to 4 weeks. Immunomodulatory therapy with cytokines is now standard therapy in chronic granulomatous disease and may be of benefit in the hyper-IgE syndrome. Bone marrow transplantation is reserved for severe immunodeficiency diseases such as severe combined immunodeficiency.

Vaccines have an important role to play in some children with recurrent infections. For example, influenza and polyvalent pneumococcal vaccines are underutilized agents that provide welcome protection against morbid childhood infections by the respective agent. These vaccines are particularly useful in the context of recurrent infections in daycare centers. The recent availability of a conjugated pneumococcal vaccine now extends protection against invasive pneumococcal infections to children below the age of 2 years and is especially useful in patients with complement component deficiency and asplenia. Live virus vaccines are contraindicated in patients with congenital or acquired agammglobulinemia or with severe combined immunodeficiency, as they are either ineffective (in the case of inactivated vaccines) or potentially deadly (as with

live or attenuated viral vaccines). They are, however, useful in select immundeficiencies including complement component deficiency, HIV-positive children, and patients with milder immunodeficiency diseases such as transient hypogammaglobulinemia of infancy and some combined immunodeficiency diseases such as ataxia-telangiectasia. In some cases, such as the DiGeorge syndrome, the decision to use live viral vaccines is dependent on the T-cell count: a CD4 count of 400 cells/μL or more heralds tolerance to vaccination with live attenuated organisms. Whenever possible, inactivated vaccines (such as the Salk polio vaccine) are to be used in immunodeficient patients and their siblings in preference to live viral vaccines. Another frequently raised issue relates to whether it is appropriate to maintain the affected child in a protective environment by such measures as withdrawal from daycare or school and social isolation. Every attempt should be made to maintain the child in his or her age-compatible environment, and isolation procedures are rarely called for save for children with severe combined immunodeficiency.

11.4   PRIMARY IMMUNODEFICIENCIES

Talal A. Chatila

Primary immunodeficiency diseases result from genetic defects affecting the development and/or the function of components of the immune system. They frequently manifest soon after birth, although some become evident later in life. Frequent infections are the hallmark of immunodeficiency syndromes, with the types of infections reflecting the nature of the defect. Autoimmune disorders and certain malignancies occur more frequently in patients with immunodeficiency diseases.

Primary immunodeficiency diseases may affect either acquired immunity, as seen in cellular and humoral deficiency diseases, or innate immunity, as seen in deficiencies of the various complement components and phagocytic cell deficiencies. This section reviews representative immunodeficiency diseases of altered development and function of T and B cells. Table 11-3 summarizes the current information on the genetic basis of immunodeficiency diseases.

These defects have served as experiments of nature to unravel the complexities of lymphocyte development and functions. Abnormalities affecting T cells alone or in combination with B lymphocytes frequently lead to states of combined immunodeficiency, the severity of which depends on the extent of the T-cell defect because of the role of T lymphocytes in supporting B-lymphocyte function. In contrast to combined immunodeficiency diseases where both T- and B-cell compartments are affected, T-cell function in isolated B-cell immunodeficiency syndromes, such as X-linked agammaglobulinemia, remains intact.

11.4.1   Severe Combined Immunodeficiency

Severe combined immunodeficiency (SCID) is at the extreme end of the spectrum of immunodeficiency states and is characterized by the breakdown of adaptive immune function, both cellular and humoral. This syndrome is caused by a heterogeneous group of genetic abnormalities that result in severe T-cell depletion (or dysfunction) with either primary or secondary B-cell dysfunction. Histologically, the thymus is very small and depleted of lympho-

TABLE 11-3
GENETIC BASES OF IMMUNODEFICIENCY DISORDERS

DISORDER	GENE	FEATURES
Severe combined immunodeficiencies		
Reticular dysgenesis	Unknown	Failure of lymphoid/myeloid lineages
$T^-B^-NK^+$	RAG1, 2 (11p13)	Absence of T and B cells
Omenn syndrome	RAG1, 2 (11p13)	Few T/B cells
$T^-B^+NK^-$	γc chain (Xq13.10)	Absent T and NK cells
	Jak3 (19p13.1)	
$T^-B^+NK^+$	IL-7Rα	Absent T cells
ADA deficiency	ADA (20q13.11)	T/B/NK-cell lymphopenia
PNP deficiency	PNP (14q13.1)	T-cell lymphopenia, variable B-cell number
Combined immunodeficiencies		
Hyper-IgM immunodefi- ciency	CD154(Xq26.3)	Ineffective T/B and T/macrophage cell interaction
MHC class II deficiency	CIITA (16p13)	Failure of isotype switching
	RFX-5 (1q21), RFXAP(13q)	CD4$^+$ T-cell deficiency; poor antibody responses
ZAP70 deficiency	ZAP70(2q12)	Absent CD8$^+$ and nonfunctional CD4$^+$ T cells; secondary B-cell dysfunction
CD3 subunit deficiency	CD3ϵ(11q23); CD3γ(11q23)	Decreased T-cell receptor expression, autoimmunity
Wiskott-Aldrich syndrome	WASP(Xp11.22)	Thrombocytopenia, eczema
Ataxia-telangictasia	ATM(11q22.3)	Radiosensitivity
Primary B-cell immunodeficiencies		
X-linked agammaglobulinemia	Bᴛᴋ(Xq24)	Agammaglobulinemia, no B cells
Autosomal recessive	μ heavy chain (14q32.3)	Agammaglobulinemia, no B cells
Agammaglobulinemia	5 surrogate light chain (22q11.22)	
Common variable immunodefi- ciency	Unknown	Hypogammaglobulinemia, normal or increased B-cell number, autoimmun- ity, malignancy
IgA deficiency	Unknown	Infections, reactions to IgA-containing blood products
Transient hypogammaglobulin- emia	Unknown	Normal B-cell number and vaccine responses of infancy
X-linked lymphoproliferative	SAP(Xq24)	Severe EBV infections, lymphoma, hypogammaglobulinemia disease

cytes and Hassall corpuscles. Peripheral lymphoid tissues are also atrophied and depleted of lymphocytes.

In its most severe forms, SCID poses the risk of imminent death from infection with virtually any pathogenic microorganism, including bacteria, viruses, fungi, and protozoa. Persistent infections of the lung, chronic diarrhea, and wasting dominate the clinical picture. Candidal infections of the oropharynx, esophagus, and skin are common early manifestations of the disease. Infections with rotavirus can be persistent and may spread to extraintestinal sites, and respiratory syncytial virus infections can result in giant-cell pneumonia. Varicella, herpes, measles, and adenoviruses can result in progressive, ultimately fatal infections. SCID patients are also susceptible to opportunistic infections caused by microorganisms that are ordinarily innocuous. Infection with *Pneumocystis carinii* and/or cytomegalovirus can lead to chronic, progressive pneumonitis. Patients with SCID may fall victim to inadvertent inoculation with live, attenuated organisms. Fatal infections have been reported following vaccination of SCID patients with live viral vaccines such as that of measles or with the mycobacterium bacillus Calmette-Guérin (BCG). Transfusion with nonirradiated blood products that contain T lymphocytes may lead to severe graft-versus-host disease (GVHD). A usually milder form of GVHD may result from maternal T cells that have crossed the placenta. Histologically, the thymus in SCID patients is usually very small and is depleted of thymocytes and Hassall corpuscles. Peripheral lymphoid tissues are commonly atrophied and depleted of lymphocytes.

Most children with SCID become acutely sick and require urgent medical attention within months after birth. However, the age at presentation and the clinical manifestations of SCID can vary widely among different patients despite similar genetic defects. Depending on the underlying abnormality, some patients with SCID may start life with seemingly normal immune function only to subsequently suffer progressive immunodeficiency.

RETICULAR DYSGENESIS

This rare form of SCID is characterized by failure of lymphoid and myeloid lineage development in the face of normal erythroid and megakaryocytic cell development. The molecular deficit underlying this disorder is unknown. Affected neonates exhibit alymphocytosis and agranulocytosis with profound immunodeficiency; these infants are susceptible to recurrent infections with a wide variety of bacterial, fungal, and viral organisms. The disease is fatal in infancy unless treated with bone marrow transplantation, which is curative.

RAG DEFICIENCY

T^-, B^-, NK^+ SCID (also known as Swiss-type SCID) is an autosomal recessive disorder originally described in Swiss infants who suffered from fatal infections associated with severe lymphopenia. It is characterized by selective failure of lymphoid cell development that results in the lack of both T and B cells at all stages of development. Natural killer cells are characteristically spared, as are nonlymphoid hematopoietic cell lineages. Bone marrow transplantation is curative. Swiss-type SCID results from mutations or deletions in the recombination activating genes 1 and 2 (RAG1 and RAG2). Both genes cooperate in initiating V(D)J recombination in T and B lymphocytes, and deficiency of either gene product abrogates this reaction. The deleterious effects of failed V(D)J recombination on lymphocyte development are explained by the failure to assemble antigen receptor complexes on the surface of developing T and B cells, which provide essential survival signals. NK cells are spared, as they do not undergo V(D)J recombination and are governed by distinct developmental pathways. The human disease is mirrored in mouse models of RAG1 and RAG2 deficiency, which exhibit identical immune deficits.

Omenn syndrome is a variant form of RAG deficiency. Patients present with intense erythroderma, protracted diarrhea, hepatosplenomegaly, and failure to thrive. Investigation typically reveals hypogammaglobulinemia, elevated IgE, and intense eosinophilia with T-cell infiltration of several organs, including the skin, gut, liver, and spleen. There is severe lymphocyte depletion from the thymus and other lymphoid organs. B cells are either markedly depressed in numbers or totally lacking, and the T cells present are severely restricted in their heterogeneity and skewed toward the Th2 phenotype, consistent with the clinical picture of high IgE and eosinophilia. Omenn syndrome patients suffer from partially inactivating mutations in either RAG1 or RAG2 genes; thus, siblings of patients with Omenn syndrome may present with a Swiss-type SCID picture.

SCID FROM MUTATIONS ALONG A COMMON CYTOKINE SIGNALING PATHWAY

SCID with selective failure of T- and NK-cell development in the face of normal or increased peripheral B-cell numbers represents the most common form of SCID and accounts for up to 25% of all new cases. In the overwhelming majority of cases the disease is transmitted in an X-linked fashion, and consequently, male infants are selectively affected (hence the designation X-linked SCID). However, autosomal recessive inheritance has been described in a few cases. As detailed below, both the X-linked and the autosomal recessive forms result from distinct defects affecting elements along the same pathway (Fig. 11-4).

In X-linked SCID, a family history of X-linked disease can be elicited in one-third of the patients. As in other X-linked disorders, most of the remaining cases result from an unrecognized X-linked carrier state in the mother or a spontaneous mutation. X-linked SCID is characterized by the total failure of T- and NK-cell development and the complete absence of host T cells from circulation and from lymphoid organs. The thymus is hypoplastic and is devoid of thymocytes and of Hassall corpuscles. Although transplacental engraftment of maternal lymphocytes can frequently result in the presence of significant numbers of circulating T cells, these maternal T cells display very poor function. The numbers of circulating B cells are usually increased, and their phenotype is normal, indicating that the defect does not appear to interfere significantly with B-cell development. However, the B cells of X-linked SCID patients are functionally abnormal in that they produce reduced amounts of immunoglobulins in vitro and appear to suffer from a block affecting their terminal differentiation. T cells of female carriers of the X-linked SCID gene display nonrandom inactivation of their X chromosome. All examined T cells appear to retain the X chromosome carrying the wild-type but not the defective X-linked SCID allele, indicating an essential role for this allele in T-cell survival.

Patients with X-linked SCID exhibit mutations in a cytokine receptor subunit, termed common γ chain or γc. This chain is a

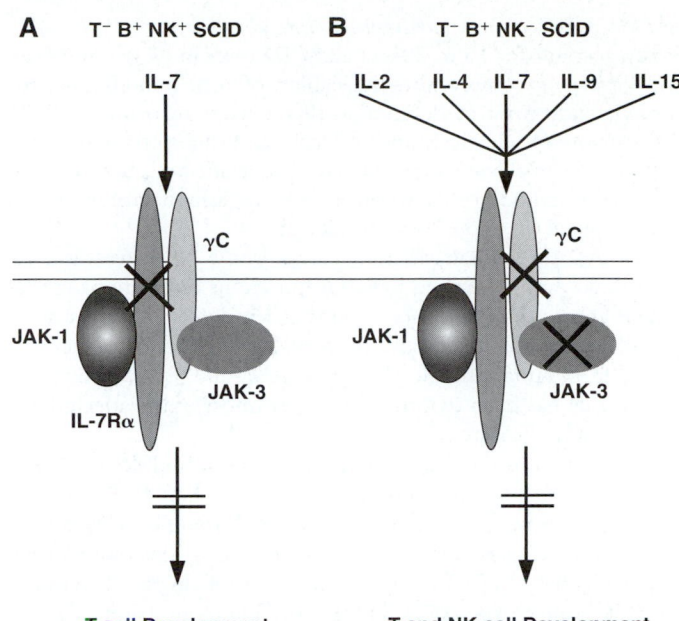

FIGURE 11-4   Schematic diagram of the mutation in IL-7Rα associated with failure of T-cell development in SCID (left side) and of the mutations in γc and JAK-3 associated with failure of T-cell and NK-cell development in SCID (right side).

component of several cytokine receptors, including those for IL-2, IL-4, IL-7, IL-9, and IL-15, and is thought to play an essential role in receptor-mediated signal transduction. Although selective disruption of other γc-containing cytokine receptors is associated with distinct forms of immunodeficiency, it appears that failure of T-cell development in X-linked SCID is related to absent IL-7 receptor function. Children with inactivating mutations in the IL-7 receptor α chain gene present with SCID and failure of T-cell development. NK-cell development is normal, indicating that another cytokine pathway mediates NK-cell generation.

Autosomal recessive T-cell-deficient SCID results from mutations in Jak3 kinase, a protein tyrosine kinase that associates with the γc chain and mediates its signaling function. The clinical presentation is identical to X-linked SCID. Hence, Jak3 kinase deficiency accounts for the majority of cases of autosomal recessive T-cell-deficient SCID, and the three defects (γc, Jak3, and IL-7 receptor) elegantly demonstrate a genetic immunodeficiency disorder resulting from disruption of sequential steps of a lymphocyte signal transduction pathway.

X-linked SCID is diagnosed by examining T lymphocytes of female carriers for nonrandom X-chromosome inactivation patterns. Confirmation of the diagnosis can be achieved by direct sequencing of affected genes (γc chain and, when indicated, Jak3 and IL-7 receptor genes). Bone marrow transplantation restores normal T-cell development and function but frequently fails to correct impaired B-cell function because donor B cells often fail to engraft. In such cases, intravenous immunoglobulin therapy is maintained indefinitely.

SCID CAUSED BY DISORDERS OF THE PURINE SALVAGE PATHWAY

Metabolic abnormalities may result in forms of SCID that are quite similar to SCID disease from intrinsic stem cell defects. Two specific disorders of the purine salvage pathway, *adenosine deaminase*

(ADA) deficiency and *purine nucleoside phosphorylase (PNP) deficiency,* account for 15 to 20% of all SCID cases in North America. *ADA deficiency* compromises the viability of both T and B cells and is particularly toxic to developing thymocytes. In contrast, *PNP deficiency* more selectively affects T cells and their progenitors, although B cells of some patients may also be affected. Both conditions are inherited in an autosomal recessive fashion with ADA deficiency being the more prevalent defect.

The ADA gene is located on chromosome 20. Most cases of ADA deficiency are caused by point mutations or deletions in the gene that result in the loss of enzyme expression or in the production of an unstable or inactive protein. Partial ADA deficiency resulting from mutations affecting the stability and/or the activity of the enzyme has been reported. However, most of the affected individuals were healthy.

ADA catalyzes the deamination of adenosine and deoxyadenosine to inosine and deoxyinosine, respectively (Fig. 11-5). Its deficiency results in the accumulation in lymphocytes of deoxyadenosine and a particularly toxic metabolite, deoxyadenosine trisphosphate (dATP), to levels 50- to 1000-fold higher than those normally found. The dATP inhibits the interconversion of ribonucleotides to deoxyribonucleotides, which is catalyzed by the enzyme ribonucleotide reductase; lack of deoxyribonucleotides (other than dATP) results in cell cycle arrest. High levels of dATP also inhibit RNA synthesis, disrupt DNA repair mechanisms, and interfere with DNA methylation by blocking the activity of the enzyme *S*-adenosylhomocysteine hydrolase.

Patients with ADA deficiency usually present within months after birth with recurrent infections, profound lymphopenia, and hypogammaglobulinemia. However, ADA deficiency may also present with a picture of progressive immunodeficiency with initial studies showing normal or near-normal immune parameters. Skeletal abnormalities, including cupping and flaring of the costochondral junctions and dysplasia of the pelvis, are frequently encountered but are not pathognomonic. The thymus is depleted of thymocytes, though changes suggestive of early thymocyte differentiation and rare Hassall corpuscles may occasionally be seen. Diagnosis is established by demonstrating low ADA activity in red blood cells in conjunction with elevated levels of deoxyadenosine and dATP in blood and urine. Prenatal diagnosis using fetal blood samples is available. In all cases, the outcome is fatal unless treatment is provided. Bone marrow transplantation is currently the only therapy that provides permanent cure for this disease. However, the peculiarly high incidence of graft failure in ADA-deficient patients following haploidentical bone marrow transplantation severely restricts the utility of this treatment modality. Enzyme replacement therapy with ethylene glycol–modified ADA provides an alternative treatment modality that is safe and relatively effective for those patients lacking a suitable bone marrow donor. Trials of gene replacement therapy are currently under way and may help provide lasting therapy for ADA-deficient patients.

Unlike ADA deficiency, PNP deficiency is frequently associated with relatively normal B-cell numbers and immunoglobulin levels in the face of profoundly depressed T-cell numbers and function. PNP is encoded by a single gene that is located on chromosome 14. The enzyme catalyzes the conversion of inosine to hypoxanthine and guanosine to guanine. PNP deficiency derives from point mutations or deletions affecting the PNP gene and results in the accumulation of PNP substrates inosine and guanosine. As in ADA deficiency, the deleterious effects of PNP deficiency on T lymphocytes are related to the accumulation of deoxyguanosine trisphosphate (dGTP) and to deoxyinosine trisphosphate, respectively, leading to inhibition of ribonucleotide reductase activity and cessation of DNA synthesis. Clinically, the patients suffer from severe bacterial and viral infections. Additionally, neurologic abnormalities are seen in upward of two-thirds of the patients, and autoimmune diseases, particularly autoimmune hemolytic anemia and thrombocytopenia, in about a third. The thymus is severely depleted of developing T cells. Bone marrow transplantation is currently the only therapeutic modality available for these children. Diagnosis is established by demonstrating low PNP activity in blood cells in conjunction with elevated levels of deoxyguanosine and dGTP in blood and urine.

11.4.2 Primary T and Combined T and B Immunodeficiencies

MHC CLASS I AND CLASS II DEFICIENCIES

Patients failing to express MHC class I or class II molecules present with specific abnormalities affecting the development and functioning of CD8+ and CD4+ T cells. In MHC class II deficiency, the development of CD4+ T cells in the thymus is markedly impaired, though not totally aborted. This is a direct consequence of the failure of CD4+ thymocytes to undergo positive selection. The available CD4+ T cells cannot mount delayed-type hypersensitivity responses, nor can they provide help to B cells to generate antigen-specific humoral responses, resulting in a combined immunodeficiency. Responses to mitogenic lectins and to allogeneic cells are usually preserved. Patients with MHC class II deficiency are prey to recurrent infections not unlike those seen in other forms of SCID. Chronic diarrhea and malabsorption are very common, and recurrent severe viral infections can be fatal. Bone marrow transplantation corrects the immune deficit.

SCID with MHC class II deficiency is an autosomal recessive disease that accounts for 5% of all cases of SCID and results from the failure to express MHC class II molecules, including HLA-DP, HLA-DQ, and HLA-DR. It is most prevalent in patients of Mediterranean ancestry. The underlying abnormalities seem to reside not in the MHC genes but in *trans*-acting regulatory factors that control the expression of these genes. At least three distinct mo-

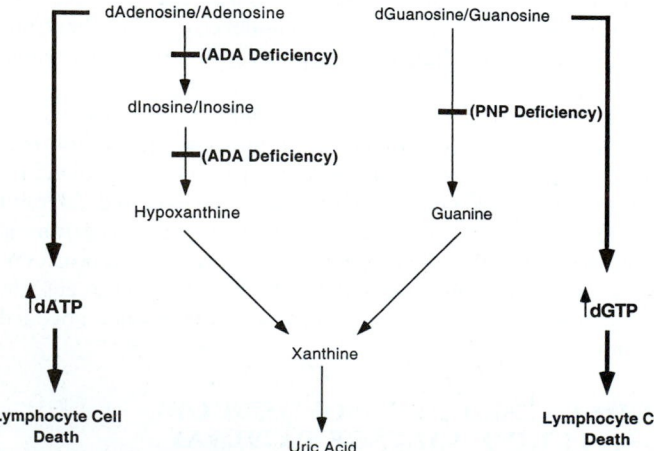

FIGURE 11-5 Diagram of the enzymatic pathways affected in SCID ascribable to adenosine deaminase deficiency or to deficiency of purine nucleoside phosphorylase.

lecular defects have been identified. The first affects a transcriptional factor termed CIITA. The other defects involve components of a transcriptional complex, termed RFX-5 and RFXAP, that binds a conserved response element (X box) in the MHC class II promoter region.

A reciprocal scenario of failure of CD8$^+$ T-cell development and function attends cases of MHC class I deficiency. These patients suffer from recurrent viral infections, and some are particularly prone to chronic lung disease. In these patients, CD8 development is impaired, and those CD8$^+$ T cells in circulation may fail to recognize antigens because antigen-presenting cells lack MHC class I molecules that present peptides. CD4$^+$ T-cell function is intact, and, unlike the case of MHC class II deficiency, antibody responses are not affected in MHC class I–deficient patients. MHC class I deficiency is also inherited as an autosomal recessive form.

CD3 DEFICIENCY

Impairment of TCR/MHC recognition can also result from point mutations in the TCR-associated CD3 subunits γ and ϵ. These mutations impair the assembly and the export of TCR chains to the cell surface. The patients' T cells have decreased responses to mitogens that act via the TCR/CD3, such as MHC-restricted antigens, lectins, or monoclonal antibodies to the various subunits of TCR/CD3. Clinically, the patients suffer from severe recurrent infections with bacteria and viruses as well as intractable diarrhea and failure to thrive.

An important consequence of impairment of TCR/MHC interaction in the thymus is the development of an enhanced propensity for autoimmunity. This is a direct consequence of derangement of negative selection in the thymus, leading to the export of autoreactive T cells to the periphery. Both MHC and TCR deficiency syndromes are associated with autoimmune phenomena (hemolytic anemia, autoimmune enteropathy, and autoantibody production). This association also includes other T-cell immunodeficiencies in which the underlying pathology may impair processes of thymic selection, such as ADA and PNP deficiency and the DiGeorge syndrome.

ZAP70 DEFICIENCY

The protein tyrosine kinase ZAP70 is selectively expressed in T lymphocytes and is activated on engagement of the T-cell receptor by antigen/MHC complexes. ZAP70 is indispensable to the program of T-cell activation and proliferation, and its deficiency renders the T cell refractory to antigenic stimulation. ZAP70 deficiency, an autosomal recessive disease resulting from insertions and mutations affecting the kinase gene, results in recurrent infections and impairment of both cellular and humoral immunity. Patients have virtually no CD8$^+$ T cells in circulation or in peripheral lymphoid organs. The thymus contains CD4$^+$, CD8$^+$ immature thymocytes but no CD8$^+$ single-positive mature thymocytes, indicative of a vital role for ZAP70 in CD8$^+$ T-lymphocyte development. Although ZAP70-deficient patients have normal numbers of CD4$^+$ T cells, these cells are unresponsive to antigens or to mitogens that act by engaging the T-cell receptor. Bone marrow transplantation successfully cures some of these patients.

LYMPHOKINE DEFICIENCY

A group of patients with combined immunodeficiency whose circulating lymphocytes are normal in number and in phenotype were found to suffer from defects in the production of T-cell lymphokines, including interleukins and interferon-γ. Notwithstanding their normal number and phenotype, T cells of these patients proliferate poorly in response to antigens and mitogens, but their proliferative responses normalize on supplementation with the lymphokine interleukin 2. The underlying molecular abnormalities appear to interfere with lymphokine gene transcription, although their precise nature remains to be established.

HYPER-IgM IMMUNODEFICIENCY

This immunodeficiency is characterized by a deficiency of IgA and IgG associated with normal or elevated serum IgM levels. The overwhelming number of patients are boys suffering from an X-linked form of this disorder, which is associated with mutations in the gene encoding CD154 (CD40 ligand), an inducible T-cell surface protein that serves as a counterreceptor for the TNF receptor family member CD40. Immunodeficiency with increased IgM may also occur sporadically as an autosomal dominant disease, as an acquired disorder, and in association with the congenital rubella syndrome.

Patients with X-linked hyper-IgM immunodeficiency are particularly susceptible to infections with bacterial pathogens commonly associated with hypogammaglobulinemia. In addition, they are highly susceptible to infections with *Pneumocystis carinii* and frequently first present with interstitial pneumonia caused by this pathogen. Some patients with milder forms of X-linked hyper-IgM immunodeficiency may also present with chronic parvovirus infection, which manifests as pure red cell aplasia. In addition to their increased susceptibility to infection, many of these patients develop neutropenia, thrombocytopenia, renal lesions, and aplastic and hemolytic anemia, presumably manifestations of autoimmune disease induced by IgM antibodies. Enlarged cervical lymph nodes and hepatosplenomegaly are frequent findings. Malignant IgM-producing B-cell lymphomas of the intestinal tract have been reported in several cases.

In X-linked hyper-IgM immunodeficiency the hypoglobulinemia appears to reflect a defect in isotype switching caused by a lack of CD40 signaling in B cells. B cells expressing IgM and IgD are present in normal numbers, but IgG- and IgA-bearing B cells cannot be found. The susceptibility to *Pneumocystis carinii* also reflects lack of engagement of CD40 on macrophages and dendritic cells by CD154 of helper T cells.

Therapy involves correcting the hypogammaglobulinemia with immunoglobulin infusion therapy and prophylaxis against *Pneumocystis carinii* infection with trimethoprim-sulfamethoxazole. Chronic parvovirus infection usually remits on immunoglobulin replacement therapy. Bone marrow transplantation has been successfully employed in severe cases.

DIGEORGE SYNDROME

DiGeorge syndrome represents a prime example of aborted T-cell development caused by the absence or disruption of the thymic microenvironment. In contrast to X-linked SCID and other disorders of lymphoid stem cells, in which the lymphoid lineages are the only tissues affected, in the DiGeorge syndrome there is aberrant development of several tissues, including those of the thymus, heart, and parathyroid glands because of the disruption of normal embryogenesis of a group of cephalic neural crest cells. The majority of patients with the DiGeorge syndrome exhibit hemizygous interstitial deletions of chromosome 22q11, and a small percentage present with chromosome 22 aneuploidy (monosomy 22 or large deletions of the long arm of chromosome 22). Deletions in the same locus are also present in the closely related velocardiofacial syndrome. Prenatal diagnosis is possible by fluorescent in situ hybridization using appropriate DNA probes. Several conditions overlap in their clinical presentation with DiGeorge syndrome in the absence of 22q11 deletions, including fetal alcohol syndrome and retinoic acid embryopathy. Most cases are not inherited, but a few manifest an autosomal dominant inheritance.

The clinical manifestations of the DiGeorge syndrome can be mild and isolated or more severe and widespread. Commonly encountered craniofacial findings include micrognathia, hypertelorism, shortened philtrum, and low-set, dorsally rotated auricles with or without malformations. Cardiac anomalies include conotruncal defects such as tetralogy of Fallot, transposition of the great vessels, double-outlet right ventricle, and ventricular septal defects, and branchial arch defects, such as interrupted aortic arch or aortic arch hypoplasia. The parathyroid glands may be absent or reduced in number, and subclinical hypoparathyroidism is frequently present. Major congenital anomalies involving the diaphragm, the eyes, the kidneys, and the central nervous system also abound. Moderate to severe mental retardation is seen in most patients.

The thymus in the DiGeorge syndrome may be absent or, more commonly, hypoplastic The spectrum of immune dysfunction observed in this condition ranges from the severe (so-called complete DiGeorge syndrome) to the subtle (partial DiGeorge syndrome). In the complete form of the DiGeorge syndrome there exists a picture of SCID. The T cells may be totally absent because of inability of committed T-cell precursors to mature in the thymus. The B cells are usually normal or increased in number, but patients nevertheless suffer from hypogammaglobulinemia and absent antigen-specific antibody responses because of lack of T-cell helper function. Far more common is the picture of partial DiGeorge syndrome, where T-cell depletion is moderate to minimal and B-cell number and function are normal. Natural killer cell activity is generally unaffected in both forms of the disease. Interestingly, older patients with DiGeorge syndrome are prone to develop some autoimmune diseases, most notably juvenile rheumatoid arthritis. This may reflect disease-related defects in thymic selection processes.

In most cases, the immunologic deficit ameliorates with time because of compensatory residual thymic tissue or extrathymic maturation of T cells. Severe immunologic deficit has been successfully managed with thymic transplant. However, because of the spontaneous improvement in immunologic function noted in most patients, this form of therapy is rarely indicated except in patients with the complete form of DiGeorge syndrome. Intravenous immunoglobulin replacement therapy may be of benefit in selected cases with severe immunologic deficits.

COMBINED IMMUNODEFICIENCIES ASSOCIATED WITH OTHER DEFECTS

In addition to the aforementioned diseases of T-cell development and activation, there are a host of other diseases that are associated with T-cell dysfunction. Two diseases of particular interest are ataxia-telangectasia and the Wiskott-Aldrich syndrome.

ATAXIA-TELANGIECTASIA AND OTHER DISORDERS OF DNA REPAIR Ataxia-telangiectasia (AT) is an autosomal recessive disease characterized by progressive cerebellar ataxia, oculocutaneous telangiectasia, immunodeficiency, high incidence of cancer, and increased sensitivity to ionizing radiation. Heterozygote carriers are estimated to constitute up to 1.4% of the United States population. A hallmark of AT is heightened sensitivity to ionizing radiation and radiomimetic agents. The responsible gene, ATM, maps to chromosome 11q22-23 and encodes a member of the phosphatidyl-

inositol 3-kinase family. The ATM protein is involved in monitoring DNA repair and coordinating DNA synthesis with cell cycle progression. ATM mutations completely abrogate protein expression or function, leading to the accumulation of DNA strand breaks. This in turn activates programmable cell death (apoptosis), leading to progressive depletion of affected cell types.

Ataxia usually manifests first as a staggering gait in infancy; its onset heralds other manifestations of neurologic dysfunction including apraxia of ocular movement and choreoathetosis. Telangiectasias are first apparent as dilatation of small blood vessels in the bulbar conjunctivae and become visible in the skin at the age of 5 years. They are most notable around the ears, the neck, antecubital fossae, and popliteal fossae. Endocrine abnormalities such as gonadal dysgenesis and insulin-resistant diabetes mellitus are frequently encountered. Recurrent sinopulmonary infections are a notable feature of the disease and reflect the underlying immunodeficiency. If untreated, they can frequently lead to bronchiectasis. The serum levels of oncofetoproteins, including serum α_1-fetoprotein and carcinoembryonic antigen, are elevated. For children 1 year of age or older, an elevated serum α_1-fetoprotein level coupled to a clinical picture of ataxia and telangiectasia confirms the diagnosis.

Immunodeficiency in AT is the result of defects in both cellular and humoral immunity. The thymus is abnormally small and is sparsely populated by lymphoid elements, and peripheral lymphoid tissues exhibit depletion of resident T cells. The number of circulating $CD4^+$ T cells may be reduced, although the population of circulating TCR^+ T cells may be expanded. Parameters of T-cell function such as proliferation in response to mitogens, ability to reject an allograft, and delayed-type hypersensitivity reactions are usually defective. B cells are usually found in normal numbers, but IgA and IgE concentrations are low because their heavy chain constant-region genes are located further downstream from the V(D)J elements. Genes more proximally located, including those encoding IgM and IgD, are unaffected. IgA deficiency is encountered in up to 70% of the affected persons and may precede the clinical manifestation of immunodeficiency by many years. IgE deficiency is similarly prevalent. IgG deficiency, which is found in up to one-half of all patients, most frequently reflects a selective decrease in the levels of IgG2 and IgG4 subclasses.

Patients with AT are at a high risk for developing malignancies, particularly those of the lymphoid system. Over 85% of the tumors reported in affected children are either acute lymphocytic leukemia or lymphomas. The incidence of tumors of epithelial origin increases progressively with age. The increased frequency of tumors in this syndrome extends to include relatives of affected patients. Chromosomal abnormalities abound and are thought to contribute to tumorigenesis. Loci of recombining immunoglobulin and T-cell receptor genes are particularly affected. Most of the chromosomal breaks are found in chromosomes 7 and 14 at sites of rearranging immunoglobulin superfamily genes. In light of their heightened sensitivity to ionizing radiation and their increased risk for developing malignancies, exposure of AT patients to x-rays should be curtailed. Similarly, radiomimetic agents should be avoided in treating these patients for malignancies.

Besides AT, other chromosomal instability disorders are also associated with immunodeficiency. *Bloom syndrome*, associated with DNA ligase I deficiency, also features telangiectasia, immunologic and central nervous system abnormalities, and a high incidence of leukemia. *Nijmegen breakage syndrome* is a rare autosomal recessive disorder associated with microcephaly with normal or near-normal intelligence, combined cellular and humoral immunodeficiency, and a high incidence of malignancy, especially lymphoid. This disease results from mutations in a gene termed *NBS1* (for Nijmegen breakage syndrome 1), whose protein product, termed nibrin, is involved in repair of double-stranded DNA breakages.

WISKOTT-ALDRICH SYNDROME Wiskott-Aldrich syndrome (WAS) is an X-linked immunodeficiency disease characterized by a triad of thrombocytopenia with small platelets, eczema, and increased susceptibility to pyogenic and opportunistic infections. A related disorder, X-linked thrombocytopenia, is characterized by isolated chronic thrombocytopenia. Between the two phenotypes are attenuated forms of WAS in which eczema and immunodeficiency are variably expressed. All three phenotypes result from mutations affecting the same gene, which maps on Xp11.22 and is referred to as WASP (Wiskott-Aldrich syndrome protein) gene. WASP is a cytoplasmic proline-rich protein that integrates diverse signal transduction pathways with the cellular cytoskeleton. Mutations that severely compromise WASP expression result in classical WAS phenotype, whereas milder mutations underlie X-linked thrombocytopenia and other attenuated forms of WAS.

Affected boys frequently present early in infancy with bleeding, including bloody diarrhea or exsanguination following circumcision. Eosinophilia, elevated IgE, and positive prick tests to common allergens frequently accompany the eczema, suggesting an underlying allergic etiology. The eczematous skin may become infected with staphylococci after excessive scratching. Immunodeficiency may manifest as persistent sinopulmonary infections and/or unusually severe childhood viral infections, including varicella. WAS patients are also at high risk of developing lymphomas and leukemia. Lymphomas commonly develop at extranodal sites, particularly in the brain and in the gastrointestinal tract. Overall, many WAS patients die of bleeding, infection, or malignancy within the first decade of life.

The platelets are invariably low in number and are small in size, the latter being a diagnostically useful feature. They display impaired aggregation in response to ADP, epinephrine, risotectin, and collagen. Thrombocytopenia is a consequence of both ineffectual thrombocytosis and, more importantly, enhanced sequestration from abnormal platelet cytoarchitecture. Splenectomy ameliorates the thrombocytopenia and normalizes the reduced platelet volume. Autoimmune thrombocytopenia may complicate the course of some WAS patients and precipitate postsplenectomy thrombocytopenia.

Immunodeficiency in WAS results from impairment of both cellular and humoral immunity. T-cell proliferative responses to mitogens and specific antigens become progressively diminished with age, and cutaneous energy is common. A characteristic morphologic abnormality of T lymphocytes, a near absence of microvilli, is apparent under electron microscopy.

Humoral abnormalities abound as a consequence of defective T-cell function. There is increased catabolism of serum immunoglobulins, whose levels have a regular pattern: the IgA and IgE are elevated, the IgM decreased, and the IgG normal. The response to isohemagglutinins and other polysaccharide antigens is absent or very diminished; as a result, the response to polysaccharide vaccines of *Haemophilus influenzae* type B (Hib) and pneumococcus is very poor. Responses to protein antigens are also defective, reflecting abnormal T-helper-cell function.

Obligate female heterozygotes exhibit skewed X-chromosome inactivation in all blood cell lines but not in other tissues such as fibroblasts. As in the case of X-linked SCID and other X-linked immunodeficiency diseases, this finding indicates that hematopoietic cells carrying the inactive WAS alleles are impaired in their development and/or survival relative to their normal counterparts. Rare cases of female WAS patients have been described which result from the presence of a mutant WASP gene on one X chromosome and a mutation in the other X chromosome.

The treatment of choice in WAS is a bone marrow transplant from an HLA-matched donor. When a donor is not available, splenectomy often has a satisfactory outcome in improving the platelet count and normalizing platelet size. However, splenectomy compounds the immunologic deficit and increases the risk of overwhelming infections with encapsulated organisms. Intravenous γ-globulin administered at intervals of 2 to 3 weeks is beneficial in preventing pyogenic infections and is indicated postsplenectomy to counter the added risk of infections.

11.4.3   Primary B-Cell Immunodeficiency Diseases

In this section we consider antibody deficiencies that feature abnormal B-cell development and function in the presence of essentially normal T-cell development and function. Patients with antibody deficiency syndromes usually present with a history of recurrent pyogenic infections of the respiratory tract or other organs and chronic gastrointestinal disease including giardiasis. The bacterial infections are mainly caused by encapsulated, pyogenic organisms such as *Haemophilus influenzae*, *Streptococcus pneumoniae*, *Staphylococcus aureus*, and *Neisseria meningitidis*. Viral infections are usually cleared normally by these patients, although they are prone to recurrent infections with the same virus because they cannot produce protective antibodies against the offending agent. Tonsils of patients with X-linked or autosomal recessive agammaglobulinemia are either hypoplastic or absent. Radiologic studies may be helpful in evaluating the size of the adenoid tissue and the thymus gland and in assessing the sinuses and lung fields. Evidence for recurrent infections such as scars from previous abscesses or chronic otitis media is often noted.

Measurement of serum immunoglobulins and IgG subclasses is an important screening test in the diagnosis of antibody deficiencies. Other screening tests for antibody production in vivo include the assessment of specific antibody formation. Isohemagglutinins should be present in all normal individuals except those with group AB red cells. Titers should be greater than 1:8 in normal subjects over the age of 3 years. Antibodies to streptolysin O and other streptococcal antigens are found in the sera of most individuals after infancy. The determination of serum antibody titers after tetanus or diphtheria immunizations or immunization with *Haemophilus influenzae* and pneumococcal vaccines provides valuable information about the ability of an individual to mount specific antibody responses. Most of the antibody response to tetanus and diphtheria resides in the IgG1 subclass (with some IgG3), whereas the antibody response to polysaccharide antigens resides in both IgG1 and IgG2 subclasses.

When a patient is found to have low immunoglobulin levels, additional in vitro tests are used to characterize the nature of the B-cell defect. Enumeration of circulating B lymphocytes is based on the presence of several surface receptors not found on T cells. These include surface immunoglobulins and B-cell–specific surface molecules such as CD19 and CD20.

X-LINKED AGAMMAGLOBULINEMIA

This disorder (XLA) is characterized by the early onset of recurrent pyogenic infections in association with low serum concentrations of all immunoglobulin classes and the virtual absence of immuno-globulin-bearing B cells in peripheral blood and lymphoid tissues. However, B-cell precursors are found at normal frequency in the bone marrow. T cells are normal in number and function.

The cellular basis of the antibody deficiency is arrested B-cell development in the bone marrow. Although B-cell numbers and their plasma cell progeny are severely deficient, pre-B cells containing intracytoplasmic μ chains are usually produced in normal numbers. The very few B cells found in the bone marrow and in the circulation display an immature phenotype as defined by cell surface markers. These cells are capable of undergoing isotype switching and plasma cell differentiation, and, surprisingly, moderately low IgG or IgA is occasionally encountered in few affected boys. However, these XLA patients are unable to respond with antibody production to immunization with antigens.

X-linked agammaglobulinemia is caused by mutations in a gene that maps to Xq22 and encodes the Bruton tyrosine kinase, or Btk, a member of the Tec family of tyrosine kinases that is expressed in the cytosol of all B-lineage cells, including pre-B cells, and in myeloid cells. Btk is critical to the development of B cells; the block in B-cell development in XLA is a direct consequence of deficient Btk function and underlies disease pathogenesis. B cells of obligate heterozygote females are normal, but their active X chromosome is exclusively the one that harbors the normal Btk allele. In contrast, other cells of other lineages, including T cells, may utilize either X chromosome, a reflection of the selective role of Btk in B-cell maturation.

Male infants with X-linked agammaglobulinemia frequently become symptomatic late in the first year of life following the consumption of placentally transferred maternal γ-globulin. However, it is important to appreciate that even affected boys of the same family may vary in the onset and severity of their disease, depending on environmental exposure, the presence of other siblings, and severity of immunoglobulin deficiency. Recurrent infections, especially with encapsulated pyogenic organisms such as staphylococci, pneumococci, streptococci, and *Haemophilus influenzae*, commonly involve the upper and lower respiratory tract causing pneumonia, otitis, purulent sinusitis, and bronchiectasis. Pulmonary disease may be caused by less virulent serotypes (eg, type 37 *S. pneumoniae*) and yet take a severe course with complications such as empyema. Additional infections include meningitis, sepsis, pyoderma, osteomyelitis, and giardiasis. Although most respond to appropriate antibiotics, they are bound to recur unless prophylactic immunoglobulin therapy is instituted. Without immunoglobulin therapy, many of these children acquire chronic progressive bronchiectasis and ultimately die of pulmonary complications.

Children with X-linked agammaglobulinemia have an increased susceptibility to infection with enteroviruses such as echovirus and polio viruses, the latter frequently precipitated by administration of live attenuated polio virus vaccine. These infections give rise to serious complications, including encephalomyelitis and paralytic polio. Patients suffering from enteroviral encephalomyelitis may respond to treatment with high doses of γ-globulins administered either intravenously or intrathecally and containing high-titer antibodies to the culprit viruses. Several patients with X-linked agammaglobulinemia have also developed syndromes resembling dermatomyositis in conjunction with disseminated echovirus infection. This complication of the disease is generally fatal despite use of steroids or antimetabolites. Chronic inflammation and swelling of the large joints, which resemble rheumatoid arthritis, develop in one-third to one-half of these children before the diagnosis is es-

tablished. This complication resolves with the institution of γ-globulin replacement.

Laboratory findings include severe deficiency in all major immunoglobulin classes, with the IgG levels usually less than 100 mg/dL and serum IgA and IgM levels less than 1% of adult values. B lymphocytes are absent from the blood and from all lymphoid tissue. Lymph nodes are small and lack germinal centers and plasma cells. Female carriers can be identified by assessing the pattern of X-chromosome utilization in their B-cell population.

The widespread availability of γ-globulin suitable for intravenous administration has vastly changed the effectiveness of treatment in XLA. The optimal dose and frequency of administration have to be determined for each patient. The minimal dose is 300 mg/kg of body weight per month, but this is rarely adequate in most cases. Some patients require as much as 600 mg/kg every 2 to 3 weeks to achieve adequate prophylaxis against infection and maintain good pulmonary function. Antibiotics should be used as appropriate for acute infections. Patients with XLA do not produce antibody responses on immunization and should not be given any live or attenuated virus vaccines.

XLA has been reported in association with growth hormone deficiency. Some patients with this presentation carry mutations in the Btk gene indistinguishable from those of patients with no growth hormone deficiency, suggesting that the latter finding is incidental. Others harbor no detectable Btk mutations, suggesting a distinct molecular defect that remains unknown.

Autosomally inherited congenital agammaglobulinemia derives from a variety of point mutations and large deletions involving the μ heavy chain gene or mutations in the genes encoding the surrogate light chain and the B-cell signal transduction adapter BLNK.

COMMON VARIABLE IMMUNODEFICIENCY

The primary feature of this disorder is deficiency of immunoglobulins of all classes in the face of apparently normal B-cell development. This disease affects both sexes and results from any one of a number of heterogeneous defects that impair the differentiation of B cells into plasma cells. Family members have a higher incidence of other immunologic abnormalities including selective IgA and/or IgG subclass deficiency and autoimmunity, consistent with a common genetic predisposition shared among these disorders. The frequent association of common variable immunodeficiency (CVID) and IgA deficiency with certain MHC haplotypes that include unusual class I, II, and III genes suggests a common susceptibility locus on chromosome 6.

Non-MHC genes or environment factors may be necessary to precipitate clinical immunodeficiency because many related individual carriers of the same haplotypes are asymptomatic. Such factors may include drugs such as phenytoin, D-penicillamine, gold, and sulfasalazine. The development of infectious mononucleosis has also been associated with common variable immunodeficiency, although occurrence of such a contingency in a male should raise suspicion of X-linked lymphoproliferative disease (discussed later in this chapter).

Most patients with common variable immunodeficiency have normal numbers of B cells that are clonally diverse, undergo clonal expansion in response to antigenic stimulation, and respond with DNA synthesis when their cell surface immunoglobulins are cross-linked by anti-IgM antibodies. The molecular basis of impaired differentiation of patient B cells into plasma cells is unclear. Hypogammaglobulinemia may result in extensive B-cell proliferation leading to hypertrophy of the spleen, lymph nodes, and intestinal lymphoid tissues. In addition to the B-cell deficiency, many of these patients have or eventually develop T-cell abnormalities. Over 50% of patients eventually exhibit cutaneous anergy.

Common variable immunodeficiency varies in its time of onset as well as in its clinical and immunologic features. Symptoms are uncommon before the age of 6 years, and in most patients the disease begins in the second or third decade of life. Recurrent and chronic respiratory tract infections, particularly paranasal sinusitis, bronchitis, and pneumonia, are prominent features. The IgG levels are usually less than 500 mg/100 mL, and IgA and IgM levels are less than 50 mg/100 mL. Patients with common variable immunodeficiency usually have low isohemagglutinin titers and a markedly reduced antibody response on challenge with a variety of antigens. Despite the immunoglobulin deficiency, patients with common variable immunodeficiency frequently manifest autoantibodies such as rheumatoid factor or anti–red blood cell antibody resulting in Coombs test–positive hemolytic anemia.

A frequent complication of common variable immunodeficiency is a sprue-like syndrome with diarrhea, malabsorption, steatorrhea, and protein-losing enteropathy occurring in up to 60% of the patients. These gastrointestinal abnormalities may be associated with heavy bacterial overgrowth, jejunal villous atrophy, or intestinal nodular lymphoid hyperplasia. *Giardia lamblia* infection is common and appears to be responsible for many of the gastrointestinal complications seen in these patients.

Another distinguishing feature of common variable immunodeficiency is the frequent occurrence of noncaseating granulomas of the lungs, spleen, liver, and skin. An infectious etiology for these lesions has not been identified, but steroids have been reported to be helpful in their treatment. Amyloidosis, hemolytic-uremic syndrome, and an increased incidence of malignancy, particularly reticuloendothelial tumors, have also been reported in these patients. Individuals with common variable immunodeficiency are at a greater risk for malignancy, chiefly lymphomas, whose incidence progressively increases with age.

Patients with common variable immunodeficiency frequently have associated hematologic disorders, including pernicious anemia, hemolytic anemia (including Coombs test–positive hemolytic anemia), anemia from folate or vitamin B_{12} malabsorption, leukopenia, and/or thrombocytopenia. These patients may also suffer from nondeforming polyarthritis and/or polyarthralgias similar to those encountered in congenital agammaglobulinemia that are similarly responsive to treatment with immunoglobulin replacement therapy. Furthermore, autoimmune disorders such as rheumatoid arthritis, systemic lupus erythematosus, and idiopathic thrombocytopenic purpura are seen in patients with common variable immunodeficiency and in their relatives at a much higher incidence than in the normal population.

Treatment of common variable immunodeficiency centers on immunoglobulin replacement and specific treatment of infectious complications with appropriate antibiotics. Autoimmunity and other disorders associated with common variable immunodeficiency respond to standard therapies for the respective disease.

X-LINKED LYMPHOPROLIFERATIVE DISEASE (DUNCAN SYNDROME)

Affected males suffer from severe, often fatal infections with Epstein-Barr virus (EBV) associated with fulminant hepatitis, B-cell lymphomas, agranulocytosis, aplastic anemia, or acquired hypogammaglobulinemia. These complications are attributed to uncontrolled polyclonal T- and B-cell expansion triggered by the EBV infection. Approximately half of the affected individuals die of fatal infectious mononucleosis. The most common cause of death is hepatic necrosis and/or bone marrow failure resulting from infiltration of these organs with cytotoxic T cells and natural killer cells. Survivors suffer from acquired hypo- or agammaglobulnemia and/or malignant lymphomas. Most of the lymphomas are extranodal, Burkitt type, many involving the ileocecum.

The underlying defect involves mutations in the *SH2D1A* gene, found on the long arm of the X chromosome (Xq25). It encodes a protein known as SAP [for signaling lymphocyte activation molecule (SLAM)-associated protein]. SAP is an SH2 domain containing a 128–amino acid peptide that is expressed in T cells and associates with SLAM, an inducible T-cell surface molecule involved in T/B-cell interaction. SAP controls signal transduction via SLAM, and failure to regulate SLAM signaling by SAP accounts for the exaggerated yet ineffective T-cell response seen in this disease.

Affected individuals have no indication of a preexisting immunologic abnormality and do not appear to suffer from increased susceptibility to other infections. Therapies such as corticosteroids, immunosuppressants, and cytotoxic agents aimed at blunting the uncontrolled T-cell activation during acute EBV infection may be useful. Immunoglobulin replacement therapy is indicated in case of hypogammaglobulinemia, and bone marrow transplant provides definite therapy if attempted early in life, ideally before EBV infection sets in.

TRANSIENT HYPOGAMMAGLOBULINEMIA OF INFANCY (THI)

The normal full-term newborn has a serum IgG level that is the same or sometimes slightly higher than that of the mother, reflecting active transport of IgG across the placenta during the last trimester of pregnancy. Normally, infants usually do not begin significant synthesis of IgG until age 2 to 3 months. Catabolism of transplacental IgG (half-life of 25–30 days) precipitates a physiological hypogammaglobulinemia between 4 and 6 months of age. In THI, there is an abnormal prolongation and accentuation of the physiological hypogammaglobulinemia of infancy resulting from delayed onset of immunoglobulin synthesis. THI affects both male and female infants and in some cases shows a familial pattern.

Affected infants usually present after 6 months of age with recurrent viral and pyogenic infections of the upper and lower respiratory tract and rarely the skin or meninges. Recurrent otitis media and bronchitis are the most common infections observed in these patients. In some cases the disorder is associated with food allergy. Nevertheless, many infants with transient hypogammaglobulinemia are free of significant infection and have been found incidentally among relatives of immunodeficient persons. Such infants usually have no specific physical findings, typically thrive, and have normal peripheral lymphoid tissue.

Patients with THI have normal numbers of B and T lymphocytes in circulation, and the T lymphocytes respond normally to mitogen stimulation. Importantly, and unlike patients with XLA or CVID, patients with THI are capable of synthesizing specific isohemagglutinins to human type A and B erythrocytes and respond with high titer antibodies to diphtheria and tetanus toxoid vaccination even though the immunoglobulin concentrations are low.

Lymph nodes from these patients display very small or no germinal centers, with marked reduction in the number of plasma cells.

Because these patients have a normal number of circulating B cells, the defect presumably involves terminal differentiation of B cells into antibody-producing plasma cells. A transient defect in T-helper-cell function has been incriminated in the pathogenesis of THI.

Patients with THI usually recover spontaneously by the age of 3 to 4 years. After the onset of normal IgG synthesis, their prognosis is excellent. The majority of patients with THI do not require immunoglobulin replacement therapy and can be followed with conservative therapy and periodic immunoglobulin level determination every 3 to 4 months. In those patients with severe recurrent infections or with dangerously low immunoglobulin levels, replacement therapy is indicated, usually for 12 to 36 months. These patients should be investigated thoroughly and followed carefully to distinguish this condition from other permanent immunodeficiencies.

IgG SUBCLASS DEFICIENCIES

There are four subclasses of human IgG (IgG1, IgG2, IgG3, and IgG4), each corresponding to a specific chain constant region gene. Approximately 67% of serum IgG is IgG1, 20 to 25% is IgG2, and 5 to 10% is IgG3. IgG4 usually comprises 5% or less of the total. IgG2 is the slowest of the subclasses to reach adult levels. The four different chains confer different effector functions. In most individuals with IgG subclass deficiency, the deficient IgG subclass is produced at low levels despite the presence of affected chain constant region gene(s).

IgG subclass deficiencies have been related to an increased susceptibility to infection, primarily involving the respiratory tract in children and adults. Recurrent otitis media and sinusitis are present in virtually all of the children with IgG2 subclass deficiency, and recurrent pneumonia is present in about 40% of them. On investigation, an underlying history of sinopulmonary infections is discovered. Many children with IgG2 subclass deficiency have bouts of recurrent diarrhea. As in other cases of hypogammaglobulinemia, the possibility of viral infection, giardiasis, and bacterial overgrowth should be considered. For a few children, the predominant symptom at presentation is recurrent diarrhea.

A clue to the diagnosis of IgG subclass deficiency is the presence of a normal or borderline IgG level (lower limit of normal range for age) in a child with a documented history of recurrent infections. Given their history of repeated antigenic stimulation by infectious organisms, these children are expected to have high serum IgG levels. Analysis of IgG subclasses and measurement of specific antibody serum titers to *Haemophilus influenzae*, *Streptococcus pneumoniae*, and *Neisseria meningitidis* are invaluable in interpreting the clinical significance of IgG subclass deficiency. Therapy for IgG subclass deficiency may involve the use of prophylactic antibiotics and, in select cases, intravenous γ-globulins.

11.5   COMPLEMENT DISORDERS

Jonathan D. Gitlin

The essential nature of the complement system, which comprises more than 30 plasma and cell membrane proteins, was first recognized more than a century ago in studies exploring the immunologic defenses against pathogenic bacteria. The many biological functions of the complement system are determined by a complex cascade of protein activation and inhibition. Genetically determined deficiencies in each component of this cascade have now been described, and these rare, inherited disorders provide unique insight into the specific functions of the individual complement proteins. The clinical presentation of affected individuals may include undue susceptibility to infection, autoimmune disease, or angioedema, depending on the specific role of the deficient component.

C3 is the most abundant complement component in plasma, and activation of this protein by both the alternative and classical pathways results in the majority of the biological activity of the complement system. Activation of C3 by the classical complement pathway is initiated by the binding of immune complexes. Because C3 may also be activated via the alternative pathway, inherited deficiency of the proteins of this early classical pathway (C1q, C1r, C1s, C2, C4) is not usually associated with recurrent infection. Instead, the absence of these proteins is usually associated with the presence of autoimmune disease such as discoid lupus, SLE, glomerulonephritis, and vasculitis, in part because of the role of these proteins in the clearance of immune complexes.

The alternative pathway of complement activation occurs independent of antibody via interaction with complex polysaccharides on the microbial surface. The activation of C3 by proteolytic cleavage results in the generation of C3b, a serum opsonin essential for the activation of phagocytic cells. As a result, deficiency of C3, the soluble components that regulate turnover of this protein (factor H, factor I), or the cofactors D, B, and properdin results in severe recurrent infections with encapsulated pyogenic organisms. Affected patients will therefore present at a young age with bacteremia, pneumonia, and sinusitis most frequently from *Streptococcus pneumoniae* or *Haemophilus influenzae*. As specific immunity develops in such individuals, the incidence of such infections becomes less, and many patients will be asymptomatic in adulthood.

The terminal complement components (C5-C9) assemble to form the membrane attack complex integral to the lysis of gram-negative bacteria. Individuals with deficiencies in these components are unduly susceptible to infection with *Neisseria* species, for which this mechanism of lysis is an essential component of host defense. As a result, affected patients often present with recurrent meningococcal meningitis or disseminated gonococcal infection.

From a practical point of view, the diagnosis of complement deficiency should be considered in any child with recurrent bacterial infection. The presence of associated rheumatologic disease in such children should increase suspicion of an abnormality in the complement cascade. With the exception of C2 deficiency, which is largely asymptomatic, these disorders are rare, being inherited as autosomal recessive or, in the case of properdin, X-linked diseases. In most circumstances, the measurement of total hemolytic complement activity in the serum of suspected patients will reveal a marked decrease, which can then be further analyzed by quantifying the individual components in specialized laboratories.

The low prevalence of the inherited complement deficiencies obviates the usefulness of screening for such disorders in children with their first systemic bacterial infection. An exception to this may be systemic meningococcal infections, where the frequency of C5 to C9 deficiency (~20%) would appear sufficient to warrant analysis of total hemolytic complement activity in such patients. There are no specific therapies for the complement deficiencies. Management of such patients often includes long-term prophylactic antibiotic treatment into adulthood. In the case of associated autoimmune disease, therapy is directed at treatment of the underlying rheumatologic disorder.

11.5.1   Hereditary Angioneurotic Edema

The activity of the first component of complement, C1, is controlled by a serine protease inhibitor in plasma termed the C1 inhibitor (C1INH). This protein inactivates active C1 and serves as a major control point in the complement cascade. Inherited deficiency of C1INH results in excessive activation of C2 and C4 with subsequent episodic, localized, and recurrent edema of the skin, gastrointestinal tract, and upper airway. C1INH deficiency is inherited as an autosomal dominant disorder. Eighty-five percent of affected patients have about 30% of the normal concentration of circulating C1INH; the remaining individuals synthesize normal amounts of inactive protein. These two groups of patients are phenotypically indistinguishable.

Affected patients may have recurrent attacks of angioedema at any time during childhood, and most patients will be diagnosed by the second decade. Nevertheless, the severity and frequency of attacks increase at adolescence, and they persist into adulthood. Most patients associate trauma or stress as antecedent precipitants; exogenous estrogens and pregnancy are also implicated. The swelling is nonpruritic and rarely painful and usually resolves within 5 days. The majority of patients experience episodes of abdominal pain, often relieved by the acute onset of emesis. These symptoms are secondary to angioedema of the bowel wall and are very characteristic for this disorder. The most life-threatening complication consists of laryngeal edema, which can lead to rapid upper airway occlusion.

Because of the inheritance pattern, most individuals will have a positive family history, helping to confirm the diagnosis. During attacks the CH50 will be reduced, as will the C2 and C4. Quantification of C1INH levels is useful for diagnosis, but activity must be measured to exclude those patients with normal but inactive protein. Neither patient history or genotype is sufficient to predict attacks, and thus, long-term prophylaxis is warranted in most patients. Attenuated androgens such as danazol and antifibrinolytics such as tranexamic acid are equally effective, but the latter may be better tolerated in children because of unwanted effects of androgens. Fresh frozen plasma or C1 esterase concentrate is effective in treating acute attacks. Acute airway management must be pursued in patients with laryngeal edema. Antihistamines, steroids, and epinephrine are of no use in such situations. The long-term outcome is favorable.

References

Cicardi M, Bergamaschini L, Cugno M, et al: Pathogenetic and clinical aspects of C1 inhibitor deficiency. Immunobiology 199:366–376, 1998
Sullivan KE: Complement deficiency and autoimmunity. Curr Opin Pediatr 10:600–606, 1998
Whaley K, Schwaeble W: Complement and complement deficiencies. Semin Liver Dis 17:297–310, 1997

11.6   FEVER IN IMMUNOCOMPROMISED PATIENTS

David B. Haslam

Care of the child with immunodeficiency presents the pediatrician with considerable challenges. Depending on the nature of the immune deficit, such children are at risk of fulminant, even fatal infections in situations that would pose minimal risk to a child with intact immunity. In order to decrease the likelihood of infection in immunodeficient children, preventive strategies often include the use of prophylactic antimicrobials and supplemental vaccines. On the other hand, vaccines containing live or attenuated viruses are often withheld from children with immunodeficiency because the risks of the vaccine itself may outweigh the likely benefit. Finally, any immunocompromised child with fever or other signs of infection must be approached with more forethought and urgency than is usually required in a child with intact immunity.

Classically, immunodeficiency most commonly had a genetic basis. Inborn defects in humoral, cell-mediated, and innate immunity have all been well described. Other genetic conditions, such as sickle-cell hemoglobinopathy, result in defects in phagocytic function. However, in the present era, immunodeficiency is most commonly iatrogenic in origin. Chemotherapy for hematologic or solid organ malignancy accounts for the majority of children with immune dysfunction. Moreover, the management of severe connective tissue disease and organ transplantation requires attenuation of the immune system. As a consequence, the incidence of severe immunodeficiency has markedly increased over previous decades.

In this section, guidelines for preventive care and an approach to fever in the immunodeficient child are presented. These guidelines are necessarily general in that deficiency in various branches of the immune system predisposes children to different opportunistic infections. For example, the child with profound neutropenia is at increased risk of bacteremia with gram-negative organisms such as *E. coli* or *Pseudomonas aeruginosa*, whereas the child with immunoglobulin subclass deficiency is more susceptible to pneumonias attributable to encapsulated bacteria such as *Streptococcus pneumoniae* or *Haemophilus influenzae*. For specific vaccination concerns the reader is referred to recommendations of the Advisory Committee on Immunization Practices and regularly updated guidelines published by the Infectious Diseases Subcommittee of the American Academy of Pediatrics. The approach to fever in individual children with immunodeficiency is best done in an anticipatory fashion, in collaboration with a pediatric immunologist or infectious disease consultant.

11.6.1   Additional Vaccines Recommended for Children with Immunodeficiency

In addition to the vaccines given to all children, some children with immunodeficiency benefit from vaccinations against organisms that are not part of the routine childhood series. This group includes pneumococcal vaccine, influenza vaccine, and passive immunization with intravenous immune globulin (IVIG). In some circumstances, immune globulin with high titers against particular organisms is available (such as varicella zoster immune globulin). These additional vaccines are provided to children with immune dysfunction, as described below.

CHILDREN WITH CONGENITAL DEFECTS OF IMMUNE FUNCTION

Children with congenital immune defects, particularly those that involve immunoglobulin synthetic defects, often do not mount a protective humoral response after infection or vaccination. Therefore, such children should receive passive immunization with regularly scheduled infusions of intravenous γ-globulin (IVIG) in order to provide protection against commonly encountered pathogens (see Sec. 11.4). The addition of other vaccines is probably of little benefit in this setting, and as described later, live-virus vaccines (OPV, MMR, varicella) should be withheld from these children. Their siblings should receive inactivated polio vaccine but may receive measles, mumps, and rubella vaccines because the vaccine strains are not transmitted person to person.

CHILDREN RECEIVING IMMUNOSUPPRESSIVE THERAPY

Children undergoing therapy for malignancy or organ transplantation may benefit from administration of the influenza vaccine, ideally before the onset of immunosuppressive therapy, because response to the vaccine during courses of chemotherapy or immunosuppression may be blunted. If immunization before immunosuppression is not possible, the vaccine should be administered at least 3 to 4 weeks after chemotherapy is discontinued and the absolute neutrophil count is greater than $1000/mm^3$. In addition to influenza vaccine, such children should receive pneumococcal vaccine, ideally before the onset of immunosuppression. Thereafter, as discussed below, only inactivated vaccines should be administered. In some circumstances, such as profound immunosupresion or prolonged courses of chemotherapy, it may be advisable to immunize passively with IVIG.

Patients with Hodgkin disease are at particular risk of pneumococcal infections and therefore should receive the pneumococcal vaccine. Ideally, the vaccine should be given at least 10 to 14 days before the onset of therapy. If this is not possible, and the child is vaccinated during chemotherapy, a booster dose should be given 3 months after discontinuing chemotherapy. The Hib vaccine should be administered at the same time, if the child had not previously been vaccinated against *Haemophilus influenzae* type b. Children with acute lymphoblastic leukemia in remission who have not previously been vaccinated or developed natural infection should be provided the varicella vaccine, as the risks of VZV infection in this situation outweigh the potential risks of vaccination. With this one exception, varicella and other live-virus vaccines are withheld from children during the course of chemotherapy or immunosuppressive therapy.

CHILDREN UNDERGOING BONE MARROW TRANSPLANTATION

Many children will acquire protective immunity against vaccine-preventable diseases from the donor. However, there are several factors that affect antibody production in the recipient, including donor's immunity, type of transplant, receipt of immunosuppressives, and graft-versus-host disease. In some situations, immunity acquired at transplantation is transient, and antibody titers fade after transplantation. In an effort to boost posttransplant immunity, donors may be immunized before transplant, and the recipient is vaccinated in the first month after transplantation. In theory, this approach could be applied to all inactivated antigens.

CHILDREN INFECTED WITH HUMAN IMMUNODEFICIENCY VIRUS

HIV-infected children should receive the regularly scheduled immunizations, with the exceptions of oral polio vaccine (OPV) and varicella vaccine, as discussed later. MMR may be administered unless the child is severely immunocompromised. In addition to the regularly scheduled vaccines, HIV-infected children should receive influenza vaccine annually and either the conjugate pneumococcal

vaccine in infancy or the 23-valent pneumococcal vaccine at 2 years of age.

ASPLENIC CHILDREN

Children with functional or anatomic asplenia, whether from congenital asplenia, hemoglobinopathies, or surgical removal, are at greatly increased risk of fulminant infection with encapsulated organisms. As a consequence, these children should receive either the conjugate pneumococcal vaccine in infancy or the 23-valent pneumococcal vaccine at 2 years of age and be revaccinated after 3 to 5 years. Similarly, asplenic children should receive the quadrivalent meningococcal vaccine at 2 years of age.

11.6.2 Contraindications to Vaccination in Children with Immunodeficiency

CHILDREN WITH CONGENITAL DEFECTS OF IMMUNE FUNCTION

As a general rule, all children with congenital immunodeficiency, particularly those with qualitative or quantitative T-lymphocyte abnormalities, should not receive live bacterial or viral vaccines. Such vaccines include BCG, oral poliovirus vaccine (OPV), measles, mumps, and rubella (MMR), and varicella vaccine. Fatal poliomyelitis and measles have occurred in children with congenital immunodeficiency after vaccination. Therefore, when an inactivated viral vaccine is available, such as inactivated poliomyelitis vaccine (IPV), this should be used in the place of a live virus.

Household contacts of individuals with congenital immunodeficiency should not receive oral poliovirus vaccine (OPV), as the vaccine strain may be transmitted to the affected child. Conversely, MMR may safely be administered to household contacts, as the vaccine strains are not transmitted from person to person. Finally, varicella vaccine may be given to household contacts. Transmission of the vaccine strain occasionally does occur to close contacts, but disease tends to be mild. In the event that the family member of a child with immunodeficiency develops a rash following varicella vaccination, there is no need to administer VZIG to the deficient child, even if contact is known to have occurred.

CHILDREN RECEIVING IMMUNOSUPPRESSIVE THERAPY

In general, children receiving chemotherapy for malignancy should not receive live bacterial or viral vaccines. The exception is varicella vaccination, which may be given judiciously to susceptible children with acute lymphoblastic leukemia when in remission if the risks of infection with the natural virus outweigh the risks of vaccination. If immunosuppressive therapy is discontinued, most experts recommend waiting at least 3 months before administering live viral vaccines to susceptible individuals. Depending on the underlying disease, the intensity of chemotherapy, or presence of ongoing radiation therapy, it may be advisable to delay vaccination longer in some instances.

Children receiving systemic corticosteroids are also at risk of developing disease from live virus vaccines. As a general guideline, any child receiving at least the equivalent of 2 mg/kg prednisone per day, daily or on alternate days, for more than 14 days is at risk and should not receive live-virus or live-bacteria vaccines. Inhaled or topical corticosteroids are not felt to place the child at increased risk. These children may therefore be immunized during therapy.

Children who have received high-dose corticosteroids for less than 14 days may be immunized when the steroids are discontinued, preferably 2 weeks after the last dose. In those children on high-dose corticosteroids for greater than 2 weeks, a minimum of 1 month should elapse from the last dose of steroids until administration of a live-virus vaccine.

CHILDREN UNDERGOING BONE MARROW TRANSPLANTATION

Live-virus and live-bacteria vaccines should not be administered to children within the first 2 years following bone marrow transplantation. Thereafter, children who have undergone bone marrow transplantation may be vaccinated with MMR. A second dose is given at least 1 month after the first unless serologic response is demonstrated after the first dose. Oral poliovirus vaccine and varicella vaccine should not be given to bone marrow transplantation patients, nor should OPV be given to household contacts. As mentioned above, varicella vaccine may be given to household contacts, as the risk of serious disease in contacts of vaccinated persons is low.

CHILDREN INFECTED WITH HUMAN IMMUNODEFICIENCY VIRUS

Vaccination of children infected with HIV must take into consideration that the disease-free survival may be prolonged with newer antiretroviral agents, and the risk from vaccination, though not absent, is small. Moreover, HIV-infected children may develop severe complications of natural viral infection, particularly measles, in which case the mortality rate among HIV-infected patients may be as high as 40%. Therefore, it is recommended that HIV-infected children receive MMR at 12 months of age or sooner during a measles epidemic. The exception is advanced disease with severe immunocompromise, in which case MMR should not be given.

Other live-virus vaccines, such as OPV and varicella, should not be given to HIV-infected individuals. As with other immunocompromised patients, OPV should not be given to household contacts, whereas varicella vaccine may be administered to household contacts of HIV-infected children.

11.6.3 Management of Fever in the Immunocompromised Child

In this section, fever in the child with profound neutropenia will be used as a paradigm for the approach to suspected infection in any child with severe immunodeficiency. Recommendations that differ substantially for other immunodeficiency states are described at the end of the chapter. The reader is reminded that these guidelines represent a generalized approach. Individualization is expected to some degree and depends on the severity of the individual's immunologic compromise, findings on physical examination, prior history of infection and antibiotic use, and local patterns of antimicrobial resistance.

Neutropenia associated with fever is a common sequel of antineoplastic therapy. Consequently, numerous clinical trials comparing various aspects of the decision-making process have been performed, allowing the development of practice guidelines, published by the Infectious Diseases Society of America. Much of the following discussion is adapted from these guidelines.

A single temperature greater than 38.3°C, or temperature >38.0°C over 1 hour in duration, is considered a febrile state. In this situation, the risk of serious infection follows an inverse

relationship to neutrophil count. A neutrophil count less than 1000/mm³ increases risk of infection only slightly. In contrast, up to 20% of patients with a neutrophil count <100/mm³ will have bacteremia, and approximately 50% will be found to have an established or occult source of infection. In addition to the absolute neutrophil count, the rate of decrease and duration of neutropenia are important considerations; rapidly decreasing counts or prolonged neutropenia confers a higher risk.

The site of infection and the responsible pathogens differ somewhat among neutropenic patients, depending on the cause of neutropenia. For example, cancer chemotherapy is often associated with disruption of mucosal and alimentary surfaces, providing a portal of entry for the organisms colonizing these sites. Patients with hereditary neutropenia, like patients with defects in neutrophil function, tend to have recurrent skin, periodontal, and upper respiratory tract infections.

INVESTIGATION OF THE FEBRILE, NEUTROPENIC CHILD

Patients with quantitative or qualitative neutrophil defects may manifest few localized signs of infection because of an impaired ability to mount an inflammatory response. Therefore, a high index of suspicion for infection must be kept in mind when evaluating these patients. Detailed physical examination should focus on the sites most likely involved, which include the oropharynx (including periodontium), the lungs, perineum (particularly the perirectal region), skin, and vascular access sites.

Laboratory investigation should include a complete blood count and at least two sets of blood cultures. When an indwelling vascular catheter is in place, cultures should be obtained from each lumen as well as from a peripheral vein. In order to determine whether the catheter is the focus of infection, some centers perform quantitative cultures and compare the number of colony-forming units isolated from the catheter versus a peripheral culture. Automated blood culture systems currently in use will detect most commonly isolated fungi and anaerobic bacteria in addition to aerobic bacteria. Nevertheless, in the setting of profound neutropenia and compromised mucosal surfaces, it is advisable to culture blood specifically for anaerobic bacteria and fungi.

In specific instances, imaging studies such as chest radiograph, ultrasound, CT, or MRI of the abdomen, sinuses, or other sites may be indicated, particularly if the fever is prolonged and no apparent source is identified.

EMPIRIC ANTIMICROBIAL THERAPY

Regardless of findings on physical examination and initial laboratory investigations, all neutropenic patients with fever should receive empiric antibiotic therapy directed at the organisms most commonly identified in this setting (Table 11-4). Whereas gram-negative organisms formerly predominated, the last several years have seen a shift to gram-positive organisms, which now account for more than 70% of isolates in children undergoing chemotherapy. Coagulase-negative staphylococci, which are the single most commonly isolated species, follow a reletively indolent course. However, some gram-positive bacteria, such as S. aureus and the viridans streptococcus S. mitis, may be associated with rapidly progressing shock, noncardiogenic pulmonary edema, and multiorgan failure such as is more commonly associated with gram-negative sepsis. The goal of empiric antimicrobial therapy is to provide coverage for those organisms likely to be associated with rapid progression and sepsis. Some centers do not include coverage for less

TABLE 11-4

MICROORGANISMS ASSOCIATED WITH FEVER IN IMMUNOCOMPROMISED PATIENTS

CONDITION	COMMON ORGANISMS
Neutropenia (including cancer chemotherapy or bone marrow transplantation).	Gram-positive cocci: *Staphylococcus aureus,* coagulase-negative staphylococci, *Streptococcus pneumoniae, Streptococcus pyogenes,* viridans group streptococci, *Enterococcus faecalis,* and *E. faecium* Gram-negative bacilli: *Escherichia coli, Klebsiella* species, *Pseudomonas* species Viruses: Respiratory syncytial virus, parainfluenza, adenoviruses, herpes simplex virus, cytomegalovirus Fungi and protozoans: *Candida* species, *Aspergillus* species *Pneumocystis carinii*
Solid organ transplantation	Bacteria: Varies with site of organ transplanted—includes gram-negative, gram-positive, and occasionally anaerobic organisms Viruses: Cytomegalovirus, Epstein-Barr virus, hepatitis B and C viruses, adenoviruses Fungi and protozoans: *Aspergillus* species, *Candida* species *Pneumocystis carinii*
Splenectomy	Bacteria: Predominantly encapsulated organisms; *Streptococcus pneumoniae, Neiserria meningiditis, Haemophilus influenzae*
Human immunodeficiency virus infection	Bacteria: *Streptococcus pneumoniae* and other encapsulated organisms, *Salmonella* species, enteric organisms, *Mycobacterium tuberculosis, Mycobacterium avium* complex Viruses: Herpes simplex, cytomegalovirus, varicella-zoster, Epstein-Barr, respiratory viruses (including measles) Fungi and protozoans: *Candida* species, *Aspergillus* species *Pneumocystis carinii*

SOURCE: Adapted from Pizzo PA: Fever in immunocompromised patients. N Engl J Med 341:893–900, 1999.

virulent organisms, such as coagulase-negative staphylococci and *Corynebacterium jeikeiu,* in initial regimens but adjust antimicrobials after the identity and sensitivity of the pathogen have been determined.

Numerous clinical trials comparing initial antimicrobial therapy have been performed in adults and children with fever and neutropenia. Many single agents or antibiotic combinations have been found to be efficacious with minimal toxicity in most settings. As a general rule the regimen should provide broad coverage for gram-negative organisms, including *Pseudomonas,* and at least some coverage for *S. aureus.* Single-agent regimens meeting these criteria include ceftazidime or imipenem, either of which may be considered standard of therapy. Although initial therapy with two agents is often used, there are no marked differences in outcome between monotherapy and duotherapy. The advantages of dual antibiotic treatment include synergistic activity against many gram-negative organisms and decreased development of antibiotic resistance. In some instances vancomycin is added to provide coverage for organisms such as methicillin-resistant *S. aureus,* coagulase-negative staphylococci, viridans streptococci, and β-lactam-resistant *Streptococcus pneumoniae.* Thus, the initial regimen may consist of either monotherapy or duotherapy; indications for addition of vancomycin should be considered. A schema incorporating these options is presented in Fig. 11-6.

The decision as to whether vancomycin should be included in the initial regimen deserves particular attention. On the one hand, an increase in the number of infections caused by gram-positive organisms that are resistant or tolerant to β-lactams, such as coagulase-negative staphylococci and viridans streptococci, suggests that vancomycin should be part of the initial regimen. This is particularly of concern because viridans streptococcal infections can occasionally be fulminant and lead to death within 24 hours in these patients. On the other hand, large comparative trials have found that addition of vancomycin to the initial regimen does not decrease the overall mortality attributable to gram-positive organisms. Additionally, there is concern that excessive use of vancomycin has led to an increase in vancomycin resistance among some highly resistant organisms, particularly enterococci. As a consequence, it is recommended that vancomycin use be restricted to situations in which there is a high likelihood that its use is warranted. Based on these observations, the Infectious Disease Society of America's recommendation is that vancomycin be added to the initial regimen if the patient has severe mucositis (which would predispose to viridans streptococcal bacteremia), known colonization with methicillin-resistant *S. aureus* or β-lactam-resistant *S. pneumoniae,* an obvious catheter-related infection (likely implicating coagulase-negative staphylococci), or hypotension or other signs of sepsis (see Fig. 11-6). Other instances in which vancomycin might be added to the empiric initial regimen include a high incidence of methicillin resistance among hospital *S. aureus* isolates and institutions in which there is a high incidence of fulminant infection with gram-positive organisms.

When vancomycin is included in the initial regimen, ceftazidime is suggested as an appropriate second antibiotic. The combination

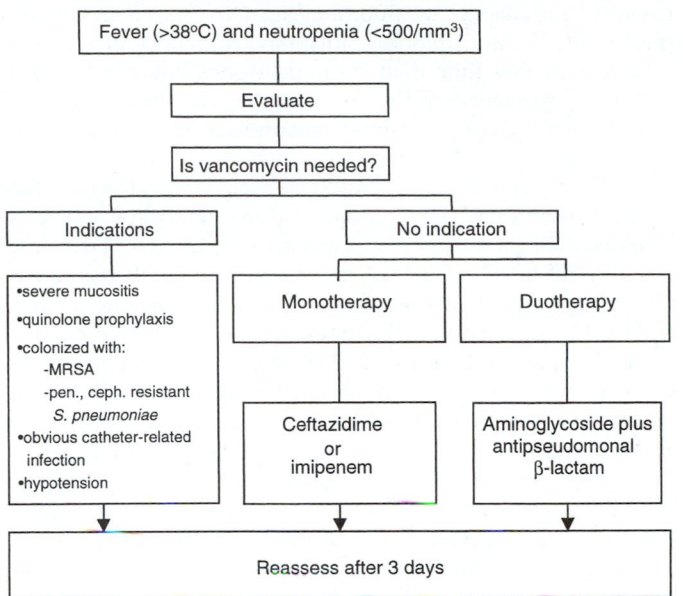

FIGURE 11-6   Guide to the initial management of the febrile neutropenic patient. See text for discussion regarding choice of antibiotics in monotherapy and duotherapy. Abbreviations: MRSA = methacillin-resistant *S. aureus*; pen. = penicillin; ceph. = cephalosporin. SOURCE: *Hughes WT, Armstrong D, Bodey GP, et al: 1997 guidelines for the use of antimicrobial agents in neutropenic patients with unexplained fever. Infectious Diseases Society of America. Clin Infect Dis 25: 551–573, 1997.*

of vancomycin plus ceftazidime has been extensively studied in neutropenic patients and has been found to be safe and efficacious. Vancomycin should be discontinued after 48 hours if the clinical course is stable and organisms requiring the use of this agent are not isolated.

ADJUSTMENT OF ANTIMICROBIAL THERAPY

The mean time to defervesence in febrile neutropenic patients is 5 days after broad-spectrum antibiotics are initiated, with a range of 2 to 7 days. Within that time, a reassessment of antimicrobial therapy should be undertaken. Isolation of a suspected pathogen from initial cultures may result in adjustment of antibiotics to provide optimal activity against the offending organisms. Nevertheless, the regimen should continue to provide broad coverage, as polymicrobial and secondary sites of infection occur. If the vascular catheter is identified as the source of infection, in most cases the infection can be treated with the catheter in place. Indications for immediate catheter removal include the presence of septic emboli, hypotension associated with catheter use, or evidence of a subcutaneous catheter tunnel infection. Relative indications for catheter removal include infection with *Bacillus, Corynebacterium, Pseudomonas, Serratia, Stentotrophomonas,* and *Acinetobacter.* Most experts urge immediate removal of the catheter if *Candida* sp. are isolated. Persistently positive blood cultures after 48 hours of appropriate antibiotic therapy may indicate an infected intravascular focus; removal of the catheter should be considered, and echocardiogram of the heart and large vessels may indicate septic foci.

At approximately the third day of therapy, regardless of whether an organism has been isolated, the condition of the patient determines further therapy, as described below.

DEFERVESCENCE WITHIN 3 DAYS   If the child demonstrates a favorable response to therapy within 3 days of admission, a change in therapy from intravenous to an oral antibiotic such as cefixime might be appropriate, assuming the following conditions are met: absence of signs of sepsis (other than fever) on admission, no evident source of infection, clinical improvement, negative cultures at >48 hours, and ANC > 100 mm³. Alternatively, such patients may be discharged from the hospital to continue parenteral antibiotics at home. Either approach assumes that the social situation is reliable and that close follow-up has been arranged. As mentioned above, if the patient is stable or improved, and no gram-positive organisms have been isolated, vancomycin should be discontinued if it was begun initially. In patients who remain afebrile after the third day, antibiotics may be discontinued after 7 days, particularly if the ANC is greater than 500/mm³ or the bone marrow is recovering. Patients in whom the ANC remains <100/mm³ on the third day, or those with ongoing mucositis or other factors that might predispose to recurrent infection, should continue parenteral antibiotics as an inpatient, even if they become afebrile (Fig. 11-7).

More recently, some centers have adopted guidelines that allow outpatient management of selected low-risk children with fever and neutropenia after a single dose of parenteral antibiotics and careful evaluation. After careful examination and obtaining a complete blood count and blood cultures, the child is given a parenteral antibiotic such as ceftazidime and then discharged on an oral antibiotic such as ciprofloxacin. Most centers do not consider initial outpatient management if the patient has hemodynamic instability or severe mucositis or is undergoing induction chemotherapy or bone marrow transplantation. As mentioned above, it is assumed that close follow-up and a reliable home situation exist.

Recently, initial management with oral antibiotics alone was found to be efficacious in low-risk patients with fever and neutropenia. These patients received amoxicillin-clavulanate plus ciprofloxacin and were observed in hospital. The use of oral antibiotics as the initial empiric therapy remains investigational but may prove to be a valid approach to the management of low-risk children with fever and neutropenia.

FEVER PERSISTS MORE THAN 3 DAYS   In neutropenic patients with continued fever after 3 days of therapy, consideration should be given to the following possibilities: (1) a nonbacterial infection,

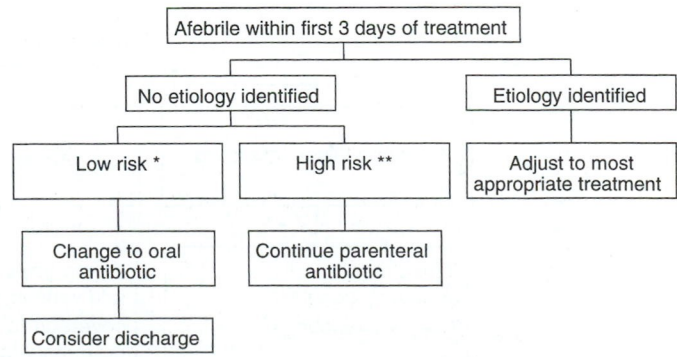

FIGURE 11-7   Management of patients who become afebrile in first 3 days of initial antibiotic therapy. * = clinically well; ** = absolute neutrophil count < 100/mm³, severe mucositis, or unstable vital signs. SOURCE: *Hughes WT, Armstrong D, Bodey GP, et al: 1997 guidelines for the use of antimicrobial agents in neutropenic patients with unexplained fever. Infectious Diseases Society of America. Clin Infect Dis 25:551–573, 1997.*

(2) presence of a organism resistant to the antibiotics in use, (3) organisms that are inaccessible to antibiotics (such as an abscess or catheter-associated infection), (4) inadequate serum levels of antimicrobials, or (5) a noninfectious source of fever (particularly drug fever). Each of these possibilities should be assessed. In particular, persistently febrile children should be examined thoroughly for the presence of a new or previously unidentified focus of infection. Blood cultures should be repeated from vascular access catheters and a peripheral site. Serum levels of aminoglycosides and vancomycin should be obtained if the patient is receiving either of these antibiotics. Consideration may be given to imaging studies of the abdomen, chest, or sinuses. Occasionally, viral cultures of blood, urine, and saliva may be useful, as might serologic testing or polymerase chain reaction to detect cytomegalovirus, Epstein-Barr virus, herpes simplex virus, or enteroviruses. In some situations testing for *Chlamydia, Toxoplasma,* or mycobacteria may be indicated. Gastrointestinal symptoms may be an indication of pseudomembraneous colitis secondary to *C. difficile.*

Depending on the condition of the patient, three options are available (Fig. 11-8). (1) Continue antibiotics without change and continue close observation. This is most appropriate if the neutropenia is expected to resolve in the near future. (2) Change or add antibiotics, particularly to broaden gram-negative coverage, and add vancomycin if a gram-positive organism is isolated that would be expected to be resistant or tolerant to β-lactams, or if the patient is demonstrating progressive or deteriorating disease. (3) Add antifungal therapy. Although fewer than one-third of patients who remain febrile after 7 days of antibiotic therapy will be found to have a fungal infection, most experts would agree that amphotericin B should be added to the regimen in such a setting.

DURATION OF ANTIMICROBIAL THERAPY

The duration of antimicrobial therapy in febrile neutropenic patients depends on neutrophil count, resolution of fever, and the presence or absence of a focus of infection. Of these, neutrophil count is most useful in deciding when to discontinue antibiotics. As mentioned previously, a patient who is afebrile and has a neu-

trophil count greater than 500/mm³ may have antibiotics discontinued after 7 days. In some situations, antibiotics may be discontinued at that time even if the neutrophil count is less than 500/mm³, particularly if the bone marrow demonstrates signs of recovery and there is no ongoing mucositis or other portal for microbial entry.

Persistent fever in patients with neutropenia is a particular challenge. As mentioned above, addition of amphotericin B should be considered for the patient who remains febrile and has a neutrophil count <500/mm³ on the seventh day of therapy. If the patient remains neutropenic and febrile after the addition of amphotericin B, broad-spectrum antibiotics and amphotericin B are continued for a minimum of 2 weeks. At that time, imaging studies of the chest, abdomen, and other sites should be considered if they have not already been performed. If these are negative, and the patient appears clinically stable, consideration may be given to discontinuing antibiotics and antifungals at that time despite the persistence of fever. Similarly, it may be reasonable to discontinue antibiotics 4 to 5 days after the ANC reaches >500/mm³, even in the presence of ongoing fever. Discontinuing antibiotics in any patient with ongoing fever, particularly those who remain neutropenic, requires that the patient be observed closely as an inpatient and undergo repeated evaluations in order to identify a focus.

OTHER TREATMENT MODALITIES

Antiviral agents are not routinely recommended for neutropenic patients unless physical examination suggests infection with herpes simplex virus, varicella zoster virus, or a respiratory virus such as influenza A. Patients with isolated neutropenia are not particularly prone to systemic CMV or HSV infections unless the neutropenia is related to bone marrow transplantation.

Granulocyte transfusions are rarely indicated in the febrile neutropenic patient because the risks generally outweigh likely benefits. Hematopoietic colony-stimulating factors such as G-CSF and GM-CSF have been demonstrated to shorten the duration of febrile episodes associated with neutropenia following chemotherapy. Nonetheless, administration of these agents is generally not recommended as adjunctive therapy for patients with fever and neu-

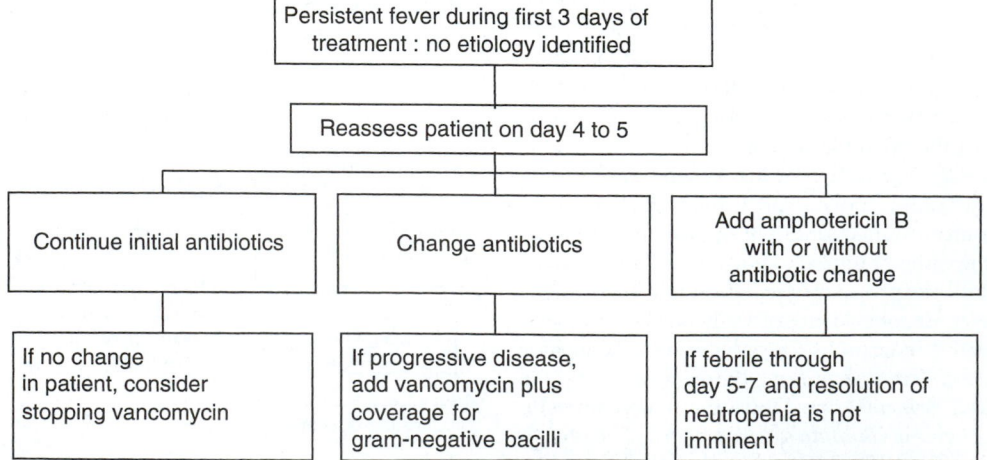

FIGURE 11-8   **Management of patients who have persistent fever after 3 days of treatment and for whom the etiology of the fever is unknown. See text for discussion of adjustment in antibiotics or the addition of amphotericin B. SOURCE:** *Hughes WT, Armstrong D, Bodey GP, et al: 1997 guidelines for the use of antimicrobial agents in neutropenic patients with unexplained fever. Infectious Diseases Society of America. Clin Infect Dis 25:551–573, 1997.*

tropenia. However, some clinicians administer colony-stimulating factors to febrile patients in whom the duration of neutropenia is known to be prolonged.

References

Anaissie EJ, Vartivarian S, Bodey GP, et al: Randomized comparison between antibiotics alone and antibiotics plus granulocyte-macrophage colony-stimulating factor (*Escherichia coli*-derived) in cancer patients with fever and neutropenia. Am J Med 100:17–23, 1996

Freifeld A, Marchigiani D, Walsh T, et al: A double-blind comparison of empirical oral and intravenous antibiotic therapy for low-risk febrile patients with neutropenia during cancer chemotherapy. N Engl J Med 341:305–311, 1999

Hughes WT, Armstrong D, Bodey GP, et al: 1997 guidelines for the use of antimicrobial agents in neutropenic patients with unexplained fever. Infectious Diseases Society of America. Clin Infect Dis 25:551–573, 1997

Mullen CA, Petropoulos D, Roberts WM, et al: Outpatient treatment of fever and neutropenia for low risk pediatric cancer patients. Cancer 86:126–134, 1999

Pizzo PA: Fever in immunocompromised patients. N Engl J Med 341:893–900, 1999

11.7   ALLERGIC DISEASES AND ATOPY

Talal A. Chatila

11.7.1   Introduction

Allergic diseases are a group of ailments that share common pathogenic mechanisms including IgE-mediated immediate hypersensitivity reactions to environmental allergens and a more fundamental pathogenic activation of TH2-type immune responses. Included among these diseases are upper and lower allergic airway diseases (rhinitis, rhinosinusitis, asthma), ocular allergic diseases, eczema, and food and drug allergies. They frequently cluster together in the same family and are transmitted vertically from generation to generation, consistent with a strong genetic component in disease pathogenesis.

An explosive increase in prevalence in this century, especially in Western societies, leads to the current estimate that up to 50% of the population of Western societies shows reactivity on skin testing to one or more environmental allergens. In some subpopulations up to one in four children suffer from asthma. This allergic disease epidemic has been linked to many factors including social affluence, changes in life style, urban residence, infant diet, and overuse of antibiotics. Suspicion has recently focused on the decline in infectious diseases as a common denominator among many risk factors. It is thought that childhood infections promote T-helper (TH)-cell differentiation toward TH1-type and away from the atopy-promoting TH2 lineage. Consistent with this hypothesis is an observed decrease in incidence of atopic diseases among children vaccinated with the mycobacterium *bacillus Calmette-Guérin* (BCG).

Allergic diseases are immunologic diseases in that their genesis and manifestations result from the functioning of components of the immune system. Disease pathogenesis is mediated by both in-

nate immune responses, involving mast cells, basophils, eosinophils, and dendritic and Langerhans cells as well as acquired immune responses involving T and B lymphocytes. Orchestrating the allergic response is the TH2 CD4$^+$ T-helper-cell lineage, which is now appreciated to play a central role in the pathogenesis of allergic diseases. TH2 cells recruit other components of the innate and acquired immune response by virtue of their production of a set of proatopic cytokines, including IL-4, IL-5, IL-10, and IL-13. They promote the production of IgE, a key trigger of immediate hypersensitivity reactions, and help sustain chronic allergic inflammation in such diseases as asthma and eczema.

The increased knowledge of allergic diseases and their pathogenesis has stimulated the development of new therapeutic approaches, including desensitization therapy with defined allergen preparations or pharmacologic interventions aimed at depleting IgE or targeting the action of mediators such as leukotrienes.

11.7.2   Immunologic Basis of Atopy

Allergic disorders develop out of a close interaction between genetic predisposition and environmental triggers. A unifying attribute of these disorders is atopy, defined as the predisposition to generate IgE antibodies on exposure to environmental antigens. Subsequent exposure to the offending antigen, or allergen, triggers an immediate-type hypersensitivity reaction. This is an IgE-mediated tissue response that is characterized by increased vascular permeability, vasodilatation, smooth muscle contraction, and local inflammation. The atopic (or allergic) trait is an intrinsic property of the host immune system. It involves pathways of acquired immune response, including specialized T helper cells and IgE-producing B cells, as well as components of the innate immune response including mast cells, eosinophils, basophils, and neutrophils. Lesions that interfere with critical components of the host immune response in atopy may attenuate or fully abrogate the atopic phenotype. For example, patients with agammaglobulinemia cannot mount IgE-dependent immediate hypersensitivity reactions.

In contrast, many adverse reactions to foods or drugs are not allergic in nature in that they proceed independently of the immune system, eg, milk intolerance from lactase deficiency, or involve nonatopic mechanisms of immune injury, such as delayed-type hypersensitivity reaction to poison ivy.

TH2 CELLS

IgE production is one feature of a more fundamental specific immune response orchestrated by the TH2 subset of CD4$^+$ TH cells. TH2 cells are critical for promoting acute hypersensitivity responses and maintaining the state of chronic and relapsing eosinophil-predominant inflammation characteristic of chronic allergic inflammation.

TH2 cells represent a separate lineage of T helper cells that arises from an uncommitted, pluripotent TH0 state. TH0 cells may differentiate toward either the TH1 or TH2 lineage, which are distinguished by their profile of cytokine production. TH2 cells produce a distinct set of cytokines necessary for the allergic response, including IL-4 and IL-13, which promote IgE production; IL-5 and GM-CSF, which promote eosinophil production in the bone marrow; and IL-10, which promotes B-cell differentiation into plasma cells. In contrast, TH2 cells do not produce IL-2 and interferon-γ. These cytokines are characteristic of TH1 cells, which reciprocally do not produce TH2-type cytokines.

ROLE OF ALLERGEN AND THE CELLULAR MILIEU

Induction of an immune response requires uptake and processing by antigen-presenting cells (APCs), which then present peptide fragments to specific T cells. The type of APC, the expression on APC of molecules that can augment T-cell stimulation, and the secretion of cytokines can all sway the TH phenotype of the resultant T-cell response.

Among the most efficient APCs are dendritic cells. After exposure to antigen, these cells residing in the mucosa migrate to regional lymphoid tissues. This anatomic translocation is accompanied by increased surface expression of MHC class II antigens and costimulatory molecules, along with the acquisition of potent antigen-presenting capabilities. There is evidence to suggest that dendritic cells are heterogeneous, with a myeloid-like dendritic cell subset more prone to stimulate TH2 differentiation. Consistent with these observations, the quantity and phenotype of dendritic cells appear altered in atopic individuals in a way that promotes TH2 responses.

Neighboring cells can influence the outcome of TH-cell differentiation. In particular, mast cells and NK1.1 cells can polarize the local cytokine milieu in ways that favor TH2 responses by virtue of their production of IL-4. Preexisting allergen-specific IgE may favor the induction of TH2 responses, both by activating mast cells to produce IL-4 and IL-13 and by facilitating B-cell antigen presentation.

ALLERGENS

The host is typically exposed to very low levels of allergens, small to medium-sized proteins that are highly soluble and are carried on desiccated particles such as pollen. On contact with the mucosa they are eluted from their carrier particles and diffuse into the mucosa. Too large a protein may not easily pass through mucosal surfaces, and proteins that are too small may not be able to crosslink IgE on mast cells.

Allegens are frequently enzymatically active. In particular, proteases feature prominently among allergens. Der p I, the major allergen of the house dust mite *Dermatophagoides pteronyssinus*, is a cysteine protease. Papain, a protease derived from the papaya fruit that is used in both industrial and medicinal applications, is a homolog of Der p I and a well-known allergen in its own right. Another industrial allergen is subtilisin, a protease that was frequently used in some laundry detergents. The reason many allergens are enzymatically active is not clear, but it is possible that the enzymatic activity may potentiate antigen uptake and/or presentation or skew the immune response toward the TH2 lineage.

REGULATION OF IgE PRODUCTION

A critical component of the atopic phenotype is IgE. The production of this antibody ensues from the interaction of antigen-presenting B cells with antigen-specific T helper cells. At the molecular level, IgE production requires active reorganization of the B-cell genome at the immunoglobulin heavy chain locus on chromosome 14. In the case of IgE, two distinct signals delivered on the interaction of naive, antigen-presenting B cells with antigen-specific TH cells are required to shift immunoglobulin production from IgM to IgE. The first signal can be provided by the cytokines IL-4 or IL-13, which are the only cytokines that can support IgE production by cultured B cells. These cytokines stimulate transcription at the Cϵ gene locus, which contains the exons encoding the constant-region domains of the IgE heavy chain.

A second signal is delivered by the interaction of a B-cell protein termed CD40 with its protein ligand, termed CD40L, that is expressed on the surface of TH cells following engagement of the T-cell receptor by peptide-MHC complexes. CD40-CD40L interaction activates the genetic rearrangement that creates a functional ϵ heavy chain and is also required for isotype switching into IgG and IgA. Patients with the X-linked hyper-IgM syndrome (XHIM) are deficient in CD40L; as a result, their B cells are unable to undergo isotype switching to produce IgE. Similarly, mice with targeted disruption of the CD40L or CD40 genes lack serum IgE.

TH2 cells provide both signals necessary for IgE production. TH2-derived IL-4 and IL-13 drive germ-line transcription at the C exons. CD4$^+$ TH2 cells also provide the second signal necessary for IgE production, CD40L, thereby promoting isotype switching to IgE. CD4$^+$ TH2 cells are present in respiratory mucosa and regional lymphoid tissues of atopic individuals, where they promote IgE production by interacting with naive B cells presenting allergen-derived peptide antigens. TH2 cells are critical to the maintenance of the allergic inflammation typical of atopic diseases such as asthma, and they can mediate the passive transfer of allergic airway responses.

IgE RECEPTORS

IgE mediates two distinct functions in the host: initiation of the immediate hypersensitivity reaction and promotion of antigen presentation leading to augmented immune responses. These functions are mediated by dedicated receptors expressed on immune cells. The first is the high-affinity IgE receptor, or FcϵRI, a multimeric receptor expressed on a variety of cells including mast cells, basophils, dendritic and Langerhans cells, and activated eosinophils and monocytes. FcϵRI binds IgE with high affinity (10^{-10} M), which exceeds by two to four logs the binding affinities of other immunoglobulin Fc receptors, and with 1:1 stoichiometry. An important consequence of the high-affinity binding of FcϵRI to IgE is that in atopic individuals with high IgE levels, virtually all FcϵRI molecules are constitutively bound by IgE.

Crosslinking by multivalent allergenic proteins of IgE bound to FcϵRI on mast cells, basophils, and activated eosinophils initiates a signal transduction cascade that results in the exocytosis of stored granules and the release of their content. It also results in the de novo synthesis by these cells of cytokines and inflammatory mediators. Because of the very high affinity of allergen-IgE and IgE-FcϵRI interactions, FcϵRI isoforms expressed on antigen-presenting cells, including dendritic, Langerhans, and activated monocytic cells, allow efficient antigen presentations at very low levels of antigen. The antigen-presenting function of FcϵRI is important for potentiation and long-term maintenance of IgE-driven allergic and inflammatory responses. This role may be especially important in chronic allergic inflammatory diseases such as eczema and asthma.

A second IgE receptor, FcϵRII or CD23, is expressed on B cells and antigen-presenting cells. Its affinity for IgE (10^{-8} M), although lower than that of FcϵRI, nevertheless remains substantially high. A major function of FcϵRII is to augment cellular and humoral immune responses in settings of recurrent allergen encounters.

IMMEDIATE AND LATE-PHASE HYPERSENSITIVITY REACTIONS

Crosslinking of IgE bound to FcϵRI on tissue mast cells or on circulating basophils triggers the release of granules containing preformed mediators including histamine, TNF-α, proteoglycans, and neutral proteases including tryptase, chymase, and carboxypeptidase. It also results in the rapid de novo synthesis of lipid-derived mediators including prostaglandin D_2, the chief prostaglandin product of mast cells, as well as platelet-activating factor and leukotrienes B_4, C_4, D_4, and E_4. The release of these mediators induces an immediate hypersensitivity reaction, which in an atopic individual can be visualized by the "wheal and flare" skin reaction on scratching of the skin with an allergenic substance. It is characterized by vasodilatation, edema, and smooth muscle contraction. A similar reaction pattern is seen in other tissues such as bronchial airways, where mediator release on allergen inhalation rapidly induces mucosal edema, mucus production, smooth muscle constriction, and reduced airflow. The immediate hypersensitivity reaction is reversible, and usually subsides within 2 hours of its initiation.

IgE-induced immediate hypersensitivity reaction is often followed by a late-phase reaction, a second wave of hypersensitivity responses occurring several hours after the acute reaction. The late-phase reaction may manifest as a second wave of decreased airflow in asthmatics or recurrence of sneezing and rhinorrhea in patients with allergic rhinitis 4 to 8 hours after the initial allergen contact. A similar recurrence of clinical symptoms occurs in other allergic diseases as well.

The late-phase reaction arises from the recruitment to the allergen challenge site of an inflammatory cellular infiltrate that includes neutrophils, T lymphocytes, and eosinophils. Eosinophil recruitment plays a central role.

IgE-DEPENDENT AND -INDEPENDENT ALLERGIC INFLAMMATION

Despite the pivotal functions of IgE in immediate hypersensitivity reactions, there are situations where mast cell degranulation may proceed by IgE-independent mechanisms. For example, the syndrome of active anaphylaxis, with mast cell degranulation and mediator release, can be induced in humans by repeated infusion of IgA-containing blood-derived product (blood, plasma, or immunoglobulin preparations) in individuals who are IgA deficient. Such infusions result in the development by these individuals of IgG (rarely IgE) anti-IgA antibodies. On rechallenge with the offending product, IgG/anti-IgA immune complexes are formed that precipitate mast cell degranulation and anaphylaxis by interaction with low-affinity Fc receptors for IgG on mast cells.

An important example of chronic allergic inflammation proceeding by IgE-independent mechanisms involves patients with so called intrinsic asthma. In contrast to the overwhelming majority of children and many adults with asthma in whom evidence of pathogenic immediate hypersensitivity can be demonstrated by skin testing, individuals with intrinsic asthma lack evidence of IgE-mediated reactions. However, airways of patients with intrinsic asthma exhibit an inflammatory infiltrate and a TH2 cytokine expression pattern that is very similar to that found in patients with allergic asthma. These findings confirm a principal function of IgE in promoting chronic allergic inflammation by triggering acute and late-phase reactions in response to minute amounts of environmental allergen. In effect, IgE dramatically lowers the threshold for chronic allergic inflammation to develop in response to perennial allergen exposure.

TARGETING THE IMMUNOLOGIC PATHWAYS OF ATOPY

The allergic response can be attenuated or even abrogated by measures aimed at modifying its underlying immune mechanisms. Foremost is scrupulous allergen avoidance, which can result not only in symptomatic relief but, if persistent long term, may result in hyposensitization. This has been most successfully demonstrated for dust mite allergy. Furthermore, early life avoidance of a dust mite–rich environment may forestall the development of respiratory allergic diseases such as asthma. Immunotherapy with allergenic extracts is also effective in hyposensitizing the allergic response.

Several therapies target specific components of the allergic response. Antihistamines target the vasoactive effects of the mast cell. They are useful in immediate hypersensitivity reactions but ineffective for the late-phase reaction or chronic allergic inflammation, which is better managed by steroids. The recent development of leukotriene receptor antagonists has provided a valuable steroid-sparing tool to combat the effect of persistent leukotriene production by eosinophils and other inflammatory cells in chronic allergic inflammation.

Novel therapies are being introduced aimed at interrupting key pathways in atopic response. Interruption of signals delivered by IL-4 and IL-13 by using soluble IL-4 receptors is also showing promise in allergic diseases such as asthma. Anti-IgE monoclonal antibodies that block binding of IgE to FcεRI without inducing immediate hypersensitivity reaction or anaphylaxis reduce IgE levels in humans by binding to IgE and removing it via immune complex formation. These antibodies attenuate both the early and late-phase responses to inhaled allergen and reduce the associated increase in eosinophils in sputum.

11.7.3 Genetic Basis of Atopy

Allergic disorders develop out of a close interaction between genetic predisposition and environmental triggers. Environmental factors such as exposure to inciting allergens play an important role in the development and sustenance of allergic diseases. However, the development of allergic disorders is also governed by strong genetic influences. The common wisdom that allergies run in families has been vindicated by numerous studies that have shown a stepwise increase in the risk for development of allergic disorders in relation to history of parental disease. Lack of parental history of allergic disorders is associated with a low disease incidence in offspring (around 10%), climbing up to 40% and 70% when one or both parents are affected. Furthermore, family history of one allergic disorder such as atopic dermatitis heightens the risk for other allergic disorders such as allergic rhinitis or asthma, giving rise to the idea of a genetically determined atopic trait that ties together diverse allergic disorders.

Both autosomal recessive and autosomal codominant inheritance with variable penetrance have been invoked in explaining the genetic transmission of allergic disorders. This is not surprising given the genetic complexity of these diseases and the multiplicity of susceptibility genes. Additionally, there appears to be a higher risk of inheritance of some allergic disorders in the context of a positive maternal history as compared to paternal history, suggesting either an imprinting effect or an immunologic interaction between mother and fetus during pregnancy.

ATOPY

Several aspects integral to the genesis of allergic inflammation have been found to be genetically determined, including the capacity to generate IgE responses (or atopy), reactivity toward specific allergens, and several disease-specific manifestations. A fundamental pathogenic mechanism common to all allergic disorders is IgE-mediated inflammation. Sufferers of allergic disorders are genetically predisposed to generate IgE antibodies to environmental allergens and to respond with immediate hypersensitivity reactions on subsequent exposure. This attribute, known as atopy, affects up to 40% of populations of Western societies, and it underlies the development of allergic diseases in susceptible individuals. It should be emphasized that atopy itself is not a malady. Rather, it is best viewed as a heritable trait that under special circumstances, such as repeated exposure to allergens and the confluence of other genetic risk factors, may give rise to allergic diseases.

ATOPY SUSCEPTIBILITY GENES

The hereditary nature of atopy together with its central role in fostering allergic disorders has led to an intensive search for predisposing genes, commonly referred to as atopy susceptibility genes. Studies employing genome-wide scans and candidate gene approaches have led to the identification of a number of candidate loci and susceptibility genes. Not surprisingly, many of these have turned out to be intimately involved in the regulation of IgE production or in mediating IgE effector functions.

A key pathway that regulates IgE production involves the cytokines IL-4 and IL-13 and a common subunit of their respective receptor complexes, the IL-4 receptor α subunit (IL-4R). All three components of this pathway have been linked to both atopy and specific allergic diseases, including asthma and atopic dermatitis. In addition, several human chromosomal regions have been associated with increased risk of atopy (Table 11-5).

OTHER SUSCEPTIBILITY GENES

Atopy susceptibility genes predispose to a general state of enhanced IgE production and responsiveness regardless of the inciting antigen. The capacity of direct IgE responses toward a specific allergen is determined by the antigen-recognizing structures of the immune system: antigen-presenting HLA class II molecules and antigen/HLA-reactive T-cell receptor (TCR) molecules. Allelic forms of both HLA class II and TCR genes are associated with reactivity to specific antigens. Among HLA class II molecules, DRB1.1501 predisposes to *Ambrosia* pollen allergens. Specific IgE responses to dust mite allergens were linked to the TCRα/δ region on chromosome 14.

Other genes have been found to promote disease-specific aspects of an allergic disorder without necessarily predisposing to atopy. These genes may promote tissue localization of a particular allergic disorder, may promote tissue inflammation, or may modulate a disease-specific manifestation such as bronchial hyperactivity. Up to 5% of patients with cystic fibrosis are susceptible to developing allergic bronchopulmonary aspergillosis, an otherwise rare disease characterized by intense allergic inflammatory reaction to airway-colonizing *Aspergillus* species. Interestingly, study of individuals who suffer from ABPA but not cystic fibrosis identified more than half of these to be hetrozygous carriers of CFTR mutations. These results indicate that mutants of the CFTR gene act to promote the development of ABPA in the context of an atopic background.

Tumor necrosis factor (TNF) and the β-adrenergic receptor provide other examples of gene-modulating aspects of allergic diseases. Alleles of TNF and the closely related lymphotoxin genes have been found at higher frequency in asthmatics than in non-asthmatics. These alleles do not seem to promote atopy but may result in enhanced production of these proinflammatory cytokines, thus contributing to the allergic inflammation. In the case of the β_2-adrenergic receptor gene, several polymorphisms in its coding region appear to modulate the manifestations of asthmatic symptoms. For example, an arginine-to-glycine polymorphism at position 16 in the extracellular domain of the β_2-adrenergic receptor is associated with nocturnal asthma, and another allele, glutamic acid 27, is associated with protection against bronchial hyperactivity.

ROLE OF THE ENVIRONMENT

The established role of genetic predisposition in allergic diseases does not deny a critical contribution of environmental influences in the evolution of these disease. Allergen exposure is one cardinal and obvious environmental contribution. However, additional environmental influences have to be invoked if one is to explain a perplexing feature of allergic diseases, namely, their rise in stature from a relatively restricted set of diseases in earlier eras into true modern epidemics. Although air pollution had earlier been a primary suspect in this spread of allergic airway diseases such as asthma, attention has now focused on the role of infectious diseases in modulating the atopic potential of the immune system. Improved hygiene in Western societies may promote the differentiation of the CD4 T lymphocytes into T helper 2 (TH2) cells, which secrete atopic disease-promoting cytokines such as those that promote IgE synthesis and mucus secretion (IL-4 and IL-13), eosinophil production (IL-5), and mast cell and basophil development (IL-3). In contrast, exposure to childhood infections may promote T-helper-cell differentiation into TH1 cells, which express a different array of cytokines including IL-2 and interferon-γ. The hygiene hypothesis, as it is known, provides a satisfactory explanation for the marked increased in the prevalence of allergic diseases in more affluent social classes, in richer countries, and in urban as compared to rural environments.

TABLE 11-5

GENETIC LOCI IMPLICATED IN HUMAN ALLERGIC DISORDERS.

LOCUS	CANDIDATE GENE(S)
5q23-q31	IL-4, IL-13, other cytokines
6p21	HLA class II, TNF, lymphotoxin
11q13	FcεRIβ chain
12q14	Interferon-gamma
13q21.3	Unknown
14q11.2	TCRα chains
16p12	IL-4Rα chain

References

Chatila TA: Genetics of atopic diseases. Curr Opin Pediatr 10:584–587, 1998

Cookson W: The alliance of genes and environment in asthma and allergy. Nature 402 (Suppl):B5–B11, 1999

Cookson WOC, Mofalt MF: Genetics of asthma and allergic diseases. Hum Mol Genet 9:2359–2364, 2000

Ono SJ: Molecular genetics of allergic diseases. Annu Rev Immunol 18: 347–366, 2000

11.8 ALLERGIC DISORDERS

Leonard Bacharier

Allergic disorders are common in childhood, with at least 25% of children being affected by some form of atopic illness. In addition, the impact of these disorders on the lives of children and their families can be extraordinary, with numerous days of restricted activities, absences from school and work, and ever-increasing costs of health care and medications. It is thereby incumbent on the pediatrician to recognize these disorders and initiate appropriate interventions aimed at minimizing symptoms and preventing complications of these disorders.

HISTORY

A central component of the history of a child with suspected allergic disease is an assessment of exposure to factors known to provoke or exacerbate symptoms. Some patients may report symptoms on a seasonal basis, and other patients have chronic year-round (perennial) symptoms. The occurrence of temporal variations in symptoms reflects the seasonal differences in the levels of many inhalant allergens. Tree pollens are most prevalent in the spring, grass pollens in the early summer, and weeds release their pollen grains in the fall. Outdoor mold spores are most prominent in the spring, summer, and fall seasons and decline to minimal levels during times of snow cover. Other factors, including geographic locale, altitude, and relative humidity, influence the patterns of allergen exposure. House dust mites, an important source of allergens, are present perennially, as are the allergens from furred pets such as cats and dogs. More recently, the clinical importance of allergens from cockroaches and molds has become evident. Cockroach allergen is perennial in its presence. Indoor molds are present year-round but may also vary according to the season, with *Alternaria* and *Cladosporium* predominating indoors during warm weather and *Penicillium* and *Aspergillus* predominating indoors during the winter months.

The occurrence of symptoms following specific exposures suggests specific allergen sensitivities. Symptoms on entering a damp basement or a barn suggest allergy to molds. Ocular pruritus and nasal congestion that develop in the home where a cat is present makes sensitivity to cat allergen likely. Symptoms of rhinitis or asthma with house cleaning, especially dusting and vacuuming, imply allergy to dust mites. In addition, patients with respiratory tract allergy also develop symptoms on exposure to nonspecific airway irritants such as tobacco smoke, perfumes, and other strong odors.

Many symptoms associated with respiratory tract allergy are nonspecific and therefore overlap with other nonallergic disorders. Nasal congestion is a common pediatric complaint, and one must differentiate between allergic rhinitis and nonallergic disorders such as viral upper respiratory tract infections (URIs) and sinusitis. The presence of nasal and ocular pruritus, clear coryza, and frequent sneezing and the absence of fever suggest allergic rhinitis, as does the yearly recurrence of similar symptoms. Purulent coryza suggests an infectious process and may represent either the normal progression of a viral URI (which resolves spontaneously over a few days) or sinusitis if symptoms are persistent. Postnasal drainage may accompany all of these processes and results in frequent clearing of the throat, sore throat, and both daytime and nocturnal cough.

Chronic or recurrent episodes of cough may be caused by asthma, especially if the cough is dry or produces clear mucus. Cough in the context of physical exertion such as sports, laughter, and crying suggests airway hyperresponsiveness typically seen with asthma. Persistent cough with purulent sputum suggests disorders such as cystic fibrosis, chronic sinusitis, and bronchiectasis.

The response to specific interventions, both medical and environmental, is also helpful in establishing a diagnosis of allergic disease. Antihistamines are widely used, and a clinical response to this form of therapy suggests underlying allergy. Response of a cough to bronchodilators suggests asthma. Significant symptomatic improvement on relocation from a specific environment where allergen exposure is present to one where such exposure is minimal (vacation, hospitalization, moving) also implicates an allergic etiology.

A detailed family history may also aid in the diagnosis of allergic disease. Children of atopic parents are at increased risk of developing allergies themselves. Seventeen percent of children born to nonatopic parents develop allergies. If one parent is atopic, this prevalence rises to 20 to 50%, and if both parents are atopic, the prevalence of atopy in their offspring rises to 50 to 70%.

PHYSICAL EXAMINATION

A careful physical examination may disclose findings that corroborate a diagnosis of allergic disease. Presence of dark circles under the eyes (*allergic shiners*) is a nonspecific finding commonly seen in children with allergic rhinitis and results from significant nasal congestion and obstruction leading to impeded blood flow and pooling in the infraorbital regions. Additional wrinkles below the eyes (*Dennie-Morgan lines*) frequently accompany allergic shiners. Frequent rubbing of the nose secondary to pruritus and coryza produces the *allergic salute* and over time may result in a *transverse nasal crease*. The nasal mucosa in allergic rhinitis is typically edematous and pale and may be accompanied by profuse clear rhinorrhea. Adenoidal and/or tonsillar hypertrophy frequently accompanies allergic respiratory tract disease and may contribute to the frequent occurrence of *mouth breathing. Cobblestoning* of the posterior oropharynx results from chronic postnasal drainage. Ocular findings of allergic (hay fever) conjunctivitis include bilateral conjunctival injection, periorbital edema, and excessive lacrimation. The presence of intense pruritus, photophobia, thick tenacious ocular discharge, and giant papillae of the superior eyelid suggests vernal conjunctivitis.

Examination of the skin may reveal findings of *atopic dermatitis,* including xerosis (dry skin), erythematous papules with excoriations, and lichenification in a typical distribution (see Atopic Dermatitis in Sec. 14.3.2). Other cutaneous manifestations of allergic disease include *urticarial lesions* (hives), *angioedema,* and *dermatographism.*

The presence of asthma may result in increased anteroposterior diameter of the chest secondary to chronic air trapping. Signs of respiratory distress, including use of accessory muscles of respiration and retraction of the chest wall, may accompany asthma, especially during an acute exacerbation. Patients with asthma typically have generalized expiratory wheezing and a prolonged time spent in the expiratory phase of the respiratory cycle. Pulse oximetry may demonstrate hypoxemia. Digital clubbing is a rare finding in asthma, and its presence should prompt an evaluation of other disorders including cystic fibrosis, bronchiectasis, and cyanotic congenital heart disease.

DIAGNOSTIC TESTING

IN VIVO TESTING If a complete medical and environmental history and physical examination findings are suggestive of underlying atopy, skin testing for immediate hypersensitivity to allergens may be helpful in identifying specific sensitivities. This procedure attempts to produce a localized IgE-mediated (type I) hypersensitivity reaction. Skin testing may be performed using extracts of allergenic materials including dust mites, pollens, animal danders, molds, insect venoms, drugs, and foods. These extracts are introduced into the skin either via a prick (epicutaneous method) or by intradermal injection. Allergic individuals are predisposed to produce IgE antibodies directed against specific allergens. These antibodies are bound to IgE receptors present on the surface of cutaneous mast cells. If an allergen is recognized by allergen-specific IgE on the mast cell surface, the mast cell IgE receptors undergo crosslinking, leading to mast cell activation and degranulation. Degranulation of the mast cell releases a multitude of biochemical mediators, including histamine. Histamine binds to the type 1 histamine receptor (H_1R) and results in local vasodilation and increased vascular permeability, producing a *wheal*. An axonal reflex is also triggered and produces an area of surrounding erythema (*flare*). The development of this wheal-and-flare reaction requires approximately 15 to 20 minutes and typically resolves rapidly. Occasionally, a highly sensitive patient may experience a more protracted local reaction, and this is more common following intradermal testing.

The interpretation of skin testing for immediate hypersensitivity may be complicated by several factors. The presence of antihistamines (such as diphenhydramine, hydroxyzine, and loratadine) may produce false-negative skin tests by antagonizing the effects of histamine at the type 1 histamine receptor. To control for this possibility, patients are asked to withhold antihistamines or drugs that possess antihistamine-like effects (such as tricyclic antidepressants) for at least 72 hours before skin testing. Some drugs, such as astemizole, have much longer half-lives and must be withheld for at least 8 weeks before skin testing can be performed. In addition, a positive control of histamine phosphate (1 mg/mL) is generally included with skin testing to confirm the absence of H_1R antagonism. Although corticosteroids do suppress delayed-type hypersensitivity skin tests, there is no evidence that short-term or prolonged use of systemic steroids interferes with immediate hypersensitivity skin testing. Patients with dermatographism may develop reactions at skin test sites because of the hyperreactive nature of their skin and not from a type 1 hypersensitivity reaction. To control for such occurrences, a negative control consisting of the diluent used for the other extracts being tested is also applied. A positive reaction to an allergen consists of a wheal-and-flare response that is 3 to 5 mm in diameter greater than the negative control.

Most extracts used in standard skin testing have been shown to lack specific irritant properties. However, some nonstandardized allergens, especially drugs and some foods, may possess irritant properties, and caution should be exercised in interpreting results of skin testing using such agents, as false-positive results may occur because of the irritant effect eliciting a wheal-and-flare–type reaction. The timing of skin testing to particular allergens, especially insect venoms and penicillin, is critical. Following a systemic reaction to insect venom or penicillin, there may be a transient state (4–6 weeks following the reaction) of decreased levels of allergen-specific IgE. Skin testing during this time period may produce false-negative results and thereby fail to diagnose the existence of a potentially life-threatening allergy. Therefore, skin testing following anaphylaxis should be postponed for 4 to 6 weeks to allow for reaccumulation of allergen-specific IgE.

The ability to demonstrate cutaneous sensitivity to an allergen is present during infancy. Atopic infants and young children typi-cally demonstrate sensitivity to food allergens, especially those patients with atopic dermatitis, but may not display cutaneous type I hypersensitivity to inhalant allergens until 3 to 5 years of age.

The presence of a positive skin test to a specific allergen does not confirm that the allergen is responsible for triggering the patient's condition. False-positive reactions are not uncommon and are more common with food allergens than with inhalant allergens. In order to confirm the contribution of a specific allergen, provocation testing may be helpful. This is particularly useful in evaluating a child for possible food allergies (see Sec. 11.10) or may involve a nasal or bronchial challenge with the allergen in question. Although the latter two modalities are generally limited to research studies, food challenges are more feasible in an office setting.

LABORATORY EVALUATION

The presence of eosinophils in the blood or secretions is a consistent finding among patients with allergic disease. Eosinophils normally represent up to 1 to 3% of peripheral blood leukocytes. Peripheral blood eosinophilia is present if the percentage of eosinophils in the peripheral blood exceeds 5% or if the total eosinophil count exceeds 350 cells per cubic millimeter of blood. Although elevated total eosinophil counts are common in atopic individuals with allergic rhinitis, asthma, and atopic dermatitis, one must exclude the multitude of nonallergic disorders associated with eosinophilia, including those listed in Table 11-6.

In addition to peripheral blood eosinophilia, many atopic disorders are characterized by the presence of eosinophils in secretions and tissues. Nasal secretions from patients with allergic rhinoconjunctivitis may contain more than 5 to 10% eosinophils as identified by Hansel stain. Asthma is associated with a chronic eosinophilic infiltrate of the airways, and presence of eosinophils is characteristic of bronchoalveolar lavage and biopsy specimens from asthmatic individuals.

The production of IgE is another characteristic of the atopic state. Serum IgE levels increase with age in both allergic and nonallergic individuals, reaching adult values by 5 to 7 years of age.

TABLE 11-6

DIFFERENTIAL DIAGNOSIS OF EOSINOPHILIA

CLASS OF DISORDER	FREQUENTLY ASSOCIATED WITH EOSINOPHILIA
Allergic	Asthma, allergic rhinitis, urticaria, atopic dermatitis
Pulmonary	ABPA, eosinophilic pneumonia (Loeffler syndrome)
Infectious	Metazoan infections (ascariasis, schistosomiasis, trichinosis, hookworm) Visceral larvae migrans Histoplasmosis, coccidioidomycosis
Dermatologic	Dermatitis herpetiformis, pemphigus vulgaris, psoraisis, atopic dermatitis
Malignant	Eosinophilic leukemia, Hodgkin disease
Vasculitic/collagen vascular	Churg-Strauss syndrome, dermatomyositis, polyarteritis nodosa
Gastrointestinal	Eosinophilic gastroenteritis, allergic colitis, inflammatory bowel disease
Drug reactions	Gold, antimicrobials, anticonvulsants, growth factors (GM-CSF)
Idiopathic	Hypereosinophilic syndrome, pulmonary infiltrates with eosinophilia

Serum IgE is present at a concentration that is significantly less than the concentrations of other serum immunoglobulins (IgG, IgA, and IgM). Many patients with allergic disease have elevated levels of IgE, but this is not a universal finding. Patients with atopic dermatitis frequently have markedly elevated levels of serum IgE. The presence of elevated serum IgE levels at birth or in infancy is suggestive of the subsequent development of allergic disease. Like eosinophilia, elevated IgE levels are also associated with nonallergic disorders, which include immunodeficiency conditions (hyper-IgE syndrome, Wiskott-Aldrich syndrome), parasitic infection (visceral larval migrans, ascariasis), neoplasia (Hodgkin lymphoma), allergic bronchopulmonary aspergillosis, and cystic fibrosis.

In addition to total serum IgE levels, the detection of allergen-specific IgE in the serum is possible. The determination of allergen-specific IgE in vitro is performed using the RadioAllergoSorbent test (RAST) or a variation of this method. The basis of this study is that a solid-phase support to which allergens are bound is incubated with patient serum. Following a washing step, a radiolabeled antihuman IgE antibody is incubated with the solid-phase support and then washed again. The proportion of radiolabel that remains bound to the support is determined and is proportional to the amount of allergen-specific IgE in the patient's serum. Recent versions of this method have employed newer solid supports and colorimetric/fluorimetric assay methods. The primary advantages of in vitro testing for allergen-specific IgE are the lack of interference of antihistamines as seen with skin testing and the lack of potential allergic reaction provoked by skin testing. However, in vitro testing is generally less sensitive and more expensive than skin testing. In addition, results are not immediately available at the time of the patient's evaluation and thus cannot be integrated into patient education on allergen avoidance. Therefore, in most clinical situations, skin testing is the preferred method for determining sensitivity to specific allergens (see below).

APPROACHES TO THERAPY

There are four major modalities available in the management of allergic disease: avoidance of specific triggers, pharmacotherapy, immunotherapy, and prevention of sensitization to allergens (Table 11-7).

TABLE 11-7
THERAPEUTIC APPROACHES TO ATOPIC DISEASE

MODALITY	SPECIFIC EXAMPLES
Minimize exposure	Dust mites: plastic zippered encasings, remove carpet, acaricides, minimize humidity
	Pollens and outdoor molds: keep windows closed, air conditioning, HEPA filters
	Indoor molds: reduce humidity, meticulous housecleaning, bleach
	Animals: remove furred and feathered pets from home
	Cockroaches: meticulous hygiene, traps
Pharmacotherapy	Antihistamines ± decongestants
Immunotherapy	Antiinflammatory agents: mast cell stabilizers, corticosteroids
Prophylaxis	Minimize exposure to aeroallergens and tobacco smoke during infancy and childhood
	Breast-feeding

AVOIDANCE OF SPECIFIC TRIGGERS Following the identification of the specific allergens to which an individual is sensitive (through history, knowledge of local patterns of allergen prevalence, and appropriate in vivo and in vitro testing), specific measures directed at minimizing exposure to such allergens are indicated. Many studies have demonstrated that strict attention to the avoidance of aeroallergens leads to significant improvement in disease control. Dust mites are the source of allergens commonly responsible for perennial allergic rhinitis and contribute to the inflammatory responses characteristic of asthma and atopic dermatitis. Dust mites are found in greatest numbers in upholstered furniture, mattresses, and other bedding, and carpeting. Covering mattresses, box springs, and pillows in impermeable zippered covers reduces the level of dust mite allergen in a bedroom several hundredfold. In addition, bedding should be washed weekly at 130°F, and carpeting should be removed to reduce reservoirs for dust mites. Upholstered furniture should be removed from the bedroom, as should heavy window coverings such as draperies. Several chemical acaricides, which kill dust mites, are available, but frequent reapplication is critical to maintain a significant reduction of dust mite allergen. Because dust mites require ambient humidity for growth, maintaining the relative humidity of a home below 50% also helps control mite growth. If carpeting cannot be removed, vacuuming should be performed on a weekly basis with a cleaner equipped with a double-thickness bag and/or a high-efficiency filter. Because little dust mite allergen is airborne, the use of air filtration systems has a negligible effect on mite allergen levels.

Cockroaches are an increasingly important source of allergen, especially in urban areas. Control of cockroach infestation is difficult and involves the use of insecticides and bait traps combined with meticulous hygienic practices. However, the efficacy of these approaches on the control of allergic disease and asthma is unclear at the present time. Reduction of visible cockroaches is attainable, but a significant reduction of cockroach allergen is difficult, likely because of large reservoirs of cockroaches and allergen in areas that are not visible or easily accessible.

Household pets are a significant source of indoor allergens. Cat allergen is generally regarded as a more potent allergen than is dog allergen, and this is reflected in the greater prevalence of sensitization to cats compared to sensitivity to dogs. The major dog and cat allergens are detectable in saliva and dander. Although the quantity of allergen recovered varies from breed to breed, all breeds produce these allergens. Both cat and dog allergens become airborne and are detected in significant amounts in schools and other locales never visited by these animals. Removal of the pet from the home is considered the most effective approach to reducing allergen burden. Even following removal of a cat from the home, cat allergen may be detectable for at least 3 to 4 months. Because cat allergen is highly sticky, even if the cat is kept outdoors, a significant amount of cat allergen will be brought into the home on family members' clothing by passive transfer. Washing of the animals results in transient decreases in skin allergen and airborne allergen levels. High-efficiency air-filtering systems (eg, HEPA) also reduce airborne cat and dog allergen levels and may serve an adjunctive role to the allergen control measures above.

Exposure to pollens from trees, grasses, weeds, and molds is difficult to avoid outdoors during the pollination seasons. Keeping doors and windows closed and using air conditioning and air filtration systems minimize the presence of these outdoor allergens inside homes. Sensitive individuals should also avoid sleeping near open windows or having a window fan in their bedrooms. Molds are present both indoors and outdoors and can be present seasonally or perennially. Outdoor molds are particularly problematic in temperate regions of the United States, especially after leaves have fallen from trees and begin to decay. Indoor molds accumulate in areas of moisture, such as damp basements and bathrooms. Interventions that are helpful in minimizing exposure to these important allergens include the use of dehumidifiers, cleansing areas of mold accumulation with antifungal agents, including bleach, and keeping windows closed.

PHARMACOTHERAPY An ever-expanding armamentarium of antiallergic drugs is available to patients with atopic diseases. Antihistamines are the cornerstone of pharmacologic therapy for allergic rhinoconjunctivitis. These drugs function by blocking the interaction between the mast cell–derived mediator, histamine, and the H_1 histamine receptor. If administered prior to allergen exposure, antihistamines will block H_1 receptors and prevent the development of the allergic symptoms typically produced by histamine, which include nasal and ocular pruritus, sneezing, and rhinorrhea. This class of medications is also effective when administered following allergen exposure. Sedation was the major limitation of the first generation of antihistamines. This resulted from their lipophilic nature and ability to readily cross the blood-brain barrier and interact not only with H_1 receptors but also with dopamine, serotonin, and acetylcholine receptors. The ability of first-generation antihistamines to interact with acetylcholine receptors also explains the occurrence of anticholinergic symptoms, such as blurry vision and dry mouth. More recently, second-generation antihistamines have been developed which possess greater selectivity for the H_1 receptor and a greatly reduced capacity to cross the blood-brain barrier. Thus, this class of H_1 receptor antagonists provides the beneficial effects of classical antihistamines without significant side effects. A listing of representative antihistamines is provided in Table 11-8. In addition to orally administered H_1R antagonists, topical antihistamines are available for the treatment of allergic rhinitis (azelastine) and allergic conjunctivitis (levocabastine).

IMMUNOTHERAPY Although antihistamines produce relief of many allergic symptoms, they do not address the underlying pathophysiological processes involved in the disease state, namely, mast cell degranulation and subsequent release of inflammatory mediators such as cytokines and chemokines, which lead to recruitment of inflammatory cells. In other words, H_1R antagonists interfere with the early phase of the allergic response without affecting the late-phase inflammatory response. Fortunately, additional classes of antiallergic drugs are capable of influencing both phases of the response to allergen. Mast cell–stabilizing agents, such as cromolyn sodium and nedocromil sodium, are effective in blocking mast cell mediator release when used as prophylactic agents before allergen exposure. Cromolyn preparations are available for ocular and nasal administration. Newer ocular agents, such as lodoxamide and olopatadine, possess both H_1R antagonist and mast cell–stabilizing properties. Corticosteroids are potent antiinflammatory agents that prevent the late phase of the allergic response and provide relief of many symptoms of allergic rhinoconjunctivitis, urticaria, and asthma. Many preparations of intranasal corticosteroids are available and do not appear to produce the systemic side effects seen with systemic steroids.

DESENSITIZATION If therapy with the combination of environmental controls and pharmacotherapy fails to provide significant symptom control, allergen immunotherapy (hyposensitization, desensitization) may be an option for some patients. This mode of therapy involves the subcutaneous administration of increasing doses of allergens to which an individual is sensitized. Although the exact mechanisms by which this modality produces clinical improvement remain unclear almost 70 years after its introduction, numerous studies have demonstrated improvement in symptom control, medication use, and quality of life of patients with allergic rhinoconjunctivitis. Similar evidence has been provided for the role of allergen immunotherapy in asthma. This form of therapy is likely to be most beneficial to patients who are sensitive to a small number of relevant aeroallergens because the effect of immunotherapy is allergen-specific. The onset of effect from immunotherapy is delayed, requiring 1 to 2 years before onset of clinical improvement. In addition, the occurrence of systemic, anaphylactic reactions is a known complication of the administration of immunotherapy. These factors must be thoroughly considered on a patient-by-patient basis in determining if immunotherapy is a reasonable therapeutic option.

It is clear that the exposure to aeroallergens during the first years of life is associated with the subsequent development of allergic disease, especially asthma. Children exposed to higher levels of dust mite allergen during the first year of life are more likely to have dust mite sensitivity and asthma than children who were exposed to lower levels of dust mite. Therefore, children at risk for the development of atopic disease should be provided a home environment with many of the environmental controls recommended for patients with known allergic disease. These should include minimization of exposure to dust mites, furred pets, and tobacco smoke in the hope that these interventions will prevent sensitization to

TABLE 11-8

H_1-RECEPTOR ANTAGONISTS

GENERIC NAME	TRADE NAME	DOSAGE	AGE INDICATION
First generation (sedating)			
Chlorpheniramine maleate	Chlor-Trimeton	0.35 mg/kg/d	≥ 12 years
Diphenhydramine HCl	Benadryl	5 mg/kg/d	≥ 6 years
Hydroxyzine HCl	Atarax	2 mg/kg/d	
Second generation (nonsedating)			
Astemizole	Hismanal	20 mg BID	≥ 12 years
Cetirizine[a]	Zyrtec	2.5–5 mg QD	2–5 years
		5–10 mg QD	≥ 6 years
Fexofenadine	Allegra	60 mg BID	≥ 12 years
Loratadine	Claritin	10 mg QD	≥ 6 years

[a] Minimally sedating.

these important allergens and thereby negatively influence the development of clinical allergy.

References

Demoly P, Michel F-B, Bousquet J: In vivo methods for study of allergy: skin tests, techniques and interpretation. In: Middleton E Jr, Reed CE, Ellis EF, et al, eds: Allergy: Principles and Practice, 5th ed, vol I. St Louis, CV Mosby, 1998:430

Simons FER, Simons KJ: The pharmacology and use of H_1-receptor antagonist drugs. N Engl J Med 330:1663–1670, 1994

11.9 ALLERGIC RHINITIS AND CONJUNCTIVITIS

Leonard Bacharier

Rhinitis is the most common manifestation of allergic disease, affecting 10 to 22% of adults and 10 to 42% of children. Symptoms frequently become apparent during the first 5 years of life and may occur in a seasonal and/or perennial (year-round) pattern. Because sensitization to individual allergens requires repeated exposures, several seasons of exposure are necessary for the development of allergy to pollens or molds. This may explain why children with allergic rhinitis under the age of 5 years are typically sensitized to perennial indoor allergens, such as dust mites and animal danders, rather than seasonal allergens such as ragweed.

The symptom complex of allergic rhinoconjunctivitis results from the biochemical mediators elaborated during a type I (IgE-mediated) hypersensitivity reaction. Following the inhalation of aeroallergens into the nose, water-soluble antigens enter and diffuse through the mucous blanket that covers the respiratory tract mucosa. Interaction of these allergens with allergen-specific IgE on the surface of mast cells initiates cellular activation, culminating in the release of a multitude of preformed and newly synthesized bioactive molecules, including histamine and prostaglandin D_2. These mediators produce symptoms shortly after allergen exposure and remit relatively quickly. However, symptoms frequently recur several hours later, coincident with a rise in many of the same mediators seen in the early response, along with a rise in cytokines (eg, IL-4 and IL-5) and the influx of helper T cells and eosinophils. This late allergic response is responsible for the inflammation seen in allergic rhinitis and contributes to the chronicity of the condition.

Nasal congestion is the most frequently reported symptom by patients with allergic rhinitis. Congestion resulting in near-total nasal obstruction may result in mouth breathing. Nasal pruritus may result in frequent wrinkling of the nose and/or rubbing of the nose with the heel of the hand, producing the allergic salute. Over time, this maneuver may lead to the formation of a transverse nasal crease. Pruritus of the palate, pharynx, and ears frequently accompanies nasal symptoms. Sneezing, often in paroxysms, is a common complaint, as is watery clear coryza. Postnasal drainage is a common problem and may result in worsening cough with recumbency. Uncomplicated allergic rhinitis is rarely associated with systemic pyrexia. Ocular symptoms may include excessive lacrimation and conjunctival injection.

Physical examination frequently discloses significant nasal congestion caused by edema of the mucosa overlying the nasal turbi-

nates. The mucosa is pale with a blue hue and may appear redundant. In adolescents and adults, nasal polyps may be present. Polyps are uncommon in younger children, and their presence should suggest an alternative diagnosis, most often cystic fibrosis. The posterior oropharynx may have a cobblestoned appearance because of lymphoid hyperplasia. Edema of the nasal mucosa impedes venous return and results in infraorbital dark circles (allergic shiners) and periorbital edema. Additional wrinkles below the eyes (Dennie-Morgan lines) frequently accompany allergic shiners. Although these findings are common among children with allergic rhinitis, none are pathognomonic of the disorder.

The diagnostic evaluation of a patient with suspected allergic rhinitis may include examination of the nasal secretions for a predominance of eosinophils, which is suggestive, but not pathognomonic, of allergic rhinitis. Peripheral blood eosinophilia and elevated serum IgE levels are common, but nonspecific, findings. Testing for specific allergen sensitivities, by either skin testing or in vitro methods, should be interpreted in the context of the patient's history in order to determine the clinical relevance of positive results.

The mucosal edema associated with allergic rhinitis is, in part, responsible for several complications of nasal allergy. Allergic inflammation may produce eustachian tube dysfunction and recurrent otitis media. Edema of the osteomeatal complex leads to impaired mucociliary clearance from the sinuses and contributes to the development of infectious sinusitis. Disturbances of olfaction and taste are quite bothersome to patients, as are interruptions of sleep by nasal obstruction and postnasal drainage. Prolonged mouth breathing may lead to disturbances in facial growth and dental malocclusion. Patients with allergic rhinitis have a higher incidence of bronchial hyperreactivity than patients without rhinitis and appear to be at increased risk for the subsequent development of asthma.

The approach to therapy in the patient with allergic rhinitis follows the treatment algorithm described above. Patient education focused on avoidance of allergens is central to the management of allergic rhinitis. Strict adherence to these principles may reduce symptoms, need for medications, and complications of rhinitis. Pharmacologic therapy is an adjunct to allergen avoidance. Antihistamines are the cornerstone of therapy for allergic rhinitis and are most effective for controlling sneezing, nasal and ocular pruritus, and coryza but provide less relief from nasal congestion.

If the combination of allergen avoidance and antihistamines does not adequately control symptoms, the addition of an antiinflammatory agent should be considered. Cromolyn sodium is available for both ocular and nasal administration and is most effective when administered before allergen exposure, such as before the onset of the spring pollen season, and continued throughout the time of exposure. Cromolyn has no appreciable side effects, but for maximal efficacy, it should be administered four to six times daily. For allergic conjunctivitis, two agents that possess both mast cell–stabilizing properties and H_1 receptor antagonist properties are lodoxamide and olopatadine. Topical nasal steroids are the most effective medication for all symptoms of allergic rhinitis and *non*allergic *r*hinitis with *e*osinophilia *s*yndrome (NARES). Agents currently available include pressurized metered dose inhalers or aqueous preparations of beclomethasone dipropionate, budesonide, flunisolide, fluticasone propionate, and triamcinolone. Once- or twice-daily administration is necessary for maximal efficacy. The most frequent adverse effects of these agents are local irritation and epistaxis. Concern surrounding the potential systemic effects of nasally applied steroids has discouraged their use in children. However, when administered at the lowest dose required to maintain their clinical effect, these agents rarely produce clinically significant side effects.

References

Meltzer EO: Treatment options for the child with allergic rhinitis. Clin Pediatr 37:1–10, 1998
Rachelefsky GS: Pharmacologic management of allergic rhinitis. J Allergy Clin Immunol 101:S367–369, 1998

11.10 FOOD ALLERGY

Leonard Bacharier

Adverse reactions to foods are common, and it is instructive to categorize these reactions on the basis of their underlying pathogenic mechanism. From a mechanistic standpoint, adverse reactions to foods may be immunologically mediated or mediated by non-immunologic mechanisms. Immune-based adverse food reactions are mediated predominantly by IgE. However, other immune mechanisms, including antigen-dependent cellular cytotoxicity, immune complexes, and cell-mediated hypersensitivity, have been implicated in other adverse reactions to foods. Nonimmunologic food intolerances are common and include enzyme deficiencies (lactase deficiency) and toxin exposure (staphylococcal, botulinal).

Adverse reactions to foods are a common complaint in pediatric practice. Large surveys have revealed that approximately 25% of parents believe their child had experienced at least one adverse reaction to a food. However, detailed investigation of these patients, including double-blind placebo-controlled food challenges, confirms an adverse reaction in only one-third of these patients, often to fruits and fruit juices. Food hypersensitivity is most commonly expressed in the first years of life, with an approximate prevalence of up to 5% in children under the age of 4 years and 1 to 2% in older children.

Food allergy mediated by IgE parallels other IgE-mediated hypersensitivity disorders. If a susceptible individual is exposed to an allergen, a humoral immune response may ensue with the eventual production of allergen-specific IgE. Mast cells bind these IgE molecules through high-affinity IgE receptors expressed on their surfaces. Exposure of these sensitized mast cells to allergen results in cellular activation and release of preformed and newly synthesized mediators. These mediators, which include histamine and products of arachidonic acid metabolism, are responsible for many physiological responses such as vasodilation, increased vascular permeability, and smooth muscle contraction. These mediators may act locally, such as within the gastrointestinal tract, to produce nausea, vomiting, and diarrhea, or they may act systemically, producing cutaneous, respiratory, and cardiovascular effects. Positive food challenges in patients with atopic dermatitis are associated with a rise in serum histamine levels, further supporting the role of mast cell mediators and other histamine-releasing factors in immediate hypersensitivity reactions to foods. In addition to allergen-specific IgE, food-specific IgG antibodies and immune complexes are detectable in individuals with food hypersensitivity. However, these are also demonstrable in normal individuals, making the role of these antibodies in the pathogenesis of these disorders unclear.

The most commonly reported symptoms of food allergy are cutaneous in nature, including pruritic macular eruptions, urticaria, and angioedema. Onset of symptoms tends to be rapid, occurring within minutes of ingestion of the offending food. Children with atopic dermatitis frequently have evidence of IgE-mediated sensitivity to a variety of foods, and may develop a flat red pruritic rash within minutes of ingestion of specific foods. They may also develop worsening dermatitis hours to days after consumption of a food to which they are sensitive. Foods are responsible for many cases of acute urticaria, but they are rarely responsible for chronic hives. Gastrointestinal complaints are common and include nausea, vomiting, and abdominal cramping. Diarrhea is less common. Although acute respiratory symptoms may be a manifestation of food-induced anaphylaxis, chronic respiratory symptoms are an uncommon manifestation of food allergy. Respiratory tract involvement may be manifested as rhinitis, sneezing, cough, wheezing, and/or laryngeal edema. It is important to recognize that asthmatic reactions may be elicited by foods without antecedent or simultaneous development of cutaneous symptoms.

Anaphylaxis is the most explosive of the adverse reactions to foods and results in several fatalities per year. Fatal reactions typically occur in a patient with a known history of allergy to a food who consumes the food outside of the home. Asthma is common among patients with fatal anaphylaxis, as are denial of symptoms and delayed administration of medications, especially epinephrine. Although allergic reactions have been reported to a wide variety of foods, a short list of foods is responsible for the majority of IgE-mediated reactions, especially anaphylaxis, in children. These include eggs, cow's milk, soy, wheat, peanuts, tree nuts, fish, and shellfish.

The food-induced enterocolitis syndrome presents during infancy with vomiting and diarrhea typically associated with cow's milk or soy proteins. These patients demonstrate poor weight gain and may have bloody diarrhea and peripheral edema. Examination of the gastrointestinal mucosa demonstrates chronic inflammation and villous injury. An IgE-mediated mechanism is not responsible for this syndrome, as the majority of patients lack milk- or soy-specific IgE. Removal of the offending protein from the diet and provision of a casein hydrolysate formula usually results in prompt symptomatic improvement. The majority of patients are able to tolerate milk and soy later in life. Allergic colitis presents during infancy with bloody diarrhea. Children with allergic colitis do not appear systemically ill and typically respond to the elimination of dietary milk and/or soy. Gluten-sensitive enteropathy is another example of non-IgE-mediated food hypersensitivity in which patients sensitive to the gluten contained in wheat, barley, oats, and rye may present with malabsorption and failure to gain weight.

A detailed history is critical for the accurate diagnosis of adverse food reactions. The timing of ingestion and onset of symptoms is useful in differentiating between IgE-mediated disease and other disease mechanisms. Other historical details include the quantity of food necessary to provoke symptoms, the method of food preparation, the interval of time since the last reaction, and any therapeutic interventions that may have been required. A detailed diary of dietary contents is occasionally helpful in identifying potential candidates for adverse food reactions. Similarly, the elimination of suspected foods for 1 to 2 weeks may be utilized in the diagnosis of food allergy, but such diets rarely provide additional information. Percutaneous skin testing with food allergen extracts is helpful in assessing for the presence of allergen-specific IgE. False-negative skin tests are uncommon, making a negative skin test with an appropriately prepared extract very effective in excluding an IgE-mediated sensitivity.

The only proven mode of therapy for food hypersensitivity is strict avoidance of the responsible food. This requires extensive education of parents, children, and other caretakers with regard to reading product labels to avoid accidental exposure to the offending allergen. Clinical sensitivity to allergens such as cow's milk and soy typically diminishes over time, and strict dietary avoidance may lead to a more rapid loss in sensitivity to these allergens. Although most children outgrow these sensitivities, allergies to peanuts, tree nuts, fish, and shellfish tend to be lifelong in nature and are associated with the majority of fatal reactions in adolescents and adults. Children with a history of anaphylaxis to foods should wear a medical identification badge and have an epinephrine self-administration kit available at all times in the event of exposure and the development of systemic symptoms. At the present time, allergen immunotherapy to foods is not a clinical option because of the high rate of systemic reactions associated with such therapy.

References

James JM, Sampson HA: An overview of food hypersensitivy. Pediatr Allergy Immunol 3:67–78, 1992

Roesler TA, Barry PC, Bock SA: Factitious food allergy and failure to thrive. Arch Pediatr Adolesc Med 148:1150–1155, 1994

Twarog FJ: Food-induced allergy in childhood. Allergy Asthma Proc 19: 219–222, 1998

11.11 LATEX ALLERGY

Robert C. Strunk

Latex is the most common cause of anaphylaxis presenting to pediatric hospital inpatient units and emergency departments, causing 27% of all episodes, more than food (25%) and drugs (16%). It is the most common cause of severe reactions that start while in hospital and the cause of most of cases that require ICU care. In some series, as many as 8 of 10 anaphylactic reactions occurring during surgery in children are caused by latex allergy. Early on in the recognition of latex as a cause of allergic reactions, it was determined that children with spina bifida and congenital urologic problems were most at risk for severe reactions. These children had multiple surgical procedures and were exposed to latex-containing products outside an operating room at regular intervals. The incidence of latex allergy may be increasing, and circumstances (patient profile, hospital location, route of exposure) in which life-threatening reactions occur appear to be broader than previously recognized. Forty percent of reactions occur in patients with a primary diagnosis outside the previously recognized high-risk groups (eg, spina bifida), and 60% of the severe reactions occur outside an operating room.

Patients with spina bifida and congenital urologic conditions requiring multiple surgeries are still the greatest risk categories. Among the spina bifida patients, sensitization to latex is most highly correlated to the number of previous operations, total serum IgE, presence of a VP shunt, and personal history of atopy. Among those spina bifida patients sensitized to latex, a clinical reaction to the latex is most highly correlated with a higher number of previous operations, personal history of atopy, and allergy by skin testing. As in studies of spina bifida patients, a number of studies find that atopy increases the risk of sensitization in other patient types by six- to 10-fold. Atopy seems to lower the threshold both to sensitization to latex and to presence of clinical reactions.

The correlation between number of past operations and sensitization and clinical reactions to latex is well established, both within high-risk groups and in general surgical patients. Recent studies have suggested that multiple surgeries place a patient at risk, even those without a high-risk disease. One study found that three surgeries produced significantly greater risk for sensitization than a single surgery. History of a surgical procedure in the first year of life may also be a risk factor, as most of the patients in a non-high-risk diagnostic category who had severe anaphylaxis from latex had had surgery before 1 year of life. Also supportive of the importance of surgery in the first year of life is the observation that adults with spinal cord injuries and multiple surgeries had no clinical reactions to latex (and only 2 of 50 such patients tested had a positive allergy test to latex).

An interesting risk factor for allergy to latex is allergy to fruits, particularly melons, peaches, and bananas. Several studies have demonstrated that these fruits contain antigens that crossreact with antigens in latex. Of 57 fruit-allergic patients, almost 90% had a positive skin test to latex; 10% had a clinical reaction to latex when challenged with a latex glove. Of 50 allergy patients without fruit allergy, only two had a positive test for latex, and neither of these had a clinical reaction when challenged.

Intraoperative anaphylactic reactions to latex can occur without prior history of a clinical reaction or presence of a high-risk diagnostic category, although the incidence of such reactions is very low. One study of 1523 patients reported only two patients with tachycardia, hypotension, and bronchospasm starting between 6 and 40 minutes after initiation of surgery. Interestingly, both of these patients had had multiple surgeries and were first exposed to latex under 1 month of age.

Latex allergy results from specific sensitization to soluble proteins remaining on the surface of latex-made products. There are a large number of proteins capable of binding to IgE antibodies, ranging in size from <10 kDa to 100 kDa. Hevein, a 4.7-kDa polypeptide and the predominant component in the fraction with latex proteins smaller than 10 kDa is a major allergen with a positive test in 81% of patients with clinical symptoms on exposure to latex products.

There are several different ways to screen for latex allergy. Questionnaires about prior problems with latex have a very high specificity for detection of latex allergy as determined by presence of a positive skin test (0.92) but a low sensitivity for the presence of antilatex IgE (0.58). Skin-prick testing with glove eluate has a very high negative predictive value (ie, if the test is negative, reactions to latex will almost certainly not occur). RAST-CAP, an in vitro test for the presence of allergen-specific IgE, also has a very high negative predictive value. However, in a patient with no history of symptoms on exposure to latex, the predictive value of IgE antibodies against latex for development of anaphylaxis during anesthesia appears to be very low.

The high prevalence of antibodies to latex in children with spina bifida, along with the strong correlation between number of operations and development of latex antibodies over time, justifies a primary prophylaxis by avoiding latex during anesthesia and surgery in all these patients. A latex-free environment appears to be an effective prophylaxis to development of allergy. Sixty-seven patients with spina bifida underwent all procedures without use of latex materials. Patients were followed up to 4.1 years. Sixty-four percent either did not develop allergy or had a decrease in IgE antibody titer during the period of observation. However, 13% had increased sensitization, and 6% became sensitized. Thus, it appears that exposure to latex during medical procedures is the main cause of new sensitization, but other forms of contact can induce sensitization. Mild sensitization can be reduced by prophylactic avoidance of latex.

Avoiding contact with latex during surgery is sufficient to avoid reactions. Some authors have suggested use of antihistamines and systemic steroids before procedures (similar to the protocol used to avoid repeat reactions from radiocontrast media administration); however, others have found that reactions can be prevented if there is simply avoidance of latex or use of latex products that have been thoroughly washed in patients known to be at risk or in patients with a history of a reaction to a latex product. Holzman studied 267 anesthetics in 167 high-risk children, many with other allergies and thus even more at risk for clinical sensitivity to latex. Only one reaction occurred, during injection of an epidural catheter with bupivacaine and fentanyl, and that may not even have been related to latex allergy.

All patients admitted to hospital, especially those to have surgery, should be questioned about latex allergy. Questions should probe for respiratory and skin symptoms on exposure to any latex product, including balloons, and the presence of allergy to fruits. Patients with a positive history should be further evaluated for latex allergy with skin test or RAST-CAP or should avoid latex during the hospitalization.

Children with a history of anaphylaxis should have home epinephrine prescribed and reviewed at regular visits, as inadvertent exposure can occur and cause severe reactions. Use of skin testing in patients without history of symptoms when exposed to latex is not established. Although one-third with sensitivity demonstrated by skin tests or RAST have no history of a clinical reaction, the risk of a reaction on exposure in these patient is very low. One study challenged 12 children with a positive skin test but without a history of sensitivity and found no reactions.

References

Dibs SD, Baker MD: Anaphylaxis in children: a 5 year experience. Pediatrics 99:E7, 1997

Theissen U, Theissen JL, Mertes N, Brehler R: IgE-mediated hypersensitivity to latex in childhood. Allergy 52:665–669, 1997

11.12 ADVERSE REACTIONS TO DRUGS

Leonard Bacharier

Adverse reactions frequently complicate pharmacologic therapies. Although the vast majority of these reactions are a consequence of pharmacologic properties of the drug, between 6 and 15% of these events are immunologic in nature. Therefore, nonimmunologic reactions predominate and include idiosyncratic reactions, drug overdose, drug-drug interactions, teratogenic effects, and side effects. This section focuses on immune-mediated adverse drug reactions.

The incidence of drug allergy in the pediatric population is less than that seen in adults and is not influenced by underlying atopic status. Individuals with allergy to one drug are, however, at greater risk for developing allergic responses to multiple drugs. Patients with HIV infection appear to have an increased rate of adverse drug reactions, likely because of dysregulation of immune response and exposure to multiple pharmacologic agents. Additional factors that predispose to adverse drug reactions include the frequency, dose, and route of drug administration. Drugs given in short frequent courses and those given parenterally induce allergic reactions more often than orally administered agents given for prolonged periods of time.

Most drugs used in clinical practice are low-molecular-weight molecules that are incapable of eliciting an immune response (haptens). However, conjugation of haptens to serum proteins or other carriers confers the capacity to generate an immunologic response. In addition to the native drugs, drug metabolites frequently act as immunogens. Immunologic responses to drugs may include one or more of the four types of hypersensitivity reactions described by Gell and Coombs. A pharmacologic agent may induce specific IgE and may, on subsequent exposure, trigger anaphylaxis. Alternatively, a drug may induce an IgG-predominant response, leading to the development of serum sickness. Binding of a drug to the surface of red blood cells may lead to antibody-mediated hemolysis. Finally, the induction of a delayed-type hypersensitivity reaction mediated by T lymphocytes and monocytes may result in the development of a contact dermatitis.

The immunologic mechanism underlying the reaction determines the timing of onset of symptoms. The intravenous administration of a drug to an individual with preexisting drug-specific IgE may elicit an immediate (within 1 hour) or delayed (up to 72 hours) reaction. Cutaneous eruptions are the most commonly reported adverse reactions to medications, with morbilliform and maculopapular eruptions predominating. Urticaria is supportive, but not pathognomonic, of an IgE-mediated process. The absence of urticaria or pruritus makes an IgE-mediated reaction unlikely but does not exclude other immunologic drug reactions. Other cutaneous manifestations of drug hypersensitivity include erythema multiforme minor and major (Stevens-Johnson syndrome), toxic epidermal necrolysis, vasculitis, fixed drug eruptions, and photosensitivity reactions. These reactions typically present more than 72 hours following the initiation of therapy.

Although cutaneous eruptions are the predominant form of pediatric adverse drug reactions, other organ systems may be involved. Anaphylaxis to medications is uncommon in childhood but, when present, may include respiratory tract involvement with laryngeal edema and wheezing and/or cardiovascular collapse. Fever, arthritis, vasculitis, and gastrointestinal and neurologic manifestations may accompany serum sickness reactions.

A careful history is essential in establishing the association between a drug and a potential adverse reaction. Identification of all pharmacologic agents used by the patient, including over-the-counter items and herbal remedies, and the temporal relationship between drug administration and symptom development are essential. Any coexisting conditions, especially viral infections, must be integrated into the assessment of these reactions because viral exanthems are more common than adverse drug reactions. Because prior exposure is generally required for an immunologic drug reaction, a history of prior exposure to the drug without adverse effects does not exclude the development of an adverse reaction on subsequent exposure.

Laboratory testing for adverse drug reactions is limited. Peripheral blood eosinophilia is supportive of an allergic process. Although immediate hypersensitivity skin testing may be performed to most agents, the validity of such studies, with the exception of penicillin, is unknown. Patients with a history of anaphylaxis, urticaria, or serum sickness associated with penicillin administration should undergo skin testing, although patients with histories of maculopapular or morbilliform eruptions appear to be at low risk for an immediate-type reaction. Skin testing with a panel of three reagents provides informative data on the risk of anaphylaxis with subsequent exposure to penicillin.

Benzylpenicillin comprises 95% of tissue-bound penicillin and is considered the major determinant of penicillin. Because benzylpenicillin is a hapten incapable of crosslinking IgE on mast cell surfaces, benzylpenicillin has been coupled to a polylysine backbone to form a multivalent antigen, which is commercially available and useful in skin testing. A positive skin test to polylysine-penicillin or benzylpenicillin indicates sensitization to penicillin and places the individual at risk of an allergic reaction upon penicillin administration. However, not all penicillin-sensitive individuals are identified using these two reagents. Metabolites of penicillin, including benzylpenicilloate and benzylpenilloate, are responsible for most cases of penicillin-induced anaphylaxis. Together, these two metabolites constitute the "minor determinants." Failure to include a minor determinant mixture in the penicillin skin test panel will result in a failure to detect up to 10% of individuals with penicillin sensitivity at risk for anaphylaxis. Another caveat in the interpretation of penicillin skin testing is that a negative response to all three reagents does not eliminate the possibility of an urticarial eruption or delayed reaction upon readministration. This skin test protocol has demonstrated that the majority of patients with a history of an adverse reaction related to penicillin administration lack penicillin-specific IgE and tolerate future administration of penicillin. The duration of time between the last reaction and skin testing is also important. Penicillin sensitivity declines over time, with more than 80% of skin test–positive individuals becoming skin test negative within 10 years. In vitro RAST testing for penicillin-specific IgE is limited to the major determinants and thus will not identify all patients with sensitivity to penicillin.

Discontinuation of the suspected agent is the first step in the therapy of an allergic reaction. If anaphylaxis is present, therapy should include epinephrine, antihistamines, and corticosteroids. If the history is highly suggestive of either an IgE-mediated reaction or Stevens-Johnson syndrome, use of alternative agents for future therapy is preferred. Choosing an alternative agent must include the recognition of crossreacting agents that may elicit a similar reaction upon administration. Clinically relevant examples include a low, but not absent, rate of crossreactivity between penicillin and cephalosporin antibiotics. Although there is a 3 to 7% rate of crossreactivity between penicillin and cephalosporins, the rate appears to be lower for second- and third-generation cephalosporins. There is a high rate of crossreactivity between penicillin and the carbopenem antibiotic imipenem, but there is minimal crossreactivity between penicillin and the monobactam antibiotic aztreonam. However, the presence of identical side chains in aztreonam and ceftazidine is responsible for the high rate of crossreactivity between these two agents.

In clinical situations where the use of an alternative agent is not applicable, desensitization to the agent of choice may be necessary. Although this procedure is frequently effective for IgE-mediated reactions, it should not be employed for non-IgE-mediated processes such as Stevens-Johnson syndrome or serum sickness. Close medical supervision by personnel skilled in the management of anaphylaxis is imperative, given the frequent occurrence of systemic reactions during desensitization. Desensitization must be repeated for each subsequent administration of the medication.

References

Patterson R, Deswarte RD, Greenberger PA, Grammer LC, Brown JE, Choy AC: Drug Allergy and Protocols for Management of Drug Allergies, 2nd ed. Providence, RI, Oceanside Publications, 1995:1–27

Roujeau JC, Stern RS: Severe adverse cutaneous reactions to drugs. N Engl J Med 331:1272–1285, 1994

11.13 ANAPHYLAXIS

Leonard Bacharier

Anaphylaxis describes an immunologically based, IgE-mediated, systemic reaction to an allergen. When a similar reaction occurs without an identifiable IgE-mediated mechanism, it is termed anaphylactoid. Anaphylaxis from any cause occurs at a rate of 0.4 cases per million individuals per year. Adults have a greater risk of anaphylactic reaction than children do. Females have an increased rate for anaphylaxis to intravenous muscle relaxants, aspirin, and latex, whereas insect sting anaphylaxis is more common in males. The risk of anaphylaxis increases with the length and frequency of encounter with a specific antigen, with repeated interrupted courses of medications conferring the highest risk. The likelihood of a second episode of anaphylaxis to a specific allergen decreases as the interval between original attack and readministration increases. The route of exposure also influences the likelihood of reaction, with parenteral administration having the greatest likelihood of precipitating a reaction. Atopy does not seem to increase susceptibility to anaphylaxis in general. However, atopic individuals have an increased incidence of latex anaphylaxis and are more likely to be receiving allergen immunotherapy.

A wide variety of allergens are capable of provoking anaphylaxis. Antibiotics, including penicillin and other β-lactam antibiotics, are a frequent cause of anaphylaxis. Latex has become an increasingly important cause of anaphylaxis, especially in children with spina bifida or urogenital malformations. Medications administered in the operating room, including induction agents (thiopental), opiates, neuromuscular blocking agents (succinylcholine), protamine, and heparin, may provoke anaphylactoid or anaphylactic reactions. Blood products, including intravenous IgG and allergen immunotherapy extracts, may induce anaphylaxis. Antisera, including antilymphocyte globulin and antitoxins raised in horses (rabies, venom), may elicit anaphylaxis. Foods are a common cause of anaphylaxis in childhood, with peanuts, tree nuts, shellfish, fish, milk, eggs, soy, and wheat triggering reactions with the highest frequencies. Hormones, including insulin, and venoms from the *Hymenoptera* genus may provoke anaphylaxis. Anaphylactoid reactions may follow the administration of aspirin, other cyclooxygenase inhibitors (NSAIDs), and radiographic contrast media. The term idiopathic anaphylaxis is applied to cases of anaphylaxis for which, despite an extensive evaluation, a causative agent cannot be identified.

Anaphylaxis is the result of massive activation of IgE-sensitized mast cells by an allergen. Following introduction of allergen, by either the parenteral, enteral, or, rarely, inhalational route, interaction of the allergen with IgE on the surface of sensitized mast cells leads to mast cell activation and release of preformed and newly formed mediators. Histamine release from mast cells is detected in the blood within 5 to 10 minutes after allergen exposure, and levels remain elevated for 30 to 60 minutes. Urinary levels of histamine (and its metabolites) remain elevated for longer periods. Tryptase, a mast cell–derived protease, reaches peak serum levels 60 to 90 minutes after the onset of anaphylaxis and remains elevated for approximately 4 hours. The interaction between histamine and the type 1 histamine receptor (H_1R) results in increased vascular permeability, vasodilation, smooth muscle contraction, exocrine gland secretion, and irritation of sensory nerves, and may result in coronary artery vasospasm. Activation of type 2 histamine receptors (H_2R) in the heart results in increased heart rate and contractility. Non-IgE-mediated reactions may involve activation of the complement pathway with generation of the anaphylatoxins C3a and C5a, which can bind to their receptors on mast cells and lead to mast cell activation. The effects of these mediators, as well as members of the kinin and coagulation pathways, include the loss of intravascular fluid volume and vasodilation. This may be followed by vasoconstriction and myocardial depression. Hypotension in anaphylaxis correlates with serum levels of histamine, tryptase, and C3a.

Symptoms of anaphylaxis typically begin 5 to 30 minutes after parenteral exposure to allergen but may be delayed up to 2 hours (or more) if the antigen is ingested. Cutaneous symptoms of urticaria and/or angioedema are the most common finding, occurring in 88% of cases. Flushing is reported by nearly one-half of patients with anaphylaxis. Respiratory tract symptoms may include dyspnea or wheezing (47% of cases), edema of the epiglottis, hypopharynx, and/or trachea (56% of cases), and/or rhinitis (16% of cases). Cardiovascular involvement may be manifested by dizziness, syncope, and/or hypotension in 33% of cases. It should be noted that cardiovascular collapse may occur in the absence of cutaneous or respiratory symptoms and may occur secondary to hypotension, dysrhythmia, or myocardial infarction. Patients often report a sense of "impending doom" during the course of an anaphylactic episode. Gastrointestinal complaints include nausea, emesis, abdominal cramping, and/or diarrhea and occur in one-third of cases. Headache is reported by 15% of patients experiencing anaphylaxis. Because the allergic response includes both an early and late phase, it is not surprising that anaphylaxis may include both an early and late phase. "Biphasic anaphylaxis" involves a recrudescence of symptoms several hours after the initial symptoms have subsided and is more common if the initial symptoms developed more than 30 minutes following allergen exposure or if the allergen was administered by mouth. Occasionally, symptoms of anaphylaxis persist for more than 24 hours (protracted anaphylaxis). Death may occur at any time following allergen exposure, even with prompt and appropriate therapy. Postmortem analysis of victims of anaphylaxis discloses acute pulmonary hyperinflation, bronchial edema, eosinophilic infiltration of the pulmonary vasculature, visceral congestion with eosinophils, and elevated serum tryptase levels. Cardiac examination varies from normal myocardium to significant myocardial damage.

TREATMENT AND PREVENTION

Because of the rapid evolution of the anaphylaxis syndrome, prompt recognition and institution of therapy are critical. Fatal episodes of anaphylaxis are often associated with delayed recognition and delayed institution of therapy. Even with timely recognition

and therapy, fatalities do result from anaphylaxis. Several deaths occur each year following the ingestion of foods, especially peanuts. Fatalities are associated with underlying asthma, eating the food away from home, and a delay in the institution of appropriate therapy, particularly epinephrine. Thus, prevention of recurrent episodes is critical. A thorough assessment for the causative agent should be performed. Skin testing is currently available for many foods, penicillin, and *Hymenoptera* venoms to confirm sensitization to these allergens. Extensive education regarding avoidance strategies is imperative. Patients with a history of anaphylaxis should wear medical identification tags and carry a self-injectable epinephrine device. Such devices allow the patient or parent to administer epinephrine immediately on development of symptoms before reaching a medical care facility.

References

Bochner BS, Lichtenstein LM: Anaphylaxis. N Engl J Med 324:1785–1790, 1991

Sampson HA, Mendelson, L, Rosen JP: Fatal and near-fatal anaphylactic reactions to food in children and adolescents. N Engl J Med 327:380–384, 1992

11.14 SERUM SICKNESS

Leonard Bacharier

Serum sickness is the prototypic immune complex (type III) hypersensitivity reaction, originally described following the administration of heterologous serum (eg, equine antitetanus). Unlike an IgE-mediated hypersensitivity reaction, serum sickness can develop following the initial exposure to an antigen and does not require prior sensitization. Because the use of heterologous serum to treat infectious and toxin-mediated diseases has declined, most cases of serum sickness now occur in association with antibiotic therapy. Agents that elicit serum sickness reactions include antimicrobial agents such as cefaclor and penicillin, immunomodulatory antibody products including antithymocyte globulin, antilymphocyte globulin, mouse antihuman OKT3 monoclonal antibodies, and *Hymenoptera* stings.

Unlike the type I (IgE-mediated) hypersensitivity reactions seen in allergic rhinitis and anaphylaxis, which result from the interaction between IgE and a foreign antigen, serum sickness follows the interaction between IgG (and occasionally IgM) and a foreign antigen. This form of hypersensitivity reaction occurs days after exposure to an antigen, following the development of an immune response toward the antigen. As the immune response against a foreign antigen progresses, high-affinity IgG antibodies are generated and combine with soluble antigen to form an antigen-antibody complex. In most situations, these complexes are cleared from the circulation by the reticuloendothelial system without adverse effects. However, if the antigen and antibody are present in sufficiently high concentrations (with moderate antigen excess), intravascular immune complexes form and deposit in blood vessel walls within joints and renal glomeruli. These immune complexes then activate the classical complement pathway, which leads to vascular wall injury and the influx of neutrophils, culminating in inflammation and tissue injury. IgE may also be detected during serum sickness reactions, especially if urticaria is a prominent component.

In primary serum sickness reactions, symptoms typically begin 6 to 12 days following exposure to the inciting agent but may be delayed as much as 3 weeks. However, if an individual has previously been exposed to the antigen, illness may arise 1 to 3 days following exposure. If the initial exposure elicited an IgE response to the antigen, anaphylaxis may occur as well. Clinical findings include a variable combination of fever, cutaneous eruption, joint complaints, lymphadenopathy, myalgia, and proteinuria. Following subcutaneous or intramuscular injection, pruritus and erythema around the injection site may precede the onset of systemic symptoms by 1 to 3 days. Cutaneous findings are always present and include pruritus, erythema, urticaria, angioedema, or other polymorphous eruptions. Administration of antithymocyte globulin to patients undergoing bone marrow transplantation has been associated with a serpiginous eruption over the palms and soles. Arthralgia, and less commonly arthritis, involves multiple joints, including both large (knees and ankles) and small (fingers and toes) joints. Following subcutaneous injection, regional lymph nodes often become enlarged and tender. Peripheral edema occurs in 33% of patients. Gastrointestinal complaints may include nausea, cramping, and diarrhea. Neurologic involvement is uncommon but, when present, may take the form of peripheral neuritis or the Guillain-Barré syndrome. Unlike serum sickness in experimental animal systems, cardiac involvement and nephritis are rare in the human disease. Symptoms usually persist 7 to 10 days and remit spontaneously.

The differential diagnosis for serum sickness reactions should include other processes that include circulating immune complexes (cryoglobulinemia), urticarial vasculitis with depressed complement levels, systemic lupus erythematosus, and acute rheumatic fever. Laboratory evaluation may be helpful in differentiating serum sickness from the above disorders. Peripheral blood leukocyte and eosinophil counts are variable. Circulating plasma cells are noted occasionally. The erythrocyte sedimentation rate may be elevated. Examination of the urine may reveal mild proteinuria. Immune complexes may be detected in the serum by the Raji cell or C1q binding assays. Serum levels of complement components C3 and C4, as well as the total hemolytic complement (CH50), are typically depressed, whereas C1q may be normal or decreased.

The initial step in the treatment of serum sickness is discontinuation of the causative agent. Because this disorder is self-limited, supportive care is generally all that is required. Nonsteroidal anti-inflammatory agents, such as ibuprofen and naproxen sodium, provide relief from fever and arthralgias. Type 1 histamine receptor antagonists, such as hydroxyzine and diphenhydramine, may relieve pruritus and urticaria. If these agents provide inadequate control of symptoms, addition of a systemic steroid such as prednisone at a dose of 1 to 2 mg/kg per day usually provides rapid relief.

The only effective method for the prevention of serum sickness is avoidance of the foreign antigen. If no alternative therapy is available, such as the administration of anti–snake venom derived from horse serum, skin testing may be performed prior to administration. Sequential intradermal injection of tenfold dilutions of horse serum, from 1:100 to 1:10,000, may identify preexisting IgE antibodies directed against horse serum. The absence of a reaction at the highest concentration of horse serum suggests that the likelihood of an IgE-mediated anaphylactic reaction is very low but does not exclude the possibility of a serum sickness reaction.

References

Bieloryl L, Gascon P, Lawley T, et al: Human serum sickness: a prospective analysis of 35 patients treated with equine antithymocyte globulin for bone marrow failure. Medicine 67:40–57, 1988

Kearns GL, Wheeler JG, Childress SH, et al: Serum sickness-like reactions to cefaclor: role of hepatic metabolism and individual susceptibility. J Pediatr 125:805–811, 1994

RHEUMATOLOGY

David N. Glass, Associate Editor

12.1 PATHOGENIC MECHANISMS IN THE INFLAMMATORY RHEUMATIC DISEASES OF CHILDHOOD

Susan D. Thompson and David N. Glass

At least 100,000 children per annum are likely to attend a pediatric rheumatology unit with musculoskeletal problems and at least as many are probably seen by other physicians, including rheumatologists with an adult practice, orthopedic surgeons, and sports medicine specialists. The majority of these children will have syndromes of short duration, some of an inflammatory nature, while other children will have one of the many pain syndromes that affect children and give rise to musculoskeletal symptomatology. A smaller portion, perhaps 20% of the whole, will have a chronic inflammatory rheumatic disease (Table 12-1). The chronic diseases, although affecting only a small number of patients, are a major cause of morbidity, and sometimes of mortality, in childhood and tend to have common pathogenic mechanisms with features of autoimmunity. Mechanisms of underlying diseases such as juvenile rheumatoid arthritis (JRA), spondyloarthropathy, juvenile onset dermatomyositis, systemic lupus erythematosus (SLE), and scleroderma are reviewed in this chapter.

AUTOIMMUNITY

A variety of demographic, genetic, and pathologic features, present in varying degrees, characterize organ-specific and systemic autoimmune diseases.

Demographic Features

Common demographic features include characteristic age of onset patterns (see Fig. 12-1), gender biases, and a tendency for quite marked ethnic differences in disease occurrence. Most autoimmune diseases save for the spondyloarthropathies have an excess occurrence in females. The majority of paraphenomena, including the detection of autoantibodies, are also much more prevalent in females than in males. Different ethnic groups appear to be differentially susceptible to autoimmune diseases, and clinical phenotypes for a given disease may show marked differences between ethnic groups. For example, early-onset pauciarticular-onset JRA is rare in non-white populations; however, the genetic and/or environmental basis for these differences remains unknown.

Genetic Features

Family History

A family history of the disease affecting the proband and of other autoimmune diseases, especially in first- and second-degree female relatives of the proband, is common. In pediatric rheumatology this is perhaps best documented in dermatomyositis. However, the pattern of inheritance is infrequently that of a traditional monogenic disease with a mendelian lineage. For example, a family history of juvenile rheumatoid arthritis is uncommon and when reported usually involves affected siblings, with a somewhat higher concordance for affected twins, although mother/daughter combinations have also been reported. Indeed, in the past, the relative rarity of the disease suggested that this familial occurrence is related to chance. An alternative view gathering substantial credence is that diseases such as JRA and SLE are complex genetic traits with multiple contributing loci throughout the genome. These loci can be divided into those that are disease-specific, which include HLA (human leukocyte antigens) loci, and those that predispose to autoimmunity in general, which include MHC (major histocompatibility complex)-linked non-HLA loci.

HLA Associations and Linkage

The HLA region spans approximately 4000 kilobases on the short arm of chromosome 6 and may contain greater than 300 genes that code for a variety of proteins required by the immune system along with the well-studied HLA class I, II, and III molecules. Linkage to HLA alleles in this large region does not necessarily implicate a particular HLA gene in pathogenesis; MHC-linked non-HLA genes may also be involved in the disease process. These non-HLA genes may regulate synthesis or removal of proteins that mediate inflammation, including cytokine genes such as those coding for tumor necrosis factor (TNF) or the complement genes, which have been implicated in predisposition to SLE.

Many HLA associations are well documented in pediatric rheumatic diseases; such associations may represent true linkage between the disease and HLA but may also represent stratification due to incomplete mixing of the population, a *founder effect*. The subtypes of JRA have their own individual HLA associations, which are of varying strengths (Table 12-2). For at least one type of JRA, pauciarticular disease, linkage has been shown by a strategy involving simplex families in a process known as the *transmission disequilibrium test*.

Non-HLA Region Genes

The involvement of genes outside the HLA locus is a credible explanation for the nonmendelian patterns of inheritance in autoimmune diseases. In JRA, candidate genes under study include the IL-10 gene, for which genotypes containing a polymorphism in the 5' flanking region associated with lower IL-10 production were significantly associated with extended oligoarthritis. Genome-wide screens in populations with pediatric rheumatologic diseases have not been completed, although data being generated in adult-onset rheumatoid arthritis and SLE are clearly applicable in some pediatric rheumatology patients.

TABLE 12-1

AUTOIMMUNE FEATURES OF PEDIATRIC RHEUMATIC DISEASE

AUTOIMMUNE FEATURE	PAUCI JRA (EARLY ONSET)	PAUCI JRA (SPONDYLO-ARTHROPATHY)	POLY JRA	SYSTEMIC JRA	JUVENILE DERMATOMYOSITIS	SCLERODERMA	SYSTEMIC LUPUS ERYTHEMATOSUS
Age of onset	0–6 years	7+ years	0–4 years 6+ years	Throughout childhood	1–13 years	Throughout childhood	Throughout childhood, increasing through puberty
Gender	F>>>M	M>>F	F>M	M=F	F>M	F>M	F>>M
Ethnicity	White	All	All	–	++	–	+++
Familial index disease	++	+++	++	+	+/–	+/–	+
Family history of other autoimmune diseases	+++	++	+++	+/–	+++	+/–	++
HLA genes	++++	++++	++	+/–	+	++	+
Non-HLA genes	+	+	+/–	–	–	–	++
Lymphocytes	++	++	++	++	++	++	++
Antigen presenting cells	+++	+++	+++	+++	++	–	
Circulating autoantibodies	ANA anti-DEK antibodies	None	Can be IgM RF+ or IgM RF–	None	ANA(+) Jo(–)	Scl 70	ANA anti-DNA
Synovial T-cell clonality	++	+	+++	+	+	?	+

JRA, juvenile rheumatoid arthritis; RF, rheumatoid factor; IgM, immunoglobulin M; ANA, antinuclear antigen.

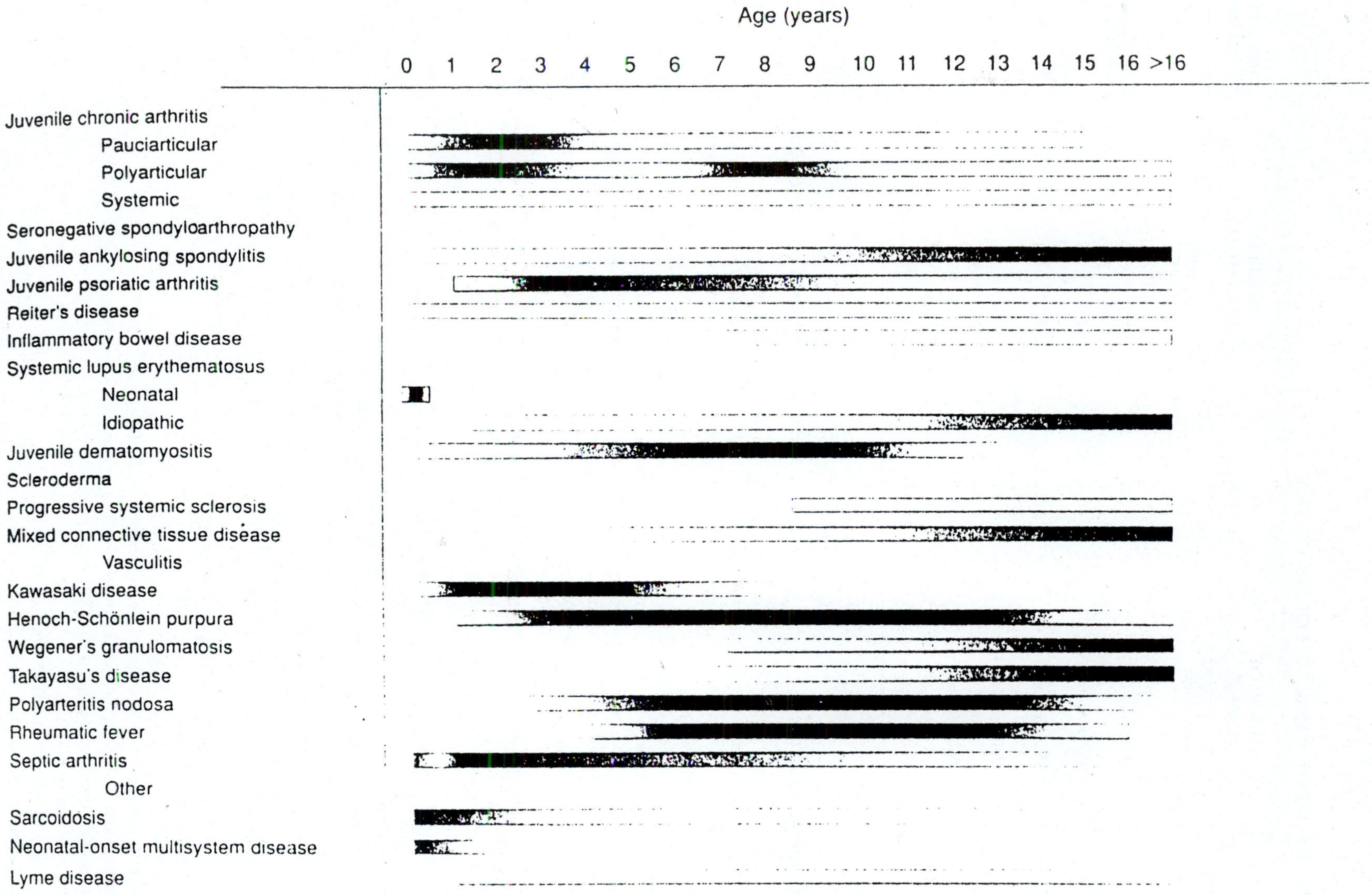

Age (years)

0 1 2 3 4 5 6 7 8 9 10 11 12 13 14 15 16 >16

FIGURE 12-1 Characteristic ages of onset of rheumatic diseases of childhood. *Petty RE: in Oxford Textbook of Rheumatology, JP Maddison, ed: 2nd ed. Oxford University Press, New York, 1998.*

BLE 12-2

LA ASSOCIATIONS WITH VARIOUS FORMS OF JRA

DISEASE ONSET TYPE	COURSE OF DISEASE	HLA TYPE	ALLELE SPECIFICITY	RELATIVE/ODDS RISK/RATIO
Pauciarticular	Pauciarticular	A2	DRA1 *0201	4.6
		DR5	DRB1 *1104	2.8–7
		DP2	DPB1 *0201	4.3
	Pauci and Poly	DR8	DRB1 *0801	4.3–10.3
		DR6	DPB1 *1301	2.8–10
	Polyarticular	DR1	DRB1 *0101	2.5
		DQ1	DQA1 *0101	2.8–4.6
	Pauciarticular	DR4	DRB1 *0401	0.3–0.02
		DR7		0.1
Systemic	Polyarticular	DR4	DRB1 *0401	2.6
		DP4	DP1 *0401	0.3
Polyarticular (RF−)	Polyarticular	DP3	DPB1 *0301	2.8
		DP8	DRB1 *0801	8.2
Polyarticular (RF+)	Polyarticular	DR4	DRB1 *0401/04	6.8

Footnote: From Dr. J. Brezinski (Unpublished).

The Chronic Inflammatory Process

The histopathologic hallmark of autoimmunity is a round-cell infiltrate composed of lymphocytes, plasma cells, and antigen-presenting cells, including dendritic cells and macrophages. Further analysis of these cells identifies phenotypes indicative of memory and activation, including the expression of CD45RO and IL-2 receptor on the T lymphocytes; products of the activation process such as the cytokines IFN-γ and TNF-α; and smaller specialized cytokines (chemokines) involved in cell trafficking, such as MCP-1, RANTES, and MIP-α, and an up-regulation of their receptors. In addition, the surface expression of adhesion molecules may provide a structural basis for the localization of cells at the site of the inflammatory process.

The cell types which may be contributing to this process in the joint extend beyond those of the immune system to chondrocytes, an important cellular component of cartilage, and to fibroblasts and monocyte-derived cells that, respectively, comprise the A and B cells of the synovial lining. All of these cells can release mediators of inflammation, which themselves contribute to cell localization and activation, as well as to angiogenesis, an important part of the inflammatory process. Proinflammatory cytokines such as TNF-α, IL-2, and IL-6 are secreted by CD4+ and CD8+ T cells. Broadly speaking, autoimmune disease may result from imbalances between these two subsets.

Autoimmune diseases arising from a delayed hypersensitivity response are associated with a proinflammatory Th1 (Tc1) or type 1 cytokine response, whereas the type 2 cytokines may depress this inflammatory response to some extent. In contrast, in immediate hypersensitivity reactions such as asthma, the type 2 cytokines, particularly IL-4 tend to sustain the disease process. In JRA, the type 1 cytokines are found much more readily.

The fact that mediators of inflammation are detected in tissues of many types of autoimmune disease can lead to common therapeutic strategies. The recent successful introduction of TNF-α-specific antibody and TNF-soluble receptor treatments for RA and JRA are striking examples of biologicals that may be used in many autoimmune diseases, including those seen by pediatric rheumatologists.

Antigen-Specific Immune Response

A defining feature of autoimmunity is the presence of autoantibodies, which are indicative of a self-reactive immunologic response in involved tissues. Although the target antigens are autologous, the inciting event leading to their generation may be a cross-reacting exogenous molecule. Detection and quantitation of these autoantibodies may have clinical utility. Evidence of T- or B-cell clonality, or the identification of multiple expanded clones that are structurally similar in the CDR3 site for antigen recognition, constitute the strongest evidence of ongoing antigen presentation in a chronically inflamed joint.

Environmental Triggers

Although no infectious agent(s) have been definitively established as the cause of JRA, an environmental component has been suggested by documented changes in the prevalence of JRA over two decades. In addition, seasonality has been described for systemic-onset disease. In pauciarticular JRA, the peak age of onset at 1 to 3 years and the rare occurrence before 6 months of age or after the seventh birthday suggest exposure to an infectious agent of early childhood during a period of immunologic vulnerability. In all likelihood, the mechanisms of pathogenesis for pediatric rheumatic disease will one day be defined on both the environmental and genetic levels where exogenous triggers result in autoimmunity only in genetically predisposed individuals.

References

Albani S: Infection and molecular mimicry in autoimmune diseases of childhood. Clin Exp Rheumatol 12 (Suppl 10):S35–41, 1994

Becker KG, Simon RM, Bailey-Wilson JE, et al: Clustering of non-major histocompatibility complex susceptibility candidate loci in human autoimmune diseases. Proc Natl Acad Sci U S A 95:9979–9984, 1998

Ginn LR, Lin JP, Plotz PH, et al: Familial autoimmunity in pedigrees of idiopathic inflammatory myopathy patients suggests common genetic risk factors for many autoimmune diseases. Arthritis Rheum 41:400–405, 1998

Glass DN, Giannini EG: Juvenile rheumatoid arthritis as a complex genetic trait. Arthritis Rheum 42(11):2261–2268, 1999

Moroldo MB, Donnelly P, Saunders J, Glass DN, Giannini EH: Transmission disequilibrium as a test of linkage and association between HLA alleles and pauciarticular-onset juvenile rheumatoid arthritis. Arthritis Rheum 41:1620–1624, 1998

Mosmann TR, Coffman RL: TH1 and TH2 cells: different patterns of lymphokine secretion lead to different functional properties. Annu Rev Immunol 7:145–173, 1989.

Petty RE, Southwood TR, Baum J, et al: Revision of the proposed classification criteria for juvenile idiopathic arthritis: Durban, 1997 [see comments]. J Rheumatol 25:1991–1994, 1998

Romagnani S: Lymphokine production by human T cells in disease states. Ann Rev Immunol 12:227–257, 1994

12.2   GENERAL APPROACH TO RHEUMATOLOGIC DISEASE IN CHILDREN AND ADOLESCENTS

Murray H. Passo

The approach to rheumatologic diseases (RD) must include a dual consideration of systemic and musculoskeletal conditions. Often, the musculoskeletal component is a small contributor to the overall symptomatology of the patient. Four categories of diseases or conditions are considered in the process of evaluation: (a) focal rheumatologic conditions related to abnormal anatomy, overuse, or localized inflammation; (b) systemic diseases with rheumatologic manifestations; (c) rheumatologic diseases with systemic manifestations; and (d) biopsychosocial conditions with musculoskeletal symptoms. Psychological contributions, either primary or secondary, enter into the patient's symptoms in virtually all cases. The physician must weigh both the subjective symptom of pain and the objective evidence of compromised function; the pediatrician also needs to assess the parents' perception of pain.

The cardinal components of the history and physical examination provide a diagnosis in the majority of cases. The interview also enables the physician to understand the behavioral, emotional, and attitudinal aspects of the situation. Table 12-3 provides a scheme for the general approach to rheumatic diseases.

Host Factors

Host factors suggest diagnostic possibilities before the patient is interviewed. With some diseases, categories may overlap, but the majority of patients cluster in the groups as listed in Table 12-4.

Hereditary Factors

The family history is helpful in providing clues or risk factors for rheumatologic conditions; particularly spondyloarthropathies; inflammatory bowel diseases; familial Mediterranean fever; psoriasis; rheumatic fever; and, to a lesser extent, immune thyroid diseases; fibromyalgia; rheumatoid arthritis; and lupus. Although not hereditary, environmental and situational factors contribute to symptoms in many cases.

History and Physical Examination

A comprehensive, scrupulous compilation of details helps to identify the features suggestive of the rheumatic diseases (see Table

TABLE 12-3

SEQUENCE OF EVALUATION FOR SUSPECTED RHEUMATIC DISEASE

Evaluate for the following:
    Any obvious host factors?
    Characterize chief complaint—location, features
    Multisystemic involvement
    Identify high-risk visceral signs and symptoms
    Functional assessment of patient
    Laboratory evaluation targeted at clues above
    Imaging strategy dictated by signs/symptoms
    Organ-specific diagnostic tests
    Compilation of data and synthesis of treatment plan

12-4). This cannot be overemphasized as the most meaningful information to obtain before moving to laboratory testing and radiologic studies.

Common Features Suggestive of Rheumatic Diseases (RD)

Rheumatic diseases overlap virtually every subspeciality area of medicine. Fever, fatigue, musculoskeletal pain, dermatologic conditions, ocular symptoms, and mucous membrane findings are common. Multisystemic involvement is suggestive of RD. Vascular manifestations, both micro- and macrovascular, such as Raynaud phenomenon, focal ischemia or infarction, hypertension, migraine, and vasculitis are common signs in RD.

Assessment of Severity

Functional Assessment

In the general approach to the RD, evaluation of patient's functional status is important in the overall assessment. Are the patient's daily activities interrupted? How has pain or immobility impacted quality of life and the ability to uphold vocational (school) and avocational (recreation, social) responsibilities? Is the patient rendered dependent on help for essential activities? Is the degree of impairment corroborated by objective findings?

Diseases Requiring Immediate Identification and Treatment

Several rheumatic diseases present with or subsequently develop life-threatening complications that require immediate intervention: (a) *acute rheumatic fever* with pancarditis or chorea; (b) *systemic JRA* with pericarditis (rarely myocarditis) and macrophage activation syndrome; (c) *systemic lupus erythematosus* (SLE) with involvement of the cardiac, pulmonary, or central nervous system; cytopenias; hypercoagulopathy; and rapidly progressive renal involvement; (d) *dermatomyositis* with gastrointestinal ischemia, profound muscle weakness with respiratory insufficiency, dysphagia, dysphonia, and cutaneous infarctions; and (e) *acute vasculitis* syndromes such as Kawasaki disease, polyarteritis nodosum (PAN), and any hypertensive or CNS crisis.

Any suspicion of infection in bone or joint, malignancy, or structural derangement such as avascular necrosis of bone or slipped capital epiphysis requires immediate consultation. Biopsychosocial rheumatic conditions that cause significant school absences and an inability to uphold responsibilities require immediate attention and

TABLE 12-4
CLUSTERING OF RHEUMATIC DISEASES BY DEMOGRAPHIC CATEGORIES

HOST FACTORS

Age*	Infant	Toddler/Preschool	Schoolage	Adolescent
	NOMID	JRA	HSP	Fibromyalgia
	Neonatal lupus	Kawasaki disease	Rheumatic fever	JRA
	Neonatal sarcoid	Growing pains	SLE	SLE
	Joint infection	Psoriatic arthritis	Hypermobility	Enthesis-related arthritis
			Dermatomyositis	Vasculitis

Gender	Female	Male
	Autoimmune diseases	Spondyloarthropathy
	JRA	Vasculitides
	Hypermobility syndrome	
	Fibromyalgia	
	Uveitis, chronic	

Race/Ethnicity	
	Native American—B27/spondyloarthropathy
	African-American—SLE, dermatomyositis, sarcoid
	Asian—Behçet, SLE, vasculitis
	White—JRA
	Jewish—Inflammatory bowel diseases, familial Mediterranean fever

* *Cassidy JT, Petty RE, eds: Textbook of Pediatric Rheumatology. Philadelphia, W.B. Saunders, 1995.*
NOMID, neonatal-onset multisystem inflammatory disease; JRA, juvenile rheumatoid arthritis; SLE, systemic lupus erythematosus, HSP, Henoch-Schönlein purpura.

expeditious intervention; included under this heading are reflex sympathetic dystrophy, psychogenic rheumatism, and fibromyalgia.

Laboratory Investigation

Laboratory testing to provide supportive evidence of rheumatic disease includes a urinalysis, complete blood count (CBC) with differential, erythrocyte sedimentation rate (ESR) or C-reactive protein, and selected chemistries. These tests are only an adjunct to signs and symptoms noted from the history and physical examination. These tests are rarely diagnostic of a specific disease; rather, they provide evidence of chronic disease, end organ dysfunction, or inflammation.

A urinalysis for protein or blood is a useful screen to glean evidence of glomerular injury as seen in SLE, subacute bacterial endocarditis (SBE), PAN, and Henoch-Schönlein purpura (HSP), for example.

A CBC with platelet quantitation and white blood cell differential is helpful in several aspects. Each component of the CBC may suggest a rheumatic disease or underlying systemic disease with rheumatic symptoms. Moderate anemia with a normochromic or hypochromic pattern and a low reticulocyte count may indicate an inflammatory process that has been present for at least several weeks. More profound anemia requires further evaluation for hemolysis, malignancy, bone marrow suppression, or blood loss. The patient with systemic-onset JRA may have severe anemia, reaching a nadir of 6 to 7 g/dL without blood loss or hemolysis after several weeks.

An elevated white blood cell (WBC) count occurs with infections, systemic-onset JRA, Kawasaki disease, and hematologic malignancies. A low WBC count may be seen in viral or postviral illnesses, SLE, or hematologic malignancies, especially in acute lymphoblastic leukemia. A high platelet count is typical of most chronic inflammatory diseases, while a low platelet count is seen in SLE, viral infection, and infiltrative processes in the bone marrow

such as leukemia. Beware of low platelet count in systemic JRA, which would herald macrophage activation syndrome (MAS) (see Sec. 12.4).

Elevated acute-phase reactants, such as the erythrocyte sedimentation rate (ESR), C-reactive protein (CRP), platelets, and fibrinogen indicate an inflammatory disease or tissue injury as opposed to a mechanical disease. Marked elevation of the ESR to greater than 100 mm/h suggests systemic-onset JRA, acute rheumatic fever, vasculitis, SLE, or malignancy. A high ESR in an ill-appearing child with thrombocytopenia suggests an infiltrative process in the bone marrow: malignancy, SLE, or infection (tuberculosis, disseminated histoplasmosis, or HIV infection). A low ESR in an ill-appearing child suggests hypofibrinogenemia seen in disseminated intravascular coagulation, a component of MAS.

Blood chemistries are ordered as indicated by the findings in the history and physical examination. Five muscle-related enzymes, including creatine kinase, aldolase, AST, ALT, and lactic dehydrogenase (LDH), are useful if muscle disease is suspected. If underlying malignancy is suspected, abnormal uric acid and LDH measurements may prompt consultation with a hematologist.

Joint aspiration is essential in a febrile child with monarticular swelling in which infection is suspected. The synovial fluid analysis includes gross appearance for turbidity, routine bacterial culture and Gram stain, WBC count with differential, and glucose concentration. In inflammatory arthritis, such as JRA, the WBC count may range from 2000 to 100,000 WBC/μL with over 25% neutrophils; glucose concentration is typically at least half that of plasma or serum glucose; and cultures for bacteria, mycobacteria, and fungi are negative. Infection is suspected when WBC count is greater than 50,000 and neutrophils exceed 90% of the differential with low glucose concentration. Exceptions include viral infection, gonococcal arthritis in which the WBC count may be lower, and a sympathetic effusion ascribable to osteomyelitis.

Serology for group A β-hemolytic streptococcus is critical for diagnosing acute rheumatic fever because the diagnosis requires evidence of a preceding streptococcal infection. Because the antistreptolysin O (ASO) titer is elevated in only 70 to 80% of people with acute rheumatic fever, the addition of a second antistreptococcal antibody, such as anti-DNase B, increases the likelihood of detecting a recent streptococcal infection to 95%.

Lyme serology and Western blot assays are helpful when a suggestive history and physical findings are present. Because false-positive Lyme enzyme-linked immunosorbent assays (ELISAs) may occur in some rheumatic diseases, a Western blot assay is required to confirm or negate the diagnosis. A high percentage of children living in areas in which *Ixodes dammini* is endemic (eg, Connecticut, Massachusetts, upper Midwest) will have positive serologies in the absence of disease attributable to the spirochete.

The antinuclear antibody (ANA) and rheumatoid factor tests are often performed to assess musculoskeletal complaints. These tests are most useful in the context of objective arthritis or multisystem disease suggestive of SLE or another connective tissue disease. Their interpretation is rarely simple, and neither test is sensitive or specific enough to be conclusive.

As many as 9% of healthy children have a low-positive ANA (1:10) and no associated disease. Studies have shown that the combination of a positive ANA test and joint pain do not predict the development of JRA or SLE. In the presence of compelling physical findings and a suggestive history, however, a positive ANA test or rheumatoid factor is valuable supportive evidence. A negative ANA test does not exclude SLE or JRA, and a positive ANA test is not diagnostic or disease-specific. A positive ANA test may be seen in any of the connective tissue diseases, SLE, mixed connective tissue disease (MCTD), systemic sclerosis, dermatomyositis, Sjögren syndrome, or JRA. JRA is much more common, whereas the other connective tissue diseases have additional features such as visceral involvement. Importantly, among patients with systemic JRA, those who have the greatest visceral involvement are usually ANA- and RF-negative. A positive rheumatoid factor test is seen in only 10% of patients with JRA and a small number of patients with SLE, Sjögren syndrome, and MCTD. Positive titers are also seen in chronic infection, such as subacute bacterial endocarditis, osteomyelitis, leprosy, and sarcoidosis. Thus, the ANA and RF must be analyzed in the context of objective abnormalities and signs/symptoms of the entire clinical condition.

The interpretation of most other assays for autoantibodies, such as SSA (anti-Ro), SSB (anti-La), and RNP (antiribonucleoprotein) is even more complex but may narrow the diagnosis to SLE, MCTD, or Sjögren syndrome. A few autoantibodies are quite specific but not very sensitive. Anti-Sm antibodies (Smith) and anti-double-stranded (or native) DNA antibodies, for example, are seen almost exclusively in SLE, but many SLE patients do not have them. Direct agglutination test (DAT) or direct Coombs test may be positive in SLE or MCTD and may not necessarily be indicative of active hemolysis.

Inherited complement deficiencies predispose children to various illnesses, including SLE. Serum levels of complement proteins C3 and C4 may be abnormally low in SLE and in some rare types of vasculitis, such as urticaria with hypocomplementemic vasculitis. In contrast, levels of complement proteins C3 and C4 are elevated in Wegener's granulomatosis, HSP, Kawasaki disease, and PAN. Levels of complement proteins provide clues to disease activity only in the context of SLE, vasculitis, and glomerulonephritis. Hypocomplementemic forms of glomerulonephritis include SLE, membranoproliferative, poststreptococcal (C3), and other chronic bacteremic infections, such as subacute bacterial endocarditis and shunt nephritis.

Quantitation of immunoglobulin levels may suggest evidence of RD in two ways: (a) Immunoglobulin A deficiency, the most common immunodeficiency, affects at least 1 in 1000 people and is associated with an increased risk for JRA-like arthritis, as well as other autoimmune diseases, such as thyroiditis, myasthenia gravis, autoimmune thrombocytopenia, and pernicious anemia. (b) Panhypogammaglobulinemia, as in Bruton disease, may be associated with a polyarthritis. Indirect evidence of RD may be seen with elevated levels of one or more immunoglobulins because of chronic immune stimulation.

Imaging Studies

The use of imaging studies in the evaluation of rheumatic diseases is growing in sophistication and availability. Initial evaluation usually includes plain-film radiographs of the involved area. Obtaining radiographs of both the affected and unaffected sides—both wrists, for example—makes it easier to assess for asymmetric changes in bone maturation and structural changes. Acute changes on plain film are seen in fractures and existing dysplasias, bone malformations, and preexisting diseases (preclinical) such as malignancy. Evidence of bony changes on plain film requires 10 to 14 days or more in osteomyelitis or avascular necrosis, and months to years in JRA.

Computerized tomography is an excellent modality to image bone detail in selected cases, such as osteoid osteoma, spondylolysis, and joint disease with bone destruction secondary to longstanding disease. Cervical vertebrae, temporomandibular joints, and sacroiliac joints are particularly difficult to evaluate by plain film and are best imaged by CT scanning. Ultrasound modalities are helpful to identify joint fluid, tenosynovitis, bursitis, and cystic structures, and are used therapeutically to aspirate or inject these structures. Doppler ultrasound is valuable in evaluation of the vasculitides with occlusive disease or aneurysm formation.

Magnetic resonance imaging (MRI) and spectroscopy are informative in identification of soft-tissue injury, marrow infiltration, and inflammation. Contrast-enhanced imaging with gadolinium provides details of synovium, intra-articular fluid, and nonbone periarticular and intra-articular structures. Intramedullary infarction, tumor, and bone marrow replacement are seen with MRI. Abnormal enhancement of inflamed muscle serves as a guide for biopsy site selection in myopathies, especially dermatomyositis. Spectroscopy will potentially provide information about metabolic abnormalities in tissues as the field expands.

Special studies are selected systematically by recommendation of the radiologists and subspecialists for evaluation of organ-specific problems, such as central nervous system imaging, high-resolution chest CT for lung fibrosis and obstructive lesions, and imaging of gastrointestinal and intraabdominal structures.

^{99m}Tc-phosphate bone scanning early in the course of disease can often localize ischemia (AVN), infection, or tumor before these lesions are apparent on plain film, thus leading to early intervention. Dual-photon dexatometry (bone densitometry) permits evaluation for osteoporosis, a common problem in JRA and in patients treated with corticosteroids.

An important concept in the evaluation of rheumatic diseases is the principle that the clinical spectrum of these dynamic diseases evolves over a period of months to years. The history, physical examination, and selective laboratory tests with imaging studies will provide the data to build the evidence for inflammatory diseases, to eliminate other diseases, and to corroborate the biopsychosocial conditions that enter into the entire spectrum of rheumatic diseases.

References

Cabral DA, Petty RE, Fung M. et al: Persistent antinuclear antibodies in children without identifiable inflammatory rheumatic or autoimmune disease. Pediatrics 89(3):441–444, 1992.

Cawkwell GD, Passo MH: Pursuing the source of musculoskeletal pain. Contemp Peds 11:7290–7294, 1994.

Graham TB, Blebea JS, Gylys-Morin V, et al: Magnetic resonance imaging in juvenile rheumatoid arthritis. Semin Arthritis Rheum 27(3):161–168, 1997.

Grassi W, Cervini C: Ultrasonography in rheumatology: an evolving technique. Ann Rheum Dis 57:268–271, 1998.

Harcke HT, Mandell GA, Cassell IL. Imaging techniques in childhood arthritis. Rheum Dis Clin North Am 23(3):523–544, 1997.

Petty RE: Children and adolescents. In: Maddison JP, ed. Oxford Textbook of Rheumatology, 2nd ed. Oxford, UK, Oxford University Press, 1998.

12.3 EVALUATION OF MUSCULOSKELETAL PAIN

Murray H. Passo

Although the majority of children who have recurrent limb pain have no demonstrable organic lesion, the evaluation of musculoskeletal pain is a common problem for the primary care physician. Reports indicate that up to 15% of school-age children have occasional limb pain and that 4.5% of children experience pain severe enough to cause interruption of normal activities for longer than 3 months. Between 5 and 10% of children have psychosomatic illnesses, and psychosomatic musculoskeletal complaints account for more than 10% of new patient referrals to pediatric rheumatology centers. Fewer than 0.1% of children, however, have juvenile rheumatoid arthritis (JRA), and a similar small percentage have pains caused by other chronic rheumatic disease. This chapter focuses on the history and physical examination, on the use of screening laboratory tests and diagnostic imaging, and on the differential diagnosis of musculoskeletal pain in childhood.

An evaluation for musculoskeletal pain must differentiate among (a) a primary musculoskeletal disease, (b) an underlying systemic disease, and (c) a "benign" syndrome with no obvious organic etiology. A psychological contribution to the pain enters, either primarily or secondarily, into almost all cases and needs to be considered.

The anatomic structures involved in the etiology of musculoskeletal pain include skin, subcutaneous fat, fascia, muscle, bone, joint capsule, ligaments, tendons, entheses, and nerves. The *enthesis* is the insertion site of the ligament, tendon, or fascia on bone, and is especially involved in spondyloarthropathies. Usually a combination of anatomic structures is involved in a single disease process. Considering infection, noninfectious inflammation, malignancy, metabolic, or traumatizing injury to these tissues permits the development of a long list of different disease processes that could be the cause of the pain.

CHIEF COMPLAINT

Pain is a subjective complaint that can only be described by the sufferer; however, in pediatrics, one has to rely on the parents' perceptions and on the behavior, altered function, and objective changes that the child exhibits. Additionally, the parents' attitude toward the child's complaints may provide insight. Previous experience with pain as well as the current emotional status of the patient may influence the intensity of the pain. The seasoned clinician recognizes that the "chief" complaint may not be what is actually bothering the patient or parents the most; often there is a "hidden agenda."

Location

The profile of pain described by Engel (1970) included the six dimensions listed in Table 12-5. The first task is to identify the location of the pain as precisely as possible. Pain can be referred from proximal or distal structures, as is the case with hip pain referred to the medial knee. It is important to determine details of the circumstances when the pain was first noticed. Have the patient describe the onset of the symptoms. Was the onset acute versus insidious? The precise details of the chronology can be extremely helpful. Mechanical problems or anatomic derangements are usually worsened by movement. Is the major symptom pain or *stiffness*? Joint stiffness should be distinguished from pain. Stiffness after long periods of immobility suggests an inflammatory arthropathy but can also be a sign of a noninflammatory condition called *fibromyalgia*.

Is a single area involved, or have sites been additive, episodic, or migratory? Migratory arthritis is defined as involvement of a few joints and subsequent involvement of other joints as the previously affected joints improve; in additive arthritis, the initial joints do not resolve, and additional joints are affected. Table 12-6 includes examples of each pattern.

Temporal Aspects

The frequency, duration, and variability of episodes are important in analyzing recurrent or intermittent bouts of pain. Knowledge of the intensity of the pain can be helpful when it correlates with objective physical findings; pain that is disproportionately severe may suggest malignancy or acute rheumatic fever when corroborated by other historical or clinical information. The qualitative aspect of the pain (ie, throbbing, aching, burning, or tingling) may be difficult for children to describe. Burning and tingling suggest nerve involvement. Nighttime pain often suggests intramedullary bone pressure seen in avascular necrosis, bone marrow replacement with malignancy, or osteoid osteoma, a benign bone tumor.

Persistent daytime and nighttime pain indicates serious disease. Does the pain interrupt sleep or daily activities, including vocational, recreational, and school participation. In addition, the phy-

TABLE 12-5

PAIN PROFILE—A DESCRIPTION OF PAIN

Aspects to be described:
1. Topographical—location as precisely as possible
2. Quantitative—intensity: negligible, tolerable, intractable, excruciating
3. Temporal—chronology, frequency, duration, variability, pattern of involvement, periodicity, course
4. Qualitative—description of what the patient feels: throbbing, aching, burning, pressure
5. Associated physiological aspects—aggravating or alleviating factors; effects of activity, rest, movement; associated symptoms
6. Behavioral and psychological—changes in life's routine, responsibility, and recreation; secondary gain; conversion mechanism; depression, anxiety, anger

TABLE 12-6

DIFFERENTIAL DIAGNOSIS OF PATTERNS OF JOINT INVOLVEMENT

MIGRATORY JOINT INVOLVEMENT	EPISODIC JOINT INVOLVEMENT	ADDITIVE JOINT INVOLVEMENT	MONARTICULAR INVOLVEMENT

• Acute rheumatic fever
• Disseminated gonococcal infection
• Leukemia
• Henoch-Schönlein purpura
• Meningococcemia, chronic
• Post-*Yersinia enterocolitica*
• Post-*Mycoplasma* pneumonia
• Inflammatory bowel disease
• Whipple disease
	• Inflammatory bowel disease
	• Leukemia
	• Recurrent rheumatic fever
	• Lyme disease
	• Crystal-induced arthritis (rare)
	• HLA-B27 arthropathies
	• Benign hypermobility syndrome
	• JEA—juvenile episodic arthritis
	• Patellofemoral compartment syndrome
		• JRA
		• Spondyloarthropathies
		• Any connective tissue disease
			• Infectious arthritis
			• Adjacent osteomyelitis
			• Pauciarticular JRA
			• Reactive arthritis
			• Other idiopathic arthritides
			• Anatomic abnormalities
			  – Osteochondritis dissecans
			  – Avascular necrosis
			  – Slipped capital femoral epiphysis
			• Villonodular synovitis
			• Primary bone tumors
			• Overuse syndromes
			• Trauma

sician should be sensitive to whether the complaint is being used for secondary gain. Is the child depressed or anxious, or seemingly unconcerned?

Complaints of swelling, limitation of motion, alterations in locomotion and usual daily activities, stiffness, fatigability, weakness, and lack of stamina are sought. One must establish whether the complaints are solely subjective or whether objective changes such as fever, weight loss, or rashes have been observed. Asking for examples is often helpful in determining the significance of the complaint. Enlarged bone contours are sometimes misinterpreted as swelling. Try to determine the duration of objective findings, particularly because some findings bear less significance if they are fleeting, lasting only a few minutes. Explore antecedent events such as travel, trauma, infections, recent activity, immunizations, exposure to hepatitis or blood products, tick bites, and current medications.

REVIEW OF SYSTEMS

Perhaps the most helpful part of the history in identifying an underlying systemic disease is the thorough review of systems, readily accomplished during the physical examination. A list of signs and symptoms with associated diseases is listed in Table 12-7. Clues from the review of systems can also provide evidence of a functional or psychosomatic disease. Some of these patients complain of pain in numerous areas, including headaches, chest pain, and abdominal pain.

The patient should be questioned explicitly about impaired growth; weight loss; alopecia; oral and genital ulcerations; gastrointestinal dysfunction; menstrual changes; Raynaud phenomenon; recurrent infection; bruising; nervousness; sleep alterations; and poor school attendance. Experiences for acquisition of sexually transmitted diseases must be explored in the age-appropriate patient with unexplained tenosynovitis, migratory polyarthritis, or acute oligoarthritis.

PAST MEDICAL HISTORY

The past medical history should include previous episodes of the same complaint. Rheumatic fever, periodic syndromes, immunodeficiencies, and other disease states often have previous episodes that are mimetic of the current complaints.

One needs to review the family medical history and the current status of the family health and social situation. Children often im-

itate pain that is present in another family member, and they may develop pain in response to family stress. The family history may be contributory if there is inflammatory bowel disease, psoriasis, spondyloarthropathies, or other autoimmune phenomena such as thyroid disease, multiple sclerosis, lupus, or rheumatoid arthritis.

What previous attempts have been made to diagnose or treat the symptom? Acquisition of old records, including laboratory and imaging results, can give some insight into the amount of attention that has been sought for this complaint. Ask about previous medical and paramedical encounters, prescribed medications, over-the-counter therapies, folk remedies, and changes in diet. Both deletions and additions to the diet may be important. The answers to these questions provide an insight into the family's approach to pain and illness, and may offer clues to a psychosomatic origin of the child's symptoms. Previous medications and response may offer clues to alleviating factors and side effects of prior treatment. NSAIDs in rheumatic fever, antibiotics in infection, and steroids in JRA, SLE, or malignancy may blunt or hide the objective measures of the disease.

PHYSICAL EXAMINATION

The physical examination of patients with musculoskeletal pain must be thorough. Examination of the extremity is not complete without a thorough inspection of the entire body to rule out systemic causes for the pain. Clues for systemic disease are listed in Table 12-7. Examination of the bones should systematically include all four extremities and the spine. Remember to include the cervical spine and temporomandibular joints in the examination; they are frequently omitted. The area of pain should be carefully examined by inspection and palpation in an attempt to identify the specific anatomic structure by careful scrutiny of the painful area. Expert palpation may isolate the involved tissue to bone, joint, bursa, enthesis, or tendon sheath. Evaluation for color change, heat, tenderness, swelling, range of motion, and symmetry are important. Measurement for evidence of swelling, atrophy, or hypertrophy is helpful, both in providing objective measures and in establishing duration and effects of the painful process. Limb-length discrepancy can be a clue to the site and to the cause of limb pain, and may give evidence for a previous chronic inflammatory process. Accelerated growth of the limb is caused by inflammation in the joint with resultant hyperemia and increased blood flow to the adjacent

TABLE 12-7

ELICITING THE REVIEW OF SYSTEMS: COMMON SIGNS AND SYMPTOMS OF SYSTEMIC CONDITIONS WITH MUSCULOSKELETAL MANIFESTATIONS AND RHEUMATOLOGIC DISEASES

SIGN/SYMPTOM	MOST COMMON ASSOCIATED ILLNESSES	SIGN/SYMPTOM	MOST COMMON ASSOCIATED ILLNESSES
Fever	Acute rheumatic fever	Shortness of breath	Scleroderma
	Infection—septic joint; osteomyelitis		Dermatomyositis
	Systemic JRA		SLE
	Malignancy—leukemia, lymphoma		JRA
	SLE	Abdominal symptoms: pain; diarrhea; vomiting	Inflammatory bowel disease
	Familial Mediterranean fever		Dermatomyositis
Weight loss, poor growth, delayed puberty	Inflammatory bowel disease		Pancreatitis
	Any chronic disease		SLE
	Hypothyroidism		Fibromyalgia
	Malignancy		Medication-induced illness
	Infectious/postinfectious disease		Henoch-Schönlein purpura
Hypertension tachycardia	SLE, PAN, HSP		Hepatitis
	Myocardial disease		Psychosomatic condition
Fatigue	All inflammatory rheumatic diseases	Genital lesions	Behçet disease; Reiter syndrome; gonococcal infection
	Fibromyalgia	Rash:	SLE (may be photosensitive)
Alopecia	SLE, dermatomyositis	Photosensitivity	Dermatomyositis (may be photosensitive)
Red eyes	Conjunctival injection: Kawasaki syndrome; Stevens-Johnson syndrome; Reiter syndrome		Infectious (parvovirus B19 is photosensitive)
			Systemic-onset JRA
Painful eyes	Iritis: sarcoidosis; spondyloarthropathies; Behçet disease; inflammatory bowel diseases; JRA (rarely symptomatic)	Evanescent	Psoriatic arthritis
		Psoriasis	Vasculitis (Kawasaki syndrome)
		Livedo reticularis	
Mouth sores	SLE	Palpable purpura	Henoch-Schönlein purpura; polyarteritis nodosa
	Inflammatory bowel disease	Ulcerations	
	Behçet disease	Urticaria	Serum sickness—urticaria
	Reiter syndrome (painless)	Erythema marginatum	Acute rheumatic fever
Red lips/tongue	Kawasaki syndrome		
	Stevens-Johnson syndrome	Erythema migrans	Lyme disease
Headache	SLE	Erythema nodosum	Sarcoidosis; inflammatory bowel disease; histoplasmosis; streptococcal infection
	Fibromyalgia		
	Central nervous system vasculitis		
	Lyme disease	Raynaud phenomenon	Scleroderma (systemic sclerosis)
	Psychosomatic condition		SLE
Trouble swallowing	Dermatomyositis		Mixed connective tissue disease
	Scleroderma	Vasomotor instability	Reflex sympathetic dystrophy
	Mixed connective tissue diseases		
Chest pain	Pericarditis/carditis: systemic-onset JRA		
Friction rubs	SLE		
	Acute rheumatic fever		
	Histoplasmosis		
Chest wall tenderness	Chest wall pain/costochondritis: fibromyalgia; JRA; spondyloarthropathies		

JRA = juvenile rheumatoid arthritis; SLE = systemic lupus erythematosus; PAIN = polyarthritis hodosa; HSP = Henoch-Schönlein purpura

physis. Atrophy can indicate disuse or neurovascular compromise. In the infant or young child, it is helpful to observe normal active motion, especially gait, to pinpoint the area involved, particularly because pain is difficult to assess or may be absent. One needs to evaluate for discoloration of a painful area. Erythema overlying joints is usually indicative of intra-articular sepsis, adjacent bone infection, crystal-induced synovitis, or acute rheumatic fever. Vasomotor instability, however, with pallor and coolness of the limb is indicative of overwhelming sympathetic response to the pain, such as reflex sympathetic dystrophy or severe pain of other etiology. In reflex sympathetic dystrophy, the skin may be hyperesthetic, eliciting exquisite pain with only light touch.

Crepitus is a palpable and often audible crunching present throughout the range of motion of an involved structure, either joint or tendon sheath. Painful crepitus indicates an intra-articular abnormality; however, popping or cracking joints that are not pain-

ful are usually innocent. The latter are frequently of concern to parents and patients.

Beware of painful loss of motion in joints, especially pseudo-paralysis suggestive of intra-articular sepsis or fracture, or the hip, which abducts and externally rotates with flexion suggestive of slipped capital femoral epiphysis. These conditions require urgent intervention.

The physical examination should emphasize inspection for several abnormalities that particularly associate with RD. Subcutaneous nodules, usually felt over extensor surfaces, suggest rheumatoid arthritis or, rarely, rheumatic fever, a vasculitic syndrome, or serum sickness. Nail changes, including clubbing, pitting, onycholysis, and splinter hemorrhages, may be seen in inflammatory bowel disease, psoriasis, or subacute bacterial endocarditis, respectively. Periungual telangiectasia, or nailfold capillary dilation, suggests possible inflammatory systemic diseases such as SLE, dermatomyositis/scleroderma, or MCTD. The eye is examined for evidence of conjunctivitis, episcleritis, or acute iritis, which can be highly suggestive of a systemic disease. Mucous membrane lesions are common in Reiter syndrome, Behçet syndrome, SLE, Sjögren syndrome, vasculitic syndromes, and inflammatory bowel diseases. Proximal muscle weakness is likely to result from a myopathic disorder such as dermatomyositis, whereas distal muscle weakness is usually secondary to a neuropathic process.

DESCRIPTION OF CLINICAL PAIN PATTERNS

The cardinal feature of inflammatory arthritis is *stiffness after inactivity,* principally manifested as immobility in the morning, after naps, and after prolonged periods of sitting. Pain is usually described as deep aching, occasionally sharp, and diffusely present throughout the joint. The pain and stiffness are aggravated by initial movement but seem to *improve* with subsequent activity. Duration of stiffness and pain may not be significant features in young children, and difficulty with locomotion may be more obvious. Swelling is almost uniformly present in these joints, although occasionally thickened synovium and limitation of motion are the only features. One will see such findings in any of the connective tissue diseases, but particularly in JRA and spondyloarthropathies. Painful, inflamed entheses are the hallmark of spondyloarthropathies such as ankylosing spondylitis, seronegative enthesopathy and arthropathy (SEA) syndrome, and Reiter disease.

Pain Aggravated by Activity

Inflammatory disorders can be distinguished from mechanical pain, which is aggravated by activity. A common example is anterior knee pain syndrome, also called patellofemoral compartment dysfunction or chondromalacia patella, which causes most patients to complain of knee pain with retropatellar grinding or a catching sensation and, occasionally, locking or buckling. The pain is aggravated by activity that loads the patellofemoral joint in flexion; for example, squatting, climbing stairs, standing from a seated position, running, and kneeling. Sitting with the knees flexed for prolonged periods of time may also aggravate the pain. Any part of the extensor mechanism of the knee may be involved, including the quadriceps insertion, patellofemoral compartment, inferior pole of the patella, infrapatellar fat pad and bursae, patellar tendon, or tibial tubercle.

On physical examination, the usual patient with the patellofemoral pain syndrome has palpable patellofemoral crepitus. The patella may be hypermobile. Knee effusion may be present; however, a tense, warm effusion is rarely seen. The medial border of the infrapatellar surface is often tender, as is the corresponding surface of the underlying femur. The differential diagnosis for patellofemoral pain must include a torn medial meniscus and osteochondritis dissecans.

Nighttime Pain

Boring, aching pain, especially pronounced at nighttime and often awakening the patient, should suggest neoplastic disease, either benign or malignant. Osteoid osteoma, a benign tumor usually occurring in the femur or tibia, causes nighttime pain but is characteristically relieved by an analgesic dose of nonsteroidal antiinflammatory drug, particularly aspirin. Radiographs are helpful in establishing the diagnosis; however, bone scan and computerized tomography may be necessary to delineate the lesion.

Nonosseous malignant neoplasms in children, chiefly acute leukemias or metastatic neuroblastoma, commonly cause osteoarticular pain that is usually severe and often disproportionate to the objective physical findings. The pain may be episodic and migratory. A careful physical examination, however, often demonstrates tenderness in the area of neoplastic infiltration. Frank arthritis has been reported in some patients. Laboratory investigations including complete blood count with differential and LDH, radiographs, and radionucleotide bone scans generally yield the proper diagnosis. Occasionally, diagnostic features lag behind the pain by weeks or months.

Refusal to Move

Infectious diseases of bone and joint are usually very painful and accompanied by conspicuous physical findings, including refusal to walk or to move the affected limb. Swelling, marked limitation of active motion, and extreme pain are the hallmarks of septic arthritis. In osteomyelitis, moderate to severe pain, systemic toxicity, and local metaphyseal bone tenderness adjacent to joint swelling are often found. Synovial fluid analysis and appropriate cultures are necessary to differentiate these infectious processes from other inflammatory and neoplastic conditions. Radiograph findings on plain film may not be visible for 10 to 14 days, but radionucleotide bone scan can localize the infection.

The child who does not want the legs, pelvis, or low back to be moved may well have discitis. This disorder, characterized by moderate to severe pain, is aggravated by any compression of the inflamed intervertebral disk. Patients often become apathetic and want to be left alone. Although the pain is often referred to the hip area, examination of the hips does not substantiate joint involvement. The spine is flattened and loses its natural curves. In older children and adolescents, pain in the lower back, at the sacroiliac joint, or over the anterior pelvis may indicate pelvic osteomyelitis. Plain film, bone scan, and magnetic resonance imaging help to establish the diagnosis.

Laboratory tests and imaging procedures useful in the evaluation of musculoskeletal pain are discussed in Sec. 12.2. It takes time to diagnose many musculoskeletal diseases, especially the chronic rheumatic diseases that evolve over several weeks or months. Patients and families may be anxious for results, but patience and careful follow-up are necessary. While it is important to identify promptly conditions that require immediate treatment, it is also important to avoid improper labeling of children, which carries potentially severe consequences for insurability and self-image.

References

American College of Rheumatology Ad Hoc Committee on Clinical Guidelines: Guidelines for the initial evaluation of the adult patient with acute musculoskeletal symptoms. Arthritis Rheum 39:1–8, 1996

Cawkwell GD, Passo MH: Pursuing the source of musculoskeletal pain. Contemp Peds 11:7290–7294, 1994

Doherty M: Introduction; and The minimum rheumatological examination. In: Doherty M, Hazleman BL, Hutton CW, Maddison PJ, Perry JD, eds: Rheumatology Examination and Injection Techniques. London, WB Saunders, 1992:1–19

Engel GL: Pain. In: MacBryde CM, Blacklawn RS, eds: Signs and Symptoms: Applied Pathologic Physiology and Clinical Interpretation, 5th ed. Philadelphia, JB Lippincott, 1970:44–61

Passo MH: Aches and limb pain. In: Symposium on Persistent Signs and Symptoms. Pediatr Clin North Am 29(1):209–219, 1982

Polley HW, Hunder GG: Interviewing to obtain the history of rheumatic disease; and Introduction to physical examination of the joints. In: Rheumatologic Interviewing and Physical Examination of the Joints. Philadelphia, WB Saunders, 1978:1–45

12.4   JUVENILE RHEUMATOID ARTHRITIS

Carol A. Wallace and David D. Sherry

Juvenile rheumatoid arthritis (JRA) is a term used in the United States for a heterogeneous group of chronic inflammatory arthritides that occur in childhood. Other terms, such as juvenile chronic arthritis or idiopathic chronic childhood arthritis, are used worldwide and encompass not only what is thought of as juvenile rheumatoid arthritis in the United States, but also spondyloarthropathy, ankylosing spondylitis, and psoriatic arthritis.

Juvenile rheumatoid arthritis is defined as the onset before age 16 of persistent synovitis in one or more joints for at least 6 weeks (3 months is preferable), with all other causes being excluded. The prevalence is 1 in 1000 and the incidence is 1.4 in 10,000 in the United States. JRA is subdivided into pauciarticular (four or fewer joints), polyarticular (more than four joints), and systemic (accompanied by spiking fevers) onset types, depending upon the presentation in the first 6 months of disease. Because these distinctions are based on the number of joints involved at onset, rather than on the biology of the inflammation, an etiologic difference, or difference in outcome, differences in the course of pauciarticular and polyarticular disease are often minimal. In the next decade, how we describe, categorize, understand, and treat childhood arthritis will undergo dramatic changes.

ETIOLOGY

A disease of persistent inflammation of the synovium, JRA has long been considered a manifestation of autoimmunity; however, intense investigation has failed to identify autoantibodies or target antigens. The contribution of HLA alleles in persistent pauciarticular JRA (DRB1* 1301, 0801) and polyarticular JRA (DPB1* 0301) is emerging as important, possibly through their effect on T-lymphocyte receptor function (see Table 12-2). It is postulated that persistence of microbial antigens initiates synovial inflammation (chronic infection), that antibodies against microbial antigens cross-react with self (molecular mimicry), or that an infection promotes the presentation of self–HLA peptides to self–T cells.

Evidence for an infectious etiology includes the arthritides seen with rubella, parvovirus, or *Borrelia burgdorferi;* the clinical features (abrupt onset, high-spiking fever, rash, hepatosplenomegaly, lymphadenopathy, and serositis); and a clustering of US and Canadian cases in the autumn. Polymerase chain reaction enables identification of microbes and their antigens in synovial tissue.

The immunologic cascade involved in JRA is thought to be initiated by presentation of antigen(s) to T lymphocytes by antigen-presenting cells (macrophages, B cells, dendritic cells, fibroblasts, and endothelial cells). Subsequent T-cell activation stimulates T- and B-lymphocyte production. Release of cytokines such as TNF-α, IL-1, and IL-6 triggers polyclonal T-cell expansion and a host of inflammatory mediators including prostaglandins, neutrophils, complement proteins, kinins, proteases, and lysosomal enzymes that promote migration of inflammatory cells into the synovial tissue and fluid, increase vascular permeability, and damage cartilage and bone.

Pathology

The histology of the inflamed synovium in all subtypes of JRA is identical to that of adult rheumatoid arthritis and is characterized by lymphocytic and plasma cell infiltration. Villous hypertrophy and hyperplasia of the synovial lining and prominent vascular endothelial cell hyperplasia with angiogenesis promote the secretion of large amounts of protein-rich synovial fluid and the migration of neutrophils, lymphocytes, and macrophages into the joint. Synovial fluid white cell counts usually range from 2000 to 30,000/mL. However, counts exceeding 50 to 100,000/mL can be seen in patients with systemic-onset JRA.

An exuberant inflammatory process leads to growth of the synovium on the articular cartilage (pannus formation). Lysosomal hydrolyses that break down proteoglycans and collagen facilitate invasion of the avascular cartilage by the pannus. Prolonged synovial inflammation causes irreparable damage to the cartilage, erosion and destruction of subchondral bone, and the formation of synovial-lined cysts.

Small areas of bone at the margins of articular cartilage (bare areas) are exposed directly to the inflamed synovium; erosions at this site provide an early radiographic clue to bony destruction in rheumatoid arthritis.

CLINICAL PRESENTATIONS

In the absence of laboratory tests specific for the diagnosis of JRA, patient history and physical examination assume critical importance. A cardinal feature in the history for synovitis is morning stiffness (or soreness) of at least 15 minutes, with improvement in movement later in the morning. Parents, other family members, or caregivers may observe changes in walking, running, climbing stairs, or eagerness to play. Children may need help with dressing, eating, bathing, toileting, and other activities that were previously performed independently. Enuresis may recur in a recently toilet-trained child, and developmental milestones may be lost.

All joints must be examined for swelling, decreased motion, tenderness, pain, decreased strength, muscle atrophy, and bony enlargement. Abnormal pupils, rash, lymphadenopathy, organ enlargement, and pericardial and pleural rubs should be noted. Occasionally, synovitis may be painless, but the diagnosis requires the physical finding of swelling due to inflammation. Indirect evidence of synovitis in those joints whose swelling cannot be visualized (ie, spine, hip, and shoulder) is decreased passive range of motion that is often manifest by the guarding of motion of the joint. Observing the child moving about in the exam room can be as important as direct examination, which may be difficult in an uncooperative, frightened toddler or infant.

Pauciarticular Onset

Pauciarticular (oligoarticular) JRA, defined as synovitis in four or fewer joints over the first 6 months of symptoms, occurs in 40 to 60% of children with JRA. The ratio of males to females is 1:6.5; the usual age of onset is 1 to 3 years. Typically, the child has few symptoms and an insidious onset. A quarter of these children will report no pain and come to medical attention after joint swelling is incidentally found. The knee is most frequently involved, followed by the ankle, and then the small joints of the hand, but almost any joint can be affected. Isolated hip or neck arthritis occurs rarely, although it may also portend evolution into ankylosing spondylitis or psoriatic arthritis.

Asymptomatic uveitis (inflammation of the uveal tract—iris, ciliary body, and choroid) develops in approximately 20% of children with pauciarticular JRA, and more frequently in patients with a positive antinuclear antibody (ANA) test. Ophthalmologic screening by slit-lamp examination every 3 to 4 months is paramount.

Seventy percent of children with pauciarticular JRA are ANA-positive, usually in low titer ($\leq$1:320). Mild elevation of erythrocyte sedimentation rate (ESR) or C-reactive protein (CRP) and mild thrombocytosis with a slight decrease in hemoglobin are possible, but these tests are usually normal, as are other laboratory tests. The rheumatoid factor test is rarely positive, but if it is, it often portends conversion to a polyarticular course. Fever, rash, night pain, weight loss, thrombocytopenia, or leukopenia are not seen in this disease, and should prompt further investigations.

Polyarticular Onset

Polyarticular JRA, defined as involvement of at least five joints during the first 6 months, is found in 30 to 40% of children with JRA. Females predominate with two peak ages of onset: 1 to 3 years of age and early adolescence. Both large and small joints can be affected; presentations vary from scattered joint involvement to symmetric synovitis of nearly all joints in the body. Involvement of the cervical spine, hips, shoulders, and temporomandibular joints (TMJ) is common. In most patients, the onset is insidious and accompanied by fatigue. Some patients have low-grade fever, weight loss, and rheumatoid nodules.

Rheumatoid factor positivity can be found in some adolescent patients. In this group, the disease closely resembles adult rheumatoid arthritis, often with the presence of rheumatoid nodules or vasculitis and occasionally Felty syndrome (splenomegaly and leukopenia). About 30% of patients with polyarticular JRA have positive ANA test results. Children with polyarticular JRA can develop asymptomatic chronic iritis but are at less risk to do so than are children with pauciarticular disease.

Systemic Onset

Systemic-onset disease, defined as the occurrence of fever and other systemic findings that often precede the onset of joint disease, affects about 10 to 20% of children with JRA. Males and females are affected equally. Age of onset peaks at 5 to 10 years but spans infancy through adulthood. The key finding is daily fever, which, although erratic, usually spikes once or twice a day, rising above 39.3°C (103°F) and falling to normal. The peak of the fever curve is often in the evening and may be accompanied by intense arthralgia and myalgia. When the temperature is normal, the child may feel quite well only to appear ill again when the fever spikes. Frequently, the fever precedes arthritis by weeks or months. Because JRA is a diagnosis of exclusion, patients with systemic-onset disease usually have an appropriately extensive evaluation to rule out infection and malignancy.

Patients with systemic-onset JRA may have a plethora of other systemic manifestations that usually precede the appearance of synovitis. A macular, evanescent, pink to salmon-colored rash exhibits discrete borders with or without central clearing; it is often best seen during the fever. The rash may be raised, is usually nonpruritic, and is migratory over the trunk, thighs, and axillae. It can be induced by mild trauma (Koebner phenomenon). The child with typical fever and rash but without arthritis may be considered to have probable systemic-onset JRA after other causes are exhaustively ex-

cluded. The diagnosis is not firm until synovitis appears. Other systemic manifestations include pericarditis; myocarditis; pleuritis; lymphadenopathy; hepatosplenomegaly; abdominal pain; fatigue; anorexia; weight loss; and, rarely, asymptomatic iritis. With time a few or many inflamed joints will appear. These tend to be markedly swollen and more painful than the arthritis of other subgroups. Nighttime pain and awakening are not unusual.

DIAGNOSIS

Laboratory abnormalities can be extensive with often dramatic leukocytosis (>40,000) and thrombocytosis (>1 million) and high CRP and serum ferritin levels. The ESR is often over 100 mm/h. Anemia, low albumin, and elevated transaminases are found frequently, but rheumatoid factor and DNA are rarely positive. During the acute phase of disease, some children become severely ill with development of leukopenia, thrombocytopenia, profound anemia, decreased sedimentation rate and fibrinogen, and elevated D-dimer—a picture consistent with diffuse intravascular coagulation. Serum transaminases may abruptly increase to >1000, the bone marrow may exhibit hemophagocytosis, and the patient can have a cardiopulmonary arrest and expire. This crisis is called *macrophage activation syndrome* (MAS); treatment with corticosteroids is effective if initiated early.

There is no radiologic study that can diagnose JRA unless the disease is so advanced that characteristic erosions and joint destruction have occurred. Bone scan may reveal increased uptake on both sides of an affected joint consistent with increased blood flow or may be entirely normal. MRI with gadolinium contrast can highlight inflamed synovium and increased joint fluid, but cannot distinguish the underlying cause.

Radiology

Plain films, bone scan, magnetic resonance imaging (MRI), and computerized tomography (CT) can all be helpful in evaluation of the child with joint pain or swelling, depending on the specific situation. Plain radiographs are useful to monitor for the possibility of joint destruction and effectiveness of treatment. The earliest radiographic change is soft-tissue swelling followed by periarticular osteopenia. In young children, joint space widening can initially be seen because of increased intra-articular fluid or synovial hypertrophy. The hypervascularity of involved joints may stimulate adjacent growth plates and result in either bony enlargement, usually knee or ankles, or premature epiphyseal closure often seen in the wrist or hip.

The intense inflammation can also stimulate periosteal new bone formation in the short tubular bones of the phalanges, metacarpals, and metatarsals, and occasionally long bones. A characteristic radiographic finding in children with JRA involving a finger is widening of the mid-portion of a phalange from periosteal new bone formation.

Joint space narrowing is found after a significant amount of cartilage has been destroyed. The temporomandibular joint (TMJ) is at particular risk for destruction because the epiphysis is immediately adjacent to a thin amount of articular cartilage. When the epiphysis is destroyed, micrognathia ensues. CT currently provides the best images for evaluation of possible joint damage in the TMJ.

Erosions and cysts form when the inflamed synovium involves subchondral bone. In late stages, these cysts may collapse, leading to marked joint irregularity. Fibrous ankylosis and bony fusion can then occur and are not uncommon in JRA, particularly in the wrist and cervical spine of patients with systemic-onset disease. Erosion of the odontoid process can lead to subluxation of C1 and C2. Children with JRA involving the neck should be followed with flexion and extension lateral radiographs of the cervical spine, especially if they are involved in gymnastics and sports. Repeat films should be done before general anesthesia.

Bone scan may be normal or may reveal increased uptake on both sides of an affected joint consistent with increased blood flow. MRI with gadolinium contrast can highlight inflamed synovium and increased joint fluid, but cannot distinguish the underlying cause. Significant damage to the cartilage and bone can be present early in the course of JRA, when the plain radiographs do not appear abnormal. Unfortunately, MRI cannot be used to evaluate possible joint damage on a routine basis at present.

DIFFERENTIAL DIAGNOSIS

A thorough and diligent evaluation to exclude other processes such as infection and malignancy must be emphasized. Table 12-6 outlines the most common diseases to consider when evaluating a child with a swollen joint (or joints). The diagnoses of pauciarticular JRA, polyarticular JRA, or postinfectious arthritis require swollen joints or other evidence of synovitis. A well child with joint pain but no swelling may have an orthopedic condition (avascular necrosis, slipped femoral epiphysis, Osgood-Schlatter disease), benign

nocturnal limb pains of childhood hypermobility, or a psychogenic pain syndrome.

TREATMENT

Goals of treatment are to prevent joint destruction, promote normal growth and development, and achieve remission of disease (ie, no joint swelling, no morning stiffness, no joint pain, and normalization of ESR, if previously elevated). The pillars of treatment are medications, physical/occupational therapy, and education of the family.

Medications

The medical treatment of JRA is hampered by the lack of known etiology and by the nonspecific actions of medications available; however, our current understanding of how quickly joint destruction can occur and the long-term outcome of JRA has led to earlier and more aggressive treatment over the last decade (Fig. 12-2). For those patients with persistent or severe disease, joint injections and use of remittive agents (medications thought to retard joint destruction) is standard practice early in the course of disease. Many patients require a combination of remittive medications to treat the progressive synovitis. All of these medications (as well as NSAIDs) have potential side effects and require ongoing laboratory moni-

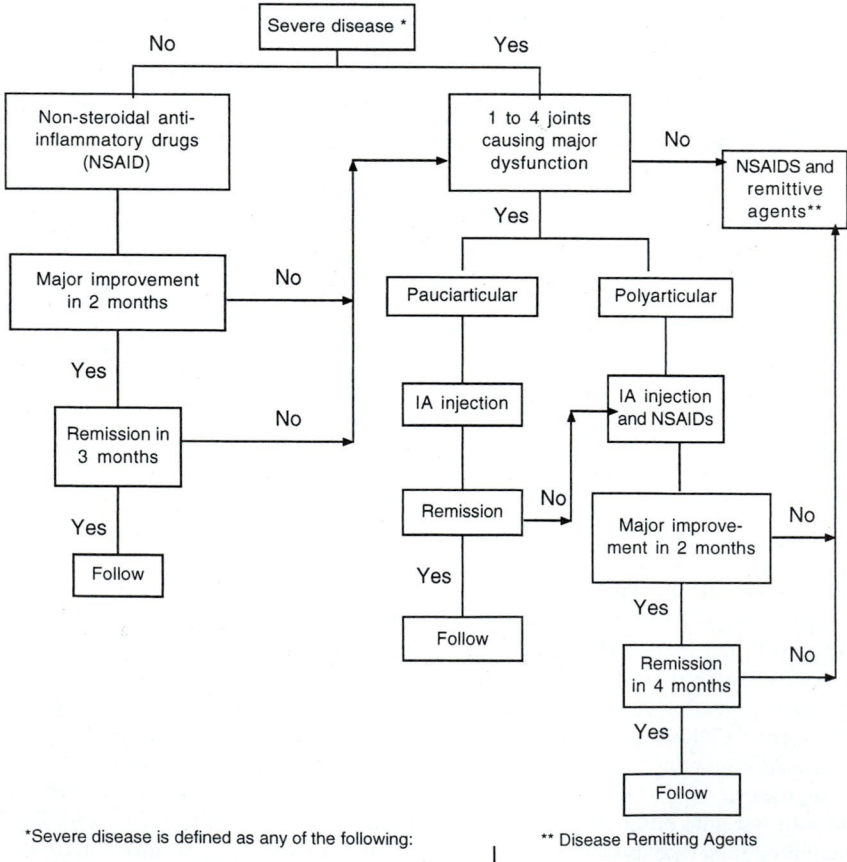

FIGURE 12-2 A protocol for treatment of pauciarticular and polyarticular JRA.

*Severe disease is defined as any of the following:

Presence of flexion contractures
Muscle atrophy
Extra-articular manifestations (fever, nodules etc.)
Pain interfering with sleep
Missing school (or preschool)
Greater than 1 hour of morning stiffness
Activities of daily living (ADLs) take >50 percent
 longer than normal
> 50 percent decrease in gross motor speed or endurance

** Disease Remitting Agents

a) Hydroxchloroquine
 Sulfasalazine
 Methotrexate (PO, SQ, IV)
 Azathioprine
 Cyclosporine
 Entanercept
b) Specific one (or combinations)
 will depend on patient and circumstances
c) Doses and routes often need adjusting

toring. Oral and IV pulse corticosteroids do not appear on the treatment algorithms but may be used for short periods in patients with very severe disease, flares of disease, or systemic manifestations. An algorithm for the treatment of systemic-onset JRA is not presented because the treatment varies considerably, ranging from NSAID to high-dose methylprednisolone and experimental drugs.

Outpatients with active JRA need to be seen every 1 to 3 months for thorough evaluation and medication adjustments. It usually takes many months, even years, to achieve remission of disease. After remission is achieved, medications are kept stable for many months to years before they are gradually tapered and discontinued. With better knowledge of the etiology of disease and development of more effective medications the algorithms presented here will undergo many changes, perhaps incorporating regimens for induction therapy early in disease (use of many medications and biologicals together) followed by maintenance therapy.

Physical Therapy

Physical and occupational therapy are an important part of treating children with JRA. The treatment goals are to maintain and improve range of motion, strength, and function. The therapist should be experienced in the treatment of JRA. Because loss of age-appropriate developmental skills can occur, functional skills need to be monitored by a therapist experienced in the treatment of JRA. Frequency of therapy visits varies considerably, but all therapy depends on a daily home program done by the child and parent. Long-term cooperation with physical and occupational therapy is difficult but is enhanced if the therapist tailors the home program to address age, extent of disease, school activities, sports, hobbies, and family dynamics. Low-impact exercise such as swimming is important for cartilage and joint health.

Nighttime splinting of the wrist, hand, knee, elbow, or ankle may decrease morning stiffness and help to prevent flexion contractures. Loss of extension can often be improved after corticosteroid injection followed by serial casting of a knee, ankle, wrist, finger, or elbow. Ice, heat, ultrasound, or a combination of these modalities can help restore motion and decrease pain due to muscle spasm. When leg-length difference is present, a shoe lift for the short limb will help to prevent contralateral knee or hip flexion contractures. Children with arthritis of the tarsals and metatarsals may ambulate more easily with shoe splints (soft orthotics).

School can present a problem for children with arthritis. Stiffness from prolonged sitting can be helped by being allowed to get up and move about the classroom. Upper-extremity involvement may make writing, drawing, working on the blackboard, and participation in class difficult. Some children will need extra time to pass from class to class. An extra set of books at home greatly lessens the load that needs to be carried to and from home. Physical education and sports can be a challenge; most children do well when allowed to participate as much as they are able. Exercise will not damage joints or worsen arthritis if bony destruction is not present. Rarely, a child may need a shortened school day, but home tutoring is almost never indicated.

In the United States, Public Law 94-142 (the Education for All Handicapped Children Act of 1975) mandates public schools to provide transportation to and from school and therapy services for those individuals with disabilities that impact their education. This applies to many children with JRA who have limitations of range, strength, and coordination that alters their function at school. Physical and occupational therapists are available in the school to treat severely involved children whose disease precludes them from meeting their educational goals in a timely fashion. These therapists work in conjunction with the patient's rheumatology team.

Education

Patient and family education is an important ongoing part of treatment. The Arthritis Foundation and the American Juvenile Arthritis Organization are excellent sources for additional information and peer support. The emotional impact of this chronic and often painful and disabling disease on the child, siblings, and parents should not be underestimated. Exacerbations of disease after a long period of remission, as well as the period of early to midadolescence, are particularly stressful for many patients and families. Most children and families do not need long-term counseling, but may benefit from short-term family or individual treatment.

Outcome

The outcome of juvenile rheumatoid arthritis is variable for all subtypes. Some patients may experience a single episode of disease lasting 3 to 6 months, while others are afflicted with continuous chronic inflammation and worsening joint destruction and disability. Children do not outgrow JRA nor does puberty alter its course. Outcome can be measured by functional ability, persistence of synovitis, or radiographic findings. Recent studies of patients followed for more than 5 years do not exist. Studies published from 1959 to 1991 reveal that severe functional disability occurs in 9 to 48% of children with JRA after a mean of 10 years of follow-up, range 5 to 25 years. When these studies are combined (weighting for number of patients), 31% of patients at long-term follow-up were unable to perform some or all activities of daily living, were using a wheelchair, or were bedridden. Ascertainment biases towards the most severe patients and a failure to distinguish between those patients treated early and late make these studies imperfect.

Another assessment of the outcome for JRA patients is the presence of persistent synovitis. Studies published from 1966 to 1991 revealed that 31 to 55% of patients with JRA continue to have active arthritis at 10 or more years of follow-up. These percentages vary little with subtype. A recently published population study from Sweden revealed that half of patients with JRA followed 10 or more years continued with active synovitis. Thus, between one-third and one-half of patients with JRA may begin their adult lives with active arthritis and be at continuing risk for joint destruction.

Radiographic changes are yet another measure of severity of disease and outcome. All patients with JRA are at risk for joint damage—it is common and can occur early in disease. Twenty-eight percent of pauciarticular-onset patients develop radiologic evidence of joint damage at a median time of 5 years, whereas half of those with polyarticular- and systemic-onset JRA develop joint damage within 2 years after onset of disease.

Mortality from JRA in North America is rare, is largely confined to children with systemic JRA, and is calculated at 0.29% of all patients with JRA, which rate greatly exceeds standardized mortality rates for American children.

References

Giannini EH, Brewer EJ, Kuzmina N et al: Methotrexate in resistant juvenile rheumatoid arthritis: results of the USA–USSR double-blind, placebo-controlled trial. N Engl J Med 326(16):1043–1049, 1992

Huang JL, Chen LC: Sulphasalazine in the treatment of children with chronic arthritis. Clin Rheumatol 17:359–363, 1998

Klein-Gitelman MS, Pachman LM: Intravenous corticosteroids: adverse reactions are more variable than expected in children. J Rheumatol 25:1995–2002, 1998

Lovell DJ, Giannini EH, Reiff A, et al: Etanercept in children with polyarticular juvenile rheumatoid arthritis. N Engl J Med 342:763–769, 2000

Mouy R, Stephan JL, Pillet P, Haddad E, Hubert P, Prieur AM: Efficacy of cyclosporine A in the treatment of macrophage activation syndrome in juvenile arthritis: report of five cases. J Pediatr 129:750–754, 1996

Padeh S, Passwell JH: Intra-articular corticosteroid injection in the management of children with chronic arthritis. Arthritis Rheum 41:1210–1214, 1998

Reiff A, Rawlings DJ, Shaham B, et al: Preliminary evidence for cyclosporin A as an alternative in the treatment of recalcitrant juvenile rheumatoid arthritis and juvenile dermatomyositis. J Rheumatol 24:2436–2443, 1997

Savolainen HA, Kautiainen H, Isomaki H, Aho K, Verronen P: Azathioprine in patients with juvenile chronic arthritis: a long-term follow-up study. J Rheumatol 24:2444–2450, 1997

See Y: Intra-synovial corticosteroid injections in juvenile chronic arthritis—a review. Ann Acad Med Singapore 27:105–111, 1998

Shaikov AV, Maximov AA, Speransky AI, Lovell DJ, Giannini EH, Solovyev SK: Repetitive use of pulse therapy with methylprednisolone and cyclophosphamide in addition to oral methotrexate in children with systemic juvenile rheumatoid arthritis: preliminary results of a long-term study. J Rheumatol 19:612–616, 1992

Wallace CA, Sherry DD: Trial of intravenous pulse cyclophosphamide and methylprednisolone in the treatment of severe systemic-onset juvenile rheumatoid arthritis. Arthritis Rheum 40:1852–1855, 1997

12.5   SPONDYLOARTHROPATHIES

David A. Cabral and Lori B. Tucker

The juvenile spondyloarthropathies have traditionally included juvenile ankylosing spondylitis (JAS), Reiter disease (RD), the arthropathy of inflammatory bowel disease (IBD), and juvenile psoriatic arthritis (JPsA). In adults, the term *spondyloarthropathy* (referring to arthritis of the spine) appropriately distinguishes a group of chronic arthritides that have axial skeletal involvement, are associated with HLA-B27, and are rheumatoid factor–negative. In children, these diseases should be distinguished from juvenile rheumatoid arthritis (JRA); however, the term spondyloarthropathy is inappropriate because most children with these diseases do not have arthritis of the spine, and inflammatory disease of the sacroiliac joints is an infrequent or late finding.

Among the features that help distinguish juvenile spondyloarthropathy from JRA, enthesitis is the most defining. *Enthesitis refers to inflammation (pain, tenderness, and swelling) of the enthesis, the site of attachment of tendon, ligament, or fascia to bone.* A pediatric task force of the International League Against Rheumatism (ILAR) has proposed a new system of classification for the idiopathic chronic arthritides of childhood. Within this scheme of classification for juvenile idiopathic arthritis, *enthesitis-related arthritis (ERA)* describes most patients previously described as having a juvenile spondyloarthropathy, SEA syndrome (syndrome of seronegative enthesopathy and arthropathy), HLA-B27-associated arthropathy and enthesopathy syndrome, pauciarticular-onset JRA type II, and JAS. *ERA* should replace all of these designations. Patients previously described as having JAS should be described as having JRA with sacroiliitis and/or spondylitis; patients with arthritis and IBD are described as having ERA with IBD. Juvenile

psoriatic arthritis is distinguished separately, and Reiter disease, or reactive arthritis, is not considered idiopathic.

12.5.1 ENTHESIS-RELATED ARTHRITIS

With a prevalence on the order of 20 per 100,000, ERA is about half as common as JRA and twice as common as JPsA. Children having ERA should be distinguished from those with these other chronic arthritides for etiologic, genetic, prognostic, and therapeutic reasons. In addition to enthesitis, other characteristic features distinguishing ERA from the other inflammatory arthritides include a high frequency of HLA-B27, late childhood onset, a male preponderance, a familial occurrence of other spondyloarthropathies, and peripheral arthritis that asymmetrically involves the lower limbs (Table 12-8).

ETIOLOGY

There is no known cause, but the strong familial tendency and the high frequency of HLA-B27 reflect a genetic predisposition. The similarity to reactive arthritis in epidemiology and gut histology implicates bacterial antigens as an additional factor. There may also be hormonal influences on the expression of the disease.

CLINICAL PRESENTATIONS

By definition, in a child with chronic arthritis, ERA can be diagnosed if there is (a) both arthritis and enthesitis, or (b) if there is arthritis or enthesitis with at least two of the following: (i) sacroiliac joint tenderness and/or inflammatory spinal pain; (ii) presence of HLA-B27; (iii) family history in at least one first- or second-degree relative of medically confirmed HLA-B27-associated disease; (iv) anterior uveitis that is usually associated with pain, redness, or photophobia; (v) onset of arthritis in a boy after 8 years of age.

Early Musculoskeletal Manifestation

Although often insidious and episodic, the onset may also be acute and may resemble septic arthritis when presenting as a monoarthritic process. Children with ERA present with morning pain and stiffness relieved by activity, predominantly in joints of the lower extremities and often in the low back and buttocks. They may also complain of pain at the entheses commonly around their heels, feet,

TABLE 12-8

COMPARISON OF JRA, ERA, AND JPsA

	JRA	ERA	JPsA
Enthesitis	Very rare	Very frequent	Uncommon
M:F	1:4	9:1	1:2.5
Mean onset age (yrs)	5	10	6
Uveitis	Asymptomatic	Symptomatic	Asymptomatic
HLA-B27-positive	15%	75%	15%
ANA-positive	60%	<10%	50%
Family history	Rare	Frequent for HLA-B27-associated diseases	Frequent for psoriasis

JRA, juvenile rheumatoid arthritis; ERA, enthesis-related arthritis; JPsA, juvenile psoriatic arthritis.

and knees. Examination may reveal evidence of oligoarthritis asymmetrically involving the knees or ankles, and sometimes the hips or small joints of the feet. (Hip joint involvement at disease onset is uncommon in JRA.) Early involvement of the midfoot (tarsitis, enthesitis, and tenosynovitis) with pain, tenderness, and swelling is less common, but if present, is very characteristic of ERA. Exquisite tenderness may be elicited by palpation of the entheses, particularly at the calcaneal insertions of the Achilles tendon and the plantar fascia, beneath the metatarsal heads and the base of the fifth metatarsal, the tibiatuberosities and the 2, 6, and 10 o'clock positions of the patella, and the ischial tuberosities. Pelvic compression and distraction or direct palpation may elicit sacroiliac joint pain. Axial involvement should be determined by history and by examining the back for range of movement and flattening of the lower back on forward flexion. Costovertebral motion can be monitored by serial measurements of maximum chest expansion. Cervical disease is not as common as in JRA and usually follows lumbar involvement; however, atlantoaxial axial instability has been reported in early disease.

Extra-Articular Manifestations

High fever with constitutional symptoms of anorexia, fever, and weight loss may occur in 5 to 10% of children with ERA; however, these findings should also alert the physician to the possibility of inflammatory bowel disease, particularly if there is growth delay. Subclinical ileocolonoscopic evidence of gut inflammation is reported to occur in up to 80% of patients, and these changes may be predictive of development of AS; this also may have etiologic significance. Acute symptomatic iritis, more commonly unilateral, may occur in 5 to 10% of children with ERA. Aortic valve insufficiency is a rare complication. Restrictive lung disease probably does not occur in childhood.

DIAGNOSIS

Patients may have nonspecific inflammatory changes with a normocytic normochromic anemia, mild leukocytosis, a thrombocytosis, and a high ESR. Immunoglobulins, and specifically immunoglobulin A, may be elevated. HLA-B27 is frequently present.

TREATMENT

As for all forms of juvenile idiopathic arthritis, the patient is best served by treatment in a multidisciplinary setting by professionals specifically trained in the treatment of childhood rheumatic diseases. The first line of therapy is regular NSAIDs: naproxen, tolmetin sodium, ibuprofen, or indomethacin. Optimal effect from these requires at least a month of continuing treatment. Intra-articular injection of triamcinolone hexacetonide (1 mg/kg/large joint) is valuable if there are a few joints that are responding poorly to NSAID therapy.

The pain of enthesitis is often difficult to treat; local injection of corticosteroids is generally unsuccessful, and patients often require use of low-dose oral prednisone. For patients in whom NSAID therapy provides inadequate disease control, sulfasalazine and methotrexate are safe and effective second-line therapies, but they require regular monitoring of blood count and hepatic transaminases. Custom-made hard orthotics to redistribute the weight from sites of painful enthesitis and heel raises to alleviate stress in the retrocalcaneal area and the knee are very useful. Physiotherapy should aim to maintain or restore muscle strength and range of

movement in and about affected joints. Special attention should be paid to range of movement of the back and chest.

Some patients have a short course of disease lasting 3 to 6 months, with pauciarticular arthritis and/or enthesitis that resolves completely. This pattern resembles *reactive arthritis*, although neither an inciting pathogen preceding gastrointestinal nor genitourinary symptoms may be identifiable. Other patients may have a course of episodic flares that lasts for years. Within about 10 years a majority of patients with a more chronic course have a high likelihood of developing symptomatic and radiologically confirmed sacroiliitis with spondylitis (previously known as JAS). They may have an intermittent or slowly progressive course with loss of lumbosacral flexion and decreasing chest expansion. At the worst degree of severity, patients progress to a symmetric erosive and ankylosing polyarthritis by adulthood, predominantly in the lower limbs, together with ankylosing disease of the back and sacroiliac joints and restrictive lung disease.

12.5.2   Arthritis of Inflammatory Bowel Disease

Inflammatory arthritis occurs in about 15% of patients with either Crohn disease or ulcerative colitis. Arthritis in the peripheral joints is twice as common as axial disease, is more frequent in girls, is not associated with HLA-B27, and usually occurs in association with flares of gut inflammation. Patients with IBD and axial involvement are predominantly males with HLA-B27. In this latter group, the course of the axial disease is more independent of the bowel inflammation.

Joint disease may precede the diagnosis of IBD by months to years. For all patients with ERA, certain features should suggest the diagnosis of IBD: prominent fatigue; weight loss; unexplained growth delay and fevers; oral ulcers; abdominal pain or tenderness; diarrhea or hematochezia; extraintestinal manifestations such as erythema nodosum, pyoderma gangrenosum, or clubbing; marked anemia; hypoalbuminemia; or a very high ESR.

Peripheral arthritis in association with a flare of bowel inflammation often responds to aggressive treatment of the bowel disease with corticosteroids, sulfasalazine, or other second-line agents. NSAIDs may also be necessary; otherwise, the principles of treatment are as for ERA.

12.5.3   Juvenile Psoriatic Arthritis

In a child with chronic arthritis, juvenile psoriatic arthritis is diagnosed by the presence of (a) arthritis and psoriasis or (b) arthritis and at least two of the following: (i) dactylitis; (ii) nail abnormalities (pitting or onycholysis); (iii) family history of psoriasis confirmed by a dermatologist in at least one first-degree relative. Arthritis may precede the skin disease by many years.

Overlapping patterns of psoriatic arthritis occurring in the adult population include asymmetric oligoarthritis, symmetric rheumatoid-like arthritis, predominant distal interphalangeal joint disease, arthritis mutilans, and spondylitis. In children with psoriatic arthritis, the predominant pattern at onset is that of asymmetric oligoarthritis of small and large joints often with dactylitis. (Asymmetric involvement of the small joints would be very atypical for JRA.) Over time, many patients develop polyarthritis. Similarly to young children with JRA, those with psoriatic arthritis are at risk of developing asymptomatic chronic anterior uveitis; they are also likely to be ANA-positive. A small minority who develop sacroiliitis has HLA-B27.

The principles of treatment are as for JRA, including the recommendation for frequent monitoring for asymptomatic uveitis with slit-lamp examinations performed every 3 months.

12.5.4   Reactive Arthritis/Reiter Disease

In the context of the "spondyloarthropathies," reactive arthritis describes a disease occurring 1 to 4 weeks following a gastrointestinal (*Yersinia enterocolitica, Y. tuberculosis, Shigella flexneri, Salmonella typhimurium, Campylobacter jejuni*) or genitourinary (*Chlamydia trachomatis* and *Mycoplasma tiny*) infection. Reactive arthritis with the extra-articular manifestations of conjunctivitis and urethritis can be referred to as Reiter disease, although this rarely occurs in children. Other forms of reactive arthritis (eg, poststreptococcal, postgonococcal) differ in pattern of involvement, course, and prognosis, and are not considered among the spondyloarthropathies.

Patients present with florid inflammation of one or two of the large weight-bearing joints; enthesitis is also common. The joints may be very hot, red, tender, and painful, and if a monarthritis, it may be clinically indistinguishable from a septic arthritis. Joint fluid aspiration with culture may be necessary to exclude septic arthritis. Cultures from the gut, urethra, and conjunctiva may reveal one of the above causative organisms. The arthritis is most often transient, lasting only a few days, but it may also last a few months, sometimes with remissions and exacerbations. Treatment with NSAIDs is usually effective. Uncommonly, a patient may develop a persistent arthritis that is indistinguishable from ERA with sacroiliitis and spondylitis.

References

Burgos-Vargas R: Ankylosing tarsitis: clinical features of a unique form of tarsal disease in the juvenile-onset spondyloarthropathies. Arthritis Rheum 34(Suppl):D196, 1991

Burgos-Vargas R, Pacheco-Tena C, Vazquez-Mellado J: Juvenile-onset spondyloarthropathies. Rheum Dis Clin North Am 23(3):569–598, 1997

Burgos-Vargas R, Vazquez-Mellado J: The early clinical recognition of juvenile-onset ankylosing spondylitis and its differentiation from juvenile rheumatoid arthritis. Arthritis Rheum 38(6):835–844, 1995

Cabral DA, Malleson PN, Petty RE: Spondyloarthropathies of childhood. [Review]. Pediatr Clin North Am 42:1051–1070, 1995

Cabral DA, Oen KG, Petty RE: SEA syndrome revisited: a long-term follow-up of children with a syndrome of seronegative enthesopathy and arthropathy. J Rheumatol 19:1282–1285, 1992

Hussein A, Abdul-Khaliq H, van der Hardt H: Atypical spondyloarthritis in children: proposed diagnostic criteria. Eur J Pediatr 148:513–517, 1989

Jacobs JC, Berdon ED, Johnston WE: HLA-B27-associated spondyloarthritis and enthesopathy in childhood: clinical, pathologic, and radiographic observations in 58 patients. J Pediatr 100:521–528, 1982

Petty RE, Southwood TR, Baum J, et al: Revision of the proposed classification criteria for juvenile idiopathic arthritis: Durban, 1997 [see comments]. J Rheumatol 25(10):1991–1994, 1998

Roberton DM, Cabral DA, Malleson P, Petty RE: Juvenile psoriatic arthritis: follow-up and evaluation of diagnostic criteria. J Rheumatol 23: 166–170, 1996

Rosenberg AM, Petty RE: A syndrome of seronegative enthesopathy and arthropathy in children. Arthritis Rheum 25:1041–1047, 1982

Southwood TR, Petty RE, Malleson PN, et al: Psoriatic arthritis in children. Arthritis Rheum 32(8):1007–1013, 1989

12.6   VASCULITIDES

Jaime de Inocencio

Vasculitis, defined as inflammation of blood vessels, is a feature of multiple rheumatic and nonrheumatic diseases in childhood. This chapter addresses only those diseases in which vasculitis plays a central role in both pathogenesis and clinical presentation. Vasculitides comprise 6 to 9% of new referrals to pediatric rheumatology clinics in North America and Europe. This number clearly underestimates the actual prevalence of vasculitis in pediatrics, because many children with the two most common types of vasculitides, Henoch-Schönlein purpura and Kawasaki disease, are followed by community pediatricians, cardiologists, or nephrologists.

Classification of vasculitis is based on the size of the blood vessels involved or the pathology of the lesions. Examples of *large-vessel vasculitis* include *temporal arteritis* (giant-cell granulomatous arteritis) and *Takayasu disease* (granulomatous arteritis). Involvement of *medium-sized vessels* occurs in *polyarteritis nodosa* and *Kawasaki disease* (both necrotizing vasculitides). *Small-vessel vasculitis* is exemplified by *Henoch-Schönlein purpura* (leukocytoclastic vasculitis), *Wegener granulomatosis* (granulomatous vasculitis), *Churg-Strauss syndrome* (granulomatous vasculitis), *microscopic polyangiitis* (necrotizing vasculitis), *essential cryoglobulinemic vasculitis* (leukocytoclastic vasculitis), and *cutaneous leukocytoclastic angiitis*. This chapter reviews these processes according to their incidence in pediatric patients (Fig. 12-3).

12.6.1   Henoch-Schönlein Purpura (Anaphylactoid Purpura)

Henoch-Schönlein purpura (HSP) is the most common form of systemic vasculitis in childhood. The main features of the disease include nonthrombocytopenic palpable purpura (present in 100% of affected children), arthritis or arthralgia (75–85%), colicky abdominal pain with or without gastrointestinal hemorrhage (60–85%), and renal involvement (10–50%). Seventy-five percent of the patients are younger than 7 years, with a mean age at presentation of 4 years. Almost entirely confined to childhood, the disease is more common in males (male:female ratio of 1.2–2:1), although sex differences are not seen in patients older than 16 years. HSP has a seasonal pattern, with peaks in winter and spring. Its annual incidence has been calculated as 13.5/100,000 children. HSP is an IgA-mediated leukocytoclastic vasculitis, characterized by neutrophil infiltration and fibrinoid necrosis in the vessel walls of arterioles, capillaries, and postcapillary venules, with deposition of IgG, IgA, and C3.

ETIOLOGY

The etiology of the disease is unknown. In about 50% of patients the disease is preceded by an upper respiratory infection. However, HSP has multiple triggers including bacterial infections (GABHS, *Legionella, Yersinia, Mycoplasma*), viral infections (Epstein-Barr, varicella-zoster, cytomegalovirus, parvovirus, hepatitis B virus), drugs (penicillin and other beta-lactam antibiotics, chlorpromazine, quinidine, thiazide diuretics), vaccines (measles, yellow fever, cholera), food additives, and insect bites.

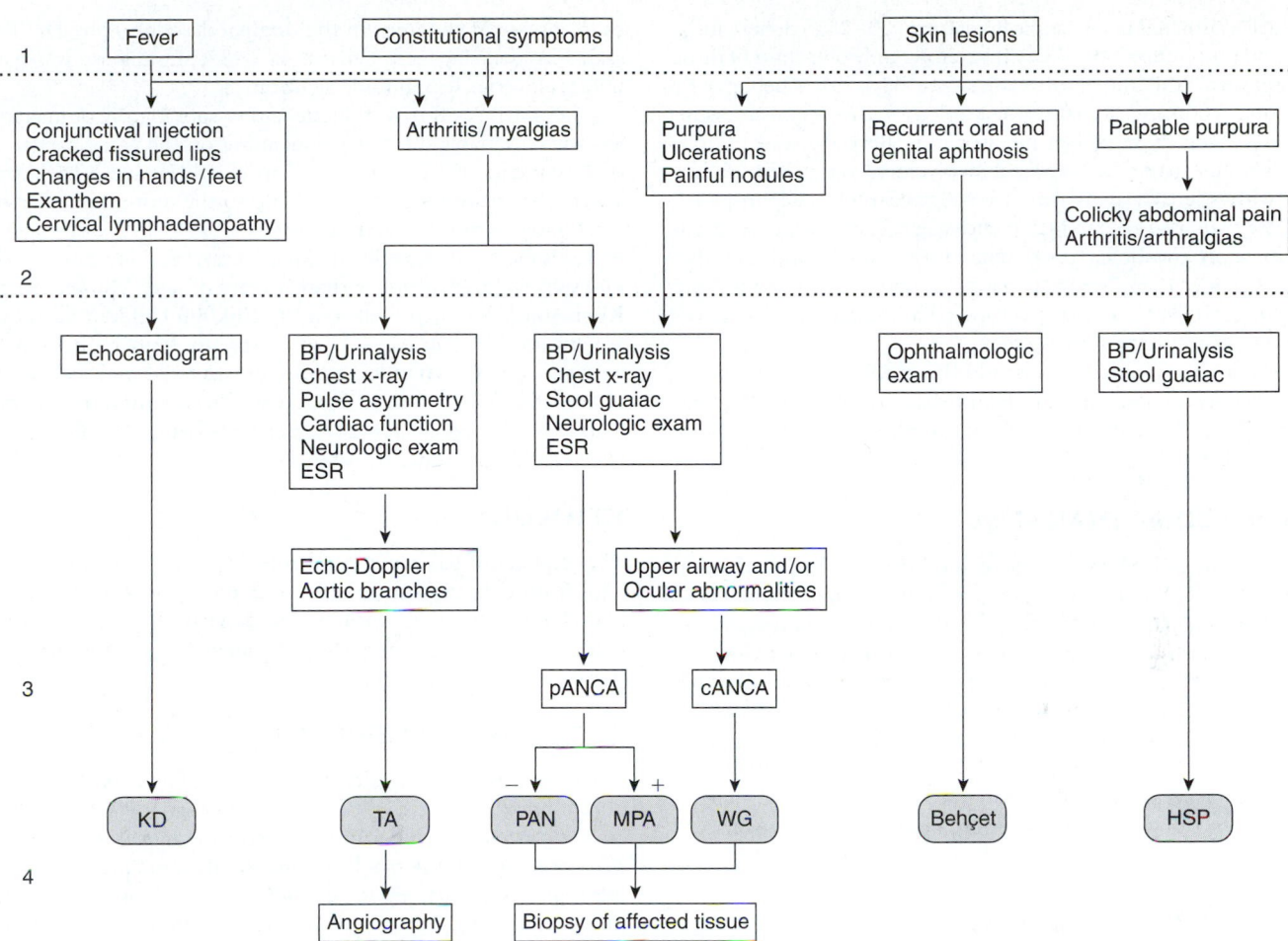

FIGURE 12-3 Pediatric vasculitides evaluation strategy. Abbreviations used: KD, Kawasaki disease; TA, Takayasu arteritis; PAN, polyarteritis nodosa; MPA, microscopic polyangiitis; WG, Wegener granulomatosis; HSP, Henoch-Schönlein purpura; cANCA, pANCA - cytoplasmic, perinuclear, antineutrophil cytoplasmic antibodies. Level 1 represents the most characteristic presenting complaints; level 2 represents associated clinical findings; level 3 represents complementary evaluations to be considered; and level 4 represents the corresponding diagnosis and confirmatory tests. Diagnosis of Kawasaki disease, Behçet disease, and HSP is based on clinical criteria.

CLINICAL PRESENTATION

Onset of HSP may be acute or subacute, with clinical features of the disease most commonly developing in an additive manner over a short time span. Skin lesions, present in all patients, are the initial manifestation in about 50% of patients. The typical rash begins as small wheals or erythematous maculopapules that evolve into petechial or purpuric lesions, more prominent on dependent and pressure-bearing areas. Although usually located over the lower extremities or buttocks, the rash may involve upper extremities, trunk, and face. In young children, HSP might present as edema and purpura involving the face and ears. Skin lesions tend to occur in crops and last from 5 days to 4 weeks. Angioedema of the scalp, perineal area, and extremities may precede the rash.

Joint involvement is the second most common manifestation of HSP, affecting more than two-thirds of children. In about 25% of patients, arthritis/arthralgias of large joints, particularly knees and ankles, are the initial symptom of HSP; this nonspecific finding confounds the diagnosis until the appearance of skin rash 24 to 48 hours later. Because joint swelling is often periarticular, there may be no true joint effusion despite significant pain on motion. Joint

symptoms typically resolve spontaneously after a few days without residual deformity, but may recur with new exacerbations of HSP.

Gastrointestinal (GI) symptoms are present in more than two-thirds of affected children. The most common complaint is colicky abdominal pain, frequently associated with vomiting. Pain may be severe enough to mimic an acute abdomen and may precede the rash in as much as 10 to 15% of patients, again confusing the clinical picture. Of those patients with HSP and abdominal pain, about 50% have occult bleeding, 30% have melena, and 15% have hematemesis, sometimes in the context of diarrhea. However, only 5% have a major GI bleed. Upper gastrointestinal series show nonspecific changes such as thickening of the bowel wall, "thumbprinting," and filling defects. On the other hand, ultrasound studies are abnormal in up to 80% of patients with GI involvement, including increased echogenicity and thickening of the wall of the second portion of the duodenum and/or hydrops of the gallbladder. These findings are not present in patients with HSP but without GI complaints. More uncommon GI complications include perforation, bowel infarct, or intussusception, usually ileoileal.

Renal involvement in patients with HSP ranges between 10 and 50% but is most commonly limited to transient urinary abnormalities such as isolated microscopic hematuria (20–25%) or hematuria plus mild proteinuria (40–45%). Therefore, only one-third of those patients with HSP and renal involvement have either nephritis or nephrotic syndrome. Renal histopathology shows lesions indistinguishable from those of IgA nephropathy (Berger disease). Prognosis for those patients with renal involvement is excellent: only 1 to 2% with severe renal involvement will have residual nephropathy, with less than 1% progressing to end-stage renal disease. A recent analysis of prognostic factors of renal disease in HSP indicates that an age of more than 7 years at onset, persistent purpura for more than 1 month, and decreased factor XIII are significant risk factors for progression of renal involvement.

Less common manifestations of HSP include acute scrotal swelling secondary to vasculitis and hemorrhage of the scrotal vessels, pancreatitis, pulmonary hemorrhage, encephalopathy, hemiparesis, and convulsions.

LABORATORY DIAGNOSIS

The diagnosis of HSP is made on clinical grounds because laboratory tests are not diagnostic. Elevations of acute-phase reactants and white blood cell count are frequent. Platelet count and coagulation studies are normal. Serum levels of IgA are frequently elevated. Hemoglobin may be depressed in the context of severe bleeding. Elements of arthritis, acute abdominal pain, or renal involvement may confuse the picture if they precede the appearance of the characteristic rash. Patients with severe abdominal pain frequently require hospital admission. Ultrasonography is the preferred imaging technique to rule out intussusception, because barium enema will miss an ileoileal intussusception, which is common in HSP.

TREATMENT

Treatment is supportive. Most children may be managed as outpatients with appropriate analgesia and hydration. Development of GI and renal complications may be monitored by assessing stool guaiac test, blood pressure, and urine dipsticks at the clinic, unless severe intestinal or renal involvement necessitates hospital admission. Nonsteroidal anti-inflammatory drugs may be used to manage severe joint pain, although they should be avoided in the setting of significant renal disease. Prednisone in a dosage of 1 to 2 mg/kg/d is helpful in the management of painful edema and scrotal swelling, and is sometimes used in children with severe abdominal pain, although its efficacy has not been proven. Treatment of HSP nephritis remains controversial. Therapies used include intravenous pulses of methylprednisolone, cyclophosphamide, and azathioprine, alone or in different combinations, as well as plasmapheresis. These patients are best managed by pediatric nephrologists with experience in HSP nephritis.

HSP is a self-limited disease that usually lasts 1 to 2 weeks. Parents should be told that the disease has a tendency to recur within an initial 6-week period but that exacerbations may occur as late as 2 years after onset. The prognosis of the disease is excellent. HSP morbidity is determined in most cases by GI complications during the acute phase and by renal involvement in the long-term.

12.6.2 Kawasaki Disease

An idiopathic process that affects children under 5 years of age nearly 80% of the time, KD is the second most common systemic vasculitis in childhood and represents the leading cause of acquired heart disease in children. In the original description by Dr. Tomisaku Kawasaki Japanese patients in 1967, the disease was named mucocutaneous lymph node syndrome.

The disease occurs worldwide, either sporadically or in epidemics, with a variable incidence depending on the racial background of the patients; children of Asian, particularly Japanese, background are preferentially affected. According to the more recent Japanese epidemiologic survey covering the years 1995–1996, the incidence of KD is increasing steadily in that country, reaching a rate of 108/100,000 children younger than 5 years of age. The incidence of KD is much lower in whites, 5–9/100,000 children in the same age group. Rates in blacks may be slightly higher. In Japan, the peak age of onset is 6 to 12 months, but 18 to 24 months in Europe and in the United States. The disease occurs more frequently in males (1.5:1) and clusters in winter and spring. About 1 to 3% of affected children suffer recurrences.

ETIOLOGY

The etiology of KD remains unclear. Many clinical and epidemiologic features of the disease suggest an infectious etiology, although efforts to identify a responsible organism have been unsuccessful to date. The hypothesis that a superantigen triggers the disease has not been confirmed by most groups.

CLINICAL PRESENTATION

The diagnosis of KD requires the presence of fever of at least 5 days duration and four of the following five criteria: *bilateral conjunctival injection* without exudate; nonvesicular *polymorphous exanthem* primarily on the trunk and frequently more prominent in the perineal region; *changes in lips and oral cavity,* including injected pharynx, injected or dry fissured lips, and strawberry tongue; *changes of the peripheral extremities,* including edema or erythema of hands and feet, or desquamation of the fingers/toes, usually beginning periungually; and nonfluctuant *cervical lymphadenopathy,* with one node at least 1.5 cm in diameter. The presence of fever is required in 100% of patients; other criteria occur in approximately 90% of patients save for cervical lymphadenopathy, which is present in only 50 to 75% of patients. Patients with fever and fewer than four criteria can be diagnosed with KD when coronary artery disease is detected by two-dimensional echocardiography or coronary angiography.

The course of the disease is divided into three phases. The *acute phase* encompasses a febrile period of 1 to 2 weeks and is characterized by fever to 104°F or higher; prolonged and remittent conjunctival injection, more intense in the bulbar than in the palpebral conjunctivae; mouth and lip changes without oral or lingual ulcerations; rash; reddening of the palms and soles and/or swelling of the hands and feet; and cervical lymphadenopathy. During this phase patients frequently exhibit extreme irritability. Less-common features include aseptic meningitis; diarrhea; hepatic dysfunction with mild obstructive jaundice and ALT/AST elevations; hydrops of the gallbladder; and sterile pyuria. Up to 30% of patients develop arthralgias or arthritis, usually polyarticular, involving knees, ankles, and hands. Synovial fluid analysis reveals polymorphonuclear cell counts over 100,000/mm³, suggesting septic arthritis. Cultures, however, are sterile. Arthritis is self-limited, resolving in 3 weeks, although it may persist for as long as 3 months. Cardiovascular involvement is discussed below.

The *subacute phase* typically begins about 10 to 25 days after onset of fever and lasts until all signs of clinical activity subside.

Although fever, rash, and lymphadenopathy typically resolve during this time, irritability and conjunctival injection may persist. Patients exhibit desquamation of the fingers and toes, thrombocytosis, and coronary artery (CA) aneurysms or dilation in 20 to 25% of untreated children or in 5 to 9% of treated children. Around the second to third week of illness patients can develop pauciarthritis involving hips, knees, or ankles. Synovial fluid analysis reveals a less-significant white cell count and fewer polymorphonuclear cells than during the acute phase. Arthritis in this phase is also self-limited.

The *convalescent phase* begins during the third or fourth week of illness, when clinical signs disappear, and continues until all parameters of inflammation normalize, usually 6 to 8 weeks after onset.

LABORATORY DIAGNOSIS

The diagnosis of KD typically requires the exclusion of other possible etiologies such as streptococcal or staphylococcal infection, serum sickness, or other vasculitic processes. The WBC count typically shows a neutrophilic leukocytosis; there may be a mild normocytic, normochromic anemia; and the platelet count is frequently elevated to >1,000,000. The sedimentation rate is often quite high. The rash of toxic shock syndrome may be confused with the morbilliform eruption or intense perineal erythema of KD, but shock and multiorgan dysfunction (liver, kidneys) do not occur in KD in the absence of cardiovascular complications.

ATYPICAL KD

Patients whose clinical presentations omit two of the six primary symptoms, particularly cervical lymphadenopathy and rash, are characterized as having atypical or incomplete KD, even though they present with prolonged fever and elevation of acute phase reactants during the first 7 to 10 days and thrombocytosis and desquamation of the fingers/toes after the first week of illness. These patients are more likely to be younger than patients with typical KD and should receive an echocardiogram because of their increased risk of cardiovascular complications.

TREATMENT

Treatment of KD during the acute phase includes aspirin at 80 to 100 mg/kg/d and intravenous gammaglobulin (IVGG), 2 g/kg as a single dose infused over 12 hours. The administration of IVGG is usually associated with rapid resolution of fever and clinical symptoms. Patients with incomplete responses to therapy or clinical rebounds can receive a second course of IVGG. Rare complications of IVGG include aseptic meningitis and polyserositis.

The role of corticosteroids in KD is controversial. This therapy was abandoned after an initial report citing increased rates of CA aneurysms associated with this therapy. More recently, however, a preliminary report of 4 children who failed therapy with IVGG after two courses of treatment (initially at 2 g/kg, then at 1 g/kg) documented clinical improvement after treatment with methylprednisolone pulses (30 mg/kg IV). Echocardiographic follow-up showed normal CA.

After the first 2 weeks, aspirin is decreased to doses of 3 to 5 mg/kg/d for another 4 to 6 weeks in order to inhibit platelet aggregation. If there are no CA abnormalities aspirin can be discontinued at this time. Long-term management guidelines for pharmacologic therapy, physical activity, follow-up, and diagnostic

testing of KD patients according to the CA abnormalities were published by the American Heart Association in 1994.

The prognosis of KD depends mostly on the development of cardiovascular complications. During the acute phase, up to 30% of patients develop pericardial effusions that resolve spontaneously and only rarely progress to tamponade. Myocarditis is common as well, and can be recognized by the presence of tachycardia disproportionate to the degree of fever, gallop rhythm, or ECG changes. Abnormalities of the coronary arteries may be detected within 3 days of onset of KD but more commonly occur from 10 days to 4 weeks after onset in 5 to 9% of treated children. Development of coronary artery aneurysms after the sixth week is considered rare. Factors associated with increased risk of coronary disease include age less than 1 year, male sex, fever for more than 16 days, cardiomegaly, arrhythmias other than first-degree heart block, and recurrence of fever after an afebrile period of at least 48 hours. Recent studies demonstrate that patients without aneurysms may develop late functional abnormalities, including myocardial perfusion defects, decreased coronary flow reserve, intimal thickening, and increased total coronary artery resistance. These results are of concern regarding long-term cardiovascular prognosis of KD.

KD recurs in approximately 1 to 3% of the patients, increasing their risk of developing cardiovascular complications. Myocardial infarction is the principal cause of death. It may occur during the illness but happens more commonly within the following year. According to the last Japanese Epidemiologic Survey, the fatality rate is 0.16% in children younger than 1 year and 0.05% in those older than 12 months, for a global fatality rate of 0.08%. Other cardiac abnormalities may be present, including valvular insufficiency (1%), aneurysm formation in other medium muscular arteries (1–2%), or the rare development of severe peripheral ischemia/gangrene.

12.6.3   Polyarteritis Nodosa

Polyarteritis nodosa (PAN) represents the classic form of focal segmental necrotizing vasculitis and is associated with aneurysmal nodules along the wall of medium-size arteries. The disease is rare in childhood. Mean age recorded in most series is 9 years, although sporadic reports involved infants younger than 1 year. When the disease occurs in childhood there is a male predominance (1.6–2.5: 1). The cause is unknown, but appearance of PAN after drug exposures and infections due to hepatitis B virus or streptococci has implicated immune complexes.

CLINICAL PRESENTATION

The main features of the disease are constitutional symptoms (fever, anorexia, and fatigue) that are present in almost 100% of affected children, together with skin and musculoskeletal involvement, which is reported in as much as 80% of patients. Cutaneous manifestations include erythematous rashes, maculopapular purpuric lesions (similar to those of HSP), painful skin nodules, livedo reticularis, cutaneous ulcers, and, rarely, digital infarction or gangrene. Arthromyalgias, arthritis, and myositis are common as well. Renal involvement manifesting as hematuria, proteinuria, hypertension, or rapidly progressive glomerulonephritis may be present in up to 60% of patients. Gastrointestinal disease (bleeding, ulcerations) and neurologic involvement (mononeuritis multiplex, peripheral neuropathy, hemiparesis, encephalopathy, stroke) are less frequent. Orchitis is a classical symptom of PAN, although it is less frequently seen in patients without concomitant HBV infection.

A subset of the disease is cutaneous PAN, characterized by skin involvement without systemic disease. Lower extremities are more commonly involved with palpable purpura, painful nodules, livedo reticularis, and ulcerations. The trunk or upper extremities can be involved as well. Skin biopsy reveals necrotizing vasculitis. The condition is treated with oral corticosteroids, and has a favorable prognosis. Relapses are common.

LABORATORY DIAGNOSIS

Diagnosis of the disease is often difficult because of the variability of presenting complaints. There are no specific laboratory tests. Acute-phase reactants are elevated, and anemia is common. Other laboratory abnormalities depend on specific organ involvement. The diagnosis is based primarily on the clinical constellation of purpura, mononeuritis multiplex, and renal involvement. Biopsy of affected tissue (skin, kidney, skeletal muscle, or sural nerve) will confirm the diagnosis.

TREATMENT

Treatment with corticosteroids and immunosuppressive drugs, particularly cyclophosphamide in IV bolus, have increased the 5-year survival rate from 10% in the 1950s to 85% at the present time. Patients with PAN and active HBV infection should receive antiviral therapy.

12.6.4   Microscopic Polyangiitis

Microscopic polyangiitis (MPA), a systemic vasculitis of small-sized vessels, is distinguished from PAN by the occurrence of rapidly progressive glomerulonephritis and pulmonary hemorrhage. The disease is rare in children. Patients frequently have perinuclear-labeling antineutrophil cytoplasmic antibodies (pANCA) targeted against myeloperoxidase (MPO). The disease has a worse prognosis than PAN with a 5-year survival rate of 60 to 65%. Patients require aggressive therapy with corticosteroids, immunosuppressive drugs, and, frequently, plasmapheresis. Relapses are common.

12.6.5   Wegener Granulomatosis

Wegener granulomatosis (WG) is a necrotizing granulomatous vasculitis of small-sized vessels characterized by the triad of upper and lower respiratory tract involvement and glomerulonephritis. Relatively mild forms of WG without renal involvement have been described. The disease is rare in children. Prior to adulthood WG usually presents during adolescence and affects females twice as often as males. The indolent nature of the disease may delay the diagnosis for months, although presentation is acute in some patients. Frequently, the initial complaints are constitutional symptoms similar to those of PAN (fever, rash, weight loss, arthralgias), which are associated in up to 75 to 90% of patients with upper airway illnesses such as cough, nasal stuffiness/mucosal ulceration, sinusitis, or earache. Nasal (saddle nose) deformity and subglottic stenosis (SGS) are more common in children than in adults (50% vs 10–15%, respectively). A high proportion of patients with SGS require surgical intervention to maintain airway patency. The development of pulmonary manifestations (infiltrates, nodules, hemoptysis, or pleuritis) usually suggests the diagnosis, although they are less common at presentation in children (20–25%) than in adults (40–50%). Ocular abnormalities, including conjunctivitis, dacry-

ocystitis, scleritis, and proptosis, may be present in 10 to 15% of children at disease onset. Proptosis, which can be present in 15% of patients during the course of the disease, is of particular concern because it may result in optic nerve ischemia and visual loss in about half the affected children. Renal involvement is even more uncommon at presentation (8–10%), although eventually as much as 60 to 70% of children develop glomerulonephritis during the evolution of the disease. Other manifestations of WG include arthritis, present in one-third of the children at presentation and two-thirds of the children at follow-up; cutaneous disease including palpable purpura, vesicles, skin ulceration, and subcutaneous nodules (10% at presentation, 50% at follow-up); pericarditis; and neurologic involvement.

The diagnosis of WG has been greatly facilitated by its association with positive cytoplasmic ANCA (cANCA) labeling. The target of these antibodies is the cytoplasmic protein proteinase 3 (PR3). Confirmation of the disease is established by the detection of granulomatous inflammation on biopsy of upper airway, lung, kidney, or skin. Remission is achieved in 90% of the patients using glucocorticoids and methotrexate or in severe cases, cyclophosphamide; however, 50% relapse.

12.6.6.   Takayasu Arteritis

Takayasu arteritis (TA), also known as *pulseless disease,* is a rare disease in children, which is characterized by granulomatous vasculitis of large vessels. The underlying pathology is a segmental arteritis of the aorta and its major branches, which can cause weak or absent pulses in the upper extremities. TA presents with coarctation of the aorta, congestive heart failure, and/or hypertension, in association with features of systemic vasculitis such as fever, constitutional symptoms, polyarthralgias/polyarthritis, and myalgias. Ischemic manifestations frequently present in adults, such as visual disturbances, neurologic deficits, or claudication, are uncommon in children. Laboratory abnormalities are nonspecific, including anemia and elevation of the ESR. Glucocorticoids constitute the initial treatment, although as much as 40 to 50% of patients require the addition of cyclophosphamide or methotrexate because of persistent disease activity. Antiplatelet agents can be added to the therapy in patients with transient neurologic deficits. Surgery is of value in the management of stenotic lesions that do not regress after medical therapy.

12.6.7   Behçet Disease

Behçet disease (BD) is a small-blood-vessel vasculitis of unknown origin characterized by the clinical triad of painful recurrent oral and genital ulcerations and inflammatory eye disease. The disease is uncommon in children, with most cases reported from the eastern Mediterranean or the Far East. The most constant clinical feature of the disease is recurrent buccal aphthosis, which is present in 96% of the patients, with a mean number of 13 attacks per year. Other features include skin lesions (92%), such as a positive pathergy test (appearance of a pustule or papule surrounded by erythema 48 hours after needle prick), erythema nodosum, or necrotic folliculitis; genital aphthosis (70%); eye lesions (61%) such as uveitis, retinal vasculitis, papilledema, or optic atrophy; arthralgias (46%) or arthritis. Less-common manifestations of the disease include venous (15%) or arterial (7%) thrombosis; neurologic involvement such as meningitis (9%); benign intracranial hypertension (4%); hemiparesis or paraparesis (4%); seizures or peripheral neuropathy (3%); pulmonary or gastrointestinal involvement.

The diagnosis is based on the criteria of the international study group for BD, which require recurrent oral ulceration observed by a physician at least 3 times over a 12-month period plus at least two of the following: recurrent genital ulceration, eye lesions, skin lesions, and positive pathergy test. Although males and females are similarly affected, BD tends to run a more benign course in females. Mortality ascribable to the disease is 3%, mostly secondary to CNS involvement, large-vessel thrombosis, or GI perforation. Corticosteroids, oral or topical, represent the initial therapy. Azathioprine can be of help in cases of severe vasculitis with large vessel, CNS, or eye involvement.

References

Athreya BH: Vasculitis in children. Pediatr Clin North Am 42:1239–1261, 1995

Dajani AS, Taubert KA, Takahashi M, et al: Guidelines for long-term management of patients with Kawasaki disease. Circulation 89:916–922, 1994

Jeannette JC, Falk RJ, Andrassy K, et al: Nomenclature of systemic vasculitides. Proposal of an international consensus conference. Arthritis Rheum 37:187–192, 1994

Kaku Y, Nohara K, Honda S: Renal involvement in Henoch-Schönlein purpura: a multivariate analysis of prognostic factors. Kidney Int 53:1755–1759, 1998

Kerr GS: Takayasu's arteritis. Rheum Dis Clin North Am 21:1041–1058, 1998

Koné-Paut I, Yurdakul S, Bababri SA, et al: Clinical features of Behçet's disease in children: an international collaborative study in 86 children. J Pediatr 132:721–725, 1998

Lhote F, Guillevin L: Polyarteritis nodosa, microscopic polyangiitis, and Churg-Strauss syndrome. Clinical aspects and treatment. Rheum Dis Clin North Am 21:911–947, 1995

Newburger JW, Takahashi M, Beiser AS, et al: A single intravenous infusion of gamma globulin as compared with four infusions in the treatment of acute Kawasaki syndrome. N Engl J Med 324:1633–1639, 1991

Rottem M, Fauci AS, Hallahan CW, et al: Wegener granulomatosis in children and adolescents: clinical presentation and outcome. J Pediatr 122:26–31, 1995

Shulman ST, De Inocencio J, Hirsch R: Kawasaki disease. Pediatr Clin North Am 42:1205–1222, 1995

12.7   PEDIATRIC SYSTEMIC LUPUS ERYTHEMATOSUS

Earl D. Silverman

OVERVIEW

Systemic lupus erythematosus (SLE) represents the prototype of a pediatric autoimmune disease with the presence of autoantibodies as its hallmark. The incidence of SLE diagnosed prior to age 18 is approximately 10 to 20 new cases per 100,000 population per year with an overall prevalence of 1 to 2 cases per 1000 people less than 18 years of age. Both the incidence and prevalence rates are higher in African-Americans, Asians, Southeast Asians, and Hispanics. The female predominance (4–4.5:1) in pediatric patients is lower than

in adults (9:1). The mean age at diagnosis is approximately 12 to 13 years, but presentation as young as 4 years of age is routinely reported. Presentation prior to 1 year of age is very rare and manifests as congenital nephrotic syndrome.

Neonatal lupus erythematosus (NLE) must not be mistaken for early-onset SLE. NLE is a disease caused by the transplacental passage of maternal autoantibodies, and the fetus/neonate is an innocent bystander with an apparently normal immune system. Early-onset pediatric SLE is a disease in which the child produces autoantibodies and the immune abnormalities are intrinsic to the child's immune system.

ETIOLOGY

Although the triggering mechanisms are not fully defined (see Sec. 12.1), the production of autoantibodies is the hallmark of SLE. These autoantibodies are usually directed against histone, nonhistone, RNA-binding, cytoplasmic, and nuclear proteins. Antinuclear antibody (ANA) occurs in most, if not all, patients with SLE. With more sensitive detection systems, ANA-negative SLE is very rare. Anti-DNA antibodies are present in approximately 70% of patients, while antibodies directed against the small nuclear ribonuclear proteins (anti-Sm and anti-70kDa RNP antibodies) occur in 40 to 70% of patients. Antibodies directed against small cytoplasmic ribonuclear proteins (anti-Ro and/or anti-La antibodies) occur in 20 to 30% of patients, anticardiolipin antibodies in 30 to 50% of patients, and rheumatoid factor 15 to 30% of patients. Antiribosomal P antibodies are present in approximately 15% of patients and are associated with psychosis and depression.

Antiphospholipid and anticardiolipin antibodies are detected in 60 to 70% of patients. These autoantibodies may be associated with the lupus anticoagulant (LAC), an antibody that reacts with phospholipids in the reagent used in the partial thromboplastin time (PTT) determination, and is often seen in conjunction with anticardiolipin antibodies. Patients with LAC do not bleed; instead, they have an increased incidence of deep vein thrombosis, thromboemboli, or, less commonly, arterial thrombosis. Antiphospholipid antibodies are associated with multiple neurologic manifestations including stroke, seizures, chorea, and other movement disorders; pseudotumor cerebri; and migraine headache; as well as with nonneurologic disorders such as thrombosis, thrombocytopenia, or recurrent abortion.

CLINICAL PRESENTATIONS

Arthritis, dermatitis, and nephritis remain the most common manifestations, but any organ may be affected (Table 12-9). The large variation in the individual clinical manifestations likely reflects patients referred to pediatric rheumatologists, nephrologists, immunologists, hematologists, or adult rheumatologists, rather than the total referral base. Systemic symptoms reflecting a generalized inflammatory process (fever, malaise, weight loss, and lethargy) are very common. In 90% of patients, a disease manifestation either occurs within the first year of diagnosis or it fails to arise. The exception is CNS disease in which only 75% of patients with CNS SLE will have their first episode of CNS disease within the first year of diagnosis.

Renal Disease

The incidence of renal involvement varies between 61 and 81% of patients. The current gold standard for the classification of renal

TABLE 12-9

CLINICAL FEATURES OF SYSTEMIC LUPUS ERYTHEMATOSUS

	AT DIAGNOSIS	AT ANY TIME
Fever	60–90%	80–100%
Arthritis	60–88%	60–90%
Skin rash (any)	60–78%	60–90%
Malar rash	22–60%	30–80%
Renal	20–80%	48–100%
Cardiovascular	5–30%	25–60%
Pulmonary	18–40%	18–81%
Central nervous system	5–30%	26–44%
Gastrointestinal	14–30%	24–40%
Hepatosplenomegaly	16–42%	19–43%
Lymphadenopathy	13–45%	13–45%

disease is the World Health Organization (WHO) morphologic classification of lupus nephritis; these criteria address severity of disease and prognosis and are extensively used in both therapeutic trials and cohort studies. The WHO classification system was modified by the Pathology Advisory Group for the International Study of Kidney Disease in Children (ISKDC) to include six major groupings, each of which may have subgroups (Table 12-10).

Patients in class I have no evidence of proteinuria, hematuria, and/or an active urinary sediment. Class II disease (mesangial lupus) generally has an excellent prognosis. Class III disease (focal proliferative lupus nephritis [FPLN]) represents a transition between class II and class IV (see below). The presence of crescentic nephritis or necrosis significantly worsens the prognosis; patients should be treated as though they had class IV nephritis. However, in the abscence of necrosis or crescents, the outcome is generally better. The most severe form of nephritis, and the form requiring the most aggressive therapy, is diffuse proliferative lupus nephritis (DPLN) or class IV nephritis. An elevated blood pressure at disease

TABLE 12-10

CLASSIFICATION OF LUPUS NEPHRITIS*

  I. **Normal**
    A. **Normal by light and electron microscopy**
    B. **Normal by light microscopy, but deposits present by electron microscopy**
  II. **Pure Mesangial Disease**
  III. **Segmental and Focal Proliferative Lupus Nephritis (FPLN)**
    A. **Active and necrotizing lesions**
    B. **Active with sclerosing lesions**
    C. **Sclerosing lesions**
  IV. **Diffuse Proliferative Lupus Nephritis (DPLN)**
    A. **Without segmental necrotizing lesions**
    B. **With segmental necrotizing lesions**
    C. **With segmental active and sclerotic lesions**
    D. **Inactive, sclerotic**
  V. **Membranous Lupus Nephritis**
    A. **Pure membranous**
    B. **Associated with lesions II (A or B)**
    C. **Associated with lesions III (A, B, or C)**
    D. **Associated with lesions IV (A, B, C, or D)**
  VI. **Advanced Sclerosing Lupus Nephritis**

* Many pathologists use only the major headings without mention of the subcategories.

presentation, prior to steroid therapy, suggests that the patient has DPLN or renovascular disease.

End-stage renal disease or death occurs in 20 to 50% of children with this form of nephritis at 10-year follow-up, as compared to an 80 to 85% 10-year survival rate for all children with nephritis. The more favorable prognosis seen in recent years may be related to more aggressive therapy. Class V (membranous nephritis) has the most variable outcome. In approximately one-third of affected patients, the disease requires minimal therapy; in one-third of the cases, there is a good response to corticosteroid therapy; and in one-third of patients, immunosuppressive therapy is required in addition to corticosteroid therapy. Class VI portends end-stage renal disease.

Accurate placement of patients in the correct WHO classification is facilitated by assessment of clinical and laboratory features, as well as by interpretation of renal biopsy by an experienced pathologist. The prognosis and treatment of renal disease vary according to the WHO classification. Although most patients with clinical evidence of renal disease should have a kidney biopsy, patients with normal renal function, a normal urinalysis, and a normal blood pressure should be monitored without biopsy until features of renal disease appear. The mainstay of therapy is corticosteroids with or without an additional immunosuppressive agent; however, the duration of corticosteroid treatment and the choice and duration of the additional immunosuppressive agent are controversial. A suggested approach to treatment follows.

Class I

No therapy for renal disease is required.

Class II Mesangial

These patients can be managed successfully with low- to moderate-dose steroids and hydroxychloroquine. Although renal flares occur, the proteinuria rarely exceeds 1 g/d, and most, if not all, patients will maintain normal renal function over two to three decades of follow-up. Side effects of corticosteroid therapy (eg, hypertension) are more likely than impairment of renal function.

Class III Focal Proliferative Lupus Nephritis

Many of these patients may be treated with low- to moderate-dose corticosteroids if the histopathologic damage on biopsy is mild. However, if the biopsy shows focal segmental necrotizing lesions in addition to focal proliferative disease, then class III lupus nephritis tends to be associated with a poorer prognosis. These patients usually require therapy with high-dose steroids (prednisone 2 mg/kg/d; maximum 60 mg/d) and cytotoxic agents.

Class IV Diffuse Proliferative Lupus Nephritis

Patients with a renal biopsy showing DPLN generally have the most serious renal pathology. The most recent meta-analysis of multiple therapeutic trials for class IV nephritis suggests that using cyclophosphamide and azathioprine in addition to corticosteroids has similar efficacy when compared to corticosteroids alone. Initial treatment should always include high-dose steroids (prednisone 2 mg/kg/d; maximum 60 mg/d), divided three times daily for 4 to 8 weeks (usually 4 weeks), consolidated to a once-daily dose for 2 weeks, and then tapered slowly over several months. At our hospital, we add azathioprine (2–3 mg/kg/d), which is initiated as soon as possible following pathologic diagnosis; other hospitals use cyclophosphamide, although its toxicities, especially malignancy and infertility, are greater than those of azathioprine. Some advocate initial use of cyclophosphamide followed by maintenance therapy with azathioprine to decrease the toxicity of cyclophosphamide.

Class V Membranous Nephritis

As described above, one-third of patients require very little therapy and another one-third of patients respond well to low or moderate doses of corticosteroids. Determining which third will have the poorest outcome is difficult. A potential clue to the development of severe membranous nephritis may be the presence of low complement levels or the presence of class IV nephritis in addition to hallmarks of class V disease on the renal biopsy. The optimal regimen for patients with lupus membranous nephropathy is unknown; however, preliminary results with cyclosporine are encouraging.

The utility of plasmapheresis requires separate attention. This therapy was initially heralded as an alternative for DPLN; however, the only controlled trial failed to demonstrate a beneficial effect on long-term outcome. Methotrexate therapy may be useful in selected patients with long-term disease that is difficult to control and should be considered for corticosteroid-dependent patients with class II, class III, or even class V disease.

Central Nervous System

CNS disease occurs in 20 to 40% of patients and is associated with significant morbidity and mortality. Both the central and/or the peripheral nervous systems may be involved with multiple syndromes and presentations (Table 12-11).

Occurring in 10 to 20% of cases, psychiatric illnesses range from mood disorders to depression to frank organic brain syndrome. Neurocognitive testing detects impairments in cognitive function or learning difficulties in a high percentage of patients, but the true incidence is unknown.

Depression secondary to active disease must be differentiated from a secondary depression arising from environmental factors or from medication side effects. Overt psychosis or organic brain syndrome occurs in approximately 10% of all patients with SLE and may be attributed to endogenous CNS disease, metabolic imbalance, or infection, the latter sometimes precipitated by steroid therapy. In most patients with psychosis or organic brain syndrome, a lumbar puncture is indicated.

Seizures, seen in approximately 10 to 20% of patients, may be the presenting sign of more significant organic brain disease, the result of an infarction, or the sole manifestation of CNS involvement. Movement disorders encompass cerebellar ataxia, hemiballismus, tremor, parkinsonian-like movements, and chorea. SLE, or antiphospholipid antibody syndrome, is currently the most common cause of chorea in developed countries.

Cranial nerve involvement is more common than peripheral neuropathy. Rarely, hemiparesis or transverse myelitis may occur. Although not studied in children, the incidence of autonomic dysfunction is 40 to 50%, is usually mild, and may lead to changes in heart rate.

A common symptom occurring in approximately 20 to 30% of cases, the typical headache responds to mild analgesia. However, a severe, unremitting headache, sometimes referred to as a lupus headache, usually reflects active disease, or it may represent cerebral vein thrombosis. In all cases of unremitting headache, appropriate investigations must be performed to rule out cerebral vein thrombosis or infection. A more benign cause of headache is pseudotumor cerebri ascribable either to the underlying disease or to steroid medication. Migraine headache may reflect active CNS SLE.

TABLE 12-11
NEUROPSYCHIATRIC LUPUS

Diffuse:	Psychosis
	Depression
	Organic brain syndrome
	Cognitive function deficits
Nondiffuse:	Seizures
	Cranial nerve palsy
	Brown syndrome
	Optic atrophy or optic neuritis
	Blindness
	Papilledema
	Parkinson-like syndrome
	Coma
	Headache—unremitting or migrainous
	Transverse myelitis
	Aseptic meningitis
	Cerebrovascular accident—infarction
	Pseudotumor cerebri
	Multiple sclerosis
	Leukoencephalopathy
Movement disorders:	Chorea
	Hemiballismus
	Cerebellar ataxia
	Tremor
	Hemiparesis
	Dystonia
Peripheral nervous system:	Peripheral neuropathy
	Guillain-Barré syndrome
	Paraparesis
	Myasthenia-like syndrome
Infection:	Bacterial
	Viral
	Fungal
	Opportunistic

Examination and culture of cerebrospinal fluid (CSF) are performed to rule out the possibility of CSF infection or hemorrhage. An elevated CSF protein and/or CSF white blood cell count in the absence of infection is suggestive of cerebritis. Neuroradiologic investigation of the central nervous system (CT or MRI scan) may demonstrate specific structural lesions such as infarction, embolus, cerebral vein thrombosis, and subdural or intracranial hemorrhage, but these modalities are generally not helpful in measuring overall CNS disease activity. Levels of complement proteins and anti-DNA antibodies, which may correlate with disease activity at other sites, may be normal with CNS involvement.

The therapy of CNS disease varies with the manifestation. Most clinicians do not treat isolated cognitive impairment. Active psychosis and/or organic brain syndrome are potentially life-threatening complications and should be treated aggressively with an immunosuppressive regimen that includes high-dose corticosteroids and azathioprine or cyclophosphamide. Psychotropic drugs serve as adjunctive, but not primary, therapy.

Dermatologic Disease

Skin involvement manifesting as malar rash, discoid rash, or photosensitivity occurs in 60 to 90% of patients. A rash in the malar area involving cheeks and nasolabial folds is quite specific; dermatomyositis is the only disease in the differential. A discoid rash is rarer than a malar rash. Although isolated discoid lupus is commonly seen in adults, all pediatric patients with a discoid rash must be followed for the development of true SLE. Many but not all patients exhibit photosensitivity, and prolonged sun exposure may lead to a flare of systemic disease. Sun-exposed areas should be protected with light clothing and a sunscreen with a high ultraviolet (UV) light protection rating against both UVA and UVB. The rash of subacute cutaneous SLE appears as an annular rash with a raised border and central sparing; it, too, has a photosensitive component and is often associated with anti-Ro and anti-La antibodies. Alopecia, listed in the original classification, occurs in 25 to 35% of patients, although it is rarely clinically significant. A vasculitic rash consisting of oral or nasal erosions or ulcers on the arms, legs, or ears may occur in up to 25% of patients and is often associated with systemic involvement.

Musculoskeletal Involvement

As many as 90% of patients exhibit joint involvement, typically a polyarticular arthritis that affects both large and small joints; severe pain and significant morning stiffness are common symptoms. Control of extra-articular sites of disease activity will usually calm the arthritis. Therapy with nonsteroidal anti-inflammatory agents and antimalarial agents may control arthritis as an isolated symptom, but low-dose corticosteroid therapy may be required in some cases.

Patients with SLE are at a high risk for the development of avascular necrosis (AVN) of many joints; this complication is likely secondary to the disease process, to antiphospholipid antibodies, and/or to the use of corticosteroids. AVN occurs in 10 to 20% of patients, who present with acute pain, joint tenderness, and synovial effusion. Septic arthritis must also be considered if a fever is present.

Hematologic Involvement

Anemia, thrombocytopenia, and leukopenia occur in 50 to 75% of patients. Only a Coombs-positive hemolytic anemia satisfies the diagnostic criteria of the American College of Rheumatology, but both normochromic, normocytic anemia, and microcytic, hypochromic anemia are more common in SLE. The Coombs test is positive in approximately 30 to 40% of patients, but less than 10% of patients have overt hemolysis. Thrombocytopenia is present in 15 to 45% and may precede the diagnosis of SLE. Leukopenia occurs in 20 to 40% of cases (lymphopenia and/or granulocytopenia).

The presence of lupus anticoagulant (LAC) in 20 to 30% of cases may have little or no effect on the PT, but the PTT is prolonged. Patients with the lupus anticoagulant do not bleed, rather, they have an increased incidence of deep vein thrombosis, thromboemboli, and, less commonly, arterial thrombosis. The risk for thrombosis appears to be related to the presence of the lupus anticoagulant and not simply anticardiolipin antibodies.

Although 20 to 30% of patients have splenomegaly on physical examination, of more importance is the presence of functional asplenia, which may increase the incidence of sepsis.

Cardiac Involvement

Although cardiac tamponade is rare, symptomatic pericarditis occurs in approximately 5 to 25% of patients and is commonly associated with pleurisy. In contrast, clinically important myocarditis or endocarditis is uncommon (10% of patients). Longer survival times and the use of corticosteroid therapy have led to an increase in atherosclerotic heart disease and myocardial infarction. Other factors predisposing to atherosclerotic heart disease include hypertension, hyperlipidemia, antiphospholipid antibodies, and coronary vasculitis. Coronary arteritis can be associated with acute myocardial infarction. Valvular cardiac involvement is commonly seen in autopsy studies, but it is rarely clinically significant.

Pulmonary Disease

The reported incidence of pulmonary involvement varies between 25 and 75% of all patients with SLE. There are protean pulmonary manifestations ranging from severe life-threatening pulmonary hemorrhage or infection to a chronic interstitial lung disease to asymptomatic abnormalities on pulmonary function tests. Decreased diffusion capacity is the most common abnormality. Abnormalities of pulmonary function tests account for the 75% incidence of lung disease. In the acutely ill patient with severe lung disease, the differential diagnosis includes acute lupus pneumonitis, pulmonary hemorrhage, or pulmonary infection, the latter even prior to steroid or immunosuppressive treatment. Pleural involvement occurs in up to 50% of cases, is commonly seen in association with pericarditis, and is usually easy to treat.

Gastrointestinal Disease

Gastrointestinal (GI) involvement occurs in 20 to 40% of patients. Abdominal pain is the most common GI symptom and can be the result of peritoneal inflammation (serositis), vasculitis, pancreatitis, and/or direct bowel wall involvement (enteritis). Peritoneal inflammation of underlying SLE must be differentiated from an infective peritonitis. Pancreatitis is a rare cause of abdominal pain in pediatric SLE and may arise from the use of corticosteroids and azathioprine.

Hepatomegaly occurs in 40 to 50% of patients. Abnormalities on liver function tests may occur in up to 25% of patients, but are usually mild and transient. When jaundice is a prominent feature in a patient with SLE, then a second disease, such as obstruction, hemolysis, or viral hepatitis, is the likely cause. Patients with SLE are at an increased risk to develop drug hepatotoxicity.

Endocrine Involvement

The thyroid is the most common endocrine organ involved in SLE with antithyroid antibodies present in 40 to 50% of patients and clinical hypothyroidism in 10 to 20%. Grave disease is much less common than hypothyroidism. Steroid-induced diabetes mellitus occurs in as much as 10% of patients, but a lower percentage require insulin treatment. Rarely, hypoparathyroidism and growth hormone deficiency have been reported.

COMPLICATIONS OF TREATMENT

Although steroids are the mainstay of therapy in patients with severe disease, side effects are frequent and include acute vascular necrosis (described above); osteoporosis with fracture or vertebral body collapse; growth failure; cataracts; glaucoma; steroid-induced diabetes mellitus; hyperlipidemia; hypertension; and premature atherosclerosis. Unfortunately, patients with pediatric-onset SLE generally require steroids more frequently and at higher doses than adults. Therefore, although steroids can be life-saving in SLE, every attempt should be made to avoid their use or to use the minimal dose required.

The rational use of cytotoxic agents is limited by the lack of good clinical studies; their use should be reserved for severe and/or life-threatening disease. Azathioprine has a good safety profile, but leukopenia and increased susceptibility to infection must be considered in all patients using this medication. In addition to all the side effects of azathioprine, long-term use of cyclophosphamide is associated with an increased risk of malignancy and infertility. Many pediatric rheumatologists will treat almost all patients with hydroxychloroquine (5–6 mg/kg/d) because studies suggest that its use is associated with fewer disease flares and an improved lipid profile. Because the major toxicity is ophthalmologic, patients require retinal examinations every 6 to 9 months.

References

Boumpas DT, Austin HA 3rd, Fessler BJ, Balow JE, Klippel JH, Lockshin MD: Systemic lupus erythematosus: emerging concepts. Part 1: Renal, neuropsychiatric, cardiovascular, pulmonary, and hematologic disease. Ann Intern Med 122:940–950, 1995

Boumpas DT, Fessler BJ, Austin HA 3rd, Balow JE, Klippel JH, Lockshin MD: Systemic lupus erythematosus: emerging concepts. Part 2: Dermatologic and joint disease, the antiphospholipid antibody syndrome, pregnancy and hormonal therapy, morbidity and mortality, and pathogenesis. Ann Intern Med 123:42–53, 1995

Cameron JS: Lupus nephritis in childhood and adolescence. Pediatr Nephrol 8:230–249, 1994

Lee LA, Weston WL: Cutaneous lupus erythematosus during the neonatal and childhood periods. Lupus 6:132–138, 1997

Lehman TJ: A practical guide to systemic lupus erythematosus. Pediatr Clin North Am 42:1223–1238, 1995

Rich MW: Drug-induced lupus. The list of culprits grows. Postgrad Med 100:299–302, 307–308, 1996

Silverman E: What's new in the treatment of pediatric SLE. J Rheumatol 23:1657–1660, 1996

12.8 MIXED CONNECTIVE TISSUE DISEASE

Earl D. Silverman

OVERVIEW

Mixed connective tissue disease (MCTD), the most controversial of the rheumatic illnesses, is the prototype of an overlap syndrome. The controversy centers around its definition and its existence as a unique, separate disease. The main reason for describing MCTD as a separate entity is its association with antibodies against an extractable nuclear antigen now called U1-RNP, but the significance of this association is questionable. Adults with very high levels of this autoantibody were said to have a unique clinical syndrome consisting of features overlapping idiopathic myositis, systemic lupus erythematosus (SLE), and progressive systemic sclerosis or scleroderma (SSc). The common features included arthritis, swollen fingers, tight skin, abnormal esophageal motility, Raynaud phenomenon, and myositis, but in contrast to SLE, anti-DNA antibodies were not detected and patients were corticosteroid responsive and free of renal disease Although circulating antibodies were thought to be specific for the RNP autoantigen, similar antibodies were found in 40% of patients with SLE and in SLE patients in whom anti-DNA antibodies were only infrequently found. The problem of diagnosis and comparing different cohorts began early because the symptoms and signs could occur in different combinations and there was no precise clinically defined disease. It is still controversial whether MCTD is a distinct disease or a disease in transition that will differentiate into a defined illness.

The pediatric literature is even more confusing than the adult literature. The earliest series described children with significant cardiac and renal involvement and thrombocytopenia in the presence of high-titer speckled ANA and anti-RNP antibodies. In this regard, pediatric patients more closely resembled the clinical and laboratory features of a subgroup of patients with SLE with anti-RNP antibodies, although some patients had myositis. Indeed, many pediatric patients will meet criteria for the diagnosis of SLE or scleroderma. Both the uniqueness of the clinical syndrome and the specificity of anti-RNP antibodies in pediatric patients are questionable. Anti-RNP antibodies have been found in as few as 50% of children with overlap symptoms; conversely, most patients with anti-RNP antibodies do not have clinical features consistent with MCTD.

EPIDEMIOLOGY

Because the definition of the disease may vary, the true incidence of pediatric MCTD is difficult to obtain. The youngest reported patient with MCTD was 5 years of age, and the number of patients increases with an increase in age. A nationwide study from Finland showed an annual incidence rate of 0.10, which compares to 0.37 for SLE, 0.05 for scleroderma, and 0.30 for inflammatory myositis in children. A surveillance questionnaire from Japan showed that the crude annual incidence rates per 100,000 at risk was 0.05 for MCTD, which compares to 0.83 for JRA, 0.47 for SLE, 0.16 for inflammatory myopathies, 0.01 for SSc, and 0.04 for SS.

Follow-up studies demonstrate either severe disease or differentiation into SSc or SLE in the majority of pediatric patients. Large prospective and retrospective studies of patients with high-titer anti-RNP antibodies in the absence of anti-Sm and anti-DNA antibodies reported that only 25 to 50% of patients followed for 7 years or more still had features of an overlap, rather than another defined rheumatic disease. The transformation occurred at a mean of 2 to 3 years, but there was a large standard deviation (3 years or more). Mortality rates as high as 25% have been reported, and the highest mortality was associated with severe Raynaud phenomenon. A large review at five large, pediatric rheumatology centers in England and the United States found only 12 patients still carried the diagnosis after follow-up of more than 5 years. The term *undifferentiated autoimmune rheumatic/connective tissue disorder* has been suggested to replace MCTD.

CLINICAL FEATURES

There is a female predominance (80%), with Raynaud phenomenon, fever, arthritis, skin rashes, and myositis the most common features. Although originally described as a relatively benign disorder, subsequent reports have described involvement of multiple internal organs. CNS involvement is rare but includes cerebral vascular disease with hemorrhage and death and transverse myelitis. Clinically significant eye involvement is very rare. Acute pericarditis and/or pericardial effusion and mitral valve prolapse are the most common cardiac features, while myocarditis and cardiomyopathy tend to be severe, progressive, and life-threatening. Pulmonary involvement is common clinically, and pulmonary function tests frequently show small airway obstruction early in the disease course, with a progressive impairment of alveolar gas exchange. A restrictive airway disease may be seen in more than 50% of patients, and pulmonary hypertension, when present, tends to be severe. The characteristic pulmonary pathologic finding is intimal proliferation and hypertrophy of the pulmonary arterioles with sparing of the interstitial areas. Gastrointestinal abnormalities similar to those found in patients with SLE, myositis, or SSc are frequent. Any area of the GI tract may be affected, but the esophagus is the most common location, with incidence rates of up to 85% for esophageal symptoms including heartburn and dysphagia, and/or abnormal esophageal function as demonstrated by manometric abnormalities. Liver disease is uncommon. GI abnormalities are not related to disease duration nor to the presence of Raynaud phenomenon. Renal involvement is seen in 45 to 50% of pediatric patients and up to 33% of adults. The lesions are consistent with membranous, membranoproliferative, or mesangioproliferative nephritis. A loss in joint function may be seen in up to one-third of the cases. Vasculitis may present with splenic vasculitis, oral, digital, GI, or genital ulceration. The development of other autoimmune diseases may occur, including Hashimoto thyroiditis, myasthenia gravis, and cold agglutinin syndrome.

Infection is the leading cause of death followed by cardiac complications or pulmonary hypertension and renal failure. The mortality rate is similar to pediatric-onset SLE and SSc.

LABORATORY DIAGNOSIS

Typical patients exhibit positive, speckled ANA, anti-RNP antibodies, rheumatoid factor, and hypergammaglobulinemia. Other laboratory abnormalities may include elevated muscle enzymes, thrombocytopenia, lymphopenia, a mild anemia, an elevated ESR, and hypocomplementemia. All patients with MCTD should have high-titer antibodies against the U1-RNP autoantigen, although anti-RNP levels determined by ELISA may fluctuate in accordance with disease activity.

HLA-DR4 has been reported to occur more frequently in patients who continue to have features of MCTD as compared with the patient groups who differentiate, although definite RA may develop in HLA-DR4-positive patients.

THERAPY

As originally described MCTD was said to be a corticosteroid-responsive illness with a good prognosis. However, more recent reports suggest that only a subgroup of patients are persistently steroid responsive, and some may require high-dose intravenous methylprednisolone. In the other patients, the outcome and therapy are directed to the disease into which the patient differentiates. The outcome in the patients who develop SLE is similar to most patients with SLE, as is the therapy. Unfortunately, the same is true for the patients who develop systemic scleroderma. These patients are usually unresponsive to therapy, although there have been reports of the efficacy of immunosuppression. However, the long-term prognosis is guarded.

References

Michels H: Course of mixed connective tissue disease in children. Ann Med 29:359–364, 1997

Mier R, Ansell B, Hall MA, et al: Long-term follow-up of children with mixed connective tissue disease. Lupus 5:221–226, 1996

Pelkonen PM, Jalanko HJ, Lantto RK, et al: Incidence of systemic connective tissue diseases in children: a nationwide prospective study in Finland. J Rheumatol 21:2143–2146, 1994

Sharp GC, Irvin WS, Tan EM, Gould RG, Holman HR: Mixed connective tissue disease—an apparently distinct rheumatic disease syndrome associated with a specific antibody to an extractable nuclear antigen (ENA). Am J Med 52:148–159, 1972

12.9   SJÖGREN SYNDROME

Earl D. Silverman

Sjögren syndrome (SS) consists of the triad of xerostomia, keratoconjunctivitis sicca (KSS), and abnormalities of the minor salivary glands. When the onset is an isolated event, the disease is referred to as primary SS; its association with another autoimmune disease is called secondary SS. Proposed criteria for pediatric-onset SS are similar to the adult criteria: (a) KSS as demonstrated by Schirmer test and rose bengal; (b) xerostomia; (c) lymphocytic infiltrate on minor salivary gland biopsy with at least two foci per 4 mm²; (d) laboratory evidence of at least one of the following: positive rheumatoid factor (RF), antinuclear antibody (ANA), or anti-Ro and/or anti-La antibodies. Children with recurrent parotitis should be screened for the presence of autoantibodies because the risk of developing either primary or secondary SS increases with age.

CLINICAL FEATURES

In primary SS, there is a female:male ratio of approximately 3:1. The most common presenting symptoms are recurrent parotitis and KSS. The pediatric syndrome tends to resemble the syndrome in adults, but is generally milder, although recurrent parotitis and immunologic abnormalities are more common. Neurologic involvement is rare in children and appears to be restricted to ophthalmologic involvement. Renal disease is common in adults with primary SS as the majority will have renal tubular acidosis; nephrotic range proteinuria and renal failure may develop. Although renal involvement is rarely mentioned in the pediatric literature, pediatric patients should be carefully watched for the development of renal disease, particularly renal tubular acidosis. Neurologic involvement is rare in children and appears to be restricted to ophthalmologic involvement. Extraglandular manifestations may be present. Hypergammaglobulinemic purpura is the most common extraglandular feature and is more frequent in children than in adults. Annular erythema, the rash associated with anti-Ro and anti-La antibodies, is also seen.

Laboratory investigations show a positive ANA, the presence of IgM RF, and hypergammaglobulinemia in most cases. Patients as young as 2 years old have been described with primary SS; patients as young as 3 years old have been described with secondary SS.

It is not clear whether primary SS or secondary SS is more common in children. However, all patients with primary SS should be monitored for the development of a secondary autoimmune disease, which development occurs in approximately 50%. The most common associated diseases are SLE and juvenile rheumatoid arthritis (JRA), but SS may also be seen in association with polyarteritis nodosa, scleroderma, thyroiditis, or polymyositis.

Long-term outcome of primary SS is generally very good, although the signs and symptoms will persist. However, patients may be at a higher risk than the general population for lymphoma and, in particular, mucosa-associated lymphoid tissue (MALT) lymphoma. As with adults, diffuse infiltrative lymphocytosis (DILS) can occur in children with HIV-1 and can resemble SS, but these patients usually have many extraglandular features. Although there have not been many HLA studies in children, the association with HLA-DR3 and DR 52 as seen in adults is maintained in children.

There is an approximately 15 to 20% fetal loss in pregnancies of women diagnosed with SS—a rate similar to the outcome of pregnancies in women with SLE. However, it must be remembered that primary SS generally occurs after age 40; therefore, most pregnancies in women with SS occur prior to the development of the SS. Children born to mothers with SS and anti-Ro and/or anti-La antibodies are at risk for the development of neonatal lupus erythematosus.

References

Anaya JM, Ogawa N, Talal N: Sjögren syndrome in childhood. J Rheumatol 22:1152–1158, 1995

Bell M, Askari A, Bookman A, et al.: Sjögren syndrome: a critical review of clinical management. J Rheumatol 26:2051–2061, 1999

Drosos AA, Tsiakou EK, Tsifetaki N, Politi EN, Siamopoulou-Mavridou A: Subgroups of primary Sjögren's syndrome. Sjögren's syndrome in male and paediatric Greek patients. Ann Rheum Dis 56:333–335, 1997

Geterud A, Lindvall AM, Nylen O: Follow-up study of recurrent parotitis in children. Ann Otol Rhinol Laryngol 97:341–346, 1988

Mikulicz J: Uber eine eignartige symmetrishce Erkrankung der Tranen und Mundspeicheldrusen. Berl Klin Wochenschrift 759, 1888

Tomiita M, Saito K, Kohno Y, Shimojo N, Fujikawa S, Niimi H: The clinical features of Sjögren's syndrome in Japanese children. Acta Paediatr Jpn 39:268–272, 1997

12.10 JUVENILE DERMATOMYOSITIS

Lisa G. Rider

Juvenile dermatomyositis (JDM), the most common clinical form of the juvenile idiopathic inflammatory myopathies (IIM), is a systemic connective tissue disease characterized by chronic skeletal muscle and cutaneous inflammation of unknown cause. Symptoms generally begin before 18 years of age. Juvenile polymyositis (JPM), which is 10- to 20-fold less common than JDM, has similar features without cutaneous involvement. Myositis overlapping with another connective tissue disease (overlap myositis) is found in similar frequency to JPM in childhood. These patients meet criteria for both IIM and a second connective tissue disease, such as systemic lupus erythematosus, scleroderma, systemic vasculitis, or juvenile rheumatoid arthritis. Other clinical forms of IIM have been described in children, including cancer-associated, focal, orbital, eosinophilic, inclusion-body, and granulomatous myositis, and dermatomyositis sine myositis, but these subsets are rarer.

The annual incidence of JDM and JPM ranges from 0.15 to 0.5 cases per 100,000 children in various countries around the world. JDM and JPM are 3.5- to 5-fold less common than adult DM and PM. JDM has a median age of onset at approximately 7 years, with a bimodal age distribution in childhood peaking at 3 to 7 years and in the early teenage years. Girls are affected 2 to 4 times more frequently than boys. The racial distribution of JDM in the United States is similar to the racial distribution of the general population. JPM and overlap myositis have a peak age of onset at approximately 9 years of age and a stronger female predilection than JDM.

ETIOLOGY

The pathogenesis of JDM is uncertain, but may involve chronic immune activation in genetically susceptible individuals following exposure to specific environmental triggers. Evidence for genetic risk factors include an increased prevalence of other autoimmune diseases in relatives of IIM patients and rare families in which more than one relative develops an IIM. The class II major histocompatibility locus HLA B8-DRB1*0301-DQA1*0501 is the major risk factor for JDM in white and Hispanic patients. The same haplotype appears to be a risk factor for JPM and overlap myositis. These disorders are polygenic, and other polymorphic loci have been suggested to be risk factors in white JDM patients, including HLA DMA*0103, the cytokine polymorphisms interleukin-1 receptor antagonist-VNTR IL1RN*1 and the tumor necrosis factor-α polymorphism TNF-2. Other immunogenetic loci are currently under investigation as possible risk factors.

Evidence supporting a role for environmental triggers in the pathogenesis of juvenile IIM includes reports of seasonal clustering of JDM onset and new cases of IIM in the same geographic location. A number of environmental stimuli are temporally associated with the onset of myositis in children. Infectious triggers of JDM or JPM include viruses such as coxsackie, echo, influenza, parainfluenza, parvovirus B19, hepatitis B, HTLV-1; bacteria, including group A *Streptococcus pyogenes, Mycoplasma pneumoniae,* and *Tropheryma whippelli;* parasites such as *Toxoplasma gondii, Trichinella spiralis, Wuchereria bancrofti,* and *Leishmania infantum;* and the spirochete *Borrelia burgdorferi.* Further support for infections in the etiopathogenesis of juvenile IIM includes the detection of some of these organisms in affected muscle by polymerase chain reaction technology, the responsiveness of the myositis to specific antimicrobial therapies or intravenous gammaglobulin, and evidence of molecular mimicry, as suggested by enhanced immune responses in JDM patients to streptococcal M5 peptides that are homologous to skeletal muscle myosin. Echovirus-induced JDM has been most often associated with X-linked agammaglobulinemia, although JDM and JPM have been seen in combination with other primary immunodeficiencies such as Wiskott-Aldrich and common variable immunodeficiency, without infectious triggers. Noninfectious exposures associated with the onset of individual cases of JDM include ultraviolet light, growth hormone, drugs (D-penicillamine and carticaine), and vaccines (hepatitis B, influenza, and MMR). One case-controlled epidemiologic study conducted in the United States, however, found no difference in exposure to infectious and noninfectious environmental factors in JDM patients within 6 months of symptom onset compared to age- and geographically matched control children.

The pathogenic process in affected muscle and cutaneous tissues appears to be chronic perivascular and perimysial inflammation, with a predominance of B cells, CD4+ T cells, and macrophages. Interleukin 1α and -β, the primary cytokines present in inflamed muscle of adult IIM patients, are produced by these inflammatory cells, as well as by ischemic muscle fibers and endothelial cells. Tumor necrosis factor-α and transforming growth factor-β, as well as a number of other pro- and anti-inflammatory cytokines, are also variably produced by affected muscle. Complement products, including the terminal C5b-9 membrane attack complex, are deposited on muscle blood vessels, resulting in endothelial damage, capillary loss, and later perifascicular atrophy and ischemic injury.

CLINICAL FEATURES

JDM patients most often present with rash followed by muscle weakness. Symptoms commonly develop over a period of weeks to months, although the disease may occasionally present acutely. Characteristic rashes include heliotrope, a faint lilac to erythematous discoloration over the eyelids that may be a accompanied by periorbital edema, and Gottron papules, erythematous plaques over the extensor surfaces, particularly involving the small joints of the hands, but also frequently the elbows, knees, and ankles. Periungual capillary changes, including dilatation, dropout, and tortuosity, are seen in over 90% of patients, and may reflect vasculopathy in other organs as well as active disease. Malar and facial erythema, and erythematous rashes involving other sun-exposed as well as nonsun-exposed areas are also common. Cutaneous ulceration, resulting from thrombosis of subcutaneous vessels, is a serious complication, but one that is seen in less than 10% of patients. Dystrophic calcification of the skin, subcutaneous tissue, and fascia is seen in up to 30% of JDM patients, and its development is associated with a delay to diagnosis and treatment. Cellulitis, skin breakdown, or ulceration may develop in the deposits. Calcinosis often resolves over an unpredictable time frame.

Muscle weakness characteristically involves the proximal limb and axial muscles, although distal muscle weakness is evident in more severely affected children. The first symptom of JDM may be decreased endurance, fatigue, or muscle pain. Involvement of the striated and smooth muscle of the gastrointestinal tract, resulting in difficulty swallowing or handling secretions, and palatal involvement leading to hoarseness and dysphonia are seen in up to 50% of JDM patients. Respiratory muscle weakness with restrictive lung disease and lower gastrointestinal tract dysmotility may also occur.

Arthritis is present in two-thirds of patients, and frequently involves the interphalangeal joints. Contractures of large joints often accompany severe, persistent muscle weakness. Vasculitis of the gastrointestinal tract, observed in less than 10% of JDM patients, may result in severe abdominal pain, gastrointestinal bleeding, or perforation. Constitutional symptoms, including fever, Raynaud phenomenon, and lymphadenopathy, are seen in as much as 25% of patients at the onset of illness. Growth failure and osteoporosis are common, resulting from prolonged treatment with glucocorticoids, as well as from active disease. Insulin resistance, in isolation or in conjunction with partial or total lipodystrophy, has been increasingly recognized in association with JDM. Other less common systemic manifestations of JDM include cardiac disease with arrhythmias, pericarditis, or myocarditis; pulmonary involvement with interstitial lung disease, pneumomediastinum, or pneumothorax; hepatitis and cholestasis; hematologic sequelae of hemolytic anemia, thrombocytopenia, and myelofibrosis; neurologic manifestations of CNS vasculitis, peripheral neuropathy, and retinopathy; genitourinary involvement with reports of myoglobinuria, testicular inflammation, ureteral necrosis of the middle segment of the renal pelvis, and hypoalbuminemia resulting in diffuse edema.

LABORATORY DIAGNOSIS

The diagnosis of JDM is often made using the classification criteria of Bohan and Peter, which requires the presence of the characteristic skin rashes of heliotrope or Gottron papules. In addition, two of the following four criteria are necessary to classify a patient as having "probable" JDM and three of the four criteria are needed to confirm "definite" JDM:

1. Symmetric proximal muscle weakness;
2. Elevation of the serum concentrations of skeletal muscle enzymes, which include creatine kinase, aldolase, lactate dehydrogenase, or transaminases;
3. Electromyographic abnormalities, including a triad of (a) small-amplitude, short-duration, polyphasic motor-unit potentials, (b) fibrillations, positive sharp waves, increased insertional irritability, and (c) spontaneous bizarre high-frequency discharges;

4. Muscle biopsy abnormalities of degeneration, regeneration, necrosis, phagocytosis, and an interstitial mononuclear cell infiltrate. Perivascular inflammatory infiltrates resulting in perifascicular atrophy may also be present.

A diagnosis of "probable" JPM requires three of the above criteria and "definite" JPM requires four criteria; the characteristic rashes are not present in JPM.

Thirty to 50% of adult IIM patients have a myositis-specific autoantibody. These are autoantibodies to cellular translational proteins found only in patients meeting diagnostic criteria for an IIM, which can be helpful in establishing a diagnosis of IIM. In a large North American registry, 8% of juvenile IIM patients have autoantibodies to aminoacyl-tRNA-synthetases, 2% have autoantibodies to signal recognition particle (all with JPM), and 4% have anti-Mi2 autoantibodies (all with JDM). Although the data in juvenile IIM is preliminary and based on small numbers of patients, the epidemiologic and clinical features, as well as therapeutic responses for each of these autoantibody subsets, appear to be distinct and to have many similarities to adult IIM patients with the same autoantibodies. Juvenile and adult IIM patients with antisynthetase autoantibodies, for example, have severe muscle weakness frequently in association with arthritis, fever, interstitial lung disease, Raynaud phenomenon, and mechanic's hands. Myositis often flares in these patients when glucocorticoids are reduced, and they often require cytotoxic therapies and have a chronic illness course. Juvenile and adult PM patients with antisignal recognition particle autoantibodies have severe proximal and distal weakness and extremely elevated serum creatine kinase. They often have a chronic illness course and require multiple cytotoxic therapies, responding poorly to most treatments.

Other immune-mediated diseases presenting with photosensitive or erythematous rashes, muscle weakness, and/or systemic features can be confused with JDM. These include systemic lupus erythematosus, scleroderma, systemic juvenile rheumatoid arthritis, psoriasis, and eczema. Echo and parvovirus infections, toxoplasmosis, and Lyme disease are infections that may result in myositis with cutaneous involvement. Drugs and toxins inducing cutaneous rashes and myopathy include mercury (contained in paints), D-penicillamine, hydroxyurea, and phenobarbital.

Children presenting with signs of a myopathy without cutaneous involvement should have other inflammatory, as well as noninflammatory, myopathies excluded prior to establishing a diagnosis of JPM. Benign acute childhood myositis is a self-limited illness presenting acutely following a prodromal infectious illness in which myalgias, distal lower extremity weakness, elevated serum muscle enzymes, myoglobinuria, and leukopenia are seen. It is associated with such infectious agents as influenza, coxsackie, varicella, adenovirus, and herpes viruses, and mycoplasma. Pyomyositis due to *Staphylococcus aureus* and group A streptococcus is a localized infection frequently involving thigh or hip muscles, and associated with fever, as well as muscle pain and tenderness. Infectious myositis from hepatitis B, HTLV-1, and parasitic infections may present with identical symptoms and biopsy findings of JPM. Noninflammatory myopathies that may mimic JPM include muscular dystrophies (Duchenne, Becker, fascioscapulohumeral, and limb girdle dystrophies, and sarcoglycan deficiencies); metabolic myopathies (glycogen storage diseases including acid maltase, myophosphorylase, and phosphofructokinase deficiencies; familial periodic paralysis; myoadenylate deaminase deficiency; and lipid storage diseases); mitochondrial myopathies; and endocrinopathies (hyper- and hypothyroidism, Cushing syndrome, Addison disease, and parathyroid disorders). Neurologic illnesses such as myasthenia gravis and Guillain-Barré syndrome, as well as drug-induced myopathies (associated with lipid-lowering agents; nonsteroidal anti-inflammatory drugs; penicillin and sulfa antibiotics; cimetidine and ranitidine; zidovudine; diuretics; and anesthetics) should also be excluded. Steroid myopathy should be considered in IIM patients treated for prolonged periods with high-dose glucocorticoids, particularly in patients experiencing an insidious progression of proximal muscle weakness of the pelvic girdle muscles who have normal serum muscle enzymes and other associated corticosteroid toxicities.

TREATMENT

A general treatment algorithm for JDM is provided in Fig. 12-4. Therapy must be tailored to each individual patient according to disease severity and prognostic factors, as well as the likelihood for adverse events from medications. Risk factors for poor prognosis include severe disease activity; ulceration; calcification; severe dysphagia; interstitial lung disease; certain myositis-specific autoantibodies (anti-aminoacyl-tRNA-synthetases and antisignal recognition particle autoantibodies); vasculopathy on biopsy; and delay to treatment. The goals of treatment include eliminating inflamma-

tion from the muscle, skin, and other involved organs; treating and preventing acute life-threatening complications; and restoring muscle strength and function; as well as preventing morbidities, such as calcinosis and osteoporosis.

Daily corticosteroid therapy is the foundation of treatment for JDM and has reduced mortality from 40% in the era prior to steroid therapy to the current mortality of 3%. Steroids are often administered in divided doses initially, and then consolidated and slowly reduced over months, as serum muscle enzymes return to normal and strength improves. Additional first-line therapies in the management of JDM include photoprotective measures such as sunscreens and sun avoidance, use of topical steroids and hydroxychloroquine for cutaneous manifestations, and the administration of supplemental calcium and vitamin D for patients with inadequate dietary intake. Physical therapy is an integral part of first-line management to maintain and to restore muscle strength and endurance, and to improve and to prevent joint contractures. With active myositis, passive range of motion exercises and pool therapy are used; for nonambulatory patients, a tilt table is also recommended. After disease stabilization, isometric exercises, later followed by isotonic and resistive exercises are suggested. The majority of JDM patients respond at least partially to first-line therapies.

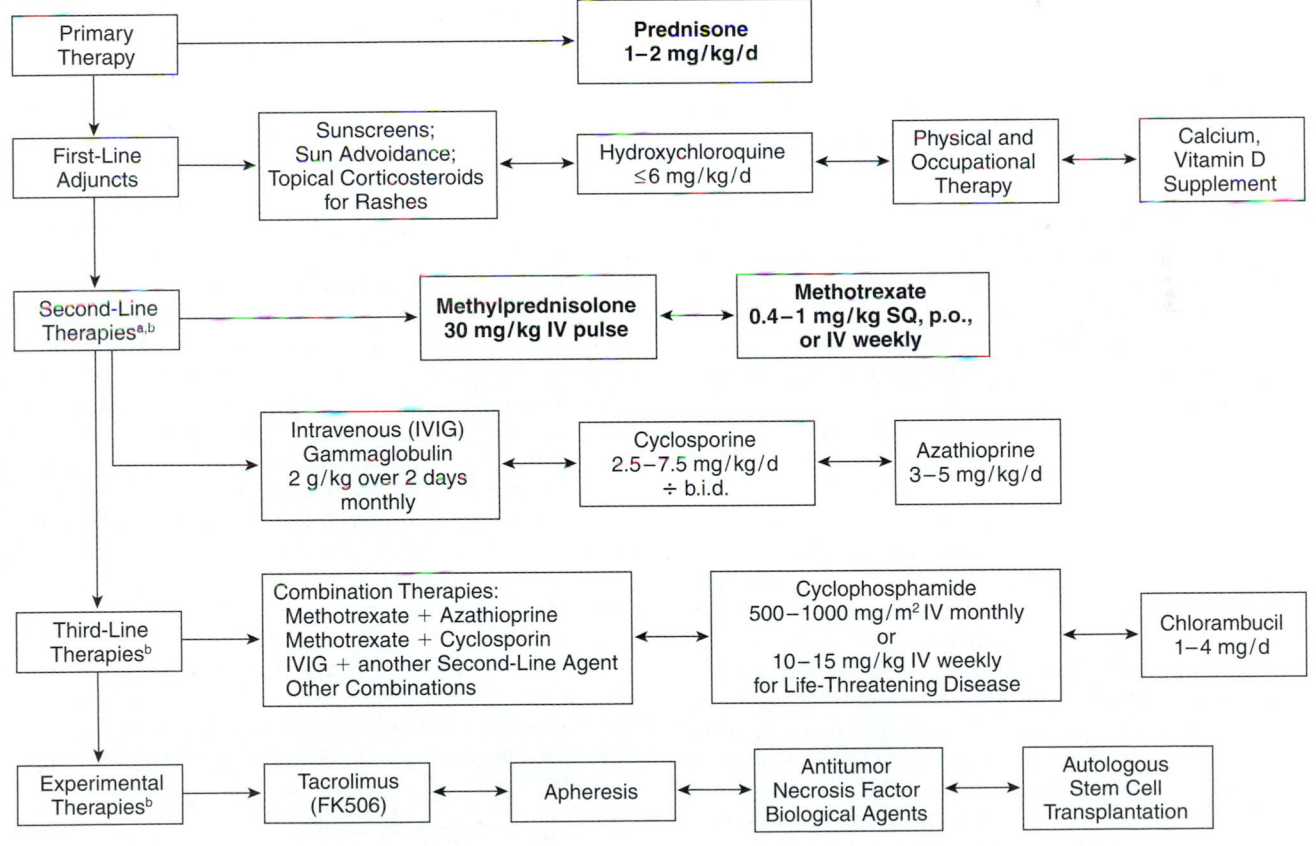

[a]Second-line therapies should be considered in steroid-refractory patients, patients with unacceptable corticosteroid toxicity, and as part of initial therapy to attempt to limit corticosteroid toxicity, or in patients with risk factors for poor prognosis. Risk factors for poor prognosis include patients with severe disease activity, ulceration, calcification, severe dysphagia, interstitial lung disease, certain myositis-specific autoantibodies (such as anti-aminoacyl-tRNA synthetase and antisignal recognition particle autoantibodies), vasculopathy on muscle biopsy, and patients with delay to treatment.

[b]Second- and third-line therapies, as well as experimental agents, should be considered in patients with life-threatening disease.

FIGURE 12-4   Therapeutic algorithm for juvenile dermatomyositis.

Second-line therapies should be considered in steroid-refractory patients, patients with unacceptable corticosteroid toxicity, and as part of initial therapy to attempt to limit corticosteroid toxicity, or in patients with risk factors for a poor prognosis. Patients with acute, life-threatening complications, such as severe dysphagia, gastrointestinal ulceration, myocarditis, or severe, early interstitial lung disease, may also benefit from high-dose intravenous pulse methylprednisolone and/or cyclophosphamide.

Intravenous pulse methylprednisolone is often used to obtain rapid control of symptoms and to reduce toxicity from long-term high-dose daily oral corticosteroids. When therapy in addition to corticosteroids is contemplated, methotrexate is preferred in children as the initial second-line agent. Treatment benefit is apparent within 4 to 8 weeks, and it may be effective for treating cutaneous disease. Intravenous gammaglobulin (IVIG) is particularly useful in acute settings in patients who are seriously ill or who are at high risk for infection. IVIG may be useful as a short-term agent in JDM, particularly in treating severe cutaneous disease or in treating certain subsets of patients with infectious triggers. Cyclosporine shows promise as a steroid-sparing agent in steroid-refractory patients, including the treatment of DM rashes. Azathioprine, which has response rates comparable to methotrexate, is often reserved for more refractory patients. Because the onset to peak treatment effect is often 2 to 4 months, azathioprine has a relatively high incidence of gastrointestinal intolerance and leukopenia, as well as a greater risk of secondary malignancy. For patients with extremely recalcitrant disease, combinations of second-line agents or third-line therapies, such as cyclophosphamide and chlorambucil, may be used. Because of chlorambucil's potential for inducing secondary malignancies, treatment should be limited to no more than 6 months duration and used only in patients refractory to other available therapies or with life-threatening disease.

Amelioration of underlying myositis disease activity is important in the prevention of calcinosis. Colchicine has been effective in reducing the acute inflammation associated with dystrophic calcification. No controlled studies have been conducted for treating calcinosis. In severe circumstances, surgical removal may be attempted when the myositis is quiescent.

PROGNOSIS

While data on long-term outcome are limited, prompt diagnosis and treatment have reduced mortality to less than 3%. Approximately one-third of JDM patients recover from illness within 2 years without clinical relapse, one-third develop a relapsing-remitting illness course, and one-third have continuously active disease without long-term improvement. Calcinosis occurs in up to 30% of recent JDM series, which may be minimal or severely debilitating. Up to 20% of patients may have residual weakness or functional disability, and a large percentage of clinically inactive patients have reduced aerobic exercise tolerance. Patients with JPM primarily have a chronic illness course, while patients with overlap myositis often have a relapsing-remittive disease course.

References

Bohan A, Peter JB, Bowman RL, Pearson CM: Computer-assisted analysis of 153 patients with polymyositis and dermatomyositis. Medicine (Baltimore) 56:255–286, 1977

Bowyer SL, Blane CE, Sullivan CB, Cassidy JT: Childhood dermatomyositis: factors predicting functional outcome and development of dystrophic calcification. J Pediatr 103:882–888, 1983

Crowe WE, Bove KE, Levinson JE, Hilton PK: Clinical and pathogenetic implications of histopathology in childhood polydermatomyositis. Arthritis Rheum 25:126–139, 1982

Pachman LM: Juvenile dermatomyositis: pathophysiology and disease expression. Pediatr Clin North Am 42:1071–1098, 1995

Pachman LM, Hayford JR, Chung A, et al: Juvenile dermatomyositis at diagnosis: clinical characteristics of 79 children. J Rheumatol 25:1198–1204, 1998

Rider LG: Assessment of disease activity and its sequelae in children and adults with myositis. Curr Opin Rheumatol 8:495–506, 1996

Rider LG, Miller FW: Classification and treatment of the juvenile idiopathic inflammatory myopathies. Rheum Dis Clin North Am 23:619–655, 1997

12.11 SCLERODERMA

Audrey M. Nelson

Scleroderma is a spectrum of disorders characterized by an abnormal accumulation of collagen in the tissues. The term *scleroderma* means *hard skin*, which is the result of this abnormal deposition of collagen. Scleroderma is divisible into two major groups: systemic sclerosis, a multisystem disorder with a generally poor prognosis, and localized scleroderma, a disorder usually confined to the skin and subcutaneous tissues with a benign self-limited prognosis. These are rare conditions. The estimated annual incidence of systemic sclerosis is between 0.45 and 1.9 per 100,000 people, with less than 3% of these being children. The annual rate of localized scleroderma including all ages is 2.7 per 100,000. Localized scleroderma is more common in childhood, particularly the linear form for which 67% of individuals are diagnosed before the age of 18.

The etiology of scleroderma is unknown and the pathogenesis is poorly understood. Common to all the types is an abnormality of regulation of fibroblasts and the production of collagen. In systemic sclerosis, vascular endothelial damage with subsequent vascular abnormalities is also a prominent component. Cytokines released by activated monocytes and lymphocytes no doubt play a role in the underlying vascular abnormalities as well as fibroblast proliferation with resulting increased collagen production. Autoimmunity, environmental factors, infection, and trauma have all been implicated in some types of scleroderma. Chronic graft-versus-host (GVH) disease from maternal transfer of cells has been implicated in systemic sclerosis, and patients with GVH from bone marrow transplant have developed cutaneous changes consistent with localized scleroderma. A number of drugs and environmental toxins have also been associated with scleroderma-like reactions.

12.11.1   Systemic Sclerosis

CLASSIFICATION

Systemic sclerosis may also be divided into two separate groups: limited cutaneous scleroderma, which includes CREST syndrome (calcinosis, Raynaud phenomenon, esophageal dysfunction, sclerodactyly, telangiectasias), and diffuse cutaneous scleroderma. The latter includes both proximal and distal skin involvement and internal organ dysfunction, particularly involving the GI tract, lungs, kidneys, and heart.

CLINICAL FEATURES

The initial manifestation of systemic sclerosis in most children is Raynaud phenomenon. The vasospastic process is usually severe and often results in fingertip ulcerations. Subsequently, there is gradual thickening and tightening of the skin starting in the distal extremities, particularly the fingertips, and slowly progressing to involve the face and trunk. Occasionally, systemic sclerosis may start with an edematous phase with associated joint pain and stiffness.

The most common sites of internal organ involvement are the lungs and the GI tract, particularly the distal esophagus. Depending upon the sensitivity of the testing utilized, the esophagus may be involved in 50 to 75% of children with systemic sclerosis, and the lung may be involved in 45 to 100%. The kidneys are affected in about 11%, and the heart in 20 to 25%. Esophageal involvement is characterized by motor abnormalities in the distal smooth-muscle portion. The most specific symptom is dysphagia. Gastroesophageal reflux is common, but is not specific for scleroderma. Children also may develop evidence of pseudo-obstruction because of motility dysfunction in the small intestine, but this is rare.

Pulmonary involvement is usually asymptomatic in the early phases. As the disease progresses, patients may complain of a dry cough without sputum production, or of mild dyspnea. These symptoms become much more severe with progressive fibrosis. Pulmonary hypertension may develop, leading to right ventricular hypertrophy and right ventricular failure. The onset of systemic hypertension may be fairly rapidly followed by proteinuria and impairment of renal function. The incidence of renal involvement has decreased, however, since the institution of aggressive treatment of hypertension with ACE inhibitors.

Early in the course of systemic sclerosis, joint complaints are frequent. Occasionally, joint swelling may occur. This usually subsides as the disease advances. As the skin becomes stiffer, the joints also stiffen, resulting in immobility and flexion contractures.

DIAGNOSIS

The diagnosis of systemic sclerosis is made from the clinical findings of sclerodactyly, nail bed capillary abnormalities, and evidence of internal organ involvement. The nail bed capillary changes include enlargement of capillary loops and disorganization of the capillary pattern as well as areas of capillary dropout. The capillaries may be viewed with a microscope or under the high-power field of an ophthalmoscope. Laboratory tests help to confirm the diagnosis. About 80% of patients have serum antinuclear antibodies and about 50% have antibodies to Scl-70 (topoisomerase I). In the fluorescent test for ANA, the most characteristic patterns are nucleolar and speckled. Anticentromere antibodies are most frequently associated with the limited (CREST syndrome) form of the disease; although this is more characteristic in adults. In children, anticentromere antibodies and Scl-70 antibodies may occur in either subtype.

Esophageal manometry is the most sensitive technique for ascertaining esophageal abnormalities; however, a barium swallow may demonstrate more severe motor dysfunction and evidence of reflux. Pulmonary manifestations may be ascertained through routine chest radiography and pulmonary function testing, particularly the carbon monoxide diffusion capacity; however, high-resolution CT of the chest is a much more sensitive imaging technique. Cardiopulmonary involvement may also be evaluated by electrocardi-ography and echocardiography, and renal involvement by urinalysis looking for evidence of proteinuria and tests of renal function such as the creatinine clearance.

TREATMENT

Treatment of systemic sclerosis is mainly supportive and aimed at specific manifestations of the disease. For mild manifestations confined to the skin, no treatment is necessary except for moisturizing agents which may help to prevent cracking and dryness of the skin. Physical therapy measures should be instituted early to help to prevent progressive flexion contractures and loss of mobility. For Raynaud phenomenon, various medications have been effective, including calcium channel blockers such as nifedipine and alpha blockers such as doxazosin. Paraffin baths and biofeedback techniques in older children also may be beneficial. In the early edematous phase with significant joint symptoms, glucocorticosteroids may be utilized. There is no role for glucocorticosteroids in more advanced disease, and in fact these are contraindicated.

D-Penicillamine has been shown to be helpful in some patients, particularly for cutaneous manifestations. Methotrexate may be of benefit for the skin and articular symptoms. Studies in adults are currently ongoing evaluating the role of cyclophosphamide for treatment of pulmonary involvement.

PROGNOSIS

The course of systemic sclerosis is one of gradual evolution and increasing impairment over several years. When internal organ involvement develops, the prognosis is poor. Patients with limited cutaneous scleroderma have a better outlook. In this subset, the disease process may plateau and not progress or may even remit.

12.11.2   Localized Scleroderma

Localized scleroderma is the most common form of scleroderma with an incidence of 2.7 per 100,000 in the overall population. The prevalence of localized scleroderma is 50 per 100,000 before the age of 18. The term *morphea* is frequently applied to this group of conditions, as it serves to separate localized scleroderma from its more severe and ominous counterpart systemic sclerosis. The most common subtypes of localized scleroderma are morphea, generalized morphea, linear scleroderma, and deep morphea.

CLINICAL FEATURES

Plaque morphea is characterized by the insidious onset of an oval or round circumscribed area of cutaneous induration with a waxy ivory color in the center surrounded by a violaceous halo. When the plaques become more extensive and involve more than two anatomic sites, the term *generalized morphea* is applied. The most common type of morphea or localized scleroderma in children is linear scleroderma. Sixty-seven percent of all patients with linear scleroderma have the diagnosis before the age of 18 years. It is characterized by linear streaks that typically involve an upper or lower extremity. When joint lines are crossed, flexion contractures usually develop. Linear scleroderma may be associated with morphea plaques in other areas of the body as well. The linear streaks become progressively more indurated and extend from the dermis through the subcutaneous tissue into muscle and underlying bone. They tend to follow a dermatomal distribution. When the linear lesion involves the scalp or face, it has been called *en coupe de sabre*.

This term was applied because the lesion is felt to be reminiscent of the depression caused by a dueling stroke from a sword. Patients with en coupe de sabre type may have associated seizures, uveitis, dental abnormalities, ocular muscle dysfunction, and progressive hemifacial atrophy.

Lesions of deep morphea are frequently more subtle and are characterized by thickening below the level of the dermis. In eosinophilic fasciitis, which is considered by some to be a deep form of morphea, the involvement is in the extremities but spares the hands and feet. The skin appearance is described as "peau d'orange" because of the irregular firmness beneath the epidermis. Associated features include eosinophilia and hypergammaglobulinemia. Symptomatic internal organ involvement is absent in localized scleroderma. Subtle abnormalities of esophageal motility and pulmonary function may be detected in some children, but these do not progress to symptomatic or functionally important impairments. Raynaud phenomenon, if present, is typically unilateral and occurs in the context of extensive involvement of the distal extremities.

DIAGNOSIS

The diagnosis of localized scleroderma is based on the typical clinical appearance of skin lesions. Occasionally, in early cases, or in the deep forms, a skin biopsy may be helpful for diagnostic confirmation. The depth of involvement in the tissues defines the various subtypes. Plaque morphea indicates superficial involvement of the dermis, whereas the deep forms of morphea involve the subcutaneous tissues. Linear scleroderma involves the dermis and extends through the subcutaneous tissues to the bone. There are no diagnostic laboratory studies; however, frequent laboratory abnormalities include eosinophilia, hypergammaglobulinemia, positive antinuclear antibody test, rheumatoid factor, antibodies to denatured DNA, and antihistone antibodies. Antibodies to centromere, Scl-70, nuclear RNP, Sm, and SSA are absent.

TREATMENT

Localized scleroderma is a benign condition that usually spontaneously begins to remit after 3 to 5 years. Any decision regarding treatment must bear this in mind. Plaque morphea lesions are of cosmetic concern only and require no therapy other than consideration of topical agents such as moisturizing lotions or topical glucocorticosteroids. However, there is significant risk for disability in patients with linear scleroderma and the deep subtypes; thus, systemic treatment may be considered. If there is active inflammation with progressive involvement, particularly with associated eosinophilia and hypergammaglobulinemia as seen in eosinophilic fasciitis, glucocorticosteroids may be required. No controlled trials have demonstrated that efficacy of any therapeutic agents; however, anecdotal reports and clinical experience have shown favorable results in some patients with methotrexate, hydroxychloroquine, and D-penicillamine. When involvement crosses a joint line, physical therapy should be initiated early to help to prevent flexion contractures.

PROGNOSIS

The prognosis in localized scleroderma is usually good; however, rare cases have been reported to progress to systemic sclerosis. The condition is characterized by an early inflammatory phase with progression to multiple or extensive lesions, then stabilization, and finally to improvement with softening of the skin and increased pigmentation. The mean duration of activity is 3 to 5 years. However, in linear scleroderma, the disease may be active for as long as 20 years. Patients who develop disability related to localized scleroderma are mainly in the linear and deep groups.

References

Blaszczyk M, Jablonska S, Szymanska-Jagiello W, Jarzabek-Chorzelska M, Chorzelski T: Immunologic markers of systemic scleroderma in children. Pediatr Dermatol 8(1):13–20, 1991

Lababidi HMS, Nasr FW, Khatib Z: Juvenile progressive systemic sclerosis: report of five cases. J Rheumatol 18(6):885–888, 1991

Peterson LS, Nelson AM, Su WPD: Subspecialty clinics: rheumatology and dermatology. Classification of morphea (localized scleroderma). Mayo Clin Proc 70:1068–1076, 1995

Uziel Y, Krafchik BR, Silverman ED, Thorner PS, Laxer RM: Localized scleroderma in childhood: a report of 30 cases. Semin Arthritis Rheum 23(5):328–340, 1994

Uziel Y, Miller ML, Laxer RM: Scleroderma in children. Pediatr Clin North Am 42(5):1171–1203, 1995

Vancheeswaran R, Black CM, David J, et al: Childhood-onset scleroderma. Is it different from adult-onset disease? Arthritis Rheum 39(6):1041–1049, 1996

12.12 PAIN SYNDROMES

Murray H. Passo

This chapter describes evolving concepts of several musculoskeletal pain syndromes seen in childhood, which syndromes were rarely included in previous pediatric textbooks. Several of these conditions have been recognized in adults for many years. Reports of these conditions affecting children have been published. A psychological contribution to these pain syndromes enters either primarily or secondarily into almost all cases. These pain syndromes can be readily diagnosed by the typical pattern of somatic and rheumatic complaints and the salient physical findings.

12.12.1 Growing Pains

Growing pains are the most common cause of recurrent limb pain in childhood. A debate concerning the entity of growing pains has been ongoing for decades. "Growing pain" is probably a misnomer because the pains are not associated with physiological growth. There appears to be no correlation between the occurrence of growing pains and the rapid phase of growth, epiphyseal closure, or hormonal changes. Perhaps this term is used because the condition occurs in growing people and does not usually occur in adulthood (after cessation of growth). An extension of the syndrome in adults may include restless leg syndrome. It appears that the prevalence of growing pains is between 4.2 and 33.6%; however, this wide range is dependent on the criteria utilized for diagnosis. The low incidence reported by Naish and Apley was indicative of their stricter criteria: recurrent pain lasting at least 3 months and causing disruption of normal daily activities.

The pathogenesis of growing pain is unknown. Many etiologies have been suggested, including orthopedic deformities, postural abnormalities, and psychosocial problems. Studies have shown that there is a familial incidence of growing pains and emotional disturbances. Oster reported that 39.2% of the children had multiple symptoms, with headache or abdominal pain in addition to the limb pain. Apley suggested that recurrent limb pains were perhaps an expression of a reaction pattern that might partly reflect an emotional disturbance or might reflect part of a familial pattern of pain reactivity.

Growing pains are characterized as deep aching located in nonarticular sites, primarily within the muscle groups. The pain is typically bilateral, usually occurring late in the day or the evening. The pain is not associated with limping or limited mobility. There is no history of trauma or infection, and objective findings are lacking on physical examination. The areas most frequently involved include the thighs, calves, popliteal fossae, and, occasionally, the forearms and trunk. Rarely the pain is located in the periarticular tissues. The complaint of intrinsic joint pain should not be misdiagnosed as growing pains, but rather should herald a thorough investigation for causes of articular pain, such as infection, neoplasm, connective tissue diseases, and orthopedic and endocrine disorders.

Growing pains may occur during the day or evening, and occasionally may awaken the child from sleep. In contrast to patients with JRA, these children are usually asymptomatic in the morning. Occasionally, the child may complain of "heaviness" in the legs on arising. Naish and Apley divided growing pains into three groups: diurnal, nocturnal, and ill-defined. The diurnal pains usually occur during the day and are aggravated by exertion. The pain may bring the child in from play. Children in this group had a strong family history of "rheumatism" or adult variants of fibromyalgia and an association with psychological problems.

The nocturnal pain group had pain that awakened them from sleep. The discomfort tended to be severe, rapid in onset, and of short duration. These children had fewer psychological problems than those in the diurnal group. The patients with ill-defined pains had no clear distinction between diurnal and nocturnal pains.

The parents report no swelling, color changes, or warmth of the affected limb. The physical examination is likewise unrevealing. Roentgenograms and laboratory tests are sometimes necessary to alleviate parental concern. These tests include erythrocyte sedimentation rate, complete blood count, muscle enzyme determination, and serologic tests that are uniformly negative.

The treatment for this condition is empirical. One may prescribe heat, massage, analgesics such as nonsteroidal anti-inflammatory agents or acetaminophen, and "a tincture of time." The parents and the child should be reassured that there is no serious organic disease and that the problem will not progress to arthritis or to other deforming conditions, despite its recurrent nature. It is helpful to explore the family situation in a search for psychosocial stress, which may give the physician insight into the family dynamics and parent–child interaction. The consensus of opinion is that growing pains have no long-term sequelae and represent a relatively benign condition.

12.12.2   Hypermobility Syndrome

Joint hypermobility is an underrecognized common etiology of joint discomfort in children and may be responsible for a variety of musculoskeletal complications including patellar subluxation, articular dislocation, premature osteoarthritis, and increased susceptibility to ligamentous injury. Most studies consider the benign hypermobility syndrome to be a distinct entity. Additional hereditary diseases that must be considered in the differential diagnosis of joint laxity include (a) Ehlers-Danlos syndrome, (b) Marfan syndrome, (c) marfanoid hypermobility syndrome, (d) osteogenesis imperfecta, (e) Williams syndrome, and (f) two inborn errors of metab-

olism—homocystinuria and hyperlysinemia. These diseases have additional features that differentiate them from the isolated joint laxity seen in the benign hypermobility syndrome.

Joint hypermobility is seen in 4 to 13% of the general population. Articular hypermobility is more common in children, and declines during the school-age years. It occurs more commonly in persons of African, Asian, and Middle Eastern descent. The affected children are usually school-aged and adolescents, although patients under 5 years old are described. Girls are affected more than boys.

The diagnosis of joint hypermobility is based on the criteria proposed by Carter and Wilkinson and modified by Beighton. These features can be demonstrated by five simple maneuvers: (a) extension of the wrist and metacarpophalangeal joints so that the fingers are parallel to the dorsum of the forearm (Fig. 12-5A); (b) passive apposition of the thumb to the flexor aspect of the forearm (Fig. 12-5B); (c) hyperextension of the elbows 10 degrees or more (Fig. 12-5C); (d) hyperextension of the knees 10 degrees or more (Fig. 12-5D); and (e) flexion of the trunk with the knees fully extended so the palms rest on the floor (Fig. 12-5E). Patients are scored on a 9-point scale, with 1 point awarded for each hypermobile site. The Beighton score of 4 or more points is considered indicative of hypermobility. Previous criteria have included exaggerated flexion and inversion of the ankle; however, this test is less used because of its subjective nature. The examiner should look for stigmata or heritable connective tissue diseases, in particular, high-arch palate, ocular and cardiac lesions, skin hyperelasticity, abnormal thin scars, velvety texture of skin, and arachnodactyly. Measurements, including height, arm span, and upper/lower segments, may be necessary to exclude a Marfan or marfanoid syndrome.

An increased incidence of a familial tendency for joint hypermobility has been reported. The parents may report that they were loose-jointed as youngsters. Many patients consider themselves "double-jointed" and participate in activities where hypermobility may be advantageous, such as ballet or gymnastics.

The symptoms attributed to the hypermobility syndrome include joint and muscular pain, transient joint effusions, and subjective stiffness. The joints most commonly involved are the knees and the joints of the hand. The ankles, feet/toes, hips, elbows, and back may also be affected. Localized areas of hypermobility may be present but not fulfill criteria for the syndrome. Joint effusions may be present; however, special consideration must be given to a concurrent inflammatory arthropathy such as juvenile rheumatoid arthritis. A high frequency (66%) of hypermobility has been described in a group of children with recurrent episodes of joint pain of unknown origin, also called *juvenile episodic arthritis/arthralgia*. Arthralgia is more common in hypermobile children when compared to nonhypermobile children. Hypermobility may coexist or predispose to fibromyalgia. Interestingly, patients with widespread, diffuse aching are often found to have laxity in their joints, which probably predisposes to the onset of the pain syndrome.

The laboratory investigation—including a complete blood count, erythrocyte sedimentation rate, rheumatoid factor, and antinuclear antibody tests—is usually negative unless there is an underlying inflammatory condition. If a joint effusion is present, a diagnostic arthrocentesis is recommended to differentiate hypermobility syndrome from an inflammatory arthropathy. Synovial fluid in JRA contains an inflammatory infiltrate of several thousand leukocytes, predominantly polymorphonucleocytes, whereas in hypermobility synovial fluid is typically noninflammatory with less than 200 leukocytes. Joint radiographs show no evidence of joint space narrowing, osteopenia, or erosive change. One should avoid invasive studies, such as arthroscopy or biopsy.

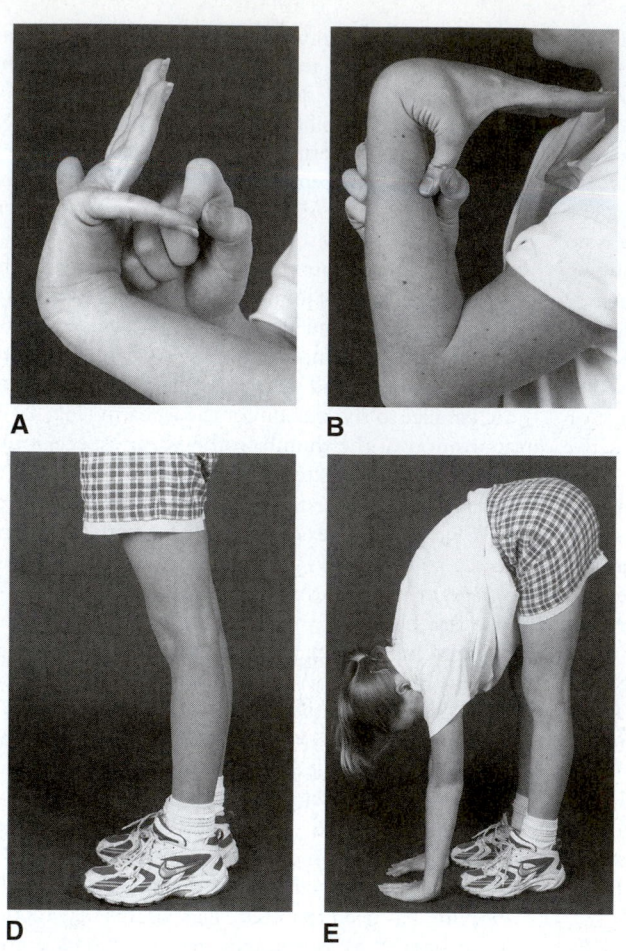
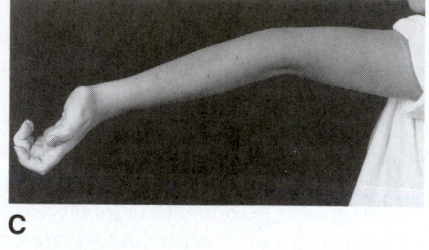

FIGURE 12-5 Beighton criteria for hypermobility. A. Hyperextension of 5th digit. B. Hyperextension of thumb. C. Hyperextension of the elbow. D. Hyperextension of the knees. E. Flexion of the trunk.

The treatment includes (a) explanation of joint laxity and mechanism of pain, with reassurance that an underlying arthritis does not exist; (b) analgesics; (c) a physical therapy program to maintain good periarticular muscle strength; and (d) avoidance of strenuous activities that aggravate the musculoskeletal pain. In most patients, the pain is relieved with nonsteroidal, anti-inflammatory agents. Heat or cold applications are suggested for relief of pain or stiffness. Swimming is strongly endorsed as a good sport to improve strength and cardiovascular endurance without excessive impact loading and strain on the supportive tissues. Psychological problems appear to be important in perpetuating symptoms in some patients. An overlap with other pain syndromes, in particular fibromyalgia, may exist. The joint laxity provides objective criteria to implicate as the source of joint pain in these patients, nonetheless, one must not overlook psychosocial features which may contribute to the pain. The rehabilitation program must address both the physical and emotional needs of the child. The prognosis is good while the patients are young; however, studies suggest that premature osteoarthritic changes may occur.

12.12.3 Reflex Sympathetic Dystrophy Syndrome

The reflex sympathetic dystrophy syndrome (RSDS) is characterized by pain, swelling, and limitation of motion in an extremity; there are associated vasomotor instability, trophic skin changes, and bony demineralization. This syndrome has been called shoulder-hand syndrome, Sudeck atrophy, causalgia, algoneurodystrophy, reflex neurovascular dystrophy, hysterical edema, and posttraumatic osteoporosis. The current nomenclature is *complex regional pain disorder*.

Disorders underlying RSDS in adult patients include infection, fracture, peripheral neuropathy, central nervous system abnormalities, cervical osteoarthritis, myocardial infarction, and trauma (mild to severe). These conditions rarely antedate pediatric RSDS. The antecedent injury or illness may be relatively minor in relation to the severity of the RSDS. In one of the first series of pediatric RSDS, Bernstein reported that only 11/24 (46%) of his cases in children had an antecedent illness or trauma.

The patient experiences a continuous burning sensation, which is augmented by light touch of the skin. Even gentle stroking of the skin causes marked discomfort and withdrawal of the limb. This hyperesthesia or "don't touch me" type of sensitivity is characteristic of RSDS. The limb is usually held in a spastic posture, and the patient refuses to move it because of pain. Passive movement of the limb is likewise resisted. There is swelling of the distal extremity, with or without pitting edema. Vasomotor changes with evidence of either vasospasm or vasodilation are present, including coolness or warmth, pallor or erythema, and accompanying hyperhidrosis. Late in the course of the illness, the patient may develop trophic skin changes, with alterations in the nails, hair, and pigmentation.

The pathophysiology of this syndrome is unknown. Jacobs suggested that this is hysterical edema. He demonstrates how anyone can reproduce the syndrome by partially flexing all the joints of the hand and then forcing the muscles into spasm in a fixed claw. Numbness, tingling, and color changes ensue, and one develops a severe degree of pain and reluctance to move the hand. This maneuver indeed reproduces the symptoms triggered by an emotional or an organic stimulus, such as trauma and/or peripheral nerve insult. Probably both stimuli interact in some cases. A complex pain mechanism explained by the gate theory through the spinal cord pathways is now suggested.

Several authors reported that in their large series of children with RSDS there were certain trends in the psychosocial background of these patients. There was a history of parental conflict, "enmeshment" with the mother, a tendency to accept responsibility beyond their years, and difficulty in expressing anger or being self-assertive. Indifference for the future function of the limb was noted. Secondary gain was evident, because the children had increased parental attention and decreased school responsibilities. Many of these children had been highly involved in school activities, sports, or social functions prior to their RSDS. Psychotherapy was included as a major therapeutic intervention in many patients.

The laboratory studies are usually negative in this syndrome. The complete blood count, erythrocyte sedimentation rate, muscle enzymes, calcium, potassium, antinuclear antibody tests, and rheumatoid factor test are negative. Electromyograms and nerve conduction studies are positive only in the cases where there has been a peripheral nerve injury. Bone radiographs in the adult patient characteristically reveal a patchy osteoporosis. Children do not uniformly have demineralization, and when it occurs there is a diffuse, mild osteopenia. Bone scintigraphy utilizing ^{99m}Tc-labeled phosphate or polyphosphates may be positive, showing diffuse uptake in the juxta-articular tissues of the distal extremity. Conversely, the affected limb may have reduced radionucleotide flow patterns. A negative bone scan, however, does not preclude the diagnosis.

Multiple treatment modalities are suggested to break the pain cycle and to reduce the sympathetic overtone. Early intervention is important to minimize duration of the pain cycle. The mainstay of treatment is physical therapy to encourage the child to use the affected limb. Immobilization is contraindicated and aggravates the pain and edema. The child and the family must understand that resuming normal activity of the limb is essential to recovery. Analgesics are usually necessary in order to allow the patient to participate more comfortably in the physical therapy. Contrast baths with cold and heat application may provide temporary pain relief. Superficial desensitization techniques, such as rubbing or massaging, are sometimes helpful. A recognized treatment in adults is sympathetic ganglion block or surgical sympathectomy. These have been effective in several children with RSDS, although according to some investigators, they are not usually necessary.

Transcutaneous nerve stimulation and electrical stimulation at acupuncture sites, as well as psychotherapy, biofeedback, and behavioral therapy, may be efficacious in children who do not have rapid resolution with physical therapy, analgesics, and desensitization techniques.

The prognosis in children is generally good, although relapses may occur at times of stress or retraumatization to the limb. Adults usually do not regain complete remineralization of their bones, but remineralization has been reported to occur in children. Several authors have also pointed out that children rarely develop the trophic skin changes or chronic contractures seen in adult patients.

12.12.4   Primary Fibromyalgia Syndrome in Childhood

Primary fibromyalgia syndrome is a common rheumatic condition with characteristic signs and symptoms, including widespread musculoskeletal aching, fatigue, stiffness, and sleep disturbance. The literature is replete with synonyms for this condition, including fibrositis syndrome; fibromyositis; universal musculoskeletal pain enhancement syndrome; myofascial pain syndrome; muscular or tension rheumatism; and monarticular rheumatism. The term fibrositis is undesirable because evidence for inflammatory process is lacking. Primary fibromyalgia is often unrecognized or misdiagnosed as rheumatoid arthritis, Lyme disease, or psychogenic rheumatism. Recognition of this condition is contingent on informing primary care physicians about its existence in children.

Skepticism and controversy over the diagnosis of fibromyalgia continue because of the paucity of abnormal laboratory, radiographic, and histologic findings. The etiology of the syndrome is not known; however, multiple hypotheses are suggested.

Fibromyalgia is most frequently diagnosed in women from 20 to 50 years old; however, in children, it is most prevalent in 13- to 15-year-old girls and has been reported in children as young as 5 years old. This pain syndrome is estimated to account for 7.5% of new patient referrals to the US pediatric rheumatology clinic disease registry in 1998. In large population-based studies, fibromyalgia or diffuse musculoskeletal pain similar to fibromyalgia is seen in 1.2 to 7.5% of children.

Fibromyalgia is characterized by chronic aching, pain, and stiffness in at least three body areas for a minimum of 3 months. This duration is necessary to distinguish this disorder from the insidious development of one of the connective tissue diseases. The pain may be described as sharp, dull, constant, intermittent, burning, heavy, or numb. The *hallmark of the physical examination is the presence of tender points,* which are well described and categorized in the literature (see Fig. 12-6). These tender points are defined by the American College of Rheumatology as one of the criteria for classification of fibromyalgia. The 18 tender points are identified by digital palpation over the following anatomic sites: the suboccipital muscle insertions; bilateral low cervical in the intertransverse spaces at C5-C7; bilateral trapezius muscle midpoint of the upper border; bilateral supraspinatus at the origin above the scapula near the medial border; bilateral second rib anteriorly at the second costochon-

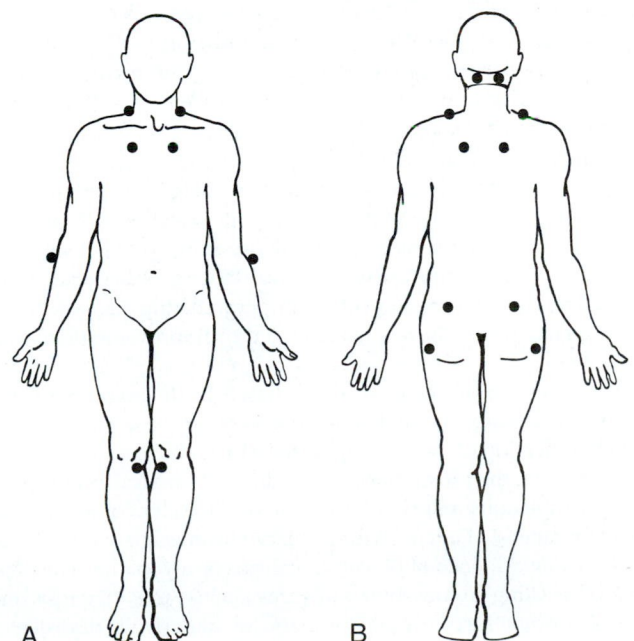

FIGURE 12-6   Fibromyalgia tender points. A. Anterior view. B. Posterior view.

dral junction; lateral epicondyle bilateral 2 cm distal to the epicondyle; bilateral gluteal in the upper outer quadrants of the buttocks; bilateral greater trochanter posterior to the trochanteric prominence; and bilateral medial fat pad of the knee. The tender points are found in specific anatomic sites in periarticular structures, including the muscles, ligaments, entheses (tendon insertion sites), bursae, subcutaneous tissues, and bony prominences. The criteria require 11 of 18 tender points; however, children and adolescents have been reported to have fewer tender points than adults. A minimum of five tender points is required in order to exclude patients who have localized myofascial pain secondary to overuse syndromes or localized trauma. These areas are significantly tender in patients with fibromyalgia; moreover, there may be tender points of which the patient is not aware. Patients are not significantly tender "all over," although their pain sensitivity is enhanced compared to normal subjects.

Patients typically complain of stiffness, especially in the morning, which is of shorter duration than in the inflammatory arthropathies. The stiffness is relieved by mild activity. Patients also report a subjective feeling of joint swelling, usually a diffuse transient puffiness in the hands and fingers; however, objective swelling is not seen by the examiner.

Other associated features of this condition include fatigue or chronic exhaustion, especially when arising in the morning and again in the evening. Patients often feel anxious, although they may not readily include this among their presenting complaints. A sleep disturbance is usual, but many patients do not recognize their sleep alterations. The parents or roommate may be aware of the sleep disorder, having noticed frequent "tossing and turning" and awakening during the night. Some patients complain that pain keeps them up at night. Studies show that adults with fibromyalgia have a significant disturbance of alpha wave activity in stage four NREM (nonrapid eye movement) sleep.

Certain factors seem typically to aggravate or relieve the symptoms of fibromyalgia. Several authors suggest modulating factors—some aggravating and some alleviating. The aggravating factors include cold or humid weather, fatigue, sedentary state, anxiety, and overactivity. Relieving factors include heat applications; moderate activity; warm, dry weather; massage, and rest, nap, or vacation time. Female patients often get worse during the premenstrual or menstrual periods. Additional associations include functional complaints of irritable bowel syndrome, migraine or tension headaches, paresthesias, Raynaud phenomenon, and dizziness. The dizziness has been attributed to neurocardiogenic orthostatic hypotension in some cases. Some of these patients have personality traits and behavior patterns, such as anxiety and depression, compulsion, overwork, and perfectionism. Psychological factors, either primary or secondary, can become important in perpetuating the syndrome. The patients have a course characterized by improvements and exacerbations.

The diagnosis of this syndrome is based on the presence of aching, pain and stiffness, the demonstration of *multiple* tender points, and identification of modulating factors. In addition to the multiple tender points, the most important finding on physical examination is the conspicuous *absence* of articular swelling, loss of motion, or muscle weakness. Patients with primary fibromyalgia syndrome do not have any evidence of objective arthritis or myopathy. The presence of swelling in any joint mitigates against this diagnosis and should prompt further evaluation for an underlying disorder. A complete blood count, erythrocyte sedimentation rate, rheumatoid factor test, antinuclear antibody test, muscle enzyme determination, and thyroid function tests are necessary in most patients to exclude other conditions. Roentgenograms are negative in fibromyalgia.

The physician must establish a supportive and understanding role with the patient in order to help guide the patient to recovery. The patient is encouraged to accept responsibility for management of his or her pain. The management of fibromyalgia includes pain relief, moderate activities, improved sleep patterns, and emotional support. The first priority is to establish the diagnosis and to tell the patient that she or he does not have arthritis and will not need to contend with the crippling or destructive complications of JRA. A detailed explanation of the nonrestorative sleep pattern, deconditioning, tender points, and pain is illustrated for the patient to understand the concepts of their condition.

Nonsteroidal anti-inflammatory agents and acetaminophen are prescribed for pain relief. Addictive narcotic analgesics should be avoided. These patients are not often "cured" and may need to develop a tolerance to a chronic level of discomfort. Heat, cold, massage, and ultrasound treatments are often helpful for local tender point treatment.

Of paramount importance is reconditioning of the patient. The child is encouraged to resume normal daily responsibilities, such as going to school. A regular physical therapy program should be recommended for muscle stretching and strengthening. An aerobic exercise program, which may include bicycling, walking, or swimming, is suggested to gradually recondition the patient. The activity enhances the patient's sense of well-being and self-esteem and reduces anxiety and muscle tension; in addition, it has some modulatory effect on sleep patterns. The rationale for aerobic exercise is based on an observation that endurance athletes do not get fibromyalgia; moreover, aerobic exercise has been demonstrated in patients with fibromyalgia to be efficacious in pain reduction compared to isometric exercise programs.

The sleep disorder is important in the pathogenesis of fibromyalgia and may require treatment with a tricyclic, such as amitriptyline or cyclobenzaprine, at bedtime. Morning drowsiness, however, may conflict with the patient's tolerance to the medication.

The emotional component of the syndrome may require counseling. Stress reduction techniques with biofeedback or self-hypnosis may be helpful in patients with resistant pain. Patients may benefit from cognitive-behavioral treatment or treatment for depression, anxiety, or stress. Psychiatric consultation is often necessary in the more complex patients.

The outcome of patients with fibromyalgia in childhood is perhaps better than the outcome in adults. After several years, most patients are improved, either in remission or with less symptomatology at follow-up.

12.12.5 Psychogenic Rheumatism

In three of the pain syndromes discussed above, there are specific physical findings: that is, joint hypermobility, tender points, or bizarre limb posturing with swelling and vasomotor changes. In addition, the patients commonly have psychological problems that contribute to the perpetuation of the pain. Thus, these conditions involve both organic and psychological abnormalities. In psychogenic rheumatism, the child also has complaints of joint pain, but objective physical abnormalities are lacking, and the complaints cannot be categorized into any established organic diagnosis. In some cases, these musculoskeletal complaints may be a manifestation of hysteria. Creak described three hysterical patterns: (a) a true conversion hysteria in which the symptoms are caused by conversion of anxiety into somatic complaints; (b) hysterical prolongation of a symptom originally part of an organically determined disease; and (c) organic disease in which psychological factors play an important part. The hypermobility syndrome, fibromyalgia, and RSDS may represent the second and third patterns of childhood hysteria.

The children with psychogenic rheumatism complain of pain in excess of what one would expect from the slight or absent physical findings. This is especially true when one considers that children with JRA, who have objective findings of inflammation, generally do not complain of excessive pain. Patients who have severe, debilitating pain associated with avascular necrosis of bone, osteomyelitis, discitis, or neoplasm have significant objective physical findings; moreover, they have positive laboratory and radiographic tests.

There are several signs and symptoms that should alert the physician to a possible psychological problem, including: (a) dramatic urgency for an appointment that is disproportionate to the magnitude of the complaints; (b) a written list of complaints and questions; (c) a lengthy portfolio of previous laboratory and radiographic studies; (d) a previous examination that shows a trivial, noncontributory abnormality that has been implicated as the cause for the pain; (e) a preoccupation with permanent disability based on anecdotal reports from friends and relatives of the family; (f) a parent who shares in the pain and suffering, for example, "we hurt here" or "we took medication," or, conversely, a completely silent parent, with the other being the sole spokesperson; (g) immediate muscular resistance during attempted passive movement on examinations; (h) exaggerated facial grimacing when objective physical findings are lacking; and (i) holding the doctor's hand or forearm for protection from pain. These signs should help the physician anticipate underlying psychological problems; however, they do *not* rule out the possibility of an organic problem.

Children with psychogenic rheumatism may have symptoms of depression, which are often attributed to the chronic pain. They do not readily admit to feelings of depression. Alternatively, the pain may *mask* the depressive mood and protect the individual from an overt primary depressive disorder. The symptoms of this depressive disorder include lack of initiative, inactivity, fatigue, withdrawal from school and social activities, poor sleep, anorexia, and depressive mood. Many of these patients are "juvenile workaholics" prior to the development of the pain syndrome—they do superior academic work and are heavily loaded with extracurricular activities. In contrast, some of the children are learning-disabled, underachieving, and have poor self-esteem. A history of a prior illness or trauma may be elicited, and for unknown reasons the patient "fails to recover" and has emotional prolongation of the symptoms. After the development of chronic pain, the child will often have a history of school absenteeism and disinterest in social activities. The continued pain causes both the patient and the parents to worry about a serious underlying condition which has not evolved fully enough to be diagnosed. This results in multiple medical consultations with endless and costly physical studies. These additional investigations, in turn, generate further concern and anxiety for the patient.

Proper recognition of this syndrome is the first step toward rehabilitation of the patient. Psychological treatment can only proceed after the physician is satisfied with the diagnosis. The physician must express to the patient that this type of pain is very real and that it is not due to an undiscovered ailment. A great disservice is done to the patient by implicating, out of frustration, that the pain is peculiar or perhaps imaginary ("all in their heads"). One can anticipate resistance to accepting this explanation, from both the patient and the parents. Parents may say that they have been told by other physicians that the problem is psychological. In addition, it has been observed that there is commonly a disagreement between the two parents. One parent perpetuates the disabling state and one parent acknowledges the psychological problem.

The management of these patients includes several steps. First, the physician must limit further investigations. Reinvestigation perpetuates the patient's anxiety and discredits the diagnosis. Second, a well-planned rehabilitation program using physical and occupational therapy should be instituted. A gradual reinstitution of normal activities is essential. Encourage the patient to return to school and to accept normal responsibilities, but discourage extracurricular activities in the beginning. We have successfully used inpatient rehabilitation and physical therapy, which have allowed our patients to "reenter with honor" when they return to school. The third component involves evaluation and treatment of the underlying psychological problems. This may require involvement of a psychiatrist, clinical psychologist, and/or social worker. Often the primary care physician has insight into preexisting family problems and can satisfactorily elicit and treat the psychological problems. The family must be instructed not to be solicitous of the pain but to be supportive of all the child's attempts to become more active. With physical reconditioning, the patient will have more energy and can add more activities. It is essential that the patient form a close relationship with the treating physician. The prognosis for the patient's recovery is good if the underlying problems are dealt with effectively. Some patients, however, are extremely difficult to manage and will abandon the proposed treatment and continue to shop around and pursue the "cure" that previous physicians could not offer.

References

Bernstein BH, Singsen BH, Kent JT, et al: Reflex neurovascular dystrophy in childhood. J Pediatr 93(2):211–215, 1978

Everman DB, Robin NH: Hypermobility syndrome. Pediatr Rev 19(4): 111–117, 1998

Gedalia A, Press J: Articular symptoms in hypermobile schoolchildren: a prospective study. J Pediatr 119(6):944–946, 1991

Gedalia A, Press J, Klein M, Buskila D: Joint hypermobility and fibromyalgia in schoolchildren. Ann Rheum Dis 52:494–496, 1993

Mikkelsson M, Sourander A, Piha J, Salminen J: Psychiatric symptoms in preadolescents with musculoskeletal pain and fibromyalgia. Pediatrics 100(2):220–227, 1997

Oster J, Nielsen A: Growing pains. Acta Paediatr Scand 61:329–334, 1972

Rotes-Querol J: The syndromes of psychogenic rheumatism. Clin Rheum Dis 5:797–805, 1979

Sherry DD, McGuire T, Elizabeth M, et al: Psychosomatic musculoskeletal pairs in childhood: clinical and psychological analyses on 100 children. Pediatrics 88:1093–1099, 1991

Sherry DD, Weisman R: Psychologic aspects of childhood reflex neurovascular dystrophy. Pediatrics 81(4):572–578, 1988

Siegel DM, Janeway D, Baum J: Fibromyalgia syndrome in children and adolescents: clinical features at presentation and status at follow-up. Pediatrics 101(3):377–382, 1998

Wilder R, Berde CB, Wolohan M, Vieyra MA, Masek BJ, Micheli LJ: Reflex sympathetic dystrophy in children: clinical characteristics and follow-up of seventy patients. J Bone Joint Surg Am 74(6):910–919, 1992

Yunus M, Masi A: Juvenile primary fibromyalgia syndrome: A clinical study of 33 patients and matched normal controls. Arthritis Rheum 28:138–145, 1985

12.13 AMYLOIDOSIS AND FAMILIAL MEDITERRANEAN FEVER

Philip J. Hashkes

12.13.1 Amyloidosis

Amyloidosis is characterized by the extracellular accumulation of protein fibrils that eventually interfere with organ function. These fibrils usually derive from soluble circulating protein precursors that undergo secondary structural changes to form insoluble fibrillar deposits. Amyloid is recognized in histologic specimens by the binding of Congo-Red with green-yellow birefringence under polarized light.

Amyloidosis is the end result of many disease processes. At least 15 different protein precursors have been identified. The most common type of amyloid seen in children is the AA type, which derives from the acute-phase reactant protein serum amyloid A (SAA). AL amyloidosis, related primarily to multiple myeloma or other B-cell dyscrasias, is rarely seen in childhood. The precursor of AL is the immunoglobulin light chain. Other types of amyloidoses derive from mutations in amyloid precursors that result in tissue deposition of abnormal proteins. The most common form is the ATTR type in which the precursor is transthyretin, a serum protein that carries thyroxin and retinol-binding protein. Most of these genetic disorders are autosomal dominant. Symptoms rarely appear before the third decade.

CLINICAL FEATURES

The deposition of AA is associated with infectious diseases and chronic inflammatory conditions such as familial Mediterranean fever (FMF; see below) and juvenile idiopathic arthritis (JIA). Amyloidosis can also be seen following long-standing inflammatory bowel disease, Behçet disease, and systemic lupus erythematosus. Chronic infections associated with amyloidosis include tuberculosis, leprosy, bronchiectasis, and chronic osteomyelitis.

Amyloidosis appears mainly in systemic-onset JIA, but can also be found in polyarticular JIA, psoriatic arthritis, and juvenile ankylosing spondylitis. The risk of amyloidosis in JIA is geographically dependent, but no consistent genetic factors have been observed. The prevalence of AA amyloidosis in European patients with JIA is between 3 and 11%, but it is almost nonexistent in the United States. In recent years, a decrease in the incidence of amyloidosis has been observed, related perhaps to the more aggressive medical therapy of JIA.

Renal disease is the dominant clinical manifestation of AA deposition. Patients typically present with proteinuria, often intermittent at first, with rapid progression to the nephrotic syndrome and eventual renal failure. In FMF, proteinuria and amyloidosis may precede the more typical manifestations and may occur in early childhood. Elevated serum creatinine level at presentation is a poor prognostic sign. Renal tubular acidosis may also be seen. Renal vein thrombosis is a common complication in patients with nephrotic syndrome. Abdominal pain and diarrhea may reflect intestinal wall edema. Spleen and/or liver enlargement is seen in 25 to 60% of patients, usually without biochemical abnormalities.

While tissue deposition is widespread in AA amyloidosis, other clinical manifestations usually appear only in long-standing amyloidosis. These include macroglossia, cardiomyopathy, peripheral neuropathies, malabsorption, weight loss, and bleeding disorders. Amyloidosis arthropathy also occurs late, is characterized by stiffness rather than pain, and can involve both large and small joints. The hereditary amyloidoses often present in the third decade of life with cardiomyopathy and/or sensorimotor and autonomic peripheral neuropathy. The clinical syndrome derived from mutations in transthyretin (TTR) is termed familial amyloidotic cardiomyopathy or polyneuropathy.

DIAGNOSIS

No blood test is diagnostic of amyloidosis. However, markedly increased erythrocyte sedimentation rate, C-reactive protein, and SAA levels with active inflammation, proteinuria, and hypoalbuminemia suggest the presence of amyloidosis.

The definitive test for amyloidosis is tissue demonstration of amyloid. Rectal or gingival biopsy or subcutaneous fat aspiration is the procedure of first choice, because internal organ biopsies are associated with a high risk of bleeding in patients with amyloidosis. The sensitivity of rectal biopsy and/or subcutaneous fat aspiration in detecting AA amyloidosis is between 64 and 97%. Rectal biopsy is preferred in FMF, because amyloid is generally not found in the subcutaneous fat of these patients. Performance of immunohistochemistry, in addition to Congo-Red staining, increases the yield of positive biopsies.

An excellent noninvasive assay for detection and quantification of AA renal amyloidosis is based on the specific binding of serum amyloid P-component (SAP) to amyloid fibrils. Radioiodinated (^{123}I) SAP is administered intravenously and is scanned with a gamma camera 24 hours later. Localized amyloid deposits, rapid plasma clearance, and increased whole-body retention are seen in patients with significant amyloid accumulation. Deposits of amyloid can be demonstrated in organs without overt clinical signs. This procedure may be useful in monitoring the effect of therapy. An algorithm for evaluation of a patient with suspected amyloidosis is presented in Fig. 12-7.

TREATMENT

Prevention is much more effective than the treatment of disease after it develops. Aggressive treatment of underlying infections, JIA and other inflammatory conditions, and colchicine therapy for FMF (see below) usually prevent the development of amyloidosis. After amyloidosis has appeared, colchicine and anti-inflammatory therapy may slow or retard the progression of disease, but usually do not reverse the process. Chlorambucil has been shown to increase life expectancy in JIA-related amyloidosis but is associated with higher risks of secondary leukemia and infertility.

The nephrotic syndrome, hypertension, and renal failure require directed therapy and may progress to a need for dialysis. Renal transplant may be an option in patients with well-controlled inflammatory processes; recurrence within 4 years has been reported in some patients. Treatment of AL amyloidosis consists of chemotherapy, mainly high-dose melphalan and prednisone. Initial studies indicate that liver transplantation may be the definitive treatment for ATTR amyloidosis.

12.13.2 Familial Mediterranean Fever

FMF is a periodic disorder with an autosomal recessive inheritance. FMF is prevalent mainly in Sephardic Jews, Armenians, Turks, and Levantine Arabs, and is rare among Northern Europeans, blacks,

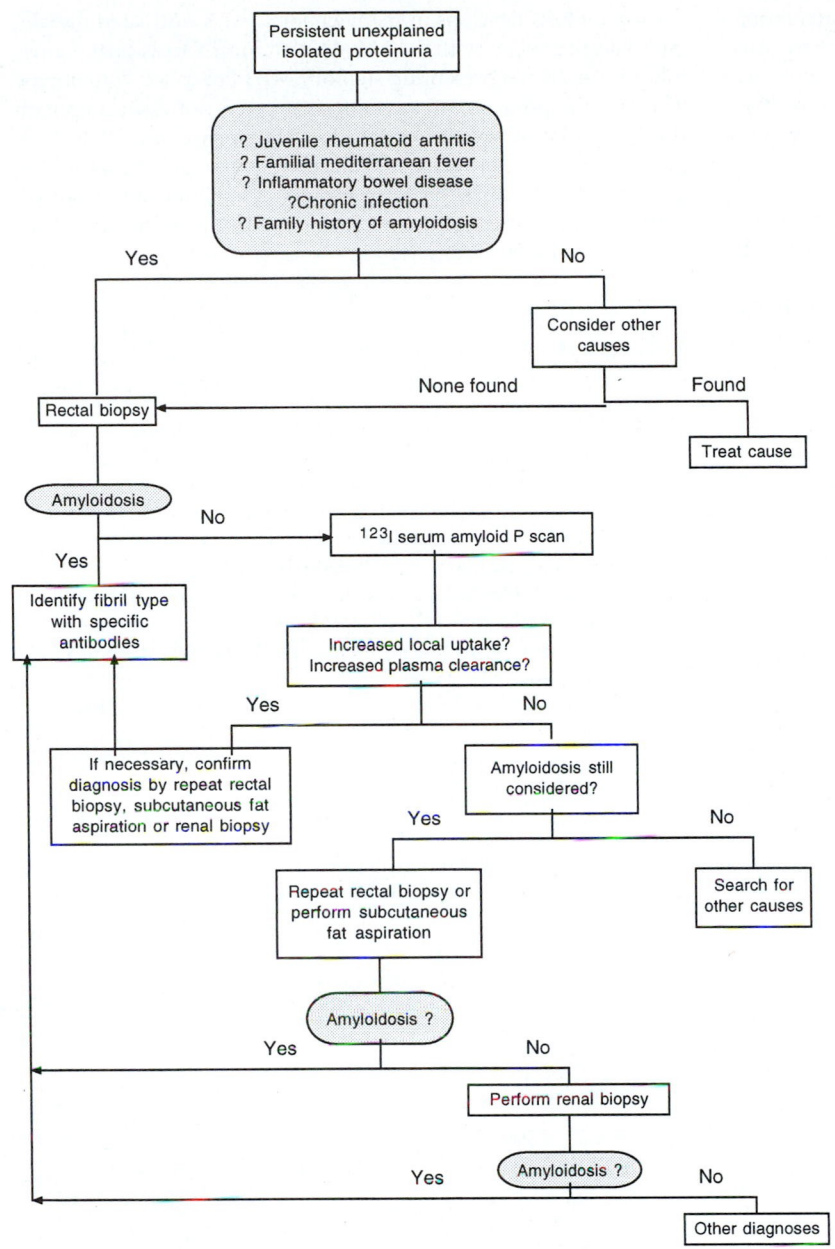

FIGURE 12-7 Algorithm for the diagnosis of amyloidosis in children.

and Chinese. Recently, the gene responsible for the development of FMF has been localized to the short arm of chromosome 16. The product of this gene is a 781-amino-acid protein termed *Pyrin,* which plays an important role in the regulation of the polymorphonuclear cell inflammatory response. More than 10 missense mutations have been identified, mainly in exon 10, of which the most common is the substitution of methionine for valine at the 694 amino acid (M694V). This mutation is prevalent especially among North African Jews and appears to be associated with the early onset of severe disease and the development of amyloidosis.

CLINICAL MANIFESTATIONS

Symptoms usually appear during the first decade of life. At irregular intervals, almost all patients have periodic febrile episodes that last between several hours and 5 days. Attacks can appear as often as several times per week or considerably less frequently, with intervals of several years between episodes. Severe abdominal pain resembling peritonitis accompanies the fever in nearly 90% of patients.

Other symptoms related to serositis include pleuritis (33–45% of patients), pericarditis, and scrotal swelling. A characteristic erysipelas-like rash around the ankles appears in 15 to 25% of patients. Arthralgias, arthritis, and myalgias are seen in 50 to 75% of patients. The most common form consists of brief episodes of extremely painful monoarthritis, mainly in the lower extremities. Nearly 10% of the patients may develop prolonged episodes of arthritis lasting more than 1 month or chronic arthritis with residual joint damage.

Less-common manifestations include episodes of protracted hyperglobulinemic febrile myalgia responsive to corticosteroid therapy, splenomegaly, Henoch-Schönlein purpura, polyarteritis nodosa, aseptic meningitis, and thyroid abnormalities.

DIAGNOSIS

Diagnostic criteria for FMF have been described based on the clinical pattern, family history, and response to colchicine therapy. Laboratory tests are nonspecific and do not contribute to the diagnosis, although acute-phase reactant levels, erythrocyte sedimentation rate, C-reactive protein, fibrinogen, and leukocyte counts are usually elevated. Because only a few of the common mutations are currently tested in the laboratory, genetic analysis cannot reliably be used to diagnose FMF. As many as 30% of FMF patients test either as heterozygote carriers or do not show any of the mutations.

The differential diagnosis includes other causes of periodic fever: cyclic neutropenia, hyperimmunoglobulinemia D syndrome, familial Hibernian fever, and Behçet disease. Autosomal dominant periodic fever syndromes have recently been associated with mutations in the tumor necrosis factor receptor 1, resulting in a 50% decrease in soluble receptor levels. A benign syndrome of periodic fever, aphthous-stomatitis, pharyngitis, and cervical adenitis (PFAPA) has been described in children less than 10 years old. Repeated throat cultures are negative for streptococcus. Episodes are usually longer than in FMF, lasting 5 to 7 days, and resolve dramatically after administration of one dose of prednisone (1–2 mg/kg).

TREATMENT

The treatment of FMF with daily prophylactic colchicine, introduced by Goldfinger in 1972, is efficacious in preventing both acute attacks and amyloidosis. Treatment is started with 1 mg/d, regardless of age, weight, frequency, and severity of attacks. This dose is effective in preventing amyloidosis in nearly all patients and preventing attacks in 65% of patients. Other patients will need doses as high as 2 mg/d in two divided doses, and 5% will not respond to the higher dose. Colchicine is generally well tolerated. The most common side effects, diarrhea and nausea, are usually transient and amenable to gradual dosage changes. No effects of colchicine on growth and development have been observed.

Amyloidosis develops in many children with untreated disease, especially in patients with the M694V mutation. Occasionally, amyloidosis can be the presenting sign of FMF (also called "phenotype 2"), and the presence of amyloidosis is often not associated with the frequency or severity of attacks. The amyloidosis of FMF is predominately nephrogenic. Colchicine therapy can retard the progress but usually does not reverse existing amyloidosis. However, marked improvement of the nephrotic syndrome following colchicine therapy has been reported in several patients.

References

David J, Vouyiouka O, Ansell BA, Hall A, Woo P: Amyloidosis in juvenile rheumatoid arthritis: a morbidity and mortality study. Clin Exp Rheumatol 11:85–90, 1993

Drenth JPH, The International Hyper IgD Study Group: Hyperimmunoglobulinemia D and periodic fever syndrome: the clinical spectrum in a series of 50 patients. Medicine 73:133–144, 1994

Gedalia A, Adar A, Gorodischer R: Familial Mediterranean fever in children. J Rheumatol 19(Suppl 35):1–9, 1992

Goldfinger SE: Colchicine therapy for familial Mediterranean fever. N Engl J Med 291:932–934, 1974

Marshall GS, Edwards KM, Butler J, Lawton AR: Periodic fever, pharyngitis and aphthous stomatitis. J Pediatr 110:43–46, 1987

The French FMF Consortium: A candidate gene for familial Mediterranean fever. Nat Genet 17:25–31, 1997

The International FMF Consortium. Ancient missense mutations in a new member of the RoRet gene family are likely to cause familial Mediterranean fever. Cell 90:797–807, 1997

Woo P: Amyloidosis in children. Baillieres Clin Rheumatol 8:691–697, 1994

INFECTIOUS DISEASES

Dennis L. Murray

13.1 GENERAL CONSIDERATIONS

13.1.1 Antibacterial Therapy

Charles G. Prober

The first antibiotic to be discovered was penicillin, a natural product of *Penicillium* mold. Innumerable microbial products have been investigated since then, and much work has been done in chemically modifying these natural products in an attempt to enhance the beneficial effects, while minimizing the undesirable effects. These modified products, termed *semisynthetic antibiotics*, increased stability and solubility, improved pharmacokinetics (ie, wider distribution and longer half-life), and increased antimicrobial activity. Minimizing the undesirable effects creates antibiotics with decreased toxicity and increased efficacy.

Unfortunately, overuse of this vast array of antibiotics now is one of our most pressing problems. Antibiotics are the most commonly prescribed drugs with sales that exceed $5 billion per year. In children antibiotics represent about 30% of all prescribed drugs. During a recent 10-year period, antibiotic production and use increased 300%, whereas the population increased by only 11%.

Misuse of antibiotics is common. Thirty to 65% of antibiotic prescriptions in hospitals are found to be irrational, inappropriate, or of questionable value. In community practice, market research data have determined that 50% of physicians prescribe antibiotics for the common cold. The reasons for this antibiotic "abuse" are multifactorial, but the desire to help patients, fear of missing a bacterial infection that might respond to antibiotics, and the ease of treating a possible bacterial infection versus considering and investigating an alternative diagnosis all contribute.

One prevalent attitude is that the risk of not treating an infection is greater than the risk of side effects from antibiotic treatment. In fact, approximately 5% of patients taking antibiotics experience side effects, and the indiscriminant use of antibiotics alters the drug-resistance patterns of isolates from the individual being treated and from the environment in general. Furthermore, a potentially more serious infection such as meningitis can be masked by incidental antibiotic therapy.

GENERAL PRINCIPLES OF ANTIBIOTIC THERAPY

Antibiotic Selection

The decision to prescribe an antibiotic is based upon proof or strong suspicion that the patient has a bacterial infection. Probable viral infectious or noninfectious processes should not be treated with antibiotics. However, in the critically ill patient in whom there is some chance that a bacterial infection may be a contributing factor, it is prudent to administer antibiotics effective against the most likely pathogens.

Whenever possible the antibiotic selection should be based upon the isolation of a pathogen, but most patients who require antibiotic therapy present with an acute problem that mandates initial empiric therapy. The specific antibiotic chosen is based upon knowledge of the pathogens likely to cause a specific infection and the likely antibiotic sensitivities in a specific host. If more than one antibiotic is active against the likely pathogens *at* the site of infection, the specific agent should be chosen on the basis of relative toxicity, convenience of administration, and cost. Table 13-1 outlines one set of suggested drugs of choice for a wide variety of childhood infections. Table 13-5 gives parenteral doses of antibiotics.

Route of Administration

Systemic antibiotic selection of the route for therapy varies depending upon factors including the ease of convenience of administration, the drug levels required for therapy, and questions of assuring compliance. Outpatient therapy is usually given orally except when a single intramuscular injection may suffice or if long-term intravenous therapy is required. In the sick hospitalized patient the intravenous route is commonly used, because it assures direct delivery of the antibiotic, and, in general, the blood concentration of antibiotic attained is higher. Patients who do not have established intravenous access can have antibiotics administered intramuscularly, unless they have a bleeding disorder or are in shock or have certain infections such as meningitis and endocarditis. If treatment is likely to be prolonged, frequent intramuscular injections are uncomfortable for the patient, and the intravenous route is preferable.

Increasingly, antibiotics are initially given by the parenteral route until the patient is stable, when the oral route is used to complete the course of therapy. This innovative treatment protocol is most common in treating osteomyelitis and septic arthritis. Compliance must be assured, the adequacy of antibiotic absorption must be assessed frequently, and the patient must have frequent clinical examinations. The advantages are self-evident: technical demands related to prolonged maintenance of an intravenous access route are reduced, as are risks of thrombophlebitis, catheter-associated infections, and the duration of hospitalization.

Duration of Therapy

The duration of antibiotic administration recommended for specific infections is often based on uncontrolled experience, not on controlled trials. Guidelines concerning the duration of therapy for most infections are outlined in this text. However, clinicians should not commit patients to a rigid duration of therapy when the infection is first diagnosed; therapy should be guided by clinical response rather than by an arbitrary number of days.

Clinical monitoring usually involves sequential physical examinations with special reference to the site originally infected and

TABLE 13-1
DRUGS OF CHOICE: A PRESCRIBING GUIDE

		RECOMMENDED ANTIBIOTIC(S)	
DIAGNOSIS	**PROBABLE PATHOGEN(S)**	**EITHER**	**OR**
Ears and sinuses			
Acute otitis media	*S. pneumoniae* *H. influenzae* (most strains not typeable) *N. catarrhalis*	Amoxicillin	Amoxicillin-clavulanate
Acute sinusitis	As above	Amoxicillin	Amoxicillin-clavulanate
Upper airway			
Pharyngitis			
Exudative	*S. pyogenes* (group A strep)	Penicillin	Cephalexin
Membranous	*Corynebacterium diphtheriae*	Erythromycin	Penicillin
Epiglottitis	*Haemophilus influenzae b**	Cefotaxime	Ampicillin + chloramphenicol
Eyes			
Cellulitis			
Preseptal			
Spontaneous	*Haemophilus influenzae b**	Cefotaxime	Ampicillin + chloramphenicol
After trauma (especially penetrating trauma near the eye, eg, insect bites, scratches)	*Haemophilus influenzae b** *S. aureus*	Cefotaxime ± nafcillin	Cefuroxime
Orbital	*Haemophilus influenzae b** *S. aureus* *S. pneumoniae*	Cefotaxime ± nafcillin	Cefuroxime
Conjunctivitis			
Neonate <5 d old	*N. gonorrhoeae*	Penicillin	Ceftriaxone
Neonate >5 d old	*Chlamydia trachomatis*	Erythromycin	Sulfonamide
Central nervous system			
Meningitis			
Neonate	Group B *Streptococcus* *Escherichia coli* *Listeria monocytogenes*	Ampicillin + gentamicin	Ampicillin + cefotaxime
Infant or child	*Haemophilus influenzae b** *S. pneumoniae* *N. meningitidis*	Cefotaxime	Ampicillin + chloramphenicol
Abscess			
Without trauma	Microaerophilic streptococci Anaerobes	Penicillin + chloramphenicol	Metronidazole
With trauma (refers to penetrating trauma, including postneurosurgery)	Microaerophilic streptococci Anaerobes *S. aureus*	Nafcillin + chloramphenicol	Nafcillin + metronidazole
Abdomen			
Peritonitis			
Primary	*S. pneumoniae* *E. coli*	Ampicillin + gentamicin	Cefotaxime
After perforation	Enterobacteriaceae Anaerobes	Clindamycin + gentamicin	Cefoxitin
CAPD (secondary to continuous ambulatory peritoneal dialysis)	Coagulase-negative staphylococci Enterobacteriaceae Anaerobes	Vancomycin + cefotaxime	Cefazolin + gentamicin
NEC (necrotizing enterocolitis in neonates)	Coagulase-negative staphylococci	Vancomycin + cefotaxime	Clindamycin + gentamicin
Kidneys			
Pyelonephritis	Enterobacteriaceae (most frequently *E. coli*)	Ampicillin + gentamicin	Cefotaxime
Cystitis and asymptomatic bacteriuria	Enterobacteriaceae (most frequently *E. coli*) *S. aureus*	Sulfisoxazole	Amoxicillin
Perinephric abscess	Enterobacteriaceae	Nafcillin + cefotaxime	Nafcillin + gentamicin

(continued)

TABLE 13-1   Continued

DIAGNOSIS	PROBABLE PATHOGEN(S)	RECOMMENDED ANTIBIOTIC(S)	
		EITHER	OR
Skin and soft tissues			
Cellulitis			
Extremity	*S. aureus*	Nafcillin + penicillin (to prevent treatment failure when *S. pyogenes* is infective agent)	Clindamycin
	S. pyogenes		
Face (buccal cellulitis)	Hib*	Cefotaxime	Ampicillin + chloramphenicol
Impetigo	*S. pyogenes*	Cephalexin	Erythromycin
	S. aureus		
Fasciitis	*S. pyogenes*	Penicillin + clindamycin	
Myositis	*S. aureus*	Nafcillin	Vancomycin
Bones (osteomyelitis)			
In neonates	Group B *Streptococcus*	Nafcillin + gentamicin	Nafcillin + cefotaxime
	S. aureus		
	Enterobacteriaceae		
Acute hematogenous	*S. aureus*	Nafcillin	Clindamycin
In children with sickle cell anemia	*S. aureus*	Nafcillin + cefotaxime	Cefotaxime
	Salmonella sp.		
After puncture wound to the foot	*Pseudomonas aeruginosa*	Ticarcillin + tobramycin	Ceftazidime
Joints			
Infections in neonates	Group B *Streptococcus*	Nafcillin + gentamicin	Nafcillin + cefotaxime
	S. aureus		
	Enterobacteriaceae		
Infections in infants and children	*S. aureus*	Cefotaxime ± nafcillin	Cefuroxime
	S. pneumoniae		
	Hib*		
Infections in adolescents	*S. aureus*	Nafcillin + penicillin	Ceftriaxone + nafcillin
	N. gonorrhoeae		
	S. pneumoniae		
Postoperative infections	*S. aureus*	Nafcillin + cefotaxime	Nafcillin + gentamicin
	Coagulase-negative staphylococci		
	Enterobacteriaceae		
Blood (septicemia/bacteremia)			
In neonates <7 d old	Group B *Streptococcus*	Ampicillin + gentamicin	Ampicillin + cefotaxime
	E. coli		
	L. monocytogenes		
Nosocomial	Coagulase-negative staphylococci	Vancomycin + cefotaxime	Vancomycin + tobramycin
	S. aureus		
	Enterobacteriaceae		
In children	*S. pneumoniae*	Cefotaxime	Ampicillin + chloramphenicol
	N. meningitidis		
	Hib*		
In adolescents	*N. meningitidis*	Penicillin + nafcillin	Cefotaxime
	N. gonorrhoeae		
	S. aureus		
Pericarditis	*S. aureus*	Cefotaxime ± nafcillin	Nafcillin + chloramphenicol

* Infections caused by *Haemophilus influenzae b* (Hib) are rare among children who have completed the full series of Hib vaccinations.

body temperature. Signs of inflammation and fever should resolve within several days after appropriate antibiotics are initiated. Laboratory monitoring may include repeat bacterial cultures to assure sterilization, and for severe infections, it may be useful to monitor the peripheral white blood cell count and acute phase reactants [eg, erythrocyte sedimentation rate (ESR) or C-reactive protein]. A lack of clinical or laboratory response to therapy may mandate a change of antibiotics.

CLASSIFICATION OF ANTIBIOTICS

Antibiotics target unique bacterial synthetic processes that differ from those in human cells. This directed attack is referred to as *selective toxicity*. Only four general categories of sites of antibacterial action have been commercially developed (Table 13-2): inhibition of cell wall synthesis, nucleic acid synthesis, protein synthesis, and folate synthesis. Antibiotics can be classified by mechanism of action or may be classified as either bacteriostatic or bactericidal. Bacteriostatic agents inhibit bacterial cell replication but require the host's immune factors to clear the infection, whereas bactericidal agents kill the bacteria. If host immunity is suppressed or the infection is in an area of poor immunologic surveillance (eg, CSF), bacteriostatic agents may not be as effective as bactericidal agents.

Chloramphenicol and erythromycin are bacteriostatic against most bacteria, although chloramphenicol is bactericidal against

TABLE 13-2

CLASSIFICATION OF ANTIBIOTICS BY MECHANISM OF ACTION

Inhibition of cell-wall synthesis	Vancomycin
	Penicillins
	Cephalosporins
	Aztreonam
	Imipenem
Inhibition of nucleic acid synthesis	Rifampin
	Quinolones
	Metronidazole
Inhibition of protein synthesis	Aminoglycosides
	Spectinomycin
	Tetracyclines
	Chloramphenicol
	Erythromycin
	Clindamycin
Inhibition of folate synthesis	Sulfonamides
	Trimethoprim

Haemophilus influenzae type b, *Streptococcus pneumoniae,* and *Neisseria meningitidis.* Bactericidal antibiotics include penicillins, cephalosporins, vancomycin, and aminoglycosides. They cause microbial death by cell lysis. Some antibiotics, such as the sulfonamides and tetracyclines, may be either bacteriostatic or bactericidal, depending on the concentration of drug, the nature of the environment, and the specific bacteria against which they are being used.

ANTIBIOTIC RESISTANCE

The development of microbial drug resistance inescapably results from the widespread utilization of a growing array of antimicrobial agents, coupled with the ability of bacteria to acquire and spread resistance and the capacity of humans to spread bacteria. Antimicrobial drug resistance represents the greatest threat to successful antibiotic therapy and is a major driving force behind the search for newer drugs. Infections caused by *S. aureus* can no longer be treated with penicillin, and an increasing number of strains are not sensitive to methicillin or related drugs (eg, oxacillin and nafcillin). The rate of ampicillin resistance among strains of *H. influenzae* type b has risen from 0% to more than 30% in the United States, and the rate of penicillin resistance among clinical isolates of *S. pneumoniae* is steadily increasing. The potential consequences of antibiotic resistance for the individual patient are an increased likelihood of hospitalization, a longer hospital stay, and about a two-fold increased death rate. Furthermore, the treatment of drug-resistant bacteria often demands the use of more toxic and expensive drugs.

Developing countries and hospitals have become the common breeding grounds and reservoirs for antimicrobial-resistant pathogens. Clinical isolates commonly are resistant to a number of antimicrobial agents. "Multiresistance" usually arises when the same mechanism confers resistance to several agents or when individual resistance genes cluster on either the bacterial chromosome or on extrachromosomal resistance plasmids (R-plasmids).

There are a limited number of mechanisms by which bacteria develop resistance to antibiotics. In very general terms, these mechanisms include (a) the production of enzymes that inactivate or modify the antibiotic; (b) decreased antibiotic uptake or an active efflux system; and (c) alteration in antibiotic target (Table 13-3). *β*-Lactamases probably are the best known inactivating enzymes produced by resistant bacteria. Bacterial resistance to penicillins and cephalosporins is often mediated by these enzymes. Alterations in outer-membrane proteins can decrease penetration of antibiotics into the bacteria. An example of an alteration of the antibiotic target may also result in resistance. Strains of penicillin-resistent *S. pneumoniae* have a markedly reduced affinity of the penicillin protein. Bacteria may develop resistance mediated by more than one mechanism.

USE OF ANTIBIOTICS IN COMBINATION

Usually a single antibiotic can be prescribed to treat an uncomplicated infection caused by a single pathogen. The most common reason for combining two or more antibiotics is to assure adequate therapy until the infecting pathogen has been identified. Combination therapy is also advisable when the infection is presumed or proved to be caused by more than one bacterium that cannot be adequately treated with a single agent. Pelvic and intraabdominal infections, usually caused by a mixture of aerobes and anaerobes, are examples.

Combining two agents may theoretically prevent or delay emergence of resistance, which justifies the use of two drugs to treat *Pseudomonas aeruginosa* or mycobacterial infections. Antibiotics are also prescribed in combination in the hope that there will be greater inhibition or killing of the pathogenic bacteria than would occur with single-drug therapy. An example is treatment of enterococcal infections with a penicillin *plus* an aminoglycoside. Disadvantages of combination antibiotic therapy include an increased incidence of superinfection and toxicity, increased cost, and potential adverse drug interactions.

GUIDANCE IN ANTIBIOTIC USE

The rational use of antibiotics requires knowledge of their spectrum of activity, certain aspects of their pharmacokinetics, their most common side effects, and their cost as compared to agents of equal safety and efficacy. The formulations available and the palatability of each are also particularly relevant in children. The seasoned clinician will depend on a small number of antibiotics that have established reliability. The newest antibiotics are not necessarily the best, although they are often among the most expensive.

The minimum kinetic knowledge required for frequently prescribed antibiotics includes the following:

TABLE 13-3

MECHANISMS OF RESISTANCE TO ANTIMICROBIAL AGENTS

ENZYME INACTIVATION	ALTERED TARGET	DECREASED ACCUMULATION
β-Lactam antibiotics	*β*-Lactam antibiotics	*β*-Lactam antibiotics
Amikacin	Spectinomycin	Chloramphenicol
Gentamicin	Streptomycin	Quinolones
Tobramycin	Erythromycin	Tetracycline
Kanamycin	Clindamycin	Trimethoprim
Netilmicin	Quinolones	Erythromycin
Chloramphenicol	Rifampin	Tetracycline
	Sulfonamides	
	Tetracycline	
	Trimethoprim	
	Vancomycin	

- The expected concentration of the antibiotic at the site of infection that will be attained after the selected dose. This implies knowledge of the serum concentrations attained and the diffusion characteristics of the antibiotic into infected tissue. The adequacy of the anticipated concentration of drug at the site of infection is determined by the antibiotic sensitivity pattern of the infecting bacterium.
- The half-life ($t_{1/2}$) of the antibiotic. In general, antibiotics should be administered every third half-life.
- The sources of pharmacokinetic variation, knowledge of which necessitates some understanding of excretion and metabolism. If an agent is excreted primarily by the kidneys or by the liver, and the patient has compromised renal or hepatic function, the dose may have to be adjusted. Some host variables that influence the kinetics of different antibiotics are outlined in Table 13-4. The use of antibiotics in infants whose organ maturity is evolving presents a special challenge to clinicians.

Dosing

Many factors determine the correct dosage of antimicrobials, including age (dosages for premature and newborn infants differ from those for older children), weight, and route of administration. Significant liver or renal disease often requires adjustments in dose. Parenteral dosages of several commonly used antimicrobials are listed in Table 13-5.

SPECIFIC ANTIBIOTICS CLASSIFIED BY MECHANISM OF ACTION

Antibiotics that Affect Cell-Wall Biosynthesis

Penicillins

Penicillin G is the "natural" or "native" penicillin; all other penicillins are semisynthetic compounds. The basic structure of penicillin consists of a 6-aminopenicillanic acid (6-APA) nucleus and a variety of side chains. The 6-APA nucleus has a thiazolidine ring connected to a β-lactam ring. The integrity of the β-lactam ring is necessary for antibacterial activity. Hence organisms that produce β-lactamases, which break the ring configuration, render the drug inactive.

The penicillins can be divided into three groups on the basis of their antibacterial spectrum.

NARROW-SPECTRUM, β-LACTAMASE-SENSITIVE PENICILLINS The prototype of this group is penicillin G. This antibiotic is active against most gram-positive bacteria with the exception of penicillinase-producing *S. aureus*. In recent years, an increasing proportion of isolates of *S. pneumoniae* have developed relative or absolute resistance to penicillin. Penicillin G is also active against most *Neisseria* species and against some gram-negative anaerobes. Penicillin G is not active against most gram-negative aerobic organisms. Bacteria sensitive to penicillin generally have a minimal inhibitory concentration (MIC) less than 0.05 mg/L.

A 100,000-IU/kg dose of penicillin G (1 IU = 0.6 µg) administered intravenously results in serum concentrations in excess of 10 mg/L, 200-fold higher than the MIC of most sensitive bacteria. This antibiotic also diffuses widely, attaining therapeutic concentrations in most body tissues. For example, up to 25% of serum concentrations are attained in the CSF during the treatment of bacterial meningitis. The $t_{1/2}$ of penicillin G is less than 1 hour and it is eliminated primarily by renal tubular secretion. This secretion can be inhibited by probenecid. Because renal dysfunction will compromise the elimination of penicillin, dosages may need to be reduced in patients with renal insufficiency. This is only necessary in the most extreme circumstances, owing to the low toxicity of penicillin.

Penicillin V, the phenoxymethyl analogue of penicillin G, is a much more stable acid than is its parent compound and therefore better absorbed from the gastrointestinal tract. A 250-mg dose of this preparation results in concentrations roughly equivalent to those attained after two doses of orally administered penicillin G. Procaine penicillin is a commonly used intramuscular preparation that produces low (3 mg/L) concentrations of drug sustained over several days. It is best suited to the single-dose outpatient treatment of very sensitive organisms (eg, penicillin-sensitive *N. gonorrhoeae*

TABLE 13-4

SOME VARIABLES THAT INFLUENCE THE KINETICS OF ANTIBIOTICS

VARIABLE	MECHANISM OF EFFECT	EXAMPLE
Age	Decreased renal function early in life and late in life	Need to decrease dose of aminoglycosides in neonates and elderly
Renal function	Important for drugs dependent on renal excretion	Need to decrease dose of aminoglycosides in patients with compromised function
Liver function	Important for drugs metabolized in the liver	Need to decrease dose of chloramphenicol in patients with compromised function, eg, premature newborns
Fever/burns	Increased excretion or increased volume of distribution of some drugs	Need to increase dose of aminoglycosides
Acetylation status	Important for drugs metabolized by acetylation	Need to increase dose of isoniazid in rapid acetylators on once- or twice-weekly regimen
Diabetes mellitus	Reduced absorption of certain drugs after intramuscular dosing	Need to increase dose of intramuscular penicillins in diabetics
Cystic fibrosis	Increased clearance and volume of distribution of some drugs	Need to increase dose of aminoglycosides and penicillins in these patients
	Altered absorption	Chloramphenicol palmitate malabsorbed because of lipase deficiency
Gastrointestinal surgery	Altered absorption of drugs in patients with short bowel, eg, ileal bypass	Ampicillin bioavailability is 15% of normal after small bowel bypass

From Kalant H and Roschlau WHE: Principles of Medical Pharmacology, 4th ed. Toronto, Canada, University of Toronto, 1985.

TABLE 13-5

PARENTERAL DOSES OF ANTIBIOTICS

ANTIBIOTICS THAT INHIBIT CELL-WALL SYNTHESIS

DRUG	$T_{1/2}$ (hours)	DAILY DOSE (kg/day)	SIDE EFFECTS*
PENICILLINS			
Natural Penicillins			
Penicillin G	0.5	100–300,000 U/kg div q4h	Hematologic—Coombs-positive hemolytic anemia; neutropenia; thrombocytopenia
			Neurologic—seizures with renal compromise
			Renal—interstitial nephritis
Procaine penicillin G	12	25–50,000 U/kg IM x1	
Benzathine penicillin G	2 weeks	600,000 U IM x1 if <27.5 kg 1.2 million U IM x1 if >27.5 kg	
Anti-Staphylococcal Penicillins			
Nafcillin	1	50–100 mg/kg div q6h	Hepatitis
Oxacillin	1	50–100 mg/kg div q6h	Hepatitis
Aminopenicillins			
Ampicillin	1.2	100–400 mg/kg div q4–6h	Rash with mononucleosis Pseudomembranous colitis
Carboxypenicillins			
Carbenicillin	1	400–600 mg/kg div q6h	Platelet aggregation defect
Ticarcillin	1	200–300 mg/kg div q6h	Hypernatremia; hypokalemia
Ureidopenicillins			
Azlocillin	1	200–300 mg/kg div q4–6h	
Mezlocillin	1	200–300 mg/kg div q4–6h	
Piperacillin	1	200–300 mg/kg div q4–6h	
Penicillin + β-lactamase Inhibitors			
Ticarcillin/clavulanate	1.2	200–300 mg/kg div q4–6h	Superinfection
Ampicillin/sulbactam	1.2	100–200 mg/kg div q6h	Superinfection
CEPHALOSPORINS			
1st Generation			
Cephalothin	1	75–125 mg/kg div q6h	Hematologic—Coombs-positive hemolytic anemia
Cephazolin	2	50–100 mg/kg div q8h	
2nd Generation			
Cefuroxime	1	100–150 mg/kg div q8h	Serum sickness
Cefoxitin	1	80–160 mg/kg div q4–6h	Coagulopathy (moxalactam, cefoperazone, cefamandole)
3rd Generation			
Ceftriaxone	8.5	50–100 mg/kg div q24h	Gall bladder sludging
Cefotaxime	1.2	100–150 mg/kg div q6–8h	
Ceftazidime	1.8	100–150 mg/kg div q8h	
GLYCOPEPTIDES			
Vancomycin	4–6	40 mg/kg div q6h	Nephrotoxicity concomitantly with aminoglycosides Histamine release ("red man syndrome")
MONOBACTAMS AND CARBAPENEMS			
Aztreonam	2	90–120 mg/kg div q6–8h	
Imipenem-cilastatin	1	40–60 mg/kg div q6h	Epileptogenic
Meropenem	1	60 mg/kg div q8h	Neurotoxicity

ANTIBIOTICS THAT INHIBIT NUCLEIC ACID SYNTHESIS

DRUG	$T_{1/2}$ (hours)	DAILY DOSE (kg/day)	SIDE EFFECTS*
Ciprofloxacin	4	20–30 mg/kg div q12h	Cartilaginous damage in animals
Metronidazole	6–14	30 mg/kg div q6h	Neurologic—peripheral neuropathy; seizures; encephalopathy; Antabuse effect with alcohol
			Neutropenia

ANTIBIOTICS THAT INHIBIT PROTEIN SYNTHESIS

DRUG	$T_{1/2}$ (hours)	DAILY DOSE (kg/day)	SIDE EFFECTS*
AMINOGLYCOSIDES			
Gentamicin	2	3–5 mg/kg div q8h	Nephrotoxicy with trough >2 μg/mL;
			Irreversible vestibular ototoxicity with sustained peak >12 μg/mL
			Neuromuscular blockade after IV push or with copious irrigation; treat with calcium
Tobramycin	2	3–5 mg/kg div q8h	Nephrotoxicity with trough >2 μg/mL Cochlear ototoxicity
Amikacin	2	15 mg/kg div q8h	Nephrotoxicity with trough >10 μg/mL Cochlear ototoxicity

(continued)

TABLE 13-5   Continued

ANTIBIOTICS THAT INHIBIT PROTEIN SYNTHESIS

DRUG	T$_{1/2}$ (hours)	DAILY DOSE (kg/day)	SIDE EFFECTS*
Chloramphenicol	3	50–75 mg/kg div q6h	Hematologic—reversible marrow toxicity with serum levels >20–25 μg/mL; aplastic anemia; "gray baby" syndrome with serum levels >25 μg/mL
Erythromycin	2–4	20–40 mg/kg div q6h	Increased levels of theophylline and anti-coagulants Torsades with Propulsid@ Cardiotoxicity with Seldane@
Clindamycin	2–4	25–40 mg/kg div q6–8h	Pseudomembranous colitis Increased transaminases Neuromuscular blockade

ANTIBIOTICS THAT INHIBIT FOLATE SYNTHESIS

DRUG	T$_{1/2}$ (hours)	DAILY DOSE (kg/day)	SIDE EFFECTS*
Trimethoprim-Sulfamethoxazole	11	8–12 mg TMP; 40–60 mg SMX/kg div q12h	Bone marrow suppression Stevens-Johnson syndrome Increased anti-coagulant effect

* Within each category, side effects are listed opposite the agent with which they are most frequently associated.
DAILY DOSES IN MENINGITIS
Ampicillin 200–400 mg/kg div q6h
Cefotaxime 300 mg/kg div q6h
Ceftazidime 150 mg/kg div q8h
Ceftriaxone 100 mg/kg div q12h
Meropenem 120 mg/kg div q8h
Vancomycin 60 mg/kg div q6h

and group A streptococci). Benzathine penicillin is another preparation given intramuscularly. Serum concentrations of less than 0.1 mg/L, sustained for as long as 3 to 4 weeks, are attained with this formulation. It is used to prevent recurrent group A streptococcal infections in patients with rheumatic fever.

The most frequent indications for the use of penicillin G and its derivatives in children are for infections caused by all species of streptococci, with the exception of group D streptococci, and infections caused by sensitive *Neisseria* species. However, in geographic areas where the incidence of penicillin-resistant *N. gonorrhoeae* exceeds 10%, empiric therapy with penicillin is not recommended.

BROAD-SPECTRUM, β-LACTAMASE-SENSITIVE PENICILLINS (AMINO-, CARBOXY-, AND UREIDOPENICILLINS) Examples of aminopenicillins include ampicillin and amoxicillin. The activity of the aminopenicillins against gram-positive bacteria is similar to that of penicillin. Aminopenicillins are, however, more active against group D streptococci, *Listeria monocytogenes,* and non-β-lactamase-producing *H. influenzae*. They are also active against some *Escherichia coli, Shigella, Salmonella,* and indole-negative *Proteus* species. The MICs necessary against gram-negative organisms are usually in the range of 1 to 5 mg/L.

The serum concentration of ampicillin after a 1-g intravenous dose is approximately 40 mg/L; after a 500-mg dose taken orally, it is approximately 4 mg/L. Concentrations of amoxicillin are usually twice those of ampicillin after an equivalent oral dose. The distribution, t$_{1/2}$, and excretion characteristics of the aminopenicillins are similar to those of penicillin.

Ampicillin and its derivatives are among the most useful antibiotics for treating children suffering from infections caused by sensitive gram-negative aerobic bacteria, enterococci, *L. monocytogenes,* and β-lactamase-negative *H. influenzae*. Amoxicillin is the favored drug for the treatment of acute otitis media.

Carboxypenicillins are represented by carbenicillin and ticarcillin; ureidopenicillins are represented by piperacillin, azlocillin, and mezlocillin. These antibiotics have a broader spectrum of gram-negative activity than do the aminopenicillins, and include activity against most strains of *P. aeruginosa*. The usual MICs of *P. aeruginosa* range from 12 to 25 mg/L, with piperacillin consistently being the most active agent. Maximum serum concentrations of these antibiotics are usually in excess of 150 mg/L, after a dose of 3 to 5 g. These antibiotics are used almost exclusively in the treatment of urinary tract, lung, and bloodstream infections caused by ampicillin-resistant enteric gram-negative pathogens.

β-LACTAMASE-RESISTANT PENICILLINS These penicillins include nafcillin, oxacillin, methicillin, cloxacillin, dicloxacillin, and flucloxacillin. The principal bacteriologic advantage of this group of antibiotics is their activity against β-lactamase-producing staphylococci. Most isolates of *S. aureus* have MICs of 0.25 to 0.5 mg/L. These antibiotics are less active than penicillin G against the other gram-positive bacteria, and they are inactive against gram-negative enteric organisms. Maximum serum concentrations after a 1-g intravenous dose of nafcillin, methicillin, or oxacillin range from 20 to 40 mg/L; whereas after a 500-mg oral dose of cloxacillin or oxacillin, they range from 4 to 8 mg/L. Dicloxacillin and flucloxacillin have an enhanced absorption after oral administration.

Serum concentrations of these agents are twice those of cloxacillin or oxacillin after an equivalent oral dose. These penicillins are used almost exclusively for the treatment of mild, moderate, and severe infections caused by *S. aureus,* including cellulitis, osteomyelitis, pneumonia, and septicemia.

Toxicity The adverse reactions of all penicillins are similar. In general, these agents are well tolerated; however, suspension formulations tend to have an unpleasant taste and aftertaste and, as a result, may be poorly accepted. All penicillins have a wide toxic-to-therapeutic ratio, although they can cause hypersensitivity reactions, neurotoxicity, nephrotoxicity, and hematologic toxicity.

Hypersensitivity reactions are relatively common and include rashes, serum sickness, anaphylaxis, nephritis, and drug fever. Urticarial skin reactions and anaphylaxis, which occur within 20 to 30 minutes after a dose, are termed *immediate reactions.* These are the most dangerous reactions and constitute absolute contraindications to future treatment with a penicillin derivative. Fortunately, the incidence of anaphylaxis is only 0.004 to 0.4% of individual courses of therapy.

Nonurticarial skin eruptions that occur several days after the initiation of a course of penicillin are relatively common and do not preclude future therapy with penicillins. Many such eruptions represent the rash of a viral infection for which an antibiotic has been inappropriately prescribed. Patients manifesting these sorts of reactions must not be labeled "penicillin-allergic."

Convulsions and other forms of central nervous system irritation may occur when high doses of a penicillin have been administered, particularly to patients with compromised renal function. Reactions are also more likely when high CSF concentrations of drug are attained, such as in patients with meningeal inflammation, or in those with the drug administered directly into their central nervous system.

Interstitial nephritis can occur during the course of therapy with any penicillin, although it is usually associated with the administration of methicillin. Hypokalemia is another renal side effect of high-dose penicillin therapy that results from penicillins acting as nonresorbable anions.

Coombs-positive hemolytic anemia may occur with any of the penicillins, as may neutropenia. Neutropenia is most common among patients receiving a β-lactamase-resistant penicillin and usually resolves when the antibiotic is stopped. Decreased platelet aggregation, which may precipitate bleeding, has been noted at high concentrations of most penicillins. It is most marked with carbenicillin and ticarcillin.

In addition to the reactions noted above, which are common to all of the penicillins, ampicillin can cause a characteristic nonurticarial maculopapular rash that does not appear to have an allergic etiology. This rash usually appears 3 to 4 days after the onset of therapy and is more frequent in patients suffering from viral infections, especially infectious mononucleosis.

Cephalosporins

The cephalosporins are currently divided into four generations with original agents being referred to as *first-generation cephalosporins,* and the most recent agents as *fourth-generation cephalosporins.* A list of representative cephalosporins from each generation is presented in Table 13-6. In general, the spectrum of activity of the cephalosporins increases with each generation because of decreasing susceptibility to bacterial β-lactamases.

TABLE 13-6

REPRESENTATIVE CEPHALOSPORINS CLASSIFIED BY GENERATION

ROUTE	FIRST	SECOND	THIRD	FOURTH
Parenteral	Cephalothin	Cefamandole	Cefotaxime	Cefapime
	Cefazolin	Cefotetan	Cefoperazone	
	Cephradine	Cefoxitin	Ceftazidime	
		Cefuroxime	Ceftizoxime	
		Cefonicid	Ceftriaxone	
Oral	Cephalexin	Cefaclor	Cefixime	
	Cefadroxil	Cefuroxime	Cefpodoxime	
		Cefprozil	Ceftibuten	

FIRST-GENERATION CEPHALOSPORINS These cephalosporins are active against most staphylococci, pneumococci, and all streptococci, with the important exception of enterococci. MICs against sensitive gram-positive organisms are usually less than 0.5 mg/L. Their activity against aerobic gram-negative bacteria and against anaerobes is limited. Maximum serum concentrations after a 500-mg dose of oral cephalexin are approximately 20 mg/L, whereas they are 50 and 100 mg/L after 1-g intravenous doses of cephalothin and cefazolin, respectively. These antibiotics distribute widely throughout the body, but do not penetrate well into the CSF. Therefore, they must not be used to treat meningitis. Their $t_{1/2}$ ranges from 30 minutes to 1.5 hours, and they are eliminated unchanged in the urine. Doses may need adjustment in the presence of renal insufficiency, although these agents have a wide toxic-to-therapeutic ratio.

The first-generation cephalosporins are rarely drugs of first choice. They may, however, be useful in patients who are intolerant to penicillins. They should not be administered to patients with a history of immediate-type hypersensitivity reactions to penicillins, as similar reactions to cephalosporins may be observed. These antibiotics are useful in the perioperative prophylaxis of surgical procedures that carry a high risk of postoperative infections caused by staphylococcal species, such as those involving the cardiovascular system and bones.

SECOND-GENERATION CEPHALOSPORINS These cephalosporins have a broader bacteriologic spectrum than do the first-generation agents. For example, cefamandole, cefuroxime, and cefaclor not only are more active against gram-negative enteric bacteria but are active against both β-lactamase-negative and -positive strains of *H. influenzae,* generally at concentrations below 2 mg/L. The major bacteriologic advantage of cefoxitin and cefotetan is their activity against a broad range of anaerobic pathogens, most anaerobes being inhibited by less than 16 mg/L. Maximum serum concentrations of cefamandole, cefuroxime, and cefoxitin after a 1-g intravenous dose are approximately 100 mg/L. Concentrations of cefaclor are approximately 10 mg/L after a 200-mg oral dose. The half-lives of the second-generation agents are similar to those of the first-generation agents. There are "long-acting" agents currently being marketed (eg, cefadroxil), but their greater cost should discourage widespread use. Excretion of second-generation cephalosporins is primarily renal, and they distribute widely. However, they do not attain sufficient concentrations in the CSF to warrant their use in the treatment of bacterial meningitis.

Second-generation cephalosporins, like the first-generation agents, are rarely drugs of first choice. Cefuroxime, because of its activity against gram-positive cocci and *H. influenzae,* has been actively promoted as a good agent for the treatment of a variety of infections in children, including cellulitis, osteomyelitis, septic arthritis, and pneumonia. However, it is no longer recommended for the therapy of bacterial meningitis, because of several reports of bacteriologic failures. Cefaclor is recommended for the outpatient management of children with infections thought to be caused by a gram-positive coccus or *H. influenzae.* The most common indication for this antibiotic is otitis media. However, other, less expensive, better tolerated, and equally efficacious agents are available. Cefoxitin and cefotetan are effective agents in the prevention and treatment of intraabdominal or pelvic infections.

THIRD-GENERATION CEPHALOSPORINS This generation is increasing in numbers at a rate that intimidates most clinicians. These agents retain much of the gram-positive activity of the first two generations, although their antistaphylococcal activity is reduced 5- to 10-fold. They are remarkably active against most gram-negative enteric isolates, with MICs usually less than 0.5 mg/L. Some third-generation cephalosporins (eg, ceftazidime and cefoperazone) also are active against most isolates of *P. aeruginosa.* Maximum serum concentrations of the third-generation agents range from 50 to 150 mg/L after a 1-g intravenous dose. In healthy subjects, their half-lives range from 1 hour (cefotaxime) to between 6 and 8 hours (ceftriaxone). These antibiotics diffuse well into most tissues, in contrast to members of the first two generations. Cefotaxime and ceftriaxone, in particular, penetrate well into the CSF. With the exception of cefoperazone, which is excreted primarily in the bile, excretion is primarily renal.

The possible indications for third-generation cephalosporins at present include empiric therapy of suspected bacterial meningitis and treatment of hospital-acquired multiple-resistant gram-negative aerobic infections and suspected infections in certain compromised hosts (eg, those with fever and neutropenia). Ceftriaxone also is the drug of choice in treating infections caused by *N. gonorrhoeae* in geographic areas with a high incidence of penicillin-resistant isolates.

FOURTH-GENERATION CEPHALOSPORINS This newest generation of cephalosporins combines the antistaphylococcal activity of first-generation agents with the gram-negative spectrum (including *Pseudomonas*) of third-generation cephalosporins. Possible indications for use include the therapy of infections suspected or proved to be caused by multiple-resistant pathogens.

Toxicity Serious, adverse reactions to the cephalosporins are uncommon. As with most antibiotics, the full spectrum of hypersensitivity reactions may occur, including rashes, fever, eosinophilia, serum sickness, and anaphylaxis. Allergic reactions are seen in approximately 5% of courses. The incidence of immediate-type allergic reactions to the cephalosporins is increased among patients known to be allergic to penicillins. The precise frequency of these cross-reactions is not known; estimates vary from 5 to 16%. Adverse reactions attributable to irritation at the site of administration are common. These reactions include local pain after intramuscular injection, phlebitis after intravenous administration, and minor gastrointestinal complaints after oral administration.

Therapy with cephalosporins leads to the development of a positive direct Coombs reaction during approximately 3% of courses. This is, however, not commonly associated with hemolytic anemia. Some of the cephalosporins are associated with dose-related neph-

rotoxicity, probably due to tubular damage (eg, cephaloridine), whereas others are associated with an interstitial nephritis (eg, cephalothin).

The third-generation drugs may cause transient elevations of liver function test results and blood urea nitrogen concentrations. They also have a profound inhibitory effect on the vitamin K–synthesizing bacterial flora of the gastrointestinal tract. In addition, agents that possess an *N*-methylthiotetrazole side chain (eg, cefoperazone) can cause hypoprothombinemia and bleeding, as well as a disulfiram-like reaction in patients who consume ethanol during therapy.

β-Lactamase Inhibitors

β-Lactamase inhibitors competively inhibit β-lactamase enzymes, restoring the original spectrum of activity to enzyme-susceptible antibiotics.

Currently marketed inhibitors include clavulanic acid in fixed combination with either amoxicillin or ticarcillin, and sulbactam in fixed combination with ampicillin. Although clavulanate-amoxicillin is effective in the therapy of such infections as otitis media, sinusitis, lower respiratory tract infections, and skin and soft-tissue infections, equally effective and less costly alternatives for these infections are generally available. However, some infections are polymicrobial and may involve anaerobes; for these the addition of a β-lactamase inhibitor might be of value. These infections include infected animal and human bites, odontogenic infections, chronic sinusitis, and intraabdominal infections.

The side effects of these agents reflect those of their parent compounds. Gastrointestinal disturbances, especially diarrhea, are common among those receiving orally administered β-lactamase inhibitors. It appears that these symptoms can be partially ameliorated by giving the drug with food and following each dose with 2 to 4 ounces of fluid.

Vancomycin

The primary activity of this cell-wall-active antibiotic is against gram-positive bacteria. With the exception of a few recent case reports, most clinical isolates of *S. aureus* and coagulase-negative staphylococci are inhibited by less than 1.6 mg/L of this antibiotic. Disturbingly, vancomycin-resistant enterococci (VRE) are being reported at an increasing rate, especially with hospital-acquired infections. Gram-positive bacilli, including *Clostridium* species, are very sensitive to vancomycin, but gram-negative bacteria are resistant.

Vancomycin is not absorbed from the gastrointestinal tract. Maximum serum concentrations after a 10-mg/kg intravenous dose are approximately 25 mg/L, six-fold higher than the MIC of the usual bacteria being treated. It diffuses quite widely throughout the body and, during meningeal inflammation, attains concentrations in the CSF approximately 10 to 20% of serum concentrations. The $t_{1/2}$ of vancomycin is approximately 4 to 6 hours in patients with normal renal function. The drug is excreted unmetabolized, almost exclusively in the urine. Doses should be reduced in patients with decreased renal function.

Vancomycin historically has had a reputation for toxicity. Many of its original adverse reactions, including ototoxicity and nephrotoxicity, were probably due to impurities in the formulation. Now that a more purified form is available, these adverse reactions are uncommon. Nephrotoxicity has been demonstrated when an aminoglycoside is used concomitantly. One of the more common side effects is the "red man" syndrome, which is characterized by fever, chills, erythema, and paresthesia. Although more likely to occur after a rapid infusion of the drug, "red man" syndrome also occurs after slow infusions and appears to be mediated by histamine.

Despite its introduction several decades ago, vancomycin only recently gained widespread use. The reasons for its revival relate to the emergence of several important pathogens. These include methicillin-resistant *S. aureus* and coagulase-negative staphylococci, multiple-drug-resistant pneumococci, and enterotoxin-producing *C. difficile*. The first three organisms are treated intravenously; the last, when associated with pseudomembranous colitis, is treated with oral vancomycin.

Aztreonam

Aztreonam is the first member of a new and unique class of antibiotics referred to as "monobactams." Although monobactams are β-lactam antibiotics, their structure is so different that cross-immunogenicity does not appear to be a problem; they can be prescribed for patients with penicillin or cephalosporin allergies. Aztreonam is resistant to a broad range of β-lactamases produced by gram-negative bacteria and therefore is active in vitro against most gram-negative organisms. *Activity against gram-positive bacteria is very limited*. In comparison with the aminoglycosides, aztreonam appears to be less nephrotoxic and ototoxic. Clinical experience in children is very limited; consequently, this antibiotic cannot currently be recommended for general use.

Imipenem and Meropenem

Imipenem and Meropenem are members of a new class of β-lactam antibiotics called *carbapenems*. Because imipenem is rapidly metabolized by renal brush-border enzymes, it is administered with cilastatin, a substance that inhibits imipenem metabolism by the kidney. Meropenem is administered alone, as it is more stable in vivo to inactivation by human renal dehydropeptidase. The carbapenems have the broadest antimicrobial spectrum of any currently available antibiotics, with activity against gram-negative and gram-positive aerobes and anaerobes. They appear to have toxicity profiles similar to that of other β-lactam agents. Imipenem is epileptogenic in high doses, whereas meropenem appears to have less neurotoxicity. Experience with these antibiotics in children is limited; consequently, they cannot currently be recommended for general use.

Antibiotics that Inhibit Nucleic Acid Synthesis

Rifampin

Rifampin is active against a wide range of gram-positive and gram-negative bacteria. It is also very active against the majority of *Mycobacterium tuberculosis* strains, with MICs under 0.5 mg/L. Rifampin is given orally and is well absorbed from the gastrointestinal tract. Maximum serum concentrations of 8 mg/L are usually attained after a 600-mg dose. Rifampin penetrates well into most body tissues and fluids, including lungs, liver, pleural and ascitic fluid, bone, tears, saliva, and CSF, even in the absence of inflammation. The $t_{1/2}$ of rifampin ranges from 2 to 5 hours. It is metabolized in the liver and excreted principally in the bile and, to a lesser degree, in the urine.

Hypersensitivity reactions include dermatitis and a flu-like syndrome, occasionally with thrombocytopenia, hemolytic anemia, and acute renal failure. Cholestatic hepatitis is another possible adverse reaction. All patients receiving this antibiotic should be advised that their bodily secretions, including urine, saliva, sweat, and tears, will develop a reddish-orange discoloration. This is especially important for patients who wear soft contact lenses, which may be permanently discolored.

Important drug interactions with rifampin have been recognized. For example, it enhances the metabolism of chloramphenicol, oral contraceptives, warfarin, propranolol, and anticonvulsants, all of which are metabolized in the liver. Doses of these concurrently administered agents may need to be increased to maintain therapeutic concentrations.

The use of rifampin as a single agent is limited by the fact that bacteria can rapidly develop resistance. It is, however, one of the first-line agents to be used in combination in the treatment of patients with most forms of tuberculosis. It also is the antibiotic of choice for the prophylaxis of contacts of patients with serious infections caused by *H. influenzae* type b and *N. meningitidis*. Rifampin has also been used to eradicate upper respiratory carriage of *S. aureus* and group A *Streptococcus*.

Quinolones

The prototype of the quinolone antibiotics is nalidixic acid. This naphthyridine derivative has been used almost exclusively as a urinary antiseptic. It is as active as ampicillin against gram-negative enteric isolates, but has no useful activity against gram-positive bacteria or against species of *Pseudomonas*. Because nalidixic acid is only partially absorbed from the gastrointestinal tract, large doses are necessary to attain therapeutic urinary concentrations. These high doses have caused side effects, including visual disturbances. An additional problem has been the rapid development of bacterial resistance during therapy. These factors have limited the use of this antibiotic.

Research directed at modifying the chemical structure of nalidixic acid has resulted in the development of an ever-growing family of fluorinated quinolone derivatives, including ciprofloxacin, enoxacin, lomefloxacin, norfloxacin, ofloxacin, pefloxacin, and trovafloxacin. The spectrum of activity of these derivatives is continually increasing and now includes most gram-positive bacteria; for example, methicillin-resistant *S. aureus* and many *Pseudomonas* organisms. In addition, when compared with nalidixic acid, most gram-negative enterics have greatly reduced MICs to the new derivatives. Most quinolones are absorbed well after oral administration, and thus represent the first agents available for the oral treatment of systemic infections caused by resistant gram-negative enteric isolates and *Pseudomonas* species. These agents are also of great value because their activity is unrelated to that of other antibiotics and resistance is not plasmid-borne. In adults, the quinolones may be preferred over alternate agents for treatment of complicated urinary tract infections, suspected bacterial gastroenteritis, osteomyelitis caused by gram-negative bacilli, and invasive external otitis. Unfortunately, because the quinolones cause cartilaginous damage to young experimental animals, their use in children at present should be limited to recalcitrant infections for which alternatives are lacking. However, recent data suggest that quinolones may be safe for administration to children, with the frequency of cartilage or joint toxicity being similar to that in adults. If this observation is confirmed in long-term studies, the use of quinolones in children may be more acceptable.

Metronidazole

The antibacterial activity of metronidazole is restricted to anaerobes, being most active against gram-negative anaerobic bacilli such as *Bacteroides* and *Fusobacterium,* most of which have MICs under 3.12 mg/L. Activity against gram-positive anaerobic cocci is less consistent, with about 75% of such strains being inhibited by 12.5 mg/L.

Metronidazole can be administered intravenously, orally, or rectally. Maximum serum concentrations after a 7.5-mg/kg dose administered intravenously are 20 to 25 mg/L. Concentrations after an equivalent oral dose are similar, and those after an equivalent rectal dose are about half. The drug diffuses well into all tissues; therapeutic concentrations can be attained in CSF, bile, bone, and abscesses. The $t_{1/2}$ of metronidazole is approximately 8 hours. It is metabolized to acid and hydroxy metabolites. Between 60 and 80% of the drug is eliminated by the kidneys, and 6 to 15% is eliminated in the feces. Hepatic insufficiency prolongs the $t_{1/2}$ of unchanged metronidazole, and doses usually have to be adjusted. Renal insufficiency usually does not necessitate dose adjustment.

Metronidazole therapy is often associated with a metallic taste and nausea. More serious but less frequent adverse reactions include a reversible peripheral neuropathy, seizures, encephalopathy, and neutropenia. A disulfiram-like reaction can occur when metronidazole is taken with alcohol. Several studies conducted in laboratory animals have indicated that prolonged use of high-dose metronidazole can be carcinogenic. However, there is no evidence that it is carcinogenic in humans.

Metronidazole has been shown to be effective in a wide variety of infections caused by anaerobes. The most common applications of this antibiotic have been in the treatment of pelvic and intra-abdominal sepsis and brain abscesses. It is also a suitable and less expensive alternative to vancomycin in the treatment of pseudomembranous colitis caused by *C. difficile.* Also, despite inconsistent in vitro activity of metronidazole against the principal etiologic agent of "nonspecific vaginitis," *Gardnerella vaginalis,* it is the antibiotic of choice for treatment of this infection.

Antibiotics that Inhibit Protein Synthesis

Aminoglycosides

The aminoglycoside group of antibiotics contains a large number of structurally related compounds. Streptomycin was the first of these agents to be discovered. Subsequently developed agents include neomycin, kanamycin, gentamicin, tobramycin, amikacin, and netilmicin. Streptomycin is primarily used to treat tuberculosis (see Sec. 13.2.21). Gentamicin, tobramycin, netilmicin, and amikacin are the most common aminoglycosides; they are discussed as a group, with only their clinically important differences emphasized.

These antibiotics are active primarily against gram-negative and limited numbers of gram-positive aerobes. They are inactive against the vast majority of anaerobes. All four of the aminoglycosides are active against most strains of *P. aeruginosa,* with tobramycin consistently demonstrating the greatest activity and netilmicin the least. Gentamicin is consistently the most active of these agents against strains of *Serratia marcescens.* Otherwise, their relative antibacterial

activities are similar, with most sensitive strains being inhibited by less than 3 to 4 mg/L.

An important aspect of aminoglycoside activity against gram-negative aerobes is the increasing resistance developed over recent years. Resistance is most often due to antibiotic inactivation by enzymes produced by the bacteria. There are at least 12 such inactivating enzymes. Gentamicin is susceptible to the largest number of these enzymes (9 of 12) and amikacin is susceptible to the smallest number (1 of 12). When widespread resistance develops to one of the aminoglycosides being used in a particular hospital, changing to an alternate agent usually results in a return to increased sensitivity.

The pharmacokinetics of all the aminoglycosides are similar. They are poorly absorbed from the gastrointestinal tract, but well absorbed after intramuscular or intravenous administration. Maximum serum concentrations of gentamicin, tobramycin, and netilmicin are 5 to 8 mg/L after unit doses of 1 to 2.5 mg/kg. Maximum serum concentrations of amikacin range from 15 to 30 mg/L after a unit dose of 7.5 mg/kg. The aminoglycosides are distributed in most extracellular fluids, but do not attain therapeutic concentrations in CSF. The main site of deposition of these drugs is the kidney, which accounts for approximately 40% of the total antibiotic in the body. The cortex accumulates approximately 85% of the load, and the resulting concentrations are more than 100-fold greater than serum concentrations. Their half-lives range from 1.5 to 2.5 hours, and they are eliminated, primarily unchanged, by glomerular filtration. The doses of the aminoglycosides must be carefully monitored and adjusted in the presence of renal insufficiency. The total daily dose is adjusted by either prolonging the dosing interval or by reducing the unit dose. Nomograms, based upon the measured or approximated glomerular filtration rate, are available to guide these adjustments. Some centers use single daily dose aminoglycoside therapy instead of multiple daily doses. In addition to the convenience of once-daily dosing, studies show that this strategy is safe and effective.

Toxicity The most important toxicities of the aminoglycosides are ototoxicity and nephrotoxicity. These toxic effects are more common in adults than in children, who generally tolerate this class of drugs well. Ototoxicity may be primarily vestibular or cochlear. The agent most commonly associated with vestibular toxicity is gentamicin, with an estimated incidence in adult populations of 2%. This ranges from mild vertigo to severe Meniere syndrome. Damage is usually permanent, but symptoms may eventually be reduced by adaptation. The agents most likely to cause cochlear toxicity are amikacin and tobramycin. Although the frequency of hearing loss following treatment with these drugs is low, it may occur without any warning and may be irreversible. Risk factors that seem to predispose to ototoxicity include cumulative dosage, advanced age, and maternal history of preexisting renal compromise or hearing loss. Controlled trials in adult patients have found little difference in the incidence of ototoxicity following treatment with gentamicin, tobramycin, or amikacin.

Early manifestations of nephrotoxicity may include hypokalemia, glycosuria, alkalosis, hypomagnesemia, hypocalcemia, and enzymuria. The enzyme excreted as an early manifestation of aminoglycoside nephrotoxicity is the lysosomal enzyme N-acetyl-β-D-glucosaminidase (NAG). Renal damage is dose related and generally reversible.

Another less common but important side effect of the aminoglycosides is a competitive type of neuromuscular blockade, seen most often after intraperitoneal administration or after intravenous push. Hypersensitivity reactions to systemically administered aminoglycosides are uncommon.

Because of their relatively narrow toxic-to-therapeutic ratio, serum concentrations of the aminoglycosides should be monitored. When using multiple daily dosing, peak concentrations of gentamicin, tobramycin, and netilmicin should not exceed 10 mg/L, and trough concentrations should be below 2 mg/L. Amikacin peak and trough concentrations should not exceed 30 mg/L and 10 mg/L, respectively. When using single daily dosing, levels approximately 8 hours after the start of dosing should be in the range of 2 to 5 mg/L for gentamicin, tobramycin, or netilmicin, and 10 to 15 mg/L for amikacin.

Indications   The most important indications for using one of the aminoglycosides are for treatment of proven or suspected gram-negative infections of the blood, bones, joints, respiratory tract, urinary tract, or soft tissues. The aminoglycosides also are valuable in the empiric therapy of febrile, neutropenic episodes in immunocompromised patients.

Tetracyclines

The tetracyclines are not frequently prescribed for children because of their age-related toxicities. They are, therefore, discussed only briefly with special attention to these toxicities.

The tetracyclines are active against a wide range of gram-positive and gram-negative bacteria, *Mycoplasma*, *Rickettsia*, and *Chlamydia*. They are also active against *Treponema pallidum* and moderately active against a wide range of anaerobes. All tetracyclines are absorbed adequately, but incompletely, from the gastrointestinal tract. They are chelated by various cations and are absorbed more completely during fasting. These antibiotics distribute widely and attain concentrations in the CSF of 10 to 50% of simultaneous serum concentrations. Most of these agents are excreted primarily by renal glomerular filtration, with lesser amounts being eliminated in the bile. Doxycycline is an exception, with 90% appearing in the feces. The half-lives of the tetracyclines range from 6 hours for tetracycline to between 18 and 22 hours for doxycycline.

Toxicity   The adverse effects of tetracyclines relate to tooth and bone deposition. Permanent binding to dental calcium can produce a dose-related, brownish, fluorescent discoloration of the teeth when the drugs are administered during the period of dental calcification (from the fifth month of gestation to approximately 8 years of age). Bone deposition may result in temporary cessation of bone growth. This effect is reversible when the drug is discontinued.

Other adverse effects of tetracyclines that are not age related include gastrointestinal disturbances, photosensitivity, hepatotoxicity, and neurotoxicity. Hypersensitivity reactions to the tetracyclines are rare.

Photosensitivity reactions may be caused by any of the tetracyclines but are most frequent with doxycycline. Unfortunately, doxycycline is frequently prescribed as a prophylactic agent against diarrhea in persons traveling to tropical, sunny climates. Hepatotoxic reactions are uncommon, but fatal liver necrosis has been described after large intravenous doses in pregnant women. The pathogenesis of this reaction is unknown.

Manifestations of neurotoxicity are observed frequently and almost exclusively with minocycline. Dizziness, weakness, vertigo, and ataxia appear within the first few days of therapy. Another neu-

rologic side effect of these agents is benign intracranial hypertension that is self-limited and resolves when the therapy is discontinued.

Indications   Indications for tetracycline therapy in adults and children over 8 years of age include infections caused by *M. pneumoniae*, Q fever, psittacosis, brucellosis, rickettsial species, ehrlichiosis, and lymphogranuloma venereum. Tetracycline is also used to treat gonorrhea and syphilis in the penicillin-allergic nonpregnant patient and is frequently prescribed to patients with acne vulgaris. Doxycycline is an effective chemoprophylactic agent against *E. coli*-induced diarrhea and against meningitis caused by *Neisseria meningitidis* or anthrax.

Chloramphenicol

Chloramphenicol is active against aerobic bacteria except *P. aeruginosa*, most anaerobes, and the majority of *Mycoplasma*, *Chlamydia*, and *Rickettsia* organisms. Most susceptible bacteria have MICs less than 5 mg/L.

Chloramphenicol is rapidly and completely absorbed from the gastrointestinal tract. The intravenous formulation of chloramphenicol is a succinate that must be hydrolyzed in vivo to biologically active free drug. Maximum serum concentrations attained after an oral or intravenous dose of 25 mg/kg range from 15 to 25 mg/L. There is, however, considerable interpatient variability. Chloramphenicol diffuses well into most body fluids and tissues. Even in the absence of meningitis, concentrations in the CSF often reach 70 to 80% of serum concentrations.

Chloramphenicol is metabolized in the liver. It is converted to a biologically inactive, water-soluble monoglucuronide. Impaired liver function can result in high serum concentrations. About 90% of chloramphenicol is excreted in the urine, but only 5 to 10% of this is in the unchanged biologically active form; dosage does not need to be adjusted in the presence of renal failure. The serum $t_{1/2}$ is approximately 3 hours.

Toxicity   The most feared adverse effect of chloramphenicol therapy is aplastic anemia. This is a nondose-related phenomenon, and the mechanism is unclear. The precise frequency of this complication is not known but is estimated to be 1 in 40,000 treatment courses. A second type of hematopoietic depression is dose related. Serum concentrations in excess of 20 to 25 mg/L invariably result in reduced iron utilization by the bone marrow. This eventually leads to anemia and, less commonly, to thrombocytopenia and leukopenia. This type of marrow toxicity is reversible when the antibiotic is discontinued.

A toxic reaction to chloramphenicol in neonates is the "gray baby syndrome." This is a form of circulatory collapse associated with excessive and sustained serum concentrations of unconjugated drug. Neonates are susceptible because of their immature hepatic drug-metabolizing enzymes.

Chloramphenicol serum concentrations should be monitored during therapy, and dosing should be adjusted if peak concentrations exceed 25 to 30 mg/L.

Indications   Chloramphenicol is effective in treating typhoid fever, rickettsial diseases, brain abscesses, and a variety of other infections in which anaerobes are usually pathogenic. In the penicillin-allergic patient, chloramphenicol is effective for infections caused by *H. influenzae*, *S. pneumoniae*, and *N. meningitidis*. Because of the availability of equally effective, less-toxic agents, oral formulations of chloramphenicol are no longer made or available in the United States; an intravenous preparation is available.

Clindamycin

Clindamycin is active against most gram-positive bacteria, both aerobic and anaerobic. It also is active against most gram-negative anaerobic rods, but it is inactive against most gram-negative aerobes. Sensitive organisms usually have MICs less than 0.5 mg/L.

Clindamycin is well absorbed from the gastrointestinal tract. An oral dose of 300 mg results in maximum serum concentrations of 4 to 5 mg/L. It may be prescribed as a capsule or as a suspension. Maximum serum concentrations after an intravenous dose are two- to three-fold higher than after an oral dose. Clindamycin distributes widely, but penetrates into CSF poorly. The drug is metabolized primarily in the liver, with less than 25% of a dose ultimately excreted in the urine. Thus, hepatic insufficiency has a more profound effect on the disposition of this drug than does renal insufficiency. The $t_{1/2}$ of clindamycin is 2 to 4 hours.

Toxicity The most important group of adverse reactions to clindamycin are gastrointestinal disturbances. Approximately 30% of patients treated with this drug develop diarrhea. This diarrhea is usually self-limited and subsides when therapy is discontinued. It may be associated with nausea, vomiting, and abdominal cramps. A more severe gastrointestinal side effect is pseudomembranous colitis, which was first described in association with this antibiotic. It is caused by gastrointestinal overgrowth of toxin-producing *C. difficile*. Almost every antibiotic has now been implicated in the pathogenesis of pseudomembranous colitis, and clindamycin is not the most frequent culprit. Furthermore, pseudomembranous colitis is much less common in children than in adults.

Minor abnormalities of liver function tests are quite common during clindamycin therapy, and cardiovascular collapse has been observed after rapid intravenous administration.

Indications The most important uses of clindamycin are in treating a variety of anaerobic infections, including those caused by *B. fragilis*. Some infections treated successfully with clindamycin, usually combined with an aminoglycoside, include intraabdominal and pelvic infections, aspiration pneumonia, infected decubitus ulcers, and periodontal disease. Clindamycin is also valuable in treating a variety of staphylococcal and streptococcal infections. Many experts recommend its use combined with penicillin in treating necrotizing fasciitis due to group A streptococci.

Erythromycin

The antibacterial activity of erythromycin is similar to that of clindamycin. It is generally active against gram-positive aerobes and anaerobes. It is inactive against most gram-negative enterics but is active against certain nonenteric gram-negative species, including *Neisseria, Haemophilus, Bordetella, Campylobacter,* and *Legionella*. The gram-negative anaerobes are not reliably sensitive. *Rickettsia, Mycoplasma pneumoniae, Ureaplasma,* and *Chlamydia* are usually inhibited by attainable concentrations of erythromycin. Most sensitive bacteria are inhibited by less than 1.0 mg/L of this antibiotic.

Erythromycin base is adequately absorbed from the gastrointestinal tract. The base is inactivated by gastric acidity, and therefore absorption can be enhanced by enclosing the antibiotic in a capsule or by administering it as a stearate or estolate derivative. Maximum serum concentrations after a 500-mg dose of base or stearate are approximately 1 mg/L. Concentrations are two- to four-fold higher after an equivalent dose of the estolate formulation. A 500-mg dose of intravenous erythromycin results in maximum serum concentrations of about 5 mg/L.

Erythromycin is distributed throughout body water. It attains only low concentrations in the CSF, even with inflamed meninges. Only a small amount of erythromycin is excreted in its original form; the remainder is metabolized. The $t_{1/2}$ is approximately 2 hours.

Toxicity Oral erythromycin formulations often result in gastrointestinal disturbances, including nausea, vomiting, diarrhea, and abdominal cramps. These adverse effects are likely to occur at high doses. A much more serious adverse reaction, fortunately rare among children, is cholestatic hepatitis. It occurs most commonly with the estolate preparation and is probably due to the propionyl ester linkage. Manifestations can include jaundice, fever, pruritus, rash, increased liver size, and eosinophilia. Resolution usually occurs when the antibiotic is discontinued.

Intravenous erythromycin is frequently associated with thrombophlebitis. Ototoxicity, manifested as tinnitus and transient deafness, is a rare adverse reaction.

Indications Erythromycin is an effective alternative to penicillin for treating streptococcal and pneumococcal infections, although many *S. pneumoniae* are becoming resistant. Erythromycin is also indicated for treating respiratory *Mycoplasma* infections, for eradicating *Bordetella pertussis* and *Corynebacteria diphtheria* from the nasopharynx, *Chlamydia* infections, Legionnaire's disease, gonorrhea or syphilis during pregnancy, and for eradicating *Campylobacter* from the stools of patients with *Campylobacter* gastroenteritis. Erythromycin should not be used alone in treating otitis media. Although it is active in vitro against the majority of bacteria responsible for this infection, middle ear concentrations are not consistently above the MIC for strains of *H. influenzae*. If used for this indication, it should be given with a sulfonamide. An erythromycin-sulfonamide fixed combination is marketed for this indication.

Azithromycin

Azithromycin is a macrolide antibiotic that is structurally related to, but distinct from, erythromycin. Its biochemical modifications result in superior oral bioavailability, a greatly extended serum and tissue half-life (both exceeding 48 hours), and excellent in vivo activity against most of the organisms susceptible to erythromycin. In addition, it has excellent activity against *C. trachomatis*, with MICs between 0.03 and 0.5 mg/L. It is particularly well suited for treating genital infections caused by *Chlamydia*. A single oral dose is as effective as a 7-day course of erythromycin or doxycycline.

Clarithromycin

Clarithromycin is another macrolide antibiotic that is similar to azithromycin. A special feature of clarithromycin is its activity against selected mycobacteria. It is particularly useful in the treatment of atypical mycobacteria, especially infections caused by *M. avium-intracellulare* in immunocompromised individuals.

Antibiotics that Inhibit Folate Synthesis

Sulfonamides

Sulfonamides were the first group of synthetic antibacterial compounds. These antibiotics originally had a wide range of activity, but this range is considerably compromised by acquired bacterial resistance. Gram-positive bacteria that are usually sensitive to sulfonamides include group A streptococci, *S. viridans*, some *S. pneumoniae*, and *Nocardia* species. Staphylococci are variably sensitive, and *S. faecalis* is resistant. The most sensitive gram-negative bacteria are *Neisseria* species, many enterobacteria, *H. influenzae*, and *B. pertussis*. *Chlamydia* and nonbacterial pathogens such as *Toxoplasma* and *Plasmodium falciparum* are also sensitive to the sulfonamides.

The sulfonamides are often classified on the basis of their half-lives, which range from 2 to 6 hours with the short-acting sulfonamides, such as sulfanilamide, sulfadiazine, and sulfisoxazole, to 150 to 200 hours with the ultralong-acting sulfonamide, sulfadoxine. Most of the sulfonamides are well absorbed from the gastrointestinal tract. Serum concentrations vary somewhat among the different agents; but after the usual recommended, orally administered doses, maximum concentrations are typically in the range of 50 to 100 mg/L. Concentrations are higher after intravenous administration. These antibiotics are distributed widely and attain therapeutic concentrations in CSF. The sulfonamides are acetylated in the liver and some also undergo glucuronidation. Free and conjugated sulfonamides are excreted by renal glomerular filtration and secretion. The longer-acting sulfonamides undergo more complete tubular resorption than do the shorter-acting agents. Minimal amounts of the sulfonamides are excreted in the bile.

Toxicity Sulfonamides may cause a variety of hypersensitivity reactions, ranging from mild rashes to life-threatening Stevens-Johnson syndrome. The latter reaction is more common with the longer-acting sulfonamides. Hematologic toxicity also may occur with sulfonamide use. Reactions include agranulocytosis, which is usually reversible upon discontinuation of the drug, and hemolytic anemia in patients with deficiency of G6PD. Renal damage was common with the older sulfonamides, which were poorly water soluble. Patients developed crystalluria, which led to urinary obstruction and hematuria. Renal damage may be a manifestation of a hypersensitivity reaction. Sulfonamides are contraindicated in the neonate and during the latter part of pregnancy, as they may displace bilirubin from protein-binding sites, possibly leading to jaundice and kernicterus. Neonates seem to be more susceptible to the potential renal toxicity of these agents.

Indications Clinical uses of the sulfonamides include the treatment of acute, uncomplicated urinary tract infections and infections caused by *Chlamydia, Nocardia, Toxoplasma*, and chloroquine-resistant *P. falciparum*. For the latter two infections the sulfonamide is administered combined with pyrimethamine. The sulfonamides are also used as prophylactic agents; for example, in children with rheumatic fever who are allergic to penicillin and in children with frequently recurring urinary tract infections. When used to reduce the incidence of recurrent urinary tract infections, the sulfonamide is usually administered in combination with trimethoprim.

Trimethoprim

Trimethoprim has a bacterial spectrum similar to that of the sulfonamides, although it generally has lower MICs against most isolates. Trimethoprim is active against enterococci, whereas the sulfonamides are not.

Trimethoprim is well absorbed from the gastrointestinal tract. Maximum serum concentrations of 2 mg/L are attained after a 160-mg dose. Tissue concentrations of this antibiotic often exceed serum concentrations except in the brain, skin, and fat. Trimethoprim is metabolized primarily in the liver. Approximately 50% of an administered dose is excreted unchanged in the urine, and the remainder is excreted as metabolites. The $t_{1/2}$ is about 11 hours.

At high dosages, trimethoprim may cause nausea and vomiting. Blood dyscrasias have occurred rarely. Because trimethoprim is an antifolate, anemia secondary to folate deficiency may occur, especially among those patients with a preexisting folate deficiency.

Trimethoprim is commonly used with another antibiotic, usually a sulfonamide. Infections treated with this combination include urinary tract infections, sinusitis, otitis media, shigellosis, nocardiasis, and *Pneumocystis carinii* pneumonitis. Systemic infections caused by gram-negative aerobes resistant to multiple antibiotics have also been treated with this antibiotic combination. In addition, the combination is effective prophylactically in patients with recurrent urinary tract infections and in immunocompromised patients at risk for pneumonia caused by *P. carinii*.

SPECIAL ISSUES IN PEDIATRIC ANTIBIOTIC THERAPY

Intravenous Infusions

Antibiotics frequently are given intravenously to hospitalized children with serious infections. Intravenous administration does not assure drug delivery. Antibiotic stability in the delivery solution and potential drug incompatibilities must be considered. As a general rule, intravenous drugs should always be given separately. If this is not possible, the compatibility of the mixed agents must be verified.

When drugs are given intravenously, the delivery system itself must also be considered. Pediatric unit doses may be so small relative to the volume in the intravenous infusion system that it becomes impossible to determine whether the dose has been completely delivered. The use of dilute solutions of the antibiotics should circumvent this problem. The use of in-line filters with infusion systems may remove certain antibiotics. In addition, certain drugs may adhere to the plastics of the infusion sets, reducing the dose delivered to the patient.

Influence of Food and Beverages on Oral Antibiotics

Major factors in achieving compliance in young children are smell and palatability. Table 13-7 indicates which antibiotics should be taken on an empty stomach and which should be taken with food.

Ingestion of beverages may also influence the bioavailability and tolerance of oral antibiotics. Table 13-8 indicates the antibiotics to which these restrictions apply.

Antibiotics and the Mother

Antibiotics that cross the placenta must be avoided if they are toxic to the fetus. Table 13-9 provides data on the approximate ratios of infant to maternal concentrations of various antibiotics.

If a breast-feeding mother is receiving an antibiotic that is excreted in breast milk, the effects of this "unprescribed" agent on the infant must be considered. Table 13-10 indicates the antibiotics that are excreted in breast milk. Information on some antibiotics is not available. If no data on breast-milk excretion of a specific agent are available and a potential exists for serious toxicity, an alternate agent should be prescribed.

TABLE 13-7

ANTIBIOTIC ADMINISTRATION AND FOOD CONSUMPTION

Antibiotics that should be taken on an empty stomach
  Most penicillins (except those listed below)
  Most tetracyclines (except those listed below)
  Erythromycin base and stearate
  Clindamycin
  Isoniazid
  Rifampin
Antibiotics that should be taken with food
  Amoxicillin
  Amoxicillin-clavulanic acid
  Penicillin V
  Doxycycline
  Minocycline
  Erythromycin estolate and ethylsuccinate
  Metronidazole
  Nalidixic acid
  Nitrofurantoin
  Sulfonamides

TABLE 13-8

ANTIBIOTIC ADMINISTRATION AND LIQUID CONSUMPTION

Antibiotics to be taken with liberal amounts of fluid
  Most penicillins
  Erythromycin base and stearate
  Sulfonamides
  Tetracyclines
Antibiotics not to be taken with milk
  Coated erythromycin base and stearate
  Tetracyclines
Antibiotics not to be taken with acidic fluids
  Most penicillins
  Erythromycin base and stearate

TABLE 13-9

DEGREE OF TRANSPLACENTAL TRANSPORT OF ANTIBIOTICS

MATERNAL CONCENTRATIONS ATTAINED IN FETUS	ANTIBIOTICS
≥50%	Aminoglycosides
	Ampicillin
	Chloramphenicol
	Methicillin
	Nitrofurantoin
	Penicillin
	Sulfonamides
	Tetracyclines
<20%	Cephalosporins
	Clindamycin
	Dicloxacillin
	Erythromycin
	Nafcillin
	Oxacillin

TABLE 13-10

ANTIBIOTIC EXCRETION INTO BREAST MILK

Antibiotics that attain substantial concentrations in breast milk
  Chloramphenicol
  Tetracycline
  Erythromycin
  Trimethoprim-sulfamethoxazole
  Aminoglycosides
  Metronidazole
  Sulfonamides
Antibiotics that are excreted in only trace amounts in breast milk
  Clindamycin
  Nitrofurantoin
  Penicillins
  Cephalosporins

TABLE 13-11

ANTIBIOTIC ADMINISTRATION IN THE PATIENT WITH IMPAIRED RENAL FUNCTION

Major dose adjustments required
  Aminoglycosides
  Vancomycin
  Trimethoprim-sulfamethoxazole
Minor dose adjustments required
  Penicillins
  Cephalosporins
  Tetracyclines
  Erythromycins
No dose adjustments required
  Clindamycin
  Chloramphenicol
  Metronidazole
  Rifampin
Avoid
  Methenamine
  Nalidixic acid
  Nitrofurantoin
  Polymyxin B
  Spectinomycin

Antibiotics and the Newborn Infant

Neonates, especially those born prematurely, present special pharmacokinetic issues. Hepatic and renal metabolism of drugs and volumes of distribution differ from older children and adults. Therapy must be guided by kinetic data derived specifically from neonates, especially for antibiotics that have a narrow toxic-to-therapeutic ratio, such as aminoglycosides and vancomycin. The daily dosages of almost all antibiotics are lower in the neonate than in the older child.

Antibiotics and Impaired Hepatic or Renal Function

Most antibiotics are excreted to some degree by the kidneys. Renal impairment often necessitates a reduction in the daily dosage. This is especially important when antibiotics with narrow toxic-to-therapeutic ratios are prescribed. The daily dosage can be reduced either by reducing the individual unit doses or by reducing the frequency of administration. The first dose usually is not altered because the prolonged $t_{1/2}$ associated with renal impairment does not affect maximum first dose concentrations. Table 13-11 provides guide-

TABLE 13-12

ANTIBIOTIC ADMINISTRATION IN THE PATIENT WITH IMPAIRED HEPATIC FUNCTION

Antibiotics that may require dose adjustment in the presence of
  hepatic impairment
  Chloramphenicol
  Clindamycin
  Doxycycline
  Erythromycin*

Antibiotics that should be avoided or used with caution because of
  possible hepatotoxicity
  Rifampin
  Tetracyclines

* With the specific exception of the estolate.

lines for altering antibiotic doses during renal impairment. These guidelines are meant to complement, not replace, the measurement of serum concentrations.

Some antibiotics are metabolized by the liver and others are excreted in the bile. Table 13-12 indicates those antibiotics for which dose adjustment may be necessary with liver disease. If possible, it is advisable to avoid antibiotics that have been associated with hepatotoxicity in patients with impaired liver function. These antibiotics include erythromycin estolate, sulfonamides, and rifampin.

The Prophylactic Use of Antibiotics

A large source of antibiotic "misuse" is attempted prophylaxis. If an antibiotic can effectively treat an infection, it is often assumed that the antibiotic should also be able to prevent the infection. Although this reasoning may appear to be logical, it is in fact erroneous. The specific situations in which antibiotic prophylaxis has proved effective are outlined in Table 13-13. Other infectious conditions in which chemoprophylaxis may be effective are enumerated in Table 13-14.

TABLE 13-13

CLINICAL SITUATIONS IN WHICH ANTIBIOTIC PROPHYLAXIS HAS PROVED EFFECTIVE

DISEASE/INFECTION	ANTIBIOTIC OF FIRST CHOICE
Leprosy	Dapsone
Close contacts of *Neisseria meningitidis* infections	Ceftriaxone
Close contacts of *Haemophilus influenzae* type b infections	Rifampin
Pneumocystis carinii pneumonia	Trimethoprim-sulfamethoxazole, pentamidine aerosol, dapsone
Rheumatic fever	Penicillin
Syphilis	Penicillin
Vibrio cholerae	Tetracycline
Recurrent urinary tract infections	Trimethoprim-sulfamethoxazole
Recurrent otitis media	Sulfisoxazole, amoxicillin
Mycobacterium tuberculosis	Isoniazid
Group B streptococcus in neonate	Ampicillin, penicillin
Neonatal gonococcal ophthalmia	Topical 1% silver nitrate, 0.5% erythromycin, 1% tetracycline Ceftriaxone

TABLE 13-14

CLINICAL SITUATIONS IN WHICH ANTIBIOTIC PROPHYLAXIS MAY BE INDICATED

DISEASE/INFECTION	ANTIBIOTIC
Asplenia	Penicillin
Diphtheria	Erythromycin
Infectious endocarditis	(For details see Sec. 13.1.10)
Pertussis	Erythromycin
Postoperative infections	*

* The specific choice of agent depends on the nature of the surgical procedure.

An important rule to follow when prescribing antibiotics prophylactically is that the duration of their administration should not be prolonged. For example, most perioperative prophylactic regimens should be prescribed for no more than 24 to 48 hours. Unfortunately, antibiotics have often been continued for more than 7 to 10 days postoperatively. This practice only serves to increase antibiotic side effects and costs, and encourages the emergence of resistant bacteria.

References

American Academy of Pediatrics: Principles of judicious use of antimicrobial agents for pediatric upper respiratory tract infections. Pediatrics 101: 163, 1998

Gold HS, Moellering RC: Antimicrobial-drug resistance. N Engl J Med 335:1445–1453, 1996

Hampel B, Hullmann R, Schmidt H: Ciprofloxacin in pediatrics: worldwide clinical experience based on compassionate use—safety report. Pediatr Infect Dis J 16:127–129, 1997

Nelson JD: Pocketbook of Pediatric Antimicrobial Therapy, 13th ed. Baltimore, MD, Williams & Wilkins, 2001

Prober CG: Cephalosporins: an update. Pediatr Rev 19:118–127, 1998

Prober CG, Stevenson DK, Benitz WE: The use of antibiotics in neonates weighing less than 1200 grams. Pediatr Infect Dis J 9:111–121, 1990

Ruff ME, Shotik DA, Bass JW, Vincent JM: Antimicrobial drug suspensions: a blind comparison of taste of fourteen common pediatric drugs. Pediatr Infect Dis J 10:30–33, 1991

Soumerai, SB, Ross-Degnan D: Drug prescribing in pediatrics: challenge for quality improvement. Pediatrics 86:782–784, 1990

13.1.2 Antiviral Therapy

Charles G. Prober

Research efforts in the field of molecular virology have resulted in a growing understanding of the unique aspects of viral replication and biochemistry, allowing the development of safe and effective antiviral agents. Effective antiviral therapy currently is available for treating infections caused by herpes simplex virus (HSV), varicella-zoster virus (VZV), cytomegalovirus (CMV), certain respiratory viruses, and human immunodeficiency virus (HIV; Table 13-15). In general, these antiviral agents should be used after the identification of a specific viral pathogen in a host likely to suffer substantial morbidity or death as a result of the infection. To maximize therapeutic effectiveness, treatment should be initiated as early in the course of the infection as possible. Finally, consideration should be given to the possibility that the virus might become resistant to the agent during the course of therapy. Although resistant viral isolates have

TABLE 13-15
DOSES OF ANTIVIRAL AGENTS*

			ANTIVIRAL AGENTS	
DRUG	**ROUTE**	**T$_{1/2}$**	**DAILY DOSE (mg/kg/day)**	**SIDE EFFECTS**
Acyclovir	IV	2.5 h	30 mg/kg div q8h for newborns 15–30 mg/kg div q8h	Neurotoxicity with impaired renal function: hallucinations, tremor
Amantadine	PO	15 h	5 mg/kg div q8–12h if 1–9 years 5 mg/kg div q24h if <40 kg 200 mg div q12h if >40 kg	
Foscarnet	IV	3 h	CMV: 180 mg/kg div q8h × 14–21 days, then 90–120 mg/kg div q24h as maintenance HSV: 80–120 mg/kg div q8–12h until resolved	
Ganciclovir	IV	3.6 h	10 mg/kg div q12h × 14–21 days, then 5 mg/kg div q24h × 5–7 days/week	
Oseltamivir	PO	—	150 mg div q12h × 5 days if >18 years	
Ribavirin	Aerosol	9.5 h	1 vial (6 g in 300 mL sterile water) Given by SPAG-2 aerosol generator over 12–18 h/d × 3–7 days	Not for use in adults; teratogenic in animals
Valacyclovir	PO	2.5 h	1–2 g div q12h; dose and duration depend on underlying disease	

* Doses listed are for the treatment of acute viral infections. Doses for prophylaxis are found in the relevant sections.
IV = intravenous; PO = by mouth; CMV = cytomegalovirus; HSV = herpes simplex virus; SPAG-2 = Small Particle Aerosol Generator model 2.

been identified, they generally have not been clinically relevant except in immunocompromised hosts.

HERPES VIRUSES

Vidarabine was the first drug found to be effective in the treatment of HSV and VZV infections, but acyclovir currently is the most useful agent for these infections. Both vidarabine and acyclovir are synthetic purine nucleoside analogues that interfere with the replication of viral DNA. Vidarabine is phosphorylated intracellularly to a triphosphate form and probably inhibits viral replication by interacting with the viral DNA polymerase. Acyclovir has specificity for the viral thymidine kinase, which phosphorylates the drug to the monophosphate form. The drug is then further phosphorylated by the host cell thymidine kinase, and the triphosphate form inhibits the viral DNA polymerase. Vidarabine and acyclovir restrict the synthesis of herpes simplex types 1 and 2 (HSV-1 and HSV-2) and VZV in vitro and in vivo. Neither drug is effective against acute CMV infection, because CMV replication does not require thymidine kinase. Acyclovir inhibits Epstein-Barr virus (EBV) in vitro, but its efficacy for treating clinical EBV disease appears to be limited. Topical antiviral agents available to treat keratoconjunctivitis caused by HSV include trifluorothymidine or vidarabine ophthalmic drops.

The decision to treat HSV-1, HSV-2, and VZV infections depends on whether the infection is primary or recurrent, clinical presentation, and host factors, including age and underlying conditions. Primary infections are more often treated than recurrent infections because of the absence of specific immunity. Because neonates infected with HSV and immunocompromised hosts infected with either HSV or VZV can suffer substantial morbidity and mortality, antiviral therapy generally is indicated.

Both vidarabine and acyclovir are safe in clinical practice, although patients should be monitored for potential side effects. Neurotoxicity (paresthesias and other neurologic symptoms such as tremor, ataxia, and hallucinations) rarely occurs during vidarabine treatment, especially in patients with impaired renal function. If acyclovir is administered with an inadequate volume of fluid or too rapidly, it can precipitate in the renal tubules, causing damage. Creatinine should be monitored in patients treated with vidarabine or acyclovir, especially if more than 5 to 7 days of therapy is anticipated. The dosage should be reduced if the creatinine concentration is above 1.5 mg/dL. Both drugs can reduce the white cell count, but neither has caused significant clinical morbidity as a result. Both drugs can cause gastrointestinal symptoms, including anorexia, nausea, vomiting, and diarrhea. Both drugs can cause extensive skin sloughs with infiltration of the intravenous dose. Acyclovir has the advantage of being available in an oral form. Because less than 20% of the oral dose is absorbed, oral administration is appropriate only for non-life-threatening infections. Acyclovir resistance of HSV isolates has been observed. It has not resulted in morbidity, except in patients infected with HIV in whom progression of infection caused by drug-resistant isolates has necessitated the use of alternate therapy, such as foscarnet. Valacyclovir and famciclovir are chemical analogues of acyclovir and ganciclovir, respectively. Their chemical modification results in enhanced oral bioavailability, but the spectrum of activity or efficacy when compared with the parent drug is unchanged. Their use in children has been limited to date.

The diagnosis of infection caused by HSV-1 or HSV-2 is an indication for intravenous antiviral therapy as discussed in Sec. 2.17.7. Antiviral therapy also is indicated for immunocompromised children with primary HSV-1 or HSV-2 infection. Although the risk of life-threatening dissemination is low even among severely compromised patients, severe local symptoms can persist for 2 weeks or longer. Herpes encephalitis is another indication for intravenous antiviral therapy. HSV encephalitis is caused by HSV-1 in children beyond the newborn period (see Sec. 13.4.6).

Acyclovir can be considered for treatment of serious HSV infections in other patients in whom the indications are less well established. Examples of such patients include otherwise healthy children with severe herpes stomatitis and those children with eczema herpeticum. If hospitalized, intravenous acyclovir may be used, but if the patient is ambulatory, oral therapy is appropriate. Acyclovir in the oral capsule formulation is licensed for treating primary and recurrent genital HSV infection, usually caused by HSV-2. The recommended dosage is 200 mg five times per day. Sexually active teenagers or abused children may present with this infection and should be treated if the clinical symptoms are significant and the child is able to take capsules. Severe primary genital HSV also can be treated with intravenous acyclovir. The topical formulation of acyclovir has limited efficacy.

VARICELLA-ZOSTER VIRUS

The indications for antiviral therapy in varicella-zoster virus infection are discussed in Sec. 13.4.11.

CYTOMEGALOVIRUS AND EPSTEIN-BARR VIRUS

Several drugs have been developed that are active against CMV. One example is the compound dihydroxypropoxymethylguanine (DHPG, or ganciclovir), which has efficacy in bone marrow and solid organ transplant recipients and in patients infected with HIV. Therapeutic trials in neonates with clinically severe, congenitally acquired CMV infections are being conducted. DHPG is also a nucleotide analogue that inhibits viral synthesis by mechanisms similar to those of acyclovir. However, its hematologic and renal toxicities may be substantial, and its use should be restricted to the most severe and otherwise untreatable CMV infections (see Sec. 13.4.7).

INFLUENZA

Amantadine and rimantadine are two antiviral compounds with known efficacy that are used as prophylaxes for influenza A virus infections. Both drugs also are effective for treating acute influenza A infection, if initiated within 48 hours of onset of illness. Unfortunately, neither amantadine nor rimantadine are active against influenza B. The mechanism of action of these tricyclic amines appears to involve early events in viral replication. As with other viral pathogens, primary influenza A virus infection is more likely to cause serious lower respiratory tract illness than are subsequent infections with closely related strains of the virus. Therefore, infants and young children are at particular risk for pneumonia caused by influenza A. In most children, the infection is self-limited. In certain high-risk populations such as children with chronic lung disease (eg, cystic fibrosis), influenza A may cause significant morbidity. The best approach to this infection is prevention by vaccination. However, if a high-risk patient has not received vaccine prior to an influenza A epidemic, amantadine or rimantadine may be useful for prophylaxis. Amantadine can be used to treat influenza A in adults and children, whereas rimantadine is FDA approved only for the treatment of influenza A in adults.

Amantadine is available as a pediatric suspension (50 mg per 5 mL) and in capsule form (100 mg). The dosage for children from 1 to 9 years of age is 4.4 to 8.8 mg/kg/d, given once or divided into two doses per day with a maximum dosage of 150 mg per day. Older children should receive 200 mg per day. Prophylaxis should be given for at least 10 days after a known exposure or up to 90 days during an epidemic. The drug should be given to symptomatic patients as soon as possible after the onset of illness and continued for 24 to 48 hours after symptoms have resolved. The dosage should be reduced for patients with impaired renal function.

The known side effects of these drugs include dizziness, ataxia, confusion, and anxiety. Rimantadine is better tolerated than amantadine.

A new class of antivirals that are neuraminidase inhibitors and active against both influenza A and B viruses reduce the duration of illness caused by these viruses in adults.

RESPIRATORY SYNCYTIAL VIRUS

Primary RSV infection often causes pneumonia or bronchiolitis, which can be particularly severe in children with chronic lung disease, in children with congenital heart disease, in infants and children with immunodeficiency or who are taking immunosuppressive medication, and in infants younger than 6 weeks of age.

Ribavirin is a nucleoside analogue that inhibits a wide spectrum of RNA and DNA viruses. It is FDA approved for administration as an aerosol to treat lower respiratory tract infections caused by RSV. The drug shortens the duration of symptoms of bronchiolitis and pneumonia, including hypoxia, caused by RSV and also may reduce the duration of mechanical ventilation and hospitalization in infants with respiratory failure as a consequence of RSV pneumonia. Criteria for the use of ribavirin in RSV-infected infants vary between institutions. The American Academy of Pediatrics criteria for use include those at high risk of serious RSV disease, such as infants or children with underlying cardiac or pulmonary disorders; those with underlying immunosuppressive diseases or therapy; and those who are severely ill as judged by blood gas determinations and lack of clinical response to other therapies. The drug must be administered with a small-particle aerosolizer, which can result in environmental exposure for health care personnel, although these units now contain a "scavenger" that decreases the amount of drug in the environment. The toxicity of aerosolized ribavirin appears to be minimal, although the drug can precipitate bronchospasm and has caused irritation of the eyes and skin of exposed health care workers. Declining use of ribavirin aerosol and development of a mechanism to decrease environmental exposure have led to decreased reports of toxicity in health care workers.

References

Balfour HH: Antiviral drugs. N Engl J Med 340:1255–1268, 1999

Committee on Infectious Diseases: The use of acyclovir in otherwise healthy children with varicella. Pediatrics 91:674, 1993

Crumpacker CS: Molecular targets of antiviral therapy. N Engl J Med 321:163–172, 1989

Mertz GJ: Herpes simplex virus. In: Galasso GJ, Whitley RJ, Merigan TC, eds: Antiviral Agents and Viral Diseases of Man, 3rd ed. New York, Raven Press, 1990

Smith DW, Frankel LR, Mathers LH, et al: A controlled trial of aerosolized ribavirin in infants receiving mechanical ventilation for severe respiratory syncytial virus infection. N Engl J Med 325:24–29, 1991

Steele RW: Antiviral agents for respiratory infections. Pediatr Infect Dis J 7:457–461, 1988

13.1.3   Infection Control in Clinics, Hospitals, and Physicians' Offices

Margaret C. Fisher

The goal of infection control programs is to protect patients and staff from acquiring or transmitting infectious diseases. Through surveillance and reporting, nosocomial infections are identified and policies are developed to limit such infections. The Joint Commission on Accreditation of Healthcare Organizations inspects hospitals and other health care delivery systems to ensure that appropriate infection control practices are being followed.

Infection control is equally important in the outpatient setting. Although less is written about outpatient clinics and offices, the practice of infection control remains an integral part of patient care in these settings. The goal is the same as for inpatients: protection of staff and patients from acquiring and transmitting infectious diseases.

TRANSMISSION

To practice infection control, one must understand the routes of transmission of infectious agents. By far the most common route of transmission is via hands. Hands come into contact with a variety of contaminated objects or body sites; organisms are moved on the hands from one person to the next and from one body site to another. Because hands are frequently implicated in the transmission of bacteria, fungi, parasites, and viruses, hand washing is central to all infection control programs.

Some pathogens are aerosolized in small or larger droplets. Small droplets can be carried by air currents and remain suspended; large droplets require relatively close contact (within a few feet) in order for the droplet to move from one person to the next. Body fluids, such as oral secretions, nasal discharge, or urine, may be common modes for transmission of infection, both among children and between child and health care worker.

SITE OF ACQUISITION

The site and frequency of infection will depend on the host and the pathogens in the environment. The hospitalized child may be exposed to other ill children in the hospital room, in the surgical or radiology suites, in hallways, and in playrooms. Procedures and examinations can expose the child to a nosocomial infection. Children at highest risk for infection are those with underlying immune problems and those who require intensive care. Infection rates vary from 1 to 3 per 100 hospital discharges in those receiving care on the pediatric ward, and from 30 to 50 per 100 discharges from newborn intensive care units.

Infection rates in outpatients have not been extensively studied. In general, children who visit doctors' offices have had better outcomes and a fewer number of infections than those who do not receive regular care. Nonetheless, the opportunity to acquire infection exists in the outpatient setting. The healthy child who comes for a routine office visit may be exposed to infectious agents while in the waiting room during play with other patients, in the examination room due to pathogens in the air or present on equipment, and during procedures including immunization or examination.

COMMON ETIOLOGIES

NOSOCOMIAL INFECTION The most common cause of infection in the hospitalized child is viral illness which is acquired from other patients, from visitors, and from the hospital staff. Nosocomial respiratory infections are most common during the winter and are due to seasonal viruses such as influenza and respiratory syncytial virus. Patients who require respiratory support are at risk for bacterial pneumonia. Endotracheal tubes bypass the normal body defenses, and drugs, such as morphine, impair pulmonary macrophage function. Tubes also occlude the orifices of the sinus ostia and the eustachian tubes and increase the risk for hospital-acquired sinusitis and otitis media.

Bacteremia is usually a complication of intravenous therapy; the site and duration of catheterization and the underlying illness of the patient are the primary factors determining the frequency of bacteremia. The convenience of intravascular catheters carries with it the concomitant risk of infection; in contrast to adults, in whom peripheral venous catheters are changed every 3 to 4 days, infants' limited vascular access often prevents routine rotation at IV sites. The risk of infection of peripheral or central venous catheters can be minimized by adhering to strict aseptic technique during catheter insertion and during manipulation of the catheter. Entry into the system should be minimized; if blood samples are taken from the indwelling catheter, all studies should be taken at a single time. Transparent dressings are not necessary, and in some studies, the use of transparent dressings was associated with higher infection rates. Changing the catheter over a wire also increases the risk for infection because it is very difficult to disinfect the skin around the indwelling catheter. Catheters inserted in the femoral area are more likely to become infected than those inserted in vessels of the hand or antecubital fossa. In the patient with a central venous catheter, blood cultures positive for organisms such as *Staphylococcus epidermidis, Staphylococcus aureus, E. coli, Klebsiella spp., Enterobacter spp.,* or *Candida spp.* should raise the question of nosocomial bacteremia.

Nosocomial urinary tract infections occur in patients who are catheterized and in those with obstruction to urine flow. Catheterization to obtain urine for analysis or culture carries with it a 1% risk of subsequent infection. Indwelling urinary catheterization is complicated by infection at a rate of 3 to 5% per day, and all long-term indwelling urinary catheters become colonized. Infection of the lower urinary tract can be complicated by spread to the kidneys and bacteremia. Common causes of infection in the urinary tract include those organisms colonizing the perineum: Enterobacteriaceae, enterococci, and *Candida spp.*

Gastrointestinal infections can be acquired nosocomially after ingestion of contaminated foods or medicines or after transfer of viruses or bacterial pathogens on hands or instruments. Outbreaks of colitis due to *Clostridium difficile* and transmission of vancomycin-resistant *Enterococcus* have been traced to use of electronic thermometers. In these cases, the thermometer box becomes contaminated during use and allows spread of the pathogen from patient to patient. Children with rotavirus infection are often asymptomatic; thus children hospitalized or visiting offices during the winter and spring may be shedding rotavirus. These viruses are transmitted from child to child by the fecal-oral route and from child to child by the unwashed hands of caregivers.

Indwelling devices placed for the management of trauma, neurosurgical processes, or monitoring can lead to infection of the central nervous system. Ventricular shunts, ventricular reservoirs, and lumbar drains are all prone to infection; manipulation increases the risk. Once infected, foreign bodies in the central nervous system typically cannot be sterilized simply with the use of antibiotics; thus, they must be removed as soon as medically feasible.

Hospital-acquired skin infections generally complicate surgery and burns. Rarely, bacterial infections, such as impetigo or ringworm, are transmitted by direct contact of one child's skin with another, or by the unwashed hands of a caregiver. Nosocomial musculoskeletal infections are uncommon; the highest risk patients are neonates and those in intensive care who suffer bacteremia, which may seed the bones or joints. Direct inoculation of muscles, bones, and joints is rare.

COMMUNITY-ACQUIRED INFECTION As with the hospitalized patient, viral illness is typically the most commonly acquired infection in outpatient offices and clinics. That many children are asymptomatic when most contagious for organisms, such as respiratory syncytial virus, chickenpox, and rotavirus, favors transmission in the outpatient setting.

The use of indwelling catheters in outpatients is now common. Sterile technique must be used for entry of the catheter. Dressing changes should be performed weekly or whenever the site becomes wet or soiled. Families must be able to contact a health care provider immediately should the catheter become dislodged or broken. Patient education is essential; the families must understand the risks and benefits of the catheter, as well as the techniques for catheter care (see Sec 17.6).

PREVENTION

Prevention of infections requires the cooperation and effort of all members of the health care team. The most important aspect of infection control is hand washing; unfortunately, this important means of infection control, although universally endorsed, is not universally practiced. Hands should be washed by rubbing the hands vigorously under running water for 15 seconds before and after every patient encounter, even if gloves have been worn. The type of soap is not of major import; antibacterial soaps are not necessary for routine care. All health care providers must be continually reminded of the importance of hand washing.

CHILDREN AS INPATIENTS

"Standard precautions" is the term applied to the precautions that should be followed when caring for hospitalized patients. The type of isolation system varies from hospital to hospital; infection control personnel should be contacted regarding room assignment and precautions to be used for contagious patients.

Many children and adults with contagious diseases are asymptomatic and thus are not identified as being infected. The caregiver must consider all body fluids as being potentially contagious and should handle them so as to avoid inadvertent transfer of pathogens from the patient to the caregiver or to another patient.

PATHOGENS TRANSMITTED BY DIRECT PERSONAL CONTACT Gloves should be worn for contact with mucous membranes or when contact with body fluids is anticipated. Gloves need not be worn for routine well-child care such as wiping a nose, changing a diaper, or examining a child. Gowns should be worn to prevent soiling of clothes with blood or body fluids. Gowns are also required as part of the isolation procedures for some hospitalized patients. Sinks with adjacent disposable towels should be conveniently located in all patient care areas. A rest room equipped with a diaper-changing area should be present for patients and families, as well as for office staff.

RESPIRATORY PATHOGENS Masks are required in many hospitals for care of children with respiratory infections; special masks (NIOSH-certified N-95 respirators) are required when caring for a patient who is suspected or confirmed to be infectious with tuberculosis. Because most children with tuberculosis do not have cavitary lesions, they typically do not transmit tuberculosis, and special masks are usually unnecessary.

BLOODBORNE PATHOGENS Goggles should be worn to protect the eyes when splashes of blood or body fluid are anticipated. Blood or body fluid spills should be cleaned up promptly by a person wearing gloves. A freshly prepared bleach solution (diluted 1:64, $\frac{1}{4}$ cup bleach to 1 gallon of water) is an effective disinfectant for cleaning environmental surfaces and instruments. Impermeable and puncture-proof needle-disposal units should be available in any area where needles or sharp instruments are used. Care must be taken to ensure that the needle boxes are out of the reach of children. There are state and local regulations for removal and incineration or sterilization of needles and sharps. Policies for dealing with needle-stick injury should be written and enforced. Each office should have a plan of action that will be taken in the event of a needle-stick injury. All employees who might encounter blood or blood-containing fluids as part of their duties should be immunized against hepatitis B virus.

CHILDREN COLONIZED WITH RESISTANT BACTERIA Judicious use of antimicrobials is an important step in reducing the emergence of resistant bacteria. Children who become colonized with resistant bacteria usually remain colonized for weeks to months. When these children are hospitalized, they are placed in contact isolation to prevent the spread of resistant bacteria to other hospitalized patients.

CHILDREN AS OUTPATIENTS

Waiting areas in offices and clinics offer the opportunity for child-to-child interactions that facilitate the transmission of infectious agents. Separate waiting areas for sick and well children should be considered. Triage can be done when the family calls for an appointment. Immunocompromised children should be moved to an examination room promptly to avoid unnecessary exposures.

Toys in the clinic, office, or hospital play areas should be cleaned on a regular basis. Ideally, cleaning should be done between use by different children; however, practically, daily cleanup is appropriate. A dishwasher can be used to clean toys at the end of the day. Toys that cannot be cleaned should not be used. Furniture and floors should be cleaned regularly and whenever soiled by body fluids or excretions. Rugs are difficult to clean and thus are not ideal floor coverings. The examination table and weighing area should be equipped with disposable paper mats.

Personal and office equipment should be cleaned between patients. Stethoscopes, pens, and computer equipment have been sampled and found to be contaminated with bacterial pathogens. Care should be taken to clean or wipe these surfaces regularly. Equipment that comes in contact with patients must be disinfected and, in some cases, sterilized. The extent of disinfection required depends on the type of contact. Equipment that enters the tissues must be sterile, whereas equipment touching intact skin need not be sterile. Blood-pressure cuffs and oximetry probes should be wiped off between patient contacts and should not be placed directly on damaged or infected skin. When economically and medically feasible, disposable equipment should be used.

Physicians should be aware of air-flow patterns within their offices. Certain infections, including varicella, measles, and tuberculosis, can be transmitted via small, aerosolized droplets circulating in the air. The air in many offices is recirculated; at times the air from the examining rooms is recirculated into the waiting room. The amount of time that infectious droplets will remain within a room depends upon the number of air exchanges per hour.

TABLE 13-16

ILLNESS IN HEALTH CARE PERSONNEL

CONDITION	WORK RESTRICTION	LENGTH OF RESTRICTION
Conjunctivitis	Restrict from direct patient care	Until discharge resolved
Common cold	Stress hand washing and use of tissues for nasal discharge	
Cytomegalovirus	None	
Gastroenteritis	Restrict from direct patient care and food preparation	Until symptoms resolve or person is deemed noncontagious
Hepatitis A	Restrict from direct patient care	Until 1 week after onset of jaundice
Hepatitis B	None unless performing procedures with a high risk of transmission of blood from provider to patient	
Herpes simplex, orofacial	Restrict from direct care of newborn infants	Until lesions dry
Human immunodeficiency virus (HIV)	None unless performing procedures considered to be at risk for transmission of blood from provider to patient	
Measles	Exclude from office or hospital	Until 7 days after onset of rash
Mumps	Exclude from office or hospital	Until 9 days after onset of parotitis
Pediculosis	Restrict from direct patient contact	Until treated
Pertussis	Exclude from office or hospital	Until treated for 5 days
Rubella	Exclude from office or hospital	Until 5 days after onset of rash
Scabies	Restrict from direct patient care	Until treated
Staphylococcal skin infection	Restrict from direct patient care	Until treated for 24 hours
Streptococcal infection, group A	Restrict from direct patient care	Until treated for 24 hours
Tuberculosis, active	Exclude from office or hospital	Until proven noninfectious
Varicella	Exclude from office or hospital	Until lesions crust
Zoster	If lesions covered, restrict from care of immunocompromised patients; if lesions cannot be covered, restrict from all patient care	Until lesions crust

Preparation of the skin prior to immunizations can be accomplished with alcohol wipes. Skin preparation for suturing lacerations, incising skin, or obtaining blood for culture requires the use of tincture of iodine or povidone-iodine.

Policies for outpatient care of children colonized with resistant bacteria have not been standardized. Bacteria such as vancomycin-resistant *Staphylococcus aureus* can be acquired from respiratory therapy equipment in children requiring home care for tracheostomies. Some experts recommend strict isolation of these patients in offices and outpatient clinics, while others feel this is necessary only during hospitalization. Other resistant bacteria, such as *Streptococcus pneumoniae,* may be frequent colonizers of the nasopharynx of otherwise well children; devising isolation procedures for these children is impractical.

Because health care workers are capable of transmitting disease, each office or hospital should have written policies regarding exclusion of staff members with contagious illnesses (Table 13-16). Respiratory infections are not usually a reason for exclusion, but yearly influenza vaccination is recommended. Emphasis should be placed on hand washing and use of tissues to prevent transmission of respiratory viruses to patients and other staff members. Skin testing for tuberculosis is recommended at the time of employment.

References

Bennett JV, Brachman PS, eds: Hospital Infections. Boston, Little, Brown and Company, 1992

Bolyard EA, Tablan OC, Williams WW, et al: Guideline for infection control in health care personnel, 1998. Infect Control Hosp Epidemiol 19:407–463, 1998

Centers for Disease Control and Prevention, Immunization of health-care workers. Recommendations of the Advisory Committee on Immunization Practices (ACIP) and the Hospital Infection Control Practices Advisory Committee (HICPAC). Morb Mortal Wkly Rep 46(RR-18):1–42, 1997

Centers for Disease Control and Prevention: Public Health Service guidelines for the management of health-care worker exposures to HIV and recommendations for postexposure prophylaxis. MMWR Morb Mortal Wkly Rep 47(RR-7):1–33, 1998

Garner JS, The Hospital Infection Control Practices Advisory Committee, Centers for Disease Control and Prevention: Guideline for isolation precautions in hospitals. Infect Control Hosp Epidemiol 17:53–80, 1996

Goodman RA, Solomon SL: Transmission of infectious diseases in outpatient health care settings. JAMA 265:2377–2381, 1991

Larson EL: APIC guideline for handwashing and hand antisepsis in health care settings. Am J Infect Control 23:251–269, 1995

Lohr JA, Downs SM, Dudley S, Donowitz LG: Hospital-acquired urinary tract infections in the pediatric patient: a prospective study. Pediatr Infect Dis J 13:8–12, 1994

Mangram AJ, Horan TC, Pearson ML, et al: Guideline for prevention of surgical site infection, 1999. Infect Control Hosp Epidemiol 20:97–132 and 250–278, 1999

Pearson ML, The Hospital Infection Control Practices Advisory Committee: Guideline for prevention of intravascular-device-related infections. Infect Control Hosp Epidemiol 17:438–473, 1996

Rutala WA: Disinfection and sterilization of patient-care items. Infect Control Hosp Epidemiol 17:377–384, 1996

13.1.4 Use of the Clinical Microbiology Laboratory

John C. Christenson and E. Kent Korgenski

If the clinician is able to determine the causative agent of an infection by recognizing the clinical syndrome with which the patient presents, no diagnostic microbiological tests are needed. Minor or self-limited infections similarly require little specialized input. Microbiological tests are useful when decisions regarding treatment, isolation, or potential complications are anticipated. Clinicians should resist the idea of ordering tests merely for "completeness." Limitations of available tests, generally expressed by their known sensitivity, specificity, and predictive values, must be considered carefully when making a decision about treatment.

COLLECTION AND TRANSPORT OF CLINICAL SPECIMENS

Better yield can be achieved by utilizing transport media that provide nutrients that allow the survival of microorganisms. Prompt transport to the laboratory is key to higher yield and recovery. Failure to collect a specimen appropriately or to use transport media may severely affect the recovery of the organism. Refrigeration of the specimen may help to ensure recovery if transport to the laboratory is delayed. When in doubt, the laboratory should be called for instructions before obtaining the specimen.

Ideally, specimens should be collected for culture before the initiation of antimicrobial therapy. When collecting clinical specimens, health care personnel need to minimize the likelihood of contamination. Thorough washing of the skin and of the caps of blood culture bottles with betadine is required for blood cultures; when obtaining urine specimens, suprapubic aspiration after betadine wash is the method with the least potential for contamination. A swab taken from the surface of unbroken skin is generally not useful in the management of soft tissue infections and should be avoided. Bedside inoculation of isolation and/or transport media is critical to assure the correct diagnosis in infections due to *Neisseria gonorrhoeae, Chlamydia trachomatis,* and *Mycoplasma pneumoniae.*

Advances in automated microbiology, molecular testing, and better nutrient media have reduced the time required to obtain a final report. However, some tests still require additional time and the need for an expert technologist. Most bacterial pathogens in blood will grow within 8 to 48 hours. Bacterial pathogens in urine usually grow within 12 to 48 hours of inoculation. With shell-vial systems, viruses such as herpes simplex and cytomegalovirus can be detected within 24 to 48 hours. While many advances have been made, the isolation of mycobacteria, most fungi other than *Candida spp.,* viruses other than HSV and CMV, fastidious bacteria, and anaerobes continues to require prolonged incubation periods.

RAPID AND MOLECULAR DIAGNOSTICS

Despite numerous advances in the field of rapid and molecular diagnostics, a simple Gram stain of a clinical specimen remains an important part of clinical microbiology. Gram stains, fluorescent stains (for acid-fast bacilli, *Bordetella pertussis,* respiratory viruses, herpes simplex, varicella-zoster virus, *Chlamydia trachomatis, Giardia,* and *Cryptosporidium*), and antigen-detection assays (for rotavirus, respiratory syncytial virus, and *Streptococcus pyogenes*) are vital in daily clinical practice. Unfortunately, use of bacterial antigen detection (BAD) assays of cerebrospinal fluid and urine has a low yield and are seldom useful clinically. These should not be ordered routinely. With appropriate training of personnel and provision of needed equipment, many rapid diagnostic tests can be performed in a clinician's office. A quality assessment program should be an integral part of office testing.

The recent introduction of molecular tests such as polymerase chain reaction (PCR) and DNA probes has significantly enhanced the clinician's ability to diagnose certain infections; these tests en-

able better understanding of the etiology of known diseases such as encephalitis and have improved our ability to treat these infections. The time necessary to diagnose herpes simplex and enterovirus central nervous system infection has improved dramatically with the introduction of PCR (see Secs. 13.4.6 and 13.4.2). The use of pulsed-field gel electrophoresis and other molecular tests have enabled epidemiologists to compare clinical bacterial isolates to prove or disprove relatedness when nosocomial infections and/ or outbreaks are suspected.

ANTIMICROBIAL SUSCEPTIBILITY TESTING

Knowledge of emerging resistance in the community is an important criterion for the selection of appropriate empiric therapy. Antimicrobial resistance among *Streptococcus pneumoniae* isolates is probably the most important problem facing clinicians who care for children. In vitro susceptibility results are usually determined by disk diffusion (Kirby Bauer), broth dilution, or automated (bioMerieux Vitek, Dade Microscan) methodology. Etest, a newer method that utilizes an antibiotic diffusion gradient and determination of the minimum inhibitory concentration (MIC) value, can be used with many different fastidious or hard to test organisms. Although all of these methods provide qualitative results—susceptible, intermediate, or resistant—broth dilution assays, automated methodologies, and Etest also enable the determination of the MIC for the organism. Many clinicians get confused when attempting to interpret MIC data: interpretation criteria may vary between the organisms and the antimicrobial agents tested. Rather than being concerned over the actual MIC value or size of the zone of inhibition, the clinician should pay attention to the interpretation provided by the laboratory and should confine comparisons to antibiotics within the same general class. For example, with nontypable *Haemophilus influenzae,* an MIC of 8 μg/mL for a cephalosporin would typically be considered "susceptible," whereas an MIC of 4 μg/mL for ampicillin would be "resistant."

References

Cockerill FR: Conventional and genetic laboratory tests used to guide antimicrobial therapy. Mayo Clin Proc 73:1007–1021, 1998

Jorgensen JH: Laboratory issues in the detection and reporting of antimicrobial resistance. Infect Dis Clin North Am 11:785–802, 1997

Paisley JW, Lauer BA: Pediatric blood cultures. Lab Med Clin North Am 14:17–30, 1994

Pfaller MA, Herwaldt LA: The clinical microbiology laboratory and infection control: emerging pathogens, antimicrobial resistance, and new technology. Clin Infect Dis 25:858–870, 1997

Tenover FC, Baker CN, Swenson JM: Evaluation of commercial methods for determining antimicrobial susceptibility of *Streptococcus pneumoniae.* J Clin Microbiol 34:10–14, 1996

Wilson ML: General principles of specimen collection and transport. Clin Infect Dis 22:766–777, 1996

13.1.5   Fever

Fever—its height, duration, and pattern—is mentioned as part of the clinical description of many infections. Often fever is the first symptom noted by parents; many parents consider the fever itself to be a serious illness that requires immediate cure. Sometimes fever is the only appreciable manifestation of the child's illness. This clinical situation is generally divided into two distinct clinical entities: fever without localizing signs and fever of unknown origin. The former refers to an infant or young child whose fever has developed acutely and who has been febrile for a relatively short time—hours or days. The young age of the infant, although a cause for concern on the part of parents and clinicians, is also the prime determinant of evaluation and management.

Fever of unknown origin is a syndrome usually involving an older child who has been febrile at least twice a week for a duration exceeding 2 weeks; findings may be more consistent with chronic illness (eg, weight loss) than with acute illness. In this instance, the prolonged duration of fever and the inability to ascertain the cause after a limited outpatient evaluation are the sources of concern.

FEVER WITHOUT LOCALIZING SIGNS IN INFANTS AND CHILDREN
Julie A. Jaskiewicz

Fever is one of the most common reasons parents seek medical advice for their children. Measurements of temperature in normal children indicate an average core temperature of a healthy infant is $37° ± 0.8°C$ ($98.6°F ± 2.1°F$). This normal temperature may be influenced by several factors, including age, environmental temperature, metabolic rate, thickness of clothing, time of day, and acute illness. Most experts agree that fever is defined as a rectal temperature of $38°C$ ($100.4°F$) or greater. Clinicians often make management decisions based upon a documented temperature elevation. For very young infants, a measured temperature elevation by a reliable care provider should be considered accurate regardless of the actual temperature recorded at the physician's facility.

Fever often forecasts the onset of an acute infectious process in children. The vast majority of these febrile illnesses are self-limited viral infections, and the children recover fully without requiring medical intervention. Occasionally, fever is associated with a potentially life-threatening bacterial infection, and prompt diagnosis and antimicrobial therapy can be life-saving. The challenge for the clinician is to identify and treat all children with serious bacterial infection and to avoid using antimicrobial therapy for the majority of children with self-limited viral diseases.

Febrile infants are at increased risk for systemic bacterial infection, including bacteremia; sepsis; meningitis; osteomyelitis; septic arthritis; skin and soft tissue infection; urinary tract infection; pneumonia; and gastroenteritis. These infections may initially present as fever without localizing signs, defined as an acute febrile illness for which the etiology of fever remains uncertain following a thorough history and physical examination. The risk for systemic bacterial infection is greatest for the febrile infant in the first few months of life, when the infant's immune system is the least mature and exposure to bacterial pathogens acquired during passage through the birth canal is greatest. These very young infants also have a limited ability to localize and contain infection and may show subtle symptoms that are easily attributable to other noninfectious causes. Therefore, the accepted management strategies are different for the very young febrile infant and the older child.

THE FEBRILE INFANT 60 DAYS OF AGE AND YOUNGER

Numerous studies of febrile infants less than 60 days of age show a prevalence of systemic bacterial infection, bacteremia, and meningitis in febrile infants of 8% (range 5–12%), 2.5%, and 1%, respectively. Group B streptococcus and *Escherichia coli* are the most frequent causes of bacteremia, meningitis, and osteomyelitis in the first 8 weeks of life. Between 4 and 8 weeks of age, *Salmonella* species, *Streptococcus pneumoniae,* and *Haemophilus influenzae* type b will also contribute to a small number of bacteremia and meningitis cases. *Listeria monocytogenes* can be an infrequent cause of bacteremia and meningitis in infants less than 60 days of age. Urinary tract infections are mainly caused by *Escherichia coli,* and *Salmonella* species are the most frequently isolated pathogens from infants with bacterial gastroenteritis.

Although not an invasive bacterial disease, the clinician should be aware that infections with herpes simplex virus type 2 and with enteroviruses can present with fever without localizing signs in young infants ≤6 weeks of age. Herpes simplex viral infections (HSV) are relatively unusual in this age group, but disseminated HSV can be a devastating illness and early identification of affected infants is essential if intervention is to be successful. Unfortunately, early diagnosis of HSV can be difficult because most infected mothers will be asymptomatic at the time of delivery and many will not recall a prior history of HSV infection. Two-thirds of HSV-infected infants will present before 2 weeks of age and nearly all will present by 1 month of age. A positive maternal history of HSV or other sexually transmitted diseases, especially with a history of unexplained fever at delivery, or the presence of vesicular lesions on the infant, increases the risk of HSV, particularly for infants less than 2 weeks old. In this situation, skin, mucous membrane, and CSF cultures for HSV should be obtained, and intravenous acyclovir is strongly recommended (see Sec. 13.4.6). Enteroviruses may cause fever in young infants, especially during the summer and fall. Most infections covered by enteroviruses have no serious sequelae and do not require specific antiviral therapy (see Sec. 13.4.2).

Evaluation

A universally accepted approach to the evaluation and management of the young febrile infant does not exist. Usually, clinicians begin their evaluation of a febrile infant with a global assessment of whether the child appears well or ill. However, even when objective criteria for clinical appearance are used, many senior, experienced clinicians will identify infants subsequently proved to have systemic bacterial infections as "well appearing" (up to 67% in one study). In addition, no single laboratory test or group of tests taken together are predictive of systemic bacterial infection in infants.

Until recently, the typical evaluation of febrile infants without localizing signs included complete blood count, urinalysis, chest roentgenogram, and cultures of blood, urine, and cerebrospinal fluid for bacterial pathogens, followed by hospitalization and parenteral antimicrobial therapy for a minimum of 48 hours. This approach assures that every febrile infant, with and without bacterial infection, will be treated. This is still the standard of care at some teaching hospitals.

In the late 1980s, an approach that identifies infants who are at *low risk for systemic bacterial infection* was proposed. The *Rochester criteria* (Table 13-17) help to identify febrile infants who are unlikely to have systemic bacterial infection and who therefore may not require parenteral antimicrobial therapy or hospitalization. When prospectively applied in a large study of febrile infants less than 60 days of age, the Rochester criteria had a negative predictive value of 99.1% (95% confidence interval equal to 97.6 to 99.7%). The minimum evaluation for all febrile infants should include a careful history and physical examination, a complete blood count, urinalysis, and cultures of blood and urine specimens for bacterial pathogens, followed by application of the Rochester criteria.

TABLE 13-17

ROCHESTER CRITERIA TO IDENTIFY INFANTS *UNLIKELY* TO HAVE SERIOUS BACTERIAL INFECTION

1. Infant appears generally well
2. Infant has been previously healthy
   - Born at term (≥37 weeks of gestation)
   - Did not receive perinatal antimicrobial therapy
   - Was not treated for unexplained hyperbilirubinemia
   - Is not receiving antimicrobial agents
   - Had not been previously hospitalized
   - Had no chronic or underlying illness
   - Was not hospitalized longer than mother
3. No evidence of skin, soft-tissue, bone, joint, or ear infection
4. Laboratory values
   - Peripheral blood WBC count 5.0–15.0 × 10^9 cells/L (5000–15,000/μL)
   - Absolute band count ≤1.5 × 10^9 cells/L (≤1500/μL)
   - ≤10 WBC per high-power field (×40) on microscopic examination of a spun-urine sediment
   - ≤5 WBC per high-power field (×40) on microscopic examination of a stool smear (only for infants with diarrhea)

The laboratory tests included as part of the Rochester criteria were selected because they can be done in most providers' offices and the results are usually obtained in a short period of time. Some clinicians include a band-to-neutrophil ratio of less than 0.2 in the definition of low-risk febrile infants. Cerebrospinal fluid evaluation is not included as part of the Rochester criteria, and none of more than 750 prospectively studied low-risk febrile infants by the Rochester criteria have had bacterial meningitis. Still, some experts recommend CSF evaluation for all febrile infants under 60 days of age. To date, there are no published data to establish the relative risk for bacterial meningitis if CSF is not obtained. Recent studies suggest that as much as 50% of urinary tract infections might be missed by urinalysis alone, therefore a bladder tap or catheterized specimen of urine should be obtained and cultured for bacteria pathogen in all febrile infants 60 days of age or less.

A chest roentgenogram is no longer considered necessary to assign infants to the low-risk group for systemic bacterial infection. More than 90% of pneumonias in infants less than 2 to 3 months of age are caused by viruses, and the majority of infants with bacterial pneumonia appear ill and/or have one or more laboratory tests that would exclude them from the low-risk group. Still, lower respiratory tract infections in young infants can be serious, and if signs of lower respiratory tract disease are present, including persistent tachypnea, grunting, cyanosis, or focal lung sounds on chest examination, then *low-risk criteria should not be applied* and a chest roentgenogram should be obtained. The decision regarding hospitalization is then made based upon an assessment of respiratory compromise; the need for supportive therapy such as supplemental oxygen, cardiorespiratory monitoring, and intravenous fluids and/or medications; and the availability of telephone, transportation, and reliable caregivers at home.

It is important to note that *the Rochester criteria apply only to well-appearing febrile infants.* Certainly, while the clinical assessment of young febrile infants remains subjective at best, any infant who appears toxic (lethargy, poor perfusion, marked hypo- or hyperventilation, or cyanosis) must be evaluated for possible sepsis with chemical analysis of CSF (glucose, protein, and cell count) and cultures of blood, CSF, and urine for bacterial pathogens. The infant should be hospitalized and given parenteral antimicrobial

therapy, including a third-generation cephalosporin, such as ceftriaxone or cefotaxime, plus ampicillin to cover the possibility of infection with *Listeria monocytogenes.* In regions in which *L. monocytogenes* infections are rare, it may be reasonable to treat an ill-appearing infant with normal CSF with only a third-generation cephalosporin. *It is never appropriate to apply low-risk criteria in the evaluation of an ill-appearing infant under 60 days of age.*

Management Guidelines

No consensus is available for the optimal management of the young febrile infant, but guidelines have been established to enable clinicians to identify treatment options for their patients depending upon clinical experience, particular parental concerns, and the reliability of caregivers to observe the infant and to maintain follow-up. Increasing data show that some febrile infants at low risk by the Rochester criteria may be adequately managed without antimicrobial therapy and/or hospitalization. These infants will avoid the cost of hospitalization and may be spared the potential iatrogenic complications that are sometimes associated with parenteral therapy and hospitalization.

After a careful history and physical examination, a complete blood count, urinalysis, and cultures of blood and urine specimens for bacterial pathogens, infants who meet the Rochester criteria do not require additional laboratory evaluation. While it is clear that the Rochester criteria will accurately identify infants without systemic bacterial infection, the criteria have missed a rare infant with systemic infection, most frequently ascribable to urinary tract infection. A normal urinalysis may not exclude the possibility of a urinary tract infection, so it is strongly recommended that urine be obtained for culture in these infants. Most experts still recommend that a specimen of blood be obtained for culture, even though the likelihood of bacteremia is less than 1% in a low-risk infant.

There are two management options for the low-risk infant: observation without antimicrobial therapy or treatment with parenteral antimicrobial agents. These options may be exercised in either the inpatient or outpatient setting. *If the clinician chooses to treat a low-risk infant with antimicrobial agents, CSF must be obtained for culture* prior to parenteral antimicrobial therapy. Infants to be managed with observation alone do not require a lumbar puncture.

The decision to hospitalize a febrile infant should be made independent of the decision to treat that infant with antimicrobial agents. Regardless of an infant's assessment of risk for bacterial infection, an infant who requires supportive care, such as oxygen or intravenous fluids, may require hospitalization. Outpatient management of a febrile infant should only be considered if: (a) the caregiver will be able to adequately observe the infant and note important changes; (b) the caregiver has easy access to a telephone and can return quickly to the medical care facility should the infant's condition change; and (c) a physician can be identified who will be available to see the infant quickly if necessary, and who will provide follow-up care within 24 hours. When these conditions cannot be adequately met, the infant should be hospitalized, although not necessarily treated with antimicrobial therapy.

An alternative approach is to complete the laboratory evaluation with specimens of blood, urine, and CSF for culture for bacterial pathogens, to administer 50 mg/kg of ceftriaxone by intramuscular route, and to provide careful follow-up. This approach has been studied in infants 60 days of age or less and in infants 28 to 89 days of age with satisfactory outcomes. Using hypothetical models, this approach was also found to be cost-effective. Two disadvantages of this strategy are the unnecessary administration of ceftriaxone to a large number of children and the necessity of performing a lumbar puncture on all low-risk infants to avoid the possibility of partially treating meningitis.

Low-risk infants with a positive blood or urine culture require immediate follow-up, repeat cultures, and hospitalization for parenteral antimicrobial therapy. Infants with only a positive urine culture who appear well and who are afebrile at follow-up require a repeat urine culture and may be considered for outpatient management with parenteral antibiotics.

The Rochester criteria have successfully identified febrile infants younger than 60 days of age who are at low risk for systemic bacterial infection, but significant controversy and physician anxiety persists regarding the care of infants less than 30 days of age. Current available data do not consistently show an increased risk for bacterial infection in infants less than 30 days of age, as compared to infants between 30 and 60 days of age. Still, some experts do not believe febrile infants younger than 30 days of age can be managed safely in the outpatient setting and will hospitalize all infants in this age group for parenteral antimicrobial therapy. An alternative to this strategy might be to hospitalize all febrile infants younger than 30 days of age for observation, with antimicrobial therapy reserved for those infants who do not meet the Rochester criteria.

Well-appearing infants who fail to meet the Rochester criteria need further evaluation with a lumbar puncture and cerebrospinal fluid examination; cultures of specimens of blood, CSF, and urine; and a chest roentgenogram if signs of lower respiratory tract illness are present. As with all ill-appearing infants, those who do not meet the Rochester criteria should be hospitalized and given parenteral antimicrobial therapy. An exception may be the well-appearing infant who does not meet low-risk criteria, but who is diagnosed with a specific viral infection, for example, respiratory syncytial virus infection with a positive rapid-antigen test. In this situation, the infant is unlikely to require parenteral antimicrobial therapy. Note, however, that if the clinician chooses to treat such a patient with antimicrobial agents, culture of blood, urine, and CSF specimens for bacterial pathogens should be done.

THE FEBRILE INFANT BETWEEN 61 AND 90 DAYS OF AGE

Febrile infants between 61 and 90 days of age should be evaluated by the Rochester criteria and managed according to the preceding guidelines. Many clinicians feel more confident observing well-appearing infants in this age group, as compared to younger infants, and they often choose to observe these infants as outpatients without antimicrobial therapy. Regardless of the management strategy chosen for a febrile infant between 61 and 90 days of age, the physician is strongly encouraged to obtain blood and urine specimens for bacterial pathogens culture and to maintain close follow-up with the infant.

THE FEBRILE CHILD 3 TO 36 MONTHS OF AGE

By 3 months of age, the likelihood that an infant will develop infection with organisms acquired during passage through the birth canal is low. The infant's immune system is more mature and the infant is more interactive with individuals and the environment. For these reasons, both parents and clinicians feel more comfortable observing the natural history of a febrile illness in children older than 3 months of age before intervening.

Children between 3 and 36 months of age are more likely than older children to have *occult bacteremia*, defined as a positive blood culture for a bacterial pathogen in a febrile child without clinical evidence of sepsis or focal infection (except otitis media). Most studies suggest that the likelihood of bacteremia increases with increasing temperature. At a temperature of 39°C (102.2°F) or higher, approximately 3 to 5% of children in this age group will have bacteremia.

Until the early 1980s, about 50% of episodes of occult bacteremia were caused by *S. pneumoniae*, 25% by *H. influenzae* type b (Hib), 7% by *Salmonella* species, and 6% by *N. meningitidis*. Although *S. pneumoniae* was responsible for most cases of occult bacteremia, about 50% of episodes of bacterial meningitis in the same age group were caused by Hib. The epidemiology of occult bacteremia and its complications was dramatically altered with the licensing of Hib conjugate vaccine for use in infants in 1990. Since 1990, there has been a tremendous decrease in invasive *H. influenzae* type b disease. Currently, more than 85% of episodes of occult bacteremia are caused by *S. pneumoniae*.

Clinicians are concerned about children with occult bacteremia because of the potential for devastating morbidity and mortality associated with complications of bacteremia, including meningitis, pneumonia, osteomyelitis, septic arthritis, cellulitis, pericarditis, persistent bacteremia, and shock. Rates of meningitis following occult bacteremia are 2%, 15%, and 50% for *S. pneumoniae*, *H. influenzae* type b, and *N. meningitidis*, respectively. Most strategies for managing febrile infants and children between 3 and 36 months of age are influenced by the likelihood of serious sequelae following occult bacteremia.

Evaluation

Clinical evaluation alone will not identify all bacteremic children. The acute illness observation scale developed by McCarthy and colleagues is only capable of detecting serious illness with a sensitivity of 74% and a specificity of 75%. Studies show that response of temperature elevation to antipyretics is not a reliable indicator of occult bacteremia. As with the younger infant, a child who appears toxic should be hospitalized and treated with antimicrobial agents.

Among laboratory tests assessed for their capability to identify children at increased risk for occult bacteremia, the single most useful test is the total white blood cell (WBC) count. A large meta-analysis of febrile children between 3 and 36 months of age without localizing signs showed that the relative risk for occult bacteremia is increased five-fold if the total WBC count is 15,000/μL or greater.

Blood cultures should be obtained whenever occult bacteremia is suspected, especially if the patient is to receive empiric antimicrobial therapy. Many physicians obtain blood cultures from children 3 to 36 months of age with temperatures in excess of 39.0°C (102.2°F) without localizing signs of infection and with WBC counts greater than 15,000/μL.

Whenever meningitis is suspected, a lumbar puncture should be performed to obtain CSF for glucose, protein, and WBC count and for culture. Urinary tract infections are present in about 7% of boys 6 months of age and younger, and in about 8% of girls 1 year of age and younger with fever without localizing signs. The absence of white blood cells in the urine as detected by microscopic examination is not sensitive enough to exclude the diagnosis of a urinary tract infection in these young children. A urine specimen obtained by bladder tap or catheterization should be cultured for bacterial pathogens in all boys younger than 6 months of age, and in all girls younger than 1 year of age. Chest roentgenograms are useful only if the febrile child has respiratory symptoms, such as cough, tachypnea, or rales. A stool specimen for culture for bacterial pathogens should be obtained if the child has bloody or mucoid diarrhea, or if there are greater than 5 WBCs per high-power field on a microscopic stool smear.

Management

Baraff et al. developed a practice guideline for the management of the febrile child between 3 and 36 months of age that is used. Although this guideline provides management strategies based upon current data and expert opinion, actual management decisions will need to be made by the clinician on an individual patient basis.

Toxic-appearing febrile children who show no localizing signs should be hospitalized and given parenteral antimicrobial therapy with a third-generation cephalosporin such as ceftriaxone or cefotaxime. Blood, urine, and CSF specimens for culture for bacterial pathogens should be obtained prior to administering antimicrobial agents.

Well-appearing children between the ages of 3 and 36 months who have no localizing signs and a temperature less than 39.0°C (102.2°F) are unlikely to have occult bacteremia and do not require further laboratory tests or antimicrobial therapy. These children may be sent home if they have a reliable caregiver and can return to the medical facility if fever persists beyond 48 hours or if their clinical condition deteriorates. Acetaminophen 15 mg/kg per dose every 4 hours is recommended for fever. The clinician should be careful to provide the caregiver with specific instructions for acetaminophen dosing to minimize the likelihood of toxicity.

Well-appearing children without localizing signs and temperature 39.0°C (102.2°F) or higher should be considered for antimicrobial therapy, and the guideline provides two treatment options. Intramuscular ceftriaxone may be administered to either all children with temperatures of ≥39.0°C (102.2°F) or to children with temperatures of 39.0°C (102.2°F) or higher and who have a peripheral blood WBC count of 15,000/μL or greater. *All children who are to be given antimicrobial therapy require a blood specimen for culture for bacterial pathogens before beginning therapy.* Urine and stool cultures and chest roentgenogram should be obtained as warranted by age and clinical situation. In the absence of physical examination findings suggestive of meningitis, a lumbar puncture for CSF culture for bacterial pathogens is not necessary prior to antimicrobial therapy. This practice may increase the likelihood of undetected, partially treated meningitis, but for infants who have had at least two Hib vaccinations, the risk of serious sequelae is low. Some experts believe that children with temperatures in excess of 39.0°C (102.2°F) can be observed carefully without treating with antimicrobial agents. Regardless of which management option is selected, some children with occult bacteremia will be undetected and untreated. For this reason, clinicians must ensure that caregivers are good observers, know what to look for if the child's condition worsens, and will reliably return to the physician for follow-up within 24 to 48 hours, or sooner if necessary.

Intramuscular ceftriaxone (50 mg/kg once daily) is the preferred antimicrobial agent for treating possible occult bacteremia in this age group. Oral antibiotics, such as amoxicillin (60–150 mg/kg daily), have also been used, but must be given in higher than usual doses in order to achieve serum levels of drug comparable to those seen with parenteral therapy. In choosing a therapeutic plan, the physician must balance the risk of antimicrobial therapy, including the potential for allergic reaction, side effects, and the development of bacterial resistance, with the benefit of preventing the complications of occult bacteremia.

Children with blood cultures positive for bacterial pathogens need timely reevaluation and a thorough physical examination to detect focal abnormalities. In the absence of focal findings, the clinician's next step is determined mainly by the child's clinical appearance and the bacterial pathogen that has been isolated. Children with blood cultures positive for *H. influenzae* type b or for *N. meningitidis* are at risk for serious complications and require a repeat blood culture, lumbar puncture and CSF culture, chest roentgenogram, hospitalization, and parenteral antimicrobial therapy with a third-generation cephalosporin. Approximately 70% of children with blood cultures positive for *S. pneumoniae* will clear the organism without antimicrobial therapy and therefore have a low risk of complicated, invasive disease. In this situation, children with bacteremia who are afebrile at the time of reevaluation and who appear well with a normal physical examination should have a repeat blood culture for bacterial pathogens and continue on outpatient antimicrobial agents (ceftriaxone or oral amoxicillin). However, those children with *S. pneumoniae* bacteremia who appear ill, or who have persistent fever at reevaluation, need repeat blood and CSF cultures, hospitalization, and parenteral antimicrobial agents.

References

Baker MD, Avner JR, Bell LM: Failure of infant observation scales to identify serious illness in febrile 1–2-month-old infants. Pediatrics 85:1040–1043, 1988

Baker MD, Bell LM, Avner JR: Outpatient management without antibiotics of fever in selected infants. N Engl J Med 329:1437–1441, 1993

Baraff LJ, Bass JW, Fleisher GR, et al: Practice guideline for the management of infants and children 0 to 36 months of age with fever without source. Ann Emerg Med 22:1198–1210, 1993

Baskin MN, O'Rourke EJ, Fleisher GR: Outpatient treatment of febrile infants 28 to 89 days of age with intramuscular administration of ceftriaxone. J Pediatr 120:22–27, 1992

Bass JW, Steele RW, Wittler RR, et al: Antimicrobial treatment of occult bacteremia: a multicenter cooperative study. Pediatr Infect Dis J 12:466–473, 1993

Dagan R, Powell KR, Hall CB, Menegus MA. Identification of infants unlikely to have serious bacterial infection although hospitalized for suspected sepsis. J Pediatr 107:855–860, 1985

Fleisher GR, Rosenberg N, Vinci R, et al: Intramuscular vs. oral antibiotic therapy for the prevention of meningitis and other bacterial sequelae in young, febrile children at risk for occult bacteremia. J Pediatr 124:504–512, 1994

Greenes DS, Harper MB: Low risk of bacteremia in febrile children with recognizable viral syndromes. Pediatr Infect Dis J 18(3):258–261, 1999

Jaskiewicz JA, McCarthy CA, Richardson AC, et al: Febrile infants at low risk for serious bacterial infection—an appraisal of the Rochester criteria and implications for management. Pediatrics 94:390–396, 1994

Lieu TA, Baskin MN, Schwartz JS, Fleisher GR: Clinical and cost-effectiveness of outpatient strategies for management of febrile infants. Pediatrics 89:1135–1144, 1992

McCarthy CA, Powell KR, Jaskiewicz JA, et al: Outpatient management of selected infants younger than two months of age evaluated for possible sepsis. Pediatr Infect Dis J 9:385–389, 1990

Sadow KB, Derr R, Teach SJ. Bacterial infections in infants 60 days and younger: epidemiology, resistance, and implications for treatment. Arch Pediatr Adolesc Med 153(6):611–614, 1999

FEVER OF UNKNOWN ORIGIN
Russell W. Steele

Fever of unknown origin (FUO) is a convenient term for classifying patients who warrant a particular systematic approach to diagnostic evaluation and management.

The definition of FUO generally requires an immunologically normal host with oral or rectal temperature 38.0°C (100.4°F) at least twice a week for more than 3 weeks, a noncontributory history and physical examination, and 1 week of outpatient investigation. Early diagnostic studies normally include a complete blood cell count; lactate dehydrogenase (LDH); uric acid; urinalysis and culture; chest roentgenogram; tuberculin skin test; erythrocyte sedimentation rate (ESR) or C-reactive protein (CRP); and, in the older child, a titer of antinuclear antibodies.

Management of patients with comorbidity factors such as acquired or congenital immunodeficiency, neutropenia, and occurrence of fever during prolonged hospital stays is not considered in the following discussion.

The greatest clinical concern in evaluating FUO is identifying patients whose fever has a serious or life-threatening etiology for whom a delay in diagnosis could jeopardize successful intervention. Cancer and severe bacterial infections are the causes most frequently discussed and most likely to influence diagnostic and management approaches. However, the vast majority of children with prolonged FUO resolve their illnesses without a diagnosis and do not exhibit long-lasting effects. Therefore, it appears appropriate for most children to delay extensive diagnostic evaluation until the child has remained febrile for at least 6 weeks.

Because of the ready availability of more sensitive serologic assays and more precise radiographic scanning procedures, the etiologies of FUO in children, as well as in adults, have changed over the past three decades (Table 13-18). The most striking change has been the virtual elimination of laparotomy as a final step in evaluation, a procedure routinely recommended in the 1970s but now eliminated due to advances in radiologic imaging technology.

Two-thirds of children who now present with FUO resolve their fever without determination of a cause, as contrasted with only 10 to 20% in series published 20 to 30 years ago. In addition, a higher percentage of children with malignancies are now definitively diagnosed earlier in their course of illness. A greater percentage of the remainder may have viral illnesses that are more difficult to diagnose, but are more likely to resolve without intervention; such cases lead to an overall reduction in total cases of FUO.

Three newly defined infectious diseases now account for a moderate number of cases: Epstein-Barr virus infection, cat-scratch disease, and Lyme disease. All three can be confirmed with serologic assays showing both IgM and, later, IgG antibodies to the respective pathogens. Cat-scratch disease also can be confirmed with compatible liver lesions documented by abdominal sonograms or CT scans.

Clinical Evaluation

An oral or rectal temperature ≥38°C (100.4°F) is two standard deviations above the average for normal children and most appropriately defines fever. Rectal recordings are preferred for younger children. Tympanic temperatures are so unreliable that they cannot be used to monitor febrile patients. Many parents think that any temperature above the average, that is 37°C or 98.6°F, is abnormal and seek consultation for these observations. Unless there are other clinical findings, either historically or during physical examination,

TABLE 13-18

ETIOLOGY OF FEVER OF UNKNOWN ORIGIN IN CHILDREN

DISEASE CATEGORY	1990–1996[a]	1980–1990[b]	1970–1980[c]
Infectious	44%	22%	38%
EBV	15%	8%	2%
Cat-scratch disease	5%	2%	0%
UTI	4%	4%	5%
Osteomyelitis	10%	1%	1%
Tuberculosis	0%	0%	2%
Others	10%	7%	29%
Autoimmune	8%	6%	17%
JRA		3%	10%
SLE		2%	2%
Others		1%	5%
Malignancy	3%	2%	9%
Leukemia		1%	5%
Lymphoma		1%	2%
Others		0%	2%
Others	2%	3%	18%
No diagnosis	43%	67%	18%

[a] Jacobs RF, Schutze GE: *Bartonella henselae* as a cause of prolonged fever and fever of unknown origin in children. Clin Infect Dis 26:80–84, 1998.
[b] Steele RW, Jones SM, Lowe BA, Glasier CM: Usefulness of scanning procedures for diagnosis of fever of unknown origin in children. J Pediatr 119:526–530, 1991.
[c] Averaged from McClung HJ: Prolonged fever of unknown origin in children. Am J Dis Child 124:544–550, 1972; Pizzo PA, Lovejoy FH Jr, and Smith DH: Prolonged fever in children: review of 100 cases. Pediatrics 55:468–473, 1975; Lohr JA, Hendley JO: Prolonged fever of unknown origin: a record of experiences with 54 childhood patients. Clin Pediatr. 16:768–773, 1977.
EBV = Epstein-Barr virus; UTI = urinary tract infection; JRA = juvenile rheumatoid arthritis; SLE = systemic lupus erythematosus.

reassurance is the only intervention warranted for temperatures less than 38°C (100.4°F).

For "subjective" fevers, usually meaning that the child feels warm to the parent or another caregiver, a diary recording of morning and afternoon rectal temperature measurements for at least 1 week should be obtained before initiating diagnostic evaluation. Children often feel warm, particularly when environmental temperatures are high enough to induce flushing or perspiration. Despite widespread public perceptions, few parents (or grandparents) can determine low-grade temperature elevations by simply touching their children's forehead. Core temperatures greater than 39.4°C (103°F) consistently produce skin temperature changes that can be recognized by most caregivers.

The number of documented febrile recordings during the 21-day observation period is arbitrarily suggested as two per week. However, cases should be individualized. Well-defined events such as otitis media or limited viral illnesses can account for some febrile periods. Conversely, antipyretic therapy might mask significant temperature spikes.

Occasionally, an observation period in the hospital is the only way to verify fever in children whose parents insist that fever exists, but in whom the observation cannot be confirmed. In cases of factitious fever (Munchausen syndrome by proxy), potential underlying family psychopathology should be assessed and managed with appropriate professional evaluation and counseling.

Although there is a natural tendency to consider unusual or exotic diseases when confronted with prolonged fever in children, common viral or bacterial pathogens that present atypically are more frequent. Therefore, epidemiologic information and history of exposure prior to illness are major components of the initial evaluation. Diagnoses quite common in one area of the country might not even be considered in other locations. Examples include Lyme disease (Northeast and certain areas of the Midwest), tularemia (Midwest and far West), coccidioidomycosis (Southwest), and tuberculosis (urban).

Age is the next critical factor. Leukemia peaks in early childhood, whereas lymphomas are unusual before age 8 years. HIV infection presenting as FUO is more prevalent during the first year of life or after adolescence. Most autoimmune disease is seen in school-age children and adolescents, so screening tests for this category would usually be limited to an older age group.

Patient history should be more detailed than that obtained for acute illnesses, carefully examining family history, previous illnesses, recent symptoms, current medications, travel, and exposure to pets or humans with potential communicable pathogens. Weight loss, failure to thrive, or decreased activity during afebrile periods are more ominous systemic signs that will usually require a more rapid diagnostic evaluation. Of all symptoms, the presence of pain is the single finding that is likely to suggest specific laboratory studies. Therefore, pain should be completely characterized by its severity, location, periodicity, precipitating factors, and response to attempted therapy. Prolonged fever and bone pain may be the only manifestations of bone tumors, leukemia, osteomyelitis, syphilis, cat-scratch disease, tuberculosis, or histiocytosis X. In the presence of documented fever and constitutional symptoms, a history of abdominal pain necessitates evaluation for autoimmune diseases, pyelonephritis, Crohn disease, and hepatitis, as well as abdominal abscesses and tumors.

Physical examination occasionally provides the first diagnostic clue, especially when directed toward areas where abscesses or solid tumors are less apparent. Thorough abdominal and rectal exams are essential, as the abdomen and pelvis represent the largest area for such masses. Bones and joints can be adequately evaluated if the child is cooperative. Transillumination of sinuses is only useful in the older child and adolescent; younger children require selective CT scans to diagnose sinusitis.

Laboratory and Radiographic Investigation

Diagnostic evaluation should begin with basic studies done during outpatient observation as summarized in Table 13-19. The complete blood count accomplishes three goals: (a) it is a screen for leukemia, anemia, and neutropenia; (b) it identifies some acute-phase reactant changes by quantitating polymorphonuclear leukocytes, immature granulocytes, and platelets; and (c) it helps eliminate some specific, although unusual, diagnostic considerations, such as eosinophilia (present in some parasitic diseases), Howell-Jolly bodies (congenital or functional asplenia), or pathogens on blood smear (malaria, relapsing fever). Additional screening for leukemia is achieved with a serum LDH and uric acid. Urinalysis and urine culture should be obtained because urinary tract infection is the second most commonly identified infectious cause of FUO. Remember that fever is second only to abdominal pain as a symptom of pyelonephritis. Chest roentgenograms may identify an unexpected pneumonia, but they are also important in screening for tumors, particularly lymphomas, and for tuberculosis. A Mantoux skin test (5 tuberculin units), rather than a multiple puncture device, should be placed to rule out tuberculosis. In older children, an antinuclear antibody (ANA) determination is beneficial for diagnosing systemic lupus erythematosus, although no single test

TABLE 13-19

INITIAL EVALUATION OF CHILDREN WITH FEVER OF UNKNOWN ORIGIN AND RATIONALE FOR SCREEN

History and physical (all causes)
Complete blood cell count (leukemia and infections)
Lactate dehydrogenase, uric acid (leukemia and lymphomas)
Urinalysis and culture (infection)
Chest roentgenogram (infections and malignancy)
Tuberculin skin test (tuberculosis)
Antinuclear antibody titer—older child (autoimmune)
ESR or CRP (all causes)

ESR = erythrocyte sedimentation rate; CRP = C-reactive protein

consistently identifies autoimmune processes. Patients with systemic juvenile rheumatoid arthritis (JRA) are most likely to present with fever alone, but JRA is rarely associated with a positive ANA response.

The initial outpatient evaluation (see Table 13-19) generally requires 1 week for completion of laboratory testing and for reporting of final results. After this time, the physician must decide whether continued observation or progressive laboratory investigation is

TABLE 13-20

PROTOCOL FOR CONTINUED EVALUATION OF CHILDREN WITH FEVER OF UNKNOWN ORIGIN

Phase 1: Outpatient (after 3–6 weeks of fever)
  Complete blood cell count (repeat)
  Erythrocyte sedimentation rate (repeat)
  Urinalysis and culture (repeat)
  Epstein-Barr virus (EBV) serology
  Bartonella henselae serology
  Chest roentgenogram (review if already obtained)
  Blood culture
  Antistreptolysin O
  Human immunodeficiency virus (HIV) antibody (if there are risk factors)
  Twice-daily temperature recordings (by parents at home)
Phase 2: Inpatient (after 6 weeks of fever)
  Hospitalize for observation
  Lumbar puncture
  Repeat blood cultures
  Sinus radiographs
  Ophthalmologic examination for iridocyclitis
  Liver enzymes
  Serologic tests
    Cytomegalovirus
    Toxoplasmosis
    Hepatitis A, B, and C
    Tularemia (in endemic regions)
    Brucellosis (with risk factors)
    Lyme disease (in endemic regions)
    Leptospirosis
    Salmonellosis
Phase 3: Inpatient (after 6 weeks of fever if condition worsens)
  Abdominal ultrasonography
  Abdominal CT scanning
  Gallium or indium scanning
  Upper gastrointestinal tract x-ray series with follow-through (older child with any abdominal symptoms)
  Bone marrow (including aspirate, biopsy, and culture)
  Technetium bone scanning

more appropriate. Decisions are based primarily on the clinical status of the child and the results of the initial evaluation. For most patients, observation is the most prudent course of action. The majority of patients will become afebrile by 6 weeks.

Once a decision is made to pursue additional testing, selection of subsequent studies is guided primarily by a knowledge of the more common etiologies. This approach takes into consideration patient age, epidemiologic and geographic information, and any positive findings from a detailed history and physical examination. In addition, testing for some less-common etiologies should be included for diseases known to progress in severity if diagnosis and treatment are delayed. Examples of the latter category include abdominal tumors, Lyme disease, and Crohn disease.

Table 13-20 summarizes a practical approach to a step-wise, yet systematic, evaluation. Earlier studies can be accomplished during continued outpatient evaluation, although hospitalization is required for those more invasive (and costly) procedures suggested during later phases of investigation. The rationale for each test should be apparent. Individual circumstances will certainly modify selection of tests to the extent that any two patients are very unlikely to have the same studies ordered.

Finally, patience on the part of the physician is required. The best test to arrive at a final etiologic diagnosis remains repeated careful clinical assessment with interim histories and physical examinations. Even under these conditions, fever will often resolve before specific causes have been delineated.

References

Jacobs RF, Schutze GE: *Bartonella henselae* as a cause of prolonged fever and fever of unknown origin in children. Clin Infect Dis 26:80–84, 1998

Kazanjian PH: Fever of unknown origin: review of 86 patients treated in community hospitals. Clin Infect Dis 15:968–973, 1992

Knockaert DC, Vanneste LJ, Vanneste SB, Bobbaers HJ: Fever of unknown origin in the 80s: an update of the diagnostic spectrum. Arch Intern Med 152:51–55, 1992

Petersdorf RG: Fever of unknown origin: an old friend revisited. Arch Intern Med 152:21, 1992

Steele RW: Fever of unknown origin (FUO). In: Steele RW (ed): A Clinical Manual of Pediatric Infectious Disease. East Norwalk, CT, Appleton and Lange, 1986

Steele RW, Jones SM, Lowe BA, Glasier CM: Usefulness of scanning procedures for diagnosis of fever of unknown origin in children. J Pediatr 119:526–530, 1991

13.1.6   Interferon and Cytokines in Infectious Diseases

Allan S.Y. Lau

Individuals infected with pathogens, including bacteria, viruses, and parasites, activate their immune system to send signaling molecules—cytokines—to mobilize different arms of host defense. Cytokines are potent, pleiotropic polypeptides that act as local and/or systemic intercellular regulatory factors. They play crucial roles in many biological processes, such as microbial infections, inflammation, immunity, and hematopoiesis, and are produced by macrophages/monocytes, lymphocytes, fibroblasts, and endothelial cells. Cytokines identified to date include interferons (IFNs), interleukins (ILs), tumor necrosis factors (TNFs), growth factors

(eg, epidermal growth factors), and differentiating factors (eg, colony-stimulating factors).

Although important in immune defense, overproduction of cytokines, such as IL-1 in rheumatoid arthritis and TNF-α in sepsis, can cause tissue injury leading to systemic pathology. Thus, inhibiting the synthesis of specific cytokines or blocking their activity may modify the progression of inflammatory diseases. The availability of purified recombinant cytokine products and their antagonists has sparked therapeutic trials of this approach.

INTERFERONS

IFNs are produced by most, if not all, vertebrates in response to viral infection. These glycoproteins possess antitumor and immunomodulatory activities in addition to their antiviral effects. IFNs can be classified into three major groups—namely, α, β, and γ. Whereas IFN-α and -β are similar in protein structure and bind to the same receptor, IFN-γ is quite distinct and has its own receptor system. The IFN-α family comprises at least 15 subtypes inducible by viruses, bacteria, and tumor cells. They are produced primarily by macrophages and null and B lymphocytes. Human IFN-β is induced by viral and other foreign nucleic acids in fibroblasts, macrophages, and epithelial cells. Produced primarily by T cells in response to foreign antigens and mitogens, IFN-γ may be more useful as an immunomodulator than an antiviral agent. Compared with other IFNs, IFN-γ is more effective in inhibiting intracellular microorganisms other than viruses [eg, some *Rickettsia*, bacteria (*Listeria*), and protozoa].

The antiviral actions of IFNs are mediated by at least two pathways: degradation of RNA via the activation of a specific ribonuclease, and induction of an IFN-regulated kinase that inactivates translation initiation factor 2α. With respect to immune effects, IFNs regulate the expression of immunoglobulin, major histocompatibility (MHC) antigens, and cytokines. In addition, IFN-γ enhances the differentiation and function of macrophages.

CLINICAL APPLICATION OF INTERFERONS With recombinant DNA technology, all three types of IFNs can now be produced in *E. coli* in large amounts, and their use has been approved for specific clinical indications in the United States since 1994. IFN-α is approved for treatment of hairy-cell leukemia, chronic myelogenous leukemia, condyloma acuminata (human papilloma virus), hepatitis B and hepatitis C virus infection (the latter as monotherapy or in combination with ribavirin), and Kaposi sarcoma in AIDS patients. The former IFN-γ is approved for prophylactic use in patients with chronic granulomatous disease to prevent recurrence of bacterial infections. Additionally, IFNs have demonstrable efficacy in laryngeal papillomatosis, early stages of HIV infection, multiple myeloma, hemangiomas, and basal cell and cutaneous squamous cell carcinoma.

Dosages of leukocyte-derived or recombinant IFN-α vary widely. The duration of therapy is also highly variable, ranging from a few weeks in condyloma acuminata to 1 year in hepatitis C. The most common side effects, found in patients receiving more than a few million units, consist of a flu-like syndrome characterized by fever, chills, fatigue, headache, myalgia, and malaise; these symptoms can be ameliorated by acetaminophen. More serious side effects, including relative leukopenia, thrombocytopenia, and hepatotoxicity, are observed in patients receiving high doses of IFNs. In general, even these changes are transient and rapidly reverse following discontinuation of IFN therapy.

COLONY-STIMULATING FACTORS

Granulocyte-macrophage colony-stimulating factor (GM-CSF) acts upon multiple steps of myeloid differentiation, as well as on precursors of megakaryocytes, mast cells, and B cells. It also has effects on neutrophil functions such as phagocytosis, migration, and metabolism. In contrast, the effects of granulocyte colony-stimulating factor (G-CSF) are largely restricted to neutrophil functions such as phagocytosis, release of superoxide, antibody-dependent cellular cytotoxicity, and migration. Both recombinant human GM-CSF and G-CSF have been used as adjunctives to augment neutrophil production and to reduce the duration of neutropenia in recipients of bone marrow transplantation and cancer chemotherapy. Similar results have been described in certain leukemias, including patients with acute myelogenous and hairy-cell leukemias, as well as patients with other diseases, including aplastic anemia, myelodysplasia, drug-induced agranulocytosis, and chronic neutropenia (see Table 13-20). In general, the recipients showed increases in peripheral-blood granulocyte counts, fewer opportunistic infections, and shorter hospital stays. Treatment appeared to be well tolerated, despite the common occurrence of mild to moderate flu-like symptoms and occasional fluid retention problems. In addition, GM-CSF and G-CSF did not appear to stimulate residual leukemic clones in patients. Thus, application of these growth factors to the bedside represents a major contribution of biotechnology to a difficult area of therapeutics in febrile, neutropenic patients.

References

Healy GB, Gelber RD, Trowbridge AL, et al: Treatment of recurrent respiratory papillomatosis with human leukocyte interferons. N Engl J Med 319:401–407, 1988

International Chronic Granulomatous Disease Cooperative Study Group: A controlled trial of interferon-γ to prevent infection in chronic granulomatous disease. N Engl J Med 324:509–516, 1991

Lau AS, Lehman D, Geertsma F, Yeung M: Biology and therapeutic uses of myeloid hematopoietic growth factors and interferon. Pediatr Infect Dis J 15:563–575, 1996

Mustafa MM, Ramilo O, Saez-Llorens X, et al: CSF prostaglandin, IL-1 β and TNF in bacterial meningitis: clinical and laboratory correlation in placebo-treated and dexamethasone-treated patients. Am J Dis Child 144:883–887, 1990

Reichman RC, Oakes D. Bonnez W, et al: Treatment of condyloma acuminata with three different interferons administered intralesionally. Ann Intern Med 108:675–679, 1988

13.1.7 Bacteremia, Sepsis, and Septic Shock

Richard F. Jacobs and Toni Darville

Children presenting with pathogenic bacteria in a blood culture (*bacteremia*) manifest a wide spectrum of clinical signs and symptoms. The continuum from bacteremia to sepsis, severe sepsis, and septic shock depends upon a complex series of interrelated events that include the specific bacterial etiology; the inoculum of bacterial organisms; strain variations or virulence factors; extracellular components or toxin production; the site of infection; the immunologic competence of the host; and the host's response to the bacterial infection. Bacteremia may be occult, a transient phenomenon not associated with a specific focus of infection, or it may result from the extension of an invasive bacterial infection originating in the genitourinary, gastrointestinal, upper or lower respiratory tracts, or integument. Specific secondary foci of infection (meningitis, osteomyelitis, pyelonephritis, peritonitis, intraabdominal abscess, or facial cellulitis) may result. Recurrent or persistent bacteremia may result from established infectious foci (endocarditis, abscess, foreign-body infection).

EPIDEMIOLOGIC CONSIDERATIONS

Epidemiologic factors that influence the incidence, specific etiology, morbidity, and mortality of bacteremia in children include the site of acquisition (maternal genital tract, community-acquired vs. nosocomial transmission), immunocompetence of the host, and the presence or absence of foreign material (umbilical, arterial/venous catheters; central venous catheters; Foley catheters; peritoneal catheters; ventriculoperitoneal shunts; and foreign material following complex congenital heart disease surgery).

Acquisition from the maternal genital tract is the cause of neonatal bacteremias from *S. agalactiae* (group B streptococcus), *E. coli, Enterococcus* species, *L. monocytogenes,* and other gram-negative enteric bacilli other than *E. coli.* Once beyond the newborn period, *S. pneumoniae, N. meningitidis, S. aureus, S. pyogenes, Salmonella* species, and nontypable *H. influenzae* are the most common microorganisms causing community-acquired bacteremia in the normal child. A dramatic decline in the incidence of *H. influenzae* type b bacteremia in children has occurred as a consequence of widespread use of conjugate vaccines. Immunocompetent children with bacteremia must be evaluated for potential extension of local tissue infections; this includes children with pneumonia (*S. pneumoniae*, nontypable *H. influenzae*), gastroenteritis (*Salmonella* species), pyelonephritis (*E. coli, Klebsiella pneumoniae*), salpingitis (*N. gonorrhoeae*), cutaneous infections (*S. pyogenes, S. aureus*), invasive group A streptococcal disease (postvaricella), and toxic shock syndrome (streptococcal). *S. aureus* toxic shock is not associated with a positive blood culture.

In patients with underlying diseases causing an immunocompromised state, the presence or absence of foreign material affects the incidence and etiology of bacteremias, most of which are nosocomial in origin. Indwelling vascular lines, urinary catheters, and endotracheal tubes, as well as other foreign material, predispose newborns and children to nosocomial infections due to coagulase-negative staphylococci (most commonly *S. epidermidis*), Enterobacteriaceae, enterococcus, fungi, and other less-common opportunistic infections. In immunocompromised children without foreign bodies (eg, intravascular devices), endogenous sources of Enterobacteriaceae, *S. aureus,* and fungi become important causes of bloodstream infections.

SEPSIS AND SEPTIC SHOCK

Sepsis and septic shock are relatively common occurrences among infants and children. In term newborns, early onset sepsis occurs in approximately 1 to 10 neonates per 1000 live births, with a mortality of approximately 20%. In premature infants, the attack rate for sepsis is 15 per 100 and mortality approaches 50%. The prevalence of sepsis in hospitalized patients increased significantly in the past decade; in some studies, the diagnosis of sepsis has accounted for more than 25% of admissions to high-acuity units, with an associated mortality approaching 10%. Advances in medical therapy and increased use of invasive medical procedures and devices are factors contributing to a growing population of immunocompromised and seriously ill patients at increased risk for sepsis. Septic shock occurred in 44.0% of immunocompromised patients admitted to our pediatric intensive care unit with an infectious disease diagnosis over a 3-year period.

Although the organisms primarily responsible for sepsis and septic shock vary among different age groups, the clinical picture is the same. It has become clear over the past 10 years that the clinical syndrome of septic shock is the result of endogenous protein and phospholipid mediators secreted by the injured host. The failure of therapeutic interventions directed at single mediators of the sepsis cascade reiterates both the complex and multifactorial nature of the process and the need to classify patients unambiguously at the outset.

Throughout this discussion, sepsis terminology established for pediatric critical care uses adaptations of the definitions for adults that were proposed by Bone and colleagues.

In current usage, the term *sepsis* implies a characteristic clinical pattern of hemodynamic and metabolic derangements arising from infection. A similar or even identical clinical syndrome can arise from noninfectious causes such as trauma, pancreatitis, and diseases of immunologic dysfunction. Therefore, the phrase *systemic inflammatory response syndrome (SIRS)* is used to describe this inflammatory process, independent of its causes (Table 13-21). When SIRS is the result of infection, it is termed *sepsis*. Infection can be a clinical diagnosis and does not depend on positive cultures. SIRS and its sequelae represent a continuum of clinical and pathophysiological severity that may result in multiple organ dysfunction and death. *Severe SIRS* or *severe sepsis* is defined as SIRS or sepsis "associated with organ dysfunction, hypoperfusion, or hypotension." Hypoperfusion abnormalities include lactic acidosis, oliguria, an acute alteration of mental status, or an increased alveolar-arterial oxygen gradient or other evidence of inadequate oxygenation.

Shock associated with SIRS is defined as "hypotension persisting despite adequate fluid resuscitation, along with the presence of hypoperfusion abnormalities or organ dysfunction." *Septic shock* is defined as shock plus clinical evidence of infection. In children, a decline in blood pressure is often a late and ominous terminal event during shock. The characteristic hemodynamic alterations in early septic shock are a low systemic vascular resistance and a normal to supranormal cardiac output. Patients in early septic shock often

exhibit a normal systemic arterial blood pressure or a normal mean arterial pressure with an increased pulse pressure. When compensatory mechanisms for diminishing vascular resistance are lost, or when sepsis-associated myocardial dysfunction ensues, the patient's status may rapidly deteriorate. Because of the rapidity of change and the possibility of catastrophic deterioration, identification of the early stage of shock is critical; in these circumstances, evidence of hypoperfusion, rather than hypotension per se, should be sought.

Immunology and Pathophysiology

Sepsis and septic shock comprise a cascade of metabolic, immunologic, and clinical changes that is initiated by a focus of infection or injury and that ends with severe endothelial damage, profound hemodynamic derangements, and, often, death. Study of the pathophysiology of septic shock initially concentrated on the interactions of endotoxin or lipopolysaccharide from the cell wall of gram-negative bacteria with various inflammatory pathways. Attention now focuses on the central role of inflammatory cells and of the cytokines released upon stimulation not only by lipopolysaccharides (LPS) but by enterotoxin, toxic-shock syndrome toxins, gram-positive or yeast cell-wall products, and viral or fungal components. The inflammatory mediators that are released include TNF, IL-1, IL-6, procoagulant mediators, and colony-stimulating factors. Although the monocyte/macrophage is a principal source of these cytokines, we know that they are also produced by a variety of other cells: epidermal cells, synovial fibroblasts, lymphocytes, vascular endothelial cells, and astrocytes/microglial cells of the brain.

Sepsis usually begins with a nidus of infection or injury. At the cellular level, it is clear that endotoxin or lipopolysaccharide components of the bacterial cell wall are responsible for most clinical manifestations of infection by gram-negative bacteria. Lipooligosaccharides, cell-wall constituents, toxic-shock syndrome toxins, enterotoxins, and other substances are also well-known modulators of the immunologic response now thought to be associated with the pathophysiology of septic shock (Fig. 13-1). After endotoxin or another stimulus gains access to the circulation, mononuclear phagocytes are stimulated to release TNF, IL-1, IL-6, and platelet-

TABLE 13-21
DEFINITIONS OF SEPSIS AND SEPTIC SHOCK

Sepsis: The systemic inflammatory response due to infection
Systemic Inflammatory Response Syndrome (SIRS): A characteristic clinical response manifested by two or more of the following conditions:

Hyper- or hypothermia	Temperature $\geq 38.4°C$ or $< 36°C$
Tachycardia	Infant heart rate > 160 bpm
	Child heart rate > 150 bpm
Tachypnea	Infant respiratory rate > 60 bpm
	Child respiratory rate > 50 bpm
Pathologic white blood cell count	$> 15,000$ cells/μL, < 5000 cells/μL, or $> 10\%$ immature (band) forms

Severe SIRS: SIRS or sepsis associated with one of the following manifestations of organ hypoperfusion:

Lactic acidosis	
Oliguria	Urine output < 0.5 mL/kg/h for 2 h
Altered mental status	
Inadequate oxygenation	A-a gradient > 40 mm Hg, $PA_{O_2} < 70$ on room air or $Sa_{O_2} < 92\%$ on room air

Severe sepsis: All of the above plus clinical evidence of infection
Shock due to SIRS: Meet the criteria for SIRS plus one of the following:

Hypoperfusion requiring > 40 mL/kg isotonic fluid (crystalloid or colloid) and/or inotropic support
Hypotension
More than one manifestation of organ hypoperfusion
Septic shock: The above criteria plus clinical evidence of infection

bpm = beats per minute

IMMUNE CELLULAR INTERACTIONS DURING SEPSIS AND SEPTIC INJURY

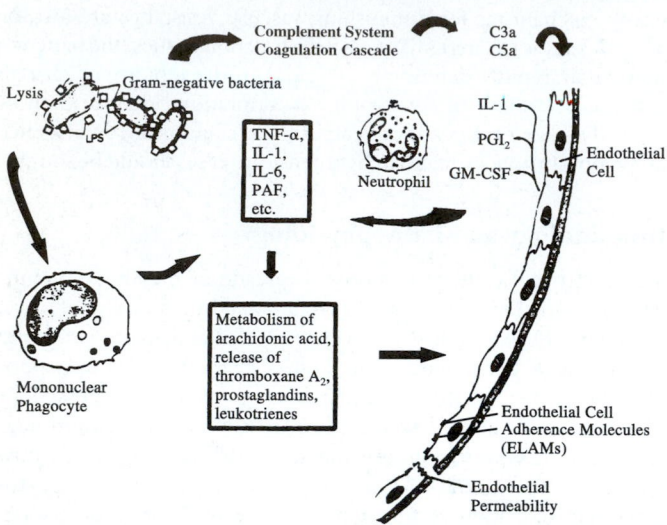

FIGURE 13-1   Inflammatory consequences of bacterial sepsis.

activating factor (PAF). These mediators stimulate metabolism of arachidonic acid to form leukotrienes, thromboxane A_2, and prostaglandins [especially prostaglandin E_2 (PGE$_2$) and prostaglandin I_2 (PGI$_2$)]. Almost all of these agents have direct effects on the vascular endothelium. Endotoxin, TNF, PAF, leukotrienes, and thromboxane A_2 each increase endothelial permeability. The vascular endothelium also seems to be one of the primary targets for IL-1-induced changes in sepsis. Endotoxin or lipopolysaccharide may also damage endothelium indirectly. The endothelium, in turn, is stimulated to synthesize and elaborate a number of secondary factors that contribute to the inflammatory process. These include endothelial-cell adherence molecules (ELAMs), tissue plasminogen activator, IL-1, PGI$_2$, and granulocyte-monocyte colony-stimulating factor (GM-CSF). The ELAMs attract neutrophils to vascular endothelium. GM-CSF enhances a number of neutrophil functions, including phagocytosis, degranulation, and cytotoxicity. Neutrophils may also be activated directly by most of the cytokines. As a result, neutrophil-induced damage may occur during degranulation (through release of free-radical oxygen species and lysosomal enzymes), during adherence to the endothelium (through vasodilatation), and during aggregation (through microemboli formation).

Activation of the complement system and the coagulation cascade contribute to the pathophysiology of septic shock. The alternative complement pathway can be activated experimentally by lipopolysaccharide and gram-positive cell-wall components. The classical pathway is mainly activated by complexes of cell-wall components and antibodies. The subsequent release of the anaphylatoxins—C3a and C5a—promote vascular abnormalities and neutrophil activation. Increased concentrations of activated complement are associated with fatal outcome in bacterial septic shock of both gram-positive and gram-negative origin.

Activation of the coagulation cascade occurs through stimulation of factor XII (Hageman factor) by microbial cell-wall components. Activated factor XII triggers both the intrinsic coagulation pathway, through activation of factor XI, and endothelial cells and macrophages to produce tissue factors that activate the extrinsic coagulation pathway. The activation of these pathways may lead to

the consumption of coagulation factors and to disseminated intravascular coagulation (DIC). TNF and IL-1 promote procoagulant activity at the endothelial surface, and PAF recruits platelets and encourages their aggregation. Several lines of investigation implicate TNF as a systemic soluble mediator that plays a central role in sepsis and septic shock.

The systemic and tissue-specific cellular mechanisms of TNF-induced pathophysiology depend on its direct effects, as well as its ability to promote the release of other soluble mediators from host cells. TNF induces IL-1 release from endothelial cells and macrophages, and then IL-1 stimulates the biosynthesis of other cytokines. IL-1 and other cytokines appear to enhance the sensitivity of tissues to the effects of TNF. Both TNF and IL-1 are potent inducers of IL-6. IL-1 and IL-6 induce some of the characteristic physiological derangements associated with injury, including fever and acute-phase protein responses. Studies in human beings show that TNF, IL-1, and IL-6 are released in the serum of patients with meningococcal septic shock, and elevated levels of IL-6 in the presence of IL-1 in these patients are most often associated with a fatal outcome. The morbidity and mortality associated with elevated levels of TNF are synergistically enhanced by even low concentrations of IL-1, so that stimulation of IL-1 biosynthesis by this cytokine serves to amplify TNF-mediated shock and tissue injury.

Clinical Presentation

The signs and symptoms of bacteremia are highly variable in children and depend on the age of the patient, the underlying disease, the duration of illness, the specific microorganism, and the host response to the infection.

Although young, immunocompetent children between the ages of 3 months and 2 years may present with fever and no focus of infection (see Sec. 13.1.5), most children of all ages will have a systemic response to bacteremia. The primary signs and symptoms of a systemic inflammatory response (SIR) include fever or hypothermia, shaking chills, hyperventilation, tachycardia, cutaneous lesions (petechiae, purpura, or both), and changes in mental status such as confusion, agitation, lethargy, obtundation, or coma. Important clinical parameters to assess in a child suspected of having bacteremia include delayed capillary refill (greater than 3 to 5 seconds), cyanosis, oliguria or anuria, or altered mental status. These, coupled with the laboratory findings of hypoxemia in the absence of pulmonary disease, acidosis, or oliguria, are definitive signs of hypoperfusion. Specific attention should be placed on accurate blood pressure measurement, as well as adequacy and characterization of peripheral pulses.

Laboratory Evaluation

The laboratory evaluation of patients suspected of having bacteremia or clinical sepsis includes blood culture, complete blood count with differential, a urinalysis and urine culture collected by suprapubic tap or sterile catheterization, and a chest roentgenogram. Depending upon the individual patient, the completion of a traditional septic work-up with lumbar puncture, to include CSF analysis with Gram stain and culture, and specific laboratory tests, including electrolytes, renal function studies, aminotransferases, prothrombin and partial thromboplastin times, and serum fibrinogen levels, should be contemplated. In patients with petechial or purpuric cutaneous manifestations of sepsis, Gram stain of scrapings of the purpuric lesions may yield the etiologic organism, increasing the positive yield of rapid diagnostic tests and confirmatory culture by up to 10% in some studies. Close examination of the peripheral blood smear may disclose evidence of splenic dysfunction (Howell-Jolly bodies) or fragmented red blood cells as seen in DIC. In patients with respiratory distress, pulse oximetry is used to evaluate oxygenation. Arterial blood gases should be obtained early as a means of evaluating acid-base status, as well as ventilatory response in patients with severe sepsis or septic shock.

Therapy

The initial selection of presumptive antibiotics for a child with bacteremia, sepsis, severe sepsis, or septic shock is based upon the clinical situation; age of the patient; underlying immunologic status; community-acquired versus nosocomial infection; secondary metastatic foci of infection; and local antibiotic resistance patterns. Monotherapy in immunocompetent children and combination therapy in immunocompromised children should be based on results of culture and susceptibility testing from cultures of sterile body fluids. Presumptive antibiotics are typically selected to cover the most serious organisms that cause bacteremia.

In the newborn, the combination of ampicillin plus gentamicin or ampicillin plus cefotaxime in standard dosages has been the mainstay of therapy. In the neonatal intensive care unit, the substitution of vancomycin for ampicillin for patients with central vascular catheters or foreign bodies (eg, ventricular shunts, cardiac patches) has been prompted by the increased incidence of coagulase-negative staphylococcal bacteremia. In the infant aged 1 to 3 months, the age-specific pathogens include those found in neonates, as well as bacterial isolates of older children. The combination of ampicillin plus cefotaxime is appropriate presumptive antibiotic coverage in these patients. In immunocompetent children over 3 months of age, third-generation cephalosporins (cefotaxime or ceftriaxone) are the standard presumptive antibiotic regimens with significant clinical success in multiple studies. With drug resistance now identified as a common problem in many areas, the use of vancomycin plus cefotaxime or ceftriaxone is standard therapy for life-threatening sepsis, sepsis with meningitis, and in patients predisposed to invasive pneumococcal sepsis.

In immunocompromised children, combination therapy using a broad-spectrum penicillin (eg, ticarcillin) monobactam, third- or fourth-generation cephalosporin (eg, ceftazidime) in combination with an aminoglycoside, is appropriate for broad-spectrum gram-negative coverage. Penicillin/β-lactamase inhibitors, carbapenems (eg, imipenem-cilastatin), or monobactams (eg, aztreonam) can prove valuable if the patient is known to harbor resistant bacteria, or if local epidemiology warrants. An intravascular catheter or other foreign material should prompt coverage for gram-positive organisms such as *Staphylococcus epidermidis, S. aureus,* or enterococci, with the addition of a semisynthetic antistaphylococcal penicillin (eg, nafcillin or oxacillin) or vancomycin where methicillin-resistant gram-positive microorganisms are found to constitute a significant percentage of confirmed infections. In patients not responding to broad-spectrum antibacterial therapy, presumptive antifungal therapy should be considered. All antibiotic or anti-infective regimens should be modified appropriately in culture-positive cases, depending on the specific organism and sensitivity testing.

Local antibiotic susceptibility patterns should always be used to select presumptive antibiotic therapy by category of patient. This is especially important in immunocompromised patients with community-acquired and nosocomial infections (patients with intravascular catheters or foreign body material). It is important to document therapeutic levels of specific antibiotics (aminoglycosides and vancomycin), especially in acutely ill patients with altered clearance and volumes of distribution that will affect antibiotic half-lives. Even before susceptibilities are known, isolation of the following bacteria in the blood culture should prompt consideration of the potential for antimicrobial resistance: penicillin- and/or cephalosporin-resistant *Streptococcus pneumoniae* (especially with concomitant meningitis); ampicillin-, gentamicin-, and/or vancomycin-resistant *Enterococcus faecium;* penicillin-resistant *Neisseria meningitidis;* and variable resistance for selected Enterobacteriaceae, as well as non-Enterobacteriaceae among gram-negative organisms.

The use of intravenous immunoglobulin (IVIG) for the prevention or treatment of sepsis remains controversial. A 1999 analysis by the Cochrane Database of Systemic Reviews concluded that there remains insufficient evidence to support routine administration of IVIG preparations investigated to date for treatment of infants with suspected or subsequently proved neonatal sepsis. However, the Cochrane Database of Systemic Reviews stated that polyclonal IVIG significantly reduces mortality among adults, despite a failure to show statistically significant results among neonates with sepsis.

Supportive management of sepsis, severe sepsis, and septic shock is directed toward restoration of adequate tissue perfusion and maintenance of efficient respiratory function. Details of fluid resuscitation and management of shock are discussed in Secs. 4.1.2 and 4.1.4.

Potential Immunotherapy

Potential immunotherapies for septic shock operate by two mechanisms: neutralization of lipopolysaccharide before it activates the cytokine cascade, and interruption of the cytokine cascade and secondary mediators of sepsis.

The outermost portion of endotoxin consists of a series of oligosaccharide side chains that are structurally and antigenically diverse and are responsible for the O serotype of gram-negative bacteria. Internal to the O side chains are core oligosaccharides, which have closely similar structures among all gram-negative bacteria, and lipid A, which is even more highly conserved. It is lipid A that is responsible for most of the toxicity of endotoxin.

In animals, antibodies against the lipid A portion of the endotoxin molecule confer protection against gram-negative infection, but results of clinical trials of polyclonal or monoclonal antibodies against endotoxin in patients with presumed sepsis or in children with meningococcal septic shock have proven disappointing. Bactericidal permeability-increasing (BPI) protein, an endogenous neutrophil protein that binds and inactivates endotoxin, is now in phase 1 clinical trials.

Gram-negative bacteria may be the most potent stimulus of septic shock, but gram-positive bacteria, viruses, and fungal pathogens are well-known inducers of TNF and IL-1 as well. A prospective, double-blind, randomized clinical trial with monoclonal antihuman TNF failed to reduce mortality in patients with sepsis. A recent study using a TNF inhibitor, a dimer of an extracellular portion of the TNF receptor, and the Fc portion of IgG, showed that mortality was increased in the treated patients. Blockade of IL-1 by administration of IL-1 receptor antagonist (IL-1ra) has also been tried in a large clinical trial, with no survival advantage seen in treated patients. Thus, anticytokine therapies have not yet altered the course of this catastrophic illness, and some level of inflammatory cytokines may well be essential to survival after infectious challenge.

Prognosis

The mortality of sepsis, severe sepsis, and septic shock depends on the initial site of infection, the presence of multiple-organ dysfunction syndrome, and the bacterial pathogen. In studies of immunocompromised children with gram-negative bacillary sepsis, the mortality may range from 40 to 60%. Otherwise normal, healthy children with proven sepsis and shock had a mortality rate of 10% (14 of 143 children). Poor prognostic signs in children include hypotension, coma, leukopenia (WBC <5000 cells/μL), thrombocytopenia (<100,000 platelets/μL), low fibrinogen level (<150 mg/dL), and evidence of multiple-organ dysfunction, including acute renal failure, adult respiratory distress syndrome, acute hepatic failure, central nervous system dysfunction, and myocardial depression. The morbidity for survivors of bacteremia, sepsis, severe sepsis, and septic shock is relatively low in children.

References

Bone RC, Fisher CJ, Clemmer TP, et al: A controlled clinical trial of high-dose methylprednisolone in the treatment of severe sepsis and septic shock. N Engl J Med 317:653–658, 1987

Darville T, Giroir BP, Jacobs RF: The systemic inflammatory response syndrome: immunology and potential immunotherapies. Infection 21:279–290, 1993

Dupont HL, Spink WW: Infections due to gram-negative organisms: an analysis of 860 patients with bacteremia at the University of Minnesota Medical Center, 1958–1966. Medicine 48:307–332, 1969

Greenman RL, Schein RMH, Martin MA, et al: A controlled clinical trial of E5 murine monoclonal IgM antibody to endotoxin in the treatment of gram-negative sepsis. JAMA 266:1097–1102, 1991

Hack CE, Nuijens HH, Felt-Bersma RJF, et al: Elevated plasma levels of the anaphylatoxins C3a and C5a are associated with a fatal outcome in sepsis. Am J Med 86:20–26, 1989

Hughes WT, Armstrong D, Bodey GP, et al: Guidelines for the use of antimicrobial agents in neutropenic patients with unexplained fever. J Infect Dis 161:381–396, 1990

Jacobs RF, Sowell MK, Moss M, et al: Septic shock in children: bacterial etiologies and temporal relationships. Pediatr Infect Dis J 9:196–200, 1990

Members of American College of Chest Physicians/Society of Critical Care Medicine Consensus Conference Committee: Definitions for sepsis and organ failure and guidelines for use of innovative therapies in sepsis. Crit Care Med 20:864–874, 1992

Tracey KJ, Lowry SF, Cerami A: Cachectin/tumor necrosis factor alpha in septic shock and septic adult respiratory distress syndrome [editorial]. Am Rev Respir Dis 138:1377–1379, 1988

Tracey KJ, Vlassara H, Cerami A: Cachectin/tumor necrosis factor. Lancet 1:1122–1126, 1989

The Veterans Administration Systemic Sepsis Cooperative Study Group: Effect of high-dose glucocorticoid therapy on mortality in patients with clinical signs of systemic sepsis. N Engl J Med 317:659–665, 1987

Waage A, Brandtzaeg P, Halstensen A, et al: The complex pattern of cytokines in serum from patients with meningococcal septic shock: association between interleukin-6, interleukin-1, and fatal outcome. J Exp Med 169:333–338, 1989

Ziegler EJ, Fisher CJ Jr, Sprung CL, et al: Treatment of gram-negative bacteremia and shock with HA-1A human monoclonal antibody against endotoxin: a randomized double-blind placebo-controlled trial. N Engl J Med 324:429–436, 1991

13.1.8   Meningitis

Jay Tureen

Meningitis, an infection of the subarachnoid space and leptomeninges caused by a variety of pathogenic organisms, continues to have a significant incidence of mortality and morbidity. *Bacterial,* or *purulent, meningitis* is the most important form in the United States in terms of incidence, sequelae, and ultimate loss of productive life. *Aseptic meningitis,* usually caused by viruses, especially enteroviruses (see Sec. 13.4.2) is more common; however, significant sequelae are rare and the disease is self-limited. *Granulomatous meningitis,* caused either by *M. tuberculosis* or fungi, is a major cause of neurologic injury and death in other parts of the world.

Meningitis is a medical emergency with urgent need for rapid diagnosis and institution of appropriate antibiotic therapy and supportive measures. One must maintain a high index of suspicion when confronted with a febrile child or one who has altered mental status, because the first few hours of care may make a critical difference in outcome.

BACTERIAL MENINGITIS

EPIDEMIOLOGY   Important aspects to consider include age, ethnicity, season, host factors, and regional patterns of antibiotic resistance among likely pathogens. The first month after birth represents the period of highest attack rate for meningitis, with likely pathogens including *S. agalactiae* (group B streptococcus), *E. coli,* other gram-negative enteric organisms, and *L. monocytogenes.* Beyond the neonatal period the most important pathogens are *S. pneumoniae* and *N. meningitidis. Haemophilus influenzae* type b (Hib) was formerly the most common pathogen causing meningitis in infants and children; however, the incidence of invasive disease has been reduced substantially by immunization with conjugate vaccines.

Bacterial meningitis is reported with increased frequency among African-Americans, Native Americans, and individuals in rural areas. Although socioeconomic factors may contribute to this increased incidence, not all investigators agree that this is the only factor.

Seasonal patterns of disease have been noted to occur, with meningitis caused by *N. meningitidis* and *S. pneumoniae* peaking in the winter months, Hib showing a biphasic distribution with peaks in the early winter and spring, and *L. monocytogenes* occurring most frequently in the summer months. The reason for these patterns may lie in the modes for acquiring the organisms, with meningococcus, pneumococcus, and *Haemophilus* spread by the respiratory route, more likely in those months with increased incidence of common respiratory diseases, and *Listeria* acquired as a result of foodborne contamination or contact with farm animals.

Host factors that predispose to infection include congenital or acquired immune deficiency states, hemoglobinopathies, asplenia, and chronic liver or renal disease. In general, individuals with these conditions show increased susceptibility to encapsulated organisms such as *S. pneumoniae. Neisseria meningitidis* occurs with increased frequency in persons with deficiencies of the terminal components of complement.

Finally, emergence of bacteria that are resistant to commonly prescribed antibiotics has changed empiric treatment of presumed bacterial meningitis. In the past decade, pneumococci with reduced sensitivity or resistance to penicillins and cephalosporins have been identified in virtually all parts of the world and, in some areas, may compromise the utility of those drugs for empiric therapy. In 1998, an average of 25% of US isolates of *S. pneumoniae* showed decreased susceptibility to penicillin. This figure varied geographically from 14 to 38%, depending on the region. The clinician must be aware of emerging patterns of resistance within the community and in the hospital setting for patients who develop illness as a secondary complication.

PATHOGENESIS Meningitis develops as a consequence of bacterial entry into the subarachnoid space either through hematogenous seeding, direct extension from a contiguous focus, or as a result of congenital, traumatic, or surgical disruption of normal anatomic barriers.

Hematogenous spread is the most common cause of infection and may occur in the setting of other foci of disease (eg, pneumonia, otitis media, cellulitis) or as a consequence of spontaneous bacteremia. For the common pathogens spread by the respiratory route, the initial event is colonization of the upper respiratory tract. The next step involves bacterial passage through or between mucosal cells to the submucosal space, with multiplication and survival. Organisms then enter the bloodstream through submucosal capillaries or lymphatic channels, and multiply because of the absence of circulating antibody and the presence of bacterial capsular polysaccharides, which permit the bacteria to resist phagocytosis. When bacteremia is present, meningeal invasion occurs in relation to the degree of bacterial density in blood, and the portal of entry to the subarachnoid space appears to be the choroid plexus. After the subarachnoid space has been invaded, bacterial growth occurs freely because of the relative paucity of defenses. The CSF contains few fixed or circulating scavenger cells to remove bacteria and has poor opsonic and bactericidal capability. The lack of an effective cellular or humoral immune response until infection is well established results in abundant bacterial multiplication, usually to the level of 10^6 to 10^7 organisms per milliliter of spinal fluid.

Nonhematogenous causes of meningitis include spread of infection from a contiguous site (otitis media, mastoiditis, sinusitis, cranial bone or vertebral osteomyelitis) and anatomic disruption (basilar skull fracture, following neurosurgical procedures, or congenital dermal sinuses along the craniospinal axis). The common feature of any cause of infection is the introduction of pathogenic bacteria into the subarachnoid space and resultant bacterial multiplication.

PATHOPHYSIOLOGY AND ETIOLOGY Many pathophysiological disturbances are present in bacterial meningitis and probably occur as a consequence of the host response to the infecting organism. These abnormalities may play a role in development of neurologic sequelae following meningitis, and an understanding of them is important to care effectively for the patient with meningitis.

After a decade of intensive study using animal models, a broad outline of the cellular and molecular basis of these pathophysiological changes has been elucidated. Once bacteria gain access to the subarachnoid space, components of the bacterial cell wall (lipopolysaccharide, lipooligosaccharide, teichoic acid) stimulate generation of proinflammatory cytokines (TNF, IL-1β, IL-6, PAF, and others). These, in turn, increase adhesion of leukocytes to cerebral vascular endothelium, promoting increased blood-brain barrier permeability and migration of leukocytes into the subarachnoid space. White blood cell– and endothelium-derived reactive oxygen species, and perhaps nitric oxide, then participate in altering cerebrovascular reactivity. This, in combination with increased intra-

cranial pressure, leads to cerebral ischemia and alterations in cerebral metabolism.

Other compounds that may cause direct cytotoxic neuronal injury include reactive oxygen and nitrogen species (oxygen radical, nitric oxide, peroxynitrite, hydroxyl radical), excitatory amino acids, caspases, and matrix metalloproteinases. Experimental studies demonstrate improved neuronal survival when specific inhibitors of these compounds are used.

Cerebral edema represents a combination of vasogenic, cytotoxic, and interstitial edema. When severe, it causes markedly increased intracranial pressure. Abnormalities of brain metabolism include hypoglycorrhachia and CSF lactic acidosis. Low CSF glucose levels occur by impaired glucose transport across the blood-brain barrier and possibly by increased cerebral glucose utilization. CSF lactic acidosis indicates anaerobic glucose utilization within the central nervous system. Cerebral perfusion is reduced in meningitis in approximately 30% of children in whom brain blood-flow studies have been performed. In addition to disordered cerebral vasoreactivity, other factors that may lead to reduced perfusion include cerebral vasculitis and arterial or venous infarcts. Increased intracranial pressure is nearly uniformly present in meningitis and not only contributes to reduced cerebral perfusion pressure but may also cause cerebral herniation. Pathogenesis of increased intracranial pressure is multifactorial and includes contributions from brain edema, increased CSF volume, and abnormalities of cerebral blood flow. The blood-brain barrier, comprising the choroid plexus, cerebral microvasculature, and arachnoid membrane, shows increased permeability in meningitis.

Although many patients with meningitis have good neurologic outcome with standard supportive measures and antibiotics, patients with more profound central nervous system disturbance require more intensive treatment. In that situation one must recognize the potential pathophysiological disturbances and employ adjunctive therapeutic modalities (eg, to reduce intracranial pressure) in conjunction with supportive care and antimicrobial therapy.

PATHOLOGY Pathologic changes in meningitis reflect the inflammatory mass in the subarachnoid space, cerebral vasculitis, cerebral edema, and cellular injury. The inflammatory mass usually begins in the basilar cisterns, spreads around the cerebellum, and then over the cerebral convexities. Those cranial nerves that traverse the subarachnoid space are particularly prone to injury in meningitis, perhaps due to the surrounding inflammation. Vasculitis of both arteries and veins occurs, particularly in meningitis caused by *S. pneumoniae*, resulting in tissue ischemia and arterial and venous infarcts. Direct cellular injury, whether a consequence of bacterial toxins, host factors, or ischemia, is frequently noted in postmortem studies. The etiologic agents responsible for meningitis are highly age-specific (Table 13-22).

CLINICAL MANIFESTATIONS The classic triad of symptoms in meningitis includes fever, headache, and stiff neck. However, in children under 2 years of age, stiff neck or other signs of meningeal irritation may be absent. Alteration of level of consciousness is usual, occurring in up to 90% of patients. The majority present with irritability, lethargy, or confusion; however, 10 to 15% present in coma, a very poor prognostic sign. Physical examination may reveal signs of meningeal irritation—stiff neck and positive Kernig and Brudzinski signs. Infants may have a bulging fontanelle. Cranial nerve abnormalities, particularly of the sixth cranial nerve, may be

TABLE 13-22

ETIOLOGY OF BACTERIAL MENINGITIS BY AGE GROUP

AGE GROUP		% OF CASES
Neonates		
	Group B streptococcus	60
	E. coli, other gram-negative enterics	30
	Listeria monocytogenes	2
	Other	8
Toddlers (1–23 mo)		
	S. pneumoniae	41
	N. meningitidis	32
	H. influenzae type b and others	5
	Other	22
Children >2yr		
	N. meningitidis	54
	S. pneumoniae	26
	Other	20

the consequence of increased intracranial pressure or of inflammation in the subarachnoid space. Focal neurologic abnormalities are uncommon early in the disease, but when present may be indicators of infarct.

Systemic signs may also be present in meningitis. The most common occur in the setting of meningococcal disease. Initially the rash in meningococcal disease is a transient erythematous, macular eruption, which presages the appearance of petechiae, ecchymoses, and purpura. When present, petechiae or ecchymoses should raise suspicion of overwhelming meningococcal sepsis, in which approximately 50% of patients will have concurrent meningitis. With this disease, and with meningitis due to gram-negative enteric organisms, hypotension, when present, is usually due to the systemic effects of endotoxin. Most other causes of meningitis—those due to *S. pneumoniae*, *H. influenzae*, and *Listeria*—are usually not accompanied by endotoxic shock. Hypotension in the setting of disease caused by these other organisms is most commonly the result of volume depletion.

DIAGNOSIS Once the diagnosis of meningitis is suspected, immediate examination of the CSF is indicated. A specific reason to

delay lumbar puncture is if there is a strong suspicion of an intracranial mass lesion. Worrisome findings include papilledema or a history of an indolent process with focal neurologic findings. In those instances, lumbar puncture can be delayed until a mass can be excluded by cranial CT or MRI scanning. CSF abnormalities include more than 6 WBCs/μL, elevated protein concentration, hypoglycorrhachia, elevated opening pressure, and organisms on Gram stain. The range of these abnormalities for different types of meningitis is shown in Table 13-23.

Pleocytosis is the rule in bacterial meningitis, with CSF WBC counts in the range of 100 to 10,000 cells/μL, although early in the disease, the WBC count may be normal. Polymorphonuclear cells predominate and usually account for more than 90% of the total. Very high WBC counts (greater than 50,000/μL) raises the possibility of an intracranial abscess that has ruptured into the ventricle.

Hypoglycorrhachia is commonly found in bacterial meningitis, with CSF glucose usually less than 50% of simultaneous serum glucose. Other causes of hypoglycorrhachia include tuberculous and fungal meningitis, subarachnoid hemorrhage, and carcinomatous meningitis.

Cerebrospinal fluid protein concentration is usually elevated, in the range of 100 to 500 mg/dL, but as elevated protein reflects an alteration in the blood-brain barrier, it is not, by itself, diagnostic of bacterial infection. Protein concentration may be significantly elevated in patients with meningitis caused by *M. tuberculosis*.

The Gram stain is positive in more than 90% of patients with untreated meningitis; however, it must be interpreted by an experienced microbiologist, as errors in interpretation are common. Pneumococci, when overdecolorized, may resemble meningococci, *Haemophilus* may be thought to be gram-negative enteric organisms or vice-versa, and debris may resemble gram-positive cocci. *Listeria* are frequently difficult to identify on direct smear.

Culture is positive in 70 to 90% of patients with untreated meningitis, but prior treatment with oral antibiotics substantially reduces this yield. In this setting, the use of antigen-detection methods such as latex particle agglutination may help in etiologic identification. These methods, when performed in the first 48 to 72 hours after oral antibiotics are given, will identify the pathogen in approximately 90% of patients.

In addition to culture and Gram stain of CSF, blood culture may also be useful in specific etiologic diagnosis. Blood cultures are

TABLE 13-23

CSF FINDINGS IN VARIOUS TYPES OF MENINGITIS

	PYOGENIC	PARTIALLY TREATED	GRANULOMATOUS	ASEPTIC	PARAMENINGEAL FOCUS[a]
Cells/mm³	200–5000	200–5000	100–500	100–700	100–500
Cytology	PMN	Mostly PMN	L	PMN → L	Variable
Glucose[b]	Low	Low	Low	Normal	Normal
Protein	High	High	High	Slightly high	Variable
Gram stain	Positive	?Positive	Negative	Negative	Negative
Culture	Positive	?Negative	Positive	Negative	Negative
CIE or LA	Positive	Positive	Negative	Negative	Variable
Lactic acid	High	High	High	Normal	Variable
Pressure	High	High	High	Normal	Variable

[a] Parameningeal focus refers to a localized focus of infection near the subarachnoid space that may spill some products of inflammation into the CSF. Such a site could be a brain abscess, an epidural abscess, sinusitis, or mastoiditis.

[b] CSF glucose concentration should be considered in relation to blood glucose concentration; normally CSF glucose is 50 to 70% of blood glucose.

PMN = polymorphonuclear neutrophil; L = lymphocyte; CIE = counterimmunoelectrophoresis; LA = latex agglutination.

positive in 40 to 75% of instances of bacterial meningitis, depending on the pathogen, and should be performed routinely.

In addition to studies aimed at making an etiologic diagnosis, other laboratory studies are indicated as well. Peripheral-blood WBC and differential are useful in assessing the likelihood of a serious bacterial infection, and leukopenia may be a poor prognostic sign, particularly in the settings of meningococcal and pneumococcal disease. Similarly, prolonged blood coagulation studies in conjunction with thrombocytopenia may indicate DIC, which is often present with serious gram-negative infection. Serum and urine electrolytes and osmolality should be measured routinely to look for the syndrome of inappropriate antidiuretic hormone secretion (SIADH), marked by hyponatremia in association with increased urine osmolality and increased urine concentration of sodium. Additional studies, such as roentgenographic examinations, are rarely needed in the diagnosis of meningitis; however, they may be useful in identifying coexisting complicating factors. Cranial CT may indicate cerebral edema early in the infection, and later may show subdural effusion or empyema.

TREATMENT Effective treatment of meningitis depends on early aggressive supportive therapy and selection of empiric antimicrobials appropriate for the likely pathogens. General supportive measures address the consequences of serious intracranial pathology. Patients who are comatose or who have impaired gag reflex should have their stomach contents emptied and should be considered for intubation to protect the airway. Hypoxia should be treated with supplemental oxygen. Hypoventilation is particularly worrisome in these patients because elevated PA_{CO_2} may cause cerebral vasodilatation and potentiate increased intracranial pressure. Hypercarbia should be considered as another indication for intubation and assisted ventilation.

Fluid management is critically important in patients with meningitis. SIADH occurs in approximately 30% of patients with bacterial meningitis, and warrants fluid restriction. However, a clinical study has documented the importance of maintaining an adequate cerebral perfusion pressure in this disease. Inappropriate fluid restriction may result in volume depletion, leading to inadequate circulating volume if carried to extremes. If SIADH is present, fluids should be limited to replacement of insensible losses plus urine output (generally around two-thirds of maintenance requirement) until ADH excess resolves; if SIADH is not present, fluids should be administered in an amount appropriate to maintenance requirements, and electrolytes should be carefully monitored.

Therapy of increased intracranial pressure must be directed at maintaining an adequate degree of cerebral perfusion pressure as in other conditions complicated by intracranial hypertension. Available modalities may include hyperventilation, withdrawal of CSF through an intraventricular catheter, or possibly the careful use of osmotic diuretic agents.

In suspected meningitis, antibiotics are routinely administered empirically while cultures are pending. The initial choice of antibiotics is based on the likely pathogens for age group, known exposures, and any unusual risk factors for the patient. The principles of antimicrobial therapy of meningitis include selection of an antibiotic that is bactericidal against the suspected pathogen and that achieves a concentration in CSF at least 10 times the minimal bactericidal concentration for the organism, as this is the concentration that has been shown in animal studies to correlate with most effective sterilization of CSF. Suggested choices for empiric therapy are listed in Table 13-24.

TABLE 13-24

EMPIRIC TREATMENT OF BACTERIAL MENINGITIS BASED ON AGE

Neonates <8 days
  Ampicillin (100 mg/kg/day div q12h)
    plus
  Aminoglycoside (5.0 mg/kg/day div q12h)
    or
  Ampicillin plus cefotaxime (100 mg/kg/day div q12h)
Neonates >7 days
  Ampicillin (150 mg/kg/day div q8h)
    plus
  Aminoglycoside (7.5mg/kg/day div q8h)
    or
  Ampicillin plus cefotaxime (150 mg/kg/day div q8h)
Infants 1–3 mo
  Ampicillin (300 mg/kg/day div q6h)
    plus
  Cefotaxime (200 mg/kg/day div q6h) or ceftriaxone (100 mg/kg/day div q12h)
    plus
  Vancomycin (60 mg/kg/day div q6h) **if** *S. pneumoniae* suspected based on positive Gram stain or positive latex agglutination. Therapy should be modified based on susceptibility data.
Infants >3 mo
  Cefotaxime (200 mg/kg/day div q6h) or ceftriaxone (100 mg/kg/day div q12h)
    plus
  Vancomycin (60 mg/kg/day div q6h) **if** *S. pneumoniae* suspected based on positive Gram stain or positive latex agglutination. Therapy should be modified based on susceptibility data.
Children >6 yr
  Penicillin G (300,000 units/kg/day div q4h) or cefotaxime or ceftriaxone at above doses
    plus
  Vancomycin (60 mg/kg/day div q6h) **if** *S. pneumoniae* suspected based on positive Gram stain or positive latex agglutination. Therapy should be modified based on susceptibility data.

Therapy should be appropriately narrowed when sensitivity data are available. In addition to antibiotic therapy, clinical studies have shown some improvement in neurologic outcome following the early institution of corticosteroid therapy, particularly in children with *H. influenzae* type b meningitis. Dexamethasone, 0.15 mg/kg per dose, is administered concurrently with the start of antibiotic treatment, and continued every 6 hours for 4 days. Duration of antibiotic therapy is 14 to 21 days for neonatal meningitis caused by group B streptococci, and a minimum of 21 days for gram-negative enteric organism. For meningitis in older infants or children, treatment should be 7 days for *N. meningitidis*, 7 to 10 days for *H. influenzae* type b, and 10 to 14 days for *S. pneumoniae*.

OUTCOME Mortality rates in bacterial meningitis vary considerably depending on the age of the patient and the pathogen. Individuals with meningococcal meningitis without overwhelming meningococcemia have a fatality rate of 12%, whereas newborns with gram-negative meningitis succumb 70% of the time. Death rates from *H. influenzae* type b and *S. pneumoniae* are approximately 3% and 6%, respectively.

Morbid sequelae occur in approximately 30% of survivors, but there is also an age and pathogen predilection, with the greatest incidence of sequelae occurring among the very young and in those infected with either gram-negative bacteria or *S. pneumoniae*.

The most common neurologic sequelae include deafness in 3 to 25% of patients, cranial nerve palsies in 2 to 7%, and severe injury, such as hemiparesis or global brain injury, in 1 to 2% of patients. More than 50% of patients with neurologic sequelae at discharge from hospital will improve with time, and recent advances in cochlear implant therapy may provide hope for the child with hearing loss.

PREVENTION   Prevention of meningitis currently takes two forms: chemoprophylaxis of susceptible individuals known to be exposed to an index patient and active immunization. Chemoprophylaxis is currently indicated for preventing secondary meningitis due to *H. influenzae* type b and *N. meningitidis* (see Secs. 13.2.15 and 13.2.23).

Active immunization against *H. influenzae* has resulted in a dramatic reduction in invasive disease, with a >95% reduction in meningitis caused by that organism. Immunization is currently recommended for infants as a three-dose series at 2, 4, and 6 months of age. Conjugate vaccines for immunization against invasive *S. pneumoniae* have shown great promise in clinical trials. They are immunogenic against the strains that cause more than 80% of cases of invasive pneumococcal disease and showed significant reduction in cases of invasive disease in a large clinical trial.

References

Kaplan S, Feigin R: The syndrome of inappropriate secretion of antidiuretic hormone in children with bacterial meningitis. J Pediatr 92:758–761, 1978

Klein JO, Feigin RD, McCracken GHJ: Report of the Task Force on Diagnosis and Management of Meningitis. Pediatrics 78:959–982, 1986

Lebel MH, Freij BJ, Syrogiannopoulos GA, et al: Dexamethasone therapy for bacterial meningitis: results of two double-blind, placebo-controlled trials. N Engl J Med 319:964–971, 1988

Peltola H, Kilpi T, Anttila M: Rapid disappearance of *Haemophilus influenzae* type b meningitis after routine childhood immunization with conjugate vaccines. Lancet 340:592–594, 1992

Pomeroy SL, Holmes SJ, Dodge PR, Feigin RD: Seizures and other neurologic sequelae of bacterial meningitis in children. N Engl J Med 323:1651–1657, 1990

Powell K, Sugarman L, Eskenazi A, et al: Normalization of plasma arginine vasopressin concentrations when children with meningitis are given maintenance plus replacement fluid therapy. J Pediatr 117:515–522, 1990

Quagliarello V, Scheld WM: Bacterial meningitis: pathogenesis, pathophysiology, and progress. N Engl J Med 327:864–872, 1992

Quagliarello VJ, Scheld WM: Treatment of bacterial meningitis. N Engl J Med 336:708–716, 1997

Rennick G, Shann F, deCampo J: Cerebral herniation during bacterial meningitis in children. BMJ 306:953–955, 1993

Saez-Llorens X, Ramilo O, Mustafa M, Mertsola J, McCracken GH Jr: Molecular pathophysiology of bacterial meningitis: current concepts and therapeutic implications. J Pediatr 116:671–684, 1990

13.1.9   Infections of Bones, Joints, and Soft Tissues

Robin B. Churchill

Bone and joint infections may occur at any age but are most common in children, where they continue to present a diagnostic and management challenge. Early diagnosis and aggressive initial treatment, the key to successful treatment and prevention of compli-

cations, requires a multidisciplinary approach that includes the pediatrician, an orthopedic surgeon experienced in the treatment of children, and frequently, an infectious disease consultant. Although disabling sequelae still occur in some cases, most children diagnosed early in the course of illness recover completely with proper management. Soft tissue infections in children, generally less difficult to diagnose and treat than skeletal infections, remain important because of their greater frequency of occurrence and the need for antibiotic therapy, occasionally in conjunction with hospitalization.

OSTEOMYELITIS

Acute Hematogenous Osteomyelitis

EPIDEMIOLOGY   Acute hematogenous osteomyelitis (AHO) is more common in young children and males. Around 50% of cases occur before 6 years of age; males are affected twice as often as females. There is often a history of some type of minor blunt trauma or intercurrent illness, such as an upper respiratory tract infection.

PATHOGENESIS   The majority of bone infections in children are of hematogenous origin. Less commonly, bony infection occurs following penetrating trauma or surgery, or by extension of an adjacent infectious process. Impaired host defense also increases the risk of skeletal infections.

The vascular anatomy of long bones in children underlies the predilection for localization of bloodborne bacteria. In children, unlike adults and young infants, the blood supply of the epiphysis is separate from the metaphysis. The nutrient artery to the metaphysis empties into a system of venous sinusoids in which sluggish flow facilitates deposition of bacteria. Infection originates on the venous side of the system and spreads to the nutrient artery, which then becomes thrombosed. The resultant ischemia prevents host defenses from reaching the area and encourages bacterial proliferation. This series of events is described as the "cellulitic phase" of acute osteomyelitis. Formation of an abscess can then occur, followed by rupture into the subperiosteal space and subsequent elevation of the periosteum, which is more loosely adherent in children than in adults. If infection is uncontrolled, purulent material may extend up and down the diaphysis and circumferentially around the bone. In areas in which the metaphysis is intraarticular, such as the hip and shoulder, the intraosseous abscess may rupture into the joint resulting in septic arthritis. In newborns and young infants, blood vessels connect the metaphysis and epiphysis, and rupture of pus into the adjacent joint space is not only more common but more likely to give rise to permanent disability.

Thrombosis of blood vessels and elevation of the periosteum deprive the bone of its blood supply, resulting in necrosis. As a result of the inflammatory process, granulation tissue forms around the dead bone, which separates from live bone and becomes a *sequestrum*. New bone growing around the dead bone is called an *involucrum*. Sinus tract formation occurs in the involucrum allowing pus to escape and eventually form sinus tracts through the skin. The involucrum is mechanically weak and may become the site of pathologic fractures.

CLINICAL MANIFESTATIONS AND DIFFERENTIAL DIAGNOSIS
Early signs of skeletal infection may be subtle, especially in the neonate who typically does not appear ill. The earliest sign of osteomyelitis in infants is failure to move the affected extremity (pseudoparalysis), pain on passive movement, or both. Older children frequently present with fever, pain at the site of infection in the

metaphysis, and refusal to use the affected extremity. Nonspecific constitutional symptoms such as nausea, vomiting, anorexia, and headache can occur, but are not prominent. There is intense tenderness over the metaphysis of the bone on palpation, and muscles of the adjacent joint are frequently in spasm. The joint is held in a position of comfort, usually mild flexion, but to a lesser degree than with septic arthritis. Soft tissue changes of swelling, erythema, and heat are generally late findings in osteomyelitis. After several days, a sympathetic sterile effusion may occasionally form in a nearby joint, presenting a problem in differentiation from septic arthritis.

Long bones are most often involved in acute hematogenous osteomyelitis in children. The most common sites of involvement are the lower femoral and upper tibial metaphyses. Next in frequency are the proximal femoral metaphysis and distal metaphyses of the radius and humerus. Long tubular bones are involved nearly 10 times as often as cuboidal bones of the wrist or ankle (5% of cases), the irregular bones of the ischium and pubis (3%), and the flat bones such as ribs, skull, sternum, or scapulae (2%).

The differential diagnosis of osteomyelitis includes cellulitis, septic arthritis, pyomyositis, malignancy, collagen vascular disease, and trauma. In differentiating cellulitis from bone infection, tenderness disproportionate to physical findings suggests osteomyelitis. Septic arthritis may be differentiated from osteomyelitis by its more discrete joint findings and its greater degree of joint immobility, in addition to a lack of metaphyseal tenderness. History, clinical scenario, and radiologic studies are helpful in differentiating skeletal infection from other diagnoses. Recovery of the causative organism is best obtained by biopsy or aspiration, which not only establishes the diagnosis, but also facilitates susceptibility testing and rules out other processes.

The predominant organism in acute hematogenous osteomyelitis in all age groups is *Staphylococcus aureus* followed by *Streptococcus pyogenes*. Table 13-25 summarizes the organisms cultured from blood or bone from 742 patients with acute hematogenous osteomyelitis in four case series. The incidence of oteomyelitis due to *Haemophilus influenzae* type b has fallen considerably in recent years because of the impact of an effective vaccine. Recent reports suggest that *Streptococcus pneumoniae* is becoming a more frequent cause of skeletal infections in children under 3 years of age. Group B streptococcus and gram-negative enteric bacteria occur almost exclusively in neonates in whom multiple foci may be affected. *Pseudomonas* infections usually occur as a result of puncture wounds to the feet. Anaerobic infections can result after puncture wounds or open fractures.

TABLE 13-25

FREQUENCY OF ORGANISMS CAUSING ACUTE OSTEOMYELITIS IN INFANTS AND CHILDREN (n = 742)

ORGANISM	PERCENTAGE OF PATIENTS
Staphylococcus aureus	44
Streptococcus pyogenes	7
Haemophilus influenzae	6
Coagulase-negative staphylococci	3
Pseudomonas	3
Streptococcus pneumoniae	2
Group B streptococcus	1
Unknown/other	34

SPECIAL CLINICAL SITUATIONS

Neonatal Osteomyelitis Diagnosis of osteomyelitis in an infant who is less than 1 month of age requires a high index of suspicion. Young infants with bone infections often lack fever and other systemic signs of illness. Symptoms may be limited to failure to move an extremity and fussiness. Predisposing factors include prematurity, preceding infection, bacteremia, exchange transfusions, and the presence of intravascular catheters. *S. aureus,* group B streptococcus, and enteric gram-negative bacteria are the most common etiologic agents. Candida must also be considered, especially in the premature infant who has had previous antibiotic therapy and placement of intravascular catheters. Neonates are more likely to have multifocal disease and decompression of pus into the adjacent joint resulting in an associated septic arthritis.

Pelvic Osteomyelitis Pelvic osteomyelitis often presents a diagnostic dilemma. Most patients present with fever, refusal to bear weight or limp, and pain that seems to be localized to the hip, groin, or buttock. Initial diagnostic impressions often include intra-abdominal pathology, other intrapelvic problems, and septic arthritis of the hip joint. In these cases, imaging studies, such as bone scans, MRI, or CT, may be particularly helpful in establishing the diagnosis.

Osteomyelitis in the Child with Sickle Cell Anemia Aseptic bone infarcts are common in children with sickle cell disease. The signs, symptoms and radiographic changes mimic those of acute osteomyelitis, making differentiation between the diagnoses difficult. Neither bone scan nor MRI reliably discriminates between the two conditions. Ultrasonography has been reported as a method assisting in differentiation between infarction and infection. Diagnostic aspiration of the site should be done in an attempt to recover the organism and confirm the diagnosis. *Salmonella* species are the most frequent cause of bone infection in the sickle cell patient followed by *S. aureus*. Aggressive surgery and prolonged parenteral therapy may be necessary for treatment of osteomyelitis in the child with sickle cell disease.

Nonhematogenous Osteomyelitis

There are a myriad of factors that can predispose to the development of nonhematogenous osteomyelitis, including, but not limited to, open fractures, decubitus or neuropathic ulcers, sinusitis, mastoiditis, dental infections, bites, and puncture wounds. These infections are frequently polymicrobial with the concomitant isolation of aerobes and anaerobes. Cultures from an associated wound or sinus tract do not predict the etiology of bone infection in most cases. In patients with osteomyelitis secondary to trauma or infected contiguous soft tissue, it is imperative to base antimicrobial therapy on results of bone cultures, not on cultures of wounds or draining sinus tracts.

Puncture wounds of the foot through sneakers or certain other types of shoes may lead to *Pseudomonas* osteochondritis. If a child did not receive prophylactic antibiotic therapy at the time of the injury, gram-positive organisms may also contribute to the infection.

DIAGNOSIS Early diagnosis and prompt, effective treatment are the most significant factors ensuring a good response to therapy and prevention of complications. The definitive diagnostic method in osteomyelitis is recovery of a pathogenic organism from the bone

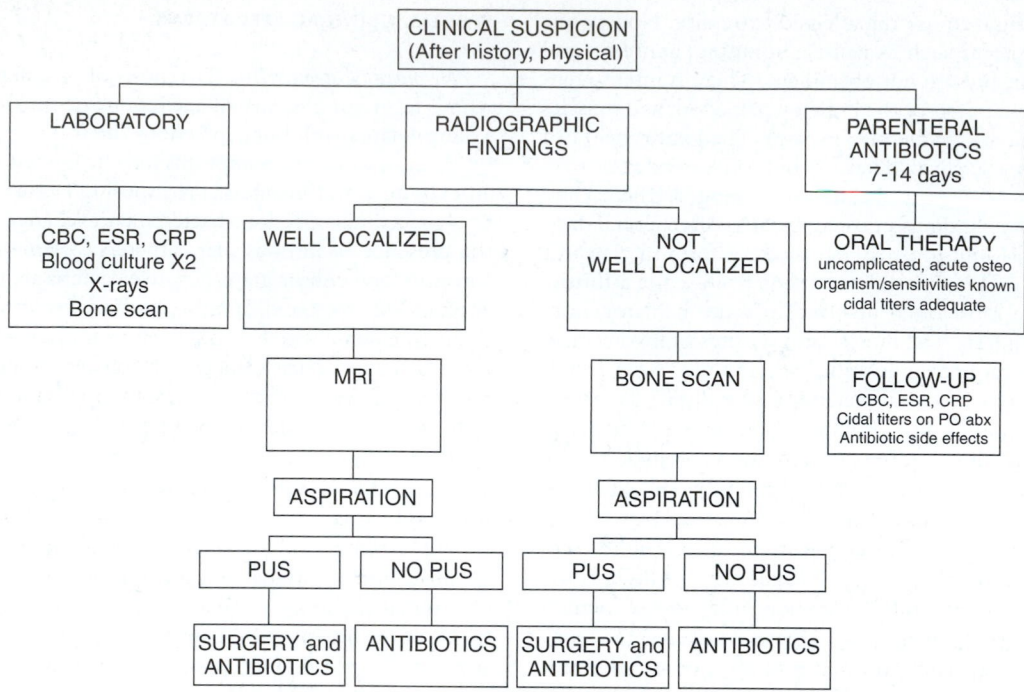

FIGURE 13-2 An algorithmic approach to the management of a patient with suspected acute hematogenous osteomyelitis. **SOURCE:** *Portions of this figure have been adapted from the Journal of the American Academy of Orthopedic Surgeons, Volume 3(4), pp. 183–193, 1995, with permission.* **CBC = complete blood count; ESR = erythrocyte sedimentation rate; CRP = C-reactive protein.**

by needle aspiration or biopsy. Aspiration of the affected bone provides material for culture, guides antibiotic therapy, and if pus is present, determines that surgical drainage will be needed. Other supporting laboratory or radiologic studies may be necessary to confirm the need for bone aspiration and, at times, to localize the area to be aspirated. Figure 13-2 outlines an approach to the diagnosis and management of a patient with suspected acute hematogenous osteomyelitis.

No specific laboratory test for the diagnosis of osteomyelitis exists, with the exception of isolation of a pathogen from the bone. Bone cultures are positive in 38 to 86% of cases and confirm the diagnosis. Blood cultures are useful, demonstrating the organism in 30 to 76% of cases. The highest diagnostic yield occurs when multiple specimens are cultured. The ability to recover an organism from blood or bone cultures decreases with prior antimicrobial therapy. Therefore, if the patient is stable and blood and bone cultures are done in a timely fashion, it is preferable to delay the initiation of antibiotics until cultures are obtained.

Other laboratory studies may be helpful but are nonspecific. Peripheral white blood count (WBC) and differential may or may not be abnormal. The erythrocyte sedimentation rate (ESR) rises slowly and initially may be normal or minimally elevated. ESR usually peaks 3 to 5 days after the initiation of therapy and returns to normal in 3 to 4 weeks. Many experts find C-reactive protein (CRP) to be a more responsive measure of the efficacy of therapy, because it rises earlier, peaks within 48 hours of onset of symptoms, and returns to normal after approximately 1 week of efficacious therapy.

Radiologic Studies

Plain Radiographs Plain films begin to show destructive changes approximately 10 to 14 days after the onset of bone infection. They may be helpful acutely in demonstrating changes in the deep soft tissue adjacent to the affected bone. To detect alterations of the soft tissue, identical views of the contralateral limb are recommended.

Radionuclide Scanning Radiophosphate bone scintigraphy using technetium (^{99}Tc) is the most commonly used test. Isotope accumulates to a greater degree in areas of increased vascularity and rapid bone turnover, resulting in a *hot spot* reflected on the scan. Conversely, infected areas may have associated compromise of the vascular supply, causing the area to appear *cold* or normal, resulting in a false-negative interpretation. Although bone scans have a high degree of sensitivity and specificity, they do not make the diagnosis of skeletal infection. Bone scans indicate abnormal areas of bone without revealing whether the abnormality is due to infection, tumor, or injury. Bone scans are not required in the diagnostic workup of every child with presumed bone infection. If the site of infection is easily localized by physical examination, a bone scan is not necessary prior to aspiration. It has been shown experimentally that aspiration of bone or joint does not compromise results of subsequent bone scans. Bone scans are particularly helpful in cases where the site of infection is not readily apparent by physical examination or when multiple sites of involvement are suspected.

Gallium scans or indium-labeled leukocyte scans are less commonly used techniques in the diagnosis of skeletal infection. Indium-labeled leukocyte scans, which reflect migration of white blood cells into areas of inflammation, are useful in diagnosis of osteomyelitis associated with trauma, recent surgery, or prosthetic devices.

Magnetic Resonance Imaging MRI is an effective modality for imaging bone and is quite sensitive and specific in diagnosis of musculoskeletal infections. It is not useful as a screening study, but can be considered when there is an indication where the pathology is localized either from physical examination or radionuclide scanning. It can be especially helpful in cases in which the spine or the pelvis is the site of infection, conflicting clinical data exists, or in planning surgical intervention.

THERAPY

Surgical Therapy The need for surgery in osteomyelitis depends on the extent of the pathologic process in individual patients. In children who present early in the "cellulitic phase," antibiotic therapy alone is likely to be sufficient. If pus is encountered during diagnostic aspiration, if a subperiosteal or intramedullary abscess is detected by ultrasound or MRI, or if a bone lesion is evident on plain films, surgical intervention is warranted. Surgical drainage and débridement remove inflammatory products more rapidly than do host defense mechanisms, providing a more effective environment for antibiotic penetration and preventing further bone necrosis. Drainage of an abscess reduces the inoculum of bacteria present, and débridement of necrotic and avascular bone eliminates areas prone to poor penetration where bacteria can persist. It is well accepted that *Pseudomonas* osteochondritis is mainly a surgical disease. When thorough curettage and débridement is achieved, 7 to 10 days of antipseudomonal therapy is usually sufficient.

Medical Therapy Initial antibiotic therapy for osteomyelitis should be based on Gram-stained specimens obtained from bone aspiration when possible. The importance of obtaining the exact bacteriologic diagnosis by blood or bone culture cannot be over-emphasized. In the absence of such data, initial therapy is empiric and must be directed at likely pathogens based on age of child and considering underlying medical conditions.

In the neonate, staphylococci and group B streptococci are the major pathogens, but coverage for enteric gram-negatives must be included. An appropriate initial therapeutic regimen includes an antistaphylococcal β-lactam plus an aminoglycoside. A third-generation cephalosporin, such as cefotaxime, is a suitable alternative to an aminoglycoside for gram-negative coverage.

Before the era of widespread use of the conjugate *H. influenzae* type b (Hib) vaccine, initial antibiotic therapy for children less than 5 years of age included coverage for gram-positive cocci, as well as *H. influenzae*. In areas of the world where Hib immunization is standard, it is reasonable to use coverage against *S. aureus, S. pyogenes,* and *S. pneumoniae* alone in the fully immunized, non-immunocompromised child. In the nonimmunized or immuno-compromised child who may still be at risk for Hib disease, the addition of a third-generation cephalosporin to an antistaphylo-coccal/streptococcal agent or the use of cefuroxime alone could be considered.

In otherwise healthy children older than 5 years of age, osteo-myelitis is nearly always caused by gram-positive cocci, so empiric initial therapy with an antistaphylococcal drug alone is used. In immunocompromised children or those with underlying medical conditions, broader-spectrum coverage may be appropriate.

There are several options for delivery of antibiotic therapy in the treatment of osteomyelitis. The entire course of therapy may be delivered parenterally through a central venous catheter, a periph-erally inserted central catheter (PICC), or a flexible, silastic, pe-ripheral intravenous line. Another common option is to initiate therapy parenterally, followed by orally administered drugs after the clinical condition has stabilized and any necessary surgical proce-dures have been done. Oral therapy usually is initiated after 5 to 14 days of parenteral therapy, and is equally efficacious when the responsible organism and its susceptibilities are defined. The se-

lected option depends on a patient's particular situation considering factors such as location, extent, and severity of disease, as well as the patient's ability to tolerate oral therapy and the likelihood of compliance. It is important to recognize that exact length of par-enteral or parenteral-oral therapy is dependent on a patient's re-sponse and may need to be extended in severe disease or in the immunocompromised patient.

If sequential parenteral/oral therapy is implemented, the oral drug chosen should be active against the identified pathogen, or if the pathogen has not been isolated, it should be identical in spec-trum of activity to the parenteral drug to which the patient has shown clinical response. Contraindications to oral therapy include the inability to swallow or retain medication, lack of an effective oral agent, and failure to demonstrate adequate clinical response to parenteral antibiotics. Some experts also feel that failure to dem-onstrate the etiologic agent and an inability to monitor the degree of drug absorption also constitute contraindications to oral therapy. Especially in young children, palatability of oral suspensions is an important feature. In general, cephalosporins are more palatable than penicillins. Clindamycin is an excellent drug for staphylococcal osteomyelitis in older children, but most young children will not tolerate the taste of the oral solution.

Dosages of oral antibiotics required in sequential intravenous-oral regimens are two to three times those used for minor infec-tions. It is desirable to monitor absorption of oral antibiotics and compliance by measurement of serum bactericidal levels against the isolated organism or measurement of antibiotic serum levels.

The minimum or optimum duration of antimicrobial therapy for acute osteomyelitis is unknown. The usual recommended du-ration for infections caused by *S. aureus* and gram-negative bacilli is 4 to 8 weeks. However, each patient must be evaluated individ-ually, taking into account the speed of clinical response, whether surgical débridement was done, normalization of CRP or ESR, and radiologic findings.

COMPLICATIONS AND PROGNOSIS The most common compli-cation in acute hematogenous osteomyelitis is chronic or recurrent osteomyelitis, which occurs in fewer than 5% of cases. Development of chronic osteomyelitis is more common following nonhemato-genous osteomyelitis. Pathologic fractures can occur but are rare. If the bone growth plate is involved, there is a risk of abnormal length of affected bone. In general, the outcome of well-managed cases of acute osteomyelitis in pediatric patients is favorable.

SEPTIC ARTHRITIS

EPIDEMIOLOGY Septic arthritis is most frequent in children under 3 years of age. In most cases, a single, large joint is involved. As with osteomyelitis, males are affected more frequently. There may be a history of trauma, or recent infection of the skin or upper respiratory tract. Underlying medical conditions such as immuno-deficiencies and hemoglobinopathies are predisposing factors.

PATHOGENESIS The anatomy of the synovial joint likely plays a role in its predisposition to infection. Lacking a basement mem-brane, synovial tissue lining the joint secretes a transudate of serum. The rest of the joint surface is composed of avascular cartilage. These components provide an environment that under certain cir-cumstances are conducive to bacterial proliferation. Bacteria enter the joint by hematogenous seeding, direct extension from an ad-jacent focus, or direct inoculation during a joint aspiration, arthrotomy, or trauma. Initially, after bacterial invasion occurs, the synovial membrane swells and produces increased amounts of fluid, distending the joint. If infection persists without treatment, pus accumulates in the area and destruction of cartilage follows. Subluxation or dislocation of the joint with increased intra-articular pressure occurs when the joint capsule is distended by purulent fluid. This increased pressure may compromise blood supply in certain areas. In the hip, this may lead to avascular necrosis of the femoral head.

CLINICAL MANIFESTATIONS   Children generally present acutely with a painful, erythematous, warm joint, and refusal to move or bear weight on the affected extremity. Fever, toxicity, and irritability are often accompanying features. The joint is held in the position of most comfort, usually mild flexion. When the hip is involved, joint swelling is generally not obvious, but the affected hip is held in a position of flexion, abduction, and external rotation. Young children may exhibit the phenomenon of "referred pain," in which symptoms from an infected hip joint are referred to the ipsilateral knee. Failure to recognize this presentation increases the risk of complications.

ETIOLOGIC AGENTS   As in osteomyelitis, etiologic agents of septic arthritis vary by age. *S. aureus* is the leading organism in all age groups. In neonates, group B streptococcus and enteric gram-negative organisms are also important to consider and may be isolated from an affected joint as a consequence of an adjacent osteomyelitis. *Staphylococcus aureus, S. pyogenes,* and *S. pneumoniae* are the most common pathogens in children less than 5 years of age. *Haemophilus influenzae* type b, the most common organism in this age group in the past, is no longer a prominent agent in septic arthritis. In children older than 5 years, *S. aureus* and *S. pyogenes* are the main pathogens.

Other organisms reported to cause septic arthritis in children include *Neisseria meningitidis, Kingella kingae, P. aeruginosa,* and enteric gram-negative organisms. *Neisseria gonorrhoeae* is a consideration in neonates and sexually active adolescents. *Salmonella* species are frequently isolated in patients with sickle cell disease.

DIAGNOSIS

Joint Aspiration   Because of the risk of long-term orthopedic complications, septic arthritis is an orthopedic emergency. Joint aspiration is the most important component of the diagnostic evaluation. Patients in whom the diagnosis is suspected should undergo immediate joint aspiration to rapidly confirm the diagnosis. Synovial fluid should be sent for gram stain, aerobic and anaerobic cultures, and cell count with a leukocyte differential. Fungal cultures may be considered in some instances. Leukocyte counts in the range of 50,000 cells/mm³, with a predominance of segmented neutrophils are suggestive of bacterial arthritis, even in the absence of a positive culture. However, it should be recognized that white blood cell counts in joint fluid can vary widely, with ranges from 2000 to 300,000 per mm³. Synovial fluid glucose and protein may be measured but are nonspecific.

Laboratory Tests   In addition to cultures of joint fluid, it is important to obtain blood cultures, which are positive 30 to 40% of the time. As in osteomyelitis, peripheral white blood count, ESR,

and CRP may be useful in the work-up of the patient with suspected joint infection, but are nonspecific. Although frequently abnormal, they do not confirm or exclude the diagnosis. CRP and ESR are valuable adjuncts in gauging response to therapy.

Radiologic Studies   Plain films may demonstrate evidence of soft tissue swelling or widening of the joint space. In the hip, lateral displacement or subluxation of the femoral head may be evident. Normal plain films do not eliminate the possibility of pyogenic arthritis of a joint. Ultrasonography is the best method of detecting joint fluid, especially in the hip. It has the advantage of being noninvasive, usually does not require sedation, and generally is more readily available than MRI. MRI is also a sensitive method for detecting joint fluid and may demonstrate abnormalities in adjacent bone or soft tissue if present. The decision on the need for MRI should be made in conjunction with the consulting orthopedic surgeon.

TREATMENT   An orthopedic surgeon experienced in treating children should be involved in the management of the child with septic arthritis. The goals of therapy are decompression of the joint space and removal of inflammatory debris by adequate drainage; sterilization of the joint through the use of appropriate antimicrobial agents; relief of pain; and prevention of joint deformity.

Drainage of the infected joint may be achieved through repeated aspiration, arthroscopic lavage, or open drainage with lavage. Repeated aspiration may be appropriate for an older child with an infection of short duration and a very sensitive organism. However some experts feel that arthroscopic or open drainage with lavage is superior to drainage by aspiration because they allow a thorough cleansing and removal of inflammatory debris that cannot be evacuated by aspiration. It is universally accepted that septic processes involving the hip should be managed by open drainage and irrigation of the joint space. Successful management of septic arthritis of the hip by arthroscopic irrigation, débridement, and drainage has been reported. Some experts also recommend open drainage for involvement of the shoulder capsule.

Antimicrobial therapy should be instituted as soon as possible after blood cultures and joint fluid samples are obtained. Empiric, initial antibiotic choice is based on the likely pathogens at various ages, the results of Gram stain of the joint aspirate, and any special considerations dictated by the patient's underlying medical problems or clinical situation.

Regimens for all age groups should include an antistaphylococcal agent. Otherwise, empiric choice of agents is similar to that recommended for osteomyelitis. If *N. gonorrhoeae* is a consideration, ceftriaxone or cefotaxime should be used. Parenteral antibiotics are used initially and continued until there is no further need for surgical intervention and the child is afebrile and clinically improving with normalization of laboratory parameters. Exact length of therapy is dependent on the clinical situation, the patient's response, and the particular organism. Therapy is usually continued for at least 2 weeks after the patient is afebrile, joint fluid accumulation has resolved, and laboratory parameters have normalized. Therefore, the usual duration of therapy in septic arthritis is 3 to 6 weeks.

PROGNOSIS AND COMPLICATIONS   Sequelae of septic arthritis include joint deformity and residual dysfunction, abnormal bone growth, and in the hip, avascular necrosis of the femoral head. Risk factors for subsequent complications include delay in drainage and institution of antibiotic therapy, age <6 months, infection of the hip or shoulder, adjacent bony involvement, and infection with *S. aureus* or gram-negative bacteria.

CELLULITIS

Cellulitis is an acute infection of the skin, involving the subcutaneous tissues. Infection usually develops associated with a breach in skin integrity or an associated skin lesion. *S. aureus* and *S. pyogenes* are the most common etiologic agents, although other organisms may be involved, especially in the immunocompromised host or after trauma. Extremities are frequent sites of infection because they are more subject to minor trauma that may go unnoticed. It is sometimes difficult to determine whether an underlying osteomyelitis or septic arthritis is present. Tenderness disproportionate to the soft tissue findings suggests involvement of deeper structures. It is very important to differentiate uncomplicated cellulitis from a more serious condition, group A streptococcal necrotizing fasciitis. Necrotizing fasciitis is characterized by severe pain, systemic toxicity, and laboratory abnormalities. A more detailed discussion of this condition is provided elsewhere (see Section 14.12).

DIAGNOSIS   The presence of cellulitis is usually easily recognized clinically by findings of erythema, warmth, and edema of an area. Fever is often present. In the past, blood cultures were frequently positive in cellulitis because of *H. influenzae*. When cellulitis is caused by other organisms, blood cultures are not as useful. If an aspirate of the area is done, it should be taken from the area of maximum inflammation.

THERAPY   Therapy in the immunocompetent child, particularly those immunized against Hib, is aimed at gram-positive organisms. In the afebrile, nontoxic child, oral therapy with a pencillinase-resistant penicillin or a first-generation cephalosporin may be adequate. Parenteral therapy should be used in the febrile patient if progression is rapid or if associated lymphangitis or lymphadenitis is present. Seven to 10 days of therapy is usually sufficient and can be achieved by sequential parenteral-oral therapy when the patient's condition warrants.

References

Burnett, MW, Bass JW, Cook BA: Etiology of osteomyelitis complicating sickle cell disease. Pediatrics 101:296–297, 1998

Churchill JA, Mazur JM: Ankle pain in children: diagnostic evaluation and clinical decision making. J Am Acad Orthop Surg 3:183–193, 1995

Faden H, Grossi M: Acute osteomyelitis in children: reassessment of etiologic agents and their clinical characteristics. Am J Dis Child 145:65–69, 1991

Luhmann JD, Luhmann SJ: Etiology of septic arthritis in children: an update for the 1990s. Pediatr Emerg Care 15:40–42, 1999

Nelson JD: Acute osteomyelitis in children. Infect Dis Clin North Am 4: 513–522, 1990

Nelson JD: Skeletal infections in children. Adv Pediatr Infect Dis 6:59–78, 1991

Scott RJ, Christofersen MR, Robertson WW, et al: Acute osteomyelitis in children: a review of 116 cases. J Pediatr Orthop 10:649–652, 1990

13.1.10   Infective Endocarditis

Janet A. Stockheim and Stanford T. Shulman

Infective endocarditis (IE) in pediatric patients is often associated with an underlying congenital heart defect. Acquired heart lesions (eg, rheumatic valvulitis disease) and structurally normal hearts, however, may also be infected. Accurate diagnosis and appropriate medical management, with surgery in some cases, are required to achieve a satisfactory outcome of this previously uniformly fatal disease.

Establishment of IE results from the interaction of several host and microbial factors. Endocardial surfaces damaged by turbulent blood flow attract platelets and fibrin, leading to the formation of a nonbacterial thrombotic lesion. Experimental animal models have demonstrated that healthy, intact endothelium is resistant to colonization by circulating microbes; in contrast, damage of endocardium with a plastic catheter leads to rapid microbial colonization. The endocardium appears to be a preferential site of microbial adherence and may have some specificity for binding with certain bacteria.

Two mechanisms, the Venturi and jet effects, combine to damage endocardial surfaces as blood is forced from an area of high pressure into a low-pressure sink. The Venturi effect deposits bacterial colonies immediately beyond the orifice that demarcates the pressure drop. Large pressure gradients are essential to these mechanisms, which explains the low risk of IE in isolated atrial septal defects and the higher risk of IE in small, rather than large, ventriculoseptal defects (VSDs).

Following endocardial damage, bacterial access to the bloodstream and adherence to endocardial surfaces are required for the establishment of IE. Although transient bacteremia is common, it infrequently results in IE, and not all bacteria are capable of initiating this process. The presence of several factors, including bacterial surface polysaccharides, endothelial binding proteins, and agglutinating antibodies that clump bacteria, promote adherence of organisms to damaged endocardial surfaces. In some cases, microbial invasiveness may be more important than host or tissue factors in initiating infection.

Many of the classic manifestations of IE are immunologically mediated. In IE patients with arthralgias and arthritis, splenomegaly, Roth spots, glomerulonephritis, and thrombocytopenia, circulating immune complex levels are significantly higher than in IE patients without those manifestations. Levels of immune complexes decline as these physical manifestations resolve.

MICROBIOLOGY   Bacteremia in patients with IE is believed to be low grade and continuous. As much as 10% of cases of IE yield consistently negative blood cultures, most often as a result of prior antibiotic therapy. Fastidious organisms with special growth requirements may be difficult to culture. Bacteria infecting right-sided heart lesions may be filtered by pulmonary phagocytes, significantly reducing the number of bacteria in a peripheral blood sample. In evaluating patients for IE, it is preferable to obtain at least three separate blood cultures over a 24- to 48-hour period if the patient is stable. Blood should not be drawn through indwelling vascular catheters because contamination may be misleading. If only one of several blood cultures is positive, IE is less likely.

Streptococci and staphylococci account for approximately 75% of cases of IE. Viridans streptococci are the most common cause of IE, although pediatric IE is increasingly associated with staphylococci and unusual gram-negative and fungal organisms. *Staphylococcus aureus* has a tendency to infect hearts with normal anatomy and is associated with persistence of bacteremia and prolonged fevers. Coagulase-negative staphylococci and *S. aureus* tend to infect prosthetic heart valves within 2 months after implantation and are significant pathogens in neonates who require intensive care and intracardiac central lines. Enterococci (especially *E. faecalis*) are well known and important IE pathogens. Gram-negative infections of the heart, although infrequent, are increasing in frequency and are most often associated with intravenous drug use, prosthetic or otherwise abnormal valves, invasive procedures, or nosocomial acquisition. HACEK is an acronym for a group of small, fastidious gram-negative coccobacilli—*Haemophilus aphrophilus, Actinobacillus actinomycetemcomitans, Cardiobacterium hominis, Eikenella corrodens,* and *Kingella kingae*. These organisms normally inhabit the upper respiratory tract and are usually associated with IE when recovered from the bloodstream. Anaerobic and microaerophilic bacteria as well as polymicrobial infections are responsible for a minority of cases of IE. In adults, these infections occur mostly among intravenous drug users or originate from oropharyngeal, gastrointestinal, or genitourinary sites. Candidal IE occurs occasionally, often associated with indwelling catheters. Aspergillus IE has been reported in children following open heart surgery. *Streptococcus pneumoniae* is a common cause of bacteremia in children, but accounts for <1% of cases of childhood IE, frequently in structurally normal hearts. Despite antibiotic therapy in many cases, 61% of the reported cases had fatal outcomes.

CLINICAL MANIFESTATIONS AND DIAGNOSIS   Fever and fatigue are common manifestations of IE in children, whereas other symptoms and physical signs occur with lower frequency (Table 13-26). The "incubation period" of IE, that is, the time from bacteremia to onset of symptoms, is generally less than 2 weeks, although the diagnosis may be delayed for weeks or months. Early manifestations may be mild or nonspecific, and patients may not seek medical attention promptly. New or changing murmurs are infrequent findings in children; difficulty in the diagnosis of IE or improper use of short courses of antibiotics for nonspecific complaints may contribute to delays in diagnosis. In a child with underlying congenital heart disease and fever, fatigue, or worsening cardiac function, the diagnosis of IE requires a high index of suspicion. Among all pediatric series, most of the classic manifestations of IE are infrequent, including Roth spots (small hemorrhagic retinal lesions with pale centers), Osler nodes (small, tender, reddish-purple nodules typically found on the digital pads), Janeway lesions (painless hemorrhagic macules on palms or soles), and splinter hemorrhages (linear streaks in nailbeds).

Several laboratory tests offer supportive evidence for the diagnosis of IE. Continuous bacteremia is typical; multiple blood cultures should be obtained over a 24- to 48-hour period. Other common laboratory findings include anemia and elevated erythrocyte sedimentation rate (ESR). The presence of rheumatoid factor is dependent on the duration of infection. When present, it offers supportive evidence for the diagnosis of IE and is useful for following the patient's response to therapy. Hematuria and associated hypocomplementemia occur in less than half of patients, and aseptic meningitis has been reported in a minority of children with IE.

Accurate diagnosis of IE based on clinical presentation and laboratory results can be challenging. Sensitive and specific diagnostic criteria would serve to ensure diagnostic uniformity among patient

TABLE 13-26

PRESENTING FEATURES IN CHILDREN WITH INFECTIVE ENDOCARDITIS

CLINICAL FEATURES	NO./TOTAL NUMBER OF CHILDREN EVALUATED	%
Fever	389/441	88
Fatigue/malaise	57/95	60
Splenomegaly	191/398	48
Gastrointestinal complaints	45/95	47
Weight loss	33/76	43
Respiratory symptoms	31/76	41
Petechiae	93/326	29
Arthralgias	34/125	27
Headache	20/76	26
Septic emboli	51/201	25
New or changing murmur	100/420	24
Neurologic signs	46/244	19
Sore throat	8/76	11
Rigors	7/76	9
Chest pain	8/95	8
Conjunctival hemorrhages	3/48	6
Splinter hemorrhages	19/299	6
Visual changes	4/76	5
Janeway lesions	11/224	5
Roth spots	13/322	4
Osler nodes	12/297	4
Stiff neck	3/76	4
Arthritis	2/76	3

LABORATORY FEATURES	NO./TOTAL NUMBER OF CHILDREN EVALUATED	%
Elevated ESR	36/48	75
Anemia	54/147	37
Hematuria	66/189	35
Rheumatoid factor positive	13/67	19

SOURCE: Dajani AS, Taubert KA, Wilson W, et al: Prevention of bacterial endocarditis. Recommendations by the American Heart Association. JAMA 277:1794–1801, 1997.

series and surveys, to identify patients requiring therapy for true IE, and to minimize unwarranted, prolonged, parenteral therapy in patients with alternative conditions. In 1994, the Duke University Endocarditis Service developed new diagnostic criteria for IE based on pathologic evidence or on a combination of clinical findings. According to the Duke criteria, clinically diagnosed definite IE must meet two major criteria, one major and three minor criteria, or five minor criteria. Major criteria are multiple positive blood cultures for typical IE organisms or evidence of endocardial involvement, either echocardiographically or by the development of a new valvular regurgitant murmur. Minor criteria are a predisposition (eg, congenital heart defect), fever, vascular phenomena, immunologic phenomena, minor echocardiographic findings, and microbiological or serologic evidence that does not meet major criteria. All of the major and minor criteria have qualifying details.

Echocardiography aids in the diagnosis of IE. Transthoracic 2D echocardiography (TTE) has resolution of approximately 2 mm, with sensitivities for diagnosis of IE from 59 to 82% in children. Transesophageal echocardiography (TEE) may improve the sensitivity of detecting vegetations and is especially useful for visualizing prosthetic valves, but it has more associated risks than does TTE in children and should not be used as a substitute for TTE. Use of

TABLE 13-27

CARDIAC CONDITIONS ASSOCIATED WITH ENDOCARDITIS

ENDOCARDITIS PROPHYLAXIS RECOMMENDED

High-risk category
  Prosthetic cardiac valves, including bioprosthetic and homograft valves
  Previous bacterial endocarditis
  Complex cyanotic congenital heart disease (eg, single ventricle states, transposition of the great arteries, tetralogy of Fallot)
  Surgically constructed systemic pulmonary shunts or conduits
Moderate-risk category
  Most other congenital cardiac malformations (other than above and below)
  Acquired valvular dysfunction (eg, rheumatic heart disease)
  Hypertrophic cardiomyopathy
  Mitral valve prolapse with valvular regurgitation and/or thickened leaflets*

ENDOCARDITIS PROPHYLAXIS NOT RECOMMENDED

Negligible-risk category (no greater risk than the general population)
  Isolated secundum atrial septal defect
  Surgical repair of atrial septal defect, ventricular septal defect, or patent ductus arteriosus (without residua beyond 6 mo)
  Previous coronary artery bypass graft surgery
  Mitral valve prolapse without valvular regurgitation*
  Physiological, functional, or innocent heart murmurs*
  Previous Kawasaki disease without valvular dysfunction
  Previous rheumatic fever without valvular dysfunction
  Cardiac pacemakers (intravascular and epicardial) and implanted defibrillators

---

* See text for further details.
SOURCE: Dajani AS, Taubert KA, Wilson W, et al: Prevention of bacterial endocarditis. Recommendations by the American Heart Association. JAMA 277:1794–1801, 1997.

TEE should be considered, however, when transthoracic views are inadequate, when right-sided lesions are suspected, or for optimal evaluation of prosthetic valves.

TREATMENT Prior to the availability of antibiotics, IE was uniformly fatal. With timely and appropriate medical therapy, IE can be cured and complications minimized. When patients are clinically stable, at least three blood cultures should be collected over a period of 24 to 48 hours before empiric antibiotic therapy is initiated. In patients with cardiac compromise related to valvular dysfunction or with clinical features highly suggestive of IE, collection of multiple blood cultures over a much shorter time period is appropriate, followed by initiation of empiric antibiotic therapy. Following identification of an infecting organism, selection of antibiotics should be based on results of susceptibility testing.

Some basic considerations apply in determining therapy for IE. A prolonged course of therapy with high-dose parenteral bactericidal antibiotics is required. In most cases, oral antibiotics are insufficient for cure. Therapy should be bactericidal rather than bacteriostatic, because the relatively avascular vegetations offer little access to host defenses. β-Lactams (including penicillins and cephalosporins) and vancomycin are used most frequently. Gentamicin is commonly added for a period of time to achieve synergy with a β-lactam or vancomycin, especially when *S. aureus*, viridans streptococci, or enterococci are the causative organisms. Rifampin is useful in combination when *S. aureus* infects prosthetic valves. High doses of antibiotics are required to exceed the minimum bactericidal concentration (MBC) for the infecting organism, and synergistic combinations are recommended in some situations to improve therapy or to shorten its duration. All antibiotic regimens are administered over several weeks, with exact durations dependent on identification and antibiotic susceptibility of the organism, choice of antibiotic or synergistic combination, and the presence or absence of prosthetic material. Generally, regimens are extended approximately 2 weeks in the presence of foreign material. Examples of treatment regimens at the extremes of the spectrum include a 2-week course of penicillin G with gentamicin for treatment of

---

TABLE 13-28

PROPHYLACTIC REGIMENS FOR DENTAL, ORAL, RESPIRATORY TRACT, OR ESOPHAGEAL PROCEDURES

SITUATION	AGENT	REGIMEN*
Standard general prophylaxis	Amoxicillin	Adults: 2.0 g; children: 50 mg/kg orally 1 h before procedure
Unable to take oral medications	Ampicillin	Adults: 2.0 g intramuscularly (IM) or intravenously (IV); children: 50 mg/kg IM or IV within 30 min before procedure
Allergic to penicillin	Clindamycin *or*	Adults: 600 mg; children: 20 mg/kg orally 1 h before procedure
	Cephalexin†, or cefadroxil† *or*	Adults: 2.0 g; children: 50 mg/kg orally 1 h before procedure
	Azithromycin or clarithromycin	Adults: 500 mg; children: 15 mg/kg orally 1 h before procedure
Allergic to penicillin and unable to take oral medications	Clindamycin *or*	Adults: 600 mg; children: 20 mg/kg IV within 30 min before procedure
	Cefazolin†	Adults: 1.0 g; children: 25 mg/kg IM or IV within 30 min before procedure

---

* Total children's dose should not exceed adult dose.
† Cephalosporins should not be used in individuals with immediate-type hypersensitivity reaction (urticaria, angioedema, or anaphylaxis) to penicillins.
SOURCE: Dajani AS, Taubert KA, Wilson W, et al: Prevention of bacterial endocarditis. Recommendations by the American Heart Association. JAMA 277:1794–1801, 1997.

TABLE 13-29

PROPHYLACTIC REGIMENS FOR GENITOURINARY, GASTROINTESTINAL (EXCLUDING ESOPHAGEAL) PROCEDURES

SITUATION	AGENTS*	REGIMEN†
High-risk patients	Ampicillin plus gentamicin	Adults: ampicillin 2.0 g intramuscularly (IM) or intravenously (IV) plus gentamicin 1.5 mg/kg (not to exceed 120 mg) within 30 min of starting the procedure; 6 h later, ampicillin 1 g IM/IV or amoxicillin 1 g orally Children: ampicillin 50 mg/kg IM or IV (not to exceed 2.0 g) plus gentamicin 1.5 mg/kg within 30 min of starting the procedure; 6 h later, ampicillin 25 mg/kg IM/IV or amoxicillin 25 mg/kg orally
High-risk patients allergic to ampicillin/amoxicillin	Vancomycin plus gentamicin	Adults: vancomycin 1.0 g IV over 1–2 h plus gentamicin 1.5 mg/kg IV/IM (not to exceed 120 mg); complete injection/infusion within 30 min of starting the procedure Children: vancomycin 20 mg/kg IV over 1–2 h plus gentamicin 1.5 mg/kg IV/IM; complete injection/infusion within 30 min of starting the procedure
Moderate-risk patients	Amoxicillin or ampicillin	Adults: amoxicillin 2.0 g orally 1 h before procedure, or ampicillin 2.0 g IM/IV within 30 min of starting the procedure Children: amoxicillin 50 mg/kg orally 1 h before procedure, or ampicillin 50 mg/kg IM/IV within 30 min of starting the procedure
Moderate-risk patients allergic to ampicillin/amoxicillin	Vancomycin	Adults: vancomycin 1.0 g IV over 1–2 h; complete infusion within 30 min of starting the procedure Children: vancomycin 20 mg/kg IV over 1–2 h; complete infusion within 30 min of starting the procedure

* Total children's dose should not exceed adult dose.
† No second dose of vancomycin or gentamicin is recommended.
SOURCE: Dajani AS, Taubert KA, Wilson W, et al: Prevention of bacterial endocarditis. Recommendations by the American Heart Association. JAMA 277:1794–1801, 1997.

highly penicillin-susceptible viridans streptococcal IE on a native valve, and 6 weeks or more of nafcillin with rifampin and gentamicin to treat *S. aureus* in the presence of prosthetic material.

Surgical intervention, in addition to medical therapy, is indicated in fungal IE or when bacteremia persists despite appropriate antibiotic therapy, when congestive heart failure (CHF) is uncontrolled by medical therapy, or when abscess of the valve annulus or the myocardium, systemic embolic events, rupture of a valve leaflet or chordae, or acute valvular insufficiency with cardiac failure supervenes. Prosthetic valve endocarditis per se is not an indication for surgery, but surgical intervention may improve the outcome, especially with staphylococcal infections. Among pediatric IE patients, the most frequent indications for surgical intervention are persistent infection, embolic events, and worsening CHF. The aortic valve is most often involved in IE that requires surgery, followed by the mitral valve. Despite the absolute need for surgery in fungal IE, more operative interventions are performed in children infected with *S. aureus* and viridans streptococci than are performed in fungal IE.

The most frequent complications of IE are congestive heart failure and arterial embolization. Intracardiac lesions that may lead to congestive heart failure include leaflet dysfunction and valvular insufficiency caused directly by vegetations or by chordal rupture, abscesses of the myocardium or valvular annulus, and myocardial infarction or conduction defects. Pericarditis may result from bacteremic spread of infection or direct extension and usually is associated with *S. aureus* IE. Arterial emboli occur most frequently when large mobile vegetations develop on valves. While vegetations slowly regress with effective therapy, sudden disappearance of a vegetation should raise the possibility of embolization.

Emboli originating from left-sided vegetations can affect vascular beds in the systemic or cerebral circulation, whereas right-sided lesions produce pulmonary emboli. Mycotic aneurysms most commonly occur at vessel bifurcations and can involve any artery. The pathogenesis of mycotic aneurysms may involve septic embol-

ization of the vasa vasorum; direct bacterial infection of the intraluminal surface of the vessels, with rupture through the wall; contiguous spread of infection; or destruction of an arterial wall by immune complex deposition. Metastatic infections are infrequent complications of IE, most often associated with staphylococcal or candidal infection. They may serve as a source of viable organisms to reinfect the endocardium and should be identified and treated appropriately, with drainage if necessary.

PREVENTION The American Heart Association's (AHA) most recent recommendations for prevention of bacterial endocarditis were published in 1997. They are based on several factors, including underlying heart condition, risk of bacteremia with specific procedures, risk of adverse drug reactions, and the cost of prophylaxis versus the benefit of preventing a life-threatening infection with potential for serious morbidity. Table 13-27 lists high- and moderate-risk cardiac conditions for which prophylaxis is recommended, as well as the cardiac conditions that carry negligible risk of infection and for which IE prophylaxis is not recommended.

The mouth appears to be the most common source for organisms responsible for IE, and bacteremia may occur frequently in the presence of poor oral hygiene even without dental manipulation. The importance of good oral hygiene and routine dental care (personal and professional) should be emphasized to all cardiac patients. Tables 13-28 and 13-29 provide the AHA's antibiotic recommendations for patients undergoing specific procedures. Normal oral flora may be altered in patients already taking antibiotic prophylaxis (eg, penicillin for rheumatic fever prophylaxis), in which case a different class of drugs (clindamycin, azithromycin, or clarithromycin) may provide more protection against the patient's own oral microbes. In a series of apparent failures of IE prophylaxis, most failures occurred following dental procedures, and prophylactic antibiotic regimens generally had been administered improperly.

The genitourinary tract is the second most common source of IE-causing bacteria, and some nonesophageal gastrointestinal tract procedures are also associated with a high rate of bacteremia. Prophylactic antibiotic regimens for high-risk genitourinary and gastrointestinal procedures are directed against enterococci, a greater threat to IE-prone endocardium than gram-negative bacilli.

References

Awadallah SM, Kavey RE, Byrum CJ, Smith FC, Kveselis DA, Blackman MS: The changing pattern of infective endocarditis in childhood. Am J Cardiol 68:90–94, 1991

Dajani AS, Taubert KA, Wilson W, et al: Prevention of bacterial endocarditis. Recommendations by the American Heart Association. JAMA 277:1794–1801, 1997

Del Pont JM, DeCicco LT, Vartalitis C, et al: Infective endocarditis in children: clinical analysis and evaluation of two diagnostic criteria. Pediatr Infect Dis J 14:1079–1086, 1995

Durack DT, Lukes AS, Bright DK: New criteria for diagnosis of infective endocarditis: utilization of specific echocardiographic findings. Am J Med 96:200–209, 1994

Martin JM, Neches WH, Wald ER: Infective endocarditis: 35 years of experience at a children's hospital. Clin Infect Dis 24:669–675, 1997

Stockheim JA, Chadwick EG, Kessler S, et al: Are the Duke criteria superior to the Beth Israel criteria for the diagnosis of infective endocarditis in children? Clin Infect Dis 24:1451–1456, 1998

Wilson WR, Karchmer AW, Dajani AS, et al: Antibiotic treatment of adults with infective endocarditis due to streptococci, enterococci, staphylococci, and HACEK microorganisms. JAMA 274:1706–1713, 1995

13.2   BACTERIAL INFECTIONS

13.2.1   Actinomycosis and Nocardiosis

Ashir Kumar

ACTINOMYCOSIS

Actinomycosis is a slowly progressive suppurative infection characterized by fistula formation. A number of gram-positive, non-spore-forming bacteria from the genus *Actinomyces* are the etiologic agents. The disease was recognized in 1877 by Bollinger as a suppurative swelling of the jaws of cattle. It is encountered worldwide in three main clinical forms: cervicofacial, thoracic, and abdominal; metastatic lesions to other sites are also reported. With appropriate therapy, most patients with cervicofacial or abdominal infection recover completely.

MICROBIOLOGY AND PATHOGENESIS *Actinomyces israeli,* the species that most commonly produces human disease, is part of normal oral flora. *Actinomyces naeslundii, A. viscosus, A. odontolyticus, A. meyeri,* and *Propionibacterium (Arachnia) propionica* are also established etiologic agents. Actinomycosis is often polymicrobial in nature, and concomitant bacterial species such as *Eikenella corrodens, Actinobacillus actinomycetemcomitans, Fusobacterium, Capnocytophaga, Staphylococcus,* microaerophilic streptococci, and Enterobacteriaceae are often isolated from actinomycotic lesions. *Actinomyces sp.* require an anaerobic or microaerophilic environment for growth and demonstrate gram-positive branching filaments, often appearing as beaded filaments. Although uncommon

in children, actinomycosis has been reported in infancy. The disease is not communicable, and is unrelated to occupation, season, or race.

A pivotal step in pathogenesis is the disruption of mucosal barriers, allowing access of these organisms to deep tissue. Once inoculated, the organism replicates and spreads contiguously in a slow and progressive manner with little respect for tissue planes. An acute inflammatory stage with painful, cellulitic reaction is occasionally seen; however, most lesions progress to a chronic stage without significant early cellulitic reaction. The lesions present as masses with characteristic "wooden" walls due to extensive fibrosis. As the lesion matures, it becomes soft and fluctuant, forming sinus tracts.

CLINICAL MANIFESTATIONS Cervicofacial disease, accounting for 60% of patients with actinomycosis, presents as an indurated swelling or mass, usually at the angle of the jaw, but it can occur anywhere on the cheek, mandible, or anterior neck. The duration of illness is typically several months. Pain is seldom prominent, and a low-grade fever may occur in as many as 50% of patients. Lymphatic spread and associated lymphadenopathy are uncommon. The skin overlying the mass may become violaceous, and sinus tract formation with spontaneous discharge often occurs. There may be associated trismus. The drainage may reveal 1-mm-diameter yellow friable masses, termed *sulfur granules,* which are actually colonies of *Actinomyces.* The diagnosis of actinomycosis should be considered in virtually any chronic mass lesion or recurrent abscess in the head and neck region. Higher prevalence of actinomycetes were found in tonsils and adenoids removed for obstructive indications.

Other sites of disease in the upper respiratory tract include maxillary and ethmoid sinusitis. Actinomycosis is an uncommon but important cause of otitis media, as untreated cases can have fatal extension into the mastoid and central nervous system. As a cause of middle ear disease, actinomycosis is characterized by numerous episodes of otitis media that transiently respond to antibiotics (conventional short-course therapy) and by resistance to myringotomy. Diagnosis can be made by microbiological examination of material from the middle ear that appears to be a cholesteatoma.

Thoracic involvement accounts for about 15% of patients with actinomycosis and results from aspiration of the organism in oropharyngeal secretions or, less commonly, from an extension of cervicofacial or abdominal disease. The most common presentation is a slowly progressive disease involving the parenchyma and pleura. As the disease progresses, the lung becomes consolidated and an abscess may form; the pleura and thoracic wall are invaded and produce empyema, rib involvement, subcutaneous abscesses, or draining sinuses. The high incidence of bacteremic dissemination has resulted in mortality rates as high as 50% in some series. Pulmonary actinomycosis must be differentiated from nocardiosis, tuberculosis, fungal infections, and cancer. Mediastinal actinomycosis is uncommon. Because of the slow progression of disease, if bone is involved, both destruction and new bone formation occur, producing wavy periostitis in the ribs or sawtooth changes in the vertebral bodies.

Abdominal actinomycosis most often begins in the ileocecal region as a complication of appendicitis or appendectomy; however, it may also arise from a perforating gastrointestinal ulcer or after the intestinal mucosa is penetrated by a sharp object such as a knife, ingested bone, or bullet. The initial symptoms are insidious and include abdominal discomfort, fever, weight loss, change in bowel habits, and malaise.

Months to years may pass from the time of the inciting event to clinical recognition of this indolent infection. Abdominal examination often reveals a mass. Unless the abscess ruptures through the abdominal wall and produces a typical draining sinus from which sulfur granules or organisms can be recovered, differentiation from appendicitis, regional enteritis, cancer, abscess, tuberculosis, amebiasis, and other intraabdominal disorders is only possible after a biopsy. The infection may extend to involve the liver, other abdominal organs, and spine, or it may penetrate the diaphragm to produce thoracic disease. Perirectal or perianal disease may result from extension of pelvic infection or abdominal disease. A recurrent fistula that fails to heal after drainage or fistulotomy is suggestive of actinomycosis. Hepatic infection occurs in 5% of cases of abdominal actinomycosis, usually by direct extension. Rarely, actinomycosis may present secondary to hematogenous spread to the liver. Renal involvement often occurs due to direct extension from pelvic or abdominal abscesses.

Pelvic actinomycosis is commonly associated with the presence of any type of intrauterine contraceptive device (IUD) and appears to occur rarely unless the IUD has been in place for at least 2 years. It has been reported months after removal of an IUD, making a history of prior use important. Presentation is that of an indolent infection, with fever, weight loss, abnormal vaginal bleeding, and pain being common. A "frozen pelvis" mimicking malignancy is ascribed to fibrosis. Tuboovarian abscess is an early presentation. Involvement of the bladder and ureters may cause hydroureter and hydronephrosis. The presence of *Actinomyces*-like organisms on Papanicolaou-stained cervical specimens associated with pain, abnormal bleeding, or discharge is an indication for removal of the IUD and a 14-day course of penicillin or tetracycline. Rarely, lesions mimicking tumors are seen in extremities, possibly secondary to traumatic inoculation.

DIAGNOSIS The diagnosis is obvious when a draining sinus in the neck, chest, or abdomen produces sulfur granules. Such granules may be seen normally in the tonsil. Rarely, other bacteria such as *S. aureus* and *Nocardia* form similar granules. Microscopic examination of such actinomycotic granules reveals gram-positive beaded filaments that are not acid-fast. The bacteriologic identification from sulfur granules or a sterile site confirms the diagnosis. *Actinomyces sp.* are easily grown below the surface in thioglycollate medium, provided the inoculum does not contain other organisms. Growth usually appears within 5 to 7 days but may take as long as 2 to 4 weeks. Because these organisms are normal flora of the oral cavity and female genital tract, in the absence of sulfur granules, isolation of the organisms is insufficient for diagnosis. Pathologic examination of a biopsied lesion will reveal a central suppurative area surrounded by chronic granulation tissue, and a thick fibrous capsule. When present, sulfur granules appear as basophilic or amphophilic masses with a radiating fringe of eosinophilic clubs. They may be yellow, white, pinkish gray, gray, or brown. Use of immunofluorescence antibody (IFA) allows species identification in fixed tissue or sulfur granules directly. Serology is not useful for diagnosis.

TREATMENT Penicillin is the drug of choice. Initially, intravenous aqueous penicillin, 200,000 U/kg per day (maximum dose: 18–24 million U/d) should be given for 2 to 4 weeks for cervicofacial disease and for 4 to 6 weeks for pulmonary and abdominal infection, depending on the extent of the disease and response to therapy. Subsequently, patients should receive oral penicillin G, 50,000 to 100,000 U/kg per day for 6 to 12 months. If the duration of treatment is not extended beyond the resolution of measurable disease, relapses will occur. Patients allergic to penicillin may be

treated with erythromycin, clindamycin, chloramphenicol, or tetracycline (minocycline). Isolates of *A. actinomycetemcomitans* are often resistant to penicillin. Accessible abscesses should be incised and drained. Because extensive fibrosis may limit antibiotic penetration of the abscess, surgical excision should be considered for lesions that respond slowly to antibiotic therapy.

NOCARDIOSIS

Nocardiosis is a localized or disseminated infection with protean clinical manifestations caused by a soil-borne aerobic actinomycete of the family Nocardiaceae acquired through the respiratory tract. Pulmonary infection occurs in 80% of affected patients and may be either acute or chronic, with frequent dissemination and death. Hematogenous dissemination involves particularly the nervous system and soft tissues. Catheter-associated nocardiosis has also been reported. Primary skin and subcutaneous disease is chronic and benign, yet disfiguring and occasionally disabling.

EPIDEMIOLOGY Human beings acquire pulmonary infections by inhaling contaminated dust particles, whereas traumatic inoculation through the skin is responsible for subcutaneous disease. There is no evidence for airborne animal-to-person or person-to-person spread. Nosocomial outbreaks have been linked to environmental sources. About 15% of all patients with nocardiosis are children. *Nocardia* is an opportunistic pathogen. More than one-half of the patients with pulmonary disease due to *Nocardia sp.* are immunocompromised hosts. There is an increased risk of nocardiosis in patients with alveolar proteinosis, dysgammaglobulinema, and chronic granulomatous disease.

Members of the family Nocardiaceae reproduce by fragmenting into bacillary and coccoid elements, but are distinguished by filamentous growth with true branching. These organisms are not commensals in human beings or animals, but are soil saprophytes often found in decaying organic material worldwide. *Nocardia asteroides* is the etiologic agent most often isolated, particularly from pulmonary lesions. *Nocardia brasiliensis* and *N. otitidis-caviarum* have been identified with increasing frequency as causes of mycetomas and the lymphocutaneous syndrome. Like *Actinomyces sp.*, these organisms appear as gram-positive branching filaments; they are, however, weakly acid-fast. *Nocardia sp.* grow readily on simple media as pigmented colonies due to rudimentary aerial mycelia.

Nocardiosis produces suppurative necrosis and abscess formation typical of pyogenic infection. In contrast to the pronounced tissue fibrosis seen in actinomycosis, nocardiosis seldom provokes more than a loose wall of granulation tissue. This absence of encapsulation accounts for the tendency of this organism to disseminate from its initial pulmonary focus. Sulfur granules are not formed by this organism except in the skin in the lymphocutaneous or mycetoma syndromes.

CLINICAL MANIFESTATIONS Symptoms of pulmonary nocardiosis resemble other chronic lung infections, with a tendency for remissions and exacerbations. Fever, night sweats, malaise, productive cough, pleuritic pain, anorexia, and weight loss are frequent. Localized infiltrates are the most common finding. Solitary lung abscess, necrotizing pneumonia, progressive nodular fibrosis, or empyema, which can form sinus tracts to the chest wall resembling actinomycosis, may be seen. The differential diagnosis includes tuberculosis, actinomycosis, fungal infections, and tumor. In high-risk patients, the diagnosis should be suspected when soft-tissue swellings or abscesses and/or central nervous system mass lesion develop in conjunction with a current or chronic pulmonary infection.

Hematogenous dissemination occurs in 30% of patients with pulmonary diseases. Central nervous system involvement presents as a brain abscess or meningitis. Metastatic subcutaneous abscesses are common, as are hepatic and renal lesions. Most children with pulmonary nocardiosis are immunocompromised; for example, they have chronic granulomatous disease, acute leukemia, or Hodgkin disease, or they are transplant recipients or are receiving steroid therapy. In immunocompromised patients the infection may be fulminant.

Mycetoma, or *Madura foot,* is a localized chronic infection of the skin, subcutaneous tissues, and bone, usually of the foot. It is characterized by swelling and sinus tracts that drain purulent material and may occasionally contain sulfur granules. Evidence of systemic disease such as fever or malaise is lacking; local pain is rare. Nocardial mycetoma occurs endemically in the tropics. Many true fungi produce the same lesion, particularly in Africa and Asia.

The lymphocutaneous syndrome is a subcutaneous nodule or abscess with lymphangitis and regional lymphadenopathy; the initial lesion may ulcerate. Lymphocutaneous infection, particularly by *N. brasiliensis,* resembles sporotrichosis and may be associated with traumatic injury. *Nocardia* skin infection may also present as cellulitis, wound infection, or superficial abscess. *Nocardia* has been reported to cause keratitis, endophthalmitis, peritonsillar abscess, ventriculitis associated with a ventriculoperitoneal shunt, and cervicofacial infection resembling actinomycosis.

DIAGNOSIS Gram stain will reveal delicate, weakly gram-positive, irregularly stained or beaded branching filaments from the clinical specimen. Retention of carbolfuchsin in a modified acid-fast stain that decolorizes with 1% sulfuric acid instead of acid alcohol will differentiate *Nocardia* from *Actinomyces.* Biopsy material should be stained by the Brown-Brenn (tissue Gram stain) and modified Fite (tissue acid-fast) stains. The diagnosis is confirmed by culture. Blood agar is a satisfactory isolation medium, but growth in liquid media produces a dry, waxy surface pellicle similar to mycobacteria and may aid in visualizing branching filaments. *Nocardia sp.* grow poorly on many inhibitory media used for fungal isolation and can be inhibited by many antibiotics. Recovery of the pathogen can be increased by the use of selective media. Cultures from sterile sites will grow in 2 to 10 days. In mixed cultures from respiratory secretions, rapidly growing bacteria may obscure small nocardia colonies, and colonial characteristics sufficient to arouse suspicion often take 2 to 4 weeks to develop. Routine serology is not available. An experimental assay in development, which detects antibody to a 55-kDa *Nocardia* antigen, is sensitive and specific; serum titers of ≥1:256 are seen in 90% of patients.

TREATMENT Sulfonamides are the most effective and best-studied drugs for the treatment of nocardiosis and are considered the drugs of choice. Sulfadiazine given at 100 mg/kg per day (maximum dose: 1.5–2.0 g divided q6h) to achieve a peak blood level of 100 to 150 μg/mL is the standard treatment. At this dose, oliguria, azotemia, and crystalluria can occur. Liberal fluid intake with the addition of sodium bicarbonate to alkalinize the urine can minimize these side effects. Trimethoprim-sulfamethoxazole (TMP-SMX) has also been used for therapy, especially when intravenous treatment is desired. Patients unable to tolerate sulfonamides may receive minocycline, ampicillin, or erythromycin. The use of drugs other than sulfonamides should be supported by in vitro susceptibility testing. Other agents with potential clinical usefulness include

amikacin, cefotaxime, ceftriaxone, amoxicillin-clavulanate, and imipenem. *N. farcinica* isolates are often resistant to several antibiotics. Treatment should be continued for 6 to 12 months. The value of and need for combination therapy is unresolved, although CNS disease usually requires a two- or three-drug combination for the first 6 to 12 months. Surgical therapy with drainage of abscesses and empyemas is useful; however, medical treatment of abscesses has been successful. Metastatic lesions have appeared after the completion of an otherwise effective course of sulfonamides, so careful long-term follow-up is mandatory.

Nocardiosis as a complication of AIDS may be underreported owing to the common use of TMP-SMX in prophylaxis and treatment of *Pneumocystis* pneumonia. Treatment of nocardiosis in transplant recipients can be hampered by the adverse pharmacologic interaction of cyclosporin and sulfonamides, causing nephrotoxicity. However, sulfonamide-containing regimens resulted in 82% survival rate among infected renal transplant patients, whereas nonsulfonamide regimens have had only a 36% survival rate. TMP-SMX may be used in the first year after organ transplantation to prevent *Nocardia* infection.

References

Actinomycosis

Apotheloz C, Regamey C: Disseminated infection due to *Actinomyces meyeri:* case report and review: Clin Infect Dis 22:621–625, 1996

Foster SV, Demmler GJ, Hawkins EP, Tillman JP: Pediatric cervicofacial actinomycosis: South Med J 86:1147–1150, 1993

Puzilli F, Salvati M, Ruggeri A, Raco A, et al: Intracranial actinomycosis in juvenile patients: case report and review of the literature: Childs Nerv Syst. 14:463–466, 1998

Smego RA, Foglia G: Actinomycosis. Clin Infect Dis 26:1255–1263, 1998

Snape PS: Thoracic actinomycosis: an unusual childhood infection: South Med J 86:222–224, 1993

Nocardiosis

Farina C, Boiron P, Goglio A, Provost F, Northern Italy Collaborative Group on Nocardiosis: Human nocardiosis in Northern Italy from 1982–1992. Scand J Infect Dis 27:23–27, 1995

Law BJ, Marks MI: Pediatric nocardiosis. Pediatrics 70:560, 1982

Smego RA Jr, Callis HA: The clinical spectrum of *Nocardia brasiliensis* infection in the United States. Rev Infect Dis 6:164, 1984

vanBurik J, Hackman RC, Nadeem SQ, et al: Nocardiosis after bone marrow transplantation: a retrospective study. Clin Infect Dis 24:1154–1160, 1997

13.2.2   Anaerobic Infections

Mobeen H. Rathore and Salman Ahmad

Anaerobic organisms alone or in combination with aerobes are responsible for a wide variety of infections ranging from superficial skin infections to intraabdominal and intracranial infections. Because of the difficulties encountered in the isolation of these pathogens, mainly avoidance of high oxygen tension and the need for sophisticated laboratory equipment, the diagnosis is often presumptive and the treatment usually empirical when the index of suspicion is high. Anaerobic infections have not been studied as well in the pediatric population and may well be less frequent than in adults. This may partially be explained by higher prevalence of chronic or debilitating conditions in adults that are risk factors for anaerobic infections. Precise data about the incidence of anaerobic infections in children are lacking; however, it is estimated that anaerobes may account for as much as 10% of bacteremias in childhood.

EPIDEMIOLOGY AND PATHOGENESIS Anaerobic organisms are widely distributed in nature; they are recovered from the soil and from the skin, mucous membranes, and the bowels of many animals. Only a very few anaerobic organisms have been identified as responsible for disease in human beings (Table 13-30).

Under normal conditions anaerobes are seldom virulent; however, with disruption of normal skin or mucous membrane barriers they can gain entry into the deeper tissues, proliferate, and cause significant infection. Although anaerobes are widely prevalent in nature, the source of infection in the majority of cases is the patients' own endogenous flora. Some of these bacteria are strict anaerobes, unable to survive in oxygen; others are facultative anaerobes, able to survive in oxygen or without oxygen. The presence of devitalized tissues, low oxygen tension, and low pH serve as major contributing factors in the pathogenesis of anaerobic infections. Host defense mechanisms, virulence factors (bacterial adherence factors), production of toxins (eg, *Clostridium* species), and presence of other bacteria polymicrobial infections all play important roles in the complex pathogenesis of anaerobic infections.

CLINICAL MANIFESTATIONS The commonly encountered diseases caused by anaerobic infections in children are listed in Table 13-31. The principal sites of anaerobic infection are deep soft-tissue infections around the mouth and oropharynx, peritonitis and peritoneal abscesses following appendicitis or bowel rupture, and brain and lung abscesses. Beyond menarche, anaerobic bacteria are part of the flora of pelvic infection, such as salpingitis, tuboovarian abscess, and others.

Clinically it is often difficult to distinguish anaerobic soft-tissue infections from aerobic infections. Anaerobic infections tend to be more foul smelling, but gas is not present unless gas-producing organisms such as *C. perfringens* are involved. The occurance of bacteremia is often associated with serious disease in neonates and immunocompromised children.

DIAGNOSIS The diagnosis of anaerobic infection is most often made on clinical grounds. The definitive diagnosis of anaerobic infections requires isolation and identification of pathogens by culture methods. This is not easily accomplished in most clinical situations because of several factors, including contamination of specimen by normal skin and mucous membrane commensals, pres-

TABLE 13-30

COMMON ANAEROBIC BACTERIA

Gram-positive
Cocci: *Peptococcus, Peptostreptococcus,* Microaerophilic streptococci
Bacilli: *Clostridium* species, *Actinomyces, Propionibacterium, Lactobacillus, Bifidobacterium, Eubacterium*
Gram-negative
Cocci: *Veillonella*
Bacilli: *Bacteroides, Prevotella, Porphyromonas, Fusobacteria*

TABLE 13-31

ANAEROBIC BACTERIAL INFECTIONS IN CHILDREN

Central Nervous System
Brain abscess, subdural empyema
Oropharyngeal and Respiratory Tract
Chronic sinusitis; chronic otitis media; mastoiditis; periodontal infections; parapharyngeal abscess; retropharyngeal abscess; tonsillar abscess; peritonsillar abscess; cervical adenitis; lung abscess; empyema; Lemierre syndrome*; aspiration pneumonia; gingivitis; Ludwig angina
Intraabdominal and Pelvic
Peritonitis; peritoneal abscess; salpingitis; intraabdominal visceral abscesses; pelvic inflammatory disease
Skin and Soft Tissue
Cellulitis; fasciitis; paronychia; animal and human bite infection
Toxin Mediated
Botulism; *C. difficile*-associated diarrhea
Miscellaneous
Bacteremia associated with gastrointestinal disease; septicemia in immunocompromised host; puerperal sepsis

---

* Soft-tissue infection of the neck caused by *Fusobacterium.*

ence of other bacteria in polymicrobial infections, need for special transport media to prevent the specimen from drying or being exposed to high oxygen tension, and the requirement for sophisticated laboratory equipment. Therefore, the presence of organisms on Gram stain and sterile culture from a specimen is strongly suggestive of an anaerobic pathogen when the clinical picture is consistent. In addition, one may also suspect anaerobic infection because of the presence of foul smell in the clinical specimen or site from which the specimen was obtained. Antimicrobial susceptibility studies for anaerobic bacteria are frequently not available from the average hospital laboratory. These studies should, however, be requested in exceptional and life-threatening cases.

TREATMENT The management of anaerobic infections requires appropriate use of antibiotics and surgical intervention when indicated. Because anaerobic organisms have a special propensity for abscess formation, it is important to identify the abscess and to drain it surgically or under radiologic guidance. The treatment of anaerobic infections is empirical in most instances. Antibiotics should be selected based on the organ system involved and the knowledge of likely pathogens. Because infections involving anaerobes are often polymicrobial, antibiotic combinations may be required. In general, with life-threatening infections such as those of central nervous system, thorax, and abdomen, the patient should be empirically started on a combination antibiotic regimen effective against both anaerobic and aerobic organisms. For oropharyngeal infections, penicillin G is still the drug of choice and is active against all anaerobes except *Bacteroides spp.* which produce β-lactamase. Metronidazole and clindamycin have excellent activity against anaerobes including the ones that produce β-lactamase. Clindamycin is superior to penicillin or metronidazole for serious lung infection. Antibiotic combinations with β-lactamase inhibitors (amoxicillin/clavulanic acid, ticarcillin/clavulanic acid, ampicillin/sulbactam, and piperacillin/tazobactam) are also useful alternatives for treatment of anaerobic infection and are being used more frequently. Among the cephalosporins, cefoxitin and cefotetan have antianaerobic activity. Chloramphenicol, imipenem, and some of the newer quinolones also have antianaerobic activity.

References

Brook I: Bacteriology of intracranial abscesses in children. J Neurosurg 54: 484, 1981

Brook I: Aerobic and anaerobic microbiology of necrotizing fasciitis in children. Pediatr Derm 13:281–284, 1996

Finegold SM, Goldstein EJ, eds: Proceedings of the First North American Congress on Anaerobic Bacteria and Anaerobic Infection. Clin Infect Dis 16(suppl 4):S161, 1993

Sener B, Hascelik G, Onerci M, Tunckanat F: Evaluation of the microbiology of chronic sinusitis. J Laryngol Otol 110:547–550, 1996

Simo R, Hartley C, Rapado F, et al: Microbiology and antibiotic treatment of head and neck abscesses in children. Clin Otolaryngol 23:164–168, 1998

CLOSTRIDIAL INFECTIONS

Mobeen H. Rathore and Marwan S. Shalabi

Clostridium difficile

Clostridium difficile is an anaerobic spore-forming gram-positive bacillus responsible for both colonization and infection. Colonization tends to be higher among hospitalized patients and young infants; as many as 50% of healthy neonates and young infants can be colonized. Colonization declines to 2 to 5% in healthy adults. Infection is frequently acquired nosocomially where the organism is transmitted by hands of personnel caring for symptomatic or colonized patients. Spores can survive outside the gut for weeks to months. Unfortunately, commonly used disinfectants are ineffective in eradicating the spores from the surfaces. This organism causes a spectrum of illnesses referred to as *Clostridium difficile–associated disease* (CDAD).

Administration of antibiotics is the most common risk factor for developing CDAD. It is thought that the offending antibiotic kills the normal flora of the gut, allowing *C. difficile* to flourish without competition. The organism produces toxins A and B that cause an inflammatory reaction leading to damage of the large intestine. Almost any antibiotic can predispose to CDAD; however, the penicillins, especially amoxicillin, are the most common offenders in childhood, followed by cephalosporins and clindamycin. Symptoms of CDAD can develop up to 6 weeks after stopping antibiotics. CDAD has also been associated with the administration of cancer chemotherapeutic agents.

CLINICAL MANIFESTATIONS Presentation of CDAD can range from asymptomatic colonization to severe, sometimes life-threatening disease. Asymptomatic colonization of the gut occurs frequently in neonates and young infants. *Clostridium difficile* can cause watery diarrhea similar to viral gastroenteritis, severe diarrhea similar to that in dysentery or colitis, and, rarely, bacteremia with distant metastatic infections. Pseudomembranous colitis is a severe form of colonic involvement causing characteristic raised yellowish plaques, which can be seen by colonoscopy. This form of colitis can be complicated by perforation, peritonitis, and abdominal abscesses.

DIAGNOSIS A high index of suspicion is most crucial in the diagnosis of CDAD. Colitis caused by CDAD may be associated with peripheral leukocytosis with a shift to the left and the presence of both white and red blood cells in a stool specimen. Isolation of the organism alone is not evidence of infection because intestinal colonization can occur. The presence of *C. difficile* toxin in the stool is diagnostic in children over 1 year of age. In younger infants sigmoidoscopy should be considered to confirm diagnosis since the toxin is not usually pathogenic due to a lack of receptors. Most cases of CDAD occur secondary to toxin B alone or combined with toxin A. A tissue culture assay for identifying the toxins is considered the gold standard. However, this assay only detects the presence of toxin B; as a result, diagnosis of toxin A–induced colitis can be missed. In addition, a tissue culture assay takes as long as 24 to 48 hours for the results to be available, thereby making it impractical. Assays such as enzyme-linked immunosorbent assays (ELISAs) and monoclonal antibody tests are rapid and more practical, but these tests are less sensitive than tissue culture assay. Use of the immunoenzyme assay is acceptable for clinical diagnosis of CDAD. Sigmoidoscopy or colonoscopy should be considered in selective cases and can be an important diagnostic tool.

TREATMENT Oral metronidazole 30 mg/kg/d divided every 6 hours for 7 to 14 days is the drug of choice for CDAD. Oral vancomycin 50 mg/kg/d divided every 6 hours for 7 to 14 days is also efficacious, but parenteral vancomycin is not efficacious. Because oral vancomycin is more expensive and its use is associated with the emergence of resistant organisms, this drug should be reserved only for instances of metronidazole failure. Metronidazole is the only drug that should be used for parenteral therapy. Clinical relapse occurs in 10 to 30% of the cases, in which case, repeating the course of antibiotics is recommended. Because the excretion of the organism and the toxin can be prolonged after clinical cure, follow-up testing for *C. difficile* or its toxins is not indicated. Oral bacitracin (25,000 units PO given every 6 hours) is another alternative.

In addition to antibiotic use, hydration should be ensured, the offending antibiotic stopped, and, where possible, antibiotics avoided for a few weeks until the normal microbial balance is reinstituted in the intestine. Probiotics, such as *lactobacillus GG*, may be useful to prevent recurrence.

PREVENTION Meticulous attention to hand washing and strict contact isolation should be emphasized as measures to prevent nosocomial transmission of *C. difficile*. Children with CDAD should be excluded from child care for the duration of the diarrhea or, if space permits, placed in a separate, protected area.

Clostridium botulinum

EPIDEMIOLOGY Botulism is an acute descending paralysis that results when a neurotoxin of *Clostridium botulinum* blocks neuromuscular transmission. *Clostridium botulinum* is an anaerobic spore-forming gram-positive bacillus commonly found in the soil. It produces seven antigenically different neurotoxins, A through G. Botulism is caused mainly by toxins A and B, and rarely by toxins E and F. Toxins C and D cause botulism in animals. There are three main forms of botulism: "infantile botulism," the most common type, was first described in 1976; "food-borne botulism," which occurs after ingestion of preformed toxin formed in inadequately preserved food; and "wound botulism," which results from contamination of wounds by spores. A fourth category called "unclassified" has been described in adults who lack evidence of wound or food source of botulism neurotoxin. Recently, "inadvertent botulism" has been described as an iatrogenic disease occurring in patients who have been treated with botulinum toxin injections for dystonia or other movement disorder.

This section focuses on infantile botulism, in which ingested spores of *C. botulinum* germinate in the infant colon and produce the neurotoxin, which is absorbed and carried by blood to the peripheral cholinergic synapses, where it binds irreversibly to them. This leads to blocking of acetylcholine release, resulting in flaccid paralysis. This toxin is the most lethal organic compound known.

Other clostridial species such as *C. baratii* and *C. butyricum* can produce clinical syndromes identical to botulism. Discovery of these organisms has increased the number of strains that may cause intestinal toxemias of infancy for which *C. botulinum* is the prototype.

CLINICAL MANIFESTATIONS Infantile botulism occurs almost exclusively in the first 6 to 12 months of life. There is no gender predilection. The youngest patient reported had an onset at 6 days of life, and the oldest patient reported had an onset at 12 months. Onset of infant botulism occurs at a significantly younger age in formula-fed infants as compared to breast-fed infants. In most cases of infant botulism, the source of spores is not identified. History of honey ingestion prior to the onset of the illness is present in only 15% of the infants. The classic presentation is constipation, progressive weakness, impaired respiratory effort, weak cry, poor feeding, and poor suck, gag, and swallow reflexes.

Infant botulism displays a spectrum of presentations. At one end of the spectrum, the infant may present with transient mild weakness and hypotonia that may go unnoticed. The other end of the picture is a fulminant, even fatal, illness; sometimes similar to sudden infant death syndrome (SIDS). The first sign of the illness is constipation. The paralysis is usually symmetric and descending, starting with the cranial nerves, and results in an expressionless face, ptosis, weak cry, and impaired gag or suck reflexes followed by generalized progressive hypotonia. Deep-tendon reflexes are normal initially but diminish later in the course of the illness. The infant is usually afebrile unless the course is complicated by secondary bacterial infection. Paresis peaks in 1 to 2 weeks and may persist for as long as 3 weeks, followed by recovery over the next few weeks. Children are hospitalized for an average of 1 month; most of them require management in an intensive care unit.

DIAGNOSIS Botulism should be suspected in any infant who presents with progressive weakness, poor feeding, and constipation. Sepsis is the most common admitting diagnosis in patients found to have infantile botulism. Other admission diagnoses include dehydration, viral syndrome, and failure to thrive. The differential diagnosis includes hypothyroidism, metabolic disorders, drug or heavy-metal poisoning, myasthenia gravis, poliomyelitis, Guillain-Barré syndrome, Hirschprung disease, and Werdnig-Hoffmann disease. Despite a sad, lethargic appearance and a feeble cry, the infant conveys a paradoxical sense of alertness because the toxin does not cross the blood-brain barrier. This clinical distinction helps to distinguish patients with infantile botulism from those with sepsis. Electromyography is a helpful bedside test, which often shows a pattern of brief, small, abundant potentials (BSAP), or fasciculation.

Diagnosis is established by isolating *C. botulinum* in the stool because this organism is not a normal inhabitant of fecal flora. Because of the associated constipation, an enema with sterile nonbacteriostatic water is often necessary for obtaining a stool specimen. Toxin can be isolated from the stool by mouse neutralization assay or ELISA. The former is the test of choice; demonstrating toxicity in the mouse after injecting it with the material obtained from the stool or serum of the patient is diagnostic. This toxic effect on the mouse can be prevented by prior injection with the specific mono-

valent botulinum antitoxin. This can also help identify the type of toxin causing the disease. In approximately 10% of the cases of infantile botulism, the neurotoxin can be detected in the blood. In cases of foodborne or wound botulism, the toxin is more likely to be detected in blood. Cerebrospinal fluid and peripheral blood count are usually normal, although some patients may show elevated protein in the spinal fluid.

TREATMENT Supportive management and anticipation of potential complications are crucial in the treatment of infantile botulism (Table 13-32). Most patients require prolonged intubation (median 21 days). Enteral feeding is preferable because stimulation of gut motility may purge the organism and reduce amounts of toxin, as well as obviate the need for indwelling venous catheters.

Specific treatment by the recently introduced human-derived botulism immune globulin (BIG) shows promising results, reducing hospital stays from 5.5 to 2.5 weeks. Treatment with BIG should be started as early as possible (for more information about BIG contact Infant Botulism Prevention Program, Health and Human Services, State of California, 510-540-2646).

Antibiotic usage may theoretically lead to lysis of *C. botulinum*, releasing further neurotoxin. Therefore, if antibiotics are required for the treatment of secondary infections (pneumonia, urinary tract infection, or otitis media), the choice should focus on antibiotics such as nalidixic acid or trimethoprim-sulfamethoxazole to which *C. botulinum* is resistant. Aminoglycosides should be avoided because they may contribute to further neuromuscular blockade and worsen the disease.

PREVENTION Although history of honey ingestion is present in a minority of cases, children younger than 12 months should not be fed honey. Isolation of the infected infant is not required, but meticulous hand washing should be emphasized. Soiled diapers should be autoclaved; staff members with open wounds should not handle the diapers. Local and state health departments and the Centers for Disease Control and Prevention should be notified.

Clostridium perfringens

EPIDEMIOLOGY *Clostridium perfringens,* an anaerobic gram-positive bacillus, is the most common cause of gas gangrene (myonecrosis), but it is also implicated in cellulitis, necrotizing fasciitis, food poisoning, and necrotizing enteritis (enteritis necroticans). Although carried in the human colon and vagina, *C. perfringens* may gain access to surgical or traumatic wounds by perforation of the abdominal viscera. Factors that may facilitate the growth of *C. perfringens* include penetration of deep tissue, presence of a foreign body, extensive tissue devitalization, tissue anoxia, polymicrobial infections, and anaerobic environment. *Clostridium perfringens* produces extracellular toxins, causing tissue necrosis, edema,

TABLE 13-32
COMPLICATIONS OF INFANT BOTULISM

Apnea
Adult respiratory distress syndrome
Necrotizing enterocolitis
Otitis media
Pneumonia
Urinary tract infection
Syndrome of inappropriate antidiuretic secretion (SIADH)

thrombosis of blood vessels, and gas gangrene, but infiltration of leukocytes is characteristically minimal.

Gas gangrene may occur after trauma, postoperatively or spontaneously in the presence of another primary pathology, such as a tumor, burn, or diabetes. Other organisms associated with gas gangrene include *C. bifermentans, C. sordellii, C. septicum, C. novyi,* and *C. histolyticum.* Food poisoning occurs after ingestion of foods heavily contaminated by a heat-labile enterotoxin produced by *C. perfringens* type A. Necrotizing enteritis occurs secondary to β-enterotoxin produced by *C. perfringens* type C.

CLINICAL MANIFESTATIONS Gas gangrene associated with a wound is heralded by sudden, persistent, and progressive pain at the site of injury; local, tense swelling; tenderness; pallor; and a thin hemorrhagic exudate. Pallor gives way to a bronze or magenta discoloration, and hemorrhagic purplish bullae appear. Soft-tissue crepitance may be present, but if the amount of gas is small, it may not be seen on plain radiography or other imaging studies. A peculiar offensive odor, sometimes described as sweet, may be noted, with a brown serosanguineous discharge. Eventually, the muscle becomes gangrenous, black, friable, and liquefied. Infection may progress to shock, multiorgan failure, and death. On the other hand, *C. perfringens* can cause a localized cellulitis similar to group A streptococcal cellulitis.

Food poisoning caused by *C. perfringens* is usually a self-limited illness, often causing outbreaks. Typically, the illness starts 8 to 12 hours after ingestion of contaminated meat and meat products. Symptoms usually last less than 24 hours and include nausea, severe abdominal pain, and profuse nonbloody diarrhea. Fever is absent and vomiting is uncommon.

Necrotizing enteritis is a rare life-threatening foodborne illness that is a major cause of death in children in some parts of the world because of its propensity to cause intestinal perforation, sepsis, and death.

DIAGNOSIS Although gas gangrene is a clinical diagnosis, early recognition is critical for successful management. Myonecrosis and crepitance are classic findings but not pathognomic because infections with other organisms may also produce gas. In one series of 49 cases of gas gangrene and myositis in which gas was reported in soft tissue, the organisms cultured, in descending order of frequency, were *Proteus, Enterococcus, E. coli, Klebsiella, Enterobacter, Staphylococcus, Streptococcus, Pseudomonas,* and *Bacterioides.* Only one case was caused by *Clostridium.*

Gram stain of the drainage may show large gram-positive bacilli, in the absence of neutrophils. In the presence of gram-positive bacilli and suspicious clinical picture, diagnosis of gas gangrene should be made until proven otherwise. Isolation of *C. perfringens* from deep tissues should be attempted, but failure to isolate the organisms does not exclude the diagnosis. On the other hand, the organism may be isolated from a traumatic wound as a contaminant. The presence of an appropriate clinical picture is important to make the diagnosis. In general, there is no satisfactory diagnostic test for gas gangrene, and one should not lose valuable time waiting for laboratory or radiologic test confirmation.

Demonstration of large number of *C. perfringens* in the implicated food and isolation of the same serotype from the stool are helpful in the diagnosis of food poisoning. Enterotoxin may also be isolated from the stool specimen.

TREATMENT Surgical intervention is critical to the management of gas gangrene. Urgent intervention may require radical débridement, drainage, and removal of foreign bodies. Decompressing fascial compartments is essential to prevent further tissue anoxia. Polyvalent gas gangrene antitoxin has no proven benefit. The antitoxin is an equine preparation, which is not available commercially, that has a 20% risk of causing serum sickness. Hyperbaric oxygen is favored by some experts as mode of therapy after surgical intervention, but access to hyperbaric oxygen treatment limits the usefulness of this application. No adequately controlled studies document the effectiveness of this therapy.

Antimicrobial therapy is an important adjunct. Broad-spectrum antibiotics are indicated until culture and sensitivity reports allow for appropriate antibiotic adjustments. Penicillin G (250,000–400,000 U/kg/d divided every 4 hours) has excellent activity against *C. perfringens* and must be included in an antibiotic regimen. However, approximately 5% of the clostridial species show variable degrees of resistance to penicillin. *Clostridium perfringens* is also susceptible to clindamycin, metronidazole, and cefoxitin. Penicillin or clindamycin may also be valuable as prophylactic agents in patients with grossly contaminated wounds.

Clostridial cellulitis is treated by incision and drainage in addition to the antibiotics. Radical débridement is usually not necessary. Treatment of food poisoning is symptomatic. Necrotizing enteritis requires use of antitoxin to the β toxin produced by *C. perfringens* type C. Use of antitoxin is of considerable benefit for this condition.

References

Clostridium difficile

Bartlet JC: *Clostridium difficile:* history of its role as an enteric pathogen and the current state of knowledge about the organism. Clin Infect Dis 18:S265–272, 1994

George WL: Clostridial intoxication and infection. In: Feigin RD, Cherry JD, eds: Textbook of Pediatric Infectious Diseases, 4th ed. Philadelphia, WB Saunders, 1998:1566–1569

Gerding DN: Diagnosis of *Clostridium difficile*-associated disease: patient selection and test perfection. Am J Med 100:485–486, 1996

Johnson S, Gerding DN, Olson MM, et al: Prospective controlled study of vinyl glove use to interrupt *Clostridium difficile* nosocomial transmission. Am J Med 88:137–146, 1990

McFarland LV, Surawicz CM, Stamm WE: Risk factors for *Clostridium difficile* infection. N Engl J Med 320:204–210, 1989

Ravizzola G, Manca N, Dima F, Signorini C, Garrafa E, Turano A: Isolation of a *Clostridium* exotoxin producer other than *Clostridium difficile* from a patient with diarrhea. J Clin Microbiol 36:2396, 1998

Wolf LE, Gorbach SL, Granowitz EV: Extraintestinal *Clostridium difficile:* 10 years experience at a tertiary care hospital. Mayo Clin Proc 73:943–947, 1998

Clostridium botulinum

Frankovich TL, Aron SS: Clinical trial of botulism immune globulin for infant botulism. West J Med 154:103, 1991

Glatman-Freedman A: Infant botulism. Pediatr Rev 17:185–186, 1996

Hatheway CL, McCroskey LM: Examination of feces and serum for diagnosis of infant botulism in 336 patients. J Clin Microbiol 25:2334–2338, 1987

Spika JS, Shafer N, Hargrett-Bean N, et al: Risk factors for infant botulism in the United States. Am J Dis Child 143:828–832, 1989

Clostridium perfringens

Afghani B, Stutman HR: Toxin related diarrheas. Pediatr Ann 23:549–550, 1994

Bessman AN, Wagner W: Nonclostridial gas gangrene. Report of 48 cases and review of the literature. JAMA 223:958–963, 1975

Cohen RF, Yourofsky LA: Gas gangrene: a postoperative complication. J Foot Surg 19:202–206, 1980

Hart GB, Lamb RC, Strauss MB: Gas gangrene. J Trauma 23:991–1000, 1983

Lund BM: Foodborne disease due to Bacillus and Clostridium species. Lancet 336:982–986, 1990

13.2.3   Anthrax

Denise Bratcher

Anthrax is an acute infectious disease caused by the gram-positive, encapsulated, nonmotile, spore-forming rod *Bacillus anthracis*. *Bacillus anthracis* is capable of producing three exotoxins—protective factor, lethal factor, and edema factor—which contribute to its virulence. Anthrax occurs most commonly in agricultural regions in the Middle East, Africa, Australia, Europe, New Zealand, South and Central America, and the Caribbean, and is rarely reported in the United States. Its potential as an agent of bioterrorism should prompt immediate notification of the local or state health department, the hospital epidemiologist, and the local and state health laboratories upon first suspicion of an anthrax-like illness.

EPIDEMIOLOGY   Anthrax most commonly occurs in herbivores, which acquire the disease by grazing in areas contaminated by *B. anthracis* spores. *Bacillus anthracis* spores can survive for prolonged periods of time. Human cases arise because of occupational exposure to infected animals or their products, and have been reported after contact with anthrax spores in imported hides, wool, goat hair, bone meal, and toys. While the discharge from cutaneous anthrax lesions is potentially infectious, no person-to-person transmission is documented. The incubation period is 1 to 7 days after contact.

CLINICAL MANIFESTATIONS   In humans, three types of anthrax infections occur: cutaneous, inhalation, and gastrointestinal.

Cutaneous anthrax is the most common naturally occurring form, appearing primarily in industrial and agricultural employees. Introduction of anthrax spores into a cutaneous abrasion results in a small erythematous papule that vesiculates and eventually forms a painless eschar. Marked edema occurs as a result of exotoxins released from *B. anthracis*. Associated lymphangitis or painful regional lymphadenopathy may be noted. Healing occurs within a few weeks; without antibiotic therapy, the mortality rate is reported to be as high as 20%.

Inhalation anthrax (woolsorter's disease) occurs after *B. anthracis* spores are deposited in alveolar spaces, usually related to industrial processing of contaminated animal products. Described as biphasic, inhalation anthrax is difficult to diagnose early. The initial nonspecific symptoms, including fever, dyspnea, chest pain, cough, headache, vomiting, abdominal pain, and weakness, are similar to symptoms of influenza. Symptoms progress over a few days to include fever, severe dyspnea, diaphoresis, hypoxemia, and shock, usually leading to death. A key finding on chest radiograph is widening of the mediastinum, consistent with lymphadenopathy. Hemorrhagic meningitis and bacteremia are common.

Gastrointestinal anthrax, never reported in the United States, occurs following ingestion of contaminated, undercooked meat. Patients present initially with nausea, vomiting, and malaise, and progress rapidly to bloody diarrhea, gross ascites, hemorrhagic lymphadenitis, and sepsis. A pharyngeal form of anthrax occurs when *B. anthracis* is directly absorbed from contaminated meat through mucous membranes; the clinical picture includes profound submental swelling, adenopathy, and systemic symptoms. Anthrax has been described in multiple forms in children, including periorbital cellulitis in a young child and meningitis acquired from a mother with septicemia in a neonate.

DIAGNOSIS   If cutaneous anthrax is suspected, a Gram stain and culture of vesicular fluid will confirm the diagnosis. *Bacillus anthracis* grows in ordinary nutrient broth. Laboratory diagnosis of anthrax is suspected when characteristic large, gram-positive, sporulating bacilli are seen on Gram stain. If inhalation anthrax is suspected, a widened mediastinum on chest radiograph in a patient with overwhelming flu-like illness is pathognomonic. Peripheral blood smears may show visible bacilli on Gram stain, and blood culture should show growth within 24 hours. Microbiology laboratories should be alerted to the possibility of anthrax when clinical suspicion warrants. Rapid diagnostic tests, such as enzyme-linked immunosorbent assay and polymerase chain reaction, are available at national reference laboratories.

TREATMENT   Although few clinical studies of the treatment of anthrax exist, high-dose penicillin is the drug of choice for all forms of anthrax. Other alternatives include doxycycline, ciprofloxacin, erythromycin, tetracycline, and chloramphenicol. For inhalation or meningeal anthrax, large does of penicillin plus streptomycin or parenteral ciprofloxacin are recommended. Natural strains of *B. anthracis* show resistance to sulfamethoxazole, trimethoprim, cefuroxime, aztreonam, and third-generation cephalosporins.

When anthrax cases occur following a terrorist attack, antibiotic resistance to penicillins and tetracyclines is possible. Empiric therapy in this scenario should begin with intravenous ciprofloxacin or other quinolones.

PREVENTION   Prevention of human disease ultimately depends upon control of animal disease and industrial contamination. Standard barrier isolation precautions should be instituted for patients with all forms of anthrax. Burning or steam sterilization of contaminated dressings or bedding is recommended. Animal and human vaccines are available.

Human anthrax vaccine (produced by the Bioport Corporation, formerly the Michigan Biologic Products Institute in Lansing, Michigan) is a sterile filtrate of an avirulent *B. anthracis* strain. Vaccine is recommended for those in contact with imported animal hides, hair, or textiles in the workplace and for those persons whose investigational or diagnostic work may bring them into contact with anthrax spores. The vaccine series of three subcutaneous injections given 2 weeks apart, followed by three additional subcutaneous injections given at 6, 12, and 18 months, plus an annual booster dose is now given to most US military personnel. The vaccine is well-tolerated, with mild erythema and tenderness occurring occasionally at the site of injection. Rarely, fever and chills occur.

References

Inglesby TV, Henderson DA, Bartlett JG, et al: Anthrax as a biological weapon. JAMA 281:1735–1745, 1999

LaForce FM: Anthrax. Clin Infect Dis 19:1009–1013, 1994

Interim recommendations for antimicrobial prophylaxis for children and breastfeeding mothers and treatment of children with anthrax. MMWR 50:1014–1016, 2001

13.2.4　*Arcanobacterium*

Dennis L. Murray

Arcanobacterium haemolyticum (formally *Corynebacterium haemolyticum*) is a gram-positive (sometimes gram-variable) bacillus that is responsible for cases of both pharyngitis and cutaneous infections. This pleomorphic, nonsporulating bacillus grows like *C. diphtheriae* on Loeffler medium, but grows poorly on tellurite media. Optimal growth is achieved on either human or rabbit blood agar, but the organism will grow on standard blood agar plates. The bacterium typically has a black opaque dot in the center of each colony. *Arcanobacterium haemolyticum* can liberate toxins, including a dermonecrotic toxin, using a mechanism similar to that for the production of erythrogenic toxin by group A streptococci (GAS).

EPIDEMIOLOGY　Humans are the primary host of *A. haemolyticum*. Peak age of illness is in the second decade of life, whereas GAS, which may cause a similar presentation, peaks in the first decade of life. No seasonal variation occurs, but studies suggest that more females than males are affected. Disease is spread person to person, presumably by respiratory droplets. The incubation period is unknown.

CLINICAL MANIFESTATIONS　Presentation of disease caused by *A. haemolyticum* is similar to GAS pharyngitis with fever, pharyngeal exudate, and lymphadenopathy, but palatal petechiae and strawberry tongue are usually absent. In up to 50% of cases, a maculopapular or scarlatiniform rash is present. Beginning peripherally and spreading centrally sparing the face, palms, and soles, the rash typically starts 1 to 4 days after symptoms of the sore throat begin and persists for more than 2 days in the majority of patients. Occasionally, the rash is accompanied by pruritus.

Skin infections, especially chronic ulceration, caused by *A. haemolyticum* occur mainly in tropical countries. Invasive infections, including sepsis, brain abscess, meningitis, osteomyelitis, and pneumonia have been reported.

DIAGNOSIS　*Arcanobacterium haemolyticum* should be suspected in adolescents and young adults complaining of sore throat who have a rash. Isolation of *A. haemolyticum* from a clinical specimen is diagnostic. Use of human or rabbit blood agar improves the culture yield for *A. haemolyticum* as compared to the yield from a standard sheep blood agar plate. Coinfection with GAS and *A. haemolyticum,* as well as Epstein-Barr virus and *A. haemolyticum,* have been reported.

TREATMENT　No prospective randomized study has established efficacy of antimicrobial treatment for *A. haemolyticum* infection. In vitro *A. haemolyticum* is sensitive to erythromycin, clindamycin, chloramphenicol, tetracycline, and vancomycin. The organism has variable sensitivity to penicillin and is usually resistant to sulfonamides and trimethoprim-sulfamethoxazole. Erythromycin is the drug of choice. Bacteriologic failure occurred when penicillin was given to treat pharyngitis from which *A. haemolyticum* was cultured. Whereas pharyngitis due to *A. haemolyticum* has resolved in the untreated patient, invasive disease caused by *A. haemolyticum* can be fatal.

References

Carlson P, Kontiainen S, Renkonen OV: Antimicrobial susceptibility of *Arcanobacterium haemolyticum*. Antimicrob Agents Chemother 38:142, 1994

Miller RA, Brancato F, Holmes KK: *Corynebacterium haemolyticum* as a cause of pharyngitis and scarlatiniform rash in young adults. Ann Intern Med 105:867, 1986

Nyman M, Banck G, Thore M: Penicillin tolerance in *Arcanobacterium haemolyticum*. J Infect Dis 161:261, 1990

Waagner DC: *Arcanobacterium haemolyticum:* biology of the organism and diseases in man. Pediatr Infect Dis J. 10:933-939, 1991

13.2.5　*Bacillus cereus*

Denise Bratcher

Bacillus cereus is a gram-positive, spore-forming, motile aerobic rod that also grows well anaerobically. A common soil saprophyte, *B. cereus* is ubiquitous in the environment, frequently isolated from plants, meat, eggs, and dairy products. It causes two different types of food poisoning: the emetic type, caused by a preformed, heat-stable toxin, and the diarrheal type, caused by toxin production from spores in the gastrointestinal tract. Although cases are likely underreported because of the relatively mild associated illnesses, it is an uncommon cause of food poisoning in the United States. Invasive disease caused by *B. cereus* is also described, especially in immunosuppressed patients, intravenous drug users, or patients with implanted devices.

EPIDEMIOLOGY　Food poisoning occurs as a result of eating either food contaminated with spores (diarrheal form) or food containing preformed toxin (emetic form). Spores of *B. cereus* are heat resistant, often surviving heating or cooking. The diarrheal type is caused by enterotoxins produced by *B. cereus* in the small intestines, and has an incubation period of 6 to 24 hours. This type is most often associated with contaminated meat or vegetables. The emetic form of food poisoning occurs after ingestion of preformed toxin, usually in contaminated fried or cooked rice, and has a much shorter incubation period of 30 minutes to 6 hours. Person-to-person transmission does not occur.

CLINICAL MANIFESTATIONS　The predominant symptoms of the diarrhea syndrome of food poisoning caused by *B. cereus* are profuse, watery diarrhea and abdominal cramps; vomiting occurs in about 25% of patients. The duration of illness is usually 12 to 24 hours. The emetic syndrome is characterized by nausea, vomiting, and abdominal cramps within hours of ingesting contaminated foods. Diarrhea also occurs in about one-third of patients and may be the result of additional enterotoxin production. The duration of illness is usually 6 to 24 hours. Both syndromes are usually mild and self-limited. Because *B. cereus* can be isolated from the stools of asymptomatic individuals, confirmation of food poisoning requires the isolation of *B. cereus* from a stool or emesis specimen in addition to its isolation from contaminated foodstuff (100,000 or more colony-forming units/g).

In recent years, *B. cereus* has emerged as a significant cause of virulent endophthalmitis following trauma, ranking as the second most common pathogen of posttraumatic ophthalmitis after *Staphylococcus epidermidis*. *Bacillus cereus* endophthalmitis typically follows a penetrating injury, usually due to a projectile foreign body. It also occurs among intravenous drug users. Severe pain develops rapidly in conjunction with a drastic reduction in visual acuity, chemosis, periorbital swelling, and proptosis. Patients often develop associated fever, leukocytosis, and malaise. Many patients require enucleation, and recovery of useful vision is rare. Management is aggressive, typically including surgical intervention, as well as parenteral, intraocular, and topical antimicrobial treatment.

Multiple other human infections caused by *B. cereus* have been reported. Although often considered contaminants, *B. cereus* and other *Bacillus* species have been increasingly identified as true pathogens. Clinically significant bacteremia due to *B. cereus* has been reported among neonates, intravenous drug users, immunocompromised patients, and those with an indwelling catheter or prosthetic device. *Bacillus cereus* is a small but significant cause of endocarditis, particularly when associated with intravenous drug use or valvular disease. Pneumonia is reported in immunosuppressed patients and neonates. Meningitis and brain abscess due to *B. cereus* have been documented, often occurring in children with ventricular shunts or neonates. The significance of isolation of *B. cereus* from wounds is often difficult to determine; the pathogenicity is supported by its presence in surgical biopsy specimens. Local disease manifests primarily in postsurgical or traumatic wounds or burn wounds. Severe deep infections such as necrotizing fasciitis and gangrene have occurred.

DIAGNOSIS   The diagnosis of invasive *B. cereus* infections is often hampered because *Bacillus* species are commonly considered contaminants. Among neonates, immunocompromised hosts, intravenous drug users, and other at-risk populations, *B. cereus* should be considered as a potential pathogen. *Bacillus cereus* grows readily on nutrient agar or peptone media at 25 to 37°C (77–98.6°F) and may require the addition of certain amino acids.

TREATMENT   *Bacillus cereus* food poisoning is self-limited and requires no antimicrobial therapy. Occasionally, severely dehydrated patients may require fluid and electrolyte replacement.

Antibiotic therapy is indicated in invasive *B. cereus* infections. While controlled clinical trials have not defined an optimal regimen, empiric therapy with vancomycin or clindamycin, with or without an aminoglycoside, is most commonly cited in the literature. *Bacillus cereus* is characterized by resistance to β-lactam antibiotics, but is usually susceptible in vitro to aminoglycosides, chloramphenicol, ciprofloxacin, clindamycin, erythromycin, imipenem, and vancomycin.

Surgical intervention is usually necessary in ophthalmic or skin infections due to *B. cereus*. Removal of prosthetic devices is typically necessary for a cure.

PREVENTION   Foodborne outbreaks of *B. cereus* can be prevented by appropriate storage and preparation of food, especially cooked rice. Bacterial growth in food may be prevented if hot food is kept above 60°C (140°F) or rapidly cooled to less than 10°C (50°F). Careful attention to aseptic technique and handwashing is necessary to prevent *B. cereus* infections among immunocompromised patients and those with indwelling devices.

References

Banerjee C, Bustamante CI, Wharton R, et al: *Bacillus* infections in patients with cancer. Arch Intern Med 148:1769–1774, 1988

Berner R, Heinen F, Pelz K, et al: Ventricular shunt infection and meningitis due to *Bacillus cereus*. Neuropediatrics 28:333–334, 1997

Cotton DJ, Gill VJ, Marshall DJ, et al: Clinical features and therapeutic interventions in 17 cases of *Bacillus* bacteremia in an immunosuppressed patient population. J Clin Microbiol 25:672–674, 1987

David DB, Kirkby, GR, Noble BA: *Bacillus cereus* endophthalmitis. Br J Ophthalmol 78:577–580, 1994

Patrick CC, Langston C, Baker CJ: *Bacillus* species infections in neonates. Rev Infect Dis 11:612–615, 1989

Sliman R, Rehm S, Shlaes DM, et al: Serious infections caused by *Bacillus* species. Medicine (Baltimore) 66:218–223, 1987

13.2.6   Brucellosis

Ralph C. Gordon

Brucella melitensis is a gram-negative coccobacillus that causes most of the human brucellosis seen in North America. This disease has been known as undulant fever, and its presentation may vary from a mild febrile illness to a major systemic disease with endocarditis, meningitis, arthritis, or osteomyelitis.

EPIDEMIOLOGY   Brucellosis is rare in the United States and infrequently seen in children. In 1997, only 20 of 98 cases reported to the Centers for Disease Control were patients aged 14 or younger. Until recently, brucellosis was primarily an occupational hazard for veterinarians and other individuals exposed to animals. This changed markedly with immunization of herds and improved sanitation in meat-processing plants so that infections ascribable to *B. abortus* (cattle) and *B. suis* (swine) have essentially disappeared. The typical patient seen in the United States now tends to be an Hispanic male from California or Texas who acquired *B. melitensis* from contaminated goat's milk or goat cheese that was imported from or ingested in Mexico.

CLINICAL MANIFESTATIONS   Because brucellosis in children is uncommon in North America, discussions of its presentation in the younger individual are often based on reports from the Middle East. Investigators in Israel found that evening or nocturnal fever, joint symptoms, and hepatomegaly and/or splenomegaly, accompanied by low white blood counts, normal to mildly elevated sedimentation rates, and elevated liver enzymes characterized most pediatric patients. Although death from brucellosis is unusual, this study found a 20% reinfection or relapse rate. A study of brucellosis in California found that children and teenagers had more gastrointestinal symptoms than did adults, and noted a low case-fatality rate of 0.1%. Similarly, only one death attributed to brucellosis was reported to the Centers for Disease Control in 1996.

DIAGNOSIS   Isolation of *Brucella* from blood cultures and use of serologic techniques are the two preferred methods of diagnosis.

Serologic assays in general use at this time are the serum agglutination test (SAT), which is positive at dilutions of 1/160 or greater, and a newer, more sensitive ELISA test reporting titers for IgG, IgM, and IgA antibodies. Both tests use *B. abortus* as the antigen in the United States, and the titers reported are based on cross-reactions. Patients with persisting bacteremia or evidence of relapse may need special radiographic studies, such as bone scans or abdominal scans, to look for specific foci of infection requiring surgical drainage or more prolonged treatment. *Brucella* titers tend to fall during treatment—a persistently high IgG titer suggests continuing infection.

TREATMENT In brucellosis, the organisms are found intracellularly in polymorphonuclear and mononuclear phagocytes. During bacteremia, organisms distribute throughout the reticuloendothelial system, localizing in the spleen and liver, as well as in other organs. The most effective antibiotics are those that penetrate into the intracellular environment. An effective regimen for adult patients has been doxycycline for 45 days, in combination with gentamicin for 7 days; or, alternatively, a combination of doxycycline and rifampin for 45 days. Ofloxacin has been found to be just as effective in combination with rifampin as a doxycycline-rifampin regimen in treatment of adults.

Treatment of the pediatric patient less than 8 years of age is difficult because of the need to avoid tetracycline; the American Academy of Pediatrics advises using trimethoprim-sulfamethoxazole for 4 to 6 weeks for younger children. For more serious infection, or in the presence of complications, a 7- to 14-day course of gentamicin can be added to the traditional regimen of trimethoprim-sulfamethoxazole and rifampin.

PREVENTION Individuals should avoid the ingestion of unpasteurized milk products and cheeses from Mexico. Goat's milk is most commonly involved in food source outbreaks of brucellosis at this time, but exposure to infected cattle and swine, or their products, can also lead to disease. Laboratory-acquired brucellosis has been reported on many occasions. There is an attenuated vaccine that can be used to immunize animals, but this product is responsible for human disease and can be hazardous to animal handlers.

References

Centers for Disease Control and Prevention: Summary of notifiable diseases, United States, 1997: MMWR Mortal Morb Wkly Rep 46:54, 1998

Chomel BB, DeBess EE, Mangiamele DM, et al: Changing trends in the epidemiology of human brucellosis in California from 1973 to 1992: a shift toward foodborne transmission. J Infect Dis 170:1216, 1994

Gottesman G, Vanunu D, Maayan MC, et al: Childhood brucellosis in Israel. Pediatr Infect Dis J 15:610, 1996

Solera J, Martinez-Alfaro E, Espinosa A: Recognition and optimum treatment of brucellosis. Drugs 53:245, 1997

3.2.7 *Burkholderia* and *Pseudomonas*

Jane L. Burns

Pseudomonas and *Burkholderia* species are nonlactose fermenting gram-negative bacilli that were classified in the same genus until recently. The name *Burkholderia* was proposed in 1992 for seven species that were previously classified as *Pseudomonas*. Because the two geni have related biochemical characteristics, *Burkholderia* may be misidentified as *Pseudomonas* or other nonfermenting gram-negative bacilli. The *B. cepacia*-complex (comprised of six subspecies, termed *genomovars*) is the most important *Burkholderia* species, causing infections in patients with cystic fibrosis and chronic granulomatous disease. *Burkholderia pseudomallei* is the etiologic agent of melioidosis, a common pediatric infection in Southeast Asia. Other *Burkholderia* species that occasionally cause human disease are *B. mallei*, the etiologic agent of glanders, a rare zoonosis seen in the Far East, and *B. gladioli*, an occasional cause of cystic fibrosis infection.

The most clinically important *Pseudomonas* species is *P. aeruginosa*, but *P. paucimobilis* has been increasingly recognized in both nosocomial and community-acquired infections. Other pseudomonads that are occasionally seen in human disease include *P. putida, P. fluorescens,* and *P. stutzeri.*

EPIDEMIOLOGY *Pseudomonas aeruginosa* is found widely in the natural environment, including in soil and water, and is also endemic in most hospital environments. It is an opportunistic pathogen that rarely causes disease in normal hosts, but it may cause serious infections in patients with underlying conditions, including neutropenia, immunodeficiency, and cystic fibrosis, and in hospitalized patients with wounds, burns, or indwelling catheters. The epidemiology of *P. aeruginosa* transmission is not well understood, but person-to-person transmissibility is suggested by studies of risk factors for colonization of young children with cystic fibrosis. However, common environmental sources cannot be excluded.

Burkholderia species are primarily plant and animal pathogens and are generally avirulent in healthy humans. Their distribution in nature appears to be somewhat more limited than pseudomonads, and they are less easily isolated from sources in either the natural or hospital environment. However, *B. cepacia*-complex, in particular, has a unique ability to grow in standard disinfectant solutions, which can result in serious nosocomial outbreaks. There is also good evidence of person-to-person transmission in cystic fibrosis.

CLINICAL MANIFESTATIONS Bacteremia with *P. aeruginosa* is commonly seen in neutropenic or burn patients who have acquired the organism nosocomially. *Pseudomonas paucimobilis* has also been recognized as a rare etiologic agent of septicemia in both immunocompromised patients and in previously well children. *Burkholderia cepacia* bacteremia has been described in cystic fibrosis patients and in patients with chronic granulomatous disease. In addition, pseudobacteremia has been reported in association with contaminated intravenous devices and solutions.

Both *P. aeruginosa* and *B. cepacia* are important causes of pulmonary infection in patients with cystic fibrosis. *Pseudomonas aeruginosa* can be isolated from the sputum of the majority of patients with cystic fibrosis. Worsening of pulmonary function is frequently associated with acquisition of the organism and/or conversion of the organism to a mucoid phenotype. Pulmonary exacerbations usually improve with antipseudomonal therapy. In contrast, *B. cepacia* is generally found in the sputum of only a small proportion of cystic fibrosis patients. However, these patients often have an exaggerated decline in pulmonary function and during their course may develop "cepacia syndrome," a systemic illness characterized by an often fatal necrotizing pneumonia.

Pneumonia is a common manifestation of both *P. aeruginosa* and *B. cepacia* infections in subpopulations of immunocompromised patients including children with hemoglobinopathies, malignancy, and human immunodeficiency virus infection. Pneumonia is also the most common manifestation of *B. cepacia* in chronic granulomatous disease.

Urinary tract infections caused by *P. aeruginosa* are associated with an indwelling urinary catheter or other foreign body, or are ascribable to obstruction of urinary drainage.

Pseudomonas folliculitis caused by immersion in contaminated hot tubs is a superficial self-limited infection in healthy hosts. Otitis externa, or "swimmer's ear," is most commonly caused by *P. aeruginosa*. *Pseudomonas aeruginosa* is also the etiology of osteochondritis associated with a puncture wound of the foot through the sole of a sneaker. Soft tissue infections caused by *P. aeruginosa* include infected decubitus ulcers and surgical wound infections. Lymph node infections caused by *P. paucimobilis* have been reported in previously healthy children and *B. cepacia* lymphadenitis has been described in chronic granulomatous disease.

Melioidosis caused by *B. pseudomallei* is a common pediatric infection in rural Southeast Asia, associated with underlying risk factors including diabetes mellitus and renal insufficiency. It may manifest as a localized infection or fulminant septicemia. Pneumonia is the most common localized presentation, but skin, bone, and soft tissue infections may also occur. In disseminated infections, patients are septicemic and hepatosplenic abscesses are occasionally seen. Relapse is common in severe disseminated disease.

DIAGNOSIS   Diagnosis of an invasive infection caused by *Pseudomonas* or *Burkholderia spp.* is based upon the isolation of the organism from a normally sterile site. In hospitalized patients, isolation of the organism may simply represent colonization, especially for patients with endotracheal tubes or tracheostomies or may be indicative of disease. However, in cystic fibrosis, pulmonary infection isolation of either *P. aeruginosa* or *B. cepacia* from oropharyngeal swab, sputum, or bronchoalveolar lavage fluid is presumptive evidence of infection and has been correlated with the presence of an antibody response. Nonaeruginosa pseudomonads and *B. gladioli* have also been isolated from cystic fibrosis sputum cultures, but their clinical significance is unclear.

Diagnosis of melioidosis can be made by isolation of the organism from the blood or other affected site. However, serologic assays and molecular diagnostic tests are currently being developed as rapid assays, because of the high mortality in septicemic disease.

TREATMENT   Both *Pseudomonas* and *Burkholderia spp.* are resistant to many antibiotics; susceptibility testing is required to determine optimum therapy. In addition, organisms can readily develop resistance after exposure to antimicrobial agents. *Pseudomonas aeruginosa* is commonly susceptible to extended-spectrum β-lactam agents (including ticarcillin with or without clavulanate, piperacillin with or without tazobactam, ceftazidime, cefaperazone, and cefepime) and aminoglycosides. Resistance to the quinolone antibiotics (including ciprofloxacin) seems to develop readily, and the carbapenem antibiotics (imipenem, meropenem) are generally reserved for resistant isolates or for use in immunocompromised patients as a single agent. For uncomplicated infection in a normal host, treatment with a single agent and removal of a foreign body, where appropriate, may be adequate therapy. However, in immunocompromised hosts or cystic fibrosis lung infection, potentially synergistic two-drug combinations are recommended (synergy testing of cystic fibrosis isolates is available through the Referral Center for Susceptibility and Synergy Studies at Columbia University, e-mail: synergy@columbia.com). *Burkholderia cepacia* is even more intrin-

sically resistant to antibiotics than *P. aeruginosa* and is uniformly resistant to the aminoglycosides and polymyxin. In addition to the quinolones and β-lactams, agents that may have activity against *B. cepacia* include doxycycline, chloramphenicol, and trimethoprim. *Burkholderia pseudomallei* is also highly resistant to antibiotics. Traditional therapies include doxycycline, chloramphenicol, and trimethoprim-sulfamethoxazole. However, in vitro studies suggest improved activity of piperacillin, amoxicillin-clavulanate, and third-generation cephalosporins; ceftazidime has demonstrated good activity in vivo.

PREVENTION   Both active and passive immunization strategies have been attempted for the prevention of *P. aeruginosa* infections in high-risk populations, including in patients with cystic fibrosis, immunocompromised patients, and following burns or major trauma. Antibiotic suppression of chronic *P. aeruginosa* infections in cystic fibrosis patients is widely practiced in Europe, and recent studies of inhaled high-dose tobramycin suggest clinical and microbiological efficacy.

References

Chaowagul W, White, NJ, Dance DAB, et al: Melioidosis: a major cause of community-acquired septicemia in northeastern Thailand. J Infect Dis 159:890–899, 1989

Fergie JE, Shema SJ, Lott L, et al: *Pseudomonas aeruginosa* bacteremia in immunocompromised children: analysis of factors associated with a poor outcome. Clin Infect Dis 18:390–394, 1994

Kosorok MR, Jalaluddin M, Farrell PM, et al: Comprehensive analysis of risk factors for acquisition of *Pseudomonas aeruginosa* in young children with cystic fibrosis. Pediatr Pulmonol 26:81–88, 1998

Ramsey BW, Pepe MS, Quan JM, et al: Chronic intermittent administration of inhaled tobramycin in patients with cystic fibrosis. N Engl J Med 340: 23–30, 1999

Saiman L, Mehar F, Niu WW, et al: Antibiotic susceptibility of multiply-resistant *Pseudomonas aeruginosa* isolated from patients with cystic fibrosis, including candidates for transplantation. Clin Infect Dis 23:532–537, 1996

13.2.8   *Campylobacter*

Guillermo Ruiz-Palacios and Larry K. Pickering

Campylobacter organisms are motile, comma-shaped, gram-negative bacilli that derive their name from the Greek words meaning "curved rod." *Campylobacter* has been recognized as a pathogen of many animal species including humans. There are 21 species of the genus *Campylobacter*, but only 12 are responsible for illness in humans: *C. jejuni, C. coli, C. fetus,* and *C. upsaliensis* are the most common species isolated from children. The species most frequently associated with acute infectious diarrhea are *C. jejuni* and *C. coli. Campylobacter jejuni* is a leading cause of bacterial enteritis. *Campylobacter upsaliensis, C. lari, C. hyointestinalis,* and *C. jejuni* subspecies *doylei* are associated with diarrhea, abdominal pain, fever, and vomiting. *Campylobacter fetus* is an infrequent cause of bacteremia and occasionally of meningitis in debilitated and immunocompromised individuals, including neonates.

EPIDEMIOLOGY   *Campylobacter jejuni* is found in the intestinal tract of turkeys, chickens, sheep, cattle, and other farm animals and birds, all of which serve as reservoirs of infection. The reservoirs for most other *Campylobacter* species also are animals. Contamination of meat, especially chickens, during slaughter may be the way bacteria enter the human food chain. The main source of *C. jejuni* and *C. coli* infection in humans is poultry, although milk, water, dogs, cats, hamsters, and ferrets are potential sources. In the United States from 1996 to 1998, *Campylobacter* was the most common organism detected by the Foodborne Diseases Active Surveillance Network (FoodNet). Because many species of *Campylobacter* other than *C. jejuni* and *C. coli* may not be detected by methods used by many microbiology laboratories, their prevalence may be underestimated.

Rates of *C. jejuni* infection in the United States peak in the summer and fall, but cases occur throughout the year. Common-source outbreaks of *C. jejuni* have occurred in school children following ingestion of unpasteurized milk. Person-to-person transmission also can occur, particularly among diapered children and in families. Outbreaks of diarrhea in childcare centers have been ascribed to person-to-person transmission, but these outbreaks are uncommon. Transmission to neonates from infected mothers can occur. Perinatal human infections due to *C. fetus* have been related to maternal infections during pregnancy or at the time of delivery. *Campylobacter fetus* also is responsible for abortion in cattle and sheep. The incubation period is usually 1 to 7 days, but it can be longer.

CLINICAL MANIFESTATIONS   Clinical manifestations of infection caused by *Campylobacter* range from absence of symptoms to fulminant sepsis and death. Manifestations depend on the species involved and characteristics of the host, such as age and immune status.

The most common clinical manifestation of *C. jejuni* and *C. coli* infection is gastroenteritis. The disease occurs in all ages but is more common in children less than 5 years of age, with a second peak at 15 to 29 years of age. Predominant symptoms include diarrhea, abdominal cramps (which occasionally are severe and sometimes mistaken for appendicitis), fever, headache, malaise, and myalgia. Diarrhea may be watery and profuse initially. After the first few days, stools contain blood in approximately 20% of individuals in developed countries, with lower rates of bloody diarrhea occurring in developing countries. Most persons recover in 5 to 7 days, but in 20%, the disease may be severe and prolonged or may recur. Severe or persistent infection in older children and adolescents can mimic acute inflammatory bowel disease.

Immunoreactive complications including reactive arthritis, Guillain-Barré syndrome, Reiter syndrome, and erythema nodosum have been associated with *C. jejuni* during the convalescent stage of infection. Serologic studies and culture results indicate that 20 to 40% of patients with Guillain-Barré syndrome are infected with *C. jejuni* in the 1 to 3 weeks prior to onset of neurologic symptoms.

Gastroenteritis due to *C. jejuni* or *C. coli* usually is not associated with bacteremia, except in neonates and immunocompromised individuals. Infection due to *C. fetus* is uncommon; when it occurs, typically in immunocompromised hosts, bacteremia and disseminated infection (including endocarditis, thrombophlebitis, and meningitis) can also be present. Bacteremia due to other species, including *C. upsaliensis, C. hypointestinalis, C. jejuni* subspecies *doylei,* and *C. concisus,* generally occurs in debilitated and immunocompromised individuals.

Perinatal infections are associated with *C. fetus,* but rarely with *C. jejuni.* The association of *C. fetus* and perinatal infection may be the consequence of the colonization of the maternal genital tract and to tropism for fetal tissue. Perinatal infections include abortion, stillbirth, premature labor, and neonatal sepsis and meningitis, each responsible for considerable morbidity and mortality.

DIAGNOSIS   Isolation of the organism from stool requires a selective enrichment medium containing antibiotics to suppress colonic microflora and a filtration method using cellulose membranes for isolation of species inhibited by antibiotics. Standard blood culture media are acceptable for the isolation of *Campylobacter* from blood and other sterile body sites, but slow growth requires that bottles be kept for at least 2 weeks. *Campylobacter fetus* generally is isolated from blood and rarely from stool.

TREATMENT   The most important aspects of therapy for gastroenteritis are rehydration and correction of electrolyte abnormalities. Most isolates of *C. jejuni* are susceptible to macrolides, quinolones, and aminoglycosides, although rapid emergence of resistance by *C. jejuni* has been documented to fluoroquinolones (eg, ciprofloxacin and ofloxacin) and less frequently to erythromycin. *Campylobacter jejuni* gastroenteritis is best treated early in the course of illness with oral erythromycin for 5 days at 40 mg/kg/day, maximum 2 g/day. When given early in the course of infection, antimicrobial therapy serves to shorten the duration of clinical symptoms and the period of excretion of the organism. Therapy given later in the course of gastroenteritis does not affect clinical signs or symptoms, but may decrease the period of excretion of the organism. HIV-infected individuals and other immunocompromised persons also should receive antibiotics for treatment of *Campylobacter* gastroenteritis. Ciprofloxacin or ofloxacin may be alternative agents in persons greater than 18 years of age. *Campylobacter jejuni* strains are almost universally resistant to cephalosporins, penicillin, vancomycin, and rifampin.

Bacteremia should be treated for 3 to 4 weeks with an antimicrobial agent to which the organism is susceptible, generally aminoglycosides, meropenem, or imipenem. The duration of therapy may need to be extended depending on clinical and microbiological response and the host's underlying immune status.

PREVENTION   Precautions against fecal-oral spread, especially hand washing, should be taken in homes and in childcare facilities. Appropriate handling, storage, and cooking of poultry should be stressed. Poultry and meat should be cooked until no longer pink in the middle [internal temperature greater than 73°C (165°F)]. Unpasteurized milk should not be ingested. HIV-infected persons should avoid animals less than 6 months of age, especially those with diarrhea. In the hospital, in addition to standard precautions, contact precautions are recommended for diapered and incontinent children for the duration of illness.

References

Allos BM, Blaser MJ: *Campylobacter jejuni* and the expanding spectrum of related infections. Clin Infect Dis 20:1092, 1995

Alterkruse SF, Stern NJ, Fields PI, Swerdlow DL: *Campylobacter jejuni*—an emerging foodborne pathogen. Emerg Infect Dis 5:28, 1999

Bourke B, Chan VL, Sherman P: *Campylobacter upsaliensis:* waiting in the wings. Clin Microbiol Rev 11:440, 1998

Pigrau C, Bartolome R, Almirante B, Planes AM, Gavalda J, Pahissa A: Bacteremia due to *Campylobacter* species: clinical findings and antimicrobial susceptibility patterns. Clin Infect Dis 25:1414, 1997

Wassenaar TM: Toxin production by *Campylobacter spp.* Clin Microbiol Rev 10:466, 1997

13.2.9   Cat-Scratch Disease

Andrew M. Margileth

Cat-scratch disease (CSD) is a benign, self-limited illness primarily ascribable to *Bartonella henselae* infection. It is characterized by chronic (≥ 3 weeks), tender, regional (cervical/axillary) lymphadenopathy, a history of cat contact with or without a scratch, and a primary skin lesion. In a healthy child, the enlarged node persists for several months and then resolves spontaneously. About 10% of patients have moderate to severe morbidity, including the oculoglandular syndrome, encephalopathy, seizures, systemic disease with blindness due to neuroretinitis, hepatosplenomegaly, prolonged fever, and, rarely, osteomyelitis or pancytopenia.

EPIDEMIOLOGY   Several thousand patients with CSD have been reported since its first description by Debre in 1950. Annually in the United States, an estimated 22,000 patients are diagnosed, with more than 2000 hospitalizations. About 80% of the cases occur in individuals under 21 years of age. The disease occurs worldwide, in all races, predominantly in males (55%). In warm, humid areas of the United States and other countries with a higher prevalence of cat fleas, there is a higher incidence of CSD. In cooler zones, CSD occurs more often during the fall and winter. Family outbreaks may occur, often involving siblings within 2 to 3 weeks of one another.

Recent studies provide both serologic and culture data to confirm a role for *Bartonella henselae* as an etiologic agent for CSD, especially in immunocompromised hosts. *Bartonella henselae* is the primary cause of clinical CSD in more than 90% of patients. *Bartonella henselae* has been isolated from cats and cat fleas and is a relatively common feline infection in young cats. *Afipia felis* rarely may cause CSD. Recently, two adults with clinical CSD, one with an extensive chest-wall abscess, were confirmed to have their illness caused by *B. clarridgeiae*. Severe CSD in individuals with AIDS manifests primarily as bacillary angiomatosis involving the skin, liver, bone, bone marrow, and spleen. Presently, there are 12 species of *Bartonella*.

CSD is transmitted by cutaneous, ocular, or mucous membrane inoculation. In most cases, the animal contact is a kitten younger than 1 year of age, although kittens may remain bacteremic with *B. henselae* for up to 2 years. Although the exact mechanism of cat to human transmission is unclear, recent studies have revealed that the cat flea, *Ctenosephalides felis,* readily transmitted *B. henselae* among cats. In the absence of fleas, transmission did not occur.

In the absence of cat contact, about 2 to 4% of patients report dog contact. Direct human-to-human transmission of *B. henselae* infection has not been reported.

An atypical presentation occurs in 10 to 14% of patients with CSD (Table 13-33). Parinaud oculoglandular syndrome is the most common, followed by encephalopathy; severe, chronic systemic disease; and neuroretinitis.

CLINICAL MANIFESTATIONS   Compilations of more than 2000 patients cite 95% with cat contact and 77% reporting cat scratches and/or a bite. A primary inoculation papule or pustule occurred in 54% of patients, an ocular granuloma in 6%, and mucous membrane ulcers were noted in 4%. Between 3 and 10 days can elapse from the time of the scratch or contact until a primary skin papule or pustule forms. Depending on the site of contact, unilateral con-

TABLE 13-33

CLINICAL MANIFESTATIONS IN CAT-SCRATCH DISEASE

CLINICAL FEATURE	NUMBER	PERCENT (%)
Typical presentation	1784	86
Inoculation lesion	1271	61
(skin, eye, mucous membrane)		
Unusual manifestations	299	14
Parinaud oculoglandular syndrome	125	6.1
Encephalopathy (radiculopathy)*	51	2.4
Systemic disease, severe, chronic	48	2.3
Neuroretinits	30	1.4
Erythema nodosum	15	0.7
Thrombocytopenic purpura	7	0.3
Hepatosplenomegaly	7	0.3
Osteomyelitis	8	0.3
Primary atypical pneumonia	3	0.1
Breast tumor	3	0.1
Angiomatoid papules	2	0.1

Findings in 2083 patients compiled by the author between 1957 and 1999.
*Complication in 14 patients with typical cat-scratch disease.

junctival granulomas occur occasionally (Table 13-34). Most primary lesions persist for 1 to 3 weeks, rarely for 6 weeks to 5 months. Within 2 weeks of the scratch (range 7–60 days), enlarged tender lymph nodes appear proximal to the inoculation site. In spite of extensive lymphadenopathy, patients usually are not ill. Only one-third of patients have fever greater than 101°F/38.3°C (range 101°–107.6°F/38.3°–42°C), usually lasting 5 to 9 days but rarely up to 2 months. Malaise, fatigue, headache, and anorexia may occur in 50% of patients. Less often, splenomegaly, sore throat, conjunctivitis, blindness, various rashes, and, rarely, arthralgias and/or parotid swelling occur. About 50% of children and adolescents have adenopathy only, whereas nearly 75% of adults develop some systemic signs or symptoms (Table 13-33).

Regional lymphadenopathy with single or multiple nodes is a hallmark of CSD. Because the upper extremities, head, and neck are the most likely sites for scratches, more than 80% of the involved nodes are in the axillary, epitrochlear, cervical, and/or supraclavic-

TABLE 13-34

CRITERIA FOR DIAGNOSIS OF CAT-SCRATCH DISEASE

Lymphadenopathy (≥ 10 mm) present ≥ 3 weeks.*

1. Cat or flea contact with or without a scratch mark or a regional inoculation lesion (skin papule, eye granuloma, mucous membrane).
2. Laboratory/radiology: Negative PPD or serology for other infectious causes of adenopathy; sterile pus aspirated from node; polymerase chain reaction assay positive for *Bartonella henselae* or *Afipia felis* (highest sensitivity). CT scan: liver/spleen abscesses.
3. Positive enzyme-linked immunoassay or immunofluorescent antibody assay serology test $>1{:}64$ for *B. henselae* or *Bartonella clarridgeiae.* Fourfold rise in titer between acute and convalescent specimens is definitive.
4. Biopsy of node, skin, liver, bone, or eye granuloma showing granulomatous inflammation compatible with cat-scratch disease; positive Warthin-Starry silver stain.

*Three of four criteria confirm the diagnosis; in an atypical case, all four criteria may be needed.

ular areas. Submandibular and preauricular lymphadenopathy also occurs. In about two-thirds of patients, the adenopathy consists of a single or several nodes in one region; the other one-third of patients have enlarged nodes in two or more anatomic sites. If adenopathy is detected in more than one area, a search should be made for additional inoculation lesions.

The majority of lymph nodes are 1 to 6 cm in diameter, but initially edema and swelling may extend 10 to 12 cm. During the first 2 weeks of illness, the nodes are usually tender. Erythema of overlying skin may occur early in the disease and resolve as the node decreases in size. Cellulitis is observed rarely.

The lymphadenopathy usually regresses over 2 to 4 months but can persist for 1 to 3 years in 1 to 2% of patients. Large lymph nodes with erythema and tenderness regress more slowly and tend to be suppurative. Approximately 15% of nodes suppurate.

Unusual clinical manifestations occurring in 14% of reported patients include: the oculoglandular syndrome of Parinaud; encephalitis; neuroretinitis; severe chronic systemic disease, with or without hepatosplenomegaly; thrombocytopenic purpura; osteomyelitis; and primary atypical pneumonia. CSD should always be considered in any patient with an ocular lesion and parotid-area swelling due to preauricular lymphadenopathy (see Table 13-33).

Children with central nervous system involvement (1–2% of patients) may develop encephalopathy, meningitis, radiculitis, polyneuritis, or myelitis with paraplegia. The onset of blindness or neurologic symptoms is usually sudden and occurs within 1 to 6 weeks of the onset of adenopathy. In 61 patients with central nervous system involvement, the frequency of major symptoms and signs found was convulsions or coma in 75%, neurologic and/or behavioral abnormalities in 97%, and fever in 50%. In 48% of the patients, cerebrospinal fluid pleocytosis, elevated protein, or both were detected.

Electroencephalograms were abnormal for one to several months in the majority of these patients. Severe manifestations have lasted 1 to 2 weeks, with gradual recovery to normal status in 1 to 12 months in all patients. Visual acuity improved greatly in 30 subjects with neuroretinitis. Recovery from thrombocytopenic purpura, osteomyelitis, pneumonitis, and Parinaud syndrome has been complete.

Although responsible for severe illness in the immunocompromised patient, CSD may be missed or confused with other clinical manifestations related to human immunodeficiency virus (HIV). Although CSD has not been reported in children with HIV, the syndrome in 49 adults was characterized by unusual lesions of skin, bone, brain, liver, and spleen as a consequence of bacillary angiomatosis and peliosis. Paradoxically, the lesions had an excellent response to antibiotic therapy. CSD patients with HIV often present with numerous generalized skin lesions, ranging from pink to deep reddish-purple papules to sessile or pedunculated nodules. The nodules are firm, indurated, and usually nontender. These nodules range in size from 1 to 6 cm. Clinically, the lesions are indistinguishable from Kaposi sarcoma, histiocytoid hemangioma, epithelioid hemangioma, and/or pyogenic granuloma. Radiographs of lesions located over bone may show bone loss and periostosis, as well as a large soft-tissue mass.

DIAGNOSIS The diagnosis of CSD is based upon clinical features and is confirmed with specific serologic studies. Performance of a *Bartonella* polymerase chain reaction (PCR) hybridization assay on lymph node and/or abscess aspirates or a biopsy specimen provides the highest diagnostic sensitivity. Although certain serologic tests for diagnosis are available from several commercial laboratories, en-

zyme-linked immunoassay (EIA) to detect IgM *B. henselae* antibodies are only 71% sensitive in patients who fulfill two or more criteria for CSD. The CDC (and some state health departments) performs a very sensitive (96–98%) immunofluorescent antibody assay (IFA) for *B. henselae* antibody. The IFA test for *B. henselae* has both high sensitivity (98%) and specificity (98%).

Lymph nodes may show distinct but nonspecific stages: reticulum cell hyperplasia followed by tubercle-like or stellate granulomas, then multiple microabscesses, and, ultimately, frank abscess formation. The pathology may be confused with tularemia, brucellosis, tuberculosis, or sarcoidosis. Small pleomorphic gram-negative bacteria are best demonstrated by the Warthin-Starry silver impregnation stain from skin lesions or lymph nodes removed during the first 3 to 4 weeks after the onset of illness. The CSD bacilli are found less frequently in stellate granulomas with suppurative or caseous centers, and when seen, the organisms are degenerating.

The CSD skin test, a delayed hypersensitivity-type skin test, is still a valuable diagnostic tool, but usually not available. The positive skin test reaction consists of a wheal or papule with 5 mm or more of induration, with or without erythema, occurring 48 to 72 hours after intradermal inoculation of 0.1 mL of antigen. Induration may persist for 5 to 6 days or longer. A positive test may be obtained for about 10 years after an episode of CSD. Although the CSD skin test is reliable, safe, and has excellent specificity (90–98%) with a sensitivity of 80 to 100%, *Bartonella* serology is readily available through commercial laboratories. Both the skin or serology tests may be negative if duration of illness is less than 3 or 4 weeks.

Eosinophilia is reported in 8 to 43% of patients. Initially, the number of polymorphonuclear cells in peripheral blood may be increased, with a mild leukocytosis. The ESR is usually elevated during the first few weeks of adenopathy, thus suggesting inflammatory lymphadenitis.

Three of the four criteria (Table 13-34) confirm the diagnosis in a typical illness. All four criteria may be necessary in an atypical illness, including a node biopsy showing histopathology consistent with CSD. The presence of pleomorphic rod-shaped bacilli on the Warthin-Starry silver stain, however, is not specific for *B. henselae*. If the diagnosis remains uncertain, a biopsy must be considered to rule out a benign tumor or lymphoma. CSD should be considered in all patients with persistent or chronic lymphadenopathy, because it is the most common cause of regional lymphadenitis in children and adolescents. The differential diagnosis includes lymphogranuloma venereum; typical or atypical tuberculosis; bacterial adenitis; tularemia; brucellosis; histoplasmosis; coccidioidomycosis; sarcoidosis; toxoplasmosis; infectious mononucleosis; and benign or malignant tumors.

TREATMENT AND PROGNOSIS The majority of patients need no active therapy. The parents and child should be reassured that the adenopathy is benign and that it will probably subside spontaneously within 2 to 4 months. Thus, management consists of reassurance, analgesics for pain, and prudent follow-up. If suppuration occurs, aspiration relieves painful adenopathy, and the patient usually becomes symptom-free within 24 to 48 hours. If fluid reaccumulates, reaspiration may be needed. Incision and drainage is not recommended because chronic (6–13 months) sinus tract drainage may result.

For the moderate to severely ill patient azithromycin (Zithromax) 5 to 12 mg/kg per day once daily, or rifampin, 20 mg/kg per day in two doses for 2 to 3 weeks, may be quite effective. For children over 12 years of age, ciprofloxacin, 20 to 30 mg/kg per day in two doses for 2 to 3 weeks, may also be effective. Oral trimethoprim-sulfamethoxazole (TMP-SMX), 10 mg TMP/50 mg SMX/kg per day, may be effective given two or three times daily for 7 to 10 days or longer, depending upon clinical response. In a severely ill patient suspected of having CSD, administration of IM or IV gentamicin may be prudent. No well-controlled, randomized clinical trials have been conducted that clearly demonstrate a clinically significant benefit of antimicrobials for the treatment of CSD.

Paradoxically, patients infected with HIV and associated systemic illness, with angiomatous skin nodules, hepatitis, involvement of the spleen, and/or lytic bone lesions as a consequence of either *B. henselae* or *B. quintana* have responded promptly to commonly used antibiotics (erythromycin, doxycycline, antimycobacterial drugs).

The prognosis is excellent; lymphadenopathy usually regresses spontaneously in 2 to 4 months. One attack appears to confer lifelong immunity. Complications and sequelae are rare and have not been reported in typical illnesses. Second attacks of CSD occurred in three adults in one study of over 2000 patients.

PREVENTION   The suspect cat need not be destroyed as it is invariably well; only 5% of family members scratched by the same cat develop CSD. The patient with CSD does not require isolation or quarantine, because there is no evidence of disease spread from human to human. Rigorous control of flea infestation in pets is essential for immunocompromised subjects. Preventative measures include declawing and regular nail clipping of young cats; keeping cats indoors; flea control; proper handling of the litter box; washing hands after close contact with a cat, especially a kitten; and washing bites and scratches with soap and water.

References

Arisoy ES, Correa AG, Wagner ML, Kaplan SL: Hepatosplenic cat-scratch disease in children: selected clinical features and treatment. Clin Infect Dis 28:778–784, 1999

Bass JW, Vincent JM, Person DA: The expanding spectrum of *Bartonella* infection: II. Cat-scratch disease. Pediatr Infect Dis J 16:163–179, 1997

Brouqui P, Lascola B, Roux V, Raoult D: Chronic *Bartonella quintana* bacteremia in homeless patients. N Engl J Med 340:184–189, 1999

Grando D, Sullivan LJ, Flexman JP, et al: *Bartonella henselae* associated with Parinaud's oculo-glandular syndrome. Clin Infect Dis 28:1156–1158, 1999

Jacobs RF, Schutze GE: *Bartonella henselae* as a cause of prolonged fever and fever of unknown origin in children. Clin Infect Dis 26:80–84, 1998

Koehler JE, Sanchez MA, Garrido CS, et al: Molecular epidemiology of *Bartonella* infections in patients with bacilliary angiomatosis-peliosis. N Engl J Med 337:1876–1883, 1997

Kordick DL, Brown TT, Shin K, Breitschwerdt EB: Clinical and pathological evaluation of chronic *Bartonella henselae* or *Bartonella clarridgeiae* infection in cats. J Clin Microbiol 37:1536–1547, 1999

13.2.10   Chancroid

Stephen J. Barenkamp

Chancroid is a sexually transmitted disease caused by the organism *Haemophilus ducreyi*. The illness is characterized by painful genital ulcers and tender inguinal adenopathy that may suppurate. Also known as "soft chancre," chancroid is one of the three major causes of genital ulcer disease among young sexually active patients in this country; the other major causes are genital herpes and syphilis. Among the patient population seen by pediatricians, chancroid is seen principally among teenagers and young adults. Because sexual contact is the only known route of transmission, sexual abuse must be strongly suspected if chancroid is diagnosed in a child.

Haemophilus ducreyi appears microscopically as a pleomorphic gram-negative rod. *Haemophilus ducreyi* was originally assigned to the *Haemophilus* genus, but more recent studies, including genetic transformation and DNA hybridization analyses, suggest that *Haemophilus ducreyi* is not related to the true haemophili and should be placed in a separate genus.

EPIDEMIOLOGY   Chancroid is a common cause of genital ulcer disease throughout the world. Although generally considered a relatively uncommon cause of disease in the United States, it continues to be diagnosed, particularly among individuals from lower socioeconomic groups. The highest incidence of disease is reported among patients, including adolescents, presenting with genital ulcer disease in large urban areas. Symptomatic disease in this country has been reported most commonly among nonwhite heterosexual males. However, symptomatic disease is not restricted to men. Female prostitutes have been implicated as important sources of infection in several of the outbreaks described in the United States. Recent data suggest that chancroid may be more common in this country than previously suspected, as it can be difficult to correctly diagnose by traditional clinical and laboratory means.

Chancroid is said to be particularly common in Africa, Asia, and Latin America, where it may be a more common cause of genital ulcer disease than is syphilis. Epidemiologic studies, primarily from Africa, demonstrate that the presence of genital ulcer disease, much of which may represent chancroid, is strongly associated with an increased risk of heterosexual transmission of human immunodeficiency virus (HIV) infection.

CLINICAL MANIFESTATIONS   The incubation period of chancroid is usually between 4 and 7 days; rarely less than 3 days or more than 10 days. Typically, the first lesion noted is a small inflammatory papule surrounded by a zone of erythema. Within 2 or 3 days a pustule forms that soon ruptures, leaving a sharply circumscribed ulcer with ragged undermined edges *without* induration. The base of the ulcer usually has a granular appearance and is always painful. In males, the most common sites for the ulcers are on the distal prepuce, the mucosal surface of the prepuce on the frenulum, or in the coronal sulcus. In females, the majority of lesions are at the entrance to the vagina. Painful tender inguinal adenopathy is present in as many as 50% of patients and is usually unilateral. The involved lymph nodes may rapidly become fluctuant and rupture, with the formation of inguinal ulcers.

The combination of a painful ulcer with tender inguinal adenopathy is suggestive of chancroid, and when accompanied by suppurative inguinal adenopathy is almost pathognomonic. However, a substantial percentage of patients with *Haemophilus ducreyi* infection may have ulcers that can be confused with other causes of genital ulcer disease such as herpes simplex virus (HSV) or syphilis. As many as 10% of patients with chancroid may be *coinfected* with *Treponema pallidum* or HSV. Thus, it becomes mandatory to establish a definitive diagnosis by laboratory means if one is to feel confident of the correct diagnosis.

DIAGNOSIS   As noted earlier, making a diagnosis of chancroid on clinical grounds alone is difficult because the clinical presentation is often not classic and many clinicians do not have a great deal of experience with the disease. Definitive diagnosis of chancroid requires isolation of the organism from a genital ulcer or from involved lymph nodes. However, the organism is quite fastidious and is difficult to isolate, even under the best of circumstances. To obtain specimens for culture, a swab should be used to obtain material from the purulent base of an ulcer or a fluctuant inguinal lymph node should be aspirated directly. Gram stain of purulent material may reveal gram-negative rods in the characteristic "school-of-fish" pattern, but this appearance is probably more characteristic of in vitro propagated organisms. Even with use of the selective media now recommended for isolation of *Haemophilus ducreyi*, it is estimated that the sensitivity of culture is no higher than 80%.

Given the low sensitivity of culture, alternative nonculture-based diagnostic tests have been evaluated. Serologic assays have been evaluated as diagnostic aids, but they lack sensitivity during the acute stages of infection and are not available commercially. Nucleotide-based diagnostic methods have also been investigated over the last few years. Perhaps most promising are the polymerase chain reaction (PCR)-based techniques. These assays demonstrate high sensitivity and, in addition, appear to identify a number of patients with chancroid, from whom bacterial cultures for *Haemophilus ducreyi* are negative. Multiplex PCR assays that can simultaneously amplify and subsequently detect DNA from *Haemophilus ducreyi*, *Treponema pallidum*, and HSV from genital ulcer specimens are undergoing field trials and show promise. PCR testing may be commercially available in the near future.

Even if chancroid is diagnosed definitively, it is recommended that patients also be tested for HIV at the time of diagnosis. In addition, it must be remembered that up to 10% of patients with chancroid may be coinfected with *Treponema pallidum* or HSV. Appropriate testing for these other pathogens should be strongly considered when a patient presents with any form of genital ulcer disease.

TREATMENT AND PROGNOSIS Successful antimicrobial treatment of genital ulcers caused by *Haemophilus ducreyi* cures infection, resolves clinical symptoms, and prevents transmission to others. However, in cases of extensive ulcerative disease, scarring may result despite successful antimicrobial therapy. The Centers for Disease Control and Prevention currently recommend one of four antibiotic regimens for treatment of chancroid: (a) azithromycin: 1 g orally in a single dose; (b) ceftriaxone: 250 mg intramuscularly in a single dose; (c) ciprofloxacin: 500 mg orally twice a day for 3 days; or (d) erythromycin base: 500 mg orally 4 times a day for 7 days. All four regimens are effective for treatment of chancroid in patients with HIV infection. A successful response to therapy is usually evident within 48 to 72 hours, as evidenced by decreased ulcer tenderness and pain. Complete healing of ulcers may take up to 28 days, but is often achieved in 7 to 14 days. Healing of fluctuant adenopathy is slower than that of the ulcers and may require needle aspiration through adjacent intact skin even during successful therapy.

Patients with HIV infection must be closely monitored, as they may require longer courses of antimicrobials than the standard regimens outlined above. Treatment failures have been observed with several of these regimens, and there is some suggestion that those individuals who are most immunosuppressed are at the greatest risk for failure of standard regimens. The erythromycin 7-day regimen appears to be most successful in HIV-infected persons.

PREVENTION To prevent further spread of *Haemophilus ducreyi* disease, it is critical to identify all sexual contacts of infected indi-

viduals. The CDC recommends that all persons who have had sexual contact with a patient with proven *Haemophilus ducreyi* infection within the 10 days before onset of the patient's symptoms should be examined and treated. The examination and treatment of contacts should be administered even in the absence of symptoms.

References

Al-Tawfiq JA, Palmer KL, Chen C-Y, et al: Experimental infection of human volunteers with *Haemophilus ducreyi* does not confer protection against subsequent challenge. J Infect Dis 179:1283–1287, 1999

Centers for Disease Control and Prevention: 1998 Guidelines for treatment of sexually transmitted diseases. Morb Mortal Wkly Rep 47(No. RR-1): 1–116, 1998

Di Carlo RP, Martin DH: The clinical diagnosis of genital ulcer disease in men. Clin Infect Dis 25:292–298, 1997

Mertz KJ, Weiss JB, Webb RM, et al: An investigation of genital ulcers in Jackson, Mississippi, with use of a multiplex polymerase chain reaction assay: high prevalence of chancroid and human immunodeficiency virus infection. J Infect Dis 178:1060–1066, 1998

Trees DL, Morse SA: Chancroid and *Haemophilus ducreyi*: an update. Clin Microbiol Rev 8:357, 1995

13.2.11   Chlamydial Infections

Mary Allen Staat

Chlamydia are nonmotile, gram-negative, obligatory intracellular bacteria that cannot produce energy. The infectious particle, known as an elementary body, attaches to the surface of a susceptible cell and is phagocytized, then transformed into a reticulate body, a larger metabolically active particle that divides by binary fission. After 48 hours, multiplication stops, and the products of division are released from the cell as elementary bodies, ready to infect new cells. *Chlamydia* can be grown in tissue culture on susceptible cells.

The four recognized species within the genus of *Chlamydia* are *C. psittaci, C. pneumoniae,* and *C. trachomatis,* all of which cause disease in humans, and *C. pecorum* which does not. *Chlamydia psittaci* is responsible for psittacosis (ornithosis), and *C. pneumoniae* causes pneumonia, pharyngitis, and bronchitis. *Chlamydia trachomatis* has up to 15 different serotypes, known as serovars (Table 13-35), that are associated with a spectrum of diseases. Serovars A to C are associated with trachoma, D to K with genital infections, and L1 to L3 with lymphogranuloma venereum. The most common infections of *C. trachomatis* are those of the genital tract—urethritis and epididymitis in the male, cervicitis and salpingitis in the female—and neonatal conjunctivitis and pneumonia in infants, who acquire the infection by passage through an infected genital tract.

Chylamydia trachomatis

Infections of the Genital Tract

Nongonococcal Urethritis Nongonococcal urethritis in the male is a common sexually transmitted infection, caused by *Chlamydia* in 35 to 50% of cases: ureaplasma and possibly other causes account for the remainder. The presumptive diagnosis is made by excluding gonorrhea by smear and culture of the purulent urethral discharge, or by rapid tests using ligase or polymerase chain reaction (PCR)

TABLE 13-35

CHLAMYDIAL INFECTIONS IN HUMANS

SPECIES	SEROVAR	CLINICAL MANIFESTATIONS
Chlamydia trachomatis	A, B, C	Trachoma
	D–K	Urethritis, epididymitis, cervicitis, pelvic inflammatory disease, inclusion conjunctivitis, infantile pneumonia
	L1–L3	Lymphogranuloma venereum
Chlamydia psittaci		Psittacosis, ornithosis
Chlamydia pneumoniae		Pharyngitis, cough, pneumonia

testing of urine. The definitive diagnosis is made by culturing *Chlamydia* from the discharge.

The treatment of choice for chlamydial urethritis is azithromycin 1 g orally in a single dose or doxycycline 100 mg orally twice a day for 7 days. Erythromycin is another alternative drug. Successful treatment requires that the sexual partners of the patient be treated as well.

Epididymitis Epididymitis, an important complication of urethritis in young men, is most likely caused by gonococcal and/or chlamydial infection and is treated with oral doxycycline for 10 days and ceftriaxone 250 mg IM in a single dose.

Female Genital Tract Infections In most women chlamydial infections are asymptomatic, but clinical manifestations include endocervical erosion, mucopurulent cervical exudate, and urethritis. Definitive diagnosis depends on demonstration of *Chlamydia* in a cervical specimen either by tissue culture or by the rapid direct slide immunofluorescent method using monoclonal antibodies. Testing the urine by lyase or PCR tests is another method by which the diagnosis can be made. *Chlamydia* is also responsible for approximately 25% of salpingitis, and therapeutic regimens should include doxycycline (or erythromycin). Sexual partners must also be treated. Chlamydial infection is a common cause of pelvic inflammatory disease in sexually active adolescent females (see Sec. 3.6).

Lymphogranuloma Venereum Lymphogranuloma venereum is a sexually transmitted chlamydial disease caused by serovars L1 to L3. The incidence of this disease has progressively declined in the United States; however, it is still quite prevalent in many developing countries. The disease is rare in children, infrequent in adolescents, and shows a marked male predominance.

The clinical course is divided into three stages. The primary lesion, transient and clinically mild, usually appears as a papule or a shallow ulcer on the penis or vaginal wall. Systemic manifestations can include fever, chills, and anorexia. Pronounced lymphadenitis or lymphadenopathy in the inguinal area represents the secondary lesion, which occurs 2 to 6 weeks later; the nodes are large and often fluctuant (buboes). This form of disease is found predominantly in males. The tertiary form (not necessarily preceded by lymphadenopathy) presents as strictures in the anal, rectal, and vaginal areas. Once suspected, the diagnosis can be best confirmed by complement-fixation or microimmunofluorescence tests, using the specific antigens. The treatment of choice is doxycycline 100 mg orally twice a day for 21 days.

Perinatally Transmitted Infections

Two to 13% of women have positive chlamydial cervical culture at delivery. Babies born through an infected birth canal are at risk of acquiring the infection and of developing inclusion conjunctivitis, pneumonia, or both.

Newborn Inclusion Conjunctivitis Acute purulent conjunctivitis in the newborn, also known as inclusion blenorrhea, affects approximately 35% of infants born through infected birth canals; the incidence appears to be 10 to 80 per 1000 live births. The incubation period is 5 to 12 days. The infant develops a watery discharge from the eyes that becomes progressively more purulent, and the eyelids become swollen. If the condition is untreated, lymphoid follicles and a membranous conjunctivitis can develop and persist for weeks or months. The conjunctivitis must be distinguished from that produced by pyogenic bacteria (*N. gonorrhoeae, S. aureus,* and others), as well as from adenovirus and herpesvirus infections and from chemical conjunctivitis resulting from silver nitrate prophylaxis. Conjunctival cultures on blood and chocolate agar media will rule out bacterial pathogens. The most useful diagnostic method is examination of Giemsa-stained conjunctival scrapings and demonstration of inclusion bodies. Because *Chlamydia* are obligate intracellular agents, the conjunctivae must be scraped rather than swabbed to get the inclusion bodies onto the slide. *Chlamydia* can also be demonstrated by culture, immunofluorescence, or ELISA. The conjunctivitis responds symptomatically to topical treatment with sulfonamides, tetracycline, or erythromycin. Optimal management, however, is to prescribe oral erythromycin, 40 to 50 mg/kg per day for 2 weeks. This regimen facilitates faster resolution of the conjunctivitis and also serves to prevent the development of chlamydial pneumonia by eradicating colonizing *Chlamydia* in the nasopharynx.

Attempts to provide prophylaxis against inclusion blenorrhea have not met with success. Neither erythromycin nor tetracycline instilled into the eyes at birth is 100% effective. Prevention can be achieved only by identifying and treating pregnant women prior to delivery.

Chlamydial Pneumonia of Infancy Chlamydial pneumonia is an important infection during the first 6 months of life; 10 to 20% of infants born through infected genital tracts will develop pneumonia. Identifying culture-positive women during the last trimester and treating them (and their sexual partners) with a 2-week course of oral erythromycin prevents disease in the newborn. The diagnosis of chlamydial pneumonia (or conjunctivitis) in a neonate is clear evidence of maternal infection, and both parents should be treated.

Trachoma

Trachoma produces chronic inflammation of the mucous membranes of the eye and is a major cause of blindness in many developing countries of the world. The disease is spread from eye to eye;

poor sanitation contributes to its prevalence. Flies can be involved as mechanical vectors.

Trachoma starts as follicular conjunctivitis. The follicles heal with necrosis, which can cause severe conjunctival scarring, which, in turn, produces lacrimal stenosis, lid distortion, and entropion, resulting in severe scarring of the cornea and blindness. The end result occurs only after many years of active disease. A World Health Organization expert committee suggested that the diagnosis of trachoma requires at least two of the following four criteria: lymphoid follicles on the upper tarsal conjunctiva; typical conjunctival scarring; vascular pannus; and limbal follicles.

Trachoma is prevalent in countries afflicted by poverty and poor sanitation. The incidence of active disease in such communities is highest among children under 10 years of age. Teenagers are less likely to be infected, and only 5% of adults show signs of active disease. The diagnosis is usually clinical; it can be confirmed by examining conjunctival scrapings with Giemsa stain or immunofluorescence demonstrating the infective particles. *Chlamydia* can also be cultured with embryonated eggs or tissue culture. Serologic tests are not very helpful clinically, but they are important epidemiologic tools. The treatment and control of trachoma are complex and involve important international health issues that are not dealt with in this section.

Chlamydia psittaci

Psittacosis (ornithosis) is contracted by human beings from infected birds such as parrots and related species (parakeets, cockatoos, finches); ornithosis is the term used for infections acquired from other birds. *Chlamydia* cause a natural infection in turkeys, pigeons, ducks, chickens, and other fowl; the birds may appear ill and may die, or they may show almost no evidence of disease. Birds transmit the disease to human beings by the respiratory route, and the incidence is higher among poultry workers and possibly pet shop workers. Person-to-person transmission is also possible, and health care personnel can acquire the disease from patients. The incidence has decreased since the implantation of importation controls of parrots into the United States. Children acquire the disease infrequently.

Clinically there are two forms of this infection: the more common form presents with fever, chills, headache, and pneumonia; less commonly, it may present like severe influenza or a mild case of typhoid fever. The incubation period is 7 to 14 days. The patient's temperature rises steadily, and there may be complaints of headache, malaise, and nausea. Mental confusion may be observed. If pneumonia is present, as it is in most patients, the cough is prominent; the sputum may be blood-streaked. Radiologically, the appearance is that of extensive interstitial pneumonia. Untreated, the disease lasts several weeks. Once it is suspected (usually as an atypical pneumonia or epidemiologically because of contact with birds), the best methods of confirmation are serologic, namely a four-fold rise in specific antibody or isolation of the infective agent in tissue culture. The treatment of choice is tetracycline for 21 days, given orally if tolerated, or otherwise parenterally. The results of therapy are not dramatic. Erythromycin is probably effective as an alternative agent.

Chlamydia pneumoniae

Within the past two decades *Chlamydia* were found to be a common and important cause of community-acquired pneumonia in older children and adults. The first two isolates from young adults were designated TW-183 and AR-39, and the agent was designated

TWAR. Since then, the agent has been found to be antigenically distinct from the other two species of *Chlamydia* and has been recognized as a third species to infect humans—*C. pneumoniae*, unlike *C. psittaci*, appears to be a primary human pathogen. Epidemiologic studies have revealed that *C. pneumoniae* is a fairly common cause of infection in children >7 years of age and in young adults; along with *Mycoplasma*, it probably is the most common cause of community-acquired pneumonia. The clinical manifestations range from very mild to severe pneumonia. Sometimes it causes bronchitis without pneumonia. Small epidemics have been described in colleges and among military recruits. This organism is difficult to culture; the diagnosis is based on serology, and is usually retrospective.

Treatment of choice is erythromycin or tetracycline; the former is preferred for children younger than 8 years. The optimal duration of therapy is not clear, but a course of up to 3 weeks may be necessary.

References

Campbell LA, Perez-Melgosa M, Hamilton DJ, et al: Detection of *Chlamydia pneumoniae* by polymerase chain reaction. J Clin Microbiol 30: 434–439, 1992

Carballal G, Mahony JB, Videla C, et al: Chlamydial antibodies in children with lower respiratory disease. Pediatr Infect Dis J 11:68–71, 1992

Centers for Disease Control and Prevention: 1998 Guidelines for treatment of sexually transmitted diseases. MMWR Morb Mortal Wkly Rep 47: (No. RR1), 1998

Grayston JT, Aldous MB, Easton A, et al: Evidence that *Chlamydia pneumoniae* causes pneumonia and bronchitis. J Infect Dis 168:1231–1235, 1993

Heggie AD, Jaffe AC, Stuart LA, et al: Topical sulfacetamide vs oral erythromycin for neonatal chlamydial conjunctivitis. Am J Dis Child 139: 564–566, 1985

Oldach DW, Gaydos CA, Mundy LM, et al: Rapid diagnosis of *Chlamydia psittaci* pneumonia. Clin Infect Dis 17:338–343, 1993

Schachter J, Grossman M, Azimi PH: Serology of *Chlamydia trachomatis* in infants. J Infect Dis 146:530–535, 1982

Schachter J, Sweet RL, Grossman M, et al: Experience with routine use of erythromycin for chlamydial infections in pregnancy. N Engl J Med 314: 276–279, 1986

Tipple MA, Beem MO, Saxon EM: Clinical characteristics of afebrile pneumonia associated with *Chlamydia trachomatis* infection in infants less than 6 months of age. Pediatrics 63:192–197, 1979

13.2.12   Cholera

Ashir Kumar

An acute life-threatening disease characterized by enormous loss of fluid and electrolytes due to profuse diarrhea and vomiting, cholera has been responsible for global scourges for centuries. The most recent pandemic of cholera started in Chennai (formerly Madras), India, by the first non-O1 *Vibrio cholerae* serogroup called O139 Bengal strain. This strain rapidly spread from Calcutta to Bangladesh, and later to Thailand. Continued spread throughout the world would represent the eighth cholera pandemic. The outbreaks caused by *V. cholerae* O139 have spread rapidly, even among the elderly who were previously exposed to cholera caused by *V. cholerae* O1. This suggests that the immunity to *V. cholerae* O1, whether from natural infection or vaccination, is not protective against *V. cholerae* O139.

EPIDEMIOLOGY Endemic cholera primarily affects children. The infection is most prevalent among children in the 2- to 4-year age group; however, *V. cholerae* O139 has been reported in newborns. Endemic cholera cases mainly occur during the summer and monsoon months on the Indian subcontinent. Imported cases of *V. cholerae* O139 has been reported in the United States. In 1992, 103 cholera cases were reported in the United States, primarily in travelers returning from Latin America, Asia, and Africa.

Strains of *V. cholerae* have been isolated from aquatic environments in areas where the disease is endemic, as well as from areas where no cases occur. The organism is well adapted to warm stagnant environments with increased salinity. Bacteria easily grow on chitinous shellfish, which explains the reports of cholera following ingestion of seafood. The classic fecal-oral paradigm is a well-known means of transmission; however, contamination of a variety of foods by food handlers or contamination of fresh fruit and vegetables by cholera-contaminated water has also been attributed to the spread of disease. Occasionally, a case is acquired from contaminated food in the United States. Healthy individuals shedding the organism also contribute by contaminating food items, as well as by contaminating the environment.

MICROBIOLOGY *Vibrio cholerae* is a gram-negative, highly mobile, curved bacillus with a single polar flagellum. There are at least 140 somatic serogroups based on somatic (O) antigens. Although nontoxigenic strains of *V. cholerae* are occasionally isolated from patients with diarrhea or sepsis, cholera is caused only by cholera toxin–producing strains of O1 or O139 serogroups. Until 1992, only strains of serogroup O1 were associated with epidemic cholera, although other non-O1 *V. cholerae* serogroups resulted in sporadic diarrhea. The *V. cholerae* O1 are further divided into three serotypes (Ogawa, Inaba, and Hikojima), based on specific antigenic determinants, and into two biotypes (classical and ElTor). *Vibrio cholerae* O139, first identified in 1993, represents a mutation of O1 antigen in a typical *V. cholerae* O1 ElTor strain.

Vibrio cholerae is oxidase-positive, a slow lactose fermenter that also ferments glucose and sucrose. It grows easily in alkaline media in the presence of bile salts and is exquisitely sensitive to acid and to drying. The organism can be isolated on a variety of culture media, but a selective medium, such as thiosulfate-citrate-bile salt-sucrose (TCBS) agar is recommended. On TCBS agar, *V. cholerae* bacilli appear as 2- to 4-mm large, smooth, round, yellow colonies with opaque centers and translucent edges that contrast with the blue-green agar. Suspicious colonies can be rapidly identified by agglutination tests utilizing specific *V. cholerae* O1 and O139 antigens.

PATHOGENESIS Persons with blood type O are more susceptible to contract cholera and typically exhibit a more severe illness. Similarly, persons with less gastric acidity are more prone to disease. Because *V. cholerae* are sensitive to acid, a large inoculum ($\geq 10^8$) is required to cause disease. Lower inoculum size may produce disease in individuals with less gastric acidity. Once in the small intestine, the rapid penetration of the intestinal mucous coat is achieved through the organism's motility, chemotaxis, and elaboration of mucinase.

Several genes are responsible for the virulence of *V. cholerae*. The toxin-coregulated pilus A gene, *TcpA*, governs effective colonization. *Vibrio cholerae* adheres to enterocytes without invading the mucosal barrier and thus avoids peristaltic expulsion. Adherent bacteria multiply and elaborate an enterotoxin, also known as choleratoxin or choleragen. This toxin is very similar to heat-labile *E. coli* enterotoxin. The toxin is composed of one A subunit, which is further divided into A1 and A2, and five B subunits.

Only epidemic strains of *V. cholerae* O1 and *V. cholerae* O139 possess the *ctxA* and *ctxB* genes that encode for enterotoxin subunits A and B. The B subunits of cholera toxin bind the toxin to G_{M1}-ganglioside receptors on enterocytes, after which the A1 subunit enters the cell. The A1 subunit irreversibly activates the adenylate cyclase system in the mucosa, leaving it in "on" position, leading to synthesis of cyclic adenosine monophosphate (cAMP), and thus increasing the intracellular concentration of cAMP. The increase in intracellular cAMP turns on electrolyte secretory pathways through activation of protein kinases. Thus, the active secretion of sodium and chloride into the gut lumen, with water following it passively, results in secretion of isotonic fluid surpassing the absorptive capacity of the colon.

CLINICAL MANIFESTATIONS The incubation period for cholera is from 6 hours to 5 days, with most cases occurring between 1 and 3 days. Toxigenic strains of *V. cholerae* serogroups O1 and O139 produce infections ranging from asymptomatic to severe fatal illness. Most infected individuals have no symptoms, approximately 25% develop mild to moderate symptoms, and less than 5% develop classic cholera. Anorexia and mild abdominal pain may precede the onset of diarrhea.

Initially there is brownish fecal matter in the liquid stools. After the diarrhea becomes copious, the stools are pale gray in color with a faint fishy smell and contain mucous flecks, giving them a classic "rice water" look. Vomiting may occur after the onset of diarrhea. The patient may be normothermic, hypothermic, or may have a low-grade fever. Because of the massive amount of fluid and electrolyte loss, occasionally exceeding 1 L per hour, severe dehydration, hypovolemia, and shock may develop within a few hours. If not treated vigorously and promptly, severe dehydration progresses to hypovolemic shock, metabolic acidosis, and anorexia leading to death within hours of the onset of symptoms.

Clinical features of severe fluid and electrolyte loss are obvious. A listless, detached mental status is common. Children may also develop seizures, hypoglycemia, and loss of consciousness. Hyponatremia and hypokalemia are more pronounced in children because of the greater loss of sodium and potassium in stools. Hypokalemia may cause severe muscle cramps, marked weakness and hypotonia, as well as ileus and cardiac arrhythmias. In pregnant women, cholera is a severe disease resulting in very high fetal mortality, especially during the third trimester.

DIAGNOSIS The clinical diagnosis of cholera is suggested by the acute onset of profuse, watery diarrhea in the absence of significant abdominal pain and systemic manifestations. A monoclonal antibody-based coagglutination test for direct detection of *V. cholerae* O1 in fecal specimens is sensitive and specific, does not require culturing of fecal specimens, and is completed in less than 5 minutes. Rapid etiologic diagnosis can also be made by dark-field or phase microscopy. Actively motile *Vibrio* organisms are seen in large numbers in stool. Specific antisera for *V. cholerae* O1 and O139 will immobilize and extinguish the characteristic "shooting star" movement of the *Vibrio*. Rectal swab or stool culture will also establish the diagnosis.

TREATMENT The primary goal of therapy is to replace fluid and electrolyte losses, usually with lifesaving results. Antibiotic therapy is of secondary importance. Patients who are unconscious, in shock, or suffering from ileus should receive rapid intravenous rehydration.

Otherwise, oral rehydration with a glucose-electrolyte solution is preferred. The success of the oral approach is predicated on the continued absorption of sodium associated with active glucose transport in the enterocytes, even in the presence of toxin-induced secretion of fluid and salt. Oral rehydration solution containing 2.0 to 2.5% glucose, 70 to 90 meq/L sodium, and 20 meq/L potassium is appropriate (a solution with similar composition can be used intravenously when indicated). Fluid volume from 40 to 74 mL/kg, depending on the estimated deficit, should be given in 4 hours. Following rehydration, an oral maintenance solution should be used to replace ongoing fluid loss. The maintenance solution differs from the rehydration solution in its lower concentration (40–60 meq/L) of sodium. The administered volume of the maintenance solution should not exceed 150 mL/kg/24h; if additional fluid is needed, water, breast milk, or other low-solute fluids should be used. Vomiting is not a contraindication for oral hydration, because small amounts of solution can also be given frequently by spoon or through a nipple.

Altered sensorium and convulsions should prompt investigation and management of hypoglycemia, hypernatremia, or cerebral edema. Replacement of potassium may be indicated, even for patients with anuria, to prevent hypokalemia-induced cardiac arrhythmias. Conservative treatment of renal failure is desired.

Antibiotic treatment for 2 to 3 days will shorten the clinical course, reduce the volume requirement for rehydration, and decrease the period of bacterial excretion. Tetracycline, 50 mg/kg/d, given every 6 hours, is the antibiotic of choice. *Vibrio cholerae* is also generally sensitive to trimethoprim-sulfamethoxazole, furazolidone, chloramphenicol, and the aminoglycosides. The recently identified *V. cholerae* O139 is susceptible to tetracycline, but has been reported to be resistant to trimethoprim-sulfamethoxazole and furazolidone. Rapid emergence of multidrug resistance isolates all over the world is of grave concern.

PREVENTION Sanitation and good personal hygiene are of primary importance in controlling cholera, but these measures are often difficult to implement in poor, developing countries.

Clinical cholera confers effective and long-lasting immunity. The protection stems from the development of local vibriocidal antibodies directed against the *V. cholerae* cell-wall lipopolysaccharide, and from antitoxin antibodies directed against the cholera toxin B subunits. Either class of antibody is protective; together they exert synergistic protective effects. Hence, the ideal vaccine should stimulate production of both types of antibody in the intestinal mucosa.

Only the inactivated whole-cell parenteral vaccine is available in the United States. It induces a short-lived (3–6 months) immunity in 50% of vaccinated individuals and has no role in the control of endemic or epidemic cholera. Oral vaccines consisting of inactivated vibrios given with or without the B subunit of *V. cholerae* toxin have been tested and have been shown to confer moderate immunity up to 3 years in adults. Young children, however, develop immunity that lasts less than 1 year. A genetically engineered vaccine, which is derived from wild-type classical *V. cholerae* O1 with 94% of the gene encoding the A subunit deleted (strain CVD 103-HgR), is immunogenic and safe; it is minimally excreted in the feces of the vaccinated children. Several placebo-controlled research trials of adults, children, and infants demonstrated the safety and immunogenicity of a single dose of CVD 103-HgR vaccine. The recent identification of *V. cholerae* O139 as another cause of epidemic cholera poses an additional hindrance in the development of the optimal cholera vaccine, because protective antibodies against *V.*

cholerae O1 do not protect against cholera caused by *V. cholerae* O139.

References

Carpenter CCJ: The treatment of cholera: clinical science at the bedside. J Infect Dis 166:2–14, 1992

Fukuda JM, Yi A, Chaparro L, et al: Clinical characteristics and risk factors for *Vibrio cholerae* infection in children. J Pediatr 126:882–886, 1995

Lacey SW: Cholera: calamitous past, ominous future. Clin Infect Dis 20:1409–1419, 1995

Levine MM: Oral vaccines against cholera: lessons from Vietnam and elsewhere. Lancet 349:220–221, 1997

Simanjuntak CH, O'Hanley P, Punjabi NH, et al: Safety, immunogenicity, and transmissibility of single-dose live oral cholera vaccine strain CVD 103-HgR in 24- to 59-month-old Indonesian children. J Infect Dis 168:1169–1176, 1993

Singh J, Bora D, Sachdeva V, et al: *Vibrio cholerae* O1 and O139 in less than five-year-old children hospitalized for watery diarrhoea in Delhi, 1993. J Diarrhoeal Dis Res 15:3–6, 1997

13.2.13   Diphtheria

Gary D. Overturf

Diphtheria, caused by *Corynebacterium diphtheriae*, occurs throughout the world. It may present at any time of the year, although it is most common during winter. The major reservoir for infection is human beings. Closeness and duration of contact with an ill person or a healthy carrier are important determinants of infection spread. As a result, attack rates in households and in crowded living conditions are high.

EPIDEMIOLOGY Nasopharyngeal carriers of *C. diphtheriae* are the principal source of new infections, but cutaneous lesions can be a reservoir as well. In temperate climates, the skin lesions of diphtheria are superficial, indolent sores that resemble impetigo. Individuals with skin lesions generally do not develop toxic manifestations. Untreated, healthy nasopharyngeal carriers can be colonized for many weeks. The rate of decline of asymptomatic carriage is about 5% per day.

The incidence of diphtheria is inversely related to the percentage of immune individuals in an area and remains a common disease in countries without effective immunization programs. The incidence of diphtheria in the United States has declined dramatically since aggressive immunization efforts were begun. Since 1980, fewer than five patients with diphtheria are reported annually. Concurrently, diphtheria has shifted from a disease of children to a disease of adults with waning immunity. The potential for outbreaks continues, however, if segments of a community are not immunized.

Corynebacterium diphtheriae are irregularly staining gram-positive, nonspore-forming, unencapsulated slender rods. Branching and clubbed ends result in a cuneiform appearance. Metachromatic granules are common. There are three phenotypes of the organism: gravis, intermedius, and mitis, differentiated by colony morphology, growth characteristics, and biochemical reactions. All are capable of elaborating a cytotoxic exotoxin, which interferes with protein synthesis in host cells. The ability of a strain of *C. diphtheriae* to produce toxin is conferred by a lysogenic bacteriophage that carries the gene for toxin production. Toxins produced by the three types are qualitatively similar, but the gravis and intermedius strains produce more toxin than does the mitis strain.

CLINICAL MANIFESTATIONS The incubation period of diphtheria is 2 to 4 days but may be as long as 1 week. The clinical signs and symptoms depend on the primary site of infection. The toxic manifestations are the same regardless of the primary site of proliferation of the organism.

The posterior pharynx, including the tonsils, is the most common site of infection. In a large series of diphtheria reported from Los Angeles County Hospital between 1940 and 1950, the sites of primary infection (number of patients) were tonsillopharyngeal (1366), nasal (27), laryngeal (20), laryngotracheobronchial (6), wound (6), ear (5), eye (3), umbilical (1), vaginal (1), and tracheobronchial (1).

Tonsillopharyngeal Diphtheria This usually has an insidious onset of symptoms, in contrast to streptococcal sore throat. There is mild sore throat with slight redness and low-grade fever. Systemic signs of illness are absent in the early stages. Within 1 or 2 days, areas of yellow or "dirty" white exudate appear, most frequently on or adjacent to the tonsils; these areas subsequently coalesce to form a light reflective, sharply outlined pseudomembrane on the mucous membranes of the pharynx, tonsils, and uvula. Pseudomembranes consist of necrotic epithelium embedded in an inflammatory, organized exudate at the surface. Less frequently, such lesions are found in the nose, larynx, and lower respiratory tract. Rarely, pseudomembranous lesions extend to the middle ear, the esophagus or the stomach, or involve the skin or mucosa of the genitalia.

Inflammatory changes in underlying epithelium may extend into the submucosa, where hemorrhage may be present. The bacilli remain in these surface lesions and rarely invade deeper structures or cause bacteremia. Diphtheria toxin is absorbed from the local lesion, causing damage in distant organs and tissues.

Persons with partial antitoxic immunity may not progress beyond the exudative stage. In those lacking immunity, the pseudomembrane may spread to the soft palate and to the posterior pharynx, but not anteriorly. There is bleeding with attempts to remove the pseudomembrane. Cervical lymph nodes may be mildly enlarged, but the single large, tender nodes characteristic of streptococcal infection are not found. With extensive membrane formation, there may be dysphagia and drooling. After approximately 5 days, the pseudomembrane changes to a grayish color secondary to hemorrhage as it loosens and sloughs. Occasionally (approximately 10% of patients) the illness has a hyperacute presentation with high fever, systemic toxicity, cerebral obtundation, and rapid proliferation of the pseudomembrane associated with marked edema of the face and neck. This phenomenon is referred to as "bull neck" diphtheria, which has a grave prognosis.

Laryngotracheobronchial Diphtheria In fewer than 5% of patients, diphtheria of the laryngotracheal area occurs in the absence of tonsillopharyngeal involvement, but in about 10% of patients, there is secondary downward spread from the pharynx. Varying degrees of hoarseness, stridor, and respiratory embarrassment occur, depending on the extent and thickness of the membrane in relation to the caliber of the airway. Young children are at higher risk of compromise because of small airways. Rarely, the membrane extends into the bronchi, resulting in a virtual cast of the airway, which is invariably fatal.

Nasal Diphtheria Primary nasal diphtheria is more common in infants and young children. The discharge is mucoid, profuse, and grayish in color. After a few days when the membrane begins sloughing there is often blood in the discharge. This is the mildest form of diphtheria and seldom has toxic manifestations.

Other Mucous Membranes and Skin Rarely, the primary site of infection is the mucous membrane of the eye, vagina, or ear. An ulcerating lesion with exudate or pseudomembrane forms, but these are self-limited lesions uncommonly associated with toxicity. Skin lesions are most often superficial, have no characteristic appearance, and are not associated with pseudomembranes. Occasionally, ulcerating or ecthymatous lesions develop. They occur in persons with preexisting antitoxic immunity or they induce immunity because they are not associated with toxic manifestations. Individual lesions heal, but new ones may form at the sites of breaks in the integrity of skin from insect bites or trauma over a period of weeks.

Effects of Toxin The heart, kidneys, and neural system are susceptible to damage by diphtheria toxin. The degree of toxic damage is determined by two factors: (a) the extent of disease at the primary site and, hence, the amount of toxin produced and disseminated hematogenously; and (b) the amount of circulating antitoxin. The latter is determined by both the preexisting antitoxin resulting from prior subclinical infection or immunization and by the therapeutic amounts of antitoxin administered. Because immunity wanes with the passing years, previously immunized persons can eventually become susceptible to toxin.

Electrocardiographic evidence of myocardial toxicity is present in many patients with diphtheria, but clinically manifest myocarditis develops in about 10% of patients. Myocarditis generally develops during the first week of illness, but can be delayed for 1 month or longer. Dysrhythmias are common. Death occurs more often from severe dysrhythmia (including complete heart block) than from heart failure. On histology, myocarditis is characterized by degenerative or "toxic" damage, rather than by inflammation. Minute hemorrhages may be present, or, in some areas, an accompanying round-cell infiltration may be seen. The conducting system frequently is involved.

Renal failure is rare, but minor injury as reflected by changes in the urinalysis (proteinuria, cylindruria, increased cells) is common. If toxic nephropathy develops, it is almost uniformly fatal. Hemolytic uremic syndrome has been reported in diphtheria. The kidneys may exhibit cloudy swelling, with swollen granular epithelial cells of the convoluted tubules. Interstitial nephritis may occur. Lesions in the adrenal cortex, similar to those present in meningococcemia, often are found in fatal infections. Hepatic function may be mildly impaired; liver cells show degenerative changes at autopsy, with scattered areas of focal necrosis.

Neural involvement is common, occurring in 5 to 10% of patients, and can be manifested as isolated peripheral nerve palsies or as a symptom complex mimicking Guillain-Barré syndrome. Contiguous muscles in the palate, pharynx, or larynx are most commonly involved and tend to be affected earlier in the disease course than the extraocular muscles, diaphragm, or muscles supplied by peripheral nerves. Paralysis can occur as early as the first week of illness, but more often develops between the second and sixth week. If the patient does not succumb to respiratory complications of paralysis, full recovery can be expected within a few weeks. Degenerative changes in the nervous system occur in nearly all fatal infections. In the spinal cord, changes are seen in the ganglion cells of the anterior horns and in the posterior root ganglia. The cranial nerves and their centers can be affected, but the cortex is spared. Other lesions encountered are degenerative changes in the spleen and lymph nodes; occasionally, subcapsular hemorrhages in these organs are seen. Subcutaneous hemorrhages are frequent.

DIAGNOSIS Many bacterial and viral pathogens can cause pseudomembranous tonsillitis, the most common being *S. pyogenes*, adenoviruses, and Epstein-Barr virus. Although there is sometimes exudate on the part of the uvula touching the enlarged tonsil in these conditions, the pseudomembrane does not otherwise extend away from the tonsil. In rare instances of laryngeal diphtheria without oropharyngeal involvement, the diagnosis is suspected if there is a history of exposure to diphtheria or when a pseudomembrane is seen at the time of laryngoscopy or bronchoscopy. Otherwise, the differential diagnosis from viral causes of croup is exceedingly difficult.

When diphtheria is suspected, attempts should be made to isolate the organism from the local lesion. It is advisable to take specimens for culture from the nasopharynx as well as the throat because the yield of positive results is 20% greater with two cultures as opposed to one culture. If transport time to the laboratory is longer than 24 hours, the swabs should be placed in laboratory-recommended commercial transport medium. Specimens should be inoculated onto recommended media (usually a Loeffler or Pai slant, a cystine-tellurite agar plate, and a 5% sheep's blood agar plate) and incubated overnight at 35°C (95°F). Growth from slants may be stained with Neisser or Loeffler methylene blue and examined for the characteristic morphologic appearance of *C. diphtheriae* (eg, metachromatic granules). Toxigenicity is usually determined using the modified Elek immunodiffusion test in reference laboratories.

The degree of leukocytosis in the peripheral blood generally reflects the severity of disease. In mild to moderate disease, the leukocyte count is between 10,000 and 20,000/μL. The likelihood of a fatal outcome rises sharply in patients with leukocyte counts higher than 25,000/μL. Thrombocytopenia and disseminated intravascular coagulation (DIC) are rare. Some patients develop mild anemia.

In postdiphtheritic paralysis, protein concentrations increase in the cerebrospinal fluid (CSF), but there is no increase in the number of cells and the glucose content is normal, as occurs in idiopathic Guillain-Barré syndrome. The protein content continues to increase during the initial weeks of neurologic symptoms and slowly returns to normal after clinical recovery.

Albuminuria is common, and in severe disease there may be cells and casts in the urine.

TREATMENT Diphtheria antitoxin neutralizes circulating toxin but has no effect on toxin that is bound to cells. It should be administered as soon as possible after onset of disease. Therefore, the decision to treat is usually made before culture results are available and is based on a compatible clinical picture in a susceptible individual. Diphtheria antitoxin is an equine serum, so tests for sensitivity must be done by instilling a 1:10 dilution into the conjunctival sac or by performing an intradermal test dose with a 1:100 dilution of the antiserum. If the patient has an immediate reaction, a desensitization procedure is done.

The dosage of antitoxin is empirical and based on the extent of disease. Dosage is not based on body weight, but on the estimated amount of toxin present. Suggested dosages are presented in Table 13-36. The antiserum is administered intravenously. Antitoxin is of dubious value for patients with cutaneous diphtheria, but some authorities recommend it because toxic manifestations have occasionally been reported.

TABLE 13-36

GUIDELINES FOR DIPHTHERIA ANTITOXIN THERAPY

STATUS OF DISEASE	DOSAGE OF ANTITOXIN
Pharyngeal, laryngeal, or nasal of >48 h duration	20,000–40,000 Units
Nasopharyngeal	40,000–60,000 Units
"Bull neck" or any disease of >48 h duration	80,000–120,000 Units
Skin lesions	None or 20,000 Units
Asymptomatic susceptible contacts	None or 5–10,000 Units

Antibiotic therapy has little or no effect on the clinical evolution of diphtheria. It is given primarily to render the patient noncontagious. *Corynebacterium diphtheriae* is susceptible to penicillin and erythromycin and probably other macrolides (eg, clarithromycin) as well. Erythromycin (40 mg/kg/d divided every 6 hours) is given by mouth. Alternatively, daily procaine penicillin G (25,000–50,000 U/kg in two divided doses) can be given intramuscularly, or aqueous crystalline penicillin G (100,000–150,000 U/kg divided in 4 doses) can be given to the patient. Treatment is given for 14 days. After completion of antibiotic therapy, the throat and nasopharynx should be cultured three times, at least 24 hours apart, to determine whether the pathogen has been eradicated. Respiratory isolation precautions are maintained until there is culture confirmation of eradication of the pathogen from the nasopharynx. Some patients with cutaneous diphtheria have asymptomatic respiratory tract colonization with *C. diphtheriae*, and thus, throat and nasopharyngeal cultures are necessary in these patients as well. If there is persistent nasopharyngeal carriage after the first course of therapy, a repeat course of erythromycin therapy should be given.

Corticosteroid therapy (to mitigate myocarditis or nephritis) is ineffective and is not recommended. Carnitine is a cofactor in the transport of fatty acids to the interior of cell mitochondria. Because fatty acids accumulate in the cytoplasm of human heart cells in patients with diphtheritic myocarditis, carnitine might be beneficial. In one study, 10% DL-carnitine (100 mg/kg/d in two divided doses for 4 days) decreased the incidence of myocarditis as compared with a control group, but this needs to be confirmed before carnitine can be recommended as routine therapy. Treatment otherwise is supportive.

A patent airway must be maintained in patients with diphtheria. Nasotracheal intubation or tracheostomy may be needed. Patients should be monitored carefully for signs or symptoms of myocarditis, nephropathy, or neuropathy. Patients should be observed closely for signs of laryngeal, pharyngeal, or diaphragmatic paralysis. If there is difficulty with swallowing, oral feedings should be withheld and parenteral nutrition provided. Respiratory paralysis is managed by standard procedures. During the stage of sloughing of the pseudomembrane, tracheal suction may be successful in removing obstructive fragments.

Exposed household and other close contacts of an index patient with diphtheria are at increased risk of becoming asymptomatic carriers or of developing disease. Immunization provides antitoxic immunity, but no immunity to infection with *C. diphtheriae*. All exposed persons should be examined promptly. Individuals with symptoms consistent with diphtheria should be investigated and treated appropriately. Cultures should be obtained from all exposed, asymptomatic persons, and they should be considered potentially contagious until the culture results are known. All close contact should be kept under surveillance for 7 days.

Previously immunized contacts should be given a booster dose of diphtheria toxoid if they have not received a booster within 5 years. Individuals who are not immunized, or whose immunization status is uncertain, should be given prophylaxis with erythromycin (40 mg/kg/d in four divided doses for 7 days) or a single intramuscular injection of 50,000 U benzathine penicillin G per kilogram (maximum 1,200,000 U). Immunization with DTaP or Td, depending on age, should be initiated. If the individual cannot be kept under surveillance, some authorities recommend giving 5000 to 10,000 U of diphtheria antitoxin intramuscularly. In most circumstances, the risk of allergic reactions makes this practice inadvisable.

PROGNOSIS Overall, the fatality rate is about 10%, but the prognosis depends on type of disease, age, and general condition of the patient, and the interval from onset of disease to receipt of antitoxin therapy. More than half the patients with bull-neck diphtheria die in spite of aggressive intensive care. If myocarditis or renal failure occurs early in the course of disease, the prognosis is grim. If the patient is managed in an intensive care facility, death from airway obstruction is unlikely, unless pseudomembrane extends into the bronchi. After recovering from the acute illness, patients remain at risk for late development of paralysis or myocarditis. There are no permanent sequelae of diphtheria unless anoxic damage has occurred.

PREVENTION Because an attack of diphtheria does not provide reliable immunity to the toxin, recovered patients should receive diphtheria toxoid. The Maloney and Schick skin tests are no longer used or available for testing immunity to diphtheria. Immunity is associated with a level of specific antibodies of 0.01 IU/mL. Newborn infants have transient immunity from maternal antibodies when the mother is immune.

Preparations of diphtheria vaccine are administered with tetanus and pertussis (eg, DTaP) antigens until age 7 years, and only with tetanus (eg, Td) thereafter. Also, diphtheria preparations given before age 7 years have 6.7 to 25 Lf (limes flocculation units) of diphtheria toxoid, indicated by an uppercase D; whereas vaccines given after the seventh birthday contain not more than 2 Lf, indicated by lowercase d. All infants should be routinely immunized according to the harmonized Recommended Childhood Immunization Schedule developed by the Advisory Committee on Immunization Practices of the Centers for Disease Control, the American Academy of Family Physicians, and the Committee on Infectious Diseases of the American Academy of Pediatrics. Booster doses of diphtheria toxoid (combined with tetanus toxoid as Td) should be given every 10 years.

References

Karzon D, Edwards K: Diphtheria outbreaks in immunized populations. N Engl J Med 318:41–43, 1988

Koopman JS, Campbell J: The role of cutaneous diphtheria infections in a diphtheria epidemic. J Infect Dis 121:239–244, 1975

Ramos ACMF, Elias PRP, Barrucand L, da Silva AF: The protective effect of carnitine in human diphtheric myocarditis. Pediatr Res 18:815–819, 1984

Thisyakorn U, Wongvanich J, Kumpeng V: Failure of corticosteroid therapy to prevent diphtheritic myocarditis or neuritis. Pediatr Infect Dis 3:126–128, 1984

13.2.14   Enterococci

Dwight A. Powell

Historically classified as group D streptococci, enterococci are now classified as a separate genus with at least 14 different species.

EPIDEMIOLOGY Only two species, *E. faecalis* and *E. faecium*, account for all but a rare case of human disease. *Enterococcus faecalis* is responsible for about 80 to 90% of human cases, but several studies show a rising proportion of cases due to *E. faecium*. These two species usually have very different antibiotic susceptibility profiles, in that resistance to vancomycin is far more common among *E. faecium*. Enterococci are facultatively anaerobic gram-positive cocci that normally inhabit the bowel. Approximately half of newborn infants have acquired colonization with enterococci by 1 week of age. These very hardy organisms grow at temperatures of 10° to 60°C (50°–140°F) and remain viable for weeks on environmental surfaces such as bed rails, sinks, faucets, and doorknobs. Human-to-human spread is common in hospital settings.

Enterococci are generally not highly invasive pathogens and are typically classified as opportunists. They lack not only the major exotoxins and endotoxins associated with virulent streptococci and staphylococci but also the enzymes that enable rapid tissue spread. Infections are most often associated with prolonged hospitalization, use of broad-spectrum antibiotics, indwelling lines, immunocompromised state, or loss of integrity of the gastrointestinal tract, urinary tract, or skin.

CLINICAL MANIFESTATIONS The three most common types of infection associated with enterococci are urinary tract infection, polymicrobial abdominal infections, and bacteremia or sepsis. Although infrequent, cases of focal organ infection, such as endocarditis, meningitis, and wound infections, may be severe. Urinary tract infections caused by enterococci almost never occur in otherwise healthy children. Enterococci are associated with indwelling urinary catheters and account for approximately 15% of nosocomial urinary tract infections in children. Enterococci may be involved in intra-abdominal polymicrobial infections following intestinal perforation such as ruptured appendix or necrotizing enterocolitis. Bacteremia or sepsis in children may not be identified with a specific focus, but common risk factors are use of broad-spectrum antibiotics or intravascular catheters in association with underlying conditions such as surgery, immunosuppression, transplants, or major organ dysfunction. Bacteremia without a focal infection may result in a self-limited illness, a low-grade infection requiring specific antibiotics, or a severe and life-threatening illness, particularly in newborns or children with underlying disease. Bacteremia is often polymicrobial with other enteric microorganisms. Mortality occurs in up to 25% of cases, but is hard to separate from the underlying health problems. In newborns, infection may present as early onset sepsis in the first several days of life, similar to early onset group B streptococcal sepsis. However, most neonatal enterococcal infections are nosocomial and occur after the second week of life, typically in the setting of bacteremia attributable to line infection or necrotizing enterocolitis. The most common presenting signs are apnea, bradycardia, fever or hypothermia, and abdominal distention.

DIAGNOSIS Enterococci are easily isolated on standard bacterial culture plates or broth media. They are distinguished from nonenterococcal catalase-negative gram-positive cocci by the PYR reaction (hydrolysis of L-pyrrolidinyl-β-naphthylamide), the ability to hydrolyze esculin, and growth in 6.5% NaCl at 45°C (113°F).

TREATMENT The most important aspect of treating enterococcal infections is determination of antibiotic susceptibility. Enterococci have an intrinsic resistance to cephalosporins, oxacillin, clindamycin, and aminoglycosides. Ampicillin is the antibiotic of choice for simple infections of the lower urinary tract with susceptible enterococci (about 98% of *E. faecalis* and 15% of *E. faecium*). Serious infections such as meningitis and endocarditis must be treated with the addition of an aminoglycoside to achieve synergistic, bactericidal activity. Unfortunately, high-level aminoglycoside resistance, which precludes synergistic activity, is increasing among enterococci. For ampicillin-resistant enterococci, vancomycin is the antibiotic of choice. However, vancomycin-resistant strains of enterococci (VRE) are increasing at an alarming rate. Data from the Surveillance Network Database—USA, from 1995 to 1997, have shown an increase in *E. faecium* VRE from 28 to 52%. *Enterococcus faecalis* VRE remained unchanged at 2%. Several hospital outbreaks of VRE have been reported in children. Antibiotic selection for treatment of VRE must depend on laboratory susceptibility profiles, because many strains are multiple-drug resistant. Prevention of further spread of VRE will depend on appropriate control measures such as active surveillance for VRE in intensive care settings, contact isolation to minimize person-to-person transmission, and restriction of the use of vancomycin and other broad-spectrum antibiotics.

References

Christie C, Hammond J, Reising S, et al: Clinical and molecular epidemiology of enterococcal bacteremia in a pediatric teaching hospital. J Pediatr 125:392–399, 1994

Das I, Gray J: Enterococcal bacteremia in children: a review of seventy-five episodes in a pediatric hospital. Pediatr Infect Dis J 17:1154–1158, 1998

Green M: Vancomycin-resistant enterococci: impact and management in pediatrics. Adv Pediatr Infect Dis 13:257–277, 1998

McNeeley DF, Saint-Louis F, Noel GJ: Neonatal enterococcal bacteremia: an increasingly frequent event with potentially untreatable pathogens. Pediatr Infect Dis J 15:800–805, 1996

Moellering RC: Vancomycin-resistant enterococci. Clin Infect Dis 26:1196–1199, 1998

13.2.15 *Haemophilus influenzae*

Mark R. Schleiss and Arnold L. Smith

Although the type of infectious diseases caused by *Haemophilus influenzae* has changed considerably in recent years as a result of the widespread implementation of routine childhood immunization against type b organisms, this organism remains an important pathogen. There are two major categories of *H. influenzae*: the unencapsulated strains and the encapsulated strains. The unencapsulated strains are responsible chiefly for infections at mucosal surfaces, including conjunctivitis, otitis media, sinusitis, and bronchitis. In contrast, one of the six antigenically distinct encapsulated strains, strain type b, is associated with invasive diseases such as septicemia, meningitis, cellulitis, septic arthritis, epiglottitis, and pneumonia. Prior to the availability of an effective vaccine, *H. influenzae* type b (Hib) was the most common cause of pediatric bacterial meningitis in the United States.

EPIDEMIOLOGY Humans are the only natural host for *H. influenzae*. Maintenance of the organism in the human population depends upon person-to-person transmission, which occurs efficiently via respiratory droplet spread. Nontypable strains colonize the upper respiratory tract of as many as 75% of healthy adults. Hib strains colonize the nasopharynx of children at a rate of 3 to 5%; the effectiveness of vaccines is related (in part) to the ability to diminish the incidence of nasopharyngeal colonization (see below). Although both nontypable and type b strains of *H. influenzae* are easily spread via person-to-person transmission, the Hib strains have historically been associated with invasive disease in children. Prior to the availability of effective immunization, nasopharyngeal acquisition of Hib occured in most children at some point in the first 5 years of life. Although nasopharyngeal colonization by Hib may be asymptomatic, breakthrough bacteremia with subsequent development of focal infection was at one time a common occurrence and a major pediatric public health problem in the United States.

In the prevaccine era, invasive Hib disease characteristically had a striking age-related incidence, with approximately 85% of disease occurring in children younger than 5 years of age. The peak incidence of the most serious form of invasive disease, meningitis, occurred between 6 and 12 months of age. Hib epiglottitis was, in contrast, predominantly a disease of older children, with more than 80% of the infections occurring in children over 2 years of age. In the prevaccine era, approximately 20,000 instances of invasive Hib disease occurred annually in the United States, affecting about 1 in 200 children under 5 years of age. Chronic illnesses associated with increased risk for invasive Hib disease include sickle-cell disease, asplenia, agammaglobulinemia, Hodgkin disease, and complement deficiencies. Increased risk has also been associated with childcare attendance, the presence of young siblings, household crowding, lower socioeconomic status, and passive smoke exposure. Breast-feeding confers some protection against disease. A bimodal seasonal disease pattern has been described, with one peak of illness in the autumn between September and December, and a second peak in the spring between March and May. Although invasive Hib infection has historically been uncommon in adults, apparently due to the gradual development of protective antibodies over time in the context of asymptomatic nasopharyngeal colonization, Hib can occasionally cause invasive infection in adult patients. Remarkably, in a post-Hib vaccine era, Hib meningitis has now become more common in adult patients than in children. It remains to be seen what effect (if any) will be conferred by routine childhood Hib immunization on the epidemiology of adult infections.

The epidemiology of invasive Hib disease has changed dramatically in recent years as a consequence of the widespread use of conjugate vaccines. In 1987, the first Hib vaccine (purified PRP) was licensed in the United States for use in children 18 months of age and older. Over the next few years, dramatic decreases in the incidence of invasive disease were seen in older children. However, because Hib meningitis had always been a more significant problem in children under 1 year of age, the most significant decline in invasive disease was not observed until late 1990, when protein-PRP conjugate vaccines were approved for use in infants, beginning at 2 months of age. In populations with high rates of vaccine coverage, the incidence of Hib disease has been reduced by more than 95%. The protective efficacy of these vaccines exceeded initial expectations because of an unanticipated decrease in nasopharyngeal carriage, ultimately leading to a decreased environmental burden of Hib and a resultant protection even of unimmunized children due to the effect of this "herd immunity." The conjugate vaccines are so effective in preventing Hib infection that the finding of invasive disease in a fully immunized child should prompt further diagnostic evaluation for the possibility of an underlying immunodeficiency.

An important aspect of Hib epidemiology is the risk it poses to contacts. Although the direct contagiousness of invasive Hib infection is limited, a significant risk for secondary disease exists among household contacts of a patient with Hib disease, particularly in the 30 days following exposure to an index patient. This is a consequence of the risk of droplet spread under conditions of continuous household exposure. Colonization rates over 70% have been noted following exposure in closed populations, such as within families or in day care centers. This becomes the rationale for chemoprophylaxis following exposure to an invasive case of Hib disease (see below).

Another less common but recently recognized route of acquisition of *H. influenzae* is vertical transmission via the maternal birth canal. This phenomenon has been manifest in recent years as an increase in bacteremia and meningitis in neonates caused by nontypable strains acquired from the mother's genital tract. These strains are genetically distinct from those colonizing the upper respiratory tract.

MICROBIOLOGY *Haemophilus influenzae* is a small gram-negative coccobacillus that may show considerable microscopic pleomorphism, necessitating careful and cautious interpretation of Gram stains of clinical specimens. Biochemical identification of *H. influenzae* is performed based on the demonstration that growth on rich media (blood agar) is dependent upon supplements; factors X and V. The X factor is a heat-stable, iron-containing protoporphyrin (hemin) essential for the function of enzymes of the electron-transport chain utilized in aerobic metabolism. The V factor is a heat-labile coenzyme nicotinamide adenine dinucleotide (NAD). Although both factors are present in erythrocytes, the V factor must be released from the cell in order to sustain growth, and hence standard blood agar is an unsatisfactory media for growth of *H. influenzae*. The V factor may be exogenously provided from lysed red blood cells, as are present in chocolate agar. The growth of *H. influenzae* is fastidious and the viability of the organism is lost rapidly, necessitating expeditious handling of clinical specimens. Following overnight incubation, gray colonies appear that are 0.5 to 0.8 mm in diameter, which are rough or granular in appearance. Encapsulated strains typically produce larger mucoid or glistening colonies.

The polysaccharide capsule of *H. influenzae* plays a central role in molecular pathogenesis and immune response. Six antigenically and biochemically distinct capsular polysaccharide subtypes (a to f) have been identified. Although type b encapsulated strains have historically been of primary clinical and immunologic importance (because of the association with invasive infection, including meningitis), the other encapsulated strains are also capable of producing invasive disease. Latex agglutination tests that identify the polyribosylribotol phosphate (PRP) capsular polysaccharide unique to type b are available for rapid diagnosis. Lipopolysaccharide (LPS) is another important component of the *H. influenzae* cell wall that contributes to pathogenesis. Although chemically different from the LPS of the Enterobacteriaceae, the biological activity of Hib LPS appears to be similar to that of other gram-negative endotoxins. Multiple adhesins target specific cells of the airway and provide redundancy for adherence to respiratory tissues. *H. influenzae* encodes three distinct IgA proteases that may play a role as virulence factors by interfering with host mucosal defenses. Another clinically important aspect of the molecular microbiology of *H. influenzae*

has been the identification of genes responsible for antimicrobial resistance. Resistance to ampicillin has become extremely common, ranging from 5 to 50% of isolates in various parts of the world. Susceptibility testing should therefore be performed on all isolates identified in invasive infections.

The molecular determinants responsible for nasopharyngeal colonization and subsequent bacteremic invasiveness of *H. influenzae* remain poorly understood. Invasive disease requires the spread of bacteria from the upper respiratory tract to the bloodstream, and subsequently to other body sites. The organism must first colonize and then invade the respiratory mucosal epithelium. The exact mode of entry of the organism into the blood vessel is unknown. The size of the bacterial inoculum and the intercurrent presence of a viral respiratory tract infection are factors that potentiate the risk of invasive disease. It is commonly believed that all *H. influenzae* can invade and transcytose respiratory epithelial cells. Those strains able to resist complement-mediated lysis (those with capsule) or opsonophagocytosis (because of a lack of "natural" antibody) can then replicate in the bloodstream, causing invasive disease. Although meningitis constitutes more than half of all recognized invasive Hib disease, other potential metastatic sites include the lungs, joint synovium, pleura, peritoneum, and pericardium.

Noninvasive or mucosal infections are much more frequent than invasive disease, particularly in the postvaccine era. Nontypable strains of *H. influenzae* seldom cause bacteremia in children beyond the neonatal period. It is therefore presumed that these infections represent extensions of *H. influenzae* from the respiratory mucosa to contiguous body sites. Noninvasive infections include otitis media, sinusitis, bronchitis, and pneumonia. Local extension of nontypable *H. influenzae* can occur via the eustachian tube, bronchi, or through the sinus passages. Disease is more likely if normal clearance mechanisms or immune function is impaired, such as after viral infection, sinus obstruction, or eustachian-tube dysfunction.

IMMUNITY Age-dependent susceptibility to Hib infections correlates with an age-dependent nature of immune response to Hib capsular polysaccharide. At the age of maximal risk for infection (when the nadir of protective transplacental immunity is reached), serum anti-PRP antibodies are low or absent. Even after recovery from illness, antibody levels in infants remain low. As a consequence, instances of second or third episodes of invasive Hib disease are well-described; thus, a previous episode of invasive infection does not obviate the need for Hib immunization. This failure to make serum anti-PRP antibodies is typical of the natural delay in immune response of infants to polysaccharide antigens. PRP stimulates B cells but does not adequately activate macrophages and appropriate T-helper cells, and therefore it is considered to be a T-cell-independent antigen. The characteristics of T-cell-independent antigens are limited immune responses, particularly in young infants; no booster response occurs with repeated antigenic stimulations, and the antibody is of low affinity and mostly IgM. The development of a Hib vaccine that was more immunogenic and protective for young infants required conversion of PRP from a *T-cell-independent antigen* to a *T-cell-dependent antigen*, using the principles of carrier-hapten linkage.

CLINICAL MANIFESTATIONS OF DISEASE CAUSED BY TYPABLE STRAINS

Meningitis   Prior to Hib vaccines, meningitis was the most common and serious manifestation of invasive disease. Disease is insidious in onset, with a preceding nonspecific febrile illness that provides no specific clues as to the underlying pathogen. The signs and symptoms can be nonspecific. Young infants may present with irritability, lethargy, anorexia, or vomiting. Only older children are likely to present with the classic findings of headache, photophobia, and meningismus. The absence of meningismus on examination is therefore not a helpful negative finding for excluding the diagnosis of meningitis in an infant. Approximately 30% of children will have seizures at some point in the course of Hib meningitis. Like patients with meningococcal disease, children with Hib bacteremia can have a petechial rash. They can also have a secondary site of infection, such as a septic arthritis or facial cellulitis (see below). Shock is present in approximately 20% of cases. Anemia is common, the result of a combination of accelerated red blood cell destruction and diminished erythropoiesis. Complications of *H. influenzae* type b meningitis include subdural effusion or empyema, ischemic or hemorrhagic cortical infarction, cerebritis, ventriculitis, intracerebral abscess, and hydrocephalus. Prompt use of intravenous antibiotics and good supportive care are the mainstays of therapy, but the mortality from Hib meningitis remains at approximately 5%, even with prompt diagnosis and appropriate supportive care. Long-term sequelae occur in 15 to 30% of survivors and are manifest as sensorineural hearing loss, language disorder, mental retardation, and developmental disorders.

Epiglottitis Acute upper airway obstruction caused by Hib infection of the epiglottis and superglottic tissues is perhaps the most dramatic and rapidly progressive form of disease caused by this organism. In contrast to the peaking of meningitis in children under 1 year of age, epiglottitis occurs primarily in older children (2 to 7 years of age) and usually has an abrupt onset with high fever, dysphagia, drooling, and toxicity. Occasional cases of Hib epiglottitis are still observed in even older children who were never fully immunized. Hib is also an important cause of epiglottitis in adult patients.

Classically, the child with Hib epiglottitis will drool, because of an inability to swallow oropharyngeal secretions. Progressive respiratory distress develops over a period of hours with tachypnea, stridor, cyanosis, and retractions. The patient may sit forward with the chin extended to maintain an open airway ("tripod" position). Few conditions produce such a striking constellation of symptoms and findings. A lateral neck radiograph is helpful if the clinical presentation is subtle, but the study should be performed cautiously and without undue delays with a physician experienced in airway management in attendance. Diagnostic studies should not delay the need for direct inspection of the epiglottis in the operating room and insertion of an endotracheal tube. The mortality rate is 5 to 10% and is invariably related to poor control of the airway early in illness.

Septic Arthritis/Osteomyelitis In the prevaccine era, Hib was the leading cause of septic arthritis in children less than 2 years of age. Approximately 8% of *H. influenzae* invasive disease presents as septic arthritis, typically affecting large joints, particularly knees, ankles, hips, or elbows. A contiguous osteomyelitis may be present, but isolated osteomyelitis without an adjacent septic joint is uncommon. Characteristically, there is a preceding nonspecific illness, followed by pain, swelling, and erythema of the involved joint. Clinical signs in children with a septic hip may be less prominent than for other joints, with findings limited to decreased range of motion of the joint or referred pain from the hip. Septic arthritis of the hip joint requires surgical drainage; the majority of cases involving the

shoulder require open drainage. There is a strong association of septic arthritis with meningitis, necessitating lumbar puncture.

Cellulitis *Haemophilus influenzae* type b cellulitis usually involves the face, head, or neck. The vast majority of cases occur in the first 2 years of life. Buccal cellulitis, seen almost exclusively in children during the first year of life, presents as a raised, warm, tender, and indurated area that progresses to a violaceous hue. The clinical presentation may mimic erysipelas. Periorbital (preseptal) cellulitis is similarly seen in young children and often occurs in the setting of contiguous sinus disease. It must be differentiated from the more serious orbital cellulitis. Hib cellulitis is a bacteremic disease, and meningitis must be excluded by lumbar puncture.

Occult Bacteremia Although the vast majority of children with Hib bacteremia present with a focus of infection, occasionally bacteremia can be the sole manifestation of disease in the febrile child. These children are usually younger than 2 years of age and have temperatures of 39°C (102.2°F) or higher. In the prevaccine era, Hib was the second leading cause of occult bacteremia, behind *S. pneumoniae*. However, there is an important distinction between Hib and pneumococcal bacteremia; whereas most episodes of untreated occult pneumococcal bacteremia resolve spontaneously without sequelae, 30 to 50% of children with occult Hib bacteremia will develop focal infections, including meningitis. Hence, in any child with a positive blood culture for Hib, the possibility of meningitis must be seriously considered.

Pneumonia Hib pneumonia is clinically indistinguishable from other bacterial pneumonias. It was estimated to cause as many as one-third of cases of documented bacterial pneumonias in the prevaccine era. Radiologically it can appear as a segmental, subsegmental, interstitial, or lobar pattern. There is a strong association with pleural effusion; 50% of cases have evidence of pleural involvement on initial radiographic examination. The best diagnostic test is the blood culture, which is positive in almost 90% of cases. Complications of Hib pneumonia include pericarditis, meningitis, and pleural empyema often requiring decortication.

Pericarditis The classic presentation of *H. influenzae* pericarditis is that of a toxic child with fever, respiratory distress, and a clear chest on examination. Associated conditions include pneumonia and meningitis. Hib pericarditis may become clinically manifest while a child is receiving antibiotic therapy and should be considered in the differential diagnosis of the child with persistent fever while on therapy for *H. influenzae* meningitis. Although the diagnosis may be suggested after careful inspection of the cardiac silhouette and jugular veins, echocardiography is the best modality for establishing the diagnosis of pericardial effusion. Pericardiocentesis is the diagnostic procedure of choice. Early pericardectomy, in conjunction with antibiotics, is the treatment of choice.

Neonatal Disease In recent years *H. influenzae* has been increasingly recognized as a cause of bacteremia and meningitis in the neonatal period. Neonatal infections are usually caused by nontypable *H. influenzae*, which can also be cultured from the maternal genital tract, the presumed source of the infection. The disease is one of early-onset sepsis, with more than 80% of cases occurring during the first day of life. Maternal-to-fetal transmission probably occurs in utero, because the infection is associated with prematurity, low birthweight, and maternal complications such as premature rupture of membranes and chorioamnionitis. Routine therapy with ampicillin and gentamicin for presumptive neonatal sepsis may not be effective if an ampicillin-resistant strain of *H. influenzae* has caused the infection.

Brazilian Purpuric Fever A nonserotypable *H. influenzae*, biogroup III (which is identical to the *H. aegyptius* group), is the etiology of Brazilian purpuric fever (BPF), recently discovered in children in southern Brazil. Following an antecedent episode of purulent conjunctivitis, children with BPF become bacteremic and present with fever, shock, and purpura fulminans. The disease may mimic meningococcemia, but has not been reported in the United States.

Other Invasive Infections Hib bacteremic disease has also been rarely associated with seeding of other body sites. Endophthalmitis, glossitis, uvulitis, thyroiditis, endocarditis, lung abscess, epididymitis, peritonitis, intraperitoneal abscesses, hepatobiliary disease, and brain abscesses have been reported.

CLINICAL MANIFESTATIONS CAUSED BY NONTYPABLE STRAINS Nontypable strains of *H. influenzae* frequently cause otitis media, sinusitis, conjunctivitis, and bronchitis. The conjunctivitis is usually bilateral and purulent, and often is associated with acute otitis media ("conjunctivitis-otitis" syndrome). Although these respiratory tract infections are common, they are rarely life-threatening and generally are not associated with bacteremia. Underlying medical conditions such as prematurity, cerebrospinal fluid (CSF) leak, congenital heart disease, and immunoglobulin deficiency may predispose to invasive disease with the nontypable strains of *H. influenzae*. The finding of nontypable *H. influenzae* systemic infection should prompt an immunologic investigation, even if these obvious risk factors are absent. Importantly, immunization with conjugate Hib vaccines does *not* confer protection against the nontypable strains: nontypable *H. influenzae* remains a major etiology of otitis media in children. The encapsulated non-Hib strains of *H. influenzae* are occasionally implicated as causes of invasive disease. A recent report of a series of cases of *H. influenzae* type f meningitis suggested that these organisms could conceivably "emerge" as important causes of invasive disease in children in the post-Hib vaccine era, although this trend has not yet become widespread.

DIAGNOSIS The primary criterion for the diagnosis of *H. influenzae* infection is isolation of the organism from the infectious focus (blood, CSF, or any other site of infection, such as joint, pericardial, or empyema fluid). Patients with epiglottitis usually have positive blood cultures; cultures from the inflamed epiglottitis should be obtained only after the airway has been secured. Whenever invasive disease is encountered, or meningitis is suspected on clinical grounds, lumbar puncture should be performed. Because the organism is fastidious, specimens should be processed immediately after they are acquired. Gram stain should be performed on any body fluid possibly infected with *H. influenzae*. Organisms are seen in about 90% of stained CSF smears in patients with meningitis, and the Gram-stain appearance of CSF has important implications in the management of pediatric meningitis. The appearance of gram-positive cocci suggests the possibility of pneumococcal meningitis, and the possible need for empirical vancomycin therapy, whereas the appearance of organisms consistent with *H. influenzae* suggests the potential usefulness of steroid therapy (see below). The CSF of a child with Hib meningitis characteristically has a marked pleocytosis, a low glucose concentration, and an elevated protein

concentration, but these findings are not specific for the diagnosis of Hib meningitis.

The type b capsular polysaccharide (PRP) can be detected in body fluids (serum, urine, joint fluid, CSF) from children with invasive disease. The three most commonly used assays are countercurrent immunoelectrophoresis (CIE), latex particle agglutination (LPA), and coagglutination (CoA). The tests are most useful when performed on CSF from children with meningitis who have been pretreated with antibiotics, because cultures may be unrevealing in this setting. Unfortunately, immunization with the Hib conjugate vaccines often results in urinary excretion of antigen for days to weeks, and such false-positive results limit the usefulness of these assays. False-positive reactions are unusual in the CSF.

For infections caused by nontypable strains of *H. influenzae*, antigen detection and blood cultures are of little diagnostic value, because bacteremia is rare. The diagnosis is usually clinical, although a microbiological diagnosis can be established for pneumonia/bronchitis by culture of sputum, for otitis media by diagnostic tympanocentesis, for sinusitis by culture of sinus aspirate, and for conjunctivitis by culture of the eye discharge.

TREATMENT

Invasive Disease Because bacteremia is central in invasive *H. influenzae* type b disease, therapy must anticipate the need for adequate central nervous system (CNS) penetration and be of sufficient duration to sterilize the primary and any secondary foci. The emergence of antibiotic resistance further necessitates that therapy of invasive infections includes β-lactamase-stable agents.

Because of the emergence of ampicillin-resistant isolates of *H. influenzae*, in the setting of proven or suspected Hib meningitis, cefotaxime or ceftriaxone are recommended until the antibiotic susceptibility of the organism is known or an alternative diagnosis is established. Both antibiotics have bactericidal activity against Hib, including β-lactamase-producing strains, and both penetrate well into infected CSF. Ceftriaxone is approved for once-daily therapy of meningitis at a dose of 100 mg/kg/d and can be administered by daily intramuscular injections if intravenous access is difficult, or used to complete a course of outpatient therapy in the patient who is clinically stable. Empiric therapy with ampicillin alone is not justified because approximately 50% of Hib isolates in the United States are resistant, although it is effective for isolates that are documented to be susceptible. Other extended-generation cephalosporins with indications for meningitis include ceftazidime and cefepime, but because of their overly broad spectrum they are not desirable choices for therapy of documented Hib meningitis. Vancomycin should be included empirically (until culture results are available) for all cases of pediatric meningitis in those areas of the United States where levels of *S. pneumoniae* resistance to penicillin are high and when *S. pneumoniae* cannot be excluded.

Meropenem is an acceptable alternative to third-generation cephalosporins with a well-established track record of efficacy for pediatric meningitis, including meningitis caused by Hib. However, meropenem does not appear to have activity for *S. pneumoniae* with high-level resistance to penicillins and therefore should not be used as single-agent therapy when pneumococcal meningitis is suspected.

Cefuroxime has good activity against *H. influenzae* and *S. aureus*, and is a reasonable choice for empiric therapy of some infections when *H. influenzae* is in the differential diagnosis, such as pneumonia, cellulitis, or bone and joint infections. However, caution must be taken with this agent if the diagnosis of meningitis has not been excluded, because cefuroxime is associated with delayed sterilization of the CSF.

Although chloramphenicol became the drug of choice for Hib infections shortly after the appearance of ampicillin-resistant strains in the 1970s, with the emergence of the third-generation cephalosporins, chloramphenicol is now rarely used because of the need to monitor serum levels to prevent toxicity. Chloramphenicol-resistant strains are becoming increasingly prevalent in some parts of the world, so local resistance patterns must be considered. However, ampicillin in combination with chloramphenicol remains a reasonable option for treatment of invasive Hib disease in the United States. Although adequate blood levels of chloramphenicol can be achieved with oral administration, it is usually advisable to initiate therapy intravenously. Oral chloramphenicol has been used successfully to complete the course of antibiotic therapy in invasive Hib disease, but the current lack of availability of oral chloramphenicol in the United States limits the usefulness of this option. Serum levels should be monitored and maintained between 10 and 20 mg/L in all patients receiving chloramphenicol. Although chloramphenicol has dose-related and reversible bone-marrow toxicity, this is usually evident only in the neonate, the child with liver disease, or after prolonged treatment. Idiosyncratic aplastic anemia in young children is very rare.

The duration of antibiotic therapy is determined by the site of infection and the clinical response. Children with uncomplicated Hib meningitis can be treated for 7 to 10 days. Children with cellulitis can be changed to oral therapy after several days of parenteral therapy, provided they have had a satisfactory clinical response and do not have meningitis. Patients with septic arthritis should receive at least 14 to 21 days of therapy, in conjunction with appropriate surgical care. Children with pericarditis, empyema, or osteomyelitis may require longer courses of intravenous antibiotic treatment (3 to 6 weeks) followed by a course of oral therapy. Children with occult Hib bacteremia should be treated initially with parenteral antibiotics, given the risk for focal infection.

Supportive therapy is also vital in the management of children with invasive Hib disease. For meningitis, adjunctive therapy with dexamethasone appears to decrease the incidence of hearing loss and neurologic sequelae. The recommended dose is 0.6 mg/kg/d divided every 6 hours for 4 days, with the first dose given just before or with the first antibiotic dose. Management of the child with meningitis requires anticipation of complications such as shock, SIADH, subdural empyema, and secondary foci of infection. Prolonged fever during treatment of Hib meningitis is common and does not imply failure of the antibody regimen, but should prompt consideration of additional foci of infection (pericarditis, subdural effusion, etc). Children treated with dexamethasone have a shorter duration of fever acutely, but are still at risk to develop secondary fevers late in the course of illness.

In children with epiglottitis, the first priority is airway management. Endotracheal intubation is optimally performed in the operating room by an experienced anesthesiologist. If it can be done safely, cultures of the epiglottis may be obtained at this time, and blood cultures should be obtained once the airway is secure. Intravenous antibiotics should be administered as soon as possible.

For patients with joint infections, subdural empyema, pericarditis, or pleural empyema, surgical consultation is required. Infected joint fluid should be aspirated from the child with septic arthritis, particularly with septic arthritis of the hip joint, to reduce pressure and to prevent avascular necrosis of the femoral head. Most orthopedic surgeons prefer open drainage of the hip.

Noninvasive Disease Numerous orally administered antimicrobials are available to treat respiratory tract infections caused by nontypable *H. influenzae*. Generally, therapy in this setting is empiric, without specific culture confirmation of *H. influenzae* as the etiology. Despite the increasing prevalence of β-lactamase-producing organisms, both among Hib strains and as nontypable *H. influenzae*, amoxicillin remains the drug of choice for empiric therapy of acute otitis media and sinusitis because of its low cost and safety. Agents with activity against β-lactamase-producing organisms should be used if amoxicillin therapy fails. Consideration must be given to performance of diagnostic tympanocentesis in such patients, particularly to exclude the possibility of high-level penicillin-resistant isolates of *S. pneumoniae*. Among the available alternative antimicrobials are amoxicillin-clavulanate, trimethoprim-sulfamethoxazole, erythromycin-sulfisoxazole, newer macrolides such as clarithromycin and azithromycin, and second- and third-generation oral cephalosporins such as cefuroxime axetil, cefixime, cefpodoxime, cefprozil, and loracarbef.

PREVENTION Two modalities are available to prevent Hib disease: chemoprophylaxis to prevent secondary disease and active immunization to prevent endemic disease. The widespread success of immunization has rendered chemoprophylaxis largely of historical interest only.

Many studies have documented the increased risk of invasive disease among household contacts in the month following onset of disease in the index case. The attack rate is a function of age, approaching 4% in children under 2 years of age. Rifampin is the most effective antibiotic for eradicating Hib from the nasopharynx, primarily because of its exquisite ability to penetrate respiratory secretions. Children under 12 years of age should receive 20 mg/kg once daily for 4 days, and adults should receive 600 mg once daily for 4 days. The quinolones may also be effective, although they have not been studied sufficiently and are not approved for use in children. Prophylaxis should be instituted as soon as possible, because the risk of secondary disease is greatest during the few days after disease onset in the index patient. Prophylaxis is recommended only if it can be given within 2 weeks of disease onset. Because therapeutic antibiotics do not consistently eradicate Hib from the nasopharynx, rifampin should also be given to the index patient prior to hospital discharge. The use of rifampin chemoprophylaxis in childcare settings remains controversial, primarily because the risk of secondary disease in this setting is not well-defined. Coordination with the local health department and consultation with an expert is warranted. Fortunately, most childcare attendees are now immunized and therefore at low risk of secondary disease.

The first vaccine used in an effort to prevent Hib invasive disease was a purified type b capsular polysaccharide vaccine, introduced in the United States in 1985. Postlicensure, the majority of studies suggested that protection afforded by this vaccine was, at best, marginal. By 1988, this vaccine was replaced by the more immunogenic *conjugate vaccines*. These vaccines covalently linked PRP (the process of "conjugation") to an immunogenic carrier protein, in the process creating a semisynthetic carrier-hapten. With these vaccines, much higher levels of antibodies are induced, particularly in infants and young children; booster responses are seen with subsequent injections; and the antibody is predominantly IgG. Four Hib-conjugate vaccines have undergone extensive evaluation in humans and have been licensed for use in infants beginning at 2 months of age. Recommendations for Hib vaccination are detailed in Sec. 1.5.2.

References

Friesen CA, Cho CT: Characteristic features of neonatal sepsis due to *Haemophilus influenzae*. Rev Infect Dis 8:777–780, 1986

Galil K, Singleton R, Levine OS, et al: Reemergence of invasive *Haemophilus influenzae* type b disease in a well-vaccinated population in remote Alaska. J Infect Dis 179:101–106, 1999

Jorgensen JH: Update on mechanisms and prevalence of antimicrobial resistance in *Haemophilus influenzae*. Clin Infect Dis 14:1119–1123, 1992

Korones DN, Marshall GS, Shapiro ED: Outcome of children with occult bacteremia caused by *Haemophilus influenzae* type b. Pediatr Infect Dis J 11:516–520, 1992

Lebel MH, Freij BJ, Syrogiannopoulos GA, et al: Dexamethasone therapy for bacterial meningitis. Results of two double-blind, placebo-controlled trials. N Engl J Med 319:964–971, 1988

Smith AL: Pathogenesis of *Haemophilus influenzae* meningitis. Pediatr Infect Dis J 6:783–786, 1987

Waggoner-Fountain LA, Hendley JO, Cody EJ, et al: The emergence of *Haemophilus influenzae* types e and f as significant pathogens. Clin Infect Dis 21:1322–1324, 1995

Wenger JD: Epidemiology of *Haemophilus influenzae* type b disease and impact of *Haemophilus influenzae* type b conjugate vaccines in the United States and Canada. Pediatr Infect Dis J 17(Suppl 9):S132–136, 1998

13.2.16 *Legionella pneumophila*

Lorry G. Rubin

Legionella pneumophila was first recognized as the etiology of an outbreak of pneumonia among attendees at a 1976 American Legion Convention. Pneumonia caused by *Legionella* species, known as Legionnaire disease or legionellosis, is a common cause of community-acquired pneumonia in adults and is a cause of nosocomial pneumonia and pneumonia in immunocompromised adults and children. *Legionella pneumophila* also causes Pontiac fever, an uncommon, short incubation, influenza-like illness that primarily affects adults with symptoms of fever, malaise, myalgia, chills, headache, and pleuritic pain.

EPIDEMIOLOGY Although approximately 40 *Legionella* species have been identified, only one-half have been isolated from humans. *Legionella pneumophila*, comprised of 14 serotypes, is the most virulent species, accounting for the majority of human infections. *Legionella pneumophila* serogroup 1 causes 50 to 90% of human infections, whereas *L. pneumophila* serogroup 6, other *L. pneumophila* serogroups, and *Legionella micdadei* cause most of the remainder of human infections. These bacilli are nutritionally fastidious, aerobic rods that, after recovery on artificial media, stain as gram-negative. *Legionella micdadei* is unique among *Legionella* species in that it can be visualized in specimens using a modified acid-fast stain.

Infection with *Legionella* results from inhalation of contaminated aerosols from environmental or aquatic sources. *Legionella* are not transmitted from person to person. *Legionella spp.* are ubiquitous in natural freshwater habitats such as lakes, rivers, and groundwater. From these sources they gain entry into water systems of buildings, including hospitals. These bacteria thrive at temperatures between 30°C (86°F) and 54°C (129.2°F) and are killed at temperatures above 60°C (140°F). *Legionella spp.* are facultative intracellular pathogens and may replicate in nature within various

protozoa, including amoeba. Community outbreaks of *Legionella* have occurred and have been linked to aerosol-generating machinery, including cooling towers, evaporative condensers, showers, respiratory therapy devices, air conditioners, ultrasonic mist machines for vegetables, whirlpool spas, and humidifiers. Nosocomial infections and hospital outbreaks also occur and are most commonly traced to the water supply, particularly the hot-water supply.

Most cases of Legionnaire disease occur in susceptible elderly or middle-aged adults. *Legionella* are responsible for 1 to 15% of community-acquired pneumonias that require hospitalization. The incubation period has been estimated to range from 2 to 10 days with an average of 7 days. The main risk factors in adults are chronic lung disease, immunosuppression, especially associated with corticosteroid treatment or organ transplantation, and cigarette smoking.

Extrapulmonary infection occurs rarely, with the heart a specific site of infection. In children, extrapulmonary infection has been found in the liver, spleen, and groin. The entry point may be bacteremic spread from the lung, and *Legionella* have been recovered in blood cultures of patients with pneumonia. The origin of localized extrapulmonary infection is more commonly a postoperative wound that was irrigated with *Legionella*-contaminated water.

Legionellosis is uncommon in the pediatric age group. Only 22 (1.7%) of 1308 cases of legionellosis reported to the Centers for Disease Control and Prevention in 1992 were in the neonate to 19-year-old age group. In pediatric legionellosis, the risk factors for serious infection are immune compromise due to cancer therapy, corticosteroid treatment, primary immune deficiency, or underlying lung disease including nosocomial infection in children on ventilators. *Legionella* pneumonia is being increasingly reported as a nosocomial pathogen of neonates in the newborn nursery or special care nursery. At least seven recent reports have documented serious or fatal *Legionella* pneumonia in newborns. Cases have occurred in both full-term and premature infants and in infants with congenital heart disease. *Legionella spp.* are probably responsible for 1 to 5% of mild-to-moderately severe community-acquired pneumonias in healthy children. These infections may resolve without antibiotic therapy effective against these pathogens. Subclinical infection probably occurs, as evidenced by serosurvey data that anti-*Legionella* antibody titers increase with age.

CLINICAL MANIFESTATIONS The most important clinical presentation of infection in both children and adults with legionellosis is acute lobar pneumonia presenting as an acute febrile illness with cough that may be accompanied by chest pain. Patients may initially have symptoms not referable to the lungs such as chills, abdominal pain, myalgias, confusion, malaise, anorexia, and watery diarrhea. However, these clinical findings are not sufficiently specific to differentiate *Legionella* pneumonia from community-acquired or nosocomial pneumonia of other etiologies. Chest radiographs show evidence of alveolar, rather than interstitial, infiltrates. Disease is most often unilateral but may progress to bilateral disease. Pulmonary nodules with or without cavitation may occur, especially in immunocompromised hosts. Pleural effusion may occur, but the incidence is not different from other bacterial pneumonias. Progressive respiratory distress, and often respiratory failure, develops over several days. Copathogens are rarely recovered. The fatality rate among previously healthy, appropriately treated individuals is about 6%. *Legionella* infection is relatively common in renal or cardiac transplant patients presenting within several weeks after transplantation with fever and pulmonary nodules on chest radiograph.

Alternatively, these patients may have prodromal symptoms of malaise, myalgias, and headache, followed by an abrupt onset of dyspnea, cough, and pleuritic chest pain indicating pneumonia.

In neonates, the clinical presentation is that of acute respiratory distress requiring mechanical ventilation. Because of the fulminant nature of the infection and/or the failure to consider this organism, the diagnosis is established in some infants only at autopsy.

DIAGNOSIS Nonspecific laboratory abnormalities commonly include leukocytosis with a left shift, hyponatremia, proteinuria, or elevation of liver function tests. Hyponatremia is significantly more frequent in the initial stage of legionellosis than in pneumonia caused by other etiologies. Specific laboratory diagnosis is established by culture of pulmonary secretions (the "gold standard"), by direct detection of organisms in pulmonary secretions, by urinary antigen detection, or by serology. A useful clue to the diagnosis is the presence of inflammatory cells without bacteria on a Gram-stained preparation of lower respiratory secretions; *Legionella* induce a polymorphonuclear leukocyte inflammatory response, but stain poorly with Gram stain. However, the absence of significant numbers of polymorphonuclear leukocytes does not exclude the diagnosis.

Legionella do not grow on ordinary laboratory media and must be cultured on special medium, most commonly buffered charcoal yeast extract (BCYE) agar enriched with L-cystine, iron, α-ketoglutarate, and N-2-acetamido-2-aminoethanesulphonic acid buffer. To inhibit overgrowth of other microorganisms present in the clinical specimen that may interfere with recognition of colonies of *Legionella*, the sputum may be washed with acid or heated prior to inoculation, and/or the enriched BCYE agar may be supplemented with antibiotics. Some commercial lots of BCYE agar have exhibited poor performance using clinical specimens. Colonies take an average of 3 days to appear.

Because of the difficulty of recovering the organism in culture, direct detection of bacteria or serology is frequently used to diagnose legionellosis. Detection of organisms on smears of respiratory secretions using specific antibodies by direct (or indirect) immunofluorescence (DFA) using polyclonal or monoclonal antibodies is a rapid and reasonably sensitive (average sensitivity approximately 60%) alternative or adjunct to culture. The specificity of DFA testing is high (95–99%) particularly when using monoclonal antibody. Detection of *Legionella* antigens in urine by radioimmunoassay or by enzyme immunoassay is an excellent test. Antigen can be detected as early as a few days after onset of infection. A commercially available test (Binax, S. Portland, ME) has a sensitivity of 80 to 90% that is superior to DFA testing of sputum and that is highly specific, but it detects only *L. pneumophila* type 1. Antigenuria is typically prolonged beyond resolution of clinical infection and should not be used to judge the adequacy of therapy. A commercial kit is available for polymerase chain reaction–based amplification and detection of *Legionella* DNA in environmental specimens; direct detection tests using *Legionella*-specific DNA probes are being developed for analysis of clinical specimens.

Serology by indirect immunofluorescence (IFA) is a useful method for retrospective diagnosis of legionellosis. A fourfold rise in antibody titer to more than 1:128 is diagnostic; a single convalescent titer of 1:256 or more in a patient with a characteristic clinical presentation is highly suggestive. Although an acute serum sometimes shows an elevated titer, not all patients seroconvert, and seroconversion may take 6 weeks or longer. Another drawback is that seroconversion is occasionally the result of serologic cross-reaction after infection with another organism, for example, *Citrobacter freundii* or *Bacteroides fragilis*. Although it has been stated that infected children younger than 1 year do not seroconvert, seroconversion has been documented in several young children with legionellosis. In summary, although culture is the gold standard, direct detection of organisms on smears of respiratory secretions or detection of antigen in urine are useful tests to diagnose infection with *Legionella*. Measurement of specific antibody titers is a complementary test to confirm infection.

TREATMENT Legionnaire disease may be fatal; therefore appropriate therapy should be instituted promptly in suspected cases. Based upon extensive but uncontrolled clinical experience, the antibiotic of choice for treatment of *Legionella* infection is intravenously administered erythromycin. Although typically prescribed at a dose of 40 mg/kg/d, doses of up to 100 mg/kg/d have been administered without difficulty. Oral erythromycin may be substituted after a definite clinical response to complete a 14- to 21-day course, with 21 days for immunocompromised patients. Experience suggests that rifampin is effective in combination with erythromycin and should be added for patients with severe infections, for those who fail to respond to erythromycin, and for severely immunocompromised patients. When treating a patient with a solid organ transplant, it is important to consider that erythromycin inhibits the metabolism of cyclosporine, and rifampin has the opposite effect.

Based on in vitro activity and clinical experience, clarithromycin may become the treatment of first choice for oral treatment because of similar or superior activity and less gastrointestinal irritation than erythromycin. Similarly, because of the availability and convenience of an intravenous formulation of azithromycin, it is likely that this will replace intravenous erythromycin. Unlike erythromycin, fluoroquinolone antibiotics, such as ciprofloxacin, are bactericidal for *Legionella* and limited clinical experience has been positive. Doxycycline and trimethoprim-sulfamethoxazole have been used successfully in some patients. In a few cases of infection with *L. micdadei*, patients who failed treatment with erythromycin responded to treatment with trimethoprim-sulfamethoxazole. Clinical experience shows that β-lactam antibiotics and aminoglycosides are ineffective in treating *Legionella* pneumonia.

PREVENTION Outbreaks in hospitals are investigated by culturing water sources in the hospital for *Legionella*. There are three accepted methods for decontaminating the water supply: hyperchlorinating the water supply; superheating the water to between 70°C (158°F) and 80°C (176°F) with flushing of the distal sites; and installing a copper-silver ionization unit in the water supply line.

References

Carlson NC, Kuskie MR, Dobyns EL, et al: Legionellosis in children: an expanding spectrum. Pediatr Infect Dis J 9:133–137, 1990

Levy I, Rubin L: *Legionella* pneumonia in neonates: a literature review. J Perinatol 18:287–290, 1998

Muder RR, Yu VL: Mode of transmission of *Legionella pneumophila:* a critical review. Arch Intern Med 146:1607–1612, 1986

Roig J, Carreres A, Domingo C: Treatment of Legionnaires' disease—current recommendations. Drugs 46:63–79, 1993

Stout JE, Yu VL: Legionellosis. N Engl J Med 10:682–687, 1997

13.2.17 Leptospirosis

Michael Katz

Leptospirosis is a multisystem disease, which was described under a variety of clinical syndromes before discovery of the causative agent unified these syndromes into one disease. Such conditions as Weil disease (occasionally used to refer to the most severe form of leptospirosis), swamp fever, and field fever in Europe; 7-day fever (nanukayami) and autumnal fever (Hasami-Netsu) in Japan; cane-field fever in Australia; and Bushy Creek fever and Fort Bragg fever in the United States, are known to result from leptospiral infections. There is ample epidemiologic evidence that swine, cattle, dogs, and rodents serve as reservoirs.

All leptospires belong to one species, *Leptospira interrogans,* which consists of two complexes, *interrogans* and *biflexa*. The pathogenic strains belong to the *interrogans* complex, and at least a dozen strains are known to infect human beings. Only three, however—the *icterohaemorrhagiae* serogroup (from rats), the *pomona* serogroup (from swine), and the *canicola* serogroup (from cattle and dogs)—do so with any frequency. The *hardjo* serovariant from cattle also has caused disease in human beings.

Leptospirosis is not common, but there is an indication that it is an emerging infection. Although only 54 patients were reported to the Centers for Disease Control in 1988, an outbreak of this infection in 1995 in Nicaragua affected several thousand people. In 1997, an outbreak in India of an epidemic febrile illness associated with uveitis was diagnosed as leptospirosis. Clinical leptospirosis is not always recognized, as evidenced by antileptospiral antibodies in individuals who have no history of leptospirosis. Active surveillance on two Hawaiian islands revealed an annual incidence rate of 128 per 100,000. Among the factors most strongly associated with this infection are household use of rainwater catchment systems and contact with animal tissues and cattle.

The reservoir animals retain leptospires in their renal tubules and shed large numbers of these organisms in the urine for months after infection. Human beings become infected through contact with animal urine, either directly or secondarily through contaminated soil or water. Leptospiras are very sensitive to acid and perish in solutions of low pH in a few hours; but in alkaline or neutral medium, they persist for weeks, provided that the temperature is above 22°C (71.6°F). Thus, during the warm seasons, stagnant waters and moist soil are common sources of infection. Infection can be acquired through cut or abraded skin, or through respiratory or conjunctival epithelium with immersion. The disease is associated with farming, abattoirs, and sewers, as well as with camping, fishing, and contact with pet dogs. It is more frequent in summer and early fall, and has a 3:1 predominance of males. Seventy percent of infections occur in individuals between 10 and 40 years of age.

CLINICAL MANIFESTATIONS   Clinical manifestations vary somewhat with the infecting serogroup. The *canicola* and *pomona* groups tend to cause less-severe disease than does the *icterohaemorrhagiae* group. Nevertheless, in an outbreak of the *hardjo* infection from cattle in Great Britain, there were four fatalities among 120 people with this infection.

In general, leptospirosis is a biphasic disease that develops after a median incubation period of 1 week, with a range of 2 to 20 days. The initial phase, lasting 4 to 7 days, is the septicemic stage. It is characterized by sudden onset of fever, headache, myalgia, and gastrointestinal disturbances, such as abdominal pain, nausea, and vomiting. During this period, the organisms multiply in monocytes.

Host defense depends on immune resistance, with the cell-mediated responses developing earlier than antibodies.

Physical examination usually reveals an acutely ill patient, who may be confused or delirious. Conjunctivitis, uveitis, pharyngeal infection, lymphadenopathy, hepatosplenomegaly, macular exanthem, and icterus may be seen. In one study, two-thirds of the patients had abnormal radiographic findings in the lungs. Small nodular densities predominated, but a few patients had larger areas of consolidation. During this stage the patient has leptospiremia and proteinuria. The fever ends by lysis. The patient may remain well and comfortable for 1 to 3 days, until the start of the second phase of the disease, which is subclinical in most patients.

In those patients who have symptoms, the second phase begins with meningitis, which may be subclinical, and with fever, which may be of a lower grade than during the first phase. CSF shows features characteristic of aseptic meningitis, with mononuclear pleocytosis, usually not exceeding 500 cells/μL, a normal glucose, and an elevated protein concentration. During this phase, the patient no longer has leptospiremia, but does have leptospiruria. Because the patient has developed antibodies to the organism by now, this phase is also sometimes referred to as the immune stage.

Ten percent of patients develop a severe form of the disease, characterized by prolonged fever, jaundice, azotemia, hemorrhage, vascular collapse, and an altered state of consciousness. The same biphasic pattern of the disease can be seen in this severe form, but the severity of symptoms and their prolongation may last well into the second phase, obscuring the signs that mark the end of the first phase. It has been suggested that this severe form is caused by a toxin elaborated by the microorganism, but no such toxin has yet been demonstrated. Thrombocytopenia and renal failure can develop and appear to be correlated, although a causal relationship has not been demonstrated. Other complications include acute acalculous cholecystitis, hydrops of the gallbladder, cholangitis, pancreatitis, and peripheral gangrene.

DIAGNOSIS   Leptospirosis must be considered in patients with aseptic meningitis, hepatitis, generalized malaise with myalgia, and fever of undetermined origin. Those who have recently returned from tropical environments and have an illness resembling hemorrhagic fever should also be suspected of having leptospirosis. Definitive diagnosis involves demonstrating leptospires in the patient's blood or urine by culture or by inoculation of guinea pigs, hamsters, or mice, but this method is laborious and prolonged. A rapid diagnosis can be made by determining the specific IgM using the DOT-ELISA method, which is accurate and inexpensive, and is therefore preferable to the older, commonly used microagglutinin test. The DOT-ELISA method is based on a series of leptospiral antigens, may be performed in a routine laboratory, and is more sensitive and easier to perform than the older method. A sensitive assay for *Leptospira spp.* by a polymerase chain reaction (PCR) has been developed. It is based on a 331–base pair sequence from a gene of the *L. interrogans* serovar *canicola*. This assay, capable of detecting as few as 10 bacteria, has been applied to human CSF and urine. It was positive in patients with leptospirosis and negative in uninfected controls. It is considered to be the most efficient and accurate diagnostic test. However, it is less effective in an epidemiologic evaluation. It can only identify the infecting organism to the genus level; it cannot distinguish a serovar. For this purpose, the microagglutination test based on the ability of the suspect serum to agglutinate live strains of *Leptospira* is the most accurate test.

TREATMENT Efficacy of antimicrobial therapy remains controversial. In one study, doxycycline was reported beneficial, especially if started early in the disease. Two prospective, randomized studies of therapy with penicillin have shown opposite results, one indicating definite benefit and the other no benefit. Because doxycycline may not be used in children less than 8 years of age or in pregnant women, penicillin is the only choice available for these patients. Based on the study that did show benefit, therapy should be given intravenously for 7 days. In a retrospective study of severely ill hospitalized children in Brazil, treatment with penicillin or ampicillin was associated with an accelerated recovery from acute renal failure and thrombocytopenia, but not other complications or the duration of fever. No human vaccine is currently available. An inactivated veterinary vaccine does not prevent leptospiruria. Therefore, vaccinated animals can still be sources of human infection.

PROGNOSIS The prognosis depends on two principal factors: virulence of the infecting organism and the age of the patient. In anicteric leptospirosis, death is virtually unknown, but in classic Weil disease with jaundice, case fatality may be as high as 20%. Mortality tends to be higher in the oldest age group and lower in children.

References

Centers for Disease Control: Outbreak of acute febrile illness and pulmonary hemorrhage—Nicaragua, 1995. MMWR Morb Mortal Wkly Rep 44:839–843, 1995

Edwards CN, Nicholson GD, Hassell TA, et al: Penicillin therapy in icteric leptospirosis. Am J Trop Med Hyg 39:388, 1988

Marotto PCF, Marotto MS, Santos DL, et al: Outcome of leptospirosis in children. Am J Trop Med Hyg 56:307–310, 1997

McLain JB, Ballou WR, Harrison SM, Steinweg DL: Doxycycline therapy for leptospirosis. Ann Intern Med J 100:696, 1984

Merien F, Baranton G, Perolat P: Comparison of polymerase chain reaction with microagglutination test and culture for diagnosis of leptospirosis. J Infect Dis 172:281–285, 1995

Watt G, Alquinza LM, Padre LP, et al: The rapid diagnosis of leptospirosis: a prospective comparison of the DOT enzyme-linked immunosorbent assay and the genus-specific microscopic agglutination test at different stages of illness. Infect Dis 157:840, 1988

13.2.18   Listeriosis

Ralph C. Gordon

Listeria monocytogenes is a nonsporulating, motile gram-positive rod that most commonly causes septicemia and meningitis. The usual pediatric patient is a young infant, whose mother ate *Listeria*-contaminated food during pregnancy in the context of the depressed cellular immunity of the gravid state. Presentations in infants include early onset or late-onset disease similar to that by the group B streptococcus. Infections may also occur following *Listeria* ingestion by children with malignancies on chemotherapy, human immunodeficiency virus infection, diabetes, or during steroid treatment of collagen-vascular disorders.

EPIDEMIOLOGY It is estimated that there are a total of about 1850 cases of listeriosis annually in the United States, in both children and adults, with around 425 deaths. Recent reports show that enteric infections may also occur in normal children from drinking tainted milk and may cause disease ranging from mild gastroenteritis to a febrile illness with bacteremia.

The organism is widely distributed in nature, and light contamination of food occurs frequently. Sources include sheep, goats, pork, cattle, and poultry, which may cause infection through direct contact with workers, contaminated milk products or meats, or soiling of vegetables with manure. Food-borne listeriosis is a public health problem in many countries, especially countries in North America and Europe.

Infection in infants occurs through transplacental infection, premature rupture of membranes, or fecal contamination from the mother at the time of birth. The high risk of infection in the compromised host, whether infant, pregnant female, or others, is related to failure of the complex mechanisms of cellular immunity, which are influenced by an immature or altered physiological state, disease, or drugs.

The highest incidence of *Listeria* meningitis occurs in infants less than 1 month of age, as demonstrated in a 1995 Centers for Disease Control survey involving more than 10 million Americans. There were 39.2 cases of *Listeria* meningitis per 100,000 population, which was approximately one-third of the rate for group B streptococcus meningitis in that same age group. All infants with *Listeria* invasive disease had meningitis, whereas streptococcal invasive disease, with or without meningitis, was considerably more common. Adults age 60 years and older comprised the group with the next highest incidence of listeriosis.

The case fatality rate for *Listeria* meningitis in all ages was 15%, second only to the 21% seen with *Streptococcus pneumoniae,* and considerably higher than meningitis caused by *Haemophilus influenzae* (6%), *Neisseria meningitidis* (3%), and group B streptococcus (7%), respectively.

CLINICAL MANIFESTATIONS AND DIAGNOSIS Although infection in the pediatric patient usually involves septicemia or meningitis, less frequently seen syndromes may include rhomboencephalitis, brain abscess, and endocarditis. In addition, the stools of infants with *Listeria* infection can pose a nosocomial hazard to other babies in the nursery. Epidemics have occurred in that setting.

Laboratory studies generally reveal a polymorphonuclear response to *Listeria* infection in the peripheral blood and cerebrospinal fluid of humans, while monocytosis is primarily seen in laboratory animals. CSF protein levels can often reach 1000 mg/dL, leading to sludging and hydrocephalus. Diagnosis is based on isolation of the organism from blood and cerebrospinal fluid, and it should be noted that Gram stains of the latter are often negative in meningitis. The laboratory must study gram-positive rods isolated from infants or compromised hosts with care before discarding them as "diphtheroids." Serologic studies in humans have some utility in the investigation of food-borne outbreaks, but have had little clinical application.

TREATMENT Optimal antimicrobial therapy of listeriosis is not well defined, although most authorities suggest 2 or 3 weeks of ampicillin given intravenously. An aminoglycoside is often added because of the synergism seen in laboratory and animal models. This plan has been used successfully for more than two decades. The need for longer treatment courses relates to the presence of meningitis or unusual conditions, such as endocarditis.

Trimethoprim-sulfamethoxazole is a highly effective combination in treatment of listeriosis. It is attractive because of its good intracellular penetration, but must be avoided in the newborn or allergic patient. Cephalosporins are not effective in the treatment of listeriosis. It is generally believed that a better outcome in listeriosis may be associated with early diagnosis and initiation of treatment, although no clinical studies exist that confirm this belief.

PREVENTION Compromised hosts, including pregnant women, should be advised of the potential risks of eating food products that have been implicated in outbreaks of listeriosis. These foods include various specialty cheeses, hot dogs, pâté, cold cuts, and other delicatessen products that may be contaminated during preparation or processing. Leftover foods and ready-to-eat food should be reheated before eating. Some experts believe that high-risk persons should avoid eating soft cheeses and delicatessen meats altogether.

References

Dalton CB, Austin CC, Sobel J, et al: An outbreak of gastroenteritis and fever due to *Listeria monocytogenes* in milk. N Engl J Med 336:100, 1997

Schuchat A, Robinson K, Wenger JD, et al: Bacterial meningitis in the United States in 1995. N Engl J Med 337:970, 1997

Slutsker L, Schuchat A: Listeriosis in humans. In: Ryser ET, Marth EH, eds: *Listeria*, Listeriosis and Food Safety, 2nd ed. New York, Marcel Dekker, 1999

St. Georgiev V: *Listeria monocytogenes.* in: St. Georgiev V, ed: Infectious Diseases in Immunocompromised Hosts. Boca Raton, FL, CRC Press, 1998

13.2.19   Lyme Disease

Michael A. Gerber

Lyme disease is the most commonly reported vector-borne illness in the United States, accounting for more than 95% of such cases. It is caused by the spirochete, *Borrelia burgdorferi,* which is transmitted to humans through the bite of an *Ixodes* tick. Lyme disease is a multisystem, multistage, inflammatory illness.

EPIDEMIOLOGY Since 1982, the number of reported cases of Lyme disease in the United States has increased about 25-fold, with a mean of approximately 12,500 cases reported annually in recent years. More than 90% of the cases of Lyme disease are reported from approximately 150 counties in 13 states located along the northeastern and mid-Atlantic seaboard and in the upper north-central region. The highest reported rates of Lyme disease occur in children 2 to 15 years of age and in persons 30 to 59 years of age. The principal risk factor for acquiring Lyme disease in endemic areas is residence in suburban or rural areas that are wooded or overgrown with brush and infested by infected vector ticks. The ticks that can transmit Lyme disease (*Ixodes scapularis,* also known as the black-legged or deer tick, in the eastern United States, and *I. pacificus,* also known as the western black-legged tick, in the western United States) are found in wooded areas, high grasses, marshes, gardens, and beach areas. Humans acquire *B. burgdorferi* from infected ticks at the time the tick takes a blood meal.

Lyme disease is not spread by person-to-person contact or by direct contact with infected animals. Although transplacental transmission of *B. burgdorferi* has been reported, the effect of such transmission on the fetus remains uncertain. Available data suggest that congenital Lyme disease occurs only very rarely, if at all. Transmission in breast milk has not been documented. Although *B. burg-*

dorferi can survive in stored blood for several weeks, the risk for transfusion-acquired Lyme disease appears to be minimal.

CLINICAL MANIFESTATIONS The clinical manifestations of Lyme disease depend on the stage of the disease—early, localized disease; early, disseminated disease; or late disease. The most common manifestation of early, localized Lyme disease, erythema migrans, appears 3 to 30 days (but typically within 7 to 10 days) after a tick bite at the site of the bite. Erythema migrans begins as a red macule or papule and usually expands over days to weeks to form a large, annular, erythematous lesion that is at least 5 cm and as much as 70 cm in diameter (median of 15 cm). The rash may be uniformly erythematous or it may appear as a target lesion with variable degrees of central clearing. It can vary greatly in shape and, occasionally, may have vesicular or necrotic areas in the center. Erythema migrans is usually asymptomatic but may be pruritic or painful, and may be accompanied by systemic symptoms such as fever, malaise, headache, myalgias, and arthralgias. Patients with early, localized Lyme disease can also present with a flu-like illness without erythema migrans.

The most common manifestation of early, disseminated Lyme disease is multiple erythema migrans. The secondary skin lesions, which usually occur from 3 to 5 weeks after the tick bite, consist of multiple annular erythematous lesions similar to, but usually smaller than, the primary lesion. Other common manifestations of early, disseminated Lyme disease are cranial nerve palsies, especially facial nerve palsy, and meningitis. Carditis, which usually is manifested by various degrees of heart block, although rare, may also occur at this stage. Systemic symptoms such as myalgias, arthralgias, headache, and fatigue are common in the early, disseminated stage.

Late Lyme disease is characterized by arthritis, which is usually monoarticular or oligoarticular, that affects the large joints, particularly the knee. The arthritis occurs weeks to months after the initial infection. Although the affected joint is typically swollen and tender, the intense pain associated with a septic arthritis is usually not present. Encephalitis, encephalopathy, and polyneuropathy are also manifestations of late Lyme disease but are rare in children.

DIAGNOSIS For patients who present with the characteristic lesion of erythema migrans, the diagnosis should be based on the clinical presentation alone. For patients who do not have erythema migrans, the diagnosis also should be based on clinical findings, but with support from laboratory testing. Methods for identifying the presence of *B. burgdorferi* in a patient (eg, culture, antigen detection, histopathology) have poor sensitivity and/or specificity and may require invasive procedures (eg, skin biopsy) to obtain an appropriate specimen for testing. Therefore, laboratory confirmation usually depends on serologic testing for antibodies to *B. burgdorferi.*

Unfortunately, serologic tests for Lyme disease have not been adequately standardized. In addition, antibodies to *B. burgdorferi* are not detectable in most patients with early, localized Lyme disease. Furthermore, some patients who are treated with antimicrobial agents early in the course of their disease never develop antibodies to *B. burgdorferi.* However, most patients with early, disseminated Lyme disease, and virtually all patients with late Lyme disease, have antibodies to *B. burgdorferi.* As with other infections, once such antibodies develop, they may persist for many years despite cure of the disease. Consequently, tests for antibodies should not be used to assess the success of treatment. Because of the poor sensitivity and specificity of the serologic testing for *B. burgdorferi* that is currently available in most commercial laboratories, testing for serum antibodies to *B. burgdorferi* should be performed in a reference laboratory whenever possible.

The enzyme immunosorbent assay (EIA) is the most commonly used test for detection of antibodies to *B. burgdorferi*. This test may give false-positive results because of cross-reactive antibodies in patients with other spirochetal infections (eg, syphilis, leptospirosis, relapsing fever), certain viral infections (eg, varicella), and certain autoimmune diseases (eg, systemic lupus erythematosus). In contrast to patients with syphilis, those with Lyme disease do not have positive nontreponemal syphilis tests such as the VDRL or RPR. In addition, antibodies directed against certain bacteria in the normal oral flora may cross-react with antigens of *B. burgdorferi* and produce a false-positive test result.

Currently, the Western immunoblot test is the most useful test for corroborating positive or equivocal EIA results; as a result, a two-test approach is recommended for confirming the diagnosis of *B. burgdorferi* infection. Sera that are positive or equivocal by a sensitive EIA should be tested by a standardized Western immunoblot for the presence of antibodies to proteins specific for *B. burgdorferi;* those that are negative by a sensitive EIA do not require immunoblot testing.

A major problem in diagnosing Lyme disease is the widespread practice of ordering serologic tests in patients with only nonspecific symptoms (eg, fatigue, arthralgia) who have a low pretest probability of having Lyme disease. Almost all positive serologic test results in such patients are false-positives. Patients with Lyme disease almost always have specific signs (eg, erythema migrans, facial nerve palsy, arthritis), and although nonspecific symptoms commonly accompany these specific signs, nonspecific symptoms are almost never the only clinical manifestation of Lyme disease.

TREATMENT Table 13-37 lists the recommended treatment for Lyme disease in children. Doxycycline is the drug of choice for treatment of early, localized disease in children 8 years of age and older. Precautions to avoid exposure to the sun (eg, the use of sunscreen) should be taken because a rash develops in sun-exposed areas in about 20% of persons who take doxycycline. Amoxicillin is recommended for those children less than 8 years of age and for those children who cannot tolerate doxycycline. For patients allergic to penicillin, alternative drugs are cefuroxime axetil and erythromycin or azithromycin, although erythromycin and azithromycin may be less effective. Most experts treat persons with early, localized Lyme disease for 21 days. Overall, clinical response to therapy is prompt and erythema migrans resolves within several days of initiating therapy. Treatment of erythema migrans almost always prevents development of later stages of Lyme disease.

Multiple erythema migrans and arthritis should be treated with orally administered antimicrobial agents. Most experts also recommend orally administered antimicrobial agents for facial nerve palsies, although some experts recommend a lumbar puncture if central nervous system involvement is suspected. If cerebrospinal fluid pleocytosis is found, they recommend parenterally administered antimicrobial therapy as for meningitis. Meningitis and recurrent or persistent arthritis should be treated with parenterally administered antimicrobial agents. However, some experts will provide a second course of an orally administered antimicrobial agent for recurrent or persistent arthritis before using a parenterally administered agent. Mild carditis is usually treated orally with doxycycline or amoxicillin. Most experts treat severe carditis with parenterally administered therapy. The optimal duration of anti-

TABLE 13-37

RECOMMENDED TREATMENT OF LYME DISEASE IN CHILDREN

DISEASE CATEGORY	DRUGS AND DOSAGES
Early, Localized Disease	
≥8 years old	Doxycycline, 100 mg twice daily for 21 days
<8 years old	Amoxicillin, 25–50 mg/kg/d, divided into two doses (maximum 2g/d) for 21 days
Early, Disseminated Disease	
Multiple erythema migrans	Same as for early, localized disease but for 28 days
Isolated facial nerve palsy	Same as for early, localized disease but for 28 days
Facial nerve palsy with evidence of central nervous system involvement	Same as for meningitis
Carditis	
Mild	Same as for early, localized disease
Severe	Same as for meningitis
Meningitis	Ceftriaxone 75–100 mg/kg IV or IM once daily (maximum 2 g/d) or penicillin 300,000 U/kg/d IV given in divided doses q4h (maximum, 20 million U/d) for 14–21 days
Late Disease	
Arthritis	Same as early, localized disease but for 28 days
Persistent or recurrent arthritis	Same as for meningitis
Neurologic disease	Same as for meningitis

microbial therapy for the various stages of Lyme disease is not well established, but there is no evidence that children with any manifestation of Lyme disease benefit from either prolonged (>4 weeks) or repeated courses of either orally or parenterally administered antimicrobial agents.

PROGNOSIS There is a widespread misconception that Lyme disease is difficult to treat successfully and that persistent or recurrent disease is common. In fact, the long-term prognosis for children who are treated with appropriate antimicrobial therapy for early or late stages of Lyme disease is excellent. The most common reason for a lack of response to appropriate antimicrobial therapy for Lyme disease is misdiagnosis (ie, the patient actually does not have Lyme disease). Approximately 10% of adults and fewer than 5% of children with Lyme arthritis develop inflammatory joint disease that does not respond to antimicrobial agents and typically affects one knee for months to years. Because of the increased frequency of certain HLA-DR4 alleles in these patients, an autoimmune mechanism has been proposed.

It is not uncommon for children with early Lyme disease to have persistence of vague, nonspecific symptoms after completing an appropriate course of antimicrobial therapy. The persistence of such symptoms is not an indication of treatment failure. Within 6 months of completing the initial course of antimicrobial therapy, these vague, nonspecific symptoms will resolve without additional antimicrobial therapy. For those unusual patients who have persistent symptoms more than 6 months after the completion of antimicrobial therapy, an attempt should be made to determine whether these symptoms are the result of active infection, a postinfectious phenomenon, or another illness.

PREVENTION In endemic residential areas, clearing brush and trees, removing leaf litter and woodpiles, keeping grass mowed, applying pesticides, erecting fences to exclude deer, and maintaining tick-free pets may reduce tick exposure. Application of tick and insect repellents that contain DEET (N,N-diethyl-m-toluamide) to the skin provides additional protection and is safe when used according to product label instructions. Repellent sprays containing permethrin are also effective when applied to clothing. Animal studies indicate that transmission of *B. burgdorferi* from infected ticks usually requires a prolonged duration of attachment ($\geq$48 hours). Therefore, careful inspection and prompt removal of ticks can substantially reduce the risk of Lyme disease. Routine use of antimicrobial agents to prevent Lyme disease following a deer tick bite, even in highly endemic areas, is not recommended. Serologic testing for Lyme disease at the time of a recognized tick bite also is not recommended. When preventive measures have failed, morbidity can be substantially reduced by detecting and treating persons with Lyme disease in the early stages.

A Lyme disease vaccine was recently licensed for persons 15 to 70 years of age. This vaccine appears to be safe and effective, but whether its use is cost-beneficial has yet to be clearly established. Decisions regarding the use of this vaccine should be based on an assessment of an individual's risk as determined by activities and behaviors relating to tick exposure in endemic areas. This vaccine should be considered an adjunct to, not a replacement for, the practice of personal protective measures against tick exposure and the early diagnosis and treatment of Lyme disease. The vaccine is not recommended for children less than 15 years of age until data concerning the safety and immunogenicity of this vaccine in this age group are available and the Food and Drug Administration has approved the vaccine for use in younger children.

References

Adams WV, Rose CD, Eppes SC, Klein JD: Cognitive effects of Lyme disease in children. Pediatrics 94:185–189, 1994

Gerber MA, Shapiro ED, Burke GS, Parcells VJ, Bell GL: Lyme disease in children in Southeastern Connecticut. N Engl J Med 335:1270–1274, 1996

Gerber MA, Zemel LS, Shapiro ED: Lyme arthritis in children: clinical epidemiology and long-term outcomes. Pediatrics 102:905–908, 1998

Nadelman RB, Wormser GP: Lyme borreliosis. Lancet 352:557–565, 1998

Reid MC, Schoen RT, Evans J, Rosenberg JC, Horwitz RI: The consequences of overdiagnosis and overtreatment of Lyme disease; an observational study. Ann Intern Med 128:354–362, 1998

Shapiro ED: Lyme disease. Pediatr Rev 19:147–154, 1998

Steere AC, Sikand VK, Meurice F, et al: Vaccination against Lyme disease with recombinant *Borrelia burgdorferi* outer-surface lipoprotein A with adjuvant. N Engl J Med 339:209–215, 1998

Warshafsky S, Nowakowski J, Nadelman RB, Kamer RS, Peterson SJ, Wormser GP: Efficacy of antimicrobial prophylaxis for prevention of Lyme disease: a meta-analysis. J Gen Intern Med 11:329–333, 1996

13.2.20 *Moraxella catarrhalis*

Basim I. Asmar

Moraxella catarrhalis, considered avirulent in the 1960s and 1970s, is now recognized as an important mucosal pathogen, particularly in otitis media and sinusitis in children, as well as in exacerbations of bronchitis in adults with chronic lung disease.

EPIDEMIOLOGY *Moraxella catarrhalis* is a normal inhabitant of the upper respiratory tract. Nasopharyngeal colonization rate is highest during infancy and early childhood and lowest in adulthood. Colonization rates of as high as 36 to 50% in infants and young children, and 5 to 7% in adults, have been reported. In one study of a large cohort of infants who were followed prospectively from birth to 2 years of age, 66% became colonized with *M. catarrhalis* by 1 year and 77.5% by 2 years of age. In the same group, nasopharyngeal colonization increased from 27% during healthy visits to 63% on visits associated with otitis media. Other studies have shown that colonization of children varies with the season and is more common in fall and winter (46%) than in spring and summer (9%). Overall, colonization was higher in children with upper respiratory tract infection (36%) than in children without (18%), and was more common in children aged 24 months (32%) than in children older than 24 months (14%). The mode of transmission of the organism is presumed to be direct contact with contaminated respiratory tract secretions and/or droplet spread.

After the oropharynx is colonized, colonization of the tracheobronchial tree can follow, which may lead to the development of bronchitis or pneumonia in adults with underlying risk factors such as smoking, intercurrent viral infection, corticosteroid treatment, or immunosuppression. In children, pneumonia may develop in those with intercurrent viral infection, underlying lung disease, prematurity, or immunoglobulin deficiency. Risk factors for development of bacterial tracheitis and pneumonia in children in an intensive care setting include endotracheal intubation and frequent suctioning. Colonization with *M. catarrhalis* is reported to be more common in asthmatic children than in normal children.

Moraxella catarrhalis is an aerobic gram-negative diplococcus that has a striking resemblance to meningococcus and gonococcus, save that it is unencapsulated. It has a tendency to resist decolonization. It grows well on blood and chocolate agars, forming small, opaque, gray-white nonhemolytic colonies. Recovery of the organism from the mixed flora of mucosal surfaces can be enhanced by using selective culture media such as modified Thayer-Martin or TV broth (Mueller-Hinton broth supplemented with trimethoprim and vancomycin).

CLINICAL MANIFESTATIONS *Moraxella catarrhalis* is the third most common cause of otitis media in children, following *Streptococcus pneumoniae* and nontypable *Haemophilus influenzae*. Several studies show that *M. catarrhalis* accounts for 3 to 20% of pathogens recovered from middle-ear fluids of children with acute otitis media, and the organism may occur as a single pathogen or in combination with other organisms. Otitis media caused by *M. catarrhalis* cannot be distinguished clinically from otitis caused by *S. pneumoniae* or *H. influenzae*. However, it is more likely to remit spontaneously than is disease caused by *S. pneumoniae* or *H. influenzae*.

Recent studies also show that *M. catarrhalis* is an important cause of acute and chronic sinusitis in children. It accounts for 20% of bacterial isolates recovered from sinus cavities and, similar to otitis media, is surpassed in frequency by *S. pneumoniae* and *H. influenzae*. The clinical manifestations of acute sinusitis caused by *M. catarrhalis* are similar to those caused by *S. pneumoniae* and *H. influenzae*.

Although bronchopulmonary infections caused by *M. catarrhalis* have generally been noted in adults with chronic lung disease, pneumonia has also been reported in children. Because sputum samples are usually not available in children, most documented pneumonia cases were severe and occurred primarily in immuno-compromised patients. In one report, five premature infants younger than 6 months with preexisting lung disease were diagnosed as having pneumonia following a 2- to 4-day prodrome of cough, tachypnea, and retractions. *Moraxella catarrhalis* was recovered from bronchial aspirations. All patients required assisted ventilation for marked hypoxia. Associated *M. catarrhalis* bacteremia has been reported in other patients with pneumonia.

Moraxella catarrhalis has also been reported as a cause of bacterial tracheitis in healthy, as well as immunocompromised, patients. Other underlying conditions associated with increased predisposition to *M. catarrhalis* infections in children include AIDS, leukemia, and immunoglobulin deficiencies. In adults, *M. catarrhalis* pneumonia is more common in patients with chronic lung disease, AIDS, and malignancy. *Moraxella catarrhalis* has been implicated as a cause of a variety of other infections including urethritis, conjunctivitis, pyogenic arthritis, shunt-associated ventriculitis, peritonitis, septal cellulitis, endocarditis, bacteremia, and meningitis. Urethritis caused by *M. catarrhalis* can be mistaken for gonococcal urethritis. Conjunctivitis caused by *M. catarrhalis* in the newborn can mimic ophthalmia neonatorum caused by *Neisseria gonorrhoeae*.

Bacteremia caused by *M. catarrhalis* is less well understood and has been reported sporadically in a variety of clinical settings, in both children and adults. The clinical severity of *M. catarrhalis* bacteremia has varied from self-limited febrile illness to lethal sepsis. Some reviews indicate that a significant proportion of children with *M. catarrhalis* bacteremia had an underlying immune defect (malignancy, AIDS, neutropenia, low IgG level) or a predisposing respiratory factor (chronic lung disease, tracheostomy, mechanical ventilation). However, some healthy, immunocompetent patients with no predisposing factors have presented with *M. catarrhalis* bacteremia. In most such patients the source of the infection was an upper airway focus (otitis, sinusitis) or pneumonia. Children with *M. catarrhalis* bacteremia may present with different clinical manifestations. Some children present with petechial or purpuric rashes resembling infection caused by *N. meningitidis*. Other patients present with nonspecific symptoms and no focus of infection, similar to patients with occult pneumococcal bacteremia. Meningitis caused by *M. catarrhalis* occasionally results from hematogenous spread or as a complication of ventriculoperitoneal shunt infection. Endocarditis is rare, and the few reported cases were associated with a high mortality rate.

TREATMENT　Before 1970, all strains of *M. catarrhalis* were susceptible to penicillin and ampicillin. However, β-lactamase-producing strains progressively increased during the 1980s. Presently almost all *M. catarrhalis* isolates are producers of β-lactamases. The β-lactamase inhibitors clavulanic acid and sulbactam are active against the enzymes produced by *M. catarrhalis*.

In vitro, *M. catarrhalis* isolates are generally susceptible to ampicillin/sulbactam and amoxicillin/clavulanic acid; erythromycin; azithromycin; clarithromycin; trimethoprim-sulfamethoxazole; chloramphenicol; tetracycline; aminoglycosides; fluoroquinolones (eg, ciprofloxacin); and both second- and third-generation cephalosporins (cefuroxime, cefaclor, cefprozil, cefpodoxime, cefixime, and loracarbef). Cefaclor is less active than cefuroxime against *M. catarrhalis*. Most β-lactamase-producing strains respond to treatment with β-lactam/β-lactamase inhibitor combination, as well as second- and third-generation cephalosporins. However, antimicro-

bial treatment should be guided by in vitro susceptibility testing, especially for invasive infections. *M. catarrhalis* strains are resistant to vancomycin, oxacillin, and clindamycin.

References

Abuhammour WM, Abdel-Haq NM, Asmar BI, Dajani AS: *Moraxella catarrhalis* bacteremia: a 10-year experience. South Med J 92:1071–1074, 1999

Berg RA, Bartley DL: Pneumonia associated with *Branhamella catarrhalis* in infants. Pediatr Infect Dis J 6:569–573, 1987

Faden H, Harabuchi Y, Hong JJ, Tonawanda/Williamsville Pediatrics: Epidemiology of *Moraxella catarrhalis* in children during the first 2 years of life: relationship to otitis media. J Infect Dis 169:1312–1317, 1994

Van Hare GF, Shurin PA, Marchant CD, et al: Acute otitis media caused by *Branhamella catarrhalis*: biology and therapy. Rev Infect Dis 9:16–27, 1987

Verghese A, Berk SL: Lower respiratory tract infections: *Moraxella (Branhamella) catarrhalis*. Infect Dis Clin North Am 5:523–538, 1991

13.2.21　Mycobacterial Infections

Mycobacterium tuberculosis
Jeffrey R. Starke

Despite important advances in its treatment over the past two decades, tuberculosis remains a major infectious disease. Approximately one-third of the world's population harbors *Mycobacterium tuberculosis* and is at risk for developing disease in the near or distant future. Many areas of the world have experienced an increase in tuberculosis incidence and prevalence over the past 15 years, caused in part by the epidemic of infection with the human immunodeficiency virus (HIV), which is a potent risk factor for the development of tuberculosis disease in adults infected with *M. tuberculosis*. The failure to control tuberculosis in both developed and developing countries represents one of our greatest public health failures.

The terminology used to describe various phases of tuberculosis can be confusing, but it follows the pathophysiology of the disease. A child is in the *exposure* stage when the child "shares the air" with an adult with contagious tuberculosis. In this stage, the child may have breathed *M. tuberculosis* into the lungs, but there are no clinical manifestations and the tuberculin skin test remains negative. Some children in this stage ultimately develop a positive tuberculin skin test if infection takes hold. Whereas adults in this stage usually do not get treated, young children are treated because progression to disease may occur rapidly.

Latent infection with tuberculosis means that replication of *M. tuberculosis* has occurred within the lungs and, perhaps, in other tissues. The tuberculin skin test is positive, but the chest radiograph is normal or shows only evidence of the initial infection. In addition, there are no signs or symptoms of disease. All children and most adults with tuberculosis infection should be treated to prevent development of disease in the future.

Tuberculosis *disease* occurs when clinical manifestations of pulmonary or extrapulmonary tuberculosis become apparent either by clinical signs and symptoms, by chest radiograph, or by other diagnostic techniques.

Two elements determine a child's risk for developing tuberculosis disease. The first is the likelihood of exposure to an individual with infectious tuberculosis, which is primarily determined by the individual's environment. The second is the ability of the person's immune system to control the initial infection and keep it clinically dormant. Without treatment, disease develops in 5 to 10% of immunologically normal adults with tuberculosis infection. In young children, the risk is greater; as many as 40% of those less than 1 year of age with untreated tuberculosis infection develop radiographic or clinical evidence of tuberculosis disease. Methods of preventing disease in infected individuals benefit children and adolescents even more than adults.

EPIDEMIOLOGY About 60% of cases of childhood tuberculosis occur in infants and children less than 5 years of age. The ages of 5 to 14 years are often called the "favored age" as children in this range may become infected but usually have the lowest rate of tuberculosis disease. The gender ratio for tuberculosis in children is about 1:1 in contrast to adults, in whom males predominate.

Children acquire *M. tuberculosis* from adults in their environment. Environmental risk factors include those characteristics that make it more likely that the child shares the air with an adult with infectious tuberculosis. Factors that increase the risk of a child being infected with *M. tuberculosis* include: (a) birth or travel/residence in a country in which tuberculosis is endemic; (b) early childhood environments with exposures to multiple caregivers, for example, orphanages; or (c) contact with high-risk adults who have had previous residence in a jail, prison, or high-risk nursing home; homelessness in some communities; use of illegal drugs; experience as a health-care worker who cares for high-risk patients; or locally defined risk factors. Factors that increase the risk of developing disease once infected include age less than 2 years; coinfection with HIV; other immunocompromising diseases or treatments; and malnutrition.

Most children are infected with *M. tuberculosis* in the home, but outbreaks of childhood tuberculosis centered in elementary and high schools, nursery schools, family daycare homes, churches, school buses, and stores have occurred in the United States. Childhood tuberculosis case rates in the United States and in other countries are strikingly higher among ethnic and racial minority groups and among the poor. In the United States, approximately 85% of tuberculosis cases in children occur among African-American, Hispanic, Asian, and Native American children.

The recent epidemic of HIV infection has two major effects on the epidemiology of childhood tuberculosis. First, HIV-infected adults with tuberculosis may transmit the infection to children, some of whom will develop tuberculosis disease. Second, children with HIV infection are at increased risk of progressing to tuberculosis disease once infected. Studies of childhood tuberculosis demonstrate increased case rates that are associated with a simultaneous increase of tuberculosis among HIV-infected adults in the community. Tuberculosis may be underdiagnosed in HIV-infected children because of the similarity of its clinical presentation to other opportunistic infections and because of the difficulty in confirming the diagnosis with positive cultures. Children with tuberculosis should have HIV serotesting because the two infections are linked epidemiologically.

Transmission of *M. tuberculosis* is virtually always by person-to-person spread via the respiratory route. Mucous droplets become airborne when the index case coughs, sneezes, laughs, or sings. Infected droplets dry and become droplet nuclei, which remain suspended in the air for hours. Environmental factors, such as poor air circulation, enhance transmission. Rarely, transmission occurs by direct contact with infected body fluids such as urine or purulent sinus tract drainage.

Of the several patient-related factors associated with transmission of *M. tuberculosis,* a positive acid-fast smear of the sputum correlates most closely with infectivity. However, adults with a negative acid-fast sputum smear may still be contagious. Extensive epidemiologic studies show that most children with typical tuberculosis disease rarely, if ever, infect other children or adults. In the absence of cavitary lesions, which are extremely rare in childhood, the bacilli are relatively sparse in the endobronchial secretions of children with pulmonary tuberculosis. When children with tuberculosis cough, they rarely produce sputum and lack the tussive force necessary to suspend infectious particles in the air. However, adolescents with reactivation forms of pulmonary tuberculosis, particularly if they have pulmonary cavities or extensive infiltrates, may be infectious to others. Many experts initially place hospitalized children with pulmonary tuberculosis in respiratory isolation, especially if their parents or adult visitors have not yet been fully evaluated for tuberculosis. However, the risk of transmission from the child is remote.

MYCOBACTERIOLOGY AND PATHOPHYSIOLOGY Mycobacteria are nonmotile, nonspore-forming, pleomorphic, weakly gram-positive rods that are typically slender and slightly bent. The cell walls contain lipid and wax that make these organisms more resistant than most others to light, alkali, acid, and the bactericidal action of antibodies. Growth is slow with a generation time of 14 to 24 hours. Acid-fastness, the capacity to perform stable mycolate complexes with certain aryl methane dyes, is the hallmark of mycobacteria. Cells appear red when stained with fuchsin (Ziehl-Neelsen or Kinyoun stain), appear purple with crystal violet, or exhibit yellowgreen fluorescence under ultraviolet light (auramine and rhodamine, as in Truant stain). Truant stain is the most sensitive method for visualizing mycobacteria in a clinical specimen.

Identification of mycobacteria species depends on their staining properties and their biochemical and metabolic characteristics. Isolation on solid media often takes 3 to 6 weeks, followed by another 2 to 4 weeks for drug-susceptibility testing. The newer automated radiometric methods using liquid broth allow isolation from clinical specimens and identification of mycobacteria within 7 to 10 days.

In more than 95% of cases, the portal of entry for *M. tuberculosis* is the lung. Small particles are inhaled beyond the normal clearance mechanisms of the lungs and multiply initially within the alveoli and alveolar ducts. The initial inflammation with polymorphonuclear leukocytes is replaced by epithelioid cell proliferation and the appearance of giant cells with lymphocytic infiltration. Macrophages ingest the bacilli but are not able to kill them. Replication of the organisms occurs within the macrophages, which carry some of the organisms through lymphatics to the regional lymph nodes.

As the initial cycle of macrophage ingestion and replication of bacilli continues, development of cutaneous hypersensitivity and cell-mediated immunity occurs most often between 4 and 8 weeks after onset of infection. During this time, the initial focus grows larger and has not yet become encapsulated. Occasionally this focus is visible on the chest radiograph, but the radiograph usually remains normal and the child is asymptomatic. If adequate immunity is established, the parenchymal portion of the primary complex heals completely by fibrosis and/or calcification after undergoing caseous necrosis and encapsulation.

During the creation of the parenchymal lesion and the accelerated caseation brought on by the development of hypersensitivity, the bacilli from the primary complex spread via the bloodstream and lymphatics to the apices of the lungs, liver, spleen, meninges, peritoneum, lymph nodes, bones, and joints. This dissemination can involve large numbers of bacilli, which lead to disseminated tuberculosis disease. More commonly, small numbers of bacilli circulate and leave microscopic foci scattered in various tissues. These metastatic foci are usually clinically inapparent, but they may be the origin of either extrapulmonary tuberculosis or reactivation pulmonary tuberculosis.

In most cases of tuberculosis infection in children, the infection is held in check locally and distantly. However, in some individuals, hilar or paratracheal lymph nodes become enlarged by the host inflammatory reaction to the tubercle bacilli. The nodes may encroach upon the regional bronchus or bronchiole. Partial obstruction caused by external compression leads to hyperinflation in the distal lung segment. Inflamed, caseous nodes may attach to the bronchial wall and erode through it, leading to endobronchial tuberculosis. Air is reabsorbed beyond this obstruction, and collapse of the segment of the lung occurs. The resulting lesion is a combination of pneumonia and atelectasis, commonly referred to as a collapse-consolidation or segmental lesion.

A fairly predictable timetable is apparent for events that may complicate the initial tuberculosis infection and complications. Massive lymphohematogenous dissemination leading to miliary or disseminated disease occurs no later than 3 to 6 months after infection. Clinically significant lymph node or endobronchial tuberculosis usually appears within 3 to 9 months. Lesions of the bones and joints usually take at least a year to develop, while disease of the genitourinary tract may be evident 5 to 25 years after infection.

CLINICAL MANIFESTATIONS

Latent (Asymptomatic) Infection The vast majority of children with tuberculosis infection develop no signs or symptoms at any time. Occasionally, the initiation of infection is marked by several days of low-grade fever and mild cough. Rarely, the child experiences a clinically significant disease with high fever, cough, malaise, and flu-like symptoms that resolve within a week. These children have a reactive tuberculin skin test, and the purpose of treating them is to prevent them from developing reactivation tuberculosis in the future.

Pulmonary The symptoms and physical signs of pulmonary tuberculosis in children are surprisingly meager considering the degree of radiographic changes often seen. The physical manifestations of disease tend to differ by the age of onset. Young infants and adolescents are more likely to have significant signs or symptoms, whereas school-aged children usually have clinically silent radiographic disease. More than 50% of infants and children with pulmonary tuberculosis have no physical findings and are discovered only via contact tracing of an adult with tuberculosis. Infants are more likely to experience signs and symptoms because of their small airway diameters relative to the parenchymal and lymph node changes that occur. Nonproductive cough and mild dyspnea or wheezing, especially at night, are the most common symptoms. Systemic complaints such as fever, night sweats, anorexia, and decreased activity occur less often. Some infants have difficulty gaining weight or develop a true failure-to-thrive presentation that does not improve significantly until after several months of treatment.

Pulmonary signs are even less common. Some young children with bronchial obstruction have signs of air trapping, such as localized wheezing or decreased breath sounds, that may be accompanied by tachypnea or frank respiratory distress. Occasionally,

these nonspecific symptoms and signs are alleviated by antibiotics, suggesting that bacterial superinfection distal to the focus of bronchial obstruction caused by tuberculosis has contributed to the clinical presentation of disease.

In chest radiography, the hallmark of pulmonary tuberculosis in infants and children is the relatively large size and importance of the hilar or paratracheal lymphadenitis as compared with the less significant size of the initial parenchymal focus (Fig. 13-3). Hilar lymphadenopathy is almost invariably present with childhood tuberculosis, but it may not be distinct on a plain radiograph when calcification is not present. Significant atelectasis and/or pulmonary infiltrate make it impossible to discern the lymph node enlargement. As the hilar or mediastinal lymph nodes continue to enlarge, partial bronchial obstruction caused by external compression from the enlarged nodes causes air trapping, hyperinflation, and even lobar emphysema. As the lymph nodes attach to and infiltrate the bronchial wall, reabsorption of air and atelectasis occur. The radiographic findings are similar to those caused by aspiration of a foreign body; in effect, the lymph node is acting as the foreign body. Multiple segmental lesions in different lobes may be apparent simultaneously, and segmental atelectasis and hyperinflation lesions can occur together. Children with tuberculosis may have the radiographic picture of lobar pneumonia without impressive or specific adenopathy. Rarely, bullous lesions occur in the lungs that can lead to pneumothorax. Enlargement of the subcarinal lymph nodes causes compression of the esophagus and, rarely, a bronchoesophageal fistula. A sign of subcarinal tuberculosis is horizontal splaying of the main stem bronchi.

Adolescents with pulmonary tuberculosis may develop segmental lesions with adenopathy or apical infiltrates with or without cavitation that are typical of adult reactivation tuberculosis (Fig. 13-4). Regional lymphadenitis is absent in the latter type of disease.

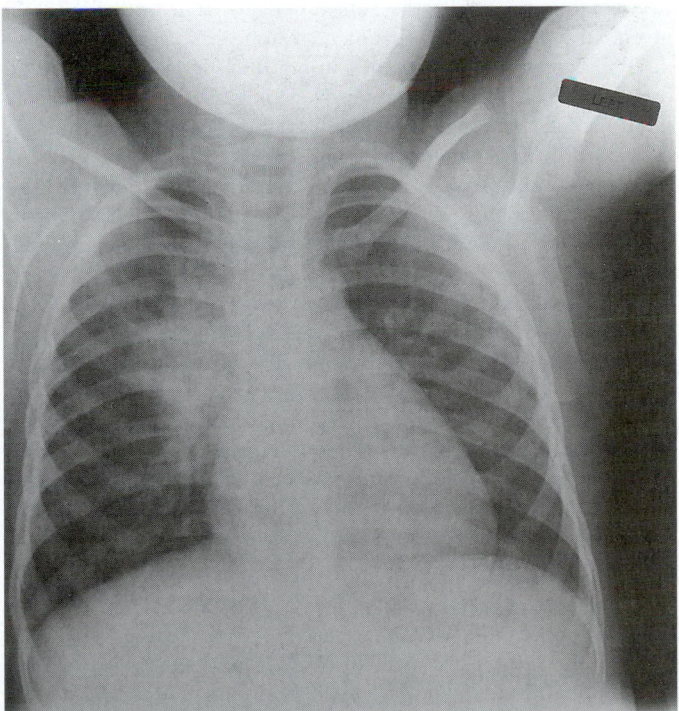

FIGURE 13-3 A chest radiograph from a child with early pulmonary tuberculosis demonstrating hilar adenopathy and perihilar infiltrate.

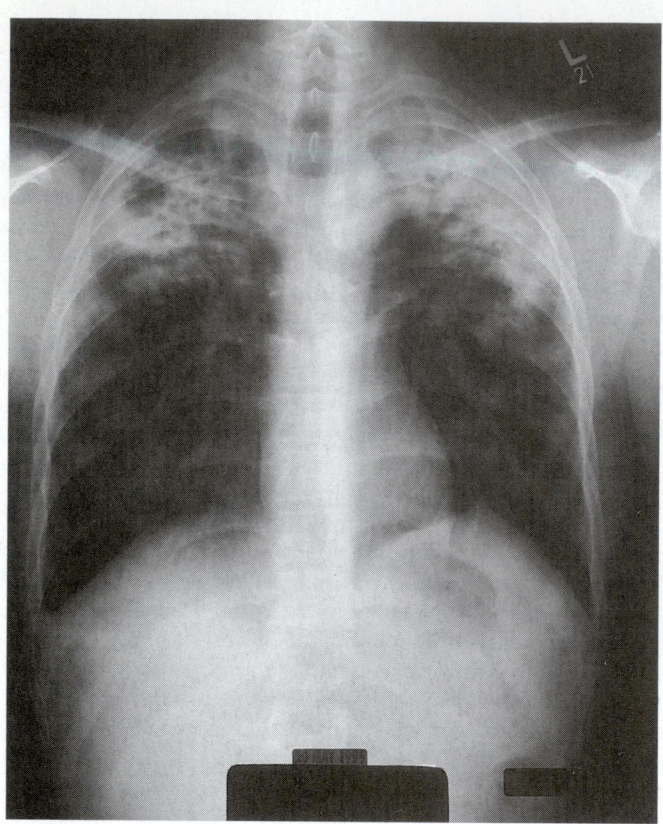

FIGURE 13-4 An adolescent with severe bilateral upper lobe tuberculosis, with cavitation on the right side.

The course of thoracic lymphadenopathy and bronchial obstruction can follow several paths if antituberculosis chemotherapy is not given. In many cases, the segment or lobe reexpands and the radiographic abnormalities resolve completely. However, these children are still at risk for developing reactivation tuberculosis later in life. In some cases, this segmental lesion resolves, but residual calcification of the parenchymal focus and regional lymph node occurs. Finally, bronchial obstruction may cause scarring and progressive contraction of the lobe or segment, which may be associated with cylindrical bronchiectasis and chronic pyogenic infection.

A rare but serious complication of tuberculosis in children occurs when the parenchymal focus enlarges and develops a large, caseous center. This progressive primary tuberculosis presents like bronchopneumonia, and may be accompanied by high fever, severe cough, dullness to percussion, rales, and decreased breath sounds. Liquefaction in the center may result in formation of a thin-walled cavity. Before the advent of antituberculosis chemotherapy, the mortality rate of this form of tuberculosis was 30 to 50%. With effective treatment, the prognosis is excellent for full recovery.

Pleural Tuberculous pleural effusions, which can be local or general, originate in the discharge of bacilli into the pleural space from a subpleural pulmonary focus or caseated subpleural lymph node. Asymptomatic local pleural effusion is so frequent in childhood pulmonary tuberculosis that it is basically a component of the primary complex. Most large and clinically significant effusions occur months to years after the initial infection. Tuberculous pleural effusion is infrequent in children younger than 6 years of age, and

rare in those below 2 years of age. Effusions are usually unilateral, but they can be bilateral. They are virtually never associated with a segmental pulmonary lesion and are rare in miliary tuberculosis.

The clinical onset of tuberculous pleurisy is usually fairly sudden. It is characterized by low to high fever, shortness of breath, chest pain on deep inspiration, dullness to percussion, and diminished breath sounds on the affected side. The presentation is similar to that of pyogenic pleurisy. The fever and other symptoms may last for several weeks after the start of ultimately effective antituberculosis chemotherapy. Although corticosteroids may reduce the clinical symptoms, they have little effect on the ultimate outcome. The tuberculin skin test is positive in only 70 to 80% of cases. The prognosis is excellent, but radiographic resolution may take months. Scoliosis rarely complicates recovery of a long-standing effusion.

Cardiac Tuberculous pericarditis occurs in only 0.4% of infected children. It arises by direct invasion or by lymphatic drainage from caseous lymph nodes in the subcarinal area. Pericardial fluid may be serofibrinous or hemorrhagic. However, tubercle bacilli rarely are found on direct smear of the fluid. Extensive fibrosis of the pericardial sac may lead to obliteration with development, usually years later, of constrictive pericarditis. The presenting systems usually are nonspecific: low-grade fever, poor appetite, failure to gain weight, and chest pain. A pericardial friction rub may be heard, or, if a large effusion already is present, distant heart sounds, tachycardia, and narrow pulse pressure may suggest the diagnosis. In the prechemotherapy era, half the patients died; now, with appropriate drugs and use of corticosteroid therapy to diminish the size of the effusion, the prognosis is excellent.

Disseminated (Miliary) The lymphohematogenous spread of bacilli that accompanies the initial infection is usually asymptomatic. Rarely, patients experience protracted hematogenous tuberculosis caused by the intermittent release of tubercle bacilli as a caseous focus erodes through the wall of the blood vessel in the lung. Although the clinical picture may be acute, more often it is indolent and prolonged, with high fevers accompanying the release of organisms into the bloodstream. Early pulmonary involvement is surprisingly mild, but diffuse lung involvement becomes apparent if treatment is not given promptly. Culture confirmation can be difficult. Bone marrow or liver biopsy with appropriate stains and cultures may be necessary and should be performed if the diagnosis is considered and other tests are unrevealing.

The most common clinically significant form of disseminated tuberculosis is miliary disease, which occurs when massive numbers of bacilli are released into the bloodstream, causing disease in at least two organs. This form of disease usually occurs within 2 to 6 months after the primary infection. The clinical manifestations are protean, depending on the number of organisms that disseminate and the focus of infection. Lesions are usually larger and more numerous in the lungs, spleen, liver, and bone marrow than in other organs. This form of tuberculosis is most common in infants and in malnourished or immunosuppressed patients. The onset of clinical disease is sometimes explosive, with the patient becoming gravely ill in several days. More often, the onset is insidious, the patient not being able to pinpoint the true time of initial symptoms. The most common signs include malaise, anorexia, weight loss, and low-grade fever. Within several weeks hepatosplenomegaly and generalized lymphadenopathy develop in about 50% of cases. About this time, the fever may become higher and more sustained, but the chest radiograph usually is normal and respiratory symptoms are few. Within several more days to weeks, the lungs become filled with tubercles, causing dyspnea, cough, rales, and wheezing. As pulmonary disease progresses, alveolar air-block syndrome may result in frank respiratory distress, hypoxia, and pneumothorax or pneumomediastinum. Signs or symptoms of meningitis or peritonitis are found in 20 to 40% of patients with advanced disease. Severe headache in a patient with miliary tuberculosis usually indicates the presence of meningitis. Abdominal pain or tenderness is usually a sign of tuberculous peritonitis. Choroid tubercles occur in 13 to 87% of patients and are highly specific for miliary tuberculosis. Unfortunately, the tuberculin skin test is nonreactive in as much as 50% of patients with advanced disease.

Central Nervous System Central nervous system tuberculosis is the most serious complication in children, and is uniformly fatal without effective treatment. This condition usually arises from the formation of a caseous lesion in the cerebral cortex or meninges that develops during the occult lymphohematogenous dissemination of the initial infection. This lesion, called a *Rich focus*, increases in size and discharges small numbers of tubercle bacilli into the subarachnoid space. The resulting exudate may infiltrate the cortical or meningeal blood vessels, producing inflammation, obstruction, and subsequent infarction of the cerebral cortex. This exudate also interferes with the normal flow of CSF in and out of the ventricular system at the level of the basal cisterns, leading to a communicating hydrocephalus. The combination of vasculitis, infarction, cerebral edema, and hydrocephalus results in severe damage that occurs gradually or rapidly. Abnormalities in electrolyte metabolism, especially hyponatremia caused by SIADH or salt-wasting, also contribute to the pathophysiology.

Tuberculous meningitis complicates about 0.3% of untreated tuberculosis infections in children. This condition is extremely rare in infants under 3 months of age because pathologic events usually need this much time to develop. It is most common in children between 6 months and 4 years of age.

The clinical progression of tuberculous meningitis may be rapid or gradual. Rapid progression occurs more frequently in infants and young children who may experience symptoms for only several days before the onset of acute hydrocephalus, seizures, and cerebral edema. More often, the signs and symptoms progress slowly over several weeks and can be divided into three stages. The first stage, which typically lasts 1 to 2 weeks, is characterized by nonspecific symptoms such as fever, headache, irritability, drowsiness, and malaise. Focal neurologic signs are absent, but infants may experience a stagnation or loss of developmental milestones. The second stage usually begins more abruptly. Lethargy, nuchal rigidity, Kernig and Brudzinski signs, seizures, hypertonia, vomiting, cranial nerve palsies relevant to a basilar meningitis, and other focal neurologic signs are apparent. This clinical picture usually correlates with the development of hydrocephalus, increased intracranial pressure, and vasculitis. The third stage is marked by coma, hemiplegia or paraplegia, hypertension, decerebrate posturing, deterioration in vital signs, and, eventually, death. The prognosis of tuberculous meningitis correlates closely with the clinical stage of illness at the time treatment with antituberculosis chemotherapy and corticosteroids begins. The majority of patients in the first stage have an excellent outcome, whereas most patients diagnosed in the third stage who survive have permanent disabilities including blindness, deafness, paraplegia, and mental retardation. It is imperative that antituberculosis chemotherapy be considered for any child who develops basilar meningitis and hydrocephalus with no other apparent eti-

ology. The key to diagnosis is often identifying the adult from whom the child acquired *M. tuberculosis.*

Another manifestation of central nervous system tuberculosis is the tuberculoma, which presents clinically as a brain tumor. Tuberculomas account for as many as 40% of brain tumors in children in some areas of the world, but they are rare in North America. These lesions, which occur most often in children less than 10 years of age, are usually singular, but they may be multiple. In adults, lesions are usually supratentorial, but in children, they are often infratentorial, located at the base of the brain near the cerebellum. The most common symptoms are headache, fever, and seizures. The paradoxical development of tuberculomas in patients with tuberculous meningitis while receiving effective chemotherapy has been recognized since the advent of computed tomography. The cause and nature of these tuberculomas are poorly understood, but their development does not require a change in the therapeutic regimen. Whenever a child with tuberculous meningitis deteriorates or develops focal neurologic findings while on treatment, this phenomenon should be considered. Corticosteroids may help alleviate the occasionally severe clinical signs and symptoms. These lesions may be very slow to resolve clinically, persisting radiographically for months or years.

Lymph Node Tuberculosis of the superficial lymph nodes is the most common form of extrapulmonary tuberculosis in children. Most cases occur within 6 to 9 months of the initial infection, although some cases appear years later. The tonsillar, anterior cervical, and submandibular nodes become involved secondary to extension of a primary lesion of the upper lung fields or abdomen. Infected nodes in the inguinal, epitrochlear, or axillary regions, which are rare in children, result from regional lymphadenitis associated with tuberculosis of the skin or skeletal system.

In the early stages of infection, the lymph nodes usually enlarge gradually. The nodes are firm but not hard, discrete, and nontender. The nodes usually feel fixed to underlying or overlying tissue. Disease is most often unilateral, but bilateral involvement may occur. As infection progresses, multiple nodes are affected, resulting in a mass of matted nodes. Systemic signs and symptoms other than low-grade fever are usually absent. The chest x-ray is usually normal, although adenopathy in the chest may be apparent. Occasionally, the illness is more acute with rapid enlargement of cervical nodes, high fever, tenderness, and fluctuance. If left untreated, the infection may resolve, but more often progresses to caseation and necrosis of the lymph node. The capsule of the node breaks down, resulting in the spread of infection to adjacent nodes. The skin overlying the massive nodes becomes thin, shiny, and erythematous. Rupture results in a draining sinus tract that may require surgical removal; if the correct diagnosis is made prior to rupture, however, the process can be cured with antituberculous therapy alone.

Skeletal Skeletal tuberculosis results from lymphohematogenous seeding of tubercle bacilli during the initial infection. Bone infection also may originate as a result of direct extension from a regional lymph node or a neighboring infected bone. The time interval between infection and clinical disease can be as short as 1 month in cases of tuberculous dactylitis, or as much as 30 months or more for tuberculosis of the hip. The infection usually begins in the metaphysis. Granulation tissue and caseation destroy bone by direct infection and by pressure necrosis. Soft-tissue abscess and extension of the infection through the epiphysis into the nearby joint often complicate the bony lesion.

Weight-bearing bones and joints are affected most commonly. Most cases of bone tuberculosis occur in the vertebrae, causing tuberculosis of the spine or Pott disease. Although any vertebral body can be involved, there is a predilection for the lower thoracic and upper lumbar vertebrae. Involvement of two or more vertebrae is common; these vertebrae are usually contiguous, but there may be skip areas between lesions. Infection in the body of the vertebrae leads to bony destruction and collapse. The infection may extend out from the bone, causing a paraspinal, psoas, or retropharyngeal abscess. The most frequent clinical signs and symptoms of tuberculous spondylitis in children are low-grade fever, irritability, and restlessness, especially at night; back pain; and abnormal positioning in gait or refusal to walk. Spinal rigidity may be caused by profound muscle spasm. Other sites of skeletal tuberculosis, in approximate order of frequency, are the knee, hip, elbow, and ankle. The degree of involvement can range from mild joint effusion without bone destruction to frank destruction of bone and restriction of the joint caused by chronic fibrosis. The tuberculin skin test is reactive in 80 to 90% of cases, and culture of joint fluid or bone biopsy usually yields the organism.

Tuberculous dactylitis is a form of bone tuberculosis that is peculiar to infants. Affected children develop distal endarteritis followed by painless swelling and cystic bone lesions in the hands.

Abdominal and Gastrointestinal   Tuberculosis of the oral cavity or pharynx is very unusual. Tuberculosis of the larynx causes chronic hoarseness and is often accompanied by upper-lobe apical pulmonary disease and sputum production in adolescents and adults. Tuberculosis of the esophagus is very rare in children and may be associated with a tracheoesophageal fistula. Tuberculous peritonitis is uncommon in adolescents and rare in young children. Whereas generalized peritonitis is caused by dissemination of organisms, most localized disease is caused by direct extension from an abdominal lymph node, intestinal focus, or tuberculous salpingitis. Initial pain and abdominal tenderness are mild. Rarely, the lymph nodes, omentum, and peritoneum become matted in children and can be palpated as a "doughy," irregular, nontender mass. Ascites and low-grade fever are common. Tuberculous enteritis is caused by hematogenous dissemination of organisms in most cases. The jejunum and ileum near Peyer's patches and the appendix are the most common sites of involvement. Mesenteric adenitis usually complicates this disease. Lymph nodes may cause intestinal obstruction or erode through the omentum to cause generalized peritonitis. This entity should be considered in any child with chronic gastrointestinal complaints and a reactive tuberculin skin test.

Genitourinary   Renal tuberculosis is rare in children, and the incubation period is several years or longer. Tubercle bacilli can be isolated from the urine in cases of miliary tuberculosis, even in the absence of renal disease. In true renal tuberculosis, small caseous tubercles develop in the renal parenchyma and release *M. tuberculosis* into the tubules. A mass may develop near the renal cortex that discharges large numbers of bacteria through a fistula into the renal pelvis. Infection can spread locally to the ureters, prostate, or epididymis. Renal tuberculosis is often clinically silent in the early stages. The only signs may be sterile pyuria and microscopic hematuria. As the disease progresses, dysuria, flank, or abdominal pain and gross hematuria develop. Superinfection by other bacteria is

frequent and may delay recognition of the underlying tuberculosis. Hydronephrosis or ureteral stricture may complicate the disease.

Tuberculosis of the genital tract is uncommon in both males and females before puberty. This condition usually originates from lymphohematogenous spread, but can complicate direct spread from the intestinal tract or bone. In adolescent girls, the fallopian tubes are most often involved, followed by the endometrium, the ovaries, and the cervix. The usual symptoms are low abdominal pain and dysmenorrhea or amenorrhea. Chronic infection usually leads to infertility. Genital tuberculosis in adolescent males is rare. Tuberculous orchitis presents as a nodular, painless swelling of the scrotum that is usually unilateral.

Other Sites   Cutaneous tuberculosis, which was more common decades ago, arises as an extension of disease from the primary infection, from hematogenous dissemination, or from hypersensitivity to the bacilli. Skin lesions associated with the initial infection can be caused by direct inoculation of the skin through an abrasion, cut, or insect bite. Regional lymphadenitis is striking, but systemic symptoms are usually absent. The most common form of hypersensitivity lesion is erythema nodosum, which is characterized by large, painful, purple-brown, indurated nodules on the shins and forearms. Scrofuloderma occurs when a caseous lymph node ruptures to the outside and leaves an ulcer or sinus tract. Papulonecrotic tuberculids are miliary lesions of the skin that appear most frequently on the face, trunk, and upper thighs. Their characteristic "apple-jelly" center is best demonstrated by placing a glass slide over the lesions. Tuberculosis verrucosa cutis is a wart-like lesion, which is most common on the arms or legs, that represents autoinoculation of bacilli in a person already sensitized to the organism.

Ocular tuberculosis is very rare in children. This condition usually involves the conjunctiva or cornea and usually results from direct inoculation. Unilateral redness and lacrimation are often associated with enlargement of the preauricular, submandibular, or cervical lymph nodes.

Tuberculosis of the middle ear results from a primary focus in neonates who aspirate infected amniotic fluid or from hematogenous dissemination in older children. The most common signs and symptoms are painless otorrhea, tinnitus, decreased hearing, facial paralysis, and perforated tympanic membrane. Enlargement of local lymph nodes may accompany infection. Diagnosis can be difficult because stain and cultures of material from the ear are frequently negative, and the histology of affected tissue usually shows acute and chronic inflammation without granuloma formation.

Congenital   True congenital tuberculosis is exceedingly rare, with fewer than 300 cases reported. *Mycobacterium tuberculosis* can pass from the placenta to the fetus through the umbilical vein. The mothers of these infected infants frequently suffer from tuberculous pleural effusion, meningitis, or disseminated disease during pregnancy or soon afterwards. However, the diagnosis of tuberculosis in the newborn often leads to the discovery of the mother's tuberculosis. Initial infection in the mother just before or during pregnancy is more likely to lead to congenital infection than previous infection. However, even massive involvement of the placenta with tuberculosis does not usually give rise to congenital infection. The tubercle bacilli first reach the fetal liver, where an initial focus develops with associated involvement of regional lymph nodes. Organisms then pass through the liver into the main fetal circulation, leading to foci in the lung and other tissues. The bacilli in the lung usually remain dormant until after birth, when oxygenation and pulmonary circulation increase significantly. Congenital tuberculosis also may occur by aspiration or ingestion of infected amniotic fluid if a caseous placental lesion ruptures directly into the amniotic cavity.

Symptoms of true congenital tuberculosis may be present at birth, but more commonly begin in the second or third week of life. The most common signs and symptoms are, in order of frequency, respiratory distress; fever; hepatic or splenic enlargement; poor feeding; lethargy or irritability; lymphadenopathy; abdominal distention; failure to thrive; ear drainage; and skin lesions. Many infants have an abnormal chest radiograph, most often a miliary pattern. Only one-third of affected infants have meningitis. This clinical presentation in newborns is similar to that caused by bacterial sepsis and other congenital infections. The diagnosis of neonatal tuberculosis should be suspected in an infant with signs and symptoms of bacterial or congenital infection whose response to antibiotic and supportive therapy is poor, and whose mother has risk factors for developing tuberculosis.

Tuberculosis and HIV Infection   In general, the clinical presentation of tuberculosis in children with HIV infection is similar to that in children without HIV infection. However, children with HIV infection more commonly have extrapulmonary tuberculosis, and pulmonary tuberculosis has a more aggressive picture, more often leading to substantial infiltrates or cavitation within the lung. Establishing the diagnosis of tuberculosis in an HIV-infected child can be difficult, the skin test is often negative and microbiological confirmation of disease is difficult to achieve in many cases. An aggressive evaluation for tuberculosis should be undertaken for any child with known HIV infection, or risk factors for HIV infection, who develops pulmonary disease or any unusual constellation of signs and symptoms.

DIAGNOSIS   There are two primary ways in which a child with tuberculosis can be discovered. The first is when tuberculosis is considered part of the differential diagnosis of a symptomatic child. Many children with tuberculosis are discovered through contact investigations of adults who are thought to have infectious tuberculosis. In these cases, children have relatively asymptomatic disease that would have progressed or escaped detection if the contact tracing had not occurred. The importance of the epidemiologic setting of the child in establishing the diagnosis of tuberculosis cannot be overemphasized. Often, the most important maneuver in determining whether the child has tuberculosis is testing the adults in close contact with the child to determine whether any adult has or recently has had infectious pulmonary tuberculosis.

General laboratory and other tests are usually unrevealing for children with tuberculosis. Screening tests such as a complete blood count and differential, erythrocyte sedimentation rate, and blood chemistries are usually normal. When considering a diagnosis of extrapulmonary tuberculosis, analysis of appropriate tissue or fluids often leads to establishing the correct diagnosis. In cases of tuberculous meningitis, the CSF leukocyte count usually ranges from 10 to 500 cells/mm³, but occasionally is higher. Polymorphonuclear leukocytes may be common initially, but in a large majority of cases, lymphocytes are predominant. The CSF glucose level is typically less than 40 mg/dL, but rarely goes below 20 mg/dL. The protein level is elevated and may be markedly high (400–5000 mg/dL) secondary to hydrocephalus and spinal block. Although the lumbar CSF is grossly abnormal, ventricular CSF may have normal chemistries and cell counts because samples are obtained proximal to the site of obstruction.

In cases of pleural tuberculosis, the pleural fluid usually yields results indicative of a mild exudate: specific gravity is 1.012 to 1.025, the protein level is usually 2 to 4 g/dL, and the glucose may be low, although it is often in the low-normal range (20–40 mg/dL). There are typically several hundred to several thousand white blood cells/mm³, with an early predominance of polymorphonuclear cells followed by a high concentration of lymphocytes. Biopsy of the pleura may show evidence of granuloma formation and the organisms.

Tuberculin Skin Testing   A positive tuberculin skin test is the hallmark of infection with *M. tuberculosis*. The definitive test is the Mantoux skin-test technique, which involves intradermal injection of 0.1 mL of purified protein derivative containing five tuberculin units. The results are interpreted as the transverse diameter of induration present 48 to 72 hours after injection. A variety of host-related factors—including very young age, malnutrition, immunosuppression by disease or drugs, viral infection, measles vaccination, and overwhelming tuberculosis—can depress tuberculin reactivity in a child infected with *M. tuberculosis*. Approximately 10% of immunocompetent children with tuberculosis disease do not react initially to a tuberculin skin test; however, most become reactive after several months of treatment, suggesting that the disease contributed to this anergy. Anergy with tuberculosis may be global or specific to tuberculin, so a positive control skin test with a negative tuberculin test never rules out tuberculosis disease. False-positive reactions to tuberculin skin tests can be caused by cross-sensitization to antigens of nontuberculous mycobacteria or, in some cases, previous immunization with bacille Calmette-Guérin (BCG) vaccine. No reliable method distinguishes tuberculin reactions caused by a BCG vaccination from those resulting from infection with *M. tuberculosis*. However, many infants who receive a BCG vaccine never develop a positive tuberculin reaction. When a reaction does occur, the induration is usually less than 10 mm and the reaction wanes after several years. One study of BCG cross-reaction in Native American children vaccinated at birth showed that all positive Mantoux reactions occurred within the first 6 months after vaccination. In general, a reactive area of 10 mm or more in a BCG-vaccinated child indicates infection with *M. tuberculosis* and necessitates further diagnostic evaluation and treatment. A history of prior BCG vaccination is never a contraindication to tuberculin testing.

The interpretation of the tuberculin reaction should be influenced by the purpose for which the test was given and the consequences of false classification. Because there is always some overlap in reactions to the Mantoux test between groups of individuals with and without infection with *M. tuberculosis*, false-positive and false-negative results always occur within a population. To try to minimize false results, reaction size limits for determining a positive result are made. Patients are then stratified by risk of infection (Table 13-38). For adults and children at the highest risk of having infection progress to disease, a reactive area of at least 5 mm is classified as a positive result. For other high-risk groups, including children less than 4 years of age, a reactive area of at least 10 mm is considered positive. For all other low-risk persons, the cutoff point for a positive reaction is raised to 15 mm. The key to this scheme is obtaining an adequate history of possible risk factors for acquiring infection with *M. tuberculosis*. Classifying children by this scheme depends on the willingness and ability of the clinician and

TABLE 13-38

AMOUNT OF INDURATION THAT DEFINES A POSITIVE MANTOUX TUBERCULOSIS SKIN TEST

REACTION SIZE	RISK FACTORS
≥5 mm	Contacts of infectious cases
	Abnormal chest radiograph
	HIV infection or other immunocompromise
≥10 mm	Birth or previous residence in a high-prevalence country
	Residence in long-term care or corrections facility
	Certain medical risk factors: diabetes mellitus, silicosis, renal disease
	Occupation in health care field; exposure to tuberculosis patients
	Member of a locally defined high-risk group
	Close contact of a high-risk adult (except health care workers)
	Age <4 years
≥15 mm	No risk factors

family to create a thorough history for the child and for the adults who are in the child's environment. In general, tuberculin skin testing of low-risk children yields few positive results, and the majority of these positive results will be false-positive.

Stains and Cultures The most important laboratory tests for the diagnosis of tuberculosis are the acid-fast stain and mycobacterial culture. The best culture specimen for pulmonary tuberculosis in a child is the early morning gastric aspirate obtained before the child has risen and before peristalsis has emptied the stomach of the pooled secretions that were swallowed overnight. In general, acquisition of these samples requires hospitalization. Unfortunately, even under optimal conditions, three gastric aspirates yield *M. tuberculosis* in fewer than 50% of cases. Therefore, negative cultures never exclude the diagnosis of tuberculosis in a child. The culture yield from bronchoscopy in children with tuberculosis is usually less than the yield from properly obtained gastric samples.

Fortunately, the need for culture confirmation in children with tuberculosis is usually small. If a child has a positive tuberculin skin test, clinical or radiographic findings suggestive of tuberculosis, and known contact with an adult case of tuberculosis, the child should be treated for tuberculosis disease. The drug susceptibility test results from the adult case can be used to determine the best therapeutic regimen for the child. Cultures always should be obtained from a child with suspected tuberculosis when the source case isn't known, or when the source case has a drug-resistant isolate.

Unfortunately, acid-fast stain of various fluids and tissues from children with tuberculosis disease is usually unrevealing. Acid-fast stain of gastric samples is positive in fewer than 10% of cases, and staining of other infected material is positive in less than 25 to 50% of cases.

Nucleic Acid Amplification The main form of nucleic acid amplification studied in children with tuberculosis is the polymerase chain reaction (PCR), which uses specific DNA sequences as markers for microorganisms. Various PCR techniques have a sensitivity and specificity of more than 90%, as compared with sputum culture, for detecting pulmonary tuberculosis in adults. However, the usefulness of PCR in childhood tuberculosis is much less. Compared with the clinical diagnosis of pulmonary tuberculosis in children, the sensitivity of PCR has varied from 25 to 83% and specificity has varied from 80 to 100%. A negative PCR result never eliminates tuberculosis as a diagnostic possibility. The major use of PCR is in evaluating children with significant pulmonary disease when the diagnosis is not established readily by clinical or epidemiologic grounds. PCR may be particularly helpful in evaluating immunocompromised children with pulmonary disease, or in children with extrapulmonary disease.

TREATMENT Mycobacteria replicate slowly and remain dormant in the body for prolonged periods. The treatment of tuberculosis is affected by the presence of naturally occurring drug-resistant organisms in large bacterial populations, even before chemotherapy is initiated. This drug resistance is caused by mutation at one of several chromosomal loci. The loci for resistance to one drug are not linked to the loci for resistance to other antituberculosis drugs. Although a population as a whole may be considered drug-susceptible, a subpopulation of drug-resistant organisms occurs at fairly predictable frequencies within the main population. The frequency for these drug-resistant organisms varies for the various drugs: streptomycin, 10^{-5}; isoniazid, 10^{-6}; rifampin, 10^{-7}. A cavity containing 10^9 bacilli will have thousands of drug-resistant organisms, whereas a caseous lesion with a much smaller population contains but few resistant organisms.

These microbiological characteristics of *M. tuberculosis* explain why single antimicrobial drugs cannot cure tuberculosis disease in adults. The major biological determinant of the success of antituberculosis therapy is the size of the bacterial population within the host. For patients with a large population of bacilli, such as adults with cavities or extensive infiltrates, many drug-resistant organisms are present initially, and at least two antituberculosis drugs must be given. Conversely, for patients with infection but no disease, the bacterial population is small, drug-resistant organisms are rare or nonexistant, and a single drug, such as isoniazid, can be given. Children with pulmonary tuberculosis and patients with extrapulmonary tuberculosis have medium-size populations in which significant numbers of drug-resistant organisms may or may not be present. In general, these patients are treated with at least two, and usually three or four, drugs.

Drugs for Tuberculosis

Table 13-39 details the first-line antituberculosis drugs used to treat tuberculosis in children.

Isoniazid Isoniazid (INH), a synthetically produced drug, is the most potent and valuable single drug in the treatment of tuberculosis. An oral dose attains a plasma concentration 20 to 80 times the usual level required to inhibit the growth of tubercle bacilli (0.02–0.05 μg/mL) within several hours, with high concentrations persisting for 6 to 8 hours in plasma and sputum. INH penetrates readily into the CSF, even in the absence of inflammation, and into caseous tissue. It is partially conjugated in the liver to an acetylated, inactive, nontoxic form. The rate and degree of acetylation are genetically determined.

The principal side effects of INH are peripheral neuritis and hepatitis. Peripheral neuritis results from competitive inhibition of pyridoxine metabolism. This is more likely to occur at higher dosages of INH (>10 mg/kg/d) in alcoholics and people who are poorly nourished. This is rarely a problem in children, although

TABLE 13-39

FIRST-LINE DRUGS USED TO TREAT TUBERCULOSIS INFECTION AND DISEASE IN CHILDREN

DRUG	DOSAGE FORMS	DAILY DOSE (mg/kg/day)	TWICE-WEEKLY DOSE (mg/kg/dose)	MAXIMUM DOSE
Ethambutol	Tablets: 100 mg 400 mg	15–25	50	2.5g
Isoniazid*	Scored tablets: 100 mg 300 mg Syrup†: 10 mg/mL	10–15‡	20–30	Daily: 300 mg Twice weekly: 900 mg
Pyrazinamide*	Scored tablets: 500 mg	20–40	50	2 g
Rifampin*	Capsules: 150 mg 300 mg Syrup: formulated in syrup from capsules	10–20	10–20	600 mg
Streptomycin (IM administration)	Vials: 1 g 4 g	20–40	20–40	2 g

*Rifamate is a capsule containing 150 mg of isoniazid and 300 mg of rifampin. Two capsules provide the usual adult (>50 kg body weight) daily dose of each drug. Rifater capsules contain isoniazid, rifampin, and pyrazinamide.
†Most experts advise against the use of isoniazid syrup because of its instability and because of a high rate of gastrointestinal adverse reaction (diarrhea, cramps).
‡When isoniazid is used in combination with rifampin, the incidence of hepatotoxicity increases when the dose exceeds 10 mg/kg/d.

precautions must be taken during adolescence, for breast-feeding babies, during pregnancy, or when the total daily dose of INH exceeds 300 mg. Pyridoxine (10 mg for each 100 mg of INH) should be given daily when indicated.

Hepatotoxicity is a problem in patients older than 35 years. In children, hepatitis is rare and mild. Concomitant use of rifampin or phenytoin increases the likelihood of hepatitis, as do INH dosage regimens in excess of 15 mg/kg/d.

Children who are taking INH need not have serum liver-enzyme testing unless they have a previous history of liver disease or predisposition to the development of liver disease. Careful questioning about symptoms should be done monthly, with warnings to report such symptoms as nausea, loss of appetitie, or right upper-quadrant pain promptly. Other infrequent side effects are convulsions, psychoses, loss of memory, allergic manifestations, and a lupus-like syndrome with arthritis and antinuclear antibodies.

Rifampin Rifampin is a semisynthetic drug that has wide antimicrobial activity against bacteria and mycobacteria. It is absorbed readily from the gastrointestinal tract after oral administration, with peak concentrations of 6 to 32 μg/mL (MIC for *M. tuberculosis* 0.5 μg/mL) occurring in 3 hours. Rifampin readily diffuses to all tissues and body fluids, including CSF; it is excreted primarily through the biliary tract and kidneys.

Rifampin is relatively nontoxic; the principal side effect is hepatitis, which occurs with a frequency of 1%. Hepatitis seems to be more common in patients who are treated with the combination of rifampin and INH. Gastrointestinal disturbances, rashes, reversible leukopenia, thrombocytopenia, and elevation of blood urea nitrogen have been reported. Rifampin potentiates the action of anticoagulants such as dicumarol. Rifampin may chemically interfere with birth control pills, making them ineffective. Administration of the drug may also impart an orange-red color to feces, urine, sputum, saliva, tears, and sweat. Rifampin should be included in

the treatment of all serious tuberculosis infections. The suggested dosage is 10 to 20 mg/kg/d (maximum, 600 mg). A liquid preparation is not commercially available, but can be prepared in community pharmacies.

Pyrazinamide (PZA) PZA is a bactericidal drug that attains a therapeutic concentration in the CSF and in macrophages. It is recommended as the third drug of a three- or four-drug regimen, particularly for the first 2 months of therapy. It should be used in treating mycobacteria with multiple-drug resistance, as well as in meningeal and miliary infections. In doses of 20 to 40 mg/kg/d (adult dose 2 g/d) it is well tolerated by children.

Streptomycin Streptomycin was the first effective antituberculosis drug. It is given intramuscularly and is rapidly absorbed into the bloodstream, reaching peak levels that are 50 to 100 times more than the MIC of 0.2 μg/mL. It diffuses readily into the pleural fluid, but does not diffuse into the CSF unless the meninges are inflamed. Streptomycin is excreted mainly in the urine, with 80% recovery within 24 hours. The principal toxic effect is eighth nerve damage, mainly of the vestibular branch, resulting in vertigo and ataxia that is usually permanent. Hearing loss is less common and usually affects the high-frequency range before affecting the lower frequencies. Children readily adjust to vestibular defect with minimal difficulty. At current dosage schedules, hearing defects are rare in children.

Ethambutol Ethambutol is an odorless water-soluble compound rapidly absorbed from the gastrointestinal tract and excreted in the urine, mainly with its form unchanged. It is bacteriostatic at the usual dose of 15 mg/kg/d. The only important toxic effect is a retrobulbar neuritis that infrequently results in loss of visual acuity, defects in visual fields, and inability to distinguish between red and green; the visual changes are completely reversible. This side effect should be monitored by monthly studies of visual acuity and visual fields and tests for green color vision. Unfortunately, the inability to monitor the toxic effect of retrobulbar neuritis by the required visual examinations limits its use in young children. It is not used routinely, but can be safely administered to children when needed. Ethambutol is used as the fourth drug in a multidrug regimen, and its major purpose is to prevent emergence of resistance to other drugs.

Other Drugs   The emergence of multidrug-resistant *M. tuberculosis* strains occasionally requires the use of secondary drugs. Ethionamide, cycloserine, capreomycin, amikacin, rifabutin, and fluoroquinolones have been used, but the experience with these agents is limited in children.

Corticosteroids   These drugs are controversial in the management of tuberculosis. They can be used only if effective antituberculosis therapy is in place. They are useful when the host inflammatory response to *M. tuberculosis* contributes to tissue damage. Generally accepted indications are for the management of tuberculous meningitis, tuberculous pleural effusion, pericarditis, and endobronchial disease.

TREATMENT OF EXPOSURE AND INFECTION   In the United States, children exposed to potentially infectious adults with pulmonary tuberculosis should be started on treatment, usually isoniazid only, if the child is younger than 5 years of age or has risk factors for the rapid development of tuberculosis disease. Failure to do so may result in the development of severe tuberculosis even before the tuberculin skin test becomes reactive; the "incubation" of disease may be shorter than that for the skin test. The child is treated for a minimum of 3 months after contact with the infectious case is broken. After 3 months, the tuberculin skin test is repeated. If the second test is positive, infection is documented and isoniazid should be continued for a total of 9 months; if the second skin test is negative, the treatment can be stopped.

Two circumstances of exposure deserve special attention. A difficult situation arises when exposed children are anergic because of HIV infection or other immunocompromise. These children are particularly vulnerable to rapid progression of tuberculosis, and it may not be possible to tell whether infection has occurred. In general, these children should be treated as if they have tuberculosis infection. The second situation is potential exposure of a newborn to a mother or other adult with possible pulmonary tuberculosis. In general, this exposure should be treated the same as for an older child. The neonate should be started on isoniazid and continued on it until tuberculosis disease in the adult can be ruled out, or for 3 months after the person with tuberculosis is no longer contagious.

The treatment of children infected with *M. tuberculosis* before they have developed disease is a mainstay of modern tuberculosis control. Many large, well-documented studies show that isoniazid is extremely effective in preventing the development of tuberculosis disease in infected children. Because isoniazid is so safe in this age group, any child or adolescent with a "positive" tuberculin skin test and no evidence of tuberculosis disease should receive treatment. In most cases, treatment is 9 months of isoniazid. Isoniazid is usually given every day by self-supervision, but can be administered twice weekly under the direct observation of a health care worker in cases of high-risk infection, particularly if an adult with active tuberculosis who also is being treated twice a week is present in the home. The optimal length of isoniazid therapy has been debated

for 40 years. The summary opinion of experts is that 9 months of therapy is the optimal length of treatment for children with tuberculosis infection.

If a child is exposed to or infected with an isoniazid-resistant but rifampin-susceptible strain of *M. tuberculosis,* rifampin should be substituted for isoniazid. If the infecting strain is resistant to both isoniazid and rifampin, usually two other drugs are used, but an expert in tuberculosis should be consulted for this situation.

TREATMENT OF DISEASE   Over the past two decades, a large number of trials of antituberculosis therapy for children with drug-susceptible pulmonary tuberculosis have demonstrated that the optimal regimen is 6 months duration, starting with at least three antituberculosis medications, usually isoniazid, rifampin, and pyrazinamide. Isoniazid and rifampin are continued for the entire 6 months, whereas pyrazinamide is used only for the first 2 months of therapy. Medications are usually given every day for the first 2 weeks to 2 months of therapy. After this time, medications can be given safely and effectively twice weekly under the observation of a health care worker. In all the reported trials for these regimens, the overall success rate for therapy was greater than 98% and the incidence of clinically significant adverse reactions was less than 2%. If the child is at risk for being infected with isoniazid-resistant tuberculosis because of previous treatment of the adult source case, or because the child has lived in an area of the world where resistance rates are high, most experts would add a fourth drug, usually ethambutol or streptomycin, to the initial regimen, until the exact drug susceptibility of either the child's isolate or the adult source case's isolate can be established.

Controlled clinical trials for treating various forms of extrapulmonary tuberculosis are almost nonexistent. Extrapulmonary tuberculosis is usually caused by fairly small numbers of mycobacteria. Most nonlife-threatening forms of extrapulmonary tuberculosis respond well to a 6-month treatment regimen using three or four drugs in the initial phase, similar to that used for pulmonary tuberculosis. One exception may be bone and joint tuberculosis, which is associated with a higher failure rate when only 6 months of chemotherapy is used, especially if surgical intervention has not been performed. Some experts recommend at least 9 to 12 months of therapy for bone and joint tuberculosis. Tuberculous meningitis usually has not been included in trials of extrapulmonary tuberculosis because of its serious nature and low incidence. Several recent trials suggest that 9 months of therapy is effective if isoniazid, rifampin, and pyrazinamide are administered during the initial phase of treatment. The official recommendation of the American Academy of Pediatrics for tuberculous meningitis is 12 months of therapy that includes at least isoniazid and rifampin and usually one or two other drugs in the initial phase of treatment. However, some experts believe that a treatment duration of 6 to 9 months is adequate if pyrazinamide is included in the initial regimen. Most experts add a fourth drug at the beginning of therapy to protect against initial drug resistance.

In general, the treatment of tuberculosis in HIV-infected children is the same as it is in children without HIV infection. Although some experts previously recommended lengthening the duration of therapy to 9 to 12 months in HIV-infected children, many trials have shown that adults with HIV infection and tuberculosis can be treated for the same length of time as adults without HIV infection who have tuberculosis.

The incidence of drug-resistant tuberculosis is increasing in many areas of the world. In the United States, approximately 10% of isolates of *M. tuberculosis* are resistant to at least one drug. Many countries in Latin America and Asia routinely report drug-resistance rates of 20 to 30%. Patterns of drug resistance among children tend to mirror those found in adults in the same population. For children in the United States, certain epidemiologic factors, such as being immigrants from Asia or Latin America, or a history of previous antituberculosis treatment in the adult source, correlate with drug resistance. Therapy for drug-resistant tuberculosis is successful only when two bactericidal drugs to which the infecting strain of *M. tuberculosis* is susceptible are given. When a child has a possible drug-resistant tuberculosis disease, at least three, and usually four or five, drugs should be administered initially, until the susceptibility pattern is determined and a more specific regimen can be designed. The specific treatment plan must be individualized for each patient, but durations of therapy of 12 to 18 months are not uncommon.

SUPPORTIVE CARE Activity does not need to be restricted in children with tuberculosis unless the child develops respiratory embarrassment or immobilization is needed for treatment, as in some cases of vertebral tuberculosis. Adequate nutrition is important, although reestablishment of weight gain may take several months. The major problem with treating tuberculosis in children and adults is nonadherence with therapy. Suspected cases of tuberculosis must be reported to the local health department so that it can compile accurate statistics, perform necessary contact investigations, and assist both patients and health care providers in overcoming barriers to adherence with therapy. In general, patients with tuberculosis disease should be treated with directly observed therapy, employing the help of a third party, such as a health department worker who observes the child and family during the administration of medication.

In general, children undergoing treatment for tuberculosis infection or disease should be seen every 4 to 6 weeks to monitor adherence, to observe for adverse reactions to medications, and to follow improvement in clinical course. Routine biochemical monitoring for adverse reactions is not necessary in asymptomatic children. Radiographic changes with intrathoracic tuberculosis occur slowly, and frequent chest radiographic monitoring is not necessary. A common practice for treating pulmonary tuberculosis is to obtain a chest radiograph at diagnosis and several months after the initiation of therapy to insure that no unusual changes have occurred. Children with tuberculosis infection do not need a repeat chest radiograph.

PREVENTION The only available vaccine against tuberculosis is BCG, which employs live attenuated bacilli. The BCG vaccines are extremely safe in immunocompetent hosts. Local ulceration and regional suppurative lymphadenitis occur in 0.1 to 1% of vaccines. These lesions usually resolve spontaneously, but occasionally require chemotherapy with either isoniazid or erythromycin. Rarely, surgical incision of the suppurative draining node is necessary, but this should be avoided rather than encouraged. Systemic complaints such as fever, convulsions, and irritability are extraordinarily rare after BCG vaccination. Rare children with undiagnosed immunocompromising conditions (such as severe combined immunodeficiency) develop systemic infection after neonatal BCG vaccination.

An accurate assessment of the efficacy of the BCG vaccines throughout the world is extremely difficult, as they have been given under various conditions in differing populations. Several controlled trials yielded greatly disparate results in protection, ranging from 0 to 80%. Apparently, BCG vaccination given during infancy has little effect on the ultimate incidence of tuberculosis among adults in a population. However, many experts feel that BCG vaccines are more effective in preventing disseminated tuberculosis among infants and young children. Retrospective studies from Europe and Asia yielded estimates of the protective effect of BCG in young children of 60 to 80%, and the effect is particularly strong for tuberculous meningitis and severe forms of disease.

BCG vaccination works well in some situations, but poorly in others. Clearly, BCG vaccination has had little effect on the ultimate control of tuberculosis throughout the world. Any protective effect created by BCG probably wanes over time. BCG vaccination has never been adopted as part of the strategy of control of tuberculosis in the United States. Its only recommended use in the United States is for children who will invariably be exposed to adults with multidrug-resistant tuberculosis due to family and other epidemiologic factors.

PROGNOSIS The prognosis of tuberculosis in infants, children, and adolescents is excellent with early recognition and effective chemotherapy. In most children with pulmonary tuberculosis, the disease completely resolves and, ultimately, radiographic findings are normal. The prognosis for bone and joint tuberculosis and for tuberculous meningitis depends on the stage of disease at the time antituberculosis medications are started. With all forms of extrapulmonary tuberculosis, the major problems usually are delayed recognition of the cause of disease and delayed initiation of treatment.

A resurgence of tuberculosis infection and disease is occurring among children in many regions of the world. As long as the conditions that promote tuberculosis, such as poverty, poor access to health care, overcrowding, and now HIV infection continue, this upward trend is likely to be sustained.

References

Centers for Disease Control and Prevention: Screening for tuberculosis and tuberculosis infection in high-risk populations. MMWR Morb Mortal Wkly Rep 44(RR-11):19–34, 1995

Chan SP, Birnbaum J, Rao M: Clinical manifestations and outcome of tuberculosis in children with acquired immunodeficiency syndrome. Pediatr Infect Dis J 15:443–447, 1996

Huebner RE, Schein MF, Bass JB: The tuberculin skin test. Clin Infect Dis 17:968–975, 1993

Hussey G, Chisolm T, Kibel M: Miliary tuberculosis in children: a review of 94 cases. Pediatr Infect Dis J 10:832–836, 1991

Lifschitz M: The value of the tuberculin skin test as a screening test for tuberculosis among BCG-vaccinated children. Pediatrics 36:624–627, 1965

Schaaf HS, Beyers N, Gie RP: Respiratory tuberculosis in childhood: the diagnostic value of clinical features and special investigations. Pediatr Infect Dis J 14:189–194, 1995

Starke JR, Correa AG: Management of mycobacterial infection and disease in children. Pediatr Infect Dis J 14:455–470, 1995

Steiner P, Rao M: Drug-resistant tuberculosis in children. Pediatr Infect Dis 4:275–282, 1993

Ussery XT, Valway SE, McKenna M, McCray E: Epidemiology of tuberculosis among children in the United States. Pediatr Infect Dis J 15:700–704, 1996

Vallejo JG, Ong LT, Starke JR: Clinical features, diagnosis, and treatment of tuberculosis in infants. Pediatrics 94:1–7, 1994

Waeker N, Connor J: CNS tuberculosis in children: a review of 30 cases. Pediatr Infect Dis J 9:539–543, 1990

Nontuberculous *Mycobacterial* Infections
Jeffrey R. Starke

The nontuberculous mycobacteria (NTM) have been collectively identified by a variety of terms including mycobacteria other than tuberculosis, atypical, nonpathogenic, unclassified, and environmental or opportunistic mycobacteria. Although grouping these organisms can be helpful, classification based on specific etiologic agent is preferable because this has implications for the predisposing factors, usual clinical course, diagnosis, and appropriate medical and surgical management of the infection.

Mycobacteria are true bacteria. They are nonmotile, nonspore-forming, slender pleomorphic rods. Their cell walls have a complex structure that includes a variety of proteins, carbohydrates, and lipids. Studies using high-pressure liquid chromatography reveal a variable species-related distribution of mycolic acids, each species having a distinct mycolic acid fingerprint that can be used for identification.

EPIDEMIOLOGY More than 50 species of *Mycobacterium* have been described, of which about half are pathogenic in humans. The most commonly encountered are *M. avium, M. intracellulare,* and *M. scrofulaceum,* which are classified together as the *Mycobacterium avium* complex (MAC).

The direct detection of NTM is similar to that for *M. tuberculosis.* All NTM are acid-fast but can be visualized in fluid and tissue samples often less than 50% of the time. Although even a single organism visualized on an entire slide is suspicious, false-positive results can be caused by contamination of stain solutions, tap water, distilled water, delivery tubes, or immersion oil. Direct detection of the various NTM by nucleic-acid amplification is advancing, but appropriate primers and reagents are not yet commercially available for most species.

Methods used for the isolation of *M. tuberculosis* from clinical samples also are useful for the isolation of NTM. All mycobacteria are obligate aerobes that grow best in the presence of 5 to 10% CO_2. Isolation on solid media of slow-growing NTM takes 2 to 6 weeks. Only the rapid growers (*M. fortuitum, M. chelonei,* and *M. abscessus*) form visible colonies in less than 10 days. Use of radiometric isolation systems usually leads to isolation of any species of NTM within 14 days. Some newly recognized species of mycobacteria cannot be cultivated but can be detected by nucleic-acid amplification. Most clinical laboratories now use high-pressure liquid chromatography (HPLC) analysis to speciate these organisms.

Determining the species of NTM causing infection is crucial to directing chemotherapy. Although drug-susceptibility testing of MAC isolates is not predictive of clinical response and does not contribute significantly to care of the patient, susceptibility testing for the rapid growing mycobacteria can be informative. For these mycobacteria, susceptibility testing to antibiotics such as amikacin, cefoxitin, doxycycline, sulfonamides, and the macrolides may be particularly helpful.

Transmission of NTM to humans occurs from environmental sources including soil, water, dust, and aerosols. NTM have been isolated from as much as 80% of soil samples, and certain strains of MAC are found in fresh and brackish waters in warmer climates. Other mycobacteria have been isolated from natural water supplies and tap water. Although mycobacteria are frequently found in animals, particularly swine and poultry, there is little evidence to suggest animal-to-human transmission. There is no evidence that person-to-person transmission occurs. Clusters and isolated cases of nosocomially acquired disease due to NTM are being reported with increasing frequency. Most common are outbreaks caused by the rapid growers, which are associated with injectors, continuous ambulatory peritoneal dialysis, contaminated skin marking, and injection solutions and hemodialysis.

The true incidence and prevalence of NTM infections are difficult to determine because there is no mandatory reporting. Isolation of the organism does not prove infection, and distinguishing among saprophytes, colonizers, and pathogenic organisms can be difficult. A survey in the 1980s estimated the prevalence of NTM disease in the United States as 1.8 cases per 100,000 population, approximately 20% of the prevalence of tuberculosis. Rates were highest for disease due to MAC, *M. kansasii,* and *M. fortuitum.* The age distribution of NTM disease varies by mycobacterial species and site of disease. Pulmonary disease is rare in children, but occurs more often in older adults. The majority of cases of NTM lymph node infection occur in children less than 5 years of age.

Clinical disease caused by NTM is common among both adults and children with AIDS and other immunosuppressing conditions. Prior to the advent of antiretroviral therapy, almost 25% of deceased patients with AIDS had autopsy evidence of widespread disease caused by MAC. In one epidemiologic survey, 7.8% of children 0 to 9 years of age with AIDS had disseminated NTM infection; MAC caused more than 90% of cases. Patients with malignancies, especially leukemia and lymphoma, appear to have a higher incidence of NTM infections than the general population in the same geographic area. NTM infections are being diagnosed more often in transplant patients, including children.

The majority of NTM that cause human disease are of low virulence. Infections in immunocompetent hosts require an unusual exposure or direct route of inoculation such as trauma. These infections are generally characterized by findings limited to the inoculation site. NTM infections do not exhibit lymphohematogenous dissemination in normal hosts. Immunocompromised hosts are at increased risk for systemic and disseminated NTM infection, but these typically occur in the setting of extreme and prolonged immunocompromise, such as in individuals with advanced AIDS. Although the portal of entry for the MAC is usually the oropharynx or respiratory tract, the pattern of disseminated disease in patients with AIDS is most consistent with an intestinal portal.

CLINICAL MANIFESTATIONS

Lymph Node The most common site of clinically significant NTM infection in children are the superficial lymph nodes of the head and neck. The vast majority of cases are caused by MAC. Lymph node infection as a result of NTM is most common in young children because of their tendency to put objects contaminated with soil, dust, or standing water into their mouths. Although NTM adenitis is more common in North America than is tuberculous adenitis, clinicians should never presume NTM to be the cause of apparent mycobacterial cervical adenitis until tuberculosis has been ruled out by a thorough epidemiologic history, evaluation of the family for tuberculosis, skin testing, and culture. The vast majority of children who develop NTM adenitis are immunologically normal.

Lymphadenitis caused by NTM usually involves a group of lymph nodes, most often located unilaterally, in the anterior cervical chain or submandibular region. Involvement of the supraclavicular lymph nodes is very unusual and suggests infection with *M. tuberculosis* or malignancy.

Lymph node enlargement usually occurs over weeks to months. Systemic signs or symptoms are rare in immunocompetent children. The involved lymph nodes are usually painless, firm, but not hard, and usually seem fixed to the underlying or overlying tissues. With further progression, the lymph nodes soften and become fluctuant and may rupture through the skin, causing drainage and formation of a sinus tract that can persist for months or years. Healing is characterized by fibrosis and scarring of the skin which can be extensive and disfiguring.

The standard tuberculin skin test may show a reaction with any NTM lymph node infection, but is more likely to cause a reaction with disease caused by *M. fortuitum* or the MAC. The greatest difficulty in differential diagnosis is usually distinguishing between adenitis caused by NTM and *M. tuberculosis*. The most important distinguishing feature is the epidemiologic setting, which determines whether children may have been exposed to *M. tuberculosis*. Lack of contact with an adult with tuberculosis, a skin test reaction of less than 10 mm, and a poor response to standard antituberculosis chemotherapy suggest the diagnosis of NTM cervical adenitis.

Cutaneous and Soft Tissue In immunocompetent hosts, the most common form of cutaneous NTM infection is the skin granuloma, frequently called swimmer's granuloma, caused by *M. marinum*. These infections are associated with aquatic activities such as swimming, boating, fishing, or even care of tropical fish. Direct trauma from contact with shrimp, barnacles, coral, or fish hooks may lead to infection. This mycobacterium can be isolated from swimming pools and natural sources of freshwater and saltwater. Cases of *M. marinum* infection usually are sporadic, although outbreaks of swimming pool granuloma involving hundreds of people have been reported. Typical skin lesions are nontender inflammatory nodules that progress to ulcerated granuloma or to chronic warty lesions over several weeks to months. The most commonly affected sites are areas where trauma is frequent such as the elbows, knees, feet, and hands. The typical lesion is 1 to 2 cm in diameter and is not accompanied by regional adenopathy. Most lesions heal spontaneously within a few months, but occasionally a nodular, sporotrichoid-like area spreads up an extremity. The clinical diagnosis is confirmed by culture of the discharge from the lesions or by biopsy. Many of these children have a highly reactive Mantoux tuberculin skin test.

In many tropical areas throughout the world, *M. ulcerans* causes an itching nodule on the arms or legs, which then breaks down to form a shallow ulcer. This lesion is referred to as a *Buruli ulcer*. Isolation of *M. ulcerans* is extremely difficult and the diagnosis is usually made on clinical grounds. Excision of the lesion usually constitutes therapy, and treatment with several different antibiotics has led to variable success.

An increasing number of mycobacterial cutaneous infections are caused by the rapidly growing mycobacteria, particularly *M. fortuitum*, *M. abscessus*, and *M. chelonei*. These localized skin or subcutaneous lesions are associated with accidental or iatrogenic trauma. Manifestations usually include cellulitis, a draining abscess that may be single or multiple, or tender nodules. Seropurulent drainage, poor wound healing, and development of sinus tracts after an operative procedure should suggest this diagnosis.

Pulmonary The most common NTM infection in adults is pulmonary disease with MAC, with or without some form of underlying chronic lung disease. The clinical presentation includes cough, production of sputum, low-grade fever, and weight loss. In addition, hemoptysis, pleuritic chest pain, and night sweats may occur. Pleural effusions caused by NTM are rare. *Mycobacterium kansasii* is the cause of lung disease most frequently in the midwestern and southwestern United States. Some patients have underlying chronic lung disease, and the infection may resemble pulmonary tuberculosis. Dissemination beyond the lung is rare in immunocompetent patients, but is common in immunosuppressed hosts.

Pulmonary infection by NTM in children is rare. Strains of the MAC are the most frequent cause of pediatric NTM pulmonary infection. The majority of infected children are immunocompetent with no underlying pulmonary disease. The most common presentation is similar to the primary tuberculosis complex. Patients have mild cough and low-grade fever with few systemic signs or symptoms. Occasionally, localized wheezing is noted and the diagnosis of an aspirated foreign body should be considered. Enlargement of hilar or mediastinal lymph nodes is common. These species can be isolated from the gastric secretions of healthy children, so diagnosis requires repeated isolation of the same mycobacterium in association with pulmonary deterioration.

Special mention should be made of the association between NTM colonization and infection and cystic fibrosis (CF). Unfortunately, a standard definition of NTM disease in CF patients, using clinical, radiographic, and pulmonary function testing results, is not possible. A single isolation of an NTM in the sputum of a CF patient who is not experiencing a decline in pulmonary function probably represents colonization, and treatment is not necessary. However, repeated isolation of the same species of NTM in association with declining pulmonary function is more suggestive, but not diagnostic, of invasive NTM disease in the lung.

Other Sites Several cases of osteomyelitis caused by the MAC have been described in children. In these cases, the bony lesions are usually the only sites of infection. The most frequent findings are lytic lesions of the long bones or lesions of the small bones of the hands, feet, skull, ribs, and sternum. In most patients, the lesions persist for several years, and then become inactive or resolve spontaneously.

Very few cases of NTM meningitis have been reported in children. The clinical presentation and laboratory values are generally similar to those commonly seen in patients with tuberculous meningitis. Before the AIDS epidemic, disseminated NTM infection had been reported in fewer than 20 children. Most of these children died. Lesions of the lungs, long bones, liver, gastrointestinal tract, and bone marrow were common.

NONTUBERCULOUS MYCOBACTERIA AND AIDS The major risk factor for NTM infection in patients with AIDS is the level of immune dysfunction, reflected by the concentration of $CD4^+$ cells in the blood. The mean concentration of $CD4^+$ cells in patients with disseminated NTM infection is less than $60/mm^3$. The most frequent causative agent of disseminated NTM infection is the MAC, but disease also results from infection with *M. kansasii*, *M. fortuitum*, *M. chelonei*, *M. xenopi*, *M. haemophilum*, and other novel, unidentified mycobacteria.

Disseminated NTM infection most commonly affects the blood, bone marrow, liver, spleen, and lymph nodes, but organisms have been recovered from virtually every organ of the body. Patients have a variety of signs and symptoms. The most common presentation is persistent fever with weight loss or failure to thrive. Gastrointestinal symptoms are common, especially chronic diarrhea, abdominal pain, and extrahepatic biliary obstruction. Radiographic imaging of the abdomen and physical examination often reveal marked hepatosplenomegaly, focal lesions in the liver or spleen, diffuse thickening of bowel walls, and enlarged mesenteric lymph nodes. Severe anemia requiring transfusion is frequent. Less commonly, cutaneous lesions, superficial lymph node enlargement, or endobronchial disease without pneumonia may occur. Many of the signs and symptoms described earlier are common in patients with AIDS and other conditions or infections; but fever, abdominal pain, diarrhea, anemia, and weight loss are significantly associated with disseminated NTM infection. Diagnosis of disseminated NTM infection is easily established by culture of a normally sterile site. Only one or two mycobacterial blood cultures are necessary to confirm the diagnosis in most cases.

DIAGNOSIS The key to diagnosis of NTM infection is a high level of suspicion based on epidemiologic factors and clinical presentation. This etiology should be especially considered in patients with chronic cervical lymphadenitis, in cases of chronic cutaneous ulcers or other skin lesions with poor wound healing, and in immunosuppressed hosts.

Nonspecific laboratory tests such as blood counts, ESR, urinalysis and serum chemistry tests are usually normal in children with NTM infections. Skin testing with purified protein derivative from *M. tuberculosis* may be helpful in the detection of infections caused by NTM. These infections are usually associated with skin test reactions less than 10 mm in diameter, but larger areas of induration may be seen. A negative tuberculin skin test never eliminates consideration of NTM infection. Of course, similar reactions may be caused by *M. tuberculosis* infection. NTM antigens for skin testing are no longer available commercially because of poor sensitivity and specificity, as well as a lack of quality control during production.

Acid-fast stains of appropriate patient samples may give an early clue to the presence of NTM infection but are frequently negative because the number of organisms is small. Histologic studies of affected tissues may be helpful if classic granulomatous changes are evident.

The most direct method for diagnosing NTM disease is culture of involved fluid or tissue specimens. Because of their ubiquity in the environment, isolation of NTM may represent colonization or infection without recognizable disease. Most experts suggest considering five clinical observations when determining whether an isolated NTM is the cause of disease:

1. Quantity of growth is usually moderate to heavy, especially in respiratory tract specimens, when disease occurs.
2. Repeated isolation of the same mycobacterium from the same site is likely to indicate true infection.
3. The site of origin of a positive specimen is important. The majority of NTM isolated from urine, gastric aspirates, and oropharyngeal secretions are contaminants, whereas NTM isolation from closed aspiration of lymph nodes or abscesses, and from deep-tissue fluids, biopsy specimens, or resected tissues usually indicates disease.
4. The species of mycobacteria is important. Isolates of NTM that rarely cause human disease should be viewed with caution.
5. Host risk factors should be considered. In the presence of predisposing conditions, the index of suspicion should be raised so that less-stringent criteria are applied to the evaluation of specimens that are culture-positive for NTM.

TREATMENT Specific treatment of NTM disease depends on the location and extent of the infected tissue, the host immune system, and the mycobacteria species involved. In general, surgery plays a more important role in the management of NTM disease than in tuberculosis, because chemotherapy is often ineffective for NTM and most NTM infections are localized and therefore amenable to surgical excision. An important initial consideration is determination that *M. tuberculosis* is not the causative pathogen. Until NTM are identified by culture, treatment is usually directed at *M. tuberculosis,* both for therapeutic reasons and for infection control.

To properly direct chemotherapy, it is important to determine the infecting species of NTM. In general, *M. kansasii, M. marinum, M. xenopi, M. gordonae, M. malmoense, M. szulgai,* and *M. haemophilum* are susceptible to some or all of the standard antituberculosis drugs. Treatment of the rapidly growing mycobacteria and most strains of the MAC require other antibiotics.

In general, excisional biopsy remains the treatment of choice for cervical lymphadenitis caused by NTM. Incisional biopsy should not be performed because it frequently leads to development of a draining sinus tract or recurrent disease. Total excision of the inflammatory mass usually precludes persistence or recurrence. However, removal of all involved lymph nodes may be impossible due to the close proximity of vital structures. Excision is best performed early, in order to improve the cosmetic outcome before extension of disease into the subcutaneous structures occurs. Chemotherapy is not generally necessary for children with NTM lymphadenitis. If tuberculosis cannot be reasonably excluded, an initial course of antituberculosis therapy should be considered. Many cases of cervical adenitis caused by the MAC resolve during treatment with standard antituberculosis medications, although no controlled trials have been reported. In these cases, the causative organisms usually are not susceptible to the chemotherapeutic agents used and spontaneous resolution may have occurred. In a small percentage of cases in which complete surgical excision is not possible, recurrence of adenitis is a problem. Chemotherapy may be helpful; the purpose is to prevent extension of recurrence so that a second surgical procedure is not necessary. The most commonly used regimen is a combination of at least two drugs, including clarithromycin, rifampin or rifabutin, and ethambutol.

Many cases of cutaneous disease caused by *M. marinum* resolve spontaneously. Acceptable chemotherapy regimens for more extensive lesions include doxycycline, or rifampin plus ethambutol, administered for a minimum of 3 months. The rate of resolution is variable, but therapy must be given for at least 3 to 4 weeks before the clinical response can be evaluated. No controlled clinical trials for treatment of cutaneous or soft-tissue disease caused by rapid-growing mycobacteria have been reported. Most isolates of *M. fortuitum* are susceptible to amikacin, cefoxitin, ciprofloxacin, clarithromycin, and imipenem. Drug susceptibility for *M. chelonei* and *M. abscessus* is more variable. For serious disease, intravenous therapy with amikacin and cefoxitin is recommended initially until clinical improvement is evident. Removal of foreign bodies is essential for resolution of infection at these sites. In cases of extensive disease, surgical excision of affected tissue may shorten the duration and morbidity of the infection.

Pulmonary infections with NTM in children are rare and no controlled therapy trials have been reported. Most isolates of MAC are resistant to antituberculosis drugs used singly. However, combination therapy with standard antituberculosis drugs generally has been successful in the treatment of adults with pulmonary MAC infection. If standard therapy is not effective, second-line drugs with significantly more side effects and greater toxicity must be used. Resectional surgery may be necessary for localized disease. Treatment of disease caused by *M. kansasii* is usually successful because it is susceptible to rifampin, ethambutol, often isoniazid, and streptomycin. The usual length of recommended combination therapy is 12 to 18 months.

Recent studies show that certain multiple-drug regimens can provide symptomatic relief, prolong life, and lead to partial clearing or reduction in the level of NTM bacteremia in patients with AIDS. However, treatment with various antimycobacterial agents may be associated with considerable toxicity. Patients with HIV infection usually have significantly higher rates of adverse reactions to most antimycobacterial drugs, just as they do to many other classes of drugs. The most commonly used drugs for patients with AIDS and disseminated MAC infection are clarithromycin, azithromycin, amikacin, ciprofloxacin, ethambutol, and rifampin or rifabutin. While ethambutol and ciprofloxacin are not usually used in children, their use is probably justified in children with AIDS because the purpose is to provide palliative therapy over a relatively short time. Although many different therapeutic regiments have been studied, recommendation of any specific drug regimen or duration of therapy for disseminated MAC disease in patients with AIDS is difficult. Most experts use the combination of clarithromycin and either rifamycin or ethambutol as initial therapy. Most experts recommend placing immunocompromised patients with AIDS who are at high risk for disseminated MAC infection with CD4$^+$ counts of less than 100 cells/mm^3 on a preventive medication such as clarithromycin or rifabutin.

References

Aitken ML, Burke W, McDonald G: Nontuberculous mycobacterial disease in adult cystic fibrosis patients. Chest 103:1096–1099, 1993

Hoyt L, Oleske J, Holland B, et al: Nontuberculous mycobacteria in children with acquired immunodeficiency syndrome. Pediatr Infect Dis J 11:354–360, 1992

Levin M, Newport MJ, D'Souza S, et al: Familial disseminated atypical mycobacterial infection in childhood: a human mycobacterial susceptibility gene? Lancet 345:79–83, 1995

Lincoln EM, Gilbert LA: Disease in children due to mycobacteria other than *Mycobacterium tuberculosis*. Am Rev Respir Dis 105:683–714, 1972

Margileth AM: Nontuberculous (atypical) mycobacterial disease. Semin Pediatr Infect Dis 4:307–311, 1993

Wolinsky E: Mycobacterial diseases other than tuberculosis. Clin Infect Dis 15:1–10, 1992

Wolinsky E: Mycobacterial lymphadenitis in children: a prospective study of 105 nontuberculous cases with long-term follow-up. Clin Infect Dis 20:954–963, 1995

Mycobacterium leprae (LEPROSY)
Wayne M. Meyers

Mycobacterium leprae, an acid-fast bacillus (AFB), was the first identified mycobacterium and the first known etiologic agent of a chronic disease in humans. Hansen discovered the leprosy bacillus in 1873, by the microscopic study of unstained tissue fluid from the skin of leprosy patients. Leprosy is present on all inhabited continents. Today, the World Health Organization (WHO) reports approximately 950,000 registered leprosy patients in the world, and estimates a total of 2 million. The annual incidence is 600,000 to 800,000. Southern Asia accounts for 75% of all patients (India alone accounts for 65%); Africa, 12%; and the Americas, 8%. In the United States, there are now approximately 6000 patients with a history of leprosy and the annual incidence is around 150, with about 20% acquired indigenously. Only Texas, Louisiana, and Ha-

waii are considered endemic states. Prevalence of leprosy seldom exceeds 5% in populations in endemic areas, and the gender ratio in children is 1:1. Children usually make up 20 to 30% of all detected cases. There are no established genetic susceptibility factors. Socioeconomic deprivation correlates well with the geographic distribution of areas with higher incidences of leprosy.

Infected humans are the usual reservoir of infection; however, naturally acquired leprosy is well known in wild armadillos in the southern United States, and in wild monkeys and chimpanzees in West Africa and probably elsewhere. Humans may acquire leprosy from infected armadillos and other zoonotic sources.

Skin-to-skin contact can transmit leprosy, but the nasorespiratory passage is thought to be the most common route. Nasal secretions of untreated lepromatous patients contain massive numbers of leprosy bacilli. Aerosols of such secretions transmit leprosy to the upper respiratory tract of contacts. Transmission by mother's milk and transplacental infection is considered uncommon. Cord blood from the placenta of some lepromatous mothers contains *M. leprae*-specific IgA and IgM antibodies, and levels of these antibodies rise in some infants after birth. Clinical leprosy in children under 1 year of age, although unusual, is well described. In a group of 49 such infants, approximately 50% of the mothers had clinical leprosy, suggesting subclinical infection with a transient bacteremia during gestation.

CLINICAL MANIFESTATIONS The classification schema for leprosy is shown in Table 13-40. An alternative simplified binomial classification devised by the World Health Organization divides patients with five or fewer skin lesions (paucibacillary; PB) from those with more than five lesions (multibacillary; MB). The incubation period is typically 2 to 5 years, but may be much longer. There are no prodromal signs. Virtually all leprosy patients have neuropathy in cutaneous nerves, and many have sensory and motor trunk involvement of peripheral nerves. Nerve damage is most frequent in borderline leprosy. Neuritis or neurotropic changes (eg, clawing of the hands, footdrop, facial palsy, or tissue damage of insensitive hands or feet) often prompt the patient to seek care.

Often the earliest manifestation of leprosy is a single skin lesion, hypopigmented in dark skin and erythematous in light skin (Fig. 13-5), that may heal spontaneously or evolve into one of the established forms. Sensory changes within the lesion are commonly slight or nondetectable. Definitive histopathologic diagnosis can only be established by finding the rare AFB in nerves.

Lepromatous leprosy involves nearly the entire skin, but infiltrations are heaviest in the cooler areas—ears, central face, extensor surfaces of extremities (Fig. 13-6). In the earliest form in children, called "juvenile leprosy," slight changes in texture of the skin may be detectable and are best seen in open sunlight. Early macules are equally difficult to see, and sensory changes are slight. Eyebrows are thinned, even absent in advanced stages. The highly anergic form called Lucio leprosy appears only in Latin American patients, especially those from Mexico and Costa Rica. This form is so diffuse that it can go unrecognized for long periods. Patients with advanced forms of Lucio leprosy often have cutaneous vasculitis with widespread punched-out ulcers (Lucio phenomenon).

The clinical course of leprosy is often punctuated by two types of acute reactional episodes that are medical emergencies. The first (type 1 reaction) represents an upgrading of the host's cell-mediated immunity. Cutaneous lesions become acutely edematous and erythematous, and one or more peripheral nerves are swollen and painful. Early anti-inflammatory treatment prevents permanent nerve damage with further disease progression. The second type of

TABLE 13-40
CLASSIFICATION OF LEPROSY

GROUP	CLINICAL FEATURES	HISTOLOGIC FEATURES
Tuberculoid (TT)	Single or few well-defined anesthetic macules or plaques. Peripheral nerve involvement common.	Granulomas, with or without giant cells. No subepidermal clear zone. Bacilli rare.
Borderline-tuberculoid (BT)	Lesions similar to TT, but more numerous. Borders less distinct. Satellite lesions around larger lesions. Nerve involvement common.	Granulomas similar to TT. Nerves infiltrated. Occasional bacilli in nerves. Subepidermal clear zone.
Borderline (BB)	More lesions than BT. Borders vague. Satellite lesions frequent. Nerve involvement common.	Epithelioid cells and histiocytes focalized by lymphocytes. Nerves with increased cellularity. Bacilli most common in nerves. Subepidermal clear zone.
Borderline-lepromatous (BL)	Lesions numerous and similar to BB. Some nerve damage.	Histiocytic infiltrations tend to evolve toward both epithelioid cells and foamy cells. Nerves have less cellular infiltration. Bacilli plentiful in nerves and histiocytes. Subepidermal clear zone.
Lepromatous (LL)	Multiple nonanesthetic macules or papules, symmetrically distributed. Neural lesions late. Madarosis, leonine facies, testicular damage late.	Foamy histiocytes with many bacilli. Bacilli in blood vessels and arrector muscles. Few lymphocytes. Subepidermal clear zone. Numerous bacilli in nerves without much intraneural cellular infiltration.
Indeterminate (I)	Vaguely defined hypopigmented or erythematous macule.	Lymphocytes and histiocytes around skin appendages and nerves. Rare bacilli in nerves.

reaction (erythema nodosum leprosum; ENL) only occurs in the lepromatous patient. It presents as a rapid onset of multiple, tender, subcutaneous nodules accompanied by fever, and sometimes synovitis and iridocyclitis. It is initiated by an immune complex reaction and is often accompanied by vasculitis and ulceration.

DIAGNOSIS The cardinal signs of leprosy are hypoesthetic skin lesions, enlarged peripheral nerves, and AFB in skin smears. In the absence of another obvious diagnosis, any one of these findings suggests leprosy.

Contact history and residence in an endemic area are important factors. Experienced observers can often render a diagnosis from clinical findings, but histopathologic confirmation is recommended. The entire skin surface should be examined, preferably in open sunlight, and peripheral nerves palpated. Unexplained damage to hands or feet or muscle weakness (eg, clawed hands or footdrop)

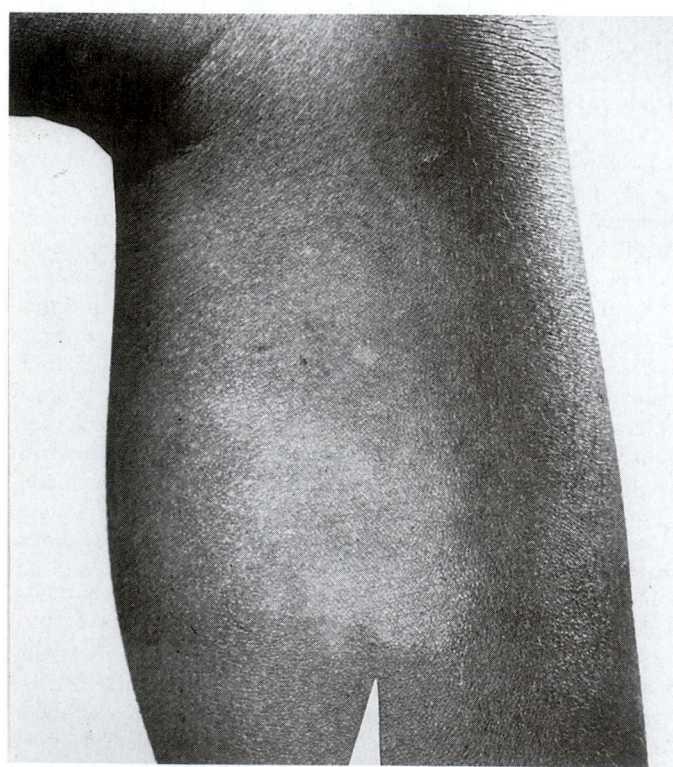

FIGURE 13-5 Indeterminate leprosy on calf of a Filipino child. Borders of this hypopigmented lesion are indistinct.

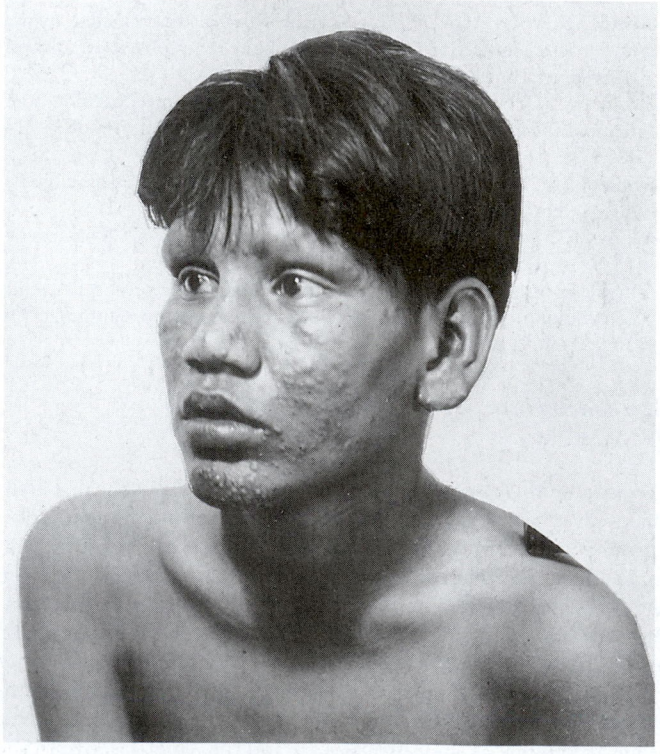

FIGURE 13-6 Lepromatous leprosy in an adolescent Filipino boy. Note loss of eyebrows, thickening of earlobes, and thickened skin with papules over the face.

suggests neuropathy. Lepromatous patients may complain of a chronic stuffy nose.

Sensory testing for changes in light touch in lesions are best performed with wisps of cotton or graded nylon fibers, and heat-cold discrimination impairment with warm and cool water in test tubes. This can be extremely difficult in children, and repeated testing is often required.

Specialists should be consulted in the taking and evaluation of skin smears for AFB. False-positive skin smears are often encountered. Serologic testing for PGL-I, a species-specific antigen, and anti-PGL-I antibodies are available, but they are little used because most PB patients are negative. DNA technology detects even small numbers of *M. leprae* in tissue sections and in skin and nasal smears, but results must be carefully correlated clinically.

TREATMENT Rifampin, dapsone, and clofazimine are the most commonly used antileprotics. Monotherapy is contraindicated because of known resistance of *M. leprae* to at least rifampin and dapsone; however, multidrug-resistant strains are rare. The antibacterial multidrug therapeutic (MDT) regimen chosen is based on the type of leprosy according to the WHO classification:

- *Paucibacillary regimen for adults:* Rifampin 600 mg once monthly plus dapsone 100 mg daily. This regimen is given for 6 months and then discontinued. The monthly dose of rifampin is given under supervision.
- *Multibacillary regimen for adults:* Rifampin 600 mg and clofazimine 300 mg once monthly, plus dapsone 100 mg daily and clofazimine 50 mg daily for at least 12 months. The monthly rifampin and 300 mg of clofazimine are given under supervision. Some clinicians continue therapy for MB leprosy until skin smears are negative.
- *MDT for children as a percentage of the adult dose:* Less than 15 kg, 25%; 15 to 30 kg, 50% 30 to 45 kg, 75%; and greater than 45 kg, 100%.

WHO recommendations have been subject to periodic changes, and clinicians are advised to consult appropriate authorities for current information.

Patients with type 1 reactions should receive analgesics and, initially, high daily doses of corticosteroids tapered to a minimal effective dose. Those with ENL should receive thalidomide if applicable; otherwise, corticosteroids are given and ophthalmologic consultation should be obtained. Patients on clofazimine tend to experience less-severe ENL.

All patients should be checked for motor and sensory losses. Even patients under optimal treatment often continue to have silent progressive neuropathy. Patients with deformities and insensitive hands and feet should be seen by specialists for appropriate care.

References

Brubaker ML, Meyers WM, Bourland J: Leprosy in children one year of age and under. Int J Lepr Other Mycobact Dis 53:517–523, 1985

Hastings RC, ed: Leprosy, 2nd ed. Edinburgh, Churchill Livingstone, 1994.

Jacobson RR: Treatment of leprosy. In: Hastings RC, ed: Leprosy, 2nd ed. Edinburgh, Churchill Livingstone, 1994

Ottenhoff THM: State of the art lectures: immunology of leprosy: lessons from and for leprosy. Int J Lepr Other Mycobact Dis 62:108–121, 1994

Ridley DS, Jopling WH: Classification of leprosy according to immunity: a five-group system. Int J Lepr Other Mycobact Dis 34:255–273, 1966

Van Brakel WH, Khawas IB: Silent neuropathy in leprosy: an epidemiological description. Lepr Rev 65:350–360, 1994

13.2.22 *Mycoplasma* Infections

Julia A. McMillan

Mycoplasma are a special class of bacteria called Mollicutes that contain both pathogenic and commensal species. They are the smallest known microorganisms ($0.2 \mu m$) able to replicate in culture media, but precursor substances (eg, peptides, native proteins, cholesterol) are required for growth. The *Mycoplasma* genome encompasses approximately one-sixth that of the common bacterium *Escherichia coli*.

Unlike other bacteria, *Mycoplasma* organisms lack rigid cell walls; this feature precludes staining with organic dyes (such as those used in the Gram stain procedure) and renders the organisms insensitive to antibiotics that inhibit wall synthesis (such as the penicillins and polymyxins).

The best-characterized human mycoplasma disease is respiratory tract infection with *M. pneumoniae*, a prominent cause of the atypical pneumonia syndrome. *Mycoplasma hominis* is associated with a variety of genitourinary and perinatal conditions, including postpartum maternal sepsis, neonatal skin infections and meningitis, and "sterile" pyelonephritis. Problems associated with *U. urealyticum*, and possibly *M. genitalium*, are pelvic inflammatory disease, salpingitis, and nongonococcal urethritis in sexually active individuals. Ureaplasmas may have a relationship to chorioamnionitis, prematurity, low birthweight, and neonatal pneumonia. Available information is ample for the recognition and appropriate treatment of *M. pneumoniae* disease. At present, no general recommendations can be made for the other problems mentioned because of incomplete clinical, epidemiologic, pathologic, and microbiological data.

Mycoplasma pneumoniae

Infections with *M. pneumoniae* occur throughout life, but the respiratory disease syndrome, often called atypical pneumonia, is most common in school children, adolescents, and young adults. It is estimated that *M. pneumoniae* is responsible for about one-fifth of all instances of pneumonia. Much more frequent than atypical pneumonia are several nonpneumonic respiratory syndromes; together these conditions contribute about six episodes per 100 population annually to the burden of human respiratory infections. The prevalence of *M. pneumoniae* disease varies greatly from year to year, with larger clusters of infections occurring in irregular 3- to 4-year cycles. The spread of infection is facilitated by prolonged close contact, such as within household units, childcare centers, college dormitories, and military barracks. Natural protective immunity is apparently limited, because repeat episodes of infection and pneumonia have been documented.

CLINICAL MANIFESTATIONS The most frequent recognizable clinical presentation of *M. pneumoniae* infection is tracheobronchitis, consisting of nonspecific systemic symptoms such as malaise, headache, low-grade fever, persistent cough, and increased respiratory secretions. Coughing can occur in paroxysms, often worse at night, and may persist for several weeks if untreated. Patients with pneumonia present similarly but show evidence of progression to pulmonary involvement by physical examination or chest x-ray after as many as 7 days of generalized symptoms. Generally, pulmonary disease is not severe, leading to the term "walking pneumonia." Other syndromes that may be seen are upper respiratory infections, pharyngitis, and illnesses associated with wheezing. Because these clinical findings are nonspecific, *M. pneumoniae* disease tends to be underdiagnosed.

The nonspecificity and usual mildness of symptomatology are often coupled with a paucity of physical findings. The patient's complaints often appear greater than is suggested by examination. The pharynx can be erythematous, with or without associated lymphadenopathy. Palpation of the trachea may stimulate a coughing paroxysm. If pneumonia is present, scattered crepitations or wheezes can be heard on inspiration, usually over one or the other lower lobes. Rarely is there sufficient pulmonary consolidation or pleural effusion to be recognized by physical examination. It should be emphasized that symptoms and signs evolve gradually over several days to 1 week or more, and repeated examinations may be necessary to suggest the correct diagnosis. Other findings that are useful in recognizing the syndrome are otitis media, evidence of sinusitis, and skin rashes (maculopapular, occasionally vesicular, rarely erythema multiforme).

The chief importance of routine laboratory tests is to exclude other conditions. Blood leukocyte levels and differential counts are usually within normal limits. Erythrocyte sedimentation rate may be elevated during the course of the disease. Subclinical hemolysis is occasionally evident. Children with sickle-cell disease often show marked polymorphonuclear leukocytosis, which complicates the interpretation of their laboratory findings.

About 75% of adult patients with pneumonia due to *M. pneumoniae* develop antibodies against the I antigen on human erythrocytes (cold agglutinin antibody) within 7 to 10 days of initial symptoms. The titer of cold agglutinin antibody, as determined by serial dilution of the patient's serum, correlates roughly with the severity of disease. A titer of at least 1:64 in a patient with pneumonia is highly suggestive of *M. pneumoniae* infection. Although this test is not specific (other bacterial and viral causes of pneumonia are infrequently associated with a positive test for cold agglutinins), a strong positive reaction coupled with a compatible clinical picture can be useful in choosing initial therapy.

Chest x-rays can document and detail the occurrence of pneumonia. Usually, infiltration appears in a bronchopneumonic pattern involving segments of one of the lower lobes. Frank consolidation (filling of alveolar spaces) is uncommon, although subsegmental areas of atelectasis are frequent. Pleural effusions are usually unilateral, small, and transient, when they occur.

DIAGNOSIS The diagnosis of *M. pneumoniae* is suggested by the clinical picture, usual patient age (5–40 years), and exclusion of other entities. Helpful adjuncts are knowledge of other individuals in families, institutions, or communities with compatible respiratory infection, and the development of cold hemagglutinins during the first or second week of symptoms. Cultures, not available in most diagnostic laboratories, may require 2 to 6 weeks to complete. Serodiagnostic testing for the complement-fixing (CF) antibody against *M. pneumoniae* depends upon a four-fold or greater titer change between an acute specimen and another specimen collected 2 to 3 weeks later. Thus, both tests offer only retrospective diagnosis. Commercially available methods for detecting IgM against *M. pneumoniae* have been developed and correlate well with CF-antibody testing. IgM antibody develops within 7 days of the onset of illness, thus diagnosis can be made using one serum sample early in the course of infection. Some research laboratories have developed polymerase chain reaction (PCR) assays that detect small numbers of *M. pneumoniae* organisms in respiratory secretions and other body fluids. This assay has allowed a more complete understanding of the role of *M. pneumoniae* in nonrespiratory-tract illness. However, because asymptomatic shedding of *M. pneumoniae* is known to persist for weeks following initial infection, the significance of a positive PCR in the absence of an associated antibody response is not known. From a practical viewpoint, diagnosis most often is based on clinical and epidemiologic features and response to empirical therapy. Severe or unusual presentations may offer greater difficulty.

Untreated infections usually run their natural course in 1 to 3 weeks, but persistent coughing and malaise may extend several weeks into convalescence. The response to proper treatment given during the acute phase of illness is relatively dramatic, with abatement of fever usually within 24 hours. Controlled antibiotic efficacy studies show significant reduction in other objective evidence of morbidity, such as hospital days and duration of pulmonary infiltration. Respiratory tract involvement may extend to contiguous sites, namely middle ears (particularly in younger children) or paranasal sinuses (recognized mainly in adults). Unusual pulmonary manifestations include perfusion defects, noncardiogenic pulmonary edema, massive pleural effusions, and lung abscesses. Complications involving nonrespiratory sites are legion; their frequency is difficult to assess accurately as many reports concern only hospitalized patients, and the precision with which etiologic diagnosis was established varies. Examples include various skin rashes, with full-blown Stevens-Johnson syndrome being most severe; single- or multiple-joint nonsuppurative arthritis; myositis and myocarditis; vascular occlusive problems and microembolic phenomena; hemolytic anemia; and many nervous system problems, such as psychoses, meningoencephalitis, infarctions, and various radiculopathies. Successful isolation by culture of *M. pneumoniae* from nonrespiratory sites is rarely reported, but its detection by PCR in cerebrospinal fluid (CSF) and blood in patients with a variety of nonrespiratory conditions suggests that direct invasion by the organism may contribute to the pathogenesis.

TREATMENT Erythromycin has been the treatment of choice for suspected *M. pneumoniae* infection in children because of its narrow antibacterial spectrum, its low toxicity (especially in children under 8 years), and its high level of in vitro activity against *M. pneumoniae*. For preadolescent children an oral dose of 30 to 40 mg/kg/d divided into four evenly spaced administrations is usually effective. Therapy should be continued for 10 to 14 days to minimize symptomatic relapses. Tetracycline is an effective alternative therapy for children older than 7 years. Adult doses of 1 to 2 g of erythromycin or tetracycline per 24 hours orally can be used in adolescents weighing more than 60 kg. Intravenous administration of erythromycin lactobionate can be used for severely ill patients. Clarithromycin and azithromycin are as effective as erythromycin in vitro, and clarithromycin's effectiveness (15 mg/kg/d in two divided doses) has been documented in a clinical study in children. Resistance of *M. pneumoniae* to erythromycin has not been recognized as a clinical problem, although resistant organisms may be isolated from patients after successful treatment and can be induced easily in the laboratory. Several of the quinolones (ciprofloxacin, ofloxacin, and sparfloxacin) demonstrate in vitro efficacy and are clinically effective in treating adults with atypical pneumonia. This class of antibiotics should not be used in prepubertal children. *Mycoplasma pneumoniae* is not affected by the penicillin antibiotic group, and there is variable sensitivity to the aminoglycosides and chloramphenicol.

Natural *M. pneumoniae* disease appears to confer limited protective immunity; reinfections have been documented as soon as 13 months after the original infection in young children, and repeated episodes of pneumonia have been seen within 4 to 10 years in older children.

Mycoplasma hominis

Both *M. hominis* and *Ureaplasma urealyticum* colonize, and in some cases infect, the human genitourinary tract. *U. urealyticum* is discussed in Sec. 13.2.36.

EPIDEMIOLOGY   *Mycoplasma hominis* is found in the genitourinary tract of 10 to 50% of apparently healthy women and is also thought to be a cause of chorioamnionitis, postpartum fever, and pyelonephritis. Not surprisingly, *M. hominis* has also been detected on the skin and mucous membranes and in gastric aspirates of newborn infants whose mothers are colonized or infected. During the 1980s and 1990s several prospective studies attempted to define a relationship between *M. hominis* and low birth weight and premature delivery, without consistent success. In both prospective studies and individual case reports, *M. hominis* was isolated from the CSF of newborns, most often without associated evidence of inflammation. In most cases, the infection had no apparent impact on the clinical course, despite the fact that no specific antimycoplasma therapy was given. *Mycoplasma hominis* has, however, been the only reported pathogen associated with a variety of conditions in predominantly premature newborns, including chronic meningitis and ventriculitis, wound infection, scalp abscess, pericardial effusion, brain abscess, lymphadenitis, and septicemia.

In older children and adults, *M. hominis* rarely causes infection outside the genitourinary tract. Bacteremia, arthritis, peritonitis, soft tissue infection, endocarditis, empyema, and meningitis have been reported, primarily in postpartum or immunocompromised patients. Hypogammaglobulinemia appears to be an important risk factor.

Neither *M. pneumoniae* nor *U. urealyticum* can be identified without the use of special media. *Mycoplasma hominis*, however, will grow on blood agar and in broth media used for the routine isolation of bacteria from blood. The laboratory should be requested to look specifically for *M. hominis* when a localized purulent infection yields no pathogen using conventional methods, particularly if the patient is a newborn or immunocompromised.

Mycoplasma hominis infection can be treated with tetracyclines or clindamycin, and it is moderately sensitive to chloramphenicol and rifampin. Unlike the other mycoplasmas that cause infection in humans, *M. hominis* is not susceptible to erythromycin. There are no prospective studies evaluating the benefit of immunoglobulin therapy, but the susceptibility of hypogammaglobulinemic patients to *M. hominis* infection suggests that immune globulin might be of benefit for patients with nongenitourinary infection.

References

Block S, Hedirack J, Hammerschlag MR, et al: *Mycoplasma pneumoniae* in pediatric community-acquired pneumonia: comparative efficacy and safety of clarithromycin vs. erythromycin ethylsuccinate. Pediatr Infect Dis J 14:471–477, 1995

Broughton RA: Infections due to *Mycoplasma pneumoniae* in children. Pediatr Infect Dis 5:71–85, 1986

Clyde WA JR: Clinical overview of typical *Mycoplasma pneumoniae* infections. Clin Infect Dis 17:S32–36, 1993

Gelfand EW: Unique susceptibility of patients with antibody deficiency to mycoplasma infection. Clin Infect Dis 17(Suppl 1):S250–253, 1993

Ieven M, Ursi D, Van Bever H: Detection of *Mycoplasma pneumoniae* by two polymerase chain reactions and role of *M. pneumoniae* in acute respiratory tract infections in pediatric patients. J Infect Dis 173:1445–1452, 1996

Wientzen RL: Genital mycoplasma and the pediatrician. Pediatr Infect Dis J 9:232–235, 1990

13.2.23   Neisserial Infections

Neisseria gonorrhoeae
Mary Allen Staat

A commonly reported infectious disease in the United States, gonorrhea is sexually transmitted and principally affects adolescents and young adults. Infants can be infected by passage through an infected birth canal. Children can acquire the disease through sexual play, molestation, and sexual abuse. The principal manifestation of the uncomplicated infection is a urethral or vaginal discharge; however, localized infections of the fallopian tubes, joints, conjunctiva, and anus, as well as disseminated infection, can occur.

The gonococcus is a gram-negative kidney-bean-shaped diplococcus, nonmotile and nonencapsulated, fastidious in its nutritional requirements, and it grows best aerobically in 4 to 10% CO_2 with increased humidity on a medium of chocolate agar with antibiotics (Thayer-Martin medium) that suppress the growth of other microorganisms. Gonococci grow in small colonies that are easily identified; they elaborate indophenoloxidase—the basis for identification by an oxidase test. However, definitive identification (required in more complicated clinical settings and for medicolegal purposes) requires the use of specific fluorescein-conjugated antibody staining or sugar fermentation.

Neisseria gonorrhoeae infects nonciliated columnar and transitional epithelial cells. Attachment to the cells is mediated by pili and the outer-membrane opacity proteins. Within 24 to 48 hours after attachment, the organism synthesizes enzymes to facilitate penetration to submucosal tissues. The host produces a neutrophil response, which results in sloughing of the epithelium, submucosal abscesses, and a purulent exudate. *Neisseria gonorrhoeae* is capable of invading the bloodstream and disseminating to other sites, such as the joints and meninges. Bacteremic spread is also more likely to occur in conjunction with menstruation, which facilitates spread to the upper genital tract (salpingitis). Deficiency of one of the terminal components of the complement system (especially factors 5, 6, 7, or 8) places the patient at increased risk of disseminated, chronic, or recurrent gonococcal disease.

EPIDEMIOLOGY   Gonococcal infection is limited to humans, and transmission is almost always sexual (genital, anal, or oral). There has been a steady decline in reported gonorrhea cases over the past two decades. The rate in children younger than 10 years of age is low; the rate for boys and girls between the ages of 10 and 14 years is 8 and 54 per 100,000, respectively. The rates for teenagers ages 15 through 19 years are 354 males and 718 females per 100,000. Sexual transmission and risk factors for gonococcal infection are further discussed in Sec 3.6.1.

CLINICAL MANIFESTATIONS   The incubation period of gonorrheal infection is varied, but symptoms usually appear within 1 week of infection. The majority of infected males present with urethritis, which has been described at all ages, even in the newborn. Most gonococcal infections in the mature female are asymptomatic, but there may be thick purulent cervical or urethral discharge and pain upon manipulation of the cervix. The following types of gonococcal infections are of particular relevance to the pediatrician.

LOCALIZED INFECTIONS

Gonococcal Ophthalmia Gonococcal ophthalmia can occur at any age, but it notoriously afflicts the newborn infant, who is infected by contact with gonococci from the birth canal. One or both eyes may be infected. The instillation of 1% silver nitrate solution into the eyes of all newborns shortly after birth greatly reduced the incidence of gonococcal ophthalmia neonatorum, but isolated failures have occurred.

The appearance of a purulent or serosanguineous discharge, typically 2 to 7 days after delivery, should prompt careful evaluation of a Gram-stained smear and culture for *N. gonorrhoeae*. Purulent discharge occurring within 48 hours of birth is most often the result of chemical conjunctivitis, and during the second week of life the likely diagnosis is *C. trachomatis*. Edema, congestion of lids and conjunctiva, periorbital swelling, and adherence of eyelashes ("matting") because of purulent exudate compose the typical clinical picture of gonococcal ophthalmia. A Gram-stained smear of the exudate shows an abundance of polymorphonuclear leukocytes, some containing intracellular diplococci. Spontaneous recovery may occur, but permanent damage, such as iridocyclitis and corneal ulceration, occurs in about one-third of untreated individuals. In view of the serious consequences of gonococcal ophthalmitis, treatment should be commenced as early as feasible, based on the results of a Gram-stained smear, without awaiting cultural confirmation. Infants with suspected gonococcal ophthalmia should have a blood culture and lumbar puncture done to evaluate for systemic disease and should be treated with antibiotics until results of the cultures are known.

Prophylaxis of ophthalmia neonatorum continues to be important because of the high prevalence of *N. gonorrhoeae* among pregnant women. The classic method described by Credé involves the instillation of 1% silver nitrate into the conjunctival sac shortly after birth. However, erythromycin (0.5%) or tetracycline (1%) ophthalmic ointment from a single-use tube or ampule appears to be equally effective and has the virtue of not producing chemical conjunctivitis.

Vulvovaginitis Approximately one-fifth of vulvovaginitis infections in preadolescent girls is caused by *N. gonorrhoeae*. Before puberty, the vaginal mucosa is more susceptible to infection than it is in the mature female. The majority of gonococcal infections in girls less than 9 years of age result from sexual abuse by an infected adult or adolescent. Typically, girls with vulvovaginitis present with a thick green or creamy vaginal discharge that is voluminous. However, asymptomatic infections consisting of labial erythema and scanty secretions have been described. Because the endocervical glands in the prepubertal female are not developed, infection rarely spreads to the fallopian tubes and upper genital tract. However, tubal infection or peritonitis occurs in about 6% of untreated patients. Septic complications, such as arthritis, have also been reported.

Cervicitis In postpubertal females, the endocervix is the primary site of infection. A mucopurulent discharge from the cervical os is frequently accompanied by severe pelvic pain upon manipulation of the cervix. In 10 to 20% of women with lower genital tract disease, the infection may ascend from the vagina or cervix to the upper genital tract to cause inflammation of the endometrium (endometritis), fallopian tubes (salpingitis), ovaries (oophoritis), or the pelvic peritoneal cavity (pelvic peritonitis).

Urethritis Infection in young men usually presents with a purulent urethral discharge; it is commonly associated with dysuria, frequency, and meatal erythema. Gonococcal urethritis occurs in preadolescent boys, in whom it is usually the result of sexual experimentation or molestation. Urethritis may also occur in women and is associated with dysuria and frequency.

Pharyngeal Infections Pharyngeal infection is increasingly common in adults and adolescents as a result of orogenital sexual practices. It has also been reported in children. The clinical findings, when present, are cryptic tonsillitis, pharyngitis, and erythema and swelling of the soft palate. When it is suspected, the infection is diagnosed by identifying the organism in culture.

Anorectal Infections Anorectal gonorrhea occurs in children who have been molested, in sexually active young men and women, and in the neonate. Symptoms include rectal pain, tenesmus, mucopurulent rectal discharge, and rectal bleeding. On inspection, the mucous membrane is friable and erythematous, and a discharge may be present.

Pelvic Inflammatory Disease (Salpingitis) Infection rarely spreads to the upper genital tract in prepubertal girls. However, with the onset of menarche and sexual intercourse, some 10 to 20% of young women with gonorrhea will develop tubal infections (see Sec. 3.6.1).

Disseminated Infections Disseminated disease constitutes only 0.1 to 0.3% of infections. Hematogenous spread of gonococci can originate from local infections and can occur at any age; there is a predisposition to dissemination during the neonatal period, during pregnancy, and at the time of menses, as well as in drug users and in patients with accompanying liver disease. Disseminated infection is strikingly frequent among asymptomatic female carriers. Disseminated gonococcemia in the neonatal period may be associated with arthritis and meningitis.

Arthritis and tenosynovitis are the most common manifestations in adolescents and adults. During the phase of bacteremia, a migratory polyarthritis is typical. All joints may be affected, but knees, ankles, and wrists prevail. Accompanying skin lesions are common and consist of clusters of erythematous or hemorrhagic lesions about 2 mm in diameter, whose centers are gray or black because of necrosis, or hemorrhage, or both. Skin lesions are found more frequently on the extremities, clustered around joints. At the time of bacteremia, cultures of joint fluid are rarely positive, but later bacteria may localize to one or more joints, at which time there may be purulent effusion containing viable gonococci.

More than 30 instances of gonococcal meningitis have been reported among newborn infants and adults. It may present as a typical pyogenic meningitis, but frequently the simultaneous presence of urethritis, arthritis, or cutaneous lesions affords clues to its cause.

DIAGNOSIS In gonococcal ophthalmia, vulvovaginitis, and urethritis, examination of a stained smear of the purulent discharge will usually reveal intracellular gram-negative diplococci. Although this finding is virtually diagnostic, confirmatory cultures are important for precise bacteriologic identification, especially for medicolegal purposes. In females, symptoms are usually insufficient evidence for presumptive diagnosis, and gram-stained smears of secretions from the vagina or endocervix are frequently negative. The presence of nonpathogenic *Neisseria* species (eg, *N. sicca*, *N. subflora*) may occasionally result in false-positive smears. Thus, at present the diagnosis of gonorrhea in females is best accomplished by culture. Specimens collected from both the endocervical canal and the rectum should be cultured.

Disseminated disease is difficult to diagnose because cultures of blood, joint fluid, or skin lesions show growth of gonococci in less than one-third of patients; even under optimal circumstances in which all three tissues are cultured, fewer than 50% of suspected cases are confirmed bacteriologically.

For best results, specimens for culture should be collected using swabs made of a synthetic fiber (eg, calcium alginate) and transported in a medium that will keep the organisms alive (eg, Transgrow agar, a modification of Thayer-Martin medium). Rapid diagnosis of gonococcal infection using DNA probes, enzyme immunoassays, and DNA amplification techniques in both urine and secretions from the vagina or endocervix may become widespread in the near future.

TREATMENT

Antimicrobial Therapy Recommended guidelines for treatment schedules are issued by the Centers for Disease Control and Prevention. The most recent guidelines (1998) emphasize the need for empirical therapy for coexistent chlamydial infections. The addition of doxycycline or azithromycin to ceftriaxone may decrease the development of antimicrobial-resistant *N. gonorrhoeae* because most gonococci in the United States are susceptible to these agents. Azithromycin 1 g orally in a single dose or doxycycline 100 mg orally twice a day for 7 days is the recommended regimen for treatment of uncomplicated genital chlamydial infection in children ≥8 years of age. For children who are <45 kg, erythromycin base in a dose of 50 mg/kg/d divided into four doses for 7 to 10 days should be prescribed. An alternative is azithromycin, 20 mg/kg in a single dose. Children ≥45 kg but <8 years of age may be given a one-time, 1-g dose of azithromycin.

Uncomplicated Gonococci Infections in Adolescents (Vaginal, Cervical, Urethral, Rectal Infections) There are a number of regimens available for treatment of the adolescent with uncomplicated gonococcal infection. Treatment with a cephalosporin is preferable in patients younger than 17 years of age because of the possible effect on immature joints. Cefixime 400 mg orally or ceftriaxone 125 mg intramuscularly in a single dose, or ciprofloxacin 500 mg or ofloxacin 400 mg orally in a single dose can be given. Fluoroquinolone-resistant cases have been reported in the United States; however, these cases comprise less than 1% of all strains evaluated in surveillance, thus fluoroquinolones may still be used.

Uncomplicated Gonococcal Infections in the Pharynx Pharyngeal infections are more difficult to eradicate than genital infections. The recommended regimens for treatment of gonococcal pharyngitis include ceftriaxone 125 mg intramuscularly in a single dose, or ciprofloxacin 500 mg or ofloxacin 400 mg orally in single doses.

Gonococcal Conjunctivitis in Adolescents The recommended treatment is a single 1-g dose of ceftriaxone and one-time lavage of the infected eye with saline solution.

Disseminated Gonococcal Infection in Adolescents The treatment of disseminated gonococcal infection is ceftriaxone 1 g intramuscularly or intravenously every 24 hours. Alternative treatments include cefotaxime or ceftizoxime 1 g intravenously every 8 hours. Ciprofloxacin, ofloxacin, or spectinomycin can be used for those who are allergic to β-lactam drugs.

These regimens should be continued for 24 to 48 hours after improvement is seen and then followed by cefixime 400 mg orally twice daily for a total of 7 days of therapy. If a fluoroquinolone is used, completion of therapy with the oral form of the drug should be continued for 7 days. The recommended therapy for meningitis and endocarditis is ceftriaxone 1 to 2 g intravenously every 12 days for a duration of 10 to 14 days for meningitis and at least 4 weeks for endocarditis.

Ophthalmia Neonatorum The key to treatment is parenteral administration of an effective antimicrobial agent. Because of the high prevalence of penicillin resistance, ceftriaxone 25 to 50 mg/kg intravenously or intramuscularly should be administered in a single dose. Although one dose of ceftriaxone is sufficient therapy for neonatal conjunctivitis, most infants receive antibiotics for 48 to 72 hours until blood and cerebrospinal fluid cultures are found to be negative.

Local treatment includes lavage of the eye with 0.9% NaCl solution and instillation of topical antimicrobial drops (chloramphenicol or tetracycline drops can be used). When iritis is present, a mydriatic drug (1% atropine) should also be used. Topical therapy alone is not sufficient for cure.

Disseminated Gonococcal Infection in Infants Treatment consists of ceftriaxone 25 to 50 mg/kg per day intravenously or intramuscularly in a single daily dose for 7 days (10–14 days if meningitis is documented). Cefotaxime 25 mg/kg intravenously or intramuscularly every 12 hours may be used instead of ceftriaxone. Cefixime has not yet been approved for the treatment of this disease in children or infants.

Treatment for Children Allergic to or Intolerant of Penicillin and Cephalosporins If the child is too young to use one of the fluoroquinolones, then treatment with spectinomycin in a single dose of 40 mg/kg (maximum 2 g) is recommended.

Other Aspects of Therapy Several other aspects of management require consideration. Gonorrhea is often accompanied by other sexually transmitted infections. The CDC recommends that all adults and adolescents treated for gonorrhea also be treated for chlamydial infection. In addition, a serologic test for syphilis is recommended, and HIV testing should be considered. Pregnancy testing in females of child-bearing age is advised. Many states have passed laws allowing minors to be treated for sexually transmitted infections without parental consent, in order to encourage teenagers to seek therapy even though they are unwilling to have their parents know that they are sexually active.

Part of management of gonorrhea is to identify and treat the sexual contacts of the patient; therefore, patients should be instructed to refer sexual partners for evaluation and treatment. There is a high probability that children who acquire gonorrhea have been sexually abused. Such cases should be reported to child protective services for a complete investigation. The laws of all states require such a report and protect the person making the report from liability. Physicians should be aware of and comply with these laws in their own states. Antimicrobial prophylaxis for known exposure is effective and shall be considered in cases of rape or sexual abuse if the perpetrator is not apprehended. A condom should be used for protection from infection with all sexual contacts.

References

Centers for Disease Control and Prevention: Summary of notifiable diseases, United States, 1997. MMWR Morb Mortal Wkly Rep 46(54), 1997

Centers for Disease Control and Prevention: 1998 Guidelines for treatment of sexually transmitted diseases. MMWR Morb Mortal Wkly Rep 47(No. RR-1), 1998

Giedinghagen DH, Hoff GL, Biery RM: Gonorrhea in children: epidemiologic unit analysis. Pediatr Infect Dis J 11(11):973, 1992

Hammerschlag MR, Cummings C, Roblin PM, Williams TH, Delke I: Efficacy of neonatal ocular prophylaxis for the prevention of chlamydial and gonococcal conjunctivitis. N Engl J Med 320:769, 1989

Schwarcz SK, Whittington WL: Sexual assault and sexually transmitted diseases: detection and management in adults and children. Rev Infect Dis 12(Suppl 6):S682, 1990

Neisseria meningitidis
Michele M. Estabrook and Janice J. Kim

The meningococcus is a normal commensal organism of the human upper respiratory tract. Colonization only infrequently leads to disseminated disease, yet the meningococcus remains a significant pathogen worldwide, particularly in children.

Meningococci (*N. meningitidis*) are gram-negative diplococci, often described as biscuit-shaped. They grow well on an enriched medium such as chocolate or Mueller-Hinton agar in a moist environment at 35°C (95°F) to 37°C (98.6°F) and an atmosphere of 5 to 10% carbon dioxide. Meningococci are identified by their ability to ferment glucose and maltose. They also contain cytochrome oxidase, giving rise to the positive "oxidase test."

EPIDEMIOLOGY The meningococci have been divided into serogroups based on antigenic differences in their capsular polysaccharides. Groups A, B, C, W-135, and Y cause most meningococcal disease. Meningococci can be further divided into serotypes and subtypes based on antigenic differences among subcapsular proteins and glycolipids. The serologic characteristics of meningococci have considerable epidemiologic and immunologic importance for studying outbreaks and transmission of disease, and in developing specific meningococcal vaccines.

Since the dramatic reduction of invasive infection due to *Haemophilus influenzae* in association with immunization, *N. meningitidis* ranks second to *Streptococcus pneumoniae* as a leading cause of bacterial meningitis in childhood in the United States. The average annual rate of invasive meningococcal disease varies in multiyear cyclical waves, from 0.5 to 2.0 cases per 100,000 population. Age groups with the highest incidence are children 2 years of age or less and young adults ages 15 to 19 years. The distribution of meningococcal serogroups in the United States has shifted in recent years. Three serogroups, B, C, and Y, each account for approximately 30% of the cases that are reported. The prevalence of me-

ningococcal disease varies seasonally, with the highest attack rate occurring in the winter and early spring.

Meningococcal disease remains a major problem in developing countries, with many areas having an endemic rate of disease of 10 to 25 per 100,000 population. Major periodic epidemics occur, with rates of 100 to 500 per 100,000 population. Group A disease, now rare in the United States, is the leading cause of meningococcal disease worldwide, especially in Asia and sub-Saharan Africa.

Transmission of meningococci from person to person occurs through inhalation of infected droplets. During nonepidemic periods, asymptomatic carriage rates vary from 2 to 30% in a normal population. During epidemics the carriage rate can approach 100% in closed populations.

Serum antibody leading to complement-mediated bacterial killing prevents dissemination of meningococci from the nasopharynx. This antibody is present in the newborn and is probably IgG of maternal origin. As maternal antibody wanes, children from 3 to 24 months of age experience the highest incidence of meningococcal disease. By adulthood, most individuals have developed natural immunity against the meningococcus.

Individuals with congenital deficiencies of the terminal complement components (C5, C6, C7, C8, and C9) as well as deficiencies of properdin have an increased risk of recurrent meningococcal and gonococcal infections. All patients with an initial systemic neisserial infection should be evaluated with a CH50 assay; approximately 20% will have a terminal component deficiency, and in these patients, the risk of subsequent meningococcal infections can be reduced by vaccination.

CLINICAL MANIFESTATIONS The spectrum of meningococcal infection is diverse, ranging from asymptomatic colonization to fulminant sepsis.

Neisseria meningitidis is usually found on the pharynx as a commensal, but has been isolated in association with clinical infections of mucosal surfaces. Patients presenting with meningococcal disease often have overt pharyngitis, and culture-positive household contacts often report recent pharyngitis. Instances of primary purulent meningococcal conjunctivitis have been reported and may lead to invasive disease. *Neisseria meningitidis* has also been isolated occasionally from the genitourinary tract of asymptomatic and symptomatic individuals, especially in homosexual populations, and may be the causal agent in some cases of urethritis, cervicitis, and proctitis.

The spectrum of invasive meningococcal disease also varies, but the most common presentation is meningococcemia with or without meningitis. Initially, symptoms may include fever, pharyngitis, arthralgias, and myalgias, but progress rapidly to meningitis and/or generalized sepsis with a hemorrhagic rash. The dominant features on examination are a toxic-appearing febrile patient with rash and signs of meningeal irritation. Skin lesions can provide an important diagnostic clue but are absent in 20 to 30% of patients with meningococcal meningitis. An evanescent maculopapular rash has been observed in some patients early in the illness. A petechial rash, a classic finding in meningococcemia, occurs in 50 to 60% of patients. These skin lesions, which represent systemic vasculitis, include minute petechiae, coalescent irregular or geographic lesions, large ecchymoses, and palpable purpuric lesions. Bullae may appear in areas of extensive ecchymosis. Erythema nodosum has also been described.

The general approach to diagnosis and treatment of acute bacterial meningitis is discussed in Sec. 13.1.8. In fulminant meningococcal disease, meningitis may be absent. Septic shock and disseminated intravascular coagulation (DIC), often heralded by spreading hemorrhagic rash, may rapidly lead to death (Sec. 13.1.7). Concomitant pneumonia, septic arthritis, purulent pericarditis, and myocarditis have been observed.

Other forms of systemic disease can occur. Unsuspected meningococcal bacteremia has been observed in infants who had blood cultures drawn during evaluation for fever. On examination, a maculopapular rash was sometimes noted, and patients were often sent home on oral antibiotics for minor infections. Meningitis developed in some of these cases. Other systemic meningococcal diseases include primary meningococcal pneumonia, septic arthritis, purulent pericarditis, endophthalmitis, and mesenteric adenitis. Chronic meningococcemia, another infrequent systemic manifestation, is characterized by prolonged fevers, migratory arthritis, and rash. The skin rash resembles the lesions of gonococcemia and often appears quite suddenly during the onset of febrile episodes. Blood cultures are often initially negative. Complications such as meningitis may develop.

DIAGNOSIS Cultures of blood and cerebrospinal fluid (CSF) should be obtained from children in whom invasive meningococcal infection is suspected. Confirmation of the diagnosis requires isolation of *N. meningitidis* from a normally sterile site such as blood, CSF, or joint fluid. Other sites that may yield the organism in the appropriate clinical setting are pericardial or pleural fluid and petechial skin lesions. The diagnosis is presumptively established if gram-negative diplococci are seen in a normally sterile site in the absence of positive cultures. The use of antigen-detection testing in blood or CSF may be of value in diagnostic evaluation. A positive antigen test for *N. meningitidis* from blood or CSF, in the absence of a positive culture, provides a probable diagnosis when the clinical features suggest meningococcal infection. Rapid antigen tests may be unreliable for group B *N. meningitidis*. Antigen-detection methods should not be used to test urine.

Differential diagnosis in children presenting with fever and a petechial rash include enteroviral infections, infectious mononucleosis with rash, atypical measles, rickettsial diseases, streptococcal infection, bacterial endocarditis, disseminated gonococcal infection, and typhoid fever. Chronic meningococcemia may be mistakenly diagnosed as Henoch-Schönlein purpura. Children with *H. influenzae* or pneumococcal infections can present with fulminant sepsis and petechiae or purpura.

TREATMENT Patients suspected of having meningococcemia with or without meningitis require prompt appropriate antimicrobial therapy. Penicillin is the drug of choice. Cefotaxime or ceftriaxone are acceptable alternatives. For patients with a history of anaphylaxis to a penicillin, chloramphenicol is the drug of choice. The minimum duration of therapy has not been established, but intravenous antibiotics for 5 to 7 days are usually sufficient. In underdeveloped countries, alternative therapies, including a single intramuscular dose of chloramphenicol in oil, have been effective. Recently, infections due to penicillin-resistant meningococci were reported in Spain, the United Kingdom, and South Africa. Resistance is chromosomally mediated and caused by a decreased affinity of a penicillin-binding protein. These isolates have remained sensitive to third-generation cephalosporins.

Shock may develop despite initiation of antibiotics. Close monitoring and supportive care to minimize hemodynamic and metabolic alterations are important (Sec. 13.1.7). The use of heparin for DIC and the use of steroids, plasmapheresis, and leukopheresis in fulminant meningococcemia remain controversial.

COMPLICATIONS Despite the availability of adequate antibiotics, mortality remains approximately 10% in the United States. Unfavorable prognostic factors in patients at presentation include absence of meningitis, hypotension, presence of petechiae for less than 12 hours, fever of 40°C (104°F) or higher, leukocyte count $<15,000/\mu L$, and platelet count $<100,000/\mu L$. High levels of circulating endotoxin and tumor necrosis factor are also poor prognostic indicators.

Arthritis, pericarditis, episcleritis, and cutaneous vasculitis may occur 3 to 5 days after initiation of therapy and appear to be immune-complex mediated. Effusions are sterile and usually respond to nonsteroidal anti-inflammatory agents. Some studies suggest a disproportionately high incidence of hearing loss (9–38%) as compared with other bacteria that cause meningitis. However, other neurologic sequelae are less common.

PROPHYLAXIS The risk of meningococcal disease is increased among close contacts (0.3–5.9%). Hence, prophylaxis for household, daycare, and other close contacts is indicated. Rifampin is given 10 mg/kg orally every 12 hours to children 1 month of age or older to a maximum of 600 mg orally every 12 hours for 2 days. In infants less than 1 month of age, each dose is reduced to 5 mg/kg. The use of ceftriaxone, given as a single intramuscular dose of 125 mg for children 12 years of age or younger and 250 mg for children older than 12 years of age and for adults, is an alternative prophylactic regimen. Ceftriaxone's efficacy in eradicating pharyngeal carriage has been documented for group A meningococci; it is unlikely that ceftriaxone's efficacy will vary by serogroup. Penicillin and related drugs do not eliminate nasopharyngeal carriage. Thus, patients with invasive meningococcal disease should receive prophylaxis before discharge from the hospital.

PREVENTION A quadrivalent vaccine composed of capsular polysaccharides of meningococcal groups A, C, Y, and W-135 is currently licensed in the United States. The vaccine is immunogenic in adults and in children 2 years of age and older. No vaccine currently is available for protection against group B disease. Because the risk of disease is relatively low and immunity is not durable, routine immunization of children with meningococcal vaccine is not recommended at this time.

Immunization is recommended for consideration as an adjunct to control outbreaks due to serogroups represented in the quadrivalent vaccine. It is also recommended for children 2 years of age or older who have anatomic or functional asplenia and those with terminal complement component or properdin deficiencies. The vaccine is administered to all US military recruits, and some colleges recommend that entering students receive immunization. It may also be of benefit for travelers to countries that have hyperendemic or epidemic disease, such as the sub-Saharan "meningitis belt" of Africa, Nepal, and Saudi Arabia.

New meningococcal serogroups A and C capsular vaccines composed of polysaccharide-protein conjugates are under development. Researchers are also investigating the use of meningococcal protein and detoxified lipooligosaccharides as potential vaccines that would confer immunity in children and would also protect against group B disease.

References

American Academy of Pediatrics: Meningococcal infections. In: Pickering LK, ed: 2000 Red Book: Report of the Committee on Infectious Diseases, 25th ed. Elk Grove Village, IL, American Academy of Pediatrics, 396–401, 2000

Diaz PS: The epidemiology and control of invasive meningococcal disease. Concise Rev Pediatr Infect Dis 18:633–634, 1999

Figueroa JE, Densen P: Infectious diseases associated with complement deficiencies. Clin Microbiol Rev 4:359–395, 1991

Sáez-Nieto JA, Lujan R, Berrón S, et al: Epidemiology and molecular basis of penicillin-resistant *Neisseria meningitidis* in Spain: a 5-year history (1985–1989). Clin Infect Dis 14:394–402, 1992

Wong VK, Hitchcock W, Mason WH: Meningococcal infections in children: a review of 100 cases. Pediatr Infect Dis 8:224–227, 1989

13.2.24   *Pasteurella multocida*

Morven S. Edwards

Infections caused by *Pasteurella multocida* may exhibit a variety of systemic manifestations, but the primary importance of this organism in pediatrics is its involvement in infections caused by animal bites. *Pasteurella multocida*, alone or as one of several organisms, is the most common cause of infected animal bites.

Pasteurella multocida is a small nonmotile gram-negative rod that grows well on standard media, including blood, chocolate, and Mueller-Hinton agars. Colonies resemble those of enterococci on blood agar plates. If *P. multocida* is suspected, the laboratory personnel should be alerted so that appropriate biochemical testing can be performed to confirm its presence.

EPIDEMIOLOGY   There are several species in the genus *Pasteurella*. The most common human pathogen is *P. multocida,* but human infection may also be a consequence of exposure to the related species *P. canis* or *P. dagmatis*. There are three subspecies of *P. multocida: multocida, septica,* and *gallicida*. More than half of human infections are caused by *P. multocida* subspecies *multocida*. Defining the subspecies aids in epidemiologic investigation, but is not necessary in the usual clinical setting.

The organism is found as a component of the oral flora of 70 to 90% of cats and 25 to 50% of dogs. Other animals that may be kept as pets, including rabbits, rats, or pigs, also may harbor the organism in the respiratory tract or oral secretions. Animals colonized with *P. multocida* are asymptomatic. The usual mode of transmission is direct inoculation from the bite or scratch of an infected animal. *Pasteurella multocida* has been implicated as causal in 50% of canine and 80% of feline bite infections.

The pathogenesis of infection caused by *P. multocida* is dependent upon the portal of entry of the organism. The three major clinical expressions of infection are focal infection of bone or joint soft tissue, pulmonary infection, and disseminated infection. Focal infection is established by direct inoculation of the organism into the subcutaneous tissue, bone, or joint space after a cat scratch or bite or a dog bite. Inoculation is likely to be deeper after a cat than a dog bite, and penetration of the periosteum, or joint space, or a tendon sheath is more often a consequence of cat than of dog bites. The organism produces endotoxin, which may promote the inflammatory reaction that is observed, often within hours after inoculation.

Pulmonary infection occurs as the result of inhalation of *P. multocida*. Animal-to-human but not human-to-human spread has been documented. The organism has low pathogenicity in the respiratory tract, and infection has been documented almost exclusively in the setting of altered host resistance from disease processes such as bronchiectasis or chronic bronchitis.

Disseminated infection occurs when hematogenous dissemination complicates primary soft tissue or pulmonary infection. Bacteremic infection is a particular risk for children with hepatic dysfunction and alteration in efficiency of reticuloendothelial clearance mechanisms.

CLINICAL MANIFESTATIONS   Focal soft-tissue infection, usually manifested as cellulitis, develops rapidly after inoculation of *P. multocida*. The average time of onset of erythema, swelling, and pain is within 24 hours after an animal bite or scratch. Infections due to *P. multocida* characteristically develop drainage that is watery gray or serosanguineous. Infection in the subcutaneous space may result in abscess formation and regional adenopathy. Infection may also present as tenosynovitis, septic arthritis, or osteomyelitis. These manifestations of infection are more likely a consequence of penetrating injury from a cat bite rather than from a dog bite. Joint stiffness with cellulitis of the hand is a finding suggestive of tendon sheath involvement.

When *P. multocida* infection is not related to an animal bite, the most common site of infection is the respiratory tract. The clinical manifestations of infection are those expected for children with exacerbations of chronic underlying conditions, such as bronchiectasis or chronic bronchitis. Several cases of pleural empyema and of lung abscess also have occurred.

Meningitis, with or without bacteremia, is the most common manifestation of disseminated childhood infection caused by *P. multocida*. Most of the children diagnosed as having *Pasteurella* meningitis have been younger than 1 year of age and most have had contact with a pet within the household. Usually these infections develop after animal contact such as licking that does not violate cutaneous barriers. The presenting features include lethargy, irritability, and fever. There are no features at presentation that distinguish *Pasteurella* meningitis from that caused by other bacterial pathogens.

Pasteurella multocida has been isolated on occasion from children with periappendiceal abscess or with peritonitis in association with appendicitis. It is not known whether these infections arise from hematogenous spread or from ingestion of the organism. There are also case reports of unusual manifestations of infection due to *P. multocida* such as tonsillitis, endocarditis, or infection of a ventriculoperitoneal shunt. Brain abscess has resulted from a dog bite that penetrated a small child's skull.

DIAGNOSIS   The organism can be isolated from the drainage of bite wounds and from other sites of focal infection, such as joint fluid or aspirate of the subperiosteum. Pleural fluid or sputum may yield the organism in patients with pulmonary infection. In disseminated infection, *P. multocida* can be isolated from cultures of blood or, with meningeal involvement, from the cerebrospinal fluid. Laboratory differentiation from morphologically similar organisms, such as *Haemophilus influenzae,* is not difficult.

TREATMENT   Penicillin or ampicillin is the drug of choice for *P. multocida* infection. Broad-spectrum oral cephalosporins such as cefixime or ceftibutin may also be effective. Because polymicrobial infection should be assumed as a consequence of an animal bite, empiric therapy consisting of oral amoxicillin-clavulanate or intravenous ampicillin-sulbactam should be initiated in this setting while culture results are pending. Parenterally administered broad-spectrum cephalosporins such as cefotaxime have good in vitro activity against *P. multocida*, but clinical studies to prove their efficacy are lacking.

In children who are allergic to β-lactam agents, the optimal treatment for *P. multocida* infection is problematic. Tetracycline is effective, but tetracyclines should not be administered to children younger than 8 years of age unless the benefits of therapy are considered greater than the risk of dental staining. Among the macrolides, azithromycin exhibits good activity against all strains of *P. multocida*. It is more than active than either erythromycin or clarithromycin, but clinical experience with its use is limited. The recommended oral alternative for empiric treatment of dog or cat bite wounds in penicillin-allergic children is an extended-spectrum cephalosporin or trimethoprim-sulfamethoxazole plus clindamycin. With this regimen, it is the trimethoprim-sulfamethoxazole that is effective against *P. multocida* as well as *S. aureus*. The clindamycin component is active in vitro against anaerobes, as well as against *S. aureus* and streptococci. This same combination of antibiotics may be employed parenterally for wounds of sufficient severity to warrant hospitalization.

The usual duration of therapy is 7 to 10 days for focal soft-tissue infections. Longer duration of therapy for septic arthritis and osteomyelitis may be required. For pulmonary or disseminated infection, including meningitis, 10 to 14 days of therapy is usually required. Débridement of infected animal bite wounds may be necessary to optimize outcome. Infected collections of fluid should be drained. Devitalized tissue should be removed. Consultation with a specialist in hand surgery is appropriate if there is involvement of a tendon sheath of the hand. Preventive treatment for rabies (Sec. 13.4.18) should be instituted only if clinical circumstances warrant.

References

American Academy of Pediatrics: Bite wounds. In: Peter G, ed: 1997 Red Book: Report of the Committee on Infectious Diseases, 24th ed. Elk Grove Village, IL: American Academy of Pediatrics; 1997:122–126

Goldstein EJC, Citron DM, Gerardo SH, Hudspeth M, Merriam CV: Activities of HMR 3004 (RU 64004) and HMR 3647 (RU 66647) compared to those of erythromycin, azithromycin, clarithromycin, roxithromycin, and eight other antimicrobial agents against unusual aerobic and anaerobic human and animal pathogens isolated from skin and soft tissue infections in humans. Antimicrob Agents Chemother 42:1127–1132 1998

13.2.25 Pertussis

Beverly L. Connelly

Despite widespread vaccine acceptance and vaccine coverage that is higher than at anytime in the past, a steady rise in the number of cases of pertussis has been reported to the Centers for Disease Control and Prevention (CDC) in the last decade. Worldwide, the World Health Organization estimates that more than 300,000 children die annually from pertussis in unimmunized populations. Pertussis occurs year-round in the United States, although the disease peaks in the summer and fall in most locations. Humans are the only reservoir for *B. pertussis,* and transmission from person to person occurs via respiratory droplets. Attack rates following household exposure are as high as 90% in susceptible contacts. Communicability is highest early in the disease, but may persist for weeks in some individuals. Immunity following clinical pertussis, as well as pertussis immunization, may not be long-lasting. Unrecognized disease serves as a reservoir for spread of infection.

EPIDEMIOLOGY Morbidity and mortality from pertussis are highest in the young infant. Passively acquired transplacental antibodies afford little protection, and vaccine-induced immunity requires multiple immunizations. Based on CDC surveillance data from the last decade, nearly 70% of infants less than 6 months of age with recognized pertussis require hospitalization and 20% develop secondary pneumonias. Seizures complicate approximately 4% of cases, and encephalopathy develops in less than 1% of cases. Mortality is greatest in infants less than 3 months of age. The frequency of complications decline with increasing age; however, subcutaneous emphysema, pulled muscles, and even broken ribs may occur in adults following paroxysmal coughing.

The prevalence of pertussis in adolescents and adults is increasing because of waning immunity after natural disease or immunization. The characteristic "whoop" is often absent in older individuals. It is not until the nagging, forceful cough has persisted for 2 or more weeks that adolescents and adults come to medical attention. Even then, diagnosis may be delayed or disease may go unrecognized because of a low index of suspicion. Adult caretakers with undiagnosed pertussis are frequently found to be the source for pertussis in infants. Nosocomial spread by health-care workers has been well documented.

Bordetella are small, fastidious, aerobic gram-negative coccobacilli that require enriched media for isolation. *Bordetella pertussis* is a respiratory pathogen of humans only and is the sole cause of epidemic pertussis. *Bordetella parapertussis* is a closely related species that accounts for less than 5% of clinical pertussis. *Bordetella bronchiseptica* occasionally causes disease in the immunocompromised host but is better recognized as a veterinary pathogen. Only *B. pertussis* elaborates pertussis toxin (PT). A variety of other components of *B. pertussis* are biologically active as well as antigenic.

Bordetella pertussis attaches to ciliated epithelial cells of the respiratory tract, induces toxin-mediated ciliary paralysis and local inflammation, and decreases clearance of secretions. *Bordetella pertussis* is not invasive. Disease is mediated through a variety of bacterial components and toxins. PT, formerly designated as lymphocyte-promoting factor, is secreted by the bacteria and induces lymphocytosis by preventing migration of lymphocytes to the area of infection. In addition, PT inhibits the function of neutrophils, macrophages, monocytes, and lymphocytes. Bacterial adenylate cyclase toxin acts on immune cells that contact the bacteria, inducing high levels of cyclic AMP, which, in turn, down-regulate many immune cell functions. Other cell-surface proteins, including filamentous hemagglutinin (FHA), pertactin (PN, a 69-kDa nonfimbrial protein), and fimbrial agglutinogens (FIM2, FIM3), are important in bacterial attachment to ciliated respiratory epithelium. Tracheal cytotoxin selectively destroys ciliated epithelial cells. Surface lipooligosaccharide has endotoxin-like properties, whereas cytoplasmic heat-labile toxin may contribute to local cell damage.

CLINICAL MANIFESTATIONS The incubation period of pertussis is usually 5 to 10 days but may be up to 3 weeks. Clinical pertussis is a protracted illness with three identifiable stages: the catarrhal, the paroxysmal, and the convalescent stages. The catarrhal stage is the most contagious phase and is indistinguishable from a common "cold." During this stage, fever is minimal or absent: rhinorrhea, sneezing, mild cough, and sometimes mild conjunctival suffusion last from a few days to a couple of weeks. In the young infant, signs and symptoms may be minimal or absent in the catarrhal stage.

Apnea, choking, or gasping may herald the paroxysmal stage in young infants. Observation in a setting in which assisted ventilation is available is prudent in the very young infant who presents with these features. Seemingly insignificant stimuli may provoke frightening episodes of coughing in the young infant, which may be sufficiently protracted to result in hypoxia and cyanosis. Forceful coughing can result in subconjunctival and scleral hemorrhages, upper-body petechiae, umbilical and inguinal hernias, subcutaneous emphysema, rib fractures, and even central nervous system (CNS) hemorrhages. The characteristic inspiratory "whoop" of pertussis occurs in toddlers and older children at the end of a paroxysm as air is finally sucked in through a partially closed glottis. Posttussive emesis is common at all ages. Feeding becomes a major problem for the young infant and may actually provoke the paroxysm; the immediate postparoxysmal period may provide a refractory period during which feeding is possible. The severity of the child's paroxysms contrasts sharply with the lack of distress seen between coughing spells. Most of the complications from pertussis occur in the paroxysmal stage, which may last from 1 to 6 weeks. Infectivity decreases during this period, although some patients may still be culture-positive 3 weeks after the onset of cough.

During the convalescent period, coughing in the young infant may actually become louder, although generally less distressing. Overall, the paroxysmal coughing gradually lessens in severity and frequency during convalescence. Paroxysms may disappear, only to reappear in a milder form during a subsequent respiratory illness over the ensuing year.

In addition to the immediate complications already mentioned, infectious and noninfectious complications of pertussis are numerous. Uncomplicated pertussis is usually an afebrile disease, so fever should prompt evaluation for a secondary bacterial infection. Otitis media and pneumonia are the most common secondary infections. Other pulmonary complications include atelectasis, emphysema, and pneumothorax. Coughing and vomiting may result in esophageal tears with hematemesis and melena. Neurologic complications include hypoxic encephalopathy, seizures, and intracranial bleeds. Nutritional compromise and resultant failure to thrive is common in young infants recovering from pertussis. Risk of death in the young infant is between 0.3 and 1.3%.

DIAGNOSIS Classical pertussis should be readily diagnosed based on clinical features. The presence of absolute peripheral lymphocytosis (>10,000 lymphocytes/mm^3) is supportive evidence for systemically active pertussis toxin. Absolute lymphocyte counts of >20,000 cells/mm^3 are not uncommon, and total white blood cell (WBC) counts >100,000 cells/mm^3 have been reported.

The chest x-ray in pertussis is often normal, although shagginess along the cardiac border, peribronchial consolidation, and atelectasis may be seen. The presence of a focal infiltrate in a febrile child with pertussis may indicate a secondary bacterial process.

Classic pertussis in the nonimmune host is difficult to confuse with other illnesses. In the immunized individual, symptoms are less likely to be characteristic. A coughing illness for greater than 2 weeks and/or posttussive emesis should arouse suspicion. In infants presenting with apnea, respiratory syncytial virus infection and serious bacterial illness need to be excluded.

Bordetella pertussis is the cause of epidemic pertussis as well as of most sporadic pertussis. *Bordetella parapertussis* may cause a similar syndrome, but which is less severe and of shorter duration. Protracted coughing illness mimicking pertussis may also be seen

with adenovirus, mycoplasma, and chlamydia. Ancillary features of the illness such as sore throat, headache, or swollen lymph nodes, as well as knowledge of epidemiologically significant local pathogens, will aid diagnostically.

A positive *B. pertussis* culture is the gold standard for the diagnosis of pertussis. Nasopharyngeal specimens should ideally be obtained within the first 2 to 3 weeks of illness. Although the yield is less, cultures beyond 3 weeks are sometimes useful, because culture confirmation may guide public health initiatives.

Because of the fastidious growth requirements for *B. pertussis*, cultures are most accurate in a laboratory experienced in *B. pertussis* isolation. Nasopharyngeal samples should be obtained by inserting a small, flexible Dacron or calcium alginate swab through the nose into the posterior nasopharynx and leaving it there for a few seconds of cough. The best bacteriologic yield is when the swab is plated on selective *Bordetella* media at the bedside. If this is not possible, the swab should be placed in *Bordetella*-specific transport media for delivery to the laboratory. Fresh Bordet-Gengou media, Regan-Lowe charcoal agar, or modified Stainer-Scholte agar and 7 or more days of incubation may be required for isolation of *B. pertussis*. Prior antibiotic therapy will markedly reduce the isolation rate. Asymptomatic carriage of *B. pertussis* is extremely rare. (Health-care workers collecting the specimens should use appropriate masks and eyewear to avoid becoming infected.)

A direct fluorescent antibody (DFA) test on secretions from a nasopharyngeal swab is useful for rapid presumptive diagnosis but requires significant technical expertise. Inexperience in performing this test results in numerous false-positive and false-negative results.

Standardized tests for serologic diagnosis are not widely available. Results of testing for antibody to selected pertussis antigens such as PT or FHA may not correlate with clinical disease and are difficult to interpret in a highly immunized population. While high titers may occur in association with recent disease, culture-proven infection may fail to produce titer rises.

Experience with polymerase chain reaction (PCR) testing on nasopharyngeal swab specimens for pertussis is increasing; however, techniques are not standardized. PCR has proven to be sensitive and specific for the diagnosis of pertussis and is an accepted alternative to culture for case confirmation of *B. pertussis* infection when performed in experienced laboratories. False-positive results from less-experienced laboratories may overestimate the incidence of disease and induce inappropriate consumption of public health resources.

TREATMENT Treatment for clinical pertussis is primarily supportive. Hospitalization is indicated for all infants and children with severe paroxysms associated with cyanosis or apnea. Infants with potentially fatal pertussis may appear amazingly well between paroxysms. Caution should be exercised when suctioning these young exhausted infants because it will precipitate a paroxysm. Admission to an intensive care setting is indicated if emergent response to paroxysms cannot be managed on the ward. Supplemental oxygen, intravenous fluids, and nutritional support are frequently required in severe and protracted disease. Cough suppressants, expectorants, mucolytic agents, bronchial dilators, and sedatives are not beneficial in treating pertussis. Young infants should remain hospitalized until nutrition is adequate, no supportive intervention is required during paroxysms, disease is unchanged or improved for at least 48 hours, and the infant's care can be safely managed at home.

Antibiotic therapy has no discernible effect on the course of the illness once the paroxysms are well established; however, they may ameliorate disease expression for those few who are treated in the catarrhal phase. *All* suspected and confirmed cases of pertussis should be treated in order to minimize secondary spread. The drug of choice is erythromycin at a dose of 40 to 50 mg/kg/d in four divided doses for 14 days (maximum, 250 mg qid); the estolate is preferred by some experts. Stomach upset is the most commonly reported side effect of erythromycin and frequently is a reason for patient noncompliance. For the erythromycin-intolerant patient, alternative regimens include clarithromycin 15 mg/kg/d in two divided doses for 14 days; or azithromycin 10 mg/kg on day one, and 5 mg/kg on days 2 to 5 as single daily doses. While microbiological data suggest the latter regimens should be efficacious, clinical experience is limited, and cost is considerably greater. Alternative agents with limited efficacy include amoxicillin and trimethoprim/sulfamethoxazole. Resistance to erythromycin has been reported but is believed to be limited at this time.

Household and daycare contacts of confirmed pertussis patients should receive antibiotic prophylaxis for 14 days after the last contact. Prophylaxis is indicated regardless of prior immunization status. Erythromycin is the drug of choice at the same dosages used for therapy. Trimethoprim/sulfamethoxazole is generally recommended as an alternative for prophylaxis; however, efficacy as a chemoprophylactic agent has not been evaluated. Likewise, use of the newer macrolides for prophylaxis has not been studied.

PREVENTION *Bordetella pertussis* is highly contagious and has been recovered from the nasopharynx of infected individuals after 5 days of erythromycin therapy has been completed. Therefore, hospitalized patients should be managed in respiratory isolation (droplet precautions) until 5 days after the initiation of erythromycin therapy. A private room is preferred; however, culture-positive cases may be cohorted. Untreated patients should remain in isolation until 3 weeks after the onset of paroxysms. Local health officials should be notified of all cases in order to assist in outbreak control within the community. Immunization for pertussis is discussed in Sec 1.5.2.

References

American Academy of Pediatrics: Pertussis. In: Peter G, ed: 1997 Red Book: Report of the Committee on Infectious Diseases: 24th ed. Elk Grove Village, IL, American Academy of Pediatrics, pp 394–407, 1997

Centers for Disease Control: Erythromycin-resistant *Bordetella pertussis*— Yuma County, Arizona, May–October, 1994. MMWR Morb Mortal Wkly Rep 43:807–810, 1994

Edwards KM: Pertussis in older children and adults. Adv Pediatr Infect Dis 13:49–77, 1997

Muller FM, Hoppe JE, von Konig W: Laboratory diagnosis of pertussis: state of the art in 1997. J Clin Microbiol 35:2435–2443, 1997

Robbins JB, Schneerson R, Bryla DA, et al: Immunity to pertussis: not all virulence factors are protective antigens. Adv Exp Med Biol 452:207–218, 1998

13.2.26 Plague

Gary D. Overturf

Plague exists worldwide as continuing enzootic sylvatic disease in rodent–flea cycles that occasionally spreads into the human population. *Yersinia pestis,* the causative organism, is a nonmotile, gram-negative, nonspore-forming, coccobacillus. Characteristic bipolar staining can be demonstrated with Giemsa staining, but not by Gram stain. The organism grows on all standard bacteriologic media. It resists drying and most other environmental factors except sunlight and thus survives for many days in sputum or in discharges from abscesses. However, the bacterium is rapidly inactivated by all commonly used antiseptics and by boiling water.

EPIDEMIOLOGY The geographic distribution of plague is largely confined to the semiarid areas of most continents, with the exception of Australia. Enzootic North America foci are the largest in the world, occurring primarily in the southwestern United States (extending east as far as Dallas, Texas) and the Pacific coastal region, extending from Coahuila, Mexico, to Alberta and British Columbia, Canada. The disease exists almost entirely in the sylvatic form with rodent–flea cycles among a number of wild rodent species. Urban plague, the cause of the epidemics of the European Middle Ages, is dependent upon the Norwegian rat and flea (*X. cheopis*), but is now quite rare. The last epidemic of urban US plague occurred in 1925 in Los Angeles. Rarely, pneumonic plague is transmissible from person to person, bypassing both the rat reservoir and the flea vector.

In the United States and Canada, the epidemiology is more complex, and involves a number of different rodent hosts and flea vectors, as well as domestic animals. Most commonly, the infection is acquired by human exposure to infected tissues or from the bites of fleas of wild rodents such as prairie dogs, ground squirrels, chipmunks, rabbits, and other wild rodent species. Contact with squirrels accounts for nearly half of the exposures. Domestic animals, especially cats, may become infected after contact with wildlife and may transmit the infection to humans. Prior to 1977, no cat-related cases had occurred, but since that time 18 cases have been reported with 28% of the cases causing direct pneumonic plague. Therefore, direct contact with wild animals or their fleas is not required for plague transmission. With the exception of cats, most other carnivores, including dogs, are relatively resistant to plague and therefore are rarely involved in plague transmission.

CLINICAL MANIFESTATIONS In the United States, most human plague cases occur from May to September and usually present as one of three primary forms: bubonic, septicemic, or pneumonic. Bubonic plague accounts for 78% of US cases, the remainder are septicemic (13.2%), pneumonic (4.4%), or meningitic/unknown (3.4%).

The incubation period of bubonic and septicemic plague is often difficult to determine and varies from 1 to 10 days, but is usually within 2 to 6 days of contact. Skin lesions are infrequently present at the site of initial infection (eg, flea bite). The first symptom usually consists of sudden onset of fever [39°C (102.2°F) or higher], often accompanied by shaking chills. Within hours to a few days, exquisitely tender, painful, often erythematous or hot lymph nodes are present; severe pain may occur prior to swelling. The most frequently involved nodes are the inguinal or femoral nodes, followed by axillary and cervical nodes, but any node may be involved. The nodes enlarge rapidly, forming the characteristic bubo. There may be erythema of the overlying skin. Buboes may vary in diameter from 1 to several centimeters. Patients presenting with septicemic plague fail to develop visible buboes. In recent years, the incidence of septicemic plague has increased, accounting for as much as 25% of cases.

Fever may be accompanied by profound malaise and severe headache, photophobia, abdominal pain, nausea, vomiting, diarrhea, restlessness, delirium, myalgias, and weakness. The fever usually peaks during the first 24 hours and then continues at slightly lower levels for 3 to 4 days, with occasional morning remissions. The temperature may then fall, sometimes achieving nearly normal levels, followed almost immediately by a second steep rise. If no complications or pulmonary disease develop, the fever again gradually declines after the seventh to tenth day of illness, often in association with spontaneous rupture of the buboes and the beginning of resorption. Although uncommon in this disease, convulsions may be attributable either to fever alone or to the presence of concomitant meningitis.

Frequent signs are marked tachycardia, tachypnea, and hypotension. The buboes, if present, increase in size over several days until they become fluctuant and the overlying skin hemorrhagic. With clinical recovery, the lymph node abscess clears slowly, often healing within 2 weeks after onset, although occasionally the process may become chronic with the formation of ulcers and draining fistulas.

Bacteremia occurs regularly during the early phase of the disease in both mild and severe forms. In some instances, the reticuloendothelial system clears the bloodstream of organisms. In other individuals these defenses are overwhelmed and a septic phase develops, during which the patient may succumb to overwhelming endotoxemia. The bacteria may spread through the blood to the respiratory system, producing secondary pneumonia with pulmonary hemorrhages, edema, abscesses, or bronchitis. In addition, other organs, such as the brain and meninges, may become infected. Hemorrhages often occur in the skin, or more massive subcutaneous bleeding may be found. The affected areas have a distinctive red or black discoloration. A disseminated intravascular coagulation syndrome leading to gangrene of the skin, appendages, and various other organs may occur in patients who survive the initial endotoxemia.

A relatively mild form of plague (*pestis minor*) occurs rarely and may remain unrecognized. These patients demonstrate minimal toxicity, a low-grade fever, and simple lymphadenitis, rather than buboes. This clinical picture is the result of infection with a strain of *Y. pestis* lacking one or more of the virulence factors.

Pneumonic plague is usually quickly fatal, whether it is acquired by inhaling infected aerosol (primary pneumonic plague) or is secondary to hematogenous infection from septic illness (secondary pneumonic plague). The incubation period of primary pneumonic disease is very short, often less than 24 hours. The bacteria multiply rapidly within the alveoli, resulting in the absorption of massive amounts of endotoxin. Hemorrhages occur in the lungs, with epithelial desquamation and bleeding into respiratory tissues. Radiologically, the process may resemble a lobar or bronchial pneumonia or a massive pulmonary edema (eg, respiratory distress syndrome). The majority of patients die within a few hours, despite appropriate therapy.

DIAGNOSIS The bubonic form is usually accompanied by significant leukocytosis up to 50,000/mm^3, whereas in the pneumonic and septicemic forms, leukopenia or leukocytosis may be found with varying proportions of young and immature polymorphonuclear leukocytes. In meningitis, the usual spinal fluid changes of bacterial disease are present (Sec. 13.1.8).

The diagnosis is established by detecting typical gram-negative organisms in blood cultures, sputum smears, or aspirates of the affected lymph nodes (buboes). These procedures by themselves do not serve to differentiate plague from tularemia. Culture of the organism is usually successful, but often is carried out only in reference or public health laboratories. A positive fluorescent antibody staining test (often directed against the F1 capsular protein) permits rapid presumptive diagnosis. Serologic tests for antibodies to *Y. pestis* are also available (eg, passive hemagglutination of anti-F1 antibodies), but a rise in antibody may not occur until 2 weeks after the initial onset of symptoms. A four-fold rise or fall or a single titer of 10 or greater is considered diagnostic.

Classic bubonic plague can be recognized readily on clinical grounds, but the signs and symptoms of the septicemic form are similar to those of other gram-negative septicemias. Tularemia, especially when tick-borne, may greatly resemble plague, but the site of the initial bite is usually more evident with tularemia.

TREATMENT Patients with suspected plague should be placed in isolation until 48 hours after starting effective antimicrobial therapy, to prevent the potential spread of infection from possible pulmonary involvement. Therapy should be initiated as soon as the diagnosis is suspected and not await definitive diagnosis. Bodily fluids, secretions, and pus should be handled with gloves. Personnel caring for patients who are coughing should wear face masks and goggles. Careful attention must be paid to waste disposal because feces often contain *Y. pestis*.

Several antimicrobial agents are useful in specific therapy, including tetracycline, streptomycin, gentamicin, chloramphenicol, and trimethoprim-sulfamethoxazole (TMP/SMX). The efficacy of TMP/SMX is probably similar to that of tetracycline, but there is considerable documented clinical experience with tetracycline. In the laboratory, *Y. pestis* is susceptible to third-generation cephalosporins such as cefotaxime, but these drugs have only rarely been used clinically. Strains resistant to streptomycin antibiotic occur in Southeast Asia, but these strains are susceptible to gentamicin. A single strain of multiple antibiotic resistance occurred in Africa, but resistance to antibiotics has been rare among plague isolates.

Gentamicin is as effective as streptomycin and is probably the most appropriate drug to use. It is uncertain whether an aminoglycoside or tetracycline, or a combination of the two, is preferable.

Aminoglycosides should be given cautiously, in a dosage of 30 mg/kg per day in three equal doses for streptomycin, or 5 to 6 mg/kg per day for gentamicin. The patient must be carefully monitored for signs of impending shock. After 5 days, tetracycline is substituted at an oral dosage of 25 to 30 mg/kg per day, divided into four equal doses for at least an additional 5 days. When used as primary therapy for severe bubonic plague, the dosage of tetracycline is 40 to 50 mg/kg per day (in four equal doses) after a loading dose of 30 mg/kg; alternatively doxycycline can be used in dosage of 4 mg/kg (day 1) and 2 mg/kg thereafter up to a maximum dose of 100 mg twice daily. After the first 24 to 48 hours of therapy, the dosage of tetracycline can be reduced to the lower dose. Treatment is generally continued for 1 week after body temperature returns to normal, or for a total of approximately 10 days. Chloramphenicol, a less desirable choice than tetracycline, is given at a dosage of 25 to 50 mg/kg per day in four divided doses (maximum of 2 g/dose). Chloramphenicol is preferred only in the treatment of known or suspected plague meningitis or when treatment with tetracycline or aminoglycosides is contraindicated or unavailable. TMP/SMX has been used in oral doses of 8 to 12 mg/kg of the trimethoprim component and can be given either orally or intravenously. Nonspecific therapy is the same as that employed for patients with other forms of gram-negative sepsis and consists primarily of the treatment of shock, seizures, respiratory problems, and high fevers.

With present management, the mortality rate of plague is 14% in the United States. Bubonic plague has a mortality of 3 to 5%; the mortality with septicemic forms may exceed 50%, and pneumonic disease is almost universally fatal. Worldwide, untreated bubonic plague is fatal 40 to 60% of the time. Complications not previously mentioned include a reactive arthritis, lung abscesses, and persisting lymphadenitis.

PREVENTION If pneumonic manifestations of the disease are noted, contacts of the patient should be quarantined and treated prophylactically with tetracycline, although no controlled data on the efficacy of this approach are available. It seems likely that TMP/SMX is also effective, but no confirmatory evidence exists. Preventive measures against the sporadic form of plague that occurs in the United States are not feasible because *Y. pestis* is so widespread. However, in those areas of the world where the disease is transmitted by the rodent–flea–human cycle, continuous flea control accompanied by rodent controls are indicated.

An inactivated whole-cell vaccine is recommended only for those persons whose occupation regularly places them at high risk. Duration of immunity following three intramuscular doses given over 6 months is probably brief, and the safety of the vaccine has only been tested in those 18 years of age or older.

References

Centers for Disease Control: Plague—United States 1991. JAMA 268: 3055, 1992

Centers for Disease Control: Summary of notifiable diseases–1996. MMWR Morb Mortal Wkly Rep 45 (no. 53), 1997

Hull HF, Montes JM, Mann JM: Septicemic plague in New Mexico. J Infect Dis 155:113–118, 1987

Perry RD, Fetherston JD: *Yersinia pestis*—etiologic agent of plague. Clin Microbiol Rev 10:35–66, 1997

13.2.27   Pneumococcal Infections

Patricia J. Chesney

The pneumococcus (*Streptococcus pneumoniae*), a normal inhabitant of the upper respiratory tract of many infants and children, is a major cause of morbidity and mortality in persons of all ages. Most susceptible are children ≤2 years of age, as well as those children with certain congenital immunodeficiencies, splenectomized children, children with sickle-cell anemia, and children infected with human immunodeficiency virus (HIV). Following the drastic reduction in the number of cases of invasive disease caused by *Haemophilus influenzae* type b (Hib) after the introduction of a highly efficacious Hib protein-conjugate vaccine, *S. pneumoniae* became the leading bacterial cause of invasive diseases such as bacteremia, meningitis, and sepsis in the United States. *Streptococcus pneumoniae* is also the leading cause of acute otitis media. Since 1993, antimicrobial resistance of *S. pneumoniae* isolates has increased dramatically. A polysaccharide protein-conjugate vaccine, licensed in early 2000, should help reduce the incidence of invasive pneumococcal disease in infants and children.

Like many gram-positive organisms, pneumococci have a cytoplasmic membrane with >500 attached surface proteins and an adjacent cell wall. The cell wall is 6 to 7 layers thick and is constructed of a single macromolecule composed of a peptidoglycan lattice supporting linear covalently attached teichoic acid and lipoteichoic acid molecules (attached to lipids in the cytoplasmic cell membrane), which project in regular sequence to the external environment. The cell is surrounded by one of 90 distinct, genetically encoded, poly-

saccharide capsules; 18 of these capsular serotypes account for most disease. Addition of type-specific anticapsular antibody to organisms results in swelling of the capsule, which can be identified microscopically as a refractile halo (quellung reaction) and can be used to serotype strains for epidemiologic purposes. Proteins and glycoproteins associated with growth and virulence are found in the cytoplasm, on the cell membrane, in the cell wall, and projecting from the cell wall.

EPIDEMIOLOGY Following respiratory droplet spread, *S. pneumoniae* adheres to epithelial cells in the nasopharynx. More than 95% of infants are colonized in the first 2 years of life, with 6 months being the mean age of first acquisition. The duration of carriage in infants is 3 weeks to 4 months, whereas duration in adults is 2 weeks. A majority of infants become colonized with at least two serotypes on different occasions and may carry up to four serotypes at a time. In 15% of infants, acquisition of a new serotype is associated with disease caused by that serotype occurring within 1 month of acquisition. The capsular serotypes that most often colonize infants <2 years of age are serotypes 6, 14, 19, and 23. These same serotypes account for most disease in infants. Worldwide, these serotypes account for >80% of penicillin-resistant strains in all ages.

Carriage rates are lower in older children (40–50%) and in adults (5–30%). Adults with children have higher carriage rates (25%) than do adults without children (5%). Colonization rates are increased in the winter, in out-of-home childcare attendees, and in infants of parents who smoke. Carriage rates are decreased in individuals receiving antibiotic prophylaxis or therapy, and following immunization with protein-polysaccharide conjugate vaccines. Colonization with antibiotic-resistant strains most often follows a course of antibiotics or close contact with an out-of-home childcare attendee who is colonized with a resistant serotype. In older children (>5 years) and adults, protective, serotype-specific antibody against capsular polysaccharide develops in association with colonization.

Circulating IgG antibody to the capsular serotype of the infecting strain, the third component of complement, and an intact, functioning spleen are the three most important immune factors determining the outcome of infection. Pneumococci are readily phagocytosed by neutrophils and macrophages when the organism has been opsonized by the binding of serotype-specific anticapsular IgG and the third component of complement. In nonimmune hosts, nonspecific ("natural") antibodies serve a similar function. The spleen serves as the primary site of clearance in the nonimmune host.

In infants less than 2 years of age, T-lymphocyte-independent antigens, such as pneumococcal polysaccharides, do not elicit a protective immune response; this age-dependent immunodeficiency can be corrected by conjugating polysaccharides to immunogenic proteins such as diphtheria or tetanus toxoids, as demonstrated by the success of the *Haemophilus influenzae* type b-conjugate vaccines in infants.

Serotype-specific anticapsular antibodies protect against mucosal colonization and subsequent invasion. In nonimmune hosts, pneumococci attached to epithelial cells are carried to the nonmucosal surface of the cell, where they may enter the lymphatics or bloodstream. Infections caused by *S. pneumoniae* thus result from local spread to the ear or sinus, or to distant organs following entry into the bloodstream.

Children bear the burden of both noninvasive pneumococcal disease (acute otitis media and sinusitis) and invasive pneumococcal disease (IPD), the latter defined as a positive culture from a normally sterile body site. Children ≤2 years of age accounted for >30% of cases of IPD with an incidence of 145/100,000 live births, even though they represented only 2.9% of the population surveyed (Fig. 13-7). The incidence of IPD for infants ≤30 days of age was 0.04/100,000 live births/year, which illustrates the protective influence of maternal antibody.

Ethnic heritage also influences the incidence of IPD: risk is increased approximately 14-fold for White Mountain Apache populations, four-fold for Alaskan natives, and 2.5-fold for African-Americans, as compared to white children.

An important risk factor for IPD in children ages 2 to 11 months is an underlying illness of the central nervous system, heart, or kidneys. Additional conditions significant as risk factors are leukemia, HIV infection, a hemoglobinopathy, an out-of-home childcare attendance in the previous 3 months, a recent antibiotic use, and a lack of breast-feeding.

Overall, it is estimated that pneumococcal infections of all types and in all age groups result in 40,000 deaths per year in the United States. The total number of cases per year include otitis media—7 million; pneumonia—500,000; bacteremia without a focus—50,000; and meningitis—3000.

For the pediatric age groups, occult bacteremia without a focus (OBWF) accounts for 58% of all pneumococcal IPD. The incidence of pneumonia with bacteremia is increased three-fold in children ≤2 years of age, as is the incidence of meningitis (Fig. 13-7). Only adults ≥65 years of age have a higher risk of death due to pneumococcal infection.

Since the initial clinical reports of penicillin-resistant strains from Australia in 1967 and from South Africa in 1977, the prevalence of penicillin- and multidrug-resistant strains has increased dramatically. Although rates of resistance may vary from one hospital or childcare center to another, even in the same city, many US cities find that 25 to 45% of pneumococcal isolates are resistant to penicillin.

Penicillin and all β-lactam drugs act on *S. pneumoniae* by inhibiting the activity of transpeptidase enzymes (also called penicillin-binding proteins), which build the peptidoglycan lattice or scaffolding of the cell wall. As a result of antibiotic overuse, many streptococcal species colonizing the nasopharynx of adults and children have become resistant. Through the process of transformation, *S. pneumoniae* in the nasopharynx acquire DNA that encodes mutated penicillin-binding proteins from other resistant streptococcal species. These changes modify the ability of the β-lactams to bind to the organism, thus creating β-lactam–resistant organisms.

For reasons not yet understood, *S. pneumoniae* organisms that are highly resistant to penicillin are usually also resistant to many other antibiotics. Resistance to these other antibiotics is mediated by transposons and does not involve penicillin-binding proteins. Infections caused by these multidrug-resistant (MDR) organisms are particularly difficult to treat.

CLINICAL MANIFESTATIONS In children, the most common infection caused by *S. pneumoniae* is acute otitis media (AOM), and *S. pneumoniae,* the most common bacterial cause of AOM, is estimated to be responsible for more than 7 million ear infections annually in the United States. Rarely, mastoiditis complicates AOM. Paranasal sinusitis and pneumonia may also be caused by local spread of *S. pneumoniae*. Outside of the upper respiratory tract, the three most common infections caused by *S. pneumoniae* are occult bacteremia without focus (OBWF), pneumonia, and meningitis.

Occult Bacteremia without a Focus OBWF occurs in febrile children of ages 3 to 36 months and is present in 3% of those children with a temperature >39°C (102.2°F). *Streptococcus pneumoniae* causes 87% of episodes of OBWF. Management of febrile infants and children is discussed in Sec. 13.1.5.

Pneumonia Although pneumonia in children is most often caused by a virus, *S. pneumoniae* is the most common cause of community-acquired bacterial pneumonia. Of all children with pneumonia, only 1 to 3% have positive blood cultures. Characteristics of pneumonia in children bacteremic with *S. pneumoniae* include a mean age of 3.6 years, a predominance of males, fever >39°C (102.2°F), respiratory or gastrointestinal symptoms, ill appearance, alveolar infiltrates on x-ray (50% lobar consolidation), white blood cells >15

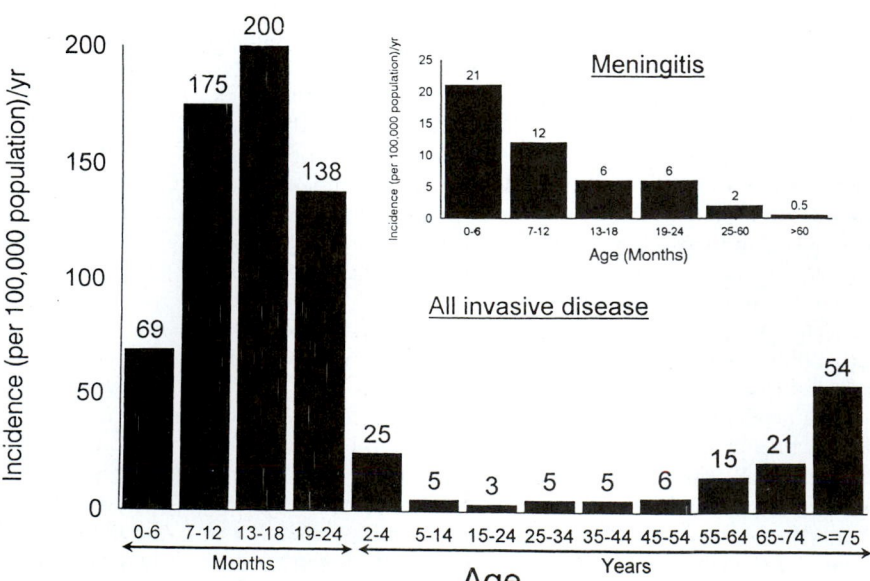

FIGURE 13-7 **Age-specific incidence of invasive pneumococcal disease, including meningitis, in southern California, April 1, 1992 to March 31, 1993. SOURCE:** *Kaiser Permanente data reprinted from the Journal of Infectious Diseases 174:752–759, 1996, with permission.*

$\times 10^3$, neutrophils >70%, CRP>60, and a history of an underlying illness. Most patients become afebrile within 24 hours of starting antibiotics. Complications are uncommon, but include necrotizing pneumonia and empyema.

Meningitis After the neonatal period, *S. pneumoniae* is the most common cause of bacterial meningitis and has the highest rate of complications. The mortality rate is 7%, and 25 to 35% of children have significant neurologic sequelae, including unilateral or bilateral hearing loss. Diagnosis and management of meningitis are discussed in Sec. 13.1.8.

Fulminant Pneumococcemia Fulminant pneumococcal infections are rare and almost always indicate an immunocompromised host. Such individuals should be carefully evaluated for asplenia, hemoglobinopathies, and deficiencies of immunoglobulins or complement proteins.

Other Invasive Diseases *Streptococcus pneumoniae* is considerably less common as an agent of cellulitis and septic arthritis than are *Staphylococcus aureus* or group A streptococci. Spontaneous pneumococcal peritonitis, which originates as an ascending infection from the vaginal tract of prepubertal females, is a puzzling, but infrequent, clinical entity. Hemolytic-uremic syndrome is another serious but rare complication of IPD.

DIAGNOSIS AND TREATMENT In the microbiology laboratory, growth of *S. pneumoniae* requires complex media containing choline, 12 amino acids, and six vitamins. Growth is enhanced in 5% CO_2 under anaerobic conditions. On Gram stain, this lancet-shaped gram-positive organism appears as single cocci, diplococci, or short chains. Rapid diagnostic tests, which can reliably and with good sensitivity detect organisms in the blood, CSF, or urine before in vitro growth occurs, are not yet available. Several polymerase chain reactions (PCR) using different antigens are being developed and appear promising.

Across the United States, the incidence of penicillin-resistant *S. pneumoniae* (PRSP) in different areas varies from 5 to 60%. Resistance is defined as intermediate (MIC = 0.1–1 μg/mL) or high level (MIC $\geq$ 2 μg/mL). Nationwide, in 1998, 25% of strains were resistant and half of those were of high-level resistance. Multidrug resistance of the highly resistant strains includes resistance to cefotaxime, erythromycin (and other macrolides), trimethoprim-sulfamethoxazole, chloramphenicol, tetracycline, and increasingly, to clindamycin and the fluoroquinolones. Vancomycin is the only drug to which no strains have yet become resistant.

Because the complications of meningitis are so serious, all patients with suspected bacterial meningitis should be treated with vancomycin at 60 mg/kg/d and cefotaxime at 200 to 300 mg/kg/d until susceptibilities of the organism are available. Ceftriaxone at 100 mg/kg/d is an acceptable substitute for cefotaxime. After susceptibilities are available, antibiotic modifications can be made as recommended in published guidelines. For susceptible organisms, aqueous penicillin G, 250,000 U/kg/d divided every 4 hours, is an appropriate regimen. Therapy is usually continued for 10 days but may extend for longer periods.

Vancomycin and complex antibiotic combinations have *not* yet been necessary to treat all other IPD in nonimmunocompromised hosts. Plasma levels of recommended agents, including the β-lactam antibiotics, are well in excess of the MICs of even the highly resistant strains isolated thus far. No clear therapeutic failures have

yet been reported for nonmeningeal invasive infections when recommended doses of systemic β-lactam agents were used in patients with normal host defenses.

Less experience is available for patients with fulminant and potentially life-threatening invasive infections, particularly in immunocompromised hosts. In these patients, the addition of vancomycin to the usual regimen for an invasive, nonmeningeal infection may be justified, providing the vancomycin is discontinued after susceptibilities reveal that therapy with β-lactam agents should be successful.

Despite the emergence of penicillin-resistant pneumococci, amoxicillin remains the drug of choice for otitis media caused by *S. pneumoniae,* as discussed in Sec. 15.1.9.

PREVENTION Penicillin prophylaxis is effective and has been recommended in the past to prevent overwhelming, fulminant pneumococcal infections in children <5 years of age with sickle-cell disease and in individuals of all ages for 1 year following a splenectomy. Infants with sickle-cell disease appear to respond well to the conjugate vaccine; therefore, future studies will be needed to determine whether chemoprophylaxis can be discontinued in vaccinated children.

Because splenectomized adults immunized with the 23-valent vaccine can still develop infection with a vaccine strain, antibiotic prophylaxis should be continued in this group. For anatomically or functionally splenectomized patients of all ages and at any time following splenectomy, those who develop fever and other non-specific signs of infection should seek medical care immediately, even if the patient has been immunized and is taking antibiotic prophylaxis. If medical care cannot be immediately accessed, patients should take a high dose of an appropriate antibiotic such as Augmentin.

A new protein-polysaccharide conjugate pneumococcal vaccine was approved for use in children in February 2000. Its use is described in Sec. 1.5.2.

References

American Academy of Pediatrics Committee on Infectious Diseases: Therapy for children with invasive pneumococcal infections. Pediatrics 99: 289–299, 1997

American Academy of Pediatrics Committee on Infectious Diseases: Recommendations for the prevention of pneumococcal infections including the use of pneumococcal conjugate vaccines and antibiotic prophylaxis. Pediatrics 106:367–376, 2000

Ghattar F, Friedland IR, McCracken GH: Dynamics of nasopharyngeal colonization by *Streptococcus pneumoniae.* Pediatr Infect Dis J 18:638–646, 1999

Kaplan SL, Mason EO, Barson WJ, et al: Three-year multicenter surveillance of systemic pneumococcal infections in children. Pediatrics 102: 538-545, 1998

Levine OS, Farley M, Harrison LH, et al: Risk factors for pneumococcal disease in children. Pediatrics 103:e28, 1999

Silverstein M, Bachur R, Harper MB: Clinical implications of penicillin and ceftriaxone resistance among children with pneumococcal bacteremia. Pediatr Infect Dis J 18:35–41, 1999

Tan TQ, Mason EO, Barson WJ, et al: Clinical characteristics and outcome of children with pneumonia attributable to penicillin-susceptible and penicillin nonsusceptible *Streptococcus pneumoniae.* Pediatrics 102: 1369–1375, 1998

Tuomanen EI, Masure AR: Molecular and cellular biology of pneumococcal infection. Microb Drug Resist 3:297–308, 1997

13.2.28   Rat-Bite Fever

Lorry G. Rubin

Rat-bite fever is an acute febrile illness that occurs after the bite of a rodent, usually a rat. Two distinct microorganisms, *Streptobacillus moniliformis* and *Spirillum minus,* cause this infection. *Streptobacillus moniliformis,* the main etiologic agent of rat-bite fever, is a fastidious, gram-negative, pleomorphic, and often filamentous and beaded, facultative anaerobic bacillus.

EPIDEMIOLOGY   In addition to rat-bite fever, *S. moniliformis* causes an overlapping syndrome, Haverhill fever, also known as erythema arthriticum epidemicum.

Sodoku, a disease reported in Asia that is currently rare in the United States, is the name given to rat-bite fever caused by *S. minus.* After an incubation period of 1 to 3 weeks, there is fever, inflammation (often accompanied by ulceration at the previously healed bite site), and regional lymphadenopathy. The fever may be intermittent and associated with rash, with afebrile intervening days. The infection responds rapidly to therapy with penicillin. *Spirillum minus* is a spirillum-like organism that cannot be grown in vitro and is identified by darkfield microscopic examination of material from an ulcer or blood smear.

Streptobacillus moniliformis is a normal inhabitant of the upper respiratory tract of rodents and may be excreted in rat urine. Humans are infected by the bite of a rat (or mouse, squirrel, cat, or weasel) or, less commonly, from a scratch from a rat; from handling a dead animal; or from contact with rat-eating carnivores. Approximately 50% of cases reported are in children. Infection may also be acquired by ingestion of milk or water contaminated with rat excreta, as occurred in epidemic form in 1916 in Haverhill, Massachusetts.

CLINICAL MANIFESTATIONS   Seven to 10 days (range 3–21 days) after a rat bite, there is an abrupt onset of fever accompanied by chills, headache, vomiting, muscle pain, and, often, asymmetric polyarthritis. Several days later there is a maculopapular and sometimes petechial rash, which is most prominent on the extremities, including the palms and soles. The bite wound has usually healed and the site exhibits no or minimal inflammation. Generalized adenopathy commonly occurs. Young children often have diarrhea and weight loss. Many of the clinical features are similar to Rocky Mountain spotted fever. Untreated, the infection follows a relapsing course lasting a mean of 3 weeks, but may have a fatal outcome or result in arthritis persistent for several months. Other reported manifestations include amnionitis, brain abscess, disseminated fatal infection in infants, endocarditis, hepatitis, meningitis, myocarditis, nephritis, and pneumonia. Patients with Haverhill fever exhibit fever, rash, and arthritis; vomiting and pharyngitis are more prominent than in patients with rat-bite fever.

DIAGNOSIS AND TREATMENT   The diagnosis is established by recovering *S. moniliformis* from cultures of blood or joint fluid, but the organism is fastidious and slow growing. Broth enriched with blood, serum, or ascitic fluid, or blood or chocolate agar incubated in a CO_2-supplemented environment should be used. Twenty-five percent of infected patients have a false-positive nontreponemal serologic test for syphilis.

Penicillin given for 10 to 14 days is the treatment of choice for rat-bite fever. The organism is susceptible to many antibiotics in addition to penicillin, including ampicillin, cefuroxime, cefotaxime, and tetracycline. Isolates are resistant to sulfonamides. For therapy of endocarditis, the addition of streptomycin to high-dose penicillin should be considered.

Because the attack rate of rat-bite fever after a rat bite is approximately 10%, individuals sustaining rat bites should be observed closely. Penicillin prophylaxis should be considered, although its efficacy is unknown.

Reference

McEvoy MB, Noah ND, Pilsworth R: Outbreak of fever caused by *Streptococcus moniliformis.* Lancet 2:1361–1363, 1987.

13.2.29   Relapsing Fever

Dennis L. Murray

Relapsing fever is a vector-borne, remittent febrile illness caused by several species of spirochetes of the genus *Borrelia,* including *B. recurrentis* and *B. hermsii,* and transmitted by lice and ticks. Louse-borne relapsing fever is caused by *B. recurrentis.* The body louse, *Pediculus humanus,* becomes infected by ingesting blood from infected humans, and the disease is transmitted when the louse is crushed and the spirochetes penetrate human skin of a new host. Epidemic *Borrelia* infection has disappeared from the United States, along with louse-borne typhus. The disease does occur in other areas of the world, particularly Africa, where epidemics occur especially among the homeless and refugee populations.

Endemic relapsing fever is transmitted by ticks of the genus *Ornithodoros.* These soft-bodied ticks are distributed worldwide and have painless bites. Most tick-borne relapsing fever in the United States occurs in the western states and is caused by *B. hermsii.* In contrast to louse-borne relapsing fever, humans are incidental hosts for the *Borrelia* causing tick-borne disease. Exposure to rodent-infested cabins or caves is important to human infection with *Borrelia* associated with tick-borne disease.

CLINICAL MANIFESTATIONS   After a variable incubation period (4–18 days, mean of 7 days), the illness starts abruptly with fever, chills, headache, myalgia, and arthralgia. Conjunctivitis, petechiae, and hepatosplenomegaly may be present. Some patients develop jaundice. This first phase of illness typically lasts 3 to 6 days and subsides spontaneously. During the next several days (5–7 days, typically), the infected patient experiences extreme fatigue and may have a diffuse maculopapular rash, but the patient is afebrile or has only a low-grade fever.

Return of fever and chills signals the relapsing phase of the disease. Several such relapses can occur, although the duration of relapses typically becomes shorter and milder over time. Relapsing fever most often resolves even among untreated patients, but increased mortality is seen during some epidemics. With appropriate therapy, case fatality rates are less than 5%.

Vertical transmission of infection can occur, resulting in abortion or severe infection of the neonate.

DIAGNOSIS AND TREATMENT   The disease is easy to diagnose during epidemic outbreaks. Relapsing fever may also be suspected, along with typhus, when body lice (*not* head lice or crab lice) are prevalent, particularly under crowded and unsanitary conditions. With the endemic form, the disease should be suspected in patients with appropriate symptoms who have had exposure to environments where *Ornithodoros* ticks are located. A definitive diagnosis is made by demonstrating the *Borrelia* on a blood smear. Spirochetes can be observed by darkfield microscopy and in Wright-, Giemsa-, or acridine orange–stained preparations of either thick or thin blood smears. Culture is an insensitive method for confirming the diagnosis, but spirochetes can be recovered from blood by using Barbour-Stoenner-Kelly (BSK) medium or by intraperitoneal inoculation of immature laboratory mice. Serologic tests are not well standardized and cross-reactions occur with other spirochetes, including the infectious agent of Lyme disease, *B. burgdorferi*.

Treatment with penicillin, tetracyclines, erythromycin, or chloramphenicol is effective. Erythromycin is considered the drug of choice for children younger than 8 years of age. Penicillin is an effective drug for the initial illness, but relapses are more common when penicillin is used. The sudden killing of many spirochetes and the release of bacterial products may produce a life-threatening Jarisch-Herxheimer reaction. For that reason the patient needs very careful monitoring and may need significant management, especially for low blood pressure, in the first 6 to 8 hours after the initial antimicrobial dose. For the febrile patient, it is safer to give as a *first* antimicrobial *low-dose* oral penicillin (7.5 mg/kg of phenoxymethyl penicillin in a single dose) or intravenous aqueous penicillin G (10,000 U/kg by infusion over 30 minutes). Following this first dose, gradual clearing of spirochetes and defervescence should occur. The patient should then receive either erythromycin or tetracycline for 7 to 10 days to prevent relapse. For afebrile patients between relapses, erythromycin or tetracycline alone can be given.

References

Barbour AG: Antigenic variations of relapsing fever *Borrelia* species. Ann Rev Microbiol 44:151–171, 1990

Spach DH, Liles WC, Campbell GL: Tick-borne diseases in the US. N Engl J Med 329:936–947, 1993

Warrell DA, Perine PL, Krause DW, et al: Pathophysiology and immunology of the Jarisch-Herxheimer reaction in louse-borne relapsing fever. Comparison of tetracycline and slow-release penicillin. J Infect Dis 147:898–909, 1983

13.2.30   *Salmonella, Shigella,* and *Escherichia coli* Infections

Andrew T. Pavia

The family Enterobacteriaceae is a large, heterogeneous group of gram-negative bacteria. Many are normal inhabitants of the GI tract of humans and other animals, but members also frequently cause disease in human beings.

Among the Enterobacteriaceae, *Salmonella, Shigella, Yersinia,* and a number of specific phenotypes of *Escherichia coli* are important causes of gastroenteritis. In addition to diarrhea, these organisms cause a variety of extraintestinal infections. Each genera includes a heterogenous group of organisms that vary in their epidemiology and clinical characteristics. Enterobacteriaceae possess three major antigenic groups that react with antisera: (a) the O or somatic antigens; (b) the H or flagellar antigens; and (c) the K or capsular antigens. Serotyping has historically been an important means of subtyping these enteric pathogens; this technique is being partially superseded by our increasing ability to identify genotypic and phenotypic markers of virulence. This chapter discusses *Sal*

monella, Shigella, and the diarrhea-causing *E. coli; Yersinia* is discussed in Sec. 13.2.37.

Salmonella

Salmonella are gram-negative, aerobic, nonlactose-fermenting, nonsporulating, flagellated bacilli. Most *Salmonella* organisms have a single, strongly agglutinating somatic antigen (the major determinant), plus one or more less-strongly reacting minor somatic antigens. Serotyping is performed by State Health Department laboratories after initial isolation of the organism. It is an extraordinarily useful tool for epidemiologic purposes. The nomenclature of *Salmonella* has been simplified recently. A serotype is now designated *S. enterica* serotype *typhimurium* or *S. enterica enteritidis,* often simplified to *S. enteritidis.* Because several serotypes represent the majority of isolates, additional epidemiologic subtyping can be useful. Plasmid profile analysis, bacteriophage typing, restriction endonuclease analysis, ribotyping, pulsed-field gel electrophoresis, and antimicrobial susceptibility have all been used as epidemiologic tools.

Identification of *Salmonella* from normally sterile sites such as blood, cerebrospinal fluid (CSF), and joint fluid does not require special media. However, selective media are necessary to identify *Salmonella* in stool, because of the vast number of other bacteria. Media range from low to high selectivity: MacConkey, deoxycholate agar, and eosin-methylene blue (EMB) agar are low-selectivity media; *Salmonella-Shigella* (SS), Hektoen enteric (HE), and xylose-lysine-deoxycholate-citrate (XLD) agar are widely used media of medium selectivity; and bismuth sulfite agar is highly selective. Stool specimens that are placed in enrichment broth prior to plating on agar media will have an increase in the yield of organisms.

EPIDEMIOLOGY   Reptiles, birds, poultry, cattle, and pigs serve as the major reservoirs for nontyphoidal *Salmonella.* In contrast, human beings are the only reservoir for *S. typhi.* The primary animal reservoir varies by serotype, and can serve as a clue to the source of contamination. For example, *S. hadar* and *S. heidelberg* are primarily associated with chickens; *S. enteritidis* with eggs; *S. choleraesuis* with pigs; and *S. marinum* and *S. urbana* with reptiles.

In the United States the highest incidence of nontyphoid *Salmonella* infection is in the first year of life, peaking in the second month at 180 cases/100,000 population per year. Thereafter, rates of isolation decline rapidly by age 5 years and remain constant throughout adulthood. *Salmonella* infections show a seasonal pattern, with a consistent peak in the summer and fall. *Salmonella typhi* infection in the United States is uncommon (approximately 400 patients per year) and rarely occurs in children less than 1 year of age. However, typhoid fever remains an important problem in many developing countries. In the United States, two-thirds of *S. typhi* infections are related to foreign travel.

Salmonella infections are acquired through ingesting the organism, most often from food, but waterborne, person-to-person and animal-to-person transmission can occur. The majority of cases are sporadic; recognized outbreaks account for a minority of cases, but provide insight into the epidemiology. Explosive or prolonged common source outbreaks have occurred as a consequence of contaminated milk, cheese, shell eggs, ice cream, and roast beef.

Since the mid-1980s, low-level contamination of the yolks of intact shell eggs with *S. enteritidis* has been an increasing problem. Recently, iguanas and other pet reptiles have emerged as an important source of infection for young children.

Sentinel county surveillance demonstrates that *Salmonella* are becoming increasingly resistant to ampicillin, chloramphenicol, streptomycin, tetracycline, kanamycin, and gentamicin. Some of these agents are rarely used in human disease, but are routinely added to animal feed as growth promoters. Substantial evidence points to antibiotic use in animal husbandry as a major source of antibiotic resistance in human isolates.

The dose necessary to cause clinical infection is estimated to be 10^5 to 10^{10} organisms, based on volunteer studies in adults. However, the number of organisms necessary to cause illness is substantially lower in other situations, including more virulent organisms, low gastric acidity, prior use of antibiotics, infants, the elderly, and defective cell-mediated immunity. Because of the relatively large number of organisms necessary to produce disease, water and person-to-person spread are less frequent sources of infection than food, which can support multiplication of the organism. Contaminated water may play a larger role in typhoid fever. Spread of *Salmonella* in childcare centers is unusual.

Following infection, nontyphoid *Salmonella* are excreted in feces for a median of 5 weeks. Excretion is more prolonged in children less than 5 years of age and for people who have had symptomatic infections. In children younger than 5 years of age, 2.6% continue to excrete nontyphoid *Salmonella* beyond 1 year, compared to fewer than 1% of patients over 5 years and older. The rate of carriage after infection is higher still in very young infants. Two to 4% of adults infected with *S. typhi* become chronic carriers, often excreting the organism for the remainder of their lives. Long-standing infection of the gall bladder plays a role in chronic carriage. Despite the large number of chronic excretors of nontyphoid *Salmonella,* carriers are rarely implicated in outbreaks or sporadic disease. In contrast, chronic carriers play a pivotal role in typhoid fever. The source of *Salmonella* is less-well understood in salmonellosis among infants. Chronic or transient asymptomatic carriage by the mother and cross-contamination during food preparation are probably important. Nursery outbreaks of salmonellosis occur. Spread of disease has been documented by contaminated medical devices such as rectal thermometers, suction equipment, and baths, but the hands of caregivers may play an important role.

PATHOGENESIS The incubation period for gastroenteritis is 6 to 72 hours (mean 36 hours); for enteric fever it is 7 to 21 days (usually 7–14 days). The incubation period is affected by the inoculum size.

There are several distinctive steps in *Salmonella* infection. Upon reaching the small intestine, the bacteria must attach to the epithelium. Chromosomally encoded long, polar fimbriae; thin, aggregative fimbriae; and plasmid-encoded fimbriae are important in this process. Deletion mutations in these genes decrease virulence after oral inoculation but not after intraperitoneal infection. *Salmonella* invade M cells (mucosal antigen-presenting immune cells) and non-phagocytic epithelial cells. Within macrophages, they may not only survive but multiply. The ability of strains to survive and reproduce in macrophages is correlated with virulence in animal models. The organism directs its own endocytosis through a complex mechanism encoded in a "pathogenicity island," a large collection of contiguous virulence genes. Interestingly, a key component of invasion is a type 3 secretion system, which is similar to systems mediating the invasiveness of *Yersinia* and enteropathic and enterohemorrhagic *E. coli*. A second pathogenicity island has been identified in some serotypes. Diarrhea is probably induced by local inflammation, induction of inflammatory mediators, and in some strains, by one or more enterotoxins or cytotoxins. When examined histolog-

ically, the organism is prominent in Peyer's patches. In some cases of nontyphoid salmonellosis, and in all cases of typhoid, the organisms reach the regional lymphatics. Bacteremia may result.

There are several important barriers to infection. The organism must survive gastric acid, which can rapidly kill *Salmonella*. Reduced gastric acidity as a result of extremes of age, medications, surgery, or *H. pylori* infection, and foods that buffer gastric acid, increases the number of organisms that reach the small intestine. Normal intestinal flora are an important barrier. Prior treatment with antibiotics, particularly those that disrupt the predominant intestinal flora, increases the risk of infection with both antibiotic-resistant and antibiotic-sensitive strains. This has been demonstrated experimentally and in outbreak investigations. The third and most complex barrier is the host immune system. Cell-mediated immunity appears to be the primary immunologic defense against *Salmonella* infections. Susceptibility appears to be highest in the first few months of life, reflecting the developing immune system. Children with HIV infection, transplant recipients and others on immunosuppressive agents, and children with advanced malignancies are at increased risk. Reticuloendothelial dysfunction is also associated with increased risk of *Salmonella* infection, including sickle cell disease, hemolytic anemias, and malaria. The available evidence suggests that humoral immunity is less important.

Bacteremia and mesenteric adenitis are the rule with *S. typhi,* and much less common with other nontyphoid *Salmonella*. However, the rate of bacteremia and extraintestinal infection varies by serotype, reflecting distinct but incompletely understood differences in virulence.

CLINICAL MANIFESTATIONS The range of clinical manifestations of *Salmonella* infection includes asymptomatic infection, gastroenteritis, bacteremia, focal infection, urinary tract infection, and enteric fever. These symptom complexes may overlap.

Gastroenteritis Diarrhea is the most common manifestation of salmonellosis. The diarrhea may be profuse and watery, reflecting predominant small-bowel involvement, or may involve smaller volume stools associated with mucous and fecal leukocytes, reflecting colonic involvement. Bloody diarrhea occurs in approximately 25% of cases. Fever, when present, tends to be highest within the initial day of onset. Headache, chills, anorexia, nausea, vomiting, and malaise may be present. Symptoms usually last 2 to 5 days, although diarrhea may be prolonged.

The most common complication of *Salmonella* gastroenteritis is dehydration and metabolic acidosis, occasionally progressing to hypovolemic shock. Infected children also may have concurrent bacteremia, may develop prolonged secretory diarrhea, or may manifest failure to thrive after acute infection.

Bacteremia Bacteremia may occur during acute *Salmonella* gastroenteritis. Factors that increase the risk include age, underlying systemic illness, hemoglobinopathy, immunosuppression, and serotype of the infecting organism.

In children with uncomplicated gastroenteritis, "silent" bacteremia occurs in 5 to 10%. The risk of bacteremia is markedly increased in infants less than 3 months of age, most likely because of the immaturity of their cell-mediated immune response. Other conditions associated with increased risk of bacteremia include malnutrition; hemolytic anemias, especially sickle-cell anemia; collagen vascular disease; schistosomiasis; bartonellosis; hematogenous or gastrointestinal tract malignancy; diabetes mellitus; previous therapy with antimicrobial agents; corticosteroids; and HIV infection.

Salmonella bacteremia is common among adults and children with AIDS. Frequently, *Salmonella* bacteremia in AIDS patients presents with fever and a paucity of gastrointestinal symptoms. The illness is often prolonged, and relapses after therapy are common. After relapse, lifetime secondary prophylaxis may be necessary.

Patients with *Salmonella* bacteremia during acute gastroenteritis cannot be readily recognized by clinical examination. Although fever usually is present and the patient appears acutely toxic, these signs may be indistinguishable from those of acute gastroenteritis without bacteremia.

Focal Infection Focal suppurative infections occur in about 10% of patients with bacteremia. *Salmonella* bacteremia can result in suppurative complication of almost any organ or tissue. Infection can result in pneumonia; empyema; pyelonephritis; abscesses of brain, liver, spleen, muscle, or other soft tissue; or endovascular infection. Endocarditis most often involves abnormal or prosthetic valves, but infection of normal valves can occur. Endovascular infections can also involve arteriovenous fistulas, preexisting aneurysms (classically atherosclerotic aneurysms), or endarteritis. *Salmonella choleraesuis* has a propensity for causing endovascular infections. Osteomyelitis caused by *Salmonella* tends to occur in injured or infarcted bone. This probably explains the predisposition of children with hemoglobinopathies, especially sickle-cell disease, to develop this complication. Meningitis is rare, occurring most often in neonates or young infants and in AIDS patients. Mortality is high, even since the advent of third-generation cephalosporins.

Enteric Fever The prototypic enteric fever is typhoid fever caused by *S. typhi*, although clinically indistinguishable enteric fever has been reported with infections by *S. paratyphi* A, *S. schottmuelleri*, *S. hirschfeldii*, and *S. choleraesuis* and less commonly by other serotypes. The enteric fever caused by nontyphoid *Salmonella* is called paratyphoid fever, and generally has less morbidity than typhoid, in that the duration of fever is briefer, patients do not appear to be as ill, and complications and relapses occur less frequently.

An average of 245 *S. typhi* isolates are reported yearly to the CDC. Three quarters of patients report international travel within the 30 days before onset of illness. The onset of enteric fever is insidious in contrast to bacteremia due to other gram-negative bacteria. The number of bacteria ingested influence attack rate and the length of the incubation period. The initial signs of infection are malaise, anorexia, headache, myalgias, and fever. The fever begins insidiously, is hectic, and gradually rises over the initial week to as high as 40°C (104°F). A relative bradycardia disproportionate to the temperature elevation is characteristic. Although diarrhea may be present during the initial stages, constipation becomes a more prominent symptom as the illness progresses. Hepatomegaly and splenomegaly, often with diffuse abdominal tenderness, are common. The abdomen may be mildly tender; but marked distension, dilated loops, or significant tenderness may indicate ileus. Leukopenia is not uncommon.

Rose spots occur in a small proportion of patients toward the second week. They are discrete (2–4 mm), palpable, erythematous lesions on the trunk. Biopsy of a rose spot reveals nests of mononuclear cells and usually yields *S. typhi*. However, rose spots are often sparse, transient, and difficult to spot on dark-skinned children. The natural course of illness is persistence of fever for 2 to 3 weeks, with slow recovery. Signs and symptoms of a chronic inflammatory process are often apparent by this time.

Complications are common. Most fatalities are the result of intestinal hemorrhage or perforation, resulting from necrosis of infected Peyer's patches. The overall mortality is 3 to 6% with treatment. Predictors of mortality include intestinal perforation, seizures, septic shock, pneumonia, delirium, and coma. Late focal infections, such as meningitis, endocarditis, osteomyelitis, and pneumonia, are rare. Relapse, a recurrence of the manifestations of typhoid fever after initial clinical response, occurred in 8 to 12% of patients who did not receive antimicrobial therapy, but may be higher in the antibiotic era. Of patients with typhoid fever, 2 to 5% become chronic carriers. The risk of becoming a chronic carrier increases with increasing age and with the presence of gall bladder disease.

Children younger than 2 years of age often have mild illness, often resembling a mild, nonspecific febrile illness. Classic typhoid fever can occur in this age group, although it is the exception.

DIAGNOSIS *Salmonella* should always be considered in a child with gastroenteritis. More severe disease; fever; headache; evidence of dysentery; immune deficiency; recent immigration from endemic areas; exposure to reptiles; undercooked meat or eggs; or an ongoing common source outbreak should increase suspicion.

The diagnosis is made by stool culture. If fresh stool cannot be obtained, a rectal swab can be cultured. The yield is higher from fresh stool, and the use of enrichment broths in the microbiology lab also improves sensitivity. Blood cultures are negative in the majority of children with *Salmonella* gastroenteritis, and agglutination tests are of no value in diagnosis. Gastroenteritis with fever, especially in a child under 2 years old, is usually an indication for obtaining a blood culture. CSF cultures should be obtained when the diagnosis is suspected in infants less than 3 months of age, even in the absence of elevated temperature, because of the increased risk in this age group.

For suspected enteric fever, serial blood cultures should be obtained. Because the concentration of organisms is low, the yield is increased by culturing larger volumes of blood and up to three specimens. In untreated patients with typhoid fever, three blood cultures during the first week have approximately a 90% yield. The yield decreases over time with a concomitant increase in positive stool cultures. Bone-marrow culture is the most sensitive procedure for recovery of *S. typhi*. Culture of bile obtained by a swallowed capsule (string test) is also sensitive, but not as sensitive as the combination of blood and bone marrow cultures.

The Widal test is problematic. It measures the titer of agglutinating serum antibodies against the O and H antigens of *S. typhi*. In untreated disease, only one-half to two-thirds of patients have a four-fold or greater increase in titer of agglutinins against typhoid O antigen. Antimicrobial therapy interferes with immunologic response. Moreover, the Widal test is not specific. In endemic areas, antibody may represent past infection, and there is cross-reactivity with antibody from nontyphoid *Salmonella* infections. In the future, PCR may increase the sensitivity and turnaround time for detection of bacteremia. Stool antigen assays are potentially attractive, but have yet to prove useful.

TREATMENT The type of illness caused by *Salmonella* directs the selection and duration of antimicrobial therapy. Uncomplicated *Salmonella* gastroenteritis requires no antimicrobial therapy; antibiotics do not shorten the clinical illness, as demonstrated in carefully conducted trials. In addition, antimicrobials may select for resistant strains and prolong *Salmonella* carriage. Antimicrobial therapy should be given to patients with enteric fever, bacteremia from nontyphoid strains, and disseminated infection with localized suppuration. Antimicrobial therapy also should be considered in infants younger than 3 to 6 months, and in patients with enterocolitis who have HIV disease or other underlying conditions that impair host resistance.

Ampicillin, chloramphenicol, and trimethoprim-sulfasoxazole (TMP-SMX) have in vitro activity and historically have been successful in treating patients with nontyphoid *Salmonella* infections (Table 13-41). Resistance to these agents has increased in recent years. A highly drug-resistant clone, *Salmonella typhimurium* DT (definitive type) 104, has spread explosively in the United States and Europe. Therefore, all isolates should be tested for susceptibility. Cefotaxime is useful for ampicillin-resistant strains and is the drug of choice for *Salmonella* meningitis. Therapy for uncomplicated bacteremia is usually given for 10 to 14 days; at least 7 days of therapy should be intravenous. Meningitis should be treated for at least 3 weeks. Fluoroquinolones have been very effective in the treatment of adults. Because fluoroquinolones are not approved for use in patients less than 17 years of age, they should be considered only as alternative agents when ampicillin, third-generation cephalosporins, and TMP-SMX cannot be used.

Ampicillin, amoxicillin, and TMP-SMX are effective therapy for typhoid fever caused by susceptible *Salmonella*. Although therapy with chloramphenicol is associated with a more rapid sterilization of blood, the rate of recurrence is somewhat higher. Multidrug-resistant *S. typhi* is a rapidly emerging problem worldwide. Ampicillin, chloramphenicol, and TMP-SMX may no longer be reasonable choices for empiric therapy, before susceptibility tests are available. Antimicrobial agents that have been used successfully in the treatment of resistant *Salmonella typhi* strains are cefotaxime, ceftriaxone, cefixime, aztreonam, ofloxacin, and ciprofloxacin. These might be predicted to work for bacteremia with resistant nontyphoid *Salmonella* as well. Short courses of oral cefixime demonstrate acceptable success rates, but the time to clinical improvement is slower than with ceftriaxone or fluoroquinolones.

Survival of patients with delirium, stupor, or coma associated with typhoid fever is improved by brief, high-dose corticosteroid therapy administered concurrently with antibiotics. Dexamethasone has been used at an initial dose of 3 mg/kg followed by eight doses of 1 mg/kg every 6 hours. Aggressive surgical intervention, together with broad-spectrum antibiotics (including anti-*Salmonella* therapy), has improved survival in typhoid fever complicated by intestinal perforation with peritonitis.

The chronic asymptomatic carriage of *S. typhi* can be extremely difficult to eradicate, especially if there is obstructive hepatobiliary disease such as gallstones. Success has been achieved with a combination of 6 weeks of ampicillin or amoxicillin with probenecid in patients who have normally functioning gallbladders without evidence of cholelithiasis. In adults, ciprofloxacin has been reasonably successful in eradicating the organism in chronic carriers. Cholecystectomy is recommended for carriers who have relapsed after therapy or who cannot tolerate antimicrobial therapy. Patients who excrete nontyphoid *Salmonella* usually do not need antimicrobial therapy. One trial of 14 days of ciprofloxacin showed disappointing results in house officers and nurses with prolonged shedding of *S. enteritidis* after a hospital outbreak.

The mortality of *Salmonella* infections ranges from 0.5 to 1.4%. Most deaths are associated with bacteremia, sepsis, or meningitis. Malnutrition, extremes of age, and underlying disease strongly influence mortality. The fatality rate for typhoid fever is less than 2% for industrialized nations, but approaches 35% for developing countries. Coma, shock, or abdominal perforation are predictors of mortality.

PREVENTION Improvements in sanitation, waste disposal, and safe drinking water led to a dramatic decrease in *Salmonella typhi* infections, but has had little impact on the control of nontyphoid *Salmonella*. Prevention of nontyphoid *Salmonella* involves many fronts. The amount of *Salmonella*, particularly antimicrobial-resistant *Salmonella*, reaching the consumer depends on practices in agriculture.

Three vaccines against typhoid fever are available for civilian use in the United States: a parenteral heat-phenol-inactivated vaccine; an orally administered, live-attenuated oral vaccine prepared from

TABLE 13-41

ANTIMICROBIAL THERAPY FOR PATIENTS WITH *SALMONELLA* INFECTIONS

SYNDROME	INFANTS	CHILDREN	HEALTHY ADOLESCENTS AND ADULTS	IMMUNOCOMPROMISED ADULTS
Gastroenteritis	Ampicillin* 200 mg/kg/d IV div q6h *or* Ceftriaxone 100 mg/kg/d IV qd *or* TMP-SMX 10 mg/kg/d IV or PO div q12h *or* Cefotaxime 200 mg/kg/d div q6h	Not indicated.	Not indicated.	Ampicillin* 1 g IV q4h *or* Ceftriaxone 2 g IV qd *or* TMP-SMX 160 mg IV or PO q12h *or* Ciprofloxacin 500 mg IV or PO q12h
Extraintestinal infection	Ampicillin* *or* Ceftriaxone *or* Cefotaxime	Ampicillin* *or* Ceftriaxone *or* Cefotaxime	Ampicillin* *or* Ceftriaxone *or* Cefotaxime	Ampicillin* *or* Ceftriaxone *or* Cefotaxime *or* Ciprofloxacin
Typhoid fever	Ceftriaxone 100 mg/kg/d for 10–14 days *or* Cefotaxime 200 mg/kg/d for 10–14 days	Ceftriaxone 100 mg/kg/d for 10–14 days *or* Cefotaxime 200 mg/kg/d for 10–14 days *or* Cefixime 8 mg/kg/d PO for 5 days	Ciprofloxacin 750 mg PO bid for 10–14 days *or* Ceftriaxone 2 g IV qd for 10–14 days *or* Cefixime 400 mg PO qd for 5 days	Ciprofloxacin 750 mg PO bid for 10–14 days *or* Ceftriaxone 2 g IV qd for 10–14 days

*Resistance is increasing worldwide. Use only for susceptible strains. TMP-SMX = trimethoprim-sulfasoxazole.

the Ty21a strain of *S. typhi;* and an injectable vaccine made from purified Vi polysaccharide. The vaccines are of roughly equal efficacy, although a published meta-analysis concluded that the efficacy of the heat-phenol-inactivated vaccine was slightly higher. However, the oral vaccine and the Vi polysaccharide cause significantly fewer side effects and are preferred. The oral Ty21a vaccine is licensed for children 6 years and older, although it is immunogenic in children 2 years and older. It requires four oral doses and must be repeated every 5 years. The Vi polysaccharide vaccine is licensed for children older than 2 years. It requires a single injection, but must be repeated every 2 years. Vaccination against typhoid fever is recommended for persons with intimate contact with a known carrier, for microbiologists, and for travelers staying in endemic areas for prolonged periods or if safe food and water cannot be assured.

Shigella

Shigella are divided into four groups and over 40 serotypes based upon serologic and biochemical reactions: *S. dysenteriae* (group A), *S. flexneri* (group B), *S. boydii* (group C), and *S. sonnei* (group D). Groups A, B, and C contain multiple serotypes, but there is only a single serotype of *S. sonnei*. *Shigella* are gram-negative, nonlactose-fermenting aerobic, nonmotile bacilli, closely related to *E. coli*. They do not survive well in the environment, and delays in plating stool specimens may significantly reduce the recovery rate. Selective media must be used to identify *Shigella* in stool to suppress routine flora and to make *Shigella* distinguishable from other Enterobacteriaceae. Several media are available, including MacConkey's bile salt, xylose-lysine-deoxycholate (XLD), and Hektoen enteric (HE). *Salmonella-Shigella* agar is also used, but it tends to be inhibitory for *Shigella* and should not be used alone. The use of two or more media improves the recovery rate, as does broth enrichment. Even optimal handling of stool specimens may not result in isolation of the organism.

EPIDEMIOLOGY   The epidemiology of shigellosis differs between developed and less-developed countries. *Shigella sonnei* is the most frequently isolated serotype in the United States and Western Europe, accounting for 60 to 80% of *Shigella* infections; *S. flexneri* is second in frequency. *Shigella dysenteriae* serotype 1 (the Shiga bacillus) is rare in developed countries, but a major problem in Sub-Saharan Africa and the Indian subcontinent.

High attack rates occur among children in childcare centers, persons in nursing homes, residents of facilities for the mentally ill, and persons living on Native American reservations. The highest attack rate for shigellosis is in children 1 to 4 years old. Breast-feeding is clearly protective. In recent years, the proportion of cases among adults has increased. Attack rates among children in developing countries are dramatically higher. *Shigella* infections show a distinct seasonal peak during July through October, but infections occur year-round.

Shigella infection is acquired through fecal oral exposure. Unlike *Salmonella* infections, however, person-to-person transmission plays a key role. In volunteer studies, as few as 10 to 100 organisms can cause disease.

Human beings are the primary reservoir of *Shigella;* higher primates can become infected, but do not play a significant role in the epidemiology. Crowding, poor sanitation, inadequate supplies of water for washing, lack of soap, and the presence of diapered children are risk factors for the spread of *Shigella*. Outbreaks of shigellosis in childcare centers are common. The spread in childcare centers plays a central role in sustaining endemic shigellosis in communities. Outbreaks have also occurred as a consequence of swimming in contaminated lakes and pools. There have been many food-borne outbreaks from an ever-expanding list of vehicles; fresh fruits and vegetables have assumed a prominent role in recent years. In developing countries, waterborne spread and close contact fuel ongoing transmission.

The role of asymptomatic carriers in the epidemiology of shigellosis is not completely understood. In one study, 17% of children excreted *Shigella* for at least 1 month after the acute illness, and 11% excreted *Shigella* for at least 2 months. In highly exposed populations, asymptomatic carriage and/or prolonged excretion may be more common.

PATHOGENESIS   The cardinal features of the pathogenesis of shigellosis are its ability to invade cells and to incite an inflammatory response. In the colon, *Shigella* bind to M cells and translocate across them. The bacteria invade macrophages within Peyer's patches and induce apoptosis with subsequent release of IL-1, migration of polymorphonuclear cells, and intense inflammatory response. *Shigella* then invade enterocytes, lyse the cytoplasmic vacuoles, and move to the cytoplasm, where they divide. The pathologic changes that accompany this include superficial ulcerations of the mucosa, hemorrhages, edema, and friability. Involvement is typically worse in the rectosigmoid and distal colon.

Shigella dysenteriae type 1 also encodes genes for Shiga toxin, a potent inhibitor of protein synthesis. Shiga toxin is responsible for the increased virulence of this organism and its association with the hemolytic uremic syndrome. Closely related toxins are produced by enterohemorrhagic *E. coli*, including *E. coli* O157:H7, which also cause hemolytic uremic syndrome. Other species of *Shigella* produce little or no Shiga toxin. There is evidence that at least some *S. sonnei* strains produce enterotoxins.

CLINICAL MANIFESTATIONS   The clinical manifestations of shigellosis vary in severity. The incubation period can be as short as 12 hours or as long as 5 days, but most often is 24 to 48 hours. Most illness begins with fever, malaise, anorexia, and occasionally vomiting or headache. Diarrhea usually begins as watery diarrhea, and may progress within hours or days to dysentery. Typical symptoms of dysentery include frequent small volume stools containing mucous and blood associated with lower abdominal cramps and tenesmus. However, the diarrhea may remain watery and copious. Asymptomatic infection also occurs.

Physical findings include fever, systemic toxicity, increased bowel sounds, and lower abdominal tenderness. The child may have signs of dehydration. Rectal prolapse may occur in 5 to 8% of patients. In general, *S. sonnei* causes milder illness with fewer complications, *S. flexneri* tends to be more severe, and *S. dysenteriae* tends to cause the most severe dysentery and extraintestinal complications. The white blood cell count is usually elevated. Leukemoid reactions with as many as 50,000 cells/μL occasionally occur in patients with *Shigella* infection.

Shigellosis is less common in neonates and young infants than in children older than 1 year, but infants and neonates are more likely to be severely dehydrated or hypothermic, are twice as likely to die, and are less likely to have classic findings such as high fever, bloody diarrhea, abdominal tenderness, and rectal prolapse. Thus, a high index of suspicion and a low threshold for obtaining stool cultures are appropriate for young infants with diarrhea.

A variety of complications of shigellosis occur. Dehydration, hypoglycemia, hyponatremia, hypernatremia, and hypokalemia can

TABLE 13-42

ANTIMICROBIAL THERAPY FOR PATIENTS WITH SHIGELLOSIS

AGENT	CHILDREN'S DAILY DOSE	MAXIMUM DOSE (USE FOR ADOLESCENTS)	COMMENTS
Ampicillin	100 mg/kg/day div q6h	500 mg qid	Resistance is very common; use only if susceptible strain
Trimethoprim-sulfamethoxazole	10 mg/kg/day (trimethoprim) div bid	160 mg bid (1 DS tablet)	Resistance is increasingly common, even in the United States
Nalidixic acid	55 mg/kg/day div q6h	1 g qid	Not licensed in the United States for this indication, but the empiric drug of choice in many regions
Cefixime	8 mg/kg/day div q12h	400 mg/d	Not licensed in the United States for this indication; poor efficacy in adults
Ceftriaxone	50 mg/day IV or IM as single dose × 3 days	1–2 g IV or IM qd	Not licensed in the United States for this indication
Ciprofloxacin	Not generally recommended	500 mg bid for 5 days	Resistance rare to date
Other fluoroquinolones	Not generally recommended	Varies	Efficacy and resistance similar to ciprofloxacin

occur; hypoglycemia and hyponatremia are associated with an increased mortality rate. Seizures are a common extraintestinal manifestation. Isolated seizures are usually not associated with any long-term neurologic sequelae. Ekiri, a severe toxic encephalopathy initially described in Japan, manifests as severe dysentery, sensory disturbances, convulsions, and rapid progression to death.

Bacteremia is uncommon in healthy children but is more common with HIV infection and severe malnutrition. Bacteremia may be associated with septicemia and disseminated intravascular coagulation. In about half of bacteremic children, there may be polymicrobial bacteremia caused by other organisms that have traversed the injured gut. Extraintestinal suppurative complications such as osteomyelitis, meningitis, septic arthritis, and splenic abscess are rare. The hemolytic uremic syndrome is an important complication of *S. dysenteriae* type 1 infection, reported in 1 to 4% of children; it is seen occasionally with *S. flexneri*. Reactive arthritis or Reiter syndrome (arthritis, urethritis, iritis in conjunction with HLA-B27) are unusual postinfectious complications of *Shigella*, usually in adolescents or adults.

DIAGNOSIS *Shigella* should be suspected in children with fever and diarrhea, particularly if there are seizures, or in those children with small-volume diarrhea with abdominal cramping, blood, or mucus in the stool. Many patients with *S. sonnei*, however, do not have bloody diarrhea. The differential diagnosis of bloody diarrhea is discussed in Sec 17.7.4.

The diagnosis hinges on the recovery of *Shigella* from a fresh stool specimen or a rectal swab. Recovery is easier early in the course of the disease. *Shigella* may not survive transportation. If rectal swabs are used, they should be placed in appropriate transport media, such as Cary-Blair media. Specimens should be processed immediately by the clinical microbiology laboratory. Even with optimal handling, false-negative cultures will occur. In volunteer studies, cultures were negative in 20% of volunteers.

Presumptive identification of *Shigella* requires at least 48 hours; definitive identification may require 72 hours. Polymerase chain reaction has been used to detect *Shigella* in stool and appears to be very sensitive, but it is not commercially available. In developed countries, the frequency of *Shigella* and *E. coli* O157:H7 infection in children with bloody diarrhea is similar. Making the distinction is critical, because shigellosis responds to antimicrobial therapy but *E. coli* O157:H7 infections do not, and some evidence suggests

that antimicrobials increase the risk of hemolytic uremic syndrome. Fortunately, new enzyme-based immunoassays for Shiga toxin allow the diagnosis of *E. coli* O157:H7 and other enterohemorrhagic *E. coli* in about 24 hours.

TREATMENT Fluid and electrolyte therapy are key components of management. Although shigellosis is a self-limited disease for most patients, antibiotic treatment during acute dysentery will reduce the duration of fever and diarrhea. Table 13-42 lists antimicrobial therapy for patients with shigellosis. Treatment of milder disease or later in the course has only modest clinical benefit but leads to more rapid cessation of shedding, usually within 1 to 2 days. This reduces the likelihood of secondary spread, and is particularly important in settings such as childcare centers and institutions. This public health benefit must be weighed against the public health risk of enhanced selection of antimicrobial-resistant disease from treating mild disease with antibiotics.

Antibiotic-resistant *Shigella* have emerged rapidly throughout the world. Strains of *S. dysenteriae* type 1 resistant to virtually all antibiotics except fluoroquinolones have spread widely in sub-Saharan Africa, the Indian subcontinent, and Latin America. Unfortunately, strains resistant to fluoroquinolones are now being reported. For other serotypes and in other regions, the situation is not as bleak but remains complex. Local resistance patterns and travel history must be taken into consideration. Ampicillin was once the drug of choice for *Shigella*, but resistance is now close to universal. Trimethoprim-sulfamethoxazole (TMP-SMX) is effective for sensitive strains. However, resistance is extremely common in Southeast and South Asia, and Latin America. In the United States, resistance to TMP-SMX has increased rapidly in many areas, and it no longer can be considered a reliable drug for empiric therapy.

Resistant strains of *S. sonnei* and *S. flexneri* are often susceptible to fluoroquinolones, nalidixic acid, ceftriaxone, cefixime, and azithromycin. Nalidixic acid is inexpensive and effective in children. A clinical trial of cefixime in children in Israel suggested good efficacy, but in a trial among adults in Bangladesh, it was not effective. Azithromycin was effective in a single trial, but the widespread use of this drug may lead to more resistance. For severe shigellosis, IV or IM ceftriaxone is effective. Although fluoroquinolones are not approved for use in children because of lingering concerns over arthropathy, two clinical trials in children with severe shigellosis suggested that ciprofloxacin or norfloxacin are safe and effective.

TABLE 13-43

CHARACTERISTICS OF *Escherichia coli* GROUPS ASSOCIATED WITH DIARRHEA

TYPE	PATHOGENESIS	EPIDEMIOLOGY
Enteropathogenic (EPEC)	Attaching and effacing lesions	Acute and chronic diarrhea in infants
Enterotoxigenic (ETEC)	Enterotoxins (LT and ST) induce accumulation of cAMP and cGMP	Watery diarrhea in infants in developing countries and in travelers
Enteroinvasive (EIEC)	Direct invasion plus exotoxins, similar to *Shigella*	Diarrhea with fever in all ages
Enterohemorrhagic (EHEC)	Attaching and effacing lesions; Shiga toxin	Hemorrhagic colitis in all ages; hemolytic uremic syndrome, generally in children
Enteroaggregative (EaggEC)	Not fully defined; enterotoxin and cytotoxin identified	Persistent diarrhea in children in developing countries and in travelers

Nalidixic acid, ceftriaxone, azithromycin, and cefixime are not FDA-approved for treatment of patients with shigellosis.

Antidiarrheal agents that reduce gastrointestinal tract motility should not be used in infants and children with diarrhea. Their use in children with shigellosis is associated with toxic megacolon and with hemolytic uremic syndrome in patients with *E. coli* O157:H7.

Shigellosis usually resolves completely in 7 to 10 days if untreated. A postdiarrheal enteropathy may occur, particularly following *S. dysenteriae* infection. Growth delay and exacerbation of malnutrition may follow shigellosis, particularly in children with preexisting malnutrition. The mortality rate depends on the setting and on the health of the child. In developed countries the mortality is less than 1%. In developing countries, the mortality can range from 10 to 30%. Risk factors for death include infection with *S. dysenteriae* type 1, malnutrition, very young age, and bacteremia.

PREVENTION Simple measures of hygiene can greatly reduce the incidence of *Shigella* infections in resource-poor settings. These measures include the provision of appropriate sanitation, safe drinking water, and soap and water for hand washing. Control of flies reduces disease. Provision of narrow-mouthed water containers that cannot be contaminated by dirty hands is a cost-effective prevention tool. Breast-feeding is a practical strategy to prevent disease in infants. These measures may be most effective for *S. dysenteriae* and *S. flexneri*, which may require a higher infectious dose.

Prevention of shigellosis in developed countries depends on control of person-to-person transmission and identification of food-borne outbreaks. Within childcare centers control measures include adequate number of sinks, methods to clean diaper-changing surfaces, prohibiting food handlers from diaper changing, cohorting of sick children, and frequent staff education. Control of spread in childcare centers is likely to impact community-wide transmission. In other institutional outbreaks, cohorting and contact isolation are important measures. Antibiotic treatment of infected persons may curtail outbreaks in closed settings. Antibiotic prophylaxis is ineffective and risks the emergence of resistance.

Both killed and live-attenuated oral vaccines have been studied but have provided only partial, transient, serotype-specific immunity. Several candidate vaccines are being tested, including polysaccharide conjugate vaccines, and molecular constructs in live vectors.

DIARRHEA-CAUSING *Escherichia coli*

Escherichia coli are gram-negative, lactose-fermenting, motile, facultative bacilli belonging to the family Enterobacteriaceae. *Escherichia coli* can be grouped by serotype, defined by the 171 somatic (O) and 56 flagellar antigens. Thus, *E. coli* O157:H7 is an example

of a specific serotype. *Escherichia coli* are the most common flora of the gastrointestinal tract and probably serve useful symbiotic functions. Most are nonpathogenic, but some possess specific virulence traits that enable them to cause meningitis, urinary tract infection, or diarrhea. The diarrhea-causing *E. coli* fall into five distinct phenotypes (Table 13-43). Each phenotype possesses unique genes encoding virulence traits, each with their own pathogenesis.

Because *E. coli* is the most common facultative organism in stool, identifying diarrhea-causing *E. coli* in stool specimens is difficult. Colonies of *E. coli* must be individually tested for specific virulence traits using bioassays, assays for specific toxins, phenotypic adherence assays, DNA probes for virulence genes, or PCR. Many of these assays are available only in research laboratories.

ENTEROHEMORRHAGIC E. COLI Enterohemorrhagic *E. coli* (EHEC) are able to cause an attaching and effacing lesion in intestinal mucosa and secrete Shiga toxin (stx). At least 12 serotypes of *E. coli* are EHEC, but one serotype, *E. coli* O157:H7 is the predominant strain in much of the world. Because it is much easier to screen for *E. coli* O157:H7, its importance relative to other serotypes of EHEC may be overestimated. Unlike most *E. coli*, *E. coli* O157:H7 ferments sorbitol slowly, which led to the development of a simple microbiologic screen, sorbitol MacConkey (SMAC) agar. With the exception of *E. coli* O157:H7, EHEC must be identified in the lab by finding evidence of stx production. Generally, this requires screening for cytotoxic activity in culture supernatants or screening 3 to 10 colonies of *E. coli* by colony-blot hybridization with DNA probes for the stx genes. Recently, enzyme immunoassays for shiga toxin have become more widely available.

ENTEROTOXIGENIC E. COLI Enterotoxigenic *E. coli* (ETEC) belong to many serotypes. They produce the enterotoxins ST and LT, which cause secretory diarrhea without invading or damaging enterocytes. They can be identified in the laboratory by detection of enterotoxin by using enzyme immunoassay or by a bioassay in which culture supernatants are added to Y1 adrenal cell or to Chinese hamster ovary cells in culture. Gene probes for the toxin genes can be applied to colony blots, a technique widely used in epidemiologic studies. PCR primes for the toxin genes have also proved sensitive.

ENTEROPATHIC E. COLI Enteropathic *E. coli* (EPEC) are an important cause of diarrhea in infants in developing countries, and were responsible for numerous nursery outbreaks in industrialized countries during the 1950s and 1960s. Traditionally defined by serotype, they are now defined by localized adherence pattern to Hep2 cells and by pathogenic characteristics. In the laboratory,

EPEC are generally identified by the presence of the EAF plasmid, which is usually detected by colony blot with the *eae* gene probe or by PCR. By definition, EPEC do not secrete Shiga toxin. Adherence assays can also be used, although they are cumbersome and require considerable expertise.

ENTEROINVASIVE E. COLI Enteroinvasive *E. coli* (EIEC) are strains of *E. coli* that closely resemble *Shigella* in their genetics, biochemical characteristics, and clinical manifestations. Identification of EIEC was traditionally performed by isolating strains of *E. coli* with a positive Sereny test (guinea pig keratoconjunctivitis). Recently, gene probes for the invasiveness genes *ipaC* have been used to screen colony blots of *E. coli* for EIEC. PCR has been used experimentally.

ENTEROAGGREGATIVE E. COLI Enteroaggregative *E. coli* (EaggEC) are the most recent phenotype of *E. coli* demonstrated to cause diarrhea. They are defined as strains that do not secrete LT or ST and that adhere to Hep-2 cells or a cover slip with a "stacked brick" pattern of adherence. This test is only available in research laboratories, is tedious, and requires care and expertise. As with other diarrhea-causing *E. coli*, it is hoped that phenotypic assays can be supplanted by newer methods based on identifying virulence genes with gene probes or PCR.

EPIDEMIOLOGY All diarrhea-causing *E. coli* are transmitted by fecal oral contact, but they differ in the infectious dose, the susceptible population, the geographic patterns, and the relative importance of food, water, and person-to-person transmission.

Escherichia coli O157:H7 and other EHEC have emerged as one of the most important enteric pathogens in developed countries. They are a relatively common cause of nonbloody and bloody diarrhea in developed countries of North and South America, Europe, and Japan. In a multicenter study in the United States, *E. coli* O157:H7 were the third or fourth most commonly identified stool pathogen. EHEC are responsible for upward of 90% of postdiarrheal hemolytic uremic syndrome (HUS) and an unknown proportion of cases of thrombotic thrombocytopenic purpura (TTP). *Escherichia coli* O157:H7 is the predominant strain in most regions. The true incidence is not known, because many laboratories do not use techniques to identify EHEC, but the Centers for Disease Control and Prevention estimates that there are more than 73,000 cases of *E. coli* O157:H7 infection annually in the United States with 60 to 250 deaths. It is not clear whether there are age-specific differences in incidence, but the complications such as HUS, TTP, and death are more frequent in young children and the elderly. *Escherichia coli* O157:H7 infections show a clear seasonal pattern with peak incidence in the summer and fall in the northern hemisphere.

The natural reservoir of EHEC is dairy cattle; however, other animals that can carry the organism include goats, sheep, pigs, deer, and elk. Outbreaks are most often the result of consumption of hamburger meat or raw milk. Several outbreaks have followed swimming in contaminated water in lakes, ponds, and swimming pools. Other outbreaks have been the result of consumption of roast beef, apple cider, unpasteurized apple juice, salami, municipal water, and produce, including leaf lettuce and alfalfa and radish sprouts. Most cases are sporadic, and consumption of undercooked hamburger is a risk factor for sporadic cases. The infectious dose for *E. coli* O157:H7 is low, estimated from one outbreak to be less than 700 organisms. Person-to-person transmission has been documented in institutions, childcare centers, homes with young children, and, rarely, in hospitals.

ETEC is an important cause of diarrhea in two groups; young children in developing countries and travelers to developing countries. In a variety of studies, ETEC accounted for 10 to 30% of diarrhea cases in infants around the time of weaning. The incidence of symptomatic ETEC disease drops sharply with age in endemic countries. However, travelers from developed countries lack immunity. Twenty to 40% of travelers' diarrhea is due to ETEC. Transmission generally results from contamination of water and food in conditions of poor sanitation, and requires a relatively high inoculum. ETEC outbreaks were once thought to be extremely rare in developed countries. However, in recent years, several outbreaks have been identified in the United States.

PATHOGENESIS

EHEC The incubation period for EHEC is usually 3 to 4 days, although it ranges from 1 to 9 days. *Escherichia coli* O157:H7 are quite acid tolerant and probably are less affected by the gastric acid barrier than other enteric pathogens. On reaching the intestine, EHEC adhere to enterocytes, primarily in the colon. A characteristic attaching and effacing lesion occurs, similar to what occurs with EPEC. Histology shows edema and submucosal hemorrhage. The defining virulence factor for EHEC is the ability to produce shigatoxin (Stx), one of the most potent protein inhibitors of protein synthesis known. Stx has been referred to in earlier publications as Shiga-like toxin because of the homology of Stx1 and Shiga toxin, and Vero toxin (a substance toxic for Vero cells and other cell lines). There are two major subtypes of Stx: Stx1 and Stx2 with numerous minor variants of Stx2. Stx is composed of an A subunit and five identical B subunits by which the toxin binds to glycolipid receptors GB3 and GB4, which facilitate endocytosis. Other putative virulence factors include a hemolysin, lipopolysaccharide (LPS), iron utilization genes, and EAST1 (discussed later in the EaggEC section). The attaching and effacing lesion is mediated by genes encoded in the LEE (locus of enterocyte effacement), a 35-kb pathogenicity island that is identical to the island found in EPEC.

The pathogenesis of hemolytic-uremic syndrome (HUS) is not fully understood, but available evidence supports the following sequence: (a) binding of EHEC to enterocytes promotes production of TNF and IL-1, which may up-regulate endothelial expression of toxin receptors; (b) Stx and LPS probably reach the systemic circulation; (c) LPS sensitizes endothelial cells to cell damage due to Stx; (d) endothelial cell damage leads to platelet aggregation, white cell activation and adherence, and microvascular damage; and (e) fibrin thrombi occur in the kidneys and potentially in many other sites, including brain, spinal cord, heart, lung, pancreas, and colon. HUS is discussed further in Sec 21.8.3.

ETEC The pathogenesis of ETEC is fairly similar to *Vibrio cholerae*. Symptoms follow an incubation period of 14 to 48 hours. ETEC colonize the surface of the small-bowel epithelium but do not invade. Binding is mediated by surface fimbriae (or pili), referred to as colonization fimbriae (CFAs). Diarrhea is caused by one of two toxins: heat-labile toxin (LT) or heat-stable toxin (ST). Strains may produce one or both toxins. LT is 80% homologous to cholera toxin at the protein sequence level, and has a similar structure and a similar function. LT induces adenylate cyclase, leading to increased levels of cyclic AMP. This activation of chloride channels results in increased chloride secretion, leading to passive efflux of water and watery diarrhea. ST binds to guanylate cyclase, a membrane-spanning enzyme, and stimulates the production of cyclic GMP.

EPEC   The incubation period for EPEC is 6 to 48 hours. EPEC adhere to the epithelial cell through a process thought to be mediated by the bundle-forming pilus, encoded in the EAF plasmid. Genes within the LEE (locus of enterocyte effacement) are activated, leading to secretion of a molecule called intimin and activation of a type III secretion system. The microvillus structure is dissolved. Intimate adherence supervenes, with activation of the cell's cytoskeleton, leading to production of a pedestal lesion. The mechanisms by which this cascade causes diarrhea are not fully understood, but may involve increased intracellular calcium and increased permeability of the tight junctions.

EIEC and EaggEC   The pathophysiology of EIEC is virtually identical to *Shigella*. It invades and divides within enterocytes, causing intense inflammation.

Much less is understood about the pathogenesis of diarrhea caused by EaggEC. Not all strains cause diarrhea in laboratory animals or in human volunteers. EaggEC adhere to small-bowel mucosa. EAST1, an enterotoxin associated with secretion, is present in about 40% of strains. Putative cytotoxins have been identified. Some data suggest that EaggEC may invade epithelial cells in vitro. Increased mucous production is seen in patients, animals, and volunteers, but the mechanism is not known.

CLINICAL MANIFESTATIONS   EHEC most often cause hemorrhagic colitis, characterized by vomiting, bloody diarrhea, and severe abdominal cramps. Fecal leukocytes may be present but are not prominent. Asymptomatic carriage and nonbloody diarrhea also occur. HUS—the triad of thrombocytopenia, hemolytic anemia, and renal failure—occurs in 5 to 10% of children infected with *E. coli* O157:H7. The rate may be lower for non-O157 strains. Risk factors for HUS include young age, use of antimotility agents, and, possibly, use of antimicrobial agents. The data implicating antimicrobial agents are based on in vitro studies that demonstrate that antimicrobial agents up-regulate toxin production. Clinical data are limited to several retrospective studies that show an association between antibiotic use and HUS or death. However, use of antibiotics as treatment for HUS worsens outcome. In adults, EHEC infection may lead to thrombotic thrombocytopenic purpura.

ETEC causes large-volume watery diarrhea. Fever and vomiting may occur, but are uncommon. The diarrhea may be mild and self-limited, or it may lead to massive fluid loss and dehydration. Blood, mucus, or fecal white cells are very uncommon. Duration is typically less than 1 week.

EPEC diarrhea typically occurs in children less than 2 years old. Diarrhea is usually watery and profuse. Vomiting and low-grade fever are common. While most cases are associated with acute disease, persistent diarrhea may occur.

EIEC causes abdominal cramps, tenesmus, fever, and small-volume stools. Blood and mucus may be present, but may be less common than with some of the more virulent strains of *Shigella*.

EaggEC most often occurs as a watery diarrhea without vomiting and with low-grade fever. Mucoid diarrhea is common, and in some series, bloody diarrhea occurs in up to one-third of patients. Of particular importance is the association of EaggEC with persistent diarrhea. In malnourished children, persistent diarrhea is associated with malnutrition and contributes to increased mortality.

DIAGNOSIS   Diagnosis of infection by diarrhea-causing *E. coli* is difficult. Techniques for the diagnosis of EHEC are widely available

in clinical laboratories, although many do not test routinely. Techniques for diagnosing the other four phenotypes are largely limited to research and public health laboratories. However, diagnosis should be vigorously pursued in outbreaks and in the evaluation of patients with persistent diarrhea, especially in the setting of foreign travel. A few commercial reference laboratories offer the Hep-2 adherence assay for diagnosing EPEC and EaggEC.

Escherichia coli O157:H7 can be identified by screening with sorbitol MacConkey agar, an inexpensive technique that should be available in all clinical microbiology laboratories. Some laboratories may routinely screen all stools during the summer and fall; the remainder of the year they screen bloody stools and those from children in whom HUS is suspected. To detect other serotypes of EHEC, methods that detect Stx are necessary. Premiere EHEC, a commercial enzyme immunoassay, was recently licensed. When used on supernatants of 24-hour broth cultures, it is highly sensitive and specific.

ETEC cannot be identified by biochemical characteristics or serotype. Definitive diagnosis is based on detection of toxin in *E. coli* colonies by bioassay in the suckling mouse assay, the Y1 adrenal cell assay, or by enzyme immunoassay. DNA probes and PCR primers directed against the genes encoding LT and ST are also used in research laboratories.

Serotyping was once the gold standard for identifying EPEC strains; it is no longer considered the primary method. According to a consensus definition, EPEC strains are those that can cause an attaching and effacing lesion in the Hep-2 adherence assay and that lack Stx. Genotypic diagnosis relies on DNA probes and PCR primers for the *eae* gene, the *bfp* gene, and the EAF plasmid.

EIEC can be diagnosed by demonstrating that an isolate with the biochemical characteristics of *E. coli* contains *Shigella* invasiveness genes. An enzyme immunoassay to detect the *ipaC* gene has been developed that can detect EIEC and Shigella. It is not yet widely available.

The gold standard for diagnosing EaggEC is the Hep-2 adherence assay, in which tested *E. coli* isolates demonstrate the stacked brick configuration. The utility of the EAC probe appears to vary by region.

TREATMENT   As for all diarrheal illness in children, the cornerstone of therapy is careful replacement of fluids and electrolytes (Sec 17.7.4). The treatment of EHEC is supportive. As noted earlier, the use of antimicrobial agents in EHEC may be associated with an increased risk of HUS. Although this remains controversial, there are no data supporting any clinical benefit, so it is prudent to avoid all antimicrobials.

Antimicrobial therapy is clearly useful in shortening the course of ETEC infections in travelers, as demonstrated in numerous studies in many settings. TMP-SMX, doxycycline, bicampicillin, furazolidine, and fluoroquinolones have demonstrated efficacy. However, resistance to TMP-SMX is common in some regions. Treatment of EPEC with TMP-SMX, oral gentamicin, and oral colistin are effective, although symptomatic therapy may suffice. Antibiotics used to treat *Shigella* can be used in EIEC, although clear data are lacking. A recent study reported prompt improvement in persistent diarrhea among HIV-infected patients with EaggEC infection when treated with ciprofloxacin 500 mg bid for 7 days. Similar studies are not available for HIV-negative persons with EaggEC infection.

Antimotility agents should be avoided in persons with inflammatory or bloody diarrhea, and in infants and children with diarrhea. Antimotility agents in low dose, and for a brief period, are safe for treating secretory diarrhea in adults. Bismuth subsalicylate reduces the severity of diarrhea in patients with ETEC infections, although salicylate absorption occurs. The general rule is that the amount of salicylate absorbed from 30 mL of Pepto-Bismol is similar to that of one 325-mg aspirin tablet.

PROGNOSIS Currently, EHEC are associated with the greatest morbidity in developed countries. Five to 10% of infected patients develop HUS; the mortality from HUS is 2 to 5%. The major complications of ETEC infection are related to dehydration and to electrolyte disturbances. Severe complications of ETEC infection should be uncommon in a setting with good rehydration facilities. However, ETEC contributes a substantial proportion of the approximately 3 million deaths that occur as a consequence of diarrhea among infants and young children in developing countries. Although several nursery epidemics caused by EPEC in the 1940s and 1950s reported mortality rates approaching 50%, the current mortality is less than 1% in developed countries. The persistent diarrhea associated with EaggEC is associated with growth failure and increased mortality. As rehydration services improve in developing countries, persistent diarrhea accounts for an increasing proportion of diarrheal mortality.

PREVENTION The most important measures for prevention of ETEC, EPEC, EaggEC, and EIEC are improvements in sanitation, including proper disposal of human waste, access to water and soap for hand washing, and clean sources of food for weaning. Breastfeeding is protective and should be encouraged. Nosocomial transmission of diarrhea causing *E. coli* occurs; therefore, careful enteric precautions should be followed.

To prevent EHEC, hamburger and other beef products should be cooked thoroughly and protected from contamination from raw meat. Unpasteurized milk and apple juice should be avoided. Because several outbreaks of *E. coli* O157:H7 were caused by diapered children in swimming pools and ponds, this is a potential area for intervention.

To prevent ETEC infection, travelers to developing countries should avoid ice, salads, and those raw fruits and vegetables without peels. They should drink only boiled or carbonated water or beverages, or bottled water from a reliable source. Infant formula should be prepared from boiled water. Routine use of prophylactic antibiotics is not recommended, particularly for children. Bismuth subsalicylate can be used for prophylaxis in adolescents and adults, but the aspirin exposure represents a relative contraindication for young children.

Because preliminary studies with inactivated ETEC vaccines prove that protective vaccines are feasible, several approaches are under active investigation.

References

General

Guerrant RL, Steiner TS, Lima AA, Bobak DA. How intestinal bacteria cause disease. J Infect Dis 179(Suppl 2):S331–337, 1999

Nataro JP: Treatment of bacterial enteritis. Pediatr Infect Dis J 17(5):420–421, 1998

Slutsker L, Altekruse SF, Swerdlow DL: Foodborne diseases. Emerging pathogens and trends. Infect Dis Clin North Am 12(1):199–216, 1998

Salmonella

Butler T, Islam A, Kabir I, Jones PK: Patterns of morbidity and mortality in typhoid fever dependent on age and gender: review of 552 hospitalized patients with diarrhea. Rev Infect Dis 13(1):85–90, 1991

Darwin KH, Miller VL: Molecular basis of the interaction of *Salmonella* with the intestinal mucosa. Clin Microbiol Rev 12(3):405–428, 1999

Mermin JH, Townes JM, Gerber M, Dolan N, Mintz ED, Tauxe RV: Typhoid fever in the United States, 1985–1994: changing risks of international travel and increasing antimicrobial resistance. Arch Intern Med 158(6):633–638, 1998

Plotkin SA, Bouveret-Le Cam N: A new typhoid vaccine composed of the Vi capsular polysaccharide. Arch Intern Med 155(21):2293–2299, 1995

Shigella

Khan WA, Dhar U, Salam MA, Griffiths JK, Rand W, Bennish ML: Central nervous system manifestations of childhood shigellosis: prevalence, risk factors, and outcome. Pediatrics 103(2):E18, 1999

Lee LA, Shapiro CN, Hargrett-Bean N, Tauxe RV: Hyperendemic shigellosis in the United States: a review of surveillance data for 1967–1988. J Infect Dis 164(5):894–900, 1991

Parsot C, Sansonetti PJ: Invasion and the pathogenesis of *Shigella* infections. Curr Top Microbiol Immunol 209:25–42, 1996

Tauxe RV, Puhr ND, Wells JG, Hargrett-Bean N, Blake PA: Antimicrobial resistance of *Shigella* isolates in the USA: the importance of international travelers. J Infect Dis 162(5):1107–1111, 1990

E. coli

Griffin PM, Tauxe RV: The epidemiology of infections caused by *Escherichia coli* O157:H7, other enterohemorrhagic *E. coli*, and the associated hemolytic uremic syndrome. Epidemiol Rev 13:60–98, 1991

Nataro JP, Kaper JB: Diarrheagenic *Escherichia coli*. Clin Microbiol Rev 11(1):142–201, 1998

Wanke CA, Gerrior J, Blais V, Mayer H, Acheson D: Successful treatment of diarrheal disease associated with enteroaggregative *Escherichia coli* in adults infected with human immunodeficiency virus. J Infect Dis 178(5):1369–1372, 1998

13.2.31   Staphylococcus

Beverly L. Connelly

Staphylococci are ubiquitous inhabitants of the skin and mucous membranes of humans and other mammals. The relationship with the host is generally benign unless there is disruption or damage to the cutaneous barriers affording an opportunity for invasion. Staphylococcal diseases may be toxin mediated or the result of direct invasion of a disrupted or damaged cutaneous barrier. Disease may be mild and self-limited, as in superficial impetigo, or severe and life-threatening, as in disseminated infection or as in toxic shock syndrome.

The term *staphylococcus* comes from the Greek staphyle meaning "a bunch of grapes." In Gram-stained specimens, they appear as gram-positive cocci in "grape-like" clusters, as well as in pairs and tetrads. Staphylococci are nonmotile, nonspore-forming bacteria that exhibit microcapsule formation. Most species are catalase-positive, facultative anaerobes, which grow best aerobically. The cell walls of staphylococci contain peptidoglycan and techoic acid, the composition of which can be used to distinguish between species. The production of coagulase, an enzyme that clots plasma, distinguishes *S. aureus* from other medically important staphylococci. The remainder of the staphylococci are taxonomically grouped as coagulase-negative staphylococci (CoNS) and represent the most common resident bacteria of humans. Selected species of CoNS, including, but not limited to, *S. epidermidis, S. haemolyticus,* and *S. saprophyticus,* are associated with human disease.

A variety of surface molecules facilitate attachment of the staphylococcal bacteria to cells or extracellular matrix material and are believed to play a role in disease pathogenesis. Coagulase binds to and activates prothrombin, inducing clot formation. Fibrinogen binding ("clumping factor") may play a role in adhesion to foreign bodies. Likewise, there are polysaccharide adhesions that are major components of CoNS "slime" or biofilm and that play a major role in adhesion of CoNS to biomedical devices. These and a variety of other adhesions have been designated *m*icrobial *s*urface *c*omponents *r*ecognizing *a*dhesive *m*atrix *m*olecules or MSCRAMMs and may facilitate staphylococcal colonization of host tissues.

Additional surface molecules, as well as secreted proteins, interfere with host defenses. Protein A on the surface of *S. aureus* binds to the Fc portion of IgG in a nonphysiological manner, inhibiting phagocytosis. Extracellular serine proteases, such as V8 from *S. aureus,* cleave and inactivate IgG, and may inactivate neutrophil defensins. Toxic shock syndrome toxin-1 (TSST-1) and enterotoxins A, B, C1-3, D, E, G, and H, act as superantigens, suppressing B cells while inducing T-cell proliferation, cytokine, and tumor necrosis factor release. The enterotoxins are responsible for the symptoms seen in food poisoning. Enterotoxins B and C are structurally very similar to TSST-1 and may be responsible for toxic shock syndrome in the absence of TSST-1. Other exogenous proteins, including hemolysins (α, β, γ, δ), phospholipase C, and hyaluronidase, enhance spreading and tissue invasion. The exfoliative toxins A and B that are responsible for erythroderma and skin separation seen in staphylococcal scalded-skin syndrome may have serine protease activity.

Colonization of the latter site may serve as a convenient location from which to spread *S. aureus* to other areas. From 20 to 50% of healthy individuals in the general population are colonized with *S. aureus*. Nasal carriage may be 50 to 85% in selected high-risk populations. Colonized individuals are at increased risk of subsequent infection, especially in the presence of significant underlying conditions such as prematurity, diabetes, intravenous drug use, or surgery, and in the presence of indwelling catheters and other foreign bodies. An underlying immunodeficiency should be considered in patients with recurrent or life-threatening staphylococcal infections.

Staphylococcus aureus INFECTIONS

Bacteria-Mediated Disease

Skin and Soft Tissue Infection Staphylococcal impetigo may appear as erythematous-crusted papules and pustules, often at the site of minor trauma such as an insect bite, and may be indistinguishable from infection caused by pyogenic streptococci. Bullous impetigo is more classically staphylococcal in origin and appears as flaccid coalescent pustules and bullae on previously undamaged skin. Furuncles occur when focal infection involves the hair follicle and surrounding tissues; carbuncles occur when multiple furuncles coalesce. Hidradenitis suppurativa is a distinct clinical syndrome of recurrent infections involving the apocrine sweat glands.

Bacteremia and Sepsis In the absence of an obvious source on physical exam, positive blood cultures for *S. aureus* should raise suspicion for an occult site such as endocarditis or osteomyelitis. Right-sided endocarditis may occur in the setting of IV drug abuse. Septic shock, disseminated intravascular coagulation, and acute respiratory distress syndrome may complicate *S. aureus* bacteremia acutely. Metastatic seeding of secondary sites may occur in as many as half of patients and may not be recognized for as long as a month after initial diagnosis of bacteremia. Catheter-associated bacteremia with *S. aureus* usually requires catheter removal.

Bone and Joint Infections *Staphylococcus aureus* is the most common cause of osteomyelitis in children. Hematogenous seeding of the metaphysis of long bones, often with a history of antecedent minor trauma, is typical. Bacteremia is present in about 50% of cases. Radiographic evidence of periosteal reaction or bone lucencies may not be apparent until well into the second week of infection.

Staphylococcus aureus is the most common cause of septic arthritis in most ages; it is the most common cause of nongonococcal arthritis in adolescents and adults. Risk factors include penetrating and nonpenetrating trauma, rheumatoid arthritis, diabetes and other chronic debilitating diseases, and immunosuppression. Presentation is usually acute. Adequate drainage of the joint, either open or closed, is essential to minimize joint destruction. Removal of any prosthetic material is usually required. Osteomyelitis and septic arthritis are discussed further in Sec 13.1.9.

Endocarditis *Staphylococcus aureus* is a leading cause of infective endocarditis (IE) in the absence of predisposing valvular disease, in association with intravenous drug abuse, and in association with prosthetic valves. *Staphylococcus aureus* IE is generally considered more fulminant than IE of other etiologies, and bacteremia may be sustained (≥ 7 days) even with appropriate antibiotics. Cardiac complications are especially common with aortic valvular involvement and include valvular destruction, myocardial abscess and fistula formation, and development of conduction abnormalities. Neurologic sequelae are common with mitral and prosthetic valve involvement. Hematogenous dissemination to any tissue may occur. Endocarditis is discussed further in Sec. 13.1.10.

Central Nervous System Infections Staphylococcal central nervous system infections are associated with neurosurgical procedures, penetrating trauma, foreign bodies, direct extension from a contiguous site, and hematogenous dissemination from a distant site. Shunt infections, meningitis, brain abscess, subdural empyema, and epidural abscesses may occur. Primary staphylococcal infection of the central nervous system (CNS) is rare. Cyanotic congenital heart disease poses a significant risk for brain abscess, due to staphylococci as well as other organisms. Because the earliest symptoms in young children are nonspecific, the diagnosis of epidural abscess is often delayed until signs of cord compression are present.

Surgical Wound Infections The risk of staphylococcal wound infection following surgery increases in the presence of underlying chronic disease, immunodeficiency, and in the presence of a foreign body. Local and systemic complications include wound dehiscence, tissue abscesses, septic thrombophlebitis, bacteremia, sepsis, and metastatic infections. Primary treatment of surgical wounds is débridement, foreign bodies involved with staphylococcal infections generally must be removed; antibiotics are adjunctive.

Foreign Bodies *Staphylococcus aureus* is a major cause of morbidity and mortality in hemodialysis patients. Local infection at the access site may progress to abscess formation and be complicated by bacteremic disease. *Staphylococcus aureus* is a leading cause of exit- and tunnel-site infections in patients on chronic peritoneal dialysis as well. Nasal carriage of *S. aureus* appears to be a major risk factor for subsequent infections in each of these patient groups. *Staphylococcus aureus* is second to CoNS as a causative agent in intravascular device-related infections in other settings.

Toxin-Mediated Syndromes

Staphylococcal Scalded-Skin Syndrome (SSSS) This is an exfoliative dermatitis mediated by exfoliatin produced by *S. aureus*. Often referred to as Ritter syndrome in young infants, SSSS may also be seen in older children. Bacteremia may or may not be present. Widespread dissemination of the toxin produces fever and tender erythema, which may rapidly progress to bullae formation. Minimal friction applied to the skin results in sloughing of the superficial layers of skin (Nikolsky sign). A less-severe syndrome resembling streptococcal "scarlet fever" may be seen in older children. The skin may be tender; however, sloughing is absent, although superficial desquamation is often seen in the convalescent phase.

Staphylococcus aureus Food Poisoning This is the most common cause of food poisoning in the United States. It is caused by the ingestion of preformed enterotoxin from contaminated foods. Foods are contaminated by toxin-producing strains of bacteria during preparation, maintained at a temperature suitable for toxin elaboration, and toxin-bearing food is then ingested by unsuspecting individuals. The incubation period for disease is short, usually less than 4 hours; nausea, vomiting, and abdominal cramps follow. Fever and headache may occasionally be present. In most individuals, the disease is self-limited, although severe dehydration and prostration may be seen in a few individuals.

Toxic Shock Syndrome (TSS) This is caused by the hematogenous dissemination of toxic shock syndrome toxin-1 (TSST-1) or the staphylococcal enterotoxins B and C. TSS has gained widespread attention because of its association with tampon use in menstruating women. As demonstrated in the numerous cases of menstrual-associated TSS during the 1980s, colonization of a mucous membrane in the nares, throat, or vagina, rather than actual invasive infection with toxin-producing strain of *S. aureus,* is often sufficient for the development of TSS. Menstrual TSS has declined dramatically and nonmenstrual TSS is currently estimated to represent half of the cases recognized. Symptoms include fever, headache, chills, vomiting, diarrhea, sore throat, and myalgias. Hypotension, capillary leak syndrome, and respiratory distress may ensue. Diffuse erythroderma resembling sunburn is often described during the course of illness, and desquamation may be a late finding. Treatment is primarily supportive. TSS must be differentiated from septic shock, streptococcal toxic shock, scarlet fever, meningococcemia, Rocky Mountain spotted fever, Kawasaki syndrome, severe drug reactions, leptospirosis, and measles.

Methicillin-Resistant *Staphylococcus aureus* (MRSA)

Since the mid 1970s, methicillin resistance among hospital-acquired *S. aureus* isolates has increased from less than 5% to more than 50% of isolates. Among these isolates, methicillin resistance is conveyed by the presence of a unique penicillin-binding protein 2a (PBP2a), the product of the chromosomal *mecA* gene, which also confers cross-resistance to other β-lactam antibiotics, including cephalosporins. In addition, these hospital-acquired MRSA are usually resistant to multiple other classes of drugs. Recognized risks associated with MRSA infections include prior antibiotic therapy and exposure to health care environments. Until recently, "community-acquired" MRSA was associated with conditions that interfaced health care, such as IV drug abuse. Truly community-acquired MRSA isolates, although β-lactam antibiotic resistant, may maintain susceptibility to a variety of other drug classes. Vancomycin is the recommended agent for treatment of MRSA until susceptibility to alternate agents other than the β-lactams can be demonstrated. More worrisome is the emergence of *S. aureus* with reduced susceptibility to vancomycin and teichoplanin, referred to as glycopeptide intermediate *S. aureus* (GISA). Patients from whom GISA have been isolated have had significant underlying diseases and had received long-term therapy for MRSA infections. The mechanism of resistance has not been established, but does not appear to be any of the mechanisms employed by vancomycin-resistant enterococcus (VRE).

TREATMENT Local care and cleansing are often sufficient therapy for impetigo. Topical bacitracin or mupirocin are useful adjunctive antibacterial therapy for these superficial infections if well circumscribed. More extensive lesions or those that cannot be differentiated from streptococci may require oral antibiotics such as dicloxacillin, cephalexin, clindamycin, or augmentin. Evaluation for potential bacteremia and treatment with systemic antistaphylococcal therapy should be considered for the neonate with bullous impetigo.

The β-lactamase-resistant penicillins—methicillin, nafcillin, oxacillin, cloxacillin, and dicloxacillin— are the mainstay of systemic treatment for staphylococcal infections. The first-generation cephalosporins, such as cephalexin and cephalothin, are useful alternative agents. Penicillins, in combination with β-lactamase inhibitors (ampicillin+sulbactam, ticarcillin+clavulanate, piperacillin+tazobactam), are also alternative agents for methicillin-susceptible staphylococci. The increasing prevalence of methicillin-resistant strains, however, has created a challenge for clinicians, especially when faced with a severely ill patient. Vancomycin is the drug of choice for treatment of serious infections caused by methicillin-resistant staphylococci; however, judicious use is warranted in order to minimize the selection for resistance. Vancomycin should not be used as a first-line therapy for methicillin-susceptible *S. aureus* infection, except in the patient with documented severe hypersensitivity to the β-lactams. Empiric use of vancomycin is appropriate pending culture results in the seriously ill patient with suspected staphylococcal infection.

For limited skin and soft-tissue infections with methicillin-susceptible staphylococcal strains, oral therapy with cloxacillin, cefadroxil, or cephalexin for 5 to 7 days is usually sufficient. Initial treatment with intravenous nafcillin or first-generation cephalosporin should be considered in patients suspected of having more serious disease. Strategies for treating minor soft-tissue MRSA infections are limited. Clindamycin is useful for selected community-acquired MRSA infections. Other strategies include topical mupirocin, oral rifampin, and oral trimethoprim/sulfamethoxasole.

Serious infections caused by methicillin-susceptible staphylococcal strains should be treated with nafcillin or a first-generation cephalosporin (eg, cefazolin). Combination therapy with an aminoglycoside (gentamicin) or rifampin may be indicated for select conditions, especially endocarditis. Vancomycin is indicated for the treatment of serious infections caused by MRSA, unless the infectious agent is clindamycin susceptible. Clindamycin should not be used in endocarditis. Combination therapy with gentamicin or rifampin may be indicated. Duration of therapy is dependent upon the nature of the infection. Septic arthritis should be treated for at least 3 weeks and osteomyelitis should be treated for at least 4 to 6 weeks. Endocarditis should be treated at least 6 weeks.

Eradication of the carrier state may be desirable in certain patients at high risk or with a history of repeated staphylococcal infections. Eradication attempts may also be indicated in order to terminate outbreaks in a health-care setting. Regimens useful for this purpose include oral rifampin for 7 to 10 days or topical mupirocin applied twice daily to the nasal vestibule for 7 to 10 days. The latter approach successfully prevents serious methicillin-susceptible *S. aureus* infections in patients undergoing peritoneal and hemodialysis and may help prevent serious postsurgical infections caused by *S. aureus*. There are no regimens that have demonstrated efficacy in eradicating MRSA carriage. Vancomycin treatment is not indicated for this purpose.

COAGULASE-NEGATIVE STAPHYLOCOCCI

CoNS are commensal skin inhabitants. Of the numerous species in this group, *S. epidermidis, S. haemolyticus,* and *S. saprophyticus* have emerged as the most widely recognized pathogens of human disease. Although *S. epidermidis* appears to be responsible for the greatest number of infections, numerous other species are now recognized in association with disease. Because of the commensal nature of the CoNS, they are often recovered from specimens when inadequate or improper collection techniques have been employed. Thus, recovery of CoNS from a normally sterile body site must be interpreted in light of the clinical circumstances of the patient. It is clear that CoNS play a major pathogenic role in selected circumstances.

DEVICE-RELATED INFECTIONS Both specific and nonspecific adhesion properties facilitate colonization of indwelling devices with CoNS, while the production of a glycocalyx slime assists the organism in evading host defenses. CoNS are responsible for approximately 40% of the cases of bacterial peritonitis in patients undergoing continuous ambulatory peritoneal dialysis (CAPD) and are the most common isolate reported in central venous catheter-associated bacteremias in pediatric intensive care settings. As many as two-thirds of the infections that occur in association with cerebrospinal fluid shunts are caused by CoNS, most often *S. epidermidis*. Contamination of the device with resident commensal organisms at the time of insertion may play a principal role in risk for subsequent infection. Breaks in sterile technique while manipulating the device may serve to introduce colonizing organisms at a time remote from insertion. The biologic characteristics of the organism and its ability to escape immune surveillance facilitate prolonged smoldering shunt infections that may manifest only as intermittent device malfunctions. As many as half of patients present without overt signs of central nervous system inflammation; thus, a high index of suspicion is required to make the appropriate diagnosis. Because CoNS is a common blood-culture contaminant when tech-

nique is poor, distinguishing the "true" catheter-related bloodstream infections can be problematic, which contributes to overuse of vancomycin.

INFECTIONS IN IMMUNOCOMPROMISED HOSTS CoNS are responsible for approximately one-third of the bacteremias in children receiving chemotherapy for childhood malignancies and are responsible for the majority of bacteremias reported in infants in neonatal intensive care units. The presence of an intravascular catheter is the predominant risk factor. In neonates, CoNS are associated with cellulitis and abscesses, omphalitis, and pneumonia, and possibly with necrotizing enterocolitis. Risks for infection include the presence of intravascular devices, loss of integrity of skin or mucosal barriers, parenteral nutrition (specifically intravenous lipid), and use of immunosuppressive drugs. It may be difficult to determine whether the culture result represents true infection.

URINARY TRACT INFECTIONS The CoNS *S. saprophyticus* represents a significant urinary pathogen in adolescent females and young women. Symptomatic urinary tract infection is the rule for *S. saprophyticus* and may involve the upper tract. Urethral trauma associated with intercourse is speculated to be a significant risk factor preceding infection in some cases. Diagnosis requires recognition that colony counts may be falsely low because of the elaboration of clumping factor. Other CoNS may be implicated in nosocomial catheter-associated urinary tract infections and should prompt catheter removal.

References

Centers for Disease Control: Four pediatric deaths from community-acquired methicillin-resistant *Staphylococcus aureus*—Minnesota and North Dakota, 1997–1999. MMWR Morb Mortal Wkly Rep 48(32): 707–710, 1999

Chambers HF: Methicillin resistance in staphylococci: molecular and biochemical basis and clinical implications. Clin Micro Rev 10:781, 1997

Jain A, Ben-Ami T, Daum RS: Staphylococcal infections in children: Part 2. Pediatr Rev 20:219, 1999

Jain A, Daum RS: Staphylococcal infections in children: Part 1. Pediatr Rev 20:183, 1999

Jain A, Daum RS: Staphylococcal infections in children: Part 3. Pediatr Rev 20:261, 1999

Kluytmans J, van Belkum A, Verbrugh H: Nasal carriage of *Staphylococcus aureus:* epidemiology, underlying mechanisms, and associated risks. Clin Micro Rev 10:505, 1997

Lowy FD: *Staphylococcus aureus* infections. N Engl J Med 339:520, 1998

Perl TM, Golub JE: New approaches to reduce staphylococcal nosocomial infection rates: treating *S. aureus* nasal carriage. Ann Pharmacother 32: S7, 1998

St. Geme JW III: *Staphylococcus epidermidis* and other coagulase-negative staphylococci. In: Long SS, Pickering LK, Prober CG, eds: Principals and Practice of Pediatric Infectious Diseases. New York, Churchill Livingstone, 1997

Smith TL, Pearson ML, Wilcox KR, et al: Emergence of vancomycin resistance in *Staphylococcus aureus*. N Engl J Med 340:493, 1999

13.2.32 Streptococcal Infections

GROUP A STREPTOCOCCUS
Mark R. Schleiss

Streptococcus pyogenes (group A streptococci) cause both superficial infections (e.g. pharyngitis, impetigo) and invasive diseases. The organism is also causally linked to systemic infections. It is also causally linked to nonsuppurative complications including acute rheumatic fever, acute glomerulonephritis, and toxic shock syndrome.

Streptococci are gram-positive cocci that tend to grow as pairs and short chains in clinical specimens. When cultured on blood agar plates, *S. pyogenes* produces β-hemolysis, in contrast to the zone of partial hemolysis (α-hemolysis) generated by *Streptococcus pneumoniae*. β-hemolytic streptococci can be divided into many groups on the basis of antigenic differences in group-specific polysaccharides located in the bacterial cell wall. More than 20 serologic groups have been identified, designated by the letters A, B, C, and so on. Of the nongroup A streptococci, group B streptococcus is the most important human pathogen (the most common cause of neonatal sepsis and bacteremia), although other groups (particularly group G) have occasionally been implicated as causes of pharyngitis.

Group A organisms can be identified more cost-effectively by a number of latex agglutination, coagglutination, or enzyme immunoassay procedures. Group A strains can also be distinguished from other groups by their sensitivity to bacitracin. A disc containing 0.04 U of bacitracin will inhibit the growth of greater than 95% of group A strains, whereas 80 to 90% of nongroup A strains are resistant to this antibiotic. The bacitracin disc test is simple to perform and interpret in an office-based laboratory, and sufficiently accurate for presumptive identification of group A streptococcus. Presumptive identification of a strain as group A can also be made on the basis of production of the enzyme L-pyrrolidonyl-β-naphthylamide (PYRase). Among the β-hemolytic streptococci isolated from throat culture, only group A isolates produce PYRase, which can be identified on the basis of the characteristic color change (red) following inoculation of a disk on an agar plate followed by overnight incubation.

The somatic cellular constituents, as well as the extracellular enzymes and toxins, of *S. pyogenes* are responsible for many of pathogenic effects observed in vivo. The major virulence factor of the organism is the M protein; more than 80 M types have been described to date. This protein, a stable dimer, is anchored to the cell membrane and transverses and penetrates the cell wall. The proximal portion of the molecule is highly conserved among group A isolates, whereas the distal portions contain type-specific epitopes localized on the tips of fibrils (fimbriae) protruding from the cell surface. *The ability of group A streptococcus to initiate disease is highly dependent upon M protein.* Strains lacking M protein are essentially nonpathogenic. Interestingly, streptococci isolated from chronic pharyngeal carriers (individuals asymptomatically colonized with *S. pyogenes*) contain little or no M protein and are also relatively avirulent.

The molecular mechanisms by which M protein mediates pathogenesis are complex. In the nonimmune host, M protein mediates an antiphagocytic effect by inhibiting activation of the alternative complement pathway. Acquired immunity to streptococcal infection is based on the development of opsonic antibodies directed against the antiphagocytic epitopes of M protein. Although such antibodies protect against infection with a streptococcus bearing homologous M protein, they, unfortunately, confer no immunity against other M types. Community outbreaks of particular streptococcal diseases tend to be associated with certain M types, and therefore M-serotyping is very valuable for epidemiologic studies.

Other streptococcal cell-wall antigens include the hyaluronic acid capsule that serves as an accessory virulence factor by inhibiting phagocytosis. Lipoteichoic acid and protein F are cell-wall constituents that play roles in the adherence of *S. pyogenes* to fibronectin on the surface of human epithelial cells, an important event in the initiation of the infectious process. Serum opacity factor (OF) is a lipoproteinase associated with M protein, which is useful in classifying strains that are not identifiable by M-typing. Another streptococcal protein, *T protein*, does not appear to be a virulence factor, but does show significant antigenic variation among clinical isolates. T-typing is therefore a useful adjunct to M-typing for epidemiologic studies of group A streptococcal outbreaks.

In addition to somatic constituents, group A streptococci produce a large variety of extracellular enzymes and toxins important in pathogenesis. The family of streptococcal pyogenic exotoxins (SPE) includes SPEs A, B, C, and F. These toxins are responsible for the rash of scarlet fever and for pyrogenicity, cytotoxicity, and enhancement of susceptibility to endotoxin. SPE B is a cysteine protease, another determinant of virulence. Group A streptococcal isolates associated with streptococcal toxic shock syndrome (see below) encode certain SPEs (A, C, and F) that are capable of functioning as superantigens. These antigens induce a marked febrile response, proliferation of T lymphocytes, and synthesis and release of multiple cytokines, including tumor necrosis factor α, interleukin-1β, and interleukin-6. This activity is attributed to the ability of the superantigen to bind simultaneously to the Vβ region of the T-cell receptor and to class II major histocompatibility antigens of antigen-presenting mononuclear cells, resulting in widespread nonspecific T-cell proliferation and increased production of interleukin-2.

Streptococcus pyogenes also elaborates two distinct hemolysins. These proteins are responsible for the zone of hemolysis observed on blood agar plates, and are also important in the pathogenesis of tissue damage in the infected host. Streptolysin O is toxic to a wide variety of cell types, including myocardium. Streptolysin O is highly immunogenic, and determination of the antibody responses engendered to this protein (ASO titer) is often useful in the serodiagnosis of recent infection. Streptolysin S targets polymorphonuclear leukocytes and subcellular organelles, although, in contrast to streptolysin O, it does not appear to be immunogenic. Other extracellular products that may play a role in tissue damage and spread of organisms through tissue planes include a family of deoxyribonucleases (DNAses A to D), hyaluronidase, and streptokinase. Nicotinamide adenine dinucleotidase (NADase), proteinase, C5a-peptidase, amylase, and esterase are also described, although the role of these proteins in pathogenesis is less clear.

EPIDEMIOLOGY Person-to-person transmission is the route by which *S. pyogenes* is primarily spread, although food- and waterborne outbreaks have occasionally been documented. Neither spread of organisms by fomites nor transmission from animals (such as family pets) appears to play a significant role in contagion. *Streptococcus pyogenes* is highly communicable and can cause disease at all ages in normal individuals who do not have type-specific immunity against the specific serotype responsible for infection. Respiratory droplet spread is the major route for transmission of strains associated with upper respiratory tract infection, although skin-to-skin spread is known to occur with strains associated with streptococcal pyoderma. Children with untreated acute infections spread organisms by airborne salivary droplet and nasal discharge. Disease in neonates is uncommon, probably due in part to the effect of protective transplacentally acquired antibody. The incidence of pharyngeal infection is highest in children over 3 years of age. *Streptococcus pyogenes* also has the potential to produce outbreaks of disease in younger children in the childcare setting.

The incubation period for pharyngitis is 2 to 5 days. Infection is most common in the northern regions of the United States, especially during winter and early spring. Children are usually not infectious 24 hours after appropriate antibiotic therapy has been started, an observation that has important implications for return to the childcare or school environment. Individuals who are streptococcal "carriers" (chronic asymptomatic pharyngeal and nasopharyngeal colonization) usually do not spread disease to others because the small reservoir of often avirulent organisms usually lack M protein.

In contrast to the epidemiology of upper respiratory tract infections, streptococcal skin infections occur most frequently during the summer, or year-round in warm climates, when the skin is exposed and abrasions and insect bites are more likely to occur. *S. pyogenes* can be present on normal skin for at least a week before lesions appear. Spread is from skin to skin, not via the respiratory tract, although impetigo serotypes may colonize the throat. Fingernails and the perianal region can harbor streptococci and play a role in disseminating impetigo. Multiple streptococcal infections in the same family are common. Both impetigo and pharyngitis are more likely to occur among children living in crowded homes and in poor hygienic conditions.

CLINICAL MANIFESTATIONS

Streptococcal Pharyngitis Acute pharyngitis represents one of the most common reasons children are seen by a pediatrician. Nevertheless, the diagnostic and therapeutic approach to the child with a sore throat remains controversial.

In general, decisions about laboratory testing and antibiotic therapy should be made only after careful consideration of epidemiologic factors and clinical findings. Children with streptococcal pharyngitis *do not* have cough, rhinorrhea, or symptoms of viral upper respiratory infection. Indeed, the diagnosis of streptococcal pharyngitis can effectively be ruled out on the basis of the clinical findings of marked coryza, hoarseness, cough, or conjunctivitis. However, although these are important exclusionary criteria, the pediatrician must be aware that the signs and symptoms of streptococcal pharyngitis may otherwise be nonspecific and vary greatly depending on the age of the patient, the severity of the infection, or the timing of the illness. There may be relatively few localizing or constitutional symptoms, such that the illness may be unrecognized (subclinical infection). Young infants will not present with classic pharyngitis. Streptococcal upper respiratory tract infections in infants and toddlers may instead be characterized by low-grade fever, anorexia, and a thick, purulent nasal discharge ("streptococcosis"). Conversely, some patients may be toxic, with high fever, malaise, headache, and severe pain on swallowing. Although rare, streptococcal toxic shock can be associated with pharyngitis. Vomiting and abdominal pain may be prominent early symptoms, simulating gastroenteritis or even acute appendicitis. Hence, streptococcal pharyngitis should be considered in the child with acute onset of abdominal pain. Because streptococcal pharyngitis is chiefly a disease of winter and spring and primarily affects children over 3 years of age, fewer throat cultures should be done in the summer and in children less than 3 years old.

Physical examination in children with group A streptococcal pharyngitis is more likely to demonstrate tonsillopharyngeal erythema, a red edematous uvula, palatal petechiae, and tender anterior cervical adenopathy than in children with pharyngitis of other etiologies. Typically, tonsils are enlarged and erythematous with patchy exudate on the surface, although the presence of exudate is not pathognomonic for streptococcal pharyngitis, and may be observed in the setting of other bacterial and viral etiologies of pharyngitis, particularly Epstein-Barr virus. The papillae of the tongue may be red and swollen ("strawberry tongue"). Cutaneous petechiae and a scarlatiniform rash may be present (see "scarlet fever," below). When the characteristic rash of scarlet fever is present, a clinical diagnosis can be made with increased confidence.

A variety of clinical scoring systems have been devised in an attempt to predict the results of subsequent throat cultures or antigen detection tests, but at best these scoring systems have no more than an 80% predictive value.

The approach to bacteriologic confirmation of a tentative diagnosis of streptococcal pharyngitis remains controversial, but despite technological improvements in rapid streptococcal testing, the throat culture remains the gold standard for the diagnosis of streptococcal pharyngitis. If performed correctly, a throat swab cultured on a blood agar plate has a sensitivity of 90 to 95% in detecting the presence of *S. pyogenes* in the pharynx. This sensitivity depends upon obtaining the specimen properly. When possible, a specimen should be obtained from the surface of both tonsils and from the posterior pharyngeal wall. Other areas of the oropharynx are not appropriate sites for culture. The culture should be examined at 24 hours postinoculation, and again at 48 hours postinoculation.

Patients who should *not* undergo throat culture include children with nasal congestion, injected conjunctiva, and cough because these features indicate the presence of acute viral pharyngitis. A positive culture in this setting reflects chronic colonization (streptococcal carrier state). Although a negative throat culture essentially rules out the diagnosis of streptococcal pharyngitis, a positive culture, unfortunately, cannot differentiate between acute infection and asymptomatic carriage. In practice, however, it is probably best to assume that all positive results in appropriately cultured patients represent streptococcal infection and to accept that some degree of overtreatment is inevitable.

Sometimes families express concern regarding the delay of 24 to 48 hours required to obtain a result of throat culture. Clinicians feel pressure to initiate therapy immediately, prior to obtaining the result of the culture. However, because treatment of group A streptococcal sore throat as long as 9 days after onset of symptoms is still effective in preventing rheumatic fever, initiation of antibiotics is seldom of urgent importance. Early antibiotic therapy may have beneficial effects in relieving symptoms and allowing an earlier return to school or childcare, but early antibiotic therapy may have disadvantages. Several controlled studies show that children receiving immediate antibiotic therapy are more likely to have symptomatic recurrences in the months following treatment than are children who delay the initiation of therapy by 48 hours. When the diagnosis of streptococcal pharyngitis seems particularly likely based on exam findings, or when social factors necessitate an immediate decision about antibiotic therapy, the use of rapid antigen-detection tests capable of identifying group A streptococci directly from the throat swab within minutes is a reasonable option.

Most kits use antibodies for the detection of group A carbohydrate antigen. Indicator systems employed are latex agglutination or enzyme immunoassay. Tests can be completed in a matter of minutes. The currently available rapid strep tests have a sensitivity of 70 to 90% as compared with standard throat cultures. In contrast to their relatively low sensitivity, the specificity of these rapid tests has consistently been 90 to 100%. Therefore, if a "rapid strep" test is positive, a culture is not necessary, and appropriate antibiotic therapy can be initiated immediately. However, when a negative rapid test is encountered, a standard throat culture has been recommended, because of the concerns about relatively low sensitivity of rapid strep test compared to culture. Recently, an improved optical immunoassay (OIA) technology was developed that is significantly more sensitive than other detection technologies used in immunoassays. OIA-based detection of *S. pyogenes* may be equivalent, or even superior, to that of traditional culture.

Scarlet Fever When a fine, diffuse erythematous rash is present in the setting of acute streptococcal pharyngitis, the illness is called scarlet fever. The rash of scarlet fever is caused by the pyrogenic exotoxins, SPE A, B, C, and F. The rash is highly dependent upon toxin expression: preexisting humoral immunity to the specific SPE toxin prevents the clinical manifestations of scarlet fever. The modes of transmission, age distribution, and other epidemiologic features are similar to those for streptococcal pharyngitis.

The rash of scarlet fever usually appears within 24 to 48 hours after onset of symptoms, although it may appear with the first signs of illness. Often noticed initially on the neck and upper chest, the rash is a diffuse, finely papular, erythematous eruption producing a bright red discoloration of the skin, which blanches on pressure. The texture is that of fine sandpaper. The flexor skin creases, particularly in the antecubital fossae, may be unusually prominent ("Pastia's lines"). The area around the mouth is pale, giving the appearance of "circumoral pallor." In severe cases, small vesicular lesions ("miliary sudamina") may appear on the abdomen, hands, and feet. Toward the end of the first week of illness, the rash begins to fade, and is followed by a desquamation over the trunk that progresses to the hands and feet. Typical scarlet fever is generally not difficult to diagnose, but it may be confused with roseola, Kawasaki syndrome, drug eruptions, and toxin-mediated *Staphylococcus aureus* infections. A history of recent exposure to another individual (eg, classroom or household contact) with streptococcal infection is a helpful clue. Isolation of *S. pyogenes* from the pharynx will confirm the diagnosis in uncertain cases, and serologic evidence of recent group A streptococcal infection may be present.

Streptococcal Skin Infections The most common form of skin infection caused by group A streptococcus is superficial pyoderma. Also referred to as streptococcal impetigo (or "impetigo contagiosa"), it occurs most commonly in tropical climates, but it can occur in northern climates, particularly in the summer months. Risk factors that predispose to this infection include low socioeconomic status, overall level of hygiene, and local injury to skin caused by insect bites, scabies, atopic dermatitis, and minor trauma. Colonization of unbroken skin precedes the development of pyoderma by approximately 10 days. This form of streptococcal infection is usually painless and the patient is usually afebrile. Streptococcal impetigo usually has the highest prevalence in young children (age 2–5 years). Infection spreads readily to other individuals directly from the skin lesions, and multiple occurrences within families are common.

Streptococcal impetigo usually appears first as a discrete papulovesicular lesion surrounded by a localized area of redness. The vesicles rapidly become purulent and covered with a thick, confluent, honey-colored crust. The appearance of the lesions of streptococcal impetigo is in contrast to the classic bullous appearance of impetigo caused by phage group II *S. aureus*. However, recent evidence indicates that many cases of nonbullous impetigo are, in fact, mixed infections containing both *S. aureus* and *S. pyogenes;* conclusions about etiology based on the clinical appearance of impetigo should be drawn with caution. The lesions are most com-

monly encountered on the face and extremities. If untreated, streptococcal impetigo is a mild but chronic illness, often spreading to other parts of the body. Regional lymphadenitis is common. The M types that give rise to streptococcal tonsillitis (types 1, 3, 5, 6, 12, 18, 19, and 24) are rarely found in streptococcal impetigo. One pyoderma-associated strain, M49, is very strongly associated with poststreptococcal glomerulonephritis (see below).

Deeper soft-tissue infections may occur following colonization of the skin with *S. pyogenes*. A deeply ulcerated form of streptococcal impetigo, *ecthyma*, may complicate streptococcal impetigo and is encountered mainly in the tropics. Streptococcal cellulitis is an acute, rapidly spreading infection of skin and subcutaneous tissue that can follow burns, wounds, surgical incisions, varicella infection, and mild trauma. Pain, tenderness, swelling, erythema, and systemic toxicity are common, and patients may have associated bacteremia. Angiitis indicates lymphatic spread. Careful serial examination is crucial, as cellulitis may progress to necrotizing fasciitis (see Fig. 13-8).

Erysipelas is a relatively rare acute streptococcal infection involving the deeper layers of the skin and the underlying connective tissue. The skin over the affected area is swollen, red, and very tender, in contrast to streptococcal impetigo, which is usually painless. Superficial blebs may be present. The most characteristic finding in erysipelas is the sharply defined, slightly elevated border, which helps to differentiate this entity from cellulitis, which has an indistinct border. At times, reddish streaks of lymphangitis may project out from the margins of the lesion. Systemic toxicity is common. For both erysipelas and cellulitis, cultures obtained by "leading-edge" needle aspirate of the inflamed area are warranted. Perianal cellulitis and vaginitis should be considered in children who complain of perineal discomfort or vaginal discharge.

Necrotizing Fasciitis Necrotizing fasciitis caused by *S. pyogenes* ("streptococcal gangrene") is an acute, rapidly progressive, severe,

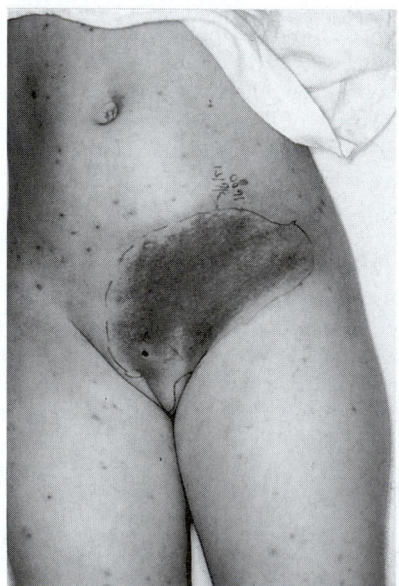

FIGURE 13-8 **Invasive soft-tissue infection due to *Streptococcus pyogenes*. This child developed fever and soft-tissue swelling on the fifth day of varicella infection. Aspiration from the leading edge of the cellulitis yielded *S. pyogenes*. Operative debridement was necessary because of the clinical suspicion of early necrotizing fasciitis.**

deep-seated infection of the subcutaneous tissue associated with extensive destruction of superficial and deep fascia. The onset is heralded by diffuse erythematous swelling, with exquisite pain at the affected site. Indeed, excruciating pain that seems inconsistent with the observed clinical findings should strongly suggest the possibility of this diagnosis. As the lesion progresses (approximately 48–72 hours), the skin becomes bluish and dusky, and bullae containing yellow or hemorrhagic fluid appear. By the fourth to fifth day, frank gangrene is present, and extensive sloughing of skin occurs. Surgical débridement of necrotic tissue is a crucial adjunct to management. The differentiation between streptococcal cellulitis and necrotizing fasciitis can be difficult, and careful serial physical examination is crucial. Consultation with a surgeon early in the course of infection is essential. If the diagnosis is uncertain, a biopsy with frozen section may be useful. Histopathology commonly reveals both microbial and neutrophilic infiltration of deep dermal and superficial fascial layers of skin, with resultant thrombosis, vasculitis, and necrosis.

Although any part of the body may be affected, streptococcal fasciitis usually begins on an extremity. It may begin at a site of trivial or inapparent trauma, or may follow cuts, burns, penetrating injuries, or blunt trauma. A major and emerging risk factor for development of streptococcal necrotizing fasciitis in recent years has been varicella-zoster virus (VZV) infection. The possibility of an association between the use of nonsteroidal anti-inflammatory drugs (NSAIDs; eg, ibuprofen) and varicella-associated necrotizing fasciitis is currently under investigation. Until more information is available, it may be prudent to avoid the use of NSAIDs in children with varicella.

Streptococcal Toxic Shock Syndrome   Streptococcal toxic shock syndrome (TSS) is characterized by hypotension and multiple organ failure. There is considerable overlap with streptococcal necrotizing fasciitis, insofar as most cases occur in association with soft-tissue infections; however, streptococcal TSS may occur in association with other focal streptococcal infections, including pharyngeal infection. Renal impairment occurs in approximately 80% of patients, and hepatic dysfunction occurs in 65%. Criteria proposed by the Working Group on Severe Streptococcal Infections for the diagnosis of streptococcal toxic shock are outlined in Table 13-44. As noted earlier, the pathogenesis of streptococcal toxic shock syndrome appears to be related in part to the ability of certain SPEs (A, C, and F) to function as superantigens.

Other Infections   Cervical adenitis, peritonsillar abscess, retropharyngeal abscess, otitis media, mastoiditis, and sinusitis still occur in children in whom the primary illness has gone unnoticed, or in whom treatment of the pharyngitis has been inadequate due to noncompliance. *Streptococcus pyogenes* is an occasional etiology of pneumonia, parapneumonic effusion, and empyema, the latter requiring drainage and frequently decortication. Acute hematogenous osteomyelitis is an important complication of streptococcal infection. Isolated bacteremia, meningitis, and endocarditis are described, but appear to be rare manifestations of acute infection. Suppurative complications from the spread of streptococci to adjacent structures were very common in the pre-antibiotic era.

NONSUPPURATIVE COMPLICATIONS   Acute rheumatic fever (ARF) and acute poststreptococcal glomerulonephritis (PSGN) are the classic nonsuppurative complications of *S. pyogenes* infections. Although the link between group A streptococcal infections and

TABLE 13-44

CRITERIA FOR DIAGNOSIS OF STREPTOCOCCAL TOXIC SHOCK SYNDROME

CASE DEFINITION OF STREPTOCOCCAL TOXIC SHOCK	
ISOLATION OF GROUP A STREPTOCOCCUS	**CLINICAL SIGNS OF SEVERITY**
From a sterile site	A. Hypotension
From a nonsterile body site	B. Two or more of the following clinical and laboratory abnormalities are required
	Renal impairment
	Coagulopathy
	Liver abnormalities
	Acute respiratory distress
	Extensive tissue necrosis (necrotizing fasciitis)
	Erythematous rash

Definite case: Isolation of group A streptococcus from a sterile site plus A. and B.
Probable case: Isolation from a nonsterile body site plus A. and B.

SOURCE: From the Working Group on Severe Streptococcal Infection (after Stevens DL: Streptococcal toxic shock syndrome: Spectrum of disease, pathogenesis and new concepts in treatment. Emerg Infect 1:69–78, 1995).

these complications has been clearly established, the mechanism or mechanisms through which the injury is produced are incompletely defined.

Acute Rheumatic Fever   During the 1960s and 1970s, this disease nearly disappeared in the United States, although it continued unabated in developing countries. Decline in incidence was attributed largely to careful disease surveillance and initiation of prompt, aggressive antibiotic therapy in primary care practice. However, in 1985, several multifocal outbreaks of rheumatic fever occurred in several parts of the United States. In contrast with earlier outbreaks in this country, most of the patients were white, middle-class children from rural and suburban communities who had good access to health care.

Rheumatic fever is most frequently observed in the age group most susceptible to group A streptococcal infections of the upper respiratory tract: children from 5 to 15 years of age. Only certain M group serotypes (1, 3, 5, 6, 18, and 24) are associated with this complication. Very mucoid strains, particularly strains of M type 18, have appeared in a number of communities prior to the appearance of rheumatic fever. The attack rate following upper respiratory tract infection is approximately 0.3 to 3% for individuals with untreated or inadequately treated infection. The latent period between the group A streptococcal infection and the onset of rheumatic fever varies from 2 to 4 weeks. In contrast to PSGN, which may follow either pharyngitis or streptococcal pyoderma, rheumatic fever occurs only after an infection of the upper respiratory tract.

The pathogenesis of ARF remains unclear. Observations that streptolysin O is cardiotoxic in animal models are provocative, but it has been difficult to link this toxicity to the valvular damage seen in ARF. Because the group A streptococcal M protein shares certain amino acid sequences with some human cardiac tissues, antibodies made against M protein may damage cardiac structures. Family predisposition and predominant HLA types reinforce the immunologic hypothesis.

There is also antigenic similarity between the group-specific polysaccharide of *S. pyogenes* and glycoproteins found in human cardiac valves, and ARF patients have prolonged persistence of these antibodies compared to controls with uncomplicated pharyngitis. Other group A streptococcal antigens appear to cross-react with cardiac sarcolemma membranes. As a result of this molecular mimicry, during the course of the host's immune response to the group A streptococci, the host's antigens may be mistaken as foreign, leading to an inflammatory cascade with resultant tissue damage. In ARF patients with Sydenham chorea, there are common antibodies to antigens found in the *S. pyogenes* cell membrane and the caudate nucleus of the brain, further supporting the concept of an aberrant autoimmune response as being responsible for ARF.

ARF is largely a clinical diagnosis that is best established by careful physical examination. The Jones criteria for the diagnosis of ARF are outlined Sec. 22.4.12. It is worth emphasizing that only a minority of patients with acute rheumatic fever will have a positive throat culture or rapid streptococcal antigen test at the time of presentation. The best evidence of an antecedent streptococcal infection is a serologic response to the organism. Serial samples should be obtained, because identification of a rising titer is particularly helpful. The most commonly used streptococcal antibody test is the ASO titer, although anti-DNase B and antihyaluronidase assays, which are measured as a part of a panel of streptococcal antibodies referred to as the "Streptozyme" panel, are also helpful. When two or more different streptococcal antibody tests are performed, an increased titer will be found within the first few months of onset in most instances of ARF.

Acute Glomerulonephritis   Glomerulonephritis can follow group A streptococcal infections of either the pharynx or the skin, and the incidence varies with the prevalence of "nephritogenic" strains of group A streptococci in the community. The clinical presentation includes hypertension, edema, proteinuria, and hematuria. M type 12 is the most frequent cause of PSGN after pharyngitis, and M type 49 is the type most commonly related to pyoderma-associated nephritis. The latent period between the group A streptococcal infection and the onset of glomerulonephritis varies from 1 to 2 weeks. The pathogenesis appears to be immunologically mediated. Immunoglobulins, complement components, and antigens that react with streptococcal antisera are present in the glomerulus early in the course of the disease, and it is postulated that antibodies elicited by nephritogenic streptococci react with renal tissue in such a way as to promote glomerular injury. In contrast to ARF, recurrences of PSGN are rare. The diagnosis of PSGN is based on clinical history, physical exam findings, and confirmatory evidence of recent streptococcal infection (see Sec. 21.8.1). Even in the absence of bacteriologic confirmation of *S. pyogenes,* the presence of skin lesions compatible with streptococcal impetigo is highly suggestive, and elevated streptococcal antibody titers in the setting of a hypocomplementemic nephritis is essentially diagnostic.

TREATMENT   Treatment approaches for group A streptococcal infections vary depending upon the clinical syndrome. Remarkably, no penicillin-resistant strains of *S. pyogenes* have yet been encountered in clinical practice. Penicillin therefore remains the drug of choice (except in penicillin-allergic individuals) for pharyngeal infections, as well as for complicated or invasive infections.

For streptococcal pharyngitis, the oral antibiotic of choice is penicillin V (phenoxymethyl penicillin). In many clinical trials, a dose of 40 mg/kg/d has been used. In general, 250 mg two or three times daily is recommended for most children. Penicillin V is preferable to penicillin G because its acid stability permits dosing without regard to meals. The most common reason for penicillin failure is noncompliance. The drug is often discontinued before the 10-day course is complete because most children appear to have recovered in 3 or 4 days. However, only the full 10-day course protects against the subsequent development of ARF. If noncompliance seems likely, parenteral therapy is indicated. A single intramuscular injection of benzathine penicillin G, 600,000 IU for patients weighing less than 27 kg (60 lb) and 1.2 million IU for those more than 27 kg, is highly effective. Because this formulation is painful when administered intramuscularly, benzathine penicillin G is often combined with procaine penicillin G to minimize discomfort at the injection site. When this combination is used in a single injection, care must be taken to ensure that an adequate amount of benzathine penicillin G is administered. The combination of 900,000 units of benzathine penicillin G and 300,000 units of procaine penicillin G is satisfactory for most children.

Even in compliant patients, recent reports suggest that penicillin fails to eradicate *S. pyogenes* from about 15% of treated patients. It is likely that many of the "failures" of penicillin therapy occur in studies in which streptococcal pharyngitis has not been rigorously defined and treatment "failure" occurred in streptococcal carriers who had viral pharyngitis at study onset.

For penicillin-allergic patients, a variety of alternative treatment options is available. Oral cephalosporins are effective in the treatment of streptococcal pharyngitis. These include cephalexin, cefadroxil, cefaclor, cefixime, cefprozil, cefuroxime axetil, loracarbef, and cefpodoxime. Oral erythromycin is also an acceptable alternative for patients allergic to penicillin or cephalosporin antibiotics. Erythromycin estolate and erythromycin ethylsuccinate are both effective, although caution must be taken to note local antibiotic-resistant rates, as up to 5% of isolates of *S. pyogenes* may be erythromycin-resistant in some regions. The newer macrolides, clarithromycin and azithromycin, have similar susceptibility profiles to that of erythromycin, but have fewer side effects. A 5-day course of azithromycin is approved by the Food and Drug Administration for the treatment of streptococcal pharyngitis, with a recommended dose of 12 mg/kg once a day for 5 days. Short-course regimens of oral cephalosporin therapy have also been studied, and offer obvious advantages from a compliance perspective. However, this needs to be balanced against the higher cost and unnecessarily broad spectrum of these agents.

The child with recurrent culture-positive pharyngitis can be a difficult management problem. It may be difficult to differentiate a streptococcal carrier with recurrent viral infection from the child with recurrent bona fide streptococcal pharyngitis. Although most streptococcal carriers do not require medical intervention, there are situations in which eradication of the carrier state is desirable. These include families in which there is an inordinate amount of anxiety about streptococci, families in which "ping-pong" spread has been occurring, or when tonsillectomy is being considered only because of chronic carriage. A course of clindamycin (20 mg/kg/d in three divided doses for 10 days) is highly effective in eradicating the carrier state and should be tried in patients with recurrent or frequent episodes of culture-proven pharyngitis. A small subset of children with recurrent streptococcal pharyngitis (seven culture-proven episodes in the preceding year) may benefit from tonsillectomy.

Antibiotic therapy for a patient with streptococcal impetigo can prevent local extension of the lesions, spread to distant infectious foci, and transmission of the infection to others. However, the ability of antibiotic therapy to prevent PSGN has not been clearly demonstrated. Patients with a few superficial, isolated lesions and no systemic signs can be treated with topical mupirocin ointment. However, if there are widespread lesions or systemic signs, oral therapy with a β-lactamase–stable agent should be administered, because mixed infections with *S. pyogenes* and *S. aureus* are common.

Patients with invasive group A streptococcal infections (necrotizing fasciitis, TSS, sepsis) should be treated with intravenous penicillin in combination with clindamycin. Because the pathophysiology of invasive group A streptococcal infection is largely toxin mediated, the use of an inhibitor of protein synthesis (such as clindamycin) improves outcome. Vigorous supportive care, including fluids, pressors, and mechanical ventilation, is also a critical aspect of management of invasive streptococcal skin and soft-tissue infections. Prompt surgical drainage, débridement, fasciotomy, or amputation may be indicated. Hyperbaric oxygen has been proposed as an adjunct to surgery for necrotizing fasciitis, although proof of efficacy is lacking. There are anecdotal reports of the successful use of intravenous gamma-globulin for streptococcal TSS, but no controlled studies demonstrate efficacy.

PREVENTION   Long-term antibiotic therapy to prevent streptococcal infections is indicated for patients with a history of acute rheumatic fever or of rheumatic heart disease. The recommended regimens are 1.2 million IU of benzathine penicillin G intramuscularly every 3 to 4 weeks, 250 mg of oral penicillin V twice a day, or 0.5 to 1 g of sulfadiazine daily.

The role of prophylaxis for household contacts of individuals with either acute streptococcal disease or nonsuppurative complications is uncertain. Some authorities recommend that all contacts should be cultured if there is a family history of rheumatic fever, or when a patient with acute glomerulonephritis is identified. An alternative approach is to treat all household contacts in the setting of acute PSGN in an effort to eradicate household transmission of nephritogenic strains. For invasive group A streptococcal infections (necrotizing fasciitis, TSS), there are limited data on which to base assessment of risk to household contacts. However, given the devastating nature of these infections and the observation that invasive disease may be caused by clonal outbreaks of more virulent strains, some experts believe that empiric antibiotic therapy of household contacts seems warranted.

Apart from rheumatic fever prophylaxis and the prevention of intrafamily spread, there are few strategies available to prevent streptococcal infection. An effective streptococcal vaccine has to provide protection from multiple serotypes. Multivalent vaccines containing multiple M-protein peptide epitopes show efficacy in animal models, but have not yet entered clinical trials.

References

Bisno AL: Group A streptococcal infections and acute rheumatic fever. N Engl J Med 325:783–793, 1991

Dajani AS: Current therapy of group A streptococcal pharyngitis. Pediatr Ann 27:277–280, 1998

Dale JB: Group A streptococcal vaccines. Inf Dis Clin North Am 13:227–243, 1999

Gerber MA: Diagnosis of group A streptococcal pharyngitis. Pediatr Ann 27:269–273, 1998

Shulman ST: Streptococcal pharyngitis: diagnostic considerations. Pediatr Infect Dis J13:567–571, 1994

Stevens DL: Streptococcal toxic-shock syndrome: spectrum of disease, pathogenesis, and new concepts in treatment. Emerg Infect 1:69–78, 1995

Stevens DL, Maier KA, Laine BM, et al: The Eagle effect revisited: efficacy of clindamycin, erythromycin, and penicillin in the treatment of streptococcal myositis. J Infect Dis 158:23–28, 1988

Tanz RR, Poncher JR, Corydon KE, et al: Clindamycin treatment of chronic pharyngeal carriage of group A streptococci. J Pediatr 119:123–128, 1991

Tsevat J, Kotagal UR: Management of sore throats in children: a cost-effectiveness analysis. Arch Pediar Adolesc Med 153:681–688, 1999

Zerr DM, Alexander ER, Duchin JS, et al: A case-control study of necrotizing fasciitis during primary varicella. Pediatrics 103:783–790, 1999

GROUP B STREPTOCOCCAL INFECTIONS
Morven S. Edwards

Group B *Streptococcus* is a common cause of infectious morbidity in the newborn and young infant. The development and implementation of guidelines for intrapartum antimicrobial chemoprophylaxis has been associated with a significant decrease in the incidence of early onset group B streptococcal infection.

Estimates of maternal colonization rates with group B streptococci during pregnancy made by using selective broth media and sampling from both the lower vagina and the rectum range from 20 to 30%. Colonization of infants occurs either vertically by the ascending route in utero or during the birth process, or horizontally after delivery. Without interruption of transmission, approximately 50% of infants delivered of a colonized mother will have mucous membrane colonization. The estimated risk for development of invasive disease among infants acquiring colonization is approximately 1%. This risk is increased when there is premature onset of labor, maternal chorioamnionitis, a prolonged interval between rupture of membranes and delivery, twin pregnancy, or maternal postpartum bacteremia, among other factors. Ongoing exposure to the organism in utero increases the risk for disseminated infection. Fetal aspiration of infected amniotic fluid may result in the development of congenital pneumonia with symptoms at birth or shortly thereafter.

The implementation of guidelines for intrapartum chemoprophylaxis of group B streptococcal infection has been associated with a significant decline in the incidence of early onset, but not of late-onset, disease.

EPIDEMIOLOGY   Group B streptococci are classified into serotypes on the basis of capsular polysaccharide antigens. The major serotypes causing invasive neonatal disease in the 1970s to 1980s were Ia, Ib, II, and III. Since 1992, a number of reports have documented the emergence of type V group B *Streptococcus*. Contemporary data indicate that serotype Ia strains now account for the greatest proportion (approximately 38%) of early onset disease isolates. The distribution of serotypes for the remaining early onset disease isolates is serotype Ib (6%), II (10%), III (31%), and V (14%), with only 1% of isolates being nontypable. Among late-onset cases of group B streptococcal infection, type III strains predominate, accounting for approximately two-thirds of infections. Serotype III strains also account for approximately 90% of isolates from infants with meningitis.

CLINICAL MANIFESTATIONS   The clinical features of early onset and later-onset group B streptococcal infections are shown in Table 13-45. Early onset infection often affects infants whose mothers

TABLE 13-45

DIFFERENTIAL CHARACTERISTICS OF EARLY VERSUS LATER-ONSET GROUP B STREPTOCOCCAL INFECTIONS IN EARLY INFANCY

CHARACTERISTIC	EARLY ONSET	LATE-ONSET	LATE, LATE-ONSET
Age at onset	<7 days (median 1 hour)	7 days–3 months (median 27 days)	>3 months
Obstetric complications	Common	Uncommon	Varies
Prematurity	Common	Uncommon	Common
Clinical presentations	Septicemia (40–45%)	Bacteremia without focus (40–50%)	Bacteremia without focus (common)
	Pneumonia (35–40%)	Meningitis (30–40%)	Bacteremia with a focus
	Meningitis (5–10%)	Osteoarthritis, cellulitis, or adenitis (5–10%)	
Infecting serotypes	Ia, Ib, II, III, V	III (~90%)	Unknown
Case-fatality rate	5–15%*	2–6%	Low

* <10% in term infants.

have had obstetric complications. However, term infants often present with no risk factors other than maternal colonization with the organism. The three common clinical presentations for early onset disease are septicemia without a focus, pneumonia, and meningitis. Regardless of the site of infection, more than 75% of these infants present with respiratory signs, including tachypnea, grunting, or cyanosis. Radiographic findings may be suggestive of respiratory distress syndrome, transient tachypnea, or congenital pneumonia. Other associated signs of early onset infection are those common to neonatal sepsis, including temperature or vascular instability, poor feeding, and lethargy. There often are no clinical signs suggesting meningeal involvement at the time of presentation, although seizures develop within 24 hours of presentation in 50% of infants with meningitis.

The three common clinical presentations for late-onset infection are bacteremia without a focus of infection, meningitis, and osteoarthritis. The onset for bacteremia without a focus may be insidious, with detection of bloodstream involvement when a sepsis evaluation is carried out for an otherwise well-appearing febrile infant. Approximately one-third of these infants have a preceding upper respiratory tract infection that may herald the development of bacteremia. For infants with meningitis, the initial signs of infection usually include fever, lethargy, irritability, poor feeding, and tachypnea. On occasion, infants with late-onset meningitis have a fulminant presentation with the development of seizures, poor perfusion, and septic shock over a matter of hours. These infants have large numbers of bacteria visible in the cerebrospinal fluid Gram stain. They usually respond poorly to supportive care and tend to have a rapidly fatal outcome or, if they survive, to have major neurologic sequelae.

The third clinical presentation for late-onset disease is focal soft-tissue infection or osteomyelitis. Group B streptococcal osteomyelitis usually has an indolent presentation and is characterized by single-bone involvement, most commonly of the proximal humerus. The signs of infection include swelling, erythema, and pain overlying the involved bone. The inflammatory signs tend to be less prominent than those of staphylococcal osteomyelitis, and group B streptococcal osteomyelitis has been misdiagnosed as Erb palsy. The hip, knee, or ankle joints are common sites of involvement for septic arthritis. Monoarticular involvement is the rule. Adenitis or cellulitis caused by group B streptococci usually is unilateral, and may involve facial or submandibular sites or the genital or inguinal region. These infants are usually bacteremic, but collections of purulence also yield the organism.

The designation "late, late-onset infection" is appropriate for infants older than 3 months of age who develop group B strepto-

coccal sepsis. In some series late, late-onset infection accounts for 20% of all late-onset disease. Those infants usually have a history of prematurity and prolonged hospitalization. Their immature host status may predispose to the development of invasive infection beyond early infancy. Bacteremia without a focus is a common presentation.

DIAGNOSIS The only way to definitively establish the diagnosis of group B streptococcal infection is by isolation of the organism from a normally sterile body site such as the blood, cerebrospinal fluid, or site of focal infection (usually bone, joint, or abscess fluid). The isolation of group B streptococci from mucous membrane sites or from a gastric washing indicates colonization only and not invasiveness. Abnormalities of the white blood cell count, such as neutropenia or elevation of the ratio of immature to total neutrophils may be found in association with group B streptococcal infection, as well as in neonatal sepsis caused by other bacterial pathogens. Antigen-detection tests are an adjunct to diagnosis but are not a substitute for appropriately performed bacterial cultures. Antigen tests of urine have produced false-positive results that can lead to inappropriate antibiotic treatment or prolonged hospitalization. Thus, the only specimens currently recommended for testing with these assays are serum or cerebrospinal fluid. Testing of infant urine to detect group B streptococcal antigen is not recommended.

TREATMENT Penicillin G is the drug of choice for the treatment of group B streptococcal infection. Initial therapy for suspected infection should consist of ampicillin and an aminoglycoside. This combination is synergistic in vitro and in vivo for killing group B streptococci and provides broad-spectrum coverage for other potential pathogens in the newborn infant. When the diagnosis of group B streptococcal infection is confirmed, penicillin G alone should be continued to complete a 10-day course of therapy for sepsis or pneumonia and a 14-day minimum course of therapy for meningitis. A 2- to 3-week course of therapy is required for the treatment of group B streptococcal septic arthritis, and 3 to 4 weeks is required for the treatment of osteomyelitis. The dose of penicillin that should be employed for the treatment of group B streptococcal sepsis (200,000 U/kg/d) is lower than that recommended for the treatment of meningitis (400,000–500,000 U/kg/d). This higher dosage is given for meningitis because the inoculum of bacteria in the cerebrospinal fluid may be as high as 10 million to 100 million colony-forming units per mL, and the goal of therapy is to exceed the minimal inhibitory concentration of the infecting isolate by a substantial margin.

A blood culture should be performed to document that antimicrobial therapy has achieved bloodstream sterility for infants with sepsis. For those with meningitis, repeat lumbar punctures should be performed after 24 to 48 hours of therapy and before discontinuing therapy. The cerebrospinal fluid findings after 14 days of therapy may suggest inadequate resolution of the inflammatory response as indicated by a proportion of polymorphonuclear cells exceeding 25% of the total, or a protein level in excess of 200 mg/dL. In this circumstance, it is appropriate to continue antimicrobial therapy for an additional week and to repeat a lumbar puncture. It is rarely necessary to continue antibiotic treatment for longer than 3 weeks.

For infants with meningitis, an enhanced computed tomographic (CT) scan of the brain should be obtained before discontinuing antibiotic therapy. This scan gives additional information about the adequacy of resolution of cerebritis or ventriculitis. On occasion, the CT scan will reveal a previously unsuspected abscess or infarct that will influence the duration of therapy or prognosis.

Provision of supportive care for infants with group B streptococcal infection includes attention to the details of fluid management, ventilation, and support of vascular volume. Seizures should be anticipated in infants with meningitis and controlled to limit brain edema and hypoxia. For infants with bone or joint infection, open or closed aspiration may be required to establish the diagnosis and to drain purulent material. A drainage procedure is required to preserve vascular supply of the hip or shoulder joints.

The mortality rate from group B streptococcal disease has declined markedly and now stands at 10 to 15% overall for early onset disease and at less than 10% for term infants. The mortality rate for late-onset disease ranges from 2 to 6%. Survivors from sepsis usually have no residua of infection. The exception is that of premature infants who have septic shock and who develop periventricular leukomalacia and attendant neurologic impairment. There are no current data for the long-term outcome of infants recovering from meningitis. Approximately one-third of infants treated for meningitis in the 1970s had serious neurologic sequelae. Infants usually recover fully from bone or joint infection, but impairment of joint function or bone growth has occurred.

PREVENTION   In 1992, the American College of Obstetricians and Gynecologists (ACOG) and the American Academy of Pediatrics (AAP) each published documents highlighting the risk factors for early onset disease and the potential benefit of intrapartum chemoprophylaxis for its prevention. The approach to selection of women differed in these two documents and neither was widely implemented. In 1996, consensus guidelines were published by the Centers for Disease Control and Prevention (CDC), ACOG, and AAP. These guidelines recommended that hospitals adopt a policy for the prevention of early onset group B streptococcal infection based on either risk factor or culture strategies. When the culture-based approach is used, all women identified as carriers of group B streptococci by cultures performed at 35 to 37 weeks' gestation are offered intrapartum chemoprophylaxis. When the risk-based method is used, those women with factors known to increase the risk for early onset infection, including onset of labor or rupture of membranes before 37 weeks' gestation, rupture of membranes 18 hours or more before delivery, or intrapartum fever are offered prophylaxis. Both strategies also target women with bacteriuria during pregnancy, as well as those women who previously delivered an infant who developed group B streptococcal infection. Penicillin G is the antimicrobial of choice and ampicillin the alternative for intrapartum chemoprophylaxis. A 53% decline in the incidence of

early onset disease has been documented since guidelines for intrapartum chemoprophylaxis became available.

The management of an infant born to a woman receiving intrapartum chemoprophylaxis is dependent upon the infant's status at birth, the duration of prophylaxis, and the gestational age of the infant. Symptomatic infants should undergo full diagnostic evaluation and empiric therapy. Limited evaluation and observation for at least 48 hours are indicated for asymptomatic infants less than 35 weeks' gestation and for those infants whose mothers received chemoprophylaxis for less than 4 hours before delivery. Observation alone is indicated for asymptomatic infants of at least 35 weeks' gestation whose mothers received chemoprophylaxis at least 4 hours prior to delivery. A comprehensive program for prevention of group B streptococcal infection awaits the licensure of protein polysaccharide conjugate vaccines now under development.

References

Centers for Disease Control and Prevention: Prevention of perinatal group B streptococcal disease: a public health perspective. MMWR Morb Mortal Wkly Rep 45:1–24, 1996

Centers for Disease Control and Prevention: Adoption of hospital policies for prevention of perinatal group B streptococcal disease—United States, 1997. MMWR Morb Mortal Wkly Rep 47:665–670, 1998

FDA Alert: Safety alert re risk of misdiagnosis of group B streptococcal infection. JAMA 277:1343, 1997

Lin F-YC, Clemens JD, Azami PH, et al: Capsular polysaccharide types of group B streptococcal isolates from neonates with early onset systemic infection. J Infect Dis 177:998–1002, 1998

Schuchat A: Group B *Streptococcus*. Lancet 353:51–56, 1999

NONGROUP A OR B STREPTOCOCCI
Dwight A. Powell

Nongroup A or B streptococci are a diverse group of gram-positive microorganisms that may be commensal or may be associated with severe, even life-threatening, infections.

EPIDEMIOLOGY   Nongroup A or B streptococci that are pathogenic for humans tend to fall into three categories: viridans streptococci, β-hemolytic streptococci groups C or G, and nonhemolytic group D. These organisms are normal resident flora of the mouth, gastrointestinal tract, or female genital tract. They are only occasionally found on the skin. Viridans streptococci, so named because of the Latin *viridis,* or green, comprise a group of at least 18 species, now subdivided into four groups: *anginosis* (previously *milleri*), *mitis, salivarius,* and *mutans.* Growth on blood agar may elicit α, γ, or occasionally β-hemolysis. β-Hemolytic groups C and G each comprise two strains, which are identifiable by colony size. Colonies >0.5 mm are considered to be in the pyogenic group of streptococci and are more likely to be pathogenic than those with colonies <0.5 mm. *Streptococcus bovis* is the only nonhemolytic group D species; it must be differentiated from enterococci, which also carry group D antigens.

Viridans streptococci do not share any of the pathogenic features of pyogenic streptococci. Their propensity to cause disease is primarily related to a high frequency of transient bacteremia following dental procedures or loss of integrity of mucosal membranes. In a study of 735 children, the rates of bacteremia following various dental procedures were: polishing teeth 24.5%, interligamental injection 96.6%, and toothbrushing 38.5%. Viridans streptococci comprised 50% of the bloodstream isolates. Some strains of viridans streptococci, particularly *S. mutans, S. sanguis,* and *S. mitis,* appear to have enhanced ability to adhere to damaged heart valves and vegetations.

Groups C and G streptococci possess in common with group A streptococci some of the pathogenic enzymes such as streptokinase and streptolysin O. Some group G organisms also contain M protein in their cell wall.

CLINICAL MANIFESTATIONS Viridans streptococci have long been recognized as a major organism causing bacterial endocarditis. In cases of endocarditis, the incidence of viridans streptococci ranges from 22 to 38%. The majority of children with bacterial endocarditis have underlying congenital heart defects and usually have undergone cardiac surgery. Rheumatic heart disease is the second most common cardiac abnormality predisposing to endocarditis.

Fever and fatigue in the background of a changing cardiac exam are the most common presenting symptoms of endocarditis. An elevated erythrocyte sedimentation rate and anemia are the most common laboratory findings. When compared to infections with *S. aureus,* those caused by viridans streptococci respond to therapy more quickly with more rapid defervescence and clearing of the bacteremia. Complications and need for heart surgery are significantly less frequent with viridans streptococcal infections. For more information on endocarditis, see Sec. 13.1.10.

Viridans streptococci are also important pathogens in some immunocompromised hosts. Bacteremia in neonates and in neutropenic patients has been described.

Group C streptococci are implicated as a cause of pharyngitis in college students. Isolation rates from the throats of students with pharyngitis as compared to controls does not vary for large-colony group C streptococci (*S. equisimilis,* 3% vs. 2.2%) or for small-colony group C streptococci (*S. anginosus,* 11.1% vs. 11%). However, the frequency of exudative tonsillitis is greater in patients with *S. equisimilis* than is the frequency in those with *S. anginosus* or with a negative throat culture. These findings suggest that while differences in colonization rates do not exist, there may still be pathogenic factors causing exudative pharyngitis in some individuals infected with large colony group C streptococci.

While reports of outbreaks of group G pharyngitis exist, a recent large study of children in Saudi Arabia failed to demonstrate any difference in isolation rates between children with or without pharyngitis. Case reports implicate group C and group G streptococci as causing a variety of pyogenic infections: pneumonia; epiglottitis; osteomyelitis; septic arthritis; pyomyositis; brain abscess; meningitis; cellulitis; endocarditis; sinusitis; urinary tract infections; bacteremia; and toxic shock syndrome. All of these occur very infrequently.

Group D streptococci (*S. bovis*) are a rare cause of disease in children. There are few reports of endocarditis (seen mainly in adults) or bacteremia, particularly in newborns.

DIAGNOSIS Streptococci are readily recovered from standard blood culture media. Complex media containing 5% sheep's blood are usually recommended for subculture of blood isolates and for the culture of streptococci from throat swabs. Colony size and hemolytic pattern determine the initial classification. There is no consensus on whether a predominance of large-colony group C or G streptococci from throat cultures should be reported. Viridans streptococci are usually differentiated from *S. pneumoniae* by a lack of optochin disk susceptibility or bile solubility, from *S. bovis* by a lack of bile esculin reaction, and from enterococci by negative PYR

hydrolysis. Speciation of viridans streptococci may be accomplished through biochemical reactions available in several commercial kits. There are limited data to support the clinical relevance of speciation at this point. It is important, however, to realize that because viridans streptococci are not common skin flora, their recovery from blood culture should be carefully scrutinized before discounting them as contaminants.

TREATMENT Groups C and G streptococci remain susceptible to penicillin; first-generation cephalosporins and erythromycin are treatment alternatives for the penicillin-allergic individual. Group D streptococci (*S. bovis*) are also generally susceptible to penicillin. An increasing incidence of penicillin resistance is emerging among viridans streptococci. Therapy must be guided by susceptibility testing, which is best performed with the E test or agar dilution. In a study of Japanese children, the recovery from throat cultures of intermediate (MIC $\geq$0.25 μg/mL) or high-level (MIC $\geq$4 μg/mL) penicillin-resistant viridans streptococci increased significantly from 62.5% to 87.5% following a short course of oral cephalosporin therapy. High-level penicillin resistance occurred in 62.5% of blood culture isolates from neutropenic children. These findings are consistent with other reports of rising penicillin resistance, particularly among blood culture isolates of neutropenic hosts. In general, these organisms remain vancomycin-susceptible. In institutions where penicillin resistance is frequent, vancomycin should be included in the broad-spectrum empiric antibiotic coverage of febrile neutropenic hosts pending antibiotic susceptibility data.

Treatment of endocarditis due to viridans streptococci or *S. bovis* is determined by antibiotic susceptibility. Utilizing guidelines from a consensus statement of the American Heart Association, highly penicillin-susceptible viridans streptococci or *S. bovis* (MIC $\leq$0.1 μg/mL) can be treated for 4 weeks with intravenous penicillin, or once daily with ceftriaxone. Gentamicin is commonly added for a period of time to achieve synergy with either a β-lactam or vancomycin. Two-week therapy with the combination of penicillin and gentamicin in adults resulted in $\geq$98% cure rates. For viridans streptococci with MIC between 0.1 and 0.5 μg/mL, penicillin and gentamicin for 2 weeks followed by penicillin for an additional 2 weeks is recommended. For viridans streptococci with MIC $\geq$0.5 μg/mL, 4 to 6 weeks of therapy is recommended with penicillin or ampicillin plus gentamicin, or with vancomycin alone.

References

Adams JT, Faix RG: *Streptococcus mitis* infection in newborns. J Perinatol 14:473–477, 1994

Mogi A, Jun-ichiro N, Yoshinaga M, et al: Increased prevalence of penicillin-resistant viridans group streptococci in Japanese children with upper respiratory infection treated by beta-lactam agents and in those with oncohematologic diseases. Pediatr Infect Dis J 16:1140–1144, 1997

Patrick C: Viridans streptococcal infections in patients with neutropenia. Pediatr Infect Dis J 18:280–281, 1999

Turner JC, Fox A, Fox K, et al: Role of group C beta-hemolytic streptococci in pharyngitis: epidemiologic study of clinical features associated with isolation of group C streptococci. J Clin Microbiol 31:808–811, 1993

13.2.33 Syphilis

Mary Allen Staat

Syphilis is a sexually transmitted disease caused by *Treponema pallidum.* The organism is a thin, delicate spirochete 5 to 20 μm long that has the appearance of a helical coil on darkfield microscopy or immunofluorescence. Human beings are the only host. The organism is readily destroyed at a temperature of 42°C (107.6°F), by soap and water, and by drying. Nearly all transmission is through sexual contact, although very close physical contact between mucous membranes might also permit transmission. Transmission by transfusion has been documented. Congenital syphilis may occur transplacentally or by passage through an infected birth canal. Long, clinically latent periods are common; the infection may persist through the patient's lifetime with a variety of clinical manifestations.

Over the past decade there has been a decline in the number of reported cases of syphilis in the United States, reflected also in the decreasing number of infants with congenital syphilis. While the national rate of syphilis has declined to the lowest level ever recorded, rates still remain high in certain US counties. Pediatricians may have to treat children or adolescents with acquired syphilis or infants with congenital syphilis, but the most common presenting problem is the management of a well-appearing infant born to a serologically positive mother.

ACQUIRED SYPHILIS

Children and adolescents who acquire syphilis follow a clinical course similar to adults. In infected children, sexual abuse must be presumed; laws require that a report be made and an investigation take place.

The incubation period is approximately 3 weeks (10–90 days) followed by the appearance of the primary stage, which is characterized by a painless indurated *chancre* that appears at the site of contact—the glans penis, the labia, or within the vagina. Primary lesions may also appear on the lips or tongue, within the anus, or on the cervix. Regional lymph nodes are usually very enlarged, hard, and painless. The chancre is usually positive for spirochetes when examined by either darkfield microscopy or immunofluorescence—the best ways to make the diagnosis. The serologic tests for syphilis (STS) may not yet be positive during the primary stage. The chancre usually disappears in 3 to 5 weeks without treatment, to be followed by the secondary stage. Secondary syphilis usually appears 6 to 10 weeks after the infection. It is characterized by malaise, fever, adenopathy, and a generalized cutaneous rash that may be macular, papular, papulosquamous, or bullous. Mucous patches are also common. Alopecia and condylomas may occur later. The patient is very infectious at this stage: the lesions are often positive for *Treponema* by either darkfield microscopy or immunofluorescence. The STSs are always positive at this stage. As the secondary stage subsides, the patient enters the latent phase. The patient continues to be seropositive without clinical manifestations. Late manifestations of syphilis (tertiary stage) are gummatous lesions, which are probably the result of hypersensitivity, as well as cardiovascular disease and neurosyphilis, both the result of longstanding vascular capillary disease and endarteritis. Tertiary syphilis is not a disease of children and thus is beyond the scope of this text.

DIAGNOSIS   The diagnosis depends on correlating clinical findings with those of the serologic tests and the results of examination of the spinal fluid.

Serologic Tests   There are two general categories of serologic tests for syphilis.

Nontreponemal antigen tests use a component of normal tissue (eg, beef-heart cardiolipin) as an antigen to measure reagin, a non-specific antibody formed by syphilitic patients. The most common nontreponemal tests are Venereal Disease Research Laboratory (VDRL) and the rapid plasma reagin (RPR) flocculation tests. Older tests that use complement fixation (Kolmer and Wassermann) are less commonly used. The VDRL test usually becomes positive 4 to 6 weeks after the infection (several weeks after the primary lesion appears) and is almost always positive at a high titer (greater than 1:32) during the secondary stage. The titer often falls during the latent phase, as it does following therapy. False-positive reactions are encountered in nonvenereal treponemal infections, and, more importantly, in a wide variety of disease states, including infectious mononucleosis, collagen vascular diseases, malaria, drug addiction, many febrile diseases, and, occasionally, in pregnancy. The RPR test is a simpler test than the traditional VDRL, capable of automation, and in all respects comparable to VDRL.

Of the treponemal antigen tests, the most widely used is the fluorescent treponemal antibody absorption test (FTA-ABS). It is both sensitive and specific for treponemal antibody and is used extensively to determine whether positive nontreponemal antigen tests are, in fact, false-positives. The test is positive in most patients with primary syphilis and in virtually all patients with secondary disease; it usually remains permanently positive despite successful treatment. False-positive tests occur rarely in mixed connective tissue and autoimmune disease and other spirochetal diseases including Lyme disease. A microhemagglutination assay for antibody to *T. pallidum* (MHA-TP) is comparable to the FTA-ABS test. These assays measure IgG and, therefore, do not distinguish disease in an infant from passively transferred maternal antibody. Antitreponemal IgM antibody testing using a method recognized by the Centers for Disease Control and Prevention as a standard may be used to determine whether an infant has congenital syphilis. These tests, however, are not yet widely available.

Other Laboratory Tests   Examination of dried smears of fluid or smears taken from syphilitic lesions can be performed by either darkfield microscopy or immunofluorescence to provide an early and specific diagnosis. The spinal fluid should be examined in selected patients because of the frequency and importance of neurosyphilis. Positive findings include an elevated cell count, an increase in the total protein and gamma globulin, and a positive reagin (VDRL) test. The VDRL is the preferred test to examine the spinal fluid; the FTA-ABS is highly sensitive but less specific (more false-positives).

TREATMENT   Early syphilis (primary, secondary, or latent of less than 1 year's duration) should be treated with a single injection of 2.4 million units of benzathine penicillin given intramuscularly for adults or teenagers. Syphilis of more than 1 year's duration should be treated with benzathine penicillin 2.4 million units intramuscularly once a week for 3 consecutive weeks. Penicillin is the best therapeutic agent and the only one shown to protect the fetus. In penicillin-allergic individuals, tetracycline given orally for 2 weeks provides an alternative. Erythromycin for a similar period of time has also been used. The treatment of neurosyphilis and that of pregnant women requires a different therapeutic approach and is not dealt with here. Penicillin treatment may be complicated by a Jarisch-Herxheimer reaction manifested by fever and an aggravated clinical picture. It is ascribed to sudden massive destruction of spirochetes and release of their toxic products. Corticosteroid treatment is helpful in ameliorating this reaction. Sexual partners should be treated. Syphilis is a reportable disease. When syphilis is diagnosed, the patient should be examined for other sexually transmitted diseases, including HIV.

CONGENITAL SYPHILIS

Congenital syphilis results from the transplacental infection of the developing fetus. An infected pregnant woman has a high probability of transmitting the infection to the fetus (90% probability during the secondary stage). Treponema organisms can cross the placenta at any stage of pregnancy, but appear to elicit little tissue response before the 15th week of gestation. Adequate treatment of the mother with penicillin protects the fetus, but the mother may become reinfected. Fetal mortality is high in this infection—25% of infected infants die in utero; another 25% die perinatally. The signs and symptoms are varied and may appear at any time between birth and 3 months of life, with 5 weeks as the median time of onset for those infants appearing normal at birth.

CLINICAL MANIFESTATIONS

Early Congenital (Prenatal) Syphilis The most severely infected infants are stillborn. Most live-born syphilitic infants have no visible lesions at birth. When lesions are present, they are most commonly on the skin and in the bones. In the first week of life, syphilis may produce bullous lesions of the skin on the palms and soles. No other syphilitic skin lesion at any age forms bullae or vesicles. The more usual pattern of skin involvement is a diffuse, symmetric, copper-colored maculopapular rash that is most intense on the face, palms, and soles. It is an infiltrative lesion that when gently scraped with a scalpel yields serum teeming with treponemas. Thus, either dark-field microscopy or direct fluorescent antibody examination may result in a rapid and definitive diagnosis. If left untreated, about 90% of syphilitic infants will eventually have some kind of skin lesion. Many varieties of papular skin rashes may occur and recur over the next months, with a high predilection for mucocutaneous sites—oral and anal. Perioral lesions may result in scarring, with fissures that persist. The recurrences become progressively less symmetric with time. The perianal condylomatous lesion (condyloma latum), so common in adults, is also seen in infancy (Fig. 13-9).

A characteristic mucous membrane lesion of infants that has no counterpart in the adult is *snuffles,* a rhinitis producing a serous discharge that frequently becomes secondarily infected. Postinflammatory scarring beneath the nose is called *rhagades.* The lesion may extend to the nasal cartilage and cause sufficient damage to result in *saddle-nose deformity.*

Congenital syphilis produces widespread lesions in the skeleton, resulting in osteochondritis at metaphyseal plates, a generalized symmetric periosteal elevation, and symmetrically occurring osteomyelitic lesions on radiographs. The humerus is the most commonly involved bone, with the tibia next; indeed, if other bones are involved, these two are almost sure to be involved as well. A bilateral moth-eaten appearance of the medial aspects of the proximal tibia that is highly characteristic of congenital syphilis has been described. More than 90% of infants with congenital syphilis show skeletal lesions. The lesions typically begin between 1 and 3 months of age; the process is usually self-limited, with healing occurring spontaneously over the next few months. The rate of healing is not noticeably affected by treatment. Radiographic findings usually disappear by 5 months of age. The bone lesions are often asymptomatic. Occasionally, there is pain, often manifested by a pseudoparalysis that may be unilateral, involving either an arm or a leg (Parrot

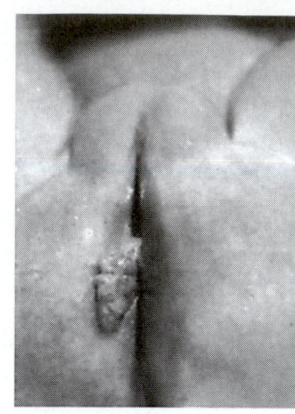

FIGURE 13-9 **Condylomata acuminata in syphilis.**

paralysis). Later in infancy, there may be recurring isolated bone lesions; dactylitis, frequently asymmetric, is a typical example.

Central nervous system involvement with abnormal cerebrospinal fluid findings are present in 40 to 60% of infants with syphilis. Jaundice as a manifestation of syphilitic hepatitis sometimes appears early in congenital syphilis and is resolved with treatment. Syphilitic pneumonitis or pneumonia alba is usually present in fatal cases, but is otherwise uncommon. Other viscera are involved less commonly. Splenomegaly and generalized lymphadenopathy are frequent manifestations of the early systemic illness. The epitrochlear nodes commonly enlarge. Involvement of the kidney, when present, takes the form of a glomerulonephritis that presents as nephrotic syndrome. Syphilis is responsible for almost half of all nephrotic syndrome in patients less than 6 months of age.

Late Congenital Syphilis Late congenital syphilis may be suspected from the stigmata, from the presence of continued active disease, or from persistently positive STSs in an asymptomatic child. In the 19th century, Hutchinson described certain complications of congenital syphilis, which are known as Hutchinson's triad: Hutchinson's incisors, interstitial keratitis, and eighth nerve deafness. The most common stigmata are Hutchinson teeth, a screwdriver or peg-shaped deformity of the upper central incisors of the second dentition (Fig. 13-10). Molars may have extra cusps that are poorly formed and that crumble under normal use. All syphilitic teeth demonstrate deficient enamel and decay more readily than normal teeth. Hutchinson incisors are visible by radiography in its preeruptive site from about 1 year of age.

Interstitial keratitis begins between 3 and 20 years of age (most commonly between 6 and 14 years). It is an intense inflammatory

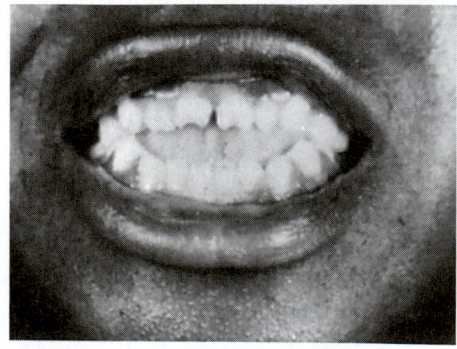

FIGURE 13-10 **Hutchinson's incisors in congenital syphilis.**

vascular infiltration of the cornea accompanied by an iritis, which may be followed by a dense cicatricial scar that produces blindness. Although usually bilateral, it may appear in one eye before it appears in the other eye. The lesion is not prevented by treatment given after the first year of disease. Early stages are characterized by marked photophobia, lacrimation, and a hazy appearance of the cornea. Later, scarring occurs.

Other active forms of late disease are gummas and osteitis, which are among the late benign syphilitic lesions. The palate and nasal septum are predilectional sites for destructive gummas, with saddle nose and perforated palatal deformities possible end results. Persistent periostitis gives rise to thickened clavicles and to a usually asymmetric saber shin. Clutton joints are symmetric synovial effusions, usually of the knees, that are sometimes painless, but which are more often warm and painful.

A more important form of active late congenital syphilis involves the central nervous system, with the most common type being meningovascular. Paresis, a potentially more dangerous form of central nervous system syphilis, occurs in juveniles, and may be detected in a preparetic state by examination of the CSF. The examination shows complement-fixing antibody, pleocytosis, and elevation of protein concentration. If untreated, parenchymal involvement may be severe and, eventually, irreversible. Juvenile tabes rarely occurs.

Any form of late congenital syphilis may have become spontaneously seronegative by the time the disease is recognized. Paradoxically, some patients become serofast, signifying an indefinitely high serologic titer unresponsive to treatment, even though therapy is otherwise successful.

DIAGNOSIS The serologic tests for syphilis were described earlier. Both treponemal and nontreponemal antibodies are transmitted from the mother to the infant. If the infant is not infected, the maternal antibodies disappear by 4 months of age. In an infected infant, a rising VDRL or RPR titer can be anticipated.

An accurate diagnosis is difficult, particularly in the first few days or weeks of life, unless *Treponema* are visible in lesions. If *Treponema* are not found, one must consider the status of the maternal infection, whether the mother has been treated, the serologic tests in the infant, the clinical findings in the infant, and the results of bone radiographs and examination of the CSF. Usually one can conclude that infection in the infant is possible, probable, or unlikely. In 1996, the CDC introduced a revised surveillance definition that also provides a good guideline for treatment (Table 13-46). Refer to the American Academy of Pediatrics Red Book for current guidelines on the treatment of congenital infection.

TREATMENT Because the probability of neurosyphilis cannot be definitively ruled out in most neonates, benzathine penicillin should not be used because it does not provide a treponemacidal level in the cerebrospinal fluid (CSF). The regimens of choice in proven or probable congenital syphilis are:

- Aqueous crystalline penicillin G, 100,000 to 150,000 U/kg/d (administered as 50,000 U/kg IV every 12 hours during the first 7 days of life and every 8 hours thereafter) for 10 to 14 days; or
- Procaine penicillin G, 50,000 U/kg intramuscularly daily in a single dose for 10 to 14 days. Adequate CSF concentrations may not be achieved with this regimen.

Follow-up is particularly important for these infants. They should be seen frequently; careful developmental evaluation, in-

TABLE 13-46

SURVEILLANCE DEFINITION FOR CONGENITAL SYPHILIS

Confirmed
  Demonstration of *T. pallidum* identified by darkfield microscopy, fluorescent antibody, or other specific stains in specimens from lesions, placenta, umbilical cord, or autopsy material.
Probable
  Any infant whose mother had untreated or inadequately treated (not with penicillin) syphilis at delivery, regardless of signs in the infant.
  Any infant (or child) who has a reactive treponemal test for syphilis plus one of the following:
    Physical signs of congenital syphilis
    Radiologic findings of congenital syphilis (long bones)
    Reactive VDRL in the CSF
    Elevated CSF cell count or protein (not otherwise explained)
    Reactive FTA-ABS-19S-IgM antibody test or IgM enzyme-linked immunosorbent assay

VDRL = Venereal Disease Research Laboratories; FTA-ABS-IgM = fluorescent treponemal antibody immunoglobulin M.

cluding vision and hearing testing, should be carried out. Nontreponemal tests should be repeated 3, 6, and 12 months after therapy. The titers are expected to decline and become nonreactive or stabilize at very low levels. In infants with congenital neurosyphilis, or in those children not evaluated for neurosyphilis, the CSF should also be examined toward the end of therapy. Repeat treatment should be considered if the STS titer increases or fails to decrease fourfold within 1 year.

Alternative Treatments When Intravenous Penicillin Is Not Available Penicillin G is the treatment of choice for congenital syphilis and neurosyphilis, and every effort should be made to treat these infections with penicillin G. Because of recent shortages of penicillin G, the CDC and American Academy of Pediatrics developed guidelines for use of alternative treatments when intravenous penicillin is not available. For infants with clinical or laboratory evidence of congenital syphilis, local sources should be sought for aqueous crystalline penicillin G. If intravenous penicillin is not available or is limited, procaine penicillin G at 50,000 U/kg/dose given intramuscularly in a single dose each day for 10 days can be given as a substitute for all or some of the doses. If neither aqueous nor procaine penicillin G is available, ampicillin may be given intravenously at 200 mg/kg/d in four divided doses for 10 to 14 days. Alternatively, ceftriaxone may be given at a dose of 75 mg/kg/d intramuscularly or intravenously for 10 to 14 days in infants <30 days; for older infants, a single dose of 100 mg/kg/d should be given. The use of ampicillin and ceftriaxone have not been well studied; thus, if these regimens are used, careful follow-up should be done to include a repeat CSF exam at 6 months of age if the initial exam was abnormal.

The recommended treatment for neurosyphilis is intravenous aqueous penicillin G. If this is not available, procaine penicillin G at 2.4 million units intramuscularly each day, plus probenicid 500 mg four times a day, for 10 to 14 days is recommended. If this regimen cannot be tolerated, then ampicillin or ceftriaxone can be used with careful clinical follow-up. It is recommended that an expert be consulted when nonstandard treatments are used.

PREVENTION Serologic tests for syphilis should be performed in all pregnant women prior to delivery and are required by law in many states. No infant should leave the hospital without the serologic status of the infant's mother having been documented at least once during pregnancy. Serologic testing also should be performed at delivery in communities and populations at risk for congenital syphilis. Serologic tests can be nonreactive among infants infected late during their mother's pregnancy. Penicillin is the only drug that, when given during pregnancy, reliably protects the fetus. If other drugs such as erythromycin are used, the infant should be treated again after birth. The infected pregnant woman's sexual partners must also be treated because the mother could become reinfected and could also reinfect her infant after penicillin therapy. Because most open lesions and possibly blood are contagious, standard precautions are recommended for all patients with suspected or proven syphilis until therapy has been administered for at least 24 hours.

References

American Academy of Pediatrics: Syphilis. In: Peter G, ed: 1997 Red Book: Report of the Infectious Diseases, 24th ed. Elk Grove Village, IL, American Academy of Pediatrics, 504–514, 1997

Centers for Disease Control and Prevention: 1998 sexually transmitted diseases treatment guide. MMWR Morb Mortal Wkly Rep 47(#RR1), 1998

Dorfman DH, Glaser JH: Congenital syphilis presenting in infants after the newborn period. N Engl J Med 323:1299–1302, 1990

Lewis LL: Congenital syphilis: serologic diagnosis in the young infant. Infect Dis Clin North Am 6:31–39, 1992

Singh AE, Romanowski B: Syphilis: review with emphasis on clinical, epidemiologic, and some biologic features. Clin Micro Rev 12:187–209, 1999

Stoll BJ, Lee FK, Larsen S, et al: Clinical and serologic evaluation of neonates for congenital syphilis: a continuing diagnostic dilemma. J Infect Dis 167:1093–1099, 1993

Zenker PN, Berman SM: Congenital syphilis: trends and recommendations for evaluation and management. Pediatr Infect Dis J 10:516–522, 1991

13.2.34 Tetanus

Gary D. Overturf

Tetanus is an acute illness caused by an exotoxin produced by the vegetative form of *Clostridium tetani*. The tetanus bacillus is an anaerobic, gram-positive, spore-forming organism. It is widely distributed in the soil in most parts of the world. *Clostridium tetani* is normally present in the intestines of horses, cattle, and other herbivora, and is found in 2 to 30% of normal human fecal flora. The highest number of colonized persons occurs in agricultural communities. A plasmid-encoded exotoxin, tetanospasmin, acts at the myoneural junction of skeletal muscles and on neuronal membranes in the spinal cord, blocking inhibitory pulses to motor neurons, producing spasms of muscles. The tetanus organism is a wound contaminant and does not cause tissue destruction or inflammation.

EPIDEMIOLOGY Tetanus in children is rare in the United States, with fewer than 20% of cases in persons less than 20 years of age. Although it has been largely eliminated from the United States, neonatal tetanus causes more than 400,000 deaths annually worldwide because of the practice of applying animal excreta to the umbilical stump for hemostasis. Neonatal tetanus is the cause of 23 to 73% of neonatal deaths and 25 to 30% in the first year of life in

developing countries. The increasing use of prophylaxis in connection with wounds of all kinds and the widespread use of active immunization have greatly reduced the incidence in older children.

Contamination of wounds by spores of the tetanus bacillus occurs without clinical signs of infection. Anaerobic conditions in the wound allow conversion of spores to the vegetative form and the subsequent production of toxin. This requires a low oxygen-reduction potential, which is achieved in deep puncture wounds, crushing injuries, and burns. Contamination with dirt, soil, or manure provides a heavy inoculum of organisms; however, *C. tetani* spores are ubiquitous, and any wound can become contaminated.

Although some toxin diffuses into the surrounding muscles, most toxin is distributed hematogenously to neural tissues. Some evidence suggests that tetanus toxin also travels along axis cylinders to reach the spinal cord and medulla. The exotoxin, tetanospasmin, consists of binding and toxin components. Tetanospasmin binding occurs to gangliosides at the myoneural junction and toxin interferes with neuromuscular transmission by inhibition of acetylcholine release. The toxin's action in the central nervous system lowers the threshold of reflexes in which the lower motor neurons are involved, and induces susceptibility to reflex spasms and convulsions. Toxin combines with high affinity to neural tissue; binding is essentially irreversible by antitoxin. Thus, only toxin circulating in the blood can be neutralized by antitoxin. Tetanospasmin also affects the sympathetic nervous system, resulting in labile hypertension, tachycardia, profuse sweating, and increased urinary excretion of catecholamines.

CLINICAL MANIFESTATIONS Two clinical forms of tetanus are observed: generalized and local. The generalized form is the result of widespread distribution of toxin; the local form is caused by distribution of toxin in the vicinity of the portal of entry. The two forms may occur simultaneously. In children, local tetanus is rare, presenting with stiffness in a single group of muscles, such as those of the jaw, the muscles of deglutition, or muscles in other parts of the body. The generalized form is more common, especially in the developing world.

Tetanus produces no characteristic pathologic changes in muscle. Various lesions may result from the violent spasms, such as hemorrhage in muscles, or even rupture of skeletal muscles and compression fractures of vertebral bodies.

Mean incubation periods are 5 to 12 days after infection. Short incubation periods (eg, ≤ 5 days) are associated with higher mortality rates, whereas long incubation periods (eg, ≥ 10 days) are associated with the lowest mortality rates. The local wound is often unremarkable and appears to be trivial. The onset is insidious, with gradually increasing stiffness of muscles, particularly those of the neck, jaw, and the large muscles of the back and lower extremities. Within 24 hours of the onset of first symptoms, the disease is generally fully evident with marked stiffness of the jaw and neck. Swallowing may be difficult, and other parts of the body musculature progressively become involved. The spasms of tetanus are quite characteristic. Cutaneous, auditory, or visual stimulation and attempts at voluntary motion initiate paroxysmal contraction of the muscles of the body as a whole that lasts for 5 or 10 seconds. During the spasm, the entire body becomes rigid; the head is retracted, the back is arched in opisthotonos, the legs and feet are extended, and the arms are outstretched, with fists clenched and thumbs adducted. The jaws are immobile, and the face assumes a tonic expression known as *risus sardonicus*. The eyebrows are raised, the palpebral fissures narrowed, the angles of the mouth drawn downward and outward, and the upper lip is pressed firmly against the teeth. Consciousness is not lost, and the patient is usually very apprehensive.

At first spasms are infrequent, with complete relaxation between episodes and only mild discomfort. With progression, spasms become more numerous, more prolonged, and painful. Relaxation between the seizures is then only partial, and a considerable degree of rigidity persists. The paroxysms may affect the respiratory muscles or those of the larynx, with fatal results. Partial or complete relaxation occurs during sleep or with anesthesia, and sedatives may afford some relief. Spasm of the sphincters with retention of urine is common. Sweating is sometimes marked; however, fever is usually absent. The duration of tetanus in fatal infections is seldom more than 3 or 4 days, and may be less than 24 hours. Death usually results from respiratory failure, the temperature sometimes showing an abrupt terminal rise. Patients who recover seldom have much fever; after several days the paroxysms gradually decrease in frequency and the muscular rigidity diminishes, although several weeks may elapse before they disappear entirely. Trismus is often the last symptom to disappear.

Tetanus Neonatorum This form of tetanus usually follows introduction of *C. tetani* into the umbilical cord, sometimes through ritualistic practices surrounding the management of the cord. The illness usually starts between the third and tenth day of life and is manifested by excessive crying and unwillingness or inability to suck. These symptoms are followed in short order by trismus, sustained tonic contractions, spasms, and convulsions. Anoxia, exhaustion, and caloric deprivation result in death.

Case fatality rates vary depending upon age, incubation period, and the availability of supportive care. Rates exceed 75% in neonates and the elderly, but may be only 15% in children with incubation periods of greater than 10 days.

DIAGNOSIS Tetanus must be diagnosed clinically. The causative organism, *C. tetani*, may not be demonstrable, but finding the organisms alone cannot confirm the diagnosis. There are few diseases with which tetanus is apt to be confused. The history of a wound, the onset with trismus, the facial expression, and the spasm accentuated by external stimuli are quite characteristic. Meningitis may be difficult to rule out without lumbar puncture. The differentiation from rabies is discussed in Sec. 13.4.18. Muscle spasms due to a dystonic reaction are easily confused with tetanus.

Local tetanus should be considered when stiffness of muscles and irritability to local mechanical stimuli develop in the neighborhood of a wound, particularly a compound fracture.

Laboratory studies are rarely specific. Cerebrospinal fluid findings are normal; leukocytosis may be present. Wounds should be débrided and cultured for *C. tetani*.

The most common and severe complications are vertebral compression fractures resulting from convulsions. Anoxia as a result of spasm of the intervertebral muscles may be a common mechanism of death. Aspiration may occur during tetanic spasms or seizures.

TREATMENT The management of tetanus includes careful supportive measures, control of spasms and seizures, prevention of complications, administration of antitoxin to prevent the binding of additional toxin, and surgical débridement where needed. Noise and unnecessary disturbance should be minimized to decrease the frequency of spasms. Maintenance of oxygenation is of prime importance. Some experts recommend routine intubation or tracheotomy and the use of assisted ventilation to reduce the risk of respiratory arrest, anoxia, and aspiration. Management of the airway includes suctioning of secretions accumulating in the pharynx and the tracheobronchial tree. Support of fluid, electrolyte, and caloric balance may be accomplished through an indwelling nasogastric tube or total parenteral nutrition.

Several classes of drugs have been used in the symptomatic management of this disease to control pain and to treat severe anxiety, seizures, spasms, and secretions. Diazepam (Valium), barbiturates, and meprobamate, in high doses given by continuous or intermittent IV administration, are useful. Most centers now manage tetanus with continuously administered neurologic blocking agents and complete support of ventilation, fluids, and nutrition.

Tetanus antitoxin in sufficient quantity may prevent unbound toxin from reaching the central nervous system but does not displace bound toxin. The dose of antitoxin should be gauged by the severity of the disease, not by the size of the patient. Human tetanus immunoglobulin in doses of 3000 to 6000 U, given intramuscularly, is recommended. If equine or bovine antitoxin must be used, the dose is 50,000 to 100,000 U. Highly purified antitoxin should be used with appropriate testing for sensitivity. In mild disease, the intramuscular route is the safest. In severe disease, one-third of the antitoxin may be given intravenously and the rest intramuscularly.

It is essential that injuries receive proper surgical care, but extensive operative intervention is neither necessary nor indicated. Although penicillin and other antibiotics will not neutralize tetanus toxin, the eradication of toxin-producing organism from the wound is achieved with antibiotic treatment. Recent data indicate that treatment with metronidazole instead of penicillin G (doses of metronidazole are 30 mg/kg/d administered in four doses intravenously and given for 10 to 14 days) improves survival and decreases disease duration.

PROGNOSIS The mortality of tetanus ranges between 30 and 50%, in spite of all therapeutic measures. Age is the single most important factor in determining outcome. The very young and the very old fare poorly. Most patients who survive 10 days of symptoms eventually recover completely. The disease leaves no sequelae.

Every patient with clinical tetanus should have roentgenography of the spine to detect thoracic or lumbar vertebrae compression fractures. Following recovery from clinical tetanus, the patient must be actively immunized against tetanus because tetanus disease does not induce immunity.

PREVENTION All age groups are susceptible to tetanus. Protection is afforded only by active or passive immunization. Recommendations for active immunization are summarized in Sec. 1.5.2. Following immunization, an antitoxin level of 0.01 IU/mL is considered protective. If an individual has completed a primary series of tetanus immunization, a booster of Td will only be needed at the time of injury for clean, minor wounds if it has been more than 10 years since the last booster; for wounds that are dirty, neglected, or where the blood supply is severely compromised, a booster of Td will be needed at the time of injury if it has been more than 5 years since the last booster.

Passive immunization is needed in addition to toxoid only if the primary series was never completed or if more than 10 years have elapsed since the previous booster. If passive immunization is needed, the product of choice is human tetanus immune globulin (TIG) 250 U intramuscularly. The human preparation provides longer protection and causes fewer adverse reactions than antitoxin of animal origin. The latter should be used only if TIG is not available and only after suitable sensitivity testing. The dose of TIG is 3000 to 5000 U intramuscularly. Td should always be given when

TABLE 13-47

SUMMARY GUIDE TO TETANUS PROPHYLAXIS IN ROUTINE WOUND MANAGEMENT

HISTORY OF ADSORBED TETANUS TOXOID	CLEAN MINOR WOUNDS		ALL OTHER WOUNDS[a]	
	Td[b]	TIG	Td[c]	TIG
Unknown or <3 doses	Yes	No	Yes	Yes
≥3 doses[c]	No[d]	No	No[e]	No

Td = Tetanus toxoid with diphtheria toxoid adsorbed; TIG = human tetanus immune globulin.

[a] Such as, but not limited to wounds contaminated with dirt, feces, soil, saliva; puncture wounds; avulsions; and wounds resulting from missiles, crushing, burns, and frostbite.

[b] For children less than 7 years old, DTaP (DT if pertussis vaccine is contraindicated) is preferred to tetanus toxoid alone. For persons ≥7 years old, Td is preferred to tetanus toxoid alone.

[c] If only 3 doses of *fluid* toxoid have been received, then a fourth dose of toxoid, preferably an adsorbed toxoid should be given.

[d] Yes, if more than 10 years since last dose.

[e] Yes, if more than 5 years since last dose. (More frequent boosters are not needed and can accentuate side effects.)

SOURCE: From Report of The Committee on Infectious Diseases, American Academy of Pediatrics, Elk Grove Village, IL. p. 566, 2000.

TIG is given, either as a booster or as the beginning of a series in the unimmunized child. If Td and TIG are given concurrently, separate syringes and sites should be used and only adsorbed toxoid is recommended in this situation.

Wound cleansing and débridement is an additional essential step in preventing tetanus. Recommendations for tetanus prophylaxis in routine wound management are shown in Table 13-47.

References

Ahmadsyah I, Salim A: Treatment of tetanus: an open study to compare the efficacy of procaine penicillin and metronidazole. Br Med J 291: 648–650, 1985

Centers for Disease Control: ACIP diphtheria, tetanus and pertussis: guidelines for vaccine prophylaxis and other preventive measures. MMWR Morb Mortal Wkly Rep 40(RR-10), 1991

Gergen PJ, McQuillan GM, Kiely M, et al: A population-based serologic survey of immunity to tetanus in the United States. N Engl J Med 332: 761–766, 1995

Saltigeral Simental P, Macias Parra M, Mejia Valdez J, et al: Neonatal tetanus experience at the National Institute of Pediatrics in Mexico City. Pediatr Infect Dis J 12:722–725, 1993

13.2.35 Tularemia

Frederic W. Bruhn

Tularemia is a zoonotic disease in which human beings are uncommon but highly susceptible hosts.

Francisella tularensis is a small pleomorphic gram-negative coccobacillus that is nonmotile and nonencapsulated. It is a fastidious organism that requires special enriched media containing cysteine or other sulfhydryl compounds for growth. Laboratory personnel should be made aware of specimens potentially infected with the organism because the potential for aerosol inhalation is high.

EPIDEMIOLOGY *Francisella tularensis* has been recovered from more than 100 species of animals. This pathogen is transmissible in numerous ways; human infections have followed bites by ticks (*Dermacentor andersoni, D. variabilis,* and *Amblyomma americanus*), deer flies (*Chrysops sp.*), as well as fleas, mites, and contact with many infected animals (including wild rabbits, sheep, squirrels, skunks, cats, and deer). Disease may occur after inhalation or intradermal injection of 10 to 50 organisms or ingestion of 100 million organisms.

Currently, most infections in the United States occur during the warm-weather months (March through September). This coincides with maximum tick activity and underscores the increasing contribution of ticks as vectors of the disease. In the past, infections with *F. tularensis* predominated during winter months and were associated with rabbits. The transmission may also occur by handling the tissues or body fluids of infected animals, insect bites, ingestion of contaminated water or inadequately cooked meat, or inhalation of contaminated particles. Human-to-human transmission has been reported only rarely and is not an epidemiologic concern.

At least five subspecies are recognized. Each has characteristic hosts, vectors, distribution, biochemical markers, and virulence for human beings and animals. Biovar *tularensis* strains (Jellison type A) tend to be more virulent, have a higher mortality, are associated with rabbit and tick vectors, and are found only in North America. Biovar *paleartica* strains (Jellison type B) are milder and rarely cause death, are commonly associated with rodents, and are not limited to North America.

Tularemia has also been reported from parts of Europe and Asia, but not south of the Tropic of Cancer. Tularemia has been reported from all the continental United States, with Arkansas, Louisiana, Oklahoma, and Texas contributing almost one-third of reported infections. The US incidence has steadily declined to less than 200 infections per year over the past decade. Children constitute approximately 20% of reported infections (third in frequency behind agricultural workers and rural housewives).

CLINICAL MANIFESTATIONS The clinical presentation may be extremely variable and includes the spectrum from low-grade fever and regional adenopathy to a fulminant fatal infection. The disease usually begins abruptly with systemic symptoms of fever, chills, malaise, weakness, and headache. A variety of skin rashes have been described. The incubation period ranges from 1 to 21 days (mean 4.5 days). Six clinical types of presentation have been described: ulceroglandular (accounting for 75% of cases), glandular (10%), typhoidal (10%), oculoglandular, oropharyngeal, and pneumonic. Children tend to exhibit fever, pharyngitis, hepatosplenomegaly, and nonspecific constitutional symptoms more often than affected adults.

Ulceroglandular syndrome This is characterized by a primary maculopapular lesion at the portal of entry; the lesion becomes pustular and then ruptures to form a painful shallow ulcer that heals slowly. The site of ulceration may reflect the source of infection; upper extremity ulcers are usually associated with mammalian vectors such as rabbits, squirrels, or cats, whereas ulcers on the lower extremities, abdomen, or back are more likely caused by exposure to ticks or deer flies. Coincidental with ulcer formation, tender, inflamed, swollen lymph nodes appear, usually in the axillary or inguinal regions. These may go on to suppurate and drain in up to 50% of infections. In the absence of specific treatment, the fever, adenitis, ulcer, and associated systemic symptoms persist for up to

1 month and beyond. Persistent bacteremia is associated with more severe infections, and seeding of other organs may occur.

Rarely reported manifestations of tularemia include pericarditis, peritonitis, meningitis, encephalitis, osteomyelitis, hepatitis, and rhabdomyolysis.

Glandular Form This form is identical to the ulceroglandular form except that the portal of entry is unknown or unrecognized.

Typhoidal Tularemia As the name implies, typhoidal tularemia presents as an acute septicemia with no localized skin lesions or adenitis. Pleuropulmonary or oropharyngeal involvement is frequently encountered (30–80%).

Oculoglandular Disease This follows conjunctival inoculation of organisms by aerosol or splashing of contaminated fluids, or by direct contact with contaminated fingers. The conjunctivae and eyelids become inflamed, and regional lymph nodes (especially preauricular) enlarge and may suppurate. Corneal ulceration may occur if untreated.

Oropharyngeal tularemia This form presents with a severe sore throat with minimal findings, ulceration, or exudation. Cervical node enlargement resembling the "bull neck" of diphtheria is associated with oropharyngeal tularemia.

Pneumonic Tularemia This is seen in laboratory workers who acquire the disease via the aerosol route. It is also seen as a companion to the typhoidal form. Pneumonia may be severe, with nonspecific symptoms of dry cough, dyspnea, and pleuritic pain. The roentgenographic features are highly variable and may mimic a variety of other atypical pneumonic processes. Absence of cutaneous ulcers or peripheral adenitis result in the diagnosis often being overlooked. The classic triad of ovoid infiltrate, hilar adenopathy, and pleural effusion is rare in children.

DIAGNOSIS Tularemia is suggested by obtaining a history of exposure (although some patients give no history of contact with any of the known vectors) or by observing the various clinical manifestations. Confirmation of the diagnosis is classically made by documenting a four-fold or greater rise in serum agglutinin titers. Titers rise after the second week of illness, reach a maximum level in 4 to 8 weeks, and may remain elevated for several years. False-positive agglutinin titers have been reported with *Brucella* or *Yersinia* infections. A single titer ≥1:160 in the presence of compatible clinical illness is consistent with the diagnosis. Recently, an outer membrane preparation of *F. tularensis* showed high sensitivity and specificity in ELISA tests for the diagnosis of tularemia. In addition, PCR tests on blood and ulcer scrapings are being developed for rapid early diagnosis.

An intradermal skin test using killed *F. tularensis* gives tuberculin-type reactions in more than 90% of patients as early as the first week. This may occur when agglutination titers are still negative. Unfortunately, the skin test may elicit an agglutinin response, and skin test antigen is currently unavailable.

The organism may be cultured from skin ulcers, lymph nodes, respiratory secretions, and gastric aspirates on cysteine-supplemented media. It is difficult to culture from the blood. *Francisella tularensis* represents a hazard in the clinical laboratory and should be handled only by informed, experienced, and immunized technicians.

Because the agglutinin titers rise relatively late and the organism is generally difficult to work with, diagnosis must often be made and treatment begun on the basis of the patient's history and clinical presentation.

TREATMENT For many years, the drug of choice was streptomycin, 30 to 40 mg/kg/d intramuscularly, divided into two doses, for at least 7 to 10 days. Failure to manifest a clinical response within 48 hours of initiation of treatment with an aminoglycoside in normal hosts makes the diagnosis of tularemia unlikely. Relapse is rare after recommended streptomycin doses. Gentamicin (5 mg/kg/d divided into three doses for at least 7–10 days) is effective. Its availability and ease of monitoring serum levels currently make gentamicin a first-line drug. Fluoroquinolones are bactericidal and show promise but are currently restricted in their use to older adolescents.

Bacteriostatic drugs, such as tetracycline and chloramphenicol, have been used in anecdotal reports but have resulted in high relapse rates, particularly when used early in the illness. If these bacteriostatic drugs are used, they should be continued for a minimum of 2 weeks. Other drugs, such as erythromycin and imipenem/cilastatin sodium, have not been studied in a controlled manner and cannot be recommended.

Reliable statistics on the mortality rate from tularemia are not available. Untreated disease prior to the beginning of the streptomycin era in 1947 had a mortality of 5 to 7%. Appropriate antibiotic therapy reduces the fatality rate to approximately 1%. Patients with typhoidal tularemia and pneumonia have a higher mortality rate. Without effective antibiotic therapy, tularemia may run a protracted course lasting weeks to months. Second attacks may occur but are usually mild.

PREVENTION A live attenuated vaccine is recommended for people who are repeatedly exposed to the organism. At present it is experimental and unlicensed, but may be obtained through the US Army, Medical Research and Material Command, Ft. Detrick, Maryland. Chemoprophylaxis has not been effective. Transmission can be prevented by appropriate care in dealing with potential sources of the organism, such as ticks (and other insect reservoirs), animals (particularly wild rabbits), and laboratory specimens.

References

Jacobs RF: Tularemia. Adv Pediatr Infect Dis 12:55–64, 1996

Gill V, Cunha BA: Tularemia pneumonia. Semin Respir Infect 12:61–67, 1997

Rodgers BL, Duffield RP, Taylor T, et al: Tularemic meningitis. Pediatr Infect Dis J 17:439–441, 1998

Sjostedt A, Eriksson U, Berglund L, et al: Detection of *F. tularensis* by PCR. J Clin Microbiol 35:1045–1048, 1997

13.2.36 *Ureaplasma urealyticum* Infections

Elaine E.L. Wang and Bernadette A. O'Hare

Ureaplasma urealyticum is one of five species in the genus *Ureaplasma* within the prokaryote family Mycoplasmataceae. The organism is oval in shape, approximately 350 μm in diameter, surrounded by a trilaminar membrane about 10 mm thick with pilus-like structures radiating from the surface. Multiplication occurs by a simple budding process. *Ureaplasma urealyticum* has at least 14 serotypes defined by serologic and biological characteristics. Their proclivity for colonization of the urogenital tract may be related to the presence of urea, their primary nutrient substrate, and the acid pH of urine.

EPIDEMIOLOGY After puberty, *U. urealyticum* colonization results from sexual contact. Seventy percent of pregnant women carry this organism in their lower genital tract. *Ureaplasma urealyticum* is transmitted from the mother to the developing fetus in one of two ways: (a) in utero, either transplacentally from the mother's blood or by an ascending route secondary to colonization of the mother's urogenital tract; (b) at delivery by passage through a colonized birth canal.

The rate of colonization of the infant is influenced by a number of factors including the gestational age, birth weight, duration of rupture of membranes, and the presence of chorioamnionitis. No infant has been found to be colonized unless the infant's mother was colonized. Although there is some evidence of nosocomial transmission, this may be the result of false-negative culture results from the mother rather than true horizontal spread.

The rate of vertical transmission varies in different studies, ranging from 22 to 65% for term infants and from 24 to 58% for preterm infants. Preterm infants were 11 times more likely to have positive ureaplasma cultures in their respiratory tract than were term infants. Colonization of the newborn infant with *U. urealyticum* appears to be inversely correlated with birth weight, although this could be biased, as very low birth weight (VLBW) infants are more likely to be tested.

Vertical transmission is not affected by the mode of delivery, but is influenced by duration of rupture of membranes. In term infants, if the membranes are ruptured for more than 1 hour, the transmission rate is doubled as compared with membrane rupture of less than 1 hour. Similarly, a lower colonization rate is observed in infants delivered by cesarean section with intact membranes versus the same delivery mode with ruptured membranes. Colonization of the neonate is also more frequent when there is clinical evidence of intraamniotic infection.

The throat, nasopharynx, and genitalia are the most frequently colonized sites. There is a difference in the rate of colonization in male (25%) and female (62%) infants, because the vagina is a common site of colonization. Comparison of colonization of individual sites (eye, nasopharynx, throat, rectum) show no significant difference. Eye and vaginal colonization fall rapidly over time, with one-third remaining positive at 15 months, but thereafter colonization remains constant for some time.

After a decline during childhood, colonization appears again when sexual activity begins.

CLINICAL MANIFESTATIONS *Ureaplasma urealyticum* is associated with a spectrum of poor reproductive outcomes including infertility, spontaneous abortion, stillbirth, prematurity, low birth weight, and neonatal morbidity. Causality, however, has not been established. No consistent relationship has been found between lower genital tract isolation and adverse pregnancy outcome. There is a consistent relationship between *U. urealyticum* with histologic chorioamnionitis and premature birth.

Ureaplasma urealyticum is recovered from the chorioamnion in 38 to 66% of patients with histologic chorioamnionitis versus only 13 to 19% of patients with normal placentas and is the single most common agent identified in chorioamnionitis. Chorioamnionitis exhibits a strong inverse correlation with gestational age at birth; it is found in 95% of pregnancies less than 25 weeks' gestation, in

40% of pregnancies between 25 and 32 weeks' gestation; and in 5% of term pregnancies.

Radiographic pneumonia is twice as frequent among LBW and VLBW babies with *U. urealyticum* in their endotracheal aspirates compared to those without. A significant increase in peripheral white blood cells has been observed in premature neonates who have *U. urealyticum* isolated in pure growth from their trachea, associated with clinical and radiographic evidence of pneumonia. Isolates from human newborns have induced pneumonia in newborn mice. Thus, present evidence suggests that *U. urealyticum* may cause pneumonia in newborns. Surfactant-deficient respiratory distress syndrome (RDS) has been observed twice as frequently in infants <34 weeks' gestation infected with *U. urealyticum*. Thus, infection may either aggravate the course of RDS or produce lung disease indistinguishable from RDS. Similarly, *U. urealyticum* infection may increase the likelihood of the development of chronic lung disease.

Ureaplasma urealyticum is a common isolate from the cerebrospinal fluid of preterm infants and may be associated with pleocytosis. The role it plays as a cause of meningitis is unclear since even untreated infants have good outcomes, and the infection appears to resolve spontaneously over several weeks.

Ureaplasma urealyticum has been recovered from the blood of babies in a neonatal intensive care unit, particularly from those babies with neonatal lung disease. A separate effect of bacteremia beyond that due to respiratory infection has not been described in this population.

It is difficult to interpret the role of *U. urealyticum* in respiratory infections in infants <1 year who may be colonized from birth, particularly as normal respiratory carriage is poorly defined. In one survey of several hundred respiratory isolates from older children, *U. urealyticum* was isolated in only 1.8% of isolates and was usually associated with other pathogens.

Hypogammaglobulinemic patients are prone to overgrowth of mycoplasma organisms at mucous membrane surfaces, presumably because the organism remains viable after phagocytosis in the absence of antibodies. Colonization of mucosal surfaces leads to hematogenous spread from the respiratory and urogenital tracts. Associated clinical syndromes include pneumonia, urinary tract infection, cellulitis, and arthritis. Between 7 and 22% of individuals with hypogammaglobulinemia develop arthritis, 20% of which is caused by *U. urealyticum*.

DIAGNOSIS The ability to diagnose *U. urealyticum* is somewhat limited. If *U. urealyticum* culture is available, it is reasonable to sample endotracheal aspirates, blood, and CSF from the premature neonate with respiratory distress or meningitis, particularly in the presence of hydrocephalus and absence of other pathogens. Culture of placental specimens may be considered after the delivery of an LBW baby. However, assignment of disease causation is difficult because of the organism's ubiquitous presence in normal persons.

These organisms are fastidious and should be transported to the laboratory in special transport media. Specimens should be refrigerated if immediate transportation is not possible. If the delay before processing is likely to exceed 24 hours, the specimen should be frozen at $-70°C$ ($-94°F$) to prevent the loss of viability and to prevent bacterial overgrowth if it was collected from a nonsterile site. *Ureaplasma urealyticum* culture involves broth, such as 10B urea broth, and agar culture, such as A8 plates.

Serologic diagnosis of ureaplasma infection in the neonate remains a research tool. Enzyme-linked immunosorbent assays

(ELISA) using a membrane protein antigen have failed to demonstrate an elevated IgM response in infected neonates.

Several polymerase chain reaction (PCR) methods are used to diagnose *U. urealyticum,* none of which is commercially available. For neonatal respiratory tract specimens, agreement between culture and PCR has been reported to be between 93 and 99%. PCR may be more sensitive. However, the lack of standardization of these PCR assays raises questions about test reproducibility in different laboratories.

TREATMENT   *Ureaplasma urealyticum* has no peptidoglycan cell wall and is therefore not susceptible to β-lactam antibiotics. *Ureaplasma urealyticum* is usually susceptible to tetracycline and erythromycin; the quinolones are showing promise.

Treatment before and during pregnancy has been attempted to reduce premature onset of labor and neonatal disease. A multicenter treatment trial, where erythromycin was initiated at the 29th week of gestation, showed no treatment benefit. In the absence of further evidence, there is no justification for empiric antibiotics to prevent pregnancy loss.

Where facilities exist, a clinically ill neonate with pneumonitis, negative bacterial cultures, and failure to respond to conventional antibiotics warrants culture or PCR of an endotracheal aspirate specimen for *U. urealyticum.* If the organism is isolated from the CSF in the absence of recovery of other etiologic agents, particularly in the presence of progressive hydrocephalus with or without pleocytosis, treatment should be considered on a case-by-case basis.

Although numerous studies have found an association between colonization of the lower respiratory tract and chronic lung disease (CLD), erythromycin treatment has not prevented development of CLD. These randomized trials can be criticized for inadequate power, but the benefits of treating colonized neonates remain to be established.

Given the in vitro susceptibilities of ureaplasmas, macrolides may be preferred for treatment. In ill preterm neonates with birth weights <1000 g, intravenous administration is usually preferred because of their poor gastrointestinal absorption. For treatment of CSF infection, the less-desirable alternative of either tetracycline or chloramphenicol must be considered because of erythromycin's poor penetration of the blood-brain barrier. However, none of these treatments can be strongly recommended in the absence of well-conducted clinical trials demonstrating that treatment is beneficial.

References

Eschenbach DA, Nugent RP, Rao AV, et al: A randomized placebo-controlled trial of erythromycin for the treatment of *Ureaplasma urealyticum* to prevent premature delivery. Am J Obstet Gynecol 164:734–742, 1991

Jonnson B, Rylander M, Faxelius G. *Ureaplasma urealyticum,* erythromycin and respiratory morbidity in high-risk preterm neonates. Acta Paediatr 87:1079–1084, 1998

Nelson S, Matlow A, Johnson G, Th'ng C, Dunn M, Quinn P: Detection of *Ureaplasma urealyticum* in endotracheal tube aspirates from neonates by PCR. J Clin Microbiol 36:1236–9, 1998

Perzigian RW, Adams JT, Weiner GM, et al: *Ureaplasma urealyticum* and chronic lung disease in very-low-birth-weight infants during the exogenous surfactant era. Pediatr Infect Dis J 17:620–625, 1998

Waites KB, Crouse DT, Cassell GH: Antibiotic susceptibilities and therapeutic options for *Ureaplasma urealyticum* infections in neonates. Pediatr Infect Dis J 11:23–29, 1992

Waites KB, Rudd PT, Crouse DT, et al: Chronic *Ureaplasma urealyticum* and *Mycoplasma hominis* infections of central nervous system in preterm infants. Lancet 1:17–21, 1988

Wang EE, Ohlsson A, Kellner JD: Association of *Ureaplasma urealyticum* colonization with chronic lung disease of prematurity: results of a meta-analysis. J Pediatr 127:640–644, 1995

13.2.37   *Yersinia enterocolitica*

Basim I. Asmar

The genus *Yersinia* is a member of the Enterobacteriaceae family that includes several important human pathogens (*Y. pestis, Y. pseudotuberculosis,* and *Y. enterocolitica*) and a number of other species that rarely cause human disease. *Yersinia enterocolitica* is a small pleomorphic gram-negative coccobacillus. It is motile at 22°C (71.6°F) to 25°C (77°F), nonmotile at 37°C (98.6°F), oxidase-negative, able to ferment glucose, and unable to ferment lactose. It grows well on all the commonly used enteric media; however, because it grows slowly and produces only pinpoint colonies at 24 hours, it is easy to overlook. Selective agar medium containing cefsulodin, irgasan, and novobiocin (CIN) enhances the growth of the organism. Isolation of the organism from specimens likely to have mixed flora, such as stools, can be enhanced by incubation in broth at lower temperatures prior to streaking on solid media. Therefore, the microbiology laboratory should be alerted to look for this organism when indicated. The organism has been classified into six biotypes and into more than 60 serotypes. The serotypes most often associated with human disease are 0:3, 0:8, and 0:9.

Yersinia enterocolitica produces a heat-stable, chromosomally encoded, enterotoxin whose role in diarrheal disease is controversial. It also produces endotoxin similar to that of other enteric organisms. *Yersinia enterocolitica* does not produce siderophores (high-affinity iron chelators), but can use those produced by other bacteria. Therefore, both iron overload and desferrioxamine (a siderophore) can increase the predisposition to systemic infection with *Y. enterocolitica.*

EPIDEMIOLOGY   *Yersinia enterocolitica* has been isolated from humans worldwide, but most commonly in cooler climates. The organism has a large animal reservoir, including cattle, sheep, swine, dogs, cats, horses, rodents, and lagomorphs. Streams, lakes, and drinking water have all been contaminated. The most common mode of transmission is ingestion of contaminated food, milk, or water. Most infections are sporadic and occur more often in winter. Occasional outbreaks have been reported within families or institutions. Common source outbreaks have been traced to raw milk, contaminated pasteurized milk, and foods prepared with contaminated water. Person-to-person transmission has not been conclusively proven but probably occurs. Because pigs are often infected, persons who eat or handle pork are at risk of getting infected. In the United States, diarrheal illness caused by *Y. enterocolitica* 0:3 in infants is associated with household preparation of raw pork intestines (chitterlings). Affected infants were probably exposed to infection by their caretakers who were cleaning the chitterlings while caring for the infants. Rarely, severe infections have been transmitted from blood transfusions. Some blood donors may occasionally have transient occult *Y. enterocolitica* bacteremia at the time of donation, and the organism can multiply to high concentrations in refrigerated blood. One instance of perinatal transmission has been reported.

The frequency of isolation of *Y. enterocolitica* from stools of patients with diarrhea is reported to be 1 to 3% in a number of studies. In one Canadian report, it was recovered in 2.8% of stool cultures from 6364 children with diarrheal illnesses over a 15-month period. It was isolated less often than *Salmonella*, but more commonly than *Shigella*, in this series. In a pediatric multicenter study in the United States, *Y. enterocolitica* was recovered from 1% of stool specimens. The yield was comparable to that of *Shigella* and *Campylobacter*, but less than that of *Salmonella*. One other study found no isolates in more than 1000 stool samples, but specimens were processed only from May to November and not during the winter months.

CLINICAL MANIFESTATIONS Infection with *Y. enterocolitica* may result in a variety of clinical presentations which, to some extent, are dependent on the age and physical state of the host. The most common clinical syndrome is acute diarrheal illness (enterocolitis) with fever (88%) and abdominal pain (65%), and is seen most frequently in children younger than 5 years of age. Vomiting occurs in at least one-third of the patients. Blood and mucus are found in the stool in approximately 25% of the children. Diarrhea may persist for 2 weeks or more. Most infections are benign and self-limited; however, intraabdominal complications occur in a small percentage of patients and include diffuse ulceration, intestinal perforation, peritonitis, intussusception, toxic megacolon, and mesenteric vein thrombosis. Rarely, patients may develop a chronic illness with intermittent diarrhea.

In older children and adolescents, *Y. enterocolitica* infection is more likely to present with pseudoappendicitis syndrome. Clinical manifestations include fever and diffuse abdominal pain that subsequently localizes to the right lower quadrant. Nausea, anorexia, and vomiting may occur. Guarding and rebound tenderness are common; leukocytosis is frequently present. Appendectomy is often performed on these patients; however, at laparotomy the appendix is normal or slightly inflamed with mesenteric adenitis and terminal ileitis. The organism can be cultured from the ileum as well as the mesenteric nodes. The pain usually resolves gradually over 1 to 2 weeks.

Adults with *Yersinia* infection are more susceptible to two manifestations that are presumed to be immunologically mediated: arthritis and erythema nodosum. In Scandinavia, reactive arthritis following *Y. enterocolitica* infection in adults occurs in about 10% of patients. The initial symptoms may include an acute diarrheal illness with fever and abdominal pain followed in 1 to 2 weeks by an aseptic arthritis. This most commonly involves the knees or ankles, but the small joints of the hands and feet can be affected. Reiter syndrome with reactive arthritis, urethritis, and conjunctivitis/uveitis is seen in 10% of these patients. The synovial fluid may contain a few hundred to 63,000 white cells per cubic millimeter with predominance of polymorphonuclear leukocytes. Cultures of the joint fluid are sterile, but *Y. enterocolitica* antigen has been detected in immune complexes within the affected joints. Reactive arthritis is more common in individuals who are HLA B27-positive. The illness lasts 1 to 4 months, but can persist for more than a year. Erythema nodosum is seen as a postinfectious syndrome primarily in middle-aged women. In Scandinavia, it occurs in 15 to 20% of patients with *Yersinia* infection. The lesions, usually located on the lower extremities, appear within a few days to several weeks after the intestinal infection and disappear within a month. Erythema nodosum may be associated with fatigue and fever.

Septicemia with *Y. enterocolitica* in children is the major complication of enteric infection in the very young and in those with iron overload syndromes. One report found that 28% of patients younger than 3 months of age with *Y. enterocolitica* enteritis developed sepsis; therefore, in those with no other underlying condition, young age may lead to bacteremia. Conditions that seem to predispose to septicemia with this organism include liver disease; hemochromatosis; diabetes mellitus; malnutrition; immunosuppressive therapy; iron overload; iron overload states such as transfusion-dependent blood dyscrasias (sickle-cell diseases, β-thalassemia, aplastic anemia); and chelation therapy. Septicemia can lead to metastatic sites of infection including hepatic and/or splenic abscesses.

Other occasional manifestations of infection with *Y. enterocolitica* include exudative pharyngitis (with or without gastrointestinal manifestations), pneumonia, lung abscess, endocarditis, urinary tract infection, cutaneous abscess, and conjunctivitis. The atypical presentations are associated with serotypes other than 0:3, 0:8, and 0:9.

DIAGNOSIS Diagnosis of *Yersinia* infection should be made by isolating the organism from appropriate clinical specimens. When infection with *Y. enterocolitica* is suspected, the laboratory should be instructed to culture specifically for this organism. The use of selective media such as CIN-containing agar is more effective than routine enteric media for recovery of the organism from stools. Cold enhancement may also increase the yield of cultures from contaminated specimens. When the organism cannot be cultured, but *Yersinia* is suspected, serologic testing may be of benefit. Tube agglutination test is the standard assay; however, enzyme-linked immunoassays (ELISA) and radioimmunoassays have also been developed. Titer determinations are available through commercial laboratories. Agglutinin titers rise 1 week after onset of symptoms and reach a peak in the second week of illness. The usefulness of serologic testing, however, is limited by cross-reactions between *Y. enterocolitica* and *Brucella abortus*, *Rickettsia*, *Salmonella sp.*, and *Morganella morganii*. Children younger than 1 year of age are also less likely to develop serologic response than are older children. In addition, some populations may have a high seroprevalence in healthy individuals. In the appropriate clinical setting, an agglutinin titer greater than 1:128 is considered presumptive evidence of infection.

TREATMENT In vitro testing indicates that *Y. enterocolitica* is susceptible to trimethoprim-sulfamethoxazole, aminoglycosides, chloramphenicol, tetracycline, third-generation cephalosporins, and the quinolones. Strains are often resistant to penicillins, ampicillin, first-generation cephalosporins, and most second-generation cephalosporins. Despite the in vitro testing, the effectiveness of antibiotics in the treatment of uncomplicated gastroenteritis or mesenteric adenitis (pseudoappendicitis syndrome) has not been established. In one pediatric trial, trimethoprim-sulfamethoxazole was compared to placebo in 34 patients with gastroenteritis; treatment did not show any significant clinical or bacteriologic benefit. However, the study was limited by the small number of patients and the initiation of treatment late in the course of the illness. Uncontrolled data suggest some benefit of therapy in patients with prolonged symptoms.

Immunocompromised patients with enterocolitis, patients with septicemia, and those with focal extraintestinal infections should be treated with antimicrobial therapy. Although there are no controlled clinical comparisons of antimicrobials in the treatment of severe *Y. enterocolitica* infections in human beings, doxycycline and gentamicin were promising in a mouse model. Trimethoprim-sulfamethoxazole (or doxycycline in older patients) can be used for focal disease. Third-generation cephalosporins, often in combination with an aminoglycoside, were shown to have successful outcome in the treatment of patients with extraintestinal infection such as septicemia. Selection of appropriate antimicrobial treatment should ultimately be guided by the clinical response of the patient and antimicrobial susceptibility results. Treatment of septicemia in patients with iron overload should include temporary discontinuation of desferrioxamine chelation therapy. Antibiotic treatment has no effect in patients with postinfectious syndromes. Recent data indicate that the third-generation cephalosporin cefotaxime is effective in the treatment of *Y. enterocolitica* bacteremia.

References

Abdel-Haq NM, Asmar BI, Abuhammour WM, Brown WJ, *Yersinia enterocolitica* infection in children. Pediatr Infect Dis J 19:954–958, 2000

Lee LA, Gerber AR, Lonsway DR, et al: *Yersinia enterocolitica* 0:3 infections in infants and children, associated with the household preparation of chitterlings. N Engl J Med 322:984–987, 1990

Lee LA, Taylor J, Carter GP, et al: *Yersinia enterocolitica* 0:3: an emerging cause of pediatric gastroenteritis in the United States. J Infect Dis 163:660–663, 1991

Naqvi SH, Swierkosz EM, Gerard J, Mill JR: Presentation of *Yersinia enterocolitica* enteritis in children. Pediatr Infect Dis J 12:386–389, 1993

Pai CH, Gillis F, Tuomanen E, et al: Placebo-controlled double-blind evaluation of trimethoprim-sulfamethoxazole treatment of *Yersinia enterocolitica* gastroenteritis. J Pediatr 104:308–311, 1984

13.3 RICKETTSIAL INFECTIONS

Gordon E. Schutze

Rickettsial infections are caused by a family of pleomorphic bacteria that contain both DNA and RNA. They are obligate intracellular parasites, have typical bacterial cell walls and cytoplasmic membranes, and divide by binary fission. Rickettsial infections have many features in common, including multiplication of the organism in an arthropod host; geographic and seasonal occurrences that are related to the arthropod life cycle, activity, and distribution; zoonotic illnesses with humans as incidental hosts (except for louse-borne typhus); fever, rash (except Q-fever and some cases of ehrlichiosis), headache, myalgias, and respiratory tract symptoms. Generalized capillary and small-vessel endothelial damage, thrombus formations, and tissue necrosis can occur and are common pathologic features. The family Rickettsiaceae is comprised of three genera that are considered important human pathogens: *Rickettsia*, *Ehrlichia*, and *Coxiella*.

Rickettsiae are obligate intracellular pathogens, most of which cause disease following replication within the endothelial lining and smooth-muscle cells of blood vessels, thus producing vasculitis. Organisms from the typhus (except scrub typhus) and spotted fever groups contain endotoxins, and most will survive only briefly outside of a host (reservoir or vector). Many of the initial symptoms and signs are referable to this pathogenesis, which may affect any organ system (Table 13-48). Progression may result in extensive vascular necrosis, vascular occlusion, and disseminated intravascular coagulopathy. This process consumes platelets and results in the characteristic thrombocytopenia. Hyponatremia, which may occur prior to this process, is the result of initial active secretion of salt into renal tubules. Subsequently, the syndrome of inappropriate

TABLE 13-48

WHEN TO CONSIDER A RICKETTSIAL INFECTION

Clinical History
　Travel to endemic area
　Exposure to vector
　Headache
　Myalgias
　Respiratory tract symptoms
Physical Examination
　Fever
　Eschar
　Characteristic rash (except Q-fever and some cases of ehrlichiosis)
General laboratory
　Hyponatremia
　Thrombocytopenia
　Leukocytosis or leukopenia
　Elevated liver function tests

production of antidiuretic hormone (SIADH) can further aggravate the hyponatremic state. Q-fever is an exception to this pathogenesis; pneumonia is the most common focus of infection; SIADH is rare, and generalized vasculitis is not seen.

Specific serum-antibody testing currently remains the most useful method of confirming the diagnosis of a rickettsial illness. A four-fold increase in antibody titer from acute and convalescent testing or a single high titer (>1:128), in conjunction with a clinically compatible illness, usually provides confirmation of the diagnosis. Many hospitals still use the Weil-Felix test for serologic testing. This method of serologic testing is insensitive and nonspecific, and is no longer an appropriate method of testing. Specific pathogen testing is now available by using various tests for detecting serum antibodies, including indirect immunofluorescence (IFA), complement fixation, microagglutination, indirect hemagglutination, latex agglutination, enzyme-linked immunosorbent assay (ELISA), radioisotope precipitation, and radioimmunoassay. Newer methods such as polymerase chain reaction performed on blood or biopsy specimens during the acute phase of the illness are specific but not widely available.

ROCKY MOUNTAIN SPOTTED FEVER

There are approximately 400 to 1200 cases of RMSF reported each year in the United States. Of these cases, approximately 90% occur between April and September. Approximately two-thirds of the cases occur in children <15 years of age, with the highest age-specific incidence occurring between 5 and 9 years of age. Although disease is rare in infants, RMSF has been described to occur in more than one family member at the same time. Today, RMSF is most common in the South Atlantic states (eg, North Carolina, South Carolina, Georgia, Virginia, and Maryland), as well as Tennessee, Mississippi, Missouri, Arkansas, and Oklahoma. Ticks that transmit the disease vary by region. In the Western United States, wood ticks (*Dermacentor andersoni*) are primary carriers and vectors of infection, whereas in the Eastern United States, the dog tick (*D. variabilis*), and in the south-central region, the Lone Star tick (*Amblyomma americanum*) represent the most common arthropod hosts. Ticks become infected by feeding on the blood of infected animals, through fertilization, or by transovarial passage. The infected tick is able to transmit the disease to humans during feeding. After attachment to humans has occurred (6–24 hours), rickettsiae are released from the salivary glands and multiply in the endothelial cells lining the small blood vessels, resulting in cell damage. For all age groups, reported risk factors include exposure to dogs, residence in a wooded area, and male sex.

CLINICAL MANIFESTATIONS The incubation period for RMSF is usually 5 to 7 days, but ranges from 1 to 14 days, depending on the size of the rickettsial inoculum. The illness is usually characterized by a short prodromal period with headache, malaise, and myalgias. The classic triad of fever, a centrifugal petechial rash, and a history of exposure to ticks is present in only 3 to 18% of patients at their initial evaluation. The onset of fever is usually abrupt and high grade [40–40.5°C (104–104.9°F)]. The skin rash, however, begins to appear on average 2 to 3 days after the onset of illness as blanching, 1- to 4-mm macules that later become petechial. The skin rash begins peripherally (eg, wrists, ankles) and spreads centrally; it is common to have involvement of the palms and soles. It is important to note, however, that only 50% of patients have a rash during the first 3 days of illness and as many as 20% of adults and 5% of children may never develop a rash. The absence of a rash should never delay the institution of appropriate antimicrobial therapy if the historical, clinical, and laboratory findings are compatible with the diagnosis of RMSF. Although physicians rely greatly on a history of tick exposure, in reported series such information was confirmed in only one-half to two-thirds of documented infections.

Other clinical manifestations include headache, mental confusion, and myalgia. The headache is described by adults and older children as being the most severe headache they have ever experienced, persisting throughout the day and unresponsive to any pain medications. Most of the major complications of this illness occur as a result of a vasculitic mechanism of injury. Complications of severe illness include encephalitis; meningitis; pulmonary edema; respiratory distress syndrome; cardiac arrhythmias; coagulopathy; gastrointestinal bleeding; hepatitis; and skin necrosis. Long-term sequelae that have been described include paraparesis; hearing loss; peripheral neuropathy; cerebellar, vestibular, and motor dysfunction; language disorders; behavioral disturbances; learning disabilities; bladder and bowel incontinence; and limb amputation. The mortality rate associated with RMSF is 20 to 25% if untreated, and 5% with appropriate antimicrobial therapy. Risk factors for an adverse outcome include nonwhite race; male gender; absence of headache; no history of tick attachment; delay in initiating therapy;

gastrointestinal symptoms; and no treatment by the fifth day of illness.

DIAGNOSIS The diagnosis of RMSF must be based only on the history and physical examination findings, because specific laboratory tests may not become positive until the second week of infection. Although laboratory abnormalities such as thrombocytopenia, hyponatremia, leukopenia, and elevated liver function tests may be present in patients with RMSF, none are specific for this illness, and therefore cannot be used to confirm a diagnosis.

Specific serologic testing should be performed to confirm a diagnosis of RMSF. This can be accomplished demonstrating a fourfold increase in antibody titer between acute and convalescent sera using one or more of the specific serologic tests as determined by a number of methods, including complement fixation, immunofluorescent assays, latex agglutination, indirect hemagglutination, or microagglutination tests. Testing is available in most state and local laboratories in highly endemic regions, as well as at the Centers for Disease Control and Prevention in Atlanta. A single titer >1:128 can also be used to confirm the diagnosis. *Rickettsia rickettsii* have been identified by immunofluorescent staining of skin biopsy specimens obtained at the site of the rash with 70% sensitivity and 100% specificity. A polymerase chain reaction assay has been developed to detect *R. rickettsii* in blood and biopsy specimens during the acute phase of illness but is not currently widely available.

Meningococcemia is an important consideration for any toxic patient with a petechial or ecchymotic skin rash. For this reason empiric therapy often includes coverage for *Neisseria meningitidis* as well as for RMSF. Other pathogens that can produce high fever and petechial rash are enteroviruses, Epstein-Barr virus, group A streptococci, measles virus, and other rickettsiae. It is important to remember that ehrlichiosis can be clinically indistinguishable from RMSF.

TREATMENT Doxycycline and tetracycline are the antimicrobial agents of choice for most rickettsial infections (Table 13-49). Chloramphenicol has been used for children younger than 9 years of age because of the side effects (eg, teeth staining) attributed to the use of tetracycline agents. The use of chloramphenicol in young children has now come into question for several reasons. Data now demonstrate that in patients with Rocky Mountain spotted fever

TABLE 13-49
THERAPY FOR HUMAN RICKETTSIAL DISEASES

GROUP DISEASE	ANTIMICROBIAL AGENT*	ALTERNATIVE AGENTS	DURATION
Spotted Fever			
Rocky Mountain spotted fever	Doxycycline	Tetracycline, chloramphenicol	7–10 days
Rickettsialpox	Doxycycline	Tetracycline, chloramphenicol	3–5 days
Typhus			
Murine typhus	Doxycycline	Tetracycline, chloramphenicol	Single dose
Epidemic typhus	Doxycycline	Tetracycline, chloramphenicol	7–10 days
Scrub typhus	Doxycycline	Tetracycline, chloramphenicol	Single dose–14 days
Ehrlichiosis			
Human monocytic ehrlichiosis	Doxycycline	Tetracycline, chloramphenicol	7–10 days
Human granulocytic ehrlichiosis	Doxycycline	Tetracycline, chloramphenicol	7–10 days
Other			
Q fever	Doxycycline	Tetracycline, chloramphenicol	7–10 days

*Doxycycline (IV): 1–2 mg/kg bid; maximum adult dose: 200 mg per day; tetracycline hydrochloride (PO): 5–12.5 mg/kg qid; maximum adult dose: 1–2 g per day; chloramphenicol succinate (IV):50–100 mg/kg/d qid; maximum adult dose: 2–4 g per day.

the mortality is higher for those treated with chloramphenicol as compared to those treated with doxycycline. Other important issues include the lack of oral preparations of chloramphenicol in the United States; the knowledge that the staining of teeth by the tetracyclines is dose related; and the lack of teeth staining with doxycyline. After informing the family of the children with life-threatening rickettsial illnesses, many experts now choose to treat patients with doxycycline regardless of the patient's age for these reasons. The optimal duration of antimicrobial therapy has not been well established for any of the rickettsial diseases because very few comparative clinical trials have examined short-course versus conventional antibiotic management. Patients should, therefore, be managed individually, reserving a briefer course for those with mild illness or for those with a rapid response to therapy. But, as a general approach for more difficult patients, therapy should be continued until patients have been afebrile for 48 to 72 hours and clinically improved.

PREVENTION Avoidance or control of arthropod vectors remains the first line of defense against rickettsial disease. If high-risk areas cannot be avoided, protective clothing that covers the arms and legs provides an excellent physical barrier to these biting arthropods. Insect repellents on skin containing N,N-diethyl-m-toluamide (DEET) or those impregnated in clothing containing permethrin become important defense mechanisms against these vectors. Avoidance of high-risk areas is still the most prudent approach for infants younger than 1 year of age because of the potential for systemic reactions with repeated applications of DEET-containing compounds. Ticks must be attached to the human host for at least 6 hours before transmitting the rickettsial organism. Rapid removal of ticks and disinfecting bedding for lice also lessens the possibility of disease transmission. The best method of removing all species of ticks is gentle traction of the attached arthropod using tweezers or similar blunt devices. After removal the site of attachment should be cleaned with alcohol. Because only a small percentage of ticks (1–10%) are infected with *R. rickettsii*, prophylactic antimicrobial agents are not indicated for asymptomatic individuals after a tick bite. Currently no licensed vaccine is available in the United States for preventing RMSF.

EHRLICHIOSIS

There are two major types of human ehrlichiosis encountered in the United States today: human monocytic ehrlichiosis (HME; *E. chaffeensis*) and human granulocytic ehrlichiosis (HGE; as yet unnamed). Other species (eg, *E. ewingii*) have also been identified as causing human disease.

There are more than 400 serologically confirmed cases reported of HME, but the exact incidence of this disease is unknown. The geographic distribution of illness closely overlaps that of RMSF, as the tick vectors are identical (*Amblyomma americanum, Dermacentor variabilis*). The majority of reported cases, however, are from Texas, Oklahoma, Arkansas, Missouri, and Georgia. The majority of children reported with this illness are white, male, and reside in a rural region. Approximately 80% of reported cases occurred during the months of May and June and 82% of reported cases have a history of tick attachment. The interval from tick exposure to the development of the illness is from 2 days to 3 weeks. White-tailed deer and dogs have been proposed as potential reservoirs of infection from which the tick feeds. Current evidence suggests that *E. chaffeensis* is introduced into the dermis of the host by the bite of

an infected tick with subsequent hematogenous spread of the organism.

Human granulocytic ehrlichiosis is closely linked to the bites from the deer tick, *Ixodes scapularis,* and the dog tick, *D. variabilis.* The majority of illness has been demonstrated in Wisconsin, Minnesota, Connecticut, and New York, but illness has also been reported in California and in other states. Although the prevalence of HGE is not known, the expanding geographic distribution of deer ticks and the predominant host, the white-tailed deer, suggests the potential for a higher prevalence of this infection in multiple geographic regions. Some serologic evidence supports a worldwide distribution. Most HGE infections are diagnosed between April and September and more than two-thirds occur in rural residents. Tick and human studies suggest a potential coinfection with comorbidity for HGE and Lyme borreliosis or babesiosis. Human granulocytic ehrlichiosis has also been demonstrated to be transmitted perinatally.

CLINICAL MANIFESTATIONS Fever, rash, headache, hepatosplenomegaly, and a systolic heart murmur are the most common abnormalities encountered on physical examination in patients with HME. The rash associated with HME is more commonly encountered in children than adults. The rash is generally distributed over the trunk or extremities and may be macular, maculopapular, petechial, or a combination of all three types. Life-threatening illness has been demonstrated in children. In one study, 25% of all patients with HME required intensive care therapy. Data on long-term morbidity and mortality in children is limited. Long-term sequelae reported to date include foot drop, speech impediment, decreased school performance, renal failure, and hypertension.

There are limited data available for the clinical presentation with HGE in children. Fever, malaise, rigors, myalgias, sweats, and headache are the most commonly described symptoms. The most important feature of HGE is a lack of abnormal findings on physical examination. Peripheral neuropathy is associated with this illness.

DIAGNOSIS The recognition of ehrlichiosis can be difficult. Patients who are evaluated during the summer with a history of tick attachment should be considered to be at risk. Elevated liver function tests, thrombocytopenia, and leukopenia [with lymphopenia (HME) or neutropenia (HGE)] are the most common laboratory abnormalities noted. Patients may also have hyponatremia, anemia, and cerebrospinal fluid abnormalities (ie, pleocytosis with a predominance of lymphocytes and an elevated total protein concentration), but none of these laboratory tests are specific for the diagnosis. Although examination of the peripheral smear looking for morulae in the monocytes (HME) or neutrophils (HGE) has been described, it is a very insensitive method for establishing the diagnosis. Likewise in vitro cultivation of the organism, immunohistologic or immunocytologic, or polymerase chain reaction are not widely available. The use of serologic testing is therefore required for confirmation in patients with compatible history and clinical findings. Human monocytic ehrlichiosis can be diagnosed with a minimum antibody titer of ≥1:64 to *E. chaffeensis* or a four-fold or greater change in antibody titers from acute and convalescent sera using indirect fluorescent antibody testing. Currently, testing for HGE requires identification of indirect fluorescent antibodies to preparations of *E. equi* or *E. phagocytophila.* A four-fold increase in titer between acute and convalescent sera or a single titer of >1:80 is required. After the causative organism for HGE is named, specific testing will become available.

If a rash is present, ehrlichiosis may be indistinguishable from RMSF. Other tick-borne infections that should be considered include tularemia, babesiosis, Lyme disease, murine typhus, and Colorado tick fever. Bacterial cultures can help exclude meningococcemia, other bacterial organisms causing sepsis, or endocarditis; while viral etiologies such as enterovirus, adenovirus, and Epstein-Barr virus can also be considered. Patients with Kawasaki syndrome are more likely to have conjunctivitis, mucous membrane involvement, and extremity changes as compared to those children with ehrlichiosis.

TREATMENT AND PREVENTION   Treatment and prevention are similar to that described above for Rocky Mountain spotted fever (see Table 13-49). There is currently no role for prophylactic antimicrobial therapy.

Q-FEVER

Cattle, sheep, and goats are the primary reservoirs for infections due to *Coxiella burnetti*. Infection in humans most often occurs after inhalation of aerosolized organisms or with ingestion of raw milk or fresh goat cheese. In urban outbreaks, infection is transmitted to humans by cats, rabbits, and dogs. Recently, several outbreaks of infection in medical research facilities occurred in individuals working with pregnant ewes. Reactivation of infection can occur in female mammals during pregnancy where high concentrations of *C. burnetti* can be found in the placenta. Animal-to-human transmission can occur during parturition of such animals by direct aerosol transmission. Tick vectors may be important in maintaining animal reservoirs, but are usually not responsible for human disease. Q-fever is endemic in virtually every country in the world, especially those areas where cattle are raised and sheep and goats are herded. Little is known about the pathologic process associated with infection because most patients recover from their illness. Evidence for human intrauterine infection has also been reported.

CLINICAL MANIFESTATIONS   The incubation period for Q-fever is usually between 14 and 22 days (range 2–6 weeks). The severity of illness in children is varied. Acute illness in older patients is usually manifested by an abrupt onset of fever, chills, weakness, headache, and anorexia. Cough and chest pain should alert the clinician to the possibility of pneumonia that occurs in approximately 50% of patients. Symptoms are exacerbated during temperature spikes, whereas patients frequently feel well during afebrile intervals. In patients younger than 3 years of age, the presentation is usually one of persistent fever without respiratory manifestations. Although pneumonitis is a hallmark of this illness, Q-fever is a systemic illness similar to the other rickettsioses. Hepatosplenomegaly and gastrointestinal manifestations (eg, vomiting, abdominal pain) are frequently noted, but rash is unusual, although it has been described in as many as 20% of patients. Most patients with Q-fever improve with or without specific antimicrobial therapy. It should be noted, however, that the initiation of therapy late in the course of illness has little effect on the course of the acute infection, and in order to prevent complications, antimicrobial therapy needs to be started within 3 days of the onset of symptoms.

A small number of patients (<1%) do not clear the organism and develop a chronic illness. The risk for developing chronic infection, however, is correlated with advancing age. Children, therefore, are infrequently diagnosed with chronic illness. Endocarditis is the major form of chronic Q-fever. Endocarditis occurs almost exclusively in patients who have had previous valvular heart disease.

Bone involvement can be demonstrated in patients with chronic Q-fever and is more prevalent among children than adults. Chronic Q-fever is difficult to treat and often ends in death.

DIAGNOSIS   Q-fever should be suspected in febrile patients who live in high-prevalence areas and who are in contact with domestic farm animals. In the United States, animal handlers and laboratory workers make up a significant portion of reported infection.

Chest roentgenographic findings for Q-fever pneumonia are nonspecific and are similar to those associated with pneumonia caused by viruses, *Mycoplasma pneumoniae*, or *Chlamydia pneumoniae*. Multiple round opacities are commonly seen even in patients who are clinically asymptomatic. Q-fever endocarditis is rare, vegetations are rarely detected, and blood cultures are usually negative. The diagnostic clue in this situation is valvular heart disease, in association with an unexplained infectious or inflammatory syndrome. Q-fever should also be considered in patients with purpuric eruptions, renal insufficiency, stroke, and unexplained hepatosplenomegaly.

Because *C. burnetti* has been transmitted with minimal exposures in laboratory settings, routine isolation by clinical laboratories for diagnostic purposes is not recommended. The approach to the diagnosis of Q-fever is serologic. Specific antiphase I and antiphase II immunofluorescent, enzyme immunoassay, complement fixation, and immune adherence hemagglutination antibody tests using paired (acute and convalescent) serum specimens is the method of choice. The ratio of phase II to phase I antibodies is >1 in acute disease, ≥1 in subacute disease, and <1 in chronic disease. Because patients with previous infection remain seropositive for prolonged periods, single positive titers cannot be used to establish a diagnosis.

TREATMENT AND PREVENTION   Treatment is similar to that of Rocky Mountain Spotted Fever as described earlier and in Table 13-49. Avoidance of contact with infected animals is the best method of disease prevention. A vaccine is currently being developed for populations considered to be at risk for the infection (eg, veterinarians, abbatoir workers). There are no specific management recommendations for exposed persons.

TYPHUS

The incidence of murine typhus has fallen from 5000 reported cases per year in 1944 to less than 50 reported cases in the year 2000. Despite this success, there still are pockets of the United States with a high prevalence of disease (eg, south Texas, southern California). Murine typhus is transmitted to human beings by infected feces from the rat flea or the cat flea. Either the flea bite or subsequent scratching by the host inoculates *Rickettsia typhi* or *R. felis* into human tissue. The incubation for murine typhus is 1 to 2 weeks, and the illness usually begins with the abrupt onset of fever. Other important signs and symptoms of infection include headache, chills, rash, nausea, myalgias, and vomiting. Compared to adult populations, children complain less frequently of headaches. The rash begins 6 to 7 days after onset of fever and is usually macular, maculopapular, or papular in appearance.

Historically, epidemic (louse-borne) typhus (*R. prowazekii*) has been a significant pathogen, causing massive epidemics of disease during periods of war and famine, accounting for thousands of deaths in prison camps during and after World War II. There have been recent outbreaks in Africa, Central and South America, but not in the United States. Epidemic typhus has an acute onset beginning 7 to 14 days after exposure to an infected louse. High fever

[39–40°C (102.2–104°F)] and headache precede by 3 to 7 days a rash, which has a central distribution, spreading to the extremities, but usually sparing the palms and soles. This rash progresses from blanching macules to papules, petechiae, and occasionally ecchymoses. Patients who have recovered from epidemic typhus may retain the organism for an extended period of time, relapsing years later with Brill-Zinsser disease, a milder illness.

Scrub typhus (*R. tsutsugamushi*) is a disease transmitted by chiggers and is endemic in Southeast Asia and the southwestern Pacific. The chigger bite results in a papule, enlarging to a bulla that rapidly sloughs, leaving a shallow ulcer. A black crust surrounded by a 1- to 2-cm erythematous raised circle then forms. At this time, other systemic symptoms begin, at first insidiously with a low-grade fever, headache, chills, and anorexia. Within 5 days, an unremitting fever to 40°C (104°F) accompanied by a severe headache is seen in virtually all patients. Generalized lymphadenopathy is the most consistent physical finding, occurring in 80 to 90% of patients. The characteristic rash of scrub typhus is maculopapular and generalized but most apparent on nonexposed skin surfaces.

Treatment for these disorders is outlined in Table 13-49.

RICKETTSIALPOX

This mild infection produced by *R. akari* has been reported primarily from New York City in the United States, but has been observed in a number of other large cities, especially during periods when large mice populations were being exterminated. Infected mite vectors of *R. akari* then attach to human beings, the most available alternative host, and produce disease. Because the skin rash resembles chickenpox, this infectious process was named rickettsialpox. Incubation is estimated at 9 to 14 days as determined by the time period following documented attachment of arthropod vectors. Initially, a red papule appears at the site of the mite bite. This lesion enlarges to form a black eschar, at which time fever is first observed. The rash begins as diffuse nonpruritic macules, progressing to maculopapules and to papulovesicles, resembling chickenpox. The palms, soles, and mucous membranes are occasionally involved, but distribution of lesions is quite variable. Fever, chills, and headache persist for about 5 days, but rarely more than 10 days. Upper respiratory and gastrointestinal symptoms are common. Untreated, recovery is still universal, but appropriate antibiotics (Table 13-49) may shorten duration of symptoms in more severe illness.

References

Abramson JS, Givner LB: Rocky Mountain spotted fever. Pediatr Infect Dis J 18:539–540, 1999

Archibald LK, Sexton DJ: Long-term sequelae of Rocky Mountain spotted fever. Clin Infect Dis 20:1122–1125, 1995

Brettman LR, Levin S, Holzman RS, et al: Rickettsialpox: report of an outbreak and a contemporary review. Medicine (Baltimore) 60:362–372, 1981

Dumler JS: Murine typhus. Semin Pediatr Infect Dis 5:137–142, 1994

Edwards MS: Ehrlichiosis in children. Semin Pediatr Infect Dis 5:143, 1994

Horowitz HW, Kilchevsky E, Haber S, et al: Perinatal transmission of the agent of human granulocytic ehrlichiosis. N Engl J Med 339:375–378, 1998

Jacobs RF, Schutze GE: Ehrlichiosis in children. J Pediatr 131:184–192, 1997

Raoult D, Marrie T: Q-fever. Clin Infect Dis 20:489–495, 1995

Ruiz-Contreras J, Montero RG, Amador JTR, Corradi EG, Vera AS: Q-fever in children. Am J Dis Child 147:300–302, 1993

Schutze GE: Prevention of tick infestation. Semin Pediatr Infect Dis 5:157–160, 1994

Schutze GE, Jacobs RF: Human monocytic ehrlichiosis in children. Pediatrics 100:E10, 1997

Thorner AR, Walker DH, Petri WA Jr: Rocky Mountain spotted fever. Clin Infect Dis 27:1353–1359, 1998

13.4   VIRAL INFECTIONS

13.4.1   Arboviruses

E. Lee Ford-Jones and Harvey Artsob

Arboviruses or arthropod-borne viruses primarily include mosquito- or tick-borne agents causing infections of the central nervous system and other febrile illnesses. Arbovirus infection should be considered in the differential diagnosis of children evaluated in the United States and Canada because:

1. Arbovirus infections can be acquired in North America; most of these infections will cause central nervous system (CNS) manifestations, with the exception of Colorado tick fever;
2. Children who have traveled abroad may be incubating viruses on arrival, manifesting signs of infection within days thereafter; and
3. There is growing concern that some arbovirus infections (eg, dengue and yellow fever) have the potential to become endemic in North America because of the establishment of relevant arthropod vectors in parts of the United States.

Most arboviruses are maintained by a nonhuman primary vertebrate (eg, birds and rodents) and a primary arthropod vector (eg, mosquito). Humans are usually only incidentally infected. The boundaries of infection are imposed by the range of the arthropod vector and the habitat of the animal reservoir, as well as various geographic and climatologic factors.

The resurgence of arboviral diseases worldwide has been facilitated by the proliferation and ineffective control of the mosquito in water supplies adjacent to an increased number of human dwellings, uncontrolled urban development, a decay in public health resources, and air travel. Of the more than 550 arboviruses recognized worldwide, only those causing the more common endemic and imported human diseases in North America are presented here.

Most important to the clinical diagnosis is the consideration of arboviral disease in children living in or returning from endemic regions, that is, recent travel history, generally within the past month. Arboviral infection is highly seasonal and occurs in specific geographic areas. Establishing a diagnosis requires a detailed clinical summary and, at a minimum, testing of paired sera. Advice can be obtained through local Infectious Diseases and Public Health consultants and at the Centers for Disease Control and Prevention, Division of Vector-Borne Infectious Diseases (970-221-6400) and Special Pathogens Branch (404-639-1115); the US Army Research Institute for Infectious Diseases (301-619-2722); and the Laboratory Center for Disease Control (204-789-2134).

ARBOVIRUSES ENDEMIC TO THE UNITED STATES AND CANADA

Of more than 60 arboviruses in the United States and Canada, the seven known to cause significant human illness are Western equine encephalitis (WEE); Eastern equine encephalitis (EEE); St. Louis encephalitis (SLE); California serogroup (CAL including LaCrosse, Jamestown Canyon, and Snowshoe hare); Venezuelan equine encephalitis; Powassan (POW); and Colorado tick fever (CTF). Except for the latter two, mosquitoes are the main vectors and epidemics often occur in years with greater rainfall. The majority of arboviral infection transmitted by mosquitoes peak during the summer and early fall in most of North America, whereas tick-borne infections may be encountered over a wider time frame, from spring to fall. See Table 13-50.

EPIDEMIOLOGY AND CLINICAL MANIFESTATIONS In selected geographic areas, WEE, EEE, SLE, POW, CAL, and VEE viruses cause febrile illnesses with central nervous system involvement, whereas CTF causes a systemic illness. During epidemics of arboviral activity, persons of all ages may be infected, but most arboviral infections are asymptomatic.

California Serogroup Encephalitis LaCrosse virus of the CAL serogroup of viruses is the most frequently reported arboviral cause of pediatric encephalitis in the United States. It occurs primarily in the upper Midwestern states between May and October, but peaks in the summer, usually in children younger than 14 years of age. The forest-dwelling mosquito vector is a daytime feeder with a very short flight range; humans are bitten when they go into the woods, possibly explaining the predominance of infection in boys.

Snowshoe hare virus is the most frequent cause of CAL serogroup encephalitis in Canada; children are the predominant age group affected. Infections due to Jamestown Canyon virus have also been documented in North America. It is not always possible serologically to distinguish which of the CAL serogroup viruses is responsible for an infection.

Fever averaging a week in duration and headache are universally reported (unless young age precludes the latter), usually after a 1- to 3-day prodrome of malaise, lethargy, and restlessness. Gastrointestinal manifestations are common, whereas respiratory findings are not. Sensorial changes from confusion to coma occur in 90% of patients, meningismus, seizures, and lethargy occur in about 50% of cases; hyperreflexia, weakness, and other neurologic findings are

highly variable. The case fatality rate of LaCrosse encephalitis is 0.5%.

St. Louis Encephalitis Sporadic cases and periodic outbreaks occur in the late summer and fall throughout the United States, including in the southeast. One large outbreak was documented in Canada in 1975. SLE virus may cause fever, headache, aseptic meningitis, or encephalitis; findings in encephalitis include confusion, lack of focal neurologic findings, seizures, and generalized weakness and tremor. The risk of illness, its severity, and the case fatality rate all increase with age. SLE is more severe in the elderly in whom there is a case fatality rate of 22%, as compared to 2% in the young. Twenty-five percent of survivors of SLE have permanent neurologic sequelae.

Eastern Equine Encephalitis EEE is the most severe, albeit rare, arthropod-borne encephalitis in North America, occurring along the Atlantic and Gulf Coasts and having a 35% case fatality rate. Infection can occur throughout the year in Florida. Risk factors include age (children <15 years old and adults >55 year old account for 70–90% of cases during outbreaks), residence, and extent of time spent in rural areas, particularly wooded areas near marshes and swamps. Infection can be either systemic (fever, chills, arthralgia, myalgia) or encephalitic, with abrupt onset of headache, confusion, focal neurologic deficits, seizures, and coma.

Western Equine Encephalitis Epidemics of WEE have occurred most frequently in North America agroecosystems west of the Mississippi River drainage, and in association with the distribution and abundance of the primary mosquito vector *Culex tarsalis*. WEE is most commonly symptomatic in the first year of life and in the elderly, although the majority of all infections are asymptomatic. Clinical presentations range from fever with headache to aseptic meningitis and encephalitis. Weakness of the extremities and altered reflexes (either hypo- or hyperreflexia) are characteristic clinical findings. The overall case fatality rate is 3 to 4%, with sequelae being common in infants.

Venezuelan Equine Encephalitis While primarily a disease of Central and South America, a VEE subtype called Everglades virus

TABLE 13-50

ARBOVIRUSES ENDEMIC TO THE UNITED STATES AND CANADA

FAMILY/VIRUS	GEOGRAPHIC AREA	VECTOR (INCUBATION PERIOD)	DISEASE SYNDROME
Togaviridae*			
Eastern equine encephalitis	Eastern Canada, eastern United States	Mosquitoes (3–10 days)	Encephalitis
Western equine encephalitis	Rural western United States, western Canada	Mosquitoes (5–10 days)	Encephalitis, fever
Flaviviridae			
Powassan	Canada, northern United States	Ticks (4–18 days)	Encephalitis
St. Louis encephalitis	Urban Midwest and southern United States; rural West, Canada	Mosquitoes (4–21 days)	Encephalitis, fever
Bunyaviridae			
California encephalitis	Western United States, western Canada	Mosquitoes (5–15 days)	Fever, encephalitis
Jamestown Canyon	United States, Canada	Mosquitoes (5–15 days)	Fever, encephalitis
LaCrosse (California serogroup)	Rural and suburban woodland exposure Midwest, eastern, southern United States	Mosquitoes (5–15 days)	Fever, encephalitis
Snowshoe hare	Canada, northern United States	Mosquitoes (5–15 days)	Fever, encephalitis
Reoviridae			
Colorado tick fever	Western United States, western Canada	Ticks (3–6 days)	Fever, myalgia

*Venezuelan equine encephalitis has also been reported in south Florida and in Texas.

SOURCE: *Modified from Calisher CH: Medically important arboviruses of the United States and Canada. Clin Microbiol Rev 7:89–116, 1994, with permission.*

is enzootic in Florida. Epizootic VEE reached into Texas in one previous outbreak. Most infected persons develop a brief, prostrating, flu-like illness, but about 5%, mostly children, develop CNS infection.

Powassan POW encephalitis occurs rarely. Since 1958, only 24 symptomatic infections have been recognized from the northeastern United States and eastern Canada; 85% of these infections occurred in persons under 20 years of age.

Colorado Tick Fever CTF symptoms include high fever; chills; arthralgia; myalgia; severe headache; ocular pain and conjunctival injection; variable hepatosplenomegaly; and transient petechial or maculopapular rash. The disease may progress to hemorrhage, aseptic meningitis, and encephalitis, and may be transmitted by transfusion. Exposure to infected ticks occurs in the western United States, and in southern Alberta and British Columbia, Canada.

DIAGNOSIS A virus-specific IgM antibody captured by enzyme-linked immunosorbent assay test from a cerebrospinal fluid (CSF) sample taken during the acute stage of illness is the most sensitive and specific means of making the diagnosis of arboviral encephalitis. A four-fold or greater change in titer is also commonly used for confirmatory diagnosis. Serologic testing of paired sera, and/or CSF, or viral nucleic acid detection is available in selected state, research, and reference laboratories. The presence of serum antibody does not confirm present or previous infection, although high-titer IgM on a single sample does provide presumptive evidence of infection. Whole-blood, serum, tissue samples, or autopsy specimens for viral isolation should be processed immediately or placed on dry ice at −70°C in consultation with the reference laboratory.

MANAGEMENT Treatment is supportive and standard isolation precautions are recommended. Person-to-person transmission does not occur, but care should be taken in handling body fluids and tissue.

PREVENTION Human vaccines to WEE and EEE are available to the US Army but not to the general public. However, the low attack rates for EEE and WEE, as well as the low morbidity of WEE, make routine preexposure vaccination impractical. A vaccine for VEE is also available.

Public health mosquito control programs may be either larvicidal (a chemically less intrusive means of controlling mosquito numbers, thus reducing the risk for disease transmission) or adulticidal (which targets adult mosquitoes during times of epidemic activity). Personal precautions to avoid mosquito bites include minimizing outdoor activity during twilight hours, repellents, protective clothing, aerosol insecticides, and screening. Permethrin applied to clothing kills adherent ticks and mosquitoes. Repellents containing DEET (*N, N*-diethyl-*m*-toluamide) should be applied to exposed skin only and used sparingly.

IMPORTED ARBOVIRAL INFECTIONS

The speed and volume of international travel have increased the risk that persons incubating arboviral diseases may arrive in the United States or Canada. Because immediate access to a specialist familiar with these diseases may not be available, all physicians must be able to recognize the possibility of travel-related disease. While rural travel is generally associated with a higher risk of arboviral infection, dengue and yellow fever occur with urban exposure. The diverse findings of infection with imported arboviruses include fever, rash, polyarthritis, meninogencephalitis, hepatitis, and hemorrhagic fever (Table 13-51).

DENGUE Hundreds of thousands of symptomatic cases of dengue are reported each year in tropical regions of the Americas, Africa, Asia, and Oceania. There was a global resurgence of dengue in the 1990s coupled with increased numbers and expanded distribution of the two relevant mosquito vectors, *Aedes aegypti* and *A. albopictus*. Dengue infections are a leading cause of hospitalization and death among children in many Southeast Asian countries.

Dengue must be considered in the differential diagnosis of a flu-like viral syndrome in all patients with a history of travel to any tropical area. The incubation period averages 4 to 7 days (range 3–14). The spectrum of illness ranges from inapparent or mild febrile illness to severe and fatal hemorrhagic disease. (See Sec. 13.4.4 for a full description of clinical manifestations.)

YELLOW FEVER This disease is endemic in South America and Africa, and the American tropics are at their highest risk of urban epidemics in over 50 years. With the expanded distribution of its vector (*A. aegypti*), there is potential for transmission. Although most cases are mild and limited to fever, headache, nausea, myalgia,

TABLE 13-51

ACUTE, FEBRILE DISEASES AND HEMORRHAGIC FEVERS CAUSED BY ARBOVIRUSES

DISEASE	GEOGRAPHIC DISTRIBUTION OF VIRUS	CLINICAL SYNDROME	INCUBATION PERIOD, d
Yellow fever	Tropical areas of South America and Africa	Febrile illness, hepatitis, hemorrhagic fever	3–6
Dengue	Tropical areas worldwide: Caribbean, Central and South America, Asia, Australia, Oceania, Africa	Febrile illness—may be biphasic with rash, hemorrhagic fever and shock	3–14
Mayaro	Central and South America	Febrile illness and polyarthritis	1–12
Chikungunya	Africa, Asia	Febrile illness, rash, and polyarthritis	1–12
O'Nyong-nyong	Africa	Febrile illness, rash, and polyarthritis	1–12
Sindbis	Africa, Scandinavia, former Soviet Union countries, Asia, Australia	Febrile illness, rash, and polyarthritis	1–12
Ross River	Australia, South Pacific	Febrile illness, rash, and polyarthritis	1–12
Oropouche fever	Central and South America	Febrile flu-like illness	2–6

All are mosquito-borne except Oropouche fever, which is midge-borne.
SOURCE: *Modified from Peter G, ed: 1997 Red Book, Report of the Committee on Infectious Diseases, 24th ed. American Academy of Pediatrics, Elk Grove, IL.*

and backache, those cases complicated by vomiting and jaundice may progress to gastrointestinal and generalized hemorrhage, encephalopathy, renal insufficiency, and myocarditis; of these cases, 25% will die. A safe, effective, and economical vaccine is recommended for those traveling to regions reporting yellow fever and to endemic zones, provided the traveler is ≥4 months of age, and preferably ≥9 months. Infants between the ages of 4 and 9 months may, under selected circumstances, be immunized.

IMPORTED ARBOVIRAL ENCEPHALITIDES More than 35,000 cases of Japanese encephalitis (JE) occur in Southeast Asia each year; children are the prime risk group. One-third of cases are fatal and one-third have permanent neurologic sequelae. An outbreak occurred in Australia. Universal childhood immunization for JE is likely to be required for control in endemic countries.

Other arbovirus infections must be considered in children with CNS manifestations who have been abroad in the previous month (eg, tick-borne encephalitis from Russia, Eastern or Central Europe, and Asia, as well as Murray Valley encephalitis from Australia). Travelers returning from Sub-Saharan Africa may present with the retinitis and encephalitis of Rift Valley fever as long as 4 weeks after infection. The fact that dengue, Japanese encephalitis, and tick-borne encephalitis are all members of the flavivirus group, which shares a common epitope on the envelope protein, means that there is considerable cross-reactivity on serologic testing, making unequivocal serologic testing difficult.

Concern has been expressed about the possible establishment of exotic arboviruses such as dengue, Japanese encephalitis, or Rift Valley fever in North America. The relatively recent establishment of the relevant mosquito vector, *A. albopictus* into at least 25 states heightens this concern, particularly for dengue and Yellow Fever viruses.

References

American Academy of Pediatrics: Arboviruses. In: 2000 Red Book, Report of the Committee on Infectious Diseases. Elk Grove, IL, American Academy of Pediatrics, 2000, pp. 170–175

Deresiewicz R, Thaler SJ, Hsu L, et al: Clinical and neuroradiographic manifestations of eastern equine encephalitis. N Engl J Med 26:1867–1874, 1997

Englund JA, Breningstall GN, Heck LJ, et al: Diagnosis of western equine encephalitis in an infant by brain biopsy. Pediatr Infect Dis J 5:382–384, 1986

Huang C, Campbell W, Grady L, et al: Diagnosis of Jamestown Canyon encephalitis by polymerase chain reaction. Clin Infect Dis 28:1294–1297, 1999

Kautner I, Robinson M, Kubnle U: Dengue virus infection: epidemiology, pathogenesis, clinical presentation, diagnosis, and prevention. J Pediatr 131:516–524, 1997

Lowry P: Arbovirus encephalitis in the United States and Asia. J Lab Clin Med 12:405–411, 1997

McFarland J, Baddour L, Nelson JE et al: Imported yellow fever in a United States citizen. Clin Infect Dis 25:1143–1147, 1997

Monath T, Tsai T: St. Louis encephalitis: lessons from the last decade. Am J Trop Med Hyg 37:40S–59S, 1987

Rust R, Thompson WH, Matthews CG, et al: La Crosse and other forms of California encephalitis. J Child Neurol 14:1–14, 1999

Steele M: Update on emerging infections from the Centers for Disease Control and Prevention—Arboviral Infections of the Central Nervous System—United States, 1996–1997. Ann Emerg Med 33:365–367, 1999

13.4.2 Enteroviruses

Harley A. Rotbart

Enteroviruses were so named because of their replication within the gastrointestinal tract. The enterovirus subgroup of the Picornaviridae (meaning small RNA viruses) family consists of nearly 70 antigenically distinct serotypes of human pathogens. Initially, antigenically related agents were characterized and designated coxsackieviruses, groups A and B, or as echoviruses, their name derived from an acronym (*e*nteric, *c*ytopathic, *h*uman, *o*rphan). New enterovirus types are now assigned consecutive serotypes (enteroviruses 68 to 72 have been identified to date) and are no longer subclassified as coxsackieviruses or echoviruses. Enteroviruses are nonenveloped, acid-stable viruses, the latter property permitting them to survive gastric secretions en route to the intestines. Enteroviruses are inactivated by ultraviolet light, chlorine, formalin, and heating to 56°C (132.8°F).

The life cycle of the enteroviruses begins with their attachment to specific receptors on susceptible host cells. One of the structural viral proteins, VP4, is dislodged from the virion, resulting in a conformational change in the virus and its penetration into the cell. Once inside, the remaining three structural proteins (VP1 to VP3) "uncoat," exposing free genomic single-stranded RNA. Changes at a single specific nucleotide may alter the secondary structure of the RNA sufficiently to result in attenuation of a neurovirulent strain of poliovirus. Very soon after uncoating, the viral RNA binds to cellular polyribosomes for translation of a single polyprotein. Cleavage of the polyprotein by cellular and viral proteases results in the formation of the four structural proteins (VP1 to VP4) and several nonstructural proteins including an RNA-dependent RNA polymerase, proteases, and a small genomic-associated protein that covalently binds to nascent viral RNA strands during replication. Replication of the viral RNA can begin as soon as the necessary proteins have been formed by the posttranslational modifications of the polyprotein noted above. A replicative intermediate RNA form, which includes a complementary negative-sense RNA strand, is generated from the genomic RNA via the action of the viral polymerase. New positive-sense RNA strands are then formed and encapsidated into 30-nm icosahedral virions by the four structural proteins. Most enteroviruses exit the cell by cell lysis and death. Certain serotypes may establish a nonlytic persistent infection state in vitro. Enterovirus infection completely shuts down host cell function with a few hours. Within 5 to 10 hours, the multiplication cycle of the enteroviruses is complete, with lytic release of as many as 10^5 virions from a single infected cell.

Despite some variability in epitopes presented by structural proteins, there is general conservation of genomic sequences among the serotypes. RNA similarities have been exploited in recent attempts to facilitate diagnosis of these infections (see below). Crystallographic structures of poliovirus and rhinovirus (another member of the picornavirus family) reveal a deep canyon on the surface of each face of the icosahedral viral capsid structure, which may accommodate receptors on host cells or antiviral agents. The receptor molecules are normal cell-surface proteins, usually used for cell-cell and cell-matrix recognition, now usurped by the viruses as docking sites for infection.

EPIDEMIOLOGY All enteroviruses have a worldwide distribution, with increased prevalence during the warm months of the year in temperate climates. Disease occurs with equal frequency throughout the year in tropical areas. Epidemics usually occur between May and October in the United States and other areas of the northern temperate zone. The seasonal prevalence of these viruses is shown in Fig. 13-11.

For all enteroviruses, person-to-person transmission occurs by the fecal-oral route without intervention of a lower animal or insect host. Symptomatic infection with these agents represents only a small proportion of the total number of infections. A majority of infected persons may excrete virus without any clinical manifestations. With paralytic poliomyelitis, spread of infection from individuals with overt paralysis is of relatively minor importance.

Enteroviruses are most often isolated from children in the first 4 years of life, with increased transmission of infection among children of lower socioeconomic status. Some serotypes are responsible for illness more often than should occur by random distribution. Echoviruses 11, 9, and 6, and coxsackieviruses B5, B2, B4, and A9, have been prominent serotypes over the past 19 years, with echovirus 11 alone accounting for 12% of all enterovirus isolates from 1970 to 1988. Any single individual is unlikely to encounter all serotypes of enteroviruses in childhood.

PATHOGENESIS Enteroviruses gain entry to the host via the oropharynx. Infection is established in the gastrointestinal tract and, to a lesser extent, the upper respiratory tract; however, the specific sites and cell types are unknown. From the intestine and/or oropharynx, virus spreads to local lymphatics and to the blood. During acute infection, enteroviruses may be recovered from both the serum and cellular fractions of blood; monocytes appear to be the most likely infected circulating cells. The patient may be asymptomatic or minimally symptomatic during the initial intestinal replication stage (1 to 5 days). The meninges, myocardium, liver, brain, and pancreas are all possible target organs; organ-specific damage consequent to a primary viremia may occur within 1 to 2 weeks following infection. Virus may also be recovered from the urine, implying either genitourinary infection or simply clearance. Enteroviruses may be excreted in the stool for as long as 6 to 8 weeks after the onset of illness, but are detectable for a shorter time in the oropharynx, usually only during the first 5 to 7 days.

CLINICAL MANIFESTATIONS Enteroviruses produce a broad spectrum of clinical findings, many of which are common to infections by different agents. The more common manifestations are discussed in the following sections.

Congenital and Neonatal Infections Group B coxsackie-viruses cause serious and often fatal disseminated disease in the newborn infant by both transplacental and postpartum transmission. This illness may include hepatitis, myocarditis, meningoencephalitis, and adrenal cortical involvement. Coxsackieviruses are an established cause of acute myocarditis of infants. The onset of illness is sudden, with loss of appetite, vomiting, coughing, cyanosis, and dyspnea. The disease may be mistaken for pneumonia, and marked pallor and tachycardia are characteristic. Hepatomegaly and cardiomegaly characteristically develop without a precordial murmur. The electrocardiogram may show lowered QRS voltage and ST- and T-wave abnormalities.

Disseminated disease caused by echoviruses may also be fatal in small infants. A predominant feature of infection is hepatic necrosis. Serologic studies show that maternal antibody appears to protect infants from severe disease, although they may acquire infection as documented by virus excretion. It is important not to induce delivery near term of a pregnant woman suspected of having an enteroviral infection because maternal antibody formation and subsequent passive transplacental transmission may protect the neonate from developing the most severe form of this infection.

Febrile Illness In young children, undifferentiated febrile illness is frequently associated with enterovirus infections. Despite the fact that the portal of entry and site of replication is the gastrointestinal tract, gastroenteritis is not common. During the months of seasonal prevalence, about seven babies per 1000 live births are hospitalized in the first 4 weeks of life because of enteroviral infection.

Rashes Large outbreaks of febrile rash disease are associated with a number of enteroviruses (particularly echoviruses 9 and 16 and coxsackieviruses A2, 4, 9, and 16, and B3, 4, and 5). Exanthemas occur more frequently in younger children. Rashes that are indistinguishable from rubella have been noted with a number of enteroviruses, and petechiae have accompanied some rashes, particularly those caused by echovirus type 9. The virus has been demonstrated in some of the skin lesions.

Hand-foot-and-mouth disease is characterized by fever with a vesicular eruption that involves primarily the buccal mucosa and tongue and less frequently the palate, gums, and lips. A maculopapular rash may appear on the hands and feet and become vesicular; it is often interdigital on the dorsum of the hands and feet and may also involve the palms and soles. The diaper area of infants may also be involved. Occasionally, disseminated vesicular rashes mimicking varicella-zoster virus infections have been observed. Rashes may be worse over eczematous areas of skin.

Coxsackieviruses A16, A5, and A10 and enterovirus type 71 are among the etiologic agents. In three such outbreaks, serious neurologic disease (aseptic meningitis, encephalitis, and/or acute flaccid paralysis) and high mortality rates have been reported, particularly among young children.

Meningitis-Meningoencephalitis Enteroviral infections of the central nervous system do not produce pathognomonic clinical manifestations. Fever, headache in older children, malaise, and signs of meningeal irritation are the predominant findings. The onset may be gradual or abrupt, with fever as high as 40°C (104°F). The fever usually lasts 3 to 5 days. Infants may have an altered

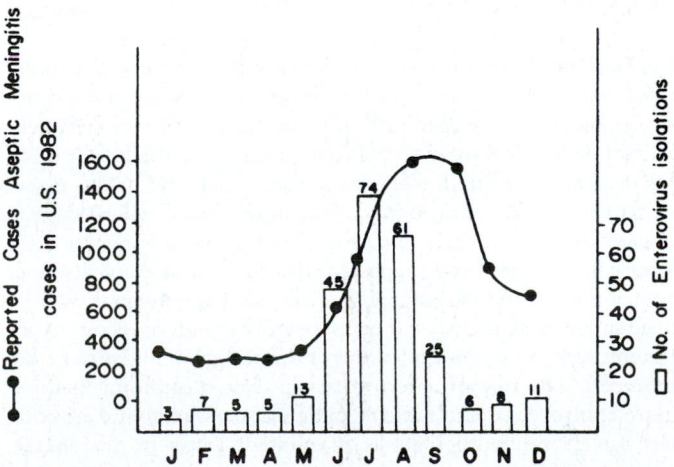

FIGURE 13-11 Seasonal incidence of aseptic meningitis and the proportion due to enterovirus.

sensorium, but meningeal signs are often absent in infants younger than 1 year of age. Focal neurologic findings are uncommon (<5% of infections). Seizures are infrequent, and only rarely is motor weakness or paralytic illness associated with enteroviruses other than polioviruses.

The CSF shows a leukocyte cell count ranging from zero to several thousand cells/μL. The cell count is usually less than 500 with a predominance of polymorphonuclear cells early in the illness; a shift to lymphocytic predominance is typically observed within 8 to 12 hours. The rapid shift to a lymphocyte predominance in a matter of hours is very unusual in bacterial meningitis, even with appropriate antimicrobial therapy.

The total protein content of the CSF is most often normal. Although the glucose content of CSF is usually normal, it may occasionally be diminished, that is, less than 50% of the simultaneous serum glucose or less than 40 mg/dL.

Viral meningitis is usually self-limited, and most patients appear to recover promptly and completely. Early studies of infants younger than 1 year of age who have had enteroviral meningitis revealed subtle neurodevelopmental abnormalities; more recent studies of larger numbers of patients and well-matched controls reveal no long-term adverse sequelae.

Enteroviral infections pose particular risks to patients with agammaglobulinemia, who are unable to eradicate enteroviruses from the central nervous system. Infections persist for years, with either recurring episodes of acute encephalitic symptoms or relentless progressive deterioration in central nervous system function. Although CSF may become intermittently culture-negative, enteroviral RNA can be continuously demonstrated by the polymerase chain reaction amplification technique. These infections may be accompanied by seizures, hemiparesis, altered sensorium, and increased intracranial pressure. There is often progressive loss of function, including focal neurologic deficits or cortical atrophy. The final phase of illness is often characterized by a dermatomyositis syndrome with virus detectable in blood and other tissues. Because children with agammaglobulinemia are at risk of contracting paralytic disease from the attenuated poliovirus vaccine strains, they and their immediate household contacts should receive only killed vaccine preparations.

Poliomyelitis   Although polioviruses, particularly type 1, are responsible for most viral paralyses, group B coxsackieviruses and enteroviruses 70 and 71 occasionally have also been associated with paralytic disease and encephalitis. The spectrum of disease caused by the polioviruses ranges from asymptomatic infection to paralytic illness. The ratio of inapparent infection to paralytic disease is estimated to range from 100:1 to 800:1. In symptomatic infection, viral meningitis occurs early. Classically, signs of acute flaccid paralysis follow after 2 to 6 days, presumably as a result of hematogenous spread of virus to the central nervous system. Characteristically, the paralysis is asymmetric in distribution, with the lower extremities and larger muscle groups more frequently involved than the upper extremities and smaller muscles. An isolated muscle group may be involved, or extensive paralysis of all extremities may occur. (A differential diagnosis of acute flaccid paralysis is presented in Sec. 13.4.17 and Table 13-59.)

Usually, as the patient's temperature returns to normal, the paralysis does not progress, and recovery occurs to a variable degree over the subsequent weeks to months. Atrophy of involved muscles becomes apparent after 4 to 8 weeks. Recovery may be extremely slow and the completeness of recovery cannot be assessed for 6 to 18 months.

The pathology of poliovirus in the central nervous system is well described. Evidence of infection is prominent in the spinal cord, medulla, pons, and midbrain. Initial cytoplasmic alteration in Nissl's substance of the motor neurons occurs, followed by nuclear changes. Pericellular infiltration of polymorphonuclear and mononuclear cells follows, and the final picture is one of destruction with neuronophagocytosis and loss of the necrotic cells.

Decades following paralytic infection, poliomyelitis victims may develop further progressive neuromuscular weakness, pain, and debilitation of the previously affected limbs or dysphagia. This manifestation, known as postpoliomyelitis muscular atrophy syndrome, is of unknown pathogenesis; immunologic mechanisms have been proposed.

Acute Hemorrhagic Conjunctivitis   Enterovirus type 70 and coxsackievirus A24 cause subconjunctival hemorrhage accompanied by swelling, redness, congestion, tearing, and pain in the eye. The prognosis is excellent, and complete recovery occurs in approximately 1 week. Rarely, a poliomyelitis-like motor paralysis has accompanied the conjunctivitis.

Herpangina   Most frequently associated with group A coxsackievirus infections, the hallmark of this infection is tiny vesicles or punched-out ulcers on the anterior pillars of the fauces, tonsils, uvula, pharynx, and edge of the soft palate. The vesicular lesions are usually 1 to 2 mm in diameter, with a surrounding red area. They may enlarge over 2 to 3 days, and as the vesicles rupture, a shallow yellow-gray ulcer remains. The illness is heralded by the sudden onset of high fever that lasts 1 to 4 days and is accompanied by loss of appetite, sore throat, and dysphagia. Approximately one-fourth of children with this illness have vomiting or abdominal pain. As with other enteroviral infections, herpangina occurs most frequently during the summer or early fall, and may also be epidemic.

Pleurodynia   An acute illness characterized by the onset of paroxysmal thoracic pain is known as *pleurodynia, Bornholm disease,* or *epidemic myalgia.* Various group B coxsackieviruses are the most common causes of this syndrome. Prodromal symptoms may include a headache, malaise, and other muscular aches. The characteristic pain is pleuritic in nature and aggravated by deep breathing, coughing, and other movement. The illness may last as long as 14 days, although 3 to 4 days is more typical.

Cardiac Involvement   Isolated *myocarditis* or *pericarditis* in older children and adults may result from group B coxsackievirus or echovirus infections. The spectrum of illness ranges from benign, self-limited pericarditis to severe, chronic, fatal myocardial disease. Virus has been isolated from pericardial fluid and heart tissue, particularly in samples obtained within the first 7 to 10 days of disease. Because illness may progress or symptoms persist for a longer time, it has been suggested that the host immune response contributes to the pathogenesis of illness. Experimental work in mice suggests that sensitized lymphocytes can indeed recognize infected tissue, although the nature of the antigen remains to be determined. The role of enteroviruses in dilated cardiomyopathy is more controversial and difficult to define; persistent viral infection has also been hypothesized as an etiologic factor in this disease. Neonatal coxsackie B virus infections may also cause a sepsis-like syndrome affecting multiple organs with predominant cardiac pathology including inflammatory infiltrates, edematous muscle with loss of striations, and occasional vasophilic granule accumulation.

DIAGNOSIS The nonspecific clinical manifestations of enterovirus infections and the potential for confusion with bacterial and other viral infections make a laboratory diagnosis desirable in many instances. Tissue culture continues to be the mainstay in laboratory methods for enteroviral diagnosis, but its relatively high cost, requirement for specially trained personnel, and long turnaround time (mean time to isolation of an enterovirus from CSF can be as long as 1 week) limit its use. Not all enteroviruses grow in tissue culture. For those serotypes, particularly the coxsackievirus A group, which grow poorly or not all, suckling-mice inoculation is required for identification—a technique too cumbersome to be widely available.

Because an antigen common to all enteroviruses has not been identified, it is impractical to screen sera for antibodies to all enteroviruses. ELISA assays are not sufficiently sensitive to replace cell culture. Nucleic acid hybridization studies using probes derived from cloned segments of poliovirus and coxsackievirus RNA have shown broad cross-reactivity with enterovirus serotypes of all subgroups. This implies evolutionary conservation of the enterovirus genome and provides a potential tool for rapid, sensitive, and specific diagnosis. Clinical trials with these reagents have been frustrated by the low titers of virus in certain infected fluids and, hence, inadequate sensitivity. The polymerase chain reaction amplification technique has been applied to enterovirus diagnosis using CSF specimens from infected patients. Sensitivity and specificity of this assay both appear to be greater than 95%. Results of colorimetric formats of this assay are available in less than 6 hours, making it potentially very useful in patient management.

When an enterovirus infection is suspected, attempts should be made to culture virus from the nasopharynx and from stool specimens, from blood, and if lumbar puncture has been performed, from CSF. The mere recovery of virus from the throat or stool does not establish it as the cause of illness. Temporal association of illness, virus recovery, and an antibody rise specific to that agent provide firmer evidence of a causative relationship. However, virus isolated from blood, CSF, pleural fluid, or myocardium certainly suggests an etiologic role. Polymerase chain reaction assays for the enteroviruses are increasingly available at academic centers and commercial reference laboratories.

TREATMENT There is currently no specific treatment for any of the enterovirus infections. Supportive measures include bed rest, antipyretics, and analgesics, as indicated. Immune globulin with specific antibody against the infecting enterovirus has been used both in newborn infants and in immunocompromised individuals, such as children with agammaglobulinemia, but its efficacy is not established. Intravenous, as well as intrathecal, administration may be necessary to ameliorate or prevent central nervous system infection in immunocompromised patients.

Bed rest is considered to be important as part of supportive care of patients with paralytic poliomyelitis, and sedatives may be an important adjunct. Such medications, however, are contraindicated in bulbar involvement or weakness of respiratory muscles. Intermittent application of moist heat seems to ameliorate the early muscle pain and spasm. Sometimes hot baths are more efficient and better tolerated, especially for small children. Physical therapy such as gentle passive movement should be used in conjunction with the moist heat to extend the range of motion and to avoid potential contractures and deformities. Rehabilitation requires intensive efforts of a physical therapy team skilled in evaluating muscle movement and able to determine when splints or supporting braces might be helpful in convalescence.

Patients with bulbar palsy may require endotracheal intubation to maintain airways and to avoid aspiration of secretions, which cannot be swallowed. Mechanical ventilation may be required with respiratory center involvement, as with diaphragmatic paralysis. The inability to void urine may require repeated emptying of the bladder by manual compression or urethral catheterization.

References

Abzug MJ, Keyserling HL, Lee ML, et al: Neonatal enterovirus infection: virology, serology, and effects of intravenous immune globulin. Clin Infect Dis 20:1201–1206, 1995

American Academy of Pediatrics, Committee on Infectious Diseases: Poliomyelitis prevention: revised recommendations for use of inactivated and live oral poliovirus vaccines (RE9853). Pediatrics 103(1):171–172, 1999

Centers for Disease Control: Death among children during an outbreak of hand, foot, and mouth disease—Taiwan, Republic of China, April-July 1998. MMWR Morb Mortal Wkly Rep 47:629–633, 1998

Jenista JA, Powell KR, Menegus MA: Epidemiology of neonatal enterovirus infection. J Pediatr 104:685–690, 1984

McKinney RE, Katz SL, Wilfert CM: Chronic enteroviral meningoencephalitis in agammaglobulinemic patients. Rev Infect Dis 9:334–356, 1987

Modlin JF: Perinatal echovirus infection: insights from a literature review of 61 cases of serious infection and 16 outbreaks in nurseries. Rev Infect Dis 8:918–926, 1986

Romero JR, Rotbart HA: Sequence analysis of the downstream 5′ nontranslated region of seven echoviruses with different neurovirulence phenotypes. J Virol 69:1370–1375, 1995

Rorabaugh ML, Berlin LE, Heldrich F, et al: Aseptic meningitis in infants younger than 2 years of age: acute illness and neurologic complications. Pediatrics 92:206–211, 1993

Rotbart HA, Ahmed A, Hickey S, et al: Diagnosis of enterovirus infection by polymerase chain reaction of multiple specimen types. Pediatr Infect Dis J 16:409–411, 1997

Rotbart HA, Kirkegaard K: Picornavirus pathogenesis: viral access, attachment, and entry into susceptible cells. Semin Virol 3:483–499, 1992

Rotbart HA, O'Connell JF, McKinlay MA: Treatment of human enterovirus infections. Antiviral Res 38:1–14, 1998

Webster ADB, Rotbart HA, Warner T, et al: Diagnosis of enterovirus brain disease in hypogammaglobulinemic patients by polymerase chain reaction. Clin Infect Dis 17:657–661, 1993

13.4.3   Viral Gastroenteritis

Paul A. Offit

Infectious diarrhea is a leading cause of disease and death worldwide. During a 1-year period (1977–1978) in Asia, Africa, and Latin America, it was estimated that 3 to 5 billion episodes of infectious diarrhea accounted for 5 to 10 million deaths. Rotaviruses; adenoviruses; small, round viruses (eg, Norwalk agent); caliciviruses; coronaviruses; and astroviruses are responsible for acute viral gastroenteritis. Rotaviruses, adenoviruses, and small, round viruses account for the majority of viral gastroenteritis in childhood.

Since their initial identification as a cause of human disease in 1973, rotaviruses have been found to be the most important cause of acute gastroenteritis in infants and young children in all countries. Studies in the United States, England, Australia, Japan, and Bangladesh found that 34 to 63% of children hospitalized with acute diarrhea were infected with rotaviruses. Rotavirus causes 3 to 4 million cases of diarrhea, 500,000 outpatient visits, 50,000 hospitalizations, and approximately 40 deaths per year in the United

States. Rotavirus-induced gastroenteritis primarily affects children 6 to 24 months of age, and most initial infections are symptomatic. The peak prevalence of the disease occurs between November and April in temperate climates, and year-round in tropical climates; infections are usually sporadic and occasionally epidemic. Rotaviruses are transmitted from person-to-person by the fecal-oral route, with an incubation period of 1 to 3 days.

Adenoviruses are probably the second most important cause of acute gastroenteritis in childhood. Disease is associated primarily with adenovirus types 40 and 41. These strains are now termed "fastidious" or "enteric" adenoviruses because they are difficult to propagate in cell culture. Similar to rotaviruses, enteric adenoviruses primarily infect children younger than 2 years of age, but unlike rotaviruses, adenovirus infections occur year-round. Although outbreaks in hospital nurseries have occurred, these viruses appear to be endemic rather than epidemic. Enteric adenoviruses have an incubation period of 3 to 10 days, which is longer than that for infection with either rotaviruses or small, round viruses.

In 1968, an outbreak of illness characterized by vomiting and fever occurred in a group of elementary school children in Norwalk, Ohio. Virus particles, 27 nm in diameter, were subsequently isolated from this outbreak by electron microscopy. Norwalk agent was the forerunner of a group of morphologically similar noncultivable agents named for the geographic location where they were found to cause disease (eg, Montgomery County agent, Hawaii agent). The morphologic similarity of a number of smaller viruses associated with gastroenteritis (including parvoviruses) led to the description of these agents as small, round viruses. Unlike rotaviruses and adenoviruses, infections with small, round viruses are usually epidemic and responsible for family and community-wide outbreaks of gastroenteritis in school-aged children, family contacts, and adults. Small, round viruses are transmitted by the fecal-oral route, with an incubation period of 1 to 2 days.

CLINICAL MANIFESTATIONS   Rotavirus infection is characterized by diarrhea, fever, and vomiting. Occasionally, congestion and coryza precede the onset of intestinal symptoms. Stools are watery and rarely contain blood, mucus, or white blood cells. Diarrhea is often associated with increased losses of sodium and chloride in the stools, isotonic dehydration, and a compensated metabolic acidosis. Vomiting often lasts 2 to 3 days and diarrhea 5 to 8 days. An encephalopathic picture occurs rarely. Subsequent rotavirus infections are progressively less likely to induce moderate-to-severe symptoms.

Infection with enteric adenoviruses is characterized by fever, diarrhea, and occasionally vomiting. Although initial symptoms of adenovirus infection in young children are generally milder than rotavirus infections, diarrhea may be prolonged, with an average duration of approximately 9 days. Similar to rotaviruses, adenoviruses may present with upper respiratory tract symptoms.

Symptoms associated with small, round virus infection are usually explosive in onset and, unlike rotaviruses and adenoviruses, last only 24 to 48 hours. Signs and symptoms include vomiting, diarrhea, abdominal cramps, nausea, headache, low-grade fever, myalgia, anorexia, and malaise.

DIAGNOSIS AND TREATMENT   Although rotaviruses, enteric adenoviruses, and small, round viruses may be detected directly in stools by electron microscopy or polyacrylamide gel electrophoresis, these procedures are not readily available in most hospitals. Fortunately, rapid diagnosis of rotaviruses and adenoviruses by solid-phase immunoassays of stool are commercially available, relatively inexpensive, and quite sensitive and specific when compared with electron microscopy. Commercial assays for the rapid detection of small, round viruses are not currently available. The treatment of acute diarrhea is discussed in Sec. 17.7.4.

PREVENTION   A rotavirus vaccine was licensed by the Food and Drug Administration on August 31, 1998, and recommended for use in all infants as a series of three doses given by mouth at 2, 4, and 6 months of age. On October 22, 1999, the Centers for Disease Control and Prevention provided evidence that the rotavirus vaccine was associated with intussusception. Infants inoculated with rotavirus vaccine were about 60% more likely to develop intussusception than infants not inoculated with rotavirus vaccine. For this reason, the rotavirus vaccine was withdrawn for use. Because intussusception in not clearly a consequence of natural rotavirus infection, the pathogenesis of intussusception following immunization remains unclear.

Alternative vaccine strategies include bovine × human reassortant rotaviruses and live, attenuated human rotaviruses. Both of these strategies are effective in preventing moderate-to-severe rotavirus infections in infants. However, large safety trials are required to demonstrate that these vaccine candidates are not also associated with intussusception.

References

Blacklow NR, Cukor G: Viral gastroenteritis. N Engl J Med 304:397–406, 1981

Centers for Disease Control and Prevention: Rotavirus vaccine for the prevention of rotavirus gastroenteritis among children: recommendation of the Advisory Committee on Immunization Practices (ACIP). MMWR Morb Mortal Wkly Rep 48:1, 1999

Christensen ML: Human viral gastroenteritis. Clin Microbiol Rev 2:51–89, 1989

Guarino A, Canani RB, Russo S, et al: Oral immunoglobulins for treatment of acute rotavirus gastroenteritis. Pediatrics 93:12–16, 1994

Jin S, Kilgore PE, Holman RC, et al: Trends in hospitalizations for diarrhea in United States children from 1979–1992: estimates of the morbidity associated with rotavirus. Ped Infect Dis J 15:397–404, 1996

Madeley CR: The emerging role of adenoviruses as inducers of gastroenteritis. Pediatr Infect Dis 5:S63–74, 1986

Offit PA: Host factors associated with protection against rotavirus disease: the skies are clearing. J Infect Dis 174:S59–64, 1996

Valazquez FR, Matson DO, Calva JJ, et al: Rotavirus infection in infants as protection against subsequent infections. N Engl J Med 335:1022–1028, 1996

13.4.4   Hemorrhagic Fevers

Ali S. Khan

The term *viral hemorrhagic fever* describes a severe, sometimes fatal, multisystem syndrome best characterized by diffuse vascular damage and dysregulation; hemorrhage does not necessarily occur and, when it does, is rarely a sufficient cause for demise. The etiologic agents of this syndrome are zoonotic, lipid-enveloped RNA viruses, and include dozens of members from four viral families (Table 13-52). These agents are localized geographically and are associated with specific vector hosts or reservoirs, although imported cases and infections caused by iatrogenic or laboratory misadventure occur outside their respective ranges. The diseases they cause are either endemic or episodic within both annual cycles and

TABLE 13-52

FEATURES OF VIRAL HEMORRHAGIC FEVERS

FAMILY	VIRUS	DISEASE	GEOGRAPHIC REGION	EPIDEMIOLOGIC DISTRIBUTION	INCUBATION PERIOD (DAYS)	RESERVOIR/VECTOR
Arenaviridae	Junin*	Argentine hemorrhagic fever	Argentina pampas	Rural	7–16	Rodent: *Calomys callosus*
	Machupo*	Bolivian hemorrhagic fever	Beni Department, Bolivia	Rural	7–14	Rodent: *Calomys musculinus*
	Guanarito	Venezuelan hemorrhagic fever	Guanarito municipality of Portuguesa state and adjacent regions of Barinas State, Venezuela	Rural	7–14	Rodent: *Zygodontomys brevicauda*
	Sabiá	Unnamed	Sao Paulo State, Brazil	Unknown; presumed rural	8	
	Lassa*	Lassa fever	Nigeria, Sierra Leone, Liberia, Guinea	Rural	7–18	Rodent: *Matomys spp.*
Bunyaviridae	Hantaan and related viruses	Hemorrhagic fever with renal syndrome	Asia & Europe (rare in Africa and the Americas)	Rural, urban *Rattus*-associated disease, and laboratory-acquired	4–42	Rodents: Arvicoline and murine genus
	Sin-Nombre and related viruses (Andes*)	Hantavirus pulmonary syndrome	Americas	Rural	4–35	Rodents: Sigmodontine genus
	Crimean-Congo hemorrhagic fever*	Crimean-Congo hemorrhagic fever	Africa, Asia, Southern Europe	Rural; contacts with ticks, domestic animals	2–7	Ticks: *Hyalomma* spp.
	Rift Valley fever	Rift Valley fever	Africa	Rural; contact with mosquitoes, domestic animals	2–7	Mosquito: *Aedes spp*
Filoviridae	Marburg*	Marburg hemorrhagic fever	Sub-Saharan Africa	Rural	3–16	Unknown
	Ebola*	Ebola hemorrhagic fever	Tropical forests, Africa (all strains except Ebola-Reston from Philippines)	Rural	3–16	Unknown
Flaviviridae	Dengue	Dengue fever/dengue hemorrhagic fever/dengue shock syndrome	Africa, Americas (excluding the northern and southern extremes)	Urban	4–7	Mosquito: *Aedes aegypti*
	Yellow fever	Yellow fever	Africa, South America	Rural, urban	3–6	Mosquito: *Aedes aegypti*
	Omsk hemorrhagic fever	Omsk hemorrhagic fever	Western Siberia	Rural agriculture, winter (muskrat and water-borne transmission)	2–4	Tick: *Dermacentor spp.*
	Kyasanur Forest disease	Kyasanur Forest disease	Karnataka State, India	Rural; man-modified forests	2–7	Tick: *Haemaphysalis spp.*

*Documented nosocomial transmission.

longer secular trends. Some are associated with high lethality and potential for person-to-person transmission.

EPIDEMIOLOGY Most arboviruses (arthropod-borne viruses) are maintained in natural cycles of infection between vector insects or ticks and vertebrate hosts. The viruses may be carried through the winter or dry months by persistence in estarating or dormant vectors, by vertical transovarial transmission in vector mosquitoes, by transtadial transmission in ticks, or in persistently infected vertebrates. In tropical locations, transmission can occur throughout the year. Human infections usually occur only in circumstances of increased viral transmission when the virus "spills over" from the enzootic cycle. Certain arboviruses, notably yellow fever and dengue, produce sufficient viremias in humans that vector-borne interhuman transmission is possible, often leading to transmission in epidemic proportions.

The arenaviruses, which cause Lassa and other hemorrhagic fevers and lymphocytic choriomeningitis, and the hantaviruses are spread from various persistently or transiently infected rodents through infected aerosols or by contact with, or ingestion of, infected excretions. In addition to vector-borne transmission, Omsk hemorrhagic fever can be transmitted from infected muskrats to trappers during skinning. Rift Valley fever and Crimean-Congo hemorrhagic fever can be transmitted from infected livestock to herders and butchers during slaughter. Person-to-person, often nosocomial, transmission of Crimean-Congo hemorrhagic fever virus and Ebola, Marburg, and Lassa viruses has led to sizable, often fearsome outbreaks.

In hyperendemic or episodic urban outbreak situations caused by either yellow fever or dengue, adults are usually solidly immune; thus, children represent the highest proportion of infected persons. Pediatric cases of Lassa fever and town-based Bolivian hemorrhagic fever confirm ample opportunity for contact between the vector/reservoir and children. The few pediatric cases noted during an outbreak of Ebola hemorrhagic fever in an otherwise susceptible population in 1995 emphasizes that this disease is not extremely infectious without direct patient contact. Not unexpectedly, children are rarely infected with the New World arenaviruses or sylvatic yellow fever that are predominantly acquired in the forest or fields.

DIAGNOSIS These diseases are geographically and ecologically limited; therefore, correctly diagnosing a patient presents an exercise in geographic medicine after accounting for the estimated incubation period. Because of the availability of specific therapy or treatment guidelines and the potential for nosocomial transmission, depending on the specific disease, these diseases should always be considered in the differential diagnosis of a patient with the appropriate clinical presentation and never generically diagnosed as a viral hemorrhagic fever.

For the most part, all of these diseases are associated with nondescript clinical presentations that include fever, myalgia, headache, and some gastrointestinal symptoms. Thus, differentiation from many other febrile illnesses can be difficult. The subsequent development of hypotension, a flushed appearance suggesting early vascular injury, and, especially, hemorrhage should trigger further diagnostic studies. Rash is a feature only in Ebola, Marburg, dengue, and Lassa fevers. The major pitfall in diagnosis among travelers is entertaining the possibility of hemorrhagic fever at the expense of performing a thorough evaluation of more common and treatable conditions, such as malaria or typhoid fever.

Overall, the disease manifestations in children resemble those in adults, with notable exceptions. Dengue shock syndrome (DSS) in the first year of life, which appears to be precipitated by maternal antibody, and the swollen baby syndrome of Lassa fever are uniquely pediatric diseases. DSS from secondary dengue virus infection also appears to be a disease that preferentially affects children for unknown reasons. (see Sec. 13.4.1).

Except in Lassa fever, thrombocytopenia is the only universal feature of these diseases. The absence of proteinuria and/or hematuria is helpful in excluding virtually all cases of arenaviral hemorrhagic fevers. Except for hantaviruses, these viruses are readily isolated from acute-phase samples under appropriate biocontainment conditions. Enzyme-linked immunosorbent assay (ELISA) techniques have proven to be sensitive and specific for rapid antigen and/or antibody detection. The older indirect fluorescent-antibody techniques remain available for many viral hemorrhagic diseases. Immunohistochemical techniques utilizing specific mono- and polyclonal antibodies have improved postmortem diagnoses using tissues and are being applied increasingly in conjunction with nucleic acid–based testing methods for direct and rapid detection of viral genome. Specific diagnostic or management questions for suspected patients can be addressed to the Special Pathogens Branch, Centers for Disease Control and Prevention, 404-639-2888.

SPECIFIC DISEASES

FILOVIRAL HEMORRHAGIC FEVERS The hemorrhagic fevers associated with Marburg and Ebola viruses are among the deadliest: case fatality rates average 26% among those with Marburg disease and 53 to 88% in outbreaks of Ebola hemorrhagic fever. Four subtypes of Ebola virus (Reston, Sudan, Zaire, and Cote d'Ivoire) may be differentiated by their associated virulence in animals and pathogenicity in humans. Little is known about the natural reservoir of these viruses, and disease spread is a function of relentless, often nosocomial, chains of person-to-person transmission. Infection manifests with an abrupt onset of prostrating fever, headache, and myalgia. Patients frequently appear restless and anxious, and they later become apathetic and exhibit other encephalopathic signs. After 3 to 8 days, a morbilliform, usually confluent, nonpruritic rash starts on the upper trunk and spreads centrifugally to involve the entire body except the face and neck. Profuse vomiting and watery diarrhea commence, accompanied by intense abdominal pain. Chest pain is a variable feature that was often noted in the Ebola-Sudan outbreak in 1976, but not in other Marburg and Ebola-Zaire outbreaks. Bleeding, chiefly from the gastrointestinal tract in the form of melena and hematemesis, but also from the vagina and gums, occurs in about 50% of patients. Multisystem failure from pneumonitis, hepatitis, pancreatitis, and tubulointerstitial nephritis combined with intractable hypotension usually leads to death. Recovery can occur within 7 to 10 days, but convalescence is prolonged.

NEW WORLD ARENAVIRAL FEVERS Junin, Machupo, Guanarito, and Sabiá viruses, the etiologic agents, respectively, of Argentine, Bolivian, Venezuelan, and Sabiá-associated hemorrhagic fevers (AHF, BHF, VHF, SHF), are maintained by specific sigmodontine rodents that are indigenous to the Americas. AHF is almost exclusively an occupational disease of agricultural workers, although more infections are being recorded among children because increasing members of the adult population have been vaccinated and children under 15 have not. Fetal infection and death have been common in pregnant women infected with Junin virus, and the virus has also been isolated from breast milk. BHF and VHF are acquired in a peridomestic setting, and cases occur in all age groups.

All four diseases present with a similar nondiagnostic history of fever, headache, myalgia, weakness, and gastrointestinal symptoms. Retroorbital pain, photophobia, and epigastric abdominal pain may occur, but complaints of pharyngitis and other respiratory symptoms are uncommon. Patients become increasingly toxic and develop a flushed appearance, conjunctival injection, and fine petechial eruptions in the oral pharynx, on the upper trunk, and especially in the axillae. Most enter into a convalescent phase after the first week of illness, but more than one-third develop neurologic complications (altered level of consciousness, ataxia, or tremors) or a hypotensive-hemorrhage phase associated with a capillary leak syndrome.

LASSA FEVER Lassa fever is a common febrile illness in West Africa, with as many as 300,000 cases and 5000 deaths annually. Lassa fever may account for as much as 10% of febrile children admitted to hospitals in disease-endemic areas. The disease is characterized by insidious onset of fever, weakness, myalgia, and generalized malaise followed by lower backache, substernal chest pain or epigastric pain, dizziness, cough, and gastrointestinal symptoms. Purulent pharyngitis, conjunctivitis, edema (particularly of the head and neck), and mucosal bleeding are highly specific signs of Lassa fever. Fulminant disease is marked by hypovolemic shock, facial and neck edema, encephalopathy, and respiratory distress from laryngeal edema, pleural effusion, pneumonitis, and pulmonary edema. Permanent sensorineural hearing loss can be a late sequela. A highly characteristic syndrome of children younger than 2 years of age caused by Lassa fever is *swollen baby syndrome*. The disorder is identified by widespread edema, abdominal distention, and bleeding.

HEMORRHAGIC FEVER WITH RENAL SYNDROME (HFRS) This syndrome is caused by four murine and arvicoline rodent-borne Old World hantaviruses. Men, particularly agricultural and forestry workers, are at greatest risk for infection in sylvatic locations. There is an unexplained paucity of cases among children, and it is possible that even symptomatic disease may be milder in children. The most severe form of HFRS is caused by Hantaan virus and is classically associated with five consecutive phases with characteristic physiological derangement: febrile, hypotensive, oliguric, diuretic, and convalescence. Hemorrhage is generally noted during the oliguric phase. However, there is considerable variation in both the incidence of various manifestations and the severity of the individual phases that may overlap.

HANTAVIRUS PULMONARY SYNDROME (HPS) This syndrome is caused by a number of New World sigmodontine rodent-borne hantaviruses indigenous to rural areas of the Americas and is a consequence of sylvatic or peridomestic transmission. Like the epidemiology of their Old World cousins, there is a relative paucity of pediatric cases. A brief nondescript febrile prodrome with chills, myalgia, malaise, diarrhea, and headache is generally followed by the precipitous onset of the characteristic cardiopulmonary phase with some degree of hypotension and progressive evidence of pulmonary edema and hypoxia as a result of capillary leak. Seventy-five percent of patients survive this phase; the remainder die of cardiovascular collapse. In South America, Andes virus infection may be associated with facial flushing, petechiae, and occasionally frank hemorrhage with person-to-person transmission. Overt hemorrhage occurs rarely in severe cases in North America. Bilateral interstitial pulmonary infiltrates in conjunction with shock are a hallmark of severe disease, as is the triad of thrombocytopenia,

immature neutrophils, and circulating immunoblasts. Atypical presentations with prominent renal insufficiency and myositis have been reported as have asymptomatic and mild infections without pulmonary involvement.

CRIMEAN-CONGO HEMORRHAGIC FEVER Crimean-Congo hemorrhagic fever is a serious tick-borne and potentially fatal illness that is acquired directly from tick bites or from contact with or aerosol transmission by blood from infected animals, but this disease also poses a significant threat for nosocomial transmission. Onset is usually abrupt with severe headache, high fever, myalgia, weakness, anorexia, back and abdominal pain, and nausea often accompanied by vomiting. There is hyperemia, which is most notable on the face, mucous membranes, and upper part of the body. The illness generally has a biphasic course: early nonspecific symptoms are followed after the sixth day of illness by hemorrhage from the nose, mouth, and gastrointestinal tract, and the appearance of large ecchymotic areas on the limbs. Most cases are apathetic or obtunded with halting speech; dizziness and mild meningeal signs are common. Elevated bilirubin and liver enzyme levels are usually present. Severe cases are delirious or comatose, and death is the consequence of circulatory collapse and disseminated intravascular coagulation.

RIFT VALLEY FEVER (RVF) Rift Valley fever is chiefly a veterinary disease of Sub-Saharan Africa, where intermittent epizootics associated with heavy rainfall cause serious losses of domestic livestock from abortions and death. Humans generally become infected in this setting by direct or aerosol-mediated contact with blood from infected animals as well as by arthropod bite. RVF usually manifests as a self-limited but severe illness characterized by fever, headache, chills, anorexia, myalgia, and prostration. The illness usually lasts 2 to 5 days, and most patients recover without complications. The disease is distinguished by three complications: (a) acute retinitis that can cause permanent decrease in vision and that occurs after the acute illness has subsided in as many as 20% of patients; (b) a severe hemorrhagic disease with hepatic involvement in fewer than 1% of patients; and (c) encephalitis associated with confusion, meningismus, paresis, hallucinations, convulsions, and recrudescence of fever in fewer than 1% of patients.

DENGUE FEVER Dengue fever is the most common arboviral infection and, in the form of dengue hemorrhagic fever (DHF), annually causes hundreds of thousands of life-threatening infections in the tropics, principally in children. Four dengue virus serotypes are predominantly transmitted by the *Aedes aegypti* mosquitoes, which are present in most tropical urban areas of the world; however, some other mosquito vectors are responsible for fairly substantial outbreaks. In the United States, these mosquitoes can be found during the summer in southeastern states, but autochthonous transmission of dengue virus occurs only in Texas. Epidemics arise in susceptible populations after the virus is introduced by viremic persons into areas with competent vectors. In areas where transmission is endemic, dengue is principally a disease of childhood. Infections occur in almost 100% of children before 8 years of age. In the absence of previous immunity, when new virus strains are introduced, or among travelers from nonendemic areas, infections occur in all age groups.

Classic dengue is a grippe-like, often biphasic illness associated with fever, muscle and joint pains, chills, headache, and lumbar back pain accompanied by anorexia, nausea, and vomiting. Facial flushing is characteristic, and in fair-skinned persons, a centrifugally spreading morbilliform rash may be detected late in the illness. Illness is self-limited and sometimes is complicated by minor hemorrhagic phenomena, such as epistaxis and minor gum, gastrointestinal, and vaginal mucosal bleeding. A positive tourniquet test, and lowered platelet, total leukocyte, and absolute monocyte and neutrophil counts reflect marrow suppression.

The above self-limited hemorrhagic phenomena should be differentiated from the hemorrhagic-shock syndrome, which is characterized by thrombocytopenia, generalized bleeding, and evidence of increased vascular permeability (eg, hemoconcentration, pleural or abdominal effusions, or hypoalbuminemia). Advanced cases are called dengue shock syndrome (DSS), which is DHF plus narrow pulse pressure and hypotension, with a case fatality rate as high as 44%. Cross-immunity among the serotypes is limited, and sequential infection, particularly when dengue 2 virus causes the second infection, increases the risk for DHF/DSS. The onset of hypotension may be precipitous and typically occurs with defervescence. The interval of vascular instability may be as brief as 24 to 48 hours and reverses spontaneously. Sensitive clinical monitoring and supportive fluid, cardiovascular support, and the exclusion of aspirin reduce DHF mortality from 25% to less than 5%.

YELLOW FEVER Yellow fever (YF) is also transmitted to humans by *Aedes spp.* with endemozoonotic circulation in Africa in a sylvatic cycle involving nonhuman primates and mosquitoes in areas of rain forests and wet savannahs. Large epidemics also can occur in urban areas infested by peridomestic *A. aegypti*, where mosquito-borne, human-to-human transmission can result. Disease in the Americas is currently limited to "jungle"-type yellow fever with sporadic infections primarily among men. However, in Africa, yellow fever has not spared children, and community-based studies show increased case fatality ratios for children.

The disease classically has been divided into three stages: infection, remission, and intoxication. Fever, headache, malaise, and musculoskeletal pain occur suddenly, often accompanied by nausea and vomiting. There are few physical signs other than conjunctivitis, flushing of the skin, and Faget's sign, a relative bradycardia. In about 10% of cases, an assumed remission is temporary, lasting only hours to a few days, when illness resumes, with the reappearance of toxicity, fever, vomiting, abdominal pain, jaundice, hematemesis (*vomito negro*), and other hemorrhaging. Patients typically are jaundiced and dehydrated with hypotension, reduced urinary output, and frequently, proteinuria. Myocarditis, azotemia, encephalopathy, progressive liver damage, and bleeding can lead to death in 30 to 50% of cases.

TICK-BORNE HEMORRHAGIC FEVERS Kyasanur Forest disease and Omsk hemorrhagic fever are tick-borne flavivirus infections that are seasonally transmitted in the areas of southern and central India and Siberia. Kyasanur Forest disease occurs mainly among villagers and lumbermen with forest contact, and Omsk hemorrhagic fever is transmitted directly from infected muskrats (as well as ticks) and may also be waterborne. These are self-limited illnesses characterized by acute fever and chills, myalgia, headache, vomiting, and diarrhea lasting 4 to 10 days in half of all cases, and hypotension, which can persist for several days. Hemorrhages tend to be minor in Omsk hemorrhagic fever and are present from the onset of illness. Neurologic signs, including depressed consciousness, neck stiffness, tremor, rigidity, pyramidal signs, and convulsions, appear in 50% of Kyasanur Forest disease cases, but are less prominent in Omsk hemorrhagic fever. Hepatitis and acute renal failure are components of both illnesses, and bronchitis, pneumonia, and

hemorrhagic pulmonary edema develop in 40% of cases; fatalities are rare.

THERAPY Recognition of and supportive therapy for shock, hemorrhage, and secondary infection are critical in cases of hemorrhagic fever. In controlled trials of adults, ribavirin reduced mortality and morbidity in Lassa fever and hemorrhagic fever with renal syndrome, and anecdotal experience suggests its efficacy in Crimean-Congo hemorrhagic fever, Rift Valley fever, and the New World arenaviral hemorrhagic fevers. Immune plasma is an effective therapy for Argentine hemorrhagic fever and immunoglobulins are available for Crimean-Congo hemorrhagic fever and for tick-borne encephalitis.

PREVENTION AND CONTROL Vector-borne infections can be prevented by avoiding at-risk locations during the seasons and/or times when risk is greatest. Simple measures include covering exposed areas of the body with clothing, avoiding outdoor activities at dusk and dawn when certain vectors are most active, and using mosquito bed nets and insecticidal room sprays. Protective clothing and repellents can reduce arthropod exposure or bites. Although repellents containing DEET are the most effective formulations, they should be used with caution on children. At least six cases of encephalopathy, three of which were fatal, have been reported in children from 17 months to 8 years of age after exposures to formulations containing as little as 10% DEET. Permethrin (0.5%, Permanone), sprayed on clothing and bed nets, effectively repels and kills mosquitoes and ticks, and impregnated material remains effective even after several washings.

Minimizing human-rodent interactions is the cornerstone of preventing infections with hantaviruses or arenaviruses. Eliminating rodent shelter, excluding rodents, and controlling rodent populations are readily accomplished in urban settings but are more difficult in the rural occupational or recreational setting. No recommendations can be made about eliminating natural infection caused by filoviruses because the host is unknown. Infections from imported nonhuman primates have been eliminated by the implementation of new quarantine regulations and reliance on captive-bred animals. Prevention of nosocomial transmission through barrier nursing methods and decontamination of clinical specimens is the most critical aspect of the strategy to minimize the risk prevention for the arenaviral and filoviral infections.

Vaccines are available for yellow fever and Argentine hemorrhagic fever. Recent cases of fatal yellow fever occurring in nonimmunized travelers underscore the importance of pretravel counseling and appropriate immunizations.

References

Bryan RT, Doyle TJ, Moolenaar RL, et al: Hantavirus pulmonary syndrome. Semin Pediatr Infect Dis 8(1):44–49, 1997

Khan AS, Ksiazek TG, Peters CJ: Viral hemorrhagic fevers among children. Semin Pediatr Infect Dis 8(1):64–73, 1997

Peters CJ, Jahrling PB, Khan AS: Management of patients infected with high-hazard viruses. Arch Virol Supp 11:1–28, 1996

Rigau-Perez JG, Clark GG, Gubler DJ, Reiter P, Sanders EJ, Vorndam AV: Dengue and dengue haemorrhagic fever. Lancet 352(9132):971–977, 1998

13.4.5   Viral Hepatitis

The topic of viral hepatitis is addressed in Sec. 18.5.1.

13.4.6   Herpes Simplex Virus Infections

Charles G. Prober

Herpes simplex virus type 1 (HSV-1) and herpes simplex virus type 2 (HSV-2) belong to a family of DNA viruses that include cytomegalovirus, varicella-zoster virus, Epstein-Barr virus (EBV), and human herpes viruses 6, 7, 8, and 9 (Table 13-53). Following primary infection, herpes simplex viruses establish a latent state; HSV-1 in the trigeminal ganglion, and HSV-2 in the sacral ganglion. From time-to-time the viruses may be reactivated, resulting in recurrent infections that may or may not be associated with symptoms. HSV-1 usually is transmitted in oral secretions, whereas HSV-2 is most often transmitted through sexual activity. HSV-1 infections occur most frequently during childhood and usually affect body sites above the waist (mouth, lips, eyes, face). HSV-2 infections occur most often during adolescence and adulthood, and involve body sites below the waist (genitalia, buttocks, thighs). The majority of infections in newborns are transmitted from the maternal genital tract and usually are caused by HSV-2.

Herpes simplex viruses are 150 to 200 nm in diameter and consist of a core of linear double-stranded DNA surrounded by an icosahedral capsid, a fibrillous tegument, and a lipid envelope. There is extensive homology between HSV-1 and HSV-2, rendering serologic distinction difficult. There are at least 60 proteins specified by the virus. Mucocutaneous epithelial cells provide the presumed initial target for viral infection, whereas neural cells in trigeminal and sacral root ganglia constitute the site of latent infection.

EPIDEMIOLOGY Humans are the only natural reservoirs of HSV. Infections caused by HSV have no seasonal predilection; however geographic location, socioeconomic status, age, and race influence the prevalence of infection. Children of lower socioeconomic classes and those from developing countries contract HSV-1 earlier in life than children of more affluent socioeconomic classes and children from developed countries. Increased direct person-to-person contact occurring in crowded living conditions probably accounts for these differences.

Primary infection with HSV-1 usually occurs in infancy or childhood, whereas primary infection with HSV-2 occurs after the onset of sexual activity. Acquisition of infection follows intimate mucocutaneous contact (eg, kissing or sexual intercourse) between a susceptible host and one shedding virus. The incubation period for most HSV infections ranges from 2 to 7 days.

As transmission and acquisition of virus often occur in the absence of symptoms, spread throughout a population may be silent, contributing to the worldwide epidemic of HSV infections. Furthermore, because infection with HSV results in lifelong latency, the prevalence of infection in any population is cumulative. Based upon multiple seroepidemiologic studies, more than 50% of young adults in the United States have been infected with HSV-1 and 20 to 30% have been infected with HSV-2.

The most devastating form of HSV infection in pediatric patients is neonatal herpes, occurring at an estimated rate of 1 in 3500 to 5000 deliveries. Genital HSV infection in pregnant women is the major source of virus for the newborn. Most infected infants contract HSV at the time of delivery through an infected birth canal.

PATHOGENESIS AND IMMUNITY Infection of the susceptible host results when HSV penetrates through abraded skin or mucosal surfaces. After minimal local replication at the site of inoculation, virus migrates along innervating axons to the sensory ganglia where infectious virus is synthesized. Visible lesions result after the virus returns to the inoculation site via peripheral sensory nerves. Vesicular lesions appear between epidermal and dermal layers and contain large amounts of virus, cell debris, and inflammatory cells. When the host is unable to limit viral replication, viremia may result in multiorgan involvement. Disseminated infection most often occurs in newborns and others with compromised immune systems.

Establishment of latency, punctuated by episodes of recrudescence, characterizes infections caused by HSV. During latency, the HSV genome is maintained in a repressed, noninfectious, "static" state. Periodic reactivation of HSV and spread down the neuraxis is associated with the development of recurrent lesions or asymptomatic viral excretion. A number of stimuli, including direct trauma to ganglia, exposure to ultraviolet lights, stress, hormonal changes, administration of immunosuppressive agents, and serious intercurrent infection are capable of precipitating recurrent infections.

The specific immunologic factors that influence the clinical course of HSV infections are not completely understood. Both an-

TABLE 13-53
INFECTIONS CAUSED BY HUMAN HERPESVIRUSES

HERPESVIRUS	SYNONYM	MANIFESTATIONS	TREATMENT
HHV-1	HSV-1	Oral mucocutaneous infection; encephalitis; keratitis; conjunctivitis; whitlow	Acyclovir
HHV-2	HSV-2	Genital mucocutaneous infection; neonatal infection; aseptic meningitis	Acyclovir
HHV-3	VZV	Chickenpox; shingles	Acyclovir
HHV-4	EBV	Infectious mononucleosis; Burkitt and B-cell lymphoma; immunodeficiency or lymphoproliferation in compromised hosts	Ganciclovir, foscarnet
HHV-5	CMV	Infectious mononucleosis; congenital infection; colitis, pneumonitis, retinitis, and hepatitis in compromised hosts	Supportive
HHV-6	Exanthema subitum	Roseola infantum, febrile illnesses, and seizures	Supportive
HHV-7		Some cases of roseola infantum	Supportive
HHV-8	KSHV	Kaposi sarcoma	Supportive

tibody- and cell-mediated immune responses are important in influencing the acquisition of disease, severity of infection, and frequency of recurrences. The important role of antibody in HSV infections is evident by investigations of neonates exposed to HSV at the time of delivery; those exposed to virus in the presence of transplacentally acquired neutralizing antibodies are significantly less likely to contract infection. Humoral immunity also influences the course of HSV infections beyond the neonatal period. For example, antibodies against HSV-1 reduce the risk of contracting HSV-2 infection by about 50%, and a first episode of genital infection caused by HSV-2 is less severe in patients with preexisting HSV-1 antibodies than in patients without antibodies.

Cellular immunity also is critical for the control of HSV infections. Clinically severe HSV infections are more common among patients with compromised cellular immunity than among normal hosts.

CLINICAL MANIFESTATIONS Most HSV infections in normal children are asymptomatic or of mild-to-moderate severity. When associated with symptoms, primary infections tend to be more severe than recurrent infections. In contrast, HSV infections in immunocompromised children, even if recurrent, may result in extensive local disease with substantial attendant morbidity. Visceral dissemination of HSV is unusual, except among neonates.

Oral Infection Herpes labialis is the most common HSV infection of childhood, with peak incidence at 1 to 5 years of age. Oral herpes infections usually are caused by HSV-1; however, oral-genital sexual practices may result in HSV-2 infection in the oral cavity. Most primary oral infections are subclinical, although careful examination may detect a few oral ulcers. When symptomatic, the severity and sites of lesions vary: buccal mucosa, tongue, palate, and fauces may be affected; the gums may also be inflamed and bleed readily. Spread of infection from the oral mucosa to the lips, skin around the mouth, and eyes may occur. Children who frequently suck their fingers may develop concomitant infections of their digits. Submandibular adenopathy, high fever, and irritability often accompany symptomatic oral infection. The most common reason for hospital admission is dehydration resulting from impaired eating and drinking.

The lips are the most common site of oral HSV-1 recurrences. Factors associated with recurrent bouts of herpes labialis (cold sores or fever blisters) include intense exposure to sun and/or wind (eg, skiing) and stressful life events. Labial herpes commonly is heralded by a burning sensation or itching for 1 to 2 days before lesions develop. In the compromised host, the lips and adjacent facial areas may be involved for prolonged periods. The usual differential diagnosis of herpes labialis includes aphthous stomatitis, herpangina, infectious mononucleosis, and impetigo. *Pharyngitis,* which cannot be distinguished clinically from other viral and bacterial causes of infection, is a common manifestation of primary HSV infection in older children.

Cutaneous Infection Primary and recurrent HSV infections may cause skin vesicles and ulcers on almost any part of the body. Primary skin infections may be accompanied by deep burning pain, edema, lymphangitis, lymphadenopathy, and fever. Vesicles may appear singly or in clusters; they tend to become pustular, crust over, and heal within a week, usually leaving no scars. *Herpetic whitlow* is an eruption that typically occurs on the fingers. It often is painful, and it is easily confused with bacterial infection. *Herpes*

gladiatorum develops in skin area abraded during the course of wrestling after contact with someone who has oral HSV infection. Skin infections also have resulted from other contact sports such as rugby.

HSV cutaneous infection can be particularly severe among patients with burns, diaper rash, or underlying eczema (eczema herpeticum). Erythema multiforme may be associated with either primary or recurrent HSV. The lesions of erythema multiforme can recur with each recrudescence of herpetic infection (see Sec. 14.6.3).

HSV infections of the skin are sometimes difficult to diagnose, particularly when the patient is not seen until the lesions are crusted or pustular, or when the affected skin area is denuded. When HSV skin lesions assume a dermatomal distribution they may be mistaken for herpes zoster.

Ocular Infection Herpetic involvement of the eye is of particular concern because it can cause loss of vision. Primary infections may be accompanied by conjunctivitis and tender preauricular nodes, with or without associated keratitis. Conjunctivitis sometimes occurs with recurrent infection, but the most common recurrent form is herpetic keratitis. This entity is readily diagnosed clinically because of the characteristic dendritic, branched, fluorescent-staining corneal ulcers. Deeper ocular involvement, including stromal keratitis and iridocyclitis, occurs occasionally. Corticosteroids, in the absence of antiviral drugs, are contraindicated because they may contribute to deeper ocular involvement.

Urogenital Infection Genital herpes infection is a common sexually transmitted disease, and at least one-third of these infections occur in people 19 years old or younger. About 75% of first-episode genital herpes and 98% of recurrent genital herpes are caused by HSV-2. Seroepidemiologic studies show that 20 to 30% of adults in the United States are seropositive for HSV-2, whereas only about 10% have histories suggestive of prior genital herpes infection. Thus, most genital herpes infections are asymptomatic. When associated with symptoms, primary infections usually are more severe than recurrent infections.

Over approximately 10 days, genital lesions associated with primary infection evolve from vesicles and pustules to ulcers, and then crust and heal during the subsequent 10 days. Lesions are distributed over the labia majora, labia minora, mons pubis, vaginal mucosa, and cervix in women. In men, lesions are typically found on the penile shaft. Local symptoms of itching and pain usually precede visible lesions by 1 to 2 days. Tender inguinal adenopathy typically appears during the second or third week of illness and tends to be the last sign to resolve. Constitutional symptoms, including headache, fever, myalgias, and backache often accompany symptomatic primary genital herpes infection. Extragenital complications of primary HSV infections include aseptic meningitis, mucocutaneous lesions beyond the genital area, pharyngitis, and visceral dissemination.

Most recurrences of genital herpes are asymptomatic. About 50% of individuals with symptomatic recurrences have local prodromal complaints for several hours to 3 days before the appearance of visible lesions. Sparse genital lesions typically increase in size over the first 3 days, reach a plateau at 6 days, and resolve rapidly. Factors implicated in precipitating recurrences include emotional stress, menses, and sexual intercourse. Of note, about 1% of individuals previously infected with HSV-2 have active viral shedding without symptoms on any given day.

Neurologic Infection   HSV infections are associated with a variety of neurologic manifestations, including encephalitis, meningitis, radiculitis, and myelitis. HSV is the most important cause of life-threatening sporadic encephalitis; almost 75% of patients die if untreated. Beyond the newborn age group, HSV encephalitis is caused by HSV-1.

Infections in Patients with Compromised Immunity   HSV infection may cause severe localized disease, contiguous infection (such as esophagitis or pneumonia in those with oral infection), or, rarely, disseminated infection in immunologically impaired persons, such as those with malignancy, congenital immunologic deficiencies, or AIDS, and in severely malnourished children. The basic defect common to all these conditions has not been ascertained, although a common denominator may be a defect in cellular immunity.

Infections in the Neonate   Herpes infections in the neonate may be localized or disseminated. At onset, about 40% of infections are localized to the skin, eyes, and mucosa (SEM), 35% are localized to the central nervous system (CNS), and 25% are disseminated.

Neonatal SEM infection typically presents during the first 1 to 2 weeks of life. Skin lesions characteristically evolve rapidly from macules to vesicles on a red base, but rapid ulceration and skin denudation may confuse the diagnosis. Skin lesions tend to appear at sites of trauma such as the site of attachment of fetal scalp electrodes, the margin of the eyes, or over the presenting body part. HSV infection should be considered whenever any vesicle appears on a neonate. Lesions of mucous membranes other than the eye are not common initial sites. Involvement of the eye may be unilateral or bilateral. Conjunctivitis, keratitis, or chorioretinitis may occur. Outcome of SEM disease is excellent if diagnosis is made promptly and antiviral therapy is administered. Recurrent skin lesions commonly occur periodically throughout the first 1 to 2 years of life.

HSV infection in the neonate is discussed in detail in Sec. 2.17.7.

LABORATORY DIAGNOSIS   The definitive diagnosis of HSV is made by viral culture. HSV can readily be isolated in a number of tissue-culture systems, and cytopathic effects can be detected within 1 to 2 days. The presence of intranuclear inclusions and multinucleated giant cells seen in Papanicolaou-stained smears, or in Tzank preparations of cells obtained by scraping the base of a suspicious lesion, support the diagnosis of HSV infection. However, because these morphologic tests are only about 67% as sensitive as virologic methods, they should not be relied upon in the management of potentially life-threatening infections. Immunofluorescence methods are much more sensitive than histologic methods for diagnosing HSV infection.

Polymerase chain reaction (PCR) is a very sensitive technique for amplifying HSV DNA from CSF and other body secretions. Laboratory standardization and false-positive reactions are potential challenges to the interpretation of PCR results.

Many serologic assays demonstrate antibodies to HSV. A primary infection is diagnosed by finding no HSV antibodies in the acute serum and a detectable HSV titer in the convalescent serum obtained after at least 1 week. A four-fold rise in titer may be observed with recurrent infections, and does not distinguish between primary and recurrent infection. Furthermore, IgM or IgA antibodies cannot be used to diagnose primary HSV infection because such antibodies also can be found with recurrent infections.

The similarity of HSV-1 and HSV-2 proteins produces extensive cross-reactivity of antibodies to these viruses in standard serologic assays. Therefore, unless research methods are used, it is not possible to differentiate HSV-1 from HSV-2 antibodies. Although commercial laboratories often report HSV-1 and HSV-2 titers separately, this practice misleads physicians who may not be aware of the cross-reactivity problem.

PREVENTION AND TREATMENT   Certain preventive measures can be used to reduce the likelihood of contracting HSV infection. For example, exposure of neonates to active maternal genital HSV infection may be reduced by cesarean delivery, especially if performed before or soon after rupture of membranes. Precautions should also be taken to prevent postnatal contact between a neonate and caretakers with nongenital herpetic lesions. Infants with suspected neonatal herpes should be isolated.

Mild gingivostomatitis requires no therapy other than maintenance of proper oral hygiene and perhaps the application of a topical anesthetic. If these infections are severe, antiviral therapy with acyclovir may be indicated (see Sec. 13.1.2). Herpetic infections on the lips, skin, and genitalia also usually require no specific therapy. Orally administered acyclovir is effective in the treatment and prevention of frequently recurrent genital HSV infections. Consultation with an ophthalmologist is advisable for children with ocular herpes. Systemic administration of acyclovir has been shown to reduce the mortality and morbidity of HSV encephalitis, neonatal herpes, and HSV infections in immunocompromised hosts. See Sec. 13.1.2 and Table 13-15 for doses and details of therapy.

References

Corey L, Spear PG: Infections with herpes simplex viruses. N Engl J Med 314:686, 1986
Prober CG: Herpes simplex virus. In: Long SS, Prober CG, Pickering LJ, eds: Principles and Practice of Pediatric Infectious Diseases. New York, Churchill Livingstone, 1997
Whitley RJ, Kimberlin DW, Roiziman B: Herpes simplex viruses. Clin Infect Dis 26:541, 1998

13.4.7   Cytomegalovirus

Mark R. Schleiss

The viral etiology of cellular inclusions first observed in 1904 was correctly postulated 16 years later by Goodpasture, who used the term *cytomegalia* to refer to the enlarged, swollen nature of the infected cells. Human cytomegalovirus was first isolated in tissue culture in 1956, and the propensity of this organism to infect the salivary gland led to its initial designation as salivary gland virus. In 1960, the virus was designated *cytomegalovirus* by Weller, and during the 1970s and 1980s knowledge of the role of CMV as an important pathogen with diverse clinical manifestations grew steadily. Although primary infection with this agent is generally asymptomatic in healthy adults, several high-risk groups, including immunocompromised organ-transplant recipients and HIV-infected individuals, are at risk of developing life- and sight-threatening CMV disease. In addition, CMV has emerged in recent years as the most important cause of congenital infection in the developed world, commonly leading to mental retardation and developmental disability.

CMV is one member of the family of eight human herpesviruses, designated as human herpesvirus 5 (HHV-5). Taxonomically, it is referred to as a *betaherpesvirus,* based on its propensity to infect mononuclear cells and lymphocytes and on its molecular phylogenetic relationship to other herpesviruses. It is the largest member of the herpesvirus family, with a double-stranded DNA genome of >240 kilobase pairs (kbp), capable of encoding over 200 potential protein products. The function of most of these proteins remains unclear. As with the other herpesviruses, the structure of the viral particle is that of an icosahedral capsid, surrounded by a lipid bilayer outer envelope.

An understanding of the process of viral replication provides insights into molecular mechanisms of antiviral therapy and protective immunity. CMV replicates very slowly in cell culture, mirroring its very slow pattern of growth in vivo (in contrast to HSV infection, which progresses very rapidly). The replication cycle of CMV is divided temporally into three regulated classes: immediate-early, early, and late. Immediate-early gene transcription occurs in the first 4 hours following viral infection, and key regulatory proteins are made to allow the virus to take control of cellular machinery. Following synthesis of immediate-early genes, the early gene products are transcribed. Early gene products include DNA replication proteins and some structural proteins. Finally, the late gene products are made approximately 24 hours after infection, and these proteins are chiefly structural proteins involved in virion assembly and egress. Synthesis of late genes is highly dependent on viral DNA replication, and can be blocked by inhibitors of viral DNA polymerase such as ganciclovir. The lipid bilayer outer envelope contains the virally encoded glycoproteins, which are the major targets of host neutralizing-antibody responses. These glycoproteins are candidates for human vaccine design (see below). The proteinaceous layer between the envelope and the inner capsid, the viral *tegument,* contains proteins that are major targets of host cell-mediated immune responses. Of these tegument proteins, the most important is the "major tegument protein," UL83 (pp65). The UL97 gene product, a phosphotransferase, phosphorylates ganciclovir.

EPIDEMIOLOGY Every mammal appears to be infected with its own species-specific cytomegalovirus, and there is no evidence for infections across species in nature. Hence, humans are the only natural host for human CMV (HCMV) infection. Although most adults eventually become infected with CMV, the epidemiology of this infection is complex, and the age at which an individual acquires CMV depends greatly on geographic location, socioeconomic status, cultural factors, and child-rearing practices. In developing countries, most children acquire CMV infection early in life, with adult seroprevalence approaching 100% by early adulthood. In contrast, in developed countries, the seroprevalence of CMV approximates 50% in young adults of middle-upper socioeconomic status. This observation has important implications for congenital CMV epidemiology, because CMV seronegative women of childbearing age are at major risk of giving birth to infants with symptomatic congenital infection if primary infection is acquired during pregnancy.

Transmission of CMV infection may occur throughout life, chiefly via contact with urine or infected respiratory secretions. Acquisition of CMV in the newborn period is common. Approximately 1% (range 0.5–2.5%) of all newborns are congenitally infected with CMV. The majority of these infections occur in infants born to mothers with preexisting immunity and are clinically silent at birth. However, long-term sequelae, including deafness, can oc-

cur (see below). The route of congenital infection is presumed to be transplacental. CMV may also be transmitted perinatally, both by aspiration of cervicovaginal secretions in the birth canal and by breast-feeding. More than 50% of infants fed with breast milk that contains infectious virus become CMV infected.

Infants who are not congenitally or perinatally infected with CMV are at high risk to acquire infection in childcare centers. The prevalence of CMV infection in childcare attendees, particularly children younger than 2 years of age, approximates 80% in some studies. Virus may be readily transmitted to susceptible children via saliva, urine, and fomites, and these children, in turn, may transmit infection to their parents.

In adulthood, sexual activity is probably the most important route of acquisition of CMV, although the observation that virus is present in saliva, cervicovaginal secretions, and semen makes it unclear which route(s) of transmission are primarily responsible for establishment of infection. Saliva alone appears to be sufficient for transmission of CMV, and this route of transmission may be responsible for those cases of heterophile-negative mononucleosis that are attributable to CMV. Kissing appears to be one way in which CMV is transmitted from toddlers to seronegative parents. Other important routes of transmission include blood transfusion and solid organ transplantation. Prior to screening of blood products, transfusion-associated CMV was an important cause of morbidity and mortality in premature infants. The routine use of CMV-negative blood products in many neonatal intensive care units has largely eliminated this problem. Posttransfusion CMV is still a risk in CMV seronegative trauma and surgery patients who often manifest CMV as hepatitis.

PATHOGENESIS AND IMMUNITY In clinical specimens, a classic hallmark of CMV infection is the cytomegalic inclusion cell. These massively enlarged cells contain intranuclear inclusions, which histopathologically have the appearance of "owl's eyes." The presence of these cells indicates productive infection, although they may be absent even in actively infected tissues.

Little is known about the molecular mechanisms responsible for the pathogenesis of tissue damage caused by CMV, particularly for congenital CMV infection. Although the major target organ for tissue damage in the developing fetus is the central nervous system, it is surprisingly difficult to culture CMV from the cerebrospinal fluid of symptomatic congenitally infected infants.

Immunity to CMV is complex and involves both humoral and cell-mediated responses. The outer envelope of the virus (which is derived from the host cell nuclear membrane) contains multiple virally encoded glycoproteins. The glycoproteins B (gB) and H (gH) appear to be the major determinants of protective humoral immunity. Antibody to these proteins is capable of neutralizing virus, and gB and gH are both targets of investigational CMV subunit vaccines.

Although important in control of severe disease, humoral responses are clearly inadequate in preventing transplacental infection, which can occur even in CMV-seropositive women. The generation of cytotoxic T-cell (CTL) responses against CMV may be a more important host immune response in control of infection. In general, these CTL involve major histocompatibility complex (MHC) class I-restricted, CD8+ responses. Although many viral gene products are important in generation of these responses, the majority of CMV-specific CTL responses target an abundant phosphoprotein in the viral tegument, pp65, the product of the CMV UL83 gene. The value of these responses has been dramatically demonstrated in passive transfer experiments in high-risk bone marrow transplant recipients, where adoptive transfer of CMV-specific CD8$^+$ T cells that target the CMV UL83 gene controls CMV disease.

Recent investigations into the molecular biology of CMV revealed the presence of many viral gene products that appear to modulate host inflammatory and immune responses. Several CMV genes interfere with normal antigen processing and generation of cell-mediated immune responses. To date, three viral gene products that inhibit MHC class I antigen presentation have been identified. One is the US11 gene product, which exports the class I heavy chain from the endoplasmic reticulum (ER) to the cytosol (rendering it nonfunctional). Another is the US3 gene product, which retains MHC molecules in the ER, preventing them from traveling to the plasma membrane. Finally, the US6 protein inhibits peptide translocation by TAP.

CLINICAL MANIFESTATIONS

Congenital CMV Infection Current estimates suggest that 30,000 to 40,000 infants in the United States are born annually with congenital CMV infection, making CMV by far the most common and important of all congenital infections. Both the likelihood of congenital infection, as well as the extent of disease in the newborn, depend upon maternal immune status. If primary maternal infection occurs during pregnancy, the average rate of transmission to the fetus is 40%, and the majority of these infants have clinical disease at birth. In the setting of recurrent maternal infection (CMV infection that occurs in the setting of preconceptual immunity), the risk of transmission to the fetus is lower, ranging from 0.5 to 1.5%, and most of these infants appear normal at birth ("silent infection"). Hence, congenital infection may be classified as symptomatic or asymptomatic in nature.

Cytomegalic Inclusion Disease Approximately 10% of congenitally infected infants have clinical evidence of disease at birth. This, the most severe form of congenital CMV infection, is referred to as cytomegalic inclusion disease (CID). CID almost always occurs in women who have primary CMV infection during pregnancy, although rare cases are described in women with preexisting immunity who presumably have reactivation of infection during pregnancy. CID is characterized by intrauterine growth retardation, hepatosplenomegaly, hematologic abnormalities (particularly thrombocytopenia), and a variety of cutaneous manifestations, including petechiae and purpura ("blueberry muffin" baby).

By far, the most significant manifestations of CID are those involving the central nervous system. Microcephaly, ventriculomegaly, cerebral atrophy, chorioretinitis, and sensorineural hearing loss are the most common neurologic consequences of CID. Intracerebral calcifications classically demonstrate a periventricular distribution and are commonly detected by CT scan. The finding of intracranial calcifications is predictive of cognitive and audiologic deficits in later life and predicts a poor neurodevelopmental prognosis. Overall, 90% of those infants who survive symptomatic CID have significant long-term neurologic and neurodevelopmental sequelae. Indeed, it is estimated that congenital CMV may be second only to Down syndrome as an identifiable cause of mental retardation in children.

Asymptomatic Congenital CMV The majority of infants with congenital CMV infection are born to women who have preexisting immunity to CMV. These infants appear clinically normal at birth. However, even though these infants appear well, they may have subtle growth retardation as compared to uninfected infants. Although asymptomatic at birth, these infants are nevertheless at risk for neurodevelopmental sequelae. The major consequence of inapparent congenital CMV infection is sensorineural hearing loss. Between 15 and 20% of these infants will have unilateral or bilateral deafness. Routine newborn audiologic screening may miss cases of CMV-associated hearing loss, because this may be a lesion that becomes evident months or years after delivery. Progression of hearing loss is quite variable.

Acquired CMV Infection

Perinatal Infection Perinatal acquisition of CMV usually occurs secondary to exposure to infected secretions in the birth canal or via breast-feeding. Most infections are asymptomatic. Indeed, breast-milk–acquired CMV has been referred to in some reviews as a form of "natural immunization." Some infants who acquire CMV infection perinatally may have signs and symptoms of disease, including lymphadenopathy, hepatitis, and pneumonitis, which may on occasion be severe. Interestingly, these infections do not appear to carry any risk of neurologic or neurodevelopmental sequelae.

CMV Mononucleosis Typical CMV mononucleosis is a disease of young adults. Although it may be acquired by blood transfusion or organ transplantation, most commonly it is acquired via person-to-person transmission. The hallmark symptoms of CMV mononucleosis are fever and severe malaise. An atypical lymphocytosis is present, as is mild elevation of liver enzymes. It may be difficult to differentiate CMV mononucleosis from Epstein-Barr virus-induced mononucleosis on clinical grounds. CMV mononucleosis is typically associated with less pharyngitis, less splenomegaly, and more posterior cervical adenopathy. As with EBV mononucleosis, the use of β-lactam antibiotics in association with CMV mononucleosis may precipitate a generalized morbilliform rash.

Transfusion-Acquired CMV Infection Posttransfusion CMV infection has a presentation similar to that of CMV mononucleosis. Hepatitis is a prominent finding. Incubation periods range from 20 to 60 days. The use of seronegative blood donors, or of frozen deglycerolized or leukocyte-depleted blood, can decrease the likelihood of transmission, and is recommended for high-risk patients (neonates, immunocompromised patients).

CMV Infections in Immunocompromised Patients CMV causes a variety of clinical syndromes in immunocompromised patients. Disease manifestations vary in severity depending upon the degree of host immunosuppression. Infection may occur as a consequence of reactivation of latent viral infection, or infection may be newly acquired via organ or bone marrow transplant from a seropositive donor. Infections may also be mixed in nature, with both donor and recipient isolates present. Viral dissemination leads to multiple-organ system involvement, with the most important clinical manifestations consisting of pneumonitis, gastrointestinal disease, and retinitis.

CMV Pneumonitis CMV is a major cause of interstitial pneumonitis in immunosuppressed children and adults. This disease may be seen in the setting of HIV infection, congenital immunodeficiency, malignancy, and solid-organ or bone marrow transplant. The mortality rate depends upon the degree of immunosuppression, with mortality rates of 90% or greater described in bone marrow transplant patients. Solid-organ transplant recipients are at risk to develop CMV pneumonitis as well, although mortality rates are lower. The illness usually begins 1 to 3 months following transplantation, with symptoms of fever and dry, nonproductive cough. It then progresses quickly, with retractions, dyspnea, and hypoxia becoming prominent. Diffuse, bilateral interstitial infiltrates are present on chest radiographs. Because the differential diagnosis of pneumonitis is extensive in immunocompromised patients, bronchoalveolar lavage or open-lung biopsy should be considered to confirm the diagnosis and direct appropriate therapy.

CMV Gastrointestinal Disease   Gastrointestinal tract disease due to CMV can include esophagitis, gastritis, gastroenteritis, pyloric obstruction, hepatitis, pancreatitis, colitis, and cholecystitis. Characteristic signs and symptoms can include nausea, vomiting, dysphagia, epigastric pain, icterus, and watery diarrhea. Stools may be hemoccult positive or frankly bloody. Endoscopy and biopsy are warranted, and characteristic cytomegalic inclusion cells may be seen in gastrointestinal endothelium or epithelium. Although CMV enteritis does not carry the same ominous prognosis as does CMV pneumonitis, antiviral therapy is warranted. It may be difficult, even with biopsy, to differentiate CMV hepatitis from chronic rejection in liver transplant patients.

CMV Retinitis   Prior to the advent of highly active antiretroviral therapy (HAART) for HIV infection, CMV retinitis was the most common cause of blindness in adult AIDS patients, with an overall lifetime prevalence of >90%. HIV-associated CMV retinitis in children has, in contrast to adults, been relatively rare, probably reflecting overall differences in CMV seroprevalence in the two populations. Retinitis is less commonly encountered in transplant patients. CMV produces a necrotic, rapidly progressing retinitis, with characteristic white perivascular infiltrates with hemorrhage ("brushfire retinitis"). Peripheral lesions may be asymptomatic, and even advanced disease does not cause pain. Strabismus or failure to fix and follow objects may be important clues to the diagnosis in children. Untreated, the disease can progress to total blindness and retinal detachment. CMV chorioretinitis is also seen in symptomatically congenitally infected infants, although it is unusual for the disease to progress to the point of vision loss. The presence of chorioretinitis in a congenitally infected infant predicts a poor neurodevelopmental prognosis.

Other CMV Syndromes   A variety of other syndromes have been attributed to CMV infection, although cause and effect relationships are often difficult to establish. Ménétrier disease is a rare disorder that is characterized by hyperplasia and hypertrophy of the gastric mucous glands, which results in massive enlargement of the gastric folds. The majority of cases appear to be CMV-associated, although the pathogenesis is unknown. In children with congenital HIV infection, coinfection with CMV appears to accelerate the HIV disease progression and HIV-associated neurologic disease. Evidence is accumulating that suggests that CMV infection may be a cofactor in the pathogenesis of atherosclerosis. In addition, the phenomena of posttransplant vascular sclerosis and postangioplasty restenosis appear to be CMV-induced lesions.

DIAGNOSIS   The most important diagnostic study in the evaluation of suspected CMV disease is the viral culture. CMV may be cultured from virtually any body fluid or organ system. Blood, urine, saliva, cervicovaginal secretions, cerebrospinal fluid, bronchoalveolar lavage fluid, and tissues from biopsy specimens are all appropriate specimens for culture. The specimen is inoculated onto human cells (usually human foreskin fibroblasts) and the cell culture monitored for the development of the characteristic CMV-associated cytopathic effect. Although culture is highly sensitive, clinical isolates of CMV may grow slowly, requiring up to 6 weeks of incubation in the virology laboratory. Hence, an adaptation of tissue culture that provides results more rapidly is the centrifugation enhancement, monoclonal-antibody culture technique, referred to as the "shell-vial" assay. In this technique, the clinical specimen is centrifuged onto a cell monolayer (in effect concentrating the specimen) and, following incubation in tissue culture, cells are stained with a monoclonal antibody to a CMV-specific antigen, usually an immediate-early gene product. A positive shell-vial culture is presumptive evidence of active CMV infection, and the test is a useful adjunct to traditional viral culture.

Caution must be exercised in the ordering and interpretation of CMV diagnostic studies, especially in infants. By definition, the diagnosis of congenital CMV infection requires identification of virus in a culture specimen acquired prior to 3 weeks of age, because perinatally acquired infections may also become detectable at this time. Hence, a positive viral culture obtained beyond 3 weeks of age may simply represent perinatal or breast-milk acquisition, and may not be interpreted as evidence of congenital CMV infection. Although theoretically helpful, CMV IgM assays are, unfortunately, too nonspecific to reliably diagnose congenital CMV. False-positives are common. It is, therefore, very difficult to make the diagnosis of congenital infection outside the immediate perinatal period. Universal screening for congenital CMV infection may be a reasonable future goal, and could enable establishment of appropriate anticipatory neurodevelopmental and serial audiologic screening programs.

Outside of the neonatal period, the major caution regarding CMV diagnosis is to use diagnostic studies appropriately to differentiate between CMV infection and CMV disease. Infants and children infected with CMV may shed virus for years, making a positive urine viral culture difficult to interpret. Immunocompromised patients often have reactivation of latent CMV with subsequent viral shedding, even in the absence of overt CMV disease. Thus, the identification of CMV by culture of urine or saliva may reflect such chronic shedding of virus and is difficult to interpret in the evaluation of patients with end-organ disease such as pneumonitis or hepatitis. In contrast to urine and saliva cultures, a positive blood culture is almost always of diagnostic importance, and is predictive of disease in immunocompromised patients. Lung biopsy or bronchoalveolar lavage may be necessary to confirm the diagnosis of CMV pneumonitis. Hepatitis may require liver biopsy for confirmation of the diagnosis, and CMV hepatitis and chronic rejection may be a difficult differential diagnosis in liver transplant patients, even with a biopsy. Newer molecular diagnostic studies, including polymerase chain reaction (PCR) and CMV antigenemia studies, are also useful and predictive in monitoring CMV disease activity in the immunocompromised.

TREATMENT   Currently, three antiviral therapies are FDA-approved for the prophylaxis and/or therapy of CMV infection. Experience with these agents is limited in children, however, and anti-CMV therapy in general should be administered only after consultation with an expert familiar with dosage and side effects. Antiviral agents may be given therapeutically for established CMV disease, or prophylactically ("preemptive" therapy) when the risk of development of CMV disease is high (such as in transplant patients).

Ganciclovir was the first compound licensed for treatment of CMV infections. It is a synthetic acyclic nucleotide structurally similar to guanine. Its structure is similar to that of acyclovir, and, like acyclovir, it requires phosphorylation for antiviral activity. The enzyme responsible for phosphorylation of ganciclovir is the product of the viral UL97 gene, a protein kinase. Resistance to ganciclovir may occur with long-term use, generally due to mutations in UL97. Ganciclovir is indicated in immunocompromised children (HIV infection, transplant recipients, other immunocompromised states) when there is clinical and virologic evidence of specific end-organ disease (pneumonitis, enteritis, etc). The usual dose is 5 mg/kg twice daily for 2 to 3 weeks, followed by 5 mg/kg once daily for the duration of therapy. Ganciclovir is myelosuppressive, an often dose-limiting toxicity in immunocompromised patients who are often on other myelosuppressive agents. Ganciclovir is also commonly used as preemptive therapy in transplant patients at high risk of developing disease (for example, a CMV-seronegative recipient of an organ from a CMV-seropositive donor). Oral or intravenous acyclovir has also been successfully used as prophylaxis in this setting, although acyclovir should never be used for therapy of active CMV disease. An oral formulation was recently approved for use in adult HIV-infected patients with CMV retinitis, but the bioavailability is poor, and there are no data supporting use in children.

There is relatively little information concerning the use of ganciclovir in the setting of congenital CMV infection. Because some of the neurologic sequelae of congenital CMV, particularly sensorineural hearing loss, progress postnatally, there is hope that ganciclovir may be a useful therapy in such infants, although definitive recommendations will have to await the completion of a current nationwide collaborative trial. Case reports suggest the efficacy of ganciclovir for acutely ill neonates with life-threatening CMV disease (eg, pneumonia), but there is no evidence at present that its use improves neurologic outcome.

Alternatives to ganciclovir include foscarnet (trisodium phosphonoformate) and cidofovir (HPMPC). Pediatric experience with these agents is limited. Although potentially useful in the setting of ganciclovir resistance, the toxicities of these antivirals are significant, and these agents should be used only in exceptional circumstances. Although they have only a modest level of activity against CMV, high-dose oral acyclovir and valacyclovir have been used for prophylaxis of CMV in high-risk individuals, but are not suitable for therapy of active disease.

Immunoglobulins have also been useful in the control of CMV disease. A CMV hyperimmunoglobulin (Cytogam) decreases the incidence of CMV disease when administered posttransplant to high-risk transplant recipients, when administered alone or in combination with nucleoside antivirals. Immunoglobulin may also be administered therapeutically for CMV disease, in combination with ganciclovir. The observation that random donor intravenous immunoglobulin (IVIG) appears to be equal in efficacy to CMV hyperimmunoglobulin suggests that the benefit may be derived from an immunomodulatory effect unrelated to virus neutralization.

PREVENTION Ultimately, control of CMV infection, particularly the devastating sequelae of congenital CID, will depend upon immunization. The major target population for a CMV vaccine is women of childbearing age. Although immunization is unlikely to prevent all congenital infection, there is hope that it would have a significant and major impact on the incidence of CID. Various vaccines are currently under development.

Until the goal of a CMV vaccine is realized, education of young women of child-bearing age about the risks of CMV and how to avoid disease transmission are the only control strategies available. Seronegative women who regularly come in close contact with large numbers of young children, particularly in childcare center environments, may be at particularly high risk. Behaviors known to be associated with transmission of infection, particularly kissing and sharing eating utensils, can be avoided, and careful hand washing after diaper changes must be emphasized.

References

Adler SP: Cytomegalovirus and child day care: evidence for an increased infection rate among daycare workers. N Engl J Med 321:1290–1296, 1989

Demmler GJ: Congenital cytomegalovirus infection and disease. Semin Pediat Infect Dis 10:195–201, 1999

Demmler GJ, Buffone GJ, Schimbor CM, et al: Detection of cytomegalovirus in urine from newborns by using polymerase chain reaction DNA amplification. J Infect Dis 158:1177–1184, 1988

Fowler KB, Dahle AJ, Boppana SB, Pass RF: Newborn hearing screening: Will children with hearing loss caused by congenital cytomegalovirus infection be missed? J Pediatr 135:60–64, 1999

Ho M: Epidemiology of cytomegalovirus infections. Rev Infect Dis 12: S701–710, 1990

Kovacs A, Schluchter M, Easley K, et al: Cytomegalovirus infection and HIV-1 disease progression in infants born to HIV-1 infected women. N Engl J Med 341:77–84, 1999

Schleiss M, Stanberry L: Herpesvirus infections of the neonatal CNS: similarities and differences between HSV and CMV. Herpes 4:74–79, 1997

Stagno S, Pass RF, Dworsky ME, et al: Congenital cytomegalovirus infection: the relative importance of primary and recurrent maternal infection. N Engl J Med 306:945–949, 1982

13.4.8   Epstein-Barr Virus Infections (Infectious Mononucleosis)

Michael T. Brady

The Epstein-Barr virus (EBV) is recognized as the major cause of heterophil-positive and heterophil-negative infectious mononucleosis. Syndromes associated with EBV range from asymptomatic infection to fulminant lymphoproliferative disease. The virus is associated with a number of malignancies, including African Burkitt lymphoma, nasopharyngeal carcinoma, Hodgkin disease, and a number of posttransplant lymphoproliferative diseases. The precise role of EBV in each of these tumors continues to be elucidated.

EBV is a member of the family Herpesviridae (gamma herpesvirus), which contains linear double-stranded DNA surrounded by a protein capsid with 162 capsomers in an icosahedral arrangement. The nucleocapsid is covered by a lipid-containing envelope derived from the nuclear membrane of the host cell. EBV infects human oropharyngeal and salivary cells (lytic infection) and human and primate B lymphocytes and epithelium of the nasopharynx (latent infection). EBV is lymphotropic for B lymphocytes and in vivo does not infect T lymphocytes. To date, the virus has been grown only in B lymphocytes of human and nonhuman primate origin, as well as in certain epithelial-lymphoid hybrid cell lines that bear EBV receptors.

Infection of lymphocytes with EBV can transform them into continuously growing lymphoblastoid cell lines containing circular genome as a plasmid. Once infected, transformed lymphoblastoid cells rarely continue to produce infectious virus in vitro, although EBV-induced antigens can be detected in the cells. The appearance of new antigens on the cell surface is thought to be responsible for the cellular immune response to the virus and for the pathogenesis of the disease produced.

EPIDEMIOLOGY To understand the epidemiology of EBV, it is important to recognize that acute primary EBV infection is not synonymous with infectious mononucleosis. Most EBV infections acquired at any age, but particularly during childhood, are asymptomatic. EBV infection is present in human populations from all parts of the world. Seroepidemiologic studies demonstrate that from 20 to 100% of children have antibodies to EBV by 6 years of age. In undeveloped areas of the world, as many as 90% of adolescents have serologic evidence of prior EBV infection. Many of these infections were acquired in the first year of life. In contrast, in the United States, only 40 to 50% of adolescents are seropositive, with higher socioeconomic groups being less likely to have evidence of prior infection. Seropositivity increases with age in all populations, so that almost all adults have serologic evidence of past EBV infection. Seroconversion is particularly high in college, where 10 to 15% of susceptibles become infected each year.

EBV is excreted in oropharyngeal secretions (low titer of virus even during acute illness) and is transmitted by contact with saliva via kissing or other mucosal contact with contaminated objects. Healthy seropositive individuals intermittently shed EBV into their oropharynx. Blood products or transplanted tissues can transmit EBV and are particularly problematic for seronegative immunocompromised transplant recipients. There is no evidence of urinary or fecal excretion. Transplacental transmission is rare. Sixty percent of immunosuppressed individuals excrete EBV. Because virus shedding is of a low titer in even immunocompromised patients, standard precautions are adequate for isolation of patients with acute or past EBV infections.

The epidemiology of infectious mononucleosis is closely related to the age of primary EBV infection; those areas where children are infected at an early age have the lowest incidence of the disease. Among susceptible adolescents and young adults, studies measuring both apparent and inapparent EBV infections indicate a clinical-to-subclinical ratio of 1:2 to 1:3. Although the ratio of clinical-to-subclinical infections in young children is not well defined, the incidence of the typical infectious mononucleosis syndrome is low. The incidence of infectious mononucleosis is approximately 50 per 100,000 persons per year, but in individuals 15 to 25 years old, the incidence doubles.

PATHOGENESIS EBV infection acquired by ingestion appears to begin in the oropharyngeal epithelial cells. The virus infects susceptible B lymphocytes within the lymphoid tissue of the pharynx. During a 30- to 50-day incubation period, virus actively replicates and disseminates throughout the entire lymphoreticular system. The EBV receptor on epithelial cells and B lymphocytes is the CD21 molecule (formerly CR2), which is also the receptor for the C3d fragment of the third component of complement. The virus elicits both humoral and cellular immune responses. Antibodies induced by the virus are directed against EBV-specific antigens, as well as to nonspecific heterophil antigens (polyclonal B cell stimulation), which cross-react with sheep and horse red-cell agglutinins, and with beef-cell hemolysins (see below).

Cell-mediated immune function is essential in the control of and recovery from EBV infection. In infectious mononucleosis induced by EBV, the initial infection of B lymphocytes is followed by an extensive proliferation of suppressor T lymphocytes (CD8$^+$-positive). These T cells are cytotoxic against EBV-infected lymphoid cells and prevent their proliferation. Associated with the absolute increase in these cytotoxic/suppressor cells is a concomitant decrease in the absolute number of T helper/inducer cells (CD4$^+$-positive lymphocytes). This results in an inversion of the CD4:CD8 ratio. Fatal infectious mononucleosis and lymphoproliferative disorders in which B-cell lymphomas develop have been identified in adults and children with defects in their cell-mediated immunity and, in particular, in their natural killer (NK) cell activity. Groups identified as developing this progressive B-immunoblastic disorder include kidney, heart, and bone marrow transplant recipients and individuals with X-linked lymphoproliferative syndrome, severe combined immunodeficiency syndrome, AIDS, ataxia-telangiectasia, and certain autoimmune diseases.

CLINICAL MANIFESTATIONS The incubation period of infectious mononucleosis syndrome is 30 to 50 days. This clinical syndrome is usually preceded by a 3- to 5-day prodrome consisting of malaise, fatigue, headache, nausea, or abdominal pain. Over the next 7 to 20 days, sore throat and fever gradually increase. The triad of fever, sore throat, and posterior cervical adenopathy occurs in more than 80% of patients with infectious mononucleosis. The sore throat is often accompanied by evidence of moderate-to-severe pharyngitis, with marked tonsillar enlargement that may be covered with shaggy gray exudate. On rare occasions, the tonsillar and peritonsillar swelling can result in airway obstruction. Fine petechiae may cover the uvula and soft palate during the initial week of illness. Throat cultures are positive for group A β-hemolytic streptococci in about 30% of patients. This may confuse the correct diagnosis of EBV mononucleosis. Fever is present in 85 to 95% of patients, is usually about 39°C (102°F), but may be as high as 40.5°C (105°F), and on average lasts 10 days. However, fever may persist for weeks in some patients with infectious mononucleosis.

Adenopathy most often involves the posterior cervical nodes, but the anterior cervical and epitrochlear nodes may also enlarge. Generalized adenopathy may also occur. The nodes are affected singly or in groups (not necessarily symmetrically) and may be very large or small (the size of grapes); they are most often firm, discrete, and moderately tender to palpation.

Splenomegaly, with the spleen palpable usually 2 to 3 cm below the costal margin, occurs in about 50% of infections. Massive splenomegaly may occur. Rupture is rare, but can be a potentially fatal complication. Hepatomegaly occurs in 10 to 30% of patients, but less than 5% of patients develop jaundice. Serum aspartate aminotransferase and serum lactate dehydrogenase (LDH) are mildly elevated in the majority of patients and may persist for weeks to months. However, chronic liver disease does not result.

Other clinical findings include bilateral supraorbital edema and rashes. A maculopapular rash occurs in about 5 to 15% of patients, but as many as 80% develop a rash if treated with ampicillin. Urticarial, bullous, hemorrhagic, and scarlatiniform rashes, as well as the Gianotti-Crosti syndrome, are also associated with infectious mononucleosis.

Neurologic complications include aseptic meningitis, encephalitis, optic neuritis, Guillain-Barré syndrome, transverse myelitis, and Bell palsy. Anemia (hemolytic or aplastic), granulocytopenia, or thrombocytopenia may occur during the acute illness or in the immediate recovery period. Respiratory and cardiac complications include interstitial pneumonia, myocarditis, and pericarditis. Laryngeal obstruction and pharyngeal edema may cause serious respiratory compromise.

In young children, infection with EBV does not usually present with typical infectious mononucleosis. Children under 4 years of age are more likely to exhibit rashes and hepatosplenomegaly. Failure to thrive, otitis media, abdominal pain, and recurrent pharyngitis are also more common in young children. Involvement of the hematopoietic system or the central nervous system, or the occurrence of prolonged fever, may be the primary or only manifestation of acute EBV infection.

EBV infection may be followed by persistent illness in adults and children with pharyngitis, lymphadenopathy, fever, headaches, arthralgia, fatigue, and psychoneurosis. The role of EBV in the persistence of these chronic manifestations is unknown.

Oral hairy leukoplakia of the tongue is a benign EBV-associated lesion commonly found in HIV-infected persons, and it is associated with few or no symptoms. Oral hairy leukoplakia is the only lesion presently known to arise as a direct consequence of the replication of the linear genome of EBV.

The x-linked lymphoproliferative syndrome (Purtillo syndrome) manifests as fatal EBV infection in males in particular families. Sporadic disease has also occurred in girls and in males with no family history of the syndrome. In these individuals, EBV infection is usually fatal and is associated with either a lymphoproliferative response, such as fatal mononucleosis, lymphoma, hemophagocytic syndrome, and B-cell immunoblastic sarcoma (seen in 75% of cases), or with an aproliferative response such as agammaglobulinemia, aplastic anemia, agranulocytosis, recurrent bacterial infections, and late malignancies (seen in 25% of cases).

EBV is also associated with a number of malignant disorders, including nasopharyngeal carcinoma, Burkitt lymphoma, leiomyosarcoma in immunocompromised patients, and, to a lesser extent, Hodgkin lymphoma (40% of Hodgkin disease in the developed world and as much as 80% of cases in the developing world).

LABORATORY DIAGNOSIS

Hematologic Findings The diagnosis of EBV-associated infectious mononucleosis is based on clinical manifestations, characteristic blood abnormalities, and positive heterophil or EBV antibodies. By the second week of infection, relative and absolute number of lymphocytes increase, with at least 10 to 20% atypical cells. Early in the disease, the atypical cells are both B and T lymphocytes. The atypical lymphocyte, or Downey cell, has a higher cytoplasm-to-nucleus ratio than a normal lymphocyte. The nucleus has coarse chromatin, and nucleoli are occasionally seen; the cytoplasm is more basophilic and vacuolated than normal. By early convalescence, the majority of the atypical lymphocytes are cytotoxic suppressor T cells (CD8$^+$). The total leukocyte count is usually 10,000 to 20,000 cells/μL, but may be as high as 50,000 cells/μL. The leukocyte abnormalities may persist for 4 to 8 weeks. An autoimmune hemolytic anemia occurs in 0.5 to 3% of infectious mononucleosis patients and is usually mediated by antibodies against the "i" antigen. A mild thrombocytopenia below 140,000 platelets/μL occurs in approximately 50% of patients. Profound thrombocytopenia with bleeding is rare.

Heterophil Antibodies Heterophil antibodies are present in as much as 90% of infectious mononucleosis cases caused by EBV in children over 4 years of age. The titer reported is the highest serum dilution at which sheep erythrocytes agglutinate after absorption of the patient's serum with guinea pig kidney. Such absorption eliminates interference caused by Forssman antibodies and by antibodies that are associated with serum sickness. Acute infectious mononucleosis also results in agglutinating antibodies to horse and bovine erythrocytes. Heterophil antibodies are directed to no

known EBV antigens. These IgM antibodies usually appear during the first or, more commonly, the second or third week of illness and become undetectable by 1 year in about 25% of individuals, using the horse red-cell agglutination test, and in 70% using sheep cell agglutinins. A number of rapid spot kits for detecting heterophil antibodies (using equine or bovine erythrocytes) are now available commercially. The correlation between results obtained by the spot and slide tests and the classic tube heterophil test is usually excellent. False-positive monospot tests have occasionally been reported in patients with lymphoma, pancreatitis, mumps, or hepatitis. False-negative tests occur most frequently in children younger than 4 years of age with EBV infectious mononucleosis and in older children tested in the first 2 weeks of illness. Only 5 to 10% of children younger than 2 years old have positive heterophil antibodies, whereas as many as 50% of children between 2 and 4 years of age will be heterophil-positive. The most accurate spot tests use horse erythrocytes, differential absorption, and reliable positive and negative controls.

EBV-Specific Antibodies The availability of specific EBV antibody tests has enabled more precise diagnosis of EBV infection. Specific antibodies detected by indirect immunofluorescence include IgG and IgM antibody to viral capsid antigen (IgG-VCA and IgM-VCA); antibodies to early antigens (EA), which consist of either a diffuse pattern (antigen present diffusely in cytoplasm and membrane), anti-D, or a restricted pattern (antigen restricted to cytoplasm only), anti-R; and antibody to EBV nuclear antigen (EBNA).

IgG antibodies to VCA are present in almost 100% of patients during the acute phase of infectious mononucleosis. Similarly, more than 95% of infectious mononucleosis patients will have demonstrable IgM-VCA on presentation, and all will have detectable antibody if tested at the appropriate time. Because IgM antibody usually lasts only 2 to 3 months, occasionally the antibody response may not be detected. Following recovery, IgG-VCA antibody remains detectable throughout life. Antibodies to early antigens are present in 70 to 80% of patients with acute infectious mononucleosis. The anti-D pattern is found predominantly in infectious mononucleosis or in reactivation syndromes, whereas the R-pattern is present in high titer in sera from patients with Burkitt lymphoma or in low levels in children younger than 2 years old with subclinical EBV infection. Antibody to the D component is a helpful marker for acute infection, as it is usually no longer detectable after 3 to 6 months. Antibodies to EBNA appear late in the course of infectious mononucleosis and remain detectable for life. Therefore, when antibody to EBNA is absent in the presence of other EBV-specific antibodies, recent infection is likely. Table 13-54 and Fig. 13-12 summarize these patterns.

Virus Identification EBV infection is most often diagnosed by clinical findings and serologic tests. DNA-DNA hybridization and, more recently, the amplification procedure of polymerase chain reaction are used to detect EBV DNA in clinical specimens; these techniques are still limited to research laboratories.

DIFFERENTIAL DIAGNOSIS The diagnosis of EBV infectious mononucleosis is straightforward in the patient who presents with sore throat, fever, posterior cervical lymphadenopathy, and malaise associated with atypical lymphocytosis and a positive heterophil test. When the heterophil test is negative, the precise etiology is more difficult to determine. Repeat heterophil antibody testing in 7 to 10 days, or the EBV-specific antibodies discussed earlier, are

TABLE 13-54

ANTIBODY PATTERNS ASSOCIATED WITH EBV INFECTION STATUS

EBV INFECTION STATUS	IgM-VCA	IgG-VCA	EBNA	ANTI-EA
No current or prior EBV infection	−	−	−	−
Acute primary EBV infection	++	++++	−	++
Recent past EBV infection (<6 mos.)	+	+++	−	++
Convalescent/post-EBV infection	−	+++	+	±
Chronic or reactivation infection	±	++++	±	+++
EBV-associated malignancies	−	++++	±	+++

EBV = Epstein-Barr Virus; VCA = viral capsid antigen; EA = early antigen; EBNA = Epstein-Barr nuclear antigen.

useful in establishing the role of the virus in the patient's illness. The most common cause of EBV-negative infectious mononucleosis is still the Epstein-Barr virus. Cytomegalovirus (CMV) is the second most common cause of heterophil-negative mononucleosis. In CMV infections, atypical lymphocytosis, fever, splenomegaly, and hepatomegaly are common. Sore throat, tonsillar exudate, and cervical lymphadenopathy occur much less commonly with CMV infection than with EBV infection and usually are less severe. Post-transfusion infection and mononucleosis are more common following CMV infection than with EBV.

Streptococcal pharyngitis may also be confused with infectious mononucleosis. Lymphadenopathy with strep throat is usually submandibular and anterior cervical. A positive throat culture for group A β-hemolytic streptococci does not eliminate the diagnosis of EBV infection because group A β-hemolytic streptococci can be isolated in 30% of patients with infectious mononucleosis.

Hepatitis A and B infection may also result in fever, lymphadenopathy, malaise, and rash associated with atypical lymphocytosis. When infectious mononucleosis is accompanied by jaundice, hepatitis A and B are frequently considered. Specific serologic tests for hepatitis A and B can help to establish the diagnosis.

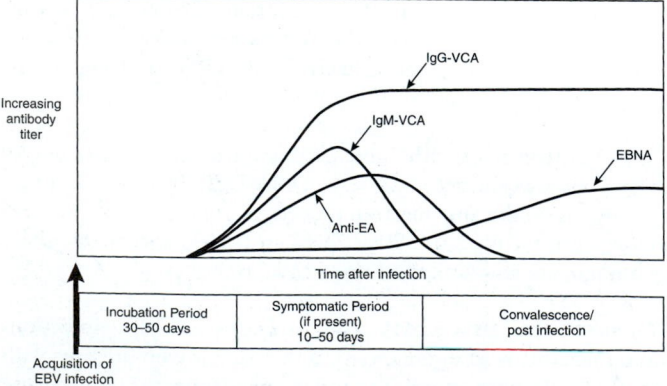

FIGURE 13-12   Typical course of serum antibody titers in infectious mononucleosis. EBV = Epstein-Barr virus; VCA = viral capsid antigen; EA = early antigen (diffuse pattern); EBNA = Epstein-Barr nuclear antigen.

Acute toxoplasmosis infection is associated with fever, fatigue, lymphadenitis, atypical lymphocytosis, and a protracted course. Exudative pharyngitis is not common with acute toxoplasmosis. Specific serologic tests and epidemiologic risk factors for toxoplasmosis are useful in differentiating between acute toxoplasmosis (see Sec. 13.6.5) and EBV infection.

Rubella and enteroviral infection occasionally result in fever, lymphadenopathy, and mild, atypical lymphocytosis. Viral cultures for rubella and enteroviruses, enteroviral RNA detection by PCR, and serologic tests for rubella can help establish the causal role of these agents.

The hematologic abnormalities associated with infectious mononucleosis accompanied by lymphadenopathy and splenomegaly may suggest the possibility of lymphoma or acute lymphocytic leukemia. The heterophil test may be helpful in differentiation. The bone marrow should be examined in any individual who has a lymphoproliferative disease without evidence of infectious mononucleosis.

TREATMENT   Currently, there is no specific antiviral therapy for EBV infection. Symptomatic care with antipyretics may be helpful. Forced rest is not helpful nor indicated. However, contact sports or other activities that may result in abdominal trauma should be avoided while the spleen is enlarged (usually 1 to 3 months). Corticosteroids are only indicated for managing potentially life-threatening complications including airway obstruction, neurologic complications, fulminant hepatitis, myocarditis or pericarditis, thrombocytopenic purpura, or hemolytic anemia. A short course of prednisone, 1 to 2 mg/kg/d given the first day in divided doses and rapidly tapered over 7 to 10 days, is usually sufficient. Longer courses may be necessary to treat hemolytic anemia and certain neurologic complications. Corticosteroids are not indicated for most patients.

If group A β-hemolytic streptococci are isolated from the throat, then appropriate antibiotic therapy is indicated. Ampicillin therapy should be avoided because of the high frequency of rashes associated with its use during infectious mononucleosis.

Specific antiviral therapy has generally not been beneficial in treating EBV infections. Acyclovir treatment of patients with infectious mononucleosis resulted in interruption of viral shedding in the throat, but had little clinical effect. Similarly, interferon-α administered prophylactically decreased the incidence of EBV shedding by kidney transplant recipients, but is not widely used for prophylaxis or treatment.

Lesions of oral hairy leukoplakia respond to oral or intravenous acyclovir, but they frequently recur in patients with HIV infection after treatment is discontinued. Aggressive, successful antiretroviral therapy frequently causes remission of lesions of oral hairy leukoplakia without specific therapy of EBV. Occasional remissions of polyclonal and monoclonal tumors have been described in persons with lymphoproliferative disorders treated with interferon-α and intravenous gamma globulin. Acyclovir is not helpful because it is active only on the lytic phase of EBV and not on the latent phase of EBV occurring in the lymphoproliferative conditions. Except for the rare occurrence of splenic rupture, severe central nervous system complications, severe hematologic problems, untreated respiratory compromise, or specific immunologic defects, the prognosis for the patient infected with EBV is excellent. Complete recovery is to be expected. During convalescence, some patients experience marked fatigue, which occasionally persists for months after the acute infection.

References

Cohen JI: The biology of Epstein-Barr virus: lessons learned from the virus and the host. Curr Opin Immunol 11:365–370, 1999

Maia DM, Garwacki CP: X-linked lymphoproliferative disease: pathology and diagnosis. Pediatr Dev Path 2:72–77, 1999

Mosier DE: Epstein-Barr virus and lymphoproliferative disease. Curr Opin Hematol 6:25–29, 1999

Okano M, Thiele GM, Davis JR, et al: Epstein-Barr virus and human diseases: recent advances in diagnosis. Clin Microbiol Rev 1:300–312, 1988

Straus SE, Cohen JI, Tosato G, Meier J: Epstein-Barr virus infections: Biology, pathogenesis and management. Ann Intern Med 118:45, 1993

Sumaya CV, Ench Y: Epstein-Barr virus infectious mononucleosis in children: I. Clinical and general laboratory findings. Pediatrics 75:1003, 1985

Sumaya CV, Ench Y: Epstein-Barr virus infectious mononucleosis in children: II. Heterophil antibody and viral-specific responses. Pediatrics 75: 1011, 1985

13.4.9   Human Herpesvirus 6

Mark R. Schleiss and David I. Bernstein

Human herpesvirus 6 (HHV-6) was isolated in tissue culture in 1986 from peripheral blood leukocytes of patients with both lymphoproliferative disorders and HIV infection. For several years after discovery it remained a "virus in search of a disease," but it is now known to be the major etiologic agent of roseola infantum and is implicated in other clinical syndromes.

HHV-6 is a prototypical herpesvirus, with a double-stranded DNA genome contained within an isosahedral capsid, surrounded by an outer envelope. Based on its molecular similarity to human cytomegalovirus, it is classified within the betaherpesvirus subfamily of the Herpesviridae. HHV-6 is further subclassified as either variant A or B, based on differences in nucleotide sequence, restriction enzyme profile, and reactivity with monoclonal antibodies. There are differences in diseases associated with each variant: HHV-6B is associated with exanthema subitum; HHV-6 has a tropism for lymphocytes, the possible site of latency. The prominent cell type infected in vivo is the mature $CD4^+$ T lymphocyte, although there is evidence from tissue culture that other cell types can be infected.

EPIDEMIOLOGY Infection with HHV-6 is ubiquitous. Virtually all children are infected by 2 to 3 years of age. There do not appear to be significant cultural, socioeconomic, or ethnic differences in incidence. Infection is seldom seen before 6 months of age, presumably because of the protective effect of transplacental antibody, and peaks between 6 and 12 months of age. Like all Herpesviridae, HHV-6 appears to cause lifelong (latent) infection, although little is known about the mechanisms or disease manifestations associated with persistence or reactivation.

HHV-6 can be found in the salivary gland and is shed in saliva of seropositive individuals, suggesting that saliva is the probable route of acquisition of infection. Primary infection in children most likely occurs via contact with HHV-6 shed in the secretions of older caregivers. HHV-6 can also be isolated from cervical secretions, suggesting that perinatal transmission is possible, but the extremely low seroprevalence of HHV-6 suggests that this observation is probably of little clinical significance. Unlike HCMV, HHV-6 is not found in breast milk.

CLINICAL MANIFESTATIONS The spectrum of disease associated with primary HHV-6 infection is broad, ranging from asymptomatic infection to fatal disseminated disease. Most commonly, however, primary infection occurs early in life and is manifest as either exanthema subitum or as an undifferentiated febrile illness. Reports of HHV-6 infection linked to other clinical syndromes must be interpreted cautiously. Because infection is ubiquitous and persistent in nature, the finding of HHV-6 antibody, or even isolation of the virus, cannot with certainty always document HHV-6 as the cause of any given clinical syndrome in older patients.

Exanthema Subitum Exanthema subitum (commonly known as roseola infantum) is a common acute febrile illness of infants and young children characterized by 3 to 5 days of fever, often accompanied by febrile seizures, followed by rapid defervescence and the appearance of an erythematous macular or maculopapular rash. This entity was at one time classified as "sixth disease" among the classic exanthematous illnesses of childhood. For many years, the cause was enigmatic, but the isolation of HHV-6 from the peripheral blood lymphocytes of four children with exanthema subitum and subsequent seroconversion indicated that HHV-6 was responsible for the observed clinical manifestations. HHV-6 is the major etiologic agent of exanthema subitum. HHV-6 viremia is transient, with virus isolation most common in the days just prior to onset of the rash. The disappearance of the culturable virus appears to correlate with the detection of neutralizing antibody.

Prior to development of the characteristic rash, there are no other clinical clues that reliably indicate that the febrile illness is caused by HHV-6, although posterior auricular adenopathy is commonly noted on physical exam. Because of fevers typically higher than 39°C (102.2°F), and a lack of differentiating clinical findings, many young infants are subjected to extensive laboratory evaluation and empiric antibiotic therapy. Defervescence followed by the onset of the characteristic rash is often misinterpreted as an antibiotic "allergy." The rash is either macular, papular, or maculopapular, and appears mainly on the trunk. The pathogenesis of the rash is unknown. Because it appears as the viremia clears and neutralizing antibody appears, it is presumed to be immune-mediated. The rash usually fades within 3 to 4 days following onset.

Fever Besides the high fever associated with exanthema subitum, HHV-6 infection is a common cause of fever *without* rash in infants. In one study, evidence for acute HHV-6 infection was identified in approximately 10% of children presenting to an emergency department for evaluation of high fever. Inflammation of tympanic membranes and a modest depression in total leukocyte count are the only other features that differentiated these children from those without HHV-6 infection. Because very young infants with high fever caused by HHV-6 infection are difficult to discriminate from those with occult empiric bacteremia, many young infants with acute HHV-6 infection are treated with antibiotic therapy (see Sec. 13.1.5).

Central Nervous System Infections Symptoms of primary HHV-6 infection usually are mild, but occasionally the infection is associated with central nervous system (CNS) complications in children with and without rash. Febrile convulsions are the most common complication associated with HHV-6 infection. In a large study of emergency room visits, HHV-6 accounted for one-third of all febrile seizures in children younger than 2 years of age. As many as 13% of all primary cases of HHV-6 infection may be complicated by febrile seizures. In some children, seizures may be prolonged or recurrent in nature. Because HHV-6 produces high fevers, it is unclear whether it is the fever itself that produces the seizures, or whether viral invasion of the central nervous system is responsible. The detection of HHV-6 DNA in the cerebrospinal fluid (CSF) has been reported in children with acute infection, suggesting that neuroinvasiveness may be a prominent feature of infection in some children. Other neurologic complications reported in acute HHV-6 infection include encephalitis, meningoencephalitis, and aseptic meningitis.

Transplant Patients Solid-organ transplant patients appear to be at increased risk for disease associated with HHV-6. It is presumed that the majority of such syndromes reflect reactivation of latent infection under conditions of immunosuppression. Rejection of kidney transplant is associated with increases in HHV-6 antibody titer and the presence of antigen in rejected kidneys. In bone marrow transplant patients, HHV-6 is implicated as a cause of interstitial pneumonitis, graft failure, and skin rashes resembling graft-versus-host disease.

Other HHV-6 Syndromes There has been some recent intriguing evidence to suggest a role for HHV-6 in the pathogenesis of multiple sclerosis (MS). These patients have a higher level of HHV-6 antibody as compared to controls, and HHV-6 DNA has been detected by polymerase chain reaction in some MS patients, but not in age-matched controls. HHV-6 is implicated as an etiology in some cases of heterophil-negative mononucleosis. Hepatitis, liver dysfunction, thrombocytopenia, thrombocytopenic purpura, hemophagocytic syndrome, chronic fatigue syndrome, and prolonged lymphadenopathy have also been described. HHV-6 is also implicated as a potential cofactor in the pathogenesis of AIDS. Both HIV and HHV-6 share a tropism for CD4[+] cells, and there is evidence that dual infection may stimulate the replication of HIV. Progression of HIV disease appears to be more rapid in children vertically infected with HIV who are also infected with HHV-6.

DIAGNOSIS The diagnosis of primary HHV-6 infection can often be made clinically in children with exanthema subitum. Primary HHV-6 infection may also be suspected in an irritable infant with high unexplained fever and no other clinical findings. Leukopenia may suggest the diagnosis, but this laboratory abnormality is non-specific. The differential diagnosis includes measles and rubella, but these are currently rare diseases in the United States. A recent history of measles immunization should be sought, because measles vaccine may produce fever and rash. The clinician should remember that enteroviruses, like roseola, may be accompanied by rashes and a febrile prodrome, but they are more likely to be seen in the late summer or early fall. Erythema infectiosum (fifth disease) is usually seen in somewhat older children. Fever is usually not as high as in roseola, and the rash is most prominent on the cheeks ("slapped-cheek" appearance). Infectious mononucleosis can produce an exanthem, particularly in those children who receive β-lactam antibiotics.

In those unusual circumstances in which specific etiologic diagnosis is necessary, the diagnosis of primary HHV-6 infection may be made by documenting a four-fold or greater rise in IgG titer. The virus can be cultured, but culture requires special techniques not available to most diagnostic virology laboratories. PCR is available, but must be interpreted cautiously, because viral nucleic acids can be detected in blood or saliva in a majority of older children and adults following acquisition of infection. The finding of HHV-6 DNA in the CSF may be helpful in the diagnostic evaluation of a child with protracted seizures.

THERAPY In immunocompetent children, primary HHV-6 infection is self-limited and no specific therapy is warranted. Data from cell culture studies suggest that, in vitro, the virus is susceptible to high doses of acyclovir, but is more sensitive to ganciclovir and foscarnet. Although there are anecdotal reports of immunocompromised patients with HHV-6 infection responding to antiviral therapy, there are no data from controlled trials.

References

Asano Y, Yoshikawa T, Suga S, et al: Clinical features of infants with primary human herpesvirus 6 infection (exanthem subitum). Pediatrics 93:104–108, 1994

Braun DK, Dominguez G, Pellett PE: Human herpesvirus 6. Clin Microbiol Rev 10:521–567, 1997

Bernstein D, Schleiss M: The growing family of Herpesviridae. Semin Pediatr Infect Dis 7:231–237, 1996

Campadelli-Fiume G, Mirandola P, Menotti L: Human herpesvirus 6: an emerging pathogen. Emerg Infect Dis 5:353–366, 1999

Hall CB, Long CE, Schnabel KC, et al: Human herpesvirus-6 infection in children: a prospective study of complications and reactivation. N Engl J Med 331:432–438, 1994

Kositanont K, Wasi C, Wanprapar N, et al: Primary infection of human herpesvirus 6 in children with vertical infection of human immunodeficiency virus type 1. J Infect Dis 180:50–55, 1999

Pruksananonda P, Hall CB, Insel RA, et al: Primary human herpesvirus 6 infection in young children. N Engl J Med 326:1445–1450, 1992

Yamanishi K, Okuno T, Shiraki K, et al: Identification of human herpesvirus-6 as a causal agent for exanthem subitum. Lancet 1:1065–1067, 1988

13.4.10 Human Herpesvirus 7 and Human Herpesvirus 8

Mark R. Schleiss

Human herpesviruses 7 (HHV-7) and 8 (HHV-8) are the newest members of the growing family of Herpesviridae. Both of these viruses were "discovered" in the 1990s. They have fundamentally different properties and produce very different disease manifestations. HHV-7 is highly related to HHV-6 and, like HHV-6, is responsible for the common childhood illness exanthema subitum (roseola infantum). HHV-8, in contrast, is strongly associated with Kaposi sarcoma, a tumor rarely encountered in childhood, but frequently observed in HIV-infected patients.

HUMAN HERPESVIRUS 7

HHV-7 is a betaherpesvirus, structurally and molecularly similar to cytomegalovirus and HHV-6. It was first isolated from CD4[+] T lymphocytes of a healthy individual. The high degree of homology with HHV-6 creates difficulty in interpretation of serologic assays, because there is considerable cross-reactivity of antibodies between HHV-6 and HHV-7 proteins.

As with HHV-6, infection with HHV-7 appears to be ubiquitous. However, HHV-7 infection appears to be acquired somewhat later in life than is HHV-6. By 2 years of age, approximately 40 to 45% of children have antibodies to HHV-7, and by 6 years of age,

70% of children are seropositive. HHV-7 can be found in the saliva, suggesting a route for person-to-person transmission.

CLINICAL MANIFESTATIONS Evidence is slowly accumulating to indicate that primary infection with HHV-7 causes clinical disease. Primary infection is clearly associated with exanthema subitum, and the rash is clinically indistinguishable from that caused by HHV-6. It is estimated that HHV-7 may be responsible for as much as 10% of episodes of exanthema subitum. Other reported clinical manifestations of primary HHV-7 infection include fever of unknown origin, simple febrile seizures, lymphadenopathy, hepatitis, and heterophil-negative mononucleosis. Table 13-55 summarizes the clinical syndromes described to date that are associated with HHV-7. Although infection is generally mild and self-limited, as with HHV-6, more severe disease is being reported.

DIAGNOSIS AND THERAPY The diagnosis of primary HHV-7 infection can be suspected in a child with exanthema subitum. Because sequential symptomatic infections with HHV-6 and HHV-7 have been described, it is important for the clinician to remember that more than one episode of "roseola" may occur in childhood. As with HHV-6, confusion may arise in children given antibiotic therapy for febrile illnesses who then develop rashes. It is seldom of importance to confirm the diagnosis of primary HHV-7 infection with laboratory tests, although for severe or complicated disease, a serologic assay that differentiates HHV-6 from HHV-7 antibodies was recently described and is available for investigational use. As with HHV-6, HHV-7 is susceptible in vitro to nucleoside antivirals, although there are no data regarding the therapeutic benefit of antivirals for this typically benign illness.

HUMAN HERPESVIRUS 8

The history of the identification of HHV-8 is unique among the Herpesviridae—indeed, among all infectious pathogens—insofar as the virus was initially "discovered" purely on a molecular biological basis using a representational difference analysis to identify disease-specific DNA sequences in tissue from HIV-infected individuals with Kaposi sarcoma (KS). Upon DNA sequence analysis, the deduced amino acid sequences were found to have strong homology to proteins from the gammaherpesvirus subfamily, which

TABLE 13-55

CLINICAL MANIFESTATIONS OF INFECTION WITH HUMAN HERPESVIRUSES 7 AND 8

Human Herpesvirus 7
- Exanthema subitum (roseola infantum)
- Fever
- Febrile seizures
- Hepatitis
- Mononucleosis syndrome
- Lymphadenopathy
- Pancytopenia

Human Herpesvirus 8
- Classical (Mediterranean) Kaposi sarcoma
- Endemic (African) Kaposi sarcoma
- Epidemic (AIDS-associated) Kaposi sarcoma
- AIDS-related body cavity-based lymphoma
- Castleman disease
- Proliferative skin lesions in immunocompromised hosts
- Multiple myeloma?

includes Epstein-Barr virus (EBV). Eventually HHV-8 was cultivated in tissue culture, proving that these DNA sequences corresponded to a bona fide infectious viral particle.

Structurally, HHV-8 consists of a prototypical enveloped particle, morphologically similar to other herpesviruses. HHV-8 appears to be tropic for B lymphocytes, especially of the CD19 subset, and also infects endothelial cells. The virus presumably establishes latent infection following primary infection, although the site(s) of latency are unknown. Evolutionarily, HHV-8 appears to have undergone considerable recombination with host genes, and the viral genome contains a variety of transduced cellular oncogenes and chemokine homologs, which are probably important in the pathogenesis of KS. It is estimated that 10% of the genes encoded by HHV-8 promote KS development due to either mitogenic, antiapoptotic, chemoattractive, angiogenic, or transforming activities. The precise contribution of these viral gene products to the pathogenesis of KS is under intense investigation in many laboratories.

The epidemiology of primary HHV-8 infection appears to vary considerably worldwide. Indeed, the routes of acquisition of infection and mechanisms responsible for person-to-person transmission remain uncertain. HIV-infected homosexual men and patients attending sexually transmitted disease clinics were found to have a higher HHV-8 seroprevalence than the general population. However, the available evidence suggests that sexual transmission of HHV-8 is probably most likely among homosexual men, with the evidence for heterosexual transmission of HHV-8 less convincing. Outside of the developed world, in contrast, nonsexual modes of HHV-8 transmission may predominate. In Africa, there is evidence accumulating for nonsexual transmission of infection in childhood, presumably a consequence of casual contact. Accordingly, KS in children, an extraordinarily rare pediatric tumor in North America, is fairly commonly encountered in children from some regions of Africa. HHV-8 has been detected by polymerase chain reaction (PCR) in salivary secretions from HIV-infected individuals, although transmission by this route is unproven. There are also reports of maternal-to-child transmission. As serologic tests become more standardized, a better assessment of the worldwide seroepidemiology of HHV-8 infection will be feasible.

CLINICAL MANIFESTATIONS There is no clinical syndrome ascribed to primary infection with HHV-8, which is probably asymptomatic. Prior HHV-8 infection appears to be necessary, but not sufficient, for the development of KS. Immunosuppression (due to HIV infection, malignancy, or chemotherapy-induced immunosuppression) is usually required for the development of KS. KS itself is a multifocal vascular neoplasm involving skin, visceral organs, and lymph nodes. KS lesions histopathologically contain distinctive proliferating cells ("spindle" cells), as well as activated endothelial cells, fibroblasts, smooth-muscle cells, and infiltrating inflammatory cells. Three variants of KS are described: "classical" KS, which is chiefly an indolent, slowly progressive form of KS seen in elderly Mediterranean men; "endemic" KS, a variant seen in Africa (including a "lymphadenopathic" form seen predominantly in young children); and "epidemic" KS, seen in HIV-infected patients. All variants are associated with HHV-8. The factors responsible for malignant transformation of HHV-8–infected endothelial cells into tumor are unknown.

Other malignant diseases have been associated with HHV-8, including multicentric Castleman disease, a lymphoproliferative syndrome associated with HIV infection, and another AIDS-associated malignancy, body cavity-based lymphoma (see Table 13-55).

Other malignancies, including skin cancer and multiple myeloma, are associated with HHV-8 in the literature, but these reports are controversial and the causal link remains unproven.

DIAGNOSIS AND THERAPY In the absence of a standardized serologic assay, serodiagnosis of HHV-8 infection is problematic. Tissue from any case of KS that is encountered in a child should probably be investigated for the presence of HHV-8 sequences, in collaboration with a reference laboratory. HIV serology should also be performed in such patients. AIDS-associated KS is reported to regress following administration of highly active antiretroviral therapy (HAART), suggesting that reversal of immunosuppression may promote resolution of the tumor. No controlled trials of specific antiviral therapy have been conducted for KS, although in a prospective analysis of ganciclovir treatment regimens for CMV retinitis in HIV-infected individuals, treatment with either oral or intravenous ganciclovir was associated with a strongly reduced risk of KS, suggesting an antiviral effect against HHV-8. Although these are intriguing data, chemotherapy and radiation therapy remain the mainstays of therapy for most cases of KS.

References

Bernstein D, Schleiss M: The growing family of Herpesviridae. Semin Pediatr Infect Dis 7:231, 1996

Chang Y, Cesarman E, Pessin MS, et al: Identification of herpesvirus-like DNA sequences in AIDS-associated Kaposi's sarcoma. Science 266: 1865, 1994

Grose C: Childhood infections with human herpesviruses types 6, 7, and 8. Adv Pediatr Infect Dis 12:181, 1996

Renne R, Zhong W, Herndier B, et al: Lytic growth of Kaposi's sarcoma-associated herpesvirus (human herpes virus 8) in culture. Nat Med 3: 342, 1996

Tanaka K, Kondo T, Torigoe S, et al: Human herpesvirus 7: another causal agent for roseola (exanthem subitum). J Pediatr 125:1, 1994

Torigoe S, Kumamoto T, Koide W, et al: Clinical manifestations associated with human herpesvirus 7 infection. Arch Dis Child 72:518, 1995

13.4.11   Varicella-Zoster Virus Infections

Beverly L. Connelly

Varicella-zoster virus (VZV) is an α-herpesvirus that infects humans almost exclusively. Like other human herpesviruses, VZV induces a primary infection (varicella), establishes a latent infection, and can reactivate to cause recurrent disease (zoster). VZV is a dsDNA-enveloped virus with the smallest genome of the human herpesviruses, encoding approximately 70 genes.

Prior to the introduction of varicella vaccine in 1995, the annual incidence of varicella in the United States approached the size of the birth cohort. An estimated 10,000 children were hospitalized annually; approximately 45 children and a slightly greater number of adults died each year from varicella and its complications between 1988 and 1995. Immunization rates in the United States have increased steadily since universal immunization was recommended in 1995; however, the CDC estimates that more than 65% of the eligible children in the United States are still unimmunized.

VZV is transmitted by the respiratory route and through close contact with cutaneous lesions of an infected individual. The incubation period for chickenpox is approximately 14 days. During this time, a primary viremia spreads the virus to the liver and possibly to other sites rich in monocytes/macrophages, where further

replication occurs. A secondary viremia involving T lymphocytes, as well as monocytes/macrophages, spreads virus to the skin where the virus replicates in the epidermis and forms the characteristic vesicular exanthem of varicella. Host humoral response is detectable within 4 days of the onset of the exanthem. Virus-specific antibody responses help inhibit VZV infection; however, it is cell-mediated immunity that is critical for limiting disease. Both nonspecific natural killer and antigen-specific T-cell responses participate in cell-mediated viral clearance. In normal hosts, antigen-specific cellular responses usually terminate secondary viremia within 72 hours. Failure to mount antigen-specific cellular responses results in progressive viral replication and dissemination with potentially fatal outcome.

Transmission may occur up to 48 hours prior to the appearance of the exanthem. Individuals remain contagious until the lesions are crusted, usually about 5 days in normal hosts. Virus is not eliminated from the host when viremia is terminated. Rather, virus becomes latent in dorsal root ganglia where it remains dormant for an extended period of time. Antigen-specific T lymphocytes are believed to be the principal gatekeepers of latent virus. Immunosuppression or natural senescence of T-lymphocyte surveillance mechanisms poses a risk for reactivation of virus and recurrent disease manifest as zoster (shingles).

Household exposure provides one of the most effective mechanisms of transmission; approximately 90% of susceptibles develop the disease within one incubation period. In the United States, varicella occurs most often in young school-aged children during the winter and early spring. This apparent "seasonality" is believed to reflect transmission facilitated by the crowded school setting. However, this "seasonality" is not exhibited in tropical climates. Children in the tropics escape infection only to remain susceptible as adults and thus are at risk for more severe disease.

VARICELLA (CHICKENPOX)

Varicella (chickenpox) is the highly communicable primary infection of VZV. Susceptible children acquire the virus from individuals with active VZV infection. The efficiency of transmission is far greater from individuals with varicella; however, individuals with zoster may also transmit the virus. Varicella may actually be most contagious just prior to the appearance of the exanthem. Following an incubation period of 10 to 21 days (up to 28 days following receipt of VZIG), individuals develop low-grade fever, headache, and malaise, followed in 24 to 48 hours by the development of the characteristic vesicular exanthem. The rash typically begins as "dew drops on rose-petals," appearing on the face, trunk, or scalp and eventually spreads to involve the entire body. The total number of lesions may vary from 50 to 500. The vesicles appear in crops for the first 3 to 5 days of the illness and may be exaggerated in areas of minor trauma or dermatitis, such as sunburn or eczema. The initial tiny vesicles evolve to larger vesicles that are filled with clear fluid that becomes cloudy with cellular debris, and finally involute with crust formation. Lesions on the skin are usually intensely pruritic but not painful. Lesions on mucous membranes become shallow ulcers, which may be painful. In the absence of secondary bacterial infection, healing occurs over 7 to 10 days without scar formation, although discrete hypo- or hyperpigmented lesions may persist for several months. Immunity following varicella is believed to be life-long; however, primary infection in circumstances in which immune responses are incomplete may predispose to a second episode of varicella. Vesicles may also be seen with infections due to herpes simplex viruses (HSV), enteroviruses (especially coxsackie), or *Staphylococcus aureus*. Occasionally, drug eruptions may be mistaken for varicella. In the neonate, vesicular eruptions may accompany congenital syphilis, congenital candidiasis, neonatal herpes, pustular melanosis, and histiocytoses. Thus, apparent second episodes of varicella may occur as a consequence of misdiagnosis of the first episode.

Varicella in the normal host is generally a benign self-limited disease. The occurrence of significant fever beyond the first 48 hours of exanthem or the progression of erythema or tenderness around crusting lesions should raise suspicion for secondary bacterial infection. Likewise, the appearance of hemorrhagic lesions, the presence of significant abdominal pain or vomiting, or altered mental status should alert clinicians to possible complications that require prompt intervention.

COMPLICATIONS The most common complications of varicella are secondary bacterial infections. *Staphylococcus aureus* and *Streptococcus pyogenes* (group A β-hemolytic streptococcus or GABHS) are the most common offenders. Secondary infections cover the spectrum from impetigo and local cellulitis to life-threatening sepsis. Progression of erythema around lesions, formation of bullae, or development of regional lymphadenitis signify secondary bacterial infection. Deep-tissue abscesses, osteomyelitis, or septic arthritis may occur. One of the most frightening secondary infections recently recognized is GABHS necrotizing fasciitis (NF). Pain in a muscle group and circumferential swelling of an extremity may be present in NF in the absence of significant overlying erythema. Magnetic resonance imaging (MRI) is useful in defining soft-tissue involvement when NF is suspected. In addition to aggressive medical management, surgical consultation is indicated for suspected NF (see Sec. 13.2.32).

Transient mild elevation in liver enzymes is common in varicella. More extensive, symptomatic hepatitis occurs with progressive disseminated varicella. Reye syndrome or acute encephalopathy with increased intracranial pressure, progressive neurologic dysfunction, and fatty degeneration of the liver was seen before the relationship between VZV and aspirin was recognized but is now a rare occurrence. Pneumonitis may be present in as many as 10% of cases of varicella. In children, lung involvement is usually mild; however, adults are at greater risk for progression to severe pneumonia and even respiratory failure.

Thrombocytopenia complicating varicella may present with hemorrhage into vesicular lesions, epistaxis, hematuria, or gastrointestinal bleeding. Thrombocytopenia may also present as a part of a coagulopathy in association with progressive varicella. Central nervous system (CNS) bleeding may rarely occur. The most common CNS complications of varicella are transient cerebellar ataxia and encephalitis. Cerebellar ataxia is generally self-limited and may occur before or after onset of the exanthem. Encephalitis may be limited or severe if associated with progressive disease. Aseptic meningitis, transverse myelitis, and Guillian-Barré syndrome have also been described.

IMMUNOCOMPROMISED HOSTS Individuals with congenital or acquired immune deficiencies that affect their ability to mount an antigen-specific T-cell response to VZV are at risk for progressive disseminated varicella, while individuals with isolated humoral immune deficiency are not. Progressive disseminated varicella involves multiple organ systems. Its onset may be heralded by severe abdominal pain or back pain before the appearance of a rash. Fever reaching to 40° to 41°C (104°–105.8°F) may persist for several days. Severe hepatitis, pneumonitis, thrombocytopenia, coagulop-

athy, encephalitis, and other organ dysfunction may all ensue. Mortality is high, even with treatment and supportive care. Individuals who have lymphoproliferative malignancies or who are stem-cell or solid-organ transplant recipients are at risk. Likewise, individuals with severe combined immune deficiencies, cartilage-hair hypoplasia, short-limbed dwarfism, Wiskott-Aldrich syndrome, or ataxia-telangiectasia are at risk. Depending on the degree of immunosuppression, individuals receiving steroids or other immunosuppressive agents for rheumatoid arthritis, systemic lupus erythematous, nephrotic syndrome, or inflammatory bowel disease may also be at risk. Because their ability to terminate viral replication is diminished, immunocompromised individuals with varicella are contagious for a longer period of time.

Individuals infected with human-immunodeficiency virus (HIV) or actual AIDS do not appear to be at the same degree of risk for progressive disseminated disease. Rather, varicella may persist for several weeks to months in HIV-infected individuals, only to reappear soon thereafter. The incidence of zoster is as high as 70%, and recurrent disease is common in this population. Episodes are usually milder than in other immunocompromised hosts, but may be severe in selected cases. Coinfection with cytomegalovirus (CMV) or Epstein-Barr virus (EBV) may increase severity, even in the otherwise normal host.

CONGENITAL AND NEONATAL DISEASE Currently, the incidence of varicella during pregnancy is quite low. However, a pregnant woman with varicella pneumonia may develop significant hypoxia and progress to respiratory failure, posing a great risk to mother and fetus. When maternal varicella occurs in the first 20 weeks of gestation, as many as 2% of fetuses may manifest findings associated with varicella embryopathy. Among the constellation of features of congenital VZV are cutaneous defects; classic cicatricial skin scarring and limb atrophy; microcephaly; cortical atrophy; seizures; chorioretinitis; microphthalmia; and significant neurologic deficits. Autonomic nervous system involvement may manifest as difficulty with sphincter control, intestinal obstruction, Horner syndrome, or other cranial nerve neuropathies. Maternal zoster does not carry this risk.

Infants born to mothers who develop varicella less than 5 days before delivery or 2 days after delivery are at risk of severe neonatal varicella because they are likely to have acquired significant virus in the absence of transplacental VZV antibody. Mothers who develop varicella more than 4 days prior to delivery synthesize VZV-specific IgG in sufficient time to permit placental transfer of antibody, which will ameliorate severe disease, but which may not protect newborns against infection. Infants whose mothers have varicella at any stage of pregnancy, or infants who acquire varicella during the first few months after birth, may manifest zoster early in life.

ZOSTER (SHINGLES)

Zoster (shingles) is recurrent disease that results from reactivated latent virus in dorsal root ganglia that replicates and spreads via the nerve to the skin. The incidence of zoster increases with increasing age, believed to be in response to declining immunity to VZV. Racial background plays a role; the lifetime incidence of zoster in African-Americans is approximately half that reported for whites. Children with malignant disorders, particularly those with lymphomas, acute lymphocytic leukemia, or AIDS, are at increased risk of developing zoster. Normal children also may develop zoster. Zoster in the first 2 years of life is usually associated with maternal gestational varicella or varicella occurring during early infancy.

Zoster appears as a unilateral process involving a single or possibly two adjacent dermatomes. Thoracic dermatomes are most often involved, followed by cranial nerve and lumbosacral regions. The lesions often appear first as patches of erythema, which then develop groups of vesicles. A few scattered lesions, remote from the dermatomes, may appear. The lesions progress over 3 to 5 days and usually dry and crust within 2 weeks. Pain or paresthesias within the involved dermatome may precede the vesicular eruption. Preeruptive thoracic pain has been mistaken for angina. Postherpetic neuralgia is relatively uncommon in pediatrics, but occurs in 50% of individuals with zoster over 60 years of age and may be severe and protracted. Zosteriform eruptions in the maxillary division of the fifth cranial nerve may occasionally be due to HSV rather than VZV.

Generalized or disseminated zoster may occur in immunocompromised hosts and mimic varicella in appearance. It can often be distinguished from varicella by a history of vesicular lesions localized to one to three dermatomes for several days prior to the generalized eruption. Multiorgan involvement may follow in the untreated immunocompromised host, as has been described for varicella in this high-risk population.

DIAGNOSIS The diagnosis of varicella and zoster is usually clinically apparent, although the child with few lesions may go undiagnosed or be misdiagnosed as "insect bites." Atypical or mild varicella may also occur in the presence of incomplete immunity. A variety of options are available when laboratory confirmation is desired.

The popular Tzanck (or Giemsa-stained) smear permits identification of giant cells and cells harboring inclusions, but does not distinguish between HSV and VZV lesions. Direct immunofluorescent antibody (DFA) staining of cells scraped from the base of a lesion using VZV-specific antibodies is a preferred technique. Where available, DFA provides a rapid and specific way to diagnose VZV infection. Viral culture of VZV requires prolonged incubation relative to other herpesviruses. The highest yield is from early lesions (clear fluid). Polymerase chain reaction (PCR) techniques for VZV are not standardized and, at this time, are principally useful as research tools for VZV.

A variety of serologic tests for VZV have been used to determine preexisting infection, susceptibility to disease, and response to immunization. The fluorescent-antibody-to-membrane-antigen, or FAMA assay, is the "gold standard" for determining biologically significant antibody; the technique, however, is cumbersome. Commercially available VZV-IgG ELISAs are often used to identify susceptible individuals who may be at risk for severe disease, such as those requiring transplantation, and to verify response to immunization in select individuals. Commercially available VZV-IgG ELISAs do not reliably identify vaccine immunity. Tests for VZV-IgM are not reliable.

TREATMENT No specific therapy is required for uncomplicated varicella. Acetaminophen is the preferred antipyretic when needed. Aspirin should be avoided in patients with varicella because of its association with Reye syndrome. Ibuprofen may be a greater risk for invasive GABHS disease complicating varicella and, therefore, should be avoided until further data are available. Daily bathing with an antibacterial soap is recommended to reduce the risk of bacterial superinfection of skin lesions. In addition, bathing provides an opportunity for careful inspection of the skin for signs of secondary infection. Fingernails should be trimmed. Pruritus can often be controlled with calamine lotion, cool compresses, or an oatmeal bath. Occasionally, systemic antipruritic agents such as diphenhydramine hydrochloride or hydroxyzine may be helpful.

Oral acyclovir (ACV) decreases the number and duration of new lesions: however, its benefit in the management of routine varicella is marginal. ACV treatment is generally not recommended for routine use in the normal host but may be considered in those patients at risk for more severe disease, for example, second case in a household, adolescents, and adults. Therapy should be started as soon as possible after disease is recognized and probably is of little benefit if started beyond the first 24 to 48 hours of exanthem. The usual dose of oral ACV for the normal host is 20 mg/kg/dose (max 800 mg/dose) four times daily for 5 days.

Intravenous ACV is indicated for the treatment of the immunocompromised child with varicella or zoster because of the potential for dissemination. The dosage of intravenous ACV is 45 to 60 mg/kg/d up to 10 kg body weight and 1500 mg/m²/d over 10 kg body weight given in three divided doses. The bioavailability of ACV following oral administration is limited and may not be adequate for these patients. If oral therapy is considered, the dosage is the same as for the immunocompetent host. Duration of therapy is usually 7 to 10 days or until lesions are crusted.

Intravenous ACV is indicated for neonates who develop varicella from their mothers and should be considered for neonates who develop varicella following household exposure. The term infant should receive 15 to 20 mg/kg/dose given every 8 hours; in premature infants, the dosing interval should be decreased to every 12 hours. Oral ACV is generally not indicated for treatment of young infants because of limited bioavailability and erratic absorption in infants.

PREVENTION

Varicella-Zoster Immune Globulin (VZIG) Passive immunoprophylaxis with VZIG should be considered for exposed *susceptible* individuals who may be at risk for severe disease. This includes immunocompromised children and pregnant women without a prior history of varicella, newborn infants whose mothers developed varicella less than 5 days before or 2 days after delivery, premature infants more than 28 weeks' gestation born to women with negative VZV histories, and premature infants less than 28 weeks' gestation regardless of maternal history when a significant exposure has occurred. Significant exposures include an active case of varicella residing in the same household or sharing the same hospital room, face-to-face indoor play with an active case of varicella, and intimate contact with a person with active zoster. VZIG should be administered as soon as possible, but within 96 hours of the exposure (0 to 10 kg = 125 IU; 10 to 20 kg = 250 IU; 20–30 kg = 375 IU; 30–40 kg = 500 IU; greater than 40 kg = 625 IU). It should be noted that VZIG may not prevent infection in these individuals and may prolong the incubation period to 28 to 35 days. VZIG has no benefit after infection is established and is not indicated in the treatment of varicella or zoster.

Live-Attenuated Vaccine The indications and contraindications for administration of varicella vaccine are discussed in Sec. 1.5.2.

Infection Control Children with varicella are usually excluded from school for the first 5 days after the appearance of rash or until the lesions are crusted. However, because children may be most contagious the day prior to the onset of the rash, this policy does not prevent the spread of varicella in school settings; immunization may be more useful. Children with active varicella or who are in the incubation period following exposure should not be admitted electively to the hospital. If admission is required for these children, appropriate isolation with airborne precautions is indicated until they are beyond the incubation period or until those who develop varicella are no longer contagious.

In the hospitalized setting, transmission of VZV from individuals with zoster to susceptible individuals has been demonstrated in the absence of intimate contact. Therefore, hospitalized patients with zoster should also be isolated to avoid inadvertent exposure of high-risk individuals.

References

Aebi C, Ahmed A, Ramilo O: Bacterial complications of primary varicella in children. Clin Infect Dis 23(4):698–705, 1996

Arvin A: Immune responses to varicella-zoster virus. Infect Dis Clin North Am 10:529–570, 1996

Brunell PA: Varicella in pregnancy, the fetus, and the newborn: problems in management. J Infect Dis 166:S42–47, 1992

Centers for Disease Control: Prevention of varicella: updated recommendations of the Advisory Committee on Immunization Practices (ACIP). MMWR Morb Mortal Wkly Rep 48(RR-6):1–5, 1999

Cohen JI, Brunell PA, Straus SE, Krause PR: Recent advances in varicella-zoster virus infection. Ann Int Med 130:922–932, 1999

Gershon AA, Mervish N, LaRussa P, et al: Varicella-zoster virus infection in children with underlying human immunodeficiency virus infection. J Infect Dis 176:1496–1500, 1997

LaRussa P, Steinberg S, Gershon AA. Varicella vaccine for immunocompromised children: results of collaborative studies in the United States and Canada. J Infect Dis 174:S320–325, 1996

Zerr DM, Alexander ER, Duchin JS, Koutsky LA, Rubens CE. A case-control study of necrotizing fasciitis during primary varicella. Pediatrics 103:783–790, 1999

13.4.12   Human Immunodeficiency Virus Type 1 Infection in Infants and Children

Michael T. Brady

Worldwide, it is estimated that 1.2 million children are infected with human immunodeficiency virus (HIV), with more than 1 million HIV-infected children in Africa alone. By the year 2000, some 3.9 million children have died from HIV infection and an additional 10 million have been orphaned as a result of HIV-related deaths of their parents. In the United States, rates of new pediatric infections increased from 1982 until 1995. Since 1995, the use of antiretroviral agents in HIV-infected pregnant women (during the pregnancy and intrapartum) and the exposed infant in the immediate postpartum period has significantly reduced perinatal transmission. Rates of new infections in children younger than 15 years of age in the United States have declined from a high of 2500 per year to approximately 400 to 600 per year. The number of HIV-infected infants and children in the United States is currently estimated to be between 10,000 and 20,000. This number has remained relatively stable because these children have an ever-increasing life expectancy. HIV was the sixth leading cause of death in children aged 1 to 4 years in 1996, and is currently the sixth leading cause of death in persons 15 to 24 years old.

Nearly 90% of HIV-infected infants and children acquire their infection vertically, during gestation or, more commonly, during labor and delivery. An increasing fraction of women with HIV contracted infection through heterosexual contact, although injection drug use by women still accounts for approximately one-third of all HIV transmission in women of childbearing age. Ethnic minorities and low-income classes are markedly overrepresented among HIV-infected women in the United States. In the United States, approximately 8% of children now alive with HIV were infected through transfusion of contaminated blood products or coagulation factors, although this fraction should continue to decline because of the effectiveness of current blood-donor screening methods. Adolescents participating in adult risk behaviors (sexual activity and injection drug use) and victims of child sexual abuse make up a few percent of the total.

The timing and mechanisms of perinatal HIV transmission are not completely understood. Evidence of HIV in fetal tissue is found in approximately 30% of first- and early second-trimester abortions by women who are HIV-infected. However, it appears likely that the majority of infants are infected in the peripartum period, either through transplacental passage of virus (late pregnancy or at the time of labor) or by exposure to HIV during birth. Postnatal transmission through breast-feeding is well documented, and this fact underlies the recommendation that mothers with HIV infection should not breast-feed if safe, alternative infant nutrition is available.

Of children born to untreated HIV-infected women, 13 to 40% will be infected. Many maternal and obstetric factors that contribute to the risk of perinatal transmission have been identified. The role of each individual factor is yet to be determined. Prematurity, advanced maternal disease, exposure to maternal blood, and higher maternal viral load are associated with higher risks for HIV transmission, but neither these factors nor other clinical or immunologic data are completely predictive of transmission. However, of all the identified risk factors, it appears that reducing the mother's viral load offers the greatest opportunity to reduce perinatal transmission. Mode of delivery (cesarean section appears to confer some protection from perinatal transmission of HIV) may also reduce the risk of perinatal transmission. HIV-infected pregnant women should be aware of the relative benefits and risks associated with a cesarean section when they and their obstetricians choose a mode of delivery.

PATHOGENESIS   HIV preferentially infects lymphocytes with the CD4 surface antigen, which, together with the cytokine cell receptor CXCR4, acts as a viral receptor. This lymphocyte subset, which includes helper lymphocytes with critical roles in maintaining immune responsiveness, also shows gradual attrition with progression of disease. The mechanism by which HIV infection causes this $CD4^+$ cell decline is not completely established, although possibilities include lytic infection of the $CD4^+$ cells themselves; induction of apoptosis through viral antigens, which may act as superantigens; destruction of infected cells by host antiviral immune mechanisms; and death or dysfunction of lymphocyte precursors or accessory cells in the thymus and lymph nodes.

HIV does infect cell types other than lymphocytes. HIV infection of monocytes, unlike that of $CD4^+$ lymphocytes, may not lead to death of the cell. Infected monocytes may act as latent but inducible reservoirs of virus and may carry virus to organs, particularly the brain, in which they become resident. Hybridization experiments demonstrate HIV viral nucleic acid in chromaffin cells of the intestinal mucosa, glomerular and tubular epithelia, and astroglia. In fetal tissue, the most consistent recovery of virus is from brain, liver, and lung. HIV-related pathology involves many organs, although it is often difficult to know whether injury is primarily a

TABLE 13-56

IMMUNOLOGIC CATEGORIES FOR HIV-INFECTED CHILDREN UNDER 13 YEARS OF AGE STRATIFIED BY AGE

IMMUNOLOGIC CATEGORY	<12 MONTHS OLD		1–5 YEARS OLD		6–12 YEARS OLD	
	CD4+ CELLS/μL	%*	CD4+ CELLS/μL	%*	CD4+ CELLS/μL	%*
1. No evidence of immune suppression	≥1500	≥25	≥1000	≥25	≥500	≥25
2. Evidence of moderate immune suppression	750–1499	15–24	500–999	15–24	200–499	15–24
3. Evidence of severe immune suppression	<750	<15	<500	<15	<200	<15

*Percent of total lymphocytes.

SOURCE: *Modified from Centers for Disease Control: Summary of 1994 revised classification system for human immunodeficiency infection in children less than 13 years of age. MMWR Morb Mortal Wkly Rep 43(No. RR-12):1, 1994.*

consequence of local virus infection, immune-mediated cytotoxic effects, or other associated infectious complications.

The hallmark stages of HIV infection in the untreated adult are an acute infection phase (seroconversion syndrome), often with flu-like symptoms, accompanied by high-grade viremia; followed by a period of immune containment of viral replication, during which the individual is usually free of symptoms; and a final period of progressive symptomatic immune compromise, with increasing viral replication. During the second asymptomatic phase, gradual and progressive abnormalities of immune function are apparent on testing. Viral load (quantification of viral particles in the plasma, representative of viral replication rate) is variable, but usually is lower than viral-load levels detected during the acute infection phase, and generally remains stable for months to years. The rapidity with which infected adults and children progress through the second (clinically stable) phase can be predicted to some degree by determining the individuals' CD4+ cell count and viral load. Lower CD4+ counts and higher viral loads are each independent predictors of more rapid disease progression. The final phase, with symptomatic immune compromise, end-organ dysfunction, and HIV-associated malignancies, is correlated with increasing viral replication and often a change in viral type (nonsyncytial → syncytial), profound attrition of CD4+ lymphocytes, and severe immune dysregulation and opportunistic infections.

Perinatal HIV infection is generally clinically silent at birth, although the "incubation period," or interval before symptoms of HIV infection become manifest, is generally shorter following perinatal infection than in adult HIV infection. During this phase, immune dysregulation is often apparent on testing, especially with regard to B-cell percentage and function; hypergammaglobulinemia with production of nonfunctional antibodies (polyclonal) is more common among HIV-infected children than among adults, typically noted as early as 3 to 6 months of age. There is an inability to respond to new antigens with appropriate immunoglobulin production. This critically affects infants without prior antigen exposure, contributing to the greater frequency and severity of invasive bacterial infections seen in pediatric HIV infection. Infants and young children have much higher absolute numbers of lymphocytes, including CD4+ lymphocytes. For this reason, depletion of CD4+ lymphocytes may not be as readily apparent in HIV-infected infants and young children, and the absolute CD4+ lymphocyte count may not be as predictive of the risk for opportunistic infections. Infants and children with HIV infection often have normal numbers of total lymphocytes, and as many as 15% of patients with pediatric AIDS may have a normal ratio of CD4+ to CD8+ lymphocytes. However, the CD4+ cell percentage is relatively similar at all ages and can frequently be used to detect CD4+ lymphocyte

abnormalities that are the result of HIV infection in infants and young children with normal absolute CD4+ lymphocyte counts. However, in infants younger than 1 year of age, neither absolute numbers nor percentage of CD4+ lymphocytes can be used to accurately identify HIV-infected infants with immune dysfunction and an associated risk for opportunistic infections, particularly *Pneumocystis carinii* pneumonia.

CLINICAL MANIFESTATIONS With few exceptions, infants with perinatal HIV infection are clinically and immunologically normal at birth. In a few instances, adenopathy may be detected in the first month of life. Clinically silent abnormalities of immune function often precede HIV-related symptoms, although the immunologic assessment of infants at risk is complicated by several unique factors. First, age-specific normal parameters for CD4+ lymphocyte count and CD4/CD8 ratio show higher absolute CD4+ numbers and wider ranges in early infancy, followed by a gradual decline over the first several years (Table 13-56). In addition, in utero exposure to illicit drugs, and possible exposure to HIV antigens without infection, may perturb lymphocyte number and function. It is thus imperative to refer to age-adjusted standards for CD4+ cell counts, and when possible, to use parameters established from observation of uninfected infants born to infected mothers.

The earliest and most common HIV-associated symptoms in infancy are rarely diagnostic. As listed by the Centers for Disease Control in the 1994 Revised Classification System, the first abnormalities detected include fever, failure to thrive, hepatomegaly and splenomegaly, generalized lymphadenopathy (defined as nodes >0.5 cm present in two or more nonbilateral sites for >2 months), parotitis, and diarrhea. Prior to the early use of aggressive combination antiretroviral therapy, approximately 90% of perinatally HIV-infected infants would manifest one or more of these symptoms in the first year of life. In the European Collaborative study of infants born to HIV-infected mothers, the conditions that best discriminated between HIV-infected and uninfected infants were chronic candidiasis, parotitis, persistent lymphadenopathy, and hepatosplenomegaly. Otitis media, rhinitis, unexplained fever, and chronic diarrhea were not significantly more common in HIV-infected infants than in uninfected infants.

Approximately 20% of HIV-infected infants present with rapidly progressive immune compromise and/or an AIDS-defining condition such as *Pneumocystis carinii* pneumonia (PCP), or serious bacterial or fungal infections within the first 3 to 6 months of life. In some infants in the first year of life, the CD4+ cell count may be normal at the time of presentation of PCP. The potential for rapid disease progression in perinatally HIV-infected children underscores the need for early identification and initiation of prophylaxis for opportunistic infection. If prenatal testing of the mother is not performed, all infants should be tested for HIV in the immediate postpartum period.

Within 2 years of birth, many HIV-infected infants, including those receiving antiretroviral therapy, have some degree of failure to thrive, linear growth failure, recurrent or chronic fever, developmental delay, persistent adenopathy, or hepatosplenomegaly. With the exception of linear growth abnormalities, most of these symptoms are less common and/or less severe with aggressive combination antiretroviral therapy. The development or worsening of these symptoms while receiving aggressive antiretroviral therapy suggests clinical failure and possible resistance to one or more of the medications in the treatment regimen.

Pneumocystis carinii **Pneumonia (PCP)**   PCP is the most common of the AIDS-indicator diseases in children and adults, and it previously affected approximately one-third of HIV-infected infants and children. The median age for presentation is approximately 9 months of age, although there is a peak at 3 to 6 months of age among rapidly progressing and previously unidentified infants. Unlike reactivation PCP in adults, this infection is usually a primary infection in HIV-infected children, presenting subacutely or abruptly with fever, cough, tachypnea, and rales. PCP may be difficult to distinguish clinically and radiologically from other pulmonary infections at this age. Because intravenous trimethoprim-sulfamethoxazole (TMP-SMX) and corticosteroids given early in the course may lead to significant improvement, diagnostic bronchoalveolar lavage should be considered early in the course of illness in the infant with a consistent clinical presentation and risk factors for HIV infection. In very young infants, PCP is associated with a high mortality rate; early studies suggested a median survival of 1 month after diagnosis. Milder disease may occur in both young infants and older children, and permits long-term survival. Prophylaxis of PCP with oral TMP-SMX is indicated for infants and children with evidence of severe immune suppression (Table 13-56), prior PCP, and in all HIV-infected infants younger than 1 year of age.

Lymphoid Interstitial Pneumonitis (LIP)   This chronic interstitial infiltration of the lungs has been described in a small number of HIV-infected adults, but is seen in 20 to 25% of HIV-infected children. There is evidence to support an association with Epstein-Barr virus infection. The condition is characterized by a chronic course with intermittent exacerbations (often during intercurrent respiratory infections). Chronic chest infiltrates seen on x-ray often suggest the diagnosis, but only open-lung biopsy is definitive. Hypoxia is seldom severe until the condition has been present for many years; improvement with corticosteroid use has been reported. As a presenting symptom of HIV infection, LIP appears to be associated with a better prognosis than other AIDS-indicator diseases, and is often seen in a symptom cluster with marked hypergammaglobulinemia, parotitis, and massive adenopathy.

Recurrent Bacterial Infections   Recurrent bacterial infections are defined as two or more episodes of sepsis, meningitis, pneumonia, internal abscesses, or bone and joint infection. Prior to aggressive antiretroviral therapy and PCP prophylaxis with TMP-SMX, recurrent bacterial infections were seen in approximately 15% of children with pediatric AIDS. The frequency of bacterial infections is far less in children receiving appropriate antiretroviral therapy and PCP prophylaxis. Less-invasive bacterial infections, such as chronic or recurrent sinus infections, otitis media, and pyodermas are somewhat more common in HIV-infected children. *Streptococcus pneumoniae* is the most frequent blood isolate in HIV-infected children, although gram-negative enterics (particularly *Salmonella*), staphylococcal, and even pseudomonal bacteremia are seen more commonly in HIV-infected children.

Prophylaxis with intravenous immunoglobulin (IVIG) may reduce the frequency and severity of serious bacterial infections. However, with appropriate antiretroviral therapy and PCP prophylaxis, the additional benefits of IVIG may be limited. IVIG use should be restricted to HIV-infected children with hypogammaglobulinemia, recurrent bacterial infections despite appropriate antiretroviral therapy, or an absence of antibodies to critical vaccine antigens following immunization, such as tetanus or *Haemophilus influenzae* type b. The conjugate pneumococcal vaccine is expected to be available in the near future. HIV-infected infants capable of mounting an immune response should receive the conjugate pneumococcal vaccine.

Progressive Neurologic Disease   Central and peripheral nervous system disease occurs more commonly and at an earlier point in HIV disease in children than it does in adults. In as many as 25% of HIV-infected infants, central nervous system (CNS) involvement manifests as a static encephalopathy, usually presenting as developmental delay in the first year of life. Many HIV-infected children will have only mild CNS disease. In approximately 33% of HIV-infected children, a progressive encephalopathy ensues, with loss of previously attained milestones and moderate to severe cognitive and motor deficits. Neuroimaging may reveal cerebral atrophy, white matter abnormalities, and/or basal ganglion calcifications, although the severity of imaging abnormalities often does not correlate with clinical findings. Because this rapidly progressive syndrome is identified less commonly in the era of combination antiretroviral therapy, it would appear that successful control of viral replication can either prohibit ongoing CNS damage from virus already present in the CNS or reduce new virus entry into the CNS.

Wasting Syndrome   Chronic failure to thrive is seen in many infants and children with advanced HIV infection, and it is nearly always multifactorial. Anorexia can result from generalized malaise and fatigue, as well as from mouth sores associated with thrush (*Candida albicans* and other yeasts), herpes simplex, and aphthous ulcers. Central nervous system deficits, including lethargy, weakness in swallowing, neuroendocrine abnormalities, malabsorption and diarrhea resulting from numerous enteric pathogens as well as primary HIV infection, and infection-induced catabolism, frequently contribute to this vexing problem. Recent combination antiretroviral therapies have resulted in better maintenance of weight gain, or in diminished weight loss. However, linear growth has not improved as dramatically (possibly because of resistance to growth hormone). In addition, combination therapies with and without protease inhibitors are associated with marked elevation of triglycerides and cholesterol and changes in fat deposition (lipodystrophy syndrome—increased fat deposition in the abdomen and upper back with loss of fat from the extremities).

Opportunistic Infections   More than a dozen specific opportunistic infections meet the AIDS definition. After PCP, the most common opportunistic infection in pediatric AIDS patients are *Candida* esophagitis and *Mycobacterium avium* complex infection. The most common infections caused by viruses are recurrent, prolonged, or disseminated infections with the cytomegalovirus (CMV), particularly of the gastrointestinal tract, and recurrent, extensive, and atypical infections with herpes simplex and varicella-zoster. Despite the long list of pathogens causing unusually severe or protracted illness in HIV-infected hosts, common respiratory viruses, including respiratory syncytial virus, seldom cause complicated illness.

Other Organ Involvement Hepatic involvement in pediatric HIV infection often takes the form of hepatomegaly with mild to moderate, fluctuating transaminitis. Less common is a severe cholestatic hepatitis seen in infected infants in the first year of life, with a poor prognosis. Liver abnormalities may be exacerbated by concomitant infection with the common viruses causing hepatitis (CMV; hepatitis A, B, and C; and the Epstein-Barr virus), by HIV infection itself, or by many of the medications used to treat HIV and its infectious complications. Renal disease is not uncommon, with proteinuria the most likely finding. Focal glomerulosclerosis and mesangial changes have been identified in children with advanced HIV infection. Cardiac abnormalities are demonstrable in as many as 50% of children at all stages of HIV disease, although the incidence of symptomatic cardiomyopathy is only 12 to 20% and it occurs late in advanced disease; ventricular dysfunction and pericardial effusion are the most commonly encountered echocardiographic abnormalities. Despite the frequency of chronic pulmonary disease in HIV-infected children, left-ventricular involvement is several times more common than is right-ventricular involvement. Direct HIV involvement, immune-mediated damage, malnutrition, and concomitant infection with myotropic viruses have all been suggested as etiologies for cardiomyopathy. Autoimmune phenomena include Coombs-positive hemolytic anemia, thrombocytopenia, and aphthous ulcers. Kaposi sarcoma and other secondary cancers are rare in HIV-infected children.

PROGNOSIS Clinical status at the time of initial presentation appears to correlate with prognosis in perinatally infected children. Approximately 15 to 20% of HIV-infected infants have an early onset of disease symptoms (average age 4 months) and progress to AIDS within 1 year if not treated appropriately. The majority of HIV-infected infants, however, have longer asymptomatic periods, averaging approximately 5 years, with approximately 8% progressing to AIDS-defining illnesses per year of life. Prior to availability of protease inhibitors the estimated mean survival for children perinatally infected, but not symptomatic in the first year of life, was approximately 9.4 years. Since the availability of protease inhibitors or nonnucleoside reverse transcriptase inhibitors and optimal opportunistic infection prophylaxis, most pediatric HIV treatment centers have documented marked reductions in both new opportunistic infections and mortality in HIV-infected children who experience immunologic improvement or stabilization following combination therapy.

Persons infected with HIV during adolescence are often not diagnosed until early adulthood, in part because pediatricians infrequently perceive adolescents as being at risk. In addition, many at-risk adolescents fail to access systems likely to provide health care, counseling, or testing.

Natural history studies in adolescents are incomplete, although HIV infection in adolescents appears to resemble the disease time course, complications, and prognosis in adults.

DIAGNOSIS Early diagnosis of the infected infant is desirable, but early recognition of the infant at risk for HIV infection may be equally as important. Only if HIV infection in the pregnant woman is identified will there be an opportunity to intervene during pregnancy with both antiviral therapy and necessary psychosocial services. Thus, HIV testing and counseling should be a routine part of pregnancy care.

The persistence of transplacentally acquired antibody to HIV in the infant complicates the use of conventional IgG antibody tests (ELISA and/or Western blot) in diagnosing HIV infection in infancy. Because such HIV antibodies may remain in uninfected infants' circulation for up to 18 months, diagnosis of HIV infection in the infant at risk requires the culture of virus from the infant (HIV culture) or the demonstration of viral nucleic acids (HIV DNA or HIV RNA detection by PCR) or HIV antigen (p24 antigen). With greater than 95% confidence, virologic testing with either HIV DNA PCR or HIV culture of peripheral blood can be expected to establish or exclude the diagnosis of HIV infection in an infant by 4 months of age. Performed appropriately, these tests have an acceptably low rate of false-positivity and can be relied upon to confirm infection at any age. The sensitivity of each is somewhat lower in the immediate perinatal period (<2 months of age), making serial testing necessary. For prospective monitoring of infants at risk, diagnostic virologic testing is recommended at least three times during the first 4 months after birth (last test at or after 4 months of age). Before parents are told that a child is infected, confirmation and review of all laboratory tests are imperative.

When infants or children without recognized risk factors for HIV infection present with findings or signs compatible with immunodeficiency, the diagnosis of HIV should be entertained along with other causes of immunodeficiency. That HIV infection is currently the leading cause of immunodeficiency in young children may prove helpful when counseling parents concerning the need to include HIV testing in any comprehensive evaluation of immunodeficiency in children.

In children from 18 months of age through adolescence, a confirmed positive serologic test for antibody to HIV (positive ELISA confirmed by Western blot or other confirmatory test) is usually sufficient to establish the diagnosis of HIV infection. Other rare pitfalls in diagnosis based upon serology alone are HIV-infected infants who produce no HIV-specific antibody (generally infants with marked immunodeficiency and associated clinical symptoms) and the unusual instance of infected infants who become seronegative when transplacental antibody disappears and before endogenous antibody is produced.

MANAGEMENT Medical care of infants at risk of HIV infection whose infection status remains uncertain requires careful prospective evaluation for early signs and symptoms of HIV infection. Because serious bacterial infection or opportunistic infections such as PCP may be the first clinical presentation associated with their HIV of infection, febrile episodes and respiratory illnesses should be aggressively managed in these infants. To reduce the risk of PCP, all HIV-exposed infants should begin PCP prophylaxis with TMP-SMX at 6 weeks of age and continue it until infection status is established. In uninfected infants, PCP prophylaxis can be discontinued. If HIV infection is proven, PCP prophylaxis must be continued through the first year of life, and longer if the child's immunologic status warrants it (evidence of severe immune suppression; see Table 13-56). HIV DNA by PCR should be performed in the first week of life, at 1 month of age, and at 4 months of age. Some experts include testing at 2 weeks of age. The HIV DNA by PCR should always be repeated if there is a positive result. HIV infection may be reasonably excluded if there are two negative tests for HIV DNA by PCR (or negative HIV cultures), with at least one of these negative tests being performed at or after 4 months of age. Because of the sensitivity and specificity of HIV DNA by PCR for diagnosis, repeat serologic testing may be postponed until 15 to 18 months of age to verify loss of passively acquired maternal antibodies. Immunization schedules for infants at risk should include inactivated polio vaccine in place of the live vaccine. Varicella vaccine may be administered to asymptomatic or mildly symptomatic HIV-infected children with no evidence of immune suppression (Immunologic Category 1). Measles-mumps-rubella (MMR) vaccine can be given to HIV-infected children without evidence of severe immune suppression (Immunologic Categories 1 and 2).

Care of children with or at risk of HIV infection requires a skilled team approach that includes medical specialists, primary care physicians, nurses, social workers, nutritionists, and developmental experts. Extensive psychosocial support is often necessary for families. Early coordination of patient management with a team skilled in the care of children with HIV infection will facilitate later care.

After perinatal HIV infection or perinatal exposure is diagnosed in an infant or child, testing should be done on siblings and on parents and their sexual partners. The initial visit of the HIV-infected or perinatally exposed child should include a thorough physical examination and laboratory evaluation as a baseline for further monitoring. This and subsequent examinations should devote particular attention to rate of growth, pulmonary symptoms and findings, location and size of enlarged lymph nodes, liver and spleen size, and neurologic and developmental assessment.

Immunologic testing (complete blood counts, CD4$^+$ cell count, and quantitative immunoglobulins) will aid in decisions regarding PCP prophylaxis, IVIG therapy, and antiretroviral therapy, and should be performed every 3 months. Quantitative HIV RNA by PCR (viral load) and CD4$^+$ cell counts are independent predictors for risk of disease progression. Probably the best global estimate of clinical well-being in pediatric HIV infection comprises rate of growth (weight, length, and head circumference growth velocities), developmental achievement, and experience with bacterial and viral infections. Following these clinical and laboratory parameters should assist in decisions concerning initiation and switching combination antiretroviral therapies, prophylaxis for opportunistic infection, nutritional interventions, and psychosocial support efforts.

***Pneumocystis carinii* Pneumonia Prophylaxis** CDC guidelines for prophylaxis of PCP in HIV-infected infants reflect age-adjusted CD4$^+$ counts and the empirical risk of PCP (evidence of severe immune suppression; Table 13-56). TMP-SMX (150 mg TMP/m^2/d, orally, 3 days per week) is the drug of choice for prophylaxis of PCP, and may also provide protection from serious bacterial infections. Alternatives to trimethoprim-sulfamethoxazole for patients who cannot tolerate this combination include dapsone, atovaquone, trimethoprim, pentamidine (aerosol or intravenous), and clindamycin plus primaquine, as single agents or in various combinations.

Intravenous Immunoglobulin (IVIG) In children with symptomatic HIV infection or with demonstrated abnormalities of immune function, administration of IVIG (400 mg/kg IV, monthly) reduces the incidence of serious bacterial infections by 25%. Mortality is not different from children receiving placebo, however, and children with greater than 200 CD4$^+$ cells/μL are most likely to benefit. For patients receiving combination antiretroviral therapy and TMP-SMX for PCP prophylaxis, the benefit of IVIG is diminished and, in most cases, not cost-effective. For this reason, only HIV-infected patients with documented defects in the production of functional antibody or a history of recurrent bacterial infections while receiving antiretroviral therapy and PCP prophylaxis should be considered for prophylaxis with IVIG.

Antiretroviral Therapy Updated information on the most current recommendations for treating HIV-infected children can be obtained by accessing the Web site of the HIV/AIDS Treatment Information Service (www.hivatis.org). Information on current pediatric clinical trials and treatment centers can be obtained by calling the AIDS Clinical Trials Group (1-800-TRIALSA).

Antiretroviral therapy for HIV-infected children has undergone a dramatic evolution over the last decade. What began as serial monotherapy with agents utilized as soon as they became available has become a more sophisticated use of combination therapies guided by careful monitoring of viral load and clinical and immunologic responses. The currently available antiretroviral agents can be divided into three distinct categories: (a) nucleoside reverse transcriptase inhibitors (NRTI); (b) nonnucleoside reverse transcriptase inhibitors (NNRTI); and (c) protease inhibitors (PI) (Table 13-57). The most effective combinations have included two nucleoside reverse transcriptase inhibitors in combination with either a protease inhibitor or a nonnucleoside reverse transcriptase inhibitor (HAART = highly active antiretroviral therapy). These three-drug regimens have been associated with dramatic reductions in viral load [(approximately 40–60% of children who adhere to these regimens reach undetectable levels of virus in their plasma (less than 400 copies/mL)] and improvements in, or preservation of, CD4$^+$ cell counts and lymphocytic function.

Because approximately one-sixth of HIV-infected children experience rapid progression beginning in the first year of life, many HIV clinicians start aggressive combination antiretroviral therapy in each child as soon as the diagnosis is established. Initiation of therapy is appropriate for all HIV-infected children identified in the first year of life. However, for children whose HIV infection status is not determined until after the first year of life, the alternatives are either to treat all HIV-infected children regardless of their clinical or laboratory status or to defer initiation of treatment until there is clinical, immunologic, or virologic evidence that disease progression is imminent. However, once a decision is made to treat, the treatment regimen should attempt to provide optimal antiviral activity consistent with that seen with the triple combination regimens. Antiretroviral regimens that do not optimally suppress viral replication are associated with poorer clinical outcomes and a higher likelihood for the development of resistance to the antiretroviral medications being administered.

Compliance is a significant problem in both HIV-infected children and adults. Durability, safety, tolerability, and adherence to antiretroviral regimens are as critical for children with HIV infection as for adults. Successful aggressive antiretroviral regimens require the administration of multiple medications with multiple doses per day. Complicating factors include lack of a liquid preparation for some of the medications (eg, ddC, d4T, delavirdine, efavirenz, indinavir, and saquinavir), poor palatability (eg, ddI and ritonavir), and the effect of food on absorption (eg, ddI and indinavir should be taken on an empty stomach; nelfinavir absorption is enhanced with a fatty meal).

Innovative measures can assist families in administering these medications to children. Children as young as 3 years of age can be taught how to take pills. Mixing medications with certain strong-tasting foods or liquids, or coating the mouth with peanut butter can help with acceptance of medications that are poor tasting. A gastrostomy tube is an effective way to avoid many of the problems

TABLE 13-57

ANTIRETROVIRAL MEDICATIONS AVAILABLE FOR TREATMENT OF HIV-INFECTED CHILDREN

MEDICATION	NEONATAL DOSE	PEDIATRIC DOSE	ADULT DOSE[a]	AVAILABLE FORMULATIONS	PRECAUTIONS/ADVERSE EVENTS
Nucleoside Reverse Transcriptase Inhibitors					
Zidovudine (ZDV or AZT)	2 mg/kg q6h	90–180 mg/m² q6–8h	200 mg q8h *or* 300 mg q12h	Syrup: 10 mg/mL Capsules: 100 mg Tablets: 300 mg Solution for injection: 10 mg/mL	Anemia, granulocytopenia, nausea, headache, myopathy, liver toxicity, macrocytosis, and xerostomia
Didanosine (ddI)	50 mg/m² q12h	90–150 mg/m² q12h *or* 180–300 mg/m² qd	<60 kg: 125 mg q12h *or* ≥60 kg: 200 mg q12h	Pediatric powder for solution: 10 mg/mL Buffered powder for solution: 100, 167, and 250 mg Chewable tablets: 25, 50, 100, and 150 mg	Diarrhea, abdominal pain, nausea, vomiting, pancreatitis, peripheral neuropathy, and retinal depigmentation
Lamivudine (3TC)	2 mg/kg q12h	4 mg/kg q12h	<50 kg: 2 mg/kg q12h *or* ≥50 kg: 150 mg q12h	Solution: 10 mg/mL Tablets: 150 mg	Headache, fatigue, diarrhea, pancreatitis, and peripheral neuropathy
Stavudine (d4T)	—	1 mg/kg q12h	<60 kg: 30 mg q12h *or* ≥60 kg: 40 mg q12h	Solution: 1 mg/mL Capsules: 15, 20, 30, and 40 mg	Headache, nausea, peripheral neuropathy, and pancreatitis, mania, and sleep disorders
Zalcitabine (ddC)	—	0.01 mg/kg q8h	0.75 mg q8h	Tablets: 0.375 and 0.75 mg Syrup (investigational): 0.1 mg/mL	Peripheral neuropathy, pancreatitis, headache, nausea, and oral and esophageal ulcers
Abacavir (ABC)	—	8 mg/kg q12h	300 mg q12h	Solution: 20 mg/mL Tablets: 300 mg	Hypersensitivity reaction (5%) (may be fatal), nausea, vomiting, headache, fever, rash, anorexia, and fatigue
Nonnucleoside Reverse Transcriptase Inhibitors					
Nevirapine (NVP)	5 mg/kg qd[b]	120–200 mg/m² q12h Note: initiate first 2 weeks of therapy at 120 mg/m² qd	200 mg q12h Note: initiate first 2 wks of therapy at 200 mg qd	Suspension: 10 mg/mL Tablets: 200 mg	Rash (may be severe; Stevens-Johnson), sedative effect, headache, diarrhea, and nausea; drug interactions are common
Efavirenz (DMP-266)	—	10–15 kg: 200 mg 15–20 kg: 250 mg 20–25 kg: 300 mg 25.5–32.5 kg: 350 mg 32.5–40 kg: 400 mg >40 kg: 600 mg All once daily	600 mg qd	Capsules: 50, 100, and 200 mg	Rash (may be severe); somnolence, insomnia, confusion, abnormal dreams, hallucinations, and agitation; teratogenic in primates; drug interactions are common
Delavirdine (DLV)	—	—	400 mg q8h	Tablets: 100 mg	Rash (may be severe; Stevens-Johnson), headache, fatigue, and nausea; drug interactions are common

TABLE 13-57 Continued

MEDICATION	NEONATAL DOSE	PEDIATRIC DOSE	ADULT DOSE[a]	AVAILABLE FORMULATIONS	PRECAUTIONS/ADVERSE EVENTS
Protease Inhibitors					
Indinavir	—	500 mg/m² q8h	800 mg q8h	Capsules: 200 and 400 mg	Hyperbilirubinemia (10%), nephrolithiasis, nausea, abdominal pain, hyperglycemia, ketoacidosis, hypertriglyceridemia, hypercholesterolemia, and lipodystrophy; drug interactions are common
Nelfinavir	—	30–40 mg/kg q8h Note: doses of 55 mg/kg or higher given q12h are being evaluated	750 mg q8h or 1250 mg q12h	Powder for oral suspension: 50 mg per 1 scoop (200 mg per level teaspoon) Tablets: 250 mg	Diarrhea (almost universal), abdominal pain, asthenia, hyperglycemia, ketoacidosis, hypertriglyceridemia, hypercholesterolemia, and lipodystrophy; drug interactions are common
Ritonavir	—	400 mg/m² q12h	600 mg q12h	Oral solution: 80 mg/mL Capsules: 100 mg	Nausea (very common), vomiting, diarrhea, anorexia, circumoral paresthesia, liver toxicity, hyperglycemia, ketoacidosis, hypertriglyceridemia, hypercholesterolemia, and lipodystrophy; drug interactions are common.
Saquinavir	—	—	Hard-gel capsules: 600 mg q8h Soft-gel capsules: 1200 mg q8h	Hard-gel capsules: 200 mg Soft-gel capsules: 200 mg	Diarrhea, headache, nausea, hyperglycemia, ketoacidosis, hypertriglyceridemia, hypercholesterolemia, and lipodystrophy; drug interactions are common
Amprenavir	—	Oral solution: 22.5 mg/kg q12h or 17 mg/kg q8h Capsules: 20 mg/kg q12h or 15 mg/kg q8h	1200 mg q12h	Oral solution: 15 mg/mL Capsules: 50 and 150 mg	Nausea, vomiting, diarrhea, circumoral paresthesia, hyperglycemia, ketoacidosis, hypertriglyceridemia, hypercholesterolemia, and lipodystrophy; drug interactions are common

[a] Adult doses are frequently used to determine the maximum dose for children as their weight or surface area increases with age. However, pharmacokinetic data for older children and adolescents have not been determined for many antiretroviral agents. In addition, when pharmacokinetic data are available, children may actually require doses that exceed the adult dose when calculated on a per kilogram or meter squared basis. When prescribing antiretroviral medications for children 10 to 18 years of age, it is appropriate to consult an HIV specialist to determine the most appropriate dose.

[b] 5 mg/kg qd for first 14 days of life; then 120 mg/m² q12h for the next 14 days; then 200 mg/m² q12h.

associated with the chronic administration of antiretroviral therapy. However, tremendous psychosocial support of the family and understanding of the difficulty with administering these medications may prove to be the most helpful in enhancing adherence with these cumbersome combination regimens.

The initial antiretroviral regimen that a child receives is the one most likely to achieve a sustained antiviral effect. Subsequent regimens are likely to be less effective because of the impact of cross-resistance to prior medications. For that reason, clinical and laboratory parameters need to be monitored carefully to detect any evidence of treatment failure (see Table 13-58). Effective antiretroviral therapy should result in maximal viral-load reduction by 12 to 16 weeks after initiation of therapy. Failure to achieve a significant viral-load reduction (approximately a two-log reduction in HIV RNA by PCR) following the use of an appropriate triple-drug combination suggests either a lack of compliance to the prescribed regimen or the presence or development of resistant virus.

Until genotypic- and phenotypic-resistance testing is evaluated in children, the decisions concerning change in antiretroviral therapy should be guided primarily by the child's prior medication history and information that will help to predict the likelihood of cross-resistance. A single agent should never be added to failing therapy. The optimal approach to changing therapy is to make a complete shift in prescribed medications, with the hope that the new regimen includes at least two medications to which the child has not been previously exposed. If the child has already received a protease inhibitor, it may be appropriate to replace the protease inhibitor with a nonnucleoside reverse transcriptase inhibitor, or vice versa. In the near future, alternate categories of antiretroviral therapy may be available (eg, fusion inhibitors, TAT inhibitors, etc), or medications in current categories may be sufficiently different from those available to make cross-resistance less likely (eg, nonpeptidic protease inhibitors).

TABLE 13-58

RECOMMENDED ANTIRETROVIRAL REGIMENS FOR INITIAL THERAPY FOR HIV-INFECTED CHILDREN

Strongly Recommended
   2NRTIs + PI
   2NRTIs + efavirenz
Alternative Regimens
   2NRTIs + nevirapine
   Zidovudine + lamivudine + abacavir
Use in Special Circumstances
   2NRTIs*
Not Recommended
   Any monotherapy (except for perinatal prophylaxis)
   Stavudine and zidovudine (antagonism)
   Zalcitabine and didanosine (similar toxicities)
   Stavudine and zalcitabine (similar toxicities)
   Zalcitabine and lamivudine (similar toxicities)

* This regimen is less effective than the Strongly Recommended and the Alternative Regimens. However, in certain patients, this may be acceptable if compliance with more complicated regimens is a concern and the viral load is not very high (<100,000 HIV copies per mL). The ease of dual NRTI therapy (particularly Combivir as one tablet twice daily) might be valuable as initial therapy of adolescents or other children just starting to take antiretroviral therapy.
NRTI = nucleoside reverse transcriptase inhibitor; PI = protease inhibitor.
SOURCE: Modified from Guidelines for the Use of Antiretroviral Agents in Pediatric HIV Infection (Web site: www.hivatis.org/guidelines/pedapril415.pdf).

PREVENTION   A solution to the worldwide HIV pandemic would be the development of a safe and effective vaccine. While many candidate vaccines are in various stages of investigation, there are still considerable obstacles impeding HIV vaccine development. Prevention of HIV infection in children entails the prevention of mother-to-infant transmission (perinatal) and prevention of transmission in adolescents who participate in adult risk behaviors. In the United States, there has been a marked reduction in perinatal HIV transmission. This reduction has been accomplished primarily by the successful administration of antiretroviral therapy to pregnant HIV-infected women. Zidovudine given to HIV-infected pregnant women starting at 14 to 32 weeks' gestation reduces perinatal transmission from 25% to 8%. More recently, many centers with the experience of managing HIV infection during pregnancy have seen their rates of perinatal transmission fall to somewhere between 1 and 3%. This continued reduction in perinatal HIV transmission has occurred because of more aggressive antiretroviral therapy and monitoring of viral loads in HIV-infected women during their pregnancies.

Shorter, less cumbersome (no intravenous zidovudine), and less expensive antiretroviral treatment regimens are efficacious in nonindustrialized nations. These regimens are appealing in areas where resources are not available for administration of the more complete regimens provided in the United States. However, they should not replace current Public Health Service recommendations because efficacy, although significantly better than placebo, does not approach the 1 to 3% perinatal HIV transmission rate commonly seen in the United States. Administration of antiretroviral agents with minimal safety data for use during pregnancy has been fairly liberal because of the obvious benefits associated with appropriate treatment of the mother's HIV infection and the reduction in perinatal transmission. It will be important to monitor both short- and long-term outcomes of infants exposed perinatally to these therapies in order to determine the impact of antiretroviral therapy during gestation. Because efavirenz is associated with central nervous system complications in primate offspring, this drug should not be used during pregnancy. Ongoing investigations will help to establish whether any of the other antiretroviral agents currently available should be withheld during pregnancy.

Numerous studies have investigated the impact of the mode of delivery on the rate of perinatal transmission. Cesarean section does appear to provide some additional protection to the infant born to the HIV-infected woman. However, in the era of highly active antiretroviral therapy and the ability to monitor viral load closely, both the risks and the benefits of cesarean section must be clearly discussed with prospective parents before any change in the mode of delivery is considered. Vitamin A supplementation is valuable for reducing perinatal HIV transmission in nonindustrialized countries where vitamin A deficiency is common. However, providing vitamin A to women who do not have vitamin A deficiency does not afford benefit. Cleansing the birth canal with microbicidal agents has been postulated as another means of reducing transmission at the time of delivery. One study that looked at chlorhexidine rinses found that the rinses failed to show a benefit. However, stronger concentrations of chlorhexidine, use of other agents, or more frequent application of the rinses may yet provide some benefit. This approach will be particularly valuable in nonindustrialized countries that do not have resources to pay for expensive antiretroviral therapy.

Breast-feeding is associated with HIV transmission. For that reason, in areas where safe alternatives to breast milk are available, breast-feeding should be prohibited. Unfortunately, in many areas of the world where HIV is particularly prevalent (eg, Sub-Saharan Africa), safe alternatives to breast-feeding are not readily available. In these areas, breast-feeding may still be essential, but should be discontinued as quickly as possible because the duration of breast-feeding appears to have implications for increasing the rate of HIV transmission.

Adolescents who participate in behaviors identified with transmission in adults (sexual promiscuity, needle-sharing for the injection of illicit drugs or anabolic steroids, etc) represent a growing population of HIV-infected children. Altering behavior is very difficult in this population. Outreach education, particularly through the use of peer counselors, has been somewhat successful in taking the message to at-risk youth.

Helpful Web Sites

1. Centers for Disease Control and Prevention www.cdc.gov
2. HIV/AIDS Treatment Information Service www.hivatis.org
3. HIV In Site (University of California at San Francisco) http://hivinsite.ucsf.edu
4. Pediatric AIDS Clinical Trials Group http://pactg.s-com/INDEX.HTM

References

Barnhart, HX, Caldwell MB, Thomas P, et al: Natural history of human immunodeficiency virus disease in perinatally infected children: an analysis from the Pediatric Spectrum of Disease Project. Pediatrics 97:710–716, 1996

Borkowsky W, Krasinski K, Pollack H, et al: Early diagnosis of human immunodeficiency virus infection in children less than 6 months of age: comparison of polymerase chain reaction, culture, and plasma antigen capture techniques. J Infect Dis 166:616–619, 1992

Centers for Disease Control and Prevention: 1995 Revised guidelines for prophylaxis against *Pneumocystis carinii* pneumonia for children infected with or perinatally exposed to human immunodeficiency virus. MMWR Morb Mortal Wkly Rep 44(RR-4):1–11, 1995

Centers for Disease Control and Prevention: Public Health Service Task Force recommendations for the use of antiretroviral drugs in pregnant women infected with HIV-1 for maternal health and for reducing perinatal HIV-1 transmission in the United States. MMWR Morb Mortal Wkly Rep 47(RR-2):1–30, 1998

Centers for Disease Control and Prevention: 1994 Revised classification system for human immunodeficiency virus (HIV) infection in children under 13 years of age. MMWR Morb Mortal Wkly Rep 43(RR-12):1–10, 1999

Connor EM, Sperling RS, Gelber R, et al: Reduction of maternal-infant transmission of human immunodeficiency virus type 1 with zidovudine treatment. N Engl J Med 331:1173–1180, 1994

Kline MW, Hollinger FB, Rosenblatt HM, et al: Sensitivity, specificity and predictive value of physical examination, culture and other laboratory studies in the diagnosis during early infancy of vertically acquired human immunodeficiency virus infection. Pediatr Infect Dis J 12:33, 1993

The International Perinatal HIV Group: The mode of delivery and the risk of vertical transmission of human immunodeficiency virus type 1—a meta analysis of 15 prospective cohort studies. N Engl J Med 340:977–987, 1999

Working Group on Antiretroviral Therapy of Children, National Pediatric HIV Resource Center: Antiretroviral therapy and medical management of pediatric HIV infection. Pediatrics 102(Suppl):1005–1062, 1998

13.4.13 Measles

Samuel L. Katz

Measles (rubeola, morbilli) was for centuries a common childhood communicable disease. Although it has become uncommon in countries where vaccine is administered widely, the disparity between developed nations and others with less available health care for infants and children is striking. The World Health Organization (WHO) estimates that nearly 1 million deaths in 1998 could be attributed to measles and its complications among children in the developing areas of the world. Prior to availability and widespread use of vaccine, the annual measles mortality exceeded 6 million.

Measles virus is a member of the genus *Morbillivirus* of the family of paramyxoviruses. Measles virus has linear negative-stranded RNA within a helical protein capsid enclosed by an outer membrane of lipid and protein. The virions are pleomorphic, with a diameter ranging from 100 to 250 nm. Six structural proteins have been identified, and their functions account for some of the known properties of the virus. Virus binds to cells expressing the CD46 complement receptor. The virus is markedly heat-labile, but is well preserved for long periods at low temperatures. Measles virus replicates in a large variety of both primary cell cultures and stable lines. The morphologic changes induced in cell cultures by measles virus are very similar to those observed in cytologic specimens prepared from respiratory tract secretions and many tissues of patients with measles.

EPIDEMIOLOGY Infection is initiated when a susceptible person inhales virus-laden droplets discharged from the nasopharyngeal secretions of an infected patient. At the portal of entry a short period of local virus multiplication and limited spread ensues, followed by a brief, low-titer, primary viremia that distributes the agent to distant sites where the virus replicates actively in lymphoid tissues, especially in monocytes. A prolonged secondary viremia occurs, associated with the onset of the clinical prodromata and the widespread dissemination of virus. From that time (about 9 to 10 days after the initial exposure) until the beginning of rash, virus can be detected throughout the body, especially in the respiratory tract and lymphoid tissues. It can also be recovered from the nasopharyngeal secretions, urine, and blood. The patient is most highly communicable to others during this 5- to 6-day period. With the onset of rash (about 14 days after initial infection), viral replication diminishes, and by 16 days it is difficult to recover virus. Coincident with the appearance of the exanthem is the detection in serum of circulating antibodies found in nearly 100% of patients by the second day of rash. Striking clinical improvement begins at this time, interrupted a few days later in a varying number of patients by secondary illness caused by bacteria that have migrated across the damaged respiratory tract lining. Sinusitis, otitis media, and bronchopneumonia develop secondary to the loss of normal local defenses.

In most countries, measles is a disease of early childhood, with peak incidence among children of preschool age and those in the early school years. The very high attack rate among exposed susceptibles results in a periodicity of epidemics at intervals of 2 or 3 years, when a new crop of susceptibles has arisen. In crowded urban areas, the 1- to 5-year-old group shows the highest incidence. The age distribution shifts to 5- to 10-year-olds in suburban and rural areas, where exposure is postponed until school attendance begins. Nearly 100% of young adults have had measles disease or measles vaccine, but a rare individual may escape the infection during childhood only to acquire it in a later decade. The epidemiology has been altered strikingly in countries where vaccine has been widely utilized.

A single attack of measles confers lifelong immunity. The immune individual whose serum antibody titer has diminished to a low or even undetectable level may develop a rapid anamnestic antibody rise after exposure or inoculation, in the absence of any symptoms or signs of infection and without detectable virus shedding. Vaccination with live attenuated measles vaccines confers comparable enduring immunity; vaccines containing inactivated antigens produce only a transient protective effect lasting 6 to 18 months.

Because virus-neutralizing IgG antibodies are transported actively across the placenta, infants born to mothers immune to measles are protected against infection for 6 to 7 months after birth. They become increasingly susceptible in the second half of the first year and may, on exposure, develop disease of varying severity. The infant of the rare mother who has never had measles or vaccine may acquire the infection at any time postnatally. Studies of secretory antibody in the IgA component of respiratory tract secretions have demonstrated measles-specific antibodies following natural infection or live vaccine, but not after vaccination using inactivated antigens.

CLINICAL MANIFESTATIONS In most patients the signs and symptoms of measles are highly characteristic, and their time of appearance and sequence are consistent. Approximately 10 days after exposure, fever and malaise signal the onset of illness. Cough, coryza, and conjunctivitis follow promptly. A gradual worsening of symptoms accompanies a steady rise in fever over the next 4 days. Two days prior to the appearance of the exanthem, Koplik spots, the classic exanthem, develop. With the onset of rash 14 days after infection, the clinical picture attains maximal severity, reaching a peak that coincides with involvement of the entire body by the eruption after 2 to 4 days. Constitutional symptoms throughout this 10-day period vary, but headache, abdominal pain, vomiting, diarrhea, and myalgia are frequent complaints. Fever reaching 40°C (104°F) to 41°C (105.8°F), often accompanied by chills, is not unusual when the rash is most florid. Febrile seizures may occur in children predisposed to them.

The conjunctivitis causes edema of the lids, increased lacrimation, and, frequently, photophobia. Sharply demarcated transverse linear injection of the lower lid margins, called a Stimson line, is present before the more generalized conjunctival inflammation obscures it. Among infants with nutritional deficiencies, especially vitamin A, more severe ocular involvement with corneal ulcers may lead to permanent scarring and loss of vision. The hacking cough is distressing, with a progressive increase in frequency and severity. With the abrupt fall in temperature, after rash has covered the entire body, the catarrhal symptoms subside dramatically, but the cough persists for another 7 to 10 days.

Koplik spots, pathognomonic of measles, appear 24 to 48 hours before the exanthem. They consist of bluish white dots about 1 mm in diameter surrounded by a rose-red areola. They tend to appear first on the buccal mucosa opposite the lower molars. Best seen in bright daylight, they are discrete and few in number initially, but within 1 day they increase rapidly and may spread to cover the entire buccal mucosa and some of the labial mucosa. With the onset of rash they fade, and frequently by the second day of the eruption they have disappeared.

Rash commences as discrete, irregular, erythematous macules behind the ears, on the neck, and along the hairline. As the rash progresses caudad over the ensuing 24 hours to involve the face, trunk, and arms, careful palpation will reveal a papular component. Involvement of the legs and feet by the end of the second day or early in the third day finds the lesions on the cheeks already coalescent; in severe infections, confluent areas of rash also appear on the trunk and extremities. The skin becomes edematous and the face swollen. Although the exanthem ordinarily blanches with pressure, a fine petechial component is often present. The exanthem fades slowly, in the same order of progression as its initial appearance; this process usually begins by the third or fourth day after onset. Subsidence of the florid eruption is followed by a fine desquamation. In children with protein deficiency, the desquamation is far more extensive and may be complicated by multiple pyogenic skin abscesses.

The marked generalized lymphadenopathy and splenomegaly that arise early in the course of the acute illness may persist for several weeks. High fever at the peak of illness may be accompanied by marked irritability, somnolence, or a state of delirium; these are transient manifestations that resolve dramatically with the disappearance of pyrexia. They do not correlate with the occurrence of subsequent central nervous system complications. Black measles, a severe form of the disease with a generalized hemorrhagic rash, bleeding from the nose, mouth, and gastrointestinal tract, and marked systemic toxicity, is rare. This form of measles was reported more frequently in the past and probably represented a form of disseminated intravascular coagulation.

DIAGNOSIS The regular sequence of prodrome, Koplik spots, and generalized rash permits a clinical diagnosis with a high degree of reliability, although physicians in highly immunized populations may now be unfamiliar with the illness. Virus isolation or antibody studies are usually unnecessary. A polymerase chain reaction (PCR) has demonstrated sensitivity and specificity in detection of measles virus sequences in clinical specimens (throat swabs, serum, CSF) before and after onset of rash. Of the available serologic tests, the measles hemagglutination-inhibition (HI) antibody determination and the enzyme immunoassay (EIA) are the most practical. Within 1 to 2 days of the onset of rash, serum antibodies to the various measles antigens are detectable; they increase rapidly thereafter to reach peak titers in the next 2 to 4 weeks. Virus-neutralizing and EIA antibodies persist indefinitely after an initial drop during the 2 to 6 months following their attainment of maximal titers. Plaque reduction antibody assays are the most sensitive tests, but are usually available only on a research basis.

Cytologic techniques for the demonstration of multinucleate giant cells in nasal secretions during the prodromal period and for the detection of inclusion-bearing cells in the urine, either at the time rash appears or soon after, have been helpful diagnostically. Less-specific laboratory findings include a low WBC count, with an absolute neutropenia and marked lymphopenia in the prodromal period and during the rash.

The differential diagnosis includes rubella, Kawasaki disease, infectious mononucleosis, roseola, scarlet fever, typhus, Rocky Mountain spotted fever, enterovirus or adenovirus exanthems, and rashes due to drug sensitivity (especially barbiturates, hydantoins, penicillins, and sulfonamides). Rubella is a far milder illness, without cough and with distinctive lymphadenopathy usually restricted to the posterior cervical, suboccipital, and postauricular nodes. Roseola (exanthema subitum) has an entirely different sequence; the rash first appears after the fever subsides. The peripheral blood count and atypical lymphocytes in infectious mononucleosis contrast with the leukopenia of measles.

COMPLICATIONS A wide variety of complications may be observed during the acute stage of measles or shortly thereafter. The respiratory tract is involved most often, but severe gastroenteritis also occurs. Acute laryngotracheobronchitis (croup) may cause sufficient airway obstruction to require tracheostomy, especially in children younger than 3 years of age. Bronchiolitis may result in severe lower airway obstruction. A rare but almost uniformly fatal interstitial pneumonia (giant cell pneumonia) has been noted in immunocompromised children, including those with AIDS, who develop a progressive persistent measles virus infection without the typical exanthem and with a unique failure to form measles-specific antibodies. The radiographic picture reveals a marked interstitial pattern emanating from both hilar regions. Measles virus can be recovered repeatedly from sputum or nasopharyngeal swabs, and typical giant cells are seen when respiratory tract secretions are stained. Attempts to prevent this complication or to treat it have been unsuccessful.

A benign asymptomatic keratoconjunctivitis that accompanies measles may persist for as long as 4 months; the lesions can be seen only by slit-lamp biomicroscopy. More severe corneal lesions occur in malnourished measles patients. Transient electrocardiographic abnormalities are common, but true myocarditis is rare. The diffuse lymphadenopathy that accompanies measles involves the mesenteric nodes and is believed to cause the abdominal pain that commonly occurs. Symptoms and signs identical to those of acute appendicitis may result in surgical intervention during the prodromal period.

Complications of bacterial origin result principally from invasion of the respiratory tract by pyogenic organisms. Otitis media and bronchopneumonia are most common; they may be caused by β-hemolytic streptococci, pneumococci, *H. influenzae* type b, or staphylococci. Peribronchitis and interstitial pneumonitis are seen in nearly all measles patients, and resolve rapidly after the development of rash and the subsidence of fever. A second fever spike, or failure of the initial spike to drop after the eruption has reached its peak, suggests a secondary bacterial infection. The appearance of peripheral leukocytosis with a shift to the left is confirmatory. A chest radiograph may disclose bronchopneumonia or a pattern of segmental or lobar involvement. Attempts at preventing secondary bacterial complications by giving "prophylactic" antibiotics during the catarrhal stage of measles have been unsuccessful. Bacterial complications are more frequent and severe in protein-deficient children.

Of those syndromes that can follow measles, the most dreaded are the various central nervous system complications. By far the most common is encephalomyelitis, but toxic encephalopathy, retrobulbar neuritis, thrombophlebitis of cerebral veins, hemiplegias from vascular infarction, and ascending paralysis with polyneuropathy have all been reported.

Toxic encephalopathy appears with striking rapidity at the peak of fever and rash; as many as 10% of patients develop a significant cerebrospinal fluid (CSF) pleocytosis, and 50% show electroencephalographic changes. More severe central nervous system manifestations become apparent after the acute illness, following a period of improvement lasting 2 days or more. Seizures, altered states of consciousness, and sudden lapse into coma mark the onset of encephalomyelitis, which occurs in only 0.1% of cases; fever returns,

and there is marked peripheral leukocytosis. Mortality ranges from 10 to 25%, and significant sequelae in the motor, intellectual, or behavioral performance occur in 20 to 50% of survivors.

During the early viremic phase of measles there is a thrombocytopenia of insufficient magnitude to cause spontaneous bleeding, but it may reflect megakaryocytic damage by the virus. Another rare and unexplained postinfectious complication, thrombocytopenic purpura, appears 4 to 14 days after the rash and may produce marked skin purpura, genitourinary and gastrointestinal bleeding, and epistaxis. Corticosteroids produce prompt relief, with cessation of bleeding and steady return of platelet counts to normal. This complication may be an autoimmune phenomenon.

Reactivation or exacerbation of tuberculosis during measles has been repeatedly documented. Loss of delayed cutaneous hypersensitivity to tuberculoprotein (and other antigens) occurs with measles and persists for several weeks thereafter, so that a previously positive reactor may give a negative skin test. Damage to the respiratory tract may explain the deterioration in some patients with cystic fibrosis. Infants with dietary protein deficiency may lapse into frank kwashiorkor during measles as a result of decreased oral intake, increased gastrointestinal losses, and the negative nitrogen balance of the infection. In contrast to these undesirable side effects, measles can sometimes induce a favorable diuresis in children with refractory nephrotic syndrome.

Gestational measles, though rare, may induce premature delivery, stillbirth, or abortion, but is not associated with an increased incidence of congenital malformations.

TREATMENT Except for general supportive measures, there is no current therapy for the patient with uncomplicated measles. For those immunocompromised patients with severe measles, intravenous ribavirin has been reported anecdotally to offer some benefit. Bed rest, avoidance of bright light if there is marked photophobia, encouragement of fluid intake, and judicious use of antipyretics for high fever and suppressants for distressing cough may be beneficial symptomatically. More specific measures, such as the use of proper antimicrobials, should be used to treat secondary bacterial complications.

Because measles apparently depletes reserves of vitamin A, resulting in a high incidence of xerophthalmia and corneal ulcers in malnourished children, the WHO recommends high-dosage vitamin A supplementation in all areas where vitamin A deficiency exists. Vitamin A supplementation decreases the frequency and severity of pneumonia and laryngotracheobronchitis due to measles virus damage of ciliated respiratory tract epithelium. For infants younger than 1 year of age, 100,000 IU, and for older patients, 200,000 IU are prescribed. The dose is given as soon as measles is recognized. A second dose is administered on the next day, if any eye signs of vitamin A deficiency appear, and repeated 1 to 4 weeks later.

PREVENTION

Passive Immunization Human immunoglobulin (IG) given soon after exposure can alter the clinical course and the antigenic effects of measles virus infection. A susceptible child should promptly be given IG, 0.25 mL/kg body weight, to prevent measles. If more than 6 days have elapsed, one cannot rely on IG either to prevent or to modify the illness. Patients with globulin-modified measles display great variations in clinical course, with prolongation of the incubation period and various expressions of signs and symptoms, but they remain a source of potential contagion to their contacts. Because of its transitory nature, passive protection should be followed in 3 months by active immunization. Because large doses of various immune globulin preparations are now administered commonly for the prevention or treatment of a number of disorders (eg, HIV infections, Kawasaki disease, immune thrombocytopenias, hepatitis B, and varicella prophylaxis) a longer interval is advised before measles virus vaccination. This will vary from 3 to 11 months depending on the product and amount of globulin administered.

Active Immunization Recommendations for administration of attenuated measles vaccines are provided in Sec. 1.5.2.

References

Centers for Disease Control: Progress toward elimination of measles from the Americas. MMWR Morb Mortal Wkly Rep 47:189–193, 1998

Centers for Disease Control: Progress toward measles elimination. MMWR Morb Mortal Wkly Rep 48:1081–1086, 1999

Committee on Infectious Diseases: Recommended timing of routine measles immunization for children who have recently received immune globulin preparations. Pediatrics 93:682, 1994

Gans HA, Arvin AA, Galinus J, Logan L, DeHovitz R, Maldonado Y: Deficiency of the humoral immune response to measles vaccine in infants immunized at age 6 months. JAMA 280:527–532, 1998

Gibbs WW: Trailing a virus (Nipah). Sci Am 8:80–87, 1999

Patterson DL, Murray PK, McCormack JG: Zoonotic disease in Australia caused by a novel member of the Paramyxoviridae. Clin Infect Dis 27:112–118, 1998

Redd SE, Markowitz LE, Katz SL: Measles vaccine. In: Plotkin SA, Orenstein WA, eds: Vaccines, 3rd ed. Philadelphia, WB Saunders, 1999

Vitek CR, Aduddell M, Brinton MJ, Hoffman RE, Redd SC: Increased protection during a measles outbreak of children previously vaccinated with a second dose of MMR vaccine. Pediatr Infect Dis J 18:620–623, 1999

Weibel RE, Caserta V, Benor DE, Evans G: Acute encephalopathy followed by permanent brain injury or death associated with further attenuated measles vaccines. Pediatrics 101:383–387, 1998

13.4.14 Molluscum Contagiosum

Lawrence F. Eichenfield

Molluscum contagiosum is a cutaneous viral infection caused by a poxvirus, *Molluscipoxvirus,* an approximately 300-nm, double-stranded DNA, brick-shaped virus. Humans are the only known source of the virus, which is spread by direct contact, including sexual contact, autoinoculation, or from contaminated fomites. The incubation period appears to be within 2 weeks to 2 months, but may be greater than 6 months. Outbreaks have been noted among wrestlers and in pools and water parks. Patients with atopic dermatitis and immunosuppressed individuals, including persons with HIV infection, tend to have more intense and widespread eruptions.

CLINICAL MANIFESTATIONS Molluscum are usually diagnosed clinically, based on morphology and distribution. Flat-topped, discrete, dome-shaped, flesh-colored lesions in excess of 1 cm can occur. Central white cores or umbilication are seen in active lesions. Molluscum lesions commonly occur on the trunk, face, and extremities, but may be generalized. Groups of lesions often occur by

body folds and intertriginous areas, secondary to skin-to-skin autoinoculation. Small, atypical, and giant lesions may be mistaken for verrucae, bacterial pustules, or cutaneous papules such as juvenile xanthogranuloma.

DIAGNOSIS Molluscum contagiosum is usually asymptomatic, although an eczematous, red, scaling patch may surround lesions in around 10% of patients, and is termed *molluscum dermatitis.* Contents of the central core, obtained by needle extraction and examined microscopically after staining with Wright's or Giemsa stain, display molluscum bodies, distinctive ovoid intracytoplasmic inclusions.

TREATMENT Molluscum contagiosum infection is usually self-limited, with the disease duration quite variable, lasting several weeks to several years. Lesions can regress spontaneously, but treatment may prevent autoinoculation and spread to other individuals. Chemical or physical destruction is commonly used to treat molluscum. Chemical treatments include cantharidin (0.7% in collodion), salicylic acid, lactic acid, and tretinoin. Physical destruction using liquid nitrogen cryotherapy or removal of the central core of each lesion usually results in resolution. EMLA (eutectic mixture of local anesthetics) cream, a topical anesthetic, may be applied 60+ minutes to 2 hours prior to needle extraction or curettage. Scarring is rare, but may occur spontaneously or secondary to treatment.

PREVENTION Children with lesions covered by clothing have a very low risk of spreading disease to others. Because infection may spread in water, families should be advised to have siblings not bathe together if an affected child has active lesions. In outbreaks (eg, among wrestlers) spread may be decreased by restricting body contact and by restricting the sharing of potential contaminated fomites (eg, towels).

References

Bugert JJ, Darai G: Recent advances in molluscum contagiosum virus research. Arch Virol Suppl 13:35–47, 1997

Choong KY, Roberts LJ: Molluscum contagiosum, swimming and bathing: a clinical analysis. Australas J Dermatol 40(2):89–92, 1999

13.4.15 Mumps

Dennis L. Murray

Mumps is a communicable, systemic viral illness usually characterized by parotitis. Mumps is caused by a paramyxovirus that is closely related antigenically to the parainfluenza virus. Virions are approximately 150 nm in diameter and contain RNA; the viral envelope has projections containing one of two structural glycoproteins, either hemagglutinin-neuraminadase or fusion.

Humans are the only known natural hosts of mumps virus, which is spread by the respiratory route. Virus can be demonstrated in respiratory secretions before and after the onset of parotid swelling. After the infection is introduced into a family, all nonimmune members are usually infected. The normal incubation period is from 16 to 18 days. Because of the variability of the parotid swelling, however, the range must be considered to be approximately 12 to 25 days. The common misconception that mumps is not as contagious as other childhood diseases stems from the substantial subclinical attack rate produced by this infection. Approximately 30%

of mumps infections go unrecognized because they do not produce parotid swelling.

The infection is most communicable from 1 to 2 days prior to parotid swelling until 5 days after parotid swelling begins. Patients are generally considered noninfectious 9 days after parotid swelling begins. The large number of subclinical infections and the fact that patients are contagious before parotitis begins make it extremely difficult to prevent infection by isolating patients. Mumps antibody is transferred across the placenta and persists during the first months of life, providing some protection to the infant.

A single attack of mumps is believed to confer permanent immunity against subsequent attack, regardless of whether parotid swelling was unilateral or even absent. It is now recognized that there are multiple causes of parotid swelling in addition to mumps. Patients immunized successfully with mumps vaccine show no evidence of losing immunity. However, because primary vaccine failure occurs at a rate of 2 to 5% with the live attenuated mumps vaccine, use of a second dose of vaccine is needed to increase population immunity and to decrease the likelihood of outbreaks of mumps disease. With the widespread use of mumps vaccine, the disease has become uncommon. In 1998, less than 1000 cases were reported, compared with more than 150,000 prior to the introduction of vaccine. In addition, there has been an upward shift in age incidence, the peak occurring in children 10 to 14 years old. Infection is most common during the late winter and early spring months. Death as a result of mumps is rare; fatalities are more frequent in persons over the age of 19 years. Virus has been recovered from multiple organs at autopsy.

CLINICAL MANIFESTATIONS A patient with mumps rarely has severe systemic manifestations. Temperatures are only moderately elevated, usually for 3 to 4 days. Symptoms such as headache, anorexia, and abdominal discomfort may precede parotid swelling by 1 to 2 days. Parotid swelling may be the first sign of illness; although it may not occur; swelling may last 7 to 10 days and be observed on one or both sides. Two or 3 days after the onset of swelling on one side, the opposite side may become involved. Sometimes swelling is only unilateral. The submandibular glands may swell along with, or in the absence of, parotid swelling. Presternal edema is sometimes present.

The entire parotid gland is swollen, including the uncinate lobe, which extends under the back of the ear lobe. The borders of the gland are usually not discrete. Pressure on the parotid gland causes pain, and trismus (spasm of the masticator muscles) may occur.

Parotid swelling produces a fair amount of discomfort. Eating or drinking acidic foods, such as orange juice, is said to elicit much discomfort. Inflammation of the orifice of the Stenson duct may or may not be present.

Anorexia is a frequent complaint. Some patients may complain of abdominal pain, which may represent involvement of the pancreas or of the ovaries in the female. Serum amylase is usually elevated during the infection. In severely ill patients, vomiting may be a significant problem.

The most feared complication of mumps in males is orchitis. Although this is seen most frequently in postpubertal males, orchitis has been reported in children as young as 3 years of age. From 14 to 35% of those who have mumps develop orchitis. The highest rate of orchitis is observed in those 15 to 29 years of age.

The onset of orchitis is usually heralded by fever toward the end of the first week of illness. There is severe pain, swelling, and tenderness. Orchitis may also occur before or in the absence of parotitis. The involvement is most often unilateral but bilateral involvement has been reported to occur. Atrophy may occur after orchitis. Unilateral atrophy will not result in sterility, but bilateral orchitis may. Development of malignancies in affected testes has been reported. Appropriate therapy for orchitis includes use of analgesics and adequate support of the testes. Application of ice has occasionally been useful.

In addition to involvement of testes, other glands are occasionally involved; oophoritis, mastitis, and pancreatitis occasionally accompany mumps. Mastitis is estimated to occur in 31% of females over 15 years of age with mumps. Oophoritis, which occurs in about 7% of postpubertal females infected with mumps virus, is usually manifested by emesis, fever, and lower abdominal pain. Involvement of the thyroid also has been reported.

Mumps virus is neurotropic. Meningitis or meningoencephalitis occurs with mumps virus infection more commonly than encephalitis. Symptoms of central nervous system (CNS) involvement typically occur 3 to 10 days after the onset of parotid gland swelling. Headache, lethargy, nuchal rigidity, and vomiting are common. Males are affected more commonly than females. CSF usually contains normal or slightly elevated protein, normal or slightly decreased glucose, and pleocytosis. Cells are usually predominantly lymphocytic with the counts ordinarily under 500 cells/μL. Counts of more than 1000/μL, however, are not rare. Virus can be isolated from CSF during the first few days of meningoencephalitis. Infection of the CNS is usually self-limited and cases of meningitis generally have a favorable prognosis. Encephalitis may result in some permanent sequelae or even death. Hydrocephalus, retrobulbar neuritis, and paralysis, developing following mumps infection, have been described.

Deafness is a complication associated with mumps. It is often unilateral. The exact frequency is difficult to ascertain. In a prospective study of hearing impairment following mumps in Finnish Army personnel, about 4% of patients had acute deafness. Most patients recovered within a few weeks. Higher tone frequencies tended to be affected most severely. Deafness is not related to central nervous system involvement.

Diabetes mellitus has been reported to occur after onset of mumps. Mumps virus may invade the pancreas and can infect beta cells in vitro. Joint involvement is an uncommon complication of mumps that is very rare in children. Large joints, especially the knees, are most frequently affected; involvement may be multiple or monoarticular. Complete recovery is usual, but symptoms may be protracted.

Mumps in pregnant women is associated with an increased rate of fetal wastage in the first trimester. There is no evidence that mumps virus infection produces congenital malformations. Although it was postulated that subendocardial fibroelastosis might be associated with fetal mumps infection, this does not appear to be so. Maternal mumps near term has resulted in transmission to the newborn infant. Mumps virus has been isolated from breast milk.

DIAGNOSIS When confronted with an infant, child, or adolescent with bilateral or unilateral parotid swellings, a differential diagnosis should include drug effects, metabolic diseases, systemic lupus erythematosus, parotid duct obstruction, and other infectious agents, both bacterial and viral. Parotid swelling has been reported in infants and children with HIV infection. Bacterial infection of the parotid gland may be accompanied by purulent discharge from the Stenson duct.

Lesions of the ramus of the mandible, such as osteomyelitis, have occasionally been mistaken for parotid enlargement. When this happens, the enlargement is usually persistent. Other causes of persistent enlargement include Sjögren syndrome, leukemia, and sickle-cell anemia. Recurrent parotitis of undetermined etiology does occur in children.

Enlarged lymph nodes in proximity to the parotid gland must be differentiated from parotid enlargement. Cervical lymph nodes are below the ramus of the mandible. Preparotid nodes are usually associated with conjunctivitis.

The mumps skin test is inaccurate and should not be used to test for immunity.

The diagnosis of mumps infection depends on either the isolation of virus in culture, demonstrating a rise in specific antibodies to mumps virus antigens, or identifying mumps-specific IgM antibody. The virus can be readily isolated from throat swabs obtained 48 hours before to 7 days after parotid swelling begins. Virus has also been isolated from urine and spinal fluid. Antibodies to parainfluenza viruses may occasionally interfere with complement fixation and hemagglutination inhibition assays for mumps antibody.

TREATMENT AND PREVENTION Conservative therapy is indicated in the treatment of mumps. Adequate attention to hydration and alimentation is essential. Patients may have difficulty with acidic foods, such as orange juice. The diet should be light, with a generous offering of fluids.

Analgesics may occasionally be necessary for severe headache or discomfort caused by parotitis. Stronger analgesics may be needed for orchitis. It is unusual for vomiting to be severe enough to require intravenous fluids. In these instances, however, electrolytes lost by vomiting should be replaced.

Hospitalized patients should be isolated for 9 days after parotid swelling begins. A similar interval of exclusion from school is recommended.

Attenuated live mumps virus vaccine is used routinely in the immunization of children, adolescents, and young adults. After a single dose of vaccine, antibodies develop in 95 to 98% of all those susceptible. Vaccine-induced immunity is long lasting. Recommendations for mumps vaccination are provided in Sec. 1.5.2.

References

Beard CM, Benson RC JR, Kelalis PP, et al: The incidence and outcome of mumps orchitis in Rochester, Minnesota, 1935–1974. Mayo Clin Proc 52:3–7, 1977

Gordon SC, Clauter CB: Mumps arthritis: a review of the literature. Rev Infect Dis 6:338–344, 1984

Hersh BS, Fine PC, Kent W, et al: Mumps outbreak in a highly vaccinated population. J Pediatr 119:187–193, 1991

Johnson CE, Kumar ML, Whitwell JK, et al: Antibody persistence after primary measles-mumps-rubella vaccine and response to second dose given at four to six vs. eleven to thirteen years. Pediatr Infect Dis J 15:687–692, 1996

Koskiniemi M, Donner M, Pettay O: Clinical appearance and outcome in mumps encephalitis in children. Acta Paediatr Scand 72:603–609, 1983

13.4.16   Human Parvovirus

Peggy Sue Weintrub

Human parvovirus (HPV) was first discovered in 1975 in serum specimens from healthy blood donors. It has subsequently been shown to be the cause of a number of clinical manifestations including erythema infectiosum (fifth disease), acute arthritis, and aplastic crises in patients with hemolytic anemias. When acquired by pregnant women, it can lead to spontaneous abortion, fetal hydrops, and stillbirths.

The Parvoviridae family includes two genera of vertebrate viruses and one genus of invertebrate viruses. Parvovirus B19 belongs to the genus *Parvovirus,* an autonomously replicating, small, single-stranded DNA virus. Only HPV B19 parvoviruses infect human beings and are known to be associated with disease.

Parvovirus infections are most commonly recognized in school-age children. Infections can be sporadic; epidemics occasionally occur, most commonly in late winter or spring. Approximately 70% of recognized infections occur in children between 5 and 15 years of age. Studies show that children younger than 5 years old have a seroprevalence of 2 to 9%; children 5 to 18 years old have a seroprevalence of 15 to 60%; and adults have a seroprevalence of 30 to 60%. Attack rates are variable and range from 10 to 60% in school outbreaks. Males and females are equally affected with erythema infectiosum; arthritis is more common in females.

Because the virus is present in respiratory secretions of viremic patients, transmission occurs via respiratory droplets. Patients with erythema infectiosum are likely to have been infectious before, not during, the rash. In contrast, patients with an aplastic crisis are likely to be most infectious at the time of the acute presentation. Parvovirus is also transmitted by transfusion of blood or, more commonly, clotting factor concentrates. Vertical transmission from mother to infant may occur.

Intranasal inoculation of HPV in human volunteers resulted in fever, malaise, and itching approximately 1 week after infection. During this period, susceptible volunteers were viremic and had respiratory shedding. During the second week of infection, IgM developed, and there was reticulocytopenia. Development of arthritis or rash during the third week of infection coincided with the development of an IgG response. Therefore, the pathogenesis in patients with erythema infectiosum or arthritis is believed to be related to immune complex disease.

CLINICAL MANIFESTATIONS

Erythema Infectiosum Erythema infectiosum (EI) is also known as *fifth disease,* one of the common childhood exanthems. It is characterized by a prodromal illness, usually consisting of malaise, pharyngitis, and a low-grade fever, followed by a rash. The classic feature of the rash is a "slapped cheek" appearance on the face, which may be accompanied by circumoral pallor or a fine desquamation. The rash then spreads to the trunk and the extremities. There it is described as erythematous and macular, often evolving into confluent areas, giving it a lattice-like appearance. The rash is pruritic in approximately 50% of patients and may come and go. It may also be precipitated by a variety of stimuli, such as heat and sun. This symptom may persist after all others have resolved. Occasionally, patients may also have an exanthem. Lymphadenopathy may be seen; in one outbreak, it was noted in almost 50% of patients in the posterior cervical chain. In general, patients feel relatively well, which may help to differentiate fifth disease from measles. Adults with EI tend to be sicker than children.

Serologic studies of acute infection during outbreaks show that as many as 50% of individuals may not have a rash and will have only nonspecific respiratory or gastrointestinal symptoms. Others may seroconvert without any symptoms.

Arthritis   Arthritis is a common syndrome associated with parvovirus B19 infection. It tends to occur more in women and in adults. It often occurs after the rash, but it may be the sole manifestation of the infection. It most often causes symmetric disease, particularly in the hands. The knees and wrists are other commonly involved joints. The symptoms are usually self-limited, but they have been reported to last for months or years. Occasionally, patients are rheumatoid factor-positive during the acute episode. Some patients meet the diagnostic criteria for rheumatoid arthritis. Occasionally, children have arthritis during infection, and one recent study suggests that HPV may be responsible for some juvenile rheumatoid arthritis.

Aplastic Crises   Parvovirus B19 is associated with aplastic crises in individuals with an underlying hemolytic anemia, including those persons with sickle-cell disease, hereditary spherocytosis, thalassemia, pyruvate kinase deficiency, autoimmune hemolytic anemia, and others. It appears to be responsible for approximately 90% of aplastic crises in these patients, although not all patients who are seropositive have experienced an aplastic crisis. Occasional reports have also been noted of patients with a pancytopenia. Parvovirus is not responsible for transient erythropenia of childhood.

B19 has a tropism for dividing red-cell precursors, leading to reticulocytopenia. Patients with an underlying hemolytic process, who have shortened red-cell survival, are unable to compensate for the erythrocyte destruction and have an abrupt decrease in hematocrit. They may present with pallor, weakness, or heart failure in severe infection. Erythropoiesis increases 6 to 8 days after the hematocrit reaches its nadir. The infection probably causes a transient aplasia in most individuals, but only those with the need for an increased rate of erythropoiesis will have clinical manifestations.

Pregnancy and Fetal Infection   A number of reports of human parvovirus B19 infections during pregnancy have been published. In the majority of maternal infections, the fetus suffers no adverse effects, although the fetus is commonly HPV-positive by IgM or polymerase chain reaction. The virus has been found in abortus tissue, and IgM antibodies to B19 have been detected in cord blood. There are reports of fetal wastage, fetal hydrops, and stillbirths following maternal infection in the first, second, and third trimesters, respectively. Two large studies show that the risk of fetal loss is 5 to 10%. In one study of infants of IgM-positive and IgG-negative mothers, 10 infants had intrauterine hydrops: four infants resolved the hydrops as documented by serial ultrasound; four had fetal death; one died immediately after an attempted intrauterine transfusion; and one premature infant died on the second day of life. There are no clinical trials that address the appropriate therapy if one identifies an HPV-induced hydropic fetus, so this series indicates that the risk-benefit of intervention must be weighed in individual patients. Another report suggests that an elevated maternal α-fetoprotein may be a marker for a poor prognosis of an affected pregnancy. There are no reports of consistent congenital abnormalities attributed to human parvovirus infection during gestation, but rare cases of hydrocephalus, intracranial calcifications, and other central nervous system structural abnormalities have been described. The precise risk of parvovirus B19 to the fetus has not been determined.

Other Manifestations   A chronic and severe anemia can be seen in patients with immune dysfunction. Other rare reported presentations are Henoch-Schönlein purpura, parvo-associated hemophagocytic syndrome, glomerulonephritis, myocarditis, numerous neurologic complications, and fulminant hepatitis.

DIAGNOSIS   The diagnoses of erythema infectiosum and aplastic crises are made primarily on clinical grounds. Under certain circumstances, such as an exposed pregnant woman, one may wish to make a specific diagnosis. Unfortunately, HPV B19 cannot be grown by using routine virologic tissue-culture techniques; it requires the use of bone marrow explant cultures. This has slowed the development of serologic testing, because it is difficult to propagate the virus to supply the needed antigen for serologic assays. At the current time, these assays are available only on a research basis or through the CDC or state health departments. The available IgM assays do show some cross-reactivity with the IgM for rubella, so it may be useful to test for both viruses when it is important to differentiate these two entities.

TREATMENT   There is currently no specific antiviral therapy for treating HPV B19. For patients with aplastic crises, supportive care, such as oxygen and, if needed, transfusions, is often life-saving. A number of reports describe an excellent response to immunoglobulin therapy in patients with immunodeficiency and/or a chronic anemia related to persistent HPV infection. There does not appear to be any role for immunoglobulin at this time for patients with erythema infectiosum or aplastic crises, as these are self-limited syndromes. There is no known role for immunoglobulin in postexposure prophylaxis for high-risk patients.

In the hospital setting, those with an aplastic crisis or chronic anemia secondary to parvovirus should be placed in isolation, and health-care workers should wear masks for droplet precautions. Pregnant women at high risk of acquiring parvovirus (teachers, childcare workers, women with young school-age children) might consider serologic testing for IgG to determine their susceptibility.

References

American Academy of Pediatrics, Committee on Infectious Diseases: Parvovirus, erythema infectiosum, and pregnancy. Pediatrics 85:131–133, 1990

Anderson MJ, Higging PG, Davis LR, et al: Experimental parvoviral infection in humans. J Infect Dis 152:257–265, 1985

Anderson MJ, Lewis E, Kidd IM, et al: An outbreak of erythema infectiosum associated with human parvovirus infection. J Hygiene 93:85–93, 1984

Kurtzman G, Frickhofen N, Kimball J, et al: Pure red-cell aplasia of 10 years' duration due to persistent parvovirus B19 infection and its cure with immunoglobulin therapy. N Engl J Med 321:519–523, 1989

Nocton JJ, Miller LC, Tucker LB, Shaller JG: Human parvovirus B19-associated arthritis in children. J Pediatr 122:186–190, 1993

Török TJ, Wang QY, Gary GE, et al: Prenatal diagnosis of intrauterine infection with parvovirus B19 by the polymerase chain reaction technique. Clin Infect Dis 14:149–155, 1992

13.4.17   Poliovirus

Roland W. Sutter and Stephen L. Cochi

Poliomyelitis is an acute infectious and communicable disease caused by poliovirus. Infection commonly results in an asymptomatic state or mild nonspecific illness. Rarely, the virus invades the central nervous system where viral replication in motor neurons causes cell destruction and permanent paralysis or weakness in the affected muscles.

Polioviruses are part of the *Enterovirus* genus (see Sec. 13.4.2) and belong to the family Picornaviridae (pico, implying small; RNA, the nucleic acid component).

In the prevaccine era, poliomyelitis was ubiquitous, with pronounced summer–early fall seasonal peaks in temperate areas, such as Europe and North America, and a more year-round pattern of transmission in tropical countries. The incubation period between exposure and first symptoms (minor illness) is 3 to 6 days, and from infection to onset of paralytic disease is usually 7 to 21 days, with a range of 3 to 35 days. Most exposures to poliovirus result in inapparent infection.

Poliovirus is transmitted by person-to-person spread via fecal-to-oral (developing countries) and oral-to-oral routes (industrialized countries) or, rarely, by a common vehicle (eg, milk, water). Persons remain most infectious immediately before and 1 to 2 weeks after onset of paralytic disease, although poliovirus replicates for substantially longer periods. It is excreted for 3 to 6 weeks in feces and for approximately 2 weeks in saliva. Secondary infection rates of susceptible household or institutional contacts are high (>90%), probably mediated by fecal-to-oral spread.

Several exposure factors occurring in association with poliovirus infection increase the risk of acquiring paralytic manifestations, including pregnancy, older age, being unvaccinated or inadequately vaccinated for poliovirus, receipt of intramuscular injections with diphtheria-tetanus toxoids and pertussis vaccine (DTP) or antibiotics, strenuous exercise, and injury such as fracture. Removal of tonsils and adenoids predisposes to bulbar poliomyelitis. Lower socioeconomic status is a risk factor for paralytic poliomyelitis in developing countries. This is most likely because children of lower socioeconomic status experience more intense exposure to poliovirus (ie, a higher virus inoculum, which has been shown in experimental studies to be a risk factor for paralytic disease). These children are also at higher risk for primary vaccine failure after trivalent oral poliovirus vaccine (OPV) because of more frequent concurrent enterovirus infections.

CLINICAL MANIFESTATIONS   Poliovirus exposure in a susceptible person results in one of the following consequences: (a) inapparent infection without symptoms; (b) minor illness; (c) nonparalytic poliomyelitis (aseptic meningitis); or (d) paralytic poliomyelitis. Inapparent infection without symptoms is the most frequent outcome (>95%). Minor illness is the most frequent form of symptomatic disease, characterized by transient illness associated with a few days of fever, malaise, drowsiness, headache, nausea, vomiting, constipation, or sore throat, in various combinations. Nonparalytic CNS involvement (aseptic meningitis), a relatively rare outcome of poliovirus infection, usually begins as a minor illness characterized by fever, sore throat, vomiting, and malaise. One to 2 days later, signs of meningeal irritation become apparent, including stiffness of the neck or back, vomiting, severe headache, pain in limbs, back, and neck. This form of the disease lasts from 2 to 10 days and recovery is usually rapid and complete. In a small proportion of these cases, the disease advances to transient mild muscle weakness or paralysis.

Paralytic poliomyelitis is a rare outcome (<1%) of poliovirus infections among susceptible persons. Its clinical course is characterized by a minor illness of several days, a symptom-free period of 1 to 3 days, followed by rapid onset of flaccid paralysis with fever and progression to the maximum extent of paralysis within a few days. After temperature returns to normal, there is usually no further progression of paralysis. If paralysis of an extremity is not com-

plete, it is more pronounced proximally. Paralysis is usually asymmetric, associated with diminished or complete loss of deep-tendon reflexes, with an intact sensory system. Paralytic manifestations in extremities begin proximally and progress to involve distal muscle groups (ie, descending paralysis). Depending on the anatomic location of motor neuron damage in the spinal cord or in the brainstem, spinal, mixed spinal-bulbar, or bulbar paralysis involving primarily respiratory muscles may be observed. The anterior horn and brainstem cells, just like other nerve cells of the CNS, cannot be regenerated or replaced, and paralysis is permanent.

The case fatality rate is variable and depends primarily on the age groups affected. The highest case fatality rates have been reported from epidemic cases in the early 20th century and among older persons, but are commonly between 5 and 10%.

DIAGNOSIS   Paralytic poliomyelitis has become a rare disease in the United States and in many other countries. Therefore, physicians may not be familiar with the disease or consider the diagnosis of poliomyelitis among more frequent causes of acute flaccid paralysis (Table 13-59). The diagnosis of paralytic poliomyelitis is dependent on: (a) clinical course; (b) virologic testing; (c) special studies; and (d) residual neurologic deficit at least 60 days after onset of symptoms.

The clinical course is helpful in assessing paralytic poliomyelitis as part of a differential diagnosis. Several studies in the developing world have attempted to assess the sensitivity and specificity of different clinical case definitions for paralytic poliomyelitis and compared the definition to the "gold standard" of virologically confirmed poliomyelitis based on poliovirus isolation from stool specimens. These studies reported similar findings. The largest study reported a sensitivity of 64% and a specificity of 82% for a case definition that included age <6 years, fever at onset, and rapid progression to maximum extent of paralysis within 4 days.

The clinical case definition for paralytic poliomyelitis requires a residual neurologic deficit at 60 days or more after onset of paralysis. Such a neurologic deficit may be apparent as complete flaccid paralysis of one or more extremities, or partial paralysis or weakness of muscles or muscle groups.

Because enteroviruses other than poliovirus and other conditions may cause acute flaccid paralysis, laboratory confirmation is critical to establishing the diagnosis of poliomyelitis. The most important is the isolation of poliovirus, which may be recovered acutely from stool, throat swabs, or, less commonly, cerebrospinal fluid taken soon after the onset of illness, and from stool specimens collected over longer periods of time, for as long as 3 to 6 weeks following paralysis onset. Isolation of poliovirus from cerebrospinal fluid (CSF) suggests a causal relationship between a poliovirus serotype and paralytic disease. Two stool samples should be collected at least 24 hours apart to confirm the diagnosis, because excretion of virus can be intermittent, and the sensitivity of isolation is <100%. It is recommended that stool specimens be collected as soon as the diagnosis of poliomyelitis is suspected, and ideally within 14 days of paralysis onset to maximize the likelihood of isolating poliovirus. After determination of serotype is accomplished, intratypic differentiation of poliovirus isolates as either vaccine-related or wild-type should be considered.

Serologic testing may be helpful in establishing the diagnosis, but sometimes causes confusion because: (a) antibody rises have already occurred by the time the first specimen has been collected; (b) antibody may be present to one or more serotypes because of previous or recent vaccination; and/or (c) heterotypic responses may be observed to one serotype after exposure to another sero-

TABLE 13-59

DISTINGUISHING FEATURES OF FOUR COMMON DIAGNOSES OF ACUTE FLACCID PARALYSIS (POLIOMYELITIS, GUILLAIN-BARRÉ SYNDROME, TRAUMATIC NEURITIS, AND TRANSVERSE MYELITIS)

FEATURE	POLIOMYELITIS	GUILLAIN-BARRÉ SYNDROME	TRAUMATIC NEURITIS (FOLLOWING INJECTION)	TRANSVERSE MYELITIS
Development of paralysis	24–48 hours onset to full paralysis	From hours to 10 days	From hours to 4 days	From hours to four days
Fever at onset	High, always present at onset of flaccid paralysis, gone the next day	Not common	Commonly present before, during, and after flaccid paralysis	Rarely present
Flaccid paralysis	Acute, usually asymmetric, principally proximal	Generally acute, symmetric, and distal	Asymmetric, acute, and affecting only one limb	Acute, lower limbs, symmetric
Progression of paralysis	"Descending"	"Ascending"		
Muscle tone	Reduced or absent in affected limb	Global hypotonia	Reduced or absent in affected limb	Hypotonia in affected limbs
Deep-tendon reflexes	Decreased or absent	Globally absent	Decreased or absent	Absent in lower limbs—early; hyperreflexia—late
Sensation	Severe myalgia, backache, no sensory changes	Cramps, tingling, hypoanesthesia of palms and soles	Pain in gluteus	Anesthesia of lower limbs with sensory level
Cranial nerve involvement	Only when bulbar involvement is present	Often present, affecting nerves VII, IX, X, XI, XII	Absent	Absent
Respiratory insufficiency	Only when bulbar involvement is present	In severe cases, enhanced by bacterial pneumonia present	Absent	Sometimes
Autonomic signs and symptoms	Rare	Frequent blood pressure alterations, sweating, blushing, and body temperature fluctuations	Hypothermia in affected limb	Present
Cerebrospinal fluid	Mild elevation of lymphocytes ~10–200/mL	Albumin-cytologic dissociation	Normal	Normal or mild in cells
Bladder dysfunction	Rare	Transient	Never	Present
Nerve conduction velocity: third week	Abnormal: anterior horn cell disease (normal during first 2 weeks)	Abnormal: slowed conduction, decreased motor amplitudes	Abnormal: axonal damage	Normal or abnormal, no diagnostic value
EMG at 3 weeks	Abnormal	Normal	Normal	Normal
Sequelae at 3 months and up to 1 year	Severe, asymmetric atrophy, skeletal deformities developing later	Symmetric atrophy of distal muscles	Moderate atrophy, only in affected limbs	Flaccid diplegia atrophy after years

SOURCE: *Adapted from Global Program for Vaccines and Immunization: Field Guide for Supplementary Activities Aimed at Achieving Polio Eradication. Geneva, World Health Organization, 1996.*

type. Paired serum specimens are required to demonstrate a four-fold or greater rise in antibody titer between acute and convalescent sera. The first serum specimen should be collected as soon as possible after onset of paralytic manifestations and the second specimen should be collected 2 to 3 weeks later. Neutralizing antibodies appear early and are usually already detectable at the time of onset of paralysis. However, if the first specimen is taken early enough, a rise in titer may be demonstrated during the course of the disease.

Nerve conduction and electromyography studies can point to the anatomic location of the paralysis—destruction of anterior horn cells in the spinal cord versus a demyelinating process in the peripheral nerves—helping to exclude the most frequent cause of acute flaccid paralysis, Guillain-Barré Syndrome (GBS). Magnetic resonance imaging (MRI) has been used infrequently, but can highlight the affected areas of the anterior column of the spinal cord. Analysis of spinal fluid may be helpful in ruling out other causes. In paralytic poliomyelitis, the CSF contains an increased number of leukocytes—usually 10 to 200 per mL, and seldom more than 500 per mL. At the onset of signs of CNS involvement, the ratio of polymorphonuclear cells to lymphocytes is high, but within a few days the ratio is reversed. The total white blood cell count slowly subsides to normal levels. The protein content of the CSF space initially is elevated only slightly. Glucose levels are usually within the normal range.

TREATMENT AND PROGNOSIS There is no specific treatment for poliomyelitis. By the time the paralytic consequences of CNS viral replication are apparent, administration of immunoglobulin or use of antiviral compounds, is not helpful. Treatment is primarily supportive; when bulbar paralysis with respiratory insufficiency ensues, respiratory support is critical. The specific objectives of therapy during the acute phase of the illness are (a) to prevent further progression of paralysis with mandatory bed rest; (b) to ensure respiratory sufficiency in cases of bulbar paralysis, if necessary, by using respirators; and (c) to relieve pain and discomfort, particularly with the application of wet heat to the affected muscles. The specific objectives during the subacute (after body temperature has returned to normal) and chronic phases (after hospital discharge) of the illness are (a) to strengthen the remaining functional muscles with physiotherapy to compensate for paralyzed or weak muscles; (b) to prevent deformities following paralysis of muscles and limbs with proper positioning of trunk and limbs, regular movements of limbs, and use of splints to ensure proper position of joints; (c) to assist with ambulation by proper use of splints, leg braces, crutches, and wheel chairs, where appropriate; and, finally, (d) to correct contracted muscles or shortened tendons with surgical procedures to ensure potential for functionality.

Antiviral compounds, particularly pleconaril, may be used under an Investigational New Drug protocol to eliminate chronic enterovirus infections that have been reported among immunodeficient patients (eg, persons with agammaglobulinemias), including persistent infections caused by poliovirus.

The prognosis in poliomyelitis depends on the severity on initial presentation (extent of weakness or paralysis), the degree of recovery achieved during the first 6 months after onset of paralysis, and the underlying medical condition. The prognosis is more guarded in patients with underlying immunodeficiency disorders. Most patients, except those with complete paralysis of a limb, are able to compensate for loss of some muscle function by strengthening the remaining functioning muscles.

The late manifestations of acute paralytic poliomyelitis (ie, postpolio syndrome) usually become apparent after an interval of 15 to 40 years, when many persons (25–40%) who contracted paralytic poliomyelitis in their childhood may experience new muscle pain, exacerbation of existing weakness, or development of new weakness or paralysis. Factors that enhance the risk of postpolio syndrome include: (a) increasing length of time since acute poliovirus infection; (b) presence of permanent residual impairment after recovery from the acute illness; and (c) female gender.

PREVENTION AND CONTROL Prevention of poliomyelitis depends on immunization with poliovirus vaccines. Vaccination recommendations are discussed in Sec. 1.5.2.

In 1988 The World Health Assembly recommended the following four strategies to be implemented in all polio-endemic countries to achieve global eradication of polio: (a) achieve and maintain high levels of routine coverage with poliovirus vaccine in infants <1 year of age to prevent accumulation of susceptible infants in this age category; (b) conduct biannual national immunization days (NIDs), targeting all children <5 years of age regardless of previous immunization history to eliminate widespread circulation of poliovirus; (c) establish sensitive systems for poliomyelitis surveillance (using acute flaccid paralysis as a screening case definition) to target supplemental immunization activities and monitor the disappearance of poliovirus; and (d) initiate "mopping-up" activities, mass campaigns that administer OPV by house-to-house visits to reach children that have been missed by the routine immunization program and NIDs.

Implementation of these strategies has resulted in an ~85% reduction in reported poliomyelitis worldwide since 1988; the certification of the Western Hemisphere as free of indigenous wild poliovirus in 1994; the elimination of wild poliovirus from the Western Pacific Region of WHO in 1997 (a region that includes China, the world's most populated country); and rapid progress toward polio eradication in virtually all polio-endemic countries. As

of 1999, poliovirus circulation was restricted to South Asia and Africa.

References

Centers for Disease Control and Prevention: Poliomyelitis prevention in the United States: Introduction of a sequential vaccination schedule of inactivated poliovirus vaccine followed by oral poliovirus vaccine. Recommendations of the Advisory Committee on Immunization Practices. MMWR Morb Mortal Wkly Rep 1997:46(RR3):1–25, 1997

Centers for Disease Control and Prevention: Progress toward global poliomyelitis eradication, 1997–1998. MMWR Morb Mortal Wkly Rep 48: 416–421, 1999

Cochi SL, Hull HF, Sutter RW, Wilfert CM, Katz SL: Status report on the global Poliomyelitis Eradication Initiative. J Infect Dis (Suppl):S1–S292, 1997

Dalakas MC, Bartfeld H, Kurland LT: The post-polio syndrome: advances in the pathogenesis and treatment. Ann N Y Acad Sci 753:1–412, 1995

Global Program for Vaccines and Immunization: Field Guide for Supplementary Activities Aimed at Achieving Polio Eradication. Geneva, World Health Organization, 1996

Paul JR: A History of Poliomyelitis. New Haven, Yale University Press, 1971

Sutter RW, Cochi SL, Melnick JL: Live attenuated poliovirus vaccines. In: Plotkin SA, Orenstein WA, eds: in Vaccines, 3rd ed. Philadelphia, WB Saunders Company, 16:364–408, 1999

13.4.18 Rabies

Moses Grossman and Peggy Sue Weintrub

Rabies is primarily a viral infection of nonhuman carnivores. It is rare in human beings; when it does occur, it is usually the result of an animal bite. Rabies presents as an acute encephalomyelitis with a very high fatality rate. The disease is characterized by restlessness, excitation, and severe intermittent spasms of the larynx and pharynx, especially on sight of food or water. The latter symptoms accounts for the synonym *hydrophobia*.

Rabies fixed virus is estimated to be 100 to 150 nm in diameter; it is an RNA virus and is classified as a rhabdovirus. It is resistant to phenol, antibiotics, and commonly used skin antiseptics, with the exception of benzalkonium chloride and other quaternary ammonium compounds. Rabies virus is quickly destroyed by ultraviolet light, sunlight, strong acids, and alkalis. Aqueous suspensions of rabies virus are inactivated in 30 minutes at temperatures of 54°C (129.2°F) to 56°C (132.8°F). Infectivity may persist for years if the virus is desiccated and kept at 4°C (39.2°F).

Bite wounds usually introduce the virus by infectious saliva; it is not known to be introduced through intact skin. The virus probably binds initially to the acetylcholine receptor and then travels centripetally, via the peripheral nerves, toward the central nervous system. After infection of the brain, virus travels via the sensory and autonomic nervous system to the eyes, salivary glands, skin, and viscera. The principal pathologic changes are confined to the central nervous system; they consist of neuronal necrosis and nonsuppurative encephalitis. Changes are most pronounced in the thalamus, hypothalamus, substantia nigra, pons, and medulla. The spinal cord and sympathetic ganglia may also show similar changes. The most distinctive histologic feature of rabies infection is the presence of pathognomonic Negri bodies, acidophilic inclusion bodies found in the cytoplasm of neurons.

The vast majority of animal rabies in the United States occurs in wildlife, not pets. Bats, skunks, wolves, coyotes, foxes, raccoons, and many other species are implicated. Rabies is not endemic in rodents or lagomorphs. For purposes of prophylaxis, bats and skunks should be considered to be rabid unless proven otherwise. Dog-associated rabies is relatively uncommon in the United States but remains a problem in many parts of Mexico, Latin America, Asia, and Africa. Dog bites continue to be a predominant reason for postexposure prophylaxis. In the United States, 40,000 individuals receive postexposure prophylaxis per year.

Annual human rabies deaths throughout the world are estimated to be in the thousands. Rabies may occur in any climate or season, and susceptibility does not seem to vary with age, sex, or race. The incidence of rabies infection is highest in children, probably because of their friendliness toward animals and their inability to defend themselves. In the United States during the past decade, approximately one-third of the reported cases of human rabies occurred in people bitten by rabid dogs outside of the United States. The remaining two-thirds of cases followed exposure to indigenous reservoirs, most commonly insectivorous bats. In almost 80% of the indigenous cases, there was no definite exposure to a rabid animal; some of these reported no animal contact and others had animal contact but no known bite or mucous membrane exposure.

The attack rate in persons bitten by rabid animals is difficult to estimate, and it depends on the location of the wound, the depth of the bite, the presence of saliva infected with virus, and the protection afforded by clothing. Administration of both active and passive immunization dramatically reduces the risk of disease in persons bitten by rabid animals.

CLINICAL MANIFESTATIONS The average incubation period is 18 to 60 days; the interval, however, can be extremely variable, as short as 5 days and as long as 6 years. It is shorter when the bite is on the head than when it is on an extremity. The illness begins with a prodrome characterized by apprehension, anxiety, insomnia, malaise, and headache. There may be pain and numbness at the site of the bite. This phase lasts 2 to 7 days and is usually followed by the onset of neurologic symptoms, initially an excitation phase, also known as "furious" rabies. The excitation phase appears rapidly; there is much apprehension and even terror. Twitching, delirium, meningismus, and mild convulsive movements are seen. When the patient attempts to swallow food or liquid, painful, violent spasms of the larynx and pharynx may occur. Later, just the sound, smell, or sight of liquid may precipitate these spasms. During these periods, cyanosis may be present, and choking and aspiration are quite common. The temperature is elevated [(39.5°C (103.1°F) to 40.5°C (104.9°F)], and generalized convulsions may occur. Maniacal behavior, such as tearing of clothes and bedding, often occurs. Intermittent periods of relative calm ensue, during which the patient is often quite lucid.

The paralytic phase appears with progressive paralysis, cessation of spasms, and coma, with death shortly thereafter. Progressive ascending paralysis may occasionally be the predominant symptom; this type of rabies being known as the dumb type. In all instances, a great many complications develop, including respiratory depression, hypoventilation, arrhythmias, and hypotension. The disease is uniformly fatal except in rare cases of individuals who contract the disease despite postexposure prophylaxis.

DIAGNOSIS AND TREATMENT When classic symptoms are present and there is a history of an animal bite, the differential diagnosis is not difficult. It is important to consider the diagnosis even without an obvious exposure, because most patients have had no known contact with rabid animals. Tetanus should be considered in the differential diagnosis. Symptoms of trismus and muscle spasms in tetanus are usually persistent, whereas they are intermittent in rabies. Other viral etiologies of encephalitis should be entertained.

Isolation of virus from the saliva, cerebrospinal fluid, lacrimal secretions, nasal secretions, and urine should be attempted. Negative results should not exclude the diagnosis, because the virus is secreted intermittently. Fluorescent antibody examination of brain tissue, skin, or corneal scrapings is fast, reliable, and accurate if done properly. Biopsy from the skin at the back of the neck, which has a heavy concentration of nerve fibers, is particularly accessible and useful for immunofluorescence. Microscopic examination of brain tissue for Negri bodies is also reliable and accurate, but it takes several days. Mouse inoculations of brain-tissue suspensions also require several days, but they allow isolation of the virus. PCR of saliva or brain has been shown to be sensitive and specific and should be attempted where the test is available.

Treatment consists of intensive supportive care, concentrating particularly on support of ventilation and circulation. Health-care providers should follow the now standard, total body-substance isolation precautions. Previous preexposure or postexposure prophylaxis had been done in the few patients who survived. There is no known role for rabies immune globulin in rabies disease, nor is there any established antiviral therapy.

PREVENTION Prevention of human infection includes general public health measures such as mandatory vaccination of dogs; quarantine for traveling pets; preexposure immunization for veterinarians, animal handlers, and any other individuals who are likely to be exposed; and most importantly, postexposure prophylaxis for those who have been bitten by animals. Wildlife rabies is a serious problem not subject to control at the present time. The most common issue involving rabies confronting the physician is whether prophylaxis should be recommended after potential exposure. Many factors influence that decision.

Species of the Biting Animal Carnivorous animals, such as skunks, foxes, coyotes, wolves, raccoons, dogs, cats, and ferrets are most likely to be infectious; bats are highly suspect. Farm animals, squirrels, opossums, weasels, muskrats, woodchucks, and mongooses may occasionally be infectious. Bites of rodents, lagomorphs, birds, and reptiles seldom require treatment.

Circumstances of the Biting Incident An unprovoked attack is more likely to occur with a rabid animal, as contrasted to the provoked attack that may ensue when children tease or bother pets while they are feeding.

Extent and Location of the Bite Severe exposures are multiple wounds, deeply penetrating wounds, or any bite on the head, neck, hands, or fingers. Mild exposures are scratches, licks, and single lacerations on the body, except the head, neck, hands, or feet.

Nonbite Exposure Open wounds or abrasions can be contaminated with infected saliva by licking. Inhalation of aerosolized rabies virus can occur in laboratory workers and spelunkers. Despite the number of patients hospitalized with rabies, there are no examples of human-to-human transmission, except by corneal transplants, in the industrialized world.

Because of the recent increase in cases without a known bite from an insectivorous bat, nonverbal individuals (eg, infants, those with altered mental status) in the same room with a bat should be considered candidates for prophylaxis.

Vaccination Status of the Biting Animal Animals whose owners can produce vaccination certificates are considered safe. If vaccination status is unknown, the animal should be considered potentially infectious.

Presence of Rabies in the Region Provided that adequate surveillance and laboratory facilities exist in an area, it is most important to know whether rabies exists in the region and in what species. This type of information can usually be provided by local public health officials.

WOUND MANAGEMENT Immediate and thorough local treatment of all bite wounds and scratches is a most important means of preventing rabies. At present, thorough washing with soap and water is believed to be best.

MANAGEMENT OF THE BITING ANIMAL Healthy-appearing dogs and cats that bite human beings should be confined and observed by a veterinarian for 10 days. Illness in the biting animal should be reported to the local health officials and the patient's physician immediately. If an animal must be killed to be captured, it should be done in a manner so as not to traumatize the head. Likewise, if the animal dies, the head should be shipped under refrigeration to a competent laboratory for diagnosis. For wildlife under suspicion, the animal should be killed and its head submitted for laboratory examination. The public health laboratory will perform an examination of the brain by the fluorescent antibody technique. If that examination is negative, one can assume that no rabies was present in the animal's saliva.

HYPERIMMUNE RABIES GLOBULIN AND VACCINE When the decision is made to initiate postexposure prophylaxis, the current recommendations of both the World Health Organization and the US Public Health Service are that both passive and active immunization be used in all instances. *Rabies immune globulin* (RIG) is prepared from the blood of patients with high levels of antibody to rabies. Each milliliter contains 150 IU. The recommended dose of RIG is 20 IU/kg. If possible, the full dose of RIG should be infiltrated around the wound; any remaining RIG should be given intramuscularly. *Equine antirabies serum* should be used only if RIG is not available. When the equine antiserum is used, the usual precautions for giving equine serum are mandatory, namely a careful history of allergy, skin, and eye tests for hypersensitivity, and careful administration with a view to prompt handling of possible anaphylaxis. The dose of this material is 40 IU/kg, and it is also given partially around the wound, with the balance intramuscularly.

Postexposure prophylaxis is also recommended for persons who report a possibly infectious exposure (bite, scratch, an open wound or mucous membrane contaminated with saliva or other infectious material) to a human with rabies. Casual contact with an infected person alone does not constitute an exposure and is not an indication for prophylaxis.

Three rabies vaccines are currently available in the United States: Human Diploid Cell Vaccine (HDCV), Rabies Vaccine Adsorbed (RVA), and Purified Chick Embryo Cell Vaccine (PCEC). All three

are safe and efficacious and can be administered intramuscularly; only HDCV can be given intradermally. Five doses are recommended, as soon as possible after exposure and again 3, 7, 24, and 28 days after the first dose. Reactions following vaccine are generally mild: nausea, abdominal pain, muscle aches, and dizziness, without the very frequent neurologic reactions that were so common with previous vaccines. Persons who need to be vaccinated in other countries may find a variety of vaccines in use.

References

Advisory Committee of Immunization Practices: Rabies prevention—United States 1999. MMWR Morb Mortal Wkly Rep 48:1–21, 1999

Bahmanyar M, Fayaz A, Nour-Salehi S, et al: Successful protection of humans exposed to rabies infection: postexposure treatment with the new human diploid cell rabies vaccine and antirabies serum. JAMA 236:2751–2754, 1976

Blenden DC, Creech W, Torres-anjel MJ: Use of immunofluorescence examination to detect rabies virus antigen in the skin of humans with clinical encephalitis. J Infect Dis 154:698–701, 1986

Kamolvarin N, Tirawatnpong T, Rattanasiwamoke R et al: Diagnosis of rabies by polymerase chain reaction with nested primers. J Infect Dis 167:207–210, 1993

Noah DL, Drenzek CL, Smith JS, et al: Epidemiology of human rabies in the United States, 1980 to 1996. Ann Intern Med 128:922–930, 1998

13.4.19 Viral Respiratory Infections

Michael T. Brady

Respiratory tract infections, which are predominantly of viral origin, are by far the most common acute infections occurring in children and adults worldwide. Infants and preschool children experience six to 10 respiratory illnesses per year, and school-age children and adolescents experience three to five illnesses annually. Fever occurs in approximately 30 to 40% of viral respiratory illnesses in preschool children and lasts an average of 3 days, with a usual maximum of 5 to 6 days. Household crowding and childcare attendance are associated with an increased risk of exposure to infected persons and, therefore, with an increased incidence of respiratory infections in infants, toddlers, and preschool children.

Acute respiratory infections are caused by a wide spectrum of viruses, which may affect all or parts of the respiratory tract from the nose to the alveoli. In general, respiratory infections are classified into upper respiratory tract infection (URI), meaning the common cold, rhinitis, pharyngitis, otitis media, and conjunctivitis; and lower respiratory tract infection, namely, croup, laryngitis, tracheobronchitis, bronchiolitis, and pneumonia. Individual viruses tend to have a predilection for particular anatomic regions within the respiratory tract and tend to be more closely associated with specific clinical syndromes. For instance, rhinovirus infections are usually confined to the upper respiratory tract and produce afebrile rhinitis; respiratory syncytial virus infection in the infant and young child commonly causes a generalized upper and lower respiratory infection and is the agent most closely associated with bronchiolitis. Parainfluenza viruses types 1 and 2 tend to cause croup. Influenza virus infections are associated with a febrile respiratory infection that causes both rhinitis and tracheobronchitis. Influenza virus is also associated with secondary bacterial infection of the lower respiratory tract.

The most frequent bacterial complication of viral respiratory infection in childhood is otitis media. Middle-ear infection is diagnosed in 30 to 35% of preschool children, with acute respiratory illnesses being evaluated in outpatient settings. The risk of otitis media varies with the particular virus responsible for the associated or antecedent viral respiratory infection. In one prospective study, the risk of developing acute middle-ear infection or effusion ranged from 15 to 30% in children with culture-proven viral infections; respiratory syncytial virus infection carried the highest risk of middle-ear disease. A large proportion of the otitis media associated with or following a viral respiratory infection is the result of a secondary bacterial infection in the middle ear. However, in many instances, aspirate cultures from middle ears of children with otitis media yield only a respiratory virus. This suggests that viruses, particularly RSV and parainfluenza viruses, may result in middle-ear disease that is clinically indistinguishable from acute purulent otitis media caused by a bacterial infection. Our knowledge of the occurrence of sinusitis during viral respiratory infections is much less clearly defined, but there is certainly evidence linking bacterial sinusitis to antecedent viral URI. Involvement of the lower respiratory tract occurs in less than 5 to 30% of viral respiratory infections, depending on the etiology of infection and the age of the child. The attack rate of lower respiratory tract infections (LRI) is highest in preschool children who are usually experiencing primary infections with the infecting virus. This section focuses primarily on lower respiratory illness occurring in children with viral infections.

Specific viral diagnosis can be achieved by viral isolation from nasopharyngeal aspirates or swabs, or by rapid viral antigen-detection tests such as immunofluorescence and ELISA, which are now available for many of the respiratory viruses. Retrospective diagnosis may be achieved using serologic methods, but the delay inherent in waiting for a convalescent serum (3–4 weeks) makes this diagnostic method less useful in clinical decision making. The advent of specific antiviral therapies, including ribavirin for respiratory syncytial virus infections and possibly influenza virus infections, amantadine and rimantadine for influenza A virus infections, and neuraminidase inhibitors (eg, zanamivir) for both influenza A and B infections, has increased the need for readily available, early, specific diagnosis.

RESPIRATORY SYNCYTIAL VIRUS

Respiratory syncytial virus (RSV) is the most important cause of viral lower respiratory tract disease in infants and toddlers. Severe illness occurs most frequently in association with primary infection, although LRI also occurs in children experiencing reinfection with the virus. When significant respiratory compromise occurs during reinfection, affected children usually have underlying compromising cardiopulmonary disease. Involvement of smaller intrapulmonary airways (bronchioles) is the hallmark of RSV lower respiratory infection. Bronchiolitis is the single most important and distinctive clinical syndrome of LRI caused by RSV.

RSV is an enveloped, single-strand RNA virus. The viral envelope is studded with spike-like projections that represent two surface glycoproteins, the fusion (F) and attachment (G) proteins. The nucleocapsid reveals helical symmetry. RSV is currently classified as a member of the Paramyxoviridae family along with mumps, measles, and the parainfluenza viruses. RSV differs from most paramyxoviruses, however, in that it lacks both a hemagglutinin and a neuraminidase. For this reason, RSV has been placed in the genus *Pneumovirus*. The virus, which matures by budding from the infected cell surface, encodes 10 viral-specific proteins. The F glycoprotein mediates fusion of viral particles to target cells and fusion of infected cells to neighboring cells. The fusion results in syncy-

tium formation. Classification of two major antigenic subgroups of RSV is based on a heavily glycosylated surface protein (G), which is responsible for attachment of the virus to target cells. Antibodies specific for both F and G proteins can neutralize viral infectivity. No other viral proteins elicit neutralizing antibody. Internal proteins appear to be major targets for cytotoxic T-lymphocyte responses, which are important in terminating established viral infections.

EPIDEMIOLOGY RSV has a worldwide distribution. Annual midwinter epidemics of RSV infection occur in temperate climates; the seasonal epidemicity of infection is less clear in the tropics or even subtropical areas (such as Florida). In the United States, epidemics may begin as early as October or as late as April and last approximately 12 to 16 weeks in larger cities. RSV is the single most common cause of infant hospitalization in industrialized nations, with 90,000 to 150,000 annual hospital admissions in the United States. In metropolitan areas, viruses of subgroups A and B frequently cocirculate, although in any given epidemic, viruses of one antigenic subgroup may predominate. During most epidemics, subgroup A viruses account for the majority of isolates.

The peak incidence of infection occurs in the first 2 years of life. Approximately 50% of children are infected with RSV by their first birthday, with a similar attack rate among previously uninfected children during the second year of life. It is difficult to identify seronegative individuals beyond the third year of life. Reinfections with RSV occur throughout life and may occur even during the same winter season. The annual risk of reinfection among school-age children is approximately 20%.

Eleven to 15% of children make outpatient physician visits with RSV LRI during the first year of life. Approximately 1 in 10 of these children requires hospitalization; more than 80% of children with more severe RSV LRI illnesses are between 4 weeks and 6 months of age. Children with compromised cardiorespiratory function, predominantly attributable to bronchopulmonary dysplasia or congenital heart disease, are at increased risk of severe illness in association with RSV infection. Children born prematurely and those with compromised immune function also experience more severe LRI with RSV infection. Persistent and progressive RSV infections can occur in children with profoundly impaired cellular immune defenses. Disease in the immediate newborn period is not common, but nosocomial outbreaks of RSV infections in neonatal units have occurred. Among seriously ill patients, boys outnumber girls by nearly two to one. Children from higher socioeconomic groups tend to have less serious disease, probably because their level of exposure to the virus is lower during the early months of life.

PATHOGENESIS AND PATHOLOGY RSV infection is first established in the upper respiratory tract; initiation of infection is most efficient following inoculation of the nose or eyes. Infection may then spread from the oropharynx and nasopharynx to the lower respiratory tract, with clinical evidence of lower tract involvement in approximately 30% of infants and toddlers experiencing their first infection. As with most respiratory viruses, RSV infects predominantly airway epithelial cells. Histopathologically, children with severe lower respiratory disease caused by RSV infection probably have coexisting bronchiolitis and interstitial pneumonia. In patients who come to autopsy, prominent histopathologic findings include airway plugging with mucus, desquamated epithelium, and inflammatory cells; necrotizing lesions of bronchial and bronchiolar epithelium; and peribronchiolar inflammation with mononuclear cell predominance. The peribronchial infiltrate may extend into the adjacent pulmonary interstitium. Patchy atelectasis and emphysema are common. Cytoplasmic inclusion bodies have been noted, but syncytium formation is not usually striking. Involvement of the lower respiratory tract decreases with increasing age and repeated infection, so that illness is usually restricted to the upper respiratory tract in school-age children.

The occurrence of severe RSV illnesses during the first 6 months of life indicates that passively-acquired maternal antibody is not adequate to ensure complete protection from RSV infection and illness. However, children with very high titers of maternally-derived neutralizing antibody are at decreased risk for infection and severe illness early in life. Experimental animal models also provide evidence of a protective role for passively administered serum antibody. These observations have led to recent strategies incorporating passive immunoprophylaxis as a method for protecting children at highest risk of severe RSV disease.

Immunity to RSV following natural infection with the virus is transient and imperfect. During epidemics, the attack rate for second infections in exposed children can range from 40 to 70%, although illness is generally not as severe. It is probable that antigenic differences in the subgroups of RSV are important in the epidemiology of reinfection with RSV, but more information is needed in this area. With subsequent exposures, reinfection attack rates decline; however, adults are readily reinfected, usually with the production of only upper respiratory symptoms.

The incubation period of RSV-induced respiratory disease is 2 to 4 days. Virus can be detected in respiratory secretions up to 4 days before the onset of symptoms and routinely for at least 7 days thereafter. In infants hospitalized with primary RSV infection, continuous viral shedding for 10 or 11 days is commonly observed; occasional children have been found to shed the virus for as long as 20 days. Person-to-person spread of RSV is usually by the droplet route or by hand-to-nose transmission; small-particle aerosols do not appear to be very important in the spread of RSV. Without careful attention to infection control procedures, nosocomial infection rates have reached 30 to 40% in children hospitalized 7 days or longer during RSV epidemics. Infection of hospital staff members with RSV is an important link in nosocomial transmission of this virus. Strict hand washing and use of gloves must be practiced routinely. Because inoculation of the eyes and nose is particularly important in acquisition of RSV infection, masks or face shields that cover the nose and eyes may provide added protection in order to prevent nosocomial acquisition of RSV by hospital staff.

CLINICAL MANIFESTATIONS RSV infection is heralded by initial symptoms indistinguishable from those of the common cold. The infant may show a nasal discharge and cough, and there may be fever. Within 1 to 2 days, the cough becomes more prominent and tachypnea may develop. With increasing severity of LRI, the work of breathing increases; substernal and intercostal retractions are noted during inspiration, and active respiratory effort is required during expiration. The expiratory phase is prolonged, and the chest is hyperexpanded and hyperresonant, providing further evidence of generalized expiratory airflow obstruction. Diffuse expiratory wheezing is usually heard, commonly with associated moist crackles.

About 40% of infants hospitalized with RSV bronchiolitis experience repeated wheezing episodes, but recurrent wheezing in these patients is frequently limited to the first 3 to 4 years of life. The reported incidence of reactive airways disease in school-age children with a history of hospitalization for RSV bronchiolitis in infancy is not substantially higher than in the general childhood population. The agent is, however, an important precipitant of wheezing in the child with reactive airways disease.

Apnea can be a relatively early manifestation of RSV infection in young infants; these infants usually have a history of premature birth. Apnea can occur associated with the respiratory tract symptoms or it may precede the respiratory symptoms and represent the initial clinical manifestation in the infant younger than 8 weeks of age. Premature infants, with or without chronic lung disease, who are still experiencing apnea may have an increase in, or a worsening of, apneic episodes when they are infected with RSV.

Radiographs of the lungs reveal hyperexpansion, increased peribronchial markings, and, frequently, areas of atelectasis or infiltrate. Clinically, densities on chest radiographs may be more striking than the degree of clinical or radiographic evidence of small airway obstruction, and these patients may be labeled as having RSV pneumonia rather than bronchiolitis, but this distinction is often arbitrary. The pulmonary densities demonstrated radiographically in RSV pneumonia are predominantly areas of atelectasis.

The vast majority of infants have a relatively mild illness and proceed to recover; some, however, may develop significant respiratory compromise. In children requiring hospitalization, hypoxemia (arterial oxygen tension averaging 50–60 mm Hg in room air) is typical, reflecting ventilation-perfusion mismatch. Arterial P_{CO_2} above 45 mm Hg despite tachypnea is indicative of impending respiratory failure and the need to prepare for ventilatory support. Fatality rates range from less than 1% to 5%, with most deaths occurring in children with underlying illnesses. Children who have underlying congenital heart diseases with pulmonary hypertension are at particular risk of death. The average duration of hospitalization for previously healthy infants without complications is approximately 2 to 3 days; full recovery may take about 2 weeks.

DIAGNOSIS RSV may be isolated by inoculating nasopharyngeal secretions into sensitive cell lines, including continuous cell lines, such as HEp-2 and HeLa. Nasopharyngeal secretions can be obtained with a small suction catheter or bulb syringe. Instillation of a small volume of preservative-free sterile saline may facilitate collection of secretions. If tracheobronchial secretions can be obtained, they may also be cultured, but nasopharyngeal secretions should be cultured simultaneously. Because RSV is quite labile at room temperature, samples of secretions should be placed in viral transport medium on wet ice at the bedside and transported directly to the laboratory for immediate inoculation to cell cultures. Under proper conditions virus growth may be detected by the appearance of syncytial cytopathic effect in 3 to 14 days, typically in 5 to 7 days. Viral isolates may be identified by use of specific antisera; when such sera are not available, the identity of the virus may be determined presumptively by observing syncytial cytopathic effect in the absence of hemadsorption of guinea-pig red blood cells to the infected monolayer. Shell-vial culture assays can be used to detect RSV with nearly 100% sensitivity within 40 hours of inoculation.

RSV infection can be diagnosed rapidly by antigen detection using immunofluorescence techniques or enzyme immunoassay (EIA); EIA is the most commonly used assay for diagnosis. The advent of monoclonal antibodies has made these techniques sensitive (85–97%), specific (88–100%), and clinically useful. Aspirated nasopharyngeal secretions are preferred for RSV antigen-detection assays. PCR detection of RSV RNA in nasopharyngeal aspirates offers another sensitive (95%) and specific (>97%) means for rapidly identifying the RSV-infected child.

RSV infection induces rises in complement fixing (CF), EIA, and neutralizing antibodies 3 to 4 weeks following the onset of illness. The overall sensitivity and specificity of diagnosing RSV serologically by using EIA on paired acute and convalescent sera is 87% and 79%, respectively.

TREATMENT Most instances of RSV bronchiolitis and pneumonia are mild and self-limited. However, because these illnesses are occasionally severe, the pediatrician should be aware of three principles in managing the disease. First, RSV bronchiolitis generally peaks in severity within 48 to 72 hours. Therefore, a previously healthy infant seen after this time is at minimal risk of developing more severe disease. Second, the complications associated with hypoxemia and CO_2 retention generally begin when the respiratory rate surpasses 60 breaths per minute. Determination of capillary blood O_2 saturation by pulse oximetry while the child is breathing room air in the outpatient department permits identification of unsuspected hypoxemia. Third, children with community-acquired RSV disease rarely have associated bacterial infections of the lower respiratory tract; antibiotic treatment for LRI is usually not indicated in these patients.

Treatment of bronchiolitis is symptomatic. Giving humidified oxygen is frequently required when managing hospitalized infants because hypoxemia is common in more severe illness. Corticosteroids are ineffective and are not specifically indicated for RSV infection without evidence of reactive airway disease. In addition, the value of inhaled β-adrenergic agonists such as albuterol is not conclusively established and remains controversial. A trial of aerosolized bronchodilator treatment may be employed in managing severely ill children, but there are no data to support the routine use of these agents.

Ribavirin delivered by small-particle aerosol hastens clinical recovery both in previously healthy children and in those children with associated compromising conditions (pulmonary hypertension, complicated congenital heart disease, bronchopulmonary dysplasia, cystic fibrosis, other chronic lung diseases, or immunocompromising conditions or therapies). Ribavirin may be considered for use in normal infants with more severe disease, in infants with underlying compromising conditions, and in previously healthy infants who are less than 6 weeks old or who were born prematurely (<37 weeks of gestation) (Table 13-60). If ribavirin is to be used, methods to establish rapid RSV diagnosis should be available.

Ribavirin is usually administered for 12 to 22 hours a day for 3 to 5 days. The concentration of ribavirin solution in the nebulizer should be 20 mg/mL of water. An alternate approach utilized 2-hour aerosol administration of a ribavirin solution of 60 mg/mL of water given three times per day. Administration of ribavirin to children requiring mechanical ventilation for RSV disease is effective, but special care must be used when the drug is administered by ventilator, as precipitation of drug in ventilator valves can occur. This may result in life-threatening ventilator malfunctions. Without special means to confine or remove ribavirin from the immediate delivery area, room air may be contaminated with ribavirin during administration. Pregnant women should be protected from environmental exposure to the drug because there is teratogenic potential in laboratory animals.

Although antibiotics are not indicated in most children with RSV infections, nosocomial bacterial infections can occur in children receiving intensive supportive care for RSV disease. Cardiorespiratory monitoring, including pulse oximetry, should be considered standard care for young infants with RSV infections. It must be remembered that demonstration of satisfactory arterial oxygen saturation by pulse oximetry does not exclude the possibility of hypoventilation and impending respiratory failure. There is a high incidence of nosocomial spread of RSV infections, and hospitals should take active preventive precautions. It is particularly important to protect immunocompromised infants, as well as infants with cardiopulmonary disease, from exposure to infants and hospital staff members with RSV infections.

The pathophysiology of apnea in RSV infection is not understood; therapy is supportive, with mechanical ventilation usually required for approximately 48 hours. Children may manifest periodic breathing for 48 to 72 hours postextubation, but recurrent apnea following RSV-associated apnea is not common, and home apnea monitoring following hospital discharge is not usually indicated.

PROPHYLAXIS A safe and effective RSV vaccine has not yet been developed. Passive immunoprophylaxis to prevent RSV infection in infants and children at increased risk for severe disease is now available using either an intravenous or an intramuscular preparation. RSV immune globulin intravenous (RSV-IGIV) is an intravenously administered polyclonal antibody preparation with high-titer RSV antibodies. It was licensed by the FDA in January 1996, for prevention of severe RSV lower respiratory tract disease in infants and children younger than 24 months of age with chronic lung disease or a history of premature birth ($\leq$35 weeks' gestation). Palivizumab (Synagis) is an intramuscularly administered monoclonal antibody (F glycoprotein of RSV—a surface protein that is highly conserved among RSV isolates) preparation. It is not derived from human immunoglobulin and, therefore, is free of potential contamination by infectious agents and can be produced more readily than RSV-IGIV. It was licensed by the FDA in June 1998, for similar indications and patient populations as RSV-IGIV.

Palivizumab or RSV-IGIV should be considered for infants and children younger than 2 years of age with chronic lung disease who require medical therapy for their chronic lung disease within 6 months of the anticipated start of the RSV season. Infants who are born prematurely at 32 weeks' gestation or earlier without chronic lung disease may still benefit from RSV immunoprophylaxis. Infants born at 28 weeks' gestation or earlier may be candidates for RSV immunoprophylaxis up to 12 months of age; infants born between 29 and 32 weeks' gestation may be candidates up to 6 months of age. Both palivizumab and RSV-IGIV are given monthly, both are very expensive, and it may be difficult to justify the use of these products on the basis of cost-effectiveness. For that reason, institutions with infants and children with chronic lung disease or significant prematurity ($\leq$32 weeks' gestation) may need to assess their local experience with RSV morbidity and hospitalizations in order to determine the optimal use of these products. RSV immunoprophylaxis should be initiated immediately prior to the RSV season, continued monthly during the RSV season, and terminated at the end. Individual practitioners should contact their health departments or diagnostic virology laboratories to determine the optimal time to initiate prophylaxis. In general, the ease of intramuscular administration and reduced concern for transmission for blood-borne pathogens makes palivizumab the preferred RSV passive immunoprophylaxis. In addition, RSV-IGIV administration requires a deferral of the live measles-mumps-rubella (MMR) and varicella vaccines for 9 months. However, because of the polyclonal nature of RSV-IGIV, it provided benefits not available from the use of a monoclonal product. Specifically, hospitalizations for non-RSV

TABLE 13-60

RECOMMENDATIONS FOR CHEMOTHERAPY OF VIRAL RESPIRATORY INFECTIONS

VIRUS	CLINICAL SITUATION	AGENT OF CHOICE	ALTERNATIVE
Respiratory Syncytial Virus	Treatment	Ribavirin 6 g/d, aerosol, either continuous aerosol of 20 mg/mL solution or intermittent aerosols of 60 mg/mL given tid over 2 h	Treatment with ribavirin is controversial
	Prophylaxis	Palivizumab 15 mg/kg, IM, once a month Duration: RSV season	RSV-IGIV 750 mg/kg, IV, once a month Duration: RSV season
Parainfluenza Virus	Treatment	None	Ribavirin (as above)
	Prophylaxis	None	None
Influenza A	Treatment	Rimantadine[a,b,c] 5 mg/kg/d, PO, every day Adult maximum: 200 mg Duration: 5–7 days	Amantadine[a,c] 5 mg/kg/d, PO, every day Adult maximum: 200 mg Duration: 5–7 days Zanamivir[d] 10 mg, oral inhalation, twice daily (aerosol solution containing 10 mg of zanamivir can be used for children 3 months to 5 years of age) Duration: 5 days
	Prophylaxis	Rimantadine[a,c] 5 mg/kg/d, PO, every day Adult maximum: 100–200 mg Duration: influenza season	Amantadine[a,c] 5 mg/kg/d, PO, every day Adult maximum: 100–200 mg Zanamivir[d] 10 mg oral inhalation, once daily Duration: influenza season
Influenza B	Treatment	None	Ribavirin (as above)
	Prophylaxis	None	None
Influenza C	Treatment	None	None
	Prophylaxis	None	None
Adenovirus	Treatment	None	Ribavirin[e]
	Prophylaxis	None	None

[a] Neither rimantadine nor amantadine is approved for children younger than 1 year of age.

[b] Rimantadine is FDA-approved for prophylaxis but not for treatment of children. However, adult data support equal efficacy of rimantadine and amantadine for treating influenza A infections. Fewer adverse events with rimantadine make it the preferable medication.

[c] Amantadine and rimantadine (following hepatic metabolism) are excreted through the kidneys. Reduced doses are required for children with significant renal impairment.

[d] Zanamivir has been approved for administration to adults and children ages 12 years and older.

[e] Anecdotal reports have suggested benefit of ribavirin administered by aerosol or intravenously to patients with severe adenovirus infections. However, similar numbers of reports have failed to show any benefit of ribavirin for treatment of adenovirus infections.

RSV-IGIV = respiratory syncytial virus immune globulin intravenous.

respiratory infections and otitis media were decreased in RSV-IGIV recipients and not those receiving palivizumab. RSV-IGIV should not be administered to children with cyanotic congenital heart disease. The safety of palivizumab in children with cyanotic congenital heart disease is not established.

PARAINFLUENZA VIRUSES

Parainfluenza viruses are common causes of acute respiratory infections in young children. Croup is the most important and epidemiologically distinctive clinical syndrome of lower respiratory disease caused by these agents. Bronchiolitis and pneumonia also occur. The initial infection usually occurs in the first few years of life; reinfections are common.

The human parainfluenza viruses are members of the Paramyxoviridae family in the genus *Paramyxovirus;* certain human viruses resemble antigenically and morphologically animal paramyxoviruses (eg, human parainfluenza virus type 1 and murine Sendai virus). The parainfluenza viruses are large (150–200 nm) enveloped viruses that contain single-stranded RNA. The nucleocapsid exhibits helical symmetry, and the viral envelope is covered with spike-like projections. These spikes contain two viral glycopeptides; the larger of these contains both the viral hemagglutinin and neuraminidase activities, whereas the smaller is responsible for hemolytic and cell-fusion properties. The virus matures by budding from the membrane of infected cells.

The human parainfluenza viruses include four serotypes (1 to 4). Each of these serotypes has a type-specific hemagglutinin (HA) antigen and a type-specific CF antigen. The former antigens are associated with the viral envelope and the latter with the nucleocapsid. There is no antigen common to all the human parainfluenza viruses, but reinfection with one parainfluenza virus serotype can lead to heterotypic serologic responses to the other types.

EPIDEMIOLOGY AND PATHOGENESIS Parainfluenza virus serotypes 1, 2, and 3 have the most important clinical effect, especially serotypes 1 and 3. Parainfluenza virus type 1 causes large outbreaks of croup, which occur in the fall months in temperate climates, frequently in alternate years. Parainfluenza virus type 2 produces smaller epidemics of croup, also in the fall months, and commonly in years when type 1 infections are not prevalent. Serotypes 1 and 2 can cause bronchiolitis and pneumonia, but not as routinely as serotype 3. Parainfluenza virus type 3 infections are usually endemic, occurring throughout the year; however, epidemics of type 3 infection also occur, most often during the fall or spring months. Parainfluenza type 3 is croup-associated, but also produces bronchiolitis and pneumonia regularly. Parainfluenza virus type 4 is widely distributed and appears to produce predominantly upper respiratory disease; its epidemiology has not been characterized as thoroughly. The incidence of croup caused by parainfluenza virus type 1 is highest in children between 6 months and 3 years of age; males are affected with croup twice as often as females. Parainfluenza virus type 1 infections may occur in the first 6 months of life, but fewer than 10% of children with croup during parainfluenza virus type 1 epidemics are younger than 6 months old, suggesting partial protection from parainfluenza virus type 1 illness by maternal antibody. When croup occurs during the first 6 months of life, an underlying airway malformation should be suspected. Parainfluenza virus type 2 epidemiology appears to be similar to that of parainfluenza type 1; however, outbreaks of croup caused by parainfluenza virus type 2 are usually less severe than those caused by parainfluenza virus type 1. Significant parainfluenza virus type 3 disease is usually limited to children under the age of 5 years. This virus is similar to RSV in that severe illness is frequently observed during the first 6 months of life, with little evidence of protection afforded by passively acquired maternal antibody. Parainfluenza virus type 3 is the second most important cause of bronchiolitis severe enough to warrant hospitalization. This virus has a high propensity to cause persistent, progressive infections in the severely immunocompromised infant host.

As with RSV, initial viral replication is in the upper respiratory tract. Subsequently, there is spread to the lower tract, where viral proliferation within airway epithelium results in cell degeneration and subsequent inflammation. Immunity to infection with parainfluenza viruses is at best incomplete. Adult volunteers with serum antibody, presumably acquired via natural infection, can readily be infected and produce URI symptoms. Available data indicate that, as with other respiratory viruses, local rather than systemic humoral immunity provides the most important defense against reinfection. Studies of hospital epidemics indicate a high attack rate and implicate shedding of virus before the appearance of symptoms.

CLINICAL MANIFESTATIONS   The clinical presentation of a child with parainfluenza virus-induced croup begins with a URI of several days' duration, followed by hoarseness and a "barking seal" croupy cough. Inspiratory stridor and marked retractions are evident in more severe infections. In most patients the temperature is elevated, frequently 38°C (100.4°F) to 40°C (104°F). While less important today than previously, it is still relevant in evaluating children with the croup syndrome to distinguish those with viral disease from those who have epiglottitis, usually caused by *Haemophilus influenzae* type b. Typically, children with epiglottitis present with the abrupt onset of high fever, sore throat, drooling, and stridor that progresses to severe airway obstruction in less than 24 hours. In contrast, children with viral croup have usually been ill for 2 to 3 days with URI symptoms progressing gradually to hoarseness, croupy cough, and inspiratory stridor. The clinical history and its tempo, and the degree of airway obstruction, provide

the most important information to the clinician attempting to differentiate between viral croup and epiglottitis. Diphtheria and bacterial tracheitis are also in the differential diagnosis of parainfluenza virus croup.

Most children with viral croup recover after 48 to 72 hours, but some children progress to severe airway obstruction; provision of an artificial airway is required in a small number of these children. When croup occurs in children younger than 6 months of age, underlying anatomic pathology of the glottis or upper trachea should be suspected. Similarly, when croup is prolonged or recurrent, anatomic contributing factors should be considered. However, recurrent "spasmodic" croup can occur in children with normal airway anatomy. The bronchiolitis and pneumonia syndromes produced by parainfluenza viruses are clinically indistinguishable from those produced by RSV.

DIAGNOSIS AND TREATMENT   Parainfluenza viruses may be cultured from nasopharyngeal secretions. These viruses are labile, and care must be taken in transporting and in rapid planting of specimens. Monkey kidney cell cultures sustain the growth of these viruses. Rapid viral diagnosis is achieved by immunofluorescent staining or EIA of nasopharyngeal aspirates with the appropriate antibody. However, the sensitivity of these methods is quite variable. PCR-based assays for detection of type-specific parainfluenza RNA should be more useful after they are available commercially. Retrospective serologic diagnosis can also be achieved by examining paired sera by hemagglutination-inhibition, neutralization, and complement-fixation techniques. Cross-reactivity among parainfluenza viruses, as well as with mumps virus, can make it difficult to diagnose infections with specific types serologically.

Treatment of parainfluenza infections of the respiratory tract is supportive, but there are special considerations for croup. These are discussed in Sec. 15.4.5. Ribavirin is effective against parainfluenza virus in vitro, but its role in clinical therapy has not been assessed systematically. Reports suggest efficacy of ribavirin in children with severe immunodeficiency and progressive parainfluenza type 3 infection, but the drug is not FDA-approved for this indication. No vaccines are available to prevent parainfluenza virus infections, although candidate attenuated virus vaccines are being developed. A passive immunoprophylaxis monoclonal antibody, similar to that used to prevent RSV, is in development.

INFLUENZA VIRUSES

Influenza is an acute, typically febrile, respiratory illness that occurs in outbreaks of varying severity, usually during winter months. During pandemics of influenza A virus infections, however, outbreaks may begin as early as late September. Influenza infection produces an illness characterized by both systemic and respiratory symptoms. This infection is often not emphasized in discussions of pediatric respiratory disease, although influenza viruses are responsible for considerable morbidity and school absences in the pediatric population. During large-scale influenza A outbreaks, rates of hospitalization for lower respiratory tract disease increase for infants and children. This is also one cause of outbreaks of unexplained fever in infants less than 2 to 3 months of age.

The influenza viruses are members of the Orthomyxoviridae family in the genus *Influenzavirus*. The type A influenza viruses are widely distributed in the animal kingdom (equine and swine viruses) and are particularly prevalent among birds. The influenza virion consists of an outer lipoprotein envelope surrounding central nucleocapsid material. The diameter of the virion is about 100 to 120 nm. The envelope is uniformly studded with spike-like projections that protrude from the viral membrane on its outer surface. The spikes are of two varieties: viral hemagglutinin (HA) and neuraminidase (NA). The inner surface of the envelope consists of the nonglycosylated viral membrane protein (M). The core ribonucleoprotein (RNP) encompasses a single-stranded RNA genome that is segmented. Each of the eight RNA fragments codes for one of eight viral polypeptides. The segmented nature of the influenza genome allows for exchange of RNA segments when two different influenza virions infect the same cell (genetic recombination). This property has great significance for the epidemiology of and control of pandemic influenza.

The sometimes confusing taxonomy of the influenza viruses is best understood in relationship to the viral polypeptides. Classification of the influenza viruses as types A, B, and C is based on the antigenic properties of the internal RNP and M proteins. In addition to type-specific antigens, influenza viruses also possess strain-specific antigens that reside in the HA and NA moieties. A standard nomenclature has been devised to classify strains of influenza A viruses according to the antigenic characteristics of their HA and NA molecules (eg, H1N1 or H3N2). Humoral immunity is conferred by strain-specific antibodies directed at the HA and NA antigens, whereas type-specific antibodies do not neutralize viral infectivity. The degree of antigenic variation among influenza B viruses is less than among type A viruses. Influenza C is biochemically distinct from both type A and B.

EPIDEMIOLOGY Winter epidemics of influenza A occur an average of 2 of every 3 years, with minor antigenic changes in the viral surface antigens of prevalent strains occurring every 1 to 2 years ("antigenic drift"). At varying intervals, major changes in the surface antigens occur ("antigenic shift"). These events, which have occurred three times during the 20th century, occur when radical alterations of the HA and/or NA antigens occur, rendering antibody to previously circulating influenza A viruses unprotective. Worldwide pandemics associated with considerable excess mortality then ensue. The antigenic alteration in influenza is an expression of genetic alteration of the viral RNA. Because the influenza RNA is broken into segments, genetic material can be exchanged when two different influenza virions infect a single cell. It is likely that the process of antigenic shift is explained by the exchange of whole RNA segments between human influenza viruses and certain animal influenza viruses. Completely novel strains capable of causing pandemics in human beings would thus be produced. Antigenic drift is manifest by both influenza A and B viruses, but antigenic shift has only been observed for influenza A.

PATHOGENESIS Influenza infection is initiated by virus inoculation in the upper or lower airways. These infections can be transmitted by the hand-to-nose route, by droplets of infectious respiratory secretions, or by small droplet aerosol. As with other respiratory viral infections, the course is determined, in part, by the presence or absence of virus-specific serum IgG and secretory IgA antibody. Antibody to the HA of the virus is apparently most important in resistance to infection, but antibody to the NA also has a contributory role. Cellular immune responses are important in terminating established infection. Respiratory mucus contains certain glycopeptides that inhibit virus attachment to the cells of the respiratory mucosa. However, these glycopeptides can be inactivated by viral NA if this enzyme is not neutralized by specific an-

tibody of the host. Virus uninhibited by antibody or mucus glycoconjugates attaches to the respiratory epithelium by interaction of the HA molecule with cell-membrane receptors. In successful infection, virus begins to replicate in the respiratory epithelium; it is then shed into the respiratory secretions, and local spread ensues. The eventual result is death of respiratory epithelial cells with desquamation. The entire airway from pharynx to alveoli may be involved. Viral infection of the alveolar epithelium can result in a diffuse pneumonia that can be life-threatening.

Viral infection remains, for practical purposes, limited to the respiratory tract; viremia is extremely rare. It is likely that inflammatory mediators synthesized and secreted by cells within the respiratory tract are responsible for the familiar systemic manifestations of the disease, but our understanding of the pathophysiology of these responses is rudimentary. Damage to the respiratory epithelium induced by influenza virus impairs mucociliary clearance of bacteria from the lower respiratory tract; neutrophil function is also impaired during influenza virus infections. These factors are probably responsible for the increased risk of bacterial superinfection observed with influenza infections.

CLINICAL MANIFESTATIONS The incubation period of influenza virus is short, generally 1 to 3 days. The most dramatic symptoms are sudden fever, chills, headache, myalgia, and prostration. Respiratory symptoms can be minimal for the first 24 hours of illness. Later, varying degrees of rhinitis and lower respiratory symptoms appear. The average duration of fever is 3 days, but occasionally fever may persist for as long as 6 days in the absence of complications. Fever reaches 39°C (102.2°F) to 40°C (104°F), routinely. There may be signs of pharyngeal and conjunctival infection, but examination of the lungs is generally negative, and positive chest radiographs are the exception. Tracheobronchitis is the most common syndrome of influenza virus LRI, but severe croup can occur during influenza A infections.

Most patients have no complications and recover after a few days. In pandemic years, however, severe illness is more likely. Three patterns of pneumonia are seen with influenza A or B virus infections: viral bronchopneumonia, secondary bacterial pneumonia, and diffuse viral hemorrhagic alveolitis. When bacterial pneumonia complicates influenza, it usually occurs after 5 to 7 days of illness; influenzal viral pneumonia typically has its onset between days 3 and 5 of illness. Although diffuse primary influenza virus pneumonia is rare, it is frequently life-threatening. Diffuse, bilateral pneumonia with a radiographic appearance suggestive of pulmonary edema or adult respiratory distress syndrome is strongly suggestive of primary hemorrhagic viral pneumonia, but may occur with overwhelming bacterial infection. Symptoms of influenza viral pneumonia include severe dyspnea, cyanosis, and the production of small amounts of bloody sputum. The clinical picture and course of hemorrhagic alveolitis due to influenza virus is analogous to the adult respiratory distress syndrome. Bacterial pneumonias in patients with influenza are caused most commonly by *Streptococcus pneumoniae* and *Staphylococcus aureus*, with *Haemophilus influenzae* and *Moraxella catarrhalis* having lesser roles. Bacterial tracheitis can also complicate influenza virus infections and may also be life-threatening. Signs of airway obstruction suggestive of croup constitute the characteristic presentation of bacterial tracheitis.

Reye syndrome has developed following infection with influenza type A and type B, usually in association with the therapeutic use of aspirin. The risk of Reye syndrome is higher with influenza B than with influenza A infections. Rarely, myocarditis has been associated with influenza A infection. Viral myositis, usually of the calves is also observed, more frequently in children with influenza B infections.

DIAGNOSIS The most satisfactory means of diagnosis is isolation of the virus. Respiratory secretions obtained by throat swab or by nasal lavage are inoculated into monkey or canine kidney cell cultures or embryonated eggs. Virus growth can be detected after 2 to 6 days by hemadsorption, hemagglutination, or on occasion by evidence of cell destruction. Specimens for viral isolation will have a higher yield when obtained in the first 72 hours of clinical illness. After that, the quantity of virus shed decreases rapidly. Rapid diagnosis may be achieved by immunofluorescent examination of exfoliated respiratory epithelial cells obtained from nasal secretions or by EIA-based viral antigen-detection assays. These rapid antigen detection techniques are generally less sensitive than viral culture and are also more likely to be successful when performed early in the course of illness. PCR-based assays for influenza RNA appear promising as a means of enhancing rapid diagnosis, as well as typing and subtyping influenza viruses.

TREATMENT In general, influenza infection in children is a self-limited condition. Supportive care directed at the major complaints of patients is usually adequate. Antipyretics other than aspirin are recommended to reduce fever and the discomfort associated with this acute febrile illness. Salicylates should not be used to treat influenza-related symptoms in children or adolescents because of the increased risk of Reye syndrome. Bed rest and maintenance of adequate fluid intake may also provide comfort.

Antiviral therapies are discussed in Sec. 13.1.2 and use in specific respiratory infections is outlined in Table 13-60. Rimantadine and amantadine are valuable for the treatment and prevention of influenza A. These medications are not yet approved for children younger than 1 year of age. Because the efficacy of rimantadine and amantadine is greatest when given within 48 hours of the onset of symptoms, they should be considered for any child who has an influenza-like illness during the time period when influenza A is known to be circulating within the community. Clinical benefit associated with amantadine or rimantadine therapy is greater for (a) children with underlying conditions that increase their likelihood for severe or complicated influenza A illness, and (b) children with severe influenza A illness. Therapy in immunocompetent children should be 2 to 5 days. Longer durations of therapy may be indicated for immunocompromised children. Epidemic strains are usually rimantadine/amantadine-sensitive. However, rimantadine/amantadine-resistant strains have been identified. These strains usually have a single amino acid change in their influenza A M2 protein. Cross-resistance (amantadine and rimantadine) is expected. Emergence of rimantadine or amantadine resistance during therapy does not appear to slow recovery, nor is it associated with an increase in viral shedding in the immunocompetent child. However, acquisition or selection of resistant virus in the immunocompromised child can result in prolonged excretion. Resistant virus can be transmitted to other susceptible individuals. Clinical response and prophylactic efficacy of antiviral therapy is reduced following transmission of rimantadine/amantadine-resistant virus.

Administration of rimantadine or amantadine for treatment of a household contact of a child at high risk for influenza morbidity might result in transmission of resistant virus to the high-risk child. For that reason, prophylaxis of the high-risk child and other household contacts without treatment of the index case is preferable in this setting to spare the child at high risk from developing influenza A morbidity.

Zanamivir and oseltamir are two neuraminidase inhibitors that are effective for both the treatment and prevention of influenza A and influenza B illness. Zanamivir is administered by an oral inhalation administration device at a dose of 10 mg twice daily in adults and children who were 5 years of age or older. For children younger than 5 years of age, 10 mg of zanamivir in solution administered by nebulizer has resulted in similar pharmacokinetic data as seen in adults. Oseltamir has been given orally to adults in doses of 75 or 150 mg twice daily for 5 days. Pediatric safety, pharmacokinetic, and efficacy data for oseltamir are not yet available. Both zanamivir and oseltamir offer greater benefit when started early (within 36 hours after onset of symptoms). Resistance to neuraminidase inhibitors can occur but is uncommon at the present time.

Both influenza A and B viruses are sensitive in vitro to ribavirin. Preliminary data in young adults with natural influenza A and B infection show modest improvements in influenza illness following therapy with ribavirin administered by aerosol. For most episodes of influenza infection in children, this approach is too costly and inconvenient. However, it might be a consideration for healthy or immunocompromised children who develop severe lower respiratory tract disease as a consequence of influenza A or B viruses. Ribavirin is not FDA-approved for the treatment of influenza infections in children or adults.

PROPHYLAXIS Immunoprophylaxis with an inactivated influenza vaccine and chemoprophylaxis using amantadine, rimantadine, and zanamivir are available measures that are effective in reducing the number of influenza virus infections and in reducing the impact of influenza disease. Since the late 1940s, the vaccination of persons at high risk each year prior to the onset of influenza season has been the most effective approach for reducing the impact of influenza. Efficacy rates associated with administration of the inactivated vaccine have ranged between 67 and 92% for reduction of influenza disease. The efficacy rates are highest when the vaccine strains and circulating strains are closely related. Currently, immunization strategies encourage the use of the influenza vaccine in persons who are most likely to experience complications following influenza or in those individuals who are at increased risk for exposure to influenza virus.

Each year, the Public Health Service Advisory Committee on Immunization Practices (ACIP) makes recommendations concerning the composition of the influenza vaccine for the next influenza season. The vaccine generally contains three virus strains (usually two type A and one type B) representing influenza viruses that are likely to circulate in the United States during the next winter. Guidelines for vaccine administration are provided in Table 13-61. The inactivated influenza vaccine is made from highly purified, egg-grown viruses that have been made noninfectious. Currently, there are three distinct preparations of the inactivated influenza vaccine: whole-virus, subvirion, and purified-surface-antigen preparations. Systemic or febrile reactions are rare with any of these antigen preparations. However, children are more likely to experience febrile reactions following influenza immunization; thus, children should receive only the subvirion or purified-surface-antigen preparations.

The duration of protection from the inactivated influenza vaccine is brief, likely less than 1 year. For children with little prior experience with influenza (<9 years of age), two doses of the influenza vaccine should be administered 1 month apart for their initial immunization in order to ensure a satisfactory antibody re-

TABLE 13-61

INFLUENZA VACCINE SCHEDULE FOR CHILDREN IN THE UNITED STATES[†]

AGE	PRODUCT	DOSE	ROUTE	NUMBER OF DOSES	
				NO PRIOR INFLUENZA VACCINE	PRIOR INFLUENZA VACCINE
6–35 mo	Subvirion or purified surface antigen (split virus)	0.25 mL	IM	2[*]	1
3–8 yr	Subvirion or purified surface antigen (split virus)	0.5 mL	IM	2[*]	1
9–12 yr	Subvirion or purified surface antigen (split virus)	0.5 mL	IM	1	1
>12 yr	Whole virus, subvirion, or purified surface antigen	0.5 mL	IM	1	1

*These two doses should be given at least 4 weeks apart.
[†]Influenza vaccines should not be administered to children with known anaphylactic hypersensitivity to eggs or any other component of the influenza vaccine.

sponse. Efficacy of current vaccines is not established in children younger than 6 months of age. Patients who have chronic diseases or immune deficiencies may develop lower postvaccination antibody titers. Some of these individuals may remain susceptible to influenza-related respiratory infections despite receiving an appropriate influenza vaccine. These patients are still candidates for influenza vaccination because their immune response to the vaccine may be adequate to prevent a more serious complication associated with lower respiratory tract involvement.

In the United States, the influenza vaccine is strongly recommended for any person ≥6 months of age who is at risk for complications of influenza or who has a high likelihood of transmitting influenza to individuals who are at high risk for complications of influenza. Children who have been identified to be at an increased risk for influenza-related complications include: (a) residents of chronic care facilities that house children with chronic medical conditions; (b) children with chronic disorders of the pulmonary or cardiovascular system including asthma; and (c) children who have required regular medical follow-up or hospitalization during the preceding year because of chronic metabolic diseases (including diabetes mellitus), renal dysfunction, hemoglobinopathies, or immunosuppression (including immunosuppression caused by medications). Influenza vaccine may be administered to any child whose parents wish to reduce the chance that their child may become infected with the influenza. Physicians, nurses, and other healthcare professionals in both hospital and outpatient care settings, employees of nursing homes and chronic care facilities, providers of homecare to persons at risk, and household members of persons in high-risk groups should be immunized yearly to reduce influenza transmission to individuals at high risk for influenza-related complications. Despite a paucity of definitive studies, influenza vaccination is considered safe during any stage of pregnancy.

Fever is the most common reaction following administration of the inactivated influenza vaccine. It typically occurs 6 to 24 hours following administration. It is more common in younger children (less than 24 months of age) and much less common following a split-virus (subvirion or purified surface antigen) vaccine. Local reactions at the inoculation site are unusual in children, but they may occur in up to 10% of adolescents following either whole- or split-virus vaccine. Currently available inactivated vaccines should not be administered to children with known anaphylactic hypersensitivity to eggs or to any other component of the influenza vaccine. Use of chemoprophylaxis with an antiviral agent (ie, amantadine or rimantadine) is a safer option for prevention of influenza A in such

children. Minor illnesses with or without fever are not contraindications to the administration of the inactivated influenza vaccine.

Rimantadine, amantadine, and zanamivir have successfully reduced influenza A infection and disease when administered prophylactically to adults or children before and during the epidemic period. These drugs have had efficacy rates of 70 to 90% in preventing illness caused by naturally occurring strains of influenza A. Only zanamivir is effective against influenza B virus.

Chemoprophylaxis may be beneficial for specific groups of children. However, chemoprophylaxis should not be considered a substitute for influenza vaccination. Children at high risk for influenza-related complications may receive chemoprophylaxis if they have not been vaccinated at the onset of an outbreak of influenza in their community. They should still receive the vaccine after the outbreak. However, the development of antibodies to the vaccine may take as long as 2 weeks after adequate immunization. This would mean that a child younger than 9 years of age who is receiving his or her first influenza vaccine may need prophylaxis for as long as 6 weeks (ie, prophylaxis for 2 weeks after the second dose of the vaccine has been received). Amantadine, rimantadine, and zanamivir do not interfere with the antibody response to the inactivated influenza vaccine. Children whose immune deficiency makes it likely that they will have an inadequate antibody response to influenza vaccine could receive chemoprophylaxis to enhance the effort to protect them from influenza-related illness. HIV-infected children and other children with immunodeficiencies are candidates for combined immuno- and chemoprophylaxis. Children who cannot be given the inactivated influenza vaccine because of a severe anaphylactic hypersensitivity to egg protein or other vaccine components may receive chemoprophylaxis throughout the influenza season. For those children for whom chemoprophylaxis is deemed appropriate, it should be instituted at the onset of the influenza virus outbreak and continued throughout the entire influenza season. In most locations, this is approximately a 6-week period.

The development of a live, mucosally administered influenza vaccine has been accomplished by cold adaptation. The cold-adapted vaccine is minimally reactigenic, with mild respiratory symptoms occurring in some recipients and with fever only rarely. Transmission of vaccine-strain virus to serosusceptible contacts of vaccine recipients has not yet been identified. Nasal secretory and serum antibodies are produced following immunization. While the serum antibody levels following vaccination with the cold-adapted strain are not uniformly as high as those produced for the inactivated vaccine, protection against experimentally induced infection and illness appears to be better in the recipients of the cold-adapted strain. A reversion from cold-adapted vaccine to wild-type virus does not appear to be a problem. Studies in children suggest that the cold-adapted vaccines may be more effective than inactivated vaccine, particularly in very young children.

Nosocomial influenza infection may be a serious concern within facilities caring for children. Transmission of influenza to children at risk for influenza-related complication can occur from contact with infected patients, infected health-care workers, and infected family members. Staff members who develop influenza illness should be required to stay home from work. Visitors, including family members with any illness consistent with influenza virus infection, should avoid or minimize contacts with patients at high risk for influenza complications. A hospital-wide visitation restriction may be necessary in certain circumstances if influenza virus activity in the community is extremely high. Any visitor who has a febrile respiratory illness should be restricted from visiting. Children identified as having an illness consistent with influenza, regardless of laboratory test results, should be isolated in single rooms or cohorted. Precautions should include droplet isolation. Hand washing is essential. Respiratory secretions should be considered infectious material. Gowns and gloves should be used when touching infected material or if soiling is likely. Because small-droplet aerosols are responsible for transmission, masks or face shields should be utilized when within 3 feet of a patient to reduce the likelihood of acquisition of influenza infection by health-care workers or by visitors. Special air handling is not required because the droplets do not remain suspended in the air. During an influenza outbreak, it may be prudent to postpone elective surgery, particularly for patients who have any symptoms of an influenza-like illness (community acquired or nosocomially acquired).

ADENOVIRUSES

The adenoviruses cause infections of the respiratory tract with the production of acute respiratory disease. Latent infections in the tonsils and adenoids are frequently established; thus recurrent shedding of adenoviruses in upper respiratory secretions of children may occur. Recurrent viral shedding is usually asymptomatic. The viruses are nonenveloped DNA viruses that are icosahedral in shape and measure 70 to 80 nm in diameter. The adenoviruses are members of the Adenoviridae family in the genus *Mastadenovirus* and can be divided into seven subgroups on the basis of the molecular characterization of their DNA. There are 41 recognized human adenovirus serotypes.

The adenoviruses account for 5 to 10% of respiratory illnesses in children, although the infection rates vary considerably. Care must be taken in associating the isolation of adenoviruses with disease entities, because recurrent excretion of the virus by children with latent infection occurs. Most children are infected with serotypes 1, 2, and 5 during the years of early childhood. Serotypes 3, 6, 7, and 21 are less frequent but important causes of respiratory infection during childhood.

CLINICAL MANIFESTATIONS

Respiratory Illness   Infants most commonly manifest upper respiratory disease symptoms: coryza, conjunctivitis, otitis media, and pharyngitis. Bronchiolitis, pneumonia, or both occur in a small percentage of children with infections caused by adenovirus serotypes 1, 2, and 5; these infections are not usually severe and are typically indistinguishable from bronchiolitis caused by RSV. In contrast, adenovirus serotypes 3, 7, and 21 may cause fulminant, progressive bronchiolitis and pneumonia, with significant long-term pulmonary sequelae (including bronchiolitis obliterans) occurring in a substantial proportion of survivors. Some children with severe adenovirus pneumonia have disseminated disease with exanthem, meningoencephalitis, hepatitis, and rhabdomyolysis. Adenovirus infection should be considered in any progressive pneumonia in infants and toddlers for which the etiology is unclear. Other adenovirus serotypes may also be associated with destructive pulmonary disease, but much less commonly. Adenoviruses have also been recovered from children with a clinical picture indistinguishable from pertussis.

Pharyngoconjunctival Fever   This syndrome, often caused by adenovirus type 3, presents after a short (3–5 days) incubation period with fever, pharyngitis, rhinitis, and cervical adenitis; conjunctivitis forms an important part of the syndrome. This syndrome is apt to occur in small epidemics in summer camps and is probably transmitted during swimming.

Epidemic Keratoconjunctivitis   This form of adenovirus infection produces corneal involvement as well as conjunctivitis and enlargement of preauricular nodes. Adenovirus serotypes 8, 19, and 37 are important causes of this syndrome.

Extrarespiratory Manifestations   The enteric adenoviruses, serotypes 40 and 41, are important causes of infant diarrhea. These agents can be identified in stool specimens by immune electron microscopy or ELISA. Adenoviruses (not necessarily the enteric serotypes) have been recovered from mesenteric lymph nodes of children with intussusception, suggesting a role for these viruses in the pathogenesis of some intussusception. Adenovirus types 11 and 21 are associated with acute hemorrhagic cystitis, producing hematuria from several days to 2 weeks' duration. Additionally, neurologic disease, principally meningoencephalitis, is attributed to adenovirus infection, and these viruses are implicated in infections of immunocompromised patients, including patients with AIDS.

DIAGNOSIS AND TREATMENT   Respiratory adenoviruses can be isolated from pharyngeal secretions, eye swabs, and feces. Primary cell lines (human embryonic kidney and lung), finite cell lines (WI-38 and MRC-5), and continuous cell lines (293, A549, and HEp-2) are all capable of supporting adenovirus replication and may be used for adenovirus detection. Using standard culture techniques, adenovirus detection by identifying characteristic cytopathic effect (CPE) may take 5 to 20 days following inoculation. Centrifugation and shell-vial culture methods yield results similar to standard culture within 5 days of inoculation. Because virus excretion from the pharynx may persist for weeks to months following adenovirus infection, the diagnostic significance of adenovirus isolation is not as strong as it is with many of the other respiratory viruses. Also, isolation of adenovirus from the pharynx is more suggestive of recent infection than is a fecal adenovirus isolate.

Rapid adenovirus antigen detection using EIA or immunofluorescence is possible, but sensitivity varies considerably with the different adenovirus serotypes and the site of infection. Multiple serologic assays are available. Complement fixation or EIA tests that detect antibodies to the common adenovirus antigen (hexon) can be used to detect recent infection by comparing paired acute and convalescent sera.

Treatment is symptomatic; there is no effective antiviral agent at this time. High doses of intravenous immunoglobulin or ribavirin (aerosol or intravenous) have been administered to children with acute, severe adenovirus pneumonia, but the efficacy of these interventions is not established. An effective, live, enteric-coated oral vaccine is available against infections caused by serotypes 4, 7, and 21. This vaccine is used routinely in military recruits, but has not been employed in civilian populations of adults or children.

RHINOVIRUSES

Rhinoviruses are small (20–30 nm), nonenveloped, icosahedral, RNA viruses. They are grouped with the enteroviruses, hepatitis A viruses, and cardioviruses to form the Picornaviridae family. They are distinguished from the enteroviruses by their acid lability. Most replicate optimally at 34°C (93.2°F) to 35°C (95°F), the temperature of the mucosa of the upper respiratory tract, and have reduced ability to replicate at or above 37°C (98.6°F). Their acid lability precludes gastrointestinal invasion. There are roughly 100 different human rhinovirus serotypes.

The association of rhinoviruses with the common cold is well known; the incidence of rhinovirus infection is greatest during the fall months. Rhinoviruses are important causes of the common cold in persons of all ages; however, the proportion of colds attributable to rhinovirus infection is higher in adults than in children. Transmission occurs primarily by the hand-to-nose route and by large-droplet spread. Hand washing and avoidance of hand contact with respiratory secretions of affected individuals reduces viral transmission.

CLINICAL MANIFESTATIONS AND DIAGNOSIS   The clinical picture of rhinovirus disease includes coryza, cough, and sore throat, usually without fever. Rhinoviruses apparently have little tendency to cause pharyngeal exudates or cervical lymphadenopathy. Healthy children occasionally develop mild cough in association with rhinovirus infections, but significant lower respiratory illness in infants and toddlers is uncommon. Rhinovirus infections are, however, important causes of wheezing exacerbations in older preschool and school-age children with reactive airways disease. Because the clinical syndrome associated with rhinoviruses is usually mild and self-evident, diagnostic evaluations are rarely indicated. Viral isolation from nasal secretions can be accomplished using sensitive cell lines (eg, human fetal kidney fibroblasts, WI-38, MRC-5, HeLa). Because of the large number of antigenic types of rhinoviruses, serologic testing is impractical. PCR-based assays may be utilized in the future to detect rhinovirus infection.

TREATMENT AND PREVENTION   No specific antiviral treatment is currently available for rhinovirus infections. Over-the-counter cough and cold preparations do not provide significant benefit for children with the common cold. Nasal obstruction may improve following nasal sprays or drops with phenylephrine (0.25%) or oxymetazoline hydrochloride (0.05%). However, most young children do not tolerate nasal sprays or drops very well. Pleconaril is a new antiviral agent with in vitro activity against picornaviruses. Efficacy and cost-effectiveness in treating the common cold are not established. Pleconaril has not yet been approved by the FDA for any indications. Vitamins (ascorbic acid), minerals (zinc), and herbal remedies (*Echinacea*) are being used with an increasing frequency for the treatment and prevention of the common cold. Controlled trials assessing the efficacy of these agents are limited. However, it is possible that these or other similar products do reduce symptoms associated with the cold. Physicians caring for children need to be aware of the widespread use of these products. In addition, they must be aware that there are inadequate data on children concerning appropriate doses and safety of most of these products.

Because of the numerous serotypes capable of causing disease and because of the uncertainties concerning the long-term persistence of even naturally acquired type-specific immunity, the control of rhinovirus infection by means of vaccines must be considered a distant possibility.

CORONAVIRUSES

The coronaviruses are enveloped, pleomorphic, RNA-containing viruses that measure about 120 nm in diameter. The surface is marked by petal-like, narrow-based projections measuring 15 to 20 nm in length. Two strains are implicated most frequently in human respiratory disease. Identification of coronavirus infection occurs chiefly in research settings. The growth of coronaviruses in tissue culture is limited; the viruses were first recovered in human tracheal organ cultures.

Coronaviruses appear capable of causing the common cold. Perhaps 3 to 5% of such illnesses in human beings are attributable to these agents, particularly in the winter months. Coronavirus epidemics have occurred. The importance of these viruses as causes of lower respiratory disease is not well defined. Diagnostic assays for human coronavirus infections are not currently commercially available. Serologic studies are generally the most useful for diagnostic and epidemiologic purposes. Treatment is symptomatic as it is for rhinovirus infections.

References

General

Denny FW, Clyde WA Jr: Acute lower respiratory tract infections in non-hospitalized children. J Pediatr 180:635–646, 1986

Denny FW, Murphy TF, Clyde WA JR, et al: Croup: An 11-year study in a pediatric practice. Pediatrics 71:871–876, 1983

Glezen F, Denny FW: Epidemiology of acute lower respiratory disease in children. N Engl J Med 288:498–505, 1973

Henderson FW, Collier AM, Sanyal MA, et al: A longitudinal study of respiratory viruses and bacteria in the etiology of acute otitis media with effusion. N Engl J Med 306:1377–1383, 1982

McIntosh K, Ellis EF, Hoffman LS, et al: Association of viral and bacterial respiratory infections with exacerbations of wheezing in young asthmatic children. J Pediatr 82:578–590, 1973

Adenoviruses

Becroft DMO: Bronchiolitis obliterans, bronchiectasis, and other sequelae of adenovirus type 21 infection in young children. J Clin Pathol 24:72, 1971

Dagan R, Schwartz RH, Insel RA, et al: Severe diffuse adenovirus 7a pneumonia in a child with combined immunodeficiency: possible therapeutic effect of human immune serum globulin containing specific neutralizing antibody. Pediatr Infect Dis 3:246–251, 1984

Pacini DL, Collier AM, Henderson FW: Adenovirus infections and respiratory illnesses in children in group daycare. J Infect Dis 156:920–927, 1987

Respiratory Syncytial Virus

Church NR, Anas NG, Hall CB, et al: Respiratory syncytial virus related apnea in infants: demographics and outcome. Am J Dis Child 138:247–250, 1984

Committee on Infectious Diseases: Reassessment of the indications for ribavirin therapy in respiratory syncytial virus infections. Pediatrics 97:137–140, 1996

Committee on Infectious Diseases and Committee on Fetus and Newborn: Prevention of respiratory syncytial virus infections: indications for the use of palivizumab and update on the use of RSV-IGIV. Pediatrics 102:1211–1216, 1998

Groothuis JR, Simoes EA, Levin MJ, et al: Prophylactic administration of respiratory syncytial virus immune globulin to high-risk infants and young children. The Respiratory Syncytial Virus Immune Globulin Study Group. N Engl J Med 329:1524–1530, 1993

Hall CB, McBride JT, Walsh EE, et al: Aerosolized ribavirin treatment of infants with respiratory syncytial viral infections. N Engl J Med 308:1443–1447, 1983

Hall CB, Powell KR, Schnabel KC, et al: Risk of secondary bacterial infection in infants hospitalized with respiratory syncytial viral infection. J Pediatr 113:266–271, 1988

MacDonald NE, Hall CB, Suffin SC, et al: Respiratory syncytial virus infection in infants with congenital heart disease. N Engl J Med 307:397–400, 1982

Influenza Viruses

Edwards KM, King JC, Steinhoff MC, et al: Safety and immunogenicity of live attenuated cold-adapted influenza B/Ann Arbor/1/86 reassortment virus vaccine in infants and children. J Infect Dis 163:740–745, 1991

Glezen WP, Paredes A, Taber LH: Influenza in children related to other respiratory agents. JAMA 243:1345–1349, 1980

Hayden FG: Amantadine and rimantadine resistance in influenza A viruses. Curr Opin Infect Dis 7:674–677, 1994

Wilson SZ, Gilbert SE, Quarles JM, et al: Treatment of influenza A (H1N1) virus infection with ribavirin aerosol. Antimicrob Agents Chemother 26:200–203, 1984

Rhinovirus and Coronavirus Infections

Fox JP, Hall CE: The Seattle virus watch. V. Epidemiologic observations of rhinovirus infections in families with young children. Am J Epidemiol 101:122–143, 1975

Gwaltney JM, Moskalski PB, Hendley JO, et al: Hand-to-hand transmission of rhinovirus cold. Ann Intern Med 88:463–467, 1978

McIntosh K, Chao RK, Krause HE, et al: Coronavirus infection in acute lower respiratory tract disease of infants. J Infect Dis 130:502–507, 1974

13.4.20 Rubella

Maria Jevitz Patterson

Rubella (German measles) is an endemic and epidemic illness, worldwide in distribution, characterized by a generalized maculopapular rash and postauricular and suboccipital lymphadenopathy. Fever and constitutional complaints are typically mild, and complications uncommon. Rubella is a disease of major significance because of the high incidence of congenital defects in children whose mothers are infected during early pregnancy. Typical anomalies caused by this congenital infection, which are known collectively as the congenital rubella syndrome (CRS), include deafness, congenital heart diseases, cataracts, and retardation.

Rubella virus is a togavirus (genus *Rubivirus*) with a single-stranded RNA genome and a lipid envelope (toga) that was first isolated in 1962. It shares other physicochemical properties with group A arboviruses. The rubella virion is roughly spherical, 60 to 70 nm in diameter, with an electron-dense core covered by a double-layered loose envelope. The virus is thermolabile; inactivation is rapid at 37°C (98.6°F) and at room temperature. However, it can be stored for short periods at −20°C (−4°F) and is relatively stable for months at −60°C (−76°F).

Direct person-to-person airborne spread by infected droplets appears to be the usual mode of transmission because of the relative instability of the rubella virus. The patient with subclinical infection is also a source of rubella virus. Patients are most contagious for a few days before and after the onset of rash, although virus may be present in pharyngeal secretions for as long as 1 week before and 2 weeks after the onset of rash. Infection acquired postnatally does not produce a chronic carrier state. In contrast, congenital rubella is characterized by chronic infection; the infants may remain contagious for months after birth. Rubella has been a notifiable disease since 1966. Prompt reporting facilitates early detection and implementation of disease control. Clinical diagnosis is confirmed by laboratory testing after reporting.

Although rubella occurs in all areas of the world, variations in epidemiologic patterns have been described from country to country. Prior to widespread use of rubella vaccines in the United States, rubella occurred primarily in children during the elementary school years. A small minority did not become infected until early adulthood.

Rubella remains an endemic illness in the United States, with a seasonal peak in the late winter and spring. Its greatest impact resulted from epidemics that in the past occurred at 6-year intervals. Following licensure of the vaccine in 1969 until 1989, the reported incidence of rubella declined more than 99% in the United States. This was followed by a resurgence in 1989 to 1991, but reported incidence from 1992 to 1996 was the lowest ever recorded, with an all-time low of 128 cases reported in 1995, and possible interruption of rubella transmission in late 1996.

Outbreaks have been confined essentially to unimmunized populations, religious communities that traditionally decline vaccination, settings in which young adults congregate, and among specific racial/ethnic groups from countries where rubella vaccine is not routinely used. Many European and Central and South American countries have yet to achieve good rubella vaccination rates, and there are limited or absent efforts in other countries. A 1995 global WHO survey showed that only 78 of 214 countries had national policies for rubella vaccination.

POSTNATAL RUBELLA

CLINICAL MANIFESTATIONS The clinical manifestations of rubella range from inapparent infection to a characteristic pattern of adenopathy, rash, and low-grade fever. The incubation period is from 14 to 21 days. A typical clinical course begins with adenopathy involving primarily the postauricular, occipital, and posterior cervical nodes, which may be slightly painful and tender. Although symptoms usually clear promptly as the rash fades, the nodes may remain palpable for several weeks. Adolescents and adults may complain of malaise, headache, a low-grade fever, sore throat, and mild coryza during a 1- to 5-day prodromal period that frequently ac-

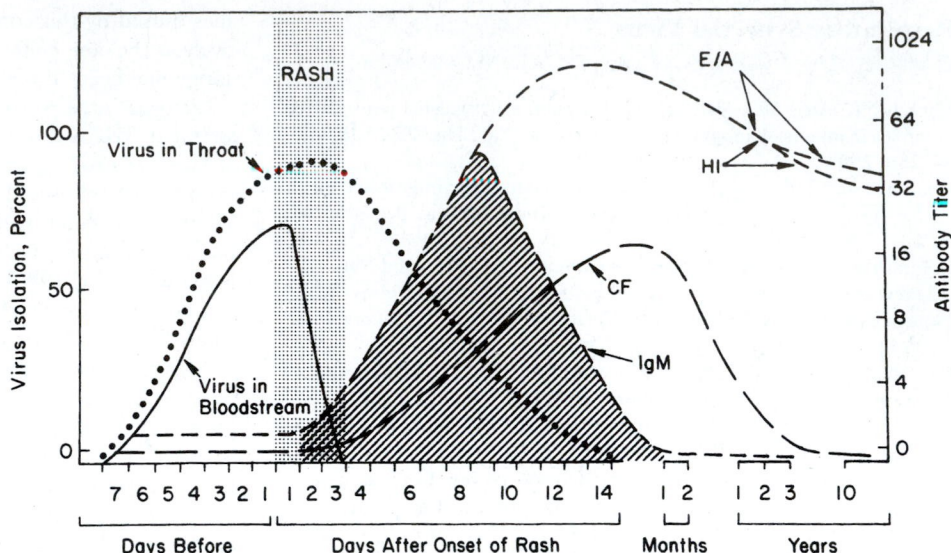

FIGURE 13-13 Schematic illustration of the natural history of rubella. SOURCE: *Adapted from Cooper LZ, Krugman S. Clinical manifestations of postnatal and congenital rubella. Arch Ophthalmol 77:434–439, 1967.* **Abbreviations: HI** = hemagglutination inhibition; **EIA** = enzyme immunoassay; **CF** = complement fixing antibodies.

companies the onset of adenopathy. In young children, the mild prodrome is usually overlooked.

The rubella rash is variable. It may be no more than a transient blush, but classically it persists for 2 to 3 days in a pattern that has been called kaleidoscopic because of its changing appearance. Initially, small irregular pink macules begin on the face and spread rapidly (usually within 24 hours) to the neck, trunk, arms, and ultimately the legs. By the next day these lesions may have coalesced, developed a maculopapular component, and become scarlatiniform. The face is frequently clearing by the time a full-blown rash is seen on the lower legs, where coalescence is uncommon. Desquamation is rare.

An enanthem consisting of punctate or slightly larger red spots on the soft palate may be present during the late prodrome and early rash phase. These lesions are not pathognomonic of rubella. Scarlet fever, infectious mononucleosis, measles, and other viral exanthems may be accompanied by similar palatal lesions.

Fever is uncommonly as high as 39°C (102.2°F) to 39.5°C (103.1°F), but may be absent in children. Polyarthralgia and polyarthritis are common manifestations of rubella among women, less common in men, and uncommon in children. Symptoms typically appear with the rash or within several days after its onset, but, rarely, they may precede the onset of rash by several days. Joint involvement, which is frequently symmetric, may range from subjective morning stiffness to full-blown arthritis characterized by swelling, redness, tenderness, and effusion. Objective signs and symptoms usually clear within several days to 2 weeks but, rarely, may persist several months. The proximal interphalangeal joints are affected most frequently, but other joints may be involved. Paresthesia, most typically numbness and tingling or "pins and needles," often accompanies, and may outlast, the joint symptoms. Joint manifestations in rubella produce no deformity. Joint symptoms are also associated with rubella vaccine, but after careful scrutiny, no causal relationship between the vaccine and persistent joint symptoms could be validated.

Postinfectious encephalitis, clinically indistinguishable from that following measles or varicella, is a rare complication of rubella that occurs less frequently than postmeasles encephalitis. Symptoms and signs of central nervous system involvement usually develop 2 to 4 days after the onset of rash. Many patients have slight decreases in platelet counts during the course of uncomplicated rubella. This thrombocytopenia usually occurs within 1 week after the onset of

rash. Presenting complaints usually include purpura, epistaxis, bleeding from the gums, hematuria, and gastrointestinal bleeding. Abnormal capillary fragility also contributes to the problem of hemostasis. Prognosis is generally excellent, but fatalities due to uncontrolled central nervous system hemorrhage do occur rarely. Most patients become symptom free within 2 weeks. The incidence of thrombocytopenia following vaccine is significantly less than after natural infection.

DIAGNOSIS Diagnosis of rubelliform rashes in acutely ill, febrile children and in young adults requires accurate historical information from parents: vaccine history, source of exposure, prodrome, progression of rash. Other childhood exanthems (human herpes virus-6, human herpes virus-7, adenovirus, enterovirus, parvovirus), as well as the possibility of primary vaccine failure, should be considered. Rubella can be diagnosed only by isolating the virus or by demonstrating rising titers of rubella antibody in the serum. Virus isolation is less practical because of relative lability of rubella virus and the complexity of the assay.

Rubella virus may be cultured from the pharynx and serum as early as 1 week before the onset of rash. Virus is promptly cleared from the serum after the rash appears, but persists in pharyngeal secretions, usually for several days after the rash and, uncommonly, for as long as 2 weeks (Fig. 13-13). Urine and stool are unreliable sources of rubella virus.

Rubella antibody may be measured in a variety of test systems based on neutralization, hemagglutination inhibition (HI), CF, latex agglutination, radial hemolysis, immunoblot, and IgM capture EIA. This wide array of reliable tests is important to provide rapid, sensitive, economical, and reliable diagnosis.

The patterns of rubella-specific IgM, HI, CF, and EIA responses during rubella are also illustrated in Fig. 13-13. Absence of rubella HI or EIA antibodies at the time of exposure indicates susceptibility to rubella. The presence of antibody at exposure confirms past rubella infection (or rubella vaccination), indicates protection from another episode of the disease, and in the pregnant woman obviates rubella-induced congenital malformation.

In patients with clinical rubella, rubella-specific IgM, HI, and EIA antibodies are detectable within 24 to 48 hours after onset of the rash, and peak titers are reached within 6 to 12 days. In subclinical rubella (primary rubella without rash), rubella-specific IgM antibodies usually reach detectable levels 14 to 21 days after exposure, a time that corresponds to the onset of rash in clinical disease.

The CF antibody response after rubella infection is slower than the HI response. Therefore it is sometimes possible to demonstrate a diagnostic rise in CF antibody with paired sera that would not show such a rise in HI antibody.

The peripheral white blood cell count is frequently characterized by a mild leukopenia with a relative lymphocytosis that may include a few atypical cells.

TREATMENT AND PREVENTION In the United States, widespread use of rubella vaccine has prevented epidemics and protected vaccine recipients from disease, with the ultimate goal of preventing fetal infection and the serious consequences of CRS. Recommendations for rubella vaccination are provided in Sec. 1.5.2.

Although immunity from rubella vaccination is long-lasting, primary vaccine failure in up to 5% of vaccines has occurred following the first dose. Determination of immune status requires documentation of 2 measles/mumps/rubella vaccines (MMR) or laboratory confirmation. Continued effort to identify and vaccinate nonimmune women of child-bearing age and effective strategies to avoid missed opportunities is critical to the United States' goal of rubella elimination. Ideally, postpubertal females should be vaccinated only after assurance that they are not pregnant and that the risk of pregnancy is essentially nil for at least 3 months after vaccination. Pregnant women should not be immunized, but should be tested for rubella susceptibility. The immediate postpartum period is an excellent time to vaccinate susceptible women. Vaccine virus has been isolated in human breast milk, but poses no hazard to the infant.

The use of gamma globulin (commercially available human immunoglobulin) in prophylaxis of rubella during pregnancy does not prevent rubella or congenital rubella in a predictable or reliable fashion.

CONGENITAL RUBELLA

Maternal infection with rubella during the first trimester of pregnancy frequently results in fetal infection. Congenital infection produces a spectrum of illness known as the congenital rubella syndrome (CRS) as a result of a viral-induced vasculitis that affects many organs and tissues.

The timing of infection is of great importance. Prospective studies after laboratory-confirmed rubella in pregnancy have documented that the rate of fetal infection is 90% after symptomatic maternal rubella during the first 12 gestational weeks; it drops to 25 to 30% during the second trimester and rises to 60 to 100% during the last weeks of gestation. Organogenesis occurs during the second to sixth week after conception, so that infection is a maximum hazard to the heart and eyes at that time. During the second trimester, the fetus develops increasing immunologic competence and no longer seems susceptible to the chronic infection characteristic of intrauterine rubella during the early weeks.

In general, earlier infection produces more extensive damage. Cardiac defects, cataracts, and glaucoma occur predominantly after maternal rubella during the first 2 months of pregnancy. Hearing loss and neurologic manifestations may occur any time during the first and, less commonly, into the second trimester. Late in pregnancy, infection does not appear to be teratogenic. Risk after reinfection, though much less than after primary rubella, has been well documented.

CLINICAL MANIFESTATIONS The consequences of rubella in utero are varied and unpredictable. Spontaneous abortion, stillbirth, live birth with anomalies (single or multiple), and normal infants are represented in this spectrum. Virtually every organ may be involved, transiently, progressively, or permanently.

During the newborn period congenital rubella may be manifested by a number of acute conditions that are self-limiting in those infants who survive. Neonatal thrombocytopenic purpura, characterized by a variable number of red purple macular "blueberry muffin" lesions, is the most common and striking of these manifestations (Fig. 13-14). It is usually associated with a high incidence of other transient lesions, such as radiolucencies in the metaphyseal portions of the long bones, hepatosplenomegaly, hepatitis, hemolytic anemia, and bulging anterior fontanelle with or without pleocytosis in the CSF. This clinical picture represents the most severe

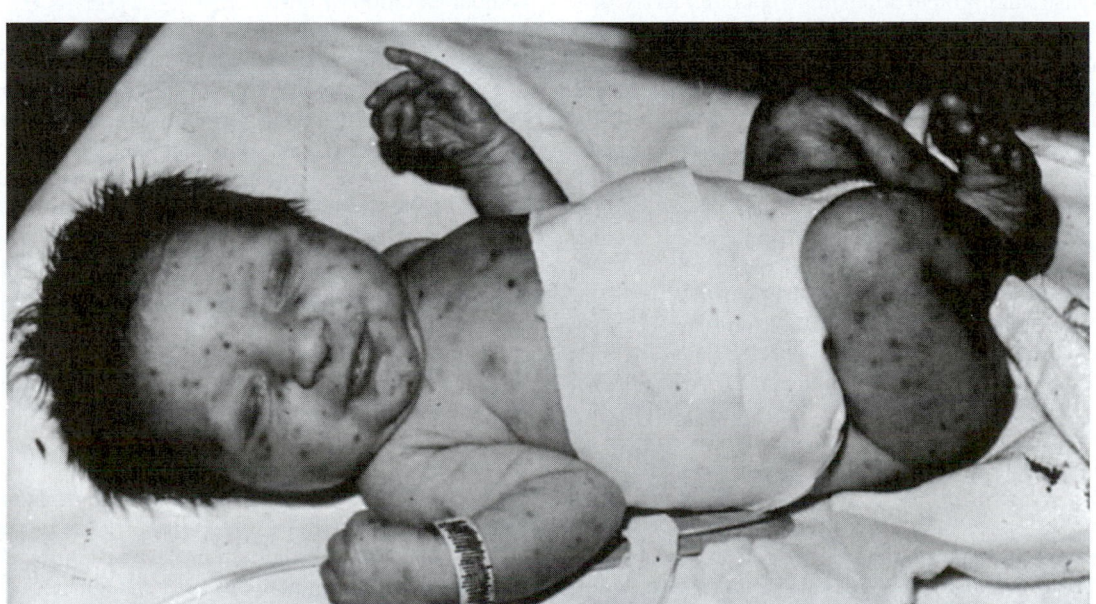

FIGURE 13-14 Infant with congenital rubella. Note "blueberry muffin" appearance with multiple petechiae.

evidence of congenital infection. Low birth weight, congenital heart disease, cataracts, deafness, and retardation with and without microcephaly frequently accompany these transient lesions.

Patent ductus arteriosus, with or without stenosis of the pulmonary artery or its branches, and atrial and ventricular septal defects are the most common cardiac lesions encountered. Permanent sensorineural deafness may be severe or mild, bilateral or unilateral. It is caused by damage to the organ of Corti. Defects in the middle-ear structures have been reported. Deafness and communication disorders may be the only overt manifestations of congenital rubella, especially if maternal infection occurs after the first 8 weeks of pregnancy.

The most characteristic ocular anomaly is a pearly nuclear cataract, unilateral or bilateral, frequently associated with microphthalmia. The lesion may be absent at birth or so small that it may not be detected without careful ophthalmoscopic examination. Congenital glaucoma, which might be present at birth, or which might develop during infancy, is clinically indistinguishable from hereditary infantile glaucoma. The cornea is enlarged and hazy, the anterior chamber is deep, and ocular tension is increased. Retinopathy, characterized by discrete, patchy black pigmentation, quite variable in size and location, is probably the most common ocular manifestation of congenital rubella. There is no evidence that this anomaly of the pigment epithelium of the retina interferes with vision. However, recognition of this lesion is a valuable aid in the diagnosis of congenital rubella.

Delayed psychomotor development during infancy is a hallmark of congenital rubella, even among many children who eventually do well. The most common consequence of the permanent brain damage from this encephalitis is mental retardation, ranging from mild to profound. Behavior disturbances and manifestations of minimal cerebral dysfunction are also common. Less common are severe spastic diplegia and autism.

Progressive rubella panencephalitis, a severe progressive neurologic deterioration beginning during the second decade of life, is a rare complication of congenital rubella. Intellectual deterioration, myoclonus, ataxia, and seizures have progressed to death over the course of several years. High rubella antibody titers in serum and CSF, elevated spinal fluid protein and gamma globulin levels, histopathologic changes of progressive panencephalitis, and isolation of rubella virus from brain biopsy add to the obvious parallel between this condition and the subacute sclerosing panencephalitis that is a rare and late sequela of measles.

Congenital rubella also poses a much greater risk of insulin-dependent diabetes mellitus (IDDM). By age 10 years, the risk is at least four times greater in CRS children than among normal children, and by adult life, the risk is 10- to 20-fold greater. In one group of adult survivors, 40% had IDDM. Patients with IDDM and congenital rubella have the same increased frequency of HLA DR3 and decreased frequency of HLA DR2 as do other patients without congenital rubella. The high prevalence of pancreatic islet cell cytotoxic or surface antibodies in congenital rubella patients with and without IDDM may reflect the in utero infection of pancreatic cells and appears to play a significant role in the pathogenesis of the IDDM in genetically susceptible individuals. More recently thyroiditis has been described.

DIAGNOSIS Despite important implications about termination of pregnancy, prenatal diagnosis suffers from inaccuracy and is not without risk. Intrauterine diagnosis at 10 weeks' gestation by reverse transcriptase-polymerase chain reaction (RT-PCR) in chorionic villous samples, at 16 weeks by amniocentesis, or at 22 weeks by cordocentesis to detect fetal IgM does not always predict fetal infection accurately. Abnormal test results should be confirmed prior to any intervention. Relying on good clinical and epidemiologic data and conventional serologic assays remains the standard. The infant with congenital rubella may remain chronically infected for many months after birth. Virus has been cultured from pharyngeal secretions, urine, CSF, cataract tissue, and virtually every organ. These infants remain a source of infection for susceptible contacts for a year or more. RT-PCR offers additional evidence for diagnosis in early infancy.

Newborn infants with congenital rubella have serum rubella antibody titers comparable to those of their mothers. Much of this antibody is transplacentally acquired IgG, but the presence of rubella-specific IgM reflects in utero antibody production by the fetus and, when present, is diagnostic of congenital rubella. In all but rare infants, by the end of 1 year IgG is usually the dominant rubella antibody. Detectable levels of hemagglutination inhibition (HI) or neutralizing antibody persist for years in most children. However, a minority, despite congenital infection, have declining titers of HI antibody beginning during the second year of life. By age 5 years approximately 20% of children with this disease have undetectable levels of antibody. Immunologic tolerance has been proposed as a mechanism for this finding. Loss of antibody cannot be correlated with severity of clinical disease. Rubella antibody that persists in infancy beyond age 6 months without evidence of postnatal infection essentially confirms the diagnosis of congenital rubella.

Cell-mediated immune responses (CMI) are impaired selectively in children with congenital rubella. Purified lymphocyte cultures from children with congenital rubella fail to respond to rubella virus antigen, as measured by lymphocyte transformation and synthesis of interferon and leukocyte migration inhibition factor. Responses to phytohemagglutinin, a nonspecific T-cell mitogen, are also depressed, but to a lesser extent. Impairment of CMI is more severe in children infected during the first 2 months than in the latter stages of gestation. Most infants with congenital rubella are no longer shedding virus and have a normal pattern of serum immunoglobulin at age 1 year. Rare infants, however, have persistent severe dysglobulinemia characterized by low levels of IgG with or without elevation of IgM.

PROGNOSIS Mortality in a group with various abnormalities due to rubella was approximately 10%. Mortality is greatest during the first 6 months of life. A surprising number of children with multisystem involvement make excellent adjustments over the years. Among a group of approximately 300 survivors of the rubella epidemic of 1963–1964 who are now adults, approximately one-third are leading relatively normal lives; one-third live with their parents and may have "noncompetitive employment"; and one-third require care in facilities with support personnel present 24 hours a day.

In a group of 58 infants with neonatal thrombocytopenic purpura, the mortality exceeded 35% after the first year of follow-up; this was not usually a consequence of bleeding but of sepsis, congestive heart failure, and general debility.

TREATMENT AND PREVENTION The optimal management of the pregnant woman with positive rubella titer exposed to rubella is unclear, but practical suggestions have been provided. Documentation of rubella immune status before pregnancy is a pivotal public health strategy, avoiding later diagnostic confusion, preventing misinterpretation of laboratory data, and allowing revaccination if the titer is low. Sadly, lack of implementation of this critical public health strategy in the United States is highlighted by documentation in late 1998 that only six states require rubella susceptibility premarital screening and no state requires subsequent vaccination.

Infants with CRS are contagious as long as they are shedding virus in their pharyngeal secretions. In general, infants who carry rubella for long periods are more severely damaged and retarded in growth and development. There is no specific therapy for congenital rubella. Early detection of auditory and visual impairment and incorporation of adequate educational therapy including parent education and counseling is important.

References

Centers for Disease Control: Rubella and congenital rubella syndrome—United States, 1994–1997. MMWR Morb Mortal Wkly Rep 46:350–354, 1997

Davidkin I, Valle M, Peltola H et al: Etiology of measles- and rubella-like illnesses in measles, mumps, and rubella-vaccinated children. J Infect Dis 178:1567–1570, 1998

Litwin CM, Hill HR: Serologic and DNA-based testing for congenital and perinatal Infections. Pediatr Infect Dis J 16:1166–1175, 1997

Mellinger AK, Cragan JD, Atkinson WL et al: High incidence of congenital rubella syndrome after a rubella outbreak. Pediatr Infect Dis J 14:573–578, 1995

Plotkin SA, Katz M, Cordero JF: The eradication of rubella. JAMA 281:561–562, 1999

Schluter WW, Reef SE, Redd SC, Dykewicz CA: Changing epidemiology of congenital rubella syndrome in the United States. J Infect Dis 178:636–641, 1998

13.5   MYCOTIC DISEASES

13.5.1   Introduction to Antifungal Therapy

Patricia M. Flynn

Antifungal agents are available in systemic and topical formulations, and some are available in both forms. Topical antifungal agents, because they are poorly absorbed, are less likely to cause toxicity and should, as a rule, be the first choice for treating skin and mucous membrane infections. However, tinea capitis and onychomycosis (fungal infection of the nails) are best treated systemically. Infections that are severe, are disseminated, or that involve the bloodstream should also be treated with systemic therapy. The availability of improved diagnostic testing and newer, safer systemic antifungal agents is expected to increase the use of these agents in the general pediatric population. Organism and disease-specific antifungal therapies are summarized in Table 13-62.

SYSTEMIC ANTIFUNGAL AGENTS

Amphotericin B

Amphotericin B is a polyene macrolide antibiotic that is active against most fungal organisms, including *Candida spp., Cryptococcus neoformans, Histoplasma capsulatum, Blastomyces dermatitidis, Coccidioides immitis,* and *Aspergillus spp.* It is the drug of choice for treating severe systemic infections caused by susceptible fungi. Amphotericin B is not active against *Pseudallescheria boydii,* some isolates of *Fusarium spp.,* and *Candida lusitaniae.* Amphotericin B acts by binding to sterols in the fungal cell membrane, causing increased cell permeability, leakage of cellular contents, and cell death. It has been reported to be both fungistatic and fungicidal, depending on the fungal organism as well as host factors.

Amphotericin B is typically administered as a 1- to 6-hour (usually 2–4-hour) daily intravenous infusion of 0.5 to 1.5 mg/kg. The dosage is dependent on the infecting organism and the extent of infection. Earlier recommendations suggested optional administration of a test dose (0.1 mg/kg) of the drug and gradual escalation to full dosage. If this practice is used, patients with severe infections should receive fungicidal doses (0.5 mg/kg) within 12 to 24 hours. Amphotericin B is highly protein bound and accumulates in tissues, especially the liver and spleen. Thus, after therapy has been established, the drug can be administered every other day or three times weekly. The drug does not penetrate into the cerebrospinal fluid, vitreous humor, or amniotic fluid. Common side effects include infusion-related fever and chills that can be treated with meperidine, antipyretics, or both. Patients who experience severe reactions can be given these agents or a hydrocortisone infusion before amphotericin B is administered. Neonates and children are less likely than adults to experience infusion-related toxicity. The frequency and severity of the infusion-related side effects often diminish with continued treatment. Nephrotoxicity (manifested by elevated serum creatinine and blood urea nitrogen concentrations), hypokalemia, and hypomagnesemia are also common, but usually reversible, side effects. Volume expansion with normal saline prior to administration of amphotericin B has reduced nephrotoxicity in adults, but there are no comparable data for children.

Amphotericin B can be administered intraventricularly in cases of meningitis; however, no data exist to suggest that intrathecal administration improves the outcome of candidal meningitis. Toxicity due to administration by this route has been reported. It can also be used as a bladder irrigant for treating uncomplicated candidal cystitis. Topical preparations (cream, ointment, and solution) can be used for mucosal and superficial skin infections.

Liposomal Preparations of Amphotericin B   Amphotericin B has been incorporated into lipid complexes, which may help to protect the kidneys from adverse effects. In general, these agents may be given at higher doses than conventional amphotericin B; however, nephrotoxicity and infusion-related symptoms remain the dose-limiting toxic effects. Three liposomal products are now commercially available: amphotericin B lipid complex (Abelcet), amphotericin B liposome (AmBisome), and amphotericin B cholesteryl sulfate (Amphotec). Each preparation achieves a higher concentration in the liver and spleen than does conventional amphotericin B. AmBisome achieves higher peak concentrations in serum and brain than does conventional amphotericin B, and Abelcet reaches higher concentrations in the lung. Concentration of the parent drug in the kidney is similar for all amphotericin B preparations. The recommended daily dosages are 3 to 5 mg/kg for AmBisome, 3 to 4 mg/kg for Amphotec, and 5 mg/kg for Abelcet. In adults use of amphotericin B lipid complex for the treatment of renal candidiasis has failed to eradicate the disease, quite possibly because the lipid complexes do not penetrate the kidney.

The liposomal preparations are indicated for patients with aspergillosis who cannot tolerate conventional amphotericin B therapy or for whom it has been unsuccessful. Abelcet and AmBisome are indicated for patients with other fungal infections if conventional therapy has failed or caused toxic effects. AmBisome is also indicated for the empiric treatment of febrile neutropenic cancer patients and for patients with visceral leishmaniasis.

TABLE 13-62

ORGANISM AND DISEASE-SPECIFIC ANTIFUNGAL THERAPY CHART

ORGANISM	DISEASE	THERAPY
Aspergillus spp.	Sinusitis	Surgical drainage. Amphotericin B 1.0–1.5 mg/kg/day. May substitute liposomal product for conventional amphotericin B if unable to tolerate conventional therapy. Itraconazole 8–10/mg/kg/day may be substituted after a good response is demonstrated to amphotericin B. The efficacy of combination therapy is unproven. Duration of therapy is undefined; suggest minimum of 6 weeks plus reversal of immunosuppression.
	Invasive or disseminated	Antifungal therapy same as for sinusitis. Surgical removal of involved tissue recommended by some experts.
	Skin	Surgical débridement. Antifungal therapy same as for sinusitis. Following adequate débridement and recovery from immunosuppression, shorter duration of therapy may be acceptable.
Blastomyces dermatitidis	Pulmonary and disseminated	Amphotericin B 0.5–1.0 mg/kg/day for moderate to severe infections. Itraconazole 4–10 mg/kg/day for mild to moderate infections. Duration of therapy is 6 months for itraconazole and 1.5–2 g total dose amphotericin B (recommended adult dosage).
Candida spp.	Oropharyngeal candidiasis (thrush)	*Infants:* Nystatin oral suspension 2 mL qid for at least 7 days. *Children:* Nystatin oral suspension 5 mL qid, swish and swallow *or* clotrimazole troche 10 mg five times daily × 7 days. *Immunocompromised or failed topical therapy:* Fluconazole IV or PO; 6 mg/kg/day loading dose followed by 3 mg/kg daily for total of 14 days.
	Cutaneous	Nystatin *or* clotrimazole *or* miconazole cream, lotion, or powder applied twice a day for at least 7 days.
	Vaginitis	Clotrimazole cream or troche *or* miconazole cream for 7 days *or* single dose of fluconazole 150 mg (adult dosage).
	Esophagitis	Fluconazole IV or PO; 6 mg/kg loading dose followed by 3 mg/kg daily for total of 14 days. For severe cases, amphotericin B 0.5–1.0 mg/kg/day × 14 days.
	Cystitis	Investigate possibility of disseminated disease. Remove catheter if possible. Fluconazole IV or PO; 6 mg/kg loading dose followed by 3 mg/kg daily for total of 14 days, *or* amphotericin B 0.5 mg/kg/day for 3–10 days, *or* amphotericin B bladder irrigation with 5 mg/100 mL water at 42 mL/h for 1–3 days.
	Peritonitis (peritoneal dialysis catheter)	5-FC 50–150 mg/kg/day divided qid, and fluconazole 6 mg/kg/day PO or IV for 4–6 weeks. Remove catheter if no improvement in 4–7 days.
	Fungemia	
	• Uncomplicated	Amphotericin B 0.5–1.0 mg/kg/day for minimum of 14 days. Fluconazole probably effective but not yet proven.
	• Catheter-related	Remove catheter. Amphotericin B 0.5–1.0 mg/kg/day for minimum of 14 days. (*C. tropicalis* and *C. parapsilosis* may require 1.0 mg/kg/day for as long as 3–4 weeks.)
	Disseminated	Amphotericin B 1.0 mg/kg/day plus 5-FC, 50–150 mg/kg/day divided qid for 4–6 weeks (may be longer if clinically severe). May substitute liposomal product for conventional amphotericin B if unable to tolerate, but renal disease demonstrates best outcome in animal models with conventional amphotericin B. Fluconazole, 12 mg/kg/day, may be an alternate, but insufficient data to recommend.
	Chronic mucocutaneous candidiasis	Ketoconazole 5–10 mg/kg/day or fluconazole 6 mg/kg/day indefinitely.
Coccidioides immitis	Nonmeningeal	No therapy in normal hosts with uncomplicated primary infection. Fluconazole, 6–12 mg/kg/day. Duration not defined; suggest 12–18 months. Amphotericin B results in similar cure rates in adults, but should be considered in severely ill or immunocompromised patients. Recommended total dose for adults is 2.5 g or higher, for children the total dose range is between 15 and 45 mg/kg/day.
	Meningeal	Same as above but duration of therapy indefinite, lifelong.

(continued)

TABLE 13-62   **Continued**

ORGANISM	DISEASE	THERAPY
Cryptococcus neoformans	Nonmeningeal	Amphotericin B 0.5–1.0 mg/kg/day with or without 5-FC, 50–150 mg/kg, divided qid. Fluconazole 12 mg/kg/day may be used for mild to moderate infections. If amphotericin B is used initially, change to fluconazole with improved clinical condition is possible after a minimum of 2 weeks. Total duration of therapy 8–12 weeks. HIV-infected patients require chronic suppressive therapy with fluconazole, 6 mg/kg/day, indefinitely.
	Meningeal	Same as for nonmeningeal but 5-FC should be used. Duration of amphotericin B plus 5-FC is 6 weeks or 8–10 weeks of fluconazole. Chronic suppressive therapy with fluconazole, 6 mg/kg/day, indefinitely.
Dermatophytes (*Trichosporum sp., Microsporum sp., Epidermophyton sp.*)	Tinea corporis, cruris, pedis	Topical clotrimazole or miconazole in cream, lotion, ointment, or powder applied twice daily for 2–3 weeks. For failures, consider other azole or allylamine preparation. Duration of therapy is 2–3 weeks.
	Tinea capitis	Griseofulvin, 10 mg/kg/day ultramicrosized or 15 mg/kg/day microsized, in 1 to 2 divided doses *or* itraconazole 3–5 mg/kg/day for 4–6 weeks.
	Onychomycosis	Itraconazole 3–5 mg/kg/day for 3–4 months *or* itraconazole pulse therapy, 3–5 mg/kg/day for 1 week per month for 2 months *or* terbinafine 250 mg (weight greater than 40 kg) or 125 mg (weight 20–40 kg) or 67.5 mg (weight less than 20 kg) for 6 weeks for fingernail and 12 weeks for toenail disease.
Malassezia furfur	Tinea versicolor	Ketoconazole cream or shampoo applied for 2 weeks *or* selenium sulfide, leave on 10 minutes daily for 7 days or 3–5 times weekly for 2–4 weeks. Successful therapy in adults with ketoconazole 400 mg single dose or 200 mg daily for 7 days.
Fusarium spp.	Fungemia or disseminated infection	Amphotericin B1.0–1.5 mg/kg/day plus 5-FC, 50–150 mg/kg/day, divided every 6 hours. May substitute liposomal product for conventional amphotericin B if unable to tolerate. Duration of therapy undetermined but 6 weeks minimum.
Histoplasma capsulatum	Pulmonary	No therapy in normal host for very mild or asymptomatic pulmonary disease. Itraconazole 4–10 mg/kg/day for mild to moderate infections, amphotericin B 0.5–1.0 mg/kg/day for moderate to severe infections, total dose of 30 mg/kg/day
	Disseminated	Amphotericin B 0.5–1.0 mg/kg/day for moderate to severe infections; total dose 30–35 mg/kg. Itraconazole 4–10 mg/kg/day for mild to moderate infections. Duration of therapy is a minimum of 3–6 months. HIV-infected patients require indefinite suppressive therapy with itraconazole.
Pseudallescheria boydii	Fungemia or disseminated infection	Miconazole 20–40 mg/kg/day divided every 8 hours. Itraconazole, 10 mg/kg/day, may be effective. Duration of therapy is undetermined but 6 weeks minimum. Amphotericin B is ineffective.
Sporothrix schenckii	Cutaneous	Itraconazole 8–10 mg/kg/day for 3 months.
Trichosporon spp.	Fungemia or disseminated infection	Amphotericin B 1.0–1.5 mg/kg/day plus 5-FC, 50–150 mg/kg/day, divided every 6 hours and fluconazole 12 mg/kg/day. May substitute liposomal product for conventional amphotericin B if unable to tolerate. Duration of therapy is undetermined but 6 weeks minimum.
Zygomycoses (*Rhizopus spp., Mucor spp., Rhizomucor spp., Cunninghamella bertholletiae*)	Rhinocerebral, pulmonary, and disseminated	Amphotericin B 1.0–1.5 mg/kg/day. Discontinuation of steroids. Surgical débridement recommended by some experts. Duration of therapy is undetermined but 6 weeks minimum.

Azoles

The azole family contains two classes of drugs: the imidazoles and the triazoles. Although the two classes are similar in their spectrum of activity and their mechanism of action, the triazoles are more commonly prescribed, because they are more slowly metabolized and have less effect on the patient's sterol synthesis. In general, the azole family of drugs has activity against *Candida albicans* and the dimorphic fungi *Histoplasma capsulatum, Blastomyces dermatitidis, Coccidioides immitis,* and *Cryptococcus neoformans*. Some species of *Candida* other than *C. albicans* are also susceptible, as are the dermatophytes. Itraconazole has activity against *Aspergillus spp.* The azoles act by inhibiting sterol 14-α-demethylase, a cytochrome P_{450} enzyme system; this inhibition results in impaired ergosterol synthesis in the fungal cell membrane. The available systemic azoles include the imidazoles (miconazole and ketoconazole) and the tri-

azoles (fluconazole and itraconazole). These agents are fungistatic. The use of azoles in combination with amphotericin B remains controversial. Some data from animal models suggest that the two agents can be antagonistic. When an azole is selected for systemic use, possible drug interactions should be carefully considered (Table 13-63).

Fluconazole This drug is effective for the treatment of esophageal, laryngeal, and vaginal candidiasis. It should also be considered in cases of oropharyngeal candidiasis unresponsive to topical therapy. The drug has successfully treated patients with systemic candidiasis when therapy with amphotericin B failed, and has been used for prophylaxis of fungal infection in adult recipients of bone marrow transplants. There are also case reports describing successful therapy for a variety of candidal infections, although fluconazole is

TABLE 13-63
AZOLE DRUG INTERACTIONS

AZOLE	COADMINISTERED DRUG	EFFECT
Fluconazole, itraconazole, ketoconazole	Terfenadine, astemizole, cisapride	Increases concentration of terfenadine, astemizole, and cisapride; may cause cardiac arrhythmia
Fluconazole, itraconazole, ketoconazole	Oral anticoagulants	Increases effect of anticoagulant
Fluconazole, itraconazole, ketoconazole	Phenytoin	Increases phenytoin concentration; decreases azole concentration
Fluconazole, itraconazole, ketoconazole	Cyclosporine	Increases concentration of cyclosporine
Fluconazole, itraconazole, ketoconazole	Rifampin, rifabutin, isoniazid	Decreases concentration of azole
Itraconazole, ketoconazole	Didanosine	Decreases absorption of azole
Itraconazole, ketoconazole	H$_2$ blockers, antacids	Decreases absorption of azole
Itraconazole, ketoconazole	Amprenavir, indinavir, nelfinavir, saquinavir	Increases concentrations of protease inhibitors
Itraconazole, ketoconazole	Ritonavir	Increases concentration of azole
Fluconazole, itraconazole, ketoconazole	Midazolam, triazolam	Increases concentrations of midazolam and triazolam
Ketoconazole	Theophyllines	Decreases concentration of theophyllines

not active against *C. krusei*. Fluconazole can be used as initial therapy for mild cases of cryptococcal meningitis in adults with AIDS and for long-term suppression of cryptococcal infection. Its usefulness in treating patients with non-AIDS–associated cryptococcal meningitis has not been defined. Fluconazole is also effective in coccidioidal meningitis and other types of coccidioidomycosis.

Fluconazole is available as an oral suspension, a tablet, and an intravenous solution. It is well absorbed from the gastrointestinal tract, and the recommended oral and intravenous dosages are identical. For patients with oropharyngeal candidiasis, a loading dose of 6 mg/kg, followed by 3 mg/kg daily for 2 weeks, is recommended. The recommended daily dosage for patients with systemic fungal infection is 400 mg for adults and approximately 12 mg/kg for children. Premature infants should receive the same dosage as older children, but the drug should be administered only once every 72 hours for the first 2 weeks of life. Fluconazole readily enters body fluids, including the cerebrospinal fluid. The drug is excreted unchanged in the urine, and the dosage must be adjusted for patients with renal impairment. The most common side effects are gastrointestinal complaints; less frequently, hepatic enzyme activity may be elevated. Drugs that interact with fluconazole are listed in Table 13-63. Development of resistance to fluconazole is reported with increasing frequency. Failure of fluconazole treatment may be attributable to resistance, especially in patients who have received chronic suppressive therapy, and to the drug's fungistatic, rather than fungicidal, effects.

Itraconazole This agent has activity similar to that of fluconazole but is also active against *Aspergillus spp*. It is indicated for the treatment of blastomycosis, histoplasmosis, aspergillosis, and onychomycosis. Recent studies show it to be effective in tinea capitis in adults and children. The oral solution of itraconazole is effective therapy for oropharyngeal and esophageal candidiasis. Currently, the agent is available as a capsule and an oral solution. The preparations are not interchangeable; the oral solution produces greater systemic drug exposure than does an equivalent dose in capsule form. Because bioavailability is affected by the acidity of the stomach, the capsules should be taken with food. The oral solution is less affected by stomach pH and should be taken while the patient is fasting. Itraconazole is highly protein bound, and very little penetrates into the cerebrospinal fluid. It is metabolized by the liver and excreted as inactive metabolites in the feces and urine. Although neither formulation is FDA approved for use in children,

reports of multiple pediatric studies describe the administration of itraconazole at dosages as high as 10 mg/kg per day for severe infections and 3 to 5 mg/kg per day for tinea capitis and onychomycosis. The duration of therapy for onychomycosis is 3 to 4 months. However, because the drug accumulates in the nail tissues, "pulse therapy" (repeated courses of 1 week of therapy followed by 1 to 3 weeks without therapy) has been reported effective for onychomycosis. As with fluconazole, gastrointestinal side effects occur most frequently. Use of itraconazole with terfenadine, cisapride, or astemizole can cause a serious drug interaction that produces life-threatening cardiac arrhythmias (Table 13-63). Itraconazole has been reported to potentiate vincristine toxicity in children undergoing concurrent chemotherapy for leukemia.

Miconazole Because they are less toxic, fluconazole and itraconazole have largely replaced miconazole as treatment for systemic fungal infections. Miconazole is still the drug of choice for systemic infections caused by *Pseudallescheria boydii*. Injectable miconazole can be administered every 8 hours at a total daily dosage of 20 to 40 mg/kg. The infusion should be administered over 2 hours to avoid infusion-related cardiac arrhythmia or anaphylactoid reaction. Other adverse reactions occur more frequently with miconazole than with the triazoles.

Ketoconazole This drug is effective therapy for candidiasis, chronic mucocutaneous candidiasis, blastomycosis, histoplasmosis, coccidiodomycosis, chromomycosis, and paracoccidioidomycosis. It is available as an oral suspension, a tablet, shampoo, and a topical cream. It is readily absorbed from the gastrointestinal tract and can be administered to children every 12 to 24 hours at a total daily dosage of 5 to 10 mg/kg. Ketoconazole is highly protein bound and does not penetrate the CNS. Gastrointestinal distress, the most frequent side effect, can be reduced if patients take the medication with food. The most severe adverse effect is rare fatal hepatotoxicity. Of all the orally absorbed azoles, ketoconazole has the greatest effect on the host endocrine system. It has the same potential serious interaction with terfenadine, cisapride, and astemizole as does itraconazole.

Other Systemic Antifungal Agents

Flucytosine Flucytosine (5-FC), a fluorinated pyrimidine related to fluorouracil, is indicated for treating serious infections caused by

Candida spp. and *Cryptococcus neoformans.* It is converted to flu-orouracil within fungal cells, where it interferes with RNA and DNA synthesis. Flucytosine is available in capsule form and is readily absorbed from the gastrointestinal tract. Because the drug is poorly protein bound and penetrates the blood-brain barrier, it is effective as adjunctive therapy for meningitis, in combination with amphotericin B. The recommended daily dosage is 50 to 150 mg/kg, divided into four equal doses. The dosage must be adjusted for patients with renal impairment and caution should be used when flucytosine is administered to patients with underlying renal dysfunction. Gastrointestinal complaints, hepatitis, and jaundice are frequent adverse effects. Plasma drug concentration should be maintained at ≤ 25 $\mu g/mL$ to avert bone marrow suppression, which is the most serious toxicity. Flucytosine should be used in combination with other antifungal agents such as amphotericin B, because pathogens rapidly acquire resistance to flucytosine when it is used alone. When used in combination with flucytosine, amphotericin B at a reduced dosage is ineffective as a treatment for *Cryptococcus.*

Griseofulvin Griseofulvin is indicated for treatment of superficial fungal infections of skin, hair, and nails that are caused by various species of dermatophytes including *Trichophyton, Microsporum,* and *Epidermophyton.* It acts by inhibiting fungal cell mitosis at metaphase and by binding to human keratin. Absorption from the gastrointestinal tract is markedly variable, but is thought to be increased by fatty meals and by the use of smaller griseofulvin crystals. Currently, formulations containing microsized and ultramicrosized griseofulvin crystals are commercially available. The daily dosage for children is approximately 10 mg/kg of ultramicrosized and 15 mg/kg of microsized griseofulvin, given as one dose or two divided doses. The duration of therapy depends on the location of the fungal infection; therapy must be continued until the infected tissue is replaced by normal tissue. Tinea corporis requires 2 to 4 weeks of therapy, tinea capitis 4 to 6 weeks of therapy, and infection of toenails at least 6 to 12 months of therapy. The safety of griseofulvin treatment is not established for children younger than 2 years of age. Griseofulvin is usually well tolerated; rash and urticaria are the most common adverse effects. Headache is also common. When given with warfarin, griseofulvin may result in decreased plasma warfarin concentration; it may also reduce the effectiveness of oral contraceptives. Phenobarbital may diminish the effectiveness of griseofulvin.

Terbinafine Terbinafine is an allylamine that acts by inhibiting fungal synthesis of ergosterol. It has been available as a topical agent for a number of years, but has only recently become available in an oral tablet form for treatment of onychomycosis. Allylamines act by inhibiting the epoxidation of squalene, thus blocking the biosynthesis of ergosterol, a component of the fungal cell membrane. The drug has not been tested in children and should be reserved for patients with refractory disease. The recommended adult regimen is 250 mg daily for 6 weeks for fingernail disease and daily for 12 weeks for toenail disease. Children who weigh more than 40 kg should receive the adult dosage. The dosage should be 125 mg/d for children who weigh between 20 and 40 kg, and 62.5 mg/d for children who weigh less than 20 kg. Gastrointestinal toxicity is observed most frequently.

TOPICAL ANTIFUNGAL AGENTS

Topical antifungal agents are available in many different preparations, including ointment, cream, solution, lotion, powder, oral and vaginal troches, and vaginal tablets. Topical agents are the treatment of choice for superficial fungal infections of the skin, mucosa, and cornea, such as dermatophytosis (tinea corporis, tinea cruris, tinea pedis), tinea versicolor, candidiasis, and fungal keratitis. Creams and lotions are generally preferable to ointments for treating diseases of the skin. Powders are used only in moist areas such as the feet, groin, or other intertriginous areas. Several of the agents used as systemic therapy are also available as topical preparations. The mechanism of action is the same, but the efficacy of the topical agents depends on their direct interaction with the fungal organisms on the surface of the skin or mucous membranes. In selecting a topical antifungal agent, consideration should be given to the type of preparation needed, the cost, and its bioavailability. Several agents now available without prescription may be used as first-line therapy for tinea corporis, with more expensive preparations reserved for resistant infection.

Polyene Antifungals

Nystatin The mechanism of action of nystatin is similar to that of amphotericin B, but nystatin is active only against superficial candidiasis. The agent is available as a cream, an ointment, a powder, a vaginal tablet, an oral tablet, a pastile, and a suspension. Nystatin suspension is the treatment of choice for oral candidiasis and should be administered four times daily. Children who are able should be instructed to swish the suspension around the mouth, and then swallow. The side effects include nausea and bad taste, but both are manageable. Topical nystatin is also frequently used for candidiasis in the diaper area and is available in combination with corticosteroids. Nystatin powder is effective for treating superficial candidiasis in skin folds, but care should be taken to prevent young infants' inhalation of the powder when it is applied to their necks.

Amphotericin B Amphotericin B is available as a cream, ointment, and oral solution. Its topical use is limited to the treatment of superficial (including oral) candidiasis.

Azoles

Multiple azole antifungal agents are available as topical preparations. They are active against *Candida spp., Trichophyton spp., Microsporum spp.,* and, in some cases, *Malassezia furfur.* The mechanism of action is that described for systemic azoles. When used as directed, topical azoles cause few side effects. Some redness and irritation can occur.

Clotrimazole is available as an oral troche, a vaginal tablet, a vaginal cream, cream, and a lotion. All but the oral troches are available over the counter. A clotrimazole and corticosteroid combination is also available, but it should be used with caution in children, who may absorb proportionally larger amounts of corticosteroid and thus be more susceptible to systemic toxicity. *Miconazole* is also available over the counter as a cream, spray, powder, lotion, and vaginal cream. These agents are readily available and inexpensive, and they should be the treatment of choice for tinea corporis (including tinea pedis and tinea cruris) and vaginal candidiasis. Topical *ketoconazole, econazole, sulconazole,* and *oxiconazole* are also available. These agents have a similar spectrum of activity but should be considered second-line agents because of cost. Ketoconazole is available as a shampoo for treatment of tinea versicolor but is ineffective therapy for tinea capitis. *Terconazole, butoconazole,* and *tioconazole* are available only as vaginal preparations.

Allylamines

Three topical allylamine agents—*terbinafine, naftifine,* and *butenafine*—are currently available. As a group, allylamines are active against the dermatophytes. These agents have not been studied in children younger than 12 years of age.

Other Topical Antifungal Agents

Tolnaftate is active against dermatophytes, but is ineffective against *Candida spp.* and is less effective than the azoles for treating tinea corporis. Many preparations of tolnaftate are available without prescription. *Halcinonide* and *ciclopirox* are topical antifungals with broad-spectrum activity against the dermatophytes, including *M. furfur.*

References

Bennett JE: Antimicrobial agents: antifungal agents. In: Hardman J, Limbird L, Molinoff P, Ruddon R, eds: Goodman & Gilman's The Pharmacological Basis of Therapeutics. New York, McGraw Hill, 1996: 1175–1190

Goodwin D, Cleary JD, Walawander CA, Taylor JW, Grasela TH: Pretreatment regimens for adverse events related to infusion of amphotericin B. Clin Infect Dis 20:755–761, 1995

Gupta AK, Hofstader SL, Summerbell RC, et al: Treatment of tinea capitis with itraconazole capsule pulse therapy. J Am Acad Dermatol 32:216–219, 1998

Howard RM, Frieden IJ: Dermatophyte infections in children. Adv Pediatr Infect Dis 14:73–107, 1999

Kintzel PE, Smith GH: Practical guidelines for preparing and administering amphotericin B. Am J Hosp Pharm 49:1156–1164, 1992

Mehta J: Do variations in molecular structure affect the clinical efficacy and safety of lipid-based amphotericin B preparations? Leuk Res 21:183–188, 1997

Namdar R, Anderson JD, Kline SS: Abelcet, amphotec, and AmBisome in the neonatal and pediatric populations: a literature review. J Pediatr Pharm Pract 3:13–28, 1998

Suarez S, Friedlander SF: Antifungal therapy in children: an update. Pediatr Ann 27:177–184, 1998

Walsh TJ, Gonzalez C, Lyman CA, Chanock SJ, Pizzo PA: Invasive fungal infections in children: recent advances in diagnosis and treatment. In: Aronoff SC, Hughes WT, Kohl S, Speck WT, Wald ER, eds: Advances in Pediatric Infectious Diseases. St. Louis, Mosby, 1996:187–290

13.5.2   Aspergillosis

Deborah Lehman

Aspergillosis, caused by any of several species of *Aspergillus,* usually manifests in immunocompromised or debilitated hosts as necrotizing cavitary pulmonary lesions or hematogenously disseminated foci in multiple organs. *Aspergillus spp.* also cause a hypersensitivity pneumonitis in immunocompetent hosts and in persons with chronic pulmonary diseases such as cystic fibrosis and asthma.

Ubiquitous in nature, *Aspergillus spp.* are commonly found in soil, water, and on decaying vegetation. Human exposure to the spores of potentially pathogenic species, particularly *A. fumigatus,* is unavoidable. *Aspergillus fumigatus* has been implicated in most of the disseminated and pulmonary infections, but *A. flavus* and *A. niger* have also been recovered as pathogens. Transmission occurs by inhalation of airborne spores that regularly contaminate the environment; human-to-human transmission or zoonotic transmission has not been documented.

Patients with immunosuppression are at greatest risk, especially those who are being treated for lymphoreticular disorders and other hematologic malignancies. Because the phagocytic functions of neutrophils and mononuclear cells appear to be the primary immune defense against invasive aspergillosis, *Aspergillus* is a common infectious etiology of death in bone marrow transplant patients. Outbreaks in transplant units have been epidemiologically linked to building demolition and construction, which releases fungal spores into the environment. There are increasing reports of invasive aspergillosis in patients with AIDS, as well as in children with chronic granulomatous disease. Aspergillosis in a patient without underlying disease is infrequent, and intensive investigation for a predisposing disorder should be undertaken. Isolated pulmonary aspergillosis may complicate underlying lung disease such as tuberculosis, bronchiectasis, lung abscess, or carcinoma.

CLINICAL MANIFESTATIONS   Infection with *Aspergillus* can manifest as three distinct syndromes; two are forms of noninvasive aspergillosis (aspergilloma and allergic bronchopulmonary aspergillosis) and one form is invasive. Aspergillomas occur when the fungus grows as a dense mass of hyphae and tissue debris in a preexistent pulmonary cavity caused by a concomitant pulmonary disease such as tuberculosis, histoplasmosis, or bronchiectasis. There is no tissue invasion, although hemoptysis may occur and may on occasion be life-threatening.

Allergic bronchopulmonary aspergillosis (ABPA) is a hypersensitivity reaction to the fungus, seen in patients with chronic pulmonary disease such as asthma or cystic fibrosis. Inhalation of fungal spores leads to hyphal colonization of the bronchopulmonary tree resulting in mucus plugging, dyspnea, wheezing, and cough. ABPA may eventually lead to large areas of bronchiectasis. There is frequently both serum and sputum eosinophilia and pulmonary infiltrates. Immunologic studies reveal elevated total IgE and *Aspergillus*-specific IgE. This form of aspergillosis is most commonly caused by *Aspergillus fumigatis,* and tissue invasion does not occur.

Invasive aspergillosis occurs in patients with profound immunosuppression resulting from therapy for hematologic malignancies and transplant procedures. Risk factors for invasive aspergillosis include prolonged neutropenia, corticosteroid therapy, and graft-versus-host disease. The disease presents as a necrotizing bronchopneumonia, with invasion of the pulmonary vessels often accompanied by thrombosis. Widespread embolization to the heart, gastrointestinal tract, skin, kidneys, and liver occurs in about one-third of patients. Invasion of the central nervous system with occlusion of cerebral vessels may lead to cerebral infarction. The mortality of invasive aspergillosis approaches 50 to 90% when the central nervous system is affected.

Aspergillus may also grow as a harmless saprophyte in the cerumen of the external auditory meatus. The paranasal sinuses, especially the maxillary sinuses, can be also be colonized by various species of *Aspergillus.* If the individual is immunocompetent, drainage or curettage usually is sufficient to cure the patient. Occasionally, the fungus becomes invasive and extends into adjoining structures. It may erode the bone and extend into the orbit or brain. This complication of *Aspergillus* sinusitis is most common in patients experiencing a relapse of acute leukemia.

Cutaneous aspergillosis manifests as erythematous macules with progressive necrosis or as a cluster of hemorrhagic bullae at sites of intravenous access. Although cutaneous aspergillosis is associated with central venous catheters and occlusive dressings in immuno-compromised hosts, it has rarely been reported after trauma in normal hosts.

In localized infection, the fungus may grow within the walls of tuberculous cavities or produce granulomatous lesions with radial proliferation of hyphae. In immunocompromised hosts *Aspergillus* hyphae may proliferate throughout the lung, and invasion of blood vessels may cause widespread dissemination. In the regions of necrotizing pneumonia, hyphae often can be identified by hematoxylin-and-eosin stain, but Gomori methenamine silver stain may be necessary to identify typical mycelial structures. The hyphae are 3 to 4 μm in diameter, septate, and reveal asymmetric dichotomous branching that may be morphologically indistinguishable from other fungi such as *Pseudallescheria boydii* or *Alternaria* species.

DIAGNOSIS Sputum can be directly examined for hyphal elements; however, a positive examination must be viewed with caution and interpreted in the context of clinical presentation. Even repeated positive sputum cultures may reflect colonization. Radiographic evidence along with evidence from direct examination may provide stronger support for the diagnosis, but lung biopsy remains the gold standard. Sputum and bronchial aspirates should be cultured on Sabouraud dextrose agar with antibiotics at temperatures above 37°C (98.6°F). Cultures of nonbiopsy bronchoscopy specimens, such as lavage fluid, sputum, and brushings, are insensitive in patients with invasive aspergillosis. However, a positive culture or smear may be indicative of disseminated infection in very-high-risk patients, such as following bone marrow or solid organ transplantation. Because invasive aspergillosis is often rapidly fatal, the finding of hyphal elements or positive cultures from superficial sites such as nasal mucous membranes should lead to a more aggressive search for deep-seated infection (eg, transtracheal aspiration, bronchopulmonary washings, bronchial brush biopsy, and open- or closed-lung biopsy). Surveillance cultures during defined high-risk periods are not useful in predicting invasive disease.

Serologic diagnosis of aspergillosis by immunodiffusion and complement fixation tests can be helpful in immunocompetent patients. Precipitins are reported in more than 90% of aspergillomas and in approximately 70% of allergic bronchopulmonary aspergillosis. Polymerase chain reaction (PCR) has been used to diagnose invasive pulmonary aspergillosis in immunocompromised patients, but this technique remains investigational.

TREATMENT Parenteral amphotericin B in doses of 1.0 to 1.5 mg/kg/d is the agent of choice; in immunocompromised hosts with invasive disease, the higher dose is recommended. In patients with lesser degrees of immunocompromise (eg, chronic granulomatous disease), after therapy is well underway and a positive response is evident, the drug can be given on alternate days, but dosage should attain 1.0 mg/kg. Duration of therapy and total optimal dose has not been ascertained, but a minimum of 6 weeks is advised. Surgical resection, in combination with antifungal therapy, is usually necessary in patients with localized aspergillomas or cutaneous aspergillosis who fail to respond to amphotericin B.

Liposomal formulations of amphotericin B may be beneficial in invasive aspergillus infections; total daily dosage can be increased as much as three to five times the conventional amount of non-liposomal amphotericin B. Itraconazole, a triazole, inhibits cell membrane synthesis and in recent studies was shown to be equivalent to amphotericin B for second-line treatment of invasive aspergillosis, as well as for long-term therapy.

Allergic bronchopulmonary aspergillosis is treated with 0.5 mg/kg/d of prednisone for 14 days, followed by alternate-day therapy for 2 months or until the patient's IgE levels show significant decline. At that point, steroids can be tapered, but relapses are common. Itraconazole may also be effective in these patients.

References

Allo MD, Miller J, Townsend T, et al: Primary cutaneous aspergillosis associated with Hickman intravenous catheters. N Engl J Med 317:1105–8, 1987

Corey JP: Allergic fungal sinusitis. Otolaryngol Clin North Am 25:225–230, 1992

Denning DW, Lee JY, Hostetler JS, et al: NIAID mycoses study group multicenter trial of oral itraconazole for invasive aspergillosis. Am J Med 9:125–44, 1994

Fraser RS: Pulmonary aspergillosis: pathologic and pathogenetic features. Pathol Ann 28 (Pt 1):231–277, 1993

Mylonakis E, Barlam T, Flanigan T, et al: Pulmonary aspergillosis and invasive disease in AIDS: review of 342 cases. Chest 114:251–62, 1998

Paterson DL, Singh N: Invasive aspergillosis in transplant recipients. Medicine 78:123, 1999

Pursell KJ, Telzak EE, Armstrong D: Aspergillus species colonization and invasive disease in patients with AIDS. Clin Infect Dis 14:141–148, 1992

Rowen JL, Correa AG, Sokol DM, Hawkins HK, Levy ML, Edwards MS: Invasive aspergillosis in neonates: report of five cases and literature review. Pediatr Infect Dis J 11:576–582, 1992

13.5.3 Blastomycosis

Dwight A. Powell

North American blastomycosis is a pulmonary or disseminated fungal infection caused by *Blastomyces dermatitidis*. Although rare in children, the infection is often difficult to detect unless considered in the differential diagnosis. *Blastomyces dermatitidis* is a dimorphic fungus that exists in the mycelial phase at room temperature and converts to a yeast phase at 37°C (98.6°F). Although isolation from natural sources has been very difficult, growth appears to occur in acidic soil in which there is decaying organic matter and high humidity. Cases of blastomycosis are reported from other countries (particularly those in central Africa), but the vast majority of cases have occurred in the Ohio and Mississippi river basins and the southeastern United States. The highest incidence of cases appears to occur in Wisconsin, Minnesota, Mississippi, and Arkansas. In endemic areas, the annual incidence of symptomatic infection is about 1 to 2 per 100,000 population. Pockets of hyperendemic regions exist where the annual incidence of symptomatic infection may approach 40 per 100,000 population.

Although it is clear that asymptomatic infections occur, the distribution and extent have not been determined, because reliable skin tests or seroepidemiologic methods are not available. When careful immunologic studies are performed in reported outbreaks of blastomycosis, as many as 50% of infected individuals are asymptomatic. Most cases of symptomatic blastomycosis occur sporadically, but there are occasional reports of small outbreaks in communities in which as many as 15 individuals may contract infection over a short period of time. The largest reported outbreak involved 46 school-aged children and two adults who were infected at a camp in Wisconsin following exposure to a beaver dam and lodge.

There is no seasonality to *B. dermatitidis* infections, and infections have been reported in all age groups including newborns. In large surveillance studies of confirmed cases of blastomycosis, pediatric patients ≤19 years old comprise ≈ 3 to 11% of all identified cases. However, the typical patient is a male, 25 to 50 years of age with an outdoor lifestyle. The incubation period from exposure to primary disease is 21 to 106 days (median 45 days). However, latency with eventual reactivation disease is probable with the finding of newly recognized infection in individuals with no exposure to endemic areas for 3 or more years. With the exception of one case of conjugal infection and two cases of intrauterine infections, human-to-human transmission is rare.

The lungs are the usual portal of entry for *B. dermatitidis* conidia. Inhaled conidia elicit an inflammatory response characterized by polymorphonuclear leukocytes (PMNs). The few conidia that survive the initial PMN phagocytosis transform to yeast, which are more resistant to phagocytosis by PMNs and alveolar macrophages. Response to the replicating yeast cells results in a mononuclear infiltrate with some granulomatous component. Spread of yeast from the lungs, although rare, may seed any body organ. Development of cell-mediated immunity is believed to be the primary mechanism in prevention of progressive blastomycosis, and lymphocyte reactivity is a marker of specific cellular immunity to *B. dermatitidis*. Most symptoms appear to result from progression of the primary infection.

CLINICAL MANIFESTATIONS Pulmonary disease is the most common manifestation of symptomatic blastomycosis. In two 10-year epidemiologic studies of confirmed cases of blastomycosis in Wisconsin and Mississippi (670 and 326 cases, respectively), 75% of the cases were isolated pulmonary disease. Pulmonary plus extrapulmonary disease occurred in 6 to 16%, whereas isolated extrapulmonary infection occurred in 9 to 18% of cases. In clinically apparent primary disease, onset is insidious, resembling a mild respiratory infection accompanied by low-grade fever, chest pain, and nonproductive cough, often with rapid resolution. These patients are usually detected only in an outbreak situation. As the symptoms increase in severity, spiking fevers, productive cough, and pleuritic chest pain develop. Subacute or chronic illness may occur with low-grade fever, productive cough, hemoptysis, weakness, anorexia, and weight loss resembling adult reactivation tuberculosis. Rarely, the illness may be fulminant and resemble adult respiratory distress syndrome. Mortality is such cases may be >50%.

Radiographic studies of the chest vary widely; there is no characteristic feature of blastomycosis that allows easy differentiation from other pulmonary infections. In acute cases, parenchymal infiltrates, lobar or segmental consolidation, and interstitial infiltrates have all been described. Large lobar infiltrates may mimic tumor. In the more chronic form of disease, air-space and interstitial infiltrates are seen, but mass-like infiltrates, pulmonary nodules, and cavitation are more common. Pleural effusions and hilar lymphadenitis occur in ≤10% of cases.

Disseminated blastomycosis is caused by hematogenous spread of the infection from the lungs to other areas of the body. Most frequently, the disease involves cutaneous and subcutaneous tissues as well as bone, the central nervous system, and the urogenital tract (only in adults). Cutaneous lesions, the most common extrapulmonary manifestation, initially appear as benign, papulopustular nodules that enlarge peripherally to form elevated, ulcerating, and verrucous granulomas. The borders are usually sharp, heaped-up, and the base commonly contains exudate. As the lesion extends

peripherally, the central area heals, leaving a soft, atrophic scar. Lytic bone lesions are the second most common extrapulmonary infection. The vertebrae, pelvis, sacrum, skull, ribs, or long bones have been reported most frequently, but essentially any bone may be involved. Granulomatous lesions of the liver and spleen are found in more than 40% of patients with disseminated disease, and the kidneys, prostate, epididymis, bladder, and testes may be involved, causing dysuria, pyuria, and hematuria.

Mortality from blastomycosis is dependent on age, immune state of the host, and the type of presenting illness. Adults >65 years of age have >10-fold higher mortality from blastomycosis than children. Although a rare infection in immunocompromised hosts when compared to histoplasmosis, cryptococcosis, and coccidioidomycosis, blastomycosis has been documented to cause severe and often fatal infections in patients with many forms of immune deficiency. Regardless of the underlying disorder, blastomycosis in immunocompromised hosts is usually an aggressive disease, often presenting with disseminated, multiple-organ involvement and a high, early mortality. Fewer than 30 patients with AIDS and blastomycosis have been reported; 90% had advanced HIV disease based on CD4 lymphocyte counts of <200 cells/mm³. Their illness was characterized by a rapidly fatal course with death usually occurring within 21 days.

DIAGNOSIS Although patients may present to a physician early in the course of infection, diagnosis is often delayed more than 30 days. Typically, patients receive one or more courses of antibiotics for bacterial pneumonia before blastomycosis is considered. Clinical diagnosis must be confirmed by laboratory studies, which include microscopic examination of smears, scrapings, aspirates, sputum, and bronchoscopic washings for the characteristic yeast-like cells. Tissue examination often helps to make the diagnosis. Caseous necrosis usually is absent. Cutaneous lesions typically reveal pseudoepitheliomatous hyperplasia and budding yeasts in pyogranulomas that are characteristic and pathognomonic. In hematoxylin-and-eosin tissue sections, one often finds the characteristic yeast cells with a thick, double-refractive cell wall, but these may be difficult to see. Therefore, routine use should be made of special stains such as the periodic acid–Schiff and Gomori methenamine silver stain, which may help to differentiate *Histoplasma* and *Cryptococcus*. Culture methods can confirm the diagnosis. The infected material should be spread on the surface of Sabouraud dextrose agar slants and incubated at room temperature or 30°C (86°F). The yeast phase may be obtained in culture by inoculating glucose blood agar medium and incubating at 37°C (98.6°F). Because of poor sensitivity and specificity, serologic methods such as complement fixation and enzyme-linked immunosorbent assay (EIA) usually are not helpful. Newer EIA tests, using more purified antigens, show sensitivities of 80 to 88% and specificities of 98 to 100% in proven blastomycosis. EIA titers of ≥1:32 support the diagnosis of blastomycosis. Cross-reactivity with antigens of other fungi, particularly *Histoplasma*, makes low titers of these serologic tests difficult to interpret. Until specific antigen or PCR methods are introduced, definitive diagnosis of blastomycosis will depend on finding the organism in tissue, body fluids, or culture.

TREATMENT The prognosis for pulmonary or disseminated disease is generally good with appropriate therapy. Untreated, widely disseminated disease always has a poor prognosis. The treatment of choice for life-threatening or severe disease is amphotericin B. Ketoconazole and itraconazole are very effective in nonlife-threatening infections in adults, but the data on pharmacokinetics, safety, and efficacy of these drugs for children are insufficient. Itraconazole has fewer side effects than ketoconazole and is probably the preferred option. Small numbers of children have been treated for 6 months with 5 to 10 mg/kg daily dose of itraconazole. However, until more data are available, patients treated with itraconazole who fail to respond within 2 to 4 weeks, who have inadequate serum concentrations, or who develop clinical deterioration, should be switched to amphotericin B (see Sec. 13.5.1 and Table 13-62 for details of anti-fungal therapy).

References

Bradsher RW: Therapy of blastomycosis. Semin Respir Infect 12:263–267, 1997

Maxson S, Miller SF, Tryka AF, Schutze GE: Perinatal blastomycosis: a review. Pediatr Infect Dis J 11:760–763, 1992

Pappas PG: Blastomycosis in the immunocompromised patient. Semin Respir Infect 12:243–251, 1997

Schutze GE, Hickerson SL, Fortin EM, et al: Blastomycosis in children. Clin Infect Dis 22:496–502, 1996

Varkey B: Blastomycosis in children. Semin Respir Infect 12:235–242, 1997

13.5.4 *Candida* Species

Patricia M. Flynn and Aditya Gaur

Candida albicans, which belongs to Fungi Imperfecti or *Deuteromycetes,* has for decades been the most recognized pathogenic species of *Candida;* however, other species of *Candida* are becoming increasingly important. *Candida tropicalis* has emerged as a pathogen in the neutropenic host that is more pathogenic than *C. albicans. C. parapsilosis* is commonly seen in infections of patients having foreign devices such as peritoneal dialysis catheters and vascular access devices and has become the second most common candidal species isolated in catheter-associated infections in the nursery.

The various species of *Candida* most frequently colonize the mouth, gastrointestinal tract, and vaginal mucosa of humans and other animal species. The incidence of colonization depends on age and other characteristics of the population studied. Hospitalized and ill children are more often colonized than are normal, healthy children. Infection occurs when the usual balance between host and colonizing organism is disrupted. *Candida* species have become important nosocomial pathogens over the last two decades. Patients in the neonatal and surgical intensive care units appear to be at greatest risk and comprise 50% of those having nosocomial fungal infections nationwide. Patients on chemotherapy and HIV infected children and adolescents are also at risk. The most frequent nosocomial fungal infection is candidemia. Surveillance of nosocomial blood stream infections (BSI) between April 1995 and June 1996 revealed that *Candida* species were the fourth leading cause of nosocomial BSI in the United States. Increasing numbers of infections are caused by species other than *C. albicans* including *C. glabrata, C. tropicalis, C. parapsilosis, C. krusei,* and other *Candida* species. The increasing frequency of candidiasis caused by species other than *C. albicans* may be influenced by multiple factors: patient population, antimicrobial therapy, cytotoxic chemotherapy, underlying diseases, and antifungal therapy.

No single factor can be implicated in increased susceptibility to *Candida* infections. In the normal human, all components of the immune system respond to *Candida* infections. T-cell defects, such as those found in patients with chronic mucocutaneous candidiasis, predispose patients to chronic *Candida* infection typically at mucous membranes of the gastrointestinal or genitourinary tract. As the number of CD4+ lymphocytes decrease in children infected with HIV, the frequency of *Candida* infections increases in these patients. Chemotherapy with associated neutropenia, as well as other neutrophil disorders, places patients at risk of mucocutaneous and disseminated infection. Premature infants, especially those weighing less than 1500 g, represent another susceptible group, and may have underlying dysfunction of both cell-mediated and humoral immunity. Breaches in the continuity of natural barriers to infection, such as those created by central venous catheters and urinary catheters can lead to *Candida* infections. Diabetes mellitus increases susceptibility to local skin, mucous membrane, and urinary tract candidiasis, but it is uncertain whether these infections result from impaired neutrophil function or increased concentrations of available glucose, which is a primary nutrient for *Candida* species. The increased concentration of glycogen that is present in the vaginal secretions of pregnant women is believed to promote increased colonization during pregnancy.

CLINICAL MANIFESTATIONS AND TREATMENT Candidiasis can be divided into two broad categories based on the findings at clinical presentation: superficial infection of the skin and mucous membranes, or systemic infections that may be associated with fungemia or invasion of internal organs. Although both types of infections occur in the immunocompromised host, only infections of the skin and mucous membranes are diagnosed in the immunocompetent child.

Infections of the Skin

Cutaneous Candidiasis Cutaneous candidiasis is benign and usually involves wet, macerated skin in such areas as the perineum in infants or diabetic patients, and intertriginous areas in obese patients. As many as 10% of infants (peak age, 2–4 months) develop this disease. *Candida* diaper dermatitis appears as a bright red eruption on intertriginous areas, with sharp borders and pinpoint satellite papules and pustules. Examination of pustule contents or potassium hydroxide–prepared skin scrapings reveals the pseudohyphae. Treatment consists of drying the region and applying topical antifungals.

Infection of the nails can be particularly indolent and persistent. Dry, heaped-up, gray granulomatous tissue appears around and on top of the infected nail. Fingernails are more often infected than are toenails. Thumbsucking is a predisposing factor. Infection of the nails is diagnosed by examination of scrapings and smears, and by cultures.

Chronic Mucocutaneous Candidiasis Chronic mucocutaneous candidiasis occurs in patients with a complex immunodeficiency syndrome characterized by immune defects of T cells and mononuclear phagocytes. Chronic mucocutaneous candidiasis is an indolent, persistent infection of the mucous membranes (eg, mouth and vagina), skin (eg, forehead and scalp), and nails. Debilitating candidal esophagitis also may occur and can be the source of secondary life-threatening bacterial infection. Although rare, other opportunistic infections may occur in these children. The *Candida* infection can be partially managed with chronic ketoconazole or fluconazole therapy.

Infections of the Gastrointestinal Tract

Oropharyngeal Candidiasis The most common presentation is acute pseudomembranous candidiasis, also called thrush. It occurs in immunocompetent infants up to approximately 5 months of age. Beyond this age, it usually occurs only in patients who are immunocompromised, including debilitated children, or in those receiving antibiotic therapy. In the absence of antibiotic use, recurrent or recalcitrant thrush warrants investigation of the immune system.

Typically, the lesions appear as pearly white plaques on the mucosal surface of the oropharynx. Attempts to remove the plaques result in spots of punctate bleeding. *Candida albicans* is by far the most common cause. Other presentations observed are acute atrophic candidiasis (glossitis) presenting frequently with a painful tongue; angular cheilosis (perleche), especially with habitual licking; and chronic hyperplastic candidiasis whose symmetric white plaques cannot be rubbed off. Sucking blisters on the digits of infants represent spread from the mouth. Treatment primarily consists of topical nystatin or clotrimazole troches except in the immunocompromised host where fluconazole is used (Table 13-62). Topical therapy with nystatin or clotrimazole is recommended for treatment of oropharyngeal candidiasis. For immunocompromised patients or cases of failed topical therapy, fluconazole is effective.

Esophagitis Immunocompromised patients are at risk of esophagitis. Approximately half of patients with esophagitis have thrush. In children and adolescents, the first symptom of esophagitis is pain in the substernal area while swallowing; in infants, the first symptoms are reduced food intake and vomiting. The lower third of the esophagus is most often affected. A specific diagnosis can be made by esophagoscopy with washings or with biopsy, smear, and culture. Results of barium swallow tests may be normal early in the illness; however, studies done later may show decreased esophageal motility and, subsequently, ulceration (ie, the "moth-eaten appearance"). These findings are not specific, because bacterial or herpes simplex virus esophagitis can produce the same results. Therapy is indicated because of the potential for significant nutritional deficit or perforation. It is reasonable to begin empiric therapy in the symptomatic immunosuppressed patient who has not been examined by esophagoscopy (see also Sec. 17.11.1).

Gastrointestinal Candidiasis In immunocompromised hosts, disease can encompass the mucosal surfaces of the gastrointestinal tract beyond the esophagus. Although diarrhea and abdominal pain have reportedly occurred in patients with gastrointestinal candidiasis, it is difficult to determine whether these symptoms are related to the *Candida* infection or to underlying conditions, such as chemotherapy-induced sloughing of mucosa. *Candida* lesions, which are often found during postmortem exams of children who died of cancer, may have served as the point of origin for more severe *Candida* infections such as fungemia and disseminated disease.

Infections of the Genitourinary Tract

Cystitis Candida infections of the urinary tract are common and usually seen in immunocompromised hosts. In addition to diabetes mellitus, an indwelling bladder catheter and prolonged antibiotic therapy are common predisposing factors to *Candida* cystitis. The cystitis usually is asymptomatic, but it may be accompanied by urethritis and dysuria. Sometimes, mucosal ulcerations and white plaques are present at the urethral meatus. Diagnosis is readily made by microscopic examination of smear and culture of the urine. Treatment options include PO or IV fluconazole, low-dose IV amphotericin B, or 1 to 3 days of amphotericin B bladder irrigation (see Table 13-62).

It is important to distinguish cystitis from candiduria associated with systemic infection. Although candiduria is not always a dependable indicator of systemic or upper tract disease, candiduria in the neonate or the neutropenic host should prompt further investigation for systemic disease. Because candiduria may be indicative of obstructive uropathy or "fungus balls" in the calyces, imaging of the kidneys by ultrasonography or computed tomography is indicated. Obstructive uropathy can occur also in patients who have indwelling bladder catheters and who have been on prolonged antibiotic therapy.

Vaginitis A self-limiting but sometimes very annoying infection, *Candida* vaginitis occurs with greater frequency in women who use birth-control pills and in women who are pregnant. Vaginitis due to *C. albicans* does not necessarily imply immunosuppression. Patients with *Candida* vaginitis usually present with pruritus and vaginal discharge. Erythema with white, cheesy exudate is typical. Diagnosis relies on microscopic examination of smears and culture. Infection by *Trichomonas sp.* should be considered and evaluated. Vaginal candidiasis can be treated with topical application of azoles; however, a single 150-mg oral dose of fluconazole has been successfully used to treat the infection in adolescents and adults. *Candida* lesions of the penis rarely occur, even in the sexual partners of women with vaginitis.

Infections of the Respiratory Tract

Laryngeal Candidiasis When severely immunosuppressed children present with hoarseness of cry or voice, laryngeal candidiasis should be considered in the differential diagnosis. This entity has also been reported in children taking inhaled corticosteroids. Typical white plaques can be seen by laryngoscopy. Systemic therapy with fluconazole or amphotericin B is indicated.

Pneumonia Primary *Candida* pneumonitis is rare and usually results from the aspiration of heavily colonized oral secretions in a very debilitated or moribund person. Secondary *Candida* pneumonitis, which is more common than primary pneumonitis is a consequence of disseminated candidemia and manifests as "fungus balls." Under these circumstances, sputum examination usually is negative and thus unreliable. Positive cultures from sputum or bronchial washes cannot differentiate between colonization and invasive disease. Most clinicians use methods other than sputum examination, including lung biopsy, to determine whether a pulmonary infiltrate is caused by *Candida sp.* Amphotericin B is the treatment of choice for both types of *Candida pneumonitis*.

Systemic Candidiasis

Candida Sepsis Candidemia, the presence of *Candida sp.* in the blood, may represent the invasion of the organism from a mucosal surface such as the gastrointestinal or urinary tract, transient fungemia related to an intravascular device, or evidence of a deep-seated or disseminated infection. The source of *Candida sp.* is often impossible to determine, but it is usually endogenous in origin. A positive blood culture may indicate disease at other sites, and clinical symptoms may be nonspecific and include fever and malaise. Because of the difficulty in determining the source of *Candida sp.*, all types of *Candida* sepsis should be treated aggressively with antifungal agents. Mortality associated with candidemia is lower among children than among adults, and candiduria rarely precedes candidemia in children.

In some patients, evidence of candidemia may be present on skin or eye exam. The typical skin lesions are discrete, firm, erythematous papules that are 0.5 to 1.0 cm in diameter and often have nodular centers and erythematous halos. The aspirate can be smeared for Gram stain and cultured; yeasts are detected in biopsy material by a methenamine silver stain. The typical retinal lesions are white, cotton-like, chorioretinal abnormalities that may extend to the vitreous. Similar manifestations of the pathologic processes can occur in internal organs.

Hepatosplenic or disseminated candidiasis is now recognized in patients undergoing myelosuppressive therapy for cancer. Typically, the patient has fever with neutropenia that is not responsive to broad-spectrum antibiotics. After recovery of the neutrophil counts, fever may continue or recur. The patient may also develop right upper quadrant pain. Computed tomography or magnetic resonance imaging may show hypodense areas representing fungal abscesses in the liver, spleen, and kidneys. Diagnosis can usually be made by this typical appearance, but definitive diagnosis requires biopsy. Although histologic analysis of lesions will indicate the presence of *Candida sp.*, cultures are usually negative. A minimum of 4 to 6 weeks of amphotericin B therapy is indicated.

Because the risk of invasive *Candida* infection or sepsis increases with prolonged fever and neutropenia, it is now common practice to begin antifungal therapy in febrile neutropenic patients with cancer who have not become afebrile while on broad-spectrum antibiotics. Clinical studies suggest that empiric antifungal therapy should be started if the infection does not respond to antibiotic therapy after 7 days, but physicians at some centers are starting therapy before this time. Therapy for fungemia is presented in Table 13-62.

Neonates Neonates represent a special population at risk of *Candida* sepsis. Severe *Candida* vaginitis in the mother, a septic picture in the setting of an intravascular catheter, or sepsis that does not respond to appropriate antibacterial therapy should suggest the possibility of neonatal *Candida* sepsis. Although the source in neonatal sepsis is often not determined, potential transmission from patient to patient and from health-care worker to patient has been observed in neonatal intensive care units. Associated meningitis or arthritis has been noted with increasing frequency.

Cutaneous evidence of *Candida sp.* may be seen in as many as half of the neonates with *Candida* sepsis. These lesions are diffuse erythroderma or vesicopustules from which the organism can be cultured. Retinal exams are an important diagnostic tool in neonates with suspected *Candida* sepsis. Central nervous system (CNS) involvement occurs in as many as one-third to one-half of cases. Autopsy findings suggest that pneumonia occurs in as many as 70% of patients with disseminated candidemia. The presence of *Candida sp.* in endotracheal specimens is not clinically significant, except to indicate that the patient is colonized. Neonates can also develop obstructive uropathy secondary to "fungal balls" in the renal pelvis. Therapy for neonatal candidiasis typically involves amphotericin as outlined in Table 13-62.

Catheter-Related Infections Candidemia can occur in patients when an intravascular catheter is colonized with *Candida* species. The distinction between catheter-related candidemia and *Candida* sepsis is not clear in the literature. Some investigators suggest the two types of *Candida* infections can be distinguished by performing simultaneous quantitative blood cultures of specimens taken from all ports of the catheter as well as from a peripheral site. If the colony count from the catheter is 10 times that from the peripheral vein, then the catheter is usually the source. The findings of many studies support the need for immediate removal of the catheter as well as antifungal therapy when candidemia is documented. If the catheter is not removed, amphotericin B infusion should be alternated through all ports. The duration of fungemia in such cases may be prolonged.

Central Nervous System Candidiasis Primary candidiasis of the brain and meninges is rare; meningitis is usually seen in neonates or immunocompromised hosts. Because of the frequent concomitant occurrence of cardiac and CNS candidiasis, patients should be evaluated for both types of lesions when one of the two is found.

Signs and symptoms of CNS candidiasis are usually subtle, but in some cases they may be fulminant. Cerebrospinal fluid (CSF) findings may be unremarkable in the neutropenic host. Definitive diagnosis is made by isolating *Candida* from CSF cultures. Treatment should include amphotericin B; the addition of 5-fluorocytosine (5-FC) improves therapy across the blood-brain barrier. Fluconazole offers promise because of its excellent penetration into the CSF, but clinical experience with this drug in the treatment of *Candida* meningitis is limited. Because intraventricular administration of amphotericin B is associated with severe toxicity, it should be used only if other options are exhausted.

Ophthalmitis A careful examination of the retina is mandatory in any patient suspected of having systemic candidiasis. The typical lesions are white, cotton-like, chorioretinal abnormalities that may extend into the vitreous. *Candida* endophthalmitis has been found frequently in patients receiving parenteral nutrition, whereas *Candida* keratitis may occur in persons who have experienced trauma to the eye or as a secondary infection in patients whose primary keratitis resulted from other causes and was treated with topical antibiotics and steroids. Endophthalmitis should be treated with systemic antifungal agents, preferably amphotericin B, as it is a manifestation of disseminated disease. Keratitis can be treated topically in conjunction with close ophthalmologic follow-up.

Cardiac Candidiasis *Candida sp.* may affect the endocardium, myocardium, or pericardium. In a review of 319 cases of fungal endocarditis, 67% of the cases were caused by *Candida sp.* Studies also indicate a temporal relation between the introduction of central venous catheters in patients with cancer and an increase in incidence of *Candida* carditis. Signs and symptoms are similar to those of endocarditis resulting from other microorganisms, except that vegetations and emboli usually are large, and large vessels, including arteries, tend to become occluded. The valves most commonly involved are the aortic and mitral valves. Treatment includes valve replacement and systemic antifungal therapy, preferably with amphotericin B for a minimum of 6 weeks following surgery.

Arthritis and Osteomyelitis   *Candida* arthritis and osteomyelitis also indicate fungemia, but the source may not be apparent. *Candida* osteomyelitis has been identified in both infants and immunocompromised patients with cancer. The knee is the most frequently affected joint. Examination and culture of the aspirates are used to diagnose *Candida* arthritis. The recommended treatment is amphotericin B for a minimum of 6 weeks, as recommended for disseminated *Candida sp.* infection.

DIAGNOSIS   A presumptive diagnosis can be made if direct microscopic examination of clinical specimens indicates the presence of pseudohyphae and budding yeast forms. Samples obtained from surface lesions of the nail or skin scrapings can be mounted in 10 to 20% potassium hydroxide to obtain a clear background. Samples from other sites or culture isolates can either be directly examined in saline or stained using periodic acid–Schiff stain, Gomori methenamine silver stain, toluidine blue stain, or Gram stain. When cultured on a solid medium, such as Sabouraud dextrose agar, *Candida sp.* appear as white or creamy colonies that are moist, pasty, and well demarcated. Cornmeal agar with Tween 80 is one of the media used for better morphologic evaluation. When suspended in human sera, *C. albicans* is identified by germ-tube production; other species are identified by biochemical fermentation and assimilation tests. Radiometric blood culture systems and lysis-centrifugation (Isolator) methods provide more rapid detection of *Candida sp.* in blood.

Serologic tests for antibodies are usually inadequate. Patients in whom *Candida* sepsis develops frequently have been so immunocompromised that they do not develop antibodies to *Candida* antigens. Furthermore, if a patient can develop antibodies, it may be in response to colonization or to an infection that does not require systemic therapy.

A variety of tests have been used to detect *Candida sp.* antigens or metabolites in blood or other body fluids. However, the clinical application of these procedures is not yet defined.

PREVENTION   Use of topical nystatin, amphotericin B, and azole agents have failed to reduce the incidence of serious *Candida* infections in patients with cancer. Results from studies of the prophylactic use of fluconazole have been mixed. Some studies report a reduction in mucous membrane and systemic fungal infections in certain populations of patients who received prophylactic antifungal agents; however, other studies also indicate a selective increase in infections with drug-resistant strains such as *C. krusei*.

The venous catheter site of any patient needing long-term intravenous alimentation requires meticulous care; such care should include changes of the dry gauze dressing every 48 hours and application of a povidone-iodine solution, which is fungistatic and bacteriostatic. Transparent dressings are associated with an increased incidence of catheter-related infections. Hand washing and attention to infection control policy are important in preventing nosocomial spread.

References

Augustin J, Lacson S, Raffalli J, Aguero-Rosenfeld ME, Wormser GP: Failure of a lipid amphotericin B preparation to eradicate candiduria: pre-

liminary findings based on three cases. Clin Infect Dis 29:686–687, 1999

Pfaller MA, Jones RN, Doern GV, et al: for the SENTRY Participant Group: International surveillance of bloodstream infections due to *Candida sp:* frequency of occurrence and antifungal susceptibilities of isolates collected in 1997 in the United States, Canada, and South America for the SENTRY program. J Clin Microbiol 36:1886–1889, 1998

Pfaller MA, Jones RN, Messer SA, et al: and the SCOPE Participant Group: National surveillance of nosocomial bloodstream infection due to species of *Candida* other than *Candida albicans:* frequency of occurrence and antifungal susceptibility in the SCOPE program. Diagn Microbiol Infect Dis 30:121–129, 1998

Stamos JK, Rowley AH: Candidemia in a pediatric population. Clin Infect Dis 20:571–575, 1995

Walsh TJ, Gonzales C, Lyman CA, Chanock SJ, Pizzo PA: Invasive fungal infections in children: recent advances in diagnosis and treatment. In: Aronoff SC, Hughes WT, Kohl S, Speck WT, Wald ER, eds: Advances in Pediatric Infectious Diseases, vol 11. St. Louis, MO, Mosby, 1996: 187–290.

13.5.5   Coccidioidomycosis

Mark R. Schleiss

Coccidioidomycosis is the infection caused by the dimorphic fungus, *Coccidioides immitis.* The life cycle of *C. immitis* demonstrates two distinct phases: a saprophytic (vegetative) phase and a parasitic phase. In soil, the organism grows as a mycelium, with branching septated hyphae. As they mature, the mycelia develop rectangular spores (arthroconidia); at this stage the hyphae become very fragile, and arthroconidia easily become airborne. When inhaled, the arthroconidia begin the parasitic phase and spherules form. Spherules are round, double-walled structures that reproduce by formation of spherical internal spores, termed endospores. A single spherule may produce thousands of endospores, and as the spherule ruptures, each endospore may, in turn, develop into a new spherule, perpetuating the parasitic phase.

Coccidioides immitis appears to be confined to the Western hemisphere. The endemic areas lie in the southwestern United States, encompassing west Texas, New Mexico, Arizona, and California. The organism can also be found in northwestern Mexico and in a few small areas of Central and South America. These endemic areas have arid climates, hot summers, few winter freezes, low altitude, and alkaline soil—ecologic conditions that favor *C. immitis.* The organism is drought resistant, and periodic increases in cases are observed when prolonged drought is followed by heavy rains. Arthroconidia may become airborne after windstorms or disruption of soil by farming or construction work. Because infection requires that arthroconidia be inhaled, person-to-person transmission does not play a role in acquisition of coccidioidomycosis.

CLINICAL MANIFESTATIONS

Primary Infection   The primary portal of entry in most patients is the lung, via the inhalation of arthroconidia, although the organism may enter through the skin. Accordingly, signs and symptoms of respiratory tract infection represent the major clinical manifestations. The majority of individuals with acute coccidioidomycosis have either asymptomatic infection or mild upper respiratory tract symptoms. Approximately 40% of patients with primary infection develop a more severe systemic illness 1 to 3 weeks after exposure, characterized by cough, malaise, fever, chills, night sweats, anorexia, and weakness. Lower respiratory tract illness may include pneumonia and parapneumonic effusion. Chest pain may be quite severe in some patients, and hemoptysis is commonly encountered in adult patients, although it is rare in children. The radiographic appearance of acute coccidioidomycosis is nonspecific. Bronchopneumonic infiltrate associated with hilar adenopathy is the most common presentation, although an interstitial pattern may be encountered. Widespread intrathoracic disease ("miliary pattern") may be encountered with disseminated infection.

An important diagnostic clue in patients with primary coccidioidomycosis is the presence of cutaneous manifestations. The most common skin manifestation of acute coccidioidomycosis is erythema nodosum—painful, tender lesions on the anterior tibial surface. The appearance of these lesions, known in California as "valley bumps," correlates with the development of cell-mediated immunity and is associated with a lower risk of dissemination. Although not specific for coccidioidomycosis, the finding of erythema nodosum in a child residing in an endemic area is highly suggestive of recent acute coccidioidomycosis. Less commonly, erythema multiforme may be present, which is also assumed to be immunologically mediated. Primary cutaneous infection with *C. immitis* is rare, with most cases being attributed to laboratory accidents. The skin may also be a target organ in the setting of disseminated infection (see below).

Disseminated Coccidioidomycosis Approximately 0.5% of patients with acute coccidioidomycosis develop disseminated infection. Dissemination is more common in men, pregnant women, and in certain ethnic groups (individuals of African, Mexican, or Filipino ancestry). Major sites of disseminated disease include bones, joints, visceral organs, and the central nervous system.

Local pain is the usual hallmark of musculoskeletal coccidioidomycosis, with warmth and swelling accompanying the systemic symptoms of infection. More than one-third of cases of disseminated coccidioidomycosis are complicated by osteomyelitis, which is unifocal in most cases. Any bone can become infected, but the most commonly involved sites are skull, metacarpals, metatarsals, spine, and tibia. Bone scans are more sensitive than plain radiographs in making the diagnosis. When present, vertebral lesions tend to be multiple and pose a high risk for central nervous system (CNS) spread. Tendinitis, synovitis, or frank arthritis may result from bloodstream dissemination. Swelling and tenderness are present, with the ankle and knee being the most commonly involved sites. Fungus can usually be cultured from the affected synovial fluid, and synovial biopsy is indicated in suspect cases.

Meningitis is a serious complication of disseminated coccidioidomycosis. It typically presents within the first 6 months following primary infection. Importantly, the signs of meningeal irritation common in bacterial meningitis are generally absent. Headache is the most common symptom. Fever, weakness, vomiting, focal neurologic deficits, and meningismus may occur, but many patients are asymptomatic; therefore, any patient with disseminated coccidioidomycosis should probably undergo lumbar puncture, irrespective of symptoms. Cerebrospinal fluid (CSF) analysis typically shows a mononuclear pleocytosis, with decreased glucose and elevated protein levels. Meningitis may be associated with parenchymal involvement evident on magnetic resonance imaging (MRI). The course of coccidioidomycosis meningitis is often chronic. Hydrocephalus is a common complication. *Coccidioides immitis* is rarely recovered from cerebrospinal fluid, but complement-fixing antibodies for coccidioidin are present in almost all cases.

Other manifestations of disseminated coccidioidomycosis may include seeding of visceral organs, genitourinary tract infection,

ophthalmic complications (chorioretinitis), and cutaneous infection. Muscle involvement may occur in disseminated cases, with occasional development of abscesses or draining sinus tracts. Pregnant women are at high risk of dissemination, and the placenta is often involved in obstetric coccidioidomycosis, although transplacental infection of the fetus appears to be relatively uncommon. Infection in the newborn may also be acquired via the birth canal. The mortality of disseminated disease is higher in neonates than in older children or adults.

Immunocompromised Patients In recent years *C. immitis* has emerged as a major pathogen in immunocompromised patients, particularly those with HIV infection. *Coccidioides immitis* also has an enhanced pathogenic potential in other immunosuppressed patients, such as organ transplant recipients, children with congenital immunodeficiencies, and patients on immunosuppressive therapies. Coccidioidomycosis in immunocompromised patients represents a mix of new and reactivated infections. Diffuse pulmonary disease is common, and lung biopsy is often required to make the diagnosis. Extrapulmonary disease may be difficult to eradicate, necessitating chronic suppressive therapy (see below). Even a remote history of residence or travel to an endemic area should be sought, because the major problem in making the diagnosis is a lack of suspicion of the possibility of coccidioidomycosis.

DIAGNOSIS Demonstration of the organism by examination and culture of clinical specimens is the most reliable way to establish the diagnosis. Sputum, joint fluid, bronchoalveolar lavage fluid, soft-tissue aspirates, and deep-tissue surgical specimens offer the best yield by culture. CSF culture is positive only about one-third of the time, and when the diagnosis of meningitis is being considered, multiple lumbar punctures may increase the diagnostic yield. It is important to remember that cultures of *C. immitis* represent a potentially severe biological hazard. Laboratory personnel should be alerted to the possibility of the diagnosis prior to processing of specimens. Microscopic examination of clinical specimens may be useful, to search for the presence of endospore-containing spherules. Fine-needle aspiration of suspect lesions in soft tissue or bone, synovial biopsies, and skin biopsies all provide suitable specimens for histopathologic evaluation.

Serology may be helpful in making the diagnosis of coccidioidomycosis. The mycelial phase antigen, coccidioidin, is the most important target of antibody response. Serum IgM antibodies ("precipitins") can be detected 1 to 3 weeks after onset of symptoms in the majority of cases and are readily identifiable by a variety of immunodiffusion, latex agglutination, or enzyme immunoassay methods. Complement-fixing serum IgG antibodies (CFA) appear later in the course of infection, and usually decline 6 to 8 months after primary infection, although antibody may continue to be detectable for years. The CFA titer is a useful marker of disease activity. Sera should be run in paired fashion (acute and convalescent) for titer comparison. Rising titers are a bad prognostic sign, whereas falling titers suggest improvement. In patients with meningitis, CFA is present in CSF in a majority of patients, and titers parallel the course of meningeal disease.

Skin tests may also be used to make the diagnosis of coccidioidomycosis. Most patients with symptomatic primary infections will have a positive test (>5-mm induration) within 1 month of disease onset. Patients with erythema nodosum may have a severe response to skin tests, because of their particularly intense delayed-type hypersensitivity response to coccidioidin antigen. Cutaneous anergy is common in individuals with disseminated coccidioidomycosis, and a negative skin test in such patients does not exclude the diagnosis.

TREATMENT The decision to initiate antifungal therapy in the setting of coccidioidomycosis depends upon the extent of disease. Although most patients with symptomatic primary infection recover spontaneously, treatment is mandated in several clinical settings. Once disease has spread outside the lung (bone, joint, and soft-tissue infections, genitourinary tract infections, and CNS involvement), antifungal therapy is almost always warranted. In certain circumstances, individuals with symptomatic primary infection should also be treated, even if disease appears to be limited to the lungs, because the risk of dissemination is high. These patients include pregnant women, young infants, the immunocompromised, and individuals with chronic or debilitating illnesses. The CFA titer at time of diagnosis is also of predictive value in making decisions regarding therapy. Disseminated disease is rarely seen if the CFA titer is 1:32 or less. Therefore, titers of >1:32 may represent an indication for therapy in symptomatic primary infection, irrespective of other clinical findings.

For severe, life-threatening infections, particularly in immunocompromised patients, amphotericin B is the drug of choice. The total dose depends on the severity of disease: most children respond to a total cumulative dose of between 15 and 45 mg/kg, although as much as 100 mg/kg has been used for severe, protracted illness. Ketoconazole has been successfully used in children with symptomatic primary infection. The dose range is from 5 to 20 mg/kg/d in a single daily dose, with a higher dose for skeletal or CNS infection. Recently, fluconazole and itraconazole have largely replaced ketoconazole as treatment alternatives to amphotericin B. *Coccidioides immitis* meningitis represents a special circumstance regarding treatment. Prior to the advent of the newer azoles, prolonged intraventricular administration of amphotericin B (via an Ommaya reservoir) was the standard treatment for meningitis. However, because of its outstanding CNS penetration and demonstrated efficacy, fluconazole has become the drug of choice for the treatment of coccidioidal meningitis. Because of the extremely high risk of relapse, the course of treatment is life-long.

References

Catanzaro A, Galgiani JN, Levine BE, et al: Fluconazole in the treatment of chronic pulmonary and non-meningeal disseminated coccidioidomycosis. NIAID Mycosis Study Group. Am J Med 98:249–256, 1995

Dewsnup DH, Galgiani JN, Graybill JR, et al: Is it ever safe to stop azole therapy for *Coccidioides immitis* meningitis? Ann Intern Med 124:305–310, 1996

Galgiani JN: Coccidioidomycosis. Curr Clin Top Infect Dis 17:188–204, 1997

Kafka JA, Catanzaro A: Disseminated coccidioidomycosis in children. J Pediatr 98:355–361, 1981

Walsh TJ, Gonzalez C, Lyman CA, Chanock SJ, Pizzo PA: Invasive fungal infections in children: recent advances in diagnosis and treatment. Adv Pediatr Infect Dis 11:187–290, 1996

13.5.6   Cryptococcosis

Deborah Lehman

Cryptococcosis is a sporadic, cosmopolitan mycotic disease that is caused by *Cryptococcus neoformans,* a yeast-like fungus that reproduces by budding and varies from 4 to 20 μm in diameter. Its mucopolysaccharide capsule aids in its identification in body fluids and tissues.

Cryptococcosis can occur in otherwise healthy people, although normal children are not frequently infected. Susceptibility to the disease is markedly increased in those with T-cell immune dysfunction, as is seen in leukemia, Hodgkin disease, HIV infections, and prolonged therapy with corticosteroids. The incidence of cryptococcal infections has been steadily increasing over the past decade as a result of the AIDS epidemic and more aggressive uses of immunosuppressive medications for organ transplantation. Cryptococcosis is now the most common life-threatening fungal infection in patients infected with HIV, occurring in approximately 5 to 10% of patients with AIDS.

Common reservoirs are soil and avian excrement. The organism withstands prolonged drying and can persist in the soil for long periods of time. Pigeons are a frequent source, but cases have been linked to other birds, including starlings. The birds themselves are probably not infected, but their excreta serve as excellent culture medium for the organisms. Most cases are avian related and are caused by *Cryptococcus neoformans* var. *neoformans.* One variant of *C. neoformans,* var. *gattii,* has been ecologically associated with eucalyptus trees in tropical regions.

CLINICAL MANIFESTATIONS Infection usually is acquired by inhaling the organisms. Disease may localize in the pulmonary parenchyma and cause an isolated pneumonitis or hematogenously disseminate to any organ of the body. The central nervous system is the most common site of infection, and cryptococcus is the most frequent cause of fungal meningitis. Other sites of infection, such as bone, joint, eye, skin, and placenta, have been reported. In HIV-infected patients, cryptococcal infections most commonly occur when the CD4 count falls below 50 cells/mm^3.

Central Nervous System Cryptococcosis Cryptococcal infection of the central nervous system is frequently indolent, presenting with nonspecific symptoms such as fever and headache. Focal neurologic deficits and altered mental status are less common and are seen in more advanced disease. Cryptococcal meningitis shares many clinical and laboratory features with tuberculous meningitis. The cerebrospinal fluid (CSF) usually reveals lymphocytosis, elevated protein levels, and reduced glucose levels. However, in AIDS patients, CSF parameters may be unremarkable. Untreated cryptococcal meningoencephalitis is generally fatal over weeks to months.

Pulmonary Cryptococcosis Pulmonary infection can be asymptomatic and discovered incidentally as a solitary nodule during radiography. When clinically apparent, however, pulmonary disease may be associated with cough productive of mucoid sputum, chest pain, fever, weight loss, night sweats, and occasional hemoptysis. Chest radiographs may show interstitial or focal infiltrates, lymphadenopathy, or, rarely, pleural effusions. Definitive diagnosis of pulmonary cryptococcosis is best made by biopsy, because asymptomatic colonization can occur.

DIAGNOSIS AND TREATMENT The demonstration of budding organisms in India ink wet preparations of the CSF establishes the diagnosis; presence of budding is essential to avoid mistaking leukocytes for yeast. The India ink preparation has an increased sensitivity for patients with AIDS as a consequence of the higher number of organisms seen in these patients. In the absence of AIDS, the sensitivity of India ink is less than 50%.

The most rapid and reliable way to diagnose cryptococcal infection is to demonstrate cryptococcal antigen in either serum or CSF. Latex agglutination tests on both cerebrospinal fluid and serum have sensitivity close to 100% in patients with AIDS, but a lower specificity as a result of some cross-reactions with other organisms. Often, the only manifestation of cryptococcosis is cryptococcal antigenemia, and the serum antigen test is useful both for screening and follow-up in symptomatic patients with advanced HIV disease.

PREVENTION AND TREATMENT Prospective controlled trials show that the oral azole agent fluconazole can reduce the incidence of cryptococcal disease in patients with advanced AIDS. However, because the incidence of cryptococcal disease is relatively low and the prophylactic therapy potentially toxic, prophylaxis is not routinely recommended. Cryptococcal meningitis currently is treated with high-dose amphotericin B (0.8 mg/kg/d) or a combination of this drug with 5-flucytosine (5-FC). Several studies demonstrated the superiority of high-dose amphotericin B in combination with 5-FC as initial therapy for cryptococcal meningitis. This regimen results in higher rates of CSF sterilization and lower mortality. The use of 5-FC in patients with AIDS can be problematic because of the concomitant use of other bone marrow suppressive drugs. Recent studies concluded that fluconazole is the preferred drug for use as consolidation and maintenance therapy following an initial 2-week induction with amphotericin B and 5-FC. Because the cure rate in central nervous system cryptococcosis does not exceed 75%, and because relapses are common, patients require lifelong suppressive therapy with an azole agent.

References

Aberg JA, Powderly WG: Cryptococcal disease: implications of recent clinical trials on treatment and management. AIDS Clin Rev 229–298, 1997–8

Dismukes WE, Cloud G, Gallis HA, et al: Treatment of cryptococcal meningitis with combination amphotericin B and flucytosine for four as compared with six weeks. N Engl J Med 317:334, 1987

Larsen RA, Bozette SA, Jones BE, et al: Fluconazole combined with flucytosine for treatment of cryptococcal meningitis in patients with AIDS. Clin Infect Dis 19:741–745, 1994

Van der Horst CM, Saag MS, Cloud GA, et al: Treatment of cryptococcal meningitis associated with the acquired immunodeficiency syndrome. N Engl J Med 337:15–21, 1997

13.5.7   Histoplasmosis

Martin B. Kleiman

Histoplasmosis, the most common endemic fungal infection in the United States, is caused by a thermal dimorphic fungus, *Histoplasma capsulatum*. The spore-bearing mold form grows at temperatures less than 37°C (98.6°F) and is commonly found in the Mississippi and Ohio River basins. The extent and degree of environmental contamination with the mold is augmented by bird droppings, which may contain spores, as well as provide factors that stimulate mold growth.

Rates of histoplasmal skin test reactivity in endemic areas increase progressively with age (Fig. 13-15). Infections occur as sporadic cases, as community-wide outbreaks when dry windy conditions facilitate aerosolization of spores, and as localized clusters caused by disturbance of heavily contaminated microenvironments.

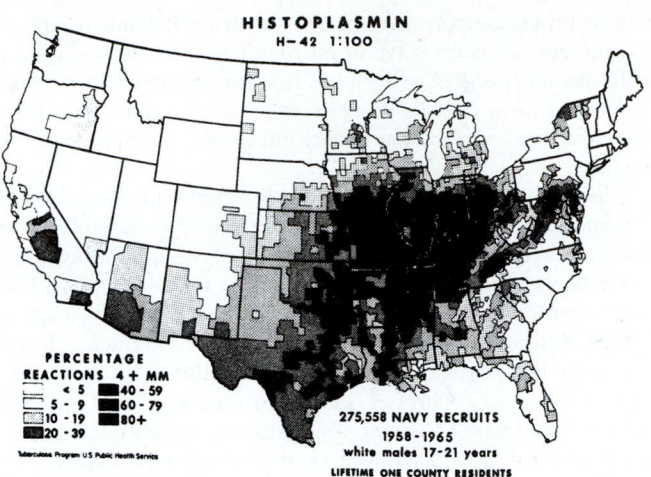

FIGURE 13-15   Geographic variation in the frequency of reactors to histoplasmin. SOURCE: *Edwards LB, Acquaviva FA, Livesay VT, et al: An Atlas of sensitivity to tuberculin, PPD-B, and histoplasmin in the United States. Am Rev Respir Dis 99:S1-132, 1969.*

Such hyperendemic foci include heavily contaminated soil, sites of bird roosts, bat-infested caves, rotting logs, and old structures.

Infection begins following inhalation of microaeruliospores, which convert in the alveoli to the yeast-like invasive forms. This results in a focus of acute pneumonitis and regional hilar adenitis. In addition to this primary focus, yeast forms also disseminate lymphohematogenously to the reticuloendothelial organs; normal cellular immune mechanisms abort further progression in the vast majority of cases. Following the development of specific cellular immunity, inflammatory changes become granulomatous with typical Langhans-type giant cells; fibrosis and calcification ensue. Although specific antibodies develop in response to infection, they do not appear to play a significant role in recovery and are not protective.

CLINICAL MANIFESTATIONS   The type and severity of symptoms reflect both the intensity of exposure and the adequacy of the host's cellular immune response. Primary infection is asymptomatic in 99% of normal hosts who are lightly exposed. Most of the remainder develop nonspecific, transient, flu-like respiratory symptoms. Infection is symptomatic in about half of otherwise normal patients who are more heavily exposed. In these patients, fever, cough, and chest pain are common; chest radiographs often show pneumonitis and/or hilar adenopathy. Symptoms are almost always self-limited and resolve within 2 weeks without treatment. Infrequently, the fever, weight loss, and fatigue persist and antifungal therapy is required. Intense exposure of immunocompetent hosts can cause severe, life-threatening illness with fever, respiratory distress, diffuse reticulonodular chest infiltrates, and sometimes progressive dissemination.

Abnormalities of cellular immune function, whether primary, acquired, or a result of relative immaturity or infancy, are risk factors for disseminating histoplasmosis. Children with AIDS are highly susceptible. Severe and disseminating infection can follow either primary disease or reactivation of a quiescent focus in these children. Illness usually begins with fever with no localizing symptoms and weight loss; if untreated, maculopapular skin lesions, pulmonary infiltrates, mucosal ulcerations, and pancytopenia may be seen. This manifestation of histoplasmosis is fatal if untreated. Histoplasmosis in patients receiving chemotherapy for neoplastic disorders or immunosuppressive therapy for nonmalignant conditions may present with fever, a syndrome of diffuse interstitial pulmonary infiltrates, and progressive hypoxia. In these children, symptoms are similar to those caused by cytomegalovirus, respiratory viruses, *Pneumocystis carinii,* or many other infectious or noninfectious etiologies.

The relative immaturity of cellular immunity in otherwise normal infants may predispose to disseminated histoplasmosis of infancy, a rare but life-threatening infection of children younger than 1 year of age. In these infants, despite what may be relatively minimal exposure to histoplasmal spores, there is heavy parasitization of the reticuloendothelial system, which further augments the cellular immune dysfunction. The humoral immune response remains intact and disease progresses, despite markedly elevated histoplasmal antibody titers. The onset of symptoms is usually insidious with only failure-to-thrive, variable fever, absent toxicity, and progressive hepatosplenomegaly. After about 4 to 6 weeks, pancytopenia and disseminated coagulopathy occur. Mucosal and gastrointestinal ulcerations and hemorrhage often accompany late symptoms; chest radiographic abnormalities may remain absent. Disseminated histoplasmosis of infancy is fatal if untreated.

Less common manifestations of histoplasmosis result either from hypersensitivity reactions to fungal antigens or from focal infections of lymph nodes or other organ systems. Focal reactions to localized infections may cause pulmonary infarction, extrinsic compression of bronchi or the hepatobiliary tract, parotitis, interstitial nephritis, focal cerebritis, or meningitis. Hypersensitivity results from a vigorous cellular immune response; arthritis, pericarditis, or erythema nodosum are most common. Hypercalcemia with nephrocalcinosis has also been a presenting manifestation. Mediastinal fibrosis which may cause stenosis/obstruction of great vessels and bronchi may be a late sequela of histoplasmosis.

DIAGNOSIS The majority of infections are subclinical or self-limited and do not require laboratory confirmation. The recognition of chest radiographic findings of typical granulomas in otherwise well patients who reside in endemic areas infrequently requires laboratory confirmation. Laboratory diagnosis is needed to evaluate patients with symptoms that may mimic those caused by other pathogens, especially symptoms caused by *Mycobacterium tuberculosis, Blastomyces dermatitidis,* or other causes of granulomatous inflammation. Laboratory diagnosis is also required to reasonably exclude a malignancy in patients with hilar or mediastinal adenopathy. Lastly, confirmation of the diagnosis is indicated for all patients who require antifungal treatment.

Specific laboratory tests used to diagnose histoplasmosis include culture, histopathologic examination of biopsy specimens, serologic testing, and antigen assay. Direct observation of typical yeast forms in tissue or body fluids and/or isolation of the fungus in culture are diagnostic. The blood, bone marrow, and urine are potential sites from which the organism can be isolated, but cultures are usually negative in mild or moderately severe infections. Disadvantages of these methods are their low sensitivities, a delay of 2 weeks required to isolate the fungus in culture, and the need for an invasive procedure to obtain tissue.

The sensitivity and specificity of antibody and antigen assays are variable, and interpretation must weigh the index of suspicion and the host's immunocompetence. Serologic tests are used most frequently for diagnosis. A single complement-fixation (CF) titer >1:16 to either the yeast or mycelial phase antigen, or the detection of H or M bands by the immunodiffusion method, strongly suggests acute or recent infection. Disadvantages of both serologic

tests are that they cross-react with other fungal antibodies, may remain elevated for 18 months following infection, or may be falsely negative in immunocompromised patients. A radioimmunoassay (RIA) that semiquantitatively detects histoplasmal antigen in urine and serum is an important rapid diagnostic test. Although insensitive in mild infections, the RIA is usually positive in serious disease, especially in progressively disseminating infections. The RIA is also used to monitor AIDS patients because they remain at considerable risk for relapse after treatment is stopped. Rising concentrations of histoplasmal urine antigen are predictive of clinical relapse. Although the histoplasmal RIA also cross-reacts with other fungal antigens, especially other dimorphic fungi, the clinical findings and the patient's exposure risk assessment usually allow accurate interpretation.

The histoplasmal skin test becomes positive 3 to 4 weeks following infection in immunocompetent hosts, and remains positive lifelong. Unless a recent conversion can be documented, it cannot distinguish recent from past infection and is therefore not useful for diagnosis. It is a convenient epidemiologic tool.

TREATMENT Most patients with histoplasmosis improve without antifungal treatment. Treatment is required for severe and/or progressively disseminating infections, for patients with prolonged symptoms (usually exceeding 2 weeks), and for patients with primary or acquired cellular immune dysfunction (see Table 13-62). Rheumatologic or hypersensitivity symptoms, such as arthritis, pericarditis, or erythema nodosum usually improve with supportive treatment. Pericarditis usually responds promptly to indomethacin.

Amphotericin B was the first antimicrobial agent found to be effective for treating histoplasmosis. It remains the recommended initial drug for treating severe infections, because it results in more rapid improvement than do newer agents, although controlled trials have not been done in children. Itraconazole is also effective for treating histoplasmosis and has the advantages of an oral route of administration and few side effects. Its chief disadvantages are its considerable cost and variable absorption. It may be used for initial treatment of nonlife-threatening infections or following induction with amphotericin B in critically ill patients. Treatment should be continued for 6 months. Absorption is improved if taken with Coca Cola Classic, and adequate serum concentrations should be confirmed (available through the Histoplasmosis Reference Laboratory, Indianapolis, Indiana). Care must be taken to avoid drug interactions (see Table 13-63). Itraconazole is also effective as secondary prophylaxis following successful treatment of histoplasmosis in patients with AIDS or in those who have had documented relapse. Secondary prophylaxis should be continued lifelong.

A brief course of steroids is often useful adjunctive treatment for patients in whom acutely inflamed lymph nodes impinge or obstruct adjacent structures. Effective antifungal agents should always be used concomitantly and the patient carefully monitored for signs of progressive infection while receiving steroids. Mediastinal fibrosis without active infection does not benefit from steroids or antifungal agents.

Prevention of infection requires avoidance of exposure. Digging at sites of bird roosts; cutting firewood; exploring bat-infested caves; cleaning/renovating basements, attics, fireplaces, or wall insulation in older homes or buildings; or being in the vicinity of excavation sites in dry or windy conditions may result in exposure to histoplasmal spores. If such activities are unavoidable, efficient, protective masks should be used, especially by those persons with compromised immune systems.

References

Fojtasek MF, Kleiman MB, Connolly-Stringfield P, et al: The *Histoplasma capsulatum* antigen assay in disseminated histoplasmosis in children. Pediatr Infect Dis J 13:801–805, 1994

Leggiadro RJ, Barrett RD, Hughes WT: Disseminated histoplasmosis of infancy. Pediatr Infect Dis J 7:799–805, 1986

Wheat LJ, Connolly-Stringfield P, Kohler RB: *Histoplasma capsulatum* polysaccharide antigen detection in diagnosis and management of disseminated histoplasmosis in patients with acquired immunodeficiency syndrome. Am J Med 87:396–400, 1989

Wheat LJ, Kohler RB, Tewari RP: Diagnosis of disseminated histoplasmosis by detection of *Histoplasma capsulatum* antigen in serum and urine specimens. N Engl J Med 314:83–88, 1986

13.5.8　Malassezia Furfur

Dwight A. Powell

The genus *Malassezia* includes two species: *M. furfur* and *M. pachydermatis. Malassezia furfur* causes superficial dermatosis, tinea versicolor, papulopustular folliculitis, and systemic infections. *Malassezia pachydermatis* is associated with systemic disease. Unlike *M. pachydermatis, M. furfur* requires lipid supplementation of standard fungal growth media for isolation. When standard fungal media is overlaid with sterile olive oil, *M. furfur* grows within 3 days.

CLINICAL MANIFESTATIONS　Tinea versicolor is a scaling dermatosis that is limited to the stratum corneum, usually involving small areas of the back or trunk, but extensive infection is possible (see Sec. 14.12.6). Lesions are characterized by slightly scaling hypopigmented or hyperpigmented patches with skip regions of normal skin in between. *Malassezia furfur* occurs as normal flora on 90 to 100% of adolescents and adults; in those who develop tinea versicolor, the yeast phase transforms to the mycelial phase. Heat, moisture, and skin occlusion favor this transformation.

Malassezia furfur is linked to seborrheic dermatitis in normal hosts, but this may not hold true for the type of seborrheic dermatitis seen in patients with AIDS. Folliculitis resulting from *Malassezia* may resemble the lesion of disseminated candidiasis. This acneiform lesion presents as follicle-limited inflammatory papules or papulopustules. It is most commonly seen over the back and chest of patients with AIDS or of those receiving broad-spectrum antibiotics or steroids. *Malassezia furfur* is reported to cause eosinophilic pustular folliculitis with pruritus in patients with AIDS, and in its papular form, this lesion is pathologically a vasculitis of the dermis. This papulopustular dermatitis responds to topical or systemic imidazole therapy. Discontinuation of steroids or antibiotics also is helpful. Recently, *M. furfur* was described as a cause of papulopustular eruptions on the face of newborns.

Malassezia furfur is a cause of culture-negative septicemia in patients receiving IV lipid feedings or total parenteral nutrition. A characteristic syndrome is noted, particularly in neonates, of fever, bilateral interstitial pulmonary infiltrates, leukocytosis, and thrombocytopenia. This syndrome also has been reported in immunecompromised adults and children with central venous catheters who were not receiving concurrent IV lipids. *Malassezia pachydermatis* is also associated with systemic sepsis in infants. At least two nursery outbreaks have been reported; in one, colonization of health-care workers by their pet dogs was believed to be a possible source of infection.

DIAGNOSIS AND TREATMENT　Diagnosis can be made by examination of skin scales (ie, scrapings) from affected areas that demonstrate hyphae and yeast forms in a characteristic "spaghetti and meatballs" pattern. In sepsis caused by contamination of lipid infusions, routine blood cultures are negative, but isolation of the organism is enhanced by culture of blood aspirates from the central catheter in lipid-supplemented media or in lysis centrifugation systems (DuPont Isolator, Wilmington, DE).

Tinea versicolor can be managed with topical 2.5% selenium sulfide, imidazole creams, or 1% terbinafine cream. Studies are pending on the use of systemic itraconazole or fluconazole. Recurrence within 1 to 2 years is common.

Ketoconazole is currently being evaluated for the treatment of seborrheic dermatitis.

For sepsis, therapy includes removal of the venous catheter that was used for alimentation and interruption of lipid feedings. A short course of therapy with amphotericin B may be indicated, particularly if a new deep line is placed. Both *M. furfur* and *M. pachydermatis* respond to amphotericin B.

References

Barber GR, Brown AE, Kiehn TE, Edwards FF, Armstrong D: Catheter-related *Malassezia furfur* fungemia in immunocompromised patients. Am J Med 95:365–370, 1993

Chang HJ, Miller HL, Watkins N, et al: An epidemic of *Malassezia pachydermatis* in an intensive care nursery associated with colonization of health-care workers' pet dogs. N Engl J Med 338:706–711, 1998

Klotz SA: *Malassezia furfur*. Infect Dis Clin North Am 3:53, 1989

Larocco M, Dorenbaum A, Robinson A, et al: Recovery of *Malassezia pachydermatis* from eight infants in a neonatal intensive care nursery: clinical and laboratory features. Pediatr Infect Dis J 7:398–401, 1988

Marcon MJ, Powell DA: Human infections due to *Malassezia spp.* Clin Microbiol Rev 5:101–119, 1992

Marcon MJ, Powell DA, Durrell DE: Methods for optimal recovery of *Malassezia furfur* from blood culture. J Clin Microbiol 245:696, 1987

Rapelonoro R, Mortureux P, Couprie B, et al: Neonatal *Malassezia furfur* pustulosis. Arch Dermatol 132:190–193, 1996

Sunenshine PJ, Schwartz RA, Janninger CK: Tinea versicolor. Int J Dermatol 37:648–655, 1998

13.5.9　Sporotrichosis

Donna M. Nobile and Martin B. Kleiman

Sporotrichosis is an uncommon, chronic mycosis caused by *Sporothrix schenckii*, a ubiquitous plant saprophyte, dimorphic fungus that grows as a mold at room temperature and as a yeast-like form in tissue. Although distributed worldwide, it is found most commonly in warm, highly humid regions and in temperate climates. Mexico, other parts of Central America, the Far East, the United States, Canada, and France are endemic areas.

Infection is characterized by isolated cutaneous or subcutaneous necrotizing nodules associated with the indolent development of suppurating nodules along the course of the proximal lymphatics. In highly endemic regions, about 10 to 25% of cases occur in children. Extracutaneous and pulmonary forms of the disease occur infrequently. The histopathologic findings of primary cutaneous disease combine features of both granulomatous and pyogenic inflammation. Granulomatous lesions consist of aggregations of epithelioid histiocytes with central areas of necrosis and neutrophils or zones of Langhan's giant cells associated with fibroblasts and lymphocytes. Occasionally, areas of microabscesses unassociated with granulomatous reaction may be seen. In chronic disease, pseudoepitheliomatous hyperplasia may be extensive and may mimic neoplasm. A common finding in sporotrichosis is the asteroid body, a round basophilic, yeast-like structure surrounded by rays of eosinophilic material thought to represent antigen-antibody complexes. The asteroid body is considered characteristic of sporotrichosis, but it is also seen in other mycoses.

Vegetable matter undergoing extensive decay is a common source of exposure. In 95% of cases, the organism is percutaneously inoculated by thorns, tree bark, or splinters, or from abrasions acquired handling hay, straw, or sphagnum moss. Fungal contamination of wounds from insect bites or inanimate objects has also been implicated in infection. Rare cases of human-to-human transmission have been reported. Sporotrichosis has been reported in many areas of the United States, but is most common along the Mississippi River Valley and in the Plains states. Most cases are sporadic, but outbreaks associated with contaminated hay bales and sphagnum moss have occurred. Infections are reported more frequently in males, but may reflect a disproportionate risk of exposure resulting from recreational or occupational activities.

CLINICAL MANIFESTATIONS The spectrum of clinical findings in sporotrichosis can be divided into lymphocutaneous, fixed cutaneous, mucocutaneous, extracutaneous (localized or multifocal), and pulmonary manifestations. Cutaneous disease is the most common manifestation of sporotrichosis in children; only rare reports document localized extracutaneous infections.

Lymphocutaneous Sporotrichosis Lymphocutaneous sporotrichosis accounts for 75% of infections. The average incubation period is about 3 weeks, but lesions may develop from 5 days to 6 months after inoculation. Infections usually involve the upper extremities, but lesions of the face and trunk are relatively common in children. The primary lesion begins as a firm, mobile, nontender subcutaneous nodule that slowly enlarges and becomes discolored. After 2 weeks, it undergoes necrosis and leaves a painless ulcer. During the next several weeks, similar nodules develop along the course of the proximal lymphatics, and these also suppurate. The intervening lymphatic channels become thickened and cord-like, and overlying cutaneous erythema develops. Lesions can persist for months to years, few heal spontaneously, and scarring often occurs at the sites of the ulcers. Constitutional and systemic symptoms are absent.

Fixed Cutaneous Sporotrichosis Fixed cutaneous disease comprises about 20 to 25% of cases. In highly endemic areas, there is a substantial incidence of skin test reactivity, presumably resulting from frequent exposure. Primary infection in these individuals appears to be limited to the site of inoculation and consists of ulcerative, plaque-like or maculopapular lesions; lymphatic abnormalities are absent. Symptoms of systemic illness sometimes occur. Fixed cutaneous lesions can resolve spontaneously, persist for years, or, after resolution, recur with differing morphology at the same site.

Mucocutaneous Sporotrichosis Although mucocutaneous lesions are most commonly seen in association with disseminated infections, they may occur as isolated lesions. The mucosal membranes of the oropharynx or nares are the most common sites of involvement. Lesions begin as erythematous, painful ulcers that can

be confused with aphthous ulcers. Regional lymph nodes usually enlarge and become firm. Lesions usually resolve spontaneously and leave nondeforming scars.

Extracutaneous Sporotrichosis Extracutaneous disease is responsible for less than 1% of reported cases of sporotrichosis, and occurs as either localized or multifocal disease. The most common site of isolated extracutaneous infection is the skeletal system. Osteoarticular manifestations include destructive arthritis, tenosynovitis, chronic osteomyelitis, and periostitis. Localized extracutaneous infections may represent metastatic foci of hematogenous origin, spread from contiguous skin lesions or from direct inoculation. The most common site of osseous involvement is the tibia, followed by the bones of the hands. Sporotrichal arthritis is slowly progressive and symptoms include joint pain, swelling, and insidious impairment of function. Osteoarticular disease usually remains localized, but can spread to contiguous structures. It rarely disseminates.

Multifocal extracutaneous disease results from hematogenous spread and is rarely described in children. It may follow cutaneous or pulmonary inoculation and occurs almost exclusively in immunocompromised patients. Predisposing conditions include AIDS, malignancy, diabetes, sarcoidosis, alcoholism, and long-term corticosteroid therapy.

Pulmonary Sporotrichosis Primary pulmonary sporotrichosis, seen almost exclusively in adults, usually results from inhalation of spores and affects the lung parenchyma or may remain localized to hilar nodes. There is usually no other extracutaneous site of infection. Apical portions of the lung are involved and chronic cavitary lesions may result. Lesions can progress and death can result. A second type of pulmonary presentation involves the hilar lymph nodes only and often mimics tuberculosis and histoplasmosis. This manifestation can remain stable for long periods and often resolves spontaneously.

DIAGNOSIS In the appropriate epidemiologic setting, typical cutaneous manifestations usually prompt consideration of sporotrichosis, especially when papulovesicular, ulcerative, or nodular lesions fail to respond to topical or systemic antibiotics. The differential diagnosis of such cutaneous lesions includes infection with *Nocardia sp., Francisella tularensis,* nontuberculous mycobacteria, tertiary syphilis, and Leishmania. Nodular lymphangitis can also be seen with infections caused by pyogenic bacteria *Pseudomonas sp., B. anthracis,* and other mycoses, including blastomycosis, chromoblastomycosis, coccidioidomycosis, cryptococcosis, and histoplasmosis. Nodular lymphangitis can be seen with mycetoma, which may be caused by bacteria or fungi. A careful travel and exposure history helps differentiate these entities. Pulmonary sporotrichosis can mimic tuberculosis, sarcoidosis, or other mycoses.

The laboratory diagnosis of sporotrichosis is difficult. Typical histopathologic findings of pyogranulomatous inflammation are not specific. Few organisms are present and the morphology of those observed may not be typical. *Sporothrix schenckii* can be isolated from fungal cultures of exudate or biopsied tissue. The organism is more readily recovered from synovial fluid than from cutaneous lesions. In cases of meningitis, the cerebrospinal fluid (CSF) typically shows a mild pleocytosis with a majority of lymphocytes, elevated protein, and hypoglycorrhachia.

Skin testing and serologic tests are not routinely available and cannot distinguish active from past infection. A sensitive and specific latex slide agglutination test that detects antibody is commercially available, but has not been widely employed. Latex agglutination may have a role in the diagnosis of pulmonary or disseminated disease when tissue samples are not readily available.

TREATMENT Iodide therapy is effective treatment of cutaneous disease. The mechanism by which iodide therapy works is unknown. Five drops of a saturated solution of potassium iodide mixed in water, milk, or juice is given three times daily; each dose is increased by five drops weekly until a maximum of 40 to 50 drops three times daily for adults and 30 drops three times daily for children is reached. Treatment continues for 6 to 8 weeks after the resolution of the lesions. Side effects include anorexia, nausea, a metallic taste, rash, fever, and swelling of the salivary glands. The extended length and inconvenience of treatment with iodide often leads to poor compliance.

Itraconazole is currently the recommended treatment for localized lymphocutaneous sporotrichosis (see Table 13-62). Response rates are excellent and side effects are few. However, treatment is expensive. Care must be taken to avoid drug interactions (see Table 13-63). Absorption is erratic and improved by taking the itraconazole with Coca Cola Classic. Serum concentrations should be documented to confirm absorption (available through the Histoplasmosis Reference Laboratory, Indianapolis, Indiana). Lesions usually resolve within 1 month of beginning treatment; treatment should be continued for several months after the lesions have healed to decrease the likelihood of relapse. Itraconazole is also the treatment of choice for isolated osteoarticular disease. Therapy should continue for 1 to 2 years. A pediatric regimen may be tailored to these recommendations.

Local hyperthermia has been effective for treating cutaneous lesions and may be considered for patients who cannot tolerate the recommended drugs. Local hyperthermia may not be readily tolerated in children. Drainage of localized lesions, particularly in osteoarticular infection, is beneficial.

Amphotericin B is used to treat progressive disseminated and pulmonary sporotrichosis. The recommended total dosage for adults is 1 to 2 g. Data in children are lacking. Itraconazole may be used for treating subacute or chronic pulmonary disease. Treatment in AIDS patients is problematic because progressive infection has been described in patients receiving amphotericin B and the relapse rate is high. Therefore, as with other systemic fungal infections in AIDS patients, lifetime prophylaxis with itraconazole is recommended. Amphotericin B is the preferred treatment for infections of the central nervous system.

References

Dooley DP, Bostic PS, Beckius ML: Spook house sporotrichosis: a point-source outbreak of sporotrichosis associated with hay bale props in a Halloween haunted house. Arch Intern Med 157:1885–1887, 1997

Hajjeh R, McDonnell S, Reef S, et al: Outbreak of sporotrichosis among tree nursery workers. J Infect Dis 176:499–504, 1997

Kauffman CA: Old and New therapies for sporotrichosis. Clin Infect Dis 21:981–985, 1995

Lynch PJ, Botero F: Sporotrichosis in children. Am J Dis Child 122:325–327, 1971

Wilson DE, Mann J, Bennett J, et al: Clinical features of extracutaneous sporotrichosis. Medicine 46:265–274, 1967

13.5.10 Zygomycosis (*Mucor* and Related Species)

Rebecca C. Brady and Judith C. Rhodes

Zygomycosis is an umbrella term for all diseases caused by fungi of the class Zygomycetes. The more common term *mucormycosis* refers to a group of invasive mycoses caused by members of the order Mucorales, within the class Zygomycetes. *Rhizopus* species are the most commonly isolated agents of mucormycosis.

The Mucorales are distributed worldwide and commonly grow in decaying organic matter. Although exposure to the airborne spores of these thermotolerant, rapidly growing fungi is universal, human disease is infrequent and is indicative of a serious underlying predisposing condition. Diabetes mellitus, particularly diabetic ketoacidosis, is the most common predisposing condition in patients with mucormycosis. Underlying disease accompanied by acidosis such as uremia, malnutrition, and congenital metabolic aciduria may also predispose to mucormycosis. Additional risk factors include neutropenia, malignancy, burns, prematurity, corticosteroid therapy, solid organ transplantation, bone marrow transplantation, and desferrioxamine therapy for management of iron and aluminum overload states.

Infection in humans most commonly occurs following inhalation of the spores of Mucorales into the respiratory tract. Spores may also be ingested or introduced directly into abraded skin. Germination of spores occurs with hyphal proliferation and invasion of tissues. Infection may spread by direct extension and hematogenous dissemination. Regardless of the tissue involved, the pathologic hallmark of mucormycosis is hyphal invasion of blood vessels with resultant hemorrhage, thrombosis, infarction, and production of black, necrotic debris. The reasons these fungi target the vasculature are unknown.

The mechanisms that account for the increased susceptibility to mucormycosis in different patient groups remain incompletely understood. Neutrophils and macrophages are important components of the host response to Mucorales, thus defects in their function likely contribute to the pathogenesis of mucormycosis. Iron is an important growth factor for these fungi; hence, interactions between iron molecules and transferrin have been postulated to play a role in predisposing deferoxamine-treated patients to the development of mucormycosis. Because these fungi metabolize ketones and grow optimally at an acid pH, the metabolic conditions encountered in ketoacidotic hosts may enhance their growth.

CLINICAL MANIFESTATIONS The clinical manifestations of mucormycosis are classified by site of involvement into rhinocerebral, pulmonary, cutaneous, gastrointestinal, disseminated, and miscellaneous infections. Rhinocerebral infection occurs most frequently and typically presents as facial pain, nasal congestion, and headache in a poorly controlled diabetic patient. From the nasal mucosa and paranasal sinuses, infection may spread to the orbit, resulting in orbital cellulitis, paresis of extraocular muscles, and proptosis. Further extension into the cerebral vasculature and brain can lead to cavernous sinus thrombosis, brain infarcts, and focal neurologic deficits.

Most cases of pulmonary mucormycosis have occurred in neutropenic hosts, especially those receiving chemotherapy for leukemia and lymphoma. Clinically, these patients present with unremitting fever and dyspnea. The chest roentgenogram may show patchy consolidation and cavity formation. Infection progresses rapidly, and hemoptysis may be a fatal complication.

Cutaneous mucormycosis usually occurs at sites of burns, trauma, and invasive procedures in immunosuppressed hosts, including premature infants. The skin lesion may begin as an area of erythema and induration that subsequently develops central necrosis. Skin lesions may also be a manifestation of disseminated infection.

Risk factors for gastrointestinal mucormycosis include malnutrition, prematurity, and underlying gastrointestinal disease. The stomach and colon are involved most frequently. Presenting findings may include nonspecific abdominal pain, hematochezia, or melena. Premature infants may experience necrotizing enterocolitis.

Disseminated infection most often follows pulmonary invasion and may spread to the brain, liver, spleen, and other tissues. Clinically, these patients have rapidly progressive multiple organ failure with a high mortality rate. Miscellaneous forms of mucormycosis include endocarditis, osteomyelitis, and pyelonephritis.

DIAGNOSIS AND TREATMENT   Mucormycosis must be differentiated from other opportunistic infections in immunosuppressed hosts. Cutaneous mucormycosis may mimic ecythyma gangrenosum, which is commonly due to *Pseudomonas aeruginosa*. Invasion of blood vessels is a major pathologic finding with *Aspergillus* infection. Not surprisingly, the pulmonary, cerebral, and cutaneous manifestations of aspergillosis are clinically indistinguishable from those of mucormycosis. The definitive diagnosis of mucormycosis requires demonstration of hyphal elements invading tissue in a biopsy specimen. Because the Mucorales may colonize body surfaces, swabs of drainage or abnormal tissue are inappropriate. Tissue biopsies, especially of black necrotic lesions, should be sent for histologic examination and for culture. Grinding of tissue should be avoided, as this may disrupt the hyphal elements. Demonstration of irregularly shaped, broad, nonseptate hyphae with right-angle branching by either hematoxylin and eosin or Grocott-Gomori methenamine silver nitrate staining is the gold standard for diagnosis of mucormycosis. The agents of mucormycosis may be difficult to isolate in culture from infected tissues. Cultures of blood, urine, and cerebrospinal fluid are rarely positive.

TREATMENT   Successful treatment of mucormycosis requires a coordinated medical and surgical approach. If possible, the underlying predisposing condition should be reversed. Metabolic acidosis should be corrected and the doses of corticosteroids and other immunosuppressive drugs should be lowered if at all possible. All devitalized tissue should be surgically removed. Often, débridement must be repeated daily for several days. Intravenous administration of amphotericin B is the mainstay of therapy for mucormycosis (see Table 13-62). Duration of therapy for antifungals is often hard to define and should be individualized for the specific location of infection in a particular patient. The currently approved azoles have no role in the treatment of this fungal infection.

References

Kline MW: Mucormycosis in children: review of the literature and report of cases. Pediatr Infect Dis 4:672–676, 1985

Mooney JE, Wanger A: Mucormycosis of the gastrointestinal tract in children: report of a case and review of the literature. Pediatr Infect Dis J 12:872–876, 1993

Rinaldi MG: Zygomycosis. Infect Dis Clin North Am 3:19–41, 1989

Robertson AF, Joshi VV, Ellison DA, Cedars JC: Zygomycosis in neonates. Pediatr Infect Dis J 16:812–815, 1997

Sugar AM: Agents of mucormycosis and related species. In: Mandell GL, Bennett JE, Dolin R, eds: Principles and Practice of Infectious Diseases, 4th ed. New York, Churchill Livingstone, 1995:2311–2321

Sugar AM: Mucormycosis. Clin Infect Dis 14(Suppl 1):S126–S129, 1992

Walsh TJ, Gonzalez C, Lyman CA, Chanock SJ, Pizzo PA: Invasive fungal infections in children: recent advances in diagnosis and treatment. Adv Pediatr Infect Dis 11:187–290, 1996

13.6   PARASITIC DISEASES

13.6.1   Antiparasitic Drug Therapy

Michael Cappello

The remarkable diversity of parasite pathogens could be expected to require a variety of drug therapies for successful treatment. However, certain broad-spectrum drugs are reasonably active against multiple closely related parasites. Mebendazole and albendazole are each effective against most intestinal nematodes, whereas praziquantel is the drug of choice for most cestode and trematode infections. Quinine sulfate remains the cornerstone of therapy for the treatment of malaria, and mefloquine or chloroquine is recommended as prophylaxis for most travelers to malaria endemic areas. Unfortunately, the current therapeutic options for American and African trypanosomiasis, as well as for leishmaniasis, are extremely limited, with regard to both efficacy and safety. Table 13-64 lists the major parasitic species that cause disease in humans along with the currently recommended drugs for therapy or prevention. Below are brief descriptions of these agents, including common side effects and toxicities. The dosing of some agents is included below, although the reader is referred to (Sec. 13.6.5) for recommended treatment regimens for malaria, trypanosomiasis, and leishmaniasis.

DRUGS FOR THE TREATMENT OF HELMINTH INFECTIONS

NEMATODES   Mebendazole (Vermox) is a broad-spectrum anthelminthic with activity against most intestinal nematode species that infect humans. It is also effective against certain filarial worms, as well as adult and larval stages of *Trichinella spiralis*. Its use may cause mild abdominal pain and diarrhea, and long-term use may lead to bone marrow suppression, alopecia, and liver toxicity. The recommended dose of mebendazole is 100 mg twice a day for 3 days (or a single 500-mg dose) for infection with the following parasites: *Ancylostoma caninum* (eosinophilic enteritis), *A. duodenale* or *Necator americanus* (intestinal hookworm), *Ascaris lumbricoides*, and *Trichuris trichiura*. For pinworm (*Enterobius vermicularis*), a single dose of 100 mg is sufficient. The dose of mebendazole for infection with *Capillaria philippinensis* is 200 mg/d for 20 days, whereas for *Mansonella perstans* infection, the recommended dose is 100 mg/d for 30 days. For trichinosis (*Trichinella spiralis*), mebendazole should be administered at a dose of 200 to 400 mg tid for 3 days, followed by 10 days of therapy at 400 to 500 mg/d. In the setting of severe symptoms caused by infection with *T. spiralis*, steroids should be given concomitantly. For visceral larva migrans caused by *Toxocara* species, mebendazole should be given at 100 mg/d for 5 days.

TABLE 13-64
DISEASE-SPECIFIC ANTIPARASITIC THERAPY

	DRUG OF CHOICE*	ALTERNATIVE AGENT(S)*
Nematode Infections		
Intestinal nematodes		
Ancylostoma duodenale, A. caninum, Necator americanus (hookworm)	Mebendazole	Pyrantel pamoate Albendazole
Ascaris lumbricoides	Mebendazole	Pyrantel pamoate Albendazole
Enterobius vermicularis (pinworm)	Mebendazole	Pyrantel pamoate Albendazole
Strongyloides stercoralis	Ivermectin *or* thiabendazole	Albendazole
Trichinella spiralis (trichinosis)	Mebendazole plus steroids	
Trichuris trichiura	Mebendazole	Albendazole
Blood and Tissue Nematodes		
Ancylostoma braziliense, A. caninum (cutaneous larva migrans, creeping eruption)	Thiabendazole (topical) *or* albendazole *or* ivermectin	
Capillaria philippinensis	Mebendazole	Albendazole
Dracunculus medinensis (guinea worm)	Metronidazole	
Mansonella ozzardi	Ivermectin	
Mansonella perstans	Mebendazole	
Mansonella streptocerca	Ivermectin *or* diethylcarbamazine	
Onchocerca volvulus (river blindness)	Ivermectin	
Toxocara canis, T. cati (visceral and ocular larva migrans)	Steroids +/− diethylcarbamazine	Mebendazole Albendazole
Wuchereria bancrofti, Brugia malayi, Loa loa (filariasis)	Diethylcarbamazine	
Cestodes		
Intestinal (Adult) Tapeworms		
Diphyllobothrium latum, Taenia saginata, T. solium, Dipylidium caninum, Hymenolepis nana	Praziquantel	
Tissue (Larval) Tapeworms		
Echinococcus granulosus, E. multilocularis	Albendazole	
T. solium (neurocysticercosis)	Albendazole *or* praziquantel	
Trematodes		
Clonorchis sinensis (Chinese liver fluke)	Praziquantel *or* albendazole	
Fasciola hepatica (sheep liver fluke)	Bithionol *or* triclabendazole (not available in United States)	
Fasciolopsis buski, Heterophyes heterophyes, Metagonimus yokogawai (intestinal flukes)	Praziquantel	
Metorchis conjunctus, Nanophyetus salmincola, Opisthorchis viverrini	Praziquantel	
Paragonimus westermani (lung fluke)	Praziquantel	Bithionol
Schistosoma haematobium, S. japonicum, S. mekongi	Praziquantel	
S. mansoni	Praziquantel	Oxamniquine
Protozoa		
Intestinal Protozoa		
Balantidium coli	Tetracycline	Iodoquinol Metronidazole
Cryptosporidium	Paromomycin	Azithromycin
Cyclospora	Trimethoprim-sulfamethoxazole	
Dientamoeba fragilis	Iodoquinol	Paromomycin Tetracycline
Entamoeba histolytica (amebiasis)		
Asymptomatic	Iodoquinol	Paromomycin Diloxanide furoate
Moderate to severe disease	Metronidazole (followed by iodoquinol)	Tinidazole
Entamoeba polecki	Metronidazole	
Giardia lamblia	Metronidazole *or* furazolidone	Paromomycin, albendazole, tinidazole
Isospora belli	Trimethoprim-sulfamethoxazole	Pyrimethamine
Microsporidiosis (Encephalitozoon intestinalis, Enterocytozoon bieneusi)	Albendazole	
Malaria	See Tables 13-67, 13-68	

(continued)

TABLE 13-64   Continued

	DRUG OF CHOICE*	**ALTERNATIVE AGENT(S)***
Other Blood and Tissue Protozoa		
Babesia spp. (babesiosis)	Clindamycin plus quinine sulfate	
Encephalitozoon hellem, Encephalitozoon cuniculi, Vittaforma corneae, Pleistophora spp. (ocular or disseminated microsporidiosis)	Albendazole	
Leishmania mexicana, L. major, L. tropica, L. braziliensis, L. donovani, L. infantum	Sodium stibogluconate *or* meglumine antimoniate *or* amphotericin B deoxycholate	Lipid-associated amphotericin B *or* pentamidine isethionate *or* paromomycin
Naegleria spp., Acanthamoeba spp. (amebic meningoencephalitis)	Amphotericin B	
Toxoplasma gondii (toxoplasmosis)	Pyrimethamine plus 1 of the following: sulfadiazine *or* clindamycin	Spiramycin
Trypanosoma brucei gambiense and *T.b. rhodesiense* (African trypanosomiasis or sleeping sickness)	Suramin sodium *or* eflornithine *or* melarsoprol	Pentamidine isethionate
Trypanosoma cruzi (American trypanosomiasis or Chagas disease)	Nifurtimox	Benznidazole
Ectoparasites		
Lice (*Pediculus humanus, P. humanus capitus, Phthirus pubis*)	1% Permethrin	
Scabies (*Sarcoptes scabiei*)	5% Permethrin	Ivermectin

*See text for recommended doses of specific agents.
SOURCE: Adapted from Drugs for parasitic infections. Med Lett Drugs Ther 40:1, 1998.

Albendazole (Albenza), also a benzimidazole, has replaced mebendazole as the drug of choice for intestinal nematode infections in many parts of the developing world. Its side effects and toxicity profile are much like mebendazole. It should not be administered to pregnant women. The dose of albendazole is a single dose of 400 mg for infection with the following nematode parasites: *A. caninum* (eosinophilic enteritis), *A. lumbricoides, E. vermicularis,* hookworm, and *T. trichiura.* For pinworm (*E. vermicularis*), the dose should be repeated in 2 weeks. The dose of albendazole for the treatment of infection with *C. philippinensis* is 400 mg/d for 10 days, and for cutaneous larva migrans (caused by dog and cat hookworms) or visceral larva migrans (*Toxocara*), the dose is 400 mg/d for 3 days.

Thiabendazole (Mintezole) is a systemically absorbed synthetic benzimidazole effective in the treatment of strongyloidiasis. However, because of its frequent side effects and toxicity, ivermectin is likely to replace it as the drug of choice for infection with *S. stercoralis.* The most common side effects of thiabendazole are gastrointestinal symptoms, although hepatotoxicity and central nervous system disorders have also been reported. The recommended dose of thiabendazole is 50 mg/kg divided in two doses (maximum dose 3 g/d) for 2 days.

Pyrantel pamoate (Antiminth), which causes neuromuscular blockade in parasites, is an effective anthelminthic agent for the treatment of the intestinal nematodes *A. lumbricoides,* hookworms (*A. duodenale* and *N. americanus*), and *E. vermicularis.* Its most frequent side effects are primarily gastrointestinal, although occasional central nervous system (CNS) effects may be seen. The recommended dose is 11 mg/kg (maximum dose 1 g) given once. For pinworm, the dose should be repeated in 2 weeks.

Diethylcarbamazine, or DEC (Hetrazan), a derivative of the older anthelminthic piperazine, has activity against many filarial nematodes. It is the drug of choice for infections caused by *Wuchereria bancrofti, Brugia malayi,* and *Loa loa.* It is also recommended for the treatment of tropical pulmonary eosinophilia. The

major side effects include gastrointestinal symptoms, headache, and myalgias. Because of severe inflammatory reactions, termed the *Mazzotti reaction,* noted in patients infected with *Onchocerca volvulus,* diethylcarbamazine is no longer recommended for treatment of onchocerciasis (river blindness). The recommended dosing for *W. bancrofti, B. malayi,* and *L. loa* is: Day 1: 1 mg/kg; Day 2: 1 mg/kg tid; Day 3: 1 to 2 mg/kg tid; Days 4 to 14 (*W. bancrofti, B. malayi*): 2 mg/kg tid; Days 4 to 21 (*L. loa*): 3 mg/kg tid. For patients without microfilaremia, the maximum dose can be given on Day 1 of treatment. The dose for tropical pulmonary eosinophilia is 2 mg/kg tid for 14 days. For visceral and ocular larva migrans, the dose of DEC is 2 mg/kg tid for 7 to 10 days.

Ivermectin (Mectizan, Stromectin) is a broad-spectrum antiparasitic agent with activity against a variety of nematodes and ectoparasites. It is the drug of choice for the treatment of onchocerciasis, and may soon become the preferred agent for the treatment of strongyloidiasis. It is also highly effective in patients with cutaneous larva migrans, and has activity against a number of intestinal nematode species. The side effects of ivermectin are primarily seen in patients treated for onchocerciasis, and may all be attributable to inflammation in response to dying microfilariae (Mazzotti reaction). The recommended dose of ivermectin for onchocerciasis (river blindness) is 150 μg/kg once, repeated every 3 to 12 months. The dose for strongyloidiasis, although not well established, is 200 μg/kg/d for 2 days. For cutaneous larva migrans, a single dose of 150 to 200 μg/kg is recommended.

CESTODE AND TREMATODE INFECTIONS Praziquantel and albendazole are the drugs of choice for nearly all infections caused by flatworms. The exception is *Fasciola hepatica* (liver fluke), which is treated with bithionol. Praziquantel (Biltricide) is a heterocyclic prazino-isoquinolin that causes rapid paralysis of intestinal cestodes and damages the tegument of trematodes. Its use is associated with primarily central nervous system and gastrointestinal side effects, which are usually mild and resolve with cessation of therapy. The concomitant use of dexamethasone, as in the treatment of neuro-cysticercosis, may decrease serum levels, whereas cimetidine and ketoconazole may increase levels of praziquantel. The recommended dose of praziquantel for the adult tapeworms *Diphyllobothrium latum, Taenia saginata, T. solium,* and *Dipylidium caninum* is 5 to 10 mg/kg given once. For infections with *Hymenolepis nana,* the dose is increased to 25 mg/kg. For the treatment of neurocysticercosis, the dose of praziquantel is 50 mg/kg/d divided tid for 15 days, usually in conjunction with steroids. The dose of praziquantel recommended for the treatment of the flukes *Clonorchis sinensis, Fasciolopsis buski, Heterophyes heterophyes, Metagonimus yokogawai, Metorchis conjunctus,* and *Opisthorchis viverrini* is 75 mg/kg/d in three divided doses for 1 to 2 days. For infections with *Paragonimus westermani,* treatment should be administered for a total of 2 days. *Nanophyetus salmincola* infections are treated with praziquantel at a dose of 60 mg/kg/d in three doses for 1 day. Praziquantal is also the drug of choice for most infections with schistosomes. Treatment consists of 20 mg/kg given bid for 1 day in *Schistosoma mansoni* and *S. haematobium,* and 20 mg/kg given bid for 1 day in *S. japonicum* and *S. mekongi.* Alternatively, oxamniquine (Vansil) can be used to treat *S. mansoni* at a dose of 10 mg/kg given bid for 1 day.

Albendazole (see nematode infections earlier) is an effective therapeutic agent for the treatment of neurocysticercosis and echinococcosis. The dose for each is 15 mg/kg/d (maximum dose 800 mg/d) divided into two doses for 8 to 30 days (neurocysticercosis) or 28 days (echinococcosis).

Bithionol (Bitin), which is available through the CDC, is the drug of choice for treatment of infections with *Fasciola hepatica.* Its side effects include gastrointestinal symptoms, photosensitivity, and urticaria. The recommended dose is 30 to 40 mg/kg on alternate days to a maximum of 2 g/d. It is also an alternative agent for treatment of the lung fluke *P. westermani* (30–50 mg/kg on alternate days for 10–15 doses).

DRUGS FOR THE TREATMENT OF PROTOZOAN INFECTIONS

INTESTINAL PROTOZOA Metronidazole (Flagyl) is a nitroimidazole that is frequently used in the treatment of infections caused by anaerobic bacteria; however, it is also effective for treatment of parasites that use an anaerobic metabolism. Most of the parasites that are sensitive to metronidazole are intestinal protozoa, including *Entamoeba histolytica, E. polecki, Giardia lamblia, Blastocystis hominis,* and *Balantidium coli.* Metronidazole is also effective against *Trichomonas vaginalis.* Because it is only active against the cyst forms of amoeba, patients with invasive disease should also be treated with an agent with activity against the trophozoite stage. Side effects include nausea, vomiting, and a disulfiram-like reaction that precludes the use of alcohol while on therapy.

The recommended dose of metronidazole is 15 mg/kg/d (maximum dose 250 mg) divided tid for infection with *G. lamblia* and *T. vaginalis.* A 5- to 10-day course is recommended for giardiasis, and 7 days is recommended for trichomoniasis. The dose of tinidazole, a related nitroimidazole, for giardiasis is 50 mg/kg once, with a maximum dose of 2 g for adults. For amebiasis, as well as for infections with *E. polecki* and *B. hominis,* the recommended dose is 35 mg/kg/d (maximum dose 750 mg) in three doses for 10 days. Of note, tinidazole is not commercially available in the United States.

Furazolidone (Furoxone) is considered by many to be the drug of choice for *G. lamblia* infections in children, although it also has activity against some bacterial pathogens. Side effects are mostly gastrointestinal, including nausea, vomiting, and a disulfiram-like reaction similar to metronidazole. The recommended dose for giardiasis is 6 mg/kg/d divided qid (maximum dose 100 mg) for 10 days.

Iodoquinol (Yodoxin) is an oxyquinolone with activity against the luminal stages of *E. histolytica, B. hominis, B. coli,* and *Dientamoeba fragilis.* It is used primarily as adjunctive therapy in amebiasis with metronidazole, in order to eradicate both the tissue stages (trophozoites) and the intestinal cysts of the parasite. The dose is 30 to 40 mg/kg/d (maximum dose 650 mg) divided tid for a total of 20 days. Side effects include nausea, diarrhea, abdominal cramps, and, less frequently, skin rash or acne.

Paromomycin (Humatin) is a poorly absorbable aminoglycoside antibiotic that is an alternative agent for the treatment of intestinal protozoa, including *G. lamblia, E. histolytica, D. fragilis,* and *Cryptosporidium* species. In patients with underlying renal insufficiency, it may cause nephrotoxicity and ototoxicity. The recommended dose of paromomycin is 25 to 35 mg/kg/d in three divided doses for 7 days.

Albendazole (see nematode infections earlier) is the drug of choice for microsporidiosis, caused by intestinal infections with *Encephalitozoon intestinalis* and *Enterocytozoon bieneusi,* as well as tissue infections caused by *E. hellem, E. cuniculi, Vittaforma corneae,* and *Pleistophora* species. The recommended dose is 400 mg, although the optimal duration of therapy is unknown.

MALARIA See Sec. 13.6.5 for a detailed discussion of drug selection and dosing for treatment of malaria.

OTHER BLOOD AND TISSUE PROTOZOA See Sec. 13.6.5 for details regarding drugs used for treatment of trypanosomiasis and leishmaniasis.

The antibiotic clindamycin is used in conjunction with quinine sulfate for the treatment of infections caused by *Babesia* species. This combination is also an alternative regimen for the treatment of chloroquine-resistant malaria. The use of clindamycin is associated with *Clostridium difficile* pseudomembranous colitis.

Pyrimethamine (Daraprim), in combination with sulfadiazine, is the drug of choice for *Toxoplasma gondii* infections. The dose of pyrimethamine is 2 mg/kg/d for 3 days, followed by 1 mg/kg/d (maximum dose 25 mg/d) for 4 weeks. The dose of sulfadiazine is 100 to 200 mg/kg/d for 3 to 4 weeks. Leucovorin should be given with each dose of pyrimethamine. Congenital toxoplasmosis should be treated for as long as 1 year. Spiramycin (50–100 mg/kg/d) is an alternative agent for the treatment of *T. gondii* infections, and is recommended for prophylactic use during pregnancy. This agent is available through the CDC.

DRUGS FOR THE TREATMENT OF ECTOPARASITE INFESTATIONS

Infestation with either lice or scabies is treated with topical permethrin (Nix, Elimite). The use of this agent is associated with pain, burning, and an erythematous rash. For lice (*Pediculus humanus, P. humanus capitus,* and *Phthirus pubis*), the concentration of permethrin is 1%, whereas for scabies infestation (*Sarcoptes scabiei*), a 5% topical solution is recommended. Although not approved by the FDA, ivermectin at 200 μg/kg is also effective in a single oral dose for the treatment of scabies.

References

Cook GC: Manson's Tropical Diseases. Philadelphia, WB Saunders, 1996

Drugs for parasitic infections: Med Lett Drugs Ther 40:1–12, 1998

Liu LX, Weller PF: Antiparasitic drugs. N Engl J Med 334:1178–1184, 1996

Pearson RD, Weller PF, Guerrant RL: Chemotherapy of parasitic diseases. In: Guerrant RL, Walker DH, Weller PF, eds: Tropical Infectious Diseases: New York, Churchill Livingstone, 1999

Wilson CM, Freedman DO: Antiparasitic agents. In: Long SS, Pickering LK, Prober CG, eds: Principles and Practice of Pediatric Infectious Diseases. New York, Churchill Livingstone, 1997

13.6.2 Diseases Caused by Nematodes or Roundworms

ASCARIASIS
Richard A. Oberhelman

Ascariasis is caused by the intestinal roundworm *Ascaris lumbricoides.* The World Health Organization has estimated that more than 1.4 billion people, or approximately one-quarter of the world's population, are infected with *A. lumbricoides,* with the largest number of infections occurring in Asia. An estimated 4 million people are infected in the United States alone, with highest infection rates among immigrants from developing countries (20–60% infected in some surveys). Young children are infected most frequently, with peak prevalence in children between the ages of 3 and 8 years living in the tropics.

Ascaris is the largest intestinal roundworm that commonly infects humans: females measure 20 to 40 cm long, and males measure 15 to 30 cm long. The female lays approximately 200,000 eggs daily; eggs are broadly ovoid and 45 to 75 μm by 35 to 50 μm. Fertilized eggs have a three-layer coat with a bile-stained, mamillated outer shell (Fig. 13-16A). Unfertilized eggs are broader and longer (ie, approximately 90 μm by 45 μm) and usually lack the mamillated outer coat (Fig. 13-16B).

Eggs are passed in the host's feces and become infective in the environment only after the first-stage larva molts within the egg (*embryonation*). The eggs are resistant to drying, low temperatures, and many chemicals. Children often infect themselves and others by playing in the same areas where they eliminate their wastes. Where human wastes are used as fertilizer (eg, the Orient), *Ascaris* infection is especially frequent.

When embryonated eggs are ingested and stimulated by enzymes in the duodenum, the larvae emerge, traverse the intestinal mucosa, and enter the mesenteric lymphatics and venules. They then enter the portal circulation and reach the pulmonary vascular bed, perforate the alveolar wall, ascend the respiratory tree to the epiglottis, and are swallowed. The vast majority of ascarids finally settle in the jejunum, where mature worms mate and females begin laying eggs in 2 to 2.5 months.

CLINICAL MANIFESTATIONS During the period of larval invasion and migration, cough, dyspnea, fever [39.5°C (103.1°F) to 40.5°C (104.9°F)], rales, and dullness to percussion of the chest may be evident. Invasion of the respiratory system by migrating larvae results in alveolar hemorrhages, and pulmonary damage may be extensive, especially with large numbers of larvae. Hemoptysis may occur, and larvae may be found in the sputum. Shifting, consolidated infiltrates and widening of the pulmonary hilum may be seen, and the eosinophil count often is very high (Löffler syndrome). During this phase, other manifestations of hypersensitivity such as urticaria and wheezing may occur with repeated infections. Larvae occasionally may traverse the pulmonary circulation and produce serious lesions in the eye, central nervous system, and kidney, resembling visceral larva migrans caused by *Toxocara* larvae.

Unless they are numerous, adult worms in the small intestine generally are associated with few symptoms. The most frequently noted symptoms in children are vague epigastric pains, nausea, vomiting, and anorexia. Severe, intermittent, colicky abdominal pain at times may result from partial intestinal obstruction. The more serious problems encountered with *Ascaris* infection result from migration of adult worms into the bile and pancreatic ducts, where they may induce biliary stone formation, pancreatitis, small intestinal perforation, and complete intestinal obstruction with intussusception. Worms occasionally may migrate cephalad and emerge through the mouth or nose (Fig. 13-17), or migrate posteriorly and pass through the rectum.

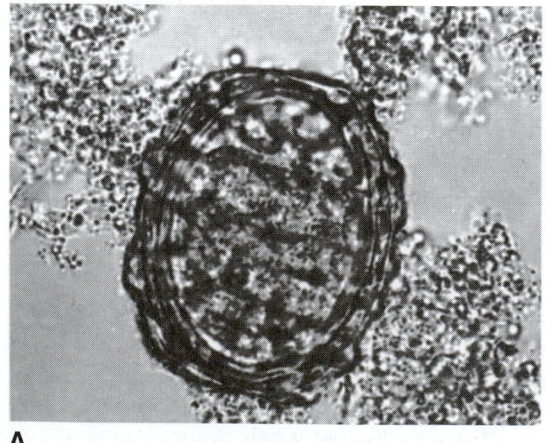
A

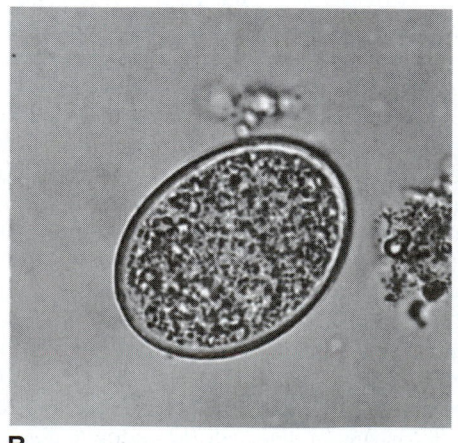
B

FIGURE 13-16   A. Fertilized egg and B. unfertilized egg of *Ascaris lumbricoides* (×448).

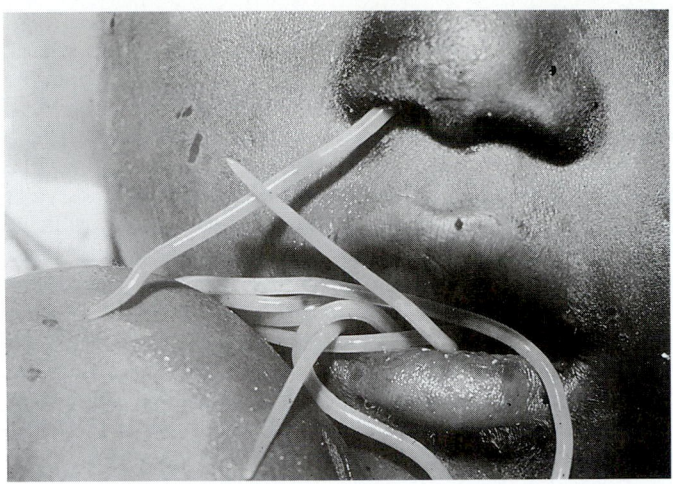

FIGURE 13-17　Adult *Ascaris lumbricoides* emerging from the nose and mouth of an infected child.

DIAGNOSIS AND TREATMENT　Generally, the diagnosis is established by identifying typical eggs of *Ascaris* in the feces. Eggs are usually abundant, and stool concentration is rarely needed to see them. However, occasionally only unfertilized or decorticated eggs are present in stool samples, and these may be difficult to recognize. If a patient brings a spontaneously passed worm to the clinic, a stool should be examined to ascertain whether any other worms remain. Because ascariasis is associated with asthma and other allergic manifestations, stools should be examined in patients with those symptoms, particularly if they are from an endemic area. Ultrasonography may be useful to diagnose biliary tract invasion. Serologic tests are rarely needed, although the bentonite flocculation test, indirect hemagglutination, and ELISA assays are useful diagnostic tests in some unusual cases.

Anthelminthic agents available to treat ascariasis are reviewed in Sec. 13.6.1. Intestinal obstruction often responds to medical management: duodenal suction, parenteral fluids, electrolyte correction, and instillation of piperazine (an anthelminthic drug that paralyzes worms) into the duodenal tube. If this fails, the obstructing worms must be removed surgically.

Strategies for control of intestinal helminth infections in developing countries, and of ascariasis in particular, are frequently based on massive country-wide anthelminthic treatment campaigns, usually using albendazole. The World Health Organization and Ministries of Health in many developing countries advocate regular (usually biannual) population-based treatment for elementary school-aged children, who statistically are at highest risk. In most cases, treatment is administered without screening stool specimens before treatment. This approach is logical in many low-income areas because rates of helminth infection and reinfection are extremely high, single-dose therapy with albendazole is highly effective and well tolerated, and poor sanitation linked with poverty makes environmental control practically and economically unfeasible.

References

Bundy DAP: Immunoepidemiology of intestinal helminth infections: 1. The global burden of intestinal nematode diseases. Trans Roy Soc Trop Med Hyg 88:259–261, 1994

Khuroo MS: Ascariasis. Gastroenterol Clin North Am 25:553–577, 1996
Muennig P, Pallin D, Sell RL, Chan MS: The cost-effectiveness of strategies for the treatment of intestinal parasites in immigrants. N Engl J Med 340:773–779, 1999
Venkatesan P: Albendazole. J Antimicrob Chemother 41:145–147, 1998

BAYLISASCARIASIS
Richard A. Oberhelman

Baylisascariasis is a potentially serious form of larva migrans that is caused by larvae of the raccoon ascarid, *Baylisascaris procyonis,* a nematode found in 50 to 80% of raccoons in North America. It also occurs in raccoons in other countries, including Germany and Japan. *Baylisascaris procyonis* is a well-known cause of larva migrans in animals, and is usually associated with central nervous system disease. Larvae of *B. procyonis* have produced fatal or severe central nervous system disease in over 45 species of mammals and birds. Other *Baylisascaris* species, including *B. melis* of badgers and *B. columnaris* of skunks, are also potential causes of human disease.

Adult *Baylisascaris* organisms are 12 to 23 cm long and reside in the raccoon's small intestine. Eggs shed with the raccoon's feces become infective in 3 to 4 weeks. Young raccoons become infected by ingesting infective eggs, while older raccoons become infected by ingesting larvae in the tissues of intermediate hosts, including rodents, rabbits, and birds.

Humans become infected with *Baylisascaris* by accidentally ingesting infective eggs from objects contaminated with the feces of wild or pet raccoons. *Baylisascaris* eggs in the soil can remain infective for years. Larvae emerge from ingested eggs and migrate to many tissues, including lung, skeletal muscles, eye, and brain. Approximately 5 to 7% of ingested larvae enter the brain, where they can produce extensive damage before they are walled off. Migrating larvae cause mechanical damage and incite vigorous host inflammatory reactions, producing eosinophilic granulomas in many tissues.

The risk of human infection with *Baylisascaris* is greatest in children younger than 4 years of age because of hygienic habits and propensity for pica and geophagia. *Baylisascaris procyonis* can produce visceral larva migrans (VLM), ocular larva migrans (OLM), and neural larva migrans (NLM), with eosinophilic meningoencephalitis, that usually presents in patients with concurrent VLM. Subclinical infection probably is most common, followed by clinical OLM, VLM, and NLM. Fatal or severe *Baylisascaris* NLM has been documented primarily in children, although the disease remains rare.

CLINICAL MANIFESTATIONS　The diagnosis of infection with *Baylisascaris* is based primarily on clinical findings, history, and serology. Clinical findings vary from mild illness to severe central nervous system (CNS) disease depending on the level and frequency of infection and the degree of CNS involvement. Signs of VLM, including hepatomegaly, eosinophilia, and elevated isohemagglutinin titers, may be present and are similar to those of toxocariasis. If enough *Baylisascaris* eggs are ingested, severe central nervous system disease can develop within 2 to 4 weeks. Clinical signs in such cases include sudden lethargy, loss of muscle coordination, decreased head control, torticollis, hemiparesis, ocular muscle paralysis, cortical blindness, and nystagmus, which may progress to coma and death. An important diagnostic finding in baylisascariasis is eosinophilic pleocytosis of the cerebrospinal fluid, especially in a patient with concurrent peripheral eosinophilia and progressive central nervous system disease. However, other parasitic pathogens, notably *Angiostrongylus cantonensis,* may also produce eosinophilic meningitis. CT and MRI findings may include marked periventricular contrast enhancement of the brain and diffuse cerebral and cerebellar atrophy. Brain biopsies have shown mixed eosinophilic inflammation and occasionally larvae.

Ocular larva migrans typically is seen in older individuals without other symptoms, and it manifests as unilateral loss of vision. Ophthalmoscopy reveals inflammation, migration tracks, and/or granulomas in the retina or choroid, or evidence of diffuse unilateral subacute neuroretinitis. If visualized, larvae are three to five times larger than *Toxocara* and measure 1.5 to 2.0 mm long.

DIAGNOSIS AND TREATMENT Serologic methods (eg, indirect immunofluorescence, ELISA, Western blotting) were developed for *Baylisascaris* and are useful in the limited number of documented cases, although patients with OLM are frequently seronegative or only weakly seropositive.

Information on effective anthelminthic treatment of this infection is limited, and the treatment of NLM is not promising. Anthelminthics that show the greatest promise include albendazole, mebendazole, thiabendazole, and levamisole. Ivermectin does not cross the blood-brain barrier well and has not proved successful in clinical cases. Even if effective drugs were available, clinical NLM caused by *Baylisascaris* has a poor prognosis because the diagnosis is usually delayed and extensive central nervous system damage has often occurred by the time diagnosis is made. In these cases, control of inflammation and supportive maintenance of the patient are both important until larvae are killed by anthelminthics or are walled off in granulomas. Ocular *Baylisascaris* has been successfully treated using laser photocoagulation.

Prevention is important because treatment is so inadequate. Keeping raccoons as pets should be discouraged, especially in households with young children. Parents should prevent access by children to known or potential areas that are contaminated with raccoon feces. Because raccoons commonly defecate on fallen timber, caution should be exercised in using it for firewood.

References

Cunningham CK, Kazacos KR, McMillan JA, et al: Diagnosis and management of *Baylisascaris procyonis* infection in an infant with nonfatal meningoencephalitis. Clin Infect Dis 18:868–872, 1994

Fox AS, Kazacos KR, Gould NS, Heydemann PT, Thomas C, Boyer KM: Fatal eosinophilic meningoencephalitis and visceral larva migrans caused by the raccoon ascarid *Baylisascaris procyonis.* N Engl J Med 312:1619–1623, 1985

Goldberg MA, Kazacos KR, Boyce WM, Ai E, Katz B: Diffuse unilateral subacute neuroretinitis. Morphometric, serologic, and epidemiologic support for *Baylisascaris* as a causative agent. Ophthalmology 100:1695–1701, 1993

Kazacos KR, Boyce WM: *Baylisascaris* larva migrans. J Am Vet Med Assoc 195:894–903, 1989

CUTANEOUS LARVA MIGRANS
Richard A. Oberhelman

Cutaneous larva migrans, or creeping eruption, is a clinical syndrome caused by nematode larvae that penetrate and migrate through the skin, causing intensely pruritic, serpiginous tracks. The disease is usually caused by the filariform larva of *Ancylostoma bra-* ziliense or *Ancyclostoma caninum* (common hookworms of dogs and cats); however, these hookworms produce a distinct clinical syndrome when infection occurs in the gastrointestinal tract. Other species of larval hookworms, such as *Necator americanus* and *Uncinaria stenocephala,* as well as larvae of *Strongyloides stercoralis* and *Gnathostoma spinigerum,* occasionally cause a similar picture. The disease is ubiquitous in the tropics. In the United States, most cases are reported from southeastern states. Infection occurs in workers, bathers, and children exposed to larvae in the soil, sand, or sandboxes where infected dogs and cats have defecated. Infection is most common in the summer or early fall.

CLINICAL MANIFESTATIONS An erythematous papule, which becomes vesicular, is frequently found at the site of larval penetration. Larvae migrate through the skin at a rate of as much as a few centimeters a day, producing highly pruritic, serpiginous tracks measuring several millimeters in width (Fig. 13-18). The major complications result from intense itching and scratching, with secondary infection by pyogenic bacteria. Larvae may migrate for weeks to months before finally dying. Lesions can occur almost anywhere, but often are found on the soles and dorsa of the feet, buttocks, face, and back. In severe cases, larvae may migrate to the lungs causing Löeffler pneumonia with shifting infiltrates. Myositis and eosinophilic enteritis are rare complications.

DIAGNOSIS AND TREATMENT The diagnosis is usually made on clinical grounds and requires no laboratory assays. Biopsy specimens may reveal an eosinophilic infiltrate, but the migrating organism is rarely seen. In rare cases with pneumonitis, larvae may be seen in sputum or gastric washings. Serologic tests for antibodies to *A. caninum* by enzyme immunoassay or Western blot may be useful if the diagnosis is uncertain.

Generally, the infection is self-limited and requires no treatment. In persistent or severe infections, topical 10% aqueous thiabendazole has been used, and oral albendazole (200 mg bid for 3 days) or thiabendazole (50 mg/kg/d in two divided doses with a maximum of 3 g/d) have been effective in reported cases. Control measures should focus on preventing skin contact or ingestion of moist soil contaminated with animal feces. Periodic anthelminthic therapy for dogs and cats may also reduce the incidence of this infection. Most puppies acquire hookworm infection in the neonatal period through the colostrum; therefore, all newly acquired puppies may be infectious and should be properly wormed.

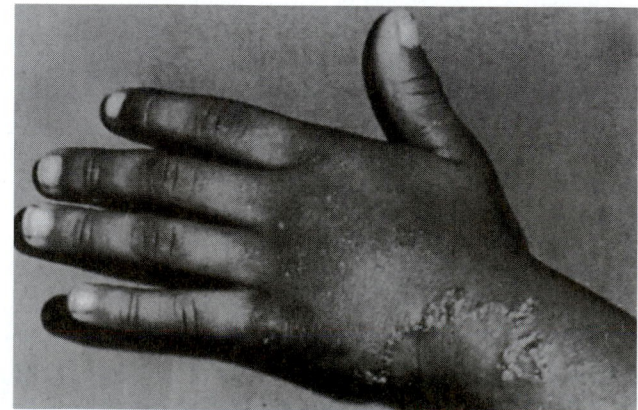

FIGURE 13-18 Typical serpiginous skin lesion of cutaneous larva migrans.

References

Despommier D: Tissue nematodes. In: Long S, Pickering L, Prober C, eds: Principles and Practice of Pediatric Infectious Diseases, 1st ed. New York, Churchill Livingstone, 1997, 1472–1476

Gilles HM: Cutaneous larva migrans. In: Cook GC, ed: Manson's Tropical Disease, 20th ed. London, WB Saunders, 1996, 1392–1394.

DRACUNCULIASIS
Richard A. Oberhelman

Dracunculiasis (dracontiasis, guinea-worm disease) is caused by infection of subcutaneous and connective tissues with the guinea worm *Dracunculus medinensis*. Once a scourge affecting thousands of people around the world, the range of this organism has been greatly reduced as a result of a global eradication program spearheaded by the Carter Center's Global 2000 program. Contemporary cases are mostly confined to certain countries in West Africa (principally Nigeria) and Sudan, the latter country accounting for more than two-thirds of the total cases reported worldwide. Currently, the Carter Center and the Centers for Disease Control and Prevention estimate that the incidence of guinea worm infection fell by 95% between 1986 and 1996.

When an individual drinks water contaminated with freshwater copepods (plankton) of the genus *Cyclops,* which contain mature guinea worm larvae, infective larvae are set free, penetrate the intestinal wall, and usually migrate to the retroperitoneal tissues, where they require about 8 to 12 months to mature. The gravid female worm, averaging 1 m in length by 1 to 2 mm in diameter, usually migrates from the deep connective tissues to emerge in the superficial subcutaneous tissues of the distal portions of the arms and legs. Following development of an indurated papule, a painful skin blister forms near the anterior portion of the worm, and infected individuals frequently immerse the affected limb into water to relieve the pain. The affected area ulcerates and when the ulcer is immersed in water, large numbers of motile larvae are discharged into the water through a ruptured prolapsed loop of the parasite's uterus. If larvae are expelled into a body of water used for drinking, such as a pond, they may be ingested by copepods and the cycle repeats.

Because of the 1-year incubation period between infection and onset of symptoms, human disease rates reflect risk factors from the previous year. In Africa, infection usually occurs during the hot, dry season when water sources are limited. Infection begins in childhood, and individuals are reinfected repeatedly throughout life. Infection is uncommon before the age of 3 years, because young children and infants seldom drink infected pond or well water.

CLINICAL MANIFESTATIONS Worms in the deep tissues usually cause no side effects. Nevertheless, migration to the skin may take many weeks or months and be accompanied by mild or severe hypersensitivity reactions such as urticaria, pruritus, erythema, and, on occasion, dyspnea and a shock-like state. Skin ulcers are most common on the ankle or between the metatarsal bones, but they have been described on almost every site. A mild-to-moderate eosinophilia usually accompanies the infection. Secondary infection of the ulcer and worm tract may provoke abscesses and septic arthritis, producing chronic deformities, contractures, and muscle atrophy. Tetanus is a common complication in inadequately immunized persons.

DIAGNOSIS AND TREATMENT Dracunculiasis can be diagnosed only when the skin ulcer appears or if the outline of the adult worm can be seen beneath the skin; immunologic tests are not reliable. Surgical removal of the worm frequently is advocated. The time-honored method of gradually rolling the worm onto a stick, a few centimeters a day, is still used today; this ancient procedure is also the inspiration for the caduceus, the symbol of medicine. However, it is important to do this when the worm first appears and to take suitable precautions to prevent sepsis. Severe inflammation and necrosis usually follow if the worm is torn during removal, and the traditional slow removal process takes an average of 89 days. Measures suggested to facilitate manual removal include killing the worm by local infiltration with acriflavine or mercuric bichloride and emptying the worm of eggs by applying a continuous water drip onto gauze-covered ulcers.

The role of chemotherapy in dracunculiasis is limited. Three antiparasitic drugs—niridazole, metronidazole, and thiabendazole—have been advocated to reduce inflammation, thereby reducing the time required for extraction. (Niridazole is not available in the United States.) Response to these drugs varies from no effect, with continued appearance of new worms, to death of the organism in the tissues associated with increased inflammation, anaphylaxis, and arthritides. No antiparasitic drug can reliably be expected to produce beneficial effects.

Establishing safe drinking water is the principal intervention needed to disrupt transmission. This may be achieved by chemical treatment with temephos (Abate), which is safe for consumption at concentrations used for water treatment, or by filtering out zooplankton using cloth or nylon filters. Together with health education and active surveillance, the global eradication program has markedly reduced the prevalence of this disease.

References

Hopkins DR, Ruiz-Tiben E, Ruebush TK: Dracunculiasis eradication: almost a reality. Am J Trop Med Hyg 57:252–259, 1997

Hunter JM: An introduction to guinea worm on the eve of its departure: dracunculiasis transmission, health effects, ecology, and control. Soc Sci Med 43:1399–1425, 1996

ENTEROBIASIS (PINWORM)
Richard A. Oberhelman

Enterobiasis is caused by the pinworm *Enterobius vermicularis,* a strictly human parasite infecting the gastrointestinal tract. Infection occurs worldwide, and clustering of cases in families is common. Infection occurs by ingestion of embryonated eggs excreted in the stool of infected persons, and may occur by hand-to-mouth transmission or by oral contact with infected fomites, such as toys, bedding, or clothing. Ingested eggs with first-stage larvae hatch in the duodenum, and the larvae develop into adults in the cecum, where they mate. The gravid female detaches from the cecal mucosa and migrates down the large bowel, usually passing out the anus onto the perianal and perineal skin, leaving a trail of eggs on the surface of the skin. Yellow-white female adult pinworms measuring 8 to 13 mm may be seen emerging from the rectum of infected children, most often around 10 or 11 p.m. In approximately 5% of patients, eggs are deposited in the bowel and may be found in feces. Generally, the worm dies after ovipositing is completed, so repeated infections are the result of autoinfection or reinfection from other environmental sources. There is no good evidence that retrograde infection occurs.

The eggs average 55 μm by 35 μm and appear flattened on one side and convex on the other. They are fully mature and infective 3 to 8 hours after being deposited, but at normal room temperature, less than 10% of eggs live for 48 hours.

In the United States, infection rates in young school children vary from 10 to 45%. Infection is unrelated to poor sanitary facilities or tropical climates. Young girls have pinworm more frequently than boys of the same age, and whites are more often infected than African-Americans. Infection is most common between early fall and late spring, perhaps related to transmission in schools. For unknown reasons, some individuals seem to be predisposed or vulnerable to reinfection. Unlike soil-transmitted helminths such as *Ascaris,* enterobiasis is more common in urban settings.

CLINICAL MANIFESTATIONS Pinworms rarely produce serious pathology, and many infections are asymptomatic. Perianal and perineal pruritus are the most common complaints. Although pruritus probably results from crawling worms, some patients with heavy pinworm infections and many worms in the rectum have little or no itching. Pruritus may provoke such severe scratching that local bleeding, secondary pyogenic infection, and lichenification can occur. Whether pinworms are a primary cause of appendicitis remains unsettled; most pathologists consider their presence in an acutely inflamed appendix to be incidental. Vaginal infection in young girls is common, and may be associated with vaginitis and discharge. Pinworms occasionally have been found in the fallopian tubes, resulting in intraabdominal ectopic migration and symptomatic granulomatous inflammation in the peritoneal cavity.

DIAGNOSIS AND TREATMENT Nocturnal perianal pruritus strongly suggests pinworm infection, especially in children. Small, creamy-white worms are often found if the perianal region is examined when the child is awakened by itching. Ova are not often seen in the stools, and the cellophane tape swab technique is the diagnostic method of choice (Fig. 13-19). A 6-cm piece of transparent (not translucent) cellophane tape is folded with its sticky side out over the end of a wooden tongue blade and then firmly applied against either side of the perianal region. Next, the tape is placed sticky side down on a microscope slide, which can be examined for pinworm ova. The swabs should be taken 2 to 3 hours after going to bed or in the morning immediately before the patient gets out of bed. Slides from specimens collected on consecutive days may be sealed and stored in the refrigerator until delivered. Neither eosinophilia nor serologic tests are useful for diagnosis.

As infection often is present in several members of a household, each family member should be examined, or the entire family should be treated simultaneously. Otherwise, reinfection may occur. Mebendazole (100 mg) or albendazole (400 mg) as a single dose given twice, initially and 2 weeks later, are treatments of choice. However, experience with these anthelminthics in children younger than 2 years of age is limited. The later dose reduces the risk of repeated infection by autoinoculation. Piperazine and pyrantel pamoate are alternatives, but these are rarely necessary because the less toxic drugs are effective.

Parents and patients should be reassured that pinworms are ubiquitous and that the infection is not a reflection of poor hygiene or the result of an unclean home. Good hand washing is the most effective means of prevention. Bed clothes, linens, and underclothes of infected children should be handled carefully and not shaken to

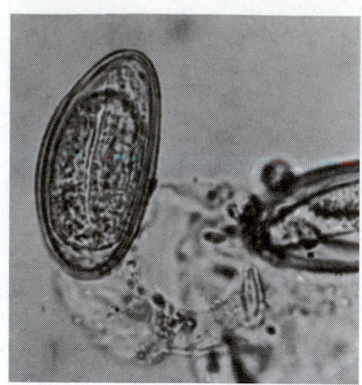

FIGURE 13-19 *Enterobius vermicularis* **ova from the stool of an infected child (cellophane tape technique) (×448).**

avoid dispersing ova into the air, and they should be laundered promptly. Control of infection in childcare centers and schools may be difficult because of high rates of reinfection, and in some cases, mass and simultaneous treatment of children and adults in institutions may be necessary.

References

Capello M, Hotez P: Intestinal nematodes. In: Long S, Pickering L, Prober C, eds: Principles and Practice of Pediatric Infectious Diseases, 1st ed. New York, Churchill Livingstone, 1997, 1465–1466

Grencis RK, Cooper ES: *Enterobius, Trichuris, Capillaria,* and hookworm, including *Ancylostoma caninum.* Gastroenterol Clin North Am 25:579–597, 1996

Hotez PJ: Parasitic infections in temperate climates. In: Katz S, Gershon A, Hotez P, eds: Krugman's Infectious Diseases of Children, 10th ed. St. Louis, Mosby-Year Book, 1998, 311–325

FILARIAL INFECTIONS
Ramya Gopinath and Thomas B. Nutman

The lymphatic dwelling parasites *Wuchereria bancrofti, Brugia malayi,* and *Brugia timori,* and the subcutaneous filarid *Onchocerca volvulus,* can cause significant morbidity in children, whereas the other filarial parasites of humans (*Loa loa, Mansonella perstans, M. streptocerca,* and *M. ozzardi*) cause minimal childhood morbidity. Each filarial parasite is transmitted by biting arthropods, either mosquitoes or flies, and all go through complex life cycles that include a slow maturation (often 3–24 months) from the infective larval stages carried by the insects, to adult worms that live associated with the lymphatics and lymph nodes (*W. bancrofti* and *Brugia* spp.) or in the subcutaneous tissues (*L. loa, O. volvulus, M streptocerca*). The offspring of these (*W. bancrofti, Brugia* spp., *M. perstans, M. ozzardi, L. loa*) adults, the microfilariae, are 200 to 400 mm in length, and either circulate in the blood (*W. bancrofti, Brugia* spp.) or migrate to the skin (*O. volvulus, M. streptocerca*) while awaiting ingestion by the insect vectors. Productive infection is usually not established, unless exposure to infective larvae is intense or prolonged. Although exposure to, and acquisition of, infection with these parasites occurs throughout childhood in endemic regions, most of the pathology associated with these infections is found in adults or older children.

Wuchereria bancrofti, *Brugia malayi*, *Brugia timori*

CLINICAL MANIFESTATIONS Lymphatic filariasis affects approximately 129 million people in Africa, Asia, India, Indonesia, the Philippines, Papua New Guinea, and focal areas of Latin America and the Caribbean. Clinical manifestations of bancroftian and brugian filariases are similar. The three most common presentations of the lymphatic filariases are asymptomatic (or subclinical) microfilaremia, acute filarial adenolymphangitis (ADL), and chronic lymphatic obstruction. Patients with asymptomatic microfilaremia may have thousands of circulating parasites/mL blood, but rarely come to medical attention except through the incidental finding of microfilariae in peripheral blood drawn between 10 p.m. and 4 a.m., reflecting their nocturnal periodicity. Many individuals with microfilaremia, however, have some degree of subclinical disease that includes microscopic hematuria and/or proteinuria or dilated (and tortuous) lymphatics when imaged. Infection with adult worms in the absence of microfilaremia can occur in 25% or more of children between the ages of 1 and 5 years, depending on the level of filarial endemicity in the community.

The most common symptomatic presentation of lymphatic filariasis in children is acute filarial adenolymphangitis (ADL), characterized by high fever, lymphatic inflammation (lymphangitis and lymphadenitis), and transient local edema. Most episodes last between 3 and 7 days, and may recur several times per year. The lymphangitis is retrograde, extending peripherally from the lymph node draining the area where the adult parasites reside, a finding that helps to distinguish filarial from bacterial lymphangitis. The upper and the lower extremities are most commonly involved with both bancroftian and brugian filariasis. Involvement of the genital lymphatics, resulting in hydrocele, occurs almost exclusively with *W. bancrofti* infection.

Regional lymph nodes are often enlarged, and the entire lymphatic channel can become indurated and inflamed. In brugian filariasis, a single local abscess may form along the involved lymphatic tract and subsequently rupture to the surface. Persistent infection and recurrent inflammation lead to dilatation and obstruction of lymphatics, resulting in elephantiasis of the limbs or breasts in both brugian and bancroftian filariasis, and hydroceles and chyluria in bancroftian filariasis. Bacterial and/or fungal superinfection of these poorly vascularized tissues becomes a significant problem. Chyluria, when it occurs, is characteristically intermittent.

Tropical pulmonary eosinophilia (TPE) occurs in an extremely small percentage of individuals infected with filarial parasites. The syndrome consists of cough and wheezing, diffuse lung infiltrates on chest x-ray, and restrictive (with or without obstructive) defects on pulmonary function testing (PFT). Extremely high levels of blood eosinophils ($>3000/mm^3$), serum IgE, and antifilarial IgG are thought to reflect an immunologic hyperresponsiveness to the parasite. Circulating microfilariae are almost never detected in these individuals. Repeated episodes of TPE or inadequate treatment can result in chronic interstitial (and irreversible) lung disease.

DIAGNOSIS Definitive diagnosis depends on demonstrating parasites directly. Adult worms can be identified on biopsy or, in bancroftian filariasis, when visualized by ultrasound in inguinal lymph nodes, scrotum, or breast. Microfilariae (except in some areas of the South Pacific where subperiodic forms are common) are found almost exclusively in the blood between 10 p.m. and 4 a.m., times that coincide with the nocturnal biting habits of the arthropod vec-

tor. Filaria-specific antibody testing is highly sensitive but cross-reactive among the filarial species. For bancroftian filariasis, detection of circulating parasite antigen (ELISA or rapid immunochromatographic testing) is highly sensitive (>98%) and specific (>99%) and antigen detection has largely supplanted microscopy, because the antigen can be detected in whole blood or serum drawn at any time of the day. Filarial DNA in whole blood can be detected by PCR, but remains largely a research technique.

Elevated total serum IgE, absolute eosinophil counts, and antifilarial antibodies provide strong supportive evidence for the diagnosis of lymphatic filariasis but are commonly elevated in many parasitic infections and therefore must be considered in conjunction with more specific tests. With the extreme elevations seen in TPE, not only should a chest x-ray and PFT be obtained for help in diagnosis, but other causes of extreme increases in IgE and eosinophils seen in children (eg, visceral larval migrans, allergic bronchopulmonary aspergillosis) must be excluded. ^{99}Tc-based lymphoscintigraphy is very useful in defining the nature and extent of lymphatic damage or dysfunction and in distinguishing lymphedema from other causes of swelling.

TREATMENT Diethylcarbamazine 9, which has both macrofilaricidal and microfilaricidal properties, remains the treatment of choice for the individual with active lymphatic filariasis (microfilaremia, antigen positivity, or adult worms on ultrasound), although albendazole (400 mg bid for 21 days) has demonstrable macrofilaricidal efficacy. Diethylcarbamazine is given in an escalating dosage schedule: day 1—1 mg/kg p.c.; day 2—1 mg/kg tid; day 3—1 to 2 mg/kg tid; day 4 and beyond—2 mg/kg tid. The duration of therapy ranges from 12 to 21 days, depending on the infecting organism. Reactions that occur after treatment consist of fever, chills, myalgias, arthralgias, headaches, nausea, and vomiting. Both the development and the severity of these reactions are directly related to the number of microfilariae circulating in the bloodstream and may represent an acute hypersensitivity reaction to the antigens being released by dead and dying parasites. These reactions may be more pronounced in brugian filariasis, usually lasting only 24 to 48 hours, and remit spontaneously.

Recently, regimens that emphasize single-dose diethylcarbamazine (DEC), ivermectin, or combinations of single doses of albendazole and DEC or albendazole and ivermectin, have sustained microfilaricidal effects. In individuals with chronic manifestations of lymphatic filariasis, treatment regimens that emphasize hygiene, prevention of secondary bacterial infections, and physiotherapy have gained wide acceptance for morbidity control. Hydroceles can be drained repeatedly or managed surgically.

Vaccine development for lymphatic filariasis is in its infancy. Single-dose combinations of albendazole with either DEC or ivermectin are now being used by filariasis control programs in many countries for annual community-wide treatment.

Onchocerca volvulus

Onchocerciasis affects approximately 18 million people, the overwhelming majority of whom live in Sub-Saharan Africa and the rest of whom live in small foci in Latin America and the Arabian peninsula. It is estimated that about 600,000 of those infected are severely visually impaired as a consequence of onchocercal eye disease (river blindness).

CLINICAL MANIFESTATIONS Skin and eye disease are the most common manifestations; both may occur in childhood, in areas of high transmission. Adult worms in subcutaneous fibrous capsules can be palpated as nodules (onchocercomas), particularly over bony prominences. The microfilariae, when in the skin, induce inflammation that manifests as intense pruritus and papular dermatitis; with long-standing cutaneous inflammation, lichenification, depigmentation ("leopard skin"), and eventual skin atrophy can occur.

Ocular pathology, very clearly related to the intensity of infection, is the most serious consequence of this infection. Inflammation around (and subsequent destruction of) microfilariae in the cornea leads to punctate keratitis. Sclerosing keratitis is common in chronic, long-standing infection, as is chronic uveitis. Posterior eye disease, including chorioretinitis, chorioretinal atrophy, and optic nerve involvement can lead to constriction of the visual field and eventual blindness.

DIAGNOSIS AND TREATMENT Microfilariae can be recovered from skin snips of the epidermis obtained as superficial (1 mm) slices using a scalpel or razor blade, or by a corneoscleral biopsy punch. The skin snips should be taken from regions with pathology, around nodules or over bony prominences of the upper or lower torso. When incubated in saline or culture medium for as long as 24 hours, microfilariae may be seen emerging from these snips in microfiladermic individuals. Six or more skin snips from these various locations are recommended for maximal diagnostic yield. Adult worms can be identified in excised nodules. Microfilariae may also be identified in the anterior chamber of the eye on slit-lamp examination. Assays to detect specific antionchocercal antibodies and PCR to detect onchocercal DNA in skin snips are now in use in specialized laboratories and are highly sensitive and specific.

The Mazzotti test is a provocative test that can be used in cases in which the diagnosis of onchocerciasis is still in doubt, providing that skin snips and the ocular examination demonstrate no microfilariae. A small dose of DEC (0.5–1.0 mg/kg) is given orally; the development or exacerbation of pruritus or rash within hours is highly suggestive of onchocerciasis.

Treatment directed at the microfilariae in the skin and ocular tissue is reviewed in Sec. 13.6.1. There is no available agent that can kill adult *O. volvulus*. Community-based administration of ivermectin every 6 to 12 months is now being used to interrupt transmission in endemic areas. This, in conjunction with vector control, has helped to reduce the prevalence of disease in endemic foci in Africa and Latin America.

References

Burnham G: Onchocerciasis. Lancet 351(9112):1341–1346, 1998

Ottesen EA, Ismail MM, Horton J. The role of albendazole in programmes to eliminate lymphatic filariasis. Parasitol Today 15(9):382–386, 1999

Rajan TV, Gundlapalli AV. Lymphatic filariasis. Chem Immunol 66:125–158, 1997

HOOKWORM INFECTION AND DISEASE

Michael Cappello

It is estimated that more than 1 billion people in the world are infected with the hookworm *Ancylostoma duodenale*, *Necator americanus*, or both. Infections with *A. duodenale* occur in the temperate regions of the world, including southern Europe, as well as the more northern regions of Africa, China, and India. *Necator americanus* is generally found in North and South America, equa-

torial Africa, and much of Southeast Asia. It is important to recognize, however, that there is significant overlap in the geographic pattern of infection and that mixed infections occur frequently. Other species of hookworm that rarely cause intestinal disease in humans include *Ancylostoma ceylanicum*, found in India and Southeast Asia, and *A. caninum*, which infects humans in Australia. At present, only rare autochthonous cases of hookworm occur in the United States.

The hookworm life cycle begins with the excretion of fertilized eggs within the feces of an infected individual. The eggs hatch to release first-stage (L1) larvae, which undergo two subsequent molts to the infective third stage (L3). These L3 hookworm larvae migrate along moisture and temperature gradients within the soil until they encounter a permissive host. When larvae contact the skin, they quickly penetrate the epidermis and dermis, ultimately invading small blood vessels and entering the venous circulation. They are then carried passively to the heart and lungs, where they lodge in the pulmonary capillaries and break through to the alveolar space. Larvae then migrate up the respiratory tree, are swallowed, and undergo their final developmental molts to the adult stage when they reach the small intestine. Once in the proximal small bowel, the adult worms attach to the mucosal surface and begin to feed. Male and female worms mate, and the female releases 10,000 to 30,000 eggs per day into the intestinal lumen. It takes approximately 6 weeks for eggs to appear in the feces of an infected individual.

Two important features of the life cycle distinguish *Ancylostoma* hookworms from *Necator*. First, *A. duodenale* can cause infection when ingested, whereas *N. americanus* can only complete its life cycle in humans following skin penetration. Second, there is epidemiologic evidence to suggest that third-stage larvae of *A. duodenale* may arrest within various tissues of their host, ultimately resuming development and completing their life cycle months to years later.

CLINICAL MANIFESTATIONS As third-stage larvae penetrate the skin a local urticarial eruption, known as ground itch, may occur. Although hookworms frequently penetrate the soles of the feet, it is important to recognize that the parasite will invade any exposed skin surface. The pulmonary migration of hookworms is rarely associated with significant clinical symptoms, although cough and wheezing may develop following infection with a large inoculum. Of note, the pulmonary phase is associated with the development of peripheral eosinophilia, and precedes the appearance of eggs in the feces.

Once in the intestine, the adult hookworms attach to the mucosa using sharp teeth (*A. duodenale*) or cutting plates (*N. americanus*) within their respective buccal capsules (Fig. 13-20). As the parasite feeds, small blood vessels in the superficial mucosa are lacerated, and blood is sucked into the worm's mouth. Hookworms have been found to secrete potent anticoagulants. It is estimated that each adult *Ancylostoma* hookworm can cause up to 0.2 cc of blood loss per day. When the plug of intestinal mucosa at the site of attachment has been digested, the worm releases and reattaches at a new site.

All of the clinically significant manifestations of hookworm infection are attributable to the loss of blood and serum proteins that are a consequence of feeding by the adult worm. In light infections, subclinical iron deficiency develops if daily iron intake cannot compensate for iron lost through intestinal bleeding. In chronic infections, significant iron deficiency leads to a microcytic, hypochromic anemia. Particularly heavy infections may also manifest as severe

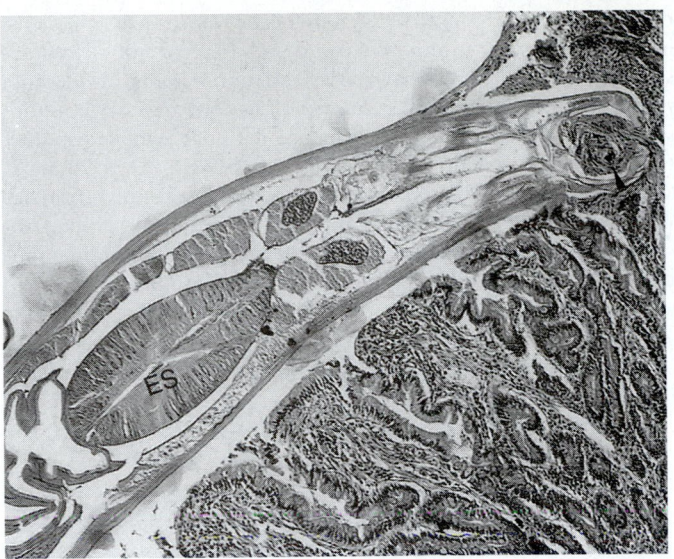

FIGURE 13-20 Adult *Ancylostoma* hookworm. Note the buccal capsule (dart), which contains teeth used to attach to the intestinal mucosa, and the muscular esophagus (ES). SOURCE: *Oribel T, Ash L: Parasites in human tissues. ASCP Press, Chicago, 1995, with permission.*

protein malnutrition, as the worm drains serum proteins in addition to red blood cells as it feeds. Rarely, high-output heart failure develops as a consequence of chronic, severe, hookworm anemia. Importantly, even children with mild infections may suffer impairment of physical and intellectual development, particularly when they also harbor other intestinal nematodes.

Intestinal infection with *A. caninum* is associated with eosinophilic enteritis, an unusual syndrome characterized by abdominal pain, tenderness, and gastrointestinal bleeding. Biopsies of the small bowel routinely show massive eosinophilic infiltrates, and occasionally a single adult canine hookworm has been identified attached to the mucosa. However, there is frequently no direct evidence of hookworm infection in patients with eosinophilic enteritis. Although the vast majority of hookworm-induced eosinophilic enteritis is reported from Australia, at least one suspected case was identified in a child from North America.

DIAGNOSIS The definitive diagnosis of hookworm infection is made by finding characteristic ova in the feces. These thin-shelled, ovoid eggs with granular-appearing contents measure 60 by 40 μm, and are generally in the two- to four-cell stage when passed in feces. It is important to recognize that many children from the developing world who are infected with hookworm frequently harbor other intestinal nematodes as well, including *Ascaris lumbricoides* and *Trichuris trichiura*, which are also associated with anemia and malnutrition. Because hookworm egg excretion can be intermittent, multiple stool examinations may be required to confirm the diagnosis. There is no microscopic means to differentiate between the eggs of *A. duodenale* and *N. americanus*, although assays using the polymerase chain reaction were developed for research purposes. In addition, there are no routinely used serum antibody or fecal antigen tests for diagnosing hookworm infection.

TREATMENT Treatment with albendazole, mebendazole, or pyrantel pamoate is reviewed in Sec. 13.6.1. Children treated for hookworm frequently experience significant catch-up growth; studies

show improvement in a number of developmental parameters following therapy. Unfortunately, in endemic areas, reinfection with hookworms occurs rapidly and the benefits of intermittent chemotherapy may be short-lived.

References

Adams, EJ, Stephenson, LS, Latham, MC, Kinoti, SN: Physical activity and growth of Kenyan school children with hookworm, *Trichuris trichiura* and *Ascaris lumbricoides* infections are improved after treatment with albendazole. J Nutr 124:1199–1206, 1994

Albonico M, Smith PG, Ercole E, et al: Rate of reinfection with intestinal nematodes after treatment of children with mebendazole or albendazole in a highly endemic area. Trans R Soc Trop Med Hyg 89:538–541, 1995

Hotez PJ: Hookworm disease in children. Pediatr Infect Dis J 8:516–520, 1989

Khoshoo V, Schantz P, Craver R, Stern GM, Loukas A, Prociv PJ: Dog hookworm: a cause of eosinophilic enterocolitis in humans. Pediatr Gastroenterol Nutr 19:448–452, 1994

Sen-Hai Y, Ze-Xiao Z, Long-Qi X: Infantile hookworm disease in China: a review. Acta Trop 59:265–270, 1995

Stoltzfus RJ, Chwaya HM, Tielsch JM, et al: Epidemiology of iron deficiency anemia in Zanzibari schoolchildren: the importance of hookworm. Am J Clin Nutr 65:153–159, 1997

STRONGYLOIDIASIS

Richard A. Oberhelman

Strongyloidiasis is an intestinal parasitosis caused by the roundworm *Strongyloides stercoralis*. *Strongyloides* has a unique ability to replicate within its host and behave as a potentially fatal opportunistic pathogen in patients who are immunocompromised, particularly in those receiving corticosteroids. The global prevalence of strongyloidiasis is estimated to be 100 million cases. *Strongyloides* infections are endemic in most tropical regions of the world, with hyperendemic areas in Brazil and central Africa. Endemic foci are also found in certain temperate areas such as the south-central United States (especially eastern Kentucky and rural Tennessee) and both Western and Eastern Europe. Most infections diagnosed in temperate climates were acquired by travel in the tropics. Humans are the principal host, but dogs, cats, and other animals may be reservoirs.

Infection is acquired when third-stage filariform larvae, which are usually found in contaminated soil or in human stool, penetrate the human skin, enter a blood or lymphatic vessel, and proceed to the lungs. Larvae break into the alveolar spaces and migrate through bronchi, trachea, esophagus, and stomach to reach the duodenum, where female worms complete their maturation. Males apparently are nonparasitic and pass with the stools after migration is completed. Adult females establish themselves in the lamina propria of the small intestine, where they lay a small number of eggs that hatch to produce sluggishly moving rhabditiform larvae. In a favorable external environment, the rhabditiform larvae molt again into the long, slender, and swift filariform larvae, which is the skin-penetrating, infective form of the parasite. While still in the intestine, rhabditiform larvae become filariform and repenetrate the colonic mucosa or perianal skin, thus starting a new parasitic generation within the same host. This endogenous cycle, known as *autoinfection*, allows the virtually indefinite persistence of the parasite in its host. In the presence of certain conditions, particularly corticosteroid therapy and profound malnutrition, the internal replication of parasites may increase dramatically (ie, hyperinfection), and large numbers of filariform larvae, as well as adults, may disseminate to extraintestinal sites and produce a fatal outcome.

CLINICAL MANIFESTATIONS Strongyloidiasis is usually characterized by marked eosinophilia, and the diagnosis should be considered in any child from endemic areas with unexplained eosinophilia. Many infections are asymptomatic. Initial skin penetration by filariform larvae may produce transient pruritic papules at the site of penetration, especially on the feet. Larval migration through the lungs may cause pneumonitis with wheezing, dyspnea, and blood-streaked sputum, resulting in Löeffler pneumonia. Like other enteric parasitoses, strongyloidiasis classically has been associated with a variety of gastrointestinal ailments, ranging from dyspepsia and postprandial bloating to diarrhea and malabsorption with a protein-losing enteropathy. Abdominal pain is particularly prevalent among pediatric patients. More severe gastrointestinal presentations have been reported, including upper and lower intestinal bleeding and perforation, emphysematous gastritis, appendicitis, granulomatous hepatitis, and eosinophilic ascites, with symptoms mimicking ulcerative colitis. Filariform larvae excreted in the stool may penetrate the skin of the perianal area, buttock, and thigh, resulting in migrating serpiginous, erythematous, and pruritic tracks called *larva currens*. Patients with strongyloidiasis receiving corticosteroids and certain other immunosuppressed patients, especially those with profound malnutrition, may develop a characteristic and usually fatal disseminated hyperinfection. Symptoms may include intractable bloody diarrhea, gram-negative sepsis, hemorrhagic pneumonitis, meningitis, brain abscess, and generalized purpura. However, disseminated strongyloidiasis has not been described as a common infection among patients with AIDS. Hyperinfection may develop even with mild corticosteroid-induced immunosuppression.

DIAGNOSIS AND TREATMENT In contrast to most helminth infections, which are diagnosed by identifying eggs in the stool, diagnosis of strongyloidiasis requires visualization of larvae in stool specimens. The most common stage of *S. stercoralis* identified in feces is the rhabditiform larva, but in occasional patients, filariform larvae, adult females, and even eggs have been seen. The sensitivity of a single stool examination performed in clinical laboratories is low (30–60%). The concentration method of Baermann allows the examination of a larger volume of feces (up to several grams) and is more sensitive than direct microscopy. Fecal culture in Petri dishes, after mixing with charcoal or peat moss, also increases the sensitivity of fecal examination. However, these procedures are rarely available for routine diagnosis in the clinical laboratory. If no special techniques are available when the diagnosis is strongly suspected on clinical grounds, careful examination of several specimens, collected on different days, is necessary before strongyloidiasis can be excluded with reasonable confidence. Although the examination of duodenal aspirate reportedly is very sensitive, this invasive method can only be recommended in pediatric patients when necessary to achieve a rapid demonstration of parasites, as in the immunocompromised child with suspected overwhelming infection. In disseminated infections, larvae and adult parasites have been found in specimens of sputum and bronchoalveolar lavage, ascitic fluid, pancreatic aspirates, and cerebrospinal fluid.

The only hematologic abnormality found in children with chronic, uncomplicated strongyloidiasis is an elevated peripheral eosinophil count, which might also be associated with elevated serum IgE. Although extremely elevated eosinophil counts (ie, >30%

of the total white count) may rarely occur, 70 to 80% of patients in most series have values between 6 and 15% (or 500–1500 eosinophils/μL), although day-to-day variation is common. Because patients with disseminated strongyloidiasis often receive immunosuppressive drugs capable of reducing the eosinophilic response, their peripheral eosinophilia might be suppressed.

Serologic tests to detect serum antibodies against filariform larvae or their antigenic products are available in a few reference laboratories. The most commonly used tests include the indirect immunofluorescence test and the enzyme-linked immunoassay, which are positive in about 85% of cases. Apparent false-positive results are found in some patients with filariasis and *Ascaris lumbricoides* infections, limiting the specificity of the assay in areas where these infections are prevalent.

The drug of choice for strongyloidiasis is thiabendazole. The recommended regimen is 25 to 50 mg/kg/d for 2 days (Sec. 13.6.1). Ivermectin, a drug for the treatment of onchocerciasis, was used successfully for the treatment of strongyloidiasis in several trials conducted in Latin America, Asia, and Africa. Recent studies suggest that ivermectin is as effective as thiabendazole for uncomplicated strongyloidiasis, but with fewer side effects. In the United States, ivermectin is not approved for the treatment of uncomplicated *S. stercoralis*, but compassionate use occasionally has been approved in patients with life-threatening disseminated infection.

References

Burke JA: Strongyloidiasis in childhood. Am J Dis Child 132:1130–1136, 1978

Genta RM: Global prevalence of strongyloidiasis: critical review with epidemiologic insights into the prevention of disseminated disease. Rev Infect Dis 11:755–767, 1989

Heyworth MF: Parastic diseases in immunocompromised hosts: cryptosporidiosis, isosporiasis, and strongyloidiasis. Gastroenterol Clin North Am 25:691–707, 1996

Mahmoud AAF: Strongyloidiasis. Clin Infect Dis 23:949–953, 1996

TOXOCARIASIS (VISCERAL AND OCULAR LARVA MIGRANS)
Richard A. Oberhelman

Visceral larva migrans (VLM) is usually caused by helminth larvae of dogs and cats that ordinarily cannot complete their life cycle in humans. Migrating larvae of zoonotic ascarids may be associated with significant pathology by wandering through extraintestinal viscera, causing tissue necrosis, and provoking eosinophilic granulomatous inflammation. Toxocariasis is more prevalent in affluent countries of North America and Europe than in the developing world.

The clinical syndrome of VLM is most commonly caused by larvae of the dog ascarid *Toxocara canis* and, less frequently, the cat ascarid *T. cati*. The disease is ubiquitous and asymptomatic infection is common. Seroprevalence surveys show presence of antibody in 16 to 30% of African-American and Hispanic children in the United States. Infection is common in both urban and rural areas.

Adult *Toxocara* live in the dog's small intestine and are 8 to 12 cm long. The ova are deposited with the dog's feces and become infective in approximately 2 weeks. If swallowed by young dogs, second-stage larvae hatch in the small intestine, penetrate the intestinal wall, and migrate to tissues, where they encyst. Some larvae return to the small intestine, where they mature, mate, and oviposit. Encystment more often occurs in female dogs than males, and the encysted larvae in tissues, including the breast and the uterus, serve as the source of perinatal and postnatal infection in puppies. In the United States, the vast majority of newborn puppies are infected and pose a health risk to those who handle them.

In humans, most infections have been reported in young children 1 to 4 years of age with a history of pica, especially geophagy. After a human ingests the embryonated egg, a second-stage larva emerges in the small intestine, penetrates the intestinal wall, and initiates somatic migration that may last for many weeks or months.

The liver is most often involved with *Toxocara*, probably because of the mesenteric venous portal drainage. Tissue granulomas consist of many eosinophils and histiocytes, with an occasional multinucleated foreign-body giant cell in an area of necrosis. A portion of a second-stage larva also may be evident. Granulomas can also be found in lung, kidney, lymph node, eyes, brain, heart, and skeletal muscle. The syndrome produced by granulomas from toxocariasis in the eye is termed *ocular larva migrans* (OLM).

CLINICAL MANIFESTATIONS Clinical presentations can vary from eosinophilia discovered by chance in an asymptomatic patient to fever, hepatomegaly, hyperglobulinemia, and marked eosinophilia. Many infections are subclinical. Some children have pulmonary symptoms (notably wheezing and rhonchi), signs of myocarditis, cutaneous nodules or urticaria, or central nervous system disease. The acute phase may last 2 to 3 weeks, and in some cases, the resolution of eosinophilia and clinical symptoms may take as long as 18 months. The most dramatic symptoms involve the retina in OLM, which is more common in older children. These include visual changes, strabismus, and retinal detachment.

DIAGNOSIS AND TREATMENT Diagnosis usually is made based on a combination of clinical features and serologic tests. Close association with a dog or cat frequently is disclosed by history, and a history of pica is commonly elicited with VLM, but not OLM. A persistently elevated eosinophil count, a moderate to high increase in gamma globulin, and elevated erythrocyte sedimentation rate all support the diagnosis. If the patient is not blood type AB, one of the antihemagglutinins (anti-A or anti-B) usually is increased, because *Toxocara* larvae contain surface antigens that stimulate isohemagglutinin production. An enzyme-linked immunoassay for *Toxocara* antibodies in serum is available through the Centers for Disease Control and Prevention (CDC) and through some private laboratories. This assay detects both IgM and IgG, and the CDC assay is reported to have a sensitivity of 85% and a specificity of 92%. Patients with visceral toxocariasis usually have elevated titers (1:1024), but those with ocular disease alone may have low or absent antibody titers.

Larvae may be detected in biopsy specimens, although most patients do not require surgical procedures for diagnosis. Occasionally, migrating larvae may also be seen in the retina.

Symptomatic VLM responds to a variety of anthelminthic drugs, including the common benzimidazole drugs mebendazole, thiabendazole, and albendazole, as well as to oral diethylcarbamazine (DEC) (see Sec. 13.6.1). DEC must be used with caution, initiated at low doses with gradual increases, because of potential toxicity from allergic responses to dying parasites. For this reason, DEC should not be used to treat ocular disease, which responds to local and/or systemic steroids in conjunction with specific anthelminthic therapy.

All dogs and cats should be dewormed periodically. Puppies and kittens should be dewormed at 2, 4, 6, and 8 weeks of age, because they usually are heavily infected and may become reinfected by breast milk.

References

Chitkara RK, Sarinas PSA: *Dirofilaria*, visceral larva migrans, and tropical pulmonary eosinophilia. Semin Respir Infect 12:138–148, 1997

TRICHINOSIS
Richard A. Oberhelman

Trichinella sp. are nematodes infecting the striated muscle of warm-blooded animals, and infection occurs by consumption of raw or insufficiently cooked infected meat. Most human infections are associated with undercooked pork, although horsemeat and wild carnivorous game, such as bear and walrus meat, may also be sources of infection. The disease occurs worldwide in both high and low income regions, with outbreaks reported from the United States, Mexico, Southeast Asia, and Europe. Because of the mode of transmission, disease is relatively uncommon in predominantly Moslem and Hindu countries where pork is rarely eaten. Most cases are linked to common source outbreaks from contaminated meat, and pork or pork products account for 75 to 80% of infections. The disease is naturally perpetuated by cannibalistic rats consumed by higher carnivores, and the practice of feeding pigs garbage containing infected meat maintains the infection in pigs.

When undercooked meat infected with *Trichinella* cysts is eaten, larvae excyst in the duodenum, invade the mucosa of the small intestine, and develop into tiny adults in 5 to 7 days. Adult nematodes mate in the intestine and fertilized eggs hatch in utero, so larvae are discharged into the gut throughout the 1 to 4 months of the adult female's life. By the second week, larvae are migrating throughout the body, and by the third week, encystment in striated muscle occurs. Here, the larvae may remain viable for years, but they usually die within 6 to 9 months and slowly calcify.

Mucosal petechiae and gastrointestinal bleeding are possible during the intestinal stage of the disease. The primary lesions are in striated muscle, where there is fiber hypertrophy, edema, and degeneration with an acute interstitial inflammatory exudate. The diaphragm is the most commonly involved muscle; infection is also common in the tongue, masseter, intercostal, extraocular, and laryngeal muscles. Eventually, larvae become trapped in an ovoid cyst. Although larvae do not encyst in the heart, their presence there during migration often causes acute myocarditis. Pathology in the central nervous system includes nonsuppurative meningitis or granulomatous inflammatory changes in the basal ganglia, medulla, and cerebellum. In the lungs, larval migration may produce a transient Löeffler pneumonitis or pulmonary edema. Eosinophilia may reach 90% during the height of larval invasion. The host's immunity is directed against both the adult and migrating larvae.

CLINICAL MANIFESTATIONS Clinical symptoms primarily depend on the number of worms ingested, number of larvae produced, and sites of invasion. During the intestinal phase, invading larvae and adult worms often cause acute gastrointestinal symptoms such as nausea, vomiting, and diarrhea, as well as fever, diaphoresis, and urticaria. These symptoms may begin within 24 hours of infection and may last up to 7 days. When larvae enter the general circulation, new symptoms may occur, including edema of the eyelids and face, conjunctivitis, splinter hemorrhages of the nailbeds, fever, and both cardiac and respiratory symptoms. Severe muscle tenderness, pain, and spasm occur during muscle invasion.

Primarily during the fourth to eighth weeks of infection, myocarditis may lead to acute congestive heart failure, and death can occur. Arrhythmias are not common, but sudden death occurring in the second to fifth weeks of infection is attributed to arrhythmias. The electrocardiogram may show ST changes and T-wave inversion. Central nervous system symptoms include headache, stiff neck, and psychoses. Ocular involvement, particularly periorbital edema and chemosis, is typical and suggests the diagnosis. With uncomplicated disease, muscle tenderness is the only persistent symptom, and it gradually diminishes in 12 to 18 months.

A rising eosinophilia beginning after 7 to 10 days and peaking at 20 to 21 days is a hallmark of this infection, with differentials that reach 20 to 60% eosinophils or higher. Leukocytosis is common. Creatine kinase and serum transaminase levels are elevated in more than 50% of patients. Hypoalbuminemia and hypergammaglobulinemia are common, and serum IgE concentration is markedly elevated.

DIAGNOSIS AND TREATMENT Unless one can elicit a history of eating raw or partially cooked pork, early diagnosis is difficult. Eosinophilia in the presence of other characteristic features, such as periorbital edema, fever, and myalgia, should suggest the diagnosis, especially if a history of recent pork consumption is elicited. Although serologic diagnosis cannot readily be used before the third week of infection, changing titers strongly suggest acute disease. Serologic tests available through regional laboratories and the Centers for Disease Control and Prevention include an enzyme-linked immunoassay, indirect hemagglutination test, a bentonite flocculation test, and a complement fixation test. Many serologic tests are not reliably positive until after the third week of infection, so testing of acute and convalescent sera may be useful. The enzyme-linked immunoassay is the most specific and most widely used of currently available immunoassays.

Muscle biopsy may be necessary in some cases to confirm trichinosis. If needed, it should be performed after the second week of infection and taken from a tender muscle mass. Muscle biopsy is necessary only when other diagnostic modalities are unable to confirm the diagnosis.

Most patients, including those with severe disease, recover completely, and trichinosis rarely is fatal. The benzimidazole drugs, such as mebendazole, thiabendazole, and albendazole, are the mainstays of therapy (see Sec. 13.6.1). Steroids generally should be avoided in uncomplicated disease, because animal studies indicate that they may increase the numbers of circulating larvae and prolong the infection. However, steroids (together with mebendazole or albendazole) are indicated for central nervous system disease and myocarditis to reduce symptoms from inflammation.

Because infection primarily results from eating raw or partially cooked pork and pork products, proper education in preparing pork and pork products is necessary. The disease can be prevented by cooking the meat thoroughly, until it is no longer pink. The thermal death point of the encysted larvae is from 62°C (143.6°F) to 70°C (158°F). *Trichinella* larvae may also be killed by freezing pork at −23.3°C (−10°F) for 10 days, although some reports indicate that *Trichinella* in Arctic wild animals can survive this procedure. The temperatures cited can generally be achieved with chest freezers, but may not reliably be achieved with upright home freezers or combination refrigerator/freezers.

Reference

Clausen MR, Meyer CN, Krantz T, et al: *Trichinella* infection and clinical disease. QJM 89:631–636, 1996

TRICHURIASIS
Poh-Lian Lim and Richard A. Oberhelman

Trichuriasis is caused by infection of the large intestine with *Trichuris trichiura*, the whipworm. Whipworm infection is cosmopolitan, but it is far more common in warm, moist climates such as the southern region of the United States, where the distribution of *Trichuris* and *Ascaris* overlap. Infection is generally acquired in childhood; whipworm ova often pollute the ground where children play. Transmission of infection occurs by ingesting embryonated eggs, which may contaminate hands or food, including fruits and vegetables, that were fertilized using human feces.

Trichuris trichiura is a distinctive nematode with a thin, whiplike anterior and a broader posterior portion. Males are 3.0 to 4.5 cm long, with a coiled posterior end; females are 3.5 to 5.0 cm long, with a blunt posterior end. The eggs are barrel-shaped, 50 μm by 22 μm, usually yellowish-brown with translucent polar plugs. Adult worms live in the cecum with their anterior portions anchored in the mucosa. The appendix and the lower ileum may also be infected. The female lays 3000 to 10,000 eggs daily, which pass out in feces. An infective-stage larva develops within the egg after 3 weeks in warm, shady, moist soil. After ingestion, the larvae hatch in the duodenum and migrate to the cecum, where they develop into mature, egg-laying adults within 1 to 3 months.

The whipworm produces an inflammatory focus at the mucosal attachment site, and ingests whole blood. Heavy infections may be associated with superficial mucosal erosions, colitis, and in young children, rectal prolapse. Heavily infected persons may develop a microcytic, hypochromic anemia from chronic blood loss. Hookworm infection often coexists with whipworm infection and may contribute to anemia. Eosinophilia of up to 25% can be found but is rare.

CLINICAL MANIFESTATIONS, DIAGNOSIS, AND TREATMENT Light infections are usually asymptomatic. Occasionally, there may be anorexia or vague abdominal discomfort. In moderate infections, abdominal pain (often in the right lower quadrant), low-grade fever, nausea, vomiting, weight loss, and pruritus are the most frequent complaints. Heavy infections may be accompanied by diarrhea, tenesmus, blood-streaked stools, and rectal prolapse, often with worms visibly imbedded in the rectal mucosa. Trichuriasis is difficult to differentiate clinically from other intestinal nematode infections or from intestinal amebiasis.

Diagnosis is made by examining the stool for the characteristic ova. Concentration techniques may increase the yield in light infections. Mebendazole (Vermox) is highly effective treatment in both adults and children (see Sec. 13.6.1). Albendazole is an excellent alternative. Problems with rectal prolapse subside with treatment.

Reference

Markell EK: Intestinal nematode infections. Pediatr Clin North Am 32: 971–986, 1995

OTHER NEMATODES
Richard A. Oberhelman

Anisakiasis

Anisakiasis is caused by several related larval nematodes, especially those of the genera *Anisakis, Phoconema,* and *Contracaecum,* that are ingested when eating raw or insufficiently cooked marine fish, as in sushi or sashimi. Most cases are associated with mackerel, but other fish, such as cod, whiting, haddock, herring, and salmon, may be infected. Human infections have been reported from Japan, the United States, and Europe.

Several clinical manifestations are seen depending on whether the worm localizes in the stomach or small intestine. In the former, acute gastritis with severe epigastric pain, nausea, and vomiting may occur, often within the first 12 hours of ingestion. More severe symptoms with fever, chills, and urticaria may develop with repeated exposure because of Arthus-type allergic reactions. Intestinal anisakiasis, however, may not become symptomatic until up to a week later. Usually, the worms are regurgitated, which terminates the episode. Invasion of the gastric or intestinal wall may be associated with a severe eosinophilic granulomatous reaction that may become chronic, causing gastric or right lower quadrant pain, eosinophilia, and fecal occult blood. Occasionally, the stomach or intestine may be perforated by the invading worm, causing an acute surgical abdomen.

Diagnosis can be difficult. Serodiagnosis generally is not available, although several experimental tests have been described to detect specific antibodies. Proper cooking of fish to at least 60°C (140°F) or freezing to −10°C (14°F) for a week will kill the worms. No chemotherapeutic agent has been found to treat anisakiasis successfully, and surgical or endoscopic removal are the only methods of treatment.

Angiostrongyliasis

Angiostrongyliasis is caused by *Angiostrongylus cantonensis,* a nematode of rodents that occasionally infects humans. This parasite, also known as the rat lungworm, is the principal cause of eosinophilic meningitis. The organism is widely distributed but most commonly found in the Pacific islands and Southeast Asia; recent cases have also been reported from Cuba and Egypt.

Humans are infected after eating raw snails, slugs, and crustacea that serve as intermediate hosts for the infective larva. The ingested larva enters the circulation and migrates by the meningeal vessels to cause a marked eosinophilic meningitis with focal neurologic signs and symptoms, including paresthesias and cranial nerve deficits. Ocular complications and neurologic sequelae are reported. Peripheral and cerebrospinal fluid eosinophilia can be as high as 90%. Angiostrongyliasis is generally a self-limited disease, but infrequent deaths occur. An ELISA test can be useful in confirming the diagnosis. Therapy with various anthelminthics, such as thiabendazole, has been attempted, but the benefit of treatment is unclear because most patients recover spontaneously. The Food and Drug Administration considers use of these drugs investigational for this indication.

Angiostrongylus costaricensis is a related parasite with a similar life cycle; it is found in South and Central America. It does not produce eosinophilic meningitis, but results primarily in gastrointestinal pathology at the site of larval penetration, including eosinophilic infiltrates with deep ulcerations and fistulae. Infection may present with a palpable mass in the right lower quadrant, and symp-toms often are misdiagnosed as acute appendicitis. Peripheral eosinophilia can exceed 60%. Young children are infected more often than adults. Treatment with thiabendazole has been recommended, but experience is limited.

References

Despommier D: Tissue nematodes. In: Long S, Pickering L, Prober C, eds: Principles and Practice of Pediatric Infectious Disease, 1st ed. New York, Churchill Livingstone, 1997, 1469–1471

Muraoka A, Suehiro I, Fujii M, et al: Acute gastric anisakiasis: 28 cases during the last 10 years. Dig Dis Sci 41:2362–2365, 1996

13.6.3 Diseases Caused by Trematodes

Hanan H. Balkhy

Trematodes belong to the phylum Platyhelminthes, also known as flatworms. Four major groups of trematodes are included in this class; blood trematode (*Schistosoma*); lung trematode (*Paragonimus*); liver trematodes (*Fasciola, Clonorchis,* and *Opisthorchis*); and intestinal trematode (*Fasciolopsis*). These parasites vary in size from 1 mm to 8 cm. Their bodies are symmetric and some are flat and leaf-like. Each adult worm has an oral and ventral sucker to allow the parasite to attach to the host. For a concise description of the various trematode diseases (including distribution, hosts, and locations), see Table 13-65.

All trematodes are digenetic, where sexual reproduction of the adult worm in the vertebrate host (definitive host) is followed by asexual reproduction in the mollusk (intermediate host). From the definitive host, eggs are excreted, and if they reach the optimal water environment, they either hatch and release miracidia or are ingested by the snail. In either case, the miracidia undergo asexual replication in the snail, releasing multiple cercariae. *Schistosome* cercariae directly penetrate the skin of humans. Some trematodes require a second intermediate host. Those of *Paragonimus* penetrate the tissues of crabs and crayfish; and those of *Opisthorchis* and *Clonorchis* involve fish, especially the carp and salmon family, to form metacercariae. After metacercariae are ingested by the final host, they migrate to their definitive habitat and develop into adult worms. Six to 12 weeks later, egg shedding begins and the life cycle is renewed.

CLONORCHIASIS

Clonorchis sinensis, also known as the Chinese liver fluke, is heavily endemic in the Far East, especially in the Chinese province of Kwantung. Children are less frequently infected than adults. Dogs, cats, badgers, and, rarely, ducks are the definitive host for the adult worm, where they commonly reside in the biliary tract. When eggs are excreted from the host, miracidia begin a rapid maturation process into cercariae, but remain in the eggshell until they are ingested by the appropriate snail. Cercariae released from the snail penetrate the flesh of freshwater fish, and metacercariae encyst under the scales of these fish. Humans are accidentally infected when consuming undercooked, contaminated fish. The larvae are released in the intestine, migrate to the liver, and mature into adults in the biliary system. In many symptomatic people, the adult worm survives up to 25 years and lays an average of 1000 eggs a day.

TABLE 13-65

SUMMARY OF DISEASES CAUSED BY TREMATODES

TYPE OF FLUKE	DISEASE	SPECIES INFECTING HUMANS	DISTRIBUTION	INTERMEDIATE HOST		LOCATION OF ADULTS
				PRIMARY	SECONDARY	
Blood	Schistosomiasis	*S. mansoni*	South America, rural Caribbean Islands, Middle East, Africa	Snails	None	Inferior mesenteric veins
		S. haematobium	Africa and Middle East, especially Egypt and Sudan	Snails	None	Vesical veins
		S. japonicum	Far East including China, Indonesia, and Philippines	Snails	None	Superior mesenteric veins
Liver	Fascioliasis	*F. hepatica*	North Africa, British Isles, Cuba	Snails	Fish	Bile ducts
	Clonorchiasis	*C. sinensis*	S. China	Snails	Fish	Bile ducts
	Opisthorchiasis	*O. felineus* *O. viverrini*	S.E. Asia, mainly Thailand	Snails	Watercress	Bile ducts
Intestine	Fasciolopsiasis	*F. buski*	S.E. Asia, mainly Thailand	Snails	Aquatic plants	Small intestine
Lung	Paragonimiasis	*P. westermani*	Far East	Snails	Crabs, crayfish	Lungs

CLINICAL MANIFESTATIONS Travelers to endemic areas develop malaise, fever, jaundice, and tender hepatomegaly when infected. Marked peripheral eosinophilia is common. Heavy infections can cause chronic symptoms of intermittent fever, abdominal pain, diarrhea, and nausea that can lead to anorexia and weight loss. Liver enzymes and bilirubin level are frequently elevated. Nonetheless, most chronically infected patients are rarely symptomatic. On occasion, irritation of the biliary ducts with subsequent epithelial hyperplasia and biliary obstruction may occur. As a result, patients may present with pyogenic cholangitis. Permanent liver damage and cholangiocarcinoma are less frequent sequelae of long-standing infections.

DIAGNOSIS AND TREATMENT In moderate to severe infections, ova are detected in the stool 3 to 5 weeks after acute symptoms. Stool concentration markedly improves the sensitivity of the test. In patients who undergo endoscopy, the adult worm may occasionally be seen.

Praziquantel 25 mg/kg three times a day for 2 days is the treatment of choice. In patients with severe biliary obstruction, surgical treatment is needed. Complete cooking of fish is strongly recommended in order to prevent disease in humans. In countries in which human feces are used as fertilizer, it is possible to break the life cycle by treating the feces with ammonium sulfate.

References

Harinasuta T, Pungpak S, Keystone JS: Trematode infections. Opisthorchiasis, clonorchiasis, fascioliasis, and paragonimiasis. Infect Dis Clin North Am 7:699–716, 1993

Lin AC, Chapman SW, Turner HR, Wofford JD Jr: Clonorchiasis: an update. South Med J 80:919–922, 1987

FASCIOLIASIS

Fasciola hepatica infects sheep, cattle, and goats. Humans are only accidental hosts. Human infections are common in major cattle and sheep-raising countries such as China, Africa, Asia, and South America. Humans become infected by eating infected raw aquatic plants such as watercress. The adult parasite measures approximately 3 cm by 1 cm and resides in the biliary tract and liver of the definitive host. Once in the biliary system, the adult worm lays eggs that are excreted in feces. In fresh water, the eggs hatch and emerging miracidia penetrate and develop within the lymph space of snails. Asexual multiplication occurs and cercariae are released; they lose their tails and encyst in the water or on aquatic plants, which are then consumed by the host. In the intestine, metacercariae excyst and emerging larvae penetrate the intestinal wall, pass through the peritoneal cavity, and migrate toward the liver. They then penetrate the liver capsule and reach their final destination in the biliary ducts, where maturity is reached in approximately 12 weeks. The adult worm may survive for up to 10 years in the definitive host.

CLINICAL MANIFESTATIONS In acute illness, symptoms include fever, diarrhea, right upper quadrant pain, and possibly liver enlargement. Leukocytosis with marked eosinophilia is usually seen with this early phase of infection. The disease is more severe in children and in those with a high infectious load. After the worms reach the biliary canaliculi, the acute symptoms subside completely.

The second phase of the illness is chronic and can cause intermittent obstruction of the biliary tract, producing symptoms similar to those of acute cholecystitis. Chronic biliary obstruction and biliary cirrhosis may develop but are extremely rare.

Halzoun is a separate clinical entity described in countries of the Middle East. People from such areas ingest raw cattle liver infected with the adult worm, which then attaches to the mucosa of the pharynx. An immediate hypersensitivity reaction develops to parasite antigens. Patients experience itchiness of the throat followed by edema of the face, lips, and conjunctiva. In more severe cases, swelling of the face and neck associated with dyspnea and asphyxia may lead to death. Symptomatic therapy and surgical removal of the parasite may be the only cure.

DIAGNOSIS AND TREATMENT Diagnosis is based on clinical symptoms, presence of eosinophilia, and detection of characteristic ova in stools or duodenal aspirates 3 to 4 months after infection. There are no readily available serologic tests, but complement fixation and skin testing using the fasciola antigen is thought to be helpful in suspected patients with a negative stool exam.

In contrast to other human trematodes, praziquantel is not effective in the treatment of fascioliasis. Bithionol (dichlorophenol) is the drug of choice at a dose of 25 mg/kg for 10 days or 30 mg/kg on alternate days for 10 to 15 doses. Bithionol may cause skin photosensitivity, nausea, vomiting, and abdominal pain. Dehydroemetine is an alternative drug; it is given as a daily IM injection of 1 mg/kg for 10 days. Infections can be avoided by thorough cooking of water plants before eating.

References

Bogitsch BJ, Cheng TC: Blood flukes. In: Human Parasitology, 2nd ed. San Diego, Bogitsch BJ, Cheng TC, eds: Academic Press, 1998, 229–248

Harinasuta T, Pungpak S, Keystone JS: Trematode infections. Opisthorchiasis, clonorchiasis, fascioliasis, and paragonimiasis. Infect Dis Clin North Am 7:699–716, 1993

FASCIOLOPSIASIS

Fasciolopsis buski is a large fluke that measures 7 cm by 2 cm and occupies the small intestine of the definitive hosts, mainly humans and the hog. The disease is prevalent in pig-raising countries, including Taiwan, Thailand, India, and Japan. Humans become infected by consuming raw or undercooked aquatic plants such as water chestnut, bamboo, and caltrop or by using teeth to peel the outer surface of plants that are contaminated with encysted metacercariae. The intermediate life cycle is identical to that of *Fasciola hepatica*. The worms reach maturity in the small intestine within 3 months and each worm is capable of releasing as many as 25,000 eggs a day.

CLINICAL MANIFESTATIONS, DIAGNOSIS, AND TREATMENT Heavy infections may present with intestinal obstruction, malnutrition, and protein-losing enteropathy that presents with generalized anasarca. In moderately infected patients, diarrhea is usually the first manifestation. Initially, this alternates with constipation; later, diarrhea predominates. Stools are foul, bulky, and occasionally bloody. Most infections, however, are asymptomatic. Diagnosis is based on identifying the ova in stools of symptomatic patients.

Treatment is with praziquantel 25 mg/kg three times a day for 1 day. A single dose of niclosamide is also effective.

OPISTHORCHIASIS

Opisthorchis felineus and *O. viverrini* are small-sized trematodes that reside in the biliary tract of cats and dogs as well as fish-eating mammals including humans. The life cycle, mode of transmission, and clinical presentation are similar to those of *Clonorchis* (also see Table 13-65).

Treatment with praziquantel at a dose of 25 mg/kg three times a day for 2 days has a cure rate that approaches 100%. Patients with heavy infectious loads may need a second course of therapy.

PARAGONIMIASIS

At least 10 *Paragonimus* species have been reported as causing human disease; *P. westermani* is by far the most common. *Paragonimus* are also known as lung flukes because the adult worm resides in the lung tissue of the definitive host, mainly dogs, cats, opossums, and, occasionally, humans. *Paragonimus westermani* is most prevalent in the Far East, Africa, and Central and South America. Other *Paragonimus* flukes such as *P. africanus*, *P. mexicanus*, and *P. kellicotti* are prevalent in Africa and North and South America.

The adult worm measures 1.5 cm by 0.8 cm. After the flukes reach maturity, they begin to lay eggs, which are released within the lung cyst and into the bronchioles and are either expectorated

with sputum or swallowed and excreted in feces. Ova that reach fresh water hatch in 2 to 3 weeks and release miracidia, which penetrate the appropriate fresh or brackish water snail, the first intermediate host. Development into cercariae takes at least 3 months. Crayfish and crabs, the second intermediate host, then ingest free-swimming cercariae or snails infected with cercariae.

The life cycle is completed when humans or other final hosts consume freshwater crustaceans infected with metacercariae. In the duodenum they excyst, emerge into the peritoneal cavity, penetrate the diaphragm, and reach their final destination in the parenchyma of lung tissue. The larvae then form a cyst in which they mature into adult worms, which survive in the host for up to 5 years. Occasionally, the larvae never reach their final habitat and form a cyst within the peritoneum, subcutaneous tissue, mediastinum, or even the central nervous system. These cysts act as space-occupying lesions and are particularly dangerous when present near vital organs.

The disease is most common in the second and third decade of life. During the acute stage of illness, constitutional symptoms are mild. Most chronically infected patients develop a cough, early morning respiratory discomfort, and occasional intermittent blood-tinged sputum accompanied by eosinophilia. Infrequently, cases are complicated by the development of lung abscesses, chronic bronchitis, and pleural effusions. In rare cases, cysts erode into bronchial arterioles with severe or even fatal consequences. As the cystic lesions age, they become calcified, the radiographic findings are easily confused with those of mycobacterial infections. Coexistence of both infections in the same host is not uncommon.

Cases of extrapulmonary paragonimiasis involve the brain, heart, liver, kidney, subcutaneous tissue, and vagina.

DIAGNOSIS AND TREATMENT In a patient with chronic cough, hemoptysis, and a history of living in or visiting an endemic area, the diagnosis can be confirmed by isolating the ova from sputum or from feces. The average size of the egg is 100 μm by 50 μm. An operculum present at one end is classic for paragonimiasis, but does not help in differentiating species. In cases of extrapulmonary disease, isolating the adult worm and/or the ova in tissue sections is ideal. Serologic tests, including complement fixation and enzyme-linked immunosorbent assay, are highly sensitive and specific in diagnosing extrapulmonary disease.

Praziquantel 25 mg/kg three times a day for 3 days is curative, and the amount of sputum production is decreased within a few weeks. In cases of cerebral disease, steroids and/or surgical treatment may be warranted.

References

Blair D, Xu ZB, Agatsuma T: Paragonimiasis and the genus *Paragonimus*. Adv Parasitol 42:113–222, 1999

Im JG, Whang HY, Kim WS, et al: Pleuropulmonary paragonimiasis: radiologic findings in 71 patients. Am J Radiol 159:39, 1992

SCHISTOSOMIASIS

This disease, also known as bilharziasis, infects more than 200 million people worldwide. The schistosomes are the only trematodes that are not hermaphrodites; they reproduce sexually in the venous bloodstream of the host. When humans are infected, five major species are involved, and the adult worms reside in a preferred venous plexus. The three most important species of the five are *S. mansoni*, which inhabits the superior mesenteric venous plexus; *S.*

haematobium, which inhabits the vesical venous plexus; and *S. japonicum,* which resides in the inferior mesenteric venous plexus. Each of these species has a distinct geographic distribution, depending on the presence of the appropriate snail intermediate host. For example, *S. mansoni* is mainly endemic in Africa, South America, and the Caribbean islands; *S. haematobium* is found in the Middle East and Africa; and *S. japonicum* is found in the Far East.

The size of the adult worm varies according to the species but on average measures 1 to 2 cm in length. Large numbers of ova are released from the female parasite every day. The fate of these eggs varies; some penetrate the venule walls to enter the lumen of intestine or bladder, where they are released to the exterior. Some are captured in the intestinal or bladder wall, and some are carried by the portal blood to be deposited in the liver or by the systemic circulation to other sites of the body. Ova present in human excreta contaminate large bodies of water, hatch, and release miracidia, which penetrate the suitable snail host. Forked-tail cercariae emerge from the snails, penetrate the skin of the definitive host, and transform into schistosomula, which enter the pulmonary venous system. After 7 to 10 days, they enter the systemic circulation through which they reach their preferred venous plexus and mature into adult male and female worms (Fig. 13-21). Patients develop symptoms at the time of ova deposition, some 4 to 6 weeks after infection. Adult worms can live for as long as 20 years in the host, although most adults probably live only 3 to 5 years.

CLINICAL MANIFESTATIONS The clinical presentation of schistosomiasis depends on many factors, including the species, load of infection, and whether the patient is a resident of an endemic area or a visitor. Schistosome dermatitis develops 1 to 2 days after cercariae penetrate the skin. The rash is pruritic and persists for 2 to 3 days, after which it spontaneously resolves. Severe forms of dermatitis are seen when cercariae of nonhuman schistosome penetrate the skin. Because humans are not the definitive host, the disease does not progress beyond this stage. The second phase of illness is most commonly seen in travelers to endemic areas. Katayama fever begins 4 to 6 weeks after exposure to cercariae, when the adult female worm begins to lay eggs. During this phase, the immune system is producing antibodies to ova and adult worm antigens.

Fever, chills, hepatosplenomegaly, and lymphadenopathy are the hallmark of this phase and tend to last for several days to several weeks.

In chronic schistosomiasis with *S. mansoni* and *S. japonicum,* patients present with abdominal pain, diarrhea, and bloody stools. Hepatomegaly is seen with significant liver involvement. With progression of disease, fibrosis associated with granuloma formation in response to ova trapped in the presinusoidal areas leads to obstruction of portal blood flow. Complications include bleeding from esophageal varices and cirrhosis of the liver. Hepatic enzymes typically remain normal and begin to rise with end-stage liver disease.

In patients with portosystemic shunts, ova may bypass the liver to embolize the lung. A chronic pulmonary inflammatory reaction can result in cor pulmonale. Ova may also embolize the central nervous system in patients with *S. japonicum* to cause transverse myelitis and seizures.

Chronic disease secondary to *S. haematobium* is associated with dysuria, terminal hematuria, and frequency. Ova deposition and granuloma formation occur in the bladder and ureter. When significant numbers of ova are deposited near the distal ureters, granuloma and fibrosis may lead to hydroureter and hydronephrosis. End-stage renal disease is seen in a small proportion of these patients, and in some endemic areas, bladder carcinoma is thought to be associated with *S. haematobium.*

DIAGNOSIS AND TREATMENT Diagnosis is made by visualizing ova in stool or urine. The eggs have a specific shape and spike that aid in species diagnosis (Fig. 13-21). Regular stool sampling for ova and parasites has a low yield. A Kato-Katz smear utilizing glycerol, which frees entrapped eggs, allows for better egg visualization. Rectal biopsies for detection of ova in the mucosa can be attempted in patients with a high index of suspicion for schistosomiasis who do not have ova in their stools.

Serologic testing using an enzyme-linked immunosorbent assay is available in commercial laboratories and is used for diagnosing recent infections in tourists to endemic areas. Because a positive test will remain positive for years, it is less useful in endemic areas.

Praziquantel is the drug of choice for treatment and is effective against all human schistosome species. A single dose of 40 mg/kg

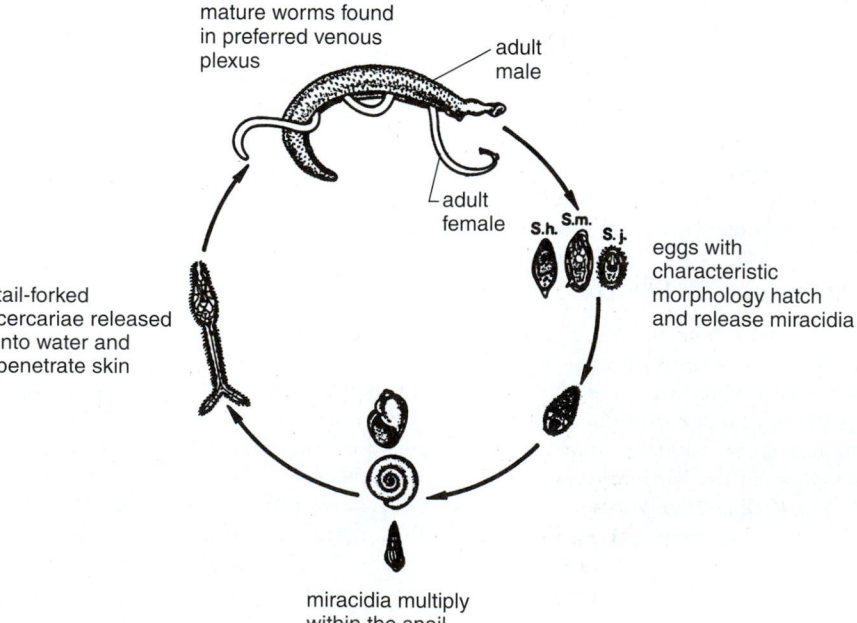

FIGURE 13-21 Life cycle of *Schistosoma* species. S.h., *Schistosoma hematobium;* S.m., *Schistosoma mansoni;* S.j., *Schistosoma japonicum.*

for *S. haematobium* and *S. mansoni* and 60 mg/kg for *S. japonicum* is curative. Visitors to endemic areas are advised against bathing and swimming in potentially contaminated ponds and streams. In areas where water sources are limited, the water should sit overnight before use.

References

Berth N, Gunderson SG, Abebe F, et al: Praziquantel side effects and efficacy related to *Schistosoma mansoni* egg loads and morbidity in primary school children in north-east Ethiopia. Acta Trop 15:53–63, 1999

Mahmoud AAF, Wahab A, Farid M: Schistosomiasis. In: Tropical and Geographical Medicine, 2nd ed. New York, McGraw-Hill, 1990, 458–473

Subramanian AK, Mungai P, Ouma JH, et al: Long-term suppression of adult bladder morbidity and severe hydronephrosis following selective population chemotherapy for *Schistosoma haematobium*. Am J Trop Med 61(6):476–481, 1999

13.6.4   Diseases Caused by Cestodes

Dennis L. Murray

The adult forms of cestodes (tapeworms) have common morphologic features that include an attachment organ, the scolex; an undifferentiated and metabolically very active neck region;, and a ribbon-like body made up of individual segments called proglottids. Each proglottid contains at least one set of male and female sex organs. Tapeworms lack a gastrointestinal tract. The proglottids absorb nutrients through their tegument. Fertilization occurs in sexually mature proglottids. An embryo, which has six hooks for burrowing into the tissues of the intermediate host, develops within each egg.

Nearly all adult tapeworms are located in the intestines of vertebrates. Humans may be accidental intermediate hosts for several species of tapeworm. Larval infections with *Taenia solium* (cysticercosis) and *Echinococcus* (hydatid disease) are the most common infections.

DIPHYLLOBOTHRIASIS

Jerrold A. Turner

Infection with fish tapeworms of the genus *Diphyllobothrium* is called diphyllobothriasis. *Diphyllobothrium latum* is the most common cause of human diphyllobothriasis. Sporadic infections are reported from many parts of the world, but the more endemic areas are the lake regions of northern Europe, Finland, Canada, and Alaska. Several other species of *Diphyllobothrium* also infect humans, especially in Alaska. Usually, other definitive hosts, such as bears, dogs, and cats, maintain the infections in nature, and humans are incidentally involved.

The adult tapeworm lives in the small intestine, where it may attain a length greater than 10 m. The proglottids are wider than they are long, hence the name "broad fish tapeworm." Gravid proglottids continuously expel eggs into the intestinal lumen through a uterine pore. More than 1 million eggs may be passed in the feces each day. The eggs measure approximately 60 µm by 40 µm and have a lid-like structure called an operculum. If the eggs reach water, a ciliated embryo develops within the egg in about 2 weeks. This ciliated stage then hatches through the opened operculum and is ingested by one of several species of copepod (water flea). In this minute crustacean, the embryo develops into a first-stage, or pro-

cercoid larva, in 2 to 3 weeks. When a freshwater fish eats the infected copepod, the larva penetrates the fish's intestinal wall and invades the muscle, where it grows into a ribbon-like plerocercoid larva (also called a sparganum) in approximately 1 month. Larger fish such as salmon, pike, perch, and trout may eat the initial fish host, and the larva again invades the muscle of the second fish. If the game fish is eaten raw or inadequately cooked, the plerocercoid larva develops in the small intestine into a mature adult after approximately 5 weeks.

CLINICAL MANIFESTATIONS   Most patients with diphyllobothriasis are asymptomatic and only recognize their infection when they pass a chain of proglottids in their stool. Gastrointestinal complaints are uncommon, but there are reports of intestinal obstruction associated with vomiting of masses of tapeworm.

In Finland and adjacent areas, as many as 2% of infected individuals may develop a megaloblastic anemia that is indistinguishable from pernicious anemia. This "tapeworm anemia" is rare in other parts of the world. This condition is the result of several factors including: (a) the location of the tapeworm high in the jejunum; (b) an affinity of the geographic strain of *D. latum* for uptake of vitamin B_{12} that is seven times that of strains from North America; and (c) a reduced level of intrinsic factor or a decreased ability to absorb vitamin B_{12} in the affected population. Neurologic complications of vitamin B_{12} deficiency may develop even in the absence of anemia. The megaloblastic anemia associated with diphyllobothriasis usually affects individuals over the age of 50, but may be seen in children as young as 9 years.

DIAGNOSIS AND TREATMENT   Fecal examination should easily reveal the characteristic eggs of *Diphyllobothrium*. The central uterine rosette and the dimensions of the proglottids are also diagnostic.

Praziquantel in a single dose of 5 to 10 mg/kg provides highly effective treatment. Patients should be informed that the drug is considered investigational by the FDA if used for this purpose. Niclosamide is also effective but is no longer available in the United States. If present, anemia should be treated concomitantly with vitamin B_{12}.

Reference

Schantz PM: Tapeworms (cestodiasis). Gastroenterol Clin North Am 25:637–653, 1996

DIPYLIDIASIS

Jerrold A. Turner

Dogs and cats are often infected with the dog tapeworm, *Dipylidium caninum*. Proglottids may actively migrate from the animal's anus or from fecal material and disintegrate, spreading tapeworm eggs in the environment. Larvae of dog and cat fleas ingest the eggs, and the tapeworm larvae mature in the flea intermediate hosts. When the dog or cat ingests an infected adult flea, the adult tapeworm develops in the animal's small intestine. Humans may acquire the infection by accidental ingestion of an infected flea. Dipylidiasis in humans is much more common in young children and infants than in adolescents and adults; infection in a 5-week old infant has been described.

CLINICAL MANIFESTATIONS, DIAGNOSIS, AND TREATMENT   The infection is often asymptomatic, but there are reports of abdominal pain, diarrhea, anal pruritus, and irritability. Eosinophilia and urticaria have also been described, but are not consistent findings. The diagnosis is made by the finding of characteristic egg packets or by identifying proglottids. Routine fecal examinations may be falsely negative. Eggs are not routinely released in the intestine and proglottids will migrate out of fresh fecal specimens. The first sign of infection is often the appearance of the proglottids on the stool or in the infant's diaper. A common error is to assume that these motile objects are pinworms or fly larvae. The parent should be asked to collect the proglottids in saline (alcohol or other fixatives make the proglottids opaque and brittle) and bring them to the laboratory. Compression of the proglottid between glass microscope slides will reveal the bilateral genital pores.

Praziquantel, given in a single dose of 5 to 10 mg/kg, is effective for treatment. The FDA has not approved the drug for this indication.

References

Schantz PM: Tapeworms (cestodiasis). Gastroenterol Clin North Am 25: 637–653, 1996

Turner JA: Cestodes. In: Feigin RD, Cherry JD, eds: Textbook of Pediatric Infectious Diseases, 4th ed. Philadelphia, WB Saunders, 1998:2513–2529

ECHINOCOCCOSIS (HYDATID DISEASE)

Jerrold A. Turner

Echinococcus granulosus, Echinococcus multilocularis, and *Echinococcus vogeli* may infect humans with their larval stages. The definitive hosts are canids. Humans become accidental intermediate hosts when the eggs from the feces of dogs, wolves, or other canids are ingested. A fourth species, *Echinococcus oligarthrus,* which has felids for definitive hosts, has been reported as a very rare infection in humans.

The adult worm of *E. granulosus* is found in the intestine of dogs, wolves, and other canids. The worm measures only about 0.5 cm in length. It has a scolex with hooks; a neck region; and one immature, one mature, and one gravid proglottid. The dog usually harbors hundreds or thousands of adult tapeworms. The eggs, which are morphologically identical to those of *Taenia spp.,* are excreted in the feces. When an intermediate host such as sheep ingests the eggs, the embryo hatches from the egg, penetrates the intestinal mucosa, and enters lymphatics or blood vessels. The host defense mechanisms destroy many embryos, but those surviving develop into expanding cystic structures called hydatid cysts. The rapidity of cyst growth is quite variable and partially dependent upon the tissue localization, but an increase in diameter of 1 cm or more per year is not uncommon. Spherical brood capsules arise from the inner germinal membrane of the cyst wall. Protoscolices, the precursors to the scolices of the adult worms, develop from the inner surface of the brood capsules and accumulate within the cyst as "hydatid sand" (Fig. 13-22). If the cyst, or a portion of it, is eaten by a suitable definitive host, adult tapeworms develop in the small intestine. Hydatid cysts are capable of developing in nearly any tissue, including the central nervous system and bone; however, 90% of them develop in either the liver or the lung, most frequently in the liver.

Human infection with hydatid cysts is most common in sheep- and cattle-raising areas such as the countries bordering the Mediterranean, Australia, New Zealand, and Argentina. In the United States, most infections are found among immigrants from endemic

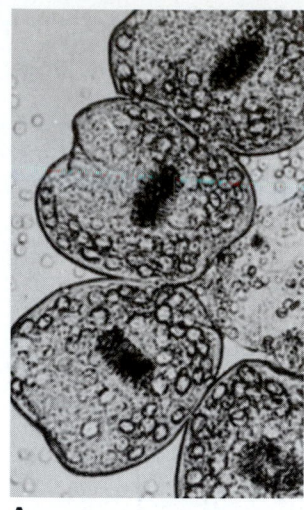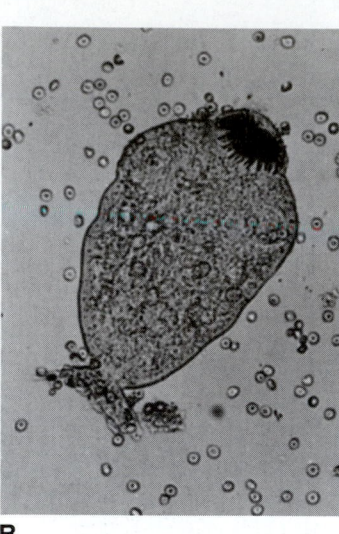

A   B

FIGURE 13-22 Hydatid sand. **A.** Scolices invaginated into cyst membrane (×140). **B.** Evaginated scolex with hooklets; stalk is present, by which the scolex is continuous with the germinal epithelium (×140).

areas. However, there have been foci of infection among Basque shepherds in California, Mormon ranchers in Utah, and Native Americans in Arizona and New Mexico. Uganda and Kenya have very high prevalence rates of human infection. In these African nations, the camel serves as an intermediate host and the population lives in very close contact with dogs.

Adult worms of *Echinococcus multilocularis* are morphologically similar to *E. granulosus,* but the larval stage in the intermediate host grows by external budding and does not produce large cystic structures. The growth of larval tissue resembles that of a malignant tumor. The condition is called *alveolar hydatid disease.* Liver tissue may be progressively destroyed and contiguous structures may be invaded. Rarely, metastatic lesions may develop in distant sites. Foxes are usually the definitive hosts and rodents are intermediate hosts. Hunters and fur traders exposed to foxes and fox fur are at risk. This infection occurs only in the northern hemisphere. It has a wide distribution in the northern midwestern states of the United States, in Canada, the former Soviet Union, Switzerland and adjacent countries, and in northern Japan. Sled dogs in Arctic villages may be sources of human infection.

Echinococcus vogeli is found in Central and South America. The definitive host is the bush dog. Rodents such as pacas and spiny rats serve as intermediate hosts. The larval stage that occasionally infects humans is called a polycystic hydatid. In this form of hydatid disease, the germinal membrane buds externally to form more vesicles and cysts, as well as to form septae that divide the original cyst into compartments. It is thought that hunting dogs become infected and are the most likely source for transmission to humans.

CLINICAL MANIFESTATIONS The majority (70%) of patients with hydatid disease caused by *E. granulosus* have single cysts. When multiple cysts are present, they are most commonly in the same organ, but they can develop in multiple sites. About 20% of children with pulmonary hydatid cysts will also have hepatic cysts. In northern Canada and Alaska, the sylvatic strain commonly causes pulmonary cysts. Both hepatic and pulmonary cysts may attain considerable dimensions without causing symptoms. It is not uncommon to find asymptomatic calcified cysts in the liver or spleen of infected adults as an incidental finding on radiologic studies or at autopsy. It takes many years for cysts to die and calcify; therefore calcifications are rarely seen in children.

Large hepatic cysts may cause pain and tenderness in the right upper quadrant. In some instances, a mass may be palpable. Biliary tract obstruction may develop, depending upon the size and location of the hepatic cyst. In adults, 5 to 15% of hepatic cysts rupture into the biliary tract causing fever, pain, and jaundice. The release of antigenic cyst fluid may cause severe allergic reactions including anaphylaxis. Patients who survive intraperitoneal cyst rupture are in danger of multiple secondary cysts developing within the abdomen.

Although pulmonary cysts often are asymptomatic, about one-third of them rupture into a bronchus or into the pleural space. Secondarily infected lung cysts appear as lung abscesses. Cysts that rupture into a bronchus may be coughed up. The patient may describe the membranes in the sputum. Complete evacuation of a pulmonary cyst results in a cure. Partial evacuation of the cyst sets the scene for bacterial growth and the production of a lung abscess.

Bone involvement may present as a bone deformity or as a pathologic fracture. The hydatid begins growth within the marrow cavity. The typical laminated membrane does not develop. Bone destruction by the parasite resembles that caused by tumor or infection. Involvement of the vertebral body causes pain and tenderness to palpation and may produce spinal cord or nerve root compression with neurologic signs and symptoms.

Intracranial hydatid cysts occur most frequently in children. The symptoms are those of an expanding mass usually causing intracranial hypertension with headache, nausea, and vomiting. Seizures may also develop.

Although alveolar hydatid disease caused by *E. multilocularis* has been described in a 5-year-old child, it is usually a disease of adults. The progressive destruction of the liver takes many years. Tender hepatomegaly, abdominal masses arising from the liver, and jaundice are common presenting findings. Extension of the parasite into large vessels may result in metastatic lesions in the lungs or brain.

Polycystic hydatid disease is a rare disease of adults. The clinical picture is similar to the findings in alveolar hydatid infections.

DIAGNOSIS A history of exposure to dogs or other canids in an area endemic for echinococcosis is very helpful. Imaging techniques such as ultrasound are effective in delineating the contents of cystic structures. The presence of daughter cysts can be diagnostic. Features noted from CT scanning or MRI may be highly characteristic septate densities. Intact pulmonary cysts appear as sharply demarcated smooth, spherical, or ovoid radiopaque "cannonball" lesions. If the cyst has ruptured, an air-fluid level may be present. A collapsed membrane on the surface of the fluid may produce the classic "water lily" sign.

Serologic testing using ELISA, immunoblots, or indirect hemagglutination tests are available through a few reference laboratories and the Centers for Disease Control and Prevention (CDC). False-negative serologic tests have been problematic, particularly in lung cysts and other sites outside of the liver. Cross-reactivity has been noted with cysticercosis and the rare infection with plerocercoid larvae of the tapeworm *Spirometra* (sparganosis).

Needle aspiration for diagnosis has been considered dangerous because of the possibility of inducing anaphylaxis or of spreading the disease by leakage into other sites. Experience shows that complications of aspiration rarely occur, and albendazole can be used after aspiration to inhibit the development of secondary spread. However, needle aspiration for diagnostic purposes should be done only after other techniques have failed.

Examination of the cyst and its contents at surgery proves the diagnosis by the presence of protoscolices and hooklets (hydatid sand), or, in cases where the cysts are sterile, by periodic acid–Schiff staining of the laminated membrane.

Alveolar hydatid disease is usually suspected when plain films of the liver show amorphous calcification surrounding 2- to 4-mm radiolucent areas. The recent development of highly sensitive and specific ELISA using an epitope, Em 18, which is not shared with *E. granulosus,* appears very promising for diagnosis and for following the response to treatment.

TREATMENT The advent of chemotherapy with benzimidazole compounds, and the success of percutaneous aspiration and injection techniques, make it necessary to carefully reassess the dominant role of surgery in the treatment of cystic hydatid disease caused by *E. granulosus.* Albendazole has replaced mebendazole as the drug of choice. Recent studies show that a combination of albendazole and praziquantel is even more successful than albendazole alone. Surgery is still considered appropriate therapy of very large liver cysts with multiple daughter cysts, superficial cysts that are subject to spontaneous or traumatic rupture, cysts communicating with the biliary tract, and infected cysts. Surgery should be preceded by albendazole treatment to decrease the likelihood of cyst rupture by decreasing pressure inside the cyst and to decrease the viability of the protoscolices. Albendazole therapy is commonly continued for 1 month or more following surgery to prevent recurrence and/or the development of secondary cysts. It is common practice to introduce a scolicidal substance such as hypertonic saline, alcohol, or cetrimide into the cyst during the surgical procedure. All of the commonly used scolicides have the potential to cause sclerosing cholangitis if there is communication between the cyst contents and the biliary tract.

Percutaneous aspiration, injection of protoscolicide, and reaspiration (the PAIR technique) coupled with albendazole therapy have replaced surgery in select cases of cystic hydatid disease in the liver, lung, and other sites. Chemotherapy alone may be effective. Smaller, uncomplicated cysts appear to respond to albendazole more readily than do larger cysts. There are reports of central nervous system lesions and muscle, vertebral, and other bone lesions resolving completely with medical therapy. As experience with albendazole and praziquantel increases, this experimental combination may become the treatment of choice for many locations of cystic hydatid disease. Because of the evolving therapy of cystic echinococcosis, consultation with CDC is advised to obtain current information (CDC Parasitic Disease Service at 770-488-7775).

Alveolar hydatid disease is treated with aggressive surgery including partial hepatectomy or lobectomy. Unfortunately, less than 30% of patients have resectable lesions at the time of diagnosis. Long-term albendazole therapy may benefit a significant number of patients with inoperable lesions. Liver transplantation has been used in select patients. However, there is the risk of regrowth and metastatic spread associated with the immunosuppression that is necessary to preserve the transplant.

Albendazole also appears to be beneficial in the treatment of polycystic hydatid disease caused by *E. vogeli.*

References

Ammann RW, Eckert J: Cestodes. *Echinococcus.* Gastroenterol Clin North Am 25:655–689, 1996

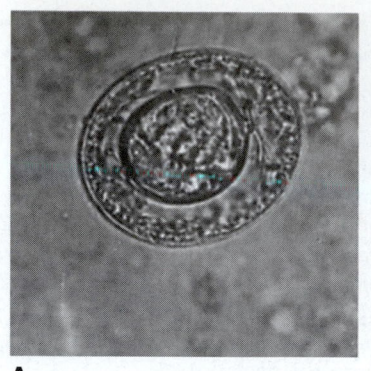
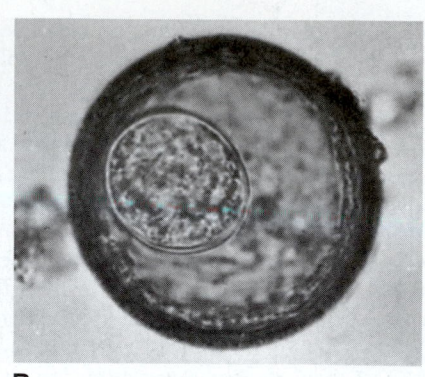

FIGURE 13-23   A. *Hymenolepsis nana* egg recovered from feces. Note polar filaments (×448). **B.** *Hymenolepsis diminuta* ovum is larger than *H. nana*, and polar filaments are absent (×448).

A   **B**

Bonifacino R, Dogliani E, Craig PS: Albendazole treatment and serological follow-up in hydatid disease of bone. Int Orthop 21:127–132, 1997

Cobo F, Yarnoz C, Sesma B, et al: Albendazole plus praziquantel versus albendazole alone as a pre-operative treatment in intra-abdominal hydatidosis caused by *Echinococcus granulosus.* Trop Med Int Health 3: 462–466, 1998

Kalaitzoglou I, Drevelengas A, Petridis A, Palladas P: Albendazole treatment of cerebral hydatid disease: evaluation of results with CT and MRI. Neuroradiology 40:36–39, 1998

Khuroo MS, Wani NA, Javid G, et al: Percutaneous drainage compared with surgery for hepatic hydatid cysts. N Engl J Med 337:881–887, 1997

Ma L, Ito A, Liu YH, et al: Alveolar echinococcosis: EM 2 plus-ELISA and EM 18—Western blots for follow-up after treatment with albendazole. Trans R Soc Trop Med Hyg 91:476–478, 1997

Mawhorter S, Temeck B, Chang R, Pass H, Nash T: Nonsurgical therapy for pulmonary hydatid disease. Chest 112:1432–1436, 1997

HYMENOLEPIASIS
Jerrold A. Turner

Infection with *Hymenolepis nana*, the dwarf tapeworm, is the most common tapeworm infection in the world. *Hymenolepsis nana* is found in 0.4% of fecal specimens submitted to state laboratories in the United States. Infections occur most frequently in warm countries. It is especially prevalent in the southern part of the former Soviet Union, the Mediterranean, the Indian subcontinent, and South America. Children are more commonly infected than adults, and high prevalence rates have been reported in institutionalized children because of fecal-oral transmission.

The adult tapeworm is usually less than 0.5 cm in length. It attaches to the mucosa of the small intestine by a scolex that has four circular suckers and a retractable structure called a *rostellum*. *Hymenolepis nana* is unique among tapeworms, because humans serve as both intermediate and definitive hosts. Eggs passed in the feces are immediately infectious for another human or for the original host (autoinfection). Ingested eggs hatch in the small intestine. The embryos penetrate the villi and transform into larval cysticercoids. After 4 or 5 days, the new adult tapeworms emerge from the tissue and attach to the intestinal mucosa. Egg production by the new worms begins about 2 to 4 weeks after infection. Eggs released from gravid proglottids in the intestine may hatch and cause internal autoinfection. Autoinfection cycles may produce hundreds or thousands of adult tapeworms in a single host.

CLINICAL MANIFESTATIONS, DIAGNOSIS, AND TREATMENT
Although well-controlled studies of clinical manifestations of *H. nana* infections are lacking, symptoms reported from several series of *H. nana* infections are anorexia or increased appetite, nausea,

vomiting, pains in the extremities, dizziness, and headache. Other reported symptoms are abdominal pain, diarrhea, restlessness, restless sleep, irritability, and nasal and anal pruritus. There are conflicting reports about correlation between the numbers of parasites and the presence of symptoms. Although a mild eosinophilia is a common finding in *H. nana* infections, it is often absent.

Routine fecal examinations using concentration techniques for ova and parasites should reveal eggs of *H. nana* (Fig. 13-23A) or *H. diminuta* (Fig. 13-23B). However, a single examination may not be adequate to rule out infection.

Praziquantel is the drug of choice for the treatment of hymenolepiasis. It is administered in a single dose of 25 mg/kg. The FDA has not yet approved praziquantel for use in this infection. Niclosamide is also effective therapy, but is no longer available in the United States. Because it is common for several individuals within a household to be infected, fecal examinations should be performed on all household members before initiating treatment. Posttreatment fecal examinations should be done after 5 weeks and again after 3 months.

References

Schantz PM: Tapeworms (cestodiasis). Gastroenterol Clin North Am 25: 637–653, 1996

Turner JA: Cestodes. In: Feigin RD, Cherry JD, eds. Textbook of Pediatric Infectious Diseases, 4th ed. Philadelphia, WB Saunders, 1998, 2513–2529

TAENIASIS AND CYSTICERCOSIS
Gary D. Overturf

The pork tapeworm *Taenia solium* and the beef tapeworm *T. saginata* are the most common tapeworms of humans. The disease has been known since ancient times, and it is found wherever insufficiently cooked pork or beef is eaten. Humans are the definitive hosts for both *T. saginata* and *T. solium*. Human infection with the pork tapeworm is uncommon in the United States and Canada, although larval infection (ie, cysticercosis) of swine may still occur. In many areas of the world, especially Mexico and parts of South and Central America, Africa, southeastern Europe, India, and China, infection with *T. solium* is relatively common. Human infection with the larval stage of *T. solium* (*Cysticercus cellulosae*), or cysticercosis, is found wherever adult *T. solium* infection is common. *Taenia saginata* infection occurs among those who eat raw or insufficiently cooked beef. Human infection with larval *T. saginata* (*Cysticercus bovis*) almost never occurs.

Humans are the mandatory definitive hosts who disseminate infection to porcine or bovine intermediate hosts. Transmission to swine usually occurs through contaminated soil, where gravid proglottids are deposited with human feces. Eggs can survive for weeks in moist soil. In cattle, grazing lands, water, or cattle feed that is contaminated with infected human feces are sources of infection. Intrauterine infection of calves has been reported.

Adult worms live in the upper small intestine, with *T. solium* measuring 2 to 8 m and *T. saginata* measuring 3 to 10 m. The scolex of the pork tapeworm is distinguished by a crown or rostellum with a double row of hooklets. The scolex of *T. saginata* is without hooks. The gravid uterus holds thousands of eggs, each with a mature six-hooked (ie, hexacanth) embryo. Eggs are 30 to 40 μm in diameter and similar in both human *Taenia* species. If the eggs are ingested by a suitable intermediate host such as swine (*T. solium*) or cattle (*T. saginata*), the embryo is liberated, penetrating the intestinal wall and disseminating via the bloodstream. The embryo of *T. solium* may invade all tissues of the body, and develops into a cysticercus or bladder worm. Cysticerci are ellipsoidal, white, translucent cysts into which the scolex is inverted.

When infected meat is eaten, the cysticercus is activated by gastric juices and bile, which stimulate evagination of the scolex. The scolex attaches to the jejunal wall, and the embryo becomes a mature tapeworm in 10 to 12 weeks for *T. saginata* and 5 to 12 weeks for *T. solium*. The adult worm seldom produces lesions, but it occasionally may cause intestinal obstruction in children because of its size. In humans, the eggs of *T. solium* are ingested, and the larval stage may develop in every tissue of the body, a condition known as *cysticercosis cellulosae*. In tissue, the larvae cause an inflammatory infiltrate of eosinophils, plasma cells, neutrophils, and lymphocytes, with eventual necrosis and fibrosis, and subsequent calcification of the parasite.

CLINICAL MANIFESTATIONS Infection with the adult *T. solium* or *T. saginata* is either asymptomatic or associated with only mild or moderate complaints. Rarely, infection can cause serious, life-threatening disease by intestinal or appendiceal obstruction, or by regurgitation and aspiration of a proglottid. Symptoms of adult *Taenia* infections include spontaneous discharge of proglottids per rectum (98%), abdominal pain (36%) or nausea (34%), weakness (25%), loss of appetite (21%) or increased appetite (17%), headache (15%), constipation (9%), dizziness (8%), diarrhea (6%), or pruritus ani (4%). Abdominal pain and nausea are most common in the morning and characteristically relieved by food. Children are more frequently symptomatic than adults. Eosinophilia occurs in 5 to 15% of cases.

Human cysticercosis with the larvae of *T. solium* is serious and sometimes fatal. Humans are accidental intermediates, acquiring the infection by inadvertently ingesting *T. solium* eggs. The larvae, which are termed *oncospheres*, escape from the egg and penetrate the duodenum, enter the lymphatic and vascular systems, and are widely disseminated throughout the body.

Cysticerci have been found in almost every tissue and organ of the body. Small numbers of cysts in muscle or subcutaneous tissue may be of little consequence, but invasion of the eye, brain, or heart may be serious. Cysts are most common (in order of frequency) in subcutaneous tissues, eyes, and brain. Except in the eye, cysts usually provoke development of a fibrous capsule.

Neurocysticercosis is highly endemic throughout the western hemisphere from Mexico to Chile. In Mexico City, it accounts for as much as 10% of neurologic admissions and more than 25% of craniotomies on the neurosurgical services; the prevalence in Mexico in the general population is approximately 4%. Cysticercosis is often observed in the United States, particularly in urban centers with large Latin American immigrant populations. Autochthonous cases of neurocysticercosis have been reported in the United States.

Neurocysticercosis in US children has been characterized by symptoms of seizure (87%), headache (32%), nausea and vomiting (32%), and altered mental status (13%). Fewer than 10% of children may present with cranial nerve palsies, gait abnormalities, papilledema, or decreased visual acuity. Sensory changes or fever are never present. Neurocysticercosis may present as a leptomeningitis, resembling tuberculous meningitis, and may cause communicating hydrocephalus. Cysticerci may be present in the ventricles (most commonly the fourth ventricle) causing obstructive hydrocephalus. Cysts that are localized at various sites in brain parenchyma can remain silent for years, only to become evident when the cysts die provoking an inflammatory response and edema. Cysts often calcify and may be discovered serendipitously. Spinal cord cysts present as transverse myelitis or arachnoiditis. Cysts may be found asymptomatically in the vitreous, but if they occur in the retina, there may be visual impairment, scotoma, or retinal detachment. Cysticerci in the myocardium may cause arrhythmias and cardiac failure.

DIAGNOSIS Observation of gravid proglottids is required for a specific diagnosis; the presence of *Taenia* eggs in the stool is insufficient. Before initiating therapy, the species of *Taenia* must be identified because disseminated cysticercosis theoretically can be caused iatrogenically in individuals with *T. solium* infection if, during therapy, they should regurgitate gravid proglottids into the upper GI tract where gastric and duodenal fluids activate the ova.

The species of the proglottid can be identified by pressing the segment between two glass microscope slides and counting the main lateral branches of the uterus. *Taenia solium* usually has 7 to 13 branches on each side; *T. saginata* usually has 15 to 20 lateral branches on each side. Fecal examination, especially with *T. saginata* infection, often is unrewarding, because intact gravid proglottids tend to be eliminated or crawl out onto the perianal area before they disintegrate and release their eggs. Thus, the perianal Scotch-tape method, similar to that used to diagnose pinworms, may be more effective for recovering *Taenia* ova.

Soft-tissue radiographic studies may reveal characteristic numerous, tiny, curvilinear calcifications in the muscle. MRI or CT will demonstrate cysts in all stages in the meninges and parenchyma (Fig. 13-24). Contrast-enhancement studies with metrizamide often are necessary to demonstrate isodense cysts in the ventricles.

In the past, ELISA has been the most frequently used diagnostic method to detect cysticercus antibodies in both serum and cerebrospinal fluid (CSF). This test can be highly sensitive, but may cross-react with other helminth antibodies, especially *Echinococcus*. The enzyme-linked immunoelectrotransfer blot (EITB) is highly specific and sensitive, although sensitivity is low when fewer than two parenchymal cysts are present. In recent series of children presenting in the United States with neurocysticercosis, fewer than 30% had positive EITB. Examination of the serum is more sensitive than the CSF. In patients with clinical and radiologic features of cysticercosis, negative serology may be an indication for biopsy, especially if the patient is from an area of low endemicity. Elevated titers in CSF are particularly useful if they exceed those in the serum. High positive titers are more often seen in those individuals with hydrocephalus or meningeal involvement.

Approximately 10% of patients with neurocysticercosis have eosinophilia. The findings on lumbar puncture are rarely helpful, and findings range from normal to isolated high protein levels with or

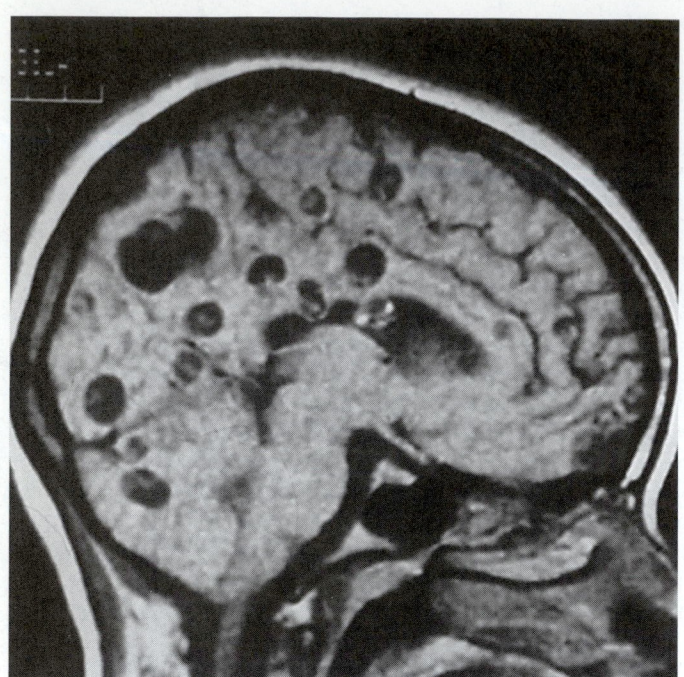

FIGURE 13-24 Neurocysticercosis. Magnetic resonance image with several cysts, some showing a punctate, dense image corresponding to the scolex. SOURCE: (*Courtesy of David Botero and J.P.S. Nobrega, University of Sao Paulo, Brazil.*)

without an inflammatory pleocytosis. Eosinophilia may be present occasionally in the CSF. A lumbar puncture should not be done in the presence of suspected increased intracranial pressure.

TREATMENT Adult tapeworm infections are treated successfully if the scolex is eliminated. An effective agent with few untoward effects is niclosamide (Yomesan). For *Taenia* infections, the single dose for adults consists of four tablets or 2 g chewed thoroughly after a light meal. For children weighing 11 to 34 kg, a single dose of two tablets (1 g) is recommended, and for those children weighing more than 34 kg, a single dose of three tablets (1.5 g) is recommended. For patients with *T. solium* infection, therapy probably should be administered in the physician's office. An antiemetic may be administered 30 minutes before the antihelminthic. If the patient does not have a bowel movement within 2 hours, a mild saline purge should be provided. Alternatively, praziquantel, an acylated isoquinole-pyrazine, is highly active against most tapeworm infections. It can be given in a single dose of 10 to 20 mg/kg in taeniasis.

Until recently, surgical intervention was the only definitive therapeutic option for the treatment of neurocysticercosis. Medical therapy remains controversial. When viable cysts are present, praziquantel or albendazole may be indicated. Currently, albendazole is the drug of choice; the daily dose is 15 mg/kg in two divided doses for 8 to 28 days. In recent studies, shorter courses have been as successful as longer courses of therapy. Corticosteroids may be given before and during therapy to ameliorate or attenuate symptoms associated with cyst death, ensuing inflammation and possible cerebral edema. Currently, therapy is recommended for children with "active" cysts, indicated on computerized tomography as ring-enhancing lesions. Some physicians prefer to treat all children rather than waiting for the natural resolution of the cyst. Others recommend that children be treated only if they are symptomatic. It is

uncertain whether children with few cysts, with or without seizures as the predominant symptom, will benefit from treatment. However, recent controlled studies show an approximately 50% reduction of cyst size at 3 months posttreatment and a three-fold reduction of seizures in albendazole-treated versus placebo-treated children. Hydrocephalus, which is a common complication of neurocysticercosis, can only be alleviated by the placement of a ventricular-peritoneal shunt. Intraventricular cysts will not respond to albendazole or praziquantel.

Anticonvulsive medication should be maintained in patients who are on specific anticysticercal therapy. Seizures are not always relieved by treatment of the cysticercosis; therefore, appropriate anticonvulsive medication may be required indefinitely.

References

Baranwal AK, Singhi PD, Khadelwal N, Singhi SC: Albendazole therapy in children with focal seizures and single small enhancing computerized tomographic lesions: a randomized, placebo-controlled, double-blind trial. Pediatr Infect Dis J 17:696–700, 1998

Rosenfeld EA, Byrd SE, Shulman ST: Neurocysticercosis among children in Chicago. Clin Infect Dis 23:262–265, 1996

St. Geme JW, Maldonado YA, Enzmann D, et al: Consensus: diagnosis and management of neurocysticercosis in children. Pediatr Infect Dis J 12:455–461, 1993

White AC Jr: Neurocysticercosis: a major cause of neurological disease worldwide. Clin Infect Dis 24:101–113, 1997

13.6.5   Diseases Caused by Protozoa

AMEBIASIS
William A. Petri, Jr.

Amebiasis denotes the disease caused by *Entamoeba histolytica*. Amebiasis occurs worldwide, but is much more common in developing nations. The preponderance of amebiasis in the developing world is a result of contaminated water and/or food leading to fecal-oral spread of the cyst. *Entamoeba histolytica* is estimated by the World Health Organization to be second only to malaria as a protozoan cause of death. For example, the 1988 Mexican national serosurvey demonstrated serologic evidence of *E. histolytica* infection in 8.4% of the population. Nearly half of the children surveyed in a refugee camp in Dhaka, Bangladesh, had evidence of infection by age 5. Amebic dysentery is most common in grade-school-age children, and amebic liver abscess in men between the ages of 20 and 50 years. In the United States, most infections are in immigrants or travelers to developing countries. Amebic liver abscess may present clinically with symptoms ≥6 months after travel to an endemic area. Residents of institutions for the mentally retarded and HIV-infected individuals are also at greater risk of *E. histolytica* infection.

Entamoeba histolytica is a protozoan with an invasive trophozoite and infectious cyst stages. The trophozoite varies in diameter from approximately 10 to 40 μm, although freshly isolated, highly motile strains sometimes reach 60 μm. Ordinarily, trophozoites reside, feed, and multiply in the lumen of the colon. After invasion occurs, trophozoites can be found at the periphery of intestinal and hepatic abscesses, and erythrophagocytosis by the trophozoites can be observed in some cases. Trophozoite galactose-containing molecules and receptors appear to regulate formation of the cyst. Cysts

(5 to 20 μm in diameter) are never found in the tissues but can survive in feces or water. After the mature cyst reaches the small intestine, the multinucleated metacystic ameba is activated and emerges through a tiny hole in the cyst wall. Almost immediately after excysting, the metacystic ameba undergoes a series of divisions, resulting in eight uninucleate amebae. These organisms do not colonize the small intestine but are usually carried to the cecum, where they may become established.

Trophozoites colonize the intestine by adhering to colonic mucin glycoproteins via a galactose and N-acetyl-D-galactosamine (Gal/GalNAc)-specific lectin. The remarkable tissue destruction for which the organism is named requires contact of the parasite with host cells via the same Gal/GalNAc lectin. Parasites that have invaded humans resist destruction by the complement arm of the innate immune system via Gal/GalNAc lectin-mediated inhibition of assembly of the membrane attack complex.

Host cells are killed via the induction of an apoptotic cascade. Host "effector" caspases are activated by the parasite immediately before destruction of the host cell. Inhibition of these human caspases blocks in vitro killing by the amebae. Trophozoites also contain a pore-forming protein, which is likely involved in the destruction of endocytosed bacteria.

Host susceptibility and resistance are likely to play an important role in this disease. For unknown reasons, amebic liver abscess is 10 times more common in men than in women. Steroid treatment and pregnancy appear to increase susceptibility to life-threatening infection. A cell-mediated immune response is likely to be important in clearing established infection through generating interferon-γ and tumor necrosis factor-α to activate macrophages and neutrophils to kill the trophozoite.

The cecal area is the most frequently involved anatomic site, followed by the rectosigmoid colon. However, any or all parts of the colon, including the appendix, may be involved. Occasionally, disease may include the terminal ileum. Initially, there may be only a few points of mucosal invasion, with little or no host reaction. Soon, however, a tiny ulcer appears on the surface and leads to a gradually expanding, underlying necrotic ulcer, the "flask-shaped" lesion. As the tissues of the mucosa are progressively destroyed by lytic necrosis, amebae continue to multiply in tissues through binary fission. Frequently, multiple microscopic lesions anastomose laterally, and ulcerations, which initially are confined to the mucosa, extend through the muscularis mucosa into the submucosa. Organisms may spread out radially, and secondary sites of invasion may occur at other levels in the colon, especially the rectosigmoid portion of the bowel. A polymorphonuclear leukocyte inflammatory response by the host may not be seen until bacterial invasion of the ulcer occurs. Often, the mucosa between ulcers appears to be normal, but it is not unusual to see a diffusely inflamed mucosa resembling that of a nonspecific ulcerative colitis. Occasionally, the pathologic process extends through the serosa and leads to perforation.

Amebomas most frequently occur in the cecum, although they have been reported in all parts of the colon. The basic lesion is a granulomatous thickening of the colon that results from lytic necrosis followed by secondary pyogenic inflammation, leading to fibrosis, proliferative granulation tissue, and focal abscesses. The lesion may be well localized and can be mistaken for a tumor, or the colonic wall may be extensively involved.

Hepatic lesions illustrate lytic destruction of the hepatic parenchyma with abscess formation. The smallest lesions can measure a few millimeters in diameter, whereas others can extend to destroy most of the liver.

CLINICAL MANIFESTATIONS　Many infections with *E. histolytica,* and all *E. dispar* infections, are without symptoms. Asymptomatic individuals are referred to as carriers or "cyst passers." It is not unusual for a child or adult carrier of *E. histolytica* to develop invasive amebiasis months later. Illness that is attributable to amebiasis can have an acute or gradual onset with mild to severe symptoms. Amebiasis occasionally can have a rapid, fulminant course. More often, there is a chronic course of a cyclical nature, consisting of mild symptoms, alternating with moderate to severe manifestations.

The clinical incubation period varies from approximately 4 days to possibly years, but is usually a week to several months. Severe disease may be characterized by the sudden onset of frequent, copious diarrhea, usually containing mucus and blood; but more often, the symptoms develop gradually, with irregular bouts of diarrhea, abdominal pain, nausea, and loss of appetite. Weight loss is seen in half of patients. Erythrophagous trophozoites can be observed in the stool in as many as one-third of cases of amebic colitis. Low-grade fever and leukocytosis are present in less than one-half of patients. If the febrile reaction is marked, or if there is considerable polymorphonucleocytosis, an amebic liver abscess should be considered. In severe intestinal disease, palpation of the abdominal wall will reveal exquisite tenderness along the portion of the involved large bowel. Colonoscopy often reveals discrete ulcers that vary in size from a pinhead to large, coalesced lesions with overhanging necrotic edges. Disease may be limited to the cecum. Barium enema examination may be normal.

Liver Abscess　Liver abscess is the most frequent complication of amebiasis. Approximately 90% of patients with amebic liver abscess are young adult males, although the male/female ratio is 1 in infants and children. About one-third to almost one-half of patients have no history of diarrhea.

Abscesses usually are found in the right lobe of the liver, although this location is not helpful for distinguishing amebic from pyogenic (bacterial) abscesses. Clinically, examination reveals an enlarged liver and tenderness in the right upper quadrant. Polymorphonuclear leukocytosis is usually greater than $12,000/\mu L$, and there is moderate anemia. The erythrocyte sedimentation rate is elevated, and chills with daily remitting fever of 39°C (102.2°F) to 40°C (104°F) are frequent. Abnormalities on routine chest radiography have been reported in 25 to 90% of patients with amebic abscesses of the liver. Frequently, the right hemidiaphragm is elevated, which is a finding of great diagnostic significance when discovered in the absence of a palpable hepatic mass. Furthermore, there may be consolidation at the base of the right lung or a right pleural effusion. At times, pain is referred to the right shoulder or the right lower quadrant of the abdomen.

Abscesses of the left lobe of the liver may present as an epigastric mass that frequently is mistaken for a neoplasm. These may rupture intra-abdominally or into the pericardial sac with dire consequences. A right hepatic abscess may extend through the diaphragm into the right chest cavity or the pulmonary parenchyma, subsequently rupturing and draining through a bronchus. Jaundice is seen in approximately 10% of amebic abscesses and usually is mild, but it can be severe with large abscesses. The serum alkaline phosphatase is moderately elevated in about two-thirds of abscesses in adults. Such elevations in children may be difficult to interpret.

Primary Amebic Abscesses of the Lung and Brain Primary amebic abscesses of the lung are rare. Lung involvement usually is secondary to hepatic abscess. Similarly, amebic brain abscesses are unusual and secondary to extraintestinal disease, especially hepatic, although several examples of direct hematogenous dissemination from the colon have been reported.

Amebiasis of the Skin Amebiasis of the skin is usually secondary to perforation of the abdominal wall after rupture of an anterior amebic abscess. It also may occur when the rectum is perforated by a fistula or sinus tract that extends to the perineal skin, or it may occur as perianal extension of amebic colitis. These lesions may be extremely painful and are likely to become secondarily infected.

DIAGNOSIS Evaluation for amebic colitis should be done in all patients in whom ulcerative colitis is being considered. Even in those patients with typical ulcers seen by colonoscopy, diagnosis should be confirmed by identifying parasites in stool or from scrapings that are obtained from an ulcer, because lesions are not pathognomonic.

Identification of *E. histolytica* in stool requires a specific antigen detection or PCR technique. Microscopy is an obsolete technique that is unable to distinguish the more frequent nonpathogenic *E. dispar* from *E. histolytica*. In addition, microscopy misses up to two-thirds of the infections detected by antigen tests or PCR. A stool antigen-detection test from TechLab (Blacksburg, VA) is the sole antigen-detection test commercially available for the specific diagnosis of *E. histolytica*. It has comparable sensitivity and specificity to PCR, but is much less cumbersome technically. The antigen-detection test takes 2 hours to perform in an EIA format, and requires fresh (not formalin- or PVA-fixed) stool samples.

Serologic tests are an important adjunct to antigen detection. Especially in the case of amebic liver abscess, in which most patients do not have detectable parasites in stool, the presence of antiamebic antibodies can be very useful in diagnosis. Tests for antiamebic antibodies are approximately 90% sensitive for amebic liver abscess and 70% sensitive for amebic colitis. The serologic tests remain positive for years after an episode of amebiasis. As a result, a substantial number (between 10 and 35%) of residents of developing countries have antiamebic antibodies detected by current serologic tests.

Colonoscopy is preferable to sigmoidoscopy for the diagnosis of amebic colitis because disease may be localized to the cecum or to the ascending colon. Wet preps of material scraped or aspirated from the base of ulcers should be examined for motile trophozoites. Biopsy specimens should be taken from the edge of the ulcers. Periodic acid–Schiff stains the parasites a magenta color and improves detection in biopsies.

Liver abscess usually is diagnosed by serologic tests in combination with a radiologic study (ultrasound, computer tomography, or magnetic resonance imaging) that demonstrates a defect in the liver. Amebic liver abscesses on CT scans are usually rounded, well-defined, and low-attenuation lesions. The wall commonly enhances with contrast. None of these characteristics are sufficiently specific to differentiate a pyogenic from an amebic liver abscess. Until more specific diagnostic techniques are developed, the diagnosis of amebic liver abscess relies on the detection of risk factors for *E. histolytica* infection, a lesion in the liver, and a positive serologic test. Presence of *E. histolytica* in stool supports the diagnosis but is not mandatory. Diagnostic aspiration under CT or ultrasonographic guidance may yield typical red-brown "anchovy paste" material, although the aspirate is more often yellow or gray-green. Typically, the aspirate is sterile (ie, no bacteria and no odor). This finding strongly suggests an amebic etiology for the abscess. Amebae are infrequently seen by direct examination, although they often can be identified in the fluid by antigen detection or PCR.

TREATMENT Asymptomatic infection with *E. histolytica* should be treated with a luminal agent alone; *E. dispar* infection does not require treatment. Oral agents effective against luminal infection include diloxanide furoate (only available through the Centers for Disease Control and Prevention), paromomycin, and iodoquinol. Duration of treatment and side effects are discussed in Sec. 13.6.1.

Invasive amebiasis (colitis, liver abscess, etc) should be treated with metronidazole for 10 days followed by a luminal agent; otherwise, patients are at risk of relapsing from residual infection in the intestine. Fever remits after 3 to 4 days of treatment with metronidazole in the majority of patients with amebic liver abscess. For the rare patient who does not respond to metronidazole alone, the addition of chloroquine and/or percutaneous drainage of the liver abscess are useful.

No vaccine is available, but prototype subunit vaccines based on the Gal/GalNAc-lectin and serine-rich protein are under study.

References

Adams EB, MacLeod IN: Invasive amebiasis. I. Amebic dysentery and its complications; II. Amebic liver abscess and its complications. Medicine 56:315–334, 1977

Lenkowski PW Jr, Eubanks AC, Dodson JM, et al: Role of the *Entamoeba histolytica* adhesin carbohydrate recognition domain in infection and immunity. J Infect Dis 179:460–466, 1999

Haque R, Ali IKM, Akther S, Petri WA Jr: Comparison of PCR, isoenzyme analysis, and antigen detection for diagnosis of *Entamoeba histolytica* infection. J Clin Microbiol 36:449–452, 1998

Haque R, Ali IKM, Petri WA Jr: Prevalence and immune response to *Entamoeba histolytica* in preschool children in an urban slum of Dhaka, Bangladesh. Am J Trop Med Hyg 60:1031–1041, 1999

Petri WA Jr, Singh U: State of the art: amebiasis. Clin Infect Dis 29:1117–1125, 1999

Ragland BD, Ashley LS, Vaux DL, Petri WA Jr: *Entamoeba histolytica*: target cells killed by trophozoites undergo apoptosis which is not blocked by bcl-2. Exp Parasitol 79:460–467, 1994

Seeto RK, Rockey DC: Amebic liver abscess: epidemiology, clinical features, and outcome. West J Med 170:104–109, 1999

Amoebiasis. Wkly Epidemiol Rec 72:97–99, 1997

BABESIOSIS

Peter J. Krause

Babesiosis is a malaria-like illness caused by intraerythrocytic protozoa that are transmitted by the bite of the same hard-bodied (Ixodes) tick that transmits Lyme disease and human granulocytic ehrlichiosis. *Babesia sp.* are parasites of mammals and birds currently classified in the subphylum Apicomplexa, together with those organisms that cause malaria (*Plasmodium sp.*) and toxoplasmosis (*Toxoplasma gondii*). More than 90 species of *Babesia* have been described. Four *Babesia* species cause disease in humans: *B. microti* from the coastal areas of southern New England and eastern Long Island and from Minnesota and Wisconsin; WA-1 from California and Washington state; MO-1 from Missouri; and *B. divergens* from Europe.

Human babesiosis is a zoonotic disease with transmission in the northeastern United States by the deer tick vector *Ixodes scapularis* (previously known as *Ixodes dammini*) from an infected animal reservoir (the white-footed mouse). Nymphal ticks feed in the late spring and summer and, if infected, transmit *B. microti* to rodents or humans. Consequently, most human cases of babesiosis occur in the summer. The white-tailed deer is an important host of the deer tick, but is not a reservoir for *B. microti*. The incidence of babesial infection is similar in children and adults. Rarely, babesiosis is acquired through blood transfusion. Transplacental-perinatal transmission of babesiosis has also been described.

CLINICAL MANIFESTATIONS The clinical manifestations of babesiosis range from subclinical illness to fulminant disease resulting in death or prolonged convalescence. Human babesiosis generally presents with mild to severe fever, fatigue, splenomegaly, and hemolysis. In clinically apparent cases, symptoms of babesiosis begin after an incubation period of 1 to 6 weeks from the beginning of tick feeding. There is often no recollection of a tick bite. Typical symptoms in moderate to severe infection include intermittent temperature to as high as 40°C (104°F) and one or more of the following: chills, sweats, myalgia, arthralgia, nausea, and vomiting. Other less-common clinical manifestations are emotional lability and depression, hyperesthesia, headache, sore throat, abdominal pain, conjunctival injection, photophopia, weight loss, and nonproductive cough. Rash seldom is noted with babesiosis, unlike other tick-borne illnesses such as Lyme borreliosis, Rocky Mountain spotted fever, or tularemia. While the number of symptoms appears to be similar in children and adults, the duration of symptoms and frequency of hospitalization is greater in adults older than 50 years of age. Children who are immunocompromised, especially those who lack a spleen, are at increased risk of life-threatening disease. *Babesia microti* may be cotransmitted with the agents causing Lyme disease and human granulocytic ehrlichiosis. Coinfection with these agents generally results in more symptoms and a longer duration of illness. Although asymptomatic babesial infections are common and usually transient, some asymptomatic people may have low numbers of circulating parasites for many months or even years. People with asymptomatic infection may experience recrudescence of disease and may be the source of transfusion babesiosis.

DIAGNOSIS The diagnosis of babesiosis should be considered in anyone with fever who has been in an endemic area, regardless of a history of tick bite, or who has received a blood transfusion. Specific diagnosis of *B. microti* infection in human hosts is best made by detecting the organism infecting red blood cells. Conventional Giemsa-stained thin films remain the most useful procedure. It is not unusual for the laboratory technician to report the ring forms of malaria on a blood smear, because there is a strong morphologic resemblance of *B. microti* and the trophozoites of *Plasmodium falciparum*. Severe cases include the presence of intense parasitemias (10–50%), red blood cells infected by multiple parasites, and extracellular parasites. Because parasitemias may be exceedingly sparse (<1%), especially early in the course of illness, other means of detection, such as amplifying the parasite number using hamster inoculation or amplifying parasite DNA using polymerase chain reaction (PCR), are often useful. In experienced hands, PCR is highly sensitive and specific. It can detect *Babesia* DNA within an afternoon, but scrupulous technique must be maintained to prevent false-positive results. Serology may quickly confirm a diagnosis of babesiosis when parasites are scarce or not detectable. Although a patient's serum often reacts at high titer (both IgM and IgG may exceed 1:2056) during the acute illness, a serologic cutoff point of 1:32 or 1:64 for *B. microti* is considered to be diagnostic. The antibody response appears to wane within a year.

TREATMENT AND PREVENTION The combination of clindamycin (20 mg/kg/d) and quinine (25 mg/kg/d) is the current therapy of choice for babesiosis. This combination first was used in an 8-week-old infant, initially thought to have malaria, who contracted babesiosis from a blood transfusion. Although this regimen leads to prompt clearing of parasitemia and resolution of clinical signs and symptoms, in most patients treatment failures have been reported, particularly in patients with HIV.

Other drug regimens have been used with varying degrees of success. Chloroquine often fails to clear parasitemia in guinea pigs and humans and is not recommended for use in babesiosis. Other antimalarial drugs, such as quinacrine, primaquine, pyrimethamine, pyrimethamine-sulfadoxine, sulfadiazine, and tetracycline, have no effect on parasitemia in animals. Pentamidine and trimethoprim-sulfamethoxazole have been used effectively to treat a case of *B. divergens*. Atovaquone and azithromycin have been used successfully for babesiosis in hamsters. Preliminary evidence suggests this drug combination is effective when used for human babesiosis.

In patients with life-threatening babesiosis, exchange blood transfusions should be used to decrease the degree of parasitemia and to remove toxic byproducts of babesial infection. Exchange transfusion only should be used in the most severe infections, such as in patients with a high parasitemia (over 5%), coma, hypotension, congestive heart failure, pulmonary edema, or renal failure. In combination with clindamycin and quinine, exchange transfusion is the treatment of choice for all cases of *B. divergens* babesiosis.

Avoidance of ticks and tick-infested areas during the transmission season is paramount. When exposure is unavoidable in endemic areas, clothing that covers the lower part of the body should be used. Tick repellants may be used on skin as directed by the manufacturer (*N,N*-diethyl-*m*-toluamide, known as DEET) or on clothing (Permanone or Duranone). DEET should be used sparingly because of rare reports of serious neurologic complications resulting from excessive application, especially to the face, hands, or abraded skin. Ticks found on people or pets should be removed as soon as possible by grasping the insect's mouth parts with tweezers, without squeezing the body. No data exist to recommend administration of prophylactic antibiotics after a tick bite to prevent babesiosis.

References

Krause PJ, Spielman A, Telford S, et al: Persistent parasitemia following acute babesiosis. N Engl J Med 339:160–163, 1998

Krause PJ, Telford SR III, Pollack RJ, et al: Babesios: an underdiagnosed disease of children. Pediatrics 89:1045–1048, 1992

Mathewson HO, Anderson AE, Hazard GW: Self-limited babesiosis in a splenectomized child. Pediatr Infect Dis 3:148–149, 1984

Meldrum SC, Birkhead GS, White DJ, et al: Human babesiosis in New York State: an epidemiologic description of 136 cases. Clin Infect Dis 15: 1019–1023, 1992

BALANTIDIASIS
Eduardo Ortega-Barria

Balantidium coli is the only common parasitic ciliate and the largest protozoan parasite of humans. The parasite has two stages in its life cycle: the trophozoite and the cyst. The cyst is the infectious stage. The cysts are spherical or ovoid with a diameter of 40 to 60 μm and remain viable at room temperature for at least 2 weeks. The motile trophozoite is the form of division. Its shape and size vary with the amount of ingested food, from 30 to 300 μm in length and 30 to 100 μm in width.

B. coli is a zoonosis and has been found in pigs, rodents, cattle, reptiles, birds, fishes, annelids, arthropods, and many simian hosts. The pig is the most common and heavily parasitized animal, in which the incidence may approach 75%. Humans appear relatively resistant to infection acquired from pigs. Once a porcine strain becomes established in the human intestine, however, the infection may spread by hand-to-mouth (via the cyst stage), and this may account for the occasional reported epidemics.

CLINICAL MANIFESTATIONS Excystation occurs in the small intestine, and the trophozoites pass to the large bowel, where they may establish themselves in the lumen; they usually fail to cause any signs or symptoms. In some patients, the trophozoites invade the mucosa and cause large ulcerative lesions similar to those produced by *Entamoeba histolytica;* however, balantidial lesions usually are larger. As the trophozoites multiply by binary fission in the mucosa and submucosa, adjacent lesions may anastomose with one another, and the ulcers often extend deeply into the muscularis. Fortunately, perforation or extraintestinal invasion rarely ensues. With invasive disease, patients may have mild to severe diarrhea with mucus and blood, abdominal pain, nausea, vomiting, and often tenesmus. The disease may be self-limiting, with spontaneous eradication and healing, or it can become chronic, with constipation alternating with diarrhea. It is not uncommon for the infection to become asymptomatic spontaneously. An occasional report of extraintestinal invasion believed to be secondary to intestinal disease has been documented.

DIAGNOSIS The diagnosis of balantidiasis rests on finding *B. coli* organisms in the patient's feces. Trophozoites are short-lived; they will disintegrate unless stool specimens are examined promptly. Cysts sometimes are found in formed stools. Irrigation over an ulcer at colonoscopy, with examination of aspirated irrigant, or biopsy, often will reveal the parasites.

TREATMENT Treatment in adults is tetracycline, 500 mg qid for 10 days; in children ($\geq$8 years of age), treatment is 10 mg/kg qid for 10 days (maximum 2 g/d). Alternatively, iodoquinol, 650 mg tid for 20 days in adults and 40 mg/kg/d in three divided doses for 20 days (maximum 2 g/d) in children, may be used. Metronidazole also has been used successfully in children and adults (35–50 mg/kg/d divided tid for up to 10 days).

References

Dorfman S, Rangel O, Bravo LG: Balantidiasis: report of a fatal case with appendicular and pulmonary involvement. Trans R Soc Trop Med Hyg 78:833–834, 1984

Esteban JG, Aguirre C, Angles R, Ash LR, Mas-Coma S: Balantidiasis in Aymara children from the Northern Bolivian altiplano. Am J Trop Med Hyg 59:922–927, 1998

Garcia-Laverde A, de Bonilla L: Clinical trials with metronidazole in human balantidiasis. Am J Trop Med Hyg 24:781–783, 1975

Blastocystis hominis INFECTION
Maria Jevitz Patterson

Although now considered a protozoan, most likely an amoeba, the exact taxonomic classification of *Blastocystis hominis* remains un-

clear. Transmission is presumed to occur by the fecal-oral route from contaminated food or water. The organism's pathogenicity is controversial, but it is thought by some to be implicated in disease, rather than colonization, when present in large numbers in the absence of other stool pathogens, especially in persons from endemic areas. Others consider *Blastocystis hominis* an enteric commensal and ascribe response to treatment as elimination of other undetected stool pathogens or resolution of noninfectious etiology.

CLINICAL MANIFESTATIONS The most commonly reported symptoms include nausea, mild diarrhea, vomiting, and abdominal cramping. Fever, weight loss, and stools with blood, mucus, or leukocytes are uncommon, but reports of invasive disease have emerged. Controlled studies fail to confirm a true pathogenic role, but it is difficult to generate valid control groups, because most stools submitted are obtained from symptomatic patients and because studies are otherwise limited. Although its role as a pathogen remains unclear, the College of American Pathologists now requires laboratories to report *Blastocystis hominis* identified by trichrome staining. Other diagnostic approaches have been used to look for organisms (indirect fluorescent antibody) and for host serologic response (ELISA), but these are not readily available.

Most patients, adult or pediatric, immunocompetent or immunocompromised, resolve symptoms spontaneously. Some experts hold that if, after thorough search for other stool pathogens (parasites, bacteria, viruses), the symptoms are protracted and *Blastocystis hominis* is found in multiple stool specimens, treatment with metronidazole or iodoquinol at standard antiprotozoan doses can be considered. Most experts would treat a patient with significant immunocompromise (eg, HIV infection).

References

Nimri L, Batchoun R: Intestinal colonization of symptomatic and asymptomatic schoolchildren with *Blastocystis hominis.* J Clin Microbiol 32:2865–2866, 1994

O'Gorman MA, Orenstein SR, Proujansky R, Wadowsky RM, Putnam PE, Kocoshis SA: Prevalence and characteristics of *Blastocystis hominis* infection in children. Clin Pediatr 32:91–96, 1993

Senay H, MacPherson D: *Blastocystis hominis:* epidemiology and natural history. J Infect Dis 162:987–990, 1990

Udkow MP, Markell EK: *Blastocystis hominis:* prevalence in asymptomatic versus symptomatic hosts. J Infect Dis 168:242–244, 1993

CRYPTOSPORIDIOSIS
Jane T. Atkins

Cryptosporidium species are related to other coccidian protozoan including *Toxoplasma, Cyclospora, Isospora, Plasmodium, Eimeria,* and *Sarcocystis. Cryptosporidium* species infect the gastrointestinal, and occasionally the respiratory, tract of a variety of warm- and cold-blooded animals. *Cryptosporidium* are tiny (2–6 μm) obligate intracellular parasites (see Fig. 13-25). Currently, there are six recognized species of *Cryptosporidium.* However, *C. parvum* is the only species associated with human disease.

The entire life cycle of *Cryptosporidium* species (see Fig. 13-26) is completed in a single host (ie, monoxenous). Humans become infected with *Cryptosporidium* by ingesting, or possibly by inhaling, the sporulated, thick-walled oocysts. Excystation occurs in the small intestine in the presence of bile salts and pancreatic enzymes, resulting in the release of four sporozoites. The sporozoites penetrate

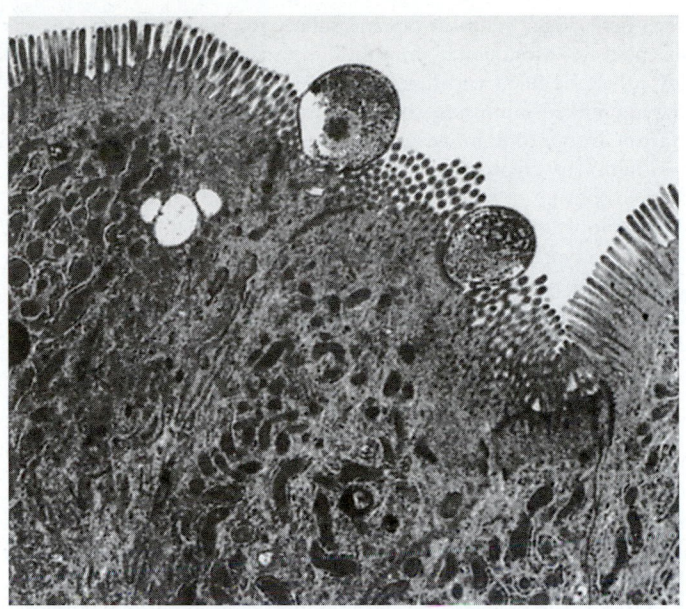

FIGURE 13-25 *Cryptosporidium* **trophozoites and merozoites in the small intestinal brush border (×10,000).**

the intestinal microvilli and differentiate into uninucleated troph-ozoites. Each trophozoite undergoes asexual replication or mero-gomy to form a type I meront. The type I meront can either au-toinfect the intestinal microvilli, producing additional type I meronts, or develop into a type II meront that undergoes game-togomy or sexual replication. Gametogomy results in the produc-tion of either a microgametocyte or macrogametocyte. These ga-metocytes fertilize to produce oocysts. The life cycle is complete when the oocysts undergo sporogomy and form the infectious spo-rozoites within the oocysts. Nearly 80% of the oocysts produced are excreted in the feces as thick-walled cysts. The remaining 20% mature into thin-walled cysts that undergo a second autoinfective stage. These two autoinfective stages (the type I meront and the thin-walled cyst) are important features in the life cycle of *Crypto-sporidium* and may account for severe disease, even when a low inoculum of oocysts are ingested, and for persistent infection in patients with AIDS.

EPIDEMIOLOGY *Cryptosporidium* species are ubiquitous. In the 1980's, *Cryptosporidium* was recognized as a significant enteric pathogen in patients with AIDS. Studies show that the incidence of AIDS-associated cryptosporidiosis has declined with the use of combination antiretroviral therapy. The true prevalence of crypto-sporidiosis in the general population is not known. Cryptosporid-iosis is more prevalent in developing countries because of unsanitary living conditions that facilitate transmission of the parasite. The seroprevalence in underdeveloped countries is reported to be nearly 65%. By contrast, in the United States and Western Europe, the seroprevalence is 25 to 35%. Cryptosporidiosis is more common in children than in adults. Children attending childcare are at high risk for cryptosporidiosis, with outbreaks reported in childcare set-tings from around the world. Secondary spread occurs in house-holds and hospitals. Travelers to developing countries are also at risk.

The principal mode of transmission of *C. parvum* is person-to-person via the fecal-oral route. *Cryptosporidium parvum* is highly infectious and is resistant to many of the standard hospital disin-fectants. In a susceptible individual who has not been exposed to *Cryptosporidium* in the past, the median infectious dose is estimated to be 132 oocysts. However, disease can occur with the ingestion of only 10 oocysts. Infected individuals may asymptomatically shed small quantities of oocysts up to 5 weeks after an acute episode.

Waterborne transmission is a common mode of spread of the organism. *Cryptosporidium parvum* is resistant to the standard con-centration of chlorine present in public drinking water and may escape the filtration system of many public water facilities. The larg-est waterborne outbreak occurred in 1993 in Milwaukee, Wiscon-sin, where an estimated 400,000 people were infected from con-taminated public drinking water. Sexual and airborne transmission also has been suggested. Occupational exposure to *C. parvum* oc-curs in farmers and animal handlers, especially those who handle cattle.

PATHOLOGY In the immunocompetent host, *Cryptosporidium* primarily infects the proximal small bowel. However, in the im-munosuppressed patient, the entire gastrointestinal tract from the pharynx to the rectum may be infected, as well as extraintestinal sites. The pathologic findings include loss of the intestinal epithe-lium, villous atrophy, and infiltration of the lamina propria with

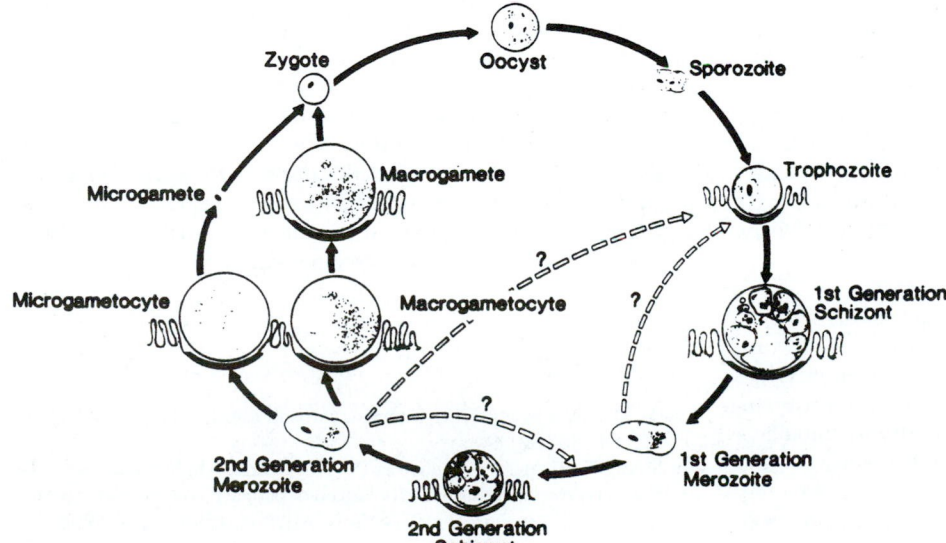

FIGURE 13-26 Proposed life cycle of *Cryptosporidium*. SOURCE: *Navin TR, Juranek DD: Cryptosporidiosis: Clinical, epi-demiologic, and parasitologic review. Rev Infect Dis 6:313–327, 1984*

mononuclear and polymorphonuclear cells. Various stages of the parasite can be seen in the villous border. The mechanism by which intestinal cryptosporidiosis causes diarrhea is not known.

Immunity to *Cryptosporidium* has not been fully elucidated. An intact cell-mediated immune system with CD4 lymphocytes and interferon is necessary for recovery from cryptosporidiosis. The presence of serum antibodies to *Cryptosporidium* does not protect against reinfection, but does decrease the severity of illness and the number of oocysts shed. Secretory antibodies appear to be beneficial. In both animal and human studies, hyperimmune bovine colostrum protects against infection with *Cryptosporidium*.

CLINICAL MANIFESTATIONS The clinical manifestations of infection with *C. parvum* range from asymptomatic infection to severe life-threatening diarrhea. The most common manifestation of infection with *C. parvum* is enteritis. Symptoms ensue approximately 2 to 14 days after ingestion of oocysts. In the normal host, cryptosporidiosis is a self-limited watery diarrhea that usually resolves in 2 weeks. The normal host who has been infected with *C. parvum* in the past may be asymptomatic or may have a mild diarrhea if exposed to a large inoculum of oocysts.

Severe cryptosporidiosis occurs in patients with immunodeficient states in addition to HIV, including individuals with cancer, hypogammaglobulinemia, severe combined immune deficiency, and bone marrow and other organ transplants. The immunosuppressed patient may have a severe life-threatening illness or intractable diarrhea that may last months, resulting in wasting. Children with underlying malnutrition who develop cryptosporidiosis tend to have a protracted, life-threatening diarrhea and prolonged shedding of oocysts. The severity of the diarrhea usually correlates with the severity of the immunosuppression of the host.

Fluid loss may be massive and weight loss is a common finding in both the immunocompetent and immunosuppressed host. Other clinical findings include fever, nausea, vomiting, crampy abdominal pain, and flatulence. Myalgia, malaise, headache, and other flu-like symptoms also have been reported.

Extraintestinal infection with *Cryptosporidium* is rare and usually occurs in the severely immunosuppressed host. Extraintestinal sites of infection with *Cryptosporidium* include the pancreas and the respiratory and biliary tracts. Infection of the respiratory tract with *Cryptosporidium* manifests as cough, shortness of breath, wheezing, croup, and hoarseness. Concomitant intestinal cryptosporidiosis does not necessarily occur with respiratory cryptosporidiosis. Patients also may have other opportunistic infections. Biliary tract cryptosporidiosis manifests as acalculous cholecystitis, sclerosing cholangitis, and hepatitis. The clinical presentation of biliary cryptosporidiosis is nonspecific and includes fever, right upper quadrant pain, jaundice, nausea, vomiting, diarrhea, and elevation of bilirubin, alkaline phosphatase, and transaminases. Radiographic abnormalities are similar to that of sclerosing cholangitis. Pancreatic cryptosporidiosis is rare and may occur with or without biliary cryptosporidiosis.

DIAGNOSIS The diagnosis of intestinal cryptosporidiosis is established by identifying the characteristic oocysts in the stool. Most clinical laboratories use the modified acid-fast stain to identify *Cryptosporidium* in the stool; however, this method lacks sensitivity. In addition, many laboratories do not routinely perform a modified acid-fast stain on all stool samples submitted for examination for ova and parasites. Thus, the potential for missing this pathogen and other coccidian parasites is high. Concentration techniques such as

Sheather's sugar solution or zinc sulfate improve the recovery of this parasite. Monoclonal immunofluorescent staining is more sensitive than modified acid-fast stain. There are commercially available enzyme-linked immunosorbent assays for detection of *Cryptosporidium* in the stool; however, they lack specificity.

Pulmonary cryptosporidiosis is established by identifying the oocysts in sputum, tracheal aspirates, and bronchoalveolar lavage, or from a biopsy of the lung and brush border. The definitive diagnosis in biliary cryptosporidiosis is established by identifying the various stages of the parasite in the biliary system on biopsy specimens. The oocysts can be found in the pancreatic duct of patients with pancreatitis. In biopsy specimens, the parasite is visualized using light microscopy stained with hematoxylin-eosin stain or electron microscopy.

TREATMENT AND PREVENTION Treatment of cryptosporidiosis remains an enigma. Fortunately, in the immunocompetent host, the diarrheal illness is self-limited and specific antimicrobial therapy is not necessary. However, in the immunocompromised host (especially in patients with AIDS), the management of intestinal cryptosporidiosis is problematic. Rehydration is essential in the management of cryptosporidiosis regardless of the immune state of the host. Peptidomimetic agents (octreotide and vapreotide) and antimotility agents (loperamide and opiates) are useful to control the diarrheal symptoms, but they do not eradicate the parasite. In the AIDS population, reconstitution of the immune system with potent combination antiretroviral therapy is the cornerstone of therapy for cryptosporidiosis.

Paromomycin, azithromycin, and nitazoxanide are the agents most active against this parasite in vivo (see Sec. 13.6.1). Paromomycin, either singly or in combination with azithromycin, is effective, but treatment failures have been reported. Hyperimmune bovine colostrum reduces clinical symptoms and shedding of oocysts, but is considered experimental therapy.

In the HIV-infected population, prevention should focus on maintaining immune function with combination antiretroviral therapy and on reducing potential exposure to oocysts in the environment, especially the water supply. In the severely immunosuppressed patient with AIDS, prophylactic use of clarithromycin for *Mycobacterium avium* complex infections inadvertently protects against cryptosporidiosis.

Prevention of waterborne outbreaks of cryptosporidiosis is a public health concern due to the resistance of *C. parvum* to standard chlorination and its ability to escape the filtration system of most public water facilities. After the Milwaukee outbreak, the Centers for Disease Control and Prevention recommended that during outbreaks all immunocompromised patients boil their water for 1 minute, use a personal filtration system that removes particles smaller than 1 μm, or use bottled water that has been distilled or purified using reverse osmotic filtration. Some experts recommend that severely immunosuppressed patients with AIDS or other immunologic disorders should avoid tap water at all times.

References

Clarke DP: New insights into human cryptosporidiosis. Clin Microbiol Rev 12:554–563, 1999

Le Moing V, Bissuel F, Costagliola D, et al: Decreased prevalence of intestinal cryptosporidiosis in HIV-infected patients concomitant to the widespread use of protease inhibitors. AIDS 12:1395–1397, 1998

Manabe YC, Clarke DP, Moore RD, et al: Cryptosporidiosis in patients with AIDS: correlates of disease and survival. Clin Infect Dis 27:536–542, 1998

Smith NH, Cron S, Valdez LM, et al: Combination drug therapy for cryptosporidiosis in AIDS. J Infect Dis 178:900–903, 1998

CYCLOSPORIASIS

Jane T. Atkins

Cyclospora is a coccidian parasite that causes acute and chronic diarrhea in immunocompetent and immunocompromised hosts. *Cyclospora* oocysts are round to oval, measuring 8 to 10 μm in diameter and variably staining with acid-fast techniques. *Cyclospora* is phylogenetically related to other coccidian parasites including *Cryptosporidium, Isospora, Toxoplasma,* and *Sarcocystis. Cyclospora ssp.* are ubiquitous, infecting a variety of animals including reptiles, insectivores, and rodents. *Cyclospora cayetanensis* is the designated name for the species that infects humans.

This organism has been recovered in the stool from inhabitants and travelers from numerous regions including North America, Central America, South America, Caribbean Islands, Eastern Europe, South Africa, Southeast Asia, and India. The organism appears to be endemic in Nepal, Peru, and Haiti. Outbreaks tend to coincide with the rainy season. There are reports of both foodborne and waterborne transmission. Person-to-person and animal-to-human transmission has not been documented. Asymptomatic carriage of *Cyclospora* has been reported. These carriers may act as a reservoir for infection. The infectious dose for *Cyclospora* is not known.

Waterborne outbreaks have been reported in Chicago and Nepal. In the United States and Canada, foodborne outbreaks associated with the consumption of raspberries imported from Guatemala were reported in the spring of 1996, 1997, and 1998. It is hypothesized that the raspberries were contaminated by water used for irrigation or diluent of pesticide spray. There also have been foodborne outbreaks of cyclosporiasis associated with the consumption of fresh basil and mesclun lettuce. In the laboratory, oocysts seeded on vegetables were not easily removed by washing. Thus, washing of fruits and vegetables may not totally eliminate the risk of infection.

CLINICAL MANIFESTATIONS *Cyclospora* infects both immunocompetent and immunocompromised patients. The incubation period is estimated to be 1 to 7 days. Infection with *Cyclospora* manifests as a prolonged diarrheal illness in both immunocompetent and immunocompromised hosts. In the immunocompetent host, the mean duration of diarrheal symptoms ranges from 9 to 43 days. Disappearance of the organism from the stool usually correlates with resolution of diarrheal symptoms. However, asymptomatic excretion of cysts may occur. In the immunocompromised host, the diarrheal illness is usually protracted, but the duration of symptoms is highly variable, ranging from a few days to several months.

Cyclosporiasis occurs characteristically with an abrupt onset of watery diarrhea accompanied by malaise, myalgia, and anorexia. Fever occurs in one-fourth of the patients. Vomiting may occur, but it is less common than diarrhea. Weight loss occurs in both immunocompetent and immunocompromised patients. In the HIV-infected patient, *Cyclospora* causes symptoms that are indistinguishable from that of Cryptosporidiosis and Isosporiasis. Acalculous cholecystitis may also occur in AIDS patients infected with *Cyclospora.*

DIAGNOSIS AND TREATMENT *Cyclospora* is visualized by light microscopy after formol-ether concentration of the stool. In fresh stool, the oocysts are unsporulated and appear as refractile spheres measuring 8 to 10 μm with a central greenish morula that contains six to nine refractile globules. The sensitivity of the wet mount is 75%. Safranin staining enhances the outline of the membrane, but does not stain internal structures. Oocysts exhibit bright-blue autofluorescence when exposed to ultraviolet light. *Cyclospora* is not visualized by Gram, Giemsa, or hematoxylin-eosin staining.

In the immunocompetent patient, the illness is self-limiting. Therapy with trimethoprim-sulfamethoxazole results in a resolution of symptoms and in a decrease in the shedding of oocysts. Agents effective against other enteric pathogens (such as norfloxacin, tinidazole, quinacrine, nalidixic acid, and diloxanide furoate) do not eradicate the oocyst of *Cyclospora.* In the HIV-infected patient, recurrent episodes are prevented using prophylaxis with trimethoprim-sulfamethoxazole 3 days a week.

References

Hoge CW, Shlim DR, Ghimire M, et al: Placebo-controlled trial of cotrimoxazole for *Cyclospora* infection among travellers and foreign residents in Nepal. Lancet 345:691–693, 1995

Ortega YR, Sterling CR, Gilman RH, et al: *Cyclospora* species—a new protozoan pathogen of humans. N Engl J Med 328:1308–1312, 1993

Pape JW, Verdier R, Boney M, et al: *Cyclospora* infection in adults infected with HIV: clinical manifestations, treatment, and prophylaxis. Ann Intern Med 121:654–657, 1994

Soave R: *Cyclospora*: an overview. Clin Infect Dis 23:429–437, 1996

Sterling CR, Ortega YR: *Cyclospora:* an enigma worth unraveling. Emerg Infect Dis 5:48–53, 1999

DIENTAMOEBIASIS

Dennis L. Murray

Dientamoeba fragilis is a protozoan parasite inhabiting the human colon that is associated with both acute and chronic gastrointestinal symptoms. Humans are likely the natural host for *D. fragilis.* Unlike most other intestinal protozoa, *D. fragilis* has no known cyst form and has not been found to invade tissues. The organism is usually 7 to 12 μm in diameter and demonstrates pointed or leaf-shaped pseudopodia. While moving actively in fresh fecal specimens, the organism quickly becomes rounded and less identifiable in stored specimens. When suitably stained, most *D. fragilis* reveal two characteristic nuclei that each contain a large karyosome with granules. Some large uninucleate forms may also be found. Because of its small size, this organism may be overlooked by inexperienced laboratory personnel.

The mode of transmission of *D. fragilis* is unknown; however, several investigators have noted a high frequency of concomitant infection with *D. fragilis* and the pinworm *Enterobius vermicularis.* It is thought that this organism infects the human host by entering and passing in pinworm eggs. Attempts to culture *D. fragilis* from pinworm eggs or larvae, however, have been consistently unsuccessful.

Dientamoeba fragilis has been found in most parts of the world. Prevalence varies widely from 1 to 38% in selected populations. Increased prevalence is seen in persons residing in crowded living conditions, such as those living in institutions and communes, and in persons traveling outside the United States.

CLINICAL MANIFESTATIONS Both acute and chronic illnesses are associated with infection caused by *D. fragilis*. Infected children and adults may present with acute watery diarrhea accompanied by abdominal pain, nausea, and vomiting. Fever, fatigue, and weakness are less common, but can occur. Stools are usually mushy or sticky, and at times may contain blood and/or mucus. *Dientamoeba fragilis* infection is most often associated with chronic abdominal pain lasting months to years. Patients may present with alternating diarrhea and constipation, flatulence, and fatigue. Some patients with chronic infection have been reported with low-grade eosinophilia. Many individuals harbor this protozoan and have no symptoms.

DIAGNOSIS AND TREATMENT This organism should be suspected in patients who have had abdominal pain and/or diarrhea for an extended period of time, particularly those patients who reside in institutions, who recently traveled outside the United States, or who are infected with pinworms. At least three stool specimens should be collected on alternate days and placed immediately in a stool preservative such as polyvinyl alcohol. Trichrome staining of stool after sedimentation concentration technique may produce the best yield of *D. fragilis* trophozoites. Interference with the detection of protozoa may occur with barium, so stool samples should be collected before radiologic studies with barium are performed. No serologic test is available.

Treatment is recommended only for symptomatic infection. Lacking clinical studies, therapy for *D. fragilis* is considered investigational by the United States Food and Drug Administration. Iodoquinol, tetracycline, and paromomycin are recommended for treatment of *D. fragilis* (see Sec. 13.6.1). Metronidazole may be effective. Adults should be treated with iodoquinol 650 mg tid for 20 days and children with 40 mg/kg/d (maximum 2 g) divided tid for 20 days. Alternatively, paromomycin 25 to 30 mg/kg/d in divided doses for 7 days may be more effective than iodoquinol, but may not be readily available. Tetracycline may be used in adults (500 mg qid for 10 days) and children ≥8 years of age (10 mg/kg qid—maximum 2 g—for 10 days).

References

Grendon JH, DiGiacomo RF, Frost FJ: Descriptive features of *Dientamoeba fragilis* infections. J Trop Med Hyg 98:309–315, 1995

Oxner, RB, Paltridge GP, Chapman BA, et al: *Dientamoeba fragilis:* a bowel pathogen? Aust N Z Med J 100:64–65, 1987

Spencer MJ, Garcia LS, Chapin M: *Dientamoeba fragilis:* an intestinal pathogen in children? Am J Dis Child 133:390–393, 1979

FREE-LIVING AMEBIC INFECTIONS
William A. Petri, Jr.

The ubiquitous, free-living amebae of the genera *Naegleria*, *Balamuthia*, and *Acanthamoeba* are the etiologic agents of rare infections of the central nervous system and eyes. *Naegleria fowleri* is the agent of primary amebic meningoencephalitis, *Acanthamoeba* and *Balamuthia* cause granulomatous amebic meningoencephalitis, and *Acanthamoeba* also can infect the eye, resulting in amebic keratitis. *Naegleria*, *Balamuthia*, and *Acanthamoeba* have trophozoite and cyst stages; for *Naegleria*, only trophozoites are found in tissues. *Naegleria* trophozoites are 10 to 30 μm in diameter and have a clear nucleus with a prominent central dense nucleolus and cytoplasmic pseudopodia. *Acanthamoeba* and *Balamuthia* trophozoites are of similar size and appearance to *Naegleria*, but the cyst

form of these parasites may also be observed in tissue. Unequivocal identification of these amebae is not routine, and specimens should be referred to a qualified protozoologist for confirmation.

Almost every example of acute primary amebic meningoencephalitis reveals a recent patient history of swimming in fresh or brackish water. The organisms probably gain access to neural tissue via the nasal mucosa and the cribriform plate. There have been several epidemics in which the same swimming facility was the focus of infection. This disease has been reported in England, the Czech Republic, Australia, Virginia, Texas, and Florida. *Naegleria fowleri* has been isolated from soil and the bottom sediment of lakes and pools from all parts of the world. It also has been reported in thermally polluted water, where it can reproduce at temperatures up to 46°C (114.8°F). Seroepidemiologic studies demonstrate that most young adults in the southern United States have agglutinating antibodies against *Naegleria*.

Granulomatous amebic encephalitis caused by *Acanthamoeba* is an illness of the immunocompromised and debilitated, whereas *Balamuthia* causes a subacute to chronic infection of both normal and immunocompromised individuals. These infections have incubation periods that exceed 1 week, and the clinical course, which usually is fatal, can last for weeks to months.

Keratitis caused by *Acanthamoeba* is most common in individuals who wear contact lenses. It is also seen as a complication of other corneal injuries. Corneal infection is associated with wearing the lenses while swimming in freshwater lakes and rivers, and with the use of homemade saline solutions to store the lenses.

CLINICAL MANIFESTATIONS Primary amebic meningoencephalitis has occurred in young, previously healthy individuals between the ages of 2 and 27 years. Most patients have been swimming in warm fresh water 2 to 5 days prior to the onset of symptoms. Very early in infection the patient may notice changes in taste or smell, followed by the abrupt onset of fever, headache, meningismus, nausea, vomiting, and a rapidly deepening coma. Death follows the onset of symptoms in approximately 1 week in most patients. Cerebrospinal fluid usually reveals large numbers of polymorphonuclear leukocytes, blood, hypoglycorrhachia, and elevated protein levels. Motile amebae can be found if the fluid is examined under high magnification on a warm stage. Most histopathologic studies show severe lytic necrosis and hemorrhage along the base of the brain in the regions of the olfactory bulbs and cerebellum.

Granulomatous amebic encephalitis predominantly is a disease of the immunocompromised, although *Balamuthia* can cause disease in the absence of identifiable immune defects. Onset is insidious, and presentation with focal neurologic deficits common. Presenting signs and symptoms include mental status abnormalities and seizures in approximately 66% of patients; fever, headache, and meningismus in 50% of patients; and ataxia or visual disturbances in 20% of patients. Skin ulcerations or nodules can be observed for months before the onset of central nervous system disease. In both subacute and chronic disease, single or multiple foci of granulomatous inflammation have been reported involving the cerebellum, midbrain, and brainstem. Examination of the spinal fluid usually reveals many mononuclear cells and is nondiagnostic. Amebae can be demonstrated in brain biopsies and in skin nodules or ulcers.

Acanthamoeba keratitis is frequently misdiagnosed as a herpes simplex virus or bacterial keratitis. Symptoms begin with a foreign-body sensation in the eye followed by severe pain, tearing, photophobia, and blurred vision. The disease progresses over days to months, with periods of temporary remission common. Signs include iritis, a distinctive corneal ring infiltrate in most patients, and an early dendriform epithelial pattern of inflammation in some patients. There may be marked inflammatory changes in the anterior and posterior chambers, and uveitis also occurs. Organisms often can be found in corneal scrapings or biopsy material.

DIAGNOSIS AND THERAPY Consider the diagnosis in a child with meningoencephalitis, a recent history of freshwater exposure, and cerebrospinal fluid (CSF) with a neutrophilic pleiocytosis and no bacteria demonstrated by CSF cultures or Gram stain. The disease can be diagnosed by finding motile amebae in the unfixed purulent cerebrospinal fluid. Therapy for *Naegleria* infection is not satisfactory. There is a single well-documented report in which early diagnosis of primary amebic meningoencephalitis was successfully treated with amphotericin B by both the systemic and intracisternal routes. It may be necessary to achieve therapeutic levels rapidly. Many other patients who were treated with this drug were not helped. Although a 9-year-old girl was treated successfully with a combination of IV and intrathecal amphotericin B and miconazole plus oral rifampin, recent use of this regimen in several other patients was unsatisfactory. In experimental *Naegleria* meningoencephalitis, tetracycline markedly potentiated the efficacy of amphotericin B. There is also little information to guide the treatment of granulomatous amebic encephalitis. There are interspecies and interstrain differences in drug susceptibility, but, in general, the diamidine derivatives (propamidine, pentamidine, dibromopropamidine), ketoconazole, paromomycin, neomycin, 5-flucytosine, and, to a lesser extent, amphotericin B are active against many isolates.

Acanthamoeba keratitis, in contrast, has been successfully treated with aggressive surgical débridement combined with the frequent (up to nine times per day) application of topical 0.1% propamidine isethionate plus neosporin or oral itraconazole plus topical miconazole. Topical polyhexamethylene biguanide also has been effective treatment for this condition in a limited number of patients.

References

Barnett ND, Kaplan AM, Hopkin RJ, et al: Primary amoebic meningoencephalitis with *Naegleria fowleri:* clinical review. Pediatr Neurol 15: 230–234, 1996

Denney CF, Iragui VJ, Uber-Zak LD, et al: Amebic meningoencephalitis caused by *Balamuthia mandrillaris:* case report and review. Clin Infect Dis 25:1354–1358, 1997

Duguid IG, Dart JK, Morlet N, et al: Outcome of *Acanthamoeba* keratitis treated with polyhexamethyl biguanide and propamidine. Ophthalmology 104:1587–1592, 1997

Ishibashi Y, Matsumoto Y, Kabata T, et al: Oral itraconazole and topical miconazole with debridement for *Acanthamoeba* keratitis. Am J Ophthalmol 109:121–126, 1990

Walker CW: *Acanthamoeba:* ecology, pathogenicity and laboratory detection. Br J Biomed Sci 53:146–151, 1996

GIARDIASIS
Scott Santibanez and Richard A. Oberhelman

Giardia lamblia is a protozoan flagellate that is the most common disease-causing parasite in the United States and the most frequently identified agent of waterborne diarrhea. Cases are especially common in areas with inadequate water and sanitation facilities. Humans are the major reservoir of infection, although other mammals, such as dogs, cats, and beavers, may be colonized and excrete cysts. Massive epidemics have occurred after the contamination of reservoirs, lakes, and streams, especially when community water supplies are not adequately filtered. In developing countries, *Giardia* infection has been reported in almost 100% of children followed prospectively from birth until age 2 years. In the United States and other developed countries, *Giardia* is prevalent in childcare centers and custodial institutions, backpackers, and in the male homosexual community. Person-to-person spread via fecal-oral route and ingestion of contaminated water are the most common modes of transmission; infection through food is less common.

Giardia cysts, present in the stool of infected persons, are the infective form. After ingestion they excyst in the small intestine, yielding trophozoites that subsequently multiply. The trophozoites remain limited to the mucosa, mucus, or lumen of the intestine and are rarely, if ever, invasive (Fig. 13-27). Encystation normally occurs prior to expulsion in the feces. Contamination of oneself and the environment with cysts is common. The number of cysts excreted varies, but it may reach as many as 10 million per gram. Infections are relatively frequent because as few as 10 cysts can infect 30% of inoculated humans.

The exact pathophysiology of the diarrhea is not known. The most severe cases are characterized by malabsorption and lactose intolerance, with varying degrees of inflammation and villous blunting. Host factors are also determinants of disease outcome; only 40% of humans infected with the same inoculum develop diarrhea. Patients with hypogammaglobulinemia frequently suffer from particularly severe cases of giardiasis. The observation that asymptomatic infections are more common in persons previously infected with *Giardia* also suggests partial immunity.

CLINICAL MANIFESTATIONS Clinical manifestations and duration of symptoms vary. Infections range from asymptomatic cases to severe, life-threatening diarrhea accompanied by malabsorption and dehydration. Infections may last from a few days to years. In naturally occurring infections, symptoms usually appear approximately 12 to 14 days after presumed exposure. Passage of cysts usually begins 7 to 10 days after inoculation (range 5 to 21 days). Symptoms include watery, foul-smelling diarrhea, which can be sudden in onset and accompanied by abdominal distension, epigastric cramping, flatus, nausea, vomiting, anorexia, and fatigue.

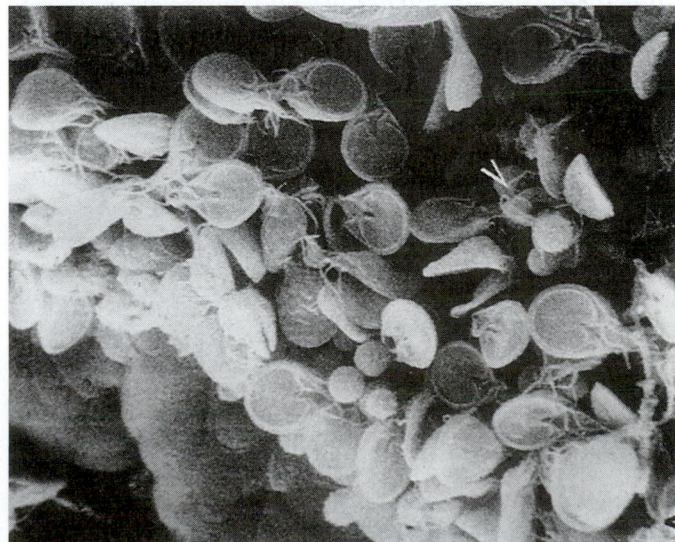

FIGURE 13-27 Trophozoites of *Giardia lamblia* attached to intestinal epithelium.

Systemic symptoms such as fever and chills are uncommon. Blood and mucus in the stools do not occur in giardiasis. Urticaria and arthritis have been anecdotally associated. In its most florid manifestations, giardiasis results in symptoms and signs associated with severe small-intestinal malabsorption and weight loss. Although some patients have severe symptoms at the onset of illness and seek medical care shortly after becoming ill, the majority who seek medical attention complain of remitting abdominal pain, nausea, or weight loss lasting weeks to months.

DIAGNOSIS   Giardiasis is confirmed by detection of the parasite or its antigens in the stool or intestinal lining. Cysts are oval, 8 to 10 μm long by 7 to 10 μm wide, and contain four nuclei. When viewed dorsally, the trophozoite has a characteristic pear shape and contains two similar nuclei. Trophozoites vary in size from 9 to 21 μm in length and 5 to 15 μm in width. Other features include four paired flagella and a ventral sucking disc with which the trophozoite attaches to the intestinal mucosa.

Cysts are the most commonly detected form in the feces, and trophozoites are almost entirely limited to liquid stools. Merthiolate-iodine-formalin (MIF) concentration improves the detection of cysts. The numbers of cysts excreted vary, and they may not be detected on any single examination. If initial stool examination is negative, three stool examinations spaced 2 days apart are recommended. Careful fecal examination detects over 90% of infected individuals but requires an experienced microscopist.

Occasionally, cysts are not detected in the feces, and sampling small intestinal fluid by intubation or by the "string test" is useful. For the string test, a capsule attached to an absorbent string is swallowed, and trophozoites attach as the capsule proceeds through the jejunum. After 4 hours the string is withdrawn and duodenal fluid on the string is examined for trophozoites. Esophagogastroduodenoscopy with biopsy may be diagnostic. Commercially available assays for detecting *Giardia* antigen in the stool may be useful when microscopy is negative. In general, these tests are more sensitive than stool examination with similar specificity, and with the added benefit of being much less time-consuming than microscopy. Antibody detection assays are rarely clinically useful, as the relationship between serum antibody and clinical disease is unclear.

TREATMENT AND PREVENTION   Because many people are asymptomatically infected, the decision to treat should be based upon presence of symptoms such as diarrhea, malabsorption, and failure to thrive. Asymptomatic cyst excreters are generally not treated except in unusual circumstances, for example, when attempting to prevent or control infections in a family with high-risk individuals such as pregnant women or patients with hypogammaglobulinemia.

Furazolidone (Furoxone) is the only anti-*Giardia* drug that is available as a suspension in the United States, thus making it particularly useful in infants and younger children. There are mixed reports on the effectiveness of furazolidone, with cure rates ranging from 77 to 92%. The dose for children is 6 mg/kg/d, divided into four doses for 7 days. Metronidazole (Flagyl) is frequently prescribed and is an effective drug for giardiasis, but it remains unlicensed in the United States for this indication. The dose is 5 mg/kg tid for 7 days for young children, whereas older children may be given the adult dose of 250 mg tid for 7 days. The most effective treatment is quinacrine hydrochloride (Atabrine), although it is no longer available in the United States because of concerns related to toxicity. Tinidazole (Fasigyn) is also effective, but it is not licensed

in the United States. Treatment failures can be treated with another drug, with longer durations of therapy, and with increased amounts of drug when metronidazole is used. Combined therapy with metronidazole and quinacrine (Atabrine) is effective in the rare patient who is refractory to multiple courses of therapy.

Food or drinks that likely are contaminated should be avoided. Hand washing and attention to personal hygiene are important preventative measures. Potentially contaminated water should be boiled or filtered, because chlorination, freezing, and disinfection by ultraviolet light are not effective against *Giardia*.

References

Aldeen WE, Carrol K, Robison A, Morrison M, Hale D: Comparison of nine commercially available enzyme-linked immunosorbant assays for detection of *Giardia lamblia* in fecal specimens. J Clin Microbiol 35(6):1338–1340, 1998

Nash TE, Herrington DA, Levine MM, Conrad JT, Merritt JW Jr: Antigenic variation of *Giardia lamblia* in experimental human infections. J Immunol 144:4362, 1990

Ortega YR, Adam RD: *Giardia:* overview and update. Clin Infect Dis 25(3):545–549, 1997

ISOSPORIASIS
Jane T. Atkins

Human isosporiasis is caused by the enteric parasite *Isospora belli*, which is phylogenetically related to the other coccidian parasites, including *Toxoplasma, Cryptosporidia, Sarcocystis,* and *Cyclospora.* *Isospora belli* is the species commonly associated with diarrheal illness in humans. After ingestion of the mature sporulated oocyst, excystation releases sporozoites in the proximal small bowel. Occasionally, sporozoites leave the intestinal tract to infect extraintestinal sites. However, typically, the sporozoites invade the enterocytes of duodenum and jejunum and mature into trophozoites. The trophozoites mature into merozoites that undergo further maturation by either asexual replication (schizogony or merogony) or sexual replication (gametogony). Gametogony produces the immature unsporulated oocyst that is passed in the stool. The form subsequently ripens in 12 to 48 hours into the infectious form or the mature sporulated oocyst, thus completing the life cycle.

Isospora belli is endemic in developing countries of Africa, Southeast Asia, and South America. In the United States, sporadic outbreaks have been reported among institutionalized patients and in the childcare setting. Isosporiasis also has been reported in travelers to endemic areas. In developing countries, isosporiasis is reported in 3 to 18% of AIDS patients. By contrast, it is reported in less than 1% of AIDS patients in the developed countries of North America and Europe.

Transmission occurs primarily by the fecal-oral route. Sexual transmission has been implied. There are no animal reservoirs. *Isospora belli* oocysts are resistant to common disinfectants and remain viable in a cool, moist environment for months. The incubation period is estimated to be 3 to 14 days and the organism is shed in the stool for up to 120 days.

CLINICAL MANIFESTATIONS   Clinically, isosporiasis is indistinguishable from cryptosporidiosis, microsporidiosis, and cyclosporiasis. The onset of the diarrhea is insidious and is associated with flu-like symptoms, including fever, headache, malaise, myalgia, and anorexia. Diffuse crampy abdominal pain, nausea, and vomiting also are present. Fecal blood and leukocytes are absent. However, Charcot-Leyden crystals and, occasionally, mucus may be present in the stool. Peripheral eosinophilia is common and patients often become dehydrated because of excessive fluid loss. Severe wasting, malabsorption, lactose intolerance, and steatorrhea have been reported, particularly in the immunosuppressed patient.

Immunocompetent children and adults typically have a protracted, but self-limited, watery diarrhea. Young infants and immunocompromised individuals typically have chronic intermittent diarrheal illness and may have a life-threatening intractable diarrhea. Individuals at risk for severe isosporiasis include patients with AIDS, α-heavy-chain disease, lymphoblastic leukemia, and human T-cell lymphotropic virus type 1–related T-cell leukemia.

Infection with *I. belli* usually remains confined to the small intestine. The histopathologic findings of the intestinal mucosa include flattening of the villi, hypertrophy of the crypts, and infiltration of the lamina propria with polymorphonuclear cells, lymphocytes, plasma cells, and eosinophils. Atypical presentations of infection with *I. belli* are rare, but have been reported in severely immunosuppressed individuals infected with HIV. Atypical sites of infection with *I. belli* include infection of the biliary tract (acalculous cholecystitis), tracheobronchial tree, mediastinum, mesenteric lymph nodes, spleen, and liver and disseminated infection.

DIAGNOSIS AND TREATMENT　　Infection with *I. belli* is established by identifying the oocyst in feces or by visualizing the intracellular stages of the parasite in biopsy specimens of the small bowel or other sites. *Isospora* can be detected in the stool by direct wet preparation; however, the organism is sparse and recovery is enhanced using concentration techniques. Modified acid-fast or auramine-rhodamine stains are commonly used to identify the oocysts of *Isospora* and other coccidian parasites found in feces. *Isospora belli* oocysts are easily distinguished from other coccidian parasites. They are large (10 times larger than *Cryptosporidium*), oval-shaped (measuring 10–20 μm by 20–33 μm), and contain one or two sporoblasts.

The treatment of choice for isosporiasis is high-dose trimethoprim-sulfamethoxazole given four times a day for 10 days, followed by low-dose trimethoprim-sulfamethoxazole given twice a day for 3 weeks. Pyrimethamine (along with folic acid) is an alternative therapy. Other agents active against *Isospora* are metronidazole and pyrimethamine-sulfadoxine. The patient's symptoms generally improve within 48 hours of initiating therapy. Relapse is common in the immunosuppressed patient infected with HIV. Thus, prophylaxis with trimethoprim-sulfamethoxazole three times a week is necessary. Other agents used for prophylaxis include pyrimethamine with or without sulfadoxine.

References

Lindsay DS, Dubey JP, Blagburn BL: Biology of *Isospora spp.* from humans, nonhuman primates, and domestic animals. Clin Microbiol Rev 10:19–34, 1997

Soave R, Johnson WD: *Cryptosporidium* and *Isospora belli* infections. J Infect Dis 157:225–229, 1988

Wittner M, Tanowitz HB, Weiss LM: Parasitic infections in AIDS patients: cryptosporidiosis, isosporiasis, microsporidiosis, cyclosporiasis. Infect Dis Clin North Am 7(3):569–586, 1993

LEISHMANIASIS
Eduardo Ortega-Barria

Leishmaniasis encompasses a group of clinical syndromes that are caused by a biologically diverse group of obligate intracellular protozoa of the genus *Leishmania*: visceral, cutaneous, and mucosal leishmaniasis. These syndromes result from the infection of macrophages throughout the mononuclear phagocyte system (eg, spleen, liver, bone marrow), of the skin, or of naso-oropharyngeal mucosae, respectively. The outcome of infection depends on the virulence and tropism of the infecting parasite and on the host's immune response. If clinically manifest but untreated, visceral leishmaniasis is life-threatening; cutaneous leishmaniasis causes chronic, but ultimately self-limited skin lesions; and mucosal leishmaniasis may cause substantial morbidity because of disfiguring lesions. An estimated 12 million people are infected worldwide.

Visceral leishmaniasis typically is caused by organisms of the *L. donovani* species complex; Old World cutaneous leishmaniasis is caused by *L. tropica, L. major,* and *L. aethiopica;* American (or New World) cutaneous leishmaniasis is caused by organisms of the *L. braziliensis* and *L. mexicana* species complexes; and mucosal leishmaniasis is caused by organisms of the *L. braziliensis* species complex. *Leishmania* species usually associated with visceral leishmaniasis can produce localized skin lesions, and species commonly found in the skin can disseminate viscerally.

In nature, leishmaniasis is transmitted by the bite of infected female phlebotomine sand flies, either of the genus *Phlebotomus* (Old World leishmaniasis) or *Lutzomyia* (New World). Leishmanial parasites have two stages in their life cycle: (a) the infective promastigote stage, which averages 15 to 20 μm in length by 1.5 to 3.5 μm in width, with a flagellum of about the same length; and (b) the nonflagellated amastigote stage, which is 2 to 5 μm in greatest diameter, found within macrophages in the mammalian host. Amastigotes multiply through binary fission within the phagolysosomes of macrophages, and spread to new host cells following destruction of earlier infected cells. Sand flies feeding on infected hosts ingest cells containing amastigotes that transform into promastigotes, multiply extracellularly in the lumen of the sand fly gut, and progressively change to infective metacyclic promastigotes. Promastigotes are introduced into the skin of the next mammalian host during a blood meal. *Lutzomyia longipalpis* sand flies have substances in their saliva that enhance the infectivity of promastigotes. Within macrophages of the mammalian host, promastigotes transform into amastigotes, and the cycle continues. The protective immune response appears to be primarily cell-mediated. CD4+ T lymphocytes, as well as T-cell and macrophage-derived cytokines (IL-2, interferon-γ) are crucial for the cure of a primary *Leishmania* infection.

Visceral Leishmaniasis

Visceral leishmaniasis is widely distributed in tropical and subtropical areas of the world. It reportedly occurs in 47 countries, but more than 50% of cases occur in Sudan and India. For native populations in some geographic areas, the disease primarily is a pediatric problem, affecting infants and young children (eg, the Mediterranean coast, China, Central and South America) or children, adolescents, and young adults (eg, Kenya, India).

Infection begins locally in the dermal macrophages at the site of the sand fly bite and disseminates throughout the mononuclear phagocyte system, particularly the spleen, liver, bone marrow, and lymph nodes. Bone marrow infiltration compromises both the erythropoietic and the granulocytic series. The spleen is markedly enlarged and congested, with hyperplasia of reticuloendothelial cells, atrophy of paracortical zones and areas of infarcts, and fibrosis. Visceral dissemination occurs in the context of anergy to leishmanial antigens, which is demonstrated by a negative leishmanin skin test and lack of lymphocyte-proliferation and interferon-γ responses to leishmanial antigens; delayed hypersensitivity also is suppressed nonspecifically to such antigens as tuberculin. Mortality of untreated persons with established disease ranges from 75 to 95%. However, studies have demonstrated that inapparent infections can outnumber clinically apparent infections by a ratio of up to 30 to 1.

CLINICAL MANIFESTATIONS The incubation period can be as long as years, but it typically ranges from weeks to months. The disease may follow a subacute, acute, or chronic course, and may be smoldering and oligosymptomatic, or floridly symptomatic. Some persons have a prolonged illness that is characterized by nonspecific clinical manifestations, which may or may not progress to classic kala-azar. Among symptomatic persons, high fever, weight loss, and cachexia are common. Reticuloendothelial-cell hyperplasia results in splenomegaly and hepatomegaly; splenomegaly can be massive. Peripheral lymphadenopathy is common in patients only in certain geographic areas (eg, Sudan).

Some patients with visceral leishmaniasis develop a syndrome called *post-kala-azar dermal leishmaniasis* (PKDL), which is characterized by skin lesions (eg, macules, papules, nodules, or patches; pigmented or depigmented) that typically are most prominent on the face. The syndrome may develop several years after therapy (eg, in India) or either during or within a few months of therapy (eg, in East Africa). Lesions may be fleeting or persistent and sometimes are associated with relapse of the visceral infection. In settings such as India, where the dermal lesions can be persistent and associated with plentiful parasites, persons with PKDL serve as chronic reservoirs of infection.

Visceral leishmaniasis has emerged as an important opportunistic infection among persons who are infected with HIV-1, and who have lived, traveled, or used IV drugs in leishmaniasis-endemic areas. Latent leishmanial infection may activate after substantial immunosuppression develops, sometimes years after leishmanial infection was acquired. The disease manifestations can be atypical and difficult to diagnose and treat.

DIAGNOSIS The diagnosis of visceral leishmaniasis is confirmed parasitologically by demonstrating the parasite in stained smears or cultures of a splenic aspirate, bone marrow aspirate, liver biopsy specimen, lymph-node aspirate or biopsy specimen, or buffy-coat preparation (see Fig. 13-28). In Indian cases of kala azar, and in HIV-infected patients, parasites may be found more frequently than usual in circulating blood monocytes. Splenic aspiration has a higher diagnostic yield than bone marrow aspiration (ie, as high as 98% vs. 80–85%) and is less painful, but it also is potentially more dangerous.

The indirect fluorescence antibody (IFA) is positive in more than 95% of patients. The enzyme-linked immunosorbent assay and the direct agglutination test have sensitivities of >90%. Except for some HIV-infected or otherwise immunocompromised persons, as well as some persons who are infected with *L. tropica,* most patients with active visceral infection have moderate to high titers of antileishmanial antibodies. In contrast, delayed-type skin-test reactivity is noted only after recovery.

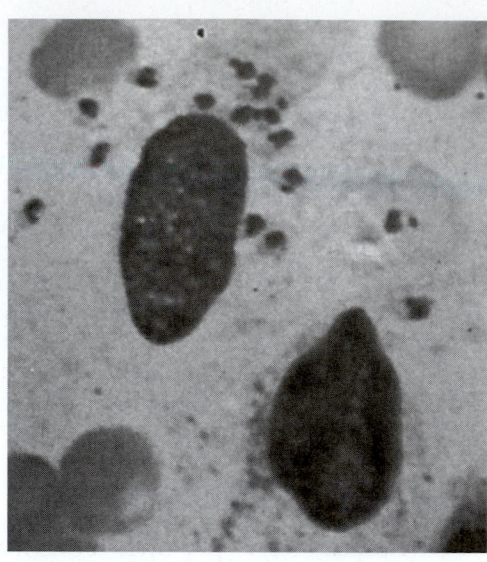

FIGURE 13-28   Amastigotes in a stained smear of a bone-marrow aspirate specimen from a patient with visceral leishmaniasis. Note the rod-shaped extranuclear kinetoplast within each amastigote.

To diagnose visceral leishmaniasis using peripheral blood rather than tissue aspirates, a PCR technique was developed for which the detection limit is one *Leishmania*-infected macrophage in 8 mL of blood. For Indian, Kenyan, or Brazilian patients with parasitologically confirmed kala-azar, this PCR procedure was highly sensitive (90%) and specific (100%). In another study, from Sudanese patients with visceral leishmaniasis, the PCR was able to detect parasite DNA in 37 of 40 (92%) blood samples.

Laboratory abnormalities include pancytopenia and a reversal of the albumin:globulin ratio because of hypergammaglobulinemia (chiefly IgG) from striking polyclonal B-cell activation and hypoalbuminemia. The transaminase values sometimes are modestly elevated. Bone marrow infiltration and hypersplenism partially explain the leukopenia and the anemia, which typically is normochromic normocytic; Coombs-positive hemolysis, bleeding, and hemodilution also can contribute to the anemia. Patients with leukopenia typically have neutropenia, marked eosinopenia, and a relative lymphocytosis and monocytosis.

The differential diagnosis includes other parasitic diseases (eg, malaria with tropical splenomegaly syndrome, African trypanosomiasis, schistosomiasis), as well as mycobacterial and bacterial (eg, miliary tuberculosis, typhoid fever, brucellosis), fungal (eg, histoplasmosis), and noninfectious diseases (eg, leukemia, lymphoma).

TREATMENT Pentavalent antimonials (Sb) are the drugs of choice. Two closely related pentavalent antimonials currently are used: sodium stibogluconate (Pentostam; Wellcome Foundation, United Kingdom) and meglumine antimonate (Glucantime; Rhône Poulenc, France). The recommended dosage of Sb is 20 mg/kg/d, without restricting the daily dose (as was previously done) to a maximum of 850 mg of Sb, for 20 to 28 days. In the United States, sodium stibogluconate is available through the CDC Drug Service (daytime: 404-639-3670; other times: 404-639-2888). Side effects are discussed in Sec. 13.6.1. Patients should be monitored weekly with serum hepatic enzyme levels, and electrocardiogram twice weekly beginning with the third week of treatment. Patients become afebrile within 4 to 5 days of therapy initiation. The various hematologic abnormalities and hypoalbuminemia usually improve substantially during therapy; reappearance of eosinophils in the peripheral blood is a good sign. However, laboratory abnormalities may take weeks to months to resolve. Likewise, regression of splenomegaly may take months. Freedom from clinical relapse for at least 6 months of follow-up is the best indicator of permanent cure. Cure rates with antimony therapy range from 80 to 95%. Relapses should be treated with the same drug for at least twice the previous duration.

Amphotericin B, 0.5 to 1.0 mg/kg daily, or every-other-day IV, for a total dose of 7 to 20 mg/kg, is considered to be very effective (98–100% success rate). AmBisome, given as a dose of 3 mg/kg on days 1 to 5 and on day 10 (total dose 18 mg/kg) cured 41 of 42 patients (98%). In another study, amphotericin B lipid complex, at a dose of 3 mg/kg administered every other day for five injections was 100% successful in patients with antimony-resistant kala-azar. A cholesterol dispersion form (Amphocil, 2 mg/kg/d for 7 or 10 days) cured 20 Brazilian patients.

Pentamidine, 2 to 4 mg/kg daily, or every-other-day IV or IM, for 15 doses, is considered to be reasonably effective; recent experience indicates that three doses per week for 5 to 9 weeks is effective and has fewer side effects. (see Sec. 13.6.1).

A combination of recombinant IFN-γ, which is a potent macrophage activator, plus antimonials has been used in some patients unresponsive to multiple courses of pentavalent antimonials alone. Aminosidine, 15 mg/kg/d IV or IM, which is the chemical equivalent of the aminoglycoside paromomycin, may be another useful adjunct. Allopurinol, which is an oral agent, has been used as an adjunct to pentavalent antimonials but with highly variable results.

Cutaneous Leishmaniasis

Cutaneous leishmaniasis is widely distributed in diverse tropical and subtropical areas of the world. More than 50% of cases occur in Afghanistan, Algeria, Brazil, Iran, Iraq, Saudi Arabia, Sudan, and Syria. This leishmanial syndrome is divided into Old World cutaneous leishmaniasis, which is caused by *L. tropica* (ie, "urban disease"), *L. major* (ie, "rural disease"), and *L. aethiopica*, and American (or New World) cutaneous leishmaniasis, which typically is caused by organisms of the *L. mexicana* and *L. braziliensis* species complexes. Leishmaniasis is endemic in the Americas, from southern Texas to most of Central and South America, as well as the Caribbean. The leishmanial species is a major determinant of the clinical course and outcome of untreated lesions.

CLINICAL MANIFESTATIONS   The first sign of clinical disease typically is a papule at the site of the sand fly bite weeks to months after the infection is acquired. Lesions generally evolve from papules to nodules to depressed ulcerative lesions with raised indurated borders (Fig. 13-29) but may be persistently nodular. Pain, pruritus, and regional adenopathy may be present. Secondary bacterial infection is common. If untreated, lesions eventually heal in months to years but leave an atrophic scar. Multiple skin lesions can result from the bites of multiple sand flies, the probing behavior of infected sand flies when feeding, or local dissemination of infection. Satellite lesions may form near a primary lesion, and may ultimately merge with the primary lesion. Sporotrichoid-like subcutaneous nodules may develop along lymphatic channels (eg, with *L. panamensis* infection).

Two unusual variants of cutaneous leishmaniasis that cause difficult-to-treat chronic disease are diffuse cutaneous leishmaniasis, which is an anergic variant with plentiful parasites, and leishmaniasis recidivans, which is a hyperergic variant with scarce parasites. Diffuse cutaneous leishmaniasis develops in some persons who are in-

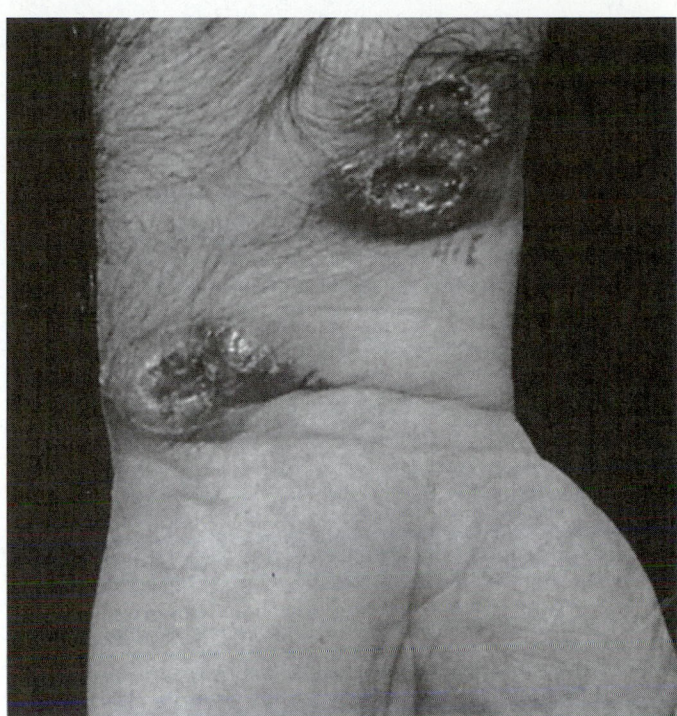

FIGURE 13-29   **Skin ulcerations in a patient with American cutaneous leishmaniasis acquired in Costa Rica. Note the raised outer border of the ulcers. This patient had sporotrichoid-like spread of lesions along lymphatic channels of his arm. SOURCE:** *(Courtesy of A. Wright.)*

fected with *L. aethiopica* or organisms in the *L. mexicana* complex who have specific anergy to leishmanial antigens. Diffuse cutaneous leishmaniasis begins as a localized papule and disseminates to cause many, persistent, nonulcerative skin lesions. The histopathology shows few lymphocytes but abundant parasites in vacuolated macrophages. Leishmaniasis recidivans is primarily found in Iran, Iraq, and neighboring areas. Recidivans lesions, which may resemble those of lupus vulgaris, slowly expand over many years, with central healing but peripheral activation and expansion.

DIAGNOSIS   Lesion scrapings, aspirates, and biopsy specimens provide useful diagnostic specimens. As lesions age, parasitologic confirmation becomes more difficult, because amastigotes become more scarce. For ulcerative lesions, one should examine multiple Giemsa-stained thin smears of lesion scrapings and obtain cultures of lesion aspirates and/or biopsy specimens. Tissue fluid should be aspirated from an active-appearing portion of the ulcer margin and inoculated in appropriate culture medium or laboratory animal (eg, BALB/c mouse or golden hamster), but it may take 2 to 3 months before the animal becomes positive. Species identification of isolated parasites with specific monoclonal antibodies, isoenzyme analysis, or use of DNA probes is available only in research laboratories or from the CDC. Specific antibodies can be demonstrated in 70 to 80% of infected individuals by IFA or EIA, but in endemic areas, antibodies fail to distinguish between previous and current infection. Delayed-type skin-test reactivity to leishmanial antigens usually is present or develops in persons with simple cutaneous or recidivans leishmaniasis, but not in persons with diffuse cutaneous leishmaniasis.

New approaches for the detection of parasites include standard DNA hybridization and the polymerase chain reaction (PCR) on skin biopsy specimens. DNA hybridization techniques have a considerable sensitivity (detecting as few as 50–100 parasites), but their potential use in routine diagnosis has been hampered by the complexity of the procedures. PCR that uses oligonucleotide primers directed to the minicircle kinetoplast DNA (kDNA) of *L. braziliensis* complex has a reported sensitivity of 87% and 100% in tests conducted under hospital and rural conditions, respectively.

The differential diagnosis includes traumatic, tropical, and stasis ulcers; fungal (eg, sporotrichosis, blastomycosis), mycobacterial (eg, cutaneous tuberculosis, *Mycobacterium marinum* infection, leprosy), and bacterial (eg, syphilis, yaws) infection; as well as other diseases (eg, sarcoidosis, neoplasms).

TREATMENT Cutaneous lesions that are large, multiple or persistent, located at cosmetically important sites, as well as those that are due to *L. braziliensis,* should be treated. Treatment is also recommended for leishmaniasis recidivans, or in diffuse cutaneous leishmaniasis. Clinically mild lesions that are known to be caused by *L. mexicana* or by *L. major* generally resolve spontaneously. The recommended treatment is 20 mg/kg body weight of pentavalent antimony once a day for 20 consecutive days (see previous discussion of visceral leishmaniasis). Clinical response, which typically begins with lesion flattening, may not be complete until weeks after the end of therapy. If the lesions have not decreased at least 75% in area by 6 weeks after the end of therapy, consider retreatment, particularly if the lesions are not progressively decreasing in size. Routinely obtaining follow-up specimens to demonstrate parasitologic response is not recommended; the persistence of some parasites is not necessarily a poor prognostic sign.

Available alternatives include various parenteral, oral, and local/topical agents. The traditional parenteral alternatives of pentamidine (eg, 3 mg/kg IV or IM every other day for four doses) and amphotericin B generally are considered to be effective, but toxic, antileishmanial agents.

Mucosal Leishmaniasis

Mucosal leishmaniasis is the metastatic complication of cutaneous leishmaniasis in which nasal, buccal, pharyngeal, and sometimes laryngeal tissues become infected because of dissemination of parasites. This syndrome is caused primarily by organisms of the *L. braziliensis* species complex, but also by *L. panamensis* and *L. guyanensis.* Mucosal disease probably develops in only a small percentage of persons who are infected with these organisms. Adequate treatment of the original cutaneous lesion(s) is assumed to further reduce the risk of developing metastatic disease. Clinically apparent mucosal disease, which develops despite the presence of antileishmanial cell-mediated immunity, usually occurs within several years, but sometimes not until decades after the original cutaneous lesion(s) healed. Development of persistent, unusual nasal symptoms such as epistaxis or symptoms of nasal obstruction should prompt consideration of the diagnosis. Untreated disease can progress to cause perforation of the nasal septum and widespread naso-oropharyngeal destruction. Parasitologic confirmation is difficult, because amastigotes typically are scarce. Therefore, the diagnosis commonly is based on the clinical manifestations and supportive laboratory data (eg, presence of antileishmanial antibodies, positive skin test). Other diagnoses to consider include paracoccidioidomycosis, histoplasmosis, rhinoscleroma, syphilis, tertiary yaws, midline granuloma, sarcoidosis, and neoplasms.

Pentavalent antimonial therapy, 20 mg Sb per kilogram body weight once a day for 28 days, is moderately efficacious against mild mucosal disease, but is less effective (because of failure to heal or relapse) for severe mucosal disease involving more than one anatomic site.

References

Andressen K, Gasim S, Elhassan AM, et al: Diagnosis of visceral leishmaniasis by the polymerase chain reaction using blood, bone marrow and lymph node samples from patients from the Sudan. Trop Med Int Health 2:440–444, 1997

Berman JD: Human leishmaniasis: clinical, diagnostic, and chemotherapeutic developments in the last 10 years. Clin Infect Dis 24:684–703, 1997

Davidson RN, di Martino L, Gradoni L, et al: Short-course treatment of visceral leishmaniasis with liposomal amphotericin B (AmBisome). Clin Infect Dis 22:938–943, 1996

Harris E, Kropp G, Belli A, Rodriguez B, Agabian N: Single-step multiplex PCR assay for characterization of New World *Leishmania* complexes. J Clin Microbiol 36:1989–1995, 1998

Herwaldt BL, Berman JD: Recommendations for treating leishmaniasis with sodium stibogluconate (Pentostam) and review of pertinent clinical studies. Am J Trop Med Hyg 46:296–306, 1992

Herwaldt BL, Stokes SL, Juranek DD: American cutaneous leishmaniasis in US travelers. Ann Intern Med 118:779–784, 1993

Nuzum E, White F III, Thakur C, et al: Diagnosis of symptomatic visceral leishmaniasis by use of the polymerase chain reaction on patient blood. J Infect Dis 171:751–754, 1995

Pearson RD, de Queiroz Sousa A: Clinical spectrum of leishmaniasis. Clin Infect Dis 22:1–13, 1996

MALARIA
Chandy C. John

Malaria is among the leading infectious causes of morbidity and mortality in children worldwide, with 300 to 500 million clinical cases occurring each year, causing between 1.5 and 2.7 million deaths, most in Sub-Saharan African children under the age of 5 years. Increasing resistance to insecticides and therapeutic agents, climatic and economic changes, population shifts, and abandonment of malaria control programs all contribute to the recent resurgence of malaria in the developing world.

Malaria in humans is caused by four species of *Plasmodium: P. falciparum, P. vivax, P. ovale,* and *P. malariae. Plasmodium falciparum* is the only *Plasmodium* species that infects all ages of red blood cells, so it generally causes a much higher level of parasitemia than the other *Plasmodium* species. *Plasmodium vivax* and *P. ovale* preferentially infect reticulocytes and tend to cause a lesser parasitemia. *Plasmodium malariae* preferentially infects senescent red cells and causes the lowest level parasitemia of the human *Plasmodium* species, but this low-level parasitemia may persist for decades.

Knowledge of the plasmodial life cycle is crucial to understanding malarial infection and disease (Fig. 13-30). Sporozoites are inoculated into the bloodstream by the *Anopheles* mosquito and migrate within minutes to the liver, where they invade hepatic parenchymal cells. Within hepatic cells, the sporozoites undergo asexual multiplication (hepatic schizogony), forming schizonts that rupture the hepatic cells and release merozoites into the bloodstream. Multiplication within the hepatic cell produces thousands of merozoites from each sporozoite-infected hepatic cell. The process of schizogony lasts from 7 to 10 days for *P. falciparum, P. ovale,* and *P. vivax,* and from 10 to 14 days for *P. malariae. Plasmodium vivax* and *P. ovale* can also produce dormant liver stages (hypnozoites) that can reactivate weeks or months after the initial infection and cause clinical relapse.

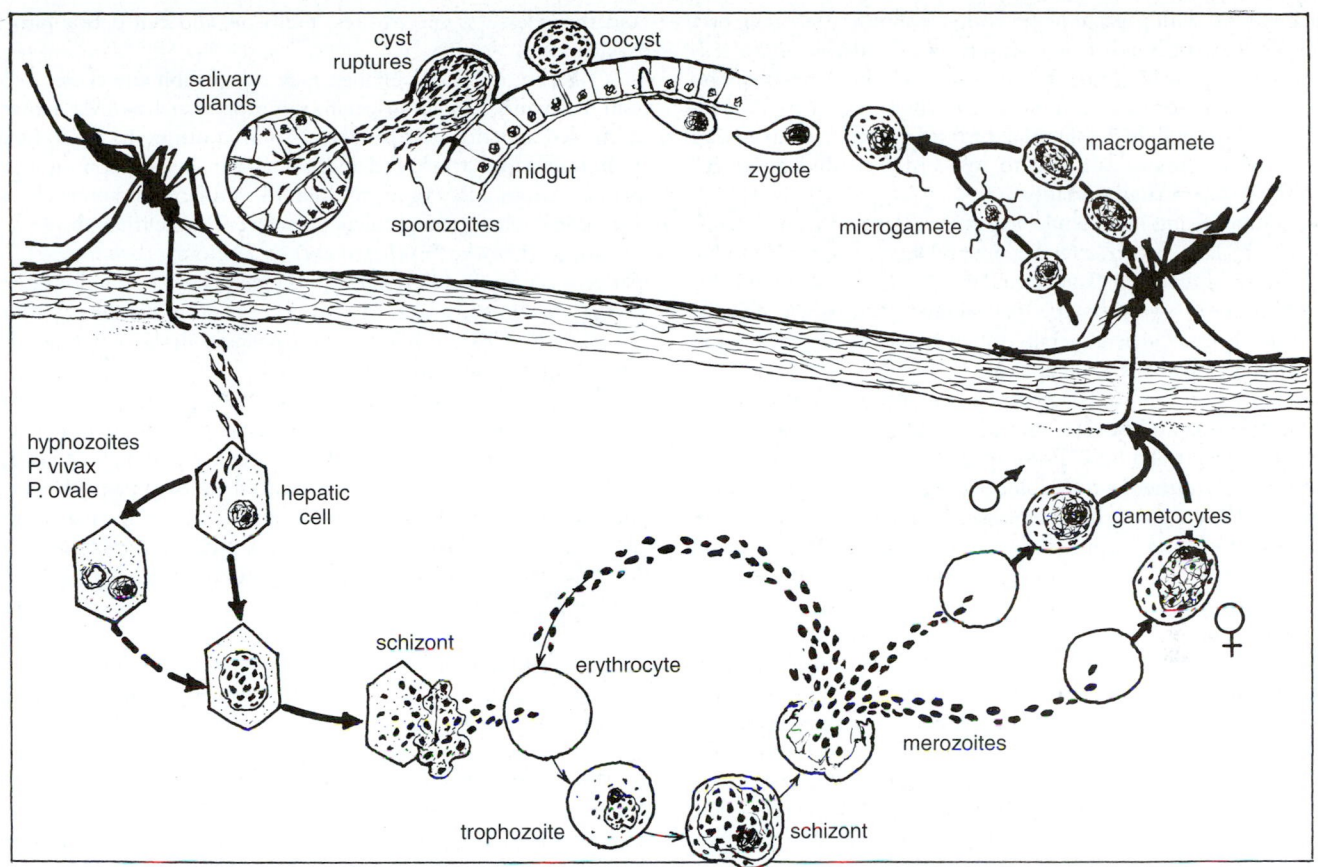

FIGURE 13-30   Life cycle of the malaria parasite in humans and in *Anopheles* mosquitoes.

Merozoites released by ruptured hepatic cells invade red blood cells, where they may either asexually multiply or undergo sexual differentiation into male and female gametocytes. Parasites established in the red blood cell (trophozoites) that asexually multiply form red blood cell schizonts. These schizonts eventually lyse the red cells containing them and release more merozoites, which continue the cycle of red cell invasion and multiplication.

Male and female gametocytes are ingested by mosquitoes with their human blood meal. In the mosquito, the male gametocyte exflagellates, releasing a microgamete that fertilizes the female macrogamete, producing a zygote. The elongated zygote, or ookinete, penetrates the stomach wall of the mosquito and forms an oocyst behind it. The oocyst grows and eventually ruptures to release numerous sporozoites, which migrate throughout the mosquito. Those that enter the salivary glands can then infect human beings bitten by the mosquito and renew the cycle of infection.

Malarial disease is caused by the blood stages of the parasite. Rupture of red cells and release of merozoites into the blood lead to the fever, chills, and malaise seen in all forms of malaria. *Plasmodium*-infected erythrocytes, opsonized with antibodies and/or complement, are less deformable than uninfected erythrocytes and are consequently trapped in the spleen, leading to splenomegaly. Anemia and thrombocytopenia are due primarily to splenic consumption of erythrocytes and platelets, but autoimmune hemolysis plays a role in the continued destruction of erythrocytes that can occur for weeks after appropriate treatment. In chronic malarial infections, dyserythropoiesis also occurs and contributes to chronic anemia.

The pathogenesis of organ dysfunction in *P. falciparum* malaria is thought to be primarily a consequence of two factors: cytoad-herence of parasitized red blood cells to capillary endothelial cells and *P. falciparum* antigen-induced cytokine production. Red cell cytoadherence in capillaries leads to sequestration of red cells and parasites in microvascular beds, and the resultant local tissue ischemia and hypoxia contributes to the renal, gastrointestinal, pulmonary, and central nervous system complications seen in falciparum malaria. TNF-α and, to a lesser extent, interferon-γ are clearly implicated in the pathogenesis of murine cerebral malaria, but the exact role of these cytokines in human malaria is less clear. Regulatory polymorphisms of cytokine genes also appear to play a role in the development of disease.

EPIDEMIOLOGY AND IMMUNITY   More than 40% of the world's population (2.5 billion people) are at risk for malaria in 90 countries in Africa, Asia, South and Central America, and Oceania. *Plasmodium falciparum* is found mainly in tropical areas, where warm weather insures the relatively constant presence of the *Anopheles* vector. *Plasmodium vivax* has the widest geographic distribution of the four species and is found in both tropical and temperate areas. *Plasmodium ovale* is found primarily in Sub-Saharan West Africa, where it appears to almost completely replace *P. vivax*. *Plasmodium malariae* can be seen in both tropical and temperate zones, but is the least common of the malaria species.

In the United States, almost all of the approximately 1000 cases of malaria that are reported annually to the Centers for Disease Control and Prevention (CDC) occur in travelers to or immigrants from malaria-endemic countries, although rare cases of local transmission have been reported. Malaria can also be acquired by direct blood exposure through blood transfusions. With present blood-screening procedures, such cases are rare in the United States. Congenital malaria, with passage of infection from mother to newborn, can also occur, although it is uncommon in endemic areas. It is seen more frequently in nonimmune women and in women who have an overt attack of clinical malaria during pregnancy. In areas where malaria is endemic, infection during pregnancy, even among semi-immune women, can lead to low birth weight and an increased risk of perinatal mortality.

Individuals living in endemic areas never develop complete immunity to malaria; rather, they become relatively tolerant to infection because of repeated exposure. These "semi-immune" individuals often have asymptomatic parasitemia, and when malarial disease does occur, it is generally much milder than that seen in nonimmune individuals.

Numerous host genetic factors also can affect susceptibility to malarial infection and disease. Heterozygous carriers of hemoglobin S (sickle-cell trait) have an 80 to 95% protection from severe malarial disease. Other hemoglobinopathies, including hemoglobin C and E and the α and β thalassemias, are also associated with some degree of protection from severe malarial disease. Alterations in erythrocyte structure or function can be protective against malarial infection and disease. The Duffy blood group antigens are required for the invasion of *P. vivax* into erythrocytes, and the almost universal absence of these antigens in West African individuals convincingly correlates with their innate resistance to *P. vivax* infection, in contrast to their susceptibility to the other three species of human malaria. Some protective effect has also been seen in individuals who carry the genes for hereditary ovalocytosis and glucose-6-phosphate dehydrogenase (G6PD) deficiency. Finally, specific human leukocyte antigens (HLA) of the major histocompatibility complex (MHC) can affect susceptibility to malarial disease. Recent studies demonstrated that Gambian children without class I antigen HLAB53 and one form of class II antigen DR13 were more likely to have severe malaria than those with these HLA types.

CLINICAL MANIFESTATIONS   The clinical presentation of malaria depends on the age and level of immunity of the infected individual, the level of endemicity, and on the *Plasmodium* species causing the illness. In areas with high endemicity, children develop severe anemia, which is seen most commonly between ages 6 months to 3 years. In areas with low- or midlevel endemicity, cerebral malaria is more common and occurs in a broader age range (6 months–6 years). In malaria-endemic areas, children younger than 6 months old, and especially those younger than 3 months old, are protected from malarial infection and disease by fetal hemoglobin and passively transferred maternal antibodies.

Children who have acquired partial immunity often present with mild, nonspecific symptoms. Asymptomatic parasitemia is common in malaria-endemic areas, so in these areas a positive blood smear for malaria does not necessarily implicate malaria as the cause of the patient's disease. Nonimmune individuals, whether children or adults, tend to present with more severe signs and symptoms than semi-immune individuals, and may develop severe disease with relatively low-level parasitemia.

Prodromal, flu-like symptoms occur during the early cycles of erythrocytic infection and may include fever (with no specific pattern), headache, malaise, myalgias, arthralgias, abdominal pain, and diarrhea. Nonimmune adults frequently exhibit the classic febrile paroxysm, which consists of three phases: a brief "cold" phase, with chills and sometimes rigors; a hot phase, with high fever, dry, flushed skin, tachypnea, and thirst; and a sweating stage, with defervescence accompanied by diaphoresis and a feeling of lassitude. The paroxysms coincide with the rupture of infected erythrocytes

and the release of merozoites, pigment, and cell debris into the circulation.

Children, especially infants, may not exhibit the classic paroxysm. In infants, more nonspecific symptoms, such as fever, lethargy, decreased appetite, and listlessness may continue to predominate. Vomiting, loose stools, and abdominal pain are very common complaints in both infants and children. Most infants and older children also have intermittent or continuous fevers, rather than the 48-hour (*P. vivax, P. ovale, P. falciparum*) or 72-hour (*P. malariae*) fever patterns classically described with these infections. Children with *P. falciparum,* in particular, may exhibit very irregular fever patterns. As many as 10% of children with malarial disease may not have documented fever during the illness.

The physical signs most frequently seen in malaria are hepatomegaly and splenomegaly, which are seen in about half of all children with acute malarial disease. In areas where malaria is highly endemic, a large percentage of children develop palpable splenomegaly over time. Malaria leads to some degree of anemia in almost all diseased individuals. Chronic anemia from repeated malarial infections can lead to growth stunting. Jaundice occurs in only 10 to 15% of malaria-infected children.

Complications from *P. falciparum* Malaria   Nonimmune children with *P. falciparum* malaria often develop complications from the disease. The World Health Organization (WHO) lists 10 defining criteria and five supporting criteria for severe malaria, as listed in Table 13-66. The most common of these complications in children are those involving the central nervous system (coma and repeated convulsions), metabolic dysfunction (hypoglycemia and acidosis), severe malarial anemia, and respiratory distress.

Cerebral Malaria   By WHO definition, cerebral malaria is present in a patient who (a) cannot localize a painful stimulus; (b) has peripheral asexual *P. falciparum* parasitemia; and (c) has no other causes of an encephalopathy. Recurrent convulsions are a frequent antecedent to subsequent impaired consciousness and coma—50 to 80% of African children with cerebral malaria by strict WHO criteria have a prior history of convulsions. Children with cerebral malaria may progress from a normal sensorium to coma within hours. Focal seizures are occasionally seen, but focal neurologic deficits are rare. Meningeal signs are usually absent. Abnormal posturing, pupillary changes, absent corneal reflexes, Cheyne-Stokes or Kussmaul respirations, and gaze abnormalities may be seen. Retinal hemorrhages have been noted in 6 to 36% of African children on admission, and papilledema, an independent

TABLE 13-66

WORLD HEALTH ORGANIZATION CRITERIA FOR SEVERE MALARIA

DEFINING	SUPPORTING
Coma	Impaired consciousness
Severe malarial anemia	Jaundice
Respiratory distress	Prostration
Hypoglycemia	Hyperpyrexia
Circulatory collapse	Hyperparasitemia
Renal failure	
Spontaneous bleeding	
Repeated convulsions	
Acidosis	
Hemoglobinuria	

indicator of poor outcome, in 2 to 12%. Children with severely increased intracranial pressure (ICP >40 mm Hg) have a very high risk of death or severe neurologic sequelae.

The mortality rate for strictly defined cerebral malaria in African children is 16 to 20%. Concurrent respiratory distress, lactic acidosis, and/or severe malarial anemia increases the mortality rate. Despite the severity of cerebral malaria, only 10% of children who survive cerebral malaria have long-term neurologic deficits.

Severe Malarial Anemia   Severe anemia is seen most often in children younger than 4 years old, and is more frequent in areas of very high *P. falciparum* transmission. Many children with malaria in endemic areas are already anemic from iron deficiency and hookworm infection. The sudden worsening of anemia caused by *P. falciparum* can lead to congestive heart failure, with subsequent respiratory distress and lactic acidosis.

Metabolic Dysfunction   Hypoglycemia (a blood glucose level of ≤2.2 mmol/L) and lactic acidosis (a plasma lactate of ≥5 mmol/L) are seen frequently in children with *P. falciparum* malaria; they are independent predictors of mortality. Blood glucose should always be measured in children on presentation with *P. falciparum* malaria since hypoglycemia is more likely than in adults.

Other Complications   Thrombocytopenia occurs frequently, but bleeding problems are rare. Children with *P. falciparum* malaria may have an elevated blood urea nitrogen and creatinine values on admission, but this is most often caused by hypovolemia and corrects with fluid administration. Renal failure from glomerulonephritis or massive intravascular hemolysis (blackwater fever) is very rarely seen in children in endemic areas and is more common in adults. Concurrent bacterial meningitis or sepsis, though infrequent, does occur in children with severe malaria and should be ruled out.

Tropical splenomegaly syndrome is a chronic complication of *P. falciparum* malaria in which splenomegaly persists after treatment of acute infection. Massive splenomegaly, hepatomegaly, anemia, and an elevated IgM level are the classic features of this disorder, which is thought to be caused by an impaired immune response to *P. falciparum* antigens. The only effective therapy for this disorder is lifelong antimalarial prophylaxis.

Nonfalciparum Malaria   In malaria caused by *P. vivax* and *P. ovale*, complications other than anemia, which is seldom as severe as that caused by *P. falciparum*, are uncommon. Nonimmune children with *P. vivax* or *P. ovale* malaria may nonetheless appear acutely ill and be profoundly fatigued during recovery from their illness. Very rarely, splenic rupture may occur after trauma. Children and adults with chronic *P. malariae* infection may develop nephrotic syndrome, caused by immune complex deposition on glomerular walls. The nephrotic syndrome caused by *P. malariae* is poorly responsive to steroids.

DIAGNOSIS   Many of the deaths caused by malaria in the United States are a result of delayed or mistaken diagnosis. Examination of Giemsa-stained thick and thin blood smears remains the primary method of diagnosis for malaria. Thick smears are more sensitive in detecting parasites, but thin smears are necessary for *Plasmodium* species identification and enable estimation of the degree of peripheral blood parasitemia. *Plasmodium falciparum* can be distinguished from the other three human malaria species by parasitemia that exceeds 2% of red cells, by red cells that contain multiple par-

asites, by the almost exclusive presence of ring forms of the parasite, by ring forms with a double chromatin dot, and by the presence of parasites in all ages of red cells. The banana-shaped gametocyte is pathognomonic for *P. falciparum* malaria. In nonimmune individuals, even low-level parasitemia may be accompanied by severe illness. Blood smear-negative cerebral malaria has been reported in individuals without prior antimalarial drug treatment.

Malaria blood smears should be repeated every 8 to 12 hours in nonimmune individuals, and several smears over a 48- to 72-hour period should be obtained before malaria is excluded as a diagnosis. Individuals have often received treatment with antimalarial medication prior to seeing a physician. If the clinical picture in these individuals is consistent with malaria, and no alternative diagnosis can be made, empiric treatment for malaria may be necessary.

No other laboratory tests are diagnostic for malaria. Findings that support the diagnosis include a normocytic, normochromic anemia, and thrombocytopenia. However, in children with concurrent hookworm infection or iron deficiency, microcytosis and hypochromia may be seen. Electrolyte abnormalities, including hyponatremia, hypokalemia, hypoglycemia, are common, and a metabolic acidosis frequently occurs in children. A mild elevation of transaminases and indirect bilirubin may be seen. The cerebrospinal fluid (CSF) in children with cerebral malaria is generally unremarkable, with fewer than 20 white blood cells, a mildly elevated protein, and a normal glucose relative to serum glucose. When elevated CSF lactate levels are seen, they are an independent predictor of mortality. Although children with cerebral malaria often have increased intracranial pressure, lumbar puncture in these children is rarely associated with neurologic deterioration.

Promising new diagnostic tests for malaria include a 10-minute immunochromatographic test for *P. falciparum* histidine-rich protein (HRP2). HRP2 is of *P. falciparum* only; it does not detect other malaria species. A second immunochromatographic test detects the enzyme lactate dehydrogenase from all four species and can distinguish between *P. falciparum* and non-*P. falciparum*. Parasite mRNA or DNA polymerase chain reaction (PCR) testing has been performed in research settings but remains a research tool.

The differential diagnosis includes typhoid, which may also present with fever, abdominal pain, vomiting, diarrhea, and malaise. The fevers of typhoid are unremittent and generally unaccompanied by chills, rigors, or diaphoresis, and the splenomegaly of typhoid is typically less marked than that of malaria. The classic typhoid "rose spot" exanthem is not seen in malaria, but it is often missing in cases of typhoid as well. In its prodromal phase, malaria can also be confused with viral or bacterial gastroenteritis, influenza, enteroviral infection, hepatitis, and other viral illnesses. Cerebral malaria can be confused with bacterial or viral meningitis or encephalitis. If blood smears are repeatedly negative for malaria parasites and antimalarial treatment does not improve symptoms, the differential diagnosis enlarges to include tuberculosis, endocarditis, brucellosis, leptospirosis, trypanosomiasis, kala-azar, histoplasmosis, and noninfectious diseases such as neoplasms.

TREATMENT   Four questions must be urgently answered in the evaluation of a child with malaria or suspected malaria: (a) Is the child semi-immune or nonimmune? (b) Does the child have *P. falciparum* malaria? (c) Was the child exposed to malaria in an area with chloroquine-resistant or chloroquine-sensitive malaria parasites? (d) Does the child have any evidence of complications from malarial disease by history, exam, or lab findings?

Children younger than 5 years old, children traveling to malaria-endemic areas but originally from a nonendemic area, and children who have been away from an endemic area for more than 6 months should be considered nonimmune. In many "malaria endemic" countries, there are large cities where little or no malaria transmission occurs, and individuals from these cities are essentially nonimmune. Children older than 5 years of age who lived continuously in a malaria-endemic area can be considered semi-immune, although the pattern of malaria transmission in their area undoubtedly makes a difference in their level of immunity.

Plasmodium falciparum malaria can be a life-threatening emergency, especially in the nonimmune individual. Any child from a malaria-endemic area with signs and symptoms of severe malaria should be treated for *P. falciparum* malaria while awaiting blood smear confirmation. Nonimmune children with documented *P. falciparum* malaria should probably be hospitalized because clinical decompensation can occur rapidly, even in children with a relatively benign initial presentation. Decisions on hospitalization of the semi-immune child with *P. falciparum* malaria depend on the child's clinical status. Nonimmune children with *P. vivax, P. ovale,* or *P. malariae* malaria generally don't develop severe complications, but they can be quite ill-appearing with the initial paroxysm.

Chloroquine-Resistant P. falciparum   From 1980 to 1995, 83% of malaria cases in the United States reported to the CDC were acquired in Sub-Saharan Africa and 7% were acquired in Asia, both areas with high-level *P. falciparum* chloroquine resistance. High-level chloroquine-resistant *P. falciparum* also occurs in South America. Individuals with chloroquine-resistant *P. falciparum* infection should be treated with oral quinine (if the patient is alert and can tolerate oral treatment) or intravenous quinidine plus either tetracycline (if the child is older than 8 years old) or pyrimethamine/sulfadoxine or clindamycin (see Table 13-67). Malaria treatment with quinine alone is associated with significant recrudescence rates, which are greatly decreased with the addition of tetracycline, pyrimethamine/sulfadoxine, or clindamycin. Children appear to tolerate oral quinine better than do adults, but its bitter taste and the side effects of cinchonism (nausea, dysphoria, tinnitus, and high-tone deafness) make compliance with a more than a 3-day regimen difficult. Children frequently vomit after receiving quinine, especially if they are febrile when receiving the drug. Acetaminophen and sponge-bathing prior to administration of oral quinine may decrease the likelihood of vomiting. If vomiting occurs within an hour, the full dose of quinine should be repeated. If vomiting occurs after 1 hour, no repeat quinine dosing is necessary.

Quinidine appears to be at least as effective as quinine at eradicating blood-stage *P. falciparum,* and in the United States, it has replaced quinine as the intravenous medication of choice for complicated *P. falciparum* malaria. The potential cardiac toxicity of quinidine necessitates that patients receive it as an intravenous infusion, never a bolus, while on continuous electrocardiographic monitoring. Infusion rates should be reduced if the QT interval is prolonged by more than 25% of the baseline value. Both quinine and quinidine can induce hyperinsulinemic hypoglycemia, which may cause lethargy or unresponsiveness that is confused with cerebral malaria, so glucose levels should be followed in severely ill patients who are on these medications. Long-term side effects from either medication are uncommon, and the cinchonism seen with quinine resolves with cessation of quinine therapy.

Alternatives to quinidine or quinine therapy in the United States are presently limited. A fixed combination of atovaquone and proguanil (marketed under the trade name Malarone by Glaxo Wellcome) is approved by the United States Food and Drug Administration (FDA) for the treatment and prophylaxis of choroquine-resistant *P. falciparum* malaria in adults and children. This combination is the alternative of choice to quinine or quinidine treatment for nonimmune individuals with mild or uncomplicated malaria. Atovaquone/proguanil should be taken with food or a milky drink, and if vomiting occurs within 1 hour of dosing, a repeat dose should be taken. All doses for treatment should be taken as a single daily dose.

Mefloquine can be used to treat chloroquine-resistant malaria, but in adults, it is associated with frequent, sometimes severe, central nervous system symptoms, including convulsions, loss of consciousness, and acute psychosis. A pediatric treatment dose is not approved by the Food and Drug Administration. If a child develops malaria while on mefloquine prophylaxis, mefloquine should not be used as treatment, because *P. falciparum* mefloquine resistance is documented in Asia (particularly Thailand), Africa, and South America. Mefloquine should not be used in conjunction with quinine or quinidine, as it may potentiate the cardiac side effects (dysrhythmias, sinus bradycardia) of quinine and quinidine.

Halofantrine, a drug similar to mefloquine, is used widely outside the United States. Prolongation of the PR and QT interval occurs in children and adults taking halofantrine, but progression to heart block or arrhythmia is rare and seems to occur primarily in those with underlying cardiac conduction defects. A severe hemolytic anemia that can mimic blackwater fever has also been reported with halofantrine, but it occurs primarily in adults who have received multiple courses of halofantrine. Absorption of halofantrine is variable, but it can be increased to potentially toxic levels if taken one hour before to two hours after meals, because food increases its absorption. Treatment failures have been reported. Given the side-effect profiles of mefloquine and halofantrine, the more limited clinical experience with these drugs in the treatment of children with malaria, and the reports of treatment failures with both drugs, quinine and quinidine are still the drugs of choice for chloroquine-resistant *P. falciparum* malaria. Artemisinin derivatives are not yet available in the United States, but they are used successfully in Asia and Africa, and large clinical trials demonstrate that they are as effective as quinine in treating severe *P. falciparum* malaria and are well tolerated.

Tetracycline and clindamycin should not be used alone in the treatment of malaria because resistance to both drugs exists and because both drugs have a delayed onset of action (approximately 48 hours). Pyrimethamine/sulfadoxine has been used as single-drug therapy for presumed malaria in travelers without immediate access to health care, but with increasing *P. falciparum* pyrimethamine/sulfadoxine resistance, first in Asia, and now in Africa and South America, it should not be used alone as primary treatment for nonimmune individuals returning from these areas.

Chloroquine-Sensitive P. falciparum Malaria and Malaria caused by P. vivax, P. ovale, and P. malariae   At the present time, chloroquine-sensitive *P. falciparum* still exists in the Middle East, Central America north of the Panama Canal, Haiti, and the Dominican Republic, but this may change. The CDC Web page (www.cdc.gov) and malaria hotline (888-232-3228) have up-to-date information on malaria drug resistance in every country. Chloroquine remains the drug of choice for chloroquine-sensitive *P. falciparum* malaria. If there is any doubt as to whether chloroquine resistance is present in the area malaria was acquired, quinine should be used. Quinine or quinidine are the drugs of choice for parenteral treatment of chloroquine-sensitive malaria.

Malaria caused by *P. vivax, P. ovale,* and *P. malariae* should also be treated with chloroquine. High-grade resistance to chloroquine

TABLE 13-67
RECOMMENDED DRUG TREATMENT OF MALARIA IN CHILDREN

MALARIA SPECIES	DRUG	ORAL DOSAGE FOR UNCOMPLICATED MALARIA	INTRAVENOUS/INTRAMUSCULAR DOSAGE FOR SEVERE MALARIA
Chloroquine-resistant *P. falciparum*	Quinine sulfate[a]	25 mg/kg/day (max 2000 mg) in 3 doses × 3–7 days	
	or Quinine dihydrochloride[b]		20 mg/kg salt (max 600 mg) over 4 h, then 10 mg/kg over 2–8 h, every 8 h, IV, until able to take oral medication or for 7 days
	or Quinidine gluconate[c]		10 mg/kg salt loading dose (max 600 mg) in normal saline over 1–2 h, IV, followed by continuous infusion at 0.02 mg/kg/min, IV, with ECG monitoring, until able to take oral medication or for 7 days
	plus Tetracycline[d] *or*	20 mg/kd/day (max 750 mg) in 4 doses × 7 days	
	Pyrimethamine/sulfadoxine (Fansidar)	Single dose on the last day of quinine therapy: <1 yr: 1/4 tablet 1–3 yr: 1/2 tablet 4–8 yr: 1 tablet 9–14 yr: 2 tablets >14 yr: 3 tablets	
	or Clindamycin	30 mg/kg/day (max 900 mg) in 3 doses × 7 days	
	Alternatives: Atovaquone/proguanil (Malarone)	Adult tabs: 250 mg atovaquone/100 mg proguanil 11–20 kg: 1 adult tab once daily × 3 days 21–30 kg: 2 adult tabs once daily × 3 days 31–40 kg: 3 adult tabs once daily × 3 days >40 kg: 4 adult tabs once daily × 3 days	
	Halofantrine[e]	8 mg/kg (max 500 mg) every 6 h × 3 doses; repeat in 1 week in nonimmune individuals	
	Mefloquine[f]	15 mg/kg base (max 1250 mg) × 1 dose, then 10 mg/kg base 8–24 h later	
	Artesunate[b,g]	4 mg/kg day 1, 2 mg/kg days 2 and 3, 1 mg/kg days 4–7 (1 tablet = 50 mg)	2.4 mg/kg first dose, then 1.2 mg/kg at 12 and 24 h, then 1.2 mg/kg daily, IV or IM, until able to take oral medication or for 7 days total
	Artemether[b,g]	Regimen same as artesunate (1 capsule = 40 mg)	3.2 mg day 1, then 1.6 mg IM daily until able to take oral medication or for 7 days total; do not give IV
	Artesunate *or* artemether *plus*	4 mg/kg daily × 3 days	
	mefloquine	15 mg/kg base (max 1250 mg), then 10 mg/kg base 8–24 h later	
All *Plasmodium* species except chloroquine-resistant *P. falciparum*	Chloroquine phosphate[h]	10 mg base/kg (max 600 mg base), then 5 mg base/kg 6 h later, then 5 mg base/kg/day × 2 days	
	Quinidine gluconate		Same as above
	Quinine dihydrochloride		Same as above
P. vivax and *P. ovale* (prevention of relapse)	Primaquine phosphate[i]	0.3 mg base/kg/day (max 15 mg) × 14 days	

[a] When quinine is used in conjunction with tetracycline or pyrimethamine/sulfadoxine, a 3-day course of quinine can be given. Travelers from Southeast Asia, those taking clindamycin, and those with persistent >1% parasitemia on day 3 should receive a 7-day course of quinine.
[b] Not available in the United States.
[c] Do not use loading dose if patient has been on mefloquine or quinine therapy in the last 24 hours.
[d] Do not use in children younger than 8 years old or in pregnant women.
[e] Halofantrine should not be taken with fatty foods, or given to patients taking drugs that prolong the QT interval, or given to those patients with preexisting cardiac conduction defects, a long QT interval, or a history of mefloquine use in the previous 28 days.
[f] High-level mefloquine resistance exists in Thailand; other medications should be used in patients acquiring malaria in Thailand.
[g] Recrudescence of infection may be decreased if single-dose pyrimethamine/sulfadoxine is given at the end of a treatment course with artesunate or artemether, as it is with quinine.
[h] Chloroquine phosphate: 250 mg of the salt = 156 mg of the base. If not available, hydroxychloroquine sulfate can be used (200 mg hydroxychloroquine base = 155 mg base).
[i] Screen for G6PD deficiency prior to giving primaquine (see text). Primaquine is given for eradication of liver stage parasites and should be given at the end of chloroquine treatment.
max = maximum; IV = intravenous; IM = intramuscular

has been reported in Oceania, but elsewhere *P. vivax* remains chloroquine-sensitive, and *P. ovale* and *P. malariae* are still chloroquine sensitive worldwide. Patients with *P. vivax* and *P. ovale* malaria should also receive a 2-week course of primaquine to eradicate dormant liver stages of these parasites. Prior to treatment with primaquine, all patients should be screened for glucose-6-phosphate-dehydrogenase (G6PD) deficiency. Individuals with the severe form of G6PD deficiency may experience an oxidant hemolysis and methemoglobinemia with primaquine administration and should not receive primaquine.

Management of Severe *P. falciparum* Malaria When a child presents with *P. falciparum* malaria, the physician must immediately assess the child's mental status and neurologic exam, hydration status, level of anemia, glucose level, acid-base status, electrolyte levels, and renal function. Antipyretics (acetaminophen) should be given to all children unless there are signs of liver failure. Acetaminophen is preferred to aspirin in the treatment of fever in malaria. Hypovolemia should be corrected with intravenous fluids or colloid. Patients with symptomatic anemia (eg, in congestive heart failure) should be transfused. Although no specific hemoglobin level is an absolute indication for transfusion in every child, most sources recommend transfusion if the hemoglobin level is 5 mg/dL or below. Hypoglycemia should be corrected with a 50% dextrose bolus, and intravenous solutions for children with severe malaria should contain at least 5% dextrose. Although it is important to correct hypoglycemia, most children, even those with severe hypoglycemia, do not respond to this correction with a rapid recovery of mental status.

Most experts recommend that lactic acidosis be treated by aggressive treatment of malarial infection, volume repletion if the patient is dehydrated, and transfusion of blood as appropriate. Lactic acidosis resolves in many children with this approach alone. Administration of sodium bicarbonate can cause a paradoxical tissue acidification, and it is generally not recommended for the treatment of lactic acidosis, although some experts suggest its use if the patient's blood pH is <7.1. Preliminary studies suggest that dichloroacetate (DCA) may ameliorate malaria-induced lactic acidosis and may reduce mortality from this condition, but larger studies are required before DCA can be recommended as standard therapy.

The role of exchange blood transfusion in malaria therapy is controversial. Most studies that have documented its usefulness have been in nonimmune individuals, often adults. Large, prospective, randomized studies have not been done and probably will not be done, especially in nonimmune individuals. The recommendations of an expert malariologist in a recent review are that exchange transfusion should be performed if there are adequate facilities, the patient is seriously ill, and the parasitemia level exceeds 15%; exchange transfusion should be considered in the patient with parasitemia in the 5 to 15% range if the patient has other signs of poor prognosis.

Prophylactic anticonvulsants have been useful in adults, but the optimal medication and dosage in children are still unclear. If convulsions do occur, they can be treated with diazepam or paraldehyde (although the latter is rarely used in the United States). Recurrent seizures should be treated with phenobarbital or phenytoin, following the standard treatment for status epilepticus.

Bacterial superinfection, including pneumonia, bacteremia, and meningitis, may occur in children with severe malaria, although it is apparently less common than in adults. In children with acute clinical deterioration, a blood glucose level should be checked,

blood cultures should be drawn, and broad-spectrum antibiotics should be initiated.

At present, the role of other interventions, such as mannitol, deferoxamine, pentoxifylline, dextran, and antibodies against tumor necrosis factor, are not clear. Corticosteroids, heparin, and cyclosporine are probably harmful and should not be used.

PREVENTION Avoidance of mosquitoes and barrier protection from mosquitoes are an important part of malaria prevention for travelers to endemic areas. The *Anopheles* mosquito feeds from dusk to dawn. Travelers should remain in well-screened areas, wear clothing that covers most of the body, sleep under a bednet (ideally one impregnated with permethrin), and use insect repellants with *N,N*-diethyl-*m*-toluamide (DEET) during these hours. Pediatric repellants with 6 to 10% DEET are available and should be used for children. Because systemic toxicity can occur in children if they absorb excessive DEET, even the pediatric repellants should be used sparingly.

Chemoprophylaxis is the cornerstone of malaria prevention for nonimmune children and adults who travel to malaria-endemic areas (Table 13-68). Weekly mefloquine is the drug of choice for malaria chemoprophylaxis in children and adults traveling to areas with chloroquine-resistant *P. falciparum*. The FDA does not approve mefloquine for children under 15 kg, but because the risks of acquiring severe malaria outweigh the risks of potential mefloquine toxicity in these children, the CDC recommends that they too receive mefloquine prophylaxis. The lack of a liquid or suspension formulation sometimes makes mefloquine administration difficult, and potential side effects include nausea and vomiting. Mefloquine is better tolerated by children if it is "disguised" in other foods. Adults have a 10 to 25% incidence of sleep disturbances and dysphoria with mefloquine, but these side effects appear to be less common in children.

A reasonable alternative to mefloquine is the fixed combination of atovaquone and proguanil (Malarone), which is approved by the FDA for the treatment and prophylaxis of chloroquine-resistant *P. falciparium* malaria in adults and children. Atovaquone/proguanil is approved for children weighing more than 11 kg. The major disadvantage of atovaquone/proguanil prophylaxis is that it must be taken every day, so it may be better suited for prophylaxis during short exposure periods.

Doxycycline is another alternative choice for prophylaxis, but it cannot be used in children younger than 8 years old, and it must be taken every day. Photosensitivity is a common side effect, and vaginal candidiasis frequently occurs in women on doxycycline prophylaxis.

Chloroquine prophylaxis alone, with pyrimethamine/sulfadoxine treatment for presumed malaria if ill, is a suboptimal regimen for children traveling to a chloroquine-resistant area. When pyrimethamine/sulfadoxine is used as a temporary measure, the child should receive medical evaluation within 24 hours. Daily primaquine and daily azithromycin are used successfully as malaria prophylaxis in adults and children in areas endemic for chloroquine-resistant *P. falciparum*, but they have not yet been studied extensively enough to be recommended as routine chemoprophylaxis for these areas. In areas where malaria remains chloroquine-sensitive, chloroquine is the drug of choice for prophylaxis. The CDC Web page (www.cdc.gov) and hotline number (888-232-3228) are useful resources for determining the current malaria prophylaxis guidelines for specific countries. No prophylaxis is completely effective, and travelers may develop malaria despite taking the recommended malaria chemoprophylaxis.

TABLE 13-68

RECOMMENDED MALARIA DRUG PROPHYLAXIS IN CHILDREN

AREA	DRUG	DOSAGE (ORAL)
Chloroquine-resistant area	Mefloquine[a]	5–15 kg: 4.6 mg base (5 mg salt)/kg/wk 15–19 kg: 1/4 tab/wk 20–30 kg: 1/2 tab/wk 31–45 kg: 3/4 tab wk >45 kg: 1 tab/wk (228 mg base)
	Doxycycline[b]	2 mg/kg daily (max 100 mg)
	Atovaquone/proguanil[c] (Malarone)	Pediatric tabs: 62.5 mg atovaquone/ 25 mg proguanil Adult tabs: 250 mg atovaquone/ 100 mg proguanil 11–20 kg: 1 pediatric tab once daily 21–30 kg: 2 pediatric tabs once daily 31–40 kg: 3 pediatric tabs once daily >40 kg: 1 adult tab once daily
Chloroquine-sensitive area	Chloroquine phosphate *plus* pyrimethamine/sulfadoxine for presumptive treatment	5 mg base/kg/wk (max 300 mg base) <1 yr: 1/4 tablet 1–3 yr: 1/2 tablet 4–8 yr: 1 tablet 9–14 yr: 2 tablets >14 yr: 3 tablets

[a]Chloroquine and mefloquine should be started 1 week prior to departure and continued for 4 weeks after last exposure.
[b]Doxycycline should be started 1 day prior to departure and continued for 4 weeks after last exposure.
[c]Atovaquone/proguanil (Malarone) should be started 1 to 2 days prior to departure and continued for 7 days after return.

References

Centers for Disease Control: Health Information for International Travel 1999–2000. Atlanta, GA, DHHS, 1999

Greenwood BM: The epidemiology of malaria. Ann Trop Med Parasitol 91:763–769, 1997

Newton CR, Krishna S: Severe falciparum malaria in children: current understanding of pathophysiology and supportive treatment. Pharmacol Ther 79:1–55, 1998

Snow R, Omumbo J, Lowe B, et al: Relation between severe malaria morbidity in children and level of *Plasmodium falciparum* transmission in Africa. Lancet 349:1650–1654, 1997

Steele RW: Malaria in children. Adv Pediatr Infect Dis 12:325–349, 1997

White NJ: The treatment of malaria. N Engl J Med 335:800–806, 1996

MICROSPORIDIOSIS

Enrique Cacaras and Jane T. Atkins

Microsporidia is a nontaxonomic term referring to an extensive group of unicellular protozoa classified in the phylum Microspora. These amitochondriate parasites are related to fungi and produce small spores with a characteristic coiled extrusion apparatus that transfers the infective sporoplasm material into the host cell. The intracellular asexual life cycle consists of a vegetative merogonic phase that reproduces the organism by binary or multiple fission (meronts) and a sporogonic phase that results in production of mature spores. Of the over 100 genera, the only 6 genera known to infect humans were *Encephalitozoon* (that includes the former *Septata intestinalis*), *Enterocytozoon, Nosema, Pleistophora, Trachipleistophora, Vittaforma,* and a group of unclassified microsporidium. During the HIV era, five new species have been described in humans: *Enterocytozoon bienusi, Encephalitozoon hellem, Encephalitozoon (Septata) intestinalis, Trachipleistophora hominis,* and *Trachipleistophora anthropophtera.*

Microsporidia are ubiquitous. The incidence, relevant reservoirs, and sources of infection are not well defined. Microsporidia that infect humans are also found in animals, including domestic mammals, but the potential for zoonotic transmission is unknown. Persistent carriage and asymptomatic infection are also described in immunosuppressed patients.

The spores are found in water sources; however, there is no direct evidence of waterborne cases or outbreaks. Microsporidia are released into the environment via stool, urine, and respiratory secretions. Person-to-person transmission is suspected but not proven. The oral route is presumably the port of entry for gastrointestinal infections, especially in the cases involving *E. bienusi,* the species that is almost exclusively found in the gastrointestinal tract. The aerosol route is an alternative presumptive route for bronchopulmonary infections with species that are rarely found in stools, such as *Encephalitozoon hellem.* Direct contact with conjunctival mucosa is postulated to be the source of isolated ocular infections. Histopathologic analysis shows invasion of some microsporidia, such as *Encephalitozoon intestinalis,* into macrophages and fibroblast of lamina propria.

CLINICAL MANIFESTATIONS Gastrointestinal disease is the most common manifestation of infection with microsporidia. However, a broad range of clinical manifestations of infection with microsporidia are reported including infection of the biliary tract, eyes, sinuses, lungs, muscles, and disseminated infections with tubulointerstitial nephritis, hepatic, cardiac, and central nervous system involvement. Microsporidia (mainly *E. bienusi* and *E. intestinalis*) cause a self-limited and chronic diarrhea in the immunocompetent host and in the non-HIV infected patient with defective cellular immunity. Immunosuppression posttransplant is a recognized risk factor for infection with microsporidia. *Encephalitozoon cuniculi* was detected in the urine and CSF from a child with seizure disorder, and serologic evidence of this same organism was found in another child with a seizure disorder and a low CD4/CD8 ratio. Keratitis and corneal ulceration are reported with infections with *N. ocularum* (parasitic primarily in invertebrates), *V. corneae* (species unique to humans, formerly known as *N. corneum*), and unclassified microsporidium. *Pleistophora spp.* have been found in patients with of myositis. Disseminated infection has been reported with *N. connor.*

Between 25 and 50% of chronic diarrhea cases of undetermined etiology in HIV-infected patients are caused by microsporidia, in particular, *E. bienusi* (the most prevalent species) and *S. intestinalis.* Microsporidia usually infect young adults with CD4 counts less than $100/mm^3$, but severely immunosuppressed children also may be infected. In some patients, microsporidiosis may be the only AIDS-defining opportunistic infection. The usual presentation is an afebrile, watery, nonbloody, nonmucoid, diarrhea with 3 to 20 bowel movements per day. The diarrhea is exacerbated by food intake and associated with progressive weight loss, anorexia, and malabsorption. Children may present with failure to thrive, intermittent abdominal pain, and chronic diarrhea. *Encephalitozoon bienusi* invades enterocytes, producing a limited inflammatory reaction with abnormalities of the villi, but rarely invades the lamina propria. Dissemination outside of the gastrointestinal tract is rare. *Encephalitozoon intestinalis* has a higher potential of dissemination. Local spread to the biliary tract results in cholangitis and acalculous cholecystitis that is indistinguishable from the AIDS cholangiopathy associated with cytomegalovirus and cryptosporidium.

Infection with microsporidia is associated with ocular, sinopulmonary, and disseminated disease in patients infected with HIV. Keratoconjunctivitis is associated with *T. homini* and all three *Encephalitozoon spp.* (*E. hellem, E. cuniculi,* and *E. intestinalis*) and is characterized by conjunctival inflammation, photophobia, blurred vision, foreign-body sensation, and decreased visual acuity. Ocular involvement is occasionally accompanied by evidence of disseminated infection with detection of the organism in the urine, sputum, and nasal mucosa. Infection with *Encephalitozoon spp.* also manifests as sinusitis with mucopurulent nasal discharge and lower respiratory tract involvement (asymptomatic or associated with bronchiolitis or pneumonia).

Disseminated infections occur in severely immunosuppressed HIV-infected patients. The pattern of distribution differs for each microsporidian species. *Encephalitozoon hellem* parasitize the keratoconjunctiva, urinary tract, nasal sinuses, and bronchial system. *Encephalitozoon intestinalis* is confined to the gastrointestinal and biliary tract, but may disseminate to the kidneys, eyes, sinuses, and, occasionally, to the respiratory tract. *Encephalitozoon cuniculi* causes widely disseminated infections involving nearly all organ systems, including the central nervous system. Recently, species of the genus *Trachipleistophora* have been described with disseminated disease.

DIAGNOSIS AND TREATMENT   A definitive diagnosis is made by identifying the organisms in the stools, body fluids (duodenal aspirate, bile, nasal secretions, sputum, bronchoalveolar lavage, urine, and conjunctival smear), or in tissue sections with light or electron microscopy. Electron microscopy is considered the gold standard for confirmation of infection and differentiation of species. It is highly specific, but it lacks sensitivity, especially when performed on stool samples. The application of molecular techniques and newer staining methods provide a reliable alternative to electron microscopy on stool samples. Concentration techniques enhance recovery of the organism in stool. Weber-modified trichrome staining using chromotrope 2R gives good resolution under oil immersion. Chemofluorescent stains, such as Uvitex 2B and Calcofluor White, are preferred by some investigators because they are highly sensitive. Sequential staining of samples in two steps may improve the sensitivity and specificity of light microscopy. Paraffin-embed-

ded tissue sections can be examined using routine histologic stains including hematoxylin-eosin, periodic acid–Schiff, silver, and Giemsa stains. Light microscopy allows diagnosis of microsporidial infection, but genus or species differentiation is uncertain with this method.

Tissue culture, immunofluorescent staining, and polymerase chain reaction are employed by research laboratories but are not readily available to most commercial laboratories. Sensitivity and specificity of serologic tests are unknown.

In several case reports albendazole administered to adults at 200 to 400 mg twice daily for 3 to 4 weeks is effective for the treatment of *Encephalitozoon spp.* infection in HIV-infected patients; however, relapses are common. *Encephalitozoon bienusi* is much more difficult to treat. The results of studies using atovaquone, furazolidone, and azithromycin are controversial. Topical fumagillin produces symptomatic improvement of ocular infections. TNP-470, a less-toxic synthetic analogue of fumagillin, holds promise as a new antimicrosporidial compound. Restoration of a patient's immune system with antiretroviral therapy improves the symptoms. In addition, a low-fat and low-residue diet reduces the volume and frequency of stools.

References

Chioralia G, Tramer T, Kampen H, Seitz HM: Relevant criteria for detecting microsporidia in stool specimens. J Clin Microbiol 36:2279–2283, 1998

Molina JM, Chastang C, Goguel J, et al: Albendazole for treatment and prophylaxis of microsporidiosis due to *Encephalitozoon intestinalis* in patients with AIDS: a randomized double-blinded controlled trial. J Infect Dis 177:1373–1377, 1998

Orenstein JM, Tanowitz HB, Weiss LM: Prevalence of microsporidiosis due to *Enterocytozoon bienusi* and *Encephalitozoon* (*septata*) *intestinalis* among patients with AIDS-related diarrhea: determination by polymerase chain reaction to the microsporidial small-subunit rRNA gene. Clin Infect Dis 23:1002–1006, 1996

Weber R, Bryan RT: Microsporidial infections in immunodeficient and immunocompetent patients. Clin Infect Dis 19:517–521, 1994

Weber R, Bryan RT, Schwartz DA, Owen RL: Human microsporidial infections. Clin Microbiol Rev 7:426–461, 1994

PNEUMOCYSTIS PNEUMONIA
Walter T. Hughes

Pneumonitis caused by *Pneumocystis carinii* occurs almost exclusively in the immunocompromised host. Both the organism and the disease it causes remain confined to the lung, even in untreated and fatal disease.

Pneumocystis carinii is found in the infected lung in both cystic and extracystic forms. The cyst is a round to oval, sometimes cup-shaped structure approximately 4 to 6 μm in diameter. Within the mature cyst are as many as eight daughter cells, referred to as *sporozoites,* that are pleomorphic and often crescent shaped. These cells eventually excyst through breaks in the cyst wall. Outside the cyst, the daughter cell, now termed a *trophozoite,* varies from 2 to 5 μm in diameter. These thin-walled trophozoites tend to cluster in masses. The exact taxonomy of *P. carinii* is not established, but recent studies on molecular structure suggest that it is more like a fungus than a protozoan.

Pneumocystis carinii infection is recognized among humans and lower animals in most countries. The natural habitat and mode of transmission are unknown. Serologic surveys show that two-thirds of normal healthy children have antibody to *P. carinii* by 4 years of age, suggesting that subclinical infection occurs frequently. Symptomatic infection occurs sporadically in immunocompromised individuals.

CLINICAL MANIFESTATIONS   Clinical features of the infection depend to some extent on the age of the host. In the infantile form, onset is insidious; with cough and mild tachypnea, usually without fever, the infection progresses over 1 to 4 weeks to a diffuse bilateral interstitial plasma-cell pneumonitis with severe tachypnea, retractions, and cyanosis. Without treatment, 50% of these infants die. The infection occurs in infants from 2 to 6 months of age who are premature or debilitated.

In children and adults, *P. carinii* pneumonitis occurs in those receiving immunosuppressive therapy for malignancies or other diseases, organ-transplant recipients, and in those with congenital and acquired immunodeficiency disorders. Onset is fairly abrupt, with fever, tachypnea, retractions, flaring of nasal alae, and cyanosis. No rales are heard. Hypoxemia can be severe. The infection progresses for several days and almost always is fatal if untreated.

In the infantile-epidemic form, there is an extensive interstitial plasma-cell infiltration with marked thickening of the alveolar septae. Organisms are found in the interstitial infiltrates as well as the alveoli. In the childhood-adult type, the disease is primarily a diffuse desquamative alveolopathy. The organisms fill the alveoli, along with reactive alveolar macrophages.

Pneumonitis develops in immunosuppressed hosts regardless of circulating *P. carinii* antibody. The incidence of the pneumonitis is greatest in individuals with impaired cell-mediated immunity. Approximately 50% of untreated infants with AIDS develop *P. carinii* pneumonitis.

DIAGNOSIS   A definitive diagnosis requires demonstrating *P. carinii* in infected lung tissue (or material from the lung) that is obtained by invasive techniques such as open-lung, transbronchial, percutaneous, or endobronchial brush biopsies. Bronchoalveolar lavage and induced sputum techniques are useful in children with AIDS. The specimen is applied to a microscope slide and stained with Gomori, toluidine blue O, and Giemsa stains (Fig. 13-31). A fluorescence-labeled antibody stain is sensitive, specific, and commercially available.

Serum antibody titers to *P. carinii* can be determined by immunofluorescent antibody and complement-fixation methods. Unfortunately, there is only a poor correlation between antibody titers and active pneumonitis. *Pneumocystis carinii* DNA has been detected in lung tissue by polymerase chain reaction, but this approach has not been studied adequately to adopt for diagnostic use.

TREATMENT   Trimethoprim-sulfamethoxazole is the drug of choice for treating *P. carinii* pneumonitis. The dosage is based on 20 mg of trimethoprim and 100 mg of sulfamethoxazole per kg per day orally, or three-fourths of this dose IV in four doses. A course of 2 weeks is usually adequate in patients without AIDS, but at least 3 weeks of treatment is needed for patients with AIDS.

Pentamidine isethionate is as effective as trimethoprim-sulfamethoxazole, but it must be administered parenterally and it is frequently associated with nephrotoxicity, hypoglycemia, and other adverse effects. The dose is 4.0 mg/kg/d as a single IV dose.

Most patients require oxygen therapy for a fairly long time. Studies in adults with AIDS show that concomitant administration of a corticosteroid, such as prednisone, reduces mortality rates in patients with an arterial-alveolar gradient of 35 mm Hg or greater.

Atovaquone is FDA approved for the treatment of mild and moderately severe *P. carinii* pneumonia in adults who cannot take or who fail to respond to trimethoprim-sulfamethoxazole. The drug is given orally and has few adverse effects.

Immunosuppressive drugs should be stopped. If hypogammaglobulinemia exists, human immune globulin (gamma globulin) should be given. Some studies suggest that dapsone, fansidar, clindamycin plus primaquine, and trimetrexate plus leucovorin may be effective in treating *P. carinii* pneumonitis.

PREVENTION   *Pneumocystis carinii* pneumonitis can be prevented by the prophylactic use of trimethoprim-sulfamethoxazole in a dosage of 5 mg of trimethoprim and 25 mg of sulfamethoxazole per kg per day. The drug is administered orally in two equally divided doses per day, one in the morning and one in the evening. Guidelines are established for prophylaxis in infants and children with HIV infection, and include HIV-infected or HIV-indeterminate infants ages 1 to 12 months; HIV-infected children ages 1 to 5 years with CD4-positive lymphocyte counts of <500/mm³ (<15%); and HIV-infected children 6 years of age and older with CD4-positive lymphocyte counts of <200/mm³ (<15%). The host is protected for only as long as the drug is administered, however, because trimethoprim-sulfamethoxazole has a static effect and does not eradicate the latent organism, even with prolonged administration. Dapsone, atovaquone, fansidar, and aerosolized pentamidine have some effect in the prevention of *P. carinii* pneumonitis.

References

Centers for Disease Control and Prevention: 1997 USPHS/IDSA guidelines for the prevention of opportunistic infections in persons infected with human immunodeficiency virus. MMWR Morb Mortal Wkly Rep 46 (No. RR-12):4–6, 1997

Hughes WT: *Pneumocystis carinii*. In: Long SS, Pickering L, Prober C, eds: Principles and Practice of Pediatric Infectious Diseases. New York, Churchill Livingstone, pp 1417–1420, 1997

Hughes WT, Anderson DC: *Pneumocystis carinii* pneumonia. In: Feigin RD, Cherry JD, eds: Textbook of Pediatric Infectious Diseases, 4th ed. Philadelphia, WB Saunders, 2490–2498, 1998

Lundgren B, Wakefild AE: PCR for detecting *P. carinii* in clinical or environmental samples. FEMS Immunol Med Microbiol 22:97–101, 1998

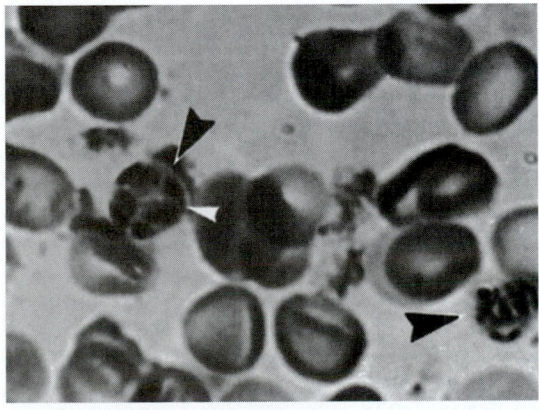

FIGURE 13-31 *Pneumocystis carinii* in bronchoalveolar lavage fluid.

TOXOPLASMOSIS
Nicole M. A. LeSaux

Toxoplasmosis is an infection of humans by the protozoan *Toxoplasma gondii,* an obligate intracellular protozoan parasite whose definitive hosts are cats and other felines. Humans are the secondary hosts. The parasite exists in three forms (a) the trophozoite or proliferative form (ie, tachyzoite); (b) the tissue cyst (ie, bradyzoite); and (c) the oocyst, which is found only in felines in which an enteroepithelial cycle occurs.

In felines, sexual reproduction in the small intestine results in the fecal excretion of a walled-off zygote known as an oocyst. Sporulation (maturation) in soil or cat litter creates a sporozoite capable of infecting another feline, a nonfeline mammal, or a bird. In the acute phase of infection, widespread infection of the secondary host tissues (muscle, brain, etc) by intracellular asexual reproduction of trophozoites (ie, tachyzoites) follows. The organisms multiply rapidly and may so distend the cell that it bursts. The released trophozoites then invade other cells. As intracellular replication rates decrease, a resting form of the tachyzoite, called bradyzoites, form in tissue cysts that are usually localized in brain, heart, and skeletal muscle. When a human ingests infected meat that contains tissue cysts, the stomach acid destroys the cyst wall and facilitates the release of bradyzoites. These transform rapidly to tachyzoites, which reside briefly in the intestinal epithelium before disseminating throughout the body and reproducing in many cell types. Primary infection with *T. gondii* acquired during pregnancy can be transmitted to the fetus by trophozoites crossing the placenta. Thus, infection can be acquired by ingesting infective oocysts from the soil or cat litter, by ingesting tissue cysts in rare or raw meat (especially pork, lamb, beef, or wild game), or by congenital transmission of tachyzoites to a fetus during acute infection in pregnancy. Contamination of water supplies with *T. gondii* oocysts has been associated with outbreaks of toxoplasmosis. Although there is no direct human-to-human transmission, acquisition by blood transfusion or organ transplantation has been reported.

Serosurveys in North America suggest that approximately 30% of the human population has been exposed to *T. gondii,* with the yearly rate of acquisition being 0.05 to 1%. About 38% of women of childbearing age in the United States are seropositive for *Toxoplasma.* The incidence of congenital toxoplasmosis is conservatively estimated to be approximately 1.3 per 1000 live births. If untreated, the transmission rate of toxoplasma infection to the fetus is estimated to be 10 to 25% if the infection occurred in the first trimester, 30 to 54% if it occurred in the second trimester, and 60% if the infection occurred in the third trimester. The risk of transmission from treated women was 6% if infection occurred at 13 weeks of gestation or earlier, 40% between 13 and 26 weeks of gestation, and 72% between 27 and 36 weeks' gestation. Maternal toxoplasmosis that is acquired during the first trimester is associated with more severe fetal disease, whereas maternal infection that is acquired late in pregnancy is associated with mild to subclinical disease.

PATHOLOGY The *T. gondii* trophozoite in peritoneal exudate or tissue culture is crescentic, measuring 4 to 7 μm by 2 to 4 μm. Masses of organisms that are seen within parasitized vacuoles of host cells superficially resemble *Leishmania* or *Histoplasma.* Pathologic lesions may affect many organs and tissues. In congenital toxoplasmosis, periaqueductal and periventricular lesions predominate. Tachyzoites invade the neurons, glial cells, ependyma, subependymal tissues, and vessels during the acute infection. A unique localized antigen-antibody reaction associated with vasculitis and necrosis occurs in the periventricular areas of the third and fourth ventricles where ependyma is absent. These necrotic areas of the brain often calcify and are visible radiologically. Hydrocephalus is a result of obstruction of the narrowest part of the ventricular system by inflammation. Glial nodules occur as a result of cellular necrosis and often contain the tachyzoite at its periphery.

Lesions of acute acquired toxoplasmosis are found principally in lymph nodes and the eye. Acute lymph node infection shows a characteristic triad of (a) reactive follicular hyperplasia, (b) clusters of epthelioid histiocytes in and encroaching on germinal centers, and (c) monocytoid B type lymphocytes in the sinuses of the lymph node. The principal inflammatory ocular lesions are located in the choroid and the sclera. There may be focal retinitis with inflammation and scarring secondary to a local immunologic response. A diffuse retinitis and secondary vitritis may occur in the presence of immune deficiency where the tachyzoites cause necrosis of three layers of the retina. Myositis is a rare manifestation of toxoplasmosis; however, myocarditis can occur and is supported by finding tachyzoites and inflammation in myocardial cells. *Toxoplasma* has been identified in testes, lungs, adrenals, pancreas, bone marrow, and other organs of patients who are immunocompromised. Tissue cysts containing bradyzoites may be identified in various organs after primary infection, and can persist for years without provoking cellular reaction or reactivating.

CLINICAL MANIFESTATIONS

Primary Infection in Immunocompetent Patients Toxoplasmosis in this population is a benign, self-limiting illness. Within several weeks to months, spontaneous resolution is to be expected, but in a minority of patients, symptoms may continue for as long as 12 months. Serologic evidence strongly suggests that as much as 75% of infections are asymptomatic. Acquired postnatal toxoplasmosis may present as a mononucleosis-like picture with fever, headache, malaise, and lymphadenopathy. The most common presentation, however, is a relatively asymptomatic localized lymphadenopathy syndrome affecting the cervical nodes. Rarely, lymphadenopathy can be generalized. There is no overlying erythema or periadenitis. Toxoplasma lymphadenopathy is estimated to account for 3 to 7% of clinically significant lymphadenopathy. The lymphadenopathy may wax and wane for months and finally resolve spontaneously. Less-common manifestations are conjunctivitis, choroiditis, splenomegaly, hepatomegaly, and rash. The incubation period is believed to be from 5 to 18 days. Circulating atypical lymphocytes may be seen as well.

Infection in Immunocompromised Patients In the immunocompromised host, primary toxoplasmosis or reactivation of toxoplasmosis sometimes can be fulminant or even fatal. Infection can involve any organ, but frequently affects the central nervous system, the lung, and the eye, causing encephalitis, pneumonitis, and chorioretinitis. Lesions frequently involve the basal ganglia. The most common manifestation of recurrent disease (90%) is a focal neurologic presentation such as seizures, speech abnormality, or hemiparesis. Such reactivation disease exhibits a ring-enhancing lesion on computed tomography. Immunosupressive illnesses such as HIV, treatment of malignancy, or organ transplantation are typical settings in which reactivation occurs.

Ocular Toxoplasmosis Retinochoroiditis caused by *Toxoplasma gondii* can occur in children and adults as a consequence of either primary or congenital infection. The principal inflammatory ocular lesions are located in the choroid and the sclera. There may be focal retinitis with inflammation and scarring secondary to a local immunologic response. A diffuse retinitis and secondary vitritis may also occur. Relapses are seen even after therapy, particularly at the onset of puberty. Immunocompromised patients may have diffuse and progressive retinal lesions. The lesions should be distinguished from those caused by cytomegalovirus or histoplasmosis.

Congenital Toxoplasmosis Congenital infection causes a spectrum of disease, from asymptomatic to fatal, depending on the fetal age at infection. If infection occurs in the first trimester, the pregnancy may terminate in abortion, or the child may be born with a typical syndrome of retinochoroiditis, encephalitis with intracerebral calcifications (typically periaqueductal and periventricular lesions predominate), microcephalus, hydrocephalus, hepatosplenomegaly, maculopapular rash, or thrombocytopenic purpura. Hypothalamic and pituitary dysfunction may occur in severe cases of toxoplasma encephalitis. Children who contract infection at a later age of gestation may have subclinical infection, or may primarily have central nervous system involvement with seizures and psychomotor disturbances. Children with subclinical infection, although appearing normal at birth, may develop visual loss, hearing deficits, delayed psychomotor development, and lower intelligent quotient scores after 4 or more years.

DIAGNOSIS Histologic identification of the trophozoite generally is indicative of acute infection. The presence of cysts reflects past infection. Detection of the *T. gondii* DNA with the use of polymerase chain reaction (PCR) may also be useful. Serologic tests must be interpreted in light of the clinical context. Many types of serologic tests are available for the diagnosis of toxoplasmosis. These include dye tests, indirect fluorescent antibody (IFA), enzyme immunoassay (EIA), direct agglutination, and immunosorbent tests for IgM.

In children and adults, *Toxoplasma*-specific IgM is usually detected within 2 weeks and peaks within 1 month of primary infection. IgM antibodies usually become undetectable within 6 to 9 months. Total IgG antibodies peak 1 to 2 months following primary infection and remain positive indefinitely. Seroconversion or a four-fold rise in specific IgG antibody titers is suggestive of recent infection. In immunodeficient hosts with serologic evidence of *T. gondii*-specific IgG, the diagnosis of clinical disease because of reactivation is established by demonstration of the organism within tissue by immunohistochemical staining, or by detecting its presence by PCR in a clinically appropriate setting.

Most cases of ocular toxoplasmosis are diagnosed clinically; serologic tests are used primarily to confirm prior exposure to *Toxoplasma gondii*, with the presence of *T. gondii*-specific IgG. Measurement of vitreous humor antibody and detection of *T. gondii* DNA by PCR is also possible, but not routinely done.

Serologically proven primary maternal toxoplasmosis during gestation should prompt testing to rule out or confirm fetal infection. Detection of *Toxoplasma*-specific IgM and IgA in fetal cord blood after 20 weeks' gestation (sensitivity of 58–77%; specificity of 96–100%, respectively) provides a definite confirmation of congenital infection. Amniotic fluid sampling to detect the parasite or its genomic material by PCR has a sensitivity of only 38 to 44% with a specificity of 97 to 100%. Both serologic and DNA tests have a low rate of false-positives. Fetal-blood sampling carries a higher risk of fetal loss as compared to amniocentesis and is not routinely used. Serial ultrasounds of the fetus to detect clinical signs of infection are also used.

If the diagnosis of congenital toxoplasmosis is suspected after birth, clinical examination focusing on ophthalmologic, auditory, and neurologic assessments, including ultrasound or computed tomography of the head, should be done. Isolation of the organism or *Toxoplasma* detection by PCR in cord or newborn peripheral blood, cerebrospinal fluid (CSF), amniotic fluid, and placental tissue confirms a diagnosis of fetal toxoplasmosis. Alternatively, the detection of *Toxoplasma*-specific IgM or IgA in the newborn blood indicates fetal infection because these antibodies do not cross the placenta. Blood should be tested at a reference laboratory that performs *Toxoplasma* IgM and IgA assays by the double-sandwich IgM EIA or the IgM immunosorbent agglutination assay. The sensitivity of the immunofluorescent and of the capture-EIA assays for IgM is insufficient for the diagnosis of congenital infection. *Toxoplasma*-specific IgE and differential agglutination tests may also be helpful in establishing a diagnosis. False-negative serologic results are possible, and persistence of *Toxoplasma*-specific IgG beyond 12 to 18 months of age is also indicative of congenital infection. Cytologic and biochemical examination of newborn CSF has poor sensitivity for the diagnosis of toxoplasmosis.

TREATMENT AND PREVENTION Immunocompetent children and nonpregnant adolescents with lymphadenopathy who have no evidence of severe organ damage do not require therapy. Spiramycin, pyrimethamine, and sulfadiazine are currently the drugs of choice for the treatment of toxoplasmosis (see Table 13-64). Spiramycin is a macrolide that concentrates in the placenta and is believed to reduce transmission of infection from mother to fetus by 50%. It does not appear to treat the fetus in utero. Spiramycin is available only as an investigational drug in the United States. Pyrimethamine and sulfonamides have marked synergistic activity against *Toxoplasma* organisms. However, encysted bradyzoites are not eliminated, leaving "treated" individuals still at risk for recurrent disease. Sulfadiazine, sulfamerazine, and sulfamethazine are also active in vitro against *T. gondii*.

In children with active chorioretinitis, treatment with pyrimethamine, sulfadiazine, leucovorin, and corticosteroids should be considered until resolution of the infection. For immunocompromised individuals, active infection (retinitis, encephalitis) should be treated. HIV-infected persons who have been treated for active toxoplasmosis should receive lifelong therapy if they have advanced disease with low CD4 counts. Daily prophylaxis with pyrimethamine and sulfadiazine is associated with the lowest relapse rate. Consideration should be given to providing suppressive therapy to pregnant HIV-positive women with low CD4 counts who are seropositive for *Toxoplasma*.

Acute Infection in Pregnant Women Pregnant women with acute infection (7 to 34 weeks' gestation) are given spiramycin orally, 1 g q8h, for 18 weeks of gestation. Antenatal diagnosis of fetal infection should be attempted. If fetal infection is excluded, spiramycin is continued until term. If fetal infection is confirmed, therapy is modified to pyrimethamine, sulfadiazine, and leucovorin. Some physicians alternate with monthly spiramycin. Infection acquired late in gestation (>34 weeks) can be treated with pyrimethamine, sulfadiazine, and leucovorin because the risk to the fetus is less. The benefits of this approach, however, are not conclusive; therapy may decrease, but does not eliminate, the possibility of fetal infection.

Congenital Infection   Congenital infection is treated in utero (as above) and for the first year of life, regardless of whether the child manifests clinical signs or symptoms of congenital infection with toxoplasmosis at birth. Early therapeutic intervention of congenital toxoplasmosis lessens neurologic sequelae, even in those infants with significant central nervous system involvement at birth. Infants with untreated or inadequately treated congenital toxoplasmosis develop psychomotor dysfunction, seizures, visual dysfunction, and hearing loss. Outcome in children with subclinical infection may manifest as low intelligence quotient and as chorioretinal lesions that may impact on development later in life.

Treatment with pyrimethamine is given to children as a loading dose of 2 mg/kg (maximum 50 mg) daily for 2 days, then 1 mg/kg (maximum 25 mg) daily for 2 to 6 months, and finally 1 mg/kg three times a week to complete a 12-month course. Sulfadiazine is given as 100 mg/kg daily in two divided doses. Folinic acid is given as 5 to 10 mg three times weekly or, if neutropenia occurs, 5 to 20 mg daily. Peripheral blood cell and platelet determinations should be obtained on a routine basis to detect bone marrow toxicity. After treatment is discontinued, retinal examinations at 3- to 6-month intervals are recommended to detect new retinal lesions.

For healthy newborns from mothers who acquired toxoplasmosis during pregnancy, the same regimen is indicated until the results of the investigations are available to rule out congenital infection. If evidence of congenital infection is present, therapy is continued for 1 year.

Prevention   Counseling of pregnant women and immunocompromised patients on avoidance measures is estimated to reduce acquisition by 50%. Eating rare or undercooked meat should be avoided; infected meat or eggs can be made safe by thoroughly heating to at least 60°C (140°F; well done). Individuals who handle raw meat should wash their hands carefully.

Because cats, which are an important source of oocysts, defecate in loose soil and sand, children must be protected from these sites. Prevention of infection in children should focus on avoiding oral contact or ingestion of soil or sand that could contain cat oocysts. Susceptible pregnant women should not handle cat litter without disposable gloves. Young domestic cats that are fed raw meat may be an important source of human infection. Cat feces should be discarded daily, before the oocysts have had a chance to sporulate (ie, 1 to 5 days) and become infective. Cat feces should be buried or flushed down a toilet.

References

Dunn D, Wallon M, Peyron F, Peterson E, Peckham C, Gildbert R: Mother-to-child transmission of toxoplasmosis: risk estimates for clinical counselling. Lancet 353:1829–1833, 1999

Hezard N, Mark-Chemla C, Foudrinier F, et al: Prenatal diagnosis of congenital toxoplasmosis in 261 pregnancies. Prenat Diagn 17(11):1047–1054, 1997

Lebech M, Joynson DHM, Seitz HM, et al: Classification system and case definitions of *Toxoplasma gondii* infection in immunocompetent pregnant women and their congenitally infected offspring. Eur J Clin Microbiol Infect Dis 15:799–805, 1996

McAauley J, Boyer KM, Patel D, et al: Early and longitudinal evaluations of treated infants and children and untreated historical patients with congenital toxoplasmosis: the Chicago collaborative treatment trial. Clin Infect Dis 18:38–72, 1994

Pratlong F, Boulot P, Villena I, et al: Antenatal diagnosis of congenital toxoplasmosis: evaluation of the biological parameters in a cohort of 286 patients. Br J Obstet Gynecol 103:552–557, 1996

TRYPANOSOMIASIS, AFRICAN (SLEEPING SICKNESS)
Eduardo Ortega-Barria

African trypanosomiasis is caused by a subspecies of the extracellular flagellate *Trypanosoma brucei* known as *Trypanosoma brucei gambiense,* which usually evolves slowly, over many years, and ends fatally if it is not treated, and *T. brucei rhodesiense,* which results in a more acute syndrome and usually kills the host in weeks or months. These diseases exist in Africa wherever the various species of *Glossina* (ie, the tsetse fly) are found.

All members of the *T. brucei* complex share a common morphology, biochemistry, and life cycle. Infective metacyclic trypomastigotes are inoculated into subcutaneous tissue of a human or another mammalian host by a bite from the tsetse fly. They are converted to the pleomorphic blood forms: long, slender forms (20–40 by 1 μm) and stumpy forms (15–25 by 3.5 μm). Within the human host, trypomastigotes multiply in blood, lymph, and extracellular spaces. The central nervous system eventually is invaded, where multiplication continues unabated. Other than humans, there is no important reservoir host for *T. brucei gambiense,* whereas *T. brucei rhodesiense* infects wild game animals. The tsetse fly is infected with ingestion of a blood meal. Trypomastigotes differentiate into procyclic forms in the midgut where they multiply by binary fission and remain for the next 2 to 3 weeks. Finally, they enter the salivary glands and transform into infective metacyclic trypomastigote forms. When the fly bites another mammal, the parasites are injected into the blood, completing the cycle of infection. Tsetse flies are long lived, both sexes take blood meals, but infection rates rarely exceed 0.1%. In endemic areas, the number of detectable infections among humans will be below 0.1%.

The inoculated metacyclic trypomastigote transform and multiply locally in the subcutaneous tissue, giving origin to a characteristic hard and sometimes painful chancre. By about the tenth day, slender forms reach the bloodstream and lymphatics, and for the next several days, their numbers increase logarithmically, spreading to several tissues. Soon thereafter, the organisms nearly disappear from the bloodstream, only to reappear later. After a variable length of time, trypomastigotes pass through the blood-brain barrier and induce a generalized meningoencephalitis.

The parasite survives in the mammalian host by periodically altering its surface antigenic coat, evading the developing immune response of the host. Each successive parasitemic wave represents a new antigenic variant that has emerged to elude the host's antibody response to the previous antigen. The parasite is covered with a variable surface glycoprotein (VSG). Each peak of parasitemia contains a predominant variable antigen type (VAT). The specific antibody response to this coat leads to the destruction of the predominant VAT or homotype. However, within each population of parasites are a number of heterotypes, one of which then becomes the next homotype that is not recognized by the host's immune response. The parasite in each successive wave of parasitemia bears a different VAT. A single trypomastigote may contain as many as 1000 genes, each encoding for a specific VSG.

A marked specific humoral antibody response (predominantly IgM) follows infection. As a result of polyclonal B-cell activation, there also are many antibodies produced to a wide variety of antigens, including red blood cells, brain, and heart. Circulating immune complexes have been reported regularly, and these may be responsible for the glomerulonephritis often accompanying acute and chronic disease.

CLINICAL MANIFESTATIONS Clinical manifestations with *T. b. gambiense* and *T. b. rhodesiense* are similar, except that Rhodesian infection causes an acute and severe disease, with few CNS symptoms, and death within a few months. Gambian infection has a milder, chronic course, with involvement of lymph nodes, CNS invasion, and a fatal outcome after several years.

In both forms, the trypanosomal chancre may be evident 2 to 3 days after the bite of the fly. Within 1 week, the lesion becomes a large, red, warm, and painful nodule that usually resolves within 3 weeks, leaving residual scarring and depigmentation. In Rhodesian trypanosomiasis, the incubation period typically is 2 to 3 weeks, whereas with Gambian infection, the onset of symptoms may be delayed for several weeks or years. Early stages are characterized by intermittent fevers, chills, headache, and generalized lymphadenopathy. The nodes are discrete, soft, nontender, and contain abundant parasites. In Gambian disease, nodes in the posterior cervical triangle may become enlarged (ie, Winterbottom sign) and, when present, strongly suggest the diagnosis. The spleen and liver may be mildly enlarged. Intermittent fevers may last for months to years with Gambian infection. Wasting and malnutrition occur, and patients often die of intercurrent infections. An irregular, circinate, evanescent rash on the trunk, shoulders, and thighs that is more evident in white persons may appear. The sedimentation rate is elevated markedly; anemia, hypoalbuminemia, and thrombocytopenia are frequent as well. Serum immunoglobulin levels (IgM), circulating immune complexes, heterophil antibodies, and rheumatoid factor are increased.

Untreated patients with Gambian disease often develop signs of central nervous system invasion. Severe headaches, insomnia, and a feeling of impending doom are typical. Next, there may be progressive mental deterioration, with patients becoming incapable of caring for themselves. Tremors, especially of the tongue, hands, or feet, as well as generalized or focal convulsions may occur. Myocarditis is particularly common and may lead to early death in the Rhodesian form of the disease. Untreated, both forms of sleeping sickness are always fatal.

The differential diagnosis includes tuberculosis, malaria, visceral leishmaniasis, brucellosis, relapsing fever, syphilis, enteric fever, and viral encephalitis.

DIAGNOSIS Definitive diagnosis depends on demonstration of the parasite from the chancre, in blood, lymph node aspirates, bone marrow, or cerebrospinal fluid (CSF). Patent parasitemia is more common during febrile episodes. It is essential to use both thick and thin Giemsa-stained blood smears, as well as to examine the buffy coat from 10 to 20 mL of citrated whole blood or the sediment from 5 mL of centrifuged cerebrospinal fluid. Because of the periodicity of the parasitemia, daily examination of blood films for 10 consecutive days is recommended. *Trypanosoma brucei rhodesiense* is found more frequently in peripheral blood, and can be shown in a single microscopic examination in 87% of cases. Examination of wet preparations of cervical lymph node aspirates help to confirm the diagnosis when trypanosomes are undetected in blood. Intraperitoneal inoculation of 0.5 mL heparinized blood or CSF into two mice is positive in 89% of *T. b. rhodesiense* cases within 2 weeks of inoculation.

The CSF should be examined to determine the stage of the disease. In advanced central nervous system disease, the CSF shows increased protein concentration; elevated cell counts, predominantly mononuclear; small number of eosinophils; and frequently trypomastigotes. In advanced untreated sleeping sickness, the IgM level in the CSF often is elevated, but it has no relationship to the presence of trypanosomes in the CSF. After successful treatment, the IgM level declines gradually, disappearing after approximately 1 year.

Immunodiagnostic methods may be helpful for epidemiologic studies and detection of latent infections. Specific antibodies can be detected after the second week of infection by indirect fluorescent antibody or EIA. The card agglutination test (CATT), a simple, direct agglutination test for stained trypanosomes, is available for the diagnosis of *T. b. gambiense*. A monoclonal antibody-based EIA for detection of trypanosome antigens in serum and CSF has a high specificity (99.9%) and sensitivity [*T. b. gambiense* (94.8%) and *T. b. Rhodesiense* (91.5%)].

TREATMENT AND PREVENTION Early treatment is essential, when the parasite is restricted to the hematolymphatic system, because the prognosis is poor once CNS involvement has occurred. Suramin and pentamidine do not penetrate the CNS adequately and are useful only in early African trypanosome infections. Pentamidine, as the isethionate salt, is used only against *T. b. gambiense*, as primary resistance of *T. b. rhodesiense* has been observed. Pentamidine is administered IM at 4 mg/kg/d for 7 to 10 doses, given daily or every second day. Both the liver and kidneys store the drug for months. Serious side effects include nephrotoxicity, hepatotoxicity, and pancreatotoxicity. Suramin, a polysulfonated naphthylamide, inhibits glycolytic enzymes of trypanosomes and a full course cures early cases of *T. b. gambiense* and *T. b. rhodesiense*. A test dose of 5 mg/kg is given and is followed by a dose of 20 mg/kg IV (maximum dose 1 g) on days 1, 3, 7, 14, and 21. Common reactions include joint pain, fever, urticaria, and paresthesia. Nephrotoxicity is the most important toxic effect; urinalysis should be done prior to administration of each dose, and the presence of casts or red blood cells in the sediment are indications for alternative therapy.

During the second stage of the disease, drugs that can penetrate into the CSF are indispensable. A lumbar puncture must be performed prior to starting therapy, periodically during treatment, 3 months after treatment, and then every 6 months for 2 to 3 years. Melarsoprol is a combination of the trivalent arsenical, melarsen oxide, and British anti-Lewisite (BAL). Melarsoprol is administered at 18 to 25 mg/kg total over 1 month, at an initial dose of 0.36 mg/kg IV, increasing gradually to a maximum of 3.6 mg/kg at intervals of 1 to 5 days for a total of 9 to 10 doses. This is the drug of choice when CNS invasion has occurred and after treatment with suramin and/or pentamidine has failed. The most serious side effect is an encephalopathy, which can occur in 1 to 10% of treated patients, with mortality in 1 to 5%. Other adverse effects include fever, headache, abdominal pain, diarrhea, vomiting, and joint pain. Difluoromethylornithine (DFMO) is a selective and irreversible inhibitor of ornithine decarboxylase, the first enzyme in polyamine synthesis of trypanosomes. Recent trials indicate that in both the hemolymphatic and central nervous system stages of *T. brucei gambiense* infection, DFMO is effective and reliable; however, effectiveness against infections with *T. b. rhodesiense* varies. The recommended dosage is 400 mg/kg/d IV in four divided doses for 14 days, followed by 300 mg/kg/d for an additional 30 days. Side effects include anemia, thrombocytopenia, diarrhea, and seizures, all of which are short-lived and reversible. A Jarisch-Herxheimer-type reaction has been reported.

Prevention of infection ideally would eliminate the vector. Tsetse flies can be controlled by using insecticides, such as chlorinated hydrocarbons and synthetic pyrethroids directed at known fly resting sites. Fly traps or screens impregnated with insecticides may be more economical and effective. Chemoprophylaxis with suramin, 0.3 to 0.7 g IV every 2 to 3 months, is reported to be highly effective. Vaccine development has been hindered by antigenic variation.

References

Control and surveillance of African trypanosomiasis. Report of a WHO Expert Committee. World Health Organ Tech Rep Ser 881:1-VI, 1–114, 1998

Croft S, Urbina JA, Brun R: Chemotherapy of human leishmaniasis and trypanosomiasis. In: Hide G, Mottram JC, Coombs GH, Holmes PH, eds: Trypanosomiasis and Leishmaniasis. Oxford University Press, Oxford, UK, 245–257, 1997

Croft S: Pharmacological approaches to antitrypanosomal chemotherapy. Mem Inst Oswaldo Cruz 94:215–220, 1999

Drugs for parasitic infections. Med Lett 37:99–108, 1995

Pentreath VW: Trypanosomiasis and the nervous system. Pathology and immunology. Trans R Soc Trop Med Hyg 89:9–15, 1995

TRYPANOSOMIASIS, AMERICAN (CHAGAS DISEASE)

Eduardo Ortega-Barria

American trypanosomiasis (ie, Chagas disease) is caused by the protozoan parasite *Trypanosoma cruzi.*

The life cycle of *T. cruzi* includes four developmental stages. The trypomastigote is found in the tissue and bloodstream of infected mammals and is responsible for the intercellular spreading of the infection. The trypomastigote is spindle shaped, measures about 20 μm, has a kinetoplast located posterior to the nucleus, and a flagellum that extends along the outer edge and reaches the anterior end of the body. In stained blood smears, trypomastigotes assume a characteristic "C" or "S" shape, with the nucleus just anterior to the middle of the cell (Fig. 13-32). The amastigote is the dividing intracellular form found in the tissues of the mammalian host. The disease is transmitted by bloodsucking insects of the family Reduvidae that become infected by ingesting trypomastigotes present in the bloodstream of infected mammals. The organisms reach the insect midgut, transform into the multiplying epimastigote stage, and change progressively to infective metacyclic

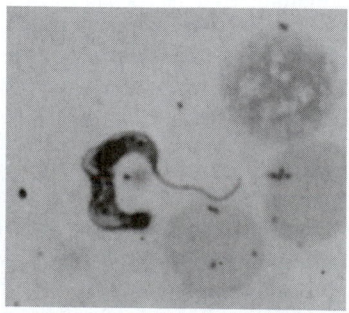

FIGURE 13-32 *Trypanosoma cruzi* **in peripheral blood smear.**

trypomastigotes until they are excreted with feces and urine during feeding. These enter the human body through an abrasion on the skin, intact mucous membrane, or the bite wound. Natural infection occurs in a wide variety of peridomestic and sylvatic animals, including birds, guinea pigs, monkeys, opossums, foxes, ferrets, squirrels, armadillos, anteaters, porcupines, rats, and mice. Domestic dogs and cats are believed to be major reservoirs for human infection. However, within the domicile, transmission from human to human through the vector is probably the most common cycle of infection.

Human Chagas disease extends from southern United States to Chile and Argentina. The Caribbean, Belize, Surinam, and Guyana are reported to be free of this infection. Approximately 16 to 18 million people are infected, with 200,000 new cases a year. The prevalence of infection is greatest in Brazil, Argentina, and Venezuela. In the United States, only three autochthonous cases of Chagas disease have been reported, but cases acquired through laboratory accidents, imported infection, and blood transfusion are reported in the United States and Canada. Congenital infection often results in spontaneous abortion, stillbirth, premature delivery, and infection in newborns. Congenital transmission occurs in only 0.7% to 2.0% of the cases in which the mother is infected, but the prognosis is poor unless antepartum therapy had been initiated. The newborns may have cardiac disorders, pulmonary edema, encephalitis, and hepatosplenic disorders. Congenitally infected children rarely survive until the age of puberty. The heart is enlarged, and thinning of the ventricular wall becomes the starting point for the formation of aneurysms. Mural thrombi may embolize systemically. The myocardium reveals focal myonecrosis, contraction band necrosis, interstitial fibrosis, and lymphocytic infiltration. In addition, the esophagus and colon are frequently affected, with dysfunction and dilatation directly related to peristaltic abnormalities or to aperistalsis caused by destruction of the ganglion cells of the muscle.

CLINICAL MANIFESTATIONS Chagas disease can be divided into three distinct phases: acute, latent, and chronic. In 95% of patients, clinical symptoms during the acute phase are either mild or absent. Shortly after penetration, parasites elicit a local inflammatory reaction at the site of entry that gives origin to the chagoma (nodular skin reaction) or the Romaña sign (unilateral periorbital edema, conjunctivitis, and preauricular lymphadenitis). Acute manifestations are usually seen in young children. Illness begins with fever, headache, anorexia, and lassitude. Cervical, axillary, and iliac lymphadenopathy; hepatosplenomegaly; vomiting; and rash are common, and occasionally, meningoencephalitis occurs.

The most common and severe manifestations of acute infection (30% of cases) are cardiovascular disturbances from myocarditis, which include cardiomegaly, functional murmurs, and conduction blocks. Examining the blood during the acute phase reveals trypomastigotes, anemia, leukocytosis with a lymphocytosis, elevated erythrocyte sedimentation rate, and increases in serum bilirubin and cardiac enzymes. During the acute phase, 5 to 10% of patients die of severe myocarditis, but in young infants with meningoencephalitis, mortality can be as high as 50%. In 2 to 3 months, the acute stage subsides, and fewer organisms are found in the peripheral blood.

The most common findings in congenital cases of Chagas disease include small size for gestational age; hepatosplenomegaly with jaundice; anemia; petechiae; edema; convulsions secondary to meningoencephalitis; and cardiovascular alterations. Many infants die during the first week of life, and those that survive may develop severe neurologic sequelae, with mental deficiency and learning disabilities.

After the acute phase, the disease enters a latent phase for 10 to 40 years or more, in which the patient may be free of clinical symptoms and appear to be in good health. There may be up to 100,000 immigrants with latent *T. cruzi* infections living in the United States. With increasing age, there is a progressive increase in the number of individuals presenting with electrocardiographic abnormalities.

Chronic cardiomyopathy is the most frequent (30–40% of patients) manifestation of chronic Chagas disease; digestive tract disorders are much less frequent (8–10%). The signs and symptoms of chronic cardiomyopathy are secondary to heart failure, arrhythmia, endomyocardial disorders, and embolic complications. Chronic cardiomyopathy may be present by the second and third decades of life; it has even been reported in teenagers and young adults. Megaesophagus and megacolon are caused by destruction of the ganglion cells of the myenteric plexus. Dysphagia, regurgitation with retrosternal burning, and paroxysmal night coughs, which presumably result from aspiration during sleep, are associated with megaesophagus. Chronic constipation, long-term fecal retention, impaction, and volvulus are seen with megacolon.

Prognosis depends on clinical stage and its complications. The acute phase is most serious in children younger than 2 years of age, and is fatal if meningoencephalitis and heart failure develop. In severe cardiomyopathy, the prognosis is poor and death usually occurs within a few years from heart failure or cardiac arrhythmia.

DIAGNOSIS Acute Chagas disease should be considered in any child who has been in an endemic area and who develops an acute febrile illness with lymphadenopathy and myocarditis. Differential diagnosis during the acute phase includes visceral leishmaniasis, malaria, brucellosis, schistosomiasis, and infectious mononucleosis. The chronic disease must be distinguished from endomyocardial fibrosis, viral myocarditis, rheumatic heart disease, and achalasia of the esophagus.

The laboratory diagnosis of Chagas disease can be made by the demonstration of the parasite by direct or indirect methods, and by serologic demonstration of specific antibodies. During the acute stage or an acute exacerbation of the chronic stage, parasites can be readily found in the blood or in leukocyte concentrates by microscopic examination. Blood culture employing NNN, LIT, or other culture media, as well as inoculation of patient's blood into laboratory animals, may aid in diagnosis at this time as well.

During chronic disease, serologic tests are the method of choice in establishing diagnosis. Antibodies appear in the blood 2 to 3 weeks after infection and persist for years. Antibodies of the IgM isotype predominate during the acute phase, with IgG appearing as the disease progresses. Complement-fixation (Machado-Guerreiro) was the first serologic procedure to be used and still is considered by many to be the most reliable immunodiagnostic method for establishing a diagnosis and evaluating specific antigens. Indirect fluorescence and ELISA tests are useful in detecting IgM or IgG antibodies, with a sensitivity of 95%. Several agglutination tests have been developed that detect the presence of antibodies, including indirect hemagglutination, direct agglutination, latex agglutination, and a flocculation test. However, patients with leishmaniasis, malaria, collagen vascular diseases, and syphilis may give false-positive reactions. In acute congenital disease, an immunofluorescence IgM test often is positive.

Blood culture and xenodiagnosis are equally useful in diagnosing chronic disease, with a sensitivity of 45% and 70%, respectively, in this phase. Xenodiagnosis is a technique whereby laboratory-reared reduviid bugs are permitted to feed on the patient; subsequently, the rectum of the bug is examined in 4 to 6 weeks for metacyclic trypomastigotes. Polymerase chain reaction (PCR) technology has been adapted to the diagnosis of acute and chronic Chagas disease. PCR is able to detect as few as one parasite in 20 mL of blood, and has a sensitivity of 96 to 100%. PCR could replace xenodiagnosis for evaluation of parasitemia in chronic chagasic patients in the near future.

TREATMENT AND PREVENTION At present, no drugs are available that can assure a complete cure of Chagas disease. Nitrofuran and nitroimidazole derivatives are effective in reducing the parasitemia and in shortening the length and severity of illness, as well as clinical symptoms, in the acute phase of the disease. The recommended dosage of nifurtimox for children 1 to 10 years of age is 15 to 20 mg/kg/d in four divided doses for 90 days; for children 11 to 16 years of age, 12.5 to 15.0 mg/kg/d in four divided doses; and for adults, 8 to 10 mg/kg/d for 120 days. Many patients develop adverse side effects, including weakness, anorexia, nausea, and vomiting. Long-term use is associated with toxic hepatitis, loss of memory, tremor, polyneuritis, and paresthesias. Benznidazole (Radanil, Roche 7-1051) (5 mg/kg/d for 30 to 120 days) is thought to act by the covalent binding of nitroreduction intermediates to macromolecules. Side effects include rash, peripheral neuritis, and granulocytopenia.

Recent studies using highly sensitive PCR detection methods, histopathology, and detailed immunologic characterization of the inflammatory process associated with chagasic cardiomyopathy indicate that effective antiparasitic treatment can stop the progression of the disease in humans, which may support treatment of patients with latent and chronic Chagas disease.

References

Gomes ML, Galvao LM, Macedo AM, Pena SD, Chiari E: Chagas' disease diagnosis: comparative analysis of parasitologic, molecular, and serologic methods. Am J Trop Med Hyg 60:205–210, 1999

Gomes ML, Macedo AM, Vago AR, Pena SD, Galvao LM, Chiari E: *Trypanosoma cruzi* optimization of polymerase chain reaction for detection in human blood. Exp Parasitol 88:28–33, 1998

Kirchhoff LV: American trypanosomiasis (Chagas' disease): a tropical disease now in the United States. N Engl J Med 329:639–644, 1993

Urbina JA: Chemotherapy of Chagas' disease: the how and the why. J Mol Med 77:332–338, 1999

Viotti R, Vigliano C, Armenti H, Segura E: Treatment of chronic Chagas' disease with benznidazole: clinical and serological evolution of patients with long-term follow-up. Am Heart J 127:151–162, 1994

Zhang L, Tarleton RL: Parasite persistence correlates with disease severity and localization in chronic Chagas' disease. J Infect Dis 180:480–486, 1999

13.7   DISEASES CAUSED BY ARTHROPODS

ARACHNIDISM

Allison Holm

Arachnids are a large group (class Arachnida) of arthropods that includes spiders, scorpions, mites, and ticks. Few of the many species of spiders are medically important, but among those that are clinically relevant are the widows (ie, *Latrodectus sp.*) that occur in both the Western and Eastern Hemispheres and the brown spiders (ie, *Loxosceles sp.*) that are found in the Western Hemisphere.

Spider Bites

Contrary to common belief, most spiders are harmless and shy, and few possess mouth parts that are sufficiently robust to penetrate human skin and inoculate venom. There are, however, several that can cause serious and sometimes fatal envenomization if they are provoked. Most notable is the black widow spider (*Latrodectus mactans*). The female is glossy black to sepia and is covered with tiny hairs. In the United States, its back or dorsum usually is black, and the underside of the abdomen has a characteristic red or crimson hourglass pattern. The average width of the abdomen is 6 mm and the overall length (with legs extended) is 40 mm. Typically, the female is found with her crude web in dark, dry habitats such as vacant rodent burrows, hollow stumps, and dark corners of barns, privies, and garages.

The bite of the female black widow spider often is not felt and resembles a pinprick. At this point of the bite, there may be slight swelling and twin, minute, red spots. Immediately after the attack, lymphatic absorption of the toxin begins, and the patient experiences local sharp, throbbing pain that increases in intensity for several hours, by which time vascular spread has occurred. Symptoms are severe and usually include diaphoresis, nausea, vomiting, hypertension, and intense, agonizing spasms, especially of the abdominal muscles. Spasticity of other muscle groups depends on the area of the bite. Severely affected individuals develop profound shock, delirium, and coma; 5% of those children who are bitten die. Usually, however, the symptoms regress, and the victim recovers.

Symptoms generally are more severe in children and the elderly than in adults. Treatment should be initiated as soon as possible with 10% calcium gluconate or methocarbamol (Robaxin, 15 mg/kg IV or intramuscularly, repeated every 6 hours) for relief of muscle spasms. An ampule of antivenin (Lyovac, Merck) should be administered by slow IV injection in 50 mL of saline, after skin testing for sensitivity to horse serum. It usually is effective within 30 minutes and may, if necessary, be repeated within 1 or 2 hours. However, use of antivenin is controversial because it is associated with serious side effects such as serum sickness and anaphylaxis. Other treatments include meperidine for sedation and relief of pain, diazepam for muscle relaxation, and systemic corticosteroids for severe reactions. Tourniquets or other procedures that are suggested for snakebites are ineffective.

Two species of brown or fiddleback spiders in the Western Hemisphere also cause serious envenomization. *Loxosceles reclusa* is found in many parts of the United States, especially in the south and central regions such as Arkansas, Missouri, and Texas. *Loxosceles laeta* is found in South and Central America. Both species of recluse spiders live indoors in houses (especially closets), where it nests in clothing and may bite when disturbed. However, they also have been found in bathrooms, bedrooms, and cellars. Recluse spiders are 10 to 15 mm in length. When well-marked, they show a violin-shaped marking on the dorsum of the cephalothorax. When disturbed, the spider bites; within 10 minutes to several hours, the site becomes painful. A local reaction can occur (necrotic cutaneous loxoscelism), a bulla may develop, and concentric areas of ischemia and erythema appear. During the ensuing 24 to 48 hours, the lesion becomes cyanotic and soon ulcerates. The necrotic ulcer slowly expands and can reach 10 to 20 cm in diameter during the subsequent weeks to months.

Viscerocutaneous loxoscelism is a systemic reaction that occurs in 25% of patients with the cutaneous reaction. It is characterized by high fever, chills, vomiting, myalgia, and even death. Treatment for the brown recluse spider bite consists of application of ice packs and elevation of the affected area, acetaminophen for relief of fever and myalgia, and antibiotics, such as erythromycin and cephalosporin, for prevention or treatment of secondary infection. Dapsone (4,4'-diaminodiophenyl sulfone) is recommended for presumed necrotic spider bites. The adult dose is 100 mg given twice daily only after confirmation that the patient has an active glucose-6-phosphate dehydrogenase enzyme.

Scorpions

Scorpions are nocturnal arachnids that hide during the day. At the terminal portion of its abdomen, the scorpion has stingers that it uses to strike its victim both swiftly and repeatedly when disturbed. Scorpions rarely attack humans, but sting by accident or in self-defense if disturbed. In the United States, the only medically important species is *Centruroides sculpturatus,* which is found exclusively in Arizona.

There are two types of scorpion venom: a relatively harmless local hemolytic material, and the often fatal neurotoxic venom that also has hemolytic and cytolytic properties. The hemolytic toxin produces a localized painful erythematous swelling that can result in severe necrosis. The neurotoxic venom produces numbness at the sting site and can cause a generalized reaction, including sweating, salivation, laryngeal edema, nausea, vomiting, abdominal cramps, and seizures. Generally, it is regarded as a good prognostic sign if the patient survives 3 hours. Death frequently occurs because of respiratory paralysis, pulmonary edema, or intractable hypotension and shock. Most of the deaths occur in infants and young children.

Treatment should be initiated as soon as possible, especially in children. Specific antiscorpion serum generally is available in those areas where these dangerous animals exist, and its administration is the single most important treatment for severe envenomization. A carefully monitored tourniquet should be applied above the wound and an ice pack placed on the area to delay absorption. Morphine is contraindicated, but seizures and shock should be managed aggressively. General supportive measures include use of antihistamines, corticosteroids, and analgesics. Care must be exercised when using barbiturates, because these may inhibit central respiration. Muscle spasm can be ameliorated with 10 mL of 10% calcium gluconate.

Mites

Mites are a ubiquitous group of Arachnida consisting of nearly 1600 genera and thousands of species. These insects are extremely minute and easily overlooked as the cause of a patient's intense pruritus. The human itch mite *Sarcoptes scabiei* and the chigger mite *Eutrombicula alfreddugèsi* are among the medically important insects infesting humans. Scabies is discussed below.

Chigger mites are approximately 0.4 mm in length and 0.25 mm in width. They are seen most commonly in the southern United States. Humans are infested when they come in contact with the larval mites when walking through underbrush or tall grass, or by sitting on mite-infested ground. The mite migrates to areas of constriction of clothing (eg, the waistband) and produces an itchy red papular eruption. After 3 to 4 days, the fully engorged chigger drops off. However, the irritating secretions remain and continue to cause intense itching.

Typically, the initial lesion is a small red macule or papule with a minute red mite in the center. By 24 hours, the lesion evolves into an intensely pruritic urticarial papule that is surmounted with a tiny vesicle containing clear fluid (Fig. 13-33). Depending on the site, the lesion can become purpuric and hemorrhagic. Symptoms can persist for days or weeks before drying up. Secondary pyogenic infection is a common consequence of excoriation.

The aim of treatment is to relieve the intense pruritus using either antihistamines or topical corticosteroids. Secondary infection should be treated with empiric antibiotics directed toward the usual causes of skin infection (*Staphylococcus aureus*, group A streptococci, etc).

Tick Bites

Both tick bites and tick-borne diseases have become more frequent, especially along the east coast of the United States. Ticks are bloodsucking ectoparasites in all of their stages, and they can be recognized easily by the organization of their mouthparts and body. They are subdivided into two major groups: the argasids, or soft ticks; and the ixodids, or hard ticks.

The female tick attaches itself to the skin by inserting its proboscis. The bite is painless, but within a few hours there is a papule at the puncture site that may be itchy and painful. The tick becomes engorged with blood for days or weeks before dropping off. The papule can progress to swelling or erythema, but usually resolves spontaneously in 2 to 3 weeks. If the papule expands to form a large (≥5 cm) annular ring with central clearing, this is a likely

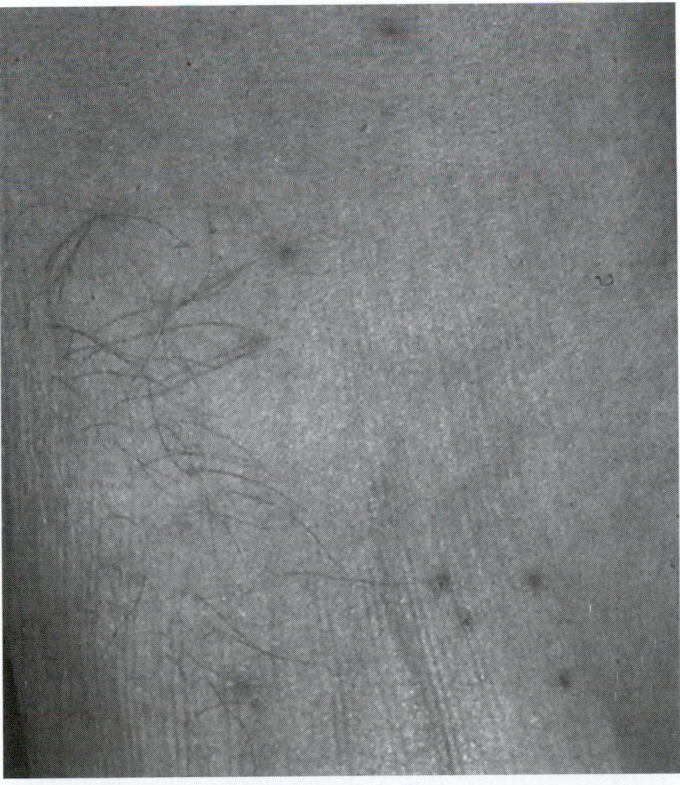

FIGURE 13-33   Multiple uninfected chigger bites of the ankle and dorsum of the foot. SOURCE: *(Courtesy of Dr. Jay Keystone, Tropical Disease Unit, Toronto Hospital, Toronto, Ontario.)*

indication of erythema migrans, the skin manifestation of Lyme disease. Erythema migrans is usually asymptomatic and resolves spontaneously in weeks to months, even in untreated patients (see Sec. 13.2.19).

Tick paralysis, which is reported to occur when female hard or soft ticks feed on domestic animals, is seen occasionally in humans, especially children. In North America, tick paralysis in humans usually is associated with species of *Dermacentor* and *Amblyomma*. Symptoms may begin with motor weakness and progress as an ascending, flaccid motor paralysis. Sensory involvement is uncommon. It often is mistaken for Guillain-Barré syndrome or poliomyelitis. Symptoms of paralysis may become evident 1 to 5 days after the bloodsucking starts, and the ascending paralysis may progress in a matter of hours to bulbar signs with facial and lingual paralysis. Patients may die of respiratory failure or aspiration pneumonia. It is believed that the female tick secretes a neurotoxin that blocks the release of acetylcholine at neuromuscular junctions. If the paralysis is not too far advanced, removal of the feeding tick is associated with prompt and often dramatic reversal of the symptoms within 24 hours.

Tick bites can produce symptoms such as fever, chills, headache, vomiting, and abdominal pain, called the *tick bite pyrexia*. Removal of the engorged tick produces resolution of symptoms within 12 to 36 hours. Ticks normally should be removed manually by gentle traction grasping the tick close to the skin with forceps and pulling straight up with steady, even pressure. The entire tick, including the mouthparts, must be removed. If mouthparts are left behind, they usually cause a severe granulomatous lesion that may not heal for months.

Prevention of tickborne disease consists of protection from exposure and prompt removal of attached ticks. Long sleeves and long pants can be worn in endemic areas, and pants should be tucked into the socks. Clothing can be treated with tick repellents such as DEET, butopyronoxyl (Indalone), or permethrin, although these are only partially effective. The skin should be checked thoroughly and ticks should be removed promptly, as the timing of tick removal appears to be critical in the prevention of disease transmission, particularly Lyme disease. Antibiotic prophylaxis following tick bites is not routinely recommended, although early disease detection and specific antibiotic treatment are key to clinical management of tick-borne diseases. [For specific tick-borne diseases see Sec. 13.2.19 (Lyme Disease), 13.2.35 (Tularemia), and 13.3 (Rickettsial Diseases).]

References

Krinsky WL: Dermatoses associated with the bites of mites and ticks (*Arthropoda: Acari*). Int J Dermatol 22:75–91, 1983
Millikan LE: Loxoscelism and other arachnid problems. In: Parish LC, Nutting WB, Schwartzman RM, eds: Cutaneous Infestations of Man and Animal. New York, Praeger, 1983, 284–295

SCABIES
Patricia J. Chesney

Scabies (sarcoptic infestation) is caused by the female mite *Sarcoptes scabiei var. hominis* (see also Sec. 14.13). Canine scabies in humans is caused by *S. scabiei var. canis*, the dog mite associated with mange.

The female mite is 0.4 mm long and has four sets of legs and a round body. The male mite is half her size. Mites are spread following direct contact with an infested individual regardless of socioeconomic class. Spread by fomites is uncommon, if it exists at all. Norwegian scabies is highly contagious by virtue of the number of mites. Norwegian scabies is primarily found in immunocompromised, debilitated, or institutionalized patients. Epidemics can occur in hospital settings.

As it takes 1 month for the allergic reaction to develop, infested individuals may be asymptomatic but contagious. Canine and avian scabies are self-limited infestations as the female cannot burrow to reproduce.

After impregnation, the gravid female exudes a keratolytic substance and burrows into the stratum corneum, forming a shallow well within 30 minutes. She gradually extends this tract by 0.5 to 5 mm/24 hours along the boundary with the stratum granulosum. As she burrows, she deposits 1 to 3 eggs per day and numerous brown fecal pellets (scybala). In 4 to 5 weeks she dies in the burrow. Eggs hatch within 3 to 5 days. The larvae move to the skin surface to molt into nymphs. The nymph matures into an adult in 2 to 3 weeks. Mating occurs and the gravid females burrow into the skin to repeat the life cycle. Symptoms are related to the presence of the mite in burrows and the ensuing immune reaction which follows about 1 month after the mite first burrows into the skin. Normal adults have 5 to 7 mites on the skin; infants and patients with Norwegian scabies have dozens of mites.

CLINICAL MANIFESTATIONS Intense and unremitting pruritus, often worse at night, is the initial manifestation. Unique features of the rash are its polymorphic appearance and distribution. Simultaneously there may be multiple types of *primary* skin lesions including small papules, pustules, vesicles, wheals, nodules, and burrows. Multiple *secondary* skin lesions are usually also present, including excoriated papules and crusted areas. The multiplicity and variety of lesions give scabies the title of "the great masquerader." Approximately 2 to 4% of patient visits to dermatologists' offices are prompted by this tiny mite.

The rash is rarely present above the neck in older children and adults. Typical areas of involvement include the flexor surfaces of the wrists, extensor surfaces of the elbows and other joints, the web spaces of the fingers, axillae, waistline, periumbilical area, buttocks in the male, areolae in the female, penis, and scrotum. In 85% of adult cases, the hands and wrists are affected. The burrows, seen only in older children and adults, are superficial, short, gray, threadlike trails of scale that are often disguised by excoriations, eczema, and impetiginization. If present, they can be diagnostic.

In infants, the face, scalp, neck, and axillae, and particularly the insteps, palms, and soles, are often affected. There is usually relative sparing of the intertriginous areas, genitals, buttocks, wrists, and extensor surfaces of joints, as compared to adults. Bullae and pustules are common, and the eruption may include wheals, vesicles, erythematous papules, and a superimposed eczematous dermatitis. In the immunocompromised host, widespread scaling and extensive crust formation is present, which may be thick over the palms, soles, nailbeds, and scalp. This nonpruritic dermatosis of hands and feet may be oozing and encrusted. Generalized lymphadenopathy and eosinophilia are often present. Ivermectin has been used as single-dose therapy, although it is not FDA approved for treatment of scabies or for any administration to children ≤5 years of age.

Untreated scabies can lead to eczematous dermatitis, impetigo, ecthyma, folliculitis, furunculosis, cellulitis, and lymphangitis. In some tropical areas, scabies is the predominant underlying focus of pyoderma.

DIAGNOSIS AND TREATMENT The diagnosis is confirmed by microscopic identification of the mite, ova, or scybala from epithelial debris. Nonexcoriated vesicles, papules, vesiculopustules, or burrows contain the mites. A drop of immersion oil can be placed on the lesion and a #15 scalpel blade used to scrape off the stratum corneum. The scraping material with the oil is placed on a glass slide and examined under low power. Actively moving mites, eggs, and/or scybala can be found in 60% of patients with a suspected diagnosis. A suspected infested caretaker could have lesions scraped before a young child, although scraping relieves the itching and children generally accept it well. If no diagnostic features are found on a scraping, an area of lesions can be painted by a felt-tipped pen and left for 10 to 15 minutes. Removal of the ink with alcohol swabs may demonstrate the burrows. Attempts should be made to confirm the diagnosis, as all close contacts should be treated simultaneously.

Although several topical acaricides are available for the treatment of scabies, 5% permethrin cream (Elimite or Acticin) is the treatment of choice for adults and children older than 2 months of age. In older children and adults, it should be applied over the entire body from the neck down with particular attention to intensely involved areas for 8 to 12 hours. In younger children, who are older than 2 months of age, because of scalp and facial involvement, it should be applied from scalp to toes, sparing the areas around the eyes, nose, and mouth. Crotamiton is another available treatment; it is applied once or twice daily for as long as 5 days. For infants younger than 2 months of age, alternative therapy includes 6% precipitated sulphur in petrolatum applied for three consecutive 24-hour periods. This product is safe but malodorous and messy, and it stains bedclothes.

Lindane (1%) cream or lotion applied for 6 to 8 hours is effective and inexpensive, but should not be used in infants, young children, pregnant women, or individuals with inflamed skin. Lindane cream and lotion are well absorbed through skin and are potentially neurotoxic if not used according to directions.

All treatments should be repeated after 1 week to treat newly hatched nymphs. Pruritus may persist for as long as 6 weeks after completion of therapy, as continued hypersensitivity to dead mite parts persists. Papular and pustular lesions generally resolve within a week. New skin lesions appearing more than 2 weeks after therapy following initial improvement suggest inadequate therapy or a reinfestation. Topical steroid creams and oral antihistamines can be used to relieve continued itching. Antibiotics should be used for secondary infections. Resistance of *S. scabiei* to lindane or permethrin has not been clearly identified.

All close contacts, including asymptomatic caregivers, should be treated simultaneously to prevent the "ping-pong" effect. Manifestations of scabies infestation can appear up to 2 months after initial exposure. Mite transmission is unlikely >24 hours after treatment, at which time children can return to school or daycare.

Although fomite transmission has not been documented, clothing and bed linens of the patient and family members can be washed or not used for 3 days after treatment.

Institutionalized or hospitalized patients with Norwegian scabies should be strictly isolated because their "mite load" is very high. Good hand washing will prevent transmission from caregivers to other patients. Simultaneous treatment of the patient and all close contacts should interrupt transmission. Retreatment after 7 to 10 days will kill newly hatched nymphs. Treating infested dogs should prevent transmission to family members.

References

Drugs for parasitic infections: Med Lett Drugs Ther 35:111, 1993

Metry DW, Hebert AA: Insect and arachnid stings, bites, infestations and repellents. Pediatr Ann 29:39–46, 2000

PEDICULOSIS OR LOUSE INFESTATIONS
Patricia J. Chesney

Human louse infestations are caused by the head louse (*Pediculus humanus var. capitis*), the body louse (*Pediculus humanus var. corporis*), and the pubic louse (*Phthirus pubis*). All belong to the order Anoplura, and are obligate ectoparasites requiring frequent daily blood meals. They require normal body temperature for growth and reproduction and can travel rapidly by crawling because they cannot fly or jump. Survival away from the host is limited to less than 24 hours, as they are dependent on the blood meal and body temperature for survival. Body and head lice are oval in appearance, with a length of 2 to 4 mm. The pubic louse is wider and shorter and has a more crab-like appearance. All lice have a stomach-associated mycetome containing symbiotic gram-positive rod bacteria. These bacteria produce nutrients necessary for the survival of the louse, and the blood meals are necessary for the survival of the bacteria.

The adult louse reaches a new host following direct contact. The female louse lays 3 to 10 eggs daily within 1 to 3 mm of the skin surface. The eggs of the head and pubic louse are attached to the hair shaft with a clear, tenacious glue from the female's accessory gland (*P. corporis* eggs are laid on cloth fibers). The small, translucent eggs have an operculum that supplies air and humidity to the developing embryo, which breathes through spiracles. After 7 to 12 days, a nymph emerges. Nymphs feed on blood, but cannot reproduce until they have undergone three molts over the next 8 to 9 days. The empty egg case (nit) remains glued to the hair shaft as the hair grows. It appears white after the embryo hatches.

Louse infestations may be asymptomatic for weeks or months. Symptoms develop when the body develops an allergy to the saliva injected by the louse during feeding. Secondary bacterial infections may result from excoriations. Only the body louse serves as a vector for human disease (typhus, trench fever, relapsing fever).

CLINICAL MANIFESTATIONS Intense pruritus is the hallmark of symptomatic pediculosis. The pruritus is initially present in a localized area without evidence of a rash. Sensitization resulting in pruritus may take 3 to 8 months to develop. Scratching results in inflammation and excoriations, which may become secondarily infected with pustules, crusting, and secondary adenopathy. Posterior or suboccipital cervical adenopathy, without obvious disease or secondary infection, is characteristic of lice. Nits are found in *P. capitis* infestations primarily in the occipital region, nape of the neck, the scalp over the ears, and at the hairline. An id reaction of erythematous plaques and patches may develop on the trunk. Head lice are most common in children ages 6 to 11 years. In the United States, it is estimated that 8 to 12 million school children have head lice. Infestation is unrelated to hygiene or hair length.

Pediculus corporis causes intensely pruritic, small, red macules or papules with a central hemorrhagic punctum located on the shoulders, trunk, or buttocks. Massive infestation may be associated with constitutional symptoms of fever, malaise, and headache. Chronic infestation may lead to "vagabond's skin," lichenified, scaling, hyperpigmented plaques primarily on the trunk. *Pediculus corporis* is rare in children, except under colder conditions when clothes are not changed frequently. The lice live under conditions of poor hygiene, in the seams of clothing and bedding, emerging onto the skin only to feed. The symbiotic bacteria of *P. corporis* produce all necessary vitamins, enabling them to live on nutritionally deficient hosts.

In *P. pubis* infestations, pruritus is less intense, excoriations are shallower, and the incidence of secondary infection is lower than for *P. corporis*. Macular ceruleae are steel-gray spots 1 to 2 cm in diameter, which may appear in the pubic area or on the chest, abdomen, or thighs. Their cause is unknown. Eyelash infestation may induce blepharitis with lid pruritus, scaling, crusting, and purulent discharge. Pubic lice are transmitted by skin-to-skin contact and represent the most contagious sexually transmitted problem. The chance of acquiring lice following one sexual exposure with an infected individual is 95%. As many as 30% of individuals with pubic lice have another sexually transmitted disease. Blacks and whites are infested equally. Pubic hair is the most common site of infestation, but *P. pubis* can spread to the perirectal hair, as well as to hair on the thighs, abdomen, chest, axillae, and beard. The infestation may spread to children's eyelashes (Phthiriasis palpebrarum) if they sleep with parents or other individuals infested with *P. pubis*. Pubic lice found in the eyelashes of younger children may be evidence of sexual abuse.

DIAGNOSIS The majority of *P. capitis* infestations involve only 1 to 10 lice. An active infestation is present only if an adult, a nymph, or an egg case containing an embryo is present. Empty egg cases alone indicate only past infection. Combing shampooed and conditioned hair in good light using a special comb with long teeth set 0.3 mm apart over a sheet of white paper is the best way to detect eggs, nits, and lice. The hair is methodically combed in 1-inch-thick sections. A magnifying glass and tweezers maybe helpful. Embryonated eggs are hard to see as they are translucent and located very close to the scalp. A brief shampoo with alcohol followed by brisk toweling may yield "a towel full of well soused lice." Distinguishing egg cases from other unrelated material attached to hair is critical and frequently inaccurate.

TREATMENT Exclusion of children from school for pediculosis leads parents and caregivers to perceive head lice as a stigmatizing and ostracizing infestation related to poor hygiene. This can lead to desperation measures on the part of parents and caregivers who may use inappropriate (head shaving, turpentine, gas, animal flea products), prolonged, frequent, and potentially dangerous "treatments." It is important to remind everyone involved that lice carry no diseases and their presence is unrelated to hygiene.

Treatment of *P. corporis* is focused on improving hygiene and cleaning clothes in hot water, or ironing clothes with a hot iron. Pediculicides are needed only if there is no access to hot water or to an iron, or if the louse is attached to body hair.

Pubic lice can be treated using any of the pediculicides used for *P. capitis* (see below). Sexual partners and bedmates should be

TABLE 13-69
TREATMENT OF HEAD LICE

MECHANISMS OF ACTION ON LICE	CLASS	AGENT	PREPARATION	RECOMMENDED USE
Neurotoxins				
Inhibits GABA function	Chlorinated hydrocarbon	Lindane* • Kwell • Scabene	 1% Shampoo 1% Lotion	•Apply for 4 minutes, rinse. •Should be used only when all other alternatives have failed.
Irreversible cholinesterase inhibitor	Organophosphate	Malathion* • Ovide	• 0.5% Lotion • 1% Shampoo	Apply to dry hair and wash out after 8–12 hours.
Disrupt Na channel in nerves	Natural pyrethrins plus piperonyl butoxide	• RID • A-200 • Pronto • R&C Shampoo	Shampoos	
Disrupt Na channel in nerves	Synthetic pyrethroids	Permethrin • NIX • Elimite† Ivermectin*†	 1% Cream rinse 5% Cream • Oral • Topical 0.8% solution	• Apply for 30–60 minutes or overnight. • Apply overnight. • Take 200 μg/kg once. • Apply once.
Kill Symbiotic Bacteria in Mycetoma	Antimicrobial agent	Trimethoprim/ sulfamethoxazole†* • Septra • Bactrim	Oral	• Standard dose for 10–14 days or • Standard dose for 3 days; repeat 1 week later.
Occlusive				
Interfere with feeding and breathing	Fat/oil based	Petrolatum, olive oil, mayonnaise, mineral oil	Topical	Apply and leave on overnight.

*Prescription only.
†Not FDA approved for this indication.

treated. For eyelash infestation, 1% mercuric oxide ointment applied four times a day for 14 days, or petrolatum used four times a day for 10 days, is effective. Nits should be removed by hand.

The pediculicides are listed in Table 13-69. Although safe when used as directed, they have the potential to affect the mammalian nervous system. They should be kept out of the reach of children. To minimize skin exposure and absorption, gloves can be used to shampoo or rinse hair, using cold water in a sink rather than a shower.

No agent is 100% ovicidal and all treatments should be repeated after 7 to 10 days in order to kill newly hatched nymphs. The synergistic natural pyrethrin plus piperonyl butoxide combinations or permethrin, which are FDA-approved formulations, should continue to be used as the first treatment of choice. If lice are detected soon after treatment (as noted above) another nonprescription pediculicide should be tried and repeated after 7 to 10 days. With continued failure, a nonprescription occlusive method could be tried, or a prescription method could be tried with physician counseling and follow-up.

Lindane has the highest potential toxicity of all the neurotoxins because it is readily absorbed through the skin and can be stored in adipose and nervous tissue. Lindane is contraindicated for premature infants and those persons with known seizure disorders or known hypersensitivity, and it should be used with caution in pregnant or nursing mothers or on inflamed skin.

Recent studies demonstrate that lice have developed mechanisms to bypass the pediculicidal activity of lindane and permethrin in this country, as well as in other countries. Lice from parts of the world where pediculicides have never been used are uniformly susceptible to these two agents. Thus, frequent and inappropriate use of these agents in addition to the sustained presence of permethrin

on hair for as long as 2 weeks may have contributed to the development of resistance. The recent approval of malathion for use and the non-FDA-approved use of TMP-SMZ, ivermectin, and occlusive materials for *P. capitis*, have developed in response to the perceived inadequate responses to traditional agents.

Bedmates should be treated prophylactically. All other close contacts should be examined and treated only if clearly infested. Fomites have not been clearly demonstrated to play a role in the transmission of head lice, as nymphs and adults require blood meals frequently and eggs require body temperature to hatch. Inactivation of lice and unhatched eggs can be achieved by washing clothes and bedding at temperatures exceeding 53.5°C (128.3°F) for 5 minutes, by dry cleaning, or by storing clothing in sealed plastic bags for 10 days, or by rinsing in a pediculicide (combs and brushes). Vacuuming floors and furniture can be used, but environmental insecticide sprays are not helpful.

Following successful treatment, continued itching or mild burning of the scalp most often represents a continued reaction of the body to louse antigens or a reaction to the topical agent and can be addressed with topical corticosteroids, oral antihistamines, and, if severe, oral steroids.

The identification of lice ≥24 hours after treatment may represent a treatment failure caused by resistance, a heavy infestation, a reinfestation, or incorrect product use. Immediate retreatment with a different agent is recommended followed by retreatment 7 to 10 days later.

Removal of nits (empty egg cases) after treatment is not necessary. If their removal is desired for aesthetic reasons, rinsing the hair with white vinegar (2.5% acetic acid) or with a commercial formic acid rinse should be followed by wrapping the hair for 30 to 60 minutes in a towel soaked in either product.

References

Chesney PJ, Burgess IF: Lice: resistance and treatment: Contemp Pediatr 15:181–192, 1998

Glaziou P, Nguyen LN, Moulia-Pelat JP, et al: Efficacy of ivermectin for the treatment of head lice (*Pediculosis capitis*). Trop Med Parasitol 45: 253–254, 1994

Gomez Urcuryo F, Zalas N: Malathion lotion as an insecticide and ovicide in head louse infestation. Int J Dermatol 25:60–65, 1986

OTHER INSECT BITES AND REACTIONS

Allison Holm

Centipedes

Centipedes (class Chilopoda) are worm-like arthropods that possess many repetitive body segments, each of which has one pair of segmented legs. Immediately below the mouth are modified legs of the first body segment (ie, the maxillipeds), which are powerful poison claws used to attack and kill prey. Although centipedes are greatly feared, they rarely bite. Usually, the pain that is caused by a bite is no more severe than the sting of a honeybee, although at times the pain can be severe, causing a marked erythematous inflammatory reaction. The pain usually diminishes rapidly and may require nothing more than a cold compress. More generalized reactions such as nausea, vomiting, and dizziness occur infrequently.

HYMENOPTEROUS DISEASE The sting of bees, hornets, yellow jackets, wasps, and fire ants introduces in nonsensitized individuals a venom that causes immediate pain, induration, and redness lasting several hours or longer. However, serious allergic reactions to these venoms, including death, may occur, especially in those who were previously sensitized to these antigens. Multiple stings may cause a profound systemic reaction such as nausea, vomiting, hypotension, loss of consciousness, and death. Approximately 8% of children develop an allergic reaction following a repeat sting. It is not clear whether subsequent experiences are associated with progressively more severe reactions. In most cases, individuals who have had local reactions continue that pattern with each sting. Systemic reactions more frequently occur in individuals who have had multiple stings, or who have been stung several times within a short period. Many advocate that venom-sensitized patients be immunized against the appropriate venoms; immunotherapy may reduce the risk of anaphylaxis to approximately 3% of patients. Children who have exhibited only cutaneous manifestations do not need immunotherapy. Allergic individuals who have not had immunotherapy should have an insect sting kit readily available that contains a syringe preloaded with epinephrine.

Treatments for local reactions include icepacks, antipruritic lotions, topical corticosteroids, and oral antihistamines for itching. Anaphylactic reactions following bee, wasp, or hornet stings, which may be life-threatening, require prompt attention. Subcutaneous injection of epinephrine 1:1000 should be administered in a dose of 0.01 mg/kg every 20 minutes; three injections may be required for severe reactions (maximum 0.3–0.5 mL). Cutaneous manifestations often can be moderated with antihistamines and glucocorticoids. In the case of honeybee stings, the stinger should be removed by gently scraping the skin with a knife blade. In severe anaphylactic shock or angioneurotic edema, IV fluids or an airway may need to be provided.

Ant stings frequently occur in the southern United States and are caused by various species of fire ants of the genus *Solenopsis*. Multiple stings and mass attacks can cause a severe reaction. Immediately after a sting, an erythematous wheal appears, which vesiculates after a few hours. A pustule forms within 24 hours; in several days to a week this ruptures, encrusts, and finally forms a small fibrous nodule or scar. Systemic reactions may occur, especially if there have been multiple stings. Localized or systemic therapy does not appear to be beneficial for ant stings, although some experts recommend symptomatic treatment of local reactions as suggested for bee and wasp stings.

MYIASIS

Allison Holm

The invasion of organs and tissues by fly larvae (maggots of the order Diptera) is termed *myiasis*. When maggot infestations are caused by species that usually are scavengers or saprophagous, the infestation is termed *accidental myiasis*. If the maggot is of a necrophagous or facultative sarcophagous species, the infestation is called a *semispecific myiasis;* infestation caused by obligatory sarcophagous species is termed *obligate myiasis*.

Accidental myiasis is caused by the ingestion of eggs or larvae of blowflies (ie, bluebottle and greenbottle flies), flesh flies, and houseflies that may be present in food or drink. These infestations are transitory, with larvae being passed in the stool without incident. Rarely, however, stubborn intestinal myiasis may result. Patients may have severe abdominal pain, nausea, and vomiting. Diarrhea and hematochezia may occur. Eventually, the larvae are expelled. Urinary myiasis has been reported, probably as a result of flies depositing their eggs about the external urethral orifice, especially in warm weather when people sleep without covers. The larvae presumably hatch and migrate into the urethra. Symptoms can be severe, with pain, blood, purulent discharge, dysuria, and frequency.

Wound myiasis is caused by flesh flies (ie, *Sarcophaga*) or blowflies (ie, *Calliphora, Phoenicia*) when the adults deposit their eggs on or about open wounds. Severe damage can result from these infestations, which usually afflict infants or the seriously injured. Cutaneous myiasis resembling furuncles may be caused by larvae of *Wohlfahrtia*. In Central and South America, as well as in Africa, cloth diapers should be ironed, because the Tumbu fly (ie, *Cordylobia*) often lays eggs on the diapers when they are hung out to dry. These hatch, and larvae penetrate the baby's skin, causing furuncular lesions similar to those caused by *Wohlfahrtia* and *Dermatobia*. Ironing kills all eggs and larvae.

Obligate myiasis, which is caused by the primary screwworms (ie, *Cochliomyia*), may cause severe and sometimes fatal suppurative nasopharyngeal and otic infestations. These flies are attracted to open wounds or nasal secretions, in which they deposit their eggs. *Hypoderma*, the eel fly, often attacks humans, with children being infested far more often than adults. The larvae actively penetrate the skin and wander for months (ie, larva migrans), causing severe pain, cramps, and general malaise. The female human botfly, *Dermatobia hominis,* deposits her eggs on the bodies of other bloodsucking flying insects, especially mosquitoes. Eggs are then transmitted to an animal host while the mosquito feeds. Larvae enter the skin through the puncture wound and produce a gradually enlarging papule or furuncle (Fig. 13-34).

Children can be protected from myiasis by proper screening or netting. Dipterous infestations should be treated promptly by surgical excision of maggots after covering the wound with 10% chlo-

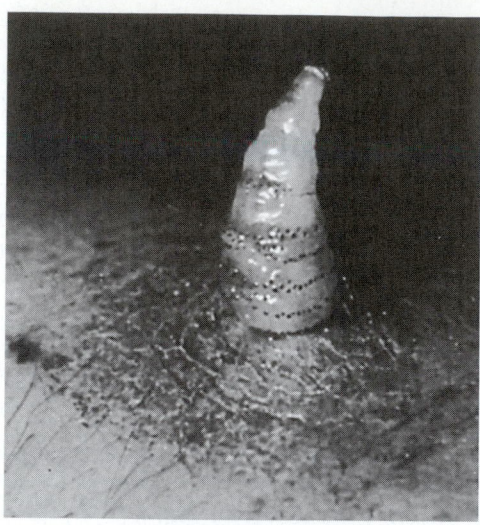

FIGURE 13-34 Myiasis caused by *Dermatobia hominis.* The posterior portion of the larva is emerging from the skin burrow. The larva matures in approximately 1 month, then drops off the host to pupate in the ground. SOURCE: *(Courtesy of Dr. Jay Keystone, Tropical Disease Unit, Toronto Hospital, Toronto, Ontario.)*

roform in vegetable oil. This should be followed by topical antibiotic therapy with polymyxin and sterile dressing.

Fleas

Fleas are small, wingless insects that jump with long, well-developed hind legs. In the United States, the most common causes of flea bites are the dog and cat fleas, *Ctenocephalides canis* and *C. felis,* respectively. Less frequently implicated is the human flea, *Pulex irritans.* Fleas are indiscriminate, and when hungry, they will feed on almost any host species. Fleas are able to jump more than 30 cm to reach their host.

Only adult fleas feed on the blood of mammals and birds, usually dropping off their temporary hosts between meals. Thus, the development of dog and cat flea eggs, larvae, and pupae occurs on mats, rags, and carpets. Because they are long-lived and can survive unfed for months to years, unoccupied houses in which dogs or cats once lived can be heavily infested.

Although flea bites may pass unnoticed in some individuals, most people (especially children) have considerable discomfort. Each bite is associated with a pruritic erythematous papule with a minute central hemorrhagic punctum. Lesions generally are clustered on the lower legs, especially around the ankles (Fig. 13-35). In the event of severe hypersensitivity to the flea's salivary secretions, papular urticaria can occur in which bullous lesions may evolve. If secondary pyogenic infection does not intervene, the lesions gradually heal.

Therapy is aimed at alleviating symptoms with oral antihistamines and topical corticosteroids. Pets should be treated with flea dips, which should be repeated periodically. Flea-infested areas may require treatment with insecticides such as malathion powder or lindane dust. Clothing sprayed with a *N,N*-diethyl-*m*-toluamide preparation (DEET) is an effective repellent.

Tungiasis

This is caused by the chigoe or sand flea *Tunga penetrans* and occurs throughout the coastal and southern United States, Central

and South America, and in tropical West and East Africa. The adult female burrows into the skin with the posterior tip of the abdomen facing out to breathe. After 2 weeks, the female has grown to approximately 1 cm in diameter, and ovipositing begins through the posterior opening into the environment where the larvae will develop to adults. The female degenerates, dies, and is sloughed in approximately 20 days, often leaving a small ulcerated site. The infection usually is found on the lower parts of the lower extremities, especially between the toes and under the toenails, which is extremely painful. Individuals who are barefoot or who wear sandals are especially vulnerable; however, almost any site can be infected. The infection generally is self-limited, but secondary infections, including tetanus, occur. Treatment is directed at removing the flea and excising lesions if necessary. Thiabendazole can be given orally for severe infestation. Antibiotics are given for secondary infection. This infection can be prevented by wearing shoes and by using insect repellents such as DEET.

Bedbugs

The common bedbug *Cimex lectularius* and the tropical bedbug *C. hemipterous* are small (ie, 4 to 5 mm by 3 mm), red-brown, dorsoventrally flattened insects that feed almost exclusively on human blood. They usually hide in crevices and cracks during the day, become active at night, and feed on individuals while they are sleeping. Nymphs take approximately 6 to 9 minutes and adults 10 to 15 minutes to engorge; then they retreat to their hiding places (eg, the mattress or behind a piece of loose wallpaper). Until hypersensitivity develops, individuals may have few complaints. The bites can be intensely pruritic. Typically, one can find several linear red urticarial or papular lesions. There often are telltale blood stains on the night clothes overlying the site of the bites. At times, bullae may be seen. Symptomatic treatment with antihistamines or topical corticosteroids may provide relief. Treatment is to eliminate the bug from the environment by using lindane, malathion, or methyl bromide.

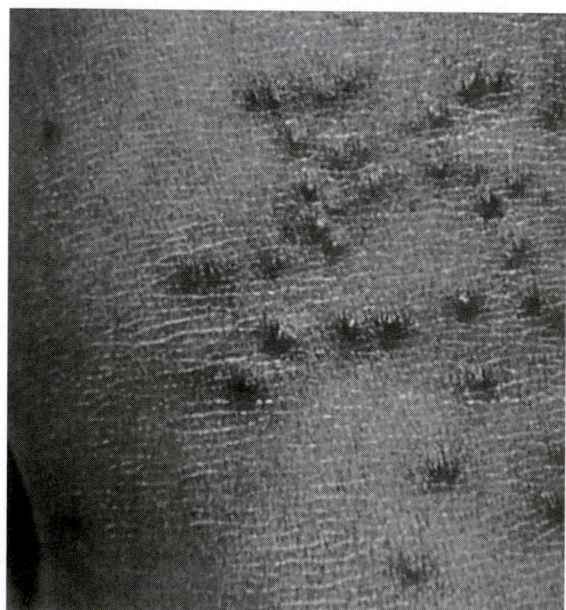

FIGURE 13-35 Numerous flea bites of the posterior aspect of the lower leg. SOURCE: *(Courtesy of Dr. Jay Keystone, Tropical Disease Unit, Toronto Hospital, Toronto, Ontario.)*

Passive Envenomization

Poison-containing hairs or spines on many caterpillars (ie, larval butterflies and moths; order Lepidoptera) can cause severe dermatitis when touched. Puss caterpillar (ie, *Megalopyge*) spines that accidentally brush the skin can cause erythema, urticaria, and intense burning, which may persist for many hours. Young children especially are prone to these severe reactions. Systemic symptoms, including nausea, vomiting, and dizziness, persisting for several hours have been reported. Poison hairs or spines that are "rubbed" onto the conjunctiva or cornea can be extremely painful. It often is possible to remove the imbedded spines by applying the sticky side of cellophane tape to the affected area. In severe cases, topical corticosteroids can alleviate the pain. If systemic signs and symptoms appear, systemic antihistamines or corticosteroids may be indicated.

When a blister beetle (order Coleoptera) such as the Spanish fly, *Lytta vesicatoria,* is crushed on the skin, a vesicating reaction occurs that is caused by cantharidin, which is a volatile terpene found in the hemolymph. This substance readily penetrates the epidermis, causing superficial, slowly evolving blisters with severe irritation and burning. If a beetle alights on the skin, the beetle should not be crushed, but it can be gently blown off.

References

Brothers W, Heckman R: Tungiasis (*Tunga penetrans*) in Utah. J Parasitol 65:782, 1979

Frazier CA: Allergic reactions to insect stings: a review of 180 cases. South Med J 57:1028–1035, 1964

Harwood RF, James MT: Entomology in Human and Animal Health, 7th ed. New York, Macmillan, 1979

Mueller HL: Further experiences with severe allergic reactions to insect stings. N Engl J Med 261:374–377, 1959

Paull BR: Imported fire ant allergy. Perspectives on diagnosis and treatment. Postgrad Med 76:155–160, 1984

Zumpt F: Myiasis in Man and Animal in the Old World. A Textbook for Physicians, Veterinarians, and Zoologists. London, Butterworth, 1965

AQUATIC ENVENOMIZATION AND DERMATITIS

Allison Holm

A large number of venomous marine animals cause mild, debilitating, or fatal envenomization. These most frequently are seen in tropical or temperate waters of North America and the Indo-Pacific region. Because of the marked increase in recreational water sports, especially diving, exposure to marine animal envenomization is more frequent.

Dermatitis

Cnidarian dermatitis and envenomization is caused by a large variety of jellyfish, sea anemones, fire corals, and Portuguese man-of-war. All of these marine animals, which are present in temperate, subtropical, and tropical environments, possess cnidae (ie, nematocysts) on the outer surface of their tentacles. These are spirally coiled, barbed, hollow threads through which toxin is forceably injected when rubbed or touched into the skin. Depending on the particular species, amount of venom injected, age of the victim, and prior sensitization, mild to severe local and/or systemic reactions may ensue. In the United States, fire corals are among the most

frequent causes of mild cnidarian stings. Immediately after contact, intense burning or a stinging sensation with central radiation appears, followed by severe pruritus and urticaria that may last for several days and leave an area of hyperpigmentation that gradually fades after several months. Hours after contact, a delayed reaction can appear, presenting as papules or hemorrhagic vesicles. At times, an erythema nodosum–like reaction can recur repeatedly over a period of several months.

Sea anemone stings usually occur in shallow water. Almost instantaneously, they produce severe burning, followed by intense itching. An area of central pallor frequently appears, surrounded by erythema and petechial hemorrhage. The envenomized area becomes edematous, and in severe envenomization, it evolves to become ecchymotic and then hemorrhagic. The lesion may ulcerate and subsequently heal after eschar formation. Milder envenomizations usually resolve uneventfully within several days.

Portuguese man-of-war (ie, *Physalia physalis* and *P. intriculus*) have long, hanging, and trailing nematocyst-containing tentacles in which an unwary swimmer can become enmeshed and severely stung. This causes an almost immediate, centripedally radiating, intense stinging sensation; subsequently, numbness or paresthesias may occur. The affected area usually has the appearance of deeply erythematous, vesicular, whip-like striations criss-crossing over one another and delineating the pattern of the tentacles on the skin. The lesions may become necrotic and ulcerate before healing and leave long-lasting, pigmented striae. The seriousness of the systemic manifestations depends largely on the extent of the area involved, previous sensitization, and age. Muscle spasm, vomiting, renal and respiratory failure, and profound hypotension can occur in severely stung individuals.

Treatment of cnidarian stings is aimed at stopping further envenomization by inactivation and/or removal of the adherent cnidae, and by treating the local and/or systemic reactions. All remaining adherent tentacles should be carefully lifted away, not brushed, with an instrument or gloved fingers, because this might discharge other cnidae. Freshwater should not be used to wash away losely adherent tentacles and cnidae, because freshwater causes their discharge. Only seawater should be used for this purpose. If available, vinegar or 3 to 10% acetic acid should be poured over the entire affected area repeatedly for at least 30 minutes or until the pain abates. This inactivates the cnidae. It remains controversial whether 40 to 70% isopropyl alcohol should be used as an alternative to acetic acid, because alcohol causes discharge of cnidae in vitro. Removal of cnidae can be a problem. Some authorities recommend applying aerosol shaving cream and then shaving off the cnidae with a safety razor. Local and systemic reactions can be treated with antihistamines or corticosteroids; anaphylaxis may require epinephrine.

Seabather's eruption is a pruritic, most often benign dermatitis that is caused by planula larvae of the phylum *Cnidaria*. When originally described, there was a history of exposure at beaches followed by the appearance of welts or "inflammatory papules," which appeared on "parts of the body . . . covered by the bathing suit." On the northeast coast of the United States, the planula larva of the sea anemone *Edwardsiella lineata* and, on the coast of Florida, the planula larva of the jellyfish *Linuche unguiculata* have been identified as the probable cause of seabather's eruption. Onset typically occurs 4 to 24 hours after exposure. Some individuals have reported a prickling sensation or develop urticarial lesions immediately, whereas others may be asymptomatic for 3 to 4 days. The duration of symptoms varies from several days to weeks. Children may have high fevers, which could lead to extensive medical studies for meningitis, sepsis, or fever of unknown origin. Treatment with antihistamines or corticosteroids may be indicated.

Toxic Seafood Poisoning

Several types of shellfish poisoning have serious and often fatal consequences. Paralytic seafood poisoning is caused by the ingestion of shellfish contaminated with saxitoxin. Saxitoxin is produced by dinoflagellates of the genus *Gonyaulax* that cause "red tide." Most cases have been reported from the northeast Atlantic coast and the Pacific Northwest, but sporadic cases have occurred in Europe, Japan, South Africa, and New Zealand. Various shellfish, including clams, mussels, scallops, and oysters, feed on these organisms and concentrate this heat-stable neurotoxin in their tissues. Following ingestion, symptoms can appear in approximately 30 minutes with circumoral and distal paresthesias that spread to the extremities. Patients frequently develop nausea, vomiting, and diarrhea. Symptoms may rapidly progress to death from central respiratory paralysis because of the toxin's effect on the respiratory and vasomotor centers. Survival for more than 12 hours is a good prognostic sign. Symptoms typically last 3 days. Presently, no specific antitoxin is available; however, supportive therapy and early airway management can be lifesaving.

Neurotoxic shellfish poisoning occurs along the coast of Florida, the Gulf of Mexico, coastal Texas, North Carolina, and New Zealand, and is caused by eating shellfish contaminated with a toxin that is produced by the alga *Ptychodiscus brevis*. The poisoning is less severe than that of paralytic seafood poisoning. Several hours after ingestion, neurologic symptoms, including paresthesias, ataxia, and gastrointestinal symptoms appear; these resolve in several days. If poisoning is diagnosed early, gastric lavage that is followed by activated charcoal and a cathartic may be helpful.

Ciguatera and Scombroid Fish Poisoning

Ciguatera fish poisoning is the most common nonbacterial illness that is associated with eating tropical reef fish such as red snapper, barracuda, amberjack, grouper, and surgeonfish that are contaminated with ciguatoxin produced by the dinoflagellate *Gambierdiscus toxicus*. Ciguatera fish poisoning occurs primarily in the Caribbean and South Pacific islands, including Australia. Toxin-contaminated fish appear to be normal in odor, taste, and texture, and the toxin is heat-stable. The toxin apparently is a mixture of agents, ciguatoxin being the most important, and acts to cause neural membrane depolarization by opening voltage-dependent sodium channels. A second toxin, maitotoxin, opens calcium channels.

Clinical manifestations of ciguatoxin poisoning are varied, affecting gastrointestinal, neurosensory, neuromuscular, and cardiovascular functions. A few minutes to several hours after eating toxin-contaminated fish, gastrointestinal symptoms occur: including nausea, vomiting, diarrhea, and abdominal pain. Symptoms may persist for several days. Neurologic symptoms may appear, including myalgias, paresthesias of the extremities and perioral region, general weakness, and, occasionally, ataxia. Characteristically, reversal of cold-hot sensation can occur. Hypotension and bradycardia can be present, although this is unusual. Symptoms may last for weeks to many months.

Generally, ciguatera fish poisoning is a clinical diagnosis, but if a piece of the suspected fish can be obtained, toxin levels can be determined by ELISA, radioimmunoassay, or bioassay. If poisoning is diagnosed early, administration of IV mannitol (1 g/kg) ameliorates the neurologic symptoms. Similarly, a calcium gluconate infusion over a 24-hour period is recommended. Persistent neuro-

logic symptoms have been treated using amitriptyline with some success.

Scombrotoxism, or scombroid fish poisoning, occurs when spoiled fish such as tuna, mackerel, bonito, and skipjack (ie, families *Scombridae* and *Scomberesocidae*) are consumed. Other nonscombroid fish such as mahi-mahi and bluefish also have been found to cause scombrotoxism. This condition occurs worldwide, and with the marked rise in fish consumption, it is frequently implicated in the United States. Symptoms occur soon after consumption of the contaminated fish; these include headache, flushing, abdominal cramps, diarrhea, tachycardia, dry mouth, and urticaria. Symptoms may last for several hours. This constellation of symptoms resembles those resulting from histamine toxicity. Some individuals report that the incriminated fish had a peppery or sharp taste. Treatment with antihistamines is indicated. Although antihistamines that are H_1 blockers bring prompt relief, administration of an H_2 blocker such as cimetidine gives simultaneous relief of peripheral, as well as gastrointestinal, symptoms. Proper refrigeration prevents scombrotoxism.

References

Auerbach PS: Marine envenomizations. N Engl J Med 325:486–493, 1991

Freudenthal AR, Joseph PR: Seabather's eruption. N Engl J Med 329:542–544, 1993

Hughes JM, Merson MH: Current concepts: fish and shellfish poisoning. N Engl J Med 295:1117–1120, 1976

Johnson R, Jonge EC: Ciguatera: Caribbean and Indo-Pacific fish poisoning. West J Med 138:872–874, 1983

Lange WR, Snyder FR, Fudata P: Travel and ciguatera fish poisoning. Arch Intern Med 152:2049–2053, 1992

Leedom J, Underman A: Diagnosing and treating ciguatera fish poisoning. Travel Med Advisor Update 3:29–30, 1993

Morrow JD, Margolies GR, Rowland J, et al: Evidence that histamine is the causative toxin of scombroid-fish poisoning. N Engl J Med 324:716–720, 1991

Perl TM, Bedard L, Kosatsky T, Hockin JC, Todd EC, Remis RS: An outbreak of toxic encephalopathy caused by eating mussels contaminated with domoic acid. N Engl J Med 322:1775–1780, 1990

Teitelbaum JS, Zatorre RJ, Carpenter S, et al: Neurologic sequelae of domoic acid intoxication due to the ingestion of contaminated mussels. N Engl J Med 322:1781–1787, 1990

Tomchik RS, Russell MT, Szmant AM, Black NA: Clinical perspectives on seabather's eruption, also known as "sea lice." JAMA 269:1669–1672, 1993

13.8 TRAVEL MEDICINE FOR CHILDREN

Michael Cappello

As international travel becomes more commonplace, questions about the appropriate preparation for family trips abroad arise more frequently. Children younger than 18 years of age should receive careful assessment of their general medical condition, as well as counseling on specific travel-associated medical and safety issues. A pretravel appointment should be made for 6 to 8 weeks prior to departure to ensure that all of the appropriate immunizations can be administered, and the necessary travel accessories can be obtained. (Table 13-70 is a checklist for international travel.) For the pediatrician, there are a number of valuable resources for information regarding current recommendations for general travel and

TABLE 13-70

CHECKLIST FOR INTERNATIONAL TRAVEL

Pretravel Office Visit (6–8 weeks prior to departure)
  Review itinerary, special health needs
  Counsel regarding safety issues, sexually transmitted diseases, food safety
  Establish need for accelerated routine immunizations, travel-specific immunizations, malaria prophylaxis
Routine Immunizations
  Measles, mumps, rubella (MMR)
  Diphtheria, tetanus, pertussis
  Polio (OPV and/or IPV)
  Haemophilus influenzae type b (Hib)
  Varicella-zoster virus
  Hepatitis B virus
Immunizations Specific for International Travel*
  Hepatitis A virus vaccine and/or immune globulin
  Meningococcal vaccine (serotypes A, C, Y, W-135)
  Typhoid vaccine (oral, Vi capsular polysaccharide, heat-phenol inactivated)
  Yellow fever virus vaccine
  Rabies virus vaccine (HDCV or RAV)
  Japanese encephalitis virus vaccine
Components of Travel Health Kit
  Names of travelers, country of origin, embassy phone number
  Significant medical conditions, allergies, blood type
  Water purification system (filter, iodine tablets)
  Sunscreen, insect repellents (permethrin, DEET)
  First aid supplies: gauze pads, tape, bandages, scissors, thermometer, antibacterial spray or ointment, oral rehydration solution
  Antihistamine (diphenhydramine), antipyretic (acetaminophen, ibuprofen)
  Prescription medications: malaria prophylaxis, antibiotics for traveler's diarrhea, currently prescribed medications

*Cholera vaccine not currently recommended.

for medical advice specific to a given region. The Centers for Disease Control of the United States Public Health Service publishes *Health Information for International Travel* (The Yellow Book), which can be ordered by telephone from the US Government Printing Office (202-512-1800). The information is also available on the Internet through the CDC Web site (www.cdc.gov/travel/travel.html).

Because accidents are the leading cause of death among international travelers, parents of young travelers must consider safety issues related to car seats (frequently not available abroad), hotel rooms or private homes, and storage of medications.

Copies of birth certificates or passports should be stored separately from the originals, in case they are lost or stolen. It is also recommended that the name, country of origin, and perhaps the telephone number of the local embassy be attached to the inside of small children's clothing. This may be useful if the child is separated from his or her parents, a particular risk in large international airports, train stations, or bus terminals. Adolescents should be counseled against sexual contact, tattooing, or body piercing abroad, all of which may carry considerable risk of acquiring infection with hepatitis viruses and HIV.

Long airplane flights can provoke anxiety for children, their caregivers, and fellow travelers. It is worthwhile to plan a variety of in-flight activities, such as reading or coloring in order to occupy the time and attention of young children, particularly toddlers. Aisle seats are preferable, in order to allow for access to lavatories and provide an opportunity to walk for short periods of time. Pre-

medication of small children with sedatives, such as diphenhydramine, prior to particularly long flights is of unclear benefit, and may result in paradoxical excitability. A recent study suggests that ear pain in children occurs commonly in association with air travel but that treatment with pseudoephedrine fails to provide significant relief of symptoms.

Routine Childhood Immunizations

Because many of the infectious diseases against which we routinely vaccinate children in the United States occur much more commonly in other parts of the world, the risk of a nonimmune individual contracting certain preventable diseases is much greater abroad. Therefore, it is important that children receive as many of the recommended doses of routine vaccines as possible prior to travel. The Advisory Committee on Immunization Practices (ACIP) of the CDC and the American Academy of Pediatrics publish accelerated dosing regimens for children who will be traveling abroad.

Infants younger than 6 months of age should not need immunization against measles because of the persistence of maternal antibody. However, because measles is endemic throughout much of the world, in particular Eastern Europe, infants older than 6 months of age should be immunized. Between the ages of 6 and 12 months, a single dose of measles vaccine, or the combined measles, mumps, and rubella vaccine (MMR), should be administered at least 1 month prior to departure. Infants vaccinated before 1 year of age will need two boosters of MMR given at least 4 weeks apart. The first should be administered at or after 12 months of age, and the second prior to starting school. All children between 12 and 15 months of age should receive MMR prior to travel, with a second dose given when they start school. The risk of serious infection with mumps or rubella in infants is low, so immunization of children younger than 1 year of age is not routinely indicated.

The ACIP currently recommends that children receive initial polio vaccination using IPV followed by OPV. Ideally, infants and children traveling outside the United States to areas where poliovirus is endemic should receive at least three doses of vaccine prior to departure. An initial IPV can be given as early as 6 weeks of age, followed by a second dose at least 4 weeks later. A single OPV can be given 4 weeks after that, with the remaining OPV administered at around school age. If departure is less than 4 weeks away, then a single dose of OPV can be given, although subsequent doses (two additional OPV immunizations at least 4 weeks apart) in the series will need to be administered while abroad.

Invasive disease caused by *Haemophilus influenzae* type b (Hib) occurs throughout the world, and the risk of acquiring this infection is presently greater abroad than in the United States. Three Hib conjugate vaccines are approved for use in infants as young as 6 weeks of age. Depending on the specific vaccine used, infants should receive either two or three doses, separated by intervals of 4 to 8 weeks, to complete the primary series. Prior to departure, an unvaccinated infant or child younger than 15 months of age should receive at least two doses of vaccine, whereas older children should receive at least one dose.

Hepatitis B vaccine should be considered in all medium- to long-term travelers, because this disease is endemic throughout most of the world. Because transmission of hepatitis B virus has been documented to occur within households, children may be at risk of acquiring infection through means other than blood transfusion or sexual contact. Infants and children residing for at least 6 months in a hepatitis B endemic area should receive at least three doses of recombinant vaccine. The first two doses should be administered 1 to 2 months apart, with the third given at least 2 months later (provided the infant is at least 6 months of age). Because sexual contact is a major risk factor for infection with hepatitis B virus, adolescents should be immunized and counseled about the need for appropriate caution and the use of condoms with all sexual partners.

Although the risk of acquiring varicella virus is not likely greater in travelers than the general population, all children 12 months of age and older should receive a single dose of varicella vaccine prior to departure. Infants younger than 1 year of age should be protected by maternal antibodies, whereas those children with prior documentation of clinical varicella are presumably already immune.

Immunizations Specific for International Travel

Hepatitis A Vaccine and Immune Globulin   Hepatitis A is endemic throughout most of the developing world, including parts of Asia, Africa, and South and Central America. Infection with the virus occurs orally, frequently through contaminated drinking water, food, or direct person-to-person contact. Although children younger than age 2 years generally experience mild forms of the disease, older children and nonimmune adults are at greater risk of developing clinically significant hepatitis. Children older than age 2 years should receive a single dose of one of the two licensed hepatitis A vaccines. A second dose should be administered 6 to 12 months later. If departure is less than 1 month away, then a single intramuscular dose of immune globulin should be given with the initial vaccination. Children younger than 2 years of age should receive only immune globulin, which provides protection against infection for 4 to 6 months.

Meningococcal Vaccine   The risk of short-term travelers acquiring infection with *Neisseria meningitidis* is relatively small. However, for those who travel to areas of high endemicity, particularly Sub-Saharan Africa, parts of South America, the Middle East, and Nepal, risk may be sufficient to warrant vaccination. The currently available tetravalent meningococcal vaccine, which covers serogroups A, C, Y, and W-135, is only recommended for children who are at least 2 years of age. The degree of vaccine-induced protection is variable for each of the different serogroups, as is the duration of immunity in children vaccinated at younger than 4 years of age. Parents should be aware that in certain instances, documentation of vaccination may be required for those traveling to Mecca during the annual Hajj.

Cholera Vaccine   The risk to travelers of acquiring infection with *Vibrio cholerae* is quite low, although the disease, when contracted, can be severe. Currently there is one cholera vaccine approved for use in the United States, with an efficacy of only about 50%. Data on the safety of this vaccine in infants younger than 6 months of age are lacking. There are currently no countries in the world that require proof of cholera vaccination for entry, making the currently available vaccine unnecessary. However, newer oral vaccines have recently been developed and some are in routine use in other countries. Preliminary studies suggest that safe alternatives may soon be available for immunizing children and adult travelers against this important global public health problem.

Yellow Fever Vaccine   Yellow fever virus, which is transmitted by mosquito bite, is endemic in Sub-Saharan Africa and tropical South America. Documentation of vaccination is required for entry into or travel from certain countries where transmission is known to occur. Parents and physicians should contact the CDC for the most up-to-date information on those countries where yellow fever transmission was recently reported. This information is available through the "Summary of Health Information for International Travel," also known as the Blue Sheet, which is published biweekly by the CDC. Because the risk of vaccine-induced encephalitis may be as high as 1% in infants, yellow fever vaccine should not be administered to infants under the age of 4 months. Infants 4 to 9 months of age should be immunized only with extreme caution, and, ideally, only if they are traveling to areas with ongoing epidemic disease transmission and adequate protection against mosquitoes cannot be guaranteed (see Table 13-68). Infants and children older than 9 months of age should be immunized if required or if they will be traveling outside of urban areas in countries endemic for yellow fever.

Japanese Encephalitis Vaccine   Japanese encephalitis (JE) virus is also transmitted by mosquito bites, and this disease occurs throughout Asia and parts of India. Despite a relatively low risk to short-term travelers, vaccination is recommended for those who will reside for at least 1 month in rural areas where JE virus transmission occurs. The three-dose vaccine regimen is administered subcutaneously on days 1, 7, and 30. For children 1 to 3 years of age, the dose of vaccine should be reduced to 0.5 mL. Unfortunately, there are little data available on the use of this vaccine in infants.

Typhoid Vaccine   Although infection with *Salmonella typhi* frequently causes severe illness in older children and adults, younger children (younger than 5 years of age) often exhibit milder forms of the disease. Children traveling to rural areas where the availability of sterile water and reliable food preparation cannot be guaranteed are at particular risk. The oral typhoid vaccine, developed from an attenuated strain of *S. typhi*, is recommended for children older than 6 years of age who will be traveling to Asia, Africa, and Latin America. The vaccine is administered in capsules given once every other day for four doses. The vaccine should be taken 1 hour before eating, and kept refrigerated prior to use. Although not routinely recommended for children under 6 years of age, there are data to suggest that the oral vaccine may be effective in children as young as 2 years of age. Alternatively, children between 2 and 6 years of age can receive the capsular polysaccharide vaccine (ViCPS), which is administered as a single intramuscular injection of 0.5 mL. Although a parenteral heat-phenol inactivated vaccine is available for children ages 6 months to 2 years, this agent is associated with significant side effects, including fever, severe local inflammation, and headache. Therefore, the parenteral vaccine should only be used in young children if the risk is felt to be prohibitively high.

Rabies Vaccine   Children who will be spending a month or more in parts of the world where rabies is endemic, which includes most of the developing countries of South and Central America, Africa, and Asia, should be considered for rabies immunization. Although the overall risk of acquiring rabies in travelers is low, young children are frequently incapable of avoiding contact with potentially infected animals, particularly dogs. Therefore, children are the group most likely to benefit most from preexposure vaccination. Immunization with either the human diploid cell rabies vaccine (HDCV) or rabies vaccine adsorbed (RVA) should be administered intramuscularly in 1-mL doses a week apart, followed by a third dose 3 to 4 weeks later. HDCV can also be given intradermally, assuming the dosing regimen will be completed at least 30 days prior to departure. However, if rabies vaccination will not be completed prior to initiation of malaria prophylaxis (chloroquine or mefloquine), the intramuscular route should be used because of potential interference of these agents with the immune response to the vaccine.

Prophylactic and Empiric Therapy

Malaria Prophylaxis The cornerstones of malaria prevention in travelers include avoidance of activities associated with mosquito contact, particularly at night; the use of appropriate insect repellents containing ≤30% DEET; and oral chemoprophylaxis; these recommendations are discussed in Sec. 13.6.5.

Traveler's Diarrhea Diarrhea affects as many as 50% of all international travelers, especially to Africa, Latin America, Asia, and the Middle East. The most frequent pathogen associated with travelers diarrhea is enterotoxigenic *E. coli,* although other bacteria (*Campylobacter jejuni* in particular), viruses, and parasites may also cause similar gastrointestinal syndromes. In most instances, the diarrhea is watery, nonbloody, and self-limited to 3 to 4 days duration. The most effective means of preventing traveler's diarrhea is avoid uncooked foods or fruits and vegetables without peels. Water that is not bottled should be boiled or treated with iodine or globaline tablets (which contain 20 mg of tetraglycine hydroperiodide, 90 mg of sodium hydropyrophosphate, and 5 mg of talc) prior to drinking or even for brushing teeth. Drinks served with ice should also be avoided, because the water used to make the ice may not have been sterilized. For infants, breast-feeding is a reliable means of reducing the risk of diarrhea and should be encouraged.

Prophylactic antibiotic therapy is not recommended for the prevention of traveler's diarrhea. Rather, expectant therapy can be used to shorten the duration of symptoms to as little as 24 hours for most travelers. In children, diarrhea can be successfully managed with aggressive hydration, even in the absence of empiric antibiotics directed at the likely pathogens. Dried packets of World Health Organization Oral Rehydration Solution (ORS) can be purchased in many developing countries. ORS should be used in addition to normal food for all children with diarrhea who show signs of dehydration. Care should be taken to ensure that the packets are mixed with the appropriate volume of bottled or sterilized water prior to administration.

For empiric therapy of traveler's diarrhea in children, trimethoprim-sulfamethoxazole (5 mg/kg trimethoprim bid) is a reasonable first-line drug, although resistance has been reported in many parts of the developing world. An alternative is ciprofloxacin (10–15 mg/kg bid), which is likely to be more effective than sulfa drugs for most bacterial causes of traveler's diarrhea. Although not approved for use in those younger than 18 years of age, there are substantial clinical data to suggest that this quinolone is safe for younger children, and liquid formulations are available. In general, antimotility agents are not recommended for children younger than 5 years of age, although in adults, they are routinely used as adjunctive therapy aimed at reducing the frequency of loose stools. If the diarrhea is bloody or associated with fever, parents should be advised to seek prompt medical attention.

Posttravel Evaluation There is no specific need to evaluate asymptomatic children returning from short-term international travel. However, children who have lived abroad for more than 6 months may need follow-up evaluation for routine immunizations and other standard health maintenance issues. Fever in the returning traveler should always be evaluated, because the differential diagnosis includes malaria, typhoid, and dengue fever, among others. Traveler's diarrhea that persists beyond 5 to 7 days should prompt a diagnostic work-up for parasites, including *Giardia lamblia, Entamoeba histolytica,* and *Cryptosporidium.* Three successive stool specimens should be sent for ova and parasites, as well as *Giardia* antigen tests. Long-term travelers should also receive a follow-up PPD skin test for tuberculosis.

References

Bienzle U, Bock HL, Kruppenbacher JP, Hofmann F, Vogel GE, Clemens R: Immunogenicity of an inactivated hepatitis A vaccine administered to two different schedules and the interference of other "travellers" vaccines with the immune response. Vaccine 14:501–505, 1996

Centers for Disease Control: Health information for international travel 1999–2000. Atlanta, GA, DHHS, 1999

Fischer PR: Travel with infants and children. Infect Dis Clin North Am 12: 355–368, 1998

Hampel F, Hulmann R, Schmidt H: Ciprofloxacin in pediatrics: worldwide clinical experience based on compassionate use—safety report. Pediatr Infect Dis J 16:127–129, 1997

Jong EC, Mcmullen R, eds: The Travel & Tropical Medicine Manual. Philadelphia, WB Saunders, 1995

Pitzinger B, Steffan R, Tschopp A: Incidence and clinical features of traveler's diarrhea in infants and children. Pediatr Infect Dis J 10:719–723, 1991

THE SKIN

Amy S. Paller, Associate Editor

14.1 FUNCTIONAL OVERVIEW

The skin, the largest organ in the body, plays many roles as the major interface with the external environment. The outer skin layer, the stratum corneum, prevents desiccation of a primarily aqueous body in a dry atmosphere. Extensive burns, drug-induced skin necrosis (toxic epidermal necrolysis), and other extensive blistering disorders, such as epidermolysis bullosa, represent situations in which the barrier is breached, leading to increased morbidity and mortality. In addition to providing a physical barrier to infection, the skin is an important component of the body's immune system. Langerhans cells provide immune surveillance, presenting antigen that activates lymphocytes. When the immune function in skin is dysfunctional, as in atopic dermatitis, the risk of infection is increased.

The skin also serves as the interface with ultraviolet light. Within the epidermis, ultraviolet B light also provides the impetus for isomerization of provitamin D to vitamin D_3, which is transported to the liver and then to the kidneys for sequential hydroxylations to form the active, 1,25-dihydroxyvitamin D_3. Exposure of normal keratinocytes to ultraviolet radiation causes mutations in tumor suppressor genes; epidermal melanin impedes transmission of ultraviolet rays. As a result, patients with albinism who have a significant decrease in epidermal melanin have an increased risk of developing ultraviolet-induced malignancies, particularly basal cell carcinomas and squamous cell carcinomas. In patients with xeroderma pigmentosum, the repair system after ultraviolet DNA damage is defective, leading to the dramatically increased risk of cutaneous sun-induced tumors in these patients (see Sec. 14.4.10).

The skin's role in thermoregulation is primarily mediated by evaporation of sweat, secreted in response to autonomic stimuli. Thermoregulation is impaired in genetic disorders of eccrine gland morphogenesis, such as hypohidrotic ectodermal dysplasia, or where eccrine ducts are obstructed by a thickened stratum corneum, as in congenital ichthyosiform erythroderma or severe atopic dermatitis. Premature infants cannot sweat well, and sweating is less even in term infants as compared with adults. During heat stress, the failure to sweat can lead to excessive body temperature, vasodilatation, and resultant hypovolemic shock. In patients with cystic fibrosis, the normally hypotonic sweat becomes hypertonic, so that thermal stress can induce dehydration.

The skin provides an important afferent limb to the nervous system in the interface with the external world through sensory perceptions of touch, pressure, itch, and pain. Skin, hair, and nails are highly visible body components, and their appearance is important for self-image and psychosocial development. Although birthmarks and acquired skin and appendageal disorders can be disfiguring, the attitude of the patient and the environment contribute greatly to the perception and resultant effect of disfigurement.

14.1.1 Skin Structure

The skin consists of three layers: epidermis, dermal-epidermal junction, and dermis. The outermost layer, the *epidermis,* is composed predominantly of ectodermally derived keratinocytes, but also contains neural crest–derived melanocytes and bone marrow–derived Langerhans cells. The epidermis is divided from the underlying dermis by the *dermal-epidermal junction,* a complex structure of particular importance in several acquired and genetic blistering diseases. The *dermis* provides the collagenous support for the epidermis and contains a network of blood vessels, lymphatics, and nerves. Below the dermis lies the subcutaneous fat, the predominant systemic energy store, which is also traversed by blood vessels and nerves.

The epidermis is a stratified, squamous epithelium composed of four major subdivisions (Fig. 14-1). Keratin tonofilaments are the predominant protein of keratinocytes and provide structural integrity. The *basal layer* of the epidermis consists of a single layer of proliferating cuboidal cells. The stem cells of the epidermis are confined to the basal layer, although the immediately suprabasal layers may also contain proliferating (transiently amplifying) cells. Above the basal layer, keratinocytes differentiate, become more flattened in appearance, and form the *spinous* (or Malphigian) *layer,* a term that derives from the microscopic appearance of their interconnections through desmosomal plaques. The number of spinous cells layers is variable, depending on body site. Increased thickening of this compartment occurs in a variety of dermatoses and is called *acanthosis.* The *granular cell layer,* which constitutes the outer one to three nucleated cell layers, is characterized by the presence of basophilic, keratohyalin granules, containing the histidine-rich protein profilaggrin. Although not seen by light microscopy, spinous and granular cells also contain an abundance of lamellar bodies, a tissue-specific, membranous organelle, enriched in lipids and lysosomal enzymes.

Above the granular cell layer, the stratum corneum is composed of multiple layers of anucleate, lipid-depleted corneocytes enclosed by a highly cross-linked protein shell, the cornified envelope, and embedded in an extracellular matrix of multiple broad lamellae enriched in lipids. These hydrophobic lipids, secreted by lamellar bodies into the intercellular space at the interface between the granular layer and the stratum corneum, form multiple membrane bilayers that impede passage of water and other substances across the stratum corneum. Normally an epidermal cell moves from the basal cell layer to the granular cell layer in about two weeks, with an additional two weeks required to exfoliate from the surface. In some hyperproliferative diseases, such as psoriasis, these transit times may be reduced to two to four days each.

The neural crest–derived melanocytes are interspersed among basal keratinocytes, where their dendrites interact with up to 36 neighboring epidermal cells. Melanocytes synthesize melanin granules that are transferred by these dendrites to epidermal cells.

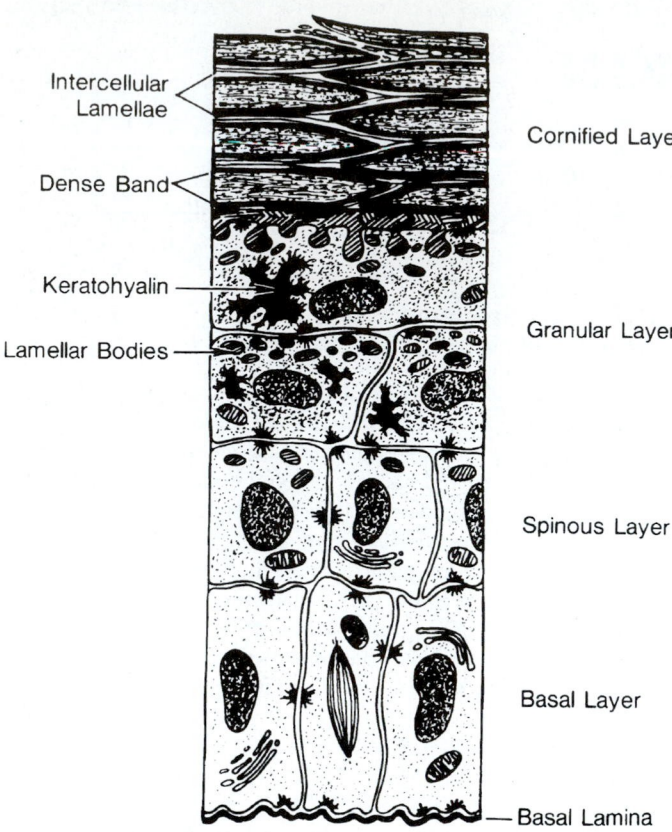

Intercellular Lamellae

Cornified Layer

Dense Band

Keratohyalin

Granular Layer

Lamellar Bodies

Spinous Layer

Basal Layer

Basal Lamina

FIGURE 14-1 **Diagrammatic view of the epidermis.** *From Williams ML: The ichthyoses: pathogenesis and prenatal diagnosis. Pediatr Dermatol 1:1–25, 1983, with permission.*

Darkly pigmented skin does not have more melanocytes, but melanin granules are larger, more heavily melanized, and persistent into higher epidermal layers. The bone marrow–derived Langerhans cells also are dendritic and interspersed among epidermal cells, but in a suprabasal distribution. On ultrastructural examination, Langerhans cells show a unique racquet-shaped organelle, the Birbeck granule. These cells can also be distinguished by their positive staining with S-100 and with the monoclonal antibody CD1. Langerhans cells participate in antigen recognition and processing, and interact with keratinocytes and T lymphocytes in immune-mediated reactions.

The dermal-epidermal junction or basement membrane zone is composed of: (1) the *plasma membrane* of the basal epidermal cell with its specialized attachment plaques, the hemidesmosomes—the hemidesmosomes include several proteins, such as bullous pemphigoid antigens, laminin 5 chains, integrins α_6 and β_4, and plectin; (2) the *lamina lucida*, which contains laminin; (3) the *lamina densa*, consisting of type IV collagen; and (4) *anchoring fibrils,* consisting of type VII collagen anchoring the basement membrane to the upper dermis. Other constituents of the basement membrane zone include fibronectin, type V collagen, entactin, and proteoglycans.

The *dermis,* which both supports the epidermis and provides the bulk and physical resilience of the skin, is a relatively acellular, fibrous tissue. Its main cellular constituent is the fibroblast, which secretes types I and III collagen, elastin, and other extracellular matrix proteins. It is divided into the outer or papillary dermis, which immediately underlies the epidermis and fills the dermal papillae, and the subjacent reticular dermis, which has a coarser pat-

tern of collagen fibers. The dermis is traversed by a network of cutaneous nerves, blood vessels, and lymphatics that transport impulses, nutrients, and immunocompetent cells to and from the skin. Perivascular mast cells and tissue macrophages are also dermal residents. The subcutaneous tissue is composed of fat cells or adipocytes surrounded by fibrous septi containing blood vessels and nerves.

Epidermal appendages are specialized structures derived from epidermis. Hair follicles arise by follicular keratinocyte growth into the dermis during the eighth to ninth week of fetal life. Hairs are classified into three types: lanugo, vellus, and terminal. *Lanugo hairs* are normally present only in fetal life, and most are shed in utero during the first portion of the last trimester. Widespread lanugo at birth is, therefore, an indicator of significant prematurity. *Terminal hairs* are the coarse, longer hairs found predominantly on scalp, eyebrows, and, after puberty, on axillae and pubis, whereas *vellus hairs* represent the finer, shorter, less pigmented hairs found on other portions of hair-bearing skin. Hair follicles undergo a cycle of several years of growth (anagen phase), followed by a brief involution phase (catagen phase), and a three-month shedding (telogen phase). Normally, hair follicle growth is asynchronous, and the duration of the anagen phase, and hence hair length, is genetically determined. But stressful events, including birth, may abruptly shunt follicles into the resting stage, producing 2 to 4 months later a marked shedding of hair (telogen effluvium). Hair growth is androgen-dependent to a varying extent, depending on body site, regulated by the conversion within the hair follicle of testosterone to its active metabolite, 5α-dehydrotestosterone.

Like hairs, nails are concretions of keratinized cells (Fig. 14-2). They arise from the nail matrix, which underlies the cuticle, and the proximal, white portion of the nail plate, the lunula. The nail bed, which underlies the distal and visible portion of the nail, is richly vascularized and innervated. The lateral edges of the nail lie free within grooves formed by the lateral nail folds. The hyponychium underlies the free edge of the nail plate, distally.

Sebaceous glands arise from the midportion of each hair follicle and secrete their fatty contents (sebum) in a holocrine manner into the follicular lumen. The function of sebum is unknown. Glands of

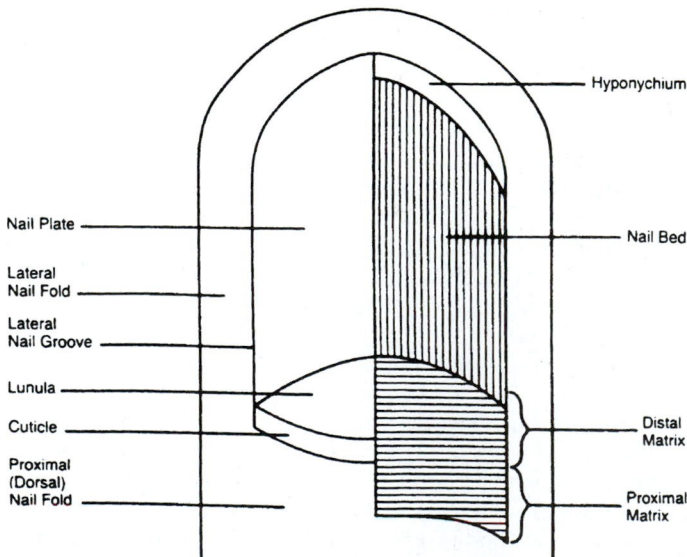

Nail Plate

Lateral Nail Fold

Lateral Nail Groove

Lunula

Cuticle

Proximal (Dorsal) Nail Fold

Hyponychium

Nail Bed

Distal Matrix

Proximal Matrix

FIGURE 14-2 **Diagrammatic view of the nail unit.** *From Karaika SJ, Scher RK: Heritable nail disorders. Dermatol Clin 5:179–191, 1987, with permission.*

the face, scalp, and upper trunk are the largest and most active. In neonates, sebaceous glands are active, owing to transplacental passage of maternal sex hormones, leading to sebaceous hyperplasia and neonatal acne. After birth, sebaceous glands involute; their subsequent enlargement and increased secretion is one of the earliest signs of puberty.

Eccrine sweat glands are composed of secretory coils located in the mid-dermis from which arise ducts that penetrate the epidermis at intervals. Two to four million eccrine glands are distributed across the skin surface, but the glands are most numerous on palms and soles. Sweating is a sympathetic autonomic response and is stimulated in response to thermoregulatory and emotional stimuli. Full-term neonates possess a full complement of eccrine glands, but function may be immature, particularly in caudal regions. Apocrine glands represent another type of sweat gland found in the axillae and perineum. These glands, whose function is probably vestigial, do not become active until puberty. Secretion is stimulated by emotions and circulating epinephrine or norepinephrine.

14.1.2   Examination of the Skin

The entire body surface should be examined in patients who have a dermatologic complaint. Primary skin lesions should be distinguished from secondary lesions.

PRIMARY LESIONS

Primary lesions occur as a direct consequence of the disease process. Macules are visually evident lesions that are flat and thus cannot be palpated. Discrete, rounded solid lesions are termed *papules* if they measure less than 0.5 cm. Larger lesions are nodules or tumors. Papules may coalesce to form plaques. Smaller primary lesions that are filled with fluid may be vesicles (clear fluid) or pustules (purulent

fluid). Larger fluid-filled lesions are termed *blisters* or *bullae*. Superficial bullae tend to be flaccid, whereas bullae in deeper locations tend to be tense. A biopsy may be required to define further the level of blistering. Other epidermal changes are scaling and lichenification. The latter change represents thickening of the epidermis with prominent skin markings, often with hyperpigmentation because of accumulated melanin. Color is another important feature to assess. Redness or erythema arises from oxygenated hemoglobin and is usually indicative of increased blood flow through the upper dermis. Blue shades may be caused by unoxygenated hemoglobin or melanin pigment deep within the dermis. Melanin in the upper dermis and epidermis produces shades between brown and black. The pigmentation from epidermal melanosis is accentuated under long-wave ultraviolet (Wood's light) illumination, whereas pigment produced in the upper dermis fades. Hypopigmentation may be owed to decreased dermal blood flow or to decreased epidermal pigmentation. Hypopigmentation and particularly depigmentation caused by loss of epidermal melanin are enhanced under Wood's light.

SECONDARY LESIONS

Secondary lesions evolve from primary lesions. When vesicles or bullae rupture, loss of all or a portion of the epidermis results in a superficial erosion. The resultant exudation forms a serous or hemorrhagic crust at the surface. Ulcerations result from loss of deeper dermal tissue either by the spontaneous evolution of primary lesions or induced by scratching (excoriations) or rubbing.

BEDSIDE PROCEDURES

POTASSIUM HYDROXIDE (KOH) PREPARATION   In a KOH preparation, scales are scraped onto a slide covered with 10% KOH and

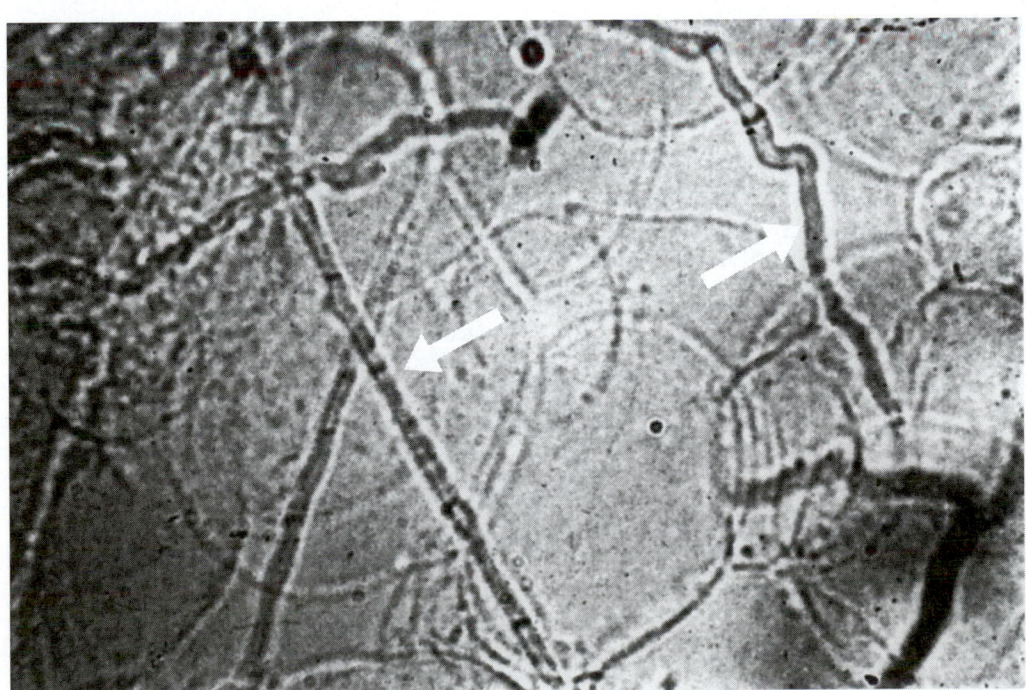

FIGURE 14-3   Potassium hydroxide preparation of scale. Note several septate hyphae overlying stratum corneum cells. Hyphae are thicker and more refractile than cell borders. (*Courtesy of Raza Aly, M.D.*)

a coverslip, and gently heated over a flame to digest keratinocyte cell walls and to preserve fungal architecture. Yeasts are identified as rounded, often budding structures. Characteristics of hyphae include parallel cell walls, periodic septae, and branching filaments that may traverse multiple cell boundaries (Fig. 14-3).

MINERAL OIL SCRAPINGS   Scabies mites and their eggs and feces are best identified under immersion oil. The highest yield results from identification and scraping of a burrow, but intact burrows are hard to find. The outer epidermis of several lesions should be removed by scraping along its length with a no. 15 surgical blade. The mite or her eggs or feces are easily recognized under low-power microscopy.

TZANCK PREPARATION   Vesicles should be ruptured and the fluid blotted away. The base is scraped gently with a no. 15 blade and streaked onto a slide, which may be stained with methylene blue, toluidine blue, and Wright or Giemsa stains. Cytopathic viruses (eg, herpes simplex, herpes zoster, vaccinia) induce formation of multinucleate giant cells with enlarged nuclei and prominent nuclear inclusions. The current availability of rapid immunologic tests from scraped material to identify herpes simplex and varicella infections has largely supplanted the use of Tzanck preparations.

SKIN BIOPSY   *Skin biopsy* is easily accomplished, in most instances, using a small manual rotary punch of 3 to 5 mm in diameter. Local anesthesia is obtained by injection of 1% lidocaine hydrochloride using a 30-gauge needle. Epinephrine is often included to enhance hemostasis but should be omitted in acral locations (eg, finger or nasal tips) and in infants and children weighing less than about 15 kg. Topical application under occlusion of a eutetic mixture of lidocaine and prilocaine can diminish the discomfort of injection of anesthesia. In some instances a larger, deeper "wedge" biopsy is needed. Scarring is expected after skin biopsy; closure with a suture will minimize the cosmetic deficit. Whether a skin biopsy is indicated and, if so, where to biopsy, requires informed judgment and, in most instances, consultation with a dermatologist.

References

Freedberg IM, Eisen AZ, Wolk K, et al: Fitzpatrick's Dermatology in General Medicine. 5th ed, New York, McGraw-Hill, 1999

Goldsmith L: Biochemistry and Physiology of Skin. New York, Oxford University Press, 1983

Holbrook KA, Sybert VP: Structural and biochemical properties of the skin of adults, children, and newborn infants. In Schachner LA, Hansen RC, eds: Pediatric Dermatology, 2nd ed. New York, Churchill Livingstone, 1995

14.2   NEONATAL DERMATOLOGY

Elaine C. Siegfried

14.2.1   Neonatal Skin Development and Physiology

The skin of a newborn infant differs from adult skin in several ways that place infants at increased risk for thermal instability, skin dam-

age, percutaneous infection, and percutaneous toxicity from topically applied agents. The neonatal body surface area-to-weight ratio is up to five times greater than that of an adult, and the thickness of infant skin is 40 to 60% less. Attenuated rete ridges, formed from comparatively fewer stem cells at the basal layer, provide a relatively limited area of surface attachment to an immature dermis, resulting in relative skin fragility. Sebaceous glands are comparatively hypertrophic for several weeks after birth, under the influence of fetal and maternal androgens, but eccrine function does not mature until after term, placing newborns at risk for hyperthermia with overbundling. The *vernix caseosa* is composed of sloughed keratinocyte and sebaceous gland lipids, with a comparatively higher proportion of glandular lipids in boys.

The most clinically significant difference between the skin of a premature and that of a term infant is the barrier function of the most superficial layer of the epidermis, the stratum corneum. Infants born before 32 weeks of gestation have a very thin stratum corneum. Although even in premature neonates the stratum corneum matures within 2 weeks after birth, during the first 2 weeks of life, premature infants suffer from significant transepidermal water loss (TEWL) with associated hypothermia and fluid and electrolyte disturbances. These problems are proportional to the degree of prematurity. TEWL is up to 15 times higher for a one-day-old infant born at 25 weeks of gestation compared to a term neonate. This can translate into fluid loss of up to 30% of total body weight in 24 hours. Barrier function rapidly improves during the first 2 weeks after birth, but at 4 weeks after gestation, TEWL from a 26-week premature infant is still twice that of a term infant. Benign clinical interventions such as barrier creams or ointments can dramatically decrease these losses. During this period cutaneous contact with chemicals that can cause neurotoxicity, such as hexachlorophene, or alter thyroid function, such as povidone iodine, should be avoided. Dessicated skin is even more susceptible to injury, providing a portal of entry for invading microbes and increasing the risk of disseminated infection.

14.2.2   Common Benign Dermatoses and Developmental Defects

NEVUS SEBACEOUS   Usually a localized lesion near the vertex of the scalp, nevus sebaceous presents at birth as a hairless plaque of coalesced yellow papules (Color Plate 1). A biopsy reveals absent to malformed hair follicles with an abundance of sebaceous glands. The 10 to 15% risk of tumor formation, especially of basal cell carcinoma, mandates that nevus sebaceous be removed by adolescence.

SEBACEOUS HYPERPLASIA   Numerous tiny, pale yellow papules representing hypertrophic sebaceous glands are seen on the nose, forehead, cheeks, and upper lip of full-term newborns. The condition resolves with waning maternal androgen levels during the first weeks of life.

MILIA   Milia are tiny cysts walled by incompletely canalized follicular or ductal epithelium and filled with sloughed keratinocyte and sebaceous debris. Milia are most common on the face of full-term newborns but may be seen on other areas. *Epstein pearls,* yellow papules often found on the hard palate, are intraoral milia. Milia usually disappear within a few weeks.

MILIARIA   Also called *prickly heat,* this common skin finding results from incomplete canalization of the eccrine ostia with resultant accumulation of sweat droplets. Two clinical variants reflect the depth of obstruction. *Miliaria crystallina* are superficial, subcorneal vesicles. *Miliaria rubra* occur within the epidermis, accompanied by focal rupture of the duct and an inflammatory response, producing erythematous papules and pustules. Miliaria is precipitated by excessive heat or bundling. Common sites include the forehead, torso, and arms. The condition is self-limited and relieved by placing the infant in a thermoneutral environment.

NEONATAL ACNE The pathognomonic comedones and small inflammatory papules and pustules of neonatal acne may be present at birth or develop within the first three months of life under the influence of maternal and fetal androgens. The condition is rarely severe enough to require treatment and usually resolves spontaneously within two to three months. Persistent or severe acne in an infant is a sign of adrenal or androgen excess in the minority of cases. Normal growth velocity and bone age are sufficient to rule out extracutaneous disease in an otherwise healthy infant. Nodulocystic acne warrants dermatologic referral for more aggressive therapy. Pustules caused by *Malassezia furfur (Pityrosporum)* contain characteristic spores and short hyphae; these resolve promptly with application of topical antifungal creams.

SUCKING BLISTERS Sucking blisters are common, transient lesions that result from intrauterine sucking. Typically, one or two blisters or erosions are present at birth on the radial forearm, wrist, or dorsal thumb or index finger. The diagnosis will usually be confirmed by observing the infant sucking vigorously on the affected area.

CUTANEOUS VASOMOTOR INSTABILITY Cutaneous vasomotor instability is common in newborns and may present as cutis marmorata, acrocyanosis, or harlequin color change. *Cutis marmorata* refers to a reticulate and mottled appearance of the skin, caused by an uneven distribution of superficial capillary blood flow. The pattern is often precipitated by exposure to cold and is more common in preterm infants. Persistent or recurrent cutis marmorata beyond the neonatal period is referred to as *livedo reticularis*. Livedo reticularis is often physiologic but can be associated with a variety of congenital and acquired pathologic conditions, including Down syndrome, trisomy 18, and the Cornelia de Lange syndrome as well as vasculopathy or frank vasculitis attributable to a wide range of infectious, inflammatory, or neoplastic processes. *Cutis marmorata telangiectatica congenita* is a congenital anomaly that approximates the reticular pattern of cutis marmorata but is fixed in a focal, often unilateral distribution. The condition may be complicated by associated skin thinning and ulceration, ipsilateral soft tissue, or even bony hypotrophy. *Acrocyanosis* results from the pooling of venous blood in the hands and feet; the deep purple color does not mark a pathologic process in an otherwise healthy infant and is reversed by warming. *Harlequin color change* is the term applied to transient erythema or duskiness of the dependent half of the body, a sharp midline demarcation, and pallor of the upper half.

NEVUS SIMPLEX Colloquially known as a *salmon patch, angel kiss* (on the glabella), or *stork bite* (on the posterior hairline), these pink-to-red blanching macules are found on the majority of newborns. They may be distributed anywhere along the midline from the brow to the nape of the neck, as well as the eyelids and alar creases. Facial lesions nearly always fade with time, but nuchal patches often persist. Nevus simplex may represent dilated superficial vessels as a result of vasomotor immaturity. These transient lesions should be distinguished from *nevus flammeus* (port wine stain), a persistent vascular anomaly that can occur on any skin site, notably within the sensory distribution of the facial nerve. Bilateral facial nevus flammeus or unilateral lesions involving all three branches of the trigeminal nerve are associated with a significantly higher risk of eye and/or CNS complications (Sturge-Weber syndrome). Large lesions on the extremities may be associated with an underlying venous varicosity ipsilateral hypertrophy (Klippel-Trenaunay syndrome).

MONGOLIAN SPOTS Mongolian spots are more common in infants with dark skin types and occur in 80 to 90% of Asian and African-American newborns. They are discussed in detail in Sec. 14.5.1.

ERYTHEMA TOXICUM NEONATORUM AND NEONATAL PUSTULAR MELANOSIS Common, transient, and innocuous eruptions of unknown etiology, erythema toxicum neonatorum and neonatal pustular melanosis may occur simultaneously and may share a common pathophysiology. *Erythema toxicum* occurs in up to 60% of term newborns, equally in boys and girls, but is uncommon in premature infants. In most infants, the onset is in the first three days. Three types of skin lesions may be present in varying proportions—erythematous macules, wheals, and vesiculopustules, usually arising from an erythematous base. Lesions can occur almost anywhere on the body, but palmoplantar and perioral sparing are diagnostic features. *Neonatal pustular melanosis* occurs in 5% of term black infants and less than 1% of white infants (Color Plate 2). The eruption is always present at birth or within the first 24 hours. Lesions evolve from noninflammatory pustules that rupture, leaving transient collarettes of scale surrounding hyperpigmented macules that may persist for several weeks. The pustular phase is evanescent and may occur in utero, leaving only pigmented macules at birth. The eruption may occur on any part of the skin but usually involves the face, neck folds, and hands and feet. The differential diagnosis of atypical eruptions is extensive and includes infectious processes that require immediate treatment (see Table 14-1). Microscopic examination of the vesicle roof prepared with potassium hydroxide is clear of yeast, whereas Wright-stained smears of the base are without the multinucleated giant epithelial cells that characterize herpesvirus infections. Pustular contents show no bacteria on Gram stain and in the case of erythema toxicum usually contain eosinophils, whereas those of transient neonatal pustular melanosis contain neutrophils. Skin biopsy is indicated if the diagnosis is uncertain.

ACROPUSTULOSIS OF INFANCY This uncommon, intensely pruritic eruption consists of vesicles and pustules confined to the palms and soles. Lesions may be present at birth or have their onset early in infancy. It is more common in males and in blacks. Lesions reoccur every two to three weeks, and fade over the next 7 to 10 days. The condition closely mimics scabies, but repeated skin scrapings are negative for evidence of mites, and empiric treatment for scabies is ineffective. Skin biopsy is not usually necessary but will reveal an intraepidermal vesicle containing eosinophils or neutrophils. Treatment with two- to four-week courses of erythromycin or oral antihistamines and potent topical steroids may relieve symptoms. The use of ultrapotent (class I) topical steroids may be justified in severe cases.

SUPERNUMERARY NIPPLES Reddish brown papules that occur anywhere along the embryologic milk lines of the chest, abdomen, or rarely the inguinal area may be accompanied by breast tissue and

TABLE 14-1

DIFFERENTIAL DIAGNOSIS OF BLISTERS AND PUSTULES IN THE NEWBORN

DISEASE	USUAL AGE	SKIN: MORPHOLOGY	SKIN: USUAL DISTRIBUTION	CLINICAL: OTHER	DIAGNOSIS/FINDINGS
Infectious causes					
Staphylococcus aureus					
Impetigo	Few days to wk	Pustules, bullae, occ. vesicles	Mainly diaper area, periumbilical	Boys > girls: occ. epidemics	Gram stains: neutrophils gram+ cocci in clusters; bacterial culture
Staphylococcal scalded skin syndrome	3 to 7 days; occ. older	Erythema; cutaneous tenderness; superficial blisters and erosions	Generalized, begins on the face; blistering and erosions in areas of mechanical stress	Irritability, fever	Skin biopsy, superficial epidermal split, bacterial cultures, blood, urine, etc.
Group A streptococcus	Few days to wk	Isolated pustules; honey-crusted lesions	No predisposed sites	Moist umbilical stump; occ. cellulitis; meningitis, pneumonia	Smear: gram+ cocci in chains; bacterial culture
Group B streptococcus	Birth or first few days	Vesicles, bullae, erosions, honey-crusted lesions	No predisposed sites	Pneumonia; sepsis	Smear: gram+ cocci; bacterial culture
Listeria monocytogenes	Usually at birth	Hemorrhagic pustules and petechiae	Generalized, esp. trunk and extremities	Sepsis; respiratory distress; maternal fever	Smear: gram+ rods; bacterial culture
Haemophilus influenzae	Birth or first few days	Vesicles and crusted lesions	No predisposed sites	Sepsis; occ. meningitis	Smear: small gram− rods; bacterial culture
Congenital syphilis	Usually at birth	Blisters or erosions on dusky or hemorrhagic base	Palms, soles, knees, abdomen, groin, buttocks	Low birthweight; hepatosplenomegaly; metaphyseal dystrophy	Darkfield or FA of involved skin; serial serology
Candidiasis					
Congenital	Birth or first wk	Erythema and fine papules evolve into pustules	Any part of body; esp. palms and soles	Prematurity	KOH: pseudohyphae, budding yeasts
Neonatal	Wk to mo	Scaly red patches with satellite papules, pustules	Diaper and intertriginous areas	Usually none; maternal intrauterine device, cervical suture; previous antibiotic therapy	KOH: pseudohyphae, budding yeasts
Herpes simplex					
Intrauterine	Birth	Vesicles, widespread bullae, erosions, scars, missing skin	Anywhere on body; skin involved in 90%	Low birth weight; microcephaly, chorioretinitis	Tzanck and FA slide tests; viral culture
Neonatal	Usual: 5 to 14 d	Vesicles, crusts, erosions; may be grouped or not	Anywhere: esp. scalp monitor sites, torso, intraoral; May follow dermatome	Signs of sepsis, irritability, lethargy; Esp. eye, CNS involvement	Tzanck and FA slide tests; viral culture
Varicella					
Intrauterine	Birth	Usually: scars, limb hypoplasia, erosions	Anywhere, esp. extremities	Maternal varicella first trimester	Tzanck and FA slide tests; viral culture
Neonatal	0 to 14 d	Vesicles on an erythematous base; may be very numerous	Generalized	Maternal varicella 4 d to 2 wk after delivery	Tzanck and FA slide tests; viral culture
Cytomegalovirus (CMV)	Birth (one case)	Vesicles	Forehead	Prematurity, jaundice, hepatosplenomegaly	Urine culture; anti-CMV IgM
Scabies	After 3 wk	Papules, nodules, vesicles, crusted lesions	Generalized, esp. palms, insteps of feet, axillae	Others in family with pruritus or rash	Scabies prep: mites, eggs, or feces

(continued)

TABLE 14-1 Continued

DISEASE	USUAL AGE	SKIN: MORPHOLOGY	SKIN: USUAL DISTRIBUTION	CLINICAL: OTHER	DIAGNOSIS/FINDINGS
Sporadic conditions: common					
Erythema toxicum neonatorum	24 to 48 h to few wk	Erythematous macules, papules, pustules	Buttocks, torso, proximal extremities; spares palms, soles	Usually term infants (birth weight >2500 g)	Smear: eosinophils, no organisms
Neonatal pustular melanosis	Birth	Pustules without erythema; hyperpigmented macules	Anywhere: esp. forehead, behind ears, neck, back	Term infants; more common in African-Americans	Smear: neutrophils, occ. eosinophils, no organisms
Miliaria crystallina	Usually first wk	Dew-drop-like vesicles, very fragile; no erythema	Esp. forehead, upper trunk, volar forearms	Warm incubator, overdressings, fever	Smear: few to no cells; no organisms
Miliaria rubra	Day to wk	Pustules on erythematous base; imposed pustules	Same as miliaria crystallina	Same as miliaria crystallina	Usually clinical: skin biopsy: intraepidermal pustule with neutrophils
Pityrosporum (Malassezia furfur) pustulosis	3 to 4 wk	Papules and pustules	Face, esp. cheeks and forehead	Resembles neonatal acne but comedones are absent	KOH: short hyphae and yeast
Sucking blisters	Birth	Flaccid bulla on nonerythematous base	Radial, forearm, wrist, hand, dorsal thumb, index finger	Infant sucks vigorously on affected areas	Clinical
Acropustulosis of infancy	Birth or first day to week	Vesicles and pustules	Hands and feet, esp. palms, soles	Severe pruritus; lesions come in crops	Clinical; skin biopsy: intraepidermal pustule with eosinophils and neutrophils
Neonatal acne	3 to 4 wk	Comedones, papules, pustules	Face, esp. cheeks, forehead	Comedones, pathognomonic	Clinical
Sporadic conditions: rare					
Langerhans cell histiocytosis	Usually birth	Papules, pustules, purpura, erosions or scars	Generalized	Lymph nodes; liver, spleen, blood may be involved	Skin biopsy: atypical S-100 CDH histiocytes
Diffuse cutaneous mastocytosis	Birth to few weeks	Bullae; thickened, yellowish skin; hives	Generalized	Wheezing, diarrhea, bleeding diatheses	Skin biopsy: mast-cell infiltrate
Maternal autoimmune bullous disease	Birth	Tense or flaccid bullae, erosions	Generalized	Maternal blistering disease	Maternal immunofluorescence biopsy
Toxic epidermal necrolysis	Birth to few weeks	Diffuse skin erythema, tenderness, erosions	Generalized	Graft-vs-host disease; *Klebsiella* sepsis, etc.	Skin biopsy: full-thickness necrosis
Erosive and vesicular dermatosis	Birth	Vesicles and erosions	Generalized, >75% of body	? Infection or placental infarctions	? Skin biopsy
Eosinophilic pustular folliculitis	Birth or later	Multiple pustules, crusted areas	Scalp, hands, feet	Often peripheral eosinophilia	Skin biopsy: folliculitis with eosinophils
Genetic and developmental causes					
Epidermolysis bullosa	Birth, rarely later	Bullae or erosions; milia, nail dystrophy; occ. cutis aplasia	Anywhere; esp. extremities, mucosa	Any epithelia (gastrointestinal, genitourinary, cornea, trachea) may be affected	Skin biopsy: electron microscopy or immunofluorescence mapping
Epidermolytic hyperkeratosis (bullous ichthyosis)	Birth	Bullae, erosions, hyperkeratoses	Generalized; blisters more on hands and feet	Family history (autosomal dominant)	Skin biopsy: abn. "keratohyalin" granules; electron microscopy
Incontinentia pigmenti	Birth or first week	Linear streaks of erythematous papules and vesicles; focal alopecia	Swirling, following Blaschko lines	Family history (X-dominant) Eye CNS abnormality	Skin biopsy: eosinophilic spongiosis and dyskeratosis

(continued)

TABLE 14-1 Continued

DISEASE	USUAL AGE	SKIN: MORPHOLOGY	SKIN: USUAL DISTRIBUTION	CLINICAL: OTHER	DIAGNOSIS/FINDINGS
Acrodermatitis entero-pathica	Week to month	Sharply demarcated, psoriasiform plaques, sometimes vesicles and bullae	Periorificial and acral	Diarrhea, irritability, alopecia, hy-peralimentation, prematurity, trial of zinc Some breast-fed infants	Low serum zinc
Hyperimmunoglobulin E syndrome	Day to week	Multiple vesicles, grouped and individual	Generalized	Recurrent *S. aureus* infection; eo-sinophilia	? Clinical (IgE not usually ele-vated in newborn period)
Aplasia cutis congenita	Birth	One or more membrane-covered depressions or ulcerations	Usually scalp	Occ. associated with epidermal nevus	Clinical; skin biopsy
Ectodermal dysplasias	Congenital or early infancy	Rarely: vesicles or bullae	Depends on specific form; acral in some	Abn. teeth, hair, nails, sweating, depends on specific form	Usually clinical
Goltz syndrome	Congenital or early infancy	Rarely: vesicles or bullae; linear bands of atrophy	Linear pattern following Blaschko lines	X-dominant, females only, limb abnormalities	Clinical
Erythropoietic porphyria	Early infancy	Vesicles or bullae	Photodistribution	Hemolytic anemia, pink urine	High porphyrins in blood, urine
Protein C deficiency	Birth or first day	Hemorrhagic bullae and skin in-farctions	May be focal or generalized	Disseminated intravascular coag-ulation	Absent protein C in blood

FA = fluorescence antibody; KOH = potassium hydroxide.

SOURCE: *Modified from table originally appearing in Frieden I: Blisters and pustules in the newborn. Curr Prob Pediatr 19:565, 1989, with permission of Year Book Medical Publishers, Inc.*

are sometimes mistaken for melanocytic nevi. Further evaluation and treatment is unnecessary. Supernumerary nipples may be electively removed by surgical excision.

APLASIA CUTIS CONGENITA The congenital absence of skin is a cutaneous anomaly most often at the scalp vertex. Sharply marginated lesions may present either singly or as multiple ulcers, bullae, or scars that measure up to several centimeters in diameter. Up to 30% have underlying skull defects. Larger defects are often deeper and may extend to the dura or meninges. These may be complicated by meningitis, hemorrhage (which has been fatal), or venous thrombosis. Aplasia cutis of the trunk and extremities is often strikingly symmetric in distribution. Histologically, aplasia cutis is characterized by absent epidermis, diminished dermis and adnexal structures or, in full-thickness lesions, the absence of all skin layers.

Several distinct subtypes of aplasia cutis have been described, based on the distribution, mode of inheritance, and associated abnormalities. Most aplasia cutis congenita occurs sporadically; autosomal-dominant and autosomal-recessive transmission have also been well documented. Associated abnormalities include cleft lip and palate, limb anomalies, cutaneous organoid nevi, and epidermolysis bullosa. Aplasia cutis may mark spinal dysraphism, omphalocele, or gastroschisis. in addition, scalp defects have been associated with specific teratogens (methimazole, intrauterine varicella, and herpes simplex) and malformation syndromes (trisomy 13, Johanson-Blizzard syndrome, amniotic band disruption complex, and the ectodermal dysplasias). Extensive aplasia cutis has been associated with elevated α-fetoprotein in maternal serum and amniotic fluid.

The cause of aplasia cutis congenita is unknown. The findings of a twin fetus papyraceous and/or a placental infarct have suggested vascular thrombosis as a cause in infants with lesions on the trunk and limbs.

Cutaneous and bony lesions heal spontaneously over a period of weeks to months. A hypertrophic or atrophic patch of alopecia remains. Lesions that fail to heal or produce cosmetically unacceptable scars can be excised with primary closure.

MIDLINE LESIONS Midline circumscribed or annular hypertrichosis, dimples, sinuses, skin tags, nodules, and cysts may be isolated skin findings or may mark underlying developmental defects. The differential diagnosis of lesions on the brow or nose includes dermoid cyst/sinus, glioma, and encephalocele. Congenital defects that present as a midline scalp nodule include encephalocele, meningocele, aplasia cutis, dermoid cyst/sinus, and heterotopic brain tissue. If the diagnosis of a midline scalp lesion is clinically uncertain, skin biopsy should be postponed until after radiographic imaging by CT or MRI. These studies may miss small associated intracranial connections. A midline pit or nodule on the neck may represent a cervical cleft or thyroglossal duct cyst/sinus. A remnant of respiratory epithelium known as a bronchogenic sinus or cyst presents at birth as a nodule or pit at the suprasternal notch. Branchial cleft anomalies, cysts or sinuses, are located along the preauricular area, pinna, and lateral neck. Aberrant branchial arch development is associated with several multiorgan syndromes including: Townes-Brocks, Treacher-Collins, Goldenhar, Hallerman-Streiff, Pierre-Robin, and branchiootorenal dysplasia. These sinuses and cysts can be watched expectantly or electively removed by surgical excision to prevent drainage or infection. A variety of midline lumbosacral skin lesions may mark occult spinal dysraphism including pits, lipomas, skin tags, hypertrichosis, hemangiomas, and nevus flammeus. Sacral dimples or sinuses are common lesions and are

only of concern when they occur superior to the gluteal cleft. In contrast, radiographic imaging is indicated for perianal hemangiomas.

AMNIOTIC BANDS Amniotic bands cause circumferential ring-like constrictions on the skin, most commonly on the extremities. They are present at the time of birth and appear to be caused by separation of the amnion from the chorion, giving rise to strands of amnion, which disrupt normal morphogenesis. Amniotic bands can cause a multitude of other abnormalities including limb amputations, syndactyly, thoracoabdominal wall defects (eg, gastroschisis, omphalocele), and craniofacial clefts.

14.2.3　Congenital Infections

Skin findings can provide a valuable clue to the diagnosis of congenital bacterial, viral, and mycotic infections. Signs that warrant prompt evaluation include vesicles and pustules, bullae and extensive erosions, erythroderma, petechiae, and purpura. The cardinal clinical and diagnostic features of infectious and noninfectious causes of blisters, pustules, and erosions in the newborn are summarized in Table 14-1.

VESICLES AND PUSTULES Many conditions cause blisters and pustules in the newborn. Vesicles are defined as small intra- or subepidermal pockets of clear fluid. If the lesions are large (>1 cm), they are referred to as *bullae*. Pustules are filled with purulent fluid. Diseases in this category range from the totally innocuous and self-limited to the severe and life-threatening. Often, initial empiric broad-spectrum systemic antimicrobial therapy is warranted, especially in unstable premature infants. A family history of blistering diseases and physical examination, including examination of the placenta, can focus the differential diagnosis. Bullae and widespread involvement should prompt a more aggressive workup.

Initial diagnostic studies for vesicles include: fluid aspirate taken from an intact pustule for Gram stain, Wright stain, fungal, viral, and bacterial cultures; KOH preparation (or Calcofluor White immunofluorescence) of the blister roof; scraping from the base of the blister for Tzanck smear (see Sec. 14.1.2). The greatest value of rapid, bedside testing is confirmation of a life-threatening infection. Congenital candidiasis and congenital herpes simplex are the most common examples. Herpes simplex can be rapidly diagnosed with a Tzanck smear that reveals viral cytopathic changes or by direct fluorescence examination using antiherpes antibodies. Vesicles on the skin of newborns tend to cluster at sites in contact with the maternal cervix; cutaneous, eye, and/or mouth lesions are presenting signs in one-third of infants. Cutaneous candidiasis is confirmed by KOH (or Calcofluor White) smear of the blister roof revealing pseudohyphae. In either case, a high index of suspicion must be maintained for the possibility of systemic disease, especially in premature infants. Malassezia folliculitis is confirmed with a KOH smear of the blister roof and contents that reveal short hyphae and spores. The diagnosis of bullous impetigo and gram-positive folliculitis is supported by a Wright stain of the blister base revealing polymorphonuclear leukocytes (PMNs) and Gram stain showing gram-positive cocci. In older children with pruritic vesicles on the palms, soles, toe or finger webs, wrists, or ankles, scrapings from vesicles can be mounted in mineral oil to detect mites, ova, and feces as confirmation of a scabies infestation.

BULLAE AND EXTENSIVE EROSIONS These may mark life-threatening diseases that may be impossible to distinguish from one another without skin biopsy. Appropriate therapy depends on correct diagnosis. Skin biopsy of staphylococcal scalded skin syndrome (SSSS) reveals a split in the superficial epidermis. Culture of blister contents is negative; the locus of infection is nasopharyngeal, perianal, focus of impetigo, or abscess. A less common condition, toxic epidermal necrolysis, can be distinguished from SSSS by histologic evidence of a split at the dermoepidermal junction. A pathognomonic feature of bullous mastocytosis, Darier's sign, is a wheal-and-flare response to stroking. Genetic disorders have variable extent of severity and long-term sequelae. Early diagnosis and genetic counseling are important aspects of management. The blisters seen in infants with a form of epidermolysis bullosa are most prominent at sites of friction. Familial forms are classified as simplex, junctional, and dystrophic, based on the skin cleavage plane. Electron microscopic analysis and/or immunofluorescence mapping are required for precise diagnosis. Vesicular skin findings that characterize incontinentia pigmenti are distributed in a linear and whorled configuration along the lines of Blaschko. This striking pattern is seen with a variety of cutaneous abnormalities, as a result of genetic mosaicism.

The cardinal clinical and diagnostic features of infectious and noninfectious causes of blisters, pustules, and erosions in the newborn are summarized in Table 14-1.

ERYTHRODERMA   Generalized redness and scaling in infancy has an alarming appearance and is often clinically and histologically nonspecific. An infant's general state of well-being and the family history provide important clues to the underlying cause. Definitive diagnosis may be possible only after a period of observation. The spectrum of disease includes common conditions limited to skin, infections, nutritional deficiencies, and immunologic disorders.

Infectious causes of erythroderma should always be considered first. The differential diagnosis includes systemic candidiasis, SSSS, syphilis, and AIDS. Congenital syphilis is uncommon, but its incidence has increased in the past decade. Also known as "the great mimicker," syphilis has a wide range of cutaneous signs. The most common cutaneous manifestation of congenital syphilis is symmetric scaling plaques of the arms and legs, especially the medial thighs, palms, and soles, sometimes present at birth, and usually within the first few weeks. The more suggestive congenital palmoplantar bullae and erosions occur in only 3% of infected infants. Mucosal lesions are also common and include superficial erosions in the mouth (mucous patches) and moist deep fissures (rhagades) around the eyes, nose, mouth, and anus. The infant's skin should be carefully examined for more specific primary skin lesions. Laboratory evaluation should include: complete blood count; KOH preparation (or Calcofluor White immunofluorescence); Tzanck smear; and surveillance cultures of the nasopharynx, rectum, umbilicus, conjunctivae, urine, and blood. Consider syphilis serology and HIV studies in epidemiologically relevant locales.

Erythroderma coupled with failure to thrive, diarrhea, and recurrent infections should prompt a search for metabolic or immunologic abnormalities with assessment of dietary history, electrolytes, protein, albumin, alkaline phosphatase, microscopic examination of hair, and a sweat test. Erythroderma in the neonate may be seen with primary immunodeficiencies (SCID, Wiskott-Aldrich, Hyper-IgE, Omenn syndrome); secondary immunodeficiencies (AIDS, graft-versus-host disease); Langerhans cell histiocytosis; neonatal lupus; and diffuse cutaneous mastocytosis. Erosive, periorificial dermatitis suggests a metabolic or nutritional disorder. Cystic fibrosis is the most common condition in this category. Other possibilities include acrodermatitis enteropathica,

biotin-dependent multiple carboxylase deficiency, prolidase deficiency, methylmalonic acidemia, maple syrup urine disease, propionic acidemia, citrullinemia, Gaucher disease, and kwashiorkor. More directed laboratory evaluation includes blood smear for leukocyte vacuoles, HIV screen, plasma zinc, and serum linoleic and arachidonic acids; amino acid and organic acid profiles; biotinidase activity; ANA, SS-A, and SS-B titers; quantitative immunoglobulins, tests of cell-mediated immunity; skeletal survey; hair examination; and skin biopsy.

Primary cutaneous conditions should be considered in thriving infants. The diagnosis may not be clear until after the neonatal period. Helpful clues to the diagnosis of atopic dermatitis are involvement of the face and extensor extremities with marked sparing of the diaper area. Seborrheic dermatitis and psoriasis frequently involve the diaper area and skin folds. The skin lesions of infantile psoriasis are often sharply circumscribed, but scale may not be prominent. Genodermatoses often present with congenital erythroderma (see Sec. 14.4). Associated abnormalities and/or skin biopsy help distinguish among the disorders categorized as ichthyoses: lamellar ichthyosis, congenital nonbullous ichthyosiform erythroderma, epidermolytic hyperkeratosis, X-linked ichthyosis, multiple sulfatase deficiency, neutral lipid storage disease, Sjögren-Larsson syndrome, trichothiodystrophy, Netherton syndrome, X-linked dominant chondrodysplasia punctata, and Keratitis-Ichthyosis-Deafness (KID) syndrome. The ectodermal dysplasias are a group of disorders with abnormalities of the skin, eccrine glands,

TABLE 14-2

DIFFERENTIAL DIAGNOSIS OF NEONATAL PURPURIC NODULES

Purpura
  Ecchymoses
  Bland thrombosis—embolization of foreign material as reported in infants receiving ECMO
  Purpura fulminans—most often associated with homozygous protein C or protein S deficiency
  Infectious vasculitis—inflammatory microemboli most commonly associated with
    Gram-negative bacterial sepsis, including *E. coli, meningococcus,* and ecthyma gangrenosum [*Pseudomonas*]
    Listeriosis
    Aspergillosis
  Leukocytoclastic vasculitis
    Cryoglobulinemia
    Acute hemorrhagic edema of infancy
  Blood dyscrasias (usually presenting with widely scattered petechiae rather than purpura, and thrombocytopenia)
    Isoimmune thrombocytopenic purpura
    Maternal ITP
    Disseminated intravascular coagulopathy
Dermal hematopoiesis
  Rubella
  Cytomegalovirus
  Syphilis
  Parvovirus B19
  Other viral infections (eg, Coxsackie B2)
  Twin transfusion syndrome
  Rh hemolytic disease of the newborn
Neoplastic-infiltrative
  Congenital leukemia
  Rhabdomyosarcoma
  Langerhans cell histiocytosis
  Neuroblastoma

hair, teeth, and/or nails. Excessive desquamation resembling post-mature skin is a characteristic finding at birth. The best-recognized form is X-linked recessive hypohidrotic ectodermal dysplasia. Infants with this disorder have a decreased ability to sweat often presenting as recurrent fever of unknown origin.

PETECHIAE AND PURPURA The differential diagnosis of non-blanching purpuric nodules is listed in Table 14-2. Skin lesions of the classic "blueberry muffin" phenotype represent extramedullary hematopoiesis and occur as a result of congenital infection with syphilis (see above section on erythroderma), rubella, cytomegalovirus, coxsackievirus, or toxoplasmosis; severe intrauterine anemia from Rh or ABO incompatibility; or twin transfusion syndrome. Skin biopsy revealing nucleated red blood cells and usually other erythroid and sometimes myeloid precursors will distinguish these lesions from the purpuric nodules associated with neoplastic infiltrates from congenital leukemia or neuroblastoma. Infectious or inflammatory vasculitis can present with clinically similar but histologically distinct skin lesions. When the cause of such skin lesions is not obvious, evaluation should include the following: complete blood count with differential, platelet, and reticulocyte counts, and blood smear examination; liver function tests; cord blood for IgM concentration; maternal and cord blood for congenital infections, including syphilis; viral cultures of the nasopharynx, rectum, and urine; and biopsy of one or more skin lesions.

References

Alper JC, Holmes LB: The incidence and significance of birthmarks in a cohort of 4,641 newborns. Pediatr Dermatol 1:58–68, 1983

Basalga E, Drolet BA, Esterly NB: Purpura in infants and children. J Am Acad Dermatol 37:673–705, 1997

Cartlidge PHT, Rutter N: Skin barrier function. In: Polin RA, Fox WW, eds: Fetal and Neonatal Physiology. Philadelphia, Saunders, 1992:771–788

Frieden IJ: The dermatologist in the newborn nursery: approach to the neonate with blisters, pustules, erosions, and ulcerations. Curr Prob Dermatol 4:143–168, 1992

Holbrook KA: Structural and biochemical organogenesis of skin and cutaneous appendages in the fetus and neonate. In: Polin RA, Fox WW, eds: Fetal and Neonatal Physiology. Philadelphia, Saunders, 1992:729–752

Howard R: Congenital midline lesions. Pediatr Ann 27(3):150–162, 1998

Lane AT: Development and care of the premature infant's skin. Pediatr Dermatol 4:1, 1987

Siegfried EC: Neonatal skin care and toxicology. In: Eichenfeld LF, Frieden IJ, Esterly NB, eds: Textbook of Neonatal Dermatology. Philadelphia, Saunders, 1999

Siegfried EC: Neonatal skin and skin care. Dermatol Clin 16(3):437–446, 1998

14.3 DISORDERS OF THE EPIDERMIS

Neil S. Prose

14.3.1 Dermatitis

Dermatitis is a term commonly used to denote inflammation of the epidermis. *Eczema* is a generic term that denotes edema within the

epidermis. In its mildest or chronic form edema is seen histopathologically as prominent tooth-like interconnections between keratinocytes (spongiosis). With more intracellular fluid accumulation, intraepidermal vesicles are formed, which are subclinical in subacute eczemas, whereas in acute eczemas, grossly evident vesicles and blisters are formed. In all these, varying degrees of epidermal acanthosis and dermal perivascular inflammation are present. Allergic contact dermatitis may be acute, as in poison oak/ivy/sumac dermatitis (Fig. 14-4), or subacute to chronic, as in nickel dermatitis. Atopic dermatitis and seborrheic dermatitis may similarly be subacute or chronic.

Seborrheic dermatitis, a common disorder of infancy, begins within two months after birth. In its mildest form, "cradle cap," patches of greasy, yellowish scale develop over the scalp vertex; in more severe cases, the scalp is erythematous, and papules spill over onto the forehead and cheeks. Intertriginous sites, particularly the axillae, neck, diaper area, and retroauricular folds, commonly show erythema and greasy scale. Rarely, the eruption may become generalized. Infantile seborrheic dermatitis is usually asymptomatic and resolves spontaneously during a period of several weeks to months. When severe, treatment with 1% hydrocortisone cream, oatmeal baths, and daily shampooing of the scalp will hasten resolution. Seborrheic dermatitis is often difficult to differentiate with certainty from atopic dermatitis. Pruritus and recurrence after therapy are usually indicative of atopic dermatitis. Histiocytosis X must be excluded by skin biopsy in all patients with unusually severe seborrheic dermatitis, particularly if clinical signs of a destructive process, such as atrophy, ulceration, or purpura, are present (Color Plate 14; Sec. 14.7). Psoriasis or a psoriasiform id reaction should be considered in patients with well-circumscribed and widespread lesions (Color Plates 3, 4).

In adolescents, seborrheic dermatitis usually manifests as dandruff, or diffuse scalp scaling which is often pruritic and may be accompanied by midfacial erythema and scaling. This dermatitis usually responds to frequent zinc or tar shampoos; with severe scalp involvement, a topical corticosteroid solution (eg, 0.025% triamcinolone or 0.01% fluocinolone) may be used. Relapse is common.

The etiology of seborrheic dermatitis is poorly understood; however, active sebaceous glands are required. Hence, seborrheic dermatitis is rarely the correct diagnosis for a scalp disorder in children between 1 and 12 years. Tinea capitis and head lice must be

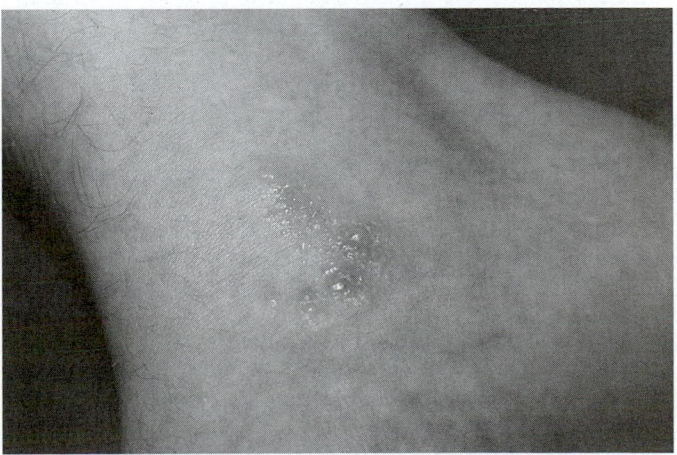

FIGURE 14-4 Poison ivy dermatitis. Mildly erythematous curvilinear collection of vesicles in a patient with early contact dermatitis to oleoresin from Rhus. (*Courtesy of Amy Paller, M.D.*)

1176   14.3   DISORDERS OF THE EPIDERMIS

excluded, and atopic dermatitis and psoriasis are the most common noninfectious causes of scalp scaling and/or pruritus in this age group. Most recently, a role for *Pityrosporum orbiculare* (a dimorphous yeast normally resident on the skin) in the pathogenesis of seborrheic dermatitis has been postulated, and clinical improvement with use of topical antifungal agents (eg, ketoconazole cream) has been noted.

Diaper dermatitis is among the most common of all pediatric disorders. In most cases, diaper rash begins as a nonallergic, irritant dermatitis caused by the combination of occlusion, friction, and wetness. Irritant diaper dermatitis is most prominent on the lower abdomen, inner thighs, and on the buttocks, and tends to spare the folds. Irritant diaper dermatitis occurs more frequently in the setting of diarrhea. The causative factors are the wetness, leading to edema of the stratum corneum and increased absorption of irritants, and stool proteases and lipases, which are most active at higher pH. Treatment involves frequent diaper changes, use of superabsorbent diapers, avoiding excessive washing, and application of a protective paste. Occasionally, a few days of application of topical hydrocortisone are necessary. *Candida albicans* commonly infects the diaper area, particularly if the irritant rash has been present for a few days or if the patient is being administered oral antibiotic therapy. Anticandidal therapy should be instituted in these settings, as well as where clinical signs, such as satellite pustules or intense erythema, suggest *Candida* dermatitis. Other common causes of dermatitis in the diaper area include seborrheic dermatitis and impetigo. Perianal streptococcal disease may present as mild erythema and scaling; it can be excluded by culture. Uncommonly, psoriasis, dermatophyte infection, and Langerhans cell histiocytosis (Sec. 14.7) may present as diaper rash.

Psoriasiform id reaction is an uncommon dermatosis that follows a severe candidal diaper dermatitis. Typically, as the diaper dermatitis is resolving, multiple well-circumscribed erythematous, scaly plaques develop over the body and particularly the scalp (Color Plate 3). Lesions evolve during one to three weeks, then slowly resolve in four to six weeks. Despite the intensity of the eruption, most infants are asymptomatic. In some, but not all, instances, candidal organisms have been recovered from distant lesions. Either atopic dermatitis or typical psoriasis will develop in a significant fraction of patients in later childhood. The diaper dermatitis or typical psoriasis is inappropriately high for this location. The distant lesions may be treated with antipsoriatic therapy (eg, triamcinolone 0.025% and liquor carbonis detergis [LCD] 5% in aquaphor); however, it is not clear that therapy shortens disease duration.

Nutritional and metabolic disorders should be considered in the infant with persistent dermatitis. *Zinc deficiency* results in a periorificial and acral dermatitis. Lesions are typically sharply marginated, eroded, and crusted plaques (Fig. 14-5) but may be psoriasiform in nature. *Candida albicans* is commonly isolated from the lesions but is a secondary invader. Dermatitis and diarrhea are usually the first signs of zinc deficiency, but with time these are accompanied by alopecia and irritability. Death from intercurrent infection is the expected outcome if zinc deficiency is not recognized or treated. Zinc deficiency may occur as an acquired or as an inherited disorder. *Acrodermatitis enteropathica.* Acrodermatitis enteropathica (see Fig. 14-5) is an autosomal-recessive trait, caused by impaired in-

testinal absorption of zinc. Symptoms of zinc deficiency usually develop after weaning from breast milk, owing to the poorer bioavailability of zinc in cow's milk. Acquired zinc deficiency is most commonly observed during prolonged total parenteral nutrition with inadequate zinc supplements but also may occur with malabsorption syndromes or chelation therapy. Premature infants are especially prone to zinc deficiency because of low stores and high requirements. Some mothers produce breast milk that is very low in zinc, and symptomatic zinc deficiency has been reported in this setting, particularly in premature infants. The diagnosis is established by a low plasma zinc concentration; care must be taken when obtaining the blood sample to avoid all contact with zinc-containing rubber materials. Response to zinc therapy (1 mg/kg/d ele-

TABLE 14-3 TOPICAL CORTICOSTEROID THERAPY

VEHICLE	COMMENTS
Creams	Best for acute eruptions
	Generally less effective than ointments
	May contain irritants or sensitizers
Ointments	Best for chronic dermatoses and palmoplantar eruption
	Generally most effective formulation
	Greasy quality may be undesirable
	Excellent emolliency
Gels	Best for hairy or greasy sites
	Generally effective formulations
	May sting on application
	Poor emolliency
Solutions	Good for hairy sites
	May sting on application

Potency of ointment vehicle (cream vehicle generally one to two classes lower)

Super*	Clobetasol propionate 0.05%
	Flurandrenolide tape
	Betamethasone dipropionate 0.05% (optimized)
	Halobetasol propionate 0.05%
Very high	Mometasone furoate 0.05%
	Diflorasone diacetate 0.05%
	Betamethasone dipropionate 0.05% (nonoptimized)
	Fluocinonide 0.05%
	Desoximetasone 0.25%
High	Triamcinolone acetonide 0.5%
	Betamethasone valerate 0.1%
	Halcinonide 0.1%
Medium-high	Fluticasone propionate 0.005%
	Triamcinolone acetonide 0.1%
	Flurandrenolide 0.05%
	Fluocinolone 0.025%
Medium	Triamcinolone acetonide 0.025%
	Desonide 0.05%+
	Alclometasone dipropionate 0.05%†
	Hydrocortisone valerate 0.2%†
	Hydrocortisone butyrate 0.1%†
	Fluocinolone acetonide 0.01%
Low	Hydrocortisone 1%, 2.5%†

* Rarely if ever indicated in children; high potential for local atrophy and systemic effects.
† Nonhalogenated; less potential for atrophy and other local effects.

CHAPTER 14 / THE SKIN

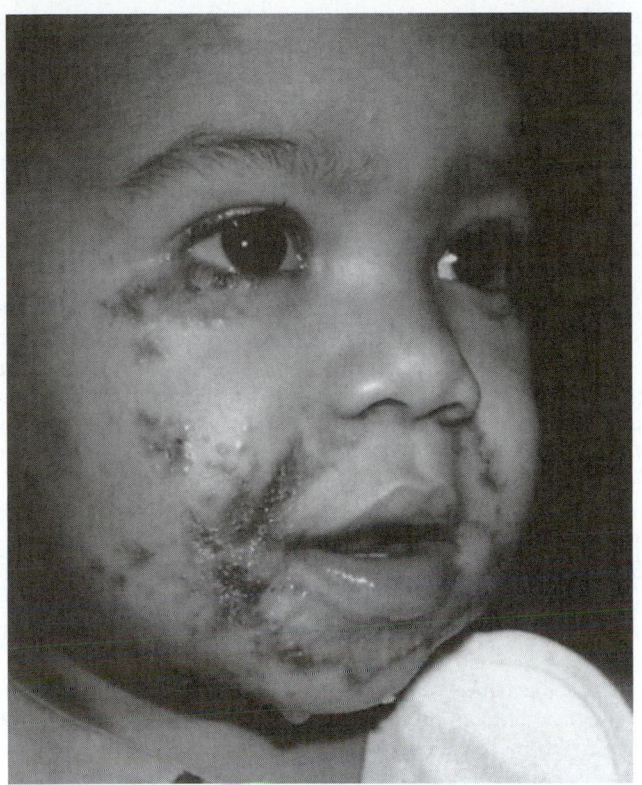

FIGURE 14-5   Acrodermatitis enteropathica. Note crusted, erosive periorificial dermatitis. (*Courtesy of Ilona Frieden, M.D.*)

mental zinc; given as zinc sulfate or gluconate) is rapid (ie, two to four days) and dramatic. A trial of zinc therapy is indicated in all infants with a suggestive clinical phenotype, even if plasma zinc concentrations are normal. The dose of zinc should be adjusted to normalize plasma zinc levels and maintain a normal growth rate. In acrodermatitis enteropathica, 10 to 45 mg elemental zinc is needed per day to overcome the absorptive defect.

Biotin deficiency may produce a cutaneous phenotype identical with zinc deficiency and occurs similarly in both acquired and genetic forms. The late infantile form of *biotin-responsive multiple carboxylase deficiency,* caused by biotinidase deficiency, commonly presents with rash and/or alopecia. Central nervous system symptoms, including ataxia, seizures, and developmental delay, and acidosis are present in most patients with time but may be episodic. Diagnosis is established by demonstration of decreased biotinidase activity in blood. Blood biotin concentrations are usually low, and urinary organic acid concentrations are increased, but values within the normal range do not exclude the diagnosis. A trial of biotin (at least 10 mg/d) is indicated for all patients with a suggestive clinical picture. Like zinc deficiency, the response is rapid and usually dramatic. Acquired biotin deficiency is rare and usually seen in patients undergoing prolonged parenteral nutrition or who ingest large quantities of egg whites that contain avidin, which binds biotin and prevents intestinal absorption.

Eczematous dermatitis has also been observed in *essential fatty acid deficiency.* Dry skin with eczematous changes in conjunction with hypopigmentation is seen in children with protein malnutrition (kwashiorkor). Periorificial dermatitis may also be the presenting sign of *cystic fibrosis,* often owing to multiple nutritional deficiencies, including zinc and essential fatty acids.

References

Boiko S: Treatment of diaper dermatitis. Dermatol Clin 17:235–240, 1999

Bosch AM, Sillevis Smitt JH, Van Gennip AH, et al: Iatrogenic isolated isoleucine deficiency at the cause of an acrodermatitis-enteropathica-like syndrome. Br J Dermatol 139(3):488–491, 1998

Darmstadt GL, Schmidt CP, Wechsler DS, Tunnessen WW, Rosenstein BJ: Dermatitis as a presenting sign of cystic fibrosis. Arch Dermatol 128: 1358–1364, 1992

Glover MT, Atherton DJ: Transient zinc deficiency in two full-term breast-fed siblings associated with low maternal breast milk zinc concentrations. Pediatr Dermatol 5:10–13, 1988

Singalavanija S, Frieden IJ: Diaper dermatitis. Pediatr Rev 16:142–147, 1995

Williams ML: Differential diagnosis of seborrheic dermatitis. Pediatr Rev 7: 204–211, 1986

14.3.2   Atopic Dermatitis

Atopic dermatitis is among the most common of all childhood skin diseases. This discussion focuses on the clinical morphology, differential diagnosis, and dermatologic management. The typical clinical finding is an ill-defined patch or plaque of scaling and erythema. Pruritus is a constant feature. Chronic scratching results in dramatic accentuation of the skin markings (lichenification), sometimes with postinflammatory hyperpigmentation, whereas the chronic eczematous process itself may result in hypopigmentation.

In infancy, lesions are most often found on the cheeks and the extensor surfaces of the extremities, but involvement of scalp and trunk is also common; in severe episodes the rash may become generalized. In school-aged children, atopic dermatitis favors the antecubital and popliteal fossae, and the posterior neck (Fig. 14-6). Ankles, wrists, and dorsa of hands and feet are also commonly involved. Occasionally disease is widespread and severe. Asians may be particularly prone to severe disease, and a papular, follicular variant of atopic dermatitis is seen in black children. Several subtle physical findings may be of help in establishing the diagnosis, including accentuation of skin markings on palms and soles; double or triple creases under the lower eyelid (Dennie-Morgan folds); conspicuous sparing of the central face ("headlight sign"); and small fissures at the base of the ear lobe. Generalized xerosis (dry

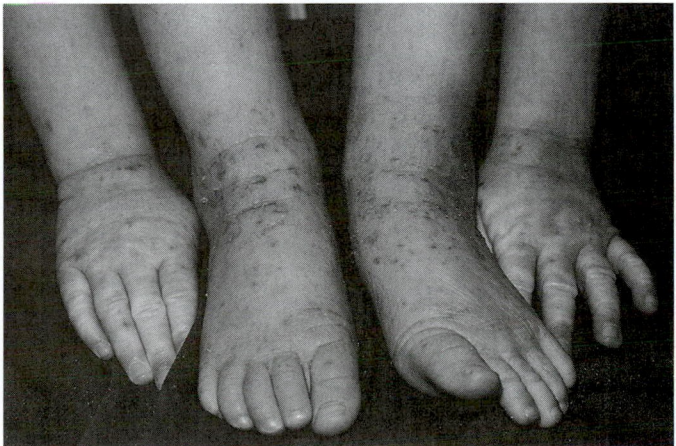

FIGURE 14-6   Atopic dermatitis. The ankle region and the dorsum of the hands and feet are covered with excoriations, and crusting from the chronic dermatitis and secondary staphylococcal infection. (*Courtesy of Amy Paller, M.D.*)

skin) is almost invariably present. The histopathology of atopic dermatitis is that of a subacute to chronic eczema, with a prominent perivascular infiltrate, often with signs of acute or chronic excoriations.

Perhaps as the result of T-cell dysfunction, atopic individuals are at risk for widespread cutaneous infection with molluscum contagiosum, and herpes simplex (eczema herpeticum). The latter presents as multiple vesicles or punched-out erosions that may be grouped or dispersed and are found on both normal and eczematized skin (Fig. 14-7). Whereas *Staphylococcus aureus* is not normally resident on skin, both uninvolved and involved areas in atopics can be colonized with *S. aureus*. Impetiginous lesions are a frequent complication of atopic dermatitis and manifest as serous crusting. Patients with severe impetigo may have fever, adenopathy, foul odor, and superficial erosions. Staphylococcal folliculitis should be considered in patients with marked pruritus and widespread excoriations. These lesions are extremely pruritic and soon excoriated; thus, a careful examination is needed to identify a follicular pustule.

Patients with atopic dermatitis also show evidence of altered autonomic function, as manifested clinically by a white rather than red flare in response to scratching or intradermal methacholine injection. This may be related to the clinical observation that, in atopic dermatitis, itching appears to precede the dermatitis and, if scratching is prevented, dermatitis will not develop.

The treatment of infants and children with atopic dermatitis must be individualized and based on disease severity. It is useful to divide therapeutic strategies into those aimed at treating the rash and those aimed at preventing future disease. Parents tend to focus on identification of "the cause." It is unusual, however, that one or a few environmental factors can be identified that, when eliminated, will lead to the hoped-for "cure." Rather, this is a condition of inherited skin "sensitivity"; that is, a variety of precipitating factors, such as dry skin (xerosis), heat, infection, specific allergens, topical irritants, and/or psychological state, may be responsible to varying degrees for a given flare of the disease. Once established, the dermatitis tends to be self-perpetuating, such that elimination of the original inciting factors may not lead to resolution of the

rash. Therefore, it is important that initial efforts be directed toward treatment of the dermatitis and its complications.

Topical corticosteroids are the mainstay in treatment of the dermatitis (Table 14-3). Because of their better emolliency and greater potency, ointments are generally preferred over creams. However, some patients with atopic dermatitis may not tolerate ointment vehicles because of increased pruritus. In general, the mildest corticosteroid that will be effective should be chosen. The prolonged use of potent corticosteroids can result in local skin atrophy, manifested by transparent skin with prominent blood vessels, telangiectasia, and cigarette-paper-like wrinkling, which is indicative of epidermal thinning. Atrophy, if unrecognized, may progress to permanent stria formation. Systemic absorption of corticosteroid, which is enhanced across dermatitic skin, can result in adrenal suppression and even iatrogenic Cushing disease. Systemic effects depend on the inherent potency of the corticosteroid, its percutaneous transport, the relative surface area treated, and the surface area–body volume ratio. "Ultrapotent" corticosteroids (class I) may readily induce local skin atrophy and adrenal suppression in adults when applied to only limited areas (eg, elbows and knees) for a few weeks. Use of agents such as clobetasol (optimized form of betamethasone dipropionate) is rarely if ever indicated in children.

Atopic dermatitis can be adequately and safely controlled with the use of a mild, nonfluorinated steroid such as 1% hydrocortisone ointment in most patients (Table 14-3). In more severe flares or on unresponsive lesions, a medium- to high-potency steroid may be indicated. As soon as possible, usually after 5 to 14 days, patients should be switched to a milder corticosteroid; thereafter, use of higher-potency steroids should be limited to focal, resistant lesions. Flexural areas are particularly prone to stria formation, and long-term high-potency steroid therapy must be strictly avoided in these regions. All fluorinated and high-potency corticosteroids should be avoided on the face and in the diaper region.

Oral antihistamines are useful adjuncts to therapy for control of pruritus. In acute flares, doses may need to be increased until sedation is achieved. Nonsedating antihistamines are for the most part

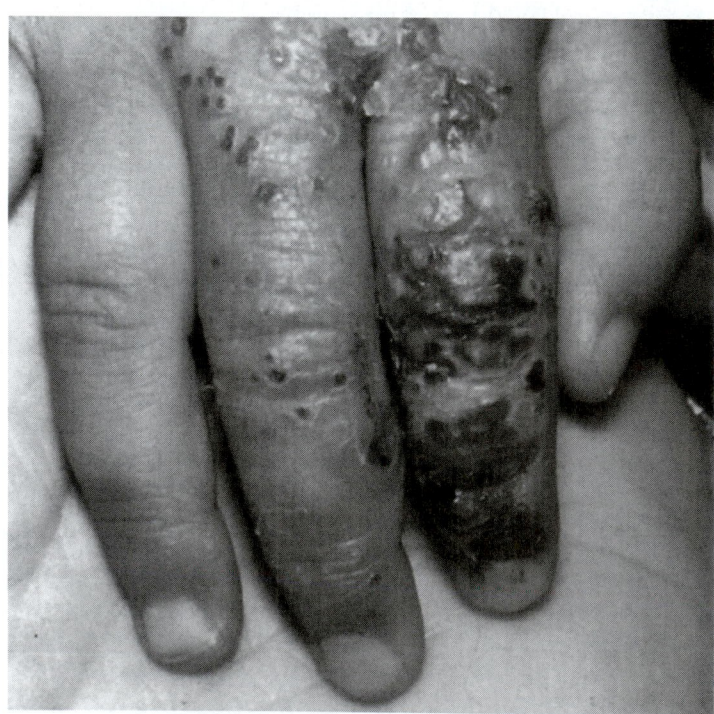

FIGURE 14-7 **Eczema herpeticum (Kaposi varicelliform eruption). Clustered erosions from ruptured vesicles, superimposed on a chronic lichenified plaque of atopic dermatitis. Widespread involvement may be associated with fever and malaise, and systemic antiviral therapy is usually indicated. (*Courtesy of Mary Williams, M.D.*)**

ineffective. With milder disease, a single night time dose is given to reduce scratching during the night. Oral antibiotics are indicated in children who show evidence of superinfection, such as serous crusting of lesions or follicular pustules, or in children who are not responding to therapy. Prophylactic antibiotic therapy is not advisable because of the potential for emergence of antibiotic resistance.

Although systemic corticosteroids almost invariably result in rapid improvement, attempts to taper or discontinue the drug are very commonly associated with a severe rebound flare. Because of this problem, and in view of the numerous side effects associated with their long-term use, systemic corticosteroids should be avoided in the management of atopic dermatitis. Most patients experiencing a severe generalized flare will respond within three to five days to a course of intensive topical therapy. Compresses using soft cotton cloths soaked in cool tap water are applied to erythematous skin for 20 minutes four to six times a day followed by application of triamcinolone 0.1% ointment or cream. Antihistamines should be given in sedative doses, and secondary bacterial, fungal, or viral infection treated. Patients in whom this regimen fails at home will invariably respond in the hospital.

Oral cyclosporine may be an effective short-term treatment option for children with disease that is unresponsive to other therapies. This medication must be used with great caution, monitoring for potential systemic side effects. Recent studies suggest that the topical application of tacrolimus ointment may be a safe and effective treatment modality for atopic dermatitis. The safety and efficacy of this medication will continue to be evaluated.

The most significant aspect of preventive therapy (Table 14-4) is decreasing skin dryness. This aim may be achieved by the liberal and frequent use of emollients (ointments are preferred to creams and particularly to lotions) and by avoidance of frequent bathing with strongly alkaline soaps. In dry environments or during the winter months, room humidification, when not contraindicated by respiratory tract mold sensitivities, is also of benefit. Attention to other factors that induce pruritus, such as woolen or synthetic fabrics, heat, sweating, and "stress," is also important in the management of atopic dermatitis. Most children respond to standard dermatologic therapy and do not require investigation of dietary triggers or food avoidance.

Atopic dermatitis is characterized by frequent remissions and exacerbations. Parents and children must understand that the treatments outlined above suppress the disease process but do not result in cure. Fortunately, the majority of children improve with age, and most are free of disease by adolescence. A national support group, the National Eczema Association for Science and Education, is available by email at *nease@teleport.com* or by telephone at 1-800-818-7546.

Several other skin disorders are more common in children with atopic dermatitis or with a familial atopic diathesis. *Pityriasis alba* is common in school-aged children and is characterized by ill-defined areas of hypopigmentation, often with a fine scale (Color Plate 5). It occurs most commonly on the cheeks, but may be seen in other locations. The pathologic process is that of a mild eczema, often caused by overdrying of the skin, which may be subclinical, and is followed by postinflammatory hypopigmentation, most evident in dark-skinned children. Vitiligo is differentiated by its sharply delineated borders surrounding totally depigmented, nonscaly macules. Tinea is distinguished by the presence of an "active border" (Color Plate 26) and a positive KOH preparation (Fig. 14-3). A mild topical corticosteroid ointment (eg, 1% hydrocortisone) may be used to treat the dermatitis; with time repigmentation will follow. Keratosis pilaris is also more common in atopic patients. Like pityriasis alba, it appears to be a manifestation of the dry skin that accompanies atopic dermatitis.

Juvenile plantar dermatosis (JPD) is a recurrent skin disorder characterized by erythema and fissuring of the weight-bearing part of the plantar surface. JPD is somewhat more common in children with atopic dermatitis and is frequently misdiagnosed as tinea pedis. The disorder occurs primarily during the winter months and is probably caused by the combined effects of hyperhidrosis and repeated wetting and drying of the feet. Occlusive shoes, such as rubber-soled sneakers, may exacerbate the condition. Treatment consists of repeated applications of petrolatum for lubrication and an absorbent powder (eg, Zeazorb). Occasionally a moderate-strength topical corticosteroid ointment (eg, 0.025% triamcinolone) is helpful.

Dyshidrotic eczema (pompholyx) is a recurrent, acute eczematous eruption involving the hands and, less commonly, the feet. The development of small, firm vesicles on the lateral borders of the finger is characteristic. The disorder is intensely pruritic, and subsequent fissuring of the fingers and palms may be painful. Control of this disorder may be achieved by the use of emollients and potent topical corticosteroids (eg, fluocinonide ointment).

TABLE 14-4
TOPICAL THERAPY FOR SCALING SKIN DISORDERS

TYPE AND EXAMPLES	COMMENTS
Emollients	
Petrolatum, lanolin, bath oils	Least irritating
	Do not remove scales
Hygroscopic agents	
10 to 20% urea	Nongreasy
	May sting on application
	Irritating
Keratolytic agents	
5 to 12% lactic acid	Most effective compounded in petrolatum
5 to 10% glycolic acid	
	May sting on application
	Irritating
	? Risk of lactic acidosis
2 to 16% salicylic acid	May sting on application
	Irritating
	Risk of salicylism with widespread application
Retinoids	
0.025 to 0.1% topical retinoic acid	Difficult to use because of irritancy
0.1 adapalene gel, solution	
0.05% to 0.1% tazarotene gel	Cream vehicle best tolerated
Synthetic vitamin D derivatives	
0.05% calcipotriene ointment	May be irritating

References

Apter AJ, Rothe MJ, Grant-Kels JM: Allergy consultation in the management of atopic dermatitis. Pediatr Dermatol 8:341–347, 1997

Berth-Jones J, Finlay AY, Zaki I, et al: Cyclosporine in severe childhood atopic dermatitis: a multicenter study. J Am Acad Dermatol 34:1016–1021, 1996

Halbert AR, Weston WL, Morelli JG: Atopic dermatitis: is it an allergic disease? J Am Acad Dermatol 33:1008–1018, 1995

Rothe MJ, Grant-Kels JM: Atopic dermatitis: an update. J Am Acad Dermatol 35:1–13, 1996

Ruzicka T, Assmann T, Homey B: Tacrolimus: the drug for the turn of the millennium? Arch Dermatol 135:574–580, 1999

14.3.3   Contact Dermatitis

Primary irritant contact dermatitis is caused by the direct effects of chemicals or physical substances on the skin. The most common primary irritants are detergents, acids, alkalis and harsh soaps, urine, and particularly feces (see discussion of diaper dermatitis, Sec. 14.3.1). *Allergic contact dermatitis* is a form of delayed or cell-mediated immunity. The induction of sensitivity occurs in three stages: formation of conjugates consisting of proteins and haptens, recognition of conjugated antigen, and proliferation of sensitized lymphocytes. The Langerhans cell, which takes up and processes the antigen, plays an essential role in this process. On cutaneous reexposure to antigen, antigen-specific effector T cells release lymphokines and recruit mononuclear cells to the area of involvement. Acute allergic contact dermatitis is characterized by intense pruritus, erythema, and vesiculation, and chronic reactions are scaly rather than vesicular. Allergic contact dermatitis is quite unusual in children younger than two years. The most common cause of contact dermatitis among children in the United States is exposure to poison ivy, oak, or sumac, all members of the genus *Toxicodendron* (formerly, *Rhus*). All portions of the plant contain the antigen. An intensely pruritic eruption begins 7 to 14 days after exposure in primary sensitization reactions and after 1 to 4 days in subsequent exposures. Rash is most common on the lower extremities but may occur at any location. The presence of a linear streak of erythema and vesiculation is a particularly helpful clinical sign (Fig. 14-4). Transfer of antigen to areas of sensitive skin (eg, face and eyelids, penis and scrotum) may result in marked dermal edema and swelling.

Treatment of mild contact dermatitis consists of cool soaks when an acute, vesicular eruption is present and of topical corticosteroid (eg, triamcinolone 0.1%) creams. When involvement is extensive and severe, a two- to three-week course of oral prednisone should be considered (eg, 2 mg/kg/d for 5 to 7 days; then 1 mg/kg/d for 5 to 7 days; then 0.5 mg/kg/d for 5 to 7 days). Children with allergy to *Toxicodendron* should be taught to recognize the plants.

Shoe allergy presents as a scaly, pruritic eruption on the dorsum of feet and toes. The antigen may be rubber or rubber accelerators, adhesives, tanning agents, dyes, or leather. Patch testing is needed to determine the cause and to develop a preventive strategy.

Nickel allergy is a common cause of chronic contact dermatitis and is usually localized to sites where earrings, bracelets, necklaces, or the metal clasp or zipper of a garment comes into contact with the skin (Fig. 14-8). Ear piercing leads to nickel sensitization in approximately 20% of individuals. This commonly presents with redness and oozing at the pierced site and can be mistaken for bacterial infection. Jewelry made of surgical stainless steel or 22K gold is usually tolerated. Other common causes of allergic contact dermatitis include **cosmetics** and **adhesives** in tapes or bandages. The worsening of any skin condition in the face of topical therapy should raise the possibility of an allergic contact dermatitis to a component of the medicament.

Neomycin and the "-caine" type of **topical anesthetics** are frequent sensitizers.

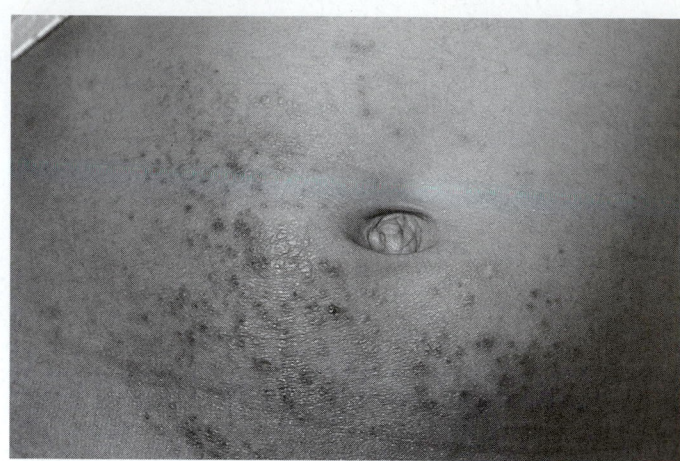

FIGURE 14-8   Subumbilical and periumbilical erythematous papules and vesicles with dryness and excoriations related to a contact dermatitis reaction to the nickel in the snap of this child's jeans. (*Courtesy of Amy Paller, M.D.*)

References

Manzini BM, Ferdani G, Simonetti V, et al: Contact sensitization in children. Pediatr Dermatol 15:12–17, 1998

Rademaker M, Forsyth R: Contact dermatitis in children. Contact Derm 20:104–107, 1989

Weston JA, Hawkins K, Weston WL: Foot dermatitis in children. Pediatrics 72:824–827, 1983

14.3.4   Psoriasis

Psoriasis is a chronic disease of exacerbations and remissions that affects approximately 1% of the population. Disease develops before the age of 20 years in 35% of patients. Although psoriasis is believed to be genetically determined, the inheritance pattern has not been defined. In 50% of affected children, a positive family history is present. The prototypic lesion of psoriasis is a uniform erythematous plaque, sharply delineated from the surrounding normal skin, and covered with tightly adherent, silvery scale (Color Plate 4). A useful diagnostic feature, the Auspitz sign, is the presence of pinpoint bleeding after the removal of scale. Lesions vary in size from pinhead-sized papules to extensive plaques and show a predilection for the elbows, knees, scalp, penis, and gluteal cleft ("gluteal pinking"). The classic, plaque form of psoriasis is seen most commonly in older children and adolescents. The development of psoriatic lesions in areas of trauma is termed the *Koebner phenomenon* or *isomorphic response* and denotes active disease. Nail involvement may take the form of numerous small pits arranged in vertical strips, detachment of the nail plate distally (onycholysis), or marked subungual hyperkeratosis.

Guttate psoriasis is particularly common in childhood and is characterized by the rapid development of numerous small scaly papules and plaques on the trunk, face, and proximal extremities. Streptococcal pharyngitis and, more recently, perianal streptococcal disease have been implicated as provocative factors for guttate psoriasis.

Psoriasis during infancy is relatively rare but may be severe and generalized. The diaper area is often the presenting site, and the persistent rash may easily be confused with candidiasis or seborrheic dermatitis. The transient psoriasiform id reaction after a severe candidal diaper dermatitis must also be distinguished (Color Plate 3). Pustular psoriasis and generalized psoriatic erythroderma are rare forms of the disease that may occur occasionally during childhood.

Although psoriasis is most often easily diagnosed on the basis of clinical appearance, skin biopsy is sometimes helpful. The most typical histologic features are acanthosis with evenly elongated rete ridges, neutrophilic spongiform pustules within the epidermis, parakeratotic stratum corneum containing neutrophils, and tortuous, dilated capillaries within dermal papillae. The epidermis is hyperproliferative in psoriasis, but the underlying cause is unknown. Although earlier investigations suggested a primary defect in epidermal maturation and/or regulation of growth and proliferation, more recent work is also supportive of a defect in immunoregulation. Some investigators have suggested that infections with microorganisms, particularly β-hemolytic streptococcus (of either the oropharynx or perianal skin) and *Candida albicans,* may be important factors in the pathogenesis of the disease. Although these infections may be clinically linked to psoriatic flares, the mechanisms whereby they induce or exacerbate psoriasis are unknown.

The natural history of psoriasis is one of remissions and exacerbations. Flares may be triggered by infection, trauma to the skin, or "stress." Although usually a lifelong disease, prolonged remissions can occur. Tar preparations and topical corticosteroids are most commonly used in the treatment of psoriasis. Anthralin (0.1 to 0.5%) creams or ointments may be applied briefly (less than 30 minutes) and then carefully washed off; care must be taken to avoid staining adjacent skin, and prolonged exposure can produce significant irritation. Monitored exposure to sunlight or to an artificial source of ultraviolet B light (suberythemagenic doses, three times a week) is a useful adjunct to tar or anthralin therapy.

Medium-to-high-potency topical corticosteroids (Table 14-3) are often used in conjunction with other therapies. In all chronic dermatoses, topical corticosteroids must be employed with caution because long-term use may be associated with local skin atrophy; widespread application may result in significant percutaneous absorption and adrenal suppression. Systemic corticosteroids are contraindicated in psoriasis because of the risk of inducing a pustular, rebound flare. Newer treatment modalities include topical calcipitriol and topical tazarotene gel. Both of these therapies are effective in some patients but may also cause significant skin irritation.

Scalp psoriasis is particularly difficult to control. The combination of a tar shampoo, topical steroid solution or gel (Table 14-4), and a salicylic acid preparation for the removal of scale (eg, Keralyt gel) may be successful. For patients with severe, erythrodermic or pustular psoriasis, psoralens and ultraviolet light (PUVA) or oral etretinate may be necessary. The potential toxicities associated with these treatments require supervision by an experienced physician. The National Psoriasis Foundation provides support for patients by email at *76135.2746@compuserve.com* or by telephone at 1-800-723-9166.

References

Atherton DJ, Cohen BL, Knobler E, et al: Phototherapy for children. Pediatr Dermatol 13:415–426, 1996

Farber EM, Mullen RH, Jacobs AH, Nall L: Infantile psoriasis: a follow-up study. Pediatr Dermatol 3:237, 1986

Honig PJ: Guttate psoriasis associated with perianal streptococcal disease. J Pediatr 113:1037–1039, 1988

Menter MA, Whiting DA, McWilliams J: Resistant childhood psoriasis: an analysis of patients seen in a day-care center. Pediatr Dermatol 2:8, 1984

Oranje AP, Marcoux D, Svensson A, et al: Topical calcipotriol in childhood psoriasis. J Am Acad Dermatol 36:203–208, 1997

Watson W, Farber EM: Psoriasis in childhood. Pediatr Clin North Am 18: 875–895, 1971

14.3.5   Other Papulosquamous Disorders

Pityriasis rosea (PR) is a common, generalized, and self-limited dermatosis. It is characterized by the progressive eruption of numerous round to oval, salmon-colored, 2- to 10-mm flat patches bearing a peripheral ring of scale. Atypical lesions may be smaller, papular, or even vesicular. Intense pruritus may occur. The lesions characteristically align along skin lines. On the back and chest, this arrangement resembles the sloping branches of a Christmas tree, but it courses horizontally in the axillary area (Fig. 14-9). The lesions favor the trunk, upper arms, legs, and, particularly, the axilla; the face is usually spared, except in young children. Involvement of palms and soles should suggest an alternative diagnosis, especially secondary syphilis, which can closely mimic PR. In sexually active adolescents, serologic testing for syphilis is mandatory. A single, larger, well-circumscribed area of erythema and scale on the trunk or extremities—the *herald patch*—may precede the generalized rash by several weeks and may be commonly mistaken for a lesion of tinea corporis or nummular eczema.

The cause of PR is unknown. Infectious etiologies suggested by the occasional temporal and geographic clustering of cases, by infrequent symptoms of fatigue or pharyngitis, and by the rarity of recurrences have not been substantiated. PR usually resolves in four to six weeks, and most patients require no treatment. Mild pruritus may be managed with emollients and oral antihistamines. More severe, symptomatic cases may benefit from suberythemagenic doses of ultraviolet light (UVB) two to three times a week.

Lichen planus is an uncommon dermatosis of unknown etiology that occurs most often in middle-aged adults; only 2% of cases develop before the age of 20. The characteristic lesions of lichen planus are intensely pruritic, violaceous, sharply defined polygonal

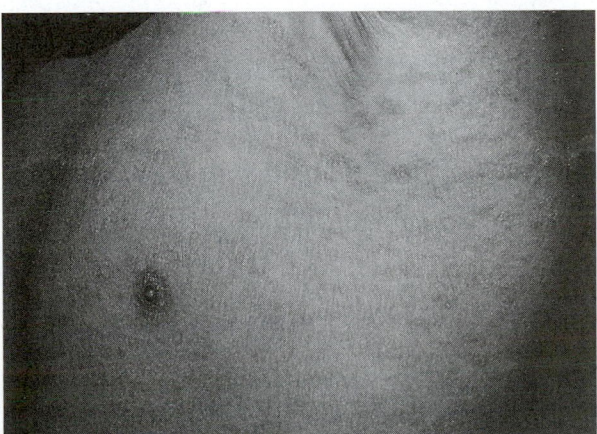

FIGURE 14-9 The trunk is covered with elliptical papulosquamous lesions with their long axis running along skin lines and thus oriented horizontally in the axillary area. Scaling tends to be largely at the periphery of lesions. (*Courtesy of Amy Paller, M.D.*)

papules on the forearms, flexor surfaces of the wrists, and extensor surfaces of the lower extremities. Oral involvement appears as a lacy array of tiny white papules on the buccal mucosa or tongue. Nail changes, which may progress from longitudinal ridging to severe nail dystrophy, are seen in 10% of patients. In rare variants of lichen planus, there may be bullous, linear, hypertrophic, or annular lesions or scarring alopecia. On biopsy, the disease is distinguished by a band-like infiltrate along the dermal-epidermal junction with partial destruction of the basal cell layer, in conjunction with hyperkeratosis and increased thickness of the granular layer. The duration of lichen planus varies from months to years, and relapses or reurrences occur in 20% of patients. Treatment consists of antihistamines, moderate potency topical corticosteroid ointments, or systemic steroids in severe or generalized cases (see Table 14-3).

Lichen striatus is a relatively common childhood skin disease, characterized by a linear array of small, violaceous, flesh-colored, or hypopigmented papules that are asymptomatic and self-limited, resolving over several months to a year (Fig. 14-10). The arms and legs are most commonly affected. Treatment is usually not required; however, a mild topical corticosteroid cream (2.5% hydrocortisone) is useful for symptomatic patients. Both lichen striatus and epidermal nevi occur in "Blaschko's lines" (Color Plate 8); however, epidermal nevi are usually more verrucous and do not involute.

Lichen nitidus is a benign, self-limited eruption composed of minute, pink-red or flesh-colored papules that may be asymptomatic or extremely pruritic. In black children, the papules of lichen nitidus are hypopigmented. Lesions favor the trunk, wrists, genitalia, and inner thighs but may be widespread. Papules tend to be grouped in patches or plaques; the presence of a linear array of papules within a scratch (the Koebner phenomenon) is a useful diagnostic finding. The skin biopsy is diagnostic, showing a discrete nest of histiocytes and lymphocytes in the upper dermis surrounded by an epidermal lip. Lichen nitidus resolves spontaneously over several months to years; the cause is not known, and there is no effective therapy.

Pityriasis rubra pilaris (PRP) is a rare skin disorder of unknown etiology. At its onset, the lesions are composed of small, tapered follicular papules that are best appreciated on the dorsal surface of the proximal phalanges or over elbows or knees. Scaling and erythema of the scalp and marked thickening of the palms and soles

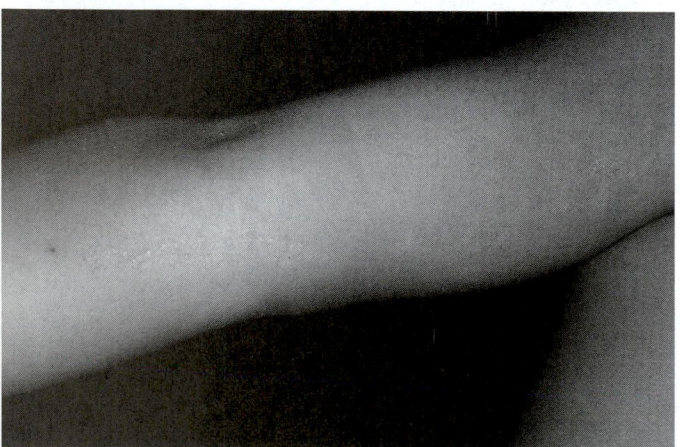

FIGURE 14-10 Streak of flat-topped, slightly erythematous papules coursing down the arm along a line of Blaschko. (*Courtesy of Amy Paller, M.D.*)

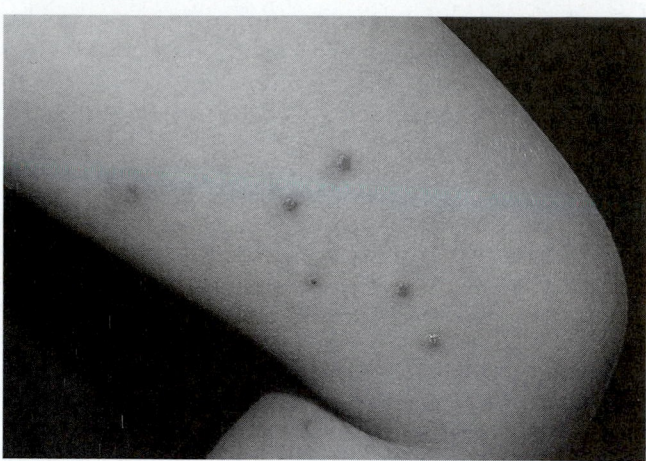

FIGURE 14-11 Pityriasis lichenoides et varioliformis acuta (PLEVA). The lesions of PLEVA are most commonly discrete papules that may be violaceous in color and erode spontaneously. They may be mistaken for bite reactions or chicken pox. (*Courtesy of Amy Paller, M.D.*)

are also characteristic. Over time, these papules coalesce into yellow to pink scaly plaques or a generalized exfoliative erythroderma that may contain islands of normal skin. The skin biopsy shows follicular plugging, perifollicular parakeratosis, and a superficial perivascular inflammatory infiltrate, features that are characteristic but not diagnostic. Disease can be either mild and localized or, rarely, severe and generalized. The majority of patients experience a complete remission within months to a few years. Topical keratolytics (Table 14-4) may be used for palmoplantar hyperkeratoses. Oral synthetic retinoids (eg, isotretinoin or etretinate) may be indicated in the severe cases. These potent drugs should be prescribed only by experienced physicians.

Pityriasis lichenoides et varioliformis acuta (PLEVA; Mucha-Habermann disease) is characterized by the rapid onset of numerous papules, macules, and papulovesicles, usually involving the trunk and extremities (Fig. 14-11). The face, scalp, palms, and soles are usually spared. The lesions of PLEVA evolve in crops, rapidly form hemorrhagic crusts, and, especially in black children, may resolve with severe postinflammatory hypopigmentation. *Pityriasis lichenoides chronica* (PLC) is a more persistent form of this disease process, and it is characterized by scaly papules and small plaques, rather than vesicles and crusts. Large plaque parapsoriasis, which is the forerunner of the cutaneous T-cell lymphoma mycosis fungoides, is a distinct entity from PLEVA and PLC and only rarely has its onset in the first two decades. Skin biopsy reveals a mononuclear perivascular infiltrate, intraepidermal extravasation of erythrocytes, vacuolization, necrosis of the basal cell layer, and, occasionally, necrosis of the entire epidermis. PLEVA may persist for weeks to months, whereas PLC persists for years. Oral erythromycin appears to shorten the course of the disease in some children. Ultraviolet light therapy (UVB) in suberythemagenic doses, two to three times per week, is also effective in some patients with PLEVA and PLC.

Reference

Drago F, Ranieri E, Malaguti F, et al: Human herpesvirus 7 in pityriasis rosea. Lancet 349:1367–1368, 1997

Gelmetti C, Rigoni C, Alessi E, Ermacora E, Berti E, Caputo R: Pityriasis lichenoides in children: a long-term follow-up of eighty-nine cases. J Am Acad Dermatol 23:473–478, 1990

Gelmetti C, Schiuma AA, Cerri D, Gianotti F: Pityriaisis rubra pilaris in childhood: a long-term study of 29 cases. Pediatr Dermatol 3:446–451, 1986

Longley J, Demar L, Feinstein RP, et al: Clinical and histologic features of pityriasis lichenoides et varioliformis acuta in children. Arch Dermatol 123:1335–1339, 1987

Taieb A, El Youbi E, Grosshans E, Maleville J: Lichen striatus: a Blaschko linear acquired inflammatory skin eruption. J Am Acad Dermatol 26: 637–642, 1991

14.4 SELECTED GENETIC DISORDERS OF THE SKIN

Amy S. Paller

During the last decade, our understanding of the molecular bases for genetic disorders of the skin has expanded tremendously. Identifying the gene mutations that lead to phenotypic manifestations facilitates prenatal diagnosis using molecular techniques. For some disorders, this information has translated into early trials of gene therapy or the development of new pharmacologic therapy based upon manipulation of gene product levels. Several support groups that provide education for patients and physicians are available and are listed for each subgroup of genetic disorders of skin. The National Organization for Rare Disorders (NORD) at 1-800-999-6673 can also help families for which there is no specific support group.

14.4.1   The Ichthyoses and Ichthyosiform Disorders

Named for the Greek term meaning "fish-like scales," this heterogeneous group of disorders is characterized by the predominant clinical feature of visible accumulation of scale. During the past decade, the underlying molecular basis for many of the ichthyotic disorders has been discovered, and many are able to be diagnosed prenatally based upon molecular analysis of genomic DNA obtained by chorionic villus sampling or amniocentesis. Rarely, ichthyosis is an acquired condition. If possible, specific diagnosis should be made as early as possible to aid in prognostication and genetic counseling. In general, therapy for these disorders is similar and is based on disease severity and tolerance rather than the specific type (Table 14-4). During the neonatal and early infantile period, however, therapy should be limited to the frequent application of bland emollients, since use of topical medications with keratolytic agents during the first 6 months of life is usually unnecessary and leads to the risk of significant absorption of potentially toxic substances (eg, absorption of lactic acid, salicylic acid).

Scaling in the genetic forms is either present at birth or has its onset within the first few years of life (with the exception of *Refsum disease,* caused by the inability to metabolize phytanic acid, in which accumulation of plant-derived branched-chain fatty acids from the diet is required for disease expression). Onset after infancy is usually indicative of an acquired ichthyosis. Causes of acquired ichthyosis include hypothyroidism, chronic renal insufficiency, malignancy (particularly lymphoma), malabsorption syndromes, essential fatty acid deficiency, sarcoidosis, and certain drugs (particularly hypocholesterolemic agents). A national support group for patients with the ichthyoses and other disorders with thickening of epidermis can be emailed at *ichthyosis@aol.com* or by calling 1-800-545-3286.

ICHTHYOSIS VULGARIS Ichthyosis vulgaris is the most common form of the ichthyoses, occuring in 1 out of 250 individuals. An autosomal-dominant trait, its onset tends to be after three months of age. Fine, white scales without erythema predominate on the exterior surfaces of the extremities, especially the legs (Fig. 14-12). There is an increased prominence of palmar-plantar markings owing to mild to moderate thickening of the palms and soles. The majority of patients with ichthyosis vulgaris show a reduced granular layer of skin with decreased filaggrin synthesis, the major protein in keratohyalin granules, but the underlying primary defect is unknown. Although most patients respond well to emollients with lactic acid, this keratolytic agent may be irritating and poorly tolerated by patients with ichthyosis vulgaris who also have atopic dermatitis.

RECESSIVE X-LINKED ICHTHYOSIS Recessive X-linked ichthyosis occurs in 1 of 2000 to 6000 boys. Scaling is often more pronounced than in ichthyosis vulgaris, and scales tend to be larger and darker; the trunk is usually involved, but palms and soles are unaffected. The antecubital and popliteal flexures are usually spared, whereas the neck and periauricular areas are affected. The disease is caused by the absence of the microsomal enzyme steroid sulfatase. Because of the deficiency of fetal placental steroid sulfatase, the first clue to diagnosis may be failure to initiate labor or of progression of labor in the pregnant mother. Abnormalities of the genitalia, particularly undescended testes, have been described in 20 to 40% of patients. Minute, asymptomatic corneal opacities are present in half of adult patients. Diagnosis can be confirmed by measurement of enzyme activity in fibroblasts, leukocytes, amniocytes, or scale, by measurement of substrate (cholesterol sulfate) accumulation in scale or blood, or by mutational (DNA) analysis. Elevated blood cholesterol sulfate levels also result in abnormal mobility of β-lipoproteins on serum lipoprotein electrophoresis. The

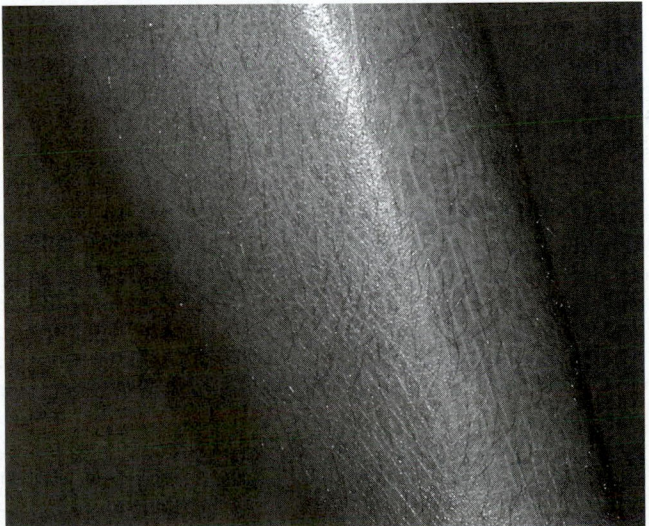

FIGURE 14-12   The scaling of patients with ichthyosis vulgaris is most severe on the lower extremities and during cold months. The palms and soles tend to be thickened as well in this autosomal-dominant common skin disorder. (*Courtesy of Amy Paller, M.D.*)

majority of cases result from deletion of the gene, and in approximately 10% of situations contiguous gene deletion occurs, leading to associated hypogonadism, anosmia, and mental retardation.

EPIDERMOLYTIC HYPERKERATOSIS Epidermolytic hyperkeratosis, or bullous congenital ichthyosiform erythroderma, is an autosomal-dominant trait caused by mutations in either the keratin 1 or keratin 10 gene encoding keratin intermediate filaments expressed in the upper layers of the epidermis. Disease may be localized and mild or generalized and severe. Large areas of denuded skin are typically present at birth, often suggesting a mechanobullous disease rather than a form of ichthyosis. However, skin biopsy sections show intracellular vacuolization and enlarged basophilic and eosinophilic granules within the spinous and granular cell layers of epidermis with overlying hyperkeratosis. Ultrastructural analysis of specimens reveals clumping of keratin tonofilaments with retraction from the cell periphery. By infancy, scaling becomes more conspicuous. Blistering occurs less frequently, is often focal, and usually is caused by secondary staphylococcal infection. Although the disorder is generalized, scaling is particularly verrucous in intertriginous areas and overlying joints. The degree of associated erythroderma and palmoplantar keratoderma is variable. Treatment of this disorder with keratolytics or retinoids is often complicated by the propensity of these agents to enhance blister formation. Irritating topical keratolytic therapies are not well tolerated. The mosaic form of epidermolytic hyperkeratosis presents as epidermal nevi with linear streaks of thickening of skin, often with increased pigmentation, following Blaschko's lines (the lines of embryologic development of skin).

LAMELLAR ICHTHYOSIS AND NONBULLOUS CONGENITAL ICHTHYOSIFORM ERYTHRODERMA Lamellar ichthyosis (LI) and nonbullous congenital ichthyosiform erythroderma (CIE) are now considered distinct disorders based upon clinical characteristics and underlying molecular basis. Both are usually autosomal-recessive conditions that almost always present at birth as a *collodion baby* (Color Plate 6), a phenotype characterized by taut, shiny skin that has been likened to cellophane (collodion). This "membrane" leads to eversion of the eyelids (ectropion) and of the lips (eclabium), digital contractures, and, rarely, restriction in respiration. In severely affected patients, the cartilaginous portions of the nose and ears may be underdeveloped. With a moist environment (such as a humidified isolette), application of emollients, and attention to the increased risks of temperature instability, fluid and electrolyte imbalance (especially hypernatremic dehydration), and infection, the membrane is shed during the first weeks of life. Although most collodion babies eventually adopt the typical characteristics of patients with either lamellar ichthyosis or CIE, some patients show a normal phenotype (lamellar exfoliation of the newborn) or other ichthyosiform disorder.

Within a few months after clearance of the collodion membrane, babies with lamellar ichthyosis show scales that are large, plate-like, and hyperpigmented, particularly in patients with darker skin. Underlying erythroderma is minimal, but ectropion and alopecia may be severe. Biopsies from patients with LI have massive thickening of the stratum corneum, mild acanthosis, and a normal granular layer. The molecular basis for LI in some families has recently been determined to be mutations in keratinocyte transglutaminase I, an enzyme that is involved in cornified envelope formation by cross-linking precursor proteins, such as involucrin. Prenatal diagnosis by molecular analysis of fetal DNA is the preferred method but is only possible in families in which the molecular defect is known.

Babies with CIE, in contrast, show scales that are lighter in color and finer than those of infants with lamellar ichthyosis. Underlying erythroderma is greater, and alopecia and ectropion may be associated. Not uncommonly, patients with CIE have associated neurologic abnormalities, and the CIE phenotype may be part of other multisystem conditions, such as the neutral lipid storage disease (Chanarin-Dorfman syndrome) or Netherton syndrome (see below). Biopsies from patients with CIE show marked acanthosis of the epidermis with a moderately thickened stratum corneum.

HARLEQUIN ICHTHYOSIS Harlequin ichthyosis is a rare, autosomal-recessive trait in which affected infants are usually stillborn or die soon after birth from massive, hyperkeratotic plates that obstruct respiratory movements and feeding. Skin tautness and massive plates of scale produce grotesque facial features with severe ectropion and eclabion and mitten-like encasement of fingers and toes. In rare survivors, the plate-like scales are shed postnatally and an intense exfoliative erythroderma ensues. The harlequin ichthyosis phenotype probably results from several underlying mutations. In general harlequin babies require vigorous supportive therapy, including a humid environment, the aggressive use of emollients, and careful monitoring of fluid and electrolyte needs. Some advocate the use of systemic retinoids for patients who survive the first few weeks of life; it should be recognized, however, that the resultant phenotype with chronic use of retinoids will continue to be that of severe CIE.

ICHTHYOSIFORM DISORDERS *Ichthyosiform disorders* occur as a component of a multisystemic disease. *Netherton syndrome* is an autosomal-recessive trait characterized by the triad of ichthyosis, brittle hair, and an atopic diathesis, especially characterized by anaphylactic reactions to food antigens. Patients usually have generalized exfoliative erythroderma during the neonatal period and early infancy, with failure to thrive, diarrhea, and hypernatremia. Later an unusual migratory annular pattern of scaling predominates, called *ichthyosis linearis circumflexa*. The underlying defect is unknown. Light microscopic examination of hairs shows a pathognomonic defect with intussusception of the hair shaft, called *trichorrhexis invaginata*, which allows the diagnosis to be made.

Patients with *trichothiodystrophy*, or sulfur-deficient brittle hair, may show a variety of associated defects, including ichthyosis, retardation, and decreased fertility. Some patients show photosensitivity, with a severe defect in DNA excision/repair that causes a type of xeroderma pigmentosum. Under polarizing microscopy, the hair from patients with this autosomal recessive disorder shows a pathognomonic banding pattern.

Sjögren-Larsson syndrome is a rare, autosomal-recessive trait characterized by the triad of ichthyosis, spasticity, and mental retardation. Ichthyosis is usually the presenting sign and begins as a pronounced postnatal desquamation. Pathognomonic retinal "glistening dots" are present in most patients by one year of age. The disorder is caused by deficiency of fatty alcohol oxidoreductase. Treatment with restriction of dietary long-chain fatty acids has been advocated.

Neutral lipid storage disease (Chanarin-Dorfman) is another autosomal-recessive disorder that results from a defect in the catabolism of triglycerides synthesized within the cell. Patients are most commonly from the Mediterranean area and show a CIE-like ichthyosis. Systemic signs include neurosensory deafness, cataracts, myopathy, fatty liver, and mild mental and growth retardation. The diagnosis can be confirmed by finding lipid droplets in circulating leukocytes. Serum triglyceride levels are normal.

The *Conradi-Hünermann syndrome* is an X-linked dominant trait that is lethal in males. At birth, patients show bands of ichthyosiform erythroderma that follow lines of Blaschko, reflecting the random activation of the mutant X chromosome. During infancy, these bands resolve, leaving follicular atrophy. Systemic signs include focal cataracts and asymmetric limb reduction defects with stippled epiphyses (chondrodysplasia punctata). Partial peroxisomal deficiency may underlie this trait. *CHILD syndrome* (Congenital Hemidysplasia with Ichthyosiform erythroderma and Limb Defects) is also an X-linked dominant trait in which the ichthyosis and limb defects with epiphyseal stippling are strictly unilateral. Peroxisomal defects have also been described in CHILD syndrome. The triad of progressive scarring *Keratitis, Ichthyosis,* and neurosensory *Deafness* characterizes *KID syndrome,* a rare disorder with dominant and recessive forms.

Darier disease is an uncommon but not rare autosomal-dominant trait. The skin eruption frequently follows intense sun exposure, most commonly between ages 5 and 15 years. Greasy keratotic papules show a predilection for seborrheic areas, face, scalp, neck, upper chest, and back, but may occur on extremities or may show a striking photodistribution. Lesions on flexural sites tend to coalesce to form erythematous, eroded plaques. Small keratotic papules are found on palms and soles. Nails are short, fragile, and may show red and white longitudinal streaks. The oral mucosa has a pebbly quality, particularly along gingival margins. The histopathology is diagnostic and shows a combination of premature and abnormal cornification of vesicles or individual epidermal cells (dyskeratosis), intraepidermal vesicles or blisters caused by desmosomal detachments (acantholysis), and parakeratosis. Topical retinoic acid (Retin A 0.05% cream) and, in some instances, brief courses of systemic retinoids (isotretinoin, acetretin) are useful (see Sec. 14.9).

14.4.2   Palmar-Plantar Keratodermas

Palmar-plantar keratodermas constitute a large group of predominantly autosomal-dominant disorders in which the disorder of cornification is predominantly limited to palms and soles. The *Unna-Thost* (nonepidermolytic) and *Vörner* (epidermolytic hyperkeratotic) types are most common and result from mutations in keratin genes. Hyperkeratosis may be diffuse or limited to papules or even linear bands, as in the *striate* form of palmoplantar keratoderma. In some forms, particularly *Vohwinkel,* constriction of the terminal digits may lead to mutilating changes. If keratoses are focal or if accompanied by erosions, *tyrosinemia* type II (Richnar-Hanhart syndrome) should be excluded. Other features of this autosomal-recessive trait are keratitis and mental retardation. Dietary restriction of tyrosine and phenylalanine is indicated. The *Papillon-Lefevre syndrome* is a recessive trait with diffuse keratoderma and periodontitis leading to premature loss of teeth. In treatment of keratoderma, keratolytics may be used followed by paring. Occasionally one of the synthetic retinoids (isotretinoin or acetretin) is indicated to preserve function.

14.4.3   Disorders of Pigmentation

OCULOCUTANEOUS ALBINISM   The genetic basis for albinism in most patients is a mutation either in the gene that codes for tyrosinase, important for melanin synthesis (*tyrosinase-negative*), or in the gene that codes for P protein (*tyrosinase-positive*), leading to abnormal transport of melanin to keratinocytes. As a result, children with this autosomal recessive group of disorders have decreased pigmentation of the skin, hair, and eyes, along with photophobia, nystagmus, and reduced visual acuity. Patients with tyrosinase-negative disease have the highest risk of ophthalmologic abnormalities and skin cancer and show no improvement with age. In contrast, tyrosinase-positive patients may have pigmentation to some degree with advancing age. Patients with all forms of oculocutaneous albinism require the consistent avoidance of sunlight, use of full-spectrum sun protectants, and wearing of protective clothing (long sleeves, brimmed hat, UV-filtering glasses) to prevent the development of cutaneous malignancy. Ophthalmologic and dermatologic follow-up are needed, and genetic counseling should be considered. The National Organization for Albinism and Hypopigmentation (NOAH) at email address *noah@albinism.org* or 1-800-473-2310 provides support for families.

HERMANSKY-PUDLAK SYNDROME   The *Hermansky-Pudlak syndrome* is a rare, autosomal recessive disorder characterized by a triad of albinism, a mild bleeding diathesis, and tissue storage of ceroid material. The platelet storage pool defect may result in epistaxis and prolonged bleeding. Deposits of ceroid-like material in lungs, gastrointestinal tract, and renal tubule cells may lead to restrictive lung disease, colitis, or renal failure, respectively. In the *Chediak-Higashi syndrome* the skin and hair assume a pigment-diluted, silvery sheen because of the accumulation of giant melanosomes with inability to transport the melanin granules to epidermal cells. The mutation in a lysosomal transport protein also leads to immunodeficiency, with the development of an "accelarated phase" by early childhood in most patients. This complication generally is triggered by Epstein-Barr viral infection, which leads to the proliferation of atypical lymphocytes and histiocytes, multiorgan infiltration, and pancytopenia. Without successful bone marrow transplantation, most patients with Chediak-Higashi syndrome die during this accelerated phase.

Children with *piebaldism* display discrete patches of depigmentation involving the central forehead, anterior trunk, and midportions of the upper and lower extremities. A midline white forelock is characteristic. Absent or grossly abnormal melanocytes are seen in the involved skin. The condition is inherited as an autosomal dominant trait owing to mutations in the *KIT* oncogene, which directs melanoblast proliferation, migration, and differentiation. *Waardenburg syndrome* is also an autosomal-dominant disorder with depigmentation of hair, skin, and irides. Its phenotypic manifestations are most commonly associated with mutations in *PAX 3,* with associated lateral displacement of the inner canthi, broad nasal root, and confluent eyebrows. Patients without the facial features may have mutations in the *MITF* gene, and patients with associated Hirschsprung disease may have mutations in three other genes encoding endothelin, endothelin receptor, or Sox 10. Sensorineural hearing loss occurs overall in 20% of patients and may depend on the role of pigment in directing development of hearing.

14.4.4   Tumor Syndromes

Pediatric patients with the autosomal-dominant type I *neurofibromatosis* (von Recklinghausen disease) usually show only multiple café au lait spots on examination. Six or more of these evenly brown-colored, sharply defined macules are present in more than 99% of patients (Fig. 14-13). Additional café au lait spots may continue to appear during the first five years of life but by definition must be larger than 0.5 cm in diameter in the child. Definitive diagnosis requires the presence of other features, such as axillary

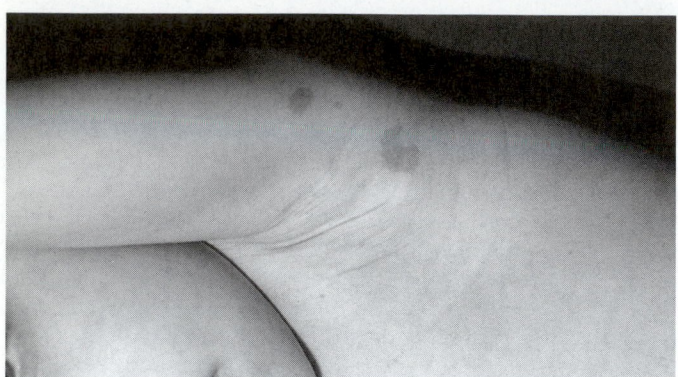

FIGURE 14-13   Young children with multiple café au lait spots have cutaneous evidence of neurofibromatosis type I. The additional finding of freckling in the axillary area, as shown here, allows the diagnosis of neurofibromatosis type I to be made definitively. (*Courtesy of Amy Paller, M.D.*)

freckling; neurofibromatosis in a first-degree relative; pseudoarthrosis; plexiform neurofibroma; or Lisch nodules, dome-shaped hyperpigmented iris hamartomas that are multiple and bilateral and present in the majority of patients of school age and older.

The causative mutation involves the gene encoding neurofibromin, a tumor suppressor gene. With one normal allele, patients have adequate tumor suppression. However, if the normal neurofibromin allele is mutated through a sporadic hit, the affected cell may show uncontrolled growth resulting in a benign or malignant tumor. The most common tumors are dermal or plexiform (deeper) neurofibromas. The plexiform neurofibromas are often manifest during infancy and early childhood as poorly circumscribed areas of induration, often with an overlying large café au lait spot. They can be deeply invasive and grow progressively and are difficult to eradicate. Dermal neurofibromas present as soft sessile or pedunculated nodules, usually first apparent during puberty. Optic gliomas occur in 15% of patients but are not treated unless they are actively growing or causing clinical problems. Defective tumor suppression increases the risk of malignancy; central nervous system tumors and nonlymphocytic leukemias may appear during childhood and neurofibrosarcomas and malignant schwannomas after 20 years of age. Perhaps the most important reason for early diagnosis is the awareness that speech and learning disabilities occur in almost a third of patients. The National Neurofibromatosis Foundation can be reached by email at *NNFF@aol.com* or by calling 1-800-323-7938.

Hypopigmented macules ranging from 1 to 4 cm in diameter are the most consistent cutaneous finding in *tuberous sclerosis,* an autosomal-dominant neurocutaneous disorder with a high incidence of spontaneous mutations and marked intrafamilial variability in the severity of phenotypic manifestations. Macules are sometimes shaped like ash leaves (*ash-leaf spots*), but they may be round, oval, irregular, or confetti-like in configuration. A Wood's lamp may be helpful to highlight subtle areas of hypopigmentation in fair-skinned patients. Together with hypopigmented macules, the presence at birth of connective-tissue nevi (slightly elevated flesh-colored plaques with a rough surface or leathery surface, particularly on the forehead [*fibrous forehead plaque*]) may allow early definitive diagnosis. Numerous skin-colored to vascularized papules and dome-shaped nodules ("adenoma sebaceum") appear on the central face during childhood in most patients with tuberous sclerosis (Color Plate 7); histopathologically these are angiofibromas. Per-

iungual, subungual, and gingival fibromas are not usually seen until puberty or adulthood. Almost all patients with tuberous sclerosis have seizures, often with onset by infancy. Two interacting genes may be mutated to cause this disorder, tuberin or hamartin. Both are involved in tumor suppression, with tumors resulting from loss of heterozygosity as described above for neurofibromatosis type I. Tumors of the central nervous system, kidneys (angiolipomas), heart (rhabdomyomas), and eyes (retinal hamartomas) occur most commonly. The National Tuberous Sclerosis Association can be contacted at 1-800-225-6872.

Basal cell nevus syndrome (Gorlin syndrome) is an autosomal-dominant disorder caused by mutations in the *patched* gene that controls cell growth and patterning. Affected patients tend to develop basal cell carcinomas during childhood or early adulthood and to display dysmorphic facies, palmoplantar pits, a variety of skeletal defects, and mental retardation. Cutaneous and visceral cysts are common, including cysts of the jaw that may become malignant. In addition to basal cell carcinomas, ovarian fibromas and carcinomas and medulloblastomas occur with increased frequency during childhood.

Peutz-Jeghers syndrome is an autosomal-dominant defect due to mutations in a serine threonine kinase. The key characteristics are gastrointestinal polyposes and hyperpigmented macules of the mucosae, perioral areas, fingers, and toes. Patients have an increased risk of malignancy of the bowel, breast, ovaries, and testes. In contrast, patients with *Gardner syndrome* (mutations in APC gene) also have gastrointestinal polyposes, but their characteristic cutaneous features are epidermal cysts and sometimes pilomatricomas. Patients with Gardner syndrome almost always develop colorectal carcinoma and have an increased risk of developing papillary adenocarcinoma of the thyroid.

14.4.5   Neurocutaneous Disorders

The most common neurocutaneous disorders, neurofibromatosis and tuberous sclerosis, are reviewed in Sec. 14.4.4. *Incontinentia pigmenti* is an X-linked dominant disorder that is thought to be lethal in males; as a result, most affected patients are female, and affected mothers may report an increased frequency of miscarriages. The cutaneous features are largely cleared by late childhood, so determination that a mother is affected may require careful review of history. Generally, three stages are described, although overlapping of stages is common. Patterned blistering that follows the distribution of the lines of Blaschko (reflecting functional mosaicism) occurs in 96% of affected patients by six weeks of age (Color Plate 8). Verrucous papules, similarly distributed, may be seen after the first several weeks and may persist for months. The hyperpigmented lines and swirls along Blaschko's lines typically appear during the first months of life and often persist for several years. Recurrence of blistering or verrucous lesions during the first decades of life has been reported. About one-fourth of patients develop a fourth stage of atrophic and/or hypopigmented streaks, which may also persist for several years. Cicatricial alopecia is a sequela of the blistering in approximately one-third of patients. The diagnosis is usually made in the neonatal period on the basis of cutaneous manifestations and examination of skin biopsy, which shows intraepidermal vesicles filled with eosinophils.

The cutaneous changes are of greatest importance as a marker for other noncutaneous abnormalities of incontinentia pigmenti. Delayed eruption of teeth, absent teeth, and malformed teeth occur in almost two-thirds of patients. Although the most common ophthalmologic abnormality is strabismus, the retinal neovascularization and detachment in patients with incontinentia pigmenti can lead to blindness in about 7% of patients. The occurrence of seizures during the neonatal period in 13% of patients, coupled with the vesicles, often leads to an erroneous diagnosis of herpes simplex infection. There is no relation between incontinentia pigmenti and incontinentia pigmenti achromians or hypomelanosis of Ito, a heterogenous group of mosaic disorders with hypopigmented streaks and swirls along Blaschko's lines (see Color Plate 9). The national support group for patients with incontinentia pigmenti can be sent email at *nipf@pipeline.com.*

Ataxia-telangiectasia is an autosomal-recessive disorder that results from mutations in *ATM,* which prevents DNA synthesis from proceeding after irradiation damage. The early ataxia in affected patients is followed by the development of telangiectasias on the bulbar conjunctival mucosae, usually beginning between two and six years of age. Telangiectasias may subsequently appear on the eyelids, nasal bridge, cheeks, ears, and flexural areas. Cutaneous granulomas that frequently ulcerate are difficult to eradicate. Other cutaneous features are loss of subcutaneous fat, sclerodermoid lesions, and cutaneous infections. Patients tend to show progressive neurologic deterioration and, variably, recurrent sinopulmonary infections related to immunodeficiency. The Ataxia-Telangiectasia Children's Project can be reached by calling 1-800-5-HELP-A-T.

Although boys with X-linked recessive *Fabry disease* (angiokeratoma corporis diffusum universale) usually present with unexplained fever, weakness, and/or acral paresthesias; the development of petechiae-like lesions or keratotic vascular papules (angiokeratomas) during adolescence may allow the diagnosis to be made. The vascular lesions are predominantly distributed between the umbilicus and knees. Due to a deficiency in alpha-galactosidase A, patients progressively deposit ceramide-trihexoside in blood vessels, leading to angina pectoris, hypertension and renal failure, and an increased risk of cerebrovascular accidents.

Menkes syndrome is an X-linked recessive disorder caused by an abnormality in copper transport. Patients have short, brittle, easily broken hairs that show pili torti (hair that twists 180°) by light microscopy. Patients show progressive neurologic deterioration with seizures and retardation and tend to die during the first years of life. The variety of other clinical manifestations reflect the need for copper as a cofactor and include pigment dilution, degenerated elastic tissue, bladder diverticula, scurvy-like bone changes, and impaired temperature regulation.

14.4.6 Epidermolysis Bullosa

This heterogeneous group of genetically determined disorders results from structural defects in the cohesive strength of skin, leading to blistering after mechanical trauma. At present, more than 15 genetically distinct forms have been recognized by their clinical features, histopathology, and inheritance patterns. EB ranges in severity from forms that are lethal in infancy or are severely disabling and deforming to localized, mild disease. A specific diagnosis should be sought to permit genetic counseling and prognostication. Prenatal diagnosis has been possible using molecular techniques if the specific DNA defect in the family is identified. Dystrophic Epidermolysis Bullosa Research Association of America (DEBRA) supports patients with all forms of epidermolysis bullosa (EB) at 1-212-995-2220.

EB is subdivided by ultrastructural and immunomapping characteristics into three major groups — *EB simplex,* in which the cleav-

age plane of the blister is through the basal epidermal cells; *junctional* or *hemidesmosomal EB,* in which the defect is in the hemidesmosome with the cleavage plane through the dermal-epidermal (DE) junction; and *dystrophic EB,* in which the cleavage plane lies below the basement membrane zone in the upper dermis. Defects in keratin genes 5 and 14, expressed in the basal layer of epidermis, cause all forms of EB simplex, and mutations in the gene encoding collagen VII, the major component of anchoring fibrils, underlie dystrophic EB. Junctional epidermolysis bullosa can result from defects in a variety of hemidesmosomal proteins, including one of the three chains of laminin 5 (EB letalis, most severe form), collagen XVII (generalized atrophic benign form), plectin (EB simplex with muscular dystrophy), and integrin subunits α 6 and β 4 (with pyloric atresia). Determination of the subtype of EB during the neonatal period is critical for prognostication and counseling but is very difficult based on clinical characteristics alone. A skin biopsy, preferably from the margin of an induced blister or a fresh blister, should be sent for immunomapping and immunomarker studies, which allow rapid diagnosis. Ultrastructural analysis may also be useful as an adjunctive test or if immunomapping is not available. In addition, other causes of widespread blistering in the newborn must be excluded (see Table 14-1 and Sec. 14.2).

EB simplex, characterized by blisters that heal without scarring or milia (small keratinaceous cysts), is almost always an autosomal-dominant disorder. Blistering may be generalized with (Dowling-Meara type) or without (Koebner type) associated mucosal and nail involvement. In the mildest cases, the blistering is limited to the hands and feet (Weber-Cockayne type), sites of maximal trauma. Although blistering may be extensive during the perinatal period (especially with the Dowling-Meara type), improvement with age is expected.

Junctional forms of EB are all autosomal recessive in inheritance. Blistering is usually severe and occurs spontaneously or after trauma. Death caused by sepsis, sometimes in conjunction with hypoalbuminemia and anemia, often occurs before six months of age. Mucous membrane involvement is often severe, and hoarseness is characteristic. Survivors tend to be growth-retarded with chronic anemia, atrophic scarring, and highly vascularized granulation tissue at sites of chronic blistering. Nails slough easily, and dental enamel is hypoplastic, requiring capping.

An autosomal dominant form of dystrophic EB is characterized by blistering at localized areas (dorsum of hands, elbows, knees in particular) that heals with scarring and milia formation. Generalized blistering resulting in extensive scarring and milia formation is the hallmark of the recessive form. Most affected patients survive the neonatal period.

Because of complex extracutaneous complications, an interdisciplinary approach encompassing pediatricians, dermatologists, nutritionists, ophthalmologists, dentists, urologists, otolaryngologists, and gastroenterologists is critical for the care of patients with recessive dystrophic EB. In addition to growth retardation, chronic anemia, and increased dental caries, intraoral scarring may lead to microstomia, ankyloglossia, loss of buccal vestibules, and occasionally laryngeal stenosis. Esophageal blisters and ulcerations cause dysphagia, which contributes to the nutritional deficiencies. Strictures form commonly in the upper (50%) or lower (25%) esophagus or at multiple sites (25%); complications include hemorrhage, perforation, esophageal web, aspiration pneumonia, and carcinoma in adulthood. In patients with esophageal stenosis, rigid adherence to an atraumatic diet of sufficient calories and nutrients may halt disease progression, but dilations may be required. Dietary treatment is preferable to repeated dilations, which are traumatic and may result in further stenosis. Patients experiencing symptoms of gastroesophageal reflux should sleep with the head of the bed elevated and use antacids at bedtime. Early placement of a gastrostomy tube is often recommended to provide additional nutrition for patients as well as to decrease the risk of esophageal trauma with eating. Painful blistering around the anal sphincter results in chronic constipation, particularly in recessive dystrophic EB. Stool softeners are essential in these patients, particularly because iron supplementation further hardens the stool; maintaining sufficient bulk in the diet is desirable but difficult to achieve. Conjunctival and corneal erosions may also occur; potential sequelae include symblepharon formation, corneal ulcerations or perforations. Recurrent urethral blistering in recessive dystrophic EB results in meatal stenosis and may lead to urinary retention and hydronephrosis.

After the first few years of life, the progressive scarring from blistering on the fingers and toes causes pseudosyndactyly ("mitten deformities") of the hands and feet (Fig. 14-14), which may result in significant functional disability. Repeated degloving procedures may be required to "correct" the hand deformities and allow an apposable thumb and palm. Squamous cell carcinomas of the skin, oral cavity, stomach, esophagus, or bronchi may develop as early as the second decade in severe recessive dystrophic EB. Persistent ulcerations should be biopsied.

To protect skin from trauma, tape and other adhesives should never be applied directly. Erosions may be covered with a nonadhesive dressing (eg, vaseline-impregnated gauze, Telfa pads) and then wrapped in soft, bulky dressings. Bandages should be soaked, never pulled off. Blisters should be decompressed daily by incision with a sterile blade to prevent lateral extension. Secondary infections, particularly with *Staphylococcus aureus,* are frequent and should be suspected if serous crusting is present. Antibacterial ointments (eg, silver sulfadiazine [contraindicated in neonates], bacitracin, or mupirocin) may be applied to erosions to discourage secondary invasion. Frankly impetiginized lesions should be cultured and treated systemically. Maintenance of adequate nutrition is an important goal in the treatment of severely affected patients. Anemia in these patients is owed both to bone marrow suppression of chronic illness and to iron, protein, and trace mineral deficiency from cutaneous losses and poor oral intake. A suboptimal response to oral or parenteral iron replacement is often observed, and trans-

fusions and/or erythropoietin may be required. Hypoalbuminemia is common in severely affected patients and may result in part from cutaneous losses. A soft diet is advisable for all patients who experience oral blisters, such as foods pureed in a blender and supplemented with vitamins and minerals. Complete liquid nutritional supplements (eg, Ensure) are helpful in maintaining adequate caloric intake.

14.4.7   Disorders of the Dermis

Ehlers-Danlos syndrome includes a group of at least 11 genetic disorders in which there is easy bruising, poor wound healing, and hyperextensibility of joints and/or skin. The skin has a soft texture and, although it is able to stretch easily, regains its normal appearance. Spread "fish-mouth" scars develop after trauma or surgery, and pseudotumor herniations of subcutaneous fat through atrophic dermal scars may be present, particularly on the lower extremities where bruising is easily seen and the thin skin leads to vessel prominence. Mutations in the gene encoding perivascular dermal collagen type V are responsible for the most common types, type I and the milder type II. Other types largely result from mutations in the synthesis of other dermal collagens. The Ehlers-Danlos Syndrome Foundation can be accessed by email at *LooseJoint@aol.com.*

Cutis laxa is a disorder of generalized decreased or absent elastic tissue that manifests both genetic (autosomal-recessive, autosomal-dominant, and X-linked recessive inheritance patterns) and acquired forms. Pendulous folds of redundant skin may be present at birth (recessive form) or may develop later (dominant form). Patients with severe involvement frequently have pulmonary emphysema, diverticula of the bladder or gastrointestinal tract, and inguinal or umbilical hernias. Mutations in elastin have been described. Acquired cutis laxa is often preceded by inflammatory skin lesions, and hypersensitivity to penicillin or isoniazid has been implicated in some instances. The disorder is usually progressive and has a poor prognosis.

Focal dermal hypoplasia (Goltz syndrome) is inherited in X-linked dominant fashion, and 90% of patients are female. Cutaneous manifestations of this functionally mosaic condition include linear and swirled areas of skin hypoplasia, ulcerations, dyspigmentation, and yellowish nodules. A number of musculoskeletal, ocular, and dental anomalies may be present. Vertical striations in the long bones (osteopathia striata) are diagnostic when present.

Lipoid proteinosis is an autosomal-recessive disorder ascribable to the deposition of hyaline material in the skin and other organ systems. The cutaneous manifestations usually develop during the first two years of life, sometimes manifesting as early erosions on the face and intertriginous areas. Waxy papules and nodules appear progressively during childhood, especially on the face and neck with diffuse thickening of the skin in other areas. A row of nodules at the free edge of the eyelid is particularly characteristic, as is thickening of the tongue. The most common systemic manifestation is hoarseness caused by vocal cord infiltration.

Pseudoxanthoma elasticum is a disorder of elastic tissue; both autosomal-dominant and autosomal-recessive forms occur. Cutaneous lesions, which begin during childhood, consist of grouped, yellowish papules that favor the axillae, groin, and neck. The areas of involvement may appear wrinkled, and their overall appearance has been likened to "plucked chicken skin." Skin biopsy is diagnostic and shows foci of basophilic, condensed, degenerating elastic fibers, and secondary calcification. Retinal angioid streaks frequently develop and may interfere with vision. Widespread arterial

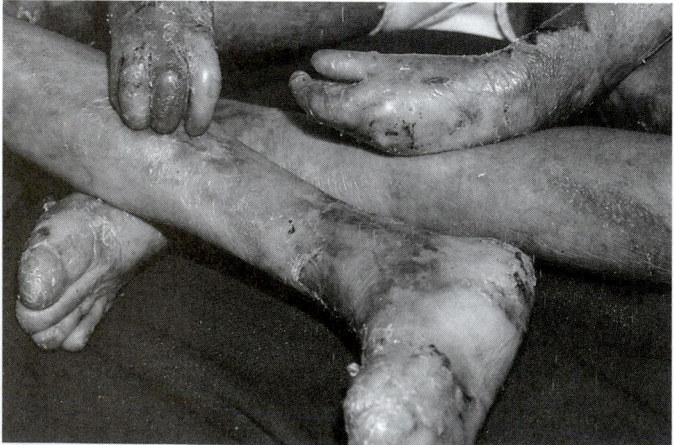

FIGURE 14-14   Generalized blistering in patients with recessive dystrophic epidermolysis bullosa results in scarring and milia formation. Patients show growth retardation and anemia and form "mitten deformities" of the distal extremities caused by scarring. (*Courtesy of Amy Paller, M.D.*)

involvement of elastic tissue degeneration and deposition of calcium may result in gastrointestinal bleeding, intermittent claudication, and angina pectoris. Support groups, the National Association for Pseudoxanthoma Elasticum, Inc. and PXE International, Inc. can be accessed by emails to *derkhn@ttuhsc.edu* and *pxe@pxe.org*, respectively.

14.4.8   Ectodermal Dysplasias and Other Primarily Ectodermal Disorders

In the ectodermal dysplasias, two or more ectodermally derived structures such as hair, nails, sweat glands, sebaceous glands, or teeth are poorly developed or absent. Although hundreds of ectodermal dysplasias have been described, the more common, well-defined disorders are briefly described here. The National Foundation for Ectodermal Dysplasias can be reached by email at *nfed1@aol.com* or *nfed2@aol.com*.

HYPOHIDROTIC ECTODERMAL DYSPLASIA This X-linked recessive trait is the most common form of ectodermal dysplasia. Phenotypic characteristics of female carriers may range from no evidence of involvement to extensive changes indistinguishable from those of affected male patients, depending on the extent of random activation of the X chromosome with the mutant gene with lyonization. The facies of patients with hypohidrotic ectodermal dysplasia are characteristic, with a frontal bossing, flat malar ridges, a depressed nasal root, thin upper lip, large pouting lower lip, small chin, and prominent ears. The mandible is underdeveloped, and partial adontia with conical or pegged teeth is common. The hair is sparse, short, and hypopigmented. Periorbital wrinkling and hyperpigmentation is usually seen. The diminished or absent sweating leads to frequent fevers of unknown origin and heat stress. Poor secretion from other glandular structures results in a progressive erosion with drainage of the nasal mucosae, poor tearing, dry mouth, and increased frequency of otitis media and pneumonia. Patients have an increased frequency of atopy, particularly atopic dermatitis and asthma. Early recognition of this disorder is key, so that parents can be taught about external cooling, such as by dowsing with cool water, and the importance of dental care by two years of age to improve mastication, facial development, speech development, and appearance.

Clinical findings in *hidrotic ectodermal dysplasia* (Clouston syndrome), inherited in an autosomal-dominant pattern, include hair and nail hypoplasia in conjunction with palmar-plantar keratoderma. Sweating is preserved. Ectodermal dysplasia of the hair and nails may also be associated with midfacial clefting in three autosomal-dominant disorders, the *Rapp-Hodgkin syndrome, ectrodactyly–ectodermal dysplasia–clefting syndrome* (with claw deformities), and *Hay-Wells syndrome* (with varying degrees of persistent eyelid fusion, or ankyloblepharon). *Dyskeratosis congenita* is a rare, usually X-linked recessive disorder. Progressive nail dystrophy, often with eventual anonychia, is generally the first sign during early childhood. Mucosal leukoplakia, particularly of the tongue and buccal mucosa, also develops during childhood and may transform into squamous cell carcinomas after the second decade of life. Reticulated hyperpigmented macules and atrophy develop in sun-exposed sites, usually during teenage years. Pancytopenia with progressive bone marrow failure develops in many patients and may require bone marrow transplantation.

In addition to EB simplex, epidermolytic hyperkeratosis, and palmoplantar keratodermas, mutations in keratin genes can cause two additional autosomal-dominant ectodermal defects. *Monilethrix* is a rare structural hair abnormality. The hair grows to 2 or 3 cm, then breaks off. With a hand lens the hair shaft is seen to undulate in width, and with light microscopy, areas of constriction lack a central medulla. Follicular prominence on the scalp and elsewhere is common. Mutations in hair keratins hHbK1 and hHbK6 have been identified. *Pachyonychia congenita* has been divided into two major subtypes, based on clinical manifestations that correlate with the underlying gene defect. In all cases, the nails are thick and dystrophic in appearance owing to distal and subungual hyperkeratosis. The surface may be rough to smooth, but the nails tend to be discolored and show increased curvature. Secondary pachyonychia resulting from *S. aureus* or *C. albicans* infection is common. Palmar-plantar keratoderma, hyperkeratotic plaques over the elbows and knees, and oral leukokeratosis, especially on the tongue, are associated features in patients with mutations in the genes encoding keratins 6a and 16, and patients with mutations in keratins 6b and 17, also expressed in adnexal structures, tend to develop myriads of sebaceous cysts (steatocystoma multiplex or vellus hair cysts) and occasionally alopecia.

14.4.9   Immunodeficiency Disorders

Primary genetic immunodeficiency disorders (Sec. 11.3) may manifest as persistent eczematous dermatitis, erythroderma, or recurrent skin infections or granulomas. In *X-linked agammaglobulinemia,* recurrent bacterial infections of the skin, particularly cellulitis and furunculosis, may be an important early sign of the disease. An atopic dermatitis-like rash occurs in many patients. Children with the *severe combined immunodeficiency syndrome* (SCID) may present in the newborn period with acute graft-versus-host disease as a result of maternal-fetal transfusion or transfusion of nonirradiated blood products. *Omenn syndrome,* a subtype of SCID, presents in infancy with scaling erythroderma associated with lymphadenopathy, hepatosplenomegaly, recurrent infections, and failure to thrive. The X-linked recessive *Wiskott-Aldrich syndrome* presents as a triad of severe eczematous dermatitis, recurrent bacterial skin infections, and thrombocytopenia with bleeding diathesis. Cutaneous manifestations of *chronic granulomatous disease of childhood,* a defect of phagocyte function inherited in both X-linked and autosomal-recessive forms, include a chronic eczematous dermatitis, perianal abscesses, and aphthous stomatitis. Abnormalities of integrin function in *leukocyte adhesion deficiency* are associated with delayed separation of the umbilical cord, recurrent cutaneous infections often with draining sinus tracts, and periodontitis. Children with the *hyper-IgE syndrome* have recurrent cutaneous staphylococcal or candidal infections in conjunction with often severe atopic dermatitis. Serum IgE levels frequently exceeding 1000 mg/dL and peripheral eosinophilia are characteristically present.

14.4.10   Photosensitivity Disorders

The *porphyrias* are a group of disorders in which accumulation of byproducts in heme metabolism lead to phototoxicity. The two forms of porphyria with cutaneous features and common onset during infancy and childhood are the rare autosomal-recessive disorder, *congenital erythropoietic porphyria,* and the more common autosomal-dominant disorder, *erythropoietic protoporphyria.* Congenital erythropoietic porphyria results from a deficiency of uroporphyrinogen cosynthetase. Exposure to ultraviolet light results in a painful, vesiculobullous eruption, with red staining of the urine and teeth during infancy. Progressive scarring and deformity of the face and acral extremities, hyperpigmentation, and facial hypertrichosis occur. Hemolytic anemia and splenomegaly are associated. Successful bone marrow transplantation may reverse the cutaneous and hematologic features. *Erythropoietic protoporphyria,* a result of ferrochelatase deficiency, usually presents during the first decade of life with an exaggerated sunburn reaction to a relatively brief sun exposure. Although frank blistering is unusual, thickened, waxy skin and scars develop on the face and dorsum of the hands with recurrent episodes. Patients need to be monitored for the development of cholelithiasis and hepatic failure, although these rarely occur. In addition to sun avoidance, the application of topical photoprotectants, and the use of sun protective clothing, administration of β-carotene may be useful in decreasing episodes. For information about the American Porphyria Foundation, call 713-266-9617.

Xeroderma pigmentosum is an autosomal-recessive disorder that usually presents in early childhood with exaggerated erythema after sun exposure. Numerous often darkly pigmented freckles and lentigines develop on sun-exposed sites, and telangiectasias are also a feature. The malignant and premalignant lesions that may appear during childhood (actinic keratoses, keratoacanthomas, squamous cell carcinomas, basal cell epitheliomas, and melanomas) result from ultraviolet light–induced cellular mutations that cannot be repaired. Death in most patients is caused by a metastatic cutaneous malignancy, and many do not survive past childhood. Early recognition and rigorous avoidance of all sources of ultraviolet light is imperative. Some genetic forms are accompanied by neurologic abnormalities, with mental and growth retardation (DeSanctis-Cacchione syndrome). The Xeroderma Pigmentosum Society can be reached by e-mail at *xps@mhv.net.*

Bloom syndrome is a rare, autosomal-recessive disorder caused by mutations in *BLM,* a DNA helicase, leading to replication-repair defects and chromosomal abnormalities including sister-chromatid exchange. Patients exhibit short stature, a severe blistering, photosensitive eruption, and an increased incidence of malignancy, especially leukemia. *Hartnup disease* is caused by abnormal tryptophan transport and absorption. The principal cutaneous manifestation is a blistering eruption at sun-exposed sites, caused by a relative niacin deficiency.

Rothmund-Thomson syndrome is a rare autosomal recessive disorder that is characterized by the development of atrophy and telangiectasia (poikiloderma), primarily of sun-exposed sites, beginning during the first year of life. Other findings include a bullous photosensitive eruption, short stature hypogonadism, cataracts, bone abnormalities, and an increased risk of sarcoma. *Cockayne syndrome* is a rare autosomal-recessive disorder with short stature, mental retardation, and prematurely senile, bird-like facies. A photosensitive eruption with scaling, erythema, and scarring begins during the first few years of life.

14.4.11   Disorders of Premature Aging

Werner syndrome is an autosomal-recessive disorder that results from mutations in *WRN,* a helicase. Signs of premature aging begin during teenage years and include cataracts, diabetes mellitus, severe vascular disease, and an increased risk of neoplasia. The most common cutaneous changes are graying of the hair (canities), shiny smooth skin (atrophy), alopecia, and distal cutaneous ulcerations related to inadequate tissue blood flow.

In *progeria* (Hutchinson-Gilford syndrome), a rare autosomal-recessive disorder, signs of premature aging can occur by one year of age. Patients experience severe growth failure, an aged appearance, and a high incidence of atherosclerosis during the late childhood and early adolescent years. The skin is thin, and subcutaneous fat is deficient, leading to venous prominence. Other cutaneous manifestations are diffuse areas of inelastic skin resembling scleroderma, total alopecia, and nail dystrophy. Patients tend to have a squeaky voice, bird-like facies, and a peculiar hunched posture with shuffling gait. Death as a teenager is common, related to cardiovascular disease.

References

Arbiser JL: Genetic immunodeficiency: cutaneous manifestations and recent progress. J Am Acad Dermatol 33:82–89, 1995

Christiano AM, Uitto J: Molecular complexity of the cutaneous basement membrane zone. Revelations from the paradigms of epidermolysis bullosa. Exp Dermatol 5:1–11, 1996

Fine JD, Bauer EA, Briggaman RA, et al: Revised clinical and laboratory criteria for subtypes of inherited epidermolysis bullosa. J Am Acad Dermatol 24:119–135, 1991

Harber LC, Bickers DR: *Photosensitivity Diseases.* Philadelphia, Saunders, 1981:154–159, 189–223, 225–257

Korf BR: Neurocutaneous syndromes: neurofibromatosis 1, neurofibromatosis 2, and tuberous sclerosis. Curr Opin Neurol 10:131–136, 1997

Landy SJ, Donnai D: Incontinentia pigmenti (Bloch-Sulzberger syndrome). J Med Genet 30:53–59, 1993

Lin AN: Management of patients with epidermolysis bullosa. Dermatol Clin 14:381–387, 1996

Micali G, Guitart J, Bene-Bain MA, Solomon LM: Genodermatoses. In: Schachner LA, Hansen RC, eds: Pediatric Dermatology. New York, Churchill-Livingstone, 1995:347–412

Orlow SJ: Albinism: an update. Semin Cutan Med Surg 16:24–29, 1997

Paller AS: Lessons from skin blistering: molecular mechanisms and unusual patterns of inheritance. Am J Pathol 148:1727–1731, 1996

Riccardi V: Von Recklinghausen neurofibromatosis. N Engl J Med 305:1617–1627, 1981

Sidhu-Malik NK, Wenstrup RJ: The Ehlers-Danlos syndrome and Marfan syndrome: inherited diseases of connective tissue with overlapping clinical features [review]. Semin Dermatol 14:40–46, 1995

Sybert VP: Genetic Skin Disorders. New York, Oxford University Press, 1997

Williams ML, Shwayder TA: Ichythyosis and disorders of cornification. In: Schachner LA, Hansen RC, eds: Pediatric Dermatology. New York, Churchill-Livingstone, 1995:413–468

Witkop CJ Jr: Inherited disorders of pigmentation. Clin Derm 3:70–134, 1985

14.5   MELANOCYTIC LESIONS AND DISORDERS OF PIGMENTATION

Seth J. Orlow

Melanocytic disorders generally present as disorders of pigmentation, although dark skin may also occur as a consequence of hyperkeratosis as seen in some epidermal disorders, particularly acanthosis nigricans. Several genetic disorders of decreased pigmentation (such as piebaldism, Waardenburg syndrome, oculocutaneous albinism, and tuberous sclerosis) and of increased pigmentation (such as neurofibromatosis) are reviewed in Sec. 14.4.

14.5.1 Nevi and Other Pigmented Lesions

FRECKLES AND LENTIGINES Freckles are small, jagged light-brown pigmented macules that most often arise in young children. These benign lesions are limited to sun-exposed areas of the skin, darken in response to sunlight, and indicate melanocytic stimulation in response to chronic, excessive sun exposure. Avoiding sun exposure during peak-intensity summer sun hours, wearing protective clothing, and using sunscreens with a high sun protective factor (SPF) rating are advisable for children with numerous freckles. Lentigines, typically darker than freckles and round or oval in shape, may arise on any part of the skin or mucous membranes as isolated findings or, when multiple, associated with various genetic syndromes.

Café au lait macules (CALM) are sharply defined, evenly pigmented macules that may occur on any part of the skin surface. Their color varies from light to medium brown, depending on the overall degree of background skin pigmentation. CALM are usually present at birth but may also arise or become evident during the first several years of life. The incidence is higher in black infants. Lesions range in size from several millimeters to more than 20 cm in diameter and on biopsy exhibit a slightly increased number of single melanocytes containing large melanosomes. The presence of more than six café au lait spots of greater than 1.5 cm in diameter in a child older than 5 years of age may be indicative of neurofibromatosis type I (Sec. 14.4.4), but CALM can also be seen in tuberous sclerosis (Sec. 14.4.4), the McCune-Albright syndrome, and a wide variety of malformation syndromes and genetic diseases.

ACQUIRED MELANOCYTIC NEVI Acquired melanocytic nevi (pigmented moles) are composed of collections or "nests" of melanocytes at the dermal-epidermal junction or within the dermis. Depending on the location of these nests, melanocytic nevi are classified as junctional, compound, or intradermal. Nevi begin to appear during the preschool years; a second wave often erupts during adolescence. By late adolescence, most individuals have 20 to 30 acquired nevi, although the number may be higher in fair-skinned children with a history of numerous or severe sunburns or in immunosuppressed children. *Junctional nevi,* in which nests are confined to the epidermis along the dermal-epidermal junction, are flat, brown-to-black, evenly pigmented macules that are found in greatest numbers on sun-exposed sites. With time, junctional nevi are believed to evolve into *compound nevi,* which are pink to dark brown in color and slightly elevated, and then *intradermal nevi,* dome-shaped or pedunculated nevi composed entirely of nests of dermal melanocytes at the dermal-epidermal junction and within the dermis. Coarse hairs may develop within compound or intradermal nevi. The appearance of new nevi and the growth of such lesions is an expected finding in children and adolescents; hence, routine removal of acquired melanocytic nevi is unnecessary, because malignant melanoma is rare in childhood. Excision in toto should be considered for nevi that ulcerate, become painful or pruritic, or change unexpectedly in size, shape, or color.

Occasionally, a ring of depigmentation develops around one or more nevi, forming a halo nevus. Histologic examination reveals a dense lymphocytic infiltrate surrounding the nevus cells. Although single and even multiple halo nevi occur commonly as an isolated condition during childhood and adolescence, *multiple halo nevi* (Fig. 14-15) are sometimes found in association with childhood vitiligo. Removal is required only when the pigmented lesion shows atypical features.

Dysplastic nevi (atypical moles) appear typically on sun-exposed sites in variegated shades of black, brown, and pink and exhibit an irregular or smudged border. Larger than ordinary acquired melanocytic nevi (ie, >5 mm in diameter), they are defined histopathologically by architectural changes (eg, extension of junctional melanocytic nests beyond the dermal component, bridging between rete ridges, fibroplasia of the papillary dermis) and by cytologic atypia. Dysplasia can be distinguished from melanoma in situ by the organization of atypical melanocytes into nests of relatively uniform size and by the absence of individual melanocytes scattered throughout the epidermis above the basal layer (*pagetoid spread*). Although the malignant potential of a solitary atypical (dysplastic) nevus is indubitably quite low, the adolescent with numerous atypical nevi is at increased risk for malignant melanoma, particularly when there is a family history. Nevus photography during regular skin examination may be useful to identify changing lesions, which should be excised.

Spitz nevus (spindle and epithelioid cell nevus) is a dome-shaped, brown to pink papule that arises commonly on the head, neck, or upper extremities. Spitz nevi are usually solitary but may be multiple and grouped. The characteristic histopathology shows pleomorphic melanocytes in well-circumscribed nests, often with acanthosis and dilated capillaries. Distinguishing Spitz nevi from malignant melanoma may be difficult even for experienced pathologists, but Spitz nevi are not malignant.

An area of light brown pigmentation similar to CALM but studded with small darker macules and/or papules is a *nevus spilus.* This benign lesion is present at birth or arises during early childhood on any part of the cutaneous surface. Histopathology demonstrates multiple, small periappendageal collections of melanocytes at the dermal-epidermal junction or within the dermis superimposed on a CALM background. No treatment is required.

Congenital melanocytic nevi, present in 1 to 2% of newborns, may cover a minute (less than 1 mm) or an enormous proportion of any part of the skin surface. Lesions vary in color from brown to black and may be flat, nodular, verrucous, or even leathery in texture. It is not unusual for congenital melanocytic nevi to become

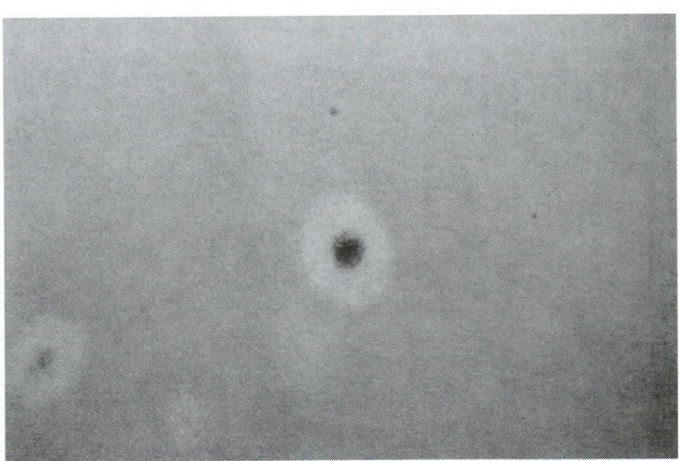

FIGURE 14-15   Several acquired pigmented nevi on the back are now surrounded by a zone of depigmentation. Two nevi have cleared clinically. (*Courtesy of Amy Paller, M.D.*)

more elevated over time and to grow long, coarse hairs. Lesions that achieve diameters of larger than 20 cm by adulthood are termed *giant congenital melanocytic nevi* (Fig. 14-16), which commonly overlie the midline of the back but may occur elsewhere, often in conjunction with numerous, widely scattered "satellite" nevi. Histologically, there are numerous melanocytes both superficially and deep within the dermis and within appendages, especially hair follicles. The presence of atypical melanocytes during the first several months of life is not indicative of malignant transformation. In addition to the potential for severe cosmetic disfigurement, congenital melanocytic nevi may be complicated by malignancy or by *leptomeningeal melanosis,* the latter seen most commonly with giant congenital melanocytic nevi involving the scalp and/ or paraspinal areas. MRI imaging with gadolinium contrast has revolutionized our ability to identify melanosis of the central nervous system. Neurologic sequelae such as seizures or mental retardation appear to be uncommon. Parents of patients with congenital nevi may wish to contact the Nevus Network Congenital Nevus Support Group, available by email at *nevusnet@bigfoot.com.* *Malignant melanoma* and other malignancies of neural crest derivation may develop in patients with giant nevi; the five-year risk may be as high as 5%. A substantial proportion of the reported fatalities have occured in the first decade of life. Melanomas arising within giant congenital nevi generally carry a poor prognosis because of difficulty in early detection; moreover the incidence of extracutaneous melanoma is at least as high.

The management of congenital melanocytic nevi is an area of considerable controversy. Excision of lesions larger than 20 cm is often advocated as a means of reducing or eliminating the risk of malignant melanoma but has no effect on the risk of neurocutaneous melanoma or melanosis. Serial excisions, skin grafting, and inflatable tissue expanders are commonly employed. Size and location of the giant nevus, as well as melanocytic extension into underlying fascia and muscle, may hinder complete eradication. Referral to a center experienced in the management of such lesions is encouraged. Careful follow-up, at three- to six-month intervals, preferably with photographs to assist in recognition of changing lesions, is mandatory for all patients with giant nevi.

Although no case of malignant degeneration of a so-called satellite nevus has been reported to date, the frequency of malignant transformation in smaller congenital nevi is not known. The routine removal of small (<1.5 cm) and intermediate (1.5 to 2.0 cm) congenital melanocytic nevi is advocated by some experts but is held to be impractical and unnecessary by others. It is prudent to examine small congenital nevi at intervals and to consider removal of problematic lesions when the child is old enough to cooperate with local anesthesia. At that time, lesions that are difficult to follow because of their location (eg, scalp or buttocks) or because they are deeply pigmented or show irregular topography (ie, where early detection of malignant transformation would be difficult) should be considered for removal.

Although the incidence of malignant melanoma within the general population has been rapidly increasing, the occurence of malignant melanoma during childhood and especially prior to adolescence remains very rare. The risk of malignant melanoma is greater in individuals with fair skin, numerous nevi (>50–100), multiple dysplastic nevi, and excessive, intense sun exposures during childhood. The familial atypical mole/melanoma syndrome, also called the *dysplastic nevus syndrome,* is believed to be an autosomal-dominant trait. When melanoma has developed in two or more family members, individuals with familial dysplastic nevus syndrome carry an exceedingly high risk for melanoma development, usually after the second decade. Children with dysplastic nevi in these kindreds should be protected from excessive sun exposures and examined at regular (6- to 12-month) intervals.

Melanoma may arise on an area of previously normal skin or less frequently in association with an acquired nevus of the banal or dysplastic type. Malignant melanoma may also arise as a rapidly growing nodule or tumor within a congenital melanocytic nevus; when the neoplasm develops deep within the dermis, clinical recognition can be delayed. Rarely, congenital malignant melanoma is acquired transplacentally. The development of pruritus, pain, or ulceration within a nevus may be a symptom of malignant transformation. Pigmented lesions that have changed rapidly and unexpectedly in size or contour, that have become irregular in color or shape, or that have developed nodules should be excised in toto for complete histopathologic evaluation.

Macular or nodular *blue nevi* may rarely be present at birth but more typically arise during childhood or adolescence. Histologically, bundles of slender, wavy melanocytes are seen deep within the dermis. The cellular blue nevus is a larger nodule (1–3 cm) most often located on the buttocks or sacrococcygeal region. Clinically typical blue nevi need not be excised, although malignant degeneration may rarely occur.

Mongolian spots (dermal melanosis) are poorly defined macular areas of blue-to-gray discoloration noted at birth, typically on the skin overlying the buttocks and sacrococcygeal region. Other areas such as the upper back, shoulders, and arms or legs may be involved, particularly in Asian infants; the palms, soles, and face are spared. The incidence of mongolian spots in newborns is generally correlated with the overall depth of pigmentation. Thus, mongolian spots occur in 90% of black, 80% of Asian, 65% of Latin American, and 5% of white newborns. Mongolian spots are caused by the persistence of migrating melanocytes within the lower dermis. These common lesions tend to disappear over the course of childhood; mongolian spots on the distal extremities may not resolve completely.

Nevus of Ota is a unilateral, mottled, blue to brown discoloration of the forehead and periorbital skin; the ipsilateral sclera may also be involved. Color depends upon the mix of dermal and epidermal involvement. *Nevus of Ito* is a comparable lesion involving the deltoid and supraclavicular regions. Most are present at birth or appear during the first year of life and persist throughout life.

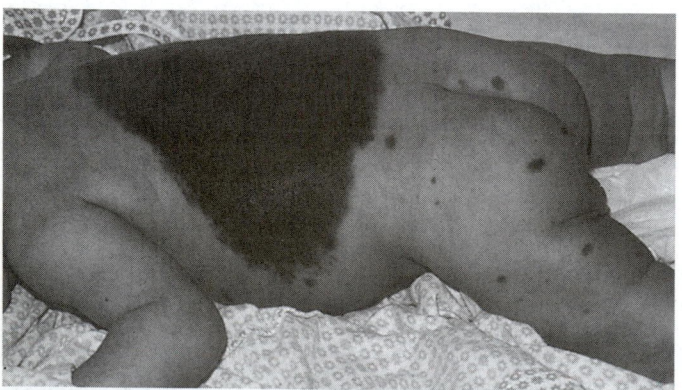

FIGURE 14-16   Giant congenital nevus involving much of the back with satellite smaller congenital pigmented nevi. Because of the location overlying the spinal column, the infant is at increased risk for having leptomeningeal melanosis as well. (*Courtesy of Amy Paller, M.D.*)

Patients with nevus of Ota may be at some increased risk for ocular melanoma during adulthood; regular fundoscopic examinations are recommended.

The *Becker nevus* is an ill-defined area of tan to brown pigmentation containing numerous coarse hairs, most commonly located on the shoulder or back of adolescent boys. Histologically, an increased melanization of the basal cell layer and increased numbers of hair follicles with prominent smooth muscle bundles are seen. Becker nevi are considered to be hair follicle hamartomas, not melanocytic nevi. The congenital smooth-muscle hamartoma is probably a variant of the Becker nevus. Patients with extensive Becker nevi should be carefully examined for associated anomalies, particularly limb and breast hypoplasias.

14.5.2   Acquired Pigmentation Disorders

Inflammatory dermatoses may result in pigmentary changes; these changes are most pronounced in patients with darker skin colors. *Postinflammatory hyperpigmentation* can originate in the epidermis from stimulation of melanin synthesis, or it can be intradermal, caused by phagocytosis of melanin granules that entered into the dermis during inflammatory disruption of the dermal-epidermal junction (pigment incontinence). Contact with furocoumarins in limes and other citrus fruits followed by exposure to sunlight may give rise to *phytophotodermatitis,* a form of postinflammatory hyperpigmentation. Intensely hyperpigmented patterns of drips or thumbprints allow the diagnosis to be made (Fig. 14-17). No treatment is necessary, but fading may be slow. *Postinflammatory hypopigmentation* is seen commonly during and after episodes of seborrheic dermatitis, atopic dermatitis, or psoriasis; the condition arises from impaired transfer of melanin granules from melanocytes to keratinocytes. Most postinflammatory pigmentary alterations resolve spontaneously, albeit slowly, over months to years.

Pigmentary disturbance may occur with several endocrine and metabolic disorders. The gradual onset of generalized hyperpigmentation in skin exposed to sunlight or repeated trauma is the most common presenting symptom of *Addison disease.* Darkening of the mucous membranes and accentuated pigmentation of previously existing scars and of the palmar creases may also be indic-

ative of adrenal insufficiency. The hyperpigmentation is caused by increased melanogenesis induced by elevated levels of proopiomelanocorticotrophic peptides. Treatment of the underlying endocrine disease results in a gradual return to normal skin color. Other disorders exhibiting hyperpigmentation include *McCune-Albright syndrome,* characterized by the combination of precocious puberty in girls, polyostotic fibrous dysplasia, and jagged, unilateral CALM with sharp and irregular margins.

Vitiligo is a common disorder characterized by complete loss of pigmentation (depigmentation) within sharply bordered areas of skin. The onset is before the age of 20 years in 50% of patients, and 30% have a family history of the disease, although the pattern of inheritance appears to be multigenic. Vitiligo may occur in association with halo nevi, with autoimmune thyroiditis, and less often with Addison disease or juvenile diabetes mellitus. Melanocyte autoantibodies may be present. The essential pathologic process is a circumscribed loss of melanocytes.

Vitiligo occurring during childhood falls into two fairly distinct clinical patterns. Segmental vitiligo, which occurs in up to 50% of childhood cases, is characterized by the loss of pigmentation limited to a segmented, quasidermatomal area of skin. Lesions are unilateral and may involve any site. Depigmentation can progress rapidly but usually remains confined to the initial segments. The development of new lesions typically ceases after the first 24 months. Segmental vitiligo is not associated with other autoimmune diseases. In contrast, generalized vitiligo (Fig. 14-18) may affect any part of the cutaneous surface and is often strikingly symmetrical in distribution. Acral (eg, distal fingers and toes) and periorificial (eg, eyes, mouth, and genitalia) surfaces are particularly common locations. Lesions tend to enlarge, and new areas of involvement may develop during many years.

Treatment of vitiligo remains problematic. Repigmentation requires cessation of ongoing melanocyte loss, stimulation of remaining melanocytes if present, or repopulation of the depigmented skin by melanocytes migrating either from peripheral uninvolved skin or from deep within unaffected hair follicles. Thus, the presence of pigmented hairs within a vitiliginous lesion is a favorable sign. Some lesions may repigment with prolonged use of a medium- to high-potency topical corticosteroid over two to four months (see Table 14-3). The topical application of psoralens followed by controlled

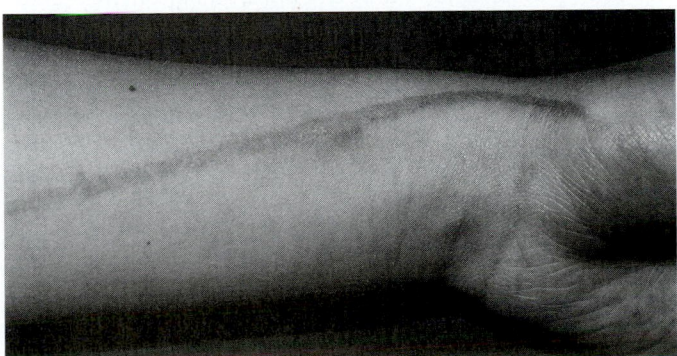

FIGURE 14-17   **Phytophotodermatitis. The patient squeezed limes while in Mexico and later developed this darkly pigmented streak on the arm. Phytophotodermatitis is a phototoxic reaction that results from cutaneous exposure to furocoumarins (as in certain fruits and vegetables) and then ultraviolet light. Although erythema and even blistering may be associated, many patients merely present with the intense pigmentation. (*Courtesy of Amy Paller, M.D.*)**

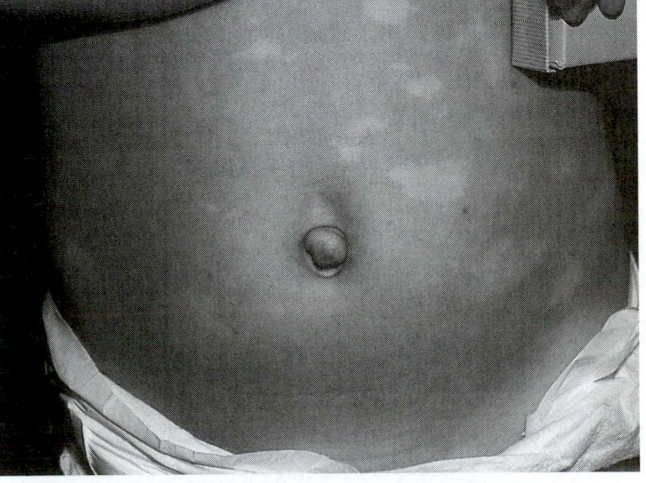

FIGURE 14-18   **Several depigmented patches located on the abdomen in this child with vitiligo. (*Courtesy of Amy Paller, M.D.*)**

exposure to sunlight or artificial sources of long-wave ultraviolet light (UVA) can be effective but requires numerous treatments over many months. Great care must be taken to avoid psoralen contact with surrounding skin because of secondary hyperpigmentation. The combination of oral psoralens and artificial, high-intensity UVA light (PUVA) also requires numerous treatments and strict compliance with the wearing of UV-screening glasses. PUVA is not recommended for children younger than 12 years or for lightly pigmented individuals of any age because of the associated long-term risk of cutaneous malignancies, especially squamous cell carcinoma. The rare association of vitiligo, uveitis, dysacousia, and aseptic meningitis is termed *Vogt-Koyanagi-Harada syndrome.* The National Vitiligo Foundation, Inc. can be reached by email at *73071.33@compuserve.com.*

The *nevus depigmentosus* is an area of circumscribed hypomelanosis that may be present at birth or develop over time. The lesions may be solitary or multiple in a pseudodermatomal distribution; some may have pigmented circular macules within their borders. Early in life, differentiation of nevus depigmentosus from the hypomelanotic macule of tuberous sclerosis may be difficult; however, other cutaneous or neurologic manifestations of tuberous sclerosis will eventually develop in most patients. Nevus depigmentosus is not associated with systemic disease.

Hypomelanosis of Ito, formerly called *incontinentia pigmenti achromians,* is an uncommon disorder characterized by a swirled pattern of hypopigmentation following Blaschko's lines (Color Plate 9). The cutaneous changes, which are the stigmata of genetic mosaicism, may be present from birth or may be progressive. They are most commonly seen in isolation but may be accompanied by a variety of musculoskeletal and neurodevelopmental disorders, including ocular hypertelorism, leg length asymmetry, seizures, and mental retardation. Evaluation should be guided by the presence or absence of abnormal findings upon careful clinical examination. Abnormal karyotypes in lymphocytes and/or fibroblasts are seen in some patients.

References

Bolognia JL, Pawelek JM: Biology of hypopigmentation. J Am Acad Dermatol 19:217–255, 1988

Chamlin SL: Moles and melanoma. Curr Opin Pediatr 10:398–404, 1998

DeDavid M, Orlow SJ, Provost N, et al: Neurocutaneous melanosis: clinical features of large congenital melanocytic nevi in patients with manifest central nervous system melanosis. J Am Acad Dermatol 35:529–538, 1996

DeDavid M, Orlow SJ, Provost N, et al: A study of large congenital melanocytic nevi and associated malignant melanomas: review of cases in the New York University registry and the world literature. J Am Acad Dermatol 36:409–416, 1997

Gallagher RP, McLean DI, Yang CP, et al: Suntan, sunburn, and pigmentation factors and the frequency of acquired melanocytic nevi in children. Similarities to melanoma: the Vancouver Mole Study. Arch Dermatol 126:770–776, 1990

Greene MH, Clark WH Jr, Tucker MA, et al: Acquired precursors of cutaneous malignant melanoma: the familial dysplastic nevus syndrome. N Engl J Med 312:91–97, 1985

Halder RM: Childhood vitiligo. Clin Dermatol 15:899–906, 1997

Nehal KS, PeBenito R, Orlow SJ: Analysis of 54 cases of hypopigmentation and hyperpigmentation along the lines of Blaschko. Arch Dermatol 132:1167–1170, 1996

Special symposia: the management of congenital nevocytic nevi. Pediatr Dermatol 2:142, 1984

14.6 IMMUNOLOGIC DISEASES

Julie Prendiville

14.6.1 Drug Eruptions

Cutaneous adverse reactions to drugs are common in pediatric practice and often present a diagnostic challenge. The pathogenesis of most drug eruptions is not well understood. With few exceptions, eg, fixed drug eruption (see below), the diagnosis cannot be based solely on the morphology of the eruption. A drug rash may manifest as urticaria, a morbilliform exanthem, erythroderma, Stevens-Johnson syndrome (SJS), toxic epidermal necrolysis (TEN), photosensitivity, lichen planus, or vasculitis, all of which have other potential causes. A high index of suspicion for drug causation is important so that an offending drug is discontinued and avoided in the future, particularly in the case of life-threatening reactions such as anaphylaxis, the drug (anticonvulsant) hypersensitivity syndrome, SJS, and TEN. Conversely, it is important not to err by labeling a child as "allergic" to a widely used medication, such as penicillin. There are no standardized laboratory investigations that are diagnostic for drug allergy, and the value of allergy testing is largely restricted to cases of IgE-mediated penicillin hypersensitivity. Therefore, a detailed history, evaluation of the morphology of the rash, consideration of a differential diagnosis, and careful clinical judgment are essential.

The timing of the reaction may be helpful. Medications begun recently, particularly within the past weeks, are more likely to be culpable than drugs taken for many months. Urticaria usually occurs within hours to one day after beginning a medication, whereas maculopapular eruptions develop 7 to 10 days into treatment unless there has been a previous exposure. Life-threatening hypersensitivity reactions to sulfonamides, carbamazepine, phenytoin, or phenobarbital characteristically occur one to four weeks after initiating therapy. Although serious adverse reactions are rare, the parents of children who are prescribed these medications should be advised to seek medical attention if a rash or fever develops within the first four to six weeks of treatment.

The morphology of the rash is an important observation. Morbilliform, "maculopapular" drug eruptions, though often extremely pruritic, are usually benign and self-limited. Some, as in the common ampicillin rash (see below) may not recur on rechallenge. These eruptions may be difficult to distinguish from viral exanthems. All patients with a morbilliform eruption, particularly those caused by sulfonamides and anticonvulsant medications, should be closely monitored during the first few days for progression to SJS, TEN, or the drug (anticonvulsant) hypersensitivity syndrome which is characterized by an erythematous exanthem, fever, hepatosplenomegaly, lymphadenopathy, hepatitis, and multiorgan disease. These life-threatening drug reactions are accompanied by fever and signs of systemic toxicity. They are sometimes initially misdiagnosed as a viral or other infectious illness.

Urticarial drug eruptions are also potentially life threatening because of the risk of airway angioedema and anaphylaxis. Acute urticaria in childhood is often associated with a viral or upper respiratory tract illness for which an antibiotic may have been administered. In such cases, it is difficult to be certain whether the cause of the urticaria is the infection, the drug, or perhaps a drug-virus interaction. It is wise to discontinue the drug and consult an allergist before considering oral rechallenge if further use of the medication is anticipated. Cefaclor causes an urticarial eruption, often associated with arthralgia, in up to 3% of children who take this antibiotic.

If urticarial reactions, the drug (anticonvulsant) hypersensitivity syndrome, vasculitis, SJS, or TEN occur as a result of drug administration, patients should be considered allergic to the medication, and the drug should not be readministered. If more than one drug is being used, all drugs that could potentially induce such a reaction, and particularly anticonvulsants, antibiotics, and sulfonamide derivatives, should be discontinued.

The most common drug reaction in childhood is the *ampicillin rash,* which occurs in up to 18% of children receiving oral ampicillin. The median time of onset is 9 days, with a range from 1 to 14 days. Lesions are fine, erythematous macules and papules that usually appear on the trunk, then spread peripherally. The mechanism of this eruption is poorly understood. In some cases it may be the result of a drug-virus interaction, such as with the Epstein-Barr virus or cytomegalovirus. It is not considered a true allergy, and if the findings are typical, readministration of the drug is not contraindicated.

The *fixed drug eruption* is characterized by one or a few discrete plaques of dusky erythema that develop hours to days after drug exposure. Central blistering is often present. The mucous membranes of the lips or penis are commonly affected, but lesions may occur on any part of the body. They typically resolve, leaving an ashy-gray postinflammatory hyperpigmentation. If the offending drug is readministered, lesions will recur in precisely the same anatomic locations. Common causative drugs include salicylates, barbiturates, phenolphthalein (found in laxatives), and tetracyclines. A nonpigmenting fixed drug eruption that presents with localized erythema and subsequently desquamates may be caused by pseudoephedrine, contained in over-the-counter remedies for upper respiratory tract symptoms.

References

Griff-Lonnevig V, Hedlin G, Lindfors A: Penicillin allergy—a rare paediatric condition. Arch Dis Child 63:1342–1346, 1988

Hebert AA, Sigman ES, Levy ML: Serum sickness-like reactions from cefaclor in children. J Am Acad Dermatol 25:805–808, 1991

Kanwar AJ, Bharija SC, Belhaj MS: Fixed drug eruptions in children: a series of 23 cases with provocative tests. Dermatologica 162:315–318, 1986

Licata AL, Louis ED: Anticonvulsant hypersensitivity syndrome. Compr Ther. 22:152–155, 1996

Penicillin allergy in childhood. Lancet 1:420, 1989

Rieder MJ: In vivo and in vitro testing for adverse drug reactions. Pediatr Clin North Am 44:93–111, 1997

14.6.2.   Hypersensitivity Reactions

Urticaria (hives) is common in children. The primary wheal is an erythematous, edematous papule or plaque produced by a sudden increase in interstitial fluid within the upper dermis. Most cases of acute urticaria result from type I, IgE-mediated hypersensitivity, but chronic urticaria may be precipitated by other pathogenetic mechanisms. The mast cell plays a central role as the effector cell in all forms of urticaria (see Sec. 11.13).

Acute urticaria is the most common form of urticaria in children. Red or pink wheals appear suddenly, persist for 2 to 12 hours, then resolve or shift to new sites. The wheals can be pale or dusky blue in the center, producing a target-like appearance that may be confused with erythema multiforme or vasculitis (Color Plate 10). Intense pruritus is usually present but may be absent. Lesions vary in size from a few millimeters to many centimeters and are often annular or geographic in configuration. The lesions may be associated with deep cutaneous edema (angioedema) or less frequently with respiratory tract involvement, producing laryngospasm or bronchospasm. The differential diagnosis includes erythema multiforme, vasculitis, exanthems, nonurticarial drug eruptions, and papular urticaria caused by insect bites. Acute urticaria can be distinguished from all these conditions by the evanescent nature of the lesions. As the wheals resolve or change shape within 12 hours, outlining lesions with ink to follow their progression or disappearance is helpful in distinguishing urticaria from erythema multiforme or urticarial vasculitis.

Assessment and management of the airway takes precedence over treatment of skin lesions. If there is evidence of respiratory distress or anaphylaxis, epinephrine in oil (Susphrine, 0.005 ml/kg, maximum 0.15 ml, given subcutaneously) is indicated. Antihistamines are the mainstay of therapy for cutaneous disease. In contrast to most other pruritic disorders, their role in urticaria is to prevent wheal formation and not simply to control pruritus. Diphenhydramine (5 mg/kg/d), hydroxyzine (2–4 mg/kg/d) or cyproheptidine (0.25–0.5 mg/kg/d) should be given in three to four divided doses. Combination therapy with two antihistamines may be required. Therapy should be continued until the child has been hive-free for at least 72 hours; thereafter the drug dosage is slowly tapered. Systemic corticosteroids are occasionally used when high doses of antihistamines are ineffective. A precipitating antigen should be searched for by a careful history, including dietary and drug history, and thorough physical examination. Most cases of urticaria in children are caused by benign viral illnesses. Specific infections such as hepatitis A and B and *Hymenoptera* stings should be considered. Foods that cause acute urticaria include shellfish, nuts, and strawberries. The most common drugs that induce urticarial reactions are penicillins, cephalosporins (especially cefaclor), and sulfonamides. These patients are at risk for anaphylaxis upon reexposure (see Sec. 11.15).

Contact urticaria occurs within minutes to a few hours after direct skin contact with a food or chemical. It is a relatively common condition and may occur at any age. Many agents including fish, tomato, and cosmetic ingredients have been causally implicated.

Chronic urticaria persisting for weeks, months, or even years may be idiopathic or caused by physical factors. Physical urticarias are precipitated by environmental factors, such as pressure, cold, ultraviolet light, and exercise. Dermographism is a common form of physical urticaria in which the pressure from "moderate" stroking results in urticarial wheals. Although sufficient stroke pressure will induce wheals on normal skin, in dermographism the threshold is much reduced. If necessary, symptoms may be minimized by preventive, antihistamine therapy (see above). *Cold urticaria* is precipitated by exposure to cold water or air, resulting in urticaria or painless swelling of exposed areas such as the face and hands. Respiratory symptoms, such as wheezing or dyspnea, may also develop. The diagnosis is confirmed with the "ice cube test," in which localized urticaria is induced by applying an ice cube to the skin for 10 minutes. Cyproheptadine, 0.25 to 0.5 mg/kg/d divided every eight hours, is usually beneficial. Because of the risk of anaphylaxis, sudden exposure to cold, such as diving into cold water, must be avoided. *Cholinergic urticaria* is a distinctive form of urticaria, relatively common in adolescents, in which multiple 1- to 2-mm wheals surrounded by macular halos of erythema are precipitated by exercise and sweating. Respiratory symptoms may also develop. Oral antihistamines are occasionally required for treatment.

Hereditary angioedema is a rare, dominantly inherited condition resulting from a deficiency or defect of C1 esterase inhibitor. Patients usually present in childhood with recurrent episodes of angioedema. These episodes differ clinically from acute urticaria in several ways: superficial wheals are absent; lesions are painful, rather than pruritic, and persistent; the swellings are unresponsive to antihistamine or corticosteroid therapy; and the family history is often positive. The diagnosis is established by finding low serum levels of C4 and C1 esterase inhibitor.

Erythema multiforme (EM), sometimes called *EM minor,* is a hypersensitivity reaction confined to the skin and/or mouth, without systemic toxicity. Infections, particularly with the herpes simplex virus, are the most common cause of EM minor, although no evidence of active herpetic lesions may be present at the time the erythema multiforme develops.

The skin lesions of EM usually have an abrupt onset but may develop during several days as crops of new lesions appear. Typical lesions begin as erythematous macules, which rapidly evolve into edematous, erythematous plaques. The central portion of the lesions may become dusky, necrotic, or blistered, with variable rings of concentric color change, including an intensification of redness at the periphery of the lesions ("target" lesions) (Color Plate 10). Multiple, symmetric lesions occur on the extremities, including the palms and soles. The face, groin, and neck are often affected as well. Lesions on the trunk are less prominent than those on the extremities (centrifugal distribution). Mucosal involvement usually begins at the same time as the skin eruption but may precede or follow it by several days. Multiple erosions, with or without overlying pseudomembranes, may develop on the lips, tongue, and palate, but these erosions do not tend to be severe.

In *Stevens-Johnson syndrome,* sometimes called *EM major,* mucosal lesions predominate, occur at more than one site, and are usually noted before cutaneous lesions (Fig. 14-19). Severe erosions of the lips and oral mucous membranes lead to marked pain. Involvement of the ocular, genital, and anal mucosae may also be severe. An extensive eruption of erythematous macules and raised lesions, often with blisters and erosions, on the face, trunk, extremities, and genitalia is associated with the mucosal lesions. Atypical target lesions and blue macules are occasionally seen as well.

Toxic epidermal necrolysis (TEN) is defined as full-thickness epidermal necrosis of more than 30% of the body surface. Many consider TEN and Stevens-Johnson syndrome to be related disorders with a similar pathomechanism; overlapping cases with manifestations that resemble both Stevens-Johnson syndrome and TEN may occur with blistering and epidermal detachment of more than 10% of the body surface area. In Stevens-Johnson syndrome with bullae or in TEN, stroking of the skin at the edge of a blister may extend it (positive Nikolsky sign). Systemic toxicity in patients with Stevens-Johnson syndrome or TEN is often severe, particularly with fever, dysphagia from esophageal erosions, tracheal and bronchial erosions, respiratory abnormalities, noninfectious hepatitis, lymphadenopathy, glomerulonephritis and acute tubular necrosis, and myocarditis. Long-term sequelae can include dyspigmentation and mucosal scarring, particularly of the eyes with resultant symblepharon, synechiae, entropion and ectropion, trichiasis, corneal opacities, and pannus formation. Strictures of the esophagus, bronchus,

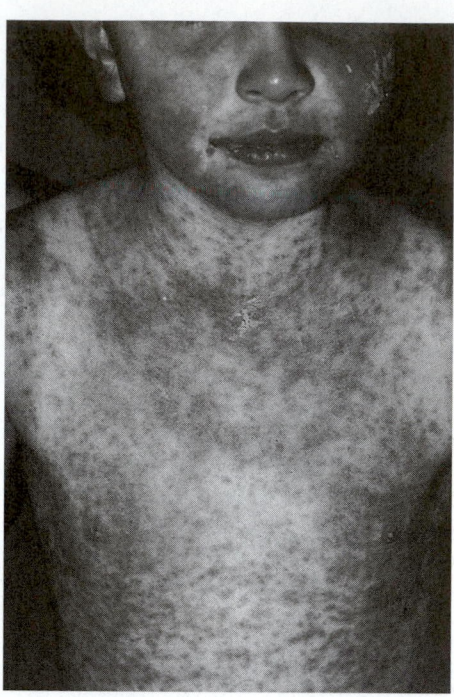

FIGURE 14-19   Stevens-Johnson syndrome. Generalized eruption of violaceous nonscaling plaques, some of which have blistered, as a reaction to administration of phenytoin. Note the oral crusting and erythema. The patient also showed conjunctivitis with crusting and erosions of the genital mucosa. (*Courtesy of Amy Paller, M.D.*)

urethra, vagina, or anus may occasionally occur. A Sjögren-like syndrome caused by damage to the lacrimal and salivary glands may also ensue. The mortality rate from massive loss of fluid and electrolytes and infection is particularly high in patients with TEN (25%).

Most cases of either Stevens-Johnson syndrome or TEN are precipitated by drugs, particularly sulfonamides and the aromatic anticonvulsants (eg, phenytoin, phenobarbital, and carbamazepine). Other drugs including penicillins, cephalosporins, and lamotrigine have also been implicated. Stevens-Johnson syndrome may also be triggered by infections, and an association with *Mycoplasma pneumoniae* is well-recognized. TEN may also develop in severe, acute graft-versus-host disease.

The differential diagnosis of EM includes urticaria, vasculitis, and other types of generalized drug eruptions or viral exanthems. SJS may be distinguished from Kawasaki disease by the presence of blistering on the lips and oral mucosa. TEN must be differentiated from staphylococcal scalded-skin syndrome (SSSS), which also presents with tender red skin. Patients with SSSS do not have mucosal blistering and do not have full-thickness epidermal detachment. If necessary, these disorders can easily be distinguished by skin biopsy (demonstrating extensive epidermal necrosis in TEN versus a subcorneal blister overlying a normal-appearing epidermis in SSSS) or by a Tzanck preparation performed on detached epidermis (demonstrating acantholytic cells in SSSS).

TREATMENT

EM minor is a self-limited process and requires no specific treatment. Symptomatic therapy including intravenous fluids may be necessary if there is severe oral mucosal involvement. Stevens-Johnson syndrome causes serious morbidity, and TEN is always life threatening. In all patients a careful history for etiologic agents should be taken, and potentially causative medications should be discontinued. Recurrent exposure to an etiologic drug must be avoided. Patients with SJS or TEN should be hospitalized for supportive care until the skin and mucosa reepithelialize. If skin loss is extensive, management in a specialized burn unit or intensive care unit may be required. Patients with respiratory distress should also be referred for intensive care. Fluid and electrolyte status must be carefully monitored, skin and blood cultures periodically taken, and patients watched closely for signs of infection. Most patients will require nutritional support in addition to fluid replacement. Pain management is also very important.

Denuded skin should be compressed with dilute (1:40) aluminum acetate (Burow) solution or saline. Protective dressings may be synthetic (eg, Vaseline gauze or Mepitel) or biological. Oral lesions can be cleansed with either clorhexidine oral solution or a sodium bicarbonate mouth wash. If conjunctival involvement is present, an ophthalmologist should see the patient on an emergency basis, because blindness is a potential complication of Stevens-Johnson syndrome. Patients with severe urethral erosions will require insertion of an in-dwelling catheter.

The use of systemic corticosteroids in the treatment of SJS and TEN is controversial. No studies have clearly demonstrated their efficacy, and they may increase the risk of infection. A recent report of successful outcome with the administration of intravenous gamma globulin, based on inhibition of Fas-mediated keratinocyte death, suggests a new treatment option that requires further testing.

References

Brice SL, Huff JC, Weston WL: Erythema multiforme. Curr Prob Dermatol 2:5–25, 1990

Mortureux P, Leaute-Labreze C, Legrain-Lifermann V, et al: Acute urticaria in infancy and early childhood. Arch Dermatol 134;319–323, 1998

Prendiville JS, Hebert AA, Greenwald MJ, Esterly NB: Management of Stevens-Johnson syndrome and toxic epidermal necrolysis in children. J Pediatr 115:881–887, 1989

Taylor JA, Grube B, Heimbach DM, et al: Toxic epidermal necrolysis: a comprehensive approach. Clin Pediatr 28:404–407, 1989

Viard I, Wehrli P, Bullai R, et al: Inhibition of toxic epidermal necrolysis by blockade of CD95 with human intravenous immunoglobulin. Science 282:490–493, 1998

Weston WL, Morelli JG: Herpes simplex virus-associated erythema multiforme in prepubertal children. Arch Pediatr Adolesc Med 151:1014–1016, 1997

Weston WL, Morelli JG, Rogers M: Target lesions on the lips: childhood herpes simplex associated with erythema multiforme mimics Stevens-Johnson syndrome. J Am Acad Dermatol 37:848–850, 1997

Weston JA, Weston WL: The overdiagnosis of erythema multiforme. Pediatrics 89:802, 1992

14.6.3   Erythema Group Reactions

Erythema annulare centrifugum (EAC) is an inflammatory disease of the skin characterized by arcuate, annular lesions most commonly involving the trunk and proximal extremities. Lesions begin as papules or small plaques and slowly expand, clearing centrally, often leaving a "trailing edge" of scale. Lesions may coalesce to form gyrate or serpiginous patterns. Lesions rarely number more than 10. Itching is usually absent or mild. Medications, tinea pedis, or indolent infections in other organs, such as urinary tract infections or dental abscesses, have been suggested as causes, but usually no etiology is found. The condition may wax and wane for months to years. The differential diagnosis includes tinea infection, erythema multiforme, annular erythema of infancy, and urticaria. The diagnosis is usually made clinically but can be confirmed by skin biopsy, which demonstrates a "tight cuff" of lymphocytes around vessels in the upper and lower dermis. Potent topical corticosteroids are occasionally helpful in treatment.

Annular erythema of infancy is characterized by recurrent arcuate skin lesions that develop early in infancy. They begin as small erythematous papules that rapidly enlarge into annular urticarial plaques. The cause of the condition is unknown. Lesions usually resolve within one year. Biopsy demonstrates a moderately dense perivascular infiltrate of eosinophils and lymphocytes. Other conditions that can cause annular erythema in young infants include neonatal lupus erythematosus, erythema annulare centrifugum, urticaria, erythema multiforme, erythema chronicum migrans, familial annular erythema, and erythema gyratum atrophicans.

Reference

Hebert AA, Esterly NB: Annular erythema of infancy. J Am Acad Dermatol 14:339–343, 1986

14.6.4   Dermatologic Manifestations of Collagen Vascular Diseases

LUPUS ERYTHEMATOSUS In lupus erythematosus (LE), the skin may be the sole organ system affected or it may be involved as a manifestation of systemic LE. Cutaneous LE is classified as (1) acute cutaneous LE (ACLE), (2) subacute chronic cutaneous LE (SCLE), or (3) chronic cutaneous LE, of which the most common variant is discoid LE (DLE). Patients with LE may also have skin findings that are not specific such as vasculitis, alopecia, mucosal ulceration, and livedo reticularis. Transient skin involvement resembling SCLE is characteristic of neonatal LE. Sunlight is an important stimulus in the initiation of cutaneous lesions in all forms of LE.

SYSTEMIC LUPUS ERYTHEMATOSUS The most common skin manifestation of systemic lupus erythematosus (SLE) (see Sec. 12.7) is acute cutaneous LE (ACLE), characterized by a transient erythematous eruption that may be localized to the malar area of the face, the "butterfly-rash," or may be more generalized. Concurrent manifestations of SLE may include musculoskeletal, renal, hematologic, or central nervous system involvement. The rash is photosensitive and may present as macular erythema, or as erythematous, edematous, scaly plaques on the malar area and nasal bridge. Similar lesions may occur elsewhere on the body especially in areas exposed to sunlight. Patients with SLE may also develop cheilitis and scarring plaques identical to those seen in DLE (see below).

Subacute cutaneous LE is characterized by a photosensitive, papulosquamous or annular-polycyclic erythema associated with positive serology for anti-Ro (SSA) or anti-La (SSB) antibodies; although usually a benign disorder with mild systemic symptoms, SCLE may sometimes occur in patients with SLE.

Nonspecific cutaneous findings are common in SLE. These include a nonscarring alopecia, mucosal ulceration (most commonly on the hard palate), and capillary loop telangiectasia of the proximal nail folds. Raynaud phenomenon, cold-induced distal acrocyanosis, or chilblain-like lesions may be associated with digital ulcerations. Cutaneous leukocytoclastic vasculitis manifested by palpable purpura or livedo reticularis with ulceration may also be seen. Rare cutaneous manifestations of SLE include urticarial vasculitis, bullous LE, and lupus panniculitis.

The histopathologic examination of biopsies of the cutaneous lesions in SLE is similar to that of DLE (see below), but the characteristic features may not all be present and are often more subtle. The immunopathology of skin lesions in SLE is also similar to DLE. Moreover, immunopathology of nonlesional, sun-exposed skin (the lupus band test) is positive in 80% of patients with SLE and may be a useful diagnostic test. Positive immunopathology in nonlesional, sun-shielded (eg, buttock) skin is less frequent but is correlated with more severe disease especially with renal involvement. Immunopathology of LE vasculitis may show IgG, IgM, and/or complement around superficial venules, in addition to deposits in basement membrane.

The severity of skin disease in SLE frequently waxes and wanes in parallel with the systemic disease. Sun avoidance and the use of broad-spectrum sunscreens are extremely important. Some cutaneous manifestations of SLE may respond to topical or intralesional corticosteroids. Antimalarials such as hydroxychloroquine or chloroquine may also be helpful. The use of systemic steroids or cytotoxic agents is determined by the activity of extracutaneous disease and is addressed in Sec. 12.7.

DISCOID LUPUS ERYTHEMATOSUS DLE is a chronic, disfiguring dermatosis that not uncommonly begins in late adolescence. The characteristic lesion is an erythematous scaly plaque that shows a triad of atrophy, telangiectasia, and follicular plugging. Hypopigmentation, depigmentation, or hyperpigmentation and scarring commonly develop with time. The scalp, face, and the pinna of the ear are the sites of predilection, but lesions may be found on other sun-exposed sites. Histopathology is usually diagnostic in DLE and shows thinning of the epidermis, degeneration of the basal cell layer, thickening of the epidermal basement membrane, a patchy lymphohistiocytic infiltrate in the dermis, and dilated follicular orifices with keratin plugs. The diagnosis of DLE may be confirmed by immunofluorescence of lesional skin, where deposition of IgG, IgM, and/or complement is observed in a broad band just below the dermal-epidermal junction. Laboratory studies including antinuclear antibodies (ANA) and anti-DNA antibodies are usually normal or negative. Only a small percentage of patients with DLE progress to SLE. However, lesions that are characteristic of DLE are seen in about 20% of patients with SLE during the course of their disease.

Treatment of DLE includes careful avoidance of sun exposure and the regular use of sunscreens with SPF of 15 or higher and efficacy in the long ultraviolet (UVA) spectrum. Potent topical (eg, fluocinonide ointment) or intralesional corticosteroids are the most commonly employed forms of therapy. Patients with disfiguring disease may benefit from antimalarials (eg, hydroxychloroquine).

NEONATAL LUPUS ERYTHEMATOSUS Neonatal lupus erythematosus (NLE) is associated with transplacental passage of maternal anti-Ro (SSA), anti-La (SSB), or anti-U$_1$RNP antibodies from mother to fetus. It is characterized most commonly by a transient skin eruption and/or permanent congenital heart block. A minority of infants have both skin and heart disease. Less common manifestations of NLE include thrombocytopenia, leukopenia, hemolytic anemia, hepatitis, hepatosplenomegaly, and pneumonitis. The skin lesions of NLE are characteristically annular, erythematous patches or plaques over the head and neck (Fig. 14-20). NLE may also present with diffuse facial erythema, particularly in a periorbital distribution referred to as "raccoon eyes," or telangiectatic lesions. Annular or macular lesions occur on the trunk and limbs and can be widespread. Lesions may be present at birth or become apparent in the first months of life. Photosensitivity appears to be a factor in precipitating NLE dermatitis, which has developed in infants receiving phototherapy for hyperbilirubinemia as well as following sun exposure.

A diagnosis of NLE is confirmed by positive serology for anti-Ro (SSA) antibodies in the mother and infant. Anti-La (SSB) antibodies are found less commonly, and NLE associated with anti-U$_1$RNP antibodies is rare. Mothers with positive serology may have SLE, but many are asymptomatic at delivery or have minor symptoms and signs of connective tissue disease. All mothers of affected infants should be carefully evaluated and followed for evidence of SLE, ACLE, or Sjögren's syndrome and advised about the risk of future affected pregnancies.

Passively transferred antibodies in the infant are lost during the first six months of life. Congenital heart block, caused by maldevelopment or scarring of the conduction system, may require the implantation of a permanent pacemaker. No treatment of the cutaneous lesions other than sun protection is required. These lesions usually resolve spontaneously by six months of age with little or no scarring. Hematologic abnormalities, hepatitis, and other systemic manifestations of NLE are also transient.

CHILDHOOD DERMATOMYOSITIS Dermatomyositis is a chronic inflammatory disease involving skeletal muscle and skin (see Sec. 12.8). It usually presents with proximal muscle weakness and a rash, but the rash may precede the onset of muscle disease. There are occasionally children who develop the typical rash of dermatomyositis with little or no associated muscle disease at onset. A purplish discoloration of the periorbital skin (*heliotrope sign*) is typical but may be subtle or absent. A diffuse macular erythema or violaceous discoloration commonly affects the malar areas of the face and may be confused with acute cutaneous LE. Erythema or erythematous scaly plaques are seen on the elbows and knees, upper back, chest, and buttocks. These lesions may resemble psoriasis but are less scaly and have ill-defined margins. Flesh-colored or erythematous papules over the metacarpophalangeal joints (*Gottron*

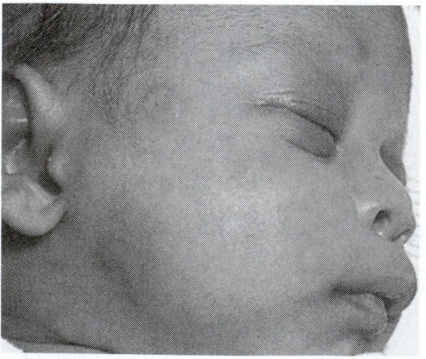

FIGURE 14-20 Neonatal lupus erythematosus. Note several annular dermal inflammatory plaques on face of young infant. (*Courtesy Ilona Frieden, M.D.*)

sign) are highly characteristic (Color Plate 11), as are capillary loop telangiectases of the periungual skin and gum margins. Vasculitis with ulceration may develop in severe disease. Subcutaneous calcifications that may ulcerate and drain develop in children with longstanding disease. The cutaneous histopathology is nonspecific and shows features of epidermal atrophy with degeneration of the basal layer and vascular dilatation. Topical therapy of skin lesions is generally ineffective. Hydroxychloroquine is reported to be of benefit but is often disappointing. Sun protection and application of broad-spectrum (UVB + UVA) sunscreens is important because the rash of dermatomyositis is often photosensitive. The decision to treat with systemic corticosteroids or other immunosuppressive agents is based on the presence of muscle disease.

SCLERODERMA Scleroderma may be localized to the skin (morphea or linear scleroderma) or may involve the skin and internal organs (systemic scleroderma) (see Sec. 12.9). Cutaneous involvement most often begins acrally. Hardening of the skin of the fingers and hands is accompanied by ulceration of the fingertips, telangiectasia, and atrophy. Raynaud phenomenon is almost always present. Facial involvement results in a taut appearance, with furrowing of the skin around the lips and restricted opening of the mouth. Facial telangiectases may be particularly prominent in the milder CREST syndrome (Cutaneous calcinosis, Raynaud phenomenon, Esophageal stenosis, Sclerodactyly, and widespread Telangiectasia), which is particularly rare in children. There is no specific therapy for the cutaneous manifestations of systemic scleroderma. Minimizing cold exposure and wearing warm clothing, gloves, and footwear will decrease the severity of vasopasm and the resultant digital ulcerations. Vasodilating agents such as the calcium channel blockers (eg, nifedipine) may be helpful.

Morphea is characterized by discrete areas of skin hardening. The indurated plaques often have a distinct violaceous border; atrophy, hypopigmentation, or hyperpigmentation may develop over time. The onset of morphea during childhood or adolescence is not uncommon. Thickening and homogenization of collagen bundles in the reticular dermis are seen on skin biopsy, but the diagnosis is usually made based on clinical characteristics. Some benefit has been reported in open label trials from the administration of prednisone in combination with methotrexate, systemic administration of calcipotriol, and application of topical calcipotriol. In the majority of children, the disease activity remits after several years. Progression from morphea to systemic scleroderma is very rare.

Linear scleroderma may occur in one or more linear bands on the face (*en coup de sabre*) or over the length of an extremity. The prognosis for linear scleroderma is less favorable than for morphea, because underlying musculoskeletal structures are often involved. Hemiatrophy of affected areas can occur and may be severely disfiguring and/or impair function of the limb. Significant antinuclear antibody (ANA) titers and anti–single-stranded DNA antibodies may be present, especially during active disease. The disease remits after three to five years. Physiotherapy is important to limit joint contractures, and massage may be of benefit. Treatment with penicillamine has been advocated in the past but has never been shown to be effective and carries a substantial risk for renal and bone marrow toxicity. In the *Parry-Romberg syndrome*, progressive linear or hemifacial musculoskeletal atrophy develops in the presence of normal or atrophic skin. Some children show mixed morphologies of linear scleroderma and facial hemiatrophy; thus, the Parry-Romberg syndrome may be a variant of linear scleroderma. These disorders may have underlying intracerebral malformations or calcifications that result in seizures or hemiparesis. *Systemic scleroderma* is rare in childhood.

Atrophoderma is characterized by depressed areas of skin that can be circumscribed (atrophoderma of Pasini and Pierini) or linear (linear atrophoderma of Moulin). The lesions have a hyperpigmented, bluish or violaceous color that resembles morphea, but there is no sclerosis or induration. Large circumscribed areas on the trunk may be difficult to distinguish from morphea, and occasionally the two conditions coexist. Linear atrophoderma on the limbs can be mistaken for linear scleroderma. The pathogenesis of atrophoderma is unknown. The histopathology is often nonspecific with subtle changes such as thinning of the dermis, edema, clumping of elastic tissue, and occasionally slight epidermal atrophy. The disease has a prolonged course, and there is no effective treatment. Atrophoderma should be distinguished from anetoderma, another condition of unknown etiology, in which there is focal loss of dermal elastic tissue. Lesions are characterized by small outpouchings of soft, shiny skin. Anetoderma may be preceded by inflammatory papules or plaques (the Jadassohn form), most common in adolescent girls, or it may arise de novo (the Schweninger-Buzzi form). Lesions tend to persist indefinitely, and no therapy is available.

Lichen sclerosus, also known as *lichen sclerosus et atrophicus* (LS&A), is an inflammatory disorder of unknown etiology that not uncommonly affects the anogenital area of prepubertal girls (Fig. 14-21). In boys, the prepuce and glans penis are the sites of predilection and may lead to phimosis or meatal obstrucion (balanitis xerotica obliterans). Affected females most often present with chronic vulvar pruritus. They may also complain of dysuria or painful defecation and constipation that result from perianal fissuring. The typical clinical appearance is a white discoloration with atrophy of the vulva and perianal area in a "figure-of-eight" pattern. The presence of purpura, telangiectasia, or erosions of the vulva or perianal skin may lead to a mistaken diagnosis of sexual abuse. Small hemorrhagic blisters can be misdiagnosed as hemangiomas. Chronic lichen sclerosis may cause adhesions and effacement of the labia minora and sometimes scarring. Extragenital lichen sclerosus is very rare in childhood. The diagnosis of genital lichen sclerosus is usually made clinically and rarely requires a skin biopsy. The characteristic histopathologic finding is a band of hyalinized collagen in the upper dermis. The course of the disease is variable but, in the majority of children, the disease appears to remit at or around puberty. Topical steroids are the most effective treatment for vulvar

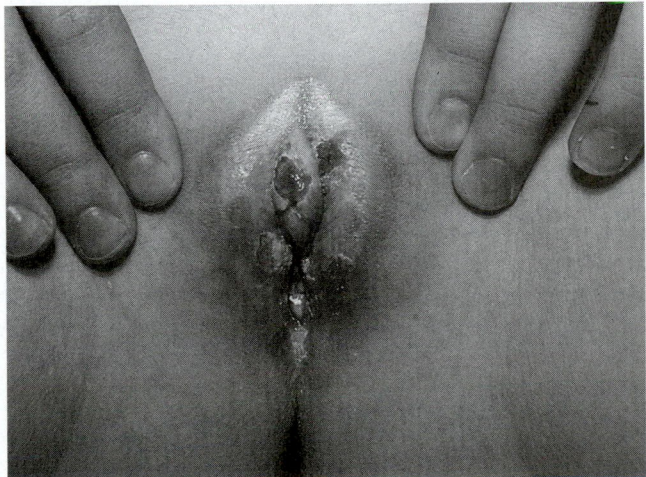

FIGURE 14-21 Lichen sclerosus et atrophicus. The labia majora and minora are covered with a coating of white scale. The entire area is reddened, and several eroded bullae are noted. The perivaginal and perianal areas are both involved. (*Courtesy of Amy Paller, M.D.*)

and perianal disease. A mid-potency steroid or application of a high-potency preparation for short periods is usually required. Surgical intervention may be necessary for boys with phimosis or meatal narrowing. There is no effective treatment for extragenital lichen sclerosus.

Eosinophilic fasciitis is characterized by painful focal or generalized skin hardening with peripheral eosinophilia. Boys are most commonly affected, and the disease is often precipitated by trauma or physical activity. Systemic corticosteroids may hasten resolution. Children with mixed connective-tissue disease (MCTD) have a combination of features of dermatomyositis, SLE, and Sjögren disease. Cutaneous findings include heliotrope sign, features of cutaneous LE, sclerodactyly, and periungual telangiectasia. Alopecia and dryness of the mucous membranes may also be present.

Vasculitis, the inflammatory destruction of blood vessels, occurs in a variety of pediatric disorders and is classified by the size of the affected vessels (see Sec. 12.6). When present, skin lesions may provide an important clinical sign for diagnosis. *Henoch-Schönlein purpura* (HSP) is a systemic leukocytoclastic vasculitis involving small vessels (venules) of the skin, joints, gastrointestinal tract, and kidneys. Rarely, it may involve the lungs and cause pulmonary hemorrhage. Skin involvement is usually the presenting sign with the development of "palpable purpura" predominantly over the lower extremities and buttocks (Color Plate 12). Early lesions may present as urticarial papules or plaques. The histopathology of HSP reveals perivascular neutrophils and their debris, fibrin deposition in vessel walls, and variable extravasation of erythrocytes. The immunopathologic demonstration of IgA deposits within vessel walls is diagnostic and may be found on nonlesional skin. HSP in most children is self-limited and requires no treatment. Because the onset of nephritis may follow that of the skin lesions by several weeks, blood pressure and urinalysis should be regularly monitored for a period of one month in all patients.

A variant of leukocytoclastic vasculitis seen in infants and toddlers that resembles HSP is termed *hemorrhagic edema of infancy,* characterized clinically by annular erythematous and purpuric plaques. Unlike HSP it commonly affects the face as well as the limbs and genitalia. Multiorgan disease is less common than in older children with HSP. Nevertheless, these infants should be evaluated for systemic involvement.

Small-vessel leukocytoclastic vasculitis, characterized clinically by palpable purpura, is seen in a number of conditions other than HSP and requires exclusion of collagen-vascular diseases. Additional causes of leukocytoclastic vasculitis are hepatitis B, cytomegalovirus, streptococcal infections, and hypersensitivity reactions to drugs such as penicillin and sulfonamide derivatives.

Polyarteritis nodosa (PAN) is a necrotizing vasculitis of small and medium-size arteries. Childhood PAN is characterized by multisystem organ involvement and the presence of painful subcutaneous nodules. Infantile PAN tends to involve more selectively the coronary arteries and is sometimes accompanied by a morbilliform eruption. This disease shares common features with Kawasaki disease (see Sec. 12.6).

References

Amitai Y, Gillis D, Wasserman D, Kochman RH: Henoch-Schonlein purpura in infants. Pediatrics 84:865–867, 1993

Krieg T, Meurer M: Systemic scleroderma. Clinical and pathophysiologic aspects. J Am Acad Dermatol 18:457–481, 1988

Lee LA, David KM: Cutaneous lupus erythematosus. Curr Prob Dermatol 1:161–200, 1989

Legrain V, Lejean S, Taieb A, et al: Infantile acute hemorrhagic edema of the skin: study of ten cases. J Am Acad Dermatol 24:17–22, 1991

Malleson PN, Prendiville J: Dermatomyositis and scleroderma in childhood B diagnosis and treatment. Curr Paediatr 5:246–251, 1995

Watson RM, Lane AT, Barnett NK, Bias WB, Arnett FC, Provost TT: Neonatal lupus erythematosus: a clinical, serological and immunogenetic study with review of the literature. Medicine (Baltimore) 63:362–378, 1984

Weston WL, Morelli JG, Lee LA: The clinical spectrum of anti-Ro-positive cutaneous neonatal lupus erythematosus. J Am Acad Dermatol 40:675–681, 1999

14.6.5   The Skin in Acquired Immunodeficiency Diseases

Genetic disorders of the immune system often present with a variety of common skin disorders, such as infection or dermatitis, or with unique manifestations that allow the diagnosis to be made (see Sec 14.4). Acquired immunodeficiency may also show cutaneous features, most commonly in patients with graft-versus-host disease or human immunodeficiency virus infection.

Graft-versus-host disease (GVHD) is a multisystem illness caused by the reaction of exogenous, immunocompetent cells against the tissues of a histoincompatible, immunosuppressed patient. Cutaneous disease is often the earliest sign of GVHD and contributes significantly to its morbidity and mortality. The clinical manifestations of GVHD are divided into acute and chronic phases. Acute GVHD develops 7 to 30 days after grafting. The rash is often an evanescent, faint eruption of erythematous macules or annular plaques resembling a viral exanthem or drug eruption. Erythema of the palms and soles around the ear lobes and the proximal nail folds is often seen. Mucosal involvement is common. In severe disease, a scarlatiniform rash begins acrally, spreads to involve the entire skin, and is rapidly followed by the development of toxic epidermal necrolysis (TEN). Most patients with TEN caused by GVHD do not survive. The characteristic skin histopathology in GVHD is that of a sparse inflammatory infiltrate at the dermal-epidermal junction and clustering of lymphocytes around individual necrotic keratinocytes (*satellite cell necrosis*). In many early or mild cases, histopathology is not diagnostic. Differentiation from a drug hypersensitivity reaction is particularly difficult. Correlation of successive biopsies with the clinical course may be required to establish the diagnosis. In chronic GVHD, mucosal and cutaneous lesions develop that mimic those seen in lichen planus. Over time, involved areas may become atrophic and show reticulate hyperpigmentation. Severe sclerodermatous changes develop in some patients with chronic GVHD.

Human immunodeficiency virus (HIV) infection in children is most commonly transmitted from an infected mother before or during birth. Pediatric HIV infection can also be transmitted by breast milk, by transfusion of contaminated blood or blood products, or, rarely, by sexual abuse. A wide variety of cutaneous manifestations of HIV infection are now recognized, although the manifestations have become less common and less severe with the advent of effective antiretroviral therapy. Most are common childhood dermatoses and infections which tend to be unusually severe, poorly responsive to therapy, and recurrent. In some children, skin disease provides the first evidence of HIV-related illness.

Mucocutaneous infection is the most common type of skin disease. Persistent oral thrush and/or candidal diaper rash occur in more than 65% of children with HIV infection. Candidal paronychia may result in destruction of the nail plate. Other fungal infections include unusual and severe patterns of tinea corporis, tinea capitis, and onychomycosis. Several cutaneous viral infections occur, especially herpes simplex, which often takes the form of chronic or recurrent gingivostomatitis or infection of the fingers (herpetic whitlow). Patients with severe HIV-related immunosuppression require intravenous therapy with acyclovir or other antiherpetic agents during herpetic episodes. Herpes zoster also occurs with increased frequency; lesions are often accompanied by severe discomfort and may eventuate in scarring. A chronic form of varicella-zoster infection has been recognized in children with HIV infection, in which multiple scattered nodular lesions may develop. Molluscum contagiosum and warts are also especially severe in HIV-infected children. Unusual patterns of human papillomavirus infection include widespread flat warts and very large and persistent condylomata acuminata. Bacterial infections of the skin occur with increased frequency as well, particularly cellulitis, impetigo, folliculitis, and ecthyma.

Several inflammatory disorders, including seborrheic dermatitis, atopic dermatitis, and psoriasis, are exacerbated by HIV infection. Drug eruptions, in many cases ascribable to trimethoprim-sulfamethoxazole, may also occur. Kaposi sarcoma, a low-grade vascular neoplasm presenting with violaceous papules and nodules in adults, is rare in pediatric HIV infection.

References

Darmstadt GL, Donnenberg AD, Vogelsang GB, Farmer ER, Horn TD: Clinical, laboratory, and histopathologic indicators of the development of progressive acute graft-versus-host disease. J Invest Dermatol 99: 397–402, 1992

Prose N: HIV infection in children. J Am Acad Dermatol 22:1223, 1990

14.6.6   Autoimmune Blistering Diseases

Autoimmune blistering diseases are mediated by circulating immunoglobulins that are deposited in the skin, resulting in inflammation and blister formation. These diseases are not common in children. The clinical features of these disorders overlap so that diagnosis requires skin biopsy specimens for histopathologic and direct immunofluorescence examinations to determine the site and type of autoantibody deposition. Indirect immunoflourescence using the patient's serum and immunoelectron microscopy may also be required to localize the autoantibody binding site within the epidermis or dermal-epidermal junction.

Linear IgA bullous dermatosis of childhood (LABD), also known as *chronic bullous dermatosis of childhood* (CBDC), usually has its onset during the first decade of life after one year of age. Typically, there is a sudden eruption of tense bullae and vesicles with clustering into annular or rosetted arrays. The scalp, face, perineum, abdomen, buttocks, and thighs are the most commonly affected sites, but the distal extremities may also be involved. Some patients have mucous membrane involvement. Scarring does not occur, but postinflammatory pigmentary changes may be pronounced. Pruritus is a variable symptom.

LABD is often initially misdiagnosed as bullous impetigo or bullous erythema multiforme. The diagnosis is established by demonstration of linear deposition of IgA and C3 at the dermal-epidermal junction on direct immunofluorescence of involved or perilesional skin. LABD usually responds to treatment with either dapsone (1.5–2.0 mg/kg/d) or sulfapyridine (60–200 mg/kg/d in divided doses). Glucose-6-phosphate dehydrogenase (G6PD) deficiency must be excluded before initiating therapy with either drug, and regular blood counts must be obtained during treatment. The addition of prednisone (1–2 mg/kg/d) may be necessary in severe cases. Episodes of remissions and exacerbations are usually followed by complete resolution within several months to a few years.

Dermatitis herpetiformis is a chronic blistering disease that is rare in childhood but characterized by intensely pruritic papules, vesicles, and occasional bullae, usually located on the elbows, knees, shoulders, neck, and sacral area. Direct immunofluorescence of perilesional skin demonstrates a granular deposition of IgA within the dermal papillae. Gluten-sensitive enteropathy can be demonstrated in 85 to 90% of cases. Although overt gastrointestinal symptoms are usually absent, jejunal villus atrophy is evident on intestinal biopsy. There is an increased frequency of HLA-B8, HLA-Dr3, and HLA-Dr7 types in these patients. The disease is usually controlled with a combination of a gluten-free diet and dapsone (1–2 mg/kg/d). Remission can often be maintained with diet alone, but spontaneous remission is unusual.

Bullous pemphigoid (BP) resembles LABD clinically but differs in that direct immunofluorescence demonstrates a linear deposition of IgG, rather than IgA, at the basement membrane zone. In the rare case in childhood, mucous membrane involvement and facial lesions are seen more frequently than in the adult form of the disease. Therapy with prednisone (1–2 mg/kg/d) is effective. Disease activity remits spontaneously in one to two years, although the course may be more prolonged.

Cicatricial pemphigoid has identical direct immunofluorescent features to BP but is characterized by severe mucous membrane involvement that may result in scarring of the conjunctival, oral, respiratory, and genital mucosa. Indirect immunofluorescence shows binding of circulating autoantibodies to the dermal component of salt-split skin, whereas in bullous pemphigoid the target antigen is epidermal. Cicatricial pemphigoid has a chronic course and may lead to blindness. Treatment entails local or systemic steroids and, in severe cases, cyclophosphamide.

Epidermolysis bullosa acquisita (EBA) presents with localized blistering on the dorsum of the hands or feet after mild trauma. Occasionally more generalized blistering resembles LABD. EBA may be associated with inflammatory bowel disease or systemic lupus erythematosus. Like bullous pemphigoid, direct immunofluorescence of a skin biopsy specimen shows linear deposition of IgG at the basement membrane zone. Patients may also have circulating IgG and anti–basement membrane zone antibodies, demonstrated by indirect immunofluorescence. The target antigen is collagen type VII, which is located in the dermis. Although the disease may respond to prednisone or cytotoxic agents, the prognosis for complete remission is poor.

In *pemphigus,* IgG autoantibodies directed against components of desmosomes (desmogleins) on the surface of keratinocytes disrupt cell-cell adhesion within the epidermis. In pemphigus vulgaris, these antibodies result in a middle to lower intraepidermal separation. In pemphigus foliaceus, the plane of cleavage is more superficial within the granular cell layer. Both diseases are rare in childhood, although a variant of pemphigus foliaceus (fogo selvagem) is endemic in certain parts of Brazil. In pemphigus vulgaris, painful oral mucous membrane erosions often precede the onset of skin lesions. Generalized, flaccid bullae and erosions measuring 5 to 20 mm are found in the scalp or intertriginous areas. Treatment with large doses of corticosteroids often in conjuction with azathioprine, or other steroid-sparing agent, is usually necessary to control the disease. Pemphigus foliaceus presents with eczematous and crusted lesions, frequently on the upper torso, and intact blisters may not be apparent. Pemphigus erythematosus is a rare form of pemphigus foliaceus associated with lupus erythematosus. Pemphigus foliaceus can sometimes be controlled with potent topical corticosteroids, but systemic corticosteroids are often necessary. With early diagnosis and adequate treatment, the prognosis for pemphigus in children is good.

NEONATAL AUTOIMMUNE BLISTERING Neonatal autoimmune blistering may result from passive transfer of IgG across the placenta from a mother affected with either pemphigus vulgaris or herpes gestationis, a bullous pemphigoid-like disease occurring during pregnancy. Blisters or erosions are usually present at birth. Neonatal blistering is self-limited, and treatment is rarely necessary. The diagnosis is usually obvious because of concurrent disease in the mother.

Reference

Rabinowitz LG, Esterly NB: Inflammatory bullous diseases in children. Dermatol Clin 11:565–581, 1993

14.7   NEOPLASTIC AND PROLIFERATIVE DISORDERS

Lawrence F. Eichenfield

Dermatofibromas (fibrous histiocytomas) are red to brown, firm nodules, ranging in diameter from a few millimeters to 2 to 3 cm. These benign lesions are often located on the lower extremities and tend to persist indefinitely. Biopsy is diagnostic and reveals irregular, intertwining bundles of collagen and histiocytes in the dermis, often with hyperplasia and hyperpigmentation of the overlying epidermis. *Dermatofibrosarcoma protuberans* is a rare, fibroblastic tumor, usually located on the trunk, that is locally invasive and may only rarely metastasize. Ten percent of cases occur during childhood. Wide local excision or Mohs surgery is indicated.

Mastocytosis is a group of disorders in which increased numbers of mast cells infiltrate tissues and organs, especially the skin. Symptoms result from degranulation of mast cells. In the most common form of cutaneous mastocytosis, *urticaria pigmentosa,* a varying number of brown to orange macules, papules, or plaques cause a cobblestone or orange peel–like appearance over any part of the skin surface (Color Plate 13). Spontaneous formation of wheals, vesiculation, or paroxysms of pruritus are not uncommon. The solitary *mastocytoma* presents as a single orange-brown nodule or plaque that may also urticate and blister with trauma, though severe pruritus is uncommon *Diffuse cutaneous mastocytosis* is a rare, severe form in which there is marked and widespread infiltration of the skin with mast cells. The skin is thickened, often with a yellow-orange hue, and widespread blistering is often present. Bone, liver, spleen, gastrointestinal tract, and other organs may also be involved. Extracutaneous disease, more common in adults than in children, may be associated with flushing and tachycardia, hypo-

tension, syncope, apnea, headache, vomiting, diarrhea, and/or abdominal pain. Mutations in the *c-kit* gene have been demonstrated in some, but not all, cases of progressive mastocytosis. The diagnosis of mastocytosis can usually be confirmed clinically by inducing an urticarial wheal-and-flare reaction by stroking a lesion (Darier's sign); however, this sign is not entirely specific to mastocytosis. Toluidine blue-stained skin biopsies demonstrate increased numbers of mast cells. The combination of H1 and H2 antihistamines is used to decrease the frequency and severity of episodes of mast cell degranulation. Patients with severe gastrointestinal symptoms may be helped by oral disodium cromoglycate. Most children with urticaria pigmentosa follow a benign self-limited course with improvement or resolution occurring during the first decade. Exposures to medications or physical factors that induce mast cell degranulation, including aspirin, alcohol, morphine, codeine, thiamine, scopolamine, polymyxin B, and very hot or cold baths or swimming pools, may provoke acute attacks of whealing, flushing, hypotension, gastrointestinal symptoms, and/or respiratory distress and should be avoided.

Several skin conditions are characterized by infiltration of cells of macrophage/monocyte lineage; these include both self-limited skin disorders and progressive infiltrative diseases that may involve multiple organ systems. Histocytic syndromes are divided into non–Langerhans cell histiocytoses and Langerhans cell histiocytoses. Non–Langerhans cell histiocytoses include sinus histiocytosis with massive lymphadenopathy, as well as indeterminate cell histiocytoses, benign cephalic histiocytosis, and juvenile xanthogranuloma. *Juvenile xanthogranuloma* (JXG) presents as one or more firm dome-shaped, yellow to orange-red papules or nodules, ranging in size from several millimeters to 1 cm or larger. The head and neck are the most common location for both single and multiple lesions, followed by the upper torso and extremities. Most JXG develops during the first year of life but is occasionally present at birth or develops later. Histologically, early lesions are composed of a monomorphous collection of ovoid cells in the dermis, whereas later ones contain foamy histiocytes, lymphocytes, and Touton giant cells. Most often, JXG resolves spontaneously within several years. Children with multiple skin lesions, children less than two years of age, and those recently diagnosed are at highest risk of intraocular JXG, which may be associated with hyphema; ophthalmologic examination should be considered. Infants with JXG should be examined for evidence of neurofibromatosis (eg, multiple café au lait spots) because of an increased incidence of myelogenous leukemia in this subset. *Benign cephalic histiocytosis* is a disorder of early childhood that is characterized by multiple 2- to 5-mm reddish-yellow papules on the head, neck, and shoulders. The lesions resolve spontaneously during several years but may leave small, atrophic scars. Skin biopsy will distinguish benign cephalic histiocytosis from fully developed JXG, because sections of the latter contain foam cells and Touton giant cells. *Sinus histiocytosis with massive lymphadenopathy* usually presents during the first decade with fever and bilateral painless cervical lymphadenopathy. Skin involvement with yellowish papules or nodules may be present. Lymph node biopsy reveals sinusoidal dilatations filled with foamy, multinucleated histocytes. The prognosis is variable.

Langerhans cell histiocytosis (LCH) refers to a group of disorders in which the basic disease process is a proliferation of Langerhans cells. LCH, also referred to as *histiocytosis X,* includes the pediatric diseases formerly referred to as Letterer-Siwe disease, Hand-Schuller-Christian disease, and eosinophilic granuloma. In acute disseminated histiocytosis (previously referred to as *Letterer-Siwe disease*), flat-topped, scaly papules in the scalp or intertriginous areas are noted at birth, infancy, or early childhood (Color Plate 14). These coalesce to form confluent, red-to-violaceous plaques. Purpuric nodules, vesicular lesions, atrophic scars, and ulcerations may also occur. LCH should be considered in infants with an intractable diaper rash or recalcitrant, severe, seborrhea-like eruption on the scalp. Skin biopsy is diagnostic and shows an infiltrate of S100, CD1+ cells, with characteristic Birbeck granules on electron microscopy. Single or multifocal bone lesions and gingival ulcerations are the most frequent extracutaneous disease, but liver, spleen, lymph node, kidney, and bone marrow are also commonly involved. Some patients with LCH present at birth with vesicles, papules, or dusky red-to-brown nodules; viscera may be involved, or the disease may be limited to the skin in the neonate. Spontaneous resolution of the neonatal disease when limited to the skin is common, but close follow-up is necessary because of recurrences. Skin may also be involved with focal lesions in the more chronic and differentiated forms of LCH, such as Hand-Schuller-Christian disease, which is defined by the classic triad of exophthalmos, diabetes insipidus, and bony lesions. The treatment of LCH is based on the severity of visceral disease. Chemotherapy is indicated in Letterer-Siwe disease with bone lesions and/or multiple organ involvement.

Lymphocytic infiltrate of Jessner is a rare cutaneous disease characterized by rapid development of reddish, firm plaques with sharp borders on the face. Biopsy reveals a dense, patchy lymphocytic infiltrate in the dermis. Lesions may resolve spontaneously but may recur.

Angiolymphoid hyperplasia with eosinophilia is an idiopathic process that manifests as red papules and nodules that occur primarily on the head and neck. The characteristic histology features both vascular proliferation and an inflammatory infiltrate composed of eosinophils and lymphoid follicles. Peripheral eosinophilia may also be present. Surgical excision or intralesional corticosteroids are suggested therapies.

Cutaneous T-cell lymphoma (mycosis fungoides, CTCL), a heterogeneous group of lymphoproliferative disorders involving the skin, are uncommon cutaneous malignancies in children and adolescents. Common cutaneous manifestations include erythematous patches and plaques, chronic papulosquamous lesions, crusted nodules, or hypopigmented papules and plaques. Chronic scaling dermatitis is a common presentation; poikiloderma may be present. Biopsy of characteristic skin or immunophenotyping to detect monoclonal rearrangement of T-cell receptor genes may be useful in diagnosis. Clinical staging (TNM classification) with assessment of extent of cutaneous and systemic involvement is appropriate. There are no treatment protocols designed specifically for children with CTCL; topical corticosteroids, topical nitrogen mustard, systemic psoralens with ultraviolet A light (PUVA) or UVB may be used for patch or plaque disease. Electron beam radiation, interferon, and systemic chemotherapy may be used for more extensive or advanced disease, but the majority of childhood patients with limited cutaneous disease have a more favorable outcome because blood or viscera are typically not involved.

References

Chang MW: Update on juvenile xanthogranuloma: unusual cutaneous and systemic variants. Semin Cutan Med Surg 18:195-205, 1999

Favara BE, Feller AC, Pauli M, et al: Contemporary classification of histiocytic disorders. The WHO Committee on histiocytic/reticulum cell proliferations. Reclassification Working Group of the Histiocyte Society. J Med Pediatr Oncol 29:157-166, 1997

Kim YH, Chow S, Varghese A, Hoppe RT: Clinical characteristics and long-term outcome of patients with generalized patch and/or plaque (T2) mycosis fungoides. Arch Dermatol 135:26-32, 1999

Koch SE, Zackheim HS, Williams ML, Fletcher V, LeBoit PE: Mycosis fungoides beginning in childhood and adolescence. J Am Acad Dermatol 17:563-570, 1987

Longacker MA, Frieden IJ, LeBoit PE, Sheretz EF: Congenital "self-healing" Langerhans cell histiocytosis: the need for long-term follow-up. J Am Acad Dermatol 31:910-916, 1994

14.8   VASCULAR TUMORS AND MALFORMATIONS

Ilona J. Frieden

CLASSIFICATION OF VASCULAR ANOMALIES

In 1982, Mulliken and Glowacki proposed a biological classification of vascular birthmarks based on natural history and biological characteristics. This classification, which has subsequently been modified, divides vascular birthmarks into *vascular tumors* (the most common being hemangioma of infancy) and *vascular malformations* (the most common being port wine stain). Although a small percentage of individuals have lesions with both malformative and neoplastic characteristics, the vast majority of vascular birthmarks can readily be classified using this schema. The major differences between hemangiomas and vascular malformations are listed in Table 14-5. In most instances, history and physical examination can achieve accurate diagnosis, but in some instances observation over time, imaging studies, or even biopsy may be required (Figs. 14-22 and 14-23).

HEMANGIOMA OF INFANCY

Clinical Manifestations and Prognosis

Hemangiomas are the most common soft-tissue tumors of infancy, occurring in up to 10% of infants by one year of age. They are more

TABLE 14-5

MAJOR DIFFERENCES BETWEEN HEMANGIOMAS AND VASCULAR MALFORMATIONS

HEMANGIOMAS	VASCULAR MALFORMATIONS
Usually either absent at birth or present as precursor lesion	Usually present at birth
Rapid growth during infancy	Static/slow growth—occasionally acceleration at puberty
Plump endothelial cells	Thin-walled, ectatic vessels
Spontaneous involution during early childhood	Persistence to adult life

SOURCE: *Adapted from Mulliken JB, Young AE: Vascular Birthmarks. Philadelphia, Saunders, 1988.*

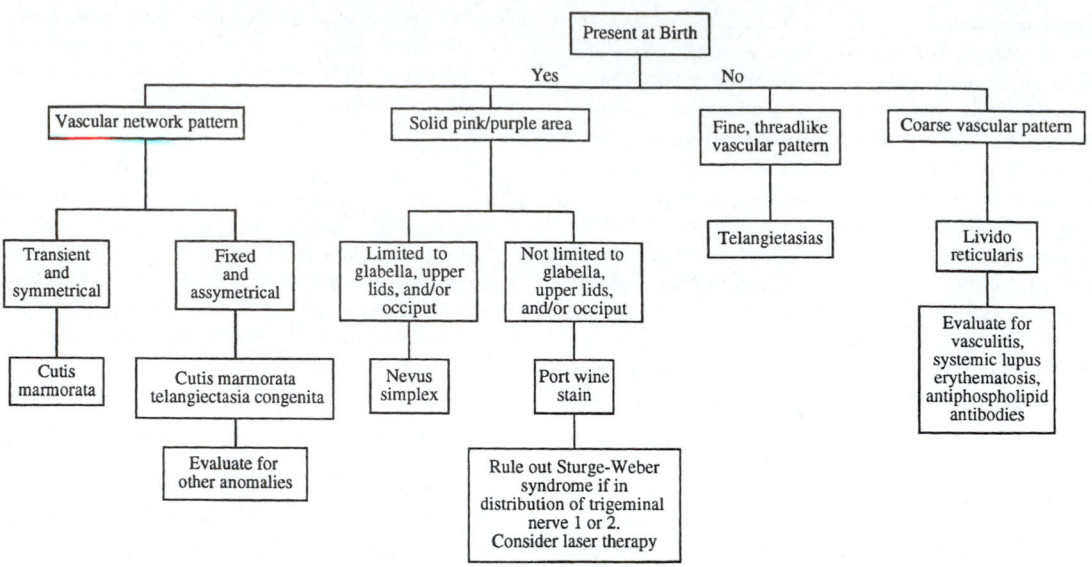

FIGURE 14-22   Flat (macular) vascular lesions.

common in girls and premature infants, especially those weighing less than 1500 grams. Single lesions predominate (85%); the head and neck (50%) and trunk (30%) are most often affected. An inherited tendency for both hemangiomas and vascular malformations has been reported, but most cases are sporadic. Hemangiomas are often absent at the time of birth or may be evident as a precursor lesion resembling a port wine stain, a bruise, or nevus anemicus. Hemangiomas present in a precursor form or completely absent at birth almost invariably go through a characteristic rapid-growth phase during the first weeks to months of life. The duration of the growth phase and ultimate size of the hemangioma is notoriously difficult to predict, particularly in early infancy. Fully formed hemangiomas present at birth are uncommon but undergo rapid involution, without a postnatal growth phase, usually within the first 18 months of life.

The clinical appearance of hemangiomas depends on the location within the skin. Hemangiomas may be composed of a superficial and/or a deep component. The clinical appearance of the superficial component (so-called strawberry hemangioma) is virtually diagnostic: a well-demarcated, elevated, bright red mass or plaque, composed of numerous coalescing papules or nodules, which blanch incompletely with pressure. The deep component, when present, is usually a soft, rubbery ill-defined subcutaneous mass, with a slightly bluish hue. In some cases hemangiomas lacking a superficial component may be difficult to distinguish from other soft-tissue growths, and ancillary studies may be necessary.

Growth Characteristics

Hemangiomas exhibit a characteristic pattern of rapid growth in the first few months of life followed by slow involution. Although the prognosis of hemangiomas as an aggregate is excellent, there is significant clinical heterogeneity: Many are innocuous and banal, but others are truly life-threatening. The majority of proliferation occurs in the first year of life, with a characteristic rapid-growth phase in the first few months followed by slower growth between

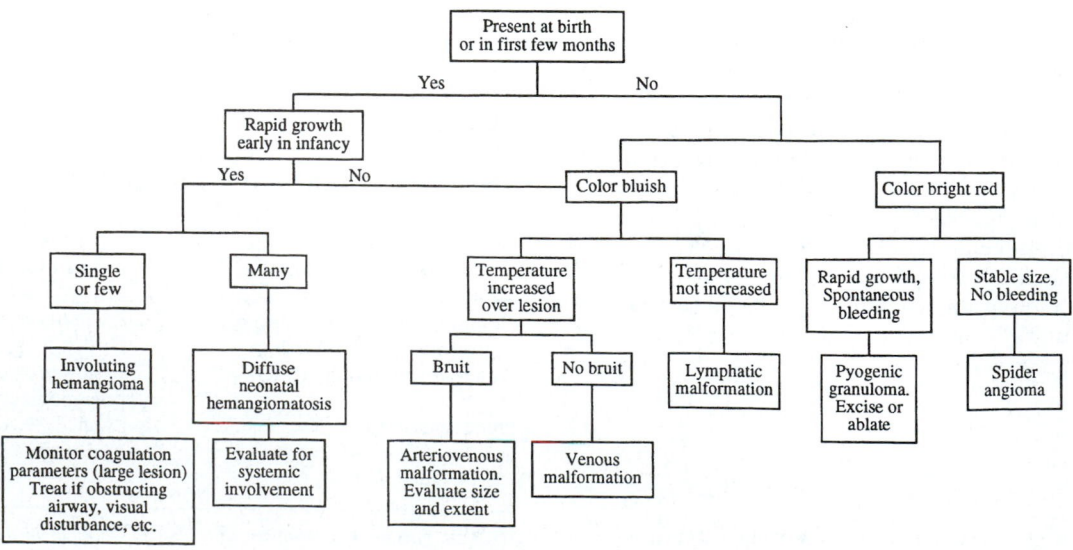

FIGURE 14-23   Palpable (nodular) vascular lesions.

6 and 12 months and cessation of growth by a year of age, although there are exceptions. Large, more biologically aggressive hemangiomas, in particular, may even continue to grow after one year of age. The timing of involution is difficult to predict in any individual case, but approximately one-third have involuted by three years of age, with a rate of involution of 10% per year thereafter. *Involution, however, does not necessarily imply resolution with completely normal skin.* Many hemangiomas do resolve with virtually normal skin, but a significant minority leave residual telangiectasias, pallor, atrophy, textural changes, or in the case of more exophytic hemangiomas, a fibro-fatty residuum (Color Plates 15A and B). Large, thick superficial hemangiomas leave significant skin alteration in approximately half of cases. Depending on the location, such residua can be either a trivial problem or a significant cause of disfigurement.

Complications

Although most hemangiomas resolve without incident, there are important exceptions. *Timing* and *location* are key elements in determining whether a complication is likely. Early in life, hemangiomas are notoriously unpredictable, and close observation is imperative. Some hemangiomas go through an extremely rapid growth phase, doubling in size in a matter of days, whereas others are more indolent. Parents should be educated about this unpredictability and the importance of reevaluation if rapid growth is occurring.

Anatomic location is critical in predicting which hemangiomas have a risk of functional problems or extracutaneous disease. Those located on the eyelid or in the periocular region can cause astigmatism and strabismus and in severe cases can lead to amblyopia. Nasal-tip hemangiomas are notoriously slow to involute and can cause permanent nasal distortion. Large hemangiomas on the pinna of the ear may deform the external ear or cause a temporary conductive hearing loss. Hemangiomas of the lip often ulcerate and even without ulceration may distort the normal lip anatomy, particularly those which involve the philtrum or cross the vermillion border. Hemangiomas overlying the mandible, chin, and upper neck have a high risk of associated airway hemangiomas, which typically have their onset between 6 and 12 weeks of age with "noisy breathing" or biphasic stridor (Color Plate 16). If airway involvement is suspected, direct visualization of the airway using a flexible fiberoptic scope should be performed. Prompt pharmacologic therapy with corticosteroids may be effective, but often tracheostomy is necessary.

Ulceration is the most common complication of hemangiomas. Most ulcerations occur in the period of rapid growth, and virtually all result in some degree of scarring. They are often extremely painful, may become infected, and rarely can cause significant hemorrhage. Hemangiomas in the perioral and perineal as well as intertriginous areas are particularly prone to ulceration, probably as a result of moisture, friction, and other local factors.

Large facial hemangiomas have been reported in association with several structural malformations, a group of associated anomalies that has recently been given the acronym *PHACE syndrome.* This acronym refers to findings including Posterior fossa defects, Hemangiomas, Arterial anomalies especially of arteries supplying the face and central nervous system, Coarctation of the aorta and cardiac defects, and Eye abnormalities such as congenital cataract, microphthalmia, and abnormal retinal vessels. Other central nervous system anomalies including absence of the corpus callosum or septum pellucidum have also been described. When sternal and/or supraabdominal clefting is present, the syndrome has been called

PHACES syndrome. The condition is much more common in girls, with an 8 to 1 ratio of females to males. Many affected individuals have only two or three of the features of the syndrome. The Kasabach-Merritt phenomenon was previously thought to be a complication of infantile hemangiomas, but it is now recognized that virtually all affected infants have other vascular tumors such as tufted angioma and Kaposiform hemangioendothelioma, not true hemangioma of infancy (see below).

Lumbosacral hemangiomas can be associated with genitourinary anomalies such as imperforate anus, renal anomalies, or with underlying spinal cord disease, especially tethered spinal cord. Hemangiomas in the lumbosacral region may be flat and telangiectatic, resembling port wine stains. Those infants with hemangiomas overlying the gluteal cleft or lumbosacral spinal should be evaluated for spinal cord abnormalities with either high-resolution ultrasound or MR imaging

Multiple hemangiomas occur in 10 to 25% of infants. When numerous lesions are present, there is an increased risk of visceral lesions, particularly liver and gastrointestinal tract, and, less commonly, brain or other sites. Careful serial physical examinations, liver ultrasound, and stool guaiac should be performed in affected infants.

The major goals of management include: preventing or reversing any life- or function-threatening complications, adequately treating ulceration, preventing permanent disfigurement left by residual skin changes, and minimizing psychosocial distress to both patient and family. An additional goal is the avoidance of overly aggressive, potentially scarring procedures for those lesions that have a strong likelihood of involution without residua. The wide range of sizes and locations of hemangiomas necessitates a flexible approach with periodic reevaluation, because the management plan may need to be modified over time depending on the age of the child and the size and location of the hemangiomas.

The uniformly hands-off approach advocated by many authorities in the past no longer seems adequate to the task. Despite the generally good prognosis of hemangiomas, parental concerns and preconceptions gathered from the internet and other sources will require discussion. Photographs demonstrating "before" and "after" examples of natural involution can be very reassuring, and serial photographs of the patient over time can also help demonstrate improvement. Discussion with parents should include a review of the natural history of hemangiomas, a plan for close observation during the period of rapid growth, a discussion of likely responses from strangers, and a promise of referral for specialty care, if this becomes necessary or if parental anxiety is unusually high.

Treatment of ulcerated hemangiomas should be directed at healing ulcers, preventing secondary infections, and decreasing pain. Large, rapidly spreading, or persistent ulcers warrant specialty referral. Superficial ulcerations may respond to application of a topical antibiotic, thick application of petrolatum, and coverage with a nonstick dressing. Nonexudative lesions may improve with a thin hydrocolloid dressing (such as Ultrathin Duoderm), if the dressing can be firmly attached on all sides. Lesions near the mouth and anus can be difficult to treat but may respond to topical metronidazole gel and application of petrolatum-impregnated gauze. Oral pain medicines such as acetaminophen or acetaminophen with codeine may be necessary. Oral antibiotics may be helpful if excessive crusting or overt secondary infection is present. Pulsed dye laser has also been shown to accelerate healing and decrease pain in ulcerated hemangiomas.

Corticosteroids are a mainstay of treatment of hemangiomas and can be given intralesionally or systemically. Intralesional injections limit the amount of medication and concentrate it in the area where it is most needed but are helpful only for small, well-localized hemangiomas. The injections have been used largely for treating periorbital hemangiomas. Potential complications include skin atrophy, infection, and systemic absorption and, for periorbital lesions, the rare complication of retinal artery occlusion.

Systemic corticosteroids are a first-line therapy for life- or function-threatening hemangiomas. Doses of 2 to 3 mg/kg per day are used routinely, and some authors advocate doses as high as 5 mg/kg per day. At least two-thirds of patients respond with either shrinkage or stabilization in the size of the hemangioma. The therapy often needs to be continued for several months, with a slow gradual taper toward the end of therapy. Many potential side effects including irritability, hypertension, immunosuppression, and growth retardation have been reported, but in most cases the treatment is well tolerated, with catch-up growth occurring after the corticosteroids are stopped.

Recombinant interferon alfa (either 2a or 2b) can be very effective in treating hemangiomas, particularly those that are resistant to corticosteroids. It is usually given as a daily subcutaneous injection of 3 million units/M^2 per day. The drug has the advantages of sparing linear growth and not causing significant immunosuppression but may have other adverse effects including irritability, neutropenia, and abnormalities of liver enzymes. The most worrisome toxicity is spastic diplegia, reported in up to 20% of cases and reversible in some. Serial neurologic examinations are imperative if the drug is used.

Several laser systems have been used to treat hemangiomas. Most widely used is the flashlamp pumped pulsed dye laser (PDL), which can be effective in treating relatively flat, superficial hemangiomas but is ineffective in treating thicker and deeper lesions because of its limited depth of penetration. Because the laser works well on flat lesions, there is a greater chance for it to be effective if patients are referred promptly at the earliest sign of hemangioma. Even so, the PDL is not effective in preventing the progression of those hemangiomas that, although appearing to be a "tiny red spot" in a very young infant, are destined to develop a deep as well as superficial component. Several treatments are necessary and the risk of scarring, although small, appears to be somewhat higher than using the same laser for treating port wine stains (see below). PDL can also be very effective in treating residual telangiectasias after hemangioma involution and can accelerate healing of ulcerated hemangiomas. Other laser systems have also been used for treating hemangiomas including Nd-YAG and other continuous wave laser systems. These lasers are more operator-dependent and have a higher risk of scarring than PDL but may be appropriate in selected cases.

Reconstructive surgical techniques are well accepted for revising permanent scars left after hemangioma involution. Earlier surgical excision is more controversial but is probably reasonable in hemangiomas with a very high likelihood of leaving a bag-like fibrofatty residual (such as pedunculated hemangiomas) or other obvious scar. If feasible, surgery is also recommended for function-threatening hemangiomas that have failed medical therapy. In those cases where the ultimate results of involution are less predictable, the risks of surgery must be carefully weighed against many factors including the rate at which involution is occurring, the reactions of the child and parents, and local specialty care resources. If significant uncertainty is present, it is usually best to delay a decision until three to four years of age and reevaluate. Multidisciplinary vascular birthmark clinics (which exist at many university medical centers) may provide helpful consultation.

OTHER VASCULAR TUMORS

Pyogenic granulomas, also known as *lobular capillary hemangiomas*, are common vascular tumors during childhood. They may develop spontaneously or in response to trauma, varying in size from a few millimeters to 1 to 2 cm. They usually grow rapidly, presenting as a red papule or nodule (Fig. 14-24) that bleeds profusely and repeatedly despite its small size. Over time lesions often have a black hemorrhagic crust and a peripheral collarette of scale. Spontaneous resolution is rare, but symptomatic lesions may be removed by shave excision or currettage, with light electrocautery of the base. Recurrences may occur despite adequate therapy, and occasionally multiple "satellite" lesions develop after removal. The differential diagnosis includes hemangioma of infancy, wart, bacillary angiomatosis, and occasionally other soft-tissue tumors.

Kaposiform hemangioendothelioma is a rare vascular tumor that can be present at birth or arise during early infancy or childhood. It is now recognized as one of the major causes of the Kasabach-Merritt phenomenon (KMP), a coagulopathy characterized by a low platelet count and decreased fibrinogen, usually with elevated fibrin split products. Clinically these lesions are often subcutaneous nodules or plaques, firm and tender with a violaceous discoloration, without overlying superficial hemangioma. As coagulopathy develops, the lesions become much more swollen with an intensely violaceous and purpuric surface. Treatment of KMP is difficult; many agents including corticosteroids, interferon alfa, aspirin, dipyridamole, vincristine, and radiation therapy have been used but without a uniform response to any one therapy.

Tufted angiomas are another cause of KMP and often have a clinical appearance indistinguishable from Kaposiform hemangioendothelioma, but plaque-type lesions of tufted angioma without associated coagulopathy have also been described. In contrast to the expected involution of infantile hemangiomas, both Kaposi-

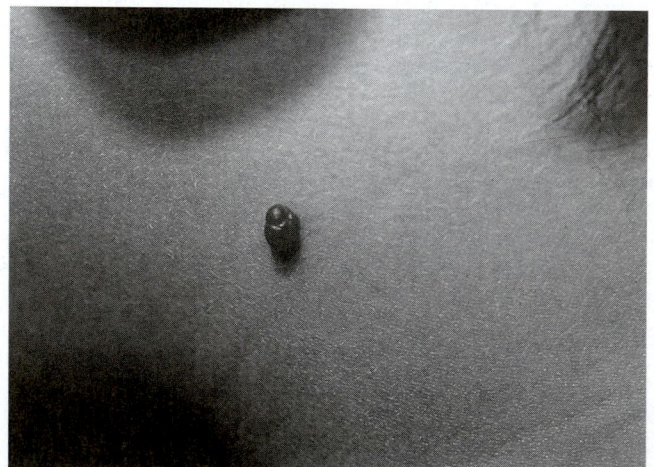

FIGURE 14-24   Pyogenic granuloma. This vascular lesion grows very rapidly after occurrence as a brightly red papule, often with a pedunculated base. Because it bleeds easily and does not often resolve spontaneously, removal is recommended. (*Courtesy of Amy Paller, M.D.*)

form hemangioendothelioma and tufted angioma can persist, even after resolution of the coagulopathy.

Spider angiomas are extremely common in children. They usually present on the face or hands as a small flat to slightly elevated red spot, often with a central red dot and small vessels radiating to a distance of 2 or 3 mm or occasionally to 10 mm or more. A history of trauma, bite, or sunburn at times predates the onset of a lesion, but many spider angiomas arise spontaneously and involute spontaneously. Others persist indefinitely. They pose no medical hazard, except for the bleeding which can occur if they are excoriated, and they can easily be removed for cosmetic reasons with either light electrocautery or pulsed dye laser. If available, the latter is the preferred modality, since the risk of scarring is somewhat less. Repeat treatments are occasionally necessary.

Angiokeratomas are vascular growths generally ascribed to a vascular malformation of the papillary dermis with overlying thickening and hyperkeratosis of the epidermis. Angiokeratomas may arise as isolated (so-called angiokeratoma circumscriptum) or multiple lesions. Scrotal angiokeratomas are very common in aging adult men but may uncommonly develop during adolescence. *Fabry disease* (angiokeratoma corporis diffusum), an X-linked recessive disorder caused by deficiency of ceramide galactosidase, may present with multiple tiny angiokeratomas grouped around the thigh, scrotum, or periumbilical region. Extracutaneous vascular disease may be evident on ophthalmologic examination and results in hypertension, cerebrovascular disease, coronary artery disease, renal disease, and vasomotor disturbances. The latter produces characteristic attacks of burning pain of the upper extremities, accompanied by suffusion or pallor and relieved by raising the arms. Diffuse angiokeratomas are also seen in fucosidosis.

VASCULAR MALFORMATIONS

The salmon patch (nevus simplex), the most common vascular anomaly of infancy, presents as a pink to red, blanchable flat area most often involving the glabella, eyelids, perinasal area, and nape. Occasionally the upper lip, scalp, or midline spine is also affected. With the exception of the nape, these lesions generally fade by two years of age, although persistence in the form of a *medial telangiectactic nevus* has occasionally been reported. Autosomal-dominant inheritance is present is some cases.

Port wine stains (PWS nevus flammeus) are congenital vascular malformations with an increased number of dilated capillaries within the upper dermis. Almost invariably present at birth, these lesions may be virtually any size and in any location. In infancy, port wine stains are often pink in color and are usually flat. Over time, the affected blood vessels become more ectatic, and the clinical appearance may change from pink to red to purple. Purple lesions may also develop a soft, multinodular texture owing to progressive vascular ectasias or develop superimposed papules, caused by the development of pyogenic granulomas within the lesion. Occasionally port wine stains are associated with underlying lymphatic or venous malformations, in which case they have a greater risk of progressive soft-tissue swelling.

The risk of extracutaneous disease depends on the distribution of the PWS. The risk of Sturge-Weber syndrome is only present if the first branch of the trigeminal nerve (V1) is involved, and even with this area affected the risk is less than 25%. Involvement of V2 or V3 dermatomes does not confer a risk of Sturge-Weber syndrome, but if gingival involvement is present, gum hypertrophy may gradually develop. Port wine stains of the extremities some-

times have associated limb hypertrophy or limb-length discrepancy, which can develop later, even if not present in infancy. Port wine stains located over the spine may, in rare instances, be associated with underlying spinal vascular anomalies and (in the case of lumbosacral lesions) tethered spinal cord.

During the past decade, effective laser therapy using the flashlamp pumped pulsed dye laser has proved safe to use even in very young children. Generally a minimum of six to eight treatments is required; results vary from complete clearance in small, blotchy lesions to fading but persistence in large lesions. Although initial studies suggested a better response in young children, size and location are probably better predictors of response than age. For unknown reasons, lesions with V2 distribution do less well, especially their most medial aspects. Other relatively negative prognostic factors to laser therapy include lesions in dark-skinned individuals, large lesions (>50 cm²), and lower-extremity involvement. Some lesions may slowly recur, necessitating periodic "touch-up" treatments. Psychosocial concerns and pain management are the most important determinants of the optimal time for treatment. Large lesions treated during childhood often require general anesthesia.

Sturge-Weber syndrome is the triad of facial port wine stain (V1 distribution), ipsilateral cerebral vascular malformation, and ophthalmologic disease (glaucoma and retinal vascular malformation). There is a high incidence of seizures and mental retardation with central nervous system angiomatosis. All patients with port wine stains involving the upper and lower eyelids require ongoing regular ophthalmologic evaluations with measurement of ocular pressure. Nevertheless, the majority of infants with port wine stains in this distribution do not have the Sturge-Weber syndrome.

The *Klippel-Trenaunay syndrome* consists of the triad of port wine stain of the skin, ipsilateral soft tissue and/or bony hypertrophy, and venous varicosities. Most patients with this syndrome actually have a combined capillary-venous-lymphatic malformation. Lesions are often restricted to one extremity, but occasionally more widespread vascular malformations are noted. Although the vascular anomalies are usually evident at birth, the soft-tissue and bony overgrowth may gradually develop; those patients with leg involvement should have limb lengths monitored regularly, since a discrepancy of more than 1 to 2 cm may require orthopedic intervention. Compression garments may be helpful in reducing progressive venous varicosities.

Venous malformations formerly called *cavernous hemangiomas* are almost always evident at birth as soft, cutaneous or subcutaneous bluish, ill-defined masses. They are usually at least partially compressible and increase when the affected area is placed in a dependent position. Many have a "bag of worms" texture caused by multiple palpable varicosities. Venous malformations may rarely be transmitted as an autosomal-dominant trait, and in some cases these have been demonstrated to result from defects in the TIE-2 receptor, which controls assembly of the smooth-muscle parenchyma surrounding the normal venous vasculature.

In *Mafucci syndrome,* multiple subcutaneous nodules combining features of spindle-cell hemangioendothelioma and venous malformations develop in association with diffuse, asymmetric enchondromatosis. The *blue rubber bleb nevus syndrome* is the association of cutaneous venous malformations with submucosal vascular anomalies of the gastrointestinal tract, particularly small intestine and distal colon, which may bleed. Occasionally liver, spleen, and central nervous system lesions may also be found.

Several types of *lymphatic malformation* (LM) (lymphangiomas) occur in infancy and childhood: cystic LMs (cystic hygroma), localized superficial lymphatic malformations (so-called lymphangioma circumscriptum), and diffuse lymphatic malformations. Cystic hygromas are usually present at birth and are most common in the neck and axilla. They present as a painless fluid-filled mass usually with attachment to deeper tissues, not to the overlying skin. Cytogenetic abnormalities such as Tumer syndrome may also be evident. *Lymphangioma circumscriptum* presents as a collection of small flesh-colored vesicular blebs ("frog spawn") clustered together, usually with focal red to black hemorrhagic areas also evident. More diffuse or mixed LMs may have firm doughy areas of soft-tissue swelling with non-pitting edema. Affected areas of the skin are prone to develop cellulitis, which can result in scarring and further lymphedema. Treatment is difficult, because even apparently well localized LMs can have inapparent, deeper extensions. Surgical excision is helpful for well-localized lesions. Surgery, sclerotherapy, laser therapy, and even liposuction have been employed as treatments, but results depend on the specific characteristics of the anomaly and are often unsatisfactory in larger lesions. The use of compression garments may be helpful in some cases.

Cutis marmorata telangiectatica congenita (CMTC) is a form of vascular malformation of capillaries and small veins, presenting at birth as a nonblanching fixed pattern of vascular mottling, which resembles livedo. Local skin atrophy or ulcerations may occur. The most common association is port wine stain, but multiple extracutaneous anomalies have been reported including seizures, glaucoma, wooly hair, cardiac defects, and limb anomalies. The cutaneous lesions may improve with time, but usually persist.

Telangiectasias represent superficial ectatic vascular channels that are seen through the surface of the skin as tiny red-to-purple, thread-like strands that blanch with pressure. Telangiectasias occur in a variety of settings and in some cases represent an early clue to an underlying systemic disease. When telangiectasias are present in association with atrophy and dyschromia (hypopigmentation and hyperpigmentation), these changes are collectively termed *poikiloderma*. Poikiloderma may develop in response to chronic actinic inflammation or following x-irradiation. It is seen in several genetic disorders, including xeroderma pigmentosum, Bloom syndrome, Rothmund-Thomson syndrome, and dyskeratosis congenita or as a feature of collagen vascular diseases, chronic GVHD, or cutaneous T-cell lymphoma. Telangiectasias may develop in response to chronic excessive topical corticosteroid usage. Cuticular telangiectasias can provide an important clue to collagen vascular disease and are commonly present in scleroderma, SLE, dermatomyositis, and mixed connective-tissue disease. Macular, often rectangular 4- to 10-mm telangiectatic mats are also seen on the face and sun-exposed sites in scleroderma, particularly in the CREST variant.

In *ataxia telangiectasia*, telangiectasias on conjunctival mucosa and sun-exposed sites on face and hands develop during preschool years and can be an early sign of the disease (see Sec. 14.4). *Hereditary hemorrhagic telangiectasia* (Osler-Rendu-Weber disease) is an autosomal-dominant disorder in which spider angiomas and telangiectasias are present on skin and the mucosa of respiratory and gastrointestinal tracts. Cutaneous lesions are not usually present in childhood. With time, multiple papules with irradiating telangiectasias develop on the lips, ears, palms and soles, and under the nails, as well as on the conjunctiva and nasal and oral mucosa.

Telangiectasias may also occur as benign phenomena localized to the skin. In unilateral nevoid telangiectasia, lesions progressively develop over one segment of the body, often one side of the torso or upper extremity. The condition is more common in females and often has its onset in early adolescence.

References

Drolet BA, Esterly NB, Frieden IJ: Hemangiomas in children. N Engl J Med 341:173-181, 1999

Enjolras O, Mulliken JB: Vascular tumors and vascular malformations (new issues). Adv Dermatol 13:375-422, 1997

Frieden IJ: Which hemangiomas to treat—and how? Arch Dermatol 133: 1593-1595, 1997

Frieden IJ, Reese V, Cohen D: PHACE syndrome: the association of posterior fossa brain malformations, hemangiomas, arterial anomalies, coarctation of the aorta and cardiac defects and eye abnormalities. Arch Dermatol 132:307-311, 1996

Golitz LE, Rudikoff J, O'Meara OP: Diffuse neonatal hemangiomatosis. Pediatr Dermatol 3:145-152, 1986

Mulliken JB, Young AE: Vascular Birthmarks. Philadelphia, Saunders, 1988

Picascia DD, Esterly NB: Cutis marmorata telangiectasia congenita: report of 22 cases. J Am Acad Dermatol 20:1098-1104, 1989

Tallman B, Tan OT, Morelli JG, et al: Location of port-wine stains and the likelihood of ophthalmic and/or central nervous system complications. Pediatrics 87:323-327, 1991

Tanner JL, Dechert MP, Frieden IJ: Growing up with a facial hemangioma: parent and child coping and adaptation. Pediatrics 101:446-452, 1998

14.9 DISORDERS OF HAIR AND HAIR FOLLICLES

Bari B. Cunningham and Sheila Fallon-Friedlander

ACNE

Acne vulgaris is the most common of all cutaneous disorders and occurs in more than 85% of adolescents. The degree of involvement is quite variable. Many individuals have mild to moderate disease of a transient nature; however, others develop severe disease which can lead to significant scarring and emotional distress. The onset of clinical disease usually occurs between the ages of 12 and 14, but mild comedonal disease may develop as early as 7 to 8 years of age and tends to occur somewhat earlier in girls than in boys. Acne generally resolves in the late teens or early 20s, but persistence into the third decade or onset in middle age, particularly in women, is not unusual. Although most acne may be thought of as physiologic, disease with unusual features such as early onset or severe recalcitrance to therapy warrants evaluation for underlying abnormalities of the adrenal or ovarian systems.

Acne is most commonly localized to areas of highest sebaceous gland concentration and activity, such as the face, chest, and upper back. Acne lesions begin with the development of the microcomedone, a small cyst plugged by accumulated sebum, desquamated epithelial cells, vellus hairs, and bacteria. The formation of closed comedones (whiteheads) and open comedones (blackheads) is initiated by abnormal cornification of the follicular orifice. The epidermal cells lining the orifice form adherent cornified sheets of cells, instead of desquamating as single cells to be carried away with the sebum flow. These cornified sheets occlude the follicular opening and lead to cystic dilatation of the follicle. Open comedones have a widely patent surface orifice.

Inflammatory lesions (ie, papules, pustules, or nodules) develop when the intradermal wall of the comedone ruptures, releasing comedonal contents into the dermis and provoking an intense, suppurative, and later a foreign-body, granulomatous-type inflammatory reaction. In cystic acne the inflammatory reaction is extreme, resulting in deep nodules, sinus tracts, and cysts.

The surge of androgen production that occurs in adolescence leads to increased sebum production. 5-Alpha-reductase, which converts testosterone to the more potent dihydrotestosterone (DHT), appears to be more highly concentrated in infrainfundibular keratocinocytes. Interleukin-1 located in the hair follicle can also stimulate hypercornification.

Sebum serves as a substrate for *Propionibacterium acnes*. This microorganism is a normal resident of the pilosebaceous unit and overgrows within the blocked sebaceous follicle. Bacterial lipases liberate free fatty acids from sebum; these lipids in turn may stimulate follicular hyperkeratosis. Other bacterial products act as irritants and as chemotactic factors that recruit neutrophils. The severity of acne appears to be genetically determined. Increased delayed hypersensitivity to *P. acnes* has been noted in patients with severe forms of acne. Systemic factors such as corticosteroid therapy and local factors, such as pore-plugging (comedogenic) cosmetics and hair tonics or external pressure from head gear, may be contributory in some patients. There is little evidence that foods or poor skin hygiene are precipitants.

The goal of acne therapy is to minimize scarring and to alleviate the psychologic distress of a disfiguring skin condition during critical years of social and sexual development. Therapy is directed toward correcting abnormal follicular keratinization, decreasing the population of *P. acnes*, and decreasing sebum production (Table 14-6). Treatment must be individualized and should be based on the severity of disease, the types of lesions, and the patient's motivation.

An important first step in the management of acne vulgaris is a careful explanation of the disease process. Many adolescents incorrectly believe that particular foods, poor personal hygiene, or even masturbation lead to acne. These beliefs can lead to unproductive behavior, such as diets or excessive face washing, and may also inhibit compliance with an effective therapeutic regimen. A strong rapport between the adolescent and the physician is essential to the successful management of this disease.

The majority of patients can be treated with topical medications of three types: benzoyl peroxide products, antibiotics, and retinoids. Each has distinct advantages, and concurrent use of these agents may have synergistic effects. Benzoyl peroxide has both bactericidal and comedolytic activities. It is available in cream, gel, lotion, and wash forms, in concentrations from 2.5 to 20.0%. Irritation evidenced by erythema and scaling is the most significant side effect; skin hypopigmentation and bleaching of clothing may also occur. This agent is particularly useful because of its bactericidal nature, and frequent use inhibits the development of bacterial resistance.

The topical retinoids (tretinoin, adapalene, tazarotene) normalize keratinocyte differentiation, decreasing the "stickiness" of the epidermal cells lining the follicular lumen. This allows the keratin plug to be expelled, thus preventing formation of comedones. Tretinoin is available in creams, gels, and liquids of varying concentrations. A microsphere formulation of the 0.1% cream appears to be better tolerated than other forms. Sustained release formulations of the 0.025% tretinoin cream and adapalene gel are also less irritating. All forms should be introduced gradually, to decrease the likelihood of adverse effects such as drying, irritation, or sun sensitivity. Daily

TABLE 14-6

THERAPY FOR ACNE VULGARIS

TYPE OF ACNE	CLASS OF MEDICATION	SPECIFIC AGENTS
Comedonal	Topicals that normalize keratinization	Tretinoin cream, gel, microemulsion Adapalene gel Tazarotene gel Azaleic acid cream
	Comedolytics	Salicylic acid Benzoyl peroxide
Inflammatory, mild	Topical antibiotic→ +/− tretinoin or adapalene +/− benzoyl peroxide	Erythromycin, clindamycin, sulfur-sulfacetamide
Inflammatory, moderate	Add systemic antibiotic	Tetracycline Doxycycline Minocycline Erythromycin
Inflammatory, moderate to severe, female	Consider adding hormonal therapy	Oral contraceptive pills
Severe, refractory +/− scarring	Systemic retinoid	Isotretinoin Close monitoring, counseling re: teratogenicity, side effects
Localized cysts	Intralesional steroids	Triamcinolone

therapy can usually be tolerated after several weeks; these agents are generally not used more than once a day.

Topical antibiotics including 2% erythromycin, 1% clindamycin, or a combination of 3% erythromycin and 5% benzoyl peroxide may be used in patients with an inflammatory component. These agents decrease colonization of the skin by *P. acnes* and may also inhibit neutrophil chemotaxis. However, resistant *P. acnes* has been documented in 20 to 60% of populations with in vitro testing. For this reason, monotherapy with topical or systemic antibiotics is discouraged. The concurrent use of topical benzoyl peroxide has been shown to inhibit and decrease resistance. Individuals with sensitive skin present a special therapeutic challenge and may benefit from sulfacetamide products or azaleic acid cream, which may also decrease postinflammatory hyperpigmentation.

The adolescent with mild to moderate acne will most often show improvement with the use of topical tretinoin or adapalene in combination with either benzoyl peroxide or a topical antibiotic. Because all these agents may cause cutaneous irritation, they are best introduced separately or on an every-other-night basis. Patients should avoid vigorous scrubbing and use a mild nonabrasive soap. Adolescents who do not respond to topical therapy or who present with a moderate to severe inflammatory form of the disease require systemic antibiotics. Tetracycline (usually 500 mg bid) is frequently prescribed because of its safety and efficacy. However, compliance may be suboptimal because the drug cannot be taken with dairy products or iron-containing foods and requires at least twice-a-day dosing. Doxycycline (50-100 mg bid) obviates these problems but is more likely to induce photosensitivity. Minocycline (usually 50-100 mg bid) may be more efficacious for some patients. Rare cases of hypersensitivity and lupus-like reactions, along with increased cost and a rare risk of dyspigmentation, argue for its use as second-rather than first-line therapy. Erythromycin (500 mg bid) is also effective and is an alternative for sexually active adolescent women because of its safety during pregnancy.

Topical therapy should be used concurrently with any oral antibiotic, and the oral antibiotic slowly tapered once significant improvement has been achieved (usually three to six months). Poor compliance and interference with tetracycline absorption by food, particularly milk, are the most common causes of treatment failures. Some patients require higher doses (eg, 500 mg tid), and long-term oral antibiotic therapy may be necessary in a small proportion of adolescents. Once patients have been using tretinoin or benzoyl peroxide regularly, comedones may be manually expressed by acne surgery.

A small subset of acne patients have a severe variant, nodulocystic acne, that is characterized by deep nodules, sinus tracts, and cysts. Repeated episodes of deep dermal inflammation frequently result in scarring. The initial treatment of cystic acne consists of topical therapy with tretinoin and topical and systemic antibiotics. Deep inflammatory nodules and cysts will resolve more quickly and with a lower risk of scarring if injected intralesionally with a dilute form of steroids (eg, 5 mg/cc of triamcinolone acetonide).

Oral isotretinoin (13-cis-retinoic acid) is a highly effective oral agent for the treatment of acne, but its expense and transient but significant side effects limit its use to patients who fail to respond to an adequate trial of conventional therapy, who understand its side effects, and who can comply with the necessary restrictions. Isotretinoin is a synthetic derivative of vitamin A that induces profound but usually temporary sebaceous gland involution; it also has anti-inflammatory and antikeratinizing effects. A 16- to 20-week course of therapy of 1.0 mg/kg per day will bring about significant and long-lasting improvement in most patients. Studies have noted that the chances of cure with this drug are higher in older teenagers when doses in excess of 100 mg/kg total dose are used. A second course of isotretinoin is required in approximately 20% of those treated.

The single most significant side effect of orally administered retinoids is their induction of severe craniofacial, cardiac, and central nervous system malformations in a high proportion of fetuses exposed in the first trimester. Effective contraception is mandatory when retinoids are used in fertile female patients. Almost all patients receiving isotretinoin develop cheilitis, xerosis, and dryness of the mucous membranes. Rarely, patients may develop depression, possibly dose-related, and families must be counseled regarding symptoms. More commonly, however, the dramatic improvement in cosmetic appearance of treated patients can ameliorate a reactive depression. Musculoskeletal pain and hair loss are less common side effects. A transient increase in serum triglyceride concentration and a decrease in high-density lipoproteins occur in 25% of patients. In rare patients, marked hypertriglyceridemia has precipitated acute pancreatitis. All patients should be screened for hypertriglyceridemia before and within one month after initiating therapy.

The oral contraceptive norgestimate plus ethinyl estradiol (Tricyclen) was approved by the Food and Drug Administration for treating inflammatory acne and may be particularly useful for girls with premenstrual flares.

Differential Diagnosis

Patients with acne should be evaluated for signs of precocious puberty or hyperandrogenism. Late onset partial congenital adrenal hyperplasia, adrenal tumors, and ovarian abnormalities, including polycystic ovarian disease, may lead to the development of premature or severe acne.

Acne rosacea is a variant that more commonly affects middle-aged patients of Celtic background and is characterized by severe inflammatory lesions of the face in the absence of comedones. *Folliculitis* of either fungal or bacterial origin may occasionally be confused with acne; culture is helpful in such cases. Folliculitis caused by gram-negative bacteria may develop in acne patients who have been administered chronic tetracycline therapy. Isotretinoin is effective therapy for this disorder. *Irritant acneiform folliculitis* may occur in athletes or others who have chin-straps or other agents occluding the face, chest, or back.

Acne fulminans is an uncommon, severe variant of acne vulgaris, most frequently seen in white male adolescents. Thought to be a severe hypersensitivity reaction to *P. acnes*, the disorder may be associated with systemic symptoms including fever, leukocytosis, hemorrhagic crusting of acne lesions, and lytic body lesions. Systemic corticosteroids are required for treatment, and isotretinoin therapy should not be instituted until severe inflammation has resolved and then only in low dose because higher doses may cause a flare of disease.

Acneiform drug eruptions are usually more monomorphous and extensive than typical acne. Possible causative agents include anticonvulsants, lithium, isoniazid, high iodine diets, and corticosteroids, including anabolic agents used by athletes.

Neonatal and Infantile Acne

Comedonal and pustular acne may be present at birth or may develop during the newborn period. The lesions are most often superficial and are usually confined to the face and upper trunk. Neonatal acne appears to result from the stimulating effect of maternal and fetal androgens on the newborn's sebaceous glands. Several studies have implicated pityrosporum (*Malassezia*) as a possible etiologic agent for some cases of neonatal acne. Complete clearing of the disease occurs within a period of one to three months. When acne develops later in infancy, benzoyl peroxide gel 2.5% may prove effective, but infants with more severe inflammatory disease, including cystic acne, may require systemic erythromycin, isotretinoin, or even intralesional or systemic corticosteroids. Unusually persistent or severe infantile acne may be indicative of abnormal androgen or cortisol production, and a complete endocrinologic workup should be considered.

References

DeGroot HE, Friedlander SF: Update on acne. Curr Opin Pediatr 10:381–386, 1998

Leyden JJ: Therapy for acne vulgaris. N Engl J Med 336:1156–1162, 1997

Lucky AW, Biro FM, Huster GA et al: Acne vulgaris in premenarchal girls. Arch Dermatol 130:308–314, 1994

Thiboutot DM: Acne: an overview of clinical research findings. Dermatol Clin 15:97–109, 1997

White GM: Recurrence rates after the first course of isotretinoin. Arch Dermatol 134:376–378, 1998

ALOPECIA

Hair is a nonliving biologic fiber found everywhere on the human body surface with the exception of the palms, soles, genitalia, and lateral digits. Deficient hair *growth* is known as *hypotrichosis*,

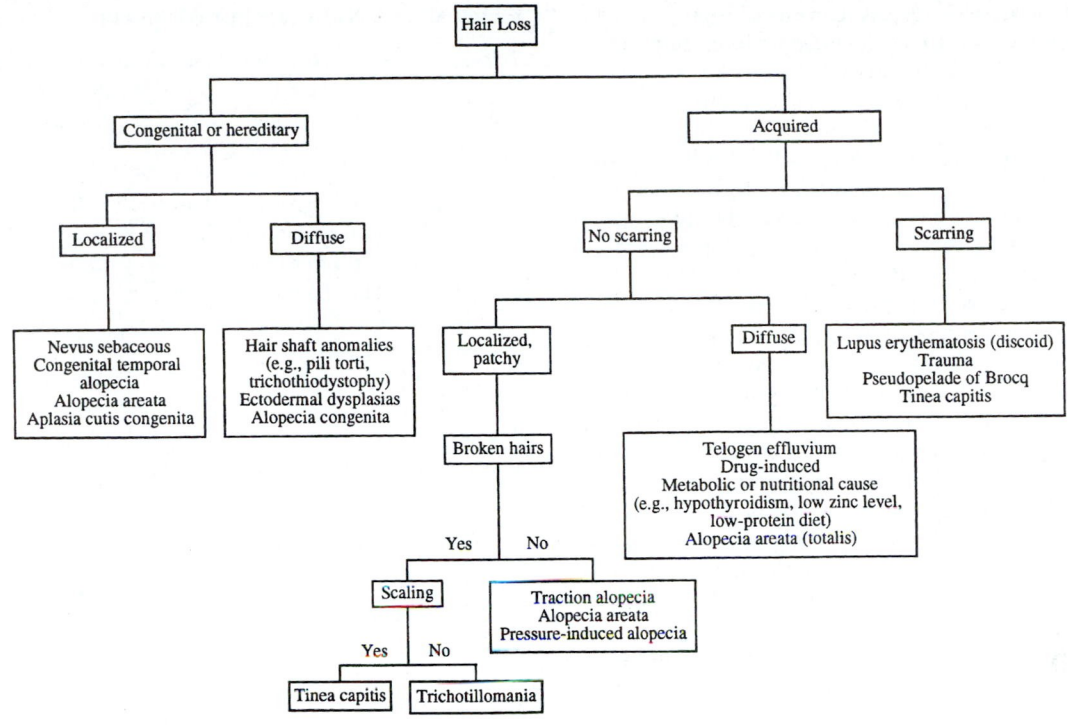

FIGURE 14-25 **Differential diagnosis of hair loss.**

whereas hair *loss* is termed *alopecia*. Alopecia is subclassified as scarring or nonscarring and as generalized or localized (Fig. 14-25). Disorders of hair in infants and children may reflect underlying biochemical or metabolic defects in addition to immunologic disease. Tinea capitis, the most common cause of hair loss in children, should be considered in any pediatric patient who presents with scaling hair loss. Untreated, longstanding tinea capitis may result in permanent scarring alopecia with serious psychological consequences.

Localized Nonscarring Alopecia

Alopecia areata is a common, idiopathic disorder characterized by the sudden appearance of round or oval patches of hair loss on the scalp as well as other body sites. The condition may have its onset as early as birth but usually appears in school-aged children. Its occasional association with autoimmune diseases such as Hashimoto's thyroiditis, myasthenia gravis, diabetes, and vitiligo has suggested an autoimmune process. Other associations include trisomy 21, chronic mucocutaneous candidiasis, adrenal disease, and atopy.

The typical lesion of alopecia areata is a smooth, shiny, hairless, round patch of the scalp that appears suddenly over the course of several days (Fig. 14-26). Scattered long hairs within the bald area or "exclamation point hairs" (hairs with a narrowed proximal diameter and often shorter length and lighter color) may be detected.

Two clinical forms of alopecia areata occur: patchy alopecia areata and alopecia totalis or universalis. In the former, a few or many patches of hair are lost and the prognosis for regrowth, either spontaneously or with treatment, is good. If patches coalesce into large areas with loss of more than 50% of scalp hair, the prognosis is generally less favorable. The presence of alopecia totalis (loss of all scalp hair) or alopecia universalis (loss of all body and scalp hair) is a poor prognostic sign, especially in children. Such hair loss re-

sponds poorly to treatment, and even if hair regrows completely, recurrent episodes of alopecia totalis are likely. Nail pitting, roughening, and loss of luster are seen in 10 to 20 percent of cases and rarely may precede hair loss. In all forms of alopecia areata, new hair growth may be lighter and finer in quality than the surrounding hair but is likely to return to its original caliber and coloration.

The diagnosis of alopecia areata is usually made clinically but can be confirmed with a scalp biopsy in atypical cases. Classically, there is a peribulbar lymphocytic infiltrate described as a "swarm of bees" while more chronic lesions may display less inflammation but fibrosis and dystrophic hair shafts.

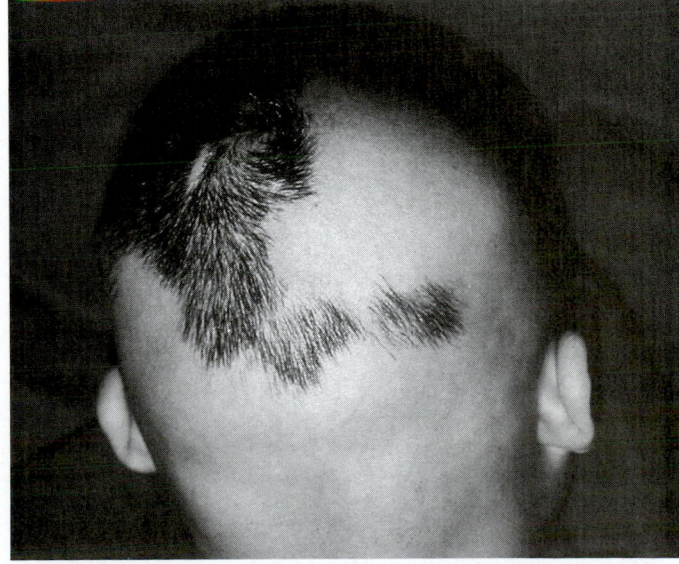

FIGURE 14-26 **The majority of the scalp is devoid of hair but appears normal without scaling or erythema in this child with alopecia areata. (*Courtesy of Bari Cunningham, M.D.*)**

Therapy for alopecia areata usually consists of topical or intralesional corticosteroids. Localized, mild disease often responds to potent (class II or I) topical corticosteroid therapy. Adolescents can often tolerate the discomfort of intralesional injections of triamcinolone acetonide (5 to 10 mg/cc) administered in three- to four-week intervals. Systemic corticosteroids can be effective in some patients, but high doses are often required to regrow hair; their discontinuation often results in recurrent hair loss. The limited benefits and undeniable risks of systemic corticosteroids preclude their use for alopecia areata in most instances.

Other therapeutic approaches include the induction of contact dermatitis with compounds such as anthralin, squaric acid dibutyl ester, or diphencyprone. Pruritus, dermatitis, and staining of clothing make this second-line therapy for the motivated patient. Treatment of the pediatric patient with alopecia areata should address the emotional needs of these children and their families. Patients with widespread, longstanding alopecia areata may experience social stigmatization and may benefit from hair prostheses. Several nonprofit companies will provide quality natural hair prostheses free of charge to patients who are in need (*www.wigsforkids.org*). The National Alopecia Areata Foundation can be accessed at *NAAF@compuserve.com*.

Trichotillomania is characterized by compulsive pulling, twisting, or breaking of hair. Affected areas of the scalp demonstrate irregularly shaped areas of partial alopecia with broken hairs of varying lengths, giving the scalp a "moth-eaten" appearance. A fringe of hair in the frontal area is usually left intact, as are inaccessible parts of the occipital scalp. The eyebrows or eyelashes may be pulled out instead of or in addition to scalp hair. The differential diagnosis includes tinea capitis, regrowing alopecia areata, and secondary syphilis. Although the diagnosis is usually made clinically, it can be confirmed with a scalp biopsy, which may demonstrate perifollicular hemorrhage, absence of significant inflammation, as well as increased catagen hair follicles. Trichotillomania may be a nervous habit analogous to nail biting in some cases but can also indicate serious psychopathology, particularly in older children.

Direct confrontation and accusation are rarely helpful. Rather than querying the patients *whether* they are engaging in hair pulling, it is helpful to ask them *when* they are pulling their hair. In addition, using the analogy to nail biting may make a frank discussion of the problem more acceptable. Behavioral modification techniques or psychiatric evaluation should be undertaken if the problem does not resolve or if other psychiatric symptoms are present. Antidepressants such as fluoxetine (Prozac) and psychotropics used for obsessive-compulsive disorder are useful adjuncts to behavioral modification, particularly in older children.

Tension or pressure on the scalp can cause hair breakage or loss, and children seem to be particularly susceptible to this problem. *Traction alopecia* is fairly common in young girls who have tight ponytails or braids. Hair thinning occurs at the scalp margin, especially in temporal areas. Folliculitis may also be present. The problem is most common in African-American girls, often exacerbated by *trichorrhexis nodosa*. If hair-styling techniques are not changed, permanent hair loss can result. *Traumatic alopecia* can result from prolonged pressure on the scalp as might occur with general anesthesia, usually near the vertex of the scalp. A "halo" of pressure alopecia can also be seen after delivery in an area corresponding to the caput succedaneum. Infants, especially those with atopic dermatitis, are particularly susceptible to *frictional hair loss* and may lose large areas of occipital and parietal scalp hair from rubbing the head against the bed.

Generalized Nonscarring Alopecia

Telogen effluvium is a form of hair loss that occurs after severe stress to the body, including birth, acute febrile illness, surgical shock, crash dieting, emotional stress, or discontinuation of oral contraceptives. Sudden stress may prematurely shift hair shafts into the resting phase (telogen growth phase). Two to three months later, when the anagen or growing phase of that hair shaft begins again, the telogen hair is shed. This form of alopecia, although alarming at times, never results in total alopecia and will resolve without intervention. The diagnosis can usually be made by careful questioning and identifying a specific trigger such as birth of a sibling or change of school.

Androgenic alopecia is inherited as an autosomal-dominant trait with variable expression. Usually the mildest and earliest feature of this alopecia is symmetrical, triangular anterior hairline recession. This pattern of hair loss is rare in the pediatric population but has been noted as early as 14 years of age. Androgenic alopecia may be seen in females, but it is generally less severe than that seen in men. In teenage girls with androgenic alopecia, as well as severe acne, hirsutism and/or menstrual irregularities, evaluation for a potential underlying endocrinologic abnormality should be undertaken.

The *loose anagen syndrome* occurs most commonly in preschool and younger school-aged girls. Characteristically the hair is fine and lighter in color than other family members' and rarely needs cutting. It is usually a sporadic condition but may be inherited in an autosomal-dominant fashion. Anagen hairs pull out easily and painlessly; on light microscopy they show distorted bulbs with a ruffled proximal hair cuticle. The condition usually improves with age. There is no therapy.

Scarring Alopecias

The scarring alopecias, rare in childhood, cause permanent pilosebaceous follicle loss and occur after trauma or infection, such as a suppurative folliculitis or a fungal *kerion* (see Sec. 14.12). In *discoid lupus erythematosus*, scarring alopecia may be preceded by erythema, hyperpigmentation, and follicular plugging. Occasionally, *pseudopelade of Brocq* may be seen in children. In this idiopathic form of scarring alopecia, multiple round to oval scarred patches of hair loss are seen. It is differentiated from alopecia areata by the presence of scarring. Hairless patches may form finger-like projections that resemble "footprints in the snow." *Folliculitis decalvans* is a rare form of scarring alopecia that is characterized by multiple inflammatory papules and pustules at the periphery of the hairless areas. *Acne keloidalis* is typically seen in postpubertal African-American males along the nape of the neck. It may represent a hypersensitivity reaction to staphylococcal organisms in individuals prone to keloidal scarring. Rarely, localized scleroderma, especially the coup de sabre form, may form linear plaques of scarring alopecia in children.

Congenital Disorders with Alopecia

A variety of congenital disorders may be associated with hypotrichosis or alopecia. *Congenital triangular alopecia* is characterized by a nonscarred circumscribed area of hypotrichosis in the frontotemporal scalp. The lesion is shaped like a triangle with the base facing the anterior edge of the hairline and may be bilateral. The condition is actually a form of hypotrichosis rather than alopecia and is identified by the presence of fine, vellus hairs within the

COLOR PLATES

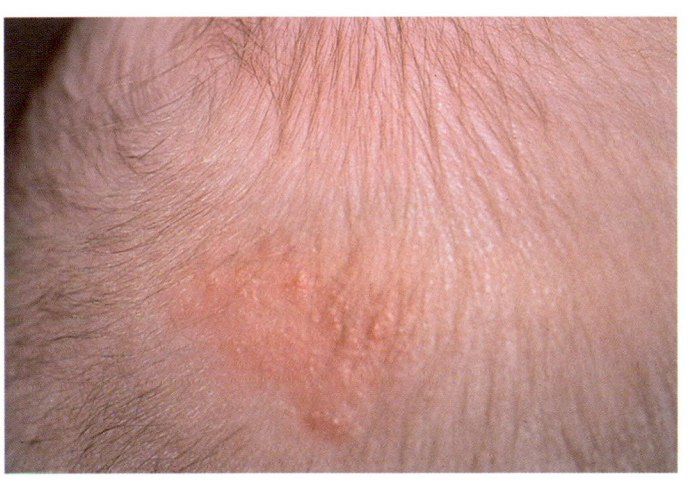

Color Plate 1. Nevus sebaceous. Note coalesced yellow papules, most commonly seen in young infants and again after puberty begins.

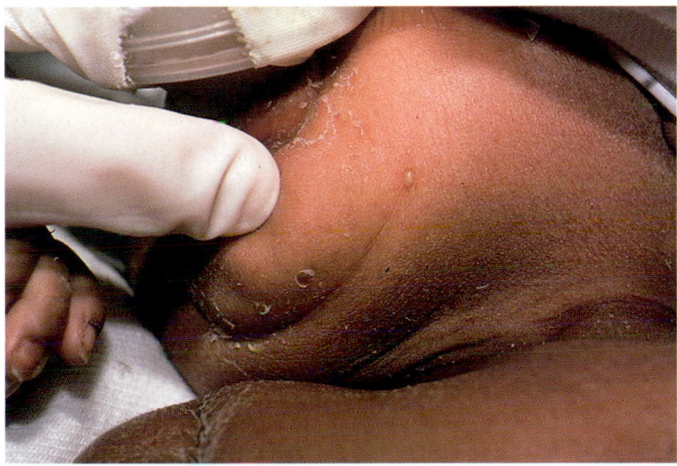

Color Plate 2. Neonatal pustular melanosis. Note superficial pustules and hyperpigmented macules, surrounded by a collarette of scale, that appear within the first 24 hours of life.

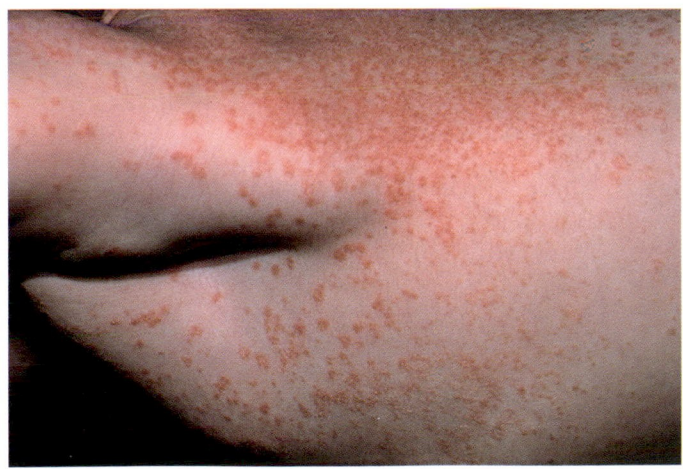

Color Plate 3. Psoriasiform id reaction after a severe candidal diaper dermatitis.

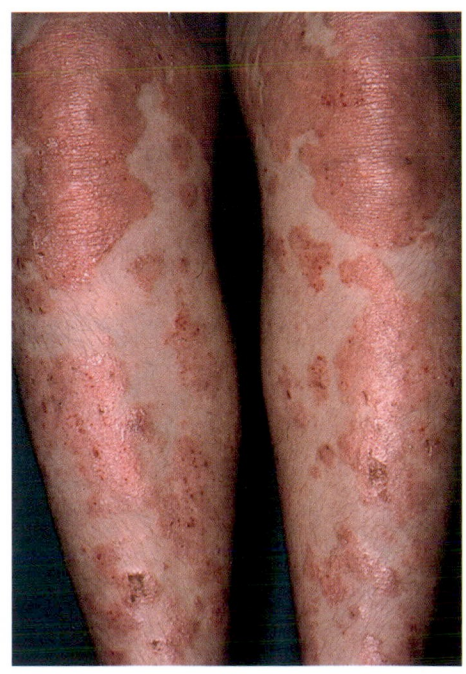

Color Plate 4. Psoriasis. Note sharp delineation from the surrounding normal skin and the tightly adherent, silvery scale.

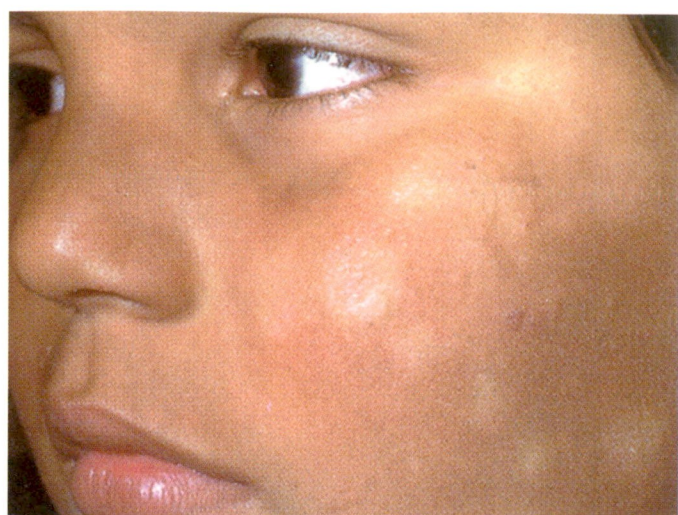

Color Plate 5. Pityriasis alba. Note ill-defined hypopigmented macules on cheek of young child. Preceding eczematous changes are also evident as erythema with slight scale.

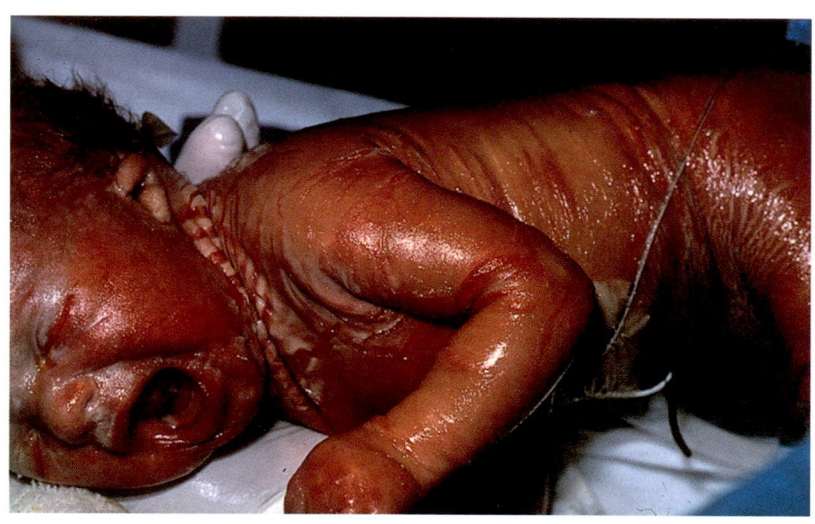

Color Plate 6. Collodion baby. Note taut, shiny skin reminiscent of cellophane, seen with lamellar ichthyosis or nonbullous congenital ichthyosiform erythroderma.

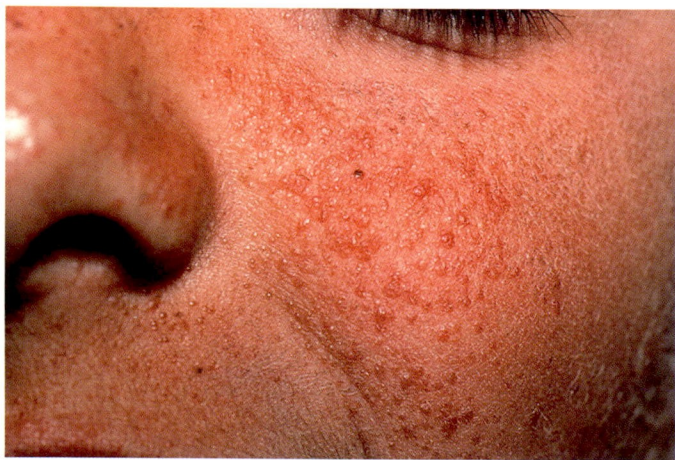

Color Plate 7. Tuberous sclerosis. Hallmarks include flesh-to pink-colored papules and nodules appearing on the central face.

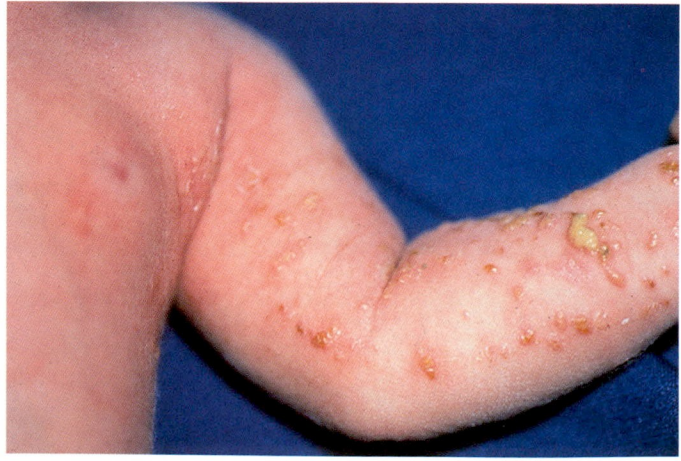

Color Plate 8. Lines of Blashko.

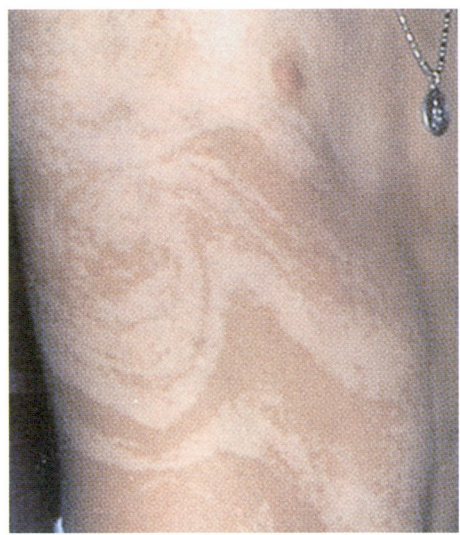

Color Plate 9. Hypomelanosis of Ito. Note linear, swirling macular bands of hypopigmentation, following the lines of Blashko.

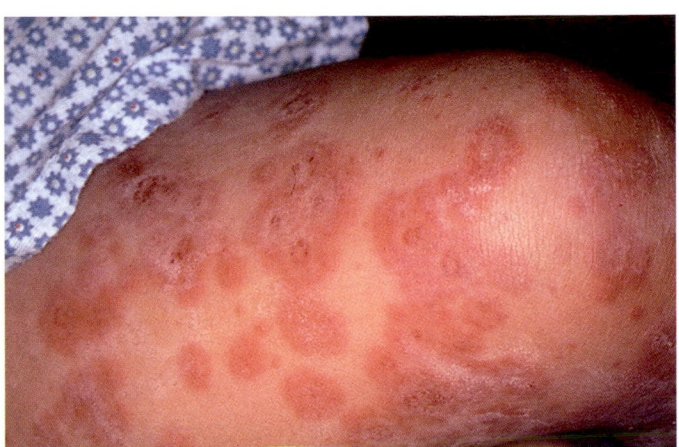

Color Plate 10. Erythema multiforme. Note target-like lesions in which the central portion is necrotic or blistered and the peripheral border is intensely erythematous.

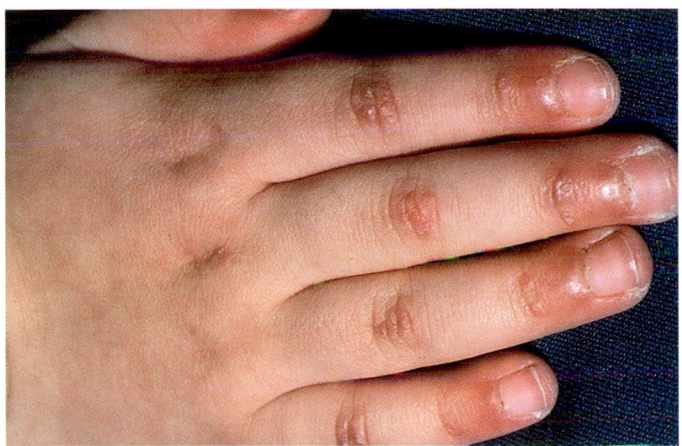

Color Plate 11. Dermatomyositis. Note erythematous papules ("Gottron sign") over the knuckles and cuticular inflammation.

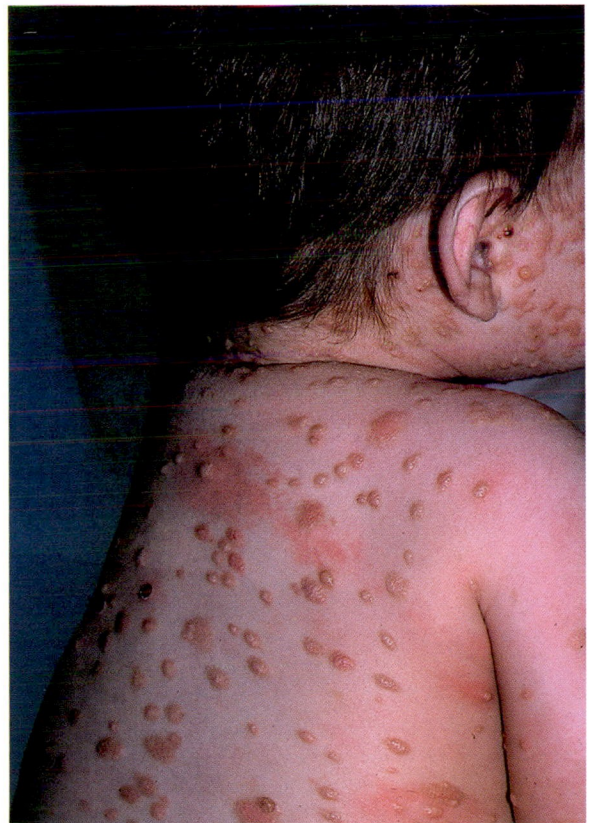

Color Plate 13. Mastocytosis. Hyperpigmented lesions are infiltrated with mast cells and urticate when traumatized (Darier sign).

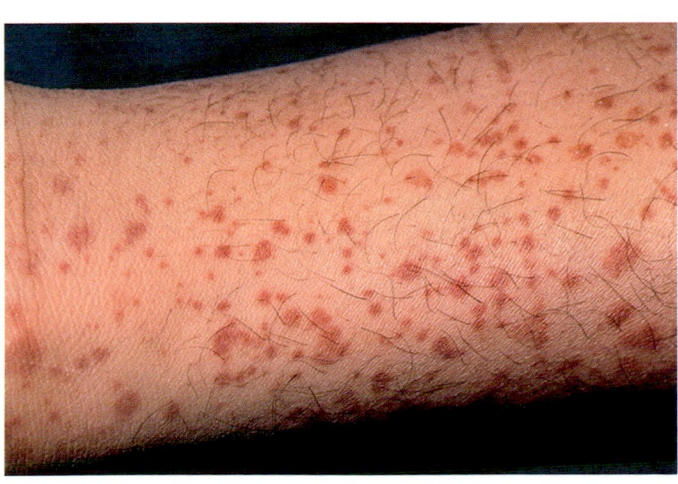

Color Plate 12. Henoch Schonlein purpura. Note erythematous, palpable, purpuric eruption on lower extremities.

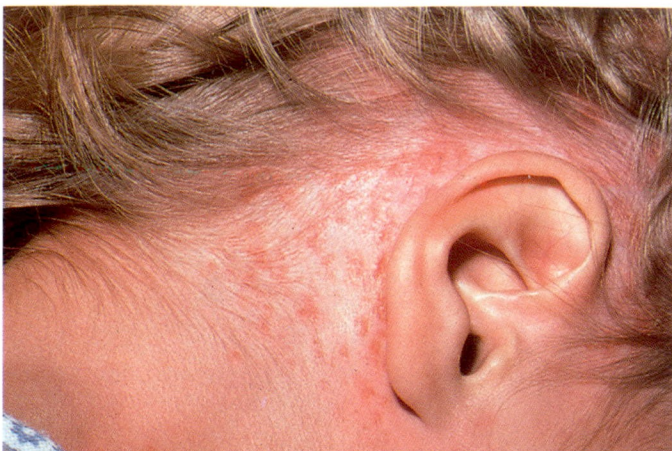

Color Plate 14. Langerhans cell histiocytosis (acute disseminated histiocytosis). Scaly papules, petechiae, or purpura on the scalp or in intertriginous areas show evidence of a destructive process and heal with atrophy and scarring.

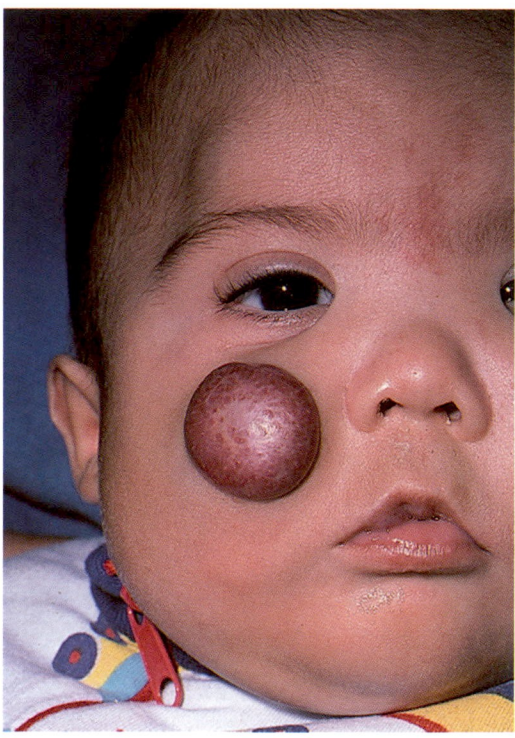 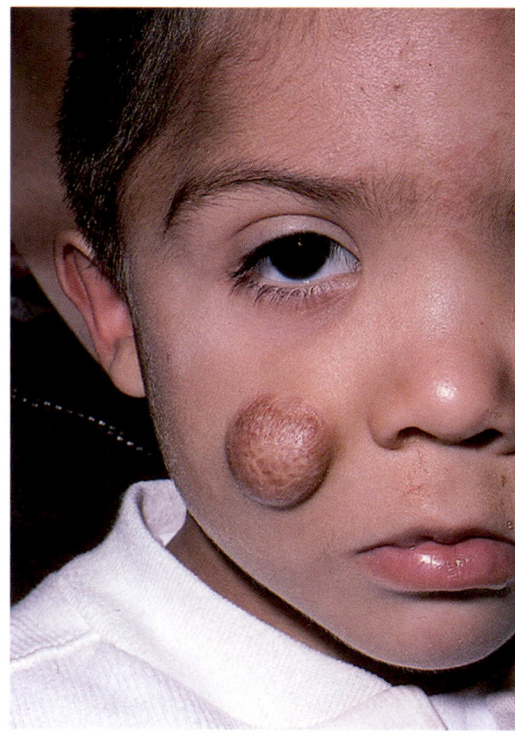

Color Plate 15A/B. Involution of hemangioma in 15A leaves residual telangiectasias and fibrous tissue.

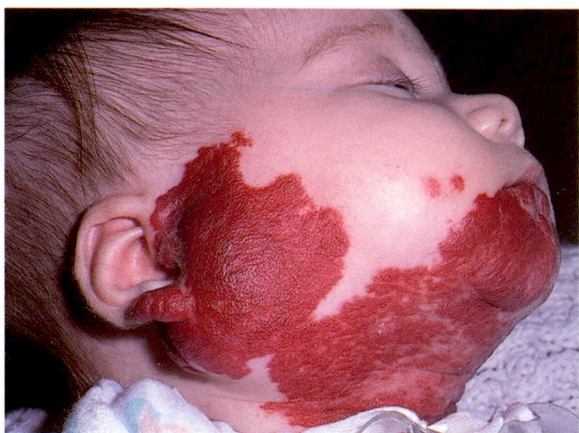

Color Plate 16. Extensive hemangiomas of the lower face are associated with hemangiomas of the airway.

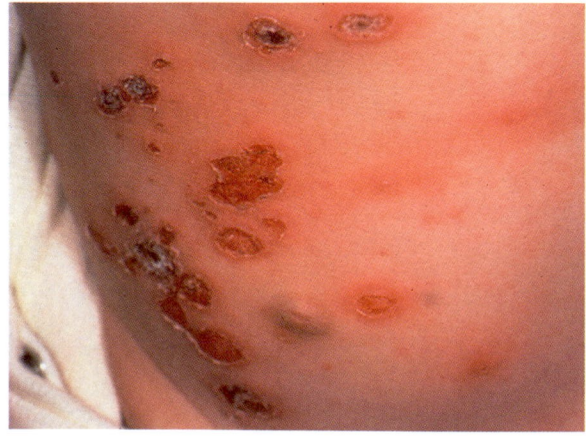

Color Plate 17. Bullous impetigo. Note both intact bullae and ruptured lesions with a collarette of scale.

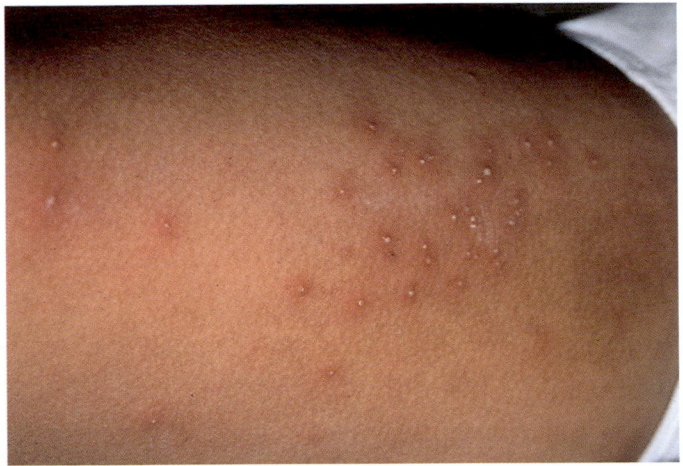

Color Plate 18. Folliculitis presents as erythematous papules and papulopustules surrounding hair follicles.

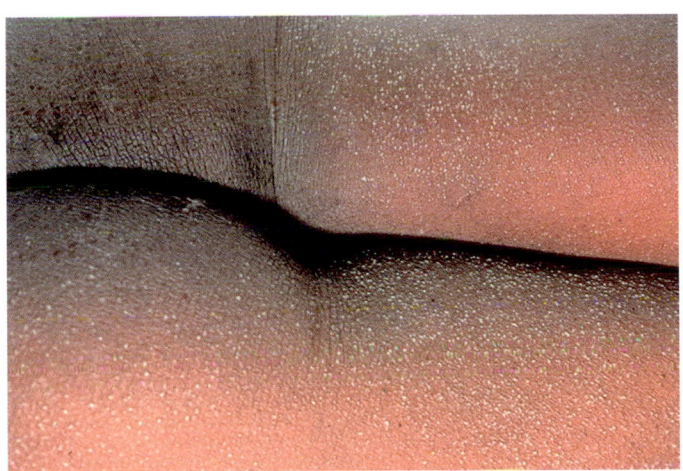

Color Plate 20. Gianotti-Crosti syndrome presents with multiple erythematous papules in symmetric distribution over the cheeks, the buttocks, or the extensor surfaces of the extremities. Multiple viruses are implicated.

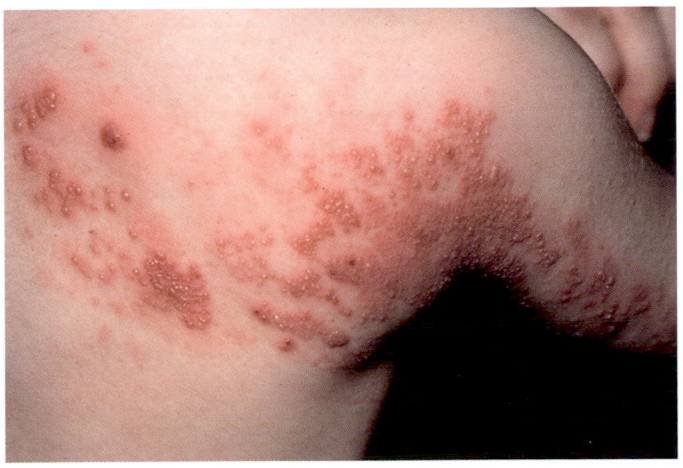

Color Plate 21. Herpes zoster. Grouped vesicles on an erythematous base follow dermatomal distribution.

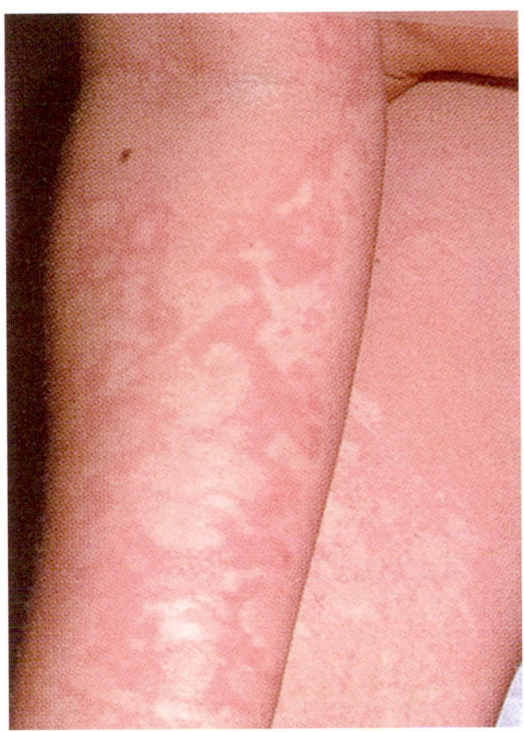

Color Plate 19. Erythema infectiosum (Fifth disease; parvovirus B19). Reticulate, lacy erythematous macules and plaques on extremities occur after the "slapped cheek" appearance.

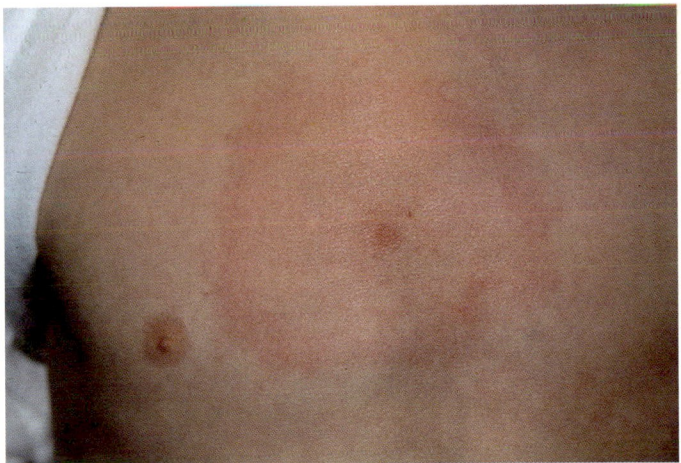

Color Plate 22. Erythema migrans of Lyme disease. Note raised border and central clearing. Lesions are usually but not always single and may show concentric rings.

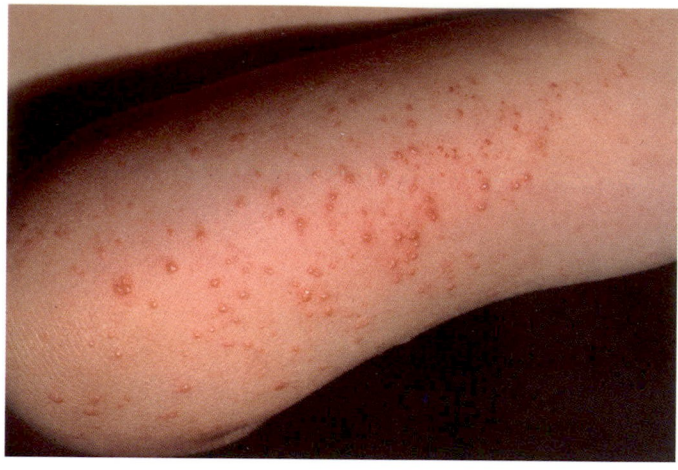

Color Plate 23. Scarlet fever. Note erythematous papules with sandpaper consistency.

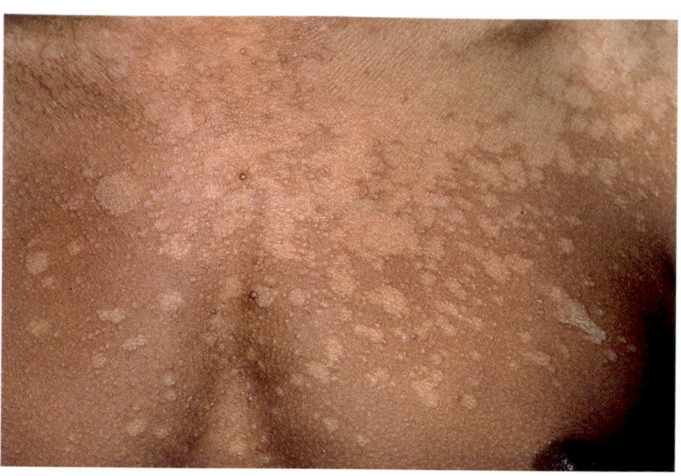

Color Plate 24. Tinea versicolor occurs on lipid-rich areas of skin and is caused by the lipophilic yeast *Malassezia furfur*.

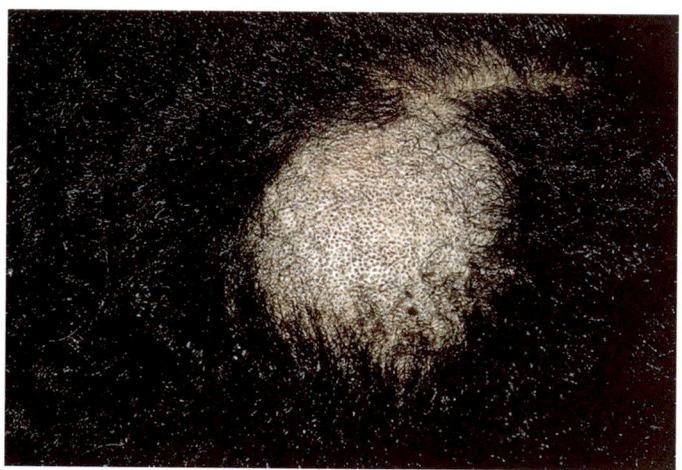

Color Plate 25. Black dot form of tinea capitis. Black dots demarcate broken hair shafts.

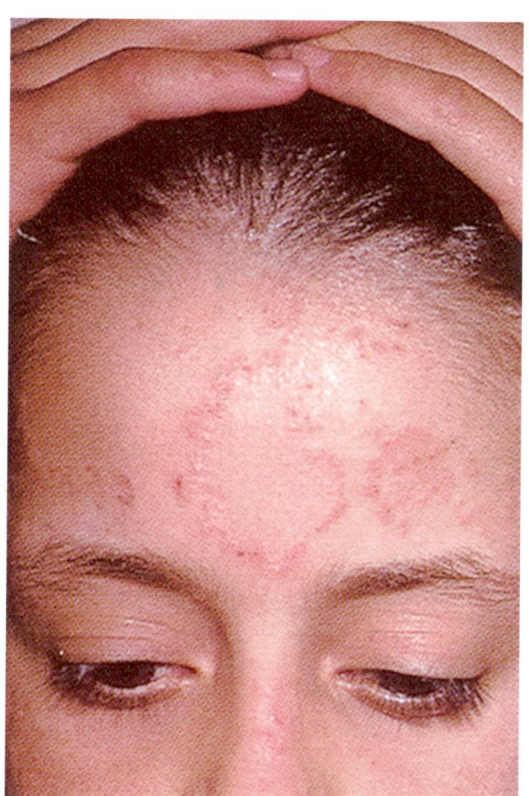

Color Plate 26. Tinea faciei. Note active, scaly border typical of dermatophyte infections.

patch. It is often erroneously attributed to forceps injury. *Hallerman-Streiff syndrome,* characterized by dwarfism, beaked nose, and brachycephaly, displays congenital alopecia most prominent over the frontal and occipital scalp, especially along suture lines. Diffuse alopecia, without structural hair abnormalities, is a feature of many hereditary disorders including hereditary trichodysplasia, oral-facial-digital syndrome, cartilage-hair hypoplasia syndrome, Coffin-Siris syndrome, trichorhinophalangeal syndrome, trichodento-osseous syndrome, and Sessenbrenner's syndrome. Several ectodermal dysplasia syndromes and syndromes of premature aging include hypotrichosis as a feature (see Sec. 14.4).

Several rare syndromes caused by X-linked dominant genes may produce patchy alopecia in affected females as a result of mosaicism. The alopecia may be linear or swirled as it follows the lines of Blaschko. These syndromes include focal dermal hypoplasia, incontinenti pigmenti, CHILD syndrome, and X-linked dominant chondrodysplasia punctata (see Sec. 14.4).

Hair Shaft Abnormalities with Hair Breakage

Trichorrhexis nodosa is the most common cause of hair breakage in African-American patients. It frequently follows chemical treatments and is believed to represent a genetic weakness in the hair shaft that is unmasked by physical or chemical injury. Although the hair is actually breaking, patients often report that the hair has stopped growing. Examination demonstrates very short (3- to 4-cm) hairs, especially on the sides of the head. Rubbing the hair between the fingers often produces broken fragments of hair. Microscopic examination demonstrates focal widening of the hair shaft with splaying of the fibers, resembling two brooms with their ends pushed together. The condition usually improves in two to four years if the hair is managed gently by avoiding further traction, excessive heat, or chemical treatments.

In *pili torti,* the hair shaft is twisted on its long axis. Early in life the hair becomes kinky and sparse and may stand on end. Pili torti is associated with several clinical syndromes. The most significant is Menkes disease, an X-linked recessive, multisystem disorder of copper metabolism caused by deficiencies in a protein believed to be a copper transporting P-type ATP-ase (see Sec. 14.4). In the Ronchese form of pili torti, keratosis pilaris and, occasionally, nail, teeth, and eye abnormalities are associated. In Bjornstad syndrome, associated sensorineural hearing loss is characteristic. Crandall syndrome consists of pili torti with hearing loss and hypogonadism.

Trichorrhexis invaginata is a distinctive hair shaft anomaly found in Netherton syndrome (see Sec. 14.4) and characterized by increased fragility, trichoschisis (transverse fractures of the hair), and low hair sulfur content. Under light microscopy some hairs may be shaped like a golf tee or canestick. With polarizing microscopy, alternating transverse bands of light and dark are seen. The typical "tiger tail" pattern of the hair shaft in trichothiodystrophy may not be evident at birth. *Monilethrix* (beaded hair) is a rare structural hair abnormality caused by mutations in hair cortex keratin. The hair is lusterless and brittle, failing to grow more than a few centimeters in length. Keratosis pilaris, mental retardation, abnormal nails and teeth, and cataracts may occur in association.

Hair Shaft Abnormalities without Breakage

Patients may display *woolly hair* which differs from that of family members or other uninvolved areas of the scalp. The hair is tightly curled, and hairs are oval in cross sections. Autosomal-dominant and -recessive forms have been described. The dominant form may be associated with keratosis pilaris atrophicans, Noonan syndrome, palmoplantar keratoderma with cardiac conduction defects, giant axonal neuropathy, and osteoma cutis. Localized areas of woolly hair represent *wooly hair nevi.* They are usually sporadic and may be associated with epidermal nevi in continuity or, more often, on another area of the body. In *uncombable hair syndrome* hair is light blonde, frizzy, and cannot be combed flat. It often glistens or is spangled in appearance. Eyebrows, lashes, and body hair are normal. Under microscopy, the hairs are triangular or kidney shaped in cross-section, although these changes are not specific for this syndrome.

Hypertrichosis

The terms *hirsutism* and *hypertrichosis* are frequently used to describe excessive hairiness, but the syndromes differ in their patterns of distribution. Hirsutism refers to an excessive growth of body hair in an androgen-dependent distribution (beard, upper lip, neck, chest, areola, linea alba, upper inner thighs). Hypertrichosis refers to a generalized or localized distribution of hair which is not androgen-dependent.

Congenital hypertrichosis may occur alone or with occasional associations. It may be diffusely distributed or localized to one area of the body. *Congenital melanocytic nevi* often have dark, coarse hair. *Becker nevi* or *smooth-muscle hamartoma* may be congenital or may develop at puberty and often present with a patch of increased hair, frequently with faint hyperpigmentation of the underlying skin. Common locations include the chest and the back. Skin biopsy usually shows an increase in perifollicular smooth muscle. A *faun-tail* in the dorsal midline of the back may be a sign of occult spinal dysraphism. Magnetic resonance imaging should be obtained with any midline congenital skin abnormality to exclude a tethered cord. Circumscribed hypertrichosis can also be caused by localized trauma such as rubbing or chronic inflammation. Cranial meningoceles, encephaloceles, and heterotopic brain tissue are often marked by a tuft of hair or by a peripheral rim of hair otherwise labeled as the *hair collai.* Hyperpigmentation and varying degrees of hypertrichosis may be seen overlying a *plexiform neurofibroma.* Similarly, a paraspinal hair whorl has been described over the thorax of a deep mediastinal plexiform neurofibroma. Localized patches of terminal hair growing from skin of normal color is not uncommon and is termed *circumscribed nevoid hypertrichosis.* Circumscribed patches of terminal hair may be seen alone or, rarely, in combination with hemihypertrophy. Tumors of the central nervous system, kidney, and adrenal gland can be associated findings. Rarely, babies may display hair in the genital region within the first three months of life without biochemical or clinical evidence of androgen excess. The condition appears to regress spontaneously. A congenital patch of hypertrichosis located on the anterior neck (cervical hypertrichosis) may be associated with retinal abnormalities or peripheral neuropathy or may be an isolated finding.

Several congenital and hereditary disorders result in hypertrichosis, including the Donohue and Lawrence-Siep forms of lipoatrophy, Cornelia de Lange syndrome, Rubinstein-Taybi syndrome, Barber Say syndrome, several forms of mucopolysaccharidoses, and the porphyrias. *Congenital hypertrichosis lanuginosa* is an autosomal-recessive form of generalized hypertrichosis. In contrast, congenital hypertrichosis with gingival fibromatosis is a familial disorder of autosomal-dominant with inheritance associated with a coarse facies and gingival hyperplasia or fibromatosis. Acquired, generalized hypertrichosis may be seen after severe head injuries or shock and in patients with anorexia nervosa, malnutrition, and hypothyroidism. Fetal alcohol syndrome may produce a small infant with generalized hypertrichosis, microcephaly, and dysmorphic facial features. Finally, medications may be associated with generalized hypertrichosis; these include phenytoin, cyclosporin, corticosteroids, diazoxide, minoxidil, psoralens, and streptomycin.

References

Baumeister FAM, Schwarz HP, Stengel-Rutkowski S: Childhood hypertrichosis: diagnosis and management. Arch Dis Child 72:457–459, 1995

Rogers M: Hair shaft abnormalities: Part I. Australas J Dermatol 36:179–184, 1995

Rogers M: Hair shaft abnormalities: Part II. Australas J Dermatol 37:1–11, 1996

Sullivan JR: Acquired scalp alopecia. Part II: a review. Australas J Dermatol 40:61–70, 1999

Sullivan JR, Kossard S: Acquired scalp alopecia. Part I: a review. Australas J Dermatol 39:207–219, 1998

Other Disorders of Hair Follicles

Keratosis pilaris, a common disorder characterized by retention of keratin scales in the pilosebaceous follicles, usually begins in childhood and often gradually resolves or improves. It is most commonly seen in patients with atopic dermatitis and may be mildly pruritic. The primary lesion is a keratotic plug that fills the follicular orifice, leading to rough horny follicular papules at the site and a rough, sandpaperlike texture to the skin. Mild to moderate perifollicular erythema is sometimes present. Rarely, marked inflammation may occur within each lesion, leading to an erroneous diagnosis of acne vulgaris or infectious folliculitis. Lesions are most common on the cheeks and extensor surfaces of the upper arms, thighs, and buttocks but may be generalized. The differential diagnosis of keratosis pilaris includes folliculitis, acne, pityriasis rubra pilaris, eruptive vellus hair cysts, syndromes with follicular inflammation and atrophy (see below), and certain rare disorders of cornification (eg, ichthyosis follicularis).

Treatment is unnecessary in mild cases. In severe or symptomatic cases, emollient therapy is particularly helpful when combined with alpha-hydroxy acids or mild topical retinoids. Urea 10 to 20% creams and/or 5 to 12% lactic acid/ammonium lactate cream or lotion can be used. Alpha glycolic creams and propylene glycol lotions are sometimes helpful. Tretinoin cream 0.1% microsphere formulation or adapalene gel may be helpful in decreasing follicular hyperkeratoses but can also irritate the treated site.

Lichen spinulosus resembles keratosis pilaris in morphology but occurs in discrete plaques 2 to 5 cm in diameter, most often located on neck, upper torso, buttocks, upper arms, or thighs. Pruritus is variable. Similar clinical findings can also occur in atopic dermatitis, follicular mucinosis, and some drug reactions.

Trichostasis spinulosa is a relatively common condition that often develops in adolescence. Hyperkeratotic papules are usually present over the shoulders or back or in the perinasal area. The plugs contain multiple vellus hairs projecting from the follicular opening and are often pigmented, incorrectly suggesting that poor hygiene is responsible for their appearance. Treatment with topical tretinoin is occasionally helpful, but many cases respond poorly to all forms of treatment.

Several rare conditions characterized by follicular inflammation followed by atrophy or scarring may occur during childhood. In *ulerythema oophyrogenes* (keratosis pilaris atrophicans), erythematous follicular papules usually begin in the eyebrows and result in partial or complete loss of eyebrow hair. The forehead, cheeks, and upper lip may also be involved, and keratosis pilaris without scarring is usually present at other sites. The condition has been associated with other ectodermal defects and congenital anomalies, including Rubenstein-Taybi and Noonan syndromes and a deletion on the short arm of chromosome 18. At least one case has responded to isotretinoin therapy. *Atrophoderma vermiculatum* is characterized by the gradual onset of erythematous follicular plugs that result in honeycomb-like atrophic and pitted scarring. The cheeks are most commonly affected, but the forehead, upper lip, and ears can also be involved. The condition can be sporadic or have autosomal-dominant inheritance. *Keratosis follicularis spinulosa decalvans* is an X-linked recessive syndrome of diffuse follicular hyperkeratosis with scarring alopecia of the scalp and, in some cases, palmar-plantar keratoderma and photophobia.

Alopecia mucinosa (follicular mucinosis) is a relatively rare inflammatory condition that results in accumulation of acid mucopolysaccharides in hair follicle epithelia. When this occurs in areas of terminal hair, a patchy alopecia may result. In other areas, scaling, mild erythema, and follicular papules coalesce to form plaques. These plaques may be relatively superficial or may have a boggy, shiny, infiltrated quality. The diagnosis is made by skin biopsy, which shows mucin between epithelial cells of hair follicles. Most cases in children regress spontaneously. Although a few cases in adolescents have been associated with Hodgkin disease or cutaneous T-cell lymphoma, the association with lymphoma generally occurs in adults. These may present as an unusual acneiform eruption. T-cell receptor gene rearrangement studies may be useful in such cases.

Several kinds of *cysts* may occur during childhood. The most common cyst in adults, the *epidermal inclusion cyst* (EIC), is relatively uncommon until puberty. These cysts most commonly present on the face, chest, or back, particularly in patients with acne. The development of multiple EICs in the absence of an inflammatory disorder suggests the possibility of Gardner syndrome, a rare autosomal-dominant disorder characterized by large bowel polyposis, desmoid tumors, and odontogenic jaw cysts. Milia, which are tiny epidermoid cysts, are very common and may occur at any time, including in the newborn period. They can develop spontaneously, after skin trauma, or in scarring forms of epidermolysis bullosa. They may also be seen in oral-facial-digital syndrome, a rare condition with abnormalities of the nose, mouth, and hands. *Pilar cysts* are virtually always located on the scalp and usually develop during adolescence. Multiple pilar cysts may be inherited as an autosomal-dominant trait. *Steatocystoma multiplex* is another dominantly inherited cystic disorder with usual onset during adolescence. Multiple small cysts varying in size from 0.5 to 2.0 cm are usually located on the chest and arms. When punctured, they drain an oily fluid. Diagnosis is confirmed by skin biopsy. *Eruptive vellus hair cysts* are an uncommon form of multiple cysts during childhood. Numerous tiny often hyperpigmented papules usually occur on the neck, upper torso, or arms. Pruritus or other symptoms are usually absent. Familial cases have been reported, possibly with autosomal-dominant inheritance.

Pilomatricomas (calcifying epithelioma of Malherbe) most frequently appear before 10 years of age and present as a deep-seated nodule fixed to the overlying tissue, with a faint blue or purple discoloration. Less commonly, lesions are dome-shaped, exophytic, and dark red in color. The lesions may feel rock-hard and angular, owing to the calcium present within the lesion. Cysts vary in size from 0.5 to 3.0 cm and are usually asymptomatic but may become inflamed and tender because of focal rupture into surrounding dermis. Ulceration of the overlying skin may also occur. Occasionally, a chalky, white material can be expressed from a central opening. Lesions are most commonly located on the face, arms, and upper torso. Somatic mutations affecting the amino-terminal segment of β-catenin, a cell adhesion protein, have been noted in most pilomatricomas that have been assessed. This protein also acts as a transcription cofactor, and the mutated form may lead to increased expression of tumorigenic genes in affected cells. Although pilomatricomas can regress spontaneously, most will persist until removed surgically. If they are asymptomatic and typical in appearance, removal can be deferred until the child is old enough to cooperate with a procedure performed under local anesthesia. Rare cases of malignant pilomatricomas have been reported, as have familial forms associated with myotonic dystrophy.

References

Arndt KA, Rand RE: Follicular syndromes with inflammation and atrophy. In: Fitzpatrick TB, Eisen AZ, Wolff K, eds: Dermatology in General Medicine, 4th ed. New York, McGraw-Hill, 1993: 766

Chan EF, Gat U, McNiff J, Fuchs E: A common human skin tumor is caused by activating mutations in β-catenin. Nat Genet 21:410–413, 1999

Cohen BA: Dermal nodules and tumors. In: Cohen BA, ed: Pediatric Dermatology, 2nd ed. London, Mosby International, 1999:120–122

Eramo LR, Esterly NB, Zieserl EJ, et al: Ichthyosis follicularis with alopecia and photophobia. Arch Dermatol 121:1167–1174, 1985

Nazarenko SA, Ostroverkhova NV, Vasiljeva EO, et al: Keratosis pilaris and ulerythema oophyrogenes associated with an 18p deletion caused by a Y/18 translocation. Am J Med Genet 85:179–182, 1999

Neild VS, Pegum JS, Wells RS: The association of keratosis pilaris atrophicans and wooly hair with and without Noonan syndrome. Br J Dermatol 110:357–362, 1984

Rand R, Baden HP: Keratosis follicularis spinulosa decalvans. Arch Dermatol 119:22–26, 1983

Wittenberg GP, Gibson LE, Pittelkow MR, el-Azhary RA: Follicular mucinosis presenting as an acneiform eruption: report of four cases. J Am Acad Dermatol 38:849–851, 1998

14.10 DISORDERS OF ECCRINE AND APOCRINE GLANDS

Lawrence F. Eichenfield

Miliaria results from obstruction of the eccrine sweat duct and its focal rupture. It is common in early infancy but can occur at any age. Miliaria crystallina is caused by superficial obstruction of the duct within the stratum corneum and is usually precipitated by a febrile illness or by a warm environment. Multiple, tiny, noninflammatory, superficial vesicles develop suddenly, commonly on the forehead and upper torso. Lesions resolve rapidly, leaving branny desquamation. The vesicles can be wiped away, and vesicular contents show no organisms and few, if any, cells. Miliaria rubra is the most common form of miliaria; it usually develops after prolonged exposure to hot, humid weather and begins a few days to weeks after exposure. The condition can also be precipitated by occlusive clothing or bandages. Small, erythematous papules or papulopustules are mostly concentrated in areas of friction from clothing, such

as the neck, waist, and thighs, or in intertriginous areas. Pruritus is common. The lesions resolve when the patient is placed in a cooler environment and looser, less occlusive clothing is worn.

Hidradenitis suppurativa is a chronic, inflammatory disease of the apocrine sweat gland, which can involve the axilla, inguinal creases, perineum, and areolae. Although children as young as four or five years of age may be affected, most cases begin during puberty. The condition is more common in women and in blacks. Hidradenitis displays some similarities with cystic acne, with primary occlusion of the follicular orifice followed by bacterial overgrowth, apocrine rupture, inflammation, and scarring. Initially, one or more tender cysts may be present in the axillae or in the inguinal area. These are easily mistaken for furuncles, but the recurrent nature of the condition and negative bacterial cultures eventually make the diagnosis obvious. In mild cases, the cysts resolve spontaneously or after drainage, and only an occasional new lesion develops. In severe cases, more and more cysts develop, suppurate, rupture, and scar, leaving sinus tracts and fistulas admixed with new inflammatory lesions. The condition can be painful and debilitating, and rarely, a rheumatologic condition characterized by joint pains, intermittent fever, elevated sedimentation rate, and normocytic anemia occurs. The condition is not caused by deodorants or antiperspirants, although these may exacerbate symptoms.

Treatment of mild cases includes topical antibiotics (eg, clindamycin), systemic antibiotics (eg, cephalexin), incision and drainage of fluctuant cysts, and intralesional injections of triamcinolone acetonide (5 to 10 mg/mL) to inflamed areas. In some instances, systemic corticosteroids may be necessary. Isotretinoin (1 mg/kg/d) is helpful in some cases, but it is usually less effective than in cystic acne; this drug should be administered only by experienced physicians. In recalcitrant cases, surgical excision of the apocrine glands may be necessary.

References

O'Loughlin S, Woods R, Kirke PN, et al: Hidradenitis suppurativa. Glucose tolerance, clinical, microbiologic and immunologic features and HLA frequencies in 27 patients. Arch Dermatol 124:1043–1046, 1988

Paletta C, Jurkiewicz MJ: Hidradenitis suppurativa. Clin Plast Surg 14:383–390, 1987

Wenzel FG, Horn TD: Nonneoplastic disorders of the eccrine glands. J Am Acad Dermatol 38:1–17, 1998

14.11 DISORDERS OF NAILS

Sheila Fallon-Friedlander

Nail abnormalities are commonly an isolated benign finding related to infection or trauma; occasionally a nail change is a manifestation of an underlying generalized skin disease, a systemic disease, or a congenital syndrome. Nail problems are often difficult to diagnose and are notoriously difficult to treat.

Most diagnoses are made clinically. The nail plate or matrix biopsy can also be performed, but the biopsy may itself cause a permanent nail dystrophy. Knowledge of nail anatomy is essential for an understanding of nail diseases (see Fig. 14-2). The nail plate is firmly attached to the vascularized, innervated nail bed by two parallel, longitudinal grooves at either side. The cuticle firmly attaches to the proximal nail plate, preventing water and bacteria from entering the area of nail synthesis, the nail matrix, that lies 2 to 3 mm proximal to the cuticle.

Onycholysis is the distal separation of the nail plate from the nail bed. It may be caused by psoriasis, trauma, certain medications (such as tetracycline), and fungal infections from yeast or tinea. Tinea infections only occasionally cause onycholysis without concomitant subungual debris; therefore, oral antifungal agents should be deferred until the causative organism is identified by culture. Obtaining a history of trauma, thumb-sucking or other chronic wet exposures, and medications is important; KOH preparations and fungal cultures are necessary for complete evaluation. Onycholysis often responds to trimming back the nail, avoidance of frequent contact with water, and use of a topical anticandidal agent (eg, clotrimazole solution).

In *koilonychia,* affected nails are concave or "spoon-shaped" rather than convex. Koilonychia may occur as an autosomal-dominant trait or in association with iron deficiency, hypothyroidism, hemochromatosis, lichen planus, keratodermas, incontinentia pigmenti, and nail-patella syndrome. When present in infancy as an isolated finding, the process resolves.

Nail pitting—punctate depressions in the nail plate—reflect an abnormality of growth in the proximal nail matrix, with imperfect nail plate formation and focal loss of hard keratin. In children, pitting is usually caused by psoriasis or alopecia areata. An occasional pit may be present as a normal variant; rarely, multiple pits occur without any apparent skin or hair disease.

Longitudinal grooves may result from any process causing inflammation in the nail matrix including trauma, lichen planus, psoriasis, alopecia areata, Darier disease, Langerhans cell histiocytosis, and graft-versus-host disease. Wide longitudinal grooves may be caused by growths (usually visible) pressing on the nail matrix, such as large periungual warts, digital mucous cysts, or the periungual fibromas of tuberous sclerosis. *Horizontal ridging* is commonly seen with inflammation of the proximal nail fold, as in candidal paronychia or atopic dermatitis. A horizontal depression, sometimes with distal nail loss (Beau's line) occurs from the abrupt cessation of nail growth with a stressful event (high fever, infection). *Median nail dystrophy* is characterized by a longitudinal groove or split in the center of the nail plate, usually the thumbnails. Splits can radiate from the central groove, resembling a fir tree. The condition can occur as a familial trait, but similar findings can also be seen in individuals who habitually pick, push back, or bite the cuticle. *Twenty-nail dystrophy* (trachyonychia) manifests with increased ridging of nails, which subsequently become dull and dystrophic with a rough, sandpaper-like quality. The condition usually develops in children and typically resolves during several years. The differential diagnosis includes psoriasis, lichen planus, alopecia areata, and pachyonychia congenita.

NAIL CHANGES ASSOCIATED WITH SYSTEMIC DISEASE

Psoriasis may cause pitting, onycholysis with or without subungual debris, nail thickening with distortion or loss of the upper surface of the nail, leukonychia, and partial or complete nail shedding. The presence of papulosquamous skin or scalp plaques allows the diagnosis to be made with certainty. It is unusual in psoriasis for all nails to be affected. Lichen planus may cause longitudinal striations, depressed ridges, nail thinning, and scarring. Pterygium formation, where the proximal nail fold and cuticle fuse with the nail plate, is an uncommon but characteristic finding in lichen planus. Oral leu-

kokeratosis and violaceous scaling skin plaques are also mainifestations of lichen planus.

Nail clubbing (acropachy), long recognized as a manifestation of cardiac and pulmonary disease, is defined as a reduction of the obtuse angle between cuticle and nail bed. In children, congenital cyanotic heart disease and cystic fibrosis are the most frequent causes. Other systemic causes include inflammatory bowel disease, thyroid disease, and chronic active hepatitis. Two kinds of autosomal-dominant clubbing can occur: isolated, familial clubbing; and pachydermoperiostosis, associated with scalp redundancy (cutis verticis gyrata) and thickening of the hands and feet. Racket nails may be confused with true clubbing. The nails are short and broad but, in contrast to clubbing, the angle formed by the proximal nail fold and nail plate is not altered. The condition may be inherited as an autosomal-dominant trait or associated with cartilage-hair hypoplasia and other skeletal dysplasias. Discoloration of the nail may also signify an underlying systemic illness (see below).

Congenital nail abnormalities may occur as isolated defects or part of a more generalized syndrome. Many neonates appear to have ingrown nails distally; these resolve without treatment. Congenital malalignment of the nail matrix is an uncommon condition in which the nail matrix of the great toenail is improperly aligned on the nail bed, resulting in medial displacement of the nail plates. Both self-limiting and persistent forms have been identified; the latter requires surgical intervention. Periodic shedding of the nails is a rare, autosomal-dominant trait. Nails are repeatedly shed, and the new nails may become progressively dystrophic.

Nail abnormalities associated with ectodermal and skeletal dysplasias may be obvious at birth or have a later age of onset. Micronychia (small nails) may be seen in the nail-patella syndrome, inherited as an autosomal-dominant trait. Other features include triangular lunulae, absent or hypoplastic patellae, renal disease (nephrosis), and occasional ophthalmologic and central nervous system abnormalities. Small nails may also occur after intrauterine exposure to alcohol, warfarin, and phenytoin, with trisomies 8, 13, and 18, and in several ectodermal dysplasias. Small or absent nails are also common in dystrophic forms of epidermolysis bullosa. Nail changes in Darier disease include white or red longitudinal streaks, distal V-shaped notching, and nail thickening. Nail dystrophy is often the first sign of dyskeratosis congenita; nail changes include splitting, pterygium formation, loss of nails, and scarring of the nail bed.

Pachyonychia congenita is transmitted as an autosomal-dominant trait. The upper surface of the nail (formed by the proximal matrix) may be thickened, with a yellow-brown discoloration and increased curvature. Distal and subungual hyperkeratosis causes thick, dystrophic-appearing nails. Associated findings may include a palmoplantar keratoderma, often with bulla formation, hyperkeratotic plaques over the elbows and knees, oral leukokeratosis, especially on the tongue, and sebaceous cysts (steatocystoma multiplex). Differential diagnosis includes onychomycosis, mucocutaneous candidiasis, and Darier disease.

DISCOLORATION OF THE NAIL

A wide variety of systemic and localized forms of nail discoloration occurs. Trauma to the nail can lead to the development of a subungual hematoma and subsequent brown-black pigmentation. Chronic trauma or pressure on toenails may also lead to similar deposition of pigment following hemorrhage within the area. Half-and-half nails consist of white discoloration of the proximal nail and red coloration of the distal portion. These nail changes have been associated with uremia, heart failure, and cirrhosis. White discoloration (leukonychia) is common. Transverse or punctate white areas are usually a result of trauma but may be familial. Longitudinal white bands are seen in Darier disease. Irregular whitening of the nails may be caused by onycholysis, with or without subungual debris. Longitudinal brown or black pigmented bands may indicate the presence of a melanocytic nevus in the nail matrix. Such bands are common in darkly pigmented races but unusual in light-skinned persons. The development of a solitary pigmented band, even in an Asian or black individual, may warrant a nail matrix biopsy to exclude a melanoma, particularly if the pigmentation involves the cuticle. Multiple pigmented nail bands may be present with oral melanotic macules and associated intestinal polyps in Peutz-Jegher disease. Nail streaks are also a feature of the Laugier-Hunziker syndrome. Brown or black pigment can also be caused by drugs, such as doxorubicin or zidovudine. The yellow-nail syndrome consists of thickened yellow nails, lymphedema, and respiratory disease. This disorder is rare in children. Yellow nails can also relate to carotene, onychomycosis, nicotine, and hyperbilirubinemia. Blue-gray nails can be associated with minocycline, phenothiazines, bleomycin, argyria, zidovudine, and congenital pernicious anemia.

References

Cohen BA: Nail disorders. In: Pediatric Dermatology, 2nd ed. Mosby International, London, 1999; 201–211

Freire-Maia N, Pinhiero M: Ectodermal Dysplasias: A Clinical and Genetic Study. New York, Liss, 1984

Samman PD: The Nails in Disease, 3rd ed. London, Heinemann Medical, 1980

Silverman R: Nail and appendageal abnormalities. In: Schachner LA, Hansen RC (eds): Pediatric Dermatology. New York, Churchill Livingstone, 1988: 613

14.12 SKIN INFECTIONS AND EXANTHEMS

Anthony J. Mancini

The treatment of common pediatric bacterial skin infections is outlined in Table 14-7.

SUPERFICIAL BACTERIAL INFECTIONS

Impetigo is a highly contagious infection of the superficial epidermis noted predominantly in preschool-age children. Although traditionally group A β-hemolytic streptococci (GABHS) were most frequently isolated in the United States, *Staphylococcus aureus* now appears to predominate. Anaerobic bacteria may be a less common cause. In general, intact skin is resistant to impetiginization, and some form of compromise of the epidermal surface is necessary to permit infection. Predisposing factors include minor abrasions and lacerations, arthropod bites, burns, varicella, and several types of dermatitis, especially atopic dermatitis. Exposed areas such as the face, arms, and legs are most commonly affected, and impetigo is most common during the summer months.

Impetigo usually presents in one of two clinical forms. *Nonbullous or crusted* impetigo, which accounts for over 70% of cases, begins with small vesicles or vesiculopustules, which rupture rapidly, leaving behind a honey-colored crust superimposed on a moist red base. Lesions are minimally symptomatic, although mild pain or pruritus may be present. Autoinoculation of the infection from scratching or digital manipulation may result in clustering and spread of multiple lesions. Associated findings include lymphadenopathy in 90% of patients, and leukocytosis may be present in up to 50% of cases.

Bullous impetigo is related to infection with a toxin-producing strain of *S. aureus*, primarily by phage group 2 or type 71, and less commonly types 3A, 3B, 3C, and 55. The initial lesions consist of flaccid bullae, which rupture easily given the superficial, subcorneal location of lysis caused by the action of the toxin on the epidermis. Patients usually present with shallow, moist, erythematous erosions with a surrounding collarette of the blister roof (Color Plate 17). Even in the absence of intact bullae, the clinical lesions are usually quite diagnostic. Lesions of bullous impetigo may have a propensity for moist, intertriginous areas such as the diaper region, axillae, and neck folds. When delivered systemically from either cutaneous or deep-tissue infection, the toxin of bullous impetigo causes the *staphylococcal scalded skin syndrome (SSSS)*.

Folliculitis is a superficial infection of the pilosebaceous unit, most typically caused by *S. aureus*. Patients present with erythematous papules and papulopustules centered around hair follicles, and most often distributed over the scalp, thighs (Color Plate 18), and/or buttocks. Warmth, moisture, and maceration predispose to folliculitis, and many cases therefore occur during the warmer summer months.

There are a variety of other types of folliculitis. *Gram-negative folliculitis*, most often caused by *Klebsiella, Enterobacter,* or *Proteus,* may be seen in patients with acne vulgaris on long-term antibiotic therapy. In these patients lesions are most common in the facial "T zones." Another form of gram-negative folliculitis, "hot tub" or *pseudomonas folliculitis,* occurs within a few days of exposure to a poorly chlorinated whirlpool or hot tub. These lesions are most common over the buttocks, legs, and arms and may be accompanied by mild constitutional symptoms such as fever and malaise. Immunocompromised patients may develop folliculitis from organisms that tend normally to be nonpathogenic, such as *Pityrosporum* or the hair follicle mite, *Demodex.* Noninfectious forms of folliculitis may also occasionally occur. *Sterile folliculitis* may occur as a result of the frequent application of exogenous agents such as hair gels, which obstruct the orifice of the pilosebaceous unit. *Eosinophilic pustular folliculitis (Ofuji disease)* occurs as recurrent pruritic follicular papules and pustules, especially on the scalp and forehead of infants. These pustules are sterile and reveal clusters of eosinophils. A similar entity has been described in adult patients with HIV infection, although there is no association with HIV in the pediatric patients.

More deeply seated infections of the pilosebaceous unit are termed *furuncles* and *carbuncles* and are usually caused by *S. aureus.* Patients with furuncles present with erythematous, painful, fluctuant nodules (*abscesses*). A carbuncle is a collection of furuncles which tends to be multiloculated and composed of interconnecting sinuses. Incision and drainage of these lesions is usually necessary, in addition to antibiotic therapy. Noninfectious causes of abscesses include those associated with acne vulgaris (as a result of follicular

TABLE 14-7

TREATMENT OF COMMON BACTERIAL SKIN INFECTIONS

THERAPY	DISORDER(S)	DOSE
Cephalexin	Impetigo/Ecthyma Folliculitis Acute paronychia	25–50 mg/kg/d po divided tid-qid
Chlorhexidine soap	Impetigo Folliculitis	Daily—bid to affected areas
Clindamycin 1% lotion	Folliculitis	bid to affected areas
Dicloxacillin	Impetigo Ecthyma contagiosum Cellulitis Folliculitis Acute paronychia	25–50 mg/kg/d po divided qid
Erythromycin*	Impetigo Ecthyma contagiosum Perianal cellulitis Blistering dactylitis	25–50mg/kg/d po divided qid
Erythromycin 2% solution	Erythrasma	bid to affected areas
Mupirocin ointment	Impetigo (localized)	tid to affected areas
Oxacillin	Cellulitis (serious infection)	100–200 mg/kg/d iv divided q 6 h
Penicillin V	Impetigo (if known GABHS) Perianal cellulitis Blistering dactylitis	25–50 mg/kg/d po divided tid-qid

GABHS = group A β-hemolytic streptococci.

* If infection with *S. aureus*, resistance may be limiting.

SOURCE: *Adapted from references for Section 3 in American Academy of Pediatrics: Staphylococcal infections/Group A streptococcal infections. In: Peter G, ed: 1997 Red Book: Report of the Committee on Infectious Diseases, 24th ed. Elk Grove Village, IL, American Academy of Pediatrics, 2000: 514–526.*

rupture and a brisk inflammatory reaction), those in response to a foreign body in the skin, or those which follow spontaneous rupture of an epidermal cyst. *"Cold" abscesses,* which are only mildly erythematous and tender, may be seen in individuals with the hyper-immunoglobulin-E (hyper IgE) syndrome.

In *blistering dactylitis* patients present with bullae on an erythematous base, usually distributed over the volar fat pad of distal phalanges, occasionally with dorsal finger or palmar involvement. More than one digit is usually involved. Gram stain and bacterial culture of blister fluid usually reveals pure growth of GABHS but occasionally yields *S. aureus* or group B streptococci. The intact blisters in blistering dactylitis, an unusual feature of streptococcal-mediated skin infections, are likely related to the thickness of the stratum corneum in the volar sites to which this condition is usually localized.

Acute paronychia, a common infection of the skin surrounding the nail, presents with erythema, edema, and tenderness of both the proximal and lateral nail folds. Small pustules or abscesses may also be present around the base of the nail. Predisposing conditions include trauma, dermatitis, frequent hand washing, and onychophagia (nail biting); *S. aureus* is most commonly isolated, although mixed infection, including anaerobic organisms, may be present. In addition to antimicrobial therapy directed against *S. aureus,* incision and drainage may be indicated.

Erythrasma is a superficial skin infection, primarily occuring in intertriginous zones, caused by *Corynebacteria minutissimum.* The clinical presentation is characterized by slightly red to tan patches with mild scaling, occuring in the toe webs, axillae, inframammary creases, groin, or gluteal crease. Lesions are symptomatic to mildly pruritic and may be confused with cutaneous fungal infections. Wood's lamp examination is helpful in confirming the diagnosis and reveals coral red fluorescence, related to the production of porphyrin compounds by the corynebacteria.

Trichomycosis axillaris is another condition caused by infection with corynebacteria. Patients present with yellow, white, red, or black concretions around hair shafts in the axillae and groin and may complain of hyperhidrosis and malodor. Microscopic examination of extracted hairs with potassium hydroxide on a glass slide reveals the organisms coating the hair shaft. *Pitted keratolysis* is also caused by corynebacteria and presents in affected patients with plantar hyperhidrosis, burning, foul odor, and small punctate pits. It is seen most commonly in males with a history of prolonged use of occlusive footwear (ie, military personnel), especially in warm, damp environments.

BACTERIAL INFECTIONS EXTENDING INTO THE DERMIS AND SUBCUTANEOUS TISSUES

Ecthyma contagiosum, caused primarily by GABHS and *S. aureus,* is a deeper cutaneous infection that extends through the epidermis into the dermis. An impetiginous crust enlarges and upon removal reveals an underlying punched-out ulcer, which may be filled with pus. The most common sites of involvement are the lower legs; if left untreated, ecthyma may progress to cellulitis or lymphagitis. Healing takes place with scar formation. *Ecthyma gangrenosum* is a cutaneous manifestation of underlying sepsis with *Pseudomonas aeruginosa.* Patients usually have an underlying serious illness such as hematologic malignancy or immunodeficiency and present with hemorrhagic papules, nodules, bullae, ulcers, and necrosis. The organism can be cultured from swabs of the lesions or biopsy tissue, and blood cultures are positive for *P. aeruginosa.* Therapy must be initiated rapidly with an aminoglycoside and synthetic penicillin and adjusted based on antimicrobial sensitivity testing.

Cellulitis is an acute infection of the subcutaneous tissues that may be caused by many different bacterial organisms. GABHS and *S. aureus* are again common etiologic agents, and the lower extremities and feet are the locations most often affected. There is frequently a history of a predisposing break in the skin barrier, such as that caused by eczema, contact dermatitis, inflammatory tinea pedis, or trauma. Associated fever, malaise, and chills may be present. In the absence of preexisting skin lesions or in the presence of fever or systemic symptoms, bacteremia should be considered, especially in very young children.

Erysipelas is a superficial form of cellulitis that presents with marked redness and pain in the affected area and often demonstrates well-demarcated, elevated borders. There may be a history of a fissured dermatitis, ulcer, or puncture wound, and GABHS is the most common etiologic agent. Although the diagnosis of both cellulitis and erysipelas is usually suggested on clinical grounds, fine-needle aspiration with Gram stain and culture may be useful in patients with immunocompromise or a suboptimal response to therapy.

Preseptal (periorbital) cellulitis is a form of cellulitis that involves the periorbital skin and soft tissues. It must be differentiated from *orbital cellulitis,* a potentially sight-threatening emergency which can occur from direct extension of preseptal cellulitis through the orbital septum, hematogenous seeding, or direct extension from infected paranasal sinuses. Preseptal cellulitis presents with erythema and edema, which tends to be fairly well demarcated. If decreased ocular movement or proptosis are present, orbital cellulitis must be considered and should be evaluated with radiologic imaging. Although *Haemophilus influenzae* type-B (HiB) has traditionally been the most frequently implicated etiologic agent, the advent of the HiB vaccine has greatly decreased the incidence of many HiB-associated childhood diseases, including preseptal and orbital cellulitis; other organisms, especially *Streptococcus* spp, are now a more frequent cause.

Perianal streptococcal cellulitis (dermatitis) occurs predominantly in children ages 6 months to 10 years and is caused most often by GABHS, and occasionally by *S. aureus.* It is characterized by sharply circumscribed, bright red perianal erythema, which may be accompanied by itching, anal fissures, constipation, and pain on defecation. Blood-streaked stools and purulent anal discharge may be present, although systemic symptoms are rare. Because similar signs and symptoms are seen with other more common dermatologic conditions, diagnosis is frequently delayed. Flares of guttate psoriasis may be associated with perianal streptococcal cellulitis; anal examination is recommended in all patients with this presentation.

Necrotizing fasciitis is a rare, rapidly progressive, and potentially fatal soft-tissue infection that develops at the level of the superficial fascia and often involves the overlying dermis, which may result in the incorrect initial diagnosis of cellulitis. Deep fascia and muscle are spared in most cases, although circumferential involvement may lead to a compartment syndrome. In most cases, a penetrating or blunt traumatic skin injury is the source of the bacterial infection. Although group A streptococci are implicated as a frequent etiologic culprit, single-organism infection is rare, and polymicrobial infection with a mix of aerobic and anaerobic organisms, including *S. aureus, E. coli, Bacteroides* spp, *Peptostreptococcus* spp, and *Clostridium* spp, is more common. Patients usually present with erythema and swelling, accompanied by exquisite tenderness and pain, usually in an extremity. This may progress to the development of clear bullae that become hemorrhagic and eventual necrosis and frank cutaneous gangrene. Fever is present in most patients, and early in the process anesthesia of the overlying skin may be a clue in the differentiation from cellulitis. Patients with invasive GABHS infection may develop associated toxic shock syndrome. Crepitance upon palpation and soft-tissue gas on plain radiography may be present in infections associated with a number of aerobes and anaerobes. Although MR or CT imaging, fine-needle aspiration, and tissue biopsy may be helpful in making the diagnosis, direct surgical inspection of fascia is the fastest and most sensitive technique. Aggressive surgical debridement, parenteral antimicrobial therapy, fluid replacement, and blood pressure support are crucial in the treatment of patients with necrotizing fasciitis and must be instituted expeditiously. Mortality is high, in the range of 30 to 70%.

References

Barzilai A, Cohen HA: Isolation of Group A streptococci from children with perianal cellulitis and from their siblings. Pediatr Infect Dis J 17: 358–360, 1998

Bass JW, Chan DS, Creamer KM, et al: Comparison of oral cephalexin, topical mupirocin and topical bacitracin for treatment of impetigo. Pediatr Infect Dis J 16:708–710, 1997

Brook I, Frazier EH, Yeager JK: Microbiology of nonbullous impetigo. Pediatr Dermatol 14:192–195, 1997

Darmstadt GL, Lane AT: Impetigo: an overview. Pediatr Dermatol 11: 293–303, 1994

Donahue SP, Schwartz G: Preseptal and orbital cellulitis in childhood. A changing microbiologic spectrum. Ophthalmology 105:1902–1906, 1998

Kokx NP, Comstock JA, Facklam RR: Streptococcal perianal disease in children. Pediatrics 80:659–663, 1987

Lewis RT: Soft tissue infections. World J Surg 22:146–151, 1998

Pichichero ME: Group A beta-hemolytic streptococcal infections. Pediatr Rev 19(9):291–302, 1998

Sadick NS: Current aspects of bacterial infections of the skin. Dermatol Clin 15:341–349, 1997

Schneider JA, Parlette HL: Blistering distal dactylitis: a manifestation of group A β-hemolytic streptococcal infection. Arch Dermatol 118:879–880, 1982

Stone DR, Gorbach SL: Necrotizing fasciitis. The changing spectrum. Dermatol Clin 15:213–220, 1997

VIRAL INFECTIONS

The treatment of warts and molluscum is outlined in Table 14-8. An extremely common condition in children, *warts* are caused by infection of the squamous epithelium of skin or mucous membranes with the human papillomavirus (HPV). More than 80 subtypes of HPV have now been described; different types may reveal specific tropisms for distinct cell types. For example, HPV types 1, 2, 4, and 7 are associated with plantar, palmar, and common warts; types 3, 10, and 28 with flat warts; and types 6, 11, 16, 18, 31, and 33 with anogenital and genital tract warts and tumors.

Common warts are found on all body surfaces and are also known as *verrucae vulgares.* They present as flesh-colored, hyperkeratotic papules, which may be solitary or multiple. Filiform lesions may occur and are characterized by a slender stalk with numerous projections distally. Common locations are the fingers, periungual regions, palms, and soles (see plantar warts below). Tiny black dots representing thrombosed capillaries may be visualized centrally, especially after manual debridement of devitalized tissue, and may be a useful diagnostic clue. Autoinoculation, presenting as lesions in a linear array, may be related to scratching and manual dissemination of the virus. Spontaneous wart regression occurs in up to 85% of lesions within two years and is believed to be related to cell-mediated immune processes. Specific anti-HPV therapies are lacking, and most effective treatments rely upon mechanical destruction of infected tissues and the resultant inflammatory response. Excessively traumatic procedures (especially in the pediatric patient) or those which result scarring are unwarranted in the treatment of warts.

Plantar warts occur most often on weight-bearing portions of the soles and may induce significant hyperkeratosis (or epidermal thickening) with resultant pain upon ambulation. Manual debridement of the hyperkeratotic surface by paring with a scalpel blade again reveals thrombosed capillaries, which may help in the differentiation from corns and calluses and may relieve discomfort. Therapy of plantar warts is more difficult given their location and endophytic nature, which is a result of weight-bearing.

Flat warts present as flat, flesh-colored to pink papules and are most commonly distributed on the face (Fig. 14-27), dorsal hands, and arms. Size usually ranges between 1 and 10 mm, and they are minimally elevated above the skin surface with absence of hyperkeratosis or scale. Treatment is usually unnecessary.

Condylomata acuminata, or anogenital warts, are more common in sexually active adolescents but may occur in infants and prepubertal children as well. They present as flesh-colored papules in perianal, genital, and perigenital tissues. The importance of iden-

TABLE 14-8

TREATMENT OF WARTS AND MOLLUSCUM CONTAGIOSUM

THERAPY	LESION(S)	REGIMEN	COMMENT
Cantharidin 0.9% in flexible collodion	MC	Apply sparingly with wooden applicator stick	Rinse in 4–6 h; do not occlude; blistering common; avoid near eyes
Cimetidine*	CW, PW	30–40 mg/kg/d po × 6 to 12 wk	Divide tid
Cryotherapy (liquid nitrogen)	CW, PW, MC	20- to 30-sec cycles × 2	Blistering and pain common; difficult in younger patients
Imiquimod 5% cream†	CA	Apply 3× per week	Rinse in 6–10 h, irritation possible
Topical immunotherapy‡	CW, PW	Following sensitization, patient applies nightly to lesions as tolerated	Irritation possible
Keratolytics (Duofilm, Occlusal, Mediplast, etc.)	CW, PW	Apply nightly; occlude	Avoid face and eyes
Manual paring	CW, PW	Debride with no. 15 blade	Should be painless; stop when pinpoint bleeding occurs
Podophyllin	CA	Apply to lesions only	Rinse in 4–8 h; most effective on moist surfaces
Tretinoin 0.1% cream	FW, MC	Apply sparingly qD	Useful for facial lesions; irritation common

CA = condylomata acuminata; CW = common wart; FW = flat wart; MC = molluscum contagiosum; PW = plantar wart.

* May be useful in some patients; non–FDA-approved indication; well tolerated.

† Approved in patients > 18 years of age.

‡ Variety of agents used, including squaric acid dibutyl ester and diphenylcyclopropenone; should be performed only under supervision of experienced dermatologist.

tifying anogenital warts in the pediatric patient lies in the possible association with a sexual mode of transmission and childhood sexual abuse. However, it is well recognized that benign modes of transmission may result in pediatric anogenital warts, and their presence is not pathognomonic of sexual abuse. A nonsexual mode of transmission may be more common in children under three years of age and may include innocent heteroinoculation or autoinoculation or passage through an infected birth canal. Anogenital warts may be caused by genital HPV types, such as 6, 11, 16, or 18, or by uncommon HPV types, such as type 2, but cause cannot be differentiated on the basis of appearance. Given the association of certain genital HPV types with anogenital carcinomas and the uncertain prognostic significance in children, periodic follow-up for anogenital dysplasia is suggested. The American Academy of Pediatrics Committee on Child Abuse and Neglect considers condylomata acuminata in infants (if not perinatally acquired) and prepubertal children "suspicious" for sexual abuse and recommends reporting to the appropriate child protective agency.

The lesions of *molluscum contagiosum,* a common skin infection caused by a poxvirus, are most common in children, although they may also occur in adults as a sexually transmitted disease or in association with immunosuppressive processes such as HIV. They are transmitted via skin-to-skin contact or autoinoculation and occasionally by fomites. Molluscum may occur at any site but are most often seen on the inner thighs, popliteal or antecubital fossae, axillae, or abdomen. Individual lesions are flesh-colored, pearly, dome-shaped papules that may reveal a central umbilication and usually range in size between 1 and 5 mm (Fig. 14-28). They may occasionally be associated with surrounding inflammation and scaling, so-called *molluscum dermatitis,* which at times is severely pruritic and improves with topical corticosteroids. The natural course of molluscum contagiosum is one of spontaneous involution, although the timing is unpredictable, and lesions may become numerous or symptomatic, necessitating therapy.

Infections with *herpes simplex virus* (HSV), a member of the Herpesviridae family, range from a mild illness (common cold sores

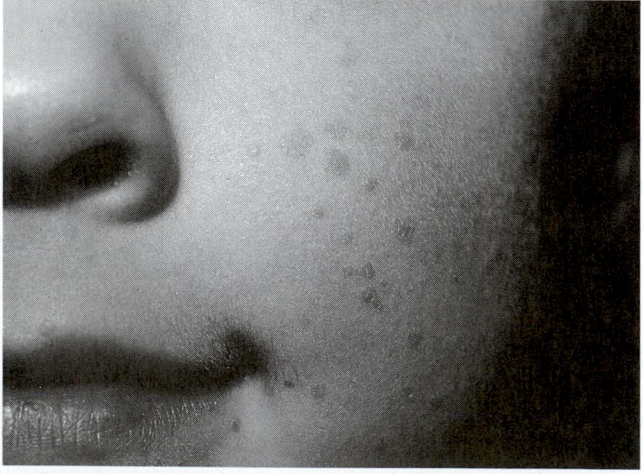

FIGURE 14-27 Flat warts (verruca plana). Numerous pink, flat-topped papules on the cheek of a four-year-old female. (*Courtesy of Anthony Mancini, M.D.*)

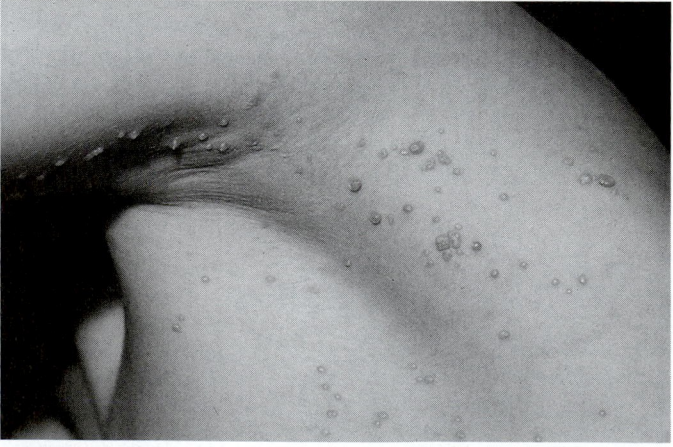

FIGURE 14-28 Molluscum contagiosum. Pearly, translucent, pink to flesh-colored papules on the inner arm, axilla, and trunk of a six-year-old male. (*Courtesy of Anthony Mancini, M.D.*)

or gingivostomatitis) to severe or life-threatening involvement (encephalitis). There are two serologic subtypes of HSV, type 1 (HSV-1) and type 2 (HSV-2). Infections of the oral cavity are most commonly ascribable to HSV-1 and may be spread to the face, conjunctivae, or cornea. Beyond the neonatal period, encephalitis is virtually always caused by HSV-1. Infection with HSV-2 in childhood may be indicative of, but is not pathogonomic for, child sexual abuse. HSV infections in the neonate are usually acquired via passage through an infected birth canal and may be limited to skin, eyes, and mucosa (SEM disease) or may be more severe and involve the central nervous system or multiple organ dissemination. HSV-2 causes approximately 75% of these illnesses. Neonatal HSV is discussed in Sec. 13.3.8.

The treatment of choice for HSV infection is acyclovir, which is available in a suspension containing 200 mg per teaspoon (5 ml). Although information regarding pediatric dosing is limited, 200 mg five times a day seems effective for children over two years of age. The decision regarding therapy of HSV is based on several factors, including severity, symptomatology, frequency of recurrences, and the immune status of the patient.

Gingivostomatitis is the most common clinical manifestation of primary HSV infection in young children. It is most commonly seen between the ages of nine months and three years, and, although self-limited over 10 to 14 days, may be associated with extreme discomfort, fever, refusal to drink, and dehydration. Patients typically present with small vesicles or erosions with erythema, which are most prominent over the gingiva, palate, lips, and tongue. Grouped vesicles or erosions on an erythematous base may be present in the perioral area. Malaise, irritability, and lymphadenopathy may also be present. Treatment is primarily symptomatic, with analgesics, antipyretics, and fluids. Some investigators advocate treatment of primary gingivostomatitis with oral acyclovir, if initiated within the first three days of illness.

Orolabial herpes or *herpes labialis,* also known as *fever blisters* or *cold sores,* most often involves the lips or perioral areas, sometimes in association with gingival lesions. These outbreaks usually represent reactivation of latent HSV and are often precipitated by sunlight or fever. Grouped vesicles or crusted erosions on an erythematous base are typical, and patients may experience a tingling or burning sensation, or "aura," one to two days prior to the onset of actual lesions.

Herpetic whitlow occurs after inoculation of HSV into the skin of the fingers and presents with erythema, pain, and, often, vesicles, pustules, or bullae. Whitlow can occur as a primary infection related to autoinoculation from another site or heteroinoculation or as reactivation of a latent infection. Acyclovir is often indicated because of extreme pain, to accelerate healing.

Eczema herpeticum, also known as *Kaposi's varicelliform eruption,* refers to HSV infection occurring in areas of skin with preexisting damage to the epidermal barrier. The most common association is in patients with atopic dermatitis. Vesicles and erosions occur in a widespread fashion over areas involved with the dermatitis (Fig. 14-7), and may be associated with fever and malaise. Secondary bacterial impetiginization may be the initial clinical impression, although grouping of the blisters or erosions may offer a subtle clue to the correct diagnosis. Mild to moderate cases can usually be adequately managed with cool compresses and oral acyclovir; toxic or immunosuppressed patients with severe involvement require hospitalization and intravenous acyclovir. Concomitant bacterial infection needs to be considered and the appropriate skin cultures and sensitivity testing performed.

References

American Academy of Pediatrics, Committee on Child Abuse and Neglect: Guidelines for the evaluation of sexual abuse of children: subject review. Pediatrics 103:186–191, 1999

American Academy of Pediatrics: Herpes simplex. In: Peter G, ed: 1997 Red Book: Report of the Committee on Infectious Diseases, 24th ed. Elk Grove Village, IL, American Academy of Pediatrics, 1997:266–276

Amir J, Harel L, Smetana Z, Varsano I: Treatment of herpes simplex gingivostomatitis with acyclovir in children: a randomized double-blind placebo-controlled study. Br Med J 314:1800–1803, 1997

Beutner KR, Tyring S: Human papillomavirus and human disease. Am J Med 102:9–15, 1997

Cohen BA, Honig P, Androphy E: Anogenital warts in children. Clinical and virologic evaluation for sexual abuse. Arch Dermatol 126:1575–1580, 1990

Obalek S, Jablonska S, Favre M, et al: Condylomata acuminata in children: frequent association with human papillomaviruses responsible for cutaneous warts. J Am Acad Dermatol 23:205–213, 1990

Orlow SJ, Paller A: Cimetidine therapy for multiple viral warts in children. J Am Acad Dermatol 28(5 Pt 1):794–796, 1993

EXANTHEMS

A summary of selected exanthems is outlined in Table 14-9.

Nonspecific Viral Exanthems

Exanthems are defined as skin eruptions occurring as a symptom of a general disease, usually infectious in origin. They are very common in children and range from nonspecific rashes to eruptions with distinct distribution or lesional morphology. A variety of infectious agents can be associated with exanthems, although viruses are by far the most common cause. Although most viral exanthematous illnesses are self-limited, the ability to differentiate them from other treatable or potentially serious disorders, such as bacterial or rickettsial infection or Kawasaki disease, is critical. The epidemiologic significance of some exanthematous illnesses, such as the risk of parvovirus B19 to developing fetuses, further highlights the importance of familiarity with these diseases.

Nonspecific cutaneous reactions to systemic viral infections are those which do not possess unique defining characteristics, such as a classic distribution, distinct lesional morphology, or associated enanthema or symptom complex. In contrast to the known causes of such classic exanthems as measles, rubella, or erythema infectiosum, the etiologic agent for these nonspecific exanthems often remains undetermined. Patients may have associated constitutional symptoms such as fever, headache, or malaise as well as respiratory or gastrointestinal complaints. Differentiation from cutaneous drug reactions may be extremely difficult and is compounded by indiscriminate prescribing of antimicrobials for patients with viral conditions. Associated symptoms, timing of the eruption, and a thorough drug intake history may be helpful in making a distinction.

Cutaneous findings in patients with nonspecific viral exanthems usually consist of blanchable erythematous macules or papules, diffusely distributed over the trunk and extremities. Less common presentations include vesicular, pustular, urticarial, or scarlatiniform lesions. Purpura is unusual, although a petechial component may be appreciated, especially when the cause is an enterovirus (see below). Common causes of nonspecific exanthems include nonpolio enteroviruses such as coxsackievirus, echovirus, and enterovirus and respiratory viruses including adenovirus, rhinovirus, parainfluenza

TABLE 14-9
SUMMARY OF SELECTED EXANTHEMS

DISEASE (CAUSE)	EXANTHEM (ENANTHEM)	ASSOCIATED FINDINGS	DIAGNOSIS	MANAGEMENT (COMMENT)
Viral				
Enteroviral exanthem (coxsackievirus, echovirus, other enteroviruses)	Red macules, papules diffusely on trunk and extremities May be petechial (Occasional oral erosions)	Low-grade fever, malaise Aseptic meningitis (with echovirus) Rarely myocarditis	Clinical, viral—esp. culture (throat, nasopharynx, rectum)	Symptomatic (If petechial, must consider meningococcemia)
Erythema infectiosum (parvovirus B19)	Bright red macular rash on cheeks, followed by reticulate lacy rash on extremities; exacerbated with sunlight or overheating	Low-grade fever, headache, coryza Arthritis (10% of children) Aplastic crises in predisposed children	Clinical, serologies	Symptomatic (Risk of fetal hydrops in exposed, susceptible pregnant women)
Measles (rubeola virus)	Erythematous macules, patches with cephalocaudad spread; heal with desquamation (Koplik spots on buccal mucosa)	Prodrome—cough, coryza, conjunctivitis, fever Toxic appearance, photophobia	Clinical, acute and convalescent serologies, virus isolation	Respiratory isolation, supportive care (Rare in United States with effective vaccination; reportable)
Mononucleosis (EBV)	Red macules, patches and papules, occasional petechiae, diffuse; rash may flare after ampicillin	Fever, respiratory symptoms, lymphadenopathy, hepatosplenomegaly, exudative pharyngitis	Heterophile antibodies, serologies Lymphocytosis in 70%	Symptomatic, activity restriction if splenomegaly
Roseola infantum (HHV-6, -7)	Pink, blanchable macules and papules, may have halo of pallor, diffuse	Prodrome—high fever precedes rash, respiratory symptoms Rarely seizures, encephalitis	Clinical	Symptomatic
Rubella (rubella virus)	Rose-pink macules, spread from face downward, fade with desquamation (Forchheimer's sign-palatal petechiae)	Prodrome—fever, malaise Lymphadenopathy (esp. postauricular, suboccipital) Arthritis	Virus isolation serologies	Respiratory isolation, supportive care (Rare in United States; reportable)
Varicella (varicella-zoster virus)	Generalized red macules with clear vesicle → crusting ("dew drop on a rose petal") (Occasional oral lesions)	Low-grade fever, malaise	Clinical, Tzanck preparation, direct fluorescence examination	Symptomatic, antihistamines, topical analgesics (Aspirin contraindicated 2° Reyes syndrome; bullae, prolonged fever with bacterial coinfection)
Bacterial				
Meningococcemia	Papules, petechiae, purpura on trunk, palms, soles	Fever, meningismus, circulatory collapse	Clinical; blood and CSF cultures	IV penicillin in ER; treatment for shock if present; contact prophylaxis
Scarlet fever (GABHS)	Red papules superimposed on diffuse erythema ("sunburn with goose pimples") (Palatal petechiae, strawberry tongue, exudative pharyngitis)	Fever, sore throat, abdominal pain, headache Pastia's lines—linear red streaks in folds Circumoral pallor	Throat culture	Penicillin
SSSS (*S. aureus*, toxin producing)	Tender erythema, blisters, peeling in sheets Early on, mostly in flexures and around nose and mouth	Fever, irritability, rhinitis	Skin biopsy, snip excision with frozen section, culture of *S. aureus*	Antistaphylococcal antibiotics, fluid & electrolyte management in severe cases
Toxic shock syndrome (*S. aureus* or GABHS)	Diffuse erythema/erythroderma Desquamation later	Fever, hypotension, shock Abnormalities in ≥3 other organ systems (see text)	Clinical, diagnostic criteria, isolation of *S. aureus* or GABHS	Fluid management, pressor support, parenteral antibiotics
Uncertain etiology				
Gianotti-Crosti syndrome (hepatitis B, EBV, enteroviruses, others)	Edematous, erythematous papules over extensor extremities, cheeks, buttocks	Occasional lymphadenopathy, hepatomegaly, splenomegaly (if hepatitis-associated)	Clinical, serologies if indicated	Symptomatic (Hepatitis association very rare in United States; exanthem may last up to 3 mo)

(continued)

TABLE 14-9   Continued

DISEASE (CAUSE)	EXANTHEM (ENANTHEM)	ASSOCIATED FINDINGS	DIAGNOSIS	MANAGEMENT (COMMENT)
Kawasaki syndrome	Polymorphous; papular, morbilliform, erythema with desquamation	Conjunctivitis, cheilitis, fever, glossitis, lymphadenopathy, peripheral edema, hydrops of gallbladder	Clinical	IVIG and aspirin
Unilateral laterothoracic exanthem (probably viral, no one agent)	Red macules, papules begin on unilateral thorax, axilla, arm and then disseminate Occasionally scarlatiniform, morbilliform, vesicular lesions	Occasional fever, conjunctivitis, pharyngitis, diarrhea	Clinical	Symptomatic (Exanthem may last up to 8 wk)

GABHS = group A beta-hemolytic streptococci; HHV-6 = human herpesvirus-6; HHV-7 = human herpesvirus-7; EBV = Epstein-Barr virus; SSSS = staphylococcal scalded skin syndrome; *S. aureus = Staphylococcus aureus.*

virus, respiratory syncytial virus, and influenza virus. In general, most summer exanthems are caused by enteroviruses and most winter exanthems by one of the respiratory viruses.

Exanthems Caused by Enteroviruses

The *nonpolio enteroviruses* include coxsackievirus group A1–A24, coxsackievirus group B1–B6, echoviruses 1–34, and enteroviruses 68–72. This group of viruses is the leading cause of exanthematous illnesses in children, especially during the summer and early fall. It is important to consider the possible association of aseptic meningitis with enteroviral infections, most notably the echoviruses. Petechiae may accompany enteroviral exanthems, especially those resulting from echovirus type 9. The presence of meningitis in a patient with a petechial enteroviral exanthem may require differentiation from other, potentially more serious infections such as meningococcemia.

Hand, foot, and mouth disease is a well-described exanthem of acral vesicular lesions combined with a vesicular and erosive enanthem. The disease is highly contagious and may occur in epidemics, especially in the summer or fall. The etiologic agent is usually a coxsackievirus, most commonly types A16, A5, or A10, although other group A as well as group B coxsackieviruses and enteroviruses have been implicated. Hand, foot, and mouth disease is most common in young children, who present with irritability and occasionally fever. Examination reveals gray-white vesicles with erythema on the palms and soles and sometimes on the buttocks. Shallow oral mucosal ulcerations also occur on the buccal surfaces, tongue, palate, uvula, gingiva, and tonsillar pillars. Therapy is supportive, and the process is generally self-limited over one week.

Herpangina is a classic enanthem caused by a variety of enteroviruses, most commonly group A coxsackieviruses. It presents clinically as tiny vesicles or erosions on the anterior tonsillar pillars, tonsils, uvula, pharynx, and soft palate, thereby resembling the enanthem of hand, foot, and mouth disease. Erosions are typically yellow-gray in color and have a surrounding rim of erythema. Patients usually have high fever and may have vomiting, dysphagia, and loss of appetite. Therapy is again supportive with bed rest, antipyretics, analgesics, and fluids.

Other Viral Exanthems

Erythema infectiosum (EI), or fifth disease, is the most common condition caused by parvovirus B19 (B19), the only member of the Parvoviridae family known to cause disease in humans. B19 may be responsible for a variety of exanthems, and recent data suggest that up to 20% of measles- and rubella-like illnesses in children may be caused by this agent. EI usually affects children between 4 and 10 years of age and is most common in late winter and spring. Transmission occurs via respiratory droplets, and patients are contagious before the rash develops. Children present initially with headache, coryza, and low-grade fever. Approximately one week after the prodrome a bright red macular rash develops on the cheeks, giving the characteristic "slapped cheek" appearance. Progression to a reticulate, lacy erythema (Color Plate 19) or an erythematous maculopapular eruption distributed primarily over the extremities and buttocks occurs within a few days. Pruritus may be present in up to 15% of patients. As the exanthem fades, temporary exacerbations may be noted with environmental triggers, including sunlight, hot baths, or physical activity. Additional manifestations of B19 infection are discussed in Sec. 13.3.16.

Infectious mononucleosis is caused by the Epstein-Barr virus (EBV). EBV is a ubiquitous virus, with up to 50% of children seroconverting by school age. The acute illness is characterized by fever, upper respiratory symptoms, and adenopathy. In addition, exudative pharyngitis and hepatosplenomegaly may also be present. The rash is fairly nonspecific, most often consisting of a diffusely distributed macular and papular eruption, occasionally associated with petechiae. The rash may acutely flare after treatment with ampicillin or other antibiotics. Serologic testing is helpful in diagnosing infectious mononucleosis. Therapy is generally supportive, although contact sports or other vigorous activities should be avoided if splenomegaly is present. Other manifestations of EBV disease are discussed in Sec. 13.3.4.

Measles, or rubeola, classically begins with a prodrome of fever, rhinitis, cough, and conjunctivitis. The characteristic enanthem, Koplik's spots, is seen during this phase and consists of punctate white-gray papules with an erythematous rim, distributed on the buccal mucosa. The exanthem appears over two to four days, begins on the head and neck, and spreads in a cephalocaudad fashion to involve the trunk and extremities. Nonpruritic, erythematous macules and papules that tend to become confluent are typical and resolve in a similar progression from head to toe over several days, leaving behind coppery-brown macules that eventually fade with desquamation. Atypical skin lesions include those with petechiae, vesicles, or palpable purpura. Measles is generally self-limited, although a number of complications can occur, including pneumonia, bronchitis, otitis, encephalitis, and myocarditis. Subacute sclerosing panencephalitis, a delayed neurodegenerative disorder, occurs in 1 in 100,000 cases. Management is primarily supportive. Measles is discussed in Sec. 13.3.13.

Papular acrodermatitis of childhood (Gianotti-Crosti syndrome) is an exanthem characterized by papules distributed symmetrically over the face, extremities, and buttocks. Described initially in 1955, an association with hepatitis B (HB) infection was noted in patients who presented with the typical skin lesions in conjunction with anicteric hepatitis and positive testing for HB surface antigen, subtype *ayw*. This association is extremely rare in the United States, where a host of viral agents have been implicated, including Epstein-Barr virus, coxsackievirus A16, parainfluenza virus, cytomegalovirus, and human herpesvirus-6. In most patients with Gianotti-Crosti syndrome, no etiologic agent is identified. The exanthem is best viewed as a distinctive cutaneous reaction to a variety of infectious agents.

Patients present with multiple erythematous, edematous papules symmetrically distributed over the extensor surfaces of the extremities (Color Plate 20), the cheeks, and the buttocks. The trunk is usually spared, and lesions are usually asymptomatic. Individual papules may be very "juicy" or "pseudovesicular," and they may occasionally be mistaken for true blisters or molluscum contagiosum. Therapy is supportive, and the process is self-limited, with spontaneous resolution over several weeks. Occasionally, the course may be delayed, with complete clearance requiring up to 3 months. Routine serologic testing for hepatitis is not indicated, but any patient presenting within the clinical spectrum of Gianotti-Crosti syndrome should have a thorough physical examination for hepatosplenomegaly and lymphadenopathy, with the appropriate evaluation if indicated.

Roseola infantum, or exanthem subitum, is a common childhood exanthem caused by human herpesvirus-6 (HHV-6) and, as more recently identified, sometimes human herpesvirus-7 (HHV-7). HHV-6 and HHV-7 are ubiquitous organisms, with seropositivity rates greater than 85 to 90% after early childhood (see Sec. 13.3.9–10). The peak age of roseola infantum is six to seven months. Patients present with a febrile illness consisting of fevers as high as 40.5°C and mild prodromal respiratory symptoms. After two to five days of fever, the patient abruptly defervesces with appearance of an exanthem consisting of pink, blanchable, discrete macules and papules distributed primarily on the trunk. The rash then fades over several days without sequelae.

Although transplacental fetal infection with *rubella* can have devastating consequences including congenital malformations, deafness, and impaired psychomotor development (Sec. 13.3.20), patients acquiring the illness postnatally commonly have a prodrome of malaise, followed by the development of fever, lymphadenopathy, and an exanthem consisting of discrete rose-pink macules that begin on the face and progress downward over one to three days. Fading followed by desquamation occurs in a rapid fashion over days. Tender postauricular and suboccipital lymphadenopathy or arthritis most commonly involving the fingers and wrists may also be present. The associated enanthem, Forchheimer's sign, occurs in one-quarter of patients and consists of petechial spots over the hard or soft palate. Rare complications of rubella include encephalitis and thrombocytopenic purpura. Therapy is supportive.

Unilateral laterothoracic exanthem is a distinct childhood exanthem that has its onset in a unilateral distribution, often over the upper thorax, axilla, or arm. Unilateral laterothoracic exanthem (ULE) occurs most often in toddlers and preschool-age children and appears to be viral in origin, although the exact etiology re-

mains unproven. The rash begins usually over the unilateral trunk or upper extremity, with progression on the ipsilateral side before eventual dissemination to a bilateral distribution. Morphologically, the lesions are usually erythematous macules or papules with a pale halo, although vesicular, morbilliform, scarlatiniform, and eczematous patterns have been reported. Even after becoming diffuse, the exanthem maintains a unilateral predominance on the initial side of involvement. Pruritus is present in up to 50% of patients. Associated symptoms that may be present include fever, conjunctivitis, pharyngitis, and diarrhea. Spontaneous resolution occurs but may be prolonged over four to eight weeks. Therapy is supportive, with topical corticosteroids relatively ineffective.

Varicella, or chickenpox, is a highly contagious disease of childhood transmitted by respiratory droplets. Although most cases are mild, severe complications such as bacterial superinfection can ensue. The causative agent is the varicella-zoster virus (VZV), a member of the Herpesviridae family of viruses. The natural epidemiology of varicella is evolving as a result of the availability of a live attenuated vaccine licensed in the United States in 1995.

Patients with varicella develop a generalized rash, which initially appears on the trunk, face, and scalp and spreads in a centrifugal fashion. Associated symptoms include low-grade fever and malaise. The skin lesions appear in crops and consist initially of an erythematous macule that quickly develops a clear vesicle, giving the classic "dew drop on a rose petal" appearance. The lesions form crusts within a few days, and the presence of lesions in all stages of evolution is characteristic. Bullous lesions are occasionally present, usually in association with superinfection with a toxin-producing strain of *S. aureus*. GABHS superinfection is one of the most common, and potentially life-threatening, complications of acute varicella and should be suspected in any child with prolonged fever (beyond four or five days) or unusually aggressive skin lesions (including induration, ulceration, or necrosis). Patients with varicella are considered contagious until all skin lesions are in the crusted stage, and treatment is primarily supportive. Systemic antiviral therapy may be useful in shortening the time to healing and reducing symptoms and is indicated in all patients at high risk for associated complications. Secondary bacterial superinfection should be promptly treated with the appropriate antimicrobial therapy.

Infection with varicella during pregnancy may lead to congenital varicella, which includes the fetal varicella syndrome (when infection is acquired earlier in gestation) or neonatal varicella (with infection acquired later in gestation). Fetal varicella syndrome is characterized by a variety of anomalies, including scarring and hypoplasia of skin in a dermatomal distribution, low birth weight, mental retardation, seizures, and a range of ophthalmological, skeletal, gastrointestinal, and genitourinary defects. The risk appears greatest with exposure prior to 20 weeks of gestation, but even in pregnancies at risk, the incidence of the syndrome is low, around 1 to 2%. Neonatal varicella results from transmission of the virus to the fetus shortly before (or in some cases, shortly after) birth. Infants at highest risk for severe disease are those who acquire the infection from a mother who develops acute varicella during the last five days of pregnancy or within two days after delivery, since protection from maternally derived antibodies is lacking. These newborns may appear normal at birth but present within the first few days of life with vesicular lesions which erupt in crops and eventually crust over. In these patients, dissemination to multiple organs may occur, and prompt recognition, diagnosis, and initiation of antiviral therapy is essential.

Herpes zoster, or *shingles,* represents reactivation of VZV, which remains dormant in the sensory root ganglia following acute infection. The incidence is low in immunocompetent children, although the risk seems to be greater in those who had either intrauterine exposure to VZV or acute varicella early in life. Herpes zoster presents with grouped vesicles on an erythematous base which are distributed within one to three sensory dermatomes (Color Plate 21). The development of lesions may be preceded by pain or paresthesias in the affected areas. The most common dermatomes to be affected are the ophthalmic (V1) branch of the trigeminal nerve and the thoracic dermatomes. Opthalmologic examination should be performed in all patients with involvement of the V1 dermatome given the possibility of associated eye involvement. Lesions of herpes zoster may be more generalized in immunosuppressed patients, and visceral involvement may be present. *Postherpetic neuralgia*, a persistent pain syndrome involving the affected dermatomes and more common in the elderly, is very rare in children. Antiviral therapy of pediatric herpes zoster is indicated in immunosuppressed patients to lower the risk of dissemination and may be beneficial in immunosuppressed patients to lower the risk of dissemination and may be beneficial in immunocompetent patients to reduce symptoms, minimize complications, and accelerate healing. A detailed discussion of other manifestations of varicella/zoster can be found in Sec. 13.3.21.

Exanthems Accompanying Bacterial Illnesses

Lyme disease, the most common vector-borne disease in the United States, is a systemic illness caused by the spirochete *Borrelia burgdorferi*. It is transmitted by ticks of the *Ixodid* species, especially the deer tick. Lyme disease affects primarily the skin, heart, joints, and nervous system. The skin lesion, which occurs at the site of the tick bite, erythema migrans (EM), occurs in two-thirds of patients and represents *early localized disease*. It presents as an expanding red patch that often shows central clearing (Color Plate 22). Epidermal changes such as scaling are absent, and vesicular or necrotic areas in the center of the lesion are present only rarely. The lesion is usually nonpruritic and may be accompanied by systemic symptoms including fever, myalgias, or malaise. A final diameter of 10 to 30 cm may be reached before fading occurs, which may take up to several weeks. The treatment of choice for early localized disease is doxycycline, or amoxicillin for children under eight years of age.

As many as one-fourth of patients develop multiple EM lesions, which are generally smaller in size than the original lesion. These secondary lesions herald *early disseminated disease*, during which time dissemination to multiple organs, including the heart and central nervous system, may occur. *Late disease* is classically manifest by arthritis, primarily of the large joints. These patients often do not have a history of preceding EM lesions. Treatment of all stages of Lyme disease is discussed in Sec. 13.2.19.

Skin lesions may be the presenting sign in 70–90% of patients with *meningococcemia*, caused by the gram-negative diplococcus *Neisseria meningitidis*. Meningococcal disease occurs most often in patients between 3 and 12 months of age but has a secondary peak in late adolescence; the infection is spread from person to person via respiratory droplets. The abrupt onset is characterized by fever, chills, malaise, and a rash that appears either purpuric or petechial in approximately half of patients; other presentations include a nonspecific macular or papular eruption, and purpura fulminans, which has a poor prognosis. Less common morphologies include pustules or bullae.

The purpuric lesions of meningococcemia are discrete, small, gray-purple papules that may be tender. The trunk and lower extremities are most commonly affected, and, left untreated, the rash progresses rapidly to purpura fulminans. Skin biopsy of purpuric lesions reveals leukocytoclastic vasculitis, with emboli containing gram-negative diplococci. Associated findings in patients with meningococcemia may include hypotension, nuchal rigidity, altered levels of consciousness, seizures, disseminated intravascular coagulation, and multiorgan failure. The progression of clinical symptoms may be very rapid, and death can occur in several hours, even with appropriate therapy. If meningococcemia is suspected, parenteral penicillin should be administered immediately, and supportive care for septic shock instituted. *Neisseria meningitidis* is also discussed in Sec. 13.2.26.

Scarlet fever, also known as *scarlatina*, is caused by toxin-producing strains of group A β-hemolytic streptococci and occurs most often in children between the ages of 4 and 10 years. The site of primary infection is usually the tonsils and pharynx, with abrupt onset of pharyngitis, fever, headache, and vomiting. The characteristic rash appears initially as tiny punctate red papules, which become confluent and spread to involve the entire body (Color Plate 23). The rash has been likened to sandpaper or "sunburn with goose pimples." Helpful diagnostic features include a perioral rim of sparing (circumoral pallor) and linear streaks of more intense erythema or petechiae in folds (Pastia's lines), including the antecubital fossae and axillae. The enanthem includes an exudative pharyngitis, posterior soft palatal petechiae, and strawberry tongue. Resolution of the disease may be associated with desquamation, especially of distal extremities and digits. Complications include glomerulonephritis and rheumatic fever. The treatment of choice for scarlet fever is penicillin V. A scarlatiniform rash in association with pharyngitis and fever may also be caused by *Arcanobacterium* (formerly *Corynebacterium*) *hemolyticum*, usually in teenagers or young adults, and may respond best to erythromycin. Diseases caused by group A streptococci are extensively discussed in Sec. 13.2.36.

Staphylococcal scalded skin syndrome (SSSS) is caused by exfoliative toxin-producing strains of *S. aureus* and occurs mainly in children, especially infants. The increased susceptibility of infants may be related to immature mechanisms of renal clearance of the toxin. Predisposing factors in adults, in whom SSSS is rare, include renal failure, immunosuppression, and HIV-1 infection. Most *S. aureus* isolates causing SSSS belong to phage group II, types 71 and 55. Patients with SSSS usually have a primary infection at sites other than the skin, such as the nasopharynx, conjunctiva, throat, or middle ear, and the toxin is hematogenously disseminated. The clinical features are related to cleavage of the epidermis in a superficial location, beneath the stratum corneum or stratum granulosum.

Patients with SSSS usually present with fever, irritability, and tender erythema of the skin, most marked in flexural areas and around the mouth and nose. Within 12 to 24 hours, extensive blisters and erosions form and may be followed by widespread superficial peeling of the skin in sheets, especially in infants. Superficial separation of the skin after rubbing (Nikolsky sign) is present. Subsequent denudation of the skin with a moist, glistening, red surface at sites of prior blistering may lead to significant cutaneous fluid losses and secondary infection with resulting sepsis. Mucosal surfaces are spared. Older children may present with more mild forms of SSSS, with more localization of lesions and less toxicity.

The differential diagnosis of SSSS in various stages may include toxic epidermal necrolysis, GVHD, scarlet fever, toxic shock syndrome, and Kawasaki disease. In most cases the history, clinical presentation, and physical examination aid in the differentiation of SSSS from these entities. Toxic epidermal necrolysis (TEN), however, may be difficult to differentiate in some patients. TEN is a rare disorder resulting in full-thickness sloughing of the epidermis, usually in response to an overwhelming drug hypersensitivity or GVHD. Skin biopsy reveals a split in the superficial epidermis in SSSS, versus full-thickness epidermal necrosis and subepidermal blister formation in TEN. A more rapid diagnostic examination can be accomplished with Wright's or Giemsa staining of a "snip excision" of a blister roof or peeled epidermal fragment, which will demonstrate the superficial versus deep blister plane and enable a distinction between SSSS and TEN. Although cultures of skin and blister fluid are characteristically negative, recovery of *S. aureus* from the blood, nasopharynx, throat, or conjunctiva confirms the diagnosis of SSSS.

Although SSSS can be a severe disease, the majority of affected children do well and recover without sequelae, and the mortality rate in children is low, around 3%. Antistaphylococcal antibiotics are a mainstay of therapy for SSSS. Older children with localized involvement and no toxicity may be managed as outpatients with oral antibiotics, but affected newborns and any patient with severe disease require hospitalization with parenteral antibiotic therapy and aggressive supportive management. Supportive measures include intravenous fluids, electrolyte management, impeccable wound care with minimal handling, and pain control.

Toxic shock syndrome (TSS) is a toxin-mediated multisystem disease defined by the presence of fever, hypotension, and a diffuse rash with desquamation as well as clinical or laboratory abnormalities in three or more organ systems. The target organ systems in TSS include gastrointestinal (vomiting or diarrhea), muscular (myalgia, elevation of creatine phosphokinase), mucous membrane (vaginal, oropharyngeal, or conjunctival hyperemia), renal (elevated blood urea nitrogen or creatinine, sterile pyuria), hepatic (elevated bilirubin or transaminases), hematologic (thrombocytopenia), and central nervous system (altered mental status). Although originally described in association with tampon use, reports of nonmenstrual-associated TSS are increasing and include cases associated with infected surgical wounds, postpartum infection, burns, and nasal packing. The cause of TSS can be either toxin-producing strains of *S. aureus* or group A streptococci. An important feature of streptococcal toxic-shock-like syndrome is the frequent association with a preceding skin or soft-tissue infection as the portal of entry for the organism. Localized swelling and erythema, usually of an extremity, are the most common findings with this presentation.

Cutaneous involvement in toxic shock syndrome presents as diffuse blanchable erythema, which may have a flexural accentuation. A papular "scarlatiniform" eruption may also be seen. Palms and soles are frequently involved and are among the most common sites for desquamation to occur, usually 1 to 2 weeks into the course of the disease. Treatment includes supportive therapy, including hydration and vasopressor support, and the administration of the appropriate antimicrobials. Initial antibiotic coverage should cover both staphylococci and streptococci, with further modification based on culture results and sensitivity testing. Identification and appropriate management of sites that serve as portal of entry for the organism are also vital. Manifestations of staphylococcal disease are discussed in Sec. 13.2.35.

Exanthems of Uncertain Etiology—Kawasaki Disease

An infectious etiology for *Kawasaki disease* seems likely, yet the association remains speculative. However, any discussion of infectious exanthems must include the disorder, given its protean cutaneous manifestations and potential for serious morbidity and mortality. Kawasaki disease is a systemic vasculitis that affects mainly children under five years of age and that is the primary cause of acquired heart disease in the pediatric patient. Characteristics of Kawasaki disease include fever for more than five days, nonpurulent conjunctival injection, oropharyngeal changes, peripheral extremity changes, cervical lymphadenopathy, and a polymorphous rash. Five of the six criteria, with fever being an absolute, must be present for diagnosis. There are multiple associated manifestations, the most concerning of which are coronary arterial aneurysms, which occurred in 15 to 25% of patients prior to therapy.

The rash of Kawasaki disease usually consists of polymorphous erythematous macules, patches, and plaques with a diffuse distribution. Desquamation is usually a feature later in the course, and is most notable over the distal extremities, hands, and feet, as well as in periungual locations. Accentuation of the eruption may be noted in the perineum and is often accompanied or soon followed by desquamation as well. Other reported patterns of the rash include morbilliform or scarlatiniform lesions and, occasionally, pustules. Blisters, epidermal changes (such as erosions or crusting), petechiae, and purpura are not characteristic of the rash of Kawasaki disease. The hands and feet often reveal edema, erythema, and induration. Treatment is with intravenous immunoglobulin and aspirin.

References

American Academy of Pediatrics: Varicella-zoster infections. In: Peter G, ed: 2000 Red Book: Report of the Committee on Infectious Diseases, 25th ed. Elk Grove Village, IL, 2000:624–638

Asano Y, Yoshikawa T, Suga S, et al: Clinical features of infants with primary human herpesvirus 6 infection (exanthem subitum, roseola infantum). Pediatrics 93:104–108, 1994

Barron KS: Kawasaki disease in children. Curr Opin Rheumatol 10:29–37, 1998

Bialecki C, Feder HM, Grant-Kels JM: The six classic childhood exanthems: a review and update. J Am Acad Dermatol 21:891–903, 1989

Cherry JD: Contemporary infectious exanthems. Clin Infect Dis 16:199–207, 1993

Heegaard ED, Hornsleth A: Parvovirus: the expanding spectrum of disease. Acta Paediatr 84:109–117, 1995

Hogan PA: Viral exanthems in childhood. Australas J Dermatol 37:S14–S16, 1996

Kakourou T, Theodoridou M, Mostrou G, et al: Herpes zoster in children. J Am Acad Dermatol 39:207–210, 1998

Mancini AJ: Exanthems in childhood: an update. Pediatr Ann 27:163–170, 1998

Manders SM: Toxin-mediated streptococcal and staphylococcal disease. J Am Acad Dermatol 39:383–398, 1998

McCuaig CC, Russo P, Powell J, et al: Unilateral laterothoracic exanthem. A clinicopathologic study of forty-eight patients. J Am Acad Dermatol 34:979–984, 1996

Resnick SD: New aspects of exanthematous diseases of childhood. Dermatol Clin 15:257–266, 1997

Shapiro ED: Lyme disease. Pediatr Rev 19:147–154, 1998

Young NS: Parvovirus infection and its treatment. Clin Exp Immunol 104(S1):26–30, 1996

FUNGAL INFECTIONS

Candida species may cause infections of mucosal epithelia, skin, and nail plates, and, although not a component of normal skin flora, they favor warm, moist regions such as the diaper region, intertriginous zones, web spaces between fingers and toes, and the corners of the mouth. The most common pathogen among *Candida* species is *C. albicans,* which is part of normal oral and intestinal flora.

Most candidal infections are noninvasive and limited, although invasive candidal infections are seen with increasing frequency in the settings of immunosuppression, HIV infection, diabetes, and prematurity. Diagnosis of cutaneous candidal infections is made on clinical grounds in conjunction with fungal culture and potassium hydroxide (KOH) examination, which reveals budding yeasts and pseudohyphae.

Diaper candidiasis may occur as a primary process or, more commonly, as a secondary infection in the setting of a primary irritant contact dermatitis. Predisposing factors may include oropharyngeal candidiasis, diarrhea, and antibiotic therapy. The earliest manifestation is an intense erythema, sometimes with maceration, distributed most commonly in the perianal region and within deep flexures. Superficial pustules develop, and spread is accomplished via "satellite lesions" of erythematous papules and papulopustules situated at the periphery of the erythema. The genitalia, inferior abdomen, inner thighs, perineum, and buttocks may all eventually be involved. In male infants, involvement of the glans penis (*candidal balanitis*) (Fig. 14-29) is common, as is involvement of the scrotum, which differentiates candidiasis from tinea cruris. Involvement of the inguinal creases helps distinguish candidiasis from irritant contact dermatitis, in which the fold regions are often spared.

Management of diaper candidiasis includes frequent diaper changes, diaper-free periods where feasible, protective barrier pastes or ointments, and topical antifungal agents, including nystatin or imidazole antifungals (miconazole, clotrimazole, ketoconazole, econazole). Low-potency topical corticosteroids, such as hydrocortisone, may be a useful adjunct to help decrease associated inflammation, but combination steroid-antifungal preparations should be avoided in the diaper area. Secondary bacterial infection may need to be considered, especially in recalcitrant cases or those with a vesiculobullous or erosive component. Although sometimes advocated because *Candida* spp. are known to colonize the intestine, the effectiveness of concomitant oral antifungal therapy, based on the hypothesis of a gastrointestinal source of acquisition of diaper candidiasis, remains unproven.

Oropharyngeal candidiasis, or *thrush,* is infection of the oral cavity with *C. albicans.* It is most commonly acquired during passage through an infected birth canal or during nursing from the skin of an infected breast. Left untreated, most cases of oropharyngeal candidiasis will resolve spontaneously, although this may require from four to eight weeks. Although frequently asymptomatic in immunocompetent children, occasionally infants with thrush may experience pain and impairment of sucking and swallowing, which may ultimately progress to candidal esophagitis and nutritional compromise.

Oropharyngeal candidiasis presents as white to gray patches, which may form "pseudomembranes" composed of epithelial cells, white blood cells, food debris, and yeast forms that cover the buccal mucosae, tongue, and gingivae. Less common sites of involvement include the soft palate, uvula, and tonsils. Removal of the patches by scraping with a tongue depressor reveals an erythematous, eroded base; a KOH examination of scrapings reveals ovoid yeast forms and pseudohyphae. Treatment consists of topical nonabsorbable antifungal agents such as nystatin, miconazole, or clotrimazole applied four times daily. Oral fluconazole has been found effective in the treatment of oropharyngeal candidiasis in immunocompromised children.

Congenital candidiasis, a rare entity, is a benign infection in the full-term infant but life-threatening systemic in the premature newborn. Organisms gain entry to the amniotic fluid from a colonized vagina; the disease presents during the first week, and usually the first few days, of life. The placenta of infected infants may reveal yellow plaques and abscesses. Invasive candidiasis, including sepsis, pneumonitis, and renal and central nervous system infection, is more likely in premature neonates and is associated with a poor prognosis.

Cutaneous lesions of congenital candidiasis, which are present in up to one-half of patients, may be diffuse, intensely erythematous macules and papules involving the trunk and extremities, sometimes with sparing of the diaper area. Erosive patches resembling a first-degree burn injury have been reported. Pustules and tiny vesicles may be present, especially over palms and soles, and the eruption resolves with significant desquamation. Bullae are rarely present. Oral thrush and nail dystrophy may also be present, and nail changes as the sole cutaneous manifestation have occasionally been reported. Topical antifungal therapy is usually sufficient for skin-limited disease, but intravenous amphotericin B is indicated in the premature infant with evidence of respiratory compromise or other signs of disseminated infection.

Chronic paronychia is a long-standing infection of the skin folds surrounding the nails that is usually caused by *C. albicans,* although a mixed infection with *Candida* spp. and bacteria may often be present. It presents with periungual erythema, cuticle loss, and transverse ridging of the nail plate. Other nail changes may include yellow discoloration and thickening. Pain, purulence, and discharge are usually absent. The diagnosis is established by the finding of budding yeasts and pseudohyphae on KOH examination or via culture. Avoidance of moisture, which favors growth of yeast cells, and application of topical antifungal creams are the mainstays of therapy. A combination steroid-antifungal cream such as triamcinolone-nystatin (Mycolog II) is also effective.

Angular cheilitis (perleche) is characterized by erythema, fissuring, and crusting at the mouth angles. Predisposing conditions include any situation that results in excessive moisture collecting in these areas, such as frequent drooling, lip licking, and use of orthodontic appliances. Entities which need to be considered in the differential diagnosis include contact dermatitis and nutritional deficiency, including deficiencies of riboflavin, zinc, or biotin. *C. albicans* is usually present, and concomitant bacterial infection may also occur. Therapy is aimed at correcting any predisposing condition as feasible, treating infection with topical antifungal (and

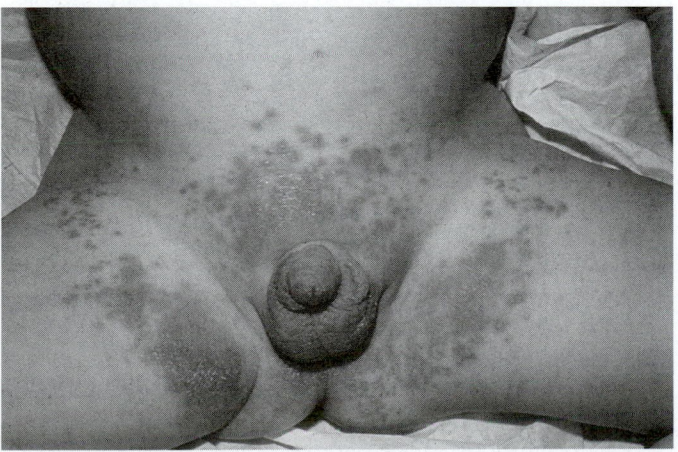

FIGURE 14-29   Diaper candidiasis with candidal balanitis. Beefy red erythematous papules and plaques with peripheral satellite papulopustules. Involvement of the glans penis (balanitis) and scrotum differentiates *Candida* from dermatophyte infection. (*Courtesy of Anthony Mancini, M.D.*)

antibacterial, if necessary) agents and applying thick barrier ointments to decrease exposure to moisture and subsequent maceration. Low-strength topical corticosteroid creams may be helpful in patients with significant inflammation.

Tinea versicolor is a superficial skin infection caused by the dimorphic lipophilic fungus *Malassezia furfur,* also known as *Pityrosporum ovale* and *P. orbiculare,* depending on the form of the yeast phase. This organism is a lipid-dependent yeast that is part of the normal human skin flora in 90 to 100% of individuals. Although most cases occur during the pubertal period, the prevalence in prepubertal children seems higher than was once believed. Infection usually localizes to areas of skin that are rich in the lipid-producing sebaceous glands, including the chest, back, and face.

Tinea versicolor occurs when the yeast form of the organism converts to the mycelial form, a transition that may be prompted by various predisposing factors, including heat, humidity, sweating, and skin occlusion. Individual host susceptibility and immunosuppression may also play a role. The most common clinical findings are sharply demarcated, hypopigmented macules and patches that may have associated fine scaling (Color Plate 24). Pruritus is occasionally present. The hypopigmented areas become more noticeable after unprotected sun exposure, caused by uneven tanning of the surrounding uninvolved skin. Other presentations include hyperpigmented or erythematous patches. The hypopigmentation seen in tinea versicolor is attributed to a product of the fungus, azalaic acid, which inhibits dopa-tyrosinase, an enzyme involved in the melanin synthetic pathway.

Differential diagnosis of tinea versicolor includes most notably pityriasis alba and vitiligo. Pityriasis alba is most common on the face, and patients often have an associated atopic diathesis. Vitiligo results in complete *de*pigmentation and is most common in periorificial regions (around the eyes, mouth, and genitalia) and over bony prominences. Scaling is usually minimal to absent in these two disorders. Other differential diagnoses include psoriasis, seborrheic dermatitis, dermatophyte infection, and confluent and reticulate papillomatosis of Gougerot and Carteaud. In darkly pigmented patients, hypopigmented lesions of cutaneous T-cell lymphoma must be considered, especially in cases with an unusual distribution or a history of recalcitrance to therapy. KOH examination of scrapings from lesions of tinea versicolor reveals numerous clusters of spores and short, stubby hyphae, the so-called pattern of spaghetti and meatballs. Culture is unhelpful since *M. furfur* is a normal skin inhabitant.

There are several treatment options, both topical and oral. Selenium sulfide 2.5% shampoo is applied to the affected areas and left on for 5 to 10 minutes prior to rinsing, for one to two weeks. Ketoconazole 2% shampoo was found effective when left on for 5 minutes prior to rinsing and used for one to three days. Topical antifungal agents may be effective but are often limited by the widespread involvement and hence required amounts of the medication. The allylamine antifungal terbinafine in a 1% spray has been approved for treatment of tinea versicolor in patients 12 years of age and older. Oral antifungal agents are quite effective and may be helpful in severe or recurrent cases of tinea versicolor. One such oral regimen is ketoconazole, which has been demonstrated effective in an adult dose of 200 mg per day for 3 to 10 days or a single, one-time dose of 400 mg, which may increase compliance and decrease the risk of associated drug toxicities, a concern in the use of oral antifungal agents. Drug delivery to the skin may be accentuated by exercise following the oral administration of ketoconazole, and showering should be avoided for 12 hours to maximize the effect.

DERMATOPHYTE INFECTIONS The treatment of dermatophyte infections is outlined in Table 14-10. *Tinea capitis* is the most common of the cutaneous mycoses in children. It occurs worldwide and in all age groups, although the most common population affected is prepubertal children over six months of age. The incidence is higher in African-Americans and Hispanics.

Tinea capitis is caused by dermatophytes in the genera *Microsporum* and *Trichophyton*. In the United States, the most common etiologic agent is the anthropophilic (human-to-human) organism *Trichophyton tonsurans,* although occasional infections are caused by the zoophilic (animal-to-human) organism *Microsporum canis,* acquired usually from infected puppies or kittens. *M. audounii,* another anthropophilic organism that was once one of the main causes of tinea capitis in this country, is now rarely implicated. The disease is spread easily from child to child as well as via infected fomites, including hair brushes, combs, furniture, and clothing. The asymptomatic carrier state is a significant problem, especially among family members of infected children, and is an important consideration in terms of reinfection of the patient and spread to other individuals.

The clinical presentation of tinea capitis is variable. Subtle scaling of the scalp without inflammation or alopecia may be confused with seborrheic dermatitis, resulting in a delay in diagnosis. Erythematous papules, plaques, and patches are common, and pustules and crusting may also be present. Some patients may have a significant pustular eruption which mimics acute bacterial pyoderma. Alopecia is frequently present; one distinct form, so-called black dot tinea, is marked by multiple tiny black dots at the skin surface, representing broken hair shafts (Color Plate 25). A marked host inflammatory reaction to the infectious agent, which is often one of the zoophilic organisms, is called a *kerion,* which presents as a boggy, tender, edematous plaque with crusting and alopecia. Secondary bacterial infection may complicate healing. Cervical or suboccipital lymphadenopathy may be present in any of the forms of tinea capitis.

Fungal culture and direct microscopic examination are most useful in diagnosing tinea capitis. Since the majority of cases are caused by the nonfluorescing endothrix (arthroconidia inside the hair shaft only) organism *T. tonsurans,* Wood's lamp examination is rarely helpful. In the occasional case caused by an ectothrix (arthroconidia inside and outside the hair shaft) organism, Wood's lamp examination reveals bright green fluorescence of the hair. Direct microscopy of removed scale or broken hairs, after addition of KOH, reveals characteristic branching, septated hyphae, and the presence of arthroconidia within or on the outside of infected hairs. Specimens for KOH examination may be obtained by gentle scraping with a no. 15 scalpel blade, gentle hair removal (preferably from an area of broken hairs) with a forceps, or the use of a moistened gauze pad to rub the scalp, with the ultimate transfer of broken hairs and scale from the gauze to the culture media with a forceps. The KOH examination may be difficult (with a fairly high percentage of false negatives) in tinea capitis and is often negative in extremely inflammatory presentations, such as kerions.

Fungal culture is the gold standard for diagnosis of tinea capitis, and specimens may be obtained by a variety of nonthreatening methods. A sterile disposable toothbrush or cytobrush (as used in cervical examinations) can be vigorously rubbed over both affected and apparently unaffected areas and plated on media. Alternatively, a standard cotton-tipped culture swab (Culturette II), as used for obtaining throat cultures, can be utilized. The material should be plated onto a commercially available fungal culture media, such as Dermatophyte Test Medium (DTM), which has a color indicator with positive cultures, or Mycosel agar. The caps are placed onto the agar bottles loosely to allow gas exchange and should be incubated for three to four weeks before deemed negative for growth.

The specifics of therapy for tinea capitis are outlined in Table 14-10. In general, topical therapy is ineffective because of involvement of hair follicles, and systemic therapy is the treatment of choice. It should be kept in mind that patients may have a clinical cure without a true mycologic cure, and therefore treatment should be continued until a repeat fungal culture is negative. Premature discontinuation of therapy is likely to lead to a relapse of infection. Because of the high contagiousness of tinea capitis, therapy should be instituted in a timely fashion and, in some cases, empirically if the clinical presentation is highly suggestive and other diagnoses seem unlikely. Lastly, as with any form of tinea, significantly inflammatory infections, or their treatment, may be associated with a diffuse, pruritic, papular eruption referred to as a *dermatophytid* (or *id*) reaction. These reactions represent immune hyperreactivity to fungal antigen and may show widespread skin involvement concomitant with the beginning of therapy. They usually respond to topical corticosteroids and oral antihistamines, and only rarely are systemic corticosteroids necessary.

Tinea corporis, or "ringworm," is a common pediatric infection which can occur on any part of the body. A variety of organisms may cause tinea corporis, including *T. tonsurans* (most common), *T. rubrum,* and *T. mentagrophytes.* It typically begins as an erythematous papule, which expands to form larger, scaly, erythematous plaque. Central clearing often occurs, resulting in annular lesions. Less common findings include vesicles, pustules, bullae, or crusting. Pruritus is variable. Lesions vary in size from a few milli-

meters to several centimeters and may range in number from one to several. Numerous lesions are uncommon, except for in the immunocompromised population. Involvement of hair follicles is referred to as *Majocchi's granuloma.* A granulomatous inflammatory response often ensues, and clinically the patients present with more discrete papular lesions, sometimes in association with the more typical annular plaques of ordinary tinea corporis. *Tinea faciei* (Color Plate 26), a dermatophyte infection of the face, may present with prominent erythema and less scaling than typical of tinea corporis. When located over hairy areas, vesicles, pustules, and crusting may develop. Diagnosis is often delayed, and oral therapy is often necessary to adequately eradicate tinea faciei.

The differential diagnosis of tinea corporis includes nummular dermatitis, psoriasis, and erythema annulare centrifugum. Erythema chronicum migrans (Lyme disease) and granuloma annulare, although they may present with annular lesions, usually lack the epidermal changes present in tinea. The herald patch of pityriasis rosea is frequently confused with tinea corporis. The subsequent appearance of the Christmas-tree pattern of secondary lesions establishes the diagnosis of pityriasis rosea; alternatively, the "trailing scale" on the inner side of the lesion may distinguish pityriasis rosea from tinea, in which case the scale is usually around the periphery and pointing outward.

Diagnosis of tinea corporis is accomplished via the demonstration of hyphae on KOH examination or by fungal culture. In obtaining the material for these examinations, the ideal site for sampling is the scale found at the advancing border of the plaques, which generally contains the highest concentration of fungal organisms.

TABLE 14-10

TREATMENT OF DERMATOPHYTE INFECTIONS (CONCENTRATION OF SUSPENSION FORMULATION, IF AVAILABLE, IN PARENTHESES)

THERAPY, COMMENT	DISORDER(S)	DOSE/REGIMEN	
Topical			
Azoles (miconazole, clotrimazole, econazole, ketoconazole, oxiconazole)	TCo, TP	Apply qd-bid × 4–6 wks	
Allylamines (naftifine, terbinafine)	TCo, TP TU*	Apply qd-bid × 2–4 wk Naftifine may be effective for distal subungual type	
Others (ciclopirox olamine, tolnaftate, butenafine)	TCo, TP	Apply qd-bid × 4–6 wk	
Systemic			
Griseofulvin	MG, TCa, TU, TCo (recalcitrant)	15–20 mg/kg/d × 6–8 wk (Suspension: 125 mg/5 ml)	Fat enhances absorption; TU may require 6 to 18 mo, may recur
Itraconazole (FDA-approved in adults only)	TCa, TU	3–5 mg/kg/d × 4–6 wk (In TU: "pulse" × 1 wk/mo × 3–4 mo) (Suspension: 10 mg/1 ml)	Beware of potential drug interactions Monitor LFTs, electrolytes
Fluconazole	TCa	6 mg/kg/d × 3–6 wk (Suspensions: 10 mg/1 ml, 40 mg/1 ml)	Beware of potential drug interactions Monitor LFTs, electrolytes
Terbinafine (FDA-approved in adults only)	TCa, TU	Dosed by weight [<20 kg: 62.5 mg/d; 20–40 kg: 125 mg/d; >40 kg: 250 mg/d] × 4–6 wk (In TU: 6–12 wk)	Less effective against *M. canis* Monitor CBC, LFTs

MG = Majocchi's granuloma; TCa = tinea capitis; TCo = tinea corporis; TP = tinea pedis; TU = tinea unguium; LFTs = liver function tests; CBC = complete blood cell count.

TINEA PEDIS   Dermatophyte infection of the feet, as well as the hands (*tinea manum*), is more common in adults but does occur in pediatric patients. The most common organism implicated is *T. rubrum*. Tinea pedis is related to the wearing of shoes, which contributes to an environment (warmth, moisture) that favors growth of dermatophyte fungi. Clinical findings vary from mild asymptomatic peeling to diffuse erythema and scaling in a "moccasin" distribution. Deep-seated vesicles may be present, and erythema and maceration of the toe web spaces are common. Bullae rarely occur and are most common in response to infection with a zoophilic organism. Tinea manum is often accompanied by tinea pedis and presents with palmar scaling and occasionally mild erythema. Finger web spaces are usually spared, and vesicles or pustules are occasionally present. When involvement of the dorsal hand occurs, the presentation is more similar to tinea corporis with well demarcated, scaly, red plaques. The diagnosis of tinea pedis or manum is established by a positive KOH preparation or fungal culture.

TINEA UNGUIUM   Tinea unguium, a type of *onychomycosis,* is a dermatophyte infection of the nail plate. It is uncommon in young children and has an increasing incidence with increasing age. Predisposing factors include nail trauma, immunosuppression, long-term therapy with corticosteroids, concomitant presence of tinea pedis, and family history of tinea unguium. The most commonly isolated organisms are *T. rubrum* and *T. mentagrophytes,* and diagnosis is confirmed either by direct microscopy with KOH examination or via isolation of the offending organism by fungal culture. The differential diagnosis of tinea unguium may include psoriasis, lichen planus, contact dermatitis, trauma, and pachyonychia congenita.

There are several presentations of tinea unguium. The *distal subungual* form is the most common and presents with onycholysis (separation of the nail plate from the nail bed) and subungual thickening with debris at the distal (free) end of the nail. In the *proximal subungual* form, subungual thickening and leukonychia (white nail discoloration) occur in the proximal (near the cuticle) portion of the nail. *White superficial onychomycosis* occurs when the fungus invades the superficial layers of the nail and results in white islands on the nail plate, which coalesce and spread with progression of the disease. *Candida* spp. may cause a chronic paronychia (see *Candida* above). Successful treatment of dermatophyte infections of the nail generally requires the administration of systemic antifungal agents, as outlined in Table 14-10.

References

Elewski B: Tinea capitis. Dermatol Clin 14:23–31, 1996

Elewski BE: Cutaneous mycoses in children. Br J Dermatol 134(S46):7–11, 1996

Fallon-Friedlander S, Suarez S. Pediatric antifungal therapy. Dermatol Clin 16:527–537, 1998

Gupta AK, Einarson TR, Summerbell RC, et al: An overview of topical antifungal therapy in dermatomycoses. A North American perspective. Drugs 55:645–674, 1998

Hoppe JE: Treatment of oropharyngeal candidiasis and candidal diaper dermatitis in neonates and infants: review and reappraisal. Pediatr Infect Dis J 16:885–894, 1997

Lange DS, Richards HM, Guarnieri J, et al: Ketoconazole 2% shampoo in the treatment of tinea versicolor: a multicenter, randomized, double-blind, placebo-controlled trial. J Am Acad Dermatol 39:944–950, 1998

Pradeepkumar VK, Rajadurai VS, Tan KW: Congenital candidiasis: varied presentations. J Perinatol 18:311–316, 1998

Sunenshine PJ, Schwartz RA, Janniger CK: Tinea versicolor. Int J Dermatol 37:648–655, 1998

EVALUATION OF THE CHILD WITH FEVER AND A RASH

The approach to the child who presents with fever and a rash must take into consideration numerous diagnostic possibilities, including infectious causes, autoimmune disorders, immune-mediated hypersensitivity reactions, and Kawasaki disease. A thorough history discussing recent travels, drug intake history, and known exposures is vital. Findings on physical examination, as well as results from the review of systems and laboratory studies, round out the evaluation and will in most cases enable a diagnosis to be made, although in some patients observation of the natural course of the disease or response to therapies may be necessary. Figure 14-30 is an algorithm of the differential diagnosis of the child with fever and a rash, with key cutaneous and extracutaneous features serving as branchpoints to narrow down the differential diagnosis.

14.13 INSECT BITES AND INFESTATIONS

Denise W. Metry and Adelaide A. Hebert

Many types of insects commonly plague children. Fortunately, local irritation from the bite or sting itself is usually the only complication. However, arthropod attacks may cause more serious consequences, including severe systemic reactions such as anaphylaxis. Insects are also important vectors of human infection and disease.

FLEAS

Domestic animals are usually responsible for bringing these insects into households from the immediate outdoors. Fleas often attack the youngest member of a household, and that child may be the only affected family member. Children are also more likely to be symptomatic, as tolerance to fleabites generally develops with age.

Typical lesions are pruritic papules that often appear in linear groups of three or four lesions, the "breakfast, lunch, and dinner" pattern (Fig 14-31). Another helpful diagnostic clue is the presence of a tiny central punctum at the center of a papule, indicative of the bite itself. Extremely sensitive individuals may develop bullous lesions. Most commonly, the majority of lesions are present below the knees, since fleas are able to jump to a height of about 18 cm. Microscopic evaluation of debris from the suspected pet's bedding material often confirms the diagnosis. Close examination of the animal may also reveal dried flea feces, crusting, or hair loss, especially over the lower back and base of the tail. Most fleabites resolve without treatment. However, pruritus should be treated with oral antihistamines, as aggressive scratching can result in secondary infection. Effective flea eradication requires treatment of both the infested animal and its living quarters. Flea larvae in the household can be controlled with insect growth regulators such as methoprene and pyriproxyfen. Similar growth regulators are available as oral medication for pets.

MOSQUITOES

The annoyance of mosquitoes is second only to their significance as vectors of disease. Mosquito bites commonly cause local allergic

FEVER and RASH		POSSIBLE DIAGNOSIS
Are petechiae present?	Yes	
	Oral mucosal petechiae	Rubella
		Group A beta hemolytic streptococci
		Arcanobacterium hemolyticum
	Skin petechiae	Epstein Barr virus, cytomegalovirus, enteroviruses
		Meningococcemia, gonococcemia
		Ehrlichiosis, leptospirosis
		Dengue
		Henoch-Shönlein purpura (HSP)
	Skin and palms/soles	Rocky Mountain spotted fever
		Rat-bite fever
Is pharyngitis present?	Yes	Epstein Barr virus
		Group A beta hemolytic streptococcus
		Arcanobacterium hemolyticum
		Gonococcemia
		Typhoid fever
		Tularemia
Blisters, erosions, or necrosis?	Yes	
	Blisters, erosions	Varicella
		Staphylococcal scalded skin syndrome
		Brucellosis
		Erythema multiforme, Stevens-Johnson
		Toxic epidermal necrolysis
		Henoch Schönlein purpura
		Graft vs. host disease (acute)
	Necrosis	Meningococcemia
		Tularemia
		Stevens-Johnson
		Toxic epidermal necrolysis
Episodic fever and rash?	Yes	Juvenile rheumatoid arthritis (systemic)
		Acute rheumatic fever
		Familial Mediterranean fever
Intense facial erythema?	Yes	Erythema infectiosum
		Systemic lupus erythematosus
		Erysipelas
		Juvenile dermatomyositis
Characteristics of Rash	Morbilliform	Measles
		Rubella
		Epstein Barr virus
		Rat-bite fever
		Kawasaki disease
		Drug eruption
	Maculopapular	Non-specific viral exanthem
		Roseola infantum
		Ehrlichiosis
		Dengue
		Leptospirosis
		Tularemia
		Epidemic or endemic typhus
		Kawasaki disease
		Drug eruption
	Urticarial	Drug eruption
		Erythema multiforme
		Serum sickness-like reaction
		Henoch-Schönlein purpura
		Urticaria
	Subcutaneous nodules	Juvenile rheumatoid arthritis
		Polyarteritis nodosa
		Acute rheumatic fever
	Erythroderma	Toxic shock syndrome
		Staphylococcal scalded skin syndrome
		Toxic epidermal necrolysis
		Drug eruption
		Graft vs. host disease (acute)
	Nail fold telangiectasia	Juvenile dermatomyositis
		Systemic lupus erythematosus

FIGURE 14-30 Fever and rash algorithm.

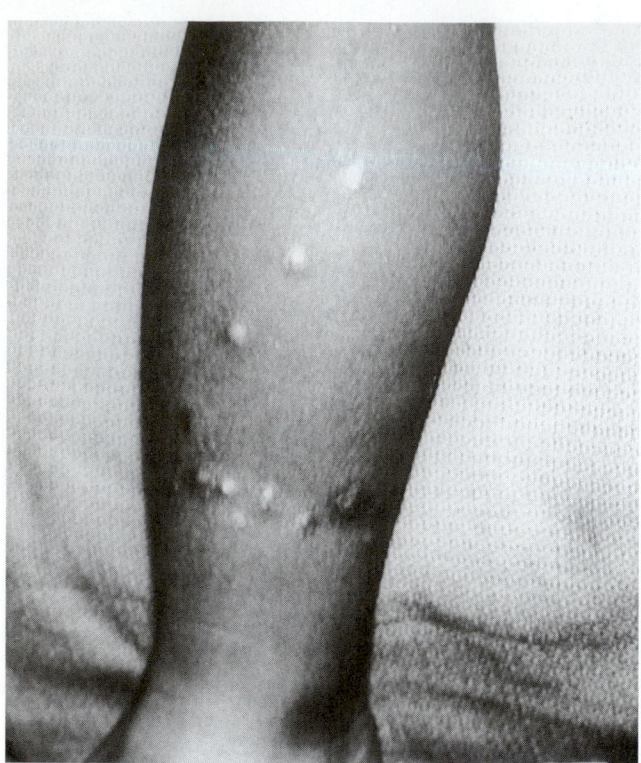

FIGURE 14-31 **Linear groups of papules characteristic of flea bites. (*Courtesy of Adelaide Hebert, M.D.*)**

reactions but may also cause severe systemic reactions in individuals susceptible to the mosquito's irritating salivary secretions, which the mosquito injects to anticoagulate its blood meal. Mosquitoes are most active during the cooler, shadier times of day and are attracted to their victims by sight, temperature, and, most important, smell. In general, they prefer men to women, blacks to whites, bright to dark clothing, and warm, sweaty skin to cool, dry skin. Mosquitoes also prefer young adults to older adults or children. Carbon dioxide released from the human breath and skin can attract a mosquito from up to 36 m away.

The best all-purpose insect repellent available is N, N-diethyl-m-toluamide, commonly known as *deet*, which is also active against biting flies, gnats, chiggers, and ticks but does not repel stinging insects, such as bees, wasps, or fire ants. Repellents containing greater than a 10% concentration of deet should not be used on a child's skin. Though rare, pediatric cardiovascular and neurologic toxicity has been reported. Most commercially available repellents advertised for children contain deet concentrations of 5 to 9%. A repellent should be applied to all exposed skin except the hands (particularly of small children), the areas near the eyes and mouth, and any broken or irritated skin. Reapplication should follow swimming or sweating. The repellent should be washed off the child with soap and water upon returning indoors. The sun protection factor (SPF) of a sunscreen is effectively reduced when used in combination with a deet-containing repellent. In such cases a higher SPF sunscreen should be applied.

The application of a topical corticosteroid will effectively reduce the swelling, redness, and pruritus of a mosquito bite. Corticosteroid use on the face or genitalia should be limited to low-potency, nonfluorinated (hydrocortisone) preparations. Over-the-counter topical antihistamines and anesthetics are popular among parents but should be discouraged because of the high incidence of asso-

ciated allergic contact dermatitis. The prophylactic use of the oral antihistamine cetirizine has proved effective in alleviating both immediate and delayed mosquito-bite symptoms.

TICKS

Ticks transmit the organisms that cause Rocky Mountain spotted fever, babesiosis, ehrlichiosis, tularemia, typhus, and Lyme disease among others (Color Plate 22) and have been implicated in certain viral encephalitides and hemorrhagic fevers. Most reports of tick bites occur in the spring and summer. Ticks have unique barbed mouthparts called *chelicerae,* which they use to attach to their victims' skin. A cement-like salivary gland substance is then secreted, which allows the insect to remain securely on the skin while feeding. Feeding occurs for approximately 7 days, until the tick is satisfactorily engorged with blood. The bite is painless.

Reactions to tick bites may result from hypersensitivity, injected toxins, or irritation to salivary gland secretions. The typical skin lesion is a solitary, erythematous papule, with or without an attached tick. In severe cases local swelling, blistering, bruising, and/or pruritus may develop as well as secondary cellulitis. Though most bites heal in two to three weeks, a persistent, hypersensitivity-type nodule, or tick granuloma, may last months to years.

A neurotoxin injected by the feeding tick causes reversible tick paralysis, more common in children. This is an acute, ascending, lower motor neuron paralysis, which may result in respiratory failure and even death. The tick must be attached at least four days for signs of paralysis to appear, and the condition will reverse itself if the tick is promptly removed by using a forceps to apply gentle, slow, reverse traction. Careless removal runs the risk of leaving the chelicerae behind in the skin, which then require surgical excision. In some cases the insect may be so firmly attached that forceps extraction is unsuccessful. In such instances it is best to infiltrate the area with local anesthesia and then superficially excise the skin underneath the area of attachment. Persistent tick granulomas may be treated surgically or with local corticosteroid injection.

The best protection available against tick bites is permethrin, which kills ticks on contact. It is recommended that permethrin repellents only be applied to a child's clothing since the safety profile of skin application has not been established. This chemical is also effective against mosquitoes, biting flies, chiggers, and scabies mites. A spray form is available, which can safely be used on clothing as well as outdoor equipment. The combined application of deet to the skin and permethrin to clothing creates a formidable barrier against many of the biting insects.

BEES, WASPS, AND YELLOW JACKETS

Notorious for their painful stings, these flying insects may also cause serious medical complications, including anaphylactic reactions. Insect stings are responsible for over 40 fatalities a year in the United States alone. Most flying insect stings occur from late spring through early fall. Although bees and wasps retaliate only when seriously threatened, yellow jackets are very aggressive scavengers who will attack without hesitation if their access to potential food (eg, an opened soda can) is impeded.

A bee dies after stinging her victim, leaving the barbed end of her stinger apparatus, or ovipositor, firmly embedded in the skin. Wasps and yellow jackets, however, retain their stingers and thus may repeatedly use them. The sting produces an immediate burning pain followed by four to six hours of intense erythema and swelling. Rarely, a delayed, serum-sickness-like syndrome may develop 7 to 14 days after a sting. Symptoms include fever, arthralgias, tender urticaria, and angioedema.

The venom of a bee, wasp, or yellow jacket is more likely than that of any other insect to produce severe hypersensitivity reactions of the immediate, IgE-mediated type. Studies in the United States suggest that up to 4% of the general population may be at risk, although the frequency of serious anaphylactic reactions appears to be less than 1%. Both the quantity of venom injected and the degree of acquired hypersensitivity determine the severity of an individual's response. Stinging insect venom includes a highly complex mixture of pharmacologically active agents, of which the acute inflammatory mediators, phospholipase and hyaluronidase, predominate. Though the venom of the wasp, bee, and yellow jacket contains genus- or species-specific antigens, antigens common to each species are also present. Thus, some patients may exhibit cross-reactivity between species.

Venom may continue to be pumped through the stinger even though the insect is no longer present; therefore, the stinger should be removed from the skin as quickly as possible by scraping rather than pinching, since grabbing the protruding end, which contains the venom sac, will only serve to squeeze more venom into the wound. Painful stings may be treated locally with ice application or lidocaine injection. Less serious systemic symptoms, such as urticaria and edema, may be treated with antihistamines and oral glucocorticoids.

Signs of anaphylaxis include the development of respiratory distress, vascular collapse, and/or shock, usually within 20 minutes of the sting. Treatment requires the emergent administration of subcutaneous epinephrine and support as necessary in an acute care setting. Children at risk should wear an identifying medical alert tag; parents should carry a sting emergency kit and be instructed in the administration of subcutaneous epinephrine (Epi-pen). Desensitization procedures are available for individuals with a history of anaphylaxis and/or positive skin testing to stimulate the development of IgG antibodies against the venom allergens; the method protects 95% of sensitive individuals.

Unfortunately, no currently available insect repellent repels the stinging insect. Neither deet nor permethrin is an effective deterrent. Children and their parents can make themselves less attractive to these insects by avoiding brightly colored clothing and sweetly scented perfumes.

FIRE ANTS

The imported fire ant, genus *Solenopsis,* is an aggressive insect common to the southern United States. These insects build their nests in the ground, preferably in recently disturbed areas such as roadsides or sidewalks. Fire ant mounds stand up to a meter high in moist soil and can usually be easily seen and avoided. Unfortunately, nests in dry, sandy soil may be quite flat. Fire ants will aggressively defend their nest and are particularly vicious because they attack in large groups.

The fire ant first uses its powerful mandibles to grip the skin, then drives its posterior stinger into its victim. The insect then rotates about its point of oral attachment to inflict additional stings in a circular pattern. The initial lesion, an edematous papule, matures over 24 hours into a sterile pustule on a red, swollen base. When such lesions are present in clusters, they are virtually diagnostic of fire ant bites (Fig. 14-32). The pustules subsequently rupture, often leaving small scars.

Fire ant venom has antigenic similarity to bee and wasp venom, and systemic hypersensitivity reactions and cross-reactivity may occur. No specific therapy or repellent exists. Systemic reactions may require systemic glucocorticoids or antihistamines. As with other stinging insects, desensitization protects against anaphylaxis.

SCABIES

Scabies is a common condition in children caused by an infestation of the *Sarcoptes scabiei* mite. Scabies is contracted by close personal contact with an infested person, therefore the acquisition and spread of scabies between children occurs with relative ease. The female mite burrows through the skin, leaving behind a trail of debris, eggs, and feces. Clinical findings result from hypersensitivity and irritation to the mite and mite products. Scabies infestation is extremely pruritic and notoriously worse at night. Frequently, other family members also complain of itching.

The distribution of scabies lesions is very helpful in making the diagnosis. In infants, the insteps of the feet are commonly affected,

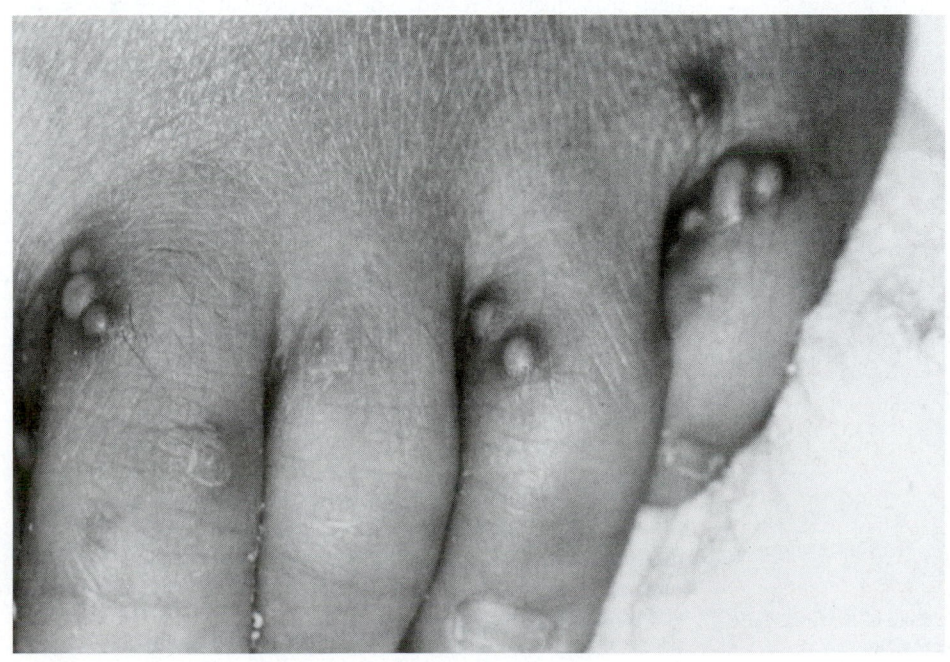

FIGURE 14-32 Grouped inflammatory pustules typical of fire ant bites. (*Courtesy of Adelaide Hebert, M.D.*)

often with vesicles or pustules (Fig. 14-33). An important diagnostic clue is an infant who is vigorously rubbing his or her feet together in an attempt to relieve itching. Unlike older children, infants commonly have involvement of the palms, axillae, and scalp. The characteristic distribution of scabies lesions at any age is wrists, finger web spaces, and waistline. Pruritic, nodular lesions of the nipples, umbilicus, axillae, or genitalia are also very suspicious for scabies. A unique clinical feature is the finding of the scabies burrow, which, although difficult to find in children, can be seen as a gray thread-like trail of scale on the skin.

Clinical variants of scabies may present diagnostic difficulties. For example, patients who bathe very frequently may have severe pruritus but only minimal skin findings. Scabies incognito occurs when treatment with topical or oral glucocorticoids masks the characteristic symptoms and signs of scabies. Lesions may be atypical in both appearance and distribution and are generally more widespread. Norwegian (crusted) scabies is a highly contagious form of scabies often seen in immunocompromised or debilitated, often institutionalized, patients. Widespread scale and crust formation is present, which may be remarkably thick over the palms, soles, and nails. Nodular scabies presents with discreet, orange-red nodules affecting the axilla and groin. Similar to the tick granuloma, nodules most likely represent a hypersensitivity reaction to retained mite parts or antigens. Lesions may persist for weeks to months and are often resistant to therapy.

The scabies preparation is a simple and rapid means of establishing the diagnosis of scabies. Using a mineral oil–coated Joseph knife or sterile scalpel blade, multiple lesions are vigorously scraped. It is ideal to perform this procedure on the child's caretaker if they have skin findings suspicious for scabies. The best lesions for diagnosis are burrows, vesicles, and nonexcoriated papules, and the best scrapings obtain the material underneath the tops and crusts of lesions. The material obtained is then transferred onto a glass slide and examined microscopically under low power. Actively moving mites, eggs, and/or feces can be found in 60% of patients in whom the diagnosis is strongly suspected. The scabies preparation, when visualized by the adult caretaker, is also an excellent means to ensure treatment compliance.

To avoid reinfestation, the patient and all close contacts must be treated simultaneously. With the diagnosis of scabies comes the (often embarrassing) task of informing all possible contacts, who must also undergo the inconvenience and expense of treatment. Therefore, a scabies preparation should always be performed to confirm the diagnosis.

The treatment of choice for scabies in adults and children is permethrin 5% cream. Permethrin has not been approved for use in infants under two months of age. Adverse reactions to permethrin most commonly result from sensory irritation and are typically mild and short-lived. However, the US preparation of permethrin also contains 0.1% formaldehyde, which is a common cause of allergic contact dermatitis. Permethrin is applied at bedtime and washed off in the morning. A repeat application should be performed after one week. In the case of Norwegian scabies, multiple applications are often necessary. The entire skin should be treated including the scalp, face (avoiding the areas around the eyes, nose, and mouth), behind the ears, between the fingers and toes, and under the nails. All clothing, bedding, and other items that have been in intimate contact with the patient must be simultaneously washed and thoroughly dried, preferably on high heat settings.

Precipitated sulfur (6%) in petrolatum applied for three successive nights is a safe alternative for children and is the treatment of choice for infants less than two months of age. Use of this product is less popular as it is malodorous and will stain clothing. The product lindane is another option, but its use has been limited by rare reports of neurotoxicity in children. Symptomatic scabies treatment includes oral antihistamines and the application of low-potency hydrocortisone creams.

Papular and pustular skin lesions generally resolve within one week following treatment, although nodular lesions may persist for months. Pruritus may continue for up to six weeks secondary to continued hypersensitivity to dead mite parts. This phenomenon must be explained to parents, who often think that their child has been inadequately treated. The development of new skin lesions more than two weeks after initial therapy, however, does suggest either reinfestation or inadequate treatment. The diagnosis of scabies carries significant social implications and requires patience, understanding, and thorough explanation by the treating physician.

HEAD LICE

Infestations with head lice are an increasing problem in the United States and other countries, because of the development of resistance. The causative organism is the *Pediculus capitis* louse. Infestation with head lice can occur at any age and within any socioeconomic group. However, the incidence is most common in female, school-aged children and is 35 times higher in whites than African-Americans. The reason for this predilection is not clear. Head lice are most commonly spread by direct head-to-head contact or from shared fomites like brushes, combs, or hats. Contrary to popular belief, infestation is not related to poor hygiene or hair length.

Lice infestation most commonly manifests as intense scalp itching, particularly of the occiput. Pruritic papules may be seen at the nape of the neck. Other common findings are secondary infection, cervical adenopathy, and fever. Close examination will reveal multiple, oval, grayish-white egg capsules (nits) that are firmly attached

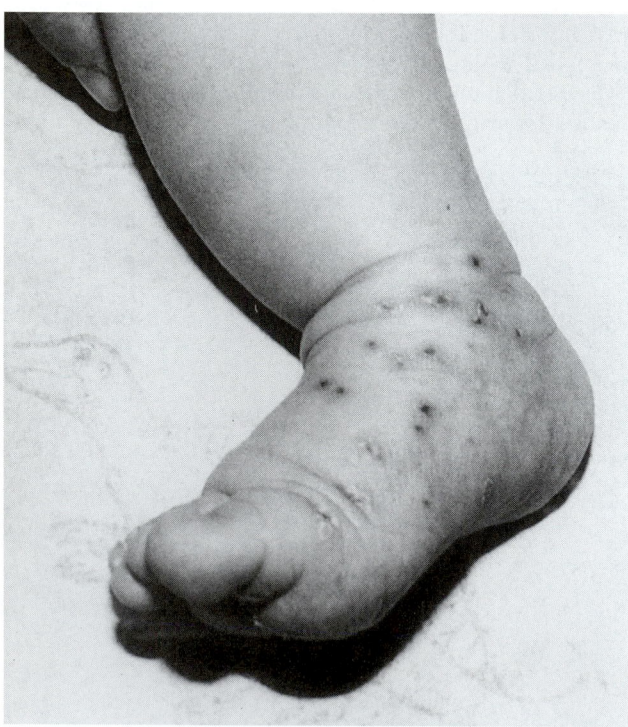

FIGURE 14-33 Pustules on the insteps of the feet are characteristic of nodular scabies. (*Courtesy of Adelaide Hebert, M.D.*)

to the hair shaft (Fig. 14-34A). The louse itself is gray, 2 to 3 mm long, and lives on the hair closest to the scalp. Diagnosis is confirmed by plucking the visibly affected hairs, which can then be examined microscopically under low power. Active infestation is based on the finding of adult lice, immature nymphs, and/or viable eggs (Fig. 14-34B). Nits are not diagnostic of active infestation.

The most effective treatment for head lice is synthetic permethrin, which is available over the counter in a 1% cream rinse. The hair is washed with a regular shampoo, rinsed with water, and towel-dried. Permethrin cream rinse is then generously applied, left on for 10 minutes, and rinsed with water. A single application is effective in over 90% of cases, but most physicians recommend a second treatment after one week. Natural (synergized) permethrin, also available over the counter, is used similarly to the cream rinse except that the hair is shampooed after the 10-minute application. Natural permethrin is not ovicidal; thus a second application after one week is mandatory.

Empty nits may be removed with either 8% formic acid or a 1:1 mixture of vinegar and water, which is applied to the hair for 15 minutes. The nits can then be removed with gentle combing of the hair using a fine-toothed comb. Similar to scabies infestation, all family members should be simultaneously treated, even if asymptomatic. Intimate fomites such as hats, towels, and pillowcases must be washed and dried on hot settings. Clothing that is not washable should be dry-cleaned. Brushes, combs, and other hair items should be washed in hot (130°F), soapy water for 10 to 20 minutes. Al-

ternatively, these items may be pretreated with a pediculide for 15 minutes and then washed in hot, soapy water. Floors, play areas, and furniture should be thoroughly vacuumed to remove any shed hairs which may have viable eggs attached.

Lindane, while once popular for the treatment of head lice, is no longer recommended because of the development of significant pediculosis resistance. Throughout the United States a growing number of treatment failures following repeated applications of permethrin have been reported. Studies involving the safety and efficacy of alternative therapies are in progress.

Body lice and pubic lice are responsible for pediculosis corporis and pediculosis pubis, respectively. The pubic louse can be distinguished from the head or body louse by its short body and longer crablike legs. Body lice are a correlate of poor hygiene, but pubic lic should be considered a sexually transmitted disease. Natural or synthetic permethrins can be used either as a 10-minute shampoo or as a lotion left on for hours. Lindane is also effective. Treatment should be repeated in one week. Sexual partners of patients with pediculosis pubis should be treated simultaneously.

SPIDERS

The two most common (and most infamous) spider species important to humans are *Lactrodectus mactans,* the "black widow," and *Loxosceles reclusa,* the "brown recluse." Both can inject harmful, potentially fatal, venom into their victims. They prefer dark, undisturbed habitats and may be found outdoors under stones and woodpiles. Indoor attacks have occurred in dark corners of garages and attics.

Lactrodectus is notorious for the scarlet red "hourglass" on its glossy, black abdomen. More potent than any snake venom, black widow venom contains a neurotoxin known as *alpha-lactrotoxin.* In the minutes following a usually painless bite, severe local pain and redness develop. Two fang marks in the skin are often evident. Over the next eight hours symptoms of profuse sweating, abdominal cramps, and leg pains reach their peak. Severe cases may eventuate in cardiac arrhythmias, internal hemorrhage, and paralysis. Approximately 1% of bites prove fatal, young children seemingly at highest risk. Initial treatment includes the application of ice and elevation of the affected extremity. The traditional administration of 10% calcium gluconate (10 ml given by iv push over five minutes) is useful for abdominal and muscle spasms. Narcotics may also be necessary for persistent pain. *Lactrodectus* antivenom produced from horse serum is also available for severe or high-risk cases but carries the significant risk of anaphylaxis.

Loxosceles reclusa, the brown recluse, is also known as the "fiddleback" spider because of the violin-shaped markings over its back. The body is typically a dull yellow or light brown color. *Loxosceles* venom contains a protein known as *sphingomy elinase D,* which functions as a platelet aggregator, neutrophil chemoattractant, and liberator of thromboxane B2. The hallmark of the brown recluse spider bite is the development of skin necrosis at the site of envenomation. Wounds at risk for necrosis are usually those that show signs of painful progression within 48 to 72 hours; less than 10% of bites lead to severe skin damage or systemic symptoms.

Characteristic *Loxosceles* skin findings include a central violaceus discoloration with blister formation surrounded by a white, ischemic halo and an outer ring of erythema. This is known as the "red, white, and blue" or "target" sign. Within a few days the center forms a black eschar, which is eventually sloughed. The most serious reported systemic complication of the *Loxosceles* bite is a syn-

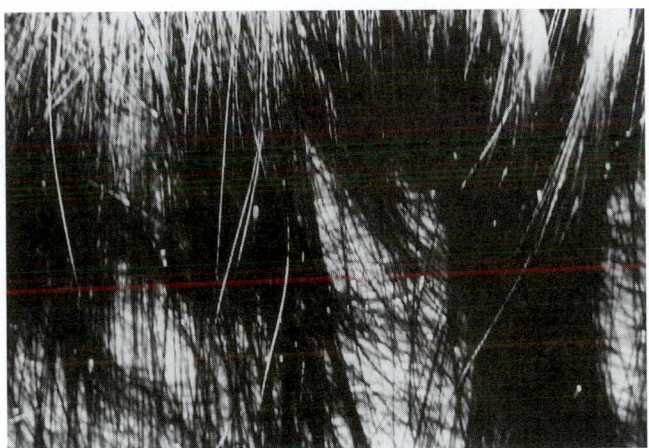

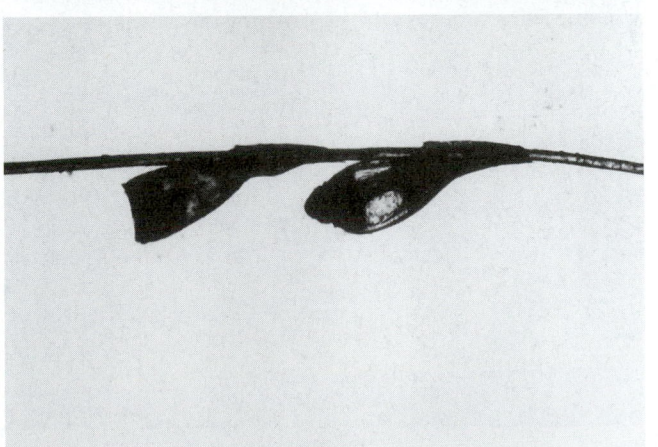

FIGURE 14-34 **(A) Nits on the hair of a patient infested with head lice. (B) Head louse nits, hatched (left) and unhatched (right).** (*Courtesy of Adelaide Hebert, M.D.*)

drome of intravascular hemolysis. Symptoms include high fever, rigors, arthralgias, and vomiting. Hematuria and petechiae may develop as well as thrombocytopenia, hemolytic anemia, and other blood dyscrasias. Laboratory evaluation for hematologic complications are indicated, especially in children in whom a *Loxosceles* bite is suspected.

The treatment of *Loxosceles* bites includes local wound care, ice compresses, and prophylactic antibiotics. The use of dapsone has been widely advocated because of its theoretically beneficial inhibition of neutrophil function. However, conclusive evidence of benefit over placebo remains limited. Systemic glucocorticoids have not proved useful for skin necrosis but are considered first-line therapy for the hemolytic syndrome. Surgical debridement is contraindicated until the wound has stabilized with medical management. Most bites may be managed with minimal medical intervention and heal without significant scarring.

References

Brown MB, Hebert AA: Insect repellents: an overview. J Am Acad Dermatol 36:243–249, 1997

Burns DA: Diseases caused by arthropods and other noxious animals. In: Champion RH, Burton JL, Ebling FJG, eds: Textbook of Dermatology, 6th ed. Oxford, Blackwell Science, 1998:1423–1481

Fradin MS: Mosquitoes and mosquito repellents: a clinician's guide. Ann Int Med 128:931–940, 1998

Hebert AA, Carlton S: Getting bugs to bug off: a review of insect repellents. Contemp Pediatr 15:85–95, 1998

Kemp ED: Bites and stings of the arthropod kind: treating reactions that can range from annoying to menacing. Postgrad Med 103:88–104, 1998

Metry DW, Hebert AA: Insect and arachnid stings, bites, infestations, and repellents. Pediatr Ann 29:39–48, 2000

Wilson DC, King LE: Arthropod bites and stings. In: Freedberg IM, Eisen AZ, Wolff K, et al, eds: Dermatology in General Medicine, 5th ed. New York, McGraw-Hill, 1999:2685–2695

14.14 MISCELLANEOUS DISORDERS

Robert Sidbury

Granuloma annulare (GA) is a common inflammatory disease of unknown etiology, characterized by oval, orange-red, firm, papulonodules located commonly on the hands and feet. There is often an "annular" appearance, with a raised, smooth, papular border surrounding normal-appearing skin, leading to a frequent misdiagnosis of ringworm (Fig. 14-35). Lesions are usually asymptomatic. Histologically, granuloma annulare is composed of histiocytes in a distinctive "palisade" surrounding collagen fibers with abundant mucin. Subcutaneous granuloma annulare is an uncommon variant in which the inflammatory process primarily involves the fat, resulting in a more macular, diffuse clinical appearance. Differentiating GA from ringworm is straightforward because of the presence of scaling in the latter. Other considerations such as rheumatoid nodules, sarcoidosis, and necrobiosis lipoidica diabeticorum can usually be eliminated based on morphology; however, skin biopsy is diagnostic. The natural history of GA is indolent growth followed by stabilization and ultimate regression over a period of years. Standard topical steroid preparations are not effective;

however, intralesional steroid injections or adhesive tape impregnated with steroids (eg, Cordran tape) can help limit progression.

Necrobiosis lipoidica diabeticorum (NLD) is an uncommon inflammatory dermatosis, typically, but not exclusively, seen in diabetic patients. NLD is rare in early childhood. Whereas only 0.3% of diabetics develop NLD, approximately 60 to 75% of patients with NLD have abnormal glucose tolerance with a higher percentage developing diabetes later. There is no conclusive evidence relating the onset of NLD to diabetic control. NLD presents as well-demarcated, often oval or elliptically shaped plaques with a distinctive red-yellow color. Telangectasias are frequently visible centrally, and lesions can ulcerate if traumatized. The pretibial region is a common site, however, upper extremities and trunk can be affected. Itching can occur, but most often lesions are asymptomatic. The etiology is not known though trauma may be a precipitating factor. Histologically, NLD is characterized by a telltale "sandwich" appearance of layered inflammatory cells around degenerating, or *necrobiotic*, collagen fibers. Cosmetic concerns typically prompt treatment with potent topical steroids; however, protection from trauma is the most useful intervention. Shin-guards are ideal protection for pretibial lesions. A thorough investigation to rule out diabetes is warranted.

Scleredema is a rare disorder of unknown etiology that presents as asymptomatic thickening of the skin primarily of the head, neck, and upper trunk. In the most common pediatric presentation, skin changes occur days to months after an acute upper respiratory infection, typically streptococcal. Symmetrical induration often begins on the neck or face, and pharyngeal involvement may lead to dysphagia. Biopsies of scleredema reveal a normal epidermis with thickness of the collagen fibers and abundant, pale-staining mucin. Scleredema can usually be differentiated from scleroderma based on the lack of epidermal atrophy and from edema because it is firm and does not pit. The natural history of classical, postinfectious scleredema is self-limited; however, some adolescent cases have a more indolent, unrelenting course that may be associated with a monoclonal gammopathy. Another subgroup of scleredema has been linked to diabetes, and appropriate evaluations should be

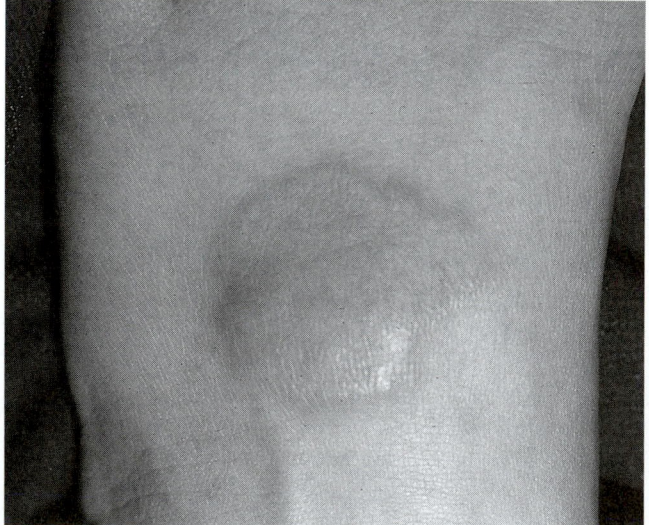

FIGURE 14-35   Annular collection of nonscaling, erythematous papules with central clearing and slight atrophy are characteristic of granuloma annulare, most commonly found on the lower extremities. (*Courtesy of Amy Paller, M.D.*)

performed. There are no uniformly effective treatments, and complications can include contractures, infection, and cardiac problems.

Scars represent fibrosis after injury to the dermis. Scars evolve in color from pink-purple to white over several months to two years. Most scars flatten after initial elevation and may even become atrophic. **Keloids** and **hypertrophic scars** are abnormal, exuberant responses to cutaneous injury and present as red-brown nodules and tumors that can be disfiguring. Precipitating events can range from diseases such as varicella and acne to exogenous agents as in piercings or surgeries. In many cases the source of injury cannot be identified. The tendency to form keloids is familial and is more common in patients with darker skin types. Keloids can be pruritic and even painful, sometimes extending beyond the margin of initial skin injury, whereas hypertrophic scars are usually asymptomatic and conform to wound boundaries. Intralesional steroid injection improves size and texture in many cases. Injections may be used independently after surgery to prevent recurrence. Other therapies aimed at reducing keloid size include silicon gel sheeting and intralesional interferon, and pulse dye laser treatment may improve discoloration.

Striae, or "stretch marks," are atrophic, linear lesions oriented perpendicularly to relaxed skin tension lines. Initially raised and pink-red in color, striae become flatter and less conspicuous with time, undergoing color changes from livid red, to pink, to white. Common associations include obesity, pregnancy, cortisol excess (eg, Cushing's syndrome), and rapid growth, as in puberty. Both systemic and topical steroid therapy can also lead to striae, which are most commonly located on the abdomen, thighs, and breasts in girls, and the outer aspect of the thighs and lumbosacral region in boys. Regardless of cause, striae are difficult to treat and can be extremely bothersome to patients. Laser therapy can effectively hasten color change, making lesions less noticeable, but there are no proven therapies for eliminating striae. Topical retinoid preparations have not proved beneficial. Reassurance that time will improve the appearance of striae is important.

Elastosis perforans serpiginosa (EPS) is a rare disorder in which dermal elastic tissue is extruded through the epidermis. Typically erythematous, keratotic papules are grouped in arciform or serpiginous lines. EPS may occur alone as an inherited trait, but it is also seen in association with Down syndrome, Ehlers-Danlos syndrome, osteogenesis imperfecta, pseudoxanthoma elasticum, Rothmund-Thompson syndrome, and after penicillamine therapy. The lesions tend to persist over years and to resolve with scarring.

Lipodystrophy is a rare disorder of fat loss that can be either localized (partial lipodystrophy) or generalized. Localized or "partial" lipodystrophy is a rare disorder of children and young adults that most commonly affects females. The disease is characterized by slowly progressive loss of subcutaneous fat usually in the upper half of the body. Facial involvement imparts a "wasted" appearance. Glomerulonephritis and complement deficiency (C3) are well-established associations. Generalized lipodystrophy, also known as *lipoatrophic diabetes* owing to its association with glucose intolerance, is a progressive, multisystem disease. The congenital form, or Lawrence-Seip syndrome, is a recessive disorder that occurs in the first two years of life. Patients present with facial dysmorphism, extensive loss of subcutaneous tissue, and other clinical expressions of endocrinologic dysregulation. Insulin resistance leads to hyperinsulinemic diabetes, hyperlipidemia, as well as other cutaneous

markers such as acanthosis nigricans. Treatment is difficult and should focus on correction of endocrinologic parameters.

Erythema nodosum (EN) is the most common, acute disorder of the fat seen in the pediatric population, although it is less common than in adults. EN presents as tender, red, warm plaques without epidermal change typically on the anterior lower extremities. Infections and medications are most often implicated, with streptococcal disease the leading culprit. Other infectious etiologies include *Yersinia* and, historically, tuberculosis, although this is increasingly rare. Sulfonamides and diphenylhydantoin are the most common medications associated with childhood EN. A clinical diagnosis is usually possible, but a deep-skin biopsy including fat reveals diagnostic septal inflammation. Differential considerations include nodular vasculitis, Henoch-Schonlein purpura, and pancreatitis, as well as other causes of panniculitis. The natural history of EN is self-limited; however, pain often mandates treatment. Oral prednisone is very effective, and nonsteroidal anti-inflammatory medications and SSKI (iodine) can be helpful. A minimum evaluation should include a complete blood count, chemistries, ASO titer, stool cultures, chest x-ray, PPD, and serologic tests for *Yersinia*.

Cold panniculitis is a form of circumscribed panniculitis caused by cold injury to the subcutaneous tissues. Classically, infants and children will present with reddish-blue, ill-defined, warm plaques on one or both cheeks, two to three days after eating a popsicle or ice cube. Prior to the development of the *Haemophilus influenzae* vaccine, cold panniculitis of the face was often mistaken for buccal cellulitis caused by *H. influenzae*. Similar lesions can occur on the extremities in children who participate in winter sports. Avoidance of further hypothermia is curative.

Subcutaneous fat necrosis of the newborn is a distinctive, self-limited condition of healthy neonates characterized by nodular, erythematous, indurated plaques most commonly on the back. The etiology is unknown; however, incidental cold exposure may contribute to the pathology. In the absence of hypercalcemia, which occurs in rare cases, reassurance is all that is necessary. Alternatively, sclerema neonatorum is a rapidly progressive, symmetrical hardening of the skin that occurs in infants with an underlying illness such as sepsis or congenital heart disease. Histologically, sclerema neonatorum is similar to subcutaneous fat necrosis of the newborn; however, the clinical setting of a gravely ill child suggests the diagnosis.

References

Berman B: Recurrence rates of excised keloids treated with post-operative triamcinolone acetonide injections or interferon alfa-2b injections. J Am Acad Dermatol 37(5 pt 1):755–757, 1997

Cron RQ, Swetter SM: Scleredema revisited: a post-streptococcal complication. Clin Pediatr 33:606–610, 1994

Hanson SG, Levy ML: Granuloma annulare. Pediatrics 103:195–196, 1999

Labbe L, Peral Y, Moleville J, Taieb A: Erythema nodosum in children: a study of 27 patients. Pediatr Dermatol 13:447–450, 1996

Laude TA: Skin disorders in black children. Curr Opin Pediatr 8(4):381–385, 1996

Moller DE, Flier JS: Insulin resistance—mechanisms, syndromes, and implications. N Engl J Med 325:938–948, 1991

Verrotti A, Chiarelli F, Amerio P, Morgasse G: Necrobiosis lipoidica diabeticorum in children and adolescents: a clue for underlying renal and retinal disease. Pediatr Dermatol 12:220–223, 1995

THE EAR, NOSE, OROPHARYNX, AND LARYNX

Robin T. Cotton, Associate Editor

15.1   THE EAR

Michael J. Rutter and Daniel Choo

15.1.1   The Normal Ear

ANATOMY

The ear is divided into the external, middle, and inner ear compartments (Fig. 15-1). The external ear consists of the auricle and the external auditory canal. The auricle is composed of cartilage that forms an intricate skin-covered framework. The primary function of the auricle is to channel sound energy toward the middle ear conducting apparatus. The lateral opening of the external auditory canal is the external meatus, which is bordered medially by the tympanic membrane. The lateral one-third of the external canal is cartilaginous, and the medial two-thirds are bony. The canal is lined by skin that possesses cerumen glands and other adnexal structures (hair follicles, sebaceous glands) in its lateral half. The external ear is innervated by branches of the trigeminal, facial, and glossopharyngeal nerves and the third cervical root (C3).

The normal tympanic membrane (Fig. 15-2) seals the opening between the external auditory canal and the middle and inner ear. The portion of the tympanic membrane inferior to the short process of the malleus (pars tensa) is a three-layered structure composed of a medial mucosal epithelium continous with the middle ear mucosa, a middle fibrous tissue layer, and finally, a lateral surface of squamous epithelium continuous with the external ear canal skin. The region of the tympanic membrane superior to the short process of the malleus (pars flaccida) does not have a middle fibrous layer, which is clinically significant because it allows the development of retraction pockets and acquired cholesteatomas.

The middle ear compartment is an aerated cavity that houses the three ossicles (the malleus, incus, and stapes), whose primary function is to focus and efficiently transmit sound energy to the inner ear. The tensor tympani and stapedius muscles are also found within the middle ear cavity and attach to the malleus and stapes bones, respectively. The middle ear is connected to the nasopharynx anterosuperiorly via the eustachian tube. This conduit is lined by a modified ciliated columnar epithelium that resembles respiratory epithelium. Posterior and superiorly, the middle ear cavity is connected to the mastoid air cell system by means of the mastoid antrum. This connection facilitates the extension of chronic middle ear disease (eg, chronic otitis media) as well as episodes of acute otitis media into the mastoid air cells, which is associated with clinical problems such as recurrent or chronic otitis media and acute, chronic, or coalescent mastoiditis.

The inner ear is arbitrarily divided into an auditory portion (the cochlea), a vestibular portion (three semicircular canals, the utricle, and the saccule), and the endolymphatic apparatus (the endolymphatic duct and sac). The cochlea is a coiled structure that houses the machinery responsible for transducing sound energy into neural impulses. The actual transducers are hair cells (one inner and three outer rows of hair cells) that are precisely arranged in the organ of Corti. The organ of Corti, in turn, rests on the basilar membrane, which resonates in response to the incoming acoustic stimuli. The cochlea maintains a very specific fluid balance, particularly in the endolymph, which has a composition more similar to intracellular fluid than extracellular fluid (ie, high potassium and low sodium), allowing the establishment of an electrochemical gradient that is critical for signal transduction and hearing. Clinical disorders that perturb this fluid homeostasis (eg, perilymphatic fistulas) result in hearing loss and/or balance dysfunction.

The semicircular canals are oriented at approximately 90° to each other, allowing detection of *angular* head motion in any given plane. Hair cells within the sensory portions of the semicircular canals (ie, the cristae) are deflected in response to head movement in a particular plane of motion. The utricle and saccule represent organs for the detection of *linear* or *gravitational* acceleration. The utricle and saccule both possess otoliths (calcium carbonate crystals) that rest on the hair cells and create an inertial mass that deflects the hair cells as a result of motion. Congenital deformities affecting only the vestibular portion of the inner ear are rare but have been reported in association with other ear anomalies such as Goldenhar syndrome. Children with congenital vestibulopathy usually present with a delay in development of motor skills (walking, coordination).

The endolymphatic duct and sac are thought to play a role in the maintenance of the specific fluid homeostasis of the inner ear. Abnormalities of the endolymphatic sac may be responsible for the hearing loss of patients with Pendred syndrome (euthyroid goiter and deafness). Further significance of the endolymphatic duct and sac is suggested by the recent recognition of enlarged vestibular aqueduct syndrome (EVAS), showing genetic linkage to the Pendred syndrome locus, as the most common bony abnormality of the inner ear (detected by computed tomography). The vestibular aqueduct serves as the bony channel that transmits the endolymphatic duct and sac. An enlarged vestibular aqueduct is associated with sensorineural hearing loss and has also been linked with hearing loss following relatively mild head trauma in children.

EMBRYOLOGY

At approximately 6 weeks of gestation, the mesoderm of the first and second branchial arches condense, giving rise to six hillocks of His. These hillocks are responsible for the formation of the auricle,

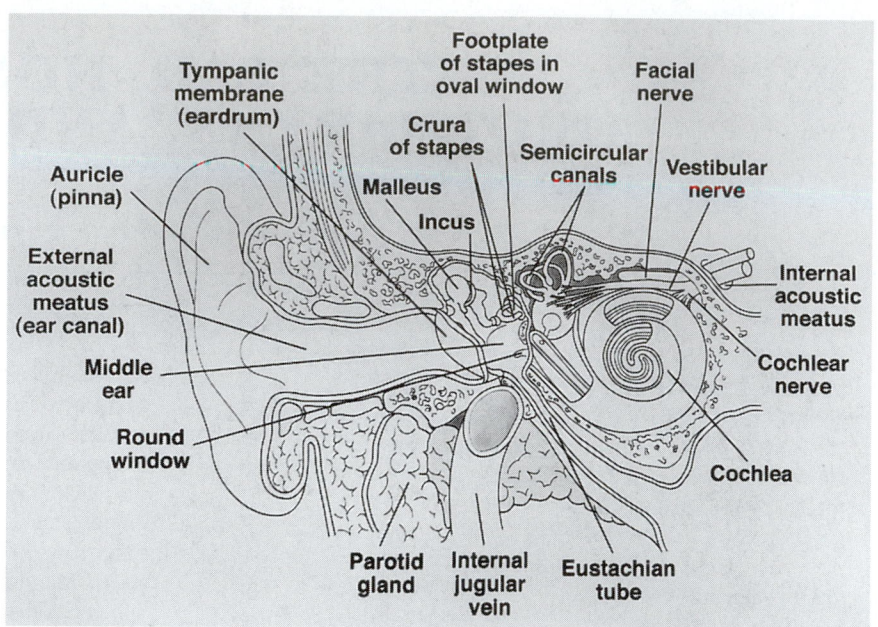

FIGURE 15-1 Anatomy of the ear: external, middle, and inner components.

which is mature in shape by 20 weeks. The external auditory canal initially is a solid core of ectoderm that invaginates medially at about 8 weeks. This core then undergoes resorption and canalization to leave a tube-like structure by 28 weeks. The most medial ectoderm remains intact to serve as the surface epithelium of the tympanic membrane. The external auditory canal does not complete ossification until approximately 3 years of age and is extremely floppy at birth, making newborn ear examinations difficult. Congenital microtia reflects an abnormal development process and is estimated to occur in up to 1 in 20,000 births. Atresia of the external auditory canal similarly points toward a development problem, typically thought to occur during the end of the first or beginning of the second trimester.

The eustachian tube forms from the space between the second arch and the first pharyngeal pouch (pharynx). The middle ear cavity then develops from an outpouching at the lateral end of the eustachian tube primordium. Pneumatization of the middle ear space begins around 10 weeks. The mastoid air cell system begins with the antrum and can be identified as early as 23 weeks. Significantly, the middle ear system is filled with mucoid mesenchyme

and secretions until close to the time of birth. The malleus and incus are derived from first and second branchial arch mesoderm and begin ossification as early as 16 weeks of gestation, when they are already of adult size. Auricular malformations (eg, microtia) are of clinical relevance. Because the auricle forms early, they may be associated with concomitant malformation of the middle ear and mastoid. In contrast, a normal auricle with canal atresia suggests a developmental defect occurring around 28 weeks, a time when the ossicles and middle ear are already formed.

The inner ear develops from a thickening of the surface ectoderm (the otic placode) that first invaginates and detaches from the surface epithelium to form the primitive otocyst (approximately 4 weeks of gestation). This otocyst forms the membranous labyrinth, including the cochlea, vestibular structures, and endolymphatic apparatus. By 6 weeks, the semicircular canals are well formed, and by 12 weeks the cochlea completes its $2\frac{1}{2}$ turns. Ossification of the inner ear structures begins at 15 weeks of gestation at multiple ossification origins and is typically complete by 23 weeks of gestation. With the exception of the endolymphatic apparatus, the inner ear is approximately adult size by the end of 24 weeks.

PHYSIOLOGY

The external ear auricle channels sound toward the ear canal and other sound transduction apparatus. The shape of the auricle also facilitates localization of sound in the environment. The length and shape of the external auditory canal imparts a particular optimal resonance frequency that affects an individual's maximum sensitivity to sound. For most people, the ear demonstrates maximum sensitivity in the range of speech frequencies. The tympanic membrane and ossicles then further refine that sound energy conduction by means of focusing the energy onto the oval window and by employing a lever mechanism that confers a mechanical advantage to the system. Once the sound energy reaches the cochlea, it causes a very specific portion of the basilar membrane to vibrate according to the frequency of the sound. This resonance of the basilar membrane then results in deflection of a specific set of hair cells and generation of an action potential. The "tonotopic" (frequency-

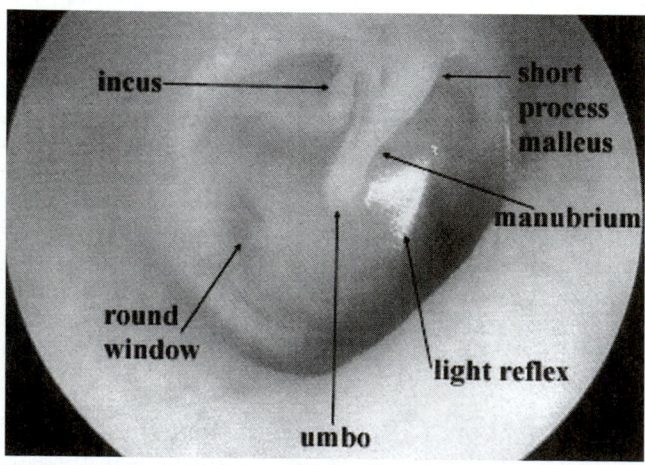

FIGURE 15-2 The tympanic membrane.

specific) arrangement of the basilar membrane and the cochlear hair cells is mirrored in the central auditory pathways, where specific neurons are activated depending on the frequency of sound detected.

In the vestibular system, deflection of hair cells again forms the basis for signal transduction. Flow of endolymph either toward (utriculopetal) or away (utriculofugal) from the vestibule causes either an increase or decrease in firing rate of vestibular sensory cells, depending on which particular semicircular canal crista is involved. This mechanism is exploited during vestibular testing. During electronystagmography (ENG), different temperature ear irrigations create a thermal gradient in the vestibular portion of the inner ear (most likely, the lateral semicircular canal). This thermal gradient creates a flow of endolymph that, in turn, stimulates a nystagmus via the vestibular-ocular reflex pathways. Cold irrigations should elicit a nystagmus toward the opposite ear. Conversely, warm irrigations are expected to elicit a nystagmus toward the ear being irrigated (see Sec. 15.1.3).

15.1.2   Molecular Genetics of Deafness

Approximately 1 in 1000 to 1 in 2000 children has a severe to profound hearing loss at birth or in early childhood. Various series estimate that upward of 50% of these cases of hearing loss result from inherited or genetic etiologies. Further subdividing this group, roughly 70% or more will have isolated hearing loss as the only phenotypic manifestation (ie, nonsyndromic hereditary hearing impairment). The remaining group has hearing loss in conjunction with other abnormalities (ie, syndromic hearing impairment). In those with nonsyndromic hereditary hearing impairment, the vast majority (~80%) will display an autosomal-recessive mode of transmission. Another 15% are estimated to have an autosomal-dominant mode of inheritance, with the remainder being X-linked or mitochondrial in nature.

Studies of large kindreds with hearing loss using linkage analysis and positional cloning techniques have identified multiple loci associated with nonsyndromic hearing impairment (Table 15-1). Fifteen autosomal dominant (DFNA1-15), 20 autosomal recessive (DFNB1-20), and eight X-linked loci (DFN1-8) have already been identified. An illustrative example of the clinical relevance of these genetic discoveries can be seen in the case of GJB2 (gap junction β-2 protein, otherwise known as connexin 26, CX 26) mutations and hereditary hearing impairment. Studying families with an autosomal recessive pattern of hearing loss identified the gene for GJB2. Linkage studies localized the candidate gene to the q arm of chromosome 13. Subsequent studies then identified a relatively common mutation involving deletion of a guanine residue at position 30 (30delG mutation). Genetic epidemiologic studies now estimate that mutations of GJB2 may account for almost half of all autosomal recessive hearing loss. In Italian, Spanish, and Israeli families, a 35delG mutation of GJB2 accounted for more than 63% of nonsyndromic autosomal recessive hearing impairment. Similarly, approximately 70% of Tunisian, French, New Zealand, and United Kingdom families show GJB2 mutations associated with nonsyndromic autosomal recessive hearing impairment. Thus, GJB2 mutations are highly significant even in general populations, and investigators are now weighing the benefits of routine screening for GJB2 mutations when evaluating hereditary hearing impairment.

TABLE 15-1

GENES ASSOCIATED WITH NONSYNDROMIC HEARING IMPAIRMENT

GENE LOCUS	GENE/LOCATION
Autosomal recessive	
DFNB1	Gap junction β-2 (GJB2)
	Connexin 26 (Cx26)
DFNB2	MYO7A
DFNB3	MYO15
DFNB4	PDS
DFNB5	OTOF
Autosomal dominant	
DFNA1	DIAPH1
DFNA2	GJB3
DFNA2	KCNQ4
DFNA3	GJB2 (Cx26)
DFNA5	DFNA5
DFNA8/12	TECTA
DFNA9	COCH
DFNA11	MYO7A
DFNA15	POU4F3
X-linked and mitochondrial	
DFN3	Xq21.1
12sRNA	1555 A>G mitochondrial
TRNA-ser	7445 A>G mitochondrial

15.1.3   Evaluation of the Auditory System

HISTORY

The evaluation of the child for possible ear or hearing pathology starts with obtaining a specific history. Behaviors such as inattentiveness, constant use of an inappropriately loud voice, excessive volume on televisions or radios, or even difficulty in classrooms can all be indicators of hearing loss. The onset and duration of hearing losses should be noted because the workup and management of congenital and acquired hearing losses differ. Associated symptoms of pain, pressure, or drainage from the ears are also significant features to note. Symptoms of dizziness in the child are often difficult to evaluate but should be pursued to rule out an inner ear vestibular disorder. Occasionally, the child with vestibular pathology will present with a developmental delay in motor skills or ambulation. A thorough history should also include inquiries into possible trauma to the auditory system. Foreign bodies in the ear canal or insertion of small objects into the ear can damage the external auditory canal, the tympanic membrane, or even the ossicular chain and produce hearing deficits. Obtaining a history of even minor head trauma (eg, a fall) in relation to hearing loss may suggest the diagnosis of enlarged vestibular aqueduct syndrome, the most common bony abnormality of the otic capsule associated with profound sudden sensorineural hearing loss.

A detailed social and family history is also significant in the evaluation of a child for potential ear and/or hearing problems. Social factors such as large institutional day care settings and exposure to second-hand smoke have been linked to an increased incidence of otitis media with effusion. A family history of hearing loss (particularly if one or more first-degree relatives display a similar hearing loss) is significant and may warrant consultation with a geneticist.

Although universal newborn hearing screening is slowly becoming the standard across the United States, a complete history for the auditory system should explore prenatal and perinatal complications such as preeclampsia, infections, premature delivery, low Apgar scores, hyperbilirubinemia, low birth weight, neonatal intensive care unit admission, and ventilatory support. All are associated with an increased risk of hearing loss. At present, most newborn hearing screening programs utilize auditory brainstem responses (ABR) and/or otoacoustic emissions (OAEs) (see below) to evaluate those children at risk. Early involvement of hearing and language specialists in the management of children with hearing deficits is important to ensure that the development of communication skills is optimized. Early identification and, if possible, corrective therapy likely results in improved outcomes.

PHYSICAL EXAMINATION

Evaluation of the auditory system begins with observation of the overall craniofacial appearance. When focusing on the auditory system, pay particular attention to the auricles. The shape of the auricle (eg, normal, "loop" ear deformities, or microtias), the position of the auricle (eg, low-set ears), or any associated skin tags or preauricular pits, suggest a possible abnormality of the auditory system. The specific examination of the ear should then focus on the external meatus and canal. One of the more mundane yet common causes of hearing loss in children is an accumulation of cerumen (or vernix caseosum in the case of the neonate). A thorough exam of the ear requires gentle removal (typically via curettage) of any debris in the external auditory canal. Pulling the auricle posteriorly and superiorly can straighten the ear canal to facilitate examination. Pain triggered by this manipulation of the auricle may suggest the diagnosis of an external otitis.

A pneumatic otoscope is used to examine all structures from the external meatus to the tympanic membrane. Careful choice of the largest speculum that can comfortably fit within the child's ear also facilitates this examination. The normal anterior canal wall of the external auditory canal demonstrates a "bulge" that obscures the anterior one-third to one-half of the tympanic membrane. In order to fully view the tympanic membrane, it is necessary to position the tip of the speculum accurately at this juncture and to angle the examiner's view in an anterior direction. Concomitantly retracting the auricle posteriorly and superiorly also makes this examination easier.

The skin of the external meatus and external auditory canal should be surveyed for erythema, edema, lesions, or drainage. A reddened and swollen external canal with clear or even purulent drainage suggests an external otitis (commonly referred to as "swimmer's ear"). The tympanic membrane should be evaluated for its overall integrity, color, vascularity, translucency, and mobility. Particularly significant areas to examine include the superior part of the tympanic membrane (pars flaccida), where retraction pockets and acquired cholesteatomas frequently originate, the anterior tympanic membrane (an area where congenital cholesteatomas are noted), as well as the remaining pars tensa (which is the most readily visualized portion of the tympanic membrane).

The tympanic membrane is normally a pale white or grayish structure. An erythematous tympanic membrane most commonly suggests an inflammatory process involving either the middle ear space (eg, otitis media) or the drum itself (myringitis). Subtle color changes in the tympanic membrane may suggest underlying vascular abnormalities of the middle ear. A bluish hue to the tympanic membrane can indicate a high jugular bulb protruding into the middle ear space, and a reddish coloration or mass seen in the tympanic membrane might raise the suspicion of an anomalous internal carotid artery in the middle ear. The vascularity of the tympanic membrane itself can also be an indicator of the status of the tympanic membrane and the middle ear space. The normal partial translucency provides some indication of the status of the middle ear structures and space. In the healthy ear, the short process, the manubrium, and the umbo of the malleus are readily visible (see Fig. 15-2). The shadow or outline of the incus and the dense bone of the promontory are also discernible. Middle ear effusions, thickening of the tympanic membrane, or other middle ear pathology such as cholesteatoma may obscure these structures. The intactness of the tympanic membrane (eg, perforated, retracted medially) should also be assessed. Finally, with a speculum that is large enough to seal off the external auditory canal, a pneumatic otoscope should be used to gently move the tympanic membrane with a puff of air. Decreased mobility of the tympanic membrane is most commonly a result of fluid in the middle ear space and can be one of the most useful clinical findings for diagnosing otitis media with effusion.

In most children (beyond the neonate stage), a very crude assessment of hearing can be performed using a simple tuning fork. In the infant, a quietly vibrating tuning fork can be placed next to the child's ear. The child with normal hearing acuity will typically turn the head toward the ear being stimulated. In the older (cooperative) child, the child's responses can provide an indication of grossly normal hearing thresholds or unilateral or bilateral hearing loss. Any abnormalities detected on examination or screening should trigger further evaluation. Audiologic evaluation, as discussed below, should be considered as an integral part in the evaluation of any child with ear or hearing abnormalities.

TESTS OF FUNCTION

Audiometry provides a quantitative measure of hearing and functionally assesses the entire auditory system. A trained audiologist uses one or more of a battery of testing techniques available, depending on the child's age and development. All children with suspected or confirmed ear pathology, suspected congenital hearing loss, or those with a delay in the development of communication skills should undergo formal audiologic testing as early as possible. No child is too young to have a hearing test.

CONVENTIONAL AUDIOMETRY For the cooperative child (typically 5 years or older), an audiometer can be used to measure the child's sensitivity to pure tones (Fig. 15-3). Tones are presented from the low frequencies (usually starting at 256 or 512 Hertz) to the high frequencies (8000 Hertz and occasionally higher) to each ear individually. The child responds when the tone is heard. In most instances, pure tones can be heard at less than 20 to 25 decibels sound pressure level. In addition to pure tone thresholds, speech audiometry can also be performed on cooperative children. The speech reception threshold (SRT) refers to the intensity required to detect *speech* (as opposed to simple pure tones). The SRT is usually similar in value to the pure tone average (the arithmetic mean of the pure tone thresholds at 500, 1000, and 2000 Hertz). The speech recognition score (or speech discrimination) refers to the child's ability to recognize and repeat a standard set of phonetically balanced words presented at an intensity that the child

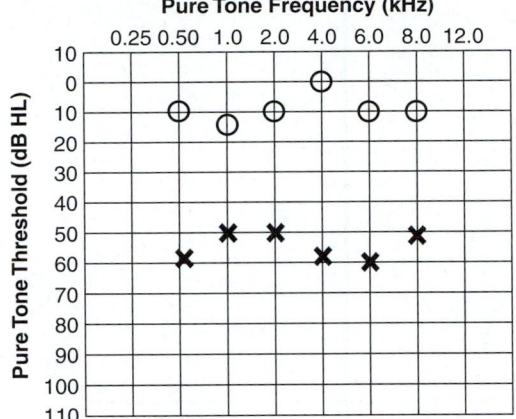

Right			Left		
SRT	Speech Recognition		SRT	Speech Recognition	
15 dB HL	100% dB HL	% dB HL	55 dB HL	70% dB HL	% dB HL

FIGURE 15-3 Conventional audiogram with left-sided hearing loss. O = right; X = left; SRT = speech reception threshold.

should be able to hear comfortably (based on pure tone thresholds and SRT). These standard tests are invaluable in documenting a child's baseline hearing level, determining whether the hearing level will affect the child's development, and providing an objective means of assessing a child's response to treatment for ear disease. For children who are too young to cooperate with these auditory techniques, behavioral testing represents a relatively inexpensive and noninvasive means of assessing a child's hearing levels. Between the ages of 18 months and 5 years, children can be motivated to participate in activities that reflect whether or not a test stimulus was heard. Visual reinforcement audiometry involves testing the child in a sound-treated room with loudspeakers positioned at each side of the child. To maintain the child's interest or to condition the child to respond when auditory stimuli are heard, a toy is typically activated near the speaker that elicited the response. By combining behavioral observation and visual reinforcement audiometry, the audiologist can usually obtain a reasonable impression of a child's auditory capabilities.

EVOKED AUDITORY BRAINSTEM RESPONSES (ABR) AND OTO-ACOUSTIC EMISSIONS (OAEs) TESTING ABR uses scalp electrodes placed on the skin to detect neural impulses following the delivery of various auditory stimuli to the ear (most commonly a broadband click). Computer-based averaging of neural activity allows for the calculation of "latencies" between distinct wave peaks. Evaluation of waveform morphology, the stimulus intensities required to elicit the response, and the latencies of the wave peaks provide a qualitative assessment of the child's auditory system.

Measurement of otoacoustic emissions (OAEs) is an emerging new method for evaluating the peripheral auditory system; it uses an extremely sensitive microphone, placed in the external ear canal close to the tympanic membrane, to measure faint sounds generated by the cochlea either spontaneously (spontaneous OAEs, SOAEs) or in response to auditory stimuli (transient evoked OAEs, TEOAEs, or distortion product OAEs, DPOAEs). Because OAEs are thought

to be generated by the hair cells of the cochlea, they may help identify or rule out the cochlear hair cells as the site of pathology in cases of sensorineural hearing loss.

IMMITTANCE AUDIOMETRY Acoustic immittance is a generic term used to refer to either the opposition (impedance) or ease (admittance) of entry of acoustic energy into the middle ear transmission system. By means of a specialized earplug that seals off the external auditory canal, it is possible to measure the acoustic immittance of the ear. Contained within the earplug are a miniature speaker, air pump, and microphone. The ear normally absorbs sound energy through the tympanic membrane and middle ear structures. Impedance provides an indirect measure of this sound absorption function by measuring the reflected sound energy. The speaker delivers sound into the external auditory canal while the pressure is varied by the air pump. The microphone then detects the sound reflected back from the ear.

In tympanometry, the reflected sound is typically measured while the pressure is varied between -300 and $+300$ cm H_2O. Several patterns of tympanograms are routinely encountered and reflect varying states of middle ear function (Fig. 15-4). A type A tympanogram is normal with the curve peaking around 0 cm H_2O. A type B tympanogram is typically flat or shows only a very shallow peak. Such tympanograms are seen in cases of otitis media with effusion or ossicular fixation. A tympanic membrane perforation can also result in a "flat" tympanogram but would usually be associated with an abnormally large canal volume (also measured routinely during tympanometry). A type C tympanogram most commonly reflects a retracted tympanic membrane and shows a curve that peaks at pressures less than -150 cm H_2O. Less reliably, otosclerosis (fixation of the stapes footplate) may be reflected in a type A_S tympanogram (for shallow). Tympanosclerosis may also show a mild decrease in an otherwise normal curve. Last, a type A_D tympanogram (for deep) shows an abnormally high peak in an otherwise normal curve and is usually associated with ossicular discontinuity or an unusually mobile or atelectatic tympanic membrane.

VESTIBULAR TESTING Several advances in the diagnosis of vestibular dysfunction have improved the diagnostic evaluation of children with dizziness. Among the more traditional tests, electronystagmography (ENG) has proven to be an extremely useful tool. ENG is performed by applying electrodes around the eyes that detect the corneoretinal potential, which assesses eye movements. The function of the inner ear vestibular apparatus is evaluated by stimulating the inner ear calorically (with warm and cold water or air irrigation), which normally produces a characteristic nystagmus based on the vestibuloocular reflex. Cold irrigations in one ear will normally cause a nystagmus in the opposite direction, whereas warm irrigations produce a nystagmus toward the ipsilateral ear. Quantification of the eye movements allows an objective measure of each inner ear's vestibular function and can provide data for discriminating between peripheral and central vestibular dysfunction. Recent improvements in ENG testing include the use of video-infrared ENG systems (video cameras mounted inside a pair of goggles "lock onto" the retina by means of a computer-controlled mechanism). Thus, eye movements can be measured without the need for a corneoretinal potential.

Computerized platform posturography also represents a significant advance in vestibular testing. By using a platform that the test subject stands on, the child's center of gravity can be recorded both

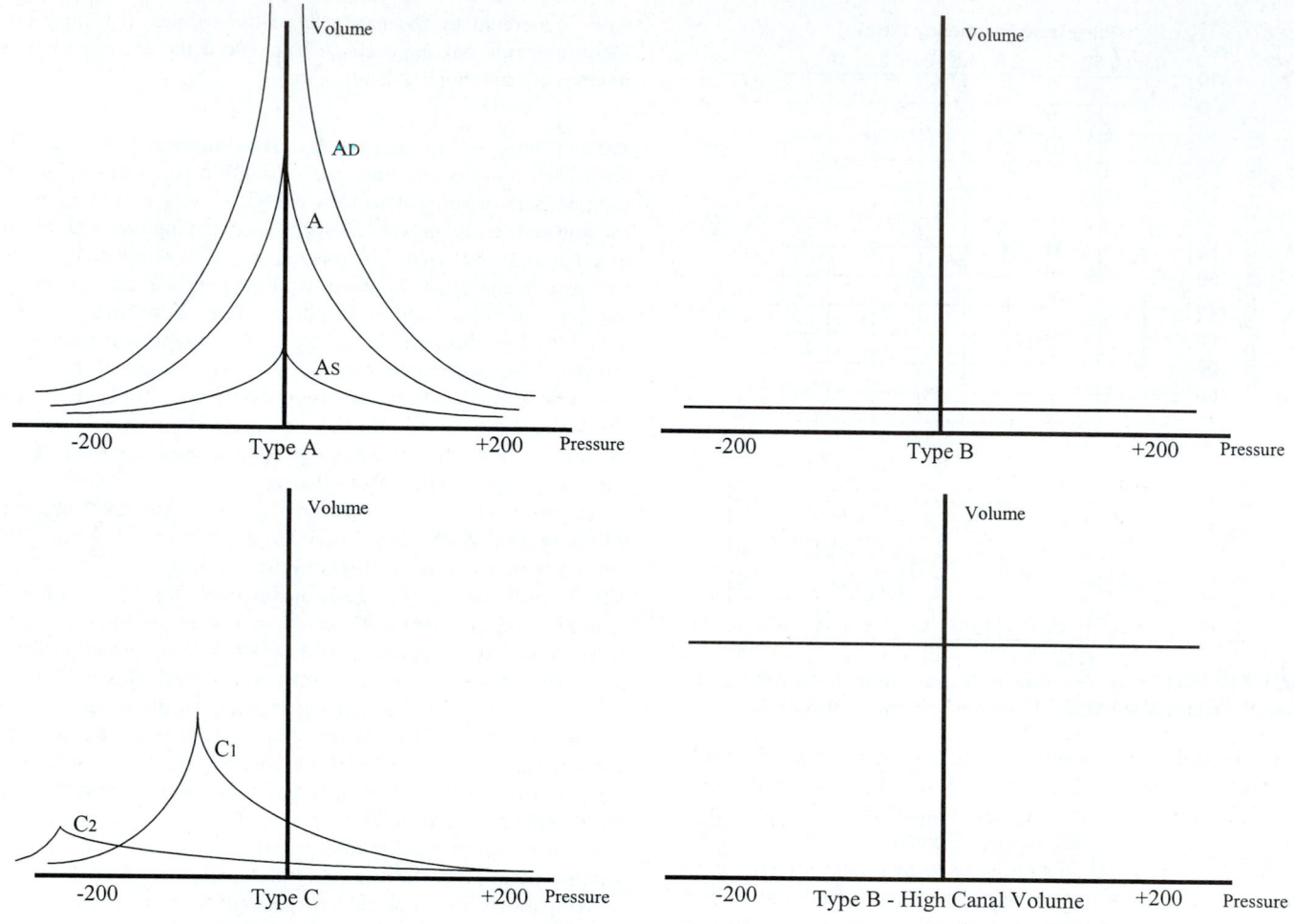

FIGURE 15-4   Illustration of various types of tympanograms. A = normal tympanogram, maximal peak (compliance) seen at 0 mm H$_2$O; A$_S$ = shallow (stiff tympanic membrane as seen with tympanosclerosis or otosclerosis); A$_D$ = deep (hypermobile tympanic membrane as seen with atelectasis or ossicular discontinuity); B = nonmobile tympanic membrane, normal canal volume (a middle ear effusion); type B high canal volume = nonmobile tympanic membrane has no pressure differential across it (tympanostomy tube or perforation); C$_1$ = mild negative middle ear pressure (eustachian tube dysfunction); C$_2$ = negative middle ear pressure below −200 mm H$_2$O (usually a middle ear effusion).

statistically as well as in response to movement of the platform. Data from such tests provide insight into the child's overall balance function, be it centrally or peripherally controlled. Certain patterns of body movements or failures to compensate for platform movement can indicate cerebellar dysfunction.

RADIOGRAPHIC EVALUATION

Imaging studies play an important role in the evaluation of the child with suspected hearing or balance dysfunction. Although plain radiographs and polytomography were once widely used to evaluate the ear, computed tomography (CT) and magnetic resonance imaging (MRI) have replaced these studies.

Optimal axial and coronal CT images of the ear using 1-mm cuts through the temporal bone identify minute pathology that can be significant in the middle ear, mastoid, and inner ear regions. Soft tissue windows are sometimes helpful in delineating soft tissue lesions or masses in the temporal bone. However, bone window images typically provide the greatest information regarding the external, middle, and inner ear regions. In the external and middle ear,

CT can demonstrate opacification of the air spaces, erosion of bony structures or ossicles, atretic plates of the external canal, and other middle ear congenital abnormalities. In the inner ear, CT can clearly show the auditory and vestibular structures of the inner ear labyrinth as well as the internal auditory canal that transmits the facial, cochlear, and vestibular nerves. CT also readily demonstrates aplasias and other malformations of the inner ear. Notably, an enlarged vestibular aqueduct is best demonstrated by CT and likely represents the most common bony abnormality of the otic capsule.

Gadolinium-enhanced MRI provides an excellent means for assessing the soft tissue structures of the ear. Lesions of the middle ear space (eg, cholesteatomas, glomus tympanicum) can often be identified on MRI. One-millimeter cuts through the temporal bone accurately visualize critical neural structures including the facial, cochlear, and vestibular nerves. With the use of gadolinium, these structures can also be evaluated for signs of inflammation or neoplastic involvement (eg, Bell palsy or neurofibroma, respectively).

Because these imaging techniques frequently necessitate sedation (particularly for the younger child), may involve ionizing radiation exposure (CT scanning), and are expensive (MRI more so than CT), the judicious use of these studies is warranted. In most cases of otitis media, for example, temporal bone imaging is not indicated. However, if complications of otitis media arise, whether intratemporal (sensorineural hearing loss, labyrinthine erosion, facial nerve paralysis) or extratemporal (meningitis, extradural abscess, sigmoid sinus thrombophlebitis), then high-resolution imaging techniques greatly facilitate diagnosis and therapeutic decision making. Imaging studies can also play a key role in the diagnosis of the child with vertigo (Sec. 15.1.5).

15.1.4 Congenital and Acquired Hearing Loss

An algorithm for suspected hearing loss is shown in Fig. 15-5. The most common causes of acquired hearing loss in children result from abnormalities of the middle ear, whereas congenital hearing loss is often a result of sensorineural deficits. Table 15-2 lists common causes of congenital hearing loss. A history of maternal "TORCH" infections [acronym for toxoplasmosis, rubella, cytomegalovirus (CMV), herpes simplex, and syphilis] during pregnancy can point toward a likely etiology for congenital hearing loss in a child. Rubella, for example, is particularly associated with cochleosaccular dysplasia and congenital deafness. Prenatal CMV infection accounts for up to 40% of congenital hearing loss. Sensorineural hearing loss is seen in 5 to 10% of children with prenatal CMV infection and in more than 50% of children with severe CMV dis-

ease. A history of maternal drug use during pregnancy may also be important. For example, isoretinoin causes congenital hearing loss with associated malformations of the cochlea, loss of auditory neurons, and general inner ear malformations. Other substances such as alcohol, cocaine, and other "recreational" drugs may also cause congenital hearing loss. Perinatal factors such as prematurity, low birth weight, low Apgar scores, and the need for neonatal intensive care unit admission have all been positively correlated with sensorineural hearing loss. Also, complicated delivery with a history of infant anoxia or severe dystocia requiring forceps delivery may provide insight into the cause of congenital hearing loss. Traumatic deliveries can cause middle ear damage that then results in conductive and/or sensorineural hearing loss.

During the very early postnatal period, routine screening of infants for problems such as hypothyroidism or phenylketonuria is now commonplace. Therefore, the likelihood of missing these etiologies is minimal. Other risk factors for hearing loss at this time include hyperbilirubinemia (typically >17.0 mg/dL), metabolic defects, as well as a wide range of hereditary congenital processes that manifest with hearing loss. The physical examination of the ear in infants should focus on identifying external and middle ear pathologies as well as features that might suggest associated inner ear anomalies. For example, stenosis or atresia of the external auditory canal associated with preauricular pits or skin tags can suggest branchiootorenal syndrome, a fairly common congenital deafness syndrome associated with malformation of the cochlea. Early audiometric testing is essential in suspected congenital hearing loss. As discussed above, accurate audiometric results can be obtained on

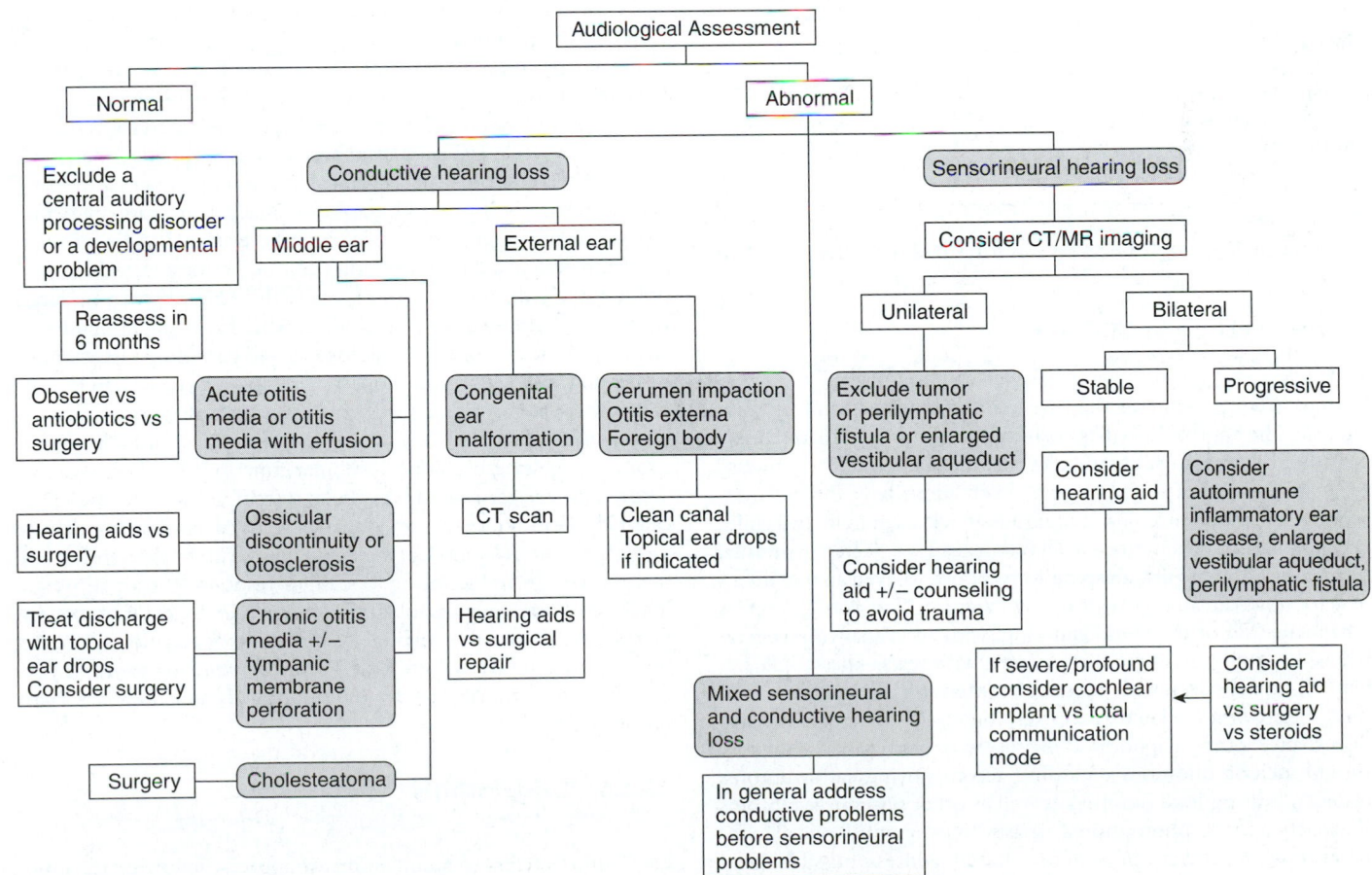

FIGURE 15-5   Algorithm for the evaluation of suspected hearing loss.

TABLE 15-2
CAUSES OF CONGENITAL HEARING LOSS

Infectious
  TORCHS infections
  HIV infection
  Otitis media with effusion
  Acute otitis media
Traumatic
  Birth canal trauma
  Forceps
Developmental defects of the ear
  Cochlear and inner ear dysplasia (eg, Mondini, Scheibe, Michel)
  Enlarged vestibular aqueduct syndrome
  Congenital stapedial footplate fixation
  Congenital aural atresia
  Microtia/anotia with or without aural atresia
  Congenital fusion of the malleus and incus
Hereditary hearing impairment syndromes
  Pendred syndrome
  GJB2 mutations
  Usher syndrome
  Waardenburg syndrome
  Crouzon syndrome
  Neurofibromatosis 2 (also NF-1)
  Alport syndrome
  Apert syndrome
  Hunter syndrome
  Hurler syndrome
  Klippel-Feil syndrome
  Jervell and Lange-Nielsen syndrome
  LEOPARD syndrome
  Goldenhar syndrome
Metabolic
  Diabetes
  Hyperbilirubinemia
  Hypothyroidism
Ototoxicity
  Aminoglycoside antibiotics

any age child through behavioral testing and/or ABR and OAE testing.

15.1.5   Vertigo in Children

Vertigo often presents to the physician with a complaint of "dizziness." The approach to diagnosis is outlined in Fig. 15-6. Differentiating the variety of experiences that may be termed "dizziness" by a child or parent is challenging. Even adults have difficulty describing the experience of a vertiginous attack accurately. In a child, vertigo may not be described at all but instead is reflected in unusual behaviors. Sudden falls, grasping for support, or even an unwillingness to move can all represent signs of vertigo. True vertigo implies a hallucination of the world spinning, with accompanying vegetative signs (pallor and vomiting, as seen with sea sickness). "Dizziness," as may be seen with postural hypotension or cardiac arrhythmias, often is not related to vertigo. Similarly, a history of visual disturbance rarely supports a diagnosis of vertigo. The history should include questions regarding accompanying ear symptoms (otalgia, hearing loss, tinnitus) as well as other systemic symptoms (headache, fever, photophobia, spastic movements, loss of consciousness). A review of systems should address possible head trauma or barotrauma (eg, extreme coughing, straining, or retching) that may result in a perilymphatic fistula, and the family history

should focus on any family members with migraine or seizure disorders.

Physical examination findings of pigmentary lesions (eg, café-au-lait spots) or neurofibromas, signs of trauma, abnormal facies, or congenital abnormalities of the external ear or eyes are meaningful. The otologic exam must rule out middle ear disease as a possible cause for the vertigo. Otitis media with effusion or evidence of acute/chronic suppurative otitis media can cause vertigo or, more frequently, a subtle compromise of balance. Cranial nerve deficits suggest possible brainstem lesions or tumor as an etiology. Abnormal visual tracking, convergence, or saccades as well as spontaneous nystagmus are all important findings in a child with vertigo. Simple tests of balance and coordination are extremely informative in children. Tasks such as hopping on one foot, performing a tandem gait, standing on a foam cushion, or simply standing from a seated position on the floor all may uncover neurologic deficits. Repeating the tasks with eyes closed helps identify those children who have compensated for vestibular deficits by relying on visual cues.

Causes of vertigo are most easily considered as being of either a central or a peripheral etiology (Table 15-3). Congenital anomalies, central nervous system infections or neoplasms, trauma, and vascular anomalies may all present with vertigo. Peripheral disorders involve the labyrinth or eighth nerve. These can either result from congenital abnormalities or may be acquired. The most common peripheral disorders causing vertigo in a child include a posttraumatic perilymphatic fistula (a leakage of inner ear fluid into the middle ear, usually from the oval or round windows), ototoxic medications, cholesteatoma, otitis media, benign positional vertigo, and benign paroxysmal vertigo of childhood. Although the underlying etiology should be addressed where possible, temporary symptomatic improvement may be obtained with vestibular suppressants such as diazepam or meclizine. This also applies in cases where the underlying etiology is unclear. Systemic steroids may be of benefit with central neoplasms and demyelinating disorders, viral labyrinthitis, vestibular neuronitis, and syphilitic inner ear disease. Based on the history and physical examination, appropriate hematologic and serologic tests, audiovestibular testing, imaging studies, or electroencephalographic studies can be performed to help pinpoint a likely diagnosis. All patients with vertigo should undergo routine audiologic testing (including ABR for younger children). Because of the anatomic, physiological, and pathologic associations of hearing loss with vestibulopathy, audiologic studies often provide either diagnostic or supportive data for a diagnosis. Electronystagmography (ENG) similarly represents a critical diagnostic tool in evaluating a child's vestibular function (see Sec. 15.1.3). The functional status of the vestibular system, as measured by ENG, can help distinguish central from peripheral etiologies, identify asymmetries in responses of a given patient's inner ears, and define the percentage reduction in vestibular response for a pathologic inner ear. Potentially useful laboratory tests include a spot glucose to rule out diabetes or hypoglycemia, electrolyte studies, thyroid function tests, and serology for HIV-1, *Borrelia burgdorferi* (Lyme disease pathogen), *Mycobacterium tuberculosis,* and *Treponema pallidum* (FTA-Abs).

15.1.6   Labyrinthitis

Labyrinthitis refers to an inflammatory process involving the inner ear (membranous labyrinth). Accordingly, the manifestations of labyrinthitis are typically vertigo, hearing loss, and tinnitus. The

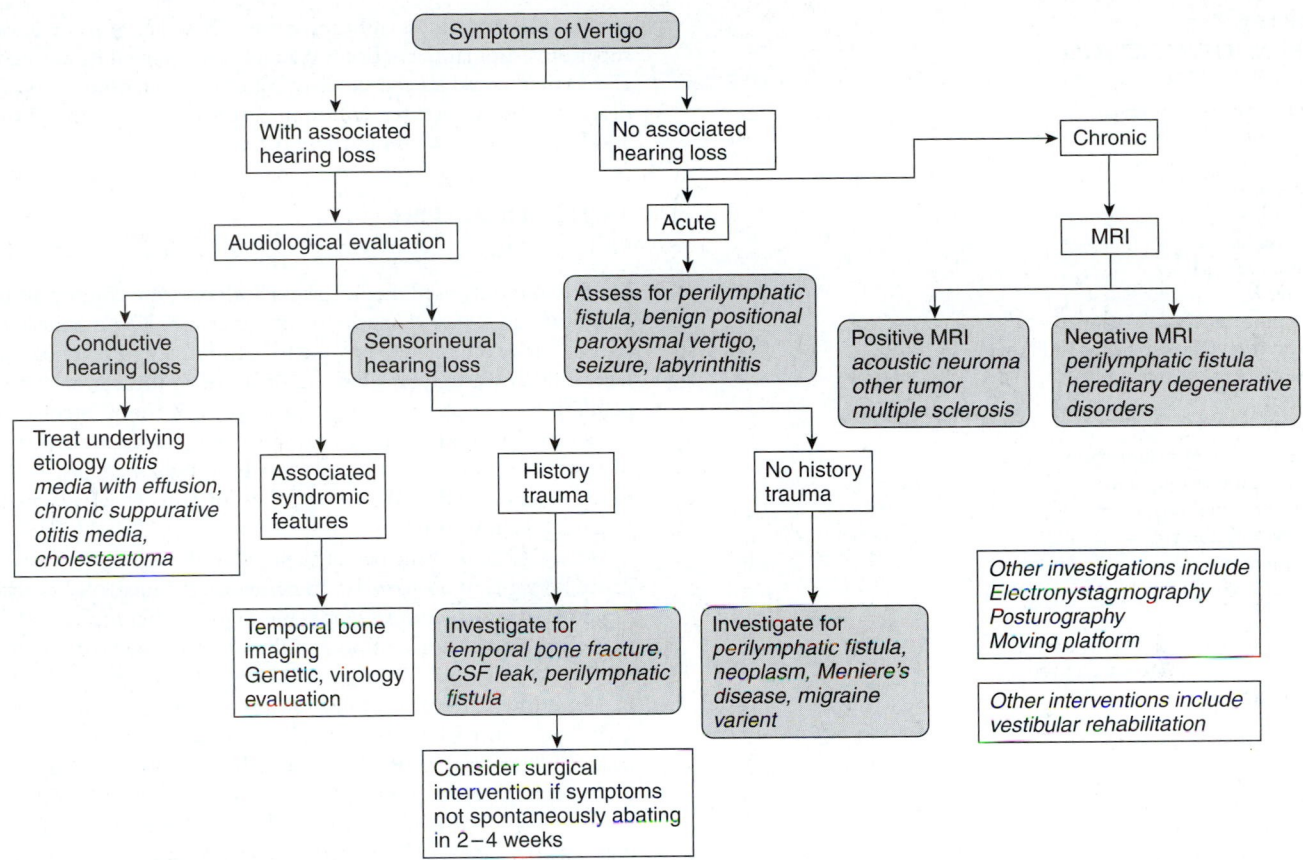

FIGURE 15-6 Algorithm for the evaluation of vertigo.

severity of symptoms correlates with the intensity and etiology of the inflammatory process in the inner ear. In cases of serous labyrinthitis, symptoms are typically mild, with the child complaining of "dizziness" without any substantial hearing loss. Most cases of serous labyrinthitis seem to be associated with concomitant acute or chronic otitis media. It has been hypothesized that the action of inflammatory cytokines through the round or oval windows may play a role in eliciting the inner ear inflammatory response.

Management of children with serous labyrinthitis is symptomatic and supportive, with treatment of the middle ear disease if present. In contrast, viral labyrinthitis is often associated with a preceding systemic viral illness or upper respiratory tract infection. Patients often report a sudden onset of vertigo or progressive dizziness. Sensorineural hearing loss is rarely a feature of viral inner ear infection in children. Systemic steroids or antiviral therapies have not been demonstrated to be beneficial. Usually, symptoms gradually abate over the course of 1 to 2 weeks. However, when viral labyrinthitis is caused by measles, mumps, rubella, and cytomegalovirus (CMV), sensorineural hearing loss is common. In the case of rubella and CMV, prenatal infection has frequently been associated with congenital deafness.

Bacterial labyrinthitis is usually a consequence of meningitis and presents as a much more acute process than serous labyrinthitis, with severe vertigo and acute hearing loss. Inoculation of the inner ear fluids by pathogenic bacteria through preformed pathways and/or the cerebrospinal fluid is the most likely mechanisms of infection. Loss of cochlear and vestibular hair cells, secondary scarring, and ossification of the labyrinth often follow bacterial labyrinthitis, which explains why spontaneous recovery of hearing is unlikely. If bacterial labyrinthitis is suspected, parenteral antimicrobial therapy

is indicated, along with antiemetics. When it is seen in conjunction with other acute infectious processes (eg, meningitis), treatment is obviously directed at the primary (as well as concurrent) pathologies.

15.1.7   Neoplasms of the Ear

Neoplasms of the ear are rare in childhood, with benign lesions being far more common than malignancy. Osteomas can present as smooth bumps or masses in the external auditory canal. These are most commonly noted in swimmers and result from cold-water exposure. Exostoses are also benign bony outgrowths in the external canal and require intervention only if they occlude the canal, causing hearing loss or other problems. Middle ear tumors such as glomus tympanicum are unusual in the pediatric population. However, "normal" anatomic variants masquerading as vascular middle ear masses do occur. Aberrant internal carotid arteries have infrequently been reported as reddish pulsatile masses as viewed through the tympanic membrane on otoscopy. Similarly, a bluish mass seen in the middle ear space by otoscopy may represent a (dehiscent) high-riding jugular bulb. Such "lesions" can cause middle ear symptoms (hearing loss, otalgia, otorrhea, etc) and should be evaluated by imaging studies (CT and/or MRI-MRA). Other lesions of the middle ear and mastoid system should be considered when otologic symptoms persist despite normal findings, routine treatment, or other interventions. Eosinophilic granuloma has been reported to manifest in the temporal bone, and other lesions such as histiocytosis, rhabdomyosarcomas, and lymphomas may also present atypically as ear disease. Leukemic or lymphomatous in-

TABLE 15-3
CAUSES OF VERTIGO

Central vertigo etiologies
Congenital
  Chiari malformations
Infections
  Meningitis
  Encephalitis
  Brain abscess
Neoplasm
  Tumors of the cerebellum
  Tumors of the cerebellopontine angle
  Tumors of the brainstem
Trauma
Vascular
  Arteriovenous malformations
  Basilar artery migraine
Demyelinating disorders
Cerebellar ataxias
Seizure disorders
Peripheral vertigo etiologies
Congenital
  Labyrinthine dysplasia/aplasia
  Stenosis of the internal auditory canal
  Congenital cholesteatoma
Genetic
  Waardenburg syndrome
  Usher syndrome
  Pendred syndrome
  Alport syndrome
  Down syndrome
Infection
  Otitis media with effusion
  Suppurative otitis media
  Cholesteatoma
  Bacterial labyrinthitis
  Viral labyrinthitis
  Syphilitic inner ear disease
  Lyme disease
  Vestibular neuronitis
Trauma
  Perilymphatic fistula
  Labyrinthine concussion
  Iatrogenic/surgical
Ototoxins
  Aminoglycosides
  Chemotherapeutic drugs
Radiation
Benign positional vertigo
Benign paroxysmal vertigo of childhood
Benign paroxysmal torticollis

volvement of the petrous apex marrow spaces has also been reported as a site of neoplastic disease in children. Treatment of these children is directed at the overall, underlying pathology with ear-specific treatments indicated only for specific sequelae (eg, facial paralysis, refractory otalgia, and otorrhea).

Inner ear tumors seen in the pediatric population most commonly involve the retrocochlear structures (eg, seventh and eighth cranial nerve complexes). Facial nerve neuromas or hemangiomas of the geniculate ganglion of the facial nerve represent temporal bone neoplasms that would likely present as facial paresis or paralysis. Vestibular schwannomas (typically as part of neurofibromatosis type II in the pediatric population), in contrast, often present with complaints of dizziness or hearing loss. These neurofibromas of the superior vestibular nerve occur bilaterally in neurofibromatosis type II and by themselves can be diagnostic. Early identification of this disease and surgical intervention may allow preservation of hearing and facial nerve function in these patients.

15.1.8   Ototoxicity

Many commonly used medications (both over the counter and prescription) can cause damage to the inner ear. The manifestations of ototoxicity can include hearing loss, tinnitus, and vestibulopathy, with different drugs causing one or more of these symptoms depending on the pharmacologic properties of the particular drug. For many drugs, ototoxicity is a well-known risk, and the benefits of treatment with any of them must be weighed against the risks to the inner ear in their use. A partial list of drugs that have ototoxic potential is shown in Table 15-4.

Several groups in the pediatric population require increased vigilance for signs of ototoxicity. In neonates, the incidence of serious gram-negative infections (sepsis, meningitis, pneumonias, etc) requires the frequent use of potentially ototoxic medications, which explains in part why children with a history of prematurity and neonatal intensive care unit admission have a higher incidence of sensorineural hearing loss and vestibular problems (including delay in head and postural control, positional nystagmus, and abnormal ENG findings such as directional preponderance and reduced caloric responses). Renal (and perhaps other organ) transplant patients also show a higher incidence of hearing and balance disorders, but in this population it is unclear whether inner ear problems result from the frequent need for ototoxic medications, previous dialysis, or more subtle metabolic abnormalities encountered in dialysis/transplant patients. Finally, children receiving chemotherapy are also at increased risk for inner ear damage from chemotherapeutic agents. Cisplatin, for example, has a well-documented effect on cochlear hair cells and is most commonly associated with a high-frequency hearing loss.

TABLE 15-4
COMMON OTOTOXIC DRUGS

Aminoglycosides
  Gentamicin
  Amikacin
Tobramycin
Streptomycin
Neomycin
Kanamycin
Chemotherapeutic drugs
  Cisplatin/carboplatin
  Nitrogen mustards
Misonidazole
Vincristine
Chlorhexidine
Erythromycin
Loop diuretics
  Ethacrynic acid
  Furosemide
Propylene glycol
Quinine
Salicylates
Vancomycin

Other drugs such as aspirin (and other salicylates) demonstrate reversible ototoxicity if stopped in a timely manner after onset of inner ear symptoms. Furosemide by itself has been reported to cause sensorineural hearing loss but has also been shown to potentiate the ototoxic effects of other drugs, such as aminoglycosides. As discussed above, the use of any potentially ototoxic medication needs to be weighed against the benefits of its therapeutic purpose. Complaints of subjective hearing loss, tinnitus, or disequilibrium may be the earliest signs of ototoxicity. Patients at high risk should undergo regularly scheduled audiologic testing before, during, and after treatment to measure and document any hearing changes. Similarly, serial ENG testing may be useful in cases of vestibulotoxicity.

Virtually all eardrops contain potentially ototoxic components, whether the active ingredients or solutes or preservatives. However, documented cases of permanent sensorineural hearing loss or vestibulopathy resulting from ototopic medications are rare. The recently introduced fluroquinolone ear drops (Floxin™, Ciloxan™) are not ototoxic and may be used safely even in the middle ear (usually via a tympanostomy tube).

15.1.9   Otitis Media

Otitis media was first described by Hippocrates, and although myringotomy and tympanocentesis have been intermittently utilized in its treatment since that time, until comparatively recently intervention had been primarily directed toward treatment of the complications of otitis media. In the preantibiotic era, the primary concern was the potential for intracranial complications of acute otitis media, which were a significant cause of mortality. Currently in the First World, mortality as a consequence of otitis media is so rare as to be occasionally (and regrettably) forgotten in the plethora of treatment guidelines available. Concern about the potential complications of acute otitis media have been supplanted by concerns about the potential long-term consequences of otitis media and the emergence of resistant organisms as a result of the liberal use of antibiotic therapies for otitis media.

Otitis media may be considered as three distinct entities: acute otitis media, otitis media with effusion, and chronic suppurative otitis media. It is estimated that in the United States alone over $5 billion is spent each year in the management of otitis media, with much of this being indirect costs such as lost parental productivity. Over 30 million prescriptions are filled each year in the United States for otitis media, accounting for 40% of all prescriptions for children under the age of 10. Otitis media is also the most common cause of visits to the doctor by children in the United States. Over 1 million sets of tympanostomy tubes are inserted each year, and between 2 and 6% of children have had at least one set of tympanostomy tubes by the age of 4.

Despite the prevalence of otitis media, there is still vigorous debate on the appropriate treatment of children with acute otitis media and otitis media with effusion. Three primary management modalities are utilized, namely, watchful waiting, antibiotic therapy, or placement of tympanostomy tubes. There have been few true advances in the care of otitis media since the reintroduction of the tympanostomy tube by Armstrong in 1954. Other forms of treatment, including antihistamines, decongestants, and tonsillectomy, have been of little or no efficacy. Limited benefit has been achieved with the use of xylitol gum and Otovent balloons. More recently newer alternatives such as vaccination and laser myringotomy have

been introduced, but their impact on the management of otitis media is not yet established.

ACUTE OTITIS MEDIA

Acute otitis media is a purulent middle ear effusion with systemic signs of illness. Acute otitis media is a disease of the young child, with the highest incidence of disease occurring in the 9-month to 4-year age group. It is estimated that 90% of children have at least one episode of acute otitis media by the age of 2 years.

ETIOLOGY The eustachian tube is shorter and narrower in children under 6 years of age than in the adult, which predisposes the child to obstruction of the eustachian tube. During a common cold the mucosal edema may cause partial or complete obstruction of the eustachian tube, and as surrounding capillaries absorb oxygen from the middle ear space, negative pressure in the middle ear space will result. Although this may in itself be enough to allow a transudate to form in the middle ear space, a viral infection of the respiratory epithelium in the middle ear space may promote an exudate in the same fashion that rhinorrhea is a consequence of the common cold. There are a variety of described risk factors, as diverse as male predisposition and positive family history, but the factor that by far outweighs any other is the common cold. Other less important risk factors include passive smoking, daycare attendance, or the presence of an older sibling in the household. The average preschool child will be exposed to as many as 10 to 12 upper respiratory tract infections each year, each carrying a significant risk of acute otitis media or otitis media with effusion.

Acute otitis media may occasionally be entirely viral in nature, but usually viral infection acts as a cofactor for a bacterial infection—a middle ear effusion is an excellent culture medium. In over 40% of cases of acute otitis media, viral particles may be isolated from the middle ear effusion, with the most common being respiratory syncytial virus (RSV). However, the most significant pathogens are bacterial, which may coexist with viral particles in the middle ear fluid. Not surprisingly, the bacteria found in middle ear fluid closely mirror the bacteria found in the nasopharynx, with recent data showing *Streptococcus pneumoniae* in 40% (of which 40% are penicillin resistant); *Hemophilus influenzae* in 25% (of which 25% are β-lactamase producers), and *Moraxella catarrhalis* in 12% (of which 100% are β-lactamase producers). In over 20% of isolates no bacteria are cultured.

Some groups of children are predisposed to acute otitis media. Neonates and children with immunodeficiency are more prone to acute otitis media with enterococci, group A β-hemolytic *Streptococcus*, and *Staphylococcus aureus*. In very rare cases there may be examples of tuberculous otitis media or otitis media complicating scarlet fever, both of which may cause extensive damage to the tympanic membrane and ossicles.

DIAGNOSIS The most common presenting symptom in acute otitis media is ear pain. In this regard children are unlike adults in that 90% of children with otalgia have an underlying otic cause for their pain, whereas the converse is true in adults. The most common nonotic causes of ear pain in the child are tonsillitis and temporomandibular joint problems. Presenting symptoms may include an associated sore throat, night restlessness, and fever. However, many children with acute otitis media (especially those less than 2 years of age) may not complain of ear pain and may not have an associated fever. It is not uncommon for the first presenting sign to be a discharging ear following tympanic membrane rupture. In the older child the classic symptoms are of the rapid onset of pain, irritability, lethargy, and fever.

A clinical diagnosis requires otoscopy and pneumatic otoscopy. The classical findings include erythema and edema of the tympanic membrane, which bulges laterally and through which a frankly purulent effusion may be seen. The normal tympanic membrane landmarks, such as the handle of the malleus, may be completely obscured. There may be associated blistering of the tympanic membrane, which should be differentiated from bullous myringitis (characterized by intense pain in the absence of an effusion). Erythema of the tympanic membrane may occur solely as a result of crying in a child, but use of pneumatic otoscopy will help establish whether an effusion is indeed present.

Tympanometry is a useful adjunct to pneumatic otoscopy, although it does not replace it. A flat (type B) tympanogram or a tympanogram with marked negative middle ear pressure (type C_2) are suggestive of a middle ear effusion (see Fig. 15-4). However, the diagnosis of acute otitis media still remains primarily a clinical one.

COMPLICATIONS In the preantibiotic era acute otitis media was a significant cause of pediatric mortality and morbidity, and this is still partly true in countries with poor access to medical resources. World Health Organization statistics from 1993 suggest that otitis media caused 51,000 deaths in children under the age of 5 in developing countries. Meanwhile, in developed countries the incidence of mortality associated with acute otitis media has plummeted since the introduction of antibiotics in the 1930s, but complications of acute otitis media are still potentially serious.

If acute otitis media is considered an abscess of the middle ear space, then the potential complications of acute otitis media can be conceptualized by considering the direction of spread of infection. The most common sequelae occur when the tympanic membrane perforates laterally, with drainage into the external ear canal. This normally causes the instant resolution of symptoms, and the perforation normally heals within 12 to 48 hours. In a small percentage of cases a permanent perforation may result. If infection is confined to the middle ear space, other complications may ensue. The long process of the incus at the incudostapedial joint is a vascular watershed, and thrombophlebitis affecting the tiny arterioles in this area may lead to avascular necrosis of the long process of the incus with an associated conductive hearing loss. The other potential complication of infection within the middle ear space is peripheral facial nerve palsy. Although the facial nerve normally travels in a bony canal in its complicated course through the middle ear, up to 55% of individuals have small areas where the bony covering is incomplete, particularly in the area of the oval window. Therefore, middle ear inflammation may cause edema of the exposed nerve, compromising its venous return within the surrounding bony canal and resulting in peripheral facial nerve palsy. Although full recovery of facial nerve function can be expected in virtually all cases, it is still recommended that the patient have insertion of a tympanostomy tube and be started on systemic antibiotic therapy. A tympanostomy tube not only serves to drain pus but also allows for antibiotic and steroid eardrops to be placed directly into the middle ear space.

If the infection spreads posteriorly, then acute mastoiditis may occur. Technically, any episode of acute otitis media has associated mastoiditis, but the term *acute coalescent mastoiditis* has commonly been reserved for bony necrosis of the septa within the mastoid air cell system and an associated subperiosteal abscess over the mastoid

process. The patient usually complains of severe pain with fever, and on examination there is inflammation and swelling behind the ear, usually with edema and bogginess over the mastoid process, causing a lateral displacement of the auricle from the head (Fig. 15-7). Otoscopically the posterior canal skin is edematous and tends to sag anteriorly, often occluding the external ear canal. Surgical treatment with cortical mastoidectomy is indicated. An associated complication is sigmoid sinus thrombosis with inflammation in the mastoid, causing thrombophlebitis of small vessels in communication with the sigmoid sinus. The sigmoid sinus not only is thrombosed but is also infected, and the clot may spread in retrograde and antegrade directions. The classic presentation with intermittent fever results from septic emboli propagating down the internal jugular vein to the lung, where cavitating abscesses may form. The treatment is again surgical, although anticoagulation may be required postoperatively. Rarely the spread of infection may be in an inferior direction with rupture of the mastoid tip, causing abscess formation medial or anterior to the sternocleidomastoid muscle (Bezold abscess). This may present with torticollis. If the spread of infection is medial, then serous labyrinthitis may result, with mild nausea or vertigo from the penetration of bacterial endotoxins into the inner ear through the round or oval windows. Very rarely acute bacterial labyrinthitis may result with severe vertigo, nystagmus, vomiting, and profound sensorineural hearing loss. This is a life-threatening condition and may require open surgical drainage of the labyrinth. In some children the mastoid air cell system may extend medially enough to pneumatize the petrous apex. Acute infection in this region presents with otitis media, deep retroorbital pain from trigeminal nerve involvement, and sixth cranial nerve paralysis (Gradenigo syndrome). This also requires surgical management.

The potentially most devastating complications of acute otitis media arise when infection travels superiorly, usually secondary to thrombophlebitis of small venae communicantes. Depending on the depth of penetration, this may present as an epidural abscess, a subdural abscess, meningitis, a cerebral abscess (usually of the temporal lobe), or very rarely otitic hydrocephalus. Even with prompt and appropriate treatment of meningitis, 10% of children will acquire permanent profound sensorineural hearing loss. Epidural and

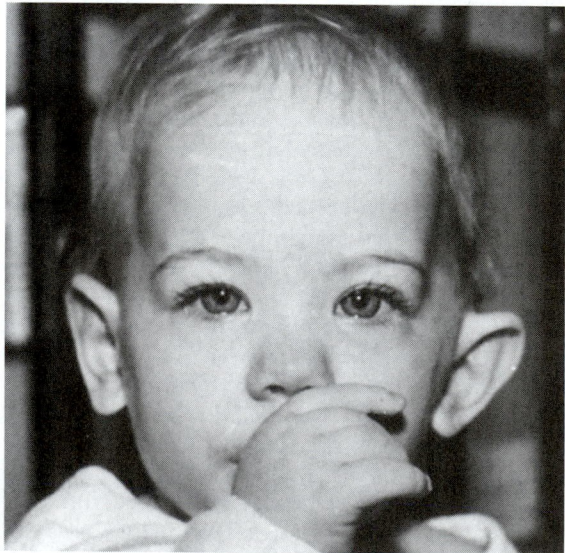

FIGURE 15-7   Child with coalescent mastoiditis. Note the downward and lateral displacement of the left auricle.

subdural abscesses may be extremely subtle on initial presentation. However, a temporal lobe abscess will classically present with complex focal seizures. Gadolinium-enhanced MRI scan is the investigation of choice, with subsequent lumbar puncture if indicated.

TREATMENT Acute otitis media resolves spontaneously in over 80% of cases. Traditionally there have been three main management options, namely, observation without the use of antibiotics, antibiotics, and tympanostomy tubes. Antibiotic treatment is the most prevalent intervention in the majority of the developed world. However, concerns about an increasing incidence of multiply drug-

resistant *Streptococcus pneumoniae* necessitates a reevaluation of this policy. A management algorithm is shown in Fig. 15-8.

The primary aim of treatment is to relieve symptoms and prevent complications. With or without antibiotic treatment, 60% of children are pain-free within 24 hours. Even after a week of treatment, antibiotic therapy is only marginally more effective in relieving symptoms than a placebo. In several parts of the world, initial non-antibiotic treatment of acute otitis media is the standard of care, yet there are few detectable differences in the overall complication rate from acute otitis media compared to countries where initial antibiotic usage is routine. If antibiotic treatment is withheld, close

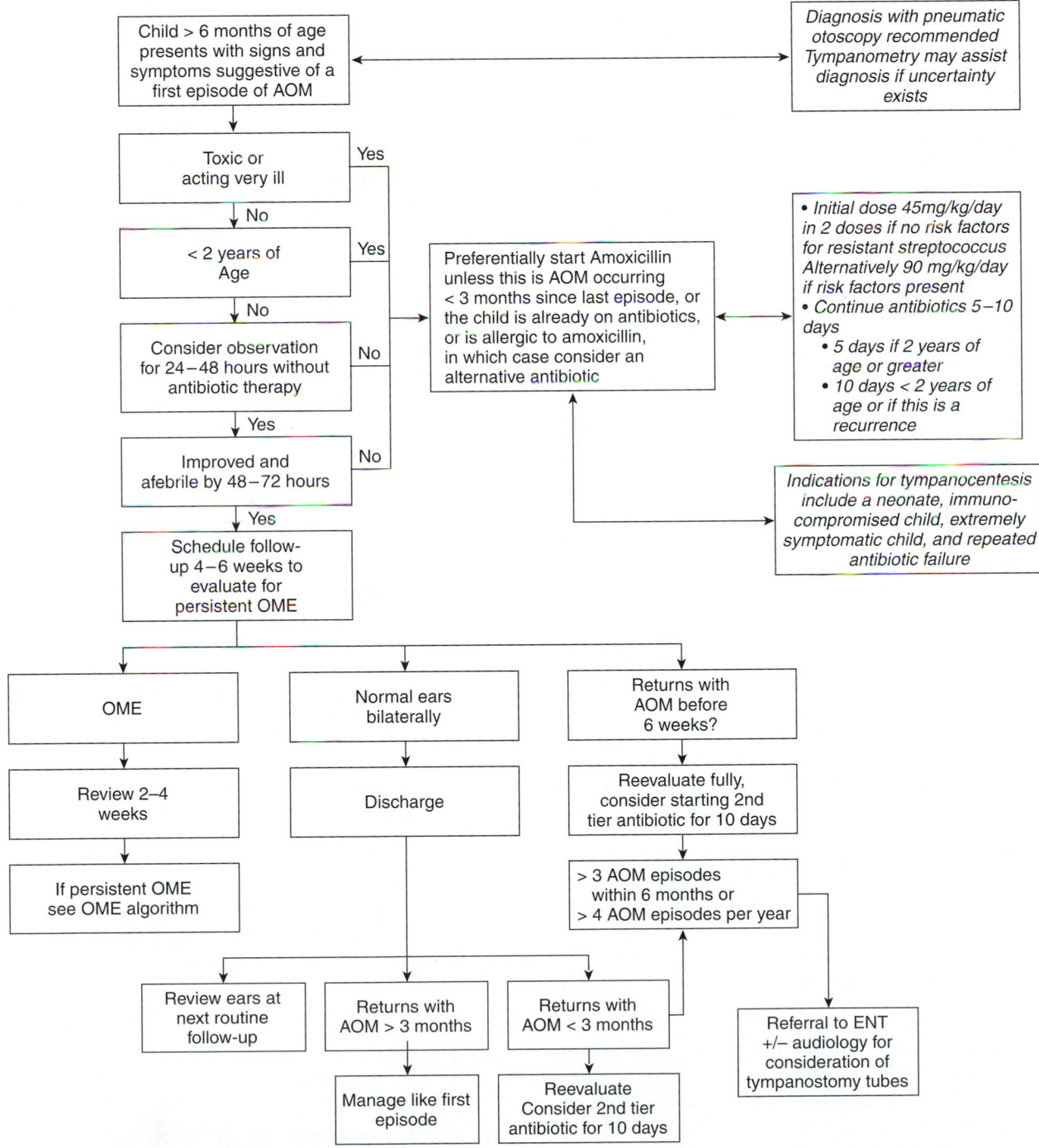

FIGURE 15-8 Management of acute otitis media. AOM = acute otitis media; OME = otitis media with effusion.

monitoring is mandatory, and if there is no improvement within 48 hours, antibiotic treatment should be instituted.

Selection of an antibiotic depends on the sensitivities of the most common bacteria causing otitis media, the concentration of the antibiotic attained in the middle ear, and the cost. The organisms that commonly cause otitis media are *Streptococcus pneumoniae, Hemophilus influenzae,* and *Moraxella catarrhalis.* Of these, in about 25% of cases β-lactamase-producing organisms are pathogenic. Therefore, the first-line choice under these circumstances remains amoxicillin, either in standard dosage (45 mg/kg/d), or in high dosage (90 mg/kg/d) for children at risk of drug-resistant *Streptococcus pneumoniae.* Amoxicillin attains very high concentrations in the middle ear, exceeding the MIC 90 of most streptococcal species. Because 80% of cases of acute otitis media resolve without antibiotic treatment, only 5% will be treatment failures because of resistance to amoxicillin. It should also be noted that although virtually 100% of *Moraxella catarrhalis* are β-lactamase producers, it remains a mildly pathogenic organism with a spontaneous resolution rate greater than 80% and a much lower complication rate than other pathogens.

There is consensus that amoxicillin is the appropriate first-line drug for acute otitis media, but there is little consensus on second- or third-line antibiotics. If amoxicillin fails, then high-dose amoxicillin plus clavulanate (ideally maintaining the standard dose of clavulanate while increasing the relative amount of amoxicillin) or, alternatively, cefuroxime or intramuscular ceftriaxone is the currently recommended alternative. In a child allergic to penicillin or cephalosporins, trimethoprim-sulfamethoxazole or a macrolide may be appropriate. Children over 2 years should be treated with antibiotics for 5 days, and children under 2 years should be treated for 10 days.

The organism most likely to cause treatment failure is multiply drug-resistant *Streptococcus pneumoniae,* and the risk factors for this include geographic prevalence, prolonged low-dose antibiotic therapy, a recent course of antibiotics, daycare attendance, age less than 2 years, and the winter season. Although an isolated episode of acute otitis media is one of the most common causes of nonwell child visits to the pediatrician and is usually easily managed, the public health implications are of concern. The current increasing incidence of multiply drug-resistant *Streptococcus pneumoniae* is in large part a result of injudicious use of antibiotics in the treatment of otitis media. It is also estimated that the total cost per episode of acute otitis media over a 3-month period is over $1300, less than 10% of this being direct cost to the patient in terms of antibiotics and doctors' fees.

Children with acute otitis media should be reassessed 8 weeks following the episode to ensure that they do not have persistent otitis media with effusion as sequelae of the acute otitis media. If a child who has failed first- or second-line treatment is extremely symptomatic or is immunocompromised, tympanocentesis or myringotomy should be considered. Tympanocentesis is reasonably straightforward. A 22-gauge spinal needle is used to puncture the anterior inferior quadrant of the tympanic membrane. However, its use is controversial because of the low but real risk of complications, including potential damage to the ossicular chain, the oval window, and rarely bleeding if there are anatomic variants such as a high-riding jugular bulb or an aberrant internal carotid artery. Therefore, it is recommended that the technique be utilized by individuals trained appropriately, and with an awareness of the relevant anatomy. A possible alternative to tympanocentesis is laser myringotomy.

RECURRENT ACUTE OTITIS MEDIA

A proportion of children have recurrent bouts of acute otitis media, occasionally with a background of otitis media with effusion. At least three episodes of acute otitis media in 6 months are required to merit a diagnosis of recurrent acute otitis media. After such a diagnosis is made, over 50% of children will have one or no further episodes in the following year no matter what treatment option is chosen. If a second episode of acute otitis media occurs more than 90 days following the first, this is not a treatment failure but an isolated new episode, and therefore first-line antibiotic therapy is appropriate if indicated.

Available treatment options include treating each episode as an isolated entity, commencing prophylactic antibiotics, or tympanostomy tube placement. Of children placed on prophylactic antibiotics, a high proportion will still have breakthrough episodes of acute otitis media, which are more likely to be caused by multiply drug-resistant organisms. Because of the current concerns about the emergence of antibiotic-resistant organisms, prophylactic antibiotic treatment seems increasingly less justifiable. Indications for tympanostomy tube placement include recurrent acute otitis media with over three episodes over a 6-month period or four episodes over a 12-month period with one having occurred recently. Tympanostomy tube placement may also be considered in children with multiple drug allergies or children who are excessively symptomatic or who respond poorly to other treatment. Alternative treatment modalities such as the use of xylitol gum, laser myringotomy, and pneumococcal vaccination are currently of only limited efficacy. Laser myringotomy is an attractive alternative to tympanocentesis or myringotomy, but limited data are available.

ACUTE OTITIS MEDIA ASSOCIATED WITH TYMPANOSTOMY TUBES

In a child with tympanostomy tubes, acute otitis media may still occur, presenting as a discharging ear, usually without pain or fever. Although this may occur as a result of contaminated water penetrating the tympanostomy tube to enter the middle ear space (eg, bath water, pool water), it is much more likely to occur as a result of a concurrent upper respiratory tract infection. Treatment with antibiotic eardrops is usually effective, although systemic antibiotics (amoxicillin ± clavulanate) may also be indicated, especially if there is a tenacious exudate that may interfere with appropriate administration of the eardrops. A recent advance has been the introduction of quinilone antibiotic eardrops (Floxin™, Ciloxan™), which are extremely effective, well tolerated, and nonototoxic. An antibiotic and steroid combination eardrop (Cipro HC™) may be utilized if desired. However, for antibiotic eardrops to be effective, they must penetrate the tympanostomy tube to reach the middle ear space. Most formulations require at least seven drops per application to penetrate into the middle ear space. Tragal pumping is important to improve penetration. A proportion of children with recurrent ear discharge may have bacterial colonization of the tympanostomy tube itself, usually because of a bacterial biofilm, which may be extremely resistant to bacterial eradication. In such circumstances removal of the tympanostomy tube may be required.

OTITIS MEDIA WITH EFFUSION

An effusion of the middle ear without evidence of an acute or systemic infection is described as *otitis media with effusion. Chronic otitis media with effusion* occurs when the effusion is present for over 3 months, whereas *persistent otitis media with effusion* may be defined as an effusion present for over a month. Synonyms include serous otitis, secretory otitis, glue ear, and middle ear catarrh. Unlike acute otitis media, otitis media with effusion is probably an underdiagnosed condition, especially if pneumatic otoscopy is not included in the diagnostic evaluation.

ETIOLOGY As with acute otitis media, the pathogenesis of otitis media with effusion involves an immature or dysfunctional eustachian tube. The highest incidence occurs in the 1- to 8-year-old age range, and the prevalence of the disorder may be as high as 20% during the winter season in this age group. Children with anatomic compromise of eustachian tube function, including those with Down syndrome, cleft palate, or any other midfacial deformity, are at increased risk, as are those with immunologic deficiency such as IgA or IgG subtype deficiencies. Upper respiratory tract infections are usually associated with the onset of otitis media with effusion and with acute otitis media, which in turn may progress to persistent otitis media with effusion. Adenoid hypertrophy may also cause eustachian tube obstruction, but it is more likely that chronic bacterial colonization of the adenoids predisposes to otitis media with effusion. Other less significant risk factors include allergy and cigarette smoke exposure and anatomic obstruction of the eustachian tube by nasogastric tubes, endotracheal tubes, or, rarely, by a nasopharyngeal carcinoma or juvenile nasopharyngeal angiofibroma.

The organisms associated with otitis media with effusion closely mirror those found on nasopharyngeal culture and those found in acute otitis media. A culture of middle ear fluid will be positive in up to 74% of cases, with *Streptococcus pneumoniae, Hemophilus influenzae,* and *Moraxella catarrhalis* present in similar proportions as seen in acute otitis media. Depending on geographic antibiotic resistance patterns, over 40% of middle ear bacterial isolates may be penicillin-resistant organisms.

DIAGNOSIS Otitis media with effusion may be silent in its presenting symptomatology and may be an incidental finding. There may be subjective symptoms such as mild balance disturbance, especially in younger children, or a change in a child's behavior. The major symptom and concern is hearing loss. Hearing can vary between a 0- and 40-decibel conductive loss with an effusion, and if the effusion is unilateral, there may be no appreciable hearing loss.

The mainstay of diagnosis is pneumatic otoscopy, which shows a retracted tympanic membrane with decreased mobility of the membrane. Fluid may be appreciated through a translucent tympanic membrane, particularly if the fluid is yellow or amber, and particularly if air bubbles or an air/fluid level is present. With eustachian tube dysfunction, the tympanic membrane may be retracted without an effusion present. Supportive testing includes tympanometry (see Fig. 15-4), acoustic reflectometry, and audiometry (see Sec. 15.1.3). Tympanometry may show a flat (type B) tympanogram or a negative-pressure (type C_2) tympanogram. Although it is possible to have a type C_2 or type B tympanogram without a middle ear effusion being present, it is very unusual to have a type A (normal peaked) tympanogram with an effusion present. Acoustic reflectometry is neither as sensitive nor as specific as tympanometry but has particular advantages with repeated measurements in an otitis-prone child, in that it is excellent in picking up a change of status of the middle ear of an individual child. This device is currently being marketed directly to families, and it may provide a useful parental guide as to when a child has otitis media.

Audiometry is the best method for checking the degree of hearing loss of a child and may be utilized at any age, as discussed in Sec. 15.1.3.

COMPLICATIONS Otitis media with effusion is the most common cause of persistent and fluctuant hearing impairment in children. A persistent effusion may cause delayed language and speech development and may place a child at a serious educational disadvantage. Some evidence suggests that prolonged auditory deprivation during critical periods of auditory imprinting could affect learning ability throughout an entire lifetime. Although it is well accepted that a bilateral 20-decibel or greater hearing loss warrants intervention, evidence now suggests that unilateral hearing loss is also disadvantageous. In children with hearing thresholds better than 20 decibels on pure tone testing, there may still be poor speech discrimination with background noise, such as may be encountered in the classroom setting.

Otitis media with effusion is associated with negative middle ear pressure, causing tympanic membrane retraction. If this persists for a prolonged period, there may be permanent weakness (atelectasis) of the tympanic membrane, and the tympanic membrane may adhere to the ossicles, causing ossicular erosion, or may adhere to the medial wall of the middle ear, causing adhesive otitis media. Prolonged retraction may cause portions of the tympanic membrane to retract deeply in the attic region or beneath the annulus, forming a bottlenecked sac that cannot clear its own desquamated epithelium. This is called a *cholesteatoma.*

TREATMENT A management approach to otitis media with effusion is shown in Fig. 15-9. Otitis media with effusion resolves completely within 2 months of diagnosis in 80% of cases. It is therefore recommended that no treatment be instigated in the initial 2 months following the onset of an effusion unless there are extenuating circumstances. If an effusion persists beyond 2 or 3 months, the chances of spontaneous resolution are substantially reduced. A trial of an antibiotic using the same antibiotic choices as with acute otitis media is appropriate. The optimal duration of treatment is debatable, with periods of treatment between 10 and 28 days being recommended. The length of treatment must be balanced against the increasing incidence of bacterial resistance. Antibiotic treatment will resolve otitis media with effusion, at least temporarily, in 50% of affected children. Other medical therapies attempted for treatment of otitis media with effusion have included systemic antihistamines, systemic or topical decongestants, and topical steroids. None are efficacious. Systemic steroids in combination with an antibiotic appear to be more effective than antibiotics alone for short-term therapy, but long-term efficacy has not been demonstrated.

If an effusion persists despite antibiotic therapy, consideration should be given to the insertion of *tympanostomy tubes.* Current recommendations are for tympanostomy tube insertion after 3 months with a bilateral effusion or 6 months with a unilateral effusion. Other indications include pathologic retraction of the tympanic membrane or chronic eustachian tube dysfunction.

There is a vast experience with tympanostomy tube insertion in children for otitis media with effusion. Tympanostomy tube insertion is the most common operation in the world, one of the safest, and one of the most effective. A general anesthetic is virtually always required in a young child. There are a plethora of different tympanostomy tubes available, and all of these balance duration of insertion against the residual perforation rate. The longer a tube remains in the tympanic membrane, the more likely a permanent perforation will result on its extrusion, requiring a further operation

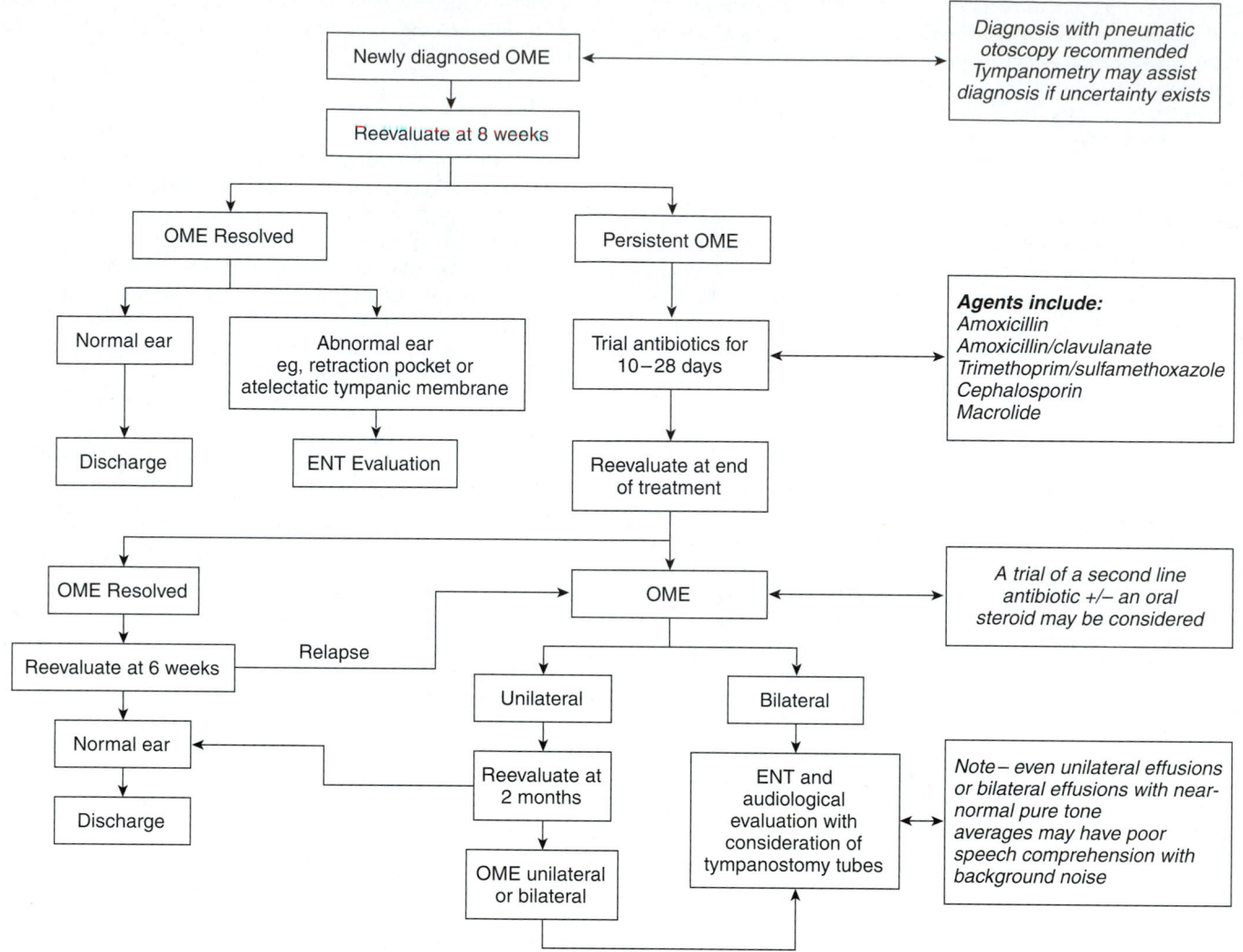

FIGURE 15-9   Otitis media with effusion algorithm. OME = otitis media with effusion.

to repair the tympanic membrane. Most children receiving a tympanostomy tube for the first time will have a short-term tube (6 to 12 months duration) inserted, with longer-term tubes being reserved for children with more chronic otitis media problems, particularly those with underlying craniofacial anomalies, and children in whom an effusion returned once the initial tympanostomy tube had extruded. The tympanostomy tube perforation rate may be as low as 1% with short-term tubes in a young child to over 10% with longer-term tubes in an older child. The purpose of a tympanostomy tube is to take over the function of the eustachian tube temporarily to aerate the middle ear, not to promote drainage of fluid from the ear. However, up to 30% of tympanostomy tubes will have middle ear drainage at some point.

Between 10% and 20% of children receiving tympanostomy tubes will ultimately require a second set of tympanostomy tubes, and in these children adenoidectomy is a consideration. Adenoidectomy serves to not only remove a source of obstruction to the eustachian tube but, more importantly, to remove a bacterial reservoir. If an adenoidectomy is performed on a child receiving a second set of tubes, it will halve the likelihood that this child will require a third set of tympanostomy tubes. Adenoidectomy should not be routinely performed in children under the age of 3, in children with cleft palates or submucous cleft palates, or in children

with velocardiofacial syndrome. The latter groups of children are at risk for developing velopharyngeal insufficiency following adenoidectomy.

CHRONIC OTITIS MEDIA

The most common form of chronic otitis media is a permanent perforation of the tympanic membrane. A less frequent variation is a perforation or retraction of the tympanic membrane with trapped epithelium that is unable to spontaneously clear desquamated debris, forming a cholesteatoma. This may occur in the presence of an intact tympanic membrane. Both perforations and cholesteatoma may be associated with recurrent foul-smelling otorrhea, termed *chronic suppurative otitis media.*

ETIOLOGY   Permanent perforations of the tympanic membrane may occur following extrusion of a tympanostomy tube or spontaneously following acute otitis media. Less commonly, a permanent perforation may result from direct or indirect trauma to the tympanic membrane.

Although a perforation may be asymptomatic, except for a conductive hearing loss, it may also be associated with recurrent episodes of discharge, usually foul smelling. The most common organisms are *Staphylococcus aureus* or *Pseudomonas aeruginosa,* with the latter often being multiply drug resistant. The profuse foul-smelling otorrhea is usually not associated with pain or fever.

DIAGNOSIS A small perforation may be asymptomatic or may be associated with a disproportionately large conductive hearing loss. Large perforations are virtually always associated with a conductive hearing loss. In some instances, small perforations may function to aerate the middle ear despite chronic eustachian tube dysfunction, in much the same way as a tympanostomy tube does. A perforation of the tympanic membrane warrants audiologic assessment both with pure tone and bone conduction audiometry to estimate the degree of conductive hearing loss. Tympanometry can confirm the presence of a perforation.

In the presence of otorrhea, particularly if this is an acute occurrence, treatment with topical antimicrobial eardrops is appropriate. The new generation of quinolone eardrops are particularly efficacious. If the otorrhea is resistant or long-standing, then obtaining a sample for culture and sensitivity is appropriate.

COMPLICATIONS A chronic perforation of the tympanic membrane is usually associated with a conductive hearing loss. This is usually related to the presence of the perforation itself, particularly if it is in the region of the round window membrane. However, there may be an underlying ossicular discontinuity, particularly if there has been erosion of the long process of the incus from atelectasis of the tympanic membrane. A sensorineural hearing loss may also occur if there has been long-term chronic suppurative otitis media. Like cholesteatoma, chronic suppurative otitis media may have the same intracranial complications seen with acute otitis media.

TREATMENT A simple perforation of the tympanic membrane without symptoms and with a minimal conductive hearing loss may not warrant intervention. However, in the presence of a conductive hearing loss or episodic otorrhea, repair of the tympanic membrane (myringoplasty) is justified. In younger children, it may be reasonable to delay repair if ongoing eustachian tube dysfunction is suspected. If the contralateral ear has an intact tympanic membrane without a middle ear effusion, it is reasonable to assume bilateral eustachian tube function.

In cases of chronic suppurative otitis media without cholesteatoma formation, eardrops to control the episodes of otorrhea are appropriate initially, before consideration of repair of the perforated tympanic membrane. If there is underlying ossicular erosion, then a simultaneous ossiculoplasty or repair of the ossicles may also be indicated. There is no role for systemic antibiotic therapy in chronic suppurative otitis media unless the infection has invaded the peri-aural tissues with associated cellulitis.

CHOLESTEATOMA

A cholesteatoma is an expanding epithelial-lined sac containing squamous debris, often infected with offensive purulent discharge. Cholesteatomas may be congenital or acquired. Congenital cholesteatomas are rare disorders characterized by a pearly-white keratin ball seen in the middle ear space behind an intact tympanic membrane. The most likely etiology is the embryologic retention of an epithelial cell rest in the middle ear space. Acquired cholesteatomas may occur as the result of perforation or severe tympanic membrane retraction. Rarely cholesteatomas may occur at the site of a tympanostomy tube insertion.

The most commonly affected areas are the attic region, superior to the short process of the malleus, and the posterior/superior quadrant of the tympanic membrane in the region of the incudo-stapedial joint. Chronic negative middle ear pressure may cause a segment of weakened tympanic membrane to retract either in the attic region or under the annulus, with a bottleneck then forming, inhibiting the natural epithelial migration of desquamated squamous debris. This may in turn become wet and infected, producing foul-smelling otorrhea and an expansile mass lesion. Cholesteatomas may secrete parathyroid hormone–like substances that promote local bony erosion. In some cases a cholesteatoma may grow quite large before becoming symptomatic.

In a patient with a history of chronic otorrhea, pneumatic otoscopy may help differentiate whether the affected portion of the tympanic membrane is a perforation or a retraction pocket. It may also be possible to observe squamous debris or granulation tissue within a perforation or a retraction pocket, suggestive of cholesteatoma. Squamous epithelium desquamating from a cholesteatoma has a classic cheesy appearance. This diagnosis is best made with otomicroscopy utilizing an operating microscope and suction debridement. If a cholesteatoma is suspected, then CT scanning of the temporal bone may provide information on the size of the cholesteatoma and the surrounding anatomic landmarks, though this is by no means mandatory. A cholesteatoma may cause a conductive hearing loss through ossicular erosion, or a sensorineural hearing loss or disequilibrium may rarely occur if a cholesteatoma has invaded the labyrinth. Cholesteatomas have the potential for central nervous system complications, and all of the potential complications of acute otitis media may occur with a cholesteatoma, particularly facial nerve palsy, meningitis, abscess formation, and sigmoid sinus thrombosis. Chronic suppurative otitis media associated with cholesteatoma requires surgical treatment, with the appropriate form of mastoid surgery dependent on the individual needs of the patient and the disease.

15.1.10   External Otitis

The healthy external ear is a self-cleaning environment with antibacterial protection. Cerumen (wax) is a protective antibacterial and waterproofing agent produced by the cerumen glands of the outer third of the external ear canal. Under normal circumstances it will slowly migrate laterally, and wax build-up or wax impaction is an abnormal consequence of manual interference with the self-cleansing action. The medial two-thirds of the external ear canal is bony with a thin layer of skin closely adherent to the bone and with no cerumen glands. The outer third of the external canal is cartilaginous with a much thicker layer of skin and fibrous tissue including extensive glandular elements.

ETIOLOGY The two most common causes of otitis externa are related to trauma and water exposure. The most common forms of trauma include cotton-tip applicators, fingernails, or foreign bodies. Organic foreign bodies are more irritating than nonorganic foreign bodies, and insects may be especially irritating. Water exposure may cause desquamation of squamous epithelium, with water absorption by retained wax predisposing to otitis externa. A patient may have a predisposition to water trapping if there are canal exostoses (bony overgrowths) partly occluding the canal, usually secondary to excessive cold-water exposure (surfer's ear). About 30% of otitis external is caused by water exposure, 30% by trauma, and in 30% there is no obvious predisposition. The remaining 10% have less common etiologies including skin disorders such as eczema or dermatitis, which may result in recurrent problems with external otitis. Occasionally there may be an infection of the sebaceous glands of the outer third of the ear canal with formation of a furuncle, a small staphylococcal abscess with symptoms disproportionate to its size. Vesicles of the tympanic membrane (bullous myringitis) may be associated with a *Mycoplasma* infection, and vesicles of the ear canal may be associated with herpes zoster infection. In Ramsey-Hunt syndrome these are associated with vesicular eruptions on the soft palate and facial nerve palsy. Rarely there may be pathologic cerumen retention with ballooning of the bony ear canal, termed keratitis obturans, which may also be associated with an underlying ciliary dyskinesia. Bacterial otitis externa is most commonly associated with *Staphylococcus aureus* or *Pseudomonas aeruginosa*. Cases resistant to treatment may have an underlying fungal or yeast infection, frequently *Candida albicans*.

DIAGNOSIS   In its initial stages, externa otitis usually presents with itching and a sensation of fullness in the ear, which rapidly progresses to severe pain and associated ear discharge. Blockage of the external ear canal will cause a conductive hearing loss. Unlike acute otitis media, movement of the pinna will greatly exacerbate the pain. There may be associated pain with chewing. Fever is unusual. On physical examination there may be frank discharge from the ear, and otoscopy may be limited by pain because of an inflamed and swollen external ear canal. In severe cases the external ear canal may be swollen completely shut. If a furuncle is present, there will be localized swelling and erythema with extreme pain on palpation of the affected area. Whenever possible it is advisable to inspect the tympanic membrane to ensure that there is no underlying cause for the discharge, such as chronic suppurative otitis media or a perforation following acute otitis media. This may not be possible at initial assessment because of edema of the external ear canal and associated pain on inspection.

Rarely a diabetic or immunocompromised patient may present with pseudomonal otitis externa that spreads via the fissures of Santorini to affect the skull base, and may present with pain and cranial nerve palsies. This condition is known as *malignant otitis externa* and carries a high mortality rate if not appropriately treated.

COMPLICATIONS   Pain and conductive hearing loss are the most common temporary symptoms associated with otitis externa. Rarely in cases with recurrent otitis externa, particularly if associated with an underlying skin condition, a canal stenosis may develop, which in turn may further exacerbate the predisposition to otitis externa. A canal stenosis is not an easily treated condition and will usually require surgical intervention.

TREATMENT   Ideally, external otitis requires prompt treatment of both the infective organism and the underlying cause. It is a great deal easier to treat this condition before the canal is so inflamed that it is swollen shut. Foreign bodies should be removed, use of cotton tip applicators should be discontinued, and swimming should cease. Debris in the ear canal should be removed with irrigation, swabbing, or suction. Antibiotic and steroid combination eardrops should be commenced that are effective against the presumed underlying organisms. The steroid component is at least as important as the antibiotic component, as this may greatly alleviate the inflammation, pain, and swelling. However, steroid drops should be discontinued in the presence of a fungal otitis externa. Eardrops should be administered several times a day in the initial

stages, and it is advantageous that the eardrops penetrate deeply into the canal. If the external canal is extremely edematous, placement of an otowick, sponge, or small piece of ribbon gauze in the external canal is useful to assure antibiotic penetrance. Systemic antibiotics are also warranted if there is surrounding cellulitis of the soft tissues adjacent to the ear or cervical adenitis. Adequate analgesia is warranted, and in severe cases narcotic administration may be justifiable.

If otitis externa is unresponsive to initial treatment, a microbiological sample for culture and sensitivity should be obtained. The most likely organisms under these circumstances are multiply drug-resistant *Pseudomonas aeruginosa* or fungi. Quinolone eardrops are usually the most effective treatment for *Pseudomonas,* and antifungal drops or cream are indicated for yeast or fungal otitis.

A furuncle may require topical and systemic antistaphylococcal antibiotics, and if the abscess is pointing, then drainage with an 18-gauge needle may dramatically alleviate the pain associated with this condition. Once the acute infection has resolved, it is prudent to reassess the ear to assure that there is no underlying predisposition to infection such as eczema or a cholesteatoma. In individuals predisposed to otitis externa, prophylactic measures may be undertaken to prevent recurrence. This may include treatment of underlying skin conditions, regular toilet of the external ear canal to prevent water trapping, surgical removal of bony exostoses, and use of alcohol ear drops after swimming to promote drainage of water from the ear.

15.1.11   Ear Trauma

EXTERNAL EAR

Blunt trauma to the auricle is a common injury sustained during athletic activities and routine childhood play. These injuries are best prevented with the routine use of bike helmets and sport-specific head protection (eg, wrestling headgear). Because of the thin skin covering and delicate perichondrium, hematomas and seromas of the auricle are common. When undiagnosed or untreated, these injuries can result in loss of auricular cartilage and subsequent auricular deformity. Appropriate treatment consists of evacuation of the fluid collection and then application of a pressure dressing to prevent reaccumulation of fluid. The child should be reevaluated at close intervals for signs of perichondritis. The use of prophylactic broad-spectrum antibiotics is generally recommended.

Penetrating trauma to the ear (most commonly bite wounds) require repair of the soft tissue defect (including reattachment of any severed portions of the auricle) and prophylactic antibiotic treatment. Perichondritis is a significant risk that can cause necrosis of cartilage and substantial auricular deformity, so careful patient follow-up is necessary. In rare cases of subtotal avulsion with extensively exposed auricular cartilage and cartilage of questionable viability, hyperbaric oxygen treatment may be considered. Frostbite injuries to the auricle are common in colder climates and should be treated by rapidly rewarming the affected area using warm sterile saline-soaked gauze. Following this, the wound should be treated similarly to a burn with topical sulfadiazine and analgesics. Again, close follow-up for signs of chondritis is essential. Burns of the auricle may require only topical treatment with sulfadiazine if superficial, but more extensive burns may require debridement, systemic antibiotics, and soft tissue reconstruction.

Trauma to the external auditory canal (EAC) usually involves foreign objects inserted into the canal. Lacerations of the canal skin may require analgesics but does not require any specific treatment. Foreign bodies in the canal can typically be removed if in the cartilaginous (lateral) portion of the canal. However, foreign bodies more medially in the canal or abutting the tympanic membrane can be difficult to remove without an operating microscope, suction, and specific otologic instruments. In general, foreign bodies should be removed as soon as possible to prevent damage to the underlying structures. Following removal of the foreign body, a complete exam of the external auditory canal and tympanic membrane is necessary to rule out any injury.

MIDDLE EAR

Traumatic injuries of the middle ear are often caused by direct mechanical trauma via the external auditory canal (eg, a foreign body inserted in the EAC or a "boxing" of the ears). The tympanic membrane may be perforated, resulting in pain, bloody drainage, and hearing loss. These traumatic perforations typically close by themselves over 3 to 4 weeks. However, such trauma can also induce a middle ear effusion and/or hemotympanum behind an intact tympanic membrane. Such middle ear effusions clear spontaneously over the course of 10 to 14 days without treatment. Careful examination and audiologic testing to rule out ossicular damage should be performed. In cases in which there is a significant and persisting conductive hearing loss, a middle ear exploration may be indicated to identify and correct an ossicular discontinuity. Very rarely, severe enough trauma results in subluxation of the stapes footplate into the vestibule of the inner ear. Such patients present with sensorineural hearing loss and vertigo and require surgical intervention.

Barotrauma to the middle ear may result from scuba diving, routine plane flights, or possibly even from excessively strong Valsalva-type maneuvers. Common findings after barotrauma are a middle ear effusion or hemotympanum. Less frequently, barotrauma may cause a leak at the oval or round windows, resulting in the leakage of perilymphatic fluid (perilymph fistula). These patients may present with sensorineural hearing loss with or without vertigo. Perilymphatic fistulas are notoriously difficult to demonstrate intraoperatively and are often treated empirically after ruling out other pathologies.

Although possible, injury to the facial nerve via middle ear trauma is exceedingly rare. For a patient presenting with a history or signs of middle ear trauma and facial paralysis, audiologic testing, temporal bone imaging, and immediate middle ear exploration are warranted.

INNER EAR

Trauma to the inner ear structures can occur in association with severe blunt head trauma and temporal bone fracture. Approximately 75% of temporal bone fractures are longitudinal (the fracture line running along the long axis of the petrous bone), with the remainder being described as transverse. Although 20% of longitudinal fractures are associated with facial nerve injuries, up to 80% of transverse fractures may be associated with facial nerve injury. Fractures through the cochlear or vestibular structures of the inner ear often cause symptoms of sudden (sensorineural) hearing loss and vertigo but are often difficult to evaluate in severely injured and often cognitively impaired patients. Longitudinal fractures are commonly associated with fracture lines that cross that EAC and/or

tympanic membrane, resulting in bloody otorrhea or hemotympanum. Conductive hearing losses secondary to ossicular disruption, CSF leak, and CSF otorrhea may also result from trauma. Management of CSF and some facial nerve injuries may require immediate middle cranial fossa and middle ear/mastoid exploration while other problems such as ossicular discontinuity and tympanic membrane perforations must wait until the patient can tolerate an elective procedure.

Barotrauma can also cause inner ear damage, as mentioned above, by inducing a perilymph fistula. Symptoms of vertigo or worsening hearing loss during times of straining or Valsalva are typical features of a patient with a perilymphatic fistula. Placing soft tissue "patches" over the oval and round windows provides a simple yet effective treatment for these patients.

References

Bess FH, Tharpe AM: Unilateral hearing impairment in children. Pediatrics 74:206–216, 1984

Bluestone CD, Klein JO: Intracranial suppurative complications of otitis media and mastoiditis. In: Bluestone CD, Stool SE, Kenna MA, eds: Pediatric Otolaryngology, 3rd ed. Philadelphia, WB Saunders, 1996: 636–645

Casselbrant ML, Mandel EM, Rockette HE, Bluestone CD: Incidence of otitis media and bacteriology of acute otitis media during the first two years of life. In: Recent Advances in Otitis Media. Proceedings of the Fifth International Symposium. New York, Decker, 1993:1–3

Eviatar L, Eviatar A: Vertigo in children: differential diagnosis and treatment. Pediatrics 59:833–838, 1977

Gates GA, Avery CA, Prihoda TJ, et al: Effectiveness of adenoidectomy and tympanostomy tubes in the treatment of chronic otitis media with effusion. N Engl J Med 317:1444, 1987

Guidelines for Audiologic Screening. Rockville, MD, American Speech-Language-Hearing Association, 1997

Hannley M: Basic Principles of Auditory Assessment. San Diego, College-Hill, 1986

Harnsberger HR, Dahlen RT, Clough S, Gray SD, Parkin JL: Advanced techniques in magnetic resonance imaging in the evaluation of the large endolymphatic duct and sac syndrome. Laryngoscope 105:1037–1041, 1995

NIH Consensus Statement: Early Identification of Hearing Loss in Infants and Young Children. Bethesda, MD, National Institutes of Health, 1993:1–24

Okumura T, Takahashi H, Honjo I, et al: Sensorineural hearing loss in patients with large vestibular aqueduct. Laryngoscope 105:289–294, 1995

Phelps PD, Lloyd GAS: Diagnostic Imaging of the Ear, 2nd ed. London, Springer Verlag, 1990

Phelps PD, Lloyd Matkin ND: Early recognition and referral of hearing-impaired children. Pediatr Rev 6:151–156, 1984

Rodrigues WJ, Schwartz RH, Akram S, Khan WN: *Streptococcus pneumoniae* resistant to penicillin: incidence and potential therapeutic options. Laryngoscope 105:300–304, 1995

Sade J, Yaniv E: Meniere's disease in infants. Acta Otolaryngol 97:33–37, 1984

Stool SE, Berg AO, Berman S, et al: Otitis Media with Effusion in Young Children. Clinical Practice Guideline, number 12. AHCPR Publication No. 94-0622. Rockville, MD, Agency for Health Care Policy and Research, Public Health Service, US Department of Health and Human Service, 1994

Todd NW: At-risk populations for hearing impairment in infants and young children. Int J Pediatr Otorhinolaryngol 29:11–21, 1994

15.2 THE NOSE AND PARANASAL SINUSES

Sally R. Shott

15.2.1 Normal Nose and Sinuses

The nose is positioned at the beginning of the respiratory tract. It is the primary organ for the sense of smell, with the fibers of the first cranial nerve coursing out of the nose through the cribriform plate to terminate in the olfactory centers in the brain. In addition, the nose modifies inhaled air. The nasal passages warm, humidify, and filter inspired air, removing 80% of particles of 5 to 10 μm in diameter and 100% of particles larger than 100 μm in diameter. The surface of the nasal mucosa is coated with mucus-secreting goblet cells and mucus glands. Cilia on the surface epithelium move the mucus at a rate of 8 to 10 mm per minute, allowing effective clearance of trapped particles. The nasal passages also participate in the initial response to inhaled bacteria, viruses, and allergens. Glycoproteins, lysozymes, and secretory IgA in nasal secretions have antimicrobial activity. Disturbances in the composition of the mucus, as in cystic fibrosis, compromise the immunologic functions of the nose and increase the number of respiratory tract infections. The nasal cavities also play a role in speech quality. Because the nasal cavity affects the resonance quality of speech, disturbances in the anatomy of the nasal passages can change speech production. For instance, if the nasal passages are blocked posteriorly by enlarged adenoids, the voice will be hyponasal. If, on the other hand, the nasal passages remain in communication with the oral cavity throughout speech production, as in the case of a cleft palate or velopharyngeal insufficiency, the speech is hypernasal.

ANATOMY AND EMBRYOLOGY

The child's nose differs from the adult nose in several ways. It has less frontal projection, and it is made primarily of cartilage. It is softer and more pliable. In the child, approximately two-thirds of the nose is cartilage, and one-third is bone. In the adult, this becomes closer to a 50-50 percentage relationship.

The external nose is made up of the two nasal bones superiorly and the upper and lower lateral cartilages inferiorly. The anterior nares are divided by a bridge of skin and cartilage called the columella, which is supported by the anteromedial aspect of the lower lateral cartilages. Inside the nasal cavity, the right and left halves are divided by the nasal septum. The nasal septum is part cartilage anteriorly, the quadrilateral cartilage, and part bone posteriorly. It courses from the columella anteriorly back to the level of the nasopharynx posteriorly (Fig. 15-10A). Inferiorly, the nasal septum communicates with the hard palate, and superiorly it ends at the cribriform plate, which separates the nasal cavity from the anterior cranial fossa.

The posterior openings of the nose, the posterior choanae, communicate with the nasopharynx, where the adenoid tissue sits. On each side of the adenoid pad, just posterior to the choanae, are the medial openings of the eustachian tubes. On the lateral walls of the nose, there are bony outgrowths called the inferior, middle, and superior turbinates (Fig. 15-10B). Between the turbinates are recesses called meatuses. Drainage ports of the lacrimal duct and the paranasal sinuses are found within these meatuses. The nasolacrimal duct opens into the inferior meatus. The frontal, maxillary, and

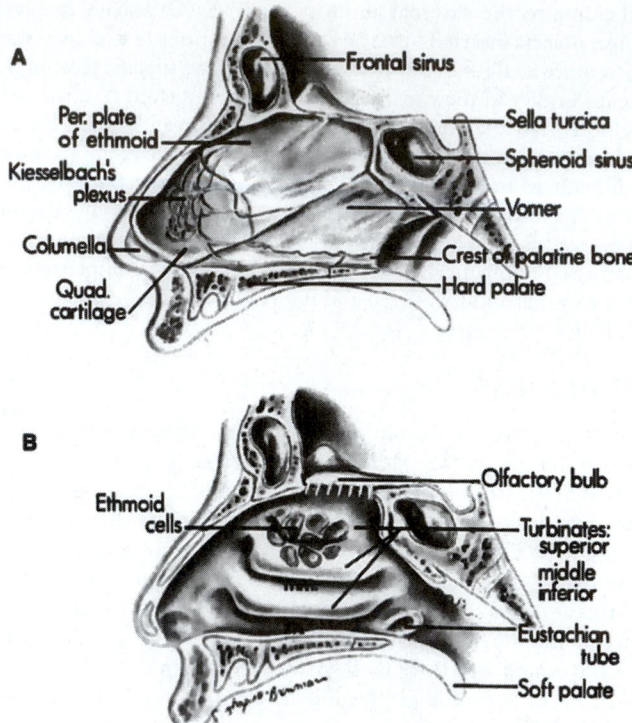

FIGURE 15-10   Internal nasal cavity. A = septum; B = lateral wall of nose (ethmoid cells are lateral to middle and superior turbinates).

anterior ethmoid sinuses drain into the middle meatus. The posterior ethmoid sinuses drain into the superior meatus. Superiorly, the nasal cavity terminates at the cribriform plate, through which olfactory fibers pass into the anterior cranium. The paranasal sinuses develop within the facial bones and include the maxillary, ethmoid, frontal, and sphenoid sinuses (Fig. 15-11). The paranasal sinuses begin as outpouchings or diverticula from the mucosal lining of the lateral nasal walls during the third and fourth month of gestation. At birth, both the maxillary and ethmoid sinuses are present. Both increase in size through adolescence. The frontal sinus develops from the anterior ethmoid air cells, and the sphenoid sinus develops from the posterior ethmoid cells. They start to develop several years after birth but are usually not visible on plain x-rays until age 5 or 6 years. Asymmetry in shape and size is more common in the frontal and sphenoid sinuses. The frontal sinus may be absent in 4 to 5% of normal adults.

They are lined with ciliated, mucus-secreting epithelium. The anterior and lateral wall of the maxillary sinus is formed by the malar bone or cheekbone. The floor of the maxillary sinus is formed by the hard palate and maxillary alveolar ridge. The tooth buds of both deciduous and permanent teeth can be found in both the anterior wall and the floor of the sinus. The maxillary sinus drains via the maxillary ostia into the nose through the middle meatus. The ethmoid sinuses are made up of two tracts of air cells, honeycombed in nature. Anteriorly, the tract drains into the middle meatus, and posteriorly, it drains in the superior meatus. The ethmoid sinuses sit between the lateral orbital walls and the upper half of the nasal septum. Superiorly sits the cribriform plate. The frontal sinuses form as outgrowths of the anterior ethmoid air cells. These sinuses sit within the frontal bone above the nose and orbits. The posterior wall separates the sinus from the anterior cranium. The size and configuration of the frontal sinuses are more variable than those of

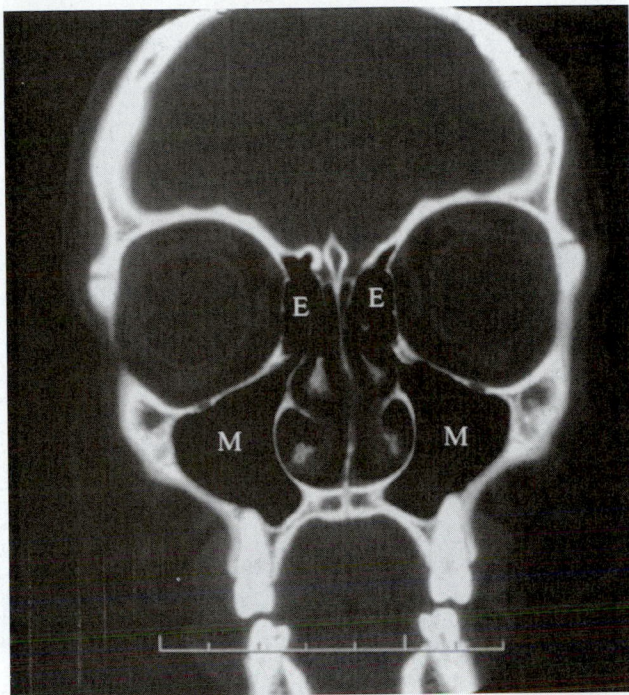

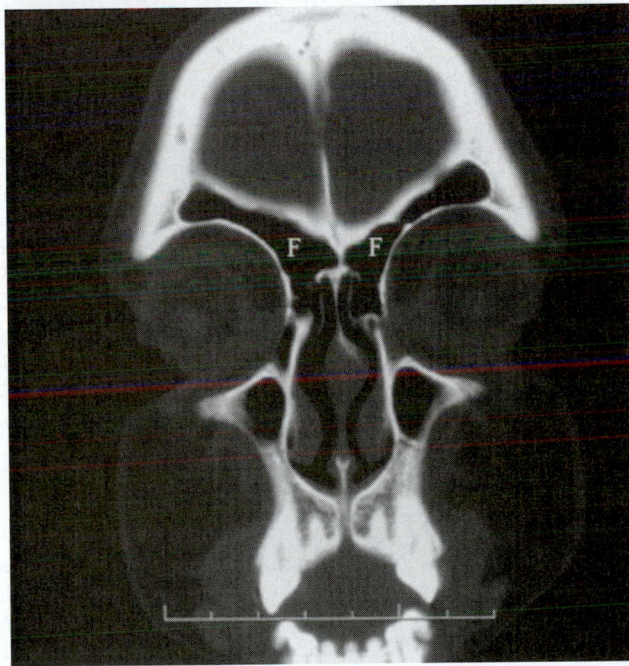

FIGURE 15-11 CT scan of the paranasal sinuses. The maxillary (M) and ethmoid (E) sinuses are visible in the anterior section (top figure). The frontal sinus (F) is visible more posteriorly (bottom figure). The sphenoid sinus is located most posteriorly within the sphenoid bone and is not visible in these sections.

the ethmoid and maxillary sinuses. There is usually a septum that divides it into right and left sides. The sides are rarely equal in size. Each side has a drainage port, called the nasofrontal duct, that drains into the middle meatus. The sphenoid sinus sits most posteriorly of all the sinuses and forms within the sphenoid bone. Lateral to the sphenoid sinus sits the cavernous sinus with contained carotid artery and cranial nerves. Superiorly, the roof of the sphe-

noid sinus is formed by the sella turcica, in which the pituitary gland sits. The sphenoid sinus is divided by a septum into right and left sides with drainage into the nasopharynx above the superior turbinates.

The blood supply to the nose is intricate and complex, coming from both the internal and external carotid arteries. The majority of the blood supply to the nose comes from the external carotid artery via the facial artery and the internal maxillary artery. Whereas the blood supply from the external carotid artery is from direct branches of the artery, the blood supply from the internal carotid artery is less direct (ie, they are off the secondary branches). The superior aspect of the nose receives its blood supply from the anterior and posterior ethmoid arteries, which are derived from the ophthalmic branch of the internal carotid artery. On the anterior nasal septum, all feeding vessels unite to form an area called the Kiesselbach plexus (see Fig. 15-10A). This area of the anterior nasal septum, called the Little area, is the most common site of anterior nasal hemorrhage. Veins closely parallel the arterial system, draining into the ophthalmic vein. The ophthalmic vein drains into the cavernous sinus. Clinically this is important because it creates a pathway by which an infection from simple skin blemishes on the external nose and surrounding facial skin can spread to the cavernous sinus.

The nerve supply to the nose and the paranasal sinuses is through sensory branches from the first and second divisions of the fifth cranial nerves. The autonomic innervation is through the vidian nerve, which carries sympathetic fibers from the carotid sympathetic chain, and through the parasympathetic fibers from the greater superficial petrosal nerve, a branch of the seventh cranial nerves. Sensory fibers originate from the specialized olfactory epithelium that perforate the cribriform plate to form the first cranial nerve.

15.2.2 Evaluation of the Nose and Sinuses

Examination of the nose in the newborn or young child can be difficult simply because of its small size. In a normal term infant an 8-French catheter should pass through each naris at birth. Inability to pass this size catheter suggests the presence of stenosis of the nasal passages or total obstruction. Other means to document patency include use of cotton wisps or fogging of a mirror.

Upward pressure applied to the tip of the nose allows examination of the anterior septum and anterior nasal passages. Use of a nasal speculum and light source allows better examination of both the anterior septum and nasal turbinates. An otoscope can also be used. Vasoconstrictors such as oxymetazoline can facilitate decongestion and provide better visualization. Examination of the more posterior aspects of the nose requires the use of fiberoptic flexible scopes or radiologic studies.

Palpation is used to examine the external nose. Nasal fractures can be diagnosed by recognizing asymmetry in the nasal bones. Nasal masses of the external nose are both easily seen and palpable. However, intranasal masses require further evaluation with radiologic studies. Although radiologic evaluation is primarily used to diagnose sinus abnormalities, palpation of the sinuses provides another diagnostic tool. Tenderness on palpation over the sinuses suggests an acute infection but is less reliable for diagnosis of chronic disease. Examination of the sinuses also needs to include assessment of the contiguous areas. Dental infections can be the source of sinus disease. Conversely, sinus tumors may erode into the alveolar ridge or hard palate in the mouth. Measurement of visual acuity and ocular mobility is important in ruling out orbital complications of sinus disease.

Plain radiographs, previously the mainstay for diagnosis of sinus disease, are readily available and can be useful in diagnosing acute sinus disease, especially in children over age 5 years when an air-fluid level is seen. The most common screening view for sinusitis is the occipitomental view or "Water view." The film is taken with the chin tilted 45° from the horizontal and provides good views of the maxillary sinuses. Computed tomography is more useful for accurate evaluation of sinus anatomy and disease and is preferred for evaluation of nasal masses and tumors and for evaluation of nasal obstruction. The CT allows visualization of both bony and soft tissue components of the sinuses and facial region. Magnetic resonance imaging (MRI) is useful in delineating vascular lesions and soft tissue masses.

15.2.3 Congenital Malformations of the Nose

Newborn infants are obligate nasal breathers. Mouth breathing is a learned behavior. Therefore, total nasal obstruction at birth can be life threatening. In addition, partial obstruction can cause varying degrees of distress including difficulties with feeding, failure to thrive, aspiration, respiratory distress, and hypoxemia. It is important to document nasal patency in all newborns.

CHOANAL ATRESIA

Choanal atresia occurs if the buccal pharyngeal membrane in the posterior nasal cavity fails to dissolve in the seventh week of gestation. Choanal stenosis occurs if there is only partial resorption. The blockage can be either unilateral or bilateral, and in 90% of cases the blockage is bony. These anomalies occur in 1 in 8000. Choanal atresia should be suspected in any newborn if suction catheters cannot be passed through the nose into the oral cavity or in those with respiratory distress relieved with crying. Classically, affected infants have intermittent cyanosis or oxygen desaturation except when crying. Eventually, they tire and will die unless an oral airway is secured by placing a small anesthetic oral airway or a large open nipple (McGovern's nipple) into the mouth. This should be taped or tied in place to assure an airway until surgical repair is performed. An orogastric tube may be sufficient to provide a means to both feed the child and also provide an open oral airway to bypass the nasal obstruction until the child learns to breathe exclusively through the mouth.

Further evaluation is best achieved by CT examination (Fig. 15-12). If CT is unavailable, an x-ray evaluation with contrast placed in the nasal passages will show failure of the contrast to pass through the blocked posterior choanae, but the CT scan delineates the atresia and allows differentiation between a bony and a membranous obstruction, which assists in surgical planning. Bilateral choanal atresia requires surgical repair within the first few days of life. A unilateral atresia repair can be delayed if the child is stable, able to eat, and is growing appropriately. Unilateral atresias are sometimes missed at birth. The child may present with unilateral chronic rhinorrhea or a unilateral sinusitis. In cases of stenosis, the need for intervention also depends on symptoms. Dilation and nasal stenting may be required, but if the stenosis is mild, observation and use of normal saline drops to keep the nasal passages clear may be all that is required. The nasal passages continue to grow after birth.

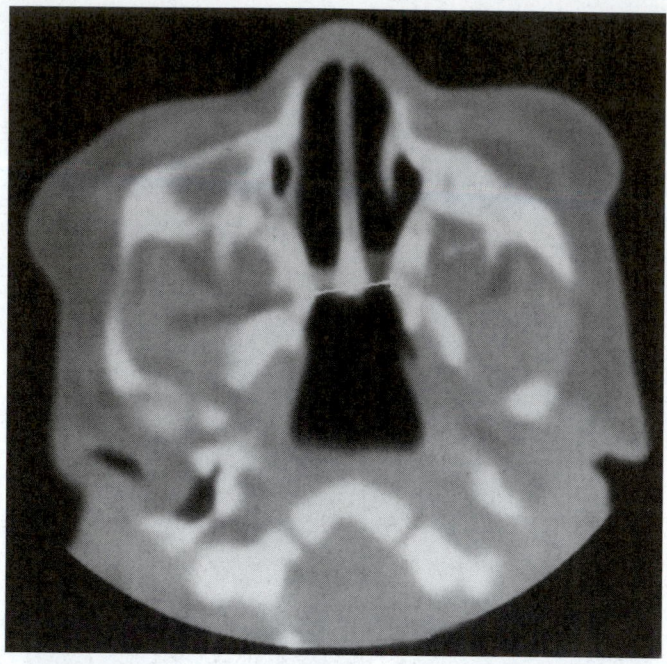

FIGURE 15-12 Computed tomography scan of an infant with choanal atresia. Note the bony and membranous tissue between the anterior nose and nasopharynx.

Before surgery it is important to rule out other congenital anomalies because up to 50% of children will have associated abnormalities as in the CHARGE syndrome (see Sec. 10.3.4). Repair of the choanal atresia can be performed by transnasal or transpalatal approaches. Simple blind puncture of the atretic plate or membrane is unwise because this can result in damage to the brain and usually closes spontaneously. Definitive surgery requires removal of the atretic plate and the posterior part of the posterior bony nasal septum or vomer with placement of nasal stents. Parents need to be trained in suctioning and care of the nasal stents, which remain in place for 4 to 6 weeks following surgery.

OTHER CAUSES OF NASAL OBSTRUCTION IN THE INFANT

Congenital masses or deformities of the nose can cause nasal obstruction in the child. *Congenital nasal septal deformity* occurs in 1% of newborns and is secondary to trauma to the nose as the child passes through the birth canal. If it is diagnosed at birth, simple reduction of the deviated septum can be done before fibrosis sets in. *Septal hematoma* can similarly be caused by birth trauma and requires immediate incision and drainage. Failure to do so can lead to septal cartilage infection and chondritis with loss of nasal septal support. Hypertrophy of the turbinates in the newborn, referred to as *"stuffy nose syndrome,"* is of unknown etiology but may be caused by transmitted maternal hormones. It usually resolves spontaneously and can be treated with saline drops to keep the nasal passages clear. Rarely, steroid nasal drops and/or stenting is needed. Following recurrent treatment with vasoconstrictor nasal drops, rebound nasal congestion and turbinate edema may occur, known as *rhinitis medicamentosa*. The use of vasoconstrictor nasal drops is contraindicated in neonates because of this and other complications including hypertension, sedation, and even coma.

A variety of congenital abnormalities may present as nasal masses. *Nasal dermoids* usually present as a midline cyst or sinus.

These epithelial-lined structures arise from trapped ectodermal tissue along lines of embryonic fusion. If they present as a sinus, only a pit or dimple may be seen on the nasal skin. Hair may extrude from the pit. They can be superficial or can course down through the nasal bone into the nasal septum. Dermoids can also communicate with intracranial structures. *Nasolacrimal duct cysts* can also present as an intranasal mass and result from failure of the lacrimal duct to perforate at the distal end in the inferior meatus. *Nasal encephaloceles* or *gliomas* result from faulty closure of the anterior cranial neuropore. Gliomas have no direct communication with the meninges, but they can contain brain tissue. Encephaloceles freely communicate with the intracranial space. CT scans are mandatory to delineate possible intracranial involvement before biopsy for all nasal masses because they can result in meningitis or cerebral spinal fluid leaks. Surgical removal may require both a nasal and an intracranial approach.

Adenoid hypertrophy is not a common cause of nasal obstruction in a newborn but may be problematic in those with craniofacial malformations. Newborns with craniofacial dysostosis, a high arch palate, or children with Down syndrome can have a contracted nasopharynx, where even mild adenoid hypertrophy can cause nasal obstruction. *Congenital hemangiomas* and *venous angiomas* may also occur in the nose and present with nasal obstruction if they are large. Surgical intervention is reserved for symptomatic cases because most will involute by 12 to 18 months of age.

15.2.4   Epistaxis

Nosebleeds are common in children. The most common site of epistaxis is from the Kiesselbach plexus on the anterior nasal septum known as the Little area (see Fig. 15-10). In this area there is a confluence of superficial, delicate vessels originating from both the external and internal carotid arteries.

In children, digital trauma (ie, nose picking) is the most common cause of epistaxis. Nosebleeds tend to be more common during the winter months, when the nasal mucosa is dryer. This lack of humidity leads to drying of the nasal secretions and formation of nasal crusts that are removed either digitally or with nasal rubbing or excessive nose blowing. The nosebleeds resolve with formation of an eschar at the bleeding site. Unfortunately, the eschar can be quite uncomfortable, and further nose picking occurs in an attempt to remove the scab, so further epistaxis occurs. Epistaxis therefore frequently occurs recurrently. Only when the child realizes the relationship of the digital manipulation with nosebleeds does this behavior stop.

Other etiologies of epistaxis include trauma to the nose from falls or sports injuries, neoplasms of the nose, and unsuspected foreign bodies. Foreign bodies are usually accompanied by unilateral bloody rhinorrhea and bad odor. Chemical irritants such as phosphorus, gasoline, and sulfuric acid can cause inflammation of the nasal mucosa with resultant hemorrhage. Mucosal irritation from cocaine abuse should be considered in older children and adolescents. Allergic rhinitis is also associated with increased epistaxis. Juvenile nasopharyngeal angiofibromas occur more commonly in male adolescents. Arteriovenous malformations, venous angiomas, and hemangiomas can occur in children and present with epistaxis. Nasopharyngeal carcinoma, rhabdomyosarcomas, and lymphomas are rare but can present initially with epistaxis. Epistaxis also may be a symptom in systemic diseases including any coagulopathy, hypertension, or renal disease. Abnormalities in blood vessel walls such as those found with vitamin C deficiency (scurvy) may also cause epistaxis.

Because epistaxis may be the harbinger of serious underlying disease, it is important to obtain a detailed history and perform a careful physical examination. If epistaxis occurs during winter months, is occuring following an upper respiratory infection, and is intermittent, it is more likely to be a benign disorder. A patient or family history of bruising or a bleeding disorder should be pursued. Medication use, especially use of nasal sprays that dry the nasal mucosa, should be considered.

The physical examination should include an overall assessment of general health. Large nosebleeds can cause hypovolemia, so the initial assessment and management are similar to those for any major hemorrhage, with assessment for tachycardia, hypotension, or orthostasis. Bruising is of particular concern because it may signify an underlying coagulopathy. Sites of bleeding can be visualized by examining the nose either using a flashlight with gentle upward pressure to the tip of the nose or using an otoscope and speculum. In older children, a nasal speculum and flashlight can be used. Examination of the more posterior aspect of the nose will require use of a flexible fiberoptic scope. If dried blood scabs or eschars are seen on the anterior aspect of the nasal septum in the area of the Kiesselbach plexus, it is very likely that digital trauma is the cause of the nasal bleeding. It is reasonable to treat assuming this to be the cause as long as appropriate follow-up is scheduled.

The approach to management of epistaxis is shown in Fig. 15-13. Appropriate initial treatment includes education about behavior changes that need to occur in regard to the nose picking and improved moisturization of the nose. If the nose is well moisturized, fewer crusts accumulate, and therefore less nose picking occurs. In addition, moisturization softens already formed eschars and allows them to remain in place until the underlying mucosal erosion has healed. Moisturization is best supplied through the use of a normal saline nose spray. It is important to use this four to five times a day to assure adequate moisturization. Placement of salves and ointments into the nose is not advisable because it may cause trauma.

Parents also require education regarding the management of further nosebleeds at home. Initially, the child should gently blow the nose, removing all blood clots in the nasal passages. Then, while in a sitting position, the nose should be pinched for 5 to 10 minutes, using the thumb and forefinger at the tip of the nose. This compresses the cartilaginous portions of the nose and applies pressure to the Kiesselbach plexus.

If bleeding continues, other therapies may be required in the physician office. These include the use of decongestant sprays and cauterization of the bleeding site with a silver nitrate stick. If the bleeding still persists, nasal packing may be needed, and the patient should be referred to an otolaryngologist. If nasal packing is required, admission for observation and monitoring for possible respiratory complications is warranted. More aggressive therapy for repeated treatment failures includes angiography, embolization of involved vessels, or arterial ligation in severe cases.

If epistaxis occurs recurrently despite conservative therapies, further evaluation is warranted. This includes coagulation and platelet studies. If warranted by the results, further consultation with a hematologist may be needed to rule out a bleeding dyscrasia, especially von Willebrand disease, one of the most common coagulopathies, in which routine coagulation studies may be normal. Measurement of von Willebrand factor antigen may be necessary. In addition, a referral to an otolaryngologist for full evaluation of the nasal passage is indicated to rule out nasal masses or other causes for the epistaxis.

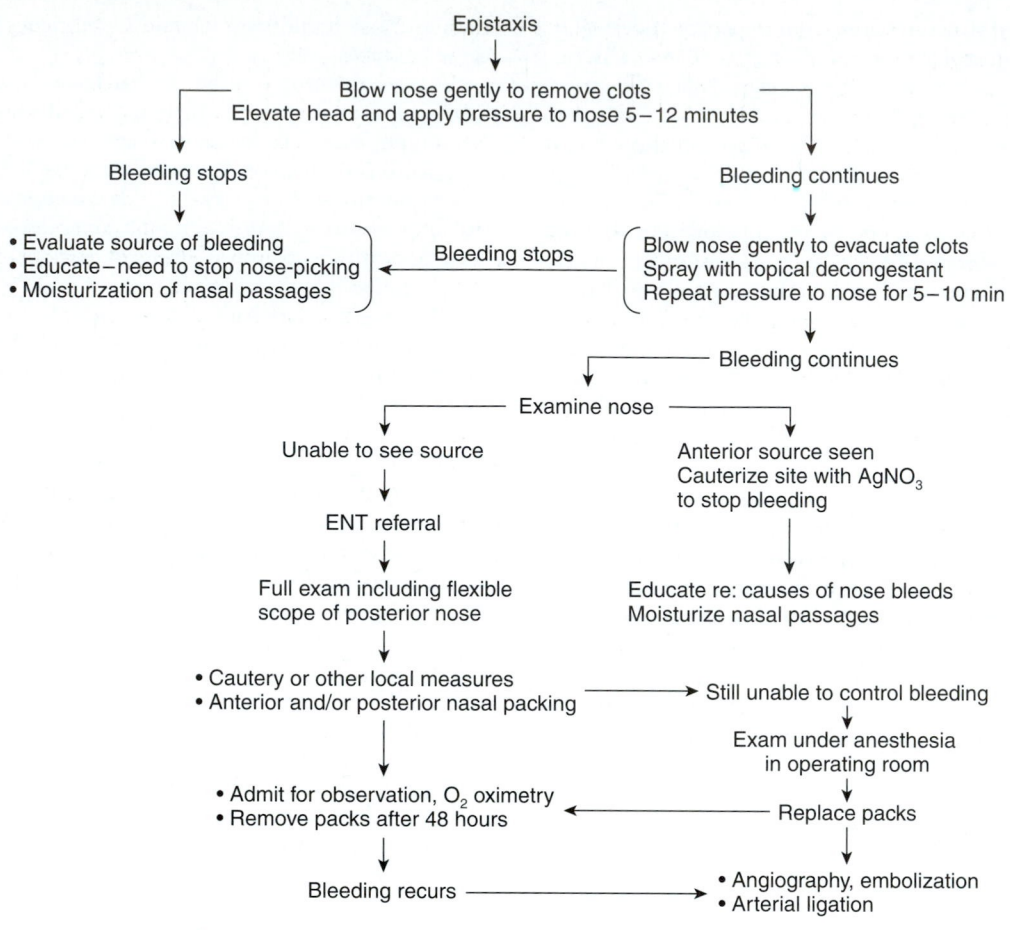

FIGURE 15-13   Treatment of epistaxis.

15.2.5   Allergic Rhinitis

Allergic rhinitis is one of the most common causes of chronic nasal obstruction in children. The causes and management approaches to allergic rhinitis are discussed in detail in Sec. 11.9. The chemical mediators released by the allergic reaction, including histamine and cytokines, cause vasodilation with nasal membrane edema. In addition, histamine stimulates the neuronally mediated sneeze reflexes and increases mucus production. When inflamed by an allergic reaction, the nasal mucosa has a characteristic appearance with edema and enlarged boggy, slightly blue turbinates.

Nasal polyps in the nose and sinuses, the most common nasal growth, usually have an allergic etiology. (The exception to this statement is nasal polyps associated with cystic fibrosis.) Allergic polyps usually originate from the middle turbinate or the ethmoid sinus.

Symptoms suggesting allergic rhinitis include nasal congestion, sneezing, rhinitis, nasal itching, and itchy eyes. Dark periorbital circles called "allergic shiners" result from the chronic venous and lymphatic stasis frequently associated with allergies, although they can also be seen with sinusitis.

In determining treatment, it is first important to determine if the child's nasal congestion and rhinorrhea are caused by allergy, have an infectious etiology, or whether there is a structural obstruction such as adenoid hypertrophy. Allergy may predispose to bacterial sinusitis, and if allergy is believed to be a contributing factor, it cannot be ignored if successful treatment is expected.

Basic tenets of treatment of allergic rhinitis include identification of allergens, avoidance of known allergens, and pharmacologic treatment. Pharmacologic interventions include the use of antihistamines in both sedating and nonsedating formulations, decongestants, and intranasal corticosteroids. Intranasal steroids can be very effective in treating allergic rhinitis and are particularly helpful for control of intermittent seasonal symptoms.

15.2.6   Infectious Disorders of the Nose and Paranasal Sinuses

VIRAL INFECTIONS

The majority of nasal and sinus infections in children are caused by viruses. Acute nasopharyngitis, the most common infection seen in children, is also referred to as an upper respiratory tract infection or a URI or the "common cold." Fever, rhinitis, congestion, and headaches are common. The same viral etiologic agents infect not only the sinuses but also the pharynx, larynx, trachea, and bronchi. Therefore, the same virus can cause mild rhinitis, croup, pharyngitis, or bronchitis in different individuals. Common viruses include rhinovirus (30% of URIs), coronavirus (10%), adenovirus, and coxsackievirus. Influenza virus is usually seen only in epidemic situations.

The course of these viral infections is usually self-limited, lasting 5 to 7 days. Treatment is supportive and symptomatic and consists of rest, antipyretics, and oral decongestants. Antihistamines are not suggested in cases of viral infections, as they decrease cilia movement and delay mucus clearance. Antihistamines also cause drying of the nasal and sinus secretions, which further impedes mucus drainage.

Excessive inflammation of the nasal mucosa from the increased mucus production associated with a viral infection can lead to ulceration of the nasal mucosa and possible complications of epistaxis or bacterial infection.

The symptoms seen in viral infections of the nose and sinuses can mimic the prodromal symptoms seen in early mumps or pertussis. Persistent unilateral rhinitis suggests the presence of a foreign body or a unilateral choanal atresia. Allergic rhinitis, also part of the differential, differs from viral rhinitis in that it is not associated with fever and is usually accompanied by other allergic symptoms such as itchy eyes and sneezing.

Topical decongestants (eg, phenylephrine hydrochloride, oxymetazoline hydrochloride) can relieve nasal congestion, but it is important to limit the use of such sprays to only 3 days to avoid tachyphylaxis and rhinitis medicamentosa. Systemic decongestants such as pseudoephedrine and phenylpropanolamine hydrochloride may also reduce congestion, but systemic effects of hyperactivity and insomnia limit their utility. Systemic decongestants should be used carefully, especially in children under 1 year of age, because of the potential side effects of cardiac stimulation, hypertension, and neurologic complications. Mucolytic agents such as guaifenesin may thin secretions, improve ciliary function, and thereby promote sinus drainage.

BACTERIAL SINUSITIS

Bacterial infections of the nose and sinuses usually occur as a complication of a viral URI. Although children 2 to 5 years of age may have six to eight URIs per year, only 5% to 10% of these develop into bacterial infections. If purulent nasal drainage is present, or if there is an associated fever, facial swelling, and headache, a bacterial infection may be present. If rhinitis persists longer than 7 to 10 days and is associated with purulent drainage, both nasal and postnasal, halitosis, and headaches, a bacterial infection must be considered. Bacterial infections can also occur secondary to nasal foreign bodies, nasal allergy, trauma, dental infections, and immunodeficiency states. Nasal obstruction from enlarged adenoids, nasal polyps, or a deviated nasal septum can predispose to bacterial infections. Chronic sinusitis is present when symptoms persist for longer than 30 days.

Children may not always complain of headache or discomfort from sinus disease. Symptoms such as cough during sleep from chronic postnasal drainage, head hitting, hair pulling, or rubbing of the head or face may be the only symptoms present. Dental pain may also be present because of the proximity of the tooth roots to the floor of the maxillary sinus.

Bacteria commonly responsible for the sinus infections include *Streptococcus pneumoniae, Moraxella catarrhalis, Staphylococcus aureus, Haemophilus influenzae,* and anaerobic species of *Peptostreptococcus, Bacteroides,* and *Fusobacterium.*

Treatment of bacterial sinusitis includes the supportive treatment used for a viral infection (see above) as well as antimicrobial therapy. As in otitis media, amoxicillin is the first drug of choice. Because of increased resistance to *S. pneumoniae,* initial doses of 80 to 90 mg/kg/d up to a maximum of 3 g/d should be used. Trimethoprim-sulfamethoxazole (TMP-SMX) is another first-line drug choice. Although the types of bacterial species causing sinusitis have not changed significantly in the last few decades, the incidence of bacterial resistance to antibiotics has changed significantly. It is

therefore important to know your regional rates of penicillin-resistant and β-lactamase-producing organisms.

The purpose of treating an acute bacterial sinusitis is to halt progression of the acute infection into a chronic infection as well as to prevent permanent sinus mucosal damage. Antibiotic therapy may also prevent serious complications of sinusitis such as orbital and periorbital cellulitis or abscesses, meningitis, brain abscess, or cavernous sinus thrombosis. If there is no improvement of symptoms after 3 to 5 days on a first-line drug, or if symptoms recur within 2 weeks of treatment, a second-line medication is indicated. Second-line antibiotics include the second- and third-generation cephalosporins, amoxicillin-clavulanate, and the macrolides. In cases of highly resistant *S. pneumoniae,* ceftriaxone, clindamycin, and/or a third-generation cephalosporin should be considered.

One of the more common controversies in antibiotic treatment of sinusitis is in regard to the length of treatment. Initial treatment is usually for 10 to 14 days. If symptoms recur, a longer course of antibiotics is indicated. Three full weeks may be needed if an infection has become chronic. Shorter courses of antibiotics have been investigated, and initial results are promising, but at this time, specific recommendations in this regard are not yet available.

Sinusitis can be complicated by the development of periorbital and orbital infections, meningitis, and intracranial infections including brain abscesses. Therefore, if a child is not responding to appropriate medical therapy, a referral to an otolaryngologist is indicated so that cultures can be obtained by diagnostic culture of the maxillary sinus to direct therapy. Cultures of the nasal secretions are not useful. Referral should also be considered if the child is immunocompromised or severely ill or toxic appearing, or if suppurative complications appear to be developing.

A referral to an allergist is appropriate if the child has symptoms and signs of allergy and/or if there is a family history of allergy. There is a strong relationship between allergy and chronic sinusitis, and successful treatment requires that both be treated. Medical and surgical treatment of sinusitis in patients with asthma has also been shown to decrease the severity of the reactive airway disease.

Complications of sinusitis can be very serious and life-threatening. The diploic vein system in the bone marrow of developing bones permits the spread of infections into contiguous areas. Infections can spread from the ethmoid sinuses into the soft tissues of the orbit, causing orbital cellulitis or abscess. Signs and symptoms suggesting an infection include periorbital inflammation and edema, proptosis, chemosis, impaired ocular mobility, as well as decreased vision. The bone and soft tissue overlying the frontal and maxillary sinus can become infected. Osteomyelitis, cellulitis, or subcutaneous abscess of the skin overlying the sinuses can occur. When this occurs over the frontal sinus, an abscess known as a "Pott puffy tumor" can occur. From the ethmoid, sphenoid, or frontal sinus, the infection can spread into the cranial cavity, causing meningitis, epidural abscess, subdural abscess, or even a brain abscess. Infections in the maxillary sinus can affect tooth growth and can cause oroantral fistulas. If any of these complications is suspected, hospitalization and CT evaluation are necessary. In addition, ophthalmologic consultation and evaluation of the cerebral spinal fluid may be required. These complications require aggressive intravenous antibiotic therapy. If there is no resolution of symptoms within 24 to 48 hours, or if the infection progresses despite antibiotic therapy and proper decongestant use, further treatment including surgical intervention is necessary. It is paramount in these situations to treat not only with antibiotics but also with topical decongestant sprays in order to decrease the sinus mucosal edema and facilitate sinus drainage.

Computed tomographic scan evaluation of the sinuses is also indicated for recurrent sinus infection. Surgical management of chronic sinusitis has been revolutionized by the development of a sinus telescope. The lateral nasal wall where the various sinus ostia drain is opened, and diseased mucosa is removed, restoring the normal anatomic drainage patterns. Nasal polyps should be removed, although in patients with cystic fibrosis and nasal polyps, the polyps are likely to recur, and revision surgery should be expected in the future.

FUNGAL SINUSITIS

Fungal infections of the nose and sinuses are uncommon except in children with alterations of their immune status such as those undergoing chemotherapy for malignancies. Fungal sinusitis can also be associated with protracted allergic rhinitis and sinusitis. *Aspergillus* and *Candida* species are most commonly seen. *Mucormycosis* infections are seen in patients with poorly controlled diabetes mellitus. Fungal sinusitis frequently presents with black, infarcted areas of the nasal turbinates or nasal septum. Fungal balls are also seen within the sinuses. Fungal disease and/or malignancies should be considered when bony erosion is observed on CT scan in association with chronic sinusitis symptoms.

NASAL INFECTIONS

Infections of the nasal skin are rare and are most commonly related to skin blemishes or to infections of the nasal hairs at the anterior choanae, resulting in a folliculitis. Digital trauma is the most common cause. Treatment consists of antimicrobial therapy against *Staphylococcus aureus,* the most common cause of these infections. Application of an antibiotic ointment to the area of the folliculitis should be performed, not with the finger, the carrier of the infection, but rather with a small cotton-tipped applicator. Twice-a-day treatment for 1 week is usually sufficient. Development of increasing erythema and cellulitis should be treated aggressively in view of the underlying potential for spread via the venous drainage of the face back to the cavernous sinus.

15.2.7   Neoplasms of the Nose and Paranasal Sinuses

Neoplasms of the nose and sinuses are uncommon. They can present as obvious mass lesions or as the underlying cause for recurrent epistaxis or recurrent sinusitis. The majority of benign neoplasms in children result from congenital anomalies of the nose and are reviewed in Sec. 15.2.3. The most common benign growths are nasal polyps caused by chronic allergic rhinitis, chronic sinusitis, and/or cystic fibrosis. Papillomas can also appear as verrucous growths within the nasal cavity, which should be excised, although recurrence is common. Fibroosseous disorders that can occur include osteomas, giant-cell granulomas, fibrous dysplasia, fibromas, and brown tumor of hypoparathyroidism. Aneurysmal bone cysts are also seen within the sinuses. After the presence of hypoparathyroidism has been ruled out, treatment by excision is indicated in order to relieve the sinus and/or nasal obstruction, curtail the local bone destruction, and rule out underlying malignancy.

Malignant tumors of the nose and sinuses in children include rhabdomyosarcoma, lymphoma, esthesioneuroblastoma (a tumor of olfactory origin), and rare metastatic lesions from primary tumors below the clavicle. Such lesions can unfortunately present no differently than the benign lesion with symptoms of recurrent epistaxis, nasal obstruction, and chronic sinus infections. Both CT scan and MRI evaluations facilitate delineation of tumor involvement. Bony erosive lesions that spread outside the confines of the nose and sinus suggest possible malignancy. Treatment depends on the specific type of tumor present and usually includes a combination of surgery, chemotherapy, and radiotherapy.

15.2.8   OLFACTORY DISORDERS

Neuroepithelial cells of the olfactory mucosa are present on the superior and middle turbinates and the upper part of the nasal septum. These olfactory chemoreceptive cells are primary neurons that project directly to the brain without synapse. One of their unique characteristics is the ability to regenerate. There are also receptors for chemical sensing on unmyelinated nerve endings in the nose as well as the oral cavity. These receptors are responsible for the burning sensation experienced in the nose when exposed to a noxious substance such as ammonia.

Loss of smell results in a marked loss of enjoyment in eating and drinking because flavor recognition is substantially dependent on smell but also causes one to lose the protective recognition of spoiled foods, smoke, or dangerous fumes.

Odor molecules must be airborne and come into direct contact with the olfactory cells. Olfactory threshold is the lowest intensity of a stimulus that can be perceived. Disorders within the nasal cavity that impede delivery of the odor molecules result in decreased smell. The most common cause of temporary anosmia is a URI. Nasal polyps, adenoid hypertrophy, or other masses in the nose can affect one's ability to smell. Intranasal tumors, such as olfactory neuroblastomas, can cause alterations of smell. Sinusitis, especially in the ethmoid sinuses, can cause smell disturbances, including anosmia and dysosmias. Head trauma in the frontal bone, the occipital area, or even severe nasal and facial trauma can cause tearing of the olfactory filaments passing through the cribriform plate.

Olfactory disturbances can suggest the presence of important illnesses and congenital anomalies. The most common congenital anomaly is Kallmann syndrome, also called hypogonadotropic hypogonadism, in which there is agenesis of the olfactory bulb and incomplete development of the hypothalamus. Other features include undescended testes, midline craniofacial abnormalities, hearing loss, and renal anomalies. Endocrine disorders have also been linked to olfactory abnormalities. Turner syndrome, hypothyroidism, and congenital adrenal abnormalities are associated with decreased smell or hyposmia. Addison disease is associated with a heightened sense of smell. Viral infections may permanently destroy the sense of smell through destruction of the chemoreceptive cells. Similarly, industrial pollutants and intranasal drug use may destroy these cells.

Intracranial tumors including meningiomas, frontal lobe gliomas, and pituitary tumors can cause abnormalities in smell. Temporal lobe tumors can cause olfactory disturbances, usually hallucinations of bad odors.

Treatment for olfactory disorders is limited. If they are caused by a URI or infection, the sense of smell usually returns once the nasal edema has resolved. Surgical intervention to remove intranasal masses is therapeutic. Vitamin A therapy may act to regenerate the olfactory cells and restore the olfactory mucosa.

15.2.9   Nasal Trauma and Foreign Bodies

Maxillofacial trauma is rare in children because the cranium and forehead are large relative to the face and protect the facial bones from injury. The pediatric facial skeleton is also more elastic and more stable, so fractures occur less often. Nasal fractures are the most common maxillofacial fracture seen in children. Nasal cartilage absorbs less of the energy of the force applied to it than the nasal bone of adults, so there tends to be more edema of the surrounding face following nasal trauma in children. There is also an increased incidence of other facial bone fractures associated with the nasal trauma in children. This increased surrounding edema, coupled with the lack of patient cooperation usually seen in this age group, sometimes makes diagnosis difficult.

Radiologic evaluation with plain x-rays is unreliable for nasal fractures in children because the nasal bones are not totally fused, and the cartilage skeleton of the nose makes fracture identification difficult. Therefore, diagnosis rests primarily on external palpation and internal examination. Initial examination may be difficult because of nasal and facial edema, so a follow-up exam may be needed 3 to 4 days following the injury. However, it is important to carefully examine the nasal septum for hematomas during the initial exam. Because of the cartilaginous skeleton, the nose tends to bend and buckle with the applied trauma instead of fracturing. The buckling of the nasal septal cartilage can result in the separation of the perichondrium from the cartilage. This results in blood accumulation between the perichondrium and the septal cartilage, a septal hematoma (Fig. 15-14). If untreated this can rapidly develop into an abscess with septal erosion from avascular necrosis and perforation of the septum with subsequent loss of nasal septal support, nasal dorsal collapse, and a saddle-nose deformity. In addition, if left untreated the infection can spread to the cavernous sinus and intracranially. If a hematoma is suspected, immediate otolaryngology consultation for drainage of the hematoma and antibiotic treatment is recommended. Packing of the nose may be necessary to reapproximate the perichondrium and nasal mucosa to the septal cartilage.

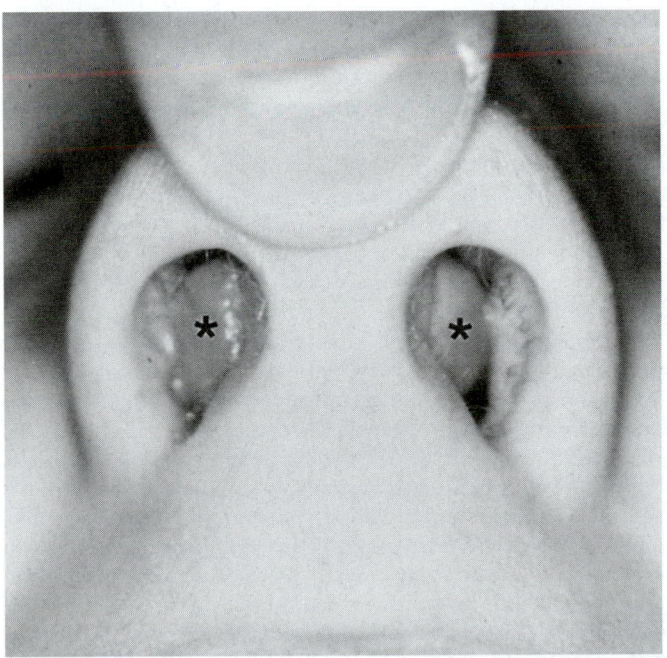

FIGURE 15-14   Nasal septal hematomas (*) are identified by unilateral or bilateral swelling of the nasal septal mucosa. The size of the swelling does not change if vasoconstrictor sprays are applied, and it is fluctuant on probing.

If a nasal fracture is present, it is best to allow as much of the edema to resolve as possible before reduction of the fracture. Repairs should be performed within 7 to 10 days in children. After that time, fibrous healing begins, and proper reduction of fracture fragments may not be possible. The goal of reduction of nasal fractures is to replace the bones in their normal position in order to allow continued growth of the bony nasal skeleton. However, there are several growth centers in the nose, and fractures frequently disrupt normal growth despite appropriate reduction. Nasal deformities may become more prominent as the child grows. In some cases formal septorhinoplasty procedures may be needed once the facial skeleton has matured.

If facial bone fractures are suspected, a CT of the facial bones should be performed to evaluate for fractures of the facial bones and paranasal sinuses. Examination should begin with assessment of patient's airway stability and severe fractures of the midface. Fractures can be associated with craniofacial dissociation and airway compromise. In these cases, an immediate tracheotomy is needed. Once the airway is stable, examination should continue with palpation of the facial bones. Fractures through the cribriform plate can cause a cerebrospinal fluid (CSF) leak or CSF rhinorrhea, which presents with clear fluid dripping from the nose. Tests for glucose content of the drainage may be misleading because nasal mucus drainage can test positive for glucose in some patients. Radionuclide imaging may be necessary to confirm and localize the defect. If there is any evidence of eye involvement, ophthalmologic consultation should be obtained. Blunt trauma to the eye, most frequently seen in sports injuries in children, can cause fracturing of the orbital floor, which is the roof of the maxillary sinus, or of the medial wall of the orbit through the lamina papyracea of the ethmoid sinus. The orbital structures, both fat and muscles, can then herniate through the fracture lines and become entrapped. Symptoms can include extraocular muscle defects, diplopia, and enophthalmos. Failure to identify such a fracture and delay in repair can result in permanent diplopia and enophthalmos.

Treatment of severe facial fractures will require several consultations (otolaryngology, ophthalmology, dental, oral surgery, neurosurgery), CT evaluations, and a well-organized plan for reconstruction. Alterations of the bony skeleton of the face can cause subsequent sinus problems related to alterations in the drainage pathways of the sinuses.

Foreign bodies in the nose are frequently seen in children. Any child presenting with unilateral rhinorrhea should be suspect. If such an object is left in place, the drainage becomes foul smelling and purulent. Examination of the nose with good lighting and suction are needed for removal. The foreign body should not be pushed into the nasopharynx, as this can put the child at risk for aspirating the object. Otolaryngology consultation is required if a foreign body cannot be easily removed. Occasionally, general anesthesia is needed for removal.

References

Brooks I, Gooch WM III, Jenkins SG, et al: Medical management of acute bacterial sinusitis: Recommendations of a clinical advisory committee on pediatric and adult sinusitis. Ann Otol Rhinol Laryngol (Suppl 182): 2–20, 2000

Cantry PA, Berkowitz RG: Hematoma and abscess of the nasal septum in children. Arch Otolaryngol Head Neck Surg 122:1373–1376, 1996

Dolan KD: Radiographic anatomy of the nasal sinus. Otolaryngol Clin North Am 4:13–24, 1971

Guarisco JL, Graham HD: Epistaxis in children: causes, diagnosis, and treatment. Ear Nose Throat J 68:522–538, 1989

Kupperberg SB, Bent JP, Kuhn FA: Prognosis for allergic fungal sinusitis. Otolaryngol Head Neck Surg 117:35–40, 1997

McGraw BL, Cole RR: Pediatric maxillofacial trauma. Arch Otolaryngol Head Neck Surg 116:41–45, 1990

Scott AE: Clinical characteristics of taste and smell disorders. Ear Nose Throat J 68:297–315, 1989

Shott SR, Myer CM, Willis R, Cotton RT: Nasal obstruction in the neonate. Rhinology 27:91–96. 1989

Sonkens JW, Harnsberger HR, Blanch GM, Babbel RW, Hunt S: The impact of screening sinus CT on the planning of functional endoscopic sinus surgery. Otolaryngol Head Neck Surg 105:802–813, 1991

Strutz J, Schumacher M: Uncontrollable epistaxis. Arch Orolaryngol Head Neck Surg 116:697–699, 1990

15.3 ORAL CAVITY AND OROPHARYNX

J. Paul Willging

15.3.1 Anatomy

The oral cavity is surrounded anteriorly by the lips. The lips are supplied with a rich sensory innervation and fine-motor control to provide a complex sphincter mechanism. The lips function to prevent the loss of saliva and food materials from the oral cavity. They close around food utensils to assist in the introduction of food materials into the mouth. The lips are also instrumental in the production of labiodental and plosive sounds for speech. The motor nerve supply is from the facial nerve. Damage to the marginal mandibular branch of the facial nerve denervates the depressor labialis, causing the lower lip to turn into the oral cavity, creating an asymmetric smile. Sensation to the lips is provided by branches of the maxillary and mandibular branches of the trigeminal nerve. Loss of sensation interferes with the protective function of the labial sphincter, often causing sialorrhea and mild feeding problems. The space between the lips and the alveolar ridge is the vestibule. It extends externally around the horseshoe-shaped dental arches. The detailed anatomy of the dental arches that support the teeth and gingival mucosa, which covers the alveolar ridges, is discussed in Sec. 16.1.1. The floor of the mouth is a horseshoe-shaped area juxtaposing the medial alveolar ridge and includes the ventral (under) surface of the tongue. The lingual frenulum divides the floor of the mouth in the midline. The geniohyoid, mylohyoid, genioglossus, and hyoglossus muscles provide support to the floor of the mouth.

THE TONGUE

The tongue is an important structure for communication and mastication. Fine-motor abilities of the tongue permit proper articulation for speech and also provide the necessary manipulation of food materials to create a finely prepared bolus for swallowing. The tongue is divided into an anterior two-thirds (which lies within the oral cavity) and a posterior one-third (which lies within the oropharynx). The division between these two areas is demarcated by the sulcus terminalis, which is the location of the circumvallate papillae that form a "V" with the apex posteriorly at the foramen cecum. The foramen cecum is the embryologic derivative of the thyroid gland. If the thyroid gland fails to descend, a lingual thyroid may be visible on the dorsum of the tongue in this area.

The mucosal covering of the tongue is composed of a mixture of papillae. The circumvallate papillae are the largest and are located posterior on the tongue. Smaller fungiform papillae are located on the lateral aspects and the tip of the tongue. The filiform papillae are the most abundant and cover the dorsum of the tongue. Taste buds are richly demonstrated on the circumvallate and fungiform papillae. The filiform papillae contain no taste buds.

The musculature of the tongue is composed of intrinsic and extrinsic muscle groups. The extrinsic muscles are the genioglossus, the hyoglossus, and the styloglossus. These muscles provide support for the tongue and assist in positioning the tongue forward and backward as well as upward and downward. The genioglossus can protrude the tongue, and its superior fibers depress the tongue tip and assist in retraction. The hyoglossus muscle flattens the tongue. The styloglossus is the primary retractor of the tongue. The intrinsic muscles of the tongue, transverse, vertical, and longitudinal muscles, are responsible for changing the shape of the tongue and are integral to both speech and swallowing.

The blood supply to the tongue is supplied by a branch of the external carotid system, the lingual artery. Sensation is supplied to the anterior two-thirds of the tongue via the lingual nerve, which is a branch of the mandibular division of the trigeminal nerve. The posterior one-third of the tongue is innervated by the glossopharyngeal nerve. Special taste afferents from the anterior tongue course through the lingual nerve to the chorda tympani nerve within the middle ear. Motor function of the tongue is controlled by the hypoglossal nerve. Injury to the hypoglossal nerve will result in a tongue that deviates to the injured side on protrusion.

PALATE, VELOPHARYNGEAL SPHINCTER, AND PHARYNX

The roof of the mouth consists of the palate. The bony hard palate is in continuity with the soft palate posteriorly. The hard palate consists of three fused bones. The paired palatine processes of the maxilla have fused in the midline and comprise the majority of the hard palate. The premaxilla is the triangular piece of bone that consists of the alveolus containing the four upper incisors. The soft palate consists of muscles that originate from the posterior edge of the hard palate and the skull base. The blood supply to the palate is from the palatine branches of the maxillary artery. Sensory innervation to the palate is supplied by branches of the maxillary division of the trigeminal nerve, whereas motor innervation is supplied through the pharyngeal plexus of the vagus nerve. Only the tensor veli palatini muscle receives innervation from the motor division of the trigeminal nerve.

The muscles of the soft palate act to create a dynamic sling. The coordinated movement of the six muscles of the soft palate allows the closure of the velopharyngeal sphincter separating the nasopharynx from the oropharynx during swallowing and speech. The levator veli palatini muscle is the primary elevator of the soft palate. The tensor veli palatini, in addition to assisting palate elevation, is the primary muscle responsible for opening the eustachian tube. Abnormalities in the orientation of this muscle or its insertion on the eustachian tube cartilage greatly predispose to chronic ear disease. The musculus uvulae is a paired muscle in the midline of the posterior soft palate. The bulk of the muscle is on the nasal surface of the soft palate, with small slips of muscle extending into the fleshy appendage hanging free from the posterior midline of the soft palate, which contracts to creat a bulge on the posterior nasal surface of the soft palate, contributing to closure of the velopharyngeal sphincter. The palatoglossus and the palatopharyngeus muscles are incorporated into the anterior and posterior tonsillar pillars, respectively. The superior pharyngeal constrictor is a paired muscle that inserts onto the midline of the posterior pharynx (median raphe) and extends around laterally to originate from the skull base. Contraction narrows the velopharyngeal sphincter.

The pharynx is a mucosally lined tube that extends from the skull base to the esophageal inlet. It is divided into three areas. The nasopharynx is located superiorly. It extends from the posterior choanae of the nasal cavity anteriorly to the level of the free edge of the soft palate inferiorly. It contains the eustachian tube and the adenoid. The oropharynx extends from the free margin of the soft palate to the vallecula. The vallecula is the space created by the junction of the tongue base with the epiglottis. The tip of the epiglottis and the lingual and fascial tonsils lie within the oral cavity. Anteriorly, the oropharynx extends to the anterior tonsillar pillars. The hypopharynx extends from the vallecula to the esophageal inlet. The larynx and pyriform sinuses are contained within the hypopharynx.

The pharyngeal constrictors are paired muscles lining the pharynx. They insert into the medial raphe on the midline of the posterior pharyngeal wall. The superior, middle, and inferior pharyngeal constrictors are responsible for the forces generated to clear materials from the pharynx during the act of swallowing. The salpingopharyngeus, stylopharyngeus, and palatopharyngeus extend from the skull base to insert into the lateral walls of the pharynx and elevate the larynx during swallowing. The innervation of all of the pharyngeal muscles is from the pharyngeal plexus of the vagus nerve except that the stylopharyngeus muscle is innervated by the glossopharyngeal nerve. Sensory innervation to the pharynx is via the glossopharyngeal nerve and pharyngeal plexus inferiorly and the maxillary division of the trigeminal nerve superiorly. The blood supply to the pharynx is from the ascending pharyngeal and superior thyroid arteries of the external carotid system.

SALIVARY GLANDS

The parotid duct (Stensen duct) enters the oral cavity through the buccal mucosa, adjacent to the second maxillary molar at the level of the gingival mucosa. The sublingual glands and the duct from the submandibular gland (Wharton duct) enter the floor of the mouth on either side of the lingual frenulum. The paired parotid glands produce the majority of the serous secretions in the mouth. The submandibular and sublingual glands produce a mucoid secretion. These glands produce secretions in response to gustatory stimuli. The majority of secretions in the mouth throughout the day are produced by minor salivary glands scattered throughout the mucosa lining the oral cavity and the pharynx.

TONSILS AND ADENOIDS

The separation between the oral cavity and the oropharynx is a line extending from the anterior tonsillar pillars (the palatoglossus muscle) across the foramen cecum of the tongue to the opposite side. The tonsils lie within the oropharynx. The faucial tonsils are paired collections of lymphoid tissue. The tonsils are bounded anteriorly by the palatoglossus muscle (anterior tonsillar pillar) and the palatopharyngeus muscle (posterior tonsillar pillar). The superior pharyngeal constrictor muscle is deep to the tonsil. The blood supply to the tonsil is from the external carotid system. The tonsillar branches of the ascending pharyngeal and lesser palatine arteries enter the superior pole of the tonsil. Tonsillar branches from the facial, lingual, and ascending palatine arteries enter the inferior pole. The nerve supply to the tonsil is via the glossopharyngeal

nerve inferiorly and branches of the lesser palatine nerves superiorly. The pharyngeal tonsil (adenoid) resides in the nasopharynx. The lingual tonsil resides in the base of the tongue. Superficial bands of lymphoid tissue connect these four masses of tonsil tissue. *Waldeyer ring* refers to this encircling mass of lymphoid (tonsillar) tissue.

The function of the tonsils (and adenoids) is to process antigens and present them to the germinal centers of the lymphoid follicles. This modulates both B- and T-cell populations within the tonsil in early childhood. With increasing age the tonsil and adenoid tissue atrophies.

EMBRYOLOGY

The oral cavity begins as a depression that invades into the developing embryo. It invaginates until the ectoderm of the stomodeum contacts the endoderm of the primitive foregut, creating the buccopharyngeal membrane. This membrane degenerates at 4 weeks of gestation, providing continuity between the ectodermally derived oral cavity and the endodermally derived oropharynx.

The five branchial arches are mesodermal condensations on the lateral cervical area of the embryo and are separated by branchial clefts externally and branchial pouches internally. The cleft is ectodermally lined, whereas the pouch is endodermally lined.

The first arch develops into the mandible, portions of the ossicles, and muscles associated with these structures. The second arch contributes to portions of the ossicles, the styloid process, portions of the hyoid bone, facial muscles, posterior belly of the digastric muscle, and the buccinator muscles. The third arch differentiates into portions of the hyoid bone and pharyngeal muscles. The fourth arch develops into the anterior/superior portions of the larynx, and the fifth arch contributes to the posterior, larynx, cricoid, and intrinsic muscles of the larynx and the inferior pharyngeal constrictor muscle.

The pharyngeal pouches give rise to a variety of structures. The first pouch becomes the middle ear cavity. The first branchial cleft gives rise to the external ear canal. The tonsils are formed from contributions from both the first and second pouches invading into the surrounding mesoderm. Lymphatic tissue then invades these primitive structures between the third and fifth months of gestation. The third pouch gives rise to the thymus gland and the inferior parathyroid glands. The fourth pouch develops into the thyroid gland and the superior parathyroids.

The hard palate is divided into a primary and secondary palate. The primary palate (containing the anterior alveolus and the four upper incisors) is derived from the medial nasal swelling. The secondary palate (the area posterior to the incisive canals) is formed by the medial growth of the lateral palatine processes of the maxilla. The primary palate has completed development by the seventh week of gestation, the secondary palate completes its fusion between weeks 10 and 12 of gestation. Clefts of the soft palate are generally associated with clefts of the secondary hard palate. Complete clefts involve the primary, secondary, and soft palate structures.

The anterior two-thirds of the tongue is derived from ectoderm, whereas the posterior one-third is derived from endoderm of the primitive foregut. Swellings begin to condense during the fourth week of gestation and are complete by the seventh week. The fungiform and filiform papillae develop by the 11th week, and the circumvallate papillae develop between weeks 8 and 20.

The floor of the mouth is a first arch derivative. The salivary glands are of ectodermal origin and are derived from the first pouch, developing between weeks 5 and 8.

15.3.2   Evaluation of the Oral Cavity and Pharynx

PHYSICAL EXAMINATION

The oral examination begins anteriorly with a systematic evaluation of structures from anterior to posterior, from left to right. The floor of the mouth is evaluated by having the patient elevate the tongue. In small children the tongue will often need to be elevated mechanically. The retromolar trigone (the area among the inferior aspect of the anterior tonsillar pillar, medial aspect of the mandible, and lateral aspect of the tongue) needs to be evaluated by pushing the lateral tongue medially to expose this region. The faucial arches need to be closely evaluated for signs of abnormality. The tonsils should be evaluated for signs of inflammatory changes as well as debris collecting within the crypts of the tonsil. Tonsillar size should be graded on a 1 to 4 scale: 4+ tonsils touch in the midline. Tonsils that are 1+ in size are contained within the tonsillar fossa; 2+ tonsils extend to the medial extent of the tonsillar pillars; 3+ tonsils extend beyond the tonsillar pillars. The oropharyngeal inlet should also be evaluated for adequacy. The tonsils may be of relatively small size but, when combined with a small oropharyngeal inlet, may be obstructing. The posterior pharyngeal wall should be evaluated for symmetry. Granular tissue may often be seen on the posterior pharyngeal wall and represent small areas of lymphoid tissue. Lateral pharyngeal bands are frequently present and represent mild inflammatory changes on the posterior pharyngeal wall secondary to nasopharyngeal drainage or other irritation of this lymphoid tissue.

The soft palate should be evaluated both at rest and in motion. The uvula deserves close attention. A bifid uvula may be a sign of a submucosal cleft of the soft palate. On phonation the soft palate should elevate. Motion of the soft palate should be symmetric. Intraoral palpation is also warranted. The floor of the mouth should be palpated for any sign of stone development within salivary ducts or a mass developing within the floor of the mouth. The hard palate should always be palpated, paying particular attention to the posterior aspect of the hard palate. A posterior projection should be apparent, signifying a normal condition. A notching of the posterior aspect of the hard palate may represent a submucous cleft palate. The buccal area should also be palpated, feeling for stones and also to express saliva from the parotid glands. The tongue should be palpated looking for abnormalities within the substance of the tongue.

ENDOSCOPIC AND RADIOLOGIC EVALUATION OF THE PHARYNX

Flexible endoscopy can be performed easily and safely in an office setting without sedation using a topical anesthetic on the nasopharynx. The nasopharynx is examined for adequacy of velopharyngeal closure, the soft palate for the presence of a submucosal cleft, the tongue base and the lingual tonsils are assessed for size and inflammatory changes, and the hypopharynx and larynx are visualized for signs of cysts, masses, or inflammation.

Radiologic evaluation often begins with a lateral neck x-ray, which provides good visualization of the nasopharynx and assesses the overall size of the adenoid pad. Retropharyngeal and inflammatory processes on the posterior pharyngeal wall may also be identified. Computed tomography and magnetic resonance imaging provide fine detail of specific abnormalities in the oral cavity and oropharynx and the relationship to surrounding structures. Sialograms are rarely performed. Sialograms require the cannulation of either the parotid duct or the submandibular duct and the installation of contrast material to visualize the ductal system within these glands. Abnormalities within the ducts (sialectasia or stones) can be identified. Infectious complications of this procedure increase in the face of active sialadenitis.

15.3.3   Congenital Malformations of the Tongue and Pharynx

CLEFT LIP AND PALATE

A cleft lip results from incomplete fusion of embryonic structures surrounding the primitive oral cavity. The clefts may be unilateral or bilateral. They are often associated with clefts of the palate (Fig. 15-15). Clefts of the palate vary greatly in their extent. Cleft palates may involve only the soft palate or may extend into the hard palate. The cleft may extend through the hard palate and the alveolar ridge and may be in continuity with a cleft of the lip. A combination of cleft lip and palate leads to significant cosmetic deformities of the nose. The structural support of the nose is not present, leading to abnormal lower lateral cartilage development and nasal septum development. Dental abnormalities are also common, as discussed in Sec. 16.8. For further discussion of cleft palate management see Sec. 10.3.4.

A submucous cleft palate may not be recognized until the child is several years of age. The muscular development of the soft palate is similar to that seen in a child with a cleft palate. The levator muscles do not attach in the midline of the soft palate but rather to the posterior edge of the hard palate. There is a mucosal covering

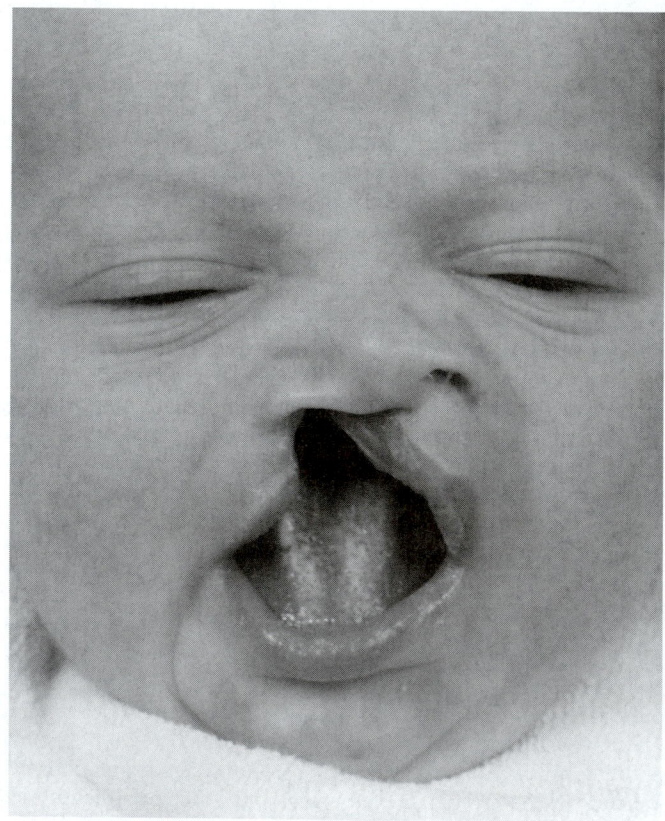

FIGURE 15-15   Clefts of the lip and alveolus create significant nasal deficiencies because of the lack of support of the nasal base.

such that there is no obvious defect of the soft palate. Palpation of the hard palate will frequently demonstrate a notch in the posterior aspect of the hard palate. Close inspection of the uvula will often demonstrate a bifid uvular structure. A blue line (zona pellucida) may be seen in the midline of the soft palate because of the lack of musculature in the midline. A notch of the posterior hard palate may also be palpable. A submucous cleft palate does not necessarily require repair, but velopharyngeal insufficiency with hypernasal speech and an increased incidence of otitis media often result.

Treatment of a child with a cleft palate requires a team approach. Craniofacial teams are generally available at major pediatric centers throughout the country. Surgical repair of the lip is generally performed at approximately 10 weeks of age, with repair of the palate being performed between 9 and 12 months of age. Early intervention with caregivers familiar with children with clefts of the palate is essential to assist the family in learning how to feed the child. Because of a cleft of the palate, a negative intraoral pressure cannot be generated for sucking. Breast-feeding is frequently unsuccessful, and bottle feeding with the conventional nipple may be difficult. Formula is essentially poured into the oral cavity at a paced rate by the feeder. Special bottle-feeding systems are commercially available to improve the oral nutrition and ease of feeding these children, but often a standard nipple can be utilized. Consultation with either an occupational therapist or speech pathologist with experience in feeding problems of children with clefts of the lip and palate is often useful.

OTHER CONGENITAL ABNORMALITIES OF THE ORAL CAVITY AND PHARYNX

Variations of the dentition and oropharyngeal mucosal lining are discussed in Sec. 16.5.

LINGUAL ANKYLOGLOSSIA This abnormality is a common disorder, also known as "tongue-tie," in which the lingual frenulum limits the movement of the anterior tongue tip. On protrusion of the tongue there is frequently a heart-shaped deformity that is created as a very short lingual frenulum tethers the midline of the tongue. The tongue frequently has difficulty protruding beyond the alveolar ridge. Infants may have difficulty attaching to the breast during breast-feeding or to the nipple of a bottle. Surgical correction of ankyloglossia is rarely necessary. The initial feeding difficulties experienced by a newborn often relate to neurologic immaturity and lack of experience of the child and mother. With time and instruction the ability to breast-feed will increase. In some cases, however, a frenulectomy is beneficial and can be performed in the newborn in an office setting. The tongue is elevated with a special retractor, and the thin lingual frenulum is divided with scissors. No anesthetic is required. Negligible bleeding is encountered. In the older child, general anesthesia is frequently required because of a lack of cooperation.

Speech difficulties secondary to ankyloglossia are quite rare. In the English language the tongue needs only to touch the upper teeth. It is more frequently the case that oromotor dysfunction is leading to the articulation errors that are being attributed to the short lingual frenulum. There are some social activities that may lead a patient to a frenulectomy, such as the inability to lick an ice cream cone. If the patient is unable to protrude the tongue, this activity can be awkward.

LINGUAL THYROID Failure of the thyroid tissue to decend into the neck from its site of origin in the tongue base may result in a raised violaceous mass that is often visible in the base of the tongue. A lingual thyroid is more common in girls, and in general, this thyroid tissue does not function normally. The size of the mass tends to increase over time. Frequently, signs of airway obstruction will lead the patient to a physician for evaluation. Thyroid hormone replacement will generally cause a reduction in size of the abnormal thyroid remnant.

THYROGLOSSAL DUCT CYSTS A thyroglossal duct cyst is a cystic mass in the midline of the neck. Occasionally, this cystic mass may present above the hyoid, within the substance of the tongue. Generally, there are no symptoms unless the cyst becomes infected, which leads to a rapid increase in size of the mass. Respiratory difficulties can ensue. Lingual thyroglossal duct cysts need to be differentiated from lingual thyroids. An ultrasound should demonstrate a thyroid gland in its normal location in the base of the neck with essentially normal structure. A nuclear medicine scan can also be utilized to identify functioning thyroid tissue. Thyroglossal duct cysts need to be surgically removed. They are generally excised through a transcervical approach, with the central portion of the hyoid bone removed when a cyst presents within the neck. Thyroglossal duct cysts remaining within the substance of the tongue can be removed endoscopically.

CLEFT TONGUE Oral-facial-digital syndrome I is an inherited X-linked dominant trait and usually includes a cleft of the tongue with multiple hyperplastic frenula, hypoplasia of the nasal alar cartilages, a medial cleft of the upper lip, an asymmetric cleft of the palate, digital malformations, and mild mental retardation. Fifty percent of these patients have hamartomas between the lobes of a divided tongue. Mohr syndrome (oral-facial-digital syndrome II) is an autosomal recessive condition associated with a conductive hearing loss, cleft lip, a high arched palate, a lobulated nodular tongue, hypoplasia of the body of the mandible, polydactyly, and syndactyly.

15.3.4 Inflammatory Disorders of the Tonsils and Pharynx

Inflammatory disorders of the oral cavity and tongue are discussed in Chap. 16. Pharyngitis presents with symptoms of sore throat, pain on swallowing, mild fever, and malaise. The pharynx and tonsils are usually erythematous on examination, and an exudate may be present over enlarged tonsils. Shotty cervical lymphadenopathy is often present. Common bacterial pathogens causing tonsillitis and pharyngitis are β-hemolytic *Streptococcus, Streptococcus pneumoniae, Hemophilus influenzae, Peptostreptococcus,* and *Diphtheroids.* The symptoms of bacterial pharyngitis are identical to infections caused by viruses. There are no reliable clinical findings that permit the differentiation of viral from bacterial pharyngitis. Throat cultures are necessary to direct treatment. Infectious mononucleosis must always be considered in cases of exudative tonsillitis with marked lymph node involvement in the posterior cervical chain. The diagnosis of mononucleosis is made by serology.

Patients with a history of recurrent adenotonsillitis (four to six bouts per year), or relapsing infection within 2 weeks of antibiotic treatment, may benefit from prophylactic antibiotic therapy for 6 to 8 weeks. Trials of an antistaphylococcal antibiotic or rifampin may be helpful in irradiating *Staph. aureus* or β-hemolytic *Streptococcus* carriage. Chronic or breakthrough infections despite adequate antibiotic therapy, infections requiring hospitalization, or complications developing from a bout of acute adenotonsillitis are indications for adenotonsillectomy. Adenotonsillectomy should not be reserved solely for recurrent streptococcal infections because repeated episodes of any bacterial infection are significant. Surgery is best performed when the acute inflammatory response has subsided, generally 6 weeks after the last infection. In some circumstances, however, a tonsillectomy is necessary during an acute infection if there are life-threatening complications such as airway compromise or spread of infection to the parapharyngeal space as a result of a peritonsillar abscess.

Infections of the tonsils invade the substance of the tonsillar tissue. These infections may extend into the surrounding tissues as well. A peritonsillar cellulitis is an infection that has extended deep to the tonsil and causes local tissue inflammation. At this stage, intravenous antibiotics usually resolve the infection. At times, the cellulitis progresses, and a coalescence of the infection leads to development of a peritonsillar abscess. The abscess collection and surrounding soft tissue edema cause medial displacement of the tonsil and asymmetry of the posterior soft palate with the uvula generally deviating away from the site of infection, and the soft palate bulges downward. Often trismus and ipsilateral otalgia are associated with a peritonsillar abscess. A characteristic muffled (hot potato) voice is heard. Treatment of a peritonsillar abscess requires drainage of the abscess. This may be accomplished in the emergency room with needle aspiration, with incision and drainage, or by tonsillectomy. A delayed tonsillectomy is generally recommended in patients with a peritonsillar cellulitis/abscess if there is a preceding history of recurring throat or tonsil infections.

Lymph nodes in the retropharynx and parapharyngeal space hypertrophy in response to infection. At times, the node becomes overwhelmed with the infection and becomes necrotic. Cellulitis may progress to abscess. Surgical drainage of the abscess in the retropharyngeal or parapharyngeal space is required. Cellulitis will generally respond to high doses of intravenous antibiotics. Peritonsillar abscess, parapharyngeal space abscess, and retropharyngeal abscess all have the potential to cause life-threatening complications if diagnosis and treatment are delayed. A mass effect can cause airway obstruction. Infection may also spread along natural tissue planes upward to the skull base, causing meningitis, or inferiorly into the mediastinum. In cases in which surgical drainage is required, intubation must be performed carefully because the act of intubation can rupture the abscess cavity with purulent material soiling an unprotected airway.

15.3.5 Adenotonsillar Hypertrophy with Airway Obstruction

Adenotonsillar hypertrophy can cause obstruction of the upper airway. Children often present with chronic snoring, interruption of airflow during inspiration, and frequently restless sleep behavior. The work of breathing increases as airway obstruction increases. Respiratory rate irregularity also increases as the work of breathing increases, but frank apnea secondary to adenotonsillar hypertrophy is uncommon in children except with severe obstruction. The evaluation and causes of sleep apnea are also discussed in Sec. 23.5.3.

Snoring is the hallmark of upper airway obstruction and may be caused by enlarged adenoid tissue or tonsils or both. When a questionable history of nighttime breathing patterns is obtained, it is often useful to have the parents record sound alone or videotape the child while sleeping to more adequately allow the physician to evaluate reports of noisy breathing, apneic episodes, and irregular breathing patterns.

Obesity is not a common feature of children with obstructive apnea. Many children present with poor weight gain because of poor eating habits. Daytime behavioral habits ranging from agitation to somnolence are often reported by parents or teachers. In severely affected children, pulmonary hypertension and cor pulmonale may develop, but these are uncommon.

If large tonsils are evident on physical examination, adenotonsillectomy is usually curative. If the tonsils are small on examination, a lateral neck radiograph may demonstrate adenoid hypertrophy. Lateral neck x-rays need to be interpreted in light of the dynamics of the upper airway. The relative size of the nasopharyngeal airway will be related to patient posture, general muscle tone, rate of air exchange, and inspiration pressures. Because static films cannot adequately capture the changing relationships of the upper airway, fluoroscopy (sometime with sedation) may provide a better evaluation in questionable cases.

Formal polysomnography is required only if neuromuscular disorders are thought to have an impact on the upper airway or in patients who exhibit central or mixed apneic episodes. Polysomnography is too expensive and time intensive for the routine diagnosis of adenotonsillar hypertrophy with airway obstruction. In those children with a convincing history of airway difficulties during sleep and enlarged tonsils or adenoids, adenotonsillectomy is usually curative. Adenoidectomy alone may resolve symptoms of obstruction in patients with small tonsils. In the presence of apnea, however, it is generally thought that both tonsillectomy and adenoidectomy should be performed.

15.3.6 Tumors of the Oropharynx

The most common benign salivary gland tumor is a mixed or pleomorphic adenoma, which generally develops within the parotid gland but can present as a mass extending from any salivary gland. Mucoepidermoid carcinoma is the most common salivary gland malignancy during childhood, most often originating in the sublingual glands. These lesions are treated by surgical excision.

Other malignant neoplasms that may involve the head and neck include rhabdomyosarcomas, Langerhans histiocytosis, and lymphoma. Extranodal tissue involvement is common in non-Hodgkin lymphomas, with approximately 25% originating in extranodal sites and one-third of these involving structures in the head and neck. Therefore, asymmetric progressive enlargement of the tonsils or adenoids should raise suspicion of a non-Hodgkin lymphoma, and tonsillectomy should be performed as a biopsy procedure. Similarly, asymmetric enlargement of the tonsils or adenoids may be caused by lymphoproliferative disease in immunosuppressed patients following solid organ transplantation.

15.3.7 Pharyngeal Trauma

The approach to oral soft tissue and tooth injuries is discussed in Sec. 16.9. Pharyngeal trauma most commonly results from a child falling while an object is in his or her mouth. The object may impale the roof of the mouth and the posterior pharyngeal wall. The internal carotid artery is adjacent to the tonsillar bed, and therefore a puncture injury at this site has the potential for devastating vascular and neurologic sequelae. If a Horner syndrome is identified at the time of initial evaluation, carotid injury should be suspected. In rare cases, the carotid intima may be injured, and delayed embolic events (up to 3 days following the injury) with stroke may occur. These objects will often impale the roof of the mouth and the posterior pharyngeal wall. Families need to be instructed to immediately seek medical attention should any alterations in mental status develop following this type of injury. Angiograms or magnetic resonance angiography are not warranted unless there is a high suspicion of carotid artery damage.

Lacerations of the soft palate rarely require repair. Large lacerations that will tend to trap food particles should be closed. Antibiotic coverage is generally not required.

References

Deutsch E: Tonsillectomy and adenoidectomy: changing indications. Pediatr Clin North Am 43:1319–1339, 1996

Gosain AK, Conley SF, Marks S, Larson DL: Submucous cleft palate: diagnostic methods and outcomes of surgical treatment. Plast Reconstruct Surg 97:1497–1509, 1996

Hollingshead W: The Pharynx and Larynx. Anatomy for Surgeons: Head and Neck, vol 1. Philadelphia, Harper & Row, 1982:389–441

McCurdy JA Jr: Peritonsillar abscess. A comparison of treatment by immediate tonsillectomy and interval tonsillectomy. Arch Otolaryngol 103:414–415, 1977

Postic WP, Shah UK: Nonsurgical and surgical management of infants and children with obstructive sleep apnea syndrome. Otolaryngol Clin North Am 31:969–977, 1998

Willging J: Paediatric head and neck tumours. In: Jones AS, Phillips DE, Hilgers FJM, eds: Diseases of the Head and Neck, Nose and Throat. New York, Oxford University Press, 1998:371–385

15.4   THE LARYNX

Robin T. Cotton

15.4.1   The Normal Larynx

The larynx is a complex evolutionary structure that permits the trachea and the bronchi to be joined to the pharynx as a common aerodigestive pathway. The larynx serves the essential functions of (1) ventilation of the lungs, (2) protection of the lungs during deglutition by its sphincteric mechanisms, (3) clearance of secretions by a vigorous cough, and (4) vocalization. The survival of the infant is predicated on the structural and neurologic integrity of the larynx, and prompt diagnostic and surgical intervention for airway management is mandatory.

The larynx is arbitrarily divided into three regions: supraglottis, glottis, and subglottis. The supraglottic larynx is composed of the epiglottis, aryepiglottic folds, arytenoid cartilages, vestibular folds (false vocal cords), and laryngeal ventricles. The glottis comprises the vocal cords. The subglottic region extends from the undersurface of the vocal cords to the base of the cricoid cartilage and represents the smallest diameter of the infant larynx. The size, location, configuration, and consistency of the laryngeal structures are all unique in the neonate.

At birth the infant larynx is approximately one-third the size of the adult larynx. The glottis of the neonate measures approximately 7 mm in the sagittal plane and 4 mm in the coronal plane. The vocal cords are 6 to 8 mm long, with the posterior aspect composed of the cartilaginous process of the arytenoid. The subglottic diameter measures approximately 4.5 by 7 mm. A diameter of less than 3.5 mm is suggestive of a subglottic stenosis.

The superior border of the larynx is located as high as the first cervical vertebra. The inferior border of the infant larynx is located at approximately the fourth cervical vertebra during infancy, and as a result, the lingual hypopharyngeal laryngeal complex sits more superiorly within the oral pharynx (see Fig. 17-24). Indeed, the hyoid cartilage can be located anterior to the thyroid cartilage. The superior location of the larynx elevates the epiglottis approximately to the level of the palate and helps to explain obligate nasal breathing over the first few months of life. An intranarial larynx creates a partially separate respiratory and digestive tract that mimics lower animal forms. This position is further enhanced in nursing, as forward thrust of the tongue causes increased elevation of the larynx. The child's and adolescent's larynx gradually lowers into the neck and enlarges this supralaryngeal region of the pharynx to better accomodate the varied sounds of human speech. Ultimately, in humans, the vocal cords have evolved the highest degree of versatility for voice production by their ability to adjust length, tension, and shape.

The configuration of the epiglottis is proportionally narrower than that of the adult and assumes either a tubular form or the shape of the Greek letter omega (Ω). The lumen of the cricoid ring is smaller than the trachea from birth to 3 years of age. Circumferential mucosal edema of 1 mm within the larynx of an infant causes the glottic area to narrow by over 60%.

15.4.2   Approach to the Child with Stridor

The evaluation of the child with stridor requires a careful history and physical examination and knowledge of the functional anatomy of the upper airway. Important points in the history and physical are summarized in Table 15-5. Symptoms vary depending on the site of obstruction, as outlined in Table 15-6. An algorithm for the evaluation of a child with stridor is shown in Fig. 15-16, and causes of stridor are listed in Table 15-7.

Clinical assessment is of the utmost importance. An immediate assessment of the urgency of the situation should be made. Age of onset and duration of stridor are important indicators as to which

TABLE 15-5

HISTORY AND PHYSICAL EXAMINATION FOR STRIDOR

HISTORY	PHYSICAL EXAMINATION
Time of onset: gradual, progressive, or sudden	Stridor, pitch, duration, and timing of the stridorous sound
Characteristics of cry	Careful inspection of the patient in the parent's arms
Relationship of stridor to feeding	Respiratory rate and degree of distress
Aspiration or reflux	
Cyanosis	Tachypnea and onset of fatigue
Previous intubation	Flaring of nasal alae and other signs of respiratory effort
Careful repeated questioning for aspirated foreign body	Auscultation of stridor

TABLE 15-6
SYMPTOMS AND THE SITE OF AIRWAY OBSTRUCTION

LOCATION	VOICE	STRIDOR	RETRACTION	FEEDING	COUGH
Laryngeal: supraglottic	Muffled "Hot potato"	Snoring Inspiratory fluttering	None until late	Difficult to impossible	Not noted
Laryngeal: subglottic	Normal Occasionally hoarse	Inspiratory-expiratory snoring	Intercostal early, then xyphoid	Normal	Barking (no other place in the airway)
Tracheal	Normal	Expiratory and wheezing	None, except in severe obstruction	Normal	Brassy

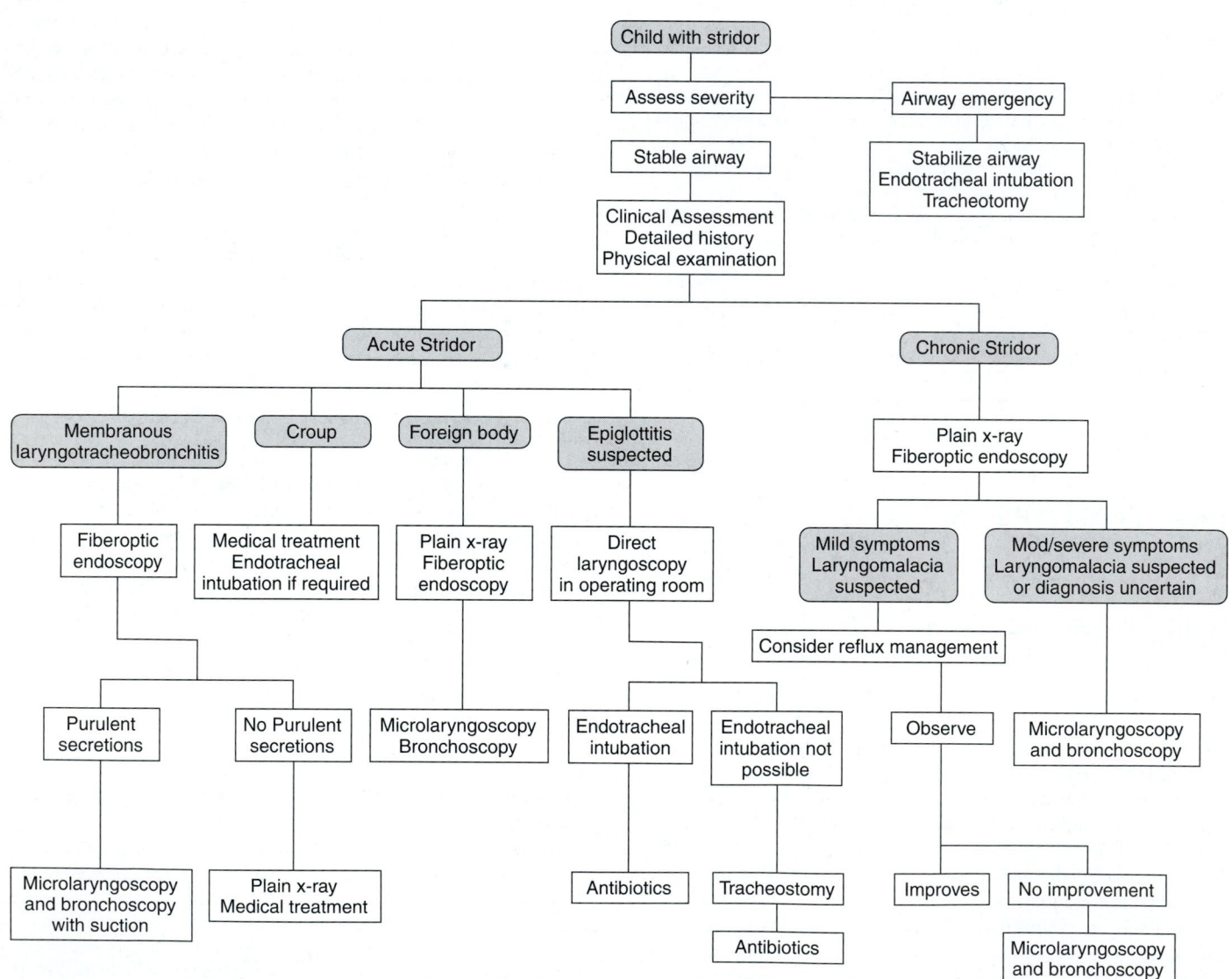

FIGURE 15-16 Algorithm for the evaluation of the child with stridor. Fiberoptic examination is performed in the awake child and provides information about cord mobility and laryngeal dynamics. It provides only limited information about structural defects below the level of the vocal cords. Rigid endoscopy using Hopkins rod lens telescopes allows detailed examination of the subglottis, trachea, and bronchi while maintaining a stable airway. The combination of fiberoptic and rigid endoscopy will accurately diagnose most congenital and acquired abnormalities of the pediatric airway.

TABLE 15-7

CAUSES OF STRIDOR IN CHILDREN

Oropharynx
  Congenital anomalies
    Lingual thyroid
    Choanal atresia
    Craniofacial anomalies (Apert syndrome, Down syndrome, Robin syndrome)
    Cysts (dermoid, thyroglossal)
  Inflammatory
    Abscess (parapharyngeal, retropharyngeal, peritonsillar)
    Allergic polyps
  Neoplasm (benign and malignant)
  Adenotonsillar hyperplasia
  Foreign body
Larynx
  Congenital anomalies
    Laryngomalacia
    Webs, cysts, laryngocele
    Cartilage dystrophy
    Subglottic stenosis
    Cleft larynx
  Inflammatory
    Croup
    Epiglottitis
    Miscellaneous; tuberculosis, diphtheria
  Vocal cord paralysis (multiple etiologies)
  Trauma
    Intubation (laryngeal or subglottic edema, subglottic stenosis)
    Neck trauma
    Foreign body
  Neoplasm
    Subglottic hemangioma
    Laryngeal papilloma
    Cystic hygroma (neck)
    Malignant (rhabdomyosarcoma, chondrosarcoma)
  Laryngospasm (hypocalcemic tetany)
Trachea and bronchi
  Congenital
    Vascular anomalies
    Webs, cysts
    Tracheal stenosis
  Foreign body (tracheal or esophageal)
  Neoplasm (benign and malignant)
    Tracheal
    Compression by neoplasm of adjacent structure (thyroid, thymus, esophagus)
  Trauma
    Tracheal stenosis secondary to intubation or tracheostomy

---

of the congenital causes of stridor is most likely. A history of intubation may indicate subglottic stenosis. Laryngomalacia is the most common cause of congenital stridor and has a characteristic history. Birth injury or neurologic abnormalities may indicate vocal cord paralysis. Acute stridor in the older child may be caused by a foreign body or acute infection.

Careful inspection of the patient is the first priority. The child should remain in the parent's arms, and the physician can judge the respiratory rate and degree of distress. The physician should look for tachypnea or the onset of fatigue that may portend respiratory collapse. Flaring of the nasal alae and the use of accessory neck or chest muscles indicate that an increased degree of respiratory effort is needed to maintain an oxygenated state. Cyanosis and air hunger, particularly from supraglottic infection or a foreign body, will cause the patient to sit with the neck hyperextended in an attempt to improve airflow. The patient should be permitted to maintain such a posture. In a gravely ill child, additional examination should not be undertaken lest it precipitate respiratory arrest. The child requires prompt transport to an appropriate hospital.

In a well-oxygenated, stable child, additional examination can proceed. An important part of the examination is auscultation that is performed both with the ear and with the aid of a stethoscope. Sequential listening over the nose, open mouth, neck, and chest can localize the probable site of obstruction, which is indicated by a heightened sound intensity. Attention is next directed to the respiratory cycle, which normally is composed of a shorter inspiratory phase and a longer expiratory phase. Laryngeal obstruction is usually associated with inspiratory noises, whereas bronchial obstruction has characteristic expiratory noises or wheezes. Similarly, in laryngeal obstruction, the time of inspiration is greatly lengthened, whereas in bronchial obstruction, expiration tends to be prolonged. Tracheal obstruction will often have both inspiratory and expiratory stridor.

The effect on the stridor of placing the infant in various positions should also be assessed. The stridors of laryngomalacia, micrognathia, macroglossia, and vascular compression diminish when the baby lies prone with the neck extended. The presence and quality of the voice or cry can help to identify laryngeal causes of stridor. A weak cry suggests vocal cord disorders or conditions with poor pulmonary function, such as neuromuscular disorders. Although laryngeal lesions are most often accompanied by voice changes, a normal voice does not rule out a laryngeal cause for stridor. For example, with bilateral vocal cord paralysis there may be a normal voice but marked airway obstruction.

Certain maneuvers can be performed to determine the nature of the obstruction. If stridor is present at birth, the first maneuver should be to open the mouth and pull the mandible and tongue forward. If the stridor lessens, the obstruction is at the level of the larynx or higher. Nasal catheters should be passed to determine the patency of the nasopharyngeal airway. In patients with choanal atresia, the placement of an oral airway will help to diagnose the disorder and to bypass the obstruction. The introduction of a laryngoscope will support the laryngeal structures and decrease the stridor of laryngomalacia but will not relieve the obstruction of vocal cord paralysis or subglottic stenosis. Pulling the mandible and tongue forward will often relieve the obstruction seen in the Robin syndrome, and emergency placement of a nasopharyngeal airway will maintain the patient until a long-term care decision can be made (see Sec. 15.3.3).

Diagnostic testing of the infant with stridor always begins with flexible fiberoptic nasopharyngoscopy while awake. This test should be performed in all patients with suspected airway pathology and can be performed in even the smallest child. Vocal cord mobility, laryngeal masses, laryngomalacia, and other laryngeal problems are easily assessed, and this test can usually be performed in an office or clinic setting. The examination begins in the anterior nasal cavity to rule out a pyriform aperture stenosis and moves posteriorly in the nose to rule out a choanal stenosis or atresia. The nasopharynx can be examined for adenoid hypertrophy or other mass lesions. Hypopharyngeal visualization will assess the hypopharyngeal tone. The epiglottis and arytenoid cartilages can be assessed for edema or erythema consistent with reflux esophagitis or infection. In addition, any evidence of laryngomalacia will be noted. Determining the mobility of the true vocal cords is an essential part of this evaluation. Occasionally a subglottic view is possible with a flexible scope, but in general only the anatomy from the true vocal cords and superior larynx can be visualized.

Radiographic evaluation provides useful information about the subglottis, trachea, and larger bronchi and therefore complements the flexible endoscopic examination. Lateral and anteroposterior plain films of the neck demonstrate the patency of the airway lumen and presence of mass lesions. The anteroposterior high-kilovoltage technique is particularly useful for depicting the upper airway, as it enhances the tracheal air column and deemphasizes the bony cervical spine. Videofluoroscopy is very helpful for evaluating dynamic airway problems such as hypopharyngeal collapse and tracheomalacia. The barium swallow is useful to detect both aspiration related to vocal cord paralysis, posterior laryngeal cleft, or H fistula and also external compression from vascular lesions. CT and MRI are useful for obtaining specific information in selected cases, eg, vascular compression of tracheobronchial tree, but are not a substitute for endoscopic evaluation.

A diagnosis is usually established by the above studies. In some cases diagnostic rigid endoscopy is still needed if (1) the diagnosis remains in question, (2) the previous evaluation suggests a subglottic lesion, and (3) a second significant distal lesion in the airway is suspected in addition to the diagnosis of a more obvious proximal lesion in the upper airway. Rigid airway endoscopy may also be necessary for therapy, eg, for removal of laryngeal papillomas.

15.4.3   Congenital Malformations

The clinical manifestations associated with congenital anomalies of the larynx include respiratory obstruction, stridor in infants or hoarseness in older children, a weakened or abnormal cry, dyspnea, tachypnea, aspiration, and sudden death. As discussed above, diagnosis is confirmed by radiologic examination, flexible endoscopy, and rigid endoscopy in select cases.

LARYNGOMALACIA

The pathogenesis of laryngomalacia, which is the most common cause of stridor in the newborn, is not completely understood. The cartilages of the infantile larynx are very flexible. As the infant inspires, the laryngeal skeleton is not stiff enough to keep the laryngeal lumen fully open. The infant epiglottis assumes a pronounced tubular or omega shape, and the aryepiglottic folds and false vocal cords are drawn into the laryngeal lumen, which results in a substantial narrowing of the lumen on inspiration. This narrowing accounts for the high-pitched stridor heard in these infants. The stridor of laryngomalacia may be present at birth but more often occurs about 2 weeks after birth. The child breathes more comfortably when relaxed and is usually more stridorous when agitated. Once other causes for stridor are ruled out, the treatment of this condition is most often close observation. As the child grows, the cartilages become more rigid and support the larynx, so the stridor resolves. Most children will outgrow the condition by 12 to 18 months. More severe laryngomalacia may cause failure to thrive secondary to airway obstruction and poor feeding or nighttime obstructive symptoms with significant oxygen desaturations. In these cases surgical trimming of the supraglottis (epiglottoplasty) is recommended.

TRACHEOBRONCHOMALACIA

Tracheomalacia is an abnormal collapse of the trachea severe enough to produce symptoms of airway obstruction. Bronchomalacia is the equivalent in the bronchi, and tracheobronchomalacia involves both. Mild tracheobronchomalacia is common and self-limited, whereas severe tracheobronchomalacia is life-threatening, and heroic measures may need to be considered, such as tracheostomy with positive-pressure ventilation. Tracheobronchomalacia may be primary or secondary to other pathology, eg, tracheoesophageal fistula, cardiac and vascular abnormalities, or cervical or mediastinal masses. Usually no treatment is required for primary tracheobronchomalacia, as the disease is self-limiting with resolution over a few years. Parents require substantial support and education, especially if the child has recurrent episodes of apnea and obstruction. Parents should be taught cardiopulmonary resuscitation. In severe cases of tracheobronchomalacia, the potential risks and benefits of any therapies need to be carefully balanced.

SUBGLOTTIC STENOSIS

Congenital subglottic stenosis can cause significant stridor in the neonate or in the early months of life. Narrowing of the subglottic airway can occur because the first tracheal ring is trapped within the cricoid cartilage, a deformity of the cricoid cartilage, or excess soft tissue within the cricoid cartilage. The diagnosis is made by rigid endoscopy under general anesthesia.

Only stenosis sufficient to produce signs of respiratory distress requires treatment. In the past, treatment often meant a tracheostomy and waiting for the subglottic space to grow with the child. Currently, if the obstruction is sufficiently severe to require a tracheostomy, early surgical correction may avoid a tracheostomy in all but the most severe cases. In contrast, acquired subglottic stenosis generally requires a tracheostomy with subsequent surgical correction to achieve decannulation. These children are often graduates of the neonatal nursery and have many other medical problems that need to be managed.

WEBS, CYSTS, AND LARYNGOCELES

Partial or complete glottic webs can occur with aberrant development of structures in and around the laryngeal inlet in the embryo. Abnormal voice and, in more severe disease, stridor and respiratory distress can be the presenting signs. Tracheostomy can be life-saving in the more complete glottic webs. Because there is an association between glottic web and velocardiofacial syndrome, children with glottic webs should have genetic testing for 22q11 gene deletions and genetic consultation.

Congenital cysts of the larynx arise from the mucus-secreting epithelium in the supraglottic region and occasionally in the subglottic space. Presenting symptoms include stridor and sometimes hoarseness. These must be distinguished from vallecular cysts that, if large, seriously interfere with swallowing and breathing. Subglottic cysts may be congenital, but they are usually secondary to prolonged or traumatic intubation. In either case, the endoscopic CO_2 laser can be used to remove the cyst.

Laryngoceles are epithelium-lined diverticula that originate from the laryngeal ventricle. They can present internally in the larynx with airway obstruction or externally as a neck mass. Total excision of the cyst by external approach is the treatment of choice, but the endoscopic CO_2 laser may be useful in selected cases. Thyroglossal duct cysts can present at birth as an obstructive lesion at the base of the tongue (see Sec. 15.3.3).

LARYNGOTRACHEOESOPHAGEAL DEFECTS

Incomplete formation of the tracheoesophageal septum can leave abnormal connections between the food and air passages. Clefts range from a slight deepening of the interarytenoid notch to a complete absence of the tracheoesophageal septum to the carina. Symptoms may vary according to the length of the cleft. The child with a significant cleft will present with recurrent aspiration, failure to thrive, or life-threatening respiratory events. Small clefts are often difficult to demonstrate radiographically or endoscopically and require a high degree of suspicion to be diagnosed early. Surgical repair is indicated for all clefts, and extensive clefts are best repaired using extracorporeal membrane oxygenation (ECMO) to permit unhindered surgical access to the entire length of the larynx, trachea, and esophagus.

15.4.4 Vocal Cord Paralysis

A list of the possible causes of vocal cord paralysis in children is presented in Table 15-8. The symptoms of unilateral vocal cord paralysis are often so mild that the disorder often goes unnoticed. Unilateral recurrent laryngeal nerve paralysis results in the affected cord assuming a midline or slightly abducted position, and the cry is weak. The cry usually returns to near normal because the unaffected vocal cord compensates for the paralyzed one. Aspiration of liquids may occur if the normal vocal cord fails to compensate for the paralyzed cord and there is incomplete laryngeal closure during deglutition. On inspiration, the normal vocal cord abducts completely to create an airway adequate for all except the most strenuous exercise. Superior laryngeal nerve injury results in paralysis of the cricothyroid muscle on the injured side. Decreased tension of the vocal cord accounts for the slight decrease in vocal range characteristic of superior laryngeal paralysis. Treatment is seldom required for unilateral vocal cord paralysis, although laryngoplasty (surgical medialization of the paralyzed cord) is occasionally performed to improve the voice or to decrease aspiration.

TABLE 15-8
CAUSES OF VOCAL CORD PARALYSIS

Congenital
  Central nervous system disease
  Birth trauma to head or neck
  Cysts (neck or chest)
Neoplasm (intracranial, cervical, thoracic)
  Benign
  Malignant
Inflammatory
  Infection (viral)
  Degenerative disease (rheumatoid arthritis)
Metabolic disease
  Diabetes mellitus
  Heavy metal poisoning (As, Pb)
Trauma (includes surgery)
  Blunt or penetrating (neck, head, chest)
  Intubation
Neurologic
  Central nervous system disease
  Neuromuscular disease (eg, myasthenia gravis)
Vascular
  Cardiovascular anomalies
  Cardiac failure (left heart enlargement)

Bilateral recurrent laryngeal paralysis is usually characterized by marked airway obstruction and a good voice; both vocal cords are paralyzed in the midline or slightly abducted position. Management of symptomatic bilateral vocal cord paralysis requires prompt airway intervention, either intubation or tracheostomy to relieve the airway obstruction. If the cause of the vocal cord paralysis is treatable, such as posterior craniotomy for Arnold-Chiari malformation, or resolves, such as Guillain-Barré syndrome, the vocal cords may regain their mobility, permitting extubation or decannulation. If the paralysis is permanent, several procedures have been advocated to create an airway adequate to allow decannulation. Partial arytenoidectomy or unilateral vocal cord lateralization by either endoscopic or external methods allows one of the vocal cords to be permanently lateralized with limited impact on the quality of the voice.

15.4.5 Inflammatory and Infective Disorders of the Larynx

VIRAL INFECTIONS

Viral laryngitis is often a component of upper respiratory infection (see also Sec. 13.4.19). Laryngeal manifestations usually include a hoarse, raspy voice, which is related to edema of the vocal cords, but airway obstruction is rare. Humidification, throat gargles, and voice rest are recommended for symptomatic relief. Laryngotracheobronchitis or croup is a common disorder of early childhood that is potentially life-threatening.

LARYNGOTRACHEOBRONCHITIS OR CROUP This disorder is easily recognized by its characteristic high-pitched, barking cough and inspiratory stridor. Viral laryngotracheobronchitis is most prevalent from age 3 months to 3 years, peaks during the second year of life, and is more common in boys than girls. Most cases occur in the late fall and early winter, reflecting the epidemiologic patterns of the various agents. Human parainfluenza virus types I and II account for most of the cases of croup in young children. Sporadic and sometimes severe cases of croup may be associated with other types of human parainfluenza virus, influenza virus types A and B, respiratory syncytial virus (RSV), measles, and a variety of other viruses. RSV is a major cause of lower respiratory tract infection in young children, and croup is its least common clinical manifestation. However, because a high percentage of young children admitted to the hospital with acute lower respiratory tract disease have high RSV isolates, this pathogen cannot be discounted as a cause of croup.

Viral upper respiratory tract infections usually affect the mucosa of the nose and nasopharynx first and then spread to involve the larynx and tracheobronchial tree. The mucosa of the subglottis of the young child is loosely attached and permits submucosal edema formation with narrowing of the airway. The barking cough and stridor characteristic of croup generally result from edema of the subglottic airway. The cricoid cartilage is normally a complete ring, and thus the airway is narrowest here, and swelling cannot occur outward. Therefore, even minimal edema can cause airway obstruction, with symptoms being more likely in young children because their small airway diameter is far more resistant to airflow.

In croup, stridor is most common on inspiration because the negative inspiratory pressure tends to collapse the already partially narrowed extrathoracic structures. Biphasic stridor occurs if the subglottis is extremely narrow. Copious secretions produced secondary to inflammation will also clog the airway, producing secondary obstruction in an already narrow region.

The differential diagnosis of viral laryngobroncheotracheitis includes spasmodic croup, bacterial croup and tracheitis, retropharyngeal abscess, angioneurotic edema, and foreign bodies of the aerodigestive tract. The most important element in evaluating children with croup is distinguishing those with croup from those with epiglottitis, although this is far less a concern in regions where *H. influenzae* vaccination has almost eliminated epiglottitis (see below). Management of croup consists of supportive treatment with cool mist. At home this can be achieved by a cool mist vaporizer or placing the child in a bathroom filled with steam from the shower or by taking the child outdoors in the cool night air. In the hospital initial management consists of hydration, cool mist with or without supplemental oxygen, and racemic epinephrine. Many physicians use a croup score, both for the initial triage of the child and to evaluate response to medical therapy. Whatever method is used, sound medical judgment is needed to predict the onset of respiratory failure, hypoxia, and hypercarbia. Most infants improve over 48 to 72 hours without further treatment, but some require intervention for impending respiratory failure.

Aerosolized racemic epinephrine (2.25%), nebulized with 100% oxygen, has become a mainstay of croup management if the patient has not had a prompt clinical response to cool mist. It acts by producing vasoconstriction and decreasing edema. The main drawback of racemic epinephrine is the rebound phenomenon, with symptom recurrence as the medication's effect wears off. The most important recent change in the medical management of croup is the use of systemic steroids. Prospective, randomized studies have demonstrated that steroid therapy decreases the length and severity of the respiratory symptoms associated with viral croup. Dexamethasone is the preparation most frequently used in doses between 0.6 and 1.0 mg/kg. The best route of administration (oral, nebulizer, intravenous), criteria for administration, and the relative effects of different steroid doses remain to be established. Sedation should either be avoided or used only in a monitored environment. Arterial pH and blood gas measurements may help in guiding treatment, but the arterial puncture may cause further agitation, exacerbating symptoms. Intubation is rarely necessary, and if it is required, the presence of an underlying congenital lesion such as subglottic stenosis or a vascular ring should be considered. Recurrent episodes of croup may occur in otherwise normal children, as discussed below.

BACTERIAL INFECTIONS

Acute epiglottitis is an infection of the larynx with rapid swelling of the epiglottis and increasing inspiratory difficulty. Since the introduction of the *Hemophilus B* vaccine, this disorder is an increasingly uncommon infection of the supraglottic larynx. *H. influenzae* still remains the most common bacterial infection of the larynx, especially in regions where vaccination is unavailable. Bacterial infections by *Streptococcus, Staphylococcus,* and others have also been implicated as causes of supraglottic infection.

Epiglottitis primarily affects children between the ages of 2 and 5 years. Bacterial laryngitis is not as common as viral laryngitis, but it may be difficult to differentiate between the two with only clinical information. Typically, children with epiglottitis present with the abrupt onset of fever, sore throat, drooling, and stridor that progresses to severe airway obstruction in less than 24 hours. The patient may sit forward with the chin extended to maintain an open airway. Few conditions produce such a dramatic constellation of

symptoms and findings, although occasionally croup or a foreign body obstruction presents similarly. However, children with viral croup are generally younger, have usually been ill for 2 to 3 days with URI symptoms progressing gradually to hoarseness, croupy cough, and inspiratory stridor. Soft tissue x-rays of the neck can help to differentiate epiglottitis and viral croup, but these are generally not required when children have typical symptoms. If epiglottitis is considered as a serious possibility, inspection of the epiglottis and hypopharynx is mandatory. This must be performed emergently but in controlled conditions where an artificial airway can be provided by skilled personnel (typically endotracheal intubation by an anesthesiologist or otolaryngologist in the operating room).

Infections such as diphtheria and tuberculosis are rare in developed countries but are still encountered in nondeveloped countries. Diphtheria is an example of a bacterial infection that can involve the larynx in addition to other areas of the upper aerodigestive tract. Tuberculosis of the larynx can occur, usually associated with a generalized pulmonary infection.

FUNGAL INFECTION OF THE LARYNX

Fungal infections of the larynx are rare in children and are usually present as a component of a more generalized disease process. Histoplasmosis and coccidioidomycosis have been identified on laryngeal biopsies or cultures in patients with a nonspecific laryngitis. Tracheostomy may be required to protect the airway in some of these patients.

OTHER INFLAMMATORY DISORDERS OF THE LARYNX

SPASMODIC CROUP In spasmodic croup, an otherwise healthy child wakes up in the middle of the night with symptoms of a barky cough and mild to severe inspiratory stridor. The condition variously responds to humidification or exposure to cold air. The next day the child appears healthy, but the cyclic episode repeats itself on two or three successive nights. The repetitive nature of this problem and its variable response to therapy are quite characteristic. The etiology is not understood. Absence of any signs of upper respiratory tract infection separates this entity from acute infectious croup and suggests an allergic origin. Gastroesophageal reflux may be a factor in some children by causing a baseline airway inflammation that, when challenged with a viral upper respiratory infection, creates additional edema to cause significant airway obstruction. Failure of typical therapies, especially in conjunction with obstructive symptoms during allergic episodes, may be cause to suspect a subglottic stenosis. Such a reduction of the already restricted subglottic space may make an otherwise normal child unable to tolerate even mild inflammation associated with allergic sensitivities.

ALLERGY The larynx is susceptible to the same allergens that affect other parts of the upper aerodigestive tract. When the mucosa of the larynx is involved, edema of the vocal cords results in a hoarse voice and a dry, scratchy feeling in the throat. The larynx may also be irritated by an allergic postnasal drip. Treatment of allergic manifestations in the larynx includes avoidance of the offending allergen, systemic antihistamines, humidification, systemic or aerosol corticosteroids, and desensitization.

ANGIONEUROTIC EDEMA Angioedema consists of localized edema of rapid onset in response to a variety of triggers including infection, drugs (especially angiotensin-converting enzyme inhibitors and aspirin), exercise, allergens, insect bites, serum sickness, collagen vascular diseases, and malignancy. It commonly affects the upper airway and can cause life-threatening obstruction. Subcutaneous epinephrine (0.01 mL/kg of 1:1000 concentration) provides rapid relief. A variety of antihistamines such as diphenhydramine provide longer-term control. Occasionally systemic steroids are required to control the problem. Hereditary angioneurotic edema is a rare disorder discussed in Sec. 17.10.4.

GASTROESOPHAGEAL REFLUX   Gastroesophageal reflux with passage of gastric contents into the pharynx is normal in infants and young children. When the anatomy and physiology of the larynx are normal, the refluxed gastric material never enters the airway. When laryngeal anatomy is abnormal, as with a laryngeal cleft, or if the normal protective reflexes are absent because of neuromuscular disease, the gastric material can impinge on laryngeal structures and may enter the airway. Even infrequent (such as once every several days) exposure can cause laryngeal inflammation and may aggravate many laryngeal and upper airway conditions in infants and children. In children with cough, oropharyngeal dysphagia, vocal cord granuloma, airway obstruction, apnea, asthma, recurrent croup, laryngomalacia, laryngitis, and subglottic stenosis, gastroesophageal reflux should be considered as an underlying etiologic factor (see Sec. 17.10.4).

15.4.6   Masses and Tumors of the Larynx

VOCAL CORD NODULES

Hoarseness can result from the formation of vocal cord nodules as a result of persistent vocal misuse or abuse by shouting, screaming, or even singing. These masses occur at the junction of the anterior and middle one-third of the vocal cords, which is the point of maximal vocal cord vibration. The size of the nodules and the resultant hoarseness usually fluctuate, depending on the child's vocal use or abuse. It is important to diagnose the cause of hoarseness in young children by performing a flexible laryngoscopy. Once the diagnosis is made, in young children a period of observation is appropriate. In older children, if the problem persists, the nodules are best managed by behavior modification and, if necessary, speech therapy. Occasionally, nodules that have fibrosed from long-standing vocal abuse may not respond to conservative management and will require endoscopic removal. If the child continues with poor speech habits, the nodules will likely recur, and therefore, speech therapy is an important adjunctive therapy.

PAPILLOMATOSIS

Although they are not considered true neoplasms, the wart-like lesions from recurrent respiratory papillomatosis are often referred to as the most common tumor of the larynx in children. The papilloma virus, especially types 6 and 11, has been shown to be the cause of the lesions, with a particular predilection for the upper aerodigestive tract, especially the larynx. The "juvenile" type of this disease usually makes its presentation at 2 to 5 years of age, causing hoarseness and marked airway obstruction in severe cases. The course of the disease is characterized by multiple cycles of growth and regression. In many cases a spontaneous remission occurs, usually around puberty. None of the recommended treatments—surgical excision, laser excision, cryotherapy, ultrasound, interferon, or topical agents—has been shown consistently to cure the disease.

The goal in treating these patients is to maintain a good voice and an unobstructed airway by repeated CO_2 laser excision of the papillomas. Not uncommonly, however, despite all efforts to keep the patient's larynx clear, rapid growth of papillomas causes airway obstruction, and a tracheotomy is required. There is an incidence of malignant transformation, making this a serious disease.

HEMANGIOMAS

These lesions may occur in the larynx, primarily in the subglottic area, and are often associated with other cutaneous hemangiomas but also occur as isolated lesions. With crying or straining, these lesions increase in size and cause significant airway obstruction. They appear as asymmetric masses on anteroposterior neck radiography, but the diagnosis must usually be confirmed by microlaryngoscopy. A primary hemangioma may be confined to the subglottic space, or it may be part of a larger mediastinal hemangioma. Occasionally, a laryngeal hemangioma may be secondary to airway invasion by a large cervicofacial hemangioma. Because many hemangiomas of infancy tend to involute after a period of growth during the first year, close observation is the initial treatment of choice. If obstructive symptoms require more aggressive therapy, dexamethasone can be administered every 72 hours aiming to limit the growth of the hemangioma while minimizing the dangers of steroid therapy in infants. If the lesion fails to decrease in size, the CO_2 laser can be used to partially remove hemangiomas without airway obstruction or hemorrhage. Increasingly, removal of the hemangiomas by external surgery followed by brief intubation is an effective and permanent solution to the problem without impacting the voice. Malignant tumors in children are very rare.

15.4.7   Trauma and Foreign Bodies

TRAUMA

Blunt or penetrating injuries may occur with sports or motor vehicle accidents. These injuries may result in mucosal laceration, laryngeal hematomas, vocal cord paralysis, or fractures of the thyroid cartilage. Patients present with various degrees of neck pain, hoarseness, hemoptysis, and airway obstruction. Physical examination may reveal anterior neck tenderness, crepitance, and absence of the normal prominence of the thyroid cartilage. Proper treatment requires recognition of the nature of the injury and protection of the airway.

Endotracheal intubation can cause mucosal lacerations, granulomas of the vocal cords, dislocation of the arytenoid cartilage, and subglottic stenosis. Subglottic stenosis is a serious complication of intubation in children. Mucosal ulcerations and pressure necrosis can occur as the mucosa is compressed by the pressure of a tight-fitting endotracheal tube against the unyielding cricoid cartilage surrounding the subglottic space; resultant chondritis or mucosal fibrosis can produce mature scar tissue that narrows the subglottic lumen significantly. A congenital smaller-than-normal airway, large endotracheal tube, inadequate fixation of the tube, prolonged intubation, mechanical ventilation, multiple intubations, infection, and cuffed endotracheal tubes all increase the risk of subglottic stenosis developing. Treatment is the same as that described for subglottic stenosis of congenital origin, relying mainly on open laryngotracheal reconstruction techniques.

FOREIGN BODY ASPIRATION

Inhalations and ingestions are common and potentially fatal pediatric accidents. In 1984, aspiration or ingestion of food or foreign objects accounted for 271 deaths in children under 5 years of age in the United States. Ninety percent of children who aspirate foreign bodies are under 3 years of age, and two-thirds are boys. Nuts, and most especially peanuts, are the most common inhaled objects. In a survey of 103 food-related asphyxiation episodes in children, the hot dog impacted in the upper airway or upper esophagus was the single most common agent in this type of death. In 1984, the National Safety Council identified foreign body aspiration or ingestion as the fourth leading cause of accidental death in this age group and as the third leading cause in infants under the age of 1 year.

The manifestations of aspiration depend on the size of the foreign body, its composition, its location, the degree of blockage, and the duration of obstruction. Except in the rare instance of impending asphyxia from an impacted laryngeal foreign body, time exists for a careful history, physical examination, and radiologic examination. History is of paramount importance in the diagnosis of foreign body aspiration because the physical examination and radiographic study can be unremarkable after the acute event. Inquiring about a characteristic history of a "spell" is critical. Serious attention should be paid to a history of respiratory difficulty being witnessed while the child was eating nuts, seeds, beans, or carrots, the primary culprits in foreign body aspiration in younger children.

Most inhaled foreign bodies travel distally into the tracheobronchial tree, but laryngeal impaction occasionally occurs. Thus, laryngeal foreign bodies account for the highest mortality in the aerodigestive tract, but survivors of transient obstruction carry a risk of hypoxic encephalopathy. Large objects such as hot dogs or balloons are apt to obstruct the glottic inlet and precipitate acute respiratory arrest. These children may survive if resuscitated by caretakers, paramedics, or emergency physicians. In the rare instance in which the child is blue and apneic, an adult should quickly look into the back of the child's throat and remove any visible object that is identified. Blind finger sweeps in the pharynx, however, are discouraged because the foreign body may easily be pushed farther into the airway during such attempts. Mouth-to-mouth resuscitation is ineffective if the upper airway is completely blocked.

Fortunately, most smaller, nonobstructing objects bypass the supraglottis, glottis, and trachea and lodge most commonly in the right main-stem bronchus. Depending on the size, location, and nature of the foreign body, local irritation produces complaints of cough, inspiratory stridor, hoarseness, wheezing, shortness of breath, and fever, symptoms that mimic the more common diseases of the respiratory tract including asthma, bronchiolitis, laryngitis, pharyngitis, and croup. Symptoms may occur within hours of the aspiration or weeks later. Thus, some aspirated foreign bodies may go unrecognized for weeks or longer.

The absence of obvious symptoms after a witnessed choking episode does not exclude the presence of a retained foreign body. Following the initial episode of paroxysmal coughing, an asymptomatic lag period occurs as the surface sensory receptors of the respiratory tract undergo normal physiological adaptations. This situation may falsely reassure the parent and the physician that the child has cleared the airway. Only two-thirds of patients seek treatment within 1 week following aspiration. Thus, the first symptoms prompting medial attention may represent a complication of foreign body impaction, such as chronic cough and fever related to recurrent or persistent pneumonia, bronchitis, or even bronchiectasis. Atypical asthma is a common misdiagnosis assigned to unsuspected airway foreign bodies.

Physical findings following aspiration are variable and dependent on the occasion and degree of luminal obstruction by the foreign

body. The child may be quiet and comfortable or exhibit signs of respiratory distress ranging from mild tachypnea to severe stridor with retractions and cyanosis. Classic physical findings in cases of foreign body aspiration consist of unilateral decreased breath sounds as a result of decreased aeration of the lung and unilateral rhonchi from partial occlusion of the bronchus. The clinical triad of wheezing, coughing, and diminished or absent breath sounds is present in only about 40% of patients, although 75% have one or more of these findings. Rapid changes in respiratory status may occur from development of edema or change in location of the foreign body. Tracheal foreign bodies are particularly treacherous in this regard, with patients alternating between periods of normality and severe obstruction.

Flexible nasolaryngoscopy may add valuable diagnostic information when inspiratory stridor is the sole physical finding and a laryngeal or hypopharyngeal foreign body is suspected by history. Laryngomalacia or inflammatory etiologies of stridor may be identified. This examination should be performed using topical anesthesia in the awake, nonsedated, upright child. It should be performed with extreme caution in small children with severe obstruction or when supraglottitis is suspected and should be performed only when airway resuscitative equipment is immediately available. When performed appropriately this procedure is very safe.

After a thorough history and physical examination, plain neck and chest radiographs should be obtained. About 10% of aspirated foreign bodies are radiopaque, making the radiographic diagnosis easy. However, the majority of foreign bodies are not obvious, and changes seen are those secondary to the obstruction of the airway by the foreign body. Anteroposterior and lateral views of the neck and chest may reveal signs of a partially obliterated tracheobronchial air column or abnormal ventilation of the affected lung. Inspiratory and expiratory views are very important. The classic radiographic abnormality is unilateral hyperlucency on an expiratory film. A ball valve effect of a partial occlusion of the bronchus allows air to enter the affected lobe or lung on inspiration but traps the air on expiration. Other studies that may demonstrate unilateral air trapping are decubitus views of the chest or chest fluoroscopy. Indirect radiologic signs include resorption atelectasis, compensatory emphysema of the contralateral lung, pneumonia, pneumothorax, and expiratory shift of the mediastinum. Late findings such as pulmonary abscess or bronchiectasis are still occasionally seen. Lobar or segmental pulmonary infiltrate from impaired clearance of respiratory secretions usually implies obstruction of days or weeks. Although radiography is useful for confirmation and localization of foreign body aspiration, up to 25% of bronchial foreign bodies, and over half of those in the trachea, yield no abnormalities on plain chest radiograph. For this reason, foreign body aspiration can never be excluded on the basis of a chest radiograph alone.

A final diagnosis is achieved only at the time of bronchoscopic examination. Because the clinical and radiographic findings can be so variable and mimic so many different pulmonary conditions, it is inevitable that a proportion of endoscopic evaluations will be performed without finding a foreign body. It is certainly preferable to perform a negative endoscopic evaluation than to leave a foreign body undiagnosed.

15.4.8 Tracheotomy

There are three major indications for long-term tracheotomy in children: airway obstruction, ventilatory support, and pulmonary toilet. Patients requiring tracheotomies for airway obstruction generally receive the procedure as young infants for either congenital laryngeal disorders or acquired subglottic stenosis. Patients requiring tracheotomy for ventilatory support are a more heterogeneous group. Respiratory failure may be associated with prematurity, central nervous system disease, or poor pulmonary reserve. Children requiring tracheotomy for pulmonary toilet generally have some degree of aspiration. This is commonly caused by discoordinated swallowing mechanisms related to neurologic disease. This group differs from the other two groups in that they have a less immediate dependence on the tracheotomy tube should accidental decannulation occur. They comprise a relatively small patient population.

The long-term outcome in children with tracheotomy has improved, mainly through advances in home care. The morbidity and mortality from tracheotomy-related events has dramatically decreased because of advances in this field. Plugging, accidental decannulation, local wound breakdown, mucosal suction trauma, and infections have been addressed by specialists in the field, giving a markedly improved quality of life for the child at home.

Comprehensive home care programs for children with tracheotomies should integrate the skills required to maintain a safe airway while promoting the child's normal development and growth (see also Sec. 6.2.1). Individualized training must be given to all caregivers to a level of basic competency. Caregivers should be able to identify proficiently when the child is having an airway-related problem and be able to perform some basic maneuvers to alleviate potential complete obstruction and cardiorespiratory arrest. The caregivers should be trained to suction and change the tracheostomy tube without difficulty. If this cannot be achieved, the child should be placed in a setting where skilled care is available, whether at home with skilled nursing or in a chronic care facility. Optimal teaching of tie securing, humidification, tracheostomy tube changing, and cardiopulmonary resuscitation are essential.

One of the most important jobs of the clinician coordinating home care for a child with a tracheostomy is to ensure that the parents or other caregivers are connected to an appropriate support network that is available at all times. The surgeon, pediatrician, nurses, speech and language pathologist, backup caregivers, and equipment providers should be easily accessible to those primarily responsible for the child's welfare.

Finally, home monitoring is controversial. Mechanical apnea monitors give an alarm with the absence of respiratory effort. They are generally used for central apnea. Cessation of respiratory effort is an extremely late sign of tracheostomy occlusion or dislodgment. Pulse oximetry, on the other hand, is associated with frequent false alarms from failure of the probe to find the pulse or from detachment. It should be stressed that no alarm system is a substitute for adequate training of responsible caregivers. There is a danger that monitoring equipment can give a false sense of security. There is no replacement for constant vigilance of the child with a tracheostomy.

References

Cotton RT: The problem of pediatric laryngotracheal stenosis: a clinical and experimental study on the efficacy of autogenous cartilage grafts placed between the vertically divided halves of the posterior lamina of the cricoid cartilage. Laryngoscope 101:1–34, 1991

Friedman E: Tracheobronchial foreign bodies. Otolaryngol Clin North Am 33:179–185, 2000

Green GE, Bauman NM, Smith RJH: Pathogenesis and treatment of juvenile onset recurrent respiratory papillomatosis. Otolaryngol Clin North Am 33:187–205, 2000

Hughes CA, Rezaee A, Ludemann JP, Holinger LD: Management of congenital subglottic hemangioma. J Otolaryngol 28:223–228, 1999

Matthews BL, Little JP, McGuirt WF, Koufman JA: Reflux in infants with laryngomalacia: results of 24-hour double-probe pH monitoring. Otolaryngol Head Neck Surg 120:860–864, 1999

Tunkel DE, Kosko JR: Vocal cord paralysis in children. Curr Opin Otolaryngol Head Neck Surg 4:419–423, 1996

Walner DL, Donnelly LF, Ouanounou S, Cotton RT: Utility of radiographs in the evaluation of pediatric upper airway obstruction. Ann Otol Rhinol Laryngol 108:378–383, 1999

15.5 EVALUATION OF HEAD AND NECK MASSES

James H. Liu and Charles M. Myer III

Head and neck masses are classified, based on etiology, as being either inflammatory or infectious, congenital, caused by vasoformative lesions, or neoplasms. The majority of lesions in children are either inflammatory or congenital in origin, but the possibility of malignancy must always be considered. The wide variety of pathologic processes can be distinguished with an organized diagnostic approach.

The history and physical examination provide initial guidance on evaluation. The age, sex, and race help narrow diagnostic possibilities. Malignant lesions are rare at birth. In infancy and early childhood, inflammatory and congenital lesions are most common. Inflammatory lesions normally have a relatively brief clinical duration and may recur at intervals, whereas congenital lesions are usually diagnosed early in life. A painless rapidly enlarging lesion is more likely to be neoplastic. A preceding upper respiratory tract infection, rash, foreign travel, tuberculosis exposure, dental procedures, previous excision of scalp or skin lesions, family history of similar lesions, or animal contacts may suggest an infectious etiology. A recent cat scratch or raw meat ingestion raises the possibility of toxoplasmosis or cat scratch as causative agents.

Midline lesions are usually benign. Posterior cervical adenopathy suggests a possible scalp infection. Cystic lesions are more likely to be benign; solid lesions are more commonly malignant. Specific characteristics of a mass, including size, surrounding edema, erythema, tenderness, and fluctuance should be considered. Enlarged lymph nodes up to 2 cm in diameter are not uncommon, especially following an upper respiratory infection. The presence of multiple small nodes bilaterally with such a history is generally of little concern. However, should there be a solitary lymph node or group of lymph nodes that is extremely hard, matted together, fixed to the skin, or demonstrating progressive enlargement without a history of associated respiratory infection, the concern regarding neoplasm becomes greater. Besides the cervical lymph nodes, one also must evaluate for the presence of generalized lymphadenopathy, hepatosplenomegaly, and fever because cervical lymphadenopathy may be a reflection of a systemic condition. The ear, pharynx, tonsils, dental structures, scalp, and skin must be evaluated thoroughly because these are possible primary sites for infection. Supraclavicular adenopathy should alert the clinician to the possibility of pulmonary or abdominal disease.

The most common head and neck mass in children is infectious lymphadenitis. Inflammatory diseases generally arise and usually are associated with overlying erythema, edema, tenderness, and fever. The possibility of a malignancy should be considered at an earlier stage if there is persistent fever, weight loss, fixation of the mass to the skin or subcutaneous tissues, or supraclavicular adenopathy. In these cases, immediate biopsy should be considered. In cases in which infectious etiologies are considered to be more likely, observation of the response to antimicrobial therapy is reasonable.

Laboratory and radiographic studies may be obtained immediately if there is a mass that suggests a possible malignancy. These could include a complete blood count (CBC) with a differential to evaluate for inflammation or a blood dyscrasia and possibly serum chemical profiles and urinalysis. If infectious etiologies are considered to be more likely, a Monospot and/or serologic tests for Epstein-Barr virus, cytomegalovirus, toxoplasmosis, tularemia, histoplasmosis, syphilis, *Bartonella hensalae* (cat scratch disease), and HIV may be considered. If a midline congenital lesion seems likely, thyroid function test and ultrasound may precede biopsy or fine needle aspiration. If malignancy is suspected, it is important to evaluate whether the mass may represent a metastatic lesion before proceeding with diagnostic biopsies. A chest radiograph or CT scan may be indicated, especially if lymphoma is being considered where mediastinal involvement is common.

Fine needle aspiration is a widely used diagnostic technique for the evaluation of head and neck mass lesions in adults, but its reliability in pediatric patients is dependent on the experience and expertise of the cytopathologist performing the investigation. It is of particular value for differentiating cystic from solid masses. Fine needle aspiration should be considered for diagnosis if there is a mass in a child less than 6 weeks of age, if the history suggests an unusual pathogen, or if the patient is immunocompromised or has fever and toxicity requiring hospitalization. If a neoplasm is suspected, an open biopsy should be considered unless a definitive diagnosis is obtained by aspiration.

INFECTIOUS MASSES

The most common causes of bacterial lymphadenitis are *Staphylococcus aureus* or group A β-hemolytic streptococci. Antimicrobial therapy should be initiated with a broad-spectrum antibiotic effective against these agents if a head and neck mass is thought to be possibly caused by an infectious etiology. In very young children, particularly those with associated periorbital inflammation, *Hemophilus influenzae* infection should also be considered. If a dental source of infection is suspected, additional anaerobic antibacterial coverage should be included in the therapeutic trial. If the mass responds to therapy (decreased erythema, tenderness, and size), therapy should be continued for several weeks. If there is no change in the size of the mass over 6 weeks, progressive enlargement of the mass over a 2-week interval, or a failure of the mass to regress over 3 months, or if the mass is fluctulent, aspiration and/or biopsy should be considered. One must recognize that shotty adenopathy may be normal in children and therefore does not require biopsy.

Other infections cause lymphadenitis. Viral lymphadenitis is generally self-limited and short in duration. Mononucleosis is generally associated with a triad of symptoms including fever, pharyngitis, and cervical lymphadenopathy. Diagnosis can be confirmed with a Monospot test for serum heterophile antibodies in 70% of cases at the end of the first week of infection and in 95% by the end of the third week of clinical symptoms, except in children less than age 4 years, where Epstein-Barr viral antibodies are more reliable tests. Toxoplasmosis is associated with cervical lymph node involvement in 80% of cases, with serology being diagnostic. Kawasaki disease may present with findings of conjunctivitis, a strawberry red tongue, lymphadenitis, and fever. Histoplasmosis may also cause lymphadenitis. Diagnosis is made by serology and/or on biopsy.

Tuberculosis infection often presents with adenopathy in the posterior cervical triangle. A PPD test and controls (to assure the patient is not anergic) should be obtained in suspect cases. Chest radiographs may also aid in confirming the diagnosis. Patients with masses caused by atypical tuberculosis caused by the organisms *M. scrofulaceum, M. avium intracellulare,* and *M. kansasii* usually have no constitutional symptoms and present with a mass with a rubbery or dull red appearance, minimal tenderness, and possibly a draining sinus. PPD is either negative or weakly positive. Actinomycosis is caused by commensal organisms of the oral cavity, usually *Actinomyces israelii*. Often the mass develops following dental extractions or infections. Diagnosis requires biopsy. Cat scratch disease is usually associated with conjunctivitis, fever, malaise, and persistent subacute lymphadenitis. The symptoms generally occur 7 to 10 days after being scratched by the animal. Serum titers for *Bartonella hensalae* are diagnostic. If cat scratch disease is suspected and the patient is very ill, a course of intravenous gentamicin should be considered. For detailed discussions of each infection see Chap. 13.

NONINFECTIOUS INFLAMMATORY MASSES

Sarcoidosis may present with masses in the lymph nodes, lungs, skin, eyes, and bones. Biopsy shows typical noncaseating granulomas. Inflammation of nonlymphoid tissue occurs in viral thyroiditis and sialadenitis.

Inflammation of the salivary glands may have various etiologies. In the newborn, especially the premature infant, sialadenitis is not uncommon and presents with swelling over one of the salivary glands. Dehydration is thought to be a contributing factor. Treatment consists of hydration and antimicrobial therapy. Viral sialadenitis secondary to mumps is almost exclusively a disease of childhood. Acute bacterial parotitis may also occur in children. This disorder may be recurrent or persistent through adolescence. If a mass undergoes enlargement associated with eating, inflammatory disease of the salivary glands should be suspected. Though there may be some generalized swelling at all times with an infected salivary gland, an increase in size is often noted specifically at the time of feeding. In cases of salivary gland disease, traditional sialography is of limited value, but a CT sialogram may be very helpful in differentiating a mass lesion from an inflammatory disorder.

Malnutrition, bulimia, obesity, and pica all may be associated with enlargement of the salivary glands. Administration of a general anesthetic may result in salivary gland enlargement from compression of the submandibular glands during positive-pressure ventilation through a mask or by a mouth gag. Similarly, wind instrument players may find salivary gland enlargement caused by pneumoparotitis, a condition in which air is forced into the salivary ductal system with resultant gland enlargement.

CONGENITAL ABNORMALITIES

Congenital abnormalities including branchial anomalies, thyroglossal duct cysts, dermoid cysts, teratomas, and laryngoceles may all present at birth or later in life as masses in the head and neck. These are discussed above (Sec. 15.3) and in Chap. 16. If prenatal ultrasonography identifies an anterior neck mass, probable lesions include teratomas, teratoid cysts, and lymphangiomas. Before delivery, plans should be made to have a high-risk team present at the birth, including a pediatric surgeon, anesthesiologist, otolaryngologist, and neonatologist. If the airway is obstructed, intubation and bronchoscopy should be performed immediately. If this is unsuccessful, tracheotomy or even extracorporeal membrane oxygenation (ECMO) may be required until further diagnostic imaging studies can be obtained to define the lesion and plan further therapy.

VASOFORMATIVE LESIONS

Hemangiomas, lymphangiomas, and hemangiolymphangiomas are found almost exclusively in children and are usually identified before the age of 2 years. Slow, progressive enlargement is common, but a rapid increase in size may be noted during periods of upper respiratory infection. In addition, hemangiomas often will demonstrate enlargement with exertion or dependency. Lymphangiomas or cystic hygromas generally are soft, compressible, and relatively diffuse, but hemangiomas may be more discrete and firm, especially when located within a muscle or the deep soft tissues.

Lymphangiomas are often located in the posterior cervical triangle and may contain multilocular cysts. About one-third of patients with lymphangiomas will originally present with signs of infection. A lymphangioma may be more discrete and firm if it has been present for many years and has undergone morphologic alterations as a result of multiple infections with secondary scarring. Cutaneous vascular changes may be indicative of hemangiomas, which are diffuse and even infiltrative. CT and MRI can allow identification of the type of lesion and define its extent.

Hemangiomas usually regress over a period of years, though surgical excision is appropriate when there is a diagnostic question, hemorrhage, repeated infections, airway compromise, high-output cardiac failure, or, rarely, significant cosmetic abnormality. Intravenous or oral steroids may be an appropriate initial alternative. Lymphangiomas rarely undergo spontaneous regression and should be managed either surgically or with sclerotherapy using an alcohol solution. Recently, several centers have used picibanil (OK-432) as a sclerosing agent. This medication is derived from *Streptococcus pyogenes* and induces the regression of macrocystic lymphangiomas. This therapy is less likely to be effective in the presence of a significant microcystic component to the lesion, massive craniofacial involvement, or following previous surgical resection.

TUMORS

Malignant and benign neoplasms are uncommon in the neonatal period and may not be accompanied by additional regional or systemic findings. Malignant neoplasms may be differentiated on occasion from benign lesions by their rapid growth, more indurated feel, and frequent attachment to skin or surrounding tissues.

Teratomas are located in or adjacent to the thyroid gland and are usually seen in newborns and young infants. Fibromatosis colli is a benign mass located in the anterior portion of the neck that presents 2 weeks or more after birth. It usually occurs following a history of birth trauma, and there is a gradual spontaneous resolution over 4 to 6 months. An ultrasound examination aids in diagnosis. Surgical excision is not indicated. Pilomatricoma, or calcifying epithelioma of Malherbe, is a benign lesion located in the intradermal or subcutaneous soft tissue that represents a hamartoma of the hair follicle. They are usually firm in consistency and attached to the skin. Surgical therapy is diagnostic and therapeutic.

Neuroblastoma and Langerhans cell histiocytosis are more common in the first several years of life. Rhabdomyosarcoma occurs most commonly between 4 and 6 years and 14 to 16 years of age. Hodgkin disease is most common in adolescents and adults, whereas non-Hodgkin lymphoma would be more common in children under age 12 years. Posttransplant lymphoproliferative disease should be suspected in immunocompromised patients following transplantation and is characterized by a discrete solid tumor or diffuse enlargement of lymphoid tissues.

References

Clary RA, Lusk RP: Neck masses. In: Bluestone CD, Stool SE, Kenna MA, eds: Pediatric Otolaryngology, vol 2. Philadelphia, WB Saunders, 1996: 1488–1496

Cunningham MJ: Congenital malformations of the head and neck. In: Cotton RT, Myer CM III, eds: Practical Pediatric Otolaryngology. Philadelphia, Lippincott-Raven, 1999:663–680

Myer CM III, Cotton RT: Lump in the neck. In: Myer CM III, Cotton RT, eds: A Practical Approach to Pediatric Otolaryngology. Chicago, Year Book Medical Publishers, 1988:212–219

Nuss RC, Cunningham MJ: Pediatric head and neck masses, cysts, sinuses, and tumors. Curr Opin Otolaryngol Head Neck Surg 1:153–160, 1993

Rosenfeld RM: Cervical adenopathy. In: Bluestone CD, Stool SE, Kenna MA, eds: Pediatric Otolaryngology, vol 2. Philadelphia, WB Saunders, 1996:1512–1524

Torsiglieri AJ Jr, Tom LW, Ross AJD, Wetmore RF, Handler SD, Potsic WP: Pediatric neck masses: guidelines for evaluation. Int J Pediatr Otorhinolaryngol 16:199–210, 1988

Tunkel DE, Baroody FM, Sherman ME: Fine-needle aspiration biopsy of cervicofacial masses in children. Arch Otolaryngol Head Neck Surg 121: 533–536, 1995

THE TEETH AND ORAL CAVITY

Murray Dock and Robert L. Creedon

16.1 GROWTH AND DEVELOPMENT

16.1.1 Oral and Dental Anatomy

HARD TISSUES

Tooth tissues grow in a manner similar to skeletal bones. Each tooth has a very specific, genetically determined shape and location (Fig. 16-1). Normal structural development requires that the tissues calcify in a manner somewhat similar to the formation of skeletal bones (Fig. 16-2). Three forms of an organic matrix calcify to varying degrees to form different components of the tooth. The tooth above the gingival margin, known as the *crown,* is covered by *enamel,* which is an organic matrix closely resembling hydroxyapatite in bone. When mature, enamel is very hard and is approximately 96% inorganic in an organic matrix. *Dentin* is the calcified tissue that makes up the bulk of the crown and root of the tooth, and dentin is only 20% organic by weight. Collagen fibers make up about 18% of this weight, and the remaining inorganic portion is in the form of hydroxyapatite crystallites. *Cementum* is the dental tissue covering the anatomic root of the tooth from the point at which the enamel layer stops. The line of demarcation is termed the *cervix* of the tooth. The density of cementum is less than that of dentin, being about 50% inorganic. Connective tissue fibers from the peridontal ligament or membrane become embedded in the forming cementum to provide the attachment of the root of the tooth to the surrounding bone.

SOFT TISSUES

The *dental pulp* is a specialized form of connective tissue filling the internal cavity of the tooth, with the pulp chamber decreasing in size with advancing age through the slow, continuous deposition of dentin. This tissue also contains nerves and vessels, which provide both sensory and nutritive functions for the tooth. Pulp can become inflamed by trauma or excessive thermal change and infected as a result of the carious process. The *periodontal ligament* is comprised primarily of white collagenous fibers which surround the tooth root and function as a suspensory ligament between the root surface and the alveolar bone.

The oral cavity is lined with varying types of mucosa in different locations. The gingivae cover an area limited to the outer surfaces of the jaws to a line termed the *mucogingival junction,* where it meets the alveolar mucosa. Gingival mucosa is pink in color, adapted to sustaining the stresses of mastication. The mucosa covering the alveolar bone of the maxilla and mandible contain numerous small vessels close to the surface resulting in red coloration.

The hard palate is covered with pink, thick mucosa that is highly keratinized and tightly bound to the periosteum covering the bone. The dorsum of the tongue is covered by specialized mucosa to accommodate its sensory function of taste. The remaining areas of the oral cavity—the lips, cheeks, soft palate, the vestibular fornix, and the floor of the mouth—are lined with relatively thin, elastic, nonkeratinized vascular mucosa.

16.1.2 Development of the Dentition

The normal sequence of tooth formation is outlined in Table 16-1. The earliest sign of the formation of teeth is seen at about the sixth week of embryonic life. The tooth buds of the primary teeth develop at 10 specific sites in the developing maxilla and mandible. The 20 succedaneous permanent teeth develop beneath the primary teeth while the permanent molars develop distally in sequential order. Calcification of the primary teeth begins at about 4 months in utero, and the enamel of all crowns is completed by 10 months after birth. The permanent teeth begin to calcify with the first molar around the time of birth, and the process is complete for all the teeth, with the exception of the third molars, by the seventh to eighth year of age.

In both the primary and permanent dentitions the process of tooth eruption correlates with root development. When the crown emerges through the gingiva, the root is usually one-half to two-thirds of its final length. Eruption continues until the antagonist in the opposing jaw is contacted in occlusion. As tooth wear takes place throughout life, eruption continues but at a much-reduced rate, keeping the teeth in occlusion. The primary cause of tooth eruption is unknown. The entire process of the eruption of both dentitions takes place from $7\frac{1}{2}$ months to 13 years of age.

Exfoliation of the primary teeth is a normal physiologic process that takes place as root development occurs in the permanent successors beneath them. The eruptive process stimulates the formation of osteoclasts, which results in the resorption of the roots of the primary teeth and their subsequent loss. The timing for exfoliation is subject to extreme variation for individual teeth. Normal exfoliation exhibits bilateral symmetry across the dental arch with the mandibular teeth preceding the maxillary teeth and anterior teeth preceding posterior teeth. Gender difference is present with girls preceding boys by 6 to 12 months.

16.1.3 Development of Dental Occlusion and Alignment

PRIMARY DENTITION The timing and sequence of each tooth taking its proper place in the dental arch follows a definite pattern. There are minor individual variations, but, in general, the maxillary

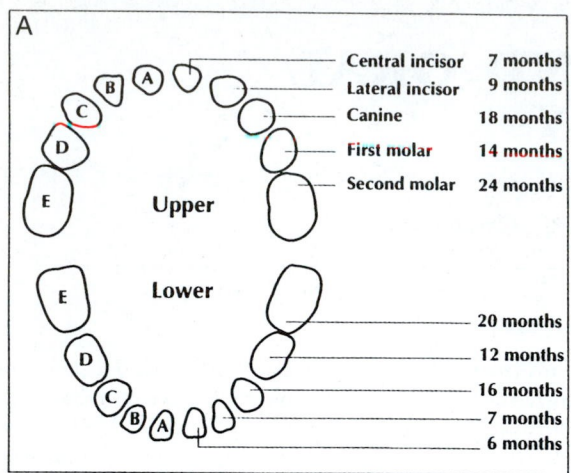

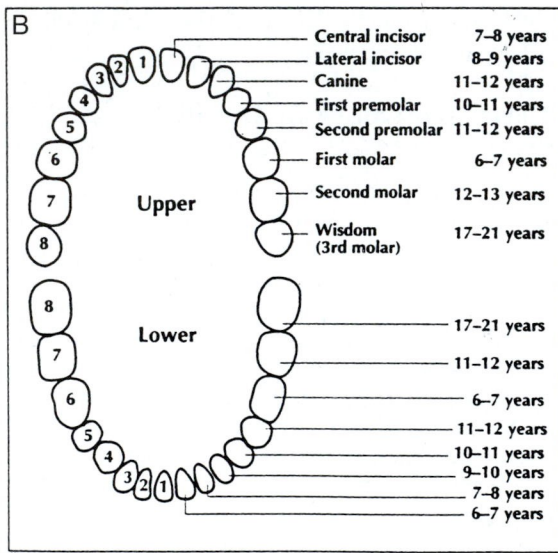

FIGURE 16-1   (A) Schematic of the primary dentition with eruption times (B) Schematic of the permanent dentition with eruption times.

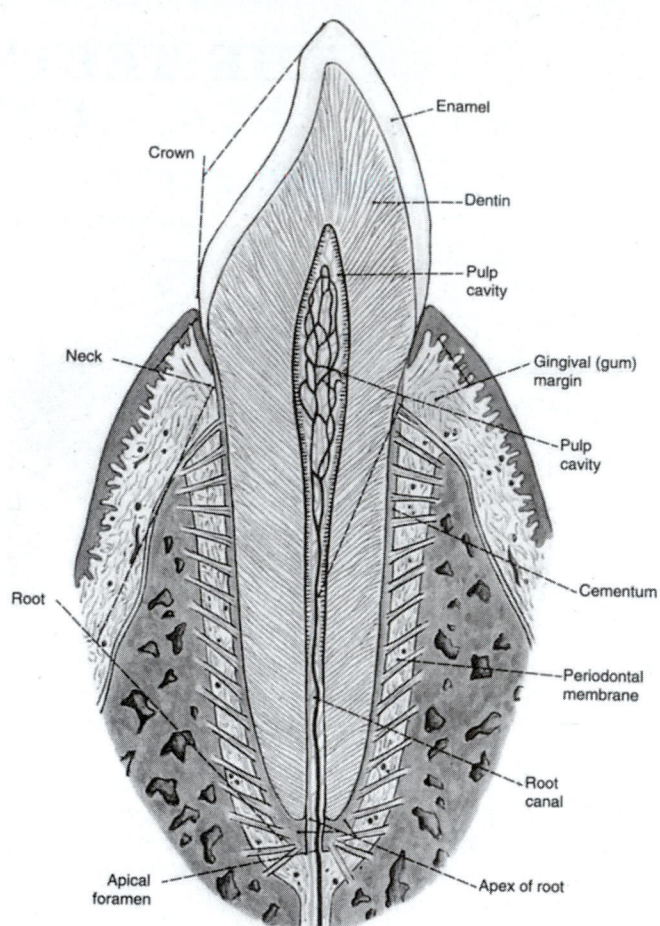

FIGURE 16-2   Schematic longitudinal section through a tooth and supporting structures.

teeth erupt about 2 months later than the corresponding teeth in the mandible. Ideally, by 3 years of age all the primary teeth have erupted and are in proper alignment with 1 to 2 mm of spacing between the anterior teeth. Proper spacing between primary teeth is desirable for favorable growth and development of the permanent dentition. Lack of spacing in the primary dentition suggests a high probability of crowding in the ensuing permanent dentition. The incisors should be upright with a minimal overbite of the anterior maxillary teeth with matching midlines of the dental arches (Fig. 16-3).

MIXED DENTITION   The first permanent molars erupt distal to the last primary molar in each arch at about 6 to $6\frac{1}{2}$ years of age. The mandibular molars usually precede the maxillary molars, and positioning is influenced by the position of the most posterior primary molars. The lower incisors begin to undergo change at about the same time. The permanent successors erupt behind or lingual to the primary incisors and will move into position as the primary incisors are lost. Often there is delay in the timely exfoliation of the primary incisors, which may result in two rows of teeth. A dental evaluation is necessary to determine whether the retained teeth require extraction. In most instances, extractions will not be required, and the primary incisors will eventually exfoliate. The lingually positioned permanent incisors typically move into proper alignment from tongue pressure. The premolars and canines erupt in that order, filling in the remaining space from incisors to the first molars. The remaining second permanent molars erupt posterior to the first molars, and the process is complete by about 13 years of age.

PERMANENT DENTITION   When the positioning of the permanent dentition is complete, ideally there should exist a well-aligned arch form in both upper and lower jaws (Fig. 16-4). The maxillary incisors should slightly overlap the lower incisors. The maxillary posterior teeth should overlap the mandibular teeth with the outside or buccal cusps of the lower teeth fitting into the occlusal depression of the upper teeth in a well-aligned fashion. The maxillary cuspid should lie between the mandibular cuspid and the first premolar or bicuspid. The eruption of third molars (wisdom teeth) is quite variable among individuals. These teeth often do not become functioning members of the permanent dentition and may require removal (see Sec. 16.2).

TABLE 16-1

CHRONOLOGY OF THE HUMAN DENTITION

TOOTH	HARD TISSUE FORMATION BEGINS	AMOUNT OF ENAMEL FORMED AT BIRTH	ENAMEL COMPLETED	ERUPTION	ROOT COMPLETED
Primary dentition					
Maxillary					
Central incisor	4 mo in utero	5/6th	1.5 mo	7.5 mo	1.5 yr
Lateral incisor	4.5 mo in utero	2/3rd	2.5 mo	9 mo	2 yr
Canine	5 mo in utero	1/3rd	9 mo	18 mo	3.25 yr
First molar	5 mo in utero	Cusps united	6 mo	14 mo	2.5 yr
Second molar	6 mo in utero	Cusp tips still isolated	11 mo	24 mo	3 yr
Mandibular					
Central incisor	4.5 mo in utero	3/5th	2.5 mo	6 mo	1.5 yr
Lateral incisor	4.5 mo in utero	3/5th	3 mo	7 mo	1.5 yr
Canine	5 mo in utero	1/3rd	9 mo	16 mo	3.25 yr
First molar	5 mo in utero	Cusps united	5.5 mo	12 mo	2.25 yr
Second molar	6 mo in utero	Cusp tips still isolated	10 mo	20 mo	3 yr
Permanent dentition					
Maxillary					
Central incisor	3–4 mo	—	4–5 yr	7–8 yr	10 yr
Lateral incisor	10–12 mo	—	4–5 yr	8–9 yr	11 yr
Canine	4–5 mo	—	6–7 yr	11–12 yr	13–15 yr
First premolar	1.5–1.75 yr	—	5–6 yr	10–11 yr	12–13 yr
Second premolar	2–2.25 yr	—	6–7 yr	10–12 yr	12–14 yr
First molar	At birth	Trace amount	2.5–3 yr	6–7 yr	9–10 yr
Second molar	2.5–3 yr	—	7–8 yr	12–13 yr	14–16 yr
Mandibular					
Central incisor	3–4 mo	—	4–5 yr	6–7 yr	9 yr
Lateral incisor	3–4 mo	—	4–5 yr	7–8 yr	10 yr
Canine	4–5 mo	—	6–7 yr	9–10 yr	12–14 yr
First premolar	1.75–2 yr	—	5–6 yr	10–12 yr	12–13 yr
Second premolar	2.25–2.5 yr	—	6–7 yr	11–12 yr	13–14 yr
First molar	At birth	Trace amount	2.5–3 yr	6–7 yr	9–10 yr
Second molar	2.5–3 yr	—	7–8 yr	11–13 yr	14–15 yr

SOURCE: *After Logan and Dronfedl: J Am Dent Assoc 20, 1933 (Slightly modified by McCall and Schour). Copyright by the American Dental Association.*

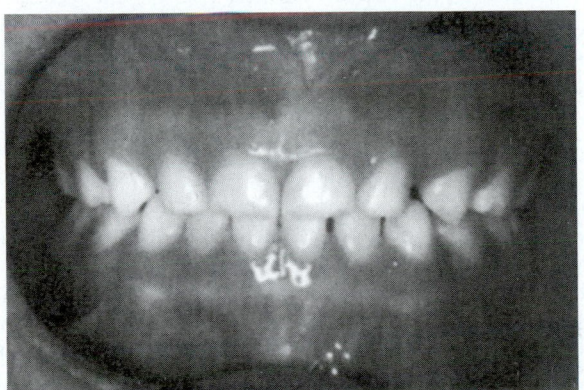

FIGURE 16-3 Normal occlusion of the primary dentition. Note that the incisors are upright with a minimal overbite of the anterior maxillary teeth with matching midlines of the dental arches.

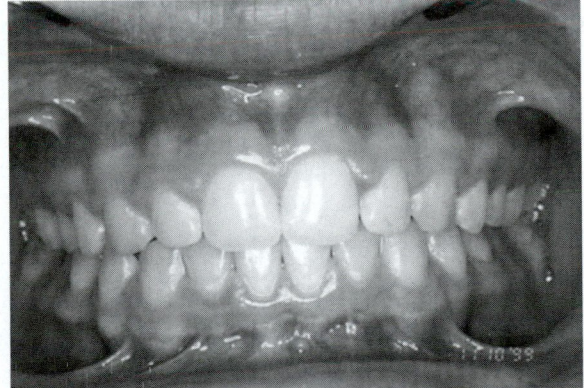

FIGURE 16-4 Normal occlusion of the permanent dentition. Note that the maxillary incisors slightly overlap the mandibular teeth with the outside of the lower teeth fitting into an occlusal depression in the maxillary teeth.

References

Bhaskar SN, ed: Orban's Oral Histology and Embryology, 10th ed. St. Louis, Mosby, 1985

Boyde A: Amelogenesis and structure of enamel. In: Cohen B, Kramer IRH, eds: Scientific Foundations of Dentistry. Chicago, Year Book, 1976

Full CA: Dental changes. In: Pinkham JR, ed: Pediatric Dentistry: Infancy through Adolescence, 2nd ed. Philadelphia, Saunders, 1994

Guidelines for management of the developing dentition in pediatric dentistry. J Pediatr Dent Special Issue: Reference Manual 1999–2000, 21–5:50

Hartsfield, JK: Premature exfoliation of teeth in childhood and adolescence. Advances in Pediatrics, vol 41. Chicago, Mosby-Year Book, 1994

McDonald RE, Avery DR: Eruption of the teeth: local, systemic, and congenital factors that influence the process. In: McDonald RE, Avery DR, eds: Dentistry for the Child and Adolescent, 7th ed. St. Louis, Mosby, 2000:180–208

Melcher AH: Biologic processes in tooth eruption and tooth movement. In: Cohen B, Kramer IRH, eds: Scientific Foundations of Dentistry. Chicago, Year Book, 1976:417–425

Symons NBB: Dentine and pulp. In: Cohen B, Kramer IRH, eds: Scientific Foundations of Dentistry. Chicago, Year Book, 1976:353–362

Tonge CH: Morphogenesis and development of teeth. In: Cohen B, Kramer IRH, eds: Scientific Foundations of Dentistry. Chicago, Year Book, 1976:325–334

16.2 DEVELOPMENTAL DISORDERS OF THE TEETH AND DENTITION

16.2.1 Abnormal Number of Teeth

HYPERDONTIA Increased numbers of teeth are most often observed as hereditary features in a family kindred. Supernumerary teeth may also be caused by physical disruptions in the embryonic dental lamina, as is frequently the case in clefts of the palate that involve the alveolar bone of the anterior maxilla. Extra teeth can be duplications of normal shape or are often dysmorphic. Most often the crowns are conical and may be reduced in size. These extra teeth are sometimes found in multiple areas of the dental arch but are more common in the maxilla. The most common example is the mesiodens, a conical, often inverted tooth in the maxillary midline between the central incisors. Supernumerary teeth can erupt into the arch in a relatively normal location, but most do not erupt and are discovered only on routine radiographic examination. Hyperdontia is associated with a variety of syndromes listed in Table 16-2.

HYPODONTIA Reduced numbers of teeth are observed in family kindreds. Third molars have the highest probability of being absent followed by the mandibular second bicuspid and then the maxillary lateral incisor. There seems to be a strong correlation between missing primary teeth and their permanent successors. Missing teeth also are observed in association with a variety of syndromes listed in Table 16-3.

16.2.2 Abnormal Tooth Morphology

MICRODONTIA Single isolated teeth may be reduced in size, or all the teeth present in an individual's total dentition may be reduced

TABLE 16-2
CONDITIONS ASSOCIATED WITH HYPERDONTIA

Cleft lip +/− cleft palate
Cleidocranial dysplasia
Crouzon syndrome
Down syndrome
Gardner syndrome
Hallermann-Streiff syndrome
Oral-facial-digital syndrome, type I
Sturge-Weber syndrome

TABLE 16-3
CONDITIONS ASSOCIATED WITH HYPODONTIA

Achondroplasia
Chondroectodermal dysplasia
Cleft lip +/− cleft palate
Crouzon syndrome
Down syndrome
Ectodermal dysplasia, hypohydrotic type
Ehlers-Danlos syndrome
Hallermann-Streiff syndrome
Incontinetia pigmenti
Reigers syndrome
Seckel syndrome

in size. In either case this finding is uniformly of hereditary etiology. Affected most commonly are the third molars and the maxillary lateral incisor. Reduced or hypoplastic lateral incisors are considered a variable expression of the gene for congenital absence of this tooth.

MACRODONTIA Apparent larger-than-normal teeth are frequently observed and in most cases result from a relative disparity in the size of the teeth and the jaw. True macrodontia however is uncommon, of unknown etiology, and usually affects isolated teeth. Unilateral macrodontia has been noted with hemifacial hyperplasia, whereas diffuse macrodontia is associated with pituitary gigantism.

GEMINATION This abnormality is produced by the incomplete division of a single toothbud, producing a bifid crown with a single pulp chamber, and is more common in the primary dentition. Gemination does not affect the number of teeth present and tends to occur in a familial pattern.

FUSION This abnormality results from the union of two embryologically developing teeth. The illusion of a tooth of increased size or a reduction in number of teeth is frequently caused by fusion that may result in impeded eruption of a permanent successor.

16.2.3 Defects of Tooth Structure

DISORDERS OF TOOTH ENAMEL Inherited defects of the structure of the enamel are broadly categorized as *amelogenesis imperfecta*, which presents with variable findings including enamel pitting, decreased thickness of enamel, brown-orange discoloration, white opaque discoloration, and/or enamel chipping. The teeth can be erroneously diagnosed as having severe dental caries. These inherited disorders are generally not associated with any syndrome, metabolic disorder, or other systemic condition and affect both the primary and permanent dentitions. However, some nutritional and systemic disorders can adversely affect the formation of enamel including vitamin A, C, and D deficiencies, exanthematous diseases, congenital syphilis, birth injury, prematurity, Rh hemolytic disease, local infection or trauma, and ingestion of chemicals, eg, fluoride and tetracycline. Disorders of tooth enamel can be treated with a variety of esthetic dental procedures.

DISORDERS OF TOOTH DENTIN *Dentinogenesis imperfecta* is an inherited disorder involving the dentinal organic matrix. There are three distinct types: Type I is found in the primary dentition in conjunction with osteogenesis imperfecta. Type II is known as *opalescent dentin* and occurs as a solitary finding in both primary and permanent dentitions. Type III has been proposed as a variation of type II occuring in the permanent teeth and is extremely rare. Clinically, the teeth have a blue to brown translucent discoloration, the opalescent dentin found in type II. Because of defects in the structure of the dentin, the enamel frequently separates, resulting in significant tooth attrition. The pulp canals tends to become obliterated, and multiple areas of periapical inflammation are common. Treatment consists of attempts to retain the teeth for as long as possible with endodontic therapy and full coverage crowns. Despite these efforts, many of these patients ultimately require full maxillary and mandibular dentures.

Dentin dysplasia may also be an inherited disorder of dentin or may be associated with systemic diseases including rheumatoid arthritis, hypervitaminosis D, and sclerosing bone disorders. The tooth crowns may appear normal or may exhibit many of the features of dentinogenesis imperfecta. Patients are at risk of periapical pathology as well as early loss of teeth due to abnormal root morphology. *Regional odontodysplasia* is characterized by the localized arrest of development of both dentin and enamel resulting from a regional vascular developmental abnormality. The enamel is thin and poorly calcified. Dentin is also poorly calcified, and the pulp chambers are excessively large. The roots of the involved teeth are short and poorly defined. Other than the vascular problem, no known etiology exists.

DISORDERS OF TOOTH CEMENTUM Defective or dysplastic cementum is rare but can result in either delayed or premature exfoliation of primary teeth. Conditions associated with cementum defects include epidermolysus bullosa, cleidocranial dysostosis, and hypophosphotasia.

16.2.4   Abnormal Tooth Color

INTRINSIC STAINING Staining of teeth can be caused by blood-borne pigments in congenital erythropoietic porphyria, cholestatic disorders, anemias, and hemolysis. Administration of drugs, particularly those of the tetracycline family, during tooth formation is a common cause of intrinsic staining. Even following the completion of tooth formation, some drugs may cause dental staining, as has been reported with minocycline, from incorporation in the deep dentinal tissue. The undesirable coloration of intrinsic stain can usually be managed by bleaching and/or other esthetic restorative procedures.

EXTRINSIC STAINING Tooth color can be affected by substances that become adherent to the teeth and/or plaque. These substances include a variety of foods, beverages, chromogenic bacteria, and iron found in infant formulas and vitamin supplements (Fig. 16-5). These problems are not developmental in nature and the stain can easily be removed with abrasive materials typically used for dental cleanings. The abrasiveness of over-the-counter toothpaste is usually insufficient to remove iron stain and other tenacious stains. Pure staining does not increase the risk of dental decay. Preventive measures include the daily removal of plaque and stain with meticulous oral hygiene.

16.2.5   Disorders of Tooth Eruption and Position

TEETHING The timing of eruption of teeth in infants can be quite variable and no interventions need to be considered to hasten the

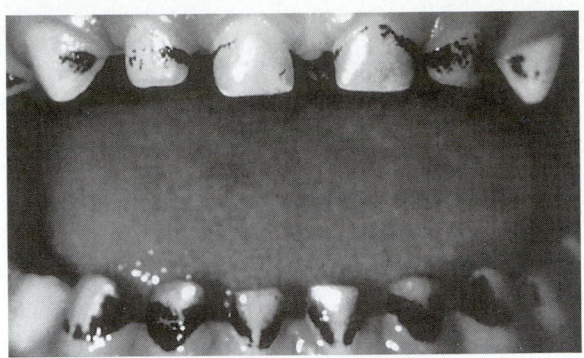

FIGURE 16-5   Iron staining of the primary dentition.

process. For primary teeth, a variation in eruption of 6 months on either side of the expected eruption (Table 16-1) is no cause for concern. Presence of bulbous gum pads provides sufficient evidence that teeth are present, with no further evaluation being indicated. At the time of eruption, commonly referred to as "teething," local discomfort may be observed. Infants may have increased drooling and mild irritability and occasionally will refuse some foods. Small amounts of localized bleeding can occur as the tooth makes its appearance sometimes preceded by a localized hematoma on the overlying gingiva. Other symptoms often attributed to teething include temperature elevation, gastric upset, and diarrhea, but there is no evidence to support these associations. Other than symptomatic treatment of pain, no treatment is required for the minor complications of tooth eruption. The gingiva should not be rubbed or cut to facilitate tooth eruption, since infection can result. Discomfort may be relieved by cool objects such as a cold wash cloth or teething ring, but frozen teething rings should be avoided because these may cause frostbite of the lips and gums. Teething powders and aspirin should be avoided. Judicious use of topical anesthetic teething preparations containing benzocaine or administration of acetaminophen may be reasonable but is usually unnecessary.

DELAYS IN TOOTH ERUPTION Marked delays in tooth eruption well beyond the usual variation can be seen in association with developmental delay, hormonal abnormalities, and as a feature of a variety of syndromes as listed in Table 16-4.

PREMATURE TOOTH ERUPTION Early emergence of one or more teeth can occur following the early loss of a primary tooth from trauma or infection, may represent precocious development, or may be unexplainable. Natal or neonatal teeth in the primary dentition erupt at or around the time of birth. These teeth are often rudimentary in form, perhaps even appearing as mere scales of enamel or shells of tooth crowns. They represent supernumerary teeth in approximately 15% of cases. Every attempt should be made to retain natal/neonatal teeth until it is possible to accurately identify whether the tooth is a normal part of the dentition. When interfering with breastfeeding, or when extremely mobile, consideration should be given to extraction. Neonatal teeth are seen frequently as a finding in several syndromes including chondroectodermal dysplasia, Hallermann-Streiff, pachyonychia congenita, and Sotos syndromes.

PREMATURE EXFOLIATION Permanent teeth do not exfoliate except in situations of localized or systemic pathology (Table 16-5). The most common reasons for early tooth loss are trauma or ex-

TABLE 16-4

CONDITIONS ASSOCIATED WITH DELAYED ERUPTION OF TEETH

Aarskog syndrome	Hunter syndrome
Acrodysostosis	Hypothyroidism
Albright hereditary osteodystrophy	Incontinetia pigmenti
Apert syndrome	Killian/Teschler-Nicola syndrome
Chrondoectodermal dysplasia	Levy-Hollister syndrome
Cleidocranial dysostosis	Maroteauz-Lamry syndrome
Cockayne syndrome	Mucopolysaccharidosis
De Lange syndrome	Miller-Dieker syndrome
Down syndrome	Osteogenesis imperfecta, type I
Dubowitz syndrome	Progeria
Frontometaphyseal dysplasia	Pyknodysostosis
Goltz syndrome	Rutherford syndrome

traction caused by caries and infection. Any other history of early loss or exfoliation would be a cause for further evaluation, especially if the child is less than 5 years of age.

DELAYED EXFOLIATION Occasionally a primary tooth will be retained beyond its normal exfoliation time and will interfere with proper eruption of the permanent successor. Delayed exfoliation requires a dental evaluation to rule out oral and/or systemic pathology. However, most cases of delayed exfoliation are idiopathic and of no consequence.

ABNORMAL ALIGNMENT OR OCCLUSION Any suspected abnormalities in the alignment of the permanent teeth or in the functional closure as the dentitions come into occlusion is sufficient reason for a consultation with an orthodontist or pediatric dentist. Depending on the malocclusion, and dental age of the patient, early correction may be the most desirable choice, often begun in the primary or early mixed dentition.

The most common disorder of alignment involves the third molars or "wisdom teeth." Occasionally these may only partially erupt, leaving a soft-tissue gingival cover (pericoronal tissue) over part of

TABLE 16-5

CONDITIONS ASSOCIATED WITH PREMATURE EXFOLIATION OF PRIMARY TEETH OR LOSS OF PERMANENT TEETH

COMMON	LESS COMMON
Hypophosphatasia	Ehlers-Danlos syndrome
Early-onset periodontitis	Hypophosphatemia
Prepubertal periodontitis	Coffin-Lowry syndrome
Juvenile periodontitis	Acatalasia
Papillion-Lefevre syndrome	Down syndrome
	Chediak-Higashi syndrome
Singleton Merten syndrome	Hyperthyroidism
	Cherubism
Hajdu-Cheney syndrome	Dentinal dysplasia, type I
	Leukemia
	Langerhans-cell histiocytoses
	Neutropenia
	Acrodynia
	Mandibuloacral dysplasia
	Metaphyseal Dysplasia with maxillary hypoplasia and brachydactyly
	Regional odontodysplasia

the crown that can easily become inflamed resulting in a pericoronitis. Gentle lavage will usually suffice as a temporary measure, but removal of the tooth or teeth is the ultimate treatment of choice. Prophylactic removal of unerupted bony impacted third molars is controversial. Proponents suggest that impacted teeth increase the risk of cyst formation and damage to adjoining structures. In addition, younger individuals have a lower incidence of postoperative complications and heal more quickly so that earlier removal may be reasonable. However, the risk of complication from impaction is relatively low and must be balanced with the risk of surgery. Many clinicians recommend that third molars not be removed unless symptoms of pain or infection develop.

References

Chiappinelli JA, Walton RE: Tooth discoloration resulting from long-term tetracycline therapy: a case report. Quintessence Int 23:539–541, 1992

Dayan D et al: Tooth discoloration—extrinsic and intrinsic factors. Quintessence Int 2:195–199, 1983

Dummet CO Jr: Anomalies of the developing dentition. In: Pinkham BS, ed: Pediatric Dentistry: Infancy Through Adolescence. Philadelphia, Saunders, 1994:57–68

Gorlin RJ, Cohen MM, Levin LS, eds: Syndromes of the Head and Neck. 3rd ed, New York, Oxford University Press, 1990

Meon R: Hypodontia of the primary and permanent dentition. J Clin Pediatr Dent 16:121–123, 1992

Parkins FM, Furnish G, Bernstein M: Minocycline use discolors teeth. J Am Dent Assoc 123:87–89, 1992

Ranta H, Lukinmma P-L, Walltimo J: Heritable dentin defects: nosology, pathology, and treatment. Am J Med Genet 45:193–200, 1993

Stewart RE, Witkop CJ, Bixler D: The dentition. In: Stewart RE, Barber TK, Troutman KC, Wei SHY, eds: Pediatric Dentistry. St. Louis, Mosby, 1982:87–134

Witkop CJ Jr: Amelogenesis imperfecta, dentinogenesis imperfecta and dentin dysplasia revisited: problems in classification. J Oral Pathol 17:547–553, 1988

16.3   DENTAL CARIES AND DENTAL CARE

16.3.1   Dental Caries

Dental caries is an infectious and transmissible disease intiated by a heterogeneous group of gram-positive bacteria present in the biofilm that forms on teeth soon after eruption. This complex community of bacteria, termed *dental plaque,* contains *Streptococcus mutans,* which is a necessary agent for the production of dental caries. *S. mutans* has been shown to be transmissible from parents or caregivers to infants at the time of tooth eruption. The dental health of direct caregivers thus becomes an important factor in the prevention of dental caries.

S. mutans bacteria produce acidic metabolic end products from dietary fermentable carbohydrates, which demineralize the enamel. This demineralization is reversible in the early stages of caries development, but as the process progresses, cavitation occurs, and bacteria further invade the mineral portion of the tooth. Once this occurs, failure to stop the process inevitably leads to loss of the tooth.

The essential components necessary for the development of dental caries are acidogenic bacteria, a susceptible host, fermentable carbohydrates, and plaque. Host characteristics that alter the susceptibility to caries include salivary composition, pH and flow rate, immunologic factors, quality of tooth maturation, and tooth morphology. Defects in any of these factors may result in increased risk of dental caries.

PATTERNS OF CARIES FORMATION Dental caries disease is usually classified by four different factors: (1) according to anatomic site of the lesion, (2) according to the severity or rate of progession of the lesion, (3) according to age patterns at which lesions predominate, and (4) according to therapies that can induce decay.

Anatomically caries will occur on the occlusal surface as pit and fissure caries or between the teeth as smooth surface caries. Root caries can also occur when gingival recession exposes the cementum to the causative bacterial agents. Linear caries describe a type of caries found predominantly in the primary dentition of children, occuring on the labial surface of the incisor teeth in areas of enamel developmental dysplasia where incremental layers have been disturbed and thus have become areas susceptible to the carious process.

Caries are classified by severity as mild, incipient, or rampant. *Arrested caries* describes any lesion that is no longer progressing because changes have occurred in the oral environment. *Recurrent* caries refers to newly developing lesions at the margins of restorations and may indicate a change in susceptibility.

Caries can occur in teeth of persons of any age, but when the disease occurs in children younger than 3 years, the condition is termed *early childhood caries*. Previously, most descriptions of early childhood caries focused on the period of nursing, giving rise to the term *nursing bottle caries*. It is now recognized that early childhood caries can be present in the absence of bottle- or breast-feeding and conversely does not always result from inappropriate bottle- or breast-feeding practices, indicating that other host susceptibility factors are involved. Early childhood caries are characterized by a very distinct pattern in which the lower primary incisor teeth are not affected, yet the damage to molars and upper incisors can be extensive (Fig. 16-6a).

Rampant caries can result not only from high dietary and/or oral hygiene risk factors but also from radiation therapy and medications used for the treatment of systemic diseases. Radiation caries an example of induced caries. Radiation involving the salivary glands can lead to xerostomia, which drastically increases caries susceptibility. For a more detailed discussion of the effects of radiation on the mouth "see Sec. 16.6." Medication caries are another example of induced caries caused by the chronic use of medication vehicles of extremely high sugar content. Patients receiving long-term oral suspensions are at particular risk and should have frequent dental visits to examine for decay and reinforce proper oral hygiene measures.

COMPLICATIONS AND TREATMENT OF DENTAL CARIES Regardless of age or circumstance, all carious lesions must be eradicated by some means. Failure to do so eventually leads to invasion of the pulp chamber of the tooth with inflammation, pain, swelling, and exudation. Since the tooth pulp is encased within a rigid structure, necrosis of the tissue within the pulp chamber occurs because of the increased pressure, which prevents blood flow. An ensuing buildup of toxic products in this space will force extension of the

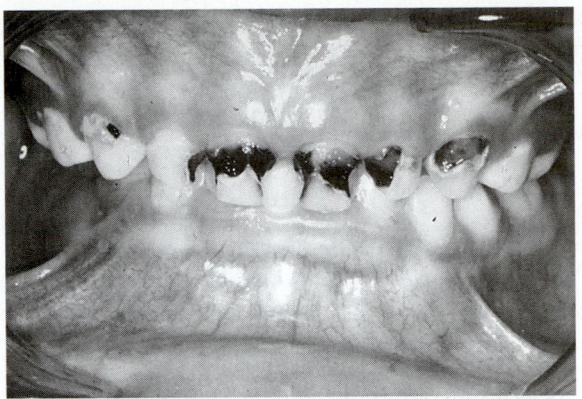

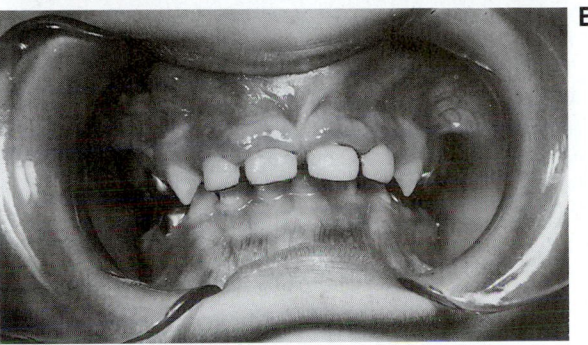

FIGURE 16-6 (A) Early childhood caries. (B) Restored early childhood caries with anterior and posterior full coverage crowns.

process into the tissue surrounding the root apices, forming an abscess within the bone. Cellulitis with acute pain ensues with swelling of soft tissues as the products drain to the outside. If the body defense mechanisms respond adequately, the infection may transiently resolve, but an acute recurrence is common.

Interruption of the caries process is the aim of any treatment with subsequent rebuilding of lost tooth structure utilizing choices from an array of methods (Fig. 16-6b). Depending on the extent to which the damage has progressed, this may involve entering the pulp chamber, cleansing and sterilizing the internal space within the crown and root, and obturating that space. A final resort is extraction of the tooth with subsequent replacement also by a variety of means. Restorative care and simple extractions in children over three years of age are readily provided using local anesthesia. Very young children, the developmentally delayed child, and those needing extensive treatment may require sedation or general anesthesia to receive the best quality of care.

PREVENTION OF DENTAL CARIES Strategies for the prevention of dental caries depend on the age of the individual. However, in general the strategies are aimed at increasing the resistance of enamel, reducing or altering the flora of the oral cavity, and changing eating habits including the content of the diet. For the very young child, preventing the initiation of early childhood caries involves regular visits to a dentist for parental counseling and support in managing the prevention plan.

The American Academy of Pediatric Dentistry recommends that infants not be put to sleep with a nursing bottle. Likewise, ad libitum nocturnal breast-feeding should be avoided. Parents or caregivers should be encouraged to have infants drink from a cup as they approach their first birthday with consumption of milk or juices from a bottle being limited to prevent the child using the bottle as a substitute pacifier throughout the day. When juice is offered, it should be from a cup to encourage more rapid consumption.

Oral hygiene measures should be implemented by the time of eruption of the first primary tooth. An oral health dental consultation visit within 6 months of the eruption of the first tooth is recommended to educate parents and caregivers and provide anticipatory guidance for the prevention of dental disease. In children older than 3 years of age, strategies focus on attempts to break the chain of events leading to dental caries. Fighting dental plaque by means of disruption with a toothbrush and floss is recommended throughout life. Fluoride use in community water supplies, application by the dental practitioner, and self-directed use as in toothpaste, coupled with dietary discretion all are effective. Modification of the diet includes reducing the quantity and frequency of between meal snacks and adherence to balanced meals daily. Snack food items that are not sticky or sugar laden but are attractive and compatible with the dietary customs of the family are very helpful. Sealants (flowable composite resin) applied to the occlusal surfaces of the teeth to block access to the deeper structures of the dentition are also very important and an effective element of any preventive program. This preventive service can be of benefit to either the primary or permanent dentition but is especially beneficial to the permanent molars.

16.3.2 Fluoride Use

Water fluoridation is the most cost effective, most convenient, and most reliable method of providing optimal fluoride benefits because it does not depend on individual compliance. Numerous studies have shown decay rates to be reduced by between 25 and 65%, depending on the population group, and water fluoridation carries minimal risk for fluorosis. For children who do not have access to optimally fluoridated drinking water or infants who are totally breast-fed, systemically administered fluoride supplements are beneficial.

To be completely effective, supplements must be taken from 6 months after birth until calcification of the permanent dentition is complete. Dosage depends on the age of the child and the existing fluoride concentration in the water supply (Table 16-6). The concentration of fluoride in the drinking water can be obtained from the water department of the municipal government. Alternatively, most state health departments will assay for fluoride for a nominal cost. Failure to ascertain this information can result in overdose and consequent dental fluorosis. When drops are used they should be given in a liquid, which, if possible, should be held in the mouth a short period before swallowing. Milk reduces the bioavailability of fluoride and should be avoided as a carrier.

Prenatal fluoride supplements are not recommended, since adequate data regarding efficacy do not exist. Milk from cows contains only 0.1 ppm, and breast milk has even less at 0.05 ppm. These facts should cause concern only if the community water concentration is less than 0.3 ppm. Infant formula that must be mixed has only the amount of fluoride imparted by the water used for reconstitution or dilution. Ready-to-feed formulas have had the fluoride removed at the point of manufacture.

For children age 6 or older, daily use of 10 ml of a 0.05% fluoride solution can reduce dental caries by as much as 35%. These products are available over the counter. Weekly mouth rinses with a 0.2% sodium fluoride solution have proved successful in large, supervised school programs. Children at high risk for caries (eg, children with orthodontic/prosthodontic appliances, with reduced salivary function, who are at dietary risks) or children who are caries active should be considered for a more intensified regimen of fluoride therapy utilizing more concentrated rinses or brush-on gels on a daily basis. If a high-caries-risk patient cannot comply with home therapy, frequent professional fluoride treatments may be substituted. Professionally applied fluoride treatments are almost always performed at periodic recall examination visits to a dental office. Fluoride-containing varnishes are another type of topically applied fluoride therapy particularly recommended for preschool-age children owing to ease of application and efficacy equal to in-office topical application systems.

COMPLICATIONS OF FLUORIDE USE There is no doubt regarding the benefits of fluoride as a caries preventive agent, but there are small associated risks. Acute toxicity is almost always a result of accidental ingestion of any fluoride product in large quantities. Preparation and dispensing errors are possible in any situation requiring dilution or reconstitution of topical solutions. To avoid accidental ingestion of large quantities, no more than 120 mg of fluoride should be prescribed at one time, and volumes of concentrated preparations should be limited to no more than 40 ml. The sequelae of ingestion over and above the recommended amount usually result in gastrointestinal irritation producing nausea, vomiting, and hypersalivation. The actual incidence of this occurrence is difficult to document, since it can result from overuse of any fluoride product, including toothpaste, and the symptoms tend to be mild, requiring no treatment. Severe acute toxicity can result in seizures and respiratory and cardiac failure and require immediate attention.

Chronic toxicity primarily manifests itself as a condition termed *fluorosis.* Dental fluorosis is defined as a disorder of tooth mineralization occurring only during tooth development. The process of maturation of the enamel in the permanent dentition is completely finished with the exception of the third molars by the age of 8 years. Any systemic effect of fluoride on increasing resistance to caries or

TABLE 16-6

DAILY DIETARY FLUORIDE SUPPLEMENTATION SCHEDULE

AGE	LESS THAN 0.3 PPM FLUORIDE IN WATER	0.3–0.6 PPM FLUORIDE IN WATER	MORE THAN 0.6 PPM FLUORIDE IN WATER
Birth–6 mo	0	0	0
6 mo–3 yr	0.25 mg fluoride	0	0
3 yr–6 yr	0.5 mg fluoride	0.25 mg fluoride	0
6 yr–16 yr	1.0 mg fluoride	0.5 mg fluoride	0

SOURCE: From American Academy of Pediatric Dentistry: Reference Manual, 1999–2000:40

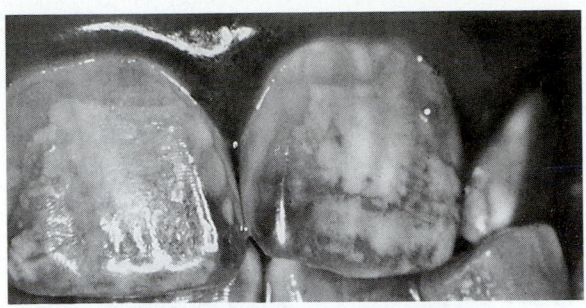

FIGURE 16-7   Moderate to severe enamel fluorosis.

creating areas of fluorosis must take place prior to this time. From this point on, all fluoride effect from whatever source is purely topical.

Incorrect dosage of supplements is the most common cause of fluorosis. Clinically, the teeth may have areas of white and/or brown discoloration, and in severe cases pitting may occur (Fig. 16-7). In most cases however, the hypoplasia is so mild that it is not considered an esthetic problem, especially in light of the obvious benefit of freedom from caries. Moderate to severe fluorosis of esthetic concern occurs when the concentration is high and of considerable duration. With newer toothpastes flavored and advertised to gain the attention of young children, there has been a noticeable increase in the incidence of fluorosis. This is directly related to swallowing of toothpaste. Parents should be encouraged to closely supervise children under the age of 6 years during brushing to limit the amount of toothpaste used and to discourage swallowing. After brushing, the mouth should be rinsed with water.

16.3.3   Prevention of Oral Injuries

The majority of orofacial injuries are the result of falls and collisions with hard surfaces. Children who participate in contact sports are at particularly high risk. Ice hockey is associated with the greatest risk of oral injury. Other high-risk sports for oral injuries include football, handball, and basketball. The use of athletic mouthguards is a simple and cost-effective measure for reducing the prevalence of oral injuries for those participating in contact sports. There are three varieties of mouthguards available: stock, mouth-formed, and custom-fitted. By far the most effective and preferred in terms of comfort is the custom-fitted (by a dentist) followed by mouth-formed guards (over-the-counter products). Stock mouthguards do not fit as well, are usually uncomfortable, and are less effective in redistributing energy from impact.

References

Adair SM: The role of fluoride mouth rinses in the control of dental caries: a brief review. J Pediatr Dent 21:101–104, 1998

Anusavice KJ: Management of dental caries as a chronic infectious disease. J Dent Educ 62:791–802, 1998

Caulfield P: Dental caries—a transmissable and infectious disease, revisited: a position paper. J Pediatr Dent 19:491–498 1997

Guidelines for fluoride use. J Pediatr Dent Special Issue: Reference Manual 1999–2000, 21-5:40

Pendrys DG, Stamm JW: Relationship of fluoride intake to beneficial effects and enamel fluorosis. J Dent Res 69:529–538, 1990

Selwitz RH, Nowjack-Raymer RE, Kingman A, Driscoll WS: Dental caries and dental fluorosis among schoolchildren who were lifelong residents of communities having either low or optimal levels of fluoride in drinking water. J Pub Health Dent 58:28–35, 1998

Shulman JD, Wells LM: Acute fluoride toxicity from home-use dental products in children, birth to 6 years of age. J Pub Health Dent 57:150–158, 1997

Stookey GK: Caries prevention. J Dent Educ 62:803–811, 1998

16.4   PERIODONTAL DISEASE

Periodontal disease encompasses disorders of the gingiva, periodontal ligament, and alveolar bone. There are multiple forms of periodontal disease and some that are unique to the pediatric population. Periodontal disease seen in children and adolescents includes gingivitis, acute necrotizing ulcerative gingivitis (ANUG), early-onset periodontitis, pericoronitis, medication-induced gingival hyperplasia, gingival fibromatosis, and systemic-disease-related gingival changes.

GINGIVITIS   Refers to inflammation limited to the gingival tissue that does not extend to the alveolar bone or periodontal ligament fibers. Inflammation leading to destruction of the periodontal ligament and bony support is referred to as *periodontitis*. Most cases of gingivitis are related to a chronic accumulation of bacteria in plaque from inadequate oral hygiene. The gingiva becomes red, there is a loss of normal stippling of the tissue, and there is bleeding with brushing. Often, gingivitis becomes worse in adolescence with associated hormonal changes as well as poorer oral hygiene practices. The condition is completely reversible with improved oral hygiene. Gingivitis is also associated with chronic mouth-breathing, and can be seen as an allergic response to local and systemic substances, as well as a feature of several systemic disorders including HIV (Table 16-7).

TABLE 16-7

SYSTEMIC CAUSES OF GINGIVAL DISORDERS IN CHILDREN

DISEASE	PERIODONTAL CHANGES
Diabetes mellitus	Generalized gingivitis
Scurvy	Generalized gingivitis
HIV	Marginal gingivitis
Lead poisoning	Blue line along marginal gingiva
Chronic bismuth exposure	Blue line along marginal gingiva
Mercury poisoning	Ulcerative gingivitis
Poor nutrition, smoking	Acute necrotizing ulcerative gingivitis/periodontitis
Mental retardation	Gingival fibromatosis
Hypothyroidism	Gingival fibromatosis
Growth hormone deficiency	Gingival fibromatosis
Epilepsy	Gingival fibromatosis
Sensorineural deafness	Gingival fibromatosis
Zimmermann-Labland syndrome	Gingival fibromatosis
Ramon syndrome	Gingival fibromatosis
Cross syndrome	Gingival fibromatosis
Rutherford syndrome	Gingival fibromatosis
Murray syndrome	Gingival fibromatosis

TABLE 16-8
SYSTEMIC CAUSES OF PERIODONTITIS

Acatalasia	Gaucher disease
Acrodynia	Hemochromatosis
AIDS	Hypophosphatasia
Blood dyscrasias	Langerhans cell histiocytosis
Agranulocytosis	Leukocyte dysfunctions
Cyclic neutropenia	Oxalosis
Leukemia	Papillon-Lefevre syndrome
Crohn disease	Sarcoidosis
Diabetes mellitus	Scurvy
Dyskeratosis congenita	Trisomy 21
Ehlers-Danlos syndrome, type VIII	

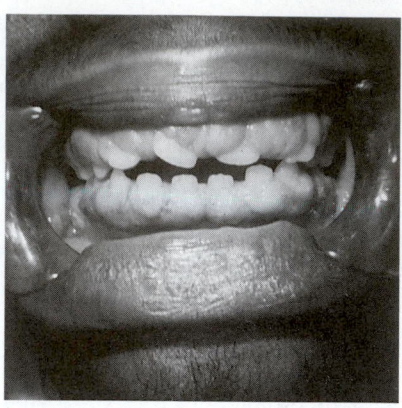

FIGURE 16-8 Phenytoin-induced gingival hyperplasia. Note the extension of the gingival mucosa over the facial surface of the teeth, almost covering the crown of the tooth.

ACUTE NECROTIZING ULCERATIVE GINGIVITIS ANUG is primarily seen in the adolescent and young adult population and is characterized by severe gingival inflammation with areas of gingival necrosis. The gingival tissue between the teeth (interdental papilla) will have a white "punched out" or crater appearance with the remaining tissue being severely inflamed producing spontaneous bleeding and a fetid odor. Patients may occasionally experience lymphadenopathy, fever, and malaise. The entire mouth is extremely painful, and patients may have difficulty with oral intake. Treatment consists of local debridement, rinsing with chlorhexidine and/or salt water and diluted hydrogen peroxide, penicillin or clindamycin for 7 to 10 days, and systemic analgesics.

PERIODONTITIS Inflammation of periodontal tissues resulting in destruction of the periodontal ligament and bony support is referred to as *periodontitis*. Clinical signs include gingival inflammation with bone loss, periodontal pocket formation, and tooth mobility. This is typically a disease of adults; however, it can occasionally be seen in children and adolescents and is referred to as *early onset periodontitis*. Early-onset periodontitis is classified as either localized or generalized with localized cases being more common. It is seen more often in males and is estimated to occur in 10% of the black population, 5% of Hispanics, and 1% of whites. A rare variant, prepubertal periodontitis, has an onset of around 4 years of age and results in the premature loss of primary teeth. Typically, with this form of periodontitis, there is little associated gingival inflammation. Often these patients have a leukocyte abnormality and an altered immune response to bacterial infections. The primary microorganism implicated as a cause of peridontitis is *Actinobacillus actinomycetemcomitans*. Periodontitis can be associated with several systemic disorders listed in Table 16-8. Treatment consists of local debridement, enhanced oral hygiene measures, and a course of antibiotics.

MEDICATION-INDUCED GINGIVAL HYPERPLASIA Several groups of medications are implicated in producing fibrous hyper-

TABLE 16-9
MEDICATIONS IMPLICATED IN GINGIVAL HYPERPLASIA

Phenytoin	Calcium channel blockers
Cyclosporin	Nifedipine
Mycophenolate mofetil	Diltiazem
Basiliximab	Felodipine
Sodium valproate (rarely)	Nitrendipine
	Verapamil

plasia of the gingiva (Table 16-9). These medications seem to sensitize gingival fibroblasts resulting in exaggerated growth especially in the presence of inflammation. Phenytoin is the best-known inducer of hyperplasia; however, many other drugs produce the same effect. The risk of hyperplasia is a factor of the medication, inherent risk, and overall oral hygiene of the patient. There is a direct correlation between the degree of hyperplasia and the level of oral hygiene. Some medications, however, will produce hyperplasia regardless of the level of oral hygiene. Phenytoin produces a generalized hyperplasia of the gingival tissues in 50% of patients. The hyperplasia begins along the interdental papilla and eventually extends over the facial surfaces of the teeth. In severe cases, the entire clinical crown may be covered (Fig. 16-8). Other drugs that are likely to produce hyperplasia include cyclosporin and nifedipine. Treatment consists of strict oral hygiene measures, the use of antibacterial agents such as chlorhexidine, and gingivoplasty or gingivectomy in severe cases. Occasionally, the patient may require substitution of another medication less likely to produce this effect. Cyclosporin-induced hyperplasia, unlike phenytoin, may spontaneously resolve upon discontinuation of the medication.

GINGIVAL FIBROMATOSIS

This type of gingival hyperplasia is typically seen in patients under the age of 20 and may be familial, syndrome related (Table 16-7), or idiopathic. Clinically, there is an increase in bulk of the gingiva, which may be localized or generalized (Fig. 16-9). The maxilla

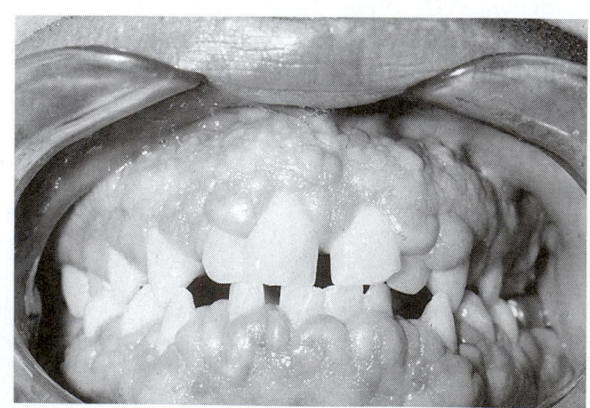

FIGURE 16-9 Gingival fibromatosis.

gingival surfaces are affected more often than the mandibular surfaces. Gingival fibromatosis is seen with greater frequency in patients with epilepsy, mental retardation, hypothyroidism, and sensorineural deafness. Treatment consists of gingivectomy along with a rigorous oral hygiene regimen. Regular follow-up is necessary, as recurrence is common.

References

Carranza FA, Newman MG: Clinical Periodontology, 8th ed. Philadelphia, Saunders, 1996

Ciancio SG: Agents for the management of plaque and gingivitis. J Dent Res 71:1450–1454, 1992

Dongari A, McDonnell HT, Langlais RP: Drug-induced gingival overgrowth. Oral Surg Oral Med Oral Pathol 76:543–548, 1993

Donly KL, Ashkenazi M: Juvenile periodontitis: a review of pathogenesis, diagnosis and treatment. J Clin Pediatr Dent 16:73–78, 1992

Hartnett AC, Shiloah J: The treatment of acute necrotizing ulcerative gingivitis. Quintessence Int 22:95–100, 1991

16.5   ORAL PATHOLOGY IN CHILDREN

16.5.1   Variations of Normal Soft Tissue

FORDYCE GRANULES Fordyce granules are yellowish-white slightly raised papular lesions found on the lips, buccal mucosa, and retromolar pad area that are usually less than 2 mm in diameter and may appear in clusters. They represent ectopic sebaceous glands, are found in 90% of the population, and increase in number after puberty. No treatment is necessary.

FISSURED TONGUE Fissured tongue or scrotal tongue is a malformation characterized by numerous small grooves or fissures radiating from a central groove on the dorsal surface of the tongue. The condition is seen in approximately 2 to 5% of the population, has a familial tendency, and is a common finding in patients with Down syndrome. Affected patients frequently have concurrent migratory glossitis. Other than encouraging the patient to clean the tongue on a daily basis, no treatment is necessary.

ANKYLOGLOSSIA Ankyloglossia describes the presence of a short lingual frenulum that can result in limited ability to move the tongue caused by the attachment of the tip of the tongue to the floor of the mouth (Fig. 16-10). Ankyglossia can be either partial or total with the tongue being completely fused to the floor of the mouth. The condition usually does not affect articulation or feeding. Depending on the site of gingival attachment, periodontal defects may rarely occur. There have been reports of an association between ankyloglossia and a more forward and anterior displacement of the larynx and epiglottis resulting in dyspnea and nursing difficulties in infants. Lingual frenulectomy should be reserved for severe cases that interfere with articulation or result in periodontal defects, dyspnea, or significant associated nursing difficulties.

MACROGLOSSIA Macroglossia is classified as *congenital, secondary,* or *relative.* Congenital macroglossia is a result of muscular hyper-

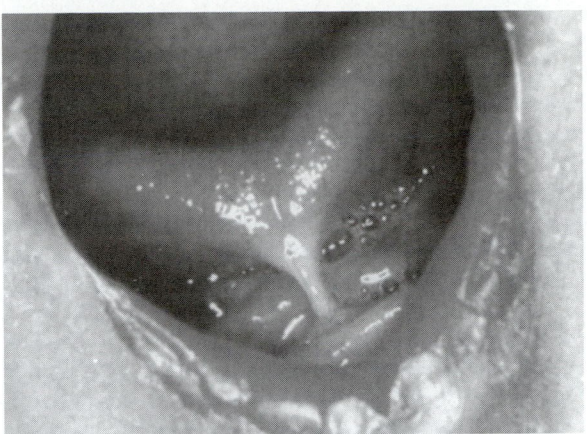

FIGURE 16-10   Lingual ankyloglossia. Depending on the degree of restriction of tongue movement, children with ankyloglossia may require surgical frenulectomy.

trophy and is seen in cases of hypothryoidism and in Beckwith-Weideman syndrome. Secondary enlargement is a result of a tumor such as lymphangioma, hemangioma, or neurofibroma. Relative macroglossia is frequently seen in syndromes including Down, Hurler, Hunter, Angelman, Treacher-Collins, and Williams. Teeth may become displaced from constant pressure of the tongue producing an anterior or lateral open bite. Additionally, the lateral borders of the tongue will often appear scalloped from pressure against the teeth. In severe situations, surgical debulking of the tongue may be necessary.

16.5.2   Benign Mucosal Lesions

Mucosal lesions are most easily classified by color and appearance. Mucosal lesions may be white or pigmented, may be ulcerated, or may have the numerous finger-like projections with a cauliflower appearance that characterizes papillary lesions. Other mesenchymal lesions, cystic lesions, and neoplasms of the jaw are also discussed in this section.

WHITE LESIONS

MIGRATORY GLOSSITIS Migratory glossitis, also known as *erythema migrans* or *geographic tongue,* is characterized by the loss of filiform papilla resulting in areas of irregular red patches surrounded by white keratotic borders on the tongue. The fungiform papillae are not affected. In addition to the dorsal areas of the tongue, the lateral aspects as well as the floor of the mouth can be affected. The condition occurs in 1 to 3% of the population, is seen twice as often in females, and tends to be familial. The cause is uncertain; however, lesions have been associated with stress or atopy and may represent an oral form of psoriasis. The lesions will quickly appear, heal, and move to other areas of the tongue. There is usually no associated pain other than when the lesion is exposed to citrus or spicy foods. Usually no treatment is required. Topical application of steroids, anesthetic agents, or retinoic acid has been used with variable results.

CANDIDIASIS Candidiasis is an opportunistic infection produced by the fungus *Candida albicans,* a normal inhabitant of the oral cavity in approximately 45% of the population. The infection is frequently seen in infants and immunocompromised patients and as an adverse effect of broad-spectrum antibiotics. Neonatal oral candidiasis occurs as a result of direct contact with vaginal micro-organisms immediately following birth. Clinically, the classic presentation is a white plaque that can easily be removed with a gauze square revealing a raw erythematous and painful surface. This is the most common form of the infection and is referred to as *pseudo-membranous candidiasis* (thrush). Erythematous candidiasis occurs as a red plaque prior to accumulation of sufficient quantities of organisms to produce the white patch. These lesions are often quite red and painful. Less commonly, *Candida* organisms can induce hyperkeratosis of the mucosa resulting in a white lesion that cannot be scraped away, producing *hyperplastic candidiasis*. It is often difficult to distinguish this form of infection from a secondary infection with *Candida* overlying other lesions such as leukoplakia or a papilloma. Any intraoral site can become infected; however, the most common sites include the buccal mucosa, tongue, and palate. The fastest and most reliable method of diagnosis is exfoliative cytology, even though a clinical diagnosis is usually made and confirmed by a response to empiric therapy. Treatment includes topical therapy with nystatin and/or systemic antifungal agents such as ketoconazole or fluconazole.

CHEWING TOBACCO LESIONS The use of smokeless tobacco often results in local irritation in the form of tissue keratosis or dysplasia. Clinically, the typical lesion is white, with a wrinkled, corrugated, and/or granular appearance with pink or red furrows. Lesions are associated with the immediate areas where the tobacco product is placed, usually in the vestibule of the mandible adjacent to the incisors and/or molars. Some lesions will involve the buccal mucosa as well as the gingiva. Upon discontinuance of the habit, most lesions will resolve spontaneously within two weeks. If lesions have a papillary appearance, have areas of ulceration or erythema, or persist after discontinuance of tobacco use, a biopsy should be performed. With continued use of smokeless tobacco, there is a significant risk of squamous cell carcinoma or verrucous carcinoma transformation.

LEUKOEDEMA Leukoedema is a common condition characterized by a grayish-white opalescent appearance of the oral mucosa. In severe cases, the tissue may appear wrinkled or corrugated. Affected areas cannot be rubbed off; however, when stretched the lesion temporarily disappears. The condition primarily affects the buccal mucosa, is asymptomatic, and usually occurs bilaterally. In rare cases, the labial mucosa, soft palate, and pharyngeal tissues may be involved. Approximately 90% of the black adult population and 50% of black children are affected. The prevalence and severity in caucasians is reported to be considerably less possibly owing to less background pigmentation allowing for more "blending" in of edematous areas. Some authorities consider leukoedema to be a normal variation of soft tissue. No treatment is necessary.

WHITE SPONGE NEVUS White sponge nevus is an autosomal-inherited disorder characterized by white, deeply folded or corrugated, spongy-appearing lesions on the buccal mucosa bilaterally. Other oral sites, including the tongue, floor of the mouth, soft palate, and alveolar mucosa, are less frequently involved. The lesions primarily appear during childhood and as early as infancy and usually do not appear after adolescence. The condition is asymptomatic, benign, and does not require treatment.

LINEA ALBA Linea alba occurs along the buccal mucosa bilaterally as a white line at the level of contact between the upper and lower teeth. It represents hyperkeratosis caused by the mucosa being pulled between the teeth. Approximately 13% of the population are affected. The condition is benign, and no treatment is required.

PIGMENTED LESIONS

ORAL MELANOTIC MACULE Melanotic macules (focal melanosis) are lesions that result from an increase in melanin deposition along the basal cell layer of the epithelium. These well-circumscribed, flat, less-than-1-cm-in-diameter lesions are usually brown, black, or bluish gray, occurring as single macules with the most common sites being the lower vermilion border extraorally and the buccal mucosa, gingiva, and palate intraorally. Oral melanotic macules are a clinical feature of Peutz-Jeghers syndrome and Addison disease. These lesions are asymptomatic, benign in nature, and require no treatment. Lesions of recent onset, enlarging lesions, or lesions of irregular pigmentation should be biopsied to rule out melanoma.

MELANOTIC NEVUS Rarely, melanotic nevus can occur on the palate and gingiva. They appear as either flat or domed-shaped lesions that are well circumscribed, ranging in color from brown to black. Treatment consists of surgical excision and biopsy to rule out early melanoma.

AMALGAM TATOO This lesion is associated with a history of amalgam restoration with the inadvertent incorporation of amalgam in open tissue. It appears on the gingiva, alveolar mucosa, or buccal mucosa as a flat, smooth bluish-gray pigmentation that is asymptomatic. Graphite tatoo is very similar in appearance and is usually found on the palate as a result of an injury with a lead pencil. No treatment is necessary; however, when the diagnosis is in doubt, a biopsy should be performed.

SUBMUCOSAL HEMORRHAGE Oral submucosal hemorrhage can present as petechiae, purpura, ecchymosis, or hematoma. Most oral submucosal bleeding is associated with trauma, but thrombocytopenia, disseminated intravascular coagulation, and viral infections (especially measles and mononucleosis) are also associated with oral mucosal hemorrhage. Additionally, persistent coughing, vomiting, and convulsions can produce petechiae and purpura along the soft palate. If the hemorrhage is not related to systemic disease, no treatment is required.

16.5.3 Vesiculo-Erosive and Ulcerated Lesions

RIGA-FEDE ULCERATION Ulcers occur on the ventral surface of the tongue in infants with a natal or neonatal tooth as a result of the infant placing the tongue over the incisal edge of the tooth while feeding or sucking. Smoothing the sharp edges of the tooth (teeth) is usually all that is necessary to promote healing.

PRIMARY HERPETIC GINGIVOSTOMATITIS Direct contact with herpes simplex results in a primary lesion, usually in children between 6 months and 5 years of age, although occasionally this occurs in older children and adults. Most often the patient is relatively asymptomatic until a recurrence, in the form of herpes labialis, occurs when the patient is older. Less frequently, initial symptoms consist of fever with lymphadenopathy and multiple vesicular lesions on the lips, gingiva, tongue, buccal mucosa, and palate. Some of the ulcers may mimic apthous ulcerations, whereas others are round or oval, usually less than 3 mm in diameter, and have a yellowish appearance. These lesions will often cluster and frequently coalesce, creating large areas of ulceration. The gingiva is typically fiery red and puffy in appearance. Typically there is an increase in salivation along with severe oral pain. The infection lasts from between 10 and 14 days with the most severe ulceration appearing between the third and seventh days. Because of the severe discomfort, patients will often limit oral intake and are at risk of dehydration. Diagnosis can be confirmed with immunofluorescence methods from a scraping of the lesion and confirmed by viral culture. Treatment consists of supportive care with topical anesthetics, encouraging oral intake to prevent dehydration, systemic analgesics, and administration of antiviral agents (swish and swallow) such as acyclovir, famciclovir, or valacyclovir. If begun within the first 3 days of onset, these agents may shorten the infectivity period as well as decrease the duration and severity of symptoms.

RECURRENT HERPES LABIALIS Recurrence of an initial oral herpes infection manifests as ulcerations primarily limited to the vermilion borders of the lips and perioral skin. The lesion consists of vesicles of clear fluid that coalesce to form a larger area of ulceration eventually developing into a brown crusted lesion leading to cracking, oozing, and occasionally bleeding. The lesion is usually unilateral but may occur bilaterally at times. Up to 45% of the population is affected with recurrent herpes labialis with intervals of recurrence varying greatly. Triggering factors include trauma, respiratory illnesses, menstruation, ultraviolet light exposure, and underlying systemic diseases. The duration of symptoms lasts between 7 and 10 days. Treatment consists of topical application of palliative creams, topical acyclovir or penciclovir cream, and/or systemic antiviral agents. Daily lysine intake may be effective in preventing recurrence.

HAND, FOOT, AND MOUTH DISEASE Coxsackie type A16, an enterovirus, causes this disorder, which is highly contagious and transferred via airborne particles or fecal-oral contamination. Children are primarily affected, although the disease can occur in adults. The lesions affect the ventral and side surfaces of the fingers and toes, the borders of the palms and soles, and the oral mucosa. The oral lesions are primarily found on the buccal and labial mucosa, tongue, and hard palate, but any oral site can be affected. The lesions begin as vesicles that eventually rupture, leaving areas of ulceration between 2 mm and 1 cm in diameter. The oral ulcerations resolve spontaneously between 7 and 10 days, and treatment is palliative consisting of systemic analgesics and topical anesthetics.

VARICELLA Oral lesions are common and may precede skin lesions. The lesions appear as small vesicles that rupture resulting in small painful ulcerations primary seen on the palate and occasionally the buccal mucosa. Gingival lesions that resemble herpetic gingivostomatitis can occur but, unlike the herpetic lesions, are usually painless.

APHTHOUS ULCERATIONS Aphthous ulcers represent the most common nontraumatic ulcer, occurring in between 20 and 60% of the population. There is a familial tendency, and females seem to be affected more than males. There are three forms of aphthous ulcerations: minor, major, and herpetiform. The differences between them are related to ulcer location, severity, and duration.

They all have a common etiology which may include trauma, stress, endocrine imbalances, allergies, nutritional deficiencies (especially vitamin B_{12}, folic acid, and iron), immunologic defects (cell mediated and humoral mediated), and bacteria (especially *L-form streptococcus*). The ulcerations are not preceded by vesicles but may be associated with prodromal symptoms of tingling or burning. Approximately 80% of all aphthous lesions are classified as *minor aphthous*, which are typically less than 1 cm in diameter and are covered by a whitish yellow fibrinous membrane surrounded by an erythematous halo. The lesions occur on nonkeratinized mucosa (buccal, labial, and vestibular mucosa, soft palate, and floor of the mouth), and typically between one and five oral sites are affected per episode. The onset is usually in childhood with a highly variable recurrence rate. Lesions are very painful, often making eating and routine oral hygiene difficult. With occasional isolated lesions, no treatment is necessary other than avoiding irritating foods. Lesions will heal spontaneously within 7 to 10 days. For more severe episodes, treatment consists of palliative creams, gels and rinses, and topical steroids. Topically applied 5% amlexanox paste has been reported to shorten the healing time and lessen the pain. Cautery with silver nitrate should be avoided to prevent tissue necrosis. Approximately 10% of aphthous lesions are classified as *major aphthous*, which are similar to minor aphthous but tend to begin after puberty with lesions being greater than 1 cm in diameter, deeper, more painful, and more likely to cause scarring than minor aphthous lesions. Because of the severe discomfort with eating, nutritional compromise is common. Treatment consists of more potent topical steroid rinses and intralesional steroids, as well as systemic steroids reserved for extremely severe episodes. The remaining 10% of aphthous ulcers are classified as *herpetiform ulcers*. Despite the implications of their name, these lesions are not associated with viral infection. Unlike the other forms of aphthous ulcers, they occur on both the keratinized and nonkeratinized mucosal surfaces of the oral cavity. The initial lesions have a somewhat herpetic appearance in that they are usually very small, less than 2 mm in diameter, and occur in clusters of up to 100 lesions that subsequently coalesce to produce large, very painful areas of ulceration that heal over 7 to 14 days. Treatment consists of palliative rinses and topical steroid rinses and gels.

BEHÇET SYNDROME Essentially all patients with Behçet syndrome will develop aphthous ulcerations. In 25 to 75% of cases, oral ulcerations are the first sign of the disease. Even though the oral lesions are aphthae, there are several clinical differences that distinguish oral lesions of this syndrome from typical aphthous lesions. Unlike typical apthae, oral lesions in Behçet syndrome frequently are observed on the soft palate and pharynx, usually with ragged borders and a larger area of surrounding erythema. Patients typically will have at least six areas of involvement. The frequency of lesions is highly variable, and the duration between 7 and 14 days per outbreak. Treatment of oral lesions is palliative. Systemic steroids and other immunosuppressive agents used to treat the underlying disease are also useful.

CROHN DISEASE Minor aphthous lesions and small granulomas along the buccal and labial mucosa may occur in patients with Crohn disease. At times, the buccal mucosa may appear fissured or lobulated. These findings may precede gastrointestinal tract lesions. Treatment of the underlying disease heals the lesions (see Sec. 17.20.2).

ERYTHEMA MULTIFORME   Up to 50% of patients with erythema multiforme have chronic or acute recurring oral lesions. Oral involvement consists of ulcers that range from aphthous-like to very large erosions with irregular borders. Typically patients will have dark hemorrhagic crusting of the lips. The buccal and labial mucosa, lips, soft palate, and tongue are most frequently affected, whereas the gingiva and hard palate are usually spared. The ulcerations are typically quite painful and in severe cases may lead to dehydration and malnutrition (see Sec. 14.6.3).

16.5.4   Papillary Oral Lesions

PAPILLOMA   Papillomas are benign lesions characterized by numerous white or pink finger-like projections similar to a cauliflower or wart in appearance. The lesions are usually pedunculated and represent a proliferation of stratified squamous epithelium. These lesions are presumed to be associated with one of the subtypes of the human papillomavirus (over 100); however, it is uncertain whether all papillomas are of viral etiology. At least 50% are linked to HPV-6 or HPV-11 subtypes. The lesions are most commonly seen on the vermilion borders of the lips as well as the palate, uvula, and dorsal of the tongue. Treatment consists of surgical excision, and recurrence is rare.

VERRUCA VULGARIS   Verruca vulgaris is associated with HPV-2, HPV-4, and HPV-6 and represents proliferation of stratified squamous epithelium. Its clinical appearance is the same as the papilloma and is usually seen on the vermilion borders of the lips. Lesions are not common intraorally but can occur on the tongue and buccal mucosa. Treatment consists of excision, cryotherapy, or electrosurgery. Occasionally, lesions will spontaneously resolve. Recurrence is rare.

CONDYLOMA ACUMINATUM   The oral lesions of this sexually transmitted disease are associated with several subtypes of human papillomavirus including HPV-6, HPV-11, HPV-16, and HPV-18, with incubation periods of 1 to 3 months following inoculation. The lesions appear identical to those in papilloma but tend to occur in clusters that coalesce, producing a broad-based lesion of up to 1.5 cm in diameter. Lesions are usually found on the palate, tongue, and labial mucosa. Treatment consists of surgical excision, cryotherapy, or electrosurgery. If the lesions occur in younger children, the possibility of sexual abuse should be investigated.

16.5.5   Benign Mesenchymal Lesions of Soft Tissue

FIBROMA   These lesions, which are caused by reactive fibrous hyperplasia in response to local irritation, are the most common oral soft-tissue tumor. They occur primarily on the lips, buccal mucosa, tongue, and palate. The surface is smooth with the color of surrounding mucosa. Borders are well demarcated, and the lesions are most often sessile and smaller than 2 cm in diameter but may be pedunculated. Treatment consists of surgical excision, and recurrence is uncommon.

PERIPHERAL OSSIFYING FIBROMA   This reactive lesion is similar to a fibroma, occurring primarily on the anterior maxillary or mandibular gingiva of teenagers, with a female predominance. It is usually a solitary lesion with a pink surface that may or may not be ulcerated and is characterized by the presence of calcified tissue in the tissue mass. Treatment consists of surgical excision.

PYOGENIC GRANULOMA   These highly vascular, rapidly growing lesions are found primarily on the gingiva and are seen most often in females, particularly during pregnancy. They may be sessile or pedunculated and may grow to several centimeters in size. The lesion is typically not painful, but surface ulceration may occur, with resultant bleeding. Treatment includes surgical excision, which should be delayed in pregnant woman until after parturition to avoid recurrence.

CONGENITAL EPULIS   The congenital epulis is a benign tumor with a pink to red smooth surface, ranging in size from a few millimeters to several centimeters, that occurs most frequently on the maxillary anterior gingival alveolar ridge of female infants. Multiple lesions develop in 10% of cases. Treatment consists of surgical excision, although small lesions may spontaneously regress.

HEMANGIOMA   Oral hemangiomas are usually dark red, blue, or purple and range from being very small to massive in size, potentially resulting in significant disfigurement. Lesions range from being flat to exophytic, and females tend to be affected more often than males. Oral hemangiomas may be observed in hemangioma syndromes such as Sturge-Weber syndrome. Small lesions may require no treatment, and larger lesions may be treated with corticosteroids, sclerosing agents, or interferon-α or may require surgical removal or debulking. Management of larger lesions is best approached in a comprehensive center with all treatment options being considered.

LYMPHANGIOMA   Oral lymphagiomas most often affect the anterior two-thirds of the tongue, producing swelling without discoloration. Superficial lesions may cause a pebbly appearance of the tongue, and deeper lesions produce localized ill-defined macroglossia. If lesions do not interfere with normal function, no treatment is necessary. Larger lesions may respond to surgical debulking or excision. These lesions do not respond to sclerosing agents.

NEUROFIBROMA   Oral neurofibromas have been reported to occur in up to 25% of cases of neurofibromatosis. Solitary lesions can occur at almost any oral site and appear as a painless, soft nodular tissue mass with the color of adjacent tissue.

16.5.6   Cysts and Pseudocysts

ORAL CYSTS OF THE NEWBORN   Between 65 and 85% of infants will develop keratin-filled cysts along the palate which are yellowish-white in color and typically are no larger than 3 mm in diameter. Cysts along the median palatal raphae arise from entrapped epithelium during fusion of the palatal shelves and are known as *Epstein's pearls*. Cysts that appear between the palatal midline and alveolar ridge are remnants of minor salivary glands and are known as *Bohn's nodules*. *Dental lamina cysts* or *gingival cysts* of the newborn appear on the alveolar ridges, often in clusters, and represent remnants of the dental lamina. All these cysts resolve spontaneously, requiring no treatment.

ERUPTION CYSTS AND HEMATOMAS   An eruption cyst develops over an erupting primary or permanent tooth as a result of fluid accumulation in the follicular space producing a soft translucent swelling of the gingival tissue. The cyst is primarily seen in children under the age of 10 and most often affects the primary mandibular molar area but can occur over any erupting tooth. It is not unusual for blood to mix with the fluid as a result of trauma, giving the cyst a bluish color. In this situation, the cyst is referred to as an *eruption hematoma*. Treatment is usually not necessary, as the tooth will erupt through the cyst with resolution of the lesion. In rare situations, when the tooth fails to erupt, simple unroofing of the cyst may be required.

MUCOCELE A mucocele is one of the most common causes of oral swelling in children and young adults, resulting from the rupture of a minor salivary gland with accumulation of mucin in the surrounding tissue. It appears as a fluctuant dome-shaped lesion, usually on the mandibular labial mucosa, ventral surface of the tongue, or buccal mucosa. There is almost always a history of trauma to the area, and the lesion will frequently increase and decrease in size. Treatment consists of surgical excision of the cyst and the associated minor salivary gland to prevent recurrence.

16.5.7 Benign Neoplasms of the Jaw

MELANOTIC NEUROECTODERMAL TUMOR OF INFANCY This neural-crest-derived tumor most commonly occurs in the anterior maxilla of infants under the age of 6 months, causing bone destruction and displacement of tooth buds. It grows rapidly, producing a smooth-surface swelling along the alveolus that may be pigmented because of the presence of melanocytes. Urinary vanillylmandelic acid levels are elevated in many patients. Treatment consists of surgical excision with a recurrence rate of 15%. Although the tumor is generally considered benign, there have been several reports of metastasis to other areas resulting in patient death.

FIBROUS DYSPLASIA Most cases of fibrous dysplasia affecting the jaws represent monostotic disease. Patients will experience an asymptomatic, slowly growing, unilateral bony expansion with the maxilla being affected more often than the mandible. As the lesion increases in size, facial asymmetry will be noted and is often the initial chief complaint. Growth of the lesion slows down and eventually ceases after the pubertal growth spurt. Males and females are affected equally. Small lesions often require no treatment, and facial recontouring can treat larger lesions resulting in cosmetic disfigurement. Malignant transformation is extremely uncommon and usually is associated with polyostotic disease.

CHERUBISM This autosomal-dominant disorder results in bilateral bony expansion of the posterior mandible and less often of the maxilla. Males are affected twice as often as females. Clinical features can be apparent as early as 1 year of age with the mean age of occurrence at 7 years. The degree of facial deformity varies greatly from very mild to severe disfigurement. Oral sequeae include displaced tooth follicles and, in severe cases, delay or failure in tooth eruption. Treatment is controversial and case-dependent. Some patients may benefit from surgical intervention, whereas others may show degrees of remission after puberty without need for any treatment.

CENTRAL GIANT CELL GRANULOMA This reactive lesion may involve oral soft tissues and bone, most often the anterior mandible. Small lesions may be asymptomatic and not apparent except on radiologic examination; larger lesions produce intraoral expansion of bone with an overlying soft-tissue mass. Treatment consists of surgical excision with curettage. The recurrence rate is between 15 and 20%.

TRAUMATIC BONE CYST These cysts of the jaw usually occur in patients between 10 and 20 years of age. The lesion usually follows trauma and is thought to be caused by resolution of an intraosseous hematoma, ischemic necrosis of bone marrow, or cystic degeneration of bone tumor. Most often the lesion is limited to the mandible, is asymptomatic, and is apparent only radiographically; however, in about 20% of cases, there will be a swelling with or without pain over the area. Treatment consists of surgical curettage to establish bleeding, which leads to rapid resolution. Recurrence is extremely rare, and the prognosis excellent.

16.6 ORAL MANIFESTATIONS OF SYSTEMIC DISORDERS

16.6.1 Oral Complications in Immunodeficiency

ACQUIRED IMMUNODEFICIENCY SYNDROME Oral manifestations include candidiasis, angular cheilitis, linear gingival erythema, aphthous ulcerations, acute necrotizing ulcerative gingivitis, hairy leukoplakia, xerostomia, parotid swelling, and Kaposi sarcoma. Oral infections often occur in HIV-infected patients up to 24 months prior to other symptoms. Lesions tend to be more severe, more widespread, and of longer duration than in immunologically normal patients. Epstein-Barr virus produces areas of hyperkeratosis forming white vertical streaks along the lateral borders of the tongue referred to as *hairy leukoplakia*. This lesion cannot be wiped off and is usually asymptomatic, only rarely being seen in pediatric patients, but if it occurs it can be treated effectively with antiviral agents or topical podophyllin resin. Severe aphthous ulceration is common in HIV-infected patients as discussed in Sec. 16.5.3. Treatment consists of topical steroid therapy. Lesions that are unresponsive should be biopsied to rule out cytomegalovirus (CMV), herpes, or deep fungal infections. Approximately 20% of adult patients will develop Kaposi sarcoma, and about 50% of these patients will develop oral lesions which are usually red to blue, may be flat or nodular, and occur singly or in multiples. Lesions typically develop on the hard and soft palate, gingiva, and tongue; however, any oral site can be affected. Lesions should be biopsied to confirm diagnosis. Treatment options include surgical removal, radiotherapy, intralesional injections with antimetabolites, and sclerosing agents (see also Sec. 13.4.12).

NEUTROPENIA Oral manifestations include mucositis and ulcerations with severity directly related to the degree of neutropenia. Nonkeratinized mucosa is primarily affected and represents an inability of the tissue to respond to trauma or infection. Oral ulcerations seen in patients with cyclic neutropenia appear identical to aphthous stomatitis. During periods of neutropenia, the gingiva can become severely inflamed with spontaneous bleeding. Oral manifestations resolve spontaneously as the neutrophil count returns to normal.

16.6.2   Oral Complications of Cancer Therapy and Bone Marrow Transplant

ORAL MANIFESTATIONS OF GVHD   Up to 75% of patients experiencing acute graft-versus-host disease (GVHD) and 80% of patients with chronic GVHD will develop oral manifestations including lichenoid hyperkeratotic lesions, buccal and labial atrophy, ulcerative lesions, and xerostomia. Patients will frequently complain of a burning sensation of the mucosa and tongue. Confirmation of GVHD can be achieved with a biopsy of the oral mucosa. Oral symptoms will usually resolve with systemic corticosteroid therapy.

CHEMOTHERAPY   Complications of chemotherapy are the result of a direct stomatotoxicity of the agents on the oral mucosa or are an indirect effect of myelosuppression with immunodeficiency. Oral adverse effects of chemotherapy include ulcerations, infections, hemorrhage, and xerostomia. Direct stomatotoxicity results from the cytotoxic action of chemotherapeutic agents on the oral mucosal cells with a decrease in the renewal rate of the basal epithelium causing atrophic thinning of the oral mucosa. Mucosal thinning is followed by a degenerative change in the supportive submucosal collagen layer, leading to the development of mucosal ulcerations. Mucositis most commonly occurs on the nonkeratinized epithelium of the mouth, such as on the buccal and labial mucosa, on the ventral and lateral surfaces of the tongue, on the soft palate, and on the floor of the mouth. The nonkeratinized mucosa apparently has a more rapid rate of cell turnover than does keratinized mucosa, increasing its susceptibility of ulceration. Treatment of mucositis is palliative. Relief of pain can be obtained by application of topical anesthetic agents, such as lidocaine, dyclonine, or benzocaine. Rinsing with a 2% solution of sodium bicarbonate in sterile saline or water may also provide relief. Chlorhexidine 2% during periods of myelosuppression may help to minimize the severity and duration of mucosal ulcers. Diet should be restricted to avoid irritating foods, and careful oral hygiene measures should be stressed. Narcotic analgesics may be necessary to relieve severe pain.

Drug-induced stomatotoxicity alters local and systemic tissue response to infection and makes the mouth exceedingly susceptible to microbial attack. Both endogenous and exogenous microorganisms are capable of producing oral infections that can become life threatening in the immunosuppressed patient. The most frequent sites of oral infection are the lips, tongue, buccal mucosa, gingiva, palate, and oropharynx. The clinical appearance of oral infections may be atypical in the myelosuppressed patient. Common fungal infections include candidiasis and aspergillosis. Bacterial infections occur in the mouth of 10 to 20% of patients being treated with antineoplastic drugs. Included among the causes of bacterial infections are species of *Klebsiella, Enterobacter, Serratia, Proteus,* and *Escherichia coli.* Oral viral infections are the result of herpes simplex virus (most common), cytomegalovirus, varicella zoster virus, and Epstein-Barr virus.

Xerostomia can occur occasionally in patients after chemotherapy, most frequently with adriamycin, although other agents have been implicated. Similarly, chemotherapy during childhood may produce changes in tooth or jaw growth and development. Management of these complications is discussed in more detail below since they are more common complications of radiation therapy.

RADIATION THERAPY   Radiation to the head and neck can result in oral mucositis, xerostomia, infections, radiation caries, periodon-

tal disease, hypogeusia and dysgeusia, trismus, alterations in growth and development of the maxilla and mandible, and defects in tooth development. Additionally, patients are at risk of developing osteoradionecrosis.

Dysfunction of the salivary gland is one of the most common sequelae of radiation to the head and neck. Irradiation primarily affects acinal function, having little effect on ductal function. Serous acinal cells are initially affected more than mucinous acinar cells. Initially, patients experience painful enlargement of the parotid gland secondary to edema and inflammatory infiltration. The saliva often becomes thick and ropy as a result of secretion of undiluted mucus. The qualitative chemical changes that occur cause a decrease in the pH from an average of 6.75 to as low as 4.05, making the patients far more prone to dental caries. The severity of dysfunction of the salivary gland is related to the radiation dose, the amount of gland included in the field of radiation, and the age of the patient. Recovery of salivary function is better in preadolescent patients owing to the increased ability of salivary tissue to regenerate in younger individuals. Patients frequently will develop sensitivity to hot, cold, and sweet foods, and therefore they limit nutrient intake. Taste is adversely affected, and swallowing becomes difficult. Occasionally, the dryness of the mouth interferes with speech and articulation. Treatment of xerostomia includes use of saliva substitutes, pilocarpine, saline irrigation, hydrogen peroxide rinses, glycerin swabs, demulcent lozenges, sugarless gum, and mouth rinses. If thick mucus is present, a 2% sodium bicarbonate mouthwash in water or saline may be useful.

Radiation therapy during childhood can produce abnormalities in tooth development as well as alterations in growth and development of facial structures. The nature and severity of impairments are related to the age of the patient and stage of development at the time of radiation. The most severe disturbances occur when radiation is administered during the early stages of tooth development. Radiation of developing teeth can cause tooth agenesis, hypoplasia, and hypocalcification. Other effects on tooth development include microdontia, shortening and blunting of roots, thinning of root structure, abnormal curvature of roots, ankylosis of the primary dentition, and failure or delays in tooth eruption. Radiation therapy also has an effect on the growth and development of facial bones as a result of irreversible damage to cartilaginous growth centers. When condylar growth centers are affected, facial asymmetry and mandibular micrognathia can occur. Maxillary hypoplasia can develop when cranial sutural growth centers have been damaged. The resulting growth disturbances can produce severe dental malocclusions, which often require surgical as well as orthodontic correction.

The most severe and most difficult to treat complication following radiotherapy to the oral region is *osteoradionecrosis.* Changes in bone that occur secondary to radiotherapy include avascularity, fatty degeneration, enlarged lacunae, microfractures, and a reduction in the number of osteocytes, osteoblasts, and osteoclasts. Blood supply to the area is often permanently altered secondary to radiation-induced fibrosis, endarteritis, and hyalinization of blood vessels. As a result of these changes, bone tissue becomes more susceptible to infection and necrosis and has a decreased ability to heal. Patients are particularly at risk of osteoradionecrosis following tooth extractions. The maxilla is less susceptible than the mandible because of greater blood supply. Prevention is aimed at limiting infection or trauma to the jaws of the irradiated patient. This is best accomplished by a pretherapy dental evaluation, with any required dental treatment being accomplished before beginning radiotherapy. Patients should also be placed on a strict oral hygiene protocol keeping the oral tissues as clean as possible. All teeth that have associated pathology and are unrestorable should be extracted. When an extraction is required after radiation therapy, systemic antibiotics should be administered. The lack of reported cases in young children seems to suggest that this age group may be unaffected or rarely affected by osteoradionecrosis.

16.6.3   Other Miscellaneous Disorders

TRISOMY 21   The oral cavity of children with Down syndrome has characteristic structural variations including abnormalities of occlusion, a small oral cavity causing a relative macroglossia, a deeply fissured tongue, and small teeth that may be hypocalcified, malformed, and more widely spaced. Tooth eruption is commonly delayed in both the primary and permanent dentitions. Dental caries are less frequent than in the general population because of the higher alkalinity of saliva in Down syndrome, but periodontal disease is more common, in part because of poorer oral hygiene. Dental treatment consists of preventive measures to include strict oral hygiene measures at home and regular dental check-ups. For high-functioning children, orthodontic treatment can be considered.

HYPOHIDROTIC ECTODERMAL DYSPLASIA   This disorder results in the abnormal development of structures of ectodermal origin. Oral findings of hypodontia include, rarely, total anodontia, hypotrophic alveolar dental ridges, protuberant lips, and hypoplasia of oral mucoserous glands. Xerostomia rarely occurs. Teeth are typically conical in shape. Females tend to show fewer and less severe dental anomalies than males. Treatment involves reshaping of conically shaped teeth and replacing missing teeth with fixed or removable prosthetics. Often, patients with many missing teeth will require complete dentures or overdentures. Pediatric patients must be monitored closely for prosthetic remakes to accommodate growth. Dental implants should be considered.

DERMATOLOGIC DISORDERS   Oral lesions occur in several forms of epidermolysis bullosa. Bullae can occur during infancy from sucking and eventually lead to significant oral scarring. Even slight abrasion from oral hygiene measures can result in bullae formation. Other oral findings include enamel hypoplasia, enamel pitting, increased susceptibility to dental caries, and delayed dental eruption. Early and frequent dental visits may help to minimize severe dental morbidity. In Papillon-Lefèvre syndrome, a recessive disorder with diffuse keratoderma, periodontitis may lead to the premature loss of teeth.

TUBEROUS SCLEROSIS   Oral manifestations of tuberous sclerosis include pitting of the enamel affecting the facial surfaces of the teeth. The permanent dentition is affected in virtually all cases, but primary teeth may or may not be affected. The enamel pits vary in size from being pinpoint and visible only with staining with disclosing solution to being quite large and apparent. The pits are primarily an esthetic concern and usually do not develop into carious lesions. Oral fibromatosis develops in up to 70% of patients with tuberous sclerosis. The fibromas usually develop in late childhood and are found primarily on the gingiva; however, the tongue, buccal and labial mucosa, and palate can be affected. In severe cases, surgical excision is indicated. Other less commonly seen oral manifestations include alveolar hyperostosis, cleft lip and palate, highly arched palate, macroglossia, and osseous fibromas of the jaws.

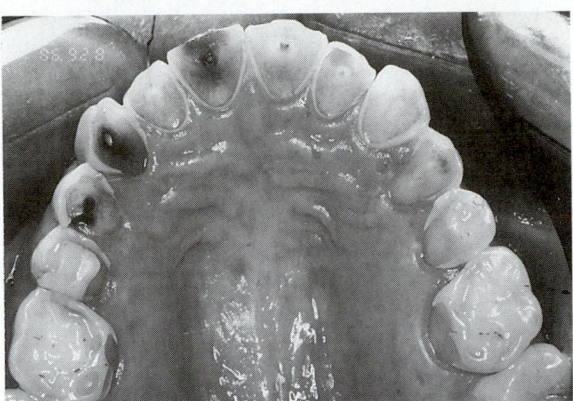

FIGURE 16-11   Bulimia-associated enamel erosion on the lingual surfaces of the permanent dentition.

DIABETES MELLITUS   Patients with juvenile-onset diabetes are more susceptible to dental caries and have a high incidence of periodontal disease. Other complications include xerostomia, with diabetic sialodenitis or nontender parotid gland enlargement, an increased susceptibility to oral candidiasis, and a higher incidence of benign migratory glossitis. Infants of diabetic mothers have a higher prevalence of enamel hypoplasia than the general population. The increased risk of dental disease demands that patients with diabetes have more frequent dental check-ups and maintain impeccable oral hygiene measures.

CHRONIC RENAL DISEASE   Chronic renal failure results in numerous oral manifestations. The oral mucosa may appear pale secondary to anemia or may have an orange color secondary to deposition of carotene-like pigments. Patients may experience xerostomia, develop parotitis, sense a metallic taste, and have an ammonia-like odor to the saliva. Uremic stomatitis characterized by generalized redness and burning of the mucosa with ulcerations can develop in severe cases of renal failure. Petechiae and ecchymoses of the gingiva and buccal and labial mucosa often occur. Patients are susceptible to periodontitis as well as acute necrotizing ulcerative gingivitis and thus should be seen frequently for dental examinations and cleanings. The developing teeth frequently are delayed in eruption and are often hypoplastic with brown discoloration.

BULIMIA   Chronic regurgitation and vomiting of gastric contents can erode tooth structures. The typical pattern of tooth loss occurs on the lingual surfaces of the maxillary teeth (Fig. 16-11). This type of erosion is also seen from consumption of excessive fruit juices or with habitual sucking on lemons and can be a feature of gastroesophageal reflux

OTHER ASSOCIATED DISORDERS   Oral ulcers are associated with Crohn disease and Behçet syndrome as discussed above. Many viral illnesses may also cause oral mucosal lesions. Dentition may be stained in cholestatic liver disease, hemolytic disease, or congenital erythropoietic porphyria, as noted in Sec. 16.2.

References

Blanchet-Bardon C, Nazarro V, Rognin C, Geiger JM, Puissant A: Acitretin in the treatment of severe disorders of keratinization: results of an open study. J Am Acad Dermatol 24:982, 1991

Eisen D, Lynch DP: The Mouth, Diagnosis and Treatment. Mosby, 1998
Neville BW, Damm DD, White DK: Color Atlas of Clinical Oral Pathology. 2nd ed, Williams and Wilkins, 1999
Regezi JR, Sciubba JJ: Oral Pathology, Clinical Pathologic Correlations. 3rd ed, Philadelphia, Saunders, 1999
Scully C, Welbury: Color Atlas of Oral Diseases in Children and Adolescents. Mosby-Year Book Europe Limited, 1994
Wood NK, Goaz PW: Differential Diagnosis of Oral and Maxillofacial Lesions, 5th ed. Mosby-Year Book, 1997

16.7 TEMPOROMANDIBULAR JOINT DISORDERS

A variety of signs and symptoms are ascribed to disorders of the temporomandibular joint, but the incidence of these disorders in children is unknown. The approach to diagnosis, the range of normal findings, and appropriate therapies remain controversial. Clearly, there can be temporomandibular joint involvement in rheumatologic disorders such as juvenile rheumatoid arthritis and when there is abnormal joint development as with hemifacial microsomia. However, the symptoms of pain, joint sounds, limited movement, and deviation of the mandible found in most cases in children are idiopathic in nature and may be normal variants. Localization and description of pain is often difficult in children, so the opportunity for mistaken diagnosis and inappropriate treatment is considerable. Therapies other than symptom relief with anti-inflammatory or analgesic medications have not been proven effective, especially those that are invasive. If temporomandibular joint pain or discomfort persists and systemic disorders are ruled out, it is most reasonable to refer the patient to a rheumatologist and/or dentist with more than occasional experience in managing children with possible temporomandibular joint disorder.

References

Doyle WA, Casamassimo PS: Temporomandibular joint disorders in children and adolescents. In: Pinkham JR, ed: Pediatric Dentistry: Infancy Through Adolescence. Philadelphia, Saunders, 1994:616–623
Guidelines for temporomandibular disorders in children and adolescents. J Pediatr Dent, Special Issue: Reference Manual 1999–2000 21/5:66–67
Kaplan AS, Assael LA: Temporomandibular Disorders: Diagnosis and Treatment. Philadelphia, Saunders, 1991
Nydell A, Helkimo M, Koch G: Craniomandibular disorders in children—a critical review of the literature. Swed Dent J 18:191–205, 1994

16.8 DENTAL MANAGEMENT OF CLEFT LIP AND/OR CLEFT PALATE

Syndromes associated with cleft lip and palate and the overall management approach are discussed in Sec. 10.3.4. An interdisciplinary team of specialists best provides management of patients with cleft lip and palate. The optimal time for initial evaluation is as soon after birth as possible. Prior to a newborn's discharge, an initial contact should be made with a craniofacial team to ensure that all medical and feeding issues are addressed. Craniofacial teams can be identified through the American Cleft Palate-Craniofacial Association (http://www.cleftline.org). The extremely important treatment timing and sequence depends on the type and severity of the cleft as well as the overall philosophy of the treatment team. Defining a long-term habilitation agenda centers around very well defined "windows of opportunity" for therapeutic interventions that optimize outcomes.

Treatment of infants with palatal clefts occurs in stages depending upon the type and severity of the cleft. Some treatment centers recommend palatal obturators to aid in feeding, but others instead instruct the caregiver to hold the infant in a more upright position during feedings and utilize bottles and nipples specifically designed for infants with clefts. In some instances, cleft segments may require repositioning through palatal orthopedic procedures prior to lip closure. Orthopedic movement can be achieved with lip taping and removable or fixed oral appliances. Alignment can be achieved over a period of 4 to 6 weeks, after which time the lip will be formally closed, usually by 3 months of age. The palate is typically closed without grafting between 9 and 12 months of age. Some centers, however, will perform primary alveolar bone grafting at the time of either lip or palate closure. The method of repairing a cleft will vary with the size and type of cleft as well as the experience and preference of the treating clinician.

Dental management of these disorders is required owing to the frequency of missing teeth as well as supernumerary teeth. Most often, the primary and permanent lateral incisors are missing. It is not unusual for teeth in the adjacent area to be malformed, hypoplastic, and rotated and to be delayed in eruption. Additionally, teeth will frequently erupt ectopically toward the midpalatal area in line with the cleft. Furthermore, children with oral clefting are more prone to dental caries and periodontal disease in the immediate area of the cleft. Dental development should be monitored by the child's dentist and orthodontist in conjunction with a craniofacial team. Patients can expect to undergo several stages of orthodontic treatment including the need for intraoral appliances to correct crossbites and possible bone grafting. It is critical that patients receive frequent and regular dental evaluations to properly time these events. If a critical event is delayed beyond optimal timing, the long-term outcome may be less favorable. After growth of the maxillofacial complex is complete and orthodontic appliances have been removed, prosthetic teeth in the form of either implants or bridges may be indicated in the area of the cleft. Additionally, patients with severe skeletal discrepancies may require orthognatic surgery to reposition the maxilla and/or mandible.

References

Millard DR, Latham R, Huifen X, Spiro S, Morovic C: Cleft lip and palate treated by presurgical orthopedics, gingivoperiosteoplasty, and lip adhesion (POPLA) compared with previous lip adhesion method: a preliminary study of serial dental casts. Plast Reconstr Surg 103(6):1630–1644, 1999
Solis A, Figueroa AA, Cohen M, Polley JW, Evans CA: Maxillary dental development in complete unilateral alveolar clefts. Cleft Palate Craniofac J 35(4):320–328, 1998
Strauss RP: Cleft palate and craniofacial teams in the United States and Canada: a national survey of team organization and standards of care.

The American Cleft Palate-Craniofacial Association (ACPA) Team Standards Committee. Cleft Palate Craniofac J 35(6):473–480, 1998

Strauss RP: The organization and delivery of craniofacial health services: the state of the art. Cleft Palate Craniofac J 36(3):189–195, 1999

Trotman CA, Ross RB: Craniofacial growth in bilateral cleft lip and palate: ages six years to adulthood. Cleft Palate Craniofac J 30(3):261–273, 1993

16.9 EMERGENCY DENTAL CARE

The majority of dental emergencies result from either trauma or infection. In all cases of orofacial trauma, a medical assessment must be completed, including a neurologic examination, and the patients' risk for tetanus should be reviewed.

TOOTHACHE

The approach to a child with a toothache is outlined in Table 16-10. Most infections in the oral cavity result from dental decay. Depending on the nature of the carious lesion, symptoms can be quite variable. Lesions can range from being quite small and totally painless to eliciting severe throbbing pain. There is not always a direct correlation between lesion size and symptoms produced. At times, very large appearing lesions may not elicit pain, whereas what may appear to be a small lesion can be excruciatingly painful. Pain elicited when exposed to cold or sweets is usually indicative of a carious lesion producing a reversible pulpitis. Treatment consists of referring the patient for dental care. Dental treatment will consist of excavation of the lesion and placing a restoration. Antibiotics are of no value, and analgesics may provide little relief.

As the decay process progresses into deeper tissues of the tooth, the pulp may develop an irreversible pulpitis with symptoms of spontaneous lingering pain that is intensified by heat or cold. The periodontal ligament may become inflamed producing pain upon

TABLE 16-10

APPROACH TO THE CHILD WITH A TOOTHACHE

Recent Trauma?
   See Tables 16-11 and 16-12, Figure 16-13
Occasional pain with cold and sweets
   Dental evaluation in 5–7 days.
   Involved teeth are typically restorable.
   Antibiotics are not indicated.
Spontaneous throbbing pain, disturbed sleep with:
   No intra- or extraoral swelling
      Dental evaluation within 24 h for extraction or root canal therapy.
      Pain medication.
   Intraoral swelling
      Dental evaluation within 24 h for extraction or root canal therapy.
      Antibiotics (penicillin or clindamycin).
      Pain medication.
   Facial swelling
      Evaluate airway stability, extent of involvement, and hydration.
      Hospitalization for intravenous antibiotics and hydration.
      Immediate dental referral for surgical drainage and/or extraction.

mastication or percussion. Treatment consists of antibiotics (penicillin VK, clindamycin, erythromycin, or a cephalosporin), analgesics, and referral for dental treatment. Dental treatment will consist of endodontic therapy (root canal therapy) or extraction. When more than one maxillary tooth, either unilaterally or bilaterally, develops similar symptoms, especially sensitivity to percussion, a maxillary sinusitis should be suspected.

Once the decay enters into pulpal tissue, the area rapidly becomes infiltrated with inflammatory cells resulting in an acute pulpitis with development of an abscess. Clinically, patients will complain of spontaneous throbbing pain especially at night. The entire pulpal tissue eventually undergoes necrosis resulting in a periapical abscess. The tooth will be tender to percussion, may exhibit mobility, and the surrounding periodontal tissue is usually inflamed. In cases where the abscess is below the muscle attachment, the infection will transgress through the least path of resistance resulting in a maxillary or mandibular facial cellulitis. Severe dental infections can lead to facial cellulitis with orbital involvement that if not aggressively treated can result in cavernous sinus thrombosis, septicemia, brain abscess, and acute airway obstruction. Treatment of localized abscesses consists of oral antibiotics (penicillin VK, clindamycin, erythromycin, or a cephalosporin) and analgesics. Severe cases of cellulitis require hospitalization for parenteral antibiotics, intravenous hydration, and surgical drainage of the infection. These patients should receive immediate dental care.

Erupting molars may cause inflammation and infection of adjacent soft tissue resulting in a pericoronitis. This is most often seen with erupting third molars. The area should be irrigated with salt-water rinses, and antibiotics should be prescribed. A dental referral should be made for evaluation of either tooth extraction or surgical removal of pericoronal tissue.

POSTOPERATIVE COMPLICATIONS

Following dental operations such as extraction, complications consist of swelling, pain, bleeding, and alveolar osteitis. *Swelling* is normal following oral surgical procedures, and extraction of impacted teeth usually will result in more swelling than extraction of nonimpacted teeth. Permanent tooth extractions usually result in more swelling than primary tooth extractions. If swelling persists beyond the third day, infection should be suspected and the patient referred for evaluation. *Pain* is expected following oral surgery and can interfere with oral intake. Mild to moderate pain can be alleviated with acetaminophen or nonsteroidal anti-inflammatory agents, while more severe pain may require narcotic analgesics. Oral *bleeding* is common following many oral surgical procedures, particularly extractions. Constant topical pressure with gauze to the area for between 30 and 60 minutes may be required to control oral bleeding. If the area continues to ooze, a wet tea bag applied to the area may help to provide relief. The tannic acid in tea bags will produce vasoconstriction of small vessels. If the area continues bleeding despite all efforts of topical pressure, the area may require curettage, the application of hemostatic agents such as a gelatin sponge or topical thrombin, and suturing. If bleeding continues beyond these measures, systemic causes should be investigated. *Alveolar osteitis* (dry socket) is caused by inflammation and delayed healing of a socket following extraction as a result of lysis of the overlying clot with exposure of underlying bone. Typically, severe often throbbing pain develops in the area 2 or 3 days following the extraction. Pain may radiate to the ear and may last for several days to weeks. Alveolitis is most often seen following extraction of mandibular third molars and is infrequently seen in children or adolescents. Treatment consists of surgical curettage of the socket to stimulate bleeding, and packing the socket with gauze and a topical anesthetic. Antibiotics are usually not of benefit as the socket rarely becomes infected.

ORAL SOFT-TISSUE INJURY

The approach to evaluation and treatment of oral soft tissue injuries is shown in Fig. 16-12. Oral lacerations should be examined carefully for the presence of foreign bodies, especially in the presence of fractured teeth. A radiograph of the lesion should be performed to rule out foreign bodies as palpation alone is usually insufficient. *Lip lacerations* require careful management to provide an esthetic closure, especially if the laceration is deep or extends through the vermilion border. Full-thickness lacerations require suturing in layers. Careful attention to anatomic alignment of the vermilion border is important. *Through and through laceration* results in communication between the skin and oral environment and is frequently contaminated. Suturing of the intraoral laceration should precede skin suturing, and the patient should be placed on a course of antibiotics effective against staphylococcal organisms. *Tongue lacerations* are commonly seen in children and usually result from a fall or blow to the chin. The tongue has a profuse blood supply, and injury can result in copious bleeding. Most tongue lacerations with approximating borders will heal without suturing; however, tears that leave unapproximated borders, such as at the tip or along the lateral borders, require suturing. *Gingival degloving* occurs when gingival tissue and periosteum is pulled away from its normal position around the tooth, exposing underlying bone. These injuries require gentle repositioning of the gingival tissue and stabilization with sutures.

TOOTH INJURIES

PRIMARY TEETH FRACTURES Fractures of hard dental tissues can be classified as enamel-only fractures, enamel-dentin fractures, enamel-dentin-pulp fractures, and root fractures. Fractures of the primary teeth are less common than in permanent teeth owing to more flexible and pliable supporting bone. Displacement rather than fracture is a more common occurrence. Small fractures limited to enamel are usually not treated. When the fracture extends into the dentin layer (slightly more yellow than enamel), the patient should be referred to a dentist for evaluation. The fractured portion may require treatment with composite bonding. When the pulp tissue has been exposed, a bright red area within the dentin layer will be evident. This type of exposure is quite painful and susceptible to infection, requiring dental evaluation within 24 hours. Depending on the severity of pulp exposure, the age of the patient, and the amount of existing root structure, treatment will consist of either extraction or immediate pulpectomy.

PERMANENT TEETH FRACTURES The approach to tooth fractures is shown in Table 16-11. Any fracture to the crown of a permanent tooth should be referred for a dental evaluation. Fractures limited to the enamel constitute a nonurgent referral, often being managed by smoothing of rough edges. Fractures that extend into the dentin, especially with symptoms of pain, should be referred for treatment as soon as possible. Treatment consists of conservative rebuilding of fractured portions with composite resin bonding materials. The prognosis is excellent for most of these teeth. Fractures involving pulp tissue are readily apparent by exposure of an area of bright red tissue within the dentin layer. These fractures require immediate referral to a dentist to cover the exposed pulp tissue. When treated promptly, the prognosis can be quite favorable. All traumatized teeth, however, are at risk of developing pulpal necrosis requiring endodontic therapy or extraction.

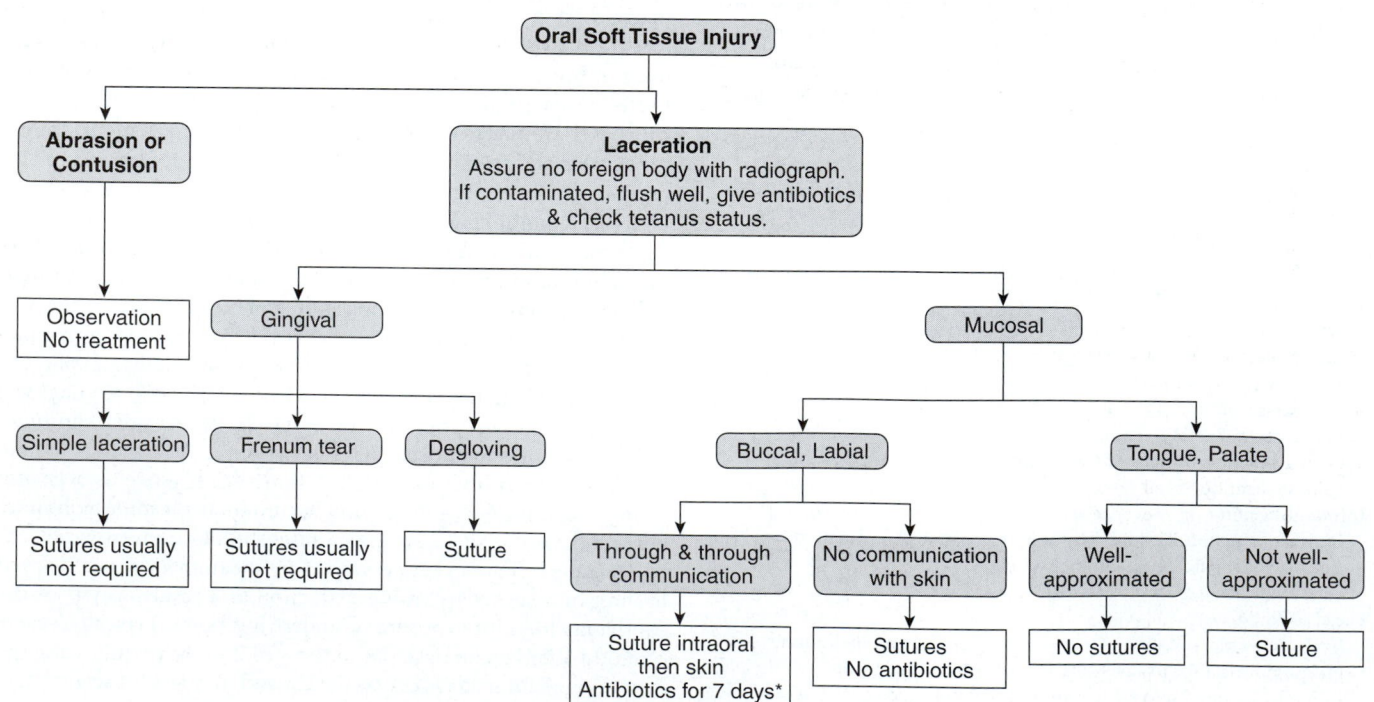

FIGURE 16-12 Algorithm for the management of oral soft-tissue injury.

TABLE 16-11

APPROACH TO THE CHILD WITH A TOOTH FRACTURE

Enamel fracture
    Dental referral in 5–7 days to smooth rough edges and restore.
Enamel and dentin fracture without pulp exposure
    Dental referral in 5–7 days for temporization or restoration.
Enamel and dentin fracture with pulp exposure
    Dental referral within 24 h for pulp therapy and temporization.
    Primary teeth may require extraction.
Complete crown severence (crown root fracture)
    Immediate dental referral.
    Remainder of tooth may require extraction.
    Root is rarely salvageable.

DISPLACEMENT OF TEETH WITHIN THE SOCKET *Intrusion* injuries consist of displacement of the tooth partially or completely into the alveolar bone, and *luxation* occurs when the tooth is displaced laterally, facially or lingually. The approach to luxation injuries is outlined in Table 16-12. Intruded primary teeth should be referred for a dental evaluation. Treatment most often consists of observation allowing for spontaneous repositioning. Teeth that remain intruded as well as teeth that have been intruded directly into the developing permanent tooth follicle will require extraction. Luxated primary teeth should be allowed to spontaneously reposition and tighten if the tooth does not interfere with occlusion. If there is functional interference or when the tooth is at risk of aspiration, extraction is indicated. Sequelae to the permanent dentition include tooth discoloration, hypoplasia, and ectopic eruption of the permanent tooth.

Intruded or luxated permanent teeth require an immediate dental evaluation. Young permanent teeth can be treated by gentle luxation, allowing the tooth to spontaneously erupt, or with orthodontic repositioning of the tooth. More mature permanent teeth are not likely to reerupt and will require orthodontic extrusion followed by endodontic therapy. Luxated permanent teeth should be treated by repositioning the tooth with conservative splinting by a dentist.

TABLE 16-12

MANAGEMENT OF TOOTH DISPLACEMENT IN THE SOCKET (LUXATION INJURIES)

Concussion: sensitive to percussion; not displaced; not loose
    Dental referral in 5–7 days to smooth rough edges and restore.
Subluxation: sensitive to percussion; not displaced; mobile
    Dental referral in 5–7 days.
    Soft diet.
Extrusion: axial displacement of the tooth, partially out of the socket
    Immediate dental referral for splinting.
    Root canal therapy may eventually be needed.
Lateral luxation: lateral displacement of the tooth in the socket; fracture of the alveolar bone
    Immediate dental referral for tooth repositioning and splinting.
    Root canal therapy may be needed.
    Primary teeth may require extraction.
Intrusion: tooth displaced into the socket
    Immediate dental referral to evaluate for either immediate repositioning, observation for natural re-eruption or orthodontic extrusion.

DISPLACEMENT OF TEETH OUT OF THE SOCKET *Avulsion* refers to displacement of the tooth out of the socket. The approach to oral trauma with tooth avulsion is shown in Fig. 16-13. Avulsed primary teeth should not be replanted. The patient should be immediately referred for a dental evaluation for a radiograph of the area to make sure that the tooth in fact was not intruded. Avulsed permanent teeth should most ideally be replanted at the site of injury. The primary determinant factor for long-term success of the replanted tooth is the length of time the tooth has been out of the socket. With delay in replantation, root resorption invariably occurs resulting in eventual loss of the tooth. Teeth replanted within 30 minutes have the best prognosis with a 90% success rate. Teeth out of the socket more than 2 hours have an extremely poor prognosis with more than 95% of these teeth experiencing total root resorption. All aspects of treatment are aimed at prevention of eventual root resorption. The following steps should be taken for immediate replantation of an avulsed tooth:

1. The tooth should always be held by the crown and not the root to avoid damage to periodontal ligament fibers.
2. If uncontaminated, the tooth is gently but firmly placed back into the socket with digital pressure. If contaminated, the tooth should be rinsed with saline before replantation. If resistance is met, the tooth should not be forced, but stored in milk or saline.
3. The replanted tooth should be stabilized by having the patient bite on gauze, or another readily available material, until seen by a dentist.
4. The patient should be transferred either to a hospital emergency room with dental staff coverage or a dental office for immediate splinting. If the tooth cannot be replanted immediately, the tooth should be placed in milk, a saline solution, or, if the patient is able, held in the mouth in the oral vestibule. Storing the tooth dry will dessicate the periodontal ligament fibers, significantly reducing the long-term prognosis.
5. Patients should be prescribed a course of antibiotics for 7 days, and tetanus immunization status of the patient should be evaluated.

Avulsed teeth will require endodontic therapy with frequent and long-term follow-up.

CHILD ABUSE

In over 50% of cases of child abuse there are injuries to the head, face, and neck with injuries to the dentition in 10% of cases. In cases of suspected child abuse most oral injuries are the result of trauma from eating utensils, objects, fingers, scalding, or caustic liquids. Typical injuries include lacerations (especially of the maxillary frenulum); fractured, luxated, or avulsed teeth; jaw and facial fractures; oral burns; oral and facial bruises; and tissue scarring from previous trauma. Teeth may be discolored or abscessed from previous trauma. Sexually transmitted oral lesions such as condyloma acuminata in prepubertal children are highly suspect for sexual abuse. It must be remembered however that these lesions can occur also from verruca vulgaris. Oral trauma from sexual abuse can also result in petechiae or bruising at the junction of the hard and soft palate.

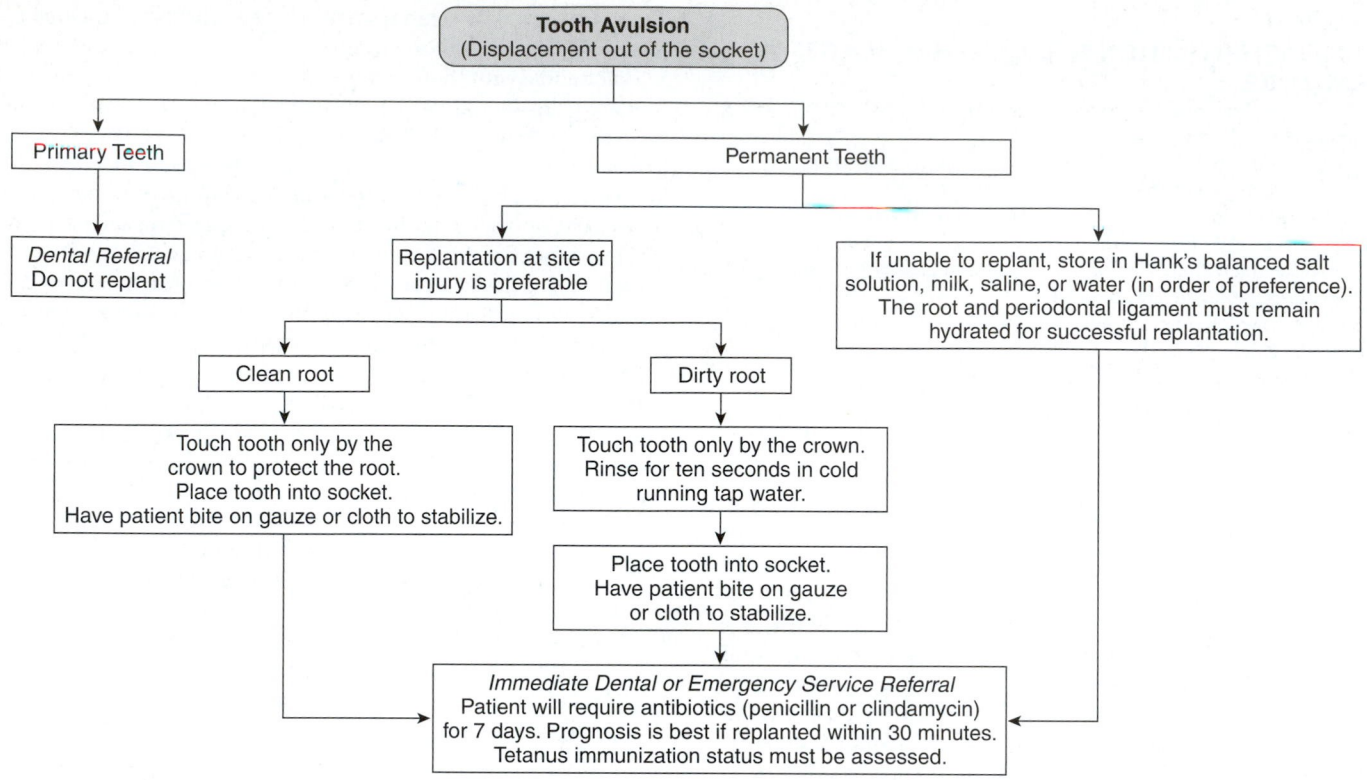

FIGURE 16-13   Algorithm for the management of tooth avulsion (displacement out of the socket).

References

Andreasen JO, Andreasen FM: Textbook and Color Atlas of Traumatic Injuries to the Teeth, 3rd ed. Copenhagen, Munksgaard, 1993

Barrett EJ, Kenny DJ: Avulsed permanent teeth: a review of the literature and treatment guidelines. Endod Dent Traumatol 13:153–163, 1997

Krasner P, Person P: Preserving avulsed teeth for replantation. JADA 123: 80, 1992

McDonald RD, Avery DR: Management of trauma to the teeth and supporting tissues. In: McDonald RE, Avery DR, eds: Dentistry for the Child and Adolescent, 7th ed. St. Louis, Mosby, 2000

GASTROENTEROLOGY AND NUTRITION

Colin D. Rudolph, Associate Editor

17.1 STRUCTURE AND DEVELOPMENT OF THE GASTROINTESTINAL TRACT

Colin D. Rudolph

17.1.1 Anatomy and Histology

The organs of the gastrointestinal (GI) tract form a continuous lumen beginning at the mouth and ending at the anus (Fig. 17-1). The major functions of the GI tract are digestion of food and absorption of the fluids and nutrients that are required for energy and as building blocks for growth. Because its lumen is contiguous with the outside world, the GI tract contains bacteria and other toxins. Therefore, it also must provide a selective barrier that permits the absorption of nutrients but prevents penetration by bacteria the other toxins. In addition, luminal contents need to be pro-

pelled through the GI tract to allow effective digestion and absorption.

The basic architecture is similar in each portion of the GI tract, with each composed of four concentric layers from the internal lumen outward (Fig. 17-2). The *mucosal layer* consists of an *epithelial lining;* a loose connective tissue known as the *lamina propria* that contains a large number of immunocompetent cells, nerves, and blood vessels; and the *muscularis mucosae,* which is a thin, circularly oriented band of smooth muscle that separates the mucosal layer from the submucosal layer. The *submucosal layer* consists of supporting collagenous fibers, blood vessels, lymphatics, nerves, ganglia, and occasional lymphoid follicles. The *muscularis propria layer* consists of two bands of smooth muscle with an intervening layer of nerves and ganglia (ie, myenteric plexus). The thicker, inner "circular layer" of muscle is oriented concentrically around the bowel lumen so that contraction results in occlusion of the lumen, whereas the outer "longitudinal layer" foreshortens the bowel. The outer *adventitial layer* consists of loose connective tissue, fat, and collagen.

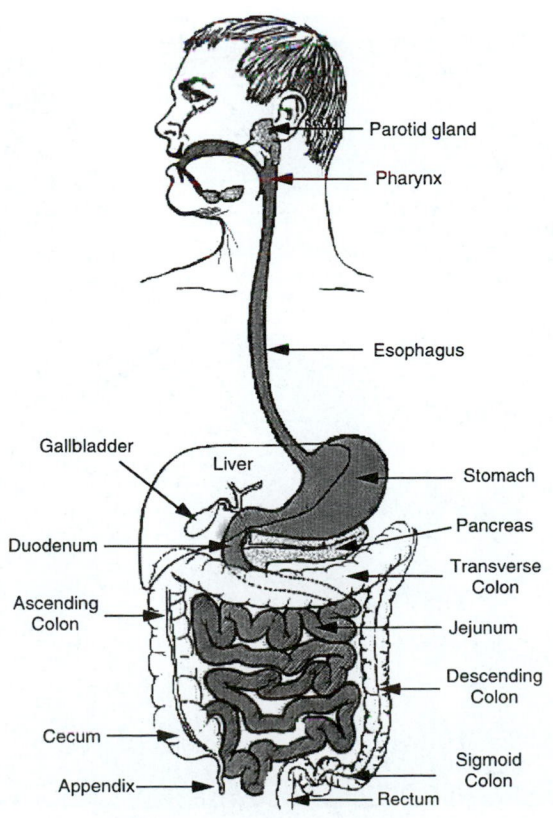

FIGURE 17-1   The gastrointestinal tract.

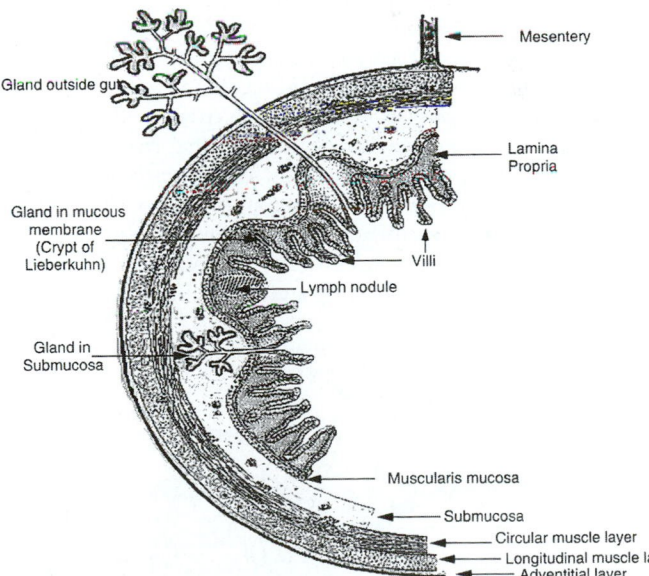

FIGURE 17-2   General organization of the gastrointestinal tract. The *mucosal layer* consists of an epithelial lining, the lamina propria, and the muscularis mucosae. The *submucosal layer* contains collagenous fibers, blood vessels, lymphatics, nerves, ganglia, and occasional lymphoid follicles. The *muscularis propria layer* consists of a circular and a longitudinal layer of smooth muscle. The outer connective tissue is the *adventitial layer.* Glands may extend into the lamina propria submucosa or outside the GI tract. SOURCE: *Harm AW, Cormack DH: Histology, 8th ed. Philadelphia, JB Lippincott, 1979.*

Invaginations of the epithelial layer form glands that may extend into the lamina propria (ie, mucosal glands), submucosa (ie, submucosal glands), or via ducts to organs outside the GI tract, including the salivary glands, liver, and pancreas. The specialized roles of each region in the GI tract largely are conferred by differences in mucosal structure and the regional expression of specific epithelial cell functions. Variations in the geometric arrangement of the muscle layers also may confer specialized contractile functions.

ESOPHAGUS

The esophagus is a tube that provides a conduit for the passage of food through the thorax to the stomach. The opening to the pharynx is closed except during swallowing; thus, air is not ingested into the GI tract during quiet respiration. Similarly, the opening into the stomach remains closed by the lower esophageal sphincter, which is a thickening of the muscularis propria situated at the diaphragm, thus preventing regurgitation of the acidic stomach contents and ingested food back into the esophagus. The mature mucosal lining of the esophagus is a simple structure that consists of nonkeratinized, stratified, squamous epithelium and submucosal glands that secrete mucins for lubrication and acid protection. The muscularis propria of the esophagus is composed of skeletal muscle fibers in the upper third and smooth muscle in the distal third. The blood supply comes from small branches of the aorta, the intercostal arteries, and esophageal branches of the left gastric artery. The veins accompany the arteries and create a connection between the portal and systemic venous circulations.

STOMACH

The stomach serves as a reservoir and mixer for ingested food. The major structural landmarks are shown in Fig. 17-3. The largest region of the stomach is the gastric *body*, which is characterized grossly by thick mucosal folds or rugae and lined by mucosa that consists of deep glands containing acid-secreting *parietal cells* and pepsinogen-secreting *chief* or *oxyntic cells.* Secreted acid serves as a barrier to bacterial colonization of the intestinal tract. Acid and pepsin initiate the digestion of proteins. Parietal cells also secrete intrinsic factor, which is necessary for the absorption of vitamin B_{12}. The gastric *antrum* is conical and extends from the incisura to the pylorus with a smooth (ie, nonrugose) mucosal surface. Antral glands largely are mucus producing and, in addition, contain spe-

cialized, slender, flask-shaped cells with slender processes extending to the luminal surface, known as *enterochromaffin cells,* that secrete hormones; the primary hormone secreted by the antrum is gastrin. The muscularis propria of the stomach consists of layers of spiral fibers that are oriented in three directions—an outer longitudinal, inner circular, and innermost oblique layer—that allow dramatic variation in stomach size and contractile patterns. The blood supply of the stomach comes from five arteries, all of which arise from the celiac axis and anastomose freely on the gastric surface. Venous return is through the portal venous system.

SMALL INTESTINE

The small intestine is the largest organ of the GI tract and is responsible for the bulk of its digestive and absorptive functions. The first portion, the *duodenum,* extends from the pylorus to the ligament of Treitz, forming a C-loop around the head of the pancreas. The common bile duct and pancreatic duct enter the duodenum at the papilla of Vater. The remainder of the small bowel is approximately 200 to 250 cm in length in the term newborn infant, and it reaches 350 to 600 cm in the adult. The proximal 40% is conventionally called the *jejunum,* and the remainder the *ileum.* There is no clear line dividing the two, but crescentic mucosal folds (ie, the valvulae conniventes) are more prominent and closely spaced in the jejunum, resulting in a feathery appearance on radiographic contrast examination compared with the ileum (Fig. 17-4). In addition, the vascular arcades through the mesentery differ in the proximal jejunum and distal ileum.

The small intestinal epithelium consists of an abundance of finger-like projections called *villi,* which increase the surface area for digestion and absorption (Fig. 17-2). At the base of the villi, in-

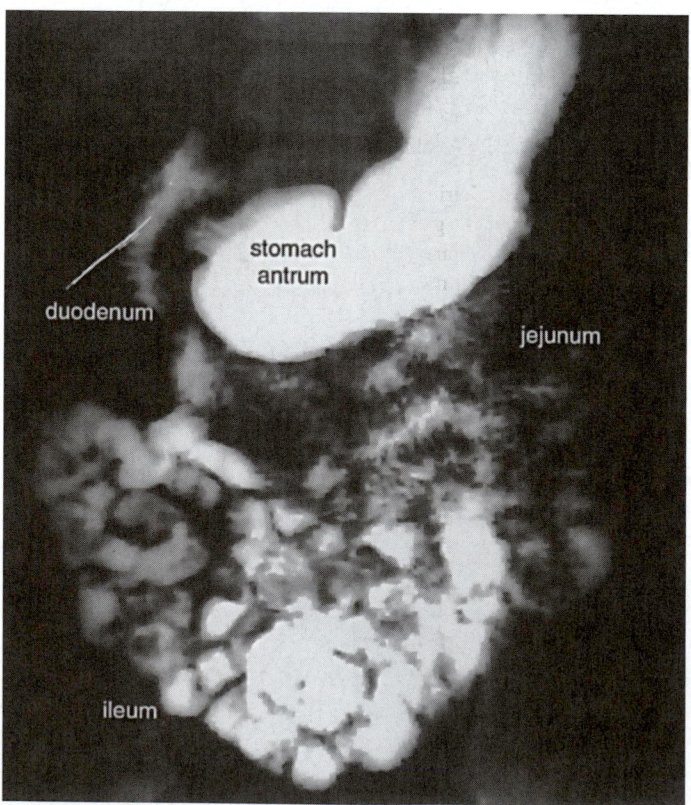

FIGURE 17-4 Radiograph of the stomach and small intestine showing different filling patterns of the jejunum and ileum.

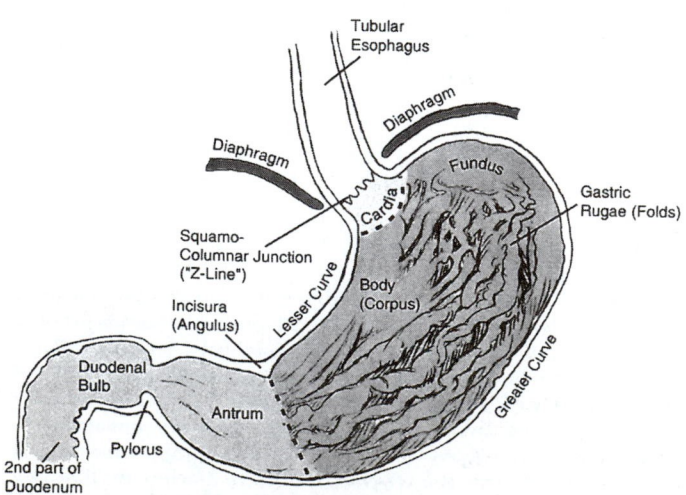

FIGURE 17-3 The anatomic regions of the stomach.

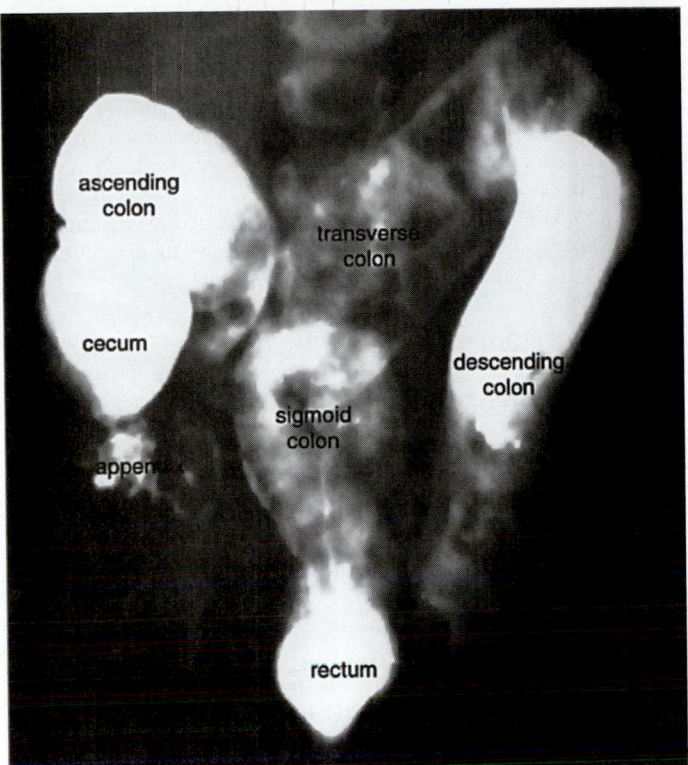

FIGURE 17-5   Radiograph of the large intestine showing major landmarks with redundancy of the sigmoid loop and transverse colon.

vaginations known as *crypts of Lieberkühn* extend to the muscularis mucosae. The villi are lined with columnar epithelial cells having a polarity of cellular membrane domains such that numerous digestive enzymes and transport proteins are located on the apical luminal surface while synthetic functions occur at the basolateral surface domain abutting the lamina propria. The villous epithelium is constantly sloughed, with new cells being generated in the crypts, so that the villous cells turn over every 7 days. Other cell types including enteroendocrine cells, immune sampling cells (ie, "M" cells), mucus-secreting goblet cells, and Paneth cells also line the epithelial surface. The lamina propria contains lymphatic vessels for fat digestion and small muscle fibers that contract, waving the villi in the gut lumen. In addition, a rich complement of lymphocytes and other immune cells are present in the lamina propria. Lymphoid aggregates penetrate through the muscularis mucosa from the submucosa. The size and number of lymphoid aggregates increase in the ileum, where they are known as *Peyer patches*. The duodenum is supplied with blood from the celiac and superior mesenteric arteries, and the remainder of the small bowel is supplied by only the superior mesenteric artery. Venous drainage is via the portal venous system.

LARGE INTESTINE

The large intestine recovers fluids and electrolytes from the gastrointestinal tract lumen before their loss in feces with undigestible materials. The major structural landmarks are shown in Fig. 17-5. The large intestine begins at the *cecum* with a narrow terminal extension called the *vermiform appendix,* and it includes the *ascending, transverse,* and *descending colons,* the *sigmoid,* and the *rectum,* ending at the anus. The epithelium consists of a smooth mucosal surface without villi but containing crescentic submucosal folds, the plicae semilunares, that project into the lumen. The epithelial lining contains polar columnar absorptive cells with microvilli on the luminal surface, which increase absorptive area. Mucosal glands (ie, crypts of Lieberkühn) have an abundance of mucus-producing goblet cells and rare endocrine cells. The lamina propria of the colon contains numerous immune cells, including macrophages and large lymphoid nodules that extend into the submucosa. The muscularis propria contains circular and longitudinal muscle layers throughout. The circular muscle is thickened adjacent to the anus, where it forms the internal anal sphincter. Three thick bundles of the longitudinal layer, known as *taeniae coli,* extend from the cecum to rectum. These bundles of muscle may shorten the colon during large bulk movements of luminal contents. The cecum as well as the ascending and proximal half of the transverse colon are supplied with blood from the superior mesenteric artery, and the remainder of the colon is supplied by the inferior mesenteric artery.

17.1.2   Embryology

The GI tract derives from an endodermal gut tube that is created by embryonic folding during the fourth week of gestation (Fig. 17-6). Animated diagrams of gastrointestinal development are available at *http://www.med.uc.edu/embryology/chapter9/animations/contents.htm.* The ectoderm and endoderm grow at different rates, which results in folding of the trilaminar germ disc to form an endoderm-lined tube internally, with ectoderm on the embryonic external surface. Mesoderm lies between the endoderm and ectoderm. The endoderm-lined tube closes completely to form the foregut and hindgut, which terminate at the buccopharyngeal membrane and cloacal membranes, respectively. The midgut portion of the tube remains open to the yolk sac until the sixth week of gestation, when the neck of the yolk sac is reduced to a slim stalk, the vitelline duct, which can persist into adult life as an outpouching of the ileum, also called a *Meckel diverticulum.*

The foregut gives rise to the pharynx, respiratory tract, esophagus, stomach, and proximal duodenum (Fig. 17-7). At approximately 3 weeks of gestation, the respiratory diverticulum or lung bud develops as a ventral outpouching of the foregut. The liver, gallbladder, and ventral pancreatic bud develop from an endodermal outgrowth appearing distal to the stomach, and the dorsal pan-

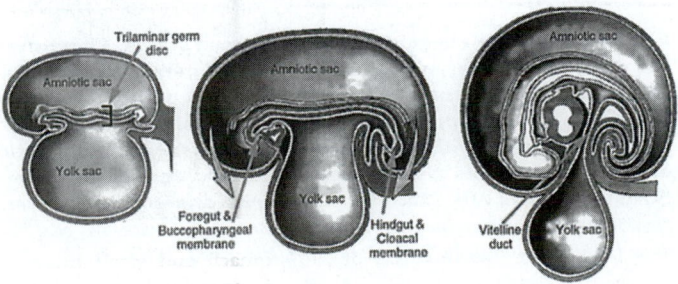

FIGURE 17-6   Process of embryonic folding during the fourth to sixth weeks of gestation. The trilaminar germ disc forms an endoderm-lined tube, which then forms the foregut and hindgut. The midgut remains open to the yolk sac until the neck is reduced to a slim stalk, the vitelline duct. SOURCE: *Larsen WJ: Human Embryology. New York, Churchill Livingstone, 1993.*

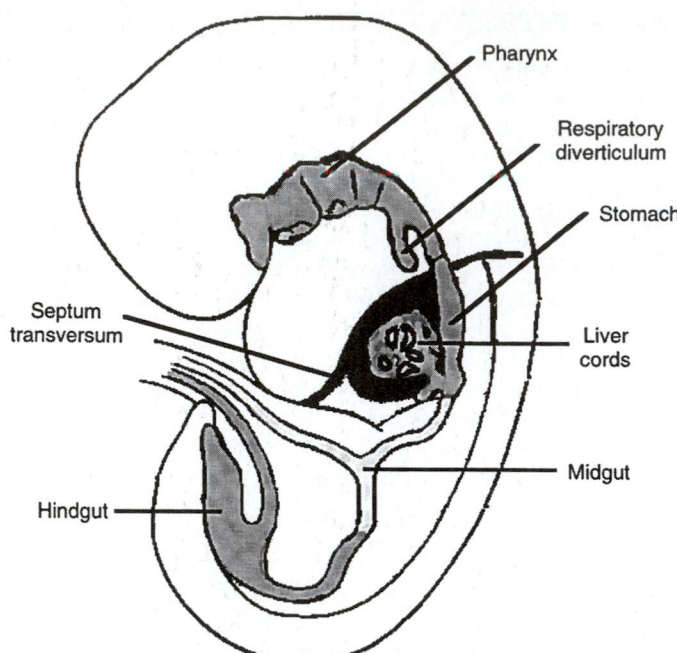

FIGURE 17-7   **The foregut (which gives rise to the pharynx, respiratory diverticulum, stomach, proximal duodenum, liver, gallbladder, and the pancreas), midgut, and hindgut in the human embryo at 4 weeks of gestation.** SOURCE: *Larsen WJ: Human Embryology. New York, Churchill Livingstone, 1993*

creatic bud arises from a different outgrowth. Rotation of the duodenum and migration of the ventral pancreatic bud result in the juxtaposition and ultimately fusion of the pancreatic buds to form a single pancreas and the unification of the pancreatic and bile ducts by the sixth week (Fig. 17-8). The distal half of the duodenum, jejunum, ileum, cecum, appendix, and proximal colon is derived from the midgut. The left one-third of the transverse colon, descending colon, and rectum is derived from hindgut.

As the gut elongates, a number of key morphologic events occur (Fig. 17-9). During the fifth week of embryonic development, the dorsal wall of the stomach grows faster than the ventral wall, expanding the stomach and forming the greater and lesser curvatures of the stomach. The stomach and liver rotate along a craniocaudal axis so that by the eighth week of gestation the greater curvature of the stomach lies to the left side and the liver to the right side of the abdominal cavity. There is insufficient space to accommodate the midgut inside the peritoneal cavity, and the gut expands into the extraembryonic coelom within the umbilical cord. During this herniation, the gut rotates 90° about the axis of the superior mesenteric artery, and on the return of the midgut to the peritoneal cavity, an additional 180° counterclockwise rotation occurs. The net result of this rotation is to position the cecum in the right lower quadrant of the peritoneal cavity by 11 weeks of gestation.

The cloaca is divided by the urogenital sinus and eventually separates into the urinary bladder and rectum, which fuses with the overlying ectoderm to form the anus. Between the fourth and sixth weeks, the lumen of the cloaca, which is derived from the end of the primitive hindgut, divides into the rectum posteriorly and the urogenital sinus anteriorly. The urogenital sinus gives rise to the bladder, urethra, and vestibule of the vagina. The rectum is contiguous with a depression in the ectoderm called the *anal pit;* this pit

breaks down to permit continuity between the endodermal lining of the rectum and the ectodermal lining of the anus.

While the gut tube lengthens, the endodermal lining proliferates, occluding the lumen by the sixth week of gestation. The maturation of mucosa proceeds in a proximal-to-distal direction as vacuoles form in the gut tube, so it is fully recanalized by week 9. Exocrine pancreatic and liver cells also arise from the endoderm. The origin of the pancreatic and gastrointestinal endocrine cells remains uncertain, but these cells probably derive from endoderm. The vasculature and muscle layers of the GI tract derive from mesoderm.

The genetic regulation of gastrointestinal development is beginning to be defined. Disruption of specific homeotic genes (*hox*) produces organ-specific gastrointestinal defects. For example, in mice disruption of the *hox c-4* gene results in esophageal obstruction, and disruption of the *hox c-8* gene causes abnormal gastric epithelial cell and muscle development. A recently identified gene expressed in epithelium of the duodenum, *pdx-1*, appears to play a crucial role in pancreatic development. A case of human congenital pancreatic agenesis was shown to result from a single nucleotide deletion in the *pdx-1* gene.

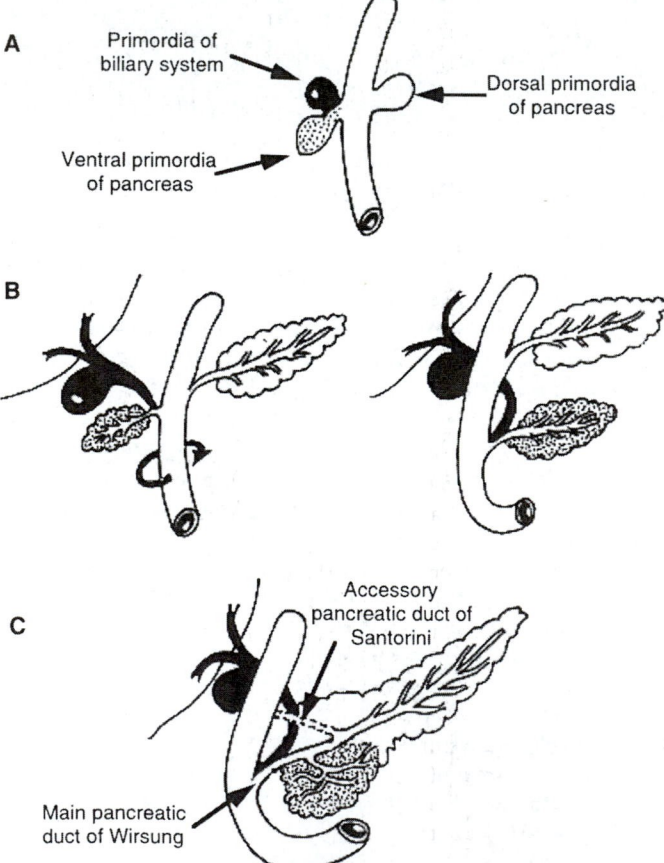

FIGURE 17-8   **A: The primordia of the biliary system. The ventral and dorsal pancreas primordia are endodermal outpouchings of the duodenum. B: The ventral pancreas rotates to a position posterior and distal to the dorsal pancreas. C: The ventral and dorsal pancreas fuse into one organ, with an anastomosis between the main pancreatic duct of Wirsung and the accessory pancreatic duct of Santorini.** SOURCE: *Hadorn HB, Much G: The exocrine pancreas: development, physiology and disease. In: Anderson CM, Burke V, Gracey M, eds: Pediatric Gastroenterology, 2nd ed. Oxford, Blackwell, 1987.*

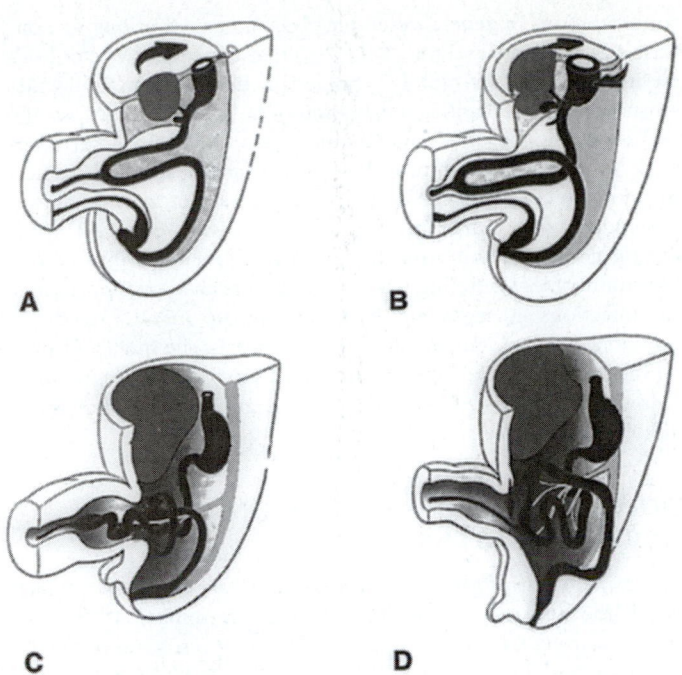

FIGURE 17-9   Elongation and rotation of the gastrointestinal tract during gestation. A: During week 5 of embryonic development, the stomach and liver rotate along a craniocaudal axis so that the greater curvature of the stomach lies to the left side and the liver to the right side of the abdominal cavity. B: By week 6, the midgut elongates and pushes into the extraembryonic coelom within the umbilical cord and then rotates 90°. C: On the return of the midgut to the peritoneal cavity at 10 to 12 weeks, an additional 180° counterclockwise rotation occurs. D: During week 11, the cecum descends to the right lower quadrant of the peritoneal cavity. SOURCE: *Larsen WJ: Human Embryology. New York. Churchill Livingstone, 1993.*

17.1.3   Neuromuscular Development and Structure

The muscle coat of the GI tract consists of the muscularis mucosa, an inner circular layer, and an outer longitudinal layer (Fig. 17-2). Layers of smooth muscle develop in the mesenchymal layer surrounding the bowel lumen in a craniocaudal pattern early during gestation, with the circular muscle layers being recognizable in the esophagus and stomach during week 5 of human gestation and in the ileum by 8 weeks. Longitudinal muscle layers are not present until 8 weeks and appear in the ileum by 10 weeks. The thickness of each muscle layer increases through gestation and after birth. The inner layer of circular muscle consists of a three- to eight-cell-thick specialized layer of fibroblasts and muscle cells containing numerous junctions between cells. This layer of *interstitial cells of Cajal* appears to generate the basic electrical rhythm, or slow waves, of the GI tract.

Neurocyte precursors migrate from the neural crest and appear in the fetal gut in a craniocaudal direction, being observed first in the stomach and duodenum at 7 weeks and reaching the rectum by 12 weeks. The congenital disorder of Hirschsprung disease results from a failure of migration by these neurocytes. The migration and maturation of enteric neural elements also is controlled by interactions between the neural crest cells and the intercellular matrix. Once the neurocytes enter the bowel, they undergo phenotypic development, with the complexity of the axonal and dendritic net-

works increasing through gestation and after birth. Neuronal intestinal dysplasias or congenital neuropathic pseudoobstruction syndromes may represent abnormalities of neurodifferentiation. The genetic mechanisms controlling the neurodevelopment of the bowel are beginning to be understood and are discussed in Sec. 17.23.3.

The enteric nervous system coordinates the spatial distribution of GI smooth muscle contractions. It consists of an intricate network of ganglia and plexuses that are capable of reflex control of GI muscle activity independent of the central nervous system (Fig. 17-10). This complex network of neural cells and fibers contains a large variety of neurotransmitters and neuromodulators similar to those that are found in the central nervous system. In addition to the intrinsic innervation, extrinsic innervation by the vagal nerve and splanchnic nerves modulates GI functions and transmits sensory information from the gut to the brain.

17.1.4   Normal Digestion and Absorption

Digestion begins with the mechanical process of lubrication and mastication in the mouth. Further mechanical grinding, mixing, lubrication, and enzymatic digestion in the stomach result in the controlled release of nutrient-containing liquid "chyme" into the lumen of the proximal small intestine. Bile and pancreatic enzymes are secreted into the intestinal lumen, where complex carbohydrates, proteins, and fats are cleaved to smaller component parts. Further digestion occurs on the mucosal surface before transport across the enterocyte into the portal bloodstream or lymph. The absorptive capacity of the small intestine normally is far in excess of needs, for 50% or more of the small intestine can be removed without deleterious effects. In diseases with inadequate digestion or diseases of the intestinal mucosa, however, the absorption of water, electrolytes, and nutrients can be so deficient as to endanger life.

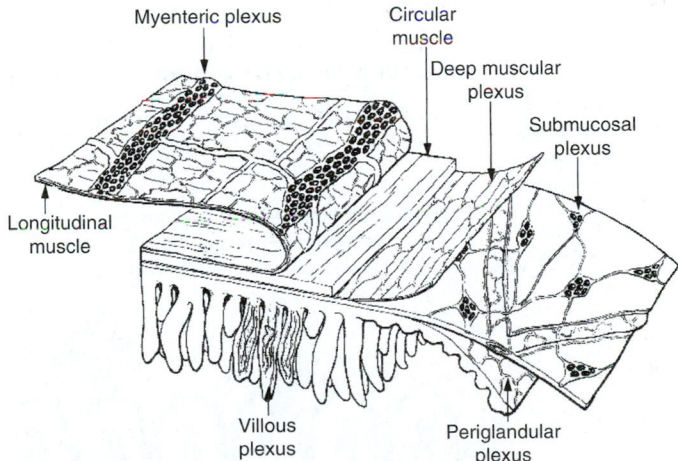

FIGURE 17-10   The enteric nervous system consists of the myenteric plexus and the submucosal plexus, which contain numerous neuronal cell ganglia. Other plexus layers consist primarily of nerve fibers extending between these nerve bodies and the muscle and the mucosal layers of the bowel wall. In addition, extrinsic nerve fibers that are supplied from the splanchnic nerves and vagus nerve enter all of these plexus layers. SOURCE: *Furness JB, Costa M: Distribution of intrinsic nerve cell bodies and axons which take up aromatic amines and their precursors in the small intestine of the guinea-pig. Cell Tissue Res 188: 527–543, 1978.*

ABSORPTION AND SECRETION OF ELECTROLYTES AND WATER

Following the ingestion of food, electrolyte- and enzyme-containing fluid is secreted into the gastrointestinal lumen. Nutrients are mechanically dispersed into this fluid, forming an emulsion in which chemical and enzymatic digestion proceeds. Most of the ingested and secreted fluid is reabsorbed before being excreted in stool (Fig. 17-11).

All water movement in the intestine is determined by osmotic gradients that are created by solute transport. The chyme that initially enters the small intestine from the stomach is typically not hyperosmotic, but as its macromolecular components are digested, the osmolarity increases dramatically, and water is pulled into the lumen. As the contents are absorbed, osmolarity decreases, and water can be absorbed. Active Na transport across the intestinal enterocyte is a two-step process that involves either channel-mediated or non-channel-mediated entry of Na into the enterocyte down an electrochemical gradient that is maintained by a basolaterally located sodium pump, the Na,K ATPase. In the small intestine, apical transporters include Na,Cl cotransporters (ie, Na,H and Cl,HCO$_3$ exchange) and nutrient carriers such as the Na,glucose (or galactose) transporter and Na,amino acid cotransporter. In the colon, Na loss is prevented by a volatile fatty acid–stimulated cotransport system and an aldosterone-sensitive Na transport mechanism that actively transport Na against a concentration gradient. The basolateral Na,K ATPase is present early during gestation in all polar epithelial cells. Expression is regulated by glucocorticoids and aldosterone. Nutrient transporters have similar ontogenic patterns, although specific regulatory elements and determinants may vary.

Secretion by the stomach, pancreas, biliary tree, and intestinal crypt cells is modulated by the active transport of electrolytes into the bowel lumen. Secretion is mediated by the electrogenic transport of Cl$^-$ or HCO$_3^-$ into the lumen. In the stomach, secretion also results from H$^+$ transport into the lumen. Na$^+$ and K$^+$ are passively transported into the small bowel lumen so that luminal concentrations in general resemble plasma concentrations. In contrast, Cl$^-$ is exchanged for HCO$_3^-$ so that concentrations of both are in the 60- to 70-mmol/L range. In the colon, an amiloride-sensitive sodium channel actively removes Na$^+$ and water, so the Na$^+$ content of stool falls to 30 mmol/L. In contrast, K$^+$ concentration increases to 75 mmol/L because of permeability characteristics of the colon and an active potassium secretory mechanism. The mucosa of the large intestine also can actively secrete Cl$^-$, producing net solute and water flow into the lumen. Various neurotransmitters, locally acting paracrine agents such as prostaglandins, and infectious agents such as bacterial enterotoxins alter the direction of net ion movement and water flow across the small and large intestine. In general, these agents act via intracellular second messengers, including cAMP, cGMP, Ca^{2+}, and inositol phosphate-diacyl glycerol.

DIGESTION AND ABSORPTION OF CARBOHYDRATES

The primary carbohydrate for breast-fed infants is lactose, which also is the principal carbohydrate in infant formulas. Other common dietary carbohydrates include fructose, sucrose, and glucose polymers (ie, glucose units linked by α-1,4 bond). More complex carbohydrates, which are termed *starch* or *amylopectins*, are characterized by having both α-1,4 and α-1,6 linkages. Nondigestible carbohydrates that comprise the structural component of plants constitute "dietary fiber." Fiber cannot be hydrolyzed by mammalian intestinal enzymes, but it is hydrolyzed in the colon by intestinal bacterial enzymes. The overall process of carbohydrate digestion begins with hydrolysis of soluble complex carbohydrates to monomeric form by luminal and brush border membrane enzymes. The monosaccharides, glucose, galactose, and fructose, are then transported across the enterocyte into the portal circulation by passive and active transport mechanisms. Abnormalities of carbohydrate absorption are discussed in Sec. 17.18.5.

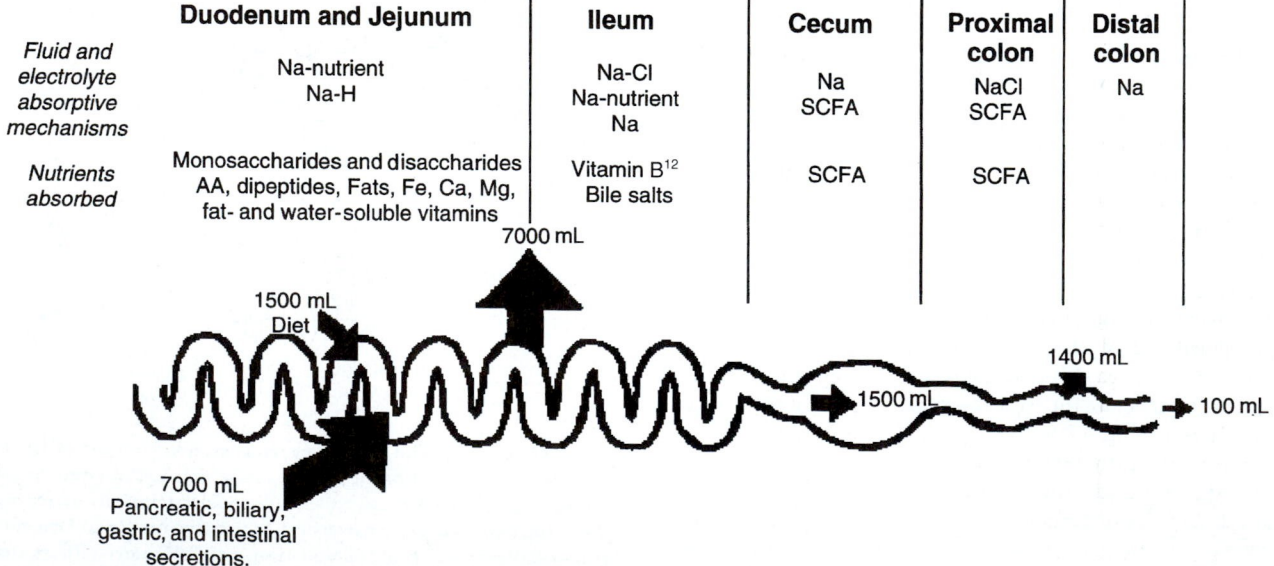

FIGURE 17-11 Overview of the intestinal fluid balance in the adult human gastrointestinal tract. Mechanisms of fluid and electrolyte absorption and the nutrients that are absorbed in various areas are listed by region. Chloride secretion is found throughout the intestine. AA-amino acids; SCFA-short-chain fatty acids. SOURCE: *Sellin JH: Intestinal electrolyte absorption and secretion. In: Sleisenger MH, Fordtran JS, eds: Gastrointestinal Disease. Philadelphia, WB Saunders, 1993:955.*

Starch is initially hydrolyzed intraluminally by salivary and pancreatic amylases to produce products that are suited for the brush border hydrolases. Both amylases have nearly identical structures, and both are potent endoglucosidases. They act at the internal α-1,4 bonds of amylose and amylopectin to produce some glucose but mainly trioses, disaccharides, and limit dextrins, which are then sequentially hydrolyzed by the brush border α-glucosidases: (1) glucoamylase, (2) isomaltase, and (3) sucrase. In the neonate, the quantitative contribution of salivary and pancreatic amylase to starch digestion is poorly defined. Salivary amylase secretion is present in the preterm infant by 34 weeks of gestation, but no pancreatic amylase secretion can be demonstrated until 4 to 6 months after birth, when starches normally are introduced into the infant diet. Salivary amylase is thought to be of minimal quantitative importance for carbohydrate digestion in the adult, but a more significant role has been postulated in the preterm infant.

The brush border enzyme glucoamylase hydrolyzes the products of amylase digestion. It has maximum activity for oligomers containing between five and nine glucose residues, and higher-molecular-weight compounds or complex carbohydrates with multiple branch points are less efficiently hydrolyzed. Glucoamylase is detectable by 20 weeks of gestation, and levels increase throughout gestation so that by 34 weeks activity is similar to that of older children. Developmental regulation and the role of diet on pancreatic amylase and intestinal hydrolase expression are now being investigated at a molecular level. Frank starch intolerance is relatively rare in infancy beyond the neonatal period.

Sucrase-isomaltase (ie, sucrase-dextrinase) is a major intestinal brush border enzyme that is first synthesized as a single-chained precursor containing active sites for sucrose and isomaltose hydrolysis. It then undergoes extensive intracellular modification before being incorporated into the brush border membrane, where it is rapidly cleaved by pancreatic proteases into the two subunits sucrase and isomaltase. Despite proteolytic cleavage, the subunits remain associated and fully active, being responsible for the hydrolysis of sucrose, isomaltose, and maltose. In the human infant, sucrase-specific activity is high by 20 weeks of gestation, being nearly equal to one-half to three-quarters the full-term infant and adult values.

Lactase is located within the microvillous membrane of the mature enterocytes at the villous tips, and it hydrolyzes lactose to glucose and galactose. Lactase-specific activity (ie, the rate of hydrolysis) is one-half to two-thirds that of the other disaccharidases, peaks at birth in term infants, and then declines to approximately 25% of term levels by 1 year of age. Low levels of lactase activity are present by 11 weeks of gestation and increase to 25% of term levels by 34 weeks. Despite the high levels of lactase activity in early infancy, the large quantities of lactose that are ingested daily (approximately, 10 to 14 g/kg) overwhelm the absorptive capacity of the small intestine, and a large amount of ingested lactose reaches the colon. Intestinal bacteria further digest the lactose to organic acids that are absorbed, salvaging nutrient calories for the infant. Thus, the rate-limiting step in lactose assimilation is hydrolysis by lactase. In contrast, the jejunal-specific activity of sucrase-isomaltase in full-term infants and adults is nearly twice that of lactase, and the rate-limiting step in the assimilation of other carbohydrates is monosaccharide absorption.

The final step in the assimilation of carbohydrates after luminal or brush border hydrolysis is absorption of the component monosaccharides. Glucose and galactose transport occur by two mechanisms: (1) simple, nonsaturable diffusion (if luminal concentration exceeds 3 mmol) and (2) active transport. The active transport mechanism is mediated at the brush border by an electrogenetic

Na^+-coupled glucose transporter, SGLT-1. The energy is provided by a Na,K ATPase localized to the basolateral membrane of the enterocyte. The facultative glucose transporter, GLUT-2, is located on the basolateral membrane. The glucose transporter is stereospecific for D-glucose and D-galactose. Active glucose transport can be demonstrated in vitro at 10 weeks of gestation, and the transporter is present throughout the entire intestine by 17 to 20 weeks of gestation, with activity increasing throughout gestation. Mutations of the SGLT-1 gene have been shown to cause glucose-galactose malabsorption, which can result in fatal diarrhea in newborn infants (see Sec. 17.18.5).

Fructose is transported either by facilitated diffusion or by a high-affinity glucose-dependent facultative transporter, GLUT-5, located on the apical membrane of the enterocyte. When large amounts of fructose are ingested without glucose, as in fruit juices, transport mechanisms may be overwhelmed, causing diarrhea.

DIGESTION AND ABSORPTION OF PROTEIN

Dietary proteins exhibit an enormous structural and biological diversity, requiring a surfeit of proteolytic enzymes and transport systems to ensure efficient digestion and absorption. As with carbohydrates, protein digestion is achieved through a series of coordinated hydrolytic steps, beginning with pepsin in the stomach and reaching completion in the intestine through the action of pancreatic proteases and peptidases. The final hydrolysis and absorption of the newly produced oligopeptides are then mediated by integral membrane hydrolases and amino acid transporters that are located within the microvillous membrane of the enterocyte.

Digestion of proteins is initiated in the stomach by the enzyme pepsin that is secreted by chief cells in concert with gastric acid production. The products of gastric digestion are large polypeptides and oligopeptides. Intraluminal proteolysis continues in the intestine and is mediated by endopeptidases and ectopeptidases that are secreted by the pancreas in precursor form. Enzyme activation requires the initial digestion of trypsinogen to trypsin by an enterokinase, a brush border enzyme. Trypsin then activates the other pancreatic enzymes. The endopeptidases act at the interior of the protein molecule to produce oligopeptides, usually of two to six amino acid residues in length, and the ectopeptidases act at the carboxyl-terminal end of the protein to remove a single amino acid. It is estimated that luminal protein digestion yields 70% oligopeptides and 30% amino acids. Peptides resulting from luminal hydrolysis are further hydrolyzed by brush border surface oligopeptidases.

Specific sodium-dependent carrier proteins of overlapping specificity actively transport amino acids into the cell. These carriers interact with all three classes of amino acids: (1) neutral, (2) acidic, and (3) basic. Other sodium-independent facilitated amino acid transport systems are present in the enterocyte on both the microvillous and basolateral membranes. In addition, proteins transport di- and tripeptides, which are further hydrolyzed by cytosolic enzymes before transport of the amino acids into the portal circulation.

The process of protein digestion and absorption is remarkably efficient, with over 95% of luminal protein being absorbed. The majority is absorbed in the duodenum and proximal jejunum; only relatively minor amounts ever reach the colon. Protein digestion and absorption are efficient even in preterm infants. Enterokinase appears relatively late in gestation (ie, 28 weeks) and reaches only 10% of adult levels by birth. In the pancreas, chymotryptic and tryptic activity have been demonstrated in vitro by 26 weeks of gestation, and a pancreatic response to secretagogues is functional at 30 weeks of gestation. The ontogeny of the brush border amino oligopeptidases as well as the dipeptide and amino acid transport systems parallel carbohydrate enzymes, although regulatory mechanisms differ. Amino-oligopeptidases are first detected immunohistochemically by 10 to 16 weeks of gestation. By 28 to 30 weeks of gestation, enzyme values are approximately one half the values that are found in term infants, so all aspects of intestinal proteolysis and transport are relatively intact, even in the preterm infant.

DIGESTION AND ABSORPTION OF FATS

Fats or lipids supply nearly 50% of the energy in human milk. The process of digestion and absorption of lipid can be divided into phases of intraluminal digestion, micellar solubilization, permeation from the lumen into the cell, reesterification in the cell, and chylomicron formation before transport out of the cell. Intraluminal digestion begins with the mechanical emulsification of the food in the mouth and the stomach. The emulsified fat is then hydrolyzed by lipase enzymes, forming fine droplets of β-monoglycerides and fatty acids.

Three major lipase enzymes are important for fat digestion. Acid-stable lipases are secreted by the body of the stomach and begin the process of fat digestion in the acid milieu of the stomach, being responsible for between 20 to 30% of the lipid digestion in infants. When nutrients enter the duodenum, mucosal hormones are released, which stimulate the pancreas to secrete pancreatic lipase and colipase. These enzymes are responsible for most fat hydrolysis in adults, being present in concentrations that are 1000-fold those required for adequate fat digestion. However, in the newborn infant (and particularly in premature infants), pancreatic secretion of lipase and bile-salt secretion are relatively inadequate, causing formula-fed infants to malabsorb 10 to 15% of dietary lipids. Breast-fed infants absorb significantly more lipid because of the presence of a unique lipase in breast milk that traverses the stomach and is then activated by bile salts in the small intestine. Breast-milk lipase may be responsible for up to two thirds of lipid hydrolysis in breast-fed infants.

The free fatty acids and monoglycerides that are produced in the intestinal lumen by lipolysis are readily solubilized into small particles, known as *micelles*, by detergent-like bile salts secreted from the liver. The micelle approaches the brush border surface of the enterocyte, and the fatty acids dissociate from the micelle and diffuse into the lipophilic cell membrane. A lack of adequate bile-salt secretion, as occurs in liver disease, results in malabsorption of fats because of inadequate solubilization. Intraluminal bile-salt concentrations are low in the newborn infant, but this does not appear to significantly limit lipid absorption.

Once the fatty acid enters the brush border luminal surface of the enterocyte, a protein with a high affinity for long-chain fatty acids, known as *fatty acid–binding protein*, transports long-chain fats to the smooth endoplasmic reticulum, where long-chain fatty acids are reesterified to form triglycerides. The resynthesized triglycerides, phospholipids, and various apoproteins form lipid-carrying particles called *chylomicrons*, which are transported through the basolateral membrane of the enterocyte and into the lymphatics. Lipoprotein synthesis and chylomicron formation are intact at birth and do not appear to limit nutrient lipid absorption postnatally in normal infants. (Specific defects in fat absorption resulting from abnormalities in the production of apoprotein B and in lym-

phatic function are discussed in Sec. 17.18.6). In contrast to long-chain fatty acids, medium-chain fatty acids are not bound by fatty acid–binding protein, and they are not reesterified before their uptake directly into the portal system. Thus, in certain disorders of fat absorption, the administration of medium-chain triglycerides provides an alternate source of energy.

17.1.5 Immunology

The GI tract is in continuity with the external environment and therefore exposed to a vast array of foreign antigens. The GI tract copes with this antigenic challenge both by creating a *barrier* that prevents antigens from crossing the epithelium and by controlling the systemic immune response to foreign antigens through a mechanism of *oral tolerance*. The GI tract wall contains a rich endowment of lymphoid tissues that are distributed diffusely through the lamina propria and in organized Peyer patches. Overlying the Peyer patches are specialized epithelia known as "M" (microfold) cells, which function in the uptake and sampling of luminal antigens. Antigens are taken up by M cells and transported into the Peyer patch, where they are processed and presented to T cells. Stimulated T and B cells migrate into the lymph and then pass into the peripheral circulation, where they "home" to the lamina propria of the gut and other exocrine tissues. The B cells mature into plasma cells and secrete IgA or IgM into the GI tract lumen.

A variety of nonimmunologic and immunologic mechanisms form a barrier to antigens and bacteria crossing the GI wall. Nonimmunologic mechanisms include the acid milieu of the stomach, proteolysis of antigens by pancreatic secretions, and peristalsis, which forces antigens and bacteria through the bowel. In addition, mucus on the epithelial surface inhibits the adhesion of bacteria and the attachment of antigens. Immunologic mechanisms that control infections resulting from extracellular organisms include antigen-independent immune responses such as polymorphonuclear leukocytes, monocytes, and complement, as well as cell- or antibody-mediated antigen-specific immune responses. Large amounts of secretory IgA, which is secreted into the intestinal lumen by the liver and intestinal mucosa, bind intraluminal microbes and antigens to inhibit their penetration across the mucosal barrier. The immune response is further enhanced through the release of cytokines, which recruit helper T cells and macrophages. Intracellular organisms such as viruses and mycobacteria are controlled by CD4 and CD8 T cells, aided by macrophages, that recognize and kill infected cells.

In the newborn, there are no reactive B-cell follicles in the Peyer patch, virtually no IgA-secreting cells in the lamina propria, and very few T cells in the gut epithelium. Within several weeks after birth, germinal centers appear, and by 3 months of age, IgA-secreting cells predominate in the lamina propria. The number of IgA-secreting cells and T cells increases with time, reaching adult numbers by 2 years of age. Despite these low cell numbers, it seems that the human mucosal immune system has all of the components to generate an immune response at birth.

Oral tolerance is an immunologic state of unresponsiveness induced by the prior feeding of an antigen and is a unique aspect of the immune system of the GI tract. Feeding of a soluble protein antigen can suppress the systemic IgM, IgG, and IgE antibody, cell-mediated immune responses to future exposures to the antigen. The selection of antigens for tolerance and the complex mechanisms involved in the development of oral tolerance have not been completely defined. However, this mechanism prevents hypersensitivity reactions to most soluble antigens that are contained in foods while maintaining active immunity to other antigens and invasive organisms. Failure to develop oral tolerance may be responsible for certain food allergies.

References

Carey MC, Hernell O: Digestion and absorption of fat. Semin Gastrointest Dis 3:189–208, 1992

Henning SJ: Functional development of the gastrointestinal tract. In: Johnson LR, ed: Physiology of the Gastrointestinal Tract, 2nd ed. New York, Raven Press, 1987:285–300

Larsen WJ: Human Embryology. New York, Churchill Livingstone, 1993

Montgomery RK, Mulberg AE, Grand RJ: Development of the human gastrointestinal tract: twenty years of progress. Gastroenterology 116: 702–731, 1999

Wershil BK: Gastrointestinal immunology. In: Gluckman PD, Heymann MA, eds: Perinatal and Pediatric Pathophysiology: A Clinical Perspective. London, Edward Arnold, 1993:414–417

17.2 NUTRITIONAL REQUIREMENTS

Neal S. LeLeiko and Miriam Horowitz

Every infant or child has a genetic potential for physical, mental, and emotional growth. Providing nutrition that fulfills all aspects of that growth potential represents optimal nutrition. When nutrition either limits growth or results in excessive body mass, either because of inadequate quality or inappropriate quantity, an individual is suffering from malnutrition (ie, undernutrition or obesity).

All published dietary requirements are guidelines that are designed to assure that most individuals will be well nourished. They are not meant to be rigidly followed by any specific individual. Precise adherence to these guidelines by any one person does not guarantee that individual will be well nourished.

17.2.1 Dietary Guidelines and the Basic Food Groups

In 1988, the first *Surgeon General's Report on Nutrition and Health* concluded that overconsumption of certain dietary components now is a major concern for Americans. The disproportionate consumption of foods that are high in fats, often at the expense of foods that are high in complex carbohydrates and fiber (eg, vegetables, fruits, and whole-grain products), increased the risk of diet-related diseases. The report reiterated the dietary guidelines issued jointly by the US Department of Agriculture (USDA) and the US Department of Health and Human Services. The recommendations of the guidelines, as revised in 1995, are summarized below.

- Eat a variety of foods
- Balance the food that you eat with physical activity
- Choose a diet with plenty of grain products, vegetables, and fruits
- Choose a diet low in fat, saturated fats, and cholesterol
- Choose a diet moderate in sugars
- Choose a diet moderate in salt and sodium

The USDA has defined a system of five basic food groups that, when combined appropriately, should provide the average American with his or her nutritional needs. These five groups are vegetables, fruits, grains (eg, breads, cereals, pastas), dairy products, and the protein group (eg, meat, poultry, fish eggs, nuts, legumes). Fats, oils, and sweets are separated, and it is recommended that they be "used sparingly."

To emphasize the concerns of the USDA regarding the importance of these dietary groups, the USDA published a "food pyramid" in 1992 as a guide to daily food choices. The pyramid emphasizes a diet based on complex carbohydrates, fruits, and vegetables. Dairy and protein serve a complementary role to assure the intake of all essential nutrients. The tip of the pyramid reinforces the need to consciously limit fats and concentrated sweets on a daily basis (Fig. 17-12). Furthermore, the pyramid illustrates the proper number of serving sizes required for most of the population.

In March 1999, the USDA released an additional food guide pyramid geared specifically to young children aged 2 to 6 years. This educational tool is part of an effort to teach children healthy eating habits from early childhood. A number of changes to the standard food guide pyramid have been made, including shortening the food group titles, depicting single serving sizes when possible, displaying the fats and sweets group on the tip of the pyramid, and stressing physical activity by showing young children engaged in exercise surrounding the pyramid. The depiction of specific foods is based on data collected through nationwide surveys. The most popular vegetables consumed included potatoes and tomatoes. Fruit juice was preferred to whole fruit. Cooked vegetables and green beans were consumed more often than green leafy vegetables. Therefore, the USDA decided to depict foods usually eaten as well as those less "popular" foods to encourage variety and an increase in fresh fruits and vegetables. Furthermore, low-fat (baked vs fried potato) and whole-grain choices are encouraged. Special attention is paid to serving sizes in an effort to guide parents in their pursuit of a properly balanced diet. Parents are instructed to provide younger children with three-fourths of the suggested serving sizes except for the milk group. Two servings of dairy are recommended for all children aged 2 to 6. However, included in the dairy group are ice cream, pudding, and cheese, which tend to be higher in fat and lower in calcium content than milk and yogurt. Therefore, special attention must be paid to the type of dairy foods eaten daily to ensure adequate daily calcium intake. Figures depicting both food pyramids and alternative food pyramids designed for vegetarian and different ethnic diets are available from the United States Department of Agriculture website: *http://www.nal.usda.gov/fnic/*.

17.2.2 Dietary Reference Intakes: the "New" Recommended Dietary Allowances

The Food and Nutrition Board (FNB) of the Institute of Medicine, National Academy of Science, has collaborated since 1992 to revise the Recommended Dietary Allowances (RDAs). In the past the RDAs, which were established for 25 nutrients in addition to energy, protein, and water, were defined as the levels of intake of essential nutrients that, on the basis of scientific knowledge, were judged to be adequate to meet the known nutrient needs of practically all healthy people. An essential nutrient is defined as a substance that must be provided by exogenous sources because it cannot be synthesized endogenously to meet the requirements of the organism. The RDAs were established with the intent to analyze and assure the adequacy of a population's intake. The FNB derived

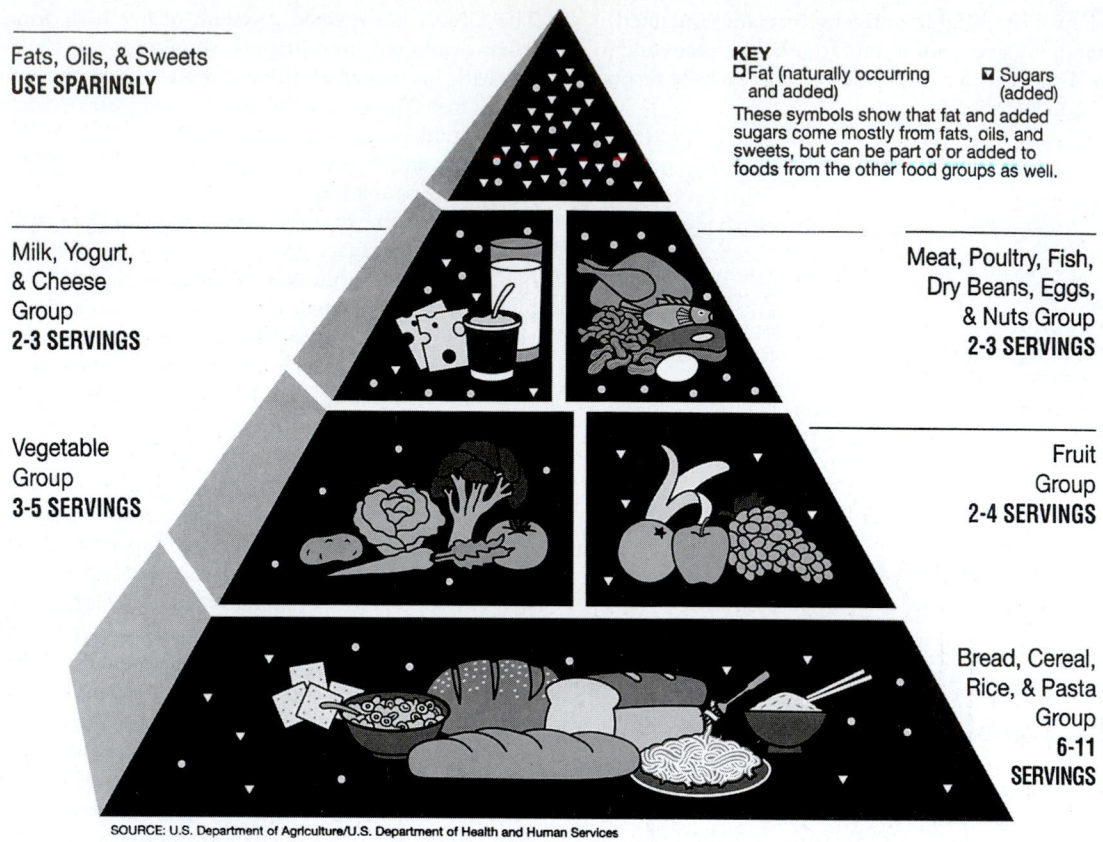

FIGURE 17-12   The food pyramid. SOURCE: *United States Department of Agriculture,* *http://www.nal.usda.gov/fnic.*

the data for the RDAs from the intakes of healthy populations. A "margin of safety" was created to include 97% of the population by adjusting upward two standard deviations from the mean on the normal distribution curve.

Following an explosion of nutrition-related scientific data, the FNB decided to replace the RDAs by *Dietary Reference Intakes* (DRIs), which broadened the focus of the FNB as well as guidelines for the United States and Canada. In addition to reviewing the current scientific literature and updating standards, the FNB took into consideration the multiple uses for which standards of intake can be applied. The DRIs were established to meet a variety of uses, those focused on the intake and adequacy of populations as well as individuals. The FNB investigated the connection between nutrient intake and the risk reduction for chronic disease. In addition, upper limits for nutrients were established, specifically addressing therapeutics and toxicities. The following are four categories that comprise the general heading of DRIs:

- **Estimated Average Requirements (EARs):** An estimated nutrient intake value that meets the requirement of half the healthy individuals in a group or population based on accepted scientific research. This level is set at the mean of the standard deviation curve. Proposed usage is to assess the adequacy of intakes of population groups. These values are utilized to establish the Recommended Dietary Allowances.
- **Recommended Dietary Allowances (RDAs):** The averaged daily dietary intake level that is sufficient to meet the nutrient requirements of virtually all (97–98%) healthy individuals in a group or population. These levels were developed based on the average requirements of a population with an adjusted factor to

cover for variability of individuals. An RDA can be set only if the Estimated Average Requirement (EAR) is known.
- **Adequate Intakes (AIs):** If the EAR is not known because of inadequate data, the RDA cannot be set. In that case an Adequate Intake (AI) is estimated. The AI is a recommended daily intake based on scientific observation or approximations of nutrient intakes of healthy group(s). The AIs are levels in which deficiency has not been observed. The AIs are to be applied to individual intake as well as to groups.
- **Tolerable Upper Limits (ULs):** The highest level of daily nutrient intake found to pose no risks of adverse effects in individuals of a healthy population. The risk of adverse effects and toxicities increases with an increase in consumption above these limits. The UL is used to guide and limit intake as well as to examine the possibility of overconsumption for the individual.

The safe range of intake is the area between the RDA and the UL. This is the area where deficiency and toxicity for the individual are most likely not to occur (Fig. 17-13). At the time of this writing, recommendations for Dietary Reference Intakes of calcium, vitamin D, phosphorus, magnesium, flouride, folate, vitamin B_{12}, and other B vitamins and choline are completed (Tables 17-1 through 17-3). Recommendations for dietary antioxidants and related compounds, trace elements, electrolytes, energy, and macronutrients and other food components are in the process of being developed and are expected to be published over the next several years.

An important distinction between the new AIs and the RDAs should be noted. The AIs do not provide the same "margin of safety" that the RDAs do for other nutrients. Therefore, these levels are only an approximation of daily dietary intake observed for

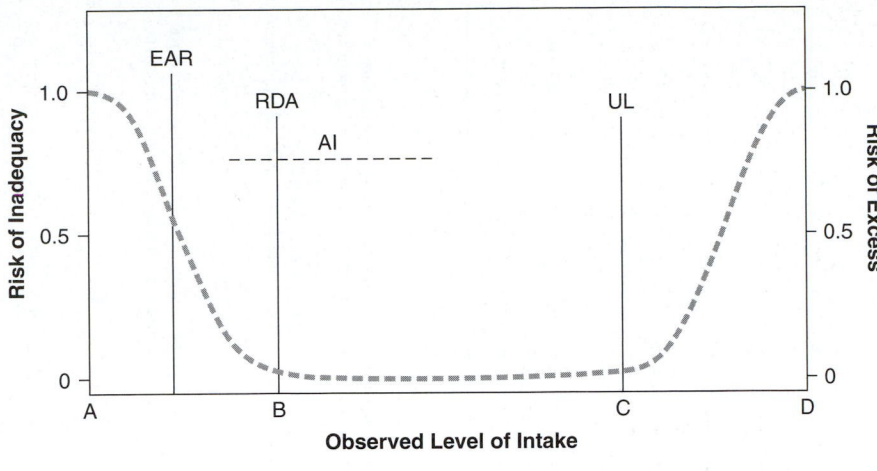

FIGURE 17-13 This figure shows that the Estimated Average Requirement (EAR) is the intake at which the risk of inadequacy is 0.5 (50%). The Recommended Dietary Allowance (RDA) is the intake at which the risk of inadequacy is very small—only 0.02 to 0.03 (2-3%). The Adequate Intake (AI) does not bear a consistent relationship to the EAR or the RDA because it is set without the ability to estimate the requirement. At intakes between the RDA and the Tolerable Upper Intake Level (UL), the risks of inadequacy and of adverse effects are both close to zero. A *dashed line* is used for AI because the actual shape of the curve has not been determined experimentally. The distances between points *A* and *B*, *B* and *C*, and *C* and *D* may differ more than is depicted in this figure. Thus, the AI may be greater or less than the RDA, if it were known. SOURCE: *Food and Nutrition Board, Institute of Medicine.*

healthy individuals. For example, despite the limited understanding of the relationship between adequate calcium intake and the risk of osteoporosis, an AI for calcium has been established. It can be inferred that inadequate scientific data exist to provide recommended daily intakes for calcium that would meet 97% of the healthy population. Furthermore, the guidelines for infants for many nutrients are AIs as well. These values are based on observations of breast-fed babies. For this population, because of limitations of reliable experimental data, the healthy breast-fed baby serves as the paradigm for adequate nutrient intake to support normal growth and development.

In addition to the nutrients found naturally in foods, the FNB took into consideration nutrients obtained from other sources, including fortification and supplementation. This is particularly true for folic acid because the bioavailability of folic acid derived from supplementation is greater than that from fortification, which is greater than that of folate ingested in folate-containing foods. Therefore, a separate measure of dietary folate equivalent (DFE) has been developed.

The above dietary guidelines are meant for healthy groups and individuals. They cannot be applied to individuals with acute or chronic disease without significant adjustment. For the ill patient, the required amounts of nutrients vary from individual to individual as a result of malabsorption, increased use, or a need to replenish decreased stores.

17.2.3   Specific Nutritional Requirements

It is useful to partition nutrients into eight major categories: (1) water, (2) energy, (3) proteins, (4) carbohydrates, (5) fats, (6) vitamins, (7) major minerals, and (8) trace elements. Each category is discussed in the context of the requirements in healthy children and considerations regarding changing requirements during illness.

WATER

Water comprises approximately 50 to 60% of body weight in young adults and 70 to 75% of body weight in infants. Total body water, expressed as a percentage of body weight, is a function of age, sex, and body composition. Total body water decreases with age and changes in body fat content. Water and electrolyte balance are exquisitely controlled, as discussed in greater detail in Sec. 21.4.

Providing adequate amounts of nutrients without adequate amounts of fluid will result in dehydration, excessive renal solute load, and inefficient use and wasting of calories. An individual's requirement for water is determined by total water losses. Water losses reflect sensible and insensible losses, renal concentrating ability, and total nutrient and water intake. Infants are especially susceptible to dehydration; their requirement for water is much greater because of insensible losses from their large surface area. They also have a higher percentage of body water, their kidneys have a limited capacity for handling solute load, they have an impaired capacity to concentrate their urine, and they are unable to consistently communicate their thirst.

In addition to the actual water in foods and liquids, oxidation of ingested foodstuffs produces water as an end product, known as metabolic water. Oxidation of 100 g of fat, carbohydrate, and protein yields 107, 55, and 41 g of water, respectively. A mixed diet produces approximately 12 mL of water per 100 calories ingested. An individual's water requirement is highly variable and quite complex. An RDA for water does not currently exist; however, a DRI is expected to be determined by the Food and Nutrition Board in the near future. Table 17-4 provides a useful method for estimating maintenance fluid requirements. Additional water must be provided when losses occur because of diarrhea, renal disease, cardiopulmonary compromise, fever, or catabolic stress.

For infants, breast milk or infant formula provides the majority of fluid requirements. Human milk and commercial formulas of standard energy density (ie, 20 kcal/oz or 0.66 kcal/mL) consist of approximately 89% water. Additional water that is produced from the oxidation of the ingested milk results in approximately 95% of the volume consumed being available as free water. In preparation of infant formula, the concentration of solutes that require excretion by the kidney must be considered. This *renal solute load* includes primarily urea formed from protein catabolism and electrolytes. The *potential renal solute load* (PRSL) in infancy is calculated as:

$$PRSL = N/28 + Na + Cl + K + P_a$$

where the units are in millimoles (or milliosmoles) except for N, which is total nitrogen in milligrams, and the term N/28 represents nitrogenous solutes. Na is sodium, Cl is chloride, K is potassium, and P_a is available phosphorus (which is assumed to be total phos-

TABLE 17-1

DIETARY REFERENCE INTAKES: RECOMMENDED INTAKES FOR INDIVIDUALS

LIFE-STAGE GROUP	CALCIUM (mg/d)	PHOSPHORUS (mg/d)	MAGNESIUM (mg/d)	VITAMIN D (μg/d)[a,b]	FLUORIDE (mg/d)	THIAMIN (mg/d)	RIBOFLAVIN (mg/d)	NIACIN (mg/d)[c]	VITAMIN B_6 (mg/d)	FOLATE (μg/d)[d]	VITAMIN B_{12} (μg/d)	PANTOTHENIC ACID (mg/d)	BIOTIN (μg/d)	CHOLINE[e] (mg/d)
Infants														
0–6 mo	210*	100*	30*	5*	0.01*	0.2*	0.3*	2*	0.1*	65*	0.4*	1.7*	5*	125*
7–12 mo	270*	275*	75*	5*	0.5*	0.3*	0.4*	4*	0.3*	80*	0.5*	1.8*	6*	150*
Children														
1–3 y	500*	460	80	5*	0.7*	0.5	0.5	6	0.5	150	0.9	2*	8*	200*
4–8 y	800*	500	130	5*	1*	0.6	0.6	8	0.6	200	1.2	3*	12*	250*
Male														
9–13 y	1300*	1250	240	5*	2*	0.9	0.9	12	1.0	300	1.8	4*	20*	375*
14–18 y	1300*	1250	410	5*	3*	1.2	1.3	16	1.3	400	2.4	5*	25*	550*
19–30 y	1000*	700	400	5*	4*	1.2	1.3	16	1.3	400	2.4	5*	30*	550*
31–50 y	1000*	700	420	5*	4*	1.2	1.3	16	1.3	400	2.4	5*	30*	550*
51–70 y	1200*	700	420	10*	4*	1.2	1.3	16	1.7	400	2.4[f]	5*	30*	550*
>70 y	1200*	700	420	15*	4*	1.2	1.3	16	1.7	400	2.4[f]	5*	30*	550*
Female														
9–13 y	1300*	1250	240	5*	2*	0.9	0.9	12	1.0	300	1.8	4*	20*	375*
14–18 y	1300*	1250	360	5*	3*	1.0	1.0	14	1.2	400[g]	2.4	5*	25*	400*
19–30 y	1000*	700	310	5*	3*	1.1	1.1	14	1.3	400[g]	2.4	5*	30*	425*
31–50 y	1000*	700	320	5*	3*	1.1	1.1	14	1.3	400[g]	2.4	5*	30*	425*
51–70 y	1200*	700	320	10*	3*	1.1	1.1	14	1.5	400	2.4[f]	5*	30*	425*
>70 y	1200*	700	320	15*	3*	1.1	1.1	14	1.5	400	2.4[f]	5*	30*	425*
Pregnancy														
≤18 y	1300*	1250	400	5*	3*	1.4	1.4	18	1.9	600[h]	2.6	6*	30*	450*
19–30 y	1000*	700	350	5*	3*	1.4	1.4	18	1.9	600[h]	2.6	6*	30*	450*
31–50 y	1000*	700	360	5*	3*	1.4	1.4	18	1.9	600[h]	2.6	6*	30*	450*
Lactation														
≤18 y	1300*	1250	360	5*	3*	1.5	1.6	17	2.0	500	2.8	7*	35*	550*
19–30 y	1000*	700	310	5*	3*	1.5	1.6	17	2.0	500	2.8	7*	35*	550*
31–50 y	1000*	700	320	5*	3*	1.5	1.6	17	2.0	500	2.8	7*	35*	550*

[a] As cholecalciferol. 1 μg cholecalciferol = 40 IU vitamin D.

[b] In the absence of adequate exposure to sunlight.

[c] As niacin equivalents (NEs). 1 mg of niacin = 60 mg of tryptophan; 0 to 6 months = preformed niacin (not NE).

[d] As dietary folate equivalents (DFEs). 1 DFE = 1 μg food folate = 0.6 μg of folic acid (from fortified food or supplement) consumed with food = 0.5 μg of synthetic (supplemental) folic acid taken on an empty stomach.

[e] Although AIs have been set for choline, there are few data to assess whether a dietary supply of choline is needed at all stages of the life cycle, and it may be that the choline requirement can be met by endogenous synthesis at some of these stages.

[f] Because 10 to 30% of older people may malabsorb food-bound B_{12}, it is advisable for those older than 50 years to meet their RDA mainly by consuming foods fortified with B_{12} or a supplement containing B_{12}.

[g] In view of evidence linking folate intake with neural tube defects in the fetus, it is recommended that all women capable of becoming pregnant consume 400 μg of synthetic folic acid from fortified foods and/or supplements in addition to intake of food folate from a varied diet.

[h] It is assumed that women will continue consuming 400 μg of folic acid until their pregnancy is confirmed and they enter prenatal care, which ordinarily occurs after the end of the periconceptional period— the critical time for formation of the neural tube.

NOTE: This table presents Recommended Dietary Allowances (RDAs) in bold type and Adequate Intakes (AIs) in ordinary type followed by an asterisk (*). RDAs and AIs may both be used as goals for individual intake. RDAs are set to meet the needs of almost all (97-98%) individuals in a group. For healthy breast-fed infants, the AI is the mean intake. The AI for other life-stage and gender groups is believed to cover needs of all individuals in the group, but lack of data or uncertainty in the data prevent being able to specify with confidence the percentage of individuals covered by this intake.

SOURCE: *The Food & Nutrition Board, Institute of Medicine, National Academy of Sciences. © Copyright 1998 by the National Academy of Sciences. All rights reserved.*

TABLE 17-2

DIETARY REFERENCE INTAKES: ESTIMATED AVERAGE REQUIREMENTS

LIFE-STAGE GROUP	PHOSPHORUS (mg/d)	MAGNESIUM (mg/d)	THIAMIN (mg/d)	RIBOFLAVIN (mg/d)	NIACIN (mg/d)[a]	VITAMIN B$_6$ (mg/d)	FOLATE (μg/d)[b]	VITAMIN B$_{12}$ (μg/d)
Children								
1–3 y	380	65	0.4	0.4	5	0.4	120	0.7
4–8 y	405	110	0.5	0.5	6	0.5	160	1.0
Male								
9–13 y	1055	200	0.7	0.8	9	0.8	250	1.5
14–18 y	1055	340	1.0	1.1	12	1.1	330	2.0
19–30 y	580	330	1.0	1.1	12	1.1	320	2.0
31–50 y	580	350	1.0	1.1	12	1.1	320	2.0
51–70 y	580	350	1.0	1.1	12	1.4	320	2.0
>70 y	580	350	1.0	1.1	12	1.4	320	2.0
Female								
9–13 y	1055	200	0.7	0.8	9	0.8	250	1.5
14–18 y	1055	300	0.9	0.9	11	1.0	330	2.0
19–30 y	580	255	0.9	0.9	11	1.1	320	2.0
31–50 y	580	265	0.9	0.9	11	1.1	320	2.0
51–70 y	580	265	0.9	0.9	11	1.3	320	2.0
>70 y	580	265	0.9	0.9	11	1.3	320	2.0
Pregnancy								
≤ 18 yr	1055	335	1.2	1.2	14	1.6	520	2.2
19–30 y	580	290	1.2	1.2	14	1.6	520	2.2
31–50 y	580	300	1.2	1.2	14	1.6	520	2.2
Lactation								
≤ 18 yr	1055	300	1.2	1.3	13	1.7	450	2.4
19–30 y	580	255	1.2	1.3	13	1.7	450	2.4
31–50 y	580	265	1.2	1.3	13	1.7	450	2.4

[a] As niacin equivalents (NEs). 1 mg of niacin = 60 mg of tryptophan; 0 to 6 months = preformed niacin (not NE).

[b] As dietary folate equivalents (DFEs). 1 DFE = 1 μg food folate = 0.6 μg of folic acid (from fortified food or supplement) consumed with food = 0.5 μg of synthetic (supplemental) folic acid taken on an empty stomach.

NOTE: This table presents Estimated Average Requirements (EARs), which serve two purposes: for assessing adequacy of population intakes and as the basis for calculating Recommended Dietary Allowances (RDAs) for individuals for those nutrients. EARs have not been established for calcium, vitamin D, fluoride, pantothenic acid, biotin, or choline, or other nutrients not yet evaluated via the Dietary Reference Intake (DRI) process. For nutrients without EARs, RDAs were not calculated. Instead, Adequate Intakes (AIs) are given. Both RDAs and AIs are designed to be used as goals for individual intake. For infants, as it is not possible to estimate average requirements, AIs are given. In this case, the AI is the mean intake observed in healthy infants fed human milk and thus must be corrected for lower levels of bioavailability of the nutrient when the nutrient is obtained from other milk or food sources.

SOURCE: *The Food & Nutrition Board, Institute of Medicine, National Academy of Sciences. © Copyright 1998 by the National Academy of Sciences. All rights reserved.*

phorus of milk-based formulas and two-thirds of the phosphorus of soy-based formula). To convert milligrams to millimoles, divide Na by 23, Cl by 35, K by 39, and P by 31.

The PRSL of commercially available milk-based formulas is about 135 mOsm/L (20 mOsm/100 kcal), and of soy protein–based formula about 160 mOsm/L (24 mOsm/100 kcal). In contrast, whole cow's milk is 308 mOsm/L (46 mOsm/100 kcal), and skim milk is 326 mOsm/L (93 mOsm/100 kcal). The use of formula with a PRSL of greater than mOsm/100 kcal places the infant at increased risk for hypertonic dehydration, whereas formulas providing 20 to 26 mOsm/100 kcal offer a margin of safety with respect to water balance and are therefore recommended. Concentrated formulas are often indicated for infants who require fluid restrictions for cardiac, pulmonary, or renal indications as well as those who have insufficient volume intake resulting in inadequate caloric intake. Formula can often be safely concentrated to 24 kcal/oz, via adding more powder/concentrate and less water, but careful attention must be paid to fluid status and hydration of the infant, particularly during times of illness with decreased fluid intake or increased losses. If higher-caloric-density formula is desired, carbohydrate or fat supplementation without additional protein or electrolyte being added to the formula is desirable.

ENERGY

Energy is required to carry out the biochemical processes of life and to perform physical work. The energy that is provided by foods is chemical energy obtained after digestion. The unit of measure for energy is either the joule or the calorie (1 joule = 4200 cal). The kilocalorie (C) is equal to 1000 calories, or the amount of heat energy that is required to raise 1 kg of water by 1°C. Energy from foods that are consumed in a child's diet derives from carbohydrate (4 kcal/g), fat (9 kcal/g), and protein (4 kcal/g). In adults (and some adolescents), calories from ethanol (7 kcal/g) also may be a contributing source of energy.

The World Health Organization defines the energy requirements of an individual as the level of energy intake from food that will balance energy expenditure when the individual has a body size and composition and level of physical activity consistent with long-term good health and that will allow for the maintenance of economically necessary and socially desirable physical activity. In children and pregnant or lactating women, the energy requirement also includes the energy needs associated with the deposition of tissues or secretion of milk.

Energy requirements are highly individualized and vary widely among healthy persons. In states of disease and activity, energy

TABLE 17-3

DIETARY REFERENCE INTAKES: TOLERABLE UPPER INTAKE LEVELS (UL[a])

LIFE STAGE GROUP	CALCIUM (g/d)	PHOS- PHORUS (g/d)	MAGNESIUM (mg/d)[b]	VITAMIN D (μg/d)	FLOURIDE (mg/d)	NIACIN (mg/d)[c]	VITAMIN B$_6$ (mg/d)	FOLATE (μg/d)[c]	CHOLINE (g/d)
Infants									
0–6 mo	ND	ND	ND	25	0.7	ND	ND	ND	ND
7–12 mo	ND	ND	ND	25	0.9	ND	ND	ND	ND
Children									
1–3 y	2.5	3	65	50	1.3	10	30	300	1.0
4–8 y	2.5	3	110	50	2.2	15	40	400	1.0
Male, female									
9–13 y	2.5	4	350	50	10	20	60	600	2.0
14–18 y	2.5	4	350	50	10	30	80	800	3.0
19–70 y	2.5	4	350	50	10	35	100	1000	3.5
>70 y	2.5	3	350	50	10	35	100	1000	3.5
Pregnancy									
≤18 y	2.5	3.5	350	50	10	30	80	800	3.0
19–50 y	2.5	3.5	350	50	10	35	100	1000	3.5
Lactation									
≤18 y	2.5	4	350	50	10	30	80	800	3.0
19–50 y	2.5	4	350	50	10	35	100	1000	3.5

[a] UL = The maximum level of daily nutrient intake that is likely to pose no risk of adverse effects. Unless otherwise specified, the UL represents total intake from food, water, and supplements. Because of lack of suitable data, ULs could not be established for thiamin, riboflavin, vitamin B$_{12}$, pantothenic acid, or biotin. In the absence of ULs, extra caution may be warranted in consuming levels above recommended intakes.

[b] The ULs for magnesium represent intake from a pharmacological agent only and do not include intake from food and water.

[c] The ULs for niacin and folate apply to synthetic forms obtained from supplements, fortified foods, or a combination of the two.

ND = Not determinable because of lack of data on adverse effects in this age group and concern with regard to lack of ability to handle excess amounts. Source of intake should be from food only to prevent high levels of intake.

SOURCE: *The Food & Nutrition Board, Institute of Medicine, National Academy of Sciences.*

TABLE 17-4

ESTIMATION OF THE DAILY MAINTENANCE FLUID REQUIREMENTS FOR INFANTS AND CHILDREN

1–10 kg	100 mL/kg
11–20 kg	100 mL plus an additional 50 mL for each kg over 10
21+ kg	1500 mL plus an additional 20 mL for each kg over 20

requirements must be further adjusted to account for additional stresses. In most clinical situations, energy requirements for children are estimated from age, with the assumption of a similarity regarding body size, physical activity, and rate of growth. Provided one recognizes that recommendations for energy requirements are based on assumptions of size and activity, the energy needs of the healthy individual may be estimated from the guidelines provided in the RDAs as listed in Table 17-5. Note that, at the time of this review, DRIs and anticipated new RDAs for energy have not been

TABLE 17-5

MEDIAN HEIGHTS, WEIGHTS, AND RECOMMENDED ENERGY INTAKES

CATEGORY	AGE (y)	WEIGHT (kg)	HEIGHT (cm)	AVERAGE ENERGY ALLOWANCE (kcal)[a] PER KILOGRAM	PER DAY
Infants	0.0–0.5	6	60	108	650
	0.5–1.0	9	71	98	850
Children	1–3	13	90	102	1300
	4–6	20	112	90	1800
	7–10	28	132	70	2000
Males	11–14	45	157	55	2500
	15–18	66	176	45	3000
Females	11–14	46	157	47	2200
	15–18	55	163	40	2200

[a] In the range of light to moderate activity, the coefficient of variation is ± 20%.

established. Therefore, the following discussion refers to the RDAs as they exist before the development of the DRIs.

For infants, the RDA recommends a mean of 108 kcal/kg/d up to 6 months of age, with 98 kcal/kg/d for infants 6 to 12 months of age. Although these numbers are based on studies of "normal intake," actual energy intakes vary widely in this range. Some researchers report intakes for healthy infants that averaged 107 kcal/kg/d at 1 month of age but that declined to only 85 kcal/kg/d by 6 months. Others report a range of 52 to 152 kcal/kg/d consumed by a group of infants studied at 3-month intervals, with total average intakes declining with age. These studies merely emphasize that RDA values provide only an estimate of caloric needs. Beyond 10 years of age, the recommended energy needs of boys and girls differ, both because of the onset of puberty and evolving activity patterns. Variability in the timing and intensity of the pubertal growth spurt as well as activity lead to substantial variation in the energy requirements of individual adolescents.

For the well-nourished, growing child, simple application of the RDAs may be sufficient as a screening evaluation of caloric adequacy. However, the RDAs are not an adequate tool for determining the energy needs of sick or malnourished children. In these instances, more precise, individualized calculations are necessary to assess a child's energy needs. For example, requirements may be significantly less than the predicted RDA values in a physically disabled or partially paralyzed child. A child with chronic illness such as cardiac disease, cystic fibrosis, spastic quadriparesis, or asthma may have daily calorie requirements substantially above the RDA. Table 17-6 shows activity and injury factors that are designed to help estimate the increase in energy requirements with various types of injury. Although these values have not been validated in pediatric patients, they have been used in the pediatric clinical setting to account for the observed differences in energy needs during illness and stress. The most reliable indicators of caloric adequacy in the sick child, however, are measurements of appropriate weight gain or loss, height, or skinfold thickness over time.

If caloric intake is consistently above or below one's actual energy requirement, a net change in body energy stores can be expected. It is important to recognize that the cumulative effect of very small changes in energy intake over a prolonged period of time can result in significant deviation from normal body composition. For example, a deviation of 150 calories in daily intake (equivalent to one can of a soft drink) could lead to a weight change of over 15 lb (7 kg) over the course of 1 year. Thus, application of various tables, "rules of thumb," or even equations that estimate resting energy expenditure are of limited value in determining the caloric requirements of any particular pediatric patient. Because the normal healthy child is in a state of positive nitrogen balance and positive

energy balance (ie, growth), even a small miscalculation will result in significant long-term deviation from the predicted outcome. Continual monitoring of growth parameters provides the only truly reliable method for determining the adequacy of energy intake. If growth is normal, it is reasonable to assume that the energy intake is adequate.

A number of methods are used to estimate the energy needs of ill children. These include indirect calorimetry, pediatric basal metabolic rate tables with appropriate activity, and growth and stress factors, as well as nitrogen balance studies. These studies are useful in the clinical setting to a certain extent. They should not be perceived as absolute values because all have a margin of error. The calculations that are products of these methods can be utilized as a guideline in which to provide adequate energy to the acutely or chronically ill child. However, as stated above, it is the growth and development of these patients that remains the gold standard of adequate energy intake or administration.

PROTEIN

Protein intake is required to supply nitrogen and amino acids for the synthesis of constituent proteins and other nitrogen-containing compounds such as polypeptide hormones. Nitrogen cannot be synthesized from fat or carbohydrate. Growth and regeneration of body components requires the constant replenishment of protein stores because of nitrogen losses from skin, hair, feces, and urine.

The term *protein quality* is used to refer to the distribution and the proportion of amino acids that the body is not capable of synthesizing in a particular protein source. A protein of high quality contains a large proportion of all essential amino acids. The required intake of protein varies inversely with the quality of the protein ingested; with intake of the higher-quality proteins, requirements will decrease. When low-quality proteins are ingested, excessive nonessential amino acids must be ingested to provide all of the essential amino acid requirement. These nonessential amino acids are either metabolized and excreted or can be deaminated and utilized as energy via gluconeogenesis. This process is not an efficient route of energy metabolism; it is both nutrient and energy consuming. Therefore, ingestion of higher-quality proteins is desirable.

Mature human milk has an average protein content of 9 g/L. A significant amount of this protein is not available for nutritional purposes. Three-quarters of the IgA in breast milk is excreted intact in the stool; additionally, both lactoferrin and lysozyme probably are not digested or absorbed. These three proteins may comprise as much as 30% of the protein in human milk, so the amount of nutritionally available human milk protein may be as low as 7.2 g/L or 1.3 g/kg/d (based on an average intake of 180 mL/kg/d). The RDA for infants is based on the amount of total protein provided in human milk. It has been estimated to be 2.0 to 2.4 g/kg/d during the first month after birth and gradually to fall to approximately 1.5 g/kg/d by 6 months of age, where it remains throughout the infant's first year. DRIs for protein have not yet been established.

Current infant formulas contain between 1.8 and 4.5 g of protein per 100 kcal, which would provide average protein intakes between 2.0 and 5.4 g/kg/d. Most nutritionists recommend intakes of less than 3.5 g/kg/d of protein for healthy infants so that renal solute load is not exceeded. Note that soy milk–based formulas contain approximately 19 g/L. This is considerably more than the protein content estimated for breast milk or in cow's milk–based formula because soy formula contains less essential amino

TABLE 17-6
GENERAL EFFECT OF ILLNESS OR INJURY ON ENERGY REQUIREMENTS

ABNORMAL STATE	ESTIMATE OF POTENTIAL CHANGE IN TOTAL DAILY CALORIC REQUIREMENT
Uncomplicated partial starvation	−20 to +20%
Postoperative state	+10 to +20%
Multiple fractures	+7 to +25%
Severe infection	+15 to +50%
Third-degree burns over more than 20% of body surface area	+35 to +100%

acids and therefore is a less efficient protein source. Therefore, it requires a higher concentration of total protein to meet nutritional needs.

As table foods replace milk, the dietary requirement of protein increases from 1.5 g/kg/d to approximately 2 g/kg/d because the quality of mixed dietary protein is about 75% that of milk protein. Dietary protein requirements beyond infancy are met relatively easily by most Western diets. There is a surprising lack of appreciation of how much (or, more accurately, how little) protein actually is necessary in the diet to meet individual needs. The RDA for a 15-year-old boy is approximately 60 g of dietary protein. A 5-oz hamburger on a bun will meet over 50% of this protein need.

Of some concern is the current popularity of so-called high-protein body-building diets, which are aggressively marketed to male adolescents. There is no proof that these high-protein diets are of any greater benefit than a normal, well-balanced diet and vigorous training for the acquisition of muscle mass. Furthermore, those diets that truly are high in protein pose a potential though unproved risk of nephrotoxicity.

CARBOHYDRATE

Dietary carbohydrate may be either digestible or nondigestible. Digestible carbohydrates provide an important source of energy for metabolism. Glucose, stored as glycogen in the liver, is the preferred energy substrate for the brain. Carbohydrates also are structural elements in glycoproteins. If adequate dietary energy is not provided, additional energy must be expended to convert protein to glucose. The converted protein loses its value as a synthetic building block, with the nitrogen being lost in urine. Another alternate means of deriving energy is via fatty acid oxidation. When carbohydrate is unavailable, fatty acids undergo β-oxidation, which results in acetyl-CoA, an intermediate of the citric acid cycle. This results in energy production. However, as in the case of gluconeogenesis, this alternate means of energy production requires energy itself. Therefore, inadequate provision of carbohydrate, which is an important source of calories, results in a net loss of body protein and fat stores, which may progress to protein-calorie malnutrition. Furthermore, inadequate energy intake from all sources can result in starvation, in which the body derives energy from ketone bodies. Carbohydrates are the predominant macronutrient in the promoted healthy diet.

Human milk provides approximately 40% of its calories as lactose, which is hydrolyzed to glucose and galactose. Fruits and vegetables contain simple sugars, including glucose and fructose; sucrose (ie, table sugar) is a combination of glucose and fructose. In the child and adult, the majority of dietary carbohydrate is consumed in the form of polysaccharides, especially plant starches. Dietary carbohydrates provide from 35 to 60% of the average American diet. Excessive intake of refined carbohydrate increases the risk of dental caries. Complex carbohydrates should be promoted, and simple and refined starches should be minimized. This will help limit the overconsumption of "empty calories" often found in foods with high concentrations of refined sugars, ie, soda, sweets, candy, and various "fruit" drinks.

Nondigestible carbohydrates, or dietary fiber, derive from plants and consist of a number of polysaccharides and lignins that are present in the cell walls of all plants. There are two forms of dietary fiber: soluble and insoluble. Soluble fiber includes pectins, gums, mucilages, and some hemicelluloses. Pectins are found primarily in fruits and vegetables. Oat bran, barley, and legumes are examples of dietary sources of soluble fiber. Insoluble fiber consisting of pre-dominantly cellulose and hemicellulose provides structure to plant cells. The major source of insoluble fiber is the bran layer of whole grains.

A number of potential benefits have been reported to result from the ingestion of high-fiber diets. Dietary increases in fiber have proven to be useful for the treatment of constipation and irritable bowel syndrome. Increasing fecal bulk by combining both soluble and insoluble fiber increases the "nondigestable" particles as well as the water-holding capacity in the colon. Furthermore, dietary fiber reduces intestinal transit time. Decreased transit time and increased volume of colonic fluids are potential mechanisms for the suggested (but unproven) beneficial effects of dietary fiber. In addition, soluble fiber has been found to lower total cholesterol and LDL-cholesterol in clinical studies along with the benefits of a low-fat diet.

Short-chain fatty acids (SCFAs) are metabolic by-products of fermented undigested carbohydrate, including fiber and lactose. Acetate, propionate, and butyrate comprise 95% of the SCFAs in the colon. These SCFAs are absorbed by the normal colon and stimulate fluid and electrolyte absorption (especially sodium transport). They are also the preferred source of energy for the colonocytes. SCFAs act to stimulate intestinal mucosal cell turnover and blood flow. Although experimental data suggest that SCFAs can act as a trophic factor for the colon, adverse effects of excessive fiber/SCFAs are real. These include gastrointestinal obstruction (especially with motility disturbances), diarrhea, bloating, gas, and a metabolic acid load.

The significance of dietary fiber for infant nutrition is unknown. Its role in the appropriate nutrition of the toddler, child, and adolescent is inferred from studies on adults. It is important that an excessive emphasis on improved high-fiber intakes does not compromise the caloric intake of children.

FAT

Fat (or lipid) provides an important, concentrated source of energy and plays a key role in the formation of the lipid "bilayer" membrane structure. In addition, the essential fatty acid arachidonic acid provides substrate for the formation of prostaglandins, leukotrienes, and thromboxanes. There are three major categories of lipids in Western diets: (1) triglycerides, (2) phospholipids, and (3) sterols. Triglycerides are the main dietary lipid. Each triglyceride consists of three esterified fatty acids that are bound to a molecule of glycerol. Triglycerides are characterized on the basis of the chain length of the bound fatty acids as short-chain fatty acids (ie, fewer than eight carbons), medium-chain fatty acids (ie, 8-12 carbons), and long-chain fatty acids (ie, >12 carbons). There are three predominant forms of phospholipid in the diet: (1) phosphatidylcholine (ie, lecithin), (2) phosphatidylserine, and (3) phosphatidylethanolamine. These are structurally similar except for the bases (ie, choline, serine, ethanolamine). The main dietary sterol is cholesterol, which is not present in foods of plant origin.

The main dietary lipid in North America is long-chain fatty acid (ie, each fatty acid contains 14, 16, 18, or 20 carbon units). The long-chain fatty acids are further classified according to their degree of saturation; that is, *saturated* (contain the maximum number of hydrogens bound to the chain), *monounsaturated* (one double bond), and *polyunsaturated* (two or more double bonds). Typical American diets contain approximately 40% each of monounsaturated and saturated fatty acids. Polyunsaturated fatty acids and glycerol account for approximately 10% each. The proportion of unsaturated to saturated fatty acids in the diet is referred to as the

P/S ratio (after the contribution of monounsaturated fatty acids has been excluded). In general, animal fats are highly saturated and have a lower P/S ratio than do vegetable fats. These distinctions are important because there is compelling evidence that links the ingestion of diets that are high in saturated fat to the development of atherosclerosis.

trans-Fatty acids are formed when manufacturers add hydrogen to liquid oils to create semisolid and more stable fats. This process results in the formation of a *trans* configuration (the *cis* configuration exists naturally in unsaturated fats). Studies have shown that consuming *trans*-fatty acids at levels similar to those in the average American diet (3% of kilocalories) will raise LDL-cholesterol and increase the risk of coronary heart disease. *trans*-Fatty acids are found in stick margarine, commercial frying fats, and high-fat baked goods. Natural sources of *trans*-fatty acids include: butter, beef and milk fats. Humans are able to synthesize most fatty acids de novo by elongation and saturation of shorter unsaturated fatty acids. However, linoleic acid (an 18-carbon fatty acid with two unsaturated bonds) and longer polyunsaturates cannot be synthesized and therefore must be provided in the diet. Linoleic acid can be lengthened to form arachidonic acid (a 20-carbon fatty acid with four unsaturated bonds), which is therefore not essential if there is adequate linoleic in the diet. Linolenic acid (an 18-carbon fatty acid with three double bonds) generally also is considered to be an essential fatty acid, although dietary deficiency is rare.

Essential fatty acid (EFA) deficiency occurs when levels of linoleic acid are too low to maintain normal fatty acid metabolism. Clinically, symptoms that are most likely to be recognized are those of a scaly dermatitis, hair loss, diarrhea, and poor wound healing. Those children who are most at risk to develop EFA deficiency include premature infants who receive inadequate linoleic acid, children with fat malabsorption from hepatobiliary or pancreatic disease, and children receiving long-term parenteral nutrition without intravenous lipid. Although the exact requirement for linoleic acid is unclear, there is general agreement that 2 to 10% of calories should be ingested as linoleic acid. The diagnosis of EFA deficiency is established by demonstrating abnormally low plasma linoleic acid levels based on analysis of either total lipid extracts or isolated phospholipids. In addition, classically there is a decrease in arachidonic acid levels and a rise in 5,8,11-eicosatrienoic acid, which reflects a high rate of conversion of oleic acid to an abnormal triene. This generally is thought to occur as a compensatory mechanism with production of more longer-chain polyunsaturated fatty acids. The increased triene and decreased arachidonic acid (ie, tetraene levels) result in a triene:tetraene ratio above 0.2, which is diagnostic of EFA deficiency.

Human milk contains 3 to 7% of calories from linoleic acid and significant amounts of linolenic acids. The actual fatty acid content varies depending on the mother's diet. Most commercial formulas derive over 10% of their calories from linoleic acid, and all contain at least some linolenic acid. Cow's milk has only approximately 1% linoleic acid, which is less than one-half of the recommended level (2.4% of calories from linoleic acid), but EFA deficiency has not been observed in healthy babies who have been fed cow's milk.

Medium-chain fatty acids comprise approximately 10% of the fatty acids in milk from the mother of a full-term infant and approximately 17% in that of the mother of a premature infant. Medium-chain triglycerides do not require bile acids to achieve solubilization and absorption. Additionally, they are absorbed directly into the portal system rather than via the lymphatic circulation. This likely explains their better absorption by premature infants compared with long-chain triglycerides. Excessive use of medium-chain

triglycerides (ie, >60% of total fat intake) as a replacement for long-chain triglycerides decreases the intake of EFAs, thus increasing the risk of EFA deficiency.

Concerns regarding excessive caloric and cholesterol intake have led to the recommendation by the Expert Panel on Blood Cholesterol Levels in Children and Adolescents that overall fat intake should be limited, because elevated cholesterol levels early in life are linked to the later development of atherosclerosis in adulthood. Therefore, they recommend that for all healthy children and adolescents over the age of 2 years, nutritional adequacy should be achieved by eating a wide variety of foods, with total fat providing no more than 30% of total calories and saturated fatty acids less than 10% of total calories. Intake of dietary cholesterol should not exceed 300 mg/d. Each of these recommendations is intended to refer to an average nutrient intake over a period of several days. The hope is that children will adopt these healthy eating habits and guidelines early in life, thereby fostering healthy eating patterns throughout life. Children who are younger than 2 years of age are specifically excluded from these recommendations because fat provides an important dietary source of energy. Therefore, emphasis on limiting fat intake can lead to inadequate caloric intake.

VITAMINS

Vitamins serve as cofactors in a wide range of vital metabolic reactions. Their biochemical actions, effects of deficiency, toxicities, and dietary sources are enumerated in Tables 17-7 and 17-8; vitamin allowances (which have not been updated since the 10th edition of the RDA, 1989) are listed in Table 17-9. Vitamins are widely used as dietary supplements. Even though vitamin supplements are a multibillion dollar industry, these supplements are of no demonstrated value for the healthy infant, child, adolescent, or adult who is consuming an adequate and varied diet. Although there is no demonstrated adverse effect to the use of a daily multivitamin supplement containing the RDA for vitamins, supplementation is expensive and unnecessary. For the otherwise well patient, use of a vitamin supplement may undermine the concept that adequate nutrition is provided through the intake of a mixed, varied diet.

During the first year after birth, breast milk from a well-nourished mother provides all of the vitamins that an infant needs, with the possible exception of vitamin D. (During the first days after birth the infant also needs vitamin K_1, which should be supplied by intramuscular injection of 0.5 to 1.0 mg or an oral dose of 1.0 to 2.0 mg at birth.) Rickets in breast-fed infants who do not receive adequate exposure to sunlight is well documented. Therefore, the Committee on Nutrition of the American Academy of Pediatrics recommends vitamin D supplementation of breast-fed infants if adequate exposure to sunlight is not assured. For the well infant who consumes over 750 mL (25 oz) of commercial formula, vitamin supplementation is not required.

MAJOR MINERALS

Approximately 98% of the body's mineral content consists of calcium, phosphorus, and magnesium, with bone containing 99% of the calcium, 80% of the phosphorus, and 60% of the magnesium. Table 17-10 outlines the principal biochemical actions, effects of deficiency, toxicity, and dietary sources of these three major minerals. Total body calcium rapidly increases during the last 2 months of gestation and during adolescence. Bone mineralization continues through the third decade, when peak bone density is achieved. The height of this peak appears to influence the development of

TABLE 17-7

SUMMARY OF CLINICALLY RELEVANT INFORMATION ON FAT-SOLUBLE VITAMINS

	BIOCHEMICAL ACTION	EFFECTS OF DEFICIENCY	EFFECTS OF TOXICITY	DIETARY SOURCES
Vitamin A	Component of retinal pigments and rhodopsin for vision in dim light, bone and tooth development, preserves integrity of epithelial cells, wound healing and growth	Night blindness, xerophthalmia, photophobia, conjunctivitis, Bitot spots, keratomalacia, hyperkeratosis of the skin and mucous membranes, poor growth, impaired resistance to infection	Carotenemia with xanthosis cutis, night sweats, dry and cracking skin, vertigo, hepatomegaly, vomiting, alopecia, increased cerebrospinal fluid pressure	Liver, fish-liver oils, milk fat, egg yolk, butter, green and deep yellow vegetables
Vitamin D	Regulates absorption and deposition of calcium and phosphorus, formation of calcium transport protein in duodenal mucosa, synthesis of calcium-binding protein in epithelial cells	*In infants and children:* rickets. *In adults:* osteomalacia	*In infants and children:* hypercalcemia, anorexia, poor growth. *In adults:* nausea, vomiting, polydipsia, polyuria, calcification of soft tissue including heart renal tubules and bronchi	Fortified milk, egg yolk, liver, salmon, butter, sardines, mackerel
Vitamin E	Antioxidant, role in red-blood-cell fragility, stabilizes cell membranes, prevents peroxidation of unsaturated fatty acids	Hemolytic anemia in premature infants, loss of neural integrity, muscle lesions, ceroid pigment deposition	Unknown	Vegetable oils, beef liver, seed oils, peanuts, soybeans, milk fat, turnip greens, eggs, butter, leafy vegetables
Vitamin K	Catalyzes prothrombin synthesis; coagulation factors II, VII, IX, X; proteins C, S, Z	Hemorrhagic manifestations	Kernicterus (water-soluble analogs only)	Vegetable oils, liver, pork, green leafy vegetables (also synthesized by normal intestinal flora)

osteoporosis later in life, emphasizing the importance of early nutrition on later health.

Milk or infant formula supplies these minerals to the infant and young child. Therefore, children with decreased intake of milk, for whatever reason, are at increased risk of dietary calcium deficiency. The ratio of calcium to phosphorus (Ca:P ratio) strongly affects net mineral absorption and varies widely in different foods. Green vegetables have a Ca:P ratio of 2.8:1, human milk of 2:1, cow's milk of 1.2:1, and meat of 0.6:1. Foods that are high in phosphates (eg, cola drinks) may predispose to bone loss. The favorable Ca:P in human milk is particularly important to assure adequate bone mineralization in infancy. Specially formulated premature and low-birth-weight formulas contain Ca:P ratios of approximately 2:1 to assure adequate bone mineralization for this high-risk population. The control of calcium metabolism is discussed in detail in Sec. 24.10.

Calcium absorption is inhibited by dietary phosphate, oxalate, fiber, alkali, and malabsorbed fat. Calcium absorption is enhanced by lactose-containing formulas and the activated form of vitamin D [1,25-$(OH)_2D_3$]. Phosphorus absorption is decreased by dietary calcium and aluminum- or magnesium-containing antacids.

TRACE ELEMENTS, IRON, AND ZINC

Trace elements constitute less than 0.0001 of the total body weight, yet many are considered to be essential for life, health, and reproduction. Trace elements serve as cofactors in enzyme reactions, components of body fluids, sites for binding oxygen, and as structural components for nonenzymatic macromolecules. Except for deficiencies of iron and iodine, which have been well known since before this century, deficiencies of other trace elements are

only beginning to be recognized as health-related problems. For example, fluoride deficiency has been linked to an increased risk of dental cavities, zinc deficiency to growth failure, chromium deficiency to glucose intolerance, copper deficiency to hypercholesterolemia, and selenium deficiency to cardiomyopathy. Adequate iron intake is a concern throughout childhood. This is especially significant in periods of rapid growth. The exclusively breast-fed infant receives adequate iron from breast milk for the first 4 to 6 months of life. It has been shown that iron from breast milk is better absorbed than from formula. However, both breast-fed and formula-fed infants should receive additional sources of iron by age 6 months. This includes iron-fortified cereals. Table 17-11 summarizes the biochemical actions, effects of deficiency, toxicity, and dietary sources of the trace elements.

17.3 FORMULAS AND NUTRITIONAL SUPPLEMENTS

Neal S. Leleiko and Miriam Horowitz

17.3.1 INFANT FORMULAS

Before the 18th century, human milk was the only available source of nutrition for a newborn infant, so milk was supplied by either the biological mother or a hired wetnurse. The development of infant formulas was a revolutionary event in the history of pediatric nutrition. No infant formula has been developed that is able to exactly mimic human breast milk, but infant formulas have been

TABLE 17-8

SUMMARY OF CLINICALLY RELEVANT INFORMATION ON WATER-SOLUBLE VITAMINS

	BIOCHEMICAL ACTION	EFFECTS OF DEFICIENCY	EFFECTS OF TOXICITY	DIETARY SOURCES
Thiamin	Combines with phosphorus to form thiamin pyrophosphate, which acts in various oxidative decarboxylations, including pyruvic acid	*Wet beriberi:* congestive heart failure, tachycardia, peripheral edema *Dry beriberi:* neuritis, paresthesia, irritability, anorexia	Unknown	Liver, meat, milk, pork, whole grains, legumes, nuts
Riboflavin	Part of the flavin coenzymes, flavin adenine dinucleotide and flavin mononucleotide, necessary for tissue oxidation and respiration and synthesis of FMN and FAD essential for growth, retinal pigment for light adaptation	Photophobia, loss of visual acuity, burning and itching of eyes, corneal vascularization, glossitis, seborrheic dermatitis, poor growth, cheilosis	Unknown	Milk, cheese, eggs, organ meats, fish, green leafy vegetables, whole and enriched grains
Niacin	Component of coenzymes I and II (NAD, NADP), cofactors in a number of dehydrogenase systems, necessary for synthesis of glycogen and breakdown of fatty acids	*Pellagra:* dermatitis, apathy, anorexia, peripheral neuropathy, encephalopathy with some degree of dementia, diarrhea secondary to atrophy of mucosa	Nicotinic acid has transient vasodilating effects, skin flushing, tingling, itching, dizziness, nausea, may induce liver abnormalities	Lean meats, poultry, peanuts, organ meats, brewer's yeast, green vegetables, enriched cereals and grains
Folate	Tetrahydrofolic acid is the active form; essential in the biosynthesis of purines, pyrimidines, and nucleoproteins; methylation reactions; one carbon acceptor	Megaloblastic anemia (should also suspect concurrent vitamin B_{12} deficiency), impaired cellular immunity, poor growth, glossitis, gastrointestinal disturbances	Unknown	Liver, leafy green vegetables, legumes, asparagus, broccoli, nuts, cheese
Vitamin B_6	Constituent of many coenzymes for decarboxylation, transamination, transsulfuration, role in hemoglobin synthesis and fatty acid metabolism	Dermatitis, cheilosis, stomatitis, peripheral neuritis (in patients on isoniazid), microcytic, hypochromic anemia, irritability, convulsions	Sensory neuropathy with progressive ataxia, altered sense of touch, pain, fever	Liver, meat, whole grains, yeast, potatoes, corn, soybeans, bananas, peanuts
Vitamin B_{12}	Essential for red-blood-cell maturation in bone marrow, coenzyme for methylmalonyl CoA mutase, transfer of one-carbon units in purine metabolism, affects central nervous system metabolism	Pernicious anemia, neurologic deterioration because of demyelination of large nerve fibers of the spinal cord, methylmalonic aciduria, homocystinuria	Unknown	Liver, organ meats, meat, eggs, cheese, fish
Biotin	Coenzyme of all carboxylases and of carbon dioxide	Lenier dermatitis, anorexia, glossitis, alopecia, nausea, anorexia, muscle pain, insomnia	Unknown	Liver, kidney, milk, egg yolk, yeast, mushrooms, banana, watermelon, strawberries, grapefruit
Pantothenic acid	Component of CoA; necessary for fat, protein, and CHO metabolism; fatty acid biosynthesis	Observed with use of antagonists, depression, hypotension, muscle weakness, nausea, sleep disturbances, abdominal pain, loss of antibody production	Unknown	Most foods
Vitamin C	Integrity maintenance of all intercellular materials, collagen biosynthesis, iron absorption and transport, metabolism of tyrosine, synthesis of corticosteroids	*Scurvy:* diffuse tissue bleeding, pinpoint peripheral hemorrhages, easy bone fracture, poor wound healing, friable bleeding gums with loose teeth	Nausea, diarrhea, cramps, massive doses may predispose to kidney stones	Citrus fruits, tomatoes, berries, green vegetables, cabbage, human milk

TABLE 17-9

FOOD AND NUTRITION BOARD, NATIONAL ACADEMY OF SCIENCES-NATIONAL RESEARCH COUNCIL RECOMMENDED DIETARY ALLOWANCES (REVISED 1989)

CATEGORY	AGE (y)	WEIGHT (kg)	HEIGHT (cm)	PROTEIN (g)	VITAMIN A (μg)	VITAMIN D (μg)	VITAMIN E (mg)	VITAMIN K (μg)	VITAMIN C (mg)
Infants	0.0–0.5	6	60	13	375	7.5	3	5	30
	0.5–1.0	9	71	14	375	10.0	4	10	35
Children	1–3	13	90	16	400	10.0	6	15	40
	4–6	20	112	24	500	10.0	7	20	45
	7–10	28	132	28	700	10.0	7	30	45
Boys	11–14	45	157	45	1000	10.0	10	45	50
	15–18	66	176	59	1000	10.0	10	65	60
Girls	11–14	46	157	46	800	10.0	8	45	50
	15–18	55	163	44	800	10.0	8	55	60

TABLE 17-10

SUMMARY OF CLINICALLY RELEVANT INFORMATION ON MINERALS

	BIOCHEMICAL ACTION	EFFECTS OF DEFICIENCY	EFFECTS OF TOXICITY	DIETARY SOURCES
Calcium	Structure of bone and teeth, activates smooth, skeletal, cardiac muscle contraction and neural transmitter release, blood coagulation	Poor mineralization of bone and teeth, osteomalacia, osteoporosis, rickets, tetany, growth impairment, possibly hypertension	*Dietary:* excessive calcification of bone, calcification of soft tissue *Parenteral:* heart block and renal stones	Cheese, milk, turnip and mustard greens, collards, kale, broccoli, canned salmon and sardines with bones, clams, oysters
Magnesium	Cofactor for many enzyme systems including ATP formation, protein synthesis, nerve impulse transmission, phosphate transfer systems, muscle contraction, principal cation of soft tissue structure of bone and teeth	Muscle tremors, convulsions, irritability, tetany, hyper/hyporeflexia	Rare dietary toxicity, toxicity more common with intravenous infusions	Whole grains, nuts, dried beans, peas, meat, milk
Phosphorus	Constituent of bones and teeth, structure of cytoplasma and nucleic acids, phospholipids, coenzyme for CHO, fat, and protein metabolism	Rickets may develop in low-birth-weight babies; neuromuscular, renal, and skeletal abnormalities	High-phosphorus infant formulas (Ca:P ratio 1:1) may contribute to hypocalcemia, tetany in early infancy	Milk, cheese, dairy products, egg yolk, meat, legumes, nuts, poultry, fish

refined to such a degree that parents who decide to bottle-feed their baby can be reasonably assured that formula-fed infants grow and develop into healthy children. Commercial formulas are appropriate for infants when a mother chooses for personal reasons not to breast-feed, when breast-feeding is medically contraindicated, or for use as a supplement when it is not practical to use stored breast milk.

During the first 4 to 6 months after birth, mother's milk and infant formula can serve as the sole source of nutrition for infants. Between 4 and 6 months, dietary iron may be inadequate, so infant formula should be iron fortified. Low-iron formulas are not adequate for infants in the first year of life. No evidence supports the rapid introduction of new foods. The nursing baby may receive adequate nutrition for most of the first year after birth from mother's milk. From 4 to 12 months, infant formulas (or mother's milk) may be supplemented with age-appropriate semisolid and solid foods that may assist in normal developmental and physiological growth. There is no developmental or nutritional rationale for the so-called "follow-up" formulas that are proposed to offer special advantages between weaning and starting cow's milk. Table 17-12 summarizes a practical and rational progression for feeding with approximate ages. It is most important to recognize that no rules apply to all infants. Each infant follows his or her own schedule of maturation, and there is wide variation from one infant to another. Table 17-12 therefore offers only a possible guideline for feeding associated with developmental milestones.

In the United States as in many other industrial countries, there are federal rules regarding how much of certain nutrients should be contained in a commercial formula. These rules were adopted because of accidents in infant formula manufacture. Presently, the Infant Formula Act of 1980 (revised in 1986) has established the minimum levels for 29 nutrients and maximum levels for nine nutrients. As a result, regardless of the manufacturer, most standard infant formulas now marketed for the healthy term infant are markedly similar with regard to most critical ingredients. Average daily requirements for vitamins and minerals are met when a minimum intake of 25 to 32 oz of standard formula (20 kcal/oz) is provided to the infant.

The standard caloric density of all term-infant formulas is the same as that of human breast milk (ie, 20 kcal/oz), and all have essentially the same osmolality (ie, 280 to 300 mOsm/kg). There are minor differences in electrolyte content, which may be important for the selection of formulas in special cases (eg, congestive heart failure, renal disease). Formulas that are available in the United States for term infants can be classified into four broad categories based on the type and nature of their protein content: (1) *cow's milk–based formulas* (eg, casein, whey protein source), (2) *isolated soy protein–based formulas,* (3) *specialized infant formulas* (which include protein hydrolysate–based formulas and amino acid–based formulas), and (4) *formulas designed specifically for the needs of premature infants* (Table 17-13). Aside from the protein source, the carbohydrate and fat components may differ in various formulas. Understanding these variations may be important in feeding infants with a variety of problems, including fat malabsorption, altered carbohydrate metabolism, and prematurity, but they are of little consequence for the normal infant.

COW'S MILK–BASED FORMULAS

Human milk protein consists of approximately 70% (human) whey and approximately 30% (human) casein. Unaltered cow's milk formulas contain approximately 18% (bovine) whey and approximately 82% (bovine) casein, although "humanized" formulas adjust this ratio to achieve approximately 60% (bovine) whey and approximately 40% (bovine) casein. Although quantitative differences exist among the whey:casein ratios of cow's milk–based term-infant formulas, the results of feeding either a casein- or whey-predominant formula to healthy, growing infants are indistinguishable.

Serum biochemical measures in infants who are fed different formulas may reflect the constituents of those different formulas.

TABLE 17-11

SUMMARY OF CLINICALLY RELEVANT INFORMATION ON TRACE ELEMENTS

	BIOCHEMICAL ACTION	EFFECTS OF DEFICIENCY	EFFECTS OF TOXICITY	DIETARY SOURCES
Chromium	Required for normal glucose metabolism, potentiates the action of insulin	Glucose intolerance, impaired growth, peripheral neuropathy, negative nitrogen balance, decreased respiratory quotient	Unknown	Meat, cheese, brewer's yeast
Copper	Necessary for red-blood-cell and hemoglobin formation, constituent of ceruloplasmin, component of key metalloenzymes, role in connective tissue biosynthesis, iron absorption	Sideroblastic anemia, neutropenia, leukopenia, depigmentation, ataxia, erythropoiesis dysfunction, anorexia, bone demineralization, increased serum cholesterol	Wilson disease, copper deposition in the cornea and liver (leading to cirrhosis), deterioration of neurologic status	Liver, oysters, kidney, shellfish, legumes, raisins, chocolate, meat, fish, nuts
Fluoride	Helps to protect against tooth decay, may minimize bone loss	Increased tendency to dental caries	Flurosis—mottled and discolored teeth, calcified muscle insertions, and exostosis	Drinking water, seafood, plant and animal foods (dependent on content in water and soil)
Iodine	Component of thyroid hormones thyroxine and triiodothyronine	Hypothyroid, simple goiter, endemic cretinism	Thyrotoxicosis, medicinally induced goiter	Iodized salt, seafood, seaweed
Iron	Structure of hemoglobin and myoglobin for O_2 and CO_2 transport, oxidative enzymes, cytochrome c and catalase	Hypochromic, microcytic anemia, growth failure	Hemochromatosis	Liver, lean meat, egg, poultry, oysters, legumes, fortified cereals, grains, dark molasses
Manganese	Cofactor for pyruvate and acetyl-CoA carboxylases, mitochondrial superoxide dismutase, and other enzymes	Weight loss, transient dermatitis, nausea and vomiting, slow hair growth, change in hair color	Neurologic changes like those of Parkinson or Wilson disease	Widely distributed, deficiency reported only with experimental diet
Molybdenum	Cofactor for xanthine, aldehyde, and sulfite oxidases	Severe brain damage, tachycardia, headache	Gout-like syndrome	Widely distributed, deficiency reported only with parenteral nutrition and genetic syndromes
Selenium	Growth factor and cofactor for glutathione peroxidase and other enzyme systems	Cardiomyopathy, muscle pain, macrocytosis	Hair loss, polyneuritis, metallic taste	Widely distributed, deficiency reported in some areas of China (Keshan) and rarely with parenteral nutrition
Zinc	Cofactor of more than 90 enzymes, including erythrocyte carbonic anhydrase and superoxide dismutase	Growth failure, hypogonadism, hypogeusia, diarrhea, dermatoses	Vomiting and diarrhea, dermatoses, copper deficiency	Widely distributed, deficiency in chronic diarrhea and parenteral nutrition

Breast-fed infants have lower serum urea nitrogen than formula-fed infants, reflecting the lower total protein and the higher quality of that protein (ie, the lower metabolic price of the high-quality protein). Infants who are fed whey-predominant formulas have higher serum threonine and branched-chain amino acids, and those fed casein-predominant formulas have higher levels of tyrosine, phenylalanine, valine, and methionine. Although these metabolic differences exist, the nutritional implications (if any) of these findings are uncertain.

SOYBEAN PROTEIN–DERIVED FORMULAS

Soybeans are the second commercial source of protein that is used in infant formula. Soy protein is the third most common type of protein found in infant formulas, casein and whey being the other

two types. Soybean milks were suggested as appropriate for infants over 50 years ago. Although there is a lack of meaningful data on the safe use of soy formulas in premature and sick infants, there is no evidence to limit their use in the well infant. Because soybean protein is of relatively low quality, it must be fortified with essential amino acids when used in infant formulas. Methionine is added to all infant soy formulas to create a protein equivalent to casein. As a result, regardless of the manufacturer, most standard infant formulas now marketed for the healthy, term infant are markedly similar with regard to most ingredients.

The Committee on Nutrition of the American Academy of Pediatrics recommends the use of soy-protein formula only in infants with:

- Vegetarian families in which animal-protein formulas are not desired.

TABLE 17-12

GUIDE FOR INFANT FEEDING IN THE FIRST 2 YEARS OF LIFE

AGE RANGE	INTRODUCTION OF NEW FEEDS	REASON FOR INTRODUCTION	DEVELOPMENTAL PATTERNS
0–2 mo	Breast milk or formula.	Meets all of the infant's nutritional needs for the first 4 to 6 months.	Rooting reflex, suck-swallow patterns, extension tongue movements.
4–6 mo	Iron-fortified, single-grain cereal mixed with milk. Rice cereal is the most hypoallergenic of the grains, and is usually introduced first.	Provides a dietary source of iron at an age when body stores from birth are depleting.	Maturation of head and neck control. Lips have muscular control to seal oral cavity. Tongue can move laterally to assist transfer of food in the mouth, and infant will draw lower lip as spoon is removed. Munching (up and down chopping motion) movements begin.
5–7 mo	Strained or pureed, single vegetables and fruits. Fruit juices by sippy cup. (Introduce vegetables first to reduce the tendency to develop a taste for sweets.)	Provides dietary sources of vitamins, minerals, and calories. Introduces new food flavors. Starts setting basis for good eating habits.	Biting reflex begins to fade. Controls sucking impulse. Opens mouth to accept spoon. Turns head freely to indicate satiety or preference.
6–9 mo	Strained or pureed meats and combination infant meals. Finger foods such as arrowroot biscuits, Cheerios, cheese sticks, small pieces of meat. Cottage cheese, plain yogurt, egg, and meat alternative such as pureed beans and lentils.	Provides additional protein, vitamins, and iron for rapid growth. Encourages chewing when teeth erupt.	Infant has ability to grasp and route food from hand to mouth, can sit with minimal support. Teeth begin to come in. Pincer grasp beginning, with voluntary release. Rotary chewing pattern develops. Increasing maturity for spoon feeding and ability to tolerate greater food textures.
9–12 mo	Chewy finger foods, bite-size meat, poultry, and fish. Soft-cooked vegetables and pieces of raw, peeled fruits. Macaroni, spaghetti, and potatoes. Gradual transition to family menu and less reliance on baby foods and formula. Variety of regular table foods. Can wean off of infant formula or breast milk and begin on whole cow's milk by age 1.	Encourages the development of hand-to-mouth coordination and proper chewing. Infant gains more independence in feeding self. Can drink from a cup and should be weaned from bottle.	Infant more mobile and may seek food on his or her own. Infant is able to spit and stick out tongue. Infant has concept of spoon and cup and becomes more proficient with their use, approximates lips to rim of the cup, and ulnar deviation of wrist develops.
12–24 mo	All daily nutritional requirements provided by a mixed table food diet. Continuing precautions to avoid foods that may pose choking hazard.	Food of high nutrient value should be offered, because intake declines with decreased rate of growth. Appetite appears to decrease.	Names food, expresses preferences, and may go on food jags. Continue to offer a balanced diet with a variety of foods, as lifelong eating habits are established.

- Galactosemia, primary lactase deficiency, or the recovery phase of secondary lactose intolerance, because these formulas are the least expensive available formulas not containing lactose.
- Potentially allergic infants (with a family history of atopy) who have not shown clinical manifestations of allergy. However, these infants should be monitored closely for allergy to soy protein.

The Committee suggested that these formulas should not be used:

- For the routine feeding of premature and low-birth-weight infants, where use should be for limited periods, if at all.
- In the dietary management of documented clinical allergic reaction to cow's-milk protein and/or soy-protein formula.
- In the routine management of infantile colic.

SPECIALIZED INFANT FORMULAS

Protein hydrolysate formulas originally were developed for infants who could not digest intact protein or were severely allergic to intact-protein formulas. These formulas consist of proteins that are hydrolyzed primarily to peptides of varying lengths and some free amino acids. They are the formulas of choice for infants with proven or presumptive allergy to cow's milk–based and/or soybean-based formulas or disorders of digestion, absorption, and metabolism. Poor taste and greater cost are significant considerations prohibiting their use.

Not all protein hydrolysate formulas are the same. The various formulas that currently are available differ in their protein source and degree of protein hydrolysis. This results in variation of the antigenicity of different formulas.

Amino acid–based formulas are the most "elemental" but not necessarily the optimal form of enteral diet that exists. These formulas are hydrolyzed to the greatest extent. Because of the highly specialized nature of these formulas, their use is limited to highly select patients. The greatest use for free amino acids is in the treatment of extreme allergy to numerous foods. Amino acid formulas are often used as the basis of an "elimination" diet to isolate the true offending antigens. Use of these formulas for short-gut syndrome is highly debatable. Utilizing free amino acids in this patient population may not be advantageous because free amino acids may not promote gut adaptation as efficiently as peptides. Furthermore, the high osmolality of these formulas may result in osmotic diarrhea. Therefore amino acid–containing diets are indicated for those patients with severe food allergies. As with the hydrolysate formulas, additional deterrents for use include great expense and poor palatability.

Premature infant formulas are discussed in Sec. 2.12.5. These formulas are generally not appropriate for use in term infants.

CARBOHYDRATE COMPONENTS OF INFANT FORMULAS

All nursing infants and 90% of formula-fed infants consume lactose as their primary source of carbohydrate. Carbohydrates supply approximately 30 to 40% of the calories in the newborn and early infant period. Corn syrup solids (ie, a mixture of glucose polymers and hydrolyzed cornstarch) are the usual source of carbohydrate in lactose-free and soy-protein formulas. The cornstarch that is used to make corn syrup is chemically modified to increase the marketability and esthetic appeal of the formula. Other carbohydrates include tapioca starch and sucrose.

Starch is more rapidly emptied from the stomach than simpler sugars are, and this may affect the choice of formula. For the infant with gastroesophageal reflux, rapid gastric emptying may be of benefit, whereas in the infant with diarrhea or who is recovering from an enteritis, the rapid emptying may be disadvantageous. These factors have not been rigorously studied in healthy infants, however. Following an acute gastroenteritis, the occurrence of secondary lactase deficiency is frequently diagnosed. Removal of lactose from the infant's diet on a temporary basis can be justified in the symptomatic infant. A lactose-free cow's milk–based formula is available. Within a few days, most infants should be able to digest a normal load of lactose; even in premature infants, there is no convincing evidence in favor of lactose exclusion for nutritional purposes. Because there is evidence that lactose appears to contribute to calcium (as well as possibly to magnesium, manganese, and phosphorus) absorption, the long-term exclusion of lactose may be contraindicated.

FAT COMPONENTS OF INFANT FORMULAS

Fat provides approximately 50% of the energy from human milk and 40 to 50% of that from formulas. Human milk contains cholesterol, whereas formulas primarily are made with vegetable-oil blends and contain little or no cholesterol. Fat blends are selected to provide a balance of saturated and polyunsaturated fatty acids. Because of the high percentage of calories from fat in both infant formulas and breast milk, there is a generous supply of the essential fatty acids linoleic acid and linolenic acid. The effect of fat and cholesterol intake during infancy on the development of coronary artery disease in later life is unknown. Specialized formulas containing medium-chain triglycerides (MCTs) as a primary source of fat (60-86%) are useful for the treatment of children with fat malabsorption resulting from hepatobiliary disease, pancreatic insufficiency, ileal resection, protein-losing enteropathy, intestinal lymphangiectasia, chylous ascites, and chylothorax. The MCT oil may enhance intestinal fat absorption without the need for pancreatic

enzymes, bile acids, or lymphatic circulation. Infants with long-term use of formulas containing a high percentage of MCT oil must be carefully monitored for essential fatty acid deficiency (see Sec. 17.2.3). There is increasing evidence that the nutritional advantages of MCT oil may require the presence of a functioning colon to facilitate absorption of unabsorbed lipid.

17.3.2 Specialized Formulas for Children and Adults

In recent years specialized enteral formulas have been developed specifically for the needs of children 1 to 6 years old. They have been designed to meet their macronutrient and micronutrient needs. Protein has been limited to adjust for renal solute load. Vitamin and mineral contents are adjusted to meet the demands of growing children. Particular attention has been paid to meeting the calcium requirements of children as well. With the provision of adequate calories and fluid, these formulas are complete diets providing all essential nutrients. Note this is not the case for the "follow-up formulas," which are marketed for children over 1 year old. There is no indication for the use of the follow-up formulas, as children without special needs should be transitioned to whole cow's milk after 1 year of life.

Specialized enteral formulas are available in many forms and varieties; they include polymeric, fiber-containing, semielemental, and elemental formulas (Table 17-13). Polymeric formulas are indicated for use as an oral supplement or as the only feeding provided by gastrostomy or jejunal feeding. The addition of fiber to a polymeric formula is sometimes useful in children receiving supplemental feedings who have either constipation or chronic diarrhea. Protein hydrolysate formulas are useful in children with cow's milk/soy allergy, malabsorption, short-bowel syndrome, inflammatory bowel disease, or pancreatic insufficiency. Free amino acid–containing formulas are most useful in children with extreme food allergies, but the high osmotic load can be problematic. Formulas with higher medium-chain triglyceride contents are of particular value in children with lympangiectasia or cholestatic liver disease. There are specific indications that may require the use of "adult" formulas for children under the age of 6. These include children who require high-calorie enteral feedings who are fluid restricted or those in end-stage renal/liver failure, who may benefit from the use of calorically dense formulas designed for adults. These formulas are concentrated to 2 kcal/cc and therefore have high osmolality. Each formula varies according to protein source, protein load, fat source, and electrolyte composition.

Children over the age of 6 can be given adult formulas prescribed to accommodate their special needs. Oral supplements designed for adults are more nutrient dense than formulas marketed for children. Often adult formulas may exceed the protein requirements of school-aged children if utilized as the sole form of nutrition support. Therefore, these very high calorie formulas would be more appropriate with the provision of additional nonprotein calories and fluid. There are over 100 adult formulas available on the market. They include formulas that are modified in macronutrients, micronutrients, and caloric/nutrient density as well as some that are disease specific, ie, renal, liver, gastrointestinal, metabolic, and allergy. Their appropriate use should be based on a rational approach to the nutritional needs of the patient and not on brand name or marketing.

TABLE 17-13

ENTERAL FEEDING PRODUCTS AVAILABLE IN THE UNITED STATES[a]

FORMULA	MANUFAC-TURER	kcal/oz	PROT. g/L	mOsm/kg	PROTEIN SOURCE	CARBOHYDRATE SOURCE	FAT SOURCE	COMMENTS
Maternal breast milk	Mom	20	10.5	290	-Mature human milk	-Lactose	-Mature human milk	-Approx 0.3 mg iron/L -Nutrient composition variable by individual
Milk-based infant formulas								
Enfamil with Iron	Mead Johnson	20	14.7	300	-Whey -Nonfat milk	-Lactose	-Soy oil -Coconut oil -Palm olein oil -High-oleic sunflower oil	-Low-iron also available (3.2 mg/L) -Nucleotides added
Follow-up	Carnation	20	17.4	350 mOsm/L	-Casein -Whey	-Corn syrup -Lactose	-Soybean oil -Coconut oil -Palm olein oil -High-oleic safflower oil	-Marketed for 6–12 months old
Gerber with iron	Gerber	20	14.7	320	-Nonfat milk	-Lactose	-Soy oil -Coconut oil -Palm olein oil -High-oleic sunflower oil	
Good Start	Carnation	20	16	265	-Partially hydrolyzed whey	-Lactose -Maltodextrin	-Soybean oil -Coconut oil -Palm olein oil -High-oleic safflower oil	-Not hypoallergenic
Lactofree	Mead Johnson	20	14.7	200	-Milk protein isolate	-Corn syrup solids	-Soy oil -Coconut oil -Palm olein oil -High-oleic sunflower oil	-Lactose-free alternative to soy formulas
Similac with iron	Ross	20	14.3	300	-Nonfat milk	-Lactose	-Soy oil -Coconut oil	-Low-iron also available (1.5 mg/L) -Nucleotides added
Similac lactose-free	Ross	20	14.5	230	-Nonfat milk	-Corn syrup solids -Sucrose	-Soy oil -Coconut oil	-Lactose-free alternative to soy formulas -Nucleotides added
Soy-based infant formulas[b]								
Alsoy	Nestle Nutrition	20	21	270	-Soy protein isolate	-Sucrose -Maltodextrin	-Soy oil	
Follow-up Soy	Nestle Nutrition	20	21	270	-Soy protein isolate	-Sucrose -Maltodextrin	-Soy oil	
Gerber Soy	Gerber	20	20.1	230	-Soy protein isolate	-Corn syrup -Sucrose	-Soy oil -Coconut oil -Palm olein oil -High-oleic sunflower oil	
Isomil	Ross Laboratories	20	16.4	240	-Soy protein isolate	-Corn syrup -Sucrose	-Soy oil -Coconut oil	
Isomil DF	Ross Laboratories	20	17.8	240	-Soy protein isolate	-Corn syrup -Sucrose	-Soy oil -Coconut oil	-Limit use to 7-10 days -Contains fiber (7.7 g/L) -For short-term use only

(continued)

TABLE 17-13 Continued

1330

FORMULA	MANUFAC-TURER	kcal/oz	PROT. g/L	mOsm/kg	PROTEIN SOURCE	CARBOHYDRATE SOURCE	FAT SOURCE	COMMENTS
Isomil SF	Ross Laboratories	20	17.8	150	-Soy protein isolate	-Glucose polymers	-Soy oil -Coconut oil	
Prosobee	Mead Johnson	20	20.1	200	-Soy protein isolate	-Corn syrup solids	-Soy oil -Coconut oil -Palm olein oil -High-oleic sunflower oil	
Premature formulas[c]								
Enfamil Premature Formula	Mead Johnson	20	20.1	260	-Whey -Nonfat milk	-Lactose -Corn syrup solids	-Soy oil -Coconut oil -MCT oil	-Available in 24 kcal/oz RTF -Low-iron also available in both concentrations
Enfamil 22	Mead Johnson	22	21	260	-Whey -Nonfat milk	-Lactose -Corn syrup solids	-High-oleic sunflower oil -Soy oil -MCT oil -Coconut oil	-For infants 1800 g through first year of life -Different home mixing instructions from other formulas -Nucleotides added
Human Milk Fortifier	Mead Johnson	1 packet + 25 mL BM = 24 kcal/oz	0.18 g/packet	1 packet + 25 mL BM increases mOsm by 60 to ~350	-Whey -Sodium caseinate	-Corn syrup solids -Lactose	-Negligible	-Vitamin, mineral, and electrolyte fortified
Similac Natural Care	Ross Laboratories	24	21.7	300	-Whey -Nonfat milk	-Lactose -Glucose polymers	-MCT oil -Soy oil -Coconut oil	-Mix with MBM or feed as alternate
Similac Neocare	Ross Laboratories	22	19.3	290	-Nonfat milk -Whey protein concentrate	-Corn syrup solids -Lactose	-Soy oil -High-oleic safflower oil -MCT oil	-For infants 1800 g through first year of life -Different home-mixing instructions from other formulas
Similac Special Care	Ross Laboratories	20	18.1	250	-Whey -Nonfat milk	-Lactose -Glucose polymers	-MCT oil -Soy oil -Coconut oil	-Available in 24 kcal/oz RTF -Low-iron also available in both concentrations
Special infant formulas								
Alimentum	Ross Laboratories	20	18.4	370	-Casein hydrolysate	-Modified tapioca starch -Sucrose	-MCT oil -Soy oil -Safflower oil	-Available as ready-to-feed -50% MCT, 50% LCT
Enfamil AR	Mead Johnson	20	16.7	230	-Nonfat cow's milk	-Lactose -Rice starch -Maltodextrin	-Palm olein oil -Soy oil -Coconut oil -High-oleic sunflower oil	-Available as a powder and ready-to-feed -Added rice -Whey:casein = 18:82

(continued)

TABLE 17-13   Continued

FORMULA	MANUFAC-TURER	kcal/oz	PROT. g/L	mOsm/kg	PROTEIN SOURCE	CARBOHYDRATE SOURCE	FAT SOURCE	COMMENTS
Neocate	SHS North America	20	24.8	342	-Free amino acids	-Corn syrup solids	-Hybrid safflower oil -Coconut oil -Soy oil	-Available as a powder -Different home-mixing instructions from other formulas
Nutramigen	Mead Johnson	20	18.7	320	-Casein hydrolysate	-Corn syrup solids -Modified cornstarch	-Corn oil -Soy oil	
Portagen	Mead Johnson	20	23.4	360	-Sodium caseinate	-Corn syrup solids -Sucrose	-MCT oil -Corn oil -Lecithin	-84% of fat is MCT
Pregestimil	Mead Johnson	20	18.7	320	-Casein hydrolysate	-Corn syrup solids -Modified cornstarch -Dextrose	-MCT oil -Corn oil -Soy oil -High-oleic safflower oil	-Available as a powder -55% MCT, 45% LCT -Extra fat-soluble vitamins, ascorbic acid, and zinc added
Similac PM 60/40	Ross Laboratories	20	15.7	280	-Whey caseinate	-Lactose	-Coconut oil -Soy oil	-Ca:PO$_4$ = 2:1 -Low Phos, K$^+$, Na$^+$ -Only available in low Fe -Available as a powder and ready-to-feed
Transitional formulas for children (1-3 years old)[d]								
Next Step	Mead Johnson	20	17.4	270	-Nonfat milk solids	-Corn syrup solids -Lactose	-Palm olein oil -Soy oil -Coconut oil -Sunflower oil	-Powder, concentrated liquid, and ready-to-feed
Next Step Soy	Mead Johnson	20	20	260	-Soy protein isolate	-Corn syrup solids -Sucrose	-Palm olein oil -Soil oil -Coconut oil -Sunflower oil	-Option for children with milk intolerance -Methionine, taurine, and carnitine added -Powder, concentrated liquid, and ready-to-feed
Formulas for children (1-10 years old)[e]								
Compleat Pediatric	Novartis Nutrition	30	37.6	380	-Beef -Caseinate	-Vegetable -Fruit -Hydrolyzed cornstarch	-MCT oil -Vegetable oil	-Unflavored -Commercial blenderized formula -Contains fiber from fruit and vegetable sources (4.4 g/L)
Kindercal (also with fiber)	Mead Johnson	30	34	310	-Casein	-Maltodextrin -Sucrose	-Canola oil -High-oleic sunflower oil -Corn oil -MCT oil	-Contains soy fiber (6.3 g/L) -Vanilla flavored
Nutren Junior (also with fiber)	Nestle Nutrition	30	30	350	-Casein -Whey	-Maltodextrin -Sucrose	-Soybean oil -MCT oil -Canola oil	-Vanilla flavored -Also available with fiber (6 g/L) *(continued)*

TABLE 17-13 Continued

FORMULA	MANUFAC-TURER	kcal/oz	PROT. g/L	mOsm/kg	PROTEIN SOURCE	CARBOHYDRATE SOURCE	FAT SOURCE	COMMENTS
Pediasure (vanilla) (also with fiber)	Ross Laboratories	30	30	310	-Sodium caseinate -Low-lactose whey protein	-Sucrose -Hydrolyzed cornstarch	-MCT oil -High-oleic safflower oil -Soy oil	-Available in strawberry, banana, chocolate, and vanilla flavors -Also available with fiber (5 g/L)
Resource Just for Kids (vanilla)	Novartis Nutrition	30	30	390	-Sodium and calcium caseinate -Whey protein concentrate	-Sucrose -Hydrolyzed cornstarch	-High-oleic sunflower oil -Soybean oil -MCT oil	-Available in French vanilla, Swiss chocolate, and creamy strawberry flavors
Special formulas for children (1-10 years old)								
Elecare	Ross Laboratories	30	30.1	596	-Free amino acids	-Corn syrup solids	-High-oleic safflower oil -MCT oil -Soy oil	-Available as a powder -Hypoallergenic
NeoCate One (powder)	SHS North America	30	30	610	-Synthetic amino acids	-Corn syrup solids	-MCT oil -Canola oil -High-oleic sunflower oil	-Orange-pineapple flavor, ready-to-feed also available -Hypoallergenic
Peptamen Junior (vanilla)	Nestle Nutrition	30	30	360	-Hydrolyzed whey	-Maltodextrin	-MCT oil -Canola oil -Soy oil	-Ready-to-feed -Flavor packets available
Vivonex Pediatric (unflavored)	Novartis Nutrition	24	24	360	-Free amino acids	-Maltodextrin -Modified starch	-MCT oil -Soy oil	-Available as a powder -Flavor packets available
Tolerex	Novartis	30	20.6	550	-Crystalline amino acids	-Glucose polymers	-Safflower oil	-Available as a powder -1% of kcal as fat -Calcium, phosphorus, and vit D inadequate for children
Other Milks[f,g]								
Evaporated whole milk	Assorted	42	70.7	N/A	-Casein -Whey	-Lactose	-Butterfat	-Inadequate vitamin A and D unless fortified; inadequate vitamin C, iron, zinc, and essential fatty acids.
Goat's milk	Assorted	30	36	N/A	-Casein -Whey	-Lactose	-Butterfat	-Inadequate vitamin D, B_6, folate, iron, and essential fatty acids

(continued)

TABLE 17-13   Continued

ADULT FORMULAS AND SUPPLEMENTS

Formula	Manufacturer	Contents	Comments
Blenderized, whole-protein supplements			
Carnation Instant Breakfast	Nestle Nutrition	Casein, egg white, whey, lactose, sucrose	Additive, high osmolality, relatively inexpensive Nutritionally incomplete
Compleat-B	Novartis	Meat- and nonfat-milk-based blenderized tube feeding	
Compleat Modified	Novartis	Meat- and caseinate-based blenderized tube feeding	
Ensure	Ross Laboratories	Lactose-free, casein, and soy proteins; 1 kcal/mL; flavored for oral use	Powder and ready-to-feed
Boost	Mead Johnson	Lactose-free, casein and soy proteins; 1 kcal/mL; flavored for oral use	Powder and ready-to-feed
High-caloric or protein-dense supplements			
Deliver 2.0	Mead Johnson	Lactose-free, casein; 2.0 kcal/mL; flavored for oral use	
Ensure Plus	Ross Laboratories	Lactose-free, casein and soy proteins; 1.5 kcal/mL; flavored for oral use	
Isocal HN	Mead Johnson	High-nitrogen feeding for volume-restricted patients	
Magnacal	Mead Johnson	High-calorie tube feeding	
Nutren 2.0	Nestle Nutrition	Lactose-free, casein; 2.0 kcal/mL; flavored for oral use	
Promote	Ross Laboratories	Lactose-free, high-protein (casein and soy) tube feeding	
Scandishake	Scandipharm	Nonfat milk, high-calorie oral feeding supplement (1.65 kcal/mL)	Nutritionally incomplete
Sustacal Plus	Mead Johnson	Lactose-free, casein and soy proteins; 1.5 kcal/mL; flavored for oral use	
TwoCal HN	Ross Laboratories	High-calorie and nitrogen (casein) for volume-restricted patients	
Elemental or protein hydrolysate			
Criticare HN	Mead Johnson	Casein hydrolysate	
Peptamen	Nestle Nutrition	Whey hydrolysate, 70% MCT	
Reabilan	Nestle Nutrition	Casein hydrolysate, 40% MCT	
Tolerex Plus	Novartis Nutrition	Free amino acids, lower nitrogen, minimal fat	Includes glutamine, arginine, branched-chain amino acids
Vital HN	Ross Laboratories	Partially hydrolyzed whey, meat, and soy, with low fat	
Vivonex TEN	Novartis Nutrition	Free amino acids, higher nitrogen, minimal fat	
Specialized formulas			
Glucerna	Ross Laboratories	High-fiber, low-carbohydrate, high-fat	For diabetics and other patients with glucose intolerance
Glytrol	Nestle Nutrition	High-fiber, low-carbohydrate, high-fat	For diabetics and other patients with glucose intolerance
Hepatic-Acid		High branched-chain amino acids	For patients with hepatic encephalopathy
Impact	Norvatis Nutrition	Increased RNA, arginine	Possible immune system modulation
Liposorb	Mead Johnson	1.35 kcal/ml; 86% MCT	For fat malabsorption
Pulmocare	Ross Laboratories	Lactose-free, high-fat, low-carbohydrate formula	Reduces CO_2 production in COPD
Respalor	Mead Johnson	Lactose-free, high-fat, low-carbohydrate formula	Reduces CO_2 production in COPD
Suplena	Ross Laboratories	High-calorie (2.0 kcal/mL), low-protein, low-electrolyte	For renal insufficiency

(continued)

TABLE 17-13 Continued

MODULAR ADDITIVES

Formula	Manufacturer	Kcal	Prot. (g)	mOsm/kg	Protein Source	Carbohydrate Source	Fat Source
Benefiber	Novartis Nutrition	16 per tbs	0	—	—		
Casec	Mead Johnson	17 per tbs	4 g per tbs	—	Casein, soy		
MCT Oil	Mead Johnson	7.67 per mL	0	—			
Microlipid	Mead Johnson	4.5 per mL	0	70			Safflower oil emulsion
Moducal Powder	Mead Johnson	3.8 per g	0	—		Maltodextrin	
Polycose Liquid	Ross Laboratories	2.0 per mL	0	900			

ᵃ Not all commercial formulas are included. Manufacturers throughout the world sell similar formulas. Formulas are listed with general characteristics. For precise constituents, check with the manufacturer because all are subject to change with minimal or no notice.

ᵇ Methionine is added to all of the soy formulas for a complete protein source.

ᶜ Except where indicated, these formulas are not appropriate for term infants.

ᵈ These formulas are marketed as alternatives to whole cow's milk. They are not necessary for a child eating a balanced diet.

ᵉ All of these formulas are ready-to-feed.

ᶠ Not recommended for infants because of increased renal solute load and poorly digestible fat.

ᵍ Increased risk of contamination and improper dilution.

LCT = long-chain triglyceride; MCT = medium-chain triglyceride; BM = breast milk.

SOURCE: *Portions of this table were provided in part from Maria Melko, RD, CSP, and Annette Stralovich, RD, Department of Nutrition and Dietetics, University of California, San Francisco.*

17.4   NUTRITIONAL ASSESSMENT

Neal S. LeLeiko and Miriam Horowitz

Assessing the nutritional status of an individual generally is referred to as "nutritional assessment," and it includes the evaluation of normal growth and health, evaluation for nutritional risk factors contributing to diseases, and the early detection and treatment of nutritional deficiencies and excesses. Complete nutritional assessment integrates a combination of subjective medical evaluations and objective measurements of the medical and nutritional history, including past and present dietary intake; physical examination, including anthropometric measurements and growth assessment; biochemical and metabolic parameters; and anticipation of future medical course (including likely complications) and effects of therapy.

Nutritional assessment in children is especially important because the single most important cause of growth retardation worldwide is undernutrition. Nutritional assessment of a disease-free infant who is seen for a health maintenance examination is a substantially different process than that for an infant with a known chronic illness. A healthy child on a routine visit to the doctor requires only a measurement of height, weight, and, for infants, head circumference (plotted on appropriate growth charts) along with a routine history and physical examination. A routine history should include a nutritional history with questions regarding family attitudes toward "health foods," "junk foods," dieting, fad diets, nutritional supplements, herbal remedies, and general nutrition. If growth is normal and there are no unusual dietary habits, further assessment is not required. The patient with poor growth or weight gain requires a more careful nutritional assessment. Any child with a history of poor growth or a chronic disorder placing him or her at risk for malnutrition should have a periodic nutritional assessment.

MEDICAL AND NUTRITIONAL HISTORY

Obtaining an accurate nutritional history is challenging. Twenty-four-hour dietary recall provides useful information, but a careful 3-day diet history that records the amount of each food or liquid that is consumed is more accurate, and 7-day diaries are preferable if feasible. Analysis of these records by a pediatric dietitian provides valuable information on caloric intake and the intake of specific nutrients. The medical history may suggest inadequate intake or malabsorption. Factors that increase energy expenditure such as fever, tachypnea, and tachycardia should be recognized.

The most useful measure of nutritional status remains the correlation of weight and height with normative values for age. Longitudinal assessment of height and weight is the best approach to monitoring nutritional adequacy in patients with chronic diseases. Slowing of growth will occur before specific indicators of malnutrition are apparent; however, the physical examination can identify signs of overt nutritional deficiency, including angular stomatitis, cheilosis, glossitis, wasting, or edema. Pubertal development is affected by nutritional status, and the Tanner stage of sexual development should be recorded. Measurements of temperature, heart rate, and blood pressure are important in the assessment of a child with severe malnutrition because hypothermia and bradycardia are grave prognostic indicators.

There are several different criteria using weight and height to classify malnutrition, and all must be judiciously applied. The most useful and widely employed are the Waterlow classification and the Gomez criteria, which are used to distinguish a chronically malnourished or "stunted" child from an acutely malnourished or "wasted" child. An expected (or predicted) weight-for-height index is employed. This assessment allows classification of the degree of stunting (ie, decreased height for age, an indicator of chronic malnutrition) and wasting (ie, decreased weight for height, an indicator of acute malnutrition). The severity of an individual's wasting and/or stunting is calculated as a percentage of the reference median value. The 50th percentile weight for that age and height for age are taken as the denominator, and the actual weight or height as the numerator. Gomez criteria assess the degree of malnutrition based upon weight for age. The actual weight is compared to the median value (50th percentile for age) for the patient's actual age. This criterion aids in the recognition of acute malnutrition. Waterlow's revised grading index for height for age and weight for height and the Gomez criteria can be found in Table 17-14.

It must be emphasized that this system of classification is useful, but it is inadequate for the complete assessment of the individual child. Chronic stunting and insufficient weight gain will result in a weight-for-height percentile that is within normal limits despite the fact that weight for age and height for age are both below the fifth percentile. This should not be interpreted as nutritionally adequate; rather, it reveals that the patient's failure to thrive is chronic.

Measurement of triceps skinfold thickness and midarm circumference provide a useful estimate of adipose tissue and lean body mass, respectively. These measurements are reliable, however, only when performed by an experienced individual such as a pediatric dietitian, and they are most useful when measured serially, being subject to intra- and interobserver variability.

BIOCHEMICAL ASSESSMENT

Several laboratory tests may reflect nutritional status, but none alone may be considered a useful parameter of nutritional assessment. Only in the correct clinical context do any biochemical measures become useful. Hemoglobin concentration, iron, total serum proteins, albumin, transferrin, cholesterol, triglyceride, and blood levels of some vitamins may be helpful in specific disease states. Measurement of visceral proteins allows some assessment of overall nutritional adequacy. Serum albumin values vary with acute infection, trauma, or stress, and they may be abnormal because of liver

TABLE 17-14

CLASSIFICATIONS OF MALNUTRITION

GRADE OF MALNU-TRITION	WEIGHT/ HEIGHT[a] (% of median)	HEIGHT/ AGE[a] (% of median)	WEIGHT/ AGE[b] (% of median)
0 degree	>90	>95	—
First degree (mild)	81-90	90-95	75-85
Second degree (moderate)	70-80	85-89	64-74
Third degree (severe)	<70	<85	<64

[a] Waterlow classification.

[b] Gomez criteria.

or renal disease. In addition to albumin, other more rapidly metabolized proteins that may be useful to monitor nutritional status include transferrin, prealbumin, fibronectin, and retinol-binding protein.

17.5 NUTRITIONAL DEFICIENCY STATES

Neil S. Leleiko and Miriam Horowitz

17.5.1 Approach to the Child with Failure to Gain Weight

The concept of failure to thrive is discussed in Sec. 1.1.2. In the broadest sense, the term *failure to thrive* is used to describe infants and children whose growth deviates from that expected for their sex and age. The initial step in evaluation is to carefully examine growth records to determine if the infant or child is failing to grow or failing to gain weight. A proportional reduction in weight and stature rarely represents acute primary malnutrition. Caloric insufficiency from inadequate intake, malabsorption, or a hypermetabolic state is suggested when weight is significantly below that expected for chronologic age with relative sparing of both head circumference and height. Causes of failure to gain weight and the approach to the evaluation of a child with poor weight gain are discussed in Sec. 1.1.2. Regardless of the cause of failure to gain weight, careful attention to nutritional rehabilitation is essential. Nasogastric tube feeding may be necessary in children who refuse adequate intake of calories. If weight gain is achieved with tube feedings, the causes of feeding disorders, including psychosocial causes, should be investigated. If weight gain is not achieved with tube feedings, causes of malabsorption or an increased caloric requirement should be considered. Cardiopulmonary disease, malignancies, hyperthyroidism, and chronic infection all may increase caloric requirements. Children who gain weight in the hospital when fed normal age-appropriate meals require referral for social services and continued close follow-up. A multidisciplinary community-based team approach involving the primary physician, nutritionist, social worker, child behavior specialist, and other community services often is the most beneficial.

17.5.2 Protein-Energy Malnutrition

The etiology of malnutrition can be primary, as when the otherwise healthy individual's needs for protein, energy, or both are not met by an adequate diet, or secondary, as a result of disease states that may lead to suboptimal intake, inadequate nutrient absorption or use, and/or increased requirements because of nutrient losses or increased energy expenditure. Protein-energy malnutrition is the most important nutritional disease in developing countries and one of the leading causes of morbidity and mortality in childhood worldwide. In the Western world primary malnutrition continues to occur with alarming frequency because of poverty. Secondary malnutrition exists as a result of chronic or acute illness.

In primary protein-energy malnutrition, calorie inadequacies generally are linked to conditions of war, social disruption, poverty, ignorance, infectious diseases, and food distribution inequalities. Therefore, socioeconomic, political, and other environmental deprivations can be considered to be the most global cause for childhood starvation with its deleterious effects on growth and development.

In the clinical setting, acute and/or chronic illness may lead to malnutrition and, if prolonged, result in failure to thrive. Although the etiology of malnutrition can be traced to an underlying pathology (ie, increased energy needs secondary to respiratory distress, fever, wound healing, or a malabsorptive state), the common pathway to a malnourished state is still a net deficiency of the nutrients that are required for an individual. Although dietary energy and protein deficiencies typically occur in concert, one may predominate, resulting in either kwashiorkor (primarily a protein-deficient state) or marasmus (primarily an energy-deficient state). Marasmic kwashiorkor also can occur and is the combination of chronic energy deprivation with a superimposed chronic or acute protein deficit. In both pathologic states, apathy, indifference, fatigue, and irritability are common.

MARASMUS

Marasmus is characterized by generalized muscular wasting and absence of subcutaneous fat. Marasmic children appear to be emaciated and very cachectic (Fig. 17-14A). They suffer with severe wasting (ie, reduced weight:height ratio) and often have linear growth stunting as well. Their skin is dry, without turgor, and appears loose and wrinkled because of the loss of subcutaneous fat. The classic appearance of a sunken or "wizened" face, resembling that of an elderly person, results from the loss of the temporal and buccal fat pads. Buccal fat pads are among the last subcutaneous adipose depots to be mobilized in starvation, and their loss reflects the duration and severity of the malnutrition. The child's hair is thin, sparse, and brittle, and lacks its normal sheen. Adaptive metabolic features such as hypothermia, slow pulse rate, and hypotension usually are present, and hypoglycemia can occur because of fasting for prolonged periods of time.

KWASHIORKOR

Kwashiorkor is caused by an insufficient intake of protein that is of adequate biological value, and it often is associated with a deficient energy intake. The term kwashiorkor comes from an African dialect on the Gold Coast meaning "the disease of the deposed baby when the next one is born." The onset of kwashiorkor typically tends to appear in young children during the weaning and postweaning phases. In areas where kwashiorkor is endemic, the main dietary staples often are a carbohydrate source that is low in protein content and quality (eg, white rice, cassava, yams). A diet of this nature may produce a fat-appearing child and, as such, has been referred to in some parts of the world as a "sugar baby."

The predominant feature of relative protein malnutrition is soft, pitting, painless edema, usually in the feet and legs but extending to the face and upper extremities in severe cases (Fig. 17-14B). Most affected children have dermatoses, including hyperkeratosis and dyspigmentation secondary to desquamation of the epidermis. Hair texture is dry, brittle, and straight, and its color changes to red or yellowish-gray. During alternating periods of adequate and poor protein intake, the hair may reflect a pattern of alternating depigmentation. This is known as the *flag sign*, where normal hair changes to depigmented hair, correlating with nutritional state. Height may be normal or stunted, depending on the duration of the protein deprivation. Although weight loss usually is appreciated, failure to gain weight appropriately often is masked by the edema. These patients typically present with pale, cold peripheral extremities and have hepatomegaly secondary to fatty infiltration.

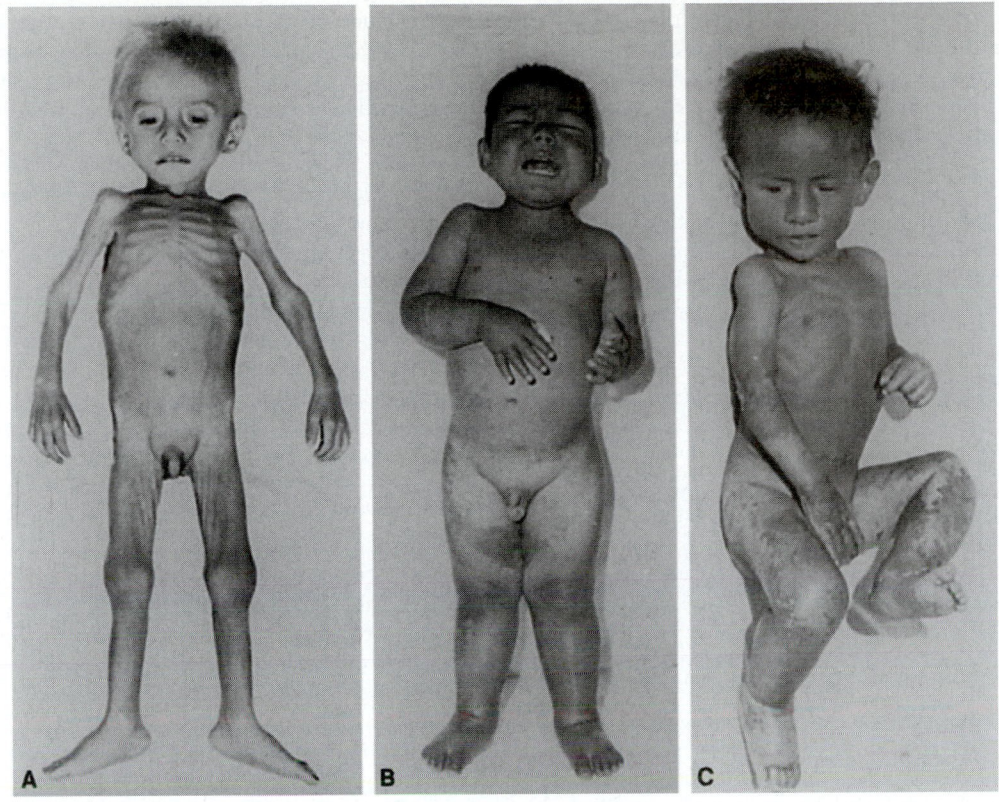

FIGURE 17-14   **A: Severe wasting in infant with marasmus. SOURCE:** *Courtesy of Dr. Benjamin Torun; from Suskind RM, ed: Textbook of Pediatric Nutrition. New York, Raven Press, 1981.* **B: Edema and skin lesions in a 3-year-old child with kwashiorkor. SOURCE:** *Courtesy of Dr. Benjamin Torun; from Shils ME, Olson JA, Shike M: Modern Nutrition in Health and Disease, 8th ed. Philadelphia, Lea & Febiger, 1990.* **C: Marasmic kwashiorkor. Note the features associated with both models of malnutrition, namely, wasting in the arms and trunk characteristic of kwashiorkor. SOURCE:** *Courtesy of Dr. Benjamin Torun; from Warren KS, Mahmoud AAF: Tropical and Geographical Medicine, 2nd ed. New York, McGraw-Hill, 1990.*

The abdomen is frequently protruding. T-cell lymphocytes and cell-mediated immune responses are blunted, making the child more susceptible to acute and chronic infections. A higher mortality rate is seen with kwashiorkor than with marasmus.

MARASMIC KWASHIORKOR

The marasmic kwashiorkor form of edematous protein-energy malnutrition is characterized by clinical features of both types of malnutrition. It can occur in prolonged protein malnutrition, when loss of subcutaneous tissue, muscle mass, and adipose stores also are prominent. The main features are the edema of kwashiorkor, with or without skin lesions, and the cachexia of marasmus (Fig. 17-14C). Marasmus, kwashiorkor, and marasmic kwashiorkor classically are described in the underdeveloped parts of the world. These specific illnesses are often influenced by local diets and intercurrent infections. Therefore, there are apparent differences from one region to another. In North America and Western Europe, problems of primary malnutrition are less common than are those of secondary malnutrition in children with other serious medical problems.

17.5.3   Refeeding Syndrome

The refeeding syndrome, which is a phenomenon first noted in postwar victims of chronic starvation, is a well-described metabolic complication of nutritional rehabilitation in severely malnourished individuals. Severe hypophosphatemia and its sequelae are the principal characteristics of refeeding syndrome. Congestive heart failure, respiratory distress, peripheral edema, convulsions, and coma have resulted from nutritional repletion after prolonged starvation. Aggressive use of total parenteral nutrition (TPN) also has accounted for refeeding syndrome catastrophes, including death in patients with anorexia nervosa or those with severe malnutrition secondary to malabsorption. Typically, patients are noted to have normal serum phosphorus levels before parenteral therapy is begun but extremely low phosphorus levels (ie, <1.2 mg/dL) at the time of decompensation.

Refeeding a malnourished individual stimulates insulin production, particularly when glucose is the predominant energy source, as in TPN. Carbohydrate repletion and insulin release together promote transport into the cell of glucose, phosphorus, water, and other predominantly intracellular ions such as potassium. The prior depletion of total body phosphorus stores during catabolism and starvation, coupled with the increased cellular influx of phosphorus during anabolic refeeding, leads to severe extracellular hypophosphatemia. Low serum phosphorus levels will eventually contribute to the intracellular depletion of phosphorylated intermediates that are necessary in intermediary metabolism and oxidative phosphorylation. Depletion of phosphorylated metabolic intermediates is thought to result in the clinical manifestations of the refeeding syndrome.

Although not classically associated with the refeeding syndrome, both hypokalemia and hypomagnesemia are well-described complications following commencement of both enteral and parenteral nutrition in severely malnourished patients. Because potassium and magnesium also are intracellular ions that are required for the synthesis of new cells, extracellular levels may fall during refeeding and therefore must be carefully monitored. The refeeding syndrome should be anticipated and phosphorus supplementation begun early in the process of nutritional resuscitation. Vigorous refeeding should be avoided during the early stages of repleting the severely malnourished patient.

17.5.4 Vegetarian Diets

Approximately 9 million Americans (approximately 4% of the U.S. population) currently consume a vegetarian diet. Children in these families likely will continue their parents' dietary habits. The American Dietetic Association and the Food and Nutrition Board of the National Research Council consider properly planned, balanced vegetarianism to be an acceptable diet alternative if it is appropriately supplemented. The groups who are especially at risk from these diets are pregnant and lactating women, infants, and children. All have in common an increased need to supply nutrition during an anabolically demanding period. The risks that are associated with vegetarianism increase in relation to the restrictiveness of the diet and/or lack of adequate planning. Children consuming a partial or semivegetarian diet are at little risk and actually are likely to be complying with recent dietary recommendations for the prevention of chronic illness.

Vegetarians typically are classified according to the types of protein they are willing to consume. *Pollovegetarians* will eat poultry (but no red meat); *pescovegetarians* will eat only fish and other seafoods; and *lactoovovegetarians* consume milk, dairy products, and eggs (but no seafood or meat). The *total* or *strict vegetarian*, or *vegan*, will not have any animal product, and he or she eats exclusively foods of plant origin. The risks of malnutrition are greatest in the strict vegetarian. Attaining caloric adequacy is the greatest problem for children consuming a vegetarian diet. To consume an appropriate energy intake with foods of low caloric density, the volume of intake must be considerably increased. This poses a much less severe problem for healthy adults than it does for growing children. Frequent meals and snacks and the use of some foods higher in fat can help vegetarian children meet their energy requirements. Adolescents may be at particular risk; dietary experimentation is part of the normal developmental process but occurs at the time of the pubertal growth spurt. Inadequate or inappropriate intake may result in decreased growth.

Vegetarian diets that contain a complete source of protein (ie, a source of protein containing the essential amino acids required by humans) such as eggs, milk, fish, or poultry can be planned for nutritional adequacy easily. Diets that contain only plant proteins that are incomplete (ie, they do not contain a full complement of essential amino acids) pose a significant planning problem. Typically, nuts, seeds, grains (ie, foods containing methionine) are combined with legumes (containing lysine) at the same meal so that adequate amounts of all essential amino acids are available for protein synthesis. This process, known as mutual supplementation, assures that there are no unduly limiting amino acids and that there is adequate dietary protein for protein synthesis. Recent research suggests that complementary proteins need not be consumed at the same meal. The consumption of essential amino acids over the course of the day should ensure adequate nitrogen retention and usage in healthy individuals. On the introduction of protein-rich foods into the infant's diet, pureed tofu, legumes, or cottage cheese is recommended.

Vitamin B_{12} is found only in products of animal origin, and this poses an important and serious risk to those vegetarians who do not consume animal products. Strict vegetarians must obtain vitamin B_{12} by using supplements or by eating vitamin B_{12}–fortified foods, including soy milk, yeast, and cereals. Although adults may take several years to develop vitamin B_{12} deficiency, infants who are breast-fed by mothers who are marginally deficient themselves are likely to be at a real and marked risk of vitamin B_{12} deficiency.

Iron, calcium, and zinc also are minerals of concern to vegetarians, especially if they do not consume animal products. Plant foods contain only nonheme iron, which is more susceptible to inhibitors of iron absorption than is heme iron (derived from meat, chicken, and fish). The vegetarian diet consists of a higher total iron content than the standard Western diet. However, iron stores in vegetarians are lower because of poor absorption of iron from plant sources. High vitamin C intake can aid in nonheme iron absorption.

Adequate calcium intake is a concern for all populations. It is of particular concern for children who consume a strict vegan diet. Foods rich in calcium should be emphasized, including calcium-fortified soy milk and calcium-fortified juices. Vegan diets tend to be vitamin D poor. Therefore, children should be exposed to sunlight and provided with vitamin D–fortified foods to meet their needs. The bioavailability of zinc from plant sources is low. As a result, vegetarians show a lower intake of zinc than nonvegetarians. It is recommended that vegetarians strive to exceed the RDAs for zinc. Supplementation of vitamins and minerals may be necessary to prevent deficiency.

The role of dietary counseling is to teach the appropriate combinations of foods that are required to achieve nutritional balance. The more restrictive the diet and the younger the child, the greater is the need for professional nutritional advice. A Food Guide Pyramid for Vegetarian Meal Planning has been developed as a guide to achieving a balanced vegetarian diet (*www.vegsource.com/nutrition/pyramid.htm*).

17.5.5 Food Fadism and Nutrition Quackery

Food fadism and quackery involve the unusual patterns of food behavior that are enthusiastically promoted and/or adopted by their adherents. Typically, nutrition fadists and quacks claim that a particular food or nutrient has a specific therapeutic value, can cure disease, or has only positive effects. They downplay or totally ignore any negative or side effects. They may claim that dietary supplements such as vitamins or special nutrients are routinely needed to achieve a healthy balanced diet or that amino acid supplements have special values unto themselves and that supplements will enhance stamina, endurance, and muscle growth. A particular regimen often is claimed to achieve particular benefits (eg, to cure obesity). Frequently, the proposed beneficial product can be purchased through only one particular company or source, and proponents discredit "conventional" sources of information as not being credible while providing testimonial evidence or a celebrity endorsement as their evidence of efficacy.

Food fadism and quackery cause harm in many ways. They cost the economy billions of dollars a year in useless expense. Sometimes, patients are harmed indirectly through delays in seeking useful treatment or advice. Direct harm ensues when a so-called alternative treatment causes death, serious injury, or unnecessary suffering. Psychological harm is inevitable when vulnerable and sometimes desperate individuals blame themselves for ineffective therapy. Surprisingly, this may result in making them even more susceptible to future deception. Finally, there is an incalculable harm to our society when the general public uses erroneous and unfounded beliefs as a foundation for unrealistic expectations about nutrition and health. These unrealistic expectations often seriously undermine confidence in the scientific approach to problems in general and to legitimate providers of health care in particular.

References

Infant Formulas

Foman SJ, Ziegler EE: Renal solute load and potential renal solute load in infancy. J Pediatr 134:11–14, 1999

Failure to Gain Weight

Farrell MK: Failure to thrive. In: Wyllie R, Hyams JS, eds: Pediatric Gastrointestinal Disease. Philadelphia, WB Saunders, 1993:271–280
Homer C, Ludwig S: Categorization of the etiology of failure to thrive. Am J Dis Child 135:848–851, 1981
Petersen KE, Washington J, Rathbun JM: Team management of failure to thrive. J Am Diet Assoc 84:810–815, 1984

Nutritional Deficiency States

Knochel JP: The clinical status of hypophosphatemia: an update. N Engl J Med 313:447, 1985
Shils ME, Olson JA, Shike M: Modern Nutrition in Health and Disease, 8th ed. Philadelphia, Lea & Febiger, 1990
Solomon SM, Kirby DF: The refeeding syndrome: a review. J Parent Ent Nutr 14:90, 1990
Viteri FE: Protein energy malnutrition. In: Walker WA, Durie PR, Hamilton JR, et al, eds: Pediatric Gastrointestinal Disease, 1st ed. Philadelphia, Decker, 1991:1596–1611
World Health Organization (WHO): Energy and Protein Requirements. FAO/WHO/UNU Expert Consultation Technical Report Series 724. Geneva, WHO, 1985

Vegetarian Diets

ADA (American Dietetic Association): Position paper on the vegetarian approach to eating. J Am Diet Assoc 77:61, 1980
American Academy of Pediatrics, Committee on Nutrition: Pediatric Nutrition Handbook. Elk Grove Village, IL, American Academy of Pediatrics, 1993
Jacobs C, Dwyer JT: Vegetarian children: appropriate and inappropriate diets. Am J Clin Nutr 48:811, 1988

Food Fadism and Quackery

Schafer R, Yetley EA: Fad diets. J Am Diet Assoc 66:129, 1975
Shils ME, Olson JA, Shike M: Modern Nutrition in Health and Disease, 8th ed. Philadelphia, Lea & Febiger, 1990

17.6 SPECIALIZED NUTRITIONAL SUPPORT: ENTERAL AND PARENTERAL NUTRITION

Melvin Heyman

Specialized nutritional support is required to provide either total or partial nutrient supplementation for patients with general undernutrition or other specific nutritional deficiencies. Nutrition support can be provided intravenously (total parenteral nutrition, TPN), enterally, or by a combination of both routes. The goal of appropriate nutrition therapy is to improve the outcome of a patient's primary illness, although data supporting this goal are typically lacking. As noted in the preceding sections, an individual's requirements for nutrients cannot be accurately predicted. Therefore, careful monitoring of the nutritional status, including evaluation of growth and developmental parameters, diet history, physical examination, anthropometric measurements, and laboratory determinations, is required at regular intervals in all patients receiving specialized nutritional support. Teams that provide pediatric nutritional support services include physicians, nurse specialists, dietitians, pharmacologists, social workers, and feeding therapists. Such teams are now available at major centers to assist or impart guidance to provide and monitor nutritional support for pediatric patients.

17.6.1 Enteral Nutritional Support

Enteral alimentation, which means supplying nutrition via the functioning gastrointestinal tract, is preferable to intravenous feeding because it is more physiological and less costly, and has far fewer and less serious complications. Nevertheless, proper caution must be exercised to avoid deleterious effects from enteral feeding.

Nutrients can be introduced into the intestinal tract by oral intake or by orogastric, nasogastric, nasoduodenal, esophagostomy, gastrostomy, jejunostomy, or gastrojejunostomy feeding tubes. The route selected depends on patient tolerance and the underlying medical condition necessitating specialized nutritional support. The orogastric route, most commonly employed in preterm infants with immature suck and swallow mechanisms, is useful to provide access for bolus feedings directly into the stomach; the tube usually is removed after each feeding. Nasogastric intubation permits more prolonged feedings, because the tube can be secured and left in position for up to several weeks. Gastrostomy feedings are implemented when the oral and nasal routes cannot be used, when patients have severe neuromuscular problems with dysphagia, or when long-term access for enteral tube feeding is necessary. Nasoduodenal or jejunostomy tubes are used in patients who may have abnormal gastric emptying or gastroesophageal reflux and aspiration. Additionally, with specially designed tubes and sometimes with the assistance of a gastroenterologist or radiologist, a gastrostomy tube can be converted into a gastrojejunostomy tube to treat these patients. Indications and contraindications for tube feedings are listed in Table 17-15.

Tube choice and route selection are two of the most important components in the delivery of enteral nutrition (see Table 17-16). Generally, the smallest size enteral tube should be chosen and the tube should be replaced only when necessary. If long-term feedings are anticipated, tubes should be polyurethane or silicone to reduce

TABLE 17-15

INDICATIONS AND CONTRAINDICATIONS FOR ENTERAL TUBE FEEDING

Indications
  Inadequate intake
    Inability to coordinate swallowing
      Prematurity
      Oropharyngeal disease
    Craniofacial trauma, especially fractured jaw
    Esophageal disorders, especially obstructive
    Central nervous system disorders
      Coma
      Severe cerebral palsy
      Cerebral trauma
      Encephalopathy
      Degenerative neurologic disorders
    Myopathies
    Anorexia
    Psychiatric disorders
      Anorexia nervosa
      Severe depression
    Inflammatory disorders (eg, collagen vascular disease, AIDS)
    Surgery
    Neoplasms
  Involuntary supplementation
    Failure to thrive associated with inadequate intake
    Transition from parenteral to enteral nutrition
    Inflammatory bowel disease
  Requiring specialized formulas
    Inherited metabolic disorders (eg, glycogen storage disease)
  Malabsorption
    Gastrointestinal disease
      Crohn disease
      Short-bowel syndrome
      Chronic diarrhea with malabsorption
      Severe gastroesophageal reflux[a]
      Pancreatitis
      Distal small intestinal fistulas
      Cystic fibrosis
  Increased Requirements
    Hypermetabolic states
      Trauma
      Sepsis
      Burns
      Severe cardiac anomalies
      Severe respiratory failure
Contraindications
  Intestinal obstruction
  Persistent emesis
  Severe respiratory distress
  Upper gastrointestinal bleeding
  Necrotizing enterocolitis

---

[a] Placement of a tube distal to the pylorus may be preferable.

the frequency of tube replacement and minimize trauma. Use of weighted tubes should be avoided to decrese the risk of bowel perforation. Gastrostomy tubes are commonly used in patients who require prolonged enteral nutritional support. Some patients are able to tolerate prolonged use of nasogastric feedings and avoid a gastrostomy; however, patients who will require tube feedings for more than 3 to 6 months should be considered for gastrostomy tube placement to avoid complications and trauma with the replacement of nasogastric tubes. This is particularly important with infants and young children, who may develop a severe feeding aver-

sion that is exacerbated by nasogastric tube irritation of the nasal passages and oropharynx. Placement of a gastrostomy tube will facilitate progression of oromotor development in some of these children even though they still depend on tube feedings for their nutrition.

Gastrostomy tubes can be placed either percutaneously, using endoscopic techniques, or surgically. Percutaneous endoscopic gastrostomy (PEG) placement, initially described by Gauderer and colleagues in 1980, is an accepted procedure that is relatively simple; a skilled endoscopist and pediatric surgeon can perform the procedure in less than 10 minutes. Although adults have the procedure performed with conscious sedation, infants and children usually require general anesthesia for PEG placement. The principal contraindications to placement of a PEG are overlying organs (eg., liver, colon), ascites, a coagulopathy, and failure to transilluminate the stomach, often resulting from a major portion of the stomach lying above the costal margin. PEG tubes have been successfully placed in patients who have undergone prior abdominal surgical procedures, including those with indwelling ventriculoperitoneal (VP) shunts, and in patients with various deformities including intestinal malrotation or severe scoliosis. Additionally, successful PEG placement has been reported in infants under 2 kg body weight. Complications of PEG tube placement include infection, which is decreased by prophylactic antibiotics before placement, pneumoperitoneum, transient fever, pain, bleeding, gastric ulceration from direct erosion of the gastric mucosa by the internal portion of the gastrostomy tube, ileus, gastric separation, gastric fistula, gastrocolic fistula, and tube extrusion. Removal of PEG devices for replacement with a standard gastrostomy tube usually is not performed for 3 months after placement to allow complete healing and maturation of the gastrostomy. Several tubes are available for use in a gastrostomy, ranging from skin-level, low-profile "buttons" to standard gastrostomy tubes (similar to Foley catheters). The choice of tube depends on the patient's and caretaker's needs and tolerance.

Pediatricians should be aware of the tubes, equipment, and resources (eg, nursing, nutritional, pharmaceutical, and home care companies) that are available in the local area because, with the current emphasis on shorter hospital stays, more patients will be discharged quickly on enteral feeding regimens and require follow-up care from their primary physicians. Management approaches for the most common complications of tube feedings are summarized in Table 17-17. These include local infections, expansion of the size of the ostomy opening with leakage around the tube, development of granulation tissue around the ostomy, inadvertent removal of the tube, movement of the tube (eg, causing pyloric obstruction), and aspiration of gastric contents.

Once a decision is made to start a patient on tube feedings, a formula must be selected; its strength, rate of infusion, and route of administration determined; and a tube selected. An *appropriate* formula must be carefully chosen by considering the patient's age, underlying disease process, and GI function. Commonly available formulas in the United States are listed in Table 17-13. Human breast milk or special premature formulas can be administered either by bolus or continuous drip to premature infants (Sec. 2.12.5). Standard infant formulas can be used for those with extraintestinal problems such as lack of oral intake secondary to anoxic brain damage. Similarly, complete formulas can be used in older children who are unable to eat because of coma, severe burns, trauma, or other reasons, or who may benefit from supplemental nutrition infused overnight.

TABLE 17-16
ENTERAL FEEDING DEVICE SELECTION

ROUTE	INDICATIONS	TUBE SELECTION
Nasogastric	For children with a functional gastrointestinal tract requiring 6 weeks or less of enteral feeding.	• Available in 5 Fr to 18 Fr • Choose the smallest tube through which formula will flow, usually 6 Fr to 8 Fr are typical • 5 Fr for infants <2.25 kg • Polyurethane and silicone are softer and longer lasting • Tube and tip are radiopaque
Nasoduodenal or nasojejunal	For children with a functional gastrointestinal tract requiring 6 weeks or less of enteral feeding. May be used postoperatively following gastric surgery.	• Available in a variety of sizes but longer than nasogastric tubes • Usually 8 Fr, 120 cm is used • Some weighted, usually with tungsten • Radiopaque
Gastrostomy	For children requiring long-term feeding longer than 6 weeks with a functional GI tract.	• Available in a variety of sizes, 12 Fr to 28 Fr • With or without disks • Tubes have an external skin disk and an internal bumper or balloon to secure placement • Balloon comes in 5-30 mL • Skin-level devices are available and are recommended for children when possible • Radiopaque
Jejunostomy	For children requiring long-term feeding longer than 6 weeks at risk for aspiration and for children whose GI tracts are compromised above the jejunum.	• Some J tubes are designed for placement through a balloon gastrostomy tube; these generally have poor gastric venting abilities • Surgically placed J tube sizes range from 12 Fr to 24 Fr • Balloon tubes are contraindicated for use in the jejunum • Radiopaque

Lactose-free, low-residue, isotonic formulas may be useful in patients with chronic diarrhea. If these are not tolerated, or a patient has lost much of his or her intestinal digestive and absorptive function, a semielemental (ie, chemically defined) formula that is specifically designed to meet the nutritional needs of infants [eg, Pregestimil (Mead Johnson), Nutramigen (Mead Johnson), or Alimentum (Ross Laboratories)] can be instituted. Under certain circumstances, including patients with severe malabsorption conditions or exquisite protein intolerance, elemental formulas may be required. Most elemental formulas provide protein as free amino acids, adequate long-chain fatty acids to meet essential fatty acid requirements, glucose and glucose polymers, minerals, vitamins, and trace elements. Neocate (SHS North America) is the first elemental formula designed to meet the nutritional needs of infants. Elecare (Ross Laboratories) and Vivonex Pediatric (Novartis Nutrition) are elemental formulas that can be used to meet the specific nutritional requirements of toddlers and children. Note that long-term effects and outcomes have not been investigated for any of these formulas. In the event that formulas are used that have been formulated to meet adult requirements [eg, Tolerex or Vivonex Plus (Novartis Nutrition) or Neocate One (SHS North America)], mineral and vitamin supplements should be provided (eg, calcium, phosphorus, vitamin D).

Modular solutions that are nutritionally complete offer the opportunity to cater the regimen to meet specific needs. As examples, fat [Microlipid (Sherwood Medical)], protein [Casec (Mead Johnson)], and carbohydrate [Polycose (Ross Laboratories)] can be added to a formula to modify its composition and meet the specific needs of selected patients. Low-residue partially (ie, semielemental) or completely (ie, elemental) digested formulas are useful during

the transition from parenteral to enteral alimentation because intestinal enzyme systems atrophy during TPN support. Considerations in choosing an enteral formula include the underlying diagnosis, nutritional status, GI function, formula osmolality, protein source and quantity, lipid content and composition, mineral, vitamin, and trace element content, feeding route, lactose (and other carbohydrate) tolerance, fiber content, and cost. Development of future formulas may lead to the addition of nutrients such as glutamine (a preferred nutrient of enterocytes), nucleotides (to augment the immune system), and growth factors.

Enteral feedings should be initiated slowly in patients with significant GI dysfunction and who are on TPN. Because hypotonic and hypertonic solutions may adversely affect gastric emptying, and using a dilute formula plus parenteral alimentation may compromise fluid status, a full-strength isotonic formula can be started at a slow, continuous rate (1 to 2 mL/kg/h). As the enteral flow rate is increased, the parenteral infusion rate can be decreased almost equally until full nutritional support by tube feeding is achieved. In patients with intact GI tracts, feedings can be initiated using a full-strength formula at a slow infusion rate or a diluted formula (eg, one-third to one-half strength) at full volume. Tolerance is continuously assessed by monitoring clinical changes such as abdominal distension, intake and output (including diarrhea and vomiting), the amount of residual food in the stomach, GI blood loss, and reducing substances and pH of the stool.

Monitoring patients who are on enteral nutrition regimens is important to determine whether the selected regimen meets the nutritional goals for each patient. Additionally, complications can be avoided by reinforcing proper preparation and administration of nutrients as well as assessing metabolic imbalances before they be-

TABLE 17-17

COMPLICATIONS OF ENTERAL FEEDINGS

PROBLEM	POSSIBLE CAUSE	SOLUTION
Mechanical problems		
Impairment of child development	1. Enteral feedings and tube interfere with feeding skill development and normal activity	1. Develop feeding schedule so that child learns association between oral activity and satiety. Establish a nonnutritive program. If possible offer small amounts of food from spoon and fluids from a cup. These offerings should be before enteral feedings. 2. Instruct family to secure tube and place child on abdomen to promote upper body development and encourage crawling. 3. Encourage normal clothing. 4. Consider skin-level device as early as possible. 5. If oral food refusal results, consult an occupational and speech pathologist.
Leaking of gastric contents onto the abdomen	Balloon or bulb of tube has slipped away from the stomach. 1. Balloon has deflated 2. Child has increased pressure in stomach from air, delayed gastric emptying, coughing, causing formula to leak 3. Tube is too small for size of stoma 4. Loss of perpendicular position 5. Frequent positioning of child onto the left side 6. Frequent pulling at tube 7. Tube's valve is defective	1. Check marking on tube and gently pull back on catheter/tube to assure that balloon is snug against stomach wall. 2. Add water to the balloon or change tube. 3. Vent tube before or after feeding. Protect skin with barrier creams. 4. Placing a larger tube is usually not recommended. Take tube out to allow stoma to shrink down. Check stoma diameter every half hour. 5. Secure tube to the abdomen to maintain the perpendicular position to the tract with minimal tension. 6. Limit the time spent on the left side after feeding. 7. Restraints or one-piece T-shirts as needed. 8. Change tube.
Redness or drainage around tube/stoma	1. Some redness and drainage are normal 2. Skin irritation results from dampness and/or leaking around tube 3. Ineffective cleaning 4. Tube has not been rotated 5. Securing device is too tight 6. Peristomal wound infection	1. Assess area more frequently. 2. Keep skin dry. Antacids or barrier creams may be necessary to protect the skin. 3. Clean area with mild soap and water. Avoid routine use of hydrogen peroxide. 4. Rotate tube once a day. 5. Loosen securing device and assess daily for ability to move slightly. (Area between the abdomen and securing device should be about the depth of a dime). 6. Antibiotic ointments or antifungals should be used only with signs of infection.

Clogged tube
  Inability to irrigate tube
  Increased formula in reflux bag
  Feedings will not flow
	1. Lack of routine flushing
	2. Aspirating gastric contents frequently
	3. Medication-formula interaction
	4. Inadequately crushed medications through the tube
	5. Gastric reflux
	6. Formula too viscous
		1. Flush tube before and after feedings and medications. Use warm water with a syringe and slight pulsating pressure every 10 minutes for 1 hour.
		2. Irrigate the tube before and after residual checks.
		3. Assess medication-formula compatibility.
		4. Crush medications finely. Use liquid when possible.
		5. Consider intestinal feedings.
		6. Use formula designed for tube diameter and change formula to one with a lower viscosity.
		7. Consider milking the tube to alleviate the obstruction.

Nasal/pharyngeal/esophageal irritation and erosion	1. Prolonged intubation with large-bore NG tube	1. Use the softest/smallest-caliber feeding tube when possible. 2. Regular assessment of nares. Moisten and clean nares every 8 hours. Lubricate lips. 3. Secure tube properly. 4. Consider gastrostomy and jejunostomy tubes for long-term feeding (> 3 months).

(continued)

TABLE 17-17   Continued

PROBLEM	POSSIBLE CAUSE	SOLUTION
Granulation tissue buildup around gastrostomy tube	1. A small amount of epithelial tissue is normal and not painful 2. Tissue may increase with increased movement 3. Some children are more prone than others	1. Skin care to prevent irritation. 2. Secure tube to minimize movement. 3. Apply silver nitrate to the tissue every other day for 1 week. 4. Cauterization may be necessary.
Bleeding	1. May occur with tube change 2. Excessive tension on the tube 3. Movement of tube against mucosa 4. Gastric ulcers or pressure necrosis	1. Lubricate the new tube well before insertion. 2. Allow slight movement in tube between the gastric and abdominal wall. 3. Secure the tube. 4. Acid inhibition, endoscopy.

Migration of tube
  Stomach to intestines (increase in stools)
  Stomach to esophagus (retching, vomiting, coughing)
  Tube into the tract (pain)
	1. Movement or migration of tube	1. Secure tube and monitor length of external tube.
		2. Restrain as necessary.
		3. Antiemetic as necessary.
		4. Stop feeding if tube position is unknown.
		5. Reposition tube.
		6. May need to verify tube position with x-ray.

Accidental removal of tube
  NG
  GT
  JT
	1. Child pulls on tube
	2. Balloon deflated
	3. Tube not secured
		1. Secure tube as instructed.
		2. Restraints may be necessary.
		3. Cover the area with a small dressing and cover with tape.
		4. Replacement should occur within 4 hours.
		5. Damaged tubes should always be replaced.
		6. If possible, consider skin-level devices.
		7. Replacement of J tubes needs to be confirmed by x-ray.

Aspiration	1. Delayed gastric emptying 2. Gastroesophageal reflux 3. Gastroparesis 4. Poor gag reflex 5. Vomiting	1. Stop feeding immediately if aspiration is suspected. 2. Never feed if child feels full or sick or is vomiting. 3. Check placement of tube. 4. Check aspirates. 5. Never feed child flat. Place on right side, sit up, or raise head of bed 30-45°. 6. Continuous feeding rather than bolus. 7. Consider antireflux medication.
Gastrointestinal problems Nausea and vomiting	1. Rapid formula administration 2. High osmolality 3. Gastric retention 4. Air in stomach 5. Tube migration from stomach to small intestine 6. Medications given with feeding 7. Child's position	1. For continuous feedings, reduce rate of administration. For bolus feedings, increase length of time for feedings. Offer smaller and more frequent feedings. 2. Select isotonic or dilute formula. Gradually increase to full-strength formula. 3. Avoid adding other food to formula (ie, strained or dehydrated baby food). Consider gastric stimulant to promote gastric emptying, continuous feedings, or postpyloric feedings. 4. Burp child during feedings or allow for short breaks. Elevate child's head during feeding and for 30 minutes after meals. Decompress routinely. 5. Stop feeding and reposition tube against stomach wall. 6. Change times of medication if possible. Check contents of medications. 7. Keep head of child elevated when feeding.

(continued)

TABLE 17-17   Continued

PROBLEM	POSSIBLE CAUSE	SOLUTION
Diarrhea	1. Rapid formula administration 2. Hyperosmolar or low-residue formulas 3. Intolerance of formula (allergy/lactose intolerance) 4. Malabsorption 5. Hypoalbuminemia 6. Bacterial contamination 7. Rapid GI transit time 8. Prolonged antibiotic therapy or other medications	1. Reduce rate of administration or initiate feedings at a low rate. 2. Rule out formula-related causes. Select isotonic or fiber-supplemented formula. Consider diluting formula concentration and gradually increase the strength. 3. Use formula lacking intolerance component (ie, lactose free). 4. Consider use of elemental or semielemental formula, MCT oil. 5. If absorptive capacity of the small intestine is compromised, consider use of hydrolyzed, peptide-based formulas or parenteral nutrition. 6. Use commercially prepared sterile formulas. Use aseptic techniques in handling and administering feedings. Avoid hanging feedings over a prolong time. Do not use a delivery set for over 24 hours. Throw away any opened formula refrigerated over 48 hours. 7. Select formula with fiber supplement. 8. Send stool for *C. difficile* toxin and culture. Monitor medications (? sorbitol content) and eliminate causative medication if possible. Check time medications are given. 9. If diarrhea persists, measure stool electrolytes and osmolality. Consider holding feedings for 24 hours and monitor effect on stool output. 10. If osmotic diarrhea persists or if secretory diarrhea is diagnosed, begin parenteral nutrition.
Cramping, gas, abdominal distention	1. Rapid administration of formula 2. Administration of cold formula 3. Malabsorption of formula	1. Reduce rate of formula administration and deliver according to patient tolerance. 2. Administer formula at room temperature. 3. Select hydrolyzed formula.
Constipation	1. Inadequate fluid 2. Inadequate fiber 3. Inadequate activity 4. Fecal impaction 5. Obstruction	1. Monitor and increase fluids. 2. Consider formula with fiber or add fiber supplement. Try prune juice. 3. Encourage activity. 4. Disimpact and add stool softeners. 5. Stop feedings.

SOURCE: *Table provided courtesy of Debby Mason, RN, PNP.*

come clinically evident. Common complications include aspiration, diarrhea, nausea, vomiting, dehydration, abdominal distention or cramps, constipation, bacterial contamination of the formula or the upper intestinal tract, nasal or skin ulcers, obstruction or infection of nasal passages, and electrolyte and mineral imbalances. Severe complications such as perforation of the posterior pharynx, esophagus, or cribiform fossa (resulting in intracranial placement of the feeding tube) are rare and generally avoidable by use of proper precautions and techniques.

17.6.2   Parenteral Nutritional Support

Parenteral nutritional support should be used for patients who are unable to maintain adequate nutritional status orally or by tube feedings via the GI tract. TPN is used when the intestinal tract cannot be used at all because of intestinal malformations or other congenital anomalies, GI surgery, suspected necrotizing enterocolitis, severe respiratory distress, pancreatitis, or other conditions in which the intestinal tract may not be able to assume the role of nutrient digestion and absorption. Supplemental parenteral nutrition is useful when the intestinal tract can assimilate some but not all of the nutrients that are necessary for normal maintenance and growth. The enhanced capability to provide defined enteral formulas with partially or completely predigested nutrients enables physicians to provide absorbable feedings; therefore, patients may require only partial supplementation of nutrients via the parenteral route. Enteral nutrients stimulate gut hormones and other secretions that may be trophic factors to the intestinal tract and, thus, may be beneficial where gut regeneration is necessary. Because prolonged use of parenteral nutrition is associated with significant complications as well as expense, careful selection of patients and judicious use of available enteral and parenteral solutions are particularly important.

As in enteral support, patient selection begins with nutritional assessment. Included in this process is a determination of whether the GI tract will be unable to absorb sufficient nutrients, in which case nutrient infusions bypassing the GI tract may be required. Indications for parenteral nutritional support are listed in Table 17-18. This list is not meant to be definitive or exhaustive; rather, it provides examples of conditions for which parenteral nutrition has been used with some success. Improved technology for and understanding of enteral nutritional support have allowed the replacement of parenteral with enteral support for some of these disorders. Each patient should be judged individually regarding needs and possible benefits versus risk of parenteral versus enteral therapy.

Parenteral nutrition may be infused via peripheral veins in patients with good venous access who require short-term (ie, <2 weeks) support and no fluid restriction. The maximum recommended concentration through a peripheral vein is 12.5% dextrose; this reduces the risk of thrombophlebitis, which occurs when the osmolality of the solution exceeds 900 mOsm/kg. Patients in whom caloric needs cannot be met by the peripheral venous route require a central venous catheter for nutrient infusion. The dextrose concentration then can be raised to 20 to 30% (ie, 2000 to 3000 mOsm/kg) or greater when infused through a central line placed appropriately, usually by an experienced pediatric surgeon, into the right atrium or superior or inferior vena cava. Percutaneous intravenous central catheters ("PICC lines") are also utilized for long-term venous access including parenteral nutrition.

After placement of a central line, the physician must always document the correct location of the catheter tip by radiography before initiating the parenteral nutrition infusion. The catheter tip should be located just proximal to the junction of the superior vena cava and right atrium. Infusion of the solution through an improperly placed catheter can be dangerous to the patient. Complications that

TABLE 17-18

CLINICAL SITUATIONS THAT MAY BENEFIT FROM PARENTERAL NUTRITION SUPPORT

Medical
  Prematurity/low birth weight
  Inflammatory bowel disease
  Major trauma
  Severe burns
  Sepsis with ileus
  Severe malabsorption syndromes
  Immune deficiency disorders (AIDS?)
  Severe respiratory distress (cystic fibrosis, ECMO)
  Short-bowel syndrome
  Necrotizing enterocolitis
  Neoplasms (adjunctive therapy)
  Radiation therapy
  Chemotherapy-induced gastrointestinal injury
  Pancreatitis
  Bone marrow transplantation
  Pseudoobstruction syndrome
Surgical
  Pre- and postoperative support
  Short-bowel syndrome
  Gastroschisis/omphalocele
  Postoperative complications (ileus, fistulas)
  Other congenital malformations

ECMO = extracorporeal membrane oxygenation.

have been associated with catheter insertion include pneumothorax, hemothorax, hydrothorax, arterial puncture, myocardial perforation, catheter embolism, air embolism, cardiac arrhythmias, cardiac tamponade, and thrombosis of the jugular or vertebral vein or in the central nervous system because of catheter malposition.

NUTRIENT SOLUTIONS

The goal of the parenteral nutritional regimen is to provide the necessary fluid and nutrients either alone or in combination with enteral nutrition for maintenance or replenishment of normal nutritional status. In children, "normal" nutritional support includes nutrients for growth. Calculations therefore must be made to infuse adequate fluid, energy, fat, protein, electrolytes, minerals, vitamins, and trace elements to meet each patient's requirements. Estimates of nutrient needs are based on oral intakes, balance studies, and "accepted" standards. Fluid and energy requirements are calculated for weight and age (see Secs. 17.2.3 and 21.2). Energy is supplied by glucose and emulsified lipid.

GLUCOSE Glucose, in the form of a dextrose monohydrate, provides 3.4 kcal/g of dextrose and can be infused safely through a central line in concentrations up to 35 g/dL (35% dextrose solution). The usual starting dose of dextrose to maintain a normal blood glucose concentration is 5 mg/kg/min. The dose can be increased as tolerated to 15 to 20 mg/kg/min; tolerance is judged by the absence of glycosuria and hyperglycemia. As noted above, the maximum recommended dextrose concentration administered via a peripheral vein is 12.5%. Premature infants often are unable to metabolize glucose at even relatively low doses and may require lower amounts and slower increases of dextrose infusions. If glucose intolerance appears in a previously stable patient, infection and sepsis must be considered; insulin may be required in selected patients to control glucose intolerance. The initial dose of insulin (usually 0.5 to 1.0 units per 10 g of dextrose in solution) may be difficult to predict accurately because the insulin binds variably to the bottle and tubing. The goal should be to have no glucose or only trace amounts in the urine, although the serum glucose concentrations may still be as high as 150 mg/dL. Adequate glucose must be provided to avoid hypoglycemia; in particular, a parenteral nutrient infusion containing a large concentration of dextrose cannot be discontinued abruptly unless another source of glucose (enteral or intravenous) is assured. High plasma insulin levels persist for 15 to 30 minutes after cessation of the glucose infusion and can lead to hypoglycemia. Problems with hypoglycemia on cessation of parenteral glucose infusions are routinely prevented by gradual tapering of the infusion rate.

LIPID Lipid emulsions in a 10% solution (1.1 kcal/mL) or a 20% solution (2 kcal/mL) are composed of triglycerides stabilized with egg phospholipids and isotonically balanced with glycerol. They provide a concentrated calorie source with relatively low osmolality. At least 1 to 2% of the total caloric intake should be essential fatty acids (as described in Sec. 17.2.3) to avoid an essential fatty acid deficiency state. The maximum recommended amount of intravenous lipid is 2.5 to 3.0 g/kg/d in adults and up to 4 g/kg/d in neonates, infants, and children. Usually, 25 to 40% of the infused calories are provided by lipids. Tolerance should be assessed by occasionally monitoring serum triglyceride concentration 4 to 8 hours after completing the lipid infusion. If the serum triglyceride level is greater than 150 mg/dL, the lipid infusion rate should be reduced. Side effects of lipid emulsion include allergic reactions (particularly in persons allergic to eggs), metallic taste, hepatomegaly, splenomegaly, transiently elevated serum transaminase (ALT, AST) concentrations, and hyperlipidemia resulting in decreased oxygenation and displacement of unconjugated bilirubin from albumin-binding sites. These last two effects are important considerations in neonates who may have pulmonary disease or indirect hyperbilirubinemia. The fat overload syndrome, which is characterized by jaundice, fever, leukocytosis, bleeding secondary to a coagulopathy, focal seizures, and possibly shock, occurs with extreme hyperlipidemia and has been reported in infants receiving lipid dosages of 4 g/kg/d or greater. Stable infants on a lipid infusion regimen may develop the fat overload syndrome in conjunction with an acquired viral or bacterial infection.

PROTEIN Protein requirements are estimated from studies of fetal nitrogen accumulation (mean nitrogen retention of 320 mg/kg/d or of 2 g/kg/d protein) or by analysis of breast-fed–infant data. Current guidelines suggest giving premature infants 2.5 to 3.5 g protein/kg/d, and term infants 2.0 to 2.5 g protein/kg/d. Increasing the nonprotein calories above a minimum of 50 to 60 kcal/kg/d appears to enhance the efficiency of protein accretion in a growing infant. The amount of protein that is necessary to attain positive nitrogen balance declines with age, so by adolescence and adulthood, the amount of protein required is 0.6 to 0.8 g/kg/d.

Most currently available amino acid solutions are not made specifically for infants and children. Newer formulations [TrophAmine (Kendall-McGaw), Aminosyn PF (Abbott Laboratories)] yield a plasma amino acid pattern resembling that seen in breast-fed infants; they possibly are preferable to the standard solutions now in general use. Addition of cysteine and other amino acids that may be essential for neonates is being considered, although evidence to support their routine use is not conclusive.

Special amino acid formulas for patients with renal or hepatic failure or sepsis also are available. However, because of their expense and lack of proven benefit in children, these solutions should not be used until their efficacy is demonstrated.

ELECTROLYTES AND MINERALS Electrolyte and mineral requirements can be met by using the guidelines listed in Table 17-19 and adjusting them as indicated for losses from vomiting, nasogastric

TABLE 17-19

RECOMMENDED ELECTROLYTE AND MINERAL REQUIREMENTS[a]

NUTRIENT	INFANT (meq/kg/d)	CHILD (mEq/d)
Sodium	2–4	2–3 per 100 kcal
Potassium	2–3	2–3 per 100 kcal
Calcium	3–4	1–2 per kg
Magnesium	0.25–0.50	0.25–0.50 per kg
Phosphate	1–2	0.3–1.0 per kg
Chloride	2–4	2–3 per 100 kcal
Acetate	To balance, adjust as indicated	To balance, adjust as indicated

[a] A pharmacist should be consulted to determine solution compatibility to avoid calcium-phosphate precipitation. To meet recommendations for premature infants, a solution containing calcium (50–60 mg/dL), magnesium (5–7 mg/dL), and phosphate (40–45 mg/dL) should be used; this solution is applicable for central parenteral infusions where the fluid intake is 120 to 150 mL/kg/d and includes 2.5 g of amino acids per deciliter.

SOURCE: *Green et al: Am J Clin Nutr 46:1324, 1986.*

suction, gastrostomy, ileostomy, colostomy, or fistula output, or diarrhea. Potassium, magnesium, and phosphorus should be monitored especially carefully when parenteral nutrition is given to a severely undernourished patient because, as the patient becomes anabolic, there is a flux of these minerals into cells (refeeding syndrome). Symptoms of hypophosphatemia, hypokalemia, and hypomagnesemia can be severe and life threatening in these patients (see Sec. 17.5.3). Potassium may be added to the solution as the acetate salt. Acetate is metabolized to bicarbonate and can be adjusted as desired to achieve acid-base equilibrium.

Precipitation of calcium phosphate in solution presents a problem in the supply of calcium and phosphorus to premature and term neonates, infants, and young children. Current solutions often do not contain adequate amounts to meet the patient's metabolic requirements for both minerals, so infants who are on long-term parenteral nutrition have a high prevalence of bone demineralization, rickets, and fractures. Recent studies also suggest that the ratio of Ca:P should be approximately 1.3:1. High concentrations of calcium and phosphorus should not be infused by peripheral vein because of the risk of the potentially caustic solution infiltrating into the soft tissues. Oral supplementation may be beneficial for selected patients.

VITAMINS AND TRACE ELEMENTS All 13 vitamins are available in a single solution to meet the guidelines established for intravenous vitamin infusions (Table 17-20). Recent shortages of intravenous pediatric vitamin preparations as a result of inadequate production have created temporary and sometimes serious problems; various vitamin (particularly thiamine and vitamin K) deficiencies have been reported because of this dilemma. In these circumstances, other formulations have been substituted and require appropriate parenteral (or enteral if feasible) supplementation of the TPN regimen. The potential toxicity of preservatives (eg, polysorbate, propylene glycol) in the vitamin preparations has been under review. Additional vitamin D (25,000 IU intramuscularly per month) may be necessary to prevent rickets in infants receiving long-term TPN. In the past, extra water-soluble vitamins have been available as an additive for intravenous solutions, and these may be necessary for patients with excess losses, such as those undergoing hemo- or peritoneal dialysis.

Several trace elements have been associated with documented deficiency states in humans. Four are routinely provided in parenteral nutrition solutions: (1) zinc, (2) copper, (3) chromium, and (4) manganese (Table 17-21). Normal excretion routes for trace elements must be considered in assessing a patient's requirements. Extra zinc may be needed in diarrheal states. Conversely, copper and manganese should be limited or totally withheld when cholestasis is present because they are both excreted mainly in bile. Selenium supplementation also may be necessary for patients on prolonged (ie, >6 weeks) TPN with no enteral intake, but excess selenium should be avoided because it can also cause significant toxicity. Selenium, chromium, and molybdenum should not be administered to patients with renal failure. Iron is provided enterally if possible or by intravenous bolus infusion of iron dextran solutions as indicated. Intramuscular injections of iron should be avoided because of complications of pain, pigmented staining of skin, and difficulties in managing allergic reactions. The addition of iron to routine parenteral nutrition solutions is controversial because it may lead to sensitization and allergic reactions. Additionally, prolonged intravenous iron administration may predispose patients to iron overload, gram-negative septicemia, or oxidant injury, especially in premature infants. Additional molybdenum and iodide may be use-

TABLE 17-20

GUIDELINES FOR VITAMINS IN PEDIATRIC PARENTERAL NUTRITION SOLUTION

VITAMIN	RDD	MVI®-PED[a]	RDD/kg PREMATURE INFANTS
A (mg)[b]	0.7	0.7	>0.2
D (μg)[b]	10	10	4
E (mg)[b]	7	7	2.8
K_1 (μg)	200	200	100
Ascorbic acid (mg)	80	80	32
Thiamine (mg)	1.2	1.2	0.48
Riboflavin (mg)	1.4	1.4	0.15
Niacin (mg)	17	17	6.8
Pyridoxine (mg)	1	1	0.18
Folic acid (mcg)	140	140	56
B_{12} (μg)	1.0	1	0.4
Biotin (μg)	—	20	8
Pantothenic acid (mg)	—	5	2
Total recommended dose	—	5 mL/d (1 vial)	2.0 mL/kg (max 5.0 mL)

[a] Multivitamin infusion for pediatrics (Armour).

[b] Vitamin A: 1 μg = 1 retinol equivalent (RE) = 3.33 IU; Vitamin D: 10 μg = 400 IU; Vitamin E: 1 mg tocopherol = 1 IU.

RDD = recommended daily dose.

ful to prevent deficiency states in patients receiving prolonged TPN, although adequate iodide appears to be provided by topical agents that are used routinely for catheter and wound care. Fluoride may be important in children with developing teeth who take no oral fluid containing fluoride, even though no data support this recommendation.

OTHER ADDITIVES TO PARENTERAL NUTRITION A variety of medications can be added safely to parenteral nutrition regimens. The compatibility of each drug with a specific solution should be checked before it is added to the solution. Common additives include heparin, H_2-receptor antagonists (cimetidine, ranitidine), and antibiotics that are compatible with the solution, which can be infused in piggyback fashion so that the parenteral nutrient infusion does not have to be discontinued. Many pharmacologic agents pre-

cipitate in parenteral nutrient solutions and therefore cannot be infused into the same venous line as the TPN solution.

CARE AND MONITORING

Careful clinical observation, laboratory assessment, and catheter technique can prevent complications that are usually associated with parenteral nutrition regimens. A pediatric nutritional support team, including a parenteral-nutrition nurse specialist designated specifically to care for these patients, has been shown to improve outcome and minimize complication rates. Complications are divided into three main categories: (1) infectious, (2) metabolic, and (3) mechanical (Table 17-22). The most common and potentially serious complications are sepsis (1 to 5% of patients), usually with *Staphylococcus, Streptococcus*, gram-negative organisms, and *Can-*

TABLE 17-21

GUIDELINES FOR DAILY AMOUNT OF TRACE ELEMENTS IN PARENTERAL NUTRITION INFUSIONS[a]

NUTRIENT	PREMATURE AND LOW-BIRTH-WEIGHT INFANTS (μg/kg/d)	INFANTS AND CHILDREN (μg/kg/d)	ADULTS
Copper	20	20	0.5–1.5 mg/d
Zinc	400	250 (<3 mo)	2.5–4.0 mg/d
		100 (>3 mo)	
		50 (child)	
Chromium	0.2	0.14–0.20	10–15 μg
Manganese	1.0	1.0	0.15–0.80 mg/d
Selenium	2.0	2.0	0.05–0.20 mg/d
Molybdenum	0.25	0.25	
Iodide[b]	1.0	1.0	
Iron[c]			
Fluoride[d]			

[a] Trace elements usually are provided as Pediatric Multiple Trace Element Solution, which contains copper, 0.1 mg/mL; zinc, 0.5 mg/mL; chromium, 1 μg/mL; and manganese, 30μg/mL. No selenium, molybdenum, iodide, iron, or fluoride is supplied in the commercially available trace element solution.

[b] Most patients appear to absorb adequate iodide through the skin from topical application.

[c] The safest approach for iron supplementation appears to be bolus infusion if oral intake is not possible.

[d] Fluoride supplementation may help dental development and have a role in bone mineral homeostasis, although no data currently support its routine use in intravenous solutions. Oral drops may be an effective alternative.

TABLE 17-22

COMPLICATIONS ASSOCIATED WITH PARENTERAL NUTRITION

Infectious
  Sepsis, bacteremia, fungemia
  Catheter site infection
Metabolic
  Fluid overaload, dehydration
  Hyperglycemia, hypoglycemia
  Hypernatremia, hyponatremia
  Hyperkalemia, hypokalemia
  Hyperchloremia, hypochloremia
  Hyperphosphatemia, hypophosphatemia
  Hypercalcemia, hypocalcemia
  Hypermagnesemia, hypomagnesemia
  Vitamin or trace element deficiency
  Essential fatty acid deficiency
  Hyperlipidemia
  Fat overload syndrome
  Amino acid imbalance
  Hyperammonemia
  Acidosis
Mechanical
  Venous thrombosis
  Superior vena cava syndrome
  Catheter occlusion because of Ca-P crystals
  Embolism
  Air embolism
  Hydrocephalus
  Extravasation of solution
  Cardiac arrhythmia
  Deep vein or myocardial perforation
  Pneumothorax
  Hydrothorax
  Hemothorax
  Catheter dislodgment
Other
  Bone demineralization
    Osteoporosis, rickets
  Hepatobiliary dysfunction
    Cholestasis, cholelithiasis
  Hepatic abnormalities
    Steatosis, fibrosis
  Renal abnormalities (decreased GFR?)
  Psychological (depression)
  Feeding problems (aversion)

GFR = glomerular filtration rate.

dida species; catheter thrombosis; and metabolic problems because of deficiencies (eg, refeeding syndrome), excesses, or imbalance of nutrients. This increased risk of sepsis requires that patients with a central line and fever be treated presumptively for infection. Clotted catheters have been successfully treated with urokinase. Long-term parenteral nutrition may lead to hepatobiliary disorders, including cholestasis or fibrosis, and skeletal demineralization. Early initiation of enteral supplementation may help to prevent the development or progression of these problems. Chronic use of loop diuretics and acid-base abnormalities especially predispose those infants receiving TPN to cholelithiasis and bone mineral loss. Increased experience with prolonged parenteral nutritional support may reveal other unrecognized nutrient deficiencies or parenteral nutrition–associated toxicities such as aluminum accumulation. Diminished renal function in patients on TPN for many (over 4) years also has recently

been reported; further studies are pending to determine the significance of this observation. Another significant problem is teaching a young child to learn to eat following a lengthy period of TPN (and even enteral tube feeding) when he or she has received no oral stimulation. Allowing a child to eat and chew minimal amounts of food material periodically may help to avoid this difficulty.

Careful observation and reassessment are paramount to the successful implementation of parenteral nutrition regimens. Proper monitoring is necessary to detect or prevent complications and to assess the efficacy and appropriateness of the solution being infused. Clinical monitoring will determine whether mechanical or infectious problems are likely to occur. Biochemical abnormalities can be uncovered by appropriate laboratory assessment before they become clinically significant. Suggested guidelines are listed in Table 17-23. The frequency of monitoring will depend on the clinical status of each patient.

SPECIAL CONSIDERATIONS IN PREMATURE INFANTS

As with older infants and children, enteral feeding should be initiated as soon as possible and is preferable to parenteral support in premature and low-birth-weight infants. Bolus feedings by orogastric tube often are satisfactory, but hourly bolus or continuous drip feedings (possibly transpyloric) may facilitate feeding tolerance and growth, particularly in the very low-birth-weight infant. The administration technique and clinical status should be reviewed if difficulties such as increased gastric residuals, severe gastroesophageal reflux, or diarrhea appear. New onset of feeding intolerance, abdominal distension, and loss of bowel sounds suggest potential sepsis or necrotizing enterocolitis, especially when accompanied by blood tinging of stools.

Parenteral access may be problematic in premature infants. Teflon peripheral catheters are preferable to scalp vein needles, and central venous catheters should be used when prolonged and total intravenous nutritional support is anticipated. Central venous access can by obtained using long catheters placed through peripheral veins, although catheters that are placed centrally by an experienced pediatric surgeon tend to have fewer mechanical problems.

Glucose usually is the first nutrient to be administered. Early hyperglycemia and glucosuria are common, in part because of immature carbohydrate metabolic pathways, inadequate insulin response and peripheral insulin resistance, and stress or infection. Supplemental insulin may be dangerous; small amounts may precipitate severe and symptomatic hypoglycemia. If supplemental insulin is used, small quantities (ie, 0.25-0.5 IU per 10 g of glucose) should be initiated with *careful* monitoring of glucose levels.

Lipid infusions are an important source of essential fatty acids and calories in premature infants, in whom fluid limitation may be problematic. Evidence for essential fatty acid deficiency appears within 1 week of lipid-free nutritional support. Careful assessment of the clinical setting is important when lipid emulsions are used in premature infants. Hyperlipidemia with elevation of triglyceride and free fatty acid levels may appear if the amount of infused lipid exceeds the infant's ability to metabolize fat. (Problems that are associated with hyperlipidemia were discussed earlier.) Although the decline in PaO_2 in infants receiving lipid emulsions appears to be minimal, it may become clinically significant when lipids are rapidly administered in high doses to infants with compromised pulmonary function. Lipid emulsions should be withheld when the unconjugated bilirubin approaches exchange levels. A minimum fat

TABLE 17-23

GUIDELINES FOR MONITORING INFANTS AND CHILDREN ON PARENTERAL NUTRITION

PARAMETER	RECOMMENDED FREQUENCY[a]
Clinical status	
Strict intake and output records	Daily
Total intake: calories, protein, lipids, fluid, other	Daily
Total output: urine, stool, other	Daily
Vital signs (temperature)	Daily, and as indicated[a]
Physical findings	As indicated
Growth measurements (anthropometrics)	
Weight	Daily
Length	Weekly
Head circumference (infants <2 y)	Weekly
Triceps skinfold	Biweekly
Midarm circumference	Biweekly

LABORATORY	INITIAL	STEADY STATE
Glucose	Every 4–6 hours[a]	As indicated[a]
Serum electrolytes (including bicarbonate)	Daily	2–3 times weekly
Blood urea nitrogen	3 times weekly	2 times weekly
Calcium, magnesium, phosphate	3 times weekly	Weekly[a]
Albumin	2 times weekly	Weekly
Alkaline phosphatase, γ-glutamyl transpeptidase	Weekly	Weekly
AST (SGOT)	Weekly	Weekly
Bilirubin (total)	Weekly, or as indicated	Weekly, or as indicated
Complete blood count with differential	2 times weekly, or as indicated	Weekly, or as indicated
Platelet count	Weekly	Weekly
Serum triglycerides	2–3 times weekly[a]	Weekly[a]
Ammonia[a]	2 times weekly	Weekly
Urine glucose (Dextrostix)	Each void	1–3 times daily[a]
Zinc	Baseline	Monthly, or as indicated
Iron/total iron-binding capacity/ferritin		Monthly, or as indicated
Copper, selenium, manganese, molybdenum		As indicated

[a] The frequency of monitoring *premature* and *low-birth-weight infants,* as well as *critically ill* older infants and children, will be guided by the clinical situation. Glucose tolerance should be monitored more frequently in these patients. Every urine voided should be tested for glucosuria, and blood levels should be obtained when the urine tests positive. Lipid tolerance in such patients also should be monitored more closely, with daily triglyceride levels obtained until the patient is on a fixed regimen and clinically stable. Premature infants require close monitoring of bilirubin levels, both conjugated and unconjugated, during parenteral nutrition infusions to assess for potential lipid interactions and hepatotoxicity. Calcium and phosphorus levels also should be checked one to three times weekly, even in stable premature infants on parenteral nutrition regimens. Ammonia levels are useful in premature infants and metabolically imbalanced patients.

amount of 0.5 g/kg/d is recommended to provide essential fatty acids. Nutritional carnitine deficiency, which may account for some cases of hyperlipidemia, has been noted in infants on prolonged TPN; however, the efficacy of carnitine supplementation remains to be demonstrated.

Protein, mineral, vitamin, and trace element solutions and recommendations are under investigation and review. Provision of several amino acids, including tyrosine, taurine, and cysteine, in parenteral solutions may be essential both for normal growth and for minimizing the complications associated with parenteral nutrition; however, further study is necessary to determine the efficacy and appropriate composition of these solutions. No parenteral protein solutions have been formulated to meet the specific needs of premature infants. Early addition of protein (ie, within 24 hours of initiating parenteral nutrition) is well tolerated and appears to enhance growth in premature infants. Mineral, vitamin, and trace element recommendations are shown in Tables 17-19 through 17-21.

Close monitoring of all patients on parenteral nutrition regimens is essential to assure optimal nutritional support and minimize complications. Guidelines are provided in Table 17-23. Low-birth-weight, premature infants require extra care and expertise in treatment to avoid complications.

17.6.3   Specialized Nutritional Support at Home

Selected stable patients who require prolonged enteral and/or parenteral nutrition support may be managed successfully in the home. An experienced team consisting of a pediatric physician specialist, pediatric nurse specialist, clinical pharmacologist, registered dietitian/pediatric clinical nutritionist, medical social worker, and, if necessary, a family therapist should be available 24 hours each day to assist the patient and family in their "hospital extension" at home. Other personnel who may be influential in helping a child at home include a feeding, occupational, or physical therapist.

Many patients receive all enteral or parenteral infusions overnight during sleep. Therefore, they are free of connecting tubes and pumps during the day and can return to fairly normal daily activities. New infusion devices (eg, pumps, connecting tubing) enable other young, preschool-aged children to receive 24-hour enteral infusions via nasogastric tube or enterostomy (eg, gastric, jejunal) wearing the equipment and solution in a lightweight backpack, thus allowing them to participate in everyday activities outside the confines of home and hospital.

When the decision is made to send a patient home, the patient (when appropriate) and family, guardian, or other caretaker must be trained and be comfortable with all equipment, in sterile/clean techniques, and in potential complications. Such training may take up to 2 weeks for parenteral nutrition regimens or as little as 1 to 3 days for home enteral support.

Access to the intestinal tract or venous system for enteral or parenteral nutrition, respectively, must be safely assured. Patients and their parents and caretakers must learn to place, secure, and maintain patency of a nasogastric tube. When enteral access is through an ostomy, care of the skin and the ostomy must be learned. Support must be available for patients should problems arise. Complications of enteral feeding, possible causes, and solutions are summarized in Table 17-17. It is useful, but not essential, that a caretaker learn to replace a gastrostomy tube should it inadvertently be pulled out; alternatively, the patient should be taken directly to a local emergency room to have the tube replaced. Otherwise, when the tube is out for more than a couple of hours, the ostomy closes and may be difficult to recannulate.

Ostomy care is relatively simple. The skin, especially around a gastrostomy, should be kept clean and dry, and it often requires no dressing if the tube is occlusive (ie, no leakage). A new stoma can be cleaned using one-fourth strength hydrogen peroxide followed by thorough drying of the area. After 2 weeks, only mild soap and water are necessary. Patients with a gastrostomy or jejunostomy can still participate in normal activities, and the use of a skin-level device (eg, Button, Gastro-Port, MIC-KEY, PeeWee, Stomate) in a gastrostomy makes the tube minimally obtrusive. The gastrostomy tube should have a snug fit yet rotate freely, and the internal portion of the tube (eg, balloon, mushroom, cross bar) should be pulled against the gastric mucosa inside the gastrostomy, which helps to prevent leakage. The amount of fluid in a balloon should be checked biweekly. A small amount tends to slowly leak out and must be replaced to avoid having the tube fall out. If gastric contents leak from the gastrostomy, the skin must be protected from acid. If significant amounts are leaking, enteral feedings may have to be discontinued until the leakage stops, and the fluids and electrolytes that are lost must be accounted for when the patient's fluid and electrolyte requirements are calculated. Often, simply removing a gastrostomy tube for a short time (eg, 1–2 hours) every day for several days will allow the gastrostomy to contract. On replacement with a similar-sized tube, the leaking ceases. Replacement with a larger tube is unlikely to achieve more than a transient improvement and may begin a cycle of recurrent "upsizing" of the tube and dilation of the gastrostomy.

Occasionally granulation tissue can cause discomfort or a small serous discharge from the gastrostomy site. Treatment with topical steroid cream (eg, triamcinolone 0.5% applied directly to the granulation tissue TID) often resolves the problem. If this is not successful, silver nitrate applied every 1 to 2 days or Kenalog 10%, 0.3 mL injected using a 1-mL tuberculin syringe, may be necessary.

An uncommon but potentially serious complication of the gastrostomy tube is a localized gastric ulcer, often diagnosed endoscopically, from direct pressure of the internal nub of the gastrostomy tube on the gastric mucosa. Antiacid therapy (H_2-receptor–blocking agent or proton pump inhibitor) and changing the tube to eliminate any internal protruding device [eg, to a Bard Button (Bard Interventional Products, Billerica, MA)] is recommended therapy.

Parenteral nutrition solutions are infused through a central venous (right atrial silastic) catheter (eg, Broviac, Hickman) that is adapted for long-term use. The catheter is tunneled under the skin and anchored by a Dacron cuff that adheres to underlying subcutaneous tissues to avoid its accidental removal. The catheter consists of material that will not be damaged by body secretions or immune mechanisms and will not lose its elasticity over time. Totally implantable venous access devices [eg, Infusa-port (Intermedics Infusaid Corporation), Port-a-cath (Pharmacia Laboratories)] also have been used, but for shorter durations (ie, <5 months) of parenteral access. PICC lines have been used for several weeks at home. To minimize the risk of thrombosis and cardiac tamponade, the catheter tip should be located just proximal to the junction of the superior vena cava and the right atrium.

Care of the patient requiring parenteral nutrition in the home involves knowledge of the necessary protocols or techniques to minimize the potential complications of this therapy. Catheter care involves clean (not necessarily sterile) technique in handling the catheter, minimizing opening or disconnection of the catheter tubing (associated with a higher rate of infection), and dressing changes (every 2 to 3 days unless otherwise indicated). Patients can infuse their parenteral nutrition during the evening and nighttime to be free of connecting tubing during the day, which allows for participation in normal everyday activities. Exercise, including swimming, is allowable with these catheters (after they are mature), but the dressing should be removed following the activity, the skin cleansed and dried, and a new dressing applied. To avoid complications that are associated with the infusion, appropriate preparation and infusion of the nutrient solution is critical. This also requires the caretaker (and patient) to be aware of any problems with the pumps or other equipment involved.

Should a catheter be torn or broken, repair kits are available for each of the long-term right atrial silastic catheters to allow splicing a new extension onto the catheter protruding from the skin. However, if the catheter breaks beneath the surface of the skin, it will need to be removed and a new catheter placed, often in a new site.

Fever or other signs or symptoms of infection always must be treated seriously. In patients with right atrial (central) catheters, fever demands immediate evaluation, and hospitalization is indicated to observe and treat a patient for presumed sepsis if no obvious source for the fever is found. Full physical examinations are performed, and laboratory screening, including complete blood counts and blood cultures (both through the line and by peripheral vein), are obtained. In most cases, and in all infants and young children, antibiotics are started until the culture results are available. Depending on the clinical setting, antibiotics may be discontinued and the patient observed for further evidence of infection if cultures are negative after 72 hours. Repeat blood cultures often are drawn through the catheter 48 to 72 hours after the antibiotics are stopped.

Monitoring is performed both in the home and during frequent clinic visits throughout the treatment period. It is important, particularly when treating patients with central lines in place, to train families to notify the physician or a member of the nutrition support team whenever unusual or abnormal symptoms or signs occur. This will help to decrease potential morbidity and mortality that are associated with these therapies.

References

Dubois J, Garel L, Tapiero B, et al. Peripherally inserted central catheters in infants and children. Radiology 204:622–626, 1997

Green HL, Hambidge KM, Schanler R, Tsang RC: Guidelines for the use of vitamins, trace elements, calcium, magnesium, and phosphorus in infants and children receiving total parenteral nutrition: report of the Subcommittee on Pediatric Parenteral Nutrient Requirements from the Committee on Clinical Practice Issues of the American Society for Clinical Nutrition. Am J Clin Nutr 48:1324–1342, 1988

Heird WC. Amino acid and energy needs of pediatric patients receiving parenteral nutrition. Pediatr Clin North Am 42:765–789, 1995

Kang A, Zamora SA, Scott RB, Parsons HG: Catch-up growth in children treated with home enteral nutrition. Pediatrics 102(4 Pt 1):951–955, 1998

Khattak IU, Kimber C, Kiely EM, Spitz L. Percutaneous endoscopic gastrostomy in pediatric practice: complications and outcome. J Pediatr Surg 33(1):67–72, 1998

Koo WW: Parenteral nutrition-related bone disease. J Parent Ent Nutr 16:386–394, 1992

Michaelis CA, Warzak WJ, Stanek K, Van Riper C: Parental and professional perceptions of problems associated with long-term pediatric home tube feeding. J Am Diet Assoc 92:1235–1238, 1992

Rombeau JL, Rolandelli RH: Clinical Nutrition: Enteral and Tube Feeding, 3rd ed. Philadelphia, WB Saunders, 1997

Wesley JR: Efficacy and safety of total parenteral nutrition in pediatric patients. Mayo Clin Proc 67:671–675, 1992

Yeung CY, Lee HC, Huang FY, Wang CS: Sepsis during total parenteral nutrition: exploration of risk factors and determination of the effectiveness of peripherally inserted central venous catheters. Pediatr Infect Dis J 17:135–142, 1998

17.7 COMMON SYMPTOMS AND SIGNS OF GASTROINTESTINAL DISEASE

17.7.1 Approach to the Child with Acute, Chronic, or Cyclic Vomiting

B. U. K. Li

Vomiting is a presenting complaint in a variety of disorders, ranging from mild gastroesophageal reflux and otitis media to small bowel obstruction or impending brainstem herniation. *Vomiting* must be differentiated from *regurgitation,* which is the effortless expulsion of gastric contents through the mouth (discussed in Sec. 17.10.4). In contrast, vomiting is a coordinated motor response of the GI tract and abdominal and thoracic muscles that results in the forceful expulsion of stomach contents. Three basic phases of vomiting can be differentiated:

1. *Nausea,* which is the sensation of impending vomiting often associated with autonomic symptoms of pallor, diaphoresis, salivation, and anorexia.
2. *Retching,* which is the spasmodic respiratory movements against a closed epiglottis.
3. *Emesis,* which is the retrograde expulsion of gastrointestinal contents through the mouth.

That these phases are distinct is supported by the observation that increased intracranial pressure can induce vomiting without nausea.

PATHOPHYSIOLOGY

Vomiting is an integrated response to noxious stimuli that is coordinated by the central nervous system. The gastric fundus relaxes and receives intestinal contents as a bolus from a single, rostral contraction of the small intestine. Antral and pyloric contractions maintain these contents within the stomach, and the lower esophageal sphincter muscle opens. Then, concerted contractions of the diaphragmatic, inspiratory intercostal, and abdominal musculature increase intraabdominal and intrathoracic pressure, which expels the gastric contents though the pharynx and out of the mouth.

The *vomiting center* is localized in the nucleus solitarius and a series of nuclei in the brainstem medulla. Stimulation not only results in the integrated motor responses discussed previously but also causes associated vasomotor activity, salivation, and bulbar responses. Afferent input to the vomiting center may arise from the posterior pharynx (eg, gagging), gastrointestinal tract (eg, distension and noxious substances), and brain (eg, dizziness and increased intracranial pressure). Humorally transmitted stimuli such as apomorphine, opiates, cytotoxins, ammonia, and ketones are mediated through the *chemoreceptor trigger zone,* which lies in the area postrema in the floor of the fourth ventricle outside the blood-brain barrier and processes most of the afferent input for the vomiting center. Receptor subtypes and neurotransmitters that are thought to play a physiological role include dopamine D_2, histamine H_1, serotonin $5\text{-}HT_3$, γ-aminobutyric acid, vasopressin, and substance P.

DIAGNOSTIC EVALUATION AND TREATMENT

An approach to the initial evaluation of a patient with vomiting is outlined in Fig. 17-15. The patient presenting with vomiting because of any etiology must first be evaluated for dehydration, and life-endangering disorders must be considered first. If bilious vomiting is described, the possibility of GI obstruction must be ruled out, as discussed in Sec. 17.7.9. If the vomitus contains blood, management and diagnosis are directed as described in Sec. 17.7.7. If the vomitus is nonbloody and nonbilious, the two most important variables that help to narrow the differential diagnosis are the child's age and the temporal pattern of vomiting. If the history is more consistent with a diagnosis of regurgitation, management should be directed as described in Sec. 17.10.4. Common causes of vomiting in various age groups are listed in Table 17-24. The duration of vomiting is either *acute,* referring to short-term episodes of abrupt onset, or *recurrent,* connoting at least three episodes over a 3-month period. Recurrent vomiting is divided into categories of *chronic vomiting,* which is associated with relatively mild vomiting episodes that occur frequently, and *cyclic vomiting,* which describes recurrent intense episodes of rapid-fire vomiting separated by asymptomatic periods.

ACUTE VOMITING Acute vomiting that is associated with fever is characteristic of gastroenteritis and systemic infections. In both the neonate and infant, a physician must be concerned with a serious systemic infection such as sepsis, meningitis, or urinary tract infection. If the evaluation for infectious causes provides no clues, possible obstruction at the gastric outlet should be excluded with upper GI radiology and/or an ultrasonographic study of the pyloric channel. If these studies still provide no etiology, then metabolic, neurologic, and endocrine causes must be considered. In the child or adolescent with a normal physical examination and who is otherwise well, acute episodes of nonbloody, nonbilious vomiting can be assumed to result from infectious etiologies unless accompanied by lethargy or altered mental status. In such cases, neurologic, endocrine, and metabolic causes of vomiting must be considered. In addition, drug and toxin screens should be considered. Diagnostic tests to evaluate acute vomiting are selected on the basis of the clinical impression of whether an infectious (eg, cultures and radiography), peptic (eg, endoscopy, pH monitoring), anatomic (eg, upper GI/small bowel follow-through radiography), or metabolic (eg, screening and definitive tests) disorder is suspected. If the etiology of vomiting can be determined, specific therapy can be provided; if the etiology remains unclear, maintenance of adequate hydration is crucial. In acute vomiting, short-term (6–12 hrs) oral rehydration usually is effective. Occasionally, however, intravenous

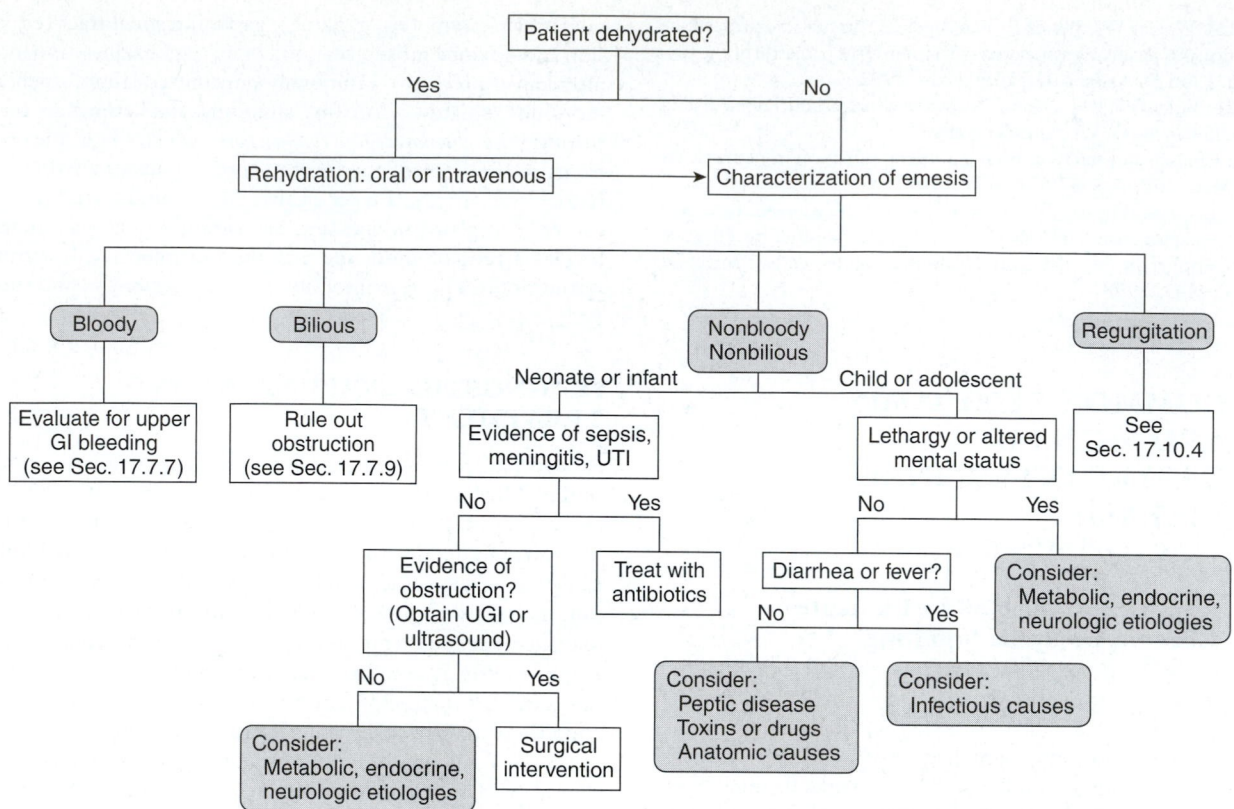

FIGURE 17-15   An approach to evaluation of the patient with vomiting. UGI-upper gastrointestinal examination; UTI-urinary tract infection. SOURCE: *Laney DW: The gastrointestinal tract. In: Rudolph AM, Kamei RK, eds: Rudolph's Fundamentals of Pediatrics. Norwalk, CT, Appleton & Lange, 2000.*

hydration is required. Pharmacologic agents are not usually indicated for the management of acute vomiting in children because they may mask the outward signs of serious disease.

RECURRENT CHRONIC VOMITING   Recurrent chronic vomiting may result from myriad causes. Infectious causes include *Helicobacter pylori* and parasitic infection (especially *Giardia lamblia*). Other GI causes include hepatitis, pancreatitis, and partial intestinal obstruction. In the infant, chronic recurrent vomiting may result from formula intolerance as well as metabolic, neurologic, or renal disease. Clues to the presence of a metabolic disorder include symptoms of lethargy, poor feeding, failure to thrive, seizure, and hyper- or hypotonia. A tense fontanelle suggests increased intracranial pressure resulting from meningitis, tumor, subdural hematoma, or vitamin A intoxication. In the older child and adolescent, the source of vomiting may lie outside the GI tract, such as in chronic sinusitis, drug intoxication, migraine, bulimia, and pregnancy.

Diagnostic evaluation of recurrent chronic vomiting is guided by the patient history and physical examination. An early morning or nocturnal occurrence is especially suggestive of gastroesophageal reflux, peptic ulcer, abdominal migraine, intracranial mass lesion, or pregnancy. Worsening on food intake is much more suggestive of upper GI tract abnormalities. Vomitus of undigested food may suggest achalasia. Projectile emesis can indicate an obstructive lesion in the stomach (eg, pyloric stenosis, antral web) or duodenum (eg, annular pancreas, duplication) or more distal intestine (eg, malrotation). Although it is uncommon, feculent vomiting sug-

gests either intestinal stasis, bacterial overgrowth, colonic obstruction, or bowel ischemia. Jaundice implicates hepatitis or gallbladder disease as an etiology for vomiting. A careful neurologic evaluation is important. Consideration of the clinical symptoms, sinus films, computed tomography, or magnetic resonance imaging of the head as well as intravenous pyelogram, toxicology screen, and pregnancy testing may be indicated. Screening tests for underlying infectious or metabolic diseases include stool examination for occult blood and parasites, complete blood count, erythrocyte sedimentation rate, electrolytes, liver transaminases, amylase, lipase, urinalysis, and culture.

If the history, physical examination, and screening tests do not provide clues to the etiology of chronic vomiting, it generally is wise to rule out obstructive lesions with upper GI contrast radiography and gallbladder disease with abdominal ultrasonography. Alternatively, upper endoscopy may be performed; radiographic studies are performed only if an etiology for vomiting is not identified. In 99 children who vomited for more than 1 month, a histologic diagnosis was found in 58% of those who underwent endoscopy. The predominant categories were peptic and infectious, including esophagitis (33%), gastritis (nonspecific and *Helicobacter pylori*, 15%), duodenitis (4%), and giardiasis (2%). Because the endoscoptist's visual impression had a sensitivity of only 33% for the underlying pathology, biopsies are essential in arriving at the proper diagnosis. Because of the high yield of diagnoses, ease of performance, and safety in an ambulatory setting, endoscopy should be mandatory in children with recurrent vomiting.

TABLE 17-24

DIFFERENTIAL DIAGNOSIS OF VOMITING BY AGE OF PRESENTATION[a]

	NEWBORN	INFANT	CHILD	ADOLESCENT
Infectious	Sepsis Meningitis Urinary tract infection	Gastroenteritis Meningitis Otitis media Respiratory infection	Gastroenteritis Otitis media Sinusitis	Gastroenteritis Sinusitus Respiratory infection

Anatomic	Atresias and webs
	Duplications
	Malrotation/volvulus
	Hirschsprung disease
	Meconium ileus
	Pyloric stenosis
		Hypertrophic pyloric stenosis
		Inguinal hernia
		Hirschsprung disease
		Intussusception
			Intussusception
			Inguinal hernia
			Bezoars
			Chronic granulomatous
			  disease
				Obstruction from peptic ulcer or
				  adhesion
				Inguinal hernia
				Bezoar
				Superior mesenteric artery syndrome

Gastrointestinal	Gastroesophageal reflux Overfeeding Pseudoobstruction syndrome	Gastroesophageal reflux Gastritis	Gastroesophageal reflux Gastritis Appendicitis Pancreatitis Hepatitis	Gastroesophageal reflux Gastritis Appendicitis Pancreatitis Hepatitis Gallbladder dyskinesia Achalasia
Neurologic	Subdural hematoma Hydrocephalus	Subdural hematoma	Neoplasm Migraine Reye syndrome	Neoplasm Migraine

**Metabolic or
  endocrine**
	Organic acidemias
	Amino acidemias
	Urea cycle defects
	Galactosemia
	Hypercalcemia
		Hereditary fructose intolerance
		Disorders of fatty acid metabolism
		  (MCAD)
		Uremia
		Congenital adrenal hyperplasia
			Diabetes mellitus	Diabetes mellitus
				Pregnancy
				Acute intermittent porphyria

Other		Pharmacologic agent Rumination	Cyclic vomiting syndrome Toxin ingestion Food poisoning Munchausen by proxy syndrome	Psychogenic Bulimia Self-induced poisoning

[a] Diagnoses are listed in the age range at which presentation with vomiting is most common. Most disorders present at other ages as well.
MCAD = medium-chain acyl dehydrogenase deficiency.

CYCLIC VOMITING Recurrent cyclic vomiting was first described by Gee in 1882. It is a syndrome with paroxysms of vomiting and intervals of complete health. The typical patient is a 6- to 7-year-old girl who develops recurrent episodes of intense vomiting (mean peak 6 emeses/h) every 2–4 weeks that begin between 1 and 7 a.m. and last 12 to 36 hours. These episodes begin and end suddenly, and they are stereotypic regarding time of onset, duration of episode, and interval between attacks. Over half of the patients develop dehydration and require intravenous rehydration. Prominently associated symptoms include lethargy, pallor, anorexia, abdominal pain, psychosocial stressors and infectious triggers, prodromal headache, and a positive family history of migraine headaches.

Cyclic vomiting remains a syndrome that is defined by its clinical pattern rather than its etiology or a defined pathophysiology. Because cyclic vomiting is a clinical symptom of multiple etiologies, extensive testing remains necessary to eliminate GI injuries and anomalies and to identify sinus, renal, metabolic, and endocrine disorders. A reasonable diagnostic approach is outlined in Table 17-25 and includes metabolic screening during the attack as well as an upper GI/small bowel follow-through radiography and con-

sideration of endoscopy with biopsies, sinus films, and brain-imaging studies.

For those children with cyclic vomiting syndrome and an identifiable underlying etiology, specific treatment is indicated. For others in whom no specific diagnosis is made, treatment remains empiric. Because nearly 80% of those with cyclic vomiting syndrome can be classified as having abdominal migraine, antimigraine approaches have been attempted both to prevent the next episode and to treat the acute one. Prophylactic use of low-dose propranolol, 10 mg BID or TID, amitriptyline, 10 to 50 mg qHS, phenobarbital 2–3 mg/kg qHS, erythromycin 20 mg/kg divided TID, and cyproheptadine, 0.25 mg/kg/d divided TID, may have efficacy in preventing or attenuating the vomiting. Although no therapy has been shown to abort an acute attack, prompt administration of intravenous glucose and fluids has been more efficacious than standard antiemetic or prokinetic agents. Anecdotal evidence is promising, but trials have been begun only recently to evaluate the efficacy of serotonergic antagonists and agonists, including ondansetron, 0.15 to 0.30 mg/kg/dose (intravenous), and sumatriptan (nasal).

TABLE 17-25

DIAGNOSTIC TESTS FOR RECURRENT CYCLIC VOMITING

SCREENING TESTS	TESTS DURING EPISODE	DEFINITIVE TESTS
Complete blood count	Serum electrolytes, pH[a]	Endoscopy
Erythrocyte sedimentation rate	Serum ammonia[a]	UGI/SBFT radiography[a]
Liver function tests	Urine δ-ALA[a]	Electroencephalogram[a]
Electrolytes	Urine organic acids[a]	Sinus films
Urinalysis	Toxicology screen[a]	Abdominal ultrasound
Urinary Ca^{2+}/creatinine ratio		Computed tomography/magnetic resonance imaging of head
		If ↓ Na^+, obtain cortisol concentration
		If ↑ anion gap, obtain lactate, pyruvate, organic acid concentrations
		If ↑ NH_3, obtain serum amino acid, urine orotic acid concentrations

[a] Greater yield if performed during an episode.

δ-ALA = δ-aminolevulinic acid; UGI/SBFT = upper gastrointestinal with small-bowel follow-through.

References

Anderson J, Lockhart J, Sugerman K, Weinberg W: Effective prophylactic therapy for cyclic vomiting syndrome in children using amitriptyline or cyproheptadine. Pediatrics 100:977–981, 1997

Fleisher DR, Matar M: The cyclic vomiting syndrome: a report of 71 cases and literature review. J Pediatr Gastroenterol Nutr 17:361–369, 1993

Gokhale R, Brady L, Huttenlocher PR, Kirschner BS: Use of barbiturates in the treatment of cyclic vomiting during childhood. J Pediatr Gastroenterol Nutr 25:64–67, 1997

Li BUK, Issenman RM, Sarna SK, eds: Proceedings of the 2nd International Symposium on Cyclic Vomiting Syndrome. Dig Dis Sci 44(Suppl):1S–120S, 1999

Li BUK, Murray RD, Heitlinger LA, Robbins JL, Hayes JR: Heterogeneity of diagnoses in cyclic vomiting. Pediatrics 102:583–587, 1998

Li BUK, Murray RD, Heitlinger LA, Robbins JL, Hayes JR: Is cyclic vomiting syndrome related to migraine? J Pediatr 134:567–572, 1999

Pfau BT, Li BUK, Murray RD, Heitlinger LA, McClung HJ, Hayes JR: Differentiating cyclic from chronic patterns of vomiting in children: quantitative criteria and diagnostic implications. Pediatrics 97:364–368, 1996

Vanderhoof JA, Young R, Kaufmann SS, Ernst L. Treatment of cyclic vomiting syndrome in childhood with erythromycin. J Pediatr Gastroenterol Nutr 17:387–391, 1993

17.7.2 Management of the Child with Acute Abdominal Pain

Richard J. Stevenson

The acute onset of abdominal pain is a common complaint in children. Approximately 10% of all children who are evaluated in emergency units have complaints referable to the abdomen. Fewer than 5% of these children will ultimately require abdominal exploration or hospital admission for observation. Thus, most causes of abdominal pain relate to medical conditions that do not require surgical management; however, differentiating abdominal pain that requires prompt surgical intervention from pain due to nonsurgical conditions often is challenging. Understanding the various types and etiologies of abdominal pain helps to identify which patient has abdominal pain that will not improve without medical or surgical intervention. In general, a careful history and repeated physical examination, combined with the selective use of diagnostic and laboratory studies, allow the examiner to discriminate the child who requires acute surgical intervention from one who will benefit from

conservative management. Occasionally, this decision cannot be made on the initial examination, and hospitalization for more intensive observation is necessary. Most acute abdominal pain resolves spontaneously. Table 17-26 lists most of the common causes of acute abdominal pain in children, and Fig. 17-16 provides an algorithm for the evaluation of the child with abdominal pain.

PATHOPHYSIOLOGY

The sensation of abdominal pain is transmitted to the central nervous system via somatic and visceral afferent fibers. The visceral afferent system innervates the visceral peritoneum and its invested structures. Visceral pain localizes poorly, but generally, pain originating in structures that derive from the foregut (eg, stomach, duodenum, pancreas) is localized to the epigastrium; pain originating in the midgut (eg, small bowel and colon to the spleen) is localized to the periumbilical region; and hindgut structure pain is felt in the hypogastrium. In contrast, pain originating from the parietal peritoneum (eg, inflammation) and abdominal wall (eg, muscle trauma) is sensed by somatic afferent fibers and is well localized. Referred pain results from the convergence of visceral and somatic pain pathways in the spinal cord or central nervous system. Pain originating in abdominal viscera therefore may be perceived as originating at a distant, well-isolated somatic location. For example, diaphragmatic irritation that is secondary to pancreatitis, a bleeding spleen, cholecystitis, or liver abscess may be interpreted as pain arising in the vicinity of the lower neck and shoulders because the diaphragm and shoulder pain pathways converge in the spinothalamic tracts at C4. Similarly, gallbladder inflammation may be sensed in the right infrascapular region, pancreatic pain may be sensed in the posterior flank, a migrating ureteral stone may be felt progressing toward the ipsilateral groin, and rectal and gynecologic discomfort may be sensed in the vicinity of the sacrum. Conversely, pain originating in somatic locations such as the right pleural surface with pneumonia may be perceived as originating in the lower abdomen because pain afferents from both regions converge at T10-11.

Pain of sudden onset more likely is associated with colic, perforations, and acute ischemia (eg, torsions, volvulus). Slower onset of pain generally is associated with inflammatory conditions such as appendicitis, pancreatitis, and cholecystitis. Colic results from spasms of a hollow muscular viscus, usually secondary to an obstructive process. The pain of colic is severe, cramping, and intermittent. Generally, there are pain-free intervals when the pain is much less intense but still subtly present. During the painful epi-

TABLE 17-26

CAUSES OF ACUTE ABDOMINAL PAIN IN CHILDREN

Infectious causes	**Abdominal trauma**
Gastrointestinal	Abdominal wall muscle bruise/strain
Appendicitis	Splenic rupture/hematoma
Meckel diverticulitis	Liver laceration or hematoma
Mesenteric adenitis	Pancreatitis or pancreatic pseudocyst
Infectious gastroenteritis	**Hematologic disease**
Food poisoning	Sickle-cell crisis
Peritonitis (especially with ascites)	Leukemia/lymphoma
Hepatitis	Hemolytic crisis
Pancreatitis	Spinal cord tumors
Nongastrointestinal	**Endocrine disease**
Pharyngitis (especially streptococcal)	Hypoglycemia
Pneumonia (especially right lower lobe)	Adrenal insufficiency
Pyelonephritis/glomerulonephritis	Diabetes mellitus (especially with ketoacidosis)
Pelvic inflammatory disease	**Vasculitic disease**
Abdominal abscess	Henoch-Schönlein purpura
Pericarditis	Periarteritis nodosa
Serositis	Mucocutaneous lymph node syndrome (Kawasaki disease)
Epididymitis	**Renal disease**
Generalized	Nephrotic syndrome
Herpes zoster	Renal colic
Mononucleosis	**Miscellaneous**
Acute rheumatic fever	Colic
Intestinal obstruction	Toxic ingestion (especially lead)
Intussusception	Testicular or ovarian torsion
Volvulus	Ectopic pregnancy
Adhesions	Inflammatory bowel disease
Hernia with incarceration	Mesenteric artery occlusion
Gallbladder	Hypokalemia
Cholecystitis	Black widow spider bite
Cholelithiasis	Acute intermittent porphyria
Hydrops	Familial Mediterranean fever

SOURCE: *Laney DW, Balisteri WF: The gastrointestinal tract. In: Rudolph AM, Kamei RK, eds: Rudolph's Fundamentals of Pediatrics. Norwalk, CT, Appleton & Lange, 1994: 349–390.*

sodes, the patient is exceedingly agitated and restless, and he or she often is pale and diaphoretic. Such patients cannot find a position of comfort. When colic is evident, one must suspect problems related to the hollow viscera (eg, biliary tree, pancreatic duct, gastrointestinal tract, urinary system, uterus, and tubes). Inflammatory pain that is secondary to peritoneal irritation usually results in a quiet, motionless, ill-appearing patient in whom pain is exacerbated by movement.

CLINICAL MANIFESTATIONS

The history often provides important clues to the etiology of pain. The time of onset, duration, and character of the pain should be determined, as well as the relationship to any inciting event such as trauma. Trauma may be associated with abdominal wall bruising or strains. More ominous diagnoses, including viscus perforation or pancreatitis with pancreatic duct laceration, also must be considered. With intestinal obstruction, pain typically precedes vomiting or other symptoms. In the event of severe colic, vomiting usually coincides with the onset of abdominal pain. If the vomiting is bilious, obstruction because of intussusception, volvulus, adhesions, or hernia is likely. In viral gastroenteritis, pain usually precedes vomiting. In appendicitis, pain is vague and poorly localized, but the pain gradually becomes more localized as the inflammation progresses and involves the peritoneal surface.

The patient's past medical history also may provide important clues. A history of a sore throat in recent weeks may suggest a diagnosis of acute rheumatic fever or mesenteric adenitis, whereas a history of previous surgery may suggest obstruction. A long history of abdominal pain and arthralgias with the acute onset of severe, localized pain and fever may suggest a diagnosis of inflammatory bowel disease with recent perforation. Arthritis may be associated with abdominal pain in Henoch-Schönlein purpura even before the typical rash appears. Coughing with pleuritic chest pain suggests pneumonia, and GI bleeding could be associated with a Meckel diverticulum, Henoch-Schönlein purpura, or intussusception. The urologic history might reveal hematuria, possibly associated with the hemolytic uremic syndrome or Henoch-Schönlein purpura. If the urine is pigmented, porphyria should be suspected. A history of polyuria and polydipsia may be consistent with diabetes.

In the female premenarcheal patient with pelvic pain, pelvic appendicitis is likely; however, a torsion or rupture of a physiological follicular cyst could be responsible for the pain. Postmenarcheal patients more likely have problems with hemorrhagic cysts, torsion of the ovary with or without tumor, or ectopic pregnancies. The patient should be questioned regarding symptoms of pregnancy and asked specifically if she is sexually active, has missed a period, or experienced vaginal bleeding with the onset of abdominal pain, which would suggest an ectopic pregnancy. In a sexually active girl,

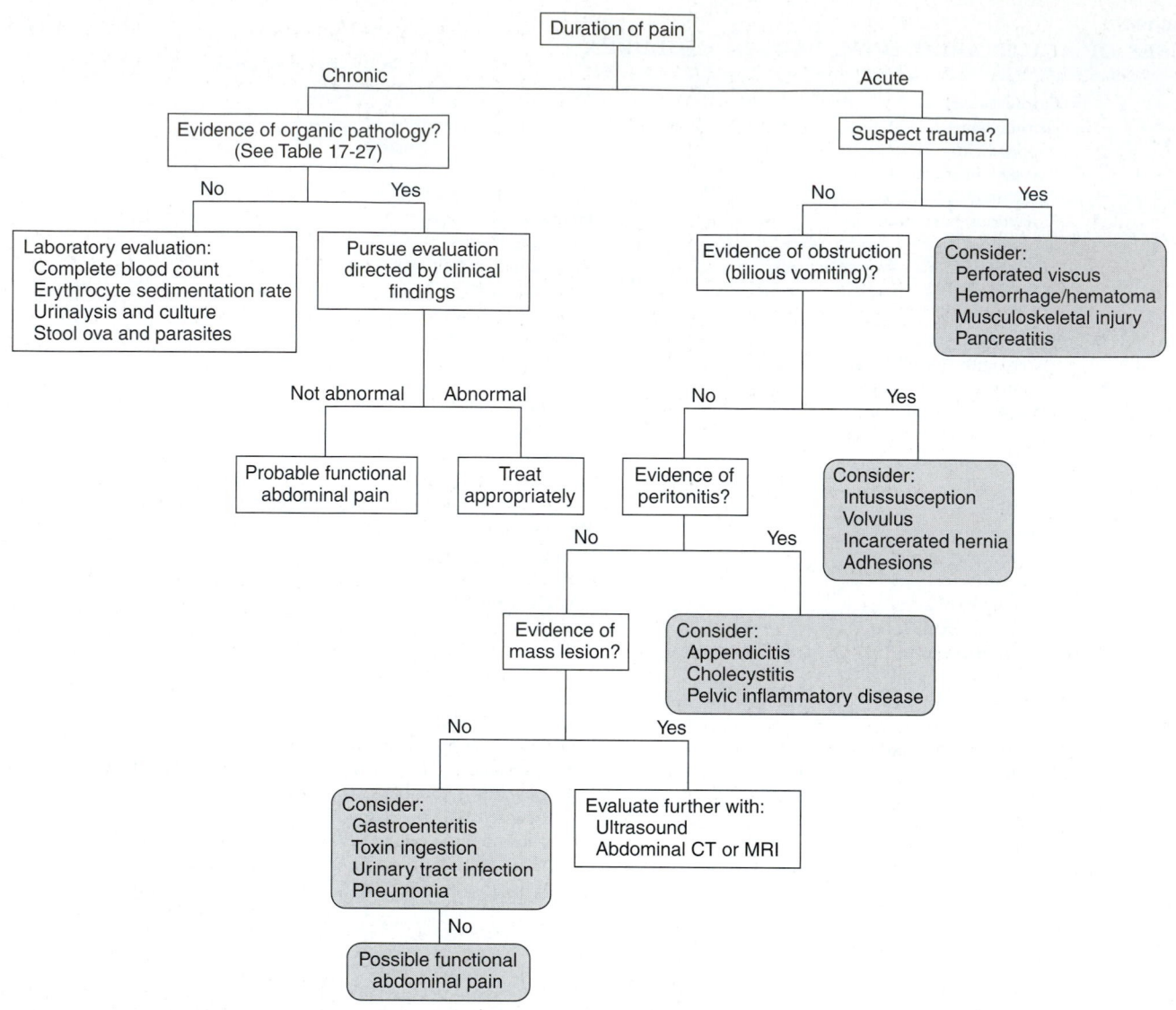

FIGURE 17-16 An approach to evaluation of the patient with abdominal pain. *Chronic pain refers to the presence of at least three discrete episodes of pain occurring over a period of 3 months or more. CT-computed tomography; MRI-magnetic resonance imaging. SOURCE: Laney DW: The gastrointestinal tract. In: Rudolph AM, Kamei RK, eds: Rudolph's Fundamentals of Pediatrics. Norwalk, CT, Appleton & Lange, 2000.*

the diagnosis of pelvic inflammatory disease should never be overlooked. If the pain occurs each month midway between periods and is unilateral, it may represent ovulatory pain or mittelschmerz. If severe pain occurs during menstruation, endometriosis should be considered. The family history might be positive for sickle-cell disease, porphyria, cystic fibrosis, or familial Mediterranean fever.

PHYSICAL EXAMINATION

The abdomen should be observed, auscultated, and palpated to evaluate distension, localized tenderness, masses, and peritonitis. The examination must be unhurried and friendly. One must take care not to frighten the patient; in selected patients, it even may be useful to administer mild sedation before the examination. One must be especially wary when examining the very obese patient, because significant, well-localized inflammation may be masked by layers of overlying fat.

If fever is significant, the patient must be thoroughly examined for an extraabdominal source. One must rule out thoracic disease (eg, pleuritic pain and pneumonia) as the source of abdominal pain. Costovertebral angle tenderness suggests pyelonephritis, but this tenderness also may accompany a high retrocecal appendicitis. The groin must be examined to exclude an incarcerated hernia/ovary or torsion of the ovary or testicle. The rectal examination is mandatory. Stool should be examined for gross blood (eg, Meckel diverticulum, ectopic gastric mucosa, polyps) or blood and mucus (eg, currant jelly stool), which suggest bowel inflammation or ischemia (eg, inflammatory bowel disease, intussusception), or for melena, which suggests upper GI bleeding. The stool must be tested for occult blood. In general, pelvic examinations may be reserved for sexually active or postmenarcheal patients. A thorough rectal examination will reveal considerable information about the cervix, uterus, adnexa, and other pelvic masses in most young girls.

DIAGNOSIS AND MANAGEMENT

Initial laboratory studies for the patient with acute abdominal pain include a complete blood count, urinalysis, and pregnancy test (for the postmenarcheal patient). Leukocytosis may indicate the presence of inflammation associated with ischemia or bowel perforation. Unfortunately, the white blood cell count may be only mildly increased with appendicitis or markedly elevated during episodes of viral illness, limiting the predictive value of this test. Thrombocytopenia may reflect severe sepsis. Consequently, physical examination remains the mainstay in diagnosing the etiology of abdominal pain, especially for appendicitis (see Sec. 17.21.7). Bacteriuria, pyuria, and a positive nitrite test suggest a urinary tract infection. An inflamed appendix lying adjacent to a ureter or bladder also may stimulate increased white and even red blood cells in the urine, so abnormal urinalysis findings do not rule out the possibility of appendicitis. In certain settings, other laboratory tests are indicated. If recent trauma is suspected, abdominal paracentesis and diagnostic lavage may be useful. Similarly, in patients with ascites, paracentesis with cell counts and culture may be necessary to rule out peritonitis.

If the physical examination and history are classic for appendicitis, little (if any) other evaluation is required before laparotomy. Abdominal radiography should be ordered selectively after the patient has been examined. Positive radiographic findings in decreasing order of frequency include bowel obstruction, calcification, ischemia (thumbprinting), and free air. A sentinel loop may be present adjacent to inflammation, as may a soft-tissue mass that displaces bowel. Calcification may represent fecaliths in the appendix or Meckel diverticulum, gallstones, renal stones, or pancreatitis, but it also may be associated with tumors, especially neuroblastoma and teratoma. Free intraabdominal air generally indicates a perforated viscus and requires surgical consultation and, usually, exploratory laparotomy. A chest film must be obtained to rule out a possible pneumothorax or pneumomediastinum with air dissected into the abdominal cavity, especially if free air is documented without being associated with significant abdominal tenderness.

Ultrasonography may be useful in patients who have not improved over hours of observation but who lack clear peritoneal signs. Ultrasonography and computer tomography have proven to be particularly useful in evaluating children with possible appendicitis. Ultrasonography also is valuable for evaluating abdominal masses and for colic other than that of GI etiology. Mass lesions that are not evident on palpation (eg, ovarian cyst, ectopic pregnancy) may be evident. Ultrasonography is mandatory in patients with a positive pregnancy test. Computed tomography is invaluable for localizing abscesses and evaluating abdominal masses, but GI and genitourinary contrast and isotope studies are more useful for the further evaluation of colic.

The diagnosis of appendicitis is confirmed in approximately 80% of children in whom peritoneal findings lead to surgical exploration. In those cases where a normal appendix is discovered, careful abdominal exploration frequently reveals another cause of pain (eg, torsion of the omentum or ovary, a bleeding ovarian cyst, Meckel diverticulum, intussusception, gallbladder disease). Other diagnoses that may not require surgery, including inflammatory bowel disease, pelvic inflammatory disease, or primary peritonitis, may be elucidated. Alternatively, the medical diagnosis becomes evident as the disease process evolves. Often, the pain resolves, and an infectious cause is presumed unless acute pain recurs; further evaluation is then indicated for anatomic causes of pain such as adhesions or volvulus or rare causes of recurrent, peritonitis-like pain such as familial Mediterranean fever or acute intermittent porphyria.

17.7.3   Approach to the Child with Recurrent Abdominal Pain

John T. Boyle

Recurrent abdominal pain (RAP) is not a diagnosis. The definition of RAP derives from the description by Apley of paroxysmal abdominal pain in children that persists for more than 3 months' duration and affects normal activity. RAP has been reported to occur in 10 to 15% of children between the ages of 4 and 16 years. At least as many children experience chronic pain but maintain normal activity and rarely come to the attention of the physician. By far, the most common cause of RAP is functional pain. The modifier "functional" is used in gastroenterology if no specific structural, infectious, inflammatory, or biochemical cause for the abdominal pain can be determined. Because the exact etiology and pathogenesis of functional pain are unknown, functional abdominal pain is too often perceived as a diagnosis of exclusion. Diagnostic criteria for functional gastrointestinal disorders have been defined recently by an International Working Team Committee. Although these definitions must be considered relatively arbitrary, given the lack of a well-defined biological basis for any of these syndromes, they provide a framework for a working diagnosis of functional pain based on the absence of alarm signals from history, physical examination, and a focused laboratory evaluation. Management of functional pain is facilitated by early diagnosis, parental education and reassurance, and the clear delineation of goals of therapy. Functional abdominal pain takes the physician out of the paradigm of cure and into the practical aspects of how to enable the patient to function and have a good quality of life despite pain. Management is best accomplished with regular return visits to monitor symptoms and changes in the physical examination and life style.

PATHOPHYSIOLOGY AND MORBIDITY OF FUNCTIONAL ABDOMINAL PAIN

There is general agreement that functional pain is genuine. The prevailing viewpoint is that the pathogenesis of the pain involves *visceral hypersensitivity* with the altered conscious awareness of gastrointestinal sensory input, with or without disordered gastrointestinal motility. Painful sensations may be provoked by physiological phenomena or concurrent physical and psychological stressful life events. Examples of physiological phenomena that may trigger pain include postprandial gastric or intestinal distension, intestinal contractions or the migrating motor complex, intestinal gas, or gastroesophageal reflux. Intraluminal physical stress factors that may trigger pain include aerophagia, simple constipation, lactose intolerance, minor noxious irritants such as spicy foods, *Helicobacter pylori* gastritis, celiac disease, or drug therapy. Systemic physical or psychological stress factors may also provoke or reinforce the pain behavior by altering the conscious threshold of GI sensory input in the central nervous system. Acute or chronic physical illness may unmask functional pain. Psychological stress factors may include death or separation of a significant family member, physical illness or chronic handicap in parents or sibling, school problems, altered peer relationships, family financial problems, or a recent geographic move.

It is not clear whether the different clinical presentations of functional abdominal pain result from a heterogeneous group of disorders or represent variable expressions of the same disorder, as suggested by the frequent occurrence of upper and lower bowel symptoms in the same patient. There appears to be a genetic vulnerability because of the high frequency of functional disorders in family members. The fact that most children "outgrow" pain symptoms also suggests that variation of neuroendocrine development may also be a factor in the pathophysiology. In some patients, associated symptoms including headache, dizziness, motion sickness, pallor, temperature intolerance, and nausea suggest a generalized dysfunction of the autonomic nervous system. Sex, intelligence, and personality traits do not distinguish patients with functional pain from those with organic pain. The majority of patients are of average intelligence. The generalization that patients with functional abdominal pain are superintellects, perfectionists, overachievers, bad mixers, or constant worriers is without foundation. However, there are some data that the incidence of functional gastrointestinal disorders may be higher in patients with mental diagnoses such as attention deficit–hyperactivity, anxiety, depression, school phobia, posttraumatic stress, bipolar, autism, and eating disorders.

The morbidity associated with functional abdominal pain is rarely physical but results from interference in normal school attendance and performance, peer relationships, participation in organizations, sports, and personal and family activities. Only one of 10 children with functional abdominal pain attends schools regularly, and absenteeism is greater than 1 day in 10 in 28% of patients. A common misconception is that pain is the direct cause of the morbidity. In fact, focus on symptom relief by parents, school, and physicians reinforces the pain behavior with attention at the time of pain, rest periods during pain, tactile stimulation and medication to alleviate pain symptoms, and absence from school on days of pain. This approach fails to reinforce nonpain responses such as normal activity. Although pain does not originate from its consequences, ongoing pain behavior is often accounted for and modified by its consequences.

ESTABLISHING AN EARLY WORKING DIAGNOSIS OF FUNCTIONAL ABDOMINAL PAIN

Primary care physicians often have difficulty making a positive diagnosis of a functional gastrointestinal disorder. One problem is that there is rarely a clear distinction between acute and chronic abdominal pain. Primary caregivers must often deal with the evolution of pain from the initial acute presentation to a chronic or recurring problem. A stepwise series of diagnostic studies to make a negative diagnosis of organic pain is usually employed (see Fig. 17-16). Empiric therapy with nonsteroidal antiinflammatory drugs, antispasmodic/anticholinergic agents, and gastric acid–reducing agents may be tried before the time criteria for RAP are met. Rather than being reassured by negative diagnosis or equivocal response to empiric therapy, parents tend to become more frustrated and anxious, particularly if they perceive that a serious disorder is being missed, or the only alternative diagnosis is an emotional or behavioral disorder. Parental uncertainty only increases the stressful environment that provokes or reinforces the pain behavior.

The diagnostic evaluation of a child with abdominal pain begins with a history to distinguish chronic from acute pain, subcategorize the clinical presentation, and address alarm signals that affect differential diagnosis. The classic criteria for RAP are met if the duration of pain exceeds 3 months and child or parents relate that the pain alters life style (Table 17-27). The 3-month time interval may be too long, as the normal course of acute pain problems is only 2 to 6 weeks. Pain behaviors include grimacing, verbalizing, sighing, visibly guarding muscles, and rubbing of the painful areas. Common life-style alterations include decreased school attendance, par-

TABLE 17-27

DIAGNOSTIC CRITERIA AND ALARM SIGNALS IN CHILDREN WITH PAROXYSMAL ABDOMINAL PAIN

Diagnostic criteria for functional periumbilical abdominal pain
    Documentation of chronicity greater than 3 months
    Compatible age range, age of onset (6 to 14 yrs)
    Characteristic features of abdominal pain
    Evidence of physical or psychological stressful stimuli
    Environmental reinforcement of pain behavior
    Normal physical examination (including rectal exam and stool occult blood)
    Normal laboratory evaluation (CBC with differential, ESR, Urinalysis, ?Stool O&P, ?UGI&SBFT)
Alarm signals that pain may have an organic cause
    Pain awakening the child at night
    Localized or persistent pain away from the umbilicus
    Involuntary weight loss or growth deceleration
    Extraintestinal symptoms (fever, rash, joint pain, recurrent aphthous ulcers, dysuria)
    Consistent sleepiness following pain attacks
    Blood in stools (guaiac-positive)
    Anemia
    Elevated erythrocyte sedimentation rate
    Positive family history of peptic ulcer disease, inflammatory bowel disease

---

CBC = complete blood count; ESR = erythrocyte sedimentation rate; O&P = ova and parasites; UGI&SBFT = upper gastrointestinal radiograph with small-bowel follow-through.

---

ticipation in age-appropriate activities, or alteration in eating behavior or sleep pattern. Children with abdominal pain may be subclassified by one of three clinical presentations: (1) abdominal pain associated with symptoms of upper abdominal distress, (2) abdominal pain associated with altered bowel pattern, and (3) isolated paroxysmal abdominal pain. The frequent occurrence of upper and lower bowel symptoms in the same patient is not uncommon. Alarm signals in the history and physical exam (Table 17-27) that raise suspicion of an underlying structural, infectious, inflammatory, biochemical, or psychogenic disorder include continuous pain, pain localized away from the umbilicus, pain or diarrhea repeatedly awakening the patient from a sound sleep, pain related to menstrual cycle, back pain, multisystem complaints, anorexia, weight loss, frequent vomiting, evidence of GI bleeding (hematemesis, melena, hematochezia, rectal bleeding, occult bleeding), profuse diarrhea, encopresis, extraintestinal symptoms (fever, rash, joint pain, recurrent aphthous ulcers), and a positive family history of inflammatory bowel disease, peptic ulcer, or migraine headache. Physical findings of linear growth deceleration, localized tenderness in the right upper or lower quadrant, localized fullness or mass effect, hepatomegaly, splenomegaly, back or costovertebral angle tenderness, perianal fissure, fistula, or soiling, and occult blood–positive stools.

In the absence of historical or physical alarm signals, the diagnosis of functional abdominal pain should be introduced into the differential diagnosis of abdominal pain persisting a month beyond the usual course of an acute disease (eg, gastroenteritis, urinary tract infection). Functional pain should be presented as a positive diagnosis and as the most common cause of all three clinical presentations of chronic abdominal pain in children. Acceptable terminologies are *functional dyspepsia* for pain with upper abdominal symptoms, *irritable bowel syndrome* for pain associated with altered bowel pattern, and *functional abdominal pain* for isolated paroxysmal pain. Parents should be told that a diagnosis of functional pain can be made when the duration of pain exceeds 3 months. A brief explanation of the concepts of an altered sensitivity to "normal" bowel activities (visceral hypersensitivity) and altered motility, the concept of stress factors, and natural history is important. They should also be told early on that functional pain is difficult to eradicate, and some continuing pain will often have to be accepted by the patient. Establishing a working diagnosis of functional pain and initiating conservative therapy before time criteria are achieved does not preclude an ongoing focused diagnostic workup when indicated by changes in the patient's history or physical examination.

DIFFERENTIAL DIAGNOSIS OF SUBCATEGORIES OF RECURRENT ABDOMINAL PAIN

ABDOMINAL PAIN ASSOCIATED WITH SYMPTOMS OF UPPER ABDOMINAL DISTRESS Symptoms of upper abdominal distress include pain or discomfort localized in the upper abdomen, pain related to eating, nausea, episodic vomiting, bloating, early satiety, and occasional heartburn and oral regurgitation. Table 17-28 lists the differential diagnosis of abdominal pain associated with symptoms of upper abdominal distress. Alarm signals such as anorexia, vomiting, weight loss, and evidence of GI bleeding (hematemesis, melena, occult bleeding) suggest an upper GI inflammatory, infectious, structural, or biochemical disorder. Focused laboratory evaluation should be performed in any patient with historical or physical alarm signals, including complete blood count with differential, erythrocyte sedimentation rate (ESR), hepatic panel, and pancreatic enzyme measurement. In cases in which recurrent vomiting is a significant part of the history, an upper GI series with small bowel follow-through and abdominal ultrasound should be considered to

TABLE 17-28
CAUSES OF RECURRENT ABDOMINAL PAIN ASSOCIATED WITH SYMPTOMS OF DYSPEPSIA

Associated with upper GI inflammation
  Gastroesophageal reflux disease (GERD)
  Peptic ulcer
  Helicobacter pylori gastritis
  NSAID (nonsteroidal antiinflammatory drug) ulcer
  Crohn disease
  Eosinophilic gastroenteritis
  Ménétrier disease
  Cytomegalovirus (CMV) gastritis
  Parasitic infection (*Giardia, Blastocystis hominis*)
  Varioliform gastritis
  Lymphocytic gastritis/celiac disease
  Henoch-Schönlein purpura
Motility disorders
  Idiopathic gastroparesis
  Biliary dyskinesia
  Intestinal pseudoobstruction
Partial small-bowel obstruction
Extraintestinal disorders
  Chronic pancreatitis
  Chronic hepatitis
  Chronic cholecystitis
  Ureteropelvic junction obstruction
  Abdominal migraine
  Psychiatric disorders

rule out gastric outlet disorder, malrotation, partial small bowel obstruction, small bowel Crohn disease, gallstones, pseudocyst, hydronephrosis secondary to ureteropelvic junction obstruction, and retroperitoneal mass. Continuous pain, especially in the context of multisystem complaints, is an alarm signal for possible psychiatric disease. Eating disorders should also be considered in any young patient with significant weight loss.

If possible, it is prudent to stop NSAIDs, iron preparations, and antibiotics such as erythromycin or tetracyclines in a patient complaining of upper abdominal discomfort. Gastroesophageal reflux disease should be suspected when heartburn, defined as a retrosternal burning discomfort that radiates toward the head or oral regurgitation of sour or bitter gastric contents, is a prominent part of the history. In the absence of peptic ulcer disease, the relationship between *H. pylori* infection and abdominal pain remains unclear. It is not unreasonable to avoid antibody testing altogether and consider treatment only in patients with endoscopically proven infection (see Sec. 17.19.2). Cholelithiasis causes biliary pain, which is typically severe, constant pain in the epigastrium or right upper quadrant that persists for hours and occurs episodically. In relapsing pancreatitis, recurrent severe epigastric pain may persist for days and often radiates to the back. Recurrent epigastric or right upper quadrant pain associated with tender hepatomegaly suggests chronic hepatitis.

Criteria for a diagnosis of functional dyspepsia include the following:

1. Persistent or recurrent pain or discomfort localized in the upper abdomen for more than 3 months.
2. Associated symptoms of nausea, episodic vomiting, early satiety, bloating, and occasional heartburn and oral regurgitation.
3. No evidence that organic disease is likely to explain the symptoms. There are no evidence-based data to support a specific diagnostic approach in a patient with no historical alarm signals and normal physical examination.

Short-term (8-week) empiric medical therapy with an H_2 blocker or proton pump inhibitor is an acceptable diagnostic test of self-limiting upper GI inflammation in patients with symptoms less than 3 months. Upper endoscopy should be considered in untreated patients with symptoms beyond 3 months, patients who fail to respond to short-term antisecretory therapy, and patients in whom symptoms recur after the end of treatment. Upper endoscopy is the gold standard to rule out inflammatory disorders in the upper GI tract and establish a firm diagnosis of functional dyspepsia. Recognizable objective findings by gross endoscopic examination include superficial erosions, ulcer, stricture, antral nodularity associated with *H. pylori* gastritis, gastric rugal hypertrophy associated with Ménétrier disease and CMV gastritis, and the small heaped-up, volcanic-like mounds, pocked with a central crater, associated with chronic varioliform gastritis. Objective histologic findings may help to diagnose reflux esophagitis, eosinophilic gastroenteritis, CMV gastritis, *H. pylori* gastritis, Crohn disease, and celiac disease. In the absence of gross ulcer or histologic evidence of *H. pylori*, superficial antral gastritis or duodenitis is of questionable clinical significance and should not dissuade a diagnosis of functional dyspepsia. There is no evidence in children that nonspecific superficial antral gastritis or duodenitis progresses to peptic ulcer. Evaluation of gastric emptying by scintigraphy to rule out gastroparesis and gallbladder function by hepatobiliary scan with ejection fraction to rule out chronic cholecystitis and biliary dyskinesia should be considered only after upper endoscopy and with consultation by a pediatric gastroenterologist. Endoscopic retrograde cholangiopancreatography is indicated only if there is biochemical or radiologic evidence of recurrent pancreatitis or biliary-type abdominal pain following cholecystectomy.

ABDOMINAL PAIN ASSOCIATED WITH SYMPTOMS OF ALTERED BOWEL PATTERN   Altered bowel pattern may include a change in frequency and/or consistency of stools (diarrhea or constipation), pain relieved with defecation, straining or urgency, feeling of incomplete evacuation, passage of mucus, or a feeling of bloating or abdominal distention. Table 17-29 lists the differential diagnosis of abdominal pain associated with symptoms of altered bowel pattern. In patients with diarrhea, focused laboratory evaluation should include a complete blood count with differential, erythrocyte sedimentation rate, stool for parasite ova, and stool for *Clostridium difficile* toxin. Lactose intolerance or malabsorption of other carbohydrates such as sorbitol (see Sec. 17.18.5) should be considered a potential primary etiology of chronic abdominal pain in the presence of diarrhea. A trial of a lactose-free diet or performance of a lactose breath hydrogen test is prudent in children with pain associated with loose bowels, bloating, and increased flatulence. Alarm signals including evidence of GI bleeding, tenesmus, pain or diarrhea repeatedly wakening the patient from a sound sleep, involuntary weight loss, linear growth deceleration, extraintestinal symptoms (fever, rash, joint pain, recurrent aphthous ulcers), positive family history of inflammatory bowel disease, iron deficiency anemia, or an elevated ESR are indications to pursue a diagnosis of inflammatory bowel disease by colonoscopy and UGI with small bowel follow-through. Diarrhea associated with encopresis suggests chronic fecal retention and megacolon. Serologic testing for celiac disease (see Sec. 17.18.2) should be considered in patients with iron deficiency anemia or secondary amenorrhea. Chronic watery diarrhea is also an indication to perform a colonoscopy to rule out microscopic inflammation that may alter colonic motility and absorptive function. The large volume of diarrhea (400 to 1200 g/d) distinguishes patients with microscopic lymphocytic, collagenous, or eosinophilic colitis from those with irritable bowel, where stool weight in excess of 300 g/day is rare.

The accuracy of colonoscopy in diagnosing inflammatory conditions of the colon is superior to the barium enema because of the direct visualization of the mucosal surface and the ability to obtain biopsy and culture specimens. Intubation of the terminal ileum can also aid in the diagnosis of Crohn disease. Recognizable objective findings by gross examination with a flexible endoscope include edema, erosions, ulceration, pseudomembranes (discrete yellow

TABLE 17-29

CAUSES OF RECURRENT ABDOMINAL PAIN ASSOCIATED WITH ALTERED BOWEL PATTERN

Idiopathic inflammatory bowel disorders
   Ulcerative colitis
   Crohn disease
Infectious disorders
   Parasitic (*Giardia, Blastocystis hominis, Dientamoeba fragilis*)
   Bacterial (*Clostridium difficile, Yersinia, Campylobacter,* TB)
Lactose intolerance
Complication of constipation (megacolon, encopresis, intermittent sigmoid volvulus)
Drug-induced diarrhea, constipation
Gynecologic disorders
Neoplasia (lymphoma, carcinoma)
Psychiatric disorders

plaques on the colonic mucosa), and polyps. Subjective gross endoscopic findings including erythema, increased vascularity, and spontaneous friability become meaningful only in the context of histology because they are subject to more interobserver variation in interpretation. Objective histologic findings include (1) cryptitis, crypt abscesses, and crypt distortion with branching and dropout, suggesting ulcerative colitis or Crohn disease, (2) noncaseating granuloma specific for Crohn disease, (3) fibrosis and histiocyte proliferation in the submucosa suggesting Crohn disease, and (4) epithelial and intraepithelial lymphocytes or eosinophils with or without subepithelial collagen thickening in lymphocytic colitis, eosinophilic colitis, and collagenous colitis, respectively. The latter should be considered specific findings only in patients with profuse diarrhea. Mild superficial increases in interstitial lymphocytes or eosinophils in the absence of crypt distortion or significant diarrhea are nonspecific and should not dissuade the physician from making a positive diagnosis of irritable bowel syndrome.

Criteria for a positive diagnosis of irritable bowel syndrome include the following:

1. Recurrent abdominal pain of at least 3 months' duration.
2. Two of the following three features:
    a. Relieved with defecation.
    b. Associated with change in the frequency of stool.
    c. Associated with the form or passage of stool.
3. No evidence that organic disease is likely to explain the symptoms.

Abnormal stool frequency may be defined as more than three bowel movements per day or fewer than three bowel movements per week. Abnormal stool form includes loose/watery stool, lumpy/hard stool, or passage of mucus with stool. Commonly patients report alternating between diarrhea and constipation. Abnormal stool passage may include straining, urgency, or feeling of incomplete evacuation. Many patients with irritable bowel also have symptoms of dyspepsia. Irritable bowel is usually associated with the same autonomic-type symptoms and signs of environmental stress and reinforcement of pain behavior described above for isolated paroxysmal pain. As in all presentations of functional bowel, associated symptoms often include headache, pallor, dizziness, and fatigue.

ISOLATED PAROXYSMAL RECURRENT ABDOMINAL PAIN   The most common pattern of isolated recurrent abdominal pain involves episodes of acute, intense midline abdominal pain lasting a few hours to several days with intervening symptom-free intervals lasting days to months. Continuous pain, especially in the context of multisystem complaints, is an alarm signal for possible psychiatric disease including malingering and conversion reaction. Behaviors associated with the pain often include grimacing, verbalizing, sighing, visibly guarding muscles, and rubbing of the painful areas. Table 17-30 lists the major differential diagnoses of recurrent paroxysmal periumbilical abdominal pain in children. It is important to try to see the patient during an attack, as it is frequently the only opportunity to assess alarm signals.

The Carnett test may help to determine whether pain is arising from the abdominal wall or has an intrabdominal origin. The site of maximum tenderness is found through palpation. The patient is then asked to cross his or her arms and assume a partial sitting position (crunch), which results in tension of the abdominal wall. If there is greater tenderness on repeat palpation in this position, abdominal wall disorders such as cutaneous nerve entrapment syndromes, abdominal wall hernia, myofascial pain syndromes, rectus

TABLE 17-30

CAUSES OF ISOLATED RECURRENT ABDOMINAL PAIN

Functional abdominal pain
Abdominal migraine
Intermittent intestinal obstruction
   Crohn disease
   Malrotation w/wo volvulus
   Intussusception with lead point
   Postsurgical adhesions
   Small-bowel lymphoma
   Eosinophilic gastroenteritis
   Angioedema
Occult constipation
Appendiceal colic
Dysmenorrhea
   Endometriosis
   Ectopic pregnancy
   Adhesions from pelvic inflammatory disease
Cystic teratoma of ovary
Musculoskeletal disorders
   Muscle pain
   Linea alba hernia
   Discitis
Vascular disorders
   Mesentertic thrombosis
   Polyarteritis nodosa
Acute intermittent porphyria
Mental disorders

sheath hematoma, or costochondritis should be suspected. Discitis, which is really an osteomyelitis of the vertebral end plate, may present as a combination of back and abdominal pain. The condition is usually associated with intermittent fever, elevated peripheral white blood cell count, and elevated erythrocyte sedimentaion rate.

Occult constipation should be suspected if a left lower quadrant or suprapubic fullness or mass effect is appreciated on abdominal exam and rectal exam reveals evidence of firm stool in the rectal vault or soft stool in a dilated rectal vault with evidence of perianal soiling. Often, a history of constipation or encopresis is unknown to the parent. Parasitic infections, particularly *Giardia lamblia, Blastocystis hominis,* and *Dientamoeba fragilis,* may present with chronic pain in the absence of altered bowel pattern. Vomiting associated with acute recurrent pain is an indication to rule out causes of intermittent intestinal obstruction including malrotation, internal hernia, intussusception, and Crohn disease. Meckel diverticulum should not be included in the differential diagnosis of chronic abdominal pain unless there are signs of obstruction suggesting intussusception or GI bleeding.

Alarm signals including pain repeatedly awakening the patient from a sound sleep, anorexia, involuntary weight loss, linear growth deceleration, evidence of GI bleeding, and extraintestinal symptoms (fever, rash, joint pain) all require evaluation for Crohn or other rare disorders such as polyarteritis nodosa, intestinal ischemia, eosinophilic gastroenteritis, and angioneurotic edema, which are indistinguishable from Crohn disease on clinical grounds. Suspicion of polyarteritis nodosa rests on evidence of extraintestinal disease, particularly renal involvement. Mesenteric vein obstruction should be considered in adolescents using oral contraceptives. Clinically, it can present gradually with progressive abdominal pain over a period of weeks. Pneumatosis is usually a late finding. The clinical presentation of eosinophilic gastroenteritis depends on the depth

of the infiltration by the eosinophilic process (Sec. 17.21.2). Submucosal disease can become manifest with abdominal pain and signs of obstruction. Angioneurotic edema can be heralded by recurrent episodes of pain in the absence of cutaneous or oropharyngeal edema. Family history is usually positive for allergy.

Recurrent fever associated with generalized abdominal pain and peritoneal signs suggests the possibility of familial Mediterranean fever. Appendiceal colic is a controversial cause of chronic abdominal pain (Sec. 17.21.7). Appendiceal colic should be suspected in patients with recurrent acute episodes of well-localized abdominal pain and tenderness, most commonly in the right lower quadrant, demonstrated on several examinations.

Dull, midline, or generalized lower abdominal pain at the onset of a menstrual period suggests dysmenorrhea. The pain may coincide with the start of bleeding or precede the bleeding by several hours. Gynecologic disorders associated with secondary dysmenorrhea include endometriosis, partially obstructed genital duplications, ectopic pregnancy, and adhesions following pelvic inflammatory disease. Cystic teratoma has been described in prepubertal patients presenting with right or left lower quadrant pain. The vast majority of such patients have a palpable abdominal mass. Benign ovarian cysts in adolescent girls do not cause recurrent abdominal pain.

Acute intermittent porphyria (AIP) is a rare disorder characterized by the temporal association of paroxysmal abdominal pain and a wide variety of central nervous system symptoms including headache, dizziness, weakness, syncope, confusion, memory loss, hallucinations, seizures, and transient blindness. AIP is often precipitated by low intake of carbohydrate or by specific drugs such as barbiturates or sulfonamides.

Criteria for a positive diagnosis of functional abdominal pain include recurrent pain over a 3-month period with no evidence of organic disease to explain the symptoms. Commonly associated symptoms include headache, pallor, dizziness, and fatigue, at least one of which is observed in 50 to 70% of cases. Although many children will claim to have pain at the time of office visits, their behavior, affect, and activity are seldom consistent with the degree of expressed discomfort. Poorly localized pressure tenderness is frequently elicited during abdominal palpation. The correct diagnosis can be established by focused diagnostic evaluation based on historical and physical alarm signals and clinical judgment. Laboratory evaluation might include CBC with differential and ESR to screen for an occult systemic inflammatory condition. The decision to do stool ova and parasite studies is dependent on incidence of *Giardia lamblia, Blastocystis hominis,* and *Dientamoeba fragilis* within the community. The most valuable diagnostic test in a patient with symptoms suggesting obstruction is an upper GI series and small bowel follow-through. Rare conditions such as lymphoma, angioneurotic edema, mesenteric vein thrombosis with ischemia, eosinophilic gastroenteritis, and pseudoobstruction will also be suggested by UGI. Abdominal ultrasound and abdominal CAT scan have low diagnostic yield for picking up appendiceal abnormalities with recurrent right lower abdominal pain. Colonoscopy and ileoscopy should be performed to rule out Crohn disease in such patients if blood work or UGI-SBFT suggests the possibility of inflammatory disease. Elective laparoscopy with planned appendectomy should be considered in patients with chronic right lower quadrant pain and negative infectious, inflammatory, and anatomic evaluation.

Abdominal migraine is a variant of functional abdominal pain. Diagnostic criteria include three or more episodes of intense acute midline pain during a 3-month period lasting several hours to days with intervening symptom-free intervals lasting weeks to months. Two of the following features are required for diagnosis: (1) headache during episodes, (2) photophobia during episodes, (3) associated classical unilateral migraine headaches, which may or may not be associated with abdominal pain, (4) family history of migraine, and (5) visual, sensory, or motor aura antedating acute pain. Associated episodes of cyclic vomiting (see Sec. 17.7.1) or diarrhea are often temporally associated with the abdominal pain. All other causes of episodic severe abdominal pain, including intermittent bowel obstruction, obstructive uropathy, relapsing pancreatitis, biliary tract disease, angioedema, and porphyria, should be considered as well as intracranial space-occupying lesions. Treatment approaches are similar to those used for cyclical vomiting.

TREATMENT AND PROGNOSIS OF FUNCTIONAL PAIN DISORDERS

TREATMENT The primary goal of treatment is resumption of normal lifestyle, not eradication of abdominal pain. A positive clinical diagnosis, reassurance, explanation, environmental modification, dietary modification, and selective pharmacologic and/or behavioral therapy constitute the mainstay of treatment for patients with all three clinical presentations. A careful explanation of the pathophysiology of the symptoms and the fact that functional pain disorders will not affect future health can have positive therapeutic effects. In many patients the symptoms spontaneously resolve or lessen after a positive diagnosis, suggesting that allaying the patient's or parent's unwarranted fears may remove a significant stress factor triggering symptoms.

The first goal is to identify, clarify, and possibly reverse physical and psychological stress factors (see above) that may have an important role in onset, severity, exacerbations, or maintenance of pain. Equally important is to reverse environmental reinforcers of the pain behavior. Parents and the school must be engaged to support the child rather than the pain. Regular school attendance is essential regardless of the continued presence of pain. In many cases it is helpful for the physician to communicate directly to school officials to explain the nature of the problem. School officials must be encouraged to be responsive to the pain behavior but not to let it disrupt attendance, class activity, or performance expectations. Within the family, less social attention should be directed toward the symptoms. Consultation with a child psychiatrist or psychologist may be indicated when there is concern about maladaptive family coping mechanisms or if attempts at environmental modification do not result in a return to a normalized life style.

It is important to address symptoms of mental disorders that may contribute to the pathogenesis of pain symptoms. Failure to treat attention deficit/hyperactivity, anxiety, or depression will adversely affect pain management. Anxiety may be primary, part of adjustment to an identifiable stress, or associated with panic disorder. Symptoms of anxiety include irritability, exaggerated startle response, poor concentration, worry, hypervigilance, motor restlessness, nervousness, difficulty sleeping, school phobia, fear of separation, and fatigability. Depressive mood is suggested by insomnia, anorexia, overeating, low energy, poor concentration, tearfulness, low self-esteem, poor concentration, feelings of hopelessness, and recurrent thoughts of death. Often there is a fine line between anxiety and depression. Many patients and parents are unable or unwilling to report feeling states or acknowledge a relationship between psychogenic stresses and pain symptoms. It is best to limit discussion of psychological issues to what the patient and family can accept and let the physician–patient/family relationship evolve

by continuing to listen actively, provide empathy, and educate about potential benefit of relaxation techniques and coping strategies. Referral for psychological treatment can be proposed as part of a multicomponent treatment package to help the patient more successfully manage the pain symptoms. It is critical that the psychologist or psychiatrist initially focus on illness behavior and expand psychotherapeutic treatments as indicated only as the patient or parents begin to see the benefits of referral.

The role of dietary modifications in the management of functional pain disorders is not established. Postprandial symptoms in functional dyspepsia may be improved by eating low-fat meals or by ingesting more frequent but smaller meals throughout the day. A high-fiber diet is recommended for both diarrhea-predominant and constipation-predominant irritable bowel and isolated functional pain. The goal for fiber intake in grams is calculated as the patient's age + 5. Excessive fiber in the diet may result in increased gas and distension and actually provoke pain. Malabsorption of dietary carbohydrates may act as a provocative stimulus in functional abdominal pain. Most often, the patient does not perceive a temporal association between ingestion of a particular sugar and the abdominal pain. Avoidance of excessive intake of milk products (lactose), carbonated beverages (fructose), dietary starches (corn, potatoes, wheat, oats), or sorbitol-containing products (vehicle for oral medication, sugar substitute in gum and candy, ingredient in toothpaste, and a plasticizer in gelatin capsules) is not unreasonable. Excessive gas in patients with IBS can be managed by advising the patient to eat slowly, to avoid chewing gum, and to avoid excessive intake of carbonated beverages, legumes, foods of the cabbage family, and foods or beverages sweetened with aspartame.

There are no evidence-based data on the effects of pharmacologic therapy in pediatric patients with functional dyspepsia. After a firm diagnosis of functional dyspepsia is established by upper endoscopy, it is not unreasonable to continue acid inhibition therapy in patients who initially responded to short-term empiric treatment but had recurrence of pain symptoms with attempts at step-down therapy. Short-term step-up therapy with a proton pump inhibitor may be tried in patients who previously did not respond to an H_2 blocker. Prokinetic therapy has been reported to provide superior symptom improvement compared to placebo in adults, especially in patients with dysmotility-like dyspepsia, where the predominant complaint is an unpleasant discomfort in the upper abdomen characterized by upper abdominal fullness, nausea, early satiety, or bloating, however, no effective agent is now available in the United States. At present, metoclopramide is the only option for treating pediatric patients and effectiveness has not been established. Metoclopramide has a significant side-effect profile, including drowsiness, dystonic reactions, and increased prolactin levels. As stated above, although *H. pylori* eradication therapy is not established to be effective in adults with functional dyspepsia, the available data clearly do not rule out the possibility. Thus, most pediatric gastroenterologists still recommend treating documented *H. pylori* in conjunction with endoscopic established functional dyspepsia. Although widely used in clinical practice, antispasmodic/anticholinergic and antinauseant drugs have not been superior to placebo in the few adult studies performed to date.

There are also no evidence-based data on the effects of pharmacologic therapy in pediatric patients with irritable bowel syndrome. Synthetic opioids such as loperamide and diphenoxylate are effective in treating IBS-associated diarrhea. Loperamide is preferred over diphenoxylate because it does not traverse the blood-brain barrier. Fiber supplements such as psyllium, methylcellulose, or polycarbophil are effective in treating both constipation and diarrhea, but their value in relief of IBS-associated abdominal pain is controversial. Nonstimulating laxatives such as mineral oil, milk of magnesia, and lactulose are effective adjuncts in treating constipation-predominant IBS. Antispasmodic/anticholinergic agents are commonly used in clinical practice to treat visceral abdominal pain, although efficacy is controversial.

Although there is a lack of formal randomized placebo-controlled trials, there has been a recent surge in the use of antidepressant and psychotropic agents to treat both diarrhea-predominant IBS and functional dyspepsia in adults. Anecdotally, this class of drugs appears to be effective in adults with or without psychiatric abnormalities, especially low-dose tricyclic antidepressants. These drugs may act as "central analgesics" to raise the perception threshold for abdominal pain or down-regulate pain receptors in the intestine. There are as yet no data on treatment of pediatric patients.

There is a recent surge in the development of novel drugs for irritable bowel syndrome in adults, including 5-hydroxytryptamine ($5-HT_3$ and $5-HT_4$)-receptor antagonists and κ-opioid agonists aimed at restoring normal visceral sensation. Significant beneficial effect of the $5-HT_3$ antagonist alosetron has been reported in diarrhea-predominant adult women with IBS; however, ischemic colitis has recently been observed as a complications of this agent, limiting its use.

Hospitalization is rarely indicated for patients with functional abdominal pain. Fifty percent of patients experience relief of symptoms during hospitalization. However, no data have been presented that the natural history of the pain is affected. Hospitalization does not enhance the fundamental goals of environmental modification. More commonly it will reinforce pain behavior.

PROGNOSIS OF RECURRENT FUNCTIONAL ABDOMINAL PAIN IN CHILDREN   There are no prospective studies of the outcome of any of the various presentations of functional abdominal pain. Once functional abdominal pain is diagnosed, subsequent follow-up rarely identifies an occult organic disorder. Interestingly, pain resolves completely in 30 to 50% of patients by 2 weeks after diagnosis. This high incidence of early resolution suggests that child and parent accept reassurance that the pain is not organic and that environmental modification is effective treatment. Nevertheless, more long-term studies suggest that 30 to 50% of children with functional abdominal pain in childhood experience pain as adults, although in 70% of such individuals the pain does not limit normal activity. Thirty percent of patients with functional abdominal pain develop other chronic complaints as adults, including headaches, backaches, and menstrual irregularities. Based on a small number of patients, Apley and Hale have described several factors that adversely influence prognosis for a lasting resolution of pain symptoms during childhood, including male sex, age of onset less than 6 years, strong history of a "painful family," and more than 6 months elapsed time from onset of pain symptoms to established functional diagnosis.

References

Apley J: The Child with Abdominal Pains. London, Blackwell Scientific, 1975

Boyle JT: Recurrent abdominal pain: an update. Pediatr Rev 18:310–321, 1997

Rasquin-Weber A, Hyman PE, Cucchiara S, et al: Childhood functional gastroinfestinal disorders. Gut 45(Suppl II): II60–II68, 1999

Walker LS, Guite JW, Duke M, Barnard JA, Greene JW: Recurrent abdominal pain: a potential precursor of irritable bowel syndrome in adolescents and young adults. J Pediatr 132:1010–1015, 1998

17.7.4   Evaluation and Treatment of the Child with Acute Diarrhea

Mitchell B. Cohen

Acute diarrhea is arbitrarily defined as a diarrheal illness lasting less than 14 days. The approach to the child with persistence of diarrhea for more than 14 days is discussed in Sec. 17.7.5, and that to the infant with intractable diarrhea in Sec. 17.18.3. Most acute diarrheal disease in children results from infectious agents. Identification of an etiologic agent is often not necessary because the disease process is self-limited and treatment is similar regardless of the cause. Rehydration and maintenance of hydration until the diarrhea resolves as well as provision of adequate nutrient intake are the mainstays of therapy (Fig. 17-17).

In several circumstances, however, identification of a pathogen alters therapy, and laboratory evaluation is therefore warranted. If leukocytes and/or gross blood is present in the stool, or the child is toxic-appearing, the likelihood of invasive bacterial infection is greater, and stool cultures should be obtained. Similarly, diarrhea in a child who is immunocompromised (see Sec. 17.17) or hospitalized requires more extensive evaluation because of the risk of opportunistic infection. Recent antibiotic treatment suggests *Clostridium difficile* as a potentially treatable cause of diarrhea. Infants younger than 2 months of age with diarrhea constitute another special category where it is important to investigate the etiology of the diarrheal illness and where the course of the illness must be followed more closely. Bacterial infections are both more common and more severe in this age group. In addition, both viral and bacterial enteropathogens can lead to a postenteritis enteropathy that requires careful nutritional monitoring; a persistent lactose intolerance that requires a temporary formula change is more common in this age group. The possibility of such sequelae dictates the need for these children to be examined and objective measures of hydration and nutrition (eg, the child's weight) established and followed during the course of the illness. An "open mind" regarding the potential of noninfectious causes of diarrhea is required in the neonate, and the diagnosis of congenital diarrheal disease, including primary malabsorption defects, transport abnormalities, and defects in brush border membrane structure, must be considered.

A number of diagnostic tests for viral, bacterial, and parasitic enteropathogens are available in most clinical laboratories. The enzyme-linked immunosorbent assay (ELISA) can identify rotavirus, and stool cultures can identify the common bacterial enteropathogens such as *Salmonella, Shigella, Campylobacter, Yersinia, Aeromonas,* and *Plesiomonas.* Special culture techniques and rapid immunoassays are available for *Escherichia coli* O157:H7 and related serotypes that cause hemorrhagic colitis. *Clostridium difficile* can be cultured and its toxins identified by immunoassay or bioassay. *Giardia* and *Cryptosporidium,* as well as other enteric parasites, can be identified by microscopic examination of stool and by rapid enzyme immunoassays or immunofluorescence assays.

ORAL REHYDRATION

Use of oral rehydration therapy (ORT) has gained worldwide acceptance because it provides rapid, safe, effective, and inexpensive therapy for diarrheal disease. Oral rehydration solutions are effec-

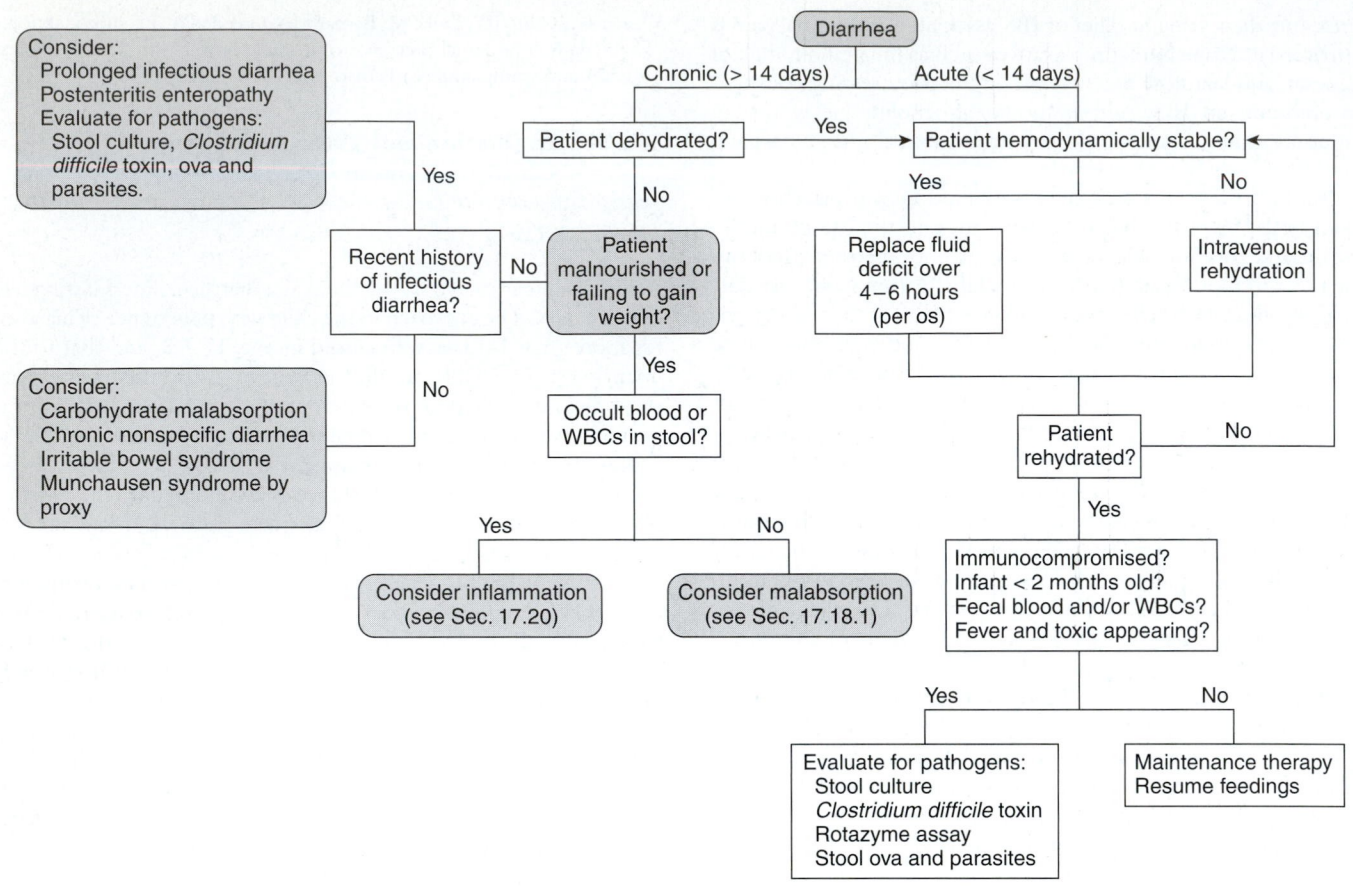

FIGURE 17-17   Management of children with diarrhea. *Acute diarrhea* is defined as diarrhea with a duration of less than 14 days; *chronic diarrhea* has a duration of more than 14 days. WBC-white blood cell.

tive in treating children regardless of the cause of diarrhea or the child's serum sodium level at the onset of therapy. The optimal oral rehydration solution should provide replacement of water, sodium, potassium, and bicarbonate, and it also should be isotonic or hypotonic. Addition of glucose to the solution augments sodium absorption by taking advantage of glucose-coupled sodium co-transport (see Sec. 17.1.4), which is maximal when glucose concentrations are no greater than 110 to 140 mmol/L (20 to 25 g/L). In cereal-based or rice syrup–based oral rehydration solutions, glucose is replaced by complex polymers that are hydrolyzed in the intestine to provide a gradual supply of both glucose and amino acids for facilitated sodium cotransport. These solutions are as effective as glucose-containing solutions for noncholera diarrhea and more effective than glucose-based solutions for treatment of cholera.

Clinical studies have shown that oral rehydration solutions with sodium concentrations of 30 to 90 mEq/L are safe and effective in the treatment of noncholera diarrhea, especially when the solutions are isotonic or hypotonic. Thus, the same solution can be used for both rehydration and maintenance therapy. However, if a rehydration solution with a high sodium concentration (ie, 75 to 90 mEq/L) is used to replace the sodium deficit during initial rehydration, a solution with a lower sodium concentration (ie, 40 to 50 mEq/L) should be used to replace ongoing losses. Table 17-31 compares the compositions of oral rehydration solutions that are commercially available in the United States with some "clear liquids." Clear liquids such as juices, soda pop, and Gatorade are

often hypertonic and contain inadequate electrolytes to replace diarrheal losses in the stool, which has electrolyte concentrations of 35 to 50 mEq/L of sodium and 15 to 40 mEq/L of potassium. Mixing oral rehydration solutions with these "clear liquids" should be strongly discouraged because this alters the concentration of sodium and/or potassium and, in most cases, increases the concentration of glucose beyond the effective range.

Oral rehydration therapy should be used for all children with mild to moderate dehydration. The fluid deficit should be replaced by offering frequent bottles, spoonfuls, or sips over an initial period of 4 to 6 hours. A child with 5% dehydration will need 50 to 75 mL/kg over the initial period to replace the deficit and keep up with ongoing losses. However, it is extremely difficult to prospectively differentiate between mild and moderate dehydration based on a physical examination alone. Therefore, a combination of clinical parameters (eg, weight gain, return of normal pulse, urine output and specific gravity, skin turgor, and overall activity level) can be used to judge the effectiveness of rehydration. Once rehydration has been accomplished, maintenance therapy should continue to replace ongoing losses with oral rehydration solution.

Contraindications to the use of ORT are shock, stool volume greater than 10 mL/kg/h, an ileus, or monosaccharide intolerance. In patients with these findings, intravenous fluid should be used for rehydration. Most other patients with true dehydration will drink oral rehydration fluids when they are offered. In patients who cannot or will not drink, oral rehydration solution can be administered via a nasogastric or gastrostomy tube. Vomiting is not a contrain-

TABLE 17-31

COMPARISON OF ORAL REHYDRATION SOLUTIONS AND CLEAR LIQUIDS

SOLUTION	SODIUM (mEq/L)	POTASSIUM (mEq/L)	CHLORIDE (mEq/L)	BASE (mEq/L)	CARBOHYDRATE mmol/L	CARBOHYDRATE g/L	OSMOLARITY (mmol/L)
Oral rehydration solutions							
WHO solution[c]	90	20	80	10	111	20	311
CeraLyte90[d]	90	20	80	10	—	40[a]	270
Rehydralyte	75	20	65	30	139	25	329
Pedialyte	45	20	35	30	139	25[b]	269
Infalyte	50	25	45	34		40[a]	approx 220
Pediatric electrolyte (generic)	45	20	35	30	139	25	269
Electrolyte ice pops	45	20	35	30	139	25[b]	269
Clear liquids							
Gatorade	20	3	17	6		58	420
Coca-Cola	2	<1		13		112	>600
Apple juice	<1	20-35				120	650-730
Kool-Aide	<1	<1				67-120	370-666
Chicken broth	250	8				0	500

[a] Proprietary rice solids or rice syrup.
[b] Flavored solutions include 20 g/L glucose and 5 g/L fructose.
[c] Jianas Brothers, Kansas City, MO.
[d] Cera Products, Columbia, MD.

dication to the use of ORT, nor does it reduce the overall success rate of ORT.

DIETARY MANAGEMENT OF ACUTE DIARRHEA

After adequate rehydration has been achieved, the next issue to address is the resumption of a normal, age-appropriate diet. Partial or complete "bowel rest" has traditionally been recommended during acute diarrhea, in part because of observations that early resumption of feeding may increase stool frequency and output. Unfortunately, this also results in malnutrition; with almost no caloric intake, children can lose 1 to 2% of body weight per day. Absorption of some nutrients may be compromised during recovery from infectious diarrhea, but on average, over 80% of dietary carbohydrate and over 50% of dietary protein and fat are absorbed. Brown and MacLean summarize: "Suboptimal absorption of some food is preferable to no malabsorption of no food." In addition, enterocyte fuels (ie, glutamine, short-chain fatty acids) may hasten repair following intestinal infection. Thus, it is clear that refeeding should be attempted promptly after rehydration.

Children who are exclusively fed breast milk and those who receive solid foods with or without human milk should resume their normal diets. Initial food choices may include readily absorbed foods such as rice and wheat noodles as well as complementary foods such as bananas (which supply potassium). Feedings that are given in small amounts and at frequent intervals also may be better absorbed. Foods containing a high sugar content (eg, fruit juices) may result in an osmotic diarrhea and should be avoided.

Those children who are exclusively or primarily fed nonhuman milk (eg, cow's milk) or commercial milk-based formula should be observed closely if they continue to consume milk. Most children will tolerate this regimen, but in some, acidosis or recurrent dehydration will occur. A delay of 24 to 48 hours in the second attempt at refeeding is warranted, and use of a lactose-free formula may be beneficial. Because of the high incidence of symptomatic,

transient lactase deficiency in very young infants who are recovering from diarrhea and not receiving human milk, it often is wise to anticipate the problem and use a lactose-free formula for the first 48 to 96 hours after rehydration in this group.

ANTIDIARRHEAL AGENTS

Four general categories of antidiarrheal agents exist: (1) adsorbents, (2) antimotility drugs, (3) antisecretory drugs, and (4) probiotics. The most widely used intraluminal agents are silicates or clay suspensions that act as adsorbents. Activated magnesium aluminum silicate (ie, attapulgite) is an adsorbent found in Diasorb, Rheaban, Donnagel, and Kaopectate. These compounds clearly alter stool consistency. Bulk-forming fibers (eg, polycarbophil, methylcellulose, psyllium seed, and soy fiber added to commercial infant formula) also are effective as hydrophilic stool normalizers. However, although both silicates and bulk-forming fibers may offer cosmetic relief, it is less clear that they are true antidiarrheals; there is no change in absolute fecal water loss. Probiotics or protective microorganisms may have immunomodulatory effects on the host and static effects on some enteropathogens, thereby altering the intestinal microflora. Two agents that alter the intestinal microflora have been shown to be effective in the treatment of diarrheal disease. *Saccharomyces boulardii*, which is a nonpathogenic yeast, can be used to treat and decrease the recurrence rate of *Clostridium difficile* enterocolitis; *Lactobacillus GG* (commercially available as Culturelle) may minimally lessen the severity of rotaviral dehydration.

Opiates, including paregoric as well as synthetic drugs such as codeine, diphenoxylate (commercially available with atropine to prevent abuse), and loperamide, are commonly used antimotility drugs for the symptomatic treatment of mild diarrhea in adults. The major side effects of opiates are sedation and intestinal ileus, but these are minimal with loperamide. Because of their side effects, antimotility drugs should not be used routinely for acute diarrhea in children and should never be used to treat bloody diarrhea. Opiate-induced ileus can cause worsening of the underlying infection, especially with dysentery, and pooling of secreted fluid in the intestine. This "third-spacing" of fluid may mislead observers into a false sense of security regarding the potential for dehydration.

Somatostatin and the synthetic analog octreotide are inhibitory (ie, antisecretory) peptides that stimulate sodium and chloride absorption and inhibit chloride secretion. Octreotide is very effective in inhibiting the secretory diarrhea that is associated with hormone-secreting tumors and in reducing the volume of AIDS-related diarrhea. Bismuth subsalicylate has both antimicrobial and antisecretory effects. Pepto-Bismol, which contains bismuth subsalicylate and a mixture of magnesium aluminum silicate clays, has been shown to be effective in treating traveler's diarrhea and as an adjunctive therapy to oral rehydration solution in decreasing the severity and duration of infantile diarrhea. Caution must be exercised in the use of bismuth subsalicylate, however, because of the possibility of acute and chronic salicylism and chronic bismuth encephalopathy resulting from overzealous administration.

References

American Academy of Pediatrics: Practice parameter: the management of acute gastroenteritis in young children. Pediatrics 97:424–435, 1996

Brown KH: Dietary management of acute childhood diarrhea: optimal timing of feeding and appropriate use of milks and mixed diets. J Pediatr 118:S92–S98, 1991

Guandalini S, Dincer AP: Nutritional management in diarrhoeal disease. Baillieres Clin Gastroenterol 12:697–717, 1996

Laney DW Jr, Cohen MB: Approach to the pediatric patient with diarrhea. Gastroenterol Clin North Am 22:499–516, 1993

Pickering LK: Therapy for acute infectious diarrhea in children. J Pediatr 118:S118–S128, 1991

Vanderhoof JA, Young RJ: Use of probiotics in childhood gastrointestinal disorders. J Pediatr Gastroenterol Nutr 27:323–332, 1998

17.7.5 Evaluation of the Child with Chronic Diarrhea

Leo A. Heitlinger

Chronic diarrhea is the passage of one or more diarrheal stools per day for a period of 2 weeks or longer. The approach to the child with chronic diarrhea is guided by several key concepts. First, both infants and young children with chronic diarrhea and failure to thrive must be evaluated with more urgency than those with loose stools and normal growth. Similarly, older children and adolescents who have maintained or gained weight despite their symptoms tend to have more benign diagnoses; therefore, they are evaluated electively. Second, chronic diarrhea that is secretory (ie, continues during fasting) rarely will be self-limited, and it may be associated with significant morbidity. Therefore, an expedited evaluation rather than a series of prolonged therapeutic trials is prudent. The causes of chronic diarrhea in infants and children with or without failure to gain weight are listed in Table 17-32; an algorithm for approaching the child with diarrhea is shown in Fig. 17-17.

HISTORY AND PHYSICAL EXAMINATION

The history of patients with chronic diarrhea provides information that allows one to focus diagnostic studies and therapeutic efforts.

The duration of diarrhea as well as the number, volume, and character of stools provide important clues. The magnitude of change from the usual bowel habit also is helpful; for example, cycles of loose stools that are interspersed with periods of constipation commonly are seen in patients with the irritable bowel syndrome. In infants, presentation in the neonatal period heralds congenital malabsorptive syndromes. Small-volume, frequent stools, tenesmus, and urgency suggest inflammation in the distal colon. Large-volume, less frequent stools suggest small bowel or proximal colonic disease. Sweet-smelling stools suggest carbohydrate malabsorption. Rancid or foul-smelling stools suggest steatorrhea. The presence or absence of blood or mucus also should be noted. The presence of blood suggests infectious or inflammatory conditions of the colon, and mucus may be seen in individuals with colitis, irritable bowel syndrome, or allergy.

Determining if the patient is adequately gaining weight is critically important. The age at which poor weight gain began may help to determine whether a congenital or acquired malabsorptive syndrome is present. Classically, cystic fibrosis results in decreased growth velocity from the newborn period. In contrast, individuals with celiac disease gain weight steadily until the introduction of gluten-containing cereals at 4 to 6 months of age. Poor growth in infants or toddlers, or weight loss in the older child or adolescent, is a warning that a malabsorptive syndrome or inadequate intake is present. Chronic diarrhea with failure to thrive is a relatively common presentation for Hirschsprung disease.

The presence or absence of associated GI or systemic symptoms also helps in determining the urgency of evaluation and identifying the appropriate diagnostic studies. For example, during infancy, chronic diarrhea or hematochezia with rash, wheezing, or vomiting often is associated with dietary protein intolerance. Although it is more important in individuals with acute than chronic diarrhea, risk factors for infection should be sought, including travel to areas endemic for diarrheal diseases (not commonly seen in temperate climates) and exposure to contaminated water supplies such as well water, streams during a camping trip, or after rural flooding. The presence of ill humans or pets in the home as well as attendance in a daycare center should be excluded. Altered immunity may be suggested by a history of recurrent respiratory, skin, or ear infections. Any family history of HIV or high-risk behaviors such as drug abuse should alert the practitioner to the possibility of diarrhea as the presenting finding in a child with HIV. A family history of inflammatory bowel disease, colonic polyps, or early colon cancer increases a child's risk of inflammatory bowel disease.

Like the history, the physical examination should be directed to several specific questions. First, does the child appear to be acutely or chronically ill? Signs of recent weight loss, abnormal growth, resting tachycardia, and the like all should be noted. Second, are there signs of global or specific nutrient deficiencies? The former would be suggested by decreased subcutaneous tissue or muscle mass, and the latter by a smooth tongue, dry and cracked lips, decreased deep tendon reflexes, and sparse hair. Third, does the child have signs of malabsorption? Distension, abnormal bowel sounds, and peripheral wasting would be suggestive of these syndromes.

DIAGNOSTIC TESTS

The importance of stool examinations in evaluating individuals with chronic diarrhea cannot be overestimated. The absence of evidence for malabsorption, infection, bleeding, or protein loss markedly narrows the differential diagnosis, and this allows one to proceed

TABLE 17-32

DIAGNOSTIC APPROACH TO CHILDREN WITH CHRONIC DIARRHEA

Normal Growth or No Weight Loss
  Infections (viral, bacterial protozoan)
    Stool culture, ova and parasites, cryptosporidium prep, *Clostridium difficile* toxin, viral studies
  Carbohydrate malabsorption (primary or secondary to mucosal damage)
    Lactose-, sucrose-, starch-restricted dietary trial or breath test, intestinal disaccharidases
  Irritable bowel syndrome (children and adolescents)
    Screening laboratory tests, avoid caffeinated beverages and fruit juices, add fiber to diet for age
  Chronic nonspecific diarrhea (infants)
    Decrease fluid intake to maintenance, avoid fruit juices, add fat and fiber to diet for age
  Munchausen syndrome by proxy
    Stool electrolytes and osmolality, magnesium
Diminished Growth, Delayed Sexual Maturation, or Significant Weight Loss
  Small intestinal mucosal damage (postinfectious enteropathy, celiac disease, allergy in infants; celiac disease, Crohn disease, eosinophilic gastroenter-
      opathy in children and adolescents)
    Qualitative fecal fat, D-xylose, fecal α_1-antitrypsin measurements, serology for celiac disease, small-bowel biopsy, UGI with small-bowel follow-
      through
  Colitis (infectious, Crohn disease, ulcerative, microscopic)
    Fecal WBC count, stool heme tests, fecal α_1-antitrypsin, colonoscopy, barium enema
  Immune deficiency (HIV, hypogammaglobulinema syndromes, neutrophil defects)
    CBC, Quantitative immunoglobulins, HIV, NBT dye test
  Structural defect (malrotation, blind loop)
    UGI radiography with small-bowel follow-through, barium enema, laparoscopy
  Pancreatic insufficiency (cystic fibrosis, Shwachman syndrome)
    Qualitative fecal fat, quantitative fecal fat, sweat electrolytes, serum immunoreactive trypsinogen, cystic fibrosis DNA analysis, duodenal intubation
  Hormone-secreting tumors (neuroblastoma, ganglioneuroma, gastrinoma, VIP-secreting tumors)
    VMA, catecholamines, VIP, gastrin assays, abdominal computed tomography

CBC = complete blood count; HIV = human immunodeficiency virus; NBT = nitroblue tetrazolium; UGI = upper gastrointestinal tract; VIP = vasoactive intestinal peptide; VMA = vanillylmandelic acid; WBC = white blood cell.

confidently with therapeutic trials. First and foremost, when patients report diarrheal stool and then either deliver stool specimens that are not consistent with their complaint or cannot deliver stools because none are passed, counseling rather than further testing is appropriate. Infectious etiologies of chronic diarrhea can be identified by stool culture (eg, *Campylobacter, Shigella, Salmonella, Yersinia*), toxin assay (eg, *Clostridium*), microscopic examination of stool for ova and parasites, and antigen detection (eg, *Giardia, Rotavirus*). Inflammatory and structural lesions within the GI tract also can be screened for by examination for white cells, occult blood, and fecal α_1-antitrypsin assay (see Sec. 17.21.6). Similarly, screening for malabsorptive disorders can be accomplished by measuring stool pH, reducing substance, and fecal fat balance (see Sec. 17.18.1).

Blood tests are used to confirm the diagnostic impression that is obtained by the history and physical examination and also to identify the presence of treatable disorders. The complete blood count is useful to determine whether anemia is present, acute-phase reactants are elevated, and neutropenia is present. Erythrocyte sedimentation rate or C-reactive protein tests also can be used as indices of inflammation that do not yield a diagnosis but rather help to direct one's approach. Quantitative immunoglobulin measurements are indicated in infants with chronic diarrhea and in children with recurrences of *Giardia* or *Cryptosporidium* infection. Serum albumin concentration is useful to determine whether protein loss is present. Similarly, measurements of liver enzymes, serum electrolytes, and creatinine levels may reveal occult liver or renal disease. If the alkaline phosphatase level is low in an individual with chronic diarrhea, the possibility of zinc deficiency should be entertained.

Other tests may be used to screen for specific malabsorptive disorders.

The role of imaging studies in the evaluation of infants and children with chronic diarrhea is limited. Upper GI/small bowel follow-through studies can be useful in eliminating the possibility of an anatomic defect (ie, malrotation, duplication, partial obstruction) or an inflammatory condition (ie, Crohn disease) from the differential diagnosis. History, physical examination, and screening laboratory studies clearly are helpful in selecting patients for this study. Barium enema generally is performed to determine the position of the cecum (to rule out malrotation), to visualize the anatomy proximal to a stricture (ie, following necrotizing enterocolitis or inflammatory bowel disease), or to rule out Hirschsprung disease. Ultrasonography rarely is indicated in the evaluation of an individual with chronic diarrhea unless one is unable to eliminate occult renal or hepatic disease as a contributing factor. At most institutions, computed tomography is a better technique than ultrasonography to rule out tumors or abscesses.

Endoscopic examinations rarely, if ever, should be the first tests in the evaluation of an infant or child with chronic diarrhea. The indications for colonoscopy in patients with chronic diarrhea include suspicion of infectious or inflammatory colitis (as evidenced by the appropriate history, physical examination, and elevated erythrocyte sedimentation rate), occult blood–positive stools, white cells in the stools, elevated fecal α_1-antitrypsin, or a combination of these. Indications for esophagogastroduodenoscopy in patients with chronic diarrhea include suspicion of celiac disease, giardiasis, postinfectious, allergic, or eosinophilic enteropathy, intestinal lymphangiectasia, or inflammatory bowel disease. Duodenal intubation for pancreatic function testing is indicated in individuals with poor growth who have neutral fat in the stool.

THERAPEUTIC STRATEGIES

The strategy for evaluating the infant or child with chronic diarrhea is to exclude the possibility of treatable organic illness. When that goal has been accomplished, treatment of toddlers with chronic nonspecific diarrhea and children with irritable bowel syndrome largely is supportive. Inadequate intake in individuals with chronic diarrhea often is iatrogenic. Prolonged use of oral rehydration solutions, clear liquids, and elimination diets may result in inadequate caloric intake and weight loss and is prevented by avoiding the administration of hypocaloric exclusion diets. Toddlers with chronic nonspecific diarrhea by definition have maintained normal growth despite diarrhea and do not have an infectious or malabsorptive cause of diarrhea. Dietary therapy of these individuals is conceptually straightforward: feed a normal diet for the child's age. Toward this end, maintenance fluid intake rather than intakes used to "avoid hospitalization," avoidance of fructose- and sorbitol-containing juices such as apple, pear, cherry, and prune, and resumption of normal fat intakes (ie, use of whole milk) should be accomplished. Should loose stool continue, use of a fiber supplement such as psyllium should be considered. Antidiarrheal agents rarely are required.

Children with irritable bowel syndrome typically exhibit cycles of diarrhea and constipation. A dietary strategy frequently employed is use of fiber supplements at a constant dose and varying fluid intake dependent on stool consistency. When stools are firm, fluid intake is increased; conversely, when stools are loose, fluid intake is decreased. Avoidance of high-fructose and sorbitol juices also should be considered when stools are loose. Once again, as a rule, antidiarrheal agents should be avoided.

References

Bhutta ZA, Molla AM, Issani Z, Badruddin S, Hendricks K, Snyder JD: Nutritional management of persistent diarrhea: factors predicting clinical outcome. Acta Paediatr Scand 381:144–148, 1992

Boyne LJ, Kerzner BK, McClung HJ: Chronic non-specific diarrhea: the value of a preliminary observation period to assess diet therapy. Pediatrics 76:557–561, 1985

Branski D, Lerner A, Lebenthal E: Chronic diarrhea and malabsorption. Pediatr Clin North Am 43:307–331, 1996

Demison GA: Fruit juice consumption by infants and children: a review. J Am Coll Nutr 15:4S–11S, 1996

Fitzgerald JF: Persistent diarrhea in a young infant. Pediatr Infect Dis J 10: 169–170, 1991

Greene HL, Ghishan FK: Excessive fluid intake as a cause of chronic diarrhea in young children. J Pediatr 102:836–840, 1983

Treem WR: Chronic non-specific diarrhea of childhood. Clin Pediatr 31: 413–420, 1992

Vanderhoof JA: Chronic diarrhea. Pediatr Rev 19:418–422, 1998

17.7.6   Approach to the Child with Constipation and Encopresis

Carlo Di Lorenzo

Constipation is defined variably on the basis of the frequency of defecation, discomfort in passing stools, delayed intestinal transit, and weight of the stools. Children complaining of constipation can describe stools that are too small, too big, too infrequent, painful or difficult to expel, or that leave a feeling of incomplete evacuation. Constipation is the chief complaint in 3% of all pediatric outpatient visits, and up to 25% of children who are referred to pediatric gastroenterologists have a disorder of defecation. The female-to-male ratio changes along the life span. Constipation is more frequent in young boys than in young girls, but after puberty, constipation is more frequent in women than in men. The incidence of constipation increases when a parent, sibling, or twin is constipated. It also is four times more common in monozygotic than in dizygotic twins.

Constipation is a symptom, not a disease or a sign, and it may be caused by many different disorders (Table 17-33). Only a minority of children have organic or anatomic causes for constipation. In the majority of children with constipation, the cause is a functional or behavioral problem. In fact, in contrast to the high incidence of constipation among the pediatric population, the incidence of Hirschsprung disease is only one in 6000 births, and Hirschsprung disease is found in fewer than 1% of children with constipation. The incidence of anorectal malformations is one in 5000. Other organic causes of constipation in children are even less common.

NONORGANIC CAUSES OF CONSTIPATION

Some breast-fed infants pass stool as infrequently as every 5 to 10 days. In the absence of vomiting, abdominal distension, or other GI symptoms, these children do not require any treatment. The frequency of bowel movements usually increases when milk formulas or solid foods are added to the diet. Some older children pass large stools at intervals of 3 or 4 days. They do not develop stool retention, do not have soiling, and have no other symptoms. They will continue to have infrequent defecation throughout their lives without any distress.

Infants who are 1 to 10 weeks of age often are brought to the pediatrician by worried parents who believe that the act of defecation is associated with great effort in their infant. These parents describe a child straining for several minutes with agonizing cries before the passage of normal stools. After defecation, the baby is comfortable again. This classical history most likely is explained by the infant being unable to increase intraabdominal pressure and relax the pelvic floor muscles in a coordinated fashion, as is required to allow the easy passage of stools. Learning this process occurs faster in some newborns than in others, but it always occurs in the first few months after birth. The use of enemas or suppositories is not indicated for this problem for several reasons. First, manipulation of the anus may be painful or frightening to a child, further discouraging defecation. Second, learning to defecate takes practice, and manipulation may delay the learning process. After repetitive manipulations of the anal area, the infant may "learn" that external intervention is required to pass stools.

The most common nonorganic cause of constipation and encopresis in children is *functional fecal retention,* which also has been called psychogenic megacolon or behavioral or idiopathic constipation. It is caused by the voluntary withholding of stool secondary to fear of defecation. Children with functional fecal retention display retentive posturing. Instead of relaxing the pelvic floor during the Valsalva maneuver, they contract the gluteal muscles in an attempt to avoid defecation. They consistently decide to postpone defecation. There are two peaks in the incidence of functional fecal retention. The first is at the time of toilet training, and the second

TABLE 17-33

CAUSES OF CONSTIPATION IN CHILDREN

Nonorganic
  Developmental
    Cognitive
    Attention-deficit disorder
  Situational
    Coercive toilet training
    Toilet phobia
    School bathroom avoidance
    Excessive parental intervention
    Sexual abuse

Organic
  Constitutional
    Colonic inertia
    Genetic predisposition
  Reduced stool volume and dryness
    Low-fiber diet
    Dehydration
    Underfeeding/malnutrition
  Anatomic malformations
    Imperforate anus
    Anal stenosis
    Anterior displaced anus
    Pelvic mass (eg, sacral teratoma)
  Metabolic
    Hypothyroidism
    Hypercalcemia
    Hypokalemia
    Cystic fibrosis
    Diabetes mellitus
    Celiac disease
  Neuropathic conditions
    Spina bifida
    Myelomeningocele
    Spinal cord trauma
    Von Recklinghausen disease
    Static encephalopathy
  Intestinal nerve or muscle disorders
    Hirschsprung disease
    Intestinal neuronal dysplasia
    Visceral myopathies
    Visceral neuropathies
  Abnormal abdominal musculature
    Prune belly
    Gastroschisis
    Down syndrome
  Connective tissue disorders
    Scleroderma
    Systemic lupus erythematosus
    Amyloidosis
  Drugs
    Opiates
    Sucralfate
    Antacids
    Antihypertensives
    Anticholinergics
    Tricyclic antidepressants
    Sympathomimetics
  Other
    Heavy-metal ingestion (lead)
    Vitamin D intoxication
    Botulism
    Cow's milk protein intolerance

is when a child begins to attend a school. Attempts to accomplish toilet training at an inappropriately early age, coercive attitudes toward rectal continence, and placement of a high love premium on a lack of "accidents" can cause the toddler to decide to "hold back." Alternatively, experience with painful passage of stool may trigger a fear of defecation; past experience with the passage of hard stools, anal fissure, or perianal infection may lead to withholding. In the older child, school, games, television, and social life can all detract from the "call to stool." Children who are accustomed to defecation at home during the morning may decide on entering school to withhold defecation until they are back in the comfort of their own home. Sexual abuse with anal penetration is another important cause of painful defecation resulting in functional fecal retention, and it should be suspected especially when there is a sudden onset of severe retentive constipation. Occasionally, there will be large fissures, patulous anus, or venereal warts that suggest, but are not diagnostic for, sexual trauma. Urinary tract infections occur in 5 to 10% of chronically constipated children, probably secondary to partial ureteral obstruction or by ascending infection from chronically soiled underwear.

When a child decides not to have a bowel movement, a fecal mass accumulates in his or her rectum. Instead of relaxing the pelvic floor muscles so that stool may pass, the child contracts the pelvic floor muscles, buttocks, and thighs. The child stands stiff, moves around on tiptoes, crossing the legs, or sits with the heels pressed against the perineum. As stools accumulate, mood and appetite deteriorate, and the child experiences abdominal pain with abdominal distension. Soiling may occur, especially during passage of flatus, because of the child's inability to control the overflow of stools. This loss of control over defecation confuses the child and often angers the parents, who believe the child is intentionally soiling his or her underwear. With increasing duration of this problem, the child develops an increasingly negative self-image.

Exclusion of most organic causes of constipation can be accomplished by history and physical examination. A careful history to uncover characteristic behaviors and a physical examination consistent with functional fecal retention may be the only evaluation that is required for diagnosis. The fecal mass filling the dilated rectum usually is appreciated by bimanual palpation. Fecal soiling is rare with Hirschsprung disease but common with functional fecal retention. Causes of painful constipation such as dermatitis, anal fissure, or a patulous anus that is suggestive of sexual abuse are evident. Anatomic disorders such as an anteriorly placed anus or a rectal mass may be palpated on rectal examination. An empty, constricted rectum in a child with chronic constipation is suggestive of Hirschsprung disease. A vascular, pigmented, or hairy patch over the lumbosacral spine may suggest occult spinal dysraphism. Light-touch sensibility in the sacral dermatomes can be tested using a wisp of cotton at the end of an applicator. Reflex contraction of the external anal sphincter in response to stroking of the perianal skin is evidence of the integrity of the sensorimotor apparatus of fecal continence.

Once functional fecal retention is considered to be likely, it is wise to treat the functional fecal retention rather than embarking on a series of tests to exclude Hirschsprung disease. There are sufficient differences between these two entities (Table 17-34) that in most cases diagnostic tests are unnecessary and only serve to reinforce the child's role as the "sick child in the family." If treatment fails, then reevaluation for an unusual condition causing the symptoms may be appropriate.

Among the strategies that have been used successfully to treat functional fecal retention are behavioral modification emphasizing

TABLE 17-34

FUNCTIONAL FECAL RETENTION VERSUS HIRSCHSPRUNG DISEASE

SIGNS AND SYMPTOMS	FUNCTIONAL FECAL RETENTION	HIRSCHSPRUNG DISEASE
Delayed passage of meconium	Never	Common
Soiling	Common	Rare
Obstructive symptoms	Rare	Common
Large-caliber stools	Common	Rare
Stool-withholding behavior	Common	Rare
Enterocolitis	Never	Possible
Localization of stools	Rectum	Extrarectal
Associated upper gastrointestinal symptoms	Never	Possible

positive reinforcement schedules, stool softeners, biofeedback training to improve rectal sensitivity and anal sphincter relaxation, cleansing enemas, prokinetic drugs, group therapy, and surgery. Functional fecal retention is best viewed as an acquired behavior in which the affected child has "forgotten" the mechanics of defecation. The physician needs to provide guidance and assure painless defecation by administering stool softeners. Parents are assigned the jobs of giving the medicine and securing private, unhurried time in the toilet for the child two or three times daily after meals (to take advantage of the gastrocolonic reflex). When sitting on the toilet, the child should press the feet firmly against the floor or a bench to facilitate defecation. The child needs to understand that responding to the defecatory urge and not holding back are key to success of the treatment. There are two phases to treatment: (1) passage of the rectal mass and (2) maintenance. Almost every fecal mass can be softened and liquefied with sufficient quantity and duration of cathartics; enemas are best avoided if possible. After elimination of the rectal mass, treatment should be continued for several months with lower-dose cathartics. Agents most commonly used in this phase include lubricants such as mineral oil, osmotic agents such as lactulose or milk of magnesia, and stimulants such as bisacodyl or senna derivatives. The dose of these drugs needs to be titrated to obtain the desired response. After experiencing months of pain- and accident-free defecation, the child will indicate there is no need for the medicine. For children older than 6 years of age who can cooperate, biofeedback can be used with success for the treatment of both constipation and encopresis. Children can learn how to relax or contract the external anal sphincter to produce evacuation or achieve continence. The role of dietary fiber in the treatment of functional fecal retention is controversial. The colonic flora contains bacterial cellulase, which converts fibers to water and short-chain fatty acids, which produce an osmotic catharsis. Increased fiber intake may allow doses of laxatives to be weaned more readily.

Treatment failures occur in approximately 20% of children with functional fecal retention regardless of the treatment. Children likely to fail are those who have suffered from functional fecal retention for many years and have developed a negative self-image, or those who find a secondary gain from the condition. In addition, children with attention deficit disorders may be very resistant to therapy because of their inability to focus and respond to the urge to defecate.

Complications requiring an acute intervention are infrequent. Rarely, the fecal accumulation is so massive that respiratory failure results from impaired diaphragmatic movement, or repeated vomiting and dehydration result from bowel obstruction. Hypertonic enemas or excessive oral phosphates may cause dehydration, shock, hyper- and hyponatremia, and hyperphosphatemia.

Not all children with encopresis are stool withholders. Some children present with a history of passage of part or an entire stool in the underclothes. The soiling tends to be sporadic and not the almost continuous seepage typical of retentive soiling. There is no history of passage of big, hard stools or cyclic pattern of retentive symptoms. The soiling seems to be impulsive rather than premeditated. In almost every case, the soiling is one of many irritating, difficult behaviors exhibited by a child who is locked in a struggle with parents over many aspects of daily living. Cathartics only make a difficult symptom worse. Nonretentive, functional soiling usually is a behavioral manifestation of emotional disturbance. It requires psychological evaluation and treatment.

ORGANIC CAUSES OF CONSTIPATION

Most organic causes of constipation are listed in Table 17-33. Anatomic abnormalities of the anus and rectum, Hirschsprung disease, and other neuropathic disorders that cause constipation are discussed in Sec. 17.23. Metabolic as well as connective tissue disorders rarely present with only constipation; other symptoms or signs generally suggest the diagnosis. Children with abnormal abdominal musculature are unable to increase intraabdominal pressure and thus have difficulty defecating. Maintaining soft bowel movements usually allows defecation. Recently, it has been suggested that in young children constipation can be a manifestation of cow's milk intolerance.

Constipation in neurologically devastated children may result from several factors. In tube-fed children, use of formulas without fiber may be constipating. The absence of normal skeletal muscle tone and abnormal coordination may result in a poor defecatory effort. There may be sensory or motor abnormalities resulting from affected enteric neurons, just as there are abnormalities in the central nervous system. Treatment approaches for constipation in children with chronic central nervous system disorders include the introduction of dietary fiber, daily administration of stool softeners, enemas, rectal irrigations, and biofeedback.

In children with spinal cord injury or dysraphism, the external anal sphincter and levator ani muscles typically are dysfunctional. Both motor and sensory function of the rectum may be affected. Fecal continence is found in only 11 to 30% of children with myelomeningocele. Biofeedback training has been helpful in patients who have preservation of some sensorimotor functions in the perianal region and who understand and cooperate in the process of training. High-fiber diets combined with a program of regular digital stimulation, suppositories, or enemas usually achieve acceptable control of soiling. Administration of antegrade colonic enemas through an appendicostomy or cecostomy has also been found beneficial in some children with myelomenigocele.

References

Agnarsson U, Warde C, McCarthy G, Evans N: Perianal appearances associated with constipation. Arch Dis Child 65:1231–1234, 1990

Anderson F: Occult spinal dysraphism: a series of 73 cases. Pediatrics 55: 826–835, 1975

Baker SS, Liptak GS, Colleti RB, et al: Constipation in infants and children: evaluation and treatment. A medical position statement of the North

American Society for Pediatric Gastroenterology and Nutrition. J Pediatr Gastroenterol Nutr 29:612–626, 1999

Gleghorn EE, Heyman MB, Rudolph CD: No-enema therapy for idiopathic constipation and encopresis. Clin Pediatr 30:669–672, 1991

Hyman PE, Fleisher D: Functional fecal retention. Practical Gastroenterol 16:29–37, 1992

Iacono G, Cavataio F, Montalto G, et al: Intolerance of cow's milk and chronic constipation in children. N Engl J Med 15:1100–1104, 1998

Loening-Baucke VA, Younoszai MK: Abnormal anal sphincter response in chronically constipated children. J Pediatr 100:213–218, 1982

Lowery SP, Srour JW, Whitehead WE, Schuster MM: Habit training as treatment of encopresis secondary to chronic constipation. J Pediatr Gastroenterol Nutr 4:397–401, 1985

Nolan T, Debelle G, Oberklaid, Coffey C: Randomized trial of laxatives in treatment of childhood encopresis. Lancet 338:523–527, 1991

Partin JC, Hamill SK, Fischel JE, Partin JS: Painful defecation and fecal soiling in children. Pediatrics 89:1007–1009, 1992

Younoszai MK: Stooling problems in patients with myelomeningocele. South Med J 85:718–723, 1992

17.7.7   Approach to the Child with Upper or Lower Gastrointestinal Bleeding

Robert H. Squires, Jr.

The clinical presentation of GI bleeding in children ranges from asymptomatic microcytic anemia to hypovolemic shock. In some children, the time from minimal symptoms to a life-threatening condition can be only a matter of minutes; therefore, a prioritized diagnostic and therapeutic approach to the child with suspected intestinal blood loss is critical. The clinician's first priority is to evaluate the patient for preshock or shock. Once the child is stable, the process of developing a diagnostic and management plan for the next few hours or days can be initiated. Causes of upper and lower GI bleeding are listed in Table 17-35.

There are three typical but often overlapping presentations of GI bleeding. Chronic and occult intestinal bleeding present with features of anemia, including pallor and fatigue. Stools are characteristically normal in color and consistency, but tests for occult blood are positive. Acute upper GI bleeding usually presents with *hematemesis,* which describes the vomiting of gross blood or coffee-ground material, or with passage of *melena,* which describes dark-colored, tarry stools that contain digested blood. An algorithm for the management of children with acute upper GI bleeding is shown in Fig. 17-18. Acute lower GI bleeding usually presents with hematochezia, which is the passage of bright red blood in the stool. Occasionally, severe acute upper GI bleeding may present with hematochezia because the blood is not altered during very rapid transit through the digestive tract. Therefore, the possibility of severe upper GI bleeding always must be included in the differential diagnosis of a child presenting with hematochezia. An algorithm for management of children with acute lower GI bleeding is shown in

TABLE 17-35

DIFFERENTIAL DIAGNOSIS OF GASTROINTESTINAL BLEEDING

ETIOLOGY	NEONATE	INFANT	CHILD	ADOLESCENT
Upper tract				
Esophagitis		++	++	++
Mallory-Weiss tear/gastric prolapse			++	++
Gastritis/duodenitis	++	++	++	++
Peptic ulcer	+	+	++	++
Duplications	+	+		
Mucosal erosion (foreign body/caustic)		+	++	++
Vascular malformation	+	+	+	+
Esophageal varices		+	++	++
Bleeding diathesis	++	+	+	+
Hematobilia		+	+	+
Nasopharyngeal bleeding		+	++	++
Swallowed maternal blood	++			
Leiomyoma	+		+	
Lower tract				
Anal fissure	+	++	+	++
Necrotizing enterocolitis	++			
Milk/soy enterocolitis	++	++		
Hirschsprung enterocolitis	+	+		
Infection	+	++	++	++
Meckel diverticulum		++	++	
Midgut volvulus	+			
Duplication	+	+	+	
Intussusception		++	++	
Polyp			++	++
Henoch-Schönlein purpura			+	+
Hemolytic-uremic syndrome		+	+	+
Inflammatory bowel disease			+	++
Bleeding diathesis	+	+	+	+
Vascular malformation	+	+	+	+
Hemorrhoids				++
Adenocarcinoma				+

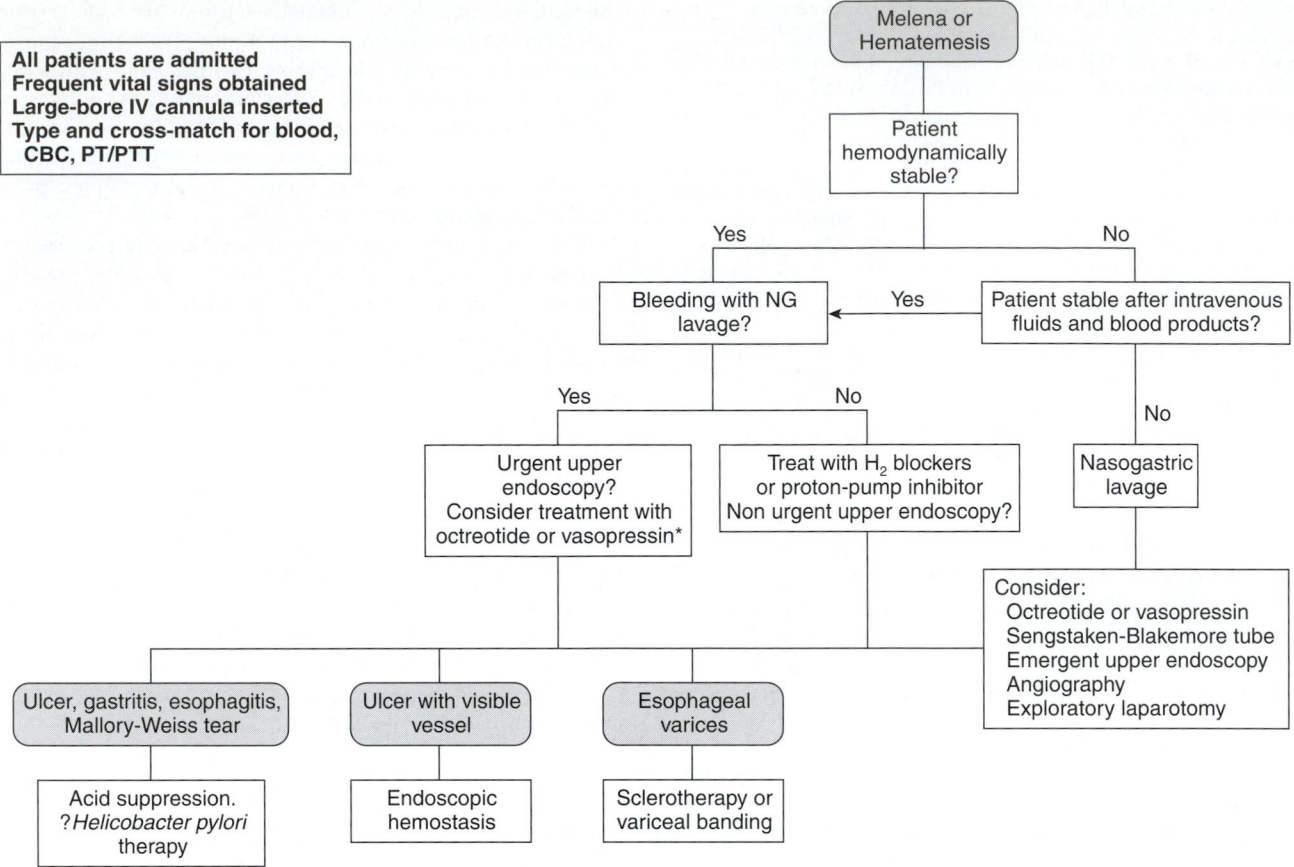

**All patients are admitted
Frequent vital signs obtained
Large-bore IV cannula inserted
Type and cross-match for blood,
CBC, PT/PTT**

FIGURE 17-18   **An approach to evaluation of the patient with upper gastrointestinal bleeding.
CBC = complete blood count; IV = intravenous; NG = nasogastric; PT/PTT = prothrombin time/
partial thromboplastin time. (Vasopressin is given as an intravenous infusion of 0.2-0.5 units/1.76
m²/min to a maximum of 0.5 units/min; octreotide is given as an intravenous bolus of 3-5 μg/kg
followed by an infusion of 3-5 μg/kg/hr.) SOURCE: *Laney DW: The gastrointestinal tract. In: Rudolph AM, Kamei RK, eds: Rudolph's Fundamentals of Pediatrics. Norwalk, CT, Appleton & Lange,
2000.***

Fig. 17-19. Children with profuse upper and lower GI bleeding can present with hypovolemia and shock.

Clues to the diagnosis of patients with intestinal bleeding are obtained with a careful history and physical examination along with focused laboratory and radiographic techniques. Historical clues to the severity and location of intestinal bleeding include the presence and duration of pallor, decreased energy, bloody or coffee-ground emesis, melena, and hematochezia. Exposure to ill contacts or contaminated food must be identified. Recent ingestion of aspirin or other nonsteroidal antiinflammatory drugs, even in appropriate doses, is associated with gastric or duodenal ulceration. The presence of substernal chest pain and bloody emesis following ingestion of a pill or tablet of any kind may result in esophageal ulceration and bleeding if the tablet fails to pass into the stomach. A Mallory-Weiss tear of the esophagus should be suspected if vomiting, retching, or a paroxysmal cough precedes hematemesis. A history of abdominal trauma may be the only clue to the presence of a hepatic laceration resulting in hematobilia. Blood that is present in a nursing mother's milk is known to manifest itself as bloody stools or emesis in her child.

Documenting that blood is indeed present in stool or emesis is an obvious first step. Ingestion of certain food colorings, iron-containing compounds, lead, or bismuth (eg, Pepto-Bismol) will produce red, black, or maroon stools or emesis. Hemoccult and He-

matest cards are simple confirmatory tests for the presence of blood, but they are not perfect. False-positive results are noted with ingestion of numerous foods, including red meat, turnips, bananas, or tomato skins. Iron and bismuth may turn the stool black and confound the reading of guaiac-based tests but do not cause a positive guaiac reaction. False-negative results are caused by ascorbic acid ingestion, a dry stool sample, or outdated reagents. The Apt-Downey test is useful in distinguishing maternal from fetal blood when intestinal hemorrhage is suspected in a newborn. Factitious bleeding has been discovered when blood (human or nonhuman) from a source other than the patient is placed in stool or emesis.

A careful physical examination reveals important clues regarding the significance and cause of bleeding. Heart rate, blood pressure, peripheral perfusion, and level of consciousnes must be monitored carefully. Tachycardia may be the only sign of intestinal hemorrhage. Skin should be inspected for evidence of pigmented discoloration of the lips, fingertips, or axilla (ie, Peutz-Jeghers syndrome), petechiae or purpura (ie, Henoch-Schönlein purpura, coagulopathy), spider angioma (ie, liver disease), and cutaneous hemangioma or telangiectasia (ie, Osler-Weber-Rendu disease). Digital clubbing is associated with chronic liver disease, esophagitis with protein-losing enteropathy, and inflammatory bowel disease. Swallowed blood originating from lesions in the oral and nasal cavity, hypopharynx, and lungs can mimic intestinal bleeding. Intus-

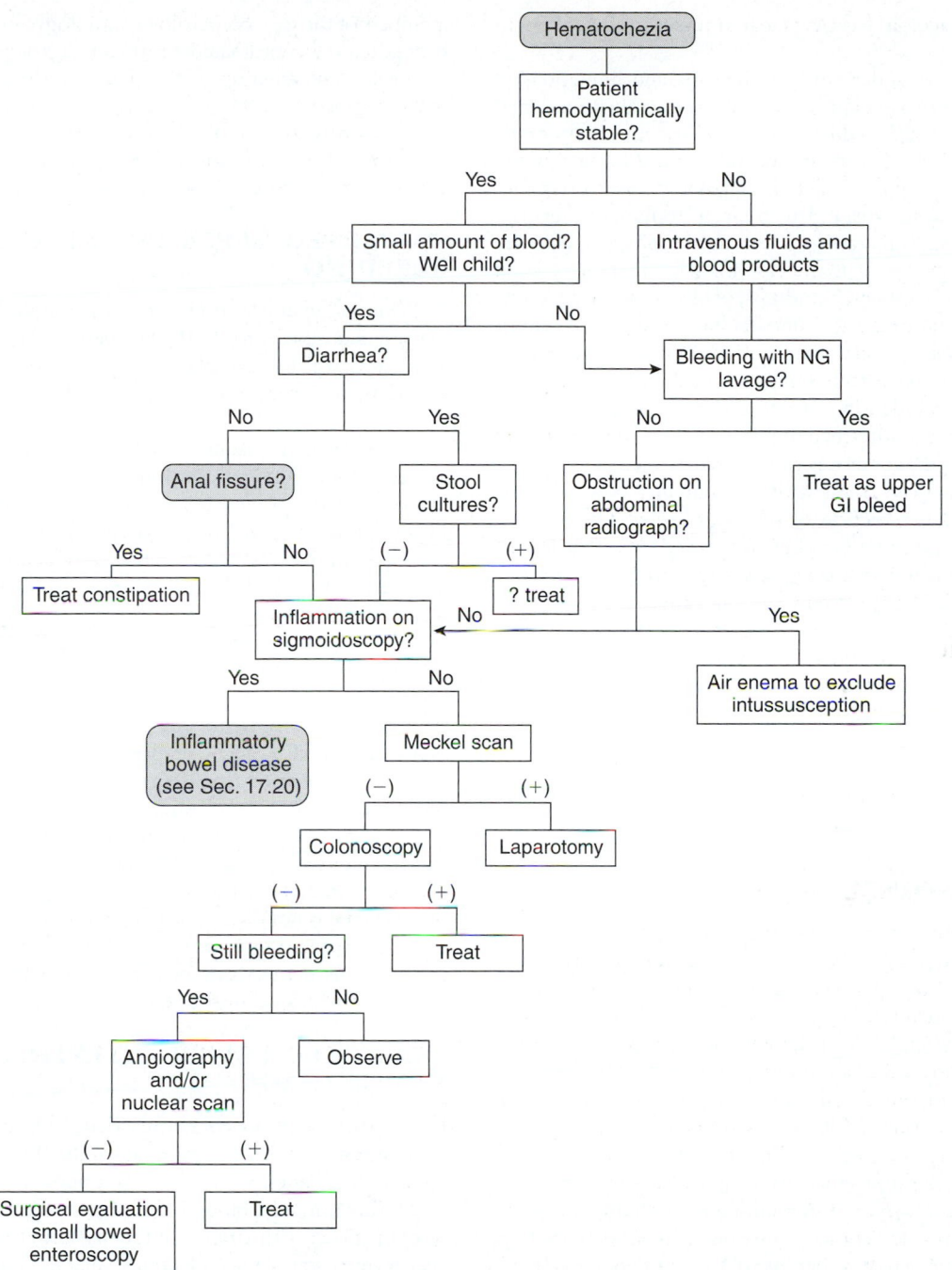

FIGURE 17-19   An approach to evaluation of the patient with hematochezia. Section 17.20 discusses the causes of inflammation of the colon, which present with hematochezia and may be visualized on sigmoidoscopic or colonoscopic evaluation. GI = gastrointestinal; NG = nasogastric.

susception, peptic ulcer disease, intestinal duplication, and inflammatory bowel disease all are associated with abdominal tenderness or mass in the right lower quadrant. An enlarged liver or spleen might suggest esophageal or gastric varices. Esophageal varices can be seen even in the absence of liver disease, as with patients having portal vein thrombosis. The perianal area must be carefully inspected and a digital rectal examination performed on all patients to look for a fissure, fistula, hemorrhoid, or rectal polyp.

Laboratory and radiographic studies are tailored to the patient's symptoms and physical findings. All patients require a complete blood count. A low mean corpuscular volume may indicate chronic blood loss. A low platelet count suggests hypersplenism, immune-mediated thrombocytopenia, hemolytic uremic syndrome, malignancy, or sepsis. Other important blood tests that may add insight to the cause of intestinal bleeding include coagulation studies and both liver and renal function tests. A blood urea nitrogen test that is disproportionately high in relation to the creatinine may suggest upper intestinal hemorrhage. Stool evaluations for white blood cells, parasites, culture (eg, *Salmonella, Shigella, Campylobacter, Aeromonas, E. coli* 0157), and *Clostridium difficile* toxin aid in the diagnosis of patients with blood in the stool. A plain-film radiograph of the abdomen should be examined for evidence of pneumatosis, toxic megacolon, gastric bezoar, intussusception, or pneumoperitoneum.

It is important to understand the benefits and limitations of additional methods that are currently available to evaluate and treat patients with intestinal bleeding. Upper endoscopy allows direct visualization of the mucosa to the second or third portion of the duodenum. Colonoscopy will detect mucosal lesions throughout the colon, including the distal 3 to 5 cm of terminal ileum. Endoscopy can be diagnostic, as is the case for esophagitis, gastritis, or colitis, or therapeutic, as is the case for sclerotherapy or band ligation of esophageal varices, hemostasis of ulcers, or polypectomy. Endoscopy also is necessary for mucosal biopsy when a diagnosis of *Helicobacter pylori* or inflammatory bowel disease is suspected. A radionuclide scan using technetium 99m (^{99m}Tc) pertechnetate (ie, Meckel scan) will identify ectopic gastric mucosa located in a Meckel diverticulum or intestinal duplication, but a negative result does not eliminate these entities as a source of bleeding. A false-positive Meckel scan can occur with inflammatory bowel disease, intussusception, or obstruction of the right ureter. Other radionuclide techniques using ^{99m}Tc sulfur colloid and ^{99m}Tc-labeled red blood cells are used to detect slow, ongoing hemorrhage or slow, intermittent bleeding, respectively. False-negative results do occur (30% in adults), however, and the study often fails to locate the bleeding site accurately. Contrast radiography is helpful in identifying patients with inflammatory bowel disease, intussusception, or stricture, but residual contrast material in the bowel will delay endoscopic or angiographic therapy. If bleeding is ongoing and brisk (ie, >0.5 mL/min), selective angiography may not only identify the site of bleeding but also provide an opportunity to embolize the offending vessel.

URGENT RESPONSE

A patient who presents with blood in emesis or in stool should be considered to be a potential emergency. The most clinically concerning findings include hypotension, orthostatic changes in pulse or blood pressure, tachycardia, an altered level of consciousness, or prolonged capillary refill. When these findings are present, the patient should be observed in an intensive care unit, where prompt, aggressive treatment can be life-saving. A common mistake is to underestimate the amount of blood loss in a hemorrhaging patient. One, but preferably two, *large-bore* intravenous catheters will allow needed fluids and blood products to be quickly administered, and these must be promptly placed. A multilumen central venous catheter provides acceptable venous access, but with severe bleeding, the increased resistance to flow because of the length of the catheter can limit the rate at which blood or fluid can be delivered, so peripheral venous access may be preferable. Supplemental oxygen should be provided. Initial blood work should include a complete blood count, serum electrolyte concentration, liver and renal function tests, coagulation studies, and a crossmatch for blood. An estimated one to two blood volumes (ie, 70 mL/kg/blood volume) of packed red blood cells or whole blood for immediate use and an additional one to two blood volumes in reserve are a reasonable estimate for the needs of children with ongoing hemorrhage. After intravenous access is secure, extracellular-like fluid in aliquots of 15 to 20 mL/kg should be infused rapidly, if necessary, to maintain perfusion until blood is available. Fresh frozen plasma is used to correct coagulation abnormalities, and platelet transfusions are given to a bleeding patient with a platelet count less than 50,000/mL. Central venous pressure and urine output should be closely monitored to guide resuscitation. Early involvement by

members of the gastroenterology, radiology, and surgery teams will strengthen the coordinated effort to treat the patient.

Ideally, investigation of the cause and location of the hemorrhage begins when the heart rate, blood pressure, and perfusion have returned to normal and the patient is stable. Occasionally, bleeding is torrential, and aggressive diagnostic and therapeutic measures must proceed in an unstable patient.

SUSPECTED UPPER INTESTINAL BLEEDING

Blood found in either vomitus or gastric aspirate confirms a bleeding site that is proximal to the ligament of Treitz. Upper intestinal endoscopy will localize bleeding in over 90% of cases and, thus, should be the procedure of choice if it is necessary to identify the site.

If the bleeding episode is not hemodynamically significant, does not require a blood transfusion, and has ceased clinically, and a mucosal erosion or ulcer is suspected, then empiric therapy with an H_2-receptor antagonist or proton pump inhibitor given in an appropriate antiulcer schedule may be initiated without diagnostic endoscopy. Upper endoscopy should be performed, however, if bleeding recurs. Diagnostic and therapeutic upper endoscopy is potentially helpful for patients with ongoing hemorrhage or if knowledge of the location of the bleeding site will alter therapy (eg, ulcer versus varices).

Upper endoscopy provides therapeutic options that were not available a few years ago. Sclerosis or banding of esophageal varices and injection and/or cautery of arterial bleeding can control bleeding where surgical intervention was once the only option. Intravenous octreotide or vasopressin can control variceal hemorrhage and is preferred by many physicians over esophageal tamponade with the potentially hazardous Sengstaken-Blakemore tube. If the bleeding site is not obvious on upper endoscopy or cannot be controlled, the decision to attempt selective angiography to identify and treat the hemorrhage before surgery should be based on the expertise at the local institution.

SUSPECTED LOWER INTESTINAL HEMORRHAGE

Hematochezia is more commonly identified with bleeding from the lower intestinal tract. However, it can be the presenting feature in up to 15% of patients with significant upper intestinal hemorrhage.

Most commonly, blood is noted in streaks on the outside of the stool or mixed with strands of mucus, and it is associated with an anal fissure, colitis (eg, infectious, allergic, chronic inflammatory bowel disease), or a colonic juvenile polyp. Visual inspection of the perianal area, careful digital rectal examination, complete blood count, and stool analysis for white cells, culture, and *Clostridium difficile* toxin are the initial diagnostic studies that should be performed. Flexible sigmoidoscopy or air-contrast barium enema is performed if symptoms persist without a diagnosis.

If bleeding is brisk and/or hemodynamically significant, flexible sigmoidoscopy is indicated early in the evaluation to identify a polyp or colitis. If the sigmoidoscopy fails to reveal a source of bleeding, a Meckel scan is useful to diagnose a Meckel diverticulum or intestinal duplication. A negative Meckel scan should prompt a full colonoscopy to the terminal ileum to identify inflammatory bowel disease, a polyp, or vascular malformation. Biopsies can be obtained at colonoscopy, even if the mucosa appears to be normal, to diagnose eosinophilic, lymphocytic, or nonspecific colitis in addition to chronic inflammatory bowel disease. If bleeding persists and the etiology remains elusive, a fourth procedure would be an upper endoscopy to identify an ulcer, esophageal or gastric varices, or vascular anomaly. Newer, smaller endoscopes allow direct visualization of the entire small bowel when looking for vascular lesions or ulcerations, but experience in children is limited. Selective angiography is useful only if bleeding is ongoing at a rate of 0.5 mL/min, and it should be considered early in the evaluation of unstable or actively hemorrhaging patients. Last, surgical inspection of the bowel combined with endoscopic visualization may be necessary in extreme cases. Early surgical intervention can be life-saving for patients with uncontrollable intestinal bleeding.

17.7.8   Evaluation of Abdominal Masses in Infants and Children

Frederick C. Ryckman

Evaluation of an intraabdominal mass requires an organized approach that considers (1) the age of the patient, (2) the location and characteristics of the mass, and (3) the initial imaging results. Diagnostic possibilities thus can be defined, and appropriate treatment options established.

The initial history is rarely of great assistance in evaluating abdominal masses in infancy. Most masses are asymptomatic and discovered unexpectedly either by the parents or during routine examinations. Some present with intestinal or urinary tract obstruction from compression by the mass. Physical findings and direct radiographic evaluation help to construct an initial differential diagnosis. The salient characteristics of the mass [eg, location, mobility, attachment to surrounding organ structures, consistency (firm to cystic)] and associated anomalies all help to identify the most likely diagnosis. Location of the abdominal mass often is the best guide to identifying the origin of the mass (Fig. 17-20). Abdominal masses exhibit great mobility if they arise from intraperitoneal structures such as the GI tract, mesentery, or omentum; retroperitoneal masses exhibit limited mobility. Inflammatory conditions promote adhesions to surrounding structures and also limit mobility. Cystic masses usually are of GI or genitourinary tract origin. Intraabdominal malignancies more often are solid in consistency and exhibit multilobular architecture. Physical assessment also should include a search for extraabdominal involvement if neoplasm is suspected.

Retroperitoneal masses include those of urinary tract, renal, adrenal, and pancreatic origin. Masses of renal origin, primarily multicystic dysplastic kidney and hydronephrosis, are the most common masses in infants and young children. Multicystic dysplastic kidney occurs as a unilateral soft cystic mass in 80% of cases, with 80% presenting by 2 years of age. Hydronephrosis or urinary tract obstruction also may present as a cystic mass. Other masses of renal origin include renal vein thrombosis, which most commonly occurs in an infant with dehydration and shock, and Wilms tumor, arising within the renal parenchyma. Wilms tumor usually presents as an asymptomatic smooth to slightly lobular abdominal mass with limited mobility at a mean age of 3.5 years; 90% present by 7 years. Mesoblastic nephroma is a benign tumor that mimics Wilms tumor in infants.

Masses of adrenal origin include adrenal hemorrhage and neuroblastoma. Spontaneous hemorrhage into the adrenal gland usually occurs in association with stress or birth trauma, producing an adrenal mass in the neonatal period. Neuroblastoma is the third most common abdominal mass in the child. It presents before 2 years of age in 50% and by 4 years in 85% as a multilobular, fixed, firm, retroperitoneal mass encasing the surrounding organs and frequently crossing the midline. Other retroperitoneal tumors include sarcomas, teratomas, lymphoma, and lipoma, which all can present with encroachment of surrounding structures or direct organ invasion or encasement. An ectopic kidney frequently is palpable in the low flank to upper pelvis.

Masses of liver origin include choledochal cysts and hepatic tumors. Choledochal cyst usually presents as a poorly defined right upper quadrant fullness in infancy with cholestatic jaundice and obstructive biliary tract symptoms, or later in childhood with right upper quadrant pain and fever from cholangitis. Hepatic tumors present as right upper quadrant to midline abdominal masses that are poorly mobile and fixed to the adjoining liver. Most are malignant (65%), with hepatoblastoma exceeding hepatocellular carcinoma by a 4:1 ratio, and present in younger children (mean 2 years vs 6 years). Splenic cysts masquerade as splenomegaly until their true nature is disclosed by ultrasonography or computed tomography.

Gastrointestinal duplication cyst is the most common mass of GI origin in the neonate, but frequently it is not identified until later childhood because of its subtle clinical presentation (see Sec. 17.13.5). Mesenteric, omental, and retroperitoneal cysts are rare cysts of lymphatic origin arising from obstruction of the draining lymphatic plexus. All are soft, cystic, multiloculated, and diffuse, often giving the suggestion on examination of ascites rather than an intraabdominal mass. Their diffuse nature and great mobility make them difficult to circumscribe. Most are asymptomatic or present with symptoms of compression of the surrounding intes-

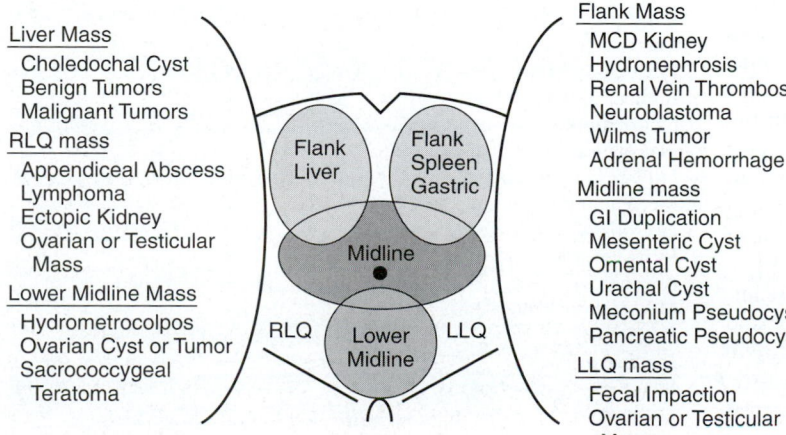

Liver Mass
  Choledochal Cyst
  Benign Tumors
  Malignant Tumors

RLQ mass
  Appendiceal Abscess
  Lymphoma
  Ectopic Kidney
  Ovarian or Testicular
    Mass

Lower Midline Mass
  Hydrometrocolpos
  Ovarian Cyst or Tumor
  Sacrococcygeal
    Teratoma

Flank Mass
  MCD Kidney
  Hydronephrosis
  Renal Vein Thrombosis
  Neuroblastoma
  Wilms Tumor
  Adrenal Hemorrhage

Midline mass
  GI Duplication
  Mesenteric Cyst
  Omental Cyst
  Urachal Cyst
  Meconium Pseudocyst
  Pancreatic Pseudocyst

LLQ mass
  Fecal Impaction
  Ovarian or Testicular
    Mass

FIGURE 17-20 Differential diagnosis of abdominal masses based on their location on physical examination. **GI** = gastrointestinal; **LLQ** = left lower quadrant; **MCD** = multicystic dysplastic; **RLQ** = right lower quadrant.

tinal viscera. Other rarer pseudocysts of the abdomen include those that are related to meconium ileus complications in the newborn or pancreatic pseudocysts most often following trauma. Both are fixed in location and inflammatory; meconium pseudocysts often contain dystrophic calcification within their walls as well. Urachal cysts present in the subumbilical region, are often inflammatory with overlying induration of the abdominal skin, and may have associated urinary tract sepsis. The palpable spleen that is associated with "wandering spleen" syndrome is very mobile, presenting in different locations at various times, has associated abdominal pain when vascular obstruction occurs, and may undergo volvulus on the narrow pancreatic pedicle.

The differential diagnosis of a midline pelvic mass includes ovarian cysts and tumors, hydrometrocolpos and hydrocolpos, and sacrococcygeal teratoma. Ovarian cysts occur in all age groups but present more commonly in adolescents. Overall, 85% of masses are cystic, most of which are benign; 15 to 20% are solid and harbor a greater likelihood of malignancy. In infants, cystic lesions are follicular and unilateral in most cases. Because of their large size relative to the small pelvis, they often are displaced into the lower abdomen. Hydrometrocolpos and hydrocolpos are masses involving the lower female reproductive tract that are complex in structural anatomy and presentation. During infancy, they present as palpable lower midline masses that can extend superiorly to the umbilicus in many cases. If the uterus is not involved (ie, hydrocolpos), it often is palpable on the top of the abdominal mass as a small nodule. Presentation may be delayed until adolescence, when the products of menstruation cannot drain, causing cyclic abdominal pain and urinary tract obstructive symptoms. Sacrococcygeal teratoma is the most common solid tumor in newborns, but it rarely presents with only a palpable abdominal mass. The mass usually is associated with an abnormal sacrum and is palpable on the ventral surface of the sacrum during rectal examination.

Other masses in the pelvis include (1) fecal collections, which are occasionally seen with Hirschsprung disease but more commonly result from functional constipation; (2) abscess collections associated with a perforated appendix or of tuboovarian origin; (3) ovarian or testicular torsion; and (4) duplications of the rectum extending in the retrorectal space. Lymphoma and ectopic kidneys also may present as right lower quadrant masses.

Radiographic investigation usually is required to establish or confirm a diagnosis. All abdominal masses in children except organomegaly and normal anatomic variants require surgical consultation. Plain-film radiographs of the abdomen are helpful as a primary screening examination, which may demonstrate calcification within the mass or associated bony abnormalities, but further imaging almost always is necessary. Abdominal ultrasonography is the primary imaging modality for the evaluation of an abdominal mass in children. The consistency of the mass (eg, solid, cystic), potential involvement of surrounding structures, and vascular invasion usually can be determined with minimal morbidity. Occasionally, the resolution of ultrasonography is limited by intestinal gas or extreme obesity. Further definition of complex intraabdominal masses, solid-tissue masses, and potential neoplasm is best obtained using computed tomography or magnetic resonance imaging because of their accuracy in characterizing the consistency and organ of origin. The three-dimensional information that is contained on these imaging studies allows characterization of both the consistency and the organ of origin for the mass, which is essential for the careful surgical planning that is required to safely remove complex masses. Magnetic resonance imaging is of particular benefit when vascular structures are involved and usually replaces angiography. Genito-

urinary tract abnormalities often require special anatomic definition with cystourethrography and genitoscopy.

References

Irish MS, Pearl RH, Caty MG, Glick PL: The approach to common abdominal diagnosis in infants and children. Pediatr Clin North Am 45: 729–772, 1998

Pearl RH, Irish MS, Caty MG, Glick PL: The approach to common abdominal diagnosis in infants and children. Part II. Pediatr Clin North Am 45:1287–1326, 1998

Quillin SP, Siegel MJ: Color Doppler US of children with acute lower abdominal pain. Radiographics 13:1281–1293, 1993

White KS: Imaging of abdominal masses in children. Semin Pediatr Surg 1: 269–276, 1992

17.7.9   Approach to the Child with Gastrointestinal Obstruction

Frederick C. Ryckman

Gastrointestinal obstruction is an important cause of morbidity and mortality in children. Early investigation employing an orderly approach is mandatory to establish the correct diagnosis and initiate appropriate treatment. Differential diagnostic pathways are best defined by the age of the patient and the level of obstruction. Table 17-36 lists potential diagnoses at different ages, and Figs. 17-21 and 17-22 provide algorithms for the evaluation of infants, children, and adolescents who present with intestinal obstruction.

EVALUATION OF THE NEWBORN INFANT WITH GASTROINTESTINAL OBSTRUCTION

The presence of intestinal obstruction often is suggested before the infant is delivered, which allows neonatal and surgical evaluation with early and planned intervention. Fetal ultrasonography may reveal maternal polyhydramnios, which occurs with disorders affecting fetal swallowing such as anencephaly, diaphragmatic hernia,

TABLE 17-36

CAUSES OF GASTROINTESTINAL OBSTRUCTION IN INFANTS, CHILDREN, AND ADOLESCENTS

DIAGNOSIS	INFANT	CHILD	ADOLESCENT
Esophageal atresia	x		
Intestinal atresia	x		
Antral web	x	x	
Duodenal web	x	x	x
Annular pancreas	x	x	
Malrotation	x	x	x
Malrotation with volvulus	x	x	x
Hirschsprung disease	x	x	x
Meconium syndromes	x	x	x
Necrotizing enterocolitis	x		
Intussusception	x	x	x
Appendicitis		x	x
Meckel diverticulum	x	x	x
Duplications	x	x	x
Inguinal hernia	x	x	x
Pseudoobstruction syndromes	x	x	x

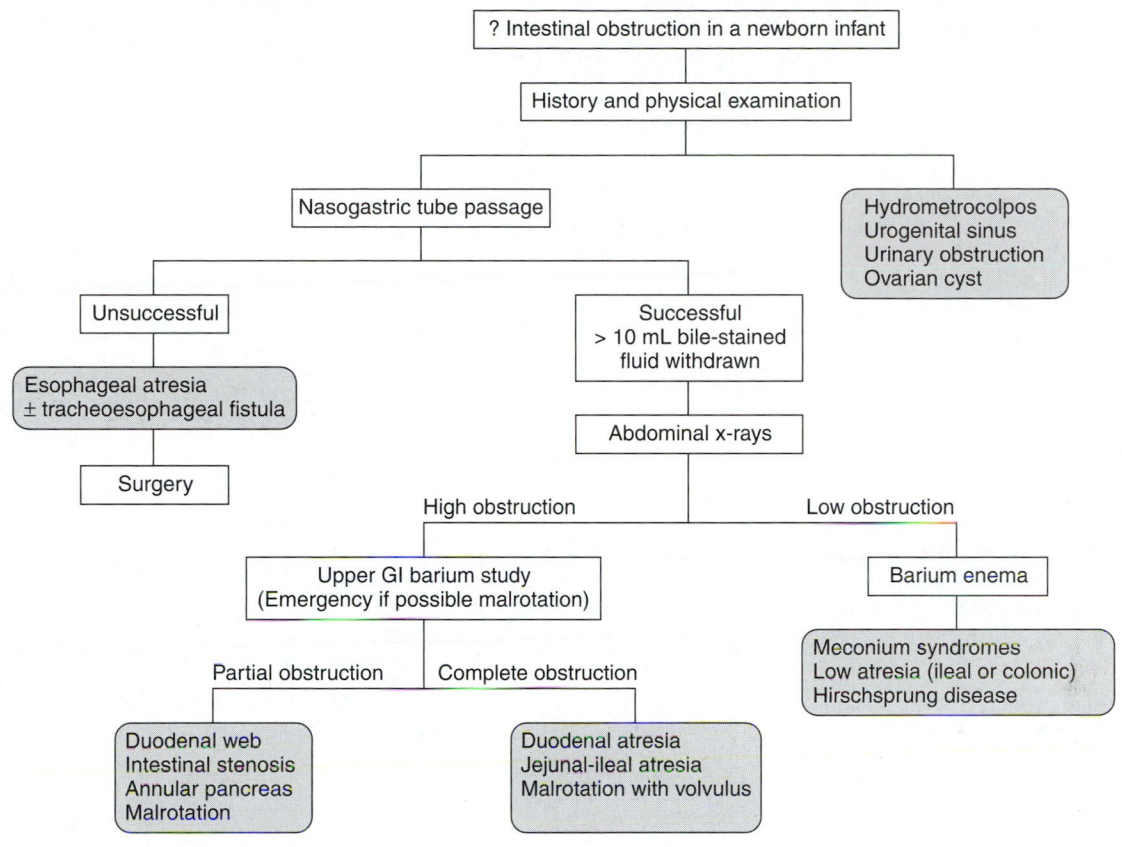

FIGURE 17-21   **Evaluation of gastrointestinal (GI) obstruction in the newborn infant.**

cystic adenomatoid pulmonary malformations, or esophageal obstruction as well as high intestinal obstruction. The presence of antenatal intestinal obstruction is suggested by the finding of a fluid-filled distended intestine, with the level of obstruction implied by the extent of the bowel distention. Meconium peritonitis, pseudocyst formation, and intraperitoneal calcifications also can be recognized by ultrasonography. The absence of a normal fluid-filled stomach suggests esophageal atresia. However, although these studies strongly suggest intestinal obstruction, they require postnatal verification before definitive treatment can be undertaken.

In the newborn, excessive salivation, vomiting, abdominal distension, or failure to pass meconium within the first 24 hours after birth may signal GI obstruction. The character of the emesis provides an important clue to defining the level of obstruction. Nonbilious emesis suggests an obstructive lesion before the ampulla of Vater, whereas bilious emesis is associated with obstruction at or beyond the ampulla. Bilious emesis, or bile-stained nasogastric tube output exceeding 10 to 15 mL on placement, requires *urgent* evaluation to exclude abnormalities requiring emergency surgical intervention such as midgut volvulus.

Infants with congenital GI obstruction often present with minimal abnormalities on abdominal examination. Upper abdominal distension is more characteristic of pyloric, duodenal, and proximal jejunal obstruction. It is not uncommon, however, for infants with high intestinal obstruction to have a scaphoid abdomen as a result of the limited amount of distended intestine. Conversely, generalized abdominal distension often accompanies distal intestinal obstruction, and loops of distended intestine may be visible or palpable. Signs of peritoneal irritation often are subtle in newborns. On palpation of the tender abdomen, the infant may grimace, cry

out, or draw the legs up toward the abdomen. Even when tenderness is elicited, significant guarding or muscular rigidity is found infrequently because of the poorly developed abdominal wall musculature in the neonate. Abdominal wall erythema may reflect underlying intraperitoneal infection in newborns, and it frequently overlies an inflammatory mass. The often subtle progression of these physical findings is best appreciated through serial examinations by the same experienced examiner. A rectal examination should be performed routinely to exclude anorectal anomalies or presacral masses and to establish the presence or absence of normal meconium.

Radiography is the cornerstone of evaluation in neonatal intestinal obstruction. Air that is swallowed by the infant serves as an excellent contrast agent to initially assess intestinal patency. In the normal newborn, air reaches the stomach in 10 to 15 minutes, the jejunum in 1 hour, and has traversed the entire small bowel in 6 hours. The colon is filled by 12 to 14 hours, and meconium is passed by 24 hours after birth. Failure of gas to progress through the entire intestine in 12 to 24 hours should raise the suspicion of intestinal obstruction; however, a severe ileus or sepsis also will mimic this radiographic picture. Although passage of intestinal gas to the rectum excludes totally obstructing lesions, it does not exclude functional obstructions resulting from Hirschsprung disease or partially obstructing lesions. Plain anteroposterior and horizontal beam radiographs often are diagnostic of complete obstructions of the intestine from duodenal atresia or jejunal-ileal atresia (see Sec. 17.13.4). In complete atresia, massive distension of the intestine occurs, and the length of distended intestine corresponds to the level of the obstruction. Incomplete obstruction allows the passage of distal gas, making prediction of the level of obstruction difficult without contrast evaluation. Duodenal obstruction with-

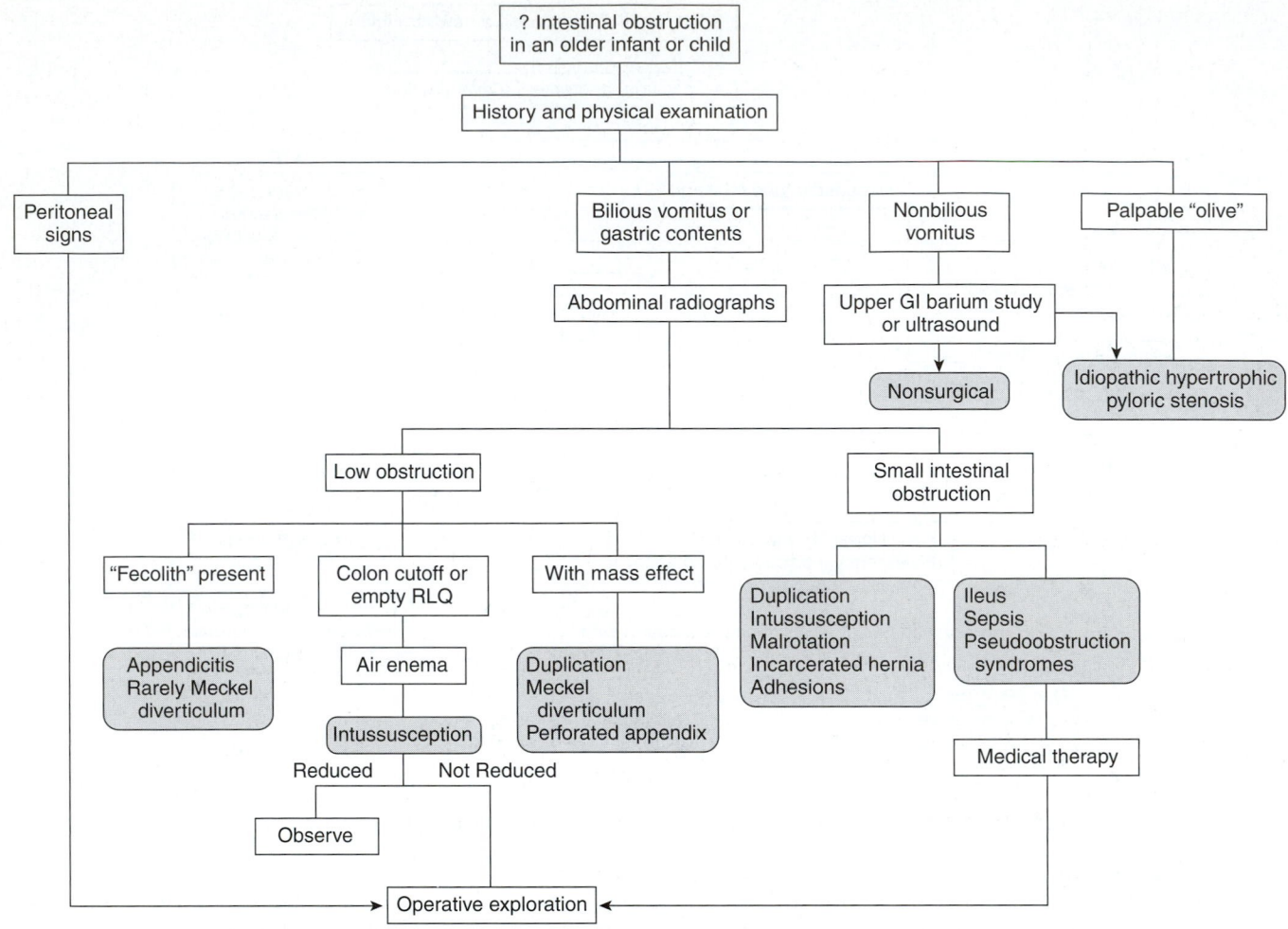

FIGURE 17-22   Evaluation of gastrointestinal (GI) obstruction in the older infant and child. RLQ = right lower quadrant; IHPS = idiopathic hypertrophic pyloric stenosis.

out dilatation or gastric distension and demonstrated distal intestinal gas are more characteristic of malrotation with volvulus. Differentiation of small from large bowel is difficult because the valvulae conniventes of the small bowel and the colonic haustra generally are not visualized in patients younger than 2 years of age. The number and length of the distended bowel loops provide the best clue to the level of obstruction. Calcification within the abdomen is characteristic of meconium syndromes with perforation (see Sec. 17.14.1) and abdominal masses. Pneumatosis intestinalis may be seen in patients with necrotizing enterocolitis. Free intraperitoneal air implies intestinal perforation.

If plain-film radiographs fail to establish a diagnosis, contrast studies may be required. High intestinal obstructions, partial obstructions, and intestinal malrotation are best defined by an upper GI contrast study. With lower obstructions, a contrast enema provides important information by identifying the site of obstruction (ie, small bowel, large bowel), location of the cecum, and presence or absence of a microcolon. Microcolon most commonly is seen in distal small intestinal obstructions, including meconium ileus and ileal atresia. Hirschsprung disease (see Sec. 17.23.3) characteristically demonstrates colonic distension with a "transition zone" at the level of aganglionosis, which must be confirmed by rectal biopsy. Additional radiographic studies rarely are indicated be-

fore definitive operative exploration and surgical correction as indicated.

EVALUATION OF INFANTS AND CHILDREN WITH GASTROINTESTINAL OBSTRUCTION

Children beyond infancy present with the classical findings of intestinal obstruction, including nausea, vomiting, colicky abdominal pain, abdominal tenderness, distension, and obstipation as the degree of obstruction progresses. The presence of nonbilious vomiting suggests either pyloric obstruction or nonobstructive etiologies such as viral or bacterial sepsis. Partial intestinal obstruction or obstruction caused by inflammatory pelvic sources often has associated diarrhea or frequent loose, low-volume stools. Bloody mucoid stools, which classically are described as "currant jelly," may occur with intussusception (see Sec. 17.14.3) or any other processes leading to intestinal ischemia. The ability to elicit localized tenderness increases with advancing age as the level of cooperation displayed by the patient improves. Specific pathologic entities may have characteristic examination findings, including the "olive" of pyloric stenosis, the "sausage-shaped" mass of intussusception, and appendiceal inflammatory masses. A history of prior abdominal surgery suggests the possibility of postoperative adhesions. An incarcerated or strangulated inguinal hernia also may cause obstruction; this is most common in premature infants or in infants during the first year of life. GI obstruction is a well-known complication of inflammatory bowel disease. Meconium ileus equivalent (ie, distal intestinal pseudo-obstruction syndrome) is an intraluminal obstruction that occurs beyond the neonatal period in patients with cystic fibrosis.

Radiographic evaluation of older infants and children is directed by their age-specific diagnostic possibilities and their clinical presentation. Supine and cross-table lateral or upright abdominal radiographs should be obtained in all patients with suspected intestinal obstruction to identify the characteristic radiographic findings of air-fluid levels and bowel distension. The absence of air in the right lower quadrant may be found with intussusception or abscess formation following appendicitis; pathologic calcifications in an appendix or Meckel diverticulum can be identified. Air may be seen within the scrotum in an incarcerated hernia. Free air within the abdomen is diagnostic of intestinal perforation.

The need for further contrast studies is dictated by the clinical findings. When peritoneal signs or complete obstruction suggests the need for laparotomy, further investigation is not warranted. The use of abdominal ultrasonography has enhanced the recognition of hypertrophic pyloric stenosis, pelvic abscesses, appendicitis, ovarian abnormalities, and intraabdominal masses causing partial intestinal obstruction. Further investigation of partial small intestinal obstruction is best undertaken using a barium upper GI series. Air insufflation enemas may be not only diagnostic but also therapeutic in cases of intussusception (see Sec. 17.14.3).

EVALUATION OF THE ADOLESCENT WITH GASTROINTESTINAL OBSTRUCTION

Intestinal obstruction in the adolescent almost always results from inflammatory disease (eg, appendicitis, pelvic inflammatory disease, inflammatory bowel disease) or adhesive bowel obstruction from prior abdominal surgery or is secondary to another intraabdominal mass. History and physical examination findings will direct the investigation toward specific organ systems. Radiographic evaluation consists of plain-film radiographs and often ultrasonography to identify contributing pathology. Complete intestinal obstructions presenting in this age group require prompt surgical intervention; partial intestinal obstructions arising from inflammatory complications of preexisting bowel disease or pelvic inflammatory sources may be managed with nonoperative treatment. Superior mesenteric artery syndrome or "cast syndrome" usually is seen with weight loss or in patients who are placed in whole-body casts. The duodenum is compressed between the superior mesenteric artery anteriorly and the aorta posteriorly. Symptoms resolve with weight gain, which is best achieved using nasojejunal tube feeding.

PREOPERATIVE MANAGEMENT

Laboratory findings in patients with intestinal obstruction rarely assist in making a definitive diagnosis, but they often identify biochemical abnormalities requiring correction before operative intervention. Disorders of acid-base balance are most common. A hypokalemic, hypochloremic metabolic alkalosis may result from excessive vomiting, whereas a metabolic acidosis may occur with hypoperfusion, necrotic bowel, or systemic sepsis. A complete blood count with differential may reveal a leukocytosis and left shift in the presence of infection or inflammation.

Hyperbilirubinemia may be present with pyloric stenosis and in up to 40% of patients with jejunal atresia. Because cystic fibrosis is commonly associated with meconium ileus (10 to 15%) and jejunoileal atresia (10 to 12%), screening genetic tests for cystic fibrosis should be obtained in these patients before their discharge from the hospital.

Once the diagnosis of GI obstruction is suspected or confirmed, aggressive fluid resuscitation should be initiated. Electrolyte abnormalities should be corrected. The patient should be placed at complete bowel rest, and a nasogastric tube should be inserted to facilitate decompression. A Foley catheter should be used when needed to monitor urine output and assess the adequacy of fluid resuscitation. Broad-spectrum antibiotics usually are begun before operative intervention in anticipation of the potential need to resect unprepared intestine.

17.8 FEEDING AND SWALLOWING

Dana Thompson Link and Colin D. Rudolph

Feeding includes food acquisition, ingestion, digestion, and absorption. This activity relieves hunger and provides multisensory stimulation, thereby providing a pleasant, rewarding experience for both the child and the caretaker. Successful feeding experiences create positive reciprocal interactions that reinforce the bonding relationship between child and caretaker. Feeding disorders disrupt this process; in addition, disruptions may prevent the infant from ingesting adequate nutrients for continued health, growth, and development.

Feeding and swallowing are complex processes that can be divided functionally into four phases, as shown in Figs. 17-23 and 17-24. The *preoral phase* is initiated when the child senses and communicates hunger. The *oral phase* is a food-processing step wherein the ingested material is formed into a bolus that can safely pass through the pharynx without entering the airway. Once the bolus enters the pharynx, the remainder of the swallowing process is involuntary and reflexive. The *pharyngeal phase* is quite rapid. It is initiated by bolus contact with the tonsillar pillars and pharyngeal wall with subsequent elevation of the larynx, vocal cord closure, and relaxation of the upper esophageal sphincter. A peristaltic wave of contraction of the pharynx propels the bolus into the esophagus.

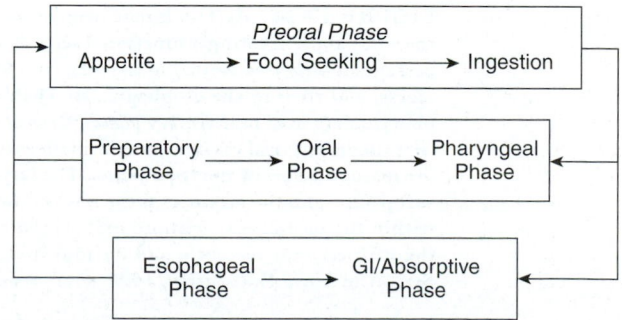

FIGURE 17-23 Model of the normal phases of feeding in infants and children. Complex interactions between phases often obscure diagnosis of the primary cause of a feeding disorder.

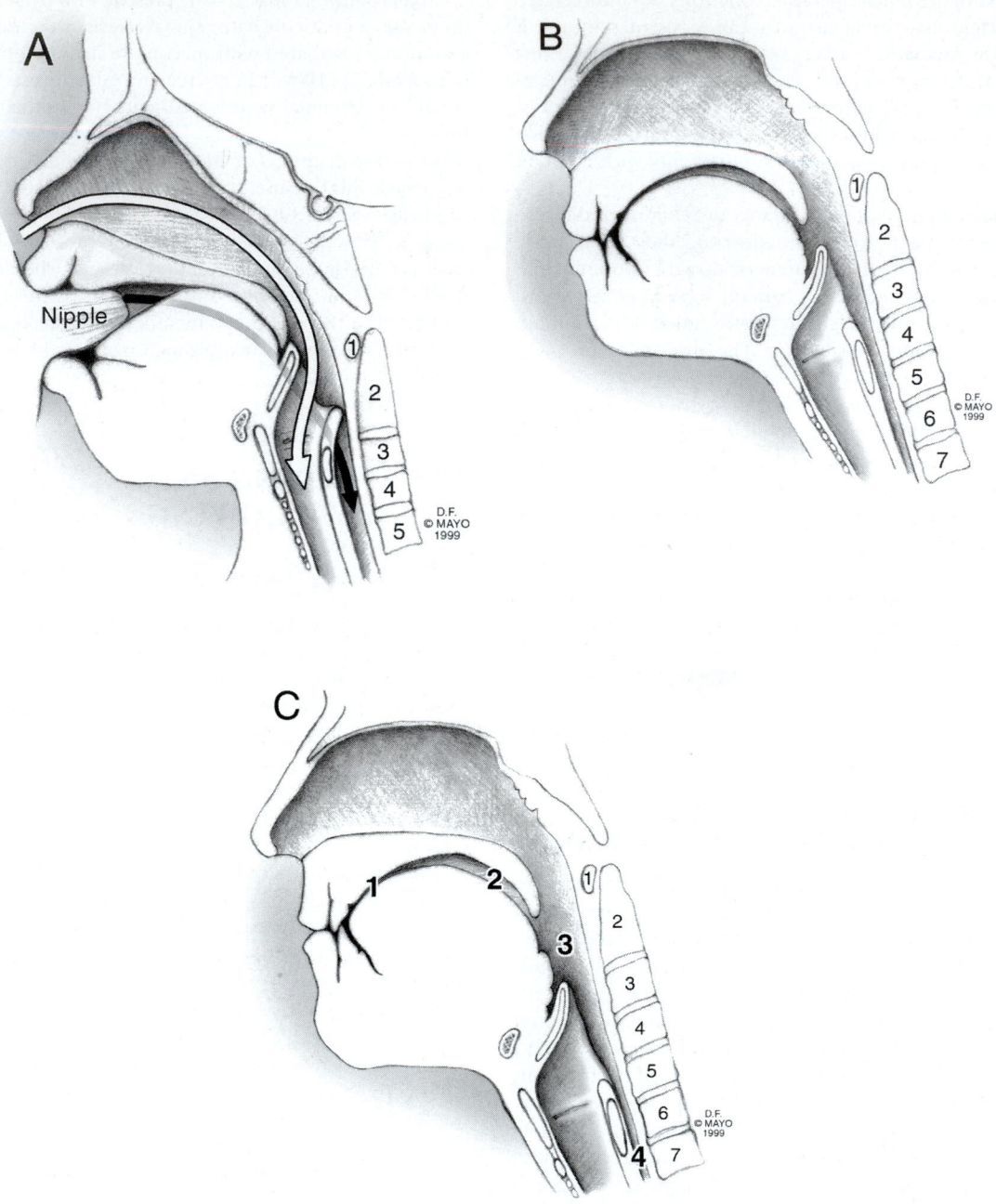

FIGURE 17-24   A: The infant oropharynx. The larynx is elevated with the epiglottis touching the soft palate, creating a functional separation between the air passages *(white arrow)* and the food passages *(black/gray arrow)* in the pharynx. Food courses around the epiglottis, into the pharyngeal recess, and then to the esophagus. **B:** The toddler (2-3 years old) oropharynx. **C:** The adult oropharynx: *(1) oral preparatory phase, (2) oral phase, (3) pharyngeal phase, (4) esophageal phase.* Note that the infant oral cavity is much smaller than the child or adult oral cavity, providing little space for manipulation of the food bolus. The larynx is elevated so that the epiglottis almost touches the soft palate, and the larynx is at the level of the first to third cervical vertebrae. The tongue is entirely within the oral cavity, with no oral region of the pharynx. In the toddler, the larynx descends to the fifth cervical vertebra, and by adulthood it descends to the sixth to seventh cervical vertebra. **SOURCE:** *Mayo Foundation, 1999, with permission.*

During passage of the bolus through the pharynx, excellent coordination between breathing and swallowing is essential to prevent aspiration. In the *esophageal phase,* the bolus is transported into the stomach. Finally, the bolus is broken down and absorbed during the digestive phase. There are developmental and maturational changes in the phases of swallowing that occur from infancy to childhood that can have a significant impact on a child's ability to feed successfully.

Symptoms of feeding and swallowing disorders in children have many manifestations and clinical presentations, anywhere from food refusal, failure to thrive, and oral aversion to recurrent pneumonia, chronic lung disease, or recurrent emesis. Swallowing and feeding disorders in infants and children are complex and can have multiple etiologies; these are listed in Table 17-37. Organic and nonorganic etiologies occur alone or in combination, making the diagnosis and treatment challenging and complicated. Feeding and swallowing can be interrupted in any phase. Successful management of the child with feeding problems begins with the identification and treatment of any correctable underlying physical cause of the feeding disorder. Identification and addressing of both parent and patient nonorganic behavioral factors occurring concurrently with a physical cause will enhance management. Only after all reasonable physical etiologies have been ruled out should a feeding or swallowing disorder be attributed to a nonorganic cause.

17.8.1   Preoral Phase

APPETITE

Centers for hunger and satiety in the hypothalamus receive afferent signals from a variety of sources. Sensory inputs that affect feeding behavior are well developed even in infants. Appetite also is affected by emotional state: infants who are not nurtured reduce their food intake and fail to thrive. Reductions in appetite are frequent in infants and children with chronic debilitating disease; however, very specific food aversions may be observed in otherwise healthy people. If ingestion of a specific food is temporally associated with a painful or uncomfortable experience, a child may refuse to ingest that food again. This type of specific aversion is observed in patients with metabolic diseases, gastroesophageal reflux, or allergies who experience nausea or discomfort after ingesting offending nutrients (eg, as seen with ingestion of sucrose in patients having hereditary fructose intolerance). More generalized feeding aversions can occur if an infant has negative experiences such as aspiration or choking during feeding. Infants who have required prolonged airway intubation or tube feeding often learn that efforts by a caretaker to approach their mouth or face likely result in discomfort, and the "oral defensiveness" can persist long after the patient is extubated.

FOOD SEEKING AND INGESTION

Preverbal infants and developmentally delayed children communicate hunger by providing behavioral cues to their provider; in turn, the caretaker must correctly interpret these cues. If the caretaker misses the cue and offers food when the child is not interested in eating, the resultant struggle can easily exacerbate the situation. In toddlers, food seeking consists of communicating hunger. Efforts to independently use a spoon and cup and, ultimately, to obtain food from the refrigerator themselves progress through development. In adults, food seeking is a complicated process that includes

most aspects of our daily lives. The mechanical process of ingestion requires the appropriate muscular coordination and sensation to bring food to the mouth. This is a learned process that evolves through normal development (Table 17-12). Neuromuscular disorders, blindness, and fatigue resulting from illness all can interfere with food ingestion.

Infants with subtle feeding disorders are less resilient in responding to difficult environments and emotional deprivation than are normal infants. Many children who have been diagnosed with nonorganic failure to thrive have subtle neuromuscular or oral-motor disorders. Successful management in this setting requires teaching caretakers how to adjust feeding techniques appropriately. Continued unsuccessful efforts to feed the child can disrupt the caretaker–child relationship even in well-adjusted families.

17.8.2   Swallowing

ORAL PHASE

The oral phase consists of bolus formation and movement of a food substance posteriorly towards the pharynx. Oral phase development begins at 15 weeks of gestation with mouthing and suckling movements. By 32 weeks, a disordered pattern of sucking bursts and pauses emerges. By 34 to 36 weeks, the fetus displays a stable pattern of rhythmic suckling and swallowing. After birth, swallowing is triggered when a certain volume of fluid occupies the oral cavity. Excellent tongue motion and coordination are needed for this phase of swallowing.

During postnatal development, there are anatomic changes that occur in the oral cavity with concurrent development and maturation of motor skills required for safe feeding (Fig. 17-12). In infancy, the oral phase of swallowing consists of the subcortically regulated process of suckling, characterized by primitive extension-retraction motion of the tongue. The small size of the mandible and oral cavity relative to the tongue and the presence of buccal fat pads facilitate suckling and provide an ideal geometry for generating suction on a nipple but leave little room or ability for manipulation of a solid bolus. Food delivery is accomplished by sealing the lips around the breast or nipple and then sealing the posterior aspect of the oral cavity with the tongue against the palate. Depressing the oral surface of the tongue creates suction pressure for bolus delivery. Suction pressures greater than 100 mm Hg are generated in the oral cavity of normal newborns, with the amount of pressure varying to adjust the flow rate to approximately 0.2 mL per suck. Too rapid a flow results in overflow of formula into the pharynx before the initiation of an organized swallow, with the potential for aspiration.

Between 3 and 6 months of age the anatomy of the oral cavity and pharynx begins to change, and infants start to suppress the suckle pattern and develop voluntary suck patterns. The anatomic changes include resorption of the buccal fat pads and the inferior and forward drop of the jaw, thus increasing the intraoral space. Tongue movements mature from extension-retraction motion of suckling to up-and-down movements of sucking, facilitating bolus manipulation and thereby allowing for a more coordinated transport of food and liquid into the oral cavity. This maturation in skill allows infants to begin eating textured food from a spoon by 8 months of age. Masticatory skills begin to develop by 6 to 8 months and continue to develop as the alveolar ridges mature and deciduous teeth erupt. At 12 months sucking patterns are minimized, and children generally transition to cup drinking and no longer use

TABLE 17-37

CAUSES OF FEEDING DISORDERS IN CHILDREN

Disorders that affect appetite, food-seeking behavior, and ingestion
Depression
Deprivation
Central nervous system disease (diencephalic syndrome)
Metabolic diseases
   Hereditary fructose intolerance
   Urea cycle disorders
   Organic acidemias
Sensory defects
   Anosmia
   Blindness
Neuromuscular disease (see below)
Oral hypersensitivity or aversion resulting from a lack of feeding experience during critical sensitive periods (long-term parenteral or enteral feeding)
Conditioned dysphagia
   Aspiration
   Oral inflammation (see below)
   Gastroesophageal reflux
   Dumping syndrome or gastric bloating after gastric surgery
   Fatigue (heart disease, lung disease)
Poverty
Anorexia nervosa

Anatomic abnormalities of the oropharynx
Cleft lip and/or palate
Macroglossia
Ankyloglossia
Pierre Robin sequence
Retropharyngeal mass or abscess
Velopharyngeal insufficiency
Tonsillar hypertrophy
Dental caries

Anatomic/congenital abnormalities of the larynx and trachea
Laryngeal cleft
Laryngomalacia
Laryngeal cyst
Subglottic stenosis
Tracheomalacia
Tracheoesophageal cleft
Tracheoesophageal compression from vascular ring/sling

Anatomic abnormalities of the esophagus
Tracheoesophageal fistula
Congenital esophageal atresia
Congenital esophageal stenosis because of tracheobronchial remnants
Esophageal stricture, web, or ring
Esophageal mass or tumor
Foreign body
Vascular rings and dysphagia lusoria

Disorders affecting suck-swallow-breathing coordination
Choanal atresia
Bronchopulmonary dysplasia
Cardiac disease
Tachypnea (respiratory rates >60/min)

Disorders affecting neuromuscular coordination of swallowing
Cerebral palsy
Bulbar atresia or palsy
Brainstem glioma
Arnold-Chiari malformation
Myelomeningocele
Familial dysautonomia
Tardive dyskinesia
Nitrazepam-induced dysphagia
Postdiphtheritic and postpolio paralysis
Möbius syndrome (cranial nerve abnormalities)
Myasthenia gravis
Infant botulism
Congenital myotonic dystrophy
Oculopharyngeal dystrophy
Muscular dystrophies and myopathies
Cricopharyngeal achalasia
Polymyositis/dermatomyositis
Rheumatoid arthritis

Disorders affecting esophageal peristalsis
Achalasia
Chagas disease
Diffuse esophageal spasm
Pseudoobstruction
Scleroderma
Mixed connective tissue disease
Systemic lupus erythematosus
Polymyositis/dermatomyositis
Rheumatoid arthritis

Mucosal infections and inflammatory disorders causing dysphagia
Adenotonsillitis
Deep neck space infections
Epiglottitis
Laryngopharyngeal reflux from GER
Gastroesophageal reflux (GER)
Eosinophilic esophagitis
Caustic ingestion
Candida pharyngitis or esophagitis
Herpes simplex esophagitis
Human immunodeficiency virus
Cytomegalovirus esophagitis
Medication-induced esophagitis
Crohn disease
Behçet disease
Chronic graft-versus-host disease

Other miscellaneous disorders associated with feeding and swallowing difficulties
Xerostomia
Hypothyroidism
Neonatal hyperparathyroidism
Trisomy 18 and 21
Prader-Willi syndrome
Allergies
Lipid and lipoprotein metabolism disorders
Neurofibromatosis
Williams syndrome
Coffin-Siris syndrome
Opitz-G syndrome
Cornelia de Lange syndrome
Interstitial deletion (13)(q21.3q31)
Globus pharyngeus
Epidermolysis bullosa dystrophica
Velocardiofacial syndrome (chromosome 22q11 deletion)

---

the suck pattern. By 18 to 24 months rotary chewing skills and increased lateral activity of the tongue contribute to more effective handling, crushing, and grinding of food.

Specific oral skills such as sucking or chewing solids are learned only at certain ages (Table 17-12). Infants who do not orally feed during these so-called "critical periods" of development have a difficult time mastering these skills later; these patients may learn how to spoon and cup feed without ever learning an effective suck. Development of the oral phase requires normal anatomy, intact sensory feedback, and normal muscle strength and coordination. Anatomic defects include cleft lip with or without cleft palate, micrognathia, and macroglossia. A weak suck may be congenital or acquired. Other causes of oral-phase dysfunction include xerostomia and temporomandibular joint pathology.

PHARYNGEAL PHASE

The pharyngeal phase of swallowing is involuntary and is triggered by bolus contact with the tonsillar pillars and pharyngeal wall. During pharyngeal swallowing the upper pharynx and soft palate close to seal the nasal cavity as the bolus enters the pharynx. The bolus is propelled to the esophagus by contraction of the pharyngeal muscles. Proprioceptive feedback adjusts this activity as needed to compensate for different types of boluses. During pharyngeal contraction, the larynx elevates, the vocal cords close, and respiration ceases to protect the lower airway from aspiration. The upper esophageal sphincter relaxes, and peristaltic contractions of the pharynx push the bolus past the displaced, closed larynx into the upper esophagus. Because the pharynx is the common chamber for the respiration and digestive pathways, important developmental changes occur to allow for safe swallowing (Fig. 17-24). In the infant, the larynx sits high in the neck at the level of vertebrae C1 to C3, allowing the velum, tongue, and epiglottis to approximate and thereby functionally separate the respiratory and digestive tracts. This allows the infant to safely breathe and feed. Even though this unique functional separation exist in infants, vigorous sucking and swallowing during feeding can cause significant reductions of minute ventilation and mild hypoxia even in normal babies. Babies with compromised cardiac or respiratory function may have serious difficulties with hypoxia during feeding.

By age 2 to 3 years the larynx descends, decreasing the separation of the swallowing and digestive tracts. Intact oral motor skills and laryngeal function are essential for coordinating the oral and pharyngeal phases of swallowing to prevent complications of aspiration. Early overflow of the bolus into the pharynx before respiration ceases may allow food to enter the trachea during inspiration. Lack of relaxation of the upper esophageal sphincter causes pooling in the piriform sinuses with resultant food overflow into the airway when the larynx descends at the end of the swallow sequence and inspiration begins. Because there is less separation of the swallowing and digestive tracts at this developmental stage, subtle anatomic or neuromuscular disorders that are not problematic in an infant can cause recurrent aspiration in a toddler.

Laryngopharyngeal sensory deficits from neurologic disorders or decreased laryngeal sensitivity from chronic extraesophageal gastroesophageal reflux predispose to problems with coordinating swallowing and increase aspiration risk. Congenital abnormalities, including laryngeal clefts or laryngomalacia, can result in dysphagia and aspiration. Myopathies, central nervous system abnormalities, tumor masses, foreign bodies, esophageal peristaltic disorders, or inflammation (Table 17-37) can disrupt the pharyngeal phase of swallowing. As noted previously, infants or children with tachypnea or cardiac compromise often have difficulty coordinating swallowing and breathing, thereby making feeding more difficult.

ESOPHAGEAL AND GASTROINTESTINAL/ABSORPTIVE PHASE

Details regarding normal esophageal physiology and disorders of esophageal motility are provided in Sec. 17.10. Abnormal peristalsis, esophageal inflammation from gastroesophageal reflux, infection, or allergy, and mechanical obstruction may all cause dysphagia. Odynophagia or postprandial pain from any GI disorder may result in the development of feeding aversions, as discussed earlier.

17.8.3   Approach to the Child with a Feeding Disorder

Symptoms of feeding disorders include refusal to eat or drink, failure to gain weight, aversions to specific food types or textures, recurrent pneumonias, and chronic lung disease. Because of the complex nature and multiple etiologies of pediatric feeding and swallowing disorders, evaluation is best achieved by an interdisciplinary team approach that includes a variety of professionals with expertise in pediatric feeding disorders. These may include speech pathologists, occupational therapists, dieticians, behavioral psychologists, nurse specialists to coordinate care, dentists, and pediatric subspecialists in gastroenterology, otolaryngology, pulmonology, radiology, and neurology or rehabilitative medicine. This approach facilitates integration of expertise from different disci-

plines to determine how organic and nonorganic factors interact in contributing to the child's swallowing disorder and overall health. The goal of a comprehensive evaluation should first be to assess the safety of oral feeding, establish the risk of aspiration, and identify anatomic, physiologic, behavioral, and psychological issues that may limit feeding. A careful developmental, medical, feeding, and dietary history and physical examination provide clues to the diagnosis and direct subsequent evaluation.

The evaluation begins with a focused feeding history including current diet, textures, and route of administration, modifications, and feeding position. A specific query into medical comorbidities that affect swallowing is made. A history of recurrent pneumonia may indicate chronic aspiration, and a history of stridor in relation to feeding may indicate a glottic or subglottic pathology contributing to feeding disorder. Specific inquiry about any previous operations involving the aerodigestive tract is important, as these factors influence the assessment.

Nutritional and psychological assessments should be undertaken early in the evaluative process. It is important to assess if caloric intake meets the metabolic needs of the child, as many patients with swallowing disorders have concurrent illness that may increase metabolic needs. Psychological assessments help to identify behavioral and parental factors that may be contributing to a feeding disorder.

A clinical oral motor assessment evaluates nonnutritive and nutritive oral motor skills. This assessment includes an evaluation of neuromuscular tone, posture, and position during feeding, patient motivation, oral structure and function, and efficiency of oral intake. The oral cavity is carefully examined for anatomic abnormalities such as ankyloglossia, cleft lip/palate, macroglossia, or very enlarged tonsils that may interfere with feeding. Poor lip closure may indicate a cranial nerve (CN) V or CN VII abnormality, and loss of gag reflex may indicate CN IX or CN X insult. The nutritive assessment involves the observation of feeding involving the patient and his or her primary feeders. The observation team notes both positive and negative interactions among the child, food, and feeder to identify primary or secondary behavior problems, which guides future structuring of treatment interventions. The oral motor assessment evaluates for obvious problems with sucking and bolus manipulation. Difficulty with oral secretions, abnormal pace of feeding, food escaping from the mouth, abnormal tongue and jaw movements, excessive swallowing, abnormal airway sounds, poor coordination of suck and/or swallow with laryngeal elevation and breathing, gagging, coughing, or emesis suggests an underlying neurologic or structural problem. Attention to articulation and voice quality also may provide useful information because the structures that are used for the oropharyngeal phases of feeding also are important for speech production. Velopharyngeal insufficiency from a structural or neurologic abnormality can present with hypernasal speech. Velopharyngeal insufficiency results in failure to adequately close the velopharynx/nasopharynx, predisposing to nasal regurgitation of food and poor pharyngeal propulsion force during swallowing.

At the end of this investigation the evaluator should have a better assessment of optimal posture for feeding efficiency and safety and optimal food consistencies and textures. This assessment will help direct other, additional studies to complete the feeding evaluation.

Anatomic disorders and other physiological disorders (Table 17-37) may manifest as a behavioral disorder and *must* be excluded before behavioral interventions are initiated. Identifying such factors is facilitated by other diagnostic tests.

DIAGNOSTIC TESTS

It often is difficult to diagnose a feeding disorder or the safety of continued oral feeding using clinical observations alone. Aspiration may occur without coughing or gagging during the clinical exam (silent aspiration). Oral, pharyngeal, laryngeal, and esophageal anatomy and function should be assessed. Three approaches are used: imaging studies, direct visualization, and occassionaly pharyngeal/esophageal manometry. Each modality provides complementary information.

Radiographic studies may reveal anatomic or structural abnormalities such as strictures, fistulas, or masses. Current evaluative radiographic studies of swallowing function are fluoroscopic imaging in the form of a videofluoroscopic swallowing study (VSS) and ultrasonography. Accessory radiographic studies are indicated in some patients with feeding and swallowing disorders, and indications are based on the clinical history and physical examination findings.

Videofluoroscopic swallowing study (VSS) evaluation should be considered in all infants and children with a feeding or swallowing disorder. A speech pathologist or occupational therapist in conjunction with a radiologist performs this examination. The advantage of this evaluation is that it provides a dynamic assessment of all phases of swallowing simultaneously, thereby providing an assessment of velopharyngeal closure, pharyngeal contraction, laryngeal penetration or aspiration, and esophageal propagation. Additionally, this evaluation can reveal any obstructive or congenital pathology that can interfere with swallowing. When performed completely (which is often problematic), the study also includes an assessment of food transit through the esophagus and can provide valuable information about potential esophageal causes of dysphagia. This is not a substitute for a more formal esophagram. Food substances given during this examination typically mirror what was determined tolerable during the oral motor evaluation. Infants are fed barium through a nipple or given a thin barium-coated puree. Children older than 12 months of age are assessed by three textures: a liquid, puree, and solid. Studying the patient in the usual and then the optimal feeding position may provide therapeutic information. The therapeutic effect of modification of bolus size and consistency, nipple, or feeding utensils can be explored. In addition, compensatory swallowing strategies can be evaluated and initiated in older children based on findings. The primary limitations of the use of VSS in children is that repeated exposure to radiation limits its use for extensive teaching of compensatory maneuvers and repeat assessment of swallowing over time to evaluate progress. Additionally, infants and children with oral aversion and feeding disorders may not ingest an adequate amount of barium to provide a meaningful study. There are other evaluative tests that can be used to overcome these limitations.

Ultrasound can capture tongue, hyoid, and palate activity and bolus transport across the tongue to the hypopharynx, thereby providing a useful evaluation of the oral phase of swallowing. It can also demonstrate the coordination of laryngeal elevation during swallowing. This test is limited in its ability to determine dysfunction of the pharyngeal phases of swallowing and lacks sensitivity for detecting aspiration. An additional limitation of this technique is its lack of standardization and varied interpretations.

Accessory imaging studies are useful in specific clinical scenarios. Any infant or child with recurrent pneumonia requires a carefully performed esophagram specifically to rule out an H-type tracheoesophageal fistula, even if aspiration is identified during a swallowing study. If there are any clinical findings suggestive of CN IX or CN X involvement, the child should have a brain MRI to identify potential brainstem, skull base, or spinal problems that can interfere with swallowing, such as Chiari malformations with tonsillar herniation, hydromyelia with myelomeningocele, and cervicomedullary junction compression by a craniovertebral junction malformation with impingement by the tip of the odontoid process. MRI evaluation of the chest is useful in patients suspected of having a vascular ring/sling cause for stridor or dysphagia and can be diagnostic, eliminating the need for endoscopy in some cases.

Flexible endoscopic evaluation of swallowing (FEES) utilizes a flexible fiberoptic laryngoscope that is passed through the nose to visualize the larynx and pharynx. With simultaneous endoscopic visualization and feeding, FEES allows for assessment of velopharyngeal closure and its impact on swallowing, pharyngeal contractility and proficiency, secretion management, laryngeal penetration, and aspiration. This test is particularly valuable for assessing the risk of aspiration in patients who are unable or unwilling to feed. Green food coloring is placed into the oral cavity to mix with the patient's own secretions. Visualization of the path of secretions and how the child handles them by spontaneous or voluntary swallows can help determine aspiration risk. Swallowing safety by modifications in food consistencies and volumes and compensatory postural changes can be assessed by the FEES examination without exposing the patient to radiation. Although anatomic abnormalities can be assessed with flexible endoscopy, a laryngeal cleft is difficult to identify except during rigid laryngoscopy. If it is suspected, flexible laryngoscopy alone is inadequate.

Manometry requires transnasal passage of a catheter that is fitted with multiple pressure ports. It is used for evaluating pharyngeal and esophageal peristalsis as well as upper and lower esophageal sphincter function. These tests are very difficult to perform in infants and children and therefore should be performed in centers with special expertise in pediatric manometry.

TREATMENT OF FEEDING DISORDERS

The careful evaluation of children with feeding disorders allows recognition and treatment of correctable lesions. Unfortunately, many children with feeding disorders have noncorrectable physical abnormalities that make oral feeding either dangerous or impossible. Some patients will need behavioral therapy to overcome secondary learned food refusal.

Decisions regarding whether to allow oral feeding depend on balancing the potential risks of aspiration and chronic lung disease with the emotional rewards and convenience of oral feeding. These decisions must be reviewed periodically because of changes in anatomic, physiological, and cognitive skill with the child's development. For example, an infant who was a "safe" feeder may develop aspiration problems when the larynx descends, and feeding will become unsafe. In contrast, a child with an anatomic abnormality of the larynx may be unsafe to feed orally as an infant, but as his or her cognitive function improves, the child may be able to learn compensatory strategies (discussed later) that allow a "safe" swallow. In some patients, the time that is required to feed orally consumes the patient's and caretaker's lives, leaving little time for other nurturing activities. Sometimes supplying a portion of the patient's nutrition by tube may be beneficial (see Sec. 17.6). Families may need counseling to help them realize that, for their child, alternate approaches to providing nutrition may be better for the child's overall well-being than persisting in efforts to feed only by mouth. The timing for aggressive behavioral intervention or the initiation of attempts at oral feeding must be decided in the context of the child's overall development and well-being.

Behavioral therapy is often required to overcome learned aversive responses to feeding. Behavioral feeding disorders and the approach to their management are discussed in Sec. 5.5. Preschool children often respond to a combination of social praise and making the availability of preferred foods contingent on eating nonpreferred foods. Patients with more severe problems may require combination treatment, which may include contingency management, "shaping" (ie, rewarding successive approximations of targeted behaviors), "positive reinforcement" (ie, rewarding the child for completing a desired behavior), and "ignoring" (ie, inattention when the child engages in inappropriate behavior). The slow advancement of goals eventually leads to full oral feeding, but success may require inpatient management.

In addition to nutritional problems, children with real or perceived feeding disorders are at risk for developing long-term psychosocial problems. Therefore, in cases of nonorganic failure to thrive, intervention should include providing access to food and parental training in compensatory approaches to feeding. In many cases, caretakers suffer tremendous emotional distress, feelings of inadequacy, and guilt that also need to be acknowledged and addressed. Family support services, respite care, and financial assistance programs should be integrated with the child's overall medical and social needs.

A variety of *therapeutic "compensatory" maneuvers* may be useful to prevent aspiration or improve the efficiency of feeding. By combining the clinical history, physical examination, and imaging studies, the therapist is able to determine the best bolus volume and texture, pace of administration, and nipples or utensils for oral feeding. Changes in body and head position also may protect the airway or allow easier passage of material through the oropharynx. For example, tilting the head forward widens the vallecular space, thereby diverting food away from the laryngeal inlet. Nipple shape, pliability, hole size, and geometry determine the rate of milk flow. More rapid milk delivery increases the frequency of swallowing and therefore decreases the time that is available for breathing between swallows. However, decreasing the flow rate increases the work of sucking, thereby increasing the total time that is required for feeding. Careful alterations often provide a useful therapeutic strategy.

Feeding an infant with an open cleft palate is particularly challenging. In this setting, mealtimes usually are most successful when a paced feeding is delivered into the infant's oral cavity and the infant is allowed to initiate swallows. Working together, a consistent feeder and the infant can learn how to coordinate the rate of formula delivery and swallows to allow oral feeding to succeed. In selected cases, prosthodontic appliances can be effective, particularly when there are anatomic abnormalities. For example, a palatal prosthesis that mechanically stimulates the pharynx during swallowing has been effective in the treatment of infants with delayed initiation of the pharyngeal phase of swallowing.

If full oral feeding cannot be achieved, then providing some oral feedings, or at least water, may be feasible. This experience will facilitate the later introduction of oral feeds and usually is rewarding for both the parents and patient. Continuing oral stimulation is important to prevent the development of aversion to oral touch, thus allowing good dental care.

References

Burklow KA, Phelps AN, Schultz JR, McConnell K, Rudolph C: Classifying complex pediatric feeding disorders. Gastroenterol Nutr 27:143–147, 1998

Darrow DH, Harley CM: Evaluation of swallowing disorders in children. Otolaryngol Clin North Am 31:405–418, 1998

Langmore SE, Terpenning MS, Schork A, et al: Predictors of aspiration pneumonia: how important is dysphagia? Dysphagia 13:69–81, 1998

Rudolph CD: Diagnosis and management of children with feeding disorders. In: Hyman P, DiLorenzo C, eds: Gastrointestinal Motility Disorders in Children. New York, Academy Professional Information Services, 1994:33–53

Willging JP: Swallowing disorders in children. Curr Opin Otolaryngol Head Neck Surg 2:504–507, 1994

17.9   ANATOMIC DISORDERS OF THE ESOPHAGUS

Joseph A. Cox and Colin D. Rudolph

17.9.1   Tracheoesophageal Fistula and Esophageal Atresia

Congenital atresia of the esophagus and tracheoesophageal fistula occur in one of every 3000 to 5000 live births. Embryologic development of the foregut of the embryo provides a basis for understanding these disorders. Approximately 3 weeks after fertilization, the cranial end of the foregut begins to become demarcated into the esophagus and trachea (see Sec. 17.1.2). A longitudinal groove separates the esophagus from the tracheal tube. As the ridges between the tracheal tube and esophageal tube proximate one another, the foregut divides into tracheal and esophageal channels. At the distal end of the trachea, the lung buds begin to develop. As the separation between the tracheal and esophageal channels continues, there also is continuing elongation of both tubes. Like the rest of the GI tract, endodermal proliferation occludes the lumen, which recanalizes by approximately 7 weeks of gestation. During the next 3 months of embryologic development, the muscle coats appear, nerve innervation takes place, and development of blood vessels occurs. In the meantime, the trachea and lung buds continue to develop and proliferate. Abnormalities of partitioning of the foregut into the esophagus and trachea and development of the esophagus at the cardiac junction lead to most anatomic esophageal anomalies.

The most common anomalies of the esophagus are shown in Fig. 17-25. Clinical presentation, diagnosis, and management are discussed below. Eighty to 90% of children with tracheoesophageal anomalies have a blind upper esophageal pouch with a fistula between a lower esophageal segment and the lower portion of the trachea in the region of the carina. Other common variations include esophageal atresia with two blind pouches, without the presence of a tracheoesophageal fistula, and an "H-type" tracheoesophageal fistula, where a fistula exists between an intact esophagus and trachea. Probably the most subtle manifestation of the entire spec-

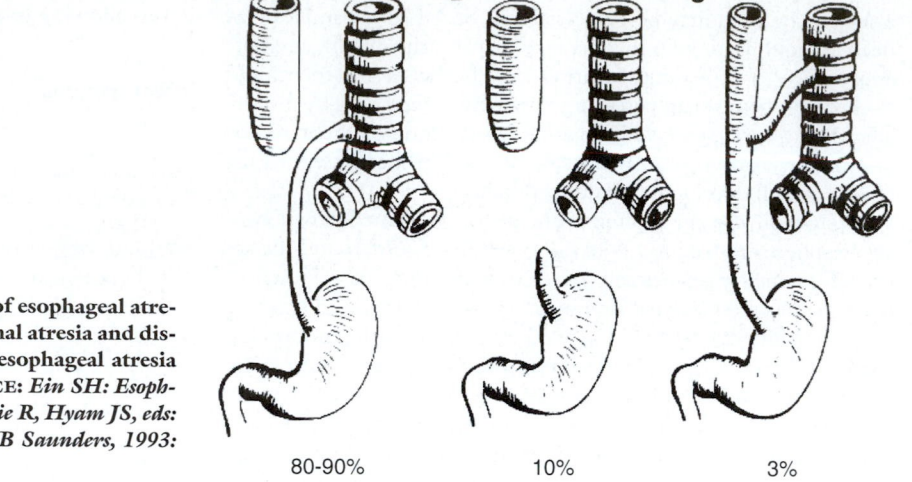

FIGURE 17-25   The three most common types of esophageal atresia and tracheoesophageal fistula (TEF). **A:** Proximal atresia and distal TEF account for 80 to 90% of cases. **B:** Pure esophageal atresia with no TEF (10%). **C:** H-type TEF (3%). SOURCE: *Ein SH: Esophageal atresia and tracheo-esophageal fistula. In: Wyllie R, Hyam JS, eds: Pediatric Gastrointestinal Disease. Philadelphia, WB Saunders, 1993: 318–336.*

trum of congenital esophageal anomalies is that of congenital esophageal stenosis, which probably results from inadequate recanalization of the esophageal lumen.

As many as 30% of infants with esophageal atresia or tracheoesophageal fistula have other congenital defects; the most common association is described by the acronym *VACTERL complex* and includes anomalies of the vertebrae (similar to those of spondylocostal dysplasia, 10%), anal atresia (10 to 15%), cardiac malformations (patent ductus arteriosus, atrial septal defect, or ventricular septal defect in 25%), tracheoesophageal fistula, renal anomalies (urethral atresia with hydronephrosis), and limb anomalies (hexadactyly, humeral hypoplasia, radial aplasia, and proximally placed thumb). Rare cases of VACTERL association in the offspring of an affected individual have been reported, but this is uncommon. Other associated anomalies include hypospadias, undescended testis, duodenal atresia (as in oculodigitalesophagoduodenal syndrome with gene defect in the 2p24-p23 region), and hydrocephalus secondary to aqueductal stenosis. Other genetic syndromes, including oculoauriculovertebral dysplasia (Goldenhar syndrome) and Opitz G syndrome, may be associated with esophageal anomalies. Polyhydramnios is present in 50% of the mothers of infants with esophageal atresia, which may lead to prenatal consideration of this diagnosis.

ESOPHAGEAL ATRESIA WITH DISTAL TRACHEOESOPHAGEAL FISTULA

The diagnosis of this most common form of a blind upper esophageal pouch with a tracheoesophageal fistula to the lower esophageal segment may be suspected in the delivery room or shortly thereafter. The infant frequently has excessive oral secretions, with episodes of choking. When an attempt is made to place a nasoesophageal gastric tube to suction the stomach, the tube cannot be passed into the stomach, and a radiograph of the chest reveals that the catheter is coiled in the blind upper esophageal pouch. The proximal pouch and stomach usually are distended with air. This constellation of findings makes the diagnosis of esophageal atresia and tracheoesophageal fistula with a high degree of certainty.

Initial management of these infants includes insertion of a soft plastic double-lumen orogastric catheter a distance of 7 cm into the blind upper esophageal pouch, taping it in this position, and connecting it to constant low negative pressure (ie, <20 cm H_2O) for continuous drainage of the pooled saliva, which prevents aspi-

ration from above. Keeping the head elevated (ie, 30°) both facilitates the drainage of secretion into the pouch for suctioning and prevents the reflux of gastric contents into the lungs. Antibiotic therapy should be initiated and surgical consultation obtained as soon as possible. Emergency gastrostomy may be required for a large-diameter tracheoesophageal fistula having acute life-threatening gastric distension with respiratory embarrassment. Rarely, some relief of acute respiratory difficulties can be achieved by judicious placement of an endotracheal tube to occlude the tracheoesophageal fistula while ventilating the patient. However, endotracheal intubation of these patients should be avoided because positive-pressure ventilation usually exacerbates acute gastric distension. In some circumstances, a contrast study of the upper pouch may be warranted not only to confirm the diagnosis of a blind upper pouch but also to investigate the possible existence of a secondary tracheoesophageal fistula to the upper segment. The possibility of aspiration of these contrast materials must be considered before this diagnostic maneuver is instituted. Evaluation for cardiac anomalies with chest radiography, electrocardiography, and echocardiography is useful before surgery because of the frequently associated cardiac anomalies.

After the patient is stabilized, there are three potential surgical approaches to this anomaly. The chosen course usually is determined by the degree of prematurity, overall clinical condition, other associated anomalies, length of the gap between the ends of the esophagus, and the surgeon's experience. Usually, the gap is 1 to 2 cm, allowing primary anastomosis of the two ends. In a healthy, full-term infant without other severe anomalies and minimal pneumonitis, primary closure of the fistula and an esophageal anastomosis can be performed within the first 24 to 72 hours after birth. In this circumstance, a gastrostomy may or may not be performed. However, if the infant has a severe pneumonia or other associated significant medical problems that increase the risk of major surgery, only decompressive gastrostomy is performed, thus allowing time for the medical problem to resolve. Head-of-bed elevation and upper pouch suction are maintained until surgery can be accomplished. In an extremely small infant with or without other severe anomalies and in whom it is apparent that surgical correction of the tracheoesophageal anomaly must be delayed, a decompressive gastrostomy, surgical closure of the tracheoesophageal fistula, and continuous suction of the upper esophageal pouch are appropriate, with the esophageal anastomosis being performed at a much later date. In the latter circumstances, a cervical diversion esophagostomy may prove to be helpful in deterring aspiration of the accumulated saliva.

Continuous intensive care is crucial in the postoperative period. Regular suction of secretions in the upper airway is crucial to prevent aspiration. Depending on the circumstances, the endotracheal tube may remain in place for a few hours to several days. Postoperative nutritional support is provided parenterally, but after 3 to 5 days, the gastrostomy tube may be used. Oral feedings usually begin within 7 to 10 days after surgery.

ESOPHAGEAL ATRESIA WITHOUT TRACHEOESOPHAGEAL FISTULA

Infants with esophageal atresia but without a tracheoesophageal fistula have excessive oral secretions with drooling and choking in the newborn period, but unlike those with a tracheoesophageal fistula, they usually have a flat, gasless abdomen. If fed, they are unable to swallow, and diagnostic studies confirm the presence of a blind upper esophageal pouch. The length of the atretic segment varies, but a wide gap usually divides the upper and lower ends of the esophagus, thus making primary anastomosis difficult or impossible.

A variety of surgical approaches have been attempted to bridge the gap between the two esophageal segments. These vary from bougienage of each segment to lengthen each segment, allowing primary repair, to exotic methods such as placing magnets in each segment to draw those segments closer. All of these surgical maneuvers are fraught with complications, and esophageal lengthening is unlikely to succeed if the gap is wider than 3 or 4 cm. If the gap exceeds 4 cm, esophageal replacement usually is necessary. Initial procedures include a gastrostomy to allow feeding and a cervical esophagostomy for diversion of the secretions. Before initiation of feeding, duodenal atresia must be ruled out, either with intraoperative instillation of fluid through the duodenum or by radiographic contrast studies. It is imperative that these infants be provided with oral motor stimulation by feeding small amounts of water to allow the normal development of feeding skills. After approximately 1 year, the gap between the two esophageal segments may be bridged with a gastric tube or a colon or small intestinal segment.

ESOPHAGEAL FISTULA WITHOUT ESOPHAGEAL ATRESIA

Infants with an "H-type" fistula may present with intermittent episodes of choking during feeding in the newborn period. Others present later with persistent choking episodes, chronic cough, recurrent aspiration-like pneumonias, or reactive airway disease. The diagnosis can be difficult; routine radiographic barium swallows often overlook the fistula. The fistula is best identified by instilling thin barium through the tip of a nasogastric tube with moderate pressure to distend the esophagus while slowly withdrawing the tube from the stomach into the esophagus. This tends to force the fistula open and allows visualization. Repeated radiography and/or esophagoscopy and bronchoscopy may be necessary before the diagnosis is recognized. Presumed congenital H-type fistulas have presented in adulthood with only mild symptoms of cough and intermittent pneumonias since childhood. Surgical division of the fistula can be achieved through a cervical approach. No gastrostomy is required, and patients usually have minimal morbidity. The fistula occasionally recurs and can be treated either surgically or endoscopically using fibrin glues or endoscopic clips.

POSTOPERATIVE MANAGEMENT AND COMPLICATIONS OF ESOPHAGEAL REPAIR

The major complication during the early postoperative period after surgical repair of esophageal atresia is leakage through the anastomosis in up to 50% of patients. Feedings are introduced very slowly because reflux into the esophagus could threaten the integrity of the anastomosis. If the infant is well for 1 week, radiographic contrast studies are performed, and if the anastomosis is intact, the infant is gradually allowed to begin oral feedings. An anastomotic leak usually presents with tachypnea and sepsis on the third or fourth postoperative day. Management usually is conservative, with antibiotics and, if necessary, placement of a chest tube. Over time, the leak usually seals, and feedings can be introduced.

Stricture formation at the site of the esophageal anastomosis frequently occurs in the first weeks to months after repair. This narrowing may require repeated dilatation either by radiographic placement of a balloon dilator or by progressive retrograde dilatation. Narrowing of the esophagus also may result in the lodging of foreign bodies or a food bolus just proximal to the stricture, thus necessitating its removal. Severe strictures require resection and secondary anastomosis. Occasionally, bronchial remnants are associated with tracheoesophageal fistula. Management of these strictures is discussed below. Peristalsis is abnormal in the lower esophageal segment, and therefore dysphagia (particularly for solids) is common. Esophagitis may be caused by lack of acid clearance from the aperistaltic segment, and peptic strictures may result. Antireflux surgical procedures may be required to prevent esophagitis. The overall prognosis after surgical repair depends on the type of anatomic abnormality and the presence of other anomalies. Most infants without other anomalies survive, but those with multiple anomalies, especially cardiac disease, have much lower survival rates.

Children who have required an esophageal replacement procedure are at even higher risk of gastroesophageal reflux with ulceration of the interposed segment. In addition, these children often have subclinical gastroesophageal reflux with silent aspiration, resulting in the development of chronic pulmonary disease. Interposed segments, particularly colonic or gastric interpositions, may distend with time, further compromising pulmonary function and occasionally requiring surgical revision.

17.9.2   Other Anatomic Anomalies of the Esophagus

Congenital esophageal stenosis and web diaphragms rarely occur (ie, one in 25,000 live births) and usually present with dysphagia when feeds are advanced to pureed or solid consistencies. Diagnosis is made by radiographic contrast studies or endoscopy. Webs and fibromuscular stenosis usually can successfully be dilated using endoscopy and/or fluoroscopy-guided balloon or bougie-type dilators. However, stenosis resulting from ectopic cartilage (ie, tracheobronchial remnant), which on endoscopy is more irregular and firmer than the fibromuscular type, should be removed by surgical resection because of the risk of esophageal perforation with dilation.

Esophageal duplications are rare lesions that present as a tubular mass in the posterior mediastinum. Secretions cause distension with pressure on contiguous structures that can cause dysphagia or respiratory symptoms. Simple surgical excision is curative.

Congenital esophageal diverticula are rare lesions with a muscle layer that usually are located just above the cricopharyngeal muscle. They may present with symptoms of choking, coughing, and dysphagia in an older child. More commonly, acquired diverticula without a muscle layer occur in neonates after traumatic efforts at airway intubation. Perforation results in infection and edema, which may cause obstruction. Antibiotic therapy and the cessation of oral feedings usually allow resolution of perforation if it is recognized early.

References

Ein SH: Esophageal atresia and tracheoesophageal fistula. In: Wyllie R, Hyams JS, eds: Pediatric Gastrointestinal Disease. Philadelphia, WB Saunders, 318–336, 1993

Martin LW, Alexander F: Esophageal atresia. Surg Clin North Am 65: 1099–1113, 1985

Nezarati, MM, McLeod DR: VACTERL manifestations in two generations of a family. Am J Med Genet 82:40–42, 1999

Randolph JG: Esophageal atresia and congenital stenosis. In: Welch KJ, Randolph JG, Ravitch MM, O'Neill JA, Rowe MI, eds: Pediatric Surgery. Chicago, Year Book, 682–697, 1986

17.10 DISORDERS OF ESOPHAGEAL MOTILITY

Colin D. Rudolph

17.10.1   Normal Esophageal Motility

The esophagus is a muscular conduit that begins in the pharynx, traverses the thoracic cavity, and ends in the stomach, which normally is located in the abdominal cavity. During inspiration, negative pressure in the thoracic cavity would promote the ingress of pharyngeal and stomach contents into the esophagus were it not for muscular sphincters at either end of the esophagus: the upper esophageal sphincter (UES) and the lower esophageal sphincter (LES). The closed UES prevents the swallowing of air during normal respiration. The pressure that is tonically maintained by the UES varies tremendously, being almost absent during sleep and increasing to over 100 mm Hg with emotional stress, straining, or when the esophagus is distended or perfused with acid fluid. The LES prevents the reflux of gastric contents into the esophagus and maintains a pressure of approximately 20 mm Hg, with values below approximately 10 mm Hg being abnormal. Two different mechanisms contribute to the generation of LES tone: a region of specialized smooth muscle at the gastroesophageal junction and skeletal muscle in the crural diaphragm that wraps around the lower esophagus as it passes through the diaphragm. With inspiration, the diaphragmatic muscles contract, thus increasing LES tone. With greater respiratory efforts, the pressure gradient between the stomach and thoracic cavity increases, but the crural diaphragm's contribution to LES tone also increases, which prevents gastroesophageal reflux. The LES tone is decreased by anesthesia, morphine, diazepam, β-adrenergic agents, dopamine, secretin, cholecystokinin, glucagon, vasoactive inhibitory peptide, progesterone and estrogen, nitrites, nifedipine, theophylline, intraduodenal fat, etha-

nol, and nicotine. Relaxation of the LES appears to be mediated by the actions of vasoactive inhibitory peptide and/or nitric oxide.

During a normal swallow (Fig. 17-26), sequential contraction of the muscles in the esophageal body is initiated by the vagus nerve, forming a pressure wave with an amplitude of 50 to 110 mm Hg that travels down the esophagus at a rate of approximately 3 cm/s. This "primary peristalsis" wave originates in the pharynx. The UES relaxes and opens before arrival of the food bolus, which passes through the UES and then down the esophagus, with muscular contraction clearing the contents of the esophagus. Similarly, with the initiation of a swallow, the LES relaxes, thus allowing the food bolus to enter the stomach. Once a person swallows, peristalsis proceeds through the entire esophagus unless a second swallow follows too closely, which will suppress the peristalsis from the original swallow. Distension of the esophageal body wall stimulates "secondary peristalsis," which is identical to primary peristalsis except that there is no swallow, pharyngeal contraction, or UES relaxation/contraction.

Relaxation of the LES that is not associated with swallowing is termed *transient lower esophageal sphincter relaxation* (TLESR). These episodes are stimulated by gastric distension, so the rate of TLESRs normally increases postprandially. These LES relaxations are accompanied by crural diaphragm relaxation, thus abolishing the tone at the gastroesophageal junction. TLESRs are an important protective mechanism, allowing belching or burping. They are suppressed when a person is supine, which is when fluid rather than air is likely to be at the gastroesophageal junction.

17.10.2   Primary Esophageal Motility Disorders

Esophageal motility disorders are classified as "primary" when they are one of a small number of isolated disorders of motility that include achalasia, diffuse esophageal spasm, nutcracker esophagus, and nonspecific esophageal motility disorders of the esophagus. In contrast, "secondary" motility disorders are associated with a known disease process. Primary esophageal motility disorders other than gastroesophageal reflux are uncommon in otherwise healthy children. Dysphagia, chest pain, or recurrent foreign-body obstruction are the usual modes of presentation, although failed esophageal peristalsis can result in spilling of residual food into the airway with symptoms of recurrent aspiration pneumonia. Diagnosis of a primary esophageal motility disorder may be suspected from observations of peristalsis on barium esophagram. Definitive diagnosis requires that either a barium study or endoscopy be performed to exclude anatomic obstruction; esophageal manometry is then performed for specific and conclusive diagnosis.

ACHALASIA

Achalasia is a motor disorder of the esophagus characterized by incomplete relaxation of the lower esophageal sphincter and a lack of normal esophageal peristalsis. Presenting symptoms include dysphagia, regurgitation, recurrent pneumonia, weight loss, and chest pain. Idiopathic achalasia appears to result from a loss of ganglion cells in the esophagus, wallerian degeneration of extraesophageal nerve fibers, and a reduction in the dorsal motor nuclei of the vagus nerve, with antibodies against the cytoplasm of the Auerbach plexus being present in many patients. Neuronal loss of CGRP-, VIP-, and NO-containing neurons is most marked. The overall incidence of achalasia is 0.4 to 0.6 per 100,000, with only about 5% of cases occurring in children, the average age of diagnosis being about 9

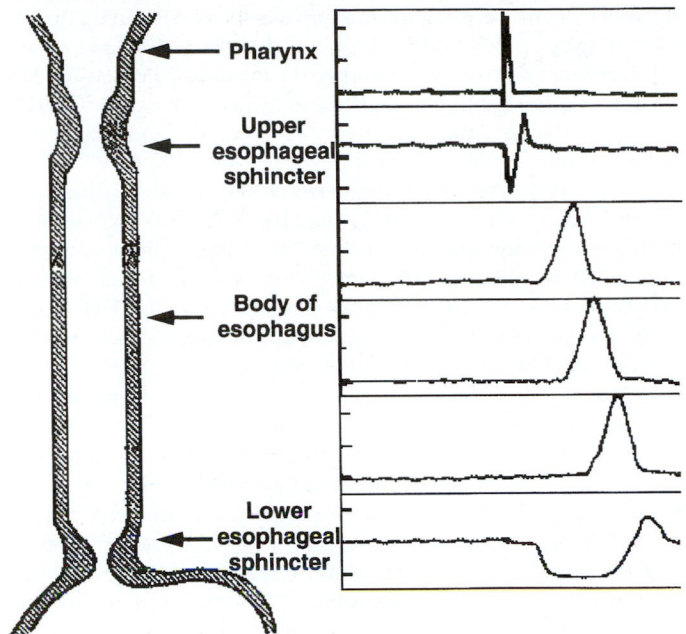

FIGURE 17-26 Before a swallow, the resting pressures of the upper and lower esophageal sphincters are elevated, thus forming a pressure barrier between the esophageal body and the pharynx or stomach, respectively. The normal swallow sequence originates as a contraction wave in the pharynx with simultaneous relaxation of the upper esophageal sphincter. The wave then progresses through the body of the esophagus. Note that the upper and lower esophageal sphincters relax before the arrival of the pressure wave, allowing the food bolus to pass through the sphincter.

years old. Achalasia may present in the first month or years after birth and then is frequently associated with an autosomal-recessive syndrome of deafness, vitiligo, short stature, and muscle weakness, or with the syndrome of alacrima and corticotropin insensitivity (Allgrove syndrome, or triple-A syndrome, which has been linked with mutations on 12q13). Rare cases of familial achalasia and of familial coexistence of achalasia and other esophageal motility disorders have been reported. Achalasia has also been associated with autoimmune polyendocrinopathy syndrome and multiple endocrine neoplasia type 2B. In Latin America, Chagas disease must be considered. Similarly, leiomyoma or other tumors of the stomach may masquerade as achalasia. Treatment with pharmacotherapy (eg, nifedipine) is variably effective and rarely provides an option for long-term management. Similarly, injection of the lower esophageal sphincter with botulinum toxin provides transient relief, but the requirement for repeated injection makes this therapy less attractive for treatment of childhood achalasia. Pneumatic balloon dilation of the LES ruptures the muscle and may provide long-term relief from symptoms. If frequent or repeated pneumatic dilation is required to prevent symptom recurrence, a Heller myotomy provides definitive surgical therapy and can be performed in children with concurrent antireflux surgery using laparascopic techniques.

OTHER PRIMARY DISORDERS OF ESOPHAGEAL MOTILITY

Diffuse esophageal spasm is characterized by prolonged (ie, >5.5 seconds) simultaneous contractions in at least 30% of the esophageal body waveforms. These contractions have multiple peaks and, often, increased amplitude. High-pressure (mean amplitude

>180 mm Hg) and prolonged (>5.5 seconds) organized peristaltic waves characterize a *nutcracker esophagus*. These disorders are rarely described in children. A variety of nonspecific esophageal motility disorders characterized by varying combinations of simultaneous contractions, abnormal waveforms, and decreased wave amplitudes are common; the pathophysiological significance of these findings remains obscure. No consistently effective treatments for esophageal motility disorders are available except in achalasia. Approaches have included calcium channel–blocking drugs, botulinum toxin injection into the esophageal muscle, and dilation with inconsistent responses.

17.10.3 Secondary Esophageal Motility Disorders

Gastroesophageal reflux disease and other inflammatory disorders of the esophagus produce motor abnormalities, including simultaneous (or slowed velocity), broad-based, multiple-peaked, low-pressure waves; aborted peristalsis; and both low or high LES pressure. Diagnosis and aggressive treatment of the reflux or other underlying disorder may normalize motility.

Esophageal dysmotility is common in connective tissue diseases, especially scleroderma, CREST syndrome, polymyositis, dermatomyositis, and mixed connective tissue disease, especially in those patients with Raynaud phenomenon. It may also occur with graft-versus-host disease following bone marrow transplant. Control of the primary disease process generally relieves the esophageal symptoms. Muscular dystrophy and diabetic neuropathy may be associated with esophageal motility disorders, as may primary disorders of GI motility such as idiopathic intestinal pseudoobstruction syndrome. Patients with esophageal atresia uniformly have aperistalsis of the distal esophagus.

17.10.4 Gastroesophageal Reflux

Gastroesophageal reflux (GER), defined as passage of gastric contents into the esophagus, is a normal physiological process that occurs throughout the day in healthy infants, children, and adults. When refluxed material passes into the pharynx and out the mouth, then "spitting up" or vomiting occurs. Half of all infants between 0 and 3 months of age and two-thirds of 4- to 6-month-old infants vomit at least once per day. The prevalence of vomiting decreases dramatically after 8 months of age. Typically infants with daily vomiting outgrow this problem by 18 to 24 months of age, and no evaluation or treatment is necessary.

In a small number of infants, GER may cause disease (GERD) characterized by chronic symptoms (Table 17-38). These include (1) malnutrition from inadequate caloric intake as a result of discomfort or calorie loss from vomiting, (2) esophageal symptoms of pain, inflammation, and bleeding, and (3) airway symptoms of hoarseness and laryngitis, cough, apnea, exacerbation of asthma, or pneumonia. Similar symptoms may occur in children over 1 year of age, but the incidence is uncertain. Some otherwise normal children continue to experience episodic vomiting with no other symptoms or problems. GERD characterized by esophagitis or airway symptoms is rarely observed in normal children, but it is frequent in disabled children with a prevalence of 6 to 30%. Other patient groups with anatomic disorders such as tracheoesophageal fistula or laryngeal abnormalities may also be more prone to GERD as a result of either inadequate esophageal clearance or defective airway protective mechanisms.

TABLE 17-38
COMPLICATIONS OF GASTROESOPHAGEAL REFLUX

Vomiting
  Parental frustration
  Iatrogenic weight loss from limitations on feeding to prevent vomiting
  Weight loss or inadequate weight gain from excessive vomiting
Esophagitis
  Dysphagia (may limit feedings, causing weight loss)
  Chest pain, heartburn
  Irritability and inconsolable crying in infants
  Hematemesis, anemia, melena
  Sandifer syndrome
  Globus sensation
  Barret esophagus
  Esophageal stricture
Respiratory disorders
  Cough, hoarseness, stridor
  Bronchospasm or wheezing
  Apnea (especially obstructive)
  Recurrent aspiration pneumonia or pulmonary fibrosis

PATHOPHYSIOLOGY

Reflux episodes occur primarily during transient lower esophageal sphincter relaxations as discussed in Sec. 17.10.1. Refluxed gastric contents are cleared by a combination of factors, including bulk clearance by gravity (when in an upright position) and peristalsis as well as neutralization of residual acid by the swallowing of alkaline saliva. During sleep, clearance mechanisms are deficient, and a single episode of gastroesophageal reflux may lead to prolonged acid exposure. Prolonged exposure to acid is associated with a higher risk of esophagitis, but extraesophageal complications of GER may occur despite esophageal acid exposure being in the normal range.

Once gastroesophageal reflux occurs, small volumes stimulate the upper esophageal sphincter (UES) pressure to increase, which prevents passage of gastric contents into the pharynx. Larger volumes of refluxed material stimulate opening of the UES, allowing the gastric refluxate to pass into the pharynx. If air is refluxed from the stomach, belching occurs. When liquid or food is refluxed, spitting up or vomiting occurs. Before the upper esophageal sphincter opens, the vocal cords close, respiration ceases, and the larynx is pulled anteriorly as the epiglottis closes over the larynx. This laryngeal closure prevents aspiration of the refluxed material, but if prolonged, it may cause apnea or laryngospasm with stridor. Following the episode of pharyngeal reflux, the material is cleared from the pharynx by either vomiting or swallowing, and breathing resumes. Abnormalities of these airway protective mechanisms will potentially result in airway symptoms from inadvertent exposure of the larynx and airway to caustic materials. The small capacity of the esophagus and recumbent posture (lack of gravity) in the infant make it more likely that refluxed material will fill the esophagus and pass into the pharynx. Thus, the infant is more likely to regurgitate or vomit when GER occurs. If an infant lacks adequate airway protective mechanisms, the more frequent reflux of gastric contents into the mouth makes him or her more likely to experience airway complications of GER than the adult.

DIAGNOSTIC TECHNIQUES

Gastroesophageal reflux is a normal physiological event; therefore, the key to evaluation and diagnosis is to determine when GER is the cause of disease. Diagnostic approaches vary depending on the presenting symptom, and in all cases, other treatable causes of the disorder must be considered during the diagnostic evaluation. No test serves as the "gold standard" for making a diagnosis of GERD. A series of tests is usually required to determine if a particular disorder is being caused by GER.

Upper gastrointestinal radiography (UGI) is often included in the evaluation of the vomiting infant. It is useful to diagnose anatomic abnormalities that present with nonbilious vomiting as with GER, such as esophageal stricture, pyloric stenosis, antral webs, or disorders of esophageal motility such as achalasia. The UGI is not useful for diagnosis of GER because reflux of ingested radiographic contrast often occurs in normal individuals.

Esophageal pH monitoring utilizes a pH sensor to record the number and duration of acid reflux episodes into the lower and/or upper esophagus. Prolonged esophageal mucosal exposure (ie, >11% of a 24-hour period in an infant and >6% in an older child) increases the risk for esophagitis, and therefore, this test is helpful to determine the risk of esophagitis. Measurement of 24-hour esophageal acid exposure should not be used as the sole determinant of whether GER is responsible for airway symptoms such as apnea, recurrent pneumonia, wheezing, or hoarsenss. Esophageal pH monitoring should be combined with a pneumogram that measures oxygen saturation and chest wall and airflow movements if one is attempting to establish a clearer cause-and-effect relationship between apnea episodes and GER; however, these time-consuming and technically challenging tests often fail to clarify if apnea is caused by GER. If esophageal pH monitoring is abnormal, there is a higher probability that GER is a contributing factor causing airway symptoms such as recurrent wheezing or pneumonia, but a normal study does not exclude GER as a potential factor.

Upper endoscopy with biopsy of the esophagus is useful to evaluate if there is esophagitis or other sequelae of chronic esophageal acid exposure such as stricture or Barrett esophagus. In addition, it allows diagnosis of other disorders such as Crohn disease and eosinophilic or infectious esophagitis.

Nuclear scintigraphy evaluates the distribution of isotope-labeled formula or food following normal feeding. Episodes of GER are monitored for up to an hour after feeding. Because GER may occur in normal individuals, documentation of these episodes is of little pathophysiological use unless aspiration into the lungs is detected. If this occurs, it is a clear indication that airway protective mechanisms are deficient.

Other tests may be utilized to evaluate children with airway symptoms. These include chest radiographs or CT scans, laryngoscopy, and bronchoscopy with alveolar lavage for lipid-laden macrophages. Often, empiric therapy may be utilized as a diagnostic test, as discussed below.

EVALUATION AND MANAGEMENT

The approach to the evaluation and management of GER varies depending on the clinical presentation. GER is a normal physiological event, so the evaluation is directed towards determining if GER is either causing or contributing to a specific disorder.

UNCOMPLICATED GER Uncomplicated GER is common in infants. A thorough history and physical examination are generally sufficient to arrive at this diagnosis, which obviates the need for any diagnostic testing. Other potential causes of vomiting should be considered in an infant with "warning signs" (Table 17-39 and Section 17.7.1) such as forceful or bilious vomiting, abdominal

TABLE 17-39

WARNING SIGNS OF DISORDERS OTHER THAN GASTROESOPHAGEAL REFLUX IN THE INFANT WITH VOMITING

Forceful or bilious vomiting
Diarrhea
Constipation
GI bleeding
Abdominal tenderness or distension
Fever or lethargy
Hepatosplenomegaly
Bulging fontanelle, macro/microcephaly, seizures
Onset of vomiting after 6 months of life

tenderness or distension, gastrointestinal bleeding, diarrhea, constipation, fever, hepatosplenomegaly, a bulging fontanelle, macro- or microcephaly, seizures, or an onset of vomiting after age 6 months. Infants with potential complications of GER such as weight loss, excessive irritability because of esophageal pain, feeding difficulties, apneic episodes, recurrent stridor, or pneumonia (Table 17-38) also require different management approaches, as detailed below. If none of these warning signals or potential complications are present, reassurance of the parents including education regarding the range of normal frequency for vomiting and the potential complications of GER is usually sufficient for management.

Some infants with cow's milk allergy have symptoms that are indistinguishable from GER. Therefore, a 1- to 2-week trial of a hypoallergenic formula may be considered. Thickening of formula with rice cereal (1-2 tbsp per ounce formula) may also be considered as an option for therapy if the vomiting is causing substantial parental angst. However, feeding with a thickened formula usually requires "cross-cutting" of the nipple and may lead to increased cough or feeding problems in some infants. Commercially available formulas with thickeners may be useful, but there are few studies that validate their efficacy.

Previously, prone positioning was recommended as a potential therapeutic approach for all infants with GER, but in otherwise well infants, prone position sleeping should not be recommended because it clearly increases the risk of sudden infant death syndrome (SIDS). Pharmacologic therapy is not indicated for the management of infants with uncomplicated GER. Vomiting usually decreases in frequency over the first year of life and resolves by 12 months of age. If symptoms worsen or do not improve by 18 to 24 months of age, the diagnosis should be reevaluated.

INFANT WITH RECURRENT VOMITING AND POOR WEIGHT GAIN An infant with recurrent vomiting and poor weight gain presents a more challenging problem. Other potential causes of poor weight gain need to be considered as outlined in Secs. 1.1.2 and 17.5.1. Often, inadequate calories are offered to the infant because the parents inadvisedly attempt to reduce the frequency or volume of vomiting. In these situations, parental education is usually sufficient to resume weight gain. If appropriate calories are consumed but vomiting is severe enough to limit weight gain, thickening of the formula or increasing the caloric density of the formula is useful. Pharmacologic therapy with a prokinetic agent, such as cisapride, may also be useful if this agent is available. Rarely, supplemental nasogastric feeding or jejunal feeding may be required to achieve weight gain. The severity of GER usually gradually decreases, and the infant can resume a more normal eating pattern by 3 to 6 months of age. Surgical therapy is almost never required to achieve good weight gain. If it is contemplated, a pediatric gastroenterologist should be consulted to consider other potential causes of vomiting.

ESOPHAGITIS Esophagitis may be caused by GER, presenting with symptoms including excessive irritability, feeding refusal, hematemesis, anemia, and atypical seizure-like movements with torsion of the neck known as Sandifer syndrome. In the older child, esophagitis may present with complaints of substernal or chest pain. The approach to the infant with feeding refusal is discussed in Sec. 17.8.3 and to the infant with GI bleeding in Sec. 17.7.7. In the infant with excessive irritability an empiric trial of aggressive antisecretory therapy may be reasonable. It is important to ensure that crying is truly excessive and to consider other potential causes of irritability because vomiting is common in infants and esophagitis is an uncommon cause of irritability. In the older child with heartburn, an empiric trial of antisecretory therapy is generally the most reasonable initial approach to therapy. If symptoms resolve, therapy can be continued for 3 months, and further evaluation is required only if symptoms recur at the cessation of therapy.

Definitive diagnosis of esophagitis requires endoscopy with esophageal biopsy. Biopsy is necessary to differentiate between other potential causes of esophagitis such as infectious etiologies or eosinophilic esophagitis (Sec. 17.11). Typical biopsies in GERD reveal thickening of the basal cell layer ($>25\%$ of mucosal thickness), increases in papillary height ($>50\%$ of mucosal thickness), and infiltration with neutrophils (>1/hpf) or eosinophils (>1 and <15 per hpf). Treatment of GER-induced esophagitis should focus on reducing the acid exposure of the esophagus. Thickening formulas may be helpful, but the most important component of management is treatment with adequate doses of antisecretory agents; either H_2-receptor blockers or proton pump inhibitors may be used. The benefit of added conventional therapies such as prone positioning is uncertain. Prone positioning is not recommended in infants because of the increased risk of sudden infant death.

Severe, prolonged erosive esophagitis can result in the development of either peptic strictures or a Barrett esophagus. Peptic strictures can be dilated, and recurrence can be prevented with either long-term, aggressive medical therapy with a proton pump inhibitor or antireflux surgery. Barrett esophagus presents with intestinal metaplasia in the distal esophagus. It is thought to represent a premalignant lesion, with evolution to esophageal adenocarcinoma over many years. There is no definitive treatment, but vigorous medical therapy or antireflux surgery is usually recommended. Because of the long-term risk of adenocarcinoma, children with this diagnosis should undergo surveillance esophagoscopy and biopsy every 3 to 5 years.

ACUTE LIFE-THREATENING EVENTS Airway symptoms may be either caused or exacerbated by GER. Acute life-threatening events (ALTEs) have been associated with GER, but may be caused by other disorders. Episodes are frightening to the observer and are characterized by a combination of apnea, change in color (cyanosis, pallor, rubra), limpness or stiffness, and choking or gagging. The first event usually occurs by 1 to 2 months of age. Those episodes associated with GER typically are obstructive in nature and occur while the patient is awake, supine, and within 1 hour of a feeding. Central apnea has not been clearly associated with GER. Diagnosis is generally best made from the typical history. Episodes occur infrequently, so even carefully performed combined 24-hour esophageal pH monitoring combined with measurements of air flow and chest wall impedance may be unable to document episodes. Therapeutic options include thickened feedings and prokinetic and acid-suppressant therapy. Position therapy with prone positioning after meals can be considered, but generally the fear of an increased potential of SIDS in an infant with previous ALTE limits the advisability of this approach. Antireflux surgery is effective, but because the episodes are self-resolving and decrease in frequency after age 6 months in most infants, surgery is very rarely indicated. Probably the most important caveat to treatment is to recognize that GER has been invoked as a cause of ALTE in infants later shown to be victims of Munchausen syndrome by proxy.

ASTHMA Asthma can be worsened by GER, and the prevalence of GER in children with asthma is about 50%. A trial of vigorous antireflux therapy (high-dose proton pump inhibitor) may provide some evidence that GER is exacerbating asthma symptoms. This approach is most reasonable in patients with coexisting symptoms of esophagitis (heartburn, dysphagia). Esophageal pH monitoring should be considered in patients with wheezing and evidence of recurrent pneumonia, those with nocturnal asthma more than once a week, and patients requiring either continuous oral corticosteroids, high-dose inhaled corticosteroids, more than two bursts per year of corticosteroids, or those with persistent asthma unable to wean medical management. If esophageal pH monitoring demonstrates an increased frequency or duration of esophageal acid exposure, a trial of prolonged medical therapy for GER should be considered. In patients who respond to therapy, a decision to consider surgical management must balance the risks of long-term medical versus surgical therapy.

RECURRENT PNEUMONIA Recurrent pneumonia may result from GER associated with aspiration, especially in children with neurologic disease or laryngeal anatomic disorders and associated poor airway protective mechanisms. Proving that GER is causing aspiration pneumonia in an individual patient is often difficult. Normal esophageal pH monitoring does not exclude GER as a cause of recurrent aspiration. Bronchoalveolar lavage with large numbers of lipid-laden macrophages suggests that aspiration occurs, but it may be difficult to determine whether aspiration occurs during swallowing or just with GER. In either case, treatment of GER is often indicated once other causes of recurrent pneumonia are ruled out. Medical therapy may be given a trial in children with only moderate pulmonary disease, but in some children with more severe pulmonary disease, antireflux surgery should be considered.

LARYNGEAL SYMPTOMS Hoarseness and recurrent croup have been associated with GER. The approach to diagnosis and treatment of GER-related laryngeal disease is unclear, but a trial of aggressive antireflux therapy with a high-dose proton pump inhibitor is reasonable. If symptoms resolve and recur with the cessation of therapy, GER is likely responsible. Decisions regarding long-term therapy must balance the risks of long-term medical or surgical therapy against the severity of underlying symptoms. Other disorders such as sinusitis, otitis media, and dental erosions have been suggested as being related to GER, but there is little evidence to support these contentions at this time.

TREATMENT OF GERD

"Conservative" therapy can be used in virtually anyone with symptoms that suggest gastroesophageal reflux. Pharmacologic therapy is used for children who are shown to have reflux disease, or in

some specific instances, it may be used empirically for a limited time. Surgery is reserved for those patients with reflux disease that is intractable to medical therapy, with symptoms too hazardous to evaluate for intractability to medical therapy, or occasionally in those whose symptoms respond well to medical therapy but who face a lifetime of such therapy because of recurrent relapses when medications are withdrawn (see Table 17-40).

CONSERVATIVE THERAPY Conservative therapy includes dietary measures (eg, small meals, thickened infant feedings, avoidance of carbonated drinks, high-fat meals, acid foods, caffeine, nicotine) and positioning. In infants, prone postioning clearly decreases the number of episodes of GER and vomiting. However, the increased risk of SIDS in the prone position needs to balanced with the potential benefits of GER treatment. In older children, elevation of the head of the bed may be useful. Treatment of obesity and the avoidance of tight clothes or bedtime snacking also may be useful.

PHARMACOLOGIC THERAPY Pharmacologic therapy consists of agents that decrease gastric acid secretion or that alter esophageal and gastric motility. Reduction in acid secretion is best achieved with either an H_2-receptor antagonist (H_2RA) or with a proton pump inhibitor (PPI). Antacids are relatively ineffective, and aluminum-containing antacids can cause toxicity if used chronically. H_2RAs and PPIs suppress gastric acid secretion via different actions on the parietal cell. The former inhibits the binding of histamine to specific (H_2) receptors on the luminal surface. Activation of these receptors by histamine stimulates the parietal cell to secrete acid by triggering a sequence of intracellular events that lead to activation

TABLE 17-40

TREATMENT OF GASTROESOPHAGEAL REFLUX DISEASE: CONSERVATIVE THERAPY/"LIFESTYLE CHANGES"

Positional changes
　Infant: supine position with head elevated (unless high risk from GER, and then consider prone)
　Older child: head of bed elevation
Nutritional therapy
　Infant
　　Trial of hypoallergenic formula for 1 to 2 weeks
　　Thicken feedings
　　　1 to 2 tbsp rice cereal/oz formula
　　　Commercial formulas with thickening agents
　　Increase caloric density of formula with concentration
　　Small frequent feeds (2.5 hours between feeds)
　Child
　　Avoid caffeinated beverages, peppermint, and chocolate
　　Weight loss if obese
　Rarely, nasogastric or nasojejunal feeding may be required
Pharmacologic therapy
　Antacids (only for relief of occasional symptoms in older children)
　Antisecretory agents
　　Histamine-2 receptor blockers (cimetidine, ranitidine, famotidine)
　　Proton pump inhibitors (omeprazole, lansoprazole, rabeprazole, pantoprazole)
　Prokinetic agents (cisapride where available)
Surgical therapy
　Nissan fundoplication
　Thal fundoplication
　Esophagogastric disconnection

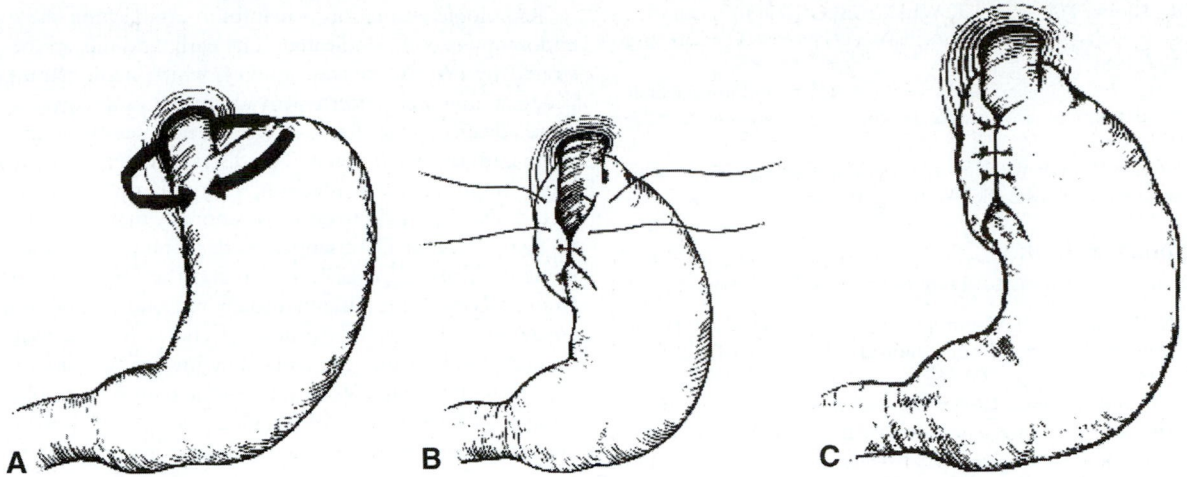

FIGURE 17-27 The Nissen fundoplication operation. A: The lower esophagus is mobilized, allowing the fundus of the stomach to be pulled up and around the lower esophagus. B and C: The fundic wrap has sutures placed to form a collar around the lower esophagus. The tightness and length of the collar vary among surgeons. SOURCE: *Schatzlein MH, Ballantine TVN, Thirunavukkarasu S, et al: Gastroesophageal reflux in infants and children. Arch Surg 114:505–510, 1979.*

of an enzyme called hydrogen/potassium adenosine triphosphatase (H^+, K^+ ATPase), which is the final step in acid production and is also known as the proton pump. Proton pump inhibitors permeate the membrane of parietal cells and accumulate in the secretory canaliculus, where they bind to and inactivate the acid-secreting proton pumps. H_2-receptor blockers need to be given at high doses, and even then, H_2RA therapy is often ineffective for treatment of erosive esophagitis or airway complications of GER. Therefore, initial PPI therapy is generally recommended for treatment of GERD in adults and adolescents. Similar recommendations are likely to follow for treatment of all pediatric patients as further experience with the administration of PPIs is garnered in infants and younger children. PPIs should be given 15 minutes before meals and usually should not be given in combination with H_2RA therapy because this can decrease efficacy. There is currently no effective prokinetic agent available for the treatment of GERD in the United States except on a compassionate use basis. Cisapride has been shown to be an effective therapy, but risks of cardiac rhythm complications resulted in withdrawal from the market. Cisapride is available in other countries and can be considered for treatment of GERD in selected cases. Bethanechol and metoclopramide are prokinetics previously used for treatment of GERD, but neither has been shown to be effective.

SURGICAL THERAPY Surgical therapy uses one of several antireflux procedures depending on the preference of the surgeon and type of patient. The most frequently performed procedure is the Nissen fundoplication (Fig. 17-27). Other variants include the Hill posterior gastropexy, the Belsey mark IV procedure, the Collis-Nissen procedure, and the Thal fundoplication. The mechanism by which these operations prevent gastroesophageal reflux is unclear; elongation of the intraabdominal segment of the esophagus likely improves the reflux barrier. In addition, there is some increase in LES tone. Children who most often require fundoplications are those with severe chronic respiratory or neurologic disease. It previously was argued that children with reflux-associated apnea and those requiring gastrostomy all needed fundoplication, but this is clearly untrue.

The operative mortality associated with Nissen fundoplication, the most commonly performed antireflux surgical procedure, is about 1%. Major complications include breakdown of the wrap, which occurs in 4 to 12%, intrathoracic herniation of the wrap, slipping of the wrap over the body of the stomach, and bowel obstruction. Other complications include gas bloat with postprandial discomfort, dysphagia, gagging, or retching. Dumping syndrome and feeding refusal may also follow antireflux surgery. In general, the risks of all complications appear to be lower in normal patients than in those patient groups most likely to require fundoplication, including patients with severe neurologic disease, esophageal atresia, and chronic lung disease caused by bronchopulmonary dysplasia, cystic fibrosis, or asthma. Laparoscopic fundoplication reduces the morbidity and shortens the hospital stay of pediatric patients undergoing antireflux surgery and is therefore preferable when available.

Gastrostomy with gastrojejunal tube feedings is an alternative to gastrostomy with fundoplication. Another recently described option for children who are at severe risk of aspiration and do not feed by mouth is esophageal-gastric separation with the creation of a Roux-en-Y to the intestine for esophageal drainage. No pediatric studies compare the long-term outcome, costs, or risks of long-term medical therapy versus surgical therapy in those children who respond to medical therapy. Recent adult studies suggest that in many instances prolonged medical therapy is more cost effective and has lower overall morbidity.

References

Esophageal Motility Disorders

Esposito C, Mendoza-Sagaon M, Roblot-Maigret B, Amici G, Desruelle P, Montupet P: Complications of laparoscopic treatment of esophageal achalasia in children. J Pediatr Surg 35:680–683, 2000

Hurwitz M, Bahr RJ, Ament ME, et al: Evaluation of the use of botulinum toxin in children with achalasia. J Pediatr Gastroenterol Nutr 30:509–514, 2000

Nakayama DK, Shorter NA, Boyle JT, Watkins JB, O'Neill JA: Pneumatic dilatation and operative treatment of achalasia in children. J Pediatr Surg 22:619–622, 1987

O'Brien CJ, Smart HL: Familial coexistence of achalasia and nonachalasic oesophageal dysmotility: evidence for a common pathogenesis. Gut 33:1421–1423, 1992

Storch WB, Eckardt VF, Wienbeck M, et al: Autoantibodies to Auerbach's plexus in achalasia. Cell Mol Biol 41:1033–1038, 1995

Gastroesophageal Reflux

Dent J, Dodds WJ, Hogan WJ, Toouli J: Factors that influence induction of gastroesophageal reflux in normal human subjects. Dig Dis Sci 33:270–275, 1988

Rudolph CD, Mazur LJ, Liptak GS, et al: North American Society of Pediatric Gastroenterology and Nutrition evidence-based guidelines for the evaluation and treatment of gastroesophageal reflux in infants and children. J Pediatr Gastroenterol Nutr 32:51–531; 2001

17.11 OTHER CAUSES OF ESOPHAGITIS

17.11.1   Infections of the Esophagus

Robert Wyllie

The most common infectious causes of esophagitis are *Candida,* cytomegalovirus, and herpes infection. These infections usually occur in patients who are immunocompromised. Classic predisposing conditions include HIV, malignancy, diabetes mellitus, and long-term therapy with corticosteroids or antibiotics. The differential diagnosis, depending on the clinical setting, includes graft-versus-host disease and radiation- or chemotherapy-induced lesions.

CANDIDA

Candida infections in the esophagus are common in patients who are immunocompromised, but they also may occur in normal infants. The most frequent symptom in children is dysphagia. Odynophagia or pain with swallowing and retrosternal burning are common. Patients may complain of nausea and vomiting, but some patients will have no symptoms. Microscopic evidence of blood loss on rectal examination is not uncommon, but melena or hematemesis is unusual. Approximately one-half of the patients will have oral thrush.

Endoscopy is the most useful way to establish the diagnosis. Visually the mucosa is hyperemic with whitish plaques, which in heavy infestation may become confluent. Brushing the affected mucosa will reveal the presence of *Candida,* but biopsies are required to demonstrate invasion. Esophageal biopsies generally are considered to be safe if the platelet count is over 50,000/mL, and brushing is safe with platelet counts as low as 15,000/mL. Histologically, biopsies demonstrate evidence of acute and chronic inflammation with ulceration. Both budding yeast and hyphae forms are usually present. Cultures of the tissue do not differentiate between commensal or infectious status for *Candida* and therefore are helpful only in determining drug sensitivity. Occasional children with *Candida* esophagitis have concomitant infection with cytomegalovirus or herpes virus.

Radiologic evaluation is helpful in establishing the diagnosis if endoscopy is contraindicated. The early findings are best demonstrated by double contrast studies, which demonstrate a shaggy, irregular mucosal pattern with abnormal esophageal motility. In more advanced cases frank ulcers and nodules producing a cobblestone pattern may be seen. The distal half of the esophagus is the most common site of infection, although any segment can be infected. Focal fungal infection occasionally may simulate neoplasm.

Symptoms usually disappear with therapy, but clinical improvement does not necessarily mean that the infection is eradicated. Immunocompetent patients usually respond to oral nystatin. Fluconazole is the usual treatment of choice for mucosal disease in immunocompromised patients. For invasive candidiasis, systemic therapy with fluconazole or amphotericin must be employed. Complications of *Candida* infection include esophageal perforation, tracheoesophageal fistula formation, and esophageal strictures.

CYTOMEGALOVIRUS

Esophagitis is usually caused by cytomegalovirus only in patients who are immunocompromised. The virus is ubiquitous and may be transmitted horizontally from person to person or vertically from mother to infant before, during, or after birth. Seropositive healthy individuals have latent cytomegalovirus, which can be transmitted through body secretions, blood products, or donor organs. Latent cytomegalovirus infection can be activated in the immunosuppressed state. The virus infects the submucosal fibroblasts and endothelial cells, but the mucosal squamous epithelium is spared. Esophageal infection usually is part of a more generalized systemic infection. Esophageal symptoms include painful swallowing, heartburn, nausea, vomiting, and anorexia. Initial lesions in the esophagus consist of serpiginous ulcers that may coalesce to form large ulcers, which characteristically are found in the middle and distal third of the esophagus.

Serology and culture of blood, urine, or stool may suggest the diagnosis of cytomegalovirus. Radiologic evaluations demonstrate nonspecific changes of esophageal irritability with abnormal motility and spasm or demonstrate deep, flat ulcerations. A specific diagnosis requires endoscopic biopsy with specimens that are taken from the ulcered areas. Histologic evaluation with routine staining demonstrates basophilic intranuclear inclusions and periodic acid–Schiff-positive cytoplasmic inclusions in the endothelial cells. More recently, monoclonal antibodies to cytomegalovirus and cytomegalovirus DNA hybridization also have aided in the diagnosis. The most reliable method of diagnosis, however, remains culture of the biopsy material.

Cytomegalovirus can be treated with antiviral drugs such as ganciclovir and foscarnet. However, symptoms may be slow to respond, and recurrence is high, if the underlying immune compromise is not corrected.

HERPES SIMPLEX VIRUS

This virus infects the squamous epithelium of the esophagus, producing discrete ulcers with raised edges. In severe infections, the ulcers may coalesce, producing a denuded mucosa. Patients present with painful swallowing, heartburn, and retrosternal pain. Children may refuse to eat or present with only nausea, vomiting, or hematemesis. The diagnosis can be suspected if herpes simplex virus infection is found in the nose or mouth. Radiologic studies demonstrate discrete ulceration with raised edges, giving a characteristic target appearance. However, radiographs are too insensitive to diagnose mild infection, and they fail to identify those patients with multiple pathogens causing their esophagitis.

Endoscopy demonstrates discrete ulcerations or a more denuded mucosa, depending on the severity of the infection. The typical vesicular lesion frequently noted on the lips or nasal passages is very rarely seen. Biopsies taken from the ulcer margin may demonstrate ballooning degeneration, ground glass–appearing intranuclear (Cowdry type A) bodies and multinuclear giant cells. Brushing and biopsy specimens should be routinely placed in special viral media for culture of herpes simplex virus because viral culture is more sensitive than histology in establishing a diagnosis. More specific techniques for the identification of herpes simplex virus, including monoclonal antibody identification of infected cells and in situ hybridization for herpes simplex virus DNA, may improve the diagnostic yield in difficult cases.

In patients with normal immune function, the natural history of esophageal herpes simplex virus infection is similar to that observed on the lips or buccal membranes. In immunocompromised patients, the infection may not resolve without therapy or the return of normal immune activity. Acyclovir is effective in treating most patients, with relief of symptoms usually occurring within the first week of therapy. Large ulcers may take longer to heal and require longer therapy. Acyclovir prophylaxis following bone marrow and solid-organ transplantation has diminished the frequency of herpes simplex virus esophagitis in the immediate posttransplant period for seropositive patients. Herpes simplex virus strains that are resistant to acyclovir have been treated with foscarnet, but foscarnet-resistant strains also have emerged. Vidarabine is an alternative treatment in these patients. Acid suppressors may be used as adjunctive therapy for symptoms of gastroesophageal reflux, but long-term therapy should be avoided, as it predisposes to esophageal fungal infection.

VARICELLA ZOSTER VIRUS

This virus, which produces chicken pox, may involve the esophagus or other parts of the digestive tract. Although rare, necrotizing esophagitis can occur in patients with herpes zoster. Vesicles can be visualized on endoscopy. Biopsy and brushing produce histologic changes that are similar to those seen in herpes simplex virus infection. Differentiation of varicella zoster virus and herpes simplex virus can be done by finding cutaneous varicelliform or zoster eruptions typical of varicella zoster infection and with immunohistologic staining of biopsy material. Cultures are of limited value because varicella zoster virus is difficult to isolate. Acyclovir in susceptible strains and foscarnet in resistant strains have been effective treatments.

OTHER INFECTIOUS AGENTS CAUSING ESOPHAGITIS

Epstein-Barr virus has been isolated from esophageal ulcers in patients with AIDS. Esophageal ulceration has also been identified with human immunodeficiency virus in the absence of any identifiable pathogen. Human papilloma virus has been identified in the esophagus, but the infection is usually asymptomatic. A number of opportunistic pathogens have been isolated from the esophagus of immunocompromised individuals, including *Cryptosporidium, Mycobacterium avium-intracellulare, M. tuberculosis,* and *Torulopsis glabrata,* which is a fungus. Bacterial esophagitis has been observed in patients with granulocytopenia, but the infection usually occurs in the face of concomitant viral or fungal infection.

17.11.2   Systemic Illness Causing Esophagitis

Robert Wyllie

A variety of systemic inflammatory disorders that are associated with esophageal disease, including Behçet disease, Crohn disease, graft-versus-host disease, sarcoidosis, and chronic granulomatous disease, are discussed in other sections of this chapter. Esophageal involvement may occur with most skin diseases that affect the oral cavity (eg, epidermolysis bullosa, Stevens-Johnson syndrome) and connective tissue diseases including scleroderma, systemic lupus erythematosus, polymyositis and dermatomyositis, and mixed connective tissue disease. The immunosuppression associated with cancer therapy increases the risk of infectious esophagitis, but mucosal inflammation commonly results from the therapy itself. Chemotherapy and radiation therapy both can cause severe esophageal inflammation with resultant esophageal stricture formation during the healing process.

17.11.3   Corrosive Esophagitis

Robert Wyllie

The Association of Poison Control Centers National Data Collection System reports approximately 2 million human exposures to poison each year. One million of these are children 6 years of age or younger; the most common age of ingestion is 1 to 3 years. Substances that most commonly are ingested include bleaches, laundry detergents, tile and toilet bowel cleaners, drain and oven cleaners, swimming pool and aquarium products, and a variety of other miscellaneous agricultural and industrial chemicals.

Caustic injury usually is caused by a strong acid or alkali. Acids cause coagulation necrosis of the mucosa, with the eschar limiting deeper injury. Acids have a disagreeable taste, usually cause immediate pain, and are rapidly expelled unless they are intentionally ingested. Acidic agents are more likely to produce injury to the stomach than the esophagus; however, acid ingestion results in esophageal injury in up to 20% of children. Ingestions in young and retarded children usually are accidental, and the volumes ingested usually are small. In older children and adolescents, ingestions are larger and often associated with attempted suicide. Acid injury to the gastric mucosa depends on the volume of food or fluid in the stomach. In the fasting child, injury is most likely to be in the body and antrum, sparing the fundus; if the stomach is full of liquid, the acidic agent will mix with the gastric contents and may cause a more diffuse injury.

Most alkaline solutions are tasteless, odorless, and are swallowed without difficulty. Alkalis produce liquefactive necrosis with intense inflammation of the surrounding tissue and thrombosis of adjacent vessels, which may result in further necrosis. Granular alkalis such as those in drain cleaners usually cause focal injury that is limited to the oropharynx or proximal esophagus, with more severe injury occurring only in 25% of children. Liquid alkali ingestion is more likely to result in severe injury to the entire esophagus and stomach. The stomach is not significantly protected by its own acid production because the neutralizing capacity of gastric acid is insignificant compared with the alkalinity of even small volumes of strong alkalis.

Infants and children with ingestions usually present with drooling, dysphagia, or abdominal pain, but they also may present with airway symptoms of stridor, retractions, and nasal flaring or hoarseness. The symptoms may develop rapidly or be delayed for several hours. The presence or absence of symptoms or oral lesions does not predict the severity of injury to the esophagus or stomach. This inability to predict the presence or severity of injury makes a careful evaluation for esophageal or gastric injury imperative. In patients with a questionable history of ingestion, no symptoms, and no physical findings, observation for several hours and documentation that the child has the ability to tolerate clear liquids usually means that additional evaluation is unnecessary. Ingestion of bleach rarely is associated with significant adverse effects, and these patients also can be observed with no further intervention. Patients with a definite history or with suspected ingestion and symptoms should undergo additional evaluation.

In the acute stages of injury, barium studies are not adequately sensitive to diagnose the extent and severity of illness, and they are not indicated. Upper endoscopy is routinely performed 12 to 24 hours after the ingestion to assess the extent of esophageal injury and gastric involvement; endoscopy within the first 12 hours may not demonstrate the full extent of esophageal injury. Caustic injury usually is graded and classified into one of three classes. First-degree burns involve only superficial injury consisting of mucosal edema or erythema. These patients tolerate feedings, and the lesions heal without scar or stricture formation. Second-degree burns are characterized by injury extending through the submucosa into the muscular layers. Endoscopically, ulcers are visualized covered by a whitish exudate. Two to three weeks following the initial injury, fibroblasts proliferate with collagen deposition. The collagen contracts over the next several weeks, with a mature scar developed by 8 weeks in most patients. If the initial ulcerations occurred circumferentially, healing with collagen contraction may result in stricture formation. Third-degree burns are associated with severe esophageal or gastric injury and accompanied by perforation. Most perforations occur within 48 hours after ingestion and are associated with symptoms of mediastinitis or peritonitis. Emergent surgical treatment for perforation is mandatory.

Initial management of caustic injury is observation. Emesis should not be induced because it may lead to additional esophageal injury. Use of neutralizing agents has been suggested, but heat production that is associated with neutralization of alkali or acid may potentiate tissue injury. The immediate dilution of acids with large volumes of milk or water within minutes of injury also has been advocated, but this increases the likelihood of emesis with poor compliance in children who have substantial esophageal or gastric irritation. Nasogastric tubes should not be passed because they may perforate a damaged esophagus or stomach. If the child has upper airway symptoms, corticosteroids may be helpful, and intubation or tracheostomy necessary.

Treatment for caustic injury with esophageal ulcers is directed at reducing the frequency of stricture formation. Many children are routinely treated with broad-spectrum antibiotics and intravenous prednisone. The rationale for antibiotics is inhibition of bacterial invasion of the esophageal mucosa. Corticosteroids inhibit the formation of strictures following alkali injury in animal models. Anecdotal reports also suggest they might be beneficial in human injury, but prospective studies in children with acid and alkali ingestion have failed to demonstrate a consistent benefit. When corticosteroids are administered, they are usually given for 3 to 4 weeks and then tapered.

More recently, collagen synthesis inhibitors including phenytoin, penicillamine, aminopropionitrite, and *N*-acetylcysteine have been shown to inhibit the formation of collagen; however, clinical studies have not been reported evaluating their efficacy in caustic ingestion. Some physicians have advocated early esophageal dilation to prevent stricture formation. Dilation is performed at frequent intervals until complete healing occurs. Early dilation carries the risk of perforation and may accentuate esophageal injury, theoretically placing the patient at risk of further esophageal injury and fibrosis. Most physicians perform dilation only after a stricture forms. More recently, investigators have placed intraluminal esophageal stents under endoscopic guidance if the initial examination demonstrates circumferential burns. This technique has not been widely adapted, however, and patients still may require dilation after the stent is removed. Use of a gastrostomy tube and string passed through the esophagus and out the gastrostomy also has been recommended for severe esophageal injury. In the event of long or multiple stricture formation, this allows guide wires and dilators to by pulled along the course of the string, thus decreasing the risk of perforation.

17.11.4   Pill-Induced Esophagitis

Robert Wyllie

Medication in pill form may occasionally lodge in the esophagus, dissolve, and cause significant inflammation. Most children have no underlying esophageal disease, but those with esophageal narrowing because of esophageal strictures, achalasia, or motility disorders are at increased risk. The most common location for pill-induced esophageal injury is the midesophagus, where the left atrium impinges on the middle third of the esophagus and there is decreased esophageal peristalsis associated with the transition from skeletal to smooth muscle. Some of the more common pills associated with esophageal irritation are tetracycline, doxycycline, aspirin, nonsteroidal antiinflammatory agents, slow-release potassium preparations, and guar gum–containing diet pills. The primary cause of injury is associated with adherence of the pill to the esophageal mucosa, with dissolution of the pill resulting in local irritation. Contributing factors include taking pills with little or no fluid, taking pills late at night when there is decreased salivation, and lying down shortly after taking a pill. Typically symptoms start shortly after ingestion and include retrosternal pain and dysphagia. A characteristic history and knowledge of the pill types that commonly are associated with pill esophagitis is usually sufficient for diagnosis. When the diagnosis is in doubt, endoscopy is the most sensitive diagnostic test and may demonstrate findings ranging from erythema to esophageal ulceration. Symptoms generally resolve within 1 to 3 weeks of discontinuing pill administration or with improved approaches to taking pills when continued ingestion of medication is necessary. Acid blockers may be helpful in patients with severe symptoms.

17.11.5   Eosinophilic Esophagitis

Colin D. Rudolph

Eosinophilic esophagitis is characterized by an intense eosinophilic infiltrate of the esophageal mucosa. Eosinophil infiltration of the esophagus is often associated with esophagitis from gastroesophageal reflux, but the density of eosinophils is generally less than 7/hpf. In contrast, eosinophil density often exceeds 15/hpf in eosinophilic esophagitis. Biopsies may otherwise be similar to those of GERD, with basal cell layer hyperplasia and papillary height increases. Presenting symptoms may be similar to those of gastroesophageal reflux disease, although dysphagia in older children or feeding refusal in infants seems to be more common than in GERD. Some children may present with esophageal stricture, presumably resulting from the chronic intense infiltration.

Diagnosis of eosinophilic esophagitis is entirely dependent on esophageal biopsy. Esophagoscopy often reveals diffuse friability with linear ulcerations throughout the entire esophagus. A subtle macroscopic indication of likely eosinophilic esophagitis is a furrowed, occasionally ringed appearance of the esophageal mucosa without erosions or other mucosal breaks. Esophageal pH monitoring may be normal, but an abnormal study does not exclude eosinophilic esophagitis because poor acid clearance may be secondary to esophageal dysmotility from inflammation. Typically, vigorous antisecretory therapy with proton pump inhibitors does not heal the esophagitis, although treatment may lead to symptomatic improvement. Allergy testing may identify likely allergic causes of eosinophilic esophagitis, which can then be treated with an elimination diet. In infants, a trial of a hypoallergenic formula is often useful. Treatment with either systemic or topical corticosteroids is usually effective, with topical therapy using agents such as fluticasone being preferable to systemic therapy. Unfortunately, multiple esophageal biopsies are often required to assure adequate therapeutic response to various therapeutic trials. For example, a child may be initially treated with proton pump inhibitors for possible GERD. When therapy fails, the diagnosis of eosinophilic esophagitis may be entertained, and an elimination diet or hypoallergenic formula trialed. If this fails, then corticosteroid therapy is attempted. Refinement of diagnostic criteria may allow for more focused treatment, but currently there is no standard diagnostic or therapeutic approach.

References

Esophageal Infections

Daveikis A: Gastrointestinal disease in immunocompromised children. Pediatr Ann 23:562–569, 1994

Heller JO, Cohen HL: Gastrointestinal manifestations of AIDS in children. Am J Roentgenol 162:387–393, 1994

Narwal S, Galeano NF, Pottenger E, Kazlow PG, Husain S, Defelice AR: Idiopathic esophageal ulcers in a child with AIDS. J Pediatr Gastroenterol Nutr 24:211–214, 1997

Caustic Ingestion

Christesen HB: Prediction of complications following unintentional casutic ingestion in children. Is endoscopy always necessary? Acta Paediatr 84: 1177–1182, 1995

Karnak I, Tanyel FC, Buyunkpamukcu N, Hicxonmerz A: Combined use of steroid, antibiotics and early bougienage against stricture formation following caustic esophageal burns. J Cardiovasc Surg 40:307–310, 1999

Litovitz TL, Klein-Schwartz W, Dyer KS, Shannon M, Lee S, Powers M: 1997 annual report of the American Association of Poison Control Centers Toxic Exposure Surveillance System. Am J Emerg Med 16:443–497, 1998

Ulman I, Mutaf O: A critique of systemic steroids in the management of caustic esophageal burns in children. Eur J Pediatr Surg 8:71–74, 1998

Pill-Induced Esophagitis

Ovartlarnporn B, Kulwichit W, Hiranniramol S: Medication-induced esophageal injury: report of 17 cases with endoscopic documentation. Am J Gastroenterol 86:748–750, 1991

Eosinophilic Esophagitis

Faubion WA, Perrault J, Burgat LJ, et al: Treatment of eosinophilic esophagitis with inhaled corticosteroids. J Pediatr Gastroenter Nutr 27:90–93, 1998

Kelly KJ, Lazenby AJ, Rowe PC, Yardley JH, Perman JA, Sampson HA: Eosinophilic esophagitis attributed to gastroesophageal reflux: improvement with an amino acid-based formula. Gastroenterology 109:1503–1512, 1995

Liacouras CA, Wenner WJ, Brown K, Ruchelli E: Primary eosinophilic esophagitis in children: successful treatment with oral corticosteroids. J Pediatr Gastroenterol Nutr 26:380–385, 1998

Ruchelli E, Wenner W, Voytek T, Brown K, Liacouras C: Severity of esophageal eosinophilia predicts response to conventional gastroesophageal reflux therapy. Pediatr Dev Pathol 2:15–18, 1999

Walsh SV, Antonioli DA, Goldman H, et al: Allergic esophagitis in children: a clinicopathological entity. Am J Surg Pathol 23:390–396, 1999

17.12 OTHER DISORDERS OF THE ESOPHAGUS

Robert Wyllie

17.12.1   Foreign Bodies of the Esophagus

Approximately 80% of all foreign-body ingestions occur in children, with a peak incidence between the ages of 6 months and 3 years. Coins are the most common foreign body that is ingested during childhood. Older children and adolescents get fish or chicken bones lodged in the esophagus or are psychiatrically impaired and swallow a variety of objects. The risk of ingestion increases following the consumption of alcohol or cold liquids because of a decrease in sensory acuity. Of the foreign bodies that come to medical attention, 80 to 90% pass without incident, but 10 to 20% require endoscopic removal. One percent or fewer require surgical removal. Gastrointestinal tract perforation following foreign-body ingestion is estimated to be less than 1%. Perforation is more common among people with congenital gut malformations or those who have had previous abdominal surgery. Once in the stomach, 95% of all ingested objects pass without difficulty through the remainder of the GI tract.

Ninety percent of children give a history of foreign-body ingestion or are observed actively swallowing an object. In some patients, the ingestions may only be inferred by the disappearance of an object followed by the onset of symptoms. Foreign bodies in children that produce symptoms most often are lodged just below the cricopharyngeal muscle. Less often, objects will become impacted at other sites of esophageal narrowing, such as the impressions made by the aortic arch and left mainstem bronchus or lower esophageal sphincter. Common presenting symptoms in young children include excess drooling, choking, and poor feeding. Older children may complain of substernal pain and dysphagia.

Occasionally, children present with only respiratory symptoms. An esophageal foreign body should be considered in infants who present with wheezing, cough, stridor, impaired speech, failure to thrive, cyanosis, or chronic pulmonary infections. The liquid and pureed diet of young children lets food slip around the object with relative ease. Respiratory symptoms arise from compression of the soft posterior tracheal wall.

DIAGNOSIS

Approximately 90% of foreign bodies are radiopaque. Radiologic examination routinely is performed to determine the location, type, and number of objects in suspected ingestion. Coins tend to lie in the coronal plane within the esophagus and in the sagittal plane within the trachea. Contrast material or fluoroscopy may be necessary to demonstrate some objects such as plastic parts or toys.

MANAGEMENT

Patients who present with evidence of respiratory compromise or who are unable to swallow their own secretions require immediate intervention. Children with an object that is identified by radiography who are able to swallow their own secretions and have no respiratory symptoms can be observed for 12 to 24 hours. Approximately one-third of the objects will pass spontaneously; the others should then be retrieved. An exception is button batteries, which, because of their potential for esophageal perforation, should be immediately removed. Button batteries that have reached the stomach usually pass through the GI tract without incident.

Fiberoptic endoscopy now is routinely employed to snare and remove objects under direct vision. Smooth, small objects that cannot be easily grasped in the esophagus can be gently pushed into the stomach. Foreign bodies greater than 10 cm in length have difficulty negotiating the duodenal sweep and should also be removed. Blind removal with Foley catheters under fluoroscopic guidance has been reported for blunt foreign bodies that are lodged in the esophagus. This technique has been particularly popular with coins, but it should be performed only by those with adequate training and experience because it has been associated with aspiration of the object into the airway.

Sharp or pointed foreign bodies in the stomach have a higher morbidity, with a perforation rate from 15 to 35%. Straight pins are the exception because they tend to pass without difficulty. Sharp objects other than straight pins are usually removed if they remain in the stomach.

Meat impaction occasionally is a problem in adolescents, and it may be an indication of underlying organic pathology, frequently being associated with either eosinophilic or reflux esophagitis. Immediate intervention is indicated in those patients who are unable to swallow their own secretions. In those patients who can swallow their own saliva, observation is indicated because the impaction often will pass spontaneously. Meat impactions have been removed with the aid of various drugs, flexible catheters, gentle pushing with a bougie or endoscope, and endoscopic share techniques. All must be performed by individuals experienced in either rigid or flexible esophagoscopy. Meat tenderizers should not be used; they have been associated with hypernatremia and esophageal perforation.

References

Conners GP, Cobaugh DJ, Feinberg R, Lucanie R, Caraccio T, Stork CM: Home observation for asymptomatic coin ingestion: acceptance and outcomes. The New York State Poison Control Center Coin Ingestion Study Group. Acad Emerg Med 6:213–217, 1999

Harned RK 2nd, Strain JD, Hay TC, Douglas MR: Esophageal foreign bodies: safety and efficacy of Foley catheter extraction of coins. Am J Roentgenol 168:443–446, 1997

Litovitz T, Schmitz BF: Ingestion of cylindrical and button batteries: an analysis of 2382 cases. Pediatrics 89:747, 1992

McGahren ED: Esophageal foreign bodies. Pediatr Rev 20:129–133, 1999

17.12.2   Perforation of the Esophagus

The most common cause of perforation of the esophagus is blunt trauma following medical instrumentation. Routine esophagoscopy carries a risk of less than one per 1000 procedures. The risk is increased in patients who are undergoing sclerotherapy, removal of foreign bodies, or esophageal dilation. Perforation also is a complication of attempted endotracheal intubation and passage of nasogastric tubes. Other causes of esophageal perforation include forceful vomiting (eg, Boerhaave syndrome), abrupt increases in abdominal pressure (as occur with falls, child abuse, automobile accidents, and during fights), foreign-body ingestion, caustic ingestion, and penetrating injuries. Medical conditions that are associated with spontaneous perforation include connective tissue disorders such as Ehlers-Danlos and Marfan syndromes.

Esophageal perforation usually is recognized by pain in the chest, abdomen, or upper back along with dysphagia and painful swallowing. There often is evidence of subcutaneous emphysema, fever, and hypotension. Immediate radiographs are abnormal in the majority of patients and may demonstrate air in the soft tissues or mediastinum, pleural effusion, or a widened mediastinum. Perforations of the cervical esophagus usually are associated with air in the soft tissues of the neck or prevertebral area. Late changes most often include abscess formation, which is best demonstrated by computed tomography. Perforation of the thoracic esophagus leads to collection of air and fluid in the right pleural space and mediastinum, whereas perforation of the distal esophagus results in abnormalities of the left pleural space, mediastinum, or abdominal cavity.

Endoscopy should not be performed when perforation is suspected. Air insufflation may cause respiratory distress in an existing perforation or extend an esophageal tear to a perforating lesion. The safest procedure is to obtain plain-film radiographs followed by the instillation of a small amount of water-soluble contrast material. If water-soluble contrast fails to show a lesion, regular barium may be needed for better visualization.

Treatment of esophageal perforation usually is surgical. Nonoperative management is considered only when the perforation has been recognized quickly, is confined to a small space, and has not been contaminated by food or gastric contents. Patients must be treated with intravenous broad-spectrum antibiotics and fed through a parenteral or enteral route bypassing the site of perforation during the healing process.

References

Engum SA, Grosfeld JL, West KW, Rescorla FJ, Scherer LR, Vaughan WG: Improved survival in children with esophageal perforation. Arch Surg 131:604–610, 1996

Panieri E, Millar AJ, Rode H, Grown RA, Cywes S: Iatrogenic esophageal perforation in children: patterns of injury, presentation, management, and outcome. J Pediatr Surg 31:890–895, 1996

Sartorelli KH, McBride WJ, Vane DW: Perforation of the intrathoracic esophagus from blunt trauma in a child: case report and review of the literature. J Pediatr Surg 34:495–497, 1999

17.13 CONGENITAL ANOMALIES OF THE STOMACH AND INTESTINE

17.13.1   Abdominal Wall Defects

Richard G. Azizkhan and Philip K. Frykman

Abdominal wall defects in infants are relatively rare embryologic anomalies occurring in one in 4000 to 5000 live births. *Omphalocele* is a central defect of the abdominal wall at the position of the umbilicus and may contain both hollow and solid visceral organs. Omphaloceles have a fascial defect greater than 4 cm in diameter and are covered by peritoneal membrane internally and amniotic membrane externally. *Umbilical hernias* are similar lesions that contain only intestine, but the fascial defects are less than 4 cm. In contrast, *gastroschisis* is a small abdominal wall defect, usually less than 4 cm in diameter, usually located to the right of the umbilical cord. Gastroschisis presents with exposed loops of bowel that are foreshortened and thickened by an inflammatory reaction of the serosa. The solid visceral organs usually remain within the abdominal cavity.

The embryology of gastrointestinal development is described in Sec. 17.1.2. During gestation, the anterior abdominal wall develops from the cephalic fold, lateral folds, and caudal fold somatopleures. By week 4 of development, there is simultaneous cranial, caudal, and lateral fusion of the embryonic folds in the midline to form the umbilical ring. During weeks 4 to 7, the somatopleures are invaded by myotomes located lateral to the vertebral column, which migrate medially, eventually becoming the three muscular layers of the abdominal wall. Parallel with abdominal wall development, the midgut undergoes elongation and herniates into the umbilical cord. During weeks 8 to 12 the myotomes differentiate to abdominal wall musculature and undergo midline fusion. By week 12 the abdominal cavity has enlarged adequately for the small intestine to reenter the abdominal cavity and undergo rotation to lie in its eventual anatomic position.

The etiology of omphalocele and gastroschisis in humans is unknown, although both anomalies have been induced experimentally in animals. Neither omphalocele nor gastroschisis is considered a hereditary defect even though they are reported to occur rarely in familial syndromes. Approximately 50 to 75% of neonates with omphalocele have associated congenital anomalies, and 20 to 35% carry major chromosomal derangements. Therefore, a detailed physical exam and systems review are imperative in a newborn with omphalocele. The embryologic events that lead to omphalocele remain controversial. Failure of the cranial, caudal, and lateral folds to fuse before myotome invasion is the most credible explanation for omphalocele development. Another proposed explanation is the failure of midgut reentry into the abdominal cavity, leaving the abdominal cavity relatively small. Omphalocele is also associated with syndromes of midline development such as the thoracoabdominal syndrome (pentalogy of Cantrell) with an upper midline omphalocele, anterior diaphragmatic hernia, sternal cleft, ectopic cordis, and cardiac anomalies and associated gene defects at locus Xq25 to q26.1. A lower midline syndrome (caudal fold defect) including bladder or cloacal extrophy, imperforate anus, colonic atresia, vesicointestinal fistula, sacrovertebral anomalies, and meningomyelocele is also associated. Other syndromes associated with omphalocele include Beckwith-Wiedemann syndrome, trisomies 13, 15, 18, and 21, and Reiger and prune-belly syndromes.

Gastroschisis is much more commonly isolated and is thought to result from a vascular disruption of the right omphalomesenteric artery. In some cases the gastroschisis may result from a small ruptured omphalocele early in gestation. Intestinal abnormalities are frequent in both gastroschisis and omphalocele, with nearly all having some degree of malrotation or lack of fixation leading to increased risk of midgut volvulus. Foreshortened bowel and intestinal atresias are found quite commonly in neonates with gastroschisis.

Omphalocele presents as a central defect of the umbilical ring with abdominal contents within a sac (Fig. 17-28). The umbilical cord is inserted in the sac, which can range in size from 4 to 12 cm. The sac often contains the stomach, loops of small and large bowel, and liver in approximately 50% of cases. A giant omphalocele presents with a large sac that may contain small and large bowel, liver, spleen, gonadal tissue, and bladder. The abdominal wall muscles are developed and are approximated in the midline in smaller omphaloceles. However, larger defects result in a smaller volume of the abdominal compartment, making reduction a challenge. Approximately 10 to 20% of omphaloceles rupture in utero. When rupture occurs early, the bowel appears thickened and matted with exudate, presenting very similarly to gastroschisis. Prenatal ultrasound may detect these lesions after 12 to 14 weeks of gestation.

Gastroschisis usually presents as a 2- to 5-cm defect to the right midline, often with the small and large bowel eviscerated, but rarely are other visceral organs involved (Fig. 17-29). There is a normal umbilical cord and occasionally a small skin bridge between the

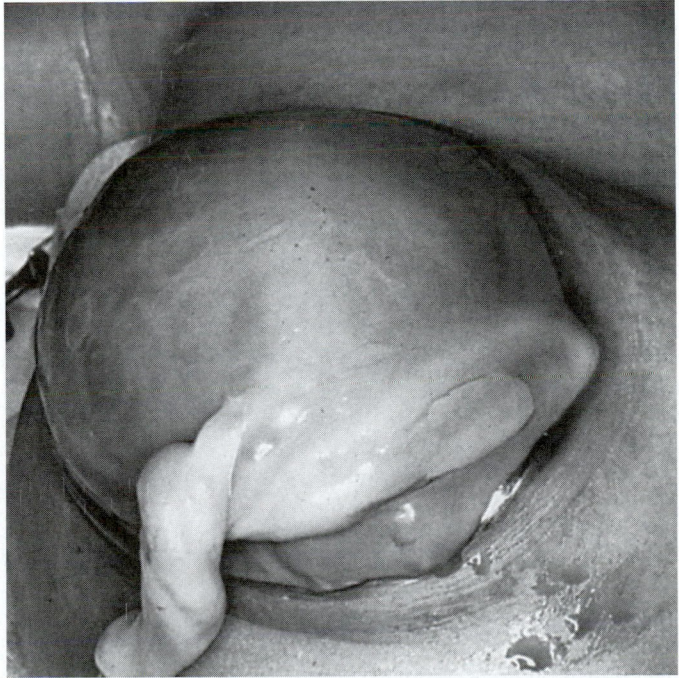

FIGURE 17-28 Moderate to large omphalocele membrane-covered abdominal wall defect. The liver is visible in the right upper quadrant through the membrane. The umbilical cord is attached to the intact membrane.

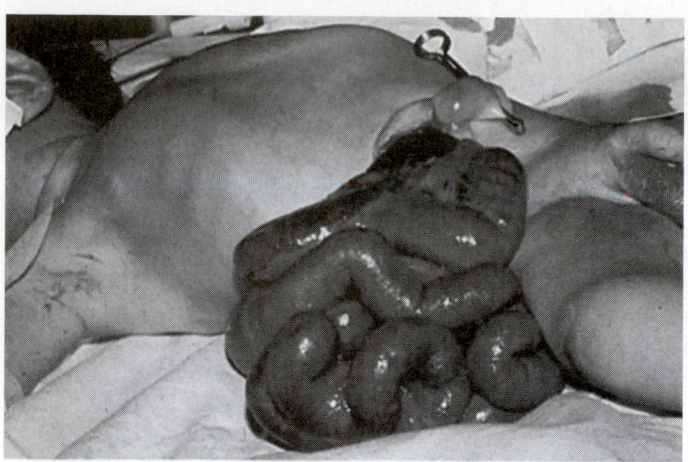

FIGURE 17-29 A right paramedian abdominal wall defect of gastroschisis. The uncovered bowel appears to be foreshortened and thickened.

umbilicus and the defect. The eviscerated bowel is often covered with a thick inflammatory peel that is presumed to result from prolonged exposure of bowel to amniotic fluid; the more normal the bowel appears, the more recently the defect is presumed to have occurred. Gastroschisis can be detected by prenatal ultrasound in the second and third trimesters.

TREATMENT

Initial management for abdominal wall defects is focused on newborn resuscitation with maintenance of hydration and temperature. Intravenous fluids need to be provided, and close monitoring of electrolytes is required because of increased fluid, electrolyte, and protein losses compared to normal neonates. Orogastric intubation with continuous low suction should be instituted to prevent vomiting or aspiration and to decompress the intestine. Exposed viscera or omphalocele membrane should be carefully covered with plastic wrap or a plastic bowel bag and warm saline-soaked gauze, with particular attention given to the prevention of angulation of the bowel, which could compromise the vascular supply. In addition, broad-spectrum intravenous antibiotics should be administered. Further management should follow careful consideration of the possible presence of associated anomalies that may alter management before surgical therapy.

Omphalocele, but not gastroschisis, can be managed nonoperatively if the physiological status of the infant is tenuous. Nonoperative management consists of the application of antiseptic agents such as silver nitrate, silver sulfadiazine cream, or povidone-iodine to initially provide a bacteriostatic eschar that subsequently is epithelialized. Once granulated, the omphalocele can accept a skin graft, which results in the creation of a ventral hernia that will require operative repair in the future.

The goal of surgical management is the reduction of abdominal viscera, approximation of fascial edges, and skin coverage. Surgical closure of the abdominal wall defect may be accomplished with a primary closure or a staged repair once the neonate is adequately resuscitated, warmed, and hemodynamically stable. Primary surgical closure is often successful in small to medium omphaloceles and gastroschisis. Reduction of abdominal viscera is attempted while intraabdominal and peak airway pressures are monitored. Elevated intraabdominal pressures (>23-25 cm H_2O) during closure can decrease vena caval blood return to the heart, which results in re-

duced cardiac output. The diaphragm can also be pushed into the thoracic cavity, causing elevated peak airway pressures with attendant risk of barotrauma and pulmonary insufficiency. Kinking of elongated hepatic veins must be prevented during reduction of the liver in omphaloceles. Associated intestinal atresias are often treated conservatively with nasogastric decompression for 4 weeks, after which time resection and primary reanastomosis are performed.

If a primary repair is not possible, a staged repair can be performed. A prosthetic silo (Silastic reinforced with Dacron) is sutured to the fascial edges to protect the eviscerated bowel. The silo is suspended upright and kept warm and moist while the bowel is progressively reduced into the abdominal cavity. Once reduction is achieved (ranging from a few days up to several weeks) without hemodynamic, respiratory, or metabolic compromise, the silo is removed, and fascia is closed. A major complication of the staged repair is the increased rate of sepsis because of the duration of open wound and use of prosthetic material.

Postoperative management includes continuation of fluid resuscitation and close monitoring of intraabdominal pressure, urine output, and airway pressures. Often bowel function will return within 2 to 3 days following primary repair of omphalocele, and enteral nutrition can be initiated. However, following gastroschisis and staged repairs, bowel function returns much more slowly, sometimes taking several weeks. Total parenteral nutrition should be started in anticipation of a prolonged period without enteral feeding.

Early postoperative complications include intestinal obstruction and necrotizing enterocolitis. Necrotizing enterocolitis is responsible for significant morbidity and mortality in patients with abdominal wall defects. Respiratory compromise from prolonged mechanical ventilation and fungal or bacterial sepsis from parenteral nutrition are potential complications, occurring weeks to months after repair. Long-term complications include ventral and inguinal hernias and growth delay.

Overall survival of infants with gastroschisis and omphalocele has steadily improved over the past two decades, and today the survival rate of infants with gastroschisis is about 95%. The survival rate of infants with omphalocele is approximately 75 to 90% and lags behind that of infants with gastroschisis, primarily because of a higher incidence of associated anomalies.

References

Cooney DR: Defects of the abdominal wall. In: O'Neill JA, Rowe RI, Grosfeld JL, Fonkalsrud EW, Coran AG, eds: Pediatric Surgery, 5th ed. St Louis, Mosby-Year Book, 1045: 1998

Novotny DA, Klein RL, Boeckman CR: Gastroschisis: an 18-year review. J Pediatr Surg 28:650, 1993

Oldham KT, Coran AG, Drongowski PJ, Wesley JR, Polley TZ: The development of necrotizing enterocolitis following repair of gastroschisis: a surprisingly high incidence. J Pediatr Surg 23:945, 1998

Swartz KR, Harrison MW, Campbell JR, Campbell TJ: Long-term follow-up of patients with gastoschisis. Am J Surg 151:546, 1986

Tracy TF: Abdominal wall defects. In: Oldham KT, Colombani PM, Foglia RP, eds: Surgery of Infants and Children: Scientific Principles and Practices. Philadelphia, Lippincott-Raven, 1083: 1997

17.13.2 Anomalies of Intestinal Rotation

Richard G. Azizkhan and Philip K. Frykman

Disorders of intestinal rotation and fixation may be asymptomatic but can present at any time during infancy or childhood, with volvulus resulting in intestinal ischemia, resultant short-bowel syndrome, and even death. The embryology of the developing intestine is discussed in Sec. 17.1.2. Failure of normal rotation results in nonrotation, incomplete rotation, paraduodenal hernia, or reverse rotation. Nonrotation is the most common anomaly, with the cecum lying on the left and small bowel on the right of the superior mesenteric artery (SMA), resulting in a foreshortened mesentery and little or no fixation of the bowel. The duodenum is frequently truncated and fused with the colon through a common mesentery around the SMA, forming a pedicle around which the midgut can rotate.

The incidence of malrotation is approximately one in 6000 live births. Malrotation is frequently associated with other anomalies and is always associated with gastroschisis and omphalocele. Often anomalies of the gastrointestinal tract such as duodenal and jejuno-ileal atresias are also associated with malrotation.

DIAGNOSIS AND TREATMENT

Clinical presentations range from chronic abdominal pain to life-threatening acute midgut volvulus. The classic presentation is the acute onset of bilious emesis in a previously healthy neonate, which results from an acute midgut volvulus. Associated symptoms may include gastric or abdominal distension, hypovolemia, and irritability, and as the bowel strangulates, the infant may become lethargic and develop septic shock. As bowel becomes necrotic, the patient will show signs of peritonitis, develop acidosis, and may have melena, hematemesis, or both. Without prompt surgical correction, midgut volvulus carries a high risk of intestinal necrosis and resultant short-gut syndrome or death. Some patients may present with duodenal obstruction as a result of kinking of a tortuous duodenum exacerbated by extrinsic compression by peritoneal (Ladd) bands. Bilious emesis with or without abdominal pain is the hallmark for this presentation and may be acute or intermittent. A small number of patients with malrotation can present in childhood with chronic or intermittent abdominal pain. Bowel distension produces crampy abdominal pain with vomiting as a result of intermittent volvulus and obstruction. Partial or intermittent volvulus results in venous and lymphatic congestion and, when long-standing, can lead to intestinal malabsorption. About half of infants with malrotation present within the first month of life, and 90% within the first year of life. Some patients with malrotation remain asymptomatic through childhood. Occasionally older children and adults present with midgut volvus.

The evaluation of the newborn with bilious vomiting is discussed in Sec. 17.7.9. In malrotation and volvulus, the abdominal radiographs may suggest a gastric outlet obstruction with large gastric bubble and paucity of distal bowel gas or a duodenal obstruction with radiographic evidence of duodenal distension. However, plain abdominal radiographs may be normal or nonspecific. Therefore, in an infant with bilious emesis, an upper gastrointestinal series is required for definitive evaluation. The upper gastrointestinal contrast study of midgut volvulus usually demonstrates a diagnostic "bird's beak" appearance of the second or third portion of the duodenum where the gut is twisted. If the duodenum is partially obstructed, a corkscrew appearance may be present.

In the older infant or child with intermittent symptoms, an upper GI contrast study may identify an abnormal location of the duodenojejunal junction (ligament of Treitz). The normal position of the duodenojejunal junction is to the left of the spine at the level of the gastric antrum and fixed to the posterior body wall. In malrotation, the ligament of Treitz is on right side, frequently inferior

to duodenal bulb, and contrast fills jejunal loops on the right side of the abdomen (Fig. 17-30). Barium enema has been used to evaluate malrotation, but it can be misleading. Malposition of the colon is frequently observed in conjunction with the duodenojejunal disorders of rotation, but approximately 15% of normal newborns have a high and mobile cecum, so the barium enema lacks specificity and sensitivity for diagnosis of rotational abnormalities. Abdominal ultrasound has been used to diagnose malrotation on the basis of superior mesenteric vessel orientation, but this should not be considered adequate for evaluation of possible malrotation.

Preoperative management of infants with malrotation and midgut volvulus includes rapid intravenous fluid resuscitation (especially in patients with protracted vomiting), nasogastric decompression, placement of a Foley catheter, and parenteral antibiotics for emergent laparotomy. A Ladd procedure is performed emergently for management of midgut volvulus with malrotation. After an incision is made in the abdominal wall, the bowel is eviscerated from the abdominal cavity to enable inspection of the mesenteric root. If a volvulus is encountered, it is untwisted in a counterclockwise direction, and the bowel is inspected for viability. Obvious necrotic areas are resected, and enterostomies are performed. In situations in which necrotic areas can be resected back to healthy tissue, primary anastomosis may be performed. Lysis of Ladd bands is performed to detach the duodenum from the colon and relieve extrinsic compression of the duodenum. The base of the mesentery is maximally widened, with the duodenum being straightened and placed in the right gutter and the cecum placed in the left side of the abdomen. An incidental appendectomy is performed to avoid future diagnostic confusion in the event of appendicitis. Question-

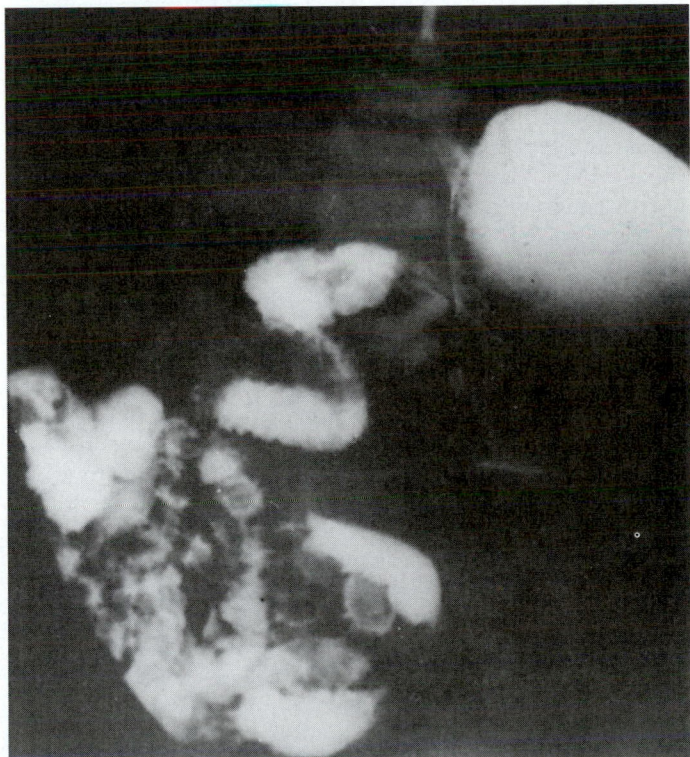

FIGURE 17-30   Upper gastrointestinal tract contrast radiograph of malrotation. The stomach is in the normal position on the left side of the abdomen. The duodenum extends across the midline to the right side, never returning to the left side of the abdomen. The proximal small bowel is located on the right side of the abdomen.

able areas of bowel viability are left in place, and a second-look procedure is performed at 12 to 36 hours to assure bowel viability.

Mortality is 5 to 10% in patients with midgut volvulus, bowel necrosis, and other anomalies. Complications following surgical repair include recurrent volvulus in 0 to 10% and bowel obstruction from adhesions. In the event of massive small bowel resection for intestinal necrosis, short-gut syndrome is a potential complication (see Sec. 17.18.7). In patients who do not require massive resection, recovery is unevenful, and long-term outcomes are excellent. In children with a serendipitous diagnosis of malrotation (usually by upper GI series), it is recommended that they undergo a prompt, elective Ladd procedure because the possibility of catastrophic volvulus exists regardless of age or manner of presentation.

References

Rescorla FJ, Shedd FJ, Grosfeld JL, et al: Anomalies of intestinal rotation in childhood: analysis of 447 cases. J Pediatr Surg 108:710, 1990

Seashore JH, Touloukian RJ: Midgut volvulus: an ever-present threat. Arch Pediatr Adolesc Med 148:43, 1994

Touloukian RJ, Smith EI: Disorders of rotation and fixation. In: O'Neill JA, Rowe RI, Grosfeld JL, Fonkalsrud EW, Coran AG, eds: Pediatric Surgery, 5th ed. St Louis, Mosby-Year Book, 1199: 1998

Warner BW: Malrotation. In: Oldham KT, Colombani PM, Foglia RP, eds: Surgery of Infants and Children: Scientific Principles and Practices. Philadelphia, Lippincott-Raven, 1229: 1997

17.13.3 Infantile Hypertrophic Pyloric Stenosis

Colin D. Rudolph

Pyloric stenosis classically presents with the gradual onset of nonbilious projectile vomiting after 3 weeks of age. However, 20% of infants are symptomatic from birth, and most are symptomatic within the first 2 months after birth. Prolonged vomiting may lead to dehydration, weight loss, and development of hypochloremic alkalosis. Hypokalemia also may occur. In fewer than 5% of patients, unconjugated hyperbilirubinemia may be observed, which is thought to result from inadequate glucose absorption and an inability to maintain glucuronyl transferase activity.

Prospective studies have demonstrated that the pyloric muscle is not hypertrophied at birth, but it appears to hypertrophy after birth, leading to gastric outlet obstruction. The pathogenesis remains unclear, but postnatal infusion of gastrin produces an identical lesion in newborn puppies, suggesting that hypergastrinemia may play an important etiologic role. Gastrin levels are known to be elevated in the newborn. In addition, prostaglandin E_2 infusion, which is used to maintain a patent ductus arteriosus in certain cardiac anomalies, has been linked to a higher incidence of infantile hypertrophic pyloric stenosis. Recent studies show a relative lack of nitric oxide (a smooth muscle relaxant) synthase innervation, decreased density of interstitial cells of Cajal, and increased synthesis of epidermal growth factor in the hypertrophied muscle, but the primary underlying cause of the disorder is still unclear.

The incidence of pyloric stenosis varies from one per 200 to one per 750 live births. Mode of inheritance is polygenic and modified by sex, with the incidence being four to six times higher in boys. Although it is believed to be more common in first-born boys, pyloric stenosis recently has been shown to be associated with smaller family size and higher socioeconomic class rather than with birth order. The incidence is two- to threefold higher in African-Americans than in whites, and it is rare in Asians.

DIAGNOSIS AND TREATMENT

The diagnosis of pyloric stenosis is best made by careful physical examination, observing visible peristalsis, and palpation of a mobile pyloric mass that is similar in size and shape to an olive. Palpation of this mass may be difficult because of an overlying dilated antrum until the stomach is emptied, either by vomiting or by passage of a nasogastric tube. Palpation of the "olive" is pathognomonic, being palpable to an experienced examiner in 60 to 80% of cases. If the diagnosis is not evident on the physical examination, ultrasonography can be used to demonstrate the thickened and lengthened pyloric muscle (Fig. 17-31). If diagnosis still remains uncertain, upper GI contrast studies provide the most definitive method for diagnosis, with characteristic findings of elongation and narrowing of the pyloric canal and partial blockage of the canal by thickened mucosa creating a double track of contrast. Upper GI study also allows the diagnosis of other causes of vomiting in infants, and it may prove to be a more direct, cost-effective approach to diagnosis when physical examination is not diagnostic. Rarely, upper endoscopy may be useful to clarify the diagnosis in equivocal cases, revealing antral fold hypertrophy or a pyloric mass.

In infants who present with dehydration, fluid resuscitation begins before diagnostic procedures are initiated. Correction of alkalosis and hypokalemia is essential before treatment, which is nonemergent and performed only after the patient is stabilized. Medical therapy with the chronic administration of atropine has been reported, but usually surgical therapy provides safe and effective treatment, with prompt relief of symptoms. The Ramstedt pyloromyotomy is the surgical procedure of choice, being curative and having mortality rates of 0.0 to 0.5% and an incidence of recurrence of 1%. A longitudinal incision divides the serosal muscle on the anterior surface of the pylorus down to the submucosa. This surgery can be accomplished using laparascopic techniques, although the benefits of this approach are not clearly evident because the incision with the open procedure is usually small. Postoperative vomiting occurs in as many as 50% of infants, but this resolves in most within 24 hours after surgery. Full oral feedings usually are administered within 2 to 3 days, and long-term prognosis is excellent. Follow-up ultrasound studies demonstrate that the pyloric muscle size regresses to a normal thickness within 12 weeks following pyloromyotomy, but follow-up studies are not routinely indicated in the otherwise thriving infant.

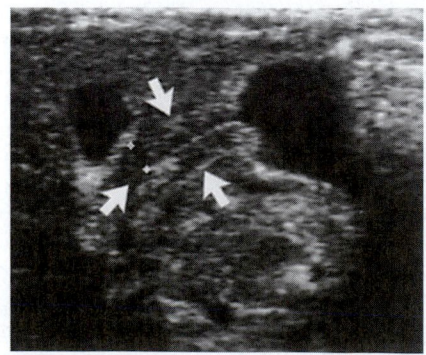

FIGURE 17-31 Hypertrophic pyloric stenosis. Ultrasonographic diagnosis shows elongated and thickened pyloric muscle *(arrows)*.

References

Forman HP, Leonida JC, Kronfeld GD: A rational approach to diagnosis of pyloric stenosis: do the results match the claims? J Pediatr Surg 25: 262, 1990

Jed MB, Melton J, Griffin MR, et al: Factors associated with infantile hypertrophic pyloric stenosis. Am J Dis Child 142:334–337, 1988

Nagita A, Yamaguchi J, Amemoto K, Yoden A, Yamazaki T, Mino M: Management and ultrasonographic appearance of infantile hypertrophic pyloric stenosis with intravenous atropine sulfate. J Pediatr Gastroenterol Nutr 23:172–177, 1996

Okorie NM, Dickson JAS, Carver RA, Steiner GM: What happens to the pylorus after pyloromyotomy? Arch Dis Child 3:1339–1340, 1988

Shima H, Ohshiro K, Puri P: Increased local synthesis of epidermal growth factors in infantile hypertrophic pyloric stenosis. Pediatr Res 47:201–207, 2000

17.13.4   Congenital Atresias, Stenosis, and Webs

Tory Meyers and Richard G. Azizkhan

Atresias of the gut occur in approximately one in 5000 live births, with the vast majority of them occurring in the duodenum or small bowel. The etiology has been attributed to a late intrauterine mesenteric vascular accident, which probably accounts for most cases of jejunoileal and colonic atresia. A lack of revacuolization of the solid cord stage during intestinal development is an alternative hypothesis and is felt to occur in duodenal atresia. Familial cases of jejunoileal and colonic atresia have also been reported, suggesting that genetic factors may play a role in the etiology. Intestinal atresias are classified into four types. Type I atresias have a normal muscular wall and an intraluminal membranous web, with or without a small fenestration. Type II atresias have a fibrous cord connecting the two ends of atretic bowel. Type III atresias are characterized by two blind-ending pouches of bowel with a wedge-shaped mesenteric defect and may be further classified into types IIIa or IIIb. Type IV atresias have multiple segments of atretic bowel, giving them the so called "string of sausages" appearance. Historical mortality reported for bowel atresias was up to 50%; however, recent studies report 85 to 100% long-term survival.

Congenital gastric outlet obstruction is exceedingly rare, occurring in fewer than one per 100,000 live births. *Pyloric webs* are the most common variety and are characterized by redundant gastric mucosa and submucosa prolapsing into the duodenum in a windsock fashion. Depending on the degree of obstruction, patients may present at any age with vague symptoms of epigastric pain, intermittent nonbilious emesis, and failure to thrive. An upper GI contrast study will demonstrate the lesion, but endoscopy is recommended before surgical repair. Neonates with complete pyloric or antral atresia present with polyhydramnios, nonbilious emesis, and an enlarged stomach with an otherwise gasless abdomen on x-ray. Upper GI shows complete gastric outlet obstruction. Treatment consists of a gastroduodenostomy or pyloroplasty with local excision, depending on the severity of the lesion. Pyloric atresia has been seen in association with junctional epidermolysis bullosa, a devastating autosomal-recessive condition in which infants develop severe vesiculobullous lesions after minimal skin friction.

Congenital microgastria is a rare anomaly that is characterized by failure of the primitive foregut to differentiate into a stomach, thus resulting in a small tubular stomach usually associated with megaesophagus and incomplete gastric rotation. Other associated anomalies include asplenia, situs inversus, and limb and cardiac abnormalities. These patients typically present with recurrent vomiting and failure to thrive. Upper GI contrast studies establish the diagnosis. The lack of a functional stomach reservoir demands that feeding be administered either as small, frequent bolus feeds or continuous jejunal feeds. Patients may develop a functional stomach after several years, so attempts at surgical intervention by construction of a jejunal reservoir in early life are ill-advised. Surgical gastric augmentation should be considered if a prolonged period of jejunal feedings and hyperalimentation does not enable sufficient gastric growth.

Duodenal atresia accounts for 50% of intestinal atresias with an incidence of more than one in 10,000 live births. Approximately 50% of patients have other associated anomalies, including cardiac, genitourinary, anorectal, or esophageal abnormalities, and nearly half will be premature. In addition, 40% of patients with duodenal atresia will have trisomy 21. Patients with complete obstruction will exhibit polyhydramnios and a dilated stomach on prenatal ultrasound. In two-thirds of the cases the obstruction is distal to the ampulla of Vater, so many patients present with bilious emesis in the neonatal period. Abdominal radiographs will show the classic "double bubble" (Fig. 17-32), and in the presence of an otherwise gasless abdomen this is sufficient to make the diagnosis. If distal gas is present, an upper GI contrast study or immediate laparotomy should be performed to differentiate this condition from malrotation with midgut volvulus. Once the diagnosis of duodenal atresia is confirmed, a thorough investigation for associated cardiac and other anomalies should be undertaken. These infants require parenteral fluid and electrolye repletion before operative correction. The surgical repair of these lesions usually entails a double diamond-shaped side-to-side duodenoduodenostomy or duodenojejunostomy to bypass the obstructed segment and minimize the chance of injury to the ampulla of Vater. A recent prospective study

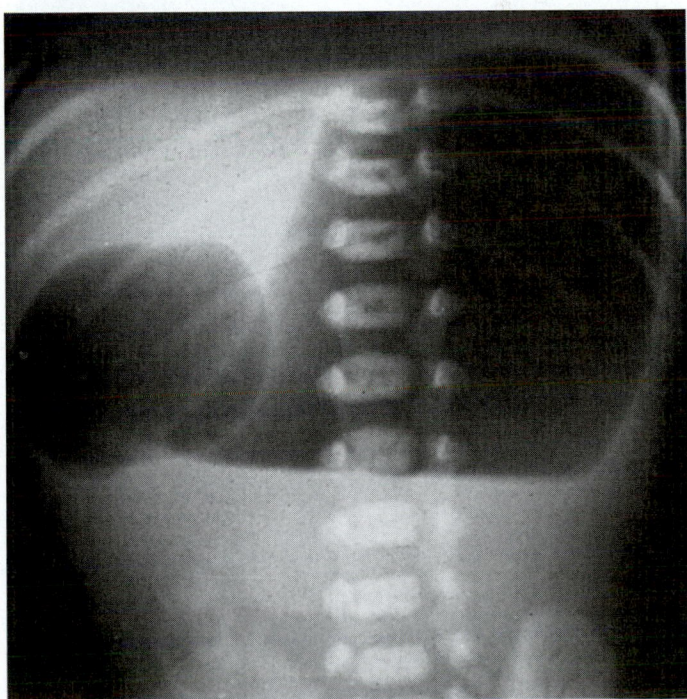

FIGURE 17-32 Duodenal atresia. Gas-filled and dilated stomach as well as gas-filled and dilated duodenum show the classic "double-bubble" appearance of duodenal atresia. No distal gas is present.

showed that nasogastric decompression rather than routine gastrostomy tube placement resulted in a more rapid return to oral feeding. Although complications such as bile duct injury, anastomotic leak, alkaline reflux, and peptic ulcer disease have been reported, the prognosis is excellent, and almost all mortalities are secondary to associated cardiac disease.

Jejunoileal atresia is usually not associated with other anomalies, in contrast to duodenal atresia. Several animal studies suggest that jejunal atresia may result from antenatal internal hernias or volvulus causing intestinal vascular compromise. The atretic segment is located in the proximal jejunum in 30% of patients, in the distal jejunum in 20%, and in the ileum in 50%. In 16% of mothers with polyhydramnios, prenatal ultrasound may detect distended fetal bowel loops and suggest the presence of intestinal obstruction. Postnatally infants with jejunoileal atresia present with abdominal distension and bilious emesis, with or without meconium stools. Abdominal radiographs demonstrate multiple dilated loops of bowel with air-fluid levels (Fig. 17-33). The diagnosis is confirmed with upper GI or lower GI contrast studies, differentiating this condition from meconium ileus secondary to cystic fibrosis. Radiographic findings of abdominal calcifications suggest in utero perforation with meconium peritonitis and portend difficulty in performing a primary anastomosis. All patients should be resuscitated, undergo nasogastric decompression, and be started on antibiotics before surgical repair. The choice of surgical repair depends largely on the pathology encountered and the length of remaining bowel. Minimizing the amount of bowel resected and performing the primary anastomosis with a tapering enteroplasty is generally preferred for management. However, in type IIIb (apple peel) atresia, the distal bowel may be extremely diminutive and have a tenuous blood supply, requiring proximal and distal stomas until bowel growth enables reanastomosis. Similarly, if there is extensive

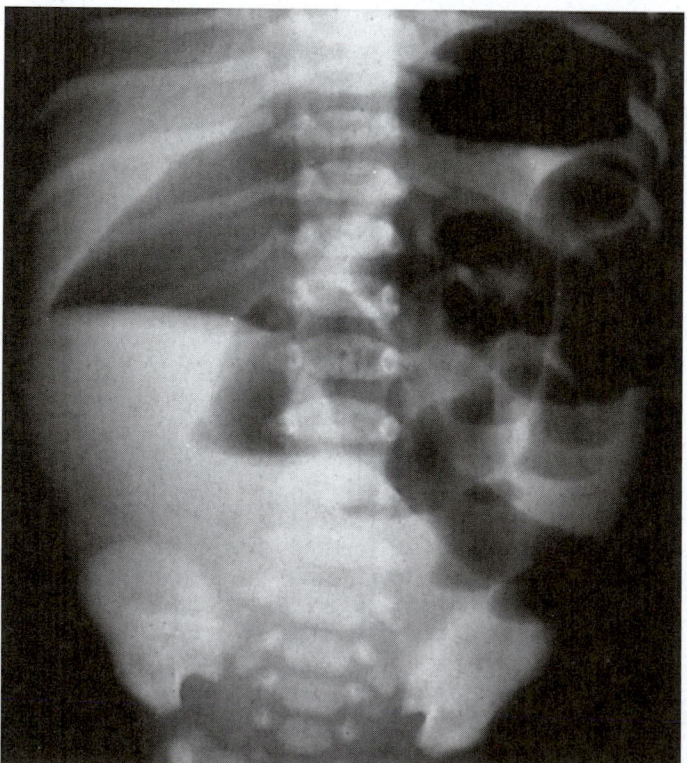

FIGURE 17-33   Ileal atresia. Dilated loops of bowel with air-fluid levels present throughout the intestine.

peritoneal soiling, an ostomy may be required. The ultimate goal of all reconstructive surgery for jejunoileal atresia is preservation of bowel length. Despite this, some patients will not have adequate bowel length and will require long-term parenteral nutrition (see Sec. 17.6) and may need bowel-lengthening procedures or small bowel transplantion. Postoperative complications after jejunoileal atresia repair include anastomotic leak (4%), prolonged adynamic ileus (9%), bacterial overgrowth in high jejunal atresia (10%), and adhesive small bowel obstruction (24%). Overall survival for patients with jejunoileal atresia today is estimated to be greater than 90%.

Colonic atresia occurs in fewer than 10% of patients with intestinal atresia. If the colonic atresia is the only segment involved, patients present with a distal bowel obstruction heralded by abdominal distension, bilious emesis, and usually a failure to pass meconium. The diagnosis is made by contrast enema demonstrating a distal microcolon and a point of obstruction. Historically these patients were treated with a diverting proximal stoma and subsequent repair. More recently, however, it has been found that primary excision and reanastomosis, even for left-sided lesions, yield good results. Survival rates approach 100%, although like jejunoileal atresia they have a significant rate of prolonged ileus (10%) and late adhesive bowel obstruction (40%).

References

Dalla Vecchia LK, Grosfeld JL, West KW, Rescorla FJ, Scherer LR, Engum SA: Intestinal atresia and stenosis; a 25-year experience with 277 cases. Arch Surg 133:490–497, 1998

Dillon PW, Cilley RE: Lesions of the stomach. In: Ashcraft KW, Murphy JP, Sharp RJ, Sigalet DL, Snyder CL, eds: Pediatric Surgery, 3rd ed. Philadelphia, WB Saunders, 391–405: 2000

Millar AJ, Rode H, Cywes S. Intestinal atresia and stenosis. In: Ashcraft KW, Murphy JP, Sharp RJ, Sigalet DL, Snyder CL, eds: Pediatric Surgery, 3rd ed. Philadelphia, WB Saunders, 406–423: 2000

Newman K: Jejunoileal atresia. In: Oldham KT, Colombani PM, Foglia RP, eds: Surgery of Infants and Children: Scientific Principles and Practice. Philadelphia, Lippincott-Raven, 1193–1200: 1997

Sato S, Nishijima E, Muraji T, Tsugawa C, Kimura K: Jejunoileal atresia: a 27-year experience. J Pediatr Surg 33:1633–1635, 1998

17.13.5   Duplications and Cysts

Rebeccah L. Brown

Intestinal duplications are rare congenital anomalies occuring in about one in 4500 (or 0.02%) autopsies. Most (60–85%) are diagnosed by 2 years of age. Intestinal duplications are defined by three common characteristics: (1) each is contiguous with and strongly adherent to some part of the alimentary tract; (2) each has a smooth muscle coat, usually of two layers; and (3) each is lined with mucosa or epithelium similar to that of the stomach, small intestine, or colon. Theories regarding the pathogenesis of intestinal duplications are numerous and include the split-notocord theory, failure of regression of embryonic diverticula, and errors of epithelial recanalization. None of these theories is sufficient to explain the pathogenesis of all duplication.

Intestinal duplications may occur anywhere from the mouth to the anus but are most common in the ileum (~50%). Three basic types have been described, including saccular or spherical cysts, intramural cysts, and tubular cysts, with spherical cystic lesions being most common. Intramural cysts project into the bowel lumen, usually at or near the ileocecal valve, and, by compression, may cause obstruction or may also result in intussusception. Communication with the normal intestinal lumen varies but is more common with tubular duplications. A common wall is shared with the adjacent intestine, and it is this relatively thick wall that differentiates intestinal duplications from thin-walled mesenteric cysts. In contrast to Meckel diverticulum, intestinal duplications are characteristically located on the mesenteric rather than the antimesenteric side of the bowel and share a common blood supply with adjacent bowel. Multiple duplications occur in 5 to 15% of patients, and as in Meckel diverticulum, about 25% have ectopic mucosa, which is gastric in most cases and occasionally pancreatic. The presence of ectopic gastric mucosa predisposes to peptic ulceration, bleeding, and occasionally perforation. If communication with the bowel exists, bleeding will be intraluminal. If not, blood may accumulate within the cyst itself, and the patient will present with a painful, rapidly enlarging mass.

The presentation of intestinal duplications depends on their type and location. The major complications arising from these lesions are obstruction, intussusception, bleeding, pain from an enlarging mass, and perforation. Abdominal pain and intermittent vomiting may be prominent symptoms. Diarrhea from bacterial overgrowth in the affected small bowel may be seen in patients with a duplication that communicates with the lumen. In some cases, an abdominal mass will be palpable. It is rare for an intestinal duplication to be diagnosed preoperatively. Indeed, most are found at laparotomy. Routine plain abdominal radiographs are rarely of value. Upper gastrointestinal contrast studies may occasionally demonstrate an extrinsic mass effect. Bleeding from gastric or duodenal duplications may occasionally be diagnosed by upper gastrointestinal endoscopy. Because of the presence of ectopic gastric mucosa in about 25% of intestinal duplications, technetium 99m pertechnetate radionuclide scanning may suggest the diagnosis, although it may be difficult, if not impossible, to differentiate a jejunoileal duplication from Meckel diverticulum with this scan. Ultrasound and computed tomography may demonstrate a cystic mass. Treatment is usually resection.

Gastric duplications account for about 5 to 7% of intestinal duplications and occur most commonly in infants, usually girls less than 1 year of age. They are usually cystic, located on the greater curvature of the stomach, and have no communication with the stomach. They tend to present with a mass effect and gastric outlet obstruction and may be confused with hypertrophic pyloric stenosis. Because the mucosal lining is often gastric and secretes acid, ulceration may occur, resulting in melena or hematemesis, perforation, or free intraperitoneal bleeding. Resection may be accomplished by dissection of the common wall between the stomach and the duplication, usually without entering the stomach. Only rarely is gastric resection required.

Duodenal duplications comprise fewer than 6% of intestinal duplications and, like gastric duplications, are usually cystic and do not communicate with the intestinal lumen. They more commonly present with obstruction rather than bleeding, with ectopic gastric mucosa identified in only about 10 to 15% of lesions. They occur most commonly in the second portion of the duodenum and may be confused with a choledochocele, congenital pancreatic cyst, or pancreatic pseudocyst. Complete surgical resection may be difficult because of the location of the cyst in proximity to the pancreaticobiliary system. Roux-en-Y drainage into the duodenum or limb of jejunum may be an acceptable alternative to resection.

Colon and rectal duplications are rare and may be associated with genitourinary malformations. Tubular lesions are most common.

Bleeding is rare because ectopic mucosa is infrequently found. Constipation, obstruction, and volvulus occur more commonly in colonic duplications. Rectal duplications may be misdiagnosed as prolapse of the rectum, hemorrhoids, fistula in ano, or perirectal abscess. Interestingly, the incidence of malignant degeneration is higher in colorectal duplications but has been noted only in adults. Surgical resection is the treatment of choice.

Mesenteric cysts are rare, occuring in about one in 100,000 hospital admissions. They are typically thin walled and may be unilocular or multilocular. They may contain serous or lymphatic fluid or may be hemorrhagic. Mesenteric cysts arise from the mesentery, anywhere from the duodenum to the rectum. Omental cysts are, by definition, confined to the lesser or greater omentum. Most mesenteric cysts arise from the small bowel mesentery. The pathogenesis is thought to be akin to a lymphatic malformation in which there is ectopic lymphatic tissue with disordered production and flow of lymph as a result of communication with the remainder of the lymphatic system. They are the abdominal equivalents of cystic hygromas of the neck. Patients will present with abdominal pain, obstructive symptoms, or a palpable abdominal mass. Plain abdominal films may demonstrate a mass effect with the appearance of ascites. Diagnosis is usually confirmed by ultrasound or computed tomography. Complete resection of the cyst is the treatment of choice. In about half of cases, there is a shared blood supply to the cyst and the bowel, making a segmental bowel resection necessary to remove the cyst.

References

Holcomb GW, Gheissari AL, O'Neill J: Surgical management of alimentary tract duplications. Ann Surg 209:167, 1989

Ildstad ST, Tollerud DJ, Weiss RG, et al: Duplications of the alimentary tract. Ann Surg 208:184, 1989

17.13.6   Meckel Diverticulum

Rebeccah L. Brown and Richard J. Stevenson

Meckel diverticulum is a remnant of the vitelline (or omphalomesenteric) duct, which connects the yolk sac to the primitive gut in the fetus. Normally, this duct is obliterated between the fifth and ninth week of gestation. Meckel diverticulum is caused by failure of obliteration of this duct. A spectrum of anomalies may result, depending on the stage of arrest of normal involution. Meckel diverticulum may remain attached in its entirety to the abdominal wall at the umbilicus or may remain attached as a fibrous cord as the distal portion involutes, but in about 75% of cases it is detached from the umbilicus. Other anomalies related to disturbance of the involution process include persistence of a patent omphalomesenteric duct or the development of an omphalomesenteric sinus or cyst. An omphalomesenteric cyst may form when both proximal and distal obliteration occur and the central portion of the duct remains patent and dilates.

Meckel diverticulum is a true diverticulum, containing all layers of the intestinal wall. The blood supply is derived from the paired vitelline arteries, of which the left involutes, and the right persists as the superior mesenteric artery. A remnant of the right vitelline artery arises directly from the mesentery to supply the diverticulum. Anatomically, the blood supply to Meckel diverticulum is unique in that the vessels to the diverticulum pass over the serosa of the ileum, terminating on the antimesenteric rather than the mesenteric side of the bowel. Ectopic tissue is identified in about half of all Meckel diverticula. Of those diverticula with ectopic mucosa, about 80% are of gastric origin, and 5% are of pancreatic origin. Ectopic gastric mucosa is identified in about 95% of Meckel diverticula resected for bleeding complications.

The "rule of twos" has often been applied to Meckel diverticulum, as it occurs in 2% of the population, is located within 2 feet of the ileocecal junction, measures about 2 inches in length and about 2 cm in diameter, has two types of ectopic mucosa—gastric and pancreatic, has a 2:1 male-to-female ratio, and is usually symptomatic before 2 years of age. Meckel diverticulum is usually clinically silent, identified either incidentally at laparotomy or at autopsy, with an estimated lifetime risk of complications from Meckel diverticulum being about 4%. Infants and children appear to be at highest risk for developing complications, with over 50% of symptomatic Meckel diverticula occurring in children less than 2 years of age. Symptomatic lesions are identified in only about 15% of children older than 4 years of age.

An increased incidence of Meckel diverticula may be seen in association with other congenital anomalies including esophageal atresia (sixfold increase), imperforate anus (fivefold increase), and various neurologic (threefold increase) and cardiovascular (twofold increase) malformations. Meckel diverticulum has also been found more commonly in patients with omphalocele, in which about 25% of patients exhibit some form of omphalomesenteric remnant. A threefold increased incidence of Meckel diverticulum has been reported in patients with Crohn disease. Interestingly, none of the Meckel diverticula resected in patients with Crohn disease contained ectopic mucosa. Rarely, carcinoid tumors have been found to arise from Meckel diverticulum. Other tumors, including sarcoma, lymphoma, adenocarcinoma, and leiomyoma, have all been reported to occur in Meckel diverticulum but have been confined mostly to adult patients.

DIAGNOSIS AND TREATMENT

The complications associated with Meckel diverticulum are bleeding, obstruction, and inflammation. The clinical presentation of Meckel diverticulum is most commonly attributable either to the presence of ectopic mucosa within the diverticulum or to fixation of omphalomesenteric duct remnants to the abdominal wall. The presence of ectopic gastric mucosa may cause ulceration that results in inflammation, bleeding, or perforation. Fixation of omphalomesenteric duct remnants may result in intestinal obstruction from torsion of small bowel loops around the point of fixation. Intussusception of Meckel diverticulum may cause intestinal obstruction and bleeding. Intestinal obstruction and infarction may occur as a result of an incarcerated internal hernia associated with a mesodiverticular band. Intestinal obstruction may also result from incarceration of a Meckel diverticulum within a hernia sac (Littre hernia). Meckel diverticulitis occurs more commonly in older patients and may be indistinguishable from appendicitis. Perforation of a Meckel diverticulum by a foreign body in the gastrointestinal tract has also been reported.

Gastrointestinal bleeding is the most common presenting symptom of Meckel diverticulum in children less than 4 years of age, occurring in 22% of all children with Meckel diverticulum and 40 to 60% of symptomatic children. The pathogenesis of gastrointestinal bleeding from Meckel diverticulum is thought to occur as a result of peptic ulceration, most often located at the base of the diverticulum at the junction of ectopic gastric mucosa and normal ileal mucosa. The mean age of children presenting with bleeding is 2.8 years. Patients most commonly present with painless rectal bleeding. Although less typical, colicky abdominal pain may accompany a brisk bleed. The color of blood may vary from bright red to dark red or maroon and may even appear as "currant jelly stool" classically described for intussusception. Black tarry stools are less suggestive of Meckel diverticulum. Bleeding may be massive, and transfusions are often required. Although bleeding may be significant, spontaneous cessation with episodic recurrences is the rule. Indeed, Meckel diverticulum is the most common cause of serious lower gastrointestinal bleeding in children. An aggressive approach to resuscitation and early diagnosis is warranted.

Right lower quadrant abdominal pain resulting from Meckel diverticulitis may be indistinguishable from that of appendicitis, usually presenting in somewhat older patients (mean 8.2 years), with diagnosis usually made at laparotomy for possible appendicitis. Similarly, obstructive symptoms, including abdominal pain, distension, and obstipation, caused by complications from Meckel diverticulum may be indistinguishable from other causes of obstruction, and the diagnosis is usually made at laparotomy.

The diagnosis of Meckel diverticulum may be elusive, and, as stated by Mayo, "Meckel's diverticulum is frequently suspected, often looked for, and seldom found." The diagnostic procedure of choice when Meckel diverticulum is suspected is the technetium 99m pertechnetate scan (or Meckel scan). The reliability of this scan is based on the observation that about 95% of bleeding Meckel diverticula contain ectopic mucosa. The high affinity of isotope for parietal cells of gastric mucosa permits the visualization of both ectopic as well as native gastric mucosa. The remainder of isotope is concentrated within the bladder. A positive scan demonstrates abnormal uptake of isotope outside of the stomach and urinary bladder. Although Meckel diverticulum is usually found in the right lower quadrant, its location may vary because of the relative mobility of the small bowel. The use of histamine H_2 blockers may enhance the diagnostic accuracy of the scan. Fasting, nasogastric suction, and bladder catheterization may also increase the diagnostic yield of the scan. If the scan is negative but the suspicion remains high, it should be repeated. The sensitivity of the Meckel scan is 85%, the specificity is 95%, and the accuracy is 90%. If the scan is negative but the clinical presentation of bleeding is strongly suggestive of a possible Meckel diverticulum, laparoscopy is reasonable.

Treatment of Meckel diverticulum depends on presenting symptoms, but in most cases aggressive fluid resuscitation and transfusion of blood products are necessary before surgery. Classically, the diverticulum is approached through a transverse right lower quadrant incision, but more recently laparoscopic-assisted resection of Meckel diverticulum has been described. When a right lower quadrant incision is utilized, an appendectomy should be performed concomitantly to prevent future diagnostic dilemmas.

If a Meckel diverticulum is found incidentally at laparotomy in an infant or very young child, most pediatric surgeons would recommend resection because of the much higher incidence of symptomatic lesions in children. Resection is clearly indicated if there is palpable ectopic mucosa, persistence of omphalomesenteric remnants with abdominal wall attachments, or history of unexplained abdominal pain. With increasing age, the risk of symptomatic complications significantly decreases. Controversy still exists regarding resection of Meckel diverticulum found incidentally at laparotomy in the older child and adult. Risks and benefits must be carefully weighed depending on the clinical situation.

References

St Vil D, Brandt ML, Panic S, et al: Meckel's diverticululm in children: a 20-year review. J Pediatr Surg 26:1289, 1991

Sfakianakis GN, Consay JJ: Detection of ectopic gastric mucosa in Meckel's diverticulum and in other aberrations by scintigraphy: indications and methods—a 10-year experience. J Nucl Med 22:732, 1981

Simms M, Corkery J: Meckel's diverticulum: its association with congenital malformation and the significance of atypical morphology. Br J Surg 67: 216, 1980

Soltero MJ, Bill AH: The natural history of Meckel's diverticulum and its relation to incidental removal. A study of 202 cases of diseased Meckel's diverticulum found in King County, Washington, over a fifteen year period. Am J Surg 132:168, 1976

Vane DW, West KW, Grosfeld JL: Vitelline duct anomalies. Experience with 217 childhood cases. Arch Surg 122:542, 1987

17.14 OTHER ANATOMIC ABNORMALITIES OF THE STOMACH AND INTESTINES

17.14.1   Meconium Diseases of Infancy

Colin D. Rudolph

Meconium ileus, meconium peritonitis, and meconium plug syndrome all present with neonatal bowel obstruction. Meconium ileus equivalent (also known as *distal intestinal pseudoobstruction syndrome* and discussed in Sec. 23.6) results from inspissated stool obstructing the ilealocecal region and occurs in patients with cystic fibrosis at any age beyond the newborn period.

Meconium ileus presents with neonatal bowel obstruction in 10 to 20% of patients with cystic fibrosis, usually within the first 24 to 48 hours after birth. Meconium ileus rarely occurs in infants without cystic fibrosis, occurring in family clusters and in infants with pancreatic ductal lesions. The secretion of hyperviscous intestinal mucus begins prenatally, resulting in thickened and inspissated meconium that obstructs the intestine in utero. The usual region of obstruction is the distal ileum. The proximal bowel is dilated from chronic obstruction, whereas the distal bowel is unused and of a small caliber, referred to as a *microcolon*. Bowel perforation because of volvulus and local ischemia occurs in approximately 50% of infants with meconium ileus. Extravasation and liquefaction of meconium can result in a giant pseudocyst formation and/or meconium peritonitis that is evident by abdominal calcifications. Bowel perforation in utero resulting in meconium peritonitis also may be caused by intestinal atresia, internal hernia, congenital peritoneal bands, or gastroschisis. In uncomplicated meconium ileus, where there is no clinical or radiologic evidence of perforation or peritonitis, administration of a hypertonic contrast enema may be therapeutic, drawing fluid into the bowel to "flush" the inspissated meconium from the colon and distal small bowel. This procedure should be performed only by a pediatric radiologist in consultation with a pediatric surgeon. Antibiotics are administered before the procedure because of the risk of bowel perforation. The hyperosmolar enema fluid can cause dehydration, so the infant should be well hydrated before the procedure. If the enema does not relieve

obstruction, or the patient has signs of peritonitis, surgical intervention is necessary. Tests should be performed to confirm the diagnosis of cystic fibrosis in all patients with meconium ileus (see Sec. 23.6).

Meconium plug syndrome is an uncommon cause of intestinal obstruction in the newborn that usually is not associated with cystic fibrosis. Instead, otherwise normal infants are unable to evacuate meconium from the colon at birth. Disorders that are associated with meconium plug syndrome include colonic inertia of prematurity and neonatal small left colon syndrome. Hirschsprung disease should be ruled out by suction biopsy. Gastrografin enema reveals a small left colon with an abrupt obstruction in the left colon or at the splenic flexure. The enema usually stimulates passage of a thick plug of meconium, and further stooling is encouraged with the administration of saline enemas. Occasionally, the Gastrografin enema needs to be repeated. Surgical therapy rarely is required.

17.14.2   Gastric Perforation

Colin D. Rudolph

Rarely, unexplained spontaneous gastric perforation, usually on the anterior portion of the greater curvature of the stomach near the cardia, occurs in the newborn during the first week after birth. Proposed etiologic factors include congenital defects of the gastric musculature, neonatal asphyxia, and hyperinflation of the stomach during mask ventilation, but no single cause has been identified. Infants present with symptoms of lethargy, poor feeding, and abdominal distension. Abdominal radiographs reveal a pneumoperitoneum. Tube decompression of the stomach, antibiotic therapy, and emergent operative therapy are usually indicated. Occasionally, diaphragmatic excursions are prevented by tense and massive abdominal distension that compromises respiration. Needle or catheter decompression of the abdomen (similar to decompression of a pneumothorax) may be necessary before surgery. Early diagnosis and prevention of sepsis improve outcome; mortality approaches 25%. In older infants and children, perforation may result from trauma or peptic ulcer disease.

17.14.3   Intussusception

Richard J. Stevenson

Intussusception occurs when one part of the intestine invaginates into the lumen of the adjoining bowel. The mesentery is dragged along with the prolapsed bowel, causing venous compression, swelling, and edema of the bowel wall. If untreated, the edema eventually will cause arterial obstruction, ischemia, and perforation. Incidence varies from one to four per 1000 live births, with a male preponderance of 3:2. Intussusception is common between 2 months and 5 years of age, with a peak incidence at 4 to 10 months.

Intussusception may result from a lead point such as a polyp or diverticulum that is pulled distally by peristaltic activity, but 95% are idiopathic. The most common lead point is a Meckel diverticulum, followed by polyp, duplication, hemangioma, suture line, appendix, tumors (ie, lymphoma), and ectopic pancreas. Idiopathic intussusception usually originates near the ileocecal junction, and it likely results from virus-induced swollen, hypertrophied Peyer patches in the ileum serving as a lead point. Henoch-Schönlein purpura and meconium ileus equivalent may be associated with intussusception, usually in the small bowel. Recently, a rotavirus vaccine was associated with episodes of intussusception leading to withdrawal from the marketplace.

DIAGNOSIS AND TREATMENT

Classically, intussusception presents with the triad of abdominal pain, vomiting, and blood in the stools. The infant awakens from sleep crying with severe, colicky abdominal pain, which is demonstrated by flexion of the knees and hips. Vomiting is common. Usually, the initial pain subsides, and the child becomes quite comfortable between episodes. A normal bowel movement often is passed with the onset of pain, but once the colon is empty and the proximal obstruction ensues, passage of stool ceases until bloody "currant jelly stools" are passed from 2 hours to several days after the pain began. Over time, pallor, diaphoresis, and apathy ensue, and the painful episodes increase in frequency. Overall, 85% of patients have pain, 75% have vomiting, and 60% pass bloody stools. The presentation rarely is painless, and occasionally, diarrhea occurs. Patients older than 2 years of age generally are brought to attention promptly, whereas infants, who cannot voice their complaints, present with lethargy, obtundation, dehydration, or even coma, thus making diagnosis more difficult. If not treated, the condition may be fatal in 2 to 5 days. Patients should be resuscitated appropriately during evaluation.

Physical examination generally reveals a soft and nontender abdomen between episodes of pain; at such times, a sausage-shaped mass may be felt in the right upper quadrant or in the mid-upper abdomen in 65% of patients. With time, the abdomen will become distended and the examination more difficult. In 75% of patients, rectal examination reveals occult blood or may precipitate passage of a bloody bowel movement. Occasionally, the intussusceptum may be palpable in the rectum.

If intussusception is suspected, an abdominal radiograph should be examined for a soft-tissue mass displacing loops of bowel. The leading edge of the intussusceptum sometimes will be outlined with air, thus establishing the diagnosis. Evidence of bowel obstruction may be present. However, a normal abdominal radiograph does not exclude intussusception. A contrast enema (preferably using air as the contrast agent) with fluoroscopic guidance is required to exclude intussusception in a patient with a suggestive history (Fig. 17-34). Surgical consultation is suggested before the enema is administered because of the risk of perforation. Although barium and water-soluble contrast media have been used in the past, the air enema has proven to be more effective in reducing intussusceptions and to cause less peritoneal cavity contamination in the unlikely event of a perforation. Successful air reduction rates of better than 90% may be anticipated. Radiologic reduction should be attempted unless the patient has evidence of peritoneal irritation, which is an absolute contraindication to radiologic reduction. Evidence of a bowel obstruction on the abdominal radiograph is a relative contraindication to air reduction, and if attempted, it should be done with caution. In the event an initial air reduction attempt is unsuccessful, it may be repeated.

The recurrence rate after radiographic reduction is 3 to 10%, and recurrences usually occur relatively soon after reduction. Consequently, the patient should be admitted for observation overnight after the reduction. Usually, stool and flatus are passed promptly. In contrast, an unsuccessful reduction or suggested perforation mandates prompt laparotomy after appropriate resuscitation. Mortality rates of less than 1% may be anticipated with the appropriate management of intussusception.

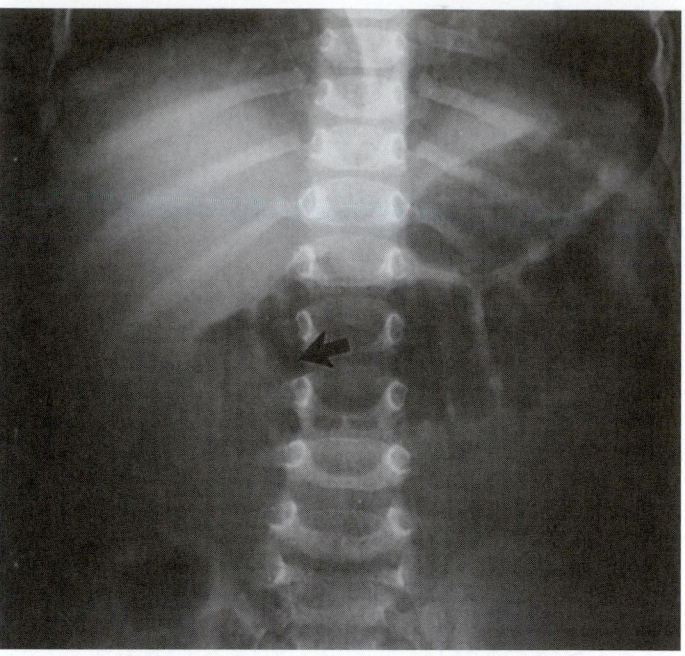

FIGURE 17-34 Air reduction of an intussusception. Note the prominent air in the descending and transverse colon. The intussusceptum in seen just below the liver *(arrow),* **clearly surrounded by air penetrating between the intussusception and the colon wall.**

Postoperative intussusception is a complication that is rare beyond the pediatric age range, with a mean age at presentation of 26 months. It is more frequent after major abdominal operations and accounts for 5 to 10% of postoperative bowel obstruction in children. The child usually presents subtly with abdominal distension and irritability and perhaps bilious emesis. Ninety percent of postoperative intussusceptions occur within 2 weeks of surgery. Severe colicky pain and bloody stools are unusual. Delay in diagnosis is common because the presentation is rather vague. Postoperative adhesive obstruction usually is suspected despite the uncommon occurrence of adhesive obstruction in the first 1 or 2 weeks after abdominal surgery. Seventy-five percent of adhesive bowel obstructions occur beyond 2 weeks postoperatively. The single most significant clue to diagnosing a patient with postoperative intussusception is the excessive amount of nasogastric aspirates compared with the expected amount for the usual patient with postoperative ileus or partial bowel obstruction. Contrast studies from above and/or below are uniformly nonrewarding. However, an abdominal ultrasound may establish the diagnosis. Air contrast enemas are virtually never therapeutic because the intussusception is confined to the small bowel in 85%. Exploratory laparotomy is required to demonstrate the intussusception, which usually is easily reduced and rarely is necrotic.

References

Mollitt DL, Ballantine TVN, Graosfel JL: Postoperative intussusception in infancy and childhood: analysis of 119 cases. Surgery 86:402–408, 1979

Palder SB, Eln SH, Stringer DA, et al: Intussusception: barium or air? J Pediatr Surg 26:271–275, 1991

West KW, Stephens B, Vane DW, et al: Intussusception: current management in infants and children. Surgery 102:781–787, 1987

17.14.4   Inguinal Hernia

Rebecca Brown and Joseph Cox

Inguinal hernias are among the most common surgical conditions of infancy and childhood. In infants, the incidence is 1 to 5%, with a male:female ratio of 9:1. Approximately 60% are on the right side, 25% on the left side, and 15% bilateral. The incidence is higher in premature infants. Children with increased intraabdominal pressure because of chronic coughing or ventriculoperitoneal shunts and those receiving peritoneal dialysis are at increased risk of inguinal hernia.

During the third month of gestation, the processus vaginalis develops as an outpouching of the peritoneum in the region of the internal ring, and it descends along the inguinal canal to the scrotum. The testis descends through the processus vaginalis into the scrotum. The processus vaginalis remains patent until birth but then is obliterated by the end of the first year. If it remains patent, a hydrocele or inguinal hernia may occur if bowel exits the peritoneal cavity and enters into the tract. If only fluid leaves the peritoneal cavity, the defect is termed a *communicating hydrocele,* which typically enlarges during crying and straining from increased intraabdominal pressure and decreases in size during sleep. Most surgeons regard communicating hydroceles as potential hernias and repair them.

DIAGNOSIS AND TREATMENT

An inguinal hernia may present asymptomatically as a bulge in the groin or scrotum. It may be made more apparent by standing and straining (eg, coughing, blowing up a balloon). Thickening of

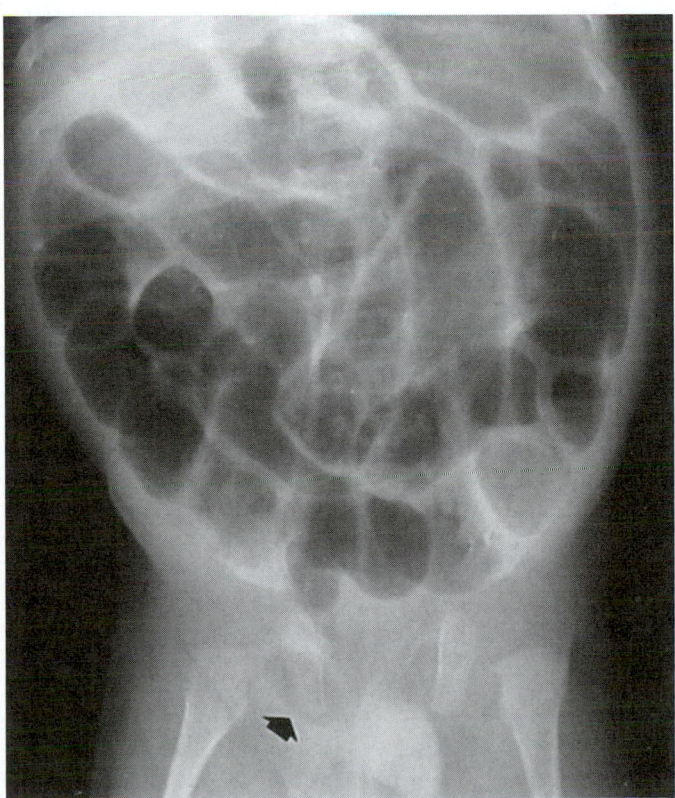

FIGURE 17-35   **Gastrointestinal obstruction with inguinal hernia. The air-filled, herniated bowel is clearly demonstrated (*arrow*).**

structures in the inguinal canal also may suggest the presence of a hernia. In women, 20 to 25% of inguinal hernias are sliding, and the ovary or tube may present in the sac. The blood supply of the ovary rarely is compromised in the hernia.

Incarcerated inguinal hernias present with the sudden onset of swelling in the groin, which gradually increases in size and becomes painful, and the child becomes increasingly irritable. On physical examination, a painful mass is noted in the groin. The differential diagnosis includes an incarcerated inguinal hernia, acute hydrocele of the cord, suppurative inguinal adenitis, or torsion of an undescended testis. Transillumination cannot reliably differentiate these diagnoses because a distended, incarcerated loop of intestine may transilluminate like a hydrocele. Vomiting, abdominal distension, and radiographic evidence of a bowel obstruction (Fig. 17-35) confirm the diagnosis of an incarcerated inguinal hernia.

An inguinal hernia requires operative repair. In a child with an incarcerated hernia and absence of peritoneal irritation or proximal small bowel obstruction, vigorous attempts usually are made at reduction. Measures that may help to reduce the hernia include sedation, elevation of the lower torso and legs, and brief exposure to a cold pack. Firm but gentle pressure usually results in hernia reduction. Subsequent repair in the near future is indicated to prevent recurrence of the incarceration. Should the incarcerated hernia be unreducible, immediate surgery is indicated. In a patient with an inguinal hernia, there is an approximately 50% chance that the processus vaginalis will be patent on the opposite side; for this reason, some surgeons suggest that both sides be explored, particularly in premature infants or those with incarceration.

References

Kapur P, Caty MG, Glick PL: Pediatric hernias and hydroceles. Pediatr Clin North Am 45:773–789, 1998

Tackett L, Breuer C, Luks F, et al: Incidence of contralateral hernia: a prospective analysis. J Pediatr Surg 34:684–687, 1999

17.15 MOTOR DISORDERS OF THE STOMACH AND INTESTINE

Carlo DiLorenzo

Movement of gut contents from one region of the GI tract to another results from coordinated contraction of the intestinal smooth muscle. GI motility is coordinated with secretory and absorptive events by complex myogenic, neural, and hormonal regulation. Most of the development of GI motility occurs between 26 and 36 weeks of gestation. Before 30 weeks, intestinal motor activity is poorly developed, with only weak, uncoordinated contractions. It is common for infants at this age to have poor gastric emptying with an inability to tolerate enteral feedings. Beyond 30 weeks postconception, newborns progressively increase the strength and coordination of their contractions; this maturation correlates with the ability to eat. By 36 weeks, GI motility is similar to that of term newborns.

Motility disorders can result from disturbances at any level of the control mechanisms, and they may involve any area of the GI tract, causing a broad spectrum of symptoms. When no obvious anatomic abnormality is found, the symptoms are considered to be part of a spectrum of *functional disorders* that result from either primary abnormalities of the nerves and muscles of the gastrointestinal tract, abnormalities of the coordination of neuromuscular activity, or abnormal sensory responses to gut stimulation. Functional disorders range in severity from recurrent abdominal pain to nonulcer dyspepsia and chronic intestinal pseudoobstruction.

Motility abnormalities have been reported in children with recurrent abdominal pain. However, their role in causing symptoms is uncertain because abnormalities are not specific and do not correlate in time with symptoms. Nonulcer dyspepsia is characterized by upper abdominal discomfort (eg, early satiety, fullness, bloating, nausea, vomiting) that is related to food intake in the absence of demonstrable structural abnormalities. It has been extensively described in adults and recently recognized in children. Many of these individuals have delayed gastric emptying of liquids and solids. Abnormal gastric and intestinal motility has been regarded as a possible factor but prokinetic drugs that improve gastric emptying rarely improve symptoms. Subtle abnormalities in GI motility are found in many children with severe nonulcer dyspepsia.

Accelerated gastric emptying rarely occurs in children, but it may follow surgery, presenting with "dumping syndrome." Increased liquid emptying rates are seen after both vagotomy and proximal as well as distal gastric resection. After fundoplication for the treatment of gastroesophageal reflux, the reservoir capacity of the fundus is lost, and gastric contents empty faster. Symptoms include abdominal discomfort, diaphoresis, pallor, lethargy, and diarrhea. Early dumping is noted during the first 30 minutes after a meal, and late dumping after 1 to 3 hours. An early and rapid emptying of hyperosmolar fluids triggers neurogenic reflexes, release of GI hormones, and a rapid fluid shift into the small bowel, which is followed by hypovolemia. Rapid glucose absorption causes hyperglycemia that is followed by reactive hypoglycemia, which is responsible for the late symptoms. Diagnosis is based mainly on symptoms and an abnormal glucose tolerance test following bolus feeding. Symptoms can be controlled by a low-carbohydrate diet, frequent small feedings, anticholinergic drugs, administration of corn starch to prevent postabsorptive hypoglycemia, and, in severe cases, infused feedings at a constant rate.

CHRONIC INTESTINAL PSEUDOOBSTRUCTION SYNDROME

This term describes a heterogeneous group of disorders that share a common constellation of symptoms and signs of mechanical bowel obstruction in the absence of physical obstruction. Many children with pseudoobstruction undergo multiple exploratory laparotomies in a futile effort to determine the anatomic cause. In pseudoobstruction abnormal GI smooth muscle and enteric nervous system function lead to ineffective GI motility. Pseudoobstruction includes both familial and nonfamilial forms. Most childhood pseudoobstruction is primary; secondary forms of pseudoobstruction are more common in adults. Table 17-41 summarizes the causes of pseudoobstruction.

The clinical manifestations of pseudoobstruction and mechanical bowel obstruction are similar. Children experience nausea, vomiting that may be bile stained, crampy abdominal pain, abdominal distension, and cessation of defecation. Chronic abdominal pain occurs in over one-half of affected children. Diarrhea is often present and can be attributed to bacterial overgrowth with steator-

TABLE 17-41

CAUSES OF CHRONIC INTESTINAL PSEUDOOBSTRUCTION SYNDROME

Primary pseudoobstruction
  Visceral myopathy
    Sporadic, familial
  Visceral neuropathy
    Sporadic, familial
Secondary pseudoobstruction
  Muscular dystrophies
  Scleroderma and other connective tissue diseases
  Neuropathy
    Postischemic
    Postviral
    Autoimmune ganglionitis
    Diabetic autonomic neuropathy
  Generalized dysautonomia
  Hypothyroidism
  Drugs: anticholinergics, opiates, calcium-channel blockers
  Severe inflammatory disease
  Post–organ transplantation
  Amyloidosis
  Chagas disease
  Fetal alcohol syndrome
  Chromosome abnormalities
  Multiple endocrine neoplasia type IIB
  Radiation enteritis
  Celiac disease
  Mitochondrial neurogastrointestinal encephalopathy (MNGIE)

rhea and bile-acid malabsorption. Approximately one-third of patients have evidence of gastric hypersecretion and peptic ulcer disease. Onset may be acute or insidious, with slow progression to more incapacitating symptoms over years. Two-thirds of patients experience symptoms at birth. During childhood, the clinical course usually is characterized by relative remissions and exacerbations. Factors such as intercurrent infections, general anesthesia and laparotomy, psychologic stress, and poor nutritional status may precipitate deterioration.

Pseudoobstruction commonly is misdiagnosed in infants and children. Despite its early and dramatic clinical presentation, the time between onset and diagnosis has averaged approximately 3 years, as symptoms mistakenly are attributed to more common conditions. The radiographic signs are those of intestinal obstruction, with dilated small intestine in one-third of children and microcolon in those with neonatal obstruction. There may be prolonged stasis of contrast material that is placed into the affected bowel. Special diagnostic testing provides information about the pathophysiology of the disease. Manometric studies are more sensitive than radiographic tests to evaluate the strength and coordination of contractions in the esophagus, gastric antrum, small intestine, colon, and anorectal area. Gastric emptying of a solid nutrient meal is the best screening test for gastroparesis. In severely affected children, there may be very delayed gastric emptying of solids or liquids and reflux of intestinal contents back into the stomach.

Failure to thrive is a consistent feature in children with serious untreated chronic intestinal pseudoobstruction. Approximately one-half of affected children require enteral tube feedings. Bolus intragastric feedings may be useful for infants and toddlers who will not suck or drink or in the administration of unpalatable nutrition supplements for older children. If gastric bolus feedings are associated with vomiting and pain, continuous drip feedings may be more successful. If there is no improvement in anorexia and early satiety after several months of optimal nutritional support, a percutaneous endoscopic or surgical gastrostomy offers the advantages of easing nutrient administration and avoiding the need for repeated nasogastric intubation. With severe gastroparesis, jejunal feedings may be indicated. Parenteral nutrition often is necessary to achieve optimal nutritional support.

Children with known pseudoobstruction syndrome may present with acute deterioration and worsening distension or pain. Abdominal radiographs may demonstrate no difference in their usual patterns of bowel obstruction. In children who had previous surgery, it is difficult to discriminate a physical obstruction that is related to adhesions from an episodic increase in the symptoms of pseudoobstruction. Conservative management usually is reasonable, but prolonged symptoms warrant investigation with radiographic contrast studies. Ninety percent of deaths in children with intestinal pseudoobstruction result from parenteral nutrition–associated complications, mainly sepsis and chronic cholestatic liver disease. Therefore, every effort should be made to maximize enteral nutritional support in parenteral nutrition–dependent children. Because growth slows and caloric requirements decrease after 5 years of age, some children can be weaned from parenteral nutrition at that time.

Prokinetic drugs such as metoclopramide, bethanechol, domperidone, and erythromycin rarely have been useful in treatment. Cisapride, which facilitates the release of acetylcholine from myenteric plexus motor neurons, is helpful in some children with less severe forms of the disease. It increases both the number and strength of contractions in the stomach and duodenum, and it accelerates GI transit. Pyridostigmine has also been reported to be beneficial in some patients. Octreotide, a long-acting somatostatin analog, has also improved symptoms and small bowel motility in some patients with pseudoobstruction. Antibiotics are intermittently administered to treat bacterial overgrowth because this is associated with steatorrhea, fat-soluble vitamin malabsorption, and malabsorption of the intrinsic factor–vitamin B_{12} complex. Constipation is treated with laxatives, suppositories, and/or enemas. An enteral lavage solution is effective in those patients with disease confined to the colon, but this will cause massive distension in children with more proximal disease.

Surgical options must be evaluated carefully. Management of acute obstructive episodes is a special challenge. Unnecessary abdominal surgery in children with pseudoobstruction should be avoided because these children often suffer from very prolonged postoperative ileus; adhesions develop, creating a diagnostic problem each time there is a new obstructive episode; and adhesions following laparotomy may distort normal tissue planes and increase the risk for bleeding and organ perforation during future surgeries. Gastrostomy reduces the number of hospitalizations by providing a quick and comfortable means to evacuate gastric contents and relieve nausea, vomiting, and pain related to gastric and bowel distension. It also can be used for enteral feeding and the administration of medications. Fundoplication rarely is indicated; following fundoplication, vomiting may be replaced by retching because of outlet obstruction at the LES. Colectomy may be curative in children with pseudoobstruction confined to the colon. Intestinal transplantation, either alone or in combination with liver transplantation, holds the promise of life-saving cure for children with chronic intestinal pseudoobstruction who depend on parenteral nutrition and have ongoing TPN-related liver damage.

References

Cucchiara S, Bortolotti M, Colombo C, et al: Abnormalities of gastrointestinal motility in children with nonulcer dyspepsia and in children with gastroesophageal reflux disease. Dig Dis Sci 36:1066–1073, 1991

DiLorenzo C: Pseudo-obstruction: current approaches. Gastroenterology 116:980–987, 1999

Dumont C, Rudolph CD: Development of gastrointestinal motility in the infant and child. Gastroenterol Clin North Am 23:655–671, 1994

Pittschieler K: Dumping syndrome after combined pyloroplasty and fundoplication. Eur J Pediatr 150:410–412, 1991

Rudolph CD, Hyman PE, Altschuler SM, et al: Diagnosis and treatment of pseudo-obstruction in children: report of consensus workshop. J Pediatr Gastroenterol Nutr 24:102–112, 1997

17.16 BACTERIA AND BOWEL FUNCTION

Robert D. Murray

17.16.1 Bacterial Colonization and Function in the Bowel

Bacteria colonize the colon because it contains elements that are critical for their growth: a warm, moist, stable environment with an abundant supply of nutrients both of exogenous (ie, dietary) and endogenous (ie, sloughed cells, mucus, secretions) origin. The resulting flora is among the most diverse in nature, incorporating over 400 different species of bacteria. It is replenished at a rate of 150 to 400 g daily, with each gram containing more than 10^{11} organisms.

Development of this complex ecosystem begins at birth. Initially, the colon is sterile and has a pH of 6.5 to 7.0. Within hours after birth, aerobes and facultative anaerobes (eg, *Escherichia coli* and *Streptococcus*) colonize to levels of 10^6 to 10^8 organisms per gram of feces. This results in an environment that is increasingly reduced in oxygen and thus favors the growth of strict anaerobes. In breast-fed infants, *Bifidobacterium* appears by day 4 to 7, reaching levels of 10^8 to 10^{11} organisms per gram. *Clostridium, Lactobacillus,* and even *Bacteroides* also may colonize at this time. The presence of these organisms is associated with an acidic luminal pH of 5.1.

It has been noted that *Bifidobacterium* produces primarily lactate and acetate via lactose fermentation. The resulting milieu has been suggested to retard the growth of pathogenic bacteria such as *E. coli* and *Salmonella* and to promote the growth of *Bifidobacterium*. In bottle-fed infants, the initial metabolic events differ. Strains of enterobacteria such as *E. coli* and *Klebsiella pneumoniae* predominate in a relatively neutral pH environment. By the end of the second week, in both breast- and bottle-fed infants, the rapid fluctuations both in bacterial numbers and in bacterial metabolic end products stabilize, and *Bifidobacterium, Eubacterium, Clostridium,* and *Lactobacillus* become the predominant species. This balance is maintained throughout adult life.

Under normal conditions, the presence of bacteria enhances colonic function. The primary nutrients for bacterial metabolism are carbohydrates, which are rapidly fermented to short-chain fatty acids (SCFAs, eg, acetate, butyrate, propionate) and gases (eg, hydrogen, carbon dioxide, methane). The SCFAs, which are the predominant colonic anions, are readily absorbed across the mucosa and indirectly coupled to sodium uptake. Water passively follows the absorption of the anions. Thus, SCFA absorption acts as a primary stimulus for colonic salt and water absorption. In addition, SCFAs comprise an essential energy resource for the colonic epithelium. Butyrate provides the primary fuel for the colonocytes, whereas acetate and propionate serve as fuels for systemic needs, thus salvaging carbohydrate energy that otherwise would be lost in feces. The lack of steady SCFA uptake and metabolism may explain the clinical condition termed *diversion colitis,* which occurs in colon pouches following creation of ostomies (see Sec. 17.21.5). The relationship between the colon and its flora is further apparent from the morphologic and physiological changes that occur when the colon is devoid of bacteria. In the germ-free state, the cecum enlarges, and the colon wall, especially the mucosal layer, thins. Whereas the normal colon is absorptive, assimilating 1.5 to 2.0 L of fluid and 275 mEq of sodium per day, the gnotobiotic colon is secretory. In the germ-free state, malabsorption of any nutrient results in brisk osmotic diarrhea. Similarly, when broad-spectrum antibiotics are administered, the normal flora can be eradicated, reducing their metabolic capacity, and this results in osmotic diarrhea.

Mounting evidence indicates that some probiotics can modify the course of infectious or "traveler's" diarrhea. The most studied probiotic has been lactobacilli, especially *Lactobacillus* GG. Lactobacilli have been noted to reduce fluid losses during rotavirus-induced diarrhea, to prevent its spread within a hospital setting, and to protect against acquisition of rotavirus in relatively malnourished toddlers. However, not all probiotics have been found to be effective in viral disease. And even those that do modify viral-induced diarrhea have failed to curb invasive bacterial diarrhea. It has been suggested that, besides differences between probiotic species in their clinical effectiveness, another reason for variability between patients is a lack of quality control. One study showed almost no correlation between package claims and actual bacterial content of the products.

The presence of bacteria in the large intestine provides a nutritional aid for the host and a barrier to pathogenic organisms, but following the administration of broad-spectrum antibiotics, the normal flora can be depleted, leading to overgrowth of opportunistic toxigenic bacteria, especially *Clostridium difficile,* which can induce a secretory and inflammatory diarrhea termed *pseudomembranous colitis.* Recent evidence also supports giving the probiotics *Lactobacillus* GG or *Saccharomyces boulardii* when antibiotics are prescribed in order to prevent subsequent bacterial overgrowth with *C. difficile,* especially in those prone to chronic *C. difficile* infection. Several other species of probiotics have demonstrated efficacy in either treating or preventing the other complications that can be associated with antibiotic use.

17.16.2   Bacterial Overgrowth

Although bacteria in the large intestine provide a nutritional aid for the host and a barrier to pathogenic organisms, excess bacteria in the upper intestine are detrimental. Bacteria in the stomach normally number fewer than 10^3 colonies per milliliter of gastric content; those of the small intestine range from 10^3 to 10^6 per milliliter. The more distal the site, the more the flora resembles that of the colon in species and number. Physiological factors that prevent bacterial overgrowth in the small bowel include: (1) gastric acidity (pH 1 to 2), (2) gastric and intestinal motility, (3) mucosal defenses such as mucus and immunoglobulins, and (4) the physical barrier

that prevents colonic reflux (ie, the ileocecal valve). Clinical conditions such as hypochlorhydria, diverticula, blind loops, strictures, inflammation, abnormal motility, and extensive surgical resection can lead to bacterial overgrowth. Conditions engendering severe protein-energy malnutrition also may result in small intestine contamination.

The clinical manifestations of bacterial overgrowth are diverse, but they primarily involve malabsorption and malnutrition. Steatorrhea is the hallmark; it is caused by deconjugation of bile salts with resultant poor micelle formation. Light microscopic examination of the mucosa generally is normal, although ultrastructural damage and disaccharidase deficiency have been identified. If severe, all types of carbohydrates are malabsorbed, resulting in profuse, watery diarrhea and, potentially, dehydration. In addition, hypoproteinemia may result from either malnutrition or loss of protein across the damaged bowel mucosa. Vitamin deficiencies, especially vitamin B_{12}, occur in certain cases. Bacterial production of D-lactate on occasion can result in metabolic acidosis. Stupor, neurologic dysfunction, and even shock may be noted clinically. Most commonly this occurs in children with short-bowel syndrome during excessive ingestion of carbohydrates. Diagnosis is by measurement of D-lactate in serum. Usually, the laboratory needs to be specifically asked to measure the D-isomer because routine lactate measurement measures only L-lactate.

The diagnosis of intestinal bacterial overgrowth can be made by culturing luminal fluid obtained at endoscopy or by breath hydrogen testing using lactulose, which is a synthetic disaccharide that cannot be digested by the brush border enzymes, as a substrate. A high fasting baseline level of hydrogen and a sudden rise in the excretion of hydrogen within several minutes of lactulose ingestion support the diagnosis, but false-negative tests are common. Empiric treatment is a reasonable option. Treatment for overgrowth consists of oral antibiotics, which may need to be given recurrently unless the underlying causative problem can be corrected. Useful agents include metronidazole (30 to 40 mg/kg/d given QID) or gentamicin (50 mg/kg/d given QID) for 7 days.

References

Harig JM, Soergel KH, Komoroski RA, et al: Treatment of diversion colitis with short-chain fatty acid irrigation. N Engl J Med 320:23–28, 1989

Perlmutter CH, Boyle JT, Campos JM, Egler JM, Watkins JB: D-Lactic acidosis in children: an unusual metabolic complication of small bowel resection. J Pediatr 102:234–238, 1983

Rhodes JM, Middleton P, Jewell DP: The lactulose hydrogen breath test as a diagnostic test for small-bowel bacterial overgrowth. Scand J Gastroenterol 14:333–336, 1979

Vanderhoof JA, Young RJ: Use of probiotics in childhood gastrointestinal disorders. J Pediatr Gastroenterol Nutr 27:323–332, 1998

17.17 GASTROINTESTINAL DISORDERS IN THE CHILD WITH IMMUNODEFICIENCY

Tien-lan Chang and Harland Winter

Children with either primary or acquired immunodeficiency have a higher risk than normal children or adults for both infectious and noninfectious complications that involve the GI tract. The major function of the immune system is to protect the host from foreign organisms or substances (see Sec. 17.1.5). The risk and severity of infection depend on the type of immunodeficiency. Individuals with deficiencies of antibody response are predisposed to extracellular bacterial infections and intestinal pathogens. For example, children with antibody deficiency have an increased incidence of *Campylobacter jejuni* enteritis. Unlike the host with an intact mucosal immune system, children with antibody deficiency often have a prolonged illness that does not respond well to antibiotics. Patients with deficiencies of T cells are predisposed to both intracellular and extracellular infections. In addition, patients with primary immunodeficiencies are more prone to develop autoimmune disorders because of their decreased ability to distinguish self-organisms from foreign organisms. Autoimmune diseases and celiac disease are more common in the IgA-deficient patient.

Gastrointestinal disorders in children with immunodeficiencies can be associated with infectious and noninfectious diseases. Infectious diseases are caused by viruses, bacteria, mycobacteria, fungi, or protozoa; noninfectious diseases can be allergic, autoimmune, or alloimmune in etiology. Dysmotility, malabsorption, and malnutrition can be associated with any of these disorders. In addition, medical treatments prescribed for children with immunodeficiencies may have significant gastrointestinal side effects.

17.17.1　Gastrointestinal Infections

The pandemic of HIV infection and AIDS has heightened our awareness of opportunistic infections, most of which have been described either in patients with primary immunodeficiencies or in immunosuppressed patients with malignancies. These infections are listed in Table 17-42 according to the sites of GI involvement. In addition to those listed, immunodeficient patients also are at increased risk for common bacterial and viral pathogens or infections with multiple organisms.

Cytomegalovirus, rotavirus, adenovirus, and *herpes simplex virus* are the most common viral agents. Cytomegalovirus is commonly identified in children with immunodeficiency and can cause inflammation or ulceration anywhere along the GI tract, including the pancreaticobiliary system. Symptoms may include diarrhea, dysphagia, vomiting, abdominal pain, and GI bleeding. Histologic identification of cytomegalovirus within the intestinal tissue is required to establish a pathogenic role because cytomegalovirus commonly is excreted in the urine or stool of asymptomatic individuals. Rotavirus is a cause of vomiting and diarrhea in immunocompro-

mised children and may disseminate into the liver parenchyma. In contrast, rotavirus rarely is a pathogen in normal or immunocompromised adults, most of whom have previously established immunity. Adenoviruses have been reported to cause colitis in adults with AIDS and fulminant hepatitis in immunocompromised children. Diagnosis of adenovirus infection depends on histologic identification, which should be confirmed by culture. Herpes simplex virus usually causes oral and esophageal lesions and produces symptoms of dysphagia and odynophagia. However, few cases have been reported in children. Other viruses such as astrovirus, picornovirus, and calicivirus have been identified in the stool of HIV-infected adults with diarrhea, and they also may have a role in pediatric patients with diarrhea. In individuals without an identifiable pathogen, HIV itself has been suggested as a cause of diarrhea and malabsorption.

Salmonella, Shigella, Campylobacter, Yersinia, Escherichia coli, and *Clostridium difficile* are the most common bacterial infections in normal or immunocompromised hosts. In the presence of bowel dysmotility, overgrowth of normal bacterial flora in the small bowel can contribute to intestinal inflammation and malabsorption. In the immunocompromised host, infections such as *Salmonella, Shigella,* and *Campylobacter* can be severe and prolonged, with a tendency to relapse and spread systemically. In one reported series of bacteremia in HIV-infected children, *Salmonella* was the second most common bacterial isolate from blood. *Clostridium difficile* probably is as prevalent among immunocompromised patients as in the immunocompetent population, with antibiotic use as the major predisposing factor. In developing countries, strains of enteropathogenic *E. coli* are important causes of diarrhea in young HIV-infected children. In the United States, gastroenteritis caused by enteropathogenic *E. coli* is rare, but it should be considered in patients with a recent history of travel.

Mycobacterium avium-intracellulare, or *M. avium* complex (MAC), accounts for the great majority of disseminated nontuberculous mycobacterial infections, involving bone marrow, liver, kidneys, and the GI tract. Approximately 12% of children with HIV infection have disseminated MAC. Although the rate of GI involvement by MAC is uncertain, 90% of children with disseminated MAC have GI symptoms such as abdominal pain, vomiting, anorexia, and diarrhea. Hepatosplenomegaly is a common physical finding. Children with disseminated MAC often have very low CD4 T-cell counts and also have a poor prognosis, with a median survival period of 9 months. *M. tuberculosis* also can infect the GI tract, usually the ileocecal region, and has been reported to cause peritonitis secondary to intestinal perforation.

Candida and *Histoplasma* are the most common fungal infections affecting immunodeficient children. *Candida* usually causes

TABLE 17-42

OPPORTUNISTIC GASTROINTESTINAL INFECTIONS

	ESOPHAGUS	STOMACH	SMALL INTESTINE	COLON
Protozoan			*Giardia lamblia*	*Giardia lamblia*
			Cryptosporidium	*Crytposproidium*
			Microsporida	*Isospora*
Fungal	*Candida*		*Histoplasma*	*Blastocystis*
Mycobacterial			*Mycobacterium tuberculosis*	*Mycobacterium tuberculosis*
			Mycobacterium avium-intracellulare	*Mycobacterium avium-intracellulare*
Viral	Herpes	Cytomegalovirus	Cytomegalovirus	Cytomegalovirus
			Adenovirus	Adenovirus

oral thrush and esophagitis. Fungal balls in the stomach can cause obstructive symptoms. *Histoplasma* has been reported to infect villi of the small intestine, resulting in abdominal pain and diarrhea. Both fungi can disseminate systemically.

Giardia is common in normal and immunocompromised children but often causes more severe diarrhea and abdominal pain and has a more protracted course in children with immunodeficiency. *Cryptosporidium* typically causes a chronic secretory diarrhea in immunocompromised patients, but the severity of the diarrhea may vary. *Cryptosporidium* also may colonize the biliary and pancreatic ducts and cause inflammation and obstruction. *Isospora* has been reported as a cause of diarrhea in immunodeficient adults, but it very rarely is a cause of diarrhea in U.S. children. *Microsporidia* are intracellular protozoan organisms that infect small intestinal epithelial cells. They are found in a significant number of HIV-infected adults with diarrhea but have yet to be reported in children.

17.17.2   Immune-Mediated Injury

Although infections are responsible for most cases of diarrhea, immunologic reactions also can play a significant role in GI symptoms. Graft-versus-host disease (see Sec. 17.21.5), an alloimmune reaction, can occur in patients with severe combined immunodeficiency from either maternofetal transfusion or transfusion of unirradiated blood; graft-versus-host disease also may result from bone marrow transplantation in older children with hematologic malignancies. Clinical signs and symptoms include skin rash, hepatitis, diarrhea, GI bleeding, or eosinophilia. Rarely, exocrine pancreatic insufficiency results from chronic graft-versus-host disease. Autoimmune mechanisms, as suggested by the presence of antiepithelial cell antibodies, may be responsible for intestinal injury in some patients with common variable immunodeficiency. Autoimmune enteropathy more commonly begins in infancy and presents with chronic diarrhea frequently requiring total parenteral nutrition (see Sec. 17.18.4). Immunologic reactions to food proteins, either cell-mediated or antibody (IgE)-mediated, also can cause intestinal inflammation and malabsorption (see Sec. 17.21.1). High titers of antigliadin and anti–milk protein antibodies have been reported with HIV infection and other intestinal diseases such as Crohn disease. The clinical relevance of these findings is unknown.

17.17.3   Medication-Induced Gastrointestinal Disorders

Medications used in the management of immunodeficiencies, whether congenital or acquired, frequently lead to nausea, abdominal pain, and vomiting. Mucosal injury, manifested by oral ulcers or diarrhea, can result from bone marrow suppression caused by agents such as methotrexate. Pancreatitis has been associated with drugs such as the reverse transcriptase inhibitors (didanosine and lamivudine), antibiotics (trimethoprim-sulfamethoxazole and pentamidine), and valproic acid. Elevated serum triglyceride and cholesterol levels, possibly caused by mitochondrial damage in the hepatocytes, have been reported in patients treated with the protease inhibitor, ritonavir. Most children with immunodeficiency are receiving multiple medications, so the evaluation of potential causes of gastrointestinal symptoms should always include a careful review of potential medication side effects.

17.17.4   Diagnosis and Management of Children with Immunodeficiency and Gastrointestinal Disorders

A child with immunodeficiency can present with any one or a combination of GI symptoms, including diarrhea, growth failure, hepatosplenomegaly, GI bleeding, abdominal pain, emesis, and dysphagia. Of these symptoms, diarrhea probably is the most common. When a child presents with diarrhea, studies on the stool should include occult blood (Hemoccult), culture (for *Salmonella, Shigella, Campylobacter, Yersinia,* and *Clostridium difficile*), immunoassays for rotavirus, *Giardia* antigen, and acid-fast stain or immunofluorescent stain for *Cryptosporidium* and *Isospora belli*. A complete blood count and blood culture should be done if there is fever. Elevated eosinophil count should raise the possibility of severe combined immunodeficiency, graft-versus-host reaction, or an allergic gastroenteritis. Testing for IgE antibody against a suspected food (eg, milk or soy protein) by a radioallergosorbent test (RAST) may be warranted. Following extensive evaluation, an identifiable cause of diarrhea can be found in 50 to 85% of patients. However, the vigor of investigation must be individualized and tempered because patients may have multiple infections, and many known infectious causes have no specific therapy. After treatable infections have been excluded, optimal management includes symptom relief and nutritional management to improve the overall quality of life.

In a child presenting with abdominal pain and vomiting, a partial bowel obstruction, cholangitis, or pancreatitis should be considered in the differential diagnosis. Serum aminotransferase levels as well as amylase and lipase concentrations should be measured. Imaging studies such as an upright abdominal radiograph to look for evidence of intestinal obstruction and abdominal ultrasonography to look for biliary/pancreatic ductal dilation or edema of the pancreas may be helpful. Radiographic evidence of intramural air in the small or large bowel (ie, pneumatosis) suggests either bacterial overgrowth or severe tissue necrosis.

Assessment of absorptive function includes testing of stool for reducing substance, pH, and fat, breath hydrogen tests, and a serum D-xylose test. A lactulose breath hydrogen test may help to diagnose small bowel bacterial overgrowth by finding an early peak of breath hydrogen after the ingestion of lactulose. Testing the stool for α_1-antitrypsin may identify patients with protein-losing enteropathy. Serum protein, albumin, prealbumin, and transferrin levels are helpful in assessing the severity of protein malnutrition in a child with poor growth.

Fiberoptic endoscopy is indicated in evaluating patients with dysphagia, upper or lower GI bleeding, or chronic diarrhea in whom no pathogen or cause has been found by other tests. Diagnosis of esophagitis caused by acid reflux, *Candida,* or cytomegalovirus can be made by esophageal biopsy. Pathogens that can be identified in biopsies of the small intestine and colon include *Cryptosporidium*, cytomegalovirus, adenovirus, *Histoplasma, Microsporidia,* and *Myobacterium avium-intracellulare*. For patients with bile duct obstruction associated with either pancreatitis or cholangitis, a biliary stent placed endoscopically can lead to significant symptomatic relief. Antibiotic prophylaxis should be considered when endoscopy is performed in patients with neutropenia or with an indwelling central venous catheter.

Both specific and supportive treatments are needed in treating a gastrointestinal disorder in a child with immunodeficiency. Specific therapy is directed at the cause of the disorder. If an infectious agent is found, appropriate therapy is initiated. Human immunoglobulin has been used in conjunction with ganciclovir to treat cytomegalovirus infection; oral human immunoglobulin has led to clearance of *Cryptosporidium* in two patients with immunodeficiency secondary to hematologic malignancies, but this therapy is not well proven. A somatostatin analog that reduces GI secretion, octreotide, has been used with some success as supportive therapy in patients with HIV infection and chronic diarrhea. Conditions that are caused by rotavirus, adenovirus, and *Microsporidia* have no known effective specific therapy. In these situations, optimizing nutritional status and controlling symptoms are of prime importance. The use of pharmacologic agents that decrease gastric acidity should be limited in duration in the immunocompromised child to reduce the risk of bacterial or fungal overgrowth that is associated with the loss of the gastric acid barrier.

The approach to nutritional management depends on the degree of intestinal injury and malabsorption. Because most diarrheal illnesses in the immunocompromised host are prolonged, after correction of fluids and electrolytes, an "elemental" diet consisting of small peptides, glucose polymers, and medium-chain triglyceride is most easily absorbed. If normal digestive and absorptive function can be documented, diet can be advanced to include more complex carbohydrates, long-chain fats, and intact proteins. Patients who are nauseous and anorectic may require placement of a gastrostomy tube for feeding and administration of medications, whereas patients who have intractable diarrhea, vomiting, GI bleeding, or pancreatitis may require total parenteral nutrition. Prolonged placement of a nasogastric feeding tube in the immunocompromised child should be limited because it increases the risk for sinusitis. In patients who require total parenteral nutrition or have prolonged diarrhea and malnutrition, serum levels of micronutrients such as selenium, zinc, vitamins, and carnitine should be determined. Deficiencies of these micronutrients can potentiate immunodeficiency. Several studies have demonstrated that megestrol acetate can stimulate appetite and improve weight gain for adults and children infected with HIV. However, the weight gain appears to be mostly in the form of body fat. Growth hormone, on the other hand, has been shown to increase lean body mass in adults with AIDS, and trials are beginning in the pediatric population. It is remarkable, but not surprising, that since the advent of HAART (highly active antiretroviral therapy) for patients with HIV infection, severe GI complications such as intractable diarrhea and wasting seem to have diminished in frequency. Although these combined antiretroviral therapies are expensive and not available in developing countries, studies have shown reduced morbidity and mortality from diarrhea in HIV-infected children who receive vitamin A supplements. Zinc supplements may also reduce the frequency, duration, and severity of diarrhea in children.

References

Bhutta ZA, Black RE, Brown KH, et al: Prevention of diarrhea and pneumonia by zinc supplementation in children in developing countries: pooled analysis of randomized controlled trials. Zinc Investigators' Collaborative Group. J Pediatr 135:689–697, 1999

Connolly GM, Forbes A, Gazzard BG: Investigation of seemingly pathogen-negative diarrhea in patients infected with HIV-1. Gut 3:886–889, 1989

Fauzi WW, Mbise RL, Hertzmark E, et al: A randomized trial of vitamin A supplements in relation to mortality among human immunodeficiency virus-infected and uninfected children in Tanzania. Pediatr Infect Dis J 18:127–133, 1999

Hirschfed S: Use of human recombinant growth hormone and human recombinant insulin-like growth factor-I in patients with human immunodeficiency virus infection. Horm Res 46:215–221, 1996

Kotler DP, Francisco A, Clayton F, et al: Small intestinal injury and parasitic diseases in AIDS. Ann Intern Med 113:444–449, 1990

Miller TL, Orav EJ, Martin SR, Cooper ER, Mcintosh K, Winter HS: Malnutrition and carbohydrate malabsorption in children with vertically transmitted human immunodeficiency virus 1 infection. Gastroenterology 100:1296, 1991

Miller TL, Winter HS, Luginbuhl LM, Orav EJ, Mcintosh K: Pancreatitis in pediatric human immunodeficiency virus infection. J Pediatr 120: 223–227, 1992

Romeu J, Miro JM, Sirera G, et al: Efficacy of octreotide in the management of chronic diarrhea in AIDS. AIDS 5:1495–1499, 1991

17.18 DISORDERS OF DIGESTION AND ABSORPTION

17.18.1 Evaluation of the Child with Malabsorption

Ivor D. Hill

Assimilation of nutrients involves a complex process of intraluminal digestion with subsequent transport of the breakdown products across the intestinal mucosa as discussed in Sec. 17.1.4. The term "malabsorption" is broadly used to characterize abnormalities of this process involving either multiple nutrients (as occurs with celiac disease) or single molecules (as found in isolated glucose-galactose malabsorption). Defects may be congenital, with onset of symptoms shortly after birth, or acquired, when the age of onset of symptoms is variable. The schema in Table 17-43 highlights the major pathogenic mechanisms of various specific malabsorptive disorders. Evaluation of the child with suspected malabsorption requires consideration of the various steps involved in digestion and absorption, together with thorough clinical assessment and selection of the most appropriate diagnostic investigations.

The nutritional consequences of malabsorption vary from mild or none to severe with malnutrition and even death. Abnormalities that impair absorption tend to have greater nutritional consequences than those impairing digestion. In general, growth is affected, manifest first by poor weight gain or weight loss and subsequently by linear growth retardation. Additional consequences involve specific nutrients causing conditions such as rickets, osteoporosis, or tetany (vitamin D and calcium deficiency), coagulation disturbances (vitamin K deficiency), or anemia (iron, folate, or vitamin B_{12} deficiency).

A detailed history is an essential part of the clinical evaluation. In most cases malabsorption is associated with chronic diarrhea, often accompanied by abdominal distension. The age of onset of diarrhea may provide clues as to the etiology. Diarrhea starting shortly after birth suggests a congenital as opposed to an acquired defect. Effort should be directed toward identifying a temporal relationship between the onset of diarrhea and dietary changes. Symptoms after changing from breast milk to formula could indicate milk protein intolerance, whereas those starting after the introduction of solid foods should raise the possibility of celiac disease.

Stool characteristics including number, fluidity, color, size, and smell may provide clues to the etiology. Carbohydrate malabsorp-

TABLE 17-43

MECHANISMS OF MALABSORPTION AND MALDIGESTION

LUMINAL PHASE	MUCOSAL PHASE	TRANSPORT PHASE
Substrate hydrolysis	**Brush border hydrolysis**	**Lymphatic**
Enzyme deficiency: cystic fibrosis, Shwachman-Diamond syndrome, chronic pancreatitis	Disaccharidase deficiency, primary and secondary	Obstruction: lymphangiectasia or secondary obstruction from cardiac, infiltrative, or inflammatory disease
Enzyme inactivation: Zollinger-Ellison syndrome		Vascular: intestinal ischemia or radiation, congenital abnormalities, or vascular disease
Rapid transit/asynchrony: post–gastric surgery, fundoplication with vagotomy		
Fat solubilization	**Epithelial transport defects**	
Impaired biliary secretions: biliary atresia with kesei procedure, cholestatic jaundice	Generalized: mucosal injury, celiac disease, eosinophilic enteropathy, tropical sprue, AIDS, infections, rotavirus and other viral infiltration, bacterial adherence, congenital defects (microvillus inclusion disease)	
Decreased bile salt synthesis; parenchymal liver disease, immaturity, inborn errors of bile acid metabolism	Isolated defects: congenital vitamin B_{12} and folate transport, amino acid transport deficiencies, carbohydrate glucose, galactose transport defect	
Bile salt deconjugation, precipitation, and binding: bacterial overgrowth, Zollinger-Ellison syndrome, drug effects		
Impaired cholecystokinin release: extensive mucosal disease		
Increased bile salt loss: terminal ileal resection or disease, cystic fibrosis		
Luminal defects in processing	**Epithelial cell processing**	
Bacterial consumption of vitamin B_{12}: bacterial overgrowth	Abetalipoproteinemia, chylomicron retention disease	

tion typically produces explosive liquid stools that are acidic and frequently cause perianal excoriation. Fat malabsorption caused by pancreatic enzyme insufficiency causes bulky, greasy, pale stools that are extremely malodorous. Intestinal mucosal abnormalities causing malabsorption (eg, celiac disease) tend to produce stools that are more loose than watery, and less greasy and malodorous than those caused by pancreatic insufficiency.

Exposure to potential infectious agents or a history of recent foreign travel should be elucidated. A past history of abdominal surgery could implicate short-bowel syndrome, a blind loop, or terminal ileum resection as the cause of malabsorption. Symptoms related to other systems should be noted. Chronic chest problems may indicate cystic fibrosis, arthritis or arthralgia can accompany inflammatory diseases such as Crohn, and a history of multiple infections raises the possibility of immune deficiency. A positive family history for cystic fibrosis, celiac disease, inflammatory bowel disease, or HIV infection should lead to consideration of these conditions in the child.

Depending on the type and severity of the problem, there may be little to find on physical examination. The more severe the malabsorption, the more pronounced the physical changes are likely to be. Growth parameters of weight, height, and head circumference must be documented and compared to the standards for age. Review of the child's growth pattern since birth may help determine the age of onset of the problem and the most likely cause. Signs of pallor (anemia), hyperkeratosis (vitamin A deficiency), bruising (vitamin K deficiency), glossitis (riboflavin deficiency), dermatitis (niacin deficiency), rickets (vitamin D and calcium deficiency), and muscle wasting with edema (protein deficiency) should be interpreted in the context of the dietary history. The abdominal examination should include inspection for distension as well as careful palpation for organomegaly or abdominal masses (tuberculous nodes or lymphoma). Examination of other systems such as the respiratory, cardiovascular, and endocrine is an integral part of the evaluation.

The choice of laboratory studies to confirm the presence of malabsorption and establish an etiology will depend on the most likely causes as determined from the history and physical examination. Table 17-44 provides a progressive approach to the diagnostic stud-

TABLE 17-44

DIAGNOSTIC STUDIES IN THE EVALUATION OF MALDIGESTION AND MALABSORPTION

Initial screening studies
 Stool examination for occult blood, leukocytes, reducing substances, and pH
 Stool examination for *Clostridium difficile* toxin, ova, and parasites, cultures for infectious bacterial and viral pathogens
 Complete blood count
 Serum electrolytes, blood urea nitrogen, creatinine, calcium, phosphorus, albumin, total protein
 Urinalysis and culture
Quantitative and qualitative tests for malabsorption
 Breath H_2 studies for carbohydrate malabsorption
 D-Xylose absorption for mucosal function
 Fecal fat studies or coefficient of fat absorption studies
 Serum iron, vitamin B_{12}, folate, carotene, prothrombin time
Specific diagnostic studies
 Sweat chloride test for cystic fibrosis
 Small intestinal biopsy for histology and mucosal enzyme
 Contrast radiographic studies: upper gastrointestinal series with small-bowel follow-through and/or barium enema
 Provocative pancreatic secretion testing
 Ultrasound for biliary tree anomalies, pancreatic mass, and stones
 Endoscopic retrogade cholangiopancreatography (ERCP) for selective evaluation of biliary or pancreatic ducts

TABLE 17-45

DIAGNOSTIC RELIABILITY OF PERORAL SMALL INTESTINE BIOPSY

Histology diagnostic; lesions diffuse; present on biopsy

Microvillus inclusion disease	Absent or abnormal microvilli, electron microscopy is diagnostic
Abetalipoproteinemia	Vacuolated, lipid-laden enterocytes with normal architecture
Agammaglobulinemia	Celiac disease–like histology with *Giardia*, serum immunoglobulins diagnostic
Mycobacterium avium-intracellulare	Acid-fast lamina propria macrophages
Whipple disease	Periodic acid-Schiff–positive lamina propria macrophages

Histology abnormal but not diagnostic; lesions diffuse; present on biopsy

Celiac disease, tropical sprue	Varying degrees of villus atrophy and crypt hyperplasia with lamina propria inflammation
Milk protein intolerance	Same as mild to moderate celiac disease
Viral enteropathy	Same as mild to moderate celiac disease
Bacterial overgrowth	Same as mild to moderate celiac disease
Cytomegalovirus enteritis	Characteristic on biopsy

Histology diagnostic; distribution patchy; therefore, may be missed on biopsy

Lymphoma	Villi widened, and lamina propria filled with malignant lymphoma cells
Lymphangiectasia	Dilated lymphatics in lamina propria and submucosa
Eosinophilic enteritis	Lamina propria infiltrated with eosinophils and neutrophils; mucosa normal to flat
Mastocytosis	Lamina propria infiltrated with mast cells and eosinophils; mucosa normal to flat
Amyloidosis	Amyloid in lamina propria and submucosa with Congo red stain; otherwise normal mucosa
Crohn disease	Varying inflammation and ulceration with subepithelial granulomas
Giardiasis, coccidiomycosis, *Strongyloides*	Mucosa normal to flat with *Giardia*, *Crytosporidium*, or *Stronglyloides* on surfaces of villi or crypts; *Eimeria*, *Isospora*, or *Microsporida* within enterocytes

Histology abnormal but not diagnostic; distribution patchy; may be missed on biopsy

Acute radiation enteritis	Celiac disease–like lesion of varying severity
Enteropathy of dermatitis herpetiformis	Celiac disease–like lesion of varying severity

SOURCE: *Trier JS: Intestinal malabsorption: differentiation of cause. Hosp Pract 23:195, 1998;* and *Trier JS: Diagnostic value of peroral biopsy of the proximal small intestine. N Engl J Med 285:1470, 1971.*

ies that may be used for this purpose. Relatively inexpensive screening tests include examination of stool for occult blood and fecal leukocytes to exclude inflammatory disorders, stool microscopy for parasites such as *Giardia*, measurement of stool pH and reducing substances to look for carbohydrate malabsorption, and a qualitative test for fecal fat globules (Sudan stain) to look for fat malabsorption. A complete blood count and differential with smear looking for anemia (iron, folate, or B_{12} deficiency), acanthocytosis (abetalipoproteinemia), eosinophilia (eosinophilic gastroenteropathy), or lymphopenia (lymphangiectasia) are useful.

If initial screening tests suggest malabsorption, more specific tests may be necessary. Hydrogen breath tests are used to confirm specific carbohydrate malabsorption. The D-xylose test assesses small intestinal mucosal integrity. It is performed by measuring the 1-hour serum xylose level or the amount of xylose excreted in a timed 5-hour urine sample after the patient ingests a standard dose of xylose based on body surface area (14.5 g/m² to a maximum of 25 g as a 10% solution). Technical difficulties associated with this test can give both false-negative and false-positive results, so it is of limited value. Low serum levels of vitamins A, D, and E occur with fat malabsorption, and folate and B_{12} deficiencies indicate proximal small intestinal and terminal ileum damage, respectively. Definitive evaluation of fat malabsorption requires a 3-day collection of stools to quantitate fat excretion and determine the coefficient of fat absorption. For this test to be meaningful, fat intake during the study

should be in the range of 2 to 3 g/kg/d (maximum 100 g/d). Determining the cause of fat malabsorption may require measurement of pancreatic enzyme levels. This is best achieved by aspirating pancreatic fluid from the duodenum after intravenous injection of secretin to stimulate pancreatic secretion. The most common cause of pancreatic insufficiency in childhood is cystic fibrosis, which requires a sweat chloride test for confirmation. The sweat test is noninvasive and should be determined in all children with suspected malabsorption before any of the more invasive tests are considered. Duodenal fluid aspirates can also be evaluated for bile acid levels in those rare cases where deficiencies cause inadequate emulsification of fats. Barium contrast studies are needed to look for conditions such as Crohn disease, malrotations, duplications, blind loops, or enteroenteral fistulas.

Establishing a specific cause for malabsorption often requires histologic examination of small intestinal mucosa. This is best obtained by means of upper gastrointestinal endoscopy with multiple biopsies. In addition to histologic evaluation, the tissue can be assayed for the intestinal disaccharidases and glucoamylase. Table 17-45 lists conditions causing malabsorption that can be identified on small intestinal biopsy.

Treatment of malabsorption disorders depends on the specific cause. In some cases simple removal of the offending agent is curative (for example, lactose elimination for lactose malabsorption and gluten-free diet for celiac disease). In others, replacement of deficiencies is possible (pancreatic enzyme supplements for cystic fibrosis). In addition to treating the underlying cause, attention should also be focused on correcting any macronutrient and micronutrient deficits that exist at the time of diagnosis in order to promote optimal growth and development of the individual. Periodic assessment of nutritional status and review of nutrient intake are mandatory in all patients with malabsorption syndromes.

References

Riley SA, Turnberg LA: Maldigestion and malabsorption. In: Sleisenger MH, Fordtran JS, eds: Gastrointestinal Disease: Pathophysiology, Diagnosis, Management, 5th ed. Philadelphia, WB Saunders, 1009–1027: 1993

Schmitz J: Malabsorption. In: Walker WA, Durie PR, Hamilton JR, Walker-Smith JA, Watkins JB, eds: Pediatric Gastrointestinal Disease: Pathophysiology, Diagnosis, Management, 2nd ed. Philadelphia, CV Mosby, 83–95: 1996

17.18.2   Celiac Disease

Ivor D. Hill

Celiac disease occurs in genetically predisposed individuals who ingest gluten from wheat products or related peptides found in barley and rye. The condition is characterized by an immunologically mediated small intestinal mucosal injury that leads to varying degrees of malabsorption of nutrients. Affected individuals have a lifelong intolerance to these dietary peptides. Removal of the offending substances from the diet leads to full clinical remission and restoration of the small intestinal mucosal damage to normality.

EPIDEMIOLOGY

The advent of serologic tests to screen individuals for celiac disease has facilitated epidemiologic studies of the condition. In many European countries celiac disease has been identified in about 1:250 of the general population. The condition has also been diagnosed in North and South America, North Africa, the Middle East countries, India, Australia, and New Zealand. It is rare or nonexistent in native Africans, Japanese, and Chinese. Recent data on the prevalence of celiac disease in Denver, Colorado suggests a prevalence similar to european countries.

PATHOGENESIS

Celiac disease is dependent on three factors: (1) a genetic predisposition, (2) exposure to specific environmental factors, and (3) immunologically mediated small intestinal mucosal damage.

GENETIC FACTORS   A specific gene has not yet been identified for celiac disease, and more than one gene may be involved. Nevertheless, there is considerable evidence for an inherited predisposition. Celiac disease occurs in 10 to 20% of first-degree relatives, and there is concordance in 30 to 40% of HLA-identical siblings and 70% of homozygous twins. The strongest evidence for genetic factors comes from HLA typing. In northern Europeans the specific HLA type DQw2 occurs in 95% of celiac patients compared to 25% of the nonceliac population. In southern European countries such as Italy, there is a strong association between celiac disease and the HLA type DR5/DR7. The primary HLA association of celiac disease seems to be with the DQ $\alpha\beta$ heterodimer encoded by the alleles DQA1*0501 and DQB1*0201. These alleles are inherited in *cis* with the DQw2 genes and in *trans* with the DR5/DR7 heterozygotes. This explains the apparent discrepancy in HLA predominant type between the northern and southern Europeans. In the small number of individuals with celiac disease who do not have either DQw2 or DR5/DR7, there is an association with the HLA type DR4.

ENVIRONMENTAL FACTORS   In addition to dietary factors causing celiac disease, there may also be other environmental trigger factors. Wheat, barley, and rye are the known dietary factors and are grains sharing a common taxonomy in the plant kingdom. Gluten is the protein portion of wheat and can be divided into an alcohol-soluble fraction called gliadin and an alcohol-insoluble fraction known as glutenin. The gliadin fraction, which is rich in glutamine and proline, contains the toxic peptides that initiate the process leading to celiac disease. Similarly, the alcohol-soluble protein fractions from barley (hordeins) and rye (secalins) contain peptides that are toxic to celiac patients. As yet the precise amino acid sequence and length of the toxic peptide causing disease are not known. Oats were thought to cause celiac disease, but this is now in dispute. Oats are more distantly related to wheat in the plant kingdom and in the pure form do not seem to initiate an immunologic response in the genetically predisposed individual. Oats are frequently contaminated by wheat flour during processing, which probably explains why they were previously believed to be toxic.

Because not all individuals with the known genetic markers develop celiac disease when exposed to the toxic dietary factors, effort has been directed toward identifying additional environmental trigger factors. Principal among these are infectious agents. A high degree of amino acid sequence homology has been found between gliadin and viruses such as adenovirus type 12 and 7, rubella, and human herpes virus 1. This raises the possibility of infection by one of these viruses triggering celiac disease, but there is still insufficient supportive evidence to confirm this. Other factors that have been considered but lack proof are stress-related events such as pregnancy.

IMMUNOLOGIC FACTORS   The small intestinal mucosal lesion is characterized by an inflammatory response consisting of increased numbers of lymphocytes, plasma cells, and macrophages in the lamina propria and increased numbers of intraepithelial lymphocytes. The precise mechanism by which exposure to the dietary toxins leads to the inflammatory response remains unknown. It is also unclear how the inflammatory response leads to the structural changes that are characteristic on small intestinal histology. These changes are characterized by a progression from inflammatory cell infiltrate to crypt depth elongation and finally to destruction of the enterocytes with flattening of the villi. Initially these changes may be patchy and confined to the proximal small bowel. With time they become more extensive and involve both the jejunum and ileum. Progressive destruction of intestinal villi leads to progressive reduction in the absorptive area.

CLINICAL FEATURES

The manifestations of celiac disease are extremely protean, and symptoms vary tremendously from patient to patient. Clinical presentations can be broadly categorized into groups, as shown in Table 17-46. The "classic" constellation of symptoms comprising malabsorptive-type diarrhea, poor weight gain, abdominal distension,

TABLE 17-46

CLINICAL MANIFESTATIONS OF CELIAC DISEASE

"Classical" gastrointestinal form
Age of onset under 2 years;
diarrhea, failure to thrive, abdominal distension,
proximal muscle wasting, irritability
Non-"classical" gastrointestinal form
Age of onset childhood to adulthood;
diarrhea intermittent or mild,
abdominal pain, bloating,
nausea, vomiting,
change in appetite,
constipation
Nongastrointestinal manifestations
  Musculoskeletal system
    Short stature, rickets, osteoporosis, dental enamel defects, arthritis/
      arthralgia, myopathy
  Skin and mucous membranes
    Dermatitis herpetiformis, atopic dermatitis, aphthous stomatitis
  Reproductive system
    Delayed puberty, infertility, recurrent abortions, menstrual irregulari-
      ties
  Hematologic system
    Anemia (iron, folate, B_{12}), leukopenia, vitamin K deficiency, throm-
      bocytopenia
  Central nervous system
    Behavioral changes, epilepsy, dementia, cerebellar degeneration
Associated conditions
  Autoimmune disorders
    Type 1 diabetes mellitus, autoimmune thyroid disease, Sjögren syn-
      drome, collagen vascular disease, liver disease (PBC), IgA glomer-
      ulonephritis
  Miscellaneous associations
    Selective IgA deficiency, Down syndrome, hyposplenism, colitis
Asymptomatic form
  Patients identified through screening studies

---

and proximal muscle wasting in the child under 2 years of age is readily recognized as a manifestation of celiac disease. With the exception of a few countries such as Sweden, this type of presentation is no longer the most common form of the disease. For reasons that are still not clear, there has been an upward shift in the age of onset of symptoms, with many patients remaining asymptomatic until late childhood, adolescence, or even adulthood. Population screening studies have demonstrated that patients can be asymptomatic despite having significant changes on their small intestinal biopsies and that mucosal damage may precede symptoms by many years.

Most symptomatic patients still have gastrointestinal symptoms as their initial manifestation of celiac disease. Diarrhea is frequently present but may be mild or intermittent for prolonged periods of time. Abdominal pain, distension, and a feeling of bloating with flatulence are fairly frequent complaints in the older child and adolescent and may be incorrectly attributed to the irritable bowel syndrome or lactose intolerance. Nausea and vomiting occur less commonly, and in rare cases, constipation has been the major complaint.

Nongastrointestinal manifestations of celiac disease are being recognized with greater frequency. Linear growth failure or delayed onset of puberty may be the only initial manifestation in the pediatric population. Dermatitis herpetiformis, characterized by extremely itchy bullous lesions on the extensor surfaces of the limbs,

trunk, and scalp, is a feature of celiac disease and can occur without any intestinal symptoms. It is more common in adults but has been described in children. Behavioral changes, fatigue, anorexia, and unexplained iron deficiency anemia are additional initial manifestations.

Celiac disease is also strongly associated with a number of conditions, many of which are of the autoimmune type (Table 17-46). Up to 6% of patients with type 1 diabetes have been found to have celiac disease, and the condition is about 50 times more common in Down syndrome than in the general population. Selective IgA deficiency occurs in about 3% of patients with celiac disease as compared to about 1:500 of the general population. Because of this strong association it is recommended that patients with any of these conditions be screened for concomitant celiac disease.

DIAGNOSIS

SEROLOGIC SCREENING TESTS   The tests most readily available through commercial reference laboratories detect antibodies to gliadin and connective tissue of smooth muscle (endomysium and reticulin). Antigliadin antibodies (AGAs) of both the IgG and IgA classes are routinely measured, whereas antiendomysium and antireticulin antibodies are usually only of the IgA type. The IgG AGAs are highly sensitive but less specific for celiac disease, whereas IgA AGAs are less sensitive but have higher specificity. Antiendomysium and antireticulin antibodies are the most sensitive and specific tests available, with claims of almost 100% sensitivity and specificity for the antiendomysium antibody test. There is a possibility that the antiendomysium antibody is less reliable as a screening test in children under 2 years of age. Both the antiendomysium and antireticulin tests are based on an indirect immunofluorescent technique that renders them subject to observer interpretation error by inexperienced technologists.

Patients with selective IgA deficiency will not produce IgA antibodies to gliadin, endomysium, or reticulin. Selective IgA deficiency occurs in a significant proportion (3%) of individuals with celiac disease. To detect such individuals through serologic screening, it is best to request a panel of tests combining IgG AGAs, IgA AGAs, and antiendomysium antibodies. All those with elevated antiendomysium antibodies are at high risk for celiac disease and should undergo small intestinal biopsy for definitive diagnosis. Patients who test positive for IgG AGAs only may be selectively IgA deficient. Such individuals should have serum IgA levels measured, and, if found to be deficient, an intestinal biopsy is recommended to exclude celiac disease.

A new serologic test showing much promise measures antibodies to tissue transglutaminase. This test is also based on an IgA-type antibody. It is probable that transglutaminase is the autoantigen against which endomysium antibodies are directed. The sensitivity and specificity of the anti–tissue transglutaminase antibody appear equal to those of the antiendomysium antibody. The anti–tissue transglutaminase assay is not based on an immunofluorescent technique and thus provides a more objective test than the antiendomysium assay. In the future the anti–tissue transglutaminase assay may replace the antiendomysium antibody as the serologic screening test of choice for celiac disease.

SMALL INTESTINAL BIOPSY   Because no serologic test is 100% reliable, small intestinal biopsy remains an essential component of the diagnosis of celiac disease. Positive serologic screening facilitates the decision to proceed to small intestinal biopsy, but if the clinical suspicion for celiac disease is sufficiently strong, a biopsy should be performed even if all serologic tests are negative. Most pathologists readily recognize a uniformly flat mucosa with villous atrophy, crypt hyperplasia, and increased numbers of intraepithelial lymphocytes as celiac disease. It requires more experience to identify patients with less severe changes who are at an early stage of the disease. The earliest findings may consist only of a mucosal inflammatory cell infiltrate with increased intraepithelial lymphocytes. Thereafter, there is progressive elongation of the crypts, an increased mitotic index, and gradual reduction in villous height. Other disorders such as autoimmune enteropathy and milk protein–sensitive enteropathy may cause flattening of the intestinal mucosa with a mucosal inflammatory cell infiltrate and could be mistaken for celiac disease.

DIAGNOSTIC CRITERIA Previously three biopsies were required to confirm the diagnosis: the first to show the characteristic histologic changes at the time of presentation, the second to demonstrate complete recovery on a gluten-free diet, and the third to show recurrent damage after reintroduction of gluten into the diet. These recommendations have been revised, and for the majority of patients there are now only two mandatory requirements for diagnosis: (1) detection of the characteristic histologic changes on small intestinal biopsy while the patient is ingesting gluten and (2) complete clinical remission on a gluten-free diet. The presence of positive celiac disease serology before biopsy, with disappearance of the antibodies after introduction of the gluten-free diet, is strong supportive evidence for the diagnosis. In a small number of cases where the initial diagnosis is in doubt, it may be necessary to revert to the three-biopsy routine in order to confirm the diagnosis. The very young child with milk protein–sensitive enteropathy can resemble celiac disease both clinically and on intestinal biopsy and is an example of such an instance.

TREATMENT

A diagnosis of celiac disease mandates lifelong dietary exclusion of gluten from wheat and related products from barley and rye. Strict adherence to such a diet is difficult and requires constant vigilance on the part of the patient. For this reason it is essential to confirm the diagnosis by means of an intestinal biopsy before starting an exclusionary diet. In the short term, dietary modification will result in rapid remission of symptoms and correction of growth and nutritional deficiencies. Long-term benefits of adhering to the diet include preventing such complications as osteoporosis and reducing the risk for intestinal malignancies. Repeating the serologic tests at intervals can help the physician and patient monitor whether gluten and related products are being adequately excluded from the diet. In those who do not have selective IgA deficiency, the antiendomysium antibody is the best test for this purpose. Persistent elevation of this antibody, or recurrence of a positive test that had previously been negative, is indicative that the patient is knowingly, or unknowingly, continuing to ingest gluten. Elevation of antiendomysium antibody levels and recurrence of significant small intestinal mucosal damage after initial recovery can precede symptoms by several years in those who do not strictly adhere to the diet.

Adherence to the diet can be particularly difficult in children, so that consultation with an experienced pediatric dietician is useful. Cookbooks and various gluten-free specialty items are available for patients with celiac disease. Information can be provided by The Celiac Disease Foundation (*www.cdf@celiac.org*), The Friends of Celiac Disease Research (*www.friendsofceliac.com*) and local support groups.

References

Murray JA: The widening spectrum of celiac disease. Am J Clin Nutr 69: 354–365, 1999

Trier JS: Celiac sprue. N Engl J Med 25:1709–1719, 1991

Troncone R, Greco L, Auricchio S: Gluten-sensitive enteropathy. Pediatr Clin North Am 43:355–373, 1996

17.18.3   Idiopathic Chronic Diarrhea of Infancy

Ivor D. Hill

Idiopathic chronic diarrhea of infancy has also been called intractable diarrhea of infancy, protracted diarrhea of infancy, severe persistent diarrhea of infancy, and prolonged diarrhea of infancy. The condition is more common in developing countries and in low socioeconomic circumstances, where it remains a major cause of morbidity and mortality. It is characterized by ongoing watery diarrhea lasting for more than 2 weeks with stool losses often greatly in excess of 30 g/kg/24 h. The initial onset of diarrhea is usually in the infant less than 3 months old, but the condition can affect the older infant as well.

ETIOLOGY AND PATHOGENESIS

As the name "idiopathic" implies, the reasons for the ongoing diarrhea in these infants are not known. In most cases the onset resembles an acute infectious episode caused by either viral or bacterial gastroenteritis. However, unlike the majority in whom acute diarrhea is a self-limiting illness, in these cases the diarrhea simply persists. This occurs even in cases where an etiology for the acute event has been identified and treated appropriately. Risk factors for diarrhea becoming chronic in infants include prematurity, early age of onset, lack of breast-feeding, poor socioeconomic circumstances, and preexisting malnutrition.

In all cases there is subtotal to total villous atrophy of the small intestinal mucosa with increased cellular infiltrate and cuboidal epithelial cells. Intestinal villous repair is ineffective for reasons that are not entirely clear. A number of mechanisms, acting individually or in combination, have been proposed to account for the ongoing mucosal damage. Loss of intestinal brush border enzymes from mucosal damage leads to secondary disaccharide intolerance, with the resultant carbohydrate malabsorption aggravating the stool losses. In severe cases the mucosal damage is so extensive there is even monosaccharide intolerance. Enterocyte destruction may result in deficiency of enteric hormones such as secretin, pancreozymin-cholecystokinin, and gastrin. This in turn may cause secondary pancreatic insufficiency and aggravate the malabsorption of fats, carbohydrates, and proteins, or hypochlorhydria, promoting small intestinal bacterial overgrowth. There is good evidence that many infants with idiopathic chronic diarrhea have an abnormal proliferation of small intestinal bacteria. These organisms may contribute directly to the ongoing diarrhea by further damaging the intestinal mucosa. Alternatively, the bacteria may be only indirectly involved through the elaboration of toxins or the deconjugation and dehydroxylation of bile acids. Unconjugated bile acids are cytopathic to enterocytes and also inhibit water and electrolyte absorption by the colon. Severe mucosal damage renders the small intestine more permeable to intact protein, causing excessive antigen uptake. The inflammatory response to such antigens may lead to further mucosal destruction and perpetuate the problem. Ultimately there is a cycle of small intestinal mucosal damage leading to further damage. The term "postenteritis enteropathy" is sometimes used to describe this state.

The progressive small intestinal mucosal damage causes malabsorption of fats, carbohydrates, proteins, vitamins, and minerals. Nutrient losses increase as the stool output increases and are cumulative as long as the diarrhea continues. In the short term the most critical losses involve water and electrolytes. Unreplaced, these result in dehydration and electrolyte imbalance, which is the cause of death in many cases. In the longer term there is progressive malnutrition with loss of subcutaneous tissue, weight loss, and ultimately extreme wasting. Hypoalbuminemia, anemia, and vitamin (A, D, and K) and mineral (zinc) deficiencies are secondary consequences. Malnutrition per se impairs the infant's ability to repair the intestinal damage and leads to both cellular and humoral immunodeficiencies, placing the infant at risk for life-threatening systemic infections.

DIFFERENTIAL DIAGNOSIS

Diagnosis of idiopathic chronic diarrhea of infancy is by exclusion. A number of specific conditions causing severe ongoing diarrhea in the very young infant have now been identified. Generalized intestinal abnormalities are discussed in Sec. 17.18.4, and conditions associated with specific congenital transport defects are discussed in Sec. 17.18.6. Primary immune deficiencies and autoimmune enteropathy have to be considered, as do metabolic conditions (acrodermatitis enteropathica) and congenital enzyme deficiencies (lactase, sucrase-isomaltase, and lipase). Cystic fibrosis and anatomic problems such as Hirschsprung disease and malrotation need to be excluded. Acquired conditions associated with chronic diarrhea in this age group include parasitic infestations (giardiasis), pseudomembranous colitis, AIDS, protein-sensitive enteropathies, and endocrinopathies (hypoparathyroidism, hyperthyroidism, adrenal insufficiency, and VIPoma). Chronic diarrhea starting after the introduction of solid foods may be indicative of celiac disease in the older infant, as discussed in Sec. 17.18.2.

MANAGEMENT

Because of the complexity involved in reaching a final diagnosis and the high mortality associated with idiopathic chronic diarrhea of infancy, these patients should be referred to a center with the facilities and expertise necessary for investigation and treatment. Initial laboratory evaluation includes determination of serum electrolytes and acid-base status, stool microscopy for leukocytes, ova, and parasites, bacterial culture, and reducing substances. Measurement of stool electrolyte content may be helpful to confirm or exclude a secretory-type diarrhea, which is characteristic of some congenital conditions causing chronic diarrhea. Other blood tests include a chemistry panel with total protein and albumin levels, a complete blood count and differential, and, where indicated, a blood culture. Urine analysis and culture should be routine, as should measurement of sweat chloride. The diagnostic workup should also include a search for immunodeficiencies including AIDS. An intestinal biopsy is essential and should include specimens for both light and electron microscopy. Before biopsy, aspiration of small intestinal fluid can be obtained for culture of both aerobic and anaerobic bacteria.

Initial treatment consists of correcting dehydration and electrolyte imbalances. Where possible the enteral route is preferred for this purpose. Often the stool losses are of such magnitude that it is not possible to maintain hydration with enteral fluids alone, and

intravenous therapy is required. Following rehydration and correction of electrolyte abnormalities, the main aim of therapy is to improve nutrition in order to promote repair of the intestinal mucosa. Factors responsible for perpetuating the diarrhea should be identified and, where possible, removed. Semielemental diets containing glucose polymers and medium-chain triglycerides are recommended to limit the antigenic exposure and minimize the potential for carbohydrate malabsorption. Administering the feeds through a nasogastric tube as a constant infusion has been helpful in decreasing stool output in some cases. Treatment of small intestinal bacterial overgrowth with a combination of oral antibiotics (gentamicin 50 mg/kg/24 h in six divided doses for 3 days and metronidazole 15 mg/kg/24 in three divided doses) and cholestyramine (0.5–1 g every 6 hours for 5 days) may be effective. Underlying vitamin deficiencies require correction.

Despite all these measures, severe diarrhea continues in some of these infants. Stool nutrient losses cannot be replaced adequately by the enteral route, and the infant becomes progressively wasted. Initiation of parenteral nutrition before this critical stage is reached has drastically reduced the mortality associated with idiopathic chronic diarrhea of infancy. This is best administered through a central venous line so that adequate nutrients can be delivered. Placing the infant NPO at this stage often markedly reduces stool output, indicating that there is a large osmotic component to the diarrhea. Because enterally delivered nutrients are trophic to the intestinal mucosa, it is essential to restart feeds as soon as it is possible to do so without compromising the infant's condition. Usually within 5 to 7 days of starting parenteral nutrition, the infant will tolerate small-volume feeds of a semielemental formula without any marked increase in stool output. The volume of formula feeds can then be slowly increased with simultaneous decrease in the amount of parenteral nutrition.

References

Hill ID, Mann MD, Househam KC, Bowie MD: The use of oral gentamicin, metronidazole and cholestyramine in the treatment of severe persistent diarrhea of infants. J Pediatr 77:477–481, 1986

Hill ID, Mann MD, Moore L, Bowie MD: Duodenal microflora in infants with acute and persistent diarrhea. Arch Dis Child 58:330–334, 1983

Mann MD, Hill ID, Peat GM, Bowie MD: Protein and fat absorption in prolonged diarrhea in infancy. Arch Dis Child 57:268–273, 1982

17.18.4   Other Generalized Mucosal Disorders Causing Malabsorption

Ivor D. Hill

In addition to celiac disease there are a number of conditions that cause a small intestinal enteropathy with malabsorption and associated diarrhea (Table 17-47). A few of these are congenital or primary and usually present early in life. Others are acquired and, with few exceptions, present more commonly in adulthood.

MICROVILLUS ATROPHY   This is also known as congenital microvillus inclusion disease and familial protracted diarrhea or Davidson disease. It is inherited in an autosomal-recessive manner and is the most commonly recognized cause of congenital diarrhea. Light microscopy of the small intestine demonstrates diffuse thinning of the mucosa with hypoplastic villus atrophy, but without crypt hypertrophy or an inflammatory cell infiltrate. Electron microscopy re-

TABLE 17-47

GENERALIZED MUCOSAL DISORDERS CAUSING MALABSORPTION

Mucosal structural abnormalities
  Microvillus atrophy
  Tufting enteropathy
  Lymphangiectasia
    Primary
    Secondary
Immune disorders
  Primary immune deficiencies
    Selective IgA deficiency
    Common variable immunodeficiency
    Severe combined immunodeficiency
    Chronic granulomatous disease
  Acquired immune deficiencies
    HIV infection
    Malnutrition
    Immunosuppressive therapy
  Autoimmune enteropathy
Food-induced enteropathy
  Protein-sensitive enteropathy
  Eosinophilic enteropathy
Infection-induced enteropathy
  Bacterial infections
    Tropical sprue
    Whipple disease
    Immunoproliferative small intestinal disease (IPSID)
  Parasitic infestations
    Giardia, Cryptosporidium, coccidiosis
Drug-induced
  Neomycin
  Colchicine
  Methotrexate
Miscellaneous
  Postinfectious enteropathy
  Lymphoma
  Sarcoid
  Radiation enteritis
  Ischemic enteritis
  Collagen vascular disorders
  Mastocytosis
  Collagenous sprue

veals mucosal surface enterocytes that lack microvilli completely or have sparse shortened villi. The apical cytoplasm of the enterocyte contains a marked increase in electron-dense secretory granules of various sizes, some of which contain glycocalyx and brush border–related material. The hallmark of the disease is the presence of microvilli within involutions of the apical membrane. The crypt epithelium is usually well preserved, as are other epithelial cells such as goblet cells, Paneth cells, and enteroendocrine cells. These structural changes are associated with a marked secretory state with respect to sodium and water and impaired glucose-coupled sodium uptake.

Affected infants present in the neonatal period with severe watery diarrhea and failure to thrive. In some cases, maternal polyhydramnios suggests diarrhea was present in utero. Fecal water losses are massive (100 to 800 mL/kg/d) and continue even when the infant is maintained on parenteral hyperalimentation and given nothing by mouth. Most tests of intestinal absorption function, such as fecal fat analysis and D-xylose uptake, are abnormal, and stool electrolyte content is consistently high in keeping with a se-

cretory-type diarrhea. The differential diagnosis includes other causes of congenital diarrhea such as congenital chloride-losing diarrhea, congenital sodium-losing diarrhea, primary bile acid malabsorption, and congenital short gut. Mortality is in excess of 80% within the first year. Treatment has been largely unsuccessful. Many dietary manipulations and medications have been tried without benefit. Therapeutic agents that have been tried include corticosteroids, antibiotics, disodium cromoglycate, prostaglandin synthase inhibitors, and cholestyramine. The long-acting somatostatin analog octreotide may decrease the stool output but does not alter the course of the disease. In nearly all cases life can be sustained only by parenteral nutrition.

SMALL INTESTINAL LYMPHANGIECTASIA This is characterized by ectasia of the enteric lymphatics. It may be congenital or primary when it is caused by malformation of the lymphatic system or secondary to diseases causing obstruction to intestinal lymphatic drainage. The primary abnormality is often associated with lymphatic abnormalities elsewhere in the body. These include hypoplasia or aplasia of the peripheral lymphatic system with lymphedema, chylous ascites, and chylothorax, or the lymphangiectasia may be part of a syndrome such as Noonan, Klippel-Trénaunay-Weber, and Turner. Diseases causing secondary obstruction to lymph flow include constrictive pericarditis, congestive heart failure, retroperitoneal fibrosis, retroperitoneal neoplasms, and mesenteric tuberculosis.

In both the primary and secondary types of lymphangiectasia there is usually diffuse involvement of the intestine. Occasionally the disorder is localized to one or more areas of the small bowel. With the exception of long-chain fatty acids and fat-soluble vitamins, small intestinal absorptive function is usually intact. However, rupture of dilated mucosal lymphatics into the intestinal lumen leads to loss of protein-rich lymph containing albumin, globulins, and lymphocytes.

Onset of symptoms in the primary form is in childhood and usually before 10 years of age. The initial presentation is often with peripheral edema and hypoproteinemia without proteinuria or hepatic dysfunction. Gastrointestinal symptoms vary from none or mild to severe. Symptoms include intermittent diarrhea, nausea, vomiting, and abdominal pain. A protein-losing enteropathy is confirmed by demonstrating elevated levels of fecal α_1-antitrypsin and, together with the presence of peripheral blood lymphocytopenia, should raise the possibility of intestinal lymphangiectasia. The diagnosis is confirmed on intestinal biopsy, which demonstrates dilated lymphatic vessels in the lamina propria and submucosa of the small intestine. There is no inflammatory cell infiltrate. The villi show no signs of atrophy but are distorted, often appearing swollen and broad. Treatment is dependent on the cause. In the small number of cases where the abnormality is localized to a section of the intestine, resection of this area is curative. When the lymphangiectasia is secondary to conditions such as constrictive pericarditis, treatment of the underlying disease will lead to resolution of the intestinal losses. In the diffuse primary form of lymphangiectasia, treatment requires limiting the amount of dietary long-chain fat to 5 to 10 g per day and providing a diet that is high in protein and medium-chain triglycerides. The medium-chain triglycerides are absorbed directly into the portal system, thereby minimizing distension of the lymphatics.

AUTOIMMUNE ENTEROPATHY This life-threatening disorder is characterized by intractable diarrhea. It usually occurs in infancy with rare reports in older children and adults. The condition may be associated with other autoimmune diseases including membranous glomerulonephritis, insulin-dependent diabetes, collagen vascular disorders, hemolytic anemia, autoimmune hepatitis, and hypothyroidism. Light microscopy of small intestinal biopsies demonstrates partial or complete villus atrophy and a mononuclear cell infiltrate in the lamina propria. The disorder appears to be autoimmune by virtue of the presence of autoantibodies to the enterocytes and other tissues (eg, antibodies to pancreatic islet cells, thyroid, parietal cells, and renal tubular epithelium). Diagnosis is dependent on (1) prolonged diarrhea with histologic features of small intestinal enteropathy, (2) lack of clinical or histologic response to an exclusion diet or a period of complete bowel rest with parenteral nutrition, and (3) the demonstration of circulating autoantibodies to gut and other tissues. A number of therapies have been attempted. Parenteral nutrition is often necessary to prevent progressive malnutrition. Corticosteroids, azathioprine, and cyclosporine have been used with varying results. Most recently the immunosuppressant tacrolimus (FK-506) has been used successfully in a small number of cases. Serial determination of enterocyte autoantibodies may be of benefit for prognostic purposes. Declining or low titers are associated with recovery, whereas persistent high titers indicate a poorer prognosis with worse outcome for the patient.

TROPICAL SPRUE This malabsorption syndrome is seen in visitors or residents of endemic tropical regions of the world. These areas include India, parts of Asia, the Philippines, the northern part of South America, Central America, some Caribbean countries, and central and southern Africa. The condition occurs in children but is more common in adults. It is most probably infectious in origin, but no specific pathogen has been identified. Damage to the intestinal mucosa progresses from the jejunum to the ileum. On small intestinal histology there is flattening of the villi, crypt elongation, and chronic inflammatory cell infiltration of the lamina propria. These changes are associated with loss of intestinal disaccharidases and malabsorption of sugars, fats, folate, vitamin B_{12}, and vitamin A. Hypoproteinemia occurs secondary to both excessive enteric losses (protein-losing enteropathy) and impaired absorption of amino acids and dipeptides. Clinical symptoms are usually insidious in onset and evolve through stages. Fatigue, weakness, anorexia, and acute diarrhea characterize the early stage. The acute diarrhea progresses to a more chronic form with steatorrhea accompanied by abdominal cramps and flatulence. Signs of nutritional deficiencies appear, including night blindness, cheilosis, glossitis, stomatitis, and hyperkeratosis. In the final stage there are muscle wasting, edema, abdominal distension, and a macrocytic anemia. These changes occur over a period of 6 months to years. On occasions the presentation is more acute, and the stages are accelerated over a few months. The condition should be suspected in patients with diarrhea and malabsorption who have lived in or recently visited an endemic area. Differential diagnosis includes parasitic infestations (*Giardia, Stongyloides stercoralis, Isospora, Capillaria philippinensis*), celiac disease, HIV infection, tuberculous enteritis, and small intestinal bacterial overgrowth syndromes. Treatment with oral administration of broad-spectrum antibiotics and nutritional supplements, including folic acid and B_{12}, usually leads to dramatic improvement.

WHIPPLE DISEASE This rare, multisystem disorder virtually always involves the small intestine, causing a severe malabsorption syndrome. Other features commonly encountered are arthritis/arthralgia, polyserositis, fever, and central nervous system symptoms.

It is caused by a gram-positive actinomycete, *Trophyrema whippellii*, a fastidious organism that has not yet been cultured. Small intestinal biopsy reveals villi that are flattened and wide. The lamina propria is extensively infiltrated with large macrophages containing PAS-positive granules representing remnants of the cell walls of degenerated phagocytosed bacilli. Numerous tiny bacilli are located in the upper epithelium, most abundantly beneath the absorptive epithelium. Mucosal and submucosal lymphatics are dilated, probably because of lymphatic obstruction by enlarged mesenteric lymph nodes. Treatment with antibiotics produces dramatic improvement, but long-term therapy is necessary.

References

Bousvaros A, Leichtner AM, Book L, et al: Treatment of pediatric autoimmune enteropathy with tacrolimus (FK506). Gastroenterology 111: 237–243, 1996

Davidson GP. Enteropathies of unknown origin. In: Walker WA, Durie PR, Hamilton JR, Walker-Smith JA, Watkins JB, eds: Pediatric Gastrointestinal Disease: Pathophysiology, Diagnosis, Management, 2nd ed. Philadelphia, CV Mosby, 862–867: 1996

Garrido JA, Sheehy TW. Tropical sprue. In: Haubrich WS, Schaffner F, Berk JE, eds: Bockus Gastroenterology, 5th ed. Philadelphia, WB Saunders, 1049–1062: 1995

Mirakian R, Richardson A, Milla PJ, et al: Protracted diarrhoea of infancy: evidence in support of an autoimmune variant. Br Med J 293:1132–1136, 1986

Phillips AD, Schmitz J: Familial microvillous atrophy: a clinico-pathological survey of 23 cases. J Pediatr Gastroenterol Nutr 14:380–396, 1992

Shifrin HD. Whipple's disease. In: Haubrich WS, Schaffner F, Berk JE, eds: Bockus Gastroenterology, 5th ed. Philadelphia, WB Saunders, 1183–1194: 1995

17.18.5   Carbohydrate Malabsorption

Ramon G. Montes

Children with carbohydrate malabsorption may be asymptomatic or present with some combination of watery diarrhea, bloating, crampy abdominal pain, or flatulence. Unabsorbed carbohydrates in the small bowel and colon exert significant osmotic pressure, which results in the secretion of fluid and electrolytes into the lumen and, in some, a watery fecal output. A portion of the carbohydrate entering the colon is fermented by colonic bacteria, with the production of lactic acid and other short-chain organic acids. These compounds may exacerbate symptoms because they also are osmotically active and, in addition, directly stimulate colonic motility. However, the colonic mucosa is capable of absorbing significant amounts of these acids, thus reducing the osmotic load and potential fluid loss in the stool. The remaining organic acids are excreted in the feces, accounting for the acidic stools that are associated with carbohydrate malabsorption. Fermentation of malabsorbed carbohydrate also results in production of the gases hydrogen, methane, and carbon dioxide. Accumulation of these gases in the colon may lead to abdominal distension and flatulence.

In addition to an individual's digestive and absorptive capacity for a given substrate, other variables such as the amount ingested, rate of gastric emptying (influenced by the accompanying meal), and the metabolic activity of the colonic flora determine whether malabsorption produces symptoms in a given patient. This explains why many individuals with primary lactase deficiency can tolerate

TABLE 17-48

COMMON CONDITIONS ASSOCIATED WITH CARBOHYDRATE MALABSORPTION

Primary or genetic
Primary lactase nonpersistence ("adult onset")
Sucrase-isomaltase deficiency
Glucose-galactose malabsorption
Congenital lactase deficiency
Ontogenetic
Lactase deficiency of the premature infant
Deficiency of pancreatic amylase in infancy
Secondary or acquired
Rotavirus infection
Giardia lamblia infection
Small-bowel bacterial overgrowth
Short-bowel syndrome
Cow's milk– and soy protein–sensitive enteropathy
AIDS
Physiological (dietary sugars)
Fructose
Sorbitol
Fiber
Vegetable oligosaccharides (eg, beans)

nutritionally significant amounts of milk without developing marked symptoms.

Malabsorption of sugars can result from primary heritable deficiencies of enzymes and transport processes that are required for their digestion or secondary to a variety of conditions such as intestinal mucosal injury. Additionally, ontogenetic forms of carbohydrate malabsorption occur during infancy secondary to the immaturity of some digestive enzymes. For example, transient lactose malabsorption is frequent in premature infants until lactase activity matures, and a degree of starch maldigestion occurs in the first year after birth because of decreased secretion of pancreatic amylase. Table 17-48 lists common examples of clinical conditions associated with carbohydrate malabsorption.

Some carbohydrates are normally malabsorbed in all individuals because of the absence of enzyme systems in humans that would be capable of their hydrolysis. Examples include structural components of plant cells (ie, dietary fiber) such as cellulose and other polysaccharides as well as indigestible oligosaccharides, including stachyose, raffinose, and verbascose, which are abundant in some cereals, legumes, and vegetables such as beans. Health-conscious parents may give inappropriately large amounts of these foods to their children, with resulting development of GI symptoms because of malabsorption with gas formation and resultant abdominal pain.

PRIMARY CARBOHYDRATE MALABSORPTION

LACTASE DEFICIENCY (LACTOSE INTOLERANCE) Lactose, a dimer of glucose and galactose, is the carbohydrate supplied in mammalian milk. Lactase, an enzyme located on the brush border near the tips of the villi, cleaves lactose, allowing absorption of its component parts. Primary lactase deficiency, also known as adult-onset lactase deficiency, is the most common of the genetically determined causes of carbohydrate malabsorption and results from a postweaning decline in intestinal lactase-specific activity. Normal infants and young children are uniformly capable of ingesting lactose-containing breast milk and other mammalian milk products. Genetically programmed down-regulation of the lactase gene in

chromosome 2q21 is detectable in children as early as the second year of life, although the onset and extent are variable. Persistence or nonpersistence of lactase activity in older children and adults is genetically determined and cannot be modulated by mantaining lactose in the diet. A genetic polymorphism acting *cis* to the lactase gene determines high or low messenger RNA expression and activity. Although persistence of lactase is genetically dominant to nonpersistence, the majority of the world's adults become "lactase deficient," except for certain Caucasian populations of northern and central European descent as well as some nomadic African tribes. The onset of symptoms usually begins after 2 years of age in blacks and Hispanics and after age 10 in most patients of northern European ancestry. In many cultures, milk products compose only a small part of the adult diet, so the symptoms of lactose intolerance are rare despite the low activity of lactase. Symptoms of diarrhea and recurrent abdominal pain occur only in those individuals with low lactase activity who ingest large quantities of lactose-containing products.

Congenital lactase deficiency presents with diarrhea shortly after birth, when lactose-containing feedings are introduced. In this very rare disorder (except in Finland), inherited as an autosomal-recessive trait, the mucosal surface is otherwise normal, and the diarrhea resolves promptly on removal of lactose from the diet.

FRUCTOSE AND SORBITOL MALABSORPTION The monosaccharides fructose and sorbitol are widely used in commercial food products, but large amounts of their monosaccharide form are not present in less-refined food products. Fructose is used extensively as an inexpensive sweetener, instead of sucrose, which is the more expensive dimer of fructose and glucose. Carbonated beverages, often consumed in significant amounts by children, contain large quantities of fructose as high-fructose corn syrup. Sorbitol is a poorly absorbed sugar that is present together with fructose in some fruits and is used in many "diet" products as a sucrose substitute. Fructose and perhaps sorbitol are absorbed across the mucosal surface by facilitated diffusion via a specific saturable carrier protein located on the apical membrane of the enterocyte (GLUT5).

Like lactose, ingested fructose and sorbitol may be malabsorbed if they are ingested in excessive quantities. Malabsorption of fructose and sorbitol has been demonstrated to be associated with clinical symptoms in otherwise healthy subjects. Approximately 70% of adults and children fail to absorb fructose completely at a dose of 2 g/kg (50 g in adults). Malabsorption of fructose frequently is associated with symptoms of diarrhea, abdominal distension, and pain. Sorbitol and fructose appear to share GLUT5 as their transport protein because malabsorption of fructose-sorbitol mixtures exceeds the sum of the malabsorbed amounts of the individual sugars. Glucose and amino acids appear to facilitate the transport of fructose across the mucosal surface, probably by increasing water flow through the apical membrane, so that when fructose is ingested as a component of sucrose or with equimolar amounts of glucose, absorption is complete in most subjects. This explains why ingestion of fruit juices with a high fructose:glucose ratio and in which sorbitol also is present (eg, apple, pear) as well as sorbitol-containing products such as chewing gum, candy, popsicles, and medications (eg, acetaminophen syrups) may cause chronic nonspecific diarrhea and recurrent abdominal pain.

Isolated fructose malabsorption is a rare autosomal-recessive disorder that has been described recently. It is distinct clinically from physiological malabsorption of fructose, but specific mutations in the GLUT5 gene located in chromosome 1p31 have not yet been identified.

SUCRASE-ISOMALTASE DEFICIENCY Sucrase-isomaltase deficiency presents later in infancy on introduction of sucrose-containing formula or fruits. The incidence is approximately 0.5% except in Canada's indigenous peoples, in whom an incidence as high as 10% has been reported. The mucosal surface has a normal structure, but the levels of sucrase activity are very low, and maltase activity is moderately decreased. These children are intolerant of sucrose and large amounts of starch, the 1,6 bonds of which require the action of isomaltase for cleavage. Thus, these children may have persistent diarrhea when they are given "elemental" formula containing corn-starch hydrolysates as a carbohydrate source. Symptoms of sucrase-isomaltase deficiency vary from severe diarrhea in infancy to intermittent, bothersome diarrhea and abdominal pain in the older child. Frequently, symptoms decrease with increasing age despite the persistence of the abnormal enzyme activity, perhaps because of colonic adaptation to malabsorbed sugar. The sucrase-isomaltase gene has been localized to chromosome 3q25-26, but its mutations have not yet been characterized. Inheritance is autosomal recessive.

GLUCOSE-GALACTOSE MALABSORPTION Glucose-galactose malabsorption results from a defect in the brush border site for sodium-linked glucose and galactose transport (SGLT1). Over 30 mutations unique to each kindred have been identified in the gene, located in chromosome 22q13.1. This rare condition is inherited as an autosomal-recessive trait, and it presents at birth with diarrhea, dehydration, and metabolic acidosis in an infant who is fed breast milk or a standard lactose-containing formula. Fructose is the only carbohydrate that can be tolerated.

SECONDARY CARBOHYDRATE MALABSORPTION

Malabsorption of carbohydrates is very common in several intestinal diseases that cause intestinal mucosal damage or atrophy (Table 17-48). Injury to the brush border by infectious agents, notably rotavirus and *Giardia lamblia*, commonly causes transient intolerance to lactose. In severe cases, malabsorption of other disaccharides, and even acquired monosaccharide intolerance, may develop. Contamination of the small bowel by bacteria, which is associated with immunodeficiency syndromes and disorders affecting intestinal motility, often leads to disaccharidase deficiencies and to impaired monosaccharide transport. In this condition, bacterial proteases and glycosidases degrade brush border enzymes, and products of bacterial metabolism, including deconjugated bile acids, interfere with glucose transport. Infants with short bowel also malabsorb carbohydrate because of insufficient surface area to which sugars may be exposed for enzymatic digestion and transport. Mucosal damage that is induced by other dietary components, as in immune-mediated cow's milk– and soy protein–sensitive enteropathy and celiac sprue, also frequently will lead to sugar malabsorption. Pancreatic insufficiency in cystic fibrosis results in maldigestion of starch because of reduced or absent pancreatic amylase. Carbohydrate malabsorption also has been reported in HIV infection, and lactase deficiency is common in children with AIDS who have diarrhea.

DIAGNOSIS AND MANAGEMENT OF CARBOHYDRATE MALABSORPTION

Neither patients nor their physicians can accurately predict lactose malabsorption based on the patient's dietary and symptom history. Attempts at empiric diagnosis are difficult, both because of the ubiquitous presence of sugars in commercial food products and because the prolonged elimination of foods (in particular, milk

products) can have serious nutritional consequences. Monitoring symptom improvement with reductions in sorbitol or fructose ingestion is more easily accomplished, but the social and psychological consequences of diet restriction often demand that a more objective diagnostic test be used. Carbohydrate malabsorption usually should be established objectively by diagnostic tests.

Measurement of reducing sugars in the stool (Clinitest) and fecal pH provide useful office or bedside screening methods. These tests require that the offending carbohydrate be in the patient's diet at the time of sampling and that a liquid stool be sampled. The sugar usually is in the aqueous portion of the stool. It may soak into the diaper, however, and ongoing fermentation destroys the carbohydrate, yielding false-negative results. Fresh stool, preferably obtained directly from the rectum, is most reliable. Unfortunately, these screening tests lack sensitivity and cannot exclude the diagnosis of carbohydrate malabsorption.

The breath hydrogen test is the most reliable diagnostic method. When carbohydrate is malabsorbed, the bacteria normally present in the colon lumen produce hydrogen gas, which is absorbed across the colon mucosa into the bloodstream and expired in breath. The breath is sampled sequentially after the patient ingests a known amount of the test carbohydrate substance. A rise of more than 10 to 20 ppm in expired hydrogen indicates that the carbohydrate is malabsorbed. An early rise in breath hydrogen suggests bacterial overgrowth. If children have recently received antibiotics, the colonic bacteria may be altered such that hydrogen is not produced, which decreases the reliability of this test. In addition, these tests do not exclude secondary causes of carbohydrate malabsorption such as celiac disease.

The definitive study for disaccharidase activity involves endoscopic biopsy with measurement of mucosal enzyme concentrations. Normal values at various age ranges are available, but this test is expensive and usually not performed unless the child is undergoing biopsy to exclude secondary causes of carbohydrate malabsorption.

Treatment of carbohydrate malabsorption requires reduction or removal of the specific sugar from the patient's diet. During infancy, malabsorption of lactose and other disaccharides usually is secondary and therefore transient, and a large variety of proprietary formulas are available to modify the infant's carbohydrate intake. For example, ontogenetic lactose malabsorption in premature infants currently is managed by using glucose polymers as the source for at least 50% of the carbohydrate in formulas designed for these babies. Congenital sucrase-isomaltase deficiency is managed with lactose-containing formulas and avoidance of sucrose-containing foods. Sacrosidase, an enzyme derived from the yeast *Saccharomyces cerevisiae* that has potent sucrase activity, has recently become available as a treatment, allowing these patients to eat an unrestricted diet. Glucose-galactose malabsorption is managed by eliminating all dietary carbohydrate except for fructose, using "modular" carbohydrate-free formulas to which fructose is added.

In older children and adults with primary lactase deficiency, avoidance of milk and other foods that are rich in lactose often is sufficient because many patients with lactose malabsorption will tolerate foods with smaller amounts of lactose (eg, cheese). Total elimination of lactose or dairy products rarely is necessary. Alternatives for patients who want to consume milk or in whom adequate calcium intake cannot be achieved by other means include drinking milk together with meals to delay gastric emptying, using prehydrolyzed milk that has been treated with microbial-derived lactase enzyme (Lactaid), or ingestion of this enzyme with milk products at mealtime. Several commercial preparations are available over the counter. These preparations in caplet or tablet form can be crushed and sprinkled over lactose-containing foods and therefore are suitable for children who cannot chew or swallow the intact product. Yogurt containing active live culture from which microbial lactase is released often is well tolerated by lactase-deficient individuals and is an alternative source of calcium.

When lactose malabsorption is diagnosed in infants and young children, restriction of dietary lactose may modify the symptoms. An underlying cause should be thoroughly sought, however, because primary lactase deficiency usually presents at a later age. If available, definitive treatment (eg, eradication of *Giardia* infestation or avoidance of gluten in celiac disease) will result in recovery of intestinal lactase activity and permit the patient to resume lactose intake. The child who is being evaluated for chronic diarrhea, gas, abdominal distension, or pain and is ingesting significant amounts of fructose or sorbitol in juices or soda may be managed initially with dietary restriction. If the symptoms subside, a diagnostic investigation seldom is required. For patients who experience flatulence following consumption of beans, legumes, and other foods containing indigestible oligosaccharides, commercial preparations of tilactase (an enzyme with α-galactosidase activity) are available.

References

Hoekstra JH, van den Aker JHL: Facilitating effect of amino acids on fructose and sorbitol absorption in children. J Pediatr Gastroenterol Nutr 23:118–124, 1996

Lloyd-Still JD: Chronic diarrhea of childhood and the misuse of elimination diets. J Pediatr 95:10–13, 1979

Martin MG: Defects in Na/glucose transporter (SGLT1) trafficking and function cause glucose-galactose malabsorption. Nature Genet 12:216–220, 1996

Montes RG, Perman JA: Lactose intolerance: pinpointing the source of nonspecific gastrointestinal symptoms. Postgrad Med 89:175–184, 1991

Smith MM, Davis M, Chasalow FI, Lifshitz F: Carbohydrate absorption from fruit juice in young children. Pediatrics 95:340–344, 1995

Treem WR, McAdams L, Stanford L, Kastoff G, Justinich C, Hyams J: Sacrosidase therapy for congenital sucrase-isomaltase deficiency. J Pediatr Gastroenterol Nutr 28:137–142, 1999

Wang Y, Harvey CB, Hollox EJ, et al: The genetically programmed down-regulation of lactase in children. Gastroenterology 114:1230–1236, 1998

17.18.6   Congenital Transport Defects

Ivor D. Hill

Congenital transport defects involving both macro- and micronutrients are listed in Table 17-47. All are uncommon, and symptoms vary from none or mild to severe with diarrhea, dehydration, and failure to thrive.

FAT TRANSPORT DEFECTS

Intraluminal lipolysis of dietary fats generates fatty acids that are passively transported into the enterocyte, where chylomicrons are formed. Chylomicrons are assembled in the endoplasmic reticulum from triglycerides, phospholipids, cholesterol esters, and apolipoproteins before transport to the Golgi apparatus. From the Golgi apparatus the chylomicrons undergo exocytosis with subsequent transport through the lymphatic system to the systemic circulation.

Apoprotein (apo) B is the major protein component of prebetalipoprotein (also called very low-density lipoprotein, VLDL) and the chylomicron. *Abetalipoproteinemia* is a rare autosomal-recessive disorder characterized by the congenital absence of apo B, which results in an inability to synthesize chylomicrons. *Hypobetalipoproteinemia* is an autosomal-dominant condition characterized by a deficiency of apo B. Homozygotes for hypobetalipoproteinemia are clinically similar to those with abetalipoproteinemia. Heterozygotes have low plasma cholesterol and low to normal triglyceride levels but are usually clinically asymptomatic. These disorders result in the accumulation of large lipid droplets in the cytoplasm of the enterocyte, as demonstrated on small intestinal biopsy. Symptoms usually begin in infancy with malodorous diarrhea and failure to thrive. Features of fat-soluble vitamin deficiencies may present after 5 years of age with night blindness, nystagmus, dysarthria, and sensory ataxia from loss of position and vibratory sensation. Retinitis pigmentosa is a constant finding. Alteration in membrane lipids leads to acanthocytosis in the peripheral blood. A very low serum cholesterol and barely detectable triglyceride level should point to the diagnosis, which is confirmed by the absence of β-lipoprotein in the blood. Treatment consists of restricting dietary intake of long-chain fats and supplementation with medium-chain triglycerides. Large doses of vitamin E and the water-soluble form of vitamins A and K should be supplied with routine monitoring of the blood levels of all fat-soluble vitamins. Adequate linoleic acid should be provided.

Chylomicron retention disease (Anderson disease) is an autosomal-recessive condition that results from defective exocytosis of chylomicrons. Clinical features are similar to those of abetalipoproteinemia. Diarrhea, steatorrhea, and decreased serum cholesterol and phospholipid levels are characteristic, but acanthocytosis, retinitis pigmentosa, and neurologic abnormalities are less severe or absent. β-Lipoprotein levels are approximately 50% of normal, and there is absence of postprandial circulating chylomicrons. Intestinal biopsy demonstrates enterocytes filled with chylomicrons.

AMINO ACID TRANSPORT DEFECTS

Congenital defects of specific amino acid transport involve both the small intestinal enterocyte and the proximal renal tubule. The clinical effects of these defects vary from none to severe life-threatening diseases.

Lysinuric protein intolerance results from a defect in transport of the dibasic amino acids lysine, ornithine, and arginine and results in massive lysinuria with inadequate urea formation and hyperammonemia after protein ingestion. *Hartnup disease* is caused by a defect in transport of free neutral amino acids. Intestinal malabsorption results in deficiency of nicotinamide synthesized from tryptophan, leading to pellagra-type manifestations. *Blue diaper syndrome* is caused by isolated malabsorption of tryptophan. *Oast-house urine disease* results from a selective defect in methionine absorption and is named for the peculiar odor imparted by the urine. *Lowe syndrome* results from malabsorption of lysine and arginine and is characterized by mental retardation, cataracts, hypotonia, renal disease, vitamin D–resistant rickets, and choreoathetosis. Defects in amino acid transport are detected by analysis of urinary amino acids. Details of clinical presentation, diagnosis, and management are discussed in Sec. 9.2.

OTHER SPECIFIC TRANSPORT DEFECTS

Congenital chloride diarrhea is an autosomal-recessive condition characterized by a selective defect in intestinal chloride transport. The defect involves the Cl^-/HCO_3^- exchange transport system in the epithelium of the ileum and colon. The dominant feature is watery diarrhea with stools that contain a high chloride and low bicarbonate concentration and a low pH. The infants are often born prematurely but are of normal size for gestational age. Polyhydramnios is a constant feature, indicative of the intrauterine onset of diarrhea. There is frequently abdominal distension with visible intestinal peristalsis that may lead one to suspect intestinal obstruction. The diarrhea rapidly causes dehydration and severe electrolyte disturbance characterized by hypochloremia, hyponatremia, and metabolic alkalosis. Treatment involves continuous replacement of the water and electrolyte losses. Initially this needs to be delivered intravenously, but very soon after birth it can be delivered via the enteral route. With treatment the prognosis is good, and most children eventually become continent for feces by 3 to 4 years of age.

Congenital sodium diarrhea is rare condition is characterized by a defect in intestinal sodium transport. The defect involves the Na^+/H^+ exchange transport system in the jejunum, ileum, and colon. Clinical features are similar to those of congenital chloride diarrhea. The pregnancy is often complicated by maternal polyhydramnios. Watery diarrhea starts at birth, and the stools characteristically have very high sodium content. In contrast to congenital chloride diarrhea, stool chloride concentration is lower than that of sodium, and the stools tend to be alkaline. The diarrhea rapidly causes dehydration and an electrolyte disturbance characterized by hyponatremia and hypochloremia, but unlike congenital chloride diarrhea there is a metabolic acidosis. Treatment involves replacing the ongoing water and electrolyte losses. Provision of sodium in the form of sodium citrate alleviates the acidosis. With treatment normal growth and development can be anticipated, and continence for feces can be expected by 3 to 4 years of age.

Acrodermatitis enteropathica is an autosomal recessive disorder of zinc absorption, likely resulting from the absence of a low molecular weight zinc-binding factor that is produced by the pancreas, binds dietary zinc and transports it into epithelial cells. It is characterized by dermatitis with bullous and pustular lesions, alopecia, ophthalmic manifestations including blepharitis, conjunctivitis and corneal opacities, diarrhea and growth retardation. Timing of the onset of symptoms during infancy depends on the duration of breast-feeding because breast milk contains the zinc binding factor. Infants that are not breast fed develop symptoms within 1 to 2 months after birth. Breast fed infants become symptomatic 2 to 3 weeks after weaning. The differential diagnosis includes exclusion of other causes of zinc deficiency that include total parenteral nutrition, cirrhosis of the liver, renal disease (nephritic syndrome, renal tubular dysfunction), other skin disorders such as psoriasis, burn injuries, and essential fatty acid deficiency, sickle cell disease and malnutrition associated with excessive alcohol intake, or ingestion of foods that contain a large amount of phosphate. Transient zinc deficiency has been reported in breast fed infants, possibly secondary to an inherited deficit of mammary zinc secretion or absent zinc binding factor in the breast milk.

Diagnosis is based on the presence of clinical findings and documentation of chronic zinc deficiency with plasma zinc concentrations below 50 μg/dL. Normal concentrations are 90 +/− 20 μg/DL (SD). Other laboratory parameters that confirm the diagnosis include decreased activity of zinc-dependent enzymes such as serum alkaline phosphatase and low red blood cell and urinary zinc levels. The gene responsible for the disorder has been mapped to chromsome 8q24.3 between D8S1713 and S8S373, thus molecular diagnostic confirmation should be possible. The treatment of choice is oral administration of 35–100 mg elemental zinc per day, in divided doses. Zinc sulfate heptahydrate (50 mg elemental zinc

in 220 mg) is commonly used, but other salts are available. This results in correction of all abnormalities. The treatment must be continued indefinitely, with adjustments of dose for growth rates and stresses such as intercurrent illnesses. Although massive doses of zinc (12 to 24 g) can result in toxicity (nausea, vomiting, lethargy, muscular incoordination, dizziness, renal failure), the safety and efficacy of zinc sulfate make it the treatment of choice for acrodermatitis enteropathica.

A number of other specific mucosal transport defects have been identified. *Congenital glucose-galactose malabsorption* is discussed in Sec. 17.18.5. Defects in absorption of vitamin B_{12} and folate present with megaloblastic anemia in infancy, as discussed in Sec. 19.2.1. Bile acid metabolism and primary bile acid malabsorption are discussed in Sec.18.4. Selective defects in the absorption of copper, causing Menke disease, is discussed in Sec. 9.11.2. Primary hypomagnesemia with secondary hypocalcemia is discussed in Sec. 24.11.5.

Reference

Desjeux JF: Congenital transport defects. In: Walker WA, Durie PR, Hamilton JR, Walker-Smith JA, Watkins JB, eds: Pediatric Gastrointestinal Disease: Pathophysiology, Diagnosis, Management, 2nd ed. Philadelphia, CV Mosby, 792–816, 1996

Wang K, Pugh EW, Griffen S et al: Homozygosity mapping places the acrodermatitis enteropathica gene on chromosomal region 8q24.3. Am J Hum Genetic 68:1055–1060, 2001

17.18.7   Short-Bowel Syndrome

Michael K. Farrell

The short-bowel syndrome is a severe, generalized malabsorptive disorder, usually resulting from congenital malformations or massive resection of the small intestine. Common antecedent causes in children include necrotizing enterocolitis, volvulus with or without malrotation, multiple atresias, and gastroschisis. Less common causes include severe meconium peritonitis, congenital short-bowel syndrome, and long-segment Hirschsprung disease. Malabsorption primarily results from the decreased mucosal absorptive surface, but other factors, including further mucosal injury, bile acid deficiency, and bacterial overgrowth, also contribute. Prognosis depends on the region and length of the resected bowel.

Total small intestinal length doubles from 26 to 38 weeks of gestation, reaching a length of between 200 and 300 cm in the normal full-term neonate. Further growth results in small bowel lengths of 600 to 800 cm in the normal adult. Hence, infants have a better prognosis because of the potential for further intestinal growth. It is difficult to quantify the minimum amount of small bowel that is required for survival without parenteral nutrition. In several series, all infants with more than 38 cm of residual small bowel survived, and all with less than 15 cm died; presence of an ileocecal valve improved survival. However, there have been numerous reports of survival with shorter lengths. The actual length is less important than the functional capacity of the residual bowel.

The anatomic location of the resection or dysfunction predicts the clinical symptoms. Duodenal resection results in decreased absorption of iron, folate, and calcium, causing anemia and osteopenia. Fortunately, the duodenum rarely requires resection. Isolated jejunal resection is well tolerated because the intact ileum adapts to absorb nutrients and excess fluid. In contrast, ileal resection has profound effects on the absorption of fluid and electrolytes; resection of more than 50% results in large water and electrolyte losses. Adaptation decreases losses. However, the absorptive reserve remains marginal, so the risk of dehydration with any stress or diarrheal illness is markedly increased. The ileum also has two specific functions: the absorption of bile salts and vitamin B_{12}. The jejunum cannot adapt to perform these functions. Ileal resection results in the malabsorption of bile salts, leading to decreased intraluminal bile salt concentrations and fat malabsorption. Vitamin B_{12} malabsorption results in the development of a macrocytic anemia. Resection of the ileocecal valve is associated with a poorer prognosis, probably because of a greater tendency for the development of bacterial overgrowth with subsequent mucosal damage.

Management of infants and children with short-bowel syndrome conventionally is divided into three phases. Phase 1 consists of the initial postoperative management and stabilization on TPN following resection. Phase 2 commences after the patient is stabilized on TPN and includes the gradual introduction of enteral feedings. Phase 3 consists of beginning a more normal diet and management of long-term micronutrient deficiencies and other complications.

After resection, compensatory mucosal growth with cellular hyperplasia and villus lengthening is primarily responsible for improved absorptive capacity. Growth and dilation of the remaining intestine occur, particularly in the preterm infant, but mucosal adaptation is the major factor determining ultimate absorptive potential. The major factor in adaptation is the presence of intraluminal foodstuff, resulting in the release of trophic factors such as epidermal growth factor and insulin-like growth factor 1.

Phase 1 is the initial phase of therapy following bowel resection, focusing on replacement of fluid and electrolyte losses. Total parenteral nutrition (TPN) is the sole source of nutrition. A central venous catheter should be inserted as soon as possible, and if feasible, a gastrostomy should be placed to provide easy access for the initiation of feeding solutions. Replacement of fluid losses must be meticulous; patients with jejunostomies, ileostomies, or high intestinal fistulas have marked water, sodium, and zinc losses. Fecal electrolyte concentrations should be measured and replaced on a volume-for-volume basis. This is most easily accomplished using "piggyback" intravenous arrays, with maintenance fluids and electrolytes provided in TPN solution and replacement solutions being adjusted to compensate for fecal or ostomy losses. Urinary electrolytes should be monitored to assess body Na^+ stores. Sodium depletion increases aldosterone secretion, which results in high urinary K^+ loss and Na^+ retention. Maintaining urinary Na^+ levels greater than K^+ levels assures that Na^+ intake is adequate. Serum electrolytes, calcium, phosphorus, and magnesium initially should be obtained at least daily. TPN laboratory studies and growth should be monitored as outlined in Sec. 17.6.2. When fluid and electrolyte losses stabilize, additional fluid and electrolytes can be added to the parenteral nutrition solutions to simplify management. Gastric hypersecretion often occurs immediately following resection. Treatment with an H_2-receptor antagonist may decrease gastric output, thus simplifying management.

Phase 2 begins when gastrointestinal motility returns and fluid and electrolytes losses are stable and predictable. The TPN provides the majority of nutrition, but enteral nutrition is begun as a continuous nasogastric or gastrostomy infusion. Initial enteral feedings are not intended to provide significant caloric intake but rather to stimulate intestinal adaptation; hence, even minimal amounts (1-2 mL/h) are beneficial. Small amounts of oral feedings should be initiated as soon as possible to prevent prolonged food refusal,

as discussed in Sec. 17.8. Enteral feedings also ameliorate parenteral nutrition-associated cholestasis. Feedings can begin despite large fluid and electrolyte losses in the stool as long as adequate replacement is provided. Stool volume, pH, and reducing substances are monitored. A marked increase in stool volume or evidence of marked carbohydrate malabsorption, manifested by a stool pH below 5.5 or the presence of moderate reducing substances, contraindicates further advancement of the enteral nutrition. Discharge planning should begin as soon as the infant is medically stable. A multidisciplinary team composed of a home care nurse, dietician, pharmacist, social worker, and pediatric gastroenterologist then should manage the infant.

During outpatient therapy, the volume of enteral feeding is slowly increased. The bowel adapts over a period of months to years, and reliance on TPN for nutritional support decreases. However, there may be a prolonged requirement for TPN; therefore, meticulous care of the intravenous catheter is essential. Limited sites are available for the placement of infusion catheters during a patient's lifetime, so aggressive treatment of potential line infections or thrombosis is mandatory before their removal is considered. The acute risk of infection must be balanced with the longer-term requirement for venous access. Other complications of TPN are outlined in Sec. 17.6.2.

The choice of formula that is best suited for therapy in short-bowel syndrome is controversial. Initially, semielemental formulas such as Pregestimil or Alimentum are preferred because the protein is partially hydrolyzed and they contain medium-chain triglycerides. In the older infant and child, the choice of formula is more difficult. Carbohydrate usually is provided as glucose polymers or sucrose because lactose is poorly tolerated. Generally, protein hydrolysates are adequately absorbed; in rare cases more elemental solutions may be required. Fat is critical because it is a potent stimulant for intestinal adaptation. Fat usually is best tolerated as medium-chain triglycerides, but sufficient long-chain fat must be administered to prevent essential fatty acid deficiency. Whatever formula is chosen, attention must be paid to the electrolyte and mineral content, with adequate compensation for any electrolyte losses. Additional fluid and electrolytes may need to be added to the enteral feeds.

If the stool volume suddenly increases, several possibilities must be considered. Intercurrent infection, bacterial overgrowth, and obstruction are all possibilities. Obstruction may result from adhesions or a narrowing or stricture of the ostomy at skin level, which is best diagnosed by digital examination and retrograde radiographic contrast study. Bacterial overgrowth can cause malabsorption and metabolic acidosis resulting from bacterial production of D-lactate in the intestine; symptoms of D-lactate acidosis include somnolence, dyspnea, and occasional encephalopathy (see Sec. 17.16.2). Cyclic treatment with antibiotics may be necessary. Bacterial overgrowth may further injure the intestinal mucosa. Carbohydrate malabsorption must be excluded.

If stool output is persistently elevated, use of an antiperistaltic agent such as loperamide may be useful; however, this may increase the risk of bacterial overgrowth. Cholestyramine may be beneficial but should be used cautiously because it will further deplete bile acid pools, thus increasing steatorrhea. Cholestyramine also nonselectively binds other nutrients, thus increasing requirements. Fiber-containing formulas may be useful. If TPN cannot be reduced or stopped after 1 year, surgical alternatives should be considered, including tapering of any dilated bowel and bowel-lengthening procedures (ie, Bianchi procedure). The risk of surgery must be carefully weighed against the benefits and long-term complications of parenteral nutrition. Intestinal transplantation should be considered in the TPN-dependent child who is developing liver disease. Before the development of liver disease, the TPN-dependent child who shows no hope of being able to survive without permanent TPN should be considered for an isolated small bowel transplant. The child should be referred to a medical center experienced in intestinal transplantation.

Phase 3 begins when the patient is weaned from enteral infusion and solid feedings begin. Micronutrient deficiencies may become evident as the intravenous supplementation of these nutrients is ceased. Bolus feedings of enteral formula are initiated and then advanced until the patient no longer requires continuous feedings. Some patients may continue to require intravenous electrolyte supplementation despite receiving adequate nutrition enterally. Vitamin B_{12} deficiency may develop 3 to 5 years later; a Schilling test should be performed, and replacement therapy initiated if necessary. Osteopenia and increased fractures are possible as a result of calcium and vitamin D malabsorption. Other complications associated with short-bowel syndrome include a colitis that is observed as enteral feedings are advanced. The cause is unclear, but treatment with sulfasalazine or similar compounds is effective. Late gastrointestinal bleeding has occurred from ulcers at anastomotic sites; treatment is resection. Renal calculi may develop; patients with ileal resection and an intact colon are particularly susceptible to oxalate stones.

References

Bueno J, Ohwada S, Kocoshis S, et al: Factors impacting on the survival of children with intestinal failure referred for intestinal transplantation. J Pediatr Surg 34:27–31, 1999

Taylor SF, Sondheimer JM, Sokol RJ, Silverman A, Wilson HL: Noninfectious colitis associated with short gut syndrome in infants. J Pediatr 119: 24–28, 1991

Thompson JS: Surgical approach to the short-bowel syndrome: procedures to slow intestinal transit. Eur J Pediatr Surg 9:263–266, 1999

Vanderhoof JA: Short bowel syndrome in children and small intestinal transplantation. Pediatr Clin 43:533–550, 1996

Vanderhoof JA, Langnas AN: Short-bowel syndrome in children and adults. Gastroenterology 113:1767–1778, 1997

Warner BW, Ziegler MM: Management of the short-bowel syndrome in the pediatric population. Pediatr Clin North Am 40:1335–1350, 1993

17.19 PEPTIC DISEASES

Eric Hassall

The term *peptic diseases* includes esophagitis, gastritis, gastropathy, peptic ulcer disease, and duodenitis. Esophagitis is not discussed in this chapter. Although this chapter provides an overview of peptic diseases, the focus is on areas of progress, especially those of importance to children, and because peptic diseases in children differ in some respects from those in adults, there are important practical implications for pediatric practitioners.

By way of introduction, the anatomic regions and major landmarks of the stomach and duodenum referred to in this section are shown in Fig. 17-3 and described in Sec. 17.1.1, and pertinent physiology is discussed as follows.

GASTRIC SECRETION

The stomach secretes acid and enzymes that initiate the digestive process and may protect the stomach and small bowel from bacterial colonization. Hydrochloric acid is secreted by parietal cells of the oxyntic mucosa of the gastric body and fundus (Figs. 17-36 and 17-37). Hydrogen ions are generated within the cell from water, or H_2O, with the OH^- being combined with cellular CO_2 to form HCO_3^- by the action of carbonic anhydrase. The HCO_3^- is exchanged for Cl^- across the basolateral membrane of the parietal cell. H^+ is exchanged for K^+ on the luminal membrane in a process that is energized by the H,K ATPase or "proton pump." K^+ and Cl^- are transported into the lumen through a Cl^- and K^+ conductance pathway. The net result of this process is secretion of H^+ and Cl^- into the lumen against a concentration gradient of more than 1,000,000:1.

In newborn humans, acidification of gastric contents to a pH of less than 4 is present almost immediately after birth. The highest acid concentrations occur within 7 to 10 days and diminish to adult levels in 60 to 90 days. The control of acid secretion in early life is unclear. During the first 2 days after birth, however, term infants fail to increase acid secretion after stimulation with pentagastrin, and the acid secretory response to betazole HCl (Histalog) is absent until 1 month of age. Basal acid output increases over the first month regardless of gestational age at birth. In response to feeds, term newborns increase acid secretion for at least 2 hours.

Acid secretion from the parietal cell is controlled by neural, endocrine, and paracrine inputs. The sight, taste, and smell of food trigger the *cephalic phase* of acid secretion, which is mediated by the release of acetylcholine and serotonin from postganglionic cholinergic fibers of the vagus nerve that stimulate mast cells to produce histamine. Food ingestion, antral dilatation, intragastric protein, and gastric pH greater than 3 stimulate secretion of the hormone gastrin from the antrum of the stomach during the *gastric phase* of

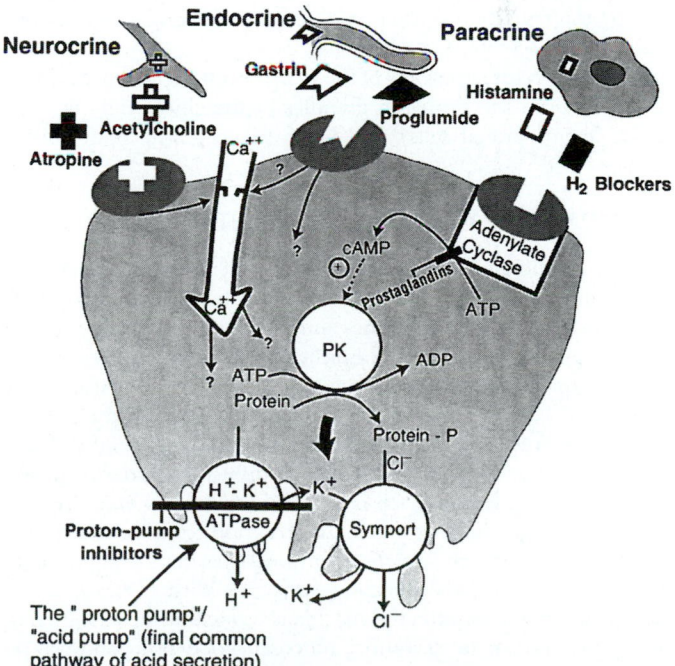

FIGURE 17-36 Representation of parietal cell, showing the secretagogue pathways for gastric acid and where various therapeutic agents work to block secretion.

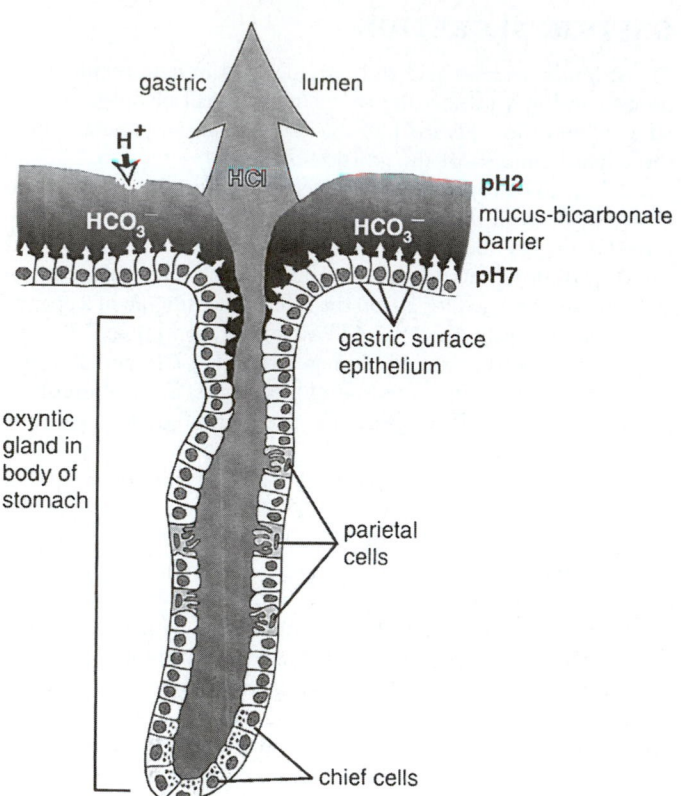

FIGURE 17-37 Representation of oxyntic gland, showing parietal cells (acid-secreting), chief cells (pepsinogen-secreting), and surface cells (mucus-secreting). The protective mucus-bicarbonate barrier between the gastric epithelium and gastric lumen also is shown.

acid secretion, which in turn stimulates further acid secretion by the parietal cells. Feedback on the stomach by neural and hormonal stimuli then inhibits further acid secretion during the *intestinal phase* of acid secretion.

Other secretory products of the gastric body include pepsinogen (secreted from the zymogen granules of the chief cells), intrinsic factor (from parietal cells), and lipase (from gastric body epithelium).

MUCUS-BICARBONATE BARRIER

Each anatomic area of the stomach has different specialized functions, but mucus is produced by all areas. Mucous synthesis is stimulated by gastrin, acetylcholine, and histamine, suggesting that it is coupled with acid secretion. Epithelial and pit cells secrete a thick (ie, 180 μm) water-insoluble mucous gel that is rich in bicarbonate (Fig. 17-37). This continuous protective layer maintains a high pH gradient between the acidic luminal pH of 1.5 to 2.5 and the neutral epithelial cell pH of 7, acting as a diffusion barrier to pepsin and HCl. Thus, the stomach is protected from autodigestion. Altered mucous synthesis or mucous destruction contributes to peptic disease; in addition, the mucus-bicarbonate barrier is compromised by ischemia, drugs, and infection, especially with *Helicobacter pylori*. Other mucosal protective mechanisms include increases in mucous and bicarbonate secretion, mucosal blood flow, and cell renewal on exposure to various noxious agents. Prostaglandin secretion appears to mediate some of these protective responses. If mucosal defenses are overcome, "back diffusion" of acid and pepsin from the lumen through the mucosal barrier occurs, with damage to the gastric epithelium and mucosa. Thus, whatever the initial

offensive factor, acid and pepsin constitute the final pathway of injury and ulceration.

17.19.1 Presentation of Peptic Diseases

In the pediatric age group, abdominal pain is a very common reason for seeking medical advice, and it is the most common presenting symptom of peptic disorders, ie, gastritis, gastropathy, duodenitis, and peptic ulcer disease. Nevertheless, these disorders (excluding esophagitis) account for fewer than 20% of children presenting with abdominal pain, even in a subspecialty practice. In addition, peptic disorders overall, including peptic ulcer disease, are far less prevalent in children than in adults.

Different peptic disorders may present with similar symptoms, and in children of 10 years or older, they may be similar to those in adults. Although epigastric pain or discomfort that is meal-exacerbated or that awakens the child from sleep often is a symptom of peptic ulcer disease in children, it is also a presenting symptom of more common disorders such as nonulcer dyspepsia and constipation. Most primary peptic ulcers in children occur between the ages of 8 and 17 years, whereas secondary ulcer disease occurs at all ages. Younger children may not be able to localize the pain to the epigastrium and may present with anorexia and irritability, especially with meals. Other presenting symptoms include anorexia, nausea, early satiety, recurrent vomiting, and anemia. Weight loss occurs less often. Gastrointestinal bleeding may occur with long-standing antecedent epigastric pain or other symptoms, but painless bleeding may be the only manifestation of ulcer disease; up to 25% of children with duodenal ulcers have this "silent" presentation, some 25% present with bleeding and antecedent pain, and the rest present with abdominal pain or recurrent vomiting. On physical examination, epigastric tenderness is an unreliable sign of gastritis or ulcer disease. Physical examination also is directed toward evaluation of whether GI bleeding has occurred (see Sec. 17.7.7).

Symptoms of gastritis or peptic ulcer can be mimicked by esophagitis, gallbladder or liver disease, pneumonia, pancreatitis, or giardiasis. Pain that is truly localized to the epigastrium is relatively uncommon in children and always requires investigation, as does upper GI bleeding with or without pain. Although presenting symptoms may lead to the suspicion that peptic disease is present, gastritis, gastropathy, duodenitis, and peptic ulcer are not clinical diagnoses; they are endoscopic and biopsy diagnoses. Suspicion also may mislead; for example, a child with hematemesis following aspirin or ingestion of nonsteroidal antiinflammatory drugs (NSAIDs) may well have bled from, for example, undiagnosed esophageal varices, a *Helicobacter pylori*–associated ulcer, or a non–*Helicobacter* ulcer, not necessarily an NSAID ulcer.

17.19.2 *Helicobacter Pylori*

Without doubt, the most exciting recent development in the area of peptic diseases has been the discovery that a bacterial infection, *Helicobacter pylori*, is a major factor in the pathogenesis of certain gastroduodenal disorders. In 1983, this organism was identified in gastric biopsies by Warren and Marshall in Australia. *H. pylori* has been causally linked to the development of chronic gastritis, peptic ulcer disease, mucosa-associated lymphoid tumors (MALT lymphoma), and gastric adenocarcinoma. The latter two disorders are exceedingly rare in children. To put the issue of *H. pylori infection* versus *disease* in context, although some 50% of the world's population is infected with the organism, the vast majority of individuals are asymptomatic, with only a mild chronic gastritis (ie, infection) and no complications thereof (ie, disease). A variety of extraintestinal disorders have been ascribed to *H. pylori,* but the evidence for an association is tenuous, at best.

H. pylori is a spiral, gram-negative highly motile bacterium that colonizes only gastric-type epithelium in the zone below the viscous layer of gastric mucus. Thus, it is largely protected from the strongly acidic intragastric milieu. It is a prodigious producer of the enzyme *urease;* this helps the organism create its own microclimate below gastric mucus and is the basis for the urea breath test, which detects its presence.

The infection is acquired primarily in childhood, with only 0.3 to 0.5% of adults becoming infected per year. The major risk factors for infection are socioeconomic status, overcrowding, absence of a hot water supply, and poor sanitation. Not surprisingly, therefore, the prevalence of infection is much higher in developing countries, where up to 90% of children are infected by age 10. In contrast, in the well-to-do in First World countries or in developing countries, the prevalence is less than 5% in this age group.

Humans appear to be the primary natural reservoir of *H. pylori* infection, the other major reservoir being water. Domestic cats can harbor *H. pylori,* but this is uncommon and may represent an infection they have acquired from humans. The organism is very difficult to culture other than from gastric biopsies, and many studies have relied on polymerase chain reaction (PCR) techniques for detection. By PCR, *H. pylori* genomic DNA has been identified in stool samples of infected children, as has bacterial antigen, even though the organism is extremely difficult to culture from feces. Almost certainly, the most likely route of transmission of *H. pylori* is person to person, by the fecal-oral or oral-oral route.

Why some individuals develop primary *H. pylori* gastritis alone (infection) and others duodenal ulcer or other sequelae (disease) is incompletely understood. However, there is evidence that the occurrence of different disorders may be determined by the interactions of different bacterial and host genotypes. For example, genetic polymorphism of interleukin-1β (IL-1β) in the host may determine why some individuals infected with *H. pylori* develop hypochlorhydria and gastric cancer and others do not; IL-1β is a potent proinflammatory cytokine that also markedly suppresses gastric acid production. The sequelae and treatment of *H. pylori* infection are discussed in Secs. 17.19.3 and 17.19.4.

17.19.3   Gastritis and Gastropathy

Gastritis is neither a clinical nor a radiologic diagnosis. Most often it is a purely histologic diagnosis made by endoscopic biopsies.

Although some conditions that injure the gastric mucosa may result in inflammation, others do not. Thus, *gastritis,* as the suffix *-itis* implies, is characterized by the presence of inflammatory cells. In contrast, *gastropathy* refers to conditions in which inflammation is not a prominent feature. Occasionally the mucosal appearance at endoscopy is typical of a particular condition, but the diagnosis of gastritis or gastropathy is usually made on the basis of biopsy findings or a combination of biopsy and endoscopic findings.

The categorization of entities into gastritides and gastropathies is an important concept and helps narrow the diagnostic possibilities in a given case. In this section, for the sake of simplicity, the term *gastritis* is often used generically to refer to both gastritides and gastropathies.

In general, gastritis may be classified by its endoscopic appearance as *erosive and hemorrhagic* or *nonerosive* (Table 17-49). Within

TABLE 17-49

CLASSIFICATION OF GASTRITIS AND GASTROPATHY

Erosive and hemorrhagic gastritis or gastropathy
  "Stress" gastropathy
  Traumatic gastropathy
  Aspirin and other NSAIDs
  Other drugs
  Portal hypertensive gastropathy
  Uremic gastropathy
  Chronic varioliform gastritis
  Bile gastropathy
  Henoch-Schönlein gastropathy
  Corrosive gastropathy
  Exercise-induced gastropathy/gastritis
  Radiation gastropathy
Nonerosive gastritis or gastropathy
  Nonspecific gastritis
  Helicobacter pylori gastritis
  Crohn disease
  Allergic gastritis and eosinophilic gastritis
  Proton pump inhibitor gastropathy
  Celiac disease
  Gastritis with autoimmune diseases
  Chronic granulomatous disease
  Cytomegalovirus
  Collagenous gastritis
  Graft-versus-host disease
  Ménétrier disease
  Pernicious anemia
  Other granulomatous gastritides
  Phlegmonous and emphysematous gastritis
  Other infectious gastritides

each of these categories, the gastritides are further classified according to specific etiology. Some conditions, eg, *H. pylori,* and Crohn disease, may present with erosions or without but are classified as *nonerosive,* as this is their most common presentation. Gastritis is much more prevalent in adults than in children; only the more common types that occur in children are discussed in any detail.

EROSIVE AND HEMORRHAGIC GASTROPATHY

Most of these entities are diagnosed endoscopically, usually in patients presenting with GI bleeding. Because inflammation is not a feature of most hemorrhagic lesions, most conditions in this category are gastropathies. Biopsies are usually not required from erosive or hemorrhagic lesions. However, there are gastritides not in the erosive/hemorrhagic category that may present with erosions or hemorrhagic lesions, and in these cases, biopsies are essential for the diagnosis, eg, *H. pylori,* Crohn disease, CMV, and allergic gastritis.

"Stress gastropathy" occurs in the seriously ill child because of physiological (not psychological) stresses such as shock, acidosis, sepsis, burns, or head injury that cause mucosal ischemia. Early lesions predominate in the fundus and proximal body, later spreading to the antrum to produce a diffuse erosive and hemorrhagic appearance. Over the last decade, the decreased incidence of perforation and major bleeding probably reflects improved cardiorespiratory and nutritional support rather than prophylactic acid-neu-

tralizing therapy. Perforation occurs more often in newborns than in older children.

Traumatic gastropathy results from forceful retching or vomiting, which produces typical subepithelial hemorrhages in the fundus and proximal body because of knuckling of the proximal stomach into the distal esophagus. This is also known as *prolapse gastropathy*. Mallory-Weiss tears of the cardia also may occur but are less common in children. Although the gastropathy and tears tend to resolve quickly, significant blood loss may occur. Showers of petechiae in the proximal stomach occur from less forceful retching. Nasogastric tubes and ingested foreign bodies are common causes of innocuous hemorrhages and erosions.

Aspirin and other nonsteroidal antiinflammatory drugs (NSAIDs) frequently cause minor erosions and hemorrhages in the body and antrum that have little clinical significance; however, more extensive ulceration with perforation and severe bleeding may be associated with NSAIDs, which produce mucosal injury by local and systemic effects.

Portal hypertensive gastropathy is a congestive gastropathy often present in children with portal hypertension resulting from any cause. Most findings are in the fundus and body, with typical "mosaic lesions" and hemorrhages.

Less common erosive/hemorrhagic gastropathies in children include *chronic varioliform gastritis* and those caused by uremia, certain drugs or alcohol, duodenogastric reflux, caustic ingestion, Henoch-Schönlein disease, exercise, or radiation.

NONEROSIVE GASTRITIS OR GASTROPATHY

Nonerosive gastritis of the antrum is by far the most common gastritis in children and adults. In nonerosive gastritis, there usually is a poor correlation between endoscopic appearance and histologic findings (ie, it usually is a purely histologic diagnosis).

Nonspecific gastritis is present in a significant number of children, and no specific cause can be identified. In these cases, the inflammation is chronic, lymphoplasmic cellular, more focal than diffuse within the biopsy, and usually superficial. It appears to be more prevalent in the antrum than the corpus, but this may reflect sampling bias.

Helicobacter pylori gastritis is the most common identifiable cause of chronic gastritis in children and does have sequelae in some patients; by far the majority of children with chronic *H. pylori* infection are asymptomatic and have no sequelae. Acute infection with *H. pylori* often is asymptomatic but may also cause nausea, vomiting, and halitosis. An acute (neutrophilic) gastritis develops with a brief period of acid hypersecretion followed by a profound hypochlorhydria. These symptoms usually resolve within about a week. Over a period of 3 to 6 months, the gastritis severity lessens, and acid secretion returns to near preinfection levels. Although spontaneous clearance of the organism occurs occasionally, the majority of adults and children develop a chronic gastritis. In the great majority of individuals this is of no consequence, and they remain asymptomatic. However, there are considerable individual and geographic variations in intensity and distribution of inflammation and in the disease associations, as described below.

When *H. pylori* causes gastritis alone, a striking diffuse nodularity of the antrum is seen in approximately 50% of cases. When *H. pylori* antral gastritis is associated with duodenal ulcer in children, this nodularity is always present; this finding does not occur in other gastritides of childhood. Definitive diagnosis of the presence of *H.*

pylori is made by gastric biopsies showing the typical gram-negative spiral rods on the surface of glandular epithelium under the mucous layer. The organism is best identified with special silver stains or Giemsa stain, with the highest diagnostic yield obtained from biopsies from the antrum, cardia, and corpus, in that order. Biopsies typically show chronic active superficial or panmucosal gastritis, often with hyperplastic lymphoid aggregates. Because the gastric mucosa appears normal at endoscopy in at least half the cases of primary *H. pylori* gastritis, biopsies should always be performed, regardless of the endoscopic appearance. The presence of *H. pylori* in biopsy specimens remains the "gold standard" for diagnosis of active, current infection.

Chronic *H. pylori* infection is also associated with different topographic distributions and severities of gastritis, including atrophic gastritis and intestinal metaplasia in some adults. Different patterns of gastritis may have prognostic implications. *H. pylori* is also associated with gastric adenocarcinoma, but the etiology of this is multifactorial, including genetic and dietary influences; *H. pylori* is but one risk factor, and then, not always. There is no evidence for a connection between early (ie, childhood) acquisition of *H. pylori* infection and gastric cancer. *H. pylori* is also associated with a rare and very slow-growing mucosa-associated lymphoid tumor (MALT) of the stomach, a diagnosis that also is made by biopsy, and usually is cured by eradication of *H. pylori* infection.

Crohn disease relatively commonly involves the stomach and duodenum. Occasionally, typical aphthous ulcers are seen endoscopically. Even in their absence, however, the histologic feature supporting a diagnosis of gastric Crohn disease is a focal, deep gastritis; diagnostic features are giant cells and granulomas. For both endoscopic and histologic findings, the antrum is the usual repository of disease.

Allergic gastritis and *eosinophilic gastritis* are discussed in detail in Secs. 17.21.1 and 17.21.2. In allergic gastritis, an eosinophilic infiltrate is present in the gastric mucosa and not deeper; endoscopy may be normal or nonspecific with swollen folds, and occasionally erosions are present. It is a benign condition, often with an identifiable allergen, and responds to antigen withdrawal. In contrast, eosinophilic gastritis can involve all layers of the gastric wall, but often there is a selective predominance of eosinophilic infiltrates in the mucosa, muscle layers, or subserosa; the disorder is less common than allergic gastritis, more severe, and often indolent. Diagnosis by endoscopic biopsy is not always possible, especially when there is limited mucosal involvement. Rarely, vomiting with swollen gastric folds is due to angioneurotic edema (see Sec. 11.5.1).

Proton pump inhibitor gastropathy results from long-term or high-dose PPI therapy with characteristic changes in the parietal cell layer. In some cases fundic gland polyps occur. The parietal cell changes, and often the polyps regress to normal some weeks after cessation of acid suppression therapy. The condition is benign.

Celiac disease can cause a lymphocytic gastritis characterized by the intraepithelial location of the lymphocytic infiltrate. Various gastritides may occur in children and adults with connective tissue diseases, scleroderma, insulin-dependent diabetes mellitus, autoimmune thyroiditis, nongoitrous juvenile hypothyroidism, and vitiligo. In *chronic granulomatous disease,* gastric involvement is common, usually presenting with symptoms of delayed gastric emptying and a narrowed, poorly mobile antrum on contrast radiography. At endoscopy, the antral mucosa often is pale, lusterless, and swollen. Mild chronic inflammation and granulomas often are present on biopsy, but the diagnostic feature is the presence of vacuolated histiocytes that are laden with brown pigmented material.

Cytomegalovirus rarely causes infection in immune-competent children, but when it does, it manifests as Ménétrier disease (see below); it is so rare in apparently immune-competent adults that its finding suggests an occult malignancy or early immune deficiency. Conversely, cytomegalovirus infection is so common in immune-suppressed patients (eg, AIDS, or post–solid organ or bone marrow transplant) that in some cases it is difficult to know whether it is a pathogen or a commensal. In such patients, this compounds the diagnostic difficulty in distinguishing between gross or histologic lesions caused by infection, graft-versus-host disease, or physiological stress, or those caused by chemotherapy. However, if the highly distinctive pattern of injury is present, it is more likely that cytomegalovirus is the cause.

Ménétrier disease is characterized by hypoproteinemia as a result of protein-losing gastropathy. Folds of the gastric fundus and body are swollen and convoluted at endoscopy. The typical childhood presentation is with upper GI symptoms and signs of edema following a viral prodome. Upper GI contrast series show swollen rugae, but this is a nondiagnostic finding. The histology is typical, with elongated, tortuous foveolae (pits), often with cystic dilatations; the lamina propria is edematous, with increased eosinophils and round cells. In the past, many children underwent open biopsy at laparotomy or partial gastric resection, but now surgery virtually never is necessary in children. The childhood form is usually caused by cytomegalovirus infection, and the natural history is one of self-resolution in weeks or months. In contrast, the adult disease usually is chronic, and partial gastrectomy is sometimes required to alleviate persistent abdominal symptoms, hypoproteinemia, and blood loss.

Collagenous gastritis is characterized by subepithelial collagen deposition and an associated gastritis. It probably is not a distinct disorder in and of itself; rather, it appears to occur as a consequence of inflammation or a local immune response in the stomach or as one histologic feature of a more diffuse disease process.

Graft-versus-host disease appears to involve the stomach much less often than the small and large bowel. When it does so, endoscopic signs of acute disease range from normal to patchy erythema to extensive mucosal sloughing. The early biopsy findings are unique to graft-versus-host disease, consisting of focal crypt cell necrosis, the remnants of which are vacuoles containing cellular debris and known as apoptotic bodies. In more severe cases, whole crypts may drop out. In advanced cases, there may be ulceration, edema, fibrosis, and perforation. Chronic graft-versus-host disease rarely involves the stomach (see Sec. 17.21.5).

Pernicious anemia is an autoimmune process causing destruction of parietal cells and atrophic fundic gland gastritis, with decreased secretion of HCl, intrinsic factor, and malabsorption of vitamin B_{12}. Endoscopically, the gastric body appears as a thin mucosa, with paucity and thinning of gastric rugae. However, these features are late and insensitive, and atrophic gastritis is a histologic diagnosis. "Juvenile" pernicious anemia is a rare condition of early childhood in which achlorhydria occurs without gastric atrophy.

Exercise-induced gastropathy/gastritis is well recognized in runners, usually presenting with blood loss anemia, with or without upper GI symptoms. Erosive gastropathy or nonerosive gastritis may occur.

Other much less common specific gastritides in children are those with other infectious causes such as tuberculosis, syphilis, actinomycosis, phlegmonous and emphysematous gastritis, herpes, candidiasis, histoplasmosis, mucormycosis, aspergillosis, cryptosporidiosis, anisakiasis, schistosomiasis, amebiasis, toxoplasmosis, and sarcoidosis.

17.19.4   Peptic Ulcer Disease

Although the term *erosion* refers to a breach of the epithelium into the mucosa, an *ulcer* extends through the muscularis mucosa into the submucosa. Strictly speaking, the difference is histologic, but in practice, the diagnosis of ulcer is made when the endoscopic appearance is that of a deep lesion. In children, duodenal ulcers are far more prevalent than gastric ulcers.

Conceptually it is useful to categorize peptic ulcer disease as "primary" or "secondary." Primary peptic ulcers generally occur in otherwise healthy individuals and are usually chronic, with fibrinopurulent debris overlying active inflammatory infiltrate, granulation tissue, and fibrosis. In contrast, secondary peptic ulcers usually are associated with or occur in the presence of systemic underlying disease; they are usually more acute in onset, often induced by physiological stress or drug ingestion, and not generally fibrotic. Primary peptic ulcers are more often duodenal, whereas secondary ulcers are more often gastric than duodenal.

PRIMARY PEPTIC ULCER DISEASE

Approximately 80% of primary, chronic duodenal ulcer disease in children is related to *H. pylori,* although only a tiny minority of children with *H. pylori* infection develop peptic ulcer disease. The mechanism by which *H. pylori* antral gastritis produces gastroduodenal disease is not certain as yet, but the cause and effect relationship between *H. pylori* and duodenal ulcer has been established in adults and children by the presence of *H. pylori* antral gastritis in most cases of duodenal ulcer and from results of treatment trials. When *H. pylori*-associated duodenal ulcers are healed by acid suppression alone, there is an ulcer relapse rate of approximately 90% by 1 year; when eradication of the *H. pylori* organism from the antrum is achieved with antibiotics, the relapse rate is less than 10%. Eradication of the organism correlates with ulcer healing, and reinfection or noneradication correlates with relapse or persistence of ulcer.

Not all primary, chronic duodenal ulcer disease is related to *H. pylori*. Approximately 20% of children with a duodenal ulcer have no *H. pylori* and an absence of gastritis. At this time, they are regarded as having "idiopathic" duodenal ulcer disease. Although the importance of psychological stressors has been overrated as an etiologic agent, they may play a role in some individuals. Also, heredity may be the major factor in the cases of non–*H. pylori* ulcer disease. Acid secretion often is somewhat higher in patients with duodenal ulcer, but there is much overlap with persons without ulcers.

Hypersecretory conditions are rare in children and usually present with ulcer disease. The best know is *Zollinger-Ellison syndrome,* in which gastrin-secreting tumors in the pancreas, duodenal wall, and other sites produce very high levels of gastrin-stimulated acid hypersecretion. This syndrome, as well as the hypersecretory disorder of *antral G-cell hyperplasia,* is very rare in children. Both typically cause multiple ulcers, often in atypical sites such as the esophagus, stomach, postbulbar duodenum, or jejunum. *Systemic mastocytosis,* a disease in which mast cells accumulate in skin, bone marrow, liver, spleen, and GI tract, also is associated with acid hypersecretion, as is hyperparathyroidism. Of note is that hypersecretory disorders do not always present with ulcer disease; even in Zollinger-Ellison syndrome, 10% of patients present with diarrhea and no ulcers, attesting to the importance of mucosal resistance as a major factor in determining whether ulceration will occur.

SECONDARY PEPTIC ULCER DISEASE

Erosions and/or ulcers can be caused by most of the conditions that cause gastropathy or gastritis, even those that are in the nonerosive category because of their more common presentation. The exceptions to this are gastropathy caused by proton pump inhibitors, portal hypertension, and pernicious anemia. Uremia and sickle-cell disease are additional causes of secondary ulcer disease.

DUODENITIS

Like gastritis, "duodenitis" is not a clinical or a radiologic diagnosis. It may be a purely endoscopic or histologic diagnosis; often it is both. Nonspecific duodenitis that is confined to the duodenal bulb with multiple duodenal erosions may occur as part of the spectrum of duodenal ulcer disease. These also may occur from physiological stress or NSAID ingestion, usually with (but occasionally without) their gastric counterparts. Duodenitis also is observed in Crohn disease and other inflammatory disorders of the small intestine, as described in portions of Secs. 17.20 and 17.21.

17.19.5   Diagnosis of Peptic Diseases

As described above, certain symptoms or signs, or a constellation thereof, may be suggestive of the presence of a peptic disease. However, in children, symptoms are a poor predictor of a specific peptic disease, so disparate peptic disorders such as esophagitis, *H. pylori* ulcer disease, non–*H. pylori* ulcer disease, and the various gastritides and gastropathies may present with similar symptoms. A positive family history of peptic ulcer disease may support a clinical suspicion of peptic disease; however, many individuals have been told they have "an ulcer" or "gastritis" on the basis of a clinical impression or a questionable barium study, without an accurate diagnosis having been made, which often makes the family history of questionable relevance.

Definitive diagnosis (or exclusion) of peptic diseases can be made only by endoscopic examination and biopsies of the appropriate areas of stomach and duodenum. In addition, in the case of an actively bleeding ulcer, endoscopy may be therapeutic as well as diagnostic in that hemostasis can be effected endoscopically. In contrast to endoscopy, upper gastrointestinal barium studies are notoriously inaccurate for the diagnosis of mucosal disease of the stomach or duodenum in children.

In recent years, considerable attention has been directed toward *H. pylori* as a pathogen. However, this is but one cause of gastroduodenal disease, and it is a very uncommon cause of symptoms in children. Because of concerns that diagnostic tests and treatments for *H. pylori* infection are being used in excess of their established benefit in the pediatric population, three consensus groups in North America and Europe have established guidelines for an approach to suspected *H. pylori* disease in children, which are different from those for adults.

Several considerations underlie the guidelines. Although *H. pylori* has an established pathogenic role for both duodenal ulcer and gastric ulcer disease, the great majority of infected individuals harbor this organism lifelong with no apparent adverse health consequences. Furthermore, although abdominal pain is a very common complaint in children, several lines of evidence indicate that *H. pylori* is very seldom the cause. Therefore, the most useful goal in the care of a child, ie, the goal of diagnostic intervention, is to determine the cause of presenting symptoms rather than the mere presence of *H. pylori* infection.

As a general principle, diagnostic tests for *H. pylori* should be employed judiciously and be reserved for those children who are most likely to derive measurable benefit, such as those who reasonably may be suspected to have peptic ulcer disease. Antibody tests utilizing whole blood, serum, or saliva are not recommended in children for clinical use. Antibody tests are of low sensitivity and specificity—the levels may remain elevated for years after eradication or resolution of infection; therefore, a positive test does not necessarily mean that infection is present at the time of testing. Urea breath tests (^{13}C or ^{14}C) are reasonably accurate for the presence of *H. pylori*. However, the mere presence or absence of *H. pylori* is not helpful in the management of a child, and this indirect testing neither determines gastroduodenal pathology nor rules out alternative or concurrent diagnoses. Urea breath tests are useful in confirming successful eradication of *H. pylori* after therapy for an endoscopically proven *H. pylori*–related ulcer. Endoscopy with biopsies provides the most accurate approach for definitive diagnosis of upper gastrointestinal mucosal diseases; therefore, an accurate diagnosis or exclusion of *H. pylori*–associated peptic ulcer disease can be made only by this means if other disorders are diagnosed or ruled out. Endoscopy is the only acceptable diagnostic test in children with upper gastrointestinal bleeding, recurrent vomiting, or persistent undiagnosed abdominal pain.

Contrast radiography has high false-positive and false-negative rates for suspected lesions of the upper GI tract in the pediatric population. Barium studies often report "poor filling of the duodenal cap," "irritability of the duodenum," or "duodenitis," and these very seldom correlate with upper gastrointestinal pathology. Even in the uncommon circumstance of an ulcer crater said to be present, radiography cannot distinguish between *H. pylori*–associated and non–*H. pylori* ulcers or ulcers of other causes. Therefore, children previously suspected to have peptic ulcer disease by an upper GI series, in whom symptoms persist or recur, should undergo endoscopy with biopsies to confirm the presence of an ulcer and to determine the presence or absence of *H. pylori* gastritis.

17.19.6   Treatment of Peptic Diseases

Although "hyperacidity" seldom is the primary problem for most of the peptic diseases, the final "erosive" pathway is acid and pepsin; therefore, acid buffering or suppression may be useful to treat symptoms as well as to heal gastritis or ulcers. However, where treatment for the underlying process or cause is available (eg, eradication of *H. pylori* when associated ulcer disease is present, or treatment of upper GI Crohn ulcers), this should be used. The most commonly used acid suppressants (see Table 17-40) block H_2 receptors on parietal cells. Ranitidine and cimetidine are available in liquid form, simplifying dosing and improving compliance. Proton pump inhibitors (PPIs) block the proton pump of the parietal cell and currently are the most potent and efficacious acid suppressants. Dosage and short-term safety of PPIs are established for erosive esophagitis in children. Antacids, which buffer gastric acid, rarely are useful because effective therapy requires that relatively large doses be administered 1 and 3 hours postprandially.

"Stress" gastritis is treated with management of the underlying hypoxemia/acidosis/sepsis and with acid suppression and antacids. Traumatic gastropathy is treated supportively and with attention to the underlying cause of forceful vomiting. Peptic disease resulting from aspirin or NSAIDs may respond to dose reduction or switching medication; in children requiring high-dose or long-term treatment with NSAIDs, concurrent treatment with a PPI may prevent ulceration and alleviate symptoms.

To attempt elimination of *H. pylori* from some 50% of the world's population is unrealistic, and there are significant negative consequences from indiscriminate use of eradication therapy. Large-scale use of antibiotics for such a task would lead to antibiotic resistance of *H. pylori* and other organisms, diminishing the usefulness of antibiotics for other infections as well. In addition, in some patients, treatment of *H. pylori* may unmask underlying GE reflux disease once the acid-suppressing effect of *H. pylori* gastritis is removed.

Eradication therapy for *H. pylori* should be given only after accurate diagnosis of *H. pylori* disease, ie, peptic ulcer disease proven to be associated with a current *H. pylori* infection, and in MALT lymphoma. Abdominal pain that is not caused by peptic ulcer disease is not an indication for eradication therapy. Those cases of true *H. pylori*–associated duodenal ulcer should be treated with triple therapy for 2 weeks with a proton pump inhibitor and two antibiotics; those currently recommended are clarithromycin and amoxicillin or clarithromycin and metronidazole. Although there is a paucity of data on the use of omeprazole and of lansoprazole in eradication regimens in children, these have been used in doses of 1 to 2 mg/kg/d, up to 40 mg per day for omeprazole, and 60 mg per day for lansoprazole. The antibiotics are administered in usual therapeutic doses. All three drugs are given in divided doses, twice daily. Because ulcers are prone to relapse, in those presenting with complications (bleeding, perforation, penetration), follow-up endoscopy is appropriate to prove healing and eradication of *H. pylori,* where that was present. Uncomplicated ulcers usually can be followed with symptom evaluation and a urea breath test to determine whether *H. pylori* has been eradicated. Urea breath tests should not be performed until 4 to 6 weeks after the end of acid suppression therapy.

There is no evidence that restrictive diets are helpful for peptic disorders other than in allergic gastropathy or when a patient anecdotally reports symptoms from a particular food. Acid-reducing operations such as vagotomy or antrectomy have a high morbidity and failure rate, and with the availability of highly effective acid-suppressing medications, these operations have become virtually obsolete in children. The current indications for surgery in peptic diseases include perforation of the stomach or duodenum, active bleeding that cannot be controlled by medical therapy or endoscopic hemostasis, gastric outlet or duodenal obstruction caused by scarring from peptic disease, or failure of medical therapy in hypersecretory syndromes; these are all rare occurrences.

References

Andersson T, Hassall E, Lundborg P, et al: Pharmacokinetics of orally administered omeprazole in children. International Pediatric Omeprazole Pharmokinetic Group Am J Gastroenterol 95:3101–3106; 2000

Dohil R, Hassall E, Jevon G, Dimmick J: Gastritis and gastropathy of childhood. J Pediatr Gastroenterol Nutr 29:378–394, 1999

Drumm B, Koletzko S, Oderda G, et al: *Helicobacter pylori* infection in children. Report of the European Paediatric Task Force on *Helicobacter pylori.* J Pediatr Gastroenterol Nutr 31:207–214, 2000

Gold BD, Abbott M, Colletti R, et al: Evidence-based guidelines for an approach to the diagnosis and treatment of *H. pylori* infection in children. J Pediatr Gastroenterol Nutr 31:490–497, 2000

Lewin KJ, Riddell RH, Weinstein WM: Gastrointestinal Pathology and Its Clinical Implications. Part 4: Stomach and Proximal Duodenum. New York/Tokyo, Igaku-Shoin, 493–587: 1992

Macarthur C, Saunders N, Feldman W: *Helicobacter pylori,* gastroduodenal disease, and recurrent abdominal pain in children. JAMA 273:729–734, 1995

Sherman P, Hassall E, Hunt RH, Fallone CA, Veldhuyzen van Zanten S, Thomson ABR: Canadian *Helicobacter* Study Group Consensus Conference on the approach to *H. pylori* infection in children and adolescents. Can J Gastroenterol 13:553–559, 1999

17.20 CHRONIC INFLAMMATORY BOWEL DISEASES

Marla C. Dubinsky and Ernest G. Seidman

Inflammatory bowel disease (IBD) refers to either ulcerative colitis or Crohn disease, disorders that are grouped together in view of similarities in their epidemiologic, immunologic, clinical, and therapeutic features. Distinguishing characteristics are listed in Table 17-50. In ulcerative colitis, the chronic inflammation is restricted to the mucosa of the large bowel. The rectum is universally involved in untreated cases. The superficial mucosal inflammation is continuous and homogeneous, with extension proximally to a varying extent along the colon. The diagnosis of ulcerative colitis usually is based on a suggestive history of bloody diarrhea and abdominal pain, which may be associated with fever. The diagnosis should be confirmed by endoscopic assessment with biopsies rather than by barium enema. Other causes of colitis in children are listed in Table 17-51.

In contrast to ulcerative colitis, the inflammatory process of Crohn disease is transmural and may involve any segment of the bowel, from the oral cavity to the anus. The asymmetric and segmental bowel involvement that characterizes Crohn disease usually facilitates its differentiation from ulcerative colitis. The terminal ileum is the site most frequently involved. Approximately two-thirds of pediatric patients with Crohn disease have some degree of colonic involvement, most often the cecum and/or ascending colon. In the 10 to 15% of patients whose disease is restricted to the large bowel, precise classification of the colitis may be difficult if no skip areas or pathognomonic granulomas are found. The presence of aphthous oral ulcerations or perianal lesions also is much more suggestive of the diagnosis of Crohn disease. Because of the myriad of intestinal and extraintestinal manifestations and the often nonspecific nature of symptoms at presentation, the diagnosis of Crohn disease is frequently difficult, resulting in diagnostic delay. Small bowel inflammatory disorders whose presentation may mimic Crohn disease are listed in Table 17-52.

Extraintestinal manifestations are present in most children with ulcerative colitis or Crohn disease. Such features may precede the intestinal symptoms by months to years. The extraintestinal manifestations associated with IBD are listed in Table 17-53.

ETIOLOGY AND EPIDEMIOLOGY

Children and adolescents account for approximately 25% of all cases of IBD. Crohn disease is primarily seen in children of school age and adolescents, outnumbering ulcerative colitis by approximately four to one. Among preschoolers, however, ulcerative colitis is about as frequent as Crohn disease. It has been suggested that the incidence of ulcerative colitis has been declining, and that of Crohn disease rising. The prevalence of Crohn disease is said to be higher among Ashkenazi Jews. Recent epidemiologic studies have suggested that the incidence of IBD is similar among African-American

TABLE 17-50

DISTINGUISHING FEATURES BETWEEN ULCERATIVE COLITIS AND CROHN DISEASE

FEATURE	ULCERATIVE COLITIS	CROHN DISEASE
Relative incidence of symptoms		
Rectal bleeding (gross)	Very common	Less common
Diarrhea	Often severe	Moderate or absent
Pain	Less frequent	Almost always
Anorexia	Mild or moderate	Can be severe
Weight loss	Moderate	Severe
Growth retardation	<10%	Approximately 40% at diagnosis
Extraintestinal manifestations	Common	Common
Involvement		
Small bowel		
Extensive	—	10%
Lower ileum	<5%	75%
Colon	100%	67%
Rectum	100%	50%
Anus	5%	45%
Distribution of lesions	Continuous	Segmental
Roentgenologic features	Superficial ulcers, loss of haustration, no skip areas, shortening	Serpiginous ulcers, thumbprinting, skip areas, string sign
Pathologic changes	Homogenous mucosal inflammation	Focal transmural disease with or without granulomas
Antineutrophil cytoplasmic antibodies	60%	10–15% (especially in those with ulcerative colitis–like disease)
Anti–*Saccharomyces cervisiae* antibodies	5%	60%

children and other children in the United States. The most important risk factor for IBD is a positive family history. There is a 5 to 20% likelihood of finding IBD in a first-degree relative of a proband in the pediatric age group. Crohn disease and ulcerative colitis may coexist in the same extended family, although strong disease concordance is usually present. There is an extremely high risk for Crohn disease (over one-third) when both parents are affected, whereas spouses, adopted children, and half-siblings are at low risk. Monozygotic twin pairs have a much stronger genetic tendency for Crohn disease than for ulcerative colitis (concordance in 44% vs 6% of unselected twin pairs). Recent genetic studies have suggested several putative disease susceptibility genes for IBD. There is also an association between IBD and other genetically determined diseases such as Hermansky-Pudlak and Turner syndromes, cystic fibrosis, and ankylosing spondylitis.

Despite intense research efforts, the etiology of IBD remains unknown. The current hypothesis suggests that the pathogenesis of IBD involves a genetically conditioned susceptibility to immune-mediated bowel injury triggered by one or more environmental factors. An imbalance in the local production of proinflammatory and down-regulatory cytokines characterizes the mucosal immune system in patients with IBD. Although there is renewed interest in searching for putative microbial pathogens, substantial clinical and experimental evidence suggests that the normal resident luminal bacterial components may be the environmental trigger.

Despite the lack of direct evidence of a role for serum antibodies in disease pathogenesis, they may serve as useful clinical markers for different types of IBD. Antineutrophil cytoplasmic antibody staining with perinuclear highlighting (pANCA) has become established as the marker most specific for ulcerative colitis, being present in approximately 60% of cases. The specificity of pANCA is imperfect for ulcerative colitis, as it has been reported to be positive in 10 to 15% of Crohn disease patients, particularly those with an ulcerative colitis–like presentation. Increased antibody titers to *Saccharomyces cerevisiae* (ASCA), a yeast organism normally found in the diet,

have been observed in the serum of the majority (60%) of patients with Crohn disease. ASCA is more specific for Crohn disease, being detectable in only about 5% of ulcerative colitis patients. Both pANCA and ASCA are generally negative in other, non-IBD forms of intestinal inflammation.

Although direct evidence for an infectious cause of IBD is lacking, infectious processes may trigger relapses. A recent viral or mycoplasmal upper respiratory tract infection commonly precedes relapses of Crohn disease, whereas an acute, infectious gastroenteritis more often precedes flares of disease activity in ulcerative colitis. Dietary factors have also been implicated; however, there is no firm evidence for a role of diet in pathogenesis of IBD. Although psychosocial stress was long implicated as playing a potential role in the pathogenesis of IBD, no causal relationship has ever been demonstrated.

17.20.1   Ulcerative Colitis

Ulcerative colitis occurs in all pediatric age groups, affecting both sexes equally with an incidence of 2 to 14 per 100,000. The mean age at diagnosis is approximately 12 years. Symptoms at presentation are usually acute, typically, bloody diarrhea mimicking an infectious colitis. In some patients, the insidious onset of chronic diarrhea without malnutrition may be present for months. The principal symptoms of ulcerative colitis are listed in Table 17-50, and the differential diagnosis is shown in Table 17-51.

At onset, only two-thirds of patients have diarrhea, and fewer than one-third have hematochezia. Tenesmus and urgency with fecal incontinence occur in one-quarter of patients. Generally, the extent of colonic involvement correlates with symptom severity. Patients with inflammation that is confined to the rectum (proctitis) usually present with the painless passage of blood-streaked stools and tenesmus. Those with more extensive colitis usually have bloody, mucoid diarrhea and cramping abdominal pain. Anorexia

TABLE 17-51

DIFFERENTIAL DIAGNOSIS OF COLITIS IN CHILDREN

Infectious
  Bacterial (*Salmonella, Shigella, Yersinia, Campylobacter jejuni, Escherichia coli* 0157)
  Parasitic (amebiasis, *Plesiomonas*)
  Viral (CMV, herpes)
  Pseudomembranous or antibiotic-associated (*Clostridium difficile*)
Chronic idiopathic
  Ulcerative colitis
  Crohn disease
  Behçet disease
  Lymphocytic colitis
  Collagenous colitis
  Intractable diarrhea (enterocolitis) of infancy
  Eosinophilic gastroenteropathy
Congenital immunodeficiencies and syndromes
  Chronic granulomatous disease
  Glycogen storage disease Ib
  Hermansky-Pudlak syndrome
Acquired immune deficiencies
  Human immunodeficiency virus–related
Allergic
  Eosinophilic colitis
Vascular
  Ischemic colitis
  Henoch-Schönlein purpura
  Hemolytic-uremic syndrome
Iatrogenic
  Radiation, chemotherapy (typhlitis)
  Diversion colitis
  Transplantation (bone marrow)
Neuromuscular
  Hirschsprung disease
  Pseudoobstruction syndromes
  Prestenotic

and nausea are common in the acute stage of moderate to severe illness, accounting for weight loss. Weight loss is often present in patients with extensive colonic involvement, but, generally, is not as severe as in Crohn disease. Exudative loss of protein through the inflamed bowel contributes to the hypoalbuminemia. Acute depletion of body water and electrolytes may occur during severe bouts of diarrhea. Fever, chills, leukocytosis, severe abdominal distension, nausea, and vomiting may indicate toxic colitis with megacolon or an impending local complication such as a free colonic perforation. Hypotension, dehydration, and altered mental status are usual in such circumstances.

Extraintestinal manifestations are listed in Table 17-53. Approximately 10% of patients have growth failure. Clubbing is common in long-standing disease. Episodes of arthralgias or arthritis coexist with colonic symptoms in 10 to 20% of affected children. A migratory, asymmetric, nondeforming arthritis affecting the large joints of the lower extremities is most common and often accompanies clinical relapses. Patients with ankylosing spondylitis can have progression of their skeletal disease independent of the colitis. Both erythema nodosum and pyoderma gangrenosum can occur with severe colitis and generally improve in parallel with the bowel disease.

Hepatobiliary complications occur in 5 to 10% of patients with IBD. Primary sclerosing cholangitis (PSC) is the most common form of chronic liver disease, occuring in approximately 3% of patients. PSC is most often associated with ulcerative colitis in that as many as 80% of adult PSC patients have ulcerative colitis. Autoimmune (chronic active) hepatitis develops in <1% of children with IBD and can be difficult to differentiate from PSC. There is no correlation between the severity or duration of the colitis and the liver disease, which may even predate the colitis.

IBD also is a risk factor for thromboembolic complications, particularly in colitis. In addition to deep-vein thromboses, repeated pulmonary emboli may occur. Ocular complications such as uveitis and episcleritis are not common in children with ulcerative colitis. However, posterior subcapsular cataracts may develop after long-term corticosteroid therapy. Regular opthalmologic evaluations are indicated.

LABORATORY FINDINGS AND DIAGNOSTIC TESTS

The diagnosis of ulcerative colitis is normally suspected on clinical grounds and confirmed by appropriate endoscopic and histologic

TABLE 17-52

DIFFERENTIAL DIAGNOSIS OF CROHN DISEASE OF THE SMALL BOWEL IN CHILDREN

Infections
  Appendicitis/appendiceal abscess
  Mesenteric adenitis
  Acute ileitis (enteritis)
    Yersinia enterocolitica
    Mycobacterium tuberculosis
    Giardia lamblia
    Entamoeba histolytica
    Campylobacter jejuni, Salmonella, Shigella (primarily colitis)
    Anisakiasis
Immunodeficiency disorders
  Congenital
  Acquired
Vascular disorders
  Hemolytic-uremic syndrome
  Henoch-Schönlein purpura
  Behçet disease
  Polyarteritis nodosum
  Systemic lupus erythematosus
  Dermatomyositis
  Systemic sclerosis
  Ischemic
Miscellaneous
  Eosinophilic gastroenteritis
  Intussusception
  Cystic fibrosis (meconium ileus equivalent)
  Chronic nongranulomatous ulcerative jejunoileitis
Iatrogenic
  Radiation
  Chemotherapy
  Transplant rejection, graft-versus-host disease
  Tumors
Obstetric and gynecologic
  Pelvic inflammatory disease
  Ectopic pregnancy
  Ovarian cysts, tumors
  Endometriosis

SOURCE: *Seidman E: Inflammatory bowel disease. In: Roy CC, Silverman A, Alagille D, eds: Pediatric Clinical Gastroenterology, 4th ed. St Louis, CV Mosby, 1995:417–493.*

TABLE 17-53

EXTRAINTESTINAL MANIFESTATIONS OF CROHN DISEASE AND ULCERATIVE COLITIS IN CHILDREN

	CROHN DISEASE	ULCERATIVE COLITIS
Fever	+++	+++
Perianal lesions	+++	
Growth failure	+++	+
Aphthous mouth ulcers	+++	+
Arthritis	++[a]	++
Ankylosing spondylitis[b]	+	+
Clubbing	++	+
Erythema nodosum	+	+
Pyoderma gangrenosum	+	+
Episcleritis, uveitis	+	+
Primary sclerosing cholangitis[b]	+[a]	+
Hepatic steatosis	+	+
Pericarditis		+
Amyloidosis	+	(+)
Thromboembolic disease	+[a]	+

[a] Primarily if the colon is involved.
[b] Unrelated to disease severity.
SOURCE: *Seidman E: Inflammatory bowel disease. In: Roy CC, Silverman A, Alagille D, eds: Pediatric Clinical Gastroenterology, 4th ed. St Louis, CV Mosby, 1995:417–493.*

findings and negative evaluation for an infectious colitis. Hypochromic, microcytic iron deficiency anemia is common. An elevated erythrocyte sedimentation rate and platelet count as well as hypoalbuminemia are frequently seen with active disease and constitute a good index of relapse. Minor, transient abnormalities of liver function tests are common; however, persistent abnormalities indicate a need to investigate for sclerosing cholangitis or autoimmune hepatitis. Positive serology for pANCA supports the diagnosis of ulcerative colitis but does not exclude Crohn colitis.

Contrast studies may be dangerous in patients with severe colitis because of the risks of perforation or precipitating toxic megacolon. These studies are contraindicated in the presence of colonic dilation. Therefore, in the acutely ill child with colitis, plain-film radiographs of the abdomen and a limited sigmoidoscopy should be done, rather than a barium enema. In severe (ie, toxic) colitis, thickening of the colonic wall usually is apparent, and "thumbprinting" can often be seen on a plain film, without contrast. Other worrisome signs of severity include colonic dilation and small bowel distention. If symptoms are mild to moderate, it is preferable to proceed directly to colonoscopy rather than to pursue barium studies, which are less sensitive and cannot distinguish between ulcerative colitis and other forms of acute or chronic bowel disorders. Although not essential because of uniform rectal involvement, colonoscopy and multiple biopsies are useful to determine the extent of the disease as well as to confirm the clinical diagnosis of ulcerative colitis. If it is thought necessary to perform a colonoscopy in patients with a history suggestive of mild to moderate colitis, preparation should be gentle, using osmotic purgatives. Colonoscopy is contraindicated in the presence of severe symptoms or inflammation. In such cases, it is optimally performed later, when the disease is better controlled.

Endoscopic findings in milder forms of ulcerative colitis typically reveal homogeneous blurring or loss of vascular pattern, along with hyperemia and edema of the mucosa. With moderate inflammation, the mucosa becomes distinctly granular and friable. More severe inflammation is associated with spontaneous bleeding and microulcerations of the mucosa. It is important for the endoscopist to note whether the mucosal involvement is diffuse, spreading proximally from the rectum. Multiple biopsies should be taken in order to map the extent of the disease, even in macroscopically normal areas. Indeed, uninvolved "skip areas" are important to document histologically, as they support a diagnosis of Crohn disease. Differentiation of ulcerative colitis and Crohn disease of the colon is often based on the presence of aphthous or linear ulcers in Crohn colitis. Mucosal biopsies may demonstrate pathognomonic granulomas of Crohn disease or may indicate active disease in regions of bowel that seemed endoscopically normal. Therefore, multiple biopsies should be obtained even when the mucosa appears to be normal. Biopsy also may help to distinguish between an acute, self-limited colitis and chronic IBD, which frequently manifests a chronic inflammatory cell infiltrate along with distorted crypt architecture, crypt atrophy, and basal lymphoid infiltrates.

MEDICAL MANAGEMENT

Ulcerative colitis is a lifelong and potentially debilitating disease, both physically and psychologically. However, with appropriate medical and surgical management and psychosocial support, almost all patients can enjoy a normal lifestyle and life expectancy. The medications employed to treat IBD act at various positions along the immune and inflammatory pathways. The commonly employed therapeutic agents and recommendations for their use are outlined below.

5-AMINOSALICYLATES   Sulfasalazine, which is composed of 5-aminosalicylic acid (5-ASA) linked by an azo bond to sulfapyridine, was used initially for rheumatoid arthritis. An unanticipated improvement in gastrointestinal symptoms was observed in patients with coexistent ulcerative colitis. Stable and poorly absorbed during passage through the small bowel, this drug is split in the colon by bacterial azoreductases. This releases the sulfapyridine moiety, which is mostly absorbed from the colon and acetylated in the liver. The 5-ASA component is poorly absorbed (10-20%) and is the active antiinflammatory moiety. Side effects of this drug (nausea, anorexia, and headache) are relatively frequent and largely related to the sulfapyridine moiety that delivers the 5-ASA to the colon. Slow acetylators or patients on higher doses of sulfasalazine are more apt to develop adverse effects.

In an effort to avoid adverse effects, equally efficacious yet more costly 5-ASA preparations have been formulated. Mesalamine preparations are enteric-coated 5-ASA, time-released when exposed to either moisture (Pentasa) or to a pH greater than 6 or 7 (Asacol, Claversal, Mesasal, and Salofalk). The development of sulfa-free aminosalicylate preparations has enabled clinicians to provide higher amounts of the pharmacologically active ingredient to the site of active bowel disease. Depending on the formulation chosen, 5-ASA is thus delivered variably to the small and/or large bowel. Olsalazine (Dipentum) links two 5-ASA molecules by an azo bond, which, like sulfasalazine, is metabolized by bacteria in the colon. Mesalamine is generally well tolerated at the therapeutic dose range employed (40-70 mg/kg/d, maximum 4.8 g). These newer preparations eliminate the side effects that are related to sulfapyridine, but they may cause diarrhea and headache. Up to 75% of patients with mild to moderate ulcerative colitis improve with 5-ASA or sulfasalazine. Once clinical remission is attained, oral mesalamine should be maintained at the same dose in the growing child in order to maintain remission. 5-ASA is also available topically in the form of rectal suppositories or enemas. There is convincing evidence that topical 5-ASA is effective for mild to moderate distal colitis. Up to 80% of patients with colitis distal to the splenic flexure will improve when treated with mesalamine enemas at doses of 1 to 4 g once or twice daily. An equivalent proportion of patients with ulcerative proctitis respond to mesalamine suppositories at doses of 500 mg twice a day. The anatomic extent and clinical severity will ultimately determine the approach to therapy. Rare cases of interstitial nephritis have been reported with chronic mesalamic usage so serum creatinine should be monitored.

CORTICOSTEROIDS Corticosteroids remain the most commonly employed agents in providing highly effective therapy for moderate to severe active ulcerative colitis. Although their actions remain incompletely understood, proposed mechanisms include the inhibition of phospholipase A_2 and cyclooxygenase, which in turn inhibit the production of inflammatory eicosanoids. The majority of patients benefit from 1 mg/kg/d of oral prednisone, to a maximum of 40 mg. Although dose-ranging trials have not been carried out in pediatrics, higher doses (2 mg/kg/d) have not been shown to produce better outcomes. In adult patients, 60 mg/d was associated with increased toxicity and with significant clinical benefit over a daily dose of 40 mg. Corticosteroids are indicated for the induction, but not the maintenance, of disease remission. Unfortunately, short-term and long-term use of corticosteroids is associated with numerous potential side effects, including hyperglycemia and glycosuria, increased vulnerability to infections, osteoporosis, osteonecrosis, myopathy, posterior subcapsular cataracts, growth retardation, behavioral and sleep disturbances, a cushingoid appearance, striae, and acne. The cosmetic side effects are frequent causes of dissatisfaction and poor adherence to therapy, particularly among adolescents. Additional complications most frequently noted during reduction in dose or withdrawal of therapy are acute adrenal insufficiency (characterized by fever, myalgias, arthralgias, nausea, and malaise) and pseudotumor cerebri. These complications significantly limit the applicability of the prolonged administration of corticosteroids in the setting of IBD.

Topically administered steroids are also beneficial in cases of distal colitis. They may be used as adjunctive therapy in patients with more proximal disease. Although hydrocortisone enemas or foam can control distal colitis, their prolonged administration can lead to adrenal suppression. Other preparations based on budesonide or fluticasone can be beneficial in such situations.

IMMUNOMODULATORY AGENTS 6-Mercaptopurine (6-MP) and its prodrug, azathioprine, constitute the most important therapeutic agents employed as steroid-sparing drugs for the long-term maintenance of remission in cases of severe ulcerative colitis and Crohn disease. These drugs are purine analogs that have both cytotoxic and immunosuppressive properties, inhibiting the proliferation and function of leukocytes. About 70% of patients respond favorably and are able to discontinue corticosteroids. Azathioprine is rapidly absorbed and converted to 6-MP, which is then metabolized further intracellularly. A favorable response to therapy significantly correlates with the intracellular levels of measured active metabolites (6-thioguanine nucleotides), and target therapeutic levels have been established recently. Because of their slow onset of action (3-6 months), 6-MP and azathioprine are not appropriate first-line therapy for patients presenting with severe active disease. Both drugs are relatively well tolerated (azathioprine, 2-3 mg/kg/d; 6-mercaptopurine, 1-1.5 mg/kg/d). Major complications are rare (<5%), but liver and pancreatic function tests as well as complete

blood counts (biweekly for 2 months, monthly for 2 months, then every third month thereafter) are mandatory. Elevated hepatic transaminases and/or leukopenia (WBC<4000/mm^3) occurs in 10 to 15% of patients, often resolving with lower doses of 6-MP. The risk of bone marrow suppression can be ascertained before initiation of therapy by testing for mutations in thiopurine methyltransferase, the catabolic enzyme that converts 6-MP into its 6-MMP metabolites. Hypersensitivity reactions characterized by skin rashes, recurrent fevers, or pancreatitis are the adverse effects most often necessitating discontinuation of 6-MP. Opportunistic infections are rare but can be potentially life threatening in any patient on immunosuppressive therapy. Despite a theoretical risk of causing increased breaks in DNA, no increased incidence of neoplasms or congenital malformations has been documented in patients receiving these drugs.

CYCLOSPORINE A Cyclosporine A (CsA) alters the immunoinflammatory cascade by inhibiting T-helper-cell production of proinflammatory cytokines. Compared to azathioprine, 6-MP, and methotrexate, CsA has a more rapid onset of action. Its use in IBD is generally restricted to patients with severe ulcerative colitis refractory to standard therapy with intravenous steroids (7-10 days), intravenous fluids, and bowel rest. Trough cyclosporine levels of 250 to 350 ng/mL of whole blood are therapeutic, with response usually seen within 7 days. Most patients (80%) improve and are able to avoid colectomy in the acute stage. However, the early relapse rate is over 40% in patients with ulcerative colitis who are on oral cyclosporine A at maintenance doses for 6 months. Use of cyclosporine A requires balancing the risks of potentially dangerous side effects (hepatotoxicity, neurotoxicity accompanied by seizures or tremors, electrolyte depletion—specifically Mg, hypertension, chronic renal damage, hirsutism, gingival hyperplasia, headaches, and paresthesias) against potential benefits, particularly in ulcerative colitis, which is a surgically curable disease.

METHOTREXATE Methotrexate is believed to act by inhibiting dihydrofolate reductase, thereby impairing DNA synthesis. It also inhibits proinflammatory cytokine production and induces T-cell apoptosis. In an uncontrolled study, methotrexate administered intramuscularly for 12 weeks showed a satisfactory clinical response in 83% of adult patients with Crohn disease and in 70% of those with ulcerative colitis. However, rates for the maintenance of remission using methotrexate orally were disappointing. Only 44% of patients with Crohn disease and 30% of patients with ulcerative colitis did not relapse within 1 year. Further uncontrolled studies have confirmed its disappointing long-term efficacy. Methotrexate is a potentially toxic drug, with leukopenia, hepatitis, hepatic fibrosis, pneumonitis, nausea, diarrhea, and hair loss among its reported side effects. In view of these results, and because of very limited experience with this drug, its use should be reserved for patients who are considered not to be surgical candidates and who have failed or not tolerated azathioprine, 6-mercaptopurine, or cyclosporine A.

ANTIBIOTICS AND OTHER DRUGS No consistent benefit has been demonstrated for antibiotic treatment in active or quiescent ulcerative colitis. Consequently, they do not have a proven role in the management unless there is a specific indication (eg, sepsis, abscess, and suspected perforation). Broad-spectrum antibiotics usually are administered to patients with signs of a toxic megacolon. A fairly high prevalence of *Clostridium difficile* toxin positivity is found in the stools of patients with severe colitis refractory to steroid therapy. A trial of oral vancomycin or metronidazole before a colectomy is considered worthwhile, in steroid-unresponsive disease is as response to therapy can be rapid and dramatic. Antidiarrheal agents are used infrequently in pediatric patients with IBD compared to adults. Loperamide is generally considered the best tolerated among these. However, such medications do not alter the inflammatory response and are contraindicated in the presence of severe disease. Similarly, opiates are useful for ameliorating pain but should be used with caution in the acute severe stages of the disease because they may alter motility and facilitate the development of toxic megacolon.

NUTRITION SUPPORT There is no evidence that bowel rest or TPN influences the outcome of ulcerative colitis. Patients requiring hospitalization for a relapse should receive parenteral nutrition if their baseline nutritional evaluation reveals that they are malnourished or if their intake is likely to be curtailed for at least 1 week. Growth failure has been reported in approximately 10% of pediatric patients with ulcerative colitis. Although much less common than in Crohn disease, this problem can significantly affect the child's self-esteem, behavior, and school performance. Nutritional support for growth failure in IBD is discussed later. A modest improvement of disease activity can be achieved by supplementing the diet with fish oils containing ω-3 fatty acids (9 g/1.73 m²/d). The magnitude of clinical benefit is likely contingent on a concomitant decrease in the ingestion of dietary ω-6 fatty acids (vegetable oils).

SURGICAL THERAPY Pancolectomy can be a life-saving procedure in the child with fulminant colitis or toxic megacolon. Ileoanal pull-through operations that preserve continence have largely replaced permanent ileostomies as the treatment of choice. Indications for surgery in the pediatric patient (Table 17-54) include urgent conditions such as massive hemorrhage, perforation, or toxic megacolon. More often, however, failure of medical therapies to control symptoms is the primary indication. Ulcerative colitis–specific and Crohn disease–specific serology (pANCA and ASCA, respectively) may not differentiate ulcerative colitis and Crohn disease before surgery when the classification remains indeterminate because those tests can lack specificity in this setting. Elective surgery should be considered in patients with steroid dependence, intolerance or complications of immunosuppressive therapy, long-standing disease, or evidence of colonic epithelial dysplasia. Growth failure that does not respond to medical and nutritional management is a less

TABLE 17-54

POSSIBLE INDICATIONS FOR SURGERY IN CHILDREN WITH ULCERATIVE COLITIS

Urgent
  Toxic megacolon
  Fulminant colitis (unresponsive to medical therapy)
  Perforation
  Hemorrhage
Elective
  Chronic active, unremitting disease
  Prolonged steroid dependence or intolerance to immunosuppressive
    medications
  High-grade dysplasia/malignancy
  Long-standing disease
  Growth failure (unresponsive to medical therapy and nutrition support

SOURCE: *Seidman E: Inflammatory bowel disease. In: Roy CC, Silverman A, Alagille D, eds. Pediatric Clinical Gastroenterology, 4th ed. St Louis, CV Mosby, 1995:417–493.*

common indication. Rarely, surgery is performed to control extraintestinal manifestations that parallel colonic activity.

A variety of pouches (J- and S-shaped) can be constructed to create a neorectum, which acts as a reservoir, reducing stool frequency and improving continence. Overall, very satisfactory results are obtained in 70 to 90% of children using the endorectal pull-through operation. The most troubling complication after pull-through is *pouchitis*, which causes an increase in stool frequency, lower abdominal pain, tenesmus, and even hematochezia. Pouchitis, which is seen in 10 to 35% of cases, has been attributed to fecal stasis, anastomotic strictures or leaks, bacterial infections, or diversion proctitis (ie, lack of short-chain fatty acids). Metronidazole has been the most effective agent in the management of pouchitis, but other therapies, including administration of probiotics such as *Lactobacillus* GG or other antibiotics such as ciprofloxacin may be useful in patients unable to tolerate metronidazole. Crohn disease that is mistaken for ulcerative colitis remains another distinct possibility in patients with chronic pouchitis.

SELECTION OF THERAPY

The various therapeutic modalities described above are selected largely on the basis of disease severity and location. Colonoscopy with biopsies can thus determine the extent of disease and direct therapy. Distal disease may benefit from topical enema or suppository therapy, whereas extensive disease or pancolitis requires orally administered or systemic medications. *Mild disease* is defined by fewer than four stools per day with or without blood, absence of systemic signs of toxicity, and a normal erythrocyte sedimentation rate (ESR). *Moderate disease* is characterized by more than four stools per day with minimal systemic symptoms. *Severe disease* is characterized by more than six bloody stools that are accompanied by fever, tachycardia, anemia, or an ESR > 30. *Toxic/fulminant colitis* is considered to be present when disease is severe with abdominal tenderness and reduced peristalsis. Such patients usually develop signs of toxicity (fever, tachycardia, leukocytosis, electrolyte disturbances, anemia) and symptoms (dehydration, mental changes, hypotension). The diagnosis of toxic megacolon is confirmed by the combination of a toxic patient with radiologic evidence of significant colonic dilatation. This complication is associated with a high risk of perforation; patients should be monitored closely with frequent physical examinations and abdominal films. A nasogastric tube should be placed to low suction, and intravenous corticosteroids and systemic broad-spectrum antibiotics administered. Lack of significant improvement within 24 to 72 hours is an indication for colonic resection.

RISK OF COLON MALIGNANCY

The long-term risk of developing colon cancer is a major concern in all patients with ulcerative colitis. The degree of risk is related to the duration as well as the anatomic extent of disease. After 10 years of having active disease, the yearly risk of developing colon cancer is 0.5 to 1.0%. The frequency of colon cancer in patients younger than 21 years of age who are diagnosed with ulcerative colitis is similarly elevated after 10 years of active disease, with incidence estimates of 9 to 20%. Adolescent patients have been seen with colon cancer as early as 7 years after diagnosis. Therefore, yearly colonoscopy with serial biopsies are indicated after about 7 years of onset of symptoms to identify signs of epithelial dysplasia, which is considered to be a precancerous lesion. If found, it is considered to be an indication for colectomy. Colon cancer that is associated with ulcerative colitis is preventable if the patient undergoes colectomy in the first decade of active disease.

17.20.2   Crohn Disease

The typical clinical and pathologic features of Crohn disease are reviewed in Table 17-50. The overall incidence is between 6 and 12 per 100,000 children younger than 18 years of age. Boys and girls are equally affected. Approximately 25% of all new cases occur in patients younger than 20 years of age, with the peak incidence during the second and third decades of life. Fewer than 5% occur in children younger than 5 years of age.

Approximately 70% of pediatric patients present with ileocolitis, usually involving the terminal ileum and cecum or right colon. Involvement limited to the colon occurs in approximately 15%. Upper endoscopy and biopsy have been shown to detect proximal GI tract involvement (ie, esophagus, stomach, and duodenum) in over 30% of pediatric patients; however, in only 1 to 2% is the disease limited to the area proximal to the ligament of Treitz.

Clinical features largely depend on the area and extent of the bowel that are affected. Not uncommonly, more than 1 year has elapsed between the onset of symptoms and diagnosis, particularly in children with primarily small bowel disease, because fewer of them present with severe or bloody diarrhea. When the small bowel is involved, patients typically present with chronic anorexia, fevers, subclinical malabsorption, and occasional vomiting. In such instances, growth failure may go unnoticed for years. Most children present with a history of chronic diarrhea. However, unlike ulcerative colitis, it is often nonbloody in nature and can be intermittent. A history of recurrent, ill-localized, crampy abdominal pain in the periumbilical region or right lower quadrant is common. This type of presentation often overlaps with symptoms of functional disorders that mimic IBD such as recurrent abdominal pain of childhood or lactose intolerance. This nonspecific presentation, if accompanied by the absence of physical findings, often leads to a delay in diagnosis. Approximately 10% of children may present initially with an acute episode mimicking an attack of appendicitis, sometimes leading to laparotomy. Others present primarily with extraintestinal manifestations or an acute onset that is indistinguishable from severe ulcerative colitis.

Many children decrease their food intake to avoid the abdominal pain that eating provokes. Loss of appetite may be severe enough to be mistaken for anorexia nervosa. Weight loss is present in approximately 75%, whereas abnormal growth velocity (<3%) is seen in almost one-half of active cases. Nausea and vomiting may indicate that the patient is acutely ill or has long-standing disease with partial or complete intestinal obstruction. Anal lesions are quite commonly overlooked in pediatric patients. However, more than one-third of children with Crohn disease present with an anal fissure, tag, abscess, and/or fistula.

Many of the extraintestinal manifestations of ulcerative colitis reviewed previously and listed in Table 17-53 also are present in patients with Crohn disease. Aphthous stomatitis and perianal lesions are particularly associated with Crohn disease. Joint complaints and perianal lesions are more common in patients with colonic involvement. Perianal lesions, including recurrent fissures, edematous skin tags, fistulas, or abscesses, may dominate the presentation. Malnutrition that is complicated by growth failure and pubertal delay may be the mode of presentation in an otherwise asymptomatic child. Growth retardation may precede clinical symptoms by years and persist despite the apparent lack of evidence of disease activity. Impaired linear growth already is present in approximately 40% of children at the time of diagnosis.

LABORATORY FINDINGS AND DIAGNOSTIC TESTS

The history and physical examination at presentation are usually highly suggestive of Crohn disease. Investigations, including radiologic and endoscopic studies, are primarily used to confirm the diagnosis and to establish the anatomic location of disease. In the presence of active disease, the sedimentation rate is usually (but not invariably) increased, and iron deficiency anemia is common. Hypoalbuminemia is present in over 60% of cases, mostly because of the protein-losing enteropathy associated with chronic inflammation. Up to 25% of children with Crohn disease may have clinically inapparent steatorrhea and increased fecal loss of bile acids. Acute-phase reactant proteins may be useful markers of disease activity. A variety of inflammatory mediators, cytokines (interleukin 6, IL-6) and cytokine receptors (soluble IL-2R) have been detected in serum in increased quantities during relapses. Stool markers of inflammation such as α_1-antitrypsin also have been widely used to determine disease activity. Indium-labeled white-blood-cell scans may identify regions of increased disease activity.

When Crohn disease is limited to the colon, its clinical and pathologic features overlap significantly with those seen in ulcerative colitis. A precise diagnosis cannot always be made in such cases of "indeterminate" colitis. The endoscopy demonstration of discrete superficial aphthous ulcerations is characteristic of Crohn disease. As the disease progresses, the ulcerations enlarge and coalesce as well as deepen. Longitudinal and transverse deep ulcerations may be interspersed by less affected mucosal islands, giving a cobblestone appearance to the involved bowel. Lesions often are discontinuous, giving rise to so-called "skip areas." Continuing inflammation results in nodular swelling and progressive fibrosis of the bowel wall, with narrowing of the lumen, which can cause complete obstruction. Eventually, a classic hose-pipe stricture may ensue, which is characterized by a rigid, edematous, fibrotic bowel wall. Transmural inflammation may result in fistulous tracts, which may cause communication between diseased loops or often with a healthy loop of bowel. Although a fistula may establish a communicating tract with other intraabdominal organs (eg, bladder, vagina) and structures (eg, perineum, abdominal wall), it most often will end blindly and form an intraperitoneal or retroperitoneal inflammatory mass (phlegmon) or a frank abscess. Microscopically, the chronic granulomatous inflammatory reaction with edema and fibrosis characteristically involves all layers of the intestinal wall. The presence of noncaseating granulomas containing multinucleated giant cells and epithelioid cells is pathognomonic, but their absence does not rule out the diagnosis of Crohn disease. As in ulcerative colitis, invasion and injury of crypts by neutrophils are frequent findings. Although cryptitis and crypt abscesses do not distinguish the type of IBD, focal crypt destruction is the most suggestive of Crohn disease.

When both the small and large bowel are involved, there is usually little doubt about the diagnosis. A tender right lower quadrant mass or fullness often is palpable. Detection of perianal disease also is very suggestive of Crohn disease. Radiologic assessments of the upper GI tract and small bowel should be confirmatory, although ulcerative colitis with "backwash ileitis" may pose a dilemma. Colonoscopy with multiple biopsies is the best approach to confirming the diagnosis when the colon is involved. The differential diagnosis of terminal ileitis includes other granulomatous inflammatory processes such as tuberculosis, histoplasmosis, amebiasis, and sarcoidosis. Lymphomas, appendicitis, adenocarcinoma, and intestinal scleroderma may mimic Crohn disease (Table 17-52). Before corticosteroid therapy is initiated, infectious and other etiologies should be excluded.

As discussed above, the diagnosis of Crohn disease is often delayed because of the nonspecific nature of intestinal and extraintestinal symptoms at presentation. Additionally, other disorders of childhood mimic IBD and are indistinguishable in the absence of invasive testing (colonoscopy with biopsies and barium studies). The presence or absence of serologic immune markers can facilitate clinical decision making in evaluating a pediatric patient presenting with nonspecific symptoms suggestive of Crohn disease in whom the physical exam is normal. Screening for Crohn disease using specific ASCA antibodies can reinforce a clinical suspicion of Crohn disease but absence does not eliminate the possibility of diagnosis of Crohn disease.

MEDICAL MANAGEMENT

In contrast to ulcerative colitis, no definitive surgical or other therapy is available for Crohn disease. Medications are employed to control symptoms and treat complications while minimizing side effects. The generally accepted strategy is that therapy should be based on symptoms rather than laboratory tests or endoscopic, histologic, or radiologic findings. Clinical remission does not imply endoscopic healing, and prolonging corticosteroid therapy on the basis of endoscopic appearance does not change the natural course of the disease. Furthermore, there is little evidence that corticosteroid maintenance therapy is effective in preventing relapses of Crohn disease.

The course of Crohn disease is highly variable and depends on the disease extent and behavior (eg, inflammatory, fistulizing, fibrostenotic). Acute fulminant episodes are less frequent than in ulcerative colitis; Crohn disease often follows a more chronic and unremitting course. Transmural inflammation may lead to intestinal obstruction (25%), blind loop syndrome, internal fistulization, and abscess formation. Massive hemorrhage is an infrequent event. Toxic megacolon is unusual. Perianal disease may occasionally precede intestinal involvement and constitute serious and disabling complications. Rectal fissures and fistulas may be associated with perirectal abscesses, perineal sepsis, rectovaginal fistulas, and varying degrees of damage to the rectal sphincters. Evaluation under anesthesia may be necessary in view of the pain. Repeat radiologic evaluations should be performed only when necessary because substantial diagnostic radiation exposure can be predicted over the patient's lifetime. Abdominal computed tomographic scans have a higher sensitivity in detecting fistulas or an abscess than do barium studies or ultrasonography.

5-AMINOSALICYLATES The utility of sulfasalazine for Crohn disease is less clear than for ulcerative colitis and depends on the site of disease activity. Randomized, controlled studies have shown efficacy for induction of remission in ileocolonic or colonic disease but not for isolated small bowel involvement. It is inferior to prednisone alone but has fewer side effects. In terms of maintenance therapy, sulfasalazine is mainly beneficial in prevention of recurrence postoperatively. As noted above, the development of sulfafree aminosalicylate formulations has enabled clinicians to employ higher doses of the active drug, directed to the site of bowel disease. Despite the heterogeneity of Crohn disease and its variable course, there is evidence that 5-ASA has a role in the induction of remission

for patients with mild to moderately active Crohn disease. There appears to be a dose-response relationship, with higher doses associated with higher remission rates. The dosage for various formulations of 5-ASA has not been established in children with Crohn disease. However, studies have demonstrated a benefit from 40 to 70 mg/kg/d. 5-ASA enemas and suppositories are effective for distal Crohn colitis and proctitis, respectively, as noted above for ulcerative colitis.

CORTICOSTEROIDS Corticosteroid therapy results in dramatic improvement in over 85% of patients with Crohn disease of the small or large bowel, often within 1 week of its initiation. The generally recommended dose of prednisone is 1.0 to 2.0 mg/kg/d (maximum 40 mg/d). Although some patients respond more favorably to 60 mg/day, the clinical efficacy is offset by the higher rate of side effects. Typically, 1 mg/kg/d is maintained for 3 to 4 weeks after remission has been achieved (for a total of 5 to 8 weeks). Gradual weaning is then attempted through decreasing the dose by 5 mg every 5 to 7 days. One-fifth of patients become steroid refractory, and over a third are steroid dependent during the first year of corticosteroid therapy. Corticosteroids are thus rarely used as monotherapy. Combination therapy with 5-ASA, metronidazole, or immunomodulatory drugs (azathioprine or 6-MP) is usually employed during the steroid-tapering period. The considerable adverse effects of conventional corticosteroids have led to the development of analogs that are systemically less active. Budesonide, the best studied among these novel steroids, has been shown to have slightly lower efficacy than prednisone in the treatment of distal ileal or ileocecal Crohn disease. Notably, budesonide has fewer glucocorticoid-associated side effects and less suppression of pituitary adrenal function than conventional steroids, but this agent is not yet available in the United States. Despite substantial evidence supporting a role for steroids in the management of active Crohn disease, there is no evidence supporting steroid maintenance therapy with either prednisone or budesonide.

IMMUNOMODULATORY AGENTS One of the most common dilemmas in moderate to severe Crohn disease is the preponderance of steroid-dependent and resistant cases. These situations constitute indications for immunomodulatory therapy. Approximately 75% of children receiving 6-mercaptopurine (6-MP) or azathioprine maintain remission off all corticosteroids. Fistulas close in 30 to 40% of patients, and perianal disease improves in the majority. The doses used in pediatric patients and the use of pharmacogenetic analysis for TPMT mutations in order to ascertain risk of myelotoxicity are discussed in section 17.20.1. One of the caveats in using these drugs is their delayed onset of action. A recent trial suggests that the intravenous administration of azathioprine does not expedite the time to response. As discussed above, intracellular levels of key metabolites, 6-TG and 6-MMP, correlate with clinical response and drug-related toxicity. The optimal duration of 6-MP therapy has not been determined. However, most pediatric patients relapse on discontinuation of therapy and are generally maintained on therapy until early adulthood.

CYCLOSPORINE A As noted for ulcerative colitis, cyclosprine A (CsA) is effective for the treatment of acute Crohn disease. Approximately 60% of steroid-refractory and fistulizing disease responds. However, a recent multicentered study on the maintenance of remission in Crohn disease failed to demonstrate any benefit from low-dose (5 mg/kg/d) CsA. Potential indications thus include chronic active disease unresponsive to corticosteroids or severe perianal and fistulous disease. Adverse effects associated with CsA include hypertension, nephrotoxicity, electrolyte imbalance (especially hypomagnesemia), hirsutism, gingival hyperplasia, paresthesias and tremors, seizures, depression, and serious opportunistic infections. Cyclosporine should thus be used for the short term as a bridge to more effective maintenance immunomodulatory therapy such as 6-MP.

METHOTREXATE A multicenter, placebo-controlled trial in adults with steroid-refractory Crohn disease revealed that parenteral methotrexate administered weekly for 16 weeks was twice as likely to allow steroid tapering and maintenance of remission (39% vs 19%). Its use in children with Crohn disease is generally restricted to patients failing to respond or those experiencing significant complications with 6-MP/AZA. A small, uncontrolled pediatric study reported an overall improvement in 64% of patients receiving subcutaneous methotrexate injections (15 mg/m²/wk), generally within 4 to 6 weeks.

ANTIBIOTICS The major indication for broad-spectrum antibiotics is intraabdominal sepsis and abscess formation. Metronidazole, the most extensively investigated antimicrobial agent for the treatment of Crohn disease, has similar efficacy (at 10-20 mg/kg/d) to sulfasalazine as primary therapy for mildly to moderately active Crohn. It is also effective for perineal lesions. However, most patients relapse when the medication is discontinued. Metronidazole has been used effectively to prevent postoperative recurrence after ileal resection. Common side effects include nausea, appetite loss, and a metallic taste. Peripheral neuropathy can occur with prolonged administration, often manifested initially as paresthesias. This complication is usually dose related but can persist for years after stopping therapy. Ciprofloxacin has recently been shown to be beneficial as an alternative to metronidazole, with efficacy similar to mesalamine. Furthermore, ciprofloxacin in combination with metronidazole is beneficial in the treatment of fistulous and perianal Crohn disease. Ciprofloxacin can potentially have adverse effects on bone growth plates and therefore should be avoided in the growing child. Among the most common side effects are myalgias and arthralgias.

BIOLOGIC THERAPIES Advances in our understanding of the immunopathogenesis of IBD have led to the development of novel biological agents genetically engineered to specifically target integral steps in the immune response cascade. Infliximab, a chimeric IgG1 monoclonal antibody directed against tumor necrosis factor (anti-TNF-α), is the first biological agent to receive FDA approval for clinical use in patients with steroid-refractory intestinal or perianal Crohn disease. Pediatric pilot studies demonstrated that anti-TNF-α is also effective for children with treatment-refractory Crohn disease. However, there are currently persistent concerns regarding long-term safety and efficacy. Therefore, use should be reserved for those patients that are refractory to other therapy.

NUTRITIONAL THERAPY Active Crohn disease responds to bowel rest with total enteral or parenteral nutrition. An elemental diet is simpler, safer, and less expensive than TPN. The diet is administered to the exclusion of other food for 1 month. There is a high early relapse rate when the diet is discontinued and a lower efficacy with distal (colonic/perianal) disease. Metaanalyses have confirmed that steroids are superior to nutrition alone in inducing remission. However, dietary therapy has no side effects and avoids the adverse effects of steroids, including growth inhibition. With flavor packets,

approximately 75% of patients are able to tolerate elemental preparations orally, avoiding the need for nasogastric infusions. Once induced, remission may be maintained by the cyclic administration of an elemental diet, 1 out of every 4 months. In addition to relapse prevention, steroid use is avoided, growth is enhanced, and bone mineralization improves.

TREATMENT OF GROWTH FAILURE Normal growth is an important indicator of disease control and therapeutic efficacy in pediatric Crohn disease. However, despite "appropriate medical therapy," Crohn disease results in permanent short stature in 20 to 35% of adults who had the disease before puberty. The nutritional impact of IBD is particularly severe in the prepubertal patient. Growth failure is a common, serious complication that is unique to the pediatric age group. There is a time limit for potential "catch-up" growth because of progressive bone maturation and eventual epiphyseal fusion. In order to be effective, therapy must therefore be initiated well before bone maturation is complete. Chronic undernutrition resulting primarily from inadequate caloric intake is by far the most important factor. Caloric intake in pediatric IBD is only 54 to 85% of estimated requirements, and anorexia often persists despite clinical remission. Intervention must be initiated early, consistently, and aggressively, assuring adequate nutritional support over a sufficient period of time in order to achieve enhanced growth. When growth is significantly impaired and the disease remains localized and nonprogressive, surgical management may be considered. In general, however, surgery is considered for growth failure only if optimal medical and nutritional therapies have failed. TPN can achieve weight gain and reverse growth arrest in Crohn disease, but metabolic and infectious complications as well as cost considerations favor the use of enteral nutritional support. Nocturnal nasogastric supplementation of an elemental or a polymeric formula (40-80 kcal/kg ideal body weight/d) effectively reverses growth failure. Compliance with high-calorie oral supplements generally is poor over the long term.

ASSESSMENT OF BONE HEALTH Osteoporosis is associated with high risk of fractures to the spine, hip, and radius and has been reported in 20 to 30% of patients with IBD. Pediatric patients are not immune to this serious complication. Decreased bone mineral density has been observed in nearly 70% of children and adolescents with Crohn disease. Although a major determinant of the development of osteoporosis, it may occur in the absence of steroid use, particularly in association with nutritional deficiencies. Bone loss can occur early in the course of disease and is often present at initial evaluation. All children with Crohn disease should have baseline and serial bone mineral density assessments. In view of the frequency of short stature and delayed bone maturation, bone mineral density results should be interpreted in terms of bone or height age, rather than chronologic age. The potential benefit of agents such as aledronate or biphosphonate for children with IBD and decreased bone mineral density has not yet been systematically evaluated.

SURVEILLANCE OF COLON MALIGNANCY Although the reported incidence of carcinoma of the colon is lower than that of ulcerative colitis, it is 20 times higher than that in the general population. Thus, patients with extensive, long-standing Crohn colitis (>10 years) warrant colonoscopic surveillance as recommended for patients with ulcerative colitis.

SURGICAL THERAPY Crohn disease cannot be cured surgically. Operative procedures should thus be reserved for complications. Up to 70% of pediatric patients require surgery within 10 years of diagnosis. Emergency surgery is indicated for massive hemorrhage, free perforation, and fulminant colitis or toxic megacolon that fails to respond to aggressive medical treatment. Elective surgery may be performed for intractability of symptoms, recurrent episodes of intestinal obstruction, or an abscess that fails to respond to conservative measures. Enteroenteric fistulas may not require surgery unless a fistula causes significant malabsorption or drains poorly.

When isolated, resection of severely involved regions of bowel (usually the terminal ileum) may allow a reduction in medication, increase well-being, and allow improved growth. Overall, 50% of pediatric patients undergoing resection for strictures or abscesses have a clinical relapse within 5 years. However, recurrence rates can be as high as 40% at 1 year postoperatively for patients with refractory and extensive ileocolonic disease. Conservative resection is recommended to prevent the potential outcome of short-bowel syndrome following multiple surgeries.

Perianal lesions sometimes heal spontaneously or with the use of antibiotics and immunomodulatory drugs. Surgical measures include abscess drainage, fistulotomy, or the use of setons. However, when severe rectal involvement is contiguous to the anal disease, fecal diversion with an ileostomy or colostomy may be required.

References

Genetics, Pathogenesis, and Epidemiology

Bennett RA, Rubin PH, Present DH: Frequency of inflammatory bowel disease in offspring of couples both presenting with inflammatory bowel disease. Gastroenterology 100:1638–1643, 1991

Binder V: Genetic epidemiology in inflammatory bowel disease. Dig Dis Sci 16:351–355, 1999

Cohen MB, Seidman E, Winter H, et al: Controversies in pediatric inflammatory bowel disease. Inflamm Bowel Dis 4:203–227, 1998

Fiocchi C: Inflammatory bowel disease: etiology and pathogenesis. Gastroenterology 115:182–205, 1998

Gilat T, Hacohen D, Lilos P, Langman MJS: Childhood factors in ulcerative colitis and Crohn's disease. An international cooperative study. Scand J Gastroenterol 22:1009–1024, 1987

Marx G, Seidman EG: Inflammatory bowel disease in pediatric patients. Curr Opin Gastroenterol 15:322–325, 1999

Satsangi J, Jewell DP, Bell JI: The genetics of inflammatory bowel disease. Gut 40:572–574, 1997

Diagnosis

Gryboski JD: Ulcerative colitis in children 10 years old or younger. J Pediatr Gastroenterol Nutr 17:24–31, 1993

Lennaerts C, Roy CC, Vaillancourt M, et al: High incidence of upper gastrointestinal tract involvement in children with Crohn's disease. Pediatrics 83:777–781, 1989

Ruemmele FM, Targan S, Levy G, Dubinsky M, Braun J, Seidman EG: Diagnostic accuracy of serological assays in pediatric inflammatory bowel disease. Gastroenterology 115:822–829, 1998

Extraintestinal Manifestations

Gokhale R, Favus MJ, Karrison T, et al: Bone mineral density assessment in children with inflammatory bowel disease. Gastroenterology 114:902–911, 1998

Herzog D, Bishop N, Glorieux F, Seidman EG. Interpretation of bone mineral density values in pediatric Crohn's disease. Inflamm Bowel Dis 4:261–267, 1998

Levine JB, Lukawski-Trubish D: Extraintestinal considerations in inflammatory bowel disease. Gastroenterol Clin North Am 24:633–646, 1995

Markowitz J, Grancher K, Rosa J, et al: Growth failure in pediatric inflammatory bowel disease. J Pediatr Gastroenterol Nutr 16:373, 1994

Passo MH, Fitzgerald JF, Brandt KD: Arthritis associated with inflammatory bowel disease in children: relationship of joint disease to activity and severity of bowel lesion. Dig Dis Sci 31:492–497, 1986

Rankin GB: Extraintestinal and systemic manifestations of inflammatory bowel disease. Med Clin North Am 74:39–50, 1990

Risk of Malignancy

Pinczowski D, Ekbom A, Baron J, et al: Risk factors for colorectal cancer in patients with ulcerative colitis: a case control study. Gastroenterology 107:117–120, 1994

Richards ME, Rickert RR, Nance FC: Crohn's disease–associated carcinoma. A poorly recognized complication of inflammatory bowel disease. Ann Surg 209:764–773, 1989

Sugita A, Sachar DB, Bodian C, et al: Colorectal cancer in ulcerative colitis. Influence of anatomical extent and age of onset on colitis-cancer interval. Gut 32:167–169, 1991

Management

Belli D, Seidman EG, Bouthillier L, et al: Chronic intermittent elemental diet improves growth failure in children with Crohn's disease. Gastroenterology 94:603–610, 1988

Dubinsky MC, Lamothe S, Yang HY, et al: Pharmacogenomics and metabolite measurement for 6-mercaptopurine therapy in inflammatory bowel disease. Gastroenterology 118:705–713, 2000

Ferguson A: Assessment and management of ulcerative colitis in children. Eur J Gastroenterol Hepat 9:858–863, 1997

Fonkalsrud EW, Loar N: Long-term results after colectomy and endorectal pull-through procedure in children. Ann Surg 215:57–62, 1992

Martin LW, Warner BW, Brockmeier M: Long-term evaluation of the endorectal Soave operation performed for ulcerative colitis or polyposis in the pediatric patient. Surgery 114:893–896, 1993

Pearson DC, May GR, Fick GH, Sutherland LR: Azathioprine and 6-mercaptopurine in Crohn's disease. A meta-analysis. Ann Intern Med 123:132–142, 1995

Present DH, Rutgeerts P, Targan S, et al: Infliximab for the treatment of fistulas in patients with Crohn's disease. N Engl J Med 340:1398–1405, 1999

Ruemmele F, Roy CC, Levy E, Seidman EG: The role of nutrition in treating pediatric Crohn's disease in the new millennium. J Pediatr 136:285–291, 2000

17.21 OTHER DISORDERS OF THE SMALL INTESTINE AND COLON

17.21.1 Gastrointestinal Manifestations of Food Protein–Induced Hypersensitivity

Peter Baehler and Ernest G. Seidman

Adverse reactions to food are defined as reproducible *food intolerances* of various etiologies. The classification includes toxic (ie, bacterial contamination), pharmacologic (ie, histamines, tyramine), metabolic (ie, disaccharidase deficiency), neuropsychological (ie, hyperactivity, irritability), and allergic (ie, immunologic) reactions.

The terms *food allergy* or *food hypersensitivity* should be reserved exclusively for reproducible adverse clinical reactions that are mediated by abnormal immune responses. Among food protein–induced allergic responses with GI manifestations, only a fraction are caused by reaginic IgE antibodies (ie, immediate type of reaction). Antigen-antibody complex formation (ie, type III reaction) and T-cell–mediated immune responses (ie, type IV reaction) also are capable of inducing symptoms in patients with a delayed-type reaction to food proteins. However, a causal relationship between a delayed-type immune response to food antigens and an adverse clinical reaction has not yet been clearly established.

During the first year after birth, cow's milk and cow's milk–based formulas are the major food antigens involved in GI allergic reactions to food proteins. There is a marked variability in the reported incidence of milk allergy, ranging from 0.3 to 7.5%, depending on the diagnostic criteria used for the study. Soy protein–based formulas are no less antigenic than cow's milk proteins; many infants who are allergic to cow's milk also will be intolerant to soy. Foods that commonly are associated with GI allergic reactions include eggs, nuts, rice, seafood, various meats (eg, chicken, beef, pork), wheat, and potatoes. Unlike cow's milk or soy protein allergy, which often is transient, nut allergy usually is lifelong and more often life-threatening. Among the 20 protein fractions in cow's milk, the whey protein β-lactoglobulin is considered to be the most antigenic.

PATHOPHYSIOLOGY OF GASTROINTESTINAL ALLERGY

Normally, the gut mucosa acts as a barrier limiting the penetration of pathogens, toxins, and foreign (ie, food) antigens into the host's internal milieu. Several defense mechanisms, both nonimmunologic and immunologic, act in concert to provide an efficient gut mucosal barrier. Among nonimmune factors are the normal bacterial flora that helps to prevent overgrowth of pathogenic organisms, the inhibition of attachment of pathogenic organisms and antigens to the epithelium by the glycoproteins in the mucous coat, and the digestive enzymes that normally hydrolyze proteins into nonantigenic peptides. Nevertheless, macromolecular antigens can escape these various lines of defense and may be absorbed intact. The absorptive epithelium and the immunocompetent cells of the lamina propria interact in the induction and regulation of immune responses to ingested antigens. Normally, food antigen exposure via the enteric route results in a local IgA response and a preferential suppression of IgG and IgE via the generation of specific T suppressor cells. This physiological phenomenon, which is referred to as *oral tolerance,* is thought to be aberrant in individuals with food allergies. A child with one or two atopic parents has a 30% or 60% chance, respectively, to develop allergic diseases. An atopic history in two first-degree relatives is associated with a slightly increased risk of a cow's milk protein allergy in infancy.

COW'S MILK PROTEIN ALLERGY

A wide variety of symptoms and clinical syndromes have been attributed to cow's milk protein allergy (Table 17-55). The majority of infants present within 3 months of exposure to cow's milk protein. Symptoms may be provoked by consumption of cow's milk–based formula, indirectly via antigen transmission through breast milk, or even by intrauterine sensitization. Gastrointestinal symptoms usually predominate in cow's milk protein allergy, but in many infants and young children, other symptoms coexist, especially eczema. Acute symptoms usually include diarrhea and projectile vomiting, thus imitating infectious gastroenteritis. Anaphylactic shock that is associated with acute severe enterocolitis is a life-threatening, although infrequent, manifestation of cow's milk protein allergy and usually occurs in the neonatal period after early sensitization. Cutaneous manifestations such as urticaria, angioedema, and acute circumoral swelling most commonly are encountered with immediate-onset (ie, type I) reactions.

The hallmark of chronic symptoms, representing delayed-type reactions, is chronic diarrhea. A variable degree of damage to the small bowel mucosa occurs, leading to malabsorption and failure to thrive (ie, cow's milk enteropathy) in more severe cases. Widespread intestinal inflammation also may cause gastritis, intestinal protein loss (ie, protein-losing enteropathy), or hematochezia because of allergic (ie, eosinophilic) colitis. Although there is some overlap between these GI manifestations, allergic colitis appears to present almost exclusively within 6 months after birth, and it generally is not associated with failure to thrive. Rarely, milk hypersensitivity may present as necrotizing enterocolitis of the newborn.

DIAGNOSIS OF FOOD ALLERGY

The standard procedure for diagnosis of food allergy, which is modified from the classical criteria of Goldman, requires a careful medical history and physical examination, elimination diet, and oral food challenge. The history may not allow differentiation between food allergy and other etiologies, but it is helpful in elucidating immediate-type reactions such as vomiting, urticaria, angioedema,

TABLE 17-55

CLASSIFICATION OF COW'S MILK PROTEIN–INDUCED GASTROINTESTINAL ALLERGIC DISORDERS

MECHANISM	ONSET	CLINICAL MANIFESTATION
IgE mediated (type I)	Immediate (0–1 h)	Gastrointestinal anaphylaxis Vomiting, diarrhea, shock, enterocolitis Atopic eczema Bronchitis/asthma Rhinitis Eosinophilic gastroenteritis Infantile colic?
Non–IgE mediated (type III or IV)	Intermediate (1–24 h) or late reactions (>24 h)	Cow's milk–induced enteropathy Diarrhea, malabsorption Eosinophilic colitis Protein-losing enteropathy Intractable diarrhea of infancy

or anaphylaxis after the ingestion of a single food. Symptoms should disappear within a few days after elimination of the suspected food(s). In chronic diarrhea, recovery may take weeks, thus making it more difficult to recognize a clear response to the restricted diet. Hypoallergenic formulas often are associated with abnormal stool character, so weight gain should be used as the main criterion for improvement. Compliance with a strict elimination diet is difficult; consultation with an experienced dietician is helpful.

A positive oral food challenge remains the definitive diagnostic hallmark for food allergy. Food challenges should always be performed under medical supervision, preferably in a hospital setting, so that any anaphylactic reactions can be managed. Patients should have been on an elimination diet from the suspected food for at least 3 to 4 weeks before the challenge. In young infants with severe symptoms, the challenge should not be done earlier than 6 months after beginning the elimination diet because of the increased risk of an anaphylactic reaction, nor should it be done in infants with malabsorption and malnutrition until nutritional rehabilitation and improved gut function have occurred. Severe intractable diarrhea requiring parenteral nutrition may ensue if a challenge is undertaken too early. An open milk challenge is adequate in children younger than 5 years of age, but in older children, a double-blind, placebo-controlled food challenge (DBPCFC), in which neither the patient and parents nor the investigator is aware of the administered food, is necessary. The offending food is administered in a graded fashion, starting with a minute quantity; the dose is doubled at intervals of 15 minutes until the patient has convincing symptoms or a standardized total dose of food has been ingested (eg, 4 oz. of milk). The absence of a reaction during the DBPCFC does not preclude the possibility of delayed-type allergic responses.

Several important practical problems are encountered with food challenges:

1. Some children are so sensitive to cow's milk protein that a challenge would impose unnecessary risks or morbidity.
2. Symptoms may change with successive challenges or differ from the patient's history, depending on the rate of food administration or the age of the child.
3. The child may have outgrown the allergy to cow's milk protein by the time of the challenge, thus incorrectly excluding the initial diagnosis of cow's milk protein allergy.
4. The adverse reaction may be caused by other factors such as lactose or sucrose intolerance or by an intercurrent acute infectious gastroenteritis.

LABORATORY TESTS

In patients with chronic diarrhea and failure to thrive or with clinical symptoms of colitis (eg, rectal bleeding), endoscopic and histologic investigations of the small bowel and/or the colon and rectum are indicated. Skin-prick testing is the most sensitive method to screen for IgE-mediated food allergies (testing local mast cell–bound antigen-specific IgE); it is equal or superior to the radioallergosorbent test determination of IgE (detecting circulating antigen-specific IgE). Its value is confined to patients with immediate-onset (ie, type I) reactions (negative predictive value >95%; sensitivity 50 to 90% with increased false positives in the eczema subgroup). Patients with delayed-onset reactions are much less often skin-test positive (ie, 15 to 20%), making this test less valuable. The diagnostic value of serum IgE concentration, peripheral eosinophilia, and circulating IgG antibodies to cow's milk protein is poor in delayed GI reactions. Assays for cellular immune response such

as the lymphocyte proliferation test generally have a low sensitivity, albeit a reasonably high specificity, thus precluding their wide applicability as screening tests.

MANAGEMENT

Treatment consists of strict elimination of the allergen from the diet. For infants and young children with cow's milk protein allergies, the appropriate choice of a cow's milk substitute should meet certain essential criteria, including no or little cross-reactivity with cow's milk protein, lower allergenicity, and nutritional adequacy. Formulas that presently are available as cow's milk substitutes for infants with cow's milk protein allergy are cow's milk protein (eg, casein, whey) hydrolysates. Soy protein formulas are not recommended in infants with cow's milk allergy because soy protein allergy frequently coexists. In older children, the poor taste of protein hydrolysate formula and high costs may seriously influence both patients' and parents' compliance. In patients with mild symptoms, a hydrolyzed formula should be used for at least 1 month to allow time for mucosal healing. In severe multiple food allergies, an amino acid–based formula may be useful.

Cow's milk protein and soy protein allergy with predominantly GI symptoms of the delayed type usually become less severe with increasing age. Most children become fully tolerant of milk by 3 years of age; however, 25% of children with IgE-mediated type I reactions to milk have not lost their hypersensitivity by this time. Reintroduction of cow's milk protein or soy protein in a previously allergic child should be performed under careful medical supervision because of the risk of anaphylaxis.

17.21.2   Eosinophilic Gastroenteritis

Peter Baehler and Ernest G. Seidman

Eosinophilic gastroenteritis is an inflammatory disease of unknown etiology that is characterized by dense infiltration of GI tract segments with eosinophils, accompanied by varying abdominal symptoms and, usually, by peripheral blood eosinophilia. The disease is relatively rare, predominantly affecting young male adults, although it may occur in children. Signs and symptoms are related to the site, extent, and layer of the GI wall involved (Table 17-56).

The most common form of eosinophilic gastroenteritis involves the mucosa of the stomach (ie, antrum), small intestine, and sometimes the colon. About one-third of pediatric patients have a history of atopic disease (eg, urticaria, eczema, asthma) and/or food allergy, with corresponding elevation of total or food-specific IgE antibodies or positive skin-prick tests. This mucosal form typically

TABLE 17-56

CLINICAL MANIFESTATIONS OF EOSINOPHILIC GASTROENTERITIS IN CHILDHOOD

Mucosal (most common, idiopathic and protein sensitive)
  Vomiting, diarrhea, failure to thrive, abdominal pain, atopy, food allergy, peripheral edema, hypoalbuminemia, anemia, occult blood loss, protein-losing enteropathy, eosinophilic colitis
Muscle Layer (idiopathic and protein sensitive)
  Vomiting, abdominal pain, weight loss, gastric outlet obstruction intestinal obstruction
Serosal (least common, idiopathic)
  Ascites

occurs in newborns and in children up to approximately 2 years of age, and it often responds well to an elimination diet.

Muscle layer involvement results in wall thickening and variable degrees of GI obstruction, with gastric outlet obstruction being most common. Vomiting is the most common symptom and may be difficult to distinguish from that of pyloric stenosis. Stenotic lesions elsewhere in the gut may mimic Crohn strictures, as will symptoms and response to therapy. Serosal involvement is rare, resulting in the insidious appearance of eosinophilic ascites, usually without significant GI symptoms. Pericardial or even pleural effusions may occur in a polyserositis-like presentation. Tissue eosinophilia also rarely may involve extraintestinal organs such as the peritoneum, gallbladder, spleen, pancreas, urinary bladder, and even pericardium.

The cause of the idiopathic disease remains unknown. Peripheral eosinophilia, seen in approximately 80% of cases, suggests an allergic etiology. Diagnosis requires the demonstration of significant tissue eosinophilia in GI biopsy specimens. Substantial overlap of the protein-sensitive form with food-protein allergy exists. Moreover, other diseases with malabsorption, protein-losing enteropathy, GI obstruction, or colitis such as Crohn disease, ulcerative colitis, parasitic infections, Ménétrier disease, chronic granulomatous disease, or idiopathic hypereosinophilic syndrome (ie, hyper-IgE syndrome) have to be distinguished from eosinophilic gastroenteritis.

Protein-sensitive forms are best managed with an elimination diet. In idiopathic forms, effective remission usually can be achieved by glucocorticoid therapy; low-dose maintenance therapy may be necessary to prevent relapse. Ketotifen has been reported to be useful in milder cases.

17.21.3 Infections of the Small Intestine and Colon

Colin D. Rudolph

Specific infectious agents, diagnosis, and treatment approaches are discussed in Chap. 13 and Sec. 17.7.4. Specific opportunistic infections of immunocompromised hosts are discussed in Sec. 17.17.1. Viral infections generally destroy the enterocytes on the villous surface of the small intestine, causing water, electrolyte, and nutrient malabsorption. Crypt enterocytes are spared, and as the infected cells are shed from the villi, immature cells migrate upward from the crypts. These immature cells are deficient in lactase and sucrase, which may contribute to a postinfection osmotic diarrhea. Histologically, there is blunting of the intestinal villi, and there may be an increased number of inflammatory cells in the lamina propria. Rotavirus typically infects children who are 6 to 24 months of age, usually during the winter months. Symptoms begin within 48 to 72 hours after exposure. Diarrhea usually lasts from 2 to 8 days, but viral shedding persists for as long as 3 weeks. Diagnosis of rotavirus is routinely achieved using ELISA methods (Rotazyme, Abbott Laboratories). Norwalk virus typically infects older children and adults during the winter and summer months; symptoms last from 12 to 48 hours. Enteric adenovirus infection most commonly infects children younger than 2 years of age. Diarrhea persists for periods as long as 2 weeks. Other known intestinal viral pathogens include calicivirus and astrovirus. Cytomegalovirus has been associated with enteritis and colitis, but almost exclusively in patients who are immunocompromised.

Bacteria damage the bowel by invasion of the mucosa, production of cytotoxins that destroy enterocytes, production of enterotoxins that cause secretion of water and electrolytes but do not destroy cells, and/or adherence to the mucosal surface with flattening of microvilli. *Salmonella* colonizes the ileum and colon as well as invades and proliferates within epithelial cells and the lamina propria, causing gastroenteritis with watery diarrhea and/or colitis with bloody diarrhea. *Shigella* invades colonocytes and produces a toxin with neurotoxic, enterotoxic, and cytotoxic effects. *Campylobacter* species may adhere to the intestinal mucosa, produce a toxin, or invade the mucosa of the terminal ileum and colon, causing symptoms that vary from mild diarrhea to frank dysentery. *Yersinia pseudotuberculosis* causes pseudoappendicitis, mesenteric adenitis, and gastroenteritis; *Y. enterocolitica* invades ileal epithelium and produces an enterotoxin. Symptoms of diarrhea, fever, and abdominal pain, which usually are associated with a marked increase in white blood cell count, generally resolve in 5 to 14 days but may persist for months. Various strains of pathogenic *Escherichia coli* cause a spectrum of disease, including traveler's diarrhea, persistent diarrhea in infants, and hemorrhagic colitis. *E. coli* 0157:H7 is associated with hemolytic uremic syndrome. *Vibrio cholerae* elaborates a toxin that causes secretory diarrhea, and *Clostridium difficile* produces toxins that may cause self-limited mild watery diarrhea lasting several days or severe pseudomembranous colitis. Classically, symptoms begin following the administration of antibiotics that reduce normal bowel flora, thus allowing an increase in *C. difficile* colonization of the bowel. *Aeromonas* usually causes acute watery diarrhea but may cause dysentery. *Plesiomonas* causes colitis-like symptoms that are associated with fever. Symptoms often persist for longer than 1 month.

Mycobacterium avium-intracellulare may cause self-limited diarrheal illness in normal hosts, but it is associated with diffuse disease involving the small bowel and colon in patients who are immunocompromised (see Sec. 17.17.1). *M. tuberculosis* may mimic inflammatory bowel disease, with disease localized to the ileocecal region. Although most cases will have pulmonary disease on chest radiographs, cutaneous tuberculin tests should be performed in all patients with Crohn disease before corticosteroid therapy is begun. Parasites, including *Entamoeba histolytica, Giardia lamblia, Isospora belli, Cryptosporidium, Blastocystis hominis, Balantidium coli, Strongyloides stercoralis, Diphyllobothrium latum,* and *Schistosoma* all may be associated with GI symptoms and disease.

17.21.4 Vascular Disease of the Small Intestine and Colon

Colin D. Rudolph

ISCHEMIC BOWEL DISEASE

Arteriosclerotic vascular disease is the major cause of ischemic bowel disease in adults, but it is extremely rare in children. Most childhood ischemic disease results from extrinsic obstruction, volvulus, or vasculitis. Systemic vasculitic diseases that affect the bowel and amyloidosis are discussed later. Extrinsic obstruction may result from any mass lesion. Symptoms of chronic mesenteric insufficiency consist of postprandial colicky periumbilical pain, with symptoms that are far worse than would be expected from physical examination of the abdomen. Chronic insufficiency also may result in protein-losing enteropathy, steatorrhea, or carbohydrate malabsorption. No specific diagnostic tests are available except for angiography, which usually is not indicated in children. Acute vascular insufficiency (eg, as occurs with volvulus or intussusception) results in more obvious findings of ileus, bilious vomiting, and mucosal necrosis with hematemesis or hematochezia.

SYSTEMIC VASCULITIS

Mesenteric vasculitis most commonly is associated with collagen vascular disorders. Degos disease is an obliterative endarteritis that affects small to medium-sized vessels and can be associated with spontaneous perforation of the bowel. Similarly, dermatomyositis often is associated with mesenteric vasculitis, intestinal ulcerations, and perforations. Other collagen vascular disorders, including polymyositis, periarteritis nodosa, and systemic lupus erythematosus, occasionally are associated with GI pain and/or bleeding.

HENOCH-SCHÖNLEIN PURPURA

Henoch-Schönlein purpura is a systemic vasculitis with deposition of IgA immune complexes in postcapillary venules throughout the body, as discussed in detail in Sec. 12.6.1. GI symptoms may be observed several weeks before onset of the "palpable purpuric" rash. Diffuse abdominal pain, vomiting, and hematochezia are common. Barium enema or upper GI series reveals a coarsening of folds and thumbprinting, as seen with ischemic disease. Endoscopy displays purpuric lesions of the small bowel and colon. Intussusception occurs in approximately 10% of children with Henoch-Schönlein purpura and abdominal pain; bowel perforation and development of bowel stricture are less common. Pancreatitis and cholecystitis have been reported. Corticosteroids may decrease the severity of GI symptoms, but treatment may mask symptoms of perforation or intussusception. The benefits of corticosteroid treatment remain controversial.

HEMOLYTIC-UREMIC SYNDROME

Hemolytic-uremic syndrome is a systemic vasculitis resulting from intravascular platelet activation, causing thrombocytopenia and renal insufficiency, as described in Sec. 21.8.3. In approximately 95% of cases, a prodromal gastroenteritis precedes the onset of systemic symptoms. In 75%, bloody diarrhea is the presenting symptom. Hemolytic-uremic syndrome may be precipitated by GI infection with *E. coli* 0157:H7, *Shigella, Campylobacter, Yersinia,* or *Salmonella*. Findings on radiographic contrast studies include thumbprinting and ulceration, which are consistent with an ischemic process. Abdominal pain may be severe enough to warrant laparotomy, and bowel perforation does occur. Late GI complications of stricture and fistula have been reported. Patients with severe GI symptoms should receive parenteral nutrition and not be fed until symptoms resolve. Pancreatitis rarely occurs.

17.21.5   Miscellaneous Disorders of the Small Intestine and Colon

Colin D. Rudolph

BEHÇET DISEASE

The usual hallmarks of Behçet disease are painful oral and perineal aphthous ulcerations. Prevalence is 1 to 10 per 100,000, with a 3:1 male predominance. The most common time for presentation is in the third decade of life, but pediatric cases are being recognized more frequently. The pathogenesis of Behçet disease remains unknown, but an autoimmune process is likely. Arthritis, erythema nodosum, iridocyclitis, and neurologic symptoms may accompany Behçet disease. GI symptoms are similar to those of Crohn disease, with involvement of the esophagus in 12%, right colon in 50%, ileum in 25%, and rectum in 25% of affected children. Fistulas and

perforation are common. Therapy with corticosteroids, thalidomide, and other immunosuppressants has achieved some success.

AMYLOIDOSIS

Accumulation of amyloid in the bowel may occur as either a primary or secondary process. In children, it usually is associated with hemodialysis, familial mediterranean fever, juvenile rheumatoid arthritis, cystic fibrosis, Crohn disease, autoimmune enteropathy, or glycogenosis. Approximately two-thirds of patients with secondary amyloidosis have GI involvement, with symptoms from obstruction, impaired motility, or ischemia resulting from infiltration around blood vessels. Biopsy of the bowel reveals submucosal and mucosal amyloid deposition, which most easily is demonstrated with special amyloid stains. Treatment with colchicine reduces the amyloid deposition in familial Mediterranean fever, but therapy with disease resulting from other etiologies is disappointing.

RADIATION ENTERITIS

Radiation therapy for malignancy often causes acute injury to the rapidly replicating bowel epithelium, and it may cause chronic damage, with submucosal fibrosis and obliteration of small blood vessels and lymphatics. Chronic radiation damage is rare in children because of the lower doses of radiation that are used in therapy for childhood tumors. Acute injury to the bowel mucosa results in malabsorption, with diarrhea and vomiting in many patients. A low-residue, low-lactose diet often is helpful in reducing symptoms during the acute phase, but if symptoms are severe, the radiation dose may need to be reduced. Acute symptoms usually resolve within 6 weeks of the completion of therapy. Chronic symptoms of dysmotility may improve on treatment of bacterial overgrowth. Local lymphatic or vascular obstruction may require limited surgical resection.

DIVERSION COLITIS

Following various surgical procedures, bowel contents are diverted through an ostomy to prevent the passage of feces into the distal colon and rectum. This may be necessary to allow healing of perianal lesions or following acute surgical interventions for bowel perforation. Occasionally, the remaining colon epithelium becomes inflamed, causing the passage of rectal blood and mucus. A deficiency of luminal short-chain fatty acids appears to be involved in the pathogenesis of diversion colitis (see Sec. 17.16). Effective therapy with the instillation of short-chain fatty acids by enema leads to the resolution of symptoms. It is important to differentiate diversion colitis from other causes of colitis such as inflammatory bowel disease because treatment of diversion colitis is by reanastomosis, and inflammatory bowel disease by medical or surgical resection.

GRAFT-VERSUS-HOST DISEASE

Graft-versus-host disease (GVHD) most frequently occurs following bone marrow transplantation. Rare cases of transfusion-acquired graft-versus-host disease have been reported in immunodeficient newborns. Following bone marrow transplantation, donor T lymphocytes mediate crypt cell lysis, with apoptosis of glandular epithelium being the most typical pathologic finding in intestinal GVHD. Acute GVHD usually starts 3 to 4 weeks following transplant. Gastrointestinal symptoms may be minimal to severe with abdominal pain, profuse watery, mucoid diarrhea, protein-losing enteropathy, intestinal bleeding, and sepsis. Generally, the severity of intestinal GVHD parallels skin and liver involvement; however, some patients have gastrointestinal symptoms with minimal if any other findings. Because gastrointestinal infection can present in a similar fashion, this must be ruled out (see Sec. 17.17). Endoscopic findings range from normal to extensive mucosal sloughing with ulceration. The most prominent changes are most frequently observed in the ileum, cecum, and ascending colon. Biopsies of normal-appearing tissue often are diagnostic, whereas biopsy of severely involved tissue may be less specific. Biopsies of the rectum may be normal if GVHD involves primarily the upper gastrointestinal tract; thus, upper endoscopy may be necessary for diagnosis. Treatment of acute intestinal GVHD includes treatment of the GVHD and supportive measures including provision of appropriate enteral or parenteral nutritional support and careful attention to fluid and electrolyte balance.

Chronic GVHD develops at 80 to 400 days after BMT and differs from acute GVHD in the time of onset, sites involved, and histologic findings in target organs. Most patients with chronic GVHD had preceding acute GVHD that either resolved or evolved into the chronic form. Gastrointestinal involvement typically includes the oral mucosa (mucositis), salivary glands (oral sicca), or esophagus. Some children present only with poor oral intake and weight loss. Esophageal findings include esophagitis (often involving the proximal and midesophagus), upper esophageal strictures and webs, and typical peptic esophagitis in the distal esophagus. Esophageal biopsies typically are infiltrated with lymphocytes, neutrophils, and eosinophils, with necrosis of individual squamous cells in the basal layer. Malabsorption may result from exocrine pancreatic insufficiency. As in acute GVHD, infectious causes of the symptoms need to be considered, including viral and fungal etiologies. Treatment consists of immunosuppressive and acid-suppressive therapy. Webs or strictures are treated with dilation.

PNEUMATOSIS INTESTINALIS

Pneumatosis intestinalis is characterized by the finding of numerous intramural gas-filled cysts involving any part of the gastrointestinal tract. In premature and newborn infants, this finding is often associated with necrotizing enterocolitis and has serious implications. In older children and adults, this rare disorder is occasionally associated with fulminant illnesses such as ischemic colitis, bowel infarction caused by midgut volvulus, or severe enteric infections. In these scenarios, pneumatosis intestinalis is commonly associated with advanced intestinal necrosis and is an ominous finding requiring intervention. However, in most cases pneumatosis intestinalis is a relatively benign disorder, being discovered incidentally during radiographic evaluation. Usually it involves the left colon. It is most often associated with chronic pulmonary diseases such as cystic fibrosis, connective tissue diseases, and gastrointestinal obstruction including chronic idiopathic intestinal pseudoobstruction. It is seen relatively frequently in patients following cancer chemotherapy or bone marrow transplantation. The pathogenesis of pneumatosis intestinalis is unknown, but several theories have been proposed. A mechanical theory suggests that gas is forced into the bowel by tracking along vascular sheaths or through mucosal breaks. Alternatively, it is proposed that gas-producing bacteria invade the bowel wall or that gas is formed from fermentation of nondigested carbohydrates. In otherwise asymptomatic patients, treatment is indicated only for associated illnesses because the lesions resolve spontaneously. Complications occur in a small minority of these cases and include penumoperitoneum, intussusception, and perforation. Antibiotic treatment with metronidazole and ampicillin,

enteral or parenteral nutrition, and bowel rest have also been successful, but it is unclear whether the lesions would resolve without therapy. Surgery is indicated in fulminant cases of pneumatosis, especially in patients with metabolic acidosis or other findings suggestive of bowel necrosis on physical examination or abdominal CT scan. A finding of mesenteric venous gas on plain abdominal radiographs or CT scan (which is more sensitive) is highly suggestive of bowel infarction.

17.21.6   Protein-Losing Enteropathy

Wallace A. Gleason, Jr.

Protein-losing enteropathy occurs when serum proteins leak into the intestinal lumen because of mucosal erosion or ulceration, rupture of lacteals from high pressure in the thoracic duct, or surface cell loss or damage with disruption of the mucosal barrier. Protein-losing enteropathy is a process with an extensive differential diagnosis (Table 17-57). Symptoms of the underlying illness, including diarrhea, abdominal pain, and allergic phenomena, may be elicited in the history. Weight for age, height for age, and weight for height can rule out malnutrition as a cause of hypoalbuminemia. Edema

TABLE 17-57

PROTEIN-LOSING ENTEROPATHY IN INFANTS AND CHILDREN

Low serum albumin
  Infectious
    Giardia lamblia
    Hypertrophic gastropathy (Ménétrier disease)
    Cytomegalovirus
    Helicobacter pylori
    Strongyloides stercoralis
  Noninfectious
    Carbohydrate-deficient glycoprotein syndrome 1b
    Congenital heparan sulfate deficiency
    Crohn disease
    Gastroesophageal reflux
    Graft-versus-host disease
    Henoch-Schönlein purpura
    Intestinal lymphangiectasia
    Posttransplant lymphoproliferative disease (PTLD)
    Primary heart disease
    Noonan syndrome
    Inflammatory bowel disease
    Nephrotic syndrome
    Multiple polyposis
    Phenobarbital hypersensitivity
    Systemic lupus erythematosus
Normal serum albumin
  Infectious
    Clostridium difficile
    Clostridium perfringens
    Measles
    Rotavirus
    Salmonella
    Necrotizing enterocolitis
  Noninfectious
    Allergic gastroenteropathy
    Cow's milk feeding
    Gluten-sensitive enteropathy
    Colonic malakoplakia
    Malnutrition

is a frequent finding, and asymmetric lymphedema may suggest an underlying malformation of lymphatic channels such as primary intestinal lymphangiectasia.

Other causes of hypoalbuminemia such as renal disease, liver disease, or malnutrition should be excluded by urinalysis and liver function studies. A reliable estimate of hepatic synthetic function is provided by the prothrombin time. Vitamin K deficiency resulting from intestinal malabsorption can lead to an abnormal result, but this should correct promptly after a parenteral dose of vitamin K. α_1-Antitrypsin excretion in the stool is the technique of choice for demonstrating protein-losing enteropathy because:

- It is a serum protein.
- It is not present in the diet, and fecal levels reflect protein originating in serum.
- Its molecular weight of 50,000 is similar to that of albumin.
- It is a protease inhibitor, resists intraluminal proteolysis, and is excreted without degradation in the stool.
- Urine contamination of the stool specimen will not invalidate the result, a feature that is particularly helpful in pediatric patients.
- Repeat samples show little variation, allowing the use of randomly obtained samples rather than a timed stool collection, and levels of fecal α_1-antitrypsin in the stool are stable, allowing transport and storage of specimens before assay.

α_1-Antitrypsin is unstable in gastric juice, so the reliability of fecal α_1-antitrypsin in detecting esophageal or gastric protein loss is questionable. Testing is not meaningful until after 1 week of age because meconium contains rather large amounts of α_1-antitrypsin.

Subclinical protein-losing enteropathy occurs in many disorders in which protein loss rarely is more than two to four times normal. This degree of loss does not lead to hypoalbuminemia, and it is of questionable significance. Forty percent of children with acute diarrheal illness have elevated levels of fecal α_1-antitrypsin. Giardiasis and strongyloidiasis, however, can cause GI protein loss in sufficient quantity to result in hypoalbuminemia and edema. These conditions are best approached by identifying the agents in stool specimens, by duodenal intubation, or by a string test such as the Enterotest.

Conditions that are associated with protein-losing enteropathy are listed in Table 17-57 and are discussed in other sections of this chapter. Fifty to sixty percent of children with Crohn disease have mild to pronounced hypoalbuminemia. Protein-losing enteropathy and finger clubbing have been reported as complications of gastroesophageal reflux. Protein-losing enteropathy with hypoalbuminemia occurs in 25% of patients after bone marrow transplantation as a result of graft-versus-host disease of the intestine. Intestinal lymphangiectasia causes protein loss, including immunoglobulins, lymphocytes, and chylomicrons, with hypoalbuminemia, lymphopenia, hypogammaglobulinemia, and steatorrhea. The intestine may be the only site of lymphatic obstruction, or it may coexist with multifocal lymphatic dysplasia (eg, Noonan syndrome). Cardiac disorders or surgical procedures in which elevated right atrial pressure is transmitted to the superior vena cava and thoracic duct, including the Fontan procedure and clinically silent constrictive pericarditis, can cause intestinal lymphangiectasia and protein-losing enteropathy. Recently, some patients have been reported to respond to steroids and low-molecular-weight heparin. Newly described entities in which protein-losing enteropathy is prominent include the carbohydrate-deficient glycoprotein syndrome 1b and congenital heparan sulfate deficiency. Intestinal lymphangiectasia

has been found in intestinal biopsy specimens of some children with idiopathic nephrotic syndrome and protein-losing enteropathy.

Although treatment of protein-losing enteropathy requires treatment of the underlying disease, octreotide injections have been anecdotally reported to be effective; oral mannose therapy is effective in treating the carbohydrate-deficient glycoprotein syndrome 1b. When specific therapy is not available, high protein intakes should be encouraged to compensate for the protein loss.

17.21.7 Appendicitis

Richard J. Stevenson

Appendicitis is the most common condition requiring emergency surgery in children. Approximately one in 15 individuals (7%) develops appendicitis. The peak incidence is 12 years of age, and it is unusual before 2 years. Boys outnumber girls by a ratio of 3:2. In one-third of cases, the appendix ruptures before operation, causing serious illness.

Luminal obstruction of the appendix is regarded as the first event leading to inflammation. Subsequent distal mucous production leads to distension of the organ and associated pain. Increasing intraluminal pressure interferes with perfusion. The resultant ischemia along with bacterial proliferation cause necrosis and ultimately perforation. Luminal obstruction may be caused by appendicoliths (calcified), fecalomas, parasites (eg, *Ascaris, Enterobius*), foreign bodies, carcinoids, old scarring, inspissated mucus associated with cystic fibrosis, or narrowing of the appendix secondary to tethering and/or kinks. In addition, the appendix is rich in lymphoid tissue, and hyperplasia theoretically may result in luminal compromise.

DIAGNOSIS

Fatigue and anorexia are frequent initial presentations of appendicitis. There may be a sensation of epigastric discomfort, which often is described as indigestion, followed by a complaint of periumbilical discomfort whether the pain is that of inflammation or colic and regardless of the location of the appendix (ie, retrocecal or pelvic). This is followed by low-grade fever (1°C above normal), nausea, and perhaps vomiting. Over several hours, the inflammation involves the parietal peritoneum, and pain localizes to the right lower quadrant. In approximately 30% of patients, the appendix may be in a location other than at the McBurney point. A pelvic appendix may result in hypogastric pain; a retrocecal appendix may irritate the psoas and obturator muscles, and a retrocolic appendix often results in pain in the right flank.

Sudden diminution of pain usually indicates perforation as the intraluminal pressure in the appendix is suddenly relieved. Peritonitis with high fever (>39.4°C), persistent vomiting, thirst, malaise, and evidence of systemic infection may ensue, or the inflammatory process may be walled off by loops of bowel and the omentum, with subsequent abscess formation and exquisite tenderness at the site of the inflammatory process. Viral or bacterial enteritis may be confused with appendicitis; on occasion, it may precede appendicitis. With this condition, nausea, vomiting, and fever usually precede the pain. Diarrhea occurs in 5 to 10% of patients with appendicitis.

When appendicitis is advanced, the patient is uncomfortable, experiences pain in walking and moving about, and may be bent at the waist. However, with early appendicitis, especially appendiceal colic, the individual may be quite active. Palpation of the abdomen should begin away from the right lower quadrant and move ventrally and carefully toward the McBurney point. Consistent localized right lower quadrant tenderness and guarding are the hallmarks of appendicitis. Voluntary guarding usually will evolve into involuntary spasm and rebound tenderness as peritonitis ensues. Rectal examination is important to check for pelvic appendicitis, which may not be evident during the abdominal examination, as well as a pelvic mass (abscess). Psoas and obturator irritation may be documented by hip extension and passive internal rotation of the thigh, respectively. Rovsing sign is positive when palpation of the abdomen in areas remote from the McBurney point results in discomfort felt in the right lower quadrant. Flank tenderness must not be overlooked. Exclusion of the other causes of lower abdominal pain, including possible right basilar pneumonia, adenopathy, testicular torsion, and hernias, is important. A pelvic examination may be deferred in the premenarcheal patient or the postmenarcheal patient if one is certain she is not sexually active, and an ultrasonography study is performed. Appendicitis can accurately be diagnosed clinically in 80%. Additional diagnostic studies are not necessary if the clinical features are characteristic. Time is of the essence because most inflamed appendices will perforate within 24 to 48 hours (65% by 36 hours) after the onset of symptoms.

Several factors make diagnosing appendicitis in children difficult. Younger children may not be able to verbalize their discomfort and progression of symptoms. Not surprisingly, 80 to 95% of patients who are younger than 2 years of age have perforated appendicitis at presentation. Because fewer than 0.2% of appendicitis cases occur before the age of 1 year, the diagnosis usually is not considered in symptomatic infants and toddlers. Abdominal distension, fever, vomiting, irritability, and lethargy should lead to the consideration of a diagnosis of appendicitis until proven otherwise. Patients beyond the neonatal period but still younger than 2 years of age usually are suspected of having acute gastroenteritis or intussusception. Patients older than 2 years of age present with appendiceal perforation 30 to 60% of the time; this incidence decreases with advancing age.

Adolescent girls are particularly difficult to evaluate, and the correct diagnosis of appendicitis may be made only 50% of the time because of other confusing issues (eg, pelvic inflammatory disease, ovarian cysts/torsion, ectopic pregnancy, and mittelschmerz). Other diagnoses that may mimic appendicitis include mesenteric lymphadenitis, urinary tract infection, midgut volvulus, choledochal cyst, intussusception, intestinal duplications, Meckel diverticulum, hemolytic-uremic syndrome, Henoch-Schönlein purpura, sickle-cell crisis, ureteral stones, gonad torsion, typhlitis, and black widow spider bite. Diagnoses in older patients are more likely to include cholecystitis, epididymitis, inflammatory bowel disease, hematocolpos, and ulcers.

Laboratory studies may support the diagnosis but usually add little to the clinical impression. A white blood cell count greater than 15,000 and a neutrophil left shift are suggestive, but even with perforated appendicitis, the count and differential may be normal. Microscopic pyuria and hematuria (not bacteriuria) may be associated with appendicitis. Other studies should be performed as indicated, but a pregnancy test (serum or urine) should never be overlooked in an ovulating woman.

The abdominal radiograph, which usually is ordered but is rarely of much value, will likely confirm the diagnosis of appendicitis if a fecalith is found. Fecalomas (noncalcified) are found in up to 25% of patients with appendicitis. If there is the slightest concern that appendectomy may be required within 8 to 12 hours, the patient should be admitted for further observation with serial examinations (preferably by the same physician) and appropriate laboratory study. If the diagnosis remains uncertain, real-time ultrasonography with graded compression can be performed. Demonstration of a nonperistalsing, noncompressible, blind-ending tubular structure more than 6 mm in diameter with a "target" appearance suggests appendicitis. The ultrasonographic study also may document complications such as abscess or other entities such as pancreatitis, cholecystitis, lymphadenopathy, uropathy, or gynecologic pathology. It has been reported that ultrasonography establishes an alternative diagnosis in 12% of cases and may change the management of the patient 18% of the time. However, in the absence of typical clinical manifestations, a positive ultrasonographic study for appendicitis is not a sufficient indication for an exploratory laparotomy. If doubt persists as to the diagnosis, a barium enema study should be considered. Persistent nonvisualization or partial visualization of the appendix, pressure indentation of the cecum, or irritability (ie, spasm) of the terminal ileum, cecum, or adjacent sigmoid colon all suggest appendicitis. A subsequent film in 8 to 12 hours may show a fecaloma outlined with barium or document a completely filled nonemptying appendix that was not visualized earlier. If the appendix fills completely without a filling defect and subsequently empties completely, it may be assumed to be normal. If an abdominal mass or abscess is suspected, computed tomography is the imaging modality of choice.

TREATMENT

The best treatment for appendicitis is early appendectomy. The patient should be prepared with rehydration, correction of electrolytes, control of fever, possible GI decompression, and administration of appropriate antibiotics. This may require several hours, but it helps to prevent untoward complications. If the appendix appears normal at laparotomy, it should be removed, and a careful search undertaken for other pathology. If the appendix is inflamed but not gangrenous or perforated, it is simply removed. The hospital stay for these patients usually is 12 to 48 hours. If the appendix is gangrenous or perforated, intraoperative anaerobic and aerobic cultures may be obtained, the peritoneum cavity irrigated, and, in the event of a well-formed abscess, drains may be placed. Broad-spectrum intravenous antibiotics are continued until the patient is afebrile and the white count is normal. The drains are gradually removed. The mortality that is associated with perforated appendicitis should be well below 1%.

Occasionally, a child presents with a history of 5 days or longer, and a mass is palpable in the right lower quadrant, which suggests appendicitis with previous perforation. If the patient is otherwise well, with little evidence of peritonitis, conservative management is indicated along with antibiotic therapy and careful observation for signs of peritonitis. Appendectomy can be performed 4 to 6 weeks later. A lack of response to antibiotics is an indication for earlier appendectomy.

Complications that occur subsequent to appendectomy may be expected in fewer than 5% of cases. The most common is wound infection, followed by intraabdominal abscess, usually associated with a gangrenous or perforated appendix. Small bowel obstruction may complicate the postoperative course and result from adhesions. Frequently, the obstruction can be relieved with nasogastric suction, but reexploration occasionally is necessary. Rarer complications include a pleural empyema or thrombophlebitis of the mesenteric and portal venous systems with subsequent pyogenic hepatic abscesses.

17.21.8   Other Disorders of the Appendix and Cecum

Richard J. Stevenson

TYPHLITIS

Typhlitis, or inflammation of the cecum, classically occurs in patients who are being treated for leukemia during periods of neutropenia, but it also may occur with other forms of neutropenia or immunodeficiency and after solid organ transplantation. This inflammatory lesion can progress rapidly to gangrene or perforation, with a high mortality rate. Most patients present with fever and right lower quadrant pain, suggesting appendicitis. The disease appears to be an infectious process, but the localization in the cecum is unexplained. Diagnosis is suggested by the symptoms and clinical setting. Plain-film abdominal radiographs may demonstrate bowel wall thickening or pneumatosis intestinalis. Computed tomography is useful in confirming the presence of cecal wall thickening. Management consists of close observation, bowel rest, fluid resuscitation, and antibiotic therapy. Granulocyte transfusions may be beneficial. Up to 80% of cases resolve without operative intervention, but if patients do not improve or perforation occurs, surgical resection is necessary. Patients are at risk for repeat episodes when they again become neutropenic following the resolution of symptoms.

CHRONIC APPENDICEAL PAIN

The appendix may be responsible for chronic right lower quadrant pain. Three varieties of chronic appendiceal pain have been recognized. Chronic appendicitis refers to the chronically inflamed appendix infiltrated by mononuclear cells. The condition is rather unusual, accounting for <1% of inflamed appendices. Recurrent appendicitis describes a once-inflamed appendix in which the inflammation resolves spontaneously without surgical intervention, resulting in focal appendiceal fibrosis. Appendiceal fibrosis may be documented in 5% of childhood interval appendectomies. The final condition is appendiceal colic, which is one cause of chronic right lower quadrant pain in children. Colic results from appendiceal cramping against an intraluminal obstruction (fecaloma, fibrosis, kink-adhesion, foreign body, parasites, carcinoid, and lymphoid hyperplasia).

Appendiceal colic is a controversial subject, with the diagnosis not being recognized as a distinct clinical entity by many pediatric surgeons. Imaging studies are generally not useful because fecalomas are usually noncalcified in children and there is usually no overt inflammation associated with appendiceal colic. Unless barium outlines a filling defect or shows marked delay in emptying from the appendix on follow-up films, barium upper and lower GI studies are often inconclusive. Appendiceal colic is, therefore, a clinical diagnosis. The patient with appendiceal colic presents as any other patient with colic. Restless and uncomfortable, they may writhe and even scream in pain. Initial anorexia and nausea will likely progress to reflexive vomiting (dry heaves) if the pain is severe. The pain often occurs in the morning on arising and after eating or drinking (5-20 minutes). On physical examination, pressure on the contracting appendix will exacerbate the pain during the episode, but there may be no pain between episodes. In this clinical setting, removal of the appendix often leads to dramatic clinical improvement with

a resolution of the recurrent symptoms. However, a recurrence of abdominal pain may occur in up to 50% of patients who underwent appendectomy for appendiceal colic, likely reflecting the imprecise nature of diagnosis.

References

Gastrointestinal Manifestations of Food Protein–Induced Hypersensitivity

Esteban MM, ed: Adverse reactions to foods in infancy and childhood, part 2. J Pediatr 121:S1–S126, 1992

European Society for Pediatric Gastroenterology and Nutrition Working Group for the Diagnostic Criteria for Food Allergy: Diagnostic criteria for food allergy with predominantly intestinal symptoms. J Pediatr Gastroenterol Nutr 14:108–112, 1992

Sampson HA: Adverse reactions to foods. In: Middleton E, Reed CE, Ellis EF, et al, eds: Allergy: Principles and Practice, 4th ed. St Louis, Mosby-Year Book, 1661–1686, 1993

Eosinophilic Gastroenteritis

Justinich C, Katz A, Gurbindo C, et al: Elemental diet improves steroid-dependent eosinophilic gastroenteritis and reverses growth failure. J Pediatr Gastroenterol Nutr 23:81–85, 1996

Whitington PF, Whitington GL: Eosinophilic gastroenteropathy in childhood. J Pediatr Gastroenterol Nutr 7:379, 1988

Ischemic Bowel Disease

Reinus JF, Brandt LJ, Boley SJ: Ischemic diseases of the bowel. Gastroenterol Clin North Am 19:319, 1990

Systemic Vasculitis

Rosenbloom ND, Winter HS: Steroid effects on the course of abdominal pain in children with Henoch-Schönlein purpura. Pediatrics 79:1018, 1987

Tarr PI, Heill MA, Clausen CR, et al: *Escherichia coli* 0157:H7 and the hemolytic uremic syndrome: importance of early cultures in establishing the etiology. J Infect Dis 162:553, 1990

Whitington PF, Friedman AL, Chesney RW: Gastrointestinal disease in the hemolytic-uremic syndrome. Gastroenterology 76:728, 1979

Radiation Enteritis

Donaldson SS, Jundt S, Ricour C, et al: Radiation enteritis in children. A retrospective, clinicopathologic correlation, and dietary management. Cancer 35:1178, 1975

Galland RB, Spencer J: The natural history and surgical management of radiation enteritis. Br J Surg 74:742, 1987

Graft-versus-Host Disease

McDonald GB, Shulman HM, Sullivan KM, Spencer GD: Intestinal and hepatic complications of human bone marrow transplantation. Gastroenterology 90:460–477, 770–784, 1986

Ponec RJ, Hackman RC, McDonald GB: Endoscopic and histologic diagnosis of intestinal graft-versus-host disease after marrow transplantation. Gastrointest Endosc 49:612–621, 1999

Pneumatosis Intestinalis

Kleinman PK, Brill PW, Winchester P. Pneumatosis intestinalis: its occurrence in the immunologically compromised child. Am J Dis Child 134: 1149–1151, 1980

Knechtle SJ, Davidoff AM, Rice RP. Pneumatosis intestinalis. Surgical management and clinical outcome. Ann Surg 212:160, 1990

Protein-Losing Enteropathy

Cohen HA, Shapiro RP, Frydman M, Varsano I: Childhood protein-losing enteropathy associated with *Helicobacter pylori* infection. J Pediatr Gastroenterol Nutr 13:201–203, 1991

Thomas DW, Sinatra FR, Merritt RJ: Random fecal α_1-antitrypsin concentration in children with gastrointestinal disease. Gastroenterology 80: 776–782, 1981

Appendicitis

Garcia Pena BM, Mandl KD, Kraus SJ, et al: Ultrasonography and limited computed tomography in the diagnosis and management of appendicitis in children. JAMA 282:1041–1046, 1999

Gorenstein A, Serour F, Katz R, et al: Appendiceal colic in children: a true clinical entity? J Am Coll Surg 182:246–250, 1996

Graff L, Radford MJ, Werne C: Probability of appendicitis before and after observation. Ann Emerg Med 20:503, 1991

Shamberger RC, Weinstein HJ, Delorey MJ, et al: The medical and surgical management of typhlitis in children with acute nonlymphocytic (myelogenous) leukemia. Cancer 57:603, 1986

Stevenson R: Chronic right-lower quadrant pain: is there a role for elective appendectomy? J Pediatr Surg 34:950–954, 1999

17.22 TUMORS OF THE GASTROINTESTINAL TRACT

Edward J. Hoffenberg

Tumors of the intestinal tract are relatively rare in children. The most common GI tumor in children is the benign juvenile polyp. However, a polyp may be the initial manifestation of an inherited polyposis syndrome associated with additional tumors and a variable risk for cancer (Table 17-58). Primary malignant tumors in children include lymphoma, adenocarcinoma, and carcinoid tumors. Other malignant tumors include those related to inflammatory bowel disease, ureterosigmoidostomies, celiac disease, HIV infection and multiple endocrine neoplasia.

17.22.1   Hereditary Polyposis Syndromes

Polyps in the gastrointestinal tract of children are most commonly benign and limited to the colon. The most common presenting symptoms are rectal bleeding or a visible polyp protruding through the anus; less common are unexplained anemia, abdominal pain, recurrent intussusception, and family history of polyposis syndrome.

JUVENILE POLYPS AND JUVENILE POLYPOSIS

Juvenile polyps are the most common type of childhood polyp, occurring in up to 1% of preschool children and accounting for 75 to 90% of all polyps in children. Juvenile polyps, also called inflammatory or retention polyps, are hamartomatous polyps, which are usually pedunculated, resembling a raspberry on a stalk, but some may be sessile, like a small bump without a stalk. The typical child with a juvenile polyp is 4 to 6 years of age, presents with intermittent painless rectal bleeding with bowel movements, has no family history suggesting a polyp syndrome, and has a single rectosigmoid polyp. Histology of the polyp shows well-differentiated, mature epithelial cells, dilated glands, and acute inflammation. Juvenile polyps are generally not thought to be neoplastic. Reactive atypia, a response to inflammation, may be difficult to distinguish from dysplasia. Focal areas of adenomatous change are seen in up to 5%. Both juvenile polyps and juvenile polyposis coli, which has a higher risk for malignancy, may have polyps in the left colon and thus may have overlapping phenotypic expression. Genetic testing may become available for discriminating between these two syndromes.

Juvenile polyposis is a term used when more than 5 to 10 juvenile polyps develop. *Juvenile polyposis coli* applies if the polyps are limited to the colon, whereas *generalized juvenile polyposis* describes the presence of polyps throughout the GI tract. Both have a significant malignant potential. Juvenile polyposis coli may be more common than was previously recognized, reportedly occurring in up to 10% of children with polyps. In juvenile polyposis coli, the polyps tend to be distributed throughout the colon rather than just in the rectosigmoid. Family members with even a single juvenile polyp should be considered to have familial juvenile polyposis, not a juvenile polyp. The familial form of juvenile polyposis coli may have a higher malignant potential than the sporadic form. A mutation of the SMAD4/DPC4 gene on chromosome 18q21 has been identified in one affected extended family. This mutation is hypothesized to alter TGF-β signaling, leading to abnormal mesenchymal development and promotion of hamartoma formation and cancer. However, because only a subset of families has this mutation, other genes may be involved in familial juvenile polyposis coli.

Generalized juvenile polyposis is extremely rare and usually presents in infancy or early childhood. Presentation includes rectal bleeding, diarrhea, anemia, hypoproteinemia, rectal prolapse, and intussusception. Hundreds of polyps carpet the stomach, small intestine, and large intestine and have a very high risk for malignancy.

Clear guidelines for evaluation and management of children with juvenile polyps and juvenile polyposis coli are not available. Some practitioners observe a rectosigmoid polyp and hope to avoid an invasive procedure if it passes spontaneously, but there is little evidence to support this approach. Recent series suggest that 10 to 15% of children with symptomatic polyps have a polyposis syndrome despite a negative family history, and these children are at increased risk for additional tumors and malignancy. Therefore, colonoscopy should be used in the initial evaluation of rectal bleeding. Colonoscopy allows both assessment of distribution and quantitation of polyps as well as removal of polyps for histology. Children with a solitary rectosigmoid juvenile polyp need no further evaluation, although additional polyps may develop in some. Children with five or more juvenile polyps, a family history of a polyposis syndrome, or with a juvenile polyp with adenomatous change should have all polyps removed and undergo surveillance colonoscopy, initially at 6 to 12 months and then every 2 years if no further polyps develop. The group of children with two to four polyps, or with any polyp proximal to the splenic flexure, has an undefined risk for colorectal cancer and could be enrolled in a surveillance program. Early colectomy should be considered if polyps show adenomatous changes.

TABLE 17-58
POLYPOSIS SYNDROMES

	MALIGNANT POTENTIAL	FEATURES
Hereditary polyposis syndromes		
Hamartomas		
Juvenile polyps (JP)	Low	<5, limited to left colon
Juvenile polyposis coli (JPC)	Moderate	>5-10, limited to colon
Generalized juvenile polyposis	High	>5-10, upper and lower GI tract
Peutz-Jeghers syndrome	Moderate	Upper and lower GI tract
PTEN (Cowdens syndrome, etc)	Low	Multiple soft tissue tumors
Adenomas: familial adenomatous polyposis related to APC gene mutations		
Familial polyposis coli (FPC)	High	Thyroid and ampulla of Vater cancer
Gardner syndrome	High	FPC plus jaw and dental anomalies, soft tissue tumors, CHRPE
Turcot syndrome	CNS cancer	FPC plus medulloblastoma, glioblastoma
Nonhereditary polyposis syndromes		
Lymphonodular hyperplasia	Low	
Inflammatory and pseudopolyps	Low	
Neurofibroma	Low	
Leiomyoma	Low	

CHRPE = congenital hypertrophy of retinal pigment epithelium; CNS = central nervous system; PTEN = protein tyrosine phosphatase gene mutation disorders.

PEUTZ-JEGHERS SYNDROME

Peutz-Jeghers syndrome describes an association of GI hamartomatous polyps and mucocutaneous hyperpigmentation. Melanosis is most common on the lips (95%) and buccal mucosa (65-85%) and less common on the nose, hands, and feet. The lesions are brown-black macules, 1 to 5 mm in diameter, and look like freckles. The number and distribution are variable, and they appear during infancy or early childhood but fade around puberty. Over 90% of patients have multiple polyps involving any part of the GI tract. The most common site is the small bowel (65–95%), followed by colon (60%) and stomach (50%). Occasionally, polyps are found in extraintestinal sites, including the bronchi and genitourinary tract. On histology, the polyps have prominent bands of smooth muscle, a feature not seen in the typical juvenile polyp.

The incidence of Peutz-Jeghers syndrome is about one in 80,000, and the inheritance pattern is autosomal dominant with variable penetrance, with no gender or ethnic predilection. Peutz-Jeghers syndrome is caused by a mutation of the STK11 gene, a serine threonine kinase, on chromosome 19p. Approximately one-third of patients with Peutz-Jeghers syndrome are diagnosed during childhood and adolescence, with the mean age of symptom onset being in the early 20s. The most common presenting complaints are intermittent, colicky abdominal pain, intestinal obstruction from intussusception, GI bleeding, and anemia. About 50% of individuals with Peutz-Jeghers syndrome develop extracolonic cancers, most commonly of the breast, cervix, ovary, testicle, and pancreas. The risk of colon cancer is 2 to 13%. Adenomatous changes are found in 3 to 6% of Peutz-Jeghers syndrome polyps.

Currently, diagnosis relies on the presence of hamartomatous polyps, characteristic skin lesions, and family history. Evaluation of the upper and lower GI tract by contrast studies or endoscopy may identify polyps. Because of the risk for malignant transformation, polyps should be removed, either endoscopically or surgically. Once the diagnosis is made, surveillance for polyps and other tumors should begin by age 10 years or sooner if symptoms develop.

Surveillance is also recommended for asymptomatic first-degree relatives beginning after age 10 years.

PTEN-MATCHS SYNDROMES

This is a new term for multiple syndromes linked to mutations in the protein tyrosine phosphatase (PTEN) gene. MATCHS derives from *m*acrocephaly, *a*utosomal dominant, *t*hyroid disease, *c*ancer, *h*amartoma, and *s*kin abnormalities. The following syndromes are probably allelic for PTEN mutations.

Ruvalcaba-Myhre-Smith syndrome is a rare entity characterized by macrocephaly, pigmented penile lesions, and hamartomatous intestinal polyps. Additional associated features include café-au-lait spots, lipomas, psychomotor retardation, and a unique lipid-storage myopathy. The intestinal polyps primarily involve the colon, although they are also found in the terminal ileum. These polyps occur during childhood, initially manifesting by rectal bleeding, edema, and abdominal pain. Some patients require colectomy.

Cowden syndrome, Bannayan-Zonana syndrome, and *Bannayan-Riley-Ruvalcaba syndrome* are allelic syndromes characterized by multiple hamartomas of skin, mucous membranes, breast, and thyroid. The mucocutaneous lesions are the most characteristic extraintestinal features of this syndrome, and they include hyperkeratotic papillomas of the lips and tongue. Multiple hamartomatous polyps may occur throughout the gastrointestinal tract but usually develop in adulthood. Symptoms include bleeding and edema secondary to protein loss. Gastrointestinal hamartomas are not malignant but may precede malignant tumors. Inheritance is autosomal dominant. A mutation of the PTEN tumor suppressor gene on chromosome 10q22-q23 has recently been identified as the cause of these syndromes.

Proteus syndrome is a rare hamartomatous disorder with prominent features of hemihypertrophy, gigantism of the extremities, angiomas, pigmented nevi, and multiple tumors, which may be lipomas or hamartomas. Polyps in the gastrointestinal tract have been reported. Because features overlap with Cowden syndrome, a PTEN mutation has been suggested to cause Proteus syndrome.

FAMILIAL ADENOMATOUS POLYPOSIS SYNDROMES

These syndromes are caused by mutations in the adenomatous polyposis coli (APC) gene on chromosome 5q21-q22 and occur in about 1:10,000 live births. They are characterized by the findings of up to hundreds of gastrointestinal adenomatous polyps. There is an autosomal-dominant inheritance but with marked variation in expression. However, about one-third of cases have no family history to suggest a familial adenomatous polyposis syndrome and represent new germ-line mutations.

The term *polyposis coli* is a misnomer because polyps occur in the upper gastrointestinal tract in 40 to 90% of cases. Adenomatous polyps usually develop by the second decade of life. They are usually small (<5 mm diameter) and may be several in number or carpet the entire colon. Additional polyps develop over time. In almost all affected individuals, polyps undergo malignant transformation by the fifth decade of life. In addition to colon adenocarcinoma, patients are at risk for cancers of the ampulla of Vater, thyroid gland, liver (hepatoblastoma), and stomach.

Traditionally, cases with prominent extraintestinal tumors were called *Gardner syndromes*. However, familial adenomatous polyposis coli and Gardner syndrome share the same APC gene mutations, and most patients with familial adenomatous polyposis coli have some extraintestinal lesions. These soft tissue tumors include desmoid tumors, sebaceous and epidermoid cysts, lipomas, and subcutaneous fibromas. Osteomas of the skull, maxilla, and mandible, supernumerary teeth, and congenital hypertrophy of the retinal pigment epithelium are also common. *Turcot syndrome* comprises rare cases of adenomatous colonic polyps plus CNS tumors, usually medulloblastoma and glioblastoma. Most, but not all, affected cases have detectable APC gene mutations, and both autosomal-dominant and -recessive inheritance have been postulated. Therefore, APC and other genes may be involved in the association of colon polyps with CNS tumors.

Diagnosis of familial adenomatous polyposis syndrome is based either on the presence of numerous adenomatous polyps in the colon or on genetic testing, which identifies about 80% of mutations. Over 100 mutations have been identified, and almost all are inactivating mutations. If an index case has an identifiable APC mutation, genetic testing can identify family members who inherited the mutation. If two or more affected members are available, linkage analysis may identify 95% of family members at risk.

Recommendations for evaluation and management are controversial. Although malignant changes rarely do occur in the first decade of life, most authorities recommend yearly screening with flexible sigmoidoscopy or colonoscopy beginning at age 10 to 12 years. Once polyps develop, colectomy should be considered because colonoscopy is not effective in identifying polyps with advanced progression toward malignancy. Total colectomy is recommended so as not to leave residual colonic mucosa. Sulindac has been reported to reduce the number and size of polyps. A selective apoptotic antineoplastic drug, derived from sulindac, is currently undergoing clinical trials for a reduction in the number of polyps. Periodic evaluation of the upper gastrointestinal tract and annual thyroid examination should be routine because of the association of thyroid carcinomas with familial adenomatous polyposis syndromes.

17.22.2 Nonhereditary Polyposis Syndromes and Benign Intestinal Tumors

CRONKHITE-CANADA SYNDROME

This noninherited syndrome is characterized by diffuse GI polyposis plus extraintestinal features of alopecia, onychodystrophy, and brown macular skin lesions. Polyps involve both the small and large intestine and are hamartomas, with histology similar to juvenile polyps. This syndrome is rare in infants and children. Prognosis is poor because of the severe malabsorption, protein-losing enteropathy, and malnutrition associated with this syndrome. GI carcinoma occurs in 5% of these patients.

LYMPHONODULAR HYPERPLASIA

This entity is characterized by submucosal, small, 1- to 5-mm, sessile lymphoid lesions that cluster in the duodenal bulb, ileocecal region, or rectosigmoid colon. Although generally considered a benign and self-limited lesion in children, colonic lymphonodular hyperplasia may cause rectal bleeding, especially in young children. In the ileum, the nodules are rare lead points for intussusception and may be seen through the teenage years without causing symptoms.

Lymphonodular hyperplasia probably represents a normal response of intestinal lymphoid tissue to an immune or inflammatory stimulus. Recognition of this entity is important to prevent confusion with lymphoma, a polyposis syndrome, or inflammatory bowel disease. Diagnosis is confirmed by the histologic features of lymphoid aggregates of mature lymphocytes, normal overlying mucosa, and a lack of tissue destruction. No therapy is required, with symptoms of bleeding usually resolving over several weeks to months.

INFLAMMATORY POLYPS OR PSEUDOPOLYPS

These are noted in severe colitis of any cause. They usually are small, less than 1 cm in diameter, but may require biopsy to differentiate from a carcinoma, especially in patients with long-standing inflammatory bowel disease. Other diseases that may give rise to inflammatory polyps include amebiasis and chronic bacterial infections.

NEUROFIBROMAS

Café-au-lait spots and neurofibromatous tumors, especially of the skin, characterize neurofibromatosis, or von Recklinghausen disease.

Tumors develop in the gastrointestinal tract in up to 25% of patients. They usually are small intramural or subserosal neurofibromas and may be found throughout the gastrointestinal tract, most commonly in the small intestine. These lesions may cause abdominal pain, bleeding, constipation, and protein-losing enteropathy. Generally, lesions are detected at endoscopy but not by radiographic studies. However, large neurofibromas may develop anywhere in the gastrointestinal tract and may require surgical removal for symptoms of bowel obstruction. Duodenal carcinoid tumors, pheochromocytomas, and mesenteric arterial vasculopathy are associated lesions.

LEIOMYOMAS

These tumors are the most common benign tumors of smooth muscle in the small intestine of adults but are rare in children, usually being found in the upper gastrointestinal tract. Small intramural lesions are incidentally found at autopsy, but larger intraluminal tumors may cause obstruction, intussusception, or intermittent intestinal bleeding. Multiple leiomyomatous lesions have been reported in children with HIV infection and are associated with Epstein-Barr virus infection. Esophageal leiomyomas often are associated with familial syndromes, including Alport disease (nephropathy, deafness, and cataracts), Carney triad (gastric stromal sarcoma, pulmonary chondroma, and extraadrenal paraganglioma), and clitoral or vulval hypertrophy associated with leiomyomas.

17.22.3 Malignant Intestinal Tumors

ADENOCARCINOMA

Primary carcinoma of the intestine is rare during childhood and adolescence. Most of these are of the mucin-producing or the signet-ring histologic varieties, which account for only 5% of tumors in adults. Carcinoembryonic antigen does not appear to be a reliable tumor marker in children, and other markers have not been identified. Risks for adenocarcinoma of the colon include familial polyposis syndrome (see above), inflammatory bowel disease (Sec. 17.20), and ureterosigmoidostomy. Colon cancer develops in 5% of patients with ureterosigmoidostomies for exstrophy of the bladder; endoscopic surveillance with biopsy should be performed every 2 to 3 years.

LYMPHOMA

The most common malignant tumors of the small intestine in children are primary intestinal lymphomas. They most frequently occur in the second decade of life and usually are non-Hodgkin lymphoma of the Burkitt type; a small number of diffuse histiocytic lymphomas, lymphoblastic lymphomas, and malignant histiocytoses of the intestine also are reported. Tumor incidence and type vary somewhat with the geographic location. Clinical findings and small bowel contrast studies may suggest an initial diagnosis of Crohn disease. Children with lymphoma may have abdominal pain, distension, vomiting, a palpable abdominal mass, and intussusception. The most common sites of involvement for all small bowel lymphomas are the terminal ileum and cecum. *Helicobacter pylori* infection is a risk factor for gastric lymphoma. Celiac disease is associated with small intestinal lymphomas. Posttransplant lymphoproliferative disease is associated with Epstein-Barr virus infection. Children frequently present with fever and lymphadenopathy. Early reduction of immunosuppression may lead to tumor regression.

CARCINOID TUMOR

The carcinoid syndrome, which is unusual in children, most often is associated with ileal tumors that have liver metastases. The neuroendocrine cells in carcinoid tumors release a number of substances, including catecholamines, bradykinins, and serotonin (ie, 5-hydroxytryptamine), that may cause diarrhea and flushing. Symptoms can be controlled with octreotide, which is a long-acting analog of somatostatin. Benign appendiceal carcinoids are discovered more frequently than malignant tumors in children. Most of these tumors are located in the distal third of the appendix and range in size from 0.1 to 2.5 cm. They usually are diagnosed incidentally at the time of surgery for appendicitis. Tumor invasion beyond the appendiceal submucosa is not unusual, but associated metastases or

recurrences have not been reported. Standard appendectomy usually is curative, although right hemicolectomy occasionally is performed for tumors larger than 2 cm. In the absence of carcinoid syndrome, the diagnosis of intestinal carcinoid in children rarely is made before surgery. Malignant carcinoid tumors are rare in children. The primary tumor may occur as a local infiltration of the intestinal wall of the ileum or colon, or rarely within a rectal duplication, and even more rarely is associated with sacrococcygeal teratomas. There can be extensive metastases to multiple organs, and surgery is not likely to be curative. Response to radiotherapy and chemotherapy with agents such as flourouracil is poor.

GASTRINOMAS

These are usually small tumors that secrete gastrin. The high levels of gastrin cause excess production of gastric acid, leading to ulcers, abdominal pain, and diarrhea, the Zollinger-Ellison syndrome. The majority of children with gastrinoma have high basal acid output and markedly elevated fasting gastrin levels, with values frequently above 500 ng/L. Diagnosis is made by measurement of an elevated fasting gastrin level and an abnormal intravenous secretin stimulation test. Secretin infusion causes serum gastrin levels to rise by at least 200 ng/L above baseline in gastrinomas but not in other conditions. Gastrinomas generally are small tumors, most commonly in the duodenum, but may be found in the pancreas or stomach. They often cannot be localized by ultrasonography or computed tomography or palpated at surgery. ^{111}In-octreotide scintigraphy may also be useful to localize the tumor or metastasis. Endoscopic ultrasonography or selective arterial secretin injection with hepatic venous sampling looking for a rise of 50% above baseline at 30 to 60 seconds may be helpful in planning surgical resection. Complications of acid overproduction are well controlled with proton pump inhibitors such as omeprazole or lansoprazole, initially at doses as high as 60 to 100 mg/d and then maintained at 20 to 60 mg/d. If oral medication is not tolerated, continuous IV infusion of H_2-receptor antagonists or intravenous pontaprazole may be titrated to achieve control of acid production. The majority of gastrinomas are malignant but slow-growing tumors. Surgical resection of gastrinomas should be performed when possible, but metastases to lymph nodes and liver are common. Liver metastases are associated with poor prognosis. There is a strong association of gastrinomas with multiple endocrine neoplasia syndrome I (MEN-I). Approximately 25% of patients with gastrinoma have MEN-I, and 50% of patients with MEN-I have gastrinoma. All gastrinoma patients should be evaluated for hyperparathyroidism and adrenal tumors.

MULTIPLE ENDOCRINE NEOPLASIA

Tumors may be associated with multiple endocrine neoplasia (MEN) syndromes, which have an autosomal-dominant inheritance. MEN-I includes abnormalities of the pancreas, anterior pituitary gland, and parathyroid gland. MEN-IIb is characterized by diffuse ganglioneuromas, lingual and buccal mucosal neuromas, medullary thyroid carcinoma, and pheochromocytoma. Pseudoobstruction and achalasia have been reported in children. In patients with MEN-IIb, yearly screening for medullary carcinoma of the thyroid should begin in infancy with measurement of morning calcitonin.

LEIOMYOSARCOMAS

These rare tumors are slow-growing tumors in children. Recurrent intestinal bleeding, abdominal pain, and palpable abdominal mass are the most common clinical features. Diagnosis may occur during surgery for obstruction or on evaluation of intussusception. Multiple leiomyosarcomatous lesions have been reported in children with HIV infection.

HEMANGIOMAS AND OTHER VASCULAR LESIONS

Bleeding is the most common manifestation of bowel hemangiomas. Intestinal obstruction or intussusception may occur with larger hemangiomas. The most common type of hemangioma contains ectatic vascular channels that involve mucosa and submucosa and protrude into the lumen. Often, children with GI hemangiomas have external manifestations suggesting the diagnosis. *Osler-Weber-Rendu syndrome* is associated with multiple skin and mucosal telangiectasias, *Klippel-Trénaunay syndrome* consists of large cutaneous and visceral hemangiomas plus skeletal and soft tissue hypertrophy. *Turner syndrome* is associated with GI telangiectasia, and *von Hippel-Lindau disease* consists of hemangioma in multiple viscera. *Blue rubber bleb nevus syndrome* is characterized by distinctive cutaneous and gastrointestinal malformations, generally presenting with gastrointestinal bleeding.

References

Chadwick EG, Connor EJ, Hanson IC, et al: Tumors of smooth muscle origin in HIV-infected children. JAMA 263:3182, 1990

Corpron CA, Black T, Herzog CE, Sellin RV, Lally KP, Andrassy RJ: A half century of experience with carcinoid tumors in children. Am J Surg 170:606–608, 1995

Cox KL, Lawrence-Miyasaki LS, Garcia-Kennedy R, et al: An increased incidence of Epstein-Barr virus infection and lymphoproliferative disorder in young children on FK506 after liver transplantation. Transplantation 59:524–529, 1995

Eng C, Ji H: Molecular classification of the inherited hamartoma polyposis syndromes: clearing the muddied waters. Am J Hum Genet 62:1020–1022, 1998

Giardello F, Hamilton S, Kern S, et al: Colorectal neoplasia in juvenile polyposis or juvenile polyps. Arch Dis Child 66:971–975, 1991

Giardello F, Hamilton S, Krush A, et al: Treatment of colonic rectal adenomas with sulindac in familial adenomatous polyposis. N Engl J Med 328:1313–1316, 1993

Giardello FM, Welsh SB, Hamilton SR, et al: Increased risk of cancer in the Peutz-Jeghers syndrome. N Engl J Med 316:1511, 1987

Hoffenberg EJ, Sauaia A, Maltzman T, Knoll K, Ahnen DJ: Symptomatic colonic polyps in childhood: not so benign. J Pediatr Gastroenterol Nutr 28:175–181, 1999

Howe J, Roth S, Ringold J, et al: Mutations in the *SMAD4/DPC4* gene in juvenile polyposis. Science 280:1086–1088, 1998

Jenne D, Reimann H, Nezu J, et al: Peutz-Jegher syndrome is caused by mutations in a novel serine threonine kinase. Nature Genet 18:38–43, 1998

Kaplan B, Benson J, Rothstein F, et al: Lymphonodular hyperplasia of the colon as a pathologic finding in children with lower gastrointestinal bleeding. J Pediatr Gastroenterol Nutr 3:704, 1984

Lamireau T, Le Bail B, Sarlangue J, Vergnes P, Lacombe D: Rectal polyps in Proteus syndrome. J Pediatr Gastroenterol Nutr 17:115, 1993

Liaw D, Marsh D, Li J, et al: Germline mutations of the PTEN gene in Cowden disease, an inherited breast and thyroid cancer syndrome. Nature Genet 16:64–67, 1997

Parkes SE, Muir KR, Sheyyab M, et al: Carcinoid tumors of the appendix in children (1957–1986): incidence, treatment, and outcome. Br J Surg 80:502, 1993

Powell S, Petersen G, Krush A, et al: Molecular diagnosis of familial adenomatous polyposis. N Engl J Med 329:1982–1987, 1993

Rustg AK: Hereditary gastrointestinal polyposis and polyposis syndromes. N Engl J Med 331:1694–1702, 1994

17.23 DISORDERS OF THE ANORECTUM

17.23.1   Congenital Anomalies of the Anorectum

Brad W. Warner

The spectrum of anorectal malformations ranges from simple anal stenosis to the persistence of a cloaca; incidence ranges from one in 4000 to one in 5000 live births and is slightly more common in boys. The most common defect in both boys and girls is an imperforate anus with a fistula between the distal bowel and the urethra in boys or the vestibule of the vagina in girls. The risk for a couple having a second child with an anorectal malformation is approximately 1%.

The embryologic development of the hindgut is discussed in Sec. 17.1.2. By 6 weeks of gestation, the urorectal septum begins to move in a caudal direction to divide the cloaca into the anterior urogenital sinus and posterior anorectal canal. Failure of the urorectal septum to form results in a fistula between the bowel and urinary tract (in boys) or the vagina (in girls). The urorectal septum divides the cloacal membrane into the urogenital and anal membranes. Complete or partial failure of the anal membrane to resorb results in an anal membrane or stenosis. The perineum also contributes to development of the external anal opening and genitalia by formation of cloacal folds that extend from the anterior genital tubercle to the anal membrane. The perineal body is formed by fusion of the cloacal folds between the anal and urogenital membranes. Breakdown of the cloacal membrane anywhere along its course results in the external anal opening being anterior to the external sphincter (ie, anteriorly displaced anus).

Management of anorectal anomalies requires that the level of the rectal pouch and presence of fistula to the urinary tract or vagina be determined; this is important in early management. Evaluating the location of a fistula can be performed at a later time.

Table 17-59 provides an anatomic classification of anorectal anomalies based on the level at which the blind-ending rectal pouch ends relative to the levator ani musculature. Traditionally, the level of the end of the rectal pouch is determined by obtaining a lateral pelvic radiograph (ie, "invertogram") after the infant is held upside-down for several minutes to allow air to pass into the rectal pouch. High lesions are above the levator and may or may not have a fistulous connection to the vagina or bladder/prostatic urethra in boys. Intermediate lesions are characterized by the rectal pouch ending within the levator, with or without a fistula to the vagina or a bulbous urethra in boys. In low lesions, the rectal pouch has completely traversed the levator musculature, and a fistula usually is evident on the skin within the midline (ie, anteriorly displaced anus). Rectal atresia refers to an unusual lesion in which the lumen of the rectum is either completely or partially interrupted, with the upper rectum being dilated and the lower rectum consisting of a small anal canal. A *persistent cloaca* is defined as a defect in which the rectum, vagina, and urethra all meet and fuse to form a single, common channel. In girls, the type of defect may be determined by the number of orifices at the perineum. A single orifice would

TABLE 17-59

CLASSIFICATION OF CONGENITAL ANOMALIES OF THE ANORECTUM

Female
  High
    Anorectal agenesis with or without rectovaginal fistula
    Rectal atresia
  Intermediate
    Anorectal agenesis with or without rectovaginal fistula
    Anal agenesis
  Low
    Anovestibular or anocutaneous fistula (anteriorly displaced anus)
    Anal stenosis
  Cloaca
Male
  High
    Anorectal agenesis with or without rectoprostatic urethral fistula
    Rectal atresia
  Intermediate
    Anorectal agenesis with or without rectobulbar urethral fistula
    Anal agenesis
  Low
    Anocutaneous fistula (anteriorly displaced anus)
    Anal stenosis

---

be consistent with a cloaca. If two orifices are seen (ie, urethra and vagina), the defect is an imperforate anus or, less commonly, a persistent urogenital sinus comprising one orifice and a normal anus as the other orifice.

From a practical standpoint, the invertogram is difficult to perform, and it is not entirely predictive of the pouch level. A crying infant may appear from the increased intraabdominal pressure and downward displacement of the gas within the pouch to have a low anomaly. Furthermore, the gas may not have traversed to the very end of the pouch, thus giving the impression of a high lesion. Inspection of the perineum alone determines the pouch level in 80% of boys and 90% of girls. Clinically, if a fistula is seen anywhere on the perineal skin of a boy or external to the hymen of a girl, a low lesion can be assumed, which allows a primary perineal repair procedure to be performed. The majority of all other lesions are high or intermediate, and they require diversion through a sigmoid colostomy that is followed by a definitive repair procedure at a later date. If required, the level of the rectal pouch can be delineated more definitively by ultrasonography or magnetic resonance imaging. Perineal ultrasonography may be useful in determining the distance between the rectal pouch and the anal skin, although ultrasonography may be subject to the same pitfalls as the invertogram. In general, a lesion can be considered to be low if the distance from the rectal pouch to the skin, as determined by ultrasonography, is less than 1 cm. Magnetic resonance imaging accurately delineates the anatomy of the pouch relative to the levator ani musculature and sphincters; it is particularly useful during postoperative evaluation of the child with continence problems after repair.

Congenital anorectal anomalies often coexist with other lesions, and the VATER or VACTERL association (see Sec. 17.9.1) must be considered. Bony abnormalities of the sacrum and spine occur in about one-third of patients with anorectal anomalies and consist of absent, accessory, or hemivertebrae and/or an asymmetric or short sacrum. The absence of two or more vertebrae is associated with poor prognosis in terms of bowel and bladder continence. Occult dysraphism of the spinal cord also may be present, and it consists of tethered cord, lipomeningocele, or fat within the filum.

Genitourinary abnormalities other than the rectourinary fistula occur in 26 to 59% of patients. Vesicoureteral reflux and hydronephrosis are the most common abnormalities, but other findings such as horseshoe, dysplastic, or absent kidney as well as hypospadias or cryptorchidism also must be considered. In general, the higher the anorectal malformation, the more frequent the associated urologic abnormalities. In patients with persistent cloacas or rectovesical fistula, the likelihood of a genitourinary abnormality is approximately 90%. In contrast, the frequency is only 10% in children with low defects (ie, perineal fistula).

Evaluation for associated anomalies should include plain-film radiography of the chest and spine to exclude abnormalities of the heart as well as the vertebrae and sacrum. If a cardiac defect is suspected, echocardiography should be performed before any surgical procedure. Ultrasonography of the spine should be obtained to exclude occult dysraphism. Before feeding, a nasogastric tube should be placed, and its presence within the stomach confirmed, to exclude esophageal atresia. Radiographic evaluation of the urinary tract should include renal ultrasonography and voiding cystourethrography; a rectourinary fistula (if present) likely will be demonstrated by the latter procedure.

SURGICAL MANAGEMENT

The newborn infant with a low lesion can have a primary, single-stage repair procedure on the perineum without need for a colostomy. Three basic approaches may be used. For anal stenosis with a normal location of the anal opening, only simple dilatation is necessary. This should be performed daily (12-Fr size for newborn infants), and the size of the dilator should be increased progressively. Over several months, the anus ultimately will admit an index finger easily, and the dilatations can be discontinued. If the anal opening is anterior to the external sphincter (ie, anteriorly displaced anus) with a small distance between the opening and the center of the external sphincter, and the perineal body also is intact, a cutback anoplasty is performed. A cut is made from the anal orifice to the central part of the anal sphincter, thus enlarging the anal opening. Alternatively, if there is a large distance between the anal opening and the central portion of the external anal sphincter, the aberrant anal opening is transposed to the correct position, and the perineal body is reconstructed.

Infants with intermediate or high lesions require a colostomy as the first part of a three-stage reconstruction. The colon is completely divided in the sigmoid region, with the proximal bowel as the colostomy and the distal bowel as a mucous fistula. Complete division of the bowel minimizes fecal contamination into the area of a rectourinary fistula, and it may lessen the risk of urosepsis. Furthermore, the distal bowel can be evaluated radiographically to determine the location of the rectourinary fistula. The second-stage procedure usually is performed 3 to 6 months later; it consists of surgically dividing the rectourinary or rectovaginal fistula with a "pull-through" of the terminal rectal pouch into the normal anal position. A posterior sagittal approach allows the central position of the anal sphincter to be identified by electrical stimulation of the perineum. An incision is made in the midline extending from the coccyx to the external sphincter. The rectum is identified, and the fistula to the vagina or urinary tract (if present) is divided. The rectum is then mobilized, and the perineal musculature (ie, levator ani and parasagittal fibers of the external sphincter complex) reconstructed. The patient is left with the protective colostomy to afford healing of the new anal anastomosis. In boys, a urinary catheter remains in place to maintain the lumen of the urethra after repair of the rectourinary fistula. The third and final stage is performed a few months after the second stage, and it consists of colostomy closure. Anal dilatations are begun 2 weeks after the pull-through procedure and continue for several months after the colostomy closure. A 12-Fr dilator is used for newborns, which is increased up to 14- or 16-Fr for older infants.

In patients with a persistent cloaca, the surgical approach generally is the same as that with high imperforate anus. The urethra is created from the tubularized old urogenital sinus, and the vagina and rectum are carefully separated and placed into the appropriate location. Often, the vagina will not reach the perineal skin, and a vaginal augmentation procedure can be performed using flaps of the perineal or labial skin or a segment of small intestine.

OUTCOME

Major morbidity in patients with anorectal malformations is related to associated anomalies. Fecal continence is the major goal regarding correction of the defect. Prognostic factors for continence include the level of the pouch and whether the sacrum is normal. The best results are seen in patients with low lesions and a normal sacrum, with incontinence reported to occur in up to 40% of patients at long-term follow-up. In patients with intermediate lesions and a normal sacrum, soiling was reported to occur in 50 to 75%. In high lesions, the rate of incontinence is nearly 100%. Despite the fairly high rate of incontinence, 84% of adult patients were satisfied with their level of cleanliness. In general, patients who have continued problems with either constipation or soiling following the repair of an anorectal anomaly should begin a bowel-training program with daily enemas. The goal of this postoperative program is to keep the lower rectum decompressed while controlling the need to defecate. Success or failure in achieving continence cannot be judged until after the age of 10 years. Anorectal biofeedback may improve continence in some children with low to intermediate lesions.

References

Hassink EA, Rieu PN, Severijnen RS, et al: Are adults content or continent after repair for high anal atresia? A long-term follow-up study in patients 18 years of age and older. Ann Surg 218:196–200, 1993
Peña A: Posterior sagittal anorectoplasty: results in the management of 332 cases of anorectal malformations. Pediatr Surg Int 3:94–104, 1988
Peña A: Imperforate anus and cloacal malformations. In: Ashcraft KW, Holder TA, eds: Pediatric Surgery, 2nd ed. Philadelphia, WB Saunders, 1993:372–392
Rintala R, Mildh L, Lindahl H: Fecal continence and quality of life in adult patients with an operated low anorectal malformation. J Pediatr Surg 27:902–905, 1992

17.23.2 Other Anorectal Disorders

Judith M. Sondheimer

HEMORRHOIDS AND ANORECTAL VARICES

Hemorrhoids are masses of vascular tissue within the anal canal. Internal hemorrhoids arise from the superior hemorrhoidal vascular plexus, lie above the pectinate line, and are covered by rectal mucosa. External hemorrhoids arise from the inferior hemorrhoidal plexus, lie below the pectinate line, and are covered by skin. Varices may be located beneath the mucosa of the rectum or in the anal

canal. They are high-pressure venous channels shunting blood from the portal venous circulation (ie, superior hemorrhoidal vein) to the systemic circulation (ie, external iliac vein) arising in response to portal hypertension.

Symptomatic hemorrhoidal disease is rare in children and almost always external hemorrhoidal. External hemorrhoids usually develop because of chronic straining or constipation. Symptoms include bright red rectal bleeding, intermittent appearance of a pearly gray or purple mass at the anal verge after defecation, and, occasionally, infection with perianal pain. Thrombosis of external hemorrhoids may occur in adolescents, producing a very painful, firm mass at the anal verge. Prolapsing hemorrhoids may be seen in childhood sexual abuse. Symptoms from hemorrhoids usually improve with treatment of underlying chronic constipation. Incision and evacuation of thrombosed hemorrhoids may be necessary, although many resolve with conservative therapy, including stool softeners, warm sitz baths, and antibiotics.

In a recent prospective study of 60 children with portal hypertension, 33% had hemorrhoids, 35% anorectal varices, and 15% only external anal varices. Only 7% of these children had symptoms that were referable to their anal vascular lesions. The development of anorectal varices relates directly to the duration of portal hypertension and possibly to antecedent sclerosis of esophageal varices. Rectal varices rarely are the source of significant bleeding. Symptomatic rectal varices may be treated by injection sclerotherapy or banding if necessary.

RECTAL PROLAPSE

This occurs when one or all layers of the rectum protrude through the anus. Mucosal prolapse is most common, and it appears as a red-purple, circular protrusion from the anus, with radial folds extending from a central lumen. Brief prolapse of a small amount of rectal mucosa is common after normal defecation. Procidentia (ie, prolapse that includes mucosal, muscular, and serosal layers of the rectum) is rare in childhood; it presents as a protrusion with circumferential folds resulting from contractions of the circular musculature of the prolapsed rectum.

Mucosal prolapse is most common under 2 years of age. The relatively flat infant sacrum and weak pelvic floor musculature are probable predisposing factors; others include constipation, acute diarrhea (including pseudomembranous colitis), malnutrition, heavy infestation with intestinal parasites (eg, trichuriasis, amebiasis), chronic cough (especially when associated with malnutrition, pertussis, cystic fibrosis), perineal muscle weakness (eg, muscular dystrophy, meningomyelocele), rectal polyp, solitary rectal ulcer syndrome, exstrophy of the bladder, and high imperforate anus repair. Massive intestinal prolapse has been reported in children sitting on unprotected swimming pool drains. Approximately 20% of patients with cystic fibrosis probably will experience rectal prolapse at some time, but cystic fibrosis is not the most common cause of rectal prolapse in childhood. In a recent study of 54 pediatric patients with mucosal prolapse, 28% had chronic constipation, 20% acute diarrhea, 11% cystic fibrosis, 24% a variety of neuromotor problems, and 16% no identifiable cause.

Most mucosal prolapses reduce spontaneously. Children learn to pinch their buttocks together on standing after defecation to reduce prolapse, and occasionally, manual assistance is needed to reduce a large prolapse. The prolapsed mucosa may bleed because of vascular congestion, and it may secrete copious mucus. A prolapse that cannot be reduced may require surgery. The anus may gape for up to 1 hour after prolapse reduction. Between episodes, the anus appears to be normal. Anorectal manometry usually is normal. In patients with prior surgical procedures on the anus or with neuromotor disorders, anal sphincter pressure may be reduced. Barium radiography may reveal the presence of a rectal polyp or rectorectal intussusception during defecation, which is thought to promote prolapse.

Treatment of underlying pathology is indicated, with special attention to the treatment of constipation and reduction of straining. Surgery rarely is needed to correct recurrent rectal prolapse. However, in resistant cases, submucosal injection of a sclerosant such as clove oil may be effective therapy.

ANAL FISSURES

These are slit-like tears of the anal canal. They usually are located on the posterior or anterior anal verge and most commonly are caused by the passage of large, constipated bowel movements. Other causes of anal fissures include crypt abscess, explosive diarrhea, perianal dermatitis or infection, inflammatory bowel disease, trauma, and sexual abuse. The most common symptoms of anal fissure are pain and bright red rectal bleeding on defecation. Anal fissure is the most common cause of rectal bleeding in infants. Inspection of the anus with gentle spreading of the buttocks usually is sufficient to reveal a fissure; occasionally, proctoscopic examination is necessary to identify fissures in the anal canal. Treatment of constipation with stool softeners, warm sitz baths, and generous lubrication of the anal skin generally are sufficient to produce healing. Anal dilation with a lubricated finger or dilator helps to relieve anal spasm and pain. A small pucker (ie, sentinel tag) may appear in the anal skin when a fissure heals. Fissures and/or tags are seen in up to 30% of older children with retentive constipation. Anal fissures that do not heal should raise the suspicion of Crohn disease; 34% of one reported group of children with Crohn disease had anal fissures or tags. Multiple anal fissures, or fissures that are associated with other signs of anal or genital trauma, must be investigated as signs of sexual abuse. In rare cases when a fissure persists, silver nitrate cauterization, perianal injection of botulinum toxin A, or surgical resection may be necessary. Surgical treatment of fissures and perianal disease secondary to Crohn disease should be avoided if possible, because healing may be very poor.

CRYPTITIS, ANAL ABSCESS, AND FISTULA

Infection of the crypts of Morgagni is common. In children wearing diapers, it most likely results from lengthy fecal exposure. In older children, it is associated with chronic diarrhea and chronic constipation; symptoms include anal itch or burning, pain on defecation, and scant rectal bleeding. Rectal examination is painful because of internal sphincter spasm. Definitive diagnosis depends on sigmoidoscopic examination in which the crypts of Morgagni appear to be deep, with swollen and hyperemic columns. Cryptitis probably is a major factor in the production of perianal abscess. Infection in crypts or the anal glands penetrates into the space between the internal and external sphincter or into the ischiorectal fossa and eventually may point on the perianal skin. The causative organisms usually are *Escherichia coli* and anaerobes or, occasionally, *Staphylococcus aureus*. Boys are affected more often than girls, especially before 6 months of age. The usual presentation is a tender, erythematous perianal lump that may cause pain on defecation, constipation, or intermittent purulent discharge. Evaluation requires a careful rectal examination and search for a fistulous tract from the abscess externally to the anal gland or crypt internally. This often

requires examination under anesthesia. Initial treatment includes warm sitz baths and stool softeners, and it may require incision and drainage. Antibiotics are optional if the initial drainage appears to be adequate. Up to 50% of abscesses will recur after the initial incision and drainage; identification of the fistula with surgical excision of both the fistula and the crypt of origin must then be undertaken. In older children, the possibility of Crohn disease must be kept in mind because treatment with metronidazole rather than surgery is indicated in such a case. The differential diagnosis also should include immune deficiency and malignancy, especially leukemia.

PRURITUS ANI

Itching of the perianal skin has many causes, the most common in childhood being perianal dermatitis or infection. Itching during and after a course of broad-spectrum antibiotics is common and probably results from overgrowth of *Candida*. Atopic dermatitis, seborrhea, contact dermatitis, perianal streptococcal infection, psoriasis, anal fissures, and lichen sclerosus et atrophicus cause significant itching. Occasionally, culture or biopsy of the perianal skin may be necessary to identify the rarer conditions when conservative therapy fails. Fecal or urinary incontinence or poor hygiene, particularly when associated with binding undergarments, may cause maceration with pruritus of perianal skin. Parasites such as pinworms, tapeworms, *Trichomonas*, scabies, and body lice may present as perianal itch. Systemic diseases such as diabetes mellitus, uremia, and obstructive liver disease also cause perineal itch, as can urinary tract infection and vaginitis. Foods containing chemical irritants or histamine releasers such as coffee, tea, wine, chocolate, colas, citrus, rhubarb, tomatoes, and chilis may cause local irritation to the perianal skin during defecation. Perianal scratching may be a symptom of anxiety. Lichenification of the perianal skin will perpetuate the sensation of pruritus.

A careful history and thorough physical examination, including a rectal examination, are key to diagnosis. Testing may include stool examination, pinworm prep, urinalysis and culture, and culture or biopsy of dermatitis. Specific treatment of pruritus ani depends on the cause, but general measures include good perianal hygiene using nondrying soaps, local emollients, loose cotton underclothing, and the prevention of scratching.

ANORECTAL DISORDERS IN SEXUAL ABUSE

Anal assault constitutes a significant proportion of all injuries resulting from childhood sexual abuse. In a recent review of 310 childhood victims of sexual abuse, abnormalities of the anus were identified in 104 children (34%). These included gaping of the anus (61 children), anal tags (44), anal fissures (33), sphincter rupture (15), condylomata acuminata (4), scarring (2), and bites (1). Other findings that are consistent with chronic anal penetration include anal vascular congestion, hemorrhoids, anal skin thickening, erythema and hyperpigmentation, and shortening of the anal canal. An understanding of the normal appearance and size of the anal aperture is important, as is an understanding of other conditions that cause anal relaxation. These latter include meningomyelocele, repair for Hirschsprung disease or imperforate anus, neuromotor conditions such as myotonic dystrophy, and inflammatory bowel disease. A recent survey of children with chronic constipation attending a gastroenterology clinic indicated that anal relaxation is a rare finding in retentive constipation. Observation of the anus is best performed in the left lateral position with gentle lateral traction on the buttocks, and measurements should be made only after allowing approximately 30 seconds for relaxation to occur.

Anogenital infections may or may not be a sign of sexual abuse. Anogenital infection with human papillomavirus may be acquired either at birth or postnatally from an infected mother. Specific typing of the virus in both the patient and caregiver may clarify the source of infection. The older the child is when genital warts appear, the higher the likelihood that they are acquired via sexual contact. Herpetic lesions may be spread from an infected caretaker or by autoinoculation from oral lesions. The simultaneous presence of anogenital warts or herpetic lesions with other sexually transmitted infections (eg, *Trichomonas,* gonorrhea, syphilis, *Chlamydia*) or physical signs of abuse increase the likelihood that sexual abuse is the cause. Perianal rashes should be cultured for sexually transmitted organisms if the history is suggestive or the rash is unresponsive to standard therapy. Several reports stress how important full evaluation of perianal rashes is to avoid overdiagnosis of sexual abuse. Examples of conditions that have been mistaken for sexual abuse because of their presentation as perianal rash include molluscum contagiosum, pemphigus, lichen sclerosus et atrophicus, psoriasis, inflammatory bowel disease, perianal *Streptococcus,* and anal stenosis.

INFECTIONS OF THE PERIANAL AREA

Many of the infections affecting the perianal area are covered elsewhere in this text. *Perianal streptococcal infection* is common during infancy and childhood. Major symptoms include a bright red confluent rash around the anal orifice, which sometimes spreads to involve the entire perineal area. Impetiginous lesions sometimes are obvious, with vesicles and honey-colored crusting. The anal canal usually is involved. Patients may experience small amounts of red rectal bleeding and considerable pain with defecation. A family history of recent streptococcal disease often is obtained, and the patient sometimes has a simultaneous streptococcal pharyngitis. Culture of the anal canal is indicated in any infant whose red "diaper dermatitis" does not heal with standard therapy. Treatment with oral penicillin is recommended, but local antibiotics are not effective. In resistant culture-proven cases, clindamycin may be used.

Anogenital warts usually result from infection with human papilloma virus types 6 and 11. Other serotypes, including type 2 (ie, the usual cutaneous wart virus), may cause perianal disease. The relationship of this infection to sexual abuse was discussed previously. Chemical removal using podophyllin is difficult in this area because isolation of the wart is not possible. Surgical removal of warts may be indicated if the involvement is extensive.

Molluscum contagiosum lesions may appear in the perianal area. The typical lesion is painless, small, gray-white, and umbilicated on a slightly erythematous base. Lesions usually are seen elsewhere on the body and most often result from autoinoculation. They may be transmitted by sexual contact. Cheesy squamous debris fills the lesion, and cytoplasmic inclusions can be seen in the expressed cells. Treatment is discussed in Sec. 13.3.14.

Candidal diaper dermatitis is the most common perianal infection in pediatrics. It is discussed in Sec. 14.3.1.

MALIGNANCY

Histiocytosis X can present as an isolated, eczematoid, perianal rash. The presence of petechiae in the rash suggests this diagnosis; biopsy is necessary to confirm the diagnosis. Although rare in childhood, malignant melanoma may develop in the anal skin. Pigmented lesions in this area should be carefully observed and biopsied if they

increase in size. Plexiform neurofibromas also may arise in the skin of the perianal area. This lesion also requires biopsy if no other signs of neurofibromatosis are present.

References

Agnarsson U, Warde C, McCarthy G, Evans N: Perianal appearances associated with constipation. Arch Dis Child 65:1231–1234, 1990

Connon AF, Davidson GP, Moore DJ: Anal size in children: the influence of age, constipation, rectal examination and defaecation. Med J Aust 153:380–383, 1990

Heaton ND, Davenport M, Howard ER: Incidence of haemorrhoids and anorectal varices in children with portal hypertension. Br J Surg 80:616–618, 1993

Heaton ND, Davenport M, Howard ER: Symptomatic hemorrhoids and anorectal varices in children with portal hypertension. J Pediatr Surg 27:833–835, 1992

Markowitz J, Daum F, Aiges H, Kahn E, Silverberg M, Fisher SE: Perianal disease in children and adolescents with Crohn's disease. Gastroenterology 86:829–833, 1984

Muram D: Anal and perianal abnormalities in prepubertal victims of sexual abuse. Am J Obstet Gynecol 161:278–281, 1989

Oriel JD: Anogenital papillomavirus infection in children. Br Med J 296:1484–1485, 1988

Piazza DJ, Radhakrishnan J: Perianal abscess and fistula-in-ano in children. Dis Colon Rectum 33:1014–1016, 1990

Vorenberg E: Diagnosing child abuse: the cost of getting it wrong. Arch Dermatol 128:844–845, 1992

Zempsky WT, Rosenstein BJ: The cause of rectal prolapse in children. Am J Dis Child 142:338–339, 1988

17.23.3 Hirschsprung Disease and Other Neuropathies

Peter J. Milla

HIRSCHSPRUNG DISEASE

Hirschsprung disease occurs in one of 5000 live births and is the most common cause of lower intestinal obstruction in neonates. It results from the absence of enteric ganglionic neurons, beginning at the anus and extending proximally for a variable distance. Sex ratios and patterns of inheritance differ with the length of aganglionic bowel. Aganglionosis is limited to the rectum and sigmoid in approximately 75% of cases; it includes the total colon in approximately 8% and occasionally may affect the whole of the intestine. The more common rectosigmoid disease shows a male predominance of about 4:1, with a sex-modified multifactorial or recessive pattern of inheritance and risk for an affected sibling of 7%. Racial distribution is equal for white and African-American infants. In longer-segment disease, the sex ratio decreases, and the sibling risk increases to as high as 20% with total colonic aganglionosis. Associated anomalies include congenital heart disease or Down syndrome in 5 to 10% of patients. Other associated syndromes include Smith-Lemli-Opitz and Waardenburg syndromes.

PATHOGENESIS Hirschsprung disease results from failure of the craniocaudal migration of neural crest cells (NCCs), which ultimately form the enteric neurons, along the GI tract during weeks 4 through 12 of gestation (see Sec. 17.1.3). It is now known that migration and differentiation of these NCCs is under the control of a variety of factors that are genetically determined. These are receptors on the migrating NCCs and neurotrophic factors secreted by mesenchymal cells, which are required by the neural crest cells for survival, proliferation, and differentiation. Expression of these molecules is probably controlled by the Hox and Sox homeobox genes. Two signaling systems have been clearly defined ret/glial-derived neurotrophic factor and endothelin receptor B/endothelin 3. In a number of families with inherited Hirschsprung disease, abnormality of the genes coding for these molecules has been detected. Further support for the role of these genes in the pathogenesis of Hirschsprung disease arises from knockout studies in transgenic mice, which create a murine form of aganglionosis. Abnormality of these genes now also has been detected in some sporadic cases of Hirschsprung disease. However, in some cases, no abnormality of these genes can be detected, and it thus is likely that other factors creating a permissive environment or in the neural crest cells themselves also play a role in the disorder. So far, knowledge of these factors has not enabled antenatal diagnosis or prognosis to be determined.

Because of the loss of intrinsic innervation of the rectum, there is an overexpression of extrinsic parasympathetic and sympathetic nerves that is particularly noticeable in the lamina propria and muscularis mucosae. The contractile action of neuropeptide Y and other agents in these nerves on the rectal smooth muscle is unopposed because of the loss of vasoactive intestinal polypeptide and nitric oxide–synthesizing enteric nerves that cause relaxation. The aganglionic segment, internal sphincter, and anal canal remain constantly contracted, thus causing obstructive symptoms with proximal dilatation and hypertrophy of the colon.

CLINICAL FEATURES Hirschsprung disease presents in one of three ways:

1. Complete intestinal obstruction, with bilious vomiting, obstipation, and massive abdominal distension
2. Delayed passage of meconium
3. Enterocolitis

A large survey performed in 1979 suggested that only 15% of infants were diagnosed within the first month after birth and that 8% were not recognized until 3 years of age or later. Currently, the diagnosis of Hirschsprung disease frequently is made in the neonatal period.

In normal full-term neonates, 90% pass meconium within 24 hours, and 99% within 48 hours. In children with Hirschsprung disease, 94% fail to pass meconium within the first 24 hours after birth. Therefore, any term infant who does not pass meconium within 48 hours should be suspected of having Hirschsprung disease. Complete intestinal obstruction can be observed in the immediate neonatal period or may occur in an older infant with only a history of constipation. Enterocolitis most often occurs during the second to fourth weeks, and it results as a consequence of delayed diagnosis. It is characterized by fever; explosive, foul-smelling, and often bloody diarrheal stools; and abdominal distension. Enterocolitis carries with it a poor prognosis, with an overall mortality rate of 4 to 33%. Enterocolitis also occurs in the postoperative period in 13% of cases. At present, the pathogenesis of enterocolitis remains unclear. Less common presentations include only constipation in approximately 5% of patients, perforation occurring during the neonatal period in 3%, fecal soiling similar to that in functional megacolon in 3%, rectal bleeding from an anal fissure in 5%, and hydroureter from urethral compression.

DIAGNOSIS Once the diagnosis of Hirschsprung disease is considered, diagnostic studies should be performed. Delayed diagnosis

increases the risk of enterocolitis as well as the potential morbidity and mortality of the disease. The most accurate and readily available diagnostic method is the suction rectal biopsy with acetylcholinesterase staining. In short-segment Hirschsprung disease, the submucosal and myenteric plexuses contain hypertrophic nerve trunks. Acetylcholinesterase staining shows their presence in the muscularis mucosae, a pattern that is pathognomonic for the disease. In total colonic aganglionosis, however, the acetylcholinesterase activity is not always increased, and the thickened nerve trunks, which are found in short-segment Hirschsprung disease, are not always present. Therefore, a normal acetylcholinesterase pattern is insufficient to exclude total colonic aganglionosis, and if the condition is clinically suspected, the biopsy must contain sufficient submucosa to reliably diagnose the absence of enteric neurons. If there is any question regarding diagnosis, a full-thickness surgical rectal biopsy allows aganglionosis in the myenteric and submucosal plexuses to be reliably recognized in 98% of cases. Barium-contrast enema is performed by inserting a small catheter just within the anal canal in a previously unprepared colon. Barium solution is slowly introduced into the rectum until an obviously dilated area becomes visible (Fig. 17-38) at the transition between the aganglionic and ganglionic bowel. Where the diagnosis remains doubtful, delayed films may show retention of contrast material. Barium enema examination is unreliable in short-segment disease and the young infant.

Anorectal manometry is technically difficult, but it can rule out Hirschsprung disease if normal relaxation of the anal sphincter is demonstrated on distension of a balloon in the rectum. Failure of

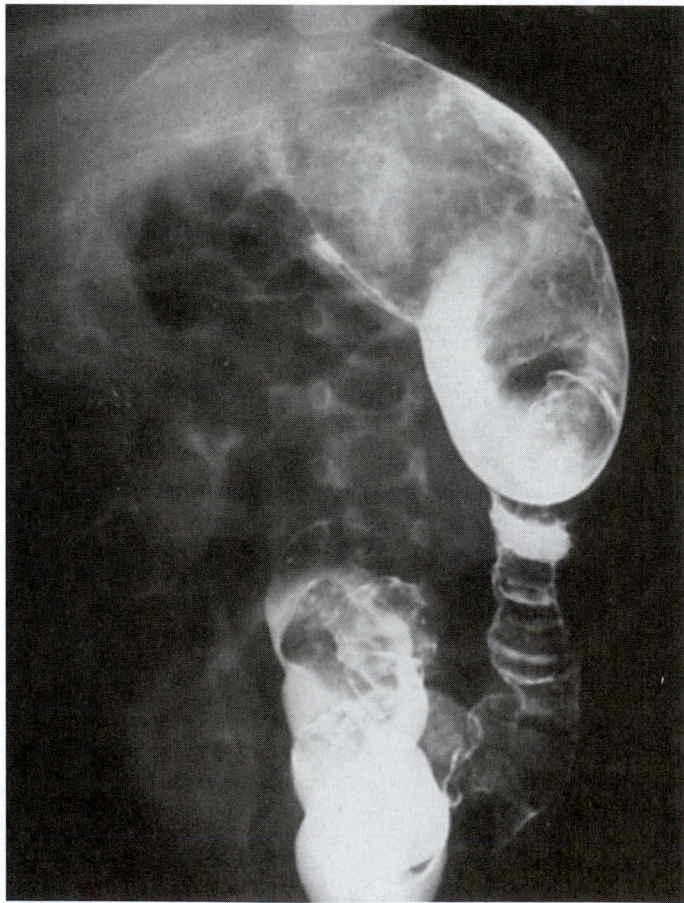

FIGURE 17-38 **Hirschsprung disease with high sigmoid colon "transition zone." Rectal biopsy is necessary to confirm the diagnosis.**

the internal anal sphincter to relax in response to distension of the rectum is diagnostic of Hirschsprung disease. Equipment that is required for manometry is not readily available in all centers, nor are individuals who are experienced with these techniques.

Syndromes that must be distinguished from Hirschsprung disease in the newborn period include meconium plug syndrome, pseudo-Hirschsprung disease with other nerve and muscle disorders of the lower colon (including intestinal neuronal dysplasia), hypoganglionosis, and hollow visceral myopathy.

MANAGEMENT During the neonatal period, obstruction (if present) is relieved through creation of a stoma that is proximal to the aganglionic segment. In total colonic disease, the stoma may have to be located high in the small bowel, leading to major problems in fluid and electrolyte imbalance. In older children, a preliminary colostomy may not be required, and definitive surgery may be performed after repeated rectal washouts and irrigation of the colon. If enterocolitis occurs, treatment consists of fluid resuscitation, broad-spectrum antibiotic coverage (including for anaerobes), nasogastric decompression, and warm saline rectal washouts to facilitate colonic decompression. A proximal colostomy is performed as soon as the patient's condition permits.

Four definitive surgical approaches have been used for Hirschsprung disease—the Swenson, Duhamel, Soave, and Boley procedures. All involve resection of the aganglionic bowel and reanastomosis of the proximal normal bowel to the normal anal canal; they differ in methods of reconstructing the bowel. Although early reconstitution of the bowel is now often favored to allow the restoration of normal bowel habit, some surgeons advise a definitive pull-through operation at 6 to 12 months of age, depending on the weight and general condition of the child. In very-short- or ultrashort-segment disease, treatment by a myectomy to transect the involved area may be effective.

The most common immediate postoperative complications are stricture or leakage at the anastomotic site following endorectal or Swenson operation and pelvic abscess may occur. Urinary incontinence or retention because of pelvic dissection generally is transient. Where there is extensive aganglionosis involving the whole colon together with part of the small intestine, continuing problems of malabsorption, fluid loss, fecal incontinence, and poor electrolyte balance are common. Even after definitive surgery, leakage and strictures may occur because of damage to the mucosa during previous episodes of enterocolitis. In addition, even if no residual aganglionic bowel remains, recurrent enterocolitis still may occur.

A few children will continue to have problems with constipation postoperatively. This usually results from residual unresected aganglionic bowel or an associated intestinal neuronal dysplasia. Investigations include contrast studies to demonstrate strictures and leaks as well as further biopsies to delineate residual aganglionic bowel or the presence of neuronal dysplasia.

VISCERAL NEUROPATHIES

A variety of disorders may affect the submucous and myenteric plexuses of the gut, and these may be limited to one area of the gut or be more widespread throughout the GI tract. Symptoms relate to both the affected length and region of the gut. It now is recognized that disordered motility may be caused by conditions other than aganglionosis of the colon or rectum. These disorders have been collectively referred to as *pseudo-Hirschsprung disease* and may result from disease of the smooth muscle coats or GI nerves.

Hypoganglionosis is a congenital or acquired disorder in which the number of myenteric neurons is reduced. The congenital form is thought to result from mechanisms similar to those producing aganglionosis, whereas acquired disease more likely results from toxic or autoimmune processes attacking neurons. The outcome of such processes is neuronal depletion. Hypoganglionosis appears to be as common a cause of severe, intractable constipation as does Hirschsprung disease, and it may affect a wide age range of patients. Presentation may not be restricted to constipation. Navarro and colleagues found that 15 of 26 patients with generalized pseudoobstruction had hypoganglionosis. Hypoganglionosis primarily is a disorder of the myenteric plexus, and it requires a full-thickness biopsy for diagnosis. The natural history of hypoganglionosis varies with its etiology. Treatment of symptoms and careful attention to nutritional status remain the mainstays of management.

Intestinal neuronal dysplasia has an incidence of less than 5% that of Hirschsprung disease. The condition may be localized or disseminated, and there are two types of dysplasia: (1) type A, in which there is sympathetic aplasia, myenteric plexus hyperplasia, and often, colonic inflammation; and (2) type B, in which the submucosal plexus is affected more and there is no sympathetic aplasia. Type B frequently presents in a manner that is indistinguishable from Hirschsprung disease. The course, however, often is benign, and conservative therapy results in spontaneous resolution of the condition. In addition to occurring in isolation, type B intestinal neuronal dysplasia commonly occurs in association with Hirschsprung disease and may be the cause of continued symptoms following surgery. Controversy has existed regarding intestinal neuronal dysplasia, but generally accepted diagnostic criteria, preferably on full-thickness biopsies, are hyperganglionosis and giant ganglia. This condition must be differentiated from transmural intestinal ganglioneuromatosis, which occurs in association with multiple endocrine neoplasia type 2B and is a marker of endocrine malignancy.

OTHER NEUROPATHIES

Other conditions causing visceral neuropathy include glial cell hyperplasia and inflammatory plexopathies, in which the myenteric plexus is infiltrated with inflammatory cells, resulting in degeneration of the neurons. Such a selective attack on the enteric neurons may result from an autoimmune process. Dysmotility also may occur because of delayed maturation of myenteric neurons, which continue to develop during the first year of life in normal infants. A systematic study of the ontogeny of enteric neurons after birth is necessary to determine the relationship between delayed morphologic development and function. A variety of toxic processes may affect myenteric neurons, resulting in their degeneration, apart from autoimmune disorders; however, these conditions are not well understood.

References

Edery P, Lyonnet S, Mulligan L, et al: Mutations of the *ret* proto oncogene in Hirschsprung disease. Nature 367:378–380, 1994

Koletzko S, Jesch I, Faus-Keβler T, et al: Rectal biopsy for diagnosis of intestinal neuronal dysplasia in children: a prospective multicentre study on interobserver variation and clinical outcome. Gut 44:853–861, 1999

Lake BD, Puri P, Nixon HH, Claireaux AE: Hirschsprung's disease. An appraisal of histochemically demonstrated acetylcholinesterase activity in suction rectal biopsy specimens as an aid to diagnosis. Arch Pathol Lab Med 102:244–247, 1978

Milla PJ: Endothelins, pseudoobstruction and Hirschsprung's disease. Gut 44:148–152, 1999

Morikawa Y, Donahoe PK, Hendren WH: Manometry and histochemistry in the diagnosis of Hirschsprung's disease. Pediatrics 63:865–871, 1979

Navarro J, Sonsino E, Boige N, et al: Visceral neuropathies responsible for chronic intestinal pseudoobstruction syndrome in pediatric practice. J Pediatr Gastroenterol Nutr 11:179–195, 1990

Swenson O, Sherman JO, Fisher JH: Diagnosis of congenital megacolon: an analysis of 501 patients. J Pediatr Surg 8:587–594, 1973

17.24 THE EXOCRINE PANCREAS

Peter R. Durie

17.24.1   Embryology and Congenital Anomalies of the Pancreas

In the fourth week of gestation, the human pancreas develops as two outpouchings of the duodenal endoderm (Fig. 17-8). A dorsal bud grows into an elongated structure that ultimately becomes the tail, body, and a portion of the head of the pancreas. The ventral sac grows more slowly but is pulled posteriorly as the duodenum rotates during normal embryologic development. It eventually fuses with the dorsal bud to create the remainder of the head of the pancreas and the uncinate process. Each bud possesses its own ductal system; the ventral duct, which arises from the common bile duct, anastomoses with the dorsal duct to form the main duct of Wirsung and opens into the ampulla of Vater. The main pancreatic duct is formed by fusion of the ventral and dorsal ducts; if present, the accessory pancreatic duct of Santorini originates from the dorsal duct. The dual embryologic origin of the pancreas provides insight into a variety of congenital anomalies that are caused by problems with migration and/or fusion of the pancreatic buds or their ductal systems (Table 17-60).

Annular pancreas probably arises from incomplete rotation of the ventral bud, and it can produce symptoms at any age. Presentation in infancy usually is characterized by high GI obstruction following polyhydramnios in utero. The "double bubble" appearance on plain-film abdominal radiographs suggests a high obstruction, of which annular pancreas is included in the differential diagnosis (see Sec. 17.7.9). In older children, partial obstruction may give rise to recurrent vomiting. Heterotopia or ectopic pancreas comprises tissue lacking any continuity with the main body of the pancreas. Most pancreatic ectopia are found in the gastric antrum. However, a small percentage can occur within the intestinal tract, and approximately 4% are extraintestinal. In most instances, this

anomaly is an incidental finding, but it occasionally may be implicated as a cause of pain, GI bleeding, or obstruction.

Complete agenesis of the pancreas is rare and usually results in severe intrauterine growth retardation and death shortly after birth. Varying degrees of pancreatic hypoplasia occur, probably resulting from defects in embryonic development. Clinical manifestations vary according to the degree of loss of the exocrine and endocrine pancreatic tissue; there may be no symptoms or variable effects of endocrine and exocrine deficiency. Pancreatic agenesis or severe hypoplasia should be considered with persisting neonatal hyperglycemia.

Defective fusion of the two pancreatic primordia leads to a number of anatomic anomalies of the pancreatic ductal system. Two anomalies with clinical implications include pancreatic divisum (ie, ventral pancreas) and anomalous junctions of the common bile duct and the pancreatic duct, or the so-called common channel. Pancreatic divisum, which is a common anomaly, arises from incomplete fusion of the dorsal and ventral pancreatic ductal systems. Association of this anatomic finding with recurrent pancreatitis is controversial. Pancreatic divisum is diagnosed by endoscopic retrograde cholangiopancreatography (ERCP). The presence of a common channel, with the pancreaticobiliary junction seen outside the duodenal wall, is associated with pancreatitis and implicated in the pathogenesis of choledochal cysts. The classic presentation is that of abdominal pain, usually in the right upper quadrant; intermittent jaundice; and, on occasion, a mass in the right upper quadrant. Occasionally cholangitis and/or sepsis may occur. Abdominal ultrasonography or computed tomography often is diagnostic, but ERCP may be required.

17.24.2   Disturbances of Exocrine Pancreatic Function

The term *pancreatic insufficiency* implies a loss of exocrine pancreatic function to the point of being unable to digest and absorb nutrients. This is reflected by clinical evidence of steatorrhea and azotorrhea. Over 98% of the pancreatic reserve must be lost before pancreatic insufficiency develops. The term *pancreatic sufficiency* has been coined to describe patients with evidence of pancreatic dysfunction in whom the reserve capacity of the pancreas remains above the threshold for developing maldigestion.

The exocrine pancreas is functionally immature at birth (see Sec. 17.1.4). Protease function probably is adequate, but lipase activity in the newborn approximates 5 to 10% of adult values and remains low throughout infancy. Amylase secretion is essentially absent at birth and remains low for the first years of life. Except possibly in times of extreme metabolic or nutritional stress, pancreatic immaturity does not appear to be of major clinical importance. Causes of pancreatic dysfunction can be divided into hereditary conditions that directly affect the exocrine pancreas or situations in which loss of pancreatic function is an acquired phenomenon. Congenital causes of pancreatic dysfunction frequently are only one manifestation of a generalized disorder.

HEREDITARY CAUSES OF EXOCRINE PANCREATIC DYSFUNCTION

CYSTIC FIBROSIS   Cystic fibrosis is by far the most common cause of disturbed pancreatic function among children. Details of inheritance patterns, genetic defect, and other manifestations of cystic fibrosis are discussed in Sec. 23.6. Pancreatic damage begins in

TABLE 17-60

CONGENITAL ANOMALIES OF THE PANCREAS

ANOMALY	CLINICAL EFFECT
Annular pancreas	Partial or complete duodenal obstruction
Ectopic pancreas	Usually none; pain or bleeding (rare)
Agenesis	Exocrine/endocrine failure; death
Hypoplasia	None; exocrine and/or endocrine failure
Ductal anomalies	
Divisum	Controversial
Common channel	Choledochal cyst; pancreatitis

utero with accumulation of proteinaceous material within the pancreatic ducts. This causes obstruction of the ductal lumina, which is followed by progressive atrophy of acini. In patients with pancreatic insufficiency, the exocrine glands are replaced by fibrous tissue and fat. Pancreatic disease may be quite variable; approximately 85% of patients have pancreatic insufficiency, with the remainder having variable degrees of pancreatic sufficiency. Regardless of their pancreatic status, all patients show evidence of impaired pancreatic fluid secretion because of the defective channel function within the pancreatic duct cells. As a group, patients with cystic fibrosis and pancreatic sufficiency experience milder symptoms, are diagnosed at a later age, and have superior survival than those with pancreatic insufficiency. Recently, it has been shown that severity of the pancreatic dysfunction strongly correlates with the type of CFTR gene mutation. Patients homozygous for δ-508 have a high likelihood of having pancreatic insufficiency. Other gene mutations are associated only with pancreatic insufficiency or with pancreatic sufficiency, but not with both. Thus, it has been possible to classify mutations as "severe" or "mild" with respect to pancreatic functional status.

SHWACHMAN SYNDROME Shwachman syndrome is the second most common cause of exocrine pancreatic dysfunction in childhood. Other features include short stature, bone marrow dysfunction, and skeletal abnormalities. An autosomal-recessive trait is suggested. Short stature with normal linear growth velocity is common. Skeletal changes include thoracic dystrophy, clinodactyly, and metaphyseal dysplasia. Bone marrow changes include neutropenia (intermittent or persistent), which is virtually universal, and less commonly anemia, thrombocytopenia, and pancytopenia. A large percentage of patients have an elevated fetal hemoglobin. Almost a third of patients, predominantly boys, develop myeloproliferative malignancies. Recurrent infections that are presumed to result from neutropenia and functional neutrophil abnormalities occasionally can result in deep tissue bacterial infections, overwhelming sepsis, and death. Pancreatic dysfunction usually is less severe than in cystic fibrosis. Most patients present with signs and symptoms of malabsorption; in at least 50%, pancreatic function improves marginally with time, with normal nutrient absorption. The pancreatic lesion clearly is one of acinar cell hypoplasia with intact function of the pancreatic ducts.

JOHANSON-BLIZZARD SYNDROME Johanson-Blizzard syndrome is a rare inherited cause of pancreatic acinar hypoplasia. The syndrome is relatively easy to detect because of agenesis of the alae nasi, hair anomalies, deafness, hypothyroidism, genitourinary defects, and delayed development. Absence of bone marrow and skeletal abnormalities differentiates it from Shwachman syndrome. The pancreatic lesion is similar to that in Shwachman syndrome, however, with acinar hypoplasia but preserved ductal function.

PEARSON PANCREATIC AND BONE MARROW SYNDROME Pearson pancreatic and bone marrow syndrome is a rare autosomal-recessive condition. Patients have macrocytic anemia with varying degrees of neutropenia and thrombocytopenia. Erythroid and myeloid precursors contain peculiar vacuolization and hemosiderosis. Nonquantitative pancreatic function assessment suggests depressed acinar and ductal function. Unlike Shwachman syndrome, there is pancreatic cell atrophy with fibrosis.

ISOLATED ENZYME DEFICIENCIES Isolated enzyme deficiencies are rare and often poorly documented. Deficiencies have been reported for amylase, trypsinogen, lipase, colipase, and also combined colipase-lipase. Enterokinase is a brush border enzyme that activates proteases by activating trypsin from the proenzyme trypsinogen. Patients with enterokinase deficiency may appear to have pancreatic insufficiency because of symptoms of malnutrition, diarrhea, protein malabsorption, and hypoproteinemia. Actual pancreatic failure resulting from malnutrition may be a complicating feature, with patients improving if they receive supplemental pancreatic enzymes. Cases of congenital pancreatic insufficiency have been described as part of the rubella syndrome and in other congenital viral infections.

ACQUIRED CAUSES OF EXOCRINE PANCREATIC DYSFUNCTION

Exocrine pancreatic disturbance may result from enteropathy, chronic pancreatitis, or surgical excision. Enteropathy that is associated with pancreatic insufficiency is best documented in celiac sprue. In most cases, pancreatic function reverts to normal with appropriate therapy that is designed to improve the cause of the enteropathy. However, irreversible pancreatic insufficiency with acinar atrophy and fibrosis is reported in adults with long-standing celiac disease, but it is a rare complication of childhood. Chronic pancreatitis from familial or idiopathic causes or from juvenile tropical pancreatitis may cause pancreatic insufficiency because of progressive accumulated damage. The manifestations and causes of chronic pancreatitis are discussed later in this section. Overt exocrine pancreatic insufficiency and diabetes mellitus are late features, often taking many years to manifest. Surgical excision may result in pancreatic insufficiency, but up to 95% of the exocrine pancreas may be excised without risk of pancreatic insufficiency. Excision may be required for hyperinsulinism (ie, nesidioblastosis), pancreatic tumors, chronic pancreatitis, or following severe trauma to the pancreas. Other causes of pancreatic insufficiency include enterokinase deficiency, congenital viral infection, and severe malnutrition.

TESTS OF EXOCRINE PANCREATIC FUNCTION

The many clinical tests of exocrine pancreatic function are summarized in Table 17-61. Almost all clinically available tests have one or more major deficiencies.

DIRECT TESTS Direct tests assess the secretory capacity of the pancreas. They involve intestinal intubation and collection of pancreatic secretions. The pancreas may be stimulated by intravenously administered exogenous hormones, a test meal, or an infusion of a duodenal stimulant such as dilute hydrochloric acid. Direct tests

TABLE 17-61

TESTS OF EXOCRINE PANCREATIC FUNCTION

DIRECT	INDIRECT	BLOOD
Exogenous[a]	Stool microscopy	Isoamylase
Secretin	Steatocrit	Trypsinogen
Cholecystokinin	Fecal fat/nitrogen	Lipase
Cerulein	Fecal enzymes	Carotene
Endogenous[b]	Panerolauryl	
Lundh meal	Breath tests	
Amino acids	Starch	
	^{14}C or ^{13}C lipids	

[a] Used singly, in combination or in sequence.
[b] Release endogenous hormones that stimulate the pancreas.

are the most sensitive because they can determine the entire range of pancreatic function, including higher levels of function within the pancreatic-sufficient range. However, they are invasive, difficult to perform, and not standardized.

INDIRECT TESTS   Indirect tests are insensitive, and many are non-specific. Those that test digestive function (eg, stool microscopy, fecal fat, fecal nitrogen) will identify a malabsorptive condition but fail to pinpoint the precise etiology. Fat absorption is best determined by quantifying fat intake and measuring fecal fat losses over 72 hours. In normal individuals, fat losses are less than 7% of intake (<15% during infancy), but in severe pancreatic insufficiency, fat losses can be as high as 30 to 60% of intake. Measurement of fecal enzymes such as chymotrypsin and elastase provides a semiquantitative assessment of pancreatic capacity.

The *bentiromide and pancreolauryl tests* assess the ability of pancreatic enzymes to digest a specific substrate. Following oral ingestion, bentiromide is hydrolyzed by chymotrypsin to yield the marker *p*-aminobenzoic acid (PABA), which is absorbed and excreted in the urine. Measurement of PABA in plasma or its urinary excretion (6 to 8 hours) indirectly reflects pancreatic function. The test is useful only for screening patients with pancreatic insufficiency. Abnormal results may occur in neonates and in patients with intestinal, hepatic, or renal disease. The principles of the pancreolauryl test are the same, but a different substrate is used.

Breath tests, based on the principle that metabolites of digestion may be exhaled during respiration, utilize a variety of ingested substrates. Starch is dependent on pancreatic amylase for digestion. In the presence of pancreatic insufficiency, undigested starch is broken down by colonic bacteria, releasing hydrogen in the breath. A two-stage starch breath test, with and without enzyme replacement therapy, is a reliable but qualitative test of pancreatic function. Breath tests utilizing substrates containing stable isotopes rely on metabolism and release of $^{13}CO_2$, which is measured in expired breath.

BLOOD TESTS   Blood tests may provide useful information regarding pancreatic function. Total serum amylase, which measures both pancreatic and salivary amylase, is not a useful test of pancreatic dysfunction; however, more specific serum assays such as pancreatic isoamylase, immunoreactive trypsinogen, or lipase may be meaningful. Low enzyme levels are recorded in patients with pancreatic insufficiency (eg, in Shwachman syndrome). Even so, in infants with pancreatic insufficiency resulting from cystic fibrosis, serum enzyme concentrations may be greatly elevated because of the ductal obstructive pathology. In older patients with cystic fibrosis and pancreatic insufficiency, the pancreas atrophies, and serum trypsinogen levels are low or undetectable. Pancreatic-sufficient patients with cystic fibrosis have normal or elevated serum trypsinogen concentrations at all ages. Elevated serum enzyme concentrations also may occur in renal failure, acute malnutrition, and acute pancreatitis.

MANAGEMENT OF PANCREATIC INSUFFICIENCY

Once the pancreatic reserve is exhausted, symptoms of maldigestion occur, often with weight loss. Ingestion of pancreatic enzymes with meals should correct the deficiency, but therapy frequently is only partially effective. Preparations with adequate potency should be selected. Pancreatic enzymes, particularly lipase, are rapidly denatured by gastric acid and pepsin. If pancreatic bicarbonate output

is reduced, low intestinal pH will reduce enzyme activity. Microencapsulated, pH-resistant enzyme preparations have been developed to provide protection from the acidic environment of the stomach. Dissolution of the protective coating occurs only when microspheres are exposed to a pH above 5.5 to 6.0. In some instances, therapy may be improved by inhibiting acid secretion, thereby creating a higher duodenal pH. Daily requirements of enzymes vary considerably from patient to patient and probably depend on the amount of food that is ingested, the intestinal milieu, and, in addition, the severity of pancreatic deficiency. Despite pancreatic enzyme supplementation, some patients have persistent fat malabsorption, requiring that fat-soluble vitamins be supplemented. Enteric-coated preparations given in excessive quantities to children with cystic fibrosis have been implicated as a cause of colonic fibrosis and stricture formation.

17.24.3   Acute Pancreatitis

Acute pancreatitis probably is more common in childhood than was previously believed. Following mechanical, biochemical, or inflammatory damage, an autodigestive process is induced because of activation of the pancreatic zymogens to active enzymes within pancreatic acinar cells. Active enzymes are released locally and into the circulation, causing a number of complications. In severe attacks, circulatory shock as well as renal and pulmonary failure may prove to be fatal. Acute pancreatitis may occur in a single episode or recur. In milder forms, there is considerable interstitial edema, but in severe cases, there are extensive peri- and intrapancreatic fat necrosis, parenchymal necrosis, and hemorrhage.

CLINICAL MANIFESTATIONS

Acute pancreatitis is a difficult diagnosis to establish; a high index of clinical suspicion must be maintained. A wide spectrum of clinical manifestations occur, many of which simulate other causes of an acute abdomen. Severe pain, often with nausea and vomiting, is an outstanding symptom. Abdominal findings are consistent with paralytic ileus. Tenderness, with guarding or rebound, often is localized to the epigastrium, and abdominal distension may be present. Ascites and fever are less frequent findings. Other nonspecific physical findings include pleural effusion, respiratory distress, coma, renal failure, and circulatory collapse.

CAUSES OF ACUTE PANCREATITIS

Acute pancreatitis may occur in children of any age. Unlike adults, in whom gallstone disease and alcohol abuse frequently are implicated, contributing factors in children are multiple and diverse (Table 17-62). No cause is found in about one-quarter of cases; in approximately one-third, pancreatitis is a feature of a multisystem disease. Traumatic cases commonly are associated with blunt abdominal injury. Metabolic factors include lipid disorders, cystic fibrosis, hypercalcemia, and a variety of organic acidopathies. With the advent of ERCP, congenital and acquired anomalies of the pancreaticobiliary ducts are more frequently identified. A large list of drugs or toxins are suspected or proven causes of acute pancreatitis.

DIAGNOSIS AND MANAGEMENT

No diagnostic gold standard currently exists. Although clinicians frequently use an elevated total serum amylase concentration as a sign of acute pancreatitis, it must be remembered that patients with normal amylase levels may have severe pancreatitis. Also, hyper-

TABLE 17-62

CAUSES OF ACUTE PANCREATITIS IN CHILDREN

PREDISPOSING FACTORS	FREQUENCY (%)	RISK OF RECURRENCE
Idiopathic	25	Common
Systemic disorders	35	Variable
Sepsis/shock		
Viral infection		
Reye syndrome		
Collagen vascular disorders		
Henoch-Schönlein purpura		
Trauma	15	Uncommon
Child abuse		
Blunt trauma		
Structural anomalies	10	Common
Pancreas divisum		
Common channel		
Stricture		
Sclerosing cholangitis		
Gallstone obstruction		
Metabolic	5	Common
Cystic fibrosis		
Hypercalcemia (TPN)		
Hyperlipidemia		
Organic acidemias		
Drugs	5	Uncommon
Familial	2	Common
Hereditary		
Sporadic		

TPN = total parenteral nutrition.

amylasemia may originate with the salivary gland, as may occur with mumps, calculi, or diabetic ketoacidosis. It also may result from other intestinal pathology or decreased amylase clearance in cases with renal insufficiency. More specific pancreatic enzyme assays, including pancreatic isoamylase, trypsinogen, or lipase, may help to confirm the diagnosis.

Imaging techniques are helpful adjunctive diagnostic tests. A plain-film radiograph of the abdomen helps to exclude other abdominal catastrophes, and a chest radiograph will identify secondary pulmonary complications. Ultrasonography directly visualizes the pancreas; increased pancreatic size, reduced density, or dilated ducts support a diagnosis of acute pancreatitis. Ultrasonography also will identify gallstones and choledochal cysts and is useful to identify and monitor pancreatic abscesses and pseudocysts. Computed tomography should be reserved for complex cases or those in whom ultrasonography yields equivocal results. ERCP is invaluable for identifying pancreaticobiliary ductal anomalies, but this invasive procedure should be limited to cases of recurrent acute pancreatitis of unknown cause. ERCP also is useful as well if surgical intervention is being contemplated, traumatic pancreatic duct laceration is suspected, or if there is associated evidence of bile duct dilation and cholestasis indicating likely obstruction by a gallstone.

There is considerable variation in the clinical course of acute pancreatitis. Some patients have a mild illness, with transient abdominal pain and few secondary complications. Others have a fulminant, rapidly progressive, and sometimes fatal course, requiring management in a critical-care setting. Patients should be observed for complications such as sepsis, shock, respiratory distress, abscess, and pseudocyst formation. Careful monitoring and management of intravascular volume, urinary output, electrolytes, acid-base balance, glucose, and calcium are essential. In cases with paralytic ileus, bowel decompression with nasogastric suction is helpful. Analgesia is achieved with narcotics, and histamine antagonists are used to reduce the acid stimulus to the pancreas. Clinical outcome depends very much on the cause of the pancreatitis and any secondary complications. Pancreatic pseudocysts frequently resolve spontaneously, but if they are infected or fail to resolve, surgical removal or drainage may be required.

17.24.4   Chronic Pancreatitis

Chronic pancreatitis is relatively rare in childhood. It usually is characterized by recurring or unremitting pain, but some patients experience no pain and may present clinically for the first time with symptoms of pancreatic failure and/or diabetes mellitus. Pathologic changes generally are irreversible and progressive, with focal or diffuse destruction of the pancreatic parenchyma, fibrotic replacement, ductal scarring, and plugging with or without calculi. Some patients with acute pancreatitis develop chronic disease as a result of residual pancreatic damage, whereas in others, the etiology of chronic pancreatitis is distinct.

HEREDITARY PANCREATITIS

Hereditary pancreatitis is the most common childhood form of chronic pancreatitis in developed countries. It is inherited in an autosomal-dominant fashion, with incomplete penetrance. The onset of pancreatitis occurs during the first two decades of life in 80% or patients, with a mean age at onset of 11 years. The diagnosis is subjective with a strong family history of chronic pancreatitis. In 1996, the molecular basis for this condition was elucidated. Mutations in the cationic trypsinogen gene cause premature trypsin autoactivation within acinar cells, which in turn causes pancreatitis through activation of other intracellular enzymes. Recurrent attacks of pancreatitis that are associated with severe abdominal pain recur at intervals of months to years. Usually, the pancreatitis is of mild to moderate severity, with severe pain resolving over 3 to 7 days, but severe hemorrhagic pancreatitis may occur. The frequency and severity of the episodes of pancreatitis decrease with age in many patients; however, some have recurrent severe pain requiring endoscopic or surgical intervention to palliate pain or relieve ductal obstruction. Pancreatic insufficiency may occur in up to 50% of patients, and diabetes mellitus in up to 25%. Pancreatic adenocarcinoma occurs with increased frequency in patients who have hereditary pancreatitis and in unaffected family members.

JUVENILE TROPICAL PANCREATITIS SYNDROME

Juvenile tropical pancreatitis syndrome is the most prevalent form of chronic pancreatitis in developing countries abutting the equator. It presents during late childhood or early adulthood, with abdominal pain and irreversible pancreatic insufficiency. Diabetes mellitus follows within 10 years. The pancreatic ducts are obstructed with inspissated secretions, which later calcify. Controversy exists regarding etiology; it has been linked with malnutrition and specific dietary deficiencies or dietary toxins. Cassava root, which is a primary source of carbohydrate in areas where tropical pancreatitis is endemic, contains cyanogenic glycosides, which cause pancreatitis in animal models. Differences in methods of food preparation, malnutrition, and genetic factors may account for the variable regional incidence of disease.

CLINICAL MANAGEMENT

Treatment of uncomplicated chronic pancreatitis usually is medical. Treatment should be conservative, with bowel rest and restriction of food and fluids by mouth when severe pain occurs. Recurring severe pain is a frequent manifestation that may result in decreased food intake, weight loss, and, in children, growth failure. Nonnarcotic analgesics should be attempted first, but if they fail, judicious use of narcotics should be contemplated. The risk of narcotic addiction is a major concern. Medical measures such as a low-fat diet and abstinence from alcohol frequently are recommended. Alternative but unproven approaches include inhibition of gastric acid secretion and feedback inhibition of pancreatic secretions by regular administration of oral pancreatic enzyme supplements.

Although surgical intervention frequently is contemplated in patients with unremitting pain, there has been little surgical experience with children. Because pain frequently remits spontaneously over a number of years, the decision to operate may be postponed, particularly when it is recognized that the outcome from surgery may not be beneficial. Prior knowledge of the pancreatic ductal anatomy by ERCP and/or computed tomography is helpful. Options include drainage procedures by ERCP or surgery, subtotal pancreatectomy, or pancreatoduodenectomy.

17.24.5   Pancreatic Tumors

Childhood tumors of the pancreas are uncommon. Pancreatic malignancy (largely carcinoma) may arise from duct, acinar, or islet cells. The most common, which carries the worst prognosis, is duct cell carcinoma. Pancreatoblastoma, which occurs only in infancy, has a more favorable prognosis. A variety of neoplasms affecting the pancreatic endocrine tissue have been described, including both benign and malignant tumors. The most common endocrine tumor is the insulinoma or islet cell hyperplasia. It may manifest at birth or any time thereafter, and it presents with symptoms of hypoglycemia, which usually is chronic, severe, and medically intractable. Medical therapy involves the provision of continuous intravenous glucose, frequent feeding to prevent hypoglycemia, and use of diazoxide to inhibit insulin secretion. Frequently, long-term medical therapy is not successful, and subtotal pancreatectomy is required. Up to 95% of the pancreatic mass may be resected without the development of pancreatic insufficiency.

References

Couper RTL: Pancreatic function tests. In: Walker WA, Durie PR, Hamilton JR, Walker-Smith JA, Watkins JB, eds: Pediatric Gastrointestinal Disease. Pathophysiology, Diagnosis, Management, 2nd ed. Philadelphia, CV Mosby, 1621–1634: 1996

Jones NL, Hofley PM, Durie PR: Pathophysiology of the pancreatic defect in Johanson Blizzard syndrome: a disorder of aciniar development. 125: 406–408; 1994

Mack DR, Forstner GG, Wilschanski M, Freedman MH, Durie PR: Shwachman syndrome: exocrine pancreatic dysfunction and variable phenotypic expression. Gastroenterology 111:1593–1602, 1996

Pitchumoni CS: Juvenile tropical pancreatitis. In: Walker WA, Durie PR, Hamilton JR, Walker-Smith JA, Watkins JB, eds: Pediatric Gastrointestinal Disease. Pathophysiology, Diagnosis, Management, 2nd ed. Philadelphia, CV Mosby, 1502–1510: 1996

Robertson MA, Durie PR: Pancreatitis. In: Walker WA, Durie PR, Hamilton JR, Walker-Smith JA, Watkins JB, eds: Pediatric Gastrointestinal Disease. Pathophysiology, Diagnosis, Management, 2nd ed. Philadelphia, CV Mosby, 1436–1466: 1996

Whitcomb DC, Gorry MC, Preston RA, et al: Hereditary pancreatitis is caused by a mutation in the cationic trypsinogen gene. Nature Genet 14:141–145, 1996

THE LIVER AND BILE DUCTS

Maureen M. Jonas, Associate Editor

18.1 MORPHOLOGY OF THE LIVER AND HEPATIC FUNCTION

Jonathan E. Teitelbaum

18.1.1 Structure of the Liver

EMBRYOLOGY OF THE HEPATOBILIARY SYSTEM

As early as the 18th day of gestation (2.5-mm stage), a thickening of the ventral floor of the distal foregut, corresponding to the future duodenum, heralds the appearance of the hepatic diverticulum. This diverticulum is formed from the proliferation of endodermal cells at the cranioventral junction of the yolk sac and foregut. Subsequently, the liver diverticulum penetrates the adjacent mesoderm and capillary plexus, known as the septum transversum. Cellular interactions between the endoderm and mesoderm result in rapid cell proliferation and the formation of hepatocytes, angioblasts, and sinusoids.

By the third and fourth weeks of gestation (3- to 4-mm stage), the growing diverticulum enlarges to form a double diverticulum and is seen as an epithelial plug projecting into the septum transversum. Division of this diverticulum into a solid cranial portion (hepatic parenchyma) and hollow caudal portion is evident by the 5-mm stage. The hepatic portion differentiates into proliferating cords of hepatocytes and intrahepatic bile ducts while the smaller cystic portion (pars cystica) forms the primordium of the gallbladder, common bile duct, and cystic duct.

The budding liver sequentially invades the viteline veins and then the umbilical (placental) veins. The vitelline veins run from the gut–yolk sac complex to the heart. As the liver invades the vitelline veins, the midsection of the veins becomes capillarized. The caudal ends persist as the primitive portal veins, and the cranial ends as the primitive hepatic veins.

The hepatocytes of the hepatic portion grow as thick epithelial sheets intermingling between branching channels of the vitelline veins within the septum transversum to form a system of connecting liver cell plates, and the capillaries become the hepatic sinusoids. The sinusoids, present by 5 weeks of gestation, act as templates for the three-dimensional growth of the hepatic cords. The liver cell plates are initially three to five cells thick; however, over time they gradually transform to one-cell-thick plates, a process that is not complete until 5 years of age. Intrahepatic bile ducts begin to form at 6 weeks of gestation within the hilum of the liver and gradually spread to the periphery until complete at 3 months.

The pars cystica is initially hollow, but epithelial proliferation obliterates the lumen early in its development. Therefore, both the primitive gallbladder and common bile duct consist of solid chords of epithelial cells directly beneath the developing liver in the 6- to 7-mm embryo. Recanalization of the common bile duct and hepatic duct occurs in the 7- to 8-mm and 10-mm embryo, respectively. At the 16-mm stage the proximal gallbladder and cystic duct are hollow. At the third month the gallbladder is fully hollow, and the intrahepatic and extrahepatic biliary structures are joined. Bile secretion into the duodenum starts by the fourth month.

In the third month the liver begins to store iron, and hematopoietic elements derived from the mesenchyme of the septum transversum localize to the extravascular component of the lobule. The liver thus becomes the major blood-forming organ of the embryo. This function is gradually transferred to the developing bone marrow so that by birth only an occasional focus of hematopoiesis remains in the liver.

MACROSCOPIC STRUCTURE

The adult liver weighs 1200 to 1500 g, representing 2% of the total adult body weight. In neonates and young infants the liver is proportionally even larger, accounting for 5% of the total body weight. The liver rests below the diaphragm, rising to the level of the nipple at the fifth intercostal space with its distal edge at or above the right costal margin. It is held in place by the falciform and triangular ligaments. During fetal life the falciform ligament conducts the umbilical vein from the umbilicus to the liver. After birth this vein atrophies to form the ligamentum teres. A thin, firm, and smooth capsule (Glissen capsule) covers the liver and is continuous with the porta hepatis where the portal vein, hepatic artery, and common bile duct enter the liver.

At the porta hepatis, the right and left hepatic ducts coalesce to form a common hepatic duct located to the right of the main hepatic artery, in front of the portal vein. The common hepatic duct is joined by the cystic duct, which drains the gallbladder at its right side to create the common bile duct. The common bile duct joins the pancreatic duct in 85 to 90% of the cases just proximil to the ampulla of Vater, which empties into the duodenum. A small percentage of cases have a longer common channel that has been associated with choledochal cysts, pancreatitis, and gallbladder carcinoma. In the remaining cases the pancreatic and common bile ducts have separate drainage into the duodenum. The ampulla of Vater is encased by the sphincter of Oddi, a complex of smooth muscle fibers that regulates the flow of bile into the intestine.

The liver has a dual blood supply. The portal vein, which is rich in nutrients as it drains the gastrointestinal tract and splenic vascular beds, carries approximately 75% of the blood to the liver. The hepatic artery, rich in highly oxygenated blood, usually arises from the second branch of the celiac artery, although this is variable. In 20% of cases the right hepatic artery arises from the superior mesenteric artery rather than branching off of the common hepatic artery. The hepatic veins that drain the liver into the suprahepatic inferior vena cava are formed by the union of the central veins.

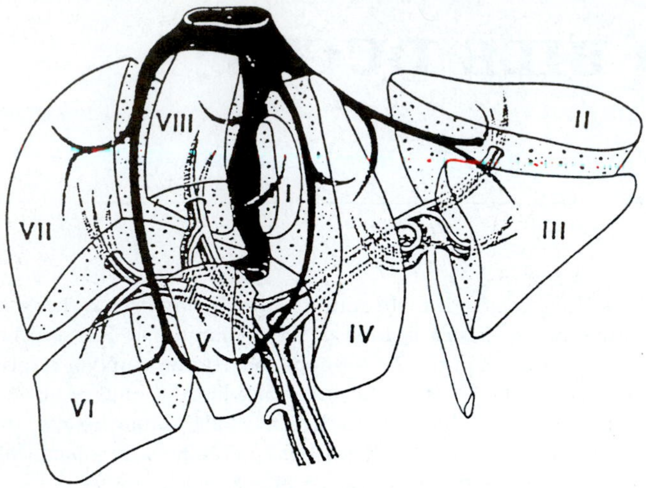

FIGURE 18-1 Functional division of the liver and the segments according to the Couinaud nomenclature. Note the separation of the left lateral lobes (II and III), which can be used for reduced-size hepatic allografts. SOURCE: Bismuth H: Surgical anatomy and anatomic surgery of the liver. World J Surg 6(1):6, 1982.

Early anatomists during the 14th century divided the liver on the basis of its lobularity. By the end of the 19th century standard divisions included right, left, quadrate, and caudate lobes. The Reidel lobe is a downward tongue-like projection of the right lobe. The left lobe is separated from the right by the attachment of the falciform ligament, the umbilical fissure, and the attachment of the ligamentum venosum. The caudate lobe is demarcated by the attachment of the lesser omentum and the porta hepatis anteriorly, the ligamentum venosum on the left and anteriorly, and the vena cava posteriorly. The right side of the caudate lobe tails out to attach to the right lobe and is called the caudate process. The quadrate lobe is defined as the bulge defined by four borders: the gallbladder and umbilical fissure, the liver edge anteriorly, and the left side of the hepatic hilum posteriorly.

Subsequently Cantie advocated dividing the liver by functional sections rather than by gross anatomy (Fig. 18-1). He injected ink into the vascular supply and identified a vascular watershed intersecting the gallbladder fossa and the vena cava fossa, dividing the liver into nearly equal halves (the right side representing 60% of the

liver volume). Each hemiliver is supplied by one portal vein, one artery, and one bile duct along the vascular watershed area. Couinaud further divided the liver into sections based on the internal anatomy of the hepatic artery and bile duct so that the left lobe contains sections 1 through 4 and the right lobe 5 through 8. This segmentation schema is clinically relevant in the context of pediatric liver transplantation, allowing transplantation of a left lateral reduced hepatic allograft. The final division of the liver into segments is based on further branching of the portal vein, hepatic artery, and bile duct.

MICROSCOPIC STRUCTURE

The microscopic anatomy of the liver had traditionally been defined as lobules with a portal tract (bile duct, branches of the hepatic artery and portal vein, along with nerves and lymphatics) and central vein. The edges of liver cells that encircle each portal tract form the limiting plate. However, in vivo microcirculatory studies revealed that the functional unit of the liver is the acinus (Fig. 18-2). This is based on the fact that the most oxygenated and nutrient-rich blood is in the portal and periportal areas, whereas the least oxygenated blood is centrilobular. Therefore, Rappaport suggested that the central vein be designated the terminal hepatic venule. He further renamed the portal area zone 1 and the hepatocytes around the terminal hepatic venule zone 3. The acinus is composed of hepatocytes arranged in plates of cells with bile canaliculi between them along with sinusoids on the vascular sides. Zone 1 cells form the most active core of the acinus and are the last to die and the first to regenerate. Zone 3 cells are the most prone to toxic, viral, or anoxic injury.

Hepatocytes represent 60% of the liver cell population and 80% of the cell volume. The organelle content within the hepatocyte varies with location in the acinar zone. Those in zone 1 are oval and oblong and have more mitochondria, whereas the zone 3 hepatocytes are round and have fewer mitochondria. Mitochondria account for 17% of the cell volume and are the most numerous of the organelles with about 2200 per hepatocyte. Peroxisomes are 1 to 2% of the hepatocyte volume and are vital in hydrogen peroxide metabolism. They are more numerous in zone 3 and play an important role in oxidation of fatty acids and detoxification. Lysosomes are electron-dense cytoplasmic organelles responsible for degrading biological material using acid hydrolases. The endoplasmic

FIGURE 18-2 Diagram of the liver acinar unit as described by Rappaport. Terminal extensions of a portal venule (TPV), hepatic arteriole (HA), terminal hepatic venules (THV), and bile ductule (BD) are labeled. SOURCE: Gumucio JJ, Miller DL: Liver cell heterogeneity. In: Arias I, Boyer J, Chisari F, Fausto N, Schachtner D, Shafritz D, et al, eds: The Liver: Biology and Pathobiology. New York, Raven Press, 1982:647–661.

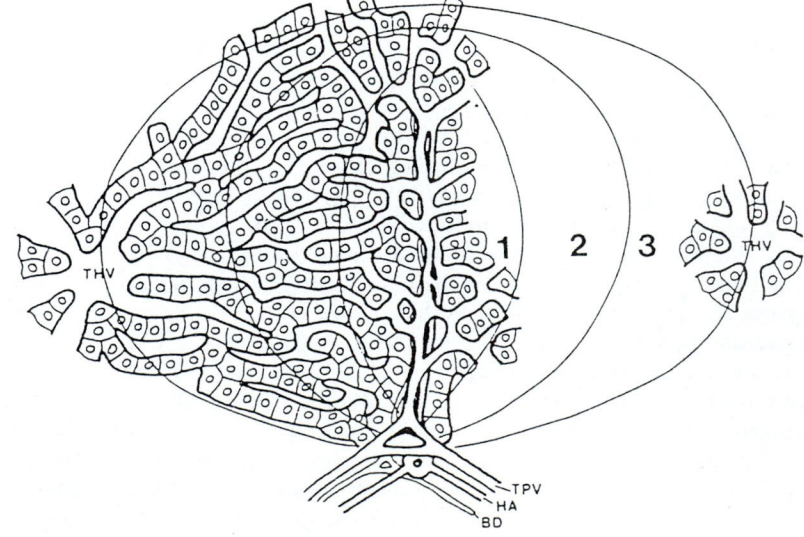

reticulum constitutes 19% of the cell volume and is the site of protein synthesis. The Golgi apparatus is responsible for processing of macromolecules.

There are four types of hepatic sinusoid lining cells whose functions include pinocytosis, phagocytosis, erythrophagocytosis, iron metabolism, clearance of immune complexes and antigens, and secretion of endogenous pyrogens, collagenase, lysosomal hydrolases, and erythropoietin. The arrangement of these sinusoid-lining cells has been clarified through the use of scanning electron microscopy and rapid freeze fixation. The endothelial cells form the wall of the sinusoid, separating the sinusoidal lumen from the subendothelial space of Disse. The sinusoidal endothelial cells lack a basement membrane and are perforated by abundant small fenestrae (average diameter 100 nm) in clusters called sieve plates, which act as blood-hepatocyte barriers. These fenestrae are denser in zone 3 than zone 1 and change in response to hormones, anoxia, and drugs. Microvilli of the hepatocytes protrude into the sinusoid through the fenestrae. The endothelial cells also express Fc receptors, suggesting a role in removing immune complexes. The space of Disse is located between the endothelial lining and the hepatocyte. As large blood cells move through the small sinusoids, they push the endothelium closer to the hepatocyte, thus promoting the circulation of plasma along the space of Disse. Lymph flow extends from the space of Disse to portal lymphatic vessels at the hilum of the liver.

Kupffer cells are hepatic macrophages most abundant in zone 1 within the sinusoidal wall, anchored to endothelial cells. These cells endocytose and destroy microorganisms, clear endotoxins and senescent erythrocytes, and can act as antigen-presenting cells. When activated they release IL-1, IL-6, TNF, TGF-β, LTB$_4$, and interferon. Stellate cells (formerly called Ito cells) are located in the space of Disse and are fat-storing cells. They store vitamin A, participate in retinoid metabolism, produce extracellular matrix proteins such as collagen I, III, IV, V, and VI, laminin, fibronectin, and proteoglycans and are thus responsible for hepatic fibrosis seen with chronic injury. Pit cells are large, granular lymphocytes attached to the sinusoidal wall that have natural killer activity. They are extrahepatic in origin and have a role in immune surveillance and hepatic antitumor defense.

Biliary drainage begins by secretion of fluid into the small biliary canaliculi formed by specialized membranes of adjacent hepatocytes. These small biliary canaliculi form channels continuous with the short duct of Hering that join the cholangioles at the limiting plate of the portal areas. These cholangioles then merge into larger bile ducts.

EVALUATION OF STRUCTURE

The macroscopic structure of the liver may be evaluated by several modalities (Table 18-1). Abdominal radiographs are of limited value for evaluation of the liver, with the only clinically relevant findings being the demonstration of calcified lesions (including some gallstones), air within the portal venous system (as seen with necrotizing enterocolitis), or air in the biliary system (as seen in gallstone ileus).

Ultrasonography uses sound waves to demonstrate changes in the echotexture of the liver. This allows for detection of cystic lesions, solid tumors, or infiltration of the hepatocytes with storage material. Biliary system abnormalities such as ductal dilatation are well visualized by ultrasonography. Choledochal cysts and gallstones are detected with an accuracy of 95 to 99%. The use of Doppler flow technology allows visualization of the vasculature associated with the liver (ie, hepatic vein, hepatic artery, portal vein) and its direction of flow.

Computed tomography (CT) enhances the spatial and density resolution of radiographic images. Images can be reconstructed along multiple planes with better ability to interpret data in three dimensions. The sensitivity is further enhanced with the use of intravenous contrast. Calcified lesions are seen with great clarity.

Magnetic resonance imaging (MRI) identifies tumors and tissue infiltrates comparably with CT, although it poorly visualizes calcium deposits. Magnetic resonance cholangiopancreatography (MRCP) is a result of recent advances in filtering of those signals within the liver that are slow moving (ie, bile) and has allowed for visualization of the bile ducts with clarity compatible to other forms of cholangiography, without the use of intravenous or intraductal contrast. Similar technology (MR angiogram) is available for the visualization of the vascular structures of the liver.

Endoscopic retrograde cholangiopancreatography (ERCP) or direct injection of contrast medium into the common bile duct through the ampulla of Vater provides excellent images of the intra- and extrahepatic biliary tree. This method also allows for endoscopic interventions including stone removal, stenting of ducts, biopsies, and papillotomy. Difficulties involve the technical expertise required in using a special side-viewing endoscope as well as the risk of pancreatitis.

Percutaneous transhepatic cholangiography (PTC) is accomplished by placing a needle into the hepatic parenchyma and injecting radiopaque contrast medium into the ductal system. This technique is often difficult in smaller children because of the small caliber of the intrahepatic ducts.

Radionuclide imaging using cholephilic radiotracers detects diffuse parenchymal abnormalities and hepatobiliary excretory dysfunction. N-Substituted iminodiacetates (IDAs) labeled with technetium-99 are used in the evaluation of infants with cholestatic liver disease based on their ability to demonstrate bile flow. Other studies can look specifically at gallbladder function and calculate the fractional percentage of bile that is ejected from the gallbladder after a fatty meal.

Liver biopsy evaluates microscopic hepatic structure and can be used to diagnose disorders, assess prognosis, determine response to therapeutic interventions, and monitor effects of hepatotoxic drugs. Analysis of the biopsy specimen can include histology, metal content, biochemical or enzyme assay, culture for viral, bacterial, or fungal pathogens, and electron microscopy. Based on the clinical setting this tissue can be obtained by different techniques.

Percutaneous liver biopsy offers a safe and relatively noninvasive means of tissue sampling. The biopsy can be performed by either an anterior, subdiaphragmatic, or right lateral approach, the last being the most commonly used. The biopsy site is typically just anterior to the right midaxillary line at about the 10th intercostal space. A single biopsy core is 2 to 3 cm in length, 1 mm in width, and weighs approximately 1 to 2 mg. Obtaining as many as three consecutive samples does not appear to increase the risk of complications. Relative contraindications to using this technique include significant coagulopathy, ascites, focal lesions (abscess, cyst, vascular lesions), and infection, infiltrate, or effusion involving the right lung. Risks of the procedure include bleeding, pneumothorax, intestinal perforation, hemobilia, and infection. Mortality is estimated at 0.009 to 0.12%. The use of ultrasound-guided biopsy allows for more specific targeting and thus an ability to sample a specific lesion and avoid vascular structures.

Transjugular liver biopsy is most commonly used when there is significant ascites or coagulopathy. It is typically performed by

TABLE 18-1

RADIOLOGIC EVALUATION OF THE LIVER AND BILIARY TRACT

PROCEDURE	COST	RADIATION EXPOSURE (RADS)[a]	PARENCHYMA	BILIARY TREE	VASCULATURE	ADVANTAGES	DISADVANTAGES
Plain films (abdomen)	+	0.03	+	+		Simple	Limited information
Ultrasound	++	None	++	+++	+++	Easy to perform, visualization of related structures (spleen, kidneys)	Relatively low specificity, operator dependent
CT	++	2.1	+++	+++	+++	Excellent sensitivity and specificity, ease of performance, permits use of contrast material	
MRI	+++	None	+++		+++	Outstanding image resolution, multiplanar views (axial, coronal, sagittal), reduced contrast media requirement; excellent for vascular anatomy	Patient immobilization and compliance limit usefulness in young children; ineffective in patients with "hardware"; insensitive to calcium deposits
MRCP	+++	None		+++		As per MRI, excellent for ductular anatomy	As per MRI
Radionuclide imaging	++	0.05 mCi/kg	++	+	+	Dynamic visualization of bile flow and gallbladder ejection	Low specificity
PTC	++	1.1[b]		+++		Excellent images; low complication rate	Ineffective in infants with biliary atresia or bile duct paucity
ERCP	+++	1.1[b]		+++		Excellent images, ability to place stents, remove stones, and biopsy	High degree of expertise needed

[a] Based on exposure to a 6- to 10-year-old.

[b] Based on 1 minute of pulsed fluoroscopy (0.9 R/min) and four spot digital films (0.05 R each).

CT = computerized tomography; MRI = magnetic resonance imaging; MRCP = magnetic resonance cholangiopancreatography; PTC = percutaneous transhepatic cholangiography; ERCP = endoscopic retrograde cholangiopancreatography.

interventional radiologists with fluoroscopic guidance. Although the amount of tissue that can be obtained is usually smaller than that obtained with a surgical or percutaneous approach, a large study in adults found that 92% of attempts were successful, and 96% of samples were of adequate size. Complications such as bleeding and arrhythmias occurred in 1.3% with an overall mortality of 0.22%.

Surgical liver biopsy obtains liver tissue via laparotomy or laparoscopy and is utilized most often in those instances when the percutaneous technique is contraindicated. The surgical methods allow for better hemostasis when the patient has a coagulopathy. This approach also allows for sampling of a larger piece of tissue or a sample from a site that is inaccessible percutaneously.

18.1.2 Normal Hepatobiliary Function

ENERGY METABOLISM

The supply of nutrients changes drastically during the transition from fetal to postnatal life. Whereas the fetus is supplied with a continuous flow of high-carbohydrate, low-fat, and high–amino acid nutrients via the placenta, the newborn is fed at intervals with a milk, high-fat, and lower-carbohydrate diet. At weaning the shift to an adult-type diet includes more carbohydrates and less fats. The liver plays a central role in these adaptations through gluconeogenesis and regulation of fat and protein metabolism. Throughout gestation the number of mitochondria and amounts of rough and smooth endoplasmic reticula increase. In addition, there is greater metabolic heterogeneity in the adult hepatocyte as compared with the fetal hepatocyte. The adult pattern develops shortly after birth as the liver's blood supply changes from one dominated by umbilical venous blood to one in which the hepatic artery plays an equally important role. This allows for the development of the functional zones within the liver, each with unique metabolic demands. Zone 1 (periportal) hepatocytes predominantly perform gluconeogenesis, β-oxidation, cholesterol biosynthesis, bile acid secretion, ureogenesis, and sulfation of drugs, whereas zone 3 (pericentral) cells perform glycolysis, lipogenesis, ketogenesis, glutamine synthesis, and glucuronidation of drugs.

CARBOHYDRATE METABOLISM

The liver plays an important role in the handling of dietary starches. This role changes as the child transitions from fetal to postnatal life and again on weaning. The first step in glucose metabolism is the phosphorylation of glucose to glucose-6-phosphate; in the fetal liver this is performed predominantly by hexokinase I, an enzyme without substrate specificity for glucose. Fetal glucose utilization approximately equals umbilical glucose uptake. Hepatic galactokinase, which phosphorylates galactose, rises rapidly in the liver near the end of gestation. Although little is known about hepatic glucose uptake in the neonate, data from the newborn lamb suggest that galactose is preferentially used by the liver for carbohydrate synthesis, whereas glucose is delivered to the peripheral tissues. At weaning two factors allow for the increase of hepatic glucose uptake. First is the presence of a high-capacity, low-affinity glucose transporter, GLUT2, that is insulin independent. The second is glucokinase, which replaces hexokinase as the predominant glucose phosphorylation enzyme within the hepatocyte, allowing for specific action on glucose and induction by insulin.

Throughout gestation the fetus actively stores some of the glucose as glycogen, so that at birth hepatic glycogen is about twice

the adult concentration at 40 to 60 mg/g of liver. The majority of this stored glycogen is utilized in the immediate postnatal period. Reaccumulation begins in the second week of postnatal life, and glycogen stores typically reach adult levels by the third week. The presumed role of this large store is to provide for the maintenance of blood glucose levels during the perinatal period, before other energy sources are available, and before the initiation of hepatic gluconeogenesis. Thus, glycogenolysis can maintain blood glucose concentrations in the normal range during fasting for as long as 10 to 12 hours.

Gluconeogenesis is the synthesis of glucose from lactate, amino acids, or other small molecules such as glycerol or proprionate. This does not appear to occur at significant rates within the fetus. Only liver and kidney have the capacity for gluconeogenesis. The rate-limiting enzyme involved in this process, phosphoenolpyruvate carboxykinase (PEPCK), rapidly rises after birth. PEPCK is a cytosolic enzyme primarily expressed in the periportal (zone 1) region. Glucose-6-phosphatase catalyzes the final step in glucose release from the liver. This enzyme, located within the microsomes, rises rapidly at term and is hormonally controlled.

PROTEIN SYNTHESIS

Protein synthesis is a major function of the liver, even in fetal life, because there is evidence that cells within the hepatic diverticulum produce albumin. The mature liver manufactures and exports most of the major plasma proteins, including albumin, lipoproteins, enzymes, coagulation proteins, and a variety of carrier proteins. Although the fetal liver is capable of synthesizing these proteins after the third month of gestation, their concentrations in fetal plasma are low. Lipoproteins increase in the first week after birth to levels maintained until puberty. Albumin reaches adult levels after several months, and there is a reciprocal decline in the primary fetal plasma protein, α-fetoprotein. Ceruloplasmin and complement factors increase to mature values during the first year. Transferrin levels are present in the low adult range at birth and slowly rise to normal adult levels thereafter.

CHOLESTEROL METABOLISM

The liver is the primary organ involved in regulating cholesterol metabolism. Newly formed cholesterol is synthesized in the endoplasmic reticulum from acetyl-coenzyme A (acetyl-CoA) through a sequence of enzymatic steps, with HMG-CoA reductase being the rate-limiting and most regulated reaction. In addition to endogenous cholesterol synthesis, the liver each day takes up several grams of cholesterol associated with all classes of lipoproteins. Chylomicron remnants, low-density lipoproteins (LDLs), and very low-density lipoproteins (VLDLs) are taken up by the LDL receptor and LDL receptor-related protein. High-density lipoproteins (HDLs) are taken up through a scavenger receptor, SR-BI. The storage form of cholesterol in the liver, cholesteryl ester, is produced by the enzymatic action of hepatic acyl-CoA cholesterol transferase on cholesterol. This substance serves as a pool for a constant supply of cholesterol through neutral hydrolase for bile acid and lipoprotein assembly in the endoplasmic reticulum.

FATTY ACID METABOLISM

Fat storage begins during fetal life, with the vast majority being in the form of triacylglycerols that contain mainly palmitic and oleic acids. The supply of fatty acids to the fetal liver is regulated by placental carnitine. Synthesis of fatty acids by the fetal liver occurs despite low levels of acetyl-CoA carboxylase, the rate-limiting step in fatty acid synthesis in the adult liver. The triacylglycerol that accumulated during fetal life is mobilized for local utilization after birth. The breakdown and oxidation of the fat by lysosomal acid lipase provides local ATP and ketone bodies for use by peripheral tissues. This intrahepatic oxidation is regulated by the availability of dietary fatty acids, enzymatic activity within the hepatocyte, and hormonal regulation. Hepatic fatty acid oxidation also plays a role in activating hepatic gluconeogenesis as long and medium chain fatty acids increase the supply of gluconeogenic precursors.

BILE ACID METABOLISM

Cholic and chenodeoxycholic acids are the two primary bile acids of humans and are synthesized from cholesterol. Studies of fetal bile reveal that bile acids are produced as early as the 10th week of gestation, with chenodeoxycholic acid being predominant. The first reaction in bile acid synthesis is catalyzed by a liver-specific microsomal cholesterol 7α-hydroxylase. This enzyme is regulated in part by negative feedback of bile acids returning by way of the portal vein during their enterohepatic recycling. However, different bile acids vary in the strength of this negative feedback, so that whereas primary bile acids successfully down-regulate synthesis, those with a 7β-hydroxy group such as ursodeoxycholic acid do not. Factors that influence cholesterol 7α-hydroxylase activity cause concomitant changes in HMG-CoA reductase, the rate-limiting enzyme for cholesterol synthesis. This allows for maintenance of a constant cholesterol pool size. After the synthesis of 7α-hydroxycholesterol, modifications to the steroid nucleus result in oxidoreduction and hydroxylation. The final step is the conjugation of cholic and chenodeoxycholic acids to the amino acids glycine and taurine within peroxisomes. Although in adults glycine is the most common conjugate, in early life more than 80% of the bile acids are taurine-conjugated because of an abundance of hepatic taurine stores. Other naturally occurring conjugates include sulfates, glucuronidide ethers and esters, glucosides, N-acetylglucosaminides, and conjugates of some drugs. These account for a relatively large amount of urine bile acids because conjugation increases the polarity of the normally hydrophobic molecules, facilitating renal excretion.

The final products, referred to as primary bile acids, are secreted in canalicular bile and stored in gallbladder bile. The gallbladder concentrates the bile and releases it into the duodenum during meals. This raises the intraluminal concentration of bile salts above the critical micellar concentration, allowing formation of micelles (macromolecular aggregates with phospholipids and cholesterol). Micelles promote solubilization of nonpolar dietary constituents and assist in the delivery of lipids to the intestinal absorptive surface. Bile acids are efficiently absorbed in the distal ileum by a carrier-mediated transport mechanism, returning to the liver by the portal vein. The total bile acid pool circulates approximately twice with each meal. Bacterial enzymes metabolize primary bile acids to secondary bile acids with different physicochemical characteristics. 7α-dehydroxylation of cholic and chenodeoxycholic acids results in the formation of the secondary bile acids deoxycholic and lithocholic acids, which are relatively insoluble and thus poorly absorbed. They make up the largest proportion of fecal bile acids. The large portion (95%) that is reabsorbed results in feedback inhibition of new bile acid synthesis.

In infants the total bile acid pool size is a fraction of that of the adult: at 32 weeks of gestation the fetus has a relative pool size one-sixth that of an adult. In a premature infant, the intraluminal bile acid concentrations may fall below the critical micellar concentration (1 to 2 mmol/L). In addition, there is less effective intestinal reabsorption of bile acids, inadequate hepatic canalicular secretion of bile acids, and inefficient hepatic uptake of bile acids from the systemic circulation. The cumulative effects of the immature bile acid metabolism and homeostasis system in newborns result in relatively inefficient absorption of dietary fats and fat-soluble vitamins and a tendency toward cholestasis.

DRUG AND TOXIN METABOLISM

Hepatic drug metabolism, or biotransformation, is divided into two broad aspects: activation (phase I) and detoxification (phase II). Different families of enzymes are important in each, and the balance between these two processes plays an important role in hepatic toxicity. The hemoprotein cytochromes of the P-450 system are associated with most phase I reactions and are particularly important in the liver, although they are found in most body tissues. These cytochromes can be detected in embryonic and fetal tissues at low levels. They catalyze diverse reactions including hydroxylation, dealkalinization, and dehalogenation. All reactions involve monooxygenation, in which one oxygen atom is inserted into the substrate. The P-450 system has overlapping substrate specificity. Twenty-eight distinct families of cytochromes of P-450 have been identified, with those in the 1A, 2C, 2D, 2E, and 3A subfamilies being particularly important in drug-xenobiotic metabolism and toxicity in humans.

Phase II detoxifying reactions are performed by different enzymes including glutathione S-transferases, glucuronosyl transferases, epoxide hydrolase, sulfotransferases, and N-acetyltransferases. These catalyze reactions to complete the transformation of hydrophobic compounds to hydrophilic ones that can be excreted into the urine or bile. Some of these enzymes are inducible, and some are polymorphic. Examples of polymorphic forms includes arylamine N-acetyltransferase 2 (NAT-2), which allows for individuals to be rapid or slow acetylators. This accounts for differences in ability to metabolize certain drugs (ie, sulfasalazine, trimethoprim-sulfamethoxazole, isoniazid). This trait has been shown to be inherited among certain ethnic groups.

EXCRETION

Hepatocytes are responsible for the excretion of numerous substances via bile, including bilirubin, drug metabolites, and heavy metals such as zinc and copper. Bile secretion starts at the beginning of the fourth month of gestation, and the presence of bile in the lumen of the intestine is responsible for the dark green color of meconium. Bile formation at the canalicular level occurs as a result of active transport of solutes followed by passive movement of water. Bile is functionally an isosmotic solution because organic constituents such as bile acids are either in mixed lipid micelles or self-aggregates and thus have less osmotic activity. Bile ductules and ducts significantly alter the volume and composition of fluid produced at the canalicular level by reabsorption and secretion of water and electrolytes. Secretin and vasoactive intestinal polypeptide (VIP) produce a bicarbonate-rich choleresis at the ductular level. In contrast, somatostatin inhibits bile flow. Bile can also be altered within the gallbladder, where it can be concentrated up to 10-fold.

Bilirubin is formed from the degradation of heme products, most notably hemoglobin, cytochromes, catalases, tryptophan pyrrolase, and muscle myoglobin. One gram of hemoglobin yields 35 mg of bilirubin. Bilirubin is formed through the cleaving of the tetrapyrrole ring of protoheme (protoporphyrin IX). Microsomal heme oxygenase reduces the iron from Fe^{3+} to Fe^{2+} and hydroxylates the α-methine carbon. The cleaved α carbon is excreted as carbon monoxide. The remaining linear tetrapyrrole is biliverdin IXα. The C-10 carbon is then reduced to form bilirubin IXα by biliverdin reductase. In healthy term infants, bilirubin is formed at a rate of 6 to 8 mg/kg/d compared to 3 to 4 mg/kg/d in healthy adults. This difference results from the increased red blood cell mass and shorter red blood cell life span in infants.

Bilirubin is poorly soluble in aqueous solvents because of extensive internal hydrogen bonding and subsequent folding, yielding a nonpolar, lipophilic molecule. The carbon-carbon double bonds at positions 4–5 and 15–16 allow for *cis* (designated Z for the German *zusammen,* meaning together) and *trans* (designated E from the German for *entgegen,* meaning opposite) forms. The naturally occurring form of bilirubin is 4Z,15Z-bilirubin IXα. The hydrophobic nature requires a carrier molecule, albumin, for transport from production in the reticuloendothelial system to excretion by the liver. The binding affinity between these two molecules is so high that at normal bilirubin levels all serum bilirubin is bound to albumin. Bilirubin is taken up by hepatocytes from the sinusoids by a plasma membrane–bound carrier called bilitranslocase. Once within the aqueous environment of the hepatocyte, bilirubin is bound to an intracellular carrier glutathione S-transferase (GST), also called ligandin or the Y protein. Bilirubin is then conjugated with glucuronic acid within the endoplasmic reticulum of the hepatocyte by bilirubin glucuronyl transferase (UDP-GT) to form both mono- and diglucuronides. Narcotics, anticonvulsants, contraceptive steroids, and bilirubin itself can increase UDP-GT activity. Alternatively, its activity may be inhibited by caloric and protein restriction.

Once conjugated, bilirubin is excreted into the bile predominantly as bilirubin diglucuronide. Infants have lower levels of UDP-GT and thus have fewer diglucuronides than adults. The rate-limiting step in bilirubin clearance is its hepatic secretion. Secretion can be enhanced by choleretic agents such as phenobarbital and inhibited by cholestatic agents such as estrogens and anabolic steroids. In pathologic conditions, bilirubin may reflux back into the circulation, causing clinical jaundice. When bilirubin conjugates enter the intestinal lumen, normal bacterial flora can hydrogenate the carbon double bonds to produce urobilinogens. Neonates lack the bacteria *Clostridium ramosum* and *Escherichia coli* and are thus more likely to absorb bilirubin from the intestine. Reduction-oxidation reactions also occur to form urobilinoids, which are not reabsorbed by the enterohepatic circulation and are thus excreted in the feces. Bilirubin can also be unconjugated by bacterial or tissue β-glucuronidase and readily absorbed from the intestine.

EVALUATION OF LIVER FUNCTION

Although commonly referred to as "liver function tests," the majority of serum tests measure the enzymes that are produced within the hepatocytes or biliary system but are not measures of physiologic function (Table 18-2). The serum levels of these enzymes are nonspecific and can be increased in numerous different pathologic processes. As described below, other common laboratory tests are more useful for the evaluation of "liver function," including measures of serum albumin, ammonia, bile acids, and coagulation studies.

Alanine aminotransferase (ALT, SGPT) **and aspartate aminotransferase** (AST, SGOT) catalyze the reversible transfer of the α-amino group of the amino acids alanine and aspartic acid to the α-keto group of α-ketoglutaric acid. This results in the formation of pyruvic acid (in the case of ALT) and oxaloacetic acid (in the case of AST) plus glutamate. Both enzymes are located within the cytosol of the hepatocytes and other tissues, and AST is also located within mitochondria. Tissue damage from trauma, ischemia, drug injury, or other mechanisms results in an increase in the serum levels of these enzymes. The degree of elevation of these enzymes often

TABLE 18-2

LABORATORY TESTS COMMONLY USED TO EVALUATE LIVER DISEASE

TEST	SOURCE	PATHOBIOLOGY	CLINICAL SIGNIFICANCE
Alanine aminotransferase (ALT, SGPT)	Liver (cytosol), minimal amounts in skeletal muscle, kidney, brain, lung, heart, and erythrocytes	Increased with necrotic or damaged hepatocytes, half-life is 18 hours	AST/ALT >2 suggests alcoholic hepatitis; level of elevation of little prognostic value
Aspartate aminotransferase (AST, SGOT)	Liver (mitochondria and cytosol), skeletal muscle, kidney, brain, lung, heart, erythrocytes	Increased with necrotic or damaged hepatocytes, less sensitive and specific indicator of hepatocellular injury than ALT, half-life is 48 hours	AST/ALT >2 suggests alcoholic hepatitis; level of elevation of little prognostic value
Alkaline phosphates (AP)	Liver (external surface of bile canalicular membrane), bone, intestine, placenta	Increased with bile duct obstruction, total ALP varies with sex and age, half-life is 7 days	Increased in cholestatic disorders; source of elevation can be determined by isoenzymes
γ-Glutamyl transpeptidase (GGT)	Liver (cellular membranes of canalicular cells); minimal amount in kidney, spleen, pancreas, heart, and brain	Can be induced by drugs (phenytoin, alcohol)	More sensitive marker for cholestasis than ALP, higher levels in premature infants
Bilirubin	Breakdown of heme	Level is influenced by formation, transport, uptake, conjugation, excretion, and enterohepatic circulation	Differential diagnosis different for conjugated versus unconjugated bilirubin
Albumin	Liver synthesis	Circulating protein, serum levels decrease with "leaks" and dilution; half-life is 21 days	Low levels can be an important prognostic feature
Prothrombin time (PT)	Coagulation factors made in liver	Half-life of factors is short, vitamin K dependent	Unresponsiveness to vitamin K may reflect advanced liver disease

SOURCE: Nelson SP, Jonas M: Clinical features of liver disease. In: Walker-Smith JA, Hamilton JR, Walker WA, eds: Practical Pediatric Gastroenterology, 2nd ed. Hamilton, BC, Decker, 1996: 110.

does not correlate with severity of disease, nor does it provide insight into the specific cause of the liver damage. Low levels of ALT and AST can be caused by B_6 (pyridoxine) deficiency because pyridoxal phosphate is a coenzyme for ALT and AST. Uremia may also cause an artificially low AST level.

Alkaline phosphatases (APs) are a group of isoenzymes that hydrolyze organic phosphate esters at alkaline pH, generating inorganic phosphate and an organic radical. Abnormally high serum values of bone isoenzyme may also be seen with increased osteoclastic activity. The liver isoenzyme is typically elevated in cholestatic conditions or biliary tract injury. Within the liver, AP is derived from the hepatocyte canalicular membrane, and elevated serum values are thought to result from increased production rather than cell necrosis. Because zinc is a cofactor for this enzyme, zinc deficiency can result in a low AP level.

γ-Glutamyltransferase (GGT) is a microsomal enzyme found in the epithelium of the small bile ductules and hepatocytes. The enzyme catalyzes the transfer of γ-glutamyl groups from glutathione and other peptides to amino acids. GGT is found in other tissues but does not rise in association with bone disease or active bone growth. The highest levels of GGT are found with biliary obstruction, but this is not specific.

Bilirubin can be measured in serum in various forms. The unconjugated form is called α-bilirubin, the monoconjugated form is called β, and the diconjugated is termed γ. That fraction of bilirubin glucuronides covalently bound to albumin is called δ-bilirubin. Virtually all serum bilirubin in the normal individual is unconjugated. Elevated bilirubin levels reflect increased production, as in hemolysis, reduced hepatic uptake, as in parenchymal liver disease, decreased conjugation, as in Gilbert disease, or decreased biliary excretion, as in bile duct obstruction. Conjugated hyperbilirubinemia (greater than 2.0 mg/dL conjugated bilirubin, or conjugated bilirubin greater than 15% of the total bilirubin) indicates hepatobiliary disease and always requires investigation. Urobilinogen is formed from the degradation of conjugated bilirubin by bacteria in the intestine. Up to 20% is reabsorbed and undergoes enterohepatic circulation. With hepatic dysfunction, more urobilinogen appears in the urine, giving it an amber hue. In complete biliary obstruction, however, urobilinogen disappears from urine as less bilirubin enters the intestinal lumen.

Bile acid levels, typically measured in serum as cholylglycine, reflect a balance of input (absorption from the intestine) and removal (uptake by the hepatocyte) of bile acids from the enterohepatic circulation. An abnormally high serum level is a sensitive indicator of cholestasis, even in the absence of jaundice. A low level may indicate an inborn error in bile acid metabolism or transport. Serum bile acid levels are usually measured in the fasting state.

Blood coagulation studies are often altered in liver disease. The liver plays three roles in the coagulation process: the synthesis of coagulation factors except for factor VIII and von Willebrand factor, the production and breakdown of factors needed for fibrinolysis such as plasminogen and plasminogen activator, and the clearance of activated clotting factors. Clotting factors II, VII, IX, and X are made in the liver from vitamin K, a fat-soluble vitamin that can be deficient in cholestatic states. The *prothrombin time* (PT) evaluates the extrinsic pathway of coagulation and is prolonged when factor I, II, V, VII, or X is deficient. Because the plasma half-lives of several of the clotting factors are short (3 to 5 hours for factor VII), the prothrombin time rapidly reflects changes in hepatic synthetic function. Hepatic dysfunction is typically associated with an increased concentration of factor VIII, which is a

product of the vascular endothelium. Consumptive states such as disseminated intravascular coagulation can also cause prolonged PT, but in this instance the factor VIII concentration would be low.

Albumin is the principal serum protein and serves to maintain intravascular colloid osmotic pressure as well as to bind and carry many compounds in the serum. It is synthesized only in the rough endoplasmic reticulum of the hepatocyte, at a rate of 150 mg/kg body weight/d. Its half-life in the serum is approximately 20 days. Decreases in serum albumin can indicate chronic impairment in hepatic synthetic function. However, decreased levels may also be the result of increased renal or intestinal losses, poor nutrition, or increased volume of distribution, as in patients with ascites. Prealbumin has a shorter half-life, so that changes in prealbumin levels represent more acute changes in hepatic synthetic function.

Ammonia concentration in the plasma represents a balance between its production and clearance. Ammonia is produced primarily by the action of colonic bacterial urease on dietary proteins. It is cleared through hepatic transformation into urea via the urea cycle. Normal hepatic function allows for the removal of 80% of portal venous ammonia in a single pass. In chronic liver disease there is impaired removal as well as shunting of portal blood to the systemic circulation, allowing ammonia and other toxins to bypass the liver and reach the central nervous system. A rise in serum ammonia may portend the onset of hepatic encephalopathy, although the absolute concentration of ammonia does not correlate with onset or degree of encephalopathy. The sample for measurement of plasma ammonia should be collected from free-flowing blood, either via an arterial source or with venipuncture without a tourniquet. Fasting serum levels more accurately reflect ammonia clearance.

Clearance tests measure the metabolism of a variety of extrinsically administered, hepatically metabolized substances to assess hepatic function. These include monoethylglycinexylidide (MEGX), *para*-aminobenzoic acid (PABA), and galactose. The rates at which the liver extracts these substances from the circulation and metabolizes them provides an indication of liver function. These tests are generally utilized only in large centers to determine the viability of donor livers or to aid in predicting impending liver failure.

Radionuclide hepatobiliary excretion scans utilize intravenously injection of ^{99m}Tc-HIDA or its derivatives. Hepatocytes promptly extract the tracer from the blood pool and secrete it into the bile canaliculi, bile ducts, and ultimately the small intestine. This test is more uniformly available than the clearance tests noted above and also assesses the liver's ability to extract a material from the blood and then excrete it via the biliary tract. This test can be used to evaluate the patency of the extrahepatic biliary tree or the functional contraction and excretion capacity of the gallbladder. Thus, it is useful in the evaluation of cholestasis, bile duct obstruction, and cholecystitis.

Enzyme analysis of hepatic tissue obtained through biopsy allows quantification of various enzyme activities, such as UDP-GT in suspected Crigler-Najjar syndrome or glycogen-degradation enzymes in suspected glycogen storage diseases.

Reference

Gourley GR: Bilirubin metabolism and neonatal jaundice. In: Suchy FJ, ed: Liver Disease in Children, 1st ed. St Louis, Mosby Year Book, 1994, 105–125

Maller ES: Laboratory assessment of liver function and injury in children. In: Suchy FJ, ed: Liver Disease in Children, 1st ed. St Louis, Mosby Year Book, 1994, 269–282

Nelson SP, Jonas M: Clinical features of liver disease. In: Walker-Smith JA, Hamilton JR, Walker WA, eds: Practical Pediatric Gastroenterology, 2nd ed. Hamilton, BC, Decker, 1996, 107–118

Schreiber RA: Hepatobiliary system structure and function. In: Walker WA, Durie PR, Hamilton JR, Walker-Smith JA, Watkins JB, eds: Pediatric Gastrointestinal Disease: Pathophysiology, Diagnosis, Management, 2nd ed. Boston, Mosby, 1996, 127–142

18.2 APPROACH TO THE PATIENT WITH HEPATOBILIARY SYMPTOMS OR SIGNS

Robert Squires and Jonathan E. Teitelbaum

Symptoms and signs of hepatobiliary disease include hepatomegaly and jaundice. In more chronic end-stage liver disease, xanthomas, spider angioma, palmar erythema, and evidence of portal hypertension, such as a *caput medusae* (portosystemic shunting via the umbilicus) or hemorrhoids, may also be observed.

Laboratory findings of cholestasis (elevated bile acids) with or without jaundice, metabolic derangements including hyperammonemia and hypoglycemia, hypoalbuminemia, coagulation abnormalities, and abnormal aminotransferase values all may provide insight into the cause and severity of liver dysfunction. Occasionally, otherwise asymptomatic patients will present with gastrointestinal hemorrhage or anemia as a result of bleeding from varices.

The approach to evaluating these findings is discussed below. The management of complications of fulminant hepatic failure and end-stage chronic liver disease is discussed in Secs. 18.12 and 18.13, respectively.

HEPATOMEGALY

An increase in the size of the liver can be detected as the edge of the liver is palpated beneath the costal margin. The presence of a generous palpable liver edge does not always mean the organ is enlarged. Flattened diaphragms, as a consequence of pneumonia or bronchial air trapping, can push the liver downward. Also, a subdiaphragmatic abscess, choledochal cyst, peritoneal cyst, or renal or adrenal mass can be mistaken for an enlarged liver.

To accurately determine if the liver is larger than normal, the liver span should be measured. This is best done along the midclavicular line, with palpation of the lower margin and percussion of the upper margin. This maneuver eliminates erroneous assumptions of hepatic enlargements in those instances in which hyperinflation of the lung results in downward excursion of the subdiaphragmatic liver. Normal values based on age and sex are shown in Table 18-3. If hepatomegaly is suggested unexpectedly by a radiologic examination, the findings should be confirmed by careful abdominal examination before extensive testing is undertaken.

Hepatomegaly may be a transient finding during systemic viral illnesses such as infectious mononucleosis, but persistent hepatomegaly is an indication for further evaluation. A firm, enlarged liver may suggest a storage disease, infiltrative process, or neoplasia. Tenderness of an enlarged liver may indicate an inflammatory process. Cystic disease of the liver may also cause hepatomegaly.

TABLE 18-3

EXPECTED LIVER SPAN (CM) IN INFANTS AND CHILDREN

AGE (Y)	MALE	SEM	FEMALE	SEM
0.5	2.4	2.5	2.8	2.6
1	2.8	2.0	3.1	2.1
2	3.5	1.6	3.6	1.7
3	4.0	1.6	4.0	1.7
4	4.4	1.6	4.3	1.6
5	4.8	1.5	4.5	1.6
6	5.1	1.5	4.8	1.6
8	5.6	1.5	5.1	1.6
10	6.1	1.6	5.4	1.7
12	6.5	1.8	5.6	1.8
14	6.8	2.0	5.8	2.1
16	7.1	2.2	6.0	2.3
18	7.4	2.5	6.1	2.6
20	7.7	2.8	6.3	2.9

SOURCE: Lawson EE, Grand RJ, Neff RK, Cohen LF: Clinical estimation of liver span in infants and children. Am J Dis Child 132:474–476, 1978.

Evaluation of hepatomegaly usually includes laboratory measurements of liver functions and an imaging study, such as an ultrasound or abdominal CT. Imaging studies can detect abnormal echotexture suggestive of fat, fibrosis, or infiltration as well as space-occupying lesions such as masses, abscess, or cysts. Liver biopsy is often required for definitive diagnosis. Disorders that should be considered in the infant or child with hepatomegaly are listed in Table 18-4.

ABNORMAL LABORATORY TESTS OF "LIVER FUNCTION"

The term "liver function tests" traditionally includes a panel of five separate measurements, including aspartate aminotransferase (AST, SGOT), alanine aminotransferase (ALT, SGPT), γ-glutamyltranspeptidase (GGT), alkaline phosphatase (AP), and measures of conjugated and unconjugated bilirubin. The biology and significance of these tests are discussed in Sec. 18.1. The text below focuses on the appropriate diagostic evaluation for abnormalities in these laboratory measurements.

Serum aminotransferase values may be elevated without other evidence of liver disease. Because the liver is a large organ with a large amount of reserve function, patients often come to clinical attention with normal hepatic function but abnormalities of serum aminotransferases. There are many disease processes that can result in elevation of these levels (Table 18-5), and the differential diagnosis is often driven by considering the clinical history, exposures to drugs and blood products, physical examination, and pattern of abnormal liver enzymes.

Elevation of serum AST and ALT values is most commonly caused by hepatocellular injury from inflammation, toxin, or passive congestion. The degree of aminotransferase elevation does not correlate with the amount of liver damage and is often of little prognostic value. The highest aminotransferase elevations are found in acute viral hepatitis, acetaminophen or other drug hepatotoxicity, and cardiovascular shock. Injury or inflammation of cardiac or skeletal muscles also causes increased AST and ALT values. Spuriously high AST has been reported in association with a "macro-AST" in which the enzyme binds to an immunoglobulin, usually IgG, re-

TABLE 18-4

DISORDERS ASSOCIATED WITH HEPATOMEGALY

Inflammation
  Viral hepatitis
  Idiopathic neonatal hepatitis
  Bile acid enzyme defects
  Canalicular bile acid transport defects
  Hepatic abscess
  Toxin and drug reaction
  Cholangitis
Kupffer cell hyperplasia
  Sepsis
  Granulomatous hepatitis
  Vitamin A toxicity
Congestion
  Congestive heart failure
  Pericardial tamponade
  Budd-Chiari syndrome
Infiltration
  Erythroblastosis fetalis
  Metastatic tumor
  Langerhans cell histiocytosis
  Leukemia
  Lymphoma
Storage
  Glycogen storage diseases
  Mucopolysaccharidoses
  Gaucher disease
  Niemann-Pick disease
  α_1-Antitrypsin deficiency
  Amyloidosis
  Hepatic porphyria
Steatosis (fatty liver)
  Malnutrition (kwashiorkor)
  Hyperalimentation
  Cystic fibrosis
  Fatty acid oxidation defects
  Diabetes mellitus
  Galactosemia
  Wolman disease
  Reye syndrome
  Steatohepatitis
  Mitochondrial enzyme defects
Tumors
  Congenital hepatic fibrosis/polycystic liver disease
  Hereditary hemorrhagic telangiectasia
  Hepatoblastoma
  Hepatocellular carcinoma

SOURCE: Walker WA, Mathis RL: Hepatomegaly: an approach to differential diagnosis. Pediatr Clin North Am 22:929–942, 1975.

sulting in decreased clearance, with serum AST measuring in the range 60 to 1100 IU/L, but ALT is normal.

Persistent aminotransferase value abnormalities in children require diagnostic evaluation because some disorders require specific therapy and others have implications for future health of the patient or family members. If aminotransferase values are acutely elevated to high levels, evaluation of liver synthetic and metabolic functions needs to be performed by measuring serum ammonia, bilirubin, albumin, and coagulation profiles. If these are abnormal, the possibility of impending liver failure needs to be considered. A history of potential inciting agents, such as toxins including acetaminophen or first exposure to fructose in an infant, should be sought. Tests for possible viral infections including hepatitis A, B, and C and EBV

TABLE 18-5

CONDITIONS ASSOCIATED WITH ELEVATION IN AMINOTRANSFERASE (AST AND ALT VALUES)

Hepatocellular inflammation (hepatitis)
Drug- or toxin-associated hepatic injury
Hypoperfusion or hypoxia
Passive congestion
  Right-sided heart failure
  Budd-Chiari syndrome
  Constrictive pericarditis
Nonhepatic disorders
  Muscular dystrophy, myopathy
  Celiac disease
  Macroenzyme of AST

should be obtained. A rising serum bilirubin with normal or near normal ALT may be an ominous sign, reflecting near complete loss of hepatocellular mass, or may indicate pure cholestasis without hepatocellular injury.

γ-**Glutamyltranspeptidase** elevation is most commonly associated with injury to bile duct epithelial cells. Such injury may result from obstruction or inflammation, with common causes listed in Table 18-6. Although marked elevation of GGT suggests a significant bile duct injury or reduced bile flow, it can be paradoxically normal with certain bile acid enzyme or canalicular transport defects such as progressive familial intrahepatic cholestasis (PFIC) syndromes types 1 and 2 (see Sec. 18.4). Some medications, especially anticonvulsants, induce synthesis of GGT and cause increased serum concentrations. It is not necessary to discontinue these medications for GGT elevations if other evidence of drug-induced liver injury is absent. GGT is found in other tissues, including the kidney, spleen, pancreas, heart, and brain; injury to these tissues may affect the serum value. If GGT is the only enzyme elevated, it is unnecessary to pursue extensive evaluations.

Serum alkaline phosphatase activity is at least twice normal in adult patients with mechanical biliary obstruction, and four times

TABLE 18-6

CONDITIONS ASSOCIATED WITH ELEVATION OF γ-GLUTAMYLTRANSPEPTIDASE (GGT)

Bile duct obstruction
  Choledochal cyst
  Biliary atresia
  Choledocholithiasis
  Cystic fibrosis
  Alagille syndrome
  Nonsyndromic paucity of intrahepatic bile ducts
  Bile duct stricture
  Pancreatitis
Cholestasis related to hepatocellular injury
  α_1-Antitrypsin deficiency
  Neonatal/giant-cell hepatitis
  Viral hepatitis
Biliary inflammation
  Sclerosing cholangitis
  Pericholangitis (associated with inflammatory bowel disease)
  Liver transplant rejection
Medications
  Phenobarbital
  Phenytoin
  Others

TABLE 18-7

CAUSES OF DIRECT HYPERBILIRUBINEMIA IN THE INFANT

Well-appearing infant
  Biliary atresia
  Choledochal cyst
  α_1-Antitrypsin deficiency
  Hepatitis B
  Alagille syndrome
  Urinary tract infection
  Idiopathic neonatal hepatitis
  Dubin-Johnson syndrome
  Total parenteral nutrition
  Progressive familial intrahepatic cholestasis type 3 (not types 1 and 2)
  Bile acid synthesis and metabolism disorders
  Bile plug syndrome
  Cystic fibrosis
Ill-appearing infant
  Sepsis
  Urinary tract infection
  Intrauterine infection
  Neonatal hemochromatosis
  Metabolic disease
    Tyrosinemia
    Galactosemia
    Fructose intolerance
    Fatty acid oxidation disorders
    Mitochondrial enzyme defects
    Carbohydrate deficient glycoprotein syndrome
  Hypopituitarism
  Idiopathic neonatal hepatitis

---

normal in over 75%. In contrast, in children elevation of alkaline phosphatase is less helpful in the assessment of cholestasis, as it may be elevated for reasons unrelated to hepatic function such as bone injury or growth. Benign elevation of serum alkaline phosphatase is an important condition to consider when faced with unexpected elevation in the range of over 1000 IU/mL. The typical clinical setting is that of an infant or toddler with an apparent viral gastroenteritis in whom alkaline phosphatase is measured. These very high levels tend to resolve spontaneously over several weeks, although familial persistent elevation of alkaline phosphatase has been described. When assayed in these settings, the serum alkaline phosphatase is usually comprised primarily of the bone isoenzyme. Treatment for this condition is reassurance and avoidance of unneeded, expensive, and invasive tests. Isolated abnormalities in serum AP of the liver isoenzyme are occasionally encountered in infiltrative processes of the liver, ie, metastatic disease or granulomatous hepatitis, or as an early indicator of primary sclerosing cholangitis in a child with underlying inflammatory bowel disease. If alkaline phosphatase and GGT are elevated, an imaging study of the hepatobiliary system should be performed. Without elevations in bilirubin, it is unlikely that an ERCP would be indicated.

Jaundice refers to the yellowish discoloration of skin, sclera, and mucous membranes caused by an excess of bilirubin in the blood. Other body fluids, such as tears, saliva, and cerebrospinal fluid, may also be tinged with yellowish hues. Jaundice is clinically evident in infants with total bilirubin levels of 4 to 5 mg/dL (68-85 μmol/L); in older children, bilirubin levels above 2 mg/dL (34 μmol/L) are usually visually evident. It is important that high bilirubin levels be further differentiated as unconjugated (indirect)

bilirubin or conjugated (direct) bilirubin. Excess levels of unconjugated bilirubin are explained by two mechanisms, an increased bilirubin load to the hepatocyte that overloads the conjugation process (eg, hemolysis, transfusion) or decreased conjugation within the liver. High conjugated bilirubin levels are caused by poorly functioning hepatocytes, obstruction of the biliary tract, or intrahepatic cholestasis.

Jaundice in newborns is common, and the challenge is identification of the child who requires further evaluation. The approach to the evaluation of the infant with jaundice is discussed in detail in Sec. 2.17.6. If the infant has conjugated hyperbilirubinemia (>2 mg/dL or greater than 15% of total bilirubin), the cause of hepatobiliary disease needs to be elucidated. Physical examination will determine whether the infant is "sick" or "well" and if clinically important features such as a pathologic rash suggestive of a neonatal infection, hepatosplenomegaly, ascites, excessive bleeding or bruising, or an altered level of consciousness are present. Disorders that need to be considered as potential causes of cholestasis in infants and diagnostic approaches are listed in Tables 18-7 and 18-8. In the well-appearing infant, disorders such as biliary atresia, choledochal cysts, α_1-antitrypsin deficiency, hepatitis B, paucity of intrahepatic bile ducts (Alagille syndrome), urinary tract infection, neonatal hepatitis, and Dubin-Johnson syndrome all should be considered. In an ill-appearing infant, metabolic disorders including tyrosinemia, galactosemia, hereditary fructose intolerance, fatty acid oxidation disorders, mitochondrial disorders, glycogen storage disease I and IV, neonatal hemochromatosis, hypopituitarism, and systemic illnesses including urinary tract infection, sepsis, or intrauterine infection all need to be considered. All of these are discussed in the sections that follow throughout this chapter.

The perinatal history may provide important clues in the identification of infants at risk for liver disease. For example, both acute fatty liver of pregnancy and the maternal HELLP (hemolysis, elevated liver tests, and low platelets) syndrome have been shown to be associated with LCHAD (long-chain 3-hydroxyacyl-CoA dehydrogenase) deficiency, a fatty acid oxidation defect, in the infant.

TABLE 18-8

EVALUATION OF THE INFANT WITH DIRECT HYPERBILIRUBINEMIA

Clinical evaluation
  Family history
  Feeding history
  Physical examination
Assessment of stool color
Fractionation of serum bilirubin
Determination of serum bile acid levels and qualitative analysis of urinary bile acid profile
Index of hepatic synthetic function (prothrombin time and albumin)
Cultures (blood, urine, spinal fluid)
Hepatitis B surface antigen and other viral and syphilis (VDRL) titers in selected high-risk patients
Metabolic screen (urine-reducing substances, urine and serum amino acids, organic acids)
α_1-Antitrypsin phenotype
Thyroxine and thyroid-stimulating hormone
Ferritin
Sweat chloride
Ultrasonography
Hepatobiliary scintigraphy
Magnetic resonance imaging (to rule out hemosiderosis)
Liver biopsy

A history of previous siblings with neonatal liver failure should raise concerns about possible neonatal hemochromatosis.

In infants after the newborn period and in older children, jaundice is much more likely to signal significant liver problems such as congenital abnormalities of the biliary tract, infections, and inborn errors of metabolism. Thus, jaundice in the older child *always* requires further investigation, which should be guided by the clinical features. Foremost is the determination of whether the child is well or ill appearing. Diagnostic evaluation is more extensive and more urgent in the ill-appearing child, as detailed in Table 18-9. Ultrasound examination may identify extrinsic obstruction from disorders such as choledochal cyst or gallstone disease. Assurance that there is not a coagulopathy, hypoglycemia, or other evidence of a life-threatening metabolic disease or fulminant hepatic failure is essential in the ill-appearing child. In many cases, liver biopsy is required to elucidate the underlying cause of liver disease.

Metabolic abnormalities such as hypoglycemia and hyperammonemia may be the presenting symptom or sign in some liver disorders. Because of the important role the liver plays in metabolic homeostasis, liver disease may present with hypoglycemia secondary to impaired gluconeogenesis or depleted glycogen stores, and hyperammonemia from the impaired detoxification ability. The evaluation of the child with hypoglycemia is discussed in Secs. 9.1.5 and 24.9. The evaluation of the child with hyperammonemia is discussed in Sec. 9.3. The finding of either hypoglycemia or hyperammonemia in a child with known liver disease suggests end-stage disease or fulminant hepatic failure with management discussed in Section 18.12.

OTHER SYMPTOMS AND SIGNS

Pruritus can be a distressing manifestation of cholestasis. Severe itching is typically generalized with the palms and soles, extensor surfaces of the extremities, face, ears, and upper trunk most severely affected. Resultant excoriation can become superinfected or can scar, causing disfiguring. The pathogenesis is poorly understood, although it is now thought that intraepidermal sensory nerve endings are activated by a circulating compound. Although there is speculation that bile acids are causative, there is no clear relationship between skin or serum levels of bile acids and itching. More recent evidence suggests a central neurogenic origin involving the opioid receptor. This hypothesis is supported by the known association of pruritus and opioids as well as by the observation that naloxone infusion can relieve itching. Treatment is generally supportive unless infection occurs. Various pharmacologic agents may be useful, including rifampin and ursodeoxycholate. Biliary diversion procedures have been helpful in specific clinical settings such as in primary familial inherited cholestasis syndromes. Pruritus can be severe enough to be a primary indication for liver transplantation.

Xanthomas are the consequence of reflux of biliary phospholipids into the plasma, which results in an increased plasma cholesterol concentration in patients with chronic cholestasis. The cholesterol is transported in blood with lipoprotein X. Cholesterol levels as high as 2000 mg/dL have been measured in this setting, which leads to its deposition in skin, mucous membranes, and arteries. There is no generally accepted treatment regimen for lowering cholesterol in patients with cholestatic diseases.

CHRONIC HEPATITIS IN THE CHILD

If an elevation of aminotransaminase levels or of other liver function tests persists for more than 3 months in a child, an aggressive attempt to define the etiology of liver injury should ensue. In adults

TABLE 18-9

EVALUATION OF THE CHILD WITH DIRECT HYPERBILIRUBINEMIA

First tier: the well-appearing child
  General
    Complete blood count, platelet count
    Electrolytes, calcium, phosphorus
    BUN, creatinine
  Assessment of hepatobiliary injury
    AST, ALT, GGT
    Bilirubin, total and direct
  Assessment of hepatocellular function
    Total protein, albumin
    Prothrombin time
    Glucose
  Studies to establish a diagnosis
    α_1-Antitrypsin level and phenotype
    Sweat chloride
    Chest radiograph for features of Alagille syndrome
    Ultrasound to identify choledochal cyst, stones, other obstruction
    Infectious disease studies
      Hepatitis A, B, C serology
      EBV serology panel
      HIV antibody
    Drug/medication history
    Liver biopsy

First tier: the ill-appearing child (in addition to those above)
  Assessment of hepatocellular function
    Ammonia
    Factors V and VII
  Studies to establish a diagnosis
    Ceruloplasmin
    24-hour urine copper excretion

Second tier: to be considered if diagnosis is not established for the child who appears either sick or well
  Urine for succinylacetone (for tyrosinemia in young patients)
  Urine for amino and organic acids
  Cortisol
  Serum and urine for abnormal bile acids
  Autoimmune markers
    Antinuclear antibody
    Antimitochondrial antibody
    Anti–smooth muscle antibody
    Anti–liver-kidney microsomal antibody
  Very-long-chain fatty acids
  Lactate:pyruvate ratio
  Carnitine (total and free) and acylcarnitine
  Cholangiography (ERCP, percutaneous, or MR)

a period of 6 months may be allowed before initiation of an aggressive evaluation, but in children several of the diseases that cause chronic hepatitis respond to specific medical therapy, and irreversible changes may occur over a 6-month period if treatment is not initiated. Causes of chronic hepatitis are listed in Table 18-10.

Chronic hepatitis can be caused by persistent viral infections, metabolic disorders, prolonged exposure to hepatotoxic drugs, or other systemic disorders. Chronic hepatitis can be mimicked by primary sclerosing cholangitis, and patients with chronic hepatitis may present with clinical and biochemical findings indistinguishable from acute hepatitis or with ascites or gastrointestinal bleeding from varices.

In a child with possible chronic hepatitis, a complete evaluation includes clinical, biochemical, and histologic assessment (Table 18-11). A careful history is necessary to assess exposure to hepatitis

TABLE 18-10
CAUSES OF CHRONIC HEPATITIS IN CHILDREN

Viral
  HBV, HCV, HDV
Autoimmune
  Type 1 autoimmune hepatitis (ANA positive)
  Type 2 autoimmune hepatitis (anti-liver/kidney microsome positive)
Disorders of copper metabolism
  Wilson disease
  Indian childhood cirrhosis
Disorders of the biliary tree
  Primary sclerosing cholangitis
Drug-associated liver disease
Metabolic liver disease
  α_1-Antitrypsin deficiency
  Glycogen storage disease III
  Cystic fibrosis
Chronic liver disease associated with systemic illness
  Chronic heart failure
  Diabetes mellitus
  Collagen vascular disease
  Obesity
  Total parenteral nutrition associated liver disease

TABLE 18-11
EVALUATION OF THE CHILD WITH CHRONIC HEPATITIS

Clinical assessment
  Nutritional assessment with focus on fat stores, muscle mass, linear growth rate, evidence for obesity
  Circulatory function to exclude primary cardiac dysfunction, hepatic outflow obstruction
  Liver function to detect evidence of portal hypertension (ascites, splenomegaly, caput medusae), cholestasis (pruritus, jaundice, fat-soluble-vitamin deficiency)
  Pulmonary function to exclude evidence of cystic fibrosis
  Assess endocrine function to exclude thyroid disease, diabetes, or adrenal insufficiency, which may be associated with elevated transaminases or with autoimmune hepatitis
  Assess risk factors for exposure to HBV, HCV, HDV
Laboratory assessment
  Biochemical assessment of liver function
    Prothrombin, serum albumin to assess synthetic function
    Serum direct and total bilirubin concentration, alkaline phosphatase to assess hepatic excretory function and biliary integrity
    Serum transaminases to assess hepatocyte inflammation
  Diagnostic evaluation
    HBsAg, anti-HbC, anti-HCV, and if needed, HCV RNA and anti-HD
    Serum ceruloplasmin
    α_1-Antitrypsin phenotype
    Sweat chloride
    ANA, anti-smooth muscle antibodies
    Abdominal ultrasound to exclude anatomic abnormality of biliary tree
    Liver biopsy
    PTC or ERCP if indicated to exclude sclerosing cholangitis

PTC = percutaneous transhepatic cholangiogram; ERCP = endoscopic retrograde cholangiopancreatography.

viruses that cause chronic hepatitis (B, C, and δ). Hepatitis A and Epstein-Barr virus do not cause chronic hepatitis. A history of exposure to potentially hepatotoxic medications such as isoniazid, nitrofurantoin, sulfonamides, and others should be determined. Features or symptoms of autoimmune disease, inflammatory bowel disease, immunodeficiency, or systemic illness should be sought. Symptoms of heart disease, obesity, or endocrine or muscle disease should be elicited because chronic elevation of serum transminases can reflect liver manifestations of systemic disease. A slit-lamp ophthalmologic examination to detect Kayser-Fleischer rings, which are suggestive of Wilson disease, may be useful.

Laboratory evaluation should include the measurement of serum levels of total and conjugated bilirubin, serum aminotransferases, alkaline phosphatase, γ-globulin, and an assessment of liver synthetic capacity by measuring albumin and prothrombin time. Serology for hepatitis B and C should be performed. Serum ceruloplasmin concentration and α_1-antitrypsin phenotype should be determined to exclude Wilson disease and α_1-antitrypsin deficiency, respectively. A screen for autoantibodies directed against smooth muscle (ASMA), nuclear components (ANA), and liver-kidney microsomes (anti-LKM) should be performed to exclude autoimmune hepatitis. Histologic examination of liver tissue is often required to elucidate the cause of liver disease or to assist in managing the patient because therapy and prognosis are based on characterization of the histologic lesion rather than on clinical or biochemical data.

References

Bergasa NV, Jones EA: The pruritus of cholestasis: potential pathogenic and therapeutic implications of opioids. Gastroenterology 108:1582–1588, 1995

Steinherz PG, Steinherz LJ, Misselbaum JS, Murphy L: Transient, marked, unexplained elevation of serum alkaline phosphatase. JAMA 252:3289–3292, 1984

Walker WA, Mathis RL: Hepatomegaly: an approach to differential diagnosis. Pediatr Clin North Am 22:929–942, 1975

Younoszai MK, Mueller S: Clinical assessment of liver size in normal children. Clin Pediatr 14:378–380, 1975

18.3 CONGENITAL ABNORMALITIES OF HEPATOBILIARY STRUCTURE

Jonathan E. Teitelbaum

SITUS INVERSUS AND HETEROTAXIA

Situs inversus and heterotaxia result in left-sided or central, respectively, location of the liver. Either may occur with other anomalies such as in the polysplenia/asplenia syndromes. Despite the altered anatomy, there have been reports of successful liver transplantation both from and into people with these anomalies.

VASCULAR ANOMALIES

There are many variations to the branching patterns of the vascular supply of the liver. In general, variations in hepatic artery anatomy do not have clinical significance except when the patient requires hepatic surgery.

Congenital anomalies of the portal vein may have clinical significance and have been associated with cardiac and urinary tract abnormalities. The presence of multiple serpiginous collateral veins surrounding a small or thrombosed portal vein is referred to as *cavernous transformation of the portal vein*. This abnormality is accompanied by portal hypertension because portal resistance is markedly elevated. It was once thought that this represented a neoplastic, hemangiomatous change. However, it is now known to represent the body's effort to maintain hepatopetal portal flow to a normal liver in the face of occlusion of the extrahepatic portal vein. The causes of portal vein thrombosis include umbilical infection (omphalitis), perinatal catheterization of the umbilical vein, pancreatitis, surgical manipulation during splenectomy, and hypercoagulable states including deficiencies of protein C, protein S, or antithrombin III, the presence of anticardiolipin antibodies, or a factor V Leiden gene mutation. Patients typically come to medical attention within the first decade of life with splenomegaly or bleeding from esophageal varices. The diagnosis is confirmed by ultrasound of the extrahepatic portal area with Doppler interrogation. Ligation or sclerosis of esophageal varices, portosystemic shunts, and, more recently, a mesenterico–left portal bypass are palliative measures. The natural history is such that over time there is a decrease in the frequency and intensity of the hemorrhagic manifestations.

Congenital absence of the portal vein has also been described. Children with this anomaly may have elevated serum ammonia, bile acids, and galactose concentrations, as they typically have formed a natural portosystemic shunt that bypasses the detoxifying ability of the liver.

18.3.1   Biliary Tract Abnormalities

CHOLEDOCHAL CYSTS

The incidence of choledochal cysts has been estimated between one in 13,000 and one in 2,000,000 live births, and they are found in girls four times more frequently than in boys. Choledochal cysts are more prevalent in Asians, specifically the Japanese. The etiology of cyst formation is unclear, although there is growing evidence that the dilatation results from an anomalous junction of the common bile duct and the pancreatic duct, resulting in a common channel that is as long as 3.5 cm, versus a normal of 5 mm. This long common channel may allow for the reflux of pancreatic proteases into the extrahepatic biliary tree, resulting in cholangitis and ste-

nosis. This hypothesis is supported by the measurement of high levels of amylase within the cysts, but the documentation of prenatal choledochal cysts suggests alternative abnormalities in the process of morphogenesis.

Most patients present within the first decade of life, with the diagnosis made in 38% in the first year of life, 34% between ages 1 and 6 years, and 28% thereafter. The classic triad of abdominal pain, jaundice, and palpable right upper quadrant mass occurs in fewer than 20% of patients. Other common symptoms are fever, nausea, and vomiting, with or without associated pancreatitis. Children may have abnormal aminotransferase, bilirubin, and pancreatic enzyme values. Ultrasound is the most valuable screening test, as it can demonstrate both intrahepatic and extrahepatic dilatation of the biliary tree. Radionuclide scanning may demonstrate the accumulation of tracer within the cyst. Endoscopic retrograde cholangiopancreatography provides better delineation of the biliary anatomy. On occasion, impacted biliary calculi within the distal biliary tree are removed, resulting in resolution of the biliary dilatation. The location of the cyst allows classification into one of five anatomic types, as described by Todani (Fig. 18-3). The overwhelming majority of choledochal cysts are of type I, diffuse enlargement of the common bile duct.

A high incidence of biliary malignancy associated with choledochal cysts is well recognized, with a reported incidence in Japan of 2.5 to 17.5%. The majority of tumors are adenocarcinomas, detected at a mean age of 35 years. The cause of the malignant transformation is unclear but may relate to the chronic reflux of pancreatic proteases as well as the mutagenic potential of secondary bile acids in a stagnant environment. This has led to the recommendation that cysts be excised with concurrent removal of the gallbladder because of the risk of neoplasia. The approach to biliary reconstruction varies depending on the cyst type, anatomy, and surgical preference; the most common procedures are hepaticoduodenostomy, hepaticojejunostomy, or jejunal interposition.

GALLBLADDER ABNORMALITIES

A variety of structural abnormalities of the gallbladder have been described. Congenital absence of the gallbladder occurs in one of 7500 to 10,000 people. Failed development of the pars cystica is the likely etiology. As an isolated abnormality this is of little clinical significance, although rarely symptoms develop because calculi form in the ductal system. In addition to extrahepatic biliary atresia, which may accompany agenesis of the gallbladder, other associations include imperforate anus, genitourinary anomalies, anencephaly, bicuspid aortic valve, and cerebral aneurysms. Hypoplasia of the gallbladder has also been described. As many as one-third of

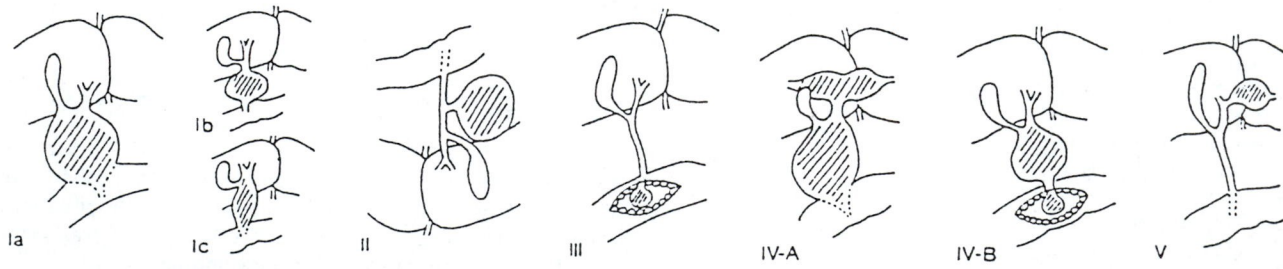

FIGURE 18-3   Types of choledochal cysts. SOURCE: Todani T, Watanabe Y, Narusue M, et al: Congenital bile duct cysts: classification, operative procedures and review of 37 cases including cancer arising from choledochal cyst. Am J Surg 134:226, 1977, with permission from Excerpta Medica, Inc.

individuals with cystic fibrosis have small, poorly functioning gallbladders. There is also an association with trisomy 18. The incidence of double gallbladder is 0.1 to 0.75 per 1000. The two cystic ducts may converge into a single duct, forming a Y-shaped structure. The accessory gallbladder may lie under the left lobe of the liver, draining into the left hepatic duct.

A "floating gallbladder" is an anatomic variant observed in up to 5% of individuals. The gallbladder lacks a peritoneal coat or supporting membrane, making the pendulous gallbladder susceptible to torsion. This presents clinically as acute, severe right upper quadrant pain with nausea and vomiting. Often the infarcted gallbladder is palpable.

EXTRAHEPATIC BILIARY ATRESIA

Extrahepatic biliary atresia is usually considered an acquired condition, as discussed in Sec. 18-9. However, there is an embryonic or fetal type of biliary atresia that comprises approximately 35% of cases and may be a true congenital biliary tract anomaly. Early onset of neonatal cholestasis and absence of bile duct remnants characterize this form. Furthermore, children with associated anomalies account for 10 to 20% of the cases. These anomalies are separated into three groups: 29% of cases have various combinations of anomalies that characterize the laterality sequence, such as polysplenia or asplenia, cardiovascular defects, abdominal organ heterotaxia, intestinal malrotation, and vascular aberrations of the portal vein and hepatic artery. A milder lateralization anomaly with intestinal malrotation is observed in 12% of cases. The remaining 59% have single or multiple anomalies of the cardiac, gastrointestinal, or urinary systems. There is speculation that this fetal form of biliary atresia has a different pathologic mechanism than the perinatal type, although this has not been proven. With increasing experience in pediatric liver transplantation and cardiac surgery, the ultimate survival rate of these patients does not appear to be significantly different than that of patients with the more common isolated form of biliary atresia.

DUCTAL PLATE MALFORMATIONS

At about the eighth week of gestation, the hepatic precursor cells that lie adjacent to the hilar portal vein vessels form a sleeve-like double layer of cells that extends toward the periphery along the smaller intrahepatic portal vein branches. This structure has been called the ductal plate. Beginning at 12 weeks of gestation and extending into the postnatal period, the ductal plate undergoes progressive remodeling. As they form, individual bile ductules are incorporated into the periportal mesenchyme that surrounds the portal vein branches. Thus, during successive periods of fetal life, ductal plate remodeling leads to the formation of the intrahepatic biliary tree. The largest ducts are formed first, followed by segmental, interlobular, and, finally, the smallest bile ductules. Arrest or derangement in remodeling leads to the persistence of primitive bile duct configurations termed ductal plate malformations. The occurrence of ductal plate malformations at different generations of the developing biliary tree gives rise to different clinicopathologic entities, such as congenital hepatic fibrosis and Caroli syndrome.

Congenital hepatic fibrosis (CHF) is the most common ductal plate malformation. It is usually associated with autosomal-recessive polycystic kidney disease (ARPKD) and occurs with an incidence of one in 6000 to 40,000 births. The hepatic lesions in ARPKD are fairly uniform and rarely give rise to macroscopically visible cysts. Microscopically the portal tracts appear enlarged by connective tissue and contain numerous somewhat dilated bile duct structures, corresponding to incompletely remodeled ductal plates. Portal tracts often lack normal interlobular ducts in the center. The abnormal dilated branching bile duct structures are in continuity with the rest of the biliary system. The renal lesion is characterized by radially arranged tubular collecting duct cysts occupying most of the large, externally smooth renal mass.

Neonates or infants who present with CHF-ARPKD usually have complications of the renal disease, whereas those who present later in childhood or in adulthood have a predominance of hepatic complications. In infants the kidneys may be enlarged and severely dysfunctional. They may be palpable on exam, and many infants will develop uremia and chronic renal failure. In these instances, hepatic fibrosis may be present but is rarely an important clinical factor. In older patients with CHF-ARPKD, the most significant abnormality is portal hypertension caused by the hepatic fibrosis and/or portal vein anomalies, such as duplication of intrahepatic branches. Hematemesis or melena is the presenting sign in 30 to 70% of patients. It may occur as early as 1 year but more typically at 5 to 13 years of age. Physical examination reveals a firm, enlarged liver, often with a prominent left lobe, and splenomegaly. In most patients the biochemical parameters of hepatic synthetic function are normal, and there is occasionally a mild elevation of aminotransferase values. There is a risk of cholangitis, which significantly contributes to morbidity and mortality.

Treatment may include portosystemic shunting for portal hypertension and aggressive antibiotic therapy for cholangitis. Alternative approaches such as variceal sclerotherapy or pharmacologic management of portal hypertension have not been well studied to date. In patients with chronic cholangitis and/or progressive hepatic dysfunction, liver transplantation may be the best treatment option.

Congenital hepatic fibrosis may also be associated with other liver malformations such as von Myenburg complexes (bile duct microhamartomas) as well as other renal lesions including autosomal-dominant polycystic kidney disease, renal dysplasia, and nephronophthisis. Presentation and management are similar to the later-onset CHF-ARPKD patients described above. Liver function tests may be unremarkable. Diagnosis is confirmed by liver biopsy, which demonstrates characteristic dysmorphic cystic structures lined with columnar biliary epithelium in the portal zones, surrounded by dense fibrous deposits. Smaller cysts are arranged along the interface between the dense plaques of connective tissue and the surrounding normally preserved parenchyma. In isolated congenital hepatic fibrosis, the prognosis is good, given the excellent preservation of parenchymal and renal function in most patients.

Caroli disease results from the congenital dilatation of the larger, segmental intrahepatic bile ducts. When this lesion is combined with the changes of congenital hepatic fibrosis, as is typically the case, the disorder is termed Caroli syndrome. Inheritance patterns are consistent with an autosomal-recessive disease. It may present at any age but is usually detected in adolescents or young adults. The clinical features reflect recurrent bouts of cholangitis and abscesses caused by bile stasis and gallstone formation within cysts, including fever, pruritus, jaundice, a tender liver, and modest elevations in serum bilirumin, alkaline phosphatase, and aminotransferase. Liver biopsy may reveal the changes of congenital hepatic fibrosis. Diagnosis is otherwise made by ultrasonography, computed tomography, percutaneous transhepatic cholangiography, or ERCP. Saccular and cystic dilation of the intrahepatic bile ducts and enlargement of the major intra- and extrahepatic biliary passages are evident. Treatment is with antibiotics to control cholangitis and partial hepatectomy for disease confined to a single lobe. These measures are only partially successful in most, and prognosis is further limited by sepsis, cholangiocarcinoma, and amyloidosis.

BILE DUCT PAUCITY SYNDROMES

Paucity of the intrahepatic bile ducts is a histologic finding defined as a ratio of interlobular ducts to portal tracts less than 0.9. Surgical biopsy is required to examine at least 20 portal tracts, the recommended sample number for definitive diagnosis. However, some authors suggest that visualization of as few as five portal tracts in a percutaneous biopsy may be sufficient in the appropriate clinical setting. Aside from syndromic paucity of the bile ducts, or Alagille syndrome, discussed below, paucity has been described in other circumstances. There is a rare nonsyndromic idiopathic paucity of the bile ducts in which patients typically present earlier in life than those with Alagille syndrome. Paucity of the bile ducts has been described in association with a wide variety of other conditions including Down syndrome, hypopituitarism, cystic fibrosis, α_1-antitrypsin deficiency, congenital infections such as cytomegalovirus, rubella, and syphilis, hepatitis B, graft-versus-host disease, chronic hepatic allograft rejection, primary sclerosing cholangitis, Zellweger syndrome, and Ivemark syndrome.

ALAGILLE SYNDROME

Eve Roberts

Alagille syndrome (arteriohepatic dysplasia, Watson-Miller syndrome, syndromic duct paucity) is a genetic disorder with autosomal-dominant transmission but highly variable expression. The incidence of Alagille syndrome is probably underestimated at one per 100,000 live births, since this is based only on those patients with disease severe enough to be readily recognized. Alagille syndrome appears to be caused by mutations in a single gene on 20p, *Jag 1*, which encodes protein ligands for NOTCH 1. This family of proteins plays a role in determining cell fate during differentiation, especially in tissues where epithelial-mesenchymal interactions are important. Inheritance is autosomal dominant, probably due to haploinsufficiency. Sporadic mutations are more common than familial occurrence. No predictable patterns of correlation between genotype and phenotype have yet been identified. In some cases Alagille syndrome may be associated with a macroscopic deletion of the short arm of chromosome 20 in some patients and with microdeletions of 20p in others.

Alagille syndrome was first described clinically as an association of congenital heart disease, usually peripheral pulmonary artery stenosis, with neonatal cholestasis. Its major clinical features include chronic cholestatic liver disease with decreased numbers of small (ie, portal, or "interlobular") intrahepatic bile ducts, structural heart disease, skeletal abnormalities including "butterfly" vertebrae and abnormal radius/ulna, posterior embryotoxon of the eye, and typical facies (see Table 18-12). Minor features include renal abnormalities, small birth size and/or poor growth, delayed puberty or hypogonadism, abnormal cry/voice ("high-pitched"), and mental retardation, learning difficulties, or antisocial behavior. Associated vascular abnormalities have been noted including decreased intrahepatic portal vein radicals, moyamoya disease, coarctation of the aorta, and anomalies of other large arterial vessels. Neurologic abnormalities described in early reports probably were not part of the syndrome itself but due instead to vitamin E deficiency from severe chronic cholestasis. Hypothyroidism and pancreatic insufficiency have also been observed in association with Alagille syndrome.

The majority of patients with clinically significant Alagille syndrome have conjugated hyperbilirubinemia in the neonatal period. Hepatobiliary scanning fails to show biliary excretion of the tracer chemical in approximately 50% of patients. Liver biopsy usually shows reduced numbers of small bile ducts with some giant-cell transformation and cholestasis. The number of portal tracts may also be reduced. In some infants, bile ductular proliferation suggesting large bile duct obstruction is found in the neonatal period, and bile duct paucity develops somewhat later. In these infants extrahepatic biliary atresia cannot be excluded simply by histologic findings. Alagille syndrome with a segmental atresia of the common hepatic duct (equivalent to type 2 biliary atresia) may occur.

TABLE 18-12

FEATURES OF ALAGILLE SYNDROME

FEATURE	EMERICK (1999) (%)	ALAGILLE (1987) (%)	DEPRETTERE (1987) (%)	WEIGHTED PERCENT OF ALL STUDIES
Bile duct paucity	85 (69/81)	100 (80/80)	81 (22/27)	91%
Chronic cholestasis	96 (88/92)	91 (73/80)	93 (25/27)	94%
Cardiac murmur	97 (90/92)	85 (68/80)	96 (26/27)	92%
Peripheral pulmonic stenosis	(49/73)	70 (66/80)		75%
Tetralogy of Fallot	(10/73)	9 (7/80)		11%
Butterfly vertebrae	51 (37/71)	87 (70/80)	33 (6/18)	67%
Characteristic facies[a]	96 (86/92)	95 (76/80)	70 (19/27)	91%
Posterior embryotoxon[b]	78 (65/83)	88 (55/62)	56 (9/16)	80%
Glomerular renal involvement	40 (28/69)	73 (17/23)		
Growth retardation	87 (27/31)	50	73 (16/23)	
Mental retardation (IQ<80)	2 (2/92)	16	0	
Developmental delay	16 (15/92)			
Pancreatic insufficiency	41 (7/17)			

[a] Facies consist of prominent forehead, moderate hypertelorism with deep-set eyes, small pointed chin, saddle or straight nose.
[b] A defect in the anterior chamber of the eye in which there is a prominence of, Schwalbe ring (this is seen in 10% of the normal population).
SOURCE: Emerick KM, Rand EB, Goldmuntz E, Krantz ID, Spinner NB, Piccoli DA: Features of Alagille syndrome in 92 patients: frequency and relation to prognosis. Hepatology 29(3):822–829, 1999.

The characteristic facies in the infant or child has the shape of an inverted triangle. The forehead is broad, and eyes are deep-set with mild hypertelorism; the nose is small and straight, and the chin is small and pointed. The facies may not be evident in the first months of life. The classic childhood appearance differs from its adult form, which may have somewhat coarse facial features, often with a long face, deep-set eyes, and prominent forehead.

The cardiac disease is usually benign (peripheral pulmonary artery stenosis), but more severe hypoplasia of the pulmonary artery branches may occur. Complex congenital heart disease such as tetralogy of Fallot has been found. Butterfly vertebrae, from failure of the anterior arches of the vertebral body to fuse, are most commonly detected in the thoracic spine. Other vertebral abnormalities have been described such as abnormalities of the interpedicular distance in the lumbar spine and spina bifida occulta. Very short distal phalanges and a short ulna have also been reported. Eye findings include posterior embryotoxon, optic disc drusen, retinal abnormalities (including abnormal pigmentation but not functional retinal degeneration), strabismus, ectopic pupil, and hypotrophic optic discs.

The renal disease associated with Alagille syndrome is highly variable. Structural abnormalities include symmetrically small kidneys or congenital single kidney. Several reports document renal cystic disease associated with Alagille syndrome. Histologic examination of kidneys in Alagille syndrome has revealed a membranous nephropathy in some cases, but the most frequent finding is lipid accumulation in the kidney (mesangiolipidosis). Nonspecific changes include azotemia, defects in concentrating urine, and nephrolithiasis. Some affected children have short stature. In addition to chronic cholestasis, pancreatic insufficiency may compromise growth.

Alagille syndrome usually has a benign course. In these patients cholestasis (including jaundice, pruritus, hypercholesterolemia with or without xanthomas, and elevated serum bile acids, alkaline phosphatase, and γ-glutamyl transpeptidase) improves or resolves over the first year of life. They do not develop cirrhosis. Severely affected children with protracted jaundice usually have a poorer prognosis and progressive liver disease. Conservative estimates put overall mortality at 20 to 25% from cardiac disease, intercurrent infection, or progressive liver disease.

Infants with Alagille syndrome should not undergo Kasai portoenterostomy. It rarely improves bile flow and renders the child in need of liver transplantation, which might otherwise have been avoided. Comparatively minor head trauma may cause significant intracranial bleeding in infants and toddlers with Alagille syndrome; mortality is significant, even in the absence of coagulopathy. Liver transplantation should be reserved for patients with hepatic failure, intolerable pruritus unresponsive to medical treatment, and severe growth failure. Liver transplantation may be more difficult because of associated heart disease, renal impairment, or vascular anomalies. Interventions to stretch the pulmonary arteries by cardiac catheterization are associated with some risk. Cardiac function should nevertheless be optimized prior to transplant. Catch-up growth after transplantation has been reported.

References

Balistreri WF, Grand R, Hoofnagle JH, et al: Biliary atresia: current concepts and research directions. Summary of a symposium. Hepatology 23:1682–1692, 1996

Desmet VJ: The cholangiopathies. In: Suchy FJ, ed: Liver Disease in Children, 1st ed. St Louis, Mosby Year Book, 1994, 145–165

Emerick KM, Rand EB, Goldmuntz E, Krantz ID, Spinner NB, Piccoli DA: Features of Alagille syndrome in 92 patients: frequency and relation to prognosis. Hepatology 29(3):822–829, 1999

Oda T, Elkahloun AG, Pike BL, et al: Mutations in the human *Jagged1* gene are responsible for Alagille syndrome. Nature Genet 16(3):235–242, 1997

18.4   METABOLIC LIVER DISEASES

Frederick J. Suchy and Benjamin L. Shneider

The liver plays a central role in the biosynthesis and degradation of carbohydrates, lipids, and amino acids. Moreover, the liver is also involved in detoxification of endogenous substrates such as bilirubin and ammonia and in the excretion of inorganic compounds such as copper and iron. Thus, the liver is involved primarily or secondarily in many inborn errors of metabolism. In this section, the focus is on those disorders that lead to acute or chronic damage to the liver. In inborn errors of metabolism such as hereditary tyrosinemia, the absence of a critical enzyme may cause an accumulation of toxic metabolites. In other disorders, progressive liver injury may occur because of failure to produce essential compounds. An example of this process is an inborn error of bile acid metabolism, which leads to progressive cholestasis because of a lack of bile acid synthesis. Severe liver injury may also result from a third mechanism, sequestration of an abnormally synthesized product within the liver, as observed in α_1-antitrypsin deficiency.

Family history, including unexplained infantile deaths or the pattern of observed symptoms, may suggest metabolic liver disease. For example, liver disease occurring after the initial ingestion of fructose should suggest a diagnosis of hereditary fructose intolerance. Clinical features of metabolic liver disease may be nonspecific and can overlap with other hepatic disorders, including viral hepatitis or drug-induced liver injury. These may include jaundice, vomiting, hepatosplenomegaly, failure to thrive, developmental delay, hypotonia, seizures, and progressive neuromuscular dysfunction (Table 18-13). Typical ages of presentation of various metabolic liver diseases are shown in Table 18-14. Initial laboratory studies are often nonspecific and include hypoglycemia, hyperammonemia, increased aminotransferase levels, acidosis, and hypoprothrombinemia. In some disorders, hepatocyte injury and loss of hepatic mass occur through the process of apoptosis rather than

TABLE 18-13

CLINICAL FEATURES ASSOCIATED WITH METABOLIC LIVER DISEASE

Coma with hyperammonemia
Hypoglycemia
Psychomotor retardation
Hepatosplenomegaly with or without liver dysfunction
Acidosis
Failure to thrive
Muscle weakness
Coagulopathy, particularly out of proportion to liver test abnormalities
Dysmorphic facial features
Cholestasis
Cardiac disease

TABLE 18-14

AGE OF PRESENTATION OF METABOLIC/GENETIC DISORDERS AFFECTING THE LIVER[a]

NEONATAL OR EARLY INFANCY	LATE INFANCY	EARLY CHILDHOOD	MID-CHILDHOOD OR ADOLESCENCE
α_1-Antitrypsin deficiency		(α_1-Antitrypsin deficiency)	
Alagille syndrome		(Alagille syndrome)	
PFIC1			
PFIC2			
PFIC3			
Primary disorders of bile acid synthesis			
Perinatal hemochromatosis			
Crigler-Najjar, type 1			
	Crigler-Najjar, type 2		
(Dubin-Johnson syndrome)			Dubin-Johnson syndrome
			Rotor syndrome
		(Wilson disease)	Wilson disease
GSD, type 4			
Hereditary tyrosinemia type 1		(Hereditary tyrosinemia type 1)	
Galactosemia			
Hereditary fructose intolerance		(Hereditary fructose intolerance)	
Zellweger syndrome			
Wolman disease			
		Cholesterol ester storage disease	
			Juvenile hemochromatosis
Niemann-Pick, type C			

[a] Parentheses indicate less frequent ages of presentation. GSD, glycogen storage disease.

liver cell necrosis. In this setting, liver function can be markedly deranged, but serum aminotransferase levels may be only modestly increased. Percutaneous or open liver biopsy, if possible, allows histologic examination and measurement of enzymatic pathways or substrate accumulation. A specific diagnosis is critically important in that it may allow effective therapy, including liver transplantation and genetic counseling.

DISORDERS OF CARBOHYDRATE METABOLISM

Galactosemia

Galactosemia is caused by a genetic defect in the normal metabolism of the monosaccharide galactose. Galactose is normally converted to glucose via three separate enzymatic reactions involving galactokinase, galactose-1-phosphate uridyl transferase, and uridine diphosphate galactose 4-epimerase. The most common severe defect involves a deficiency of galactose-1-phosphate uridyl transferase. A variety of mutations in the gene located on chromosome 9p13 have been identified in affected individuals. Inheritance is in an autosomal-recessive fashion. Inactivity of this enzyme results in the accumulation of toxic metabolites including galactose-1-phosphate and galactitol (see also Sec. 9.5.2).

The clinical presentation of galactosemia can be quite severe in the newborn period, and rapid recognition and treatment are critical. Early manifestations include lethargy, vomiting, acidosis, cataracts, failure to thrive, and jaundice. Indirect hyperbilirubinemia is commonly seen and can be accompanied by coagulopathy. Urinary tract infection and/or sepsis, typically with gram-negative species, is also a common presenting problem. Untreated disease is likely to result in severe neurologic injury.

State programs screen newborns for galactosemia in most of the United States, but clinicians should not rely on these programs for diagnosis in patients with suggestive symptoms. Urine reducing

substances are detected in infants fed galactose-containing formulas, although urine glucose dipsticks are negative. Secondary galactosemia can be seen in severe liver disease because of a lack of hepatic galactose clearance, and urinary screening may be inaccurate in this circumstance. Therefore, enzymatic assays for galactose-1-phosphate uridyl transferase should ultimately be performed using red blood cells in all cases.

Treatment consists of strict elimination of galactose from the diet. This should be initiated as soon as the diagnosis is suspected in order to prevent liver failure. This will normally reverse the hepatopathy associated with galactosemia. The long-term efficacy of dietary therapy is not perfectly successful. This is partly the result of difficulties in completely eliminating galactose from the diet and from endogenous conversion of glucose into galactose via reversal of the normal enzymatic pathways for galactose metabolism. Long-term complications often include growth failure, developmental delay, and ovarian failure despite vigilant adherence to a galactose-free diet.

Hereditary Fructose Intolerance

Hereditary fructose intolerance is an autosomal-recessive disorder caused by a genetic deficiency in the enzyme fructose-1,6-biphosphate aldolase (aldolase B), which is expressed in liver, kidney, and intestine. The classical presentation occurs in infants on the initial presentation of fructose-containing foods with the acute onset of vomiting, hypoglycemia, and hypophosphatemia preceding the development of hepatomegaly with steatosis, jaundice, and ascites. A more chronic presentation is now recognized with presenting signs and symptoms of hepatomegaly, abnormal liver enzymes, and fatty liver. Chronic exposure to fructose causes poor feeding, failure to thrive, vomiting, irritability, and poor growth. Many affected individuals evolve an eating behavior with avoidance of fructose, thus minimizing the acute manifestations of the disease. Some individuals have not been diagnosed until challenged with fructose as adults. Therefore, this disease needs to be considered in children with unexplained hepatomegaly and steatosis.

The pathophysiology of the disease involves metabolic effects of the accumulation of fructose-1-phosphate in affected individuals. This leads to the sequestration of inorganic phosphate as fructose-1-phosphate with resulting activation of AMP deaminase, which catalyzes the irreversible deamination of AMP to IMP (inosine monophosphate), a precursor of uric acid. In the cytoplasm, AMP, ADP, and ATP are maintained in a state approaching equilibrium. Depletion of tissue ATP occurs through massive degradation to uric acid and impairment of regeneration by oxidative phosphorylation in the mitochondria because of inorganic phosphate depletion. Thus, serum uric acid may be increased and phosphate decreased with acute disease. The depletion of tissue ATP causes symptoms. Sorbitol is converted to fructose and thus can lead to a similar pathologic process in these patients.

Several methods are available to make the diagnosis of hereditary fructose intolerance. A high index of suspicion is crucial because the presenting signs and symptoms can be subtle. An intravenous fructose challenge test has been described but is associated with potentially significant complications and should be avoided given current alternative diagnostic approaches. Aldolase B activity can be readily measured from liver tissue. Three different specific mutations in the aldolase B account for the disease in a large number of affected individuals. DNA diagnostic assays (including allele-specific oligonucleotide hybridization) utilizing peripheral leukocytes should be considered.

Treatment involves strict avoidance of fructose, sorbitol, and sucrose. Partial adherence to this difficult diet can ameliorate many of the acute manifestations of this disease but not the chronic problems such as growth failure. It is imperative to remember that certain intravenous solutions and oral medications can contain fructose and/or sorbitol. Patients should be informed of these risks and be proactive with their health-care providers to avoid potentially dangerous exposure (see also Sec. 9.5.3).

Glycogen Storage Diseases

The glycogen storage diseases include a wide range of clinical phenotypes that are the result of abnormalities in glycogen metabolism. Clinical manifestations can be the result of inability to utilize glycogen stores, accumulation of glycogen within the liver and/or other tissues, and the toxic effects of certain abnormal types of glycogen. Only the disorders that affect the liver are discussed in this section. Glycogen storage diseases are discussed in more detail in Sec. 9.5.1.

Fasting hypoglycemia is the hallmark of forms of glycogen storage disease in which there is an inability to utilize glycogen stores to produce glucose. Type I glycogen storage disease typically has fasting hypoglycemia as one of its early manifestations. A number of forms of type I disease exist, including deficiencies in glucose-6-phosphatase (von Gierke disease, type Ia) and various deficiencies in glucose and glucose metabolite transport (glucose-6-phosphate transport, type Ib; microsomal phosphate transport, type Ic; microsomal glucose transport, type Id). In all of these diseases fasting hypoglycemia can be life threatening, and the inability to break down glycogen can lead to significant hepatomegaly. Type Ib disease has also been associated with abnormal leukocyte function and inflammatory bowel disease. Significant hypoglycemia may also be seen in glycogen storage disease types III (debranching deficiency or Cori disease) and VI (liver phosphorylase deficiency or Andersen disease).

Inability to utilize glycogen normally leads to its accumulation in hepatocytes. Significant hepatomegaly becomes a common feature of glycogen storage disease type I but can also be seen in types III, IV (branching deficiency), and VI, where normal glycogen breakdown is impaired. Long-term glycogen deposition can increase the risk of hepatic adenomas, which are a significant risk in young adults with glycogen storage disease type I.

A very different clinical presentation can be observed in those disorders that lead to hepatic accumulation of toxic forms of glycogen. The best example of this is glycogen storage disease type IV, in which there is a deficiency of the glycogen-branching enzyme. Glycogen that accumulates in this disease has long chains of glucose in a 1-4 linkage and resembles plant starch or amylopectin. This form of glycogen is relatively insoluble and presumed to be toxic, leading to hepatocellular injury. Progressive liver disease thus becomes a major distinguishing feature of glycogen storage disease type IV. Portal hypertension and hepatic failure can develop in early childhood. The toxic amylopectin-like glycogen also appears to predispose to the development of hepatocellular adenomas.

Diagnosis of the specific type of glycogen storage disease is critical for proper treatment and for prediction of prognosis and potential complications. Specific enzymatic assays and DNA diagnostic tests are available in specialty laboratories for each of the disorders. Diagnostic assays can be performed on a number of tissues including liver, muscle, leukocytes, and fibroblasts. Careful assessment of historical information and physical and biochemical findings will often suggest a specific diagnosis.

Treatment in many of these disorders is directed at maintaining normal blood sugar levels. Frequent feeding of high-carbohydrate-containing foods and nocturnal administration of slow-release glucose polymers, such as uncooked cornstarch, are utilized. This prevents the development of hypoglycemia and also limits incorporation of excess dietary glucose into glycogen. Liver transplantation has been successfully performed for treatment of glycogen storage disease type IV. It is important to remember that these are systemic diseases that have variable degrees of involvement of both skeletal and cardiac muscle.

HEREDITARY TYROSINEMIA

Hereditary tyrosinemia type I is an autosomal-recessive disorder caused by deficiency of fumarylacetoacetate hydrolase (FAH), the last enzyme in the tyrosine degradation pathway (see also Sec. 9.2.1). The FAH gene has been mapped to chromosome 15 and cloned; over 25 mutations have been associated with the phenotype of type 1 tyrosinemia. Metabolites of tyrosine that accumulate proximal to the enzymatic block, such as succinyl acetate, succinyl acetone, fumaryl acetoacetate, and maleylacetoacetate, are highly reactive electrophilic toxic compounds that bind to sulfhydryl groups, often leading to tissue injury. Many secondary enzymatic and biochemical defects occur in tyrosinemia as a result of the accumulation of these precursor compounds. For example, succinyl acetoacetate can inhibit enzymes such as porphobilinogen synthase, leading to the accumulation of 5-aminolevulinic acid and symptoms of acute, intermittent porphyria. Deficiency or immaturity of several enzymes in the tyrosine degradation pathway can also lead to hypertyrosinemia as in *transient neonatal hypertyrosinemia*, a self-limiting condition primarily of premature infants, probably caused by an immaturity of tyrosine aminotransferase activity. Vitamin C is helpful in enhancing the activity of this enzyme. Hypertyrosinemia also occurs with severe hepatic injury, usually in association with high serum methionine levels.

Type 1 hereditary tyrosinemia occurs in acute and chronic forms that may be manifest in the same family. The acute form presents in infancy with severe liver dysfunction including jaundice, hepatosplenomegaly, failure to thrive, anorexia, ascites, coagulopathy, and rickets. The disorder may actually begin in utero as evidenced by the presence of cirrhosis and regenerative nodules at the time of presentation. The chronic form is observed later in childhood with cirrhosis, renal tubular dysfunction, rickets, and hepatocellular carcinoma. Episodes of severe peripheral neuropathy occur in patients surviving infancy, leading to morbidity from severe pain and even mortality from respiratory failure.

Laboratory studies indicate more compromise of hepatic synthetic function than would be indicated by standard liver biochemical tests. There are often hypoalbuminemia and a decrease in vitamin K–dependent coagulation factors. Serum aminotransferase values are mildly to moderately increased. Total and direct bilirubin concentrations are variably increased. Hypoglycemia is common, particularly in infants. Hemolytic anemia may be present. Renal tubular dysfunction producing a Fanconi syndrome may occur with hyperphosphaturia, glucosuria, proteinuria, and aminoaciduria. Serum tyrosine and methionine concentrations are markedly elevated. Phenolic acid byproducts of tyrosine metabolism, including p-hydroxyphenyl lactic acid, p-phenoxyphenyl pyruvic acid, and p-hydroxyphenyl acetic acid are detected in the urine. Succinylacetone and succinylacetoacetate in the urine are typical and diagnostic of this disorder. Serum α-fetoprotein concentrations are often significantly elevated in affected infants and in cord blood, suggesting prenatal onset of liver disease.

Histologic examination of the liver reveals fatty infiltration, iron deposition, varying degrees of hepatocyte necrosis, and pseudoacinar formation. Significant fibrosis may be present early in life with gradual evolution to multinodular cirrhosis. Regenerative nodules mimicking neoplasms may be present in some patients. Hepatocellular carcinoma may be found in older patients with cirrhosis. Livers of patients with hereditary tyrosinemia type 1 often contain discrete nodules containing FAH activity. This mosaicism of enzymatic reactivity is caused by somatic reversion to a normal genotype in these nodules. Molecular studies confirm correction of one of the disease-causing alleles in these nodules. These studies and other work in animal experiments suggest a strong selective advantage for FAH-expressing cells in an FAH-deficient liver. This information may be exploited in the future for gene therapy of hereditary tyrosinemia type 1.

The acute form of type 1 tyrosinemia is usually fatal in the first year of life without therapy. Treatment with a diet restricted in phenylalanine, methionine, and tyrosine does not prevent progression of the liver disease or development of hepatocellular carcinoma. Liver transplantation is the only therapy that reverses hepatic, neurologic, and most renal manifestations of the disease. Patients demonstrating cirrhotic nodules on imaging studies should undergo transplantation because of the high risk of developing carcinoma. Early liver transplantation is also indicated in patients with severe neurologic crises. Medical therapy with 2-(nitro-4-trifluromethylbenoy1)-1,3-cyclohexanedione (NTBC) has shown promise in reversing the metabolic abnormalities in hereditary tyrosinemia type 1. NTBC treatment reduces the flux through the tyrosine degradation pathway preventing the formation of metabolites that are toxic to liver and kidney. In the small number of patients who have been reported to date, toxic metabolites and serum α-fetoprotein levels decreased, and there was marked improvement in liver synthetic function. However, whether NTBC will prevent development of hepatocellular carcinoma and obviate the need for liver transplantation remains uncertain.

DISORDERS OF BILE ACID METABOLISM

Biosynthesis and transport of bile acids are critically important for normal liver function. Bile acids are one of the primary driving forces for bile flow, and any impairment in bile acid biosynthesis or transport can result in cholestasis. In addition, many of the intermediates in bile acid biosynthesis are hepatotoxic, so that abnormalities in bile acid synthesis can also lead to significant hepatotoxicity and cholestasis. Bile acid biosynthesis is the result of a complex series of hepatic-based enzymatic steps that convert cholesterol into the primary bile acids cholic and chenodeoxycholic acid. Secondary and tertiary metabolism of these bile salts can lead to a more complex range of bile salts.

Primary defects in bile acid biosynthesis generally present with cholestasis, although chronic hepatitis has also been observed (Table 18-15). However, in contrast to other disorders associated with cholestasis, impaired synthesis of bile salts results in a condition that may not be associated with either pruritus or elevated serum bile salt concentrations because the normal end products are not synthesized. A high index of suspicion for these disorders needs to be maintained because their presentations may be protean, and diagnosis requires relatively specialized testing. The possibility of a primary abnormality in bile acid biosynthesis should be entertained in any child with chronic cholestasis or hepatitis for which a clear etiology cannot be identified. Screening assays for these defects include gas chromatography and fast atom bombardment mass spectrometry of urine, serum, and/or bile. Confirmatory enzymatic and molecular assays exist for some of the defects.

Inborn errors in bile acid transport lead to primarily cholestatic liver dieases. Molecular transporters of bile acids are found on both the canalicular and basolateral hepatocyte membranes. Canalicular excretion of bile salts is mediated by the bile salt excretory protein, BSEP (also know as the sister gene of p-glycoprotein). Primary genetic defects in BSEP result in a progressive form of cholestasis that is characterized by severe pruritus, markedly elevated serum bile acid concentration, normal serum cholesterol concentration, and normal GGT values. Biliary bile acid concentrations are extremely low. Liver histology early in the course of the disease may reveal giant cell transformation and ductular proliferation. Cirrhosis and end-stage liver disease can evolve relatively quickly. Differentiation of this disease from Byler disease (see below) may be difficult but is critically important because primary defects in canalicular trans-

TABLE 18-15

INBORN ERRORS OF BILE ACID METABOLISM

ENZYME DEFICIENCY	LIVER DISEASE	TREATMENT
Δ^4-3-Oxosteroid 5β-reductase	Neonatal cholestasis	Cholic and chenodeoxycholic acid
3β-Hydroxy-C_{27}-steroid dehydrogenase	Cholestasis	Ursodeoxycholic acid
Oxysterol 7-hydroxylase	Neonatal cholestasis	Liver transplantation
Sterol 27-hydroxylase	None (neurologic disease)	Chenodeoxycholic acid

port of bile acids may be cured by liver transplantation, but Byler disease may not. Defects in basolateral transport of bile salts have not been definitively identified, although this is suspected to be the cause of a relatively rare form of cholestatic liver disease characterized by isolated elevations of serum bile salts and severe pruritus.

Secondary disorders of bile acid metabolism are observed in peroxisomal disorders such as Zellweger syndrome (cerebrohepatorenal syndrome), neonatal adrenoleukosdystrophy, and infantile Refsum disease (see Sec. 9.10).

DISORDERS OF BILIRUBIN METABOLISM AND EXCRETION

Jaundice is a common presenting feature of a wide range of pediatric disorders. In most circumstances the jaundice results from increased bilirubin load and/or toxic effects on the relatively immature bilirubin conjugation/excretory system that is found in the newborn liver. Neonatal hyperbilirubinemia is discussed in Sec. 2.17.6, and the evaluation of an infant or child with jaundice and direct hyperbilirubinemia is discussed in Sec. 18.2. Occasionally jaundice is the result of a primary abnormality in the liver's capacity to conjugate or transport bilirubin. Normal hepatic clearance of bilirubin includes glucuronidation and carrier-mediated transport of bilirubin at the basolateral and canalicular membranes of the hepatocyte. Hyperbilirubinemia is seen in primary genetic abnormalities of these processes; Crigler-Najjar and Gilbert syndromes result from defects in glucuronidation, and Dubin-Johnson syndrome results from defects in canalicular excretion of conjugated bilirubin.

Gilbert syndrome is the most benign of these disorders and probably represents a relatively common genetic phenotype as opposed to a distinct disease entity. Estimates indicate that 2 to 10% of individuals have Gilbert syndrome. The syndrome is the result of an alteration in the promoter for the bilirubin uridine diphosphate glucuronyl transferase (UDP-GT) gene. The altered promoter is transcriptionally less active and leads to a relative deficiency of the enzyme. Clinically this translates into a condition characterized by mild indirect hyperbilirubinemia (typically <5 mg/dL) without associated hemolysis or hepatocellular/canalicular injury. This may manifest with jaundice during times of stress and fasting. In addition, Gilbert syndrome may explain many cases of prolonged "physiological" jaundice in the newborn period. This entity has not been associated with any specific morbidity or mortality and does not require treatment.

Crigler-Najjar syndrome exists in two forms, types I and II. Type I is the more severe, the result of a complete absence of bilirubin UDP-GT activity. This disease presents in the newborn period with severe indirect hyperbilirubinemia, necessitating continuous phototherapy and/or exchange transfusions. Analysis of bile reveals no bilirubin conjugates. Kernicterus is a serious potential complication for children with Crigler-Najjar syndrome type I and can occur at any time in their lives. Specific DNA testing can be performed to confirm a diagnosis of Crigler-Najjar type I and can be utilized for prenatal testing. Phototherapy is the mainstay of therapy. Liver transplantation can be curative, although risk-benefit decisions for this approach are complex. Preliminary reports of hepatocyte transplantation for this disorder have been disappointing. Gene therapy may ultimately be an attractive means of curing this disease.

Crigler-Najjar type II is the result of genetic abnormalities in the bilirubin UDP-GT gene that lead to partial activity. Hyperbil-

irubinemia of <10 mg/dL is usually observed, and this is typically responsive to cytochrome P450-inducing compounds such as phenobarbital. Long-term treatment with phenobarbital is generally not recommended because it results in a cosmetic improvement but is associated with potential neurodevelopmental complications.

Dubin-Johnson syndrome is the result of a genetic deficiency in the *cMOAT/MRP2* gene, which encodes the canalicular transporter of conjugated bilirubin. The disease is manifest by relatively mild conjugated hyperbilirubinemia (3 to 8 mg/dL) with no evidence of significant hepatocellular or canalicular injury. Analysis of urinary coproporphyrins reveals a preponderance of the isoform I. Like Gilbert syndrome and Crigler-Najjar type II, this is a disease that is not associated with specific morbidity and mortality and as such does not require treatment.

DISORDERS OF FATTY ACID OXIDATION OR METABOLISM

Abnormalities in fatty acid metabolism can lead to severe forms of acute liver injury as a result of both energy deprivation and the accumulation of highly toxic intermediary metabolites of fatty acid oxidation. Normal fatty acid metabolism in the liver is a highly complex process that involves fatty acid transport into hepatocytes and mitochondria and a series of distinct enzymatic steps that generate energy from an orderly oxidation of fatty acids. At least 22 different clinical entities have been ascribed to distinct abnormalities in fatty acid oxidation. A range of clinical presentations has been described including sudden infant death, cardiomyopathies, skeletal myopathies, hepatopathy, and life-threatening hypoglycemia (Table 18-16). For further discussion of these disorders refer to Sec. 9.4. Hepatopathy has been described in two-thirds of these disorders with at least six involving relatively severe liver disease (long-chain fatty acid transport defect, carnitine palmitoyltransferase deficiency, long-chain hydroxyacyl-CoA-dehydrogenase deficiency, α and β trifunctional protein defects, and short-chain hydroxyacyl-CoA-dehydrogenase deficiency).

The typical case of severe liver disease resulting from an abnormality in fatty acid oxidation presents with acute liver disease characterized by markedly elevated serum aminotransferase levels with variable degrees of cholestasis and coagulopathy. Nonketotic hypoglycemia is a hallmark feature of these disorders. Variable degrees of myopathy (skeletal and/or cardiac) may be an accompanying feature. Some form of stressor that includes fasting typically precedes the onset of the hepatopathy. Manifestations and biochemical abnormalities may be intermittent.

Prompt recognition of defects in fatty acid metabolism is paramount for proper treatment. Diagnostic assays that examine intermediate metabolites of fatty acid oxidation need to be performed during illness, as many of the metabolites will clear with treatment. Testing in suspected fatty acid oxidation defects includes both non-

TABLE 18-16

CLINICAL FEATURES SUGGESTIVE OF INBORN ERRORS IN FATTY ACID OXIDATION

Infantile Reye-like syndrome
Recurrent Reye syndrome
Hepatic steatosis
Unexplained hepatic failure (may be recurrent)
Nonketotic hypoglycemia
Skeletal or cardiac myopathy

specific screening assays and more specific enzymatic and DNA diagnostic tests. Initial evaluation should include assays of plasma carnitine, acylcarnitines, free fatty acids, urine organic acids, and acylglycines. Liver biopsy, when feasible, may reveal steatosis. Acylcarnitines in bile can also be informative. These screening assays are typically followed up by specific enzymatic assays in fibroblasts, with DNA diagnostic confirmatory tests in those defects where specific assays exist. Fatty acid transport studies must be performed with fibroblasts when a fatty acid transport defect is suspected.

Typically treatment is directed at stopping ongoing fatty acid oxidation by halting fat catabolism. This often can be achieved by intravenous administration of 12 to 15 mg/kg/min of glucose. Subsequent avoidance of fasting is crucial. The benefits of carnitine administration and specific dietary fat restrictions or supplementation are controversial. In many circumstances a diagnosis cannot be made before the development of irreversible hepatic injury. Liver transplantation can be considered, but care must be taken to insure that there is no evidence of severe systemic or neurologic disease that would not improve following hepatic replacement.

PRIMARY MITOCHONDRIAL HEPATOPATHIES

Inherited defects of mitochondrial oxidative phosphorylation are often associated with liver disease. Neonatal and early childhood hepatic failure have been associated with defective activity of respiratory chain complexes and oxidative phosphorylation, but liver disease of varying severity at different ages has also been reported. Neonatal liver failure occurs in association with deficiency of complex IV (cytochrome c oxidase) and of complexes I and III. Evidence of liver synthetic failure is particularly prominent with hypoglycemia, hypoproteinemia, hyperbilirubinemia, hyperammonemia, and coagulopathy. Lethargy, hypotonia, vomiting, and poor feeding may be present from birth. Prenatal onset is suggested in some patients by the occurrence of fetal hydrops and congenital ascites. A key diagnostic feature in these patients is the presence of lactic acidosis and an elevated molar ratio of plasma lactate to pyruvate (normal <20:1).

Histologic features of the liver include microvesicular and macrovesicular steatosis with abnormally increased mitochondrial density and swelling. Cholestasis, bile ductular proliferation, and fibrosis or even cirrhosis may be present. Activities of mitochondrial respiratory chain enzymes can be measured in affected tissues.

There may be varying degrees of neuromuscular involvement in these patients, such as seizures and hypotonia. Because heteroplasmy for mitochondrial DNA (mtDNA) mutations is not uniform in all tissues, patients may present exclusively with liver disease or with variable involvement of other organ systems. This issue is critically important because patients may undergo successful liver transplantation only to have later onset of severe neuromuscular disease. The spectrum of respiratory chain disorders is sufficiently broad that some patients are now being recognized with a more chronic course or onset later in infancy or childhood. Alper disease is one such disorder; it is characterized by progressive neuronal degeneration and cirrhosis of the liver in childhood.

Point mutations in mitochondrial or nuclear DNA have been detected in some patients with neonatal liver failure caused by respiratory chain defects. Deletions and rearrangements of mtDNA have also been observed. Some patients presenting with severe liver disease have been found to have the mtDNA depletion syndrome, in which there is a generalized reduction of otherwise normal mitochondrial DNA molecules in affected organs. Autosomal-reces-

sive, maternal, and possibly X-linked modes of inheritance have been observed or proposed.

The prognosis for patients with acute liver failure secondary to a mitochondrial disorder is extremely poor. There is no proven medical therapy, although supplementation with mitochondrial cofactors such as coenzyme Q_{10} and antioxidants theoretically may be beneficial. Liver transplantation has been successful in patients whose disease is restricted to the liver.

REYE AND REYE-LIKE SYNDROMES

Reye syndrome is a systemic illness characterized by acute liver disease and hyperammonemic encephalopathy. This disorder had a peak incidence in the 1960s and 1970s; only rare cases have been reported since 1985. Although the cause of this disease was never fully elucidated, the stereotypic presentation after routine childhood illnesses such as varicella and influenza, and the association with aspirin ingestion, raised the possibilities of immune-mediated and/or toxic pathogenesis. The reasons for the decreasing incidence of Reye syndrome are not clear but may in part be related to the avoidance of aspirin administration to children with viral illnesses.

Children with Reye syndrome develop vomiting within a few days of the antecedent illness; the vomiting is not caused by gastrointestinal upset but more likely by the earliest stages of encephalopathy. In the mildest cases, the vomiting is associated with minimal neurologic changes such as lethargy and resolves spontaneously or with intravenous glucose. In the more severe cases, vomiting is followed quickly by progressive obtundation and the stages of metabolic coma. When the diagnosis is suspected, serum AST and ALT values should be measured; they are typically moderately to markedly elevated. Prolonged prothrombin time is common, but, in contrast to fulminant hepatitis, jaundice is not noted. Hyperammonemia is usually found at presentation; the average value is about 35 μg/dL, but the level does not correlate with the severity of the encephalopathy. The liver is enlarged but not firm; it is characterized histologically by extensive accumulation of microvesicular fat, but inflammation and cellular necrosis are absent. Electron microscopy reveals an increase in the amount of smooth endoplasmic reticulum and peroxisomes, and mitochondrial changes are described in more advanced disease. The hepatopathy resolves over the first several days of the illness, and the prognosis is determined by the central nervous system component of the illness. Treatment is directed at maintaining metabolic homeostasis with glucose administration and minimizing intracranial hypertension with maneuvers such as hyperventilation and mannitol infusion.

There are pediatric disorders that may mimic Reye syndrome with manifestations of liver disease and encephalopathy. Children who present sporadically with vomiting, lethargy with progressive coma, and biochemical evidence of hepatocellular injury may have systemic viral infections with multisystem involvement, toxin exposure, or inborn errors of metabolism. The genetic/metabolic disorders that are most likely to be confused with Reye syndrome are fatty acid oxidation defects and urea cycle defects. These should be suspected in very young children or those who have had recurrent episodes of hepatopathy and encephalopathy, especially if preceded by periods of fasting or other metabolic stress.

α_1-ANTITRYPSIN DEFICIENCY

α_1-Antitrypsin deficiency can be associated with progressive liver disease in infants, children, and adults. α_1-Antitrypsin is the principal serum inhibitor of proteolytic enzymes such as neutrophil elastase. Patients with homozygous deficiency or the protein inhibitor ZZ phenotype (PiZZ) have low serum α_1-antitrypsin activity, usually in the range of 10 to 15% of normal values. The incidence of the most common deficiency phenotype, PiZZ, is one in 2000 to 4000 live births. α_1-Antitrypsin concentration and phenotype should be measured in any child or adult presenting with chronic liver disease. Measurement of α_1-antitrypsin concentration alone is unreliable because the protein is an acute-phase reactant and may be elevated as the result of an illness. Heterozygotes with the SZ and MZ phenotypes have a less severe reduction in serum α_1-antitrypsin concentration. The association with clinical disease is less clear.

Liver disease associated with α_1-antitrypsin deficiency may present in various forms including neonatal cholestasis, juvenile cirrhosis, chronic hepatitis, and hepatocellular carcinoma. Cholestatic jaundice occurs in approximately 10 to 15% of infants with the PiZZ phenotype. Hepatomegaly and acholic stools may occur. Patients rarely may present with signs of advanced liver disease such as ascites or gastrointestinal bleeding. Although asymptomatic, another 40 to 50% of homozygous infants have abnormal liver biochemical tests in the first months of life.

Giant-cell hepatitis is a typical histologic finding in the neonate. Bile ductular proliferation may be observed initially; occasionally, paucity of bile ducts is found later. Periodic acid–Schiff-positive, diastase-resistant inclusions within hepatocytes, especially in the periportal region, represent the abnormal α_1-antitrypsin accumulation. These are a hallmark of the disorder but are not prominent before 4 months of age. Variable degrees of fibrosis may be present. Cirrhosis has been reported as early as the neonatal period, but progression to this stage is quite variable. α_1-Antitrypsin deficiency can present later in life with clinical features similar to autoimmune hepatitis. α_1-Antitrypsin deficiency is associated with emphysema in young adulthood.

The reason that only 10 to 15% of neonates with the homozygous deficiency manifest liver disease is unclear. The PiZZ defect is caused by substitution of a lysine for a glutamate at position 342, leading to misfolding of the protein and its retention in the endoplasmic reticulum. Studies in transgenic mice expressing the abnormal human protein indicate that retained α_1-antitrypsin is toxic to hepatocytes. Recent studies have shown that mutant α_1-antitrypsin molecule polymerizes in the ER by a novel loop-sheet insertion mechanism. A subpopulation of α_1-antitrypsin-deficient individuals may be susceptible to liver injury because they have another trait that reduces the efficiency with which the mutant α_1-antitrypsin protein is degraded in the endoplasmic reticulum.

The outcome of neonatal liver disease related to α_1-antitrypsin deficiency is variable. Patients presenting with cirrhosis may deteriorate within the first months of life. However, in most infants, the jaundice clears by 4 months of age. Patients may present with cirrhosis later in childhood and are at risk for hepatocellular carcinoma. Of 27 PiZZ patients identified by neonatal screening in one study of 200,000 births, 12% developed neonatal cholestasis, and another 7% had clinical evidence of liver disease in infancy. On follow-up at 18 years of age, five PiZZ patients had died, but the majority of remaining patients had normal liver biochemical tests and were free of clinical liver disease. There is no specific treatment for α_1-antitrypsin deficiency. Liver transplantation is curative for patients progressing to end-stage liver disease; the recipient assumes the Pi type of the donor organ.

WILSON DISEASE

Wilson disease (hepatolenticular degeneration) is an autosomal-recessively inherited disorder of copper metabolism. The clinical manifestations of Wilson disease result from the excessive deposition of copper in the liver, brain, kidneys, and eyes. This excessive accumulation results from disturbed incorporation of copper into ceruloplasmin and reduced biliary copper excretion. The gene for Wilson disease, mapped to the long arm of chromosome 13 and designated ATP7B, encodes a copper-transporting P-type ATPase expressed predominantly in hepatocytes. Over 60 disease-specific mutations of ATP7B have now been reported in individuals with Wilson disease. Ongoing studies on the structure and function of the ATP7B protein support its role as a copper transporter involved in intracellular trafficking of copper in the liver cells. The protein is localized predominantly in the *trans*-Golgi network, to a vesicular compartment, and possibly in mitochondria. There is also substantial information to indicate defective synthesis of the copper-binding protein ceruloplasmin. The mechanism of copper toxicity likely includes the generation of free radicals, lipid peroxidation of membranes and DNA, inhibition of protein synthesis, and reduced levels of cellular antioxidants. Hepatocellular necrosis and apoptosis may be triggered by copper-induced cellular injury. When the storage capacity of the liver for copper is exceeded, or when liver-cell necrosis results in release of cellular copper into the systemic circulation, the concentration of non-ceruloplasmin-bound copper in the circulation becomes elevated. The extrahepatic deposition of this metal in sites such as the brain is probably derived from this circulating pool of copper.

Wilson disease should be considered in any child with an unexplained hepatic, neurologic, or psychiatric illness. The natural history of Wilson disease begins with the asymptomatic accumulation of copper in hepatocytes. The clinical presentation is highly variable. Although patients as young as 2 have presented with liver disease, symptoms are rarely evident before 5 years of age. Younger children, identified by family screening or after evaluation of abnormal liver biochemical tests, are often asymptomatic. Patients less than 20 years of age tend to present predominantly with hepatic manifestations. Asymptomatic hepatomegaly or an illness mimicking acute hepatitis may occur. Hepatic insufficiency associated with cirrhosis may evolve slowly or be manifest at the time of initial diagnosis with variceal hemorrhage, ascites, edema, and stigmata of chronic liver disease. A fulminant form of the disease most often occurs in the second decade of life with the abrupt onset of liver failure associated with nonimmune hemolytic anemia. The latter complication likely results from oxidative injury to red blood cells as massive amounts of copper are released from hepatocytes.

Older patients may present with predominantly neurologic and psychiatric dysfunction. Findings initially may be quite subtle and include deterioration in school performance, behavioral changes, slurred speech, and tremors. If untreated, severe dysarthria and dystonia result, sometimes leading to psychiatric hospitalization. Kayser-Fleischer rings, copper deposits on the inner surface of the Descemet membrane, are invariably found in patients with a neurologic presentation. They are often absent in younger patients presenting only with liver disease.

Abnormalities of other organ systems are sometimes present in Wilson disease. Copper toxicity in the kidney may induce nephrocalcinosis, hematuria, and aminoaciduria. Arthritis, arthralgias, and premature osteoarthritis may also occur. Cardiomyopathy and arrhythmias may result from copper accumulation in the myocardium.

Routine laboratory studies demonstrate variable elevation in serum aminotransferase values and conjugated and unconjugated serum bilirubin concentrations. Serum alkaline phosphatase levels tend to be normal or even low. The serum copper concentration is usually low but may be elevated during episodes of hemolysis. Serum ceruloplasmin, an α_2-globulin involved in copper transport, is typically low, although this serum protein may also be reduced in other disorders associated with acute or chronic hepatic insufficiency. Urinary copper excretion, normally less than 40 to 60 μg per 24 hours, is usually more than 100 μg per 24 hours in Wilson disease. Urinary copper excretion may be elevated in other forms of liver disease, such as chronic hepatitis or fulminant hepatic necrosis.

Hepatic copper content remains the gold standard for the diagnosis of Wilson disease. The typical diagnostic concentration is more than 250 μg per gram dry weight of liver, commonly more than 1000 μg per gram. Histologic examination may show fatty infiltration, glycogen accumulation, glycogenated nuclei, and enlarged Kupffer cells. However, sometimes there are findings indistinguishable from those of chronic active hepatitis. Significant hepatic fibrosis or even cirrhosis may be a presenting feature. Distinctive mitochondrial changes may be found even at an early stage of the disease, including enlargement, separation of the inner and outer membranes, widening of the intercristal spaces, and increased density and granularity of the matrix or replacement by large vacuoles. Histochemical stains for copper may be useful when positive but are not reliable in excluding copper overload.

The most striking neuropathologic changes in Wilson disease are found in the lenticular nuclei, which may manifest atrophy, cystic degeneration, and discoloration. The thalamus, the subthalamus, and even the cerebral cortex may be involved.

Without treatment, Wilson disease is uniformly fatal. The mainstay of treatment involves chelation therapy with the copper-binding agent D-penicillamine. This preparation is administered orally in increasing doses to approximately 1 g per day in adults and 0.5 to 0.75 g/d for younger children. Chelating agents remove copper from potentially toxic sites within cells and detoxify the remaining copper. Urinary copper excretion markedly increases on initiation of therapy with D-penicillamine. Later, urinary copper excretion stabilizes, reflecting a new steady state of copper balance. A low-copper diet must also be instituted to maintain a daily intake below 1 mg per day. Foods containing high amounts of copper, such as liver, chocolate, nuts, and shellfish, should be avoided. Water sources should also be assayed for copper content. With effective chelation therapy, there is usually improvement of hepatic and neurologic function and regression of Kayser-Fleischer rings. Chelation therapy must be maintained for life. For patients who are intolerant to D-penicillamine because of hypersensitivity reactions or bone marrow suppression, therapy with an alternative chelating agent, triethylene tetramine dihydrochloride, is equally effective. Tetrathiomolybdate is another chelating agent potentially useful in patients with neurologic disease in whom D-penicillamine therapy may be associated with an initial worsening of symptoms. Several studies have indicated that zinc administration may maintain a negative copper balance in patients with Wilson disease, but zinc should be considered as a primary therapy only in patients unable to tolerate standard chelating agents. Zinc acts to prevent intestinal absorption of copper, rather than as a chelating agent.

For patients with end-stage liver disease unresponsive to chelation therapy, and for most patients with the fulminant form of Wilson disease, liver transplantation may be life saving. Various degrees of regression of neurologic and psychiatric abnormalities have been described following liver replacement.

Siblings of patients with Wilson disease should be screened carefully for the disorder, and D-penicillamine therapy should be instituted as soon as the diagnosis is confirmed in asymptomatic patients. The abundance of disease-specific mutations and their locations at multiple sites have limited molecular genetic diagnosis to kindred of known patients. Thorough evaluation by well-established clinical and biochemical tests remains essential.

NEONATAL HEMOCHROMATOSIS

Neonatal hemochromatosis is a form of neonatal liver failure characterized by an early in utero onset and associated hepatic and extrahepatic hemosiderosis. Whether this disease represents a single pathophysiologic entity or is a common pathologic endpoint of a number of diseases that lead to in utero liver failure is not known. This entity is unrelated to hereditary hemochromatosis and does not appear to be the result of a primary abnormality in fetal iron metabolism. Infants with neonatal hemochromatosis have an expected mortality of more than 90% unless prompt treatment and/or liver transplantation is undertaken.

The initial clinical presentation of neonatal hemochromatosis can be subtle and can be confused with other pathologic conditions commonly seen in the newborn. The finding of cholestatic jaundice with coagulopathy and/or ascites at birth should prompt diagnostic evaluations for neonatal hemochromatosis. Supporting biochemical features include hypoalbuminemia, hypoglycemia, hyperammonemia, and high iron saturation and serum ferritin levels. Diagnosis is dependent on documentation of hepatic insufficiency and extrahepatic siderosis with no other apparent etiology of the liver failure. Extrahepatic siderosis can be demonstrated by either biopsy of a minor salivary gland or magnetic resonance imaging of the pancreas and/or heart. Analysis of both of these studies requires assessment by a specialist experienced in these uncommon applications of the diagnostic tests. Liver histology, when available, reveals nonspecific findings with evidence of chronic hepatic insufficiency, well-established fibrosis or cirrhosis, significant hepatocellular loss, and reactive bile ductular proliferation.

Early recognition of neonatal hemochromatosis is a requisite for successful treatment. Sepsis often leads to significant morbidity and mortality in these infants because they are immunocompromised on the basis of both age and decompensated cirrhotic liver disease. Immediate referral of infants with neonatal hemochromatosis to a center experienced in liver transplantation in infants is advised. Medical therapy consists of a combination of antioxidants (vitamin E in the form of tocopheryl polyethylene glycol succinate, selenium, and N-acetyl cysteine), membrane stabilizers (prostaglandin E_1), and iron chelators (deferoxamine). The efficacy of medical therapy alone has been questioned, but it appears at a minimum to stabilize infants in preparation for liver transplantation. Liver transplantation has been successfully utilized in very small infants with neonatal hemochromatosis. Recurrence of the disease posttransplant has not been reported, although apparent iron toxicity has been observed in an infant who did not undergo chelation before transplantation.

The inheritance of neonatal hemochromatosis is complex and in many circumstances is associated with a recurrence rate that exceeds that expected for either an autosomal-recessive or -dominant pattern. For these reasons, ascertainment of a diagnosis of neonatal hemochromatosis is of critical importance for family counseling and for monitoring of future pregnancies.

HEREDITARY HEMOCHROMATOSIS
Colin Rudolph

Hereditary hemochromatosis is an inherited disorder of iron metabolism leading to progressive iron loading of parenchymal cells of the liver, pancreas, and heart. The most common form of this disease is caused by homozygosity for the C282Y mutation in the *HFE* gene. Not all patients with this genetic mutation have phenotypic expression. Other mutations have been described, but their prevalence is low. Hereditary hemochromatosis is not a disorder of childhood, but iron studies may be abnormal in children, leading to early diagnosis of children with affected parents.

Symptoms include nonspecific findings such as weakness, fatigue, and weight loss. More specific symptoms and signs include arthralgias, diabetes, hepatomegaly, amenorrhea, and congestive heart failure. Once a proband with hereditary hemochromatosis is identified, family screening is recommended for all first-degree relatives. In children of an affected parent, it is useful to perform *HFE* mutation analysis on the spouse to accurately predict the genotype in the children. If the spouse has either mutation, then the children will also need to undergo *HFE* mutation analysis, although the value of genetic testing in children is still being evaluated. In a child at risk, serum iron studies should be periodically evaluated and therapeutic phlebotomy considered if liver function tests are elevated and ferritin level is greater than 1000 ng/mL. This is unlikely until after the second decade of life.

CONGENITAL GLYCOSYLATION DISORDERS

Congenital glycosylation disorders (CGDs) are a group of hereditary multisystem disorders that result from abnormalities in the glycosylation of glycoproteins. A spectrum of clinical presentations occur, with most disorders being associated with severe psychomotor and mental retardation and with blood coagulation abnormalities causing thrombosis, bleeding, and stroke-like episodes. Carbohydrate-deficient glycoprotein syndrome Ib is caused by a deficiency of phosphomannose isomerase and is different from other CGD disorders in that patients do not have psychomotor retardation but present instead with a gastrointestinal disorder characterized by a protein-losing enteropathy. Some other case reports describe patients presenting with vomiting and diarrhea, hypoglycemia, congenital hepatic fibrosis, and coagulation factor deficiencies. These patients may be treatable with oral mannose therapy. Transferrin isoelectric focusing is the most readily available test for diagnostic screening.

PROGRESSIVE FAMILIAL INTRAHEPATIC CHOLESTASIS
Eve Roberts

The term "progressive familial intrahepatic cholestasis" (PFIC) denotes a group of inherited disorders of bile formation. Various disorders of enzymes in the bile production apparatus, usually enzymes in the bile canalicular membrane of the hepatocyte, have been identified in patients with PFIC (Table 18-17). PFIC1 and PFIC2 are characterized by normal serum γ-glutamyl transpeptidase (GGT), discordant with the severe cholestasis. In PFIC3 serum γ-glutamyl transpeptidase is elevated.

PFIC1

Patients with PFIC1, also known as *Byler disease,* present with conjugated hyperbilirubinemia in the first 3 months of life or often a little later, around 4 to 6 months old. The degree of jaundice may vary. Fat-soluble vitamin deficiencies, may be severe, resulting in rickets and vitamin K deficiency. Pruritus is severe, may be the most prominent symptom, and is refractory to most treatment. Growth retardation may not be evident initially. Liver biopsy shows little inflammation but has canalicular bile plugs with a characteristic granular appearance on electron microscopy. Portal small duct paucity may be present. Although the child appears to have severe cholestasis, the serum GGT is repeatedly normal, as is serum cholesterol. The total serum bile acid concentration is elevated. However, the concentration of chenodeoxycholic acid in bile from these patients is extremely low. Children with Byler disease have persistent diarrhea with fat malabsorption and protein loss, bouts of pancreatitis, and poor growth leading to short stature. Sweat chloride may be elevated.

Cirrhosis usually develops in early childhood and liver transplantation is required. After liver transplant, pancreatitis may still occur, and the diarrhea may get worse. Biliary diversion is an alternative treatment strategy, which decreases pruritus in most patients and may slow the progression of liver damage, if this surgical procedure is performed before cirrhosis has developed.

Patients with PFIC1 have a mutation in the gene *FIC1,* on chromosome 18q21-22, identified recently by positional cloning. This gene codes for a P-type ATPase, which probably participates in transferring aminophospholipids from the outer leaflet to inner leaflet of cell membranes. In the liver a defect in this process is predicted to interfere with biliary secretion of bile acids. The *FIC1* gene is also highly expressed in extrahepatic organs including the

TABLE 18-17

DISORDERS IN THE PROGRESSIVE FAMILIAL INTRAHEPATIC CHOLESTASIS (PFIC) GROUP (PFIC1 AND PFIC2 PREVIOUSLY GROUPED WITH BYLER DISEASE)

	PFIC1	PFIC2	PFIC3
Genetic transmission	AR	AR	AR
Pruritus	++++	++++	++
Serum GGT level	Normal	Normal	Elevated
Bile composition	Low primary bile acid concentrations	Low primary bile acid concentrations	Low phospholipid concentration
Gene	*FIC1*	*SPGP*	*MDR3*
Gene product	P-type ATPase	Bile salt excretory pump (BSEP)	MDR3 P-glycoprotein
Cellular location	Bile duct epithelial cell (?)	Hepatocyte-canalicular membrane	Hepatocyte-canalicular membrane
Functional defect	Bile acid disposition	Bile acid secretion	Phospholipid secretion

AR, autosomal recessive.

lungs, small intestine, pancreas, and kidneys. This may account for some of the clinical diversity of PFIC1.

Benign recurrent intrahepatic cholestasis (BRIC), also associated with mutations in *FIC1*, rarely presents in infancy: a few infants presented with pruritus, not jaundice, at 1 to 4 months old. Episodes of jaundice with pruritus may occur during childhood. Why mutations in the same gene produce two dissimilar clinical diseases is not yet known.

PFIC2

Some children with intrahepatic cholestasis and normal serum GGT do not have a mutation in *FIC1*. Instead they have a mutation in a gene found on chromosome 2q24. These children differ from children with PFIC1 in some important respects: those with PFIC2 do not develop pancreatitis or diarrhea, but they do have prominent inflammation with giant-cell hepatitis, fibrosis, and ductular proliferation on liver biopsy. Like children with PFIC1, children with PFIC2 have severe pruritus. They appear to have more rapidly progressive liver disease than is found in PFIC1. The gene (*SPGP*) that is abnormal in PFIC2 encodes a transporter initially called "sister of P-glycoprotein" but currently identified as the canalicular bile salt export pump (BSEP). This gene is expressed only in the liver, and its gene product is an ATP-dependent bile acid transporter. Since most mutations appear to lead to a nonfunctional protein, the consequent accumulation of bile acids inside the hepatocyte may lead to severe liver damage.

PFIC-3

A further group of children have been identified with progressive intrahepatic cholestasis but elevated serum GGT. In these children jaundice may be less prominent than pruritus; despite the clinical appearance of biliary tract obstruction, imaging reveals a normal biliary tree. On liver biopsy portal fibrosis and inflammation with bile ductular proliferation may be found early in the course of the disease; biliary cirrhosis develops later. In general patients with PFIC3 present at a somewhat older age and have a more slowly progressive chronic liver disease than those with PFIC1 or PFIC2. The gene which is abnormal in PFIC3 is *MDR3*. This gene encodes the P-glycoprotein MDR3, which is a phospholipid translocator found mainly in the bile canalicular membrane. MDR3 is responsible for biliary phospholipid secretion. Liver damage in PFIC3 may occur because phospholipids are not present in bile to protect bile duct epithelial cells from the toxicity of bile acids or other components of bile.

Other ethnic clusters of cholestatic disease, such as Aagenaes syndrome, Greenland Eskimo cholestasis, and Navajo neuropathy, may be part of the PFIC spectrum. An important differential diagnostic point is that neonatal cholestatic disease with normal serum GGT and normal serum bile acids may also be due to inborn errors of bile acid synthesis.

References

Galactosemia

Hsia DYY, Walker FA: Variability in the clinical manifestations of galactosemia. J Pediatr 59:872–883, 1961

Levy HL, Sepe SJ, Shih VE, Vawter GF, Klein JO: Sepsis due to *Escherichia coli* in neonates with galactosemia. N Engl J Med 297:823–826, 1977

Waggoner DD, Buist NRM: Long-term prognosis in galactosemia: results of a survey of 350 cases. J Inher Metab Dis 13:802–808, 1990

Hereditary Fructose Intolerance

Ali M, Rellos P, Cox TM: Herediary fructose intolerance. J Med Genet 35:353–365, 1998

Cross NCP, De Franchis R, Sebastio G, et al: Molecular analysis of aldolase B genes in hereditary fructose intolerance. Lancet 335:306–310, 1990

Odievre M, Gentil C, Gautier M, Alagille D: Hereditary fructose intolerance in childhood. Am J Dis Child 132:605–611, 1976

Glycogen Storage Diseases

Chen Y-T, Cornblath M, Sidbury JB: Cornstarch therapy in type I glycogen storage disease. N Engl J Med 310:425–425, 1984

Howell RR, Stevenson RE, Ben-menachem Y, Phyliky RL, Berry DH: Hepatic adenomata with type I glycogen storage disease. JAMA 236:1481–1484, 1976

Selby R, Starzl TE, Yunis E, Brown BI, Kendall RS, Tzakis A: Liver transplantation for type IV glycogen storage disease. N Engl J Med 324:39–42, 1991

Hereditary Tyrosinemia

Croffie JM, Gupta SK, Chong SK, Fitzgerald JF: Tyrosinemia type 1 should be suspected in infants with severe coagulopathy even in the absence of other signs of liver failure. Pediatrics 103:675–678, 1999

Holme E, Lindstedt S: Diagnosis and management of tyrosinemia type I. Curr Opin Pediatr 7:726–732, 1995

Paradis K: Tyrosinemia: the Quebec experience. Clin Invest Med 19:311–316, 1996

Poudrier J, Lettre F, Scriver CR, Larochelle J, Tanguay RM: Different clinical forms of hereditary tyrosinemia (type I) in patients with identical genotypes. Mol Genet Metab 64:119–125, 1998

Disorders of Bile Acid Metabolism

Bjorkhem I: Inborn errors of metabolism with consequences for bile acid biosynthesis. Scand J Gastroenterol [Suppl] 204:68–72, 1994

Jacquemin E, Setchell KDR, O'Connell NC, et al: A new cause of progressive intrahepatic cholestasis: 3β-hydroxy-C27-steroid dehydrogenase/isomerase deficiency. J Pediatr 125:379–384, 1994

Setchell KDR, Schwarz M, O'Connell NC, et al: Identification of a new inborn error in bile acid synthesis: mutation of the oxosterol 7α-hydroxylase gene causes severe neonatal liver disease. J Clin Invest 102:1690–703, 1998

Setchell KDR, Suchy FJ, Welsh MB, Zimmer-Nechemias L, Heubi J, Balistreri W: δ-3-Oxosteroid 5β-reductase deficiency described in an identical twin neonatal hepatitis. J Clin Invest 82:2148–2157, 1988

Disorders of Bilirubin Metabolism

Jansen PLM: Genetic disease of bilirubin metabolism: the inherited unconjugated hyperbilirubinemias. J Hepatol 25:398–404, 1996

Kartenbeck J, Leuschner U, Mayer R, Keppler D: Absence of the canalicular isoform of the MRP gene-encoded conjugate export pump from the hepatocytes in Dubin-Johnson syndrome. Hepatology 23:1061–1066, 1996

Ritter JK, Yeatman MT, Ferreira P, Owens IS: Identification of a genetic alteration in the code for bilirubin UDP-glucuronosyltransferase in the UGT1 gene complex of a Crigler-Najjar type I patient. J Clin Invest 90: 150–155, 1992

Disorders of Fatty Acid Metabolism

Al-Odaib A, Shneider BL, Bennett MJ, et al: A defect in the transport of long-chain fatty acids associated with acute liver failure. N Engl J Med 339:1752–1757, 1998

Rinaldo P, Raymond K, Al-Odaib A, Bennett M: Clinical and biochemical features of fatty acid oxidation disorders. Curr Opin Pediatr 10:615–621, 1998

Sewell AC, Bender SW, Wirth S, Munterfering H, Ijlist L, Wanders RJA: Long-chain 3-hydroxy-CoA dehydrogenase deficiency: a severe fatty acid oxidation disorder. Eur J Pediatr 153:745–750, 1994

Primary Mitochondrial Hepatopathies

Morris AA, Taanman JW, Blake J, et al: Liver failure associated with mitochondrial DNA depletion. J Hepatol 1998; 28:556–563, 1998

Sokol RJ, Treem WR: Mitochondria and childhood liver diseases. J Pediatr Gastroenterol Nutr 28:4–16, 1999

Taanman JW, Bodnar AG, Cooper JM, et al: Molecular mechanisms in mitochondrial DNA depletion syndrome. Hum Mol Genet 6:935–942, 1997

Treem WR, Sokol RJ: Disorders of the mitochondria. Semin Liv Dis 18: 237–253, 1998

Wilson Disease

Gollan JL, Gollan TJ: Wilson disease in 1998: genetic, diagnostic and therapeutic aspects. J Hepatol 1:28–36, 1998

Schaefer M, Gitlin JD: Genetic disorders of membrane transport. IV. Wilson's disease and Menke's disease. Am J Physiol 276:G311–G314, 1999

Neonatal and Hereditary Hemochromatosis

Bacon BR. Hemochromatosis: diagnosis and Management: Gastroenterology 120:718–725, 2001

Knisely AS, O'Shea PA, Stocks JF, Dimmick JE: Oropharyngeal and upper respiratory tract mucosal-gland siderosis in neonatal hemochromatosis: an approach to biopsy diagnosis. J Pediatr 113:871–874, 1988

Muiesan P, Rela M, Kane P, et al: Liver transplantation for neonatal hemochromatosis. Arch Dis Child 73:F178–F180, 1995

Sigurdsson L, Reyes J, Kocoshis SA, Hansen TWR, Rosh J, Knisely AS: Neonatal hemochromatosis: outcomes of pharmacological and surgical therapies. J Pediatr Gastroenterol Nutr 26:85–89, 1998

Congenital Glycosylation Disorders

Freeze HH. New diagnosis and treatment of congenital hepatic fibrosis. J Pediatr Gastroent Nutr 29:104–106, 1999

Niehuse R, Hasilik M, Alton G, et al: Carbohydrate-deficient glycoprotein syndrome type 1b: phosphomannose isomerase deficiency and mannose therapy. J Clin Invest 101:1414–1420, 1998

Oren A, Houwer RH: Phosphomannoseisomerase deficiency as the cause of protein-losing enteropathy and congenital liver fibrosis. J Pediatr Gastroenterol Nutr 29:231–232, 1999

Progressive Familial Intrahepatic Cholestasis

Bull LN, van Eijk MJ, Pawlikowska L, et al: A gene encoding a P-type ATPase mutated in two forms of hereditary cholestasis. Nature Genet 18:219–224, 1998

de Vree JM, Jacquemin E, Sturm E, et al: Mutations in the *MDR3* gene cause progressive familial intrahepatic cholestasis. Proc Natl Acad Sci USA 95:282–287, 1998

Jacquemin E, Hadchouel M: Genetic basis of progressive familial intrahepatic cholestasis. J Hepatol 31:377–381, 1999

Strautnieks SS, Bull LN, Knisely AS, et al: A gene encoding a liver-specific ABC transporter is mutated in progressive familial intrahepatic cholestasis. Nature Genet 1998; 20:233–238, 1998

18.5   INFECTIONS OF THE LIVER

Regino P. Gonzalez-Peralta and Christopher Jolley

18.5.1   Viral Infections of the Liver

Viral hepatitis is a global health problem affecting millions of children and adults worldwide. There are five known human viruses that primarily infect the liver and cause hepatitis: hepatitis A, B, C, D, and E viruses. The clinical consequences of viral hepatitis vary widely, from asymptomatic infection to overt fulminant liver failure, with a high mortality rate. Hepatitis B, C, and D virus infections commonly result in chronic hepatitis with its attendant long-term sequelae, including cirrhosis and hepatocellular carcinoma. Rapid developments in molecular techniques during recent years have had a tremendous impact on the ability to diagnose and understand the pathobiology of these important human pathogens. The enhanced understanding had led to the development of effective antiviral therapy and, in some cases, successful vaccine strategies.

Many other viruses, including Epstein-Barr virus, cytomegalovirus, human herpes viruses, parvovirus B19, and paramyxoviruses, can cause hepatitis but usually do so as part of a generalized multi-organ infection. Accordingly, the liver-related aspects of these viruses are briefly presented here, as these pathogens are fully reviewed in Chapter 13.

HEPATITIS A

Hepatitis A virus (HAV) is a nonenveloped, single-strand, positive-sense RNA virus that is classified as a picornavirus, based on its genomic organization and replication strategy. HAV is a highly contagious agent that is primarily transmitted via the fecal-oral route. However, there is a brief phase of viremia during HAV infection, and parenteral transmission has been reported in illicit intravenous drug users and following the transfusion of contaminated blood or blood products. HAV infection is more common among those of low socioeconomic status, where crowded living and suboptimal sanitary conditions are likely to facilitate viral spread through close personal contact. Outbreaks of HAV have also been traced to day care centers, where unsanitary practices involving young infants and children have been implicated in viral transmission. HAV infection may be acquired by the ingestion of contaminated water, milk, or foods, particularly raw or undercooked shellfish (such as mussels, oysters, and clams but not shrimp, lobster, or crabs), fresh fruits, or raw vegetables.

Following ingestion, HAV replicates in the small intestine, migrates to the liver via the portal circulation, and infects hepatocytes through interactions with membrane-bound receptors. Mature HAV virions are then excreted into bile and feces, where viral particles can usually be detected by electron microscopy within 4 weeks after infection. The incubation period before clinical symptoms of HAV manifest is short, between 2 and 6 weeks (average 4 weeks). HAV infection begins with a prodromal stage characterized by generalized malaise, fatigue, fever, chills, arthralgia, myalgia, nausea, vomiting, diarrhea, and anorexia. The prodrome lasts a few days and is followed by overt manifestations of liver disease including jaundice, hepatomegaly (which may be tender), splenomegaly, dark urine, and light-colored stools. Variable but consistent elevations of biochemical indices of liver injury such as elevated serum aminotransferase, alkaline phosphatase values, and hyperbilirubinemia are evident in nearly all affected individuals. The severity of disease caused by HAV infection is inversely correlated to age; icteric HAV infection occurs in only approximately 10% of children younger than 5 years but in up to 80% of adults.

The diagnosis of HAV infection relies on the demonstration of specific serologic markers. Antibody to HAV (anti-HAV) of the IgM type, which is detected early after infection and is present by the onset of clinical disease, serves as the indicator of acute viral infection or recent exposure to HAV (Fig. 18-4). The level of anti-HAV IgM peaks shortly after infection and then gradually declines and becomes undetectable by 8 to 12 weeks. In contrast, IgG-type anti-HAV gradually rises and presumably persists indefinitely. This test is used to determine past infection or immunization. Sensitive molecular techniques are available that reliably detect HAV RNA but are not generally available or useful in clinical practice.

In young patients hepatitis A virus infection is usually a self-limited disease that does not become chronic and rarely results in death. Thus, management is generally supportive during the acute illness. Hospitalization may be necessary for intravenous hydration in children with severe vomiting and anorexia. Severe liver dysfunction with coagulopathy, marked cholestasis, or encephalopathy is rare in the pediatric age group but more common in adolescents

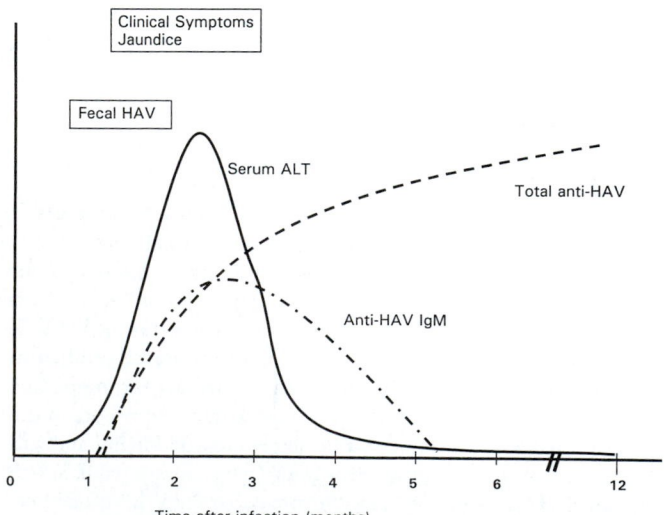

FIGURE 18-4 Time course of symptoms, ALT elevation, and serum antibodies in acute hepatitis A infection. Fecal shedding of HAV occurs before clinical illness.

TABLE 18-18

PREVENTION OF HEPATITIS A INFECTION

TYPE OF PROPHYLAXIS	DOSE (VOLUME)	DOSING SCHEDULE
Preexposure		
Intramuscular immuno-globulin	0.02 mL/kg (protects for 1–2 months)	Single dose
	0.06 mL/kg (protects for 3–5 months)	Single dose
Hepatitis A vaccine		
Vaqta (Merck)		
Children 2–17 years	25 U[a] (0.5 mL)	Initial and 6–12 months later
Persons >17 years	50 U (1.0 mL)	Initial and 6–12 months later
Havrix (SmithKline-Beecham)		
Children 2–18 years	720 EU[b] (0.5 mL)	Initial and 6–12 months later
Persons >18 years	1440 EU (1.0 mL)	Initial and 6–12 months later
Postexposure		
Immunoglobulin (in addition to HAV vaccine, if >2 years)	0.02 mL/kg Same as for preexposure	Single dose Same as for preexposure

[a] 1 U is equivalent to 1 mg of viral protein.
[b] EU = enzyme units (units used to measure viral protein).
SOURCE: American Academy of Pediatrics. Hepatitis A. In: Peter G, ed. 1997 Red Book: Report on the Committee on Infectious Diseases, 24th ed. Elk Grove Village, IL, American Academy of Pediatrics, 1997:237–246; and Centers for Disease Control and Prevention: Prevention of hepatitis A through active or passive immunization: recommendations of the Advisory Committee on Immunization Practices (ACIP). MMWR 48:1–54, 1999.

and adults. HAV infection can be particularly severe and debilitating in older patients and immunocompromised hosts. In a small proportion of patients, HAV infection can have a protracted course characterized by prolonged, intermittent, and unremitting fever, pruritus, and cholestasis that may last for months after acute infection.

Improved sanitation methods and personal hygiene are the most effective methods of preventing propagation of HAV. Preexposure prevention of HAV infection can be accomplished by the administration of immunoglobulin as passive immunization or by administration of one of the currently licensed vaccines for active immunization (Table 18-18). Passive immunization is indicated for those traveling to endemic areas whose time schedules preclude completion of the vaccine series. Immunoglobulin is also recommended to prevent viral infection in infants younger than 2 years in whom vaccine efficacy and safety have not been adequately determined. Intramuscular immunoglobulin is efficacious and safe but may interfere with the immunologic response to several live-virus vaccines including mumps, measles, rubella (administered individually or in combination), and varicella. Accordingly, mumps, measles, and rubella immunization should be delayed by 3 months and varicella vaccination by 5 months after the administration of immunoglobulin.

The administration of immunoglobulin as soon as possible, but within 2 weeks, after exposure to HAV effectively prevents infection. Postexposure prophylaxis is recommended for susceptible personal contacts of an HAV-infected individual, such as household member or sexual or needle-sharing partner. In addition, day care and nursing home staff and attendees in close contact with an HAV index case should receive passive immunization. Administration of immunoglobulin is not routinely indicated for exposures arising in school, hospital, or other workplace. Because the diagnosis of HAV infection cannot be reliably made solely on its clinical and epidemiologic features, postexposure prophylaxis should be accomplished only after serologic confirmation of HAV in index cases.

There are currently two licensed inactivated HAV vaccines. HAV immunization is currently recommended for individuals at high risk for infection, including those traveling or working in endemic areas, homosexual men, illegal drug users, and persons with clotting factor disorders or chronic liver disease. Routine vaccination is also currently recommended for children in the United States who live in "endemic" areas (rates of HAV infection twice the national average, ie, >20 cases/100,000 population), and should be considered for those living in areas of "intermediate" incidence (rates of HAV infection 10–20 cases/100,000 population).

HEPATITIS B

Hepatitis B virus (HBV) is an enveloped circular DNA virus that infects only humans and primates. HBV and the phylogenetically similar woodchuck, ground squirrel, and duck hepatitis viruses comprise the hepadnavirus family. HBV is primarily transmitted parenterally, via blood and other body fluids such as semen, cervical secretions, and saliva. Individuals at risk of HBV infection are infants born to infected mothers, intravenous drug users, homosexuals and heterosexuals with multiple partners, health-care workers, and those born in endemic areas such as Southeast Asia, the Pacific Islands, China, and Alaska. Although the prevalence of HBV infection is low in the United States (0.1–0.2%), there are an estimated 1 million HBV carriers in this country.

The clinical course and natural history of HBV infection are variable and depend on the age at which infection occurs. HBV infection during the perinatal period, infancy, and early childhood is rarely symptomatic, whereas adolescents and adults commonly develop anorexia, fatigue, myalgia, arthralgia, low-grade fever, jaundice, and hepatosplenomegaly. Variable elevations of serum aminotransferase, bilirubin, and alkaline phosphatase levels are noted. HBV acquisition during infancy results in the development of a chronic carrier state in more than 90% of cases, characterized by persistence in serum of hepatitis B surface antigen (HBsAg), high-level HBV DNA, and minimal biochemical or clinical evidence of liver disease. In contrast, acute HBV infection gradually resolves without chronic sequelae in over 90% of infected adults. Although the precise mechanisms that underlie these age-related differences in the natural history of HBV infection are unknown, experimental evidence suggests that immune tolerance to viral antigens may play an important role. In fewer than 5% of cases, HBV infection results in fulminant liver failure. Extrahepatic manifestations of HBV infection, which are primarily related to deposition of antigen-antibody complexes, include serum-sickness syndrome, glomerulonephritis, papular acrodermatitis (Gianotti-Crosti syndrome), and polyarteritis nodosa.

The diagnosis of HBV infection relies on the serologic detection of specific viral antigens and antibodies in the appropriate clinical setting (Fig. 18-5). HBsAg is usually detected early in the course of infection, even before the onset of clinical symptoms. It gradually disappears over weeks to months. In the subset of patients who develop chronic infection, HBsAg persists over extended periods,

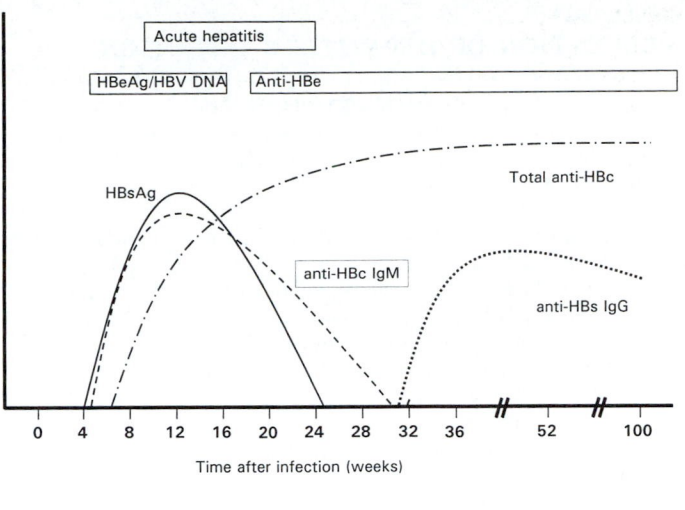

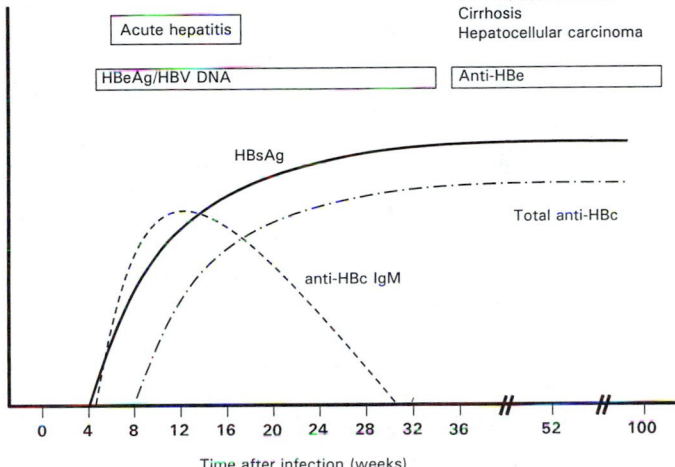

FIGURE 18-5 A. Time course of the acute symptoms and serum HBV antigens and antibodies in the typical case of acute hepatitis B infection. B. Time course of clinical features and HBV antigens and antibodies in chronic hepatitis B infection.

typically many years. Rarely, as HBsAg wanes, antibody to the hepatitis B core antigen, of the IgM class (anti-HBc IgM), may be the only marker of HBV infection. Hepatitis Be antigen (HBeAg), related to the viral core protein, and HBV DNA can be identified in serum during the acute infection. These markers, which reflect active viral replication, disappear with resolution of acute infection but persist in chronic infection. The disappearance of HBeAg and the development of anti-HBeAb indicate cessation of viral replication. In parallel with these virologic events, patients who clear the virus gradually develop anti-HBsAb. Anti-HBsAb persists indefinitely and confers life-long immunity.

Unique HBV variants have been described with stop mutations in the precore region of the virus; "precore" mutants are unable to synthesize HBeAg. Consequently, patients infected with these HBV mutants may exhibit evidence of active viral replication, determined by elevated HBV DNA levels, despite the absence of HBeAg in serum. HBV with mutations in the HBsAg has also been reported and has been associated with vaccine failure.

The management of acute HBV infection is generally supportive, with hospitalization reserved only for cases of severe disease. Effective antiviral therapies are available for chronic hepatitis B and include interferon-α and nucleoside analogs. Only the former has

TABLE 18-19

PREVENTION OF HEPATITIS B INFECTION

TYPE OF PROPHYLAXIS	DOSE (VOLUME)	DOSING SCHEDULE
Preexposure		
Hepatitis B vaccines		
Engerix-B (Merck)[a]		
Infants (born to HBV-positive or -negative moms) through 19 years	10 µg (0.5 mL)	Initial, 1 and 6 months later
Adults >20 years	20 µg (1.0 mL)	
Adults on dialysis or immunocompromised	40 µg (2.0 mL)	
Recombivax-HB (SmithKline-Beecham)		
Infants born to HBV-negative mothers	2.5 µg (0.25 mL)	Initial, 1 and 6 months later
Infants born to HBV-positive mothers	5 µg (0.5 mL)	
Children <19 years	5 µg (0.5 mL)	
Adults >20 years	10 µg (1.0 mL)	
Adults on dialysis or immunocompromised[b]	40 µg (1.0 mL)	
Postexposure		
HBIG[c] (in addition to HBV vaccine, as above)	0.02 mL/kg	Single dose

[a] Engerix-B can be given at an optional four-dose schedule: initial, 1, 2, and 6–12 months later.
[b] Special concentrated formulation for these patients.
[c] HBIG = hepatitis B immunoglobulin.
SOURCE: American Academy of Pediatrics: Hepatitis B. In: Peter G, ed. 1997 Red Book: Report on the Committee on Infectious Diseases, 24th ed. Elk Grove Village, IL, American Academy of Pediatrics, 1997:247–260.

thus far been licensed for use in children. Interferon-α induces sustained viral remission (disappearance of serum HBV DNA and HBeAg) in 25 to 40% of children and adults with chronic hepatitis B. Factors that have been associated with response to interferon include active liver disease (elevated serum aminotransferase values and active histologic inflammation), low pretreatment HBV DNA levels, female gender, short duration of disease, and absence of infection with hepatitis D virus or human immunodeficiency virus. Interferon-α is generally well tolerated by children; the most common adverse event described is a flu-like syndrome characterized by fever, headaches, chills, and myalgias, which generally resolve within the initial two to three doses. Other reported side effects include bone marrow suppression, neuropsychiatric disorders (depression and anxiety), fatigue, diarrhea, and anorexia and weight loss. Strategies to enhance response rates such as using prednisone before interferon (increasing hepatocyte HBV antigen expression) have been generally disappointing.

Lamivudine is a cytosine analog that effectively inhibits HBV replication in adults as measured by rapid and marked reduction of HBV DNA during therapy. Clinical trials are under way to determine the safety and efficacy of lamivudine therapy in children with chronic hepatitis B. Several other nucleoside analogs that are undergoing clinical testing include adefovir, lobucavir, dideoxyfluorothiacytidine (FTC), D-diaminopurindixolane (DAPD), and L-fluromethylarabinosyluracil (L-FMAU).

Although infants and children who are chronic HBV carriers have little clinical and histologic evidence of liver disease, they are at highest risk to develop cirrhosis and hepatocellular carcinoma. Because children have minimal liver disease, they often do not benefit from currently available antiviral therapy. Although screening strategies to detect early hepatocellular carcinoma are evolving, periodic determinations of serum α-fetoprotein and serial abdominal sonography, as recommended for adults, seem reasonable approaches for children with chronic HBV infection.

HBV infection can be effectively prevented after exposure by administration of hepatitis B immunoglobulin (HBIG). This preparation, with a high titer of anti-HBs, is indicated in the prevention of perinatal transmission from HBV-infected women and should

be given to neonates in the first hours of life. Completion of immunoprophylaxis in this setting is accomplished with active immunization with one of the two licensed HBV vaccines. Following the initial failure of immunization strategies, which targeted high-risk individuals, vaccination is now recommended for all newborns, all preadolescent children, and adults at high risk.

HBV vaccination is the most effective strategy to prevent HBV infection. However, postexposure prophylaxis can be achieved by the administration of hepatitis B immunoglobulin (HBIG) (Table 18-19). HBIG is particularly useful for neonates born to HBV-infected mothers and for susceptible sexual partners of acutely infected persons. HBIG can also be use to prevent HBV infection after accidental exposure.

Plasma-derived HBV vaccines have been replaced in the United States by products made by recombinant DNA technology. Because initial vaccine programs targeting high-risk individuals were ineffective in reducing the rate of HBV-related disease, universal immunization of children and adolescents is currently recommended. Recent concerns about mercury exposure in neonates and young children by thimerosal (used as vaccine preservative) prompted the development of preservative-free formulations, which are currently available. Recommendations for vaccination against HBV infection are detailed in Table 18-19.

HEPATITIS D

Hepatitis D virus (HDV, formerly called the δ agent) is a small, single-strand, negative-sense RNA virus that is phylogenetically related to plant virions. HDV is a rare cause of hepatitis in the United States but is endemic in various parts of Africa, Europe, and the Amazon basin. HDV is a defective virus that is intimately dependent on HBV, as it requires HBsAg for complete virus assembly and propagation. As such, HDV infection can occur only in individuals infected with HBV, and its pattern of transmission mimics that of HBV.

HDV infection occurs either as a coinfection, in which HDV and HBV are acquired simultaneously, or as a superinfection, in which an HBV-infected individual acquires HDV from a subsequent exposure. Coinfection rarely results in chronic hepatitis, whereas superinfection is commonly associated with chronic disease with risk or progression to cirrhosis. HDV infection should be suspected and carefully sought in cases of fulminant HBV infection or in HBV-infected individuals who experience a sudden worsening of their liver disease.

The diagnosis of HDV infection is made by the detection of anti-HDV antibody, HDV antigen, or HDV RNA in serum. Antiviral therapies are generally ineffective in chronic HBV/HDV infection. Thus, prevention or treatment of HBV is at present the best method to successfully reduce and eliminate HDV-related liver disease.

HEPATITIS C

Hepatitis C virus (HCV) is an enveloped, single-strand, positive-sense RNA virus. It is the major causative agent of non-A, non-B hepatitis. HCV is genetically heterogeneous and has been classified into six types and multiple subtypes. HCV type 1 is the most prevalent worldwide and accounts for 70% of infections in the United States. Within infected patients, HCV exists as highly heterogeneous populations of closely related genomes (quasispecies); this has turned out to have important pathobiological implications.

In the United States, the estimated prevalence of HCV infection in children ≤18 years of age is 0.1 to 0.2%, as compared to 1.8% in adults. Thus, there are approximately 150,000 children and 3 million adults chronically infected with HCV in the United States. Because HCV is a parenterally transmitted pathogen, children at risk include infants born to HCV-infected mothers and recipients of transfusions of blood and blood products before 1992 (Table 18-20). The routine screening of blood for HCV has resulted in a dramatic decline in transfusion-associated infection, and perinatal exposure has become the major mode of transmission to children.

Acute HCV infection is clinically asymptomatic in the majority of patients; occasionally fatigue, anorexia, myalgia, and manifestations of liver disease such as jaundice and hepatomegaly may be experienced during the acute phase (Fig. 18-6). The importance of HCV infection lies in its propensity to cause insidiously progressive liver damage. The natural history and pathobiology of HCV infection in infants and children is incompletely understood, but HCV infection leads to chronic liver disease in some children. It is gen-

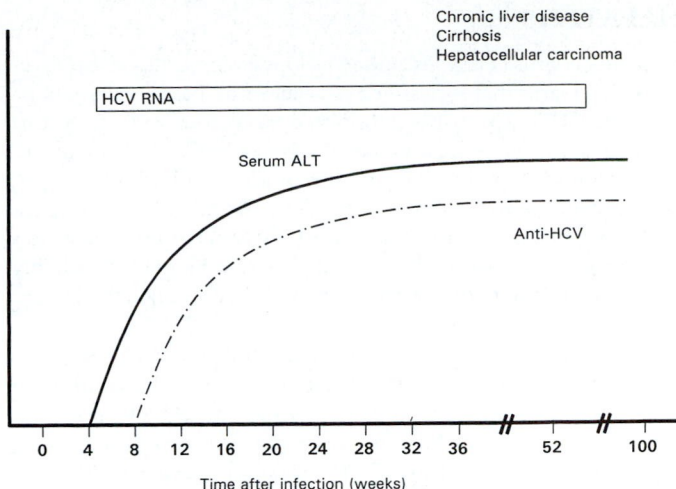

FIGURE 18-6   Time course of ALT elevation (which may be very mild), antibody to HCV, and HCV RNA in chronic hepatitis C infection. Note that there are often no symptoms until complications of chronic hepatitis develop after many years.

erally mild, although aggressive liver disease with fibrosis and even cirrhosis can occur. Extrahepatic manifestations commonly seen in adults, such as cryoglobulinemia, membranoproliferative glomerulonephritis, leukocytoclastic vasculitis, thyroiditis, and idiopathic thrombocytopenia, are seldom reported in children.

The diagnosis of HCV infection is based on the detection of antibody to HCV (anti-HCV) in serum. Confirmatory testing with a more complex recombinant immunoblot assay (RIBA) may be considered for low-risk groups such as "healthy" volunteer blood donors who are discovered to be anti-HCV positive during routine screening. Anti-HCV–positive individuals with known risk for HCV infection should be further tested for the presence of virus in serum with the polymerase chain reaction (PCR) technique. Although current immune-based assays that detect anti-HCV are accurate and reliable, PCR assays are required to identify viral infection in infants born to infected mothers, as anti-HCV antibodies present in newborns are typically derived from maternal serum. Liver biopsy is rarely indicated in acute HCV infection but may be valuable in the chronic stage. Histologic findings of chronic hepatitis C in children are similar to those in adults and include variable degrees of portal and lobular chronic inflammation, damage of small bile duct epithelia, and microvesicular and macrovesicular steatosis. Lymphoid aggregates, which suggest immunologic activation, are also frequently noted in chronic hepatitis C.

If, when, and how to treat children with chronic hepatitis C are at present uncertain and controversial, but spontaneous viral remission is unusual, and liver disease may progress silently in children. Accordingly, antiviral therapy may be of benefit but is not yet licensed in the pediatric population. Interferon-α therapy has been generally disappointing in adults, with sustained virologic response achieved in only 10 to 15% of cases. Significantly better results have been obtained with combination interferon-α and ribavirin, a synthetic nucleoside analog with sustained virologic responses observed in 40 to 50% of those treated. The use of multiple treatment regimens in mostly small and uncontrolled clinical trials of interferon-α in children with chronic hepatitis C makes direct comparison to the adult data difficult. Sustained responses to interferon-α therapy are better in children (30–60%) than in adults but still suboptimal in the small uncontrolled studies reported.

TABLE 18-20
PEDIATRIC GROUPS AT HIGH RISK FOR HCV INFECTION

GROUP	VIRAL PREVALENCE RATE
Infants born to HCV-infected mothers	
HIV-negative mothers	0–12% (average 6%)
HIV-positive mothers	0–36% (average 16%)
Recipients of multiple blood products	
Hemophilia	50–80%
Thalassemia	40–80%
Cancer survivors	10–50%
Hemodialysis	20–45%
Sickle-cell disease	10–25%
Post–extracorporeal membrane oxygenation	8%
Non-A, non-B hepatitis	80%

HEPATITIS E

Hepatitis E virus (HEV) is a nonenveloped, single-strand, positive-sense RNA virus that is classified as a calicivirus, based on its genetic structure. HEV is primarily transmitted via the fecal-oral route, usually in association with contaminated water. HEV infection is rare in the United States but is responsible for large epidemics and sporadic hepatitis in parts of Asia, Africa, the Middle East, and Mexico. The recent demonstration of anti-HEV in pigs in Midwestern states and in rats in Maryland, Hawaii, and Louisiana raises the possibility that these animals could be reservoirs of this infection in the United States.

Although childhood HEV infection is usually an acute self-limited disease, severe hepatitis and fulminant liver failure with high mortality can occur, particularly in young adults and pregnant women, although this difference in severity is not explained. After a variable incubation period (2–10 weeks), some patients develop a prodrome of fever, generalized malaise, fatigue, and anorexia. Overt manifestations of liver disease including jaundice, abdominal pain, and hepatomegaly are also common. Severe cholestasis, coagulopathy, and changes in mental status herald the development of liver failure, which can be rapidly fatal. The diagnosis of HEV infection relies on the detection of anti-HEV antibody in the appropriate clinical setting. HEV RNA can be detected with sensitive molecular techniques but this is seldom clinically indicated. Symptomatic HEV-infected children are usually managed conservatively and supportively. Because pregnant women are more likely to develop severe hepatitis, they should be carefully monitored during the illness.

EPSTEIN-BARR VIRUS

Epstein-Barr virus (EBV) is a DNA virus that is transmitted primarily by close person-to-person contact with infected secretions, particularly saliva. After initial replication in epithelial cells of the oropharynx, EBV disseminates throughout the reticuloendothelial system by propagating in B lymphocytes. In immunocompetent patients, clinical illness is typically characterized by fever, myalgia, fatigue, pharyngitis, generalized lymphadenopathy, variable lymphocytosis, and atypical lymphocytes on blood smear. Liver involvement is common in childhood EBV infection; it is manifested by hepatosplenomegaly, which may be tender, modestly elevated aminotransferase values, and, occasionally, jaundice. The course of liver disease is usually mild and self-limited but occasionally can be severe and protracted, particularly in immunocompromised hosts. Although liver biopsy is generally not indicated in EBV infection, it should be considered in severe cases with atypical features. Characteristic histologic findings that support the diagnosis of EBV include varying degrees of portal and lobular inflammation and sinusoidal infiltration by mononuclear cells.

The diagnosis of EBV usually relies on the detection of specific host-derived antibodies produced in response to viral infection (Sec. 13.4.8). Management of EBV hepatitis is usually supportive, although short courses of prednisone may be indicated in selected children with severe or prolonged illness. Antiviral agents have no proven benefit in the treatment of EBV infection in immunocompetent patients.

OTHER VIRUSES ASSOCIATED WITH HEPATITIS

Other human herpes viruses, including cytomegalovirus and human herpes virus (HHV) types 1, 2, and 6, may be associated with liver disease, predominantly in neonates and infants. The clinical course of these infections can be severe in neonates and immunocompromised children. *Congenital cytomegalovirus* presents with a clinical picture that resembles idiopathic neonatal hepatitis. Rising titers of CMV-specific IgG and IgM antibodies and urinary cultures establish the diagnosis. Characteristic cytoplasmic inclusions in biliary epithelium and hepatocytes are observed in fewer than 5% of patients, but in situ hybridization will increase yields. Cytomegalovirus causes chronic inflammation and fibrosis, distorting the lobular architecture, and can lead to cirrhosis. *Parvovirus B19* is a small single-strand DNA virus that causes erythema infectiosum and has been associated with hydrops fetalis and aplastic anemia. Although liver involvement is seldom seen in these conditions, parvovirus B19 infection has recently been implicated in fulminant liver failure in children and acute hepatitis in adults. Infections with *paramyxoviruses,* such as mumps and measles, very occasionally involve the liver and usually in the context of generalized disease. A paramyxo-like agent has been implicated in an adult with syncytial giant-cell hepatitis.

GB viruses (GBV-A, GBV-B, and GBV-C) are a newly discovered group of infectious agents that are phylogenetically related to HCV. GBV-A and GBV-B are naturally occurring viruses in tamarins, and humans are the natural host for GBV-C. This virus has also been referred to as hepatitis G virus (HGV). Initial studies correlating HGV with hepatitis and chronic liver disease have not been subsequently confirmed. Similarly, a novel transfusion-related DNA virus, TTV, has not been directly linked to liver disease. Other rare causes of childhood hepatitis include the yellow fever and dengue viruses, which are endemic in tropical and subtropical areas, and enteroviruses, which account for some cases of neonatal liver failure.

18.5.2 Other Infections of the Liver

PYOGENIC ABSCESS

Pyogenic abscesses may arise by contiguous spread after hepatobiliary surgery or trauma or by bacterial migration through the hepatic circulation. They are a recognized complication of chronic inflammatory bowel disease and appendicitis. Pyogenic abscesses more commonly involve the right lobe of the liver. Symptoms are usually mild and nonspecific and include fever and abdominal pain, although hepatomegaly, tenderness in the right upper quadrant of the abdomen, and jaundice may also occur. Leukocytosis with immature white blood cells, elevated sedimentation rate, and hyperbilirubinemia should alert the clinician to the possibility of bacterial infection involving the liver. The presumptive diagnosis of liver abscess rests on the demonstration of characteristic lesions by abdominal imaging studies such as ultrasonography, computerized tomography, and magnetic resonance. Analysis of fluid (Gram stain and culture) obtained by percutaneous aspiration, if possible, provides bacteriologic diagnosis. In children, gram-positive bacteria are most frequently implicated, although gram-negative and anaerobic pathogens are also frequently encountered. Amebic abscess can be indistinguishable in clinical presentation from pyogenic abscess, but aspirated fluid is sterile and odorless in comparison (see Sec. 13.6.5). Initial treatment of pyogenic abscess includes broad-spectrum antibiotics, which can be narrowed based on results of bacteriologic sensitivities. Percutaneous or surgical drainage should also be considered.

BACTERIAL CHOLANGITIS

Bacterial cholangitis is encountered in children with underlying hepatobiliary disease such as biliary atresia, cholelithiasis, Caroli syndrome, and other cystic diseases of the liver. The clinical manifestations include fever, jaundice, and right upper quadrant tenderness (Charcot triad) in addition to leukocytosis, hyperbilirubinemia, and elevated serum aminotransferase and alkaline phosphatase levels. Specific bacterial pathogens may be recovered by peripheral blood culture in approximately 50% of cases. Liver biopsy is rarely indicated for the diagnosis of cholangitis but should be considered in cases of prolonged, refractory infection or in immunocompromised children (particularly after liver transplantation), where the identification of specific bacterial pathogens or exclusion of other hepatobiliary problems may be critical. Histologic features of cholangitis include neutrophilic infiltration of bile duct epithelia, portal expansion, and varying degrees of bile ductular proliferation. *Escherichia coli* and other gram-negative organisms are most frequently identified in bacterial cholangitis, but anaerobes and enterococci are also commonly recovered. Thus, as for pyogenic abscesses, initial broad-spectrum antimicrobial therapy is recommended, with subsequent tailoring dictated by bacteriologic sensitivity testing. Obstructive processes that predispose to the development of bacterial cholangitis, such as bile duct stones or strictures, require specific endoscopic or surgical therapy.

OTHER BACTERIAL INFECTIONS

Other infections that involve the liver include cat-scratch disease, gonococcal perihepatitis (Fitz-Hugh–Curtis syndrome), syphilis, leptospirosis, tuberculosis, typhoid fever, brucellosis, and Lyme disease. These infections usually affect the liver as part of a generalized process and are discussed elsewhere in the text.

FUNGAL INFECTIONS OF THE LIVER

Candida species and other fungi, including *Cryptococcus neoformans, Coccidiodides immitis, Histoplasma encapsulatum,* and *Aspergillus* species, occasionally infect the liver. Fungal infections of liver are more common in immunocompromised individuals, especially those being treated for hematologic malignancy, and usually arise as part of a disseminated process, rarely as the primary infection. Clinical manifestations include fever, abdominal pain, and symptoms related to the underlying disease. Laboratory findings that alert the clinician to the possibility of fungal infection are nonspecific and include leukocytosis or leukopenia, anemia, thrombocytopenia, hyperbilirubinemia, and elevated serum aminotransferase and alkaline phosphatase values. Diagnosis relies on a high index of suspicion and meticulous serologic and radiographic evaluation. Liver biopsy may be crucial in the identification of specific fungal pathogens. Therapy includes prompt and judicious use of antifungal therapy; surgical drainage or removal of fungal abscesses, if present, may be warranted.

References

Alter MI, Kruszon-Moran D, Nainan OV, et al: The prevalence of hepatitis C virus infection in the United States, 1988 through 1994. N Engl J Med 341:556–562, 1999

American Academy of Pediatrics: Hepatitis B. In: Peter G, ed: 1997 Red Book: Report on the Committee on Infectious Diseases, 24th ed. Elk Grove Village, IL, American Academy of Pediatrics, 1997:247–260

Centers for Disease Control and Prevention: Prevention of hepatitis A through active or passive immunization: recommendations of the Advisory Committee on Immunization Practices (ACIP). MMWR 48:1–54, 1999

Chusid MJ: Pyogenic abscess in infancy and childhood. Pediatrics 62:554–558, 1978

Francis DP, Hadler SC, Prendergast TJ, et al: Occurrence of hepatitis A, B, and non-A/non-B in the United States. CDC sentinel county hepatitis study I. Am J Med 76:69–74, 1984

González-Peralta RP: Hepatitis C virus infection in pediatric patients. Clin Liver Dis 1:691–705, 1997

González-Peralta RP, Galasso GJ, Poynard T, Schalm S, Thomas HC, Wright TL: Summary of the first international symposium on viral hepatitis. Antivir Res 42:77–96, 1999

Gottrand F, Bernard O, Hadchouel M, et al: Late cholangitis after successful surgical repair of biliary atresia. Am J Dis Child 145:213–215, 1991

Hadler SC, McFarland L: Hepatitis in day care centers; epidemiology and prevention. Rev Infect Dis 8:548–557, 1986

Hadziyannis SJ: Hepatitis D. Clin Liver Dis 3:309–325, 1999

Hoofnagle JH: Therapy of viral hepatitis. Digestion 59:563–578, 1998

Jonas MM: The treatment of hepatitis C in pediatric patients. Clin Liver Dis 3:855–867, 1999

Krawczynski K, Aggarwal R: Hepatitis E: In: ER Schiff, MF Sorrell, WC Maddrey, eds: Schiff's Diseases of the Liver. Philadelphia, Lippincott-Raven, 1999

McQuillan GM, Coleman PJ, Kruszon-Moran D, Moyer LA, Lambert SB, Margolis HS: Prevalence of hepatitis B virus infection in the United States: the National Health and Nutrition Examination Surveys, 1976 through 1994. Am J Public Health 89:14–18, 1999

Novak DA, Dolson DJ: Bacterial, parasitic and fungal infections of the liver. In: Suchy F, ed: Liver Diseases in Children. St Louis, Mosby-Year Book, 1994

Piñneiro-Carrero VM, Andres JM: Morbidity and mortality in children with pyogenic abscess. Am J Dis Child 143:1424–1427, 1989

Pizzo PA, Rubin M, Freifels A, et al: The child with cancer and infection. II. Nonbacterial infections. J Pediatr 119:845–857, 1991

18.6   TOXIN-ASSOCIATED LIVER DISEASES

Regino P. Gonzalez-Peralta and Christopher Jolley

TOTAL PARENTERAL NUTRITION–ASSOCIATED LIVER DISEASE

Total parenteral nutrition (TPN) may cause liver injury in both pediatric and adult patients. Indications, monitoring, and nonliver complications of TPN are discussed in Sec. 17.6.2. The liver damage associated with TPN may be reversible; however, in situations in which prolonged TPN is required, cirrhosis and eventually liver failure have occurred. In fact, end-stage liver disease has replaced catheter-related sepsis and malnutrition as the leading cause of death in TPN-dependent infants with short bowel syndrome.

Infants, particularly those born preterm, are most susceptible to hepatic injury from TPN. The most common feature of this injury is TPN-associated cholestasis, which is generally accepted to be related to multiple factors. Premature infants will often rely solely on parenteral nutrition for long periods of time because of bowel immaturity. Necrotizing enterocolitis or congenital malformations of the gut with or without surgical resection often make prolonged use of TPN a necessity. Younger gestational age, lower birth weight, and a longer duration of TPN are associated with increased likelihood of TPN-associated cholestasis. Comorbid conditions

TABLE 18-21
DRUGS CAUSING LIVER INJURY

DRUG	TOXICITY[a]	PREDOMINANT CLINICAL PATTERN[b]	DRUG	TOXICITY[a]	PREDOMINANT CLINICAL PATTERN[b]
Analgesics			*Estrogens:*		
Acetaminophen (Tylenol)	D	A,CAH,F	Ethinyl estradiol	D	Ch,A
Acetylsalicylic acid (aspirin)	D	A	Methylestranolone	D	Ch,A
Propoxyphene (Darvon)	H	Ch	*Progestins:*		
Anesthetics			Norethindrone (Norlutin)	D	A
Halothane (Fluothane)	H	A,F	**Antithyroid agents**		
Antibiotics			Methimazole (Tapazole)	H	Ch
Erythromycin estolate	H,D	Ch	Propylthiouracil	H	A
Griseofulvin	H,D	Ch	Thiouracil	H	Ch,A,F
Isoniazid	H,D	A,CAH,F	Thiourea	H	A
Nitrofurantoin (Furadantin)	H	Ch	**Hypoglycemic agents**		
Oxacillin (Prostaphlin)	H	Ch	Carbutamide	H	A
Quinacrine (Atabrine)	H	A,F	Chlorpropamide (Diabinese)	H,D	Ch
Rifampin	H,D	Ch	Metahexamide (Euglycin)	H	Ch,A,CAH
Sulfonamides	H,D	A,CAH,F	Tolbutamide (Orinase)	D,H	Ch
Tetracyclines	D	CAH	**Psychopharmacologic agents**		
Anticonvulsants			*Phenothiazines:*		
Phenytoin (Dilantin)	H	A,Ch,F	Chlorpromazine (Thorazine)	D,H	Ch
Phenacemide Phenurone)	H	A,Ch	Mepazine (Pactal)	H,D	Ch
Trimethadione (Tridione)	H	A	Perphenazine (Trilafon)	H,D	Ch
Valproate	H	F	Prochlorperazine (Compazine)	H	Ch,A,CAH
Diuretic agents			Promazine (Sparine)	H	Ch
Chlorothiazide (Diuril)	H	Ch	Thioridazine (Mellaril)	H	Ch
Methyldopa (Aldomet)	H,D	A,CAH	*Monoamine oxidase inhibitors:*		
Quinethazone (Hydromox)	H	Ch	Iproniazid (Marsalid)	H	A,CAH
Cytotoxins and immuno-suppressants			Isocarboxazid (Marplan)	H	A
Azathioprine (Imuran)	D	A	*Other psychopharmacologic agents:*		
Chlorambucil (Leukeran)	H	A	Chlordiazepoxide (Librium)	H	Ch
6-Mercaptopurine	D	A,F,C	Diazepam (Valium)	H	Ch
Methotrexate	D	C	Ethchlorvynol (Placidyl)	H	Ch
Urethane	D	A,F,C	Imipramine (Tofranil)	H	Ch,A
Hormones and metabolic agents			Meprobamate (Equanil)	H	Ch
Androgens:			**Miscellaneous**		
Methyltestosterone	D	Ch,A	Topical copper sulfate	D	A
Norethandrolone	D	Ch,A	Ferrous sulfate	D	A,CAH
			Trimethobenzamide (Tigan)	H	Ch
			Tripelennamine (Pyribenzamine)	H	Ch

[a] D = dose-dependent liver damage; H = dose-independent liver damage due to hypersensitivity or idiosyncratic response.
[b] A = acute hepatitis; CAH = chronic active hepatitis; F = fulminant hepatitis; Ch = cholestasis; C = cirrhosis.
SOURCE: *Zimmerman H: Hepatotoxicity. The Adverse Effects of Drugs and Other Chemicals on the Liver. New York, Appleton-Century-Crofts, 1979.*

such as sepsis, hypoxia, or immature hepatic function are commonly encountered in the preterm infant, but TPN-related factors such as taurine or carnitine deficiency may also play important roles in the development of cholestasis and subsequent hepatic disease.

The onset of TPN-associated cholestasis (TPN-AC) is usually insidious. Hepatomegaly and conjugated hyperbilirubinemia raise the suspicion of likely TPN-associated cholestasis, but other etiologies of cholestasis must be considered (see Sec. 18.2). Because TPN-AC is often a diagnosis of exclusion, the evaluation includes ultrasonography and possibly hepatobiliary scintigraphy, which may identify an obstructive lesion. Other considerations are inborn errors of metabolism and congenital infection. A liver biopsy may help to exclude disorders such as storage diseases; however, the histopathology seen with TPN-associated cholestasis includes portal inflammation, cholestasis, and frequently fibrosis, which are suggestive but not diagnostic findings.

Because the specific cause of liver disease associated with TPN has not been determined, the treatment remains ill defined. Provision of at least some enteral nutrition has been shown to improve cholestasis and slow the development of liver injury. Agents such as phenobarbital and ursodeoxycholic acid are frequently used to improve bile flow. Other treatment modalities involve preventing photooxidation of the TPN solution, cycling the parenteral nutrition, and modifying its composition. In its early stages, TPN-associated liver disease may be reversible if enteral nutrition can be instituted.

In older children, adolescents, and adults, TPN-associated liver injury is more likely to present with steatosis (fatty liver) than cholestasis and inflammation. The pathophysiological process responsible for the steatosis is not completely understood, but possible mechanisms include an excessive calorie-to-nitrogen ratio, an excessive glucose infusion rate, and carnitine deficiency. As with cholestatic liver injury in infants, cessation of TPN usually results in a normalization of liver enzymes. Administration of some enteral nutrition is also useful.

DRUG HEPATOXICITY

Adverse drug reactions in children are uncommon. Nevertheless, drug-induced hepatotoxicity, when it occurs, must be promptly recognized, and the offending agent discontinued, although cessation does not always result in rapid recovery. Delays may contribute significantly to morbidity, resulting in a need for liver transplantation or in death.

The role of the liver in the processing or biotransformation of xenobiotics (foreign substances) is discussed in Sec. 18.1. Mechanisms of hepatotoxicity vary, as they depend on the drug, dosage, and patient factors such as age, gender, nutrition, and genetic predisposition. In general, medicinal and environmental agents known to have hepatotoxicity have been characterized as predictable (intrinsic) or unpredictable (idiosyncratic) hepatotoxins. The patterns of liver injuries are clinically and histopathologically diverse (Table 18-21).

Hepatotoxins that are commonly prescribed for the pediatric population include analgesics (acetaminophen), anticonvulsants, and antibiotics. Acetaminophen is a predictable or intrinsic hepatotoxin, and acetaminophen overdose has been recognized as the most common cause of liver failure in the United Kingdom. Specific therapy for acetaminophen overdose is available. *N*-Acetylcysteine, when provided in the first hours or days after overdose, replenishes glutathione stores and enables the liver to metabolize acetaminophen without generating toxic metabolites (see Sec. 4.3.3).

Examples of idiosyncratic hepatotoxic reactions are those associated with phenytoin, an anticonvulsant, and sulfasalazine, used in the treatment of inflammatory bowel disease. These drugs may cause an illness that resembles a hypersensitivity reaction, with lymphadenopathy, fever, sore throat, and peripheral as well as tissue eosinophilia. Other idiosyncratic reactions may depend on drug metabolism and are not necessarily associated with this clinical picture.

Commonly prescribed antibiotics such as erythromycin have been associated with hepatic injury, although antibiotic-associated hepatotoxicity appears to be more common in adults. Nevertheless, fulminant hepatic failure has been reported in a child receiving trimethoprim-sulfamethoxazole. Minocycline, frequently used in the treatment of adolescent acne, has been associated with the development of autoimmune hepatitis. The loss of intrahepatic bile ducts or "vanishing bile duct syndrome" has been associated with synthetic penicillins and the anticonvulsant carbamazepine. Pemoline, a stimulant used in the treatment of attention deficit disorder, has been reported to cause hepatic necrosis. Oral contraceptives have been associated with hepatic vein thrombosis (Budd-Chiari syndrome) and liver tumors. Recreational drugs of abuse are increasingly reported as causes of hepatic injury in adolescents.

It is mandatory that a history of prescribed, over-the-counter, or illicit drug usage be sought in any child who presents with evidence of hepatic dysfunction. The treatment of drug-induced liver injury depends largely on timely recognition, which may be evident by increased serum aminotransferase values, conjugated hyperbilirubinemia, coagulopathy, jaundice, or more systemic side effects such as fever, lymphadenopathy, and rash. Once a drug-induced liver injury is identified, therapy is mainly supportive, but withdrawal of the offending agent is critical to minimize hepatotoxicity.

With the exception of acetaminophen overdose, no specific therapies exist.

ENVIRONMENTAL HEPATOTOXINS

There are several types of environmental hepatotoxins. These include herbal preparations used as nutritional or health aids, contaminated food (fungicide-treated wheat), and household items such as pesticides or cleaning products. Occasionally, liver toxicity results when these toxins are ingested either as a form of drug abuse (inhalants) or as a suicide attempt.

As discussed for pharmaceutical agents, the mechanisms of hepatotoxicity of environmental toxins vary. Ingestion of poisonous mushrooms, eg, *Amanita phalloides*, results in fatty liver (steatosis) and hepatocyte necrosis that is often severe, rapidly progressive, and fatal. Venoocclusive liver disease has been reported with certain herbal teas such as comfrey, taken as a nutritional supplement.

Treatment of liver toxicity secondary to environmental agents is comparable to that for drug-induced liver injury. Avoidance or withdrawal of the offending agent is crucial, and this usually depends on an accurate historical account. Therapy is usually supportive, but there are a few exceptions. Toxicity from iron overdose is treated with chelation therapy.

References

Balistreri WF, Bove KE: Hepatobiliary consequences of parenteral alimentation. In: Popper H, Schaffner F, eds: Progress in Liver Disease. Philadelphia, WB Saunders, 1990:567–601

Briones ER, Iber FL: Liver and biliary tract changes and injury associated with total parenteral nutrition: pathogenesis and prevention. J Am Coll Nutr 14:219–229, 1995

Lee WM: Review article: drug-induced hepatotoxicity. Aliment Pharmacol Ther 7:477–485, 1993

McKenzie MW, Marchall GL, Netzloff ML, Cluff LE: Adverse drug reactions leading to hospitalization in children. Pediatrics 89:487–490, 1976

Sze G, Kaplowitz N: Drug hepatotoxicity as a cause of acute liver failure. In: Lee WM, Williams R, eds: Acute Liver Failure. Cambridge, Cambridge University Press, 1997:19–31

Zimmerman HJ: Drug-induced liver disease. In: Schiff ER, Sorrell MF, Maddrey WC, eds: Schiff's Diseases of the Liver. Philadelphia, Lippincott-Raven, 1999:973–1064

18.7 AUTOIMMUNE HEPATOBILIARY DISEASE

Regino P. Gonzalez-Peralta and Christopher Jolley

AUTOIMMUNE HEPATITIS

Formerly called autoimmune chronic active hepatitis, the term *autoimmune hepatitis* represents a variety of distinct immune-mediated liver diseases that differ both clinically and serologically. These diseases are inflammatory in nature and may overlap with immune-mediated diseases of the bile ducts, specifically primary biliary cirrhosis and primary sclerosing cholangitis. Although autoimmune hepatitis is uncommon in comparison to infectious hepatitis, early diagnosis is critical because the timely initiation of therapy can prevent or defer liver failure or end-stage chronic liver disease.

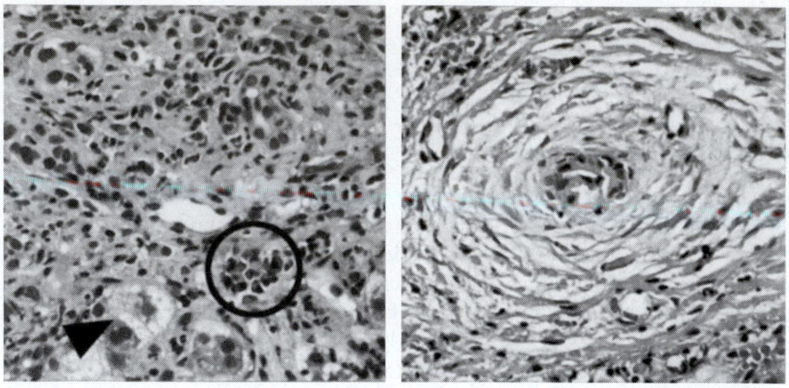

FIGURE 18-7 **A.** Photomicrograph of the liver demonstrating typical features of autoimmune hepatitis including mixed inflammatory infiltrate and a cluster of plasma cells (*circle*). **B.** Photomicrograph of the liver demonstrating the periductular fibrosis characteristic of primary sclerosing cholangitis.

The cause of autoimmune hepatitis is unknown, but genetic predisposition is believed to play a major role because autoimmune hepatitis frequently occurs in individuals with other autoimmune diseases or in families with these disorders. Research efforts have focused on the major histocompatibility complex, particularly the HLA DR region, which has been associated with genetic susceptibility to other autoimmune disorders. Predisposition alone or in conjunction with an insult such as a viral infection or drug exposure may initiate the immune-mediated cascade that results in a progressive inflammatory process within the liver. Certain viruses may exhibit molecular similarities with liver tissue, resulting in the cross-recognition of hepatic tissue as nonself and subsequent immunologic attack. Viruses that have been implicated include the hepatotropic viruses A, B, and C as well as EBV and HSV. Minocycline, pemoline, and other drugs have also been associated with the development of autoimmune hepatitis.

Autoimmune hepatitis has been characterized into three types. *Type 1 autoimmune hepatitis* is the "classic" form associated with the presence in serum of smooth muscle and/or antinuclear antibody (SMA/ANA). This form more commonly affects females and exhibits two incidence peaks, at 10 to 20 and 45 to 70 years. *Type 2 autoimmune hepatitis* is characterized by liver-kidney microsomal-1 antibody (anti-LKM-1) in serum. It tends to occur in younger children, presenting with more severe or advanced liver disease than in type 1, and there is no clear gender predilection. A less common form of autoimmune hepatitis is associated with Coombs-positive hemolytic anemia and is histologically characterized by giants cells (postinfantile giant-cell hepatitis). ANA, SMA, and LKM antibodies are not found in the serum. Rarely, "seronegative autoimmune hepatitis" is encountered, in which the histologic features of autoimmune hepatitis are recognized, and no other causes of liver disease are identified, but none of the typical autoantibodies are identified.

The clinical presentation of autoimmune hepatitis is highly variable. The onset is often insidious, with only malaise, weight loss, or anorexia. Complications of cirrhosis and portal hypertension such as variceal bleeding may be the first sign of liver disease, and jaundice can vary from nonexistent to severe. Occasionally patients can present in fulminant hepatic failure. A family history of immune-mediated diseases such as thyroiditis, arthritis, or inflammatory bowel disease should raise suspicion when one is considering autoimmune hepatitis.

The diagnosis of autoimmune hepatitis usually depends on the presence of specific serologic markers as well as liver histology. Typically patients will have elevated serum aminotransferase values in conjunction with an elevated serum total protein as a result of hypergammaglobulinemia. Viral hepatitis needs to be excluded, particularly HCV infection, which can be accompanied by either ANA or LKM autoantibody. Other causes of hepatitis, such as Wilson disease and α_1-antitrypsin deficiency, must also be considered. Confirmation of a diagnosis of autoimmune hepatitis is generally accomplished by histologic examination, although coagulopathy at presentation may preclude percutaneous biopsy. Characteristic findings include portal lymphoplasmacytic infiltrates that can extend to the surrounding hepatic lobule (Fig. 18-7A) and varying degrees of interface hepatitis, hepatocellular necrosis, and bridging fibrosis. These histologic features can also be seen with primary sclerosing cholangitis, which may need to be excluded as the primary diagnosis.

The treatment for autoimmune hepatitis is immunosuppression. Corticosteroids are typically the initial therapy and are highly effective in these disorders. Other options include azathioprine, cyclosporine, and tacrolimus. Steroid therapy is reduced gradually, but withdrawal can result in a recurrence of hepatitis. Azathioprine may be used as long-term management, alone or with continued corticosteroids if necessary. Patients presenting with liver failure may require liver transplantation, but autoimmune hepatitis may recur following transplantation.

PRIMARY SCLEROSING CHOLANGITIS

Chronic fibrosing inflammation of the intra- and extrahepatic bile ducts is the typical lesion of sclerosing cholangitis. This inflammatory process has been characterized as either primary or secondary. Secondary sclerosing cholangitis may be caused by choledocholithiasis, postoperative stricture, or toxin-induced bile ductular injury, or can be associated with other disorders such as acquired immunodeficiency syndrome and Langerhans-cell histiocytosis. The cause of primary sclerosing cholangitis (PSC) is unknown. The association between PSC and inflammatory bowel disease, as well as the occasional presence in serum of autoantibodies such as antineutrophil cytoplasmic antibody (ANCA), strongly suggests an immunologic cause. Although adults, particularly men, are the most commonly affected, PSC has been reported in the adolescent, childhood, and neonatal age groups.

The diagnosis of PSC relies on the clinical presentation, serologic examination, hepatic histopathology, and cholangiography. The clinical presentation of PSC is widely variable. Neonates with jaundice resembling that of biliary atresia have been described. Older children can be asymptomatic or present with nonspecific symptoms such as fatigue, vague abdominal pain, and/or pruritus.

Cirrhosis and portal hypertension may be the earliest indicators. PSC should be considered in any patient with inflammatory bowel disease, especially ulcerative colitis, who exhibits physical or biochemical evidence of hepatobiliary dysfunction. Hepatosplenomegaly is a common physical finding, and excoriation secondary to pruritus may be present.

Laboratory studies typically reveal elevated serum alkaline phosphatase and γ-glutamyltranspeptidase values. Circulating autoantibodies nonspecific to PSC, such as anti-smooth-muscle or anti-liver-kidney microsomal antibody, are occasionally present. The histopathologic picture of bile ductular proliferation and inflammation is also nonspecific. The classic "onion-skin lesion," concentric periductal fibrosis (Fig. 18-7B), is often absent but, when present, is virtually pathognomonic. Cholangiography is considered the best means of confirming the diagnosis of PSC. Percutaneous transhepatic cholangiography and endoscopic retrograde cholangiopancreatography (ERCP) allow visualization of the macroscopic biliary tree and in typical instances demonstrate alternating normal, strictured, and dilated portions of the biliary tree, giving it a "beaded" appearance.

There is no specific treatment for PSC. Although several agents have been tried, including corticosteroids, D-penicillamine, and bile acid sequestrants, none have proven to be helpful. Hepatobiliary drainage surgery does not appear to slow the progression toward end-stage liver disease, and colectomy in those patients with ulcerative colitis has no effect on this progressive liver injury. Supportive management includes the administration of fat-soluble vitamin supplements and antipruritic agents. Although it has not been unequivocally substantiated in double-blind controlled trials, there may be some benefit from ursodeoxycholic acid or methotrexate treatment. Complications of cholangitis may require courses of antibiotics and drainage or dilatation procedures. Once cirrhosis and portal hypertension have been established, liver transplantation may become necessary.

AUTOIMMUNE HEPATITIS/PRIMARY SCLEROSING CHOLANGITIS OVERLAP SYNDROME

The term "overlap syndrome" represents a heterogeneous mix of immune-mediated diseases affecting the hepatobiliary system. Patients with overlap syndrome will have clinical and laboratory features common to both autoimmune hepatitis and primary sclerosing cholangitis. Although the exact classification of such patients is still controversial, there are clearly patients whose illnesses share aspects of each disease. The immune mechanisms responsible for the injury as well as the clinical presentations and responses to therapy are variable.

Jaundice is often present, and typical laboratory abnormalities include hypergammaglobulinemia and elevated serum aminotransferase and alkaline phosphatase values. Circulating autoantibodies (antinuclear, anti–smooth muscle) are frequently detected. Histologically, there may be exuberant inflammation and necrosis consistent with autoimmune hepatitis as well as bile ductular injury and periductular onion-skin fibrosis suggestive of primary sclerosing cholangitis. Cholangiography may demonstrate segmental dilations or "beading" of the biliary tree.

Patients demonstrating overlap are frequently given a trial of immunosuppressive therapy. Unfortunately, as with PSC, many patients do not respond to this therapy. Liver transplantation may be the only option available, and immune-mediated relapse following transplant is a possibility.

References

Ben-Ari Z, Dhillon AP, Sherlock S: Autoimmune cholangiopathy: part of the spectrum of autoimmune chronic active hepatitis. Hepatology 18: 10–15, 1993

Debray D, Pariente D, Urvoas E, Hadchouel M, Bernard O: Sclerosing cholangitis in children. J Pediatr 124:49–56, 1994

Gregorio GV, Portmann B, Reid F, et al: Autoimmune hepatitis in childhood: a 20-year experience. Hepatology 25:541–547, 1997

Johnson PJ, McFarlane IG: Meeting report: international autoimmune hepatitis group. Hepatology 18:998–1005, 1993

Lee Y-M, Kaplan MM: Primary sclerosing cholangitis. N Engl J Med 332: 924–933, 1995

McNair AN, Moloney M, Portmann BC, Williams R, McFarlane IG: Autoimmune hepatitis overlapping with primary sclerosing cholangitis in five cases. Am J Gastroenterol 93:777–784, 1998

18.8 MISCELLANEOUS DISORDERS OF THE LIVER

Maureen M. Jonas

IDIOPATHIC NEONATAL HEPATITIS (GIANT-CELL HEPATITIS)

Idiopathic neonatal hepatitis is a descriptive term applied to liver injury in newborns in whom known infectious and metabolic disease have been excluded. It is probably a syndrome that is a phenotype common to several as yet undiscovered disorders. The liver disease is characterized by variable numbers of multinucleated "giant cells," which may be also observed in a variety of other neonatal liver diseases (Secs. 18.4 and 18.5). Idiopathic neonatal hepatitis accounts for 35 to 45% of infants with cholestasis. It occurs with a higher frequency in premature and small-for-gestational-age babies, but this may be a reflection of the increased susceptibility of the immature liver to minor insults. The familial recurrence, in some cases, is consistent with either autosomal-recessive inheritance or environmental factors such as maternal infection.

Jaundice usually appears in the first week after birth but may first be observed at 1 to 3 months. Poor feeding and vomiting are relatively uncommon but, if present, suggest a metabolic disease. Cholestasis is manifested by the intermittent passage of acholic (gray or clay-colored) stools and dark urine. The liver is almost always enlarged with a smooth soft surface, and splenomegaly is noted in nearly half the patients. Serum bilirubin concentrations rise to 8 to 12 mg/dL, with the direct-reacting fraction accounting for more than 50% of the total. The serum aminotransferase values are notably variable, the alkaline phosphatase concentration is only modestly elevated, and the prothrombin time is slightly prolonged or normal. The serum albumin and γ-globulin concentrations typically remain in the normal range throughout the course. Hepatobiliary scintigraphy reveals delayed excretion of radionuclide and patent biliary ducts.

Diagnosis is made by the exclusion of other causes of neonatal liver disease and typical liver biopsy findings. Extensive giant-cell transformation, predominantly around the central veins, is the hallmark of neonatal hepatitis. Giant cells are often filled with inspissated bile pigment; the canaliculi are usually empty.

No specific therapy is available for idiopathic neonatal hepatitis. It is important to be sure that there are no treatable causes of disease (Tables 18-7 and 18-8). Treatment is directed toward management of the nutritional consequences of cholestasis including supplementation of fat-soluble vitamins (see Table 18-27) and use of medium-chain triglyceride–containing formulas to improve absorption of calories during the cholestatic phase of the illness. Treatment with phenobarbital or corticosteroids is not indicated. Complete recovery should be expected within 6 to 8 months in 70 to 80% of patients. Chronic liver disease and portal hypertension develop in the remainder, usually in those with substantial periportal inflammation and fibrosis in their initial biopsy.

HEREDITARY RECURRENT INTRAHEPATIC CHOLESTASIS WITH LYMPHEDEMA (AAGENAES SYNDROME)

This is an extremely rare autosomal recessive disorder that has been described in Norwegian families. The disease begins with severe cholestasis in the neonatal period. Hypoalbuminemia is an occassional early finding, associated with conjugated hyperbilirubinemia and elevated pre-β- and β-lipoproteins, alkaline phosphatase, and aminotransferases. Lymphedema of the lower extremities caused by anomalous lymphatic drainage develops in the prepubertal period. The histologic appearance of the liver in Aagenaes syndrome resembles idiopathic (giant-cell) neonatal hepatitis. Cholestasis gradually improves during early childhood. Adults with the disease experience recurrent episodes of cholestasis, and cirrhosis may develop as a rare, late complication.

NEONATAL HEPATITIS ASSOCIATED WITH HYPOPITUITARISM

Infants with hypopituitarism may present with cholestatic liver disease. Associated findings include hypoglycemia, microphallus, and optic nerve hypoplasia with wandering nystagmus. Liver biopsy reveals giant-cell hepatitis, indistinguishable from idiopathic neonatal hepatitis. The pathogenesis of this disorder is unclear. The prognosis of the liver disease is excellent if recognized promptly with appropriate management of the endocrine deficiencies.

References

Aagenaes O, van der Hagen CB, Refsum S: Hereditary recurrent intrahepatic cholestasis from birth. Arch Dis Child 43:646–657, 1968

Herman SP, Baggenstoss AH, Cloutier MD: Liver dysfunction and histologic abnormalities in neonatal hypopituitarism. J Pediatr 87:892–895, 1975

Thaler MM, Gellis SS: Studies in neonatal hepatitis and biliary atresia. I. Long-term prognosis of neonatal hepatitis. Am J Dis Child 116:257–261, 1968

18.9 ACQUIRED DISORDERS OF THE BILIARY TRACT

Regino P. Gonzalez-Peralta and Christopher Jolley

EXTRAHEPATIC BILIARY ATRESIA

Biliary atresia (BA), although not a common disorder, is the most common indication for pediatric liver transplantation. Current surgical intervention and medical management have dramatically improved the prognosis for this disease since its discovery in 1817. The developments of the hepatoportoenterostomy (Kasai) procedure and liver transplantation have changed biliary atresia from a universally fatal disease to a survivable condition.

Biliary atresia results from inflammatory and progressive destruction of bile ducts, both extra- and intrahepatic, leading to fibrosis, biliary cirrhosis, and eventual liver failure. Biliary atresia has been classified into several types depending on the location and degree of atresia (Fig. 18-8). The cause of BA is unknown, but the most common form is felt to be acquired rather than congenital. Infections, intrauterine and perinatal, metabolic disorders, genetic predisposition, and environmental exposures have all been implicated as potential causes, and each may be contributory in some cases. Biliary atresia also occurs in association with a variety of other congenital anomalies, as discussed in Sec. 18.3. In these cases, the condition is presumed to result from abnormalities in morphogenesis and is therefore not considered an acquired lesion.

The most consistent clinical feature of biliary atresia is cholestatic jaundice that appears in the second or third week of life, although some infants will be jaundiced from birth. Hypopigmented or acholic stools and darkened urine are strongly suggestive of biliary atresia. An enlarged and hard liver may be evident at the time of diagnosis, and with further progression of biliary cirrhosis, splenomegaly, ascites, and bruising from coagulopathy will occur.

The evaluation of an infant suspected of having biliary atresia is the same as that for an infant with neonatal cholestasis (see Table 18-8). Frequently, the jaundiced infants will have a mixed hyper-

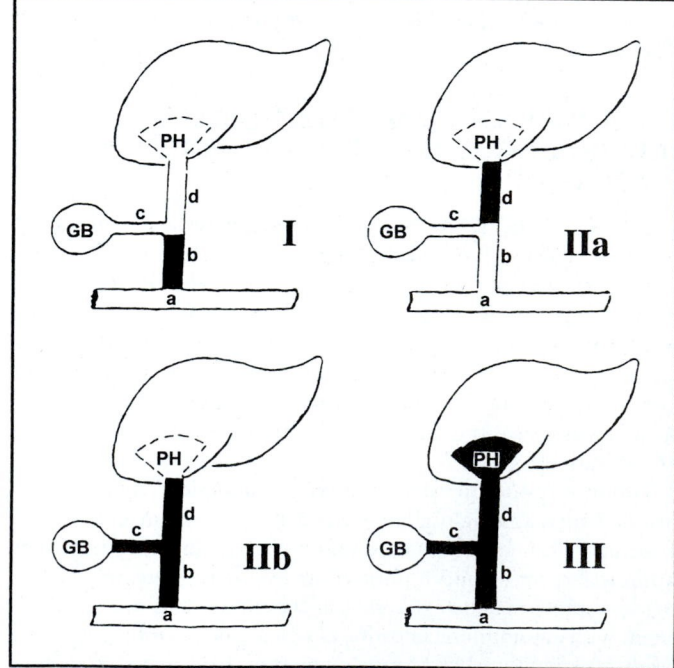

FIGURE 18-8 Patterns of involvement of the extrahepatic and intrahepatic biliary tree in biliary atresia: a, intestine; b, common bile duct; c, cystic duct; d, common hepatic duct. PH = porta hepatis; GB = gallbladder. Type I has been referred to as "correctable" biliary atresia. Types IIa and IIb are the most common. Type III, with involvement of the intrahepatic ducts of the porta hepatitis, may have the worst prognosis after portoenterostomy.

bilirubinemia with elevated serum alkaline phosphatase, GGT, and aminotransferase values. The absence of a gallbladder on sonography should raise suspicion of BA, although some affected infants will have a gallbladder. Radionuclide scans are often used to determine the presence or absence of biliary patency. Failure of excretion of radioisotope is an indication for liver biopsy and cholangiogram. Bile ductular proliferation and cholestasis are typical histopathologic findings; variable degrees of inflammation, giant-cell formation, and fibrosis are noted. The diagnosis of BA is confirmed by cholangiogram, usually intraoperatively but sometimes by ERCP.

The bile drainage procedure is a hepatoportoenterostomy or "Kasai procedure" after Morio Kasai, who developed the operation in 1968. In this operation, a loop of intestine is attached to the porta hepatis in an attempt to reestablish bile flow from the liver. Recognition of biliary atresia and the timely establishment of biliary drainage via the portoenterostomy are critical. After 3 months of age, the liver injury may be severe enough to make portoenterostomy very unlikely to be of value. Therefore, awareness of biliary atresia and early referral for diagnostic evaluation are essential. In one-third of infants treated with portoenterostomy, jaundice never resolves, and hepatic injury progresses rapidly. In approximately another one-third, jaundice resolves over several months, but cirrhosis is already established or develops over the next several years. In these children, liver transplantation is the only other treatment option, although supportive measures such as fat-soluble vitamins, choleretic agents, and nutritional therapy are useful before transplantation. Children that have undergone a Kasai procedure are at increased risk for ascending cholangitis (see Sec. 18.5.2) and therefore need prompt therapy with intravenous antibiotics if they have fever associated with increasing jaundice or other indications of worsening liver disease.

CHOLELITHIASIS

Cholelithiasis (gallstones) is now more frequently recognized in children because of improved detection with techniques such as sonography. The prevalence of pediatric cholelithiasis is unknown, largely because many infants and children with gallstones are asymptomatic.

When symptoms do occur, they usually include right upper quadrant abdominal pain, vomiting, and occasionally jaundice. The pain may or may not be associated with meals, and spontaneous resolution of the pain, presumably following passage of the obstructing stone, is not uncommon. Several conditions have been associated with gallstone formation in children (Table 18-22). Hemolytic disease, total parenteral nutrition, short bowel syndrome,

TABLE 18-22
CONDITIONS ASSOCIATED WITH CHOLELITHIASIS IN CHILDREN

Hemolytic disease
  Sickle-cell disease
  Hereditary spherocytosis
  Thalassemia major
  Hemolytic-uremic syndrome
Total parenteral nutrition
Ileal disease/resection
Pregnancy
Sepsis
Idiopathic

and adolescent pregnancy are responsible for the majority of cases. Complications of cholelithiasis include cholecystitis, cholangitis, and perforation; all are more common in adults. Pancreatitis caused by obstruction of the pancreatic duct by a stone or stones in the common bile duct is the most common complication in children.

Gallstones are typically found by ultrasonography, although stones with high calcium content may be seen on plain radiographs. Hepatobiliary scans may provide both anatomic and functional information by demonstrating the degree of gallbladder visualization and/or emptying. ERCP has therapeutic as well as diagnostic value, although it carries risks such as pancreatitis. Therapy depends on several factors including severity of symptoms, type of gallstone, and patient factors. This may range from expectant management in asymptomatic patients to cholecystectomy for those who have clinically apparent biliary colic, cholangitis, cholecystitis, or an episode of pancreatitis. Endoscopic sphincterotomy with or without stone retrieval is used in the management of bile duct stones and should be considered as urgent therapy when gallstone obstruction causes pancreatitis or elevations in liver function texts, indicating hepatic damage. Dissolution therapy using oral bile acids is not effective for pigment stones, which represent a significant proportion, if not the majority, of childhood gallstones. Lithotripsy has not been adequately studied in children.

CHOLECYSTITIS

Inflammation of the gallbladder, or cholecystitis, may result from obstruction of bile flow as with gallstones or may occur in the absence of stones, when it is called acalculous cholecystitis. Physical findings consistent with cholecystitis include right upper quadrant pain, which may radiate to the back, and localized tenderness on palpation over the gallbladder, which is worse with inspiration (Murphy sign). The differential diagnosis includes hepatitis, hepatic abscess, tumor, gonococcal perihepatitis (Fitz-Hugh–Curtis syndrome), pancreatitis, appendicitis, peptic ulcer disease, pneumonia, pyelonephritis, and renal stones. Laboratory findings often include leukocytosis, often mild increases in bilirubin and aminotransferase levels, and elevated amylase levels (even without pancreatitis). Marked elevation of the bilirubin, alkaline phosphatase, or γ-glutamyltransferase levels suggest that a stone is obstructing the biliary tree. Ultrasonography can demonstrate gallstones or a thickened gallbladder wall. Hepatobiliary scan will demonstrate poor or no visualization of the inflamed gallbladder. Calculous cholecystitis, when severe, can lead to empyema and necrosis of the gallbladder, perforation, and bile peritonitis. Hospitalization for administration of intravenous fluids, cessation of oral feeding, and administration of analgesia are appropriate. Gastric decompression may be helpful, especially if the patient has vomiting. Antibiotics are not needed in mild cases, but if fever ensues or tenderness worsens, administration of antibiotics with broad coverage for enteric organisms is reasonable. Complications of perforation, abscess, or empyema formation occur in 30% of children presenting acutely. Cholecystectomy is the procedure of choice for calculous cholecystitis. In children with sickle-cell disease, hypertransfusion should be performed before surgery.

Acalculous cholecystitis has been characterized as acute (less than 1 month duration) or chronic. Acute acalculous cholecystitis shares the clinical features of calculous cholecystitis except that there are no demonstrable gallstones. This form of cholecystitis frequently follows a severe stress such as a life-threatening illness, trauma, or burn. Congenital anomalies of the biliary system may predispose affected children to obstruction of bile flow and subsequent cholecystitis in the absence of gallstones. Chronic acalculous cholecystitis, also known as biliary dyskinesia, is a poorly understood disease that may actually represent several problems such as sphincter of Oddi dysfunction or early gallstone disease. The best approach to evaluation and treatment remains controversial, varying from observation to recommendations for laparoscopic cholecystetomy.

HYDROPS OF THE GALLBLADDER

A massively dilated gallbladder without evidence of gallstones or inflammation is termed *hydrops of the gallbladder*. The exact cause of hydrops is unknown, but there is frequently an antecendent or concurrent illness. Acute hydrops of the gallbladder has been reported in association with streptococcal infections, Kawasaki syndrome, and Henoch-Schönlein purpura. Patients vary in age from newborns to adolescents.

Symptoms include right upper quadrant pain and often an enlarged, tender, palpable gallbladder. Laboratory findings include elevated liver enzymes, making differentiation between gallbladder hydrops and cholecystitis difficult. The best means of diagnosis is ultrasonography, which will reveal a distended and thin-walled gallbladder with no stones, normal bile ducts, and no evidence of inflammation such as a thickened gallbladder wall. Spontaneous recovery is typical and surgical intervention is usually not necessary.

References

Balistreri WF, Grand R, Hoofnagle JH, et al: Biliary atresia: current concepts and research directions. Hepatology 23:1682–1692, 1996

Bishop WP, Kao SC: Prolonged postprandial abdominal pain following Kawasaki syndrome with acute gallbladder hydrops: association with impaired gallbladder emptying. J Pediatr Gastroenterol Nutr 13:307–311, 1991

Gamba PG, Zancan L, Midrio P, et al: Is there a place for medical treatment in children with gallstones? J Pediatr Surg 32:476–478, 1997

Mowat AP: Biliary atresia into the 21st century: a historical perspective. Hepatology 23:1693–1695, 1996

Otte J, Goyet JV, Reding R, et al: Sequential treatment of biliary atresia with Kasai portoenterostomy and liver transplantation: a review. Hepatology 20:41S–48S, 1994

Reif S, Sloven D, Lebenthal E: Gallstones in children. Am J Dis Child 145:105–108, 1991

Rescorla FJ: Cholelithiasis, cholecystitis, and common bile duct stones. Curr Opin Pediatr 9:276–282, 1997

Rumley TO, Rodgers BM: Hydrops of the gallbladder in children. J Pediatr Surg 18:138–140, 1983

18.10 TUMORS OF THE HEPATOBILIARY SYSTEM

Regino P. Gonzalez-Peralta and Christopher Jolley

Tumors of the hepatobiliary system are uncommon in children and comprise approximately 1 to 4% of all childhood solid tumors. They are most common in young children and usually occur in the right hepatic lobe. Because the liver is comprised of different cell types including hepatocytes, bile duct epithelium, vascular endothelium, and reticuloendothelial cells, a myriad of hepatobiliary tumors can occur. Benign lesions such as hemangiomas and hemangioendotheliomas, adenomas, focal nodular hyperplasia, and mesenchymal hamartomas are more frequent than malignant tumors such as hepatoblastomas, hepatocellular carcinomas, and cholangiocarcinomas. In general, liver tumors are asymptomatic and are discovered during routine examination as an abdominal mass. Although clinical and radiologic features may suffice to diagnose specific tumors, confirmation by examination of histologic material is usually required.

HEMANGIOMAS AND HEMANGIOENDOTHELIOMAS

These lesions arise from vascular endothelium and are the most common benign tumors of the liver in children. These lesions are generally asymptomatic, but larger or numerous tumors can be associated with hepatomegaly, abdominal pain, bruit, and/or jaundice. Clinically apparent heart failure from arteriovenous shunting within the liver or thrombocytopenia from sequestration of platelets within the tumor, termed Kasabach-Merritt syndrome, is sometimes seen. Liver hemangiomas may be discovered during evaluation of infants with multiple skin hemangiomas. Histologically, the lesions consist of dilated vascular spaces, usually lined by single rows of epithelium, which can occasionally exhibit branching and tufting. The management of smaller, asymptomatic lesions consists of careful observation, as these tumors can undergo involution after an initial proliferative phase. Systemic or intralesional steroids, interferon-α, and laser therapy have been used with some success to treat clinically significant hemangiomas, but controlled clinical trials have not been reported. Arterial embolization may be feasible in solitary, segmental lesions; liver transplantation may be the only option for extensive hepatic hemangiomatosis.

HEPATIC ADENOMAS

Hepatic adenomas are usually large, encapsulated, solitary masses commonly found in young women. Although liver adenomas have been linked to estrogen use in adults, glycogen storage disease, galactosemia, diabetes mellitus, and tyrosinemia are more important conditions associated with this lesion in children. Large tumors may exhibit evidence of central hemorrhage and necrosis, which can be detected reliably with computerized tomography. The prognosis of hepatic adenomas is generally excellent, but malignant transformation has been reported. Treatment includes discontinuation of estrogens, if used; surgical removal should be entertained in symptomatic or complicated cases such as those with hemorrhage.

FOCAL NODULAR HYPERPLASIA

This lesion is a small, unencapsulated, and generally solitary lesion that is frequently noted in young girls or women but occurs in both genders and at any age. Histologically, it is characterized by a central scar, from which fibrous septa emanate and surround hyperplastic nodules of liver cells. These distinctive histologic features can be seen after prolonged ischemia, which has led to speculation that focal nodular hyperplasia may be the result of unrecognized vascular occlusion and is not a true "tumor." The prognosis is excellent, and malignant transformation has not been reported. Treatment is conservative unless the diagnosis is in question or the mass effect is causing problems, in which case surgical excision may be warranted.

MESENCHYMAL HAMARTOMAS

Mesenchymal hamartomas are large and multilobulated tumors that are commonly palpable during abdominal examination. Like most hepatic lesions, mesenchymal hamartomas are asymptomatic unless the size of the mass is large, causing abdominal pain or jaundice from compression. Histologically, these tumors are comprised of a meshwork of hepatocytes, bile duct epithelia, and mesenchymal cells, intermixed with cystic dilations within a dense fibrous stroma. The prognosis is excellent, and malignant transformation has been reported only once. Conservative observation is usually indicated, although excision may be necessary for problematic lesions.

HEPATOBLASTOMA

Hepatoblastoma is the most common malignant liver tumor in the pediatric age group. Hepatoblastomas are single, lobulated masses that are usually discovered during infancy. These tumors may occur in association with Beckwith-Weideman syndrome, hemihypertrophy, and familial adenomatous polyposis. Serum α-fetoprotein levels are almost universally elevated in children with these tumors; this test is therefore valuable in establishing the diagnosis and can be used to monitor disease recurrence after therapy. Prognosis is fair, with overall survival rates of approximately 50% depending on the stage of the disease. The lungs and contiguous abdomen are common sites for metastasis. Treatment should be aimed at complete resection with pre- and postoperative chemotherapy. Liver transplantation has been successfully used in cases in which complete tumor resection cannot be accomplished.

HEPATOCELLULAR CARCINOMA

Hepatocellular carcinoma is the most frequent malignant tumor in adults and is often causally related to chronic viral hepatitis, genetic hemochromatosis, or alcoholic cirrhosis. In the United States, childhood hepatocellular carcinoma may occur in an otherwise healthy liver or in association with cirrhosis; the incidence is exceedingly high in hereditary tyrosinemia. Hepatocellular carcinoma may be clinically silent or present with generalized symptoms such as anorexia, fatigue, abdominal pain, and weight loss. Complications such as rupture, hemorrhage, or metastasis are rarely the initial clinical manifestations in children. Although biochemical dysfunction including elevated aminotransferase and alkaline phosphatase values, hyperuricemia, hypoglycemia, and hyperlipidemia may be present, these are usually mild and nonspecific. As in hepatoblastomas, serum α-fetoprotein may be of diagnostic and prognostic value. The prognosis is generally poor unless total excision of early tumors is possible because sustained response is rarely achieved with aggressive chemotherapy, radiotherapy, or embolization. Liver transplantation may be considered for small, localized, unresectable tumors.

References

Stocker JT: Hepatic tumors in children. In: Suchy F, ed: Liver Diseases in Children. St Louis, Mosby-Year Book, 1994

Weinberg AG, Finegold MJ: Primary tumors of childhood. Hum Pathol 14:512–537, 1983

18.11 THE LIVER IN SYSTEMIC DISORDERS

Regino P. Gonzalez-Peralta and Christopher Jolley

THE LIVER IN DISORDERS OF CIRCULATION

Ischemic hepatitis mimics toxic or infectious hepatitis and occurs in association with congestive heart failure, shock, cardiorespiratory arrest, asphyxia, prolonged seizures, or severe dehydration. Ischemic hepatitis is characterized by a marked and rapid elevation of serum aminotransferases within 24 to 48 hours after the insult. Ischemic hepatitis is distinguished from viral or toxic hepatitis by a rapid decrease in aminotransferases occurring within days of the initial insult without increasing bilirubin or worsening coagulopathy. Complications of chronic liver disease rarely develop, and the prognosis for children with ischemic hepatitis depends on the response of the underlying disorder to therapy.

Budd-Chiari syndrome is defined as noncardiogenic hepatic venous outflow obstruction. It results in ascites and liver enlargement. Mild or minimal serum bilirubin and aminotransferase elevation are present. Venous outflow obstruction caused by concentric narrowing of terminal hepatic venules without associated abnormalities of the hepatic veins or inferior vena cava is classified as venoocclusive disease and occurs most frequently following bone marrow transplantation (see below). Other forms of hepatic outflow obstruction occur rarely in childhood and are caused by occlusion of the hepatic veins or suprahepatic vena cava. Medical treatment of thrombotic occlusion of the hepatic veins or suprahepatic vena cava has not been successful. Surgery to relieve the obstruction is well tolerated by patients in whom there is no evidence of cirrhosis. Patients with evidence of progressive liver disease should be considered as candidates for liver transplantation. Children with Budd-Chiari syndrome should undergo an evaluation for hypercoaguability, which may predispose to this condition.

THE LIVER IN CYSTIC FIBROSIS

Cystic fibrosis is an autosomal-recessive disorder caused by mutations in the gene encoding a transmembrane receptor, cystic fibrosis transmembrane conductance regulator (CFTR), and it is discussed in detail in Sec. 23.10. In the liver, CFTR is expressed primarily in biliary epithelium. Largely because of prolonged patient survival and increased awareness, liver disease is now recognized in up to 50% of patients with cystic fibrosis.

The most common hepatobiliary manifestation of cystic fibrosis is hepatic steatosis. This abnormal accumulation of fat within hepatocytes is likely related to malnutrition and is generally reversible. Other conditions, including neonatal cholestasis, inspissated bile syndrome, and biliary tract anomalies such as microgallbladder, cystic duct atresia, and bile duct stenosis can also occur.

Although the precise pathogenetic effects of the CFTR defect are unknown, it results in the production of thick, tenacious secretions in the hepatobiliary system with resultant formation of "sludge" and potential gallstone formation. Over time, these abnormalities in bile lead to persistent focal microscopic or macroscopic obstructions in the intrahepatic biliary tree, resulting in a lesion of *focal biliary cirrhosis*. The clinical spectrum of liver disease in cystic fibrosis is wide, ranging from asymptomatic biochemical abnormalities to overt cirrhosis with its attendant complications, including ascites, esophageal varices, coagulopathy, and hypersplenism.

The evaluation of liver disease in children with cystic fibrosis is dictated by the clinical presentation and may include ultrasonography or other imaging modalities such as ERCP. Other causes of liver disease should be excluded. Specific management of cystic fibrosis–related liver disease depends on clinical manifestations and includes assessment of appropriate caloric intake and pancreatic enzyme supplementation. Ursodeoxycholic acid therapy (10–20 mg/kg/d in divided doses) results in normalization of aminotransferase values in most affected children with cystic fibrosis–related liver disease, presumably by enhancing bile flow. However, its long-term benefit, particularly in preventing cirrhosis, remains to be determined. Liver transplantation has been successfully used in those with decompensated liver disease.

THE LIVER IN COLLAGEN VASCULAR DISEASES

Clinical evidence of liver dysfunction is common in children with collagen vascular disorders such as systemic lupus erythematosus and juvenile rheumatoid arthritis. In these conditions, liver injury can be the result of primary hepatic involvement in the underlying disease, drug therapy (such as aspirin, methotrexate, and gold), or other unrelated liver disorders (for example, viral hepatitis). Symptoms of liver disease are often absent or mild and include hepatomegaly, splenomegaly (particularly in systemic-onset juvenile rheumatoid arthritis), and varying degrees of biochemical abnormalities. Evaluation should be directed at excluding other potential causes of liver disease. Liver biopsy may be of value in assessing extent and degree of liver damage. Discontinuation of potentially hepatotoxic drugs, if possible, should be considered.

THE LIVER IN HUMAN IMMUNODEFICIENCY VIRUS INFECTION

The development of effective antiretroviral therapy in recent years has greatly improved the prognosis of human immunodeficiency virus (HIV) infection, but it remains an important childhood disease. Although varying degrees of hepatosplenomegaly are common in children with HIV infection, overt manifestations of liver dysfunction are rare. The most common liver abnormality identified in pediatric HIV infection is hepatic steatosis, which has been reported in up to 90% of cases and is generally not considered clinically important. Other common causes of liver dysfunction in childhood HIV infection include opportunistic infections and drug therapy. Highly aggressive antiretroviral therapy, referred to as HAART, may be associated with serious hepatic injury. Biliary abnormalities such as bile duct stricture, papillary stenosis, and sclerosing cholangitis, which are commonly seen in adults, are occasionally noted in children. The management of HIV-related liver dysfunction in children includes the meticulous exclusion of opportunistic infections and discontinuation of potentially hepatotoxic drugs. The clinical utility of liver biopsy in this setting is somewhat controversial, but histologic evaluation may be the only means to detect or confirm the presence of specific pathogens and should be performed in cases in which results may alter clinical management. ERCP may provide the opportunity to culture bile for opportunistic pathogens, such as cytomegalovirus, cryptosporidia, and isospora, as well as to treat lesions such as papillary stenosis.

LIVER DISEASE AFTER BONE MARROW TRANSPLANTATION

Bone marrow transplantation is an effective therapeutic modality for many childhood malignancies and immunodeficiency syndromes. Hepatobiliary complications are common and include venoocclusive disease (VOD), graft-versus-host disease (GHVD), gallbladder disease, and viral, bacterial, and fungal infections of the liver.

Venoocclusive disease correlates in frequency to the intensity of pretransplant ablative therapy and occurs early after transplantation, usually within 30 days. VOD occurs more commonly in patients with pretransplant liver dysfunction. The pathogenesis of VOD is incompletely understood but likely involves direct toxic effects of preconditioning therapy on the terminal hepatic venules. Clinical manifestations of VOD vary but most typically include gradual weight gain, abdominal discomfort, ascites, jaundice, and varying degrees of liver dysfunction including direct hyperbilirubinemia and elevated aminotransferase values. Evidence of severe liver disease including coagulopathy, encephalopathy, and marked cholestasis is occasionally seen. The diagnosis of VOD can usually be made on the basis of clinical presentation, but sonography and other imaging modalities may be necessary to exclude gallbladder disease. Although liver biopsy may be of value to confirm the diagnosis of VOD, it is frequently contraindicated in these ill patients with significant coagulopathy and ascites. If required, liver tissue is best obtained through the transjugular approach or at laparotomy in these cases. Management is supportive; recombinant plasminogen activator, with or without heparin, may be considered in severe or refractory cases. Preliminary results in adults with difibrotide, a thrombolytic polynucleotide, are encouraging; this agent is being tested in children. The prognosis varies with severity.

Graft-versus-host disease is the result of immunologic attack by donor cytotoxic lymphocytes upon the marrow recipient. GVHD is a multiorgan disease that primarily involves the skin, gastrointestinal tract, hepatobiliary system, and lungs. Hepatobiliary manifestations of GVHD are nonspecific and typically accompany other symptoms of the disorder such as erythematous rash and profuse, usually bloody diarrhea; liver involvement alone is uncommon but occurs. The clinical presentation usually suffices to suggest the diagnosis of GVHD; skin, rectal, and rarely liver biopsy can be used to confirm the diagnosis. Treatment is directed at immunologic suppression with high-dose steroids, cyclosporine, tacrolimus, or antithymocyte globulin. The prognosis is generally good, but a proportion of patients develop a chronic form of the disease.

Other hepatobiliary complications after bone marrow transplantation include cholecystitis, which is frequently acalculous, drug-related hepatotoxicity, parenteral nutrition–associated liver disease, and infections of the liver.

LIVER DISEASE ASSOCIATED WITH OBESITY

Steatosis refers to the abnormal accumulation of fat within hepatocytes, and steatohepatitis to those cases with associated liver inflammation. In adults, steatohepatitis is commonly related to consumption of alcohol, exposure to other hepatotoxic drugs, and diabetes mellitus, but obesity probably plays a more important role in children (Table 18-23). The hepatic disorder is called nonalcoholic steatohepatitis (NASH). Steatohepatitis is usually a clinically silent disease that is commonly discovered when liver test abnormalities are discovered incidentally. However, the clinical spectrum

TABLE 18-23
COMMON CAUSES OF STEATOSIS AND STEATOHEPATITIS IN CHILDREN

Nutritional disorders	Obesity
	Malnutrition syndromes
	Prolonged fasting
Pharmacologic agents	Glucocorticosteroid
	Estrogen
	Aspirin
	Acetaminophen
	Vitamin A
	Asparaginase
	Methotrexate
	Tetracycline
Metabolic disorders	Diabetes
	Cystic fibrosis
	Wilson disease
	Glycogen storage disease
	Galactosemia
	Tyrosinemia
	Fructose intolerance
	Urea cycle defects
	Disorders of fat metabolism
Hepatotoxic agents	Alcohol
	Total parenteral nutrition
	Organic solvents
	Carbon tetrachloride
Miscellaneous	Pregnancy
	Reye syndrome

SOURCE: Roy CC, Silverman A, Alagille D: Clinical Gastroenterology. St Louis, CV Mosby, 1995.

of disease is wide, with findings of chronic liver disease occasionally evident at the time of diagnosis. The frequency of progression to cirrhosis is not known. Laboratory abnormalities in steatohepatitis are mild and nonspecific, and the diagnosis is one of exclusion. Disorders such as Wilson disease, glycogen storage disease, and cystic fibrosis may be associated with hepatic steatosis but usually have other recognizable features. Some drugs cause fat accumulation in the liver. Hepatic steatosis may be suggested by abdominal sonography or computerized tomography but should be confirmed histologically. In obese children, weight loss with hypocaloric diets and exercise leads to improvement in or resolution of liver dysfunction, but this may be difficult to achieve.

References

Albisetti M, Braegger CP, Stallmach T, Willi UV, Nadal D: Hepatic steatosis: a frequent non-specific finding in HIV-infected children. Eur J Pediatr 158:971–974, 1999

Bonancini M: Hepatobiliary complications in patients with human immunodeficiency virus infection. Am J Med 92:404–411, 1992

Diehl AM: Nonalcoholic steatohepatitis. Semin Liver Dis 19:221–229, 1999

Franzese A, Vajro P, Argenziano A, et al: Liver involvement in obese children. Ultrasonography and liver enzyme levels at diagnosis and during follow-up in an Italian population. Dig Dis Sci 42:1428–1432, 1997

Miller MH, Urowitz MB, Gladman DD, et al: The liver in systemic lupus erythematosus. Q J Med 2311:401–409, 1984

Sale GE: Hepatic complications of bone marrow transplantation. Prog Clin Biol Res 309:349–356, 1989

Schaller J, Beckwith B, Wedgewood RJ: Hepatic involvement in juvenile rheumatoid arthritis. Pediatrics 58:730–736, 1976

Sokol RJ, Durie PR: Recommendations for management of liver and biliary tract disease in cystic fibrosis. Cystic Fibrosis Foundation Hepatobiliary Disease Consensus Group. J Pediatr Gastroenterol Nutr 28:S1–S13, 1999

Wolford JL, McDonald GB: A problem-oriented approach to intestinal and liver disease after marrow transplantation. J Clin Gastroenterol 10:419–433, 1988

18.12 LIVER FAILURE

Robert Squires

Hepatic failure is a well-defined clinical syndrome in adults, comprised of encephalopathy, coagulopathy, and evidence of hepatic dysfunction without an antecedent liver disease. However, a specific definition is lacking for pediatric patients who may not fulfill all the adult criteria (Table 18-24). In particular, encephalopathy in its early stages is difficult to define in infants and children and, when it can be identified, may appear late in the course. Therefore, a working definition for children is evidence of liver injury and an uncorrectable coagulopathy in the absence of underlying chronic liver disease. Causes of acute hepatic failure in children are listed by age group and type of disease in Table 18-25. The diagnostic evaluations for most of these disorders have already been discussed above.

Essential requirements for the management of acute liver failure in children include the following: (1) establishment of an accurate diagnosis, (2) provision of intense, comprehensive medical support, and (3) availability of liver transplantation to those patients who are unlikely to recover. Complications are common and can involve every organ system (Table 18-26). The child is best served if these complications are anticipated and prevented. Careful management of fluid and electrolytes and prevention of hypoglycemia, along with meticulous attention to the detail of multisystem management, may prevent the devastating consequences of progressive encephalopathy and cerebral edema. Potentially reversible factors that precipitate hepatic encephalopathy include hypoglycemia, hypoxemia, gastrointestinal bleeding, acid-base disturbances, electrolyte abnormalities, sedative drugs, and infection. Death is usually attributable to cerebral edema with or without herniation, massive hemorrhage of the upper intestinal tract from stress injury, sepsis, or multisystem organ failure.

The child should be cared for in a quiet environment with little stimulation to minimize increased intracranial pressure but also needs close serial observation. Sedatives should be avoided. Unless the patient has increased fluid losses (eg, hemorrhage), mild fluid restriction in the range of 85 to 100% of maintenance fluids is indicated. Overzealous use of diuretics, used to treat edema or ascites, may precipitate hepatorenal syndrome. Continuous venovenous hemofiltration (CVVH) is used for patients with renal insufficiency. A central catheter is needed to provide the 15 to 20% dextrose usually required to maintain serum glucose between 110 and 130 mg/dL and to monitor central venous pressure. Gastric pH is maintained above 4.0 with an H_2-receptor antagonist to prevent gastrointestinal bleeding. Correction of the coagulopathy with fresh frozen plasma is reserved for the child who is bleeding or for whom invasive procedures are anticipated. Vitamin K supplementation should be administered to any patient with coagulopathy.

TABLE 18-24
STAGES OF HEPATIC ENCEPHALOPATHY

STAGE	CLINICAL	REFLEXES	NEUROLOGIC SIGNS	EEG CHANGES
0	None	Normal	None	Normal
I	*Infant/child:* Inconsolable crying, inattention to task	Normal or hyperreflexic	Difficult or impossible to test adequately	
	Adult: Confused, mood changes, altered sleep habits, forgetful	Normal	Tremor, apraxia, impaired handwriting	Normal or diffuse slowing to theta rhythm, triphasic waves
II	*Infant/child:* Inconsolable crying, inattention to task	Normal or hyperreflexic	Difficult or impossible to test adequately	
	Adult: Drowsy, inappropriate behavior, decreased inhibitions	Hyperreflexic	Dysarthria, ataxia	Abnormal generalized slowing, triphasic waves
III	*Infant/child:* Somnolence, stupor, combativeness	Hyperreflexic	Difficult or impossible to test adequately	
	Adult: Stuporous, obeys simple commands	Hyperreflexic, (+) Babinski	Rigidity	Abnormal, generalized slowing, triphasic waves
IV	*Infant/child:* Comatose, arouses with painful stimuli (IVa) or no response	Absent	Decerebrate or decorticate	
	Adult: Comatose, arouses with painful stimuli (IVa) or no response	Absent	Decerebrate or decorticate	Abnormal, very slow, δ activity

Susceptibility to infection is common and is a result of poor host defenses. Fever and leukocytosis may be absent; therefore, cultures of the blood and urine are obtained with any significant changes in clinical condition. Although indiscriminate use of antibiotics is avoided, the empiric use of antimicrobials may be justified if sepsis is suspected. Infections may be caused by gram-positive or gram-negative bacteria or fungus and may go unrecognized. An infant with multisystem organ failure and liver failure may have herpes simplex infection and should be treated with acyclovir until results of viral cultures are known.

Nutritional support must continue for these critically ill patients. Phosphorus requirements are high, and frequent supplemental in-

TABLE 18-25
CONDITIONS ASSOCIATED WITH ACUTE LIVER FAILURE AT DIFFERENT AGES

	INFECTIONS	DRUGS/TOXIN	CARDIOVASCULAR	METABOLIC/IMMUNE
Infant	Herpes simplex Echovirus Adenovirus EBV CMV Hepatitis B Parvovirus Measles HHV-6 Others		Hypoplastic left heart Asphyxia Myocarditis ECMO	Galactosemia Tyrosinemia Iron storage disease Fructose intolerance Fatty acid defects Mitochondrial defects Hemophagocytic syndrome Neiman Pick type II Others
Child	Hepatitis A, B, C, D Leptospirosis EBV CMV Others	Valproic acid INH Halothane Acetaminophen Phosphorus ASA Vitamin A Others	Heart surgery Cardiomyopathy Budd-Chiari Myocarditis	Fatty acid defects Reye syndrome Leukemia Autoimmune disease α_1-Antitrypsin deficiency
Adult	Hepatitis A, B, C, D Yellow fever Non-A to -E hepatitis Dengue fever Lassa fever Other	Mushroom poisoning Acetaminophen MAO inhibitor FIAU *Bacillus cereus* toxin Tetracycline Ethanol	Budd-Chiari Congestive heart failure Heat stroke Shock	Wilson disease Fatty liver of pregnancy Autoimmune disease Protoporphyria

EBV = Epstein-Barr virus; CMV = cytomegalovirus; HHV-6 = Human herpes virus 6; IHN = isoniazid; ASA = 5-amino salicylic acid; MAO = monoamine; FIAU = fialuridine; ECMO = extracorporeal membrane oxygenation.

TABLE 18-26
COMPLICATIONS IN ACUTE HEPATIC FAILURE

Metabolic
   Hypoglycemia
   Hypophosphatemia
   Hypokalemia
   Hyponatremia
Acid-base disturbance
   Respiratory alkalosis
   Metabolic acidosis
Hematologic
   Aplastic anemia
   Coagulopathy
   Disseminated intravascular coagulopathy
Ascites
Neurologic
   Encephalopathy
   Cerebral edema
   Seizures
   Intracranial hemorrhage
Multiorgan dysfunction
   Pancreatitis
   Pulmonary edema/hemorrhage
   Shock
   Acute tubular necrosis
   Hepatorenal syndrome
   Respiratory failure
   Sepsis

---

fusions are needed to maintain the serum level in the normal range. Initial protein intake should not exceed 1 g/kg/d. However, prolonged protein restriction may be unnecessary, and greater amounts of protein are used if the serum ammonia is in an acceptable range. Hyperammonemia is associated with the development of encephalopathy that may respond to lactulose at a dose that results in one to two loose stools per 8 hours. Mechanical ventilation is initiated for hypoxia or if the child demonstrates evidence of progressive coma and respiratory compromise.

The mortality rate is high for patients with acute liver failure. Although complete recovery may occur, patients with a factor V level less than 17%, a factor VII level less than 8%, or international normalized prothrombin ratio (INR) greater than 4.0 have a poor prognosis and will likely require liver transplantation to avoid death. As a bridge to transplantation, experimental treatment strategies have included growth hormone, plasmapheresis, antioxidants and other cytoprotective agents, along with temporary "bioartificial" liver support. The latter includes perfusion of plasma through a matrix of hepatocytes derived from human or porcine cell lines or hepatocyte transplantation. The use of auxiliary grafts, living related donors, and split livers may help improve the outcome for children with liver failure.

References

Alonso EM, Sokol RJ, Hart J, Tyson RW, Narkewicz MR, Whittington PF: Fulminant hepatitis associated with centrilobular hepatic necrosis in young children. J Pediatr 127:888–894, 1995

Bhaduri BR, Mieli-Vergani G: Fulminant hepatic failure: pediatric aspects. Semin Liv Dis 16:349–355, 1996

Hoofnagle JH, Carithers RL, Shapiro C, Ascher N: Fulminant hepatic failure: summary of a workshop. Hepatology 21:240–252, 1995

Plervris JN, Schina M, Hayes PC: Review article: the management of acute liver failure. Aliment Pharmacol Ther 12:405–418, 1998

Rivera-Penera T, Moreno J, Skaff C, McDiarmid S, Vargas J, Ament ME: Delayed encephalopathy in fulminant hepatic failure in the pediatric population and the role of liver transplantation. J Pediatr Gastroenterol Nutr 24:128–134, 1997

Russell GJ, Fitzgerald JF, Clark JH: Fulminant hepatic failure. J Pediatr 111:313–319, 1987

18.13 COMPLICATIONS OF END-STAGE LIVER DISEASE

Robert Squires

End-stage liver disease is characterized by progressive deterioration of numerous hepatic functions, resulting in a complex clinical picture of hypoproteinemia, coagulopathy, portal hypertension, fluid and sodium retention, and other metabolic derangements. Care of children with end-stage liver disease requires understanding of and meticulous attention to these processes.

MALNUTRITION AND SPECIFIC NUTRIENT DEFICITS

Malnutrition is virtually universal in children with severe liver disease. The etiology is multifactorial and includes anorexia, decreased nutrient intake, malabsorption, and altered utilization of nutrients. Physical conditions such as organomegaly, abdominal distension, ascites, and recurrent infections contribute to early satiety and reduced caloric intake. Decreased concentrations of intraluminal bile acids and some medications (eg, cholestyramine and antibiotics) predispose the patient to malabsorption of fat and fat-soluble vitamins. Altered protein metabolism and substrate utilization are manifested by hyperammonemia, hypoalbuminemia, reduced clotting factors, and hypoglycemia.

Nutritional therapy should maximize enteral caloric intake. Patients often require 100 to 150% of the calculated daily caloric requirement but are often unwilling or unable to consume adequate calories. Nasogastric tube feedings can ensure sufficient caloric intake, if needed. A formula containing medium-chain triglyceride (MCT) will increase fat absorption in the patient with cholestasis.

Deficiencies of fat-soluble vitamins and minerals occur in patients with chronic liver disease, and serum levels should be monitored periodically to assess the need for supplementation as detailed in Table 18-27. Vitamin E deficiency causes mild hemolysis and neuroaxonal dystrophy. Less common manifestations include skeletal or cardiomyopathy and a pigmented retinopathy. Treatment of vitamin E deficiency has improved substantially with the use of D-α-tocopheryl polyethylene glycol-1000 succinate (TPGS), absorption of which is enhanced by the formation of mixed micelles. This form of vitamin E may be mixed with other fat-soluble vitamins to enhance their absorption as well. Vitamin A deficiency is associated with night blindness, xerophthalmia, and increased mortality when patients contract measles. Vitamin K is indicated for those patients with a coagulopathy. Measurement of 25-OH-vitamin D is used to assess vitamin D sufficiency, and supplements are often required. Water-soluble vitamins and minerals given as a multivitamin preparation are useful.

TABLE 18-27

VITAMIN AND MINERAL DEFICIENCIES IN CHRONIC LIVER DISEASE

NUTRIENT	MONITOR	MANAGEMENT
Vitamins		
A	Retinol	10,000 to 15,000 IU/day
D	25-OH-Vitamin D	Vitamin D_2, 5000 to 8000 IU/d, or 25-OH-cholecalciferol, 3–5 μg/kg/d
E	Vitamin E	TPGS,[a] 15–30 IU/kg/d
K	Prothrombin time, INR	Mephyton, 2.5 to 5 mg every other day
Minerals		
Zinc	Zinc level	1% Zinc sulfate; 1–2 mg elemental Zn^{2+}/kg/d
Phosphorus	Phosphorus	Oral: 5–8 mmol phosphorus two or three times a day IV: 0.1–0.3 mmol phosphorus/kg/dose and follow serum phosphorus
Calcium	Calcium or ionized calcium if albumin is low	50 mg elemental Ca^{2+}/kg/d

[a] TPGS = tocopheryl polyethylene glycol-1000 succinate.

ASCITES

Ascites is the pathologic accumulation of fluid in the peritoneal cavity. Ascitic fluid may be noninflammatory, chylous, or inflammatory (Table 18-28). Noninflammatory ascitic fluid occurs with hepatic venous outflow obstruction (Budd-Chiari or venoocclusive disease), cirrhosis, heart failure, nephrosis, and cancer. Chylous ascites occurs with congenital lymphangiectasia or surgical trauma to lymphatic vessels. Inflammatory ascites occurs with a ruptured intraabdominal viscus or pancreatitis. Although urine, biliary fluid, and pancreatic fluid are sterile, they elicit an inflammatory response in the peritoneal cavity.

Diagnostic abdominal paracentesis should be performed to evaluate the patient with new-onset ascites. A diagnostic paracentesis in which 10 to 20 mL of ascitic fluid is withdrawn can be safely performed even in patients with coagulopathy. Ascitic fluid should be inspected visually. Chylous ascites has a milky appearance and elevated triglyceride content. The ascitic fluid should be collected to measure cell count, albumin, total protein, and amylase and for direct inoculation in blood culture media at the bedside. An increased cell count (>250 neutrophils/mm³) is associated with bacterial peritonitis. An elevated ascitic fluid amylase indicates pancreatic ascites or gut perforation. Ascites fluid in heart failure tends to a high protein concentration. Urine leakage into the peritoneal cavity can be differentiated from ascitic fluid by the high urea concentration.

In liver disease, the ascitic fluid is a transudate that develops as a result of an increased portal venous pressure, which results in increased intraluminal pressures in the mesenteric capillaries and a resultant net fluid loss into the peritoneal cavity. When hypoalbuminemia ensues, the decreased colloid osmotic pressure in the capillary potentiates the net fluid losses into the peritoneal cavity, and the body's homeostatic mechanisms respond by increasing renal sodium and water retention following activation of the renin-angiotensin-aldosterone system, sympathetic nervous system, and circulating levels of vasopressin.

Development of ascites is a poor prognostic sign in children with chronic liver disease. It may be associated with abdominal distension and discomfort and predisposes to peritonitis. For this reason, a diagnostic peritoneal tap is indicated in a patient with ascites who develops fever, worsening ascites in the face of adequate medical therapy, or acute abdominal pain. The ascitic fluid is evaluated with culture, Gram stain, cell count, and measurements of albumin, total protein, glucose, lactate dehydrogenase, and amylase. Fluid with a predominance of neutrophils is likely infected, and treatment with a nonnephrotoxic broad-spectrum antibiotic is indicated pending the results of cultures.

Treatment of ascites is accomplished with a slow gradual diuresis and mild fluid restriction. The goal of treatment is to achieve weight loss of approximately 10 mL/kg/d. This is achieved by limiting sodium intake to 0.5 g/d or 1 to 2 mEq/kg/d and enhancing urinary sodium excretion with diuretics. Severe water restriction is unnecessary unless there is profound hyponatremia (< 125 mEq/L). The diet required for severe sodium restriction is unpalatable for many patients and may contribute to decrease in intake of more important nutrients. Pharmacologic treatment, if needed, usually is begun with spironolactone (3–6 mg/kg/d divided TID or BID; adult dose 25–50 mg PO BID), a postassium-sparing diuretic that blocks the effect of aldosterone on the distal renal tubules. One to three weeks of spironolactone therapy may be needed to achieve a steady state. Therefore, a combination of spironolactone and furosemide may be used initially. The response to diuretic therapy can be monitored by measuring urinary sodium. Sodium excretion can be estimated by the product of urine sodium concentration and urine volume. Assuming that sodium is the major extracellular cation and that extracellular sodium concentration is 130 to 140 mEq/L, a negative sodium balance of 25 to 30 mEq will result in approximately 200 g weight loss. If weight is not decreasing, negative sodium balance has not been achieved. Overly aggressive use of diuretics is associated with serious complications such as encephalopathy, hypokalemia, hepatorenal syndrome, and other electrolyte disturbances. Slow weight reduction is safer and preferable.

In cases of diuretic-resistant ascites, or when there is respiratory compromise as a result of ascites, therapeutic paracentesis is indicated. Removal of 50 mL/kg can be safely performed if volume expanders are administered concomitantly in order to prevent a

TABLE 18-28

CAUSES OF ASCITES

Noninflammatory
   Heart failure
   Hepatic vein thrombosis
   Cirrhosis
   Portal vein thrombosis
   Budd-Chiari syndrome
   Venoocclusive disease
   Malignant infiltration of hepatic sinusoids
   Cancer
Chylous
   Surgical disruption of lymphatic vessels
   Congenital lymphangiectasia
Inflammatory
   Intestinal perforation
   Pancreatitis
   Biliary tract perforation
   Bacterial peritonitis

reduction in cardiac output. Most patients with ascites return to normal water and electrolyte balance. After stabilization, ascites can be subsequently managed at home with a maintenance regimen consisting of a low-sodium diet and diuretic therapy for excessive weight gain.

PORTAL HYPERTENSION AND VARICEAL BLEEDING

Portal hypertension results from a variety of causes and can be classified as postsinusoidal, intrahepatic, or presinusoidal, as outlined in Table 18-29. Clinical manifestations include splenomegaly, prominent superficial abdominal vessels, and hypersplenism. This is defined as sequestration of white blood cells and platelets within the spleen, resulting in low peripheral counts. The most significant consequence of portal hypertension is the development of varices, dilated veins, at various sites along the intestinal tract. Rupture of these varices may cause life-threatening hemorrhage. Esophageal varices are likely to develop when the pressure within the portal venous system reaches 10 to 12 mm Hg.

Signs and symptoms of variceal bleeding include melena, hematemesis, hematochezia, dizziness, pallor, and weakness. Patients and families of children with portal hypertension should be educated that if any of these symptoms or signs are observed, evaluation and treatment at the closest emergency room may be life-saving. Treatment for bleeding from esophageal varices is summarized in Table 18-30. If bleeding is confirmed, measures to establish adequate venous access and provide appropriate fluid resuscitation are initiated immediately. Initial laboratory studies will include a type and cross for red blood cell replacement, prothrombin time, and a complete blood count. A nasogastric tube is placed to empty gastric contents and reduce the risk of aspiration. Gastric lavage with normal saline removes clots from the stomach and improves visualization of the stomach if upper endoscopy becomes necessary. Blood transfusions may be needed to keep the hematocrit near 30%, but overtransfusion may precipitate further bleeding. The child should be transferred to an intensive care unit for more definitive management, which may include administration of octreotide (1 to 5 μg/kg IV bolus up to 100 μg, followed by 1–2 μg/kg/h up to 25 μg/kg/h infusion), a long-acting analog of somatostatin, along with endoscopic therapy such as variceal sclerosis or band ligation. If octreotide is administered, complications of hypoglycemia or hyperglycemia can occur, so blood glucose should be monitored.

In refractory cases, variceal decompression is achieved surgically by creation of a total or partial shunt between the portal and sys-

TABLE 18-29

MAJOR CAUSES OF PORTAL HYPERTENSION IN CHILDREN

Postsinusoidal portal hypertension
  Elevated right atrial pressure secondary to right-sided heart failure, congenital heart disease, constrictive pericarditis
  Budd-Chiari syndrome
  Venoocclusive disease
  Hepatic vein thrombosis
Intrahepatic
  Cirrhosis
Presinusoidal
  Cavernous transformation of the portal vein
  Congenital hepatic fibrosis
  Schistosomiasis
  Portal vein thrombosis

TABLE 18-30

TREATMENT OF BLEEDING FROM ESOPHAGEAL VARICES

Stabilization of circulatory status
  Correct coagulopathy (platelets and vitamin K)
  Restore intravascular volume with blood products
Control active variceal bleeding
  Endoscopy to confirm the site of bleeding
  Vasopressin or octreotide infusion for persistent bleeding
  Endoscopic sclerotherapy or banding
  Sengstaken-Blakemore tube if bleeding is uncontrollable
Prevent further bleeding
  Sclerotherapy or variceal banding
  Shunting procedure or transjugular intrahepatic portal systemic shunt (TIPS)
  Orthotopic liver transplantation

temic venous circulation to divert portal blood flow from the liver. Transjugular intrahepatic portal systemic shunt (TIPS), a new technology performed by experienced interventional radiologists, creates a shunt between a branch of the intrahepatic portal vein and the inferior vena cava via a hepatic vein. It is less invasive than a surgical shunt and technically successful in over 90% of adult patients, but experience in children varies among centers. Complications associated with any shunt include stenosis or thrombosis and an acceleration of hepatic encephalopathy.

For a child with established cirrhosis and portal hypertension but without variceal hemorrhage, optimal management is not established. Preventive medical management (propranolol) or endoscopic treatment (sclerotherpy or band ligation of varices) before the first bleeding episode has been considered in adults, but indications in children are unclear. If liver transplantation is likely to be required because of impending liver failure, shunt procedures may be contraindicated with earlier liver transplantation being preferable.

In presinusoidal obstruction caused by cavernous transformation of the portal vein, optimal management is controversial. Observation and variceal sclerotherapy or banding has been advocated unless severe thrombocytopenia results from splenomegaly. Many patients avoid surgical portal systemic shunts with this approach but advances in surgical shunt procedures have led some experts to advocate for earlier shunting to avoid potential complications from splenomegaly.

HEPATIC ENCEPHALOPATHY

Hepatic encephalopathy in children with cirrhosis and portal hypertension results from the failure of the liver to clear and detoxify intestinal toxins. In contrast to the hepatic encephalopathy that occurs in children with fulminant hepatic failure, hepatic encephalopathy in end-stage liver disease is not associated with cerebral edema, being characterized instead by changes in mental status ranging from altered performance in mental skills, such as arithmetic, to coma.

Hepatic encephalopathy is precipitated by infection, circulatory compromise from hemorrhage or diuretic therapy, sedatives, tranquilizers, or anesthetic agents, increased delivery of nitrogen to the liver associated with excessive intake or catabolism, surgical trauma, and fluid imbalance. Therapy of hepatic encephalopathy is directed toward correcting precipitating factors and eliminating bacteria and their products, including ammonia and the "false neurotransmitters" β-phenylethanolamine and octopamine. Dietary protein intake should be decreased to 1 g/kg/d during the acute phase of encephalopathy. Hypoglycemia should be corrected, and sufficient nonprotein calories should be administered to prevent catabolism. Correction of fluid and electrolyte imbalance and treatment of infection, hemorrhage, seizures, and respiratory depression should be started. Control of ammonia-producing bacteria is achieved with administration of the poorly absorbed antibiotic neomycin (50 to 100 mg/kg/d divided in three to four doses) and the nonabsorbable synthetic disaccharide lactulose (10 to 15 mL three to four times daily titrated to achieve loose stools and a stool pH <5). Lactulose inhibits colonic organisms active in formation of ammonia and lowers colonic pH, thus favoring conversion of ionized ammonia to nonionized ammonium. Ammonium is not absorbed across the intestinal mucosa and may be utilized by fecal bacteria as a source of nitrogen.

Extracorporeal hepatic perfusion may permit short-term improvement in mental status in patients awaiting liver transplantation. Several additional strategies for control of hepatic coma have been attempted, but their results have been unimpressive. Treatment with exchange transfusion, plasmapheresis, peritoneal dialysis, and corticosteroids has not altered the mortality of approximately 20% associated with hepatic encephalopathy in patients with cirrhosis and portal hypertension.

References

D'Amico G, Pagliaro L, Bosch J: The treatment of portal hypertension: a meta-analytic review. Hepatology 22:332–354, 1995

Grace ND, Groszmann RJ, Garcia-Tsao G, et al: Portal hypertension and variceal bleeding: an AASLD single topic symposium. Hepatology 28: 868–880, 1998

18.14 LIVER TRANSPLANTATION

Robert Squires

Over the last 20 years, orthotopic liver transplantation has become an important therapeutic option for children with chronic or fulminant liver disease. In the early years of liver transplantation, patient referral was delayed until signs of malnutrition, ascites, encephalopathy, and uncorrectable coagulopathy developed, placing the patients in a high–surgical risk category. Now, with an increasing donor pool, advances in medical and surgical care, and earlier referral to transplant centers, children are healthier at the time of transplant and thus better able to tolerate the operation with shorter hospital stays.

The indications for orthotopic liver transplantation in children are listed in Table 18-31, but the optimal timing in an individual case is difficult to determine. Early referral to a transplant center facilitates the coordination of care between the transplant team and referring pediatrician. Unfortunately, liver transplantation is not possible for all children with end-stage liver disease. Absolute and relative contraindications to liver transplantation are listed in Table 18-32. Children with metabolic diseases provide a unique challenge. Hepatic transplantation in patients with metabolic defects that involve but are not limited to the liver (eg, Alpers syndrome, mitochondrial DNA deletions or mutations) interrupts the pro-

---

TABLE 18-31

INDICATIONS FOR LIVER TRANSPLANTATION IN INFANTS AND CHILDREN

Obstructive biliary disease
  Extrahepatic biliary atresia
  Sclerosing cholangitis
  Choledochal cyst
Intrahepatic cholestasis
  Idiopathic neonatal hepatitis
  Alagille syndrome
  Nonsyndromic paucity of intrahepatic bile ducts
  Byler syndrome
  Familial intrahepatic cholestasis
Metabolic disease
  α_1-Antitrypsin deficiency
  Tyrosinemia
  Glycogen storage disease type, I, III, and IV
  Wilson disease
  Neonatal iron storage disease
  Galactosemia
  Hyperlipoproteinemia types 2 and 4
  Crigler-Najjar syndrome type 1
Fulminant hepatic failure
Chronic active hepatitis
  Viral
  Autoimmune
  Idiopathic
Tumor
  Hepatoblastoma
  Hepatocellular carcinoma
  Hemangioendothelioma
  Sarcoma
Miscellaneous
  Cryptogenic cirrhosis
  Congenital hepatic fibrosis
  Caroli disease
  Cystic fibrosis
  Cirrhosis related to prolonged TPN

TABLE 18-32

CONTRAINDICATIONS TO LIVER TRANSPLANTATION

Absolute
  Uncontrolled systemic sepsis not confined to the liver
  Extrahepatic malignancy with liver metastasis
  No source for portal inflow
  Irreversible extrahepatic organ system failure
  Acquired immunodeficiency syndrome
  Unresectable hepatic malignancy
  Progressive, terminal nonhepatic disease
  Complex, uncorrectable heart disease
  Irreversible neurologic injury
Relative
  Hepatic encephalopathy (stage IV)
  Partially treated systemic infection
  Significant psychosocial problems
  Portal and mesenteric venous thrombosis
  Pulmonary hypertension
  Significant intrapulmonary shunt

gressive liver disease, but patients often succumb to their condition because of the systemic nature of the disease.

Important surgical innovations have increased the donor pool. The reduced-size liver transplant, in which a portion of an adult organ, typically the left lateral segments, can be implanted into an infant or child, was the first important innovation. Next, development of the split-liver technique allowed a single donated liver to be used for two recipients. The right lobe typically goes to a small or medium-sized adult or adolescent, and the left lateral segments to an infant or small child. Finally, living related donation allows an adult relative to donate a portion of his or her liver to an infant or small child. Newer transport solutions for the donor organ contain nonionic osmotic agents and antioxidants to minimize cold storage injury and allow the organ to be maintained for up to 24 hours before irreversible damage to the liver occurs.

Survival rates range from 60 to 90% 5 years following liver transplants. Factors that negatively impact survival include age less than 1 year, weight less than 10 kg, care in the ICU before transplant, and a diagnosis of fulminant hepatic failure.

18.14.1 Complications of Liver Transplantation

Complications of liver transplantation are listed in Table 18-33. Vascular complications are the most common cause of early postoperative allograft loss and are more likely to occur if the patient weighs less than 10 kg, receives a reduced-size graft, develops hypotension during or shortly after the procedure, or has a hypercoagulable state. Hepatic artery thrombosis is three to four times more frequent in children than in adults and occurs most often within the first 30 days following transplant. The most devastating consequence following hepatic artery thrombosis is loss of the graft with the need for immediate retransplantation. If the graft survives, the long-term sequelae include progressive bile duct stenosis and occasionally allograft necrosis. Portal vein thrombosis is uncommon.

Primary nonfunction of the allograft requires immediate retransplantation before irreversible coagulopathy and cerebral edema occur. Various factors involving the donor, the transplant procedure, and the recipient influence the likelihood that primary nonfunction will develop.

Biliary complications develop in approximately 10% of liver transplant recipients. Late complications following primary duct-to-duct biliary reconstruction include stricture, biliary sludge formation, and recurrent cholangitis. Whole and reduced-size allografts have equivalent risks of biliary complications.

Acute cellular rejection occurs in approximately two-thirds of patients. Treatment is successful in 75 to 80% of cases. Chronic rejection occurs in 5 to 10% of patients and results in a decreased number of portal bile ducts and gradual development of fibrosis. Retransplantation is nearly always required, and, unfortunately, development of chronic rejection in the second allograft is common.

Infectious complications are the most common source of morbidity and mortality following transplantation. Bacterial infections are uncommon but may occur in the immediate postoperative period, usually caused by gram-negative enteric organisms, enterococci, or *Streptococcus* species. Prophylactic antibiotics are administered in the immediate postoperative period and then discontinued to prevent the development of resistant organisms. Because fungal infections carry a high mortality in the immunosuppressed host, many centers begin antifungal prophylaxis before

---

TABLE 18-33

COMPLICATIONS ASSOCIATED WITH LIVER TRANSPLANTATION

Postoperative
  Vascular thrombosis
    Hepatic artery
    Portal vein
  Primary nonfunction
  Biliary complications
Rejection
  Acute cellular rejection
  Chronic rejection
Infection
  Cytomegalovirus
  Epstein-Barr virus
  Varicella
  Pneumocystis carinii
  Fungal infections
Hypertension
Posttransplant lymphoproliferative disease

---

transplant and continue treatment for at least 6 months following transplant.

Members of the herpes virus family, in particular Epstein-Barr virus (EBV), cytomegalovirus (CMV), and herpes simplex virus (HSV), cause the majority of early and severe viral infections. Patients who are seronegative for CMV and receive an organ from a

TABLE 18-34

GENERAL PEDIATRIC CARE OF THE CHILD WITH A LIVER TRANSPLANT

Well-child care
  Immunizations
    No live virus vaccine
      Measles, mumps, rubella (MMR)
      Oral polio vaccine (OPV)
      Varicella
    Permitted vaccines
      Diphtheria, pertussis, tetanus (DPT)
      Injectable polio vaccine (IPV)
      Haemophilus influenzae B (Hib)
      Hepatitis A
      Hepatitis B
      Flu shots
  Common exposures
    Measles
      γ-Globulin
    Varicella
      Varicella-zoster immune globulin (VZIG) within 96 hours of exposure
      Acyclovir if lesions develop
  Anticipatory guidance
    No restrictions from day-to-day activities; common sense prevails
    Encourage participation in extracurricular activities
    Improved appetite and energy level may be experienced
Sick-child care
  Observe for lack of suspected response to treatment
  Vomiting and diarrhea
    May affect absorption of cyclosporine
    For unusual or prolonged symptoms, consider:
      Giardia
      Cryptosporidium
      Clostridium difficile

seropositive donor are at greatest risk for development of either CMV or EBV infection. Intravenous γ-globulin given in combination with acyclovir or ganciclovir decreases the incidence of symptomatic EBV and CMV infection. Treatment of CMV with anti-CMV immunoglobulin and ganciclovir is successful in most cases. HSV infections are more likely to respond to acyclovir. The clinical manifestations of EBV infection may include a mononucleosis-type syndrome, hepatitis simulating rejection, and extranodal lymphoproliferative disease, especially involving the bowel. High-dose intravenous acyclovir or ganciclovir is indicated for clinically significant EBV infection. Oral acyclovir should be continued until symptoms and lymphadenopathy have resolved. Posttransplant lymphoproliferative disease (PTLD) is a potentially fatal abnormal proliferation of B lymphocytes and can occur in any immunosuppressed host. PTLD is seen in up to 15% of all EBV-naive organ transplant recipients.

18.14.2 Well-Child Care in the Liver Transplant Recipient

Every child with a liver transplant should have a primary care pediatrician to oversee care (Table 18-34). Communication between the transplant team and the pediatrician is critical throughout the entire transplant process. Because of the potential for complications following transplantation, the pediatrician and transplant team usually partner in the care of the patient both before and after trans-

plantation. Adjustments in immunosuppressive medications are usually supervised by the transplant team. The pediatrician provides anticipatory guidance, reassurance, and encouragement, such as is given to any family with a child with a chronic illness. In addition, the pediatrician usually treats normal childhood illnesses and administers immunizations. No live virus vaccines should be administered, but other childhood immunizations should be given as in the normal child (see Table 18-34). Following common exposures, such as measles or varicella zoster, prophylactic regimens are recommended. When the child becomes ill, vomiting and diarrhea can affect the absorption of immunosuppressive agents, and therefore levels may need more careful monitoring. It is reasonable to contact the transplant center for guidance when this occurs. If symptoms exceed the usual expected course for an illness, other disorders that are more common in the immunosuppressed host need to be considered. The transplant team works with the primary pediatrician to direct an appropriate evaluation.

References

Alonso MH, Ryckman FC: Current concepts in pediatric liver transplant. Semin Liver Dis 18:295–307, 1998

Broelsch CE, Emond JC, Whitingtin PF, Thistlethwaite JR, Baker AL, Lichtor JL: Application of reduced-size liver transplants as split grafts, auxiliary orthotopic grafts, and living related segmental transplants. Ann Surg 212:368–375, 1990

BLOOD AND BLOOD-FORMING TISSUES

Howard A. Pearson, Associate Editor

19.1 DEVELOPMENTAL CHANGES IN RED BLOOD CELL PRODUCTION AND FUNCTION

Peter R. Dallman, Kevin Shannon, and Howard A. Pearson

19.1.1 Sites of Blood Formation

The anatomic sites of hematopoiesis undergo developmental changes during embryonic and fetal life. Red blood cell formation can be observed within the developing blood vessels of the yolk sac at 2 weeks of gestation. By 8 weeks of gestation, the site of red cell formation begins to shift to the sinusoids of the liver, where granulocyte precursors and megakaryocytes are also seen. Hematopoiesis in the liver is maximal at about 5 months and declines thereafter. Hematopoiesis in the bone marrow is evident by the fifth month of gestation, and this becomes the predominant site of hematopoiesis during the rest of gestation and later. Fetal hematopoietic development appears to be regulated by a number of genes including *GATA-1,* which induces genes that are responsible for transition of early erythroid cells, and the *c-myc* protooncogene, which plays a role in the proliferation and maturation of both early myeloid and erythroid precursors. Erythropoietin, produced in the fetal liver, also regulates fetal erythropoiesis.

BONE MARROW

During the last third of gestation, blood cells are produced almost exclusively in the marrow. In the newborn and during early infancy, hematopoietic marrow fills the bony cavities of the entire axial skeleton, the long bones, and many membranous bones. With advancing postnatal age, hematopoietic tissue gradually moves to the vertebrae, sternum, pelvis, scapulae, and proximal ends of the long bones, the rest of the marrow space becoming fatty.

In hemolytic anemias such as hereditary spherocytosis, the normal rate of red cell production can increase eightfold, and in thalassemia major erythropoietic tissue may expand 30-fold. Hematopoietic marrow tissue expands from the ends of the long bones toward the middle of the shafts, replacing the fatty marrow and resulting in loss of trabeculae and thinning of the bony cortex. In some diseases of the marrow such as myelofibrosis, and in a few, but not all, severe hemolytic anemias, blood production may extend into extramedullary sites, particularly the liver and spleen.

19.1.2 Rate of Production and Normal Values

THE FETUS

The mean hemoglobin level is 100 g/L at 12 weeks of gestation, increases to 140 g/L at 24 weeks, and by term averages 165 g/L. The RBC count increases from about 1.5×10^{12}/L at 12 weeks of gestation to 4.7×10^{12}/L at term. A marked reduction in mean corpuscular volume (MCV) occurs from a mean of 180 femtoliters (fL) at 12 weeks to 108 fL at term, an MCV that is decidedly macrocytic when compared to older individuals. Reticulocyte counts of term infants average 5.0%, and circulating nucleated red blood cells are present.

THE NEWBORN

During the first few days after birth, there are significant differences between hemoglobin levels in venous and capillary blood, with capillary hemoglobin levels about 20 g/L and hematocrits about 6% higher. The higher capillary values reflect a relative hemoconcentration because of loss of plasma from the capillaries. The rise in hemoglobin, hematocrit, and red blood cell counts that occurs between birth and 3 days of age results from a postnatal decrease in plasma volume.

The RBC production in the bone marrow is regulated by the erythrocyte-stimulating hormone erythropoietin (EPO). During fetal life and early in postnatal life, EPO is predominantly produced in the liver and switches to the kidney after birth. EPO binds to a high-affinity receptor expressed on the surface of erythroid progenitor cells called burst-forming units–erythroid (BFU-E) and colony-forming units–erythroid (CFU-E) and induces division and differentiation. EPO production is regulated by tissue oxygenation. At birth the concentration of hemoglobin averages 170 g/L. The relative polycythemia of the newborn is attributable to the low arterial PaO_2 levels in utero that stimulate erythropoietin production in the fetus and result in a high rate of erythropoiesis. After birth, PaO_2 rises, and EPO levels and the rate of erythropoiesis decrease, reflected by a decline in erythroid precursor cells in the bone marrow from an average of 35 to 15% after 1 week. The decreased production of red cells is reflected in the disappearance of nucleated red blood cells and a fall in the reticulocyte count, which continues for 6 to 8 weeks after birth. During this period, the red cell life span is about 90 days compared with 120 days in adults. As a consequence of decreased production and increased destruction, hemoglobin values in term infants decrease steadily during the first weeks of life, which is termed the *physiological anemia of infancy*, and a nadir of about 110 g/L of hemoglobin is reached at about 2 months of age. After 6 to 8 weeks, red cell production resumes, as indicated by a rise in reticulocyte count and an increase in hemoglobin level (Fig. 19-1). The rate of production is sufficient to maintain a stable mean hemoglobin concentration of about 125 g/ L despite the threefold increase of blood volume and weight that occurs during the first year of life.

HEMOGLOBIN CONCENTRATION IN PRETERM INFANTS AND THE ANEMIA OF PREMATURITY

In the preterm infant, the postnatal fall in hemoglobin concentration is more marked than in the term infant, even with optimal nutrition. The smallest infants have the greatest decline in hemoglobin concentration. By 2 months of age, values fall to a mean of about 95 g/L in infants with birth weights between 1500 and 2000 g, to 90 g/L in those with birth weights between 1000 and 1500 g, and even lower in very-low-birth-weight infants (Fig. 19-1). This decline in hemoglobin concentration is called the *early anemia of prematurity* and represents an exaggerated physiological anemia. Premature infants have levels of EPO that are inappropriately low for the degree of anemia, perhaps because hepatic production of EPO is less sensitive to reduced tissue oxygenation compared to that in the kidney. EPO treatment of preterm infants increases the reticulocyte counts if supplemental iron medication is concurrently given. However, most recent studies have shown that EPO treatment in premature infants over 1250 g does not reduce red blood cell transfusion requirements during the first months of life. The clinical benefit of EPO therapy is controversial because inappropriately low EPO levels are only one of several factors that lead to the need for transfusions. Other factors that contribute to the anemia of prematurity include a very large expansion in blood volume secondary to rapid growth, an even shorter red cell survival, and especially the relatively large amounts of blood removed for laboratory tests in sick infants.

CHILDHOOD AND ADOLESCENCE

In the preschool and preadolescent child, erythropoiesis more than keeps pace with growth, and mean hemoglobin concentrations gradually rise (Fig. 19-2, Table 19-1). Values in boys and girls first begin to diverge in adolescence with the onset of puberty, boys having higher hemoglobin levels. The higher hemoglobin values in mature men, as compared to women, result from the erythroid-stimulating effects of androgenic hormones. Figure 19-2 depicts the mean hemoglobin levels from birth to adult life.

MEAN RED BLOOD CELL VOLUME

The mean MCV at birth is 108 fL, substantially greater than the normal mean MCV of 90 fL in the adult. During the first 6 months of life, MCV continues to decrease and reaches a low of 77 fL between 6 and 12 months of age. Age-appropriate values must be used to identify both macrocytosis and microcytosis during childhood. The MCV values increase gradually throughout childhood and adolescence (Table 19-1).

RETICULOCYTES

Reticulocytes are found in large numbers in the peripheral blood of the fetus, reflecting active erythropoiesis. In the term newborn

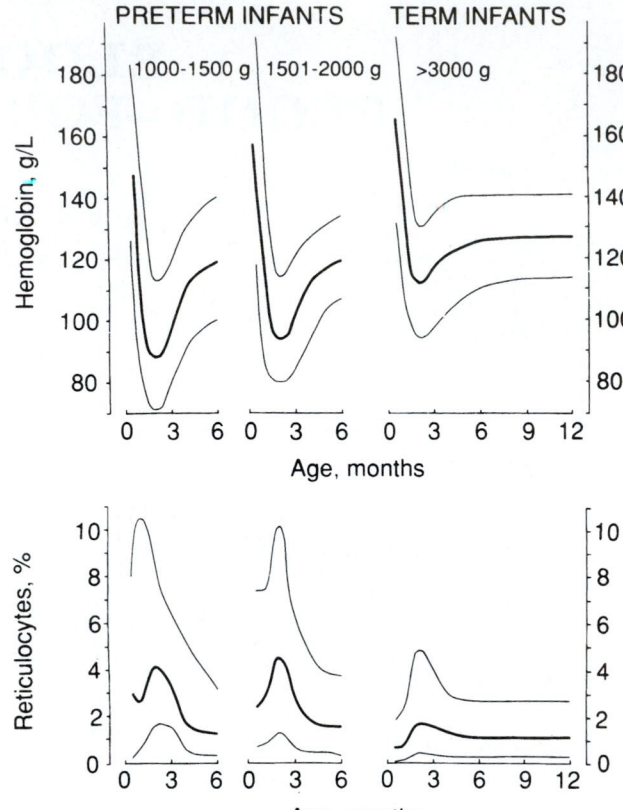

FIGURE 19-1 **Hemoglobin concentration and reticulocyte count in preterm and term infants. Median values and 95% confidence limits are indicated for each of three birthweight categories. SOURCE:** *Hemoglobin values from Ludström et al: J Pediatr 91:878, 1977; and Saarinen, Siimes: J Pediatr 92:412, 1978; reticulocyte values from unpublished data on the same infants from whom hemoglobin values were derived.*

infant, the reticulocyte count averages about 300×10^9/L, or 5% of total red cells. The reticulocyte count remains high during the first 3 days, then drops rapidly to average values below 2% by 7 days after birth. At about 2 months of age, a transient increase in

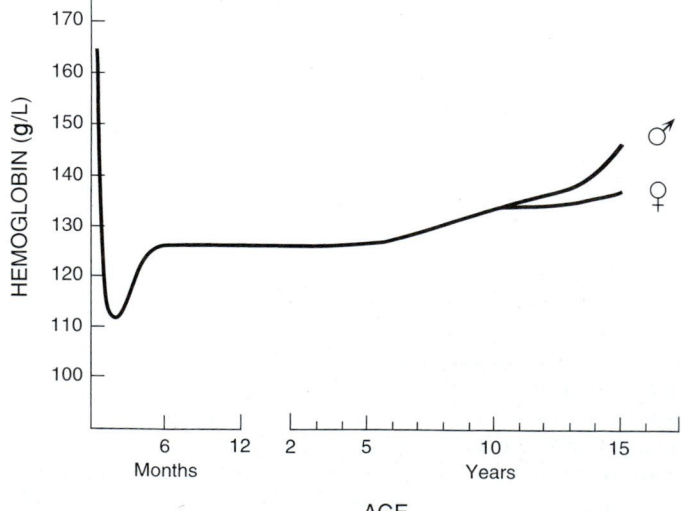

FIGURE 19-2 **Developmental changes in mean hemoglobin levels 0–15 years.**

TABLE 19-1

ESTIMATED NORMAL MEAN VALUES AND LOWER LIMITS OF NORMAL (95% RANGE) FOR HEMOGLOBIN, HEMATOCRIT, AND MCV AND MCH

AGE (Y)	HEMOGLOBIN (g/L)		PACKED CELL VOLUME (%)		MCV (fL)		MCH (pg)	
	MEAN	LOWER LIMIT	MEAN	LOWER LIMIT	MEAN	LOWER LIMIT	MEAN	LOWER LIMIT
0.5–4	125	110	36	32	80	72	28	24
5–10	130	115	38	33	83	75	29	25
11–14F	135	120	39	34	85	77	29	26
11–14M	140	120	41	35	85	77	29	26
15–19F	135	120	40	34	88	79	30	27
15–19M	150	130	43	37	88	79	30	27
20–44F	135	120	40	35	90	80	31	27
20–44M	155	135	45	39	90	80	31	27

Note: Hemoglobin and MCH were obtained by Coulter counter, packed cell volume was obtained by centrifugation, and MCV was obtained from packed cell volume divided by the Coulter red cell count. All data are based on venous blood in whites after excluding individuals with laboratory evidence of iron deficiency or inflammatory disease. Hemoglobin values are rounded out to the nearest 5 g/L. Red cell indices are calculated from combined data for both sexes because of the relatively minor difference in values. MCV = mean corpuscular volume; MCH = mean corpuscular hemoglobin.

reticulocytes coincides with increased erythropoietic activity during the recovery from physiological anemia (Fig. 19-1). Reticulocyte counts are higher in premature infants, with values as high as 10% at birth, followed by a rapid fall to values averaging below 3% between 1 and 4 weeks of age. After 4 months of age, the average reticulocyte count remains below 2% ($60–75 \times 10^9/L$).

NUCLEATED RED BLOOD CELLS (NRBC)

NRBC average about $0.5 \times 10^9/L$ in term infants and 1.0 to 1.5 $\times 10^9/L$ in preterm infants, being higher in less mature infants. Equivalent values, expressed as percentage of white cell count, are 3% in term and 6 to 9% in premature infants. After birth, the number of NRBC decreases about 50% every 12 hours, and circulating NRBC are not normally present after the first week of life.

BLOOD VOLUME

After the initial postnatal adjustments, blood volume maintains a relatively constant relationship to body weight throughout most of life. In term newborn infants, the average blood volume is 85 mL/kg, and premature infants have an average blood volume of 90 mL/kg body weight. The blood volume increases to a mean of 105 mL/kg during the first few days after birth and then decreases during the first few months. The average blood volume of infants after 6 months of age is 75 to 77 mL/kg, similar to that of older children and adults.

19.1.3   Embryonic, Fetal, and Adult Hemoglobins

Hemoglobin is a complex molecule made up of iron-containing heme groups and a protein moiety, globin. Hemoglobin accounts for more than 95% of the total protein and for about 90% of the dry weight of the red blood cell. Hemoglobin is a spherical molecule that has a molecular weight of 68,000 and is a tetramer made up of two pairs of globin chains, each of which is attached to an iron-containing porphyrin ring (heme). The type of globin chain is designated by a Greek letter followed by a subscript indicating the

number of chains per molecule. Thus, normal adult hemoglobin, which contains two pairs of α and β chains, is represented as $\alpha_2\beta_2$. The α and β polypeptide chains are chemically different, and their synthesis is directed by different genes on different chromosomes (Fig. 19-3).

Within the red cells of the embryo, the embryonic hemoglobins Gower-1, Gower-2, and Portland are demonstrable. These primitive hemoglobins contain ζ and ϵ chains. In embryos at 4 to 8 weeks of gestation, the Gower and Portland hemoglobins predominate, but by 8 to 12 weeks they have disappeared.

Fetal hemoglobin (HbF) contains α and γ polypeptide chains and can be represented as $\alpha_2\gamma_2$. HbF is resistant to denaturation by strong alkali, a property that can be used for quantification. After the eighth week of gestation, HbF is the predominant hemoglobin and at 6 months accounts for about 90% of the total (Fig. 19-3). The percentage of HbF then declines at a rate of 3 to 4% per week as adult hemoglobin synthesis progressively increases. At birth, HbF averages about 70%. Measurement of hemoglobin synthesis in cord blood reticulocytes by isotopic techniques indicates that rates of production of HbA and HbF are roughly equal. The apparent discrepancy between rate of synthesis and the total amount present is explained by the fact that most of the hemoglobin present in the newborn was synthesized weeks to months earlier, during the period when production of HbF predominated. At the time of birth there is an abrupt decrease in γ chain synthesis. The production of HbF after birth continues, but at a markedly reduced rate, resulting in a decreasing proportion of HbF. By 4 months of age, HbF is less than 20%, and at 1 year, values are less than 2%, the level seen in older children and adults. In individuals with major β-chain hemoglobinopathies and thalassemias, the rate of decline in fetal hemoglobin is slower, and elevated values may be present throughout life. Other conditions in which fetal hemoglobin may be elevated include hereditary persistence of fetal hemoglobin, D-trisomy syndrome, and aplastic anemia.

Small amounts of normal adult hemoglobin (HbA) can be detected even in embryonic life. By the sixth month of gestation there is about 5 to 10% HbA present, and a steady increase in HbA follows, which reaches about 30% at term. The production of the minor adult hemoglobin HbA_2 ($\alpha_2\delta_2$) begins in late gestation and makes up a small fraction of the total hemoglobin, and it accounts

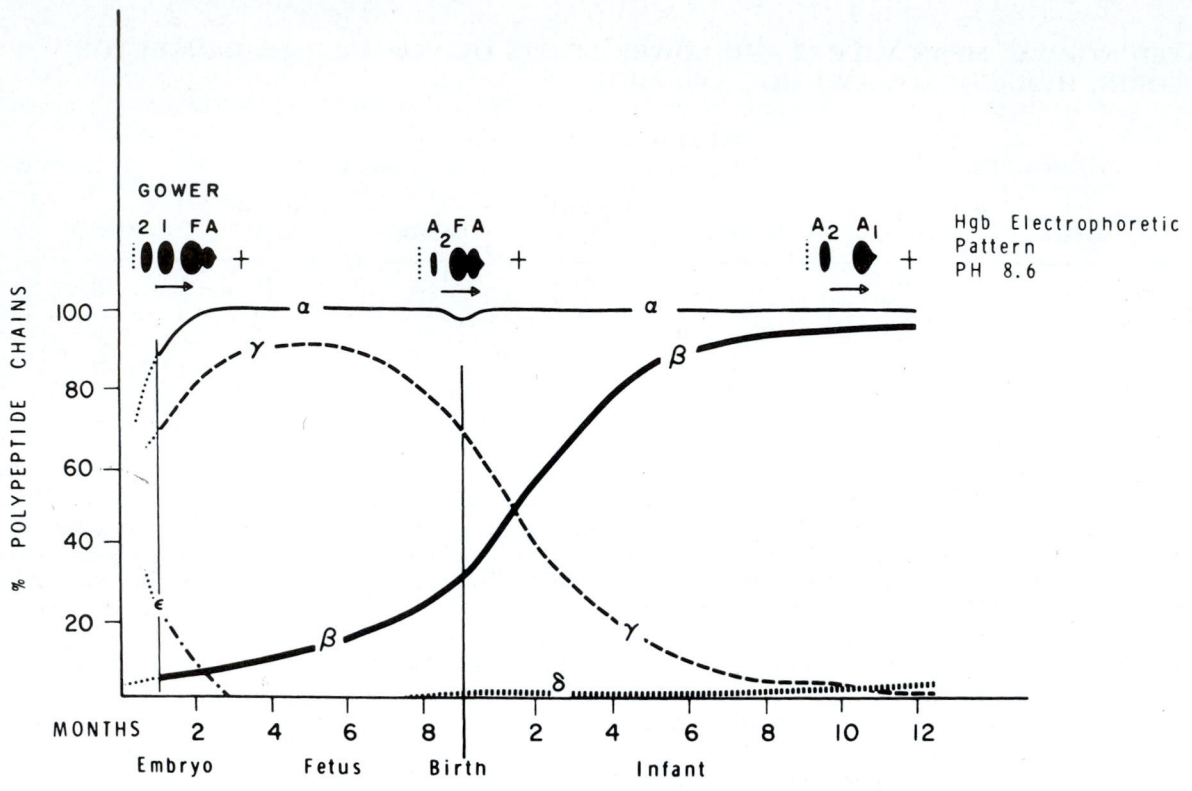

FIGURE 19-3 **Globin polypeptide chains and hemoglobins in embryonic, fetal, and postnatal periods. SOURCE: *Modified from Pearson HA: J Pediatr 69:466, 1966.***

for about 2 to 3% of total hemoglobin after the first few months postnatally. HbA_2 is diagnostically elevated in β-thalassemia trait (Sec. 19.4.7).

19.1.4 Oxygen Delivery

OXYGEN TRANSPORT DURING DEVELOPMENT

The function of hemoglobin is to combine reversibly with oxygen, allowing red blood cells to pick up oxygen from the lungs and deliver it to the tissues. This function can be depicted in quantitative terms by the oxygen dissociation curve (see Chapter 4). The oxygen saturation of a red cell suspension is plotted against the oxygen tension, and the tension at which hemoglobin becomes 50% saturated is designated as P_{50}. In the adult, the P_{50} averages 27 mm Hg (Fig. 19-4).

In the fetus and newborn the P_{50} is about 20 mm Hg, favoring the extraction of oxygen from the maternal circulation; thus, an oxygen saturation of 70% can be attained in the fetal placental veins despite a relatively low PO_2 of 30 mm Hg. Although the high oxygen affinity of fetal blood suits the conditions of the intrauterine environment, it limits the proportional release of oxygen to tissues after birth. A P_{50} that is more favorable for extrauterine conditions is not reached for 2 to 3 months after birth.

2,3-DIPHOSPHOGLYCERATE (2,3-DPG)

The postnatal shift of the oxygen dissociation curve to the right occurs because organic phosphates, especially 2,3-DPG, can decrease the affinity of the HbA for oxygen by competing with oxygen

for binding sites. HbF reacts less with 2,3-DPG and so is able to bind oxygen more tenaciously, accounting for the left-shifted oxygen dissociation curve at birth. The postnatal shift of the oxygen dissociation curve to the right is largely attributable to the decreas-

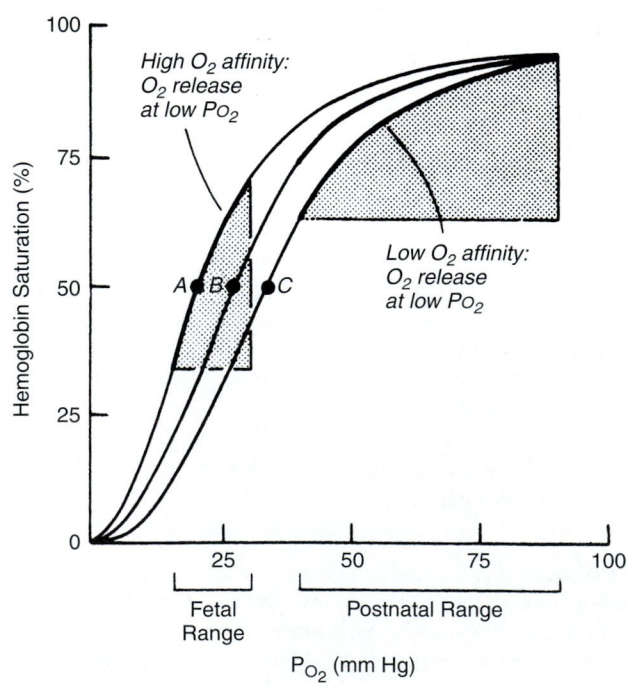

FIGURE 19-4 **Oxygen dissociation curve in the newborn *(A)*, the normal adult *(B)*, and the adult exposed to chronic hypoxia *(C)*. See text for explanation.**

ing level of HbF and its replacement by HbA. The rapid shift of the oxygen dissociation curve to the right in response to high altitude exposure and anemia results primarily from an increase in the red cell concentration of 2,3-DPG.

References

Bunn HF: Human hemoglobins: normal and abnormal. In: Nathan DG, Orkin SH, eds: Nathan and Oski Hematology of Infancy and Childhood, 5th ed. Philadelphia, WB Saunders, 1998:729–761

Dallman PR, Siimes MA: Percentile curves for hemoglobin and red cell volume in infancy and childhood. J Pediatr 94:26, 1979

Erslev AJ, Adamson JW, Eschbach JW, Winearls CG, eds: Erythropoietin: Molecular, Cellular, and Clinical Biology. Baltimore, Johns Hopkins Press, 1991

19.2   ANEMIA: DIAGNOSIS AND CLASSIFICATION

Howard A. Pearson and Peter R. Dallman

Anemia is defined as a lower than normal value for the related measurements of hemoglobin, hematocrit, and number of RBC. The lower limit of the normal range is set somewhat arbitrarily at two standard deviations below the mean at any given age. There are age-related differences in the "normal" hemoglobin level during the first decade of life and after puberty, and gender-related differences also (see Fig. 19-2). These differences must be considered in making a diagnosis of anemia. Some laboratories use only adult values and will erroneously report levels of hemoglobin that are normal in childhood as low. Defining anemia as two standard deviations below the normal mean hemoglobin results in 2.5% of normal children being classified as being anemic. Such individuals tend to track at their own low level over extended periods of time. Conversely, some individuals have hemoglobin values in the lower part of the normal range that may increase after treatment with hematinics or after the resolution of an infection or inflammatory process. Age-related normal means and lower limits of normal hemoglobin, hematocrit, and mean corpuscular volume (MCV) are shown in Table 19-1. Figure 19-2 depicts the pattern of normal mean hemoglobin levels from birth to adult life.

19.2.1   Approaches to Diagnosis

HISTORY

Historical data to be obtained include diet, infection or chronic disease, medications and other environmental exposures, and ethnicity. The diet during infancy is particularly relevant to iron deficiency. Infants who have been fed only whole cow's milk or non–iron-fortified cow milk formulas are at risk for developing iron deficiency. Although the iron present in human milk appears to be better absorbed than that in cow's milk, it is insufficient to meet the requirements for growth, and infants consuming only breast milk may develop iron deficiency after 9 to 12 months of age. Vitamin B_{12} deficiency may occur in breast-fed babies of strict vegetarian mothers (vegans). Infants exclusively fed goat's milk are at risk for developing folic acid deficiency.

The age of the child at recognition of anemia may be diagnostically important. Intrinsic abnormalities of the red cell membrane and red cell enzymopathies may present in the newborn period with anemia and jaundice, whereas major β-globin chain hemoglobin disorders such as sickle cell disease and thalassemia major usually have normal hematologic values in the neonatal period and do not become evident until 3 to 6 months of age or later. The age of onset also may be important for differentiating an acquired from a congenital disorder.

Many hemolytic anemias are genetically determined. An inherited anemia such as hereditary spherocytosis may be suggested by a family history of neonatal hyperbilirubinemia, anemia, jaundice, splenomegaly, splenectomy, or gallstones. A family history indicating dominant inheritance suggests a defect of the erythrocyte membrane or a hemoglobinopathy, whereas recessive inheritance is characteristic of many enzymopathies.

In the differential diagnosis of anemia in children, the relative frequencies of various etiologies should be considered. Iron deficiency and the anemia of acute and chronic infections are by far the most common causes of anemia in children. Next in frequency are genetic conditions such as hereditary spherocytosis. Sickle-cell diseases are prevalent in African-Americans, and thalassemia is common in people of Mediterranean or Southeast Asian ethnicity. Other causes of anemia are relatively unusual.

PHYSICAL EXAMINATION

The most important physical finding of anemia is pallor, but this is often a subtle finding that is evident only when the degree of anemia is relatively severe (Hb < 70–80 g/L). Anemia is best appreciated by pallor of the mucous membranes and conjunctivae, particularly in dark-skinned children. The red color of the lines in the palms of the hand disappears when the hemoglobin falls below 70 to 80 g/L.

Children tolerate even fairly severe anemia quite well when it develops slowly. Some children with iron deficiency anemia have few symptoms even when the hemoglobin is 50 to 60 g/L. Children with sickle cell anemia who chronically have hemoglobin levels of 65 to 80 g/L often have normal activity and few symptoms. Tachycardia is present only when anemia is severe or of sudden onset. Jaundice, best appreciated as yellow sclerae, suggests a hemolytic process, although some children with chronic hemolytic anemias are not clinically jaundiced. Lymphadenopathy, hepatosplenomegaly, and signs and symptoms of systemic diseases should be ascertained.

LABORATORY DIAGNOSIS

HEMOGLOBIN, HEMATOCRIT, AND RED CELL INDICES Modern electronic cell counters accurately measure white blood cells, red blood cells, and platelet numbers as well as hemoglobin (Hb) level, MCV (mean corpuscular volume), and MCH (mean corpuscular hemoglobin). The hematocrit (Hct) and mean corpuscular hemoglobin concentration (MCHC) are computer-derived values. Many electronic cell counters also measure red cell distribution width (RDW), which assesses the variability of size of the red cells, evident as anisocytosis on the peripheral blood smear. Hemoglobin can also be measured by spectrophotometers, which must be periodically calibrated, and Hct can be easily measured by microcentrifuges. Hematocrit values can be estimated by multiplying the Hb value by 0.3, and Hb level is estimated by dividing Hct by 0.3.

The MCV, directly measured by electronic counters, provides a basis for deciding whether the red cell population is macrocytic, normocytic, or microcytic. However, age-related norms must be employed to make this decision because RBC of the fetus and new-born are very macrocytic, whereas during the first 2 to 3 years of life they are distinctly microcytic compared to adult values (Table 19-1). The MCH reflects red cell hemoglobin content and gives a quantitative assessment of hypochromia evident on the blood smear. Because most microcytic anemias are also hypochromic, MCH is usually proportional to the MCV and may be even more sensitive than the MCV in the diagnosis of mild iron deficiency. The MCHC is a derived rather than a directly measured value and is not useful in assessing hypochromia. A high value of MCHC, however, is characteristic of spherocytosis.

RETICULOCYTE COUNT   The number of reticulocytes in peripheral blood reflects the rate at which new RBC, which contain stainable RNA, are being produced and released from the erythroid bone marrow. A high reticulocyte count can be expected when there is polychromatophilia on the blood smear and may sometimes be accompanied by an increased MCV because reticulocytes are larger than mature red cells. Reticulocyte counts can be done on a blood smear stained with new methylene blue by counting the percentage of RBC with visible blue staining of reticulum mesh. Normal RBC live for about 100 days, so about 1% are removed from the circulation each day, and in the steady state, about 1% new red cells are released from the bone marrow each day. New RBC contain stainable reticulum for about $1\frac{1}{2}$ days, so the normal reticulocyte count is 1.0 to 2.0%. The rather tedious manual method is increasingly being replaced by an automated fluorescent reticulocyte count performed by programmed electronic counters that provides an accurate absolute reticulocyte count. The normal absolute reticulocyte count is $40–75 \times 10^9/L$. Low values ($<40 \times 10^9/L$) indicate erythroid underproduction, and increased values ($> 100 \times 10^9/L$) suggest erythroid marrow hyperplasia often associated with hemolysis. Transiently high reticulocyte counts are seen after acute blood loss and after institution of specific therapy for iron, folic acid, or vitamin B_{12} deficiency.

MEASURES OF HEMOLYSIS   *Hemolysis* refers to an increased rate of RBC destruction leading to a survival time that is less than the normal 100 to 120 days. In acute hemolysis with a rapid onset of anemia, a compensatory increase in RBC production mediated by erythropoietin (EPO) takes several days before reticulocytosis occurs. In chronic hemolytic states, anemia is usually present because the rate of RBC destruction and production are not balanced. However, in some patients, the degree of hemolysis is fully compensated by increased RBC production, resulting in a normal hemoglobin level. Such patients will, however, have an elevated reticulocyte count.

In most chronic hemolytic states, RBC are destroyed *extravascularly* in the reticuloendothelial (RE) tissues of the spleen, liver, and bone marrow. Within the RE cell, hemoglobin is catabolized to iron, amino acids, and the heme metabolite bilirubin. Most patients with chronic severe hemolysis often have elevated serum levels of unconjugated (indirect) bilirubin, and many are jaundiced. However, hepatic conjugation and clearance of bilirubin may result in normal serum bilirubin levels, and hyperbilirubinemia and clinical jaundice should not be considered essential findings to consider a diagnosis of hemolysis. Chronically increased rates of bilirubin metabolism and biliary excretion, characteristic of congenital and chronic hemolysis, often result in gallstones, which are composed of calcium bilirubinate and are usually multiple, faceted, and radiopaque.

Primarily *intravascular hemolysis* is characteristic of some hemolytic anemias that are immune mediated, drug induced, or microangiopathic. Free hemoglobin is liberated into the plasma, where it combines with haptoglobin. The haptoglobin-hemoglobin complex is then cleared by RE tissues. When the rate of clearance exceeds the rate of hepatic haptoglobin synthesis, the level of serum haptoglobin decreases below the normal range (20–200 mg/dL), and patients with hemolysis are often anhaptoglobinemic. Low or absent levels of serum haptoglobin are also seen in hemolytic states where red cell destruction is primarily extravascular. In acute intravascular hemolysis the binding capacity of haptoglobin for hemoglobin may be exceeded, and unbound, free hemoglobin is excreted by the kidney, resulting in hemoglobinuria as indicated by a positive test for occult blood without RBC in the urinary sediment; in chronic hemolytic states, hemosiderin may be present in the urinary sediment.

BONE MARROW ASPIRATION AND BIOPSY

Bone marrow examination is painful and should not be undertaken for trivial reasons. For example, in sickle cell anemia, hereditary spherocytosis, and thalassemia, bone marrow examination provides little information that cannot be obtained from studies of peripheral blood. Measurement of serum ferritin levels and other iron studies almost always obviates the need for bone marrow aspiration to assess reticuloendothelial iron stores (hemosiderin).

Bone marrow aspiration may be necessary for the diagnosis of pure red cell anemias and neutropenias. The bone marrow should usually be evaluated when a diagnosis of leukemia is considered or when metastatic malignancy, bone marrow failure, or storage diseases such as Gaucher and Niemann-Pick disease are suspected. Overall cellularity, morphology, and maturation of the hematopoietic cell lines can be evaluated. Needle biopsy, which can be done at the same time as aspiration of the bone marrow, provides a large, intact specimen and is especially useful for assessing marrow architecture and cellularity. Marrow aspiration is often indicated in thrombocytopenic states to assess the numbers of megakaryocytes, an indicator of platelet production (Sec. 19.7). The most notable bone marrow finding in infants and young children, compared to older patients, is a predominance of mature lymphocytes.

19.2.2 Classification and Diagnosis of Anemia

An *erythrokinetic classification of anemia* is based on the fact that the steady-state level of hemoglobin reflects a balance between production of red cells by the bone marrow and the rate of their peripheral destruction. Thus, most anemias can be classified as production problems or hemolytic conditions.

A *morphologic classification of anemia* is based on RBC size (MCV) and morphology. A number of childhood anemias are associated with characteristic RBC appearance, and examination of RBC morphology on peripheral blood smears is an essential component of diagnosis (Fig. 19-5). A diagnostic algorithm based on both erythrokinetic and morphologic criteria is shown in Fig. 19-6.

In the workup of a child with presumed anemia, it is necessary to determine that anemia is actually present according to age-appropriate standards. Hemoglobin concentrations in blacks are

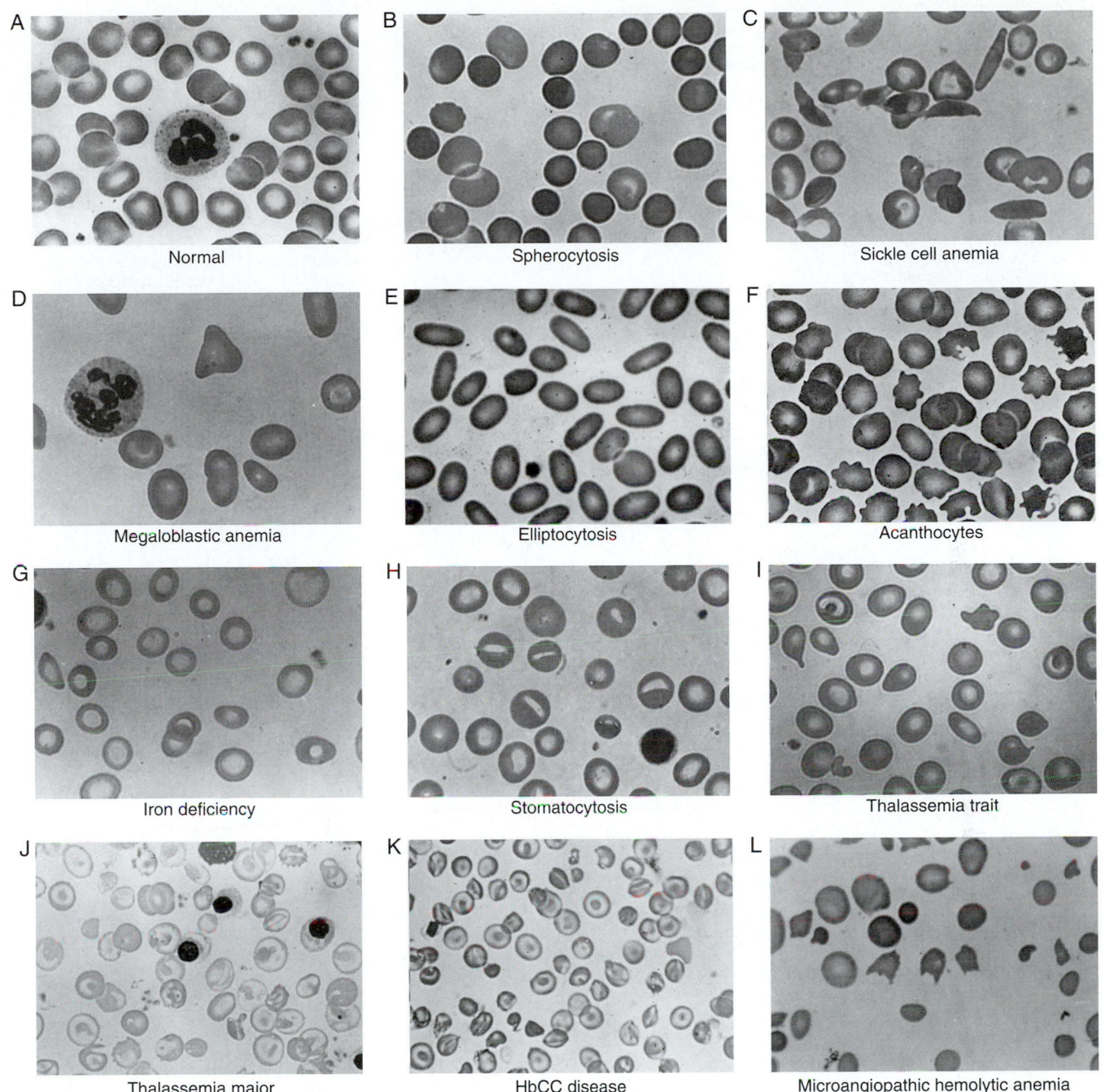

A Normal
B Spherocytosis
C Sickle cell anemia
D Megaloblastic anemia
E Elliptocytosis
F Acanthocytes
G Iron deficiency
H Stomatocytosis
I Thalassemia trait
J Thalassemia major
K HbCC disease
L Microangiopathic hemolytic anemia

FIGURE 19-5   RBC Morphology in various conditions.

about 5 g/L lower than in whites, a difference that is not explained by iron deficiency or thalassemia.

Next, an evaluation is made of whether the anemia is a result of decreased red cell production (aregenerative) or increased destruction (hemolysis). This is most easily assessed by the reticulocyte count. Because reticulocytosis reflects increased erythroid activity of the bone marrow, a sustained reticulocytosis is very suggestive of a hemolytic process, whereas reticulocytopenia is characteristic of an aregenerative process. Next, the average size and hemoglobin content of the red blood cells should be determined by measuring the MCV and mean corpuscular hemoglobin (MCH) using electronic cell counters. Finally, the actual morphology of the red blood cells should be assessed on a stained peripheral blood smear (Fig.

19-5). These readily available determinations permit a presumptive diagnosis of most anemias in children.

19.3 NUTRITIONAL ANEMIAS

19.3.1 Iron Deficiency

Kenneth R. Bridges and Howard A. Pearson

Iron deficiency anemia is the most common hematologic disease of infancy and childhood. Despite the fact that iron is the second most

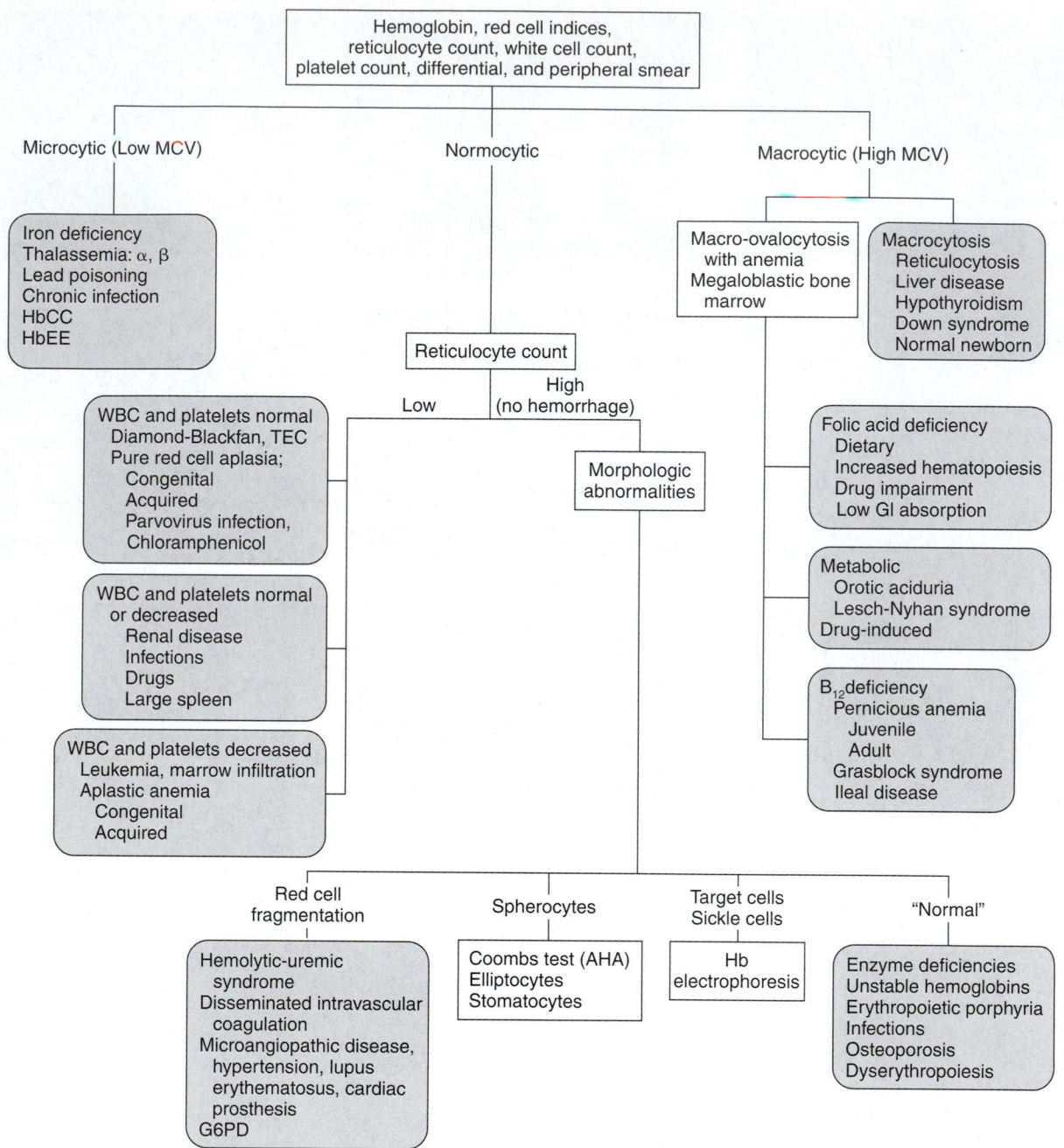

FIGURE 19-6   Algorithm diagramming the laboratory of anemia. AHA = autoimmune hemolytic anemia; GI = gastrointestinal; G6PD = glucose-6-phosphate dehydrogenase; Hb = hemoglobin; WBC = white blood cell count. SOURCE: *Modified from Hastings and Lubin, Rudolph's Fundamentals of Pediatrics, Stamford: Appleton and Lange, 2nd Edition p. 469, 1998.*

abundant metal in the earth's crust, iron is the most prevalent single nutrient deficiency worldwide. The newborn infant has about 0.25 to 0.5 g of total body iron, most in the circulating hemoglobin. An adult has up to 5.0 g of body iron, so that about 4.5 g of iron, or about 0.5 mg/d, must be absorbed during childhood. During periods of maximal growth—infancy and adolescence—the iron requirements for expanded blood volume and muscle mass may exceed the rate of iron accrual. In addition to the growth requirement, an additional 0.2 to 0.5 mg/d of absorbed iron is required to balance losses from desquamation of epithelial cells of the gas-

trointestinal tract. Because only about 10% of dietary iron is absorbed, the child's diet must contain 10 to 15 mg of iron to maintain a positive iron balance. During infancy, when only small amounts of iron-rich foods may be consumed, this level of iron intake is difficult to attain unless iron-fortified foods are provided. Infants and children from low-income families continue to have iron deficiency despite a decline in the incidence of the condition over the past 30 years. To prevent iron deficiency, the Committee on Nutrition of the American Academy of Pediatrics has recommended:

1. Breast milk should be used for at least 5 to 6 months when possible. Elemental iron supplementation of 1 mg per kilogram per day should be provided to infants who are exclusively fed breast milk beyond 6 months of age.
2. Infants who are not breast-fed should receive an iron-supplemented formula (12 mg of elemental iron per liter) for the first year of life.
3. Iron-enriched cereals should be among the first solid foods introduced.
4. Whole cow's milk should be avoided during the first year of life to prevent occult GI bleeding.

Premature infants are particularly susceptible to iron deficiency as a result of a reduced iron endowment at birth because of their small blood volume coupled with the dilutional effect of rapid growth. Iron supplementation or iron-fortified formulas should be started by 1 to 2 months of age and continued for at least 1 to 2 years.

IRON ABSORPTION

Its low aqueous solubility at neutral pH makes the acquisition of iron for metabolic use a major challenge. Gastric acidity assists conversion to the absorbable ferrous (Fe^{2+}) form, but the efficiency of this process is limited. The use of histamine H_2 blockers or acid pump inhibitors to treat peptic gastroesophageal reflux can impair iron absorption (see Sec. 17.10). Many plant products contain iron, but absorption is limited both by low solubility and by dietary chelators, such as phytates, that bind ambient iron. Heme or organic iron present in animal food products is the most readily absorbed form of iron, and its absorption occurs by a different mechanism than that of inorganic iron and is independent of gastric pH. About 10% of iron is absorbed from a mixed diet. The scarcity of meat products in the diet is the major cause of endemic iron deficiency anemia in much of the Third World. Some clinical disorders disrupt the integrity of the enteric mucosa and hamper iron absorption. Inflammatory bowel disease, particularly Crohn disease, can damage the jejunum and duodenum, where most iron absorption occurs, and gastrointestinal bleeding may exacerbate the problem. Both tropical and nontropical sprue (celiac disease) can also interfere with iron absorption.

Rarely, malabsorption of iron without a structurally defective intestine occurs as an inherited syndrome related to genetic defects of the bowel absorption factors. Iron malabsorption can be assessed by obtaining a serum iron level 1 to 2 hours after an oral dose of 1 to 2 mg/kg of elemental iron. Failure to observe a significant increase over baseline level is consistent with iron malabsorption.

BLOOD LOSS

Chronic blood loss from gastrointestinal lesions commonly causes iron deficiency. Peptic ulcer disease with chronic blood loss may present as iron deficiency anemia. Meckel diverticulum, a persistent omphalomesenteric duct that may contain ectopic gastric mucosa, is the most common congenital defect of the gastrointestinal tract that causes chronic blood loss in children. Other structural defects such as hereditary hemorrhagic telangiectasia (the Osler-Weber-Rendu syndrome) are much less frequent. Whole cow's milk contains proteins that can irritate the lining of the gastrointestinal tract in some infants, resulting in chronic blood loss and iron deficiency.

The world's leading cause of gastrointestinal blood loss is hookworm infection, caused by *Necator americanus* or *Ancylostoma duo-denale,* which is endemic in much of the world. *Trichuriasis,* or whipworm infection, and *schistosomiasis,* very common in tropical areas, may be associated with chronic blood loss and iron deficiency anemia in children. Occasionally, bleeding into the urinary tract causes iron deficiency, but gross urinary blood is usually sufficiently alarming that patients seek medical attention before iron deficiency develops. Patients with chronic intravascular hemolysis, such as occurs with intracardiac prostheses and paroxysmal nocturnal hemoglobinuria, may develop iron deficiency because of urinary excretion of large amounts of hemosiderin deposited into the renal tubules. Pulmonary blood loss sufficiently severe to produce iron deficiency can occur in idiopathic pulmonary hemosiderosis characterized by recurrent bleeding into the lungs, hemosiderin-laden macrophages in the sputum, and iron deficiency anemia (see Chapter 23).

NONHEMATOLOGIC EFFECTS OF IRON DEFICIENCY

Iron deficiency, with or without anemia, may affect growth and cognitive function in children as young as 9 to 12 months of age, and prevention of iron deficiency during infancy is imperative. Epithelial changes such as atrophy of the papillae of the tongue and spooning of the fingernails can be seen in adults with iron deficiency anemia but are unusual in children. Pica occurs variably in patients with iron deficiency anemia who may eat laundry starch, ice, and clay, which bind iron in the gastrointestinal tract. Some studies have shown that iron treatment improves the symptom of pica. Iron deficiency increases the gastrointestinal absorption not only of iron but also of a number of heavy metals, including lead, that share the same absorption pathways. Chronic exposure to environmental lead exacerbates iron deficiency by competitive inhibition of iron absorption. The cause of iron deficiency anemia in infants and adolescent girls is usually inadequate dietary intake, but GI blood loss and excessive menstrual loss must always be considered.

LABORATORY DIAGNOSIS

Iron deficiency anemia is associated with microcytic, hypochromic anemia, and the blood smear shows microcytic, hypochromic RBC (see Fig. 19-5G), and MCV and MCH are low. Because iron deficiency anemia results in an uneven red cell size (anisocytosis), an increased RDW is found. A diagnosis of iron deficiency anemia is not tenable if the red cell indices are normal. Thrombocytosis is usually present with platelet counts $>450 \times 10^9$/L, but rarely significant thrombocytopenia may be present. Reticulocyte count is low or normal. Recently measurement of reticulocyte MCH has been suggested as an early test because iron-deficient erythropoiesis in newly formed RBC can be detected.

Serum iron is low, and serum iron-binding capacity is increased, resulting in a low transferrin iron saturation ($<16\%$). When serum-transferring saturation is $<16\%$, iron can not be efficiently transferred into the developing RBC in the bone marrow.

Serum ferritin levels reflect the iron stores in the reticuloendothelial system. Low levels ($<10-15$ ng/mL) indicate that there are essentially no iron stores. Greatly elevated levels (>1000 ng/mL) occur in iron overload states such as transfusional hemosiderosis. Serum ferritin levels are increased as an acute-phase reactant during infection or inflammation and are also increased by hepatocellular diseases, somewhat limiting the diagnostic value of serum ferritin levels in these situations.

TABLE 19-2
STAGES OF IRON DEFICIENCY

	NORMAL	PRELATENT	LATENT	IRON DEFICIENCY ANEMIA
Iron stores	Present	Decreased	Absent	Absent
Serum ferritin (ng/mL)	>40	<20	<10	<10
Transferrin saturation (%)	35	35	<16	<16
Free erythrocyte protoporphyrin (ng/100 mL blood)	10	10	>35	>35
Hemoglobin (g/dL)	12	12	12	<11
MCV (fL)	80	80	80	<70

Another marker of iron status is the serum transferrin receptor (TR) level (normal <8.5 mg/L). Transferrin receptors are found on all cells except mature erythrocytes and are the primary physiological mechanism of iron uptake by developing normoblasts. Iron deficiency increases the serum TR level, apparently by release from iron-poor normoblasts in the bone marrow. Although it is not specific for iron deficiency, measurement of serum TR levels can help to distinguish iron deficiency from the anemia of chronic inflammation.

The ultimate step of heme formation is the insertion of an iron molecule into the porphyrin ring. If iron is not available to complete this step, there is an increase in the level of blood preheme porphyrins, collectively designated as free erythrocyte porphyrins (FEP) or zinc protoporphyrins (ZPP) (normal <35 mg/100 mL of whole blood). An elevation of FEP is an indication of iron-deficient erythropoiesis. Marked elevations in FEP are also seen in lead poisoning (see Chapter 4).

Progressive iron deficiency has several stages that are defined by laboratory values (Table 19-2).

Prelatent iron deficiency occurs when tissue iron stores are decreased as indicated by a low (but still >15 ng/mL) serum ferritin level. There is no anemia. Serum iron levels and TIBC are normal. *Latent iron deficiency* is characterized by low serum ferritin, low serum iron, increased TIBC, and a transferrin saturation <16% without anemia or increased FEP. In *iron deficiency anemia*, all of the measures of iron status are abnormal, and significant microcytic anemia is present.

The *β- and α-thalassemia traits* are often confused with iron deficiency because both are associated with microcytosis and hypochromia. In β-thalassemia trait, the Mentzer Index (MCV/RBC) is usually >12 in iron deficiency and <11 in thalassemia. Iron deficiency alters red cell size unevenly, whereas in contrast, thalassemia trait produces uniformly small erythrocytes. The RDW is normal in patients with thalassemia trait but is increased in iron deficiency anemia. Basophilic stippling and target cells are seen in thalassemia trait. Laboratory studies of iron metabolism are normal in thalassemia. The anemia of thalassemia trait is unresponsive to iron therapy.

TREATMENT Treatment of iron deficiency should always be coupled to diagnosis and correction of the cause when possible. Oral iron therapy is almost always sufficient to correct anemia and replace iron stores. The dose of oral iron is 2 to 6 mg of elemental ferrous iron/kg/d, given as a single or divided dose. The iron should not be mixed with milk or taken with food. GI intolerance and constipation are unusual in children. Oral iron may cause staining of the teeth, but this is temporary and can be avoided by rinsing the mouth or brushing the teeth after the medication is given. Response to iron therapy is signaled by a reticulocytosis beginning 3

to 5 days and peaking 7 to 10 days after starting therapy. An increase in hemoglobin of at least 10 to 20 g/L after 1 month is diagnostic of iron deficiency. Lack of response usually indicates noncompliance with the medication or another diagnosis. Parenteral iron (iron-dextran) is rarely indicated in children with nutritional iron deficiency but can be given by intravenous or intramuscular routes if indicated. An iron-saccharide complex for parenteral treatment of iron deficiency in adults has recently been licensed.

The *anemia of chronic inflammation* is associated with a number of pediatric diseases such as juvenile rheumatoid arthritis and other collagen vascular diseases, chronic infections, and inflammatory bowel disease. Chronic disorders that lack an inflammatory component do not produce this type of anemia. The cause of the anemia of chronic inflammation is multifactorial and includes reduced red cell survival, impaired marrow response to EPO, reduced EPO production, and impaired mobilization of iron from tissue stores.

The anemia is mild to moderate (Hb 80 to 110 g/L). Reticulocyte count is not increased; MCV is normal or slightly decreased; the RDW is slightly increased. Plasma ferritin levels are almost uniformly elevated (400 to 800 ng/mL). Inappropriately low but normal levels of serum ferritin (20–50 ng/mL) in a patient with active inflammatory disease may indicate concomitant iron deficiency. Bone marrow hemosiderin is increased, indicating defective mobilization and release from tissue stores. Serum iron level is low, but the increased TIBC characteristic of iron deficiency does not occur. A low serum iron level in the face of an elevated plasma ferritin distinguishes the anemia of chronic inflammation from iron deficiency, where both values are low. Serum transferrin receptors are normal in the anemia of inflammation but elevated in iron deficiency. Patients with the anemia of chronic inflammation have inappropriately low plasma erythropoietin levels for the degree of anemia because inflammatory cytokines suppress erythropoietin production.

Treatment of the anemia of chronic inflammation hinges on control of the underlying inflammatory or infectious process. Erythropoietin in very large doses can ameliorate the degree of anemia somewhat, but the improvement is usually modest, and EPO is rarely indicated. Despite the low levels of serum iron, iron medication is ineffective.

19.3.2 Copper Deficiency

Kenneth R. Bridges and Howard A. Pearson

Copper, like iron, is essential for normal cell growth and metabolism and is toxic in excess. Nutritional copper deficiency is rare, occurring under circumstances of extreme dietary deficit including inadvertent omission of copper from intravenous hyperalimentation, treatment of malnourished patients with a diet deficient in copper, and impaired copper absorption as a result of excess amounts of dietary zinc. The condition has also been described in small premature infants with very rapid growth rates receiving cow's milk formulas.

Copper deficiency and iron deficiency produce many similar laboratory abnormalities: microcytic, hypochromic anemia and low serum iron concentration. In copper deficiency, however, iron stores are normal, as indicated by normal levels of serum ferritin. The anemia of copper deficiency reflects impaired transport of transferrin-bound iron to the bone marrow. Leukopenia with marked neutropenia is often present, and vacuolated white cell precursors may be present in the bone marrow. Osteoporosis occurs occasionally in severe cases. Serum copper levels are <70 μg/dL. Oral treatment with 0.1 to 0.3 mg/kg of elemental copper per day (two or three times the estimated daily requirement) corrects the anemia and neutropenia. The dietary imbalance that produced the deficiency should be corrected.

19.3.3   Vitamin E Deficiency

Kenneth R. Bridges and Howard A. Pearson

Vitamin E is the most important antioxidant, free radical–scavenging substance of the lipid-soluble compartment. Vitamin E levels increase in the third trimester of fetal development, coinciding with the increase of fetal fat. Premature infants are especially susceptible to vitamin E deficiency, a condition that develops 6 to 8 weeks after birth. Addition of vitamin E and reduction of the proportion of polyunsaturated fatty acids in infant formulas have greatly reduced the frequency of this deficiency. Children with fat malabsorption syndromes, including cholestasis and cystic fibrosis, may develop vitamin E deficiency.

Vitamin E deficiency is characterized by hemolytic anemia and reticulocytosis, thrombocytosis, and generalized edema. Echinocytes and acanthocytes may be present on the peripheral blood smear (see Fig. 19-5F). Low serum levels (< 0.8 mg/g) of vitamin E or a therapeutic response to supplemental vitamin E establish a diagnosis. Effective response is obtained by treatment with 10 mg per day of oral vitamin E. Repeated intravenous administrations of large doses of vitamin E are not necessary for correction of the anemia but have been used as experimental treatment of retinopathy of prematurity or bronchopulmonary dysplasia.

References

American Academy of Pediatrics Committee on Nutrition: Iron supplementation for infants. Pediatrics 58:765–768, 1976

Andrews NC: Medical progress: disorders of iron metabolism. N Engl J Med 341:1986–1995, 1999

Lin C, Lin J, Chen S, Jiang M, Chiu C: Comparison of hemoglobin and red blood cell distribution width in the differential diagnosis of microcytic anemia. Arch Pathol Lab Med 116:1030–1032, 1992

Oski F: Iron deficiency in infancy and childhood. N Engl J Med 329:190–193, 1993

19.3.4   The Megaloblastic Anemias

Rudy Allen and Barton A. Kamen

The megaloblastic anemias are characterized by megaloblasts, large abnormal red cell precursors, in the bone marrow and macrocytes in the peripheral blood. Almost all instances of megaloblastic anemia are attributable to a deficiency of folic acid (folate) or vitamin B_{12} (cobalamin). Megaloblastic anemia is often suspected on the basis of an elevated MCV. The characteristic megaloblastic morphology seen in extreme deficiencies of these vitamins has become much less common (see Fig. 19-5D). Diagnosis is now often made when hematologic findings are relatively subtle.

FOLATE DEFICIENCY

The chief function of the folates is to serve as cofactors in metabolic reactions that involve the transfer of single carbon units, such as the conversion of deoxyuridylate to thymidylate, the nucleotide that is unique to DNA. Erythroblast maturation is arrested following DNA synthesis in the S and G_2 phases of the cell cycle, leading to an accumulation of large polychromatophilic megaloblasts in the bone marrow.

An adequate supply of folate from the mother is particularly critical during early fetal life. Folate supplementation during the first trimester decreases the prevalence of neural tube defects (NTD) in the fetus, and it is now recommended that all women of childbearing age take folate supplements. Infant formulas and breast milk provide adequate folate for term and for most low-birth-weight infants.

Folate deficiency can result from inadequate dietary intake, increased physiological demand, malabsorption, and drug interactions. Deficiency can develop relatively rapidly because little folate is stored in body tissues. Decreased intake is of particular concern in malnourished patients and those with poor diets. Increased physiological demand for folate is seen in conditions with rapid cell growth such as infancy, particularly in preterm infants, pregnancy, and lactation.

Increased requirements for folate have been invoked in patients with severe hemolytic anemias. Many hematologists recommend folic acid supplementation, 1 to 5 mg/d, for patients with sickle cell disease and other hemolytic disorders despite a number of studies that have not shown efficacy in pediatric patients. A recent report found that plasma homocysteine levels, a very sensitive marker of a folate deficiency, are not increased in patients with sickle cell anemia who were not receiving folate.

The recommended intake of folate for infants is 25 to 35 μg/d, about 3 to 5 μg/kg/d. Although folate is abundant in green vegetables and liver, milk is a relatively poor source of this vitamin. Breast milk contains about about 35 μg/L, which is sufficient to avoid folate deficiency. Cow's milk has about the same content, but powdered and evaporated milks are deficient. Heat treatment or sterilization of milk or home-prepared formula decreases the folate content by half. The heat lability of folate is not as marked in proprietary formulas, in which the vitamin is stabilized by ascorbic acid. Goat's milk is a very poor source of folate, and severe megaloblastic anemia may result if this is used as the major component of an infant's calories. Intestinal bacteria synthesize folate, absorption of which augments dietary intake. Folate-containing bacteria reside mainly in the colon, and reduction of intestinal bacterial colonization by broad-spectrum antibiotics may be associated with folate deficiency, particularly in debilitated patients.

Folate deficiency in infancy may be associated with chronic diarrhea and malabsorption states. Diarrhea may result in a depletion of intestinal γ-glutamyl hydrolase (conjugase), so that the conjugated polyglutamate forms of dietary folate can not be broken down to the monoglutamate, the absorbable form. Rare instances of congenital malabsorption of folate have been recognized in infants who developed severe megaloblastic anemia early in life.

Folate analogues such as methotrexate and antibiotics such as trimethoprim react with dihydrofolate reductase and interfere with the conversion of dihydrofolate substrates to active tetrahydrofolate. Clinical folic acid deficiency may also occur in association with anticonvulsant therapy with hydantoin as well as oral contraceptive use.

The amino acid homocysteine is derived exclusively from dietary methionine and is present in plasma at low concentrations (>2.7 ng/mL). Both folate and cobalamin deficiencies are associated with an increased plasma homocysteine level comparable to that seen in congenital homocystinuria. Hyperhomocysteinemia is associated with increased cardiac, cerebral, and peripheral vascular abnormalities including atherosclerosis and thrombosis. Increased levels of plasma homocysteine can be reduced by folate supplementation.

DIAGNOSIS   A sequence of biochemical changes occur in progressive folate deficiency. First, there is an increase in the plasma homocysteine level (>15 μm/mL). Next, serum folate levels fall below the lower limit of normal (2.7 ng/mL). Then, hypersegmented neutrophils appear in the blood (see Fig. 19-5D). RBC folate levels then become subnormal (<140 ng/mL). Finally, anemia and morphologic changes of megaloblastic anemia become evident. Macroovalocytes, large oval RBC, neutropenia, and thrombocytopenia are often present. Macrocytosis may be obscured by concomitant microcytic anemia.

Megaloblastic changes in the bone marrow affect all cell lines and are similar in both folate and vitamin B_{12} deficiency. Erythroid precursors are larger than normal and have nuclei with an open, finely granular chromatin pattern and prominent nucleoli. The cytoplasm has the eosinophilic staining of hemoglobin and appears too mature for the nucleus (nuclear-cytoplasmic dissociation). Myelocyte precursors are also enlarged and have immature nuclei.

TREATMENT   A therapeutic dose of folic acid (1.0 to 5.0 mg/d) should be given when a diagnosis of folate deficiency is established, especially in children with malabsorption syndromes. A low-dose therapeutic trial (0.1 mg/d) should be considered if specific diagnostic studies cannot be done to exclude vitamin B_{12} deficiency, and this produces a prompt reticulocyte response and an increase in hemoglobin level in folate deficiency that does not occur in vitamin B_{12} deficiency. Larger doses of folate may produce a hematologic response in vitamin B_{12} deficiency but can aggravate neurologic manifestations. After initial correction of anemia, 0.4 mg of folate, which is present in some multivitamin tablets, is an adequate daily maintenance dose.

VITAMIN B_{12} DEFICIENCY

Diagnosis of vitamin B_{12} deficiency in children is important because of the danger of irreversible neurologic damage including subacute posterior and lateral column demyelinization in the spinal cord with paresthesias, sensory deficits, and loss of deep tendon reflexes (Chapter 25). This can occur even in the absence of anemia or macrocytosis. Most deficiencies result from defects in absorption of vitamin B_{12}.

The usual diet contains a considerable excess of vitamin B_{12} over the recommended dietary allowances of 2 μg/d in the adult and 0.3 to 0.5 μg/d in infants. Animal products are the main dietary sources of vitamin B_{12}, but microorganisms also synthesize this vitamin. A minimum of 3 years is required for depletion of hepatic

stores, so dietary deficiency is rare except in strict vegetarians who avoid all animal products, including milk and eggs (vegans). Megaloblastic anemia with neurologic changes may occur in these individuals and also in their breast-fed babies.

The absorption of physiological amounts of vitamin B_{12} is dependent on the vitamin forming a complex with a specific protein, intrinsic factor (IF), produced by parietal cells of the stomach. The complex is taken up specifically in the distal ileum. Vitamin B_{12} then dissociates from the complex and is released into the circulation. In the plasma, vitamin B_{12} is bound to both the glycoprotein transcobalamin I and to a β-globulin transport protein, transcobalamin II. Cobalamin is metabolized in mitochondria to adenosylcobalamin, which is required for the metabolism of methylmalonic acid.

Most vitamin B_{12} deficiency states result from the absence or an abnormality in IF secretion by the gastric mucosa or from interference with absorption of the vitamin B_{12}-IF complex in the terminal ileum.

The term *pernicious anemia* is restricted to pathophysiological states associated with a deficiency of IF secretion. Two types of pernicious anemia have been described in children, and in both types, malabsorption of vitamin B_{12} can be corrected by administration of exogenous IF.

Congenital pernicious anemia occurs in patients with megaloblastic anemia and failure to thrive before 3 years of age. Gastric histology and acid secretion are normal, but IF is absent in the gastric secretions. There are no antibodies to intrinsic factor or associated endocrinopathies. An autosomal recessive inheritance pattern is suggested by a high incidence of consanguinity.

Juvenile pernicious anemia occurs in older children and is similar to pernicious anemia in adults. Gastric atrophy and decreased secretion of acid and pepsin are commonly associated with antibodies to IF or to parietal cells. Endocrinopathies such as hypoparathyroidism and hypothyroidism, chronic moniliosis, and immunodeficiencies such as selective IgA deficiency or abnormal lymphocyte function may occur.

Other causes of vitamin B_{12} deficiency should not be called pernicious anemia because IF is normal. These include utilization of the vitamin in the intestinal lumen by the fish tapeworm *Diphyllobothrium latum* or bacterial consumption of vitamin B_{12} in intestinal diverticuli or blind loops. Regional enteritis and surgical excision of this terminal ilium can result in B_{12} malabsorption.

Imerslund-Gräsbeck syndrome is a congenital autosomal recessive disorder with a selective ileal vitamin B_{12} malabsorption associated with proteinuria which presents in the first 2 years of life as megaloblastic anemia and failure to thrive.

Vitamin B_{12} malabsorption and transport are also decreased in a rare inherited deficiency of transcobalamin II. Serum B_{12} levels are usually normal because most of the vitamin is bound to transcobalamin I in the serum. Megaloblastic anemia, pancytopenia, failure to thrive, weakness, and diarrhea may present in the first few months of life.

DIAGNOSIS   Hematologic findings seen in vitamin B_{12} deficiency are indistinguishable from those seen in folate deficiency. However, neurologic findings that may precede anemia are found only in vitamin B_{12} deficiency. Vitamin B_{12} deficiency can be diagnosed when serum vitamin B_{12} levels are less than 100 pg/mL in the presence of a normal serum folate concentration. Serum methylmalonic acid (MMA) levels are increased in B_{12} deficiency and are normal in folate deficiency. The combination of elevated serum MMA and normal homocysteine levels is 95% sensitive in detecting cobalamin deficiency, even when only mild hematologic abnormalities are present.

Assessment of vitamin B_{12} absorption (Schilling test) is rarely used. The diagnosis of pernicious anemia can usually be established by the presence of anti-IF antibodies in the blood in association with low B_{12} levels and high MMA levels.

TREATMENT Most conditions resulting in vitamin B_{12} deficiency are related to inadequate absorption and require parenteral treatment throughout life. Once a diagnosis is established, monthly subcutaneous injections of 1 mg of cyanocobalamin or hydroxycobalamin should be given. If transcobalamin II is missing or nonfunctional, a cellular deficiency of the vitamin occurs even though the serum B_{12} level is normal. Large (1000 μg) doses of vitamin B_{12} given once or twice a week are required.

CANCER CHEMOTHERAPY AND INBORN ERRORS OF METABOLISM

The most common cause of macrocytosis and megaloblastic anemia is treatment with cancer chemotherapeutic drugs, not only with folate antagonists such as methotrexate but with a variety of other cytotoxic drugs as well. Genetic conditions associated with megaloblastic anemia include inborn errors of pyrimidine (orotic aciduria) or purine metabolism (Lesch-Nyhan syndrome).

References

Cortes HR, Griener JC, Hyland K, et al: Plasma homocysteine levels and folate status in children with sickle cell anemia. J Pediatr Hematol Oncol 21:219–223, 1999

Kamen BA, Meyers P: Megaloblastic anemias. In: Miller DR, Baehner RL, eds: Blood Diseases in Infancy and Childhood. St Louis, CV Mosby, 1997:220–240

Whitehead VM, Rosenblatt DS, Cooper BA: Megaloblastic anemias. In: Nathan DG, Orkin SH, eds: Nathan and Oski's Hematology of Infancy and Childhood, 5th ed. Philadelphia, WB Saunders, 1998:385–422

19.4   ABNORMALITIES OF HEMOGLOBIN STRUCTURE AND FUNCTION

19.4.1   Sickle Cell Diseases

Kwaku Ohene-Frempong

Sickle cell disease (SCD) is the collective designation of a group of disorders characterized by the presence of ≥50% sickle hemoglobin (HbS) in the red cell and varying degrees of hemolytic anemia. HbS, a variant of normal HbA, results from a mutation in the sixth codon of the β-globin gene, which is located on the short arm of chromosome 11. The adenine nucleotide of the normal codon, GAG, which codes for glutamic acid, is replaced by thymidine, producing GTG, a codon for valine. Replacement of a hydrophilic glutamic acid by hydrophobic valine introduces an intermolecular contact point that results in polymerization of deoxygenated HbS. Fibers of polymerized HbS make the red cells rigid and distort their round shape into characteristic sickle cells. Sickled red cells in the circulation and their increased adherence to the vascular endothelium are the ultimate causes of the many manifestations of SCD.

In decreasing order of clinical severity, four common types of SCD are recognized: HbSS, HbSβ^0, HbSC, and HbSβ^+ thalassemia. Less common types in the United States include HbSD and HbSO$_{Arab}$ diseases. Sickle cell hemoglobinopathies occur worldwide, are not restricted to dark-skinned people, and are found in diverse populations including those of African, Mediterranean, Middle Eastern, and Asiatic Indian ethnicity. In the United States, approximately 1 in 4000 newborns and 1 in 375 African-American newborns has SCD. The sickle cell trait (HbAS) is much more prevalent and occurs in about 7 to 8% of African and Caribbean-Americans.

Red blood cells that contain mostly HbS go through cycles of sickling and unsickling on oxygenation and deoxygenation as they pass through the circulation. The tendency of the individual RBC to sickle is influenced by several factors. These include the presence of other hemoglobins that may inhibit or enhance the polymerization of deoxy-HbS, the degree to which the HbS is deoxygenated, and RBC deformability and hydration. When a solution of HbS is deoxygenated, there is a characteristic delay time during which no polymerization occurs, followed by a phase of rapid polymerization. In vivo, the delay time allows most HbS-containing RBC to traverse the capillary beds before polymerization and sickling occur. A small percentage of RBC remain permanently sickled, even when fully oxygenated. Sickled red cells become dehydrated through loss of potassium and water, which enhances polymerization. Hemoglobins such as F and A within the red cell inhibit polymerization of HbS. Tissues with sluggish blood flow such as the spleen and bone marrow sinusoids, and areas with hypertonicity and high acidity such as the renal medulla, are especially susceptible to damage resulting from sickling.

Hemolysis and vasoocclusion are the two major pathophysiological consequences of intravascular sickling Intravascular hemolysis results from damage caused by repeated sickling and unsickling as well as by the microvascular trapping of rigid and stiff sickled RBC. These abnormal cells are more rapidly destroyed, and the mean RBC life span in HbSS disease is only 10 to 20 days compared with the 100 to 120 days of survival of normal red cells. Sickled RBC also adhere to and damage endothelial layers of small and large blood vessels. Microvascular occlusion leads to tissue ischemia and infarction and ultimately results in chronic organ failure. Vasoocclusion with ischemia and tissue damage are also the major causes of the episodic acute painful episodes that are the clinical hallmarks of SCD.

LABORATORY DIAGNOSIS

Laboratory evaluation of SCD should include a complete blood count with red cell indices, reticulocyte count, and evaluation of RBC morphology (see Fig. 19-5C). Table 19-3 lists the usual hematologic findings in HbSS and HbSC diseases. Quantitative hemoglobin electrophoresis at pH 8.6 and 6.2 or other hemoglobin separation methods such as isoelectric focusing and high-performance liquid chromatography (HPLC) establish the diagnosis. Establishment of the genotype of a patient may require family testing, but DNA diagnostic methods are also available in a few laboratories.

In the steady state, patients with HbSS disease have a chronic hemolytic anemia. Unconjugated hyperbilirubinemia and scleral icterus are usual. After the first or second year of life, the peripheral blood smear in HbSS disease shows variable numbers of irreversibly

TABLE 19-3

LABORATORY VALUES AND Hb IN SS AND SC DISEASES

	HbSS (RANGE)	HbSC (RANGE)
Hemoglobin	75	115
(g/L)	(60–90)	(95 – 125)
Reticulocytes	9	3.0
(%)	(5–19)	(1.5–4.5)
Irreversibly sickled RBC	+ to 4+	±
Bilirubin	2.5	<1.5
(mg/dL)	(1–5.0)	

sickled cells—a nearly specific finding in HbSS disease (see Fig. 19-5C): polychromatophilic cells, poikilocytes, target cells, and Howell-Jolly bodies. The mean cell volume (MCV) is in the normal range, and a low MCV usually indicates concomitant β- or α-thalassemia. Granulocyte and platelet counts are usually moderately increased. In HbSC disease, target cells are numerous. When both HbA and HbS are present on electrophoresis, the relative amounts of HbS and HbA have diagnostic importance. In sickle cell trait (HbAS), HbA predominates (>60–70%) in contrast to HbSβ^+ thalassemia, where there is more HbS than HbA. Hemoglobins D and G also migrate in the S position on alkali electrophoresis but have different mobility from HbS on acid agar gel electrophoresis. These hemoglobins can also be distinguished by the solubility test, which gives an abnormal result with HbS but a normal result with both HbD and HbG.

CLINICAL COURSE

The clinical course of SCD has been described by a longitudinal study between 1977 and 1995 of nearly 5000 American patients (the Cooperative Study of Sickle Cell Disease, CSSCD). Episodic acute events that interrupt the steady state and chronic organ damage account for most of the morbidity and mortality of the disease. Some of the acute complications are associated with more severe degrees of anemia, but the others are primarily attributable to vaso-occlusive phenomena. Acute events are similar in all types of SCD but occur earlier, more frequently, and often more severely in HbSS and HbSβ^0 thalassemia.

At birth, newborns with HbSS disease have normal birth weight and are not anemic. Anemia and reticulocytosis usually appear after 2 to 6 months of age. Acute vasoocclusive manifestations are unusual before 6 months of age. The first painful events are often sickle cell dactylitis, a symmetric, painful swelling of the hands and feet (hand-foot syndrome) that occurs in about 30% of patients.

Chronic disease manifestations include slow growth, and most young children are short and thin. Sexual development is delayed. Ankle ulceration, retinal disease, gallbladder disease, and, in older patients, renal, liver, and cardiac failure occur. The course of the disease does not improve with age, and median life expectancy for American patients is now 42 years for men and 48 years for women. In many Third World countries, 90% of children with HbSS disease do not survive beyond 5 years of age, and *falciparum* malaria is the leading cause of death.

ACUTE EPISODES

INFECTIONS Until recently, infections were the major cause of mortality in young children with HbSS and HbSβ^0 thalassemia.

Streptococcus pneumoniae sepsis caused death in 15 to 20% of children in the first 5 years of life. The infections were often fulminant, with hyperpyrexia, shock, and death less than 24 hours from onset of illness. The major factors contributing to this unusual vulnerability to severe pneumococcal sepsis are the early loss of splenic reticuloendothelial function (functional hyposplenia) combined with a lack of circulating antibodies against polysaccharide-encapsulated bacteria. In early life, the spleen, although often clinically enlarged, loses reticuloendothelial function (see Sec. 19.8). Chronic transfusion therapy or bone marrow transplantation can reverse functional hyposplenia in early childhood. The enlarged spleen gradually becomes small and fibrotic from autoinfarction and is rarely palpable after 6 years of age. The second reason for susceptibility to severe pneumococcal sepsis is the lack of circulating antibody directed against pneumococci. As a normal developmental phenomenon, young children cannot efficiently produce antibodies to polysaccharide antigens such as those present in the capsule of the pneumococcus (see Chapter 11). When circulating antipneumococcal antibodies are lacking, the spleen is almost exclusively responsible for the clearance of pneumococci that gain entrance to the circulation. The combination of lack of antibody plus hyposplenia accounts for the clinical features and high mortality of pneumococcal infections in young children with HbSS and HbSβ^0. A national placebo-controlled study by the CSSCD showed that oral penicillin prophylaxis reduced the incidence of invasive pneumococcal infections by 84% in HbSS children less than 5 years of age. Neonatal testing for hemoglobinopathies, education of families, and careful follow-up of affected infants has been implemented in 40 US states, and most infants with SCD are now diagnosed at birth. The hemoglobin patterns and diagnoses that can be established by neonatal screening are listed in Table 19-4. With early diagnosis and institution of penicillin prophylaxis, deaths from pneumococcal infection have markedly decreased in the United States. A second CSSCD study did not show effectiveness of continuing penicillin prophylaxis after 5 years of age, and many centers discontinue prophylaxis after this age.

Osteomyelitis may occur in patients with SCD. About half of cases are caused by *Salmonella*, and most of the rest by staphylococci.

SPLENIC SEQUESTRATION In young children in whom autoinfarction has not as yet occurred, the spleen may become acutely enlarged and engorged with blood sequestered from the systemic circulation, with resultant hypovolemia, severe anemia, and massive splenic enlargement. Recognition of the signs and symptoms of more severe anemia and acute splenic enlargement is important for early diagnosis and management to prevent a fatal outcome. Parents can be taught how to palpate the spleen size and recognize sudden enlargement. Treatment of shock by blood and fluid replacement is an essential feature of management. Splenic sequestration is often repetitive, and splenectomy is often advocated after recovery from a severe episode. Because the spleen is usually not functional, splenectomy does not appear to increase the risk of infection. Minor episodes characterized by only slight decreases of hemoglobin (10–20 g/L) associated with only modest increases in spleen size may be associated with viral infections and usually require only careful observation.

ACUTE RED CELL APLASIA ("APLASTIC CRISIS") Because of the very short, 10- to 20-day RBC survival, patients with HbSS disease are able to maintain their low but steady hemoglobin levels by markedly increasing red blood cell production by the bone marrow.

TABLE 19-4

INTERPRETATION OF RESULTS OF NEWBORN SCREENING FOR MOST COMMON HEMOGLOBINOPATHIES

SCREENING RESULT[a] (HEMOGLOBINS DETECTED IN ORDER OF PROPORTION)	PROBABLE GENOTYPE
FA	Normal; β-thalassemia trait cannot be excluded
FAS	Sickle cell trait; HbD and G traits must be excluded
FSA	HbSβ$^+$ thalassemia
FS	HbSS disease. HbSβ^0 thalassemia and HbS-hereditary persistence of HbF
FSC	HbSC disease
FAC	HbC trait
FC	HbCC disease; HbCβ^0 thalassemia must be excluded
FCA	HbCβ$^+$ thalassemia
FAE	HbE trait
FE	HbEE disease; HbEβ^0 thalassemia must be excluded
FEA	HbEβ$^+$ thalassemia
FF	Homozygous β-thalassemia; homozygous HPFH must be excluded

[a] The presence of small amounts of the fast-migrating Hb$_{Barts}$ (γ_4) indicates α-thalassemia, which may be present with any of the above neonatal hemoglobin patterns.

If this increased production is compromised for even a short time, a rapid drop in hemoglobin level occurs. The usual cause of severe red cell aplasia is infection by parvovirus B19, a virus that destroys early red cell precursors in the bone marrow, causing an abrupt interruption of red cell production (see Chap. 13). The severe aplastic crisis is characterized by much lower hemoglobin levels than usual, falling as low as 10 to 20 g/L, a very low reticulocyte count (<1%), and reduced levels of serum bilirubin. Thrombocytopenia may be present. Acute red cell aplasia is transient and self-limited. Production of IgM antibodies against parvovirus limits the infection, and RBC production spontaneously resumes within 1 to 2 weeks, heralded by a brisk reticulocytosis. Before recovery, RBC transfusion is indicated when the reticulocyte count is still very low and the patient is severely anemic. During early recovery, because of severe anemia and a high reticulocyte count, a hyperhemolytic state may be mistakenly diagnosed. During other viral infection, erythropoiesis may be temporarily reduced, resulting in a moderate decrease of the usual hemoglobin level associated with a reduced reticulocyte count, but rarely as severe as in parvovirus infection.

VASOOCCLUSIVE EPISODES (PAINFUL CRISES) Episodic attacks of pain are the most characteristic feature of SCD and the most common reason for medical consultation and hospitalization. The pain is thought to be a result of inflammation from tissue ischemia caused by acute vasoocclusion. The earliest physical manifestation of HbSS is often the hand-foot syndrome or sickle cell dactylitis, a painful often symmetric swelling of the hands and feet that occurs in about 30% of children in the first 3 years of life. As the child gets older, painful episodes involve the long bones, vertebrae, sternum, ribs, lower back, and abdomen. Precipitating events can not usually

be identified. Although painful events severe enough to require hospitalization are infrequent (<2–3/year) for most patients, less severe painful events occur often. A few children with HbSS disease have frequent, debilitating pain episodes, and other children with the same disease have infrequent painful events. The reasons for this clinical variability are largely unknown.

Therapy for painful crises is symptomatic, and management of pain must be individualized. Moderate pain unassociated with high fever or other signs of severe illness can usually be managed at home with hydration, analgesics, and rest. However, some pain episodes are so severe that hospitalization for intravenous hydration and parenteral narcotics is necessary. Management of acute pain should be based on assessment of the degree of pain, prior therapy, and outcome. A combination of nonsteroidal anti-inflammatory drugs and opioid analgesics is usually necessary to achieve adequate pain relief, with gradual weaning of these medications as the pain resolves. Unfortunately, because of exaggerated concern over addiction to opiate analgesics, inadequate therapy for pain relief may be given to these children.

ACUTE CHEST SYNDROME The development of new pulmonary infiltrate, often accompanied by fever, chest pain, tachypnea, and hypoxia, defines the acute chest syndrome. This may be a result of pulmonary infarction, infection, atelectasis, or fat embolism secondary to bone marrow infarction. Acute chest syndrome often starts as a small infiltrate in one lobe that sometimes progresses rapidly to involve multiple lobes, resulting in respiratory distress severe enough to require intubation and ventilatory support. Acute chest syndrome is a leading cause of death in adolescents and adults. Management includes oxygen therapy when necessary, careful hydration at maintenance levels, and RBC transfusions or exchange transfusions. An infectious etiology is often not determined; however, antibiotics to cover pneumococcus, *Mycoplasma*, and *Chlamydia* are usually employed.

STROKE

Stroke, a common complication of SCD, has an overall prevalence of approximately 5% in HbSS and HbSβ^0 thalassemia patients. Stroke occurs at an annual rate of 0.6% with a peak of nearly 1.0% in the 2- to 9-year age group. The reason for the high incidence in young children is unknown. There are three clinical presentations of stroke: cerebral infarcts and hemorrhage, which result in weakness and paralysis, aphasia, and seizures, and transient ischemic attacks (TIA). TIA are likely to be missed in young children. All three presentations can occur at any age, but hemorrhagic stroke is less common in patients under 20 years of age. Computerized tomography or magnetic resonance imaging (MRI) can be used to diagnose cerebral hemorrhage and infarction. In young children, obstruction of the large intracerebral blood vessels is the usual cause. Acute management includes stabilization of vital signs, careful intravenous hydration, exchange transfusion, and control of seizures. Stroke has a high risk of recurrence, and computerized tomography or magnetic resonance imaging (MRI) can be used to rule out hemorrhage. Chronic RBC transfusion therapy to decrease the percentage of the patient's HbSS RBC to below 30 to 40% decreases the rate of recurrence. Transcranial Doppler ultrasonography and magnetic resonance imaging arteriography can detect areas of stenosis of the major cerebral arteries and can identify children at high risk for overt stroke. The risk of first occurrence of stroke can be reduced in these children by chronic transfusion therapy. Approximately 20% of children with HbSS disease with no history of overt stroke have silent infarcts and brain atrophy identifiable on MRI. A significant percentage of children with these "silent infarcts" have neuropsychometric deficits.

PRIAPISM

Priapism is a prolonged painful erection that occurs in about 10% of boys with HbSS. This complication requires rapid intervention to prevent chronic damage to the penis including impotence. Management includes hydration, pain control, and transfusion including exchange transfusion. Early aspiration of the corpora cavernosa and irrigation with a dilute solution of epinephrine have been shown to be rapidly effective in many cases.

CHRONIC ORGAN DAMAGE

In addition to splenic dysfunction, progressive functional abnormalities occur with increasing age in the kidneys, eyes, lungs, heart, and liver. Renal complications include hyposthenuria, papillary necrosis and hematuria, nephrosis, nephritis, and renal failure. Occlusion of retinal vessels may lead to proliferative retinopathy, retinal detachment, and loss of vision. Progressive pulmonary infarction may lead to pulmonary hypertension and hypoxemia and right-sided heart failure. High-output left-sided heart failure may occur in patients with more severe degrees of anemia. Liver enlargement and failure may occur as a result of infarction, bile stasis, or infection. Cholelithiasis secondary to chronic hemolysis can occur as early as 3 to 4 years of age, and more than half of adults with HbSS have gallstones. Cholecystectomy is the most common surgical procedure performed in patients with SCD.

Growth retardation is commonly observed during childhood, but normal adult height is almost always eventually achieved. The onset of puberty and development of secondary sex characteristics are usually delayed by 2 to 3 years.

NEW THERAPIES

Some progress has been made in the development of new therapies for the management of SCD. Hydroxyurea, a cytotoxic agent that increases levels of HbF, decreases the WBC, reduces the frequency of painful crises, acute chest syndrome, and transfusions about 50% in adults and in initial studies in children. However, the long-term safety of hydroxyurea in patients with SCD of any age, and especially those under 5 years of age, has not been established. Other agents that can increase fetal hemoglobin include butyrate analogues, and other short-chain fatty acids are being investigated.

Bone marrow transplantation (BMT) from an HLA-matched sibling is the only curative therapy (see Chapter 20). In Europe and the United States, about 100 to 150 cases of BMT for SCD have been reported. In North America, the usual indication has been stroke or cerebrovascular disease. Overall, there is a disease-free cure rate of 80 to 85%, a mortality rate of 5 to 8%, a rejection rate of about 5%, and graft-versus-host disease occurred in about 5% of cases. BMT has been infrequently chosen by American patients.

SICKLE CELL β-THALASSEMIA

Sickle cell β^0-thalassemia has similar hematologic features as HbSS disease except for microcytosis of the RBC (CV < 70 fL). The electrophoretic pattern shows predominantly HbS, variable amounts of HbF, and elevated levels of HbA_2 (>3.5%). Vasoocclusive and other clinical events are similar to HbSS. Sickle cell β^+-thalassemia is characterized by a hemoglobin electrophoretic pattern that shows 60 to 70% HbS, 30 to 40% HbA, variable amounts

of HbF, and >3.5% HbA_2. Vasoocclusive episodes are usually infrequent and mild, and the diagnosis is often made incidentally in the evaluation of the usually mild anemia.

SICKLE CELL TRAIT

Sickle cell trait (SCT) is the heterozygous inheritance of a $Hb\beta^s$ globin gene. The prevalence of SCT in African-Americans is 1 in 12. The proportion of HbA is always >50 to 60%. The predominance of HbA within the SCT RBC prevents sickling under normal oxygen tensions. The CBC, peripheral blood smear, red cell indices, and reticulocyte count are normal. People with SCT have very few HbS-related medical problems and have normal life expectancy, but rarely, under conditions of extreme physical exertion or low oxygen tension, complications have been described. Splenic infarction has occurred in individuals with SCT flying in unpressurized aircraft at altitudes over 7000 feet, but modern commercial air travel does not pose a risk. Hypoxia accompanying anesthesia, if prolonged, may also induce sickling. Deaths have been described in physically unconditioned military recruits with SCT undergoing strenuous basic training, presumably as a result of dehydration, metabolic acidosis, and rhabdomyolysis. Increased numbers of deaths have not been recognized in individuals with SCT participating in high school, college, or professional sports. Hyposthenuria and renal papillary necrosis with gross hematuria are the most common medical complication of SCT. The hypertonicity and relative acidosis in the renal medulla can induce sickling, even in SCT RBC.

Although prenatal testing and genetic counseling have been offered to couples both of whom have SCT because of their 25% risk of having a child with HbSS, only a small number have participated. However, adolescents and adults of childbearing age with SCT should be offered education and nondirective genetic counseling.

HEMOGLOBIN SC DISEASE

Patients with SC disease are less anemic (Hb 100 g/L) and usually have less severe hemolysis than those with HbSS (see Table 19-3). Hemoglobin electrophoresis shows equal amounts of HbS and HbC, and there is no HbA. The blood smear does not show irreversibly sicked cells, but microcytosis and many target cells are present. Vasoocclusive events are usually less frequent and severe than in HbSS disease, and growth is usually normal. Functional splenectomy occurs later, and splenomegaly is usually present in adolescents and adults. There is a relatively high risk of retinal disease and aseptic necrosis in adolescents.

19.4.2 Hemoglobin C

Hemoglobin C is characterized by the substitution of a lysine for the glutamic acid residue in the 6 position of the β-globin chain. Hemoglobin C originated in West Africa and occurs in about 2.5% of African-Americans. The trait (HbAC) has no hematologic abnormalities except for increased numbers of target cells on the peripheral blood smear and the presence of 30 to 40% slowly migrating HbC on electrophoresis. Homozygotes for HbC (HbCC disease) have a mild hemolytic anemia and splenomegaly but do not have vasoocclusive symptoms. The RBC are microcytic, and the blood smear shows large numbers of target cells (Fig. 19-5K). HbCβ thalassemia is similar to HbCC disease.

19.4.3   Hemoglobin E Disorders

Hemoglobin E results from the substitution of a glycine residue for the normal glutamic acid residue in the 26 position of the β-globin chain and is very prevalent in Southeast Asia, especially Thailand and Cambodia. Hemoglobin E trait individuals (HbAE) are hematologically normal except for 40% HbE on electrophoresis and target cells on the blood smear. Homozygous HbEE disease is characterized by a mild microcytic anemia with large numbers of target cells (Fig. 19-5K). HbEβ thalassemia disease is associated with moderate to severe anemia and may be transfusion dependent. Bony abnormalities and splenomegaly resemble thalassemia intermedia (see Sec. 19.4.7).

19.4.4   Unstable Hemoglobins

Unstable hemoglobins are structurally abnormal hemoglobins that oxidize spontaneously to methemoglobin and denature and precipitate within the RBC, forming Heinz bodies. Heinz bodies make the cells relatively rigid, leading to trapping in the spleen. The inheritance pattern of unstable hemoglobins is autosomal codominant. More than 100 mutations, mostly single amino acid substitutions involving the β-globin more frequently than the α-globin chain, are responsible for unstable hemoglobinopathies. Clinical manifestations vary depending on the degree of instability of the hemoglobin. In more severe forms, chronic hemolytic anemia is seen in the heterozygote. Most of the affected patients are heterozygous for a β-globin mutation, suggesting that homozygous forms are probably incompatible with life. Neonates with unstable α-hemoglobins may develop hemolytic anemia. Fever, infections, and oxidative drugs, including those that induce hemolysis in patients with G6PD deficiency, can greatly enhance the oxidation of unstable hemoglobins and lead to hemolytic crises. Because of the loss of heme groups, dipyrrol-methenes impart a dark color to the urine. Physical findings are variable and may include jaundice and splenomegaly.

The clinical profile of patients with unstable hemoglobins depends on the degree of instability and the oxygen affinity of the unstable hemoglobin. In Hb$_{Köln}$ ($\alpha_2\beta_2^{98\ Val\rightarrow Met}$), the most common unstable hemoglobin, an increase in oxygen affinity results in mild tissue hypoxia, which stimulates EPO production and increases the hemoglobin level; anemia, if present, is usually mild. In contrast, patients with Hb$_{Hammersmith}$ ($\alpha_2\beta_2^{42\ Phe\rightarrow Ser}$), a variant associated with spontaneous denaturation and decreased oxygen affinity, have severe hemolytic anemia, with reticulocyte counts of 20 to 50%. With Hb$_{Poole}$ ($\alpha_2\gamma_2^{130\ Trp\rightarrow Gly}$), a γ-chain variant, hemolysis is noted only in the first few months of life, when HbF is predominant.

The peripheral blood smear may be normal or may show variations in size and shape and basophilic stippling. Heinz bodies can sometimes be demonstrated after a brief incubation of blood with methyl violet. However, in patients with intact spleens, longer incubation may be required before Heinz bodies are demonstrable. The isopropanol precipitation test is a screening test for unstable hemoglobins and consists of incubation of a solution of hemoglobin with 70% isopropanol at 37°C for 1 hour, which breaks the weak hydrophobic bonds in the unstable hemoglobin molecule, and the dissociated globin chains precipitate. Only about half of the unstable hemoglobins are demonstrable by electrophoresis.

Treatment of patients with unstable hemoglobins is supportive. Splenectomy, which may reduce but does not eliminate hemolysis, is reserved for patients with severe hemolytic anemia. As in other hemolytic anemias, patients with unstable hemoglobins may have parvovirus-induced red cell aplasia and may, on rare occasions, require transfusion.

19.4.5   Hemoglobins with Altered Oxygen Affinity

Hb$_{Chesapeake}$ ($\alpha_2^{92\ Arg\rightarrow Leu}\beta_2$), an α-globin variant, has a higher affinity than normal for oxygen, which causes tissue hypoxia and compensatory erythrocytosis. The differential diagnosis of erythrocytosis includes disorders in which there is either an inappropriate increase in erythropoietin production, as in neoplastic renal lesions, or an appropriate erythropoietin increase in response to chronic hypoxia such as cardiac or pulmonary disease or high altitude.

More than 50 structurally abnormal hemoglobins with high oxygen affinity have been discovered. The structural defects involve amino acid substitutions at either the contact point between the α- and β-globin chains, or at the C-terminal end of the β-globin chain. Both of these sites are critical for stabilization of hemoglobin in either oxy- or deoxy-states and for interaction with 2,3-DPG. The hemoglobin concentration may be as high as 200 g/L; red cell morphology and white cell and platelet counts are normal.

In contrast, other hemoglobin variants have an amino acid substitution that decreases oxygen affinity. One example, Hb$_{Kansas}$, releases oxgygen to the tissues and is not fully saturated even in arterial blood. Although EPO level and the hemoglobin concentration are low in affected patients, from a functional perspective (tissue oxygen delivery), anemia is not present.

The diagnosis of hemoglobins with altered affinity is based on a determination of the P_{50} value from the hemoglobin-oxygen dissociation curve. Under physiological conditions, normal adult hemoglobin is half-saturated at an oxygen tension (P_{50}) of about 26 mm Hg. High-affinity oxygen hemoglobins have a low P_{50} value and a left-shifted curve, whereas low-affinity hemoglobins have a high P_{50} value and a right-shifted curve. The RBC 2,3-DPG levels should be determined to rule out the possibility that alterations in oxygen affinity may be secondary to a defect in red cell metabolism. Electrophoresis may identify variants when the substitution results in a difference in net charge; however, a normal electrophoretic pattern does not rule out a hemoglobin with altered oxygen affinity. Most patients with these hemoglobin variants require no treatment.

19.4.6   The M Hemoglobins

Rarely, cyanosis is caused by a primary structural defect in hemoglobins. The hemoglobin Ms have amino acid substitutions adjacent to the heme moiety (usually replacement of histidine with tyrosine), which enhances the oxidation of iron and formation of methemoglobin. The M hemoglobins do not denature spontaneously and therefore do not result in hemolysis. M hemoglobins affecting the γ-globin (HbFM$_{Osaka}$, HbFM$_{Fort\ Ripley}$) cause neonatal cyanosis. Unlike patients with acquired methemoglobinemia or those with defects in methemoglobin reductase, cyanosis is usually mild, and symptoms rarely develop. There are no medications that reduce methemoglobin levels.

References

Agency for Health Care Policy and Research: Sickle Cell Disease: Screening, Diagnosis, Management, and Counseling in Newborns and Infants

(AHCPR Publication No. 93-0562). Clinical Practice Guideline, 1993 Washington DC

Bunn HF: Human hemoglobins: normal and abnormal. In: Nathan DG, Orkin SH, eds: Nathan and Oski's Hematology of Infancy and Childhood, 5th ed. Philadelphia, WB Saunders, 1998:729–761

Charache S, Terrin ML, Moore PD, et al: Effect of hydroxyurea on the frequency of painful crises in sickle-cell anemia. N Engl J Med 332: 1317–1325, 1995

Dacie J: The Haemolytic Anaemias, 3rd ed, vol 2. Edinburgh, Churchill Livingstone, 1988:322–386

Embury SH, Hebbel RP, Mohandas N, Steinberg MH, eds: Sickle Cell Disease: Basic Principles and Clinical Practice. New York, Raven, Press 1994

Wajcman H, Galacteros F: Abnormal hemoglobins with high oxygen affinity and erythrocytosis. Hematol Cell Ther 38:305–312, 1996

Walters MC, Patience M, Leisenring W, et al: Bone marrow transplantation for sickle cell disease. N Engl J Med 335:369–377, 1996

19.4.7   Thalassemia

Howard A. Pearson

Thalassemia was first defined in 1925 when Dr. Thomas B. Cooley described five young children with severe anemia, splenomegaly, and unusual bone abnormalities and called the disorder erythroblastic or Mediterranean anemia because of circulating nucleated red blood cells and because all of his patients were of Italian or Greek ethnicity. In 1932 Whipple and Bradford coined the term thalassemia from the Greek word *thalassa*, which means the sea (Mediterranean) to describe this entity. Somewhat later, a mild microcytic anemia was described in families of Cooley anemia patients, and it was soon realized that this disorder was caused by heterozygous inheritance of abnormal genes that, when homozygous, produced severe Cooley anemia.

The thalassemias are a group of hereditary anemias that result from diminished synthesis of one of the globin chains that combine to form adult hemoglobin (HbA, $\alpha_2\beta_2$). Unlike the hemoglobinopathies, no chemically different hemoglobins are present. Normal HbA contains both α and β polypeptide chains, and the most important thalassemias can be designated as either α- or β-thalassemia.

β-THALASSEMIA

The β-thalassemia syndromes are caused by abnormalities of the β-gene complex on chromosome 11. More than 150 different mutations have been described, and most of these are small nucleotide substitutions within the β gene complex. Deletions and mutations that result in abnormal cleavage or splicing of β-globin RNA may also result in thalassemia characterized by absent (β^0) or reduced (β^+) production of β-globin chains.

The β-thalassemia genes are widely distributed throughout the world but are especially prevalent in southern Italy and Greece, with a gene frequency of 2 to 5% or more. A high prevalence of β-thalassemia also occurs in the Mideast, the Indian subcontinent, Pakistan, southern China, and Southeast Asia. It is rare in persons of north European ancestry but is found in about 0.5% of African-Americans. The high prevalence of thalassemia in tropical areas is believed to be a result of increased resistance of heterozygotes to malaria (balanced polymorphism).

THALASSEMIA MINOR (THALASSEMIA TRAIT) Heterozygosity for a β-thalassemia gene results in a mild reduction of β-chain synthesis and, therefore, a reduction in HbA and mild anemia. Hemoglobin levels are 10 to 20 g/L lower than that of normal persons of the same age and gender, but the anemia may worsen during pregnancy. This mild anemia usually produces no symptoms, and longevity is normal. Thalassemia trait is almost always accompanied by familial microcytosis and hypochromia of the red blood cells. Target cells, elliptocytes, and basophilic stippling are seen on the peripheral blood smear (Fig. 19-5I). Almost all individuals with β-thalassemia trait have MCVs less than 75 fL, and mean MCV is 68 fL. In thalassemia trait the MCV is disproportionately low for the degree of anemia because of a red blood cell count that is normal or increased. The RDW is normal in thalassemia trait. The ratio of MCV/RBC (Mentzer index) is <11 in thalassemia trait but >12 in iron deficiency. Iron studies are normal. In an individual with microcytic red blood cells, a diagnosis of β-thalassemia trait is confirmed by an elevated HbA$_2$ ($\alpha_2\delta_2$) level. The normal level of HbA$_2$ is 1.5 to 3.4%, and HbA$_2$ >3.5% is diagnostic of the most common form of β-thalassemia trait. Levels of HbF ($\alpha_2\gamma_2$) are normal (<2.0%) in about half of individuals with classical thalassemia trait and moderately elevated (2.0 to 7%) in the rest.

Less common forms of β-thalassemia trait include $\beta\delta$-thalassemia trait, characterized by familial microcytosis, normal levels of HbA$_2$, and elevated levels of HbF (5–15%), and Lepore hemoglobin trait, characterized by the presence of 5 to 10% Hb$_{Lepore}$, a hemoglobin that migrates electrophoretically in the position of HbS. Lepore hemoglobin is a fusion product resulting from an unequal crossover between β and δ genes and associated with decreased β-chain synthesis. Occasionally a *silent carrier* is identified on the basis of being a parent of a child with severe thalassemia but slight or no microcytosis or elevations of HbA$_2$ or HbF.

The importance of establishing a diagnosis of β-thalassemia trait is to avoid unnecessary treatment with medicinal iron and to provide genetic counseling. Two individuals with β-thalassemia trait face a 25% risk with each pregnancy of having a child with homozygous β-thalassemia. Populations with a high prevalence of thalassemia trait can be screened to provide genetic counseling. In at-risk pregnancies, prenatal diagnosis can be performed as early as 10 to 12 weeks of gestation using fetal DNA obtained by chorionic villus biopsy. Prenatal detection has greatly reduced the incidence of new cases of β-thalassemia major in Italy and Cyprus as well in the Greek- and Italian-American communities in the United States.

HOMOZYGOUS β-THALASSEMIA (THALASSEMIA MAJOR, COOLEY ANEMIA) Homozygosity for β-thalassemia genes is usually associated with severe anemia because of a marked reduction of synthesis of the β-globin chains of HbA. However, reduction of HbA synthesis does not explain the hemolysis and ineffective erythropoiesis that are a consequence of *unbalanced* globin chain synthesis. In homozygous β-thalassemia, α-globin chains are produced in normal amounts and accumulate, denature, and precipitate in the RBC precursors in the bone marrow and circulating RBC. These precipitated α-globin chains damage the RBC membrane, resulting in destruction within the bone marrow (ineffective erythropoiesis) and in the peripheral blood.

The fetus and the newborn infant with homozygous β-thalassemia are clinically and hematologically normal. In vitro measurements demonstrate reduced or absent β-chain synthesis. Increasingly, homozygous β-thalassemia is being diagnosed in the United States by neonatal electrophoretic hemoglobin screening that shows only HbF and no HbA (see Table 19-4).

Symptoms of β-thalassemia major develop gradually in the first 6 to 12 months after birth, when the normal postnatal switchover from γ-chains to β-chains results in a decreased level of HbF (see

Fig. 19-3). By the age of 6 to 12 months, most affected infants show pallor, irritability, growth retardation, jaundice, and hepatosplenomegaly as a result of extramedullary hematopoiesis. By 2 years of age, 90% of infants are symptomatic, and progressive changes in the facial and cranial bones develop. The hemoglobin level may be as low as 30 to 50 g/L at the time of diagnosis.

LABORATORY The red cell morphology is very abnormal, with marked hypochromia and many microcytes, bizarre poikilocytes, and target cells (Fig. 19-5J). The RBC may contain irregular inclusions, which are aggregates of precipitated α-globin chains that can be identified by supravital stains. Nucleated red cells are invariably present. The reticulocyte count is moderately elevated at 5 to 8%. The white blood cell count, corrected for nucleated RBC, is moderately elevated. The platelet count is normal or increased but may be low if the spleen is enlarged. After splenectomy, thrombocytosis and increased numbers of nucleated RBC are seen. Conjugated bilirubin levels are elevated.

The hemoglobin electrophoretic pattern is predominantly HbF. Hemoglobin A is absent in homozygous β^0-thalassemia and is present but in small proportions in homozygous or doubly heterozygous β^+-thalassemia. Hemoglobin A_2 levels are of little diagnostic value.

TRANSFUSION THERAPY More than 80% of children with homozygous β-thalassemia require regular RBC transfusions by 1 to 2 years of age because of severe anemia. Life expectancy with untreated thalassemia major is less than 5 years. Before 1970, hemoglobin levels at the time of transfusion were permitted to fall as low as 40 to 60 g/L. The clinical features and outcomes of these patients with poorly transfused thalassemia major reflected severe anemia and compensatory hypertrophy of medullary and extramedullary erythroid tissue to attempt to compensate for the anemia. At these low hemoglobin concentrations, irritability, fatigability, listlessness, and anorexia were prominent symptoms. Cardiomegaly, flow murmurs, scleral icterus, and gallstones were common. Growth of these children was markedly retarded, and puberty was unusual.

The extremely ineffective erythropoiesis in poorly transfused thalassemia major evoked massive expansion of the erythroid tissue (as much as 30-fold). Marrow expansion in the maxilla and facial bones resulted in severe cosmetic deformity with overgrowth and protrusion of the upper jaw and malocclusion and jumbling of the teeth. The malar eminences were prominent, giving the eyes a mongoloid slant. These children had a striking resemblance to each other. Expansion of the marrow cavity of the cranial bones caused enlargement of the skull with frontal and parietal bossing. Radiographs showed widened diploë with perpendicular bone trabeculae giving a classic hair-on-end appearance. Expansion of the marrow cavities of the long bones resulted in marked cortical bone thinning, and pathologic fractures were common. Extramedullary hematopoiesis in the liver and spleen caused abdominal enlargement from progressive hepatosplenomegaly, and paraspinal masses of extramedullary hematopoiesis sometimes developed.

The average age of death was 15 to 20 years, and few patients survived into the late twenties. Poor survival could be attributed not only to the severe anemia but especially to a progressive increase in the body iron burden, largely a consequence of transfusions. Each unit of transfused blood results in deposition of about 250 mg of iron into the tissues, and there is no physiological means of iron excretion. Large accumulations of iron in the liver, pancreas, endocrine glands, and heart result in fibrosis and permanent tissue damage. Failure of sexual development is frequent as a result of early damage to the hypothalamic-pituitary-gonadal axis. Diabetes mellitus, hepatic fibrosis, and endocrinopathies including hypothyroidism and hypoparathyroidism may occur as result of iron deposition in these organs. Myocardial siderofibrosis develops in the second decade of life and is manifested by cardiac tachyarrhythmias and ultimately by refractory congestive heart failure, which is the usual cause of death.

Beginning in the 1970s, more vigorous transfusion programs designed to maintain a minimum hemoglobin level of 100 g/L ("hypertransfusion") were instituted to decrease the consequences of severe anemia and marrow hypertrophy. Hypertransfusion has significant advantages over a limited transfusion regimen and should be utilized whenever possible. Activity, exercise tolerance, and sense of well-being are improved. The deforming cosmetic features are reduced. Osteoporosis of the long bones and pathologic fractures are decreased, and growth is enhanced. The iron accumulation of patients receiving hypertransfusion is not significantly greater than with earlier minimal transfusion programs. Hypertransfusion does not appear to increase longevity in thalassemia major, but considerable improvement in the quality of life is achieved. By the second decade of life, massive body iron accumulation occurs, as indicated by markedly increased levels of serum ferritin (>2500 ng/mL) and by increased amounts of tissue iron, quantified by liver biopsy.

SPLENECTOMY In the past, minimally transfused patients developed splenomegaly, sometimes leading to splenectomy in early life. In children on hypertransfusion, massive splenomegaly is unusual. However, many patients ultimately develop increasing transfusion requirements exceeding 200 mL of RBC/kg/y, and splenectomy is often considered to improve survival of transfused RBC. There is an increased risk of bacterial sepsis following splenectomy, especially in young children (see Sec. 19.8).

IRON CHELATION To effect reduction of increased body iron, iron-chelating compounds that result in urinary and biliary iron excretion have become an essential component of modern therapy. The only approved iron chelator in the United States is deferoxamine (Desferal, DF). Deferoxamine is effective and nearly specific with low toxicity, and for maximal effectiveness 40 to 59 mg/kg of drug is injected subcutaneously over 8 to 10 hours during sleep using a battery-driven infusion pump 5 or 6 nights each week.

Side effects of DF include frequent hard, painful swellings at the injection sites, which have led to use of permanent venous access devices such as the Portocath. Less commonly visual and auditory neurotoxicity and osteoporosis may occur. The most important complication of DF therapy is patient nonadherence with the complex, very expensive, and often uncomfortable regimen.

Regular use of DF prevents endocrine, cardiac, and hepatic abnormalities and significantly extends life expectancy. A life expectancy to age 35 years or beyond can be expected, whereas noncompliant patients usually die during their teens or early 20s from the complications associated with iron toxicity in the heart. The difficulty of compliance to DF therapy has led to a search for other chelating agents, especially ones that could be administered orally, but at present there is no alternative to DF in the United States.

BONE MARROW TRANSPLANTATION Thalassemia can be cured by allogeneic bone marrow transplantation, and this therapeutic approach should be considered if a histocompatible marrow donor, usually a sibling, is available (see Sec. 20.4). More than 500 transplants have been done worldwide, most in Italy. For well-chelated children without evidence of liver disease, event-free survival 3 years after transplantation exceeds 80%. Results in patients with hepatic disease and in most adults are considerably worse. The relatively high immediate mortality associated with transplantation stands in contrast to the many years of reasonably normal life that can be obtained with appropriate transfusion and chelation therapies, making the decision to accept transplantation difficult for many families.

CHANGING PROFILE OF THALASSEMIA MAJOR AND PRENATAL DIAGNOSIS The advent of modern transfusion and chelation therapy has substantially changed the profile of thalassemia major in the United States by greatly extending the lives of these patients into adult life, making it increasingly a disease of adults. Widespread screening of individuals from populations with high prevalence of β-thalassemia has enabled prenatal diagnosis of affected fetuses. In Greek- and Italian-American communities the number of affected infants has sharply decreased. However, the recent large numbers of immigrants from Southeast Asia have been accompanied by many births of affected infants in these ethnic groups who have not as yet availed themselves of these procedures.

β-THALASSEMIA INTERMEDIA About 10% of patients with two β-thalassemia genes (homozygous or doubly heterozygous) are able to maintain a hemoglobin level between 60 and 90 g/L without regular transfusions and are designated as having thalassemia intermedia. These patients are either homozygous for a mild thalassemia gene (as occurs in African-Americans) or are doubly heterozygous with inheritance of one severe and one mild thalassemia gene. The homozygous inheritance of two severe β-thalassemia genes may also be influenced by the concurrent inheritance of a gene for α-thalassemia, which may reduce globin chain imbalance.

Some patients with thalassemia intermedia do reasonably well, but others have symptoms of anemia or develop severe cosmetic changes and bone disease. Transfusion therapy may be necessary to prevent these complications and massive enlargement of the spleen.

α-THALASSEMIA

The α-thalassemia syndromes are prevalent in people from Southeast Asia and usually result from deletion of one or more of the four α-globin genes on chromosome 16. In general, the severity is proportional to the number of α-globin genes deleted which can be quantitated by DNA analysis.

SILENT CARRIER (α_2-THALASSEMIA TRAIT, $-\alpha/\alpha\alpha$) Individuals with a single α-globin gene deletion are clinically and hematologically normal, but they may be identified at birth by the presence of small amounts (1–3%) of the fast-migrating Barts hemoglobin (γ_4) by neonatal hemoglobin electrophoresis (see Table 19-4). In later life, the diagnosis can be established only by determining the number of α-globin genes by DNA analysis.

α_1-THALASSEMIA TRAIT ($-\alpha/-\alpha$ OR $--/\alpha\alpha$) Individuals in whom two of four α-globin genes are deleted have mild microcytic anemia. At birth, relative microcytosis with 5 to 8% of Hb_{Barts} is present. Barts hemoglobin disappears by 3 to 6 months of age, and the hemoglobin electrophoresis becomes normal. After the newborn period, a definitive diagnosis may be impractical in this mild disorder, and the diagnosis is usually suspected when other causes of microcytic anemia, such as β-thalassemia trait or iron deficiency, are ruled out.

α_1-Thalassemia trait can occur in two ways: a *cis*-deletion in which the two deleted α genes are on the same chromosome 16, and a *trans*-deletion in which one α-gene is deleted from each of the 16 chromosomes. The *cis*-deletion is usual in Southeast Asian populations, whereas the *trans*-deletions are usual in people of African ethnicity. Thus, although α-thalassemia commonly occurs in African people, a maximum of only two genes can be deleted in any individual because of the *trans*-configuration. Consequently, the more severe α-thalassemia syndromes associated with three and four α-deletions are not seen.

HEMOGLOBIN H DISEASE ($--/-\alpha$) Three α-globin gene deletions result in hemoglobin H disease, which is associated with a marked imbalance between α- and β-globin chain synthesis. Excess free β chains accumulate and combine to form an abnormal hemoglobin, a tetramer of β chains (β_4) called HbH. HbH is unstable and precipitates within red blood cells, leading to chronic microcytic, hemolytic anemia. Laboratory findings include a moderately severe microcytosic anemia (Hb 60–100 g/L with evidence of hemolysis). Precipitated HbH can be demonstrated in the red blood cells with supravital stains. On hemoglobin electrophoresis, HbH has a fast mobility and accounts for 10 to 15% of the total hemoglobin.

FETAL HYDROPS SYNDROME ($--/--$) Deletion of all four α-globin genes results in a syndrome of hydrops fetalis with stillbirth or immediate postnatal death. In the absence of α-chain synthesis, such fetuses are incapable of synthesizing embryonic hemoglobins. At birth, hemoglobin electrophoresis shows predominantly Barts hemoglobin (γ_4) and small amounts hemoglobin H (β_4) as well as embryonic hemoglobins. The high oxygen affinity of Barts hemoglobin makes it oxygen transport ineffective, leading to the intrauterine manifestations of severe hypoxia, out of proportion to the degree of anemia. A number of infants with this syndrome who have been identified prenatally and treated with intrauterine and postnatal transfusions have survived. These infants are transfusion dependent, but some are developing normally. As in thalassemia major, the only curative therapy is bone marrow transplantation. Termination of the pregnancy is often recommended because of a high frequency of severe maternal toxemia associated with a hydropic fetus.

19.4.8 Hereditary Persistence of Fetal Hemoglobin

Hereditary persistence of fetal hemoglobin (HPFH) is characterized by persistent high levels of HbF after infancy. HPFH in persons of African ethnicity have large genetic deletions adjacent to the γ genes on chromosome 11. In the heterozygous state, anemia is not present, but 20 to 30% of the hemoglobin is HbF, evenly distributed within the RBC. Persons homozygous for deletional HPFH are healthy with red blood cells that are slightly microcytic and contain 100% HbF.

A second form of HPFH results from nondeletional point mutations in the promoter regions of the γ genes. The levels of HbF are variable from 3 to 30%, and the distribution may be either pancellular or heterocellular.

Both forms of HPFH may moderate the effect of a sickle cell gene. Double heterozygotes for HbS and HPFH have no hemolytic anemia or vasoocclusive symptoms despite a hemoglobin pattern with 60 to 70% HbS and 20 to 30% HbF. HbS-HPFH must be considered in the differential diagnosis of newborns whose electrophoretic pattern shows HbFS (see Table 19-4).

References

Forget BG, Pearson HA: Hemoglobin synthesis and the thalassemias. In: Hamdin RI, Lux SE, Stossel TB, eds: Blood: Principles and Practice of Hematology. Philadelphia, Lippincott, 1995:1500–1590

Lucarelli G, Galimberti M, Polchi P, et al: Marrow transplantation in patients with thalassemia responsive to iron chelation therapy. N Engl J Med 329:840–844, 1993

Olivieri NF: The beta-thalassemias. N Engl J Med 341:99–109, 1999

Pearson HA, Giardina P, Cohen A: The changing profile of thalassemia major. Pediatrics 97:352–356, 1996

19.5   THE HEMOLYTIC ANEMIAS

William C. Mentzer, Jr.

19.5.1   Inborn Abnormalities of the Red Blood Cell Membrane/Cytoskeleton

The red cell membrane is a lipid bilayer formed of phospholipids and unesterified cholesterol and is in dynamic equilibrium with plasma lipids, so that membrane lipid composition reflects plasma lipid levels. Phospholipids cannot be synthesized de novo by erythrocytes, but an acylation reaction that requires adenosine triphosphate (ATP) allows their synthesis from plasma lysophospholipids and free fatty acids. Thus, to a limited extent, the red cell membrane is capable of self-renewal and self-modification in lipid composition.

A variety of glycoproteins and other proteins are also found on or within the lipid bilayer. Red cell blood group antigens, exposed on the external membrane surface, are glycoproteins or glycolipids. Active transport of Na^+ and K^+ and the passive entry of anions and water into the cell are through charged pore-like channels.

The erythrocyte membrane skeleton is an assembly of proteins that lies on the inner aspect of the lipid bilayer. The major components of the membrane cytoskeleton are α and β spectrins (MW 220,000 to 240,000), actin (MW 42,000), and protein 4.1 (MW 78,000 to 80,000). In the intact erythrocyte these cytoskeletal proteins form an intricate scaffold that covers the entire inner aspect of the lipid bilayer and are attached to the lipid bilayer through a connecting protein, ankyrin. At the tail end of the spectrin β chain, there is a binding site for protein 4.1, which, with adjacent aggregates of actin, must be present for the full development of the membrane skeletal complex. The various skeletal attachments are not rigid and immutable but are thought to break and re-form under the influence of certain effectors, providing a mechanism for modulation of membrane cytoskeletal dynamics.

The state of the RBC membrane is an important determinant of cell volume, shape, and plasticity. Inherited abnormalities in the plasma lipid environment, in the structure or function of cytoskeletal proteins, or in the pathways of membrane lipid renewal may lead to abnormalities in erythrocyte shape that are usually apparent on peripheral blood smear and are often accompanied by hemolysis. Inheritance of disorders of the RBC membrane or cytoskeleton is almost always autosomal dominant. Usually, abnormalities of cation transport and cell content of cations or cell water content result in abnormalities of the red cell size (MCV), hemoglobin concentration (MCHC), and the osmotic fragility test. Abnormalities of plasma lipids, membrane phospholipids, or cholesterol content may be present as well.

HEREDITARY SPHEROCYTOSIS

Hereditary spherocytosis (HS) is the most common congenital hemolytic anemia in populations of northern European origin and occurs less frequently in other ethnic groups. The incidence of HS in the United States is approximately 1 in 5000. HS is caused by a structural or functional abnormality of cytoskeleton proteins, spectrin, ankyrin, band 3, or protein 4.2. Erythrocyte spectrin deficiency is found in most individuals and is particularly severe in the occasional patient with the recessively inherited, very severe form of the disease. In some families, a deficiency of ankyrin accompanies spectrin deficiency; in others, a deficiency in protein 4.2 or band 3 is the sole abnormality of the membrane skeleton. Defective spectrin–protein 4.1 binding has also been described in a few patients. The permeability of spherocytic red cells to Na^+ is two to three times greater than normal, which was once thought to be the primary defect but is now considered to be a secondary phenomenon.

Reticulocytes in patients with HS are not spherocytic. Transformation to the spherocytic shape takes place by gradual splenic conditioning of the abnormal erythrocytes. Normal erythrocytes traversing the splenic pulp must be sufficiently deformable to pass through pores in the splenic sinusoids with diameters of 2 μm or less. Spherocytes are more rigid than normal cells and are less able to pass through these pores and so are detained within the splenic pulp. The abnormal Na^+ permeability of spherocytes must be offset by an increase in active transport of Na^+ out of the cell if cation balance is to be maintained. Active transport requires energy in the form of ATP, which in the mature erythrocyte is generated only through glycolysis. Because the acidic, hypoglycemic environment of the spleen inhibits glycolysis, the increased ATP requirements of spherocytes can not be met. Continued consumption of energy to support active cation transport leads to metabolic depletion, which in the spherocyte results in susceptibility to loss of membrane lipid and thus membrane surface area. Because the loss of red cell membrane occurs without a reduction in cell volume, the cell becomes increasingly spherical. With assumption of the spherical shape, the cell becomes even less deformable and subject to further metabolic depletion and lipid loss and ultimately to lysis within the spleen. The importance of the spleen in the pathogenesis of hemolysis in HS is demonstrated by the abolition of hemolysis that follows splenectomy. However, after splenectomy spherocytes may be more numerous, indicating that, although erythrocyte survival is improved, the underlying membrane defect is not altered.

GENETICS Autosomal-dominant inheritance is present in most HS pedigrees, but in 10 to 25% of patients, the family history is negative. Family members should be studied by examination of the blood smear, reticulocyte count, and osmotic fragility test when an index case of spherocytosis is discovered. If no abnormality is found in either parent, spherocytosis may reflect either a new mutation or a recessive disease. The mutations responsible for spherocytosis are located on chromosome 1 (q22-q23, α-spectrin), 8 (p11.2, ankyrin), 14 (q23-q24, β-spectrin), 15 (q15-q21, protein 4.2), or 17 (q21-qter, band 3).

CLINICAL MANIFESTATIONS The characteristic features of chronic hemolytic anemia, jaundice, reticulocytosis, and splenomegaly, are present to various degrees. Hemolysis may be fully compensated, without anemia or jaundice, and reticulocytosis may be the only manifestation of increased red cell production and destruction. During the neonatal period, hyperbilirubinemia is the most prominent finding and may be severe enough to require exchange transfusion, but the disease may be mild enough to escape detection until later. During the first few months of life, the severity of anemia may require RBC transfusion, but the degree of anemia is usually moderate, and hemoglobin levels below 80 g/L are unusual. The clinical severity of HS varies widely from family to family but tends to be consistent within an individual family. Gallstones may occur as early as 3 to 5 years of age and may be the first clinical indication of the disease.

LABORATORY DIAGNOSIS An essential diagnostic feature is the presence of spherocytes on the peripheral blood smear. Small, dense, spherical cells that lack normal biconcavity (see Fig. 19-5B) may be abundant or may comprise less than 5% of the total RBC population. Polychromasia, reflecting reticulocytosis, is usually evident. The MCHC may be as high as 37 to 38%. The RDW is increased. The tendency of spherocytes to hemolyse when they are suspended in hypotonic saline solutions in vitro is the basis of the osmotic fragility test. The incubated osmotic fragility study, in which red cells are tested after 24 hours of sterile incubation at 37°C, is more sensitive and may be diagnostic even when the osmotic fragility test of fresh blood is normal or equivocal. In addition to HS, spherocytes and abnormal osmotic fragility may be present in newborns with ABO hemolytic disease and in patients with autoimmune hemolytic anemia. A diagnosis of HS may be obscured by hepatobiliary obstruction in which increases of plasma lipids and cholesterol lead to an increase in red cell surface area, converting a previously abnormal osmotic fragility test to normal.

TREATMENT Splenectomy can eliminate transfusion requirements in severe HS and virtually eliminate anemia and hemolysis in milder cases. When possible the operation should be deferred until at least the age of 5 to 6 years to minimize the risk of postsplenectomy sepsis (see Sec. 19.8). If significant hemolysis persists after splenectomy, the preoperative diagnosis of HS was probably incorrect. Although partial splenectomy may improve the rate of hemolysis, with time the splenic remnant undergoes hypertrophy with a return of more severe hemolytic anemia. In addition, partial splenectomy does not protect against the development of gallstones or aplastic crises. Occasionally, an accessory spleen overlooked at the time of splenectomy may hypertrophy and produce a late recurrence of hemolysis. In such instances, the presence of residual splenic tissue should be investigated (see Sec. 19.8). Patients with HS have been thought to have an increased requirement for folic acid because of an accelerated rate of erythropoiesis, and many hematologists recommend 1 mg of oral folic acid daily, although the need for this in children has been challenged (see Sec. 19.3.4).

HEREDITARY ELLIPTOCYTOSIS

The incidence of hereditary elliptocytosis (HE) is approximately 1 per 2500 in the United States. HE is even more heterogeneous than HS at both the clinical and molecular level. HE can be clinically classified into two broad morphologic categories: (1) common HE, which has uniformly elliptical RBC but no other hematologic abnormalities (see Fig. 19-5E); and (2) hemolytic HE, in which there are many spherocytes as well as elliptocytes. During the neonatal period, large numbers of pyknocytes and fragmented forms

may be more striking than elliptocytes, and characteristic elliptocytic morphology may become apparent only after a few months. Neonatal hemolysis and hyperbilirubinemia may require exchange transfusion even though these children have mild disease later in life. This extreme, transient infantile poikilocytosis may be the consequence of dissociation of an already defective HE membrane skeleton by the unusually large amount of free 2,3-DPG because of the inability of hemoglobin F to bind to 2,3-DPG in the neonatal period.

The majority of spectrin defects described in elliptocytic red cells involve the α-spectrin subunit and are located at the head end of the molecule, in the vicinity of the dimer-dimer binding site. Defects in β-spectrin and abnormalities of other components of the membrane cytoskeleton have occasionally been associated with elliptocytosis. The clinical heterogeneity of elliptocytosis has not been completely explained on a molecular level, and some patients have no detectable abnormalities of the cytoskeleton.

TREATMENT The role of the spleen in the pathogenesis of hemolysis in HE is similar to that in HS, and splenectomy eliminates or reduces hemolysis in most severely affected patients.

HEREDITARY STOMATOCYTOSIS AND RELATED ABNORMALITIES OF CATION PERMEABILITY

Stomatocytes are RBC that have a slit-like area of central pallor when examined on the peripheral blood smear and a cup or bowl shape in wet preparations (see Fig. 19-5H). Stomatocytosis may be the predominant morphologic abnormality in certain hereditary hemolytic anemias. In most instances hemolysis is mild and characterized only by moderate reticulocytosis, but in a small number of patients anemia is more severe. Sodium and potassium permeability is markedly increased in RBC from such patients, leading to alterations in their cation content. When the RBC cation content is increased, the concurrent obligate osmotic movement of water causes swelling. When net cation content is decreased, cell water is lost, resulting in a shrunken, dehydrated, rigid RBC. Either water excess or deficiency may predominate in the red cells of hereditary stomatocytosis syndromes. The abnormalities in cell cations and water content are reflected in the RBC and osmotic fragility. Swelling that results from excess water, termed *hydrocytosis,* is associated with an increase in the MCV, a decrease in the MCHC, and an increase in osmotic fragility. Conversely, shrinkage from water loss, called *xerocytosis,* results in a normal or low MCV, an increase in MCHC, and a decrease in osmotic fragility. In both types of stomatocytes, erythrocyte glycolysis may be accelerated to supply energy for the increased active transport of cations. As in HS, such metabolically hyperactive cells are unable to maintain an adequate supply of ATP in the acidic, hypoglycemic splenic environment. Splenectomy usually decreases but does not eliminate the hemolysis in stomatocytosis.

References

Gallagher PG, Forget BG, Lux SE: Disorders of the erythrocyte membrane. In: Nathan DG, Orkin SH, eds: The Hematology of Infancy and Childhood, 5th ed. Philadelphia, WB Saunders, 1998:544–664

Mentzer WC, Lubin BH: Red cell membrane abnormalities. In: Lilleyman JS, Hann IM, Blanchette VS, eds: Pediatric Hematology, 2nd ed. London, Churchill Livingstone, 1999:285–306

19.5.2   Abnormalities of RBC Metabolism

Because it lacks a nucleus and organelles such as mitochondria, the mature RBC cannot replicate, synthesize proteins, or generate ATP via oxidative pathways. Limited requirements for ATP are met entirely by glycolysis (Fig. 19-7). ATP is needed to initiate the first several reactions in the glycolytic sequence, to maintain cell shape and flexibility, to renew membrane phospholipids, for active transport of cations, and for the synthesis of pyridine nucleotides, glutathione, and flavin adenine dinucleotide. Glycolysis also recycles NAD to NADH, an essential cofactor in the enzymatic reduction of methemoglobin. Approximately 95% of the glucose metabolized by the red cell passes directly through the Embden-Meyerhof pathway. The remaining 5% is diverted through

the hexose monophosphate shunt, the sole source of NADPH in the mature erythrocyte (Fig. 19-7).

The reduction of oxidized glutathione, catalyzed by the enzyme glutathione reductase, requires NADPH and provides a continuing source of reduced glutathione, essential for protecting cell constituents such as hemoglobin, enzymes, and membrane from oxidative damage. The shunt is also a source of ribose pyrophosphate, utilized in the synthesis of ATP. Oxidative threats to red cell integrity are countered by three different mechanisms, each involving glutathione. Reduced glutathione may deactivate an exogenous oxidant directly or may return an oxidized cellular component, such as hemoglobin, to a reduced state. Reduced glutathione also participates in the glutathione peroxidase–mediated conversion of hydrogen peroxide to water. In both reactions, glutathione is oxidized. Subsequent recycling of oxidized glutathione to the reduced

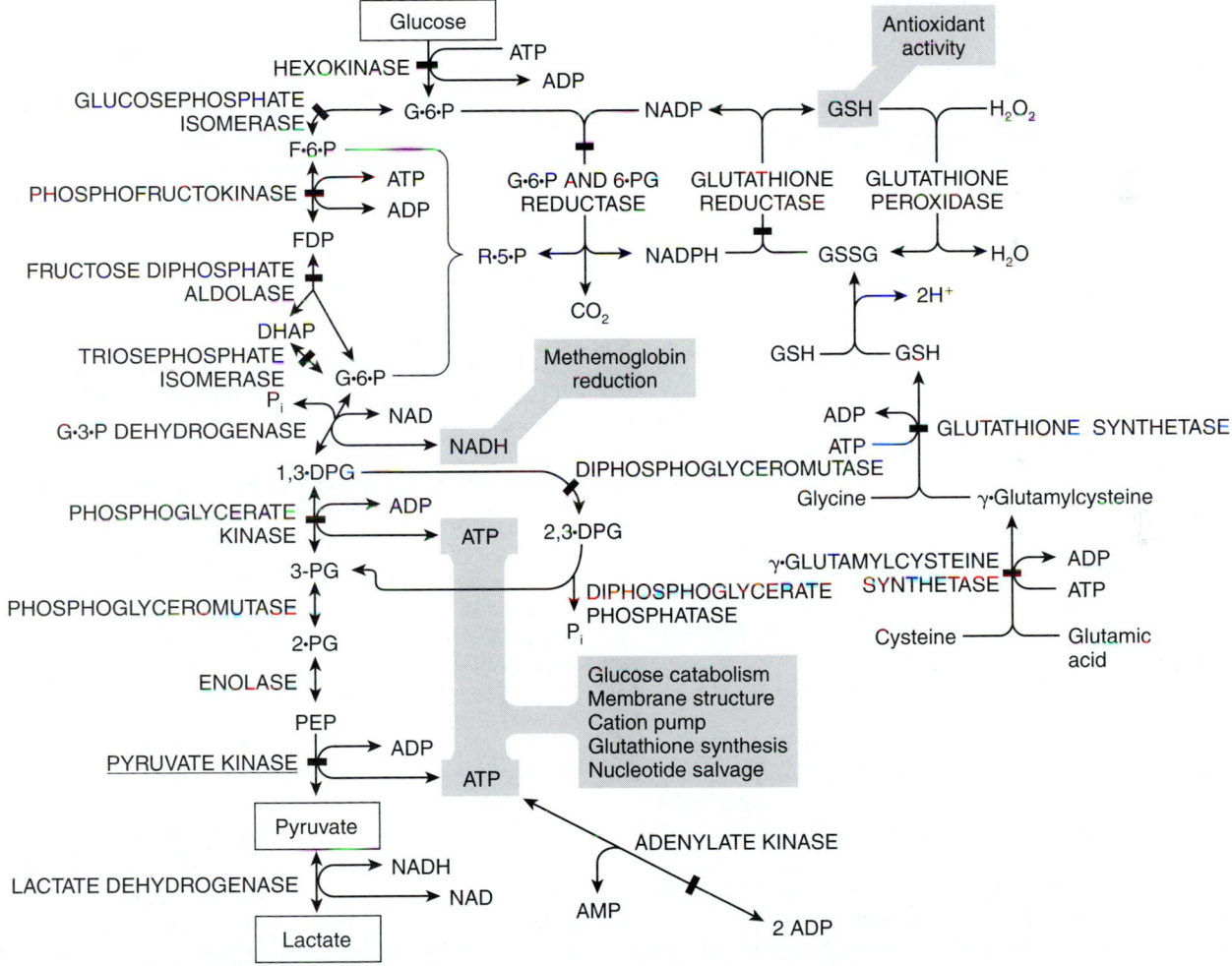

FIGURE 19-7   Glucose metabolism in mature erythrocytes. The hexose monophosphate shunt and glutathione metabolism are shown within the shaded area. Reactions involved in the synthesis of glutathione are indicated at the lower right. Solid bars indicate enzymatic deficiencies, the association of which with hereditary hemolytic disorders is well established. ADP = adenosine diphosphate; AMP = adenosine monophosphate; ATP = adenosine triphosphate; DHAP = dihydroxyacetone phosphate; DPG = diphosphoglycerate; FDP = fructose diphosphate; F-6-P = fructose-6-phosphatase; G-3-P = glucose-3-phosphate; G-6-P = glucose-6-phosphate; GSH = glutathione (reduced); GSSG = glutathione (oxidized); NAD = nicotinamide-adenine dinucleotide; NADH = reduced NAD; NADP = nicotinamide-adenine nucleotide (oxidized); NADPH = nicotinamide-adenine nucleotide (reduced); PEP = phosphoenolpyruvate; PG = phosphoglycerate; P_i = inorganic phosphate; R-5-P = ribose-5-phosphatase. SOURCE: *Modified from Hastings and Lubin, Rudolph's Fundamentals of Pediatrics, Stamford: Appleton and Lange, 2nd Edition p. 450, 1998.*

state requires a normally functioning hexose monophosphate shunt.

Enzyme proteins of the Embden-Meyerhof and hexose monophosphate shunt pathways are degraded as erythrocytes age, and a gradual loss of enzyme activity is a normal feature of erythrocyte aging. An enzymatic defect in any of the pathways of glucose metabolism can result in serious metabolic deficiencies, leading to impairment of cellular function and shortening of the cell life span.

DISORDERS OF THE HEXOSE MONOPHOSPHATE SHUNT AND METABOLISM OF GLUTATHIONE

Enzyme deficiencies of the hexose monophosphate shunt or of the pathway leading to the production of reduced glutathione can cause premature destruction of erythrocytes from oxidative damage. When the enzymatic deficiency is mild, little or no hemolysis may occur. However, when increased activity is needed (such as exposure to oxidant drugs or hydrogen peroxide), a severe hemolytic episode may occur.

GLUCOSE-6-PHOSPHATE DEHYDROGENASE DEFICIENCY More than 100 million people throughout the world are deficient in glucose-6-phosphate dehydrogenase (G6PD). The deficiency can occur in any ethnic group, although it is uncommon in North Europeans. The prevalance of G6PD deficiency exceeds 10% of the male population in Italy and Greece and is even higher in other Mediterranean, Middle-Eastern, and sub-Saharan African countries. Approximately 5% of Southern Chinese and 10% of African-American men and 2% of women are G6PD deficient.

PATHOPHYSIOLOGY The variable clinical manifestations of G6PD deficiency result from biochemically distinct mutant forms of G6PD, which can be distinguished on the basis of their different enzyme kinetics, the pH of optimal enzyme activity, their electrophoretic mobility, and stability in vitro. These mutations are almost always results of single amino acid substitutions.

The B form of G6PD is the normal or wild type in all populations. The A+ variant enzyme, present in about 30% of African-Americans, has nearly normal activity and is not associated with drug-related hemolysis. The A variant is associated with drug-related hemolysis, and another variant, designated as the A− variant whose electrophoretic migration is identical to that of the A+ enzyme also has abnormally low enzyme activity and is associated with drug-associated hemolysis variant. The form of severe G6PD deficiency prevalent in Mediterranean ethnic groups is associated with a G6PD variant designated B−.

Hemolysis in G6PD deficiency results from a failure to generate sufficient NADPH to recycle the reduced glutathione that is essential for protecting cellular components from oxidation. In the presence of an oxidant, hemoglobin forms denatured globin-glutathione complexes, which eventually precipitate as insoluble inclusions (Heinz bodies). The presence of Heinz bodies, as well as oxidative damage to the RBC membrane, leads to irreversible damage and hemolysis. Heinz bodies, detected by crystal violet staining of blood smears, may be present only early in an episode of hemolysis because red cells containing these inclusion bodies are rapidly destroyed.

Because the gene encoding G6PD is located on the X chromosome, G6PD deficiency has a sex-linked recessive pattern of inheritance. Clinical manifestations of the deficiency are usually encountered only in male hemizygotes or female homozygotes. In female heterozygotes both enzyme-replete and enzyme-deficient red cells are present because either the normal or the mutant X chromosome may be active through random X-chromosome inactivation (lyonization) in embryonic life. Some heterozygotes may have large numbers of enzyme-deficient red cells and resemble deficient male hemizygotes, whereas others may have few enzyme-deficient cells and are indistinguishable from normal. Because cells with normal enzyme activity and enzyme-deficient cells are both present, distinguishing heterozygotes from normal by the use of screening tests or quantitative assays of enzyme activity may be difficult.

CLINICAL MANIFESTATIONS The most common clinical manifestation of G6PD deficiency is episodic acute hemolysis, usually following infections or the ingestion of certain drugs or other hemolytic agents (see Table 19-5). Rarely, a patient with G6PD deficiency will exhibit chronic, lifelong, nonspherocytic hemolytic anemia, jaundice, and splenomegaly. Administration of hemolytic agents to such individuals may accelerate the rate of hemolysis.

Hemolytic episodes are characterized by increasing pallor, jaundice, dark urine, back pain, and, in the most severe disease, shock, cardiovascular collapse, and death. Between hemolytic episodes, anemia is absent, and erythrocyte survival may be normal. In African-American men who have the A− G6PD mutation, enzyme activity is nearly normal in reticulocytes and young erythrocytes, but because the enzyme is unstable, activity declines rapidly as cells age, resulting in a population of older, enzyme-deficient cells that are

TABLE 19-5

SOME AGENTS REPORTED TO PRODUCE HEMOLYSIS IN PATIENTS WITH G6PD DEFICIENCY

Drugs and chemicals clearly shown to cause clinically significant hemolytic anemia in G6PD deficiency

Acetanilide	Pentaquine
Methylene blue	Sulfanilamide
Nalidixic acid	Sulfacetamide
Naphthalene	Sulfapyridine
Niridazole	Sulfamethoxazole
Phenylhydrazine	Thiazolesulfone
Primaquine	Toluidine blue
Pamaquine	Trinitrotoluene (TNT)

Drugs probably safe in normal therapeutic doses for G6PD-deficient individuals (without nonspherocytic hemolytic anemia)

Acetaminophen	Phenylbutazone
Acetophenetidine	Phenytoin
Acetylsalicylic acid (aspirin)	Probenecid
Aminopyrine	Procaine amide hydrochloride
Antazoline	Pyrimethamine
Antipyrine	Quinidine
Ascorbic acid (vitamin C)	Quinine
Benzhexol	Streptomycin
Chloramphenicol	Sulfacytine
Chlorguanidine	Sulfadiazine
Chloroquine	Sulfaguanidine
Colchicine	Sulfamerazine
Diphenhydramine	Sulfamethoxypyridazine
L-Dopa	Sulfisoxazole
Menadione sodium bisulfite	Trimethoprim
Menaphthone	Tripelennamine
p-Aminobenzoic acid	Vitamin K

SOURCE: *Beutler E: Hemolytic Anemia in Disorders of Red Cell Metabolism. New York, Plenum, 1978.*

susceptible to hemolysis, while younger, enzyme-replete cells remain intact. Following administration of a hemolytic agent, an abrupt fall in hematocrit, associated with hemolysis of older, enzyme-deficient red cells, is followed by reticulocytosis and a gradual return of the hematocrit to normal levels, even with continued administration of the hemolytic agent. A period of equilibrium is subsequently reached in which anemia is absent and only minimal evidence of continued hemolysis is present. The laboratory diagnosis of G6PD deficiency during the recovery and equilibrium periods may be difficult because only young, enzyme-replete RBC remain in the circulation. In the more severe Mediterranean B− form of G6PD deficiency, both young and old RBC are enzyme deficient and are thus susceptible to hemolysis.

G6PD deficiency is often associated with neonatal jaundice in Asian and Mediterranean infants, even in the absence of exposure to a recognized hemolytic agent. In African-Americans, an increased incidence of jaundice is seen in premature but not in mature G6PD-deficient infants. In the Mediterranean and Asia, RBC from certain G6PD-deficient individuals are susceptible to hemolysis when raw fava beans, a dietary staple, are ingested. The hemolytic agent of fava beans can also be transmitted through breast milk.

LABORATORY DIAGNOSIS   During acute hemolytic episodes, morphologically abnormal RBC including spherocytes and fragmented cells may be present. Definitive diagnosis of G6PD deficiency can be made by quantitative assay of enzyme activity. Screening tests, which measure the ability of the erythrocyte to generate NADPH in vitro, are also available. Screening tests for G6PD may be used to identify susceptible individuals to avoid agents known to produce hemolysis (see Table 19-5). G6PD-deficient individuals should be provided with a list of such agents and counseled regarding the possible risk associated with their use. Some of these drugs produce

hemolysis only in severe deficiencies such as the B− variant or G6PD-deficient nonspherocytic hemolytic anemia. The A− variant common in African-Americans does not develop hemolysis unless potent oxidant drugs such as primaquine or naphthylene are ingested.

OTHER ABNORMALITIES OF THE HEXOSE MONOPHOSPHATE SHUNT   Inherited deficiencies of the two enzymes involved in the synthesis of glutathione, glutamyl cysteine synthetase and glutathione synthetase, may result in either episodic or chronic hemolysis. Unlike G6PD deficiency, these disorders are rare and have an autosomal-recessive pattern of inheritance. Diagnosis requires quantitative assay of red cell enzyme activity in vitro or the detection of reduced levels of erythrocyte glutathione.

Flavin adenine dinucleotide (FAD) is a required cofactor for activation of erythrocyte glutathione reductase. Dietary riboflavin deficiency, which can produce FAD deficiency, may result in diminished glutathione reductase activity, and measurement of erythrocyte glutathione reductase activity provides a convenient assay for dietary riboflavin deficiency.

DISORDERS OF GLYCOLYSIS (EMBDEN-MEYERHOF PATHWAY)

Inherited deficiencies of Embden-Meyerof glycolytic pathway enzymes are often associated with chronic hemolytic anemia (see Fig. 19-7). Inadequate glycolytic synthesis of ATP is the common denominator responsible for shortened red cell survival in these disorders. Unique features that are associated with particular glycolytic enzymopathies are highlighted in Table 19-6. The clinical manifestations, genetics, and treatment of these enzymopathies are similar, and they can be described as a group rather than individually.

TABLE 19-6
ENZYME DEFICIENCIES OF THE EMBDEN-MEYERHOF PATHWAY

ENZYME	GENETICS	TISSUES INVOLVED	CLINICAL FEATURES	RED CELL METABOLITES		OTHER REMARKS
				ATP	2,3-DPG	
Hexokinase	AR	RBC	CNSHA	↓	↓	Increased hemoglobin O_2 affinity, decreased exercise tolerance for degree of anemia
Glucose phosphate isomerase	AR	RBC, WBC, skin fibroblasts	CNSHA	↓, N	N	Spiculated microspherocytes sometimes observed
Phosphofructokinase	AR	RBC, muscle	CNSHA, myopathy (muscle glycogen storage disease)	↓	↓	
Aldolase	AR	RBC	CNSHA	N	↑	Fructose-1,6-diphosphate accumulates in RBC
Triosephosphate isomerase	AR	RBC, WBC, muscle, serum, CSF	CNSHA, severe progressive neurologic disorder	↓	—	Dihydroxyacetone phosphate accumulates in RBC, increased susceptibility to infection
Phosphoglycerate kinase	Sex-linked	RBC, WBC	CNSHA, mental retardation, myopathy	N	N, ↑	
2,3-DPG mutase	AR, AD	RBC	?CNSHA or polycythemia	N, ↑	↓	Increased hemoglobin O_2 affinity
Pyruvate kinase	AR	RBC, liver	CNSHA	N, ↓	↑	Decreased hemoglobin O_2 affinity, increased exercise tolerance for degree of anemia

AR, autosomal recessive; AD, autosomal dominant; CNSHA, congenital nonspherocytic hemolytic anemia; N, normal.

PATHOPHYSIOLOGY In pyruvate kinase deficiency, ATP depletion causes a defect in membrane cation permeability, and K⁺ is lost from the cell more quickly than Na⁺ is gained. Because ATP is unavailable for the active transport of cations to restore normal cation gradients, progressive K⁺ loss occurs, producing a reduction in cell cation content accompanied by an obligate osmotic loss of cell water, and the ATP-depleted RBC becomes a crenated sphere. Dehydrated, stiff, ATP-depleted red cells are susceptible to sequestration by the spleen. The acidic, hypoglycemic, hypoxic environment of the spleen may produce further metabolic depletion. In general, reticulocytes are resistant to this sequence of events if an alternate source of ATP synthesis, such as oxidative phosphorylation, is available. However, because reticulocytes have greater metabolic requirements for ATP than mature erythrocytes, they may be particularly vulnerable to metabolic depletion. Inhibition of oxidative phosphorylation by hypoxia also compromises ATP synthesis in reticulocytes with defective glycolysis. Sequestration of reticulocytes within the spleen, which is hypoxic as well as acidic and hypoglycemic, leads to their rapid destruction.

Deficient enzyme activity along the Embden-Meyerhof pathway results in an altered concentration of glycolytic intermediates above and below the site of deficient enzymatic function (Fig. 19-7). In particular, the concentration of 2,3-DPG may be greatly altered. Because 2,3-DPG is an important regulator of hemoglobin oxygen affinity, changes in its concentration may have implications for oxygen transport, and the clinical effects of anemia are modified to a significant degree by the intracellular concentration of 2,3-DPG characteristic of each glycolytic enzymopathy. Anemia may result in few or no symptoms in pyruvate kinase deficiency, where 2,3-DPG levels are high, enhancing oxygen transport. In contrast, in hexokinase deficiency, the same degree of anemia may be severely symptomatic because 2,3-DPG levels are subnormal.

The lower hemoglobin levels of children compared to adults has been attributed to a higher level of inorganic phosphate. In uremia, where serum phosphate and, as a consequence, red cell organic phosphate concentrations may rise, a decrease in oxygen affinity may occur. Conversely, in hypophosphatemia, such as that sometimes seen during parenteral hyperalimentation, an increase in oxygen affinity may result from the fall in red cell organic phosphate levels. When the serum phosphate drops below 0.5 mg/dL, ATP depletion may be so extreme as to result in hemolytic anemia, which can be corrected by administration of phosphate.

INCIDENCE AND GENETICS Glycolytic enzymopathies are rare but are most frequently encountered in individuals from northern Europe. Inheritance is autosomal recessive except for phosphoglycerate kinase deficiency, which is sex linked. Anemic individuals are either homozygotes or compound heterozygotes. In the latter, family studies may be useful in determining the biochemical nature of the two enzyme variants that, inherited together, have caused anemia.

CLINICAL MANIFESTATIONS Jaundice, reticulocytosis, and splenomegaly are found in most anemic patients. The severity of hemolysis varies depending on the degree to which erythrocyte glycolysis is impaired. Hemolysis and jaundice may be present in the newborn. Gallstones and anemic crises from transient erythroid hypoplasia may occur in the more severely anemic patients.

LABORATORY FINDINGS RBC morphology is usually normal, except for polychromatophilia of reticulocytosis. After splenectomy, a variable number of contracted, spiculated cells may be found. The unincubated osmotic fragility curve is normal, but after incubation, a "tail" of osmotically fragile RBC may be present. The autohemolysis of RBC incubated under sterile conditions in saline for 48 hours is increased and is usually improved by the addition of glucose to the incubation medium. Diagnosis of RBC glycolytic enzymopathies is based on quantitative enzyme assay. Comprehensive assays are available in reference laboratories, but commercial screening tests are widely available for the more common enzymopathies, including those of pyruvate kinase (PK), glucose phosphate isomerase, and triosephosphate isomerase deficiencies.

The clinical variability of these disorders is a consequence of biochemically distinct variant forms of the defective enzyme. In PK deficiency, several isozymes have nearly normal activity at the artificially high substrate concentrations used in the usual in vitro assay but are inactive at the lower substrate concentrations that occur in vivo. In addition, contamination by leukocytes may affect the results. Modification of the usual assay to exclude WBC and to include measurement of enzyme activity at low substrate concentrations will help to identify such variants.

TREATMENT Splenectomy, although not curative, usually decreases the intensity of hemolysis in severely anemic patients. In patients with mild anemia, splenectomy seldom results in significant improvement. Blood transfusions may occasionally be required, particularly after transient bone marrow aplasia.

References

Beutler E: The molecular biology of enzymes of erythrocyte metabolism. In: Stammatoyannopoulos GW, Neinhuis AW, Majerus PW, Varmus H, eds: The Molecular Basis of Blood Diseases, 2nd ed. Philadelphia, WB Saunders, 1994:331–350

Mentzer WC: Pyruvate kinase deficiency and disorders of glycolysis. In: Nathan DG, Orkin SH, eds: Hematology of Infancy and Childhood, 5th ed. Philadelphia, WB Saunders, 1998:665–703

19.5.3 Methemoglobinemia

Methemoglobin is a form of hemoglobin in which heme iron has been oxidized to the ferric state and can no longer reversibly bind oxygen. Several mechanisms enzymatically reduce methemoglobin and prevent the accumulation of levels greater than 1 to 2% of total hemoglobin. Under normal circumstances, NADPH-dependent methemoglobin reductase (NADH–cytochrome b_5 reductase) accounts for nearly all methemoglobin reduction. NADPH flavin reductase can be utilized as an alternate pathway when NADPH methemoglobin reductase is deficient but normally contributes little to the reduction of methemoglobin. Methemoglobin reductase activity in cord blood is only about 70% of that of adults, and the level of activity in fetal blood is even lower. Normal adult values are reached between 7 weeks and 6 months after birth.

An increase in the concentration of methemoglobin in the blood (methemoglobinemia) occurs when a disturbance in the balance between oxidation and reduction of heme iron occurs and can result from inherited abnormalities of hemoglobin (the M hemoglobins) or red cell enzymes or from exposure to drugs or toxins (Table 19-7). Blood methemoglobin concentrations above 15 g/L impart a chocolate brown appearance to the blood and a slate gray cyanotic hue to the skin and mucous membranes. With higher percentages of methemoglobinemia, hypoxia may occur.

TABLE 19-7

TABLE 19-7

OXIDANTS REPORTED TO CAUSE METHEMOGLOBINEMIA

Analgesics: Acetaminophen, phenacetin, pyridium
Anesthetics: Benzocaine (topical, rectal), prilocaine, lidocaine
Aniline derivatives: Marking dyes (topical)
                           Disinfectants (topical)
                           Crayons
Antimalarials: Dapsone, primaquine, pamaquine
Nitrites: Nitrate contamination of well water
                Bismuth subnitrate
                Nitroglycerin
                Nitrate food additives
                Butyl nitrite inhalants
Sodium nitroprusside
Sulfonamides
Vitamin K analogues
Potassium permanganate, chromates, chlorates, copper
Naphthalene
Gum asafetida

METHEMOGLOBIN REDUCTASE DEFICIENCY

An inherited deficiency of NADPH-methemoglobin reductase may result in either intermittent or chronic methemoglobinemia. The disorder is rare, is inherited in an autosomal-recessive pattern, and appears with greatest frequency in inbred populations. Homozygotes have lifelong cyanosis and usually have methemoglobin levels of 10 to 25%, but levels may be increased by exposure to oxidant drugs (Table 19-7). Despite the presence of methemoglobinemia, these patients have a normal life span and usually have few symptoms. About 12% of homozygotes have cognitive difficulties, and these individuals have a deficiency of methemoglobin reductase in cells, involving microsomal as well as soluble forms of the enzyme. Heterozygotes do not normally have methemoglobinemia, which may, however, develop on exposure to oxidant drugs (Table 19-7). Spontaneous methemoglobinemia may occur in the newborn period because enzyme deficiency in the heterozygote accentuates the normally low neonatal levels of methemoglobin reductase.

A number of electrophoretic variants of methemoglobin reductase have been discovered, but not all variants are associated with reduced enzyme activity and susceptibility to methemoglobin formation. NADPH flavin reductase deficiency has also been described. Because the major burden of methemoglobin reductase is borne by NADH methemoglobin reductase, methemoglobinemia is not a feature of NADPH flavin reductase deficiency. The amino acid substitutions that result in the HbM hemoglobinopathies lead to a marked increase in the rate of spontaneous oxidation of hemoglobin to methemoglobin (Sec. 19.4.6). In contrast to congenital methemoglobinemia, these hemoglobinopathies exhibit an autosomal-dominant pattern of inheritance.

TOXIC METHEMOGLOBINEMIA

A variety of drugs and chemicals may increase the rate of oxidation of hemoglobin and produce methemoglobinemia (Table 19-7). Newborns are particularly susceptible to such agents because hemoglobin F is more readily oxidized to methemoglobin than is hemoglobin A and because levels of NADH methemoglobin reductase are low. Diarrheal dehydration and acidosis induced by in-

fection or milk intolerance in infants 2 to 8 weeks of age may cause methemoglobinemia even in the absence of identifiable toxins or hereditary defects.

DIAGNOSIS   If a freshly obtained blood specimen is chocolate brown in color and does not become red when oxygenated, a presumptive diagnosis of methemoglobinemia can be made. Spectrophotometric analysis of the concentration of methemoglobin is required to confirm the diagnosis. When methemoglobinemia is acute in onset, exposure to chemicals or drugs should be suspected. The diagnosis of NADH methemoglobin reductase deficiency can be confirmed by measuring activity of the enzyme in the patient's RBC.

TREATMENT   The first step in treatment is to remove oxidant drugs or chemicals suspected of initiating methemoglobinemia. If methemoglobin levels exceed 40% or clinical symptoms are present, rapid conversion of methemoglobin to hemoglobin can be achieved by intravenous infusion of 1% solution of methylene blue in saline at a dose of 1 to 2 mg/kg body weight. The reduction of methemoglobin by methylene blue is mediated by NADPH methemoglobin reductase and requires an intact hexose monophosphate shunt as a source of NADPH. Patients should be screened for G6PD deficiency before the use of methylene blue. This drug not only is ineffective for treating methemoglobinemia but may cause hemolytic anemia in patients with G6PD deficiency. Methemoglobin levels exceeding 50% of total hemoglobin may cause serious complications or death. Exchange transfusion in addition to intravenous methylene blue therapy may be indicated. Chronic methemoglobinemia caused by NADH methemoglobin reductase activity is treated by daily oral administration of methylene blue (1.5 to 5 mg/kg in divided doses) or ascorbic acid (5 to 8 mg/kg in divided doses).

References

Mansouri A, Lurie AA: Concise review: methemoglobinemia. Am J Hematol 42:7–12, 1993
Murray KF, Christie DL: Dietary protein intolerance in infants with transient methemoglobinemia and diarrhea. J Pediatr 122:90–92, 1993

19.5.4   Destruction of Red Blood Cells Caused by Abnormalities of the Vasculature or Plasma

DRUG-ASSOCIATED IMMUNE HEMOLYTIC ANEMIA

Drug-induced immune hemolytic anemias are rare in children. Some drugs may complex with plasma proteins, evoking formation of an antibody to the drug–protein complex that adheres nonspecifically to the red cell membrane, leading to complement fixation and hemolysis. Binding of a drug directly to the red cell membrane may act as a hapten, and the complex may stimulate antibody formation. Alterations in T- and B-lymphocyte interactions by drugs may contribute to autoantibody production and subsequent immune hemolysis. *Hemolytic anemia* has been reported with phenacetin, antihistamines, sulfonamides, insulin, quinine, and other agents. In rare cases, penicillin, when given in very large doses, can bind to the red cell membrane and evoke the formation of an IgG antibody directed against the red cell membrane–penicillin complex. Antibody can be detected on the patient's red cells with the direct antiglobulin (Coombs) test, but the indirect Coombs test is usually negative unless the red cells are first incubated with penicillin.

Approximately 15% of patients receiving α-methyldopa (Aldomet) develop a dose-related positive antiglobulin test within 3 to 6 months after treatment has been initiated because the drug induces an autoantibody that reacts directly with the RBC membrane. Hemolysis occurs in fewer than 1% of those who develop antibodies and subsides rapidly when the drug is discontinued, although the positive Coombs test may remain positive for a year or more.

Cephalothin (Keflin) therapy can result in a false-positive Coombs test by nonimmunologic adsorption of plasma proteins to the surface of the red cell. Although not antibodies, these proteins are detected by the antiglobulin tests used during blood crossmatching. This reaction is dose dependent, occurs in 3% of patients, and is not associated with hemolysis. Rarely, cephalothin may act as a hapten, similar to penicillin, and a hemolytic anemia may develop.

AUTOIMMUNE HEMOLYTIC ANEMIA

PATHOGENESIS Autoimmune hemolytic anemia (AHA) can result when antibody, antibody-complement complex, or complement alone binds to the membrane of the RBC. RBC coated with antibody and/or complement are immunologically recognized and are either totally engulfed by macrophages or lose part of their membrane. Loss of surface area without a change in cell volume produces spherocytes, which are then trapped and destroyed in the liver and spleen. An alternate mechanism for red cell destruction involves the activation of complement, which directly damages the RBC membrane, resulting in intravascular hemolysis. RBC autoantibodies may arise in several ways. Infectious or other agents may interact directly with the RBC membrane to create neoantigens or with plasma proteins to form immune complexes. The immune dysregulation seen in autoimmune diseases such as lupus erythematosus may generate antierythrocyte antibodies. Finally, immune responses to drugs may lead to crossreactions with red cell membrane antigens.

CLINICAL COURSE There are two clinical forms of AHA in children: a severe, *acute-onset* form, and a more insidious, *chronic* form. Acute-onset AHA occurs in the first 4 years of life and is generally characterized by an explosive onset and rapid remission. Although a viral etiology is frequently suspected, identification of an underlying etiology is usually nonproductive. The usual presenting clinical features include acute onset of pallor, jaundice, splenomegaly, and often hemoglobinemia and hemoglobinuria. Severely anemic patients may develop congestive heart failure and hypoxemia.

Chronic AHA usually has an insidious onset, although a viral illness may be the precipitating event. Anemia is less severe than in acute-onset disease. Patients with chronic AHA should be investigated for underlying immune or neoplastic diseases. Rarely, immune hemolysis can be the first clinical indication of HIV infection. Reticulocytosis is usually present, and thrombocytopenia and neutropenia are occasionally observed. The combination of AHA and immune thrombocytopenia is designated Evans syndrome. The spleen is often enlarged, and hepatomegaly may be found.

LABORATORY DIAGNOSIS In acute AHA, hemoglobin concentration can drop to extremely low values (<20 g/L) but are usually between 40 and 60 g/L at the time of presentation. The reticulocyte count is usually elevated but may be low during the first few days, before the bone marrow responds. The platelet count is typically normal, and WBC is often increased. The serum concentration of unconjugated bilirubin and the plasma hemoglobin level are often elevated, and the serum haptoglobin level is low or absent. The peripheral blood smear may show rouleau formation, intense microspherocytes, polychromasia, and nucleated RBC.

Immune hemolytic anemias are diagnosed by the direct Coombs test to detect antibody or complement on the surface of the red cell and the indirect Coombs test, which detects free antibody in the plasma. The polyvalent rabbit antihuman reagents used by most laboratories contain both anti-IgG and anticomplement (anti-C_3d) antibodies.

The RBC autoantibodies that have highest activity at 37°C are called warm antibodies, are usually IgG, and do not cause spontaneous agglutination of red cells unless Coombs antiserum is added (incomplete antibodies). In contrast, antibodies with maximal activity at 4°C are usually IgM and are called complete antibodies because agglutination of RBC occurs without addition of Coombs antiserum.

The *Donath-Landsteiner* antibody is sometimes found in acute postinfectious autoimmune hemolytic anemia; this unusual biphasic antibody binds to the surface of the RBC and fixes complement at 4°C. When the temperature is then raised to 37°C, complement is activated, and hemolysis ensues. The Donath-Landsteiner antibody is also found in paroxysmal cold hemoglobinuria in which exposure of an affected person to cold temperature causes antibody fixation to red cells, and hemolysis occurs on rewarming. If clinical and laboratory findings suggest immune hemolysis but both the direct and indirect Coombs tests are negative, specific complement fixation techniques may be used to detect small numbers of IgG antibody molecules on the surface of the red cell. Such complement-fixation techniques are sensitive below the lowest levels that can be detected by the standard Coombs tests.

TREATMENT Treatment with corticosteroids is the mainstay of therapy of acute AHA. The rate of hemolysis usually decreases in response to treatment with 2 to 10 mg/kg/d of prednisone in divided doses, and most patients are clinically stable within 1 to 2 months. Intravenous corticosteroids should be given to severely anemic patients. Prednisone rapidly decreases red cell destruction by the reticuloendothelial system and then gradually diminishes antibody production. Patients with severe anemia and cardiorespiratory compromise may require blood transfusion or partial exchange transfusion. In a critically ill patient, transfusions may be life saving despite laboratory incompatibility. A compatible crossmatch is often impossible because of the positive direct and indirect Coombs reactions characteristic of AHA. Group O, Rh-negative cells with the most compatible crossmatch should be administered slowly, and no more should be given than necessary to stabilize cardiovascular function. Blood hemoglobin levels should be monitored, and a brisk diuresis should be initiated to minimize the risk of acute tubular necrosis (see Sec. 21.7). When a cold-reacting antibody is present, blood should be warmed to 37°C before transfusion. Splenectomy is rarely indicated for acute-onset AHA. Intravenous γ-globulin therapy is rarely effective. The dose of prednisone should be slowly tapered when hemolysis has subsided. If prednisone therapy is discontinued too rapidly, hemolysis may recur. The direct

Coombs test may remain positive for as long as 1 year. The decision to continue or discontinue steroid treatment should be based on the degree of hemolysis, not on a positive Coombs test.

Patients with *Mycoplasma pneumoniae* or *Epstein-Barr virus* infections (infectious mononucleosis) sometimes develop a positive antiglobulin test (see Chapter 13). The autoantibody associated with these two illnesses has maximal activity at 4°C. However, because some activity exists at 37°C, hemolysis can occur when the antibody titer is very high. In *Mycoplasma* infections, the antibody is usually directed against the RBC surface antigen I, whereas in EBV infections, the antibody is directed against the i-surface antigen. Patients who develop hemolytic anemia during the course of these infections usually have a brief, mild clinical course that usually requires no treatment.

In *chronic AHA,* the response to corticosteroids is generally poor. Relapses are common and may warrant a 6- to 8-week trial of immunosuppressive agents, such as azathioprine or cyclophosphamide. If severe chronic hemolysis continues, splenectomy should be considered and usually decreases the rate of hemolysis. Thymectomy has been successful in a few instances of severe chronic immune hemolytic anemia refractory to other forms of therapy.

MECHANICAL INTRAVASCULAR HEMOLYSIS

Destruction of red blood cells may result from RBC contact with abnormal surfaces, turbulent blood flow, or shearing of RBC by fibrin strands or platelet-fibrin aggregates. Mechanical fragmentation of red blood cells leads to the formation of spherocytes, microcytes, and especially schistocytes, cells with an irregular shape and one or more pointed protrusions (see Fig. 19-5L). The degree of reticulocytosis parallels the rate of hemolysis, and serum haptoglobin is low or absent. Serum hemoglobin levels may be elevated, and hemosiderin is often present in the urine. When hemolysis is of long standing, loss of urinary iron as hemosiderin may superimpose iron deficiency anemia on the chronic hemolytic process. Thrombocytopenia and reduced levels of coagulation factors may be present in giant hemangioma syndrome (see Sec. 19.7). Mechanical intravascular hemolysis within large vessels *(macroangiopathic hemolytic anemia)* is associated with abnormal turbulent blood flow over the surface of a damaged heart valve, a defective valve prosthesis, or a patch used to close an intracardiac defect. With mild degrees of hemolysis, a compensated state can often be maintained, but hemolysis may be increased by the increased cardiac output associated with physical activity. If the degree of hemolysis is severe and chronic, surgical replacement of the defective valve or prosthesis and iron therapy to replace urinary losses may be necessary.

Microangiopathic hemolytic anemia, or mechanical intravascular hemolysis within small blood vessels, occurs in disseminated intravascular coagulation (DIC) (see Sec. 19.10), localized intravascular coagulation as in hemolytic-uremic syndrome, thrombotic thrombocytopenic purpura, cavernous hemangioma (Kasabach-Merritt syndrome), or malignant hypertension. Thrombocytopenia and clotting factor deficiencies may be found as well.

LIVER DISEASE

The lipid composition of the red blood cell membrane may be altered by changes in plasma lipids induced by either hepatocellular disease or biliary obstruction. Target cells are frequently observed in liver disease and are the morphologic consequence of excess membrane lipid. Rarely, severe hepatocellular disease may be associated with hemolysis and spur cells, a type of acanthocyte, on the peripheral smear (see Fig. 19-5).

PAROXYSMAL NOCTURNAL HEMOGLOBINURIA

Paroxysmal nocturnal hemoglobinuria (PNH) is an acquired disorder in which the RBC are abnormally susceptible to complement-mediated lysis. The underlying defect is an abnormality in the synthesis of membrane glycosylphosphatidylinositol, which normally serves as an anchor for numerous red cell surface proteins including CD55 and CD59, components of the complement regulatory system. Complement-mediated lysis is the consequence of the absence of these regulatory proteins on the surface of the red cell. Hemolysis is intravascular, resulting in hemoglobinemia, hemoglobinuria, and hemosiderinuria. Hemolysis is often accentuated by decreased pH during sleep. Indirect diagnostic tests for PNH, including the acid-lysis (Ham) and the sucrose hemolysis test, are being replaced by direct measurements of the RBC membrane CD55 and/or CD59 by flow cytometry. Leukopenia and thrombocytopenia are commonly encountered in PNH; the disorder often resembles aplastic anemia and may terminate in leukemia.

Therapy consists of treatment of iron deficiency resulting from urinary iron loss and RBC transfusion as necessary. Major thromboses may require anticoagulation. Androgens and corticosteroids may be beneficial in patients in whom marrow failure rather than hemolysis predominates. A few patients have been treated successfully by BMT.

INFANTILE PYKNOCYTOSIS

This is a poorly defined syndrome characterized by hemolytic anemia that occurs during the first weeks of life and then resolves spontaneously. Although not recognized at the time of the original description, many cases may have been a result of vitamin E deficiency (see Sec. 19.3). Dense, contracted, spiculated erythrocytes, or pyknocytes, and thrombocytosis are present, and the Coombs test is negative.

References

Buchanan GR, Boxer LA, Nathan DG: The acute and transient nature of idiopathic immune hemolytic anemia in childhood. J Pediatr 88:780, 1976

Bull BS, Kuhn IN: The production of schistocytes by fibrin strands (a scanning electron microscope study). Blood 35:104, 1970

Habibi B, Hamberg J, Schaison G, Salmon C: Autoimmune hemolytic anemia in children—a review of 80 cases. Am J Med 56:61–85, 1974

Rosse WF, Ware RE: The molecular basis of paroxysmal nocturnal hemoglobinuria. Blood 86:3277–3286, 1995

19.6   WHITE BLOOD CELLS

Mitchell S. Cairo and Francisco Bracho

Pluripotent hematopoietic stem cells arising from the bone marrow or, during fetal development, from the liver and marrow space undergo proliferation and differentiation to give rise to all lineages of peripheral white blood cells. Lymphocytes, monocytes, dendritic cells, and polymorphonuclear leukocytes (neutrophils, basophils, and eosinophils) are all derived from pluripotent hematopoietic stem cells (see Secs. 19.9 and 20.4).

DEVELOPMENTAL CHANGES IN WHITE BLOOD CELL NUMBERS

The number of white cells and the proportion of each cell type in the circulating blood are helpful in the diagnosis and management of many illnesses. There are marked changes in normal values with age (Table 19-8). The mean white blood cell count (WBC) at birth is high, with a broad range of normal. A brief rise in the mean value occurs at 12 hours after birth, followed by a rapid fall until the end of the first week, after which values remain stable until 1 year of age. Subsequently, a slow, steady fall in WBC throughout childhood is seen until the values of adult life are reached.

WBC differential counts indicate the relative proportions of different kinds of leukocytes in the blood. Neutrophils account for about one-half the WBC at birth. A transient rise occurs within 12 hours, followed by a decrease between 1 month and 1 year. Neutrophil percentages as low as 20% are common in normal infants; after infancy, the proportion of neutrophils increases slowly, reaching parity with lymphocytes at 5 years of age, and then further increases to the mean adult value of 60%.

Lymphocytes account for about 30% of the WBC in the newborn. The proportion of lymphocytes increases rapidly in the first month and remains at about 60% until 2 years of age; a count of 75% lymphocytes is not unusual in children of this age. During infancy, some of the lymphocytes are large and may contain nucleoli.

The absolute count of each cell type is obtained by multiplying the total WBC by the percentage of that cell type in the differential count and is expressed as a multiple of 10^9/L. Absolute values for neutrophils and lymphocytes are more clinically relevant than percentage values. The absolute neutrophil count (ANC) decreases rapidly from a mean of about 10×10^9/L during the first day of life and then maintains a value near 3.5×10^9/L for 2 years and reaches the adult mean of 4.4×10^9/L at about 3 years of age.

African-Americans have slightly lower ANC than other races. A few metamyelocytes and even myelocytes are common in the peripheral blood of the newborn. In premature infants, more of these immature neutrophils and even myelocytes and blast cells may occasionally be seen. The absolute lymphocyte count (ALC) in early infancy is more than twice that found in the adult, 5.6 compared with 2.5×10^9/L. The ALC then increases further, to reach a peak of about 7.0×10^9/L between 6 months and 12 months of age. The ALC then gradually decreases during early childhood to a value of 3.5×10^9/L at age 6 years and a slower subsequent decline to the adult value. ALC below 1.2×10^9/L may be associated with immunodeficiency syndromes.

Monocytes, basophils, and eosinophils are relatively abundant in the first weeks after birth and then gradually decline to the lower adult values

NEUTROPHIL KINETICS

The bone marrow contains a common committed progenitor cell for the monocyte/macrophage and granulocyte pathways called the colony-forming unit: CFU-GM. Specific glycoprotein hormones termed colony-stimulating factors (M-CSF and G-CSF) induce the differentiation of a progenitor cell into monoblasts, which mature to monocytes or myeloblasts, which mature to granulocytes.

Maturation of the neutrophil through the myeloblast, promyelocyte, and myelocyte stages entails three to five cell divisions and occurs over 4 to 7 days. After this initial proliferative period, maturation proceeds through the nondividing metamyelocyte, band, and segmented stages over the following 5 to 7 days. Mature neutrophils (bands and segmented cells) in the bone marrow constitute a compartment known as the neutrophil storage pool (NSP); cells from this compartment can enter the vascular space, where about half circulate freely and the other half marginate along the endothelial surface of small veins. Marginated cells can be mobilized with exercise or administration of β-adrenergic agonists and cause transient neutrophilia. Bacterial and viral infections shift circulating cells into the marginating pool, where exposure to chemotactic factors leads to the migration of neutrophils into tissues within 2 to 4

TABLE 19-8
NORMAL LEUKOCYTE COUNTS[a]

AGE	TOTAL LEUKOCYTES		NEUTROPHILS[b]			LYMPHOCYTES			MONO-CYTES		EOSINO-PHILS	
	MEAN	RANGE	MEAN	RANGE	%	MEAN	RANGE	%	MEAN	%	MEAN	%
Birth	—[c]	—	4.0	2.0–6.0	—	4.2	2.0–7.3	—	0.6	—	0.1	—
12 h	—	—	11.0	7.8–14.5	—	4.2	2.0–7.3	—	0.6	—	0.1	—
24 h	—	—	9.0	7.0–12.0	—	4.2	2.0–7.3	—	0.6	—	0.1	—
1–4 wk	—	—	3.6	1.8–5.4	—	5.6	2.9–9.1	—	0.7	—	0.2	—
6 mo	11.9	6.0–17.5	3.8	1.0–8.5	32	7.3	4.0–13.5	61	0.6	5	0.3	3
1 y	11.4	6.0–17.5	3.5	1.5–8.5	31	7.0	4.0–10.5	61	0.6	5	0.3	3
2 y	10.6	6.0–17.0	3.5	1.5–8.5	33	6.3	3.0–9.5	59	0.5	5	0.3	3
4 y	9.1	5.5–15.5	3.8	1.5–8.5	42	4.5	2.0–8.0	50	0.5	5	0.3	3
6 y	8.5	5.0–14.5	4.3	1.5–8.0	51	3.5	1.5–7.0	42	0.4	5	0.2	3
8 y	8.3	4.5–13.5	4.4	1.5–8.0	53	3.3	1.5–6.8	39	0.4	4	0.2	2
10 y	8.1	4.5–13.5	4.4	1.8–8.0	54	3.1	1.5–6.5	38	0.4	4	0.2	2
16 y	7.8	4.5–13.0	4.4	1.8–8.0	57	2.8	1.2–5.2	35	0.4	5	0.2	3
21 y	7.4	4.5–11.0	4.4	1.8–7.7	59	2.5	1.0–4.8	34	0.3	4	0.2	3

[a] Numbers of leukocytes are in $\times 10^9$/L or thousands per mm³, ranges are estimates of 95% confidence limits, and percentages refer to differential counts.
[b] Neutrophils include band cells at all ages and a small number of metamyelocytes and myelocytes in the first few days of life.
[c] Insufficient data for a reliable estimate.

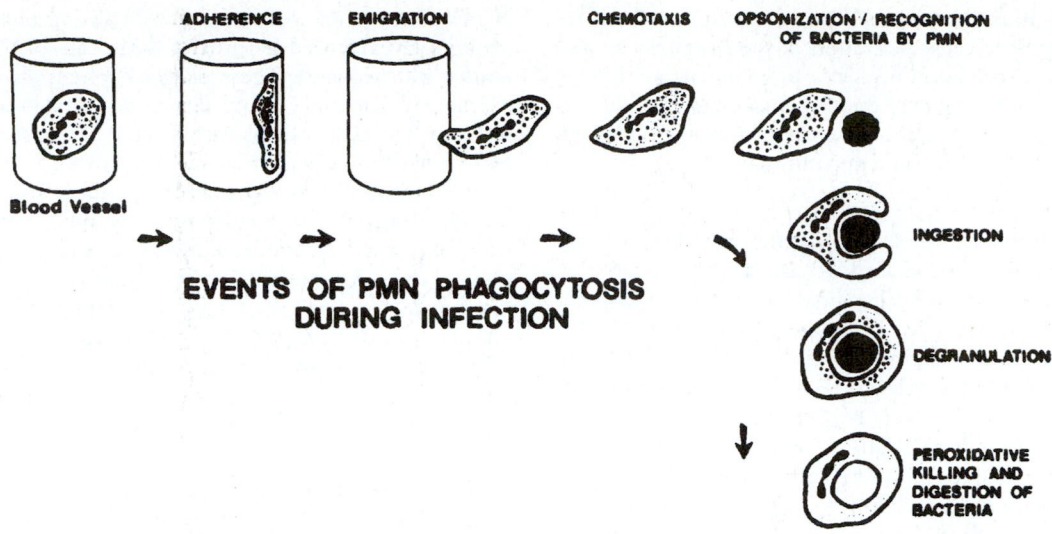

FIGURE 19-8   The events in neutrophil phagocytosis. PMN = polymorphonuclear leukocytes.

hours. Neutrophils normally spend about 12 hours in the circulation before moving either into the tissues or into areas in direct contact with the external environment, including the respiratory and GI epithelia. Neutrophils survive in the tissues for 1 to 4 days.

The size of the NSP in healthy adults is 10 times that of the circulating pool and can augment the supply of circulating neutrophils in response to an infection. The marrow responds to infection with a more rapid division of myeloid precursors. Severe infections cause increased utilization of neutrophils, and neutropenia may ensue before a compensatory increase in myeloid production can occur. Corticosteroids, endotoxin, and G-CSF accelerate the release of neutrophils from the marrow, leading to neutrophilia.

Maturation from the monoblast to mature monocyte occurs over about 6 days. Newly formed mature monocytes may remain in the bone marrow for up to 1 day, and no bone marrow reserve for this cell line exists. Monocytes circulate in the peripheral blood with a half-life of approximately 3 days. A subpopulation of monocytes migrates to different tissues after leaving the bone marrow to become distinct tissue macrophages including Kupffer cells, microglia, and alveolar macrophages. Dendritic cells are recently characterized immune cells that are derived either from a myeloid lineage or from lymphoid precursors and account for <1% of circulating mononuclear cells. These dendritic cells enter tissue and capture foreign antigens and then migrate to central lymphoid areas, where the primary immune response to antigen is initiated.

NEUTROPHIL MORPHOLOGY

The most striking morphologic features of the mature neutrophil are the multilobulated nucleus and the abundance of cytoplasmic granules in the cytoplasm. Neutrophil granules are of two types: azurophilic or primary granules and specific or secondary granules. Azurophilic granules arise during the promyelocyte stage of maturation and function as specialized lysosomes containing proteins with digestive, microbicidal, and cytotoxic properties, which include acid hydrolases, serine proteases (cathepsin G), myeloperoxidase, and acid mucopolysaccharides. Defensins, arginine- and cysteine-rich antimicrobial cationic peptides, are also constituents of the azurophilic granules and represent 5 to 7% of the cellular protein in human neutrophils. Specific granules arise during the myelocyte stage of neutrophil maturation and subsequently increase in number. These granules contain lysozyme, lactoferrin, vitamin B_{12}

transport protein, CD18/CD11c, collagenase, and receptors for laminin. In the mature neutrophil, specific granules outnumber azurophilic granules by a ratio of 2:1.

The neutrophil cytoplasm is surrounded by a cell membrane that can form pseudopods that enable cell movement and phagocytosis in response to chemical signals from the environment. Changes in cell shape are mediated by a cytoskeleton of microtubules, and pseudopod formation is facilitated by microfilaments.

NEUTROPHIL FUNCTION

Neutrophils are the circulating cells primarily responsible for eradicating pyogenic bacteria and fungi from extravascular sites in the host. The events of phagocytosis can be considered in sequential steps (Fig. 19-8).

ADHERENCE   Within minutes of tissue damage or pathogenic invasion, neutrophils marginate and then adhere to the endothelial surface of the vessel. The adherence of neutrophils is a complex phenomenon that is at least partly dependent on integrins and selectins. Adhesion molecules, particularly LFA-1, participate in the mobilization of leukocytes to infected or inflamed tissues. Neutrophils then pass through blood vessel walls by projecting pseudopods between the vascular endothelial cells and streaming out into the intracellular space of the connective tissue in a process known as diapedesis.

CHEMOTAXIS   The directed attraction of cells toward certain substances and sites of infection is termed chemotaxis and occurs within a few hours after an inflammatory stimulus. Chemotactic factors include components of complement activation, bacterial peptides, or products of macrophages or neutrophils at the site of invasion. A group of partially related compounds known as chemokines have recently been characterized as chemotactic agents.

OPSONIZATION   Opsonins are humoral factors that coat foreign antigens and allow phagocytes to selectively recognize foreign antigens. Phagocytic cells have cell surface receptors for the Fc portion of the immunoglobulin G molecule as well as the complement component C3b, both well-described opsonins. Antibodies that enhance phagocytosis are primarily immunoglobulin G, containing both the Fab and Fc portions of the molecule. The Fab portion adheres specifically to the bacteria, while the Fc portion adheres to receptors on phagocytic cells. Activation of the complement system, resulting in the formation of C3b, can be initiated either by the bacteria themselves via the alternate complement pathway or by the interaction of specific antibody with microbial antigen and activation of the classical complement pathway.

PHAGOCYTOSIS (INGESTION) Once an opsonized microbe and neutrophil establish contact, the sequential interaction between opsonins and membrane receptors leads to activation of neutrophil contractile microfilaments, resulting in the flow of pseudopods completely around the microbe. The opposed membranes of the pseudopods fuse and then invaginate, enclosing the pathogen in an internalized vacuole called a phagosome. Ingestion of the foreign particle is an active process that requires ATP, glycolysis, glycogenolysis, and oxidative phosphorylation. After the phagosome is formed, degranulation begins, and cytoplasmic azurophilic and specific granules fuse with the phagosome. The granules then rupture and discharge into the phagosome.

BACTERIAL KILLING Bacterial killing occurs within minutes after phagocytosis. Killing is initiated by two interrelated processes, degranulation with the release of granule contents into the phagosome and the respiratory burst. The respiratory burst consists of a series of reactions, all of which depend on the activity of respiratory burst oxidase, a complex system that catalyzes the one-electron reduction of oxygen to O_2^- at the expense of reduced NADPH. The respiratory burst is accompanied by a severalfold increase in oxygen consumption and a 10-fold increase in glucose utilization by activation of the hexose monophosphate (HMP) shunt. The respiratory burst results in the production of and release of large quantities of superoxide (O_2^-) and hydrogen peroxide (H_2O_2) by the phagocytes. Most of the O_2^- is rapidly converted to H_2O_2 by dismutation, either spontaneously or enzymatically by superoxide dismutase (SOD):

$$2O_2^- + 2H^+ \xrightarrow{\text{SOD}} H_2O_2 + O_2$$

NADPH consumption rises because of the O_2^--forming reaction as well as the detoxification of some of the H_2O_2 by NADPH in a glutathione-dependent process. The oxidation of glucose via the HMP shunt (see Fig. 19-7) is stimulated by the NADPH consumption and leads to the replenishment of NADPH.

The respiratory burst produces microbicidal compounds, the most potent of which are derived from O_2^- and H_2O_2, reacting in the presence of iron to form hydroxyl radical and possibly singlet oxygen. In the best-defined microbicidal system, *myeloperoxidase* derived from the azurophilic granules catalyzes H_2O_2 in combination with chloride or bromide (or other halide) to form HOCl or HOBr. These reactive species halogenate bacterial cell walls, resulting in cell death. Oxidizing radicals such as O_2^- also contribute significantly to bacterial killing. Microorganisms vary relatively little in their susceptibility to these oxygen-dependent antimicrobial systems.

Much more variability occurs in the susceptibility of microorganisms to the oxygen-independent antimicrobial systems of the neutrophil, such as those involving lysozyme, lactoferrin, defensins, and acid hydrolase.

DEVELOPMENTAL CHANGES IN NEUTROPHIL KINETICS AND FUNCTION

The production of neutrophils under homeostatic and stress situations changes with development. Mature neutrophils can be found

in the bones of 11-week fetuses. Circulating hematopoietic progenitors, as evidenced by either $CD34^+$ cells or CFU, are high in fetuses and neonates. These progenitor cells also have increased regenerative capacity compared to those found in adults, and cord/placental blood stem cells can be used as alternative sources for bone marrow transplantation (see Sec. 20.4).

In newborns, and especially premature newborns, decreased functional capacity of circulating neutrophils may predispose the neonate to bacterial infection. Neonatal neutrophil deficiencies include decreased movement, deformability, and chemotaxis, abnormal adherence and expression of receptors including CD18/CD11c, reduced phagocytosis and bacterial killing, and altered oxidative metabolism. These abnormalities in effector neutrophil function are further exacerbated during times of stress, especially during overwhelming bacterial infection.

19.6.1 Neutrophils

NEUTROPENIA

Absolute neutrophil counts between 1.0 and 1.5×10^9/L are classified as mild neutropenia, between 0.5 and 1.0×10^9/L moderate neutropenia, and below 0.5×10^9/L severe neutropenia. Patients with severe neutropenia are at risk for serious bacterial infections, and those with less severe neutropenia often develop skin infections, otitis media, adenitis, and stomatitis. Neutropenia can be a result of abnormalities of bone marrow stem-cell maturation, acquired or secondary suppression of neutrophil production, or increased destruction in the peripheral blood. Neutropenia in the newborn is often associated with overwhelming bacterial sepsis and a high mortality. Decreased CFU-GM and NSP pools, a near-maximal proliferative capacity of myeloid progenitors, and accelerated neutrophil utilization during infection all predispose the neonate to significant neutropenia, especially during bacterial sepsis.

Granulocyte transfusions have appeared to benefit some neonates with neutropenia and overwhelming bacterial sepsis (see Sec. 19.11). G-CSF therapy may prevent and improve neonatal neutropenia; however, it does not improve survival or reduce the risk of nosocomial infections in high-risk neonates.

NEUTROPENIA ASSOCIATED WITH ABNORMALITIES OF STEM-CELL DEVELOPMENT *Reticular dysgenesis* is a severe intrinsic defect of the uncommitted stem cell, leading to absent production of all the myeloid cells, but RBC and platelet production are normal. Associated abnormalities include hypogammaglobulinemia, thymic aplasia, and lymphopenia. Death usually occurs in early infancy from overwhelming bacterial or viral infection. G-CSF or GM-CSF therapy is ineffective. Stem-cell transplantation may be curative. Disorders associated with abnormal T- and B-lymphocyte function may also be related to intrinsic uncommitted stem-cell failure. Some patients with hypogammaglobulinemia have neutropenia.

Cyclic neutropenia is characterized by defective maturation of uncommitted stem cells. Patients present with episodes of fever, aphthous stomatitis, cervical lymphadenitis, and gastroenteritis occurring regularly every 21 ± 3 days, corresponding with a low ANC. At the nadir of the neutrophil count an absolute monocytosis occurs. Infections can be severe, and deaths from sepsis during the neutropenic phase have been reported. In about one-third of cases, cyclic neutropenia is inherited as autosomal dominant, although the underlying genetic defect is not known. Cyclic neutropenia may also be acquired in patients with immunologic or oncologic diseases. Diagnosis requires serial blood counts two to three times a week that demonstrate the cyclic pattern. G-CSF treatment prevents the episodic neutropenia and reduces infectious complications. Rigorous oral hygiene and judicious use of antibiotics at the nadir of the ANC are indicated. No predisposition to hematologic malignancies has been reported.

Chronic benign neutropenia is probably several disorders that are characterized by a persistently low ANC (0.2 to 1.5×10^9/L) without serious infection that may be sporadic or an autosomal-dominant trait. The exact pathogenesis is poorly understood. Clinical manifestations include mild infections of the skin and mucous membranes. Management includes careful hygiene of the skin and mouth and antibiotics for infections.

Familial severe neutropenia (Kostmann syndrome) is an autosomal-recessive condition in which the ANC is consistently below 0.2×10^9/L, with an associated monocytosis and eosinophilia. These patients are predisposed to life-threatening bacterial infection and early death. Impaired neutrophil maturation is seen in the bone marrow, where only early myeloid elements, promyelocytes, and myelocytes are present. G-CSF administration has dramatically improved the outcome of patients with Kostmann syndrome by increasing the ANC and reducing lethal infections. Some patients may acquire a mutation in the G-CSF receptor followed by transformation to malignancy, but G-CSF therapy does not appear to play a significant role in the pathogenesis of leukemia. Rare patients who do not respond to G-CSF (5 to 100 μg/kg/d) therapy may be successfully treated by allogeneic stem-cell transplant.

Shwachman-Diamond syndrome is an autosomal-recessive syndrome of neutropenia, recurrent infections, failure of exocrine pancreatic function, short stature, and metaphyseal dysostoses. These patients have failure to thrive as a result of chronic malabsorption in addition to recurrent infections. Defects of neutrophil function may also be present in some patients. A propensity for monosomy 7–related hematologic disorders including myelodysplastic syndrome and acute myelogenous leukemia (AML) occurs. Correction of nutritional deficiencies with pancreatic enzyme replacement is essential. G-CSF can be used in patients who have serious infections, and bone marrow transplantation can be curative.

Cartilage-hair hypoplasia (see Chapter 10) is an autosomal-recessive form of short-limb dysostosis characterized by fine and sparse hair found mainly in the Amish population. Moderate neutropenia and/or lymphopenia occur in about one-fourth of cases. Life-threatening infections have been noted, particularly in association with varicella zoster (VZV). Stem-cell transplantation is the treatment of choice for patients with severe recurrent infections.

Myelokathexis (Greek for "marrow retention") is a rare condition in which impaired release of mature neutrophils from the bone marrow results in neutrophil degeneration in the marrow and release of low numbers of abnormal-appearing neutrophils into the circulation. Patients have hypercellular marrows and a lifelong history of recurrent bronchopulmonary infections. Transient elevation of neutrophil counts has been reported in association with infections and therapy with G-CSF or GM-CSF.

Dyskeratosis congenita is an X-linked recessive disorder characterized by nail dystrophy, leukoplakia, and reticulated hyperpigmentation of the skin. Approximately one-third of patients have neutropenia associated with marrow hypoplasia.

ACQUIRED NEUTROPENIAS

Bone marrow failure resulting in neutropenia associated with anemia and thrombocytopenia may occur with marrow replacement or in marrow failure syndromes including aplastic anemia (see Sec. 19.9). Nutritional neutropenia may occur during starvation and with deficiencies of vitamin B_{12}, folate, and copper. Drugs may produce neutropenia either by depression of bone marrow synthesis or by evoking production of antineutrophil antibodies. Marrow production of neutrophils usually resumes within a few weeks after the offending drug is discontinued. Cytotoxic chemotherapeutic agents cause severe neutropenia. The severity of infection during these drug-related episodes is more frequent than with chronic neutropenia, and G-CSF therapy is being increasingly used to reduce the degree and duration of postchemotherapeutic neutropenia (see Sec. 19.11).

Infection, both bacterial and viral, may result in transient neutropenia by decreasing marrow production, depleting marrow reserves, or increasing neutrophil margination. Neutropenias associated with overwhelming bacterial infections have been treated with granulocyte transfusions, G-CSF, and intravenous γ-globulin (IVIG) with variable success.

Neonatal isoimmune neutropenia (NIN) is a self-limited condition, often discovered coincidentally when a CBC is performed in the newborn period, and occurs in an estimated 1/1000 live births. NIN is similar to Rh disease in that maternal antibodies result from maternal sensitization to neutrophil antigens shared by the fetus and the father but absent on the mother's neutrophils. These maternal IgG antineutrophil antibodies cross the placenta, resulting in rapid destruction of fetal neutrophils, and a neutropenia that is usually self-limited ensues. The infant should be closely monitored and infections aggressively treated with appropriate antibiotics. The infant's ANC recovers after 6 to 12 weeks, depending on the maternal antibody load. Subsequent infants are at risk for the same condition.

Autoimmune neutropenia of infancy (ANI) occurs in the first 1 to 2 years of life and is characterized by moderate to severe neutropenia but only mild infections, usually of the skin. ANI is often discovered incidentally by a routine blood count. Median age at diagnosis is 8 months with a range from 2 months to 3 years. Antibodies against neutrophil antigen 1 (NA1) or antigen 2 (NA2) can be detected in approximately one-third of patients. The disease is mild and self-limited, with 95% of children having a normal neutrophil count in 6 to 24 months. Corticosteroids have an inconsistent effect, but IVIG can rapidly, albeit transiently, increase the neutrophil count. G-CSF therapy has had the most consistent response.

Autoimmune neutropenia can also arise as a consequence of more extensive autoimmune disease such as systemic lupus erythematosus (SLE). Successful treatment of SLE may result in disappearance of the antibodies and resolution of the neutropenia.

Viral- or drug-related immune neutropenia may be acquired at any age. During viral illnesses, an antiviral antibody that crossreacts with the neutrophil may be produced, whereas in the case of a drug, the drug attaches to the neutrophil and acts as a hapten to stimulate antibody production. Drugs that have been implicated in immune neutropenias include anticonvulsants, antithyroid medications, phenothiazines, NSAIDs, cardiovascular drugs, antihistamines, sulfonamides, and synthetic penicillins. The ANC is not usually low enough to predispose to serious infection, and spontaneous recovery usually occurs when the drug is discontinued.

Mild to moderate neutropenia in addition to anemia and/or thrombocytopenia may result from trapping of the neutrophils in the expanded blood pool of an enlarged spleen. Activation of the complement pathway by infection, inflammation, or hemodialysis can cause neutropenia by increasing marginated neutrophils along endothelial surfaces or through formation of leukoemboli, especially in the lungs.

DIAGNOSTIC APPROACH

The diagnostic approach to neutropenia is influenced by whether the child is clinically ill. If neutropenia is discovered incidentally on a routine CBC, in an otherwise healthy child who has no history of recurrent infections, the most likely diagnoses are chronic benign neutropenia of infancy or cyclic neutropenia. A careful history should include current health, ill contacts, recent infections and medications, and family history of ill children or early death. Physical exam should note growth and development, hepatosplenomegaly, and lymphadenopathy.

The morphologic characteristics of the neutrophils may be diagnostic. Hypersegmented neutrophils (five or six lobes) may suggest megaloblastic anemia (see Fig. 19-5D). Giant granules are present in Chédiak-Higashi syndrome, and myelokathexis is characterized by nuclear lobulation and cytoplasmic vacuolization. Complete blood counts twice a week for 6 weeks will determine whether the neutropenia is transient, cyclic, or chronic, and whether other cell lines are involved. If the neutropenia is cyclic or chronic, blood counts on family members may suggest a familial disorder. Isolated neutropenia is an unusual presentation of malignancy, and a bone marrow aspirate is not necessary if the child is otherwise well. ANA, quantitative immunoglobulins, and an assessment of T- and B-cell function should be performed to define a possible immunologic deficiency. Specific tests of neutrophil kinetics include (1) the epinephrine stimulation test to determine excessive neutrophil margination, (2) the corticosteroid or endotoxin test to assess the marrow NSP, and (3) the Rebuck window test to determine whether there is abnormal neutrophil migration in response to injury or inflammation (see Table 19-9).

TREATMENT

Children with an ANC between 1.0 and 1.5×10^9/L usually require no specific treatment, and their risk of serious infection is small. Children with an ANC $<0.5 \times 10^9$/L are at an increased risk of developing moderate to severe bacterial and/or fungal infections and should be treated based on the clinical status and evidence of infection and not on the ANC alone. Children with $<0.5 \times 10^9$/L have a propensity for infection and should be isolated from individuals with obvious infection, maintain good personal hygiene, and be closely observed for development of infection. Children with severe neutropenia suspected of having infection should have appropriate bacterial and fungal cultures, and broad-spectrum antibiotics should be administered. Temperatures and medications per rectum should be avoided. A febrile, neutropenic patient should be hospitalized and placed on parenteral broad-spectrum antibiotics until fever subsides. Patients with chronic neutropenia often require prolonged antibiotic administration.

Granulocyte transfusions may be beneficial in neutropenic patients with severe infections that do not respond to antibiotics (see Sec. 19.11). Disorders, such as Kostmann syndrome or cyclic neutropenia, should be treated initially with G-CSF. HLA-matched allogeneic stem cell marrow transplantation may be curative in some of the severe, chronic disorders.

DEFECTS OF NEUTROPHIL FUNCTION

Children with primary defects of neutrophil function usually have recurrent infections such as aphthous ulcers or stomatitis, otitis media, cutaneous abscesses, and regional lymphadenopathy during the early months of life. The disorders of phagocyte function can be grouped into abnormalities of adherence, chemotaxis, phagocyto-

TABLE 19-9
EVALUATION OF NEUTROPHIL FUNCTION

FUNCTION	TEST	COMMENT
Chemotaxis	*Rebuck window:* Migration of cells into dermal abrasion[a]	Provides qualitative evaluation of inflammatory response in vivo
	Boyden chamber: Migration of cells through filter in response to chemotactic stimuli	May evaluate abnormal cell movement and deficient chemotactic serum factors, difficult to standardize
Opsonization	Quantitate serum opsonins: *Quantitative immunoglobulins, hemolytic complement*[a]	Establishes diagnosis of immunoglobulin or complement deficiencies
Phagocytosis and degranulation	Phagocytosis may be assessed by opsonization of particle and observing phagocytosis by vital staining PMNs; phagocytosis is quantitated by radiolabeling or using stained particles before ingestion	Quantitative methods are most sensitive measures of ingestion; slide tests fail to differentiate definitely particle adherence to PMNs from internalization
	Morphologic evaluation of degranulation[a]	Identifies large granules (Chédiak-Higashi syndrome), deficiency of granule enzymes (MPO deficiency), or bilobed neutrophil nuclei and absence of granules (specific-granule deficiency)
Bacterial metabolic burst	*Nitroblue tetrazolium dye test* (NBT): Quantitates reduction of NBT (clear) to NBTH (blue) dye[a]	Depends on generation of O_2; excellent screening for CGD
	O_2 consumption: Quantitates release of univalent reduced oxygen from PMNs	Diagnoses CGD
	H_2O_2 generation: Quantitates release of peroxide from PMNs	Diagnoses CGD and severe leukocyte G6PD deficiency
Microbicidal function	Quantitates bactericidal, fungicidal capacity of cells	Identifies microbicidal, fungicidal disorders of phagocytes (CGD): can be performed with organisms isolated from patients

[a] Studies that may be performed by most clinical laboratories.
PMNs, polymorphonuclear leukocytes; CGD, chronic granulomatous disease; MPO, myeloperoxidase.

sis, degranulation, or bacterial killing. The laboratory evaluation for these disorders is based on specific tests of neutrophil function (Table 19-9). Workup should include neutrophil count and morphology, followed by a test for the respiratory burst, such as the nitroblue tetrazolium (NBT) dye test. Clinical disorders of neutrophil function are summarized in Table 19-10.

Treatment of children with functional neutrophil abnormalities is largely supportive, but the recent use of γ-interferon has resulted in a significant improvement in both morbidity and mortality. Early diagnosis coupled with the prompt treatment of bacterial pathogens has prolonged life. Bone marrow transplantation (BMT) has resulted in partial reconstitution of normal neutrophil function. Understanding of the molecular basis for neutrophil functional abnormalities is rapidly increasing and has provided insights into the mechanisms that mediate normal function and provide protection from invasive infection.

Congenital leukocyte adherence deficiency 1 (LAD1) is a rare autosomal recessive disorder affecting adherence-related functions of neutrophils, monocytes, and lymphocytes. Children with this disorder have an increased neutrophil count in the peripheral blood because of a lack of margination but depressed inflammatory responses and failure to accumulate neutrophils at sites of infection. Delayed separation of the umbilical cord is frequently reported as well as frequent skin infections, severe periodontitis and gingivitis resulting in the loss of teeth, and intermittent life-threatening pneumonia from severe bacterial or fungal infections. Many children die during infancy from overwhelming bacterial infection. The defect in these patients results from mutations in the gene encoding CD18 located on chromosome 21 that result in a lack of adhesion molecules LFA-1, Mac-1, and CD18/CD11c. The ability of the phagocytic cells to kill intracellular microorganisms is normal, but because the cells cannot be mobilized to the sites of infection, there is a lack

of phagocytic function. Patients with <0.5% of normal CD11/18 usually die of overwhelming microbial infections within the first few years of life, whereas those with 3 to 10% have a better prognosis.

Diagnosis can be made by fluorescent cytometry of activated neutrophils and by decreased accumulation of tissue neutrophils documented by the Rebuck skin window technique. BMT is the preferred treatment because the disorder often is fatal by age 2 years, but supportive care and the use of prophylactic trimethoprim-sulfamethoxazole is indicated when BMT is not possible.

Hyperimmunoglobulin E syndrome (HIE, Job syndrome) is characterized by an at least 10-fold increase in serum IgE level, defective chemotaxis, dermatitis, and recurrent infections. Abscesses lack redness, heat, and pain and are called "cold abscesses." The principal organism responsible for infections is *Staphylococcus aureus,* although other polysaccharide-encapsulated organisms are also seen. The cellular and molecular bases for HIE are not known. Phagocytosis and bacterial killing are normal. The elevated serum IgE levels and chronic dermatitis may reflect a T-cell immunoregulatory abnormality. Antibiotic therapy is indicated for specific bacterial infections. Trimethoprim-sulfamethoxazole prophylaxis, cyclosporine A, and IVIG have been reported to be of benefit in a few cases. The prognosis is uncertain, but many patients survive into adulthood.

Impaired opsonization of microorganisms is observed in patients with deficiencies of complement components or antibodies and also in newborns.

Defective degranulation disorders have abnormal killing of anaerobic bacteria, a function dependent on the contents of both azurophilic and specific granules. Specific granule membranes contain CD18/CD11c as well as components of phagocyte oxidase system. Therefore, abnormal specific granule content, mobilization, or fusion with phagosomes also results in an abnormal respi-

TABLE 19-10
CLINICAL DISORDERS OF NEUTROPHIL FUNCTION

DISORDER	FUNCTIONAL DEFECT	INHERITANCE	GENETIC DEFECT	DIAGNOSTIC FINDINGS AND TESTS	CLINICAL
LAD1	Adherence	AR	CD18	Absent CD18 on activated neutrophils	Increased WBC, abscesses
LAD2	Adherence	AR	?Fucose	Rebuck skin window, Bombay blood type	Increased WBC, abscesses
HIE	Chemotaxis	AD	Unknown	↑ IgE, Boyden chemotaxis, dermatitis	Dermatitis, *Staph.* infections, pneumonia
SGD	Degranulation	AR	Unknown	Neutrophil morphology	Infections
CHS	Degranulation	AR	CHS gene	Albinism and neutrophil morphology	Albinism, neuropathy, infection, accelerated phase
Griscelli syndrome	Degranulation	AR	Unknown	Albinism, abnormal melanocytes	Albinism, neuropathy, infection, accelerated phase
MPO deficiency	Bacterial killing	Multiple	MPO def	Histochemistry for MPO	Mild candidal infections
G6PD deficiency	Respiratory burst	X-linked	G6PD def	Enzyme levels	Infection with catalase-negative organisms
CGD	Respiratory burst	X-linked, AR	Phox def: Gp91 kDa, p47 kDa, p22 kDa, p67 kDa	NBT, oxygen consumption, genotyping	Infection with catalase-negative organisms

LAD1, -2, leukocyte adherence deficiency 1, 2; HIE, hyperimmunoglobulin E syndrome; SGD, specific granule deficiency; CHS, Chédiak-Higashi syndrome; MPO, myeloperoxidase; G6PD, glucose-6-phosphate dehydrogenase; CGD, chronic granulomatous disease; AR, autosomal recessive; AD, autosomal dominant; NBT, nitroblue tetrazolium dye test.

ratory burst and bacterial killing. Children with these disorders have the early onset of recurrent, severe bacterial and fungal infections of the skin and deep tissues.

Specific granule deficiency (SGD) is a rare, probably autosomal recessive disorder. Patients have depressed inflammatory responses and recurrent bacterial and fungal infections of the skin and deep tissues. No specific granules are present on stained smears of the blood. Nuclear abnormalities are seen, and azurophilic granules are also decreased. Abnormalities of neutrophil function include defective chemotaxis and bacterial killing in vitro. Intravenous antibiotic therapy is indicated for bacterial infections, and prompt surgical drainage of abscesses is essential. Most patients survive into adult life.

Chédiak-Higashi syndrome (CHS) is an autosomal recessive disorder characterized by partial oculocutaneous albinism characterized by "silvery" hair, the presence of giant granules in all granule-containing cells, neutropenia, prolonged bleeding time, natural killer cell dysfunction, and frequent bacterial infections. Most patients eventually develop an "accelerated phase" of lymphohistiocytic infiltration characterized by hepatosplenomegaly, lymphadenopathy, and pancytopenia culminating in death. The onset of the accelerated phase often coincides with infection by Epstein-Barr virus. Accelerated phases can occur in young infants and may be the presenting finding of CHS. The diagnosis of CHS is confirmed by the presence of giant granules in neutrophils and eosinophils.

The CHS gene is a large gene the function of which is unknown but may involve an inability to properly sort and compartmentalize proteins into lysosomes and other organelles or promote granule and phagosome fusion.

Infections during the stable phase are treated with antibiotics. Treatment of the "accelerated phase" includes corticosteroids and VP16 or vincristine, which may induce a temporary remission. Before the onset of the accelerated phase, bone marrow transplantation has resulted in successful reconstitution of the hematopoietic and immune systems.

Griscelli syndrome is an autosomal recessive disorder with similar clinical presentation of CHS and a lethal accelerated phase but without the characteristic morphologic neutrophil granule abnormalities.

CHRONIC GRANULOMATOUS DISEASE

Chronic granulomatous disease (CGD) is usually a severe form of neutrophil dysfunction related to a defect in the respiratory burst. CGD is inherited primarily as an X-linked trait but may also be inherited in an autosomal recessive manner. Clinical features are usually noted during infancy, but occasional patients remain well until adolescence. Different subgroups are associated with abnormalities of various components of the phagocyte oxidase system, each of which results in a complete absence of the respiratory burst of the phagocytic cell.

The neutrophils of patients with CGD can ingest bacteria normally, but the oxidative processes that lead to superoxide anion formation, hydrogen peroxide production, and bacterial killing are impaired. Failure of stimulated phagocytic cells to generate superoxide anion radicals results in the loss of components of the neutrophil oxidase system and leads to absent respiratory burst activity and markedly deficient killing. Bacteria that do not produce catalase, such as *Streptococcus pneumoniae*, generate enough H_2O_2 to sustain halogenation within the phagocytic vacuoles and do not cause infections. Serious infections result from microorganisms that

produce catalase, such as staphylococci, *E. coli*, *Serratia marcescens*, *Salmonella*, and *Candida*.

CLINICAL MANIFESTATIONS   CGD is characterized by repeated infections. Cervical and inguinal adenopathy is often associated with granulation tissue containing increased pigmented histiocytes. Pulmonary disease may be fatal unless appropriate therapy is instituted. Cutaneous and perirectal infections, liver abscesses, and osteomyelitis are common. Patients with CGD often have infections caused by unusual bacteria. The isolation of *S. epidermidis*, *Serratia marcescens*, *Candida*, or *Aspergillus* from an osteomyelitic or pulmonary infection should suggest the possibility of CGD.

DIAGNOSIS   A useful screening assay is the quantitative NBT dye reaction (see Table 19-9). The diagnosis is confirmed by failure to induce an oxidative metabolic burst during phagocytosis and by the demonstration of a defect in leukocyte microbicidal activity against catalase-producing organisms. The female carrier in sex-linked CGD can be diagnosed by quantifying the number of NBT-positive leukocytes after stimulation with endotoxin. Over 90% of neutrophils are NBT-positive in normal individuals; no NBT-positive neutrophils are seen in CGD patients; and an intermediate number of NBT-positive cells are present in hemizygous female carriers.

Documentation of the molecular basis for the abnormal respiratory burst is important. Patients with absent p22-phox, p47-phox, or p67-phox have autosomal recessive inheritance, whereas those with absent gp91-phox have the X-linked form of the disease. Prenatal diagnosis is possible using fetal blood sampling.

TREATMENT   Early diagnosis and aggressive antibiotic therapy have resulted in considerable improvement in prognosis. The prophylactic use of both trimethoprim-sulfamethoxazole and interferon-γ reduces the incidence of serious infections and improves survival. In patients with infections, intravenous antibiotic therapy directed at the most likely infectious organisms should be instituted until results of cultures are available. Prolonged parenteral antibiotic therapy is needed for most deep-seated infections. Infections may be associated with severe anemia, and blood transfusions may be necessary. Genetic linkage between gp91-phox and the very rare Kell null blood phenotypes poses a potential transfusion hazard. The Kell phenotype should be determined to avoid the risk of sensitization.

About 50% of CGD patients survive to 10 years of age or longer. BMT has successfully reconstituted phagocytic function in some patients. However, because many CGD patients have indolent bacterial infections that would be exacerbated by preparation for BMT, this procedure should probably be reserved for children who fail to respond to interferon-γ therapy.

Patients with *neutrophil glucose-6-phosphate dehydrogenase (G6PD) deficiency* in whom the activity of the enzyme in leukocytes is severely reduced (<5% of normal) may have recurrent infections with catalase-positive organisms. Individuals with the very common types of G6PD deficiency that occur in those of Mediterranean and African descent (see Sec. 19.5.2) have neutrophil G6PD activity >20% of normal values, normal neutrophil function, and no increased risk of infection. However, a few patients with chronic nonspherocytic hemolytic anemia associated with mutations of the gene encoding for G6PD have profound reduction in this enzyme in their neutrophils (see Sec. 19.5.2). Because the HMP shunt is the major source of reduced NADPH required for activity of phagocyte oxidase, failure to maintain pyridine nucleotide substrate results in absence of the respiratory burst and impaired killing. The diagnosis may be established by quantifying the G6PD activity in leukocytes.

MYELOPEROXIDASE DEFICIENCY

Complete absence of the enzyme myeloperoxidase (MPO) from azurophilic granules in neutrophils is the most common neutrophil disorder, occurring in approximately 1 in 2000 individuals, and is inherited as an autosomal recessive trait. Most patients are asymptomatic or experience only mild infections. The diagnosis is established by the histochemical demonstration of an absence of neutrophil MPO. The neutrophils can be distinguished from those of patients with CGD because of normal or elevated values for oxygen consumption. Microbicidal activity is only modestly depressed.

19.6.2.   Eosinophils

Eosinophils resemble neutrophils but are bilobed and contain distinctive red staining granules. Eosinophils develop and mature in the bone marrow, have a relatively brief transit time in the blood, and ultimately migrate to and function in tissue sites. The normal absolute eosinophil count is 0.2×10^9/L, corresponding to 2 to 3% of the WBC (see Table 19-8). The ratio of blood to tissue eosinophils is normally about 1:100, with the epithelium of the intestine, especially the colon, being the most densely populated site. The most common cause of eosinophilia in developed countries is allergy. In developing countries, parasitic infections are more common. Helminthic infestations induce greater degrees of eosinophilia than do protozoan infestations. Eosinophilia may also be seen in Hodgkin disease and in the very rare eosinophilic leukemia.

In response to allergens or multicellular tissue parasites, eosinophils become stimulated in part by way of surface receptors for IgG and IgE and CD18/CD11b/c. The stimulated eosinophils then migrate to tissues, such as the respiratory epithelium or the intestinal wall, where they degranulate, releasing potent mediators including eosinophil major basic protein (MBP), believed to be a major cause of tissue damage. In parasitic infestation, the mediators released by eosinophils may kill the parasite.

Hypereosinophilic syndrome (HES) is an acquired syndrome characterized by chronic eosinophilia without a definable cause and tissue infiltration by eosinophils. Löffler syndrome is characterized by endocardial fibrosis and mural thrombi associated with HES. Treatments with corticosteroids, hydroxyurea, or hematopoietic stem-cell transplantation have been effective.

19.6.3   Monocytes/Macrophages

Macrophages are important in cellular immunity and the processing of specific antigens to lymphocytes. Similar to neutrophils, macrophages ingest and kill invading organisms. The normal absolute monocyte count in the blood is 0.4 to 0.6×10^9/L. Monocytosis is commonly seen in acute and chronic infection, particularly with intracellular organisms. Monocytosis also occurs in chronic neutropenic disorders including cyclic neutropenia.

19.6.4   Basophils and Mast Cells

Basophils account for fewer than 1% of circulating leukocytes and nucleated cells of the bone marrow. Basophil granules are rich in histamine and heparin. Mast cells, which differentiate independently from basophils, are tissue effector cells involved in hypersensitivity reactions. Basophilia occurs in chronic myelogenous leukemia and may be seen with ulcerative colitis and myxedema. Mastocytosis is a dermatologic disorder characterized by skin infiltration by mast cells. Darier sign, urticaria induced by rubbing, is suggestive, and biopsy is diagnostic. In systemic mastocytosis, mast cells infiltrate liver, bone marrow, spleen, and gut, and the prognosis is poor.

References

Boxer LA, Blackwood RA: Leukocyte disorders: quantitative and qualitative disorders of the neutrophil, parts 1 and 2. Pediatr Rev 17:19–50, 1996

Brown CC, Gallin JI: Chemotactic disorders. Hematol Oncol Clin North Am 2:61–79, 1988

Cairo MS: The use of granulocyte transfusion in neonatal sepsis. Transfus Med Rev 4:14–22, 1990

Coates T, Baehner R: Leukocytosis and leukopenia. In: Hoffman R, Benz E, Shattil S, Furie B, Cohen H, Silberstein L, eds: Hematology: Basic Principles and Practice, 2nd ed. New York, Churchill Livingston, 1995: 769–784

Grimbacher B, Holland SM, Gallin JI, et al: Hyper-IgE syndrome with recurrent infections—an autosomal dominant multisystem disorder. N Engl J Med 340:692–702, 1999

19.7   DISORDERS OF PLATELETS

Melvin H. Freedman

Platelets arise from cytoplasmic fragmentation of bone marrow megakaryocytes. After leaving the marrow, approximately one-third of the platelets are distributed to the spleen, and the other two-thirds circulate for 7 to 10 days. Megakaryocyte production and maturation are regulated by a specific growth factor designated thrombopoietin (TPO), also called the mpl ligand. C-mpl, the cellular receptor for TPO, is present on platelets as well as on the megakaryocyte and precursor cells. The balance between TPO and its receptors maintains a constant number of circulating platelets, and the normal blood platelet count is 150.0 to 400.0×10^9/L with no age-related differences. A reduction in platelets increases the level of circulating TPO, which then can bind to receptors on the megakaryocyte precursor cells, stimulating an increase in number, size, and ploidy. Hypertrophy of the megakaryocyte compartment results in an increase in the release of platelets into the circulation. Interleukin (IL)-3, -6, and -11 also stimulate platelet production, and recombinant forms of interleukin as well as TPO have been synthesized.

Platelet structure includes a bilipid membrane and a number of structural glycoproteins. The cytoplasm has granules, the most important of which are the dense granules, which contain serotonin, ADP, and ATP, and the more numerous α-granules, which contain a mixture of biologically active proteins including coagulation factors. The role of the platelet in hemostasis is discussed in Sec. 19.10.

19.7.1   Thrombocytopenia

There are three general mechanisms for thrombocytopenia: (1) increased destruction, (2) decreased production, and (3) increased pooling in an enlarged spleen. In a specific clinical situation, more than one mechanism may be operative. The etiology of thrombocytopenia can usually be determined by a detailed history and physical examination and a complete blood count including the morphology and size of the platelets on the peripheral blood smear. The mean platelet volume (MPV) is measured by many electronic cell counters; however, this may not be accurate in severe thrombocytopenia. The number of the megakaryocytes in the bone marrow aspirate is often used to differentiate between thrombocytopenias related to production and to destruction. Normal or increased numbers rule out a production problem. It is also important to attempt to determine whether the disorder is acquired or congenital and inherited. An approach to the child with thrombocytopenia is shown in Fig. 19-9.

IDIOPATHIC (IMMUNE) THROMBOCYTOPENIC PURPURA (ITP)

ITP is the most common cause of thrombocytopenia in children and is a result of immunologically mediated increased platelet destruction, which is usually acute and self-limiting but may be a recurrent or chronic disorder. Acute ITP is believed to be a consequence of a disordered immune response during recovery from a viral infection that evokes the formation of antibodies that cause platelet destruction. An alternative hypothesis implicates immune complexes derived from primary or underlying disease processes that nonspecifically adsorb to the surface of platelets, resulting in their opsonization and rapid destruction. The most common platelet antigenic glycoproteins that can evoke antibody formation are designated GPIIb-IIIa, GPI-IX, and GPV. A number of tests for measuring antiplatelet antibodies in ITP have been described, in-

cluding the measurement of the amount of platelet-associated IgG (PAIgG) and direct assay of specific platelet antibodies. However, these tests lack both specificity and sensitivity in acute ITP of childhood.

CLINICAL FEATURES   Acute ITP affects both sexes equally and has a peak incidence between 2 and 5 years of age; chronic ITP is more frequent in adolescents and young adults. ITP is more common in white than black children, perhaps because of the difficulty in recognizing cutaneous petechiae and bruising in dark-skinned children. There is frequently a history of a nonspecific or specific viral illness or of live virus immunization 1 to 6 weeks before the onset of bleeding manifestations. Acute bleeding occurs abruptly in a previously healthy child with no HIV risk factors and a negative family history. Physical findings include cutaneous petechiae and purpuric lesions, which occur spontaneously or after minor trauma. The liver, spleen, and lymph nodes are not enlarged. Severe mucosal bleeding, hematuria, and menorrhagia in girls may occur when platelet counts are $<10 \times 10^9$/L. Intracranial hemorrhage occurs in 0.5 to 1% of children with ITP and is fatal in one-third of cases. The risk appears to be greatest during the initial days of ITP, when the platelet count is very low, but it can occur at any time.

LABORATORY FEATURES   Isolated thrombocytopenia of varying severity is the major hematologic finding. The few circulating platelets may be quite large (megathrombocytes). The number of recently released, young platelets that contain RNA can be determined by flow cytometry. Increased numbers of "reticulated" platelets indicate increased production. White blood cell count and morphology are normal. Hemoglobin values are normal unless there has been prolonged bleeding. Although the necessity of doing

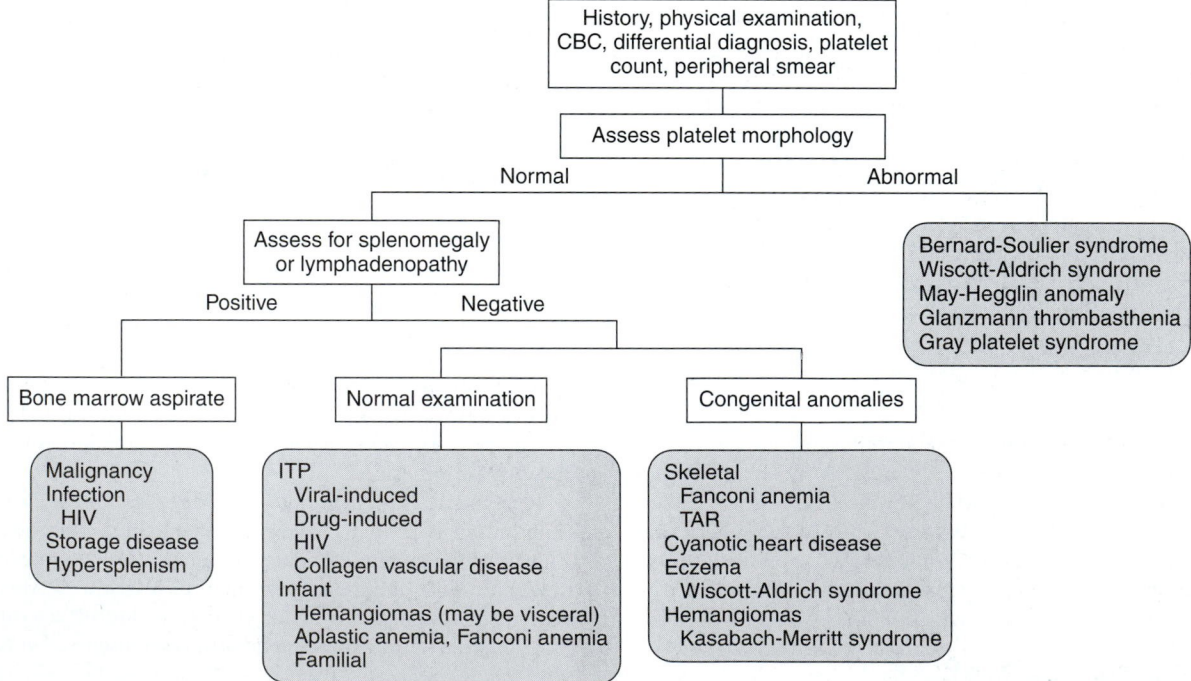

FIGURE 19-9   **Algorithm diagramming the approach to the management of the child with isolated thrombocytopenia. CBC = complete blood count; ITP = idiopathic thrombocytopenic purpura; TAR = thrombocytopenia-absent radius syndrome. SOURCE:** *Modified from Hastings and Lubin, Rudolph's Fundamentals of Pediatrics, Stamford: Appleton and Lange, 2nd Edition p. 480, 1998.*

a bone marrow study has frequently been questioned, bone marrow examination is often done and reveals normal or increased numbers of megakaryocytes, indicating that platelet production is normal and that thrombocytopenia results from increased platelet destruction. Normal marrow morphology excludes amegakaryocytic thrombocytopenias, aplastic anemia, acute leukemia, lymphoma, and replacement by malignant cells.

Giant platelets are suggestive of an inherited platelet disorder. Thrombotic thrombocytopenic purpura, hemolytic-uremic syndrome, and disseminated intravascular coagulation are associated with microangiopathic hemolysis (Figs. 19.5L and 19.9).

CLINICAL COURSE Complete remission of ITP occurs in 80 to 90% of children by 6 to 9 months after onset. The 10 to 20% of children who do not go into spontaneous remission by 9 months are classified as having chronic ITP, and most are more than 7 years of age. Treatment in the initial phase of the disease does not influence the number of chronic cases. Recurrent ITP, defined as multiple episodes of acute thrombocytopenia separated by periods of normal platelet counts, occasionally occurs.

TREATMENT Salicylate-containing medications, antihistamines, and nonsteroidal anti-inflammatory drugs that interfere with platelet function increase the risk of bleeding and should be avoided. Therapy is indicated if there is extensive cutaneous and particularly mucosal bleeding and a platelet count $<20 \times 10^9/L$. No treatment is usually indicated for patients with platelet counts $>50 \times 10^9/L$. Three treatments for acute ITP are available: intravenous immunoglobulins (IVIG), corticosteroids in various doses, and intravenous anti-Rh(D) immunoglobulin for Rh-positive patients. Mechanisms of action of these agents have been identified: (1) IVIG is believed to block the Fc receptors of the RE phagocytes, preventing them from binding and destroying IgG antibody-coated platelets; (2) corticosteroids have a rapid, dose-dependent action that reduces RE destruction of antibody-coated platelets and also more slowly reduces antibody production; (3) anti-Rh immunoglobulin produces a mild hemolytic anemia that saturates the Fc receptors of the phagocytic elements of the RE system, permitting increased survival of antibody-coated platelets. The immediate goal of therapy is to increase the platelet count to a safe level, usually $>20.0 \times 10^9/L$, in the hope of reducing the risk of severe hemorrhage. The reported percentages of ITP patients who achieve this level 72 hours from the start of therapy are: (1) IVIG, 0.8 g/kg, one dose only, or 1.0 g/kg/d for 2 days, 94 to 97%; (2) oral prednisone, 2 to 4 mg/kg/d, 79%; (3) IV anti-Rh(D), 25 μg/kg for 2 days, 82%; and (4) no therapy, 56%. Corticosteroid therapy is usually continued for about 1 month and then tapered and discontinued unless severe thrombocytopenia or spontaneous hemorrhage recurs. About a third of children who initially respond to any of these therapies have recurrent thrombocytopenia, but usually not as severe as initially and not associated with spontaneous bleeding.

Platelet transfusions are ineffective in acute ITP because the exogenous platelets are rapidly destroyed. However, in life-threatening situations, especially intracranial hemorrhage, platelet transfusions or continuous infusions should be given in combination with IVIG or high-dose IV corticosteroids.

Children with chronic ITP who have mild or recurrent bleeding are sometimes treated with intermittent courses of IVIG or high-dose corticosteroids. Other treatments that have been used in adults with chronic ITP include α-interferon, danazol (a synthetic androgen), ascorbic acid, cyclosporine, and a variety of immuno-

suppressive drugs including vinca alkaloids, azathioprine, and cyclophosphamide. No large studies of these agents have been described in children with chronic ITP, and they may have immediate and long-term toxicities.

Splenectomy is often beneficial in children with chronic, symptomatic ITP. Even children who do not have increased bleeding are at risk during surgery or accidents, and most should not participate in contact sports. About 70% of patients with chronic ITP achieve a complete remission following splenectomy, and most of the others show some improvement in platelet counts.

NEONATAL THROMBOCYTOPENIAS
(Table 19-11)

MATERNAL AUTOIMMUNE NEONATAL THROMBOCYTOPENIA Mothers with ITP may deliver a baby with neonatal thrombocytopenia. The risk is greatest if the mother is thrombocytopenic during the last trimester of pregnancy. However, any mother with a history, even a remote history, of ITP can have an affected infant. Thrombocytopenia in the infant results from passive transplacental transfer of maternal IgG antiplatelet antibodies into the fetal circulation, which cause rapid destruction of fetal platelets. The thrombocytopenia lasts up to 1 to 2 months, reflecting the survival of maternal IgG in the infant. Intracranial hemorrhage occurs in about 1 to 2% of severely affected babies, and the risk appears to be greatest in infants whose mothers (1) had a history of a previously affected infant, (2) had perinatal thrombocytopenia, and (3) were splenectomized previously for ITP. IVIG therapy is often recommended in the third trimester for mothers with thrombocytopenia, particularly if associated with active maternal bleeding.

Maternal ITP must be distinguished from a syndrome of gestational or "incidental" thrombocytopenia, which is not immunologic and occurs in as many as 5% of pregnant women at term. In gestational thrombocytopenia, maternal thrombocytopenia is not severe, and infants are not affected.

TABLE 19-11
NEONATAL THROMBOCYTOPENIAS

Maternal factors
  Immune thrombocytopenia
    Neonatal alloimmune thrombocytopenia
    Maternal autoimmune thrombocytopenia
  Intrauterine infections (TORCH syndromes)
    Toxoplasmosis, rubella, cytomegalovirus, herpes simplex, other (including HIV and parvovirus B19)
  Preeclampsia/hypertension
  Maternal drugs
Infant factors
  Disseminated intravascular coagulation, microangiopathic hemolytic anemias; giant hemangioma (Kasabach-Merritt syndrome)
  Rare bone marrow diseases
    Transient abnormal myelopoiesis of Down syndrome, osteopetrosis, congenital leukemia
    Metastatic neuroblastoma
    Congenital amegakaryocytic thrombocytopenia
    TAR syndrome
    Wiscott-Aldrich syndrome

SOURCE: *Smith OP: Inherited and congenital thrombocytopenia. In: Lilleyman US, Hann IM, Blanchette VS, eds: Pediatric Hematology, 2nd ed. Churchill Livingston, London, 1999: 419–435.*

To determine whether a fetus is affected, prenatal platelet counts can be obtained through percutaneous umbilical blood sampling (PUBS) or intrapartum from a fetal scalp vein after cervical dilatation, but these procedures have a risk of bleeding. A platelet count should be performed immediately after birth and repeated periodically. If the newborn's platelet count is <20.0 × 10⁹/L, IVIG should be given. If intracranial hemorrhage is present, combination treatment with IVIG, corticosteroids, and platelet transfusions should be considered.

NEONATAL ALLOIMMUNE (ISOIMMUNE) PURPURA (NATP) Neonatal alloimmune thrombocytopenia is a rare syndrome caused by alloimmunization of pregnant women to fetal platelet antigens absent in the mother. These IgG alloantibodies cross the placenta and attach to fetal platelets, causing rapid destruction. A number of human platelet alloantigens (HPA) are expressed on membrane glycoproteins and may produce NATP. Incompatibility of HPA-1 (also called the Pl^{A1} or Zw^a antigen) accounts for almost all cases of alloimmunization. More than 98% of people are HPA-1 positive. Therefore, the 2% of women who are HPA-1 negative have a high probability of having an HPA-1–positive spouse and are at risk of being immunized and having an affected infant. Firstborn children are affected in about 50% of cases, suggesting that antigenic exposure occurs early in the course of pregnancy. Pre- or intrapartum central nervous system hemorrhage may result in death or neurologic sequelae including hydrocephalus in 10 to 20% of cases.

A tentative diagnosis of NATP can be suspected in an otherwise normal newborn with isolated thrombocytopenia whose mother has no history of ITP and a normal platelet count. If thrombocytopenia is severe, treatment should be initiated before laboratory confirmation because of the risk of intracranial bleeding. Transfusion of HPA-1–negative platelets produces an immediate increase in platelet numbers and is the treatment of choice, but because only 2% of the population is HPA-1 negative, the most available HPA-1–negative donor is usually the mother. In preparing maternal platelets the maternal plasma should be removed by gentle washing to eliminate maternal antibody. Maternal platelet concentrates should be irradiated. If HPA-1–negative platelets are not available, transfusion of random-donor platelets or exchange transfusion should be considered if there is suspected intracranial or other severe bleeding. IVIG usually improves the platelet count and should also be given, especially if a delay in obtaining HPA-1–compatible platelets is anticipated. Corticosteroid therapy is of unproven benefit. NATP is self-limited, and the platelet count usually returns to normal in 2 to 3 weeks.

Nearly all subsequent infants of a sensitized mother who have HPA-1–positive platelets will also have NATP, and the severity of antenatal and perinatal hemorrhage may increase in later pregnancies. Antiplatelet antibody titers during pregnancy are not predictive, but platelet counts done on blood obtained by PUBS can indicate if the fetus is affected. IVIG should be given to the mother of an affected fetus beginning in midgestation and continuing until delivery. Cesarean section should be considered to protect the fetal head during delivery. HPA-1–negative platelets should be available for administration to the baby immediately after delivery.

AMEGAKARYOCYTIC THROMBOCYTOPENIA WITH ABSENT RADII (TAR) The TAR syndrome is an autosomal recessive bleeding disorder that has affected all ethnic groups and often presents as bleeding in the neonatal period. Thrombocytopenia is severe, but other blood elements are normal. Bone marrow megakaryocytes are usually absent. Chromosome breakage studies are normal. Patients have absent radii, but the thumbs are normal. Deaths can occur from bleeding during the first year, and platelet transfusions may be necessary. However, most survivors have spontaneous improvement of their platelet counts. There are no associated blood disorders. Prenatal diagnosis can be made by fetal ultrasound.

AMEGAKARYOCYTIC THROMBOCYTOPENIA This is a rare nonimmune, usually X-linked, thrombocytopenia secondary to an absence of megakaryocytes and megakaryocyte precursors in the bone marrow. There are no associated physical abnormalities. About half of these patients subsequently develop pancytopenia and hypocellular bone marrows, and some progress to leukemia. The median survival is less than 5 years. Cytokinins such as IL-3 to IL-6 and IL-11 may increase the platelet level, and BMT has been successful in a few cases.

WISKOTT-ALDRICH SYNDROME The Wiskott-Aldrich syndrome is a rare X-linked disorder characterized by thrombocytopenia and small-sized platelets that may present in the newborn period. The associated findings of eczema and immunodeficiency appear later in life. Patients with X-linked thrombocytopenias without the other features of Wiscott-Aldrich syndrome have also been described. *May-Hegglin syndrome* is a dominantly transmitted thrombocytopenia with large platelets and blue Döhle bodies in the neutrophils.

CONGENITAL INFECTIONS A number of severe systemic infections of the newborn, collectively designated the TORCH syndrome, are associated with neonatal thrombocytopenia. These are usually very ill infants who have jaundice and hepatosplenomegaly.

GIANT HEMANGIOMA AND THROMBOCYTOPENIA (KASABACH-MERRITT SYNDROME) This syndrome is caused by platelet destruction within benign hemangiomas of the skin, liver, or spleen. Some patients have evidence of a consumptive coagulopathy with low fibrinogen levels and elevated D-dimers and microangiopathic hemolysis. If the hematologic abnormalities are not severe, it may be possible to wait for spontaneous involution of the hemangioma. However, if the bleeding is severe, intervention may be necessary. Surgical excision and embolization of the hemangioma are usually not feasible because of collateral blood vessels. Radiation therapy can reduce the size of the hemangioma but has long-term risks. Medical therapies include high-dose corticosteroid therapy, which is occasionally effective. Interferon-α in a dose of 3 million units/m²/d inhibits angiogenesis and accelerates involution but may have serious neurologic toxicity.

THROMBOCYTOPENIA AND CYANOTIC CONGENITAL HEART DISEASE Patients with uncorrected cyanotic congenital heart disease who have extreme erythrocytosis may develop hyperviscosity and thrombocytopenia and bleeding. This may be improved by therapeutic phlebotomy so that the hematocrit is <55 to 60%.

19.7.2 Abnormalities of Platelet Function

A diverse group of disorders are characterized by abnormal platelet function with a normal or decreased number of platelets. Platelet function is assessed with the bleeding time and platelet aggregation and adhesion studies (Table 19-12).

TABLE 19-12

INHERITED THROMBOCYTOPENIAS

DISORDER	INHERITANCE	PLATELET FEATURE	PLATELET SIZE	OTHER FINDINGS
Bernard-Soulier syndrome	AR	Aggregation to ristocetin	Large	Qualitative and/or quantitative defect in platelet glycoprotein Ib
Pseudo-von Willebrand disease	AD	Aggregation to ristocetin	Normal	Spontaneous platelet binding of vWF
Type 2b von Willebrand disease	AD	Aggregation to ristocetin	Large	Spontaneous vWF binding to platelets
Montreal syndrome	AD	Spontaneous aggregation	Large	Calpain defect, pale-staining platelets
Gray platelet syndrome	AR	α-Granule defect	Normal	Bone marrow fibrosis
Paris-Trousseau syndrome	AD	Giant α-granules	Normal	Chromosome 11 [del(11)(q23.3;qter)]
Wiskott-Aldrich syndrome	X-linked	Dense granules in some	Small	*WASP* mutations at Xp11.22-11.23, infections
X-linked thrombocytopenia	X-linked	Dense granules in some	Small	*WASP* mutations at Xp11.22-11.23

Bernard-Soulier syndrome is an autosomal recessive disorder with mild thrombocytopenia associated with giant abnormal platelets that do not agglutinate with ristocetin and a prolonged bleeding time. There is a deficiency of platelet glycoprotein Ib, which is the receptor for von Willebrand factor; this results in poor platelet aggregation. *Glanzmann thrombasthenia* is a recessively transmitted bleeding disorder in which the platelet count is normal but platelet function is abnormal, as indicated by platelet aggregation studies. The basic defect is an absence of glycoproteins GPIIb-IIIa in the platelet membrane.

Functional abnormalities of the platelets occur in several inherited diseases caused by a deficiency or malfunction of the granules of the platelets and are designated storage pool defects. *Hermansky-Pudlak syndrome* is a recessively transmitted bleeding disorder characterized by decreased platelet dense granules and oculocutaneous albinism. It is relatively common in Puerto Ricans. Platelet dysfunction may also be present in *Chédiak-Higashi disease* where there are large and dysfunctional dense granules. *Gray platelet syndrome* is a very rare disorder in which α-granules are absent. Other syndromes of abnormal platelet granulation have been described.

DRUG-INDUCED PLATELET DYSFUNCTION

A number of drugs interfere with platelet function and may be associated with bleeding, especially in patients with another hemostatic abnormality. Aspirin (acetylsalicylic acid) irreversibly inactivates platelet cyclooxygenase and alters platelet function for the entire life span of the platelet. Other nonsteroidal anti-inflammatory drugs may also affect platelet function, but less severely than aspirin.

19.7.3   Thrombocytosis

Platelet counts exceeding 500×10^9/L are designated as thrombocytosis and may be primary, caused by myeloproliferative disorders, or secondary to another process. Most children with elevated platelet counts have a reactive thrombocytosis secondary to acute and chronic infections, inflammatory disorders, iron deficiency, or acute blood loss. Thrombocytosis is a common feature of Kawasaki

disease. Asplenic patients usually have moderate thrombocytosis as a result of elimination of the splenic pool.

Essential thrombocythemia is a rare myeloproliferative disorder associated with persistently elevated platelet counts $>1000 \times 10^9$/L. The platelets appear large and dysmorphic, and leukocytosis is often present. Paradoxically, thrombosis and hemorrhage occur commonly, and platelet function may be abnormal. Treatment includes platelet aggregation inhibitors such as acetylsalicylic acid or platelet-lowering drugs such as hydroxyurea.

19.7.4   Inherited Vessel Wall and Connective Tissue Disorders

Hereditary hemorrhagic telangiectasia (Osler-Weber-Rendu disease) is an autosomal dominant disorder in which bleeding occurs from small vascular lesions on the skin, nasal and oral mucosa, and gastrointestinal tract. Severe epistaxis is a common problem, and chronic GI blood loss may result in iron deficiency. *Marfan syndrome* is characterized by skeletal anomalies, cardiovascular abnormalities, and dislocation of the ocular lens. The syndrome is inherited as an autosomal dominant trait (see Chapter 10). Affected individuals experience easy bruising and may bleed excessively at surgery. *Ehlers-Danlos syndrome* is a disorder of type III collagen in connective tissues characterized by hyperextensible skin, hypermobile joints, a bleeding tendency consisting of subcutaneous hematomas, bruising, bleeding from gums after dental extraction, and gastrointestinal bleeding (see Chapter 10). *Pseudoxanthoma elasticum* is a rare autosomal disorder of elastic tissues with spontaneous hemorrhage into the skin and tissues resulting from defective blood vessels. *Henoch-Schönlein purpura* is a generalized vasculitis characterized by purpuric skin lesions, nephritis, and gastrointestinal bleeding (see Sec. 12.6.1 and Plate 12).

References

Beardsley DS, Nathan DG: Platelet abnormalities in infancy and childhood. In: Nathan DG, Orkin SH, eds: Nathan and Oski's Hematology of Infancy and Childhood, 5th ed. Philadelphia, WB Saunders, 1998: 1585–1630

George JN, Woolf SH: Idiopathic thrombocytopenic purpura: practice guidelines developed by explicit methods for the American Society of Hematology. Blood 8:3–35, 1996

19.8   THE SPLEEN

Howard A. Pearson

The primitive spleen can be identified as early as 5 weeks of gestational age, and by midtrimester it has become an active center of fetal hematopoiesis. The mean splenic weight at birth is 11 g; at 6 years of age 55 g; and by adult life 125 g.

The spleen is a complex organ with several anatomic compartments. The white pulp consists of germinal centers, which are dense collections of lymphocytes, plasma cells, and macrophages grouped around a central arteriole. The red pulp, which is the largest part of the organ, consists of endothelial cords that interdigitate with the macrophage-lined splenic sinuses.

The spleen normally receives about 6% of total cardiac output. Splenic blood passes through the small central arteries of the white pulp, where perpendicular branches skim off plasma and particulate material, which is thought to facilitate antigen processing and antibody production. The somewhat concentrated blood then flows into the red pulp. About 10% goes directly into the splenic sinuses, and the rest is forced into the splenic cords. Within the cords, red cells must pass through narrow endothelial apertures before entering the splenic sinuses. Blood cells then enter the splenic veins and from there enter the portal circulation.

HEMATOPOIESIS

The spleen is an active site of fetal hematopoiesis in the first and second trimesters. Splenic hematopoiesis subsequently decreases, and at term most blood cells are produced by the bone marrow. However, the spleen remains capable of resuming hematopoiesis, and extramedullary hematopoiesis, usually associated with splenomegaly, may occur in conditions associated with bone marrow failure syndromes such as osteopetrosis and myelofibrosis or with extreme erythropoietic stress as in thalassemia major (see Secs. 19.4.7 and 19.9).

RED BLOOD CELL DESTRUCTION

In a normal individual the spleen is the principal site of destruction of senescent RBC, which are rigid and nondeformable and cannot traverse the splenic cords. RBC destruction may be greatly exaggerated in states associated with abnormally rigid red cells such as spherocytes or in immune hemolytic anemias, where RBC are coated by antibody (Secs. 19.4 and 19.5).

RESERVOIR

The spleen normally contains about 50 mL of blood and about 30% of the circulating platelet pool. In individuals with splenomegaly, the splenic reservoir may be greatly increased, resulting in an apparent anemia, neutropenia, and thrombocytopenia.

"PITTING" OF RBC INCLUSIONS AND MEMBRANE VESICLES

The spleen performs a unique pitting role by removing a variety of intraerythrocytic inclusions including siderocytes, Howell-Jolly (H-J) and Heinz bodies, and membrane vesicles that resemble surface craters (RBC pocks). When RBC bearing these noncompressible inclusions are forced through the narrow endothelial apertures of the spleen, the inclusions are selectively retained and removed without destruction of the cell. Absence of the pitting function in persons with anatomic or functional asplenia results in the appearance of circulating H-J bodies and increased numbers of pocked red blood cells in the blood.

IMMUNOLOGIC FUNCTION

The spleen provides an important defense against infection by acting as a phagocytic filter for infectious organisms in the blood and is also a major source of production of IgM and properdin as well as formation of antibodies against particulate intravenous antigens. During the first few years of life, when specific circulating antibodies against polysaccharide-encapsulated organisms such as *S. pneumoniae* and *H. influenzae* have not developed, phagocytosis of these organisms during bacteremia occurs almost exclusively in the spleen. The spleen may also play an important role in the production of autoantibodies, in ITP, and in autoimmune hemolytic anemia. In these diseases, surgical splenectomy may be beneficial (see Secs. 19.5 and 19.7).

ASSESSMENT OF SPLENIC SIZE AND SPLENOMEGALY

The tip of the spleen is palpable on deep inspiration in 3 to 5% of normal children and adolescents. Occasionally, some difficulty in differentiating an enlarged spleen from other left upper-quadrant abdominal masses may occur. A useful clue suggesting splenomegaly is the downward movement of the spleen with inspiration. The spleen can be imaged by ultrasonography, CT scan, MRI, and ^{99m}Tc radionuclide scans. Ultrasonography can be used to quantify splenic enlargement and to differentiate splenomegaly from other left upper-quadrant abdominal masses. CT scan is often used to evaluate splenic trauma and to identify and characterize focal splenic pathology.

Splenomegaly occurs in a wide variety of disorders (Table 19-13). The cause of the splenomegaly can often be ascertained by history and physical examination combined with relatively inexpensive and readily available laboratory tests. In general, splenomegaly may be caused by underlying hemolytic anemias with resultant work hypertrophy, by infiltration of malignancies or storage diseases, by underlying systemic infections and inflammations, and by congestion secondary to portal or splenic vein obstruction.

A history of fever, malaise, weight loss, recent sore throat, rash, arthralgia and/or myalgia, and bone pain may suggest underlying inflammatory, infectious, or malignant processes. A history of recent travel suggests infections such as malaria. Unexplained neonatal jaundice and a family history of anemia, jaundice, splenomegaly, splenectomy, or cholelithiasis would make a congenital hemolytic anemia likely. A history of neonatal omphalitis or umbilical vein catheterization may indicate portal vein thrombosis.

The physical examination will determine whether the splenomegaly is isolated or part of a generalized hyperplasia of lymphoid and reticuloendothelial tissues. Rash, mucosal ulcerations, and/or arthritis may suggest a collagen vascular disorder. Petechiae or purpura may be manifestations of thrombocytopenia secondary to bone marrow infiltration. An underlying hemolytic process causing splenomegaly can often be ascertained by a complete blood count, including a reticulocyte count, and examination of the peripheral

TABLE 19-13

SOME CAUSES OF SPLENOMEGALY IN CHILDREN

Hemolytic Anemias (work hypertrophy)
  Congenital hemolytic anemias, hemoglobinopathies, thalassemia major
Extramedullary hematopoiesis
  Thalassemia major, osteopetrosis
Neoplasms
  Leukemia, lymphoma
Storage and infiltrative processes
  Lipidoses, glycogen storage diseases, mucopolysaccharidoses, histiocy-
    toses, sarcoid
Congestive splenomegaly
  Hepatic fibrosis, cirrhosis, portal vein thrombosis (Banti syndrome),
    splenic vein thrombosis, chronic congestive heart failure
Infections
  Bacterial: Bacterial endocarditis
  Protozoal: Malaria, toxoplasmosis
  Viral: Epstein-Barr virus, cytomegalic inclusion disease
Systemic inflammation
  Lupus erythematosus
Benign Lesions
  Hemangiomas, hamartomas, splenic cysts

blood smear. Anemia, reticulocytosis, and abnormal RBC morphology such as spherocytes, target cells, or sickle cells can identify many hemolytic anemias (see Figs. 19-5 and 19-6).

Anemia without other indicators of hemolysis often accompanies chronic infectious, inflammatory, or malignant disorders. Atypical lymphocytes are seen in infections with Epstein-Barr virus, cytomegalovirus, or toxoplasmosis.

ASSESSMENT OF SPLENIC FUNCTION

The presence of H-J bodies on the peripheral blood smear suggests splenic dysfunction or asplenia. However, the numbers of H-J bodies may be very small, and other hematologic conditions such as megaloblastic anemias may be associated with H-J bodies. Quantification of the percentage of pocked red blood cells or radionuclide scanning following injection of ^{99m}Tc sulfur-colloid or tagged heat-damaged RBC assesses splenic reticuloendothelial function and may also aid in locating accessory splenic tissue or splenosis.

19.8.1   Congenital Asplenia and Polysplenia

Congenital asplenia, polysplenia, and heterotaxia are rare, genetically determined conditions that are usually associated with congenital heart disease. These disorders are associated with genes that determine cardiac looping and left-right development in the embryo. In congenital asplenia (Ivemark syndrome), situs inversus and bilateral right sidedness of the paired viscera occur. Associated cardiac anomalies include single ventricle, pulmonary stenosis or atresia, transposition of the great vessels, atrioventricular canal defects, and abnormalities of the pulmonary veins. H-J bodies are present on the peripheral blood smear, and pocked red cells are increased. These infants are at high risk for fulminant bacterial septicemia and should be treated with prophylactic antibiotics in the first 5 years of life.

Congenital polysplenia is a syndrome of bilateral left sidedness associated with multiple spleens, which are usually found along the greater curvature of the stomach. The stomach may be on the right

side of the abdomen, and both lungs may be bilobed. Cardiac anomalies, when present, are usually less severe than seen in congenital asplenia. These children often develop biliary atresia but are not at increased risk of severe infections.

Isolated congenital asplenia without heterotaxia or heart defects is a rare recessively transmitted condition, usually discovered incidentally in the workup of a child with episodes of severe sepsis. A mutation of a homeobox gene designated as HOX11 that regulates embryonic splenogenesis may be the cause of this rare disorder.

Accessory spleens, usually located in the splenic hilus, are found in as many as 10 to 15% of individuals. Hypertrophy of these may be associated with recurrence of ITP or autoimmune hemolytic anemia after an initially successful splenectomy.

FUNCTIONAL ASPLENIA AND HYPOSPLENIA

Children with sickle cell anemia develop functional asplenia during infancy and early childhood because of alterations in splenic circulation caused by intrasplenic sickling. Despite clinical enlargement, splenic function is greatly reduced as evidenced by circulating H-J bodies and increased numbers of pocked RBC. These children are at high risk of severe bacterial infections, especially in the first 5 years of life. Children with sickle cell anemia develop anatomic asplenia in the second decade of life as a result of autoinfarction (see Sec. 19.4).

Functional hyposplenia has been described in a number of conditions, especially gastrointestinal disorders such as sprue and celiac disease and several systemic immune disorders.

19.8.2   Hypersplenism

The term *hypersplenism* has been used to describe patients with splenomegaly, peripheral cytopenia or cytopenias, and normal or increased bone marrow production of the affected blood cell, which resolves following splenectomy. In hypersplenism, the spleen is often assumed to be responsible for increased destruction of RBC, neutrophils, and/or platelets. Excluded from the definition of hypersplenism are conditions in which splenic enlargement and peripheral blood destruction occur in response to intrinsic abnormalities of the blood cells such as in congenital hemolytic anemias or autoimmune cytopenias. Hypersplenism occurs most commonly with congestive splenomegaly but is observed in other disorders as well. The severity of the cytopenias varies widely. In some instances of presumed hypersplenism, an expanded reservoir for leukocytes and platelets in a greatly enlarged spleen rather than increased destruction may cause the cytopenia, which is usually mild, and infections or bleeding does not occur. Splenectomy may not be indicated solely on the basis of the blood count.

19.8.3   Splenic Cysts

There are two types of splenic cysts. Pseudocysts result from intrasplenic infarction or hemorrhage with subsequent liquefaction of splenic tissue and blood within a fibrous capsule. Epidermoid splenic cysts contain clear fluid and have an epidermal lining.

19.8.4   Splenectomy

Indications for splenectomy can be conveniently divided into medical (hematologic) and surgical categories (Table 19-14). Medical

TABLE 19-14
COMMON INDICATIONS FOR SPLENECTOMY[a]

Medical (hematologic) indications
  Congenital hemolytic anemias
    Hereditary spherocytosis; other severe congenital hemolytic diseases
      Sequestration crisis of sickle cell anemia
  Acquired immunohematologic diseases
    Chronic idiopathic thrombocytopenic purpura; autoimmune hemo-
      lytic anemia
  Hypersplenic syndromes:
    Gaucher disease, thalassemia major and intermedia; congestive
      splenomegaly
Surgical indications
  Cysts, tumors
  Exposure, shunting for portal hypertension
  Relief of mechanical symptoms because of size
  Trauma

---

[a] These indications are not absolute and must be individualized for each specific patient.

---

indications include congenital hemolytic anemias (see Sec. 19.5). In storage diseases such as Gaucher disease the spleen enlarges and may be a mechanical burden. Partial splenectomy is feasible, but its effectiveness in the management of these diseases is controversial.

Surgical splenectomy is obviously associated with a total loss of splenic function. The risk of postsplenectomy sepsis is related to the patient's age at the time of surgery and to the underlying condition. The young child, especially <5 years of age, has a high risk of postsplenectomy sepsis, but any age group may be affected. Patients who have undergone splenectomy for trauma and for benign hematologic conditions such as ITP and hereditary spherocytosis are at less risk than patients with malignancies, thalassemia, or those with Wiskott-Aldrich syndrome.

19.8.5   Splenic Injury

Laceration and rupture of the normal spleen may occur with blunt trauma to the abdomen or follow relatively minor trauma in children with splenomegaly, especially the acute enlargement that occurs in infectious mononucleosis. Massive internal hemorrhage may result in hypovolemic shock. Physical findings include persistent and increasing abdominal pain and peritoneal signs including rebound tenderness and abdominal muscle spasm. Diaphragmatic pain may be referred to the left shoulder. Blunt splenic trauma can be diagnosed by ^{99m}Tc scan, CT scan, or ultrasound, which may show a wide range of injuries from subcapsular hemorrhage to total fracture and maceration of the spleen. Almost all children with blunt splenic trauma can be managed conservatively with inpatient observation, bed rest, and transfusions as necessary to maintain circulatory stability. A small number of children with blunt splenic trauma who cannot be clinically stabilized and those with multiple organ injury require surgery. In some circumstances, splenic repair or partial splenectomy may be possible. Long-term follow-up of children treated nonoperatively for blunt splenic trauma have not revealed significant numbers of late complications. A significant proportion of children whose spleens are removed for trauma develop splenosis.

Enlarged spleens that are not protected by the rib cage are at increased risk of splenic trauma. Children with splenomegaly should avoid contact sports and other physical activities associated with significant risk of abdominal trauma.

19.8.6   Management of Children with Asplenia and Hyposplenia

Prophylactic therapy with penicillin or an equivalent antibiotic is strongly recommended for infants or young children who have hyposplenia or asplenia. In a prospective double-blind trial of sickle cell anemia children less than 5 years old with functional hyposplenia, oral penicillin prophylaxis was shown to reduce the incidence of bacteremia by 84%. A second controlled study showed no significant benefit of penicillin prophylaxis after 5 years of age. The emergence of penicillin-resistant pneumococci may reduce the effectiveness of penicillin prophylaxis.

Children with asplenia or splenic dysfunction should be immunized with vaccines against *S. pneumoniae, H. influenzae,* and *N. meningitidis.* The 23-valent pneumococcal polysaccharide vaccine is inconstantly effective in children <5 years of age, but the seven-valent conjugate polysaccharide vaccine is immunogenic in infants. The conjugate *H. influenzae* vaccine has virtually eliminated severe disease caused by this pathogen. If a child requires an elective splenectomy, these immunizations should be given in advance of surgery but are also effective when given after splenectomy.

Parents of children with splenic dysfunction must be educated to regard significant febrile illnesses (>102°F) as signaling a potentially life-threatening situation and mandates prompt evaluation by a physician. After a blood culture has been obtained, parenteral broad-spectrum antibiotics, currently third-generation cephalosporins, should be administered. Although the risk of postsplenectomy sepsis is greatest in young children in the first few years after splenectomy, severe infections have occurred decades after splenectomy. A syndrome of severe and frequently fatal infection by *Capnocytophaga canimorsus* acquired from a sometimes trivial dog bite has been reported, and asplenic patients should be treated empirically with amoxicillin/clavulanic acid after dog bites. Asplenic patients also appear to be at increased risk of serious infections with *Bartonella bacilliformis.*

References

American Academy of Pediatrics: Active and Passive Immunization: Asplenic Children. Report of the Committee on Infectious Diseases (1997 Red Book), 24th ed. Elk Grove Village, IL, AAP, 1997:56–538.

American Academy of Pediatrics, Committee on Sports Medicine: Recommendation for participation in competitive sports. Pediatrics 81:737, 1988

Bowers PN, Bruekner T, Yost HJ: The genetics of left-right development and heterotaxia. Semin Perinatol 6:577–588, 1996

Pearson HA: The spleen and disturbances of splenic function. In: Nathan DG, Oski FA, eds: Hematology of Infancy and Childhood, 5th ed. Philadelphia, WB Saunders, 1998:1051–1068

19.9   BONE MARROW FAILURE SYNDROMES

Blanche P. Alter and Jeffrey Michael Lipton

NORMAL HEMATOPOIESIS

The development of in vivo and in vitro clonal assays for pluripotent and committed hematopoietic progenitors and the characterization of hematopoietic cell surface antigens by flow cytometry have resulted in the developmental model of hematopoiesis (see Fig. 19-10). This model describes the proliferation and differentiation of pluripotent hematopoietic stem cells that can populate the entire marrow with nucleated RBC, WBC, and platelet precursors. The immediate offspring of the stem cells are the committed progenitors of the lymphocyte (CFU-L, colony-forming unit-lymphocyte) and the multipotent hematopoietic or myeloid progenitor, the CFU-GEMM, that gives rise to committed progenitors of the granulocyte, erythrocyte, monocyte/macrophage, and megakaryocyte as well as eosinophil and basophil populations. These progenitors appear as immature, undifferentiated mononuclear cells and are present in small numbers in the bone marrow. In addition to the hematopoietic components of the system, a complex array of growth factors in addition to support elements or stroma and accessory lymphocytes, macrophages, fibroblasts, endothelial cells, and adipocytes create a regulatory milieu that interacts with differentiating hematopoietic cells. Hematopoietic cell differentiation is controlled by intrinsic transcriptional regulators within niches in the

bone marrow. Specific receptor-ligand relationships within the microenvironment support the proliferation and differentiation of specific cell types and provide a scaffold on which blood-forming cells, accessory cells, and growth factors may interact at close range.

Cell culture and recombinant DNA technology have led to the identification and ultimate cloning of the genes for many specific hematopoietic growth factors or cytokines as well as EPO. In some circumstances these factors may also influence the function of the terminally differentiated cell. In addition, an array of growth antagonists provide feedback inhibition.

The hematopoietic bone marrow has been compared to a garden. Stem cell "seeds" are anchored by receptor-ligand "roots" nurtured in stromal "soil" by growth factor and nutrient "fertilizers" to give rise to a beautiful and complex hematopoietic garden. Thus, a number of mechanisms can lead to bone marrow failure, which could result from faulty stem/progenitor cells (seeds), defective stroma and accessory cells (soil), or immunologic weeds. The hematopoietic garden concept provides a model for under-

The Progenitor Basis of Hematopoiesis

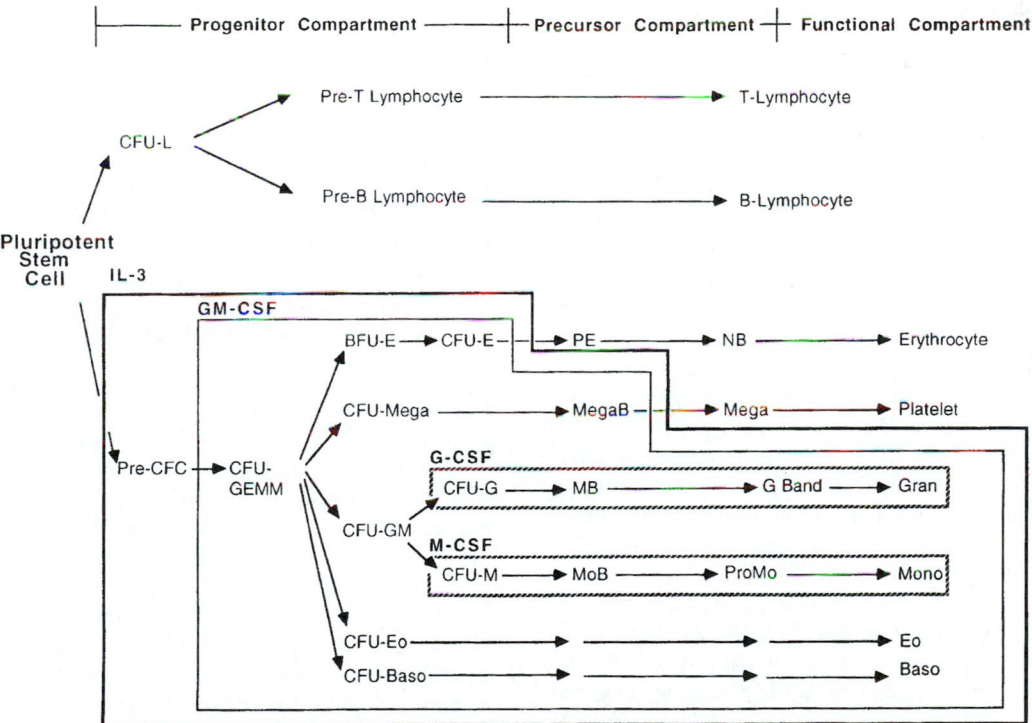

FIGURE 19-10 **The progenitor basis of hematopoiesis. Schematic diagram as defined by clonal assays and flow cytometric analysis in the human and murine systems and studies in diseases of clonal proliferation. Enclosed areas define the effect of the colony stimulating factors IL-3 (interleukin-3). GM-CSF (granulocyte, macrophage-colony stimulating factor), G-CSF (granulocyte-colony stimulating factor), and M-CSF (macrophage-colony stimulating factor). The hierarchy of hematopoietic cell differentiation proceeds from the pluripotent stem cell through the progenitor compartment, cells that are not morphologically identifiable but have undergone commitment to the morphologically identifiable precursor compartment. CFU-L, colony forming unit-lymphocyte; pre-CFC, pre-colony forming cell; CFU-GEMM, colony forming unit-granulocyte, erythrocyte, megakaryocyte, macrophage; BFU-E, burst forming unit-erythroid; CFU-E, colony forming unit erythroid; PE, proerythroblast; NB, normoblast; CFU-Mega, colony forming unit-megakaryocyte, Mega B, megakaryoblast; Mega, megakaryocyte; CFU-GM, colony forming unit-granulocyte, macrophage; CFU-G, colony forming unit-granulocyte; MB, myeloblast; G Band, granulocytic band; Gran, Granulocyte; CFU-M, colony forming unit-macrophage; MoB, monoblast; ProMo, promonocyte; Mono, monocyte; Eo, eosinophil; Baso, basophil.**

standing the pathophysiology of aplastic anemia and the other bone marrow failure syndromes observed in children.

19.9.1   Aplastic Anemia

The term *aplastic anemia* describes pancytopenia, not just anemia. Onset is often insidious, with complaints of fatigue, pallor, thrombocytopenic bleeding, bruising, and epistaxis. Infections are usually a late complication. Acquired aplastic anemia has an annual incidence of about two to six per 10^6 population, one-10th the incidence of leukemia. There is no racial or gender propensity and no peak age in childhood.

Some exposures such as radiation, cytotoxic drugs, and organic solvents regularly induce aplasia in a dose-related manner, whereas others, such as certain antibiotics and other drugs and chemicals, do so only sporadically and idiosyncratically. The antibiotic chloramphenicol, which is associated with both dose-related and idiosyncratic aplasia, warrants special mention because it may cause severe aplasia. Viruses and specific immune diseases may be implicated in some cases. Drug or viral exposures may have occurred weeks or months before the clinical presentation. Genetic propensity for a specific environmental factor and inherited familial predispositions have been described. Nonetheless, more than half of all cases remain "idiopathic."

The diagnosis requires reduction in three cell lines—anemia, thrombocytopenia, and neutropenia—as well as a hypocellular bone marrow. Physical examination may show pallor and bruising, but hepatosplenomegaly or lymphadenopathy is not present.

The diagnosis of aplastic anemia requires a complete blood count and assessment of the bone marrow for morphology and cellularity. Most patients have anemia and thrombocytopenia before granulocytopenia. The differential diagnosis includes malignant marrow infiltrations by leukemia, lymphoma, metastatic tumor, or granulomas and ineffective hematopoiesis, as in myelodysplasia.

Acquired aplastic anemia is further classified as moderate or severe. In severe aplastic anemia, the patient is pancytopenic: platelets $<20 \times 10^9/L$; neutrophils $<0.5 \times 10^9/L$; and absolute reticulocytopenia $<40 \times 10^9/L$. "Stress" erythropoiesis may be reflected by macrocytosis (MCV >100 fL), increased fetal hemoglobin, and fetal i antigen on RBC membranes. The bone marrow is hypocellular with increased fat, and more than 70% of the marrow cells are nonhematopoietic: lymphocytes, reticulum cells, mast cells, and plasma cells. Megakaryocytes are markedly reduced in number. Patients with moderate aplastic anemia do not meet these criteria for severe disease but have pancytopenia and hypocellular bone marrow. Categorization of the patient has prognostic implications because the "severe" group does poorly.

PATHOPHYSIOLOGY

Hematopoietic progenitors in blood and marrow are very low in number and respond poorly to hematopoietic stimuli, suggesting that the most primitive stem cells are absent. As primitive cells mature, the potential for self-renewal is lost, and entry into a pathway for terminal differentiation is likely. Two mechanisms of hematopoietic cell damage giving rise to aplastic anemia have been postulated (Fig. 19-11). The most primitive stem cells are mitotically quiescent. Type I damage is random, striking both immature and mature cells but most notably affecting the immature and perhaps nonmitotic cells that require many mitoses for maturation. The

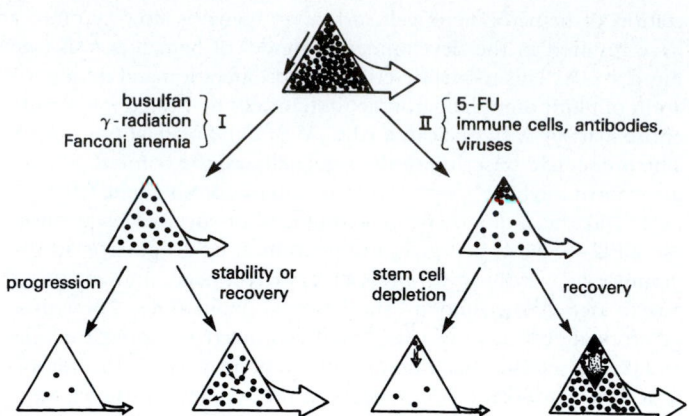

FIGURE 19-11   Mechanisms of stem cell compartment damage. **SOURCE:** *Young NS, Alter BP: Aplastic Anemias: Acquired and Inherited. Philadelphia, Saunders, 1994:37.*

mechanism may involve direct injury to DNA by irradiation or alkylating agents (busulfan). A permanent effect might be depletion of stem cell number and self-renewal capacity. Type II damage occurs in the more mitotically and metabolically active compartment of differentiating cells, which have distinct antigenic phenotypes. Cell cycle–specific chemotherapeutic agents, viral infection, or immune mechanisms may be involved, and stem cell depletion occurs as cells differentiate and are vulnerable to damage. Response of some patients to immune therapy (immunomodulation) with antithymocyte globulin or cyclosporine suggests that type II damage is relevant. With either type of damage, recovery of hematopoiesis may occur from a very small number of stem cells and thus be "clonal."

TREATMENT AND OUTCOME

Definitive treatment of the aplastic anemia is required because patients receiving only supportive care have a 50% mortality within the first 6 months and a long-term survival rate of <25%.

The optimal and curative treatment for severe aplastic anemia is stem cell transplantation (BMT) (see Sec. 20.4). About 80% of patients will have a complete or partial response to immunosuppressive therapy, most commonly antilymphocyte globulin (ATG or ALG) and cyclosporine. Corticosteroids, to prevent serum sickness from ATG or ALG, and growth factors G- or GM-CSF to increase the neutrophil count are usually included. Sustained neutrophil responses may appear within 1 month, and RBC and platelet responses by 2 to 3 months. Immunomodulatory therapy is indicated for patients with severe aplastic anemia without an HLA-matched sibling donor but may not be a long-term success because of a substantial risk of developing a clonal hematopoietic disorder such as paroxysmal nocturnal hemoglobinuria, myelodysplasia, or acute myelocytic leukemia. Even patients who recover spontaneously develop clonal disease because of intrinsic problems in immune surveillance or in the stem cell itself.

Androgen treatment may have a role in the management of moderate but not severe aplastic anemia. Supportive management is critical. Bleeding can be prevented or treated with platelet transfusions, which may be required long term in unresponsive patients. The development of alloantibodies, usually to HLA-A or -B antigens, may limit effectiveness (Sec. 19.11). The platelet count should be maintained above $5 \times 10^9/L$, although higher counts may be necessary to prevent serious hemorrhage. Practical measures include good dental hygiene, avoidance of trauma, and suppression of menses. An antifibrinolytic agent such as ϵ-aminocaproic acid may be helpful during acute oral bleeding episodes.

Neutropenia is associated with a risk of bacterial and fungal infections. Local sites such as catheter insertions require meticulous care. Febrile episodes should be treated empirically with broad-spectrum parenteral antibiotics. Prophylactic antibiotics predispose to resistant bacteria or fungi and are not recommended.

Anemia is readily treated with transfusions of packed RBC to maintain a hemoglobin >70 g/L. Development of alloantibodies may be avoided by the use of phenotypically matched blood. Iron overload will occur after a large number of transfusions. Because all patients with aplastic anemia are considered to be potential candidates for BMT, family members should not be used as donors of blood products.

Blood products should be leukocyte-depleted to reduce sensitization to leukocyte antigens and reduce the number of lymphocytes that may contain cytomegalovirus. Blood products should be irradiated to prevent graft-versus-host disease (see Sec. 19.11).

19.9.2   Inherited Bone Marrow Failure Syndromes

What appears to be "acquired" aplastic anemia may occur in individuals who are heterozygous, hemizygous, or homozygous for genes associated with marrow failure. The precise incidences of the inherited syndromes (Table 19-15) are not known. In large series, 25 to 30% of children with marrow aplasia may have an inherited disorder, resulting in 300 to 1000 new cases annually in the United States. Because of the familial association, as well as the frequency of congenital anomalies in some of the syndromes, patients may be diagnosed before the development of marrow failure, and prenatal testing is available for some conditions. Most of the diagnoses are based on clinical findings (Table 19-15) and not on specific laboratory tests. Absence of anomalies does not exclude a diagnosis, but the presence of characteristic findings suggests an inherited syndrome. Specific diagnoses have prognostic and therapeutic impli-

cations, and these patients may be at increased risk for developing malignancies (see Chapter 10 and Sec. 19.2).

FANCONI ANEMIA

Fanconi in 1927 described several siblings who had congenital anomalies, short stature, and aplastic anemia. Fanconi anemia (FA) is an autosomal recessive disorder in which about 75% of patients have major or minor congenital anomalies. More than 90% develop aplastic anemia at a mean age of 8 to 9 years, ranging from birth to 48 years. About 3% of cases are diagnosed in the first year of life, and 10% after age 16 years. The "classical" phenotype includes short stature, absent or abnormal thumbs and abnormal radii, microcephaly, café-au-láit and hypopigmented spots, dark pigmentation, and renal anomalies. The sex ratio is equal, and all ethnic groups are affected.

At least eight FA mutations have been identified. The genes for two of these have been cloned: *FANCA* and *FANCC*, which account for more than 75% of cases. The usual diagnostic test for FA involves the identification of DNA repair abnormalities in cultured peripheral blood lymphocytes, including a high proportion of metaphases with breaks, gaps, rearrangements, exchanges, endoreduplication, and triradials. These abnormalities are increased when cells are cultured with a DNA-damaging agent such as diepoxybutane (DEB) or mitomycin C (MMC). Chromosome breakage analyses have been used for prenatal diagnosis of FA.

PRESENTATION AND CLINICAL COURSE   Single cytopenias, particularly thrombocytopenia, may precede the development of pancytopenia. Macrocytic erythrocytes with increased fetal hemoglobin are often present before anemia develops. When pancytopenia develops, the bone marrow is usually hypocellular and fatty, but occasionally dyserythropoiesis and dysmyelopoiesis are found. Marrow examination, including chromosome analyses, should be performed periodically to detect malignant transformation. Cultures of marrow and blood demonstrate decreased numbers of stem cell progenitors, which correlates with hematologic abnormalities. Mean survival in FA is now in the mid-30s, with most deaths re-

TABLE 19-15

PHYSICAL ABNORMALITIES IN INHERITED BONE MARROW FAILURE SYNDROMES

FANCONI ANEMIA	DIAMOND-BLACKFAN ANEMIA	DYSKERATOSIS CONGENITA	KOSTMANN SYNDROME	SHWACHMAN-DIAMOND SYNDROME	THROMBO-CYTOPENIA ABSENT RADII	AMEGAKARYO-CYTIC THROMBO-CYTOPENIA
Skin-pigmented, café-au-lait	Facies characteristic	Skin—reticular pigmentation	Short Retardation	Short Malabsorption	Radii absent, thumbs present	Normal or CNS anomalies
Short radii and/or thumb anomalies	Thumb anomalies	Nail dystrophy		Retardation	Humeri short	Retardation
Hypogonads	Short	Leukoplakia			Fingers abnormal	Congenital heart disease
Microcephaly	Eyes—glaucoma, other	Eyes—epiphora			Leg anomalies	
Eyes—small, strabismus	Renal anomalies	Teeth bad			Skeletal anomalies	
Renal anomalies	Hypogonads	Retardation				
Low birth weight	Neck—web, short	Skeletal anomalies				
Retardation	Skeletal anomalies	Short				
Deafness	Congenital heart disease	Hyperhidrosis				
Hyperreflexia	Retardation	Hair loss				
Skeletal anomalies		Urethral stenosis				
		Esophageal anomalies				

sulting from infections and hemorrhage. Supportive care is important.

TREATMENT Unlike acquired aplastic anemia, a favorable response to androgens occurs in more than 50% of patients with FA. Most responders require continued treatment, and eventually most become unresponsive. Synthetic androgens may cause peliosis hepatis and liver tumors, and patients should be monitored regularly by ultrasonography.

Stem cell transplant is the only cure for the aplasia, but patient preparation must be modified because immunosuppression regimens that include cyclophosphamide and radiation are very toxic to nonmarrow dividing cells, which cannot repair DNA damage. The short-term survival following transplant from HLA-matched related donors is >75%. Stem cells obtained from placental blood have been used successfully to reconstitute FA patients. Ten to fifteen percent of FA patients develop acute myelogenous leukemia, and some did not have preceding aplastic anemia. Because of the DNA repair defect, most patients tolerate chemotherapy poorly, and bone marrow transplantation conditioning must use special, less myeloablative protocols. Several patients have been described with pancytopenia and myelodysplasia, with abnormal bone marrow dysplastic changes despite normal or increased cellularity. A clonal cytogenetic abnormality, possibly preleukemic, has been seen in some of these patients. FA patients are at increased risk of hepatic malignancy, which is enhanced by androgen treatment. About 5% of FA patients have developed other malignancies.

DYSKERATOSIS CONGENITA

More than 200 cases of dyskeratosis congenita (DC) have been reported, representing all racial and ethnic groups. About 80% of cases have X-linked recessive inheritance; the rest are autosomal recessive or dominant. The X-linked condition has been linked to Xq28, and the gene *DKC1* encodes the protein dyskerin, which makes prenatal diagnosis possible. The diagnostic triad of DC includes (1) dystrophic finger- and toenails, (2) reticulated mottled hyperpigmentation of the skin, and (3) mucous membrane leukoplakia. Less frequent physical findings include blocked lacrimal ducts, dentition problems, hyperhidrosis, and keratosis (Table 19-15). Approximately half the patients develop aplastic anemia with pancytopenia, macrocytosis, and increased HbF. Bone marrows are usually hypocellular. The median survival age is in the mid-30s, with most deaths resulting from complications of pancytopenia or malignancies. The average age for the development of aplasia is 15 years, and for malignancies 30 years.

TREATMENT Pancytopenia responds to androgen therapy in about 50% of patients. Supportive care is important. BMT has cured about 25% of a small number of patients, but procedure-related deaths are not infrequent because of the increased tissue sensitivity to chemotherapy. GM-CSF or G-CSF therapy may have a therapeutic role. Myelodysplasia and acute myelogenous leukemia have been reported in patients with DC.

19.9.3   Single Cytopenias

ACQUIRED RED CELL APLASIA

The differential diagnosis of acquired pure red cell aplasia (PRCA) is shown on Table 19-16. Acquired PRCA of the adult type may

TABLE 19-16

CLASSIFICATION OF SINGLE-LINEAGE CYTOPENIAS

ACQUIRED	INHERITED
Pure red cell aplasia (PRCA)	
Idiopathic	Diamond-Blackfan anemia
Drugs and chemicals	
Immune	
Thymoma	
B19 parvovirus	
Transient erythroblastopenia of childhood (TEC)	
Neutropenia	
Drugs, toxins	Kostmann syndrome
Idiopathic	Shwachman-Diamond syndrome
Tγ lymphoproliferative disease	Reticular dysgenesis
Thrombocytopenia	
Idiopathic amegakaryocytic thrombocytopenia	Thrombocytopenia with absent radii
Drugs, toxins	
Immune	

SOURCE: *Young NS Alter BP: Aplastic Anemia: Acquired and Inherited. Philadelphia, WB Saunders, 1994:9.*

be idiopathic or related to drugs, particularly phenytoin and chloramphenicol. Immune-mediated PRCA occurs in many idiopathic cases as well as those with thymoma, systemic lupus erythematosus, and chronic lymphocytic leukemia. In vitro erythroid colony assays may reveal the presence of serum lymphocyte inhibitors of erythropoiesis, and about two-thirds will respond to immunosuppression or cytotoxic agents. RBC transfusions are the primary treatment.

B19 parvovirus infects erythroid progenitors and causes transient or chronic RBC aplasia. The chronic type occurs because of persistence of parvovirus in immunodeficient patients who cannot produce neutralizing antibody. The patients have severe transfusion-dependent anemia, and bone marrows show reduced erythroid precursors. The few RBC precursors are giant pronormoblasts. Diagnosis requires demonstration of parvovirus genome (DNA) in serum, blood, or bone marrow cells. Treatment with intravenous γ-globulin (IVIgG) is usually effective.

Transient aplastic crisis (TAC) caused by parvovirus occurs only once in patients with underlying hemolytic anemias (see Sec. 19.5). Occasionally, neutrophils and platelets will also be decreased. Diagnostic levels of IgM antibody appear in the first week after infection. In utero infection with parvovirus results in up to 10% fetal death during the first and second trimesters, and neonatal hydrops fetalis occurs occasionally.

Transient erythroblastopenia of childhood (TEC) is an acquired condition in previously hematologically normal children and usually involves only anemia, reticulocytopenia, and marrow erythroblastopenia. The mean age of diagnosis is 26 months, with the majority between 1 and 3 years of age. Although many patients have had an antecedent viral illness, no specific virus has been implicated, and parvovirus has usually been excluded. Pallor and tachycardia are the only relevant findings. The anemia may require one or two transfusions, but patients usually recover spontaneously within 1 to 2 months. Bone marrow shows erythroid hypoplasia, and cultures show decreased colony-forming units-erythroid (CFU-E). Serum or cellular inhibitors of erythropoiesis are often identified. TEC has an excellent prognosis, and later hematologic complications have not been reported. TEC can be distinguished from Diamond-

Blackfan anemia because TEC patients are usually older than 1 year and have normocytic red cells, levels of HbF normal for age, no excess membrane i antigen, and no congenital anomalies.

Diamond-Blackfan anemia (DBA; *congenital hypoplastic anemia*) is characterized by macrocytic anemia and reticulocytopenia (pure red cell anemia). The bone marrow is normocellular, but erythroid precursors are markedly reduced or absent. Ninety percent of patients are diagnosed under 1 year of age, although a few cases with later onset have been described. Most of the more than 500 reported cases are white, but blacks and Asians have been affected. Three-quarters of cases are sporadic, but both dominant and recessive pedigrees have been described. One DBA gene has been cloned and mapped on chromosome 19, and at least two additional DBA genes may exist.

Approximately one-third of patients have abnormal physical findings (see Table 19-15). An increase in RBC adenosine deaminase (ADA) activity is present in 90% of cases, and chromosome breakage is not increased.

Approximately 80% of patients improve on corticosteroid therapy, maintain normal hemoglobin levels without transfusions, and can be managed on small alternate-day doses, but some require prohibitively toxic levels, and some respond initially and then become refractory, resulting in an overall response rate of only about 50%. Spontaneous remissions occur in about 25% of cases independent of steroid responsiveness (steroid responders and nonresponders). Bone marrow transplantation was curative in 25 of 35 reported cases. Non–steroid responsive patients require chronic transfusion therapy and inevitably develop iron overload that requires chelation (Sec. 19.4.7).

The current median survival is about 40 to 45 years because of improved transfusion and chelation therapy. A few patients have developed aplastic anemia (see Table 19-15), and about 5% have developed leukemia or myelodysplasias. Thus, DBA may be a myeloid premalignant condition.

Inherited single neutropenias—*Kostmann syndrome* (KS), *infantile genetic agranulocytosis, Schwachman syndrome,* and *cartilage hair syndrome*—are discussed in Sec. 19.6. Inherited thrombocytopenia, the TAR syndrome, and amegakaryocytic thrombocytopenia are discussed in Sec. 19.7.

Pearson syndrome is characterized by refractory macrocytic sideroblastic anemia with vacuolization of bone marrow myeloid and erythroid precursors, exocrine pancreatic deficiency with malabsorption, and metabolic acidosis. Ringed sideroblasts, which are iron-laden mitochondria, are present, and there are decreased numbers of progenitors. Patients have evidence of mitochondrial cytopathies, including metabolic acidosis and abnormalities of oxidative phosphorylation. Large deletions of mitochondrial DNA can be demonstrated. The inheritance of mitochondrial diseases is maternal because only ova and not sperm have mitochondria, and all of the approximately 50 reported cases have been sporadic. Most patients die in infancy. In children who survive, there is hematologic improvement, but they may develop the neurologic abnormalities of Kayne-Sayres disease (see Chapter 25).

19.9.4 Myelophthisic Anemia

Peripheral cytopenias caused by marrow replacement by disorders not intrinsic to the marrow lead to *leukoerythroblastosis* (anemia with nucleated RBC and immature white cells), which must be distinguished from *leukemoid reactions,* in which there is a reactive leukocytosis with an orderly progression of immature through mature cells, and a *leukemic hiatus,* in which there are both immature and mature cells but a gap with a lack of intermediate cells.

The major causes of myelophthisic disease in children are marrow invasion by metastatic tumor, granulomas, myelofibrosis, or osteopetrosis. *Osteopetrosis,* or marble bone disease, can be a benign autosomal dominant or severe autosomal recessive disease characterized by dense fragile bones caused by abnormal osteoclasts that do not resorb bone normally. The patients have craniomegaly and hepatosplenomegaly because of extramedullary hematopoiesis, blindness, deafness, cranial nerve palsies, and fractures. Macrocytic leukoerythroblastic anemia occurs, and bone marrow biopsies show small constricted medullary cavities, hypocellularity, and fibrosis. Cytopenias result from decreased production and increased splenic pooling. BMT can be curative, because osteoclasts are derived from marrow stem cells. α-Interferon may stimulate bone resorption, and M-CSF may augment osteoclast activity. Prenatal ultrasonography can detect increased bone density and fractures.

References

Alter BP: Fanconi's anemia: current concepts. Am J Pediatr Hematol Oncol 14:170, 1993

Alter BP, Young NS: The bone marrow failure syndromes. In: Nathan DG, Orkin SH, eds: Hematology of Infancy and Childhood, 5th ed. Philadelphia, WB Saunders, 1998:237

Drachtman RA, Alter BP: Dyskeratosis congenita. Dermatol Clin 13:33, 1995

Lipton JM, Alter BP: Diamond-Blackfan anemia. In: Feig SA, Freedman MH, eds: Clinical Disorders and Experimental Models of Erythropoietic Failure. Boca Raton, CRC Press, 39:179–186, 1993

Young NS, Alter BP: Aplastic Anemia: Acquired and Inherited. Philadelphia, WB Saunders, 1994

19.10 HEMOSTASIS

Marilyn J. Manco-Johnson

Hemostasis is a complex physiological process that functions to stop hemorrhage and repair vascular injury without compromising blood flow. Hemostasis involves interactions among elements of the blood vessel wall and subendothelial supporting structures, circulating blood platelets, and plasma coagulation proteins. Although, in vivo, all components of this system interact in a dynamic, coordinated fashion, the initiating event in hemostasis is platelet-vessel interaction followed by formation of the fibrin clot. Clot propagation is regulated and cleared by physiological fibrinolysis.

PLATELET-VESSEL INTERACTION

A series of reactions involved in the formation of a hemostatic plug is the primary means by which bleeding is arrested at the level of small blood vessels. Vascular injury exposes subendothelial collagen fibrils and provides a site for adhesion of platelets. Platelet adhesion requires the interaction of platelet membrane with the damaged endothelium via the von Willebrand protein, which binds both to subendothelial collagen and to glycoprotein Ib of activated platelets. Aggregation of additional platelets is facilitated by agonists in the area of vascular injury including thrombin, epinephrine, collagen, and ADP, which are released from other platelets. Stimulation of the platelet membrane causes activation of phospholipids, which release arachidonic acid, which is converted to prostaglandin endoperoxides by the enzyme cyclooxygenase. In turn, these endoperoxides are converted to thromboxane A_2. A similar pathway of prostaglandin metabolism in the endothelial cell produces prostacyclin, which is a potent vasodilator and an inhibitor of platelet aggregation.

PLUG FORMATION AND CONSOLIDATION

Platelet adhesion results in a fragile platelet plug. After activation, platelets undergo a change from their disc-like shape to form long pseudopods emanating from globular centers. The fibrinogen receptor is formed from two heterodimers, glycoproteins IIb and IIIa, which link platelets via fibrinogen, fibronectin, thrombospondin, and the von Willebrand protein. At the same time, tissue factor is released as a result of tissue injury, and the release of platelet phospholipid promotes the formation of thrombin, which coverts fibrinogen to fibrin and forms a tight hemostatic plug. The formation of the platelet plug is independent of the plasma coagulation system. Hence, the bleeding time, which measures platelet plug formation, is normal in most hemophiliac patients. The platelet plug begins to disintegrate physiologically after 24 to 48 hours.

COAGULATION AND ITS REGULATION

The coagulation process involves a complex, repetitive series of reactions in which a protease binds to a regulatory cofactor on a membrane surface (Fig. 19-12). This protease/cofactor combination then cleaves an inactive precursor (zymogen) to form a new enzyme. This new enzyme then combines with another cofactor, and the sequence is repeated to generate a "cascade" of reactions. The endpoint of the coagulation cascade is the generation of thrombin and the ultimate conversion of fibrinogen to fibrin.

Coagulation can be initiated by either of two pathways (Fig. 19-12). The *contact* or *extrinsic pathway* of coagulation, which is important in normal hemostasis, is initiated when tissue factor binds

the enzyme factor VIIa on membrane surfaces. This complex can activate factor X forming a membrane-bound complex that activates factor X to Xa. Factor Xa formed by the tissue factor/VIIa complex then interacts with factor Va to form another complex that converts prothrombin to thrombin. Thrombin then converts fibrinogen to fibrin, the ultimate step in hemostasis. The extrinsic system is assessed by the prothrombin time (PT). The *intrinsic system,* believed to be less physiologically important, is initiated by the binding of factor XII to foreign surfaces such as glass in vitro. The bound factor XII is cleaved by kallikrein and converted to factor XIIa, which in turn activates factor XI to XIa, which is identical to the factor XIa generated in the extrinsic system. The intrinsic system is assessed by the activated partial thromboplastin time (aPTT). The subsequent steps of conversion of prothrombin to thrombin and fibrinogen to fibrin are common to both extrinsic and intrinsic pathways. The fibrin clot that finally results is stabilized by a crosslinking enzyme, factor XIII.

The coagulation mechanism is regulated by a number of natural anticoagulants. Protease inhibitors neutralize activated coagulation proteins and dampen the coagulation cascade. Factors VIIa, IXa, Xa, and thrombin are neutralized by antithrombin III (ATT III), forming irreversible complexes that are cleared by the liver. Kallikrein and XIIa are inhibited by α_1-protease inhibitor. Factor VIIa is regulated by the extrinsic pathway inhibitor EPI. The protein C and protein S regulatory mechanism is directed at inhibiting factors Va and VIIIa.

FIBRINOLYSIS

The fibrinolytic system helps to limit formation of excessive clot at the site of injury and is activated simultaneously with coagulation. The system consists of an inactive proenzyme, plasminogen, that can be converted to enzymatically active plasmin by plasma and tissue activators released by endothelial cells. Plasmin degrades fibrin into soluble degradation products, so-called fibrin split products (FSP). Impaired action of the fibrinolytic system results in thrombotic diseases from impaired activation and hemorrhagic diseases from excessive activation.

DIAGNOSTIC APPROACH TO BLEEDING TENDENCY

The personal and family history are the best predictors of a bleeding tendency (Fig. 19-13). Individuals who have experienced excessive bleeding at circumcision, surgery, or following suture removal or dental procedures may have a congenital bleeding disorder. Anatomic causes of local bleeding and acquired bleeding disorders related to drugs, infections, or medical disorders must be excluded. The family history may suggest an inherited condition. X-linked traits include factors VIII and IX as well as Wiskott-Aldrich syndrome; heterozygous bleeding disorders include deficiencies of von Willebrand factor, factor XI, fibrinogen, and disorders of platelet number and function; bleeding tendencies caused by deficiencies of factors XIII, X, V, VII, II, and α_2-antiplasmin are usually homozygous or compound heterozygous traits.

Disorders of factors VIII, IX, and XI (the hemophilias) present with recurrent bleeding in skin and soft tissue, muscles, and joints. Bleeding may be severe and protracted after dental extraction. Persons with mild coagulation factor deficiencies may bleed only after trauma or surgery. Disorders of von Willebrand factor, fibrinogen,

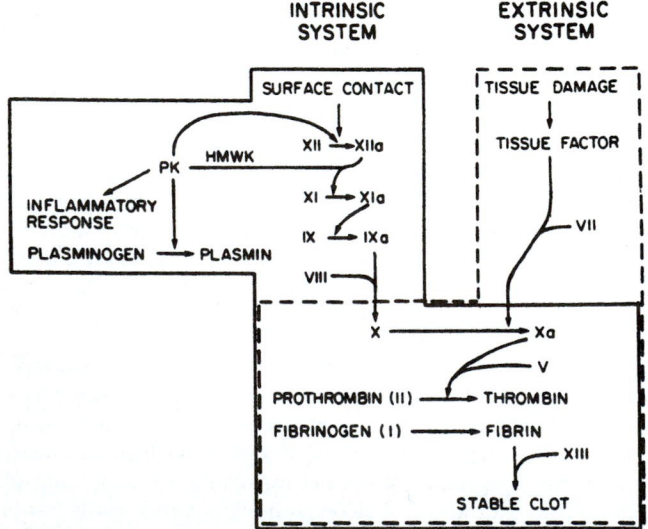

FIGURE 19-12   Scheme of blood coagulation. The suffix "a" denotes the activated factor with enzyme activity. PK = prekallikrein; HMWK = high-molecular-weight kininogen.

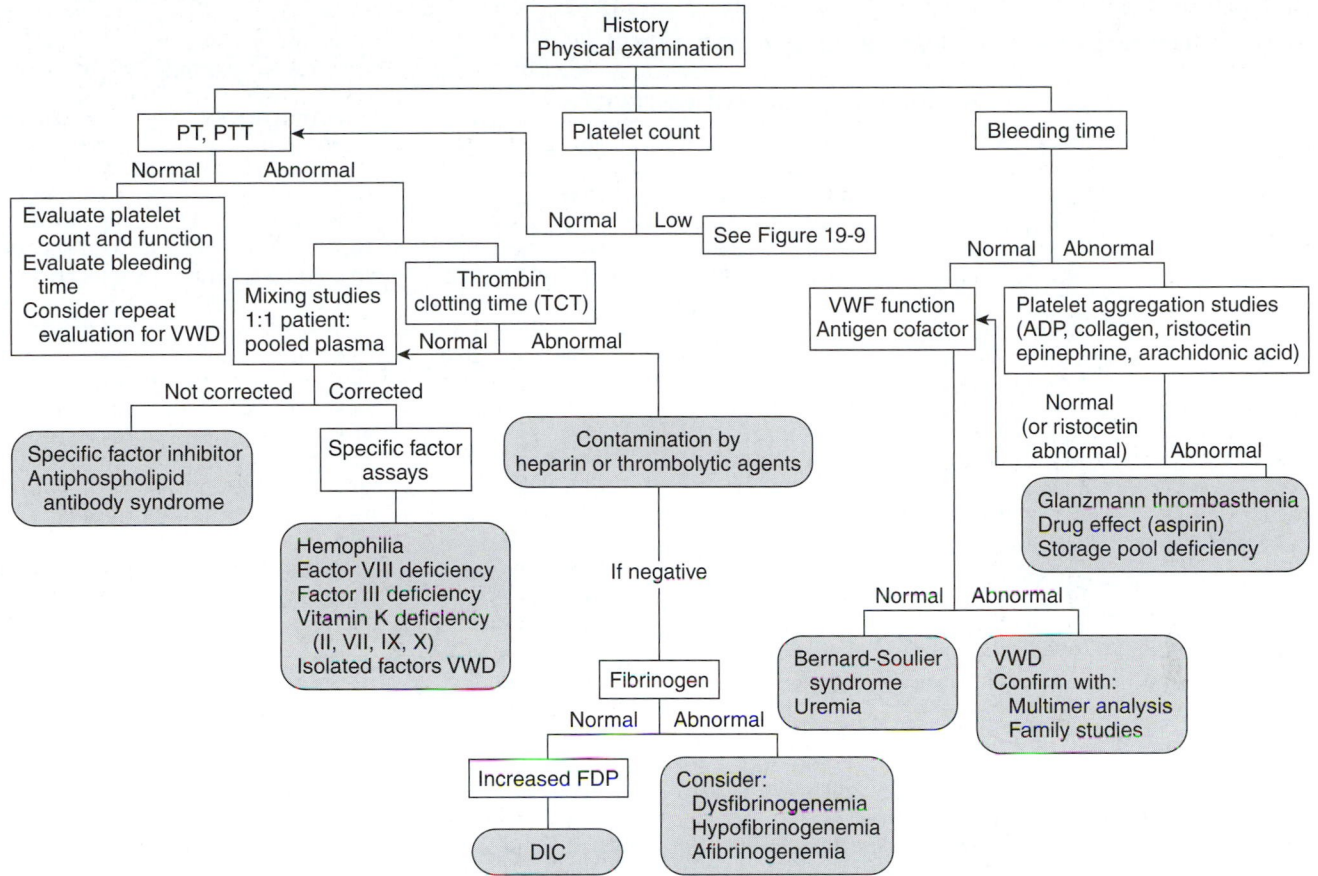

FIGURE 19-13 **Algorithm diagramming the laboratory evaluation of the child with bleeding.** **ADP** = adenosine diphosphate; **DIC** = disseminated intravascular coagulation; **FDP** = fibrin degradation products; **PT** = prothrombin time; **PTT** = partial prothrombin time; **VWD** = von Willebrand disease; **VWF** = von Willebrand factor. **SOURCE:** *Modified from Hastings and Lubin, Rudolph's Fundamentals of Pediatrics, Stamford: Appleton and Lange, 2nd Edition p. 486, 1998.*

platelet number, or platelet function present primarily with skin and mucous membrane bleeding including nosebleeds, menorrhagia, gastrointestinal bleeding, and bleeding with dental procedures. Children with a personal or family history suggestive of a bleeding disorder should receive a full hemostatic evaluation.

TESTS OF THE HEMOSTATIC MECHANISM

Three screening tests of coagulation are generally employed. (1) In the activated partial thromboplastin time (aPTT), which tests the intrinsic system, a contact-acting surface such as kaolin, calcium, and a platelet phospholipid are added to citrated plasma, and time to clot formation is measured in seconds. The normal aPTT is about 35 seconds. (2) In the prothrombin time, which tests the extrinsic system, tissue factor and calcium are added to citrated plasma, and time to clot formation is measured in seconds. The normal PT is about 12.5 seconds. (3) In the thrombin clotting time (TCT), thrombin is added to plasma, and the time to clot formation is measured in seconds. The TCT measures the conversion of fibrinogen to fibrin and is normally about 13 seconds. The platelet count is a reliable test for thrombocytopenia. The bleeding time is a global but not too accurate or specific test of platelet number and function. Special tests to measure the levels of most of the coagulation factors are available.

DEVELOPMENTAL ASPECTS OF HEMOSTASIS

Values for coagulation screening tests and specific factor assays in term and preterm infants are compared with results for adults in Table 19-17. The concentrations of many coagulation factors are decreased in premature infants and neonates. Of greatest clinical significance are the vitamin K–dependent factors (II, VII, IX, X, protein C, and protein S), which are present at 30 to 50% of adult concentration. Low plasma levels of vitamin K are common for 3 to 5 days following birth, which compounds decreased hepatic synthetic function. Prophylactic vitamin K at delivery is recommended for all infants. Plasma concentrations of the vitamin K–dependent factors do not reach adult levels for weeks to months postnatally. Factors XI, XII, prekallikrein, and kininogen are all moderately reduced at birth. In contrast, fibrinogen, factor V, factor VIII, von Willebrand factor, and factor XIII are above the normal adult range except in very small preterm infants. The decreased concentrations of coagulation factors explain the altered coagulation screening tests commonly found in neonates. Contact factor deficiencies account for the prolonged aPTT found in preterm infants. Decreased concentrations of factors II, VII, and X result in the slight prolongation of the PT found in healthy infants. Although the concentration of fibrinogen is normal in the neonate, a fetal form of fibrinogen that includes increased phosphorus and carbohydrate may

TABLE 19-17

COAGULATION SCREENING TESTS AND FACTOR LEVELS[A]

PARAMETER	PREMATURE (WEEKS OF GESTATION)			NEWBORNS (N = 60)	ADULTS (N = 40)
	19–23 (N = 20)	24–29 (N = 22)	30–38 (N = 22)		
PT (s)	32.5 (19–45)	32.2 (19–44)[†]	22.6 (16–30)[†]	16.7 (12.0–23.5)[*]	13.5 (11.4–14.0)
PT (INR)	6.4 (1.7–11.1)	6.2 (2.1–10.6)[†]	3.0 (1.5–5.0)[*]	1.7 (0.9–2.7)[*]	1.1 (0.8–1.2)
aPTT (s)	168.8 (83–250)	154.0 (87–210)[†]	104.8 (76–128)[†]	44.3 (35–52)[*]	33.0 (25–39)
TCT (s)	34.2 (24–44)[*]	26.2 (24–28)[*]	21.4 (17.0–23.3)	20.4 (15.2–25.0)[†]	14.0 (12–16)
Factor					
I (g/L von Clauss)	0.85 (0.57–1.50)	1.12 (0.65–1.65)	1.35 (1.25–1.65)	1.68 (0.95–2.45)[†]	3.0 (1.78–4.50)
I Ag (g/L)	1.08 (0.75–1.50)	1.93 (1.56–2.40)	1.94 (1.30–2.40)	2.65 (1.68–3.60)[†]	3.5 (2.50–5.20)
IIc (%)	16.9 (10–24)	19.9 (11–30)[*]	27.9 (15–50)[†]	43.5 (27–64)[†]	98.7 (70–125)
VIIc (%)	27.4 (17–37)	33.8 (18–48)[*]	45.9 (31–62)	52.5 (28–78)[†]	101.3 (68–130)
IXc (%)	10.1 (6–14)	9.9 (5–15)	12.3 (5–24)[†]	31.8 (15–50)[†]	104.8 (70–142)
Xc (%)m	20.5 (14–29)	24.9 (16–35)	28.0 (16–36)[†]	39.6 (21–65)[†]	99.2 (75–125)
Vc (%)	32.1 (21–44)	36.8 (25–50)	48.9 (23–70)[†]	89.9 (50–140)	99.8 (65–140)
VIIIc (%)	34.5 (18–50)	35.5 (20–52)	50.1 (27–78)[†]	94.3 (38–150)	101.8 (55–170)
XIc (%)	13.2 (8–19)	12.1 (6–22)	14.8 (6–26)[†]	37.2 (13–62)[†]	100.2 (70–135)
XIIc (%)	14.9 (6–25)	22.7 (6–40)	25.8 (11–50)[†]	69.8 (25–105)[†]	101.4 (65–144)
PK (%)	12.8 (8–19)	15.4 (8–26)	18.1 (8–28)[†]	35.4 (21–53)[†]	99.8 (65–135)
HMWK (%)	15.4 (10–22)	19.3 (10–26)	23.6 (12–34)[†]	38.9 (28–53)[†]	98.8 (68–135)

[a] Values are the mean, followed in parentheses by the lower and upper boundaries including 95% of the population.
Abbreviations: Ag = antigenic value; c = coagulant activity. [*]P < .05. [†]P < .01.
SOURCE: *Reverdiau-Moalic P, Delahousse B, Body G. et al: Evaluation of blood coagulation activators and inhibitors in the healthy human fetus. Blood 88:900, 1996.*

account for the mild prolongation of the TCT. Fetal forms of fibrinogen, von Willebrand factor, and others have been described. In addition to physiological alterations in coagulation, falsely abnormal coagulation studies can result from heparin contamination if blood is drawn through a catheter. Small amounts of heparin have a profound effect on the TCT time, a smaller effect on the aPTT, and least effect on the PT.

Despite prolongations of the aPTT, PT, and TCT, as well as the deficiencies of clotting factors, the whole blood of the preterm or term infant clots more quickly than the whole blood of children and adults. This paradoxic hypercoagulability has been attributed to a deficiency of naturally occurring anticoagulants or protease inhibitors such as protein C or AT-III. Fibrinolytic activity is increased in cord blood but rapidly decreases to adult levels, and FSP are not significantly elevated in normal infants.

19.10.1   Disorders of Coagulation

THE HEMOPHILIAS

Hemophilia is a clinical syndrome characterized by frequent and excessive bleeding caused by genetic deficiency or dysfunction of one of the coagulation proteins. The hemophilias manifest variably and are usually mild phenotypes when inherited as heterozygous traits and have severe symptoms when homozygous, compound heterozygous, or X-linked recessive hemizygous. The most common hemophilia, hemophilia A, is caused by a deficiency of factor VIII and accounts for 75% of hemophilia patients. Fifty percent of men with severe hemophilia A share a single mutation that consists of a p22 inversion on the X chromosome that forms a nonfunctional pseudogene, which can be detected using a PCR-based assay. The other 50% of affected men, including all those with mild hemophilia, have diverse mutations including insertions, deletions, and base pair substitutions that often require gene sequencing to detect.

Hemophilia B is caused by a deficiency of factor IX and is approximately one-fourth as common as hemophilia A. The genes for factors VIII and IX are located on the X chromosome; all of the other coagulation factors are encoded on autosomal chromosomes. Severe factor XI deficiency, also known as hemophilia C, is rare. Other proteins whose genetic deficiencies result in bleeding disorders include fibrinogen, factors II, V, VII, X, and XIII, α_2-antiplasmin, and plasminogen activator inhibitor (PAI-1). Deficiencies of components of the "contact activation cascade," including high-molecular-weight kininogen (HMWK), prekallikrein (PK), and factor XII, do not result in excessive bleeding even though marked prolongations in the aPTT occur. The von Willebrand factor (vWF), genetically distinct from factor VIII, circulates in plasma in association with factor VIII and stabilizes it. Mild to moderate deficiencies of vWF are found in approximately 1% of the population, making it the most prevalent genetic bleeding disorder.

The clinical severity of the hemophilias is classified on the basis of the level of the affected coagulant in comparison to a pool of normal individuals: severe is <1%, moderate is 1 to 5%, and mild is 5 to 30%. For most coagulation proteins, the lower limit of normal is 50 to 60%. Bleeding with activities of 30 to 50% is variable. Persons with severe deficiencies often bleed without apparent provocation, whereas persons with mild deficiencies experience excessive bleeding only with major trauma or surgery.

FACTOR VIII DEFICIENCY (CLASSIC HEMOPHILIA, HEMOPHILIA A)

The incidence of factor VIII deficiency is 1 in 7500 live male births. One-half of boys with severe hemophilia manifest excessive bleeding after neonatal circumcision. Affected infants commonly present between 6 and 12 months of age with mucous membrane bleeding after minor trauma or erupting primary teeth and soft-tissue bruising. Individuals with mild hemophilia commonly present later in childhood or adult life, often after trauma or surgery. Carrier girls with <50% plasma factor VIII activity can manifest clinical bleeding related to menses, dental procedures, surgery, and trauma. Hemophilia is suspected in a child with bruising or bleeding when the screening aPTT is prolonged and corrects with addition of an equal volume of normal plasma (see Fig. 19-13). The PT, TCT, fibrinogen concentration, and platelet count are normal. The bleeding time is prolonged in only 10% of persons with severe hemophilia. Diagnosis requires confirmation with specific assay of factor VIII activity. Assays of the von Willebrand factor are also warranted in the initial diagnosis of hemophilia A because the diagnosis of severe type III vWD or combined hemophilia A and type I vWD would otherwise be missed. A rare variant of vWD called vWD Normandy mimics the phenotype of hemophilia A and requires genetic or collagen-binding studies for accurate diagnosis. The differential diagnosis of factor VIII deficiency includes an acquired inhibitor to factor VIII or an artifact in sample processing and handling. Acquired factor VIII inhibitors are most common in women during or after pregnancy or in the elderly but rarely occur in children. An inhibitor can be excluded by determination of the factor VIII activity or aPTT before and after incubation at 37°C of a 1:1 mix of patient plasma with pooled normal plasma (see Fig. 19-13).

Prenatal determination of factor VIII activity can be performed on blood obtained by periumbilical cord blood sampling (PUBS) after 18 weeks, when fetal factor VIII levels are within the adult range. About 30% of diagnoses of hemophilia A are made in children with a negative family history, and carrier testing may be helpful. Because an important minority of female carriers have a clinical bleeding tendency, testing should be done before invasive procedures or surgery. A standard functional carrier-testing technique utilizes the ratio of factor VIII activity to the vWF antigen, which in normals is 1. A ratio of <0.8 confers a 90% chance of a hemophilia carrier, whereas a ratio of >0.9 gives a 90% chance that she is not a carrier. However, functional carrier testing does not discriminate carriers from noncarriers completely and has not been standardized for women during pregnancy. Restricted fragment length polymorphism (RFLP) is noninformative in at least 10% of families and is no longer the procedure of choice. Rarely, a female child is diagnosed with severe factor VIII deficiency. An assay of vWF must be performed to exclude type III vWD or vWF Normandy, and acquired antibodies to factor VIII must be excluded. If a girl has severe factor VIII deficiency, karyotype analysis should be performed to exclude the coexistence of a factor VIII mutation in a patient with XO Turner syndrome. If the karyotype is 46,XX, the low factor VIII level may be a result of random X inactivation according to the Lyon hypothesis or a condition known as "nonrandom X inactivation," in which one X-chromosome is selectively chosen over the other, a trait also transmitted independently on an X chromosome.

CLINICAL MANIFESTATIONS Bleeding in persons with severe hemophilia is usually internal, most often into skin, muscles, and joints, except in neonates with severe hemophilia, who may bleed from heel puncture and circumcision. Many infants with severe hemophilia A do not manifest a bleeding tendency until they become toddlers, with the minor traumas that occur with walking and climbing. Soft-tissue bleeds on the forehead, shins, and buttocks are first noticed, as well as protracted bleeding after trivial gum and tongue trauma. Multiple bruises of different ages may raise concerns about child abuse, especially if family history is negative.

Children begin to develop hemarthroses at a mean age of 2 years, which may be caused by minor trauma or may be sponta-

neous. The large joints, ankles, knees, and elbows are most frequently affected, and many children have one or two joints that are repeatedly affected. Early signs of joint bleeding include pain and tingling, abnormalities in gait and weight-bearing, and limitation of movement. Visible swelling and warmth are signs of late and severe hemarthrosis. After multiple episodes of bleeding into a single joint, hemosiderin deposition with synovial hyperplasia and bony overgrowth may occur. If recurrent bleeding is not prevented or arrested quickly, damage to cartilage, bone demineralization, cyst formation, erosion and narrowing of the joint surface, and degenerative arthritis may ensue.

Muscle hemorrhages are common in children with hemophilia A. Large amounts of blood can collect quickly in the iliopsoas and thigh muscles. Because muscles do not have a rigid casing to tamponade, hemorrhage into a large muscle can result in anemia and require weeks of therapy for complete resolution. Hemorrhages into the forearm and calf can cause compartment syndromes, which are limb-threatening emergencies.

Bleeding in the stool or vomitus usually results from rupture of a gastrointestinal mucosal hematoma. Hematuria can originate from any level of the genitourinary system. Life-threatening hemorrhages including intracranial or retroperitoneal hemorrhages occur in 10% of children with severe hemophilia A. After an initial episode, the risk of recurrence is increased. Children with severe hemophilia A are at risk for bleeding from any invasive procedure and should be pretreated with factor VIII before invasive procedures.

TREATMENT Factor VIII produced by recombinant technology is the product of choice for pediatric patients. The aim of treatment of bleeding is replacement of the deficient coagulation factor to attain a hemostatic level and stop bleeding. The dose and dose frequency are determined by the factor concentration required for hemostasis, the volume of distribution, and the plasma disappearance time of the factor. Factor VIII has a volume of distribution equivalent to the plasma volume (about 40 mL/kg). One unit (U) of any coagulant factor is defined as the amount present in 1 mL of normal, pooled plasma. One U/kg of factor VIII will raise the plasma concentration by 2%. The plasma half-life of factor VIII is approximately 12 hours.

Life-threatening hemorrhages should be treated immediately with 50 U/kg, which will raise the factor VIII level to 100%. In a suspected intracranial or retroperitoneal hemorrhage or major trauma, factor replacement should precede diagnostic tests or procedures. If an intracranial or retroperitoneal hemorrhage is confirmed, continuous infusion of factor VIII should be instituted to maintain a plasma level of 80 to 100% (4–6 U/kg/h). When the patient is stable and the hemorrhage is controlled, intermittent infusion therapy can be instituted. The child should be treated for 10 to 14 days. Neurosurgical intervention to evacuate a hematoma is rarely required.

Immediately before surgical procedures, a child should be given a bolus of 50 U/kg of factor VIII to raise the level to 100%. If a surgical procedure extends beyond 4 hours, an additional bolus of 25 U/kg should be given. Immediately after surgery, factor VIII activity should be determined, and a continuous infusion of 4 U/kg/h should be started. The factor VIII assay is used to adjust the rate of continuous infusion with a goal of maintaining a level of factor VIII of 80 to 100%. The continuous infusion is preferred because a constant plasma level without peaks and troughs is achieved. The infusion may be continued for one to several days, and thereafter factor VIII is administered by bolus infusion every 12 hours for the first 5 postoperative days, then every 1 to 2 days for the duration of wound healing. In orthopedic procedures, replacement infusions are usually required before each physical therapy session for 6 weeks.

Therapy of acute joint hemorrhages with a single infusion of factor VIII at a dose of 20 U/kg is usually associated with resolution of acute pain and joint limitation. However, single-infusion therapy is ineffective in preventing chronic joint degeneration and is not recommended. Alternative therapy for acute hemarthrosis includes infusion of multiple doses of factor VIII for each episode of joint hemorrhage, giving 40 U/kg of factor VIII immediately on recognizing a joint hemorrhage, with infusions of 20 U/kg at 24 and 72 hours and then continuing every other day until the joint is pain-free and has no swelling and full range of motion.

The optimal management to prevent joint damage in children with hemophilia is controversial. Because the severity of chronic hemophilic arthropathy can be related to the number of episodes of hemarthrosis, prophylactic therapy has been employed. In a long-term study in Sweden, children with severe hemophilia were treated with routine replacement infusions of factor VIII every other day for 30 years. This prophylactic regimen was effective in reducing (but not eliminating entirely) joint hemorrhages and in greatly reducing (but not eliminating entirely) physical and radiologic signs of joint damage. A major disadvantage of prophylactic therapy is cost, which can exceed $250,000/year for an adolescent, and the need for central venous access devices (VADs), which have a high risk of infections. Currently a prospective randomized clinical trial in the United States is in progress, comparing prophylactic infusions with the multiple-dose regimen for each hemarthrosis. Muscle hemorrhages usually respond clinically to 20 to 40 U/kg of factor VIII. Large muscle hemorrhages should be treated with higher doses and multiple infusions to prevent compartment syndromes and muscle atrophy. Soft-tissue hemorrhages are usually treated with a single infusion of 20 to 30 U/kg of factor VIII. Small hematomas may be treated with ice alone. Children with lacerations requiring sutures should receive factor VIII infusions at the time of suturing and again at the time of suture removal. Despite apparently adequate control of surgical bleeding, the wound will often break down unless infusions are given for both procedures. Fractures require factor replacement at the time of reduction and casting, after which the external cast compression is usually adequate to prevent bleeding. However, when the cast is removed, the atrophied limb is susceptible to hemorrhage after even minor trauma. Factor VIII should be infused at the time of cast removal and before each physical therapy session until the limb regains strength.

Gross hematuria is not uncommon in children with hemophilia. Factor infusions are ineffective and usually unnecessary. Hematuria is treated with bed rest and and hydration. If bleeding does not lessen over several days, a short course of prednisone, 1 to 2 mg/kg/d, is anecdotally helpful.

Desmopressin acetate (DDAVP) is a synthetic arginine vasopressin that releases stores of factor VIII and vWF from endothelial cells. Typically, factor VIII activity will rise three- to fivefold after administration of DDAVP. Hemophiliacs with a baseline factor VIII concentration of 10 to 20% can often use DDAVP instead of factor VIII concentrates for minor hemorrhages and surgery. A factor VIII assay 1 hour after DDAVP challenge is recommended before use of this product alone. Persons with mild factor VIII deficiency may be able to alternate use of DDAVP with factor VIII

concentrate following major surgery. DDAVP may be administered intravenously in a dose of 0.3 μg/kg. A high-potency nasal spray may be used in children old enough to inhale the drug. One puff in a single nostril is adequate for children less than 50 kg; two puffs, one in each nostril, is used for larger children. Therapeutic efficacy must be documented before use because mucosal inflammation or thickening may limit absorption.

Aminocaproic acid and tranexamic acid, fibrinolytic inhibitors, are useful adjunctive therapy for bleeding involving the teeth, tongue, and gums. Topical coagulants, including topical thrombin and fibrin gel, are useful to control diffusely oozing surfaces. Vitamin K replacement is not indicated.

GENERAL CARE FOR CHILDREN WITH HEMOPHILIA After a diagnosis of hemophilia has been established, families should be offered immediate and ongoing education and support to adjust to the diagnosis and begin to form a healthy and realistic view of the wellness of their child. Routine immunizations, including hepatitis A and B, should be given using small-bore needles. Prophylactic dental care is very important to avoid the need for oral surgery later. Physical exercise and fitness must be emphasized early to develop optimal musculoskeletal strength. In school years, full physical education, swimming, bicycling, and hiking are encouraged. Preactivity infusions may be necessary for participation in soccer, baseball, and similar sports. Contact sports are not recommended for children with hemophilia.

Home infusions, with or without the use of an indwelling venous access device, reduce the trauma of repeated emergency room visits and permit a child to accept hemophilia as a manageable disorder. Parents require comprehensive initial education and continuing support to maintain home infusion therapy successfully.

FACTOR VIII INHIBITORS Neutralizing antibodies to factor VIII develop in 25 to 30% of persons with hemophilia A. These antibodies, called inhibitors, are more frequent in children with severe factor VIII deficiency and are IgG_4 subtype. Inhibitor development requires exposure to factor VIII, with a median of nine exposures before antibody detection. If an inhibitor has not developed after 50 exposures to factor VIII, the probability of future antibody formation is very low. Persons with a positive family history of inhibitor formation are at greater risk. Inhibitors are quantified by their ability to inactivate factor VIII in serial dilutions of normal pooled plasma and are reported in Bethesda Units (B.U.). Inhibitors are classified as high titer ($\geq$10 B.U.) versus low titer ($<$10 B.U.) and as high responding (marked increase in inhibitor titer following reexposure to factor VIII) versus low responding (little or no increase in inhibitor titer following reexposure to factor VIII).

A new-onset inhibitor can be treated by inducing immune tolerance to factor VIII by continuous antigen exposure. A standard regimen for inducing immune tolerance is 100 U/kg of factor VIII given once a day by intravenous bolus. Other schedules have reduced the inhibitor level, and the most medically and cost-effective regimen has not yet been determined. Immune modulation with suppressive agents such as cytoxan and IVIG have been infrequently evaluated in children.

FACTOR IX DEFICIENCY (CHRISTMAS DISEASE, HEMOPHILIA B)

Factor IX deficiency is inherited as an X-linked recessive disorder. It tends to be a clinically milder disorder than hemophilia A, even at comparable levels of factor activity. In general factor IX–deficient children experience fewer joint hemorrhages and fewer arthritic joints than children with factor VIII deficiency. Inhibitors develop in approximately 5% of persons with factor IX deficiency.

Hemophilia B is diagnosed by assay of factor IX coagulant activity. Approximately 10% of hemophilia B patients manifest a dysproteinemia with a discrepancy between the factor IX activity and antigen assay. Some female carriers have factor IX activities as low as 10% and have clinically significant bleeding signs, and so potential factor IX carriers should be assessed for factor IX level. No functional carrier test for factor IX exists, but direct gene sequencing is possible. The factor IX gene defect should be determined in hemophilia B families to facilitate carrier testing and prenatal diagnosis.

TREATMENT The volume of distribution for factor IX is approximately twice the plasma volume. Therefore, 1 U/kg of factor IX concentrate increases the plasma concentration by 1%. The plasma half-life of factor IX is approximately 24 hours. A recombinant factor IX product is commercially available and is similar to the native plasma-derived factor IX except that it is not sulfated. Plasma recovery of this product is variable, with increases of plasma factor IX activity from 0.3 to 1% per 1 U/kg infused. Determining plasma recovery is important to establish proper dosing. Human plasma-derived factor IX concentrates, which are highly purified by monoclonal antibody affinity or chromatographic techniques, are effective and safe products. Intermediate-purity factor IX products, which contain significant amounts of factors II, VII, and X, are inappropriate for use in surgery or severe hemorrhages because of their intrinsic thrombogenicity.

Aggressive treatment of joint hemorrhages consists of initial treatment with 80 U/kg of factor IX, followed by 40 U/kg at 48 hours. Prophylactic infusions to prevent hemorrhages can be accomplished using twice-a-week infusions of 40 U/kg for a 3-day interval and 60 U/kg for a 4-day interval. Life-threatening hemorrhages should be treated with 100 U/kg of factor IX. Preoperative replacement should provide 80 to 100 U/kg of factor IX. Because of the long half-life, continuing therapy can be given as a bolus once a day. Factor IX activity assays should be used to monitor postoperative therapy.

VON WILLEBRAND DISEASE

von Willebrand disease (vWD) is caused by a decrease in the plasma concentration or function of the vWF protein. The vWF is encoded on chromosome 12, and the gene product is assembled as a dimer with a molecular mass of approximately 270 kDa. This dimer forms multimers ranging from 540 to 2000 kDa. vWF is synthesized in megakaryocytes and endothelial cells and is stored in subcellular compartments in the endothelial cells and the α-granules in platelets, from which regulated release occurs. Following release into the plasma, very large-molecular-weight multimers of vWF are proteolyzed to smaller multimers. When secreted into the plasma, vWF associates with and stabilizes factor VIII. The complex dissociates when factor VIII is activated in the coagulation cascade. The vWF binds to membrane GPIb on the platelet surface and to subendothelial cell collagen, supporting primary platelet adhesion. Larger molecular multimers are more effective in supporting platelet–vessel interactions, and all sized multimers stabilize factor VIII activity. The vWF antigen levels can be determined immunologically and are reflected in ristocetin-induced platelet aggregation.

PRESENTATION AND DIAGNOSIS The prevalence of vWD in the population is approximately 1%, making it the most common genetic bleeding disorder. von Willebrand disease is inherited as an autosomal dominant with incomplete penetrance. Three different forms of vWD have been described: types I, II, and III. The condition is characterized clinically by bruising, epistaxis, menorrhagia, hemorrhage after tonsillectomy and dental procedures, and gastrointestinal bleeding. Women with vWD often have menometrorrhagia, and about 15% of women with excessive uterine bleeding have vWD.

Coagulation screening tests show a normal PT, a normal or prolonged aPTT, and a normal or prolonged bleeding time. A full evaluation of vWF activity, antigen, and multimers; factor VIII activity; and blood type is necessary to characterize the disorder; (see Fig. 19-13). Populations of healthy individuals with type O blood have a range of vWF concentration that is lower than persons with types A or B. Few molecular abnormalities have been identified in the vWF gene sequence of most individuals with type I vWD. In type I vWD the decreases in factor VIII activity and vWF antigen are similar. The aPTT prolongation is proportional to the decrease in assayed factor VIII activity.

Type II vWD is a dysproteinemia with variable degrees of bleeding. The vWF antigen level may be normal. Type IIa is characterized by an absence of large and intermediate-sized multimers. Type IIb typically shows a decrease in large multimers, but these result from increased turnover of excessively large multimers. Several other type II vWD and gene mutations have been identified.

Type III vWD is an autosomal recessive disorder usually associated with severe bleeding; vWF activity and antigen and factor VIII activity are <5% of normal.

Compound heterozygotes have been described combining the various types of vWD.

TREATMENT Most patients with type I vWF can be treated with slow, intravenous infusions or with intranasal DDAVP, as in mild hemophilia A. The response of persons with type II vWD to DDAVP therapy is variable, and thrombocytopenia and thrombosis may occur in association with DDAVP therapy. Individuals with type III vWD are very unlikely to respond to DDAVP.

Human plasma-derived viral-inactivated vWF concentrates are available for replacement therapy for persons with types II or III vWD or moderate type I vWD undergoing surgery or with major hemorrhage. There are no recombinant vWF products available for clinical use. Cryoprecipitate is no longer recommended.

ϵ-Aminocaproic acid (Amicar) and tranexamic acid are especially useful to treat minor mucosal bleeding and may be given as an oral rinse that prevents local fibrinolysis. ϵ-Aminocaproic acid has been used to treat menorrhagia. Many women with vWD use oral contraceptive agents to help control menstrual bleeding.

FACTOR XI DEFICIENCY (HEMOPHILIA C)

Deficiency of factor XI is inherited as an autosomal trait and has been reported most frequently in persons of Ashkenazi Jewish ancestry. Homozygous deficiency is associated with traumatic and spontaneous hemorrhages that are generally milder than factor VIII or IX deficiencies. Heterozygotes have a 50% chance of bleeding with surgery or significant trauma. Infusions of 1 mL/kg of fresh-frozen plasma (FFP) achieves a 1% increase of plasma factor XI. The plasma half-life of factor XI is approximately 3 days.

PROTHROMBIN, FACTOR V, FACTOR VII, AND FACTOR X DEFICIENCY

Deficiencies of factors II, V, VII, and X are rare autosomally inherited disorders. Factor VII deficiency is associated with an isolated prolongation of the PT. Factor II, V, and X deficiencies prolong both aPTT and PT. Specific assays for each of these factors are available. Persons with homozygous deficiencies have mild to moderate bruising, nosebleeds, menorrhagia, bleeding associated with surgery, as well as muscle and joint hemorrhage. Heterozygous carriers may have bruising and surgical bleeding. A dose of 1 mL/kg of FFP increases plasma factor V level 2% and factors II, VII, and X 1%. The plasma half-life of factor II is 3 days, factor VII 4 to 6 hours, and factors V and X 20 hours. Factors II, VII, and X are present in variable concentrations in specific plasma-derived, viral-inactivated prothrombin complex concentrates.

AFIBRINOGENEMIA, HYPOFIBRINOGENEMIA, AND DYSFIBRINOGENEMIA

Persons with deficient or defective fibrinogen may have variable bleeding symptoms similar to those seen in platelet disorders, including epistaxis, mucous membrane bleeding, menorrhagia, and bruising. Intracranial hemorrhages can also occur, but joint and muscle hemorrhages are rare. In afibrinogenemia the aPTT, PT, and bleeding time are prolonged. The disorder can be suspected by a prolongation of the TCT. Confirmatory tests include both functional and immunologic assays of fibrinogen. Rarely, dysfibrinogenemia manifests as thrombosis secondary to impaired endogenous lysis of the abnormal fibrin clot.

DEFICIENCIES OF FACTORS OF THE INTRINSIC SYSTEM

Deficiencies of the intrinsic or contact factors, prekallikrein, high-molecular-weight kininogen, and factor XII are not associated with clinical bleeding, and contact factors may be more important in initiation of fibrinolysis and inflammation. Although factor XII deficiency may predispose to thrombosis, several large studies have not confirmed this. Disorders of the intrinsic system are suggested by a marked prolongation of the aPTT, often detected on routine preoperative screening, in a person without a bleeding disorder. Heterozygous deficiencies of high-molecular-weight kininogen and factor XII but not of prekallikrein are associated with a prolonged aPTT. The diagnosis is confirmed by specific factor assay.

CONGENITAL FACTOR DEFICIENCIES ASSOCIATED WITH NORMAL COAGULATION SCREENING TESTS

Deficiencies of factor XIII, α_2-antiplasma, and plasminogen activator inhibitor (PAI-1) do not result in prolongations of the screening tests, including aPTT, PT, TCT, or bleeding time, and require specific assay for diagnosis. These disorders should be suspected in persons with a positive bleeding history in whom all coagulation screening tests are normal (see Fig. 19-13).

FACTOR XIII DEFICIENCY After activation by thrombin, factor XIII causes clot stabilization. Homozygous factor XIII deficiency is a rare autosomal recessive disorder characterized by delayed bleeding and poor wound healing secondary to unstable clot formation. Most affected individuals have bleeding and delayed separation of the umbilical cord. Carrier mothers frequently have a history of spontaneous abortion, and liveborn babies have a 25% risk of spontaneous intracranial hemorrhage, which may be recurrent. All term infants with intracranial hemorrhage should be evaluated for factor XIII deficiency. Skin bruising and occasional joint hemorrhages may occur in these patients. Heterozygotes are asymptomatic. Quantitative fluorometric, spectrometric, or immunologic assays are available for confirmation of the deficiency. Because the plasma half-life of factor XIII is about 10 days, and only a 1% plasma level of factor XIII is adequate to maintain hemostasis, homozygous patients may receive prophylactic replacement infusions of factor XIII on a monthly schedule.

α_2-**ANTIPLASMIN AND PAI-1 DEFICIENCIES** α_2-Plasmin is involved in the regulation of fibrinolysis and plasmin inactivation, resulting in dysfunctional clot lysis and bleeding. Patients with homozygous α_2-antiplasmin deficiency have mucous membrane, skin, and soft tissue bleeding and delayed bleeding into surgical sites. Deficiency of PAI-1 is clinically similar and results in mouth, mucous membrane, skin, and soft tissue bleeding, and intracranial hemorrhage has been reported. PAI-1 deficiency can be treated with antifibrinolytic agents and plasma infusions.

VITAMIN K DEFICIENCY

Factors II, VII, IX, and X, protein C, and protein S require vitamin K to be fully functional. Posttranslation carboxylation of 9 to 12 γ-glutamic acid residues in this group of proteins is necessary for calcium-dependent surface binding. The vitamin K cycle utilizes three hepatic enzymes, vitamin K carboxylase (also known as epoxidase), epoxidase reductase, and vitamin K reductase, and two cofactors in addition to exogenous vitamin K_1 or phylloquinone. Rare genetic deficiencies of this pathway, which are autosomal recessive disorders, present with combined deficiencies of all vitamin K–dependent proteins. Much more common is acquired vitamin K deficiency associated with fat malabsorption and cholestasis and rarely poor dietary intake. Children at high risk because of malabsorption can be treated with 1 mg of parenteral vitamin K each month or 10 mg orally per week. Coumadin-type oral anticoagulants inhibit the vitamin K cycle.

Vitamin K deficiency bleeding (VKDB) in childhood occurs in three clinical syndromes. (1) Early VKDB presents during the first hours after birth with skin, intracranial, or gastrointestinal hemorrhage and is related to decreased placental transfer of maternal vitamin K; the maternal:fetal ratio of plasma vitamin K levels is 10:1. Maternal Coumadin therapy may result in peripartum bleeding of the infant. (2) Classic VKDB (hemorrhagic disease of the newborn) presents during the first week, usually in breast-fed infants. Human breast milk contains only 1.5 mg/L of vitamin K compared to 15 mg/L in cow's milk. VKDB can be prevented with a single dose of 1 mg of vitamin K_1 given intramuscularly at birth or 3 to 5 mg of vitamin K given orally in one to three daily doses. (3) Late VKDB may present up to 2 months of life and is particularly common in Asian children because of continuing poor intake and perhaps other factors. VKDB after infancy is usually caused by fat malabsorption.

In vitamin K deficiency states, the PT and aPTT are prolonged, and the TCT, fibrinogen concentration, and platelet count are normal. Assays of individual vitamin K–dependent factors show a moderately decreased antigen level with a disproportionately greater decrease in functional activity. Noncarboxylated forms of vitamin

K–dependent proteins can be measured in the plasma and confirm the diagnosis. Treatment with 1 mg of parenteral vitamin K produces a decrease in the PT within 4 to 6 hours and normalization by 24 hours. Larger doses are unnecessary. Parenteral vitamin K alone is almost always sufficient to treat vitamin K–deficient bleeding, but in severe critical bleeding, FFP infusions can correct the abnormality.

LIVER DISEASE

Severe liver disease can result in a complex coagulopathy caused by decreased clotting factor synthesis, pathologic fibrinolysis, acquired dysfibrinogenemia, platelet destruction and dysfunction, and often vitamin K deficiency (see Chapter 18). Abnormalities of coagulation screening tests include prolongations of the aPTT, PT, and TCT, decreased concentrations of fibrinogen and platelets, and elevated fibrin(ogen) split products. Bleeding emergencies or invasive procedures including liver biopsy often require replacement with plasma, cryoprecipitate, viral-inactivated concentrates of vitamin K–dependent proteins and platelets, fibrinolysis inhibitors, and DDAVP.

DISSEMINATED INTRAVASCULAR COAGULATION (DIC)

DIC is a clinical syndrome in which thrombin is generated, resulting in deposition of fibrin in small blood vessels and consumption of coagulation factors and platelets (see Sec. 4.1). The deposition of fibrin strands in the blood vessels leads to RBC fragmentation and microangiopathic hemolytic anemia (see Fig. 19-5L). Both hemorrhage and thrombosis may occur. DIC may be precipitated by severe infection, massive trauma, hypoxia, and shock. A broad range of laboratory tests of hemostasis are abnormal, including prolonged PT, aPTT, and TCT as well as hypofibrinogenemia and FSP.

Therapy is directed at correcting the underlying disease process with antibiotics and ventilatory and circulatory support. Coagulation abnormalities are treated with infusions of FFP and platelets. Low-dose heparin is sometimes used in conjunction with FFP and platelet replacement.

19.10.2   Thrombotic Disorders

GENETIC THROMBOTIC DISORDERS

Thrombophilia, a clinical syndrome characterized by recurrent thrombotic events caused by genetic deficiencies in one or more of the coagulation regulatory and fibrinolytic proteins, affects approximately 1:1000 individuals. Thrombotic events usually present after puberty but may occur during the neonatal period or in childhood. About 10% appear during the first 10 years of life. Venous thromboses are most frequent, but arterial events including stroke may also occur. Thrombophilia is often triggered by factors such as indwelling catheters, surgery, trauma, treatment for systemic disease, or oral contraceptive therapy. Such underlying conditions do not exclude genetic thrombophilia in a patient with a thrombotic episode. Most genetic thrombophilias are inherited as autosomal dominant traits with variable penetrance, and homozygotes and compound heterozygotes are severely affected. Type I defects are caused by hypoproteinemias, whereas type II defects are caused by dysproteinemias.

Factor V Leiden (Arg506→Gln) is a genetic mutation in the procoagulant factor V molecule that induces resistance to inactivation by the physiological inhibitor activated protein C. This trait is found in 3 to 10% of whites, but it does not occur in blacks or in Asians. Factor V Leiden increases the background risk of venous thrombosis in heterozygotes by sevenfold, in homozygotes by 80-fold, and is additive to factors that predispose to thrombosis. Factor V Leiden trait is suggested by increased resistance to activated protein C in a functional clotting assay and is confirmed with a PCR-based assay. Approximately 20% of individuals with resistance to activated protein C on functional testing lack the factor V Leiden mutation and may have another mutation or an acquired abnormality.

Protein C is the zymogen of activated protein C, which downregulates cofactors Va and VIIIa by enzymatic cleavage. Heterozygous protein C deficiency occurs in 0.3% of the population and increases the risk of thrombosis sevenfold. Homozygous protein C deficiency is usually lethal. At least 160 different protein C mutations have been identified.

Deficiency of protein S, the nonenzymatic cofactor for protein C, is about one-half as prevalent as protein C deficiency. Type I deficiency of protein S is identified by a decrease in the total immunologic concentration of protein S in the plasma. Type II or dysproteinemic protein S is determined in a functional clotting assay. Type III protein S deficiency is characterized by a decrease in the immunologic concentration of free protein S in the presence of normal total protein S antigen. Sixty mutations have been associated with protein S deficiency and thrombosis.

Antithrombin III deficiency is found in 0.05 to 0.1% of the population and increases the risk of thrombosis fivefold. No infants with homozygous antithrombin III deficiency have been described, attesting to a critical role in thrombin regulation. Women with antithrombin III deficiency have a high incidence of thrombosis when taking oral contraceptive agents and have an almost 100% rate of thrombosis during pregnancy or postpartum. At present 79 antithrombin III mutations have been reported.

A high level of apparently normal factor VIII (>150%), with concomitant increases in vWF, is a risk factor for venous thrombosis. This high level is present in 10% of the population and increases the risk of venous thrombosis 2.5-fold.

Hyperhomocysteinemia increases the risk of thrombosis and arterial disease 2.5-fold. Hyperhomocysteinemia is associated with a polymorphism in the methyl tetrahydrofolate reductase gene as well as dietary deficiencies of vitamins B_6, B_{12}, and folate (see Sec. 19.3.4).

A prothrombin mutation that results in increased levels of prothrombin is found in about 2% of the white population and results in a 2.8-fold risk of venous thrombosis.

NEONATAL MANIFESTATIONS AND TREATMENT Children with severe deficiencies of protein C or protein S, sometimes combined with other thrombophilic traits, may develop purpura fulminans and severe DIC in the newborn period. Many of these infants have had in utero thromboses of the brain, eye, or kidney or other central venous thromboses. Assay of protein C or protein S show levels <0.05 U/mL. Most affected infants are compound heterozygotes rather than homozygotes unless a history of consanguinity is present. The diagnosis must be established so that replacement of the missing protein can be done as soon as possible. Protein C is available for compassionate use as a human plasma-derived viral-inactivated concentrate. Lifelong oral anticoagulation with Coumadin is necessary, and, with this treatment, a small number of children have survived to adolescence. Some individuals with low plasma concentrations of protein C have deep vein thrombosis during adolescence followed by recurrent episodes of DIC and purpura fulminans.

ANTIPHOSPHOLIPID ANTIBODY SYNDROMES

Antiphospholipid antibodies include the lupus anticoagulant and anticardiolipin antibodies. Lupus anticoagulants are IgG, IgM, or IgA antibodies that interfere with phospholipid-based clotting assays. Thrombosis in association with lupus anticoagulants may occur in diverse conditions including systemic lupus erythematosus, the primary antiphospholipid antibody syndrome, leukemia, other malignancies, or after infections. Children with primary antiphospholipid antibody syndrome have a high prevalence of other autoantibodies. Thrombosis associated with a lupus anticoagulant may be venous or arterial, and pulmonary emboli and recurrent thrombosis are common. About a third of children with stroke have an IgG, IgM, or IgA antibody directed against cardiolipin. Children positive for a persistent lupus anticoagulant should be maintained on long-term Coumadin anticoagulation.

Diagnosis of the lupus anticoagulant is made by prolongation of one or more functional clotting assays that does not correct with addition of normal pooled plasma but that corrects with addition of excess phospholipid (see Fig. 19-13). The anticardiolipin antibody is usually detected in an ELISA assay.

ACQUIRED THROMBOEMBOLIC DISEASES

Deep vein thromboses (DVT) are rare in children. Lower extremity DVT are manifested by pain and swelling, and Homan sign is frequently positive. Pulmonary embolism may occur. When the upper extremities are involved, DVT is almost always associated with central venous lines (CVL) that are placed for intensive care, total parenteral nutrition, cancer chemotherapy, or hemodialysis. DVT may also complicate L-asparaginase therapy in leukemia. Clinical symptoms of acute CVL-related DVT include swelling, pain, discoloration of the involved extremity, and line blockage. The risk of DVT associated with CVL may be decreased by prophylactic flushes with heparin. Routine prophylactic therapy with Coumadin for children with CVL is not advocated but should be considered if there is recurrent DVT or pulmonary embolism. A possible associated thrombophilia should be considered.

ANTICOAGULATION   There are two major types of anticoagulant therapy. Heparin enhances the activity of antithrombin III, forming complexes with prothrombin and factors IXa and Xa, which inhibit their activity. An intravenous loading dose of 75 U/kg followed by a maintenance dose of 20 U/kg/h should maintain adequate anticoagulation, as indicated by a prolonged aPTT to $1\frac{1}{2}$ to 2 times baseline. Low-molecular-weight heparin, which can be administered subcutaneously every 12 hours, has become the treatment of choice in children; the usual dose is 1.0 mg/kg every 12 hours. Monitoring must use an anti–factor Xa assay, not the aPTT.

Oral anticoagulation is accomplished by the use of warfarin (Coumadin) therapy. Adequacy of anticoagulation is assessed by the INR, which assesses the drug-induced prolongation of the PT. The initial loading dose is 0.2 mg/kg, followed by daily maintenance doses adjusted to maintain an INR of 2.0 to 3.0.

References

Esmon CT: Blood coagulation. In: Nathan DG, Orkin SH, eds: Nathan and Oski's Hematology of Infancy and Childhood, 5th ed. Philadelphia, WB Saunders, 1998:1531–1556

Montgomery RR, Gill JC, Scott JP: Hemophilia and von Willebrand disease. In: Nathan DG, Orkin SH, eds: Nathan and Oski's Hematology of Infancy and Childhood, 5th ed. Philadelphia, WB Saunders, 1998: 1631–1660

White GC II, Marder VJ, Coleman RW, Hirsh J, Salzman EW: Approach to the bleeding patient. In: Hemostasis and Thrombosis: Basic Principles and Clinical Practice, 3rd ed. Philadelphia, JB Lippincott, 1994

19.11 USE OF BLOOD AND BLOOD PRODUCTS

Susan A. Galel and J. Lawrence Naiman

Since the advent of the HIV/AIDS epidemic in the early 1980s, physicians have become increasingly aware that blood transfusions should be used only when the benefits clearly exceeded the risks. Use of only volunteer donors, improved viral screening of donated blood, the availability of safer plasma derivatives, and better systems for removal of unwanted leukocytes have greatly reduced the risks of transmitting infection, acute reactions to transfusion, and refractoriness in patients requiring frequent transfusions. RBC components in common use and clinical indications are summarized in Table 19-18. One "unit" of a blood component is defined as that derived from one whole blood donation, which is 450 to 500 mL collected into an anticoagulant-preservative solution. Components such as red blood cells, plasma, and platelets are separated by dif-

TABLE 19-18

BLOOD COMPONENTS USED TO IMPROVE OXYGEN DELIVERY

BLOOD COMPONENT	VOLUME (mL)	HCT (%)	SHELF-LIFE	INDICATIONS AND DOSE
Red blood cells, adenine-saline added	300–400	55–65	42 days	For increasing red cell mass in symptomatic anemia 10 mL/kg raises Hct by 8 percentage points
Packed red cells CPDA-1	200–300	65–80	5 days	Indications same as above 10 mL/kg increases Hct by 10 percentage points
Whole blood	500	35–40	35 days[a]	For hypovolemic anemia and for massive transfusion or exchange in infants

[a] Shelf-life is reduced to 28 days after irradiation (citrate, phosphate, dextrose, adenine anticoagulant).

ferential centrifugation and stored separately under conditions that optimize preservation of function. One whole-blood donation represents 10 to 15% of an adult's blood volume, and one unit of a blood component should constitute an approximately 10% replacement for an adult patient. Proportional replacement in infants and children can be calculated on the basis of an estimated blood volume of approximately 75 to 80 mL/kg.

19.11.1 Red Blood Cells

Packed RBC are prepared by centrifugation of one unit of whole blood with removal of most of the plasma and are resuspended in an additive solution for storage in the refrigerator.

The usual indication for RBC transfusion is to increase the oxygen-carrying capacity of blood in patients with anemia. A decision about when to transfuse an anemic child should be based on several factors, including (1) the presence or absence of symptoms or signs of anemia, such as tachycardia, tachypnea, lethargy, and exercise intolerance; (2) the actual level of hemoglobin/hematocrit; (3) whether the anemia is acute or developed slowly; and (4) the presence of coexisting cardiopulmonary problems or infections that might impair the patient's ability to tolerate the anemia.

WHOLE BLOOD

With the advent of component therapy, whole blood has become generally unavailable. Reconstituted whole blood can be prepared by adding fresh-frozen plasma to packed RBC. A common indication for use of whole blood is exchange transfusion or massive transfusion in neonates. For exchange transfusion, the albumin in plasma facilitates bilirubin binding and removal, and coagulation proteins minimize any dilutional coagulopathy. In infants undergoing open-heart surgery, postoperative bleeding may be reduced by using whole blood that is not more than 24 to 48 hours old.

CHANGES IN BLOOD DURING STORAGE

Donor blood is collected in a mixture of a citrate anticoagulant and a preservative solution that maintains adenosine triphosphate (ATP) for RBC viability and neutral pH. Following transfusion, stored RBC regenerate 2,3-DPG, resulting in restoration of hemoglobin function within 24 hours, so that adverse effects of storage on hemoglobin function are of consequence only in patients with acute hypoxia and those receiving large volumes of stored RBC. With increasing storage, potassium accumulates in the plasma, which can cause hyperkalemia when large volumes are infused over a short time.

Whole blood stored for over 24 hours has reduced levels of platelets and labile clotting factors (V and VIII). Correction of hemostatic defects is better achieved with specific components such as platelet concentrates, fresh-frozen plasma, or recombinant coagulation factor preparations (see Secs. 19.7 and 19.10).

LEUKOCYTE-REDUCED RBC

Leukocytes in RBC products serve no useful purpose and may have deleterious effects, including febrile reactions in frequently transfused patients who have developed antileukocyte antibodies, HLA-induced alloimmunization resulting in refractoriness to platelet transfusions, and transmission of WBC-associated viruses such as cytomegalovirus (CMV). These risks can be minimized with the use of high-efficiency filters that remove over 99% of the leukocytes.

Leukocyte-reduced RBC are indicated for patients with a history of febrile transfusion reactions and for those who may require repeated transfusions. For patients at risk of CMV or possible candidates for bone marrow transplantation, leukocyte-reduced RBC are an acceptable alternative when CMV-seronegative blood is unavailable. Current leukocyte removal methods are inadequate for preventing transfusion-related graft-versus-host disease in immunocompromised recipients, and blood products should be irradiated.

FROZEN RBC

RBC that have been preserved with a cryoprotective agent, usually glycerol, may be stored at $-65°C$ for up to 10 years. Thawing requires special washing procedures to remove the glycerol as well as virtually all of the plasma, platelets, and leukocytes. The product must be transfused within 24 hours after thawing. Frozen RBC of rare blood groups can be stockpiled and obtained from national blood reference agencies for patients who have developed antibodies against high-frequency antigens.

IRRADIATION OF BLOOD PRODUCTS

Cellular blood products, including RBC, whole blood, platelets, and granulocytes, contain lymphocytes and must be irradiated to prevent graft-versus-host (GVH) reaction in susceptible recipients, including fetuses receiving intrauterine transfusion of red cells or platelets, neonatal transfusions, and patients with immunodeficiencies. Irradiation increases cellular potassium leakage and shortens RBC survival; it should be performed shortly before administration.

RED CELL SUBSTITUTES

Artificial oxygen-carrying RBC substitutes ("artificial blood") have been developed, and a few have undergone clinical trials in adults. The most promising of these is a polymerized human hemoglobin solution that is not generally available and will probably be limited to short-term emergency maintenance of oxygen-carrying capacity during acute hemorrhage and in critically ill patients with severe anemia who cannot be easily provided with compatible RBC.

ADMINISTRATION OF RBC AND WHOLE BLOOD

The most important safety factor in blood transfusion is the compatibility of RBC with any preformed antibodies in the recipient's circulation. Plasma-containing blood components, such as FFP and platelets, contain antibodies of donor origin and must be compatible with the recipient's RBC. Table 19-19 describes ABO compatibility choices for RBC and plasma transfusion. The ABO antigens are carbohydrate antigens expressed on the surface of most cells throughout the body. The cells of group O individuals bear only a precursor molecule with no A or B antigen on it. During the first year of life, exposure to A- and B-like carbohydrate antigens in the environment stimulates production of IgM antibodies against A and B antigens. Thus, group O infants produce anti-A and anti-B antibodies; group A infants produce anti-B; and group B infants produce anti-A. These so-called "naturally occurring" IgM antibodies, or isohemagglutinins, are complement-fixing and can cause immediate intravascular destruction of transfused RBC that bear the offending antigen. Plasma-containing products such as FFP and platelets may contain donor isohemagglutinins, but compatibility testing is not usually performed. Products containing

TABLE 19-19

SELECTION OF ABO-COMPATIBLE BLOOD PRODUCTS

RECIPIENT CELL TYPE	RECIPIENT ANTIBODIES	COMPATIBLE RED CELLS	COMPATIBLE PLASMA
O	Anti-A and anti-B	O only	Any
A	Anti-B	A or O	A or AB
B	Anti-A	B or O	B or AB
AB	None	Any	AB only

less than 5 mL/kg of incompatible plasma are well tolerated, but large infusions of incompatible plasma should not be given.

In general, patients produce antibodies to Rh and other non-ABO red cell surface antigens only after specific exposure by transfusion or pregnancy. These antibodies are usually IgG, are not complement-fixing, and do not cause acute intravascular hemolysis, but incompatible RBC have shortened in vivo survival (delayed transfusion reaction). The most immunogenic of the non-ABO antigens is the Rh (D) antigen. About 15% of the white population are Rh-negative and may make anti-Rh antibodies if exposed to Rh-positive RBC, and precautions to prevent exposure to this antigen are important. Although there are many other red cell antigens that induce antibodies after exposure, sensitization to these is relatively rare.

PRETRANSFUSION LABORATORY TESTING

Testing must be performed before RBC are transfused to ensure that the transfused RBC are compatible with any preexisting antibodies in the recipient and to avoid stimulation of new anti-Rh antibodies. *Typing* determines the ABO and Rh (D) type of the patient's cells. *Screening* is performed on the patient's serum to determine whether the patient has IgG antibodies to non-ABO RBC antigens. If the antibody screen is positive, further testing must be performed to identify the antibodies. Before cells are released to the patient, a *crossmatch* is performed to confirm that the donor RBC selected for transfusion are compatible with any preformed antibodies in the patient's plasma. In patients with a negative antibody screen, the crossmatch procedure may be limited to verification of ABO compatibility. In emergencies, O, Rh-negative ("universal donor"), RBC can be used if there is insufficient time to type the patient, or ABO- and Rh-compatible RBC may be given if the patient's blood type is known but there is insufficient time to perform a screen and crossmatch. However, the antibody screen should be completed as soon as possible, and, if positive, compatible RBC should then be provided.

BLOOD ADMINISTRATION

The most common cause of fatal transfusion reactions is the administration of ABO-incompatible blood because of misidentification of the patient, either at the time the sample for typing is drawn or when the blood is administered. Reconfirming that the blood is correctly labeled for the intended recipient is mandatory. RBC and other components must be filtered before infusion to remove particles that may have formed during storage. Administering RBC under pressure through small-bore needles may cause hemolysis.

In normovolemic anemic patients the volume and rate of RBC infusion are determined by the patient's ability to tolerate additional blood volume. In general, RBC transfusions should be limited to 10 to 15 mL/kg given over 2 to 3 hours and should be administered more slowly during the first 15 minutes to enable early detection of immediate transfusion reactions before the recipient has received a large volume. The patient should be monitored throughout the infusion for signs or symptoms of intolerance. Patients with severe anemia and heart failure should receive smaller total volumes of RBC, infused at a slower rate (2 mL/kg/h). Concomitant intravenous administration of a rapidly acting diuretic may help minimize the effects of volume overload. Alternatively, a partial exchange transfusion can be carried out, replacing a portion of the patient's low-hematocrit blood with packed RBC. With acute hemorrhage and hypovolemia, RBC or whole blood should be infused rapidly in sufficient amounts to restore intravascular volume. RBC infusions must be completed within 4 hours after the product has been removed from refrigeration to minimize the risk of bacterial growth.

SPECIAL CONSIDERATIONS

PRETERM INFANTS   Transfusions may be given in the neonatal period to sick preterm infants who require frequent blood sampling. However, frequent small transfusions to replace blood used for laboratory studies exposes infants to multiple donors. Transfusions should be given only when clinically necessary, and the number of donors should be limited by dedicating a full or half unit of RBC to an individual infant. Transfusions of additive RBC are safe and effective treatment for anemia in neonates. To prevent transmission of cytomegalovirus, preterm infants who weigh less than 1200 g should receive RBC obtained from CMV-seronegative donors or RBC processed through high-efficiency leukocyte reduction filters. RBC to be given to premature infants should be irradiated to prevent transfusion-related GVHD.

CHRONIC TRANSFUSION-DEPENDENT ANEMIA   Patients with chronic, severe anemias often require repeated RBC transfusions. In addition to the cumulative risk of transmitting infectious agents, chronic transfusion therapy may be complicated by alloimmunization to minor RBC antigens and iron overload. Alloantibodies to non-ABO red cell antigens such as C, Kell, Duffy (Fy), and Kidd (Jk) result in shortened survival of transfused cells. Patients with sickle cell disease and those from Southeast Asia with thalassemia who receive blood from the predominantly white donor population, which has a higher frequency of RBC antigens such as C, E, Kell, and Kidd, are at risk of developing alloantibodies to these antigens. Once alloantibodies are recognized, subsequent transfusions must employ RBC lacking the offending antigen. With the development of multiple antibodies or antibodies against antigens that are common in white donors, obtaining compatible blood may be difficult. To attempt to reduce the frequency of severe alloimmunization, extended typing for antigens likely to evoke antibodies and the prophylactic use of antigen-negative red cells have been recommended. An acceptable alternative is to use phenotypically matched RBC only for those few patients who become sensitized. Alloantibodies to leukocyte antigens are common in multiply transfused patients and result in febrile reactions, so leukocyte-reduced blood products are recommended. Iron overload is a problem in chronically transfused patients with disorders such as thalassemia, in which iron accumulates (see Sec. 19.4).

MASSIVE TRANSFUSION

When the administered volume of blood products is equivalent or greater than the patient's estimated blood volume (75 to 80 mL/kg), complications may occur, including (1) hypothermia from the rapid infusion of cold blood products. Blood should be warmed just before infusion, using a certified blood warmer to avoid hemolysis caused by excessive heating. (2) Depletion of hemostatic elements occurs after replacement of 1 to 2 blood volumes, as indicated by prolonged PT/PTT and thrombocytopenia. (3) Hypocalcemia results from citrate anticoagulants that bind free calcium and may require administration of calcium. (4) Hyperkalemia may occur because potassium leaks out of stored RBC, particularly after irradiation. All of these complications of massive transfusion may occur with extracorporeal membrane oxygenation (ECMO) and cardiopulmonary bypass.

19.11.2   Platelet Transfusion

Concentrates of platelets are prepared from one unit of donated whole blood by first removing the RBC and then concentrating the platelets. The concentrated platelets are resuspended in 50 mL of plasma, constituting a one "unit-equivalent" for dosage estimation (Table 19-20). Automated collection devices can be used to prepare "apheresis" platelets, which contain about 6 unit-equivalents of single donor platelets. Apheresis platelets are used to provide HLA-matched platelets because a full therapeutic dose can be obtained from a single donor. Platelets must be stored at room temperature to maintain viability, and shelf-life is limited to 5 days. Transfusion of platelets should be reserved for patients with counts <10 to 20×10^9/L or in surgical settings $<50 \times 10^9$/L. Bleeding may occur at higher platelet counts in patients with concurrent coagulopathy, platelet dysfunction, or vascular injury, and platelet transfusion may be indicated. Premature infants on ventilatory support are at risk for intraventricular hemorrhage, and some centers maintain platelet counts above 50×10^9/L. In patients with autoimmune or consumptive thrombocytopenia as in ITP or DIC, transfused platelets are rapidly consumed and are of questionable benefit (see Secs. 4.1 and 19.7).

One unit-equivalent of platelets per 10 kg increases the recipient's platelet count by 20 to 30×10^9/L when measured 1 hour after the infusion and is usually sufficient to achieve hemostasis. Failure to achieve the expected posttransfusion increment usually indicates the presence of platelet antibodies, often directed against HLA antigens. If anti-HLA antibodies are present, platelets compatible with the patient's antibodies should be used for further transfusions. Patients who do not have anti-HLA antibodies will not benefit from the use of HLA-matched platelets. Following transfusion, the platelet count decreases linearly over 5 to 10 days. A good immediate increment with rapid subsequent drop in platelet count is commonly associated with clinical factors such as infection, fever, or DIC.

19.11.3   Granulocyte Transfusion

Granulocyte concentrates have been used in severely neutropenic patients with life-threatening bacterial or fungal infections not responsive to antibiotic therapy after 24 to 48 hours. Because of more effective antibiotic therapy and the use of G-CSF to accelerate neutrophil recovery following myeloablative chemotherapy, granulocyte transfusions have declined. Granulocytes obtained by apheresis of a single CMV-negative, ABO- and Rh-compatible donor pretreated with corticosteroids or G-CSF are the preferred preparations. Adverse reactions include fever, chills, and dyspnea with pulmonary infiltrates. The dose is 1.0 to 2.0×10^9 granulocytes/kg/d repeated for at least 4 days.

19.11.4   Fresh-Frozen Plasma

Fresh-frozen plasma (FFP) is plasma separated and rapidly frozen to $-18°C$ or less. About 180 to 250 mL of plasma is obtained from a single unit of blood, and aliquots can be prepared for infants and small children. Shelf life is 1 year. The usual indication for FFP is to arrest or prevent bleeding from multiple coagulation factor deficiencies, including (1) vitamin K deficiency or Coumadin overdose when serious bleeding precludes waiting for a response to parenteral vitamin K, (2) liver disease, (3) DIC, (4) massive blood transfusions or exchange transfusions, and (5) correction of deficiencies of coagulation factors for which specific concentrates are not available (see Sec. 19.10). FFP is not subjected to viral inactivation procedures and should not be used if there is a safer alternative. The solvent-detergent method to inactivate lipid-enveloped viruses is now being used in a pooled plasma product designated FFP-SD, but hepatitis A and parvovirus are not inactivated by this

TABLE 19-20
BLOOD COMPONENTS USED FOR HEMOSTASIS[a]

BLOOD COMPONENT	VOLUME (mL)	SHELF LIFE	INDICATIONS AND DOSE
Platelet concentrate	50	5 days	Thrombocytopenia or thrombocytopathy; 1 unit/10^9 kg raises count by $20–30 \times 10^a$/L
Plateletpheresis	250–350	5 days	Indications same as platelet concentrate. Therapeutic effect similar to 6 units of platelet concentrate
Fresh-frozen plasma	200–250	1 year	For deficiency of multiple clotting factors, or a single factor for which no viral-inactivated or recombinant product is available; 10 mL/kg raises factor levels by approximately 10%
Cryoprecipitate	15	1 year	For hypofibrinogenemia or deficiencies of factor VIII, von Willebrand factor, or factor XIII; 1 unit/5 kg raises factor levels by 20–40%

[a] A variety of concentrated coagulation factor products, some prepared by recombinant DNA technology, are available (see Sec. 19.10).

technique. The usual initial dose of FFP for treating coagulopathies is 10 to 15 mL/kg. Allergic reactions such as hives and urticaria are common with FFP infusions.

19.11.5   Cryoprecipitate

Cryoprecipitate is formed when FFP is thawed, and each bag contains about 150 mg of fibrinogen and 80 units of factor VIII. Cryoprecipitate has been largely replaced by factor VIII concentrates in the treatment of hemophilia A. The major indication for cryoprecipitate is correction of hypofibrinogenemia, congenital factor XIII deficiency, and for DIC (see Sec. 19.10).

19.11.6   Transfusion Reactions

Non-infectious complications are summarized in Table 19-21.

Febrile reactions to blood product infusions are common, especially in patients who have received multiple transfusions, and are usually caused by antibodies in the recipient against leukocytes in the blood product or by cytokines generated by leukocytes during product storage. Cytokine accumulation is a concern in platelet products, which are stored at room temperature. Symptoms may occur immediately or as late as 1 hour after completion of the infusion. Chills are followed by fever and occasionally headache, nausea, and vomiting. Most symptoms respond to antipyretic medication. The use of leukocyte-reduced blood products prevents most febrile reactions.

Allergic reactions occur in 1 to 2% of all transfusions. Itching and urticaria start shortly after transfusion is begun and may or may not recur with subsequent transfusions, but severity does not generally increase. These reactions are probably related to immunologic reactions to constituents in plasma, but specific causes cannot usually be identified. If itching and urticaria respond promptly to antihistamines, the transfusion can be resumed safely. Giving an antihistamine (oral diphenhydramine, 1 mg/kg) before subsequent transfusions may prevent recurrences.

Anaphylactic reactions are associated with bronchospasm, angioedema, and/or hypotension. Some IgA-deficient patients have anti-IgA antibodies that react with the IgA in the blood product, but, in most cases, a cause cannot be identified. Treatment with antihistamines, epinephrine, corticosteroids, and other supportive measures is indicated. After occurrence of a severe anaphylactic reaction, administration of plasma-containing blood products should

be avoided when possible. Cellular blood products should be washed to remove plasma. IgA-deficient patients with anti-IgA should receive only washed blood cells.

Acute hemolytic reactions are usually a result of ABO incompatibility because of errors in patient identification, which can be largely avoided by clear and accurate labeling of the patient's pretransfusion blood sample and by assuring that the information on the unit of blood matches that on the patient's wristband before a transfusion is begun. When IgM anti-A or anti-B isohemagglutinins in the patient's plasma react with their corresponding antigen on the donor's RBC, intravascular hemolysis, activation of coagulation, and release of vasoactive amines occur. Symptoms include fever, chills, nausea and vomiting, chest or back pain, and anxiety. If the transfusion is stopped promptly, before many RBC have been given, severe complications may not occur, but when large volumes of incompatible blood have been given, acute renal failure, DIC, shock, and death may ensue. Acute hemolysis may also result from physical or thermal injury to donor red cells during storage or transfusion, including exposure of RBC to inappropriate temperatures, mixture of RBC with hypotonic fluids, and administration of RBC under pressure through fine-gauge needles.

Delayed transfusion reactions are caused by antibodies to non-ABO antigens that are usually IgG and do not usually bind complement or cause acute intravascular hemolysis but cause extravascular hemolysis, primarily in the spleen. Delayed transfusion reactions may occur when amnestic antibody production is stimulated by transfused RBC antigens and these antibodies react with transfused cells 1 to 2 weeks after transfusion. Patients are usually asymptomatic, but a delayed hemolytic reaction should always be considered if an unexplained fall in hemoglobin level occurs 1 to 2 weeks after a transfusion. A delayed reaction is confirmed by a positive direct Coombs test and a positive antibody screen.

The appearance of clinical and roentgenographic signs of *acute pulmonary edema* during transfusion usually signifies intravascular overload and congestive heart failure. If fluid overload is unlikely, and the heart is not enlarged, one must consider an immunologic reaction known as noncardiogenic pulmonary edema or transfusion-associated acute lung injury, which is related to leukocyte antibodies that lead to leukocyte agglutinates that lodge in the pulmonary circulation. Management includes stopping the transfusion and administering oxygen, diuretics, epinephrine, and corticosteroids. The transfusion service should be notified to initiate an appropriate investigation.

EVALUATION OF ACUTE TRANSFUSION REACTIONS

All febrile reactions or suspected acute hemolytic transfusion reactions to RBC (Table 19-22) should be evaluated as follows: (1) verification that the unit was intended for the patient, (2) reconfirming ABO/Rh types of the patient and the unit, (3) visual inspection of the color of the recipient's plasma for free hemoglobin, and (4) performance of a direct Coombs test on the recipient's posttransfusion RBC. If plasma hemoglobin concentration is not elevated and the direct Coombs test is negative, an acute hemolytic transfusion reaction is unlikely. The possibility of bacterial contamination must always be considered in every febrile transfusion reaction and is characterized by a fever spike shortly after the start of the infusion, followed by hypotension, shock, DIC, and even death. Bacterial contamination is most common in platelet products because these are stored at room temperature. If the patient shows signs of infection or endotoxin-mediated shock, cultures must be

---

TABLE 19-21

NONINFECTIOUS COMPLICATIONS OF TRANSFUSION

Hemolysis
   Recipient antibodies to transfused RBC
   Osmotic, thermal, or mechanical lysis of cells before infusion
Nonhemolytic febrile reactions
   Recipient antibodies to WBC in blood product
   Cytokines in blood product
   Bacteria in blood product
Allergic
   Recipient sensitivity to plasma in blood product
   Anti-IgA (in IgA-deficient recipient)
Pulmonary edema
   Volume overload
   Anti-WBC antibodies in blood product or recipient

TABLE 19-22

WORKUP OF ACUTE TRANSFUSION REACTIONS

Transfusionist
   Stop transfusion; treat patient symptomatically; document symptoms
      on report form; draw posttransfusion specimens; send specimens,
      unit, and report form to transfusion service

Transfusion service
  A. All reactions
     Verify that the unit was intended for recipient
  B. Febrile reactions to RBC
     Recheck recipient and unit ABO/Rh type
     Perform direct antiglobulin test (DAT) on recipient RBC
     Visually inspect recipient's plasma for free hemoglobin
     If DAT positive or free hemoglobin present, repeat serologic
       crossmatch on unit
     If serologic incompatibility or hemolysis is found, perform testing
       to identify specificity of antibody
     If hemolytic workup is negative, consider WBC-mediated reac-
       tion.
     If patient shows signs of sepsis that were not present before trans-
       fusion, culture unit and patient
  C. Febrile reactions to platelets
     Perform posttransfusion platelet count
     If poor rise in platelet count, consider testing patient for anti-
       HLA antibodies
     If good increment, consider other WBC-related or cytokine reac-
       tions
     If patient shows signs of sepsis that were not present before trans-
       fusion, Gram stain and culture unit and patient
  D. Allergic reactions
     Mild symptoms: no testing indicated
     Severe (eg, hypotension, angioedema): test patient and/or donor
       for IgA deficiency and anti-IgA antibodies
  E. Pulmonary edema
     Consider fluid overload
     Consider testing patient or donor for anti-WBC antibodies
       (transfusion-related acute lung injury)

---

obtained from the patient and blood product, intravenous antibiotics begun, and blood pressure support provided.

TRANSMISSION OF INFECTIOUS DISEASES BY BLOOD

The HIV and hepatitis B and C viruses are the most important
infectious agents transmissible by blood transfusion (Table 19-23).
Human immunodeficiency virus (HIV-1), identified in 1984 as the
causative agent of AIDS, entered the blood supply in the early
1980s before a diagnostic test became available in 1985. Current
tests used in the United States detect both antibody to HIV and
p24 HIV antigen. As a result of these tests, the risk of transmitting
HIV per unit of blood fell from approximately 1 in 2000 in 1985
to approximately 1 in 700,000 in 1996. Before 1985, HIV was
frequently transmitted by coagulation factor concentrates derived
from pooled plasma. Careful donor screening, newer manufactur-
ing methods that include virus-inactivation processes, and especially
the use of recombinant coagulation factors have markedly decreased this risk. Improved screening of donors and testing for
HBV surface antigen has made HBV transmission very rare, with a
current estimated risk of approximately 1/63,000 units.

Until 1990, posttransfusion hepatitis (PTH) was usually caused
by the hepatitic C virus (HCV). The introduction of a donor
screening test for antibodies to HCV in 1990 resulted in a decrease
from approximately 1/100 per unit transfused to less than

1/100,000 today. The introduction of viral nucleic acid testing for
HIV, HBV, and HCV will further reduce the risk of transfusion-
related viral infections.

After a cytomegalovirus (CMV) infection, the virus can persist
in lymphocytes for years and can be transmitted by cellular blood
products. Serious illness can occur in CMV-seronegative patients
with impaired immunity. Low birth weight infants, patients with
congenital or acquired immunodeficiency syndromes, bone marrow transplant recipients, and patients who are receiving immunosuppressive therapy may develop a severe and life-threatening
CMV infection after transfusion. To prevent transmission of CMV,
RBC, platelets, and granulocytes to be administered to CMV-
seronegative immunocompromised recipients should be from
CMV-seronegative donors. Leukocyte reduction filters also appear
to be effective.

Parvovirus B19, the cause of "fifth disease" or erythema infectiosum, can cause erythroid suppression and occasionally chronic
pancytopenia in immunocompromised recipients. Fetuses of pregnant women infected with parvovirus are at risk of severe anemia
and hydrops fetalis. In recipients with chronic hemolytic anemias,
parvovirus may cause aplastic crises (see Sec. 19.5). Parvovirus is
rarely transmitted by single-donor blood products but may be
transmitted by products made from multiple-donor pooled plasma.

Human T-cell leukemia virus type I (HTLVI) is a retrovirus
endemic in Japan, Africa, South America, and the Caribbean and
can cause adult T-cell leukemia/lymphoma or spinal paresis. The
virus can persist in the lymphocytes of infected persons and may
possibly be transmitted by blood transfusion. Screening for this
agent has been conducted in the United States since 1989.

Malaria and other parasitic diseases such as babesiosis, Chagas
disease, and trypanosomiasis can be transmitted by transfusion of
cellular blood products. The only way to reduce the risk of transmission is by exclusion of donors who have a history of residence
or travel in endemic areas. Despite donor questioning, there are
approximately three cases of transfusion-transmitted malaria reported each year in the United States.

Jakob-Creutzfeldt disease (JCD) is a rare slow virus infection of
the central nervous system. A disease similar to JCD occurs in cows.
It is transmitted by feeds containing bovine tissues and can be transmitted to humans who consume infected beef. Although transmission by blood transfusions has not been documented, the American
Red Cross has recently decided to reject donors who resided in the
United Kingdom and Western Europe after 1980.

TABLE 19-23

INFECTIOUS AGENTS TRANSMISSIBLE BY BLOOD

Viruses
   Hepatitis B, C
   Retroviruses: HIV-1 and HIV-2, human T-cell leukemia viruses, types
     I and II (HTLV-I/II)
   Cytomegalovirus (CMV), parvovirus, and Epstein-Barr virus (EBV)
     (mainly in immunosuppressed recipients)
Bacteria
   Associated with asymptomatic bacteremia in blood donors (*Yersinia
     enterocolitica, Salmonella*, and other gram-negative organisms)
   Caused by contamination during collection (skin flora) or processing of
     blood
Syphilis
Parasites
   Malaria, babesiosis, *Trypanosoma cruzi*, leishmaniasis

DIRECTED (RECIPIENT-DESIGNATED) DONATIONS

Designated donations from family members or friends that are dedicated for a specific recipient are often prompted by fear of AIDS, but no evidence of their increased safety exists. Families requesting such donations should be informed that current testing is not perfect and that personal history provided by donors is a mainstay of screening. Designated donors may be reluctant to reveal risk behaviors for HIV or other agents. Other indications for directed donations include antigen-negative family members of patients alloimmunized to high-frequency RBC antigens and maternal HPA-1 antigen-negative platelets for neonates with alloimmune thrombocytopenia (see Sec. 19.7.2). However, platelet or granulocyte transfusions from family members may predispose to engraftment by viable lymphocytes following parental transfusion to immunocompromised infants and children, leading to graft-versus-host disease (GVHD), and blood products from relatives should be irradiated. Women who receive transfusions from their spouses can be sensitized by "minor" red cell antigens that they lack, which might lead to a risk of hemolytic disease of the newborn in subsequent pregnancies.

References

American Association of Blood Banks: Technical Manual, 13th ed. Bethesda, American Association of Blood Banks, 1999

American Association of Blood Banks: Blood Transfusion Therapy—A Physician's Handbook, 6th ed. Bethesda, American Association of Blood Banks, 1999

Goodnough LT, Brecher ME, Kanter MH, et al: Medical progress: transfusion medicine and blood transfusion. N Engl J Med 340:438–447, 1999

Strauss RG, Blanchette VS, Hume H, et al: National acceptability of American Association of Blood Banks Pediatric Hemotherapy Committee guidelines for auditing pediatric transfusion practices. Transfusion 33: 168–171, 1993

ONCOLOGY

Alan L. Schwartz, Associate Editor

20.1 INTRODUCTION

Alan L. Schwartz

According to *Vital Statistics of the United States,* cancer is the second leading cause of death among children beyond the neonatal period. It is second only to trauma (Table 20-1). Among children in the United States 1 to 14 years of age in 1995, approximately 1500 deaths were attributed to cancer (10% of all deaths). Approximately 6000 deaths were caused by accidents (40% of all deaths). Cancer accounts for a death rate of 2.8/100,000 population among children 1 through 14 years of age. According to data from the National Cancer Institute Surveillance Epidemiology and End Results (SEER) Program, there were approximately 1,200,000 new cases of cancer in the United States during 2000 (exclusive of carcinoma in situ and nonmelanoma skin cancer). Of these, approximately 9100 (less than 1%) occurred among children younger than 15 years.

Since the introduction of the first successful chemotherapy for acute leukemia among children and the development of modern multimodality therapy, in large part attributed to multicenter comprehensive cancer programs for treatment of children, a substantial decline in the mortality rate from pediatric cancer has occurred. This trend is anticipated to continue into the 21st century. Pediatric cancer can be controlled, and cure likely is a goal that can be reached. More than 70% of children in whom cancer developed in 2000 are expected to survive the disease. This dramatic improvement in outcome among children with many pediatric cancers over three decades is shown in Fig. 20-1. These 1998 SEER data are presented as 5-year relative survival rates. The overall survival rates for all sites increased from 56% (1974 through 1976) to 74% (1989 through 1994). The 5-year survival rates for Hodgkin disease and Wilms tumor exceed 90%; the rate for acute lymphoblastic leukemia (ALL) is approximately 80%.

Historically, the two main cooperative groups for the treatment of children with cancer in the United States were Pediatric Oncology Group (POG) and the Children's Cancer Study Group (CCSG). In 2000, these groups were integrated into a single pe-

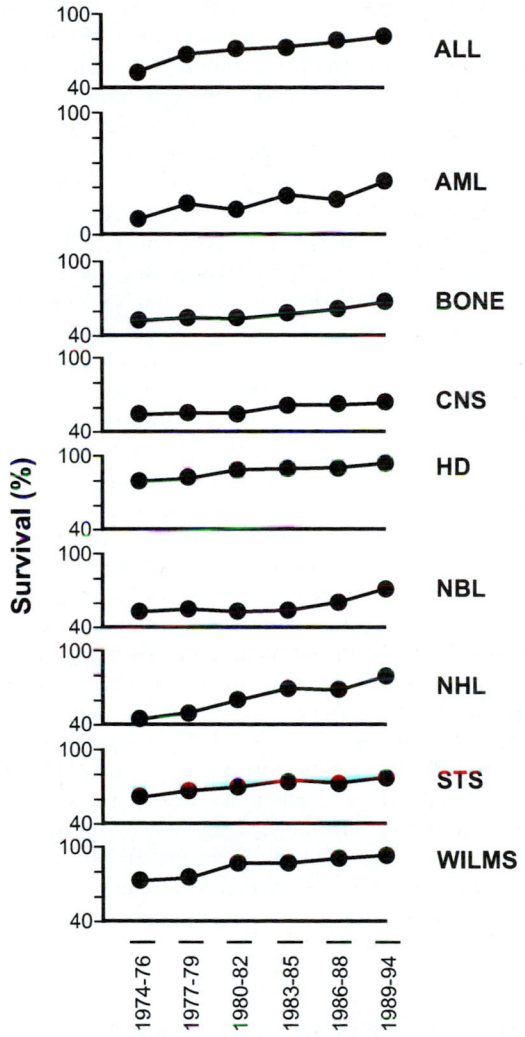

FIGURE 20-1 Trends in cancer survival among children younger than 15 years in the United States, 1974 to 1994.

TABLE 20-1

LEADING CAUSES OF DEATH AMONG CHILDREN 1–14 YEARS OF AGE, UNITED STATES, 1995

RANK	CAUSE OF DEATH	NO. OF DEATHS	DEATH RATE PER 100,000 POPULATION	PERCENTAGE OF TOTAL DEATHS
	All Causes	14,989	27.3	100.0
1	Accidents	5824	10.7	38.9
2	Cancer	1514	2.8	10.1
3	Congenital anomalies	1144	2.0	7.6
4	Homicide	1014	1.8	6.8
5	Heart disease	545	1.0	3.6

SOURCE: *Data from: Vital Statistics of the United States, 1998.*

diatric cooperative group. For the past two decades, POG and CCSG have provided data on pediatric diagnosis and treatment for approximately 95% of all children with cancer in the United States. This has allowed a close and integrated approach to patient care and clinical research and provides the platform on which substantive advances in childhood cancer cures are being made.

The incidence and frequency of various types of childhood cancers vary with age and site (Table 20-2). Neuroblastoma and soft-tissue sarcoma are the most common tumors of infancy, followed by leukemia, brain tumors, and retinoblastoma. By 1 to 2 years of age, the usual pattern of early childhood has emerged in which leukemia is the most common cancer followed by brain tumors, neuroblastoma, Wilms tumor, lymphoma, soft-tissue sarcoma, and retinoblastoma. By 10 years of age, neuroblastoma and Wilms tumor become less common, although there is an increase in the incidence of bone sarcoma, Hodgkin lymphoma, and other cancers.

Slight differences in cancer incidence by sex are found. Prepubertal white children have a male:female ratio of 1.2:1, largely because of the increased risk of ALL, lymphoma, and medulloblastoma among young boys. In addition to sex differences, a 25% higher incidence of cancer among white than black children in the United States is a result of the relative lower frequency of acute leukemia and Ewing sarcoma among black children.

It is apparent from the statistics that pediatric cancer is relatively rare. Several important advances have culminated in our current state of understanding these diseases. First, in an effort to improve the outlook among these children, leaders in pediatric oncology two and three decades ago developed cooperative clinical trials to optimize use of data on this small number of patients available for clinical trials. Note that pediatric cancer is approximately 1/100 as common as adult cancer. Second, biostatistics became an important adjunctive discipline. Prognosis often is determined biostatistically with life-table methods for estimating probability, such as Kaplan-Meier life-table analysis. Survival times have been estimated with two main endpoints—relapse or recurrence and death. Such estimates are extremely useful for discussing prognosis with parents and patients and for planning future studies. Another prominent development in pediatric oncology has been identification of clinical prognostic factors through Cox stepwise regression analysis of data on large groups of patients from the pediatric oncology clinical trials. As a consequence for many pediatric malignant tumors, children can be classified as being at good risk or poor risk. Additional

prognostic factors often include clinical stage, histopathologic features, patient age, disease stage at diagnosis, and a variety of biological factors. Such analysis has allowed clinical investigation to proceed with the use of treatments which minimize toxicity. As Teresa Vietti, founder of the POG, has emphasized, "therapy is the greatest single prognostic factor in childhood cancer."

Survival and cure can be attained in almost every type of pediatric cancer. Biological cure of pediatric cancer has been defined by Pinkel as completion of all cancer treatment with continuous freedom from clinical and laboratory evidence of cancer coupled with minimal or no risk of relapse. One must recognize that restoration of physical and mental health as well as normal functioning is the optimal goal. On occasion, however, many tumors have recurred more than 5 years after cessation of therapy, often representing delayed metastatic disease. However, second primary tumors also, although rarely, occur. The risk of second malignant tumor, different from the primary tumor, has been a concern with improved therapy for and survival of pediatric cancer. Primary care providers must be ever vigilant in long-term surveillance of patients who survive childhood cancer.

As the diagnosis and management of cancer among children have become increasingly successful, the large numbers of survivors seek to complete their education, enter the work force, secure adequate health and life insurance, and reproduce. The diseases and therapies, however, may produce side effects that limit achievement of these goals. In addition to physical sequelae such as late cardiotoxicity of doxorubicin or reproductive limitations caused by chemotherapy or radiation therapy, emotional and psychological trauma sustained by both survivor and family must be addressed.

References

Farber S, Diamond LK, Mercer RD, Sylvester RF, Wolff JA: Temporary remissions in acute leukemia in children produced by folic acid antagonist, 4-aminopteroyl-glutamic acid (aminopterin). N Engl J Med 238:787–793, 1948

Green DM, D'Angio GJ, eds: Current Clinical Oncology: Late Effects of Treatment for Childhood Cancer. New York, Wiley-Liss, 1992

Pediatric Oncology Group: Progress against childhood cancer: The Pediatric Oncology Group experience. Pediatrics 89:597–600, 1992

TABLE 20-2

APPROXIMATE FREQUENCY OF NEW CASES OF CANCER AMONG CHILDREN

SITE/TYPE	AGE <15 YR		NUMBER OF CASES PER 10⁶ BY AGE		
	NUMBER OF CASES PER 10⁶	%	0–4 YR	5–9 YR	10–14 YR
All sites	129	100			
Leukemia[a]	40	31	66	34	23
Central nervous system	25	19	26	25	22
Lymphoma[a]	16	13	7	14	20
Neuroblastoma	11	8	28	4	1.5
Soft-tissue sarcomas	8	6	9	7.5	7.5
Wilms tumor	7.8	6	18	5.7	1.1
Bone	6.3	5	1.6	4	12.1
Retinoblastoma	3.3	3	9.5	0.5	—

[a] All types.

SOURCE: *From rates for white children. Adapted from Young JL, Gloeckler R, Silverberg E, et al: Cancer incidence, survival, and mortality for children younger than age 15 years. Cancer 58(I):598–602, 1986.*

Surveillance Epidemiology and End Results. Available at:
    http://www-seeroims.ncl.nih.gov
Vital Statistics of the United States. Available at:
    www.cdc.gov/nchs/products/pubs/pubd/vsus/vsus/htm

20.2   CANCER GENETICS

Jill P. Ginsberg and Frederic G. Barr

20.2.1   Cancer as a Genetic Disease

The recognition of cancer as a genetic disease has provided a fundamental paradigm for understanding the mechanisms underlying tumorigenesis and for designing molecular strategies to diagnose and manage cancer. A malignant tumor is viewed as the outcome of a progressive series of DNA alterations. Each alteration involves a cellular gene and results in altered expression or function of the encoded product. In the context of the environmental conditions of the target cell, alteration in gene expression or function leads to phenotypic changes that provide advantageous properties for the growing cell. Subsequent DNA alterations occur within the selected clone to provide additional properties for further clonal outgrowth. The constellation of expression or functional changes resulting from this series of DNA alterations produces a complex set of growth and motility behaviors that characterize cancer.

The genes mutated in the process of tumorigenesis encode products that normally function in cellular pathways and transmit signals for growth and other relevant behaviors. The genes encoding these signaling molecules can be divided into two general categories—oncogenes and tumor suppressor genes (Table 20-3). The products of oncogenes provide signals that promote cellular growth as well as other tumorigenic behaviors. In contrast, tumor suppressor genes encode products that inhibit growth signaling pathways or promote alternative pathways leading to differentiation or cell death. The mutations of oncogenes and tumor suppressor genes that occur in cancer lead to an overall gain in growth-promoting signals by activating or increasing oncogene function and inactivating or decreasing tumor suppressor function.

ONCOGENE MUTATIONS IN CANCER

Three principal types of alterations are associated with oncogene activation—point mutation, amplification, and chromosomal translocation. The *point mutations* consist of gain or loss of one or a few nucleotides in critical functional regions of oncogenes. For example, specific mutations of RAS genes (*HRAS*, *KRAS*, and *NRAS*) have been detected in pediatric cancers such as leukemia and rhabdomyosarcoma, as well as in malignant tumors that affect adults. These mutations modify the function of RAS signaling proteins and result in increased autonomy of growth-promoting pathways from environmental control.

In the process of *amplification*, the copy number of certain oncogenes and the surrounding genomic region is aberrantly increased. The increase in copy number leads to higher transcription levels resulting in increased oncogene messenger RNA (mRNA) and protein product expression. For example, in 40% of cases of glioblastoma, amplification of the epidermal growth factor receptor gene is observed. This gene encodes a membrane-bound cell surface receptor for epidermal growth factor, which stimulates growth and motility when bound to its receptor. Another well-characterized example occurs in neuroblastoma, in which the *MYCN* gene, which encodes a growth-promoting transcription factor, is amplified 10-fold to 300-fold in 25% of cases.

In *chromosomal translocations,* aberrant DNA recombination events cause juxtaposition of genes from discontinuous genomic regions. The two potential consequences of these oncogenic translocation events are altered expression by situating an oncogene in the vicinity of regulatory elements from another genomic locus or generation of a novel oncogenic product by means of fusing protein coding regions from two separate genes (chimeric fusion protein). An example of the former scenario is Burkitt lymphoma, a B-cell malignant tumor in which the 8;14 chromosomal translocation dysregulates *MYC* expression by placing the *MYC* oncogene on chromosome 8 under control of regulatory elements of the immunoglobulin heavy chain locus on chromosome 14. An example of formation of a chimeric fusion protein is the 11;22 translocation of Ewing sarcoma, in which portions of the *EWS* gene on chromosome 22 and the *FLI1* gene on chromosome 11 are joined to produce a chimeric *EWS-FLI1* gene that encodes an oncogenic chimeric transcription factor.

At the cellular level, only one copy of a mutated oncogene is necessary to generate the gain of growth-promoting activity. This dominant genetic behavior explains the residual presence of wild-type versions of these genes in tumors with activating oncogene mutations and the effects on transfected cells. Transfer of an activated oncogene into a model recipient cell line such as NIH 3T3 murine fibroblasts converts these cells to a transformed phenotype in vitro and often a tumorigenic phenotype in vivo.

ALTERATIONS OF TUMOR SUPPRESSOR GENES IN CANCER

Unlike those of oncogenes, mutations of tumor suppressor genes decrease expression or function of growth-limiting signaling products, cause the cell to bypass inhibitory signals, and allow reentrance into the cell cycle and uncontrolled growth. Because of the need to completely remove the growth-inhibiting influence exerted by these proteins, both cellular copies of the tumor suppressor gene become defective during tumor development through several mutagenic mechanisms. Alterations of the *RB1* gene in retinoblastoma and osteosarcoma represent a *deletion* that removes functional or regulatory elements (see Sec. 20.3). A second set of inactivating alterations are *point mutations*, including *missense mutations* that inactivate expression elements or functional domains and *nonsense* and *frameshift mutations* that result in truncated or aberrant protein products. A gene often altered by point mutations in many

TABLE 20-3
GENES INVOLVED IN TUMORIGENESIS

	ONCOGENES	TUMOR-SUPPRESSOR GENES
Normal function	Growth stimulation	Growth suppression
Mutations in tumors	Point mutations Translocations Amplifications	Point mutations Deletions Allelic loss
Effect of mutations	Increase or gain of function	Decrease or loss of function
Genetics	Dominant	Recessive
Transfection	Mutant transforms normal cells	Wild type reverts tumor cells

tumor types is *TP53,* in which mutations frequently inactivate transcriptional function of the wild-type p53 protein. Finally, a very common mechanism for one of the two mutational steps is *allelic loss,* in which the wild-type tumor suppressor gene and variable amounts of the surrounding genomic region are lost to large deletions, chromosome loss, or mitotic recombination. These allelic loss events often are detected in a tumor by loss of heterozygosity of polymorphic alleles in the genomic region surrounding the associated tumor suppressor locus. For example, although the responsible tumor suppressor locus is not fully established, allelic loss localized to chromosomal region 11p15.5 often is found in Wilms tumor and embryonal rhabdomyosarcoma.

From a genetic standpoint, tumor suppressor genes behave in a recessive manner. One normal allele is sufficient to provide the needed growth restraint, whereas inactivation or loss of both alleles eliminates this negative function and predisposes to oncogenic outcomes. Tumor suppressor genes are defined by the effect of their absence. When transfected, the wild-type gene suppresses or reverts the aberrant growth characteristics of tumor cells.

20.2.2   Hereditary Cancer Predisposition

Although most mutations occurring in pediatric cancers are somatic events and the proportion of these cancers that have a strong hereditary component is relatively small, several childhood tumors occur in association with hereditary syndromes. In most hereditary cases, a mutant tumor suppressor gene is present within the germ line. Therefore one of the two tumor suppressor alterations is transmitted to every somatic cell. For genes that provide necessary developmental functions, the continued function of the wild-type allele and the silent nature of the mutant allele allow relatively normal development. In accord with the Knudson two hit model, germline carriers with mutations need only one somatic event to initiate oncogenesis. The apparent paradox of the Knudson model is that the pattern of inheritance of cancer predisposition follows a mendelian dominant pattern. At the cellular level, however, the mutant genes act in a recessive manner. The classic example of these principles is retinoblastoma, in which the first *RB1* gene mutation is inherited and the second event occurs somatically. In contrast, sporadic retinoblastoma occurs after two somatically acquired *RB1* mutations. Because of the higher probability of acquiring a single somatic *RB1* mutation, tumors in the hereditary setting tend to manifest earlier and often are multifocal, unlike the later presentation of a single lesion in the sporadic setting.

In a smaller subset of cancer susceptibility syndromes, the inherited locus is a mutant oncogene. A prime example is multiple endocrine neoplasia type 2 in which mutations occur in the *RET* gene, which encodes a cell surface protein with tyrosine kinase activity. In vitro assays that show transforming capability of the mutant *RET* genes and mutational studies that do not generally detect alteration of the second *RET* allele support the premise that the inherited mutant *RET* alleles are dominant-acting oncogenes. In these cases, inheritance of an activated oncogene is compatible with normal embryonic development and, together with subsequent collaborating genetic events, results in endocrine tumors among affected individuals.

Elucidation of the molecular basis of inherited cancers has enhanced clinical diagnosis and counseling. For patients with these tumors and the accompanying nonneoplastic manifestations, detection of a germ-line mutation indicates a hereditary cancer susceptibility. Such a patient is at high risk of additional tumors and

nonneoplastic conditions and of conceiving affected children. These persons and their families need regular evaluations and counseling. An important goal in the care of predisposed persons is to identify environmental factors that can increase the risk of development of the associated cancers and ultimately to minimize these exposures.

20.2.3   Role of Molecular Diagnosis in Oncology

Advances in cancer genetics are affecting the clinical management of neoplastic diseases, including diagnosis, prognosis, and assessment of minimal disease. Certain genetic alterations occur consistently within specific tumor categories and thus provide genetic markers for differential diagnosis. Many types of pediatric solid tumors are difficult to diagnose on the basis of morphologic features because of the lack of discernible architectural or cytologic features of differentiation. For many of the tumor categories that present as small round cell tumors, such as alveolar rhabdomyosarcoma, Ewing sarcoma, desmoplastic small round cell tumor, and synovial sarcoma, the consistent associations of specific translocations and the corresponding gene fusions have provided a panel of molecular markers.

Other genetic alterations, although not consistently present within a tumor category, allow identification of subsets of patients with differing clinical outcomes. For example, a subset of neuroblastoma is associated with deletions of chromosomal region 1p and amplification of *MYCN.* These two factors are predictive of an aggressive tumor that responds poorly to conventional chemotherapy. In the category of ALL, *TEL-AML1* gene fusion is predictive of a favorable outcome of standard chemotherapy regimens. In contrast, the *BCR-ABL* and *MLL-AF4* gene fusions in ALL are associated with high risk of failure of conventional chemotherapy regimens and a frequent requirement for stem cell transplantation.

Development of molecular strategies that allow highly sensitive detection of genetic alterations has provided new opportunities for monitoring submicroscopic disease. Strategies (see Sec. 8.1) using polymerase chain reaction have been devised to detect genetic alterations such as gene fusions in as few as one tumor cell per one million normal cells. These strategies are being studied for clinical usefulness at the time of diagnostic staging to examine grossly uninvolved sites for tumor spread, during treatment to evaluate the efficacy of therapeutic interventions, and after therapy to predict early relapse.

FUTURE THERAPEUTIC PERSPECTIVES

Malignant transformation is a multistep clonal evolution process involving sequential alterations of oncogenes or tumor suppressor genes. Even with pediatric malignant tumors that occur decades earlier than the common adult malignant tumors, multiple genetic alterations are present generally in a single tumor. A series of genomic events is needed for a cell to evolve to the full malignant phenotype. Any single mutation occurring within a cancer may be requisite, but not sufficient, for the malignant behavior of that cancer. Moreover, tumor cells can acquire additional mutations after malignant transformation that can affect other phenotypic features, such as invasiveness, metastatic potential, or drug resistance. Although a single alteration may not be sufficient to cause the full malignant phenotype, interfering with any step may provide a therapeutic opportunity. Advancement of the functional genomics of cancer and continued investigation of molecular changes during tumorigenesis are crucial for further development of rational cancer therapies.

References

Johnson PW, Burchill SA, Selby PJ: The molecular detection of circulating tumour cells. Br J Cancer 72:268–276, 1995

Lasko D, Cavenee W, Nordenskjold M: Loss of constitutional heterozygosity in human cancer. Ann Rev Genet 25:281–314, 1991

Rabbits TH. Chromosomal translocations in human cancer. Nature 372: 143–149, 1994

20.3   CELL CYCLE CONTROL

David F. Crawford

Actively growing eukaryotic cells replicate and then segregate their genetic material to produce two genetically identical daughter cells (see Chap. 10). This coordinated sequence of events, referred to as the *mitotic cell cycle,* regulates cell proliferation. Dysregulation of the cell cycle is a common feature of cancer cells.

A schematic of the cell cycle is shown in the Fig. 20-2. For cells to divide, they must duplicate their entire genome during S (the DNA synthesis) phase of the cell cycle. The duplicated DNA is distributed to the progeny during M phase (mitosis). Between the M and S phases are two gap phases: G1 follows M phase and G2 follows S phase. Important commitments are made during G1 and G2, including whether to differentiate, to remain in G1 or G2, or to continue to divide. The duration of the cell cycle and its phases varies widely among mammalian cells. However, a typical proliferating mammalian cell divides approximately once every 24 hours. The average durations of G1, S, G2, and M phases are approximately 12, 6, and 6 hours and 30 minutes, respectively.

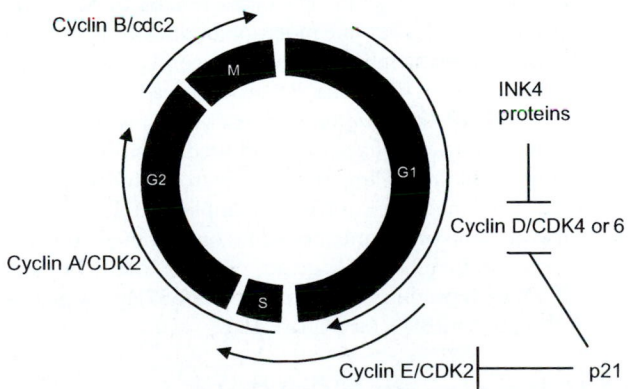

FIGURE 20-2   Schematic of the eukaryotic cell cycle. Cells duplicate their DNA during S and divide it equally between the two daughter cells during M. G1 and G2 phases intervene between S and M phases. Each of the four phases is represented by a *thick line.* The phases proceed according to the *clockwise* direction in this figure. The cyclin to cyclin-dependent kinase complexes that control progression through the cell cycle and transition points are indicated by *arrows* at the cell cycle phase where their effects are exerted. The inhibitory action of cyclin-dependent kinase inhibitors is represented by ⊢—.

The passage of cells through the cell cycle is controlled by protein kinase complexes composed of cyclins and cyclin-dependent kinases (CDKs). These complexes are inhibited by cyclin-dependent kinase inhibitors (CKIs) and modulated by the action of other proteins. Cyclin-dependent kinases control progression through particular cell cycle phases by phosphorylating other proteins, leading to activation or inactivation. For example, CDKs 2, 4, and 6 control progression through G1 and entry into S, and CDK1 (also known as *cdc2*) regulates entrance into mitosis.

Association with specific cyclins, which are controlled in a cell-cycle-dependent manner, is required for activation of CDKs. Cyclin B binds to and promotes activation of CDK1, whereas cyclins D, E, and A regulate the actions of the G1 through S CDKs. Essential regulators of the mitotic cell cycle, the CKIs inhibit the kinase activity of cyclin-CDK complexes. In some cases, cell cycle arrest, entrance into a quiescent state, or cell differentiation is mediated by up-regulated expression of CKIs. Seven CKIs have been identified and can be divided into two families — p21 and INK4. Cyclin-dependent kinases are further activated and inactivated by phosphorylation and regulated by subcellular localization.

Passage through G1 and entry into S requires cyclin D–CDK complexes. Synthesis of cyclin D depends on growth factors, or mitogens, in the extracellular environment. Withdrawal of mitogens leads to a rapid decrease in the amount of cyclin D. When activated, the cyclin D–CDK complexes phosphorylate target proteins, including RB (the product of the gene mutated in the hereditary form of retinoblastoma). Phosphorylation of RB relieves transcriptional repression of genes that promote entrance into the S phase. Cyclin-dependent kinase inhibitors from both the p21 and the INK4 families inactivate the cyclin D–CDK complexes. In this way, the presence of mitogens is linked to the cell cycle through cyclin D, CDKs, CKIs, and RB in a signaling pathway called the *RB pathway* (Fig. 20-3).

20.3.1   Cell Cycle Checkpoints Maintain the Integrity of the Genome

Signaling pathways that regulate cell cycle progression are called *cell cycle checkpoints.* They recognize a problem, such as damaged DNA, and transmit a signal to the cell cycle machinery to cause cell cycle arrest. Checkpoints detect DNA damage, DNA replication, and the spindle assembly.

Mammalian cells delay progression of the cell cycle in G1, G2, and S after damage to DNA. This allows time for repair of the damaged DNA and prevents propagation of mutations. Agents that damage DNA include environmental and therapeutic radiation, environmental toxins, and chemotherapeutic agents. Detection of DNA damage during G1 requires several proteins, including ATM (*a*taxia-*t*elangiectasia *m*utated), which is the protein encoded by the mutated gene in ataxia-telangiectasia. After recognition of DNA damage, the protein kinase function of ATM is activated, and phosphorylation of other proteins occurs. This signal leads to accumulation of a transcription factor known as p53 (Fig. 20-3). p53 up-regulates expression of many genes, including the CKI known as p21. Increased expression of p21 inactivates cyclin-CDK complexes that regulate the G1-S transition and cause G1 arrest.

During G2, as in G1, DNA damage is detected and the signal is transmitted by way of ATM. This leads to activation of p53, but G2 arrest occurs even in the absence of p53. During G2, the arrest

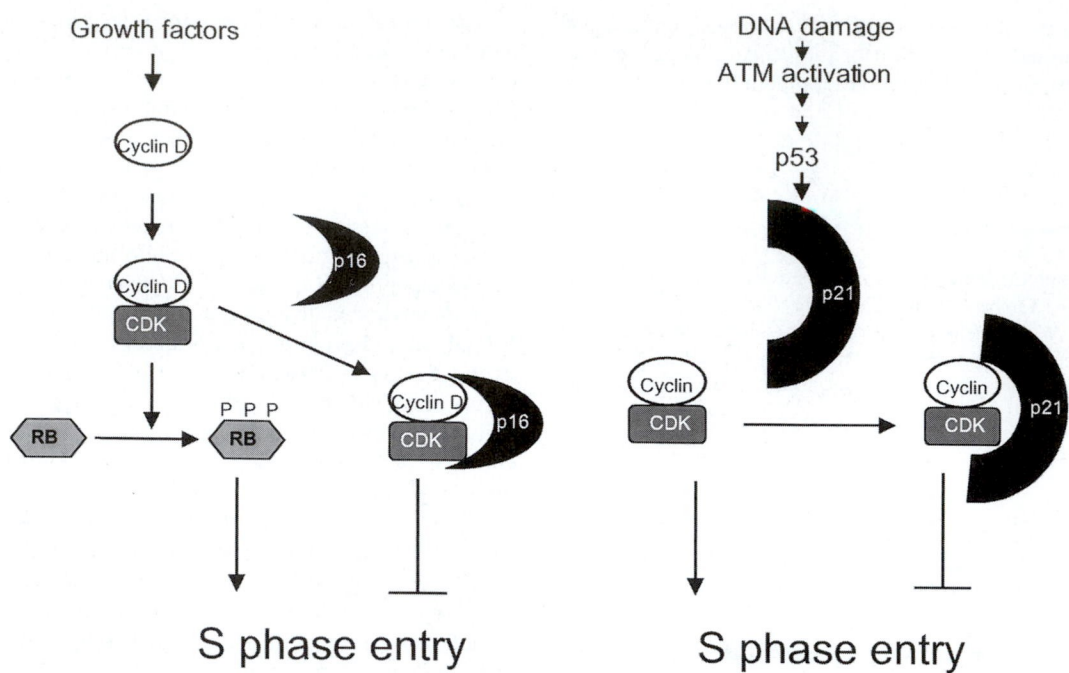

FIGURE 20-3   RB pathway: Sequence of events leading to entrance into S and the action of p16NK4a (and other INK4 proteins) to block entrance into S. Synthesis of cyclin D requires growth factors in the extracellular environment. Cyclin D and CDK4 (or 6) associate and become activated. The protein complex initiates sequential phosphorylation of RB, which relieves the transcriptional repression imposed by RB and promotes entrance into S phase. If p16 binds the cyclin-CDK complex, p16 is inactivated and RB is not activated and cells do not enter S. p53 pathway: If the DNA of cells is damaged, the p53 pathway is activated first through activation of ATM, which leads to accumulation of p53 and transcriptional up-regulation of p21. p21 binds and inactivates cyclin-CDK complexes that promote entry into S, which is similar to the role of p16 in the RB pathway.

of DNA damage is mediated by a signaling pathway that involves protein kinases and phosphatases. It culminates in phosphorylation and functional inactivation of Cdc25C. Cdc25C is a protein phosphatase that activates cyclin B–cdc2, the cyclin-CDK complex that controls the transition from G2 to M. As with G1 arrest, DNA damage during G2 leads to inactivation of a cyclin-CDK complex, but the mechanisms are different.

Mammalian cells also have checkpoints that ensure that DNA replication is completed before initiation of mitosis (the DNA replication checkpoint) and that chromosomes are properly attached to the mitotic spindle before completion of mitosis (the spindle assembly checkpoint). These checkpoints maintain the integrity of the genome. Defects in these checkpoints may contribute to the tendency of cancer cells to segregate their genetic material inaccurately, which is known as *genomic instability*.

20.3.2   Cell Cycle Gene Mutations Cause Pediatric Diseases

Four pediatric diseases have been attributed to germ-line mutations in cell cycle and checkpoint genes. *Ataxia-telangiectasia* is a rare disease characterized by cerebellar degeneration, recurrent infections, telangiectasias, and a predisposition to malignant disease, primarily leukemia and lymphoma. The mutated gene in this syndrome, which is known as *ATM*, encodes a protein that has a role in recognition of DNA damage and activation of the DNA damage checkpoints (Fig. 20-3). *Li-Fraumeni syndrome* is a genetic syndrome that predisposes affected persons to malignant disease, especially sarcoma and breast cancer. The majority of cases of Li-Fraumeni syndrome are a result of germ-line mutations that inactivate p53. *Retinoblastoma* is a malignant tumor of the retina that occurs in both sporadic and inherited forms (see Sec. 20.2). The inherited form of this illness is characterized by bilateral tumors. It is caused by a germ-line mutation in one of the two copies of the RB gene. Somatic mutations of the second copy of the gene leave the cells devoid of functional RB protein, leading to cell transformation. *Beckwith-Weidemann syndrome* (BWS) is characterized by hemihypertrophy, omphaloceles, and predisposition to embryonal tumors, including Wilms tumor, hepatoblastoma, and neuroblastoma. The inheritance of BWS is complicated. It results from abnormal expression of a number of genes on chromosome 11p15, including one of the p21 family genes, p57kip2. Many of the features of BWS are reproduced in mice that lack p57kip2, suggesting a role of this gene in BWS (see Chap. 10).

20.3.3   Derangements in Cell Cycle Regulation Contribute to Tumorigenesis

Defects in components of the checkpoint and cell cycle regulatory pathways are common in malignant cells. These alterations often allow cancer cells to grow with decreased dependence on mitogens, to proliferate in the presence of DNA damage, and to display genomic instability.

In nontransformed cells, the RB pathway is a regulator of cellular proliferation, but mutations in components of this signaling pathway are common in cancer cells. One of the INK4 family members, p16INK4a, is frequently mutated in malignant tumors among humans. Another protein, known as ARF, encoded at the p16INK4a locus, also plays a role in checkpoint control by modulating the stability of p53. Germ-line mutations in p16INK4a have been linked to the hereditary form of melanoma. Somatic mutations of the gene are frequent in sporadic cancers, including ALL among children and at least one type of brain tumor. Mutations that lead to overexpression of one of the cyclin D genes, cyclin D1, are common in human malignancies but are infrequent in cancers in children. Mutations in RB have been found in many different sporadic malignant tumors, including pediatric osteosarcoma. RB functions as a tumor suppressor by repressing the action of proteins that promote entry into S. Papillomaviruses that cause cancer use a viral protein, E7, to inactivate RB and circumvent its role in control of cell proliferation.

Most tumor cells in humans have mutations in the p53 pathway (Fig. 20-3), which transmits the DNA damage signal to the cell cycle machinery. Although the role of ATM as a tumor suppressor is evident from the disease ataxia-telangiectasia, infrequent mutations occur in sporadic cancers. p53 has a central role in controlling cell fate after DNA damage by regulating both cell cycle arrest and apoptosis (cell suicide), which may also be induced by DNA damage. Papillomaviruses that transform cells use a viral protein, E6, to inactivate p53. Signaling pathways that control the cell cycle may serve as therapeutic targets in therapy for cancer.

References

Bates S, Vousden KH: p53 in signaling checkpoint arrest or apoptosis. Curr Opin Genet Dev 6:12–8, 1996

Harper JW, Elledge SJ: Cdk inhibitors in development and cancer. Curr Opin Genet Dev 6:56–64, 1996

Hartwell LH, Weinert TA: Checkpoints: controls that ensure the order of cell cycle events. Science 246:629–634, 1989

Morgan DO: Cyclin-dependent kinases: engines, clocks, and microprocessors. Annu Rev Cell Dev Biol 13:261–91, 1997

Quesnel S, Malkin D: Genetic predisposition to cancer and familial cancer syndromes. Pediatr Clin North Am 44:791–808, 1997

Rudner AD, Murray AW: The spindle assembly checkpoint. Curr Opin Cell Biol 8:773–780, 1996

Sherr CJ. Tumor surveillance via the ARF-p53 pathway. Genes Dev 12: 2984–2991, 1998

20.4   STEM CELL TRANSPLANTATION

Robert J. Hayashi

Thirty years have passed since the first bone marrow transplantation was performed on a human patient. Since that initial breakthrough, numerous advances have enhanced the understanding of the biologic aspects of transplantation and improved technical skills for implementation. More than 40,000 stem cell transplantations are performed each year worldwide. The basic concepts of transplant biology are presented, and various components of the transplantation procedure are elaborated to emphasize the vast potential for future endeavors.

20.4.1   Historical Perspective

The origins of transplantation began with an interest after World War II in the complications and management of radiation-induced bone marrow failure. Simple experiments shielding various organs from radiation exposure showed that the spleen and subsequently the bone marrow contained essential elements that could protect animals from aplastic anemia. Critical experiments with both rats and dogs further delineated the conditions that would allow reconstitution of blood cell production. Although animals could be effectively treated in this manner, almost all of them died of the second disease, which was ultimately characterized and named graft-versus-host disease (GVHD). These observations coincided with independent studies of the HLA system and its relation to immune responses that ultimately provided the framework for defining the barriers to transplantation in the treatment of humans.

The first successful bone marrow transplantations were performed on humans in 1969; however, almost 10 years passed before consistent survival was achieved. Steady improvements in all aspects of transplantation medicine, including management of infection, transfusion, GVHD, and stem cell processing, have brought patient survival to its current levels and made stem cell transplantation a viable modality.

The late 1980s gave rise to the development of stem cell mobilization and peripheral stem cell transplantation, which further reduced morbidity and the costs of autologous stem cell rescue. This period also marked the beginning of the development of transplantation registries, through which allogeneic transplantation became available to a larger fraction of the population. Additional advances include development of cord blood transplantation, improvements in supportive care, and improvements in the control of GVHD. These advances have improved patient survival. Current regimens can provide survival rates of 60 to 70% for acute leukemia. Success rates as high as 80 to 90% have been obtained for nonmalignant diseases such as aplastic anemia, immunodeficiency, and thalassemia.

20.4.2   Strategies in the Use of Stem Cell Transplantation

Consideration of a patient for stem cell transplantation must first address the goals of therapy. Table 20-4 lists some of the accepted uses of stem cell transplantation for a pediatric patient. A common use is to achieve control of malignant tumors. This strategy capitalizes on the ability of stem cell infusion to reestablish normal hematopoiesis and thus allow dose intensification in therapy for the primary tumor that would otherwise cause life-threatening myelosuppression. Such high-intensity therapy administered at the beginning of the procedure is called the *preparative regimen*. Its function in this instance is to allow greater magnitude of tumor destruction in the hope of improving survival. If dose intensity is the primary consideration for therapy, facilitating rapid recovery of normal bone marrow function and minimizing life-threatening side effects of the preparative regimen, such as mucositis, bleeding, and infection, become the primary factors influencing the choice of stem cell source. Autologous stem cell transplantation fulfills this criterion, and autologous peripheral stem cells can be used to maximize the rate of recovery and minimize morbidity.

Unlike therapy for solid tumors, control of some malignant hematopoietic diseases can be improved with infusion of immuno-

TABLE 20-4
STRATEGY OF TRANSPLANTATION

GOAL OF PROCEDURE	GOAL OF PREPARATIVE REGIMEN	GOAL OF STEM CELL SOURCE	TYPE OF TRANSPLANT	LIMITATION	DISEASE
Eradication of refractory tumor	High intensity	Rapid hematopoietic reconstitution	Autologous	Preparative regimen acute toxicity Resistance to chemotherapy	Neuroblastoma Ewing sarcoma Wilms tumor Acute leukemia
Management of malignant hematopoietic disease	Tumor cytoreduction Preparation for engraftment	Hematopoietic reconstitution Graft-versus-tumor effect	Allogeneic	Preparative regimen acute toxicity Graft-versus-host disease Resistance to chemotherapy Immunologic resistance	Acute leukemia Chronic myelogenous leukemia High-grade lymphoma Myelodysplasia
Replacement of a defective hematopoietically derived cell	Preparation for engraftment	Establishment of normal function before irreversible toxicity develops	Allogeneic	Preparative regimen acute toxicity Graft-versus-host disease Rejection	Aplastic anemia Hurler disease Immunodeficiency Osteopetrosis Sickle-cell anemia Thalassemia

competent cells from an allogeneic donor. These cells attack the cancer in the host. This *graft-versus-tumor effect* can influence disease-free survival and may make allogeneic bone marrow transplantation a preferred modality over autologous transplantation. This procedure can still be performed to retain the high-intensity preparative therapy needed to maximize tumor kill and retain the benefits of autologous transplantation. The benefits of allogeneic transplantation must be weighed against the risks of life-threatening complications of allogeneic transplantation, such as GVHD, and the likelihood of recurrence of a refractory malignant lesion.

In the management of nonmalignant diseases, the considerations are different from those in therapy for malignant disease. If reestablishment of a normal hematopoietic system is the goal, allogeneic transplantation with infusion of normally functioning cells is the appropriate strategy. In this case, the preparative regimen should be less intensive to minimize long-term toxicity without compromising engraftment. This is a modest challenge in the case of immunodeficiencies in which the immunologic barriers to engraftment are compromised. It can be a formidable challenge in the management of diseases such as aplastic anemia, in which chronic transfusions can sensitize the host to reject donor stem cells. This category covers a broad spectrum of diseases, some acquired and others inherited. The ability to cure a particular patient must take into account not only theoretic efficacy but also the status of the individual patient. Studies of conditions such as thalassemia and sickle-cell anemia have shown that careful patient selection is critical for a successful outcome. Patients with severe organ damage before transplantation may be at increased risk of death from the procedure. A minimally affected patient is of even greater importance in conditions such as lysosomal storage diseases. In this instance, the success of the procedure depends on the newly infused hematopoietically derived cell to clear toxic accumulations of metabolites in the periphery at a sufficient tempo to prevent clinical deterioration and irreparable damage. Carefully designed studies with thorough follow-up evaluation will ultimately determine the criteria for transplantation for a particular disease.

SOURCES OF STEM CELLS FOR HEMATOPOIETIC RECONSTITUTION

The hematopoietic stem cell (HSC), a pluripotent cell, is the source of all of the mature blood cells that circulate through the body (see Chap. 19). Although the exact nature of the stem cell has remained elusive, reagents are now available to identify cell populations enriched with this valuable commodity. The surface phenotype of an HSC expresses specific markers that can be used to identify this cell population from the other inhabitants of the bone marrow—CD34 and Sca-1 with low expression of Thy-1 and Lin. The number of HSCs in a product used for transplantation has been shown to correlate with the rate of hematopoietic recovery. Each stem cell source can be distinguished by means of collection and by potential for hematopoietic reconstitution.

BONE MARROW Bone marrow has been the traditional source of stem cells. It was the sole source in the early development of transplantation. Recent studies indicate that HSCs constitute only 0.05% of the entire bone marrow population. Because of their pluripotent nature, few cells are needed to establish normal hematopoietic function after myeloablation. As few as 100 cells are needed to reconstitute normal marrow function. Although the bone marrow can reliably reconstitute normal blood production, the low number of HSCs often can result in slow engraftment.

PERIPHERAL STEM CELLS In the mid-1980s it was appreciated that stem cells could be obtained from peripheral blood and could be used to help patients recover from high-dose chemotherapy. Because stem cells represent only 0.002% of the mononuclear leukocyte population, a large volume of blood had to be collected to obtain a sufficient number of cells for hematopoietic reconstitution. The practical use of this modality arose when it became apparent that the number of stem cells in the bloodstream increased during hematopoietic recovery from chemotherapy. Further studies showed that the use hematopoietic growth factors such as granulocyte colony-stimulating factor, granulocyte-macrophage colony-stimulating factor, and others can enhance release of stem cells into the periphery, making them accessible for collection by means of leukopheresis. The development of reagents to measure stem cell markers further improved the efficiency of this process. The ability to measure stem cell content optimized the conditions for stem cell collection.

The use of peripheral stem cells for allogeneic transplantation showed that growth factors such as granulocyte colony-stimulating factor can be administered safely to normal adult donors and that sufficient numbers of stem cells can be collected with conventional pheresis techniques. Use of this stem cell source allows rapid engraftment, and the rate of acute GVHD appears to be no higher than when bone marrow is used. Studies are underway to assess the use of this technology in the care of pediatric patients.

UMBILICAL CORD BLOOD   In studies more than 15 years ago it was found that umbilical cord blood is a rich source of HSCs. Cord blood has higher numbers of hematopoietic progenitors and a greater proliferative capacity in response to cytokine administration compared to bone marrow cells. More than 10 years have passed since the first umbilical cord blood transplantation procedure. After more than 1000 transplantation procedures, it is clear that under the right conditions umbilical cord blood can be an effective stem cell source. Studies have shown that GVHD occurs less frequently with umbilical cord blood than with bone marrow transplantation.

This observation has allowed the use of mismatched cord blood products for transplantation, increasing the versatility of this stem cell source for patients who do not have a matched donor. Relatively immature or tolerant immune cells can be obtained from cord blood. Although this poses a potential advantage for cord blood over bone marrow transplantation, the immature immune system of this stem cell source has limitations. Difficulties with engraftment lead to a higher rate of rejection than occurs with conventional bone marrow transplantation. Slower rates of recovery in neutrophil and platelet production have been observed than with use of either bone marrow or peripheral stem cells. The size of the patient may be a limiting factor in use of umbilical cord blood. The number of mononuclear cells infused per kilogram of recipient body weight has been shown to be an important variable in determining the rate of hematopoietic recovery and possibly of survival. Additional studies are needed to determine the exact role of umbilical cord blood transplantation.

COURSE AND COMPLICATIONS OF TRANSPLANTATION

The clinical course of typical stem cell transplantation can be divided into distinct stages accompanied by different sets of medical challenges (Fig. 20-4). The initial phase entails administration of the preparative regimen—the intensive chemotherapy or radiation therapy given before the stem cell infusion. The nature of the pre-

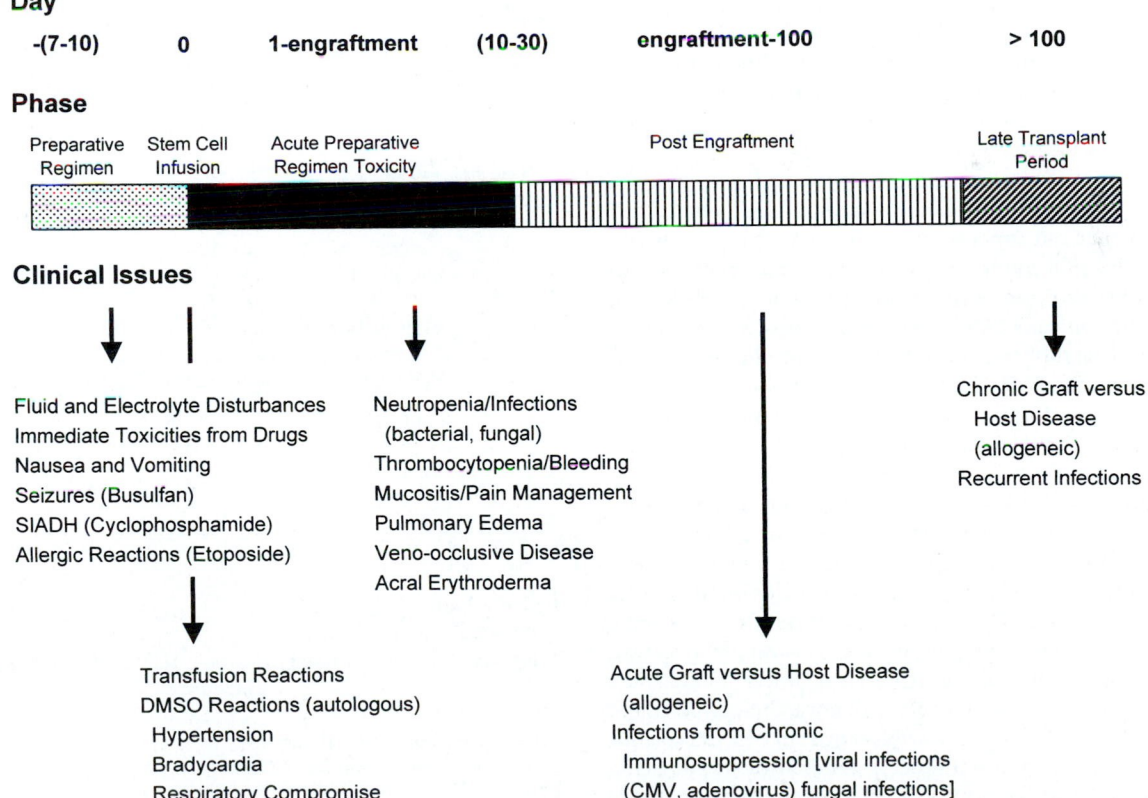

FIGURE 20-4   Transplant course and complications. The medical course of stem cell transplantation is plotted over time. The time interval from the infusion of cells (0) is indicated by *day*. The course is divided into five arbitrary periods or phases, and some of the typical medical problems encountered in each interval are indicated (*clinical issues*). In general, postengraftment and late transplantation periods are clinical issues restricted to allogeneic transplantation and are a consequence of the prolonged immunosuppression and the development of graft-versus-host disease. SIADH = syndrome of inappropriate antidiuretic hormone secretion.

parative regimen varies with various transplantation protocols and is dictated by the goal of the procedure. Administration of the chemotherapy often is at very high doses, which can cause toxic side effects not often encountered with these drugs at lower doses. Careful attention to fluids, electrolytes, renal function, and other values is needed to promote efficient clearance of drugs and to identify early signs of acute side effects.

After administration of the preparative regimen and after an appropriate rest period to ensure clearance of all of the drugs, the stem cells are infused on day 0. Medical management varies according to the nature of the stem cell product. Freshly harvested products from either bone marrow or leukopheresis can be infused with little difficulty directly into a patient who has a blood type compatible with that of the donor. In the case of blood group mismatches, the number of erythrocytes has to be decreased to avoid complications of acute red cell hemolysis. Frozen stem cell products are stored in DMSO, which has side effects such as hypertension, bradycardia, and respiratory compromise. Close monitoring and prompt management of each condition ensures that the complication rate remains minimal.

After stem cell infusion, the primary focus of care is managing the complications of the high-intensity preparative regimen. During this period, patients have little or no marrow function and depend on transfusions for maintaining erythrocytes and platelets at acceptable levels. Because of the prolonged period of neutropenia, the patients are at risk of life-threatening infection, particularly from bacterial pathogens. The mucositis caused by the preparative regimen provides an ample portal of entry for pathogens through the disrupted gastrointestinal lining. It presents challenges in pain control, bleeding, and edema of the upper airway. There are many other complications in this phase of transplantation, including venoocclusive disease, fluid retention, pulmonary edema, and acral erythroderma.

The rate of engraftment is a function of the preparative regimen, the nature and dose of stem cells infused, and the administration of medications that can suppress recovery. Engraftment, typically defined as a neutrophil count greater than $500/mm^3$ and a platelet count of $20,000/mm^3$ can occur as soon as 10 days to as long as several weeks after infusion. Once engraftment occurs, the mucous membranes heal rapidly and recovery is prompt. In general, this marks the end to the acute phase of autologous transplantation because few additional acute complications typically are encountered. In allogeneic transplantation, however, GVHD may manifest at this stage.

Graft-versus-host disease is a clinical syndrome that affects recipients of allogeneic stem cell transplants. It is a manifestation that the engrafting immune system is responding to the new environment of the host. Occurrence of this disease depends on the activity of donor T lymphocytes. The severity is a function of the degree of disparity between the donor and the recipient. An identical twin who receives a stem cell infusion from an identical sibling has a *syngeneic* transplant. Because of genetic identity, there is no risk of GVHD. Nonidentical twins have *allogeneic* stem cell transplants, and the risk of acquiring severe disease varies with the degree a relative is compatible at the HLA locus. Among full siblings, those who inherit the same HLA haplotypes from both parents and are thus identical at the HLA locus have the best odds of avoiding severe GVHD. The likelihood of having such a matched sibling, however, is only one in four. Parents and siblings who do not completely match with a patient convey a high risk of severe GVHD if they act as donors. Relatives who share only one identical haplotype with the patient are called *haploidentical* donors. Their donation

of stem cells has been limited because of the high graft failure rates and severe GVHD that substantially increase the risk of the procedure. *T-cell depletion*, a process that removes the source of GVHD from the graft, has made this transplantation modality feasible in some clinical situations.

The clinical manifestations of GVHD are reflected in the staging classification in Table 20-5. The rash, often the first sign of GVHD, can manifest as either erythroderma or a macular papular rash that typically involves the hands and feet and may progress from the top of the scalp down toward the torso. Progressive disease can lead to exfoliation, bulla formation, and disruption of the epithelial barrier that protects the host from infection. The gastrointestinal manifestation of GVHD is diarrhea, which is graded by volume of stool per day. The diarrhea typically is associated with abdominal cramping. It can be severe with bleeding and disruption of the mucosal barrier, which increases the infection rate. The hepatic manifestations of GVHD are more difficult to diagnose because cholestasis and elevated levels of transaminases immediately after transplantation arise from several sources.

Management of GVHD includes both preventive measures and control of progressive disease. Identifying the most optimally matched donor for a patient results in the lowest risk of severe disease. Prophylaxis against development of GVHD can be achieved by means of eliminating the offending T-cell population

TABLE 20-5

CLASSIFICATION OF GRAFT-VERSUS-HOST DISEASE

Acute

Stage	Skin Involvement	Gastrointestinal	Liver (bilirubin level)
1	<25% surface area	500–1000 mL/day diarrhea	2–3 mg/dL
2	25–50% surface area	1000–1500 mL/day diarrhea	3–6 mg/dL
3	Generalized	>1500 mL/day diarrhea	6–15 mg/dL
4	Desquamation	Pain +/− ileus	>15 mg/dL

Grade	Skin (stage)	Gastrointestinal (stage)	Liver (stage)
1	1–2	0	0
2	1–3	1	1
3	2–3	2–3	2–3
4	2–4	2–4	2–4

Chronic

Limited

Either or both
  Localized skin involvement
  Hepatic dysfunction caused by chronic graft-versus-host disease

Extensive

Either
  Generalized or localized skin involvement
  or hepatic dysfunction caused by chronic graft-versus-host disease
Plus
  Liver histologic evidence of chronic aggressive hepatitis, bridging necrosis, or cirrhosis
or
  Involvement of the eye
  Involvement of minor salivary glands or oral mucosa found at labial biopsy
  Involvement of any other target organ

before stem cell infusion or by means of administration of immunosuppressants, such as cyclosporine, methotrexate, or prednisone. Management of progressive disease primarily consists of the use of high-dose glucocorticoids. It is effective in the care of fewer than one half of the patients with advanced disease. Other treatments, such as antithymocyte globulin or other immunosuppressants, typically are successful for only a small fraction of patients. All of these treatments profoundly compromise the immune system and place the patient at high risk of opportunistic infection. The diagnosis of GVHD must be differentiated from multiple other causes of rashes, diarrhea, or cholestasis. Biopsies typically are performed to help differentiate GVHD from other processes to avoid the unnecessary use of immunosuppressive medication to treat patients who do not have GVHD.

Graft-versus-host disease can occur in a chronic form that has distinct clinical features. This condition often develops insidiously. Progressive destruction of epithelial tissues and glandular structures causes the clinical manifestations.

LONG-TERM TOXICITY

Numerous late side effects can occur any time after transplantation, necessitating continuous medical follow-up care of these patients. In general, the clinical conditions can be classified into three basic categories: (1) toxicity from the preparative regimen, (2) toxicity from GVHD, and (3) toxicity from long-term immunosuppression (Table 20-6).

Toxicity from the preparative regimen varies with the nature of the treatment. The high intensity of chemotherapy and radiation

potentially places any organ at risk of irreversible damage. For pediatric patients, careful monitoring of growth and a thorough review of systems often direct specific investigations, although some clinical complications occur more frequently than others (Table 20-6). The effect of radiation on growth is relatively common and can be a result of a multitude of factors. Disruption of production of growth hormone is the most common; however, the effects of radiation on thyroid function, gonadal function, and bone growth also can contribute. Thyroid dysfunction is a relatively common complication. Yearly evaluation of thyroid function often shows early signs of disease. Other toxicities from radiation include cataracts, azospermia, and gonadal failure. Many of these toxicities overlap with the toxicities of high-dose chemotherapy.

Chronic GVHD can cause severe cumulative effects on the body. Disruption of normal glandular function can result in chronic disease. Drying of the eyes can cause corneal injury; decreased salivary gland production can cause severe dental caries. Chronic inflammation of the intestine can lead to strictures and webs which can cause severe morbidity. The skin manifestations take two basic forms. One is a dry maculopapular rash indistinguishable from lichen planus. The other is a sclerodermatous condition that can extend to all parts of the body and cause fibrosis of the underlying subcutaneous tissues and fascia. The result is restriction of movement and contractures. Continuous monitoring with aggressive physical therapy can maintain function among patients who ultimately respond to immunosuppression.

Long-term administration of chronic immunosuppressive drugs, although it controls GVHD, can cause toxicity that hampers quality

TABLE 20-6

LONG-TERM TOXICITY OF STEM CELL TRANSPLANTATION

CATEGORY	SOURCE	COMMON	RARE
Preparative regimen	Total-body irradiation	Cataracts Growth impairment Oral and dental growth impairment and decay Thyroid dysfunction Infertility	Gonadal failure Restrictive lung disease Renal dysfunction Posttransplantation malignant tumors
	Chemotherapy BCNU Busulfan Cyclophosphamide	Restrictive lung disease Restrictive lung disease Gonadal failure infertility	Renal dysfunction Growth failure Bladder scarring Heart failure
	Carboplatin	Ototoxicity Renal dysfunction	Renal failure
Graft-versus-host disease	Persistent chronic graft-versus-host disease	Alopecia Chronic pain Dental caries Ocular dryness Scleroderma Recurrent infections	Bronchiolitis obliterans Cirrhosis Esophageal strictures or webs
Therapy for graft-versus-host disease	Long-term glucocorticoid therapy	Glucose intolerance Growth failure Hypertension Osteopenia Recurrent infection	Avascular necrosis of the femoral head Cataracts Recurrent fractures
	Cyclosporine	Hypertension Hypomagnesemia Recurrent infection Renal dysfunction	Seizures Renal failure

BCNU = carmustine.

of life. These toxicities include hypertension, glucose intolerance, weight gain, growth failure, avascular necrosis of the femoral head, and chronic osteopenia that leads to recurrent fractures. Cyclosporine, for example, can cause a constellation of toxicities, including hypertension, seizures, hypomagnesemia, microangiopathic hemolytic anemia, and chronic renal insufficiency. Long-term administration of this and other immunosuppressive agents can lead to recurrent infections, such as bacterial, fungal, cytomegalovirus, and adenovirus and varicella zoster (see Sec. 21.15).

20.4.3   Future Directions

The use of allogeneic stem cell transplantation for patients who do not have an HLA-matched sibling requires the use of alternative donors. Reduction of long-term toxicity of the therapy and improved control of GVHD are essential to increase the appeal of stem cell transplantation for patients with chronic diseases such as sickle-cell anemia and thalassemia, who can currently survive into adulthood with less aggressive supportive measures. Advances on the more distant horizon will include the use of gene therapy to correct genetic disease with autologous stem cell sources, which may ultimately eliminate the need for allogeneic transplantation among this patient population.

References

Anasetti C, Amos D, Beatty PG, et al: Effect of HLA compatibility on engraftment of bone marrow transplants in patients with leukemia or lymphoma. N Engl J Med 320:197–204, 1989

Cairo MS, Wagner JE: Placental and/or umbilical cord blood: an alternative source of hematopoietic stem cells for transplantation. Blood 90:4665–4678, 1997

Kessinger A: Utilization of peripheral blood stem cells in autotransplantation. Hermatol Oncol Clin North Am 7:535–545, 1993

Lazarus HM, Vogelsang GB, Rowe JM: Prevention and treatment of acute graft versus host disease: the old and the new—a report from the Eastern Cooperative Oncology Group (ECOG). Bone Marrow Transplant 19:577–600, 1997

Morrison SJ, Uchida N, Weissman IL: The biology of hematopoietic stem cells. Annu Rev Cell Dev Biol 11:35–71, 1995

Sanders JE: Bone marrow transplantation for pediatric malignancies. Pediatr Clin North Am 44:1005–1020, 1997

Thomas ED, Storb R: The development of the scientific foundation of hematopoietic cell transplantation based on animal and human studies. In: Thomas ED, Blume KG, Forman SJ, eds: Hematopoietic Cell Transplantation, 2nd ed. Malden, MA, Blackwell Science, 1999: 1–11

Weaver CH, Hazelton B, Birch R, et al: An analysis of engraftment kinetics as a function of the CD34 content of peripheral blood progenitor cell collections in 692 patients after the administration of myeloablative chemotherapy. Blood 86:3961–3969, 1995

Winston DJ, Gale RP, Meyer DV, Young LS: Infectious complications of human bone marrow transplantation. Medicine 58:1–31, 1979

20.5   ACUTE LYMPHOBLASTIC LEUKEMIA

C. Philip Steuber and David G. Poplack

Fifty years ago it was unusual for any child with ALL to live more than a few months after diagnosis. Currently more than 70% of

children with ALL are expected to survive the disease provided they receive appropriate modern therapies. This dramatic improvement in prognosis is the result of the development and use of effective antileukemia agents in combination regimens, use of CNS preventive therapy, identification of clinically and biologically defined disease subgroups, and evolution of treatment strategies tailored to risk group and disease subtype. Advances in supportive care, including antiinfective agents, blood banking practices, and nutritional support capabilities, have improved treatment of children with ALL. Clinical trials conducted under the auspices of the National Cancer Institute have been important in the genesis of effective therapies for ALL. The complexity of diagnostic methods and the intensive nature of current treatment and supportive care requirements of children with ALL necessitate that evaluation and management be provided in an established multidisciplinary pediatric cancer facility.

CLINICAL FEATURES

With a peak incidence between 2 and 5 years of age, ALL is the most common childhood malignant disease. It accounts for approximately 30% of all cases of malignant disease among children. Each year 2000 to 3000 children and adolescents in the United States receive the diagnosis of ALL. More than 80% of patients are younger than 10 years at diagnosis (Table 20-7). Children with Down syndrome, Bloom syndrome, Fanconi anemia, and ataxia-telangiectasia are at particular risk of ALL. Siblings, especially twins, of children with leukemia are approximately twice as likely to have leukemia than is the general population. Some cases of childhood ALL may be related to hereditary or acquired mutations in the p53 gene (see Sec. 20.2 and Sec. 20.3). Taken in total, however, these

TABLE 20-7

INCIDENCE OF CLINICAL AND LABORATORY CLASSIFICATION VARIABLES IN CHILDHOOD ACUTE LYMPHOBLASTIC LEUKEMIA

CATEGORY	INCIDENCE (%)
Leukocyte count	
$<10,000/\mu L$	50
$10,000–49,000/\mu L$	32
$>50,000/\mu L$	18
Age (yr)	
1–9.99	83
>10	17
FAB category	
L1	85
L2	14
L3	1
Immunophenotype	
B precursor	84
T-cell lineage	14
Mature B cell	2
Cytogenetics	
(B-lineage acute lymphoblastic leukemia)	
DI > 1.16	27
Trisomies 4 and 10	21
t(12;21)	16–18
t(1;19)	5–6
t(9;22)	3–5
t(4;11)	2

FAB = French-American-British Cooperative Working Group Classification.
DI = DNA index.

predisposing circumstances or relationships account for only a small proportion of cases.

The early manifestations of ALL are protean and reflect uncontrolled growth of the malignant cell population invading the bone marrow, lymphoid organs, and various extramedullary sites. Panmyelophthisis causing a failure of normal hematopoiesis results in varying degrees of anemia, thrombocytopenia, and neutropenia. The "4 Ps," a tetrad of *pallor* (65% of cases), *pyrexia* (61% of cases), *purpura* (48% of cases), and *pain* (23% of cases), comprise the most common presenting symptoms. Vague symptoms such as fatigue or loss of appetite may have been present from days to months before diagnosis. Fever can be caused by concomitant infection or the disease itself. Pallor reflects the severity of anemia. Bleeding manifestations, including the appearance of petechiae and purpura, usually are proportional to the degree of thrombocytopenia. Bone pain is a common presenting feature, particularly among young children with ALL, whose first symptom may be the onset of a limp or refusal to walk. Abdominal pain may result from liver and spleen distension caused by disease involvement. The differential diagnosis frequently includes infection, rheumatoid disease, bone marrow failure states, and other malignant diseases that can involve the bone marrow.

Findings at initial physical examination commonly are nonspecific. Asymptomatic lymphadenopathy and hepatosplenomegaly occur among more than one half of patients. Lymphadenopathy usually is generalized. Massive nodal and organ enlargement, although an imprecise measure of tumor burden, has been associated with a poor prognosis.

After liver, spleen, and lymph node involvement, the most commonly affected extramedullary sites of disease are the CNS, testes, and kidneys. Central nervous system involvement at diagnosis is relatively uncommon; the incidence of less than 5% usually is not associated with symptoms. However, when symptoms occur, the clinical features can include headache, nausea and vomiting, lethargy, and irritability. Patients may have nuchal rigidity and papilledema. The diagnosis of CNS leukemia is made by means of evaluation of cerebrospinal fluid (CSF) obtained through lumbar puncture. Cerebrospinal fluid findings at diagnosis in children with ALL are classified into three groups: CNS 0, in which there are fewer than 5 leukocytes per microliter of CSF and no blasts; CNS 2, in which there are fewer than 5 leukocytes per microliter of CSF but blasts are present; and CNS 3, in which there are more than 5 leukocytes per microliter of CSF and blasts are present. The clinical implication of CNS 2 is uncertain. Patients with CNS 3 disease are considered to have high-risk disease. Cranial nerve palsy is rare as a manifestation of CNS leukemia at diagnosis, but persons with this symptom would be considered to have CNS 3 findings. The most commonly affected cranial nerves are the facial (eighth), oculomotor (third), trochlear (fifth), and abducens (sixth). Kidney enlargement at diagnosis is common but of itself is not associated with adverse prognosis. Renal dysfunction caused by leukemic infiltrates in the absence of the development of uric acid nephropathy is rare. Testicular enlargement caused by leukemic infiltrates is rare at diagnosis.

LABORATORY FEATURES

More than 90% of patients with ALL have a peripheral blood count at presentation that is abnormal in at least one of the three cell lines. Normocytic, normochromic anemia and reticulocytopenia are present in approximately 80 to 85% of cases. The presenting leukocyte count ranges from severe leukopenia to extreme leukocytosis. Eighty percent of patients have a leukocyte count less than $50,000/\mu L$; among 50% the leukocyte count is less than $10,000/\mu L$ (Table 20-7). In spite of normal leukocyte counts, many patients are agranulocytic and are at risk of severe bacterial infection. Thrombocytopenia is extremely common; 75% of patients have platelet counts less than $100,000/\mu L$, and approximately 25% have a platelet count less than $20,000/\mu L$ at diagnosis. Although petechiae and purpura are present in many patients, severe bleeding is unusual at presentation, even when the platelet count is less than $20,000/\mu L$, unless there is a complicating event such as infection.

Although the diagnosis of acute leukemia may be suspected from the changes in the peripheral blood, a bone marrow aspirate is obtained for definitive diagnosis. Once the diagnosis of leukemia is confirmed, meticulous laboratory assessment of the malignant cell population is crucial if appropriate treatment is to be delivered.

Other Laboratory Studies

In addition to the changes in peripheral blood cell count, other laboratory abnormalities often are detected among patients with ALL. Patients may have elevated serum uric acid levels, the degree of elevation reflecting the extent of tumor burden. High uric acid levels occur among patients with markedly elevated leukocyte counts and extensive extramedullary disease. Renal dysfunction can occur among patients with hyperuricemia (see Sec. 21.7). Serum lactate dehydrogenase level frequently is elevated; the degree of elevation appears to correlate with tumor burden.

A variety of electrolyte abnormalities, particularly elevated serum levels of calcium, phosphorus, and potassium, may be observed in patients with newly diagnosed ALL. As with hyperuricemia and elevated lactate dehydrogenase levels, these aberrations are more frequently encountered among patients with a high leukocyte count and extensive tumor burden. Hypercalcemia is commonly thought to result from extensive leukemic infiltration of bone. It also has been found that leukemic lymphoblasts may release a parathormone-like substance. Hyperphosphatemia can accompany the extensive destruction of tumor cells. It occurs as a consequence of ineffective leukopoiesis or of chemotherapy-induced tumor lysis (see Sec. 21.7). Hyperkalemia can be caused by extensive leukemic cell lysis.

Low levels of immunoglobulin in the serum at diagnosis have been found among as many as 30% of children with ALL and have been associated with a poor prognosis. Severe coagulation abnormalities are not a typical feature of ALL at diagnosis. Although disseminated intravascular coagulation can occur, it is infrequent. Changes in results of tests of hepatic function are uncommon, even among patients with a high leukocyte count and extensive hepatomegaly.

DIAGNOSIS

For most patients with ALL, examination of the peripheral blood smear usually reveals leukemic lymphoblasts. Definitive diagnosis, however, usually requires examination of the bone marrow. The posterior iliac crest is the preferred site for marrow aspiration in the care of children. When aspiration does not yield sufficient material for evaluation, bone marrow biopsy is performed.

In ALL, the marrow usually is hypercellular and infiltrated with leukemic lymphoblasts. More than three fourths of patients have more than 50% lymphoblasts in the bone marrow at initial presentation. By convention, at least 25% blast cells are required to render a final diagnosis of acute leukemia.

Morphologic and Histochemical Classification

The cells of ALL can be subclassified on the basis of differences in appearance under a light microscope. The most widely used system, developed by the French-American-British Cooperative Working Group (FAB), divides lymphoblasts into three categories: L1 lymphoblasts are small and have scanty cytoplasm and inconspicuous nucleoli; L2 lymphoblasts are generally larger, although the size can vary, and have more prominent nucleoli and abundant cytoplasm; and L3 lymphoblasts are large, have deep cytoplasmic basophilic and prominent cytoplasmic vacuolation, and are identical cytomorphologically to the cells of Burkitt lymphoma. The L1 morphologic features occur in approximately 85% of cases of childhood ALL (Table 20-7). Lymphoblasts of the L3 type are characteristic of only 1 to 2% of cases of ALL. Although no apparent correlation between the FAB L1 and L2 morphologic types and immunologic cell surface markers exists, cells of the L3 variety possess cell surface immunoglobulin and other B-cell markers. Histochemical stains are used to differentiate the leukemic cell populations. The periodic acid–Schiff, acid phosphatase, and acid α-naphtyl acetate esterase stains are commonly performed as diagnostic adjuncts. The periodic acid–Schiff reaction is positive in approximately 50% of cases of ALL and often shows a characteristic pattern of block positivity. A positive acid phosphatase correlates with the presence of T-cell markers.

Immunophenotypic Characterization

Immunophenotyping has an important role in the diagnosis of acute leukemia. The use of monoclonal antibodies specific for various stages of B-cell, T-cell, and myeloid differentiation antigens enables the clinician to determine more definitively the origin of leukemic cells. In many cases of ALL, immunophenotyping also allows assignment of the relative stage in the process of B- or T-cell differentiation from which the leukemic clone is believed to have arisen.

Approximately 80 to 85% of cases of childhood ALL are believed to develop from monoclonal proliferation of B-cell precursors. In contrast, 15 to 17% of cases are of T-cell origin. The other 1 to 2% of cases manifest surface immunoglobulin and are classified as mature B-cell ALL (Table 20-7). A risk-based stratification system devised by the POG separates childhood ALL into T-cell, B-cell, and B-cell precursor disease and establishes treatment selection (Table 20-8).

Approximately one third of patients with B-cell precursor ALL have demonstrable cytoplasmic immunoglobulin (designated pre-B-cell ALL). Although at one time these patients were considered to have a worse prognosis, current data suggest that the poor outcome is specifically associated with a high incidence (25%) of t(1;19) translocation in this subset of patients. Specific testing for this structural rearrangement has eliminated routine testing for the presence of cytoplasmic immunoglobulin.

Although most cases of ALL express surface antigens and molecular markers that characterize them as arising from a specific lineage, there are cases of mixed lineage or biphenotype wherein markers of more than one cell type are detected on the same leukemic cell population. Simultaneous expression of lymphoid and myeloid markers occurs in ALL. In cases of childhood ALL, detection of myeloid antigens may occur in 15 to 25% of cases (see Sec. 20.6).

TABLE 20-8

RISK GROUP DEFINITIONS ACCORDING TO UNIFORM AGE AND LEUKOCYTE COUNT CRITERIA FOR B PRECURSOR ACUTE LYMPHOBLASTIC LEUKEMIA

RISK GROUP	DEFINITION	PERCENTAGE OF PATIENTS	4-YEAR EVENT-FREE SURVIVAL RATE (%)
Standard	Age 1 to 9 yr and leukocyte count <50,000/μL	68	80.3
Higher	Age ≥10.0 years or leukocyte count ≥50,000/μL	32	63.9

Additional prognostic factors
    DNA index (DI; ploidy)
    Cytogenetics
    Immunophenotyping (B lineage, T lineage)
    Central nervous system status
        CNS 1 (no blasts)
        CNS 2 (leukocyte count <5/μL, blasts present)
        CNS 3 (leukocyte count ≥5/μL, blasts present)
    Early treatment response
        Marrow at day 7 or 14
        Blood at day 7

Cytogenetic Findings

With current methods, more than 90% of cases of childhood ALL demonstrate cytogenetic abnormalities either in number (ploidy) or structure (see Chap. 10). Approximately 40% of cases are pseudodiploid; another 40% are hyperdiploid including 27% with more than 50 chromosomes. Fewer than 2% of cases are hypodiploid (fewer than 45 chromosomes). Among the structural abnormalities, translocations are the most common and occur in 40% of cases. They are detected most often in the pseudodiploid and hypodiploid groups. The most common translocations are the t(12;21), t(1;19), t(9;22), and t(4;11) (Table 20-7).

PROGNOSTIC FACTORS

Although treatment may be the single most important determinant of outcome, a number of clinical and laboratory features evident at diagnosis have value for predicting the duration of responses among patients treated for ALL and in influencing selection of therapy. Identification of these prognostic factors has provided a means of stratifying patients into risk groups and tailoring treatment so that the risk of adverse treatment-related events is balanced with the expectation for outcome. Risk-group assignment is a standard feature of treatment protocols for children and adolescents with ALL.

Multivariate analysis is helpful in assessing the relative prognostic value of any feature, whether it functions as an independent or a dependent prognostic determinant. Advances in technology, especially in molecular genetics, have led to more precise definition of some risk factors. Changes in treatment strategies may alter the relative importance of previously identified risk factors. Patient age and leukocyte count at diagnosis have universal acceptance as prognostic indicators.

Leukocyte count at diagnosis has proved to be an important

prognostic factor in almost all cases of childhood ALL. In general, the prognosis is inversely related to leukocyte count. The 20% of patients with ALL who have initial leukocyte counts greater than $50,000/\mu L$ have a particularly poor prognosis. The relation between leukocyte count and prognosis appears to be linear and continuous.

Age at diagnosis also has prognostic importance. Patients younger than 1 year and those older than 10 years tend to have a worse prognosis. Infants younger than 12 months have the poorest prognosis. Among infants ALL has a number of unique biologic features that in part may explain the relative resistance to therapy. The consensus statement developed at a 1993 meeting convened by the National Cancer Institute recommends that these age and leukocyte count criteria be incorporated into a uniform approach to risk-based assignment (Table 20-8). In addition to defining age and leukocyte count criteria, the National Cancer Institute Risk Classification Workshop recommended that certain studies always be performed at the time of the diagnosis of ALL. These include cytogenetic factors, DNA index, and immunophenotype.

Cytogenetic analysis provides important prognostic information. The association between number of chromosomes and prognosis is well characterized. Patients with hyperdiploidy (more than 50 chromosomes or DNA index greater than 1.16) have a favorable prognosis. Investigators in the POG found that among patients with hyperdiploidy, combined trisomy of chromosomes 4 and 10 is independently predictive of favorable outcome in B-precursor ALL. Patients with hypoploidy (fewer than 45 chromosomes) and pseudodiploidy fare less well. Near tetraploidy also appears to be associated with a poor prognosis, although this may not be an independent factor, because many patients with this abnormality also have T-cell disease.

In addition to variations in number of chromosomes, structural chromosomal abnormalities convey important prognostic information. A number of chromosomal translocations are associated with both a high rate of induction failure and early relapse. These include the t(8;14) translocation associated with B-cell ALL, the t(9;22) in Philadelphia chromosome–positive ALL, the t(1;19) in B-precursor ALL, and the t(4;11) translocation that occurs most frequently among infants. In the past, the presence of any translocation generally was associated with poorer outcome. Recent technical advances have led to identification of a previously unappreciated, prognostically significant rearrangement, the t(12;21) translocation. This translocation causes rearrangement of the *TEL* gene, which is present in at least 16 to 18% of cases of B-cell precursor ALL and has been associated with improved outcome.

In addition to providing diagnostic information, immunophenotype correlates with prognosis. In some studies, patients with ALL with malignant cells that express either mature B-cell or T-cell immunophenotypes have a worse prognosis than patients with B-precursor ALL, and they need different and more aggressive therapy. The prognostic influence of T-cell phenotype is less striking after adjustment for association with high initial leukocyte count. Intensity of treatment appears to influence the degree to which T-cell phenotype influences prognosis. In some recent, more intensive treatment protocols, the prognostic influence of T-cell phenotype has not been evident. Patients with mature B-cell leukemia continue to be treated with separate protocols.

In approximately 15 to 25% of cases of ALL, in addition to lymphoid characteristics, the malignant cell population expresses one or more myeloid antigens in at least 20% of the cells. The occurrence of these myeloid features does not appear to be an adverse indicator, although this topic is controversial.

Other Prognostic Factors

In the context of the FAB classification system, a relation between morphologic subtype and prognosis has been found. The FAB L1 subtype is associated with a more favorable outcome. The FAB L3 subtype, which is associated with B-cell ALL, conveys a poor prognosis. In some studies of childhood ALL, the L2 subtype has also been associated with a poor prognosis. This finding has not been universal, however, and may not be a helpful distinction.

Sex influences outcome. Girls with ALL have a more favorable prognosis. This appears to be related in part to the effect of testicular relapse and to the higher incidence of T-cell disease among boys, but these differences are also occur among populations of patients with early B-lineage ALL. Recommendations for duration of therapy may be influenced by sex. Boys need longer treatment courses.

Ethnicity is an important prognostic determinant. African-American and Hispanic patients have lower remission induction rates and a higher likelihood of bone marrow relapse. The reasons for this poorer outcome are related in part to the higher incidence of initially severe leukocytosis, mediastinal masses, and L2 morphologic features in these populations. Even when adjusted for age and initial leukocyte count, increased risk of treatment failure among nonwhite patients still appears. At this time, however, no treatment assignment criteria based solely on race are used.

Degree of extramedullary disease can be used as an indirect measure of tumor burden. In numerous studies, hepatomegaly, splenomegaly, and the presence of a mediastinal mass have been found to have prognostic importance, although on multivariate analysis these findings are found to correlate with initial leukocyte count. Despite this, some investigators use assessment of hepatomegaly and splenomegaly for assignment of risk group. For example, the Berlin-Frankfurt-Münster Study Group uses a risk factor index, computed with initial leukocyte count and measurement of hepatosplenomegaly, to define groups for therapy for childhood ALL. Low serum levels of immunoglobulin, particularly low IgM levels, have been associated with poor event-free survival rate.

Based on results of the pretreatment clinical and laboratory evaluation, risk group is assigned, and appropriate therapy is begun. An additional prognostic factor becomes response to the initial induction treatment. Patients who do not have complete remission after an initial course of induction therapy have markedly low durations of remission and survival. Even the rapidity of initial response appears to be extremely important. Patients with residual leukemia on day 7 or 14 of induction therapy have shorter event-free survival periods than do patients with marrow that shows no evidence of residual disease at those times.

THERAPY

Patients are treated according to their relative risk of failure. Patients with high-risk features are treated with more intensive, and usually more toxic, therapies. Those with lesser risk characteristics are treated with more established effective and less toxic therapies in an effort to minimize therapy-related morbidity and mortality without compromising expectations for outcome.

The standard of care of children with leukemia involves participation in a clinical trial. Such trials are designed to address treatment issues for the various risk groups. By design, improved treatment strategies are intended to reduce the impact of a given adverse prognostic factor or enhance the influence of a favorable one. Use of different prognostic factors for stratification of risk groups and treatment assignment has lead to difficulty in comparing the results of different approaches to therapy. A workshop at the National Cancer Institute resulted in a proposal for a uniform, basic approach to risk factor assessment based on a combination of clinical and laboratory criteria (Table 20-8). Using these parameters, approximately 70% of patients will be classified as standard risk and the remaining patients are high risk.

For most children and adolescents with ALL, treatment protocols are divided into four principal elements: induction therapy, intensification or consolidation therapy, continuation or maintenance therapy, and CNS preventive therapy. With the exception of the 1 to 2% of ALL patients with B-cell ALL, the duration of therapy for children and adolescents with ALL ranges from 24 to 36 months. The recommended duration of treatment of patients with standard-risk ALL may be shorter than that for patients at high risk. Girls with ALL may need less therapy. Patients with B-cell ALL are treated for a much shorter period, usually 6 to 8 months, albeit with highly aggressive and toxic regimens.

Induction Therapy

The initial phase of every ALL treatment regimen is directed at induction of remission. In general, remission is characterized as the resolution of the abnormal disease-related findings present at diagnosis on both physical examination and laboratory studies. Peripheral blood values must be returning to normal and bone marrow examination with a light microscope should show normal cellularity and less than 5% lymphoblasts. Although these are the standard criteria for defining remission on completion of induction therapy, subclinical or occult leukemia remains present and can be detected with a variety of laboratory methods.

In most clinical trials, remission induction regimens include the use of vincristine and a glucocorticoid with the addition of one or two agents, commonly L-asparaginase or an anthracycline. Three-drug regimens for patients with standard-risk ALL and four-drug regimens for those at high risk are common practice. With such therapies, after 4 weeks of treatment, the complete response rate is approximately 95%. The mortality during induction therapy is approximately 3%. Few failures of induction therapy caused by resistant disease occur among children and adolescents with ALL. The rate of response to induction therapy is in itself a prognostic indicator and patients' peripheral blood changes and bone marrow findings frequently are reassessed before completion of the induction regimen. Patients who respond slowly have lower cure rates, and plans for therapy after induction can be modified under such circumstances. Although the use of additional agents before or during standard induction therapy may not improve the already favorable induction response rate, such practices can improve overall duration of remission and affect event-free survival rates.

Postremission Therapy

After attainment of remission, substantial subsequent therapy is necessary to further reduce the malignant cell population and prevent relapse. In addition to CNS-directed therapies, postremission management usually involves two therapeutic phases—consolidation or intensification therapy and maintenance or continuation therapy.

Consolidation or intensification therapy is a period of intensified treatment that usually begins soon after induction therapy. It involves the introduction of new, non-cross-resistant drugs and drug combinations selected for different and often synergistic mecha-

nisms of action to reduce the risk of emergence of drug resistance. The agents most commonly used in these regimens include cytarabine, anthracyclines, methotrexate, cyclophosphamide, and epipodophyllotoxins. The extended use of epipodophyllotoxins is under scrutiny because of observations linking administration of these agents to the development of secondary malignant myeloproliferative disorders, particularly acute myeloid leukemia (see Sec. 20.6).

Some or all of the agents previously used during induction therapy can be readministered during consolidation therapy, often in a cyclic schedule alternating with new combinations. Another intensification therapeutic strategy involves administration of one or two aggressive multiagent treatment courses given 4 to 6 months after induction of remission—a practice designated delayed intensification. Repeated use of such aggressive therapy sequences interspersed with relatively less toxic therapy is known to improve outcome for ALL patients with high-risk features. Substantial morbidity is a consequence of aggressive consolidation or intensification therapies, but the pronounced improvements in cure rates, particularly among ALL populations at high risk, support use of these treatments.

Consolidation or intensification therapy usually is completed within the first 6 to 12 months after induction. Thereafter the patient receives maintenance therapy for an additional 18 to 24 months. The most common maintenance therapy programs involve daily oral 6-mercaptopurine and weekly methotrexate given orally or intramuscularly. Many maintenance regimens incorporate periodic pulses of additional agents such as vincristine and a glucocorticoid. In the care of patients at high risk, more intensive combinations can be included.

Central Nervous System Preventive Therapy

Although fewer than 5% of patients have CNS leukemia at diagnosis, without directed therapy, a large number of patients will have CNS involvement soon after diagnosis. A CNS relapse indicates that the patient is at increased risk of bone marrow relapse and ultimate treatment failure. Every therapeutic program for childhood ALL consequently includes some form of CNS preventive therapy, CNS prophylaxis, CNS sanctuary therapy, or presymptomatic CNS therapy.

For most patients with ALL, in the context of modern systemic therapy, a series of lumbar punctures with single-agent intrathecal therapy with methotrexate is effective at reducing the occurrence of CNS leukemia to less than 10% overall and less than 5% among patients at standard risk. Other effective intrathecal therapy regimens for ALL entail methotrexate combined with cytarabine or a glucocorticoid. Central nervous system preventive therapy begins during the induction phase and continues through the entire treatment program, usually decreasing in frequency with time.

Patients with overt CNS leukemia at diagnosis (CNS 3) or those at particular risk of development of CNS leukemia are candidates for CNS radiation in addition to more intensive systemic and intrathecal therapies.

OUTCOME

Current data indicate that the overall event-free survival rate among children with ALL exceeds 70%. Patients with standard-risk features at diagnosis are more than two thirds of the ALL population and have reported 4-year event-free survival rates of 80 to 85% (Table 20-8). The remaining one third of patients with ALL, those with high-risk prognostic indicators, have 4-year event-free survival rates of 60 to 65%. A variety of values have been used to characterize lesser or higher risk among patients with ALL. For example, patients with ALL with standard-risk age and leukocyte count criteria at diagnosis who have combined trisomies of chromosomes 4 and 10 have been reported to have an event-free survival rate of 95%.

Relapse

For the 25 to 30% of patients with ALL who have relapses, the main site of failure is the bone marrow. The duration of the first remission is a predictive indicator for both attainment and duration of a second remission. That is, the longer the first remission, the more likely it is the patient will achieve a sustained second remission. Patients who have relapses while undergoing the initial therapy fare less well than those who have relapses more than 3 months after completion of treatment. The prognosis among patients who have relapses after completion of therapy is directly related to the length of time from discontinuation of initial therapy to relapse. The nature and intensity of the initial therapy also influences responsiveness after relapse. Patients who undergo unsuccessful intensive multiagent regimens are less likely to reach or sustain a second remission.

Approximately 70 to 75% of patients who have marrow relapses have a second remission with induction therapy almost identical to the initial regimen. Selection of subsequent treatment depends on previous therapy, including reinduction response. In general, salvage therapies are intense, incorporating intensive use of drugs previously administered and new agents when possible. With aggressive rescue chemotherapy regimens, only approximately 20% of patients who have relapses while still receiving therapy have a prolonged (more than 24 months) second remission. Forty percent of those who have relapses more than 3 months after completion of the initial program may have a prolonged second remission.

Because rescue therapy for patients receiving chemotherapy alone will more likely fail than succeed, bone marrow transplantation (BMT) is commonly explored as a therapeutic option to intensify treatment. Overall disease-free survival rates for patients in second remission undergoing allogeneic BMT range from 40 to 60% (see Sec. 20.4).

Extramedullary relapse in either the CNS or the testes occurs as an isolated event or with simultaneous marrow relapse. As with marrow relapse, the later in the clinical course the extramedullary relapse occurs, the more likely it is the patient will have a favorable response to rescue therapy. Isolated CNS relapse occurs among 5 to 10% of patients. Current management of CNS leukemia involves several months of intensive parenteral systemic therapy and intrathecal therapy followed by craniospinal radiation and additional systemic therapy for 1 to 2 years. Overall long-term responses range from 25 to 70% and depend on previous therapy, particularly whether the initial CNS preventive therapy regimen included CNS radiation.

Testicular relapse probably occurs among fewer than 10% of patients. It usually manifests as painless unilateral testicular enlargement. The testes are the most frequent site of late relapse after cessation of therapy. When relapse is suspected, bilateral testicular wedge biopsy always is indicated because of the high incidence of involvement of the contralateral testis. As with CNS relapse, isolated testicular relapse usually heralds marrow relapse, so intensified systemic treatment in addition to local radiation must be recommended. Both testes should be irradiated. In some centers orchiec-

tomy is performed to remove the grossly involved testes, but the entire scrotal and inguinal canal region should be irradiated. Outcome varies with time from original diagnosis to detection and previous therapy. Approximately 50 to 70% of patients with isolated testicular relapse respond to aggressive rescue therapy.

Late Effects of Treatment

With growing numbers of survivors of childhood leukemia, increasing attention must be given to adverse late effects of treatment. Of particular concern are delayed complications of CNS preventive therapy. Both early and late neurotoxicity from CNS preventive therapy regimens occur whether intrathecal therapy is used alone or is given with radiation. Acute adverse CNS events, often seizures, occur among 5 to 15% of patients treated with state-of-the-art ALL regimens. Late neurologic sequelae can manifest as cerebral atrophy, necrotizing encephalopathy, or microangiopathy. These sequelae can cause functional CNS impairment of varying severity. Patients who undergo CNS radiation therapy are at particular risk of these events. Cranial radiation is associated with neuroendocrine abnormalities and spinal radiation with growth retardation. Newer treatment regimens no longer include radiation therapy for most children and adolescents with ALL. Means of reducing the intensity of intrathecal therapies are explored instead.

A variety of other adverse sequelae have been observed. Hepatotoxicity is associated primarily with intensive antimetabolite therapy, and cardiomyopathy can result from anthracycline exposure. Infertility can be a consequence of aggressive chemotherapy regimens, particularly among postpubescent patients. Epipodophyllotoxins to manage ALL are being scrutinized after the appearance of reports linking use of these agents to an increased incidence of second malignant tumors.

FUTURE TRENDS

Although advances have been made in the understanding and management of ALL, current therapy fails among 25 to 30% of patients. Most patients who had relapses had been classified classified as at high risk at diagnosis and received maximum-intensity therapy. In an effort to prevent relapse, it is unlikely that initial therapy for patients at high risk can be further intensified with current agents and regimens. Future improvements in outcome await better understanding of the cellular and molecular mechanisms of disease, new supportive care modalities to allow more intensive treatment, development of new strategies for the use of established agents, and the discovery of new drugs and biologic agents.

References

Camitta BM, Pullen J, Murphy S: Biology and treatment of acute lymphocytic leukemia in children. Semin Oncol 24:83–91, 1997

Crist W, Shuster J, Look T, et al: Current results of immunophenotype-, age- and leukocyte-based therapy for children with acute lymphoblastic leukemia: a Pediatric Oncology Group study. Leukemia 6:162–167, 1992

Margolin J, Poplack D: Acute lymphoblastic leukemia. In: Pizzo P, Poplack D, eds: Principles and Practice of Pediatric Oncology, 3rd ed. Philadelphia, JB Lippincott, 1997:409–462.

Pui CH, Crist W, Look A: Biology and clinical significance of cyotgenetic abnormalities in childhood acute lymphoblastic leukemia. Blood 76: 1449–1463, 1990

Smith M, Arthur D, Camitta B, et al: Uniform approach to risk classification and treatment assignment for children with acute lymphoblastic leukemia. J Clin Oncol 14:18–24, 1996

van Eyes J, Pullen J, Head D, et al: The French-American-British (FAB) classification of leukemia: the Pediatric Oncology Group experience with lymphocytic leukemia. Cancer 57:1046–1051, 1986

20.6   ACUTE AND CHRONIC MYELOID LEUKEMIA

Howard J. Weinstein

Acute myeloid leukemia (AML) accounts for about 20% of cases of acute leukemia among children and 80% of cases of acute leukemia among adults. Unlike those of ALL among children, cure rates of AML have improved only modestly over the past 20 years. The long-term survival rate is approximately 40% among children treated with chemotherapy alone. It is somewhat better for those undergoing histocompatible BMT early in first remission. Recent insights into stem cell physiology and the molecular basis of AML have greatly improved understanding of these forms of leukemia, shown their heterogeneity, and are beginning to provide new therapeutic strategies. The chronic myeloid forms of leukemia are extremely rare among children. These myeloproliferative syndromes include the adult type of Philadelphia chromosome–positive chronic myelogenous leukemia (CML) and juvenile myelomonocytic leukemia (JMML). The clinical course, biologic characteristics, and molecular pathogenesis of CML and JMML are quite different. Allogeneic BMT from either a related or an unrelated donor is the management of choice of both diseases.

20.6.1   Acute Myeloid Leukemia

EPIDEMIOLOGY

The annual incidence of AML among children is quite constant throughout the first 10 years of life, and there is a slight peak in adolescence. Approximately 400 of the 2600 cases of acute leukemia among children newly diagnosed each year in the United States are AML. In Japan and several countries in Africa, the incidence of AML is higher than that of ALL among children.

The cause of AML is unknown, and most children have no known predisposing factors. Known risk factors include exposure to high-dose ionizing radiation, previous chemotherapy (especially with alkylating agents and epipodophyllotoxins), Down syndrome, congenital bone marrow failure syndromes (Diamond-Blackfan anemia and Kostmann agranulocytosis [see Chap. 19]), and several other genetic disorders, such as Fanconi anemia and neurofibromatosis. The increased concordance of leukemia among sets of identical twins (approximately 15%) appears to result from transplacental transfer of a single leukemic clone rather than from a genetic predisposition.

Children with Down syndrome have a greater than 15-fold increased risk of leukemia. During the first 3 years of life, AML, especially FAB M7, predominates, but thereafter the ratio of ALL to AML follows the usual childhood distribution. Besides being at risk of acute leukemia, children with Down syndrome or trisomy 21 mosaicism are at risk of *transient myeloproliferative syndrome* (TMS) (see Chap. 10). This syndrome usually is diagnosed during the first several weeks of life and cannot be differentiated from con-

genital leukemia. Infants with TMS often have elevated leukocyte counts (more than $50,000/\mu L$) with circulating blasts and hepatosplenomegaly. Bone marrow aspirates from these children usually have a lower blast count than does peripheral blood. Unlike congenital leukemia, TMS usually resolves spontaneously within several weeks to months without cytotoxic therapy. The blasts from several infants with TMS have been shown to be clonal, and most have cell surface antigens characteristic of megakaryoblasts. Retrospective surveys show that as many as 30% of infants with TMS will have AML before 3 years of age.

Children with neurofibromatosis are at increased risk of malignant disease, including myelodysplastic and myeloproliferative syndromes. The *NF1* gene may function as a tumor suppressor allele because it has been shown to be homozygously deleted in blasts from children with NF1 and AML leukemia (see Chap. 10).

The risk of secondary AML among children and adults previously treated with alkylating agents and topoisomerase-II inhibitors, especially epipodophyllotoxins, is well established. Leukemia associated with use of an alkylating agent occurs within 4 to 10 years after initial therapy, is associated with abnormalities of chromosomes 5 and 7, and carries a grave prognosis. Leukemia associated with use of an epidophyllotoxin (etoposide and teniposide) has a shorter latency (2 to 4 years) and usually is of the FAB M4 or M5 subtype with chromosomal translocations involving 11q23 with rearrangement of the *MLL* gene. Children with the latter forms of leukemia often achieve complete remission with chemotherapy but invariably have a relapse and die unless they are treated by means of BMT.

CLONALITY AND PATHOGENESIS

The clonal origin of AML has been demonstrated with several methods, including cytogenetic analysis and assays with X-linked polymorphisms. During a morphologic remission, the clone is no longer detectable except with molecular methods. During hematologic relapse, the original clone reappears. The transforming event in AML could occur at any point in hematopoiesis from the pluripotent stem cell to a committed precursor, such as the myeloblast or erythroblast. Unlike the situation for myeloproliferative disorders, little evidence suggests that the target of leukemic transformation in AML is the pluripotent stem cell. Both animal and human data, however, implicate a primitive myeloid stem cell or progenitor as the likely target.

Most AML blasts maintain the requirement for hematopoietic growth factors for sustained in vitro growth, although a small number undergo spontaneous growth. The principal defect in AML is arrest of the differentiation pathway of myeloid stem cells or their precursors. The molecular mechanisms that lead to a block in differentiation are mostly unknown. In the case of acute promyelocytic leukemia, the block in differentiation is caused by 15;17 chromosomal translocation, which fuses the *PML* and retinoic acid receptor α genes to yield a fusion protein. Pharmacologic doses of all *trans*-retinoic acid induce terminal differentiation of leukemic blasts and complete remission among almost 90% of patients with acute promyelocytic leukemia (FAB M3). It appears that retinoic acid induces degradation of the fusion protein through mechanisms that involve caspases and the proteasome pathway.

CLASSIFICATION

Precise diagnosis and classification are essential to successful management and biological investigation of childhood leukemia. The FAB classification includes eight subtypes of AML (Table 20-9) and

TABLE 20-9

SUBTYPES OF AML AND THEIR ASSOCIATED CHROMOSOMAL ABNORMALITIES AND CLINICAL FEATURES

FAB SUBTYPE	PROPORTION OF CASES (%)	CHROMOSOMAL ABNORMALITY	CLINICAL OR LABORATORY FEATURES
M0 (large, agranular blasts)	2	del(5), del(7)	Blasts express at least one myeloid antigen (CD13, CD33) negative cytochemistry
M1 (myeloblasts)	10–18		
M2 (myeloblasts with differentiation)	27–29	t(8;21) (q22;q22) t(6;9) (p23;q34)	Myeloblastoma, especially orbital
M3 (promyelocytes)	5–10	t(15;17) (q22;q21)	Disseminated intravascular coagulation
M4eo (myeloblasts and monoblasts with dysplastic eosinophils)		inv(16) (p13;q22) or t(16;16) (p13;q22)	Central nervous system leukemia, eosinophilia
M4 (myeloblasts and monoblasts)	16–25	t(9;11) (p22;q23) t(11;19) (q23;p13.1) t(10;11) (p12;q23)	Age younger than 2 yr, extramedullary leukemia
M5 (monoblasts)	13–22	t(9;11) (p22;q23) t(11;19) (q23;p13.1) t(10;11) (p12;q23)	Age less than 2 yr, extramedullary leukemia, secondary leukemia after epipodophyllotoxins
M6 (erythroblasts)	1–3		
M7 (megakaryoblasts)	4–8	t(1;22) (p13;q13)	Infant onset (before 1 year of age), Down syndrome, myelofibrosis
All types		+8	Previous myelodysplastic syndrome
		−5 or del(5) (q11-35)	Older adults, toxic exposure, previous myelodysplastic syndrome
		−7 or del(7) (q22-q36)	Older adults, toxic exposure, previous myelodysplastic syndrome

differentiates AML from myelodysplastic syndromes by requiring at least 30% blasts in a marrow sample for the diagnosis of leukemia. Approximately 80% of patients younger than 2 years with AML have either the FAB M4 or M5 subtypes. The distribution of FAB subtypes among older children is similar to that among adults younger than 50 years with AML. Infants and toddlers with AML are also more likely than older patients to have greatly elevated leukocyte counts at diagnosis and extramedullary leukemia, especially involving the skin and CNS. The M7 subtype cannot be recognized with morphologic or cytochemical analysis alone and is the most common subtype of AML among children with Down syndrome.

With a combination of monoclonal antibodies that recognize myeloid antigens, several immunophenotype-based classifications of AML have been proposed. They do not provide prognosis or treatment-related information beyond that of the FAB system. Immunophenotyping has been helpful in assigning lineage to the 10 to 15% of cases of acute leukemia that cannot be characterized with morphologic or cytochemical results and in identifying M7 AML with antibodies that react against platelet antigens. In several large pediatric studies, the blasts from approximately 10 to 15% of patients with AML had lymphoid antigen expression. And in these cases the disease is considered mixed lineage or biphenotypic leukemia, but this finding does not have prognostic importance.

GENETIC FEATURES

High-resolution banding techniques have helped identify nonrandom chromosomal abnormalities among more than 70% of children with AML. Many of these abnormalities are unique to AML and are sometimes specific for a particular FAB subtype (Table 20-9). The most common chromosomal abnormalities among children and young adults with AML include inv16, t(15;17), t(8;21),

and t(9;11). Monosomy of chromosomes 5 and 7 and trisomy 8 are generally not associated with a specific FAB type and are considerably more frequent among older patients with AML.

The molecular events associated with many of the structural chromosomal changes have now been elucidated (see Chap. 10). Many of the genes cloned at the breakpoints of the chromosomal translocations or inversions are transcription factors. Polymerase chain reaction–based assays (see Sec. 8.1) are available for diagnostic purposes and can detect as few as one in one million leukemic cells in a blood or bone marrow sample. Studies are underway with these assays to determine the clinical significance of finding minimal numbers of leukemic cells during or after a course of treatment.

CLINICAL AND LABORATORY FEATURES

The initial signs and symptoms among most children with AML reflect anemia, thrombocytopenia, and neutropenia caused by bone marrow infiltration with leukemic blasts and decreased production of normal cells. These include pallor, fatigue, epistaxis or gum bleeding, petechiae or purpura, and fever or infection that has not responded to antibiotic therapy. Children with AML may have bone or joint pain, but these symptoms occur more often among children with ALL. Bulky peripheral lymphadenopathy is not a common finding, and massive hepatosplenomegaly is rare except among infants with AML. Extramedullary leukemia can manifest as gingival hyperplasia, CNS leukemia (headache, cranial nerve palsy), and skin nodules. Neonates and infants with AML typically have leukemia cutis characterized by a papular or nodular rash that is salmon or bluish to slate gray. Clinical findings of CNS leukemia at diagnosis are rare. They include signs of increased intracranial pressure or cranial nerve palsy, seventh nerve palsy being the most common. Fewer than 5% of patients with AML have myeloblastoma (also known as *granulocytic sarcoma* or *chloroma*) during the course of the illness. These are solid tumors of blasts and immature myeloid cells that typically occur in the bones and soft tissues of the head and neck (often the orbits) or in intracranial or epidural sites.

The peripheral blood counts at diagnosis among children with AML can be quite varied. The leukocyte count ranges from less than 1000/μL to more than 500,000/μL. Approximately 15 to 20% of children have an initial leukocyte count greater than 100,000/μL. Higher leukocyte counts are associated with the FAB M4 and M5 subtypes, whereas lower leukocyte counts (<5000/μL) are found in M3 or APL. Most patients have normocytic anemia (median hemoglobin concentration of 7 g/dL in one series), and approximately 50% of patients have platelet counts less than 50,000/μL. Disseminated intravascular coagulation is extremely common among almost all patients with acute promyelocytic leukemia and some infants with M5 AML.

The characteristic bone marrow findings include a hypercellular specimen with more than 30% blasts (usually 70 to 90% blasts). Bone marrow biopsy infrequently shows myelofibrosis (except for M7), and occasionally dysplastic changes in the myeloid precursors are present.

In most cases of AML, the diagnosis is straightforward after examination of the peripheral blood sample and a bone marrow aspirate. Other conditions that can cause diagnostic difficulty include the myeloproliferative disorders such as JMML, myelodysplastic syndromes, and sepsis that causes a leukemoid reaction or neutropenia caused by maturation arrest in granulocytic-monocytic precursors. In the sepsis situation the bone marrow findings may suggest acute promyelocytic leukemia because of a promyelocyte arrest with toxic granulation. However, normal granulocytic maturation ensues within a few days with resolution of the infection. Acute myeloid leukemia among infants with Down syndrome is difficult if not impossible to differentiate from TMS.

MANAGEMENT OF NEWLY DIAGNOSED ACUTE MYELOID LEUKEMIA

Substantial improvement in survival rate from less than 10% to approximately 40% among children with AML has occurred during the past 20 years. The improvement is the result of a higher percentage of children entering complete remission, a decrease in relapse rate because of more effective postremission strategies, including BMT, and improvements in supportive care. Most children with AML should be referred to pediatric oncology centers and treated in clinical trials.

Induction of Remission

The most widely used remission-induction regimen includes treatment with an anthracycline (usually doxorubicin) and cytarabine with or without thioguanine or etoposide. With this regimen, 75 to 85% of children with AML enter complete remission after receiving one to two cycles of chemotherapy. Because the remission-induction phase of therapy is associated with prolonged cytopenia (3 to 5 weeks), 5 to 10% of patients die of infectious or hemorrhagic complications. Deaths during the first several days after diagnosis are rare and often are caused by leukostasis or disseminated intravascular coagulation. Leukostasis, or plugging of blasts in vessels, is associated with elevated peripheral blast counts (more than 100,000/μL) and can cause hemorrhagic infarction of the brain or other organs. A greatly elevated leukocyte count is a medical emergency, and measures should immediately be taken to decrease the leukocyte count with chemotherapy (e.g., hydroxyurea) with exchange transfusion or leukopheresis if the patient has symptoms, such as hypoxemia or somnolence. Intensifying chemotherapy during the remission-induction phase of treatment has not increased the percentage of children achieving complete remission but has resulted in a decrease in relapse rates and improvement in overall survival rates.

All-*trans*-retinoic acid has been shown to be a very effective drug for inducing remissions in patients with acute promyelocytic leukemia. All-*trans*-retinoic acid used alone is not curative but when all-*trans*-retinoic acid is combined with standard AML induction chemotherapy, the combination is effective (75% survival) and is the recommended treatment of patients with APL.

Supportive care measures during all phases of therapy for AML are critical. They include providing indwelling central venous access, antiemetic agents, psychosocial support for the child and family, monitoring for the metabolic consequences of leukemic cell lysis (tumor lysis syndrome), empiric therapy for fever and neutropenia with broad-spectrum antibiotics, prophylactic platelet transfusion, administration of allopurinol, and prophylaxis of *Pneumocystis carinii* pneumonia and fungal infection. Use of hematopoietic growth factors has not increased remission rates or overall survival rates among children with AML. In some studies, use of these factors has been associated with slightly less infectious morbidity during periods of neutropenia. All blood products should be irradiated to prevent transfusion-associated GVHD.

Central Nervous System Therapy

Unlike therapy for ALL, management of occult CNS leukemia with intrathecal chemotherapy alone or combined with cranial irradiation has not been shown improve overall survival among children with AML. Most AML protocols, however, include intrathecal chemotherapy because isolated CNS disease has been found among approximately 20% of children who receive no CNS-directed therapy. About 10% of children with AML have blasts in the cerebrospinal fluid at diagnosis and are treated with weekly intrathecal chemotherapy until the cerebrospinal fluid is cleared of blasts. In some protocols this is followed by cranial irradiation. The presence of CNS leukemia at diagnosis does not appear to have an adverse impact on prognosis.

Treatment in Remission

Unlike therapy for ALL, the use of modestly myelosuppressive combination chemotherapy after remission has been achieved has little effect on reducing the relapse rate among patients with AML. With intensification or consolidation chemotherapy with high doses of cytarabine 5-year leukemia-free survival rates increase from 10 to 40%. The optimal intensity and duration of postremission chemotherapy remain under active investigation. The use of novel treatment approaches, including strategies to reverse the multi-drug-resistant phenotype of leukemic blasts or enhance the host immune response against leukemia, is being pursued.

Bone Marrow Transplantation

The use of marrow ablative doses of chemotherapy with or without total body irradiation followed by BMT from a histocompatible family donor in the care of children with AML in initial remission was first attempted in the mid-1970s (see Sec. 20.4). Although the cumulative pediatric experience shows a statistically significant sur-

TABLE 20-10

PROGNOSTIC FACTORS IN CHILDHOOD ACUTE MYELOID LEUKEMIA

ADVERSE FACTORS	FAVORABLE FACTORS
High leukocyte count ($>100,000/\mu$L)	FAB M1 and M2 with Auer rods
Secondary acute myelogenous leukemia or previous myelodysplastic syndrome	t(8;21)
	inv 16/M4Eo subtype
Monosomy 7 (7q-)	t(15;17)
More than one cycle to achieve complete response	Down syndrome

vival advantage for allogeneic BMT compared with chemotherapy (55 to 70% versus 40 to 50% disease-free survival rate), fewer than 25% of patients have a suitable family donor. Bone marrow transplantation is associated with more severe long-term toxicity, such as infertility and growth impairment, than is chemotherapy. With continued improvement in the efficacy of chemotherapy, some pediatric oncology groups reserve allogeneic BMT in first remission to patients at high risk only (Table 20-10). In several large, prospectively randomized pediatric trials, investigators concluded that autologous BMT is not superior to intensive chemotherapy in the first remission of AML.

Prognostic Factors

Several clinical and laboratory factors have been consistently related to prognosis among children with AML (Table 20-10). A leukocyte count greater than $100,000/\mu$L at diagnosis, monosomy 7, and secondary AML are associated with lower remission rates. Favorable factors for achieving remission include M1 and M2, disease with Auer rods, cytogenetic findings of inv(16), t(8;21), t(15;17), and Down syndrome. In some studies, the M4 and M5 subtypes, chromosome translocations involving 11q23, and need for more than one induction cycle to enter remission were found to have an adverse effect on duration of remission. Favorable features for predicting a lower likelihood of relapse include Down syndrome, FAB M1 and M2 disease with Auer rods, acute promyelocytic leukemia, and the presence of inv(16) or t(8;21).

MANAGEMENT OF REFRACTORY ACUTE MYELOID LEUKEMIA

The prognosis is poor for children who do not enter remission with an anthracycline-cytarabine regimen or who have a relapse. Allogeneic or autologous BMT offers these patients the best chance for long-term survival. Because of the high rate of relapse after autologous BMT, allogeneic BMT with alternative sources of donor stem cells (see Sec. 20.4) is being investigated in the care of these children.

De novo or acquired drug resistance is the main cause of treatment failure among patients with AML, and several mechanisms of drug resistance have been elucidated. Increased expression of the multidrug resistance gene (*mdr1*) or its product, p-glycoprotein, has been detected in blasts from approximately 40 to 60% of children and adults with relapses of AML. Increased expression of p-glycoprotein promotes the cellular efflux of many natural-product drugs, including anthracyclines and etoposide, and is associated with in vitro resistance. Several drugs, including cyclosporine and verapamil, are capable of reversing the *mdr* phenotype in vitro

through direct interaction with p-glycoprotein. Clinical trials of these drugs are in progress in an attempt to reverse multidrug resistance in vivo.

20.6.2 Chronic Myeloid Leukemia

Chronic myeloid leukemia accounts for approximately 2 to 4% of cases of leukemia among children and it includes the adult type of Philadelphia chromosome–positive CML and a rare hematopoietic malignant disease of childhood called *juvenile myelomonocytic leukemia* (formerly juvenile CML). Philadelphia-positive CML is a malignant clonal disorder of the pluripotent stem cell defined by t(9;22) translocation, which results in the *bcr-abl* fusion gene and an abnormal protein product. Chronic myeloid leukemia is characterized initially by a chronic phase (splenomegaly and extreme leukocytosis with full granulocytic maturation) that lasts 2 to 3 years followed inevitably by a blast crisis. Allogeneic BMT during the first year of the chronic phase is the best treatment and leads to cure rates among approximately 80% of children and young adults with CML.

A number of clinical and laboratory features and a very different course of disease differentiate JMML from adult-type CML. Juvenile myelomonocytic leukemia most often manifests before the age of 5 years and is commonly associated with massive splenomegaly, modest leukocytosis with monocytosis, thrombocytopenia, and elevated levels of fetal hemoglobin. Many children have skin rashes that include xanthoma, café-au-lait spots, and eczematous lesions. The bone marrow karyotype never shows the t(9;22) and is often normal, but sometimes has monosomy 7. Juvenile myelomonocytic leukemia rarely evolves into a blast crisis. The 5-year survival rate without BMT is less than 10%, most patients dying during the first year.

A number of unique biologic features have been identified in JMML, including selective hypersensitivity of granulocyte-monocyte colony-forming units to the growth factor, granulocyte-macrophage colony-stimulating factor, and spontaneous growth of peripheral blood granulocyte-monocyte colony-forming units. Children with NF1 are at increased risk of JMML. Although many chemotherapeutic agents can decrease leukocyte count and spleen size for most children with JMML, none has been shown to prolong survival. The current treatment recommendation for children with JMML is allogeneic BMT with or without pretransplant splenectomy. Unlike the situation for Philadelphia-positive CML, interferon-α has no demonstrated efficacy in JMML. Interestingly, *cis*-retinoic acid has induced some durable hematologic responses in the case of children with JMML and is undergoing further evaluation.

References

Ebb DH, Weinstein HJ: Diagnosis and treatment of childhood acute myelogenous leukemia. Pediatr Clin North Am 44:847–862, 1997

Giorgini G, Bozzola M, Locatelli F, et al: Role of busulfan and total body irradiation on growth of prepubertal children receiving bone marrow transplantation and results of treatment with recombinant growth hormone. Blood 86:825–831, 1995

Greaves M: A natural history for pediatric acute leukemia. Blood 82:1045–1051, 1993

Kantarjian HM, O'Brien S, Anderlini P, et al: Treatment of chronic myelogenous leukemia: current status and investigational options. Blood 87:3069–3081, 1996

Pui CH, Ribeiro RC, Hancock ML, et al: Acute myeloid leukemia in children treated with epipodophyllotoxins for acute lymphoblastic leukemia. N Engl J Med 325:1682–1687, 1991

Ravindranath Y, Abella E, Krischer J, et al: Acute myeloid leukemia (AML) in Down's syndrome is highly responsive to chemotherapy: experience on Pediatric Oncology Group AML Study 8498. Blood 80:2210–2214, 1992

Ravindranath Y, Yeager A, Chang M, et al: Autologous bone marrow transplantation versus intensive consolidation chemotherapy for acute myeloid leukemia in childhood. N Engl J Med 334:1428–1434, 1996

Robinson LL, Buckley JD, Bunin G: Assessment of environmental and genetic factors in the etiology of childhood cancers: the Children's Cancer Group Epidemiology Program. Environ Health Perspect 103(Suppl 6): 111–116, 1995

Tallman M, Anderson J, Schiffer C, et al: All-trans-retinoic acid in acute promyelocytic leukemia. N Engl J Med 337:1021–1028, 1997

Tenen D, Hrumas R, Licht J, Zhang D: Transcription factors, normal myeloid development, and leukemia. Blood 90:489–519, 1997

Woods W, Kobrinsky N, Buckley J, et al: Timed-sequential induction therapy improves post-remission outcome in acute myeloid leukemia: a report from the Children's Cancer Group. Blood 87:4979–4989, 1996

20.7   NON-HODGKIN LYMPHOMA

Sheila Weitzman

Pediatric lymphoma accounts for 10% of cases of malignant disease among children. It is the third most common malignant disease among North American children. Approximately 60% of cases of pediatric lymphoma are non-Hodgkin lymphoma; the others are Hodgkin disease. Unlike Hodgkin disease, non-Hodgkin lymphoma can occur even among infants, and the incidence rises steadily with increasing age. The male to female ratio is 3:1. As many as 10% of children with congenital or acquired immunosuppression have non-Hodgkin lymphoma, the highest incidence being in ataxia-telangectasia and Wiskott-Aldrich syndrome. Immunosuppression of patients receiving T-cell depleted bone marrow or solid organ transplants has resulted in a high incidence of Epstein-Barr virus (EBV)–related posttransplantation lymphoproliferative disease. Epstein-Barr virus infection early in childhood together with chronic antigen stimulation by malaria is thought to be associated with the high incidence of Burkitt non-Hodgkin lymphoma in central Africa, where it accounts for almost one half of all cases of pediatric cancer. Epstein-Barr virus DNA is present in the tumor cells in 95% of endemic cases of Burkitt non-Hodgkin lymphoma but only 15 to 20% of sporadic cases of Burkitt non-Hodgkin lymphoma in North America. Among patients with human immunodeficiency virus infection, CNS lymphoma is invariably associated with EBV infection.

ETIOLOGY AND PATHOLOGY

Most pediatric cases of non-Hodgkin lymphoma are diffuse, aggressive, high-grade lymphomas that tend to originate in extranodal lymphoid tissue such as thymus or Peyer patches. Only 10 to 15% of childhood non-Hodgkin lymphoma manifests as primary peripheral nodal disease. Some cases of non-Hodgkin lymphoma manifest in extralymphatic tissue such as bone, skin, lung, and gonad. Follicular lymphoma occurs rarely among adolescents, and patients younger than 16 years tend to have localized disease.

The spectrum of pediatric non-Hodgkin lymphoma is considerably narrower than that of non-Hodgkin lymphoma among adults. Most childhood cases of non-Hodgkin lymphoma are limited to three major categories. According to the new Revised European-American Lymphoma (REAL) classification system, approximately 50% of North American children with non-Hodgkin lymphoma have Burkitt or Burkitt-like lymphoma, 30 to 40% have lymphoblastic non-Hodgkin lymphoma, and 15 to 25% have diffuse large cell disease. Included in the REAL system as subtypes of large cell non-Hodgkin lymphoma are diffuse large B-cell non-Hodgkin lymphoma and anaplastic large cell lymphoma (ALCL), which account for most cases of pediatric large cell disease (Table 20-11).

BURKITT LYMPHOMA   Despite a similar histologic appearance, the sporadic and endemic forms of Burkitt lymphoma differ in clinical presentation. In North America and Europe, Burkitt lymphoma

TABLE 20-11

CHARACTERISTICS OF THREE MAIN FORMS OF PEDIATRIC NON-HODGKIN LYMPHOMA

	BURKITT (SPORADIC)	LYMPHOBLASTIC	LARGE CELL
Grade	50% high	30–40% high	15–25% most high, occasionally intermediate
Genetics	t(8;14)	Most none	ALCL t(2;5) (50%)
	t(8;22)	t(10-14),t(1;14)	
	t(2;8)	t(11-14)	
Immunologic features	B cell	T cell (80%) Early B (20%)	B cell (large cell B) T cell, null (ALCL)
Site	Abdominal (80%) Pharyngeal	Anterior mediastinum (50–70%) Lymph nodes supradiaphragmatic	Abdomen, mediastinum, lymph nodes, skin, bone, lung
Spread	Bone marrow CNS ++	Bone marrow CNS+	Occasionally bone marrow CNS uncommon
Survival rate (%)			
Localized	>90	>90	>90
Advanced	>80	65–80	>80

ALCL = anaplastic large cell lymphoma; CNS = central nervous system.

originates most commonly from relatively mature B cells in Peyer patches within the gastrointestinal tract, most commonly at the ileocecal junction. In 10% of cases, the disease originates from B lymphocytes within the Waldeyer ring (tonsil and adenoid). Eighty percent of patients have an abdominal mass or abdominal pain, abdominal distension, nausea, and vomiting. Localized Burkitt non-Hodgkin lymphoma can be the lead point for an intussusception, and the tumor often is diagnosed during surgery for "acute appendicitis." Involvement of tonsils or adenoids can cause airway obstruction, commonly associated with nontender cervical adenopathy. Jaw involvement occurs among only 15% of patients with sporadic Burkitt non-Hodgkin lymphoma. Patients with endemic (African) Burkitt non-Hodgkin lymphoma commonly have jaw tumors (approximately 70%) as well as involvement of the gastrointestinal tract and kidneys. Peripheral lymph node involvement is unusual. Patients with endemic Burkitt lymphoma more commonly have CNS disease (leptomeningeal, cranial nerve palsy, and paraplegia), whereas bone marrow disease occurs more frequently among patients with sporadic Burkitt lymphoma. Burkitt and Burkitt-like lymphomas are of B-cell phenotype and express surface immunoglobulin and B-cell-specific surface antigens (CD19, CD20, CD22).

Burkitt non-Hodgkin lymphoma has characteristic cytogenetic changes that involve translocation of the c-*myc* oncogene on chromosome 8 (see Sec. 20.2) to the immunoglobulin heavy chain gene locus on chromosome 14 (80%) or to one of the light chain genes on chromosomes 22 or 2. Burkitt lymphoma is the fastest growing malignant tumor among humans. The doubling time is 2 to 3 days, and the rate of spontaneous cell death is high. Patients may have hyperuricemic nephropathy even before therapy is started, and these tumors have the highest risk of tumor lysis syndrome after initiation of therapy (Sec. 21.7). The survival rate among patients with Burkitt non-Hodgkin lymphoma was poor until the design of chemotherapy protocols was based on the rapid cell cycling.

LYMPHOBLASTIC LYMPHOMA One third of cases of pediatric non-Hodgkin lymphoma are lymphoblastic lymphoma (Table 20-11). The tumor consists of cells morphologically indistinguishable from lymphoblastic leukemia. These diseases are thought to represent a spectrum of a single disease, reflected in the designation of T- or B-precursor leukemia-lymphoma in the REAL classification. Eighty percent of lymphoblastic lymphoma cases are of thymic T-cell origin and manifest commonly as an anterior mediastinal mass that may be associated with nontender supradiaphragmatic lymphadenopathy (cervical, supraclavicular, and axillary) and infiltration of liver, spleen, or kidney. The most common presenting features are caused by compression of the trachea and main bronchi. Other complications include superior vena caval compression, right ventricular outflow tract obstruction, and pleural or pericardial effusion. The lesions are high-grade lymphomas, and tumor lysis syndrome may occur, especially if renal infiltration is present. Urgency in diagnosis and therapy is mandatory.

T-cell lymphoblastic lymphoma is derived from thymic T cells, all of which express the pan-T antigen CD7 as well as other markers of immature T cells. Twenty percent of lymphoblastic lymphoma is of early B-cell lineage and expresses the phenotype of common childhood ALL (CD10, CD19, CD22, HLA-DR). B-lineage lymphoblastic lymphoma often is localized and may manifest as disease in unusual sites such as skin and bone. Translocations in lymphoblastic lymphoma usually involve translocation of a protooncogene

to one of the T-cell receptor genes on chromosome 7 or 14. These translocations do not appear to be of prognostic significance.

LARGE CELL NON-HODGKIN LYMPHOMA Large cell non-Hodgkin lymphoma (Table 20-11) is a heterogenous group of tumors in which the cells contain nuclei larger than those of the surrounding histiocytes. Subtypes include diffuse, large B-cell disease and the anaplastic Ki-1 (CD30) positive large cell lymphomas (ALCL). Large cell non-Hodgkin lymphoma can manifest anywhere and may present with abdominal disease similar to Burkitt disease or a mediastinal mass similar to lymphoblastic non-Hodgkin lymphoma. Large cell non-Hodgkin lymphoma often manifests at unusual sites, such as bone, skin, and lung. Bone marrow is less frequently involved than in the other types of non-Hodgkin lymphoma, and CNS disease is uncommon. Anaplastic large cell lymphoma commonly involves skin, peripheral lymph nodes, and bone. It may occur with manifestations such as diffuse pulmonary disease that usually do not occur with the other forms of lymphoma. Unlike the other forms of lymphoma, lymphadenopathy caused by ALCL can be tender to palpation and is more commonly associated with constitutional symptoms such as fever, night sweats, or weight loss, a high leukocyte count, and thrombocytosis, all of which are thought to be caused by excess cytokine production by lymphoma cells. Anaplastic large cell lymphoma must be included in the differential diagnosis of persistent fever and lymphadenopathy. Most large cell lymphomas are of B-cell origin. However, ALCL expresses the CD30 antigen (recognized by the Ki-1 antibody) and usually is of T-cell or occasionally null cell origin. The only characteristic cytogenetic changes occur in ALCL; approximately 50% of cells carry a translocation t(2;5) that results in production of a fusion protein ALK, which is absent from normal lymphocytes. Positive immunocytochemical results for ALK are specific for t(2;5) and helpful in differentiating ALCL from Hodgkin disease (see Sec. 20.8).

DIAGNOSIS AND STAGING

The aggressive nature of most cases of pediatric non-Hodgkin lymphoma underlies the urgency to obtain a diagnosis and begin therapy. Correct diagnosis requires morphologic examination, cytochemical analysis, genetic study, and immunophenotyping. If possible, biopsies should be performed at oncology referral centers. When a biopsy is too risky, diagnosis can sometimes be made by means of examination of pleural or pericardial fluid obtained through aspiration. Before undergoing biopsy, patients with large abdominal tumors need to be evaluated for gastrointestinal obstruction or perforation and for renal impairment caused by renal infiltration, obstruction, or hyperuricemia. Patients with an anterior mediastinal mass need urgent evaluation for airway or superior vena caval compression, pleural fluid, and cardiac tamponade. These patients should not be put into a supine position for the investigations. The studies should be performed with the patient prone or lying on the side. No patient with airway obstruction should be sedated for a procedure.

In pediatric non-Hodgkin lymphoma, staging systems reflect tumor volume. The most widely used is the St. Jude's staging system (Table 20-12), which is applicable to all three major subtypes and separates patients with localized disease (stages I and II) from those with advanced disease (stage III). Stage IV non-Hodgkin lymphoma consists of bone marrow involvement with less than 25% blasts or with CNS disease; more than 25% tumor cells in the bone

TABLE 20-12

ST. JUDE'S STAGING SYSTEM FOR PEDIATRIC NON-HODGKIN LYMPHOMA

STAGE	CHARACTERISTICS
I	Single tumor (extranodal) or single anatomic area (nodal) with exclusion of the mediastinum or abdomen
II	Single tumor (extranodal) with regional node involvement
	Two or more nodal areas on the same side of the diaphragm
	Two single (extranodal) tumors with or without regional node involvement on the same side of the diaphragm
	A primary gastrointestinal tract tumor, usually in the ileocecal area, with or without involvement of associated mesenteric nodes only, grossly completely resected
III	Two single tumors (extranodal) on opposite sides of the diaphragm
	Two or more nodal areas above or below the diaphragm
	All primary intrathoracic tumors (mediastinal, pleural, thymic)
	All extensive primary intraabdominal disease, unresectable
	All paraspinal or epidural tumors, regardless of other tumor sites
IV	Any of the above with initial central nervous system or bone marrow involvement

marrow is by convention called leukemia. Accurate staging is essential because of the differences in therapy and prognosis for patients with localized and advanced non-Hodgkin lymphoma.

TREATMENT AND PROGNOSIS

Chemotherapy is the mainstay of management of non-Hodgkin lymphoma. Surgery is needed to obtain biopsy material and to deal with complications such as intussusception or intestinal perforation. Localized abdominal tumors diagnosed at laparotomy often are easily resected, and the prognosis is excellent with a short course (6 weeks) of chemotherapy. Surgery should not be performed for the purpose of resection, however, and surgical intervention that delays the onset of chemotherapy should be avoided if possible.

Radiation therapy does not improve outcome and can be omitted except in the care of patients with CNS disease. Possibly because of rapid cell cycling, radiation given in single daily fractions is ineffective in the management of Burkitt disease. Before the start of therapy, measures must be taken to prevent *tumor lysis syndrome,* which is caused by release of potassium, urate, and phosphate from dying cells (see Sec. 21.7). Allopurinol to prevent urate production or uricase to promote urate metabolism should be instituted before chemotherapy.

The use of multiagent, intensive chemotherapy regimens has markedly improved survival among children with non-Hodgkin lymphoma. The selection of chemotherapeutic regimen is based on morphologic findings or on B-cell or T-cell immunophenotype. Intensity and duration of therapy vary markedly for localized and advanced disease. Localized Burkitt and localized large cell lymphoma have a cure rate of 90% with as little as 6 weeks of chemotherapy. Advanced stage Burkitt and B-cell ALL are managed with a short duration (3 to 6 months) of intensive multiagent chemotherapy. The addition of high-dose antimetabolite therapy such as high-dose methotrexate and high-dose cytosine-arabinoside to the

intrathecal therapy has been shown to be successful in prophylaxis and management of CNS disease. With this approach, the event-free survival rate for advanced Burkitt disease and B-cell ALL is more than 80%. Most relapses occur within the first 8 months after diagnosis. Patients with Burkitt disease who survive disease free for 10 months are likely to be cured. Both the German (BFM) and French (SFOP) study groups have obtained event-free survival rates of more than 80% for advanced stage B-cell large cell non-Hodgkin lymphoma using the same short duration, intensive protocol as for Burkitt disease. In two consecutive BFM studies, no significant differences in event-free survival rate were found among the distinct subsets of large cell lymphoma, including ALCL.

Lymphoblastic lymphoma has been shown to respond best to protocols designed for ALL. Duration of therapy usually is 18 to 24 months. With ALL therapy, the event-free survival rate approaches 90% for localized lymphoblastic lymphoma and 65 to 80% for advanced disease. The survival of children with non-Hodgkin lymphoma of all three subtypes has dramatically improved; most patients with pediatric lymphoma are now being cured. This improvement can be attributed to the enrollment of patients onto cooperative group protocols. Children with non-Hodgkin lymphoma should be treated at pediatric cancer centers.

POSTTRANSPLANTATION LYMPHOPROLIFERATIVE DISEASE
The use of T-depleted grafts for mismatched stem cell transplants and the use of drugs that deplete T cells to prevent rejection after solid organ transplants result in severe deficiencies of cytotoxic T cells. This deficiency allows growth of EBV-transformed B cells and results in posttransplantation lymphoproliferative disease (PTLPD). Lymphoma usually is of the B-cell large cell subtype, although Burkitt disease can occur. The incidence of PTLPD is higher among children, probably because of a higher incidence of EBV seronegativity at transplantation. Risk factors include the EBV status of the patient and donor at the time of transplantation (a positive donor and negative recipient represent the highest risk factor), the type of transplantation (1 to 5% of renal and liver transplants, 5 to 15% of heart and heart-lung), and the type and dose of immunosuppressive drugs. Therapy for PTLPD includes surgery for localized tumors, reduction of immunosuppression, and antiviral therapy with gancyclovir and high-titer cytomegalovirus gamma globulin, which contains high titers of antibody against EBV. If the disease progresses despite these measures, chemotherapy, interferon-α, and anti–B-cell antibody therapy can be tried. The mortality of PTLPD after solid organ transplantation remains 40 to 60%.

References

Büyükpamukçu M: Non-Hodgkin's lymphomas. In: Voute PA, Kalifa C, Barrett A, eds: Cancer in Children: Clinical Management, 4th ed. New York, Oxford University Press, 1998:119–136

Magrath IT, ed: Non-Hodgkin's Lymphomas, 2nd ed. London, Arnold, 1997

Perkins SL, Segal GH, Kjeldsberg CR: Classification of non-Hodgkin's lymphomas in children. Semin Diagn Pathol 12:303–313, 1995

Reiter A, Schrappe M, Parwaresch R, et al: Non-Hodgkin's lymphomas of childhood and adolescence: results of a treatment stratified for biologic subtypes and stage-a report of the Berlin-Frankfurt-Munster Group. J Clin Oncol 13:359–372, 1995

20.8   HODGKIN DISEASE

Melissa M. Hudson

Hodgkin disease is a hematopoietic malignant disease with unique epidemiologic features that vary geographically. Progression of Hodgkin disease initially occurs along functionally contiguous lymph nodes. If the patient is not treated, extranodal involvement eventually results from hematogenous dissemination of neoplastic cells to the liver, lungs, bones, bone marrow, and other tissues. The most common clinical presentation is painless lymphadenopathy previously attributed to infectious or inflammatory causes. Other signs and symptoms vary on the basis of the involved nodal sites and their compression of adjacent organs and tissues. Cytokine production by malignant cells causes constitutional symptoms, including anorexia, pruritus, weight loss, night sweats, and fever among some patients. Treatment with multiagent chemotherapy or combined-modality therapy including chemotherapy and radiation cures most children and adolescents with Hodgkin disease. As a consequence, contemporary treatment approaches have been focused on reducing treatment of patients with favorable presentations to avoid late treatment toxicity such as growth impairment, second malignant tumors, and organ dysfunction.

ETIOLOGY AND EPIDEMIOLOGY

The epidemiologic, clinical, and histologic features of Hodgkin disease are different in economically developed and developing countries. Epidemiologic studies support three distinct forms of Hodgkin disease attributable to interactions of environmental and host factors. The childhood form (14 years or younger) is characterized by a high incidence of the mixed cellularity histologic subtype among children living in poor socioeconomic environments. The young adult form (15 to 34 years) shows a predominance of the nodular sclerosing histologic subtype among white adolescents and young adults in developed countries. An older adult form (55 to 74 years) produces the characteristic bimodal distribution of incidence of the disease in industrialized countries. In developing countries, the early peak occurs before adolescence.

Hodgkin disease is more common among boys and men than among girls and women in all parts of the world. The sex ratio varies from 2:1 in Europe and North America to more than 3.5:1 in Asia. The male predominance is most marked among patients younger than 10 years. Among adolescents, the sex difference in incidence is less conspicuous, particularly for the nodular sclerosing histologic subtype. Hodgkin disease is rarely diagnosed among children younger than 5 years in economically developed countries.

A genetic predisposition to Hodgkin disease is suggested by the incidence variation among racial and ethnic groups, familial aggregation of the disease, and association with specific human leukocyte antigens. In some groups, race and ethnicity appear to predict the risk of Hodgkin disease independent of socioeconomic status. For example, Asians consistently have lower incidence rates despite the marked international differences in socioeconomic conditions. Conversely, even after control for social class differences, Jews in the United States have a higher risk of Hodgkin disease than do other religious groups. Many investigators have observed concordance of Hodgkin disease among first-degree relatives, including sibling and parent-child pairs. In studies of concordant monozygotic twins, the elevated risk of Hodgkin disease ranges from threefold among first-degree relatives to sevenfold among siblings.

Hodgkin disease also develops more frequently among persons with congenital or acquired immunodeficiency, leading to the speculation that an inherited subtle immune abnormality may predispose to the development of the disease by increasing the risk of malignant transformation induced by environmental factors.

Characteristic epidemiologic features, including the bimodal age-incidence and socioeconomic influences, prompted speculation that an infectious agent may contribute to the pathogenesis of some types of Hodgkin disease. Epstein-Barr virus was indirectly implicated in epidemiologic studies that showed an excess risk of Hodgkin disease after infectious mononucleosis and higher anti-EBV titers among patients with Hodgkin disease than among healthy controls. More compelling evidence of an association between EBV infection and Hodgkin disease is localization of viral genomes in the Reed-Sternberg cells, expression of EBV latent gene products in the tumor specimens, and demonstration of clonal infection. Clear differences exist with expression of EBV-associated antigens in cases of Hodgkin disease with respect to histologic subtype, geographic region, and age. Hodgkin disease associated with EBV infection occurs more frequently among children in developing countries who have mixed cellularity histologic features. These data suggest that EBV may be a cofactor in the pathogenesis of some cases of Hodgkin disease.

Herpesviruses have been considered alternative candidate viruses because they are ubiquitous and can establish persistent infection. Results of seroepidemiologic studies do not support involvement of herpes simplex, varicella zoster, cytomegalovirus, or human herpesvirus-7. However, human herpesvirus-6 has been linked with clusters of nodular sclerosing Hodgkin disease among young persons. Thus far, herpesvirus-6 genomes have not been detected within Reed-Sternberg cells, indicating that the contribution of herpesvirus-6 to the pathogenesis of Hodgkin disease is less direct than that of EBV.

PATHOLOGY

Hodgkin disease is histologically characterized by the presence of Reed-Sternberg cells within an inflammatory infiltrate of normal lymphocytes, histiocytes, plasma cells, eosinophils, and neutrophils. The neoplasm is unusual because the acknowledged malignant Reed-Sternberg cells usually represent less than 5% of the cellular infiltrate. Evidence suggests that these large, bizarre, binucleate cells originate from B lymphocytes in germinal centers of lymphoid tissue. Occasionally they appear to be of T-cell lineage. The lymphoid lineage of the Reed-Sternberg cells is supported by demonstration of clonal immunoglobulin gene and T-cell receptor rearrangements. Unlike those of other lymphoid neoplasms, cytogenetic abnormalities characteristic of Hodgkin disease have not been identified.

The Rye classification, the most accepted morphologic classification scheme for Hodgkin disease, defines four histologic subtypes: lymphocytic predominance, mixed cellularity, lymphocytic depletion, and nodular sclerosing. All histologic subtypes are responsive to therapy. Historically, prognosis for the first three histologic classes was related to the ratio of lymphocytes to abnormal cells. Histologic assignment has less prognostic significance since the development of highly effective contemporary treatment regimens, but subtyping is valuable because of its association with clinical findings such as sites of involvement, stage at presentation, and systemic symptoms.

Hodgkin disease is included in the REAL classification system, which defines the relation between lymphoid malignant tumors and normal stages of differentiation with a categorization scheme based on morphologic, immunologic, and molecular techniques. In addition to the groups designated by the Rye classification, the REAL classification includes a provisional entity, lymphocyte-rich classic Hodgkin disease, which comprises cases of diffuse lymphocytic predominance and lymphocyte-predominant mixed cellularity type.

CLINICAL MANIFESTATIONS

The most common presentation of Hodgkin disease is asymptomatic cervical or supraclavicular lymphadenopathy. Two thirds of these patients also have involvement of mediastinal lymph nodes, which can produce a nonproductive cough or other symptoms of tracheal or bronchial compression (Fig. 20-5). In rare instances patients have life-threatening cardiovascular or respiratory decompensation as a result of tumor infiltration of the pericardium, obstruction of superior vena caval blood flow, or airway compression by bulky mediastinal lymphadenopathy. Children less frequently have axillary or inguinal lymphadenopathy. Primary subdiaphragmatic nodal involvement is rare and occurs among fewer than 10% of patients. In some cases, extension of enlarged retroperitoneal lymph nodes through neural foramina produces pain and para- or quadraparesis from spinal cord compression.

Approximately 30% of children have constitutional symptoms (fever, drenching night sweats, and unexplained weight loss within the previous 6 months) which have a negative effect on prognosis because of their association with more disseminated disease. Pel-Ebstein fevers typically are associated with Hodgkin disease and are characterized by periodic febrile episodes (with or without night sweats) that last for several days and are followed by afebrile periods

of days or weeks. Less commonly reported systemic symptoms such as pruritus and alcohol-induced pain do not influence outcome.

LABORATORY FINDINGS

Nonspecific abnormalities of hematologic values may be present at diagnosis. Peripheral blood changes include neutrophilic leukocytosis, lymphopenia, eosinophilia, and monocytosis. Elevations of erythrocyte sedimentation rate, serum level of copper, or ferritin reflect activation of the reticuloendothelial system and can be used to monitor disease activity if they are abnormal at diagnosis. Anemia usually indicates the presence of advanced disease and most commonly is caused by impaired mobilization of iron stores. Coombs-positive hemolytic anemia associated with reticulocytosis and normoblastic hyperplasia of the bone marrow has also been described at presentation. Abnormalities of chemical values are infrequent in Hodgkin disease. Levels of lactate dehydrogenase in the serum are occasionally elevated at diagnosis. Elevation of serum levels of alkaline phosphatase beyond that expected for age may be associated with the presence of bony metastasis. Results of liver function studies are generally unreliable indicators of hepatic disease.

Hodgkin disease has been described in association with several autoimmune diseases, including immune thrombocytopenic purpura, nephrosis, and hemolytic anemia. Of these, immune thrombocytopenic purpura is most frequently observed and response to therapy is related to the status of the underlying Hodgkin disease. Immune thrombocytopenic purpura that manifests during remission of Hodgkin disease lacks prognostic significance. Patients with Hodgkin disease also have immune system abnormalities at diagnosis that may persist after therapy. These include abnormalities of cell-mediated immunity resulting from enhanced sensitivity to suppressor T lymphocytes and reduction of natural killer cell cytotoxicity. After treatment, humoral immunity may be transiently depressed.

Other inflammatory causes of lymphadenopathy, especially those with an indolent course, such as atypical mycobacterial or toxoplasma infections, should be considered in the differential diagnosis of lymphadenopathy (see Chap. 13). Infectious agents that produce lymphadenopathy often can be differentiated from Hodgkin disease by their characteristic clinical presentations. Non-Hodgkin lymphoma may have similar presenting signs and symptoms (see Sec. 20.7) but is typically associated with a more rapid growth of affected lymph nodes. Children with non-Hodgkin lymphoma more frequently have elevations of serum levels of uric acid and LDH (see Sec. 20.7). Although lymphadenopathy caused by bacterial or viral infection is more common than lymph node enlargement from malignant infiltration, biopsy should be performed if lymphadenopathy persists longer than 3 to 4 weeks. The site (eg, supraclavicular region) and character (eg, firm, fixed painless lymphadenopathy) may indicate the need for immediate biopsy. In such cases, excisional lymph node biopsy is preferred to establish a diagnosis because it allows evaluation of the entire nodal architecture.

CLINICAL STAGING

Staging evaluations are needed to determine the anatomic extent of disease and to plan therapy. The Ann Arbor staging classification has been the internationally accepted staging system for Hodgkin disease since 1971 (Table 20-13). This system defines three stages of disease extent based on regions of lymph node involvement and their relation to the diaphragm. Extranodal involvement is desig-

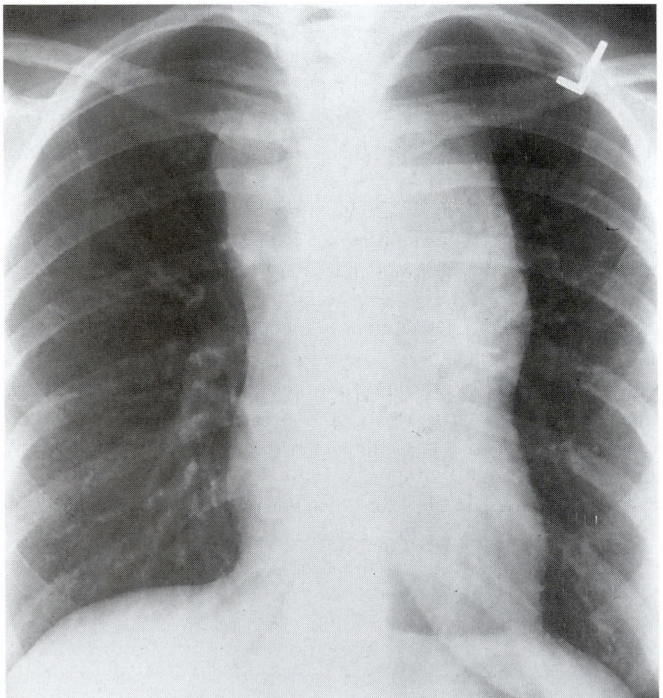

FIGURE 20-5   Chest radiograph shows a mediastinal mass in a teenage patient with nodular sclerosing Hodgkin disease. Airway patency should be assessed before such a patient is referred for anesthesia.

TABLE 20-13

ANN ARBOR STAGING CLASSIFICATION FOR HODGKIN DISEASE

STAGE	CRITERIA FOR EXTENT OF DISEASE
I	Involvement of a single lymph node area (I) or a single extralymphatic site (I_E)
II	Involvement of two or more lymph node areas on the same side of the diaphragm (II) or localized involvement of one extralymphatic organ or site and one or more lymph node regions on the same side of the diaphragm (II_E)
III	Involvement of lymph node regions on both sides of the diaphragm (III), which may also include localized extralymphatic involvement (III_E), splenic involvement (III_S), or both (III_{ES})
IV	Diffuse or disseminated involvement of one or more extralymphatic sites with or without lymph node involvement, including all patients with liver or bone marrow involvement

All stages are subclassified A or B to indicate absence or presence of unexplained fever, night sweats, or unexplained loss of 10% or more of body weight in the preceding 6 months.

nated stage IV. Substage A indicates asymptomatic disease. Substage B is appended if the patient has a fever exceeding 38°C for 3 consecutive days, drenching night sweats, or an unexplained weight loss of 10% of body weight in the preceeding 6 months. Substage E denotes localized extranodal extension of disease.

Throughout the 1970s, staging laparotomy including splenectomy was routinely recommended for newly diagnosed disease because of the need to define accurate radiation treatment fields. The following factors led to the widespread use of clinical staging in the 1980s: (1) advances in diagnostic imaging technology allowed more accurate evaluation of abdominal and pelvic lymph node involvement; (2) the increasing use of systemic chemotherapy in the case of most children obviated confirmation of microscopic retroperitoneal nodal disease; and (3) the recognition of surgical complications, overwhelming infection, and increased risk of leukemia after splenectomy motivated the desire to maintain intact splenic function (see Chap. 19). Surgical staging is recommended for children only if the findings will greatly alter the treatment plan.

THERAPY

Dramatic progress has been made over the past 30 years in the development of curative treatment of children and adolescents with Hodgkin disease. Contemporary treatment protocols for pediatric Hodgkin disease produce long-term disease-free survival for 70 to 90% of patients with advanced disease and 85 to 100% of patients with localized disease. Most children (60 to 80%) with extranodal disease also are cured of the disease. Appreciation of treatment sequelae has prompted refinements in therapy designed to reduce growth impairment, infertility, second malignant tumor, and life-threatening organ dysfunction. Current treatment strategies have focused on reducing therapy for patients with favorable presentations and have reserved intensive treatment for patients with relapsed or refractory disease.

Treatment options for children and adolescents with Hodgkin disease are radiation therapy, multiagent chemotherapy, or combined modality therapy with chemotherapy and radiation therapy. Treatment with radiation alone is effective therapy for localized

Hodgkin disease when standard tumoricidal doses of 35 to 44 Gy are applied to extended treatment volumes. Staging laparotomy is required at most centers if this option is pursued, because radiation represents local-regional rather than systemic therapy. The desire to avoid radiation-induced growth inhibition of bones and soft tissues and induction of secondary solid malignant tumors has resulted in limited use of radiation therapy as a single modality in the care of children with Hodgkin disease.

Multiagent chemotherapy is largely derived from the original non-cross-resistant mechlorethamine, vincristine, prednisone, and procarbazine (MOPP) and doxorubicin, bleomycin, vinblastine, and dacarbazine (ABVD) regimens. The MOPP combination produces long-term, disease-free survival for approximately 50% of patients. Treatment sequelae after MOPP pose increased risk of acute myeloid leukemia (see Sec. 20.6) and infertility, which has been correlated with the cumulative dose of alkylating agents. The risk of secondary leukemia can be reduced by means of limiting the total dose of alkylating agents and substituting other less leukemogenic drugs, such as cyclophosphamide, for mechlorethamine. Preservation of fertility is possible when MOPP treatment is limited to no more than three cycles for young men. Most young women maintain or resume menses after MOPP therapy, but the use of this combination confers a risk of premature menopause, particularly when MOPP is used in combination with abdominopelvic radiation.

Therapy with ABVD is effective for Hodgkin disease that does not produce an excess risk of secondary leukemia or infertility. Used initially as salvage therapy in the care of patients with MOPP-resistant disease, ABVD was later established to be more effective than MOPP, which has resulted in adoption of this regimen as standard front-line treatment of many adults with Hodgkin disease. However, concerns regarding dose-related cardiac and pulmonary toxicity attributable to doxorubicin and bleomycin have limited its use of these drugs in pediatric regimens. As a result, ABVD and similar hybrid combinations are commonly used in treatment regimens of fewer cycles of chemotherapy for patients with favorable presentations or alternated with regimens containing alkylating agents, such as MOPP or COPP, in the care of patients with advanced or unfavorable disease.

Several trials have established the efficacy of treatment with non-cross-resistant chemotherapy alone for pediatric Hodgkin disease. Protocols of chemotherapy alone offer advantages for children treated in centers lacking radiation facilities, trained personnel, or diagnostic imaging modalities needed for clinical staging. This treatment also avoids the risk of long-term growth inhibition, organ dysfunction, and solid tumor induction associated with high-dose, extended-field radiation. On the other hand, protocols of chemotherapy alone usually have higher cumulative doses of alkylating agents, which may produce acute and late treatment morbidity from myelosuppression, gonadal injury, and secondary leukemia. As a result, many pediatric oncologists prefer a combined modality approach, which has been associated with excellent treatment outcomes and reduced treatment sequelae because it limits cumulative dose exposures of radiation therapy and chemotherapy.

PROGNOSIS

Most children and adolescents with Hodgkin disease enjoy long-term, disease-free survival. Ongoing clinical trials are focusing on two primary objectives: (1) maintaining cure rates and reducing treatment sequelae among patients with favorable presentations;

and (2) identifying biologic and clinical characteristics of patients at high risk of treatment failure, for whom treatment must be further intensified to improve outcome. Because of the paucity of novel antineoplastic approaches with safe toxicity profiles, alterations in the currently effective treatment strategies must proceed cautiously to assure that disease-free survival is not compromised.

References

Goldsby RE, Carroll WL: The molecular biology of pediatric lymphomas. J Pediatr Hematol Oncol 20:282–296, 1998

Hudson MM, Donaldson SS: Hodgkin's disease. Pediatr Clin North Am 44:891–906, 1997

Hudson MM, Poquette CA, Lee J, et al: Increased mortality after successful treatment for Hodgkin's disease. J Clin Oncol 16:3592–3600, 1998

Segal GH, Perkins SL, Kjeldsberg CR: Benign lymphadenopathies in children and adolescents. Semin Diagn Pathol 12:288–302, 1995

Stiller CA: What causes Hodgkin's disease in children? Eur J Cancer 34:523–528, 1998

20.9   OSTEOSARCOMA

Holcombe E. Grier

Osteosarcoma (formerly called *osteogenic sarcoma*) is the most common malignant tumor of bone among children and adolescents. The disease peaks among adolescents, also occurs among younger children and young adults, and may occur among older adults, usually in association with Paget disease. The cause of osteosarcoma is not known. Most cases appear to occur spontaneously. However, rare cases of osteosarcoma may be associated with a germ-line mutation in the p53 gene which is linked to the Li-Fraumeni syndrome (see Sec. 20.2 and Sec. 20.11). Osteosarcoma also can be caused by irradiation.

CLINICAL PRESENTATION

Osteosarcoma classically manifests as the cardinal symptoms of pain and swelling at the site of the primary tumor. Unlike Ewing sarcoma (the second most common malignant bone tumor) systemic signs and symptoms are nearly always absent. The most common location is at the ends of long bones, especially around the knee (distal femur or proximal tibia), and in the proximal humerus.

DIAGNOSIS AND STAGING

Radiographs of involved bones usually show a permeating infiltrating process with poorly defined borders. Excess calcium deposits usually are present (blastic lesion). A soft-tissue mass extending from the bone is common, and the blastic nature of the soft-tissue mass produces the classic sunburst appearance on plain radiographs (Fig. 20-6). Evaluation includes establishing the extent of the primary lesion, best done with magnetic resonance imaging, and evaluation for possible metastasis. The most common site of metastasis is the lung, and computed tomography of that organ is critical. In rare instances, the tumor metastasizes to bones and necessitates a staging bone scan.

Definitive diagnosis is established with biopsy. Selection of biopsy site is important because inappropriate placement of the biopsy site can make future resection difficult. The biopsy material

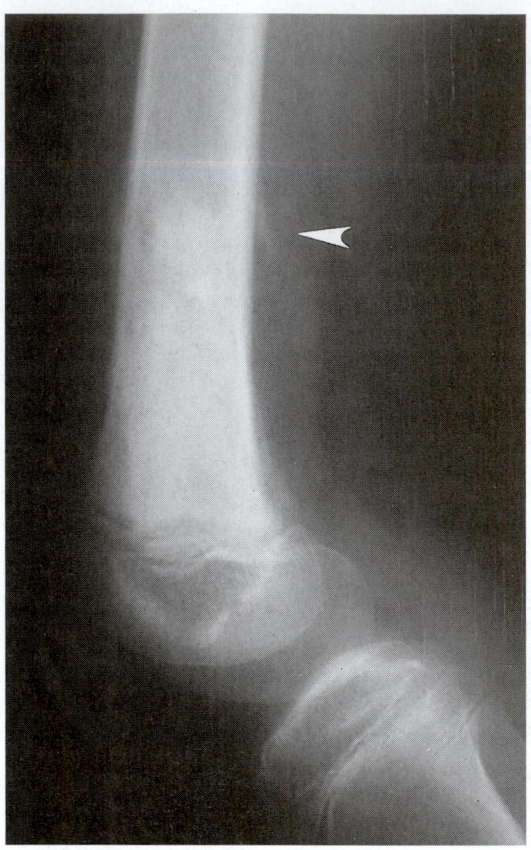

FIGURE 20-6   Radiograph shows osteosarcoma. Image shows a sclerotic lesion in the left distal femur with a poorly defined zone of transition to the proximal normal bone. The periosteum is elevated by the associated soft-tissue mass, which produces a Codman triangle (*arrow*) typical of rapidly growing bone tumors.

should be processed for the immunohistochemical analysis needed to ensure accurate diagnosis of malignant tumors in childhood.

The histologic features of osteosarcoma are sarcoma cells intermixed with malignant osteoid. In rare instances, low-grade osteosarcoma occurs, often limited to the cortex of the bone with little soft-tissue mass (parosteal and periosteal osteosarcoma). Therapy for these lower-grade tumors is controversial. The cytogenetic features of osteosarcoma, unlike those of Ewing sarcoma, are complex; multiple trisomies usually are present.

PROGNOSTIC FACTORS

The most important prognostic factor in osteosarcoma is presence or absence of metastasis at presentation. Other clinical factors associated with poor outcome include size of primary tumor and lack of lymphocytic infiltration of the tumor. Tumors associated with poor prognosis have either amplification of p-glycoprotein (the protein product of *mdr* [multiple drug resistance] gene that increases efflux of chemotherapeutic drugs from the cells) or increased erb-b2 receptors on the cell surface. However, the prognostic factor best established in osteosarcoma is the histologic response of the primary tumor to chemotherapy.

TREATMENT

Therapy for osteosarcoma requires therapy at the site of the primary tumor (local control) and therapy to irradicate any metastatic lesions. For patients without detectable metastasis, randomized trials have clearly established that chemotherapy is needed to control the micrometastasis almost certainly present. Sixty-five to 70% of patients with nonmetastatic osteosarcoma are cured with initial chemotherapy followed by surgical removal of the tumor and adjuvant chemotherapy. Treatment of the 20% of patients with metastasis results in only approximately a 25% long-term survival rate. Patients with metastasis to bone fare even worse than those with the more common metastasis limited to the lung parenchyma. Effective drugs in the management of osteosarcoma include doxorubicin, cisplatin, and high-dose methotrexate. Ifosfamide is clearly effective in the care of many patients with relapses of osteosarcoma.

Although the primary tumor in osteosarcoma may respond to radiation therapy, surgical removal of the tumor almost always is needed for cure. Limb salvage operations frequently are performed by means of replacement of diseased bone with allografts from bone banks or with metal prostheses. Retrospective comparisons have shown limb salvage operations, when feasible and with adequate margins, have outcomes comparable with those of amputation. The uncommon nonextremity osteosarcoma frequently is difficult to remove surgically and is thus associated with much worse outcome.

Treatment after relapse osteosarcoma is difficult. Some hope for success exists when the metastatic lesions are limited to the lung. Outcome improves with increasing time from initial therapy. Improved outcome is associated with smaller numbers of metastatic lesions and lesions that do not involve the pleural surface of the lung. Surgical removal of mestastatic lesions often is performed with systemic chemotherapy.

FUTURE DIRECTIONS

The next national trial in the United States will be an investigation of whether further intensification of the current chemotherapeutic agents can improve outcome for patients with osteosarcoma. Hope lies in interfering with the unique biologic features of osteosarcoma.

References

Goorin A, Perez-Atayde A, Gebhardt M, et al: Weekly high dose methotrexate and doxorubicin for osteosarcoma: the Dana Farber Cancer Institute/The Children's Hospital Study III. J Clin Oncol 5:1178–1184, 1987

Kesselring F, Penn W: Radiological aspects of "classic" primary osteosarcoma: value of some radiological investigations. Diagn Imaging 51:78–92, 1982

Meyers PA, Heller G, Healey JH, et al: Osteosarcoma with clinically detectable metastasis at initial presentation. J Clin Oncol 11:449–453, 1993

20.10 EWING SARCOMA AND PRIMITIVE NEUROECTODERMAL TUMOR

Holcombe E. Grier

Ewing sarcoma is the second most common primary malignant tumor of bone (after osteosarcoma) among children and adolescents.

Two moderately distinct pathologic patterns exist—classic Ewing sarcoma and primitive neuroectodermal tumor (PNET). Peripheral PNET is a completely different tumor from the CNS tumors with the same name. Most pathologists now consider Ewing sarcoma and PNET to be one tumor type with varying degrees of differentiation.

Ewing sarcoma–PNET can occur in soft tissue, often mimicking rhabdomyosarcoma. The annual incidence in the United States is approximately 2 cases per 1 million children. The disease peaks in the 10- to 20-year age range, but rarely occurs among infants and clearly occurs among adults. The disease is extremely rare among black children and children of Asian genetic backgrounds. Approximately 60% of children with nonmetastatic Ewing sarcoma are cured with current multimodal therapy. Success is more difficult to achieve among patients with metastasis. The cause of Ewing sarcoma is not known. The disease does not appear to be inherited or caused by exposure to toxins or radiation.

CLINICAL PRESENTATION

Ewing sarcoma–PNET can occur in almost any bone of the body. Most patients have pain and swelling. In some instances, especially among patients with large primary tumors or with metastatic disease, the presentation includes systemic signs and symptoms, such as fever, weight loss, and an increased erythrocyte sedimentation rate. Unlike osteosarcoma, which usually involves the ends of long bones, Ewing sarcoma–PNET more frequently occurs in flat bones such as the bones of the pelvis and ribs or in the midshaft of long bones.

DIAGNOSIS

Plain radiographs of involved bones usually have a permeative infiltrating process with poorly defined borders. A soft-tissue mass extending from the bone is common. The classic radiologic appearance in long bones is "onion skinning," or multiple layers of periosteum laid down in reaction to the tumor's breaking through the cortex. Children believed to have malignant bone tumors or soft-tissue tumors need referral to a large pediatric care center. Establishing the extent of the primary tumor, best done with MRI, and evaluation for possible metastasis are essential. The metastatic evaluation includes a bone scan, chest CT, and bone marrow aspiration and biopsy.

Definitive diagnosis is established with tumor biopsy. Selection of the biopsy site is important because inappropriate placement of the biopsy site can make future resection or radiation therapy difficult. The biopsy specimen should be processed for immunohistochemical analysis, solid tumor cytogenetic study, and molecular diagnostic study to ensure accurate diagnosis.

The histologic basis of Ewing sarcoma–PNET is unknown, but the tumor cells characteristically stain for a ubiquitous cell membrane component, the protein product of the *MIC2* gene, also known as CD99. Although heavy surface staining for CD99 is not definitive for Ewing sarcoma, such a positive staining result is much less commonly present in other small round cell tumors of childhood, such as rhabdomyosarcoma. In most cases, the tumor cells contain a translocation, usually between chromosome 11 and chromosome 22. This translocation juxtaposes two genes: a unique gene called *EWS* on chromosome 22 and an *ets*-like oncogene, *FLI-1*, on chromosome 11. Alternative translocations connect other *ets*-like oncogenes with the *EWS* gene. Molecular detection of these translocations helps secure the diagnosis of Ewing sarcoma–PNET.

STAGING AND PROGNOSTIC FACTORS

No widely accepted staging system exists for Ewing sarcoma. The most important prognostic factor in Ewing sarcoma is the presence or absence of clinically detectable metastatic lesions. Among patients without metastasis, those with large primary tumors do worse than those with smaller tumors. Other negative prognostic variables are older age and poor radiologic or histologic response to induction chemotherapy.

THERAPY

Management of Ewing sarcoma entails therapy at the site of the primary tumor (local control) and therapy to erradicate any metastatic lesions. For patients without detectable metastatic lesions, chemotherapy is needed to manage the micrometastasis almost certainly present. Chemotherapy also shrinks the primary tumor, frequently allowing delayed surgery or reduction in the final cone downfield of radiation therapy. A combined CCSG/POG trial showed that a five-drug combination (vincristine, doxorubicin, and cyclophosphamide alternating with ifosfamide and etoposide) provided the best results in the care of patients with nonmetastatic Ewing sarcoma. The 5-year tumor-free survival is 65 to 70% with these drugs. The results for the 20 to 25% of patients with metastasis when they come to medical attention are poorer; the 5-year tumor-free survival rate is approximately 20%. Treatment after relapse is difficult unless the patient is several years from initial diagnosis. In that circumstance, cure is possible, and intensive therapy is indicated.

Management of the primary tumor can be accomplished either with radiation therapy, surgery, or a combination of both. Trials that compare the two modalities are retrospective and do not account for the fact that smaller tumors are more frequently approached surgically. Radiation therapy for Ewing sarcoma–PNET can cause second cancers within the radiation field for 10 to 25% of patients after 30 years of follow-up study. For this reason, surgery often is used for local control when the operation will not cause functional deficits.

FUTURE DIRECTIONS

The most recent national trials have investigated whether further intensification of the current chemotherapeutic agents can improve outcome for patients with Ewing sarcoma–PNET. The unique translocation that occurs among almost all these tumors may provide a target for future therapy.

References

Dehner LP: Neuroepithelioma (primitive neuroectodermal tumor) and Ewing's sarcoma: at least a partial consensus. Arch Pathol Lab Med 118:606, 1994

Delattre O, Zucman J, Melot T, et al: The Ewing family of tumors: a subgroup of small-round-cell tumors defined by specific chimeric transcripts. N Engl J Med 331:294, 1994

Hudson TM, Hamlin DJ, Enneking WF, et al: Magnetic resonance imaging of bone and soft tissue tumors: early experience in 31 patients compared with computed tomography. Skeletal Radiol 13:134, 1985

Kuttesch JF Jr, Wexler LH, Marcus RB, et al: Second malignancies after Ewing's sarcoma: radiation dose-dependency of secondary sarcomas. J Clin Oncol 14:2818, 1996

20.11 RHABDOMYOSARCOMA

Philip P. Breitfeld and Holcombe E. Grier

Rhabdomyosarcoma represents approximately 5% of all cancers among children. It is the most common soft-tissue tumor. Approximately 250 new cases are diagnosed each year in the United States, for an annual incidence of 5 to 6 per million children younger than 15 years. Two thirds of patients are 10 years or younger. Nevertheless, adolescents and young adults can have rhabdomyosarcoma, and they appear to be underrepresented in national clinical trials sponsored by the National Cancer Institute. Approximately 70% of children with rhabdomyosarcoma can be cured with current multimodal therapy. The cause of rhabdomyosarcoma is not known. However, there is an association between rhabdomyosarcoma and germ-line mutations of the p53 gene, especially among children younger than 3 years. The association in families between maternal breast cancer, sarcoma among children, adrenocorticocarcinoma, and germ-line mutations in p53 is called *Li-Fraumeni syndrome* (see Sec. 20.2).

CLINICAL PRESENTATION

Rhabdomyosarcoma can originate in any location where there is striated muscle. Sites of presentation are most often the head and neck, including the orbit and parameningeal sites, genitourinary system, extremities, and trunk. The location of the tumor greatly influences the clinical presentation. Tumors of the neck manifest as an enlarging mass. Orbital masses can cause proptosis and ophthalmoplegia. Parameningeal tumors can cause cranial nerve dysfunction and nasal, sinus, and eustachian tube obstruction. Genitourinary tumors can manifest as a pelvic mass or with urinary

TABLE 20-14
RHABDOMYOSARCOMA PRESURGICAL STAGING SYSTEM

STAGE	SITE	T STATUS	SIZE	N STATUS	M STATUS
1	Orbit, head and neck, genitourinary other than bladder or prostate	T1 or T2	a or b	Any	M0
2	Bladder, prostate, extremity, parameningeal, other	T1 or T2	a	N0 or NX	M0
3	Bladder, prostate, extremity, parameningeal, other	T1 or T2	a	N1	M0
		T1 or T2	b	Any	M0
4	All	T1 or T2	a or b	N0 or NX	M1

T1 = tumor confined to anatomic site of origin; T2 = extension or fixation to surrounding tissue; a = ≤ 5 cm in diameter; b = >5 cm in diameter; N0 = regional nodes not clinically involved; N1 = regional nodes clinically involved; NX = node status unknown; M0 = no distant metastasis; M1 = metastasis present.

obstruction. Extremity and trunk tumors manifest as an enlarging mass.

DIAGNOSIS AND STAGING

A child with a soft-tissue mass that may be malignant needs a careful physical examination to define the size of the primary mass and to assess whether regional lymphatic spread is present. An evaluation must define the full extent of the local tumor, the presence of any regional spread to lymph nodes, and the presence of metastatic disease. Computed tomography or MRI of the primary site is performed to assess the local and regional extent of disease. To assess the risk of metastatic disease, chest CT, bone scan, and bone marrow examination are recommended. Definitive diagnosis is established with a biopsy or attempt at complete resection of the primary mass. Material obtained is processed for standard histologic evaluation, immunohistologic staining, electron microscopic examination, and molecular diagnostic study.

Rhabdomyosarcoma is a tumor of striated muscle. Detection of cross-striations, Z-band material, and expression of muscle-specific proteins helps establish the diagnosis. Rhabdomyosarcoma is histologically classified as botryoid, embryonal, or alveolar. Even a small component of a tumor that has alveolar histologic features establishes the diagnosis as alveolar rhabdomyosarcoma. The most common translocation of the alveolar histiotype is t(2;13), followed by t(1;13). These represent translocations of a *PAX* gene (either *PAX3* or *PAX7*) and the *FKHR* gene. Detection of one of these translocations helps secure the diagnosis of alveolar rhabdomyosarcoma. The embryonal histiotype is not currently known to be associated with a specific translocation but is associated with loss of heterozygosity in the region of 11p15. Although not formally classified as rhabdomyosarcoma, biologically undifferentiated sarcoma (no evidence of myogenic differentiation) behaves clinically as alveolar rhabdomyosarcoma. Children with undifferentiated sarcoma are treated as if they have rhabdomyosarcoma.

Current treatment of a child with rhabdomyosarcoma depends on complete presurgical and surgical staging, because both are used to assign risk-adapted therapy. Presurgical stage is determined from

TABLE 20-15

RHABDOMYOSARCOMA POSTSURGICAL GROUP

GROUP	DEFINITION
I	Localized disease, completely resected
II	Microscopic residual disease
III	Gross residual disease
IV	Distant metastasis not resected

the results of the initial radiologic evaluation for local, regional, and distant disease. The staging system used includes standard TNM (tumor-nodes-metastasis) criteria but stage also depends on site (Table 20-14). A surgical staging system has been developed by the Intergroup Rhabdomyosarcoma Study Group (IRSG) (Table 20-15) and is primarily based on the extent of initial surgical resection.

PROGNOSTIC FACTORS

Factors that most influence success of therapy include presurgical stage, postsurgical group, site, and nodal status. The IRSG has combined these prognostic factors to establish three risk groups (Table 20-16). Children with low-risk rhabdomyosarcoma have an 80 to 90% chance of long-term survival, children with intermediate-risk rhabdomyosarcoma have a 60% chance of long-term survival, and children with high-risk rhabdomyosarcoma have less than a 40% chance of long-term survival.

CHEMOTHERAPY

Systemic chemotherapy is indicated in the care of all children with rhabdomyosarcoma. For patients with nonmetastatic rhabdomyosarcoma undergoing initial complete surgical resection, the goal of chemotherapy is to control any micrometastatic disease. For tumors that are unresectable at diagnosis, chemotherapy is used to shrink the primary tumor to maximize the likelihood of complete resection with a second surgical procedure. With such an approach, the IRSG and international cooperative groups have found im-

TABLE 20-16

INTERGROUP RHABDOMYOSARCOMA STUDY GROUPS

RISK	STAGE	GROUP	SITE	SIZE	NODES
Low	1	I	Favorable	a or b	Any
	1	II	Favorable	a or b	N0
	1	III	Favorable[a]	a or b	Any
	2	I	Unfavorable	a	N0
Intermediate	1	II	Favorable	Any	N1
	1	III	Favorable[b]	Any	Any
	2	II, III	Unfavorable	a	N0
	3	I	Unfavorable	b	N0
	3	II	Unfavorable	a	N1
				b	Any
	3	III	Unfavorable	Any	Any
High	4	Any	Any	Any	Any

[a] Orbit or eyelid sites only.
[b] Excluding orbit or eyelid sites.

Favorable = orbit or eyelid, head and neck (excluding parameningeal), genitourinary (not bladder or prostate); Unfavorable = bladder, prostate, extremity, parameningeal, other (trunk, retroperitoneal, etc); a = ≤5cm in diameter; b = >5 cm in diameter; N0 = regional nodes not clinically involved; N1 = regional nodes clinically involved; NX = node status unknown.

pressive improvement in survival rates over the last 20 to 30 years. For most patients, chemotherapy involves use of vincristine, actinomycin D, and high-dose cyclophosphamide (VAC). Some patients with favorable sites, such as the orbit or head and neck, or patients with stage II and completely resected tumors can be treated with vincristine and actinomycin D because the outcome is so favorable. Standard chemotherapy for metastatic disease includes VAC.

MANAGEMENT OF PRIMARY TUMOR

Management of the primary tumor mass includes radiation therapy and surgical excision. The role of each depends on the site and extent of disease. Initial complete surgical resection is recommended for tumors when this can be accomplished without great risk of loss of function. For example, complete resection of a primary lesion of the bladder or prostate rarely is indicated if there is substantial risk of loss of bladder function. In contrast, some tumors in sites such as the extremities can be easily resected with complete preservation of function.

For most patients with rhabdomyosarcoma, the decision regarding the proper use of radiation therapy depends on the extent of tumor resection. The general approach involves managing the primary site with a generous volume of surrounding normal tissue. The dose administered is maximal in the care of patients with bulky tumor after surgery, and the dose is reduced in the care of patients with complete resection or with microscopic residual disease. For a few selected favorable sites, such as the orbit and head and neck, when initial complete resection is accomplished, no radiation therapy is recommended.

OUTCOME OF THERAPY

For patients with nonmetastatic disease more than 70% of patients are long-term survivors but only approximately one third of patients with metastatic disease survive. The long-term consequences of therapy among children who survive are of considerable importance. Because most children with rhabdomyosarcoma have not completed growth, current doses of conventional radiation therapy can impair growth of muscle and bone if included in the treatment volume. The long-term sequelae of surgery depend on the site. The long-term effects of VAC chemotherapy include hemorrhagic cystitis and secondary leukemia.

FUTURE DIRECTIONS

Additional new agents are needed if patients with metastatic disease are to have improvement in long-term survival. Most patients who have relapses eventually die of the disease. Better markers are needed to define which patients are likely to have successful treatment. Reductions in long-term toxicity will be aided by radiation technique that spares normal tissue, especially in young children.

References

Barr F: The role of chimeric paired box transcription factors in the pathogenesis of pediatric rhabdomyosarcoma. Cancer Res 59:1711, 1999

Diller L, Sexsmith E, Gottlieb E, Li F, Malkin D: Germline p53 mutations are frequently detected in young children with rhabdomyosarcoma. J Clin Invest 95:1606, 1995

Malkin D, Li F, Strong L, et al: Germline p53 mutations in a familial syndrome of breast cancer, sarcomas, and other neoplasms. Science 250: 1233, 1990

McHugh K, Boothroyd A: The role of radiology in childhood rhabdomyosarcoma. Clin Radiol 54:2, 1999

Pappo A, Shapiro D, Crist W: Rhabdomyosarcoma: biology and treatment. Pediatr Clin North Am 44:953, 1997

20.12 WILMS TUMOR

Daniel M. Greene

Wilms tumor is the most common primary malignant renal tumor of childhood and is the paradigm for multimodal management of a pediatric malignant solid tumor. Developments in surgical techniques and postoperative care, recognition of the sensitivity of Wilms tumor to irradiation, and the availability of several active chemotherapeutic agents have led to a dramatic change in the prognosis for most patients with this once uniformly lethal malignant disease.

EPIDEMIOLOGY

The incidence of Wilms tumor is 10 cases per million among white children younger than 15 years, and the male to female ratio is low. The incidence is approximately three times higher for blacks in the United States and Africa than for eastern Asians. The rates for white populations in Europe and North America are intermediate between these extremes. The mean age at diagnosis for patients with unilateral tumors is 42 months among boys and 47 months among girls. The mean age at diagnosis for patients with bilateral tumors is 30 months for boys and 33 months for girls.

Children with Wilms tumor may have associated anomalies, including aniridia, hemihypertrophy, cryptorchidism, and hypospadias. Children with pseudohermaphroditism or renal disease who have Wilms tumor may have Denys-Drash syndrome, and those with Wilms tumor, aniridia, genitourinary malformation, and mental retardation have the WAGR syndrome (see Chap. 21). Hemihypertrophy may occur as an isolated abnormality, or as a component of Beckwith-Wiedemann syndrome, which includes macroglossia, omphalocele, and visceromegaly (see Chap. 10).

GENETICS AND MOLECULAR BIOLOGY

The development and progression of Wilms tumor may involve a number of genetic loci, including the Wilms tumor suppressor gene (*WT1*) at 11p13, a second gene at 11p15.5, and one or more familial Wilms tumor genes that have other loci. Rapid progress in uncovering both genetic and epigenetic (imprinting) alterations is facilitating a better understanding of the disease and providing new prognostic factors for determining the intensity of therapy.

PATHOLOGY

Wilms tumor is characterized by tremendous histologic diversity. It is composed of, or thought to be derived from, primitive metanephric blastema. In addition to expressing a variety of cell types and aggregation patterns of normally developing kidney, these neoplasms often contain tissues not present in the normal metanephros, such as skeletal muscle, cartilage, and squamous epithelium. These heterotopic cell types may reflect the primitive developmental potential of metanephric blastema that does not occur in normal nephrogenesis. The classic nephroblastoma is made up of varying proportions of three cell types—blastemal, stromal, and epithelial.

Biphasic patterns (eg, blastemal and stromal cells) are frequently encountered. Some specimens consisting predominantly or exclusively of one cell are included in the Wilms tumor category if the cell type is one present in more conventional Wilms tumors.

The most frequent histologic characteristic of poor prognosis is the presence of anaplasia, indicated by the presence of gigantic polyploid nuclei within the tumor sample. Anaplastic changes may be either focal or diffuse and are rare (approximately 2% of renal tumors) among patients younger than 2 years. The rate of anaplastic changes increases to a relatively stable 13% among those 5 years or older. Anaplastic changes are considerably more frequent among black than among white patients.

Two additional histologically distinct renal tumors may be confused clinically with Wilms tumor. *Clear cell sarcoma of the kidney,* is associated with a higher rate of relapse and death than is Wilms tumor with favorable histologic features and has a strikingly high risk of metastasis in the brain and bone. *Rhabdoid tumor of the kidney* was identified for the first time in 1978, occurs more frequently among male infants, and is associated with both brain metastasis and apparently separate PNET of the brain.

Two distinct lesions that may be precursors of Wilms tumor have been identified. These small, usually microscopic clusters of blastemal cells, tubules, or stromal cells, called *nephrogenic rests,* generally are situated at the periphery of the renal lobe. The lesion that occurs within the deeper cortex or medulla has been called an *intralobar* nephrogenic rest in contrast to the more commonly encountered *perilobar* nephrogenic rest. One or both of these variants are encountered in the renal parenchyma of approximately 30% of patients with Wilms tumor and are present in about 1% of random perinatal postmortem examinations. The presence of nephrogenic rests in a nephrectomy specimen identifies that the patient is at great risk of tumor development in the contralateral kidney.

CLINICAL PRESENTATION

Most children with Wilms tumor are brought to medical attention because of abdominal swelling or the presence of an abdominal mass. This usually is noticed by a parent while bathing or dressing the child. Abdominal pain, gross hematuria, and fever are other frequent findings at diagnosis. Hypertension, present in about 25% of cases, has been attributed to an increase in renin activity.

Wilms tumor must be differentiated from splenomegaly and neuroblastoma. The latter often arises in the celiac axis or extends across the midline because of lymph node involvement. A varicocele caused by obstruction of the spermatic vein may be associated with the presence of a tumor thrombus in the renal vein or inferior vena cava. The presence of any signs of a Wilms tumor associated syndrome, such as aniridia, partial or complete hemihypertrophy, and genitourinary abnormalities such as hypospadias, cryptorchidism or ambiguous genitalia should be documented.

Imaging studies are restricted to those necessary to establish the presence of an intrarenal space-occupying lesion. They are used to determine whether the opposite kidney is involved with tumor and to ascertain the presence and extent of intravascular tumor thrombus. Contrast-enhanced CT of the abdomen, performed to evaluate the nature and extent of the mass, may suggest apparent extension of the tumor into adjacent structures, such as the liver, spleen, or colon. Most children considered to have invasion of the liver at CT are found at the time of surgical exploration to have hepatic compression rather than hepatic invasion. Small lesions, which may be nephrogenic rests or Wilms tumor in the opposite kidney, should be delineated. The patency of the inferior vena cava may be de-

picted with ultrasonography. The results of radiographic studies and ultrasonography provide sufficient information on which to make a decision about laparotomy in the care of most children.

Plain chest radiographs are obtained to determine whether pulmonary metastasis is present. Marked interobserver variability in the interpretation of CT scans of the chest and the excellent prognosis for children with pulmonary nodules identified only at CT of the chest who are treated according to the stage of the renal tumor limit the usefulness of pretreatment CT of the chest in the care of children with Wilms tumor. A radionuclide bone scan and radiographic skeletal survey are performed postoperatively for all children with clear cell sarcoma of the kidney. Brain imaging with MR imaging or CT is performed for all children with clear cell sarcoma of the kidney or rhabdoid tumor of the kidney.

STAGING

Table 20-17 describes the staging system currently used by the National Wilms Tumor Study Group.

PROGNOSTIC CONSIDERATIONS

The histologic features of Wilms tumor are the most important determinant of prognosis. Tumor size, age of the patient, presence

TABLE 20-17

NATIONAL WILMS TUMOR STUDY GROUP STAGING SYSTEM

STAGE	CHARACTERISTICS
I	Tumor limited to the kidney and completely excised. Renal capsule has an intact outer surface. Tumor not ruptured and biopsy not performed before removal (fine-needle aspiration biopsy is excluded from this restriction). The vessels of the renal sinus are not involved. There is no evidence of tumor at or beyond the margins of resection.
II	Tumor extends beyond the kidney but is completely excised. There may be regional extension of tumor (penetration of renal capsule or extensive invasion of the renal sinus). The blood vessels outside the renal parenchyma, including those of the renal sinus, may contain tumor. Biopsy is performed (except for fine-needle aspiration), or there is spillage of tumor before or during surgery that is confined to the flank and does not involve the peritoneal surface. There must be no evidence of tumor at or beyond the margins of resection.
III	Residual nonhematogenous tumor present and confined to the abdomen. Any one of the following may occur:
1	Lymph nodes within the abdomen or pelvis are involved by tumor (renal hilar, paraaortic, or beyond).
2	The tumor has penetrated through the peritoneal surface.
3	Tumor implants are found on the peritoneal surface.
4	Gross or microscopic tumor remains postoperatively (eg, tumor cells are found at the margin of surgical resection on microscopic examination). The tumor is not completely resectable because of local infiltration into vital structures. Tumor spill not confined to the flank occurs either before or during surgery.
IV	Hematogenous metastasis (lung, liver, bone, brain,) or lymph node metastasis outside the abdominopelvic region.
V	Bilateral renal involvement at diagnosis. An attempt is made to stage each side according to the foregoing criteria on the basis of extent of disease before biopsy or treatment.

of lymph node metastasis, and local features of the tumor, such as capsular or vascular invasion, have in the past been predictive of risk of tumor recurrence or progression. Recent research has focused on identification of additional prognostic factors for further stratification of therapy according to risk of recurrence. In a study of 232 children with Wilms tumor, loss of heterozygosity of 16q markers, which was present in tumor tissue from 17.2% of those with unfavorable or anaplastic histologic features of Wilms tumor, was associated with statistically significantly poorer 2-year relapse-free and overall survival percentages.

GENERAL SURGICAL PRINCIPLES

Surgical removal of the primary tumor remains the cornerstone of Wilms tumor therapy. Assessment of tumor spread at surgery is essential for accurate staging and for subsequent determination of the need for radiation therapy and administration of the appropriate chemotherapeutic regimen. Every effort must be made to remove the tumor without causing spread or spill.

Preoperative chemotherapy is administered to patients who have intravascular extension of tumor thrombus to the intrahepatic vena cava or more proximally, including the right atrium. Tumor shrinkage usually follows and makes the standard transabdominal approach feasible. Thoracoabdominal incisions, cardiac bypass, and other maneuvers necessary to extract the tumor from the heart thus can be avoided. The incidence of synchronous bilateral Wilms tumor is 4.4 to 7.0%. The management recommended is initial bilateral renal biopsy with staging of each kidney. After chemotherapy, a reevaluation is performed to determine whether there has been sufficient response of the tumors to allow tumor resection with preservation of a substantial amount of normal renal tissue.

RADIATION THERAPY

The National Wilms Tumor Studies have shown that patients with stage I and II tumors and favorable histologic findings who receive vincristine and actinomycin D do not need postoperative irradiation. A dose of 1000 cGy is sufficient for local control of Stage III disease and a tumor with favorable histologic findings if chemotherapy with vincristine, actinomycin D, and doxorubicin also is administered. Whole-lung irradiation (1200 cGy) is recommended for patients with pulmonary metastatic lesions visible on plain chest radiographs. Chemotherapy doses given immediately after completion of whole-lung irradiation are decreased 50%.

CHEMOTHERAPY

According to National Wilms Tumor Study Group findings, the chemotherapy regimens recommended for children with favorable histologic findings of Wilms tumor depend on tumor stage: stage I or II, vincristine and actinomycin D for 18 weeks; stage III or IV, a combination of vincristine, actinomycin D, and doxorubicin for 21 weeks. The relapse-free survival percentages for patients with favorable histologic findings are stage I, 94.9%; stage II, 85.9%; stage III, 91.1%; stage IV, 80.6%. For patients with clear cell sarcoma of kidney in stages I through IV, the survival percentage is 84.1%.

RECURRENT DISEASE

Children with favorable histologic features of Wilms tumor who have relapses have a variable prognosis. Favorable prognostic factors include no previous treatment with doxorubicin, relapse more than 12 months after diagnosis, and subdiaphragmatic relapse in a patient not previously given abdominal irradiation.

Children in this more favorable group should be treated aggressively because a good response to retrieval therapy can be achieved. Although surgical excision of pulmonary metastasis does not diminish the risk of a second relapse, biopsy or excision of lesions should be performed for histologic confirmation of the presence of recurrent disease, to document the site of relapse, and in the case of intraabdominal recurrence, to reduce the tumor burden before initiation of radiation therapy and chemotherapy. The optimal chemotherapy regimen has not been defined.

Patients who have had relapses after treatment with a regimen that included doxorubicin or who have a recurrence in the abdomen, including the liver, after previous irradiation have a poor prognosis. The combination of etoposide and ifosfamide has rarely produced prolonged responses in the care of these children. Several centers have suggested that a more aggressive approach, including autologous bone marrow transplantation, should be used.

FUTURE CONSIDERATIONS

The use of biological markers, such as loss of heterozygosity (LOH) for 16q, to determine which patients have greater risk of tumor recurrence must be evaluated. The role of whole-lung irradiation in the treatment of patients with stage IV disease and favorable histologic findings and the efficacy of chemotherapeutic agents other than anthracyclines in combination with vincristine and actinomycin D in the treatment of patients with stage III or IV disease and favorable histologic features with a high risk of relapse must be studied. Other problems to be carefully evaluated include the use of surgical procedures that spare the renal parenchyma in the treatment of patients with bilateral Wilms tumor. Finally the availability of techniques to identify mutations within the *WT1* gene make possible screening of persons who may be at increased risk of Wilms tumor, such as patients with aniridia, cryptorchidism, and hypospadias.

References

Breslow N, Olshan A, Beckwith JB, Green DM: Epidemiology of Wilms tumor. Med Pediatr Oncol 21:172–181, 1993

Breslow N, Sharples K, Beckwith JB, et al: Prognostic factors in nonmetastatic, favorable histology Wilms' tumor: results of the Third National Wilms' Tumor Study. Cancer 68:2345–2353, 1991

Coppes MJ, Haber DA, Grundy PE: Genetic events in the development of Wilms tumor. N Engl J Med 331:586–590, 1994

Faria P, Beckwith JB, Kishra K, et al: Focal versus diffuse anaplasia in Wilms tumor: new definitions with prognostic significance—a report from the National Wilms Tumor Study Group. Am J Surg Pathol 20:909–920, 1996

Green DM, Breslow NE, Beckwith JB, Moksness J, Finklestein JZ, D'Angio GJ: The treatment of children with clear cell sarcoma of the kidney: a report from the National Wilms Tumor Study Group. J Clin Oncol 12:2132–2137, 1994

Grundy PE, Telzerow PE, Breslow N, Moksness J, Huff V, Paterson MC: Loss of heterozygosity for chromosomes 16q and 1p in Wilms tumors predicts an adverse outcome. Cancer Res 54:2331–2333, 1994

Meisel JA, Guthrie KA, Breslow NE, Donaldson SS, Green DM: Significance and management of computed tomography detected pulmonary nodules: a report from the National Wilms Tumor Study Group. Int J Radiat Oncol Biol Phys 44:579–585, 1999

20.13 NEUROBLASTOMA

Garrett M. Broudeur and John M. Maris

Neuroblastoma, a tumor of the postganglionic sympathetic nervous system, is the most common solid tumor in childhood. Some infants with metastatic disease can have complete regression without therapy. Among some older patients, the tumor matures into a benign ganglioneuroma. Most patients have metastatic disease that progresses relentlessly despite even the most intensive multimodality therapy. Despite dramatic improvements in the cure rate of other common pediatric neoplasms, improvement in the overall survival rate among patients with neuroblastoma has been relatively modest. Advances in understanding of the biological mechanisms of neuroblastoma have provided considerable insight into the genetic and biochemical mechanisms underlying these seemingly disparate behaviors.

EPIDEMIOLOGY, GENETICS, AND BIOLOGY

Neuroblastoma accounts for 7 to 10% of all childhood cancers and is the most common malignant tumor among infants. The prevalence is approximately one case per 7000 live births, and approximately 600 new cases occur each year in the United States. This corresponds to an incidence of 10.5 per million per year among white children and 8.8 per million per year among black children younger than 15 years. This incidence is consistent throughout the world, at least among industrialized nations. The tumor is slightly more common among boys than girls with a male to female ratio of 1.2:1 in most large studies. The median age at diagnosis is 22 months, and only about 3% of cases are diagnosed after the patient is 10 years of age.

The cause of neuroblastoma is unknown in most cases, but it appears unlikely that environmental exposure has a major role. No prenatal or postnatal exposure to drugs, chemicals, or radiation has been strongly or consistently associated with an increased risk of neuroblastoma. Neuroblastoma has been reported among patients with neurofibromatosis type 1 and patients with Hirschsprung disease, suggesting that it may be part of a spectrum of disorders involving neural crest development. Most cases of the simultaneous occurrence of neuroblastoma and other disorders probably can be accounted for by chance alone. A variety of other congenital anomalies and genetic syndromes have been reported in association with neuroblastoma, but no specific abnormality has been identified with increased frequency. An increased prevalence of neuroblastoma among patients with Turner syndrome and a decreased prevalence among patients with Down syndrome has been observed, but the reasons are unclear.

Some patients have a predisposition to neuroblastoma, and this predisposition follows an autosomal dominant pattern of inheritance. As many as one fourth of all neuroblastomas may be caused by a germinal mutation (see Sec. 20.2). Results of the analysis of families with hereditary neuroblastoma are consistent with the two-mutation hypothesis proposed by Knudson for the origin of childhood cancer (see Sec. 20.2). The median age at diagnosis of familial neuroblastoma is 9 months, in contrast to a median age of 22 months in the general population. At least 20% of patients with familial neuroblastoma have bilateral adrenal or multifocal primary tumors. Evidence from a genetic linkage study showed that a predisposition locus for neuroblastoma is present at 16p12-13.

Several types of genetic change have been identified in subsets of neuroblastoma. *MYCN* amplification, 1p deletion, and 17q gain are associated with more advanced stage and a worse outcome, whereas hyperdiploidy with whole chromosome gains is associated with a good outcome. It is unclear whether *MYCN* overexpression in nonamplified tumor has biological or prognostic significance. The presumptive tumor-suppressor genes deleted from 1p, 11q, and 14q have not been identified. Genetic changes leading to DNA rearrangement or instability or to development of whole chromosome gains are unknown (see Sec. 20.2.3).

Neuroblastoma cells are derived from sympathetic neuroblasts and frequently have features of neuronal differentiation. Neuroblastoma can undergo spontaneous or induced differentiation to ganglioneuroblastoma or ganglioneuroma (see Chap. 25). Thus the factors responsive for spontaneous malignant transformation may be caused in part by failure to differentiate. Regression of neuroblastoma in infants is not understood but may involve the neurotrophin receptor pathways (TrkA, TrkB, and TrkC). The primary ligands for each of these receptors are nerve growth factor, brain-derived neurotrophic factor (BDNF), and neurotrophin-3, respectively.

There is now clear evidence that high TrkA expression in the tumor is associated with younger age, lower stage, and a favorable outcome. There is an inverse correlation between TrkA expression and *MYCN* amplification, so both factors may affect overall survival. Favorable tumors are characterized by expression of TrkA with or without TrkC, but unfavorable tumors express TrkB and its ligand BDNF. The pattern of expression of the neurotrophin receptors may have an important role in the behavior of neuroblastoma, including the likelihood that a tumor may undergo spontaneous regression or differentiation.

The genetic features of neuroblastoma are highly predictive of clinical behavior. One model proposes three distinct but interrelated subsets based on genetic and biological features, such as *MYCN* copy number; DNA content (ploidy); patterns of allelic loss on chromosomes 1p, 11q, and 14q; gain of 17q; and Trk gene expression. These subsets correspond to tumors associated with an excellent, intermediate, and poor outcome, respectively. Whether a tumor from a less aggressive type ever converts to a more aggressive type is unknown, but current evidence suggests distinct genetic differences.

CLINICAL FEATURES

Approximately one half of all neuroblastomas originate in the adrenal medulla; 30% occur in nonadrenal abdominal sites in the paravertebral ganglia, pelvic ganglia, or organ of Zuckerkandl; and 20% occur in the paravertebral ganglia of the chest or neck. Most primary tumors cause symptoms such as abdominal mass or pain. However, because of the paraspinal location of many tumors, invasion of the spinal canal through neural foramina can occur. Consequent compression of the spinal cord in the thoracic or upper lumbar region can cause paraplegia, whereas lower lumbar invasion causes a cauda equina syndrome with loss of bowel or bladder function. Midline tumors can displace or compress other structures such as the trachea or esophagus or cause obstructive symptoms. Involvement of the superior cervical ganglion can produce Horner syndrome.

Most neuroblastomas are metastatic at diagnosis. Frequent sites of metastasis are the regional or distant lymph nodes, cortical bone, bone marrow, liver, and skin. Among infants younger than 1 year, a characteristic pattern of a small primary tumor with dissemination limited to the liver and skin (with or without minimal marrow involvement) is associated with a favorable outcome. This pattern is referred to as stage 4S. However, among patients 1 year or older, the pattern of dissemination frequently involves bone marrow and cortical bone, particularly of the skull and orbits. In rare instances, disease may spread to lung and brain parenchyma, usually as a manifestation of relapsing or end-stage disease. The outlook among patients with metastatic disease older than 1 year at diagnosis is poor, even with intensive multimodality therapy.

Several paraneoplastic syndromes have been associated with neuroblastoma, although each occurs among only 1 to 3% of patients. Intractable secretory diarrhea and abdominal distension, sometimes associated with hypokalemia and dehydration, is a manifestation of secretion of vasoactive intestinal peptide (VIP). The VIP syndrome usually is associated with ganglioneuroblastoma or ganglioneuroma, and these symptoms usually resolve after eradication of the tumor.

Opsomyoclonus (also called *myoclonic encephalopathy*) consists of myoclonic jerking and random eye movement, sometimes associated with cerebellar ataxia or other neurologic disorders. These symptoms may diminish or even disappear with eradication of the tumor, and these patients usually have a favorable outcome from the oncologic perspective. However, many patients have residual neurologic abnormalities. Opsoclonus syndrome may be caused by antineuronal autoantibodies. The symptoms may vary in severity, especially worsening in association with intercurrent illnesses, and may respond to immune modulation, such as plasmapheresis or administration of glucocorticoids.

Increased secretion of catecholamines is rare, but it causes tachycardia, palpitations, profuse sweating, and flushing. This syndrome is more common among patients with pheochromocytoma.

EVALUATION AND DIFFERENTIAL DIAGNOSIS

Confirmation of a diagnosis of neuroblastoma usually requires histologic evidence of neural origin or differentiation at light microscopic, electron microscopic, or immunohistologic examination. Because the bone marrow frequently is involved, some patients are considered to have neuroblastoma because of the presence of "compatible" clumps of tumor cells involving the bone marrow and accompanied by increased levels of catecholamine metabolites in the urine. Although different groups have used different diagnostic criteria, a proposal has been made to establish international criteria to confirm a diagnosis of neuroblastoma.

When sensitive assays are used, 90 to 95% of tumors produce sufficient catecholamines to increase urinary metabolites. This provides a great advantage in confirming the diagnosis of neuroblastoma, as well as in following disease activity in the care of patients with secreting tumors. The two enzymes primarily responsible for the catabolism of catecholamines are catechol-*O*-methyl transferase and monoamine oxidase. Dopa and dopamine are converted primarily to homovanillic acid, whereas norepinephrine and epinephrine are converted primarily to vanillylmandelic acid. Most laboratories involved in neuroblastoma diagnosis measure levels of both homovanillic acid and vanillylmandelic acid in the urine.

Because of the varied clinical presentation, neuroblastoma can be confused with other neoplasms as well as nonneoplastic conditions. Diagnosis of the 5 to 10% of tumors that do not produce catecholamines is particularly difficult, as is that of the 1 % or so in which the primary tumor is not obvious. Vasoactive intestinal pep-

tide syndrome can be confused with inflammatory bowel disease, and opsoclonus-myoclonus and ataxia syndromes can resemble a primary neurologic disorder. At histologic examination, neuroblastoma tissue from primary or metastatic sites can be quite undifferentiated and can be confused with other embryonal pediatric cancers, such as rhabdomyosarcoma, Ewing sarcoma, neuroepithelioma, lymphoma, or even leukemia, especially megakaryoblastic leukemia. Molecular, biochemical, and immunologic characterization usually can help differentiate these diagnostic entities.

A standard set of recommended tests to define the clinical stage or extent of disease has been established. The more tests performed, the greater is the likelihood of finding disseminated disease. This applies particularly to the number of bone marrow aspirates and biopsies performed and the manner in which marrow disease is detected. The conventional diagnostic imaging modalities include plain radiography, bone scintigraphy, CT, and MRI. The potential specificity and sensitivity of meta-iodobenzylguanidine (MIBG) scintigraphy for evaluation of bone and soft-tissue involvement of neuroblastoma are attractive.

The three classic histopathologic patterns of neuroblastoma, ganglioneuroblastoma, and ganglioneuroma reflect a spectrum of morphologic and biochemical differentiation from immature small blue cells to completely mature ganglion cells (surrounded by Schwannian stroma). Although there are several pathologic classification systems for neuroblastoma, the Shimada classification is the most clinically useful in predicting outcome, and it is the most commonly used system. This system takes into consideration the amount of Schwannian stroma, number of mitotic figures, presence of karyorrhexis, and age of the patient.

The distribution of patients by stage or extent of disease differs depending on age at diagnosis. For example, only approximately one third of patients younger than 1 year have unresectable or metastatic disease; approximately two thirds of older patients have advanced stages of disease, which explains in part the generally better outcome among infants with neuroblastoma than among their older counterparts. Biological differences between the tumors in the two age groups appear to be important. The International Neuroblastoma Staging System (INSS) has been developed based on clinical, radiographic, and surgical evaluation of children with neuroblastoma (Table 20-18). Modifications have been proposed in this system to clarity definitions of stages as well as criteria for diagnosis and response to treatment. Biological risk groups have been proposed that incorporate clinical and laboratory variables in determining prognosis.

PROGNOSTIC CONSIDERATIONS: CLINICAL AND BIOLOGICAL MARKERS

The overall prognosis for a good outcome among patients with stage 1, 2, and 4S disease is greater than 90%. Patients with stages 3 and 4 disease have a 2-year disease-free survival rate of 20 to 40%. The outcome among infants younger than 1 year is substantially better than that among older patients with the same stage of disease, particularly those with more advanced stages of disease. However, infants with stage 4 disease and *MYCN* amplification have a poor outcome. A variety of biological variables (pathologic features of the tumor, serum markers, genetic features, gene expression patterns) appear to have predictive value as independent prognostic markers among patients with neuroblastoma. No study to date, however, has examined all variables in a large set of patients, so it is difficult to say which single variable or combination of variables,

TABLE 20-18

INTERNATIONAL NEUROBLASTOMA STAGING SYSTEM

STAGE	CHARACTERISTICS
1	Localized tumor with complete gross excision, with or without microscopic residual disease; representative ipsilateral lymph nodes negative for tumor microscopically (nodes attached to and removed with the primary tumor may be positive).
2A	Localized tumor with incomplete gross excision; representative ipsilateral nonadherent lymph nodes negative for tumor microscopically.
2B	Localized tumor with or without complete gross excision, with ipsilateral nonadherent lymph nodes positive for tumor. Enlarged contralateral lymph nodes must be negative microscopically.
3	Unresectable unilateral tumor infiltrating across the midline,[a] with or without regional lymph node involvement; *or* localized unilateral tumor with contralateral regional lymph node involvement; *or* midline tumor with bilateral extension by infiltration (unresectable) or by lymph node involvement.
4	Any primary tumor with dissemination to distant lymph nodes, bone, bone marrow, liver, skin, or other organs (except as defined for stage 4S).
4S	Localized primary tumor (as defined for stage 1, 2A, or 2B), with dissemination limited to skin, liver, or bone marrow[b] (limited to infants younger than 1 year).

Multifocal primary tumors (eg, bilateral adrenal primary tumors) should be staged according to the greatest extent of disease, followed by a subscript M (eg, 3_M).

[a] The midline is defined as the vertebral column. Tumors originating on one side and crossing the midline must infiltrate to or beyond the opposite side of the vertebral column.

[b] Marrow involvement in stage 4S should be minimal, that is, fewer than 10% of total nucleated cells identified as malignant at bone marrow biopsy or marrow aspiration. More extensive marrow involvement is considered stage 4. Findings at MIBG scan (if performed) should be negative in the marrow.

SOURCE: *Reproduced with permission from Brodeur GM, Pritchard J, Berthold F, et al. Revisions of the international criteria for neuroblastoma diagnosis, staging and response to treatment. J Clin Oncol 11:1466, 1993.*

in addition to patient age and stage, is the most powerful predictor of outcome.

Most current studies of the treatment of patients with neuroblastoma are based on risk groups in which various biological features in addition to patient age and INSS stage are considered. Preliminary data, adjusted for age and stage, suggest that analysis of DNA content of infants and *MYCN* copy number of all patients allows more precise determination of risk. Histopathologic classification of the tumor with the Shimada system is an important independent prognostic marker, at least for certain subsets of patients. Assessing tumors for TrkA expression, 1p LOH, or 17q gain also appears promising (Fig. 20-7). Judging the prognostic effect of other biological variables, such as 11q LOH, *HRAS* expression, *MRP* expression, telomerase expression, or others, must await the results of prospective therapeutic and biological studies.

THERAPEUTIC APPROACHES

The role of surgery, chemotherapy, and radiation therapy is determined in individual cases. Stage, age at diagnosis, and biological features are considered. For patients who need therapy beyond surgery, chemotherapy remains the backbone of multimodality treatment.

Surgery has a pivotal role in the management of neuroblastoma. Depending on the timing, operative procedures can have diagnostic and therapeutic value. The goals of a primary surgical procedure are to establish the diagnosis, to provide tissue for prognostic biological studies, to excise the tumor if feasible, and to stage the tumor surgically. In delayed primary or second-look surgery, response to therapy is evaluated and residual disease is removed. Surgery can also have palliative benefit in the management of recurrent or progressive disease. For most patients with INSS stages 1 and 2 disease, surgery is the only treatment needed for cure.

Chemotherapy is the predominant modality of management of neuroblastoma. A number of effective drugs have been identified. Cyclophosphamide, ifosfamide, cisplatin, carboplatin, doxorubicin, and the epipodophyllotoxin etoposide yield complete and partial response rates of 25 to 50% and have become the cornerstone of multiagent regimens. Drug combinations have been developed that take advantage of drug synergism, mechanisms of cytotoxicity, and differences in side effects. Treatment of children with advanced-stage neuroblastoma by use of these combinations improves response rates with minimal increase in toxicity. Agents under evaluation include topotecan, anti-G_{D2} antibodies, differentiating agents such as 13-*cis*-retinoic acid and fenretinide, and angiogenesis inhibitors.

Neuroblastoma is considered a radiosensitive tumor, and radiation therapy is effective in achieving local control or palliation. However, long-term control of neuroblastoma seldom is achieved with radiation therapy alone because of the propensity of this tumor to widespread metastasis. Historically, radiation has been used in the multimodality management of residual neuroblastoma and bulky unresectable tumors. The role of radiation therapy for neuroblastoma continues to be refined with the addition of targeted radiotherapeutic approaches, such as radiolabeled MIBG or anti-G_{D2} antibodies.

Attempts have been made to improve on the modest gains of intensive, combined-modality therapy by increasing the intensity of therapy with BMT. Allogeneic BMT appears to offer little if any advantage and has greater toxicity than purged autologous BMT.

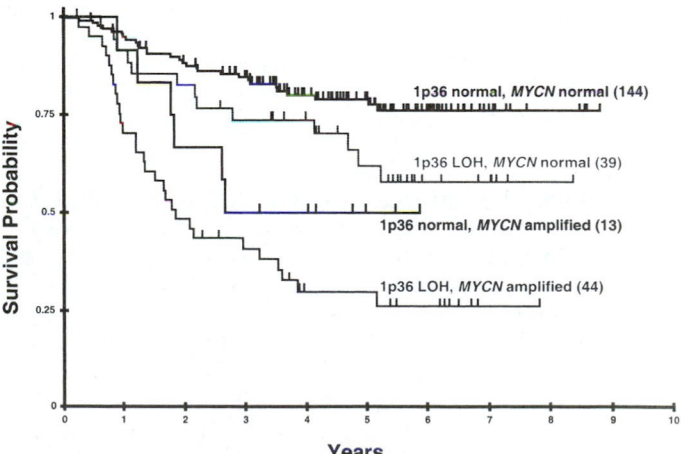

FIGURE 20-7 *MYCN* **amplification, 1p allelic loss, and survival among children with neuroblastoma. Survival of children with tumors that have** *MYCN* **amplication only, allelic loss only, both, or neither. (Source:** *Maris JM, White PS, Beltinger CP, et al. Significance of chromosome 1p loss of heterozygosity in neuroblastoma. Cancer 55: 4664, 1995.***)**

Many centers use peripheral blood stem cells (with or without CD34+ selection) as the source of progenitor cells for marrow rescue (see Sec. 20.4).

The use of dose-intensified chemotherapy combinations, with or without autologous stem cell rescue, has produced better immediate disease control in neuroblastoma, but has not translated into durable remissions among children with high-risk tumors. Future treatment strategies will address (1) the identification of novel drugs or drug combinations, (2) the use of biological agents that selectively induce apoptosis in neuroblastoma cells, (3) agents that induce differentiation, such as retinoic acid or nerve growth factor, (4) antiangiogenesis therapy, and (5) gene-targeted therapy or other approaches.

FUTURE CONSIDERATIONS

In addition to the aforementioned improvements and prospects for future therapy, areas in which the treatment of patients with neuroblastoma may improve include (1) identification of persons with a genetic predisposition to this disease, (2) development of sensitive and specific markers in serum or urine to confirm a diagnosis or to follow tumor response to treatment, (3) better biological characterization of tumors for diagnosis, classification, and prognosis, and (4) biologically based therapy targeted to the genes, proteins, and pathways responsible for initiation or maintenance of the malignant state.

References

Ambros PF, Brodeur GM: The concept of tumor genesis in neuroblastoma. In: Brodeur GM, Sowada T, Tsuchida Y, Voute PA, eds: Neuroblastoma. New York, Elsevier, 2000:521–532

Brodeur GM: Clinical and biological aspects of neuroblastoma. In: Scriver CR, Beaudet AL, Sly WS, Valle D, Vogelstein B: The Metabolic and Molecular Basis of Human Diseases, 8th ed. New York, McGraw-Hill, 1999

Brodeur GM: The concept of tumorigenesis in nemoblastoma. In: Brodeur GM, Sawada T, Tsuchida Y, Voute PA, eds: Neuroblastoma. Amsterdam, Elsevier Science, 1999 Chapter 3 entitled, "The Concept of Tumor Genesis in Neuroblastoma" by Ambros PF, Brodeur GM, Eds.: Brodeur, Sawada, Tsuchida, Voute, In: Neuroblastoma, pgs. 521–532, Amsterdam, New York, Elsevier, 2000.

Brodeur GM, Seeger RC, Schwab M, Varmus HE, Bishop JM: Amplification of N-myc in untreated human neuroblastomas correlates with advanced disease stage. Science 224:1121, 1984

Look AT, Hayes FA, Shuster JJ, Douglass EC, Castleberry RP, Brodeur GM: Clinical relevance of tumor cell ploidy and N-myc gene amplification in childhood neuroblastoma: a Pediatric Oncology Group study. J Clin Oncol 9:581, 1991

Maris JM, Matthay KK: Molecular biology of neuroblastoma. J Clin Oncol 17:2264–2279, 1999

Meister A, Larsson A: Gluthathione synthetase deficiency and other disorders. In: Scriver CR, Beaudet Al, Sly WS, Valle D: Metabolic and Molecular Basis of Inherited Disease, 7th ed. New York, McGraw-Hill, 1995:1461–1477

Nakagawara A, Arima-Nakagawara M, Scavarda NJ, Azar CG, Cantor AB, Brodeur GM: Association between high levels of expression of the TRK gene and favorable outcome in human neuroblastoma. N Engl J Med 328:847, 1993

20.14 LIVER TUMORS

Philip P. Breitfeld

A liver tumor in an infant, child, or adolescent manifests primarily as a painless abdominal mass. Approximately 70% of liver masses are malignant tumors. The probability that a lesion is malignant is related to the patient's age. Malignant lesions are almost always hepatoblastoma among children younger than 3 years, whereas hepatocellular carcinoma is progressively more common among older children. Of the benign lesions, hemagioendothelioma is most common and usually occurs among infants younger than 2 years. Liver tumors occur with a frequency of approximately 3 per million white children younger than 15 years.

EVALUATION AND DIFFERENTIAL DIAGNOSIS

Although usually painless, a liver mass can cause jaundice, weight loss, anorexia, or fever. A child with a right upper quadrant mass needs an ultrasound examination or CT with intravenous contrast medium to establish the source of the lesion. Additional clinical and laboratory variables, such as age at presentation, serum α-fetoprotein (AFP) level, and whether multiple lesions are present in the liver, aid the clinician in focusing on a limited set of diagnoses (Table 20-19). For example, a child younger than 6 months with multiple liver lesions and a normal serum AFP level most likely has hemangioendothelioma. In contrast, an 8-year-old child with a solitary mass and an elevated serum AFP level most likely has hepa-

TABLE 20-19
DIFFERENTIAL DIAGNOSIS OF A LIVER MASS IN A CHILD

DIAGNOSIS	AGE	DISTRIBUTION OF LESIONS	α-FETOPROTEIN LEVEL
Benign			
Hemangioendothelioma	<6 mo	Single or multiple	Normal
Mesenchymal hamartoma	<2 yr	Single	Normal
Inflammatory	Any	Single or multiple	Normal
UVC-related	Infant	Single	Normal
Malignant			
Hepatoblastoma	<3 yr	Single	Elevated
Hepatocellular carcinoma	>3 yr	Single or multiple	Elevated
Undifferentiated sarcoma	6–10 yr	Single	Normal
Metastatic	Any	Single or multiple	Normal

UVC = umbilical vein catheter.

tocellular carcinoma. Special clinical circumstances may suggest other specific diagnoses. For example, a female adolescent using oral contraceptives who has a hepatic mass may have an adenoma, or a neonate with a malpositioned umbilical cord catheter may have hepatic hematoma.

DEFINITIVE EVALUATION OF A LIVER MASS

Once an ultrasound or CT scan unequivocally establishes the presence of a liver mass, precise definition of the anatomic features of the liver by means of MRI or CT is essential because management of many hepatic tumors, benign and malignant, relies on surgical resection. Because both hepatoblastoma and hepatocellular carcinoma can produce AFP, all patients with a hepatic tumor need serum AFP analysis. If AFP level is elevated, the tumor usually is malignant (Table 20-19). Among infants younger than 6 months, the normal values of AFP are much higher than among older children (see Sec. 20.15), and are age dependent. Thus AFP levels measured for infants younger than 6 months should be compared with age-adjusted normal values.

For any child with a liver mass, a referral to a large pediatric center with pediatric surgeons and oncologists is recommended. The incidence of liver tumors is low (3 per million), and even the largest pediatric oncology programs care for only 5 to 8 children per year with malignant tumors of the liver.

Special circumstances can arise during the evaluation of a child with a liver mass. Hemangioendothelioma is the most likely diagnosis if the child is younger than 2 years, has normal AFP level, and imaging studies show punctate calcification. When this lesion is associated with consumptive coagulopathy, it is called *Kasabach-Merritt syndrome* (see Sec. 19.7 and Sec. 19.10). When multiple liver lesions are found and the AFP level is normal, the possibility that the lesions represent metastatic disease from a primary tumor outside the liver should be considered. The liver is the site of metastatic disease more commonly than it is the site of primary malignant disease. Metastatic disease of the liver among young children is most often from neuroblastoma. After 2 years of age, metastatic disease in the liver can be from lymphoma, sarcoma, or Wilms tumor.

DIAGNOSTIC PROCEDURES

The specific diagnosis of a liver tumor usually is made by means of resection of the entire mass if possible or by means of biopsy, either open or closed. The exception is circumstances in which hemangioendothelioma or cavernous hemangioma is suspected, and no diagnostic procedure is needed or recommended unless complete resection is possible. If the disease of the liver is thought to be metastatic, resection or biopsy is performed on the primary site of tumor rather than the disease in the liver. If the lesion is unresectable and closed biopsy is entertained, thorough evaluation of the coagulation system is performed because the patient may be at high risk of bleeding because of defective liver synthesis of clotting factors or because of consumptive coagulopathy. Correction of a substantial defect followed by open biopsy is recommended.

TREATMENT AND OUTCOME

Therapy and prognosis for liver tumors depend on the diagnosis. Complete resection is a mainstay of therapy for most benign and all primary malignant tumors of the liver.

Benign Tumors

The most common benign liver tumor is hemangioendothelioma, or cavernous hemangioma. These vascular lesions can be associated with cutaneous lesions and can cause high-output cardiac failure. When this lesion is suspected, biopsy is not recommended. Solitary lesions can be easily resected. If the lesion is unresectable (very large or multifocal) or if marked consumptive coagulopathy is present, medical therapy may be necessary. Prednisone usually is the initial therapy; however, interferon-α has recently been shown to shrink lesions that are unresectable or do not respond to prednisone. The course of these lesions is eventual regression. If the patient has no symptoms, therapy is not indicated.

Mesenchymal hamartoma is a benign tumor of the liver cured by means of complete surgical resection. The mass usually is multicystic and asymptomatic. At pathologic examination, hepatocytes, biliary epithelium, and mesenchymal elements are found. These lesions occur primarily among children younger than 2 years.

Focal nodular hyperplasia is suspected when imaging studies demonstrate a mass with a central scar with branching. This lesion commonly occurs among adolescents. Surgical resection is curative and is recommended because the mass can spontaneously rupture and bleed.

Liver cell adenoma is most likely among female adolescents taking oral contraceptives. The lesion usually is solitary and consists of an encapsulated mass of normal hepatocytes. Complete surgical resection is recommended because rupture and bleeding can occur.

Malignant Tumors

The most common primary malignant lesion of the liver is hepatoblastoma. It usually occurs among children younger than 3 years. These tumors usually are solitary, but they can be multicentric. α-Fetoprotein level is elevated. The frequency is higher among children with hemihypertrophy and Beckwith-Wiedemann syndrome and among patients with germ-line mutation of the adenomatous polyposis coli gene. Sporadic hepatoblastoma has been found in association with somatic mutations in the adenomatous polyposis coli gene. The tumor is composed of cells that resemble immature liver tissue. Lesions can be divided into fetal and embryonal subtypes. The pure fetal subtype is associated with a better prognosis. If possible, complete resection is recommended. Once the diagnosis is established after resection or biopsy, the possibility of metastatic disease should be evaluated with CT of the lung. When the primary tumor can be completely removed surgically, adjuvant chemotherapy (usually cisplatin, 5-FU, and vincristine) is recommended. If surgical excision is not possible, neoadjuvant chemotherapy is used to shrink the tumor, and second-look surgical resection is recommended as soon as feasible. The disease-free survival rate for all patients except those with initial metastatic disease exceeds 70%. Factors that favorably influence prognosis include complete surgical resection (either initial or delayed) and a rapid decrease in AFP levels in response to chemotherapy.

Hepatocellular carcinoma is the most common primary malignant tumor of the liver among children older than 3 years. The histologic features resemble those of hepatocellular carcinoma among adults. Levels of AFP are elevated among approximately 50% of patients, and approximately 30% of patients have concurrent cirrhosis. This tumor is closely associated with hepatitis virus infection, especially hepatitis B. Surgical resection is the only known curative option. As many as two thirds of tumors are unresectable. Unresectable tumors are poorly responsive to chemotherapy, and no benefit to adjuvant chemotherapy has been found. Hepatic artery chemoembolization is being tried to improve the poor prognosis of this tumor.

Undifferentiated (embryonal) sarcoma is the third most common malignant tumor of the liver. The lesions are pathologically solid, although CT or MRI may suggest a cystic nature. At ultrasound examination, the lesions appear solid. The disease can be cured only if the lesion is surgically resectable. Adjuvant or neoadjuvant chemotherapy with sarcoma-like therapy (vincristine, doxorubicin, dactinomycin, and cyclophosphamide) is indicated.

References

Chang MH, Chen CJ, Lai MS, et al: Universal hepatitis B vaccination in Taiwan and the incidence of hepatocellular carcinoma in children. Taiwan Childhood Hepatoma Study Group. N Engl J Med 336:1855–1860, 1997

Debaun M, Tucker M: Risk of cancer during the first four years of life in children from The Beckwith-Wiedemann Syndrome Registry. J Pediatr 132:398–400, 1998

Van Tornout JM, Buckley JD, Quinn JJ, et al: Timing and magnitude of decline in alpha-fetoprotein levels in treated children with unresectable or metastatic hepatoblastoma are predictors of outcome: a report from the Children's Cancer Group. J Clin Oncol 15:1190–1197, 1997

von Schweinitz D, Hecker H, Harms D, et al: Complete resection before development of drug resistance is essential for survival from advanced hepatoblastoma: a report from the German Cooperative Pediatric Liver Tumor Study HB-89. J Pediatr Surg 30:845–52, 1995

20.15 GERM CELL TUMORS

Markku Heikinheimo and David B. Wilson

Germ cell tumors originate early in life from preinvasive precursors, which transform into overt tumors during infancy, adolescence, or young adulthood. These neoplasms comprise 3% of all tumors diagnosed among children and adolescents, with an annual incidence of approximately 5 per million. Whereas 90% of germ cell tumors diagnosed during adult life are gonadal, two thirds of childhood germ cell tumors are extragonadal. The age distribution for childhood germ cell tumors is bimodal, with a peak at 3 years of age and a second peak during adolescence. One third of germ cell tumors of childhood are malignant. Most neonatal germ cell tumors, irrespective of location, are benign. With advancing age, the proportion of malignant germ cell tumors increases.

ORIGIN OF GERM CELL TUMORS

The teratoid, or monster-like, appearance of germ cell tumors reflects the abnormal development of tissues derived from pluripotent stem cells. According to one widely accepted theory, germ cell tumors arise from activated germ cells situated in the gonad or in ectopic locations. During normal development, primordial germ cells, the precursors of the gametes, migrate from their origin in the yolk sac and combine with the somatic component of the gonad in the urogenital ridge. Growth factors and extracellular matrix components have been shown to affect primitive germ cell survival, proliferation, and directional control during migration. Disruption of normal primordial germ cell migration or imbalance in the hormonal milieu of the developing gonad, in particular abnormalities in sex hormone production, can render early germ cells prone to neoplastic transformation.

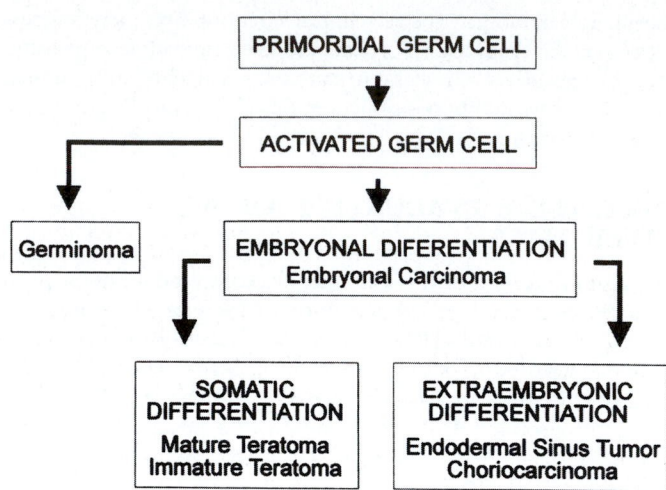

FIGURE 20-8   Schematic shows the histiogenesis of germ cell tumors.

The generally accepted histogenesis of germ cell tumors is depicted in Fig. 20-8. Germ cells may give rise to tumors at any point in their migration path or at any stage of differentiation. The pluripotential cells can differentiate into various embryonic or extraembryonic tissues, which can be either benign or malignant. An admixture of benign and malignant components is common in germ cell tumors, lending support to the notion that different classes of germ cell tumors have a common progenitor. Although there is little doubt that gonadal germ cell tumors are derived from pluripotent descendants of activated germ cells, the origin of extragonadal germ cell tumors is controversial. Cytogenetic studies suggest that such extragonadal tumors may arise from either misplaced pluripotent embryonic tissue or activated germ cells.

CLASSIFICATION

A simplified classification for germ cell tumors is depicted in Table 20-20.

TERATOMA The term *teratoma* is used to describe both benign and malignant tumors composed of haphazardly intermixed tissues that originate from pluripotent stem cells, which are foreign to the anatomic site in which they arise. The traditional belief is that tissue components from all three embryonic germ layers—endoderm, mesoderm, and ectoderm—should be represented in a teratoma. However, tumors both foreign to the site at which they arise and consisting of more that one embryonic layer can be classified as teratoma. At histologic examination teratomas are subclassified into mature teratoma, composed of well-differentiated adult-type tissues, and immature teratoma, which contains embryonic tissues, such as neural rosettes, endochondral ossification foci, or metanephric blastema. Teratoma can occur in combination with one or more of the malignant germ cell tumors, such as germinoma, embryonal carcinoma, endodermal sinus tumor, and choriocarcinoma. The most common locations for teratoma are the sacrococcygeal region and the gonads.

GERMINOMA This malignant neoplasm once was designated *dysgerminoma* when it occurred in the ovary, *seminoma* when it involved the testes, and *germinoma* when it arose at extragonadal sites. Because the histopathologic features are the same regardless

TABLE 20-20

CLASSIFICATION OF GERM CELL TUMORS AMONG CHILDREN

TUMOR	COMMON LOCATION	MARKERS	
		AFP	β-hCG
Teratoma			
Mature	Sacrococcyx, ovary, testes, anterior mediastinum	−	−
Immature	Sacrococcyx, especially with abdominal extension	+/−	−
Germinoma	Ovary, testes, anterior mediastinum, intracranial	−	−
Embryonal carcinoma	Testes	+/−	+/−
Endodermal sinus (yolk sac) tumor	Infantile testes, ovary, sacrococcyx	+++	−
Choriocarcinoma	Ovary, anterior mediastinum, intracranial	−	+++
Gonadoblastoma	Dysgenetic gonads	−	−

AFP = α-fetoprotein; β-hCG = β-human chorionic gonadotropin.

of tumor origin, these older designations have been replaced by the all-encompassing term *germinoma*.

EMBRYONAL CARCINOMA Embryonal carcinoma comprises primitive malignant cells and generally occurs in the pelvic or genital regions.

ENDODERMAL SINUS (YOLK SAC) TUMOR This is the most common malignant form of childhood germ cell tumors. These neoplasms occur most commonly in the pelvis or testes but can occur in other locations.

CHORIOCARCINOMA This malignant tumor, characterized by the presence of syncytiotrophoblast tissue, can be intermixed with other malignant germ cell tumors, such as testicular endodermal sinus tumor. Pure choriocarcinoma among children is rare but may be encountered occasionally in intracranial sites, the mediastinum, or gonads.

GONADOBLASTOMA This tumor occurs almost exclusively in dysgenetic gonads. Most of the affected persons have either a 46XY or 46XY/45XO karyotype, and 80% have the female phenotype. This tumor can occur in association with cryptorchidism. Gonadoblastoma is regarded as cancer in situ and has a low propensity for spread. However, gonadoblastoma frequently occurs in combination with germinoma, which can metastasize.

CLINICAL FEATURES

The most common clinical manifestations of germ cell tumors are signs and symptoms related to the specific location of the tumor and compression of adjacent tissues. Sacrococcygeal teratomas are frequently detected at birth as a mass in the region of the sacrum or buttocks, sometimes accompanied by obstruction of the rectum or urinary tract. These tumors most often are postsacral but occasionally are presacral. Vertebral anomalies can occur among patients with sacrococcygeal teratoma. Testicular germ cell tumors usually manifest as a painless scrotal mass. Patients with ovarian germ cell tumors typically have pain, nausea, vomiting, or other signs of an acute abdomen because of torsion of the ovary caused by the tumor. Mediastinal tumors can produce a combination of symptoms that are manifestations of tracheal compression or secondary infection, such as dyspnea, cough, wheezing, fever, or chest pain. Intracranial germ cell tumors in the midline cause signs of increased intracranial pressure, ataxia, or diabetes insipidus.

TUMOR MARKERS

The embryonic and extraembryonic components of germ cell tumors produce secreted or intracellular antigens useful in diagnosis and surveillance. The two most commonly used germ cell tumor markers in serum are AFP and the β-subunit of human chorionic gonadotropin (β-hCG). Malignant yolk sac endoderm cells within endodermal sinus tumors produce elevated serum levels of AFP, and syncytiotrophoblast tissue in choriocarcinomas produces elevated serum levels of β-hCG (Table 20-20). α-Fetoprotein is developmentally regulated, so age must be taken into consideration when judging serum AFP concentrations. β-Human chorionic gonadotropin can be detected occasionally in the cerebrospinal fluid of patients with intracerebral germinoma. Levels of several other tumor markers, including the carbohydrate antigens CA 125 and CA 19-9, may be elevated in certain germ cell tumors. Serum markers are useful for differentiating gonadal germ cell tumors from sex cord–derived tumors. For example, an elevated serum level of estradiol is associated with granulosa cell tumors, whereas the level of the bioactive peptide inhibin is elevated in the serum of patients with Sertoli cell tumors.

TREATMENT AND FOLLOW-UP CARE

The mainstay of therapy for germ cell tumors, irrespective of histologic features or location, is surgery. For benign or immature teratoma, surgery is the only therapy needed. During resection of sacrococcygeal teratoma, the coccyx is removed to minimize the risk of recurrence. Because 15% of ovarian germ cell tumors are bilateral, examination or biopsy of the contralateral ovary is indicated at surgical resection. Malignant germ cell tumors are prone to apoptosis and are therefore extremely sensitive to both radiation therapy and chemotherapy. Regimens of vinblastine, actinomycin D, cyclophosphamide, bleomycin, cisplatin, and etoposide have been used with excellent success. Late relapses as long as decades after the primary treatment have been reported. Careful long-term follow-up care of patients with germ cell tumor is warranted.

PROGNOSIS

Location and histologic features affect the biological behavior of germ cell tumors. Teratoma at any location typically has an excellent outcome. Immature teratoma has a prognosis comparable with that of mature teratoma, provided the tumor can be totally excised. In the case of sacrococcygeal teratoma, prematurity, perioperative hemorrhage, and other postoperative events result in a 10 to 20% risk of mortality. Endodermal sinus tumors of the infant testis have

TABLE 20-21

SEX CORD–STROMAL TUMORS OF THE OVARY AND TESTES

Leydig cell tumor
Sertoli cell tumor
Sertoli-Leydig cell tumor
Granulosa cell tumor
   Juvenile type
   Adult type
Mixed sex cord–stromal tumor

a better prognosis than do those at later ages and other locations including the ovary. As many as 80% of patients with malignant germ cell tumors can be cured.

Long-term survivors of germ cell tumors may have a variety of sequelae. Functional anorectal and urinary impairment occur among as many as 25% of patients with sacrococcygeal teratoma. Growth hormone deficiency or other pituitary problems may follow treatment of intracranial germinomas with surgery or radiation therapy. Among older male adolescents, testicular dysfunction after chemotherapy is common. However, fertility problems have occurred among patients with a history of teratoma treated with surgery alone, suggesting that an underlying germ cell defect may contribute to infertility.

SEX CORD TUMORS

Although not true germ cell tumors, sex cord tumors deserve mention because they are in the differential diagnosis of gonadal tumors. Sex cord tumors arise from the supportive, often hormonally active cells within the ovary or the testis. These rare tumors can be associated with multiple neoplasia syndromes, including Carney complex and Peutz-Jeghers syndrome (Table 20-21).

ACKNOWLEDGMENTS

The authors thank Pekka Lahdenne, MD, PhD, for his work on germ cell tumors (Developmental and clinical studies on germ cell tumors in childhood, Thesis, University of Helsinki, 1991) and his valuable suggestions during the writing of this chapter.

References

Castleberry RP, Cushing B, Perlman E, Hawkin EP: Germ cell tumors. In: Pizzo PA, Poplack DG: Principles and Practice of Pediatric Oncology, 3rd ed. Philadelphia, Lippincott-Raven, 1997

Lahdenne P, Kuusela P, Siimes MA, Rönnholm KAR, Salmenperä L, Heikinheimo M: Biphasic reduction and concanavalin A binding properties of serum alpha-fetoprotein in preterm and term infants. J Pediatr 118: 272–276, 1991

Mutter GL: Teratoma genetics and stem cells: a review. Obstet Gynecol Surv 42:661–670, 1987

Wylie C: Germ cells. Cell 96:165–174, 1999

20.16 HISTIOCYTOSIS

Frederick Huang and Robert J. Arceci

Histiocytosis is an incompletely understood, heterogeneous group of diseases characterized by abnormal proliferation of cells of the reticuloendothelial or mononuclear phagocytic system. These cells, generically called *histiocytes,* can be divided into two main types— dendritic cells and macrophages. Both are derived from a common hematopoietic stem cell (see Chap. 19), but mature dendritic cells and macrophages have distinct immunohistochemical, ultrastructural, and immunophenotypic differences. Functionally this class of cells serves to phagocytose and kill pathogens, process and present antigens to lymphocytes, assist in wound repair and tissue maintenance, and have important roles in antitumor immunity.

The nomenclature and classification of histiocytosis have a complex history, which began at the turn of the century. The first comprehensive classification system was introduced by the Histiocyte Society in 1987. The current organizational scheme represents a revision of that initial classification system, and more accurately reflects the different types of histiocytes and their biologic features (Table 20-22). The prototypical disorders of dendritic cell and macrophage origin, Langerhans cell histiocytosis (LCH) and hemophagocytic lymphohistiocytosis (HLH), are the focus of this chapter.

LANGERHANS CELL HISTIOCYTOSIS

The inclusive term *Langerhans cell histiocytosis* collectively refers to all of the various manifestations and degrees of severity and involvement of this highly variable disorder.

Epidemiology

Langerhans cell histiocytosis affects approximately 4 per 1 million persons per year. The male to female ratio is nearly 2 to 1. The peak age at onset is 1 year, and there appears to be an inverse relation between degree of involvement and age. Fifty percent of cases of unifocal LCH (previously eosinophilic granuloma of bone) occur among children older than 5 years. In contrast, multifocal LCH (previously Hand-Schüller-Christian disease) most commonly affects children 2 to 5 years of age, whereas systemic LCH

TABLE 20-22

CLASSIFICATION OF HISTIOCYTIC DISORDERS

Disorders of varied biological behavior
  Dendritic cell phenotype
    Langerhans cell histiocytosis
    Juvenile xanthogranuloma
    Solitary histiocytoma with dendritic cell phenotype
    Secondary dendritic cell disorders
  Macrophage phenotype
    Hemophagocytic syndromes
      Primary hemophagocytic lymphohistiocytosis
      Secondary hemophagocytic lymphohistiocytosis
        Infection-associated hemophagocytic syndrome
        Malignancy-associated hemophagocytic syndrome
    Rosai-Dorfman disease (sinus histiocytosis with massive lymphadenopathy)
    Solitary histiocytoma with macrophage phenotype
Malignant disorders
  Leukemia
    Monocyte phenotype
  Sarcoma
    Monocyte phenotype
    Dendritic cell phenotype
    Macrophage phenotype

SOURCE: *Adapted from Favara BE, Feller AC, Pauli M, et al: Contemporary classification of histiocytic disorders. Med Pediatr Oncol 29:157–166, 1997*

(previously Letterer-Siwe disease) usually afflicts children younger than 2 years. The incidence of familial LCH is less than 2%. There is no evident geographic or seasonal distribution of LCH.

Several factors may predispose to the development of LCH, including a family history of benign tumor, parental exposure to solvents, maternal urinary tract infection during pregnancy, feeding difficulties, antibiotic use (most commonly penicillin), and blood product transfusions. Associations between LCH and a patient or family history of thyroid disease, infection, vomiting or diarrhea, antibiotic use, exposure to solvents, and underimmunization have been reported.

There is a growing body of evidence that suggests a genetic basis of or predisposition to LCH. The evidence includes (1) a greater than expected incidence of malignant disease, such as acute lymphoblastic leukemia preceding the onset of LCH, (2) a younger age at onset and shorter time to diagnosis for identical twins with LCH than for other family pairs, (3) the finding of monoclonality of the pathologic Langerhans cell in LCH, and (4) the presence of various cytogenetic abnormalities. Although a clear pattern of alterations has not been identified, the description of a patient with an LCH lesion containing a t(7;12) translocation is intriguing because of the possible involvement of the *tel* gene, which is located on chromosome 12 and has a putative role in the development of myeloid and lymphoid malignant disease (see Sec. 20.6 and Sec. 20.7).

Pathology and Pathogenesis

The lesions of LCH consist primarily of increased numbers of pathologic Langerhans cells accompanied by lymphocytes, macrophages, granulocytes, eosinophils, and multinucleated giant cells. Histologic examination of Langerhans cells reveals indented nuclei with fine chromatin and clear to eosinophilic cytoplasm with a low ratio of nuclear to cytoplasmic content. Normal Langerhans cells have cytoplasmic extensions or dendrites, whereas pathologic Langerhans cells lack this morphologic feature. Langerhans cells stain positively for peanut agglutinin, in a characteristic perinuclear and cell surface pattern, as well as for S-100 protein. They also express the cell surface markers HLA-DR and CD1a. Birbeck granules, racket-shaped cytoplasmic structures the exact function of which is not known but probably relates to antigen processing, can be seen in Langerhans cells with an electron microscope. Langerhans cells lack the attributes more typical of macrophages, including acid phosphatase and nonspecific esterase positivity and CD14 and CD68 cell surface expression. Although any of these features can lend support to a diagnostic consideration of LCH, only demonstration of CD1a by means of immunophenotyping or Birbeck granules at electron microscopic examination can establish a definitive diagnosis.

The monoclonality of the pathologic Langerhans cells in LCH has been conclusively shown. This disease should be considered a monoclonal neoplastic disorder with variable clinical manifestations. Elaboration of cytokines by the abnormally proliferating pathologic Langerhans cells and activated lymphocytes, as well as accumulation and infiltration into organs, causes both localized tissue destruction and systemic symptoms.

Clinical Manifestations

The highly variable clinical presentation of LCH is a hallmark of this disease. The degree of involvement and severity in any given patient can coincide with a broad spectrum of signs and symptoms that ranges from painless involvement of a single bone to consid-

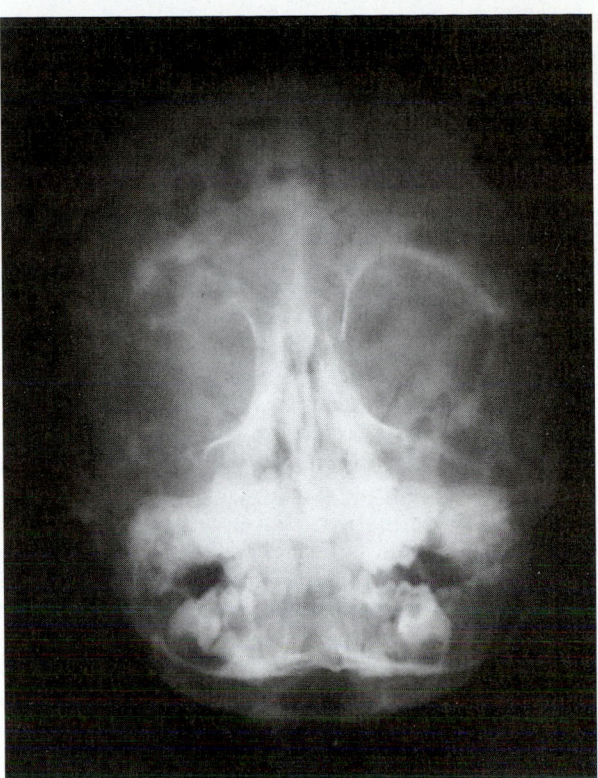

FIGURE 20-9   **Skull radiograph shows the lytic, punched-out defects typical of osseous involvement in Langerhans cell histiocytosis.**

erable morbidity from multiorgan involvement of the brain, lungs, liver, spleen, intestines, lymph nodes, bone marrow, bones, or skin.

Eosinophilic granuloma typically manifests as a solitary lesion of the bone, although multifocal bone disease is not uncommon. The calvarium is most frequently affected, but other common osseous sites include the vertebrae, mandible, ribs, ilia, scapulae, and femurs. The small bones of the hands and feet usually are spared. The lesions often cause pain and swelling of the overlying soft tissues. Because of their lytic nature, lesions usually appear as a punched-out defect on a radiograph, which is the imaging modality of choice in the initial evaluation of osseous disease (Fig. 20-9).

Skull lesions, diabetes insipidus, and exophthalmos comprise the classic triad of Hand-Schüller-Christian disease. However, disease involvement often extends to the other bones as well as the oral cavity, skin, and lymph nodes, and less commonly the brain, lungs, or liver. Infiltration of the posterior pituitary fossa usually manifests clinically as diabetes insipidus with polyuria and polydipsia (see Chaps. 21 and 24). Magnetic resonance imaging commonly reveals the absence of a normal area of high signal intensity in the posterior pituitary gland or thickening of the pituitary stalk. Diabetes insipidus can occur before the diagnosis of LCH is made and during or after therapy. The reported prevalence has been quite variable, ranging from 5 to 50%. Encroachment of the posterior pituitary fossa can perturb other pituitary and hypothalamic functions, leading to growth hormone deficiency and abnormal pubertal development. Mass lesions in the retroorbital spaces can cause exophthalmos.

Erosion of the lamina dura of the tooth, premature eruption of teeth, gingival hemorrhage, and oral mucosal ulceration can cause some of the first manifestations of LCH, especially among infants. Biopsy of oral involvement can be performed with relative ease and allows definitive diagnosis without a major surgical procedure. A seborrheic rash of the scalp, posterior auricular, intertriginous, or groin regions is common. Involvement of the external auditory canals usually results in chronic otitis externa. Chronic otitis media may be part of disease of the mastoid and temporal bone.

Headache, vertigo, seizures, paresis, nystagmus, dysphagia, clonus, ataxia, dysmetria, dysdiadochokinesia, or dysarthria suggests involvement of the brain, although some of these neurologic signs can reflect involvement of the inner ear or mastoid bone instead. Magnetic resonance imaging is the preferred radiologic modality for evaluation of the CNS and may reveal distinct lesions of any parts of the brain or changes related to atrophy or therapy. Although direct involvement of various parts of the brain, including the leptomeninges, by LCH has been extensively documented, the cause of symmetric gliotic changes commonly observed in the cerebellum remains unclear.

Signs and symptoms of pulmonary LCH include cough, hemoptysis, dyspnea, or pain. Involvement may be evident on a chest radiograph or CT scan as a micronodular and reticular pattern. Ruptured pulmonary cysts or bullae can cause pneumothorax. Hepatic involvement can be progressive and terminate in chronic insufficiency and failure with sclerosing cholangitis, cirrhosis, and portal hypertension.

Letterer-Siwe disease is the most extensive and severe manifestation of LCH and can manifest at birth. The prognosis among severely affected infants remains poor, with mortality as high as 40 to 50%. Infants with the worst prognosis frequently have involvement of the lungs, liver, or bone marrow. Patients with systemic disease often have persistent fever, irritability, anorexia, failure to thrive, and a purpuric rash that can erode and cause superinfection. Intestinal involvement can cause diarrhea. Pancytopenia with life-threatening sepsis and hemorrhage is caused by bone marrow infiltration or hypersplenism. Infants with more limited involvement may have spontaneous regression of disease over a period of weeks to months.

Prognosis and Treatment

Overall reduction in morbidity and mortality has occurred even as therapy has become more conservative and been focused on minimization of permanent sequelae. This is largely the result of improved understanding of the disease and accumulated experience with various treatment approaches from recent cooperative trials of chemotherapy for multifocal and systemic LCH.

Observation of an isolated, asymptomatic osseous lesion is appropriate, especially because it can regress spontaneously. Painful lesions that are easily accessible can be managed with curettage at the time of a diagnostic biopsy. Lesions that immediately threaten to compromise function, such as spinal cord compression from extension of a vertebral mass (but not vertebra plana alone), are managed with low-dose radiation therapy. Therapeutic options for a symptomatic recurrent or new lesion include a multiweek course of oral nonsteroidal antiinflammatory drugs, such as ibuprofen or naproxen, or radiographically guided intralesional injection of glucocorticoids.

Solitary cutaneous disease may resolve spontaneously or after use of topical glucocorticoids. Severe or resistant cases may necessitate topical treatment with 20% nitrogen mustard, which carries a carcinogenic risk. Singular involvement of a lymph node or group of lymph nodes can be managed with excisional biopsy with the caveat that extensive surgical intervention be avoided.

A critical principle in therapy for multifocal and systemic LCH has been modulation of treatment intensity according to careful risk stratification. Assignment of risk is based on an inverse correlation between extent of organ dysfunction and prognosis. Patients with no organ dysfunction have a better prognosis than those with one or more involved organs. Patients with a favorable prognosis can achieve an equally complete and durable response with a chemotherapeutic regimen containing fewer agents. For example, LCH-I, the first prospective, randomized trial of chemotherapy for LCH showed that children 2 years of age without pulmonary, hepatosplenic, or hematopoietic involvement had a good outcome. The rate of response to therapy was 90%, and the survival rate was 100%. The converse is not always true. A large number of patients with an unfavorable prognosis do not achieve an adequate response with the addition of conventional drugs or an increase in dose. In LCH-I, this group of patients had a mortality of 47%; the overall mortality was 18%. These patients may be candidates for novel therapeutic strategies, such as use of newer chemotherapeutic agents, cyclosporine, and other immunosuppressive drugs, or stem cell transplantation.

Chemotherapeutic agents that have known activity against LCH include glucocorticoids, vinblastine, etoposide, methotrexate, mercaptopurine, and doxorubicin. Although these drugs can effect, with varying success, a measurable response, efficacy must be considered in the context of possible sequelae, such as secondary malignant disease (etoposide) and cardiac dysfunction (doxorubicin).

The management of new-onset diabetes insipidus is controversial. Although spontaneous resolution can occur, polyuria and polydipsia usually persist in the absence of therapeutic intervention. The results of chemotherapy or radiation therapy are variable and often are transient. Low-dose radiation therapy may be indicated if administered soon after the onset of signs and symptoms. For long-standing diabetes insipidus caused by LCH, symptomatic control with oral or intranasal vasopressin is recommended (see Chap. 24).

HEMOPHAGOCYTIC LYMPHOHISTIOCYTOSIS

The term *hemophagocytic lymphohistiocytosis* encompasses several entities with similar clinical features but distinct pathophysiologic triggers in which the patients often have an inherited or acquired immunodeficiency. Primary HLH, formerly called *familial erythrophagocytic lymphohistiocytosis*, is inherited as an autosomal-recessive disorder; secondary HLH includes all of the other forms, such as infection-associated hemophagocytic syndrome (IAHS) and malignancy-associated hemophagocytic syndrome (Table 20-22).

Epidemiology

Primary HLH has an incidence of approximately 1.2 cases per 1 million persons per year and an equal sex distribution. The age at onset frequently is younger than 1 year, and there is a strong association with consanguinity. Age at onset is later for secondary forms of HLH, such as IAHS. Approximately 20% of cases are diagnosed before the patient is 1 year of age. Infection superimposed on immunodeficiency or immunosuppression is the classic prelude to development of IAHS. Viruses, especially EBV, are most often implicated, but infection with bacteria and other pathogens has been reported.

Pathology and Pathogenesis

Lesions of HLH contain activated macrophages and lymphocytes with hemophagocytosis, which is the pathological signature of this macrophage activation disease. The liver, spleen, lymph nodes, bone marrow, and CNS are commonly involved. In contrast to the pathologic Langerhans cells of LCH, no evidence for the monoclonality of these macrophages or lymphocytes exists.

Natural killer cells and cytolytic T lymphocytes usually are absent or impaired. In addition, characteristic systemic hypercytokinemia involves interleukin-2 (IL-2), IL-6, IL-10, IL-12, interferon-γ, and tumor necrosis factor-α. Although the exact relation between these immunologic findings remains unclear, hypercytokinemia is thought to be caused by a defect in the ability of the immune system to regulate critical pathways of activation and this constitutive hyperactivation, particularly of IL-12, IL-2, and interferon-γ, leads to uncontrolled proliferation of macrophages and lymphocytes in HLH.

Clinical Manifestations

The initial presentation of HLH is fever, hepatosplenomegaly, lymphadenopathy, and a nonspecific rash. Some infants may have signs and symptoms of CNS involvement, especially seizures, as the first manifestation of HLH. These signs and symptoms can be referred to meningeal inflammation, cortical and cerebellar involvement, or increased intracranial pressure. Pallor and purpura from pancytopenia are caused by bone marrow infiltration or splenic sequestration. Pulmonary insufficiency may be present. Constitutional findings, especially anorexia and failure to thrive, are common.

Pancytopenia, hypertriglyceridemia, and hypofibrinogenemia compose the classical triad of laboratory abnormalities. Cerebrospinal fluid findings include increased cell numbers with pleocytosis. Elevated serum transaminase and bilirubin values indicate extensive hepatic involvement. Hyperferritinemia may be part of the acute inflammatory process. All of these laboratory values are useful as indirect indicators of HLH status and usually normalize when remission occurs.

Diagnosis

To make a definitive diagnosis of HLH, all of the following criteria must be present: fever, splenomegaly, peripheral blood cytopenia involving two or more lineages, hypertriglyceridemia or hypofibrinogenemia, and hemophagocytosis without evidence of malignancy in bone marrow, spleen, or lymph nodes. For primary HLH, a family history also is needed.

Strict fulfillment of these criteria can be difficult. For example, a family history of HLH is not always present. Therefore, ready differentiation of primary and secondary forms may not be possible. This difficulty complicates administration of the most appropriate therapy. In certain cases, therapy may have to be initiated on the basis of strong clinical suspicion, even if all of the criteria have not been satisfied, to prevent permanent sequelae and optimize the chance for a good outcome.

Prognosis and Treatment

If the patient is not treated, primary HLH is fatal within a few months and thus represents a medical emergency. Several therapies, including chemotherapeutic and immunomodulatory agents, have been successful in prolonging survival. The first and only curative treatment modality is BMT (see Sec. 20.4). In 1994, the Histiocyte Society consolidated these various approaches into a uniform protocol, HLH-94, for the management of HLH. Initial therapy consists of combination chemotherapy for 8 weeks. For patients with unresponsive CNS disease, intrathecal administration of methotrexate is recommended. Continuation therapy includes additional chemotherapeutic agents. If clinical remission is achieved and a suitable bone marrow donor is available, patients with primary HLH need BMT at the start of continuation therapy. Although bone marrow from an HLA-identical sibling is preferred, stem cell transplantation from an unrelated donor can be successful. Even partial engraftment of the donor bone marrow may be sufficient for durable remission in the treatment of patients with HLH.

For patients with IAHS and other forms of secondary HLH, initial therapy with the HLH-94 protocol approach is appropriate. For patients who attain clinical remission, no further therapy is indicated. Continuation therapy is reserved for patients who have persistent or relapsed disease. Bone marrow transplantation is not recommended for these patients. Minimization of immunosuppression, antimicrobial therapy, and supportive care also can be useful.

References

Arceci RJ, Brenner MK, Pritchard J: Controversies and new approaches to treatment of Langerhans cell histiocytosis. Hematol Oncol Clin North Am 12:339–357, 1998

Arico M, Janka G, Fischer A, et al: Hemophagocytic lymphohistiocytosis: report of 122 children from the international registry—FHL study group of the Histiocyte Society. Leukemia 10:197–203, 1996

Baker KS, Delaat CA, Steinbuch M, et al: Successful correction of hemophagocytic lymphohistiocytosis with related and unrelated bone marrow transplantation. Blood 89:3857–3863, 1997

Egeler RM, Shapiro R, Loechelt B, Filipovich A: Characteristic immune abnormalities in hemophagocytic lymphohistiocytosis. J Pediatr Hematol Oncol 18:340–345, 1996

Osugi Y, Hara J, Tagawa S, et al: Cytokine production regulating Th1 and Th2 cytokines in hemophagocytic lymphohistiocytosis. Blood 89:4100–4103, 1997

William CL, Busque L, Griffith BB, et al: Langerhans'-cell histiocytosis (histiocytosis X): a clonal proliferative disease. N Engl J Med 331:154–160, 1994

KIDNEY AND URINARY TRACT

Norman J. Siegel

21.1 RENAL MORPHOGENESIS

Daniel R. Cherñavvsky and R. Ariel Gómez

Kidney morphogenesis is achieved by the ontogenic recapitulation of three kidneys: the pronephros, the mesonephros, and the metanephros. The first two are transient, although necessary, structures for the formation of the definitive kidney, the metanephros. Until recently most of our knowledge of kidney morphogenesis was limited to beautiful descriptions of anatomic-embryologic development. Advances in molecular biology are providing a better understanding of the complex mechanisms underlying the structural (and functional) development of the kidney.

21.1.1 Nephrogenesis

The kidney derives from intermediate mesoderm. In humans the pronephros is a rudimentary kidney that appears around the third week of gestation, regresses between the fourth and fifth weeks of gestation, and has no known function. The pronephros appears in the cervical region at a level located between the second and sixth somites and consists of five to seven nephric vesicles, each connected to a tubule that drains into a pronephric duct that eventually becomes the mesonephric duct and gives rise to the ureteric bud, which is essential for metanephric development. If the pronephros fails to develop, renal agenesis will ensue, sometimes accompanied by ipsilateral adrenal and lung agenesis. The mesonephros is the second transient kidney in humans and other higher vertebrates and appears between the third and fourth weeks of gestation. Mesonephric nephrons develop structures similar to filtering glomeruli constituting the first renal functional unit in the human embryo. From the fifth to the 12th week of gestation, approximately 40 mesonephric nephrons drain into the mesonephric duct (also called wolffian duct). The mesonephros degenerates in a cephalocaudal direction while the mesonephric duct gives rise to portions of the epididymis and the ductus deferens, and the mesonephric tubules form the efferent ductules in the area of the gonad in boys. In girls, part of the mesonephric duct regresses, but vestigial structures such as the epoophoron, oophoron, and Gartner duct remain. In girls, a normal mesonephric duct is necessary for the development of the müllerian ducts, and inadequate mesonephric development results in ipsilateral ureteral-renal agenesis, agenesis of the fallopian tube, and contralateral uterus unicornis and vaginal atresia.

The metanephros, the definitive kidney of mammals, appears around the fifth week of gestation. Development of the metanephros is initiated by the coinductive interaction between the ureteric bud, a branch of the caudal mesonephric (wolffian) duct, and the mesenchymal cells of the nephrogenic blastema. In the human embryo, the ureteric bud extends dorsally into the most caudal portion of the nephrogenic cord and accompanies the nephrogenic blastema in a cranial direction. The ascendent movement of the metanephric blastema from a pelvic position to its final lumbar localization is completed between the eighth and ninth week of gestation. In addition to upward migration, the metanephros undergoes a 90° rotation, allowing the renal hilum to reach a final medial position. The factors that control the ascendent migration and rotation of the metanephros are still unknown. The ureteric bud is responsible for the formation of the kidney and urinary collecting system, and the migration and division pattern determine the elaborate three-dimensional branching of the human kidney. The specific induction of the nephrogenic blastema by the ampullary portion of the ureteric bud results in the formation of nephrons, a process known as nephrogenesis.

Nephrogenesis (Fig. 21-1) is a complex process that includes the differentiation and directional growth of different cell types, resulting in the formation of nephrons. The ureteric bud induces the mesenchyme to differentiate into tubular and glomerular epithelium. In turn, the induced mesenchyme induces the ureter to grow and branch into renal mesenchyme. Around the tip of each ureteric branch, the mesenchymal cells group tightly together, a process called condensation (Fig. 21-1B). After condensation, each group of about 100 cells forms a vesicle that evolves into a comma- and then an S-shaped glomerulus (Fig. 21-1 C,D). As a result of the nephrogenic process, the metanephric mesenchyme differentiates into glomeruli, proximal tubules, loops of Henle, and interstitial fibroblasts, whereas the ureteric bud and its branches give origin to the epithelia of the collecting duct. In the human embryo glomerulogenesis is completed by week 35 of gestation. Postnatally no new nephrons form. Nevertheless, each tubule continues to mature for several months, as evidenced by elongation of the loop of Henle in the direction of the medulla and increased convolutions of the proximal tubule.

MOLECULAR REGULATION OF NEPHROGENESIS

The spatial assembly and differentiation of different cell types during nephrogenesis are governed by complex interactive signals between the differentiating cells and their milieu.

GDNF–c-RET AND GDNFR-α-RECEPTOR CASCADE Glial-derived neurotrophic factor/GDNF-α/RET signaling complex generates the major signal for outgrowth of the ureteric bud into the metanephric mesenchyme. GDNF expression in the metanephric mesenchyme spatially restricts the origin of the ureteric bud to the mesonephric duct and is also responsible for ongoing branching of the ureteric bud within the metanephric mesenchyme. In animals with targeted deletion of the GDNF, mesonephric tubules develop, and the wolffian duct forms normally, but the ureteric bud is absent. Because of the lack of ureteric induction, eventually the meta-

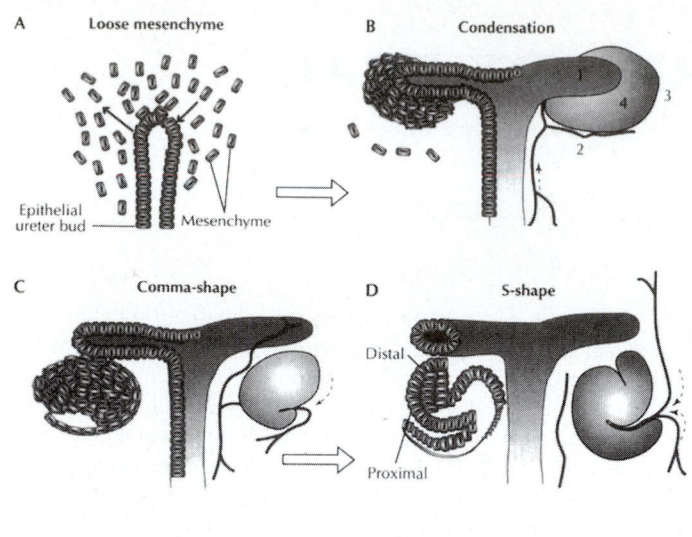

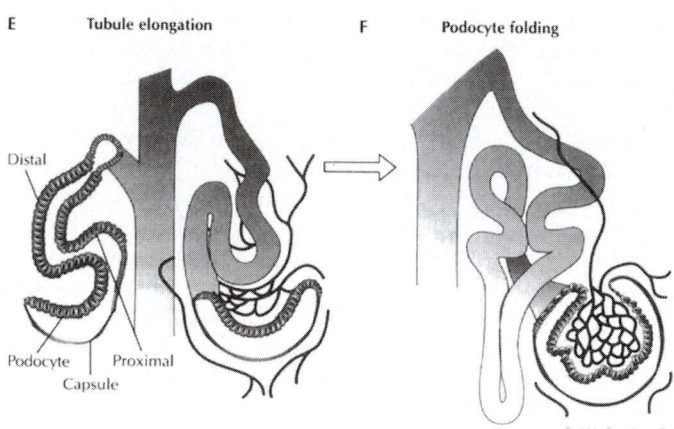

FIGURE 21-1 Schematic representation of nephrogenesis. A: The branching ureteric epithelium interaction with loose metanephric mesenchyme results in condensation of the mesenchyme in B. Cell lineages shown include (1) ureteric epithelium, (2) vasculature, (3) undifferentiated mesenchyme, and (4) condensed mesenchyme differentiating into epithelia. C and D: These stages are followed by infolding of the primitive glomerular epithelium to form comma- and S-shaped bodies. E: Elongation of the proximal and distal tubular elements subsequently occurs along with further infolding of the glomerular epithelium and vascular structures to form the mature glomerular capillary network seen in F. The initial phases of glomerular vascularization are believed to occur during the early stages of glomerular differentiation in C and D. SOURCE: *Ekbolm P: Basement membrane proteins and growth factors in kidney differentiation. In: Trelstad RL, ed: Role of Extracellular Matrix in Development. New York, Alan R. Liss, 1984:173–206.*

nephric blastema undergoes apoptosis, resulting in defective kidney development or agenesis.

PAX-2 The *Pax* gene family of transcription factors shares a DNA-binding domain named the paired box. In both mice and humans, several *Pax* genes have been shown to have relevant functions during kidney development. Two members of this family, *Pax-2* and *Pax-8,* are expressed in an overlapping fashion within the developing kidney. *Pax-2* is expressed in the mesonephric duct, the ureteric bud, and the metanephric mesenchyme. *Pax-8* distribution is similar to *Pax-2* and is expressed at a slightly later stage in the renal vesicles and in the S-shaped body.

Pax-2 mutations in humans result in kidney hypoplasia. This gene has a semidominant character: even heterozygous mutations could show phenotypic alterations, a characteristic known as haploinsufficiency. A mutation in the *Pax-2* gene leads to a human autosomal dominant syndrome of renal dysplasia, vesicoureteral reflux, and colobomas.

WT-1 The Wilms tumor suppressor gene (*WT-1*) is a transcription factor with zinc-finger binding domain involved in the mesenchymal signals that stimulate ureteric budding from the mesonephric duct. This gene is first expressed in condensing mesenchymal cells, next to the inducing bud cells, but not in the ureteric bud, and continues to be expressed through the S-shaped body stage. *WT-1* acts as a negative regulator of several growth factors, including IGF-II and PDGFA. *WT-1* is up-regulated at the beginning of condensation and prevents excessive proliferation of mesenchymal cells. Thus, in the absence of *WT-1,* blastemal growth could progress unchecked. In humans, mutations of the WT-1 gene have been associated with Wilms tumor, Denys-Drash syndrome, and Frasier syndrome (see Secs. 20.12 and 21.9).

***WNT* GENE FAMILY** Wnt proteins induce the transformation of metanephric mesenchyme into epithelium. *Wnt-11* expression is found in the developing wolffian duct as it elongates, but becomes restricted to a small region in the duct exactly at a position adjacent to the metanephric blastema. When the ureteric bud emerges, *Wnt-11* expression is found in the tip but not the stalk, and the gene is always expressed at the ends of the growing ureteric tips. *Wnt-4* is required for epithelial transformation of the induced metanephros.

EMX2* AND *BF2 The homebox gene *Emx2* is required for branching morphogenesis. In *Emx2* mutant mice, the ureteric bud elongates and contacts the mesenchyme but fails to branch. *BF2* is initially expressed in mesenchymal cells adjacent to cells that express *Pax-2.* *BF2*-expressing cells are destined to be stromal cells, and *Pax-2*-expressing cells are destined to the epithelial-nephrogenic lineage. In *BF2* mutant mice, stromal/interstitial cells persist throughout cortical and medullary morphogenesis. In these mice branching morphogenesis is greatly reduced.

INTEGRINS AND ADHESION MOLECULES Integrins are heterodimeric polypeptides composed of single α and β chains and are the major family of receptors for the extracellular matrix. $\alpha3\beta1$ and $\alpha8\beta1$ are relevant to kidney development. When $\alpha8\beta1$ integrin is absent, the ureteric bud is formed, but growth toward the metanephric mesenchyme and branching morphogenesis are inhibited. $\alpha3\beta1$-Integrin expression is found in the ureteric bud, collecting ducts, and glomerular endothelial and glomerular visceral epithelial cells.

The findings in mice carrying targeted deletion of the $\alpha3\beta1$ integrin suggest a role in glomerular visceral epithelial cell development, glomerular basement membrane organization, and branching morphogenesis.

Cell adhesion molecules (CAMs) are glycoproteins that are involved in cell-cell adhesion, and some of them, such as L-CAM (liver CAM) and N-CAM (neural CAM), are expressed in the kidney. Interactions between CAMs and extracellular matrix (ECM) glycoproteins are key events that are mediated by the integrins and appear to have a segment-specific distribution during different stages of embryonic nephrogenesis. Other molecules potentially important in kidney development include laminins, proteoglycans, and ECM-degrading enzymes.

GROWTH FACTORS Growth factors or cytokines are morphogens produced in the embryonic kidney that modulate cell survival, proliferation, differentiation, and morphogenesis. The list of potential signaling molecules, including many secreted factors and their receptors, which are either expressed in embryonic kidney or can affect its development in vitro, continues to evolve.

When insulin-like growth factor 1 (IGF-1) is blocked, marked atrophy of metanephroi occurred. Exposure to IGF-1 induced a trophic response in vitro, and in vivo studies have demonstrated that IGF-1 could reverse the kidney abnormalities induced by blocking the renin-angiotensin system. Epidermal growth factor (EGF) is a peptide produced mainly by salivary glands and kidneys. EGF binds to a putative tyrosine kinase receptor, which also binds transforming growth factor α (TGF-α). TGF-α may be an embryonic form of EGF. Expression of EGF is high in postnatal life, and expression of the TGF-α is higher in embryonic life. Inclusion of EGF in the metanephric culture model results in hypertrophy of the fetal kidney and cyst formation, but the formation of the glomeruli is inhibited. Exposure to TGF-α antibodies results in aberrant ureteric branching and poor metanephric growth.

Transforming growth factor β (TGF-β) is a superfamily that includes a large number of bifunctional regulatory proteins, such as TGF-$\beta_{1\text{-}5}$, bone morphogenetic proteins (BMPs), GDNF, and other growth activators and inhibitors. Addition of TGF-β to the metanephric culture medium inhibits metanephric growth and glomerular differentiation and arrests development of the proximal tubules and collecting ducts. BMP7-null mutant mice show either hypogenesis or agenesis of the kidneys, eye, and skeletal system. Epidermal growth factor, hepatocyte growth factor, fibroblast growth factors, and transforming growth factor and their receptors participate in branching morphogenesis and tubulogenesis.

APOPTOSIS

Programmed cell death (apoptosis) is an important mechanism for appropriate kidney morphogenesis. Most mesenchymal cells are destined to die by apoptosis unless epithelial transformation occurs.

Several growth factors including EGF and bFGF are able to protect blastemal cells from apoptosis. Several oncogenes regulate growth by modulating apoptosis (see Sec. 20.2). For example, WT-1 binds p53, inhibiting p53-induced apoptosis. WT-1–deficient mice have mesenchymal apoptosis. Gain-of-function mutations on the p53 gene result in oligonephronia and apoptosis. The additional protooncogene bcl-2 is expressed in condensing mesenchyme and ureteric bud and is down-regulated in differentiated epithelial cells. Bcl-2–deficient mice have hypoplastic cystic kidneys and massive apoptosis.

21.1.2   Vascular Kidney Development

Development of the kidney vasculature occurs simultaneously with nephrogenesis. Although traditionally the renal vessels have been assumed to originate from branching of preexisting extrarenal vessels by a process called angiogenesis, recent studies showed that renal vessels can originate from within the kidney by a process called vasculogenesis (Fig. 21-2).

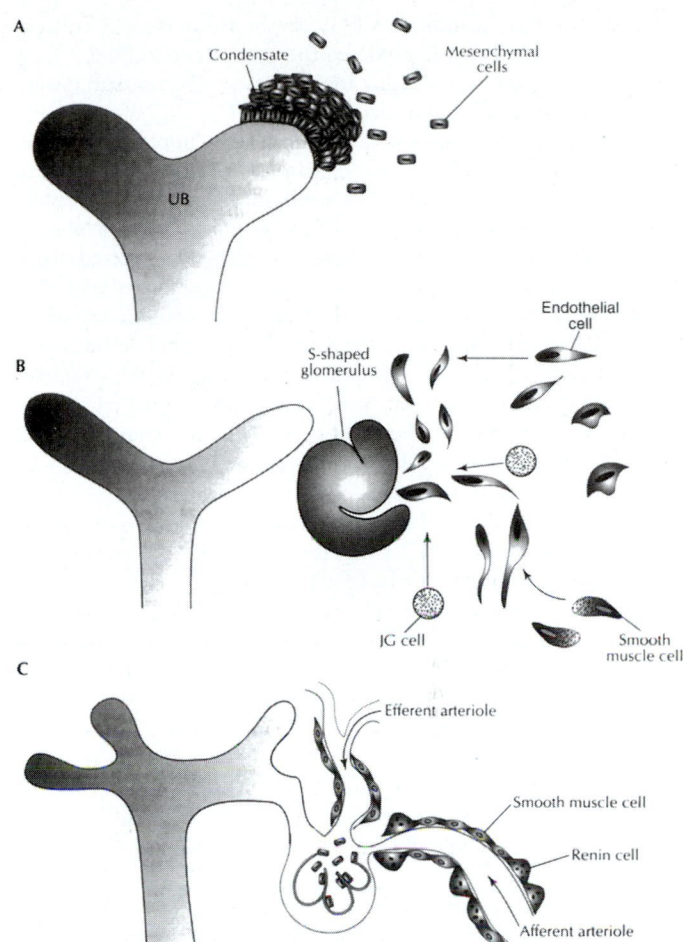

FIGURE 21-2 Major steps in vascularization of the nephron. **A:** The ureteric bud (UB) has induced the mesenchyme, which condenses around the ureteric tip and eventually differentiates into epithelial segments of the nephron. Mesenchymal cells around the condensate are not easily distinguishable from one another. However, many of these cells are precursors for endothelial, smooth muscle/mesangial, or renin-producing cells. **B:** The condensate has evolved through the stages of vesicle and comma-shaped glomerulus (not shown) to the S-shaped glomerulus shown here. The lower cleft of the glomerulus is being penetrated by endothelial cell precursors, which align to form the endothelial lining of the arteriole and also attract (or induce to differentiate into) smooth muscle, mesangial, and juxtaglomerular (JG) cell precursors. These precursors form the coating of the arterioles and the mesangial cells of the glomerulus. **C:** The glomerulus has acquired its arterioles containing smooth muscle and renin-synthesizing cells. Early in gestation, renin-containing cells are abundant along the arterioles. Glomerular capillary loops have also formed, and mesangial cells have already penetrated the glomerulus. JG, juxtaglomerular; UB, ureteric bud. SOURCE: *Gómez RA, Norwood VF: Recent advances in renal development. Curr Opin Pediatr 11:135– 140, 1999. Reprinted with permission.*

REGULATION OF VASCULAR DEVELOPMENT

Vascular endothelial growth factor (VEGF) and its receptors (Flk-1, Flt-1) have been shown to play a crucial role in kidney vascularization by promoting endothelial cell differentiation, capillary formation, and maintenance of the fenestrated endothelium phenotype. Interestingly, the growth of kidney vessels seems to depend on the regulation of VEGF by the tissue oxygen concentration. In the relative hypoxia of the embryonic kidney, VEGF synthesis is increased, inducing angioblasts to differentiate, proliferate, and assemble into endothelial tubes.

Ephrins are glycosylphosphatidylinositol-anchored proteins located either on the cell surfaces (ephrin A) or across the cell membrane (ephrin B). These membrane-bound ligands bind receptors of the tyrosine kinase family called Eph (erythropoietin-producing hepatocellular receptor), which have an extremely restricted distribution and specificity. Ephrins may mediate targeting of endothelial cells after they have acquired their differentiated phenotype.

Another system involved in vascular development is the angiopoietin system, composed of angiopoietin-1 (Ang-1), which signals through a tyrosine kinase receptor (Tie-2/Tek) expressed only on endothelial cells and early hematopoietic cells, and angiopoietin-2 (Ang-2), which also binds Tie-2, antagonizing Ang-1. Ang-2 may be synergistic with VEGF, collaborating with the invading vascular sprouts by blocking a stabilizing or maturing function of Ang-1, whereas in the absence of VEGF, the inhibition of a constitutive Ang-1 signal can contribute to vessel regression.

The Ets family of transcription factors regulates a cascade of genes involved in hematopoiesis (*CSF-1, CDD18*), renin transcription, endothelial cell differentiation (*VEGF, Flk-1, Flt-1*), and protease activity (*MMP-1, u-PA*). Severe abnormalities in the glomerular capillaries have been described in mice with targeted null mutations of the *Ets-1* gene.

Platelet-derived growth factor (PDGFβ) is probably involved in mesangial cell differentiation because mice carrying a null mutation of either *PDGFβ* or *PDGFRβ* fail to develop mesangial cells and glomerular capillary tufts.

Although significant advances have been made in our understanding of glomerular capillary morphogenesis, the formation of the renal arterioles is not as clear, and the mechanisms involved in arteriolar assembly are unknown. Numerous studies have shown a temporal and spatial relationship between renin-containing cells and branching of renal arterioles, and the renin-angiotensin system participates in the branching of the renal arterioles. Treatment of rats with inhibitors of the renin-angiotensin system leads to arrested branching of the renal arterioles, which are shorter and thicker with concentric accumulation of smooth muscle cells, suggesting that lack of angiotensin leads to immature development of smooth muscle cells, which proliferate excessively in a concentric arrangement as if the immature cells have lost their proper orientation. Similar vascular abnormalities have been observed when angiotensin-converting enzyme, angiotensin receptors, and the angiotensinogen genes are deleted by gene targeting. Interestingly, the aberrant vessel development is accompanied by a variety of histologic abnormalities including delayed glomerular development, cyst formation, and generalized architectural disarrangement. The alterations resemble those found in infants whose mothers were treated prenatally with angiotensin-converting enzyme inhibitors.

References

Baker L, Gómez RA: Embryonic development of the ureter. Semin Nephrol 18:569–584, 1998

Gómez RA: Role of angiotensin in renal vascular development. Kidney Int 54(Suppl 67):S-12–S-16, 1998

Gómez RA, Norwood VF: Recent advances in renal development. Curr Opin Pediatr 11:135–140, 1999

Lipschutz J: Molecular development of the kidney: a review of the results of gene disruption studies. Am J Kidney Dis 31:383–397, 1998

21.2 DEVELOPMENT OF RENAL FUNCTION

Michel Baum

One of the major functions of the kidney is to protect against changes in the extracellular milieu. The adult kidney maintains a precise balance matching fluid and electrolyte excretion to intake. However, the growing child must be in positive balance for a number of solutes to promote growth, and the challenge to the kidney during development is even greater. Although the full complement of nephrons is present at 34 weeks of gestation, functional renal development is far from complete at birth. Postnatal changes occur in renal blood flow, glomerular filtration, and tubular function.

21.2.1 Developmental Changes in Renal Blood Flow and Glomerular Filtration

The mature kidney receives 20% of the cardiac output, whereas the fetal kidney receives only 2% of the cardiac output from midgestation to term. Even when corrected for body surface area, neonates have only 15 to 20% of the adult renal blood flow. The postnatal increase in renal blood flow results in part from an increase in cardiac output, but predominantly from a decrease in renal vascular resistance as a result of intrinsic changes in the renal vasculature. The response of the renal vascular bed to vasoconstricting and vasodilating substances also changes with maturation but plays a minor role in the maturational decrease in renal vascular resistance.

Renal vascular resistance and perfusion pressure determine renal blood flow (RBF). The RBF is maintained constant over a wide range of blood pressures in both adults and neonates, which serves to preserve renal function during hypotension. The maintenance of RBF and glomerular filtration rate (GFR) at a constant level despite a decrease in blood pressure is termed autoregulation and is mediated by a decrease in renal vascular resistance when blood pressure falls. Because neonates and children have lower blood pressures than adults, the range of blood pressure over which autoregulation is maintained is lower in neonates and increases with age. There is autoregulation of the GFR in adults, whereas neonates have a significant fall in GFR with hypotension. Angiotensin II is thought to mediate much of the efferent arteriolar vasoconstriction, which preserves the GFR in adults during hypotension. The secretion of angiotensin II and its effect on efferent arteriolar resistance are less in neonates than in adults, which accounts for the developmental difference in autoregulation.

Glomerular filtration commences in the metanephric kidney at about 9 to 12 weeks of gestation. The GFR is lower in neonates than in adults even when corrected for body surface area. A premature neonate with a postconceptional age (the sum of gestational and postnatal age) between 28 and 34 weeks has a creatinine clearance of only 0.5 mL/min, which increases to 1 mL/min by 37 weeks postconception and to 2 mL/min in full-term neonates. Corrected for an average adult body surface area of 1.73 m², this would be only 30 mL/min/1.73 m². The GFR increases significantly in the first months of life and reaches a value comparable to

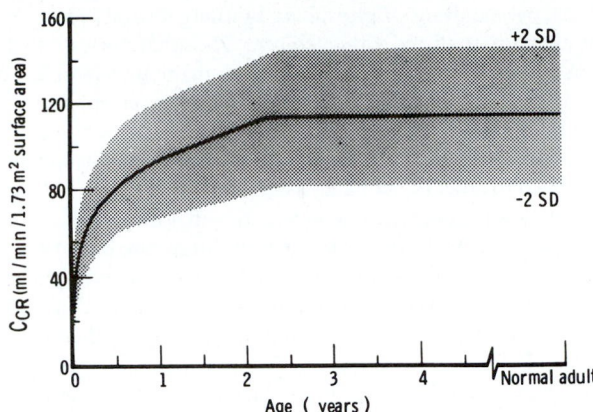

FIGURE 21-3 **Maturational changes in creatinine clearance (in mL/min/1.73 m² body surface area). The *solid line* is the mean, and the *stippled area* includes two standard deviations.**

adult (100–120 mL/min per 1.73 m²) at 1 to 2 years of age (Fig. 21-3).

A number of factors contribute to the maturational increase in GFR. Glomerular filtration is driven by the difference between the hydraulic and oncotic pressures across the glomerular capillary bed. Net filtration pressure changes along the length of the glomerular capillary. At the arteriolar end the net hydraulic pressure (the difference between the arteriolar pressure and that in Bowman's space) is far greater than the glomerular capillary oncotic pressure, resulting in a positive pressure of about 15 mm Hg favoring glomerular filtration. As protein-free filtrate is produced, the oncotic pressure of plasma rises as the protein concentration in the glomerular capillary increases, and a small decrease in the glomerular hydraulic pressure occurs as blood transverses along the capillary. The point where the pressures favoring and opposing filtration are equal and glomerular filtration ceases is termed filtration pressure equilibrium. The GFR is determined by the product of the net ultrafiltration pressure along the glomerular capillary and K_f, the ultrafiltration coefficient of the glomerular capillary. K_f is the product of the glomerular capillary surface area and the hydraulic water permeability of the glomerular capillary.

Homeostatic mechanisms that protect against changes in GFR include primary myogenic regulation of the afferent arteriolar resistance, where an increase in systemic blood pressure results in vasoconstriction of the afferent arteriole. Changes in GFR are also influenced by tubuloglomerular feedback. The macula densa of the thick ascending limb is in juxtaposition with the afferent and efferent arterioles and the glomerulus of the same nephron. An increase or decrease in glomerular filtration results in a concomitant change in sodium delivery to the macula densa, which results in a reciprocal change in GFR. The homeostatic control that maintains GFR at a constant level is in part mediated by angiotensin II.

During postnatal maturation, an increase in ultrafiltration pressure and renal blood flow contribute to the postnatal increase in GFR. However, the most important factor responsible for the maturational increase in GFR is the postnatal change in the ultrafiltration coefficient. Although the hydraulic water permeability or "porosity" of the glomerular capillary does not change significantly after birth, the glomerular capillary surface area increases markedly, and this increase in glomerular capillary surface area is the predominant factor accounting for the postnatal increase in GFR.

At birth, neonates have a serum creatinine equivalent to that of their mother as a result of the placental transfer of creatinine. Thus,

serum creatinine (S_{Cr}) does not reflect neonatal renal function. Approximately 48 to 72 hours after birth, the S_{Cr} reflects both muscle mass, which produces creatinine, and GFR. Because the muscle mass of a neonate is relatively small, S_{Cr} should decrease to 0.3 to 0.5 mg/dL. The rate which serum creatinine falls in the perinatal period is determined by the GFR, which is dependent on the gestational age of the neonate. Accurate assessment of renal function in neonates is quite difficult. Neonates usually have a urine output of 1 mL/kg/h. However, urine volume is dependent on a number of factors besides the glomerular filtration rate (see Sec. 21.7), and a decrease in urine output does not necessarily correlate with a reduction in GFR. Sequential measurements of S_{Cr} is often the best way to assess changes in neonatal renal function.

21.2.2   Maturation of Tubular Function

PROXIMAL TUBULE

The glomerular ultrafiltrate is delivered to the proximal tubule, where two-thirds of the fluid is reabsorbed. The proximal tubule reabsorbs all of the filtered glucose and amino acids and 80% of the filtered bicarbonate and phosphate. Most solute entry across the apical membrane is sodium dependent (Fig. 21-4). The low intracellular sodium generated by the basolateral Na⁺,K⁺-ATPase provides a driving force for sodium-dependent transport across the apical membrane of the proximal tubule and along the nephron. Inhibition of Na⁺,K⁺-ATPase with ouabain results in total inhibition of transport in both adult and neonatal proximal tubules. The maturational changes in Na⁺,K⁺-ATPase activity in several nephron segments are shown in Fig. 21-5. The postnatal changes in solute transport in each nephron segment, by and large, parallel the maturational changes in Na⁺,K⁺-ATPase activity. The rate of neonatal

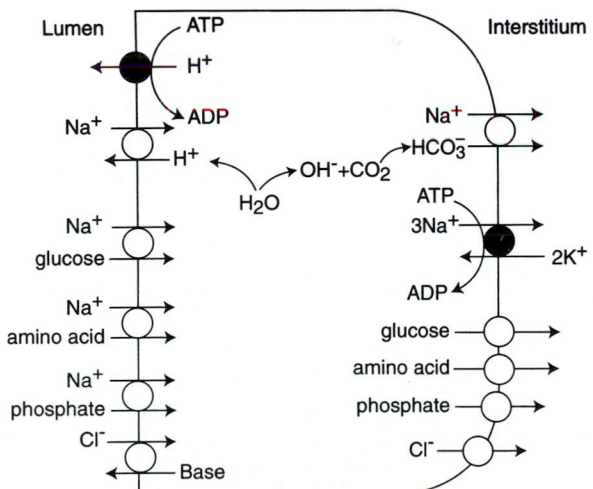

Proximal Tubule Cell

FIGURE 21-4 **Proximal tubule cell showing the transporters on the apical and basolateral membrane. Solute entry across the apical membrane is sodium dependent for most solutes. The low intracellular sodium concentration in the cell is generated by the basolateral membrane Na,K ATPase activity, which provides a driving force for sodium-dependent solute transport. Basolateral membrane solute exit is by and large via facilitated diffusion through sodium-independent transporters.**

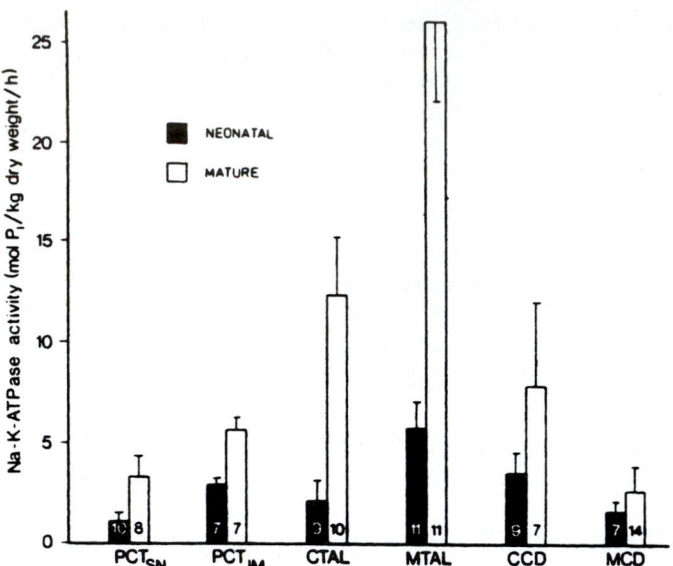

FIGURE 21-5   Na,K ATPase activity in neonatal and adult rabbit nephron segments. Abbreviations: PCT_{SN} = **superficial proximal convoluted tubule;** PCT_{JM} = **juxtamedullary proximal convoluted tubule;** CTAL = **cortical thick ascending limb;** MTAL = **medullary thick ascending limb;** CCD = **cortical collecting tubule;** MCD = **medullary collecting tubule. SOURCE:** *Schmidt U, Horster M: Na-K–activated ATPase: activity maturation in rabbit nephron segments dissected in vitro. Am J Physiol 233:F55–F60, 1977.*

proximal tubule volume and sodium reabsorption is approximately one-third that of the mature proximal tubule.

The postnatal increase in GFR is paralleled by the postnatal increase in proximal tubular transport in term neonates, so that the fraction of glomerular filtrate reabsorbed by the proximal tubule remains constant. This concordant maturational change in glomerular filtration and proximal tubular reabsorption is termed glomerulotubular balance. In premature neonates the filtered load of many solutes delivered to the kidney exceeds the tubular reabsorptive capacity.

Glucose and amino acids are reabsorbed by the proximal tubule via a Na-glucose and a number of different Na–amino acid cotransporters on the apical membrane (Fig. 21-4). Both glucose and amino acids exit across the basolateral membrane of the cell by facilitated diffusion. The rates of Na-glucose and Na–amino acid cotransport as well as the basolateral Na^+,K^+-ATPase are all less in neonatal than in mature proximal tubules.

The plasma concentration at which a solute such as glucose appears in the urine is termed the renal threshold for that solute. Below the threshold, all of the filtered solute is reabsorbed. If the plasma concentration exceeds the threshold, then the filtered load delivered exceeds the reabsorptive capacity of the tubules, and the solute is excreted in the urine. In adults glucosuria is not detected in the urine unless the serum glucose concentration is above 200 mg/dL. In neonates born before 30 weeks of gestation, glucosuria is frequently observed in the absence of hyperglycemia. Before 34 weeks of gestation, only 93% of the filtered glucose is reabsorbed by the immature kidney, but by 34 weeks of gestation over 99% of the glucose is reabsorbed, and glucosuria is not detected unless the infant has hyperglycemia. A similar maturational pattern is present for amino acids.

The renal handling of phosphate by the neonatal kidney is different than that of any other solute. Phosphate is essential for growth and development. Whereas adults maintain a neutral phosphate balance by excreting the same amount of phosphate as they absorb by the gastrointestinal tract, neonates and growing children are in positive phosphate balance. Only 60% of the phosphate absorbed from the diet in neonates is excreted in the urine. The serum phosphate level is higher in neonates than in adults, which is not a manifestation of the lower glomerular filtration rate but of a higher proximal tubular reabsorptive capacity of phosphate when factored for GFR. Phosphate is the only solute that is transported at a higher rate by the neonatal kidney than the mature kidney when factored for the GFR.

Neonates and adults respond to dietary phosphate deprivation and hypophosphatemia with an increase in the number of apical membrane Na-phosphate transporters. A high-phosphate diet causes a decrease in renal phosphate reabsorption in adults. In spite of a high-phosphate diet, neonates maintain high rates of phosphate transport, and hyperphosphatemia ensues. In addition, the phosphaturia induced by parathyroid hormone in adults is markedly attenuated in neonates. These factors are, in part, responsible for the observation that neonates may develop hyperphospatemia with reciprocal hypocalcemia when fed whole cow's milk or other formulas that are high in phosphate.

Approximately half of the filtered sodium chloride is reabsorbed by the proximal tubule. The preferential reabsorption of organic solutes and bicarbonate over chloride ions in the early proximal tubule leaves the luminal fluid with a higher chloride concentration and lower bicarbonate concentration than that in the peritubular plasma. This high lumen to peritubular chloride concentration gradient provides a driving force for passive paracellular chloride diffusion. Approximately half of the proximal tubule NaCl transport is via passive diffusion, and half is active transport. Transcellular NaCl transport is mediated by the parallel operation of the apical membrane Na^+/H^+ exchanger and a Cl^-/base exchanger (see Fig. 21-4). A significant fraction of Cl^-/base exchange is via a Cl^-/OH^- exchanger. The parallel operation of Na^+/H^+ and Cl^-/OH^- exchangers will result in the net movement of NaCl into the cell, and water will be secreted. Other Cl^-/base exchangers likely participate in active proximal tubule NaCl transport. The rates of both Na^+/H^+ and Cl^-/base exchangers are far less in the neonatal proximal tubule than in the mature segment. The rate of passive NaCl transport is also lower in the neonatal proximal tubule than that in the mature tubule. Unlike the adult proximal tubule, which has a high paracellular chloride permeability, the neonatal proximal tubule is impermeable to chloride ions. Maturational changes in both the paracellular pathway and active transport affect proximal tubule reabsorption.

As solutes are reabsorbed by the proximal tubule, concomitant reabsorption of water occurs so that the osmolality of the tubular fluid remains nearly the same as that of blood. Almost all adult tubular water flow is transcellular through water channels (aquaporin-1) on the apical and basolateral membrane. Although there are few aquaporin-1 channels on both apical and basolateral membranes, water permeability is higher in the neonatal tubule. In the neonate a significant amount of water is reabsorbed through the lipid bilayer, which has a greater fluidity than that in the mature tubule, and the resistance to water flow through the cytoplasm is less in immature tubules.

Glucocorticoids and thyroid hormone may play an important role in postnatal maturational changes in glomerular filtration rate and tubular transport. In the perinatal period, serum glucocorticoid and thyroid hormone levels increase and coincide with the maturational changes in transporter activity. Some of the transporters, which change in activity with maturation, have either glucocorticoid or thyroid response elements in their promoter regions, which affect the rate of gene transcription when these hormones are present. Administration of either glucocorticoids or thyroid hormone results in an acceleration of the maturation of several tubule transport processes.

THICK ASCENDING LIMB AND DISTAL CONVOLUTED TUBULE

The thick ascending limb reabsorbs approximately one-third of the filtered NaCl in both adult and neonate. The thick ascending limb is impermeable to water so that the fluid leaving this segment has an osmolality of 50 mOsm/kg water. An electroneutral $Na^+/K^+/2Cl^-$ cotransporter mediates sodium chloride transport across the apical membrane of the thick ascending limb (Fig. 21-6). The potassium that is reabsorbed diffuses back across the apical membrane via a potassium channel, which results in a lumen-positive transepithelial potential difference that provides the driving force for the reabsorption of calcium and magnesium across the paracellular pathway. The $Na^+/K^+/2Cl^-$ cotransporter is the transporter that is inhibited by loop diuretics such as furosemide. Furosemide not only inhibits NaCl transport but also decreases the lumen-positive potential, impairing the paracellular reabsorption of magnesium and calcium. Chronic administration of loop diuretics in neonates results in hypercalciuria, which can cause nephrocalcinosis and renal injury. The rate of NaCl transport by the neonatal thick ascending limb is less than that of the mature segment and is, at least in part, related to the lower basolateral Na^+,K^+-ATPase activity in the immature nephron (see Fig. 21-5).

The distal convoluted tubule reabsorbs about 5% of the filtered NaCl. A NaCl cotransporter on the apical membrane mediates transport in this nephron segment. The distal convoluted tubule also reabsorbs a significant amount of calcium. Thiazide diuretics inhibit NaCl transport in this segment but stimulate calcium reabsorption. For this reason, thiazide diuretics are frequently used to lower urinary calcium excretion in patients predisposed to forming calcium-containing renal stones. The relative rates of NaCl transport in neonatal and mature distal convoluted tubules have not been compared directly.

COLLECTING TUBULE

The cortical collecting tubule only reabsorbs 1 to 2% of the filtered sodium. However, the cortical collecting tubule plays a critical role in regulation of sodium and potassium homeostasis because it is responsible for the final modulation of urinary sodium and potassium excretion (see Sec. 21.4). In principal cells of the cortical collecting tubule (Fig. 21-6), sodium reabsorption is mediated by an apical membrane sodium channel. The reabsorption of sodium results in a lumen-negative transepithelial potential difference, which provides a driving force for either luminal potassium or luminal proton secretion or paracellular chloride reabsorption. Potassium is secreted across an apical membrane through a potassium-selective channel. Protons are secreted by an H^+-ATPase pump in adjoining intercalated cells (Fig. 21-6). The rates of sodium absorption, potassium secretion, and proton secretion are all increased by aldosterone.

There are profound maturational changes in transport in the cortical collecting tubule. The rate of sodium absorption is far less in the neonatal than in the mature segment because of the smaller numbers of sodium channels on the apical membrane and Na^+,K^+-ATPase pumps on the basolateral membrane of the neonatal segment. Also, the sodium channels that are present have a lower probability of being open to allow apical sodium entry.

The neonate and growing child must be in positive potassium balance for growth. Most of the filtered potassium is reabsorbed in the proximal tubule and thick ascending limb. The cortical collecting tubule is the nephron segment that makes the final adjustments to the potassium composition of the urine. In adults, the amount of potassium excreted is dependent on sodium delivery to the cortical collecting tubule and the serum aldosterone concentration. However, the neonatal cortical collecting tubule has a paucity of apical potassium secretory channels, and, even in the face of adequate sodium delivery to the distal nephron and high serum aldos-

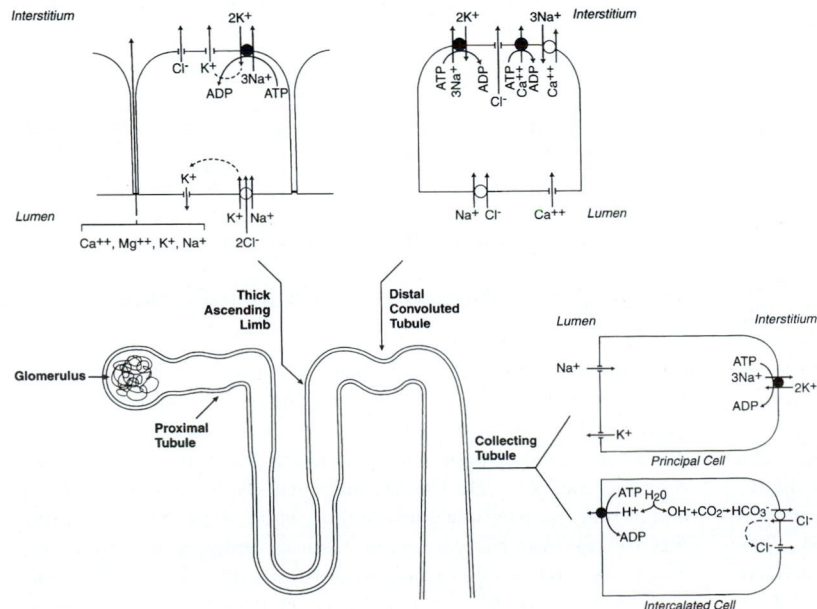

FIGURE 21-6   Main transporters on the apical and basolateral membrane of the thick ascending limb, distal convoluted tubule, and cortical collecting tubule.

terone levels, the neonate may not increase potassium excretion. This limited capacity to excrete potassium predisposes premature and term neonates to develop hyperkalemia.

MATURATIONAL CHANGES IN RENAL ACIDIFICATION

The neonatal and adult kidney must reabsorb all of the filtered bicarbonate and excrete the acid load that is generated from metabolism, which is approximately 1 meq/kg per day in adults. Growing children have a higher rate of acid generation from metabolism and also generate acid with new bone formation. Neonates have a serum bicarbonate of approximately 19 meq/L, and premature neonates can have normal serum bicarbonate levels as low as 15 meq/L. This lower serum bicarbonate concentration reflects a lower threshold for bicarbonate in the immature kidney. Tubular immaturity resulting in lower rates of bicarbonate reabsorption is the predominant contributor to the lower rate of bicarbonate reabsorption by the immature kidney, which predisposes the neonate to develop severe metabolic acidosis when there is bicarbonate loss such as occurs with diarrhea.

In the adult proximal tubule two-thirds of luminal proton secretion is mediated by the apical membrane Na^+/H^+ exchanger, and one-third of proton secretion is via an apical membrane H^+-ATPase. The protons secreted into the luminal fluid titrate the luminal bicarbonate to form H_2CO_3. Carbonic anhydrase, located on the apical membrane and in the cytosol, facilitates the interconversion of H_2CO_3 to CO_2 and H_2O. The luminal CO_2 diffuses into the proximal tubule cell, where it is converted into bicarbonate (see Fig. 21-4).

Most of the filtered bicarbonate is reabsorbed by the proximal tubule. The rate of bicarbonate reabsorption by the neonatal proximal tubule is approximately one-third that measured in the adult segment. Proximal tubule acidification mechanisms are depicted in Fig. 21-4. Both the apical Na^+/H^+ exchanger and H^+-ATPase function at slower rates in the neonatal kidney, which is the primary factor accounting for the lower rate of proximal tubule bicarbonate transport. The basolateral membrane sodium bicarbonate cotransporter functions at a comparatively high rate in the neonatal segment and does not limit proximal tubule acidification. There are maturational changes in carbonic anhydrase, but whether this limits the rate of bicarbonate transport is unclear. The lower rate of proximal tubule bicarbonate reabsorption is the predominant factor responsible for the lower bicarbonate threshold in neonates.

The adult cortical collecting tubule can either absorb or secrete bicarbonate, depending on the acid-base status. Proton secretion is mediated by the α-intercalated cell (see Fig. 21-6). Bicarbonate secretion is mediated by a β-intercalated cell, which has a Cl^-/HCO_3^- exchanger on the apical membrane and a H^+-ATPase on the basolateral membrane. The number of both α- and β-intercalated cells increase with maturation. Distal to the cortical collecting tubule is the medullary collecting tubule, which also has intercalated cells. The number of intercalated cells and rate of proton secretion by this segment is comparable in adults and neonates.

The secretion of acid from metabolism and bone formation in children is dependent on the proton secretory capacity of the distal nephron. Neonates maintain acid-base balance, in part, by the ingestion of alkali in the diet. Ammonia and titratable acids, such as phosphate, buffer the protons secreted by the distal tubule. Premature and full-term neonates for the first several days of life have a limited capacity to excrete acid because of lower rates of both titratable acid and ammonium excretion. The proximal tubule production of ammonia from glutamine is lower in neonates, which results in lower delivery of ammonia to the distal nephron. Titratable acid excretion is limited in breast-fed neonates, where the phosphate content of milk is lower than that in cow's milk formulas. In addition, neonates, unlike adults, function at near-maximal capacity of acid excretion and are thus unable to increase ammonium and titratable acid excretion and thus proton secretion in response to acidosis.

CALCIUM

Two-thirds of filtered calcium is reabsorbed by the proximal tubule in neonates and adults, predominantly by passive diffusion across the paracellular pathway and by a minor active component. The thick ascending limb reabsorbs 25% of the filtered calcium across the paracellular pathway, driven by the lumen-positive potential difference in this segment. Neonates reabsorb less calcium in this segment than adults because of tubular immaturity. Most of the remaining calcium is reabsorbed by the distal convoluted tubule. Calcium transport in this segment is active and transcellular (see Fig. 21-6).

Parathyroid hormone increases calcium transport in the cortical thick ascending limb and distal convoluted tubule. In both segments this effect is mediated by cyclic AMP. Serum parathyroid hormone levels are very low in cord blood. The secretion of parathyroid hormone is stimulated by low ionized calcium levels, and neonates respond to the physiological nadir of serum calcium with higher serum parathyroid hormone levels than those measured in adults. However, the tubule response to parathyroid hormone is markedly attenuated compared to that of adults.

A urinary Ca/Cr ratio greater than 0.2 is abnormal in a child or adult, but premature and term neonates can have a ratio that normally exceeds 1.0. The higher urinary calcium/creatinine ratio results from tubular immaturity resulting in lower rates of calcium absorption. The higher baseline urinary Ca/Cr ratio is an important factor predisposing neonates to develop nephrocalcinosis when treated with loop diuretics, which further increase urinary calcium excretion.

Citrate is the predominant urinary solute that increases urinary calcium solubility and prevents nephrolithiasis. Citrate is freely filtered by the glomerulus and partially reabsorbed by the proximal tubule via a Na-citrate cotransporter. The rate of proximal tubule citrate transport is increased in hypokalemia and acidosis, which reduce urinary citrate excretion and account for the nephrocalcinosis seen in patients with distal renal tubular acidosis. Urinary citrate levels are much higher in neonates and children than in adults. This relative hypercitruria prevents renal calculi in spite of the high rates of calcium excretion in neonates and explains why children with hypercalciuria rarely develop renal stones.

21.2.3   Concentration and Dilution of Urine

Formation of urine with an osmolality greater than that of plasma is dependent on the generation of a hypertonic medulla and the ability of the collecting tubule to alter its water permeability so that the tubular fluid can come into osmotic equilibration with the hypertonic medulla. The hypertonic medulla is generated by the countercurrent multiplication system, where the active transport of NaCl in the water-impermeable thick ascending limb results in a progressive increase in osmolality as tubular fluid reaches the bend of the loop of Henle. The anatomy of the nephron with the hairpin turn of the loop of Henle and the collecting tubule running in parallel allows the countercurrent system to create a progressively hypertonic medulla (see Fig. 21-6).

The fluid exiting the proximal straight tubule is isotonic to plasma. The thin descending limb is permeable to water but impermeable to NaCl and urea. As water is abstracted from the thin descending limb, the tubular fluid osmolality increases as the luminal sodium and urea concentrations rise until the bend of the loop, at which point the osmolality is 1200 mOsm/kg of water in the adult. The thin and thick ascending limbs are water impermeable but highly permeable to sodium and urea. Sodium leaves the thin ascending limb by passive diffusion. The medullary urea concentration is higher than that of fluid in the thin ascending limb, and urea diffuses into the tubular lumen. In the thick ascending limb, NaCl is actively transported (the only energy-requiring step in urinary concentration and dilution), leaving the luminal fluid with an osmolality of 50 mOsm/kg of water by the end of the segment. The medullary collecting tubule, unlike the cortical collecting tubule, is permeable to urea. The medullary collecting tubule urea permeability is further increased by antidiuretic hormone (vasopressin). The delivery of urea to the medulla raises medullary tonicity. Thus, urea is recycled from the medullary collecting tubule into the thin ascending limb. The accumulation of urea in the medullary interstitium plays an important role in the generation of hypertonic urine.

The final concentration of urine is dependent on whether antidiuretic hormone is present. Antidiuretic hormone is secreted in response to an increase in plasma osmolality or a reduction in the effective intravascular volume. In the absence of antidiuretic hormone, the hypotonic urine generated by the thick ascending limb and early distal tubule is excreted unchanged. Antidiuretic hormone causes the insertion of water channels (aquaporin-2) in the apical membrane of the collecting tubule. In the presence of antidiuretic hormone, the water permeability of the collecting tubule increases, and water diffuses into the hypertonic medullary interstitium, resulting in a concentrated urine.

The maximal urinary osmolality of an adult is 1200 mOsm/kg water. By comparison, the term neonate can concentrate the urine to only 600 to 800 mOsm/kg water. Adult urinary concentrating ability is achieved at 12 to 18 months of age. The limited ability to excrete hypertonic urine makes neonates more prone to develop dehydration and hypernatremia than adults.

In response to an increase in plasma osmolality or volume depletion, the neonate secretes antidiuretic hormone (vasopressin) to serum levels comparable to those of adults, but the renal response to vasopressin is attenuated. There are a number of factors that limit the ability of the neonate to excrete concentrated urine. Maximal urinary concentration is dependent on a hypertonic medulla, which is limited in neonates because of relatively low protein intake and urea generation and a reduced capacity of the neonatal thick ascending limb to reabsorb NaCl and maximize the countercurrent multiplication system. Anatomic factors such as shorter papillae, increased interstitial material, and poorly developed vasa recta impair diffusion of urea and water in the neonatal kidney. In response to vasopressin, the neonatal collecting tubule does not have an increase in water permeability comparable to that of the adult.

The neonate consumes mother's milk, which is a hypotonic fluid. Neonates are able to excrete the excess free water to maintain a plasma osmolality of 290 mOsm/kg water. The urine osmolality in both adults and neonates can be as low as 50 mOsm/kg of water. Adults with a normal urinary diluting capacity have an enormous ability to excrete free water, and rarely are able to drink enough water to decrease serum sodium concentration (see Sec. 21.4). Neonates have a limited capacity to excrete free water, and excess hypotonic fluid intake results in hyponatremia.

21.2.4 Maintenance of Extracellular Fluid Volume

The kidney plays a vital role in the transition from fetal to extrauterine life. The late-gestation fetus has a urine flow rate of 10 mL/kg per hour and excretes 5 to 10% of the filtered sodium, which reflects a glomerular tubular imbalance despite the very low glomerular filtration rate in the fetus. The high intrauterine urine flow rate can produce mild dilatation of the renal pelvis, which may be detected on a prenatal sonogram but does not always signify a pathologic abnormality.

The enormous fetal urinary loss of salt and water would not be compatible with extrauterine life. Within hours of birth the term neonate excretes less than 1% of the filtered sodium despite a concomitant increase in the glomerular filtration rate. Premature neonates have relative tubular immaturity and may excrete up to 5% of the filtered sodium for the first few days after birth. In a premature neonate, replacement of urinary losses with sodium-free solutions will result in hyponatremia. Within days the sodium losses by the premature infant diminish as the tubular sodium reabsorptive capacity increases.

There is a paucity of sodium in mother's milk and most infant formulas, yet neonates must be in positive sodium balance for growth. Thus, the neonatal kidney must be able to conserve sodium despite the relatively low sodium transport rates. This inherent conservation of sodium explains the failure of neonates to respond to a volume or sodium challenge with a natriuresis comparable to that seen in adults. For example, infusion of isotonic saline equal to 10% of an adult's weight over 30 minutes will result in excretion of 50% of the sodium load within 2 hours, whereas neonates will excrete less than 10% of the infused saline during that time.

The factors that mediate this avid sodium retention are unclear, but there are differences between the ways the adult and neonatal kidneys respond to hormones that modulate sodium transport. Plasma renin activity and aldosterone concentrations are severalfold higher in both the premature and term neonate than in the adult. Plasma renin and aldosterone levels increase in response to volume depletion in term neonates, but the effect of aldosterone to increase distal tubule sodium absorption and potassium secretion is attenuated in the neonate compared to the adult. Aldosterone has a profound effect in decreasing the urinary Na/K ratio in adults, but this effect is blunted in neonates. Premature neonates have a higher plasma renin activity than term neonates but have a somewhat limited ability to secrete aldosterone in response to volume depletion. The tubular response to aldosterone is also impaired in premature neonates, which limits their ability to excrete potassium and conserve sodium, in part because there are fewer potassium and sodium channels in the immature cortical collecting tubule. Plasma angiotensin II levels are higher in the neonate than in the adult, and augmented sodium transport in response to angiotensin II may be an important factor mediating sodium conservation by the growing neonate.

Catecholamines and renal nerves appear to play less of a role in regulating GFR and tubular sodium transport in neonates than in adults. Renal nerves contribute to the decrease in sodium excretion that occurs in the transition from fetal to extrauterine life. The urine volume and sodium excretion rates are greater with renal denervation; however, the increase is small and present for only the first

24 hours after birth. Thus, other factors such as the renin-angiotensin system likely play a greater role regulating neonatal sodium transport.

An attenuated response to volume expansion can also be caused by a blunted response to natriuretic hormones such as atrial natriuretic peptide (ANP), which is produced primarily by the cardiac atria in adults but also by the ventricles in the fetus. This peptide acts to suppress the renin-angiotensin-aldosterone axis and reduce peripheral vascular resistance. Atrial natriuretic peptide has direct renal effects to promote sodium excretion. ANP increases GFR and inhibits tubular sodium transport by blocking the angiotensin II–mediated increase in sodium reabsorption in the proximal tubule and by directly inhibiting sodium transport in the collecting tubule. The vasopressin-mediated increase in collecting tubule water transport is also antagonized by ANP.

Although the basal levels of atrial natriuretic peptide are higher in the fetus and comparable to adult levels in the neonate, the increase in plasma levels is attenuated with volume expansion in both the neonate and fetus. In addition, infusion of atrial natriuretic peptide in neonates does not increase GFR and produces a blunted increase in sodium excretion compared to adults. Thus, the neonate does not have the same capacity to respond to volume depletion or volume expansion as the adult.

References

Baum M, Quigley R: Ontogeny of proximal tubule acidification. Kidney Int 48:1697–1704, 1995

Horster MF, Zink H: Functional differentiation of the medullary collecting tubule: influence of vasopressin. Kidney Int 22:360–365, 1982

Neiberger RE, Barac-Nieto M, Spitzer A: Renal reabsorption of phosphate during development: transport kinetics in BBMV. Am J Physiol 257:F268–F274, 1989

Robillard JE, Segar JL, Smith FG, Jose PA: Regulation of sodium metabolism and extracellular fluid volume during development. Clin Perinatol 19:15–31, 1992

Satlin LM: Postnatal maturation of potassium transport in rabbit cortical collecting duct. Am J Physiol 266:F57–F65, 1994

Schmidt U, Horster M: Na-K–activated ATPase: activity maturation in rabbit nephron segments dissected in vitro. Am J Physiol 233:F55–F60, 1977

Shah M, Quigley R, Baum M: Maturation of rabbit proximal straight tubule chloride/base exchange. Am J Physiol 274:F883–F888, 1998

Winberg J: The 24-hour true endogenous creatinine clearance in infants and children without renal disease. Acta Paediat. 48:443, 1959.

21.3 RENAL DEVELOPMENTAL DISORDERS OF THE FETUS AND NEWBORN

Victoria F. Norwood and Robert L. Chevalier

During the period of active morphologic and functional development of the kidney (see Secs. 21.1 and 21.2), any number of insults may lead to a wide variety of abnormal kidney phenotypes. Inherited genetic mutations, in utero toxins, infections, obstructions, vascular events, or the disruption of normal developmental programming and patterning can individually or in combination cause a number of renal developmental abnormalities. Regardless of the nature of the initiating insult, the end result is a reduction in the normal complement of functioning nephrons and varying degrees of renal dysfunction. Bilateral abnormalities have a more ominous prognosis and commonly result in renal insufficiency. In fact, 40% of the children requiring dialysis or transplantation for end-stage renal disease have some form of renal developmental abnormality.

21.3.1 Assessment of Renal Function in the Newborn

To accurately determine the physiological effects of any renal developmental anomaly in the newborn or infant, it is important to understand that the varied functions of the kidney are not mature until after several years of life (see Sec. 21.2). Careful examination of a variety of renal functions and knowledge of appropriate norms for age will allow accurate evaluation of the immediate situation and avoid inappropriate interventions or prognostications. Age-appropriate normal values for a number of renal functions are shown in Table 21-1.

Glomerular filtration rate (GFR) is a function of intraglomerular pressure and capillary filtration and increases with increasing gestational and postnatal age (see Sec. 21.2). In clinical conditions, GFR is estimated using clearance methodologies. Renal "clearance" of a solute is defined as the volume of plasma from which the solute is completely cleared by the kidney in a given period of time (see Sec. 21.5). Of special importance in pediatrics is that clearances should be corrected to account for body surface area.

The most accurate clearance measurements are obtained using inulin, iothalamate, or radiotracer infusions, but because of the cumbersome nature of controlled, timed intravenous infusions, GFR is most commonly estimated by measuring clearance of endogenous creatinine. Because a healthy infant at steady state produces approximately 15 mg creatinine per kilogram body weight per 24 hours, this amount of creatinine should be present in a 24-hour urine collection and may be used to document completeness of the collection. Because of the difficulties collecting timed urine samples in newborns and infants, several modifications of standard clearance techniques have been developed to estimate GFR in the small child (see Sec. 21.5). Nuclear imaging by renal scintigraphy provides another method for determination of renal function in infancy. The low GFR in early childhood and the diffusibility of the compounds decrease the sensitivity and increase the background of technetium scans (^{99m}Tc-DTPA or ^{99m}Tc-MAG3), and normal maturation will inevitably result in "improvement" in function over time.

Along with rapid changes in renal blood flow and GFR during the early postnatal period, maturing kidneys undergo normal developmental advances in sodium handling, acid-base control, and urinary concentrating capacity (see Sec. 21.2). The fractional excretion of sodium (FE_{Na}) is high in newborn infants and more so in premature babies. High urine sodium losses, present in all neonates in the first several days of life, are most pronounced and prolonged in the preterm neonate and are aggravated by low sodium intake. In these situations, commonly seen in neonatal intensive care units, an infant can become hyponatremic and suffer neurologic consequences unless sodium supplementation is provided.

In a similar fashion to immature renal handling of sodium, newborns and young infants have altered acid-base homeostasis (see Sec. 21.2). Because of a reduced capacity to excrete an acid load, most newborns have a lower plasma total CO_2 concentration,

TABLE 21-1

NORMAL VALUES OF RENAL FUNCTION

AGE	GFR (mL/min/1.73 m²)	RENAL BLOOD FLOW (mL/min/1.73 m²)	MAXIMAL URINE OSMOLALITY (mOsm/kg)	SERUM CREATININE (mg/dL)	FRACTIONAL EXCRETION OF SODIUM (%)
Newborn					
Premature	14 ± 3	40 ± 6	480	1.3	2–5
Full term	21 ± 4	88 ± 4	800	1.1	<1
1–2 weeks	50 ± 10	220 ± 40	900	0.4	<1
6 mo–1 yr	77 ± 14	352 ± 73	1200	0.2	<1
1–3 yr	96 ± 22	540 ± 118	1400	0.4	<1
Adult	118 ± 18	620 ± 92	1400	0.8–1.5	<1

SOURCE: *Ellis D, Avner ED: Fluid and electrolyte disorders in pediatric patients. In: Puschett JB, ed: Disorders of Fluid and Electrolyte Balance: Diagnosis and Management. New York, Churchill Livingstone, 1985, with permission.*

which should not be confused with renal tubular acidosis unless the concentration of H_2CO_3 falls below 15 meq/L in the first 2 weeks of life.

The immature human kidney has limited concentrating capacity (see Sec. 21.2). The infant's difficulty in achieving a highly concentrated urine becomes clinically important in two different scenarios: (1) to excrete any given solute load, the smaller child requires a greater intake of fluid and a larger production of urine; (2) infants deprived of adequate fluid intake or suffering from enhanced fluid losses will become dehydrated more rapidly than older children and should be more aggressively managed.

Age-dependent differences in tubular reabsorptive capacity for sodium and urinary concentrating ability must be used in evaluating a neonate for fluid and electrolyte abnormalities (see Sec. 21.4). Whereas the normal term infant should be able to achieve a urine sodium concentration <10 meq/L and a urine osmolality > 500 mOsm/kg in the face of renal hypoperfusion, the preterm infant may not lower urinary sodium concentration <30 meq/L and may not increase urine osmolality above 350 to 400 mOsm/kg. Therefore the use of urinary indices to evaluate oliguric states or electrolyte disorders in the preterm infant requires careful attention to these differences to allow accurate diagnoses (see Sec. 21.4 and Table 21-7).

21.3.2 Abnormalities of Renal Size and Composition

RENAL AGENESIS

Complete absence of the kidney, *agenesis,* implies an insult at the earliest stages of kidney differentiation (3–5 weeks of gestation in the human) at or before the time of branching of the ureteric bud into metanephric blastema (see Sec 21.1). In the absence of the initial induction process, subsequent differentiation events fail to occur, and the kidney does not form. Other causes of "agenesis" include atrophy and regression of a severely affected ischemic or multicystic dysplastic kidney. Most commonly renal agenesis is unilateral and occurs in 1 of 500 to 1000 live births. The remaining kidney undergoes adaptive growth, and single nephron hyperfiltration occurs such that overall kidney function is maintained at more than 80% of that provided by two kidneys. Although the majority of patients with isolated unilateral agenesis are asymptomatic, when

the abnormality is detected it is important to insure that no other anomalies are present. The exact incidence is unclear, but other abnormalities such as dysplasia, obstructive lesions, malpositions, or vesicoureteral reflux may be present in the solitary kidney. Unilateral agenesis is also a common finding in a number of multiple malformation syndromes including VATER and CHARGE associations, Turner syndrome, Rokitansky-Mayer-Küster-Hauser syndrome (vaginal atresia), and many others (see Chap. 10). Evaluation should include ultrasonography of the entire urinary tract, electrolytes, BUN, and creatinine as well as a urinalysis looking for signs of infection or proteinuria suggesting preexisting glomerular damage. Because dysplastic changes may be focal, intermittent assessment of the interval growth and function of the remaining kidney should be done. A normal single kidney should increase to >95th percentile of kidney length for age by 2 years of life. Failure to achieve or maintain renal hypertrophy should be of concern relative to long-term outcome.

Fortunately, bilateral agenesis is uncommon, occurring in approximately 1 in 6000 deliveries. The lack of fetal urine production inevitably results in severe oligohydramnios and fetal or neonatal fatality. The characteristic "Potter facies" and associated dysmorphisms seen in these infants are the result of fetal compression from chronic oligohydramnios and include flattened facies, low-set ears, positional clubbed feet and hands, and pulmonary hypoplasia. Stillbirth occurs in 40% of these infants, and the others are often delivered prematurely and die of untreatable pulmonary insufficiency.

The recurrence risk of renal agenesis can be estimated, although exact inheritance patterns for the majority of these disorders are not defined. When agenesis is associated with other anomalies or syndromes for which an inheritance pattern or recurrence risk is known, a similar risk for subsequent pregnancies is expected. First-degree relatives of infants with nonsyndromic bilateral renal agenesis also have an increased prevalence of unilateral agenesis/dysplasia or other urogenital anomalies (approximately 9% as opposed to 0.5% in the general population). The recurrence risk of urinary tract anomalies in families with nonsyndromic unilateral agenesis is unknown. If first-degree relatives are normal, it can be considered to be less than 3%.

RENAL HYPOPLASIA

Renal hypoplasia is defined as a reduction in the number of nephrons and/or a decrease in nephron size without functional or differentiation abnormalities of the remaining nephrons. Therefore, isolated hypoplasia may be relatively asymptomatic, and the only feature may be small kidneys found on incidental renal ultrasonography. Hypoplasia may be either unilateral or bilateral, and when bilateral, is usually associated with renal insufficiency. Importantly, hypoplasia is frequently associated with dysplasia of the remaining renal parenchyma, and therefore, children with small kidneys should be followed carefully for signs of salt wasting and renal insufficiency.

A unique form of hypoplasia is oligomeganephronia. Usually isolated, this abnormality may occasionally be associated with other anomalies and may be inherited. These patients have very small kidneys with dramatic reductions in nephron number (as few as 20% of the normal complement). The remaining nephrons are very large, with increased glomerular diameter and dramatically lengthened tubule segments. These patients usually have polyuria, salt wasting, glucosuria, profound growth failure, and early progression to end-stage renal disease.

DYSPLASIAS

Renal dysplasia is defined as abnormal differentiation of metanephric tissue involving glomerular, tubular, and interstitial lineages resulting in poorly formed, largely nonfunctional nephrons. Although areas of dysplasia are common in the classic renal cystic diseases, and cysts are very commonly seen in dysplastic kidneys, these developmental renal anomalies should be considered as distinct entities. Most importantly, renal dysplasia is commonly associated with other urinary tract anomalies and mandates thorough evaluation of the genitourinary tract whenever renal dysplasia is detected. Dysplasia can result from a large number of genetic and environmental insults, including obstruction, occurring at variable phases of the developmental program (see Sec. 21.1). Indeed, the morphologic differences seen in individual dysplastic kidneys likely reflect the numerous possibilities by which normal nephrogenesis may be disrupted. Classically, renal dysplasia includes diffuse structural disorganization, primitive glomeruli and tubular structures surrounded by disrupted supporting stroma and vasculature, and occasional cartilaginous dysplasia. Dysplastic abnormalities can be diffuse or focal, unilateral or bilateral. The end result includes kidneys that are variably solid, cystic, small, large, functional, or nonfunctional.

One of the most commonly encountered presentations of renal dysplasia is the multicystic dysplastic kidney (MCDK). Often suspected through antenatal ultrasound or presenting as an abdominal mass in the newborn period, the MCDK consists of multiple cysts of varying sizes thoroughly distorting all normal renal structure. The ureter is often atretic. Microscopically, these kidneys are abnormal throughout, containing only primitive nephron structures. The differential diagnosis of MCDK includes severe hydronephrosis (usually from ureteropelvic junction obstruction) and occasionally autosomal dominant polycystic kidney disease (see Sec. 21.10). These entities can be discriminated by imaging studies. Ultrasound examination can often detect a rim of normal renal parenchyma in obstructed kidneys, and the inherited kidney diseases have bilateral, although not always symmetric, abnormalities. Nuclear imaging will confirm complete nonfunction of the MCDK, and obstructed or cystic kidneys will usually exhibit residual, although likely diminished, function. Bilateral MCDK is uncommon and, if no functional parenchyma exists, is a fatal defect. Unilateral MCDK is estimated to occur in approximately 1 in 4000 births. Usually detected as an incidental diagnosis on prenatal ultrasound or the

finding of a flank mass, MCDK can also present as urinary tract infection, hematuria, proteinuria, or (rarely) vomiting or respiratory compromise. The management of children with unilateral MCDK must include complete functional and anatomic evaluation of the contralateral kidney and the lower urinary tract. Approximately half of patients with a MCDK will have associated urologic abnormalities, most commonly vesicoureteral reflux and contralateral ureteropelvic junction (UPJ) obstruction. The incidence of contralateral focal dysplasia in the presence of MCDK is not known because the diagnosis of small areas of dysplasia is difficult. However, because the MCDK is largely nonfunctional, evaluation of the remaining kidney is critical, and any appropriate surgical or medical management issues must be addressed to maximize the functional potential of the remaining kidney. Postnatally, the diagnosis should be confirmed by ultrasonography, and any associated anomalies should be detected. Although routine voiding cystourethrogram (VCUG) has been recommended, recent studies have suggested that VCUG may not be mandatory if MCDK is unilateral and no other anomalies of the urinary tract are present. Follow-up through childhood should at a minimum include intermittent ultrasounds to follow the growth of the contralateral kidney and involution of the affected kidney. Failure of the expected hypertrophy should raise suspicions of dysplasia within the contralateral kidney.

Along with the spontaneous dysplasias, similar developmental renal pathologies can result from prenatal use of angiotensin-converting enzyme (ACE) inhibitors and nonsteroidal anti-inflammatory drugs (NSAIDs). ACE inhibitor fetopathy results from the use of these agents in the second and third trimester, while the majority of renal differentiation is progressing. Abnormalities include fetal hypotension, oligohydramnios/oligoanuria, growth failure, renal tubular dysplasia with renal insufficiency or failure, growth anomalies of the calvarium, and increased fetal or neonatal mortality. The effects of long-term NSAID use during the second half of pregnancy for the prevention of preterm labor and management of polyhydramnios include fetal renal dysplasia of all nephron segments and resultant functional insufficiency or failure. Unlike the usually reversible alterations in renal function caused by these agents in the mature kidney, the disruption of normal renal development results in permanent kidney damage.

Presumably as the result of tubular disarray and malfunction, dysplastic kidneys often exhibit abnormally low sodium reabsorption, acid and potassium excretion, and urinary concentrating capacities. Consequently, infants with bilateral MCDK are even more susceptible to dehydration and electrolyte abnormalities than normal infants. The combination of salt loss, metabolic acidosis, and reduced renal function result in poor growth, and hyperkalemia may be persistent.

21.3.3   Migrational Abnormalities

A number of kidney abnormalities may be considered defects in migration of the entire renal unit or imperfections in the early branching processes of the ureter (see Sec. 21.1).

These abnormalities are often isolated but are also quite common in a number of multiorgan-system syndromes. Ectopic kidneys result from abnormal ascent of the kidneys from the pelvis and may be unilateral or bilateral. In rare cases, thoracic ectopic kidneys have been reported, although most commonly the kidneys remain in the pelvis or may cross the midline to form a *crossed fused ectopia* in which both kidneys are joined. *Horseshoe kidney* refers to an abnormality in which both kidneys are fused at the lower pole by a connecting band of fibrous tissue or renal parenchyma. Duplicated ureters or collecting systems result from aberrant branching of the ureteric bud. Early branching can result in a completely duplicated kidney with a separate collecting system, ureter, and vesicoureteral junction. Later duplication may result in a single renal unit with two collecting systems drained by two ureters that may join at some point before entry into the bladder (see Sec. 21.16). Many of these defects are silent and are detected only incidentally or during evaluation of the urinary tract following infection. However, the incidence of dysplasia, obstructive lesions, vesicoureteral reflux, and stones may be higher in these kidneys. Therefore, when identified, children with these anomalies require thorough evaluation.

VATER AND CHARGE ASSOCIATIONS

Although a large number of genetic syndromes and associations include anomalies of the urinary tract, VATER and CHARGE associations are both relatively common and very often include renal or lower tract defects (see Chapter 10). VATER describes the association of *v*ertebral anomalies, imperforate *a*nus, *t*racheo*e*sophageal fistula, and *r*adial and *r*enal anomalies and can be expanded to VACTERL to include *c*ardiac and *l*imb anomalies. Although it most commonly consists of concurrent defects without a unifying genetic diagnosis, VATER association can also be seen as part of some chromosomal disorders and genetic syndromes and some teratogenic exposures such as fetal alcohol syndrome (see Sec. 10.3). The most common renal anomalies are agenesis, ectopy, dysplasia, and obstructive lesions. Vertebral anomalies and high imperforate anus defects may be associated with neuromuscular bladder dysfunction, which may be severe.

CHARGE describes the association of *c*oloboma of the retina, iris, or choroid; *h*eart defects; choanal *a*tresia; *r*etardation of growth and development; *g*enital anomalies; and *e*ar abnormalities. The most common renal anomalies are agenesis, ectopy, dysplasia, and ureteric lesions.

21.3.4 Obstructive Disorders

Urinary tract obstruction in children is most commonly congenital, although acquired lesions occasionally occur (see Sec. 21.16). The consequences of urinary tract obstruction during development are quite serious and may lead to lifelong complications (Table 21-2). Obstructive lesions may occur alone or in conjunction with other organ system malformations such that infants with urinary tract anomalies should be carefully examined for the presence of other

TABLE 21-2
CONSEQUENCES OF URINARY TRACT OBSTRUCTION DURING DEVELOPMENT

Renal insufficiency or failure
Oligohydramnios
  Potter sequence
  Pulmonary hypoplasia
Fluid and electrolyte abnormalities
  Sodium wasting
  Urinary concentrating defects
  Hyperkalemia
  Renal tubular acidosis
Hypertension
Infection
Growth failure

abnormalities. The widespread use of prenatal ultrasonography frequently detects obstructive lesions before delivery, including prenatal hydronephrosis with or without bladder enlargement. Because of very high fetal urine flow rates (see Sec. 21.2), many infants suspected of having prenatal hydronephrosis are actually not found to have significant obstruction on postnatal ultrasound. Signs of urinary tract obstruction in the early postnatal period include an abdominal mass or distension, failure to pass urine within the first 24 hours after birth, or a poor urinary stream in boys. In later infancy and childhood, urinary tract obstructions most commonly present with infection, abdominal masses with or without abdominal pain, voiding dysfunction, polyuria, or failure to thrive.

The UPJ is the most common site for congenital obstructions, accounting for approximately 65% of these types of lesions. UPJ obstructions may be unilateral or bilateral and, when unilateral, may be associated with other abnormalities such as multicystic dysplasia or vesicoureteral reflux. Mechanical or functional obstruction at the ureterovesical junction (UVJ) accounts for approximately 15% of cases of obstructive uropathy and can also occur unilaterally or bilaterally and in association with other urinary tract lesions. The most frequently seen cause of UVJ obstruction is a ureterocele, a congenital cystic dilation of the distal ureter that protrudes into the bladder. Posterior urethral valves (PUV), although relatively uncommon (2% of cases of obstructive uropathy), are the most devastating because these children (almost exclusively male) have bilateral hydronephrosis and long-term renal insufficiency. Prune belly syndrome, also known as the Eagle-Barrett triad, includes a constellation of abnormalities—deficient abdominal musculature, cryptorchism, and urinary tract anomalies (most commonly megacystis with hydroureteronephrosis). Although the etiology of prune belly syndrome remains elusive and may not be obstructive in origin, the end result usually includes some degree of permanent renal damage. Myelodysplasia and other congenital or acquired spinal cord abnormalities often have associated bladder outflow dysfunction and may result in symptoms of obstructive uropathy. Acquired obstructions, although much less common in children than in adults, occasionally occur. Tumors (including Wilms tumor, lymphoma, neuroblastoma, rhabdomyosarcoma, or other pelvic/retroperitoneal neoplasms), inflammatory masses (appendiceal abscesses, Crohn disease, tuberculosis), trauma, or stricture formation from previous instrumentation can all cause obstruction of the previously healthy urinary tract.

Evaluation of children with urinary tract obstruction should include detection of other organ system anomalies or acutely treatable complications such as urinary tract infection. To define anatomic abnormalities, ultrasound of the kidneys and bladder should include evaluation of bladder wall thickness and residual urine volume after voiding, ureteral size, and localization of any obvious transition zones, presence and degree of hydronephrosis, estimates of renal cortical thickness, and documentation of cysts or other abnormal echogenicity consistent with dysplastic changes. In addition, in cases of unilateral hydronephrosis, the length of the contralateral kidney should be measured carefully because compensatory growth begins in utero. Radioisotopic studies (usually ^{99m}Tc-DTPA or ^{99m}Tc-MAG3) may be used to estimate GFR and tubular function of each kidney. The intravenous injection of furosemide 20 to 30 minutes after injection of the isotope enhances detection of obstruction and may be quite helpful in evaluating possibly obstructive lesions. An excretion time > 20 minutes for one-half of the isotope activity indicates obstruction to urine flow. A voiding cystourethrogram will detect vesicoureteral reflux and evaluate bladder wall thickness, posterior urethral size, and voiding dysfunction. Serum electrolytes, BUN, and creatinine should be obtained as part of the initial evaluation for obstructive uropathy, although values obtained within 24 hours of birth are mostly reflective of maternal renal function (see Table 21-1). Urinalysis is also informative in that specific gravity, proteinuria, bacteriuria, or cellular elements are reflective of renal damage or intercurrent infection.

Growth failure of the obstructed kidney is unique to the pediatric population and of paramount concern regarding treatment options (see Sec. 21.16). Unfortunately, no exact formula can predict the severity of renal damage from a particular degree of obstruction occurring at any specific time during development. Although the presence of severe bilateral obstruction undoubtedly requires intervention, the indications for surgical repair of moderate unilateral obstruction are more controversial (see Sec. 21.16). The most conservative approach is to consider early surgical correction to avert renal damage to the developing kidney. Alternatively, careful observation for any progression of hydronephrosis, sustained renal growth and function, as well as increasing compensatory growth by the contralateral kidney is feasible without undue risk.

21.3.5   Vesicoureteral Reflux

The flap-valve mechanism at the UVJ prevents backflow of urine from the bladder into the upper tracts and undergoes developmental migration and maturation during fetal life. Thus primary vesicoureteral reflux (VUR) is congenital and not associated with neuromuscular or obstructive processes (see Sec. 21.6). Secondary VUR is the consequence of underlying bladder pathology such as urethral obstruction, neuromuscular defects, or voiding dysfunction. Although the genetic mechanisms behind VUR remain incompletely understood, the process may be familial, with one-fourth to one-third of siblings of index patients affected. The importance of VUR in developmental nephrology relates to the high incidence of renal scarring and dysplastic changes that develop in the maturing kidney. Whether these changes are the result of a primary developmental defect (aberrant ureteric bud branching and subsequent induction failure and dysplasia), hydrostatic damage from sterile reflux, or infective/immunologic responses to intrarenal reflux of infected urine remain debated (see Sec. 21.6). Very likely, all of these may affect the developmental programming of the growing kidney, resulting in permanent nephron loss during susceptible periods.

21.3.6   Cystic Disease in the Newborn

The polycystic kidney diseases, autosomal dominant (ADPKD) and autosomal recessive (ARPKD), are clearly developmental in origin (see Sec. 21.10). Classically, ARPKD presents in the neonatal period with enlarged, diffusely echogenic kidneys, hypertension, renal insufficiency, and varying degrees of biliary fibrosis. Macroscopic cysts are *not* seen within the kidney parenchyma. The differential diagnosis of these patients includes bilateral renal vein thrombosis, congenital leukemia/lymphoma, and a variety of genetic syndromes associated with cystic malformations of the kidneys.

ADPKD is commonly thought of as "adult" PKD because of its predominant presentation in the third to fifth decades of life (see Sec. 21.10). However, ADPKD has been diagnosed in the fetus, newborn, and throughout childhood. The clinical expression of ADPKD in newborns includes bilateral flank masses, hypertension, renal insufficiency, UTIs, hematuria, and cystic involvement of

other organ systems. Although usually silent or mild in childhood, these manifestations may occasionally be severe in the newborn period and can even present with a Potter phenotype and pulmonary hypoplasia.

21.3.7   Infantile Nephrotic Syndrome

Infantile nephrotic syndrome is defined as proteinuria present prenatally or at birth that leads to the clinical consequences of nephrotic syndrome within 3 months of age. Infantile nephrotic syndrome may be secondary to congenital infections (syphilis, HIV, TORCH), and these entities must be evaluated in any infant presenting with heavy proteinuria and edema. The most common form of infantile nephrotic syndrome is the Finnish-type congenital nephrotic syndrome (CNF) (see Sec. 21.9).

Diagnosis of CNF includes severe proteinuria with evidence of intrauterine onset (serum albumin <1.0 g/L at birth) in the absence of secondary infectious or inflammatory causes. Fetal proteinuria causes extremely elevated maternal serum or amniotic fluid α-fetoprotein levels (>2.5 multiples of the mean) (see Sec. 21.9).

An important syndrome associated with congenital nephrotic syndrome is Denys-Drash syndrome, which was initially defined as the combination of XY gonadal dysgenesis (male pseudohermaphroditism), glomerulopathy, and Wilms tumor, although a few phenotypic XX patients have been described, and not all manifestations are always present (see Sec. 21.9).

21.3.8   Fetal Intervention

Modern technologies such as ultrasonographic diagnosis of congenital anomalies, amniotic fluid testing, and chorioamnionic villus sampling now allow accurate prenatal diagnosis of a variety of developmental renal disorders. These technical advances in diagnosis provide new opportunities for fetal therapy. Although early genetic testing for single gene mutations such as AD- or ARPKD and CNF allow for counseling regarding prognosis and potential termination of pregnancy in severely affected fetuses, at the present time genetic therapies are not yet available. Recent advances in understanding the molecular mechanisms of these and other renal developmental processes should eventually allow for replacement of abnormal genes or specific molecular pharmacologic approaches.

TABLE 21-3

CRITERIA FOR PRENATAL INTERVENTION FOR FETAL HYDRONEPHROSIS

1. Singleton fetus
2. Progressive bilateral renal disease (bladder outlet obstruction)
3. No other organ anomalies or karyotypic anomaly
4. Unequivocal oligohydramnios
5. Serial sonograms to document persistent obstruction
6. No evidence of dysplasia (cysts)
7. Parents must give informed consent and recognize the experimental nature of the treatment
8. Performed only at an experienced institution with a qualified team including pediatric urologist, perinatal obstetrician, sonographer, and neonatologist.

SOURCE: *Chevalier RL: What management would you currently advise for a fetus who is found to have hydronephrosis on ultrasound examination during pregnancy? Pediatr Nephrol 5:102, 1991, with permission.*

Current treatment options for infants with severe urinary tract lesions include (1) urinary diversion or surgical correction postnatally, (2) termination of the pregnancy, (3) preterm delivery of the fetus with postnatal correction, and (4) in utero diversion or correction. In utero procedures for congenital urinary tract obstruction are experimental at this time and should be considered only if the criteria in Table 21-3 are met and the likelihood that the child would survive ex utero because of severe prematurity is remote. Fetal renal function is also used by some centers to predict potential successful outcomes. In a single aspiration of the fetal bladder, the findings of urine sodium <100 meq/L, urine chloride <90 meq/L, and urine osmolarity >210 mOsm/L suggest the possibility of adequate neonatal renal function.

References

Chevalier RL: Developmental renal physiology of the low birth weight preterm newborn. J Urol 156:714–719, 1996

Chevalier RL: Pathophysiology of obstructive nephropathy in the newborn. Semin Nephrol 18:585–593, 1998

Feldenberg RL, Siegel NJ: Clinical outcome for children with multicystic dysplastic kidneys. Pediatr Nephrol 14:1098–1101, 2000

Holmberg C, Antikainen M, Rönnholm K, Ala-Houhala M, Jalanko H: Management of congenital nephrotic syndrome of the Finnish type. Pediatr Nephrol 9:87–93, 1995

Kestilä M, Lenkkeri U, Männikkö M, et al: Positionally cloned gene for a novel glomerular protein—nephrin—is mutated in congenital nephrotic syndrome. Mol Cell 1:575–582, 1998

Limwongse C, Clarren SK, Cassidy SB: Syndromes and malformations of the urinary tract. In: Barratt TM, Avner ED, Harmon WE, eds: Pediatric Nephrology. Baltimore, Lippincott Williams & Wilkins, 1999:427–452

Lorenz HP, Adzick NS, Harrison MR: Open human fetal surgery. Adv Surg 26:259–273, 1993

21.4   FLUIDS, ELECTROLYTES, AND ACID-BASE

Norman J. Siegel

In *From Fish to Philosopher,* Homer Smith put forth the intriguing hypothesis that mankind has evolved cognitive functions and complex interactions by virtue of the ability of the kidney to maintain an internal environment independent of the sea. Claude Bernard, the renowned 19th century physiologist, noted that we live either in air or in water: the plasma or liquid part of the blood that bathes all our tissues and elements is combined air and water. Fluid therapy and correction of electrolyte disorders is essential to sustain this internal environment from which a free and independent life, physically and intellectually, is achieved.

21.4.1   Parenteral Fluid Therapy

Parenteral fluid therapy, the provision of fluids and electrolytes intravenously, was conceived in 1831 to replace water and salt lost during cholera epidemics. In the 20th century interest in intravenous (IV) fluid therapy was revived, and pediatricians assumed a leading role in advancing our understanding of the pathophysiology of fluids and electrolytes. Howland and Marriot noted that acidosis occurred as a consequence of dehydration, and Gamble

conceived the compartmentalization of body fluids, which continues to be a fundamental concept.

Diffuse interest in this area led to many systems and formulations, yet no single approach has been shown to be markedly superior. In the final analysis, the majority of these systems are empiric, based on clinical experience, and quite interchangeable. Basic principles that actually are common to the majority of different approaches to parenteral and enteral fluid therapy include:

1. A cookbook approach is dangerous and specific therapy must be individualized for each patient.
2. Calculations of fluid or electrolyte requirements are estimates based on subjective observations and cannot be assumed to be definitive.
3. The clinical response to therapy is the ultimate determinant of the effectiveness of a prescribed program for volume replacement to achieve euvolemia.
4. The safety and efficacy of fluid therapy is dependent on clear and simplified design and execution.

Parenteral fluid therapy is divided into three major components: maintenance therapy designed to sustain euvolemia; deficit therapy to replace losses of salt and water that occurred before the assessment of the patient; and replacement therapy, which reconstitutes losses that occur during a therapeutic intervention.

MAINTENANCE FLUIDS

The concepts inherent to maintenance therapy illustrate the basic principles and provide a reference point for parenteral fluid therapy in infants and children. Conceptually, adequate replacement of the water and electrolytes that are lost under ordinary homeostatic conditions during which the patient is relatively inactive and afebrile should "maintain" the patient in a euvolemic state. The volume of fluid is calculated so that minimal renal compensation is required but assumes that an isotonic urine (specific gravity 1.010 or osmolarity 280 to 310 mOsm/L) can be achieved. Fluid requirements for maintenance therapy were derived from the metabolic rate and energy expenditures of children. Holiday and Segar observed that the rate of caloric expenditure was relatively linear for infants and children in three weight categories: 100 calories/kg for 1 to 10 kg, 50 calories/kg for 11 to 20 kg, and 20 calories/kg for 21 to 80 kg. After two endogenous sources of water, water of oxidation and preformed water, have been taken into account, fluid requirements are 100 mL of exogenous water for every 100 kcal of energy expended. Thus, a single sliding scale can be used to calculate an estimate of both caloric expenditure and total maintenance fluid volume (Table 21-4). For example, in a child who weighs 14 kg, an estimate of caloric expenditure or maintenance fluid requirement would be 1000 mL for the first 10 kg plus 50 mL/kg for the next 4 kg or 200 mL, for a total of 1200 mL/d, or similarly, a caloric expenditure of about 1200 kcal/day. By the same

TABLE 21-4

CALCULATION OF CALORIC EXPENDITURE AND MAINTENANCE FLUID VOLUME[a]

WEIGHT	kcal OR mL/kg/d	mL/kg/h
1–10 kg	100	4
11–20 kg	1000 + 50 per kg > 10	40 + 2 per kg > 10
21–80 kg	1500 + 20 per kg > 20	60 + 1 per kg > 20

[a] Assumes patient is minimally active and afebrile.

TABLE 21-5
COMPONENTS OF BASIC PARENTERAL FLUIDS

	Na (meq/L)	Cl (meq/L)	K (meq/L)	LACTATE (meq/L)	OSMOLARITY (mOsm/L)
Normal saline (NS)	154	154	0	0	308
Half-normal saline (0.5 NS)	77	77	0	0	154
"Quarter"-normal saline (0.2 NS)[a]	30	30	0	0	60
Ringer lactate	130	109	4	28	271

[a] The term "quarter" normal saline is technically inaccurate but commonly used for convenience. The solution is actually one-fifth normal saline.

approach, the hourly rate of fluid therapy would be 40 cc/h (for the first 10 kg) plus 2 cc/h for next 4 kg or 48 cc/h. For patients weighing more than 80 kg, the relationship of body weight and water distribution diverges significantly, so that this sliding scale calculation is likely to overestimate fluid requirements.

Maintenance fluids provide for losses from only evaporative (insensible) sources and urinary losses. Loss of fluids and electrolytes from other sources are termed third-space losses and, if they occur, must be added to maintenance fluids to sustain euvolemia.

Solute-free water that evaporates from the skin and lungs is termed insensible water loss (IWL) because losses from these sites were not readily appreciated. Water is evaporated from the lungs for thermal regulation and to humidify inspired air and from the skin to regulate core body temperature by means of convection and conduction. Skin losses are not ordinary sweat. In the usual environment, and under ordinary conditions, IWL amounts to about one-third of the calculated maintenance fluids. IWL will be slightly greater, approximately 40%, in infants and smaller, 25%, in adolescents. Ambient temperature and humidity have a significant effect on the volume of IWL. Increased IWL should be anticipated when children are hyperthermic or tachypneic, are placed under a radiant warmer, or otherwise are exposed to a dry or particularly hot environment. Hyperthermia greater than 38°C increases IWL by 12.5% per °C. In contrast, evaporative fluid losses are reduced when children receive humidified air or become hypothermic. The proportion of IWL is about two-thirds via skin and one-third via lungs.

Maintenance fluid volume is predicated on the ability of the kidney to excrete isosthenuric urine (specific gravity 1.010; urine osmolarity 280–310 mOsm/L). Urinary losses are assumed to account for two-thirds of maintenance volume. For younger children urine output is anticipated at approximately 2 cc/kg/h. In clinical situations in which concentrating ability is altered (diabetes insipidus, prematurity, sickle-cell disease) or the renal solute load (administration of total parenteral nutrition) is increased, a more dilute urine or increased isotonic volume of urine should be anticipated, and the amount of maintenance fluids should be increased. Alternatively, clinical situations that are associated with persistently concentrated urine (excessive ADH secretion or CHF) require that the volume of maintenance fluids be decreased.

The composition of maintenance fluids must account for electrolytes (Na, K, and Cl) as well as energy needs. Based on empiric studies, 3 meq of sodium and chloride and 2 meq of potassium are required for each 100 kcal expended or for each 100 mL of fluid lost. These electrolytes will maintain homeostasis and allow for new cell growth. The addition of 5 g of dextrose in each 100 mL of fluid provides sufficient calories to avert ketosis and minimizes endogenous protein catabolism. Therefore, the parenteral fluid solution recommended for maintenance fluid therapy contains 30 meq/L of sodium and chloride, 20 meq/L of potassium, and 50

g/L of dextrose: D5 0.2 NS plus 20 meq/L KCl. Because potassium is usually added as KCl, the chloride content will exceed the maintenance requirement but is well tolerated. The sodium and chloride composition of fluids relative to normal saline is given in Table 21-5.

After a judicious calculation has been made and an appropriate fluid administered, evaluating the adequacy of maintenance fluids is essential and is based on changes in body weight, serum sodium (S_{Na}) concentration, and the overall status of the patient. Because maintenance therapy provides for only 20% of the caloric expenditure, patients can be anticipated to lose 0.5% to 1% body weight per day. If the volume of fluid being administered is less than full maintenance volume, and the concentration of glucose in that fluid is not increased, the loss of body weight will be even greater. If adequate fluids and electrolytes to meet the ongoing losses are provided, the S_{Na} concentration should remain between 130 and 140 meq/L. Increased weight combined with a fall in S_{Na} or the development of peripheral edema suggests overhydration. If not, iatrogenic factors that could have reduced either IWL or urine volume losses must be determined. In contrast, a very rapid loss of weight, combined with increased S_{Na} and/or a persistent tachycardia, would suggest inadequate fluids, and assessment of factors that might be increasing fluid losses must be undertaken. This assessment of children receiving parenteral fluid therapy is an ongoing and dynamic process that requires vigilance.

DEFICIT THERAPY

The limited ability of the kidney to maximally concentrate the urine combined with relatively larger surface area from which fluid is evaporated makes infants and young children particularly susceptible to dehydration (from common abnormalities such as gastroenteritis, diarrhea, vomiting, and excessive fluid losses). The limited urinary concentrating ability is the result of decreased urea deposition in the medullary portion of the kidney, which lowers the concentrating gradient and is a reflection of the normal development of renal function and the fact that young children generate less urea because protein is used for anabolic processes (see Sec. 21.2). Consequently, a narrow margin of reserve exists for these children when exposed to third-space (non-IWL or urinary) losses such as vomiting or diarrhea, and a state of dehydration ensues.

Three essential components must be assessed in the evaluation of a child with dehydration: (1) estimate the degree or severity of the dehydration, (2) determine the type of deficit, and (3) develop and implement a plan to repair the deficit.

The degree or severity of dehydration is estimated from the patient's history and clinical condition at the time of initial presentation. *No* piece of laboratory data (other than a documented change in body weight) can predict the degree or severity of de-

DEGREE OR SEVERITY OF DEHYDRATION
Percent Decrease in Body Weight

	MILD	MODERATE	SEVERE	EXTREME
Infants	1%_____ ⇨	5%_____ ⇨	10%_____ ⇨	15%_____ ⇨
Older Child	1%_____ ⇨	3%_____ ⇨	6%_____ ⇨	9%_____ ⇨

History of Losses	**Poor skin turgor**	**Orthostatic Hypotension**	**Shock**
Minimal Signs	**Sunken Eyes/Fontanel**	**Tachycardia**	
Decreased Frequency	**Lack of Tears**	**Oliguria**	
of Urination	**Lethargy**	**Decreased Sensation**	

FIGURE 21-7   Clinical features used to estimate degree of dehydration.

hydration. This estimation must be based on clinical observations. Numerous signs and symptoms have been evaluated to help make this clinical estimate more quantitative. In large part, a few easily remembered parameters will suffice (Fig. 21-7). Care must be taken not to overinterpret capillary refill because this sign is highly susceptible to environmental conditions such ambient temperature.

With *mild* (1–5%) dehydration, the findings are largely historical, ie, history of 12 to 24 hours of vomiting/diarrhea, etc, with minimal findings on physical examination. With *moderate* (6–10%) dehydration the patient has a history of abnormal fluid and electrolyte losses plus physical findings that include tenting of skin, sunken eyes and fontanel, slight lethargy, and dry lips and mouth. With *severe* (11–15%) dehydration, the patient will usually develop findings of cardiovascular instability (mottling of skin, tachycardia, hypotension) and neurologic involvement (extreme irritability, coma). Dehydration over a protracted period may be more severe than clinically evident. This initial assessment is almost always subjective unless a change in body weight has been documented. Although the evaluation of a specific patient by several skilled observers may produce widely varying estimates of the degree of dehydration, this assessment is essential and provides one of the key elements for developing a plan for deficit fluid therapy.

The type of deficit that is present can best be estimated from the patient's electrolyte values at the time of presentation. In large part, the type of dehydration is defined by the tonicity of the patient's serum. On this basis, states of dehydration are commonly referred to as *isotonic* (serum osmolarity 270–300; serum Na 130–150), *hypotonic* (serum osmolarity <270; serum Na <130), and *hypertonic* (serum osmolarity >310; serum Na >155). Serum osmolarity is related to BUN and glucose concentration:

$$\text{serum osmolarity} = 2\,(\text{Na meq/L}) + \frac{\text{BUN (mg/dl)}}{2.8} + \frac{\text{Glucose (mg/dl)}}{18}$$

Therefore, if BUN and glucose are in the normal ranges, the serum osmolarity may be estimated by 2 (Na). For clinical purposes these terms are used to define a type of dehydration, but the patient's serum electrolyte levels are actually a mirror image of the type of losses that have occurred. For example, in a patient who has hypotonic dehydration (ie, $S_{Na} < 130$ meq/L), the losses have consisted of more sodium than water, or the replacement fluid has contained an excess of free water. Because the pathophysiological adaptation to dehydration limits water excretion, the patient who takes in a great deal of fluid free of electrolytes will become hypo-

tonic. Similarly, in hypertonic dehydration ($S_{Na} > 155$ meq/L), the fluid that was lost consisted of more water than electrolytes, as occurs in certain types of diarrhea in which the electrolyte losses may be very low but the water losses quite high, or when IWL is increased because IWL does not contain electrolytes. Patients with isotonic or hypotonic dehydration are treated quite similarly, whereas patients with hypertonic dehydration require special attention because of serious complications during rehydration. From a practical perspective, calculations are based on the patient's weight at presentation, not the estimated normal weight.

Many approaches to the repair of fluid deficits exist, and each system has proponents, but in the final analysis, most of these programs are interchangeable; no one approach is superior to any other, and all share common principles. Initially concern should be focused on the reasonably rapid restoration and preservation of cardiovascular function to improve the perfusion of the brain and kidneys and to allow the adaptive mechanisms to reestablish intravascular volume. This first phase of therapy (frequently called the bolus) should consist of the rapid infusion of a relatively isotonic fluid such as normal saline or Ringer lactate. If a child predominantly has vomiting (eg, the infant with pyloric stenosis), Ringer lactate should not be used because the lactate will exacerbate the metabolic alkalosis associated with loss of gastric acid. Most oral rehydration fluids contain some buffer, which could exacerbate alkalosis in young children with severe vomiting. For mild or moderate dehydration, infusion of 10 to 20 mL/kg (1–2% body weight) over 1 to 2 hours should be done. If the patient is severely dehydrated, 30 to 50 mL/kg/h should be given and continued until cardiovascular signs are stable. This initial rapid infusion of isotonic fluid serves several purposes: (1) it provides time to obtain and assess the initial laboratory data; (2) it prevents the patient from becoming increasingly dehydrated; and (3) it allows the development of a comprehensive plan for replacement of fluid deficits. The quantity of fluid administered during this initial bolus therapy is not taken into account in subsequent calculations.

The second phase of therapy is designed to replace the deficit of fluids and electrolytes that has occurred. Basic principles pertain to many different plans. (1) Total body repair occurs over a relatively prolonged period in all types of dehydration. (2) Total body potassium losses cannot be replaced immediately because potassium is predominantly an intracellular ion, and rapid infusion of concentrated solutions of potassium are of little value and potentially quite dangerous. Therefore, potassium is added to the rehydration solution only after the patient has voided twice and then in concentrations that generally do not exceed 40 meq/L or a rate of infusion of 0.5 meq/kg/h. (3) Half-normal saline (77 meq Na and Cl) serves well to replace the deficits in both salt and water because this solution provides more sodium than standard maintenance fluids and more water, proportional to sodium, than is contained in plasma.

As examples of specific approaches to repair of deficits, two plans are presented (Table 21-6). In plan I, no provision is made for maintenance fluid requirements during the period of deficit repair. The infusion rate is calculated and adjusted to replace all of the estimated deficit in 6 to 8 hours. This program has the advantage of allowing the therapist to concentrate on one aspect (ie, deficit therapy) of the patient's need at one time and to consider the other aspects of fluid therapy separately. In some cases, plan I requires the relatively rapid infusion of large volumes of fluid and, therefore, is less feasible for use in adolescents, patients with diabetic keto-acidosis, infants with hypertonic dehydration, or children with more than 10% dehydration. In these circumstances and in older children, plan II is preferable. Plan II provides a slower and more prolonged repair of the deficit. In this program, provision is made for estimated maintenance needs during the period of deficit repair. As in plan I, this also provides a physiological approach to the repair of deficits but requires slightly more complex computations. The rate of infusion is calculated as maintenance rate plus sufficient fluid to replace half of the deficit over 8 hours. In children who weigh 10 kg or less, the volume of fluid to be administered will be quite similar in both plans I and II. For example, a 10-kg child who is 10% dehydrated would have an estimated deficit of 1000 ml. In plan I replacing the entire deficit (1000 ml) in 8 hours would give an infusion rate of 125 ml/h. In plan II, half the deficit (500 ml) is replaced over 8 hours (62.5 ml/h), and maintenance fluids are given (40 ml/h, see Table 21-4) for a total infusion rate of 102 ml/h. Either of these approaches is quite satisfactory for the re-hydration of patients with isotonic or hypotonic dehydration but not for infants or children with hypertonic dehydration.

Children with hypertonic dehydration represent a very special and complex problem that necessitates careful assessment and a

TABLE 21-6
AN APPROACH FOR REPAIR OF DEFICITS[a]

Phase 1 (bolus)

Rapid restoration of intravascular volume
Rate: 10–30 mL/kg/h
Fluid: isotonic solution
Duration: 1–2 hours depending on degree of dehydration and initial response

Phase 2 Replacement of deficit

Plan I	Plan II
Isotonic/hypotonic patients <25 kg	Hyperosmolar patients or weight >25 kg
Rate: replace entire deficit	Half of deficit plus maintenance
Fluid: D5 0.5 NS + 20 meq/L KCl[b]	D5 0.5 NS + 20 meq/L KCl[b]
Duration: 6–8 hours, less if clinically improved	6–8 hours, less if clinically improved

Phase 3 Maintenance needs plus ongoing losses

Rate: maintenance calculation (Table 21-4) plus third-space losses
Fluid: D5 0.2 NS plus 20 meq/L KCl[b]
Duration: as needed depending on clinical situation

[a] For patients with hypertonic dehydration ($S_{Na} > 155$ meq/L), see text.
[b] Add KCl only after patient voids twice.

change in the rapidity of deficit repair. The usual signs of dehydration (see Fig. 21-7) tend to underestimate the degree of dehydration. Because the deficit of Na is less than in other forms of dehydration, a lower concentration of Na in the repair fluid would seem appropriate. However, a very dilute solution given rapidly will cause water shifts into dehydrated hypertonic cells and can cause cerebral edema. Consequently, the rate of fluid administration is the primary concern, and either D5 0.2 NS or D5 0.5 NS may be used. The estimated deficit should be replaced over 24 to 48 hours (and maintenance fluids should be given concomitantly). The rate of fluid infusion should be adjusted so a fall in S_{Na} of 0.5 meq/L/h or approximately 12 meq/L/d is desirable. Hypertonic dehydration may be complicated by hypocalcemia, which occurs infrequently, or hyperglycemia. If the patient is symptomatic, calcium gluconate can be given IV very slowly with the aid of a cardiac monitor. Hyperglycemia occurs because of reduced insulin secretion and decreased cell sensitivity to insulin. In evaluating the rate of decline in S_{Na}, the effect of hyperglycemia must be taken into account. The measured S_{Na} is suppressed by 1.6 meq/L for each 100 mg/dL the serum glucose is above 100 mg/dL. For example, a S_{Na} of 170 meq/L with a serum glucose of 600 mg/dL is an effective S_{Na} of 178 meq/L (600 − 100 = 500; 500 × 1.6/100 = 8).

In all types of dehydration, this second phase of deficit therapy must be monitored carefully. Because the initial estimate of the degree of dehydration is based on subjective criteria, the patient's clinical response indicates the adequacy and duration of therapy. For example, the urine normally will be quite concentrated initially (specific gravity between 1.020 and 1.030), and a progressive decrease in the urine specific gravity and a progressive increase in the frequency of urination are expected. Although a specific rate of infusion may have been chosen to deliver a calculated amount of fluid over a fixed period, adjustments according to the patient's clinical response should occur. If the patient has persistent tachycardia and continues to demonstrate the signs of dehydration, the degree of dehydration may have been underestimated initially, or the ongoing losses have been more substantial than anticipated. In such circumstances, the rate of fluid administration will need to be increased, or an additional bolus of fluids given. In situations in which the patient's clinical condition improves rapidly, urine output is brisk, urine specific gravity is decreasing progressively, and the signs of intravascular volume depletion are diminished, the duration of the second phase of deficit repair may be curtailed, and the patient switched to maintenance fluids.

The third phase of deficit therapy is essentially maintenance fluids combined with replacement of ongoing third-space losses.

REPLACEMENT THERAPY

Fluids designed to replenish ongoing losses, other than IWL or urine output, are termed replacement therapy. The electrolyte composition in body fluids can vary considerably from patient to patient and is sufficiently different from the fluids used for maintenance or deficit therapy or for intravenous alimentation. When third-space losses continue for a significant period, the electrolyte content of those fluids should be determined, and replacement fluids that contain appropriate electrolytes should be administered on a volume-for-volume basis. If ongoing losses are replaced with parenteral alimentation, significant derangement of serum electrolytes may occur because the renal solute load presented will challenge the concentrating capacity and may obligate sufficient intracellular water to be used for the excretion of excessive solutes. In such circumstances, the patient clinically becomes increasingly dehydrated despite large volumes of fluid being given and large volumes of urine being excreted. If patients have an ileus, ascites, burns, or open wounds, judging the magnitude of third-space loss is difficult, and monitoring central volume for a more accurate estimate of these ongoing losses and more judicious planning for replacement therapy will be required.

ORAL HYDRATION

The oral administration of specific fluids and electrolytes to correct fluid deficits has been of interest for the past 40 years. Traditionally, a number of commercially available products have been used for initial rehydration for children with gastroenteritis. The electrolyte content of these products is highly variable, but the safety of this approach is probably related to the short duration of episodes of viral gastroenteritis. Because of untoward side effects of "home brews," particularly the development of hypernatremia, considerable concern about the appropriate sodium concentration for oral rehydration ensued. Most likely the use of ordinary kitchen utensils for the preparation of these solutions frequently led to aberrant electrolyte contents. However, the critical factor for the development of hypernatremia turned out to be the volume of fluid administered, not the sodium concentration. A number of commercially available nonprescription oral rehydration solutions are available. All of them contain (per liter): glucose/carbohydrate 20 to 30 g; Na 45 to 50 meq; Cl 35 to 80 meq; K 20 to 25 meq; citrate 30 to 34 meq; and 200 to 330 mOsm. The efficacies of these solutions are similar when administered appropriately. Basic principles for oral rehydration include the following:

1. High concentrations of carbohydrate may result in water losses and prolonged diarrhea because of the rapid transit time, bacterial overgrowth of the small intestine, and disaccharidase deficiencies. Early oral rehydration products should contain 2 to 3 g of carbohydrate per 100 mL of solution to maximize absorption, and fluids specifically designed for oral hydration, not common beverages or home brews, should be prescribed.
2. The total amount of fluid ingested is more critical than the sodium concentration. Because diarrhea is hypotonic fluid and IWL is also hypotonic, the S_{Na} will progressively rise if an inadequate volume of hypotonic fluid is given or retained.
3. Oral rehydration is most feasible in children with less than 10% dehydration. If patients are hemodynamically unstable, have large stool losses (> 10 cc/kg/h), or have an ileus, intravenous fluids will be required.
4. Oral rehydration is personnel-intense and requires that the child be given small volumes of fluid at very regular intervals; it must be planned and monitored as closely as parenteral fluid therapy.

21.4.2   Basic Concepts in Assessment of Fluid and Electrolyte Disorders

The assessment of infants, children, and adolescents who present with abnormalities in the volume of urine being excreted or the electrolyte composition of serum can be confusing and unnecessarily complex unless a systematic approach is undertaken. The first step is a careful determination of the patient's hydration or volume status. Patients with volume depletion or dehydration may exhibit classical clinical signs (see Fig. 21-7), but in many circumstances, more subtle findings such as increased pulse without fever or diminished peripheral perfusion will be important to detect. If a decrease in body weight is documented, particularly over a short in-

terval, depletion of extracellular volume can be assumed. Patients who are euvolemic generally manifest few clinical signs, and their weight should be stable. The development of generalized edema can be assumed to represent an increase in total body salt and water and will inevitably be accompanied by an increase in body weight. After a patient's volume status has been ascertained, the reabsorption of sodium and water by the kidney can be used as an index of renal perfusion and intravascular volume/tonicity.

The intact kidney responds to diminished renal perfusion in a reasonably predictable and consistent manner (Fig. 21-8). Initially, glomerular filtration rate (GFR) is maintained because of afferent arteriolar vasodilatation and constriction of the efferent arteriole (see Sec. 21.2). Because renal plasma flow is diminished, the postglomerular capillaries have an increase in protein concentration, which results in enhanced peritubular capillary reabsorption in the proximal tubule and a nearly maximal reabsorption of sodium at this site. Because aldosterone secretion has been stimulated in response to angiotensin II produced by increased renin secretion, sodium reabsorption in the distal tubule and early collecting duct is also maximized. Together, these forces result in a nearly maximal retention of the filtered load of sodium. Concomitantly, release of ADH in response to volume depletion increases the permeability of the collecting ducts, and enhanced water reabsorption in this final segment of the nephron results in an increase in urinary osmolality. Thus, when renal perfusion is diminished, the physiological sequence of events that affect both salt and water reabsorption combine to increase intravascular volume. Consequently, if the patient is volume depleted (such as dehydrated from gastroenteritis), this sequence of events will restore intravascular volume, but if the patient is volume replete (such as in CHF), edema occurs. Likewise, if renal perfusion is increased or intravascular volume is expanded, a decrease in sodium and water reabsorption would be anticipated. Of importance, these expected physiological responses of the kidney are reliable only if the kidney is intact and unaffected by pharmacologic manipulations, principally diuretic administration.

From a clinical perspective, the assessment of urinary sodium and water excretion can be used to define and evaluate disorders of urine volume and serum electrolytes (Table 21-7). Urinary sodium

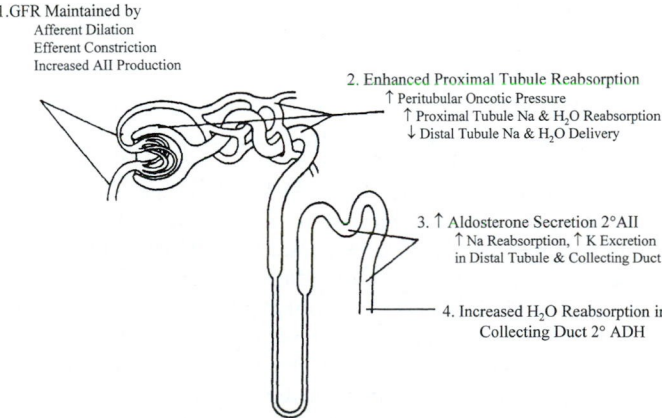

FIGURE 21-8   **The renal response to decreased perfusion results in maximal reabsorption of Na and H_2O. In states of dehydration, these adaptive mechanisms restore intravascular volume. In states of excess extracellular volume (CHF, nephrotic syndrome, etc), edema formation results. These responses are the basis of the interpretation of urinary indices for evaluation of fluid and electrolyte disorders (Table 21-7). GFR = glomerular filtration rate; AII = angiotensin II; Na = sodium; K = potassium; ADH = anti-diuretic hormone.**

TABLE 21-7

BASIC CONCEPTS IN ASSESSMENT OF FLUID AND ELECTROLYTE DISORDERS

CONDITIONS ASSOCIATED WITH STABLE OR INCREASED BODY WEIGHT	RENAL REABSORPTION		CONDITIONS ASSOCIATED WITH DECREASED BODY WEIGHT
	SODIUM	WATER	
Hypoalbuminemia (nephrosis, cirrhosis, malnutrition, enteropathy)	Maximal	High	Diarrhea, vomiting, cystic fibrosis
Congenital heart failure			
Acute glomerulonephritis			
Acute volume expansion (water intoxication, excess IV fluid)	Increased	Low	Diabetes insipidus (central or nephrogenic)
Acute renal failure (sepsis, shock, nephrotoxin)	Decreased	Impaired	Adrenal insufficiency, salt-losing nephropathy (interstitial nephritis), cystic disease, or obstructive nephropathy
Nonphysiological ADH secretion (SIADH)	Decreased	High	Diabetic ketoacidosis, osmotic diuretics

For children 1 year of age or older

Maximal sodium reabsorption: $U_{Na} < 20$ meq/L or $FE_{Na} < 1\%$

Decreased sodium reabsorption: $U_{Na} > 50$ meq/L or $FE_{Na} > 2\%$

High water reabsorption: $U_{Osm} > 500$ mOsm/L or $U/P_{Osm} > 1.5\%$

Low or impaired water reabsorption: $U_{Osm} \leq 300$ mOsm/L or $U/P_{Osm} < 1.2\%$

processing is reflected by sodium concentration in the urine (U_{Na}). In some circumstances, particularly hyponatremic states, fractional excretion of sodium (FE_{Na}) is a more accurate reflection of the renal handling of sodium. FE_{Na} can be simply calculated by the urine-to-plasma ratio of sodium divided by the urine-to-plasma ratio of creatinine and can be obtained on a spot urine. Sodium excretion reflects renal perfusion *independent* of the S_{Na} concentration. Thus, if the urinary sodium excretion is low, renal perfusion is expected to be decreased unless there is a tubular defect in sodium handling. Likewise, if urinary sodium excretion is high, renal perfusion should be increased unless there is an intrinsic or pharmacologic abnormality in the renal tubule handling of sodium. Thus, if urinary sodium excretion is elevated in a clinical circumstance associated with volume depletion or reduced body weight, a reabsorptive defect in sodium by the kidney must be identified.

Water reabsorption by the kidney is reflected in urinary osmolarity or the ratio of urinary osmolality to plasma osmolality (U/P Osm). If the U_{Osm} is elevated at least 1.5 times the S_{Osm}, ADH must be acting on the collecting duct irrespective of absolute value of the U_{Osm}. Consequently, absolute values of urine osmolality may not be an accurate reflection of ADH release in patients with significant or severe hypotonic serum: If S_{Osm} is 240 mOsm/L, U_{Osm} of only 360 mOsm/L would be indicative of an ADH effect. Because the physiological stimuli for ADH release are either an increase in S_{Osm} or S_{Na} or a decrease in intravascular volume, determining whether or not ADH is causing water reabsorption is an important component of evaluating fluid and electrolyte disorders. If U_{Osm} is high or U/P Osm > 1.5 without evidence of increased S_{Osm} or decreased intravascular volume, ADH is being secreted in a nonphysiological manner irrespective of urine volume. Combining an assessment of the patient's hydration status with an evaluation of the urinary indices can be extremely helpful in identifying specific causes for abnormalities of urine volume or derangements in serum electrolytes.

21.4.3 Disorders of Urine Volume

In euvolemic patients receiving adequate fluids, a urine output of 1.5 to 3 mL/kg/h would be expected. The assumption that changes in urine output are a direct reflection of renal function is an oversimplification of complex renal physiology. In most circumstances, the kidney maintains intravascular volume and plasma tonicity by balancing the processes of filtration, reabsorption, and secretion. If GFR is about 100 mL/min, an initial filtrate of 144 L contains 20,160 meq (460 g) of sodium entering the proximal tubule each day. The renal tubule and collecting duct reabsorb 98 to 99% of this filtrate, resulting in a final urine output of about 2 L/d, which contains 4 g of sodium.

Thus, urine volume alone is not a direct reflection of GFR. For example, if the reabsorptive processes are enhanced, increased tubule fluid is reabsorbed, and urine output may fall while glomerular filtration rate remains normal. Alternatively, GFR could be reduced severely, but a concomitant reduction in tubular fluid reabsorption would result in what would appear to be a normal urine volume. Thus, urine volume should not be interpreted as a measure of GFR, which must be estimated from serum values of creatinine and BUN (see Sec. 21.5). Either oliguria or polyuria can be assessed best by using the systemic approach outlined in Table 21-7.

ASSESSMENT OF OLIGURIA

Oliguria is defined as less than half of the expected urine volume (less than 0.8 mL/kg/h). Determining prerenal, renal, and postrenal causes, although seemingly logical, does not follow physiological principles and, at times, can be misleading and inaccurate. The causes of oliguria are understood better if considered in terms of anatomic and pathophysiological abnormalities. Anatomic abnormalities are uncommon because obstruction or occlusion of renal arteries, renal veins, or ureters must be bilateral to cause oliguria. The compensatory changes in the contralateral unaffected kidney will compensate physiologically within minutes, and unilateral obstruction at any of these anatomic sites will not produce a perceptible decrease in urine output. On the other hand, bladder outlet obstruction will cause significant oliguria and should be evaluated particularly in male infants, who may have posterior urethral valves. An obstructed bladder is usually palpable and can easily be detected with a renal ultrasound examination.

The pathophysiological causes of oliguria include decreased intravascular volume or impaired renal perfusion, acute tubular necrosis, and inappropriate ADH secretion (SIADH). Oliguria that occurs because of diminished intravascular volume or diminished renal perfusion results from maximally enhanced reabsorption of sodium and water in all nephron segments including the collecting duct (ie, ADH has been released physiologically in response to baro-receptors). Consequently, the urinary sodium concentration or FE_{Na} should be quite low (usually less than 20 meq/L or 1%, respectively), and the urinary osmolarity or U/P Osm should be high (> 500 mOsm/L or > 1.5, respectively). For children less than 1 year of age comparable values would be $U_{Na} < 30$ meq/L, $FE_{Na} < 2\%$, UOsm > 400 mOsm/L, and U/P Osm > 1.25. The term prerenal azotemia is used to denote a BUN-to-creatinine ratio greater than 20. In patients with decreased intravascular volume or diminished renal perfusion, the increase in BUN in relation to serum creatinine is a reflection of maximized reabsorption of solute including urea. Because creatinine is impermeable to the tubule epithelium and is not affected by the forces driving enhanced reabsorption, the BUN-to-creatinine ratio rises. Intravascular volume depletion occurs in conditions associated with dehydration or reduced weight, and diminished renal perfusion occurs in congestive heart failure, hypoalbuminemic states, and acute glomerulonephritis (see Table 21-7). In the latter condition, the inflammatory reaction in the glomerulus causes diminished perfusion in the postglomerular capillary bed, which invokes the same hemodynamic response as is encountered in patients with volume depletion.

Oliguria that occurs in patients with acute tubule necrosis (ATN) results from the abrupt loss of glomerular filtration because of severe renal vasoconstriction, back-leak of fluid from the tubular lumen to the capillaries, and intratubular obstruction from sloughed injured epithelial cells (see Sec. 21.7). Clinically, both the BUN and the serum creatinine concentrations increase, and tubule function is significantly diminished. The term acute tubular necrosis, although inappropriate from an anatomic perspective, is a very good reflection of tubular function in patients with an acute established renal insult, and the urinary indices are characterized by diminished sodium reabsorption, U_{Na} usually usually greater than 50 meq/L and FE_{Na} usually greater than 2%, and impaired water reabsorption (U_{Osm} 280–300 mOsm/L and U/P Osm ≤ 1.0). The small amounts of urine produced are isotonic to plasma, and a dilute urine would be as unexpected as a concentrated urine in patients with ATN. A low U_{Na} may occur when ATN follows the administration of contrast media.

Because ADH has a powerful effect on water reabsorption from the collecting duct, a significant decline in urine output and oliguria may occur when the hormone is active. Under homeostatic conditions secretion of this hormone from the posterior pituitary is regulated closely by osmolar and volume receptors. A 2% increase in plasma osmolarity will result in the release of enough ADH to produce antidiuresis, whereas a 1 to 2% decrease in plasma osmolarity will suppress ADH secretion. Baroreceptors modulate the release of ADH in response to changes in intravascular volume. If evidence of stimulation of either osmolar or volume receptors is lacking, secretion of this hormone is termed inappropriate or nonphysiological (SIADH). Patients with SIADH have a persistently concentrated urine ($U_{Osm} > 500$, U/P Osm > 1.5) in association with decreasing plasma osmolarity and expansion of intravascular volume. The water reabsorbed from the collecting duct enters the plasma and produces a dilution of the electrolytes, BUN, and uric acid ($S_{Na} < 135$ meq/L, BUN < 15 mg/dL, and uric acid < 2 mg/dL). Expansion of the intravascular space with water reabsorbed from the collecting duct results in diminished sodium reabsorption reflected by $U_{Na} > 50$ meq/L or $FE_{Na} > 2\%$ (see Table

21-7). The findings of concentrated urine despite a fall in the S_{Na} level associated with an elevated U_{Na} is considered diagnostic of SIADH. The condition is considered nonphysiological or inappropriate because the osmolar receptors have not been stimulated (S_{Na} is declining) and the baroreceptors should not have been stimulated (the increased U_{Na} indicates replete intravascular volume). This persistently concentrated urine cannot be accounted for by the known physiological regulators of ADH release.

After appropriate laboratory studies from both blood and urine have been completed, a specific cause for oliguria may not be evident. If, on clinical examination, the patient does not have overt evidence of fluid overload, a volume challenge of isotonic fluid may be indicated (20 mL/kg/h). Because the fluid being administered is isotonic, hyponatremia, which may be associated with ATN or SIADH, would not be exacerbated, and if the oliguria is secondary to volume depletion, an increase in urine output may result. Alternately, a potent loop-acting diuretic such as furosemide (4 mg/kg intravenously) would produce a diuresis even in patients with volume depletion, which might exacerbate the clinical situation if the urine formed is not replaced adequately. Diuretics would be unlikely to produce a diuresis in patients with established acute renal failure. Both of these manipulations will invalidate the use of urinary sodium and osmolarity as a diagnostic index (see Table 21-7).

ASSESSMENT OF POLYURIA

Polyuria, more than 4 mL/kg/h of urine output, arises in response to the excretion of a volume load or a tubular defect in salt or water reabsorption. During the excretion of a volume load, patients will appear well hydrated and have either a stable or a slightly increased body weight. The indices of renal salt and water reabsorption will depend on the type of fluid ingested or administered and the duration of diuresis. In the early phases of volume diuresis intravascular volume is expanded, the sodium reabsorption is diminished (U_{Na} and FE_{Na} are elevated), and as the diuresis progresses, sodium reabsorption will reflect the type of fluid given. Most often, volume overload occurs secondary to overzealous parenteral fluid therapy in attempts to promote good urine output or to protect the kidney from nephrotoxins such as chemotherapeutic agents or antibiotics. All sources of fluid should be accounted for in polyuric patients, including enteral, intraoperative, and blood products. The simplest therapy is to restrict additional fluid intake until the urine output returns to expected rates.

Polyuria also may arise when the GFR exceeds the tubular reabsorptive capacity. Patients in whom there is a tubular defect in sodium or water reabsorption generally will appear dehydrated or have a decrease in body weight. In a euvolemic state the tubule normally reabsorbs 142 L of fluid and 458 g of sodium, so even a small decrease in tubular reabsorptive capacity will result in a marked diuresis. Defects in tubular reabsorption occur in interstitial nephritis, cystic disease of the kidney, or obstructive nephropathy, and despite evidence of intravascular volume depletion, urinary sodium reabsorption is decreased (elevated U_{Na} and FE_{Na}), and water reabsorption is impaired ($U_{Osm} \leq 300$ mOsm/L and U/P Osm < 1.2). Usually, these renal disorders will be apparent from other clinical findings, but some patients with nonoliguric ATN will actually have polyuria, especially with aminoglycoside toxicity.

Finally, diabetes insipidus, in which there is either a lack of ADH secretion by the posterior pituitary or a failure of the collecting duct to respond to this hormone, invariably presents with a marked increase in urine output (see Sec. 21.11). Because the tubule reabsorptive capacity for sodium is intact, the marked diuresis is almost purely a water diuresis, and the U_{Na} and FE_{Na} are low because of intravascular volume depletion. Without ADH, the renal reabsorption of water is markedly impaired, and U_{Osm} and U/P Osm are low. Classically, these patients have a dilute urine despite a rise in S_{Na} and a decrease in intravascular volume, the two stimuli for ADH release.

21.4.4   Electrolyte Disorders

SODIUM DISORDERS

Total body sodium content is carefully controlled by two physiological processes. The S_{Na} and extracellular concentration are modulated largely through the regulation and excretion of *water*. Osmoregulatory processes, including thirst and secretion of ADH, have a major effect on the concentration of Na in serum. The renal handling of sodium (see Sec. 21.2 and 21.4.2) is a reflection of renal perfusion independent of S_{Na}. The kidney responds to subtle changes in intravascular volume by altering the reabsorption of sodium in both the proximal and the distal portions of the nephron. Thus, the S_{Na} is controlled by the interplay of total body sodium and total body water. Consequently, alterations in S_{Na} may be caused by abnormalities in sodium intake or water excretion: too much or too little salt, too much or too little water (Figs. 21-9 and 21-10).

HYPONATREMIA Hyponatremia, defined as S_{Na} less than 130 meq/L, is a common electrolyte abnormality (Fig. 21-9). A low S_{Na} may be an artifact if the blood sample was drawn through an indwelling catheter that was not cleared adequately or was proximal to a rapidly infusing hypotonic intravenous fluid. Significant hyperlipidemia may cause an increase in serum solids, and a low S_{Na} value will be reported unless the laboratory is aware of the lipid abnormality when the sample is processed. In patients with hyperglycemia the S_{Na} does not reflect the effective sodium concentration (see Sec. 21.4.1, Deficit Therapy). If the S_{Na} value is not an artifact, a systematic approach outlined in Fig. 21-9 will lead to a specific diagnosis based on an assessment of the patient's state of hydration combined with urinary indices.

In patients whose weight has decreased, loss of salt from urine, sweat, tears, or the gastrointestinal tract is the likely cause of hyponatremia. Except in situations in which renal salt loss occurs, the U_{Na} should be reduced (usually less than 20 meq/L) and U_{Osm} increased (usually greater than 500 mOsm/L). In patients with vomiting or diarrhea, the source of salt loss is obvious. In infants and young children with cystic fibrosis, however, the loss of sodium in sweat can be substantial and may not be evident, but concomitant losses of chloride in these infants frequently result in hypochloremic metabolic alkalosis without a history of vomiting.

When hyponatremic patients have clinical evidence of volume depletion but an elevated U_{Na} concentration, either an intrinsic or an extrinsic renal defect should be suspected: multicystic dysplastic kidney, polycystic kidney disease, acute interstitial nephritis, urinary tract obstruction, or acute tubular necrosis. Adrenal insufficiency or chronic diuretic therapy may cause hyponatremia because of renal sodium losses. Clearly, the combination of hyponatremia and hyperkalemia suggests a diagnosis of adrenal insufficiency in children and adolescents. In newborn infants, both congenital adrenal hyperplasia and urinary tract obstruction present with the same electrolyte abnormalities.

For patients with stable or increased weight and hyponatremia, a primary defect in water excretion must be considered. Defects in any of the five components of free water excretion can be associated with specific clinical conditions. First, diminished or limited GFR will impede the rate at which plasma can be cleared of excess water. Except in premature and very young infants, a defect in GFR is unlikely to cause hyponatremia unless GFR is reduced severely because maximal free water excretion is 10 mL for every 100 mL of GFR. Consequently, in a patient with a GFR of 100 mL/min, excess water can be cleared at a rate of 600 mL/h, and for hyponatremia to result simply from the intake of free water would require the ingestion of more than 1 L/h of electrolyte-free fluid. In healthy children with hyponatremia from excess fluid ingestion, forced water intake as a component of child abuse must be suspected. In contrast, premature and young infants have an intrinsically low GFR (10–30 mL/min) and concomitantly low free water clearance (1–3 mL/min), which contributes substantially to their propensity to develop hyponatremia. If excess fluid intake is the primary cause of hyponatremia, both the U_{Na} and U_{Osm} would be expected to be low if the patient were in the midst of a water diuresis.

The second major component of free water excretion is the delivery of fluid to the diluting segment of the nephron, the ascending limb of the loop of Henle. Consequently, if proximal reabsorption is enhanced, diminished free water excretion will result. In patients who are euvolemic or edematous, augmented proximal reabsorption occurs when effective renal blood flow is decreased in conditions such as congestive heart failure, cirrhosis, or nephrosis. In each of these settings, the U_{Na} would be low, and U_{Osm} would be elevated.

The third step in water excretion involves reabsorption of electrolytes in the diluting segment with water free of electrolytes remaining in the tubule lumen. Loop-acting diuretics and intrinsic renal disease will diminish free water excretion and result in increased U_{Na} and limited U_{Osm}.

Fourth, maximal free water excretion is dependent on corticosteroids and thyroxine. Finally, any condition that causes secretion of ADH will diminish free water excretion because water will be removed from the dilute fluid that has reached the collecting duct. In hyponatremic patients with stable or increased weight, ADH should not be released because the plasma is hypotonic and extracellular volume is replete (ie, neither the baro- nor the osmoreceptors should be activated). Therefore, if clinical evidence suggests ADH release (increased U_{Na} and U_{Osm}), SIADH syndrome is likely. Because SIADH syndrome is associated with overhydration of both the extracellular and the intracellular space along with a shift of sodium ion distribution, edema is uncommon.

Determining whether hyponatremia is from sodium loss or water excess is essential for designing effective therapy. For those patients with hypotonic volume depletion, replacement of salt and water losses by the administration of parenteral or enteral fluids is indicated (see Sec. 21.4.1). In euvolemic or edematous patients with a primary defect in free water excretion, fluid restriction so that free water intake and excretion are matched is the therapeutic goal.

Severe hyponatremia (usually $S_{Na} < 120$ meq/L) may be associated with a clouded sensorium or seizures. These CNS signs appear to be related to the rate of development of hyponatremia. Increasing the S_{Na} level to approximately 125 meq/L by the infusion of hypertonic sodium chloride will diminish or abolish CNS signs. It is not necessary and may be dangerous to rapidly increase S_{Na} above 125 meq/L. Although the amount of sodium needed to

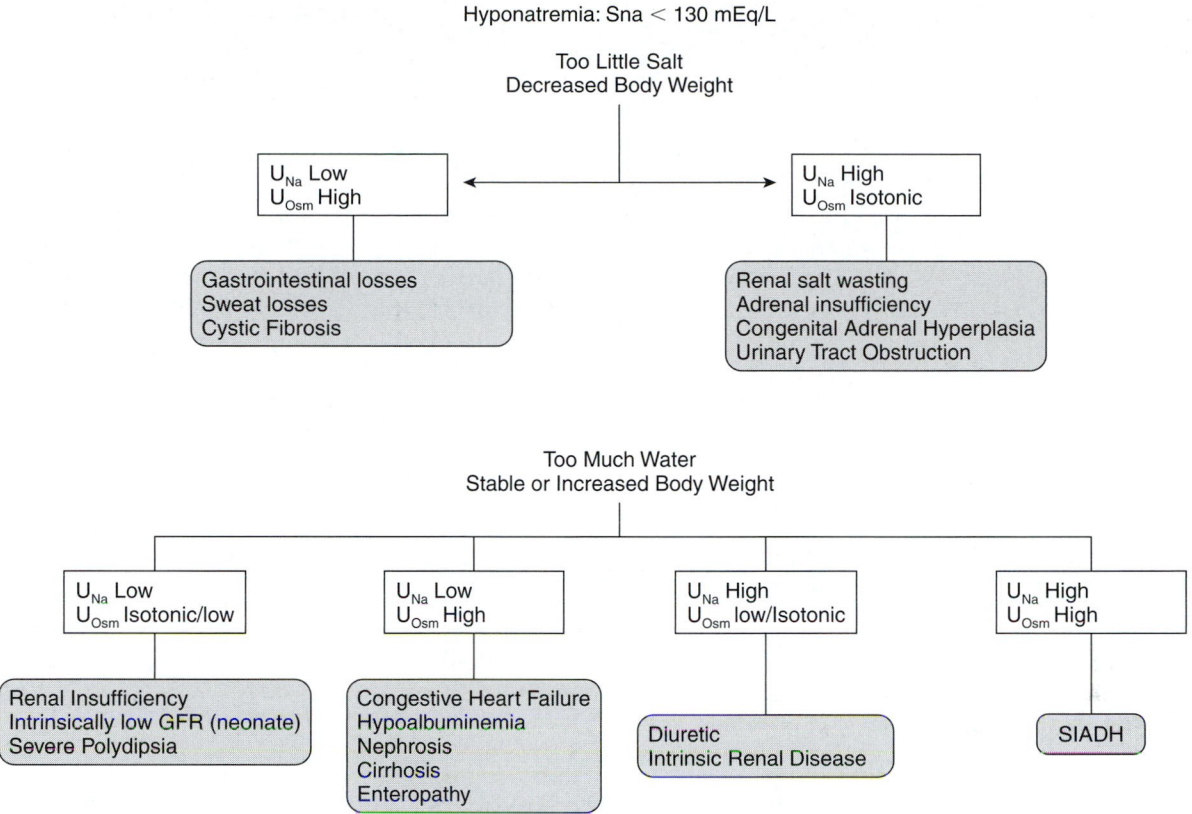

FIGURE 21-9   **Algorithm for assessment of hyponatremia (U_{Na} = urinary sodium concentration;
U_{Osm} = urinary osmolarity).**

correct the S_{Na} can be calculated, the infusion of 12 mL/kg of a
3% saline solution can be estimated to raise the S_{Na} level about 10
meq/L. For those patients with severe hypoalbuminemia and significant or symptomatic hyponatremia, infusion of intravenous albumin to increase effective renal perfusion and enhance free water
excretion may be required. For patients with particularly severe
SIADH and persistent hyponatremia despite fluid restriction, administration of a loop-acting diuretic will increase solute delivery
to the collecting duct, which produces increased urine output, and
replacement of the urine volume with isotonic saline will increase
S_{Na}.

HYPERNATREMIA   Hypernatremia, defined as S_{Na} greater than 150
meq/L, may be caused by too little water or too much salt (Fig.
21-10). The patient's state of hydration is helpful in assessing the
potential causes for hypernatremia. If a patient's body weight is
unchanged or increased slightly, hypernatremia has resulted from
a net increase in total body sodium that has not been accompanied
by an appropriate amount of water. Normally, increased sodium
intake results in transient hypertonicity of plasma, stimulation of
our thirst mechanism, and release of ADH. Acting together these
physiological factors act to restore plasma tonicity to relatively normal values. Patients who receive large quantities of hypertonic so-
dium-containing solutions (such as sodium bicarbonate, which
contains 1 meq/mL) or small children who receive formula with
inadvertently high sodium chloride content, a state of euvolemic
hypernatremia may occur. An elevated S_{Na} would be maintained
only if the offending agent was not recognized or the patient was
unable to request or obtain additional free water. Unless the period
of salt poisoning has been prolonged, eliminating the source of

sodium and providing adequate free water to restore plasma tonicity is appropriate therapy. In unusual and rare patients, extreme
hypernatremia may be related to central hypodipsia because of resetting of the osmolar receptors. Usually these children have had
significant central nervous system insults.

More often, hypernatremia is encountered in the setting of hypovolemia or dehydration: fluid that is hypotonic relative to plasma
is lost with severe gastroenteritis, excessive sweating, or after the
administration of diuretic agents. In these clinical settings, hypernatremia may occur if adequate free water has not been available
or provided to the patient (see Sec. 21.4.1). Following the administration of a diuretic, urine that contains 75 to 100 meq/L of
sodium is usually excreted. Therefore, if little or no fluid intake
occurs, the net effect of the diuretic agent would be an increase in
S_{Na} with weight loss. Similarly, the risk of hypernatremia during
oral hydration is related to adequacy of fluid intake and not to the
sodium content of the rehydration solution.

Excess free water losses occur because of enhanced IWL or the
inability of the kidney to retain water. If the amount of evaporative
water that is lost from the skin and lungs is increased because of
fever, tachypnea, or a dry environment, hypernatremia may develop
because these fluids are electrolyte-free. Because of their proportionately large surface area, premature infants cared for on radiant
warmers are particularly susceptible to the development of hypernatremia. A lack of ADH secretion by the posterior pituitary (central diabetes insipidus) or resistance of the collecting duct to respond to ADH (nephrogenic diabetes insipidus) will be manifested
as polyuria with low U_{Osm} despite significant dehydration (see Sec.
21.4.3). Central diabetes insipidus will not have a definable cause
in approximately half of patients, and the remainder will have a

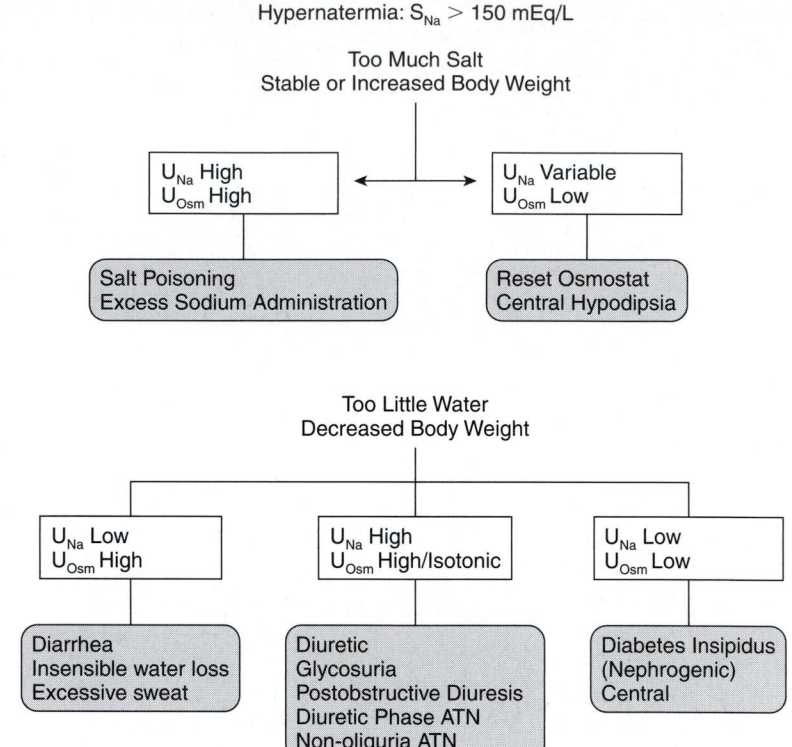

FIGURE 21-10 **Algorithm for assessment of hypernatremia (U_{Na} = urinary sodium concentration; U_{Osm} = urinary osmolarity).**

suprasellar mass, postinfectious encephalopathy, trauma with subsequent anoxic encephalopathy, cerebral edema, or, rarely, either vascular malformations or Langerhans cell histiocytosis (see Sec. 20.16). Nephrogenic diabetes insipidus may be (1) congenital, with onset in infancy manifested by episodes of fever, vomiting, and dehydration combined with a persistently hypotonic urine, or (2) acquired in association with intrinsic renal disease or pharmacologic insults such as lithium, methoxyflurane, and demeclocycline. Similarly, children with sickle cell disease have hyposthenuria and diminished response to ADH (see Chapter 19.4).

The appropriate treatment for hypernatremia in association with volume depletion has been controversial (see Sec. 21.4.1). Nuclear magnetic resonance spectroscopy of the brain has demonstrated that specific osmolytes (trimethylamines, betaine, and phosphoglycerocholine) are produced in response to chronic hypertonic volume depletion. The accumulation of these intracellular osmolytes, which are related to sorbitol and aldose reductase metabolism, may be responsible for the paradoxic cerebral edema that is associated with rapid correction of hypernatremia. Because these intracellular osmolytes neither are generated nor are dissipated rapidly, a patient would have to sustain a prolonged period of hypernatremia, probably greater than 24 hours, for these products to be produced and to be at risk for CNS complications during rehydration. Accordingly, a slow and cautious rehydration program extended over several days would allow for a progressive decrease in these compounds as extracellular tonicity is returned to normal (see Sec. 21.4.1).

For patients with central diabetes insipidus, treatment with ADH or the synthetic analog 1-deamino-8D-arginine vasopressin can result in effective water reabsorption (see Sec. 24.3). Therapy for patients with nephrogenic diabetes insipidus is more complex and may require the use of chronic thiazide diuretics, a low-salt diet, and other attempts to manipulate renal tubular reabsorption (see Sec. 21.11). For children with congenital or inherited nephrogenic diabetes insipidus, early recognition of this condition and prevention of repeated episodes of hypertonic dehydration may be of crucial importance in preventing developmental delays and learning disabilities.

POTASSIUM DISORDERS

Potassium is the most abundant intracellular cation and plays a fundamental role in cellular homeostasis. Total body potassium is maintained at about 50 meq/kg of body weight, and 98% total body potassium is intracellular, which provides a large sink to accommodate wide fluctuations in potassium intake and excretion. Although the kidney is the primary organ responsible for maintaining potassium balance, extrarenal adaptive mechanisms contribute significantly to dissipation of acute loads of potassium and include insulin secretion, catecholamines (particularly β agonists), mineralocorticoids, and acid-base balance.

Potassium handling by the kidney is complex and influenced by a number of both intrinsic and extrinsic factors. About 80% of filtered potassium is reabsorbed in the proximal tubule and will be altered markedly by osmotic diuretics, such as mannitol, which inhibit both salt and water movement in the proximal tubule. Potassium is secreted in the descending limb of Henle, with net reabsorption occurring in the thick ascending limb, which results in trapping of potassium in the medulla secondary to the countercurrent mechanism and some recycling of potassium in this deeper medullary region. The major potassium-secreting segments that can have marked effects on S_K are the late distal tubule and the collecting duct. Net movement of potassium in this region is affected by urinary flow rate, plasma potassium concentration, luminal potassium concentration, delivery of sodium and chloride, availability of nonreabsorbable anions such as sulfate or phosphate, and, finally, diuretic agents.

In evaluating patients with disorders of potassium, it must be remembered that the S_K concentration is only a very small portion of total body potassium and that alterations in the S_K may not be a reflection of overall total body potassium balance. Unfortunately, a practical and effective method for determining total body potassium status is not available, and the appearance of U waves on the electrocardiogram is a relatively crude and late-developing index of potassium balance.

HYPOKALEMIA Hypokalemia, defined as S_K less than 3.5 meq/L, requires an evaluation based on four potential sources.

Shifts of potassium from extracellular to intracellular space. In patients with alkalosis, hypokalemia occurs because of movement of potassium into cells as hydrogen ions move out of cells to buffer the extracellular alkalinity. The plasma potassium level will drop between 0.2 and 0.4 meq/L for each 0.1-unit increase in plasma pH. Although this represents a relatively mild change, hypokalemic alkalosis in children usually occurs because of vomiting, and the concomitant stimulation of aldosterone secretion will add to potassium losses. Similarly, insulin will drive potassium into cells from the extracellular fluid and result in an apparent hypokalemia. During the course of rehydration and correction of hyperglycemia after an episode of diabetic ketoacidosis, severe hypokalemia can occur in part as a result of loss of potassium from glucose-induced osmotic diuresis and the effect of insulin administration. The release of catecholamines results in increased potassium movement into skeletal muscle. Of note, β-adrenergic agonists, which are used to treat bronchospasm and reactive airway disease, can produce transient hypokalemia because of the stimulation of K movement into cells. Similarly, hypokalemia has been associated with hypothermia, barium ingestion, and periodic paralysis.

Inadequate potassium intake. Because the kidney can reduce urinary potassium excretion to less than 20 meq/L within 7 days and to less than 10 meq/L in 10 days, the intake of potassium must be drastically reduced over a prolonged period to induce total body potassium deficiency and hypokalemia.

Excessive nonrenal losses (low U_K). Because the intestines preferentially secrete potassium bicarbonate into the lumen and reabsorb sodium chloride, chronic or long-term diarrhea may produce significant potassium depletion. This mechanism is also responsible for the hypokalemic acidosis associated with augmention of the bladder with a portion of bowel. Although sweat contains only about 10 meq/L of potassium, the profound hypokalemia associated with heavy exercise and profuse sweating is contributed to by volume depletion and activation of aldosterone secretion as well as by release of catecholamines.

Excessive renal potassium losses (high U_K). Because the distal nephron is the final regulatory site for potassium homeostasis, an increase in flow through this nephron segment will increase potassium secretion. The concentration of potassium in the urine may be very low in polyuric conditions, but the high flow rate will result in significant potassium losses. Potassium secretion in this segment also is affected by sodium and chloride content. Diuretic agents, which increase flow in the distal nephron, will stimulate potassium secretion by several mechanisms: increased distal flow rate, increased luminal sodium and chloride concentration, and stimulation of aldosterone secretion. Similarly, tubule toxins such as amphotericin or ifosphamide produce a leak of potassium into the tubule fluid, and persistent, refractory hypokalemia results. Finally, either primary or secondary mineralocorticoid secretion or the administration of exogenous steroids with mineralocorticoid effects will stimulate sodium reabsorption in exchange for potassium and hydrogen. Primary hyperaldosteronism and Cushing syndrome are both relatively rare in children. Aldosterone secretion secondary to hyperreninemia from renal artery stenosis will result in hypokalemia and hypertension. Congenital adrenal hyperplasia has been associated with hypokalemia, although hyperkalemia is much more common. Finally, the rare disorders of Bartter and Gitelman syndromes, which are characterized by growth failure, muscle weakness, poor feeding, vomiting, polyuria, constipation, and normal blood pressure, must be considered in patients who have severe and continuing hypokalemic metabolic alkalosis (see Sec. 21.11). Hypokalemia cannot be corrected rapidly, and the infusion of solutions with high potassium concentration ("k-runs") are ineffective and of little use.

HYPERKALEMIA Hyperkalemia, defined as S_K greater than 6.5 meq/L, is potentially life-threatening. Although the kidney is the primary site for potassium disposal, nonrenal adaptive mechanisms, including insulin secretion and catecholamines, function to minimize the effects on S_K in response to acute ingestions. These adaptive mechanism respond to rapid infusion of potassium and dispose of the vast majority of the infused potassium. Chronic ingestion of a high-potassium diet induces additional adaptive factors, including an increase in Na,K-ATPase activity, which allows an even greater tolerance for potassium loads. Thus, hyperkalemia signals a breakdown in both acute and long-term adaptive mechanisms and requires very careful evaluation.

Release of potassium from intracellular to extracellular fluid. Hemolysis of red blood cells that are injured during venipuncture will increase the S_K significantly. Determination of S_K from a serum sample obtained from clotted blood can be associated with lysis or breakdown of cells during the clotting process, especially if marked leukocytosis or thrombocytosis is present. Finally, cellular shifts of hydrogen and potassium ions in response to acid-base disorders can be significant because for every 0.1-unit reduction in the arterial pH, an approximate 0.2- to 0.4-meq/L increase in the S_K may occur. Patients with diabetic ketoacidosis may have markedly elevated S_K, but total body potassium will have been depleted secondary to the osmotic diuresis induced by the hyperglycemia. A spurious cause for hyperkalemia should be suspected when a significantly elevated S_K is unassociated with any change in the patient's clinical condition and no notable changes are present on the electrocardiogram. Significant hyperkalemia is associated with a decrease in muscle strength and the development initially of peaked T waves on the electrocardiogram. Substantial and life-threatening arrhythmias can be induced by hyperkalemia (Fig. 21-11).

Increased potassium intake or endogenous potassium from tissue catabolism. If renal function, urine output, and the other adaptive mechanisms are intact, the development of hyperkalemia on the basis of an acute potassium load is rare. Thus, with an intact kidney, an acute potassium load from either oral or parenteral fluids can be excreted relatively efficiently and should not induce a significant sustained increase in S_K. When the rate of tissue breakdown is extremely rapid or is combined with a mild degree of renal dysfunction, hyperkalemia may result from the rapid hemolysis of red blood cells that is associated with autoimmune hemolytic anemia or an incompatible blood transfusion, the administration of cytotoxic agents to patients with malignant lymphomas, severe tissue damage from trauma or rhabdomyolysis, or the inadvertent administration of potassium-containing antibiotics to small children. Patients with extensive trauma, neuromuscular disease, or burns may be particularly sensitive to the depolarizing effects of the muscle relaxant succinylcholine and develop rhabdomyolysis with hyperkalemia.

Primary defects in potassium excretion. Patients with renal insufficiency are particularly susceptible to hyperkalemia, and patients with nonoliguric renal failure will tolerate potassium intake considerably better than those with oliguria. The plasma level of S_K in

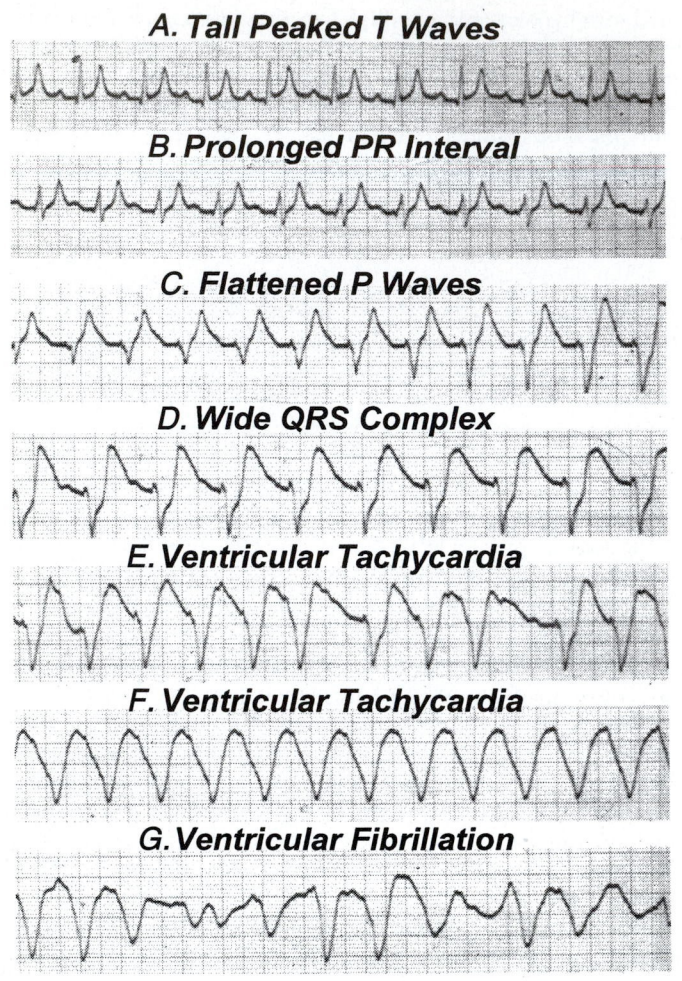

A. Tall Peaked T Waves

B. Prolonged PR Interval

C. Flattened P Waves

D. Wide QRS Complex

E. Ventricular Tachycardia

F. Ventricular Tachycardia

G. Ventricular Fibrillation

FIGURE 21-11   Electrocardiographic changes associated with hyperkalemia.

patients with renal failure also is related to the degree of metabolic acidosis, which is a common feature of chronic renal failure. Renal disorders with damage predominantly to the distal part of the nephron, such as multicystic dysplastic kidneys, reflux nephropathy, and sickle-cell disease, are particularly susceptible to the development of hyperkalemia. Moreover, although patients with chronic renal insufficiency are able to achieve potassium balance, the adaptive reserve in response to acute potassium loading is reduced signifi-

cantly. A reduction in aldosterone production or end-organ unresponsiveness to aldosterone will lead to the development of hyperkalemia. In addition, pseudohypoaldosteronism has been described in infants who have been characterized as having sodium wasting, hyperkalemia, and markedly elevated levels of renin and aldosterone (see Secs. 21.11 and 24.4). Also, the administration of competitive inhibitors of aldosterone such as spironolactone to spare potassium losses in association with diuretic administration may make patients more susceptible to hyperkalemia, particularly if an acute potassium load is given.

Similarly, drugs that impair the renin-angiotensin-aldosterone sequence may cause hyperkalemia. β-Blocking agents that inhibit plasma renin activity and the production of angiotensin II have been associated with mild hyperkalemia that is rarely clinically significant. Angiotensin-converting enzyme inhibitors (ACE-I) are known to cause hyperkalemia because of the diminished production of angiotensin II and consequent reduced aldosterone secretion. Finally, the prostaglandin inhibitors such as nonsteroidal anti-inflammatory drugs also have been associated with diminished aldosterone synthesis and the induction of hyperkalemia. In the majority of these situations, the hyperkalemia is transient and will dissipate once the offending drug has been withdrawn.

Severe volume depletion also may be associated with hyperkalemia. When renal perfusion has been diminished markedly, as in severe diarrhea or intractable congestive heart failure, delivery of sodium to the distal site will be decreased significantly. Because potassium secretion is dependent, to some extent, on exchange for sodium in the lumen of the distal tubule, the diminished delivery of sodium to this segment will decrease the rate of potassium secretion and result in hyperkalemia.

Nonfactitious hyperkalemia must be treated promptly and aggressively because of the depolarizing effect of elevated S_K on excitable tissues such as the myocardium. Figure 21-11 demonstrates the sequence of changes that occur on the ECG in association with hyperkalemia. The severity of these changes is related to the rate of rise in S_K rather than to a specific serum level of potassium. Therapeutic interventions for the treatment of hyperkalemia may take advantage of adaptive mechanisms that promote the cellular uptake of potassium, act to stabilize the excitable membrane, or actually remove excess potassium (Table 21-8). Early mild changes such as those illustrated in Fig. 21-11A may be treated with the administration of β agonists or correction of acidemia. Caution must be taken when infusing sodium bicarbonate because rapid changes in serum pH may adversely affect ionized calcium concentrations and

TABLE 21-8

THERAPEUTIC INTERVENTIONS IN HYPERKALEMIA

AGENT	MECHANISM	DOSE[a]	PRECAUTIONS/ COMPLICATIONS
β Agonist	Cell uptake	5–20 mg nebulizer	Tachycardia, hypertension
Glucose and insulin	Cell uptake	Glucose 0.5 g/kg insulin 0.1 U/kg IV over 30 minutes	Hypoglycemia, hypophosphatemia
Sodium bicarbonate	Cell uptake	0.5 meq/Kg IV over 10–15 minutes	Hypernatremia, alkalosis, hypocalcemia, tetany
Calcium gluconate	Stabilizes membrane irritability	1 mL/kg of 10% solution IV over 3–5 minutes	Bradycardia, hypercalcemia
Sodium polystyrene resin	Exchange K^+ across colonic mucosa	1–2 g/kg PO or PR in sorbitol	Hypernatremia, constipation

[a] All doses are initial starting recommendations and must be carefully adjusted for individual patients and confounding clinical situations.

cause tetany, especially if patients are hyperphosphatemic or have renal insufficiency. Although the administration of glucose and insulin also promotes cellular uptake of potassium, this therapy can be complex and lead to other metabolic abnormalities. If more ominous ECG changes appear (Fig. 21-11 C–E), stabilization of the irritable myocardium is necessary and can be achieved with the infusion of calcium gluconate, which requires careful and continuous monitoring. The sodium polystyrene sulfonate resin (Kayexalate) results in net potassium removal by exchanging potassium for sodium across the gastrointestinal mucosa and can be used to effect net potassium removal. However, this compound requires several hours of contact with the mucosa to be effective and, therefore, is indicated only if there are no substantial ECG changes or after stabilization of the ECG has been achieved. Complications of therapy with exchange resins include sodium retention and fecal impaction. In cases of significant or profound renal failure, dialysis will be required to achieve substantial removal of potassium.

CHLORIDE DISORDERS

Because the reabsorption of tubular fluid must be isoelectric (ie, for each positively charged ion, a negatively charged ion also must be reabsorbed to maintain electric neutrality across the tubule epithelium), chloride and bicarbonate have been assumed to move passively in response to the active transport of sodium and potassium. Actually chloride is the dominant and actively transported species in the ascending limb of the loop of Henle, and a number of bicarbonate-linked transporters have been described as well. Moreover, the obligatory relationship between chloride and bicarbonate reabsorption inevitably results in acid-base disorders as a consequence of or concomitant with disordered chloride metabolism. When serum chloride (S_{Cl}) is elevated, a decrease in bicarbonate reabsorption occurs, and a hyperchloremic metabolic acidosis results. Similarly, when S_{Cl} is depleted, a compensatory increase in bicarbonate reabsorption occurs, particularly in the setting of volume depletion, and a hypochloremic metabolic alkalosis develops.

HYPOCHLOREMIA Hypochloremia, generally defined as S_{Cl} less than 95 meq/L, may develop in a variety of clinical situations either from the loss of chloride or from its inadequate intake. In either situation the pathophysiological response is similar, and children with pyloric stenosis represent the prototype of this disorder. Persistent vomiting, the hallmark of pyloric stenosis, results in the loss of fluid and HCl from the stomach. The production of the hydrogen ion that is lost in gastric secretions has resulted in the production of a bicarbonate ion, which enters the blood. Because the bicarbonate ion entering the blood is unbuffered, the serum bicarbonate and pH increase, and a metabolic alkalosis is initiated. In a euvolemic state, the hyperbicarbonatemia would be corrected rapidly because the kidney would maintain a normal bicarbonate threshold and the excess bicarbonate would be excreted in the urine. However, if the vomiting results in a decrease in intravascular volume, an increase in proximal tubule reabsorption and stimulation of the renin-aldosterone system ensue. Enhanced proximal tubule reabsorption results in increased bicarbonate reabsorption because chloride is depleted in the tubular filtrate, bicarbonate can be produced at that site by the action of carbonic anhydrase, and angiotensin II stimulates sodium-proton exchange. However, the rise in the serum bicarbonate level cannot completely compensate for the fall in the S_{Cl}, and a small excess of sodium is displaced into the distal nephron. Concomitantly, the distal tubule is working under the influence of a high level of aldosterone, which promotes the

excretion of potassium and hydrogen ions in exchange for sodium, which exacerbates the metabolic alkalosis by producing hypokalemia and increasing bicarbonate reabsorption at this site. This pathophysiological sequence of events results in the development of hypokalemic/hypochloremic metabolic alkalosis in the setting of chloride depletion. From a clinical perspective, any condition in which S_{Cl} is depleted culminates in a hypokalemic metabolic alkalosis: persistent vomiting or nasogastric drainage (gastrointestinal chloride loss), loop-acting diuretics (inhibition of active chloride transport in the ascending limb), cystic fibrosis (chloride losses in sweat), congenital chloridorrhea (chloride is lost in the stool), and Bartter syndrome (genetic defects in renal chloride reabsorption).

Inadequate intake of chloride without volume depletion in patients who have received adequate volumes of parenteral fluids deficient in chloride or infants who were fed a chloride-deficient formula has been reported to cause a significant hypochloremic, hypokalemic metabolic alkalosis. In this clinical situation, diminished chloride delivery to the thick ascending limb of the loop of Henle and the macula densa may result in enhanced renin release and increased secretion of aldosterone. In addition, the reduced distal delivery of chloride could promote increased bicarbonate reabsorption as well.

For those patients who have decreased S_{Cl} associated with a metabolic alkalosis and volume depletion, volume expansion with fluids that contain acetate or lactate would be inappropriate because, with an intact liver, acetate and lactate are converted to bicarbonate and would enhance the metabolic alkalosis. Both parenteral (Ringer lactate) and oral rehydration solutions (usually citrate) contain base equivalents that may be detrimental in patients with hypochloremia (see Sec. 21.4.1). Replacement of the chloride ion with concomitant correction of intravascular volume will have a dominant effect to diminish the pathophysiological response that is perpetuating the electrolyte and acid-base abnormalities. Although potassium is an important part of the rehydration fluid regimen, high concentrations of potassium are not required. With replacement of the chloride deficit and repletion of intravascular volume, the metabolic alkalosis will be corrected, and infusion of weak acids is rarely needed. If the period of volume depletion has been excessive, the exchangeable pool of intracellular potassium may be depleted, and, under the influence of aldosterone, the distal tubule will exchange hydrogen ion for sodium, resulting in a paradoxic aciduria (ie, an acid urine in the face of an alkaline plasma). Paradoxic aciduria indicates that total body potassium stores have been depleted to a critical level and is a metabolic emergency.

HYPERCHLOREMIA From a clinical perspective, hyperchloremia, defined as S_{Cl} greater than 109 meq/L, is seen almost inevitably in combination with non–anion gap metabolic acidosis. Excessive chloride ions in extracellular fluid suppress bicarbonate reabsorption and lead to the development of metabolic acidosis. This sequence of events can be complicated further if S_{Cl} increased concomitant with intravascular volume expansion, which also decreases bicarbonate reabsorption.

Hyperchloremic metabolic acidosis generally is seen in three clinical settings: increased chloride intake, enhanced chloride reabsorption from the gastrointestinal tract, and renal tubular acidosis. Excessive chloride administration (eg, if a child were to receive normal saline as a sole hydrating solution) inevitably results in a hyperchloremic metabolic acidosis. Identification of the offending substance or reduction of the chloride content of parenteral fluid should be accomplished.

The epithelial cells of the gastrointestinal tract function to reabsorb sodium chloride and excrete potassium bicarbonate. Consequently, diarrhea is the most common cause of hyperchloremic acidosis. However, similar electrolyte abnormalities occur with fluid stasis in the bowel: small-bowel, biliary, and pancreatic drainage or fistulas, ureterosigmoidostomy, an ileal loop, or with use of bowel to augment the bladder. In the latter circumstances, urine is retained in the bowel lumen, and the exchange of electrolytes results in a hypokalemic/hyperchloremic metabolic acidosis unless the contact time between the bowel mucosa and the urine is limited. Therefore, increased S_{Cl} in a patient with a urinary diversion or bladder augmentation suggests the presence of an obstruction or a delay in emptying.

Finally, hyperchloremic metabolic acidosis without an anion gap that is persistent is a hallmark of renal tubular acidosis (see Sec. 21.11). An assessment for the presence of renal tubular acidosis is difficult in the presence or immediately following an episode of diarrheal dehydration because maximal hydrogen ion secretion by the kidney requires repletion of total body stores of sodium and potassium, which takes several weeks to achieve.

21.4.5 Disorders of Acid-Base Balance

In essence, acid-base disorders represent abnormalities in hydrogen ion (H^+) concentration in plasma. Acid generated from metabolism is approximately 1 meq/kg/d in adults and even greater in growing children. The H^+ concentration of extracellular fluid is maintained in a reasonably narrow range by a complex system of buffers (both extracellular and intracellular), the lungs, whereby volatile acids can be excreted, and the kidneys, which are responsible for the excretion of nonvolatile acids (see Sec. 21.2). The principal buffer of the extracellular fluid is the bicarbonate/carbonic acid system. From a practical perspective H^+ concentration is usually expressed as pH, which is derived from the equation: pH = pK_a + log (base/acid). The pK_a of carbonic acid is 6.1, and the ratio of bicarbonate to carbonic acid is usually 20:1, which results in a normal plasma pH of 7.35 to 7.45. In the clinical setting, the equation that relates pH to log (base/acid) is largely determined by the ratio of serum bicarbonate to PCO_2. Because the kidney is predominantly responsible for bicarbonate concentration of plasma and the lung is the primary organ that excretes PCO_2, the pH of plasma is then dependent on the interactions between these two organs. Alterations in serum pH that are largely attributable to changes in bicarbonate are referred to as metabolic, and those that relate primarily to changes in PCO_2 are referred to as respiratory.

The evaluation of acid-base disorders may seem unduly complex and is further complicated by semantics. The pH of the serum determines the patient's acid-base status. If pH is below normal, the patient has an acid*emia;* if pH is above normal, the patient is considered to have an alkal*emia.* The process by which the serum pH is altered is referred to as either an acid*osis* or alka*losis.* Thus, an alteration in serum pH (acidemia or alkalemia) is actually the result of two "osis" (see Table 21-9), one of which is primary and has been responsible for the disturbance, while the other is secondary and represents the physiological attempt to counterbalance the primary abnormality (ie, balance the relationship of HCO_3/PCO_2). Because the serum pH (emia) is a balance between a metabolic "osis" and a respiratory "osis," a primary metabolic disturbance (ie, change in bicarbonate) elicits predictable respiratory responses, and primary respiratory abnormalities elicit metabolic compensation. Although the compensatory process will attempt to correct the se-

TABLE 21-9

ASSESSMENT OF ACID-BASE DISORDERS[a]

pH	P_{CO_2}	"EMIA"	PRIMARY "OSIS"	SECONDARY "OSIS"
↓	↓	Acidemia	Metabolic acidosis	Respiratory alkalosis
↓	↑	Acidemia	Respiratory acidosis	Metabolic alkalosis
↑	↓	Alkalemia	Respiratory alkalosis	Metabolic acidosis
↑	↑	Alkalemia	Metabolic alkalosis	Respiratory acidosis

[a] The pH determines whether the patient has acidemia or alkalemia; the compensatory process (secondary "osis") never overshoots and rarely returns the pH to normal.

rum pH by balancing the ratio between metabolic and respiratory "osis," the serum pH is rarely returned to normal values and never overcompensates. The simplest way to assess the primary disorder is to compare the serum pH and PCO_2 (see Table 21-9). If a patient is acidemic (serum pH below 7.35) and the PCO_2 is also low, the primary disorder must be a metabolic acidosis (because a primary respiratory acidosis would require an increase in PCO_2), and the low PCO_2 represents a compensatory (secondary "osis") change because of the stimulation of the respiratory center of the brain by the acidemia. When the serum pH is low and the PCO_2 is elevated, the primary defect is diminished respiration causing retention of CO_2 and a respiratory acidemia. The secondary compensatory component would be a metabolic alkalosis because the kidney enhances bicarbonate reabsorption in an attempt to balance the relationship between bicarbonate and PCO_2. Similarly, if the patient is alkalemic (serum pH > 7.45) and the PCO_2 is low, the primary defect is excessive respiratory excretion of the volatile acid CO_2, resulting in a respiratory alkalosis. The kidney attempts to compensate for the low PCO_2 by diminishing bicarbonate reabsorption, and, therefore, a metabolic acidosis occurs as a secondary process. Similarly, when the serum pH is elevated but the PCO_2 is also elevated, the primary process must have been a metabolic alkalosis in which the retention of bicarbonate has suppressed the respiratory drive and resulted in retention of CO_2. The evaluation of acid-base abnormalities may lead to the establishment of specific diagnoses, particularly in children with unsuspected metabolic disorders (see Sec. 9.2).

METABOLIC ACIDOSIS

By far the most common acid-base abnormality encountered in children is metabolic acidosis, defined as pH < 7.35, PCO_2 < 35 mm Hg, and serum bicarbonate < 20 meq/L. The clinical hallmark of metabolic acidosis is an increase in both the rate and depth of respiration as the lungs attempt to compensate by the excretion of CO_2. When the acidemia is profound, the patient may develop deep pauseless breathing, termed *Kussmaul* respirations. In mild forms of metabolic acidemia, alterations in the respiratory rate will not be clinically evident. Because the maximal decrease in PCO_2 is approximately 20 mm Hg, the respiratory compensation cannot maintain the serum pH above 7.0 if the serum bicarbonate is less than 5 meq/L. The adequacy of the respiratory compensation in response to a metabolic acidemia can be most easily judged by evaluating the level of PCO_2. If the serum pH is above 7.0, the PCO_2 should approximate the two numbers following the decimal point in the pH. For example, if the serum pH is 7.25, one would anticipate a PCO_2 between 23 and 27 mm Hg if the pathophysiological compensatory mechanisms are intact.

Metabolic acidemias are derived from either the retention of acid or the loss of bicarbonate. The anion gap, which is calculated as $S_{Na} - (S_{Cl} + S_{HCO_3})$, is used to classify metabolic acidemia. Normally the anion gap is 6 to 12 meq/L and is composed of negative charges on protein (largely albumin), phosphates, sulfates, and organic anions. Conditions in which an unmeasured anion is retained result in a fall in serum bicarbonate and the development of a metabolic acidemia associated with an increased anion gap. Ketones and ketoacids are generated in patients with insulin deficiency or inadequate carbohydrate intake, lactic acid may be derived from tissue hypoxia or inborn errors of metabolism, and decreased renal function is associated with the retention of phosphate and sulfate. Some intoxicants are also associated with an anion gap acidemia and include salicylate (acetylsalicylic acid), methanol (formic acid), ethylene glycol (glyoxylic acid), paraldehyde (acetic acid), and organic acids associated with metabolic disorders (see Chapter 9).

A non–anion gap metabolic acidemia will develop in clinical situations in which a fall in serum bicarbonate is accompanied by retention of chloride. This group of disorders is frequently referred to as hyperchloremic metabolic acidosis (see hyperchloremia in Sec. 21.4.4). In general, hyperchloremic acidemia is usually associated with excessive fluid losses in the GI tract, drugs such as acetazolamide, the infusion of large quantities of chloride, or renal tubular acidosis (see Sec. 21.11).

METABOLIC ALKALEMIA

Metabolic alkalemia, defined by pH > 7.45, bicarbonate > 25 meq/L, and $P_{CO_2} > 40$ meq/L, is also frequently encountered in infants and children. The most common clinical presentation is persistent vomiting. In rare cases the suppression of respiratory drive by the alkalemia may be severe enough to cause apnea in infants. The adequacy of the respiratory compensation can be estimated on the basis of an anticipated rise in P_{CO_2} of 0.7 mm Hg for each 1 meq the serum bicarbonate is elevated above normal values.

Metabolic alkalemia derives (1) from clinical conditions associated with total body chloride depletion referred to as saline sensitive and characterized by a urinary chloride less than 10 meq/L, and (2) from conditions that are associated with increased mineralocorticoid activity that is not physiologically regulated. Hypochloremic metabolic alkalemia secondary to chloride losses occurs in patients with persistent vomiting, diuretic use, congenital chloridorrhea, and posthypercapnia (see Hypochloremia Sec. 21.4.4). These conditions will respond to the infusion of large quantities of chloride, and the metabolic disorder will resolve as total body chloride is repleted. Patients with hyperaldosteronism, Cushing syndrome, or exogenous stimulation of mineralocorticoid production as occurs with licorice ingestion will also develop a metabolic alkalemia but will not be responsive to the infusion of chloride, as these disorders are driven by the persistent effect of mineralocorticoid on the distal nephron. Mineralocorticoids enhance ammonia (NH_3) synthesis, which leads to hydrogen ion excretion and retention of bicarbonate as well as to stimulation of the hydrogen-ATPase pump, which also enhances hydrogen ion excretion with bicarbonate reabsorption. Therefore, resolution of the metabolic defect in these disorders requires elimination or inhibition of the mineralocorticoid effect. Finally, syndromes in which there is a genetic defect in chloride reabsorption, such as Bartter or Gitelman syndrome, will also present with metabolic alkalemia (see Sec. 21.11).

RESPIRATORY ACIDEMIA

Respiratory acidemia, defined as a pH < 7.35 and $P_{CO_2} > 40$ mm Hg, is not commonly encountered in children. When respiratory acidemia occurs acutely, minimal renal compensation is evident, and the serum bicarbonate is usually 23 to 25 meq/L. However,

when P_{CO_2} is retained on a chronic or long-term basis, the renal compensatory mechanisms are such that bicarbonate will be retained, and, in fact, an increase in serum bicarbonate may be a clue to the chronicity of the respiratory acidemia. In chronic conditions the serum bicarbonate will increase by 0.3 meq/L for each 1 mm Hg that the P_{CO_2} is elevated (ie, a P_{CO_2} of 50 mm Hg would be associated with a bicarbonate of 28–30 meq/L). The low serum pH in respiratory acidemia will not be corrected but may actually be worsened by infusion of bicarbonate because the CO_2 produced by the interaction of H^+ and HCO_3 cannot be excreted and will further contribute to the level of retained CO_2.

Acute respiratory acidemia usually results from asphyxiation or the suppression of respiratory drive for the muscles of respiration by drugs such as sedatives or morphine, traumatic injury, or lesions in the central nervous system. Chronic conditions in which persistent hypoventilation occurs are associated with the development of a chronic respiratory acidemia and include cystic fibrosis and bronchopulmonary dysplasia, disorders of respiratory muscles such as muscular dystrophies, massive obesity, and sleep apnea. If the CO_2 retention is relieved in patients with a respiratory acidemia, the underlying metabolic alkalemia (ie, the retained bicarbonate) will be unmasked, and the patient will appear to develop a metabolic alkalemia. This posthypercapnic metabolic alkalemia occurs because the retained CO_2 can be dissipated much more rapidly than the bicarbonate can be excreted.

RESPIRATORY ALKALEMIA

Respiratory alkalemia, defined as a pH > 7.40 with a $P_{CO_2} < 32$ mm Hg, is uncommonly diagnosed because the presenting symptoms are not usually obvious. In severe or extreme cases, acute changes in the blood pH can result in muscle contractures or tetany as a result of the effect of alkalemia on ionized calcium. The acute fall in P_{CO_2} is not compensated effectively by renal mechanisms, and little change in the serum bicarbonate will occur. However, if the respiratory rate is increased persistently, the serum bicarbonate level will decrease approximately 0.5 meq/L for each 1 mm Hg the P_{CO_2} is below normal. Because a low serum bicarbonate is thought to be the hallmark of metabolic acidemia, the acid-base disorder may not be properly diagnosed in patients with respiratory alkalemia unless the pH and P_{CO_2} are carefully assessed (see Table 21-9).

In patients with an unsuspected respiratory alkalemia, careful evaluation for potentially serious causes of increased ventilation should be undertaken. One of the first responses to mild hypoxemia is an increase in respiratory rate and a fall in P_{CO_2}. Similarly, hyperammonemia, which may be the by-product of an inborn error of metabolism or decompensation of liver function, should be evaluated. Interestingly, one of the early and subtle findings in patients with bacteremia is an increase in respiratory rate and the development of a respiratory alkalemia. Finally, drugs (most notably salicylate) may stimulate the respiratory center and produce a respiratory alkalemia. In fact, in patients with salicylate intoxication, one finds evidence of both a metabolic acidosis, the increased anion gap, and a respiratory alkalosis, a P_{CO_2} lower than that expected from the degree of acidemia because of the direct stimulation of the respiratory center by the drug.

References

Gamble JL: Chemical Anatomy, Physiology and Pathology of Extracellular Fluid. Cambridge, MA, Harvard University Press, 1950

Holliday MA: Gamble and Darrow: Pathfinders in body fluid physiology and fluid therapy for children, 1914–1964. Pediatr Nephrol 15:317–324, 2000

Holliday MA, Segar WE: Maintenance need for water in parenteral fluid therapy. Pediatrics 19:823, 1957

Rose BD, ed: Clinical Physiology of Acid-Base and Electrolyte Disorders, 4th ed. New York, McGraw-Hill, 1994

Schrier RW, ed: Renal and Electrolyte Disorders, 5th ed. Philadelphia, Lippincott-Raven, 1997

Smith HW: From Fish to Philosopher. Boston, Little, Brown, 1953

21.5 CLINICAL PRESENTATION OF RENAL DISEASE

John W. Foreman

Children with renal disorders present in a variety of ways, and historic information concerning the amount, frequency, and color of the urine is important, as are symptoms such as pain on urination (dysuria), urgency (difficulty holding urine in the bladder), or incontinence and characteristics of the urinary stream in boys. Pain is not typical of most renal diseases, but flank pain is common with renal stones and pyelonephritis. Pain from renal stones also radiates from the flank to the groin as the stone is passed and is quite excruciating (see Sec. 21.12). Loin pain is sometimes noticed by patients with acute glomerulonephritis, and edema is common in many renal diseases and often is the presenting complaint. On the other hand, recurrent dehydration is a clue to renal disorders that affect water reabsorption and sodium retention, such as tubular disorders, obstructive uropathy, and renal dysplasia. A history of maternal oligohydramnios is an important clue to poor renal function in utero.

Although a history of abnormal amounts and color of urination easily alerts the interviewer to the presence of renal disease, renal disorders can present with complaints that do not seem related to the kidney because of kidney-related functions that are independent of eliminating waste products and maintaining water balance. Children with renal disease may present with signs and symptoms of anemia because of the lack of erythropoietin production by the kidney. Failure to thrive and poor growth are also common presenting complaints in children with renal disease, and symptoms suggestive of heart failure as a consequence of hypertension and fluid overload may also arise. Similarly, children with severe hypertension (frequently related to renal disorders) can present with seizures and changes in mental status. Chronic renal failure commonly presents with nonspecific signs such as fatigue, sleep disturbances, headaches, nausea, and anorexia. The family history is sometimes informative in children with heritable kidney disorders such as Alport syndrome, hypercalciuria, cystinosis, and polycystic kidney.

The presence of hypertension, periorbital edema, abdominal masses, and genital abnormalities on physical examination would suggest a renal disease. The kidneys are easily palpated in the first week of life, and renal abnormalities such as multicystic dysplasia, hydronephrosis, and agenesis can be detected at this time by abdominal palpation.

21.5.1 Examination of Urine

Urinalysis is one of the most useful procedures in evaluating patients who have suspected renal disease. Although the utility of routine urinalysis on well patients is questionable, a high value for cost in detection of suspected renal disease exists. However, a number of children will have transient abnormalities on a urinalysis, and so repeated urinalyses are often useful to avoid more extensive and expensive evaluation.

COLLECTION OF URINE

The most informative urine to examine is the first morning specimen, as this often will be the most concentrated and acidified, and possible increases in urine protein associated with an upright posture will be minimized. The disadvantage is that a significant delay occurs between the time the urine is collected and examined. Routine cleansing of the external genitalia is helpful, especially in girls, to minimize extraneous material such as vaginal cells. Careful cleansing is imperative for a urine culture. The choice of cleansing agent is important because some, such as betadine, may interfere with the dipstick reagents. The usual agent is benzalkonium. Female patients should be instructed to wipe front to back to minimize skin flora, to spread the labia while voiding, and to collect the urine after some has been passed to minimize bacterial contamination. Sitting backwards on a standard toilet is helpful in keeping the labia separated. Boys should be instructed to retract the foreskin and cleanse the glans before voiding. For children unable to void on command, the urine is obtained by placing an adherent plastic bag over the genitalia. Stroking the paraspinal area (Perez maneuver) can stimulate voiding in a prone infant.

The urine should be examined within 30 to 60 minutes of passage because a rise in the pH, lysing of red cells, dissolution of casts, and logarithmic increases in bacterial counts occur if the urine is unrefrigerated.

Suprapubic bladder puncture and urethral catheterization are the most accurate methods of collecting urine for culture but should almost never be used for routine examination as either procedure can introduce blood. Both techniques carry some risk, although it is quite low in experienced hands. Suprapubic aspiration should be reserved for children under 2 years of age, as the bladder is an abdominal organ in this age group and easily accessible for puncture. Suprapubic bladder aspiration is best done after a period of time has elapsed from the last void or when percussion or palpation can demonstrate a full bladder. Urethral catheterization, especially in girls, is another relatively sterile way of obtaining urine for culture and is often more successful than suprapubic aspiration.

URINE TESTING

Dipsticks with small pads containing various reagents that form a specific color depending on the concentration of the substance analyzed have become a standard part of the routine urinalysis. Dipstick pads are available to determine the presence of blood, pH, the specific gravity, and the concentration of protein, ketones, glucose, nitrite, leukocyte esterase, and urobilinogen in the urine. Some tests are more accurate than others, and all are subject to interference by substances and conditions commonly found in urine. However, urine dipsticks, because of their low cost and rapid results, are quite useful in spite of these limitations but must be interpreted carefully.

URINE COLOR

Urine typically varies in color from nearly colorless to dark amber depending on the concentration. The yellow color of normal urine is mainly from urochrome. Other pigments such as carotene, urobilin, and bilirubin can impart an orange appearance. White, milky appearing urine from precipitated calcium-phosphate is seen in normal children, especially if the urine is refrigerated, and rarely from chyluria. Pinkish sediment in infant urine is common secondary to precipitated urates. Precipitated urates can also cause "brick dust" staining in the diaper. Unusual colors often come from dyes or foods but can be associated with pigments excreted in various diseases. Urine in acute glomerulonephritis typically has the appearance of tea and is variously described as rusty to cola colored. With frank bleeding the urine varies from a light rosé color to grossly red. Table 21-10 lists some of the causes of abnormal urine color.

CONCENTRATION

Beyond 6 months of age, the urine osmolality (the number of osmotically active particles) varies from 50 to 1200 mOsm/kg H_2O. Urine osmolality is the more precise way of describing urine concentration or dilution but requires special laboratory testing. Specific gravity (the weight of 1 cc of urine compared to 1 cc H_2O) can easily be measured and correlates roughly with osmolality. Glycosuria and heavy proteinuria increase the specific gravity out of proportion to the osmolality. The assessment of specific gravity by dipstick is not influenced by glucose or contrast media but is affected by protein. Specific gravity ranges from 1.001 to >1.030. If specific gravity above 1.030 is detected, a nonphysiological substance such as contrast media may be present in the urine.

URINE PH

Urine pH varies from 4.5 to 8 and is dependent on the composition of the diet (the higher the protein content the lower the urine pH), acid-base status of the child, and the time from collection to testing. An acid urine (pH < 6) is more likely to be observed after an overnight fast than after a meal. Urine pH rises with standing, especially at room temperature. An alkaline urine (pH > 6) with systemic acidosis is suggestive of, but not diagnostic of, an impairment of bicarbonate reclamation or hydrogen ion excretion. A

urine pH indicator is commonly found on the dipstick but gives only an approximation of the true urine pH. More precise measurements using a pH meter are required for the diagnosis of renal tubular acidosis (see Sec. 21.11.2).

PROTEIN

Urine normally contains a small amount of protein (<100 mg/m^2/d), of which 40% is albumin, 40% Tamm-Horsfall protein secreted by the tubule, 15% immunoglobulins, and 5% other plasma proteins. Urine protein is commonly detected by a change in the color of tetrabromophenol blue impregnated on a dipstick pad and is reported as 0 to +4. This reaction is influenced by the urine concentration and pH (markedly alkaline urine will give a false-positive reaction). Chemically measuring the protein in a timed collection of urine, typically over 24 hours, is a more precise way of determining protein excretion but is difficult in young children. The urine protein-to-creatinine ratio can be used to screen for abnormal protein excretion without the necessity of an accurately timed urine collection. Normal children under 2 years of age have a urine protein/creatinine (mg/mg) ratio that is less than 0.5, and older children and adults have a ratio that is less than 0.2. The urine protein/creatinine ratio can estimate the 24-hour urine protein excretion [24-hour urine protein excretion = 0.63 × urine protein/urine creatinine (mg/mg)] and is especially useful for following children with proteinuria in whom repetitive 24-hour urine collections are cumbersome.

Immunochemical methods can detect concentrations of urine albumin (microalbuminuria) below the threshold of standard chemical methods. Microalbumin excretion rates on an overnight urine (normal <30 μg/min or <20 mg/g creatinine) have been used to detect early renal disease, especially that associated with diabetes mellitus.

Transient increases in urine protein excretion can be seen with fever and vigorous activity. A positive reaction of +1 or greater is seen in healthy children transiently, especially if the urine is concentrated. Therefore, several urines should be examined for protein to confirm the persistence of proteinuria before an otherwise healthy child is further evaluated. Children with persistent proteinuria should first be tested for postural or orthostatic protein. If the diagnosis of postural protein is excluded, then the amount of protein excreted over 12 to 24 hours should be quantified either by an estimate or by an actual timed collection to determine the magnitude of the proteinuria.

GLUCOSE

Normally, except in premature infants, the presence of detectable amounts of glucose in the urine is abnormal. The standard dipstick method of examining urine for glucose utilizes the glucose oxidase reaction and can detect 75 to 125 mg/dL of glucose; it is quite specific for glucose. Another method is the Benedict test (Clinitest), which is based on the reduction of copper. The reagents in the Benedict test will react with all reducing substances, including glucose, and is useful for screening for inborn errors of sugar metabolism, such as galactosemia (see Chapter 9). Glycosuria most commonly arises from hyperglycemia with spillover into the urine and can occur rarely as a consequence of an inherited defect in the renal transport of glucose or a part of the global proximal tubule disorder, Fanconi syndrome (see Sec. 21.11). Very premature infants can have glycosuria because of renal tubular immaturity (see Sec. 21.2).

TABLE 21-10
CAUSES OF DISCOLORED URINE

COLOR	ASSOCIATED WITH DISEASE	ASSOCIATED WITH FOOD OR DRUGS
Red, pink, rosé, tea-colored	RBCs (hemoglobin) Myoglobin (porphyrins, porphyria) Urates in newborn	Aminopyrine, anthrocyanin, azo dyes, beets, blackberries, phenolphthalein, rifampin
Orange, yellow-brown	Urobilinogen, bilirubin	Nitrofurantoin, phenytoin, pyridium
Dark brown, black	Homogentisic acid (alkaptonuria), melanin	Methyldopa, metronidazole, phenols, phenothiazines
Blue, green	*Pseudomonas* sepsis, blue diaper syndrome	Amitriptyline, methylene blue, methocarbomal
Whitish, milky	Chyle, nephrotic syndrome, pus Calcium phosphate precipitation	

NITRITE

The nitrite test is used to detect bacteriuria (Griess test). Typically, nitrate but not nitrite is present in urine. Gram-negative organisms reduce nitrate to nitrite, but this process takes several hours. Thus, this test is dependent on the presence of nitrate in the urine, a significant number of bacteria, and time to produce nitrite. A negative result does not exclude bacteriuria, and a high level of ascorbic acid interferes with a positive reaction.

LEUKOCYTE ESTERASE

Leukocyte esterase is used to detect pyuria. Contamination of the urine with a vaginal discharge will give a positive reaction that is not indicative of a UTI or pyuria. Positive reactions should be confirmed with standard urine microscopy.

HEMOGLOBIN, MYOGLOBIN, RBCS

Hemoglobin and myoglobin will react with the reagents to form a green to blue color, depending on the concentration. The pad also lyses intact RBCs to allow the intracellular hemoglobin to react with the reagents. The sensitivity of the reaction is reported as being 5 to 20 RBCs/hpf or 0.015 mg/dL of hemoglobin. Trace reactions are very common and rarely correlated with disease. Positive reactions should be correlated with microscopy. The absence of RBCs on microscopy of the urinary sediment may indicate that the positive reaction is secondary to free hemoglobin or myoglobin but usually simply means that the urinary RBCs lysed before the microscopic examination.

MICROSCOPY

Careful microscopic examination of the urinary sediment is quite useful in the diagnosis and management of individuals with renal disease. However, routine microscopic examination of the urinary sediment from healthy individuals with a negative dipstick for blood, leukocyte esterase, and protein is of limited value. One problem with the examination of the urinary sediment is the lack of standardization of the procedure.

After being centrifuged, a drop of urine sediment is placed on a slide with a coverslip, and the area under the coverslip is scanned, especially at the edges, where casts tend to congregate. After an overall impression is gotten with low-power magnification, a number of fields are examined with high-power (400×) magnification. The number and types of cells, casts, and crystals are counted and expressed per high-power field (hpf). A supravital stain, such as the Sternheimer-Malbin stain, can be used to help identify structures but should be added before centrifuging the urine. The examination of the urinary sediment is at best a semiquantitative procedure. Variations in the amount of urine centrifuged, the initial concentration of the urine, time and speed of centrifugation, and the volume of urine in which the sediment is resuspended influence the number of cells per high-power field. In clinical practice, however, these variables are relatively unimportant, as changes in management are rarely made on whether there are 15 or 50 RBCs/hpf. Examination of the sediment can be likened to viewing abstract painting. Fine details may not be as important as the overall impression.

Red and white cells in the urine may come from anywhere in the urinary tract. Normal centrifuged urine contains fewer than three RBCs/hpf. Eumorphic red blood cells in urine resemble those in blood films, but in hypotonic urine RBCs swell and lose their typical biconcave shape. RBCs that are dysmorphic with variations in size

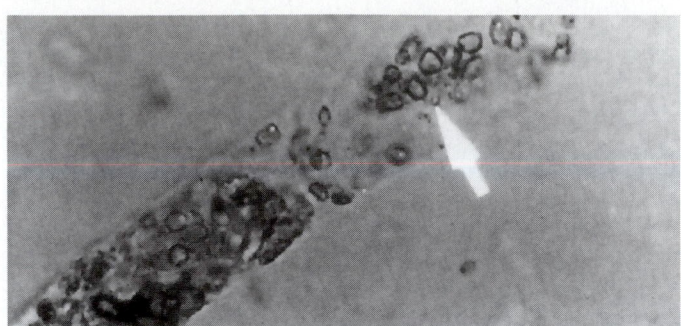

FIGURE 21-12 Red blood cell cast containing a group of dysmorphic RBCs *(arrow)*. Note the blebs on the RBC membrane of the dysmorphic cells.

and, especially, blebs like "Mickey Mouse ears" on their outer cell membrane suggest a glomerular origin (Fig. 21-12). Normal urine contains fewer than five WBCs/hpf. Increased numbers of urinary WBCs may indicate infection, but pyuria can also be seen in noninfectious inflammation of both the glomerulus and the interstitium, with fever, and with dehydration.

Casts are formed in the tubule and consist of a proteinaceous matrix with or without cells. Hyaline casts are the most common and are nearly transparent; they can be seen in normal urine, after exercise, with dehydration, and with proteinuria. Red cell casts (Fig. 21-12) are almost pathognomonic of glomerulonephritis, although they can be seen with renal infarction, renal trauma, and renal vein thrombosis. RBC casts appear yellow-brown in color, rather than red. WBC casts in the setting of a UTI are indicative of pyelonephritis; they are also seen in other causes of interstitial inflammation and can be difficult to distinguish from epithelial cell casts (broad brown casts) that are seen with tubule injury. Granular casts and fatty casts are observed in nephrotic syndrome, and waxy casts are seen in renal failure.

Crystals are commonly observed in urinary sediment and often have little clinical significance. Uric acid can form a variety of shapes, such as diamonds and needles. Calcium oxalate crystals are octahedrons that appear as a square with an X through the center. Triple phosphate or magnesium ammonium phosphate crystals are prisms that have been likened to "coffin lids" and can be seen in normal urine that is alkaline but are also seen in abundance with UTIs from urea-splitting organisms such as *Proteus*. Cystine crystals, which are flat hexagons, are pathognomonic for cystinuria.

Bacteria can be observed in the sediment but are very hard to distinguish from amorphous phosphates and urates without a Gram stain. Urinalysis reports commenting on the number of bacteria per hpf are usually questionable. The diagnosis of a UTI should rest on bacterial culture results and not on the urinalysis (see Sec. 21.6).

21.5.2 Assessment of Renal Function

An assessment of renal function should be done in anyone suspected of having a renal disorder. Longitudinal assessment of renal function is important for following children with known kidney disease to follow the effect of therapy and determine when to intervene in the failing kidney. Measurement of renal function is also useful before and after potentially nephrotoxic therapies such as chemotherapy and certain antibiotics and may be necessary for dosing drugs that are eliminated through the kidney. However, routine screening of renal function in healthy children is not advised or cost-effective.

GLOMERULAR FUNCTION

A rough assessment of glomerular function can easily be obtained by the simple measurement of serum urea and creatinine, whereas precise measurements are difficult and time consuming. This is further complicated by the ability of the normal kidney to alter its glomerular function in response to the workload much as the lung and heart do. With protein loading, normal individuals can increase the glomerular filtration rate (GFR) by 50 to 100%. An increased GFR is typically seen in newly diagnosed diabetics and children with sickle cell disease. The capacity for unaffected nephrons to increase their single-nephron GFR and compensate for diseased nephrons allows the maintenance of relatively normal function until there is significant nephron loss, initially masking the severity of the renal disease.

BUN is the abbreviation for blood urea nitrogen (actually a serum measurement), and the levels of BUN reflect glomerular function. However, BUN is also influenced by numerous factors other than the GFR. BUN levels are the net balance of production from catabolism of both endogenous and dietary protein, filtration by the glomerulus, and reabsorption by the distal nephron. Increased protein catabolism from stress or drugs such as corticosteroids and tetracycline will raise BUN independent of renal function. Whereas urea easily passes through the glomerular capillary wall, extensive reabsorption occurs in the tubule, and this reabsorption rate is flow dependent. Thus, BUN is not a good marker of glomerular function. Further, extracellular volume changes can alter urea reabsorption and BUN without significantly affecting the GFR (see Sec. 21.4 and Fig. 21-8). Dehydration alone can raise BUN. Because serum urea is influenced by dietary protein intake, BUN decreases in children with renal failure placed on low-protein diets, yet their renal function has not changed. The rise in BUN with declining GFR is curvilinear, so that only small changes occur until 50 to 60% of function is lost and then BUN rises steeply with a further decline in function. The advantage of using BUN as a marker of renal function is that it is widely available, easy to measure, and gives reproducible results from laboratory to laboratory. However, because of all the caveats already mentioned, BUN is at best only a rough guide to renal function.

Creatinine is the nonenzymatic end product of creatine metabolism. It is freely filtered by the glomerulus and also secreted by the tubule. This secretion is concentration dependent such that about 5% is excreted by tubular secretion when the creatinine is normal and as much as 50% when the serum creatinine is 10 mg/dL. Serum levels are essentially independent of the diet, which is a major advantage over BUN as marker of GFR. However, creatinine levels also correlate to lean body mass because creatinine comes from muscle creatine. Muscle wasting lowers serum creatinine levels independent of renal function. Because of this association with muscle mass, serum levels rise with age. After the age of 4 years, boys have a higher serum creatinine level than girls, although this difference is not significant until after puberty. Serum creatinine is traditionally measured using the Jaffé reaction with picric acid, which also measures noncreatinine chromagens that falsely elevate the measured level. A number of clinically relevant substances can interfere with this reaction and alter the true serum level, including bilirubin, which can lower the level, and ketones, which can raise the level. Recent methods analyze creatinine enzymatically and are not influenced by noncreatinine chromagens, ketones, or bilirubin.

Newborns, especially premature infants, have higher creatinine levels than older children, and these levels are inversely correlated to gestational and postnatal age (see Table 21-1). Serum creatinine levels fall rapidly over the first weeks of life with the postnatal increase in the GFR (see Table 21-1).

Like BUN, serum creatinine rises in an exponential curvilinear pattern with a decline in GFR, not in a linear fashion, so that minimal increases occur until 50 to 60% of function is lost. The serum creatinine doubles for each halving of GFR, so that a serum creatinine of 0.8 mg/dL that increases to 1.6 mg/dL would indicate that GFR had decreased by 50%.

Recently serum levels of cystatin C, which is a low-molecular-weight protein produced by all nucleated cells, has been proposed as a better marker of renal disease than creatinine. At present, the measurement of this protein is not available in routine clinical laboratories.

Clearance is the classical method of describing renal function and is the volume of plasma completely cleared of a given substance per unit time. Mathematically, clearance is the excretion rate of that substance divided by its plasma or serum concentration:

$$C_x = (U_x V) / P_x$$

where U_x is the urine concentration of x, V is the urine flow rate, and P_x is the plasma concentration. Substances that are freely filtered across the glomerular capillary wall and are not reabsorbed or secreted by the renal tubule can be used to determine the GFR. Traditionally, inulin, a polymer of fructose, has been the reference method for measuring GFR. However, inulin clearance measurements are difficult and are done only in specialized renal units.

The creatinine clearance (C_{cr}), on the other hand, is the most widely used method to estimate GFR. Because creatinine is secreted by the tubule, C_{cr} overestimates the GFR, and this overestimate increases with decreasing GFR. At normal levels of GFR the C_{cr} is about 10 to 20% above the actual GFR, but at a GFR below 10 mL/min, the creatinine clearance is nearly twice the inulin clearance, although this difference may not be so important in clinical practice. C_{cr} requires a complete collection of urine over a specified time period, usually 24 hours, to minimize collection and timing errors. However, in spite of this, creatinine clearances are often inaccurate. Completeness of the urine collection can be assessed by comparing the measured creatinine excretion with the expected excretion, which is approximately 10 to 20 mg/kg/d. Postpubertal girls excrete 1 g/d, and boys excrete 2 g/d of urinary creatinine. Because of the difficulties in performing timed urine collections, estimates of C_{cr} have been devised based on the child's height, which is better correlated with creatinine excretion than weight, and serum creatinine. One such formula for estimating C_{cr} is:

creatinine clearance $(mL/min/1.73m^2)$
$$= k \times Ht \ (cm)/S_{Cr} \ (mg/dl)$$

where $k = 0.55$ for children and adolescent girls, 0.7 for adolescent boys, 0.45 in term infants, and 0.33 in low-birth-weight infants. Although such estimates are easy to obtain and provide an approximation of the GFR, an overestimate of GFR is obtained, especially at lower GFR values. Nonetheless, in the clinical setting in which GFR is being followed over time in the same patient, this estimate of GFR is both practical and helpful in tracking the course of renal function.

Another method of determining GFR is the constant-infusion technique, which takes advantage of the fact that the urine excretion of a substance ($U_x V$) is the same as the infusion rate when the serum concentration of the infused substance is in steady state. Iothalamate clearances use this technique and are quite accurate but are not routinely available. Single-injection techniques are another way of determining GFR without collecting urine. Provided the injected material is not metabolized and eliminated only by glomerular filtration, the disappearance of the substance from the plasma is related to the GFR. The radioisotope DTPA nearly completely meets these criteria and has the advantages of being readily available and easily measured.

The GFR rises rapidly and curvilinearly over the first year of life and then increases gradually until puberty (see Fig. 21-3). After 2 years of age, the GFR or creatinine clearance, when expressed per unit surface area (typically 1.73 m²), is relatively constant. Before 2 years of age, knowledge of the different values for GFR for each conceptual and gestation age is necessary (see Table 21-1).

TUBULAR FUNCTION

Although glomerular function can simply be described in terms of the GFR, tubular function and its assessment is more complex (see Sec. 21.2). The tubule can be divided into the proximal and distal portions, although this is a gross oversimplification. The proximal nephron reabsorbs the bulk of the filtered load, and the distal nephron "fine-tunes" the final urine. The proximal nephron reabsorbs virtually all the filtered glucose and amino acids, 60 to 80% of the filtered sodium and phosphate, and 85% of the filtered HCO_3. The distal nephron is responsible for net H^+ion secretion and urine concentration in addition to adjusting the final excretion of other electrolytes and solutes.

Tubular function is usually described in terms of the clearance of a solute that is handled by a specific segment of the nephron or the overall clearance of a solute that is handled in a number of sites along the nephron, which is the case for most solutes. Another way of describing tubular function is to compare the clearance of a solute to the GFR, usually estimated by the creatinine clearance, and this is termed the fractional excretion (FE) of that solute. The FE of any solute x can be determined by the ratio of the urine concentration of x to the plasma concentration of x, divided by the ratio of urine creatinine concentration to the plasma concentration:

$$U_x / P_x \div U_{cr} / P_{cr}$$

This is usually multiplied by 100% to get the percent fractional excretion. Subtracting the %FE from 100% will give the percent tubule reabsorption.

PROXIMAL TUBULE FUNCTION   Disorders of the proximal tubule can vary from excess loss of a single solute, such as renal glucosuria, to global loss of virtually all solutes reabsorbed in the proximal nephron, the Fanconi syndrome (see Sec. 21.11).

DISTAL NEPHRON FUNCTION   Although the distal nephron has many functions other than concentrating and acidifying the urine, these two measures are often used to assess distal nephron function. The maximal urine-concentrating ability can usually be determined by measuring the urine concentration after an overnight fast. A normal response is a urine specific gravity above 1.020 or a urine osmolality greater than 800 mOsm/kg. This test should be done only in a closely monitored setting if the child typically drinks fluid during the night or if there is a strong possibility of diabetes insipidus (see Sec. 21.11).

A urine pH of less than 5.5, either spontaneously or after an acid load, indicates that the distal nephron can generate an acid urine, ruling out the diagnosis of type I distal RTA. Other methods

of testing the distal nephron acidification mechanisms are measuring the urinary titratable acid excretion, ammonium excretion, and the concentration of CO_2 in alkaline urine (see Sec. 21.11). A positive urinary ion gap, $U_{Cl} - (U_{Na} + U_K)$, can be used to infer intact ammonium excretion; a negative urinary ion gap suggests inadequate ammonium generation. Subjects with normal distal nephron hydrogen ion pumps are able to raise the urine P_{CO_2} above 60 mm Hg, as measured with a standard blood gas instrument. This test requires an excess of urinary bicarbonate. Individuals with absent or impaired H^+ion pumps cannot raise the urinary P_{CO_2}.

21.5.3   Diagnostic Studies

URINARY TRACT IMAGING (see Sec. 8.3)

The intravenous pyelogram (IVP) is the classic method of imaging the kidneys, ureters, and bladder, but it does require the intravenous injection of radiocontrast and a bowel relatively free of stool for good images. Poorly functioning kidneys will not visualize because sufficient contrast will not accumulate. Thus, one limitation of the IVP is the need for a moderate amount of renal function in order to obtain adequate images. The contrast also can give rise to allergic reactions and is potentially nephrotoxic. The patient also receives some gonadal irradiation in the course of the study.

The voiding cystourethrogram (VCUG) is useful for imaging the urethra and bladder and is the only reliable method of determining the presence of vesicoureteral reflux (VUR). Using radiocontrast allows imaging of the urethra, which is especially important in boys, as urethral abnormalities are much more common.

Ultrasonography has largely supplanted the IVP for imaging the kidneys and bladder. The advantages of renal ultrasonography over an IVP are that ultrasonography does not require any renal function to image a kidney, is not painful, involves no ionizing radiation, and is not associated with allergic or toxic reactions. The only disadvantage to ultrasonography is that the quality of the images is operator dependent. However, renal size, position, and pelvic dilatation can be easily determined. Increased sound wave return, termed increased echogenicity, indicates abnormalities of the renal tissue, such as dysplasia or inflammation. Tumors, cysts, and stones can be easily recognized. With the color Doppler technique, renal vessels can be identified, and information about their flow characteristics can be obtained. ultrasonography is also useful for imaging abnormalities of the bladder and determining bladder wall thickness and postvoid residual. Ureters, unless dilated, are not routinely seen. Gross renal scarring from infection can be detected with ultrasonography, but subtle scars are usually missed.

Radionuclide imaging of the kidneys can be done with a variety of isotopes but mainly is confined to technetium-99m mercapto acetyltriglycine (MAG3) and dimercaptosuccinic acid (DMSA). MAG3 is used to give a dynamic image of the kidneys with the first seconds indicating blood flow to each kidney, then the extraction of the nuclide by the glomerulus and proximal tubule, and later excretion of the nuclide from the kidney. A MAG3 scan provides information on the blood flow to each kidney, the relative but not absolute function of each kidney, and the drainage of each kidney, and such information may be useful in deciding when to operate on children with obstructive uropathy (see Sec. 21.16). DMSA, on the other hand, gives a static but clearer image of the kidneys because it binds to renal tissue but is not useful for imaging the ureters or bladder. DMSA may be useful for imaging focal renal scars and acute renal infections.

Computed tomography (CT) gives good images of the genito urinary system, especially if done with intravenous radiocontrast. CT scanning is the modality of choice for renal trauma and often for renal tumors. CT scanning is also useful for detecting nephro calcinosis and small renal stones. Spiral CT scanning with com pu ter-enhanced reconstruction of the arterial phase of renal per fusion after an intravenous bolus injection of radiocontrast can give rela tively good images of the renal arteries, avoiding aortic cathe teri zation. Spiral CT has been used to evaluate patients with sus pected renal artery stenosis and for kidney transplant donors.

Magnetic resonance imaging (MRI) has not been particularly useful for renal imaging.

Renal arteriography is reserved for patients in whom precise def inition of the renal arterial system, such as those with renal artery stenosis or renal tumors, is necessary. Balloon dilatation of the ste notic renal artery can often be done during the same procedure, avoiding the need for surgical correction. Renal arteriography can be useful to localize a site of renal bleeding.

RENAL BIOPSY

The renal biopsy has become a very useful tool for determining the histopathology of childhood renal diseases. In most instances, a percutaneous biopsy is accomplished using a spring-loaded biopsy needle that is guided with ultrasonography. In older children the procedure can be done with sedation, but young and uncooperative children may require general anesthesia. The procedure is relatively safe in experienced hands, although rarely life-threatening bleeding can occur. The tissue obtained is processed with standard histo chemical stains and examined by light microscopy; it can also be reacted with antibodies to human γ-globulin and complement components that have been conjugated with fluorescein and then examined by fluorescence microscopy for the presence of these im mune reactants. Electron microscopy is routinely done to examine the ultrastructure and to detect electron-dense deposits. With this information a specific pathologic diagnosis can be made, and the severity and chronicity of the lesion evaluated (see Sec. 21.9 and Table 21-14). Although no standard criteria for renal biopsy exist, the usual indications are children with steroid-resistant nephrotic syndrome, heavy proteinuria without the nephrotic syndrome, glo merulonephritis other than poststreptococcal, recurrent gross he maturia with significant proteinuria, reduced renal function unex plained by renal imaging or the patient's history, and family history of progressive nephropathy.

21.5.4　Evaluating the Child with Hematuria

Hematuria is a common sign of urinary tract disease but is also a common finding in otherwise healthy children. Vigorous exercise commonly causes transient microscopic hematuria. Whether the hematuria is intermittent or persistent, microscopic or gross, painful or painless is quite useful in determining the cause. Other important clues include the presence of a family history of hematuria or renal disease. The urine color is another helpful sign. Brown or tea-col ored urine is common in glomerulonephritis, whereas red or ob viously bloody urine suggests postglomerular bleeding. Glomeru lonephritis is commonly associated with other abnormalities of the urine such as proteinuria and cellular casts as well as hypertension, edema, and reduced renal function. Table 21-11 lists a simple mne monic for the causes of hematuria throughout the urinary tract.

The incidence of microscopic hematuria, defined as the presence of a positive urine dipstick for blood and more than five RBCs/hpf

TABLE 21-11
CAUSES OF HEMATURIA

T	umor rauma uberculosis
I	nfection nflammation, nephritis
C	ongenital anomaly ystic disease alciuria
S	tones ickle hemoglobin omewhere else[a]

[a] Lesions may occur anywhere in the urinary tract from renal parenchyma to bladder.

on centrifuged urine, has been assessed in epidemiologic studies. Approximately 1% of school-age children will have hematuria on at least one urine sample, and about 0.5% will continue to have he maturia on two of three samples, and only a third have hematuria on all three samples. Microscopic hematuria is twice as common in girls as in boys, and fewer than one-third had hematuria when tested again a year later. Only a very small number of children with microscopic hematuria had significant renal or urologic disease. Thus, microscopic hematuria is common in school-age children and in the majority of cases is benign.

Hypercalciuria, defined as more than 4 mg urinary calcium/kg/d, has been found in significant numbers of children with microscopic hematuria. This association is even stronger if there is a family his tory of stone disease or the occurrence of gross hematuria. The calcium-to-creatinine ratio can be used to screen for hypercalciuria (see Sec. 21.2) and for children or adolescents a urinary Ca/Cr ratio greater than 0.2 is abnormal.

The value of urinary tract imaging in children with microscopic hematuria is controversial. The yield of routine IVP or ultrasound is low, and reported findings are frequently of little clinical signifi cance. Decisions must be made on an individual case if microscopic hematuria persists for several months. Voiding cystourethrograms and cystoscopy are rarely helpful and are not indicated for the rou tine evaluation of children with either microscopic or gross hema turia.

Gross hematuria is much less common than microscopic he maturia and usually warrants a more thorough investigation (see Fig. 21-13). Trauma should be considered, especially if the urine contains clots. If trauma is a likely cause, the urinary tract should be imaged by CT scan promptly. Similarly, if a palpable flank mass is noted, a renal tumor must be considered. Brown or tea-colored urine, especially with cellular casts and protein, suggests glomeru lonephritis. The presence of dysuria and/or fever suggests hem orrhagic cystitis, which can be caused by both bacterial and viral agents. Sickle cell hemoglobinopathies are associated with recurrent gross hematuria that at times can be quite severe. Nephrolithiasis is associated with abdominal pain and nausea. Hypercalciuria, even in the absence of a demonstrable stone, is a common cause of gross hematuria. Renal cysts, especially those in ADPKD, occasionally rupture and cause gross hematuria. Coagulopathies are an ex tremely rare cause of gross hematuria and are almost always asso ciated with bleeding elsewhere. Rare causes include obstructive uropathy, tumors, and vascular malformations.

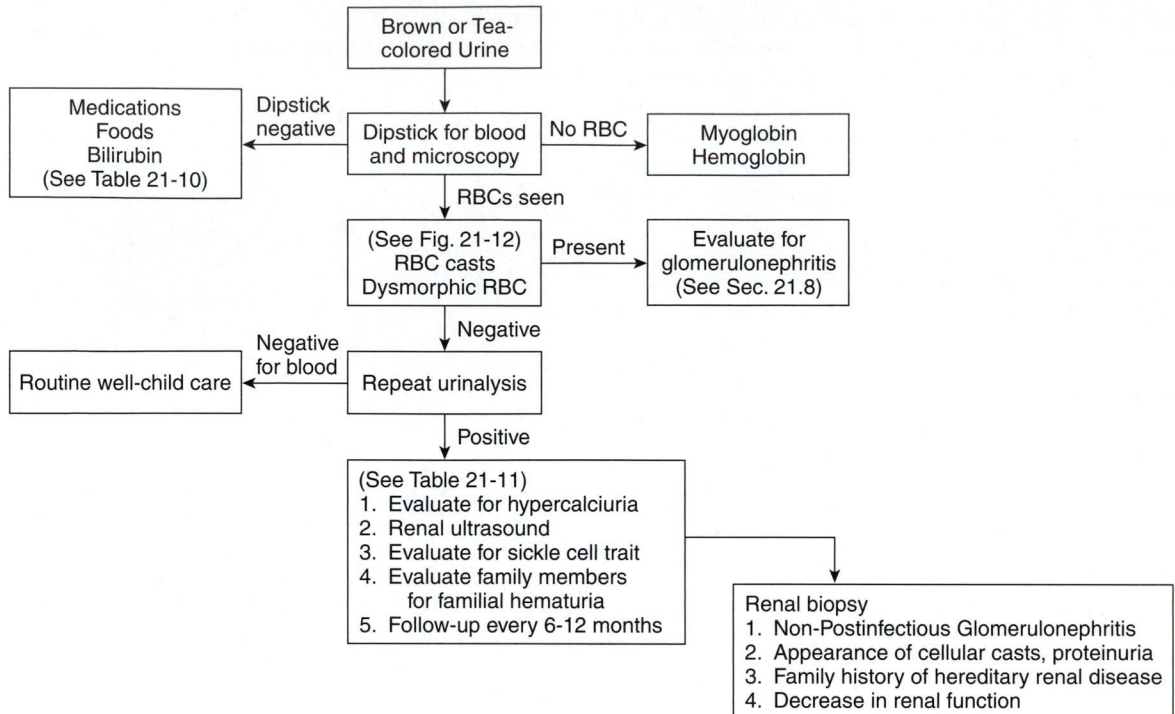

FIGURE 21-13   **Evaluation of children with brown or tea-colored urine.**

21.5.5   Evaluating the Child with Proteinuria

Most children appear to excrete urine free of protein when measured with the semiquantitative dipstick method. Proteinuria is not an uncommon finding in otherwise healthy children an approach to proteinuria is diagrammed in Fig. 21-14. If the proteinuria is associated with other signs of renal disease, such as edema, hematuria, hypertension, growth failure, or elevated serum creatinine, then a more extensive evaluation is indicated (see Sec. 21.8).

Proteinuria can be transient, orthostatic, or fixed. Transient proteinuria, defined as disappearance of proteinuria on several occasions after a positive test, accounts for 80% of patients with isolated proteinuria and occurs in conjunction with fever, exercise, cold exposure, heat stress, and emotional distress. In an otherwise healthy child, transient proteinuria is not associated with renal disease.

Orthostatic proteinuria, defined as proteinuria only in an upright position, is the next most common cause and occurs commonly in adolescents. To evaluate for orthostatic proteinuria the patient should empty the bladder before going to bed at night and then check the first urine passed on waking. A second sample is obtained later, after the patient has been upright for several hours, and tested for protein. Urine protein can be detected by dipstick, urine protein/creatinine ratio, or quantitative collection. If the recumbent urine is negative for protein and the upright urine has protein, the patient is considered to have orthostatic proteinuria. Because of a 22 to 54% false-negative rate for protein if dipsticks are used, this determination most be repeated several times, usually daily for 5 to 7 days. A more precise method is to measure the urine protein/creatinine ratio in the recumbent and upright urine samples or to quantify protein in each position. In orthostatic proteinuria, the recumbent ratio will be <0.2, but the upright sample will have an increased ratio, or the recumbent sample will have <100

mg protein/12 h and the upright sample will have 300 to 900 mg/12 h. If quantitative protein excretion exceeds 1.0 g/d, the diagnosis of orthostatic proteinuria is unlikely.

Orthostatic proteinuria is usually transient, remitting after some time, but can be persistent. Long-term studies in adults have shown orthostatic proteinuria to have a favorable outcome and not be associated with renal disease, but strict criteria, including normal renal function, blood pressure, and serum competent levels, must be used to exclude patients with other renal diseases. Patients with orthostatic proteinuria should be seen at least yearly for several years to be certain that this is not the harbinger of more serious renal disease.

Proteinuria that occurs in both upright and recumbent positions and is persistent should be evaluated more thoroughly (Fig. 21-14). Protein excretion should be quantified in a timed collection, renal function assessed using serum creatinine, and a serum C3 complement level should be obtained. If the serum creatinine and C3 complement are normal and the protein excretion rate is <40 mg/m²/h (<3 g/d), then the patient may be followed every 6 to 12 months. If these results are abnormal, then more extensive testing should be done, possibly including a renal biopsy.

EVALUATING THE CHILD WITH HEMATURIA AND PROTEINURIA

The presence of both hematuria and proteinuria more strongly suggests serious renal disease than either in isolation, especially if other abnormalities such as cellular casts, edema, hypertension, and azotemia are present Fig. 21-15. To evaluate these children, serum creatinine, C3 complement, streptococcal antibody titers (usually ASO and DNase B), and possibly ANA titer should be obtained. The urine protein excretion rate should be evaluated, and if edema is present, serum albumin should be obtained. A renal biopsy may

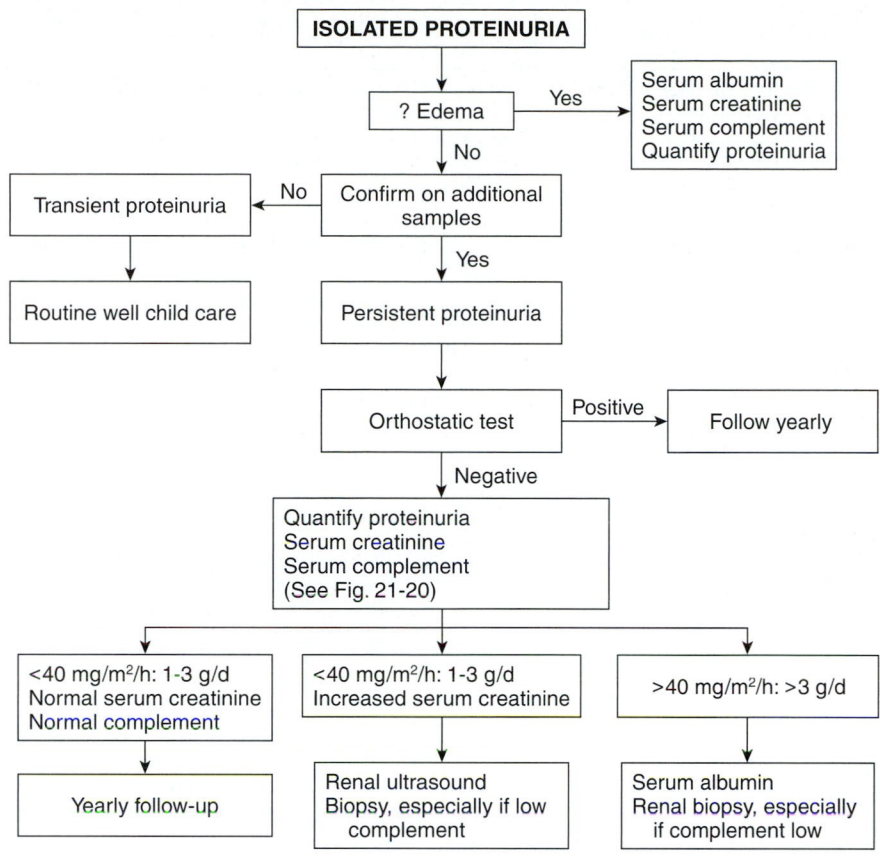

FIGURE 21-14 **Evaluation of children with isolated proteinuria.**

also be indicated, especially if the diagnosis of poststreptococcal glomerulonephritis is excluded. The decision to perform a renal biopsy is influenced by the magnitude of the proteinuria, the presence of other signs and symptoms, and the inability to establish a specific diagnosis. Patients who have a combined nephritic (hematuria, hypertension, azotemia) and nephrotic (proteinuria, low albumin, edema) syndrome are likely to have a systemic disease (SLE, HSP, vasculitis) or progressive primary glomerulopathy (mesangiocapillary disease). In children with proteinuria, hematuria, or both, a low C3 complement level suggests one of four di-

agnosis: postinfectious glomerulonephritis, SLE nephritis, mesangiocapillary glomerulonephritis, or nephritis associated with chronic infection (see Sec. 21.8 and Fig. 21-20).

21.5.6   Evaluating the Child with Edema

Edema in children can occur as a consequence of nonrenal disorders, but renal disease is the most common cause, especially if persistent (Fig. 21-16). Cardiac disease leading to heart failure may

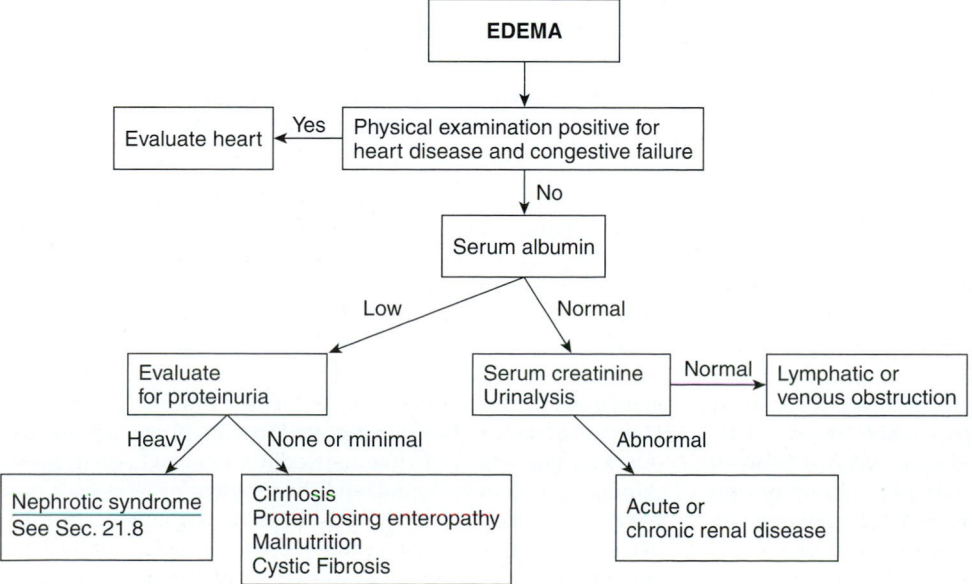

FIGURE 21-16 **Evaluation of children with edema.**

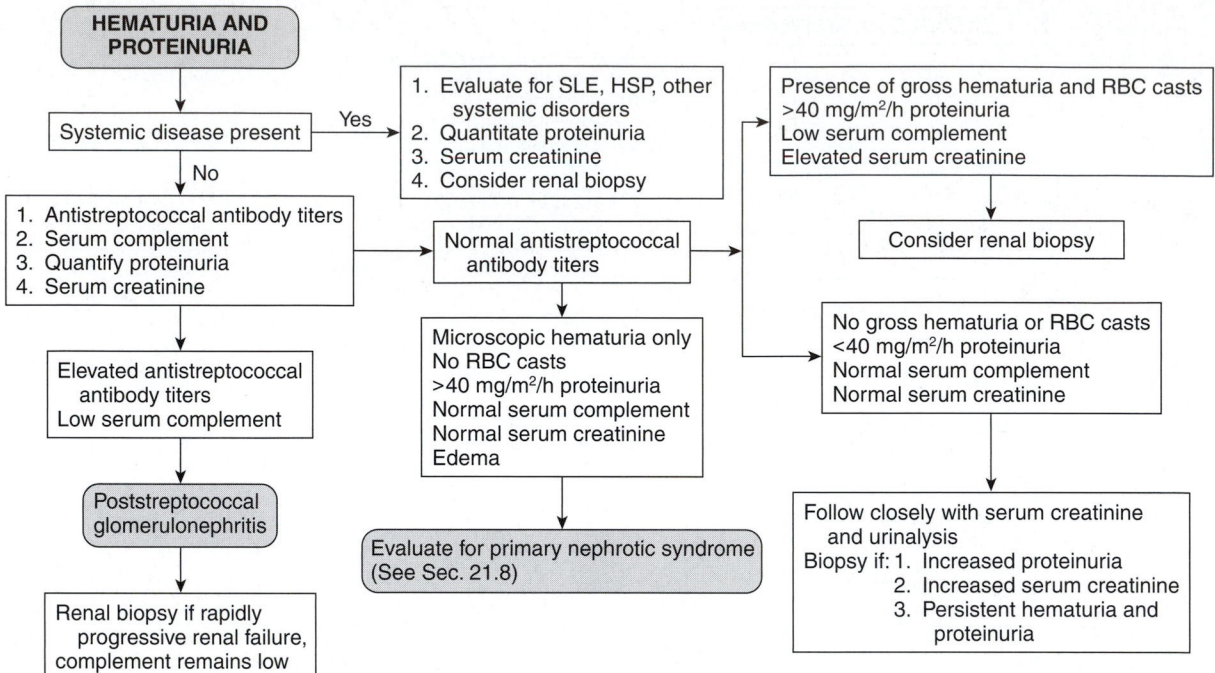

FIGURE 21-15   Evaluation of children with hematuria and proteinuria.

cause edema in children, and allergic disorders can occasionally have edema, but usually transiently and often associated with other signs such as urticaria. Hypoalbuminemia from decreased hepatic synthesis or, rarely, from protein-losing enteropathy will cause generalized edema. A careful history, physical examination, and a few laboratory tests, such as a serum albumin and urinalysis, will usually elucidate the cause of the edema.

Edema in the child with renal disease is most evident in places where tissue resistance is low, such as the periorbital tissue, abdomen, scrotum, and labia, or the hydrostatic pressure is high, such as the lower extremities. Early in renal disease the only place edema may be noticeable is in the periorbital tissue on arising. Edema from acute glomerulonephritis is usually caused by a decreased GFR with enhanced tubular reabsorption of sodium and water. In patients with nephrotic syndrome, marked proteinuria combined with hypoalbuminemia (<2.5 g/dL) lead to decreased plasma oncotic pressure, decreased sodium and water excretion, and edema. With severe or long-standing renal disease, the GFR can be reduced so much that the urine output is less than the fluid intake even with a high fractional excretion of sodium, and edema occurs.

21.5.7 Evaluating the Child with Pyuria

Pyuria is usually defined as more than five WBCs/hpf on centrifuged urine. The most common cause of pyuria is a urinary tract infection, especially if associated with other signs of infection such as fever and dysuria. The reported range of the sensitivity and specificity of pyuria for the diagnosis of a UTI is quite broad, depending on the skill of the microscopist, the rapidity with which the urine is examined after passage, and the study population (see Sec. 8.4). The true positive rate for a UTI in a child with pyuria is between 30 and 70%. On the other hand, about 30% of UTIs are not associated with pyuria. Thus, the diagnosis of a UTI rests on the growth in cultured urine of >100,000 colonies/mL of a single organism (see Sec. 21.6). Pyuria may also be the result of a viral,

mycobacterial, or a fungal infection of the urinary tract, pelvic inflammatory disease, or peritonitis..

Pyuria also occurs as a consequence of fever and dehydration. SLE and interstitial nephritis, usually from a drug reaction, are unusual causes of pyuria. Pyuria in SLE is part of a multisystem disorder and indicates that there is renal involvement. Interstitial nephritis may occur from a drug reaction, often in association with the presence of eosinophils in the urine (sometimes with eosinophilia) or in association with uveitis, the tubular interstitial nephritis uveitis syndrome. The first step in evaluating children with pyuria is to culture the urine for bacteria. If the urine culture is negative, then several additional urinalyses should be obtained to determine if pyuria is persistent. Transient pyuria in an otherwise healthy child requires no further evaluation. Persistent pyuria should be investigated, and the direction of the investigation is based on the history, physical examination, and presence of other abnormal elements in the urinalysis such as eosinophils, casts, and proteinuria.

21.5.8 Evaluation of the Child with Urination Frequency and Urgency

Children between the ages of 5 and 12 years void about four to eight times a day. Frequency refers to a pattern of increased number of voidings each day. Some children with frequency will urinate small amounts several times an hour. Urinary tract infections are the most common cause, especially if accompanied by dysuria and fever. Frequency may persist for weeks after resolution of the infection. Other causes include urethral irritation from vulvovaginitis in girls or meatitis in boys, trauma, foreign body, or bubble baths. Hypercalciuria has also been reported to cause frequency and dysuria. In a number of children, especially younger children, no discernible cause can be found, and the problem resolves with time. On occasion, anticholinergic agents, such as oxybutynin, are useful in reducing the number of voidings. Usually little evaluation is necessary beyond a history, physical examination, urinalysis, and urine culture. Imaging studies of the bladder and urethra are rarely indicated.

References

Abitbol C, Zilleruelo G, Freundlich M, Strauss J: Quantitation of proteinuria with urinary protein/creatinine ratios and random testing with dipsticks in nephrotic children. J Pediatr 116:243–247, 1990

Carlisle EJF, Donnelly SM, Halprin ML: Renal tubular acidosis (RTA): recognize the ammonium defect and pHorget the urine pH. Pediatr Nephrol 5:242–248, 1991

Dodge WF, West EF, Smith EH, Bunch H III: Proteinuria and hematuria in school children: epidemiology and early natural history. J Pediatr 88:327–347, 1976

Feld LG, Meyers KEC, Kaplan BS, Stapleton FB: Limited evaluation of microscopic hematuria in pediatrics. Pediatrics 102:e42–e47, 1998

Houser MT: Characterization of recumbent, ambulatory, and postexercise proteinuria in the adolescent. Pediatr Res 21:442–446, 1987

Schwartz GJ, Haycock GB, Spitzer A: Plasma creatinine and urea concentration in children: normal values for age and sex. J Pediatr 88:828–830, 1976

Vehaskari VM, Raploa J, Koskimies O, et al: Microscopic hematuria in school children: epidemiology and clinicopathologic evaluation. J Pediatr 95:676–684, 1979

21.6   URINARY TRACT INFECTION

Thomas Kennedy

Urinary tract infections (UTIs) are common throughout infancy, childhood, and adolescence. Nevertheless, significant uncertainty and controversy remain regarding important aspects such as localization of the site of infection to the kidneys or bladder, the need and extent of evaluation following a UTI, optimal duration of treatment, and outcome. The importance of UTI in children is related not only to frequency of occurrence but also to its significant morbidity and potentially severe long-term consequences such as hypertension and chronic renal failure. Renal scarring, the prelude to these sequelae, occurs mainly as the result of parenchymal infections in the first 2 to 4 years of life. Thus, the challenge is to diagnose and treat UTI promptly and accurately in infants and young children at an age when symptoms are most vague and the collection of urine for culture is technically most difficult.

UTI is usually defined as a bacterial infection at any level of the urinary tract, including the bladder (cystitis), renal pelvis (pyelitis), or renal parenchyma (pyelonephritis). Infections of the urethra (urethritis) and reproductive tract (eg, epididymitis, prostatitis) are much less common, most often occur as a sexually transmitted disease (see Sec. 21.16). Much of the attention and controversy regarding UTI in childhood focus on vesicoureteral reflux (VUR), defined as the retrograde flow of urine from the bladder into the ureters and/or collecting systems, which is commonly present in infants and very young children with febrile UTI.

21.6.1   Incidence and Etiology

The incidence of UTI in childhood is not known precisely because it is not a reportable disease, and many cases, especially in infants, are probably underdiagnosed or misdiagnosed. Furthermore, the definitions and criteria for diagnosis vary considerably, for example, including or excluding children with asymptomatic bacteriuria, diagnosis based on results of bagged specimens, or the requirement for bacterial growth of $>10^5$ colonies/mL. This variability notwithstanding, one large study found the incidence between birth and 12 years to be 1.3% for boys and 3.7% for girls. Although other studies support these figures, several reports in school-age girls find the incidence to be three to five times higher. The incidence of UTI in girls is usually found to be three to seven times greater than in boys. Only in the neonatal period do boys with UTI outnumber girls, probably on the basis of obstruction from posterior urethral valves and other congenital urinary tract anomalies. Although the incidence of UTI in uncircumcised boys is 10 times that of circumcised boys, this is not a justification to perform circumcision in the newborn. Statistical analysis demonstrates that almost 100 circumcisions must be done to prevent one UTI, casting serious doubt on circumcision as a public health, infection-control measure. In older boys, UTI is so uncommon that recurrent infection should raise the suspicion of self-instrumentation, a common cause in at least one study.

Recurrence of UTI is common and in some studies is as high as 80% with an approximate attrition rate of 20% following each subsequent infection. Most recurrences develop within 6 months of the previous infection and are caused by a different organism or serotype.

The majority of UTIs in the pediatric age group are caused by *E. coli*, which account for 90% of infections in most surveys. Other gram-negative organisms associated with UTI are *Klebsiella, Enterobacter, Proteus,* and *Pseudomonas.* The gram-positive organisms occasionally encountered are *Enterococcus,* group B *Streptococcus* in the neonatal period, and *Staphylococcus saprophyticus* in sexually active adolescents.

The incidence of ampicillin-resistant *E. coli* is now high enough that identification of the organism and antibiotic sensitivity testing are mandatory in all cases. Specifically, presumptive identification of the organism by dip-slide screening cultures followed by empiric therapy is no longer adequate. One important qualification on sensitivity testing of urinary pathogens is that antibiotic levels achieved in urine and renal parenchyma are so high that successful eradication of an infection using an antibiotic to which the organism is "resistant" on standard microbiological testing is possible.

21.6.2   Pathogenesis

Most UTIs occur as a result of ascending bacterial infection: from the urethra to the bladder in cystitis and from the ureter to the kidney in pyelonephritis. This route of infection occurs in all pediatric age groups, including neonates. Hematogenous spread to the kidney is the exception, but this may occur in neonates with *Staphylococcus aureus* sepsis. On the other hand, bacteremia as a result of UTI is more common, especially in neonates.

The ascending route of infection helps explain the gender difference because the shorter female urethra increases the frequency in girls. Bacteriostatic effects of prostatic fluid also play a protective role in pubertal boys.

The pathogenesis of UTI is an interplay of host defense and bacterial properties. For host defenses to function optimally, intermittent complete emptying of the bladder must occur. Both humoral and cellular components of the immune system are involved, including local IgA and IgG as well as polymorphonuclear leukocytes and mononuclear cells. Additionally, bactericidal secretions from uroepithelial cells and glycoproteins that inhibit bacterial adherence are present. Urine is an excellent culture medium, however, and persistent residual urine in the bladder not only promotes bacterial growth but also interferes with local host defenses.

Bacterial characteristics that help determine infection include resistance factors that protect against phagocytic killing, toxins that disrupt normal ureteral peristalsis, and adhesion factors. The adhesion factors, fimbriae or pili, diminish bacterial washout with voiding and permit bacteria to ascend the ureter even in the absence of vesicoureteral reflux (VUR). Clinically, the adherence properties of the causative organism vary directly with the incidence of pyelonephritis. For example, fimbriated *E. coli* were found in 94% of girls with pyelonephritis but in only 19% of those with cystitis. The pili are often called P-fimbriae because of their affinity for the P1 erythrocyte antigen, which illustrates the role of host susceptibility because the incidence of the P1 antigen in girls with UTI is significantly greater than that in the general population.

Once established in renal parenchyma, infection results in an intense inflammatory response that not only is important to control the infection but also causes many of the systemic signs and symptoms such as fever, clinical toxicity, and CVA tenderness common in pyelonephritis. This inflammatory response contributes to the scarring that may occur with parenchymal infection.

21.6.3   Diagnosis

Diagnosis of UTI is generally based on isolating a single, common urinary tract pathogen in culture at a concentration greater than 100,000 colonies per milliliter. However, cultures with more than one organism cannot be discounted, and lower colony counts may also be significant, depending on the rate of urine flow and the interval between micturitions. Any growth of bacteria in a properly done bladder catheterization or suprapubic aspirate is significant. These methods of urine collection are mandatory for the accurate diagnosis of UTI in infants not yet toilet trained. Clean-bagged specimens are not reliable, except to exclude the diagnosis if negative. In older children, clean-catch midstream collection is commonly used. Girls should be asked to sit backward on the toilet so they straddle the seat and exclude the possibility of contamination by urethral–vaginal reflux.

The initial evaluation for UTI is usually the urinalysis (see Sec. 21.5.1). The dipstick can identify the presence of blood by the hemoglobin test strip, white cells through the detection of leukocyte esterase, and gram-negative bacteria through the conversion of urinary nitrates to nitrites. Studies to determine sensitivity and specificity of the dipstick to diagnose UTI vary widely, but generally there is a higher sensitivity (~90%) than specificity (~70%) with a lower positive predictive value (~30%) (see Sec. 8.4). All tests perform better when evaluated in a population of patients in which the incidence of UTI is increased, such as febrile children, those with previous UTI, or anomalies of the urinary tract. Pyuria, as reflected by leukocyte esterase or microscopy, is neither sensitive nor specific (see Sec. 21.5.7). Sensitivity is decreased largely because pyuria may be intermittent and because of the significant occurrence of asymptomatic bacteriuria, which may be an incidental finding in a febrile child. Specificity is low because pyuria may be present in many conditions other than UTI, including any form of glomerulonephritis or tubulointerstitial nephritis, as well as acute febrile illnesses associated with volume depletion. The nitrite determination is very specific, but not very sensitive because the test is time-dependent, requiring exposure of urine to bacteria for approximately 4 hours. Therefore, a first morning urine is desirable. The nitrate conversion occurs only by gram-negative organisms. Thus, gram-positive pathogens such as group B *Streptococcus*, *Enterococcus*, and *Staphylococcus* will be missed. Microscopic hematuria is an almost universal concomitant of UTI but is too nonspecific to be helpful. Asymptomatic microscopic hematuria is almost never a presenting sign of UTI. Gross hematuria with UTI is rare in children but more common in older adolescents and adults (see Table 21-11).

Microscopic examination of a freshly voided specimen can confirm the presence of white and red cells but is inexact (see Sec. 21.5). Additionally, assessment of bacteria in the unstained sediment is unreliable and is never considered significant. Gram stain of the urine, however, is a very useful and reliable screening tool with a positive predictive value of 80% when done by experienced personnel.

The two commonly used culture media for identification of urinary pathogens, McConkey and sheep blood agar, will readily support the growth of bacteria most likely to cause UTI. However, occasionally, UTI will be caused by organisms such as *Hemophilus* and *Gardnerella*, anaerobes and fastidious aerobes that require more time or special media (eg, in the case of *Hemophilus*, chocolate agar) to grow. This explanation or the possibility of pretreatment with one or more doses of antibiotics must be kept in mind in a child who clinically appears to have a UTI but whose culture is sterile. *The gold standard for the diagnosis of UTI remains the urine culture.*

OTHER LABORATORY TESTS

There are several laboratory studies that may be helpful in differentiating upper from lower tract infection, but none are diagnostic. Leukocytosis with a left shift is frequently present in pyelonephritis and is unexpected in cystitis. Elevation of the sedimentation rate, often marked, is commonly seen in parenchymal infection but is not specific. Elevation of the BUN and creatinine usually reflects volume depletion and dehydration. Acute renal insufficiency is very unusual in pyelonephritis. The most common derangement in renal function is impaired urine-concentrating capacity, although this is rarely clinically important. Other tests of tubular injury, such as excretion of β_2-microglobulin and *N*-acetyl glucosaminidase, are used in some centers as an adjunct to diagnose pyelonephritis.

21.6.4   Associated Conditions

Any condition that interferes with complete bladder emptying poses a risk for UTI. These include constipation (very important because of frequency and successful treatment), neurogenic bladder (eg, meningomyelocele), and voiding dysfunction. The last is often overlooked, and a history of abnormal voiding patterns, especially those associated with urgency and enuresis, should be sought (see Sec. 21.16). Anatomic abnormalities of the urinary tract, including posterior urethral valves, ureterocele, and, most commonly, vesicoureteral reflux are also important risk factors. Conditions associated with chronic perineal irritation, for example, from soaps, bubble bath, pinworms, or chronic perineal trauma such as that experienced by dirt bikers or equestrians, may also predispose to infection. Other children at risk include those with nephrolithiasis; nephrotic syndrome; cocaine-exposed infants; inner-city, low-birth-weight infants; and uncircumcised boys. Bladder catheterization is an iatrogenic risk factor, particularly when the catheter is indwelling. Finally, sexually active, adolescent girls are at risk and should be advised to void following intercourse.

An important risk for UTI with resistant organisms is recent and/or recurrent use of antibiotics, whether for acute infection such as otitis media or for continuous prophylaxis. Antibiotics may convert normal periurethral flora, usually lactobacilli, to coliforms, which are found in a high percentage of girls with UTI.

Nephronia refers to acute focal bacterial pyelonephritis affecting one or more renal lobules. *Acute lobar nephronia* is being recognized more frequently and can be detected by sonography, DMSA, and CT scan. The symptoms are the same as those of diffuse pyelonephritis, although the incidence of bacteremia, even in older children, is as high as 30%. *E. coli* is the most common causative organism. Because of the small risk of abscess formation, treatment with 1 to 2 weeks of parenteral therapy has been advocated. Follow-up studies to demonstrate resolution are recommended.

Everything about *asymptomatic bacteriuria,* from definition to significance, is uncertain because what constitutes "asymptomatic" is unclear. The prevalence of asymptomatic bacteriuria in preschool-age girls is 2%, and it can be identified at routine health maintenance visits through detection of nitrites on a urine dipstick. Although the value of screening urinalyses is a topic of controversy, routine screening cultures for UTI are *not* recommended. Some data suggest that asymptomatic bacteriuria may not be a totally benign condition. However, compelling evidence from several sources suggests that children with asymptomatic bacteriuria need not and should not be treated because treatment actually increases the incidence of symptomatic infections.

Viral UTIs are very uncommon. Although viruria is often detected during acute illness, actual renal involvement and/or inflammation is poorly characterized and quite unusual. Hemorrhagic cystitis caused by adenovirus 11 and 21 is well documented in children but also very infrequent. Fungal UTI, especially with *Candida* species, usually occurs in children who are immunocompromised, on continuous antibiotics, have an indwelling catheter, or have some combination of these.

Xanthogranulomatous pyelonephritis is rarely seen in children. This form of chronic renal parenchymal infection is most often caused by *Proteus,* although other organisms, including anaerobes, have been involved. Symptoms include fever, weight loss, and abdominal or flank pain. Nephrolithiasis or another obstructing lesion is common. The best imaging study for diagnosis is CT scan, and if it is diagnosed early, treatment with antibiotics may be effective; if not, nephrectomy is required.

Cystitis cystica, also called *follicular cystitis,* is an unusual entity that is more a complication of chronic or recurrent bacterial infection of the bladder than a separate form of UTI. In this condition, lymphoid aggregates form nodules on the bladder wall that frequently go undiagnosed unless the bladder is imaged or directly visualized on cystoscopy. The changes are reversible with resolution of infection. Cystitis cystica has also been reported in girls with no urinary tract symptoms.

Interstitial cystitis is a controversial and poorly understood chronic condition that is extremely unusual in childhood, occurs mostly in girls, and is characterized by symptoms of bladder inflammation including pain, frequency, and urgency, but no infectious etiology can be identified. Episodes of hematuria may occur. Biopsy reveals superficial inflammation with petechial hemorrhage. There is no known consistently successful therapy, although a report in children found that hydrodistension therapy was very effective in relieving symptoms.

21.6.5   Clinical Manifestations

Although the definitive diagnosis of UTI is based on culture results, the decision to obtain a culture is based on clinical signs and symptoms that are often vague and nonspecific and vary with age. Therefore, a high index of suspicion for UTI is essential. In neonates, lethargy, irritability, poor feeding, vomiting, diarrhea, apnea, fever or hypothermia, and prolonged jaundice are all frequent findings. Although very nonspecific and often more suggestive of acute gastroenteritis than UTI, the diagnosis is rarely missed, since a urinalysis and urine culture are routinely part of the "rule out sepsis" evaluation performed in this age group (see Chapter 13). In the first 90 days of life, the same symptoms are common, and the evaluation for "fever, rule out sepsis" usually identifies a UTI if present. The incidence of UTI in infants in this age group with fever and no localized findings is 5 to 10%.

Infants older than 90 days and less than 2 to 3 years present the largest diagnostic challenge because the evaluation of fever in this age group does not involve a protocol in which urine is routinely examined or cultured. Fever secondary to a viral illness is the most common diagnosis in this age group, and consideration of UTI is frequently overlooked, at least initially. Fever, constitutional complaints, abdominal discomfort, and GI symptoms are common in pyelonephritis, whereas frequency and irritability on micturition are often the only indicators of cystitis.

In older children who are both verbal and toilet trained, the diagnosis becomes more straightforward. With cystitis, all or some combination of the classic signs of dysuria, frequency, urgency, suprapubic discomfort, daytime or noctural enuresis, and perhaps low-grade fever are present. With pyelonephritis, high fever, clinical toxicity, vomiting, and abdominal and/or flank pain are most common. These "upper tract" symptoms may or may not be accompanied by lower tract complaints, and surprisingly, up to one-third of children with clinical pyelonephritis have no symptoms of cystitis. The absence of CVA tenderness to percussion (Murphy test) is not reliable to exclude parenchymal infection in young children. However, when present it is helpful and should be performed as part of the physical examination of all children suspected of UTI.

Localizing the site of infection remains a clinical diagnosis. Despite claims to the contrary by supporters of renal scintigraphy, there is no "gold standard" test to differentiate renal parenchymal from a bladder infection. In many cases, differentiation is easy. For example, a 3-year-old with a 104°F fever, shaking chills, vomiting, abdominal pain, and pyuria is not a diagnostic challenge. Likewise, an afebrile 7-year-old with frequency, dysuria, foul-smelling urine, and pyuria has cystitis. The child with a 101.3°F fever, abdominal pain, and urgency, however, is less clear but should be presumed to have parenchymal infection.

21.6.6   Imaging

The first goal of imaging the urinary tract is to discover abnormalities that either may be risk factors for UTI or may preclude prompt response to therapy. These risk factors include vesicoureteral reflux or voiding dysfunction, and factors that complicate therapy include partial ureteropelvic junction obstruction or cystic kidney disease. The second goal of imaging is to monitor renal growth and detect scarring.

Determining which children to evaluate, which tests are most appropriate, and when to obtain studies is critical to develop a rational and consistent approach to this controversial component of UTI.

For a long time, majority opinion favored imaging evaluation of the upper and lower urinary tract in every child following a well-documented first UTI. Currently, a more selective approach is recommended (Fig. 21-17):

(1) All patients with documented UTI should have ultrasound to assess integrity of the urinary tract;

(2) VCUG should be obtained in all patients less than 3 years of age and all patients with or suspected of having pyelonephritis;

(3) No further studies if ultrasound is normal in children older than 3 years or with minimal symptoms at presentation.

There are several reasons for routinely imaging *infants* and young children with UTI: (1) a high incidence of VUR is found in this age group, approaching 35 to 50% (70% in children <1 year); (2) renal scarring following infection is most likely to occur in the first 2 to 4 years of life; and (3) symptoms are so vague that differentiation between upper and lower tract infection is usually impossible.

Once a decision to image the urinary tract has been reached, the choice of studies must be made.

Cystoscopy, although not an imaging study, directly visualizes the bladder, urethra, and ureteral orifices, but it is extremely invasive, generally requires general anesthesia in children, and offers little advantage over cystography in the evaluation of a child with UTI. Cystoscopy in girls with recurrent cystitis to diagnose "urethral stenosis," a condition whose existence is seriously questioned, is not indicated.

The intravenous pyelogram (IVP) has largely been replaced by sonography (see Secs. 21.5.3 and 8.3). Ultrasonography of the kidney and/or the bladder is simple and easy to carry out. Neither radiation exposure nor pain is involved, and it provides very accurate images and information on kidney size, shape, location, and texture (see Sec. 8.3). Echogenicity of the kidney may be altered with inflammation, either diffusely (as occurs in pyelonephritis) or focally (as is seen in acute lobar nephronia). Ultrasonography cannot assess renal function, reliably diagnose or exclude VUR, or demonstrate mild scars. Well-established scars can be detected, and renal growth can be documented with repeated studies over time. Assessment of renal growth is an important component of the follow-up of infants and children with VUR (Fig. 21-17). Color Doppler sonography may permit the evaluation of VUR without

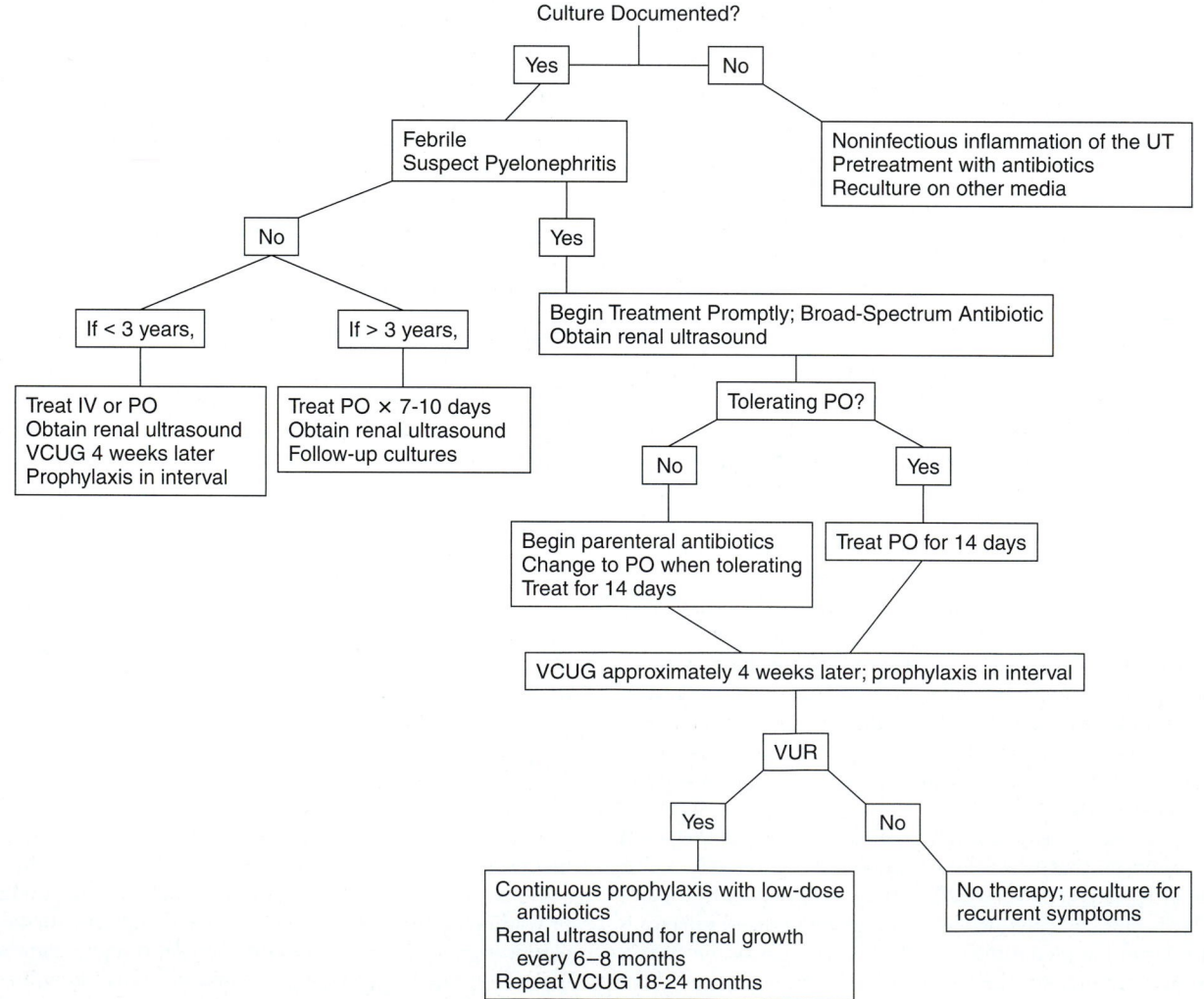

FIGURE 21-17   **Algorithm for evaluation of the child with symptoms of urinary tract infection.**
UT = urinary tract; VCUG = voiding cystourethrogram; IV = intravenous; PO = orally.

invasive catheterization or radiation exposure in the future. Ultrasonography of the bladder is limited by the requirement for a distended bladder. Information is provided on bladder wall thickness, capacity, and residual volume.

Radionuclide imaging of the kidney provides both functional and anatomic information. Renal images demonstrating "cold" spots indicate areas of tubular dysfunction and/or decreased intrarenal blood flow because DMSA is taken up mainly from peritubular blood vessels, and abnormalities may occur in the course of acute parenchymal infection or in areas of scarring, a fact that may result in errors in interpretation of the scan. Because results in animal studies have shown excellent correlation between DMSA scans and anatomic infection, and because no other reliable diagnostic study is available in children, DMSA has been touted as a "gold standard" for the localization of infection and recommended by some as a routine initial study in children with febrile UTI. Unfortunately, during the acute phase of infection, false positives and false negatives as well as a disturbingly high number of equivocal scans are reported. A sensitivity of 50 to 85% and a specificity of 45 to 90%, along with high cost and concerns regarding prolonged radiation exposure to the renal cortex, dampen enthusiasm for routine use of DMSA scars, but for the detection of renal scars in specific circumstances it may be helpful.

Voiding cystourethrography (VCUG) is performed by catheterizing the bladder and instilling radiocontrast material to distend it. Although the primary goal is to demonstrate or exclude the presence of VUR, the VCUG also provides information on the anatomy, capacity, and function of the bladder. The voiding phase is important to assess completeness of voiding and residual urine and, in boys, to look for urethral valves. If VUR is present, the severity of reflux can be assessed and graded. The disadvantages of a VCUG include its "emotional" invasiveness, the requirement for fluoroscopic x-ray exposure, and the risk of either allergic reaction or iatrogenic UTI. The radionuclide VCUG is similar but involves less gonadal radiation exposure because it avoids fluoroscopy. Although at least as sensitive as contrast cystography in detecting mild degrees of reflux, its assessment of the bladder and urethra is less precise. Because of this limitation but lower radiation exposure, a reasonable approach is to perform the radiocontrast cystogram initially and hold the radionuclide cystogram for subsequent studies if indicated.

Computed tomography (CT) of the kidney provides much the same information as a well-done ultrasound but may be useful in the evaluation of the rare child with suspected renal or perinephric abscess.

The younger the infant with UTI, the more likely an anatomic abnormality of the urinary tract will be found. Therefore, young or febrile children should have an ultrasound carried out promptly because an obstructed, infected kidney is at extremely high risk for damage (pyonephrosis). In an older child, especially if treated as an outpatient, the ultrasound can be done at a more convenient time. DMSA scanning may be done acutely if determination of parenchymal infection is warranted but if detection of scarring is the objective, this study should be delayed 6 months to 2 years and obtained only if urgently indicated. The best time for the VCUG has long been debated and remains unsettled. A UTI may interfere with normal ureteral peristalsis and result in transient dilatation and/or VUR. Therefore, to avoid mistaking mild, temporary reflux for chronic VUR, most VCUGs are delayed until the acute infection has been treated and inflammation has been resolved, generally 4 to 8 weeks, although there are no special data to make a firm recommendation. Because of the need for bladder catheterization at the time of the study, the VCUG should be scheduled at an opportune time for a culture, which should routinely be obtained.

21.6.7   Vesicoureteral Reflux

Much of the controversy regarding the significance, the extent of evaluation, and the outcome of UTI in childhood relates to the presence, the severity, and the natural history of vesicoureteral reflux (VUR). Review of the sizable medical literature on VUR yields a confusing conundrum of inconclusive and contradictory data. Moreover, the relationship between reflux and renal scarring is inconclusive. Although very little about VUR elicits total acceptance, general agreement on several aspects is clear.

Primary reflux is a congenital abnormality of the normally oblique insertion of the ureter through the bladder wall at the ureterovesical junction and is not associated with urinary tract or other congenital anomalies. Primary VUR usually resolves spontaneously during the first decade. Although the likelihood of resolution exceeds 80% when the VUR is mild, discovered in the first year of life, and unilateral, even the most severe reflux has a 40 to 50% spontaneous resolution rate. Patients with primary reflux rarely develop significant clinical sequelae such as proteinuria, hypertension, or renal insufficiency.

Secondary reflux develops from elevated intravesicular pressure that may result from abnormal voiding patterns or anomalies, including urinary tract obstruction. In one cause of secondary reflux, known as Hinman syndrome or psychological nonneuropathic bladder (see Sec. 21.16), apparently functional incoordination between detrusor contraction and relaxation of the external sphincter is acquired and leads to incomplete voiding, incontinence, and elevated intravesicular pressures culminating in VUR, hydronephrosis, and reflux nephropathy. Resolution of secondary VUR is less predictable and based on treating the underlying cause. Patients with secondary reflux are at greatest risk for long-term renal sequelae.

The true incidence of reflux in the general population is unknown, but limited data suggest 1 to 2%. In addition to a decreasing incidence with age, the rate in whites is about 10 times greater than that in African-Americans. Genetic predisposition is suggested by an increased incidence in siblings of children with a history of VUR. The risk for siblings is as high as 50% depending on the age of the child. Some clinicians recommend performing a VCUG on all siblings of a child with VUR. A less invasive approach is to be certain the parents and care providers are aware of the risk and promptly obtain urine cultures from the siblings for any unexplained febrile illness. Other abnormalities of the urinary tract that are associated with an increased incidence of secondary VUR include multicystic dysplastic kidneys, ureteropelvic junction obstruction, and the prune belly syndrome (see Secs. 21.3 and 21.16). A genetic abnormality may be responsible for both VUR and the cellular mechanisms responsible for scar formation.

Antenatal ultrasound appears to provide an important clue regarding the presence of reflux. In a recent study, 22% of fetuses with evidence of dilatation of the renal pelvis on ultrasound were found to have VUR after birth. VUR was the most common abnormality, about five times greater than the presence of either ureteropelvic junction obstruction or dysplasia and three times greater than isolated hydronephrosis. Of the infants with VUR, 60% had a normal postnatal ultrasound, emphasizing that ultrasonography cannot accurately assess reflux. On the other hand, the significance of asymptomatic primary reflux in this population is unclear.

The incidence of reflux in children with UTI is approximately 35%, although this overall rate does not consider that VUR decreases with age (eg, present in 70% of children with UTI <1 year but in only 5% of adolescents). On the other hand, only one-half of children with clinical and DMSA scintigraphy evidence of parenchymal infection will have VUR, demonstrating that reflux is not a prerequisite for pyelonephritis, which develops in the presence of ascending, adherent bacteria.

The relationship between VUR and renal scarring is controversial. In children with UTI and VUR, 20 to 40% will develop renal scars, but the cause-and-effect relationship of this association is not proven. Although scars may be present in the absence of VUR, they do not preclude the possibility of VUR in the past. Much of the uncertainty regarding VUR and renal scarring relates to the role of infection in the occurrence and progression of scarring. *Reflux nephropathy* has replaced "chronic pyelonephritis" to describe the association of renal scarring, proteinuria, hypertension, and renal insufficiency that is frequently associated with focal glomerulosclerosis on renal biopsy. The term reflux nephropathy implies that VUR alone can injure the kidney and is responsible for the scars, although this remains unproven. Therefore, another term, *postinfectious nephropathy,* has begun to appear and may be descriptively more correct. There is agreement that reflux with infection, as well as infection alone, can cause renal damage. Current thinking is that reflux associated with high pressure (ie, secondary reflux) is capable of causing injury, but not sterile or primary reflux alone.

Furthermore, the presence of VUR is not as important as the presence of *intrarenal reflux* (IRR), in which there is "pyelotubular backflow" of urine into renal papillae. IRR is best demonstrated by contrast cystography, but this imaging modality almost certainly does not demonstrate all instances of IRR. Although IRR is most commonly associated with more severe grades of VUR, it need not be. The critical feature of IRR is the presence of compound papillae whose orifices are flat and permit reflux of infected urine into renal parenchyma. The other form of papilla has convex, nonrefluxing orifices and predominates in most human kidneys. In kidneys with IRR, compound papillae are most frequently found in the bipolar region, the same area where scarring is common. Patients with primary reflux, which includes IRR, may be at risk for renal scarring.

Whether renal scars that develop in children with UTI (with or without VUR) are acquired or congenital remains unresolved. The high incidence of VUR in patients with UTI may be causative or merely result from a detection bias (see Sec. 8.4.) because investigations to detect VUR are usually initiated in response to a preceding UTI. The possibility of an underlying cellular or molecular basis for both renal scars and VUR is suggested by (1) the observation that scarring occurs most frequently in secondary reflux that is associated with other developmental anomalies of the kidney and urinary tract (MCDK, prune-belly syndrome, posterior urethral valves, meningomyelocele); (2) the association of segmental renal dysplasia, reflux, and hypertension found in patients with an Up-Askmark kidney; (3) the failure of prophylactic antibodies or surgical intervention to reduce the incidence or progression of scars in children with UTI and VUR; and (4) the inherently complex nature of renal morphogenesis in which primordial elements of both the parenchyma and collecting system must interact and are influenced by molecular processes (see Sec. 21.1).

In the final analysis, both VUR and renal scars may be the result of a defect in renal development such as aberrant ureteric bud branching on induction failure (see Sec. 21.1) or a genetically controlled molecular process as yet undetermined. Nonetheless, young infants are at greatest risk for long-term sequelae.

21.6.8   Treatment

The treatment of UTI begins with prevention, mainly by the identification and removal of risk factors that often are not evident until after an episode of UTI has occurred, and focused questions may reveal a history of constipation, abnormal voiding pattern, etc. For example, children with recurrent UTIs who drink small amounts and void twice a day should be encouraged to increase their intake and void more frequently. Children at statistically higher risk for VUR and UTI, including the siblings of children with reflux and infants with evidence of renal pelvis dilatation on antenatal ultrasound, should be identified and promptly examined, and culture of the urine obtained in the presence of an unexplained fever.

Antibiotic therapy is often begun empirically on the basis of signs, symptoms, and an abnormal urinalysis before culture and sensitivity results are available. Even before an antibiotic is chosen, a decision must be made whether to administer the antibiotic orally or parenterally. Because antibiotics are excreted by glomerular filtration and/or tubular secretion, extremely high concentrations are achieved in the kidneys and urine. Therefore, oral doses are sufficient to treat infection, even in cases of febrile UTI, when parenchymal infection is likely. A major qualification is that frequently the child or infant is quite ill and vomiting with no guarantee that an oral antibiotic will be tolerated. Furthermore, because the organism and its antibiotic sensitivity are initially unknown, parenteral therapy will provide broader coverage for young or very ill children.

The large majority of UTIs will be caused by *E. coli,* which previously have been sensitive to amoxicillin and/or trimethoprim-sulfamethoxazole. More recently, many medical centers are finding significant and increasing resistance to these antibiotics, and initial empiric therapy should be a third-generation cephalosporin. Subsequent therapy is directed by sensitivity testing of the organism, using amoxicillin if possible, because it is much less expensive and has a narrower spectrum.

The ideal duration of therapy is not known precisely. Studies investigating so-called "short course" therapy (eg, single-dose or 1- to 3-day therapy) in children have yielded contradictory and inconclusive results, and this approach is not recommended. For uncomplicated cystitis, 7 to 10 days of therapy is sufficient, whereas 14 days of therapy is indicated for children who have, or are suspected of having, pyelonephritis. Symptoms, including fever, often resolve quickly but may persist for several days. If symptoms persist for more than 48 hours, a repeat culture should be done. A follow-up culture may be done more than 72 hours after antibiotic therapy is complete.

Prophylactic therapy should be begun in infants awaiting a VCUG following a UTI and continued until normal anatomy is demonstrated. Prophylaxis is usually given continuously to young children known to have VUR, partial obstruction, or voiding dysfunction. Likewise, prophylaxis is also effective to break the cycle of infection in children with recurrent UTI who have anatomically normal urinary tracts. Choice of therapy ideally should be limited to those drugs that are effective in UTI prevention in clinical trials, including trimethoprim-sulfamethoxazole, nitrofurantoin, or sulfisoxazole. Tmp-Smx is contraindicated in infants less than 2 months. Because nitrofurantoin has a high rate of gastrointestinal intolerance, and sulfisoxazole must be administered four times daily, amoxicillin is frequently used in very young infants and is well tolerated, but its effectiveness is unproven, and infection with resistant organisms may occur. The duration of prophylactic therapy must be individualized. For example, in a child with VUR, prophylaxis should be continued until a VCUG shows resolution of reflux or for a minimum of 1 to 2 years, the intervals during which reflux is likely to resolve. In some cases, parents are reluctant to submit children to repeat VCUG, and empiric cessation of prophylactic antibiotics can be undertaken with a plan for repeat VCUG if UTI recurs. In a child without reflux but with recurrent UTI, 4 to 6 months free of infection is desirable and may be achieved with prophylactic antibiotics. Compliance with long-term medication is a major concern, and close follow-up with encouragement is important.

Reimplantation of the ureter(s) (ureteroneocystotomy) is very successful in correcting VUR. However, data do not demonstrate convincingly a reduction in either the incidence of UTI or the risk for progression of renal scarring. Surgical repair of VUR should be limited to children with the most severe grades of reflux (grade V) and those who have repeated UTIs despite antimicrobial prophylaxis. Surgery may also be considered in children 12 years or older who have persistent reflux and recurrent episodes of pyelonephritis because spontaneous resolution of VUR after this age is unlikely and may predispose females to UTI during pregnancy.

21.6.9   Outcome

The risk of recurrence following an acute UTI is significant. Studies vary, but rates of 30 to 80% are expected, and most occur within the first 6 months of the initial infection. Recurrence is highest in children with UTI risk factors such as incomplete bladder emptying but may occur in otherwise healthy children with normal voiding patterns. The risk of subsequent recurrences is more than 50%, and in some children with frequent recurrences, use of prophylactic antibiotics is warranted for several months. In the absence of obstruction or severe reflux, the long-term outcome of children with recurrent UTI is no different than those with only one infection.

The long-term outcome of UTI in the pediatric age group is very good despite the high incidence of VUR and the fact that 20 to 30% of children with febrile UTI have renal scarring during childhood. The major concerns are progressive scarring, hypertension, and renal insufficiency. Fortunately, these sequelae occur uncommonly and are usually predictable based on azotemia, hypertension, associated congenital renal abnormalities, and/or severe scars present at initial assessment. Approximately 10% of children with renal scarring will develop elevated blood pressure. The contribution of UTI, reflux, and renal scars to the development of end-stage renal disease (ESRD) is unclear, but they are probably not a major cause, independent of other associated anomalies. Nevertheless, patients with secondary reflux or scars must have long-term follow-up to monitor blood pressure, protein excretion, renal function, and renal growth. Children with renal scarring who have significant proteinuria and/or hypertension are more likely to develop progressive renal insufficiency.

Overall, the long-term outlook for children who have UTIs and are closely followed and promptly treated is excellent, especially if associated renal abnormalities are detected early. The challenge is identification of children at risk for renal sequelae and their prevention.

References

Committee on Quality Improvement, Subcommittee on Urinary Tract Infection: Practice parameter: the diagnosis, treatment, and evaluation of the initial urinary tract infection in febrile infants and young children. Pediatrics 103:843–852, 1999

Dillon MJ, Goonasekera CDA: Reflux nephropathy. J Am Soc Nephrol 9: 2377–2383, 1998

Greenfield SP, Wan J: Vesicoureteral reflux: practical aspects of evaluation and management. Pediatr Nephrol 10:789–794, 1996

Hoberman A, Wald ER, Hickey RW, et al: Oral versus initial intravenous therapy for urinary tract infections in young febrile children. Pediatrics 104:79–86, 1999

Roberts JA: Factors predisposing to urinary tract infections in children. Pediatr Nephrol 10:517–522, 1996

Smellie JM, Prescod NP, Shaw PJ, Risdon RA, Bryant TN: Childhood reflux and urinary infection: a follow-up of 10-14 years in 226 adults. Pediatr Nephrol 12:727–736, 1998

21.7   ACUTE RENAL FAILURE

Norman J. Siegel

Acute renal failure (ARF) is the sudden and unexpected loss of renal function characterized by a fall in glomerular filtration rate (GFR) and usually detected by a rise in serum creatinine (S_{Cr}). In children and adolescents, the most common cause of ARF is acquired renal disease, usually acute glomerulonephritis or hemolytic uremic syndrome, but on some occasions acute interstitial nephritis presents as ARF as well (Fig. 21-18). Acute glomerulonephritis and hemolytic uremic syndrome present with systemic signs (hematuria, proteinuria, hypertension, and edema) and can generally be differentiated from one another by the classical triads of hematuria, hypertension, and azotemia as the presenting findings in acute glomerulonephritis and of microangiopathic hemolytic anemia, thrombocytopenia, and reduced renal function in hemolytic uremic syndrome (see Figs. 21-19 and 21-26 in Sec. 21.8). Patients with acute interstitial nephritis usually do not have systemic symptoms and will present in a more occult fashion, including fever, rash, and eosinophilia.

For patients without systemic findings, particularly critically ill children, the hallmark for ARF is oliguria, defined as a urinary output of <0.8 mL/kg/h (see Sec. 21.4). A careful and systematic evaluation of patients presenting with oliguria will determine whether the decrease in urine output is caused by anatomic abnormalities or pathophysiological causes (Fig. 21-18 and Sec. 21.4). Oliguria and/or ARF will result only from the obstruction of the renal artery, vein, or ureter of a single kidney when the contralateral kidney is either absent or nonfunctional. Therefore, the anatomic causes of ARF are rare but must always be considered. The classical presentation of renal artery occlusion includes severe hypertension, hematuria, and flank pain. Renal vein thrombosis is associated with an enlarging flank mass, concomitant with the onset of hematuria, proteinuria, thrombocytopenia, and intravascular coagulopathy. Except in newborn patients who are severely dehydrated or born to mothers with diabetes mellitus, renal vein thrombosis is a rare occurrence. Acute ureteral occlusion from renal stones or malignancies can cause abdominal pain, vomiting, and classical renal colic that may radiate into the groin (see Sec. 21.12). In male infants, bladder outlet obstruction must be considered because of the development of posterior urethral valves. In these infants, the bladder is usually easily palpable, can extend to the umbilicus, and may be mistaken for an abdominal mass. Retroperitoneal ultrasound examination using both static images and Doppler flow assessment should allow for detection of each of these anatomic lesions.

Of the pathophysiological causes of oliguria [diminished renal perfusion, nonphysiological ADH secretion (SIADH), and an es-

Acute Renal Failure
Sudden Unexpected Loss of Renal Function

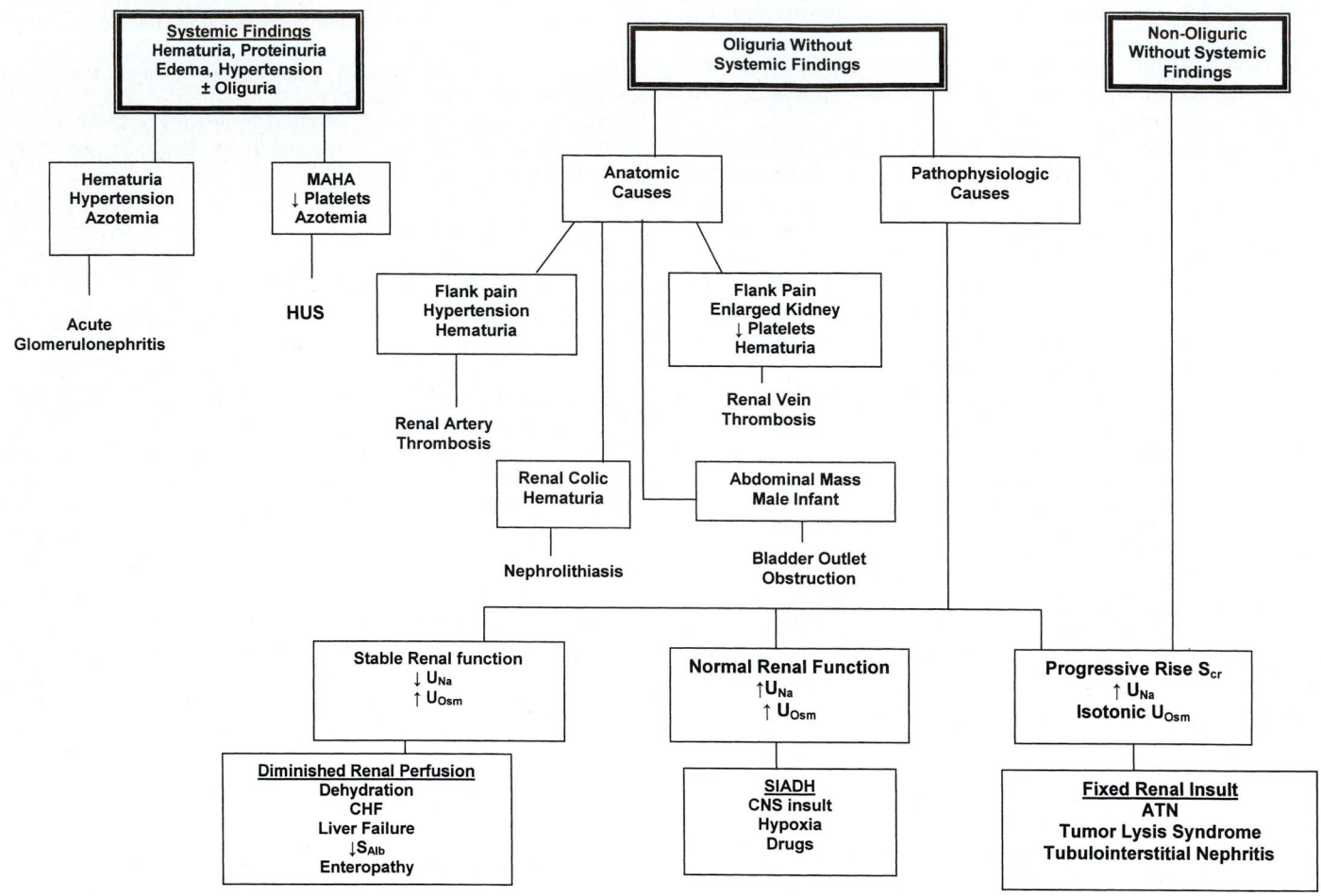

FIGURE 21-18 Algorithm for assessment of ARF. MAHA, microangiopathic hemolytic anemia; HUS, hemolytic uremic syndrome; U_{Na}, urinary sodium concentration; U_{Osm}, urinary osmolarity; S_{Alb}, serum albumin concentration; SIADH, syndrome of inappropriate antidiuretic hormone secretion; ATN, acute tubular necrosis.

tablished renal insult (acute tubular necrosis, ATN)], only one is associated with a substantial loss of renal function. The insult that produces a fixed renal injury (ATN) characteristically causes severe vasoconstriction of both the afferent and efferent arterioles, which, in turn, reduces glomerular capillary hydrostatic pressure and GFR. In addition, injury to the renal epithelium results in the sloughing of cells from the tubular basement membrane, which causes intratubular obstruction and the backleak of tubular fluid across the debrided membrane. Taken together, these pathophysiological events reduce GFR to negligible levels almost instantaneously. Moreover, this precipitous loss of GFR is not immediately reflected in the S_{cr} because the S_{cr} is a net reflection of the rate of creatinine production and excretion. Thus, in patients with ATN, the S_{cr} will rise by 0.5 to 1.5 mg/dL/d on a regular and ongoing basis until the value reaches a steady state. This relationship is important from several perspectives: (1) it clearly distinguishes ATN from the other pathophysiological causes of ARF (Fig. 21-18); (2) S_{cr} is not a reflection of GFR in patients with ATN and therefore cannot be used to calculate drug doses (the GFR should be assumed to be <10% of normal irrespective of the S_{cr} value); and (3) timing of the insult

that resulted in the development of ATN can be estimated from the S_{cr} at the time of presentation (the number of days that it would have taken for the S_{cr} to rise at 1 mg/dL/d). In contrast, for some patients with severely diminished renal perfusion, the level of renal blood flow will fall below the level that can be compensated by autoregulation (see Sec. 21.2), GFR will decrease, and the S_{cr} will rise but remain stable at a new steady state level. Thus, in patients with severe congestive heart failure, the S_{cr} may be elevated but remain at a stable and consistent value, rather than rising on a progressive daily basis as occurs with ATN. In patients with SIADH, the S_{cr} is generally low because of the hemodilution (see Sec. 21.4). Thus, an evaluation of oliguric patients without systemic symptoms that includes the urinary indices (see Table 21-7) as well as an assessment of renal function should allow a clear discrimination between these entities (Fig. 21-18).

21.7.1 Causes

ATN may be caused by a number of different factors but generally is related to renal ischemia, cellular toxins, or nephrotoxic drugs.

Systemic hypotension or transient declines in renal blood flow may lead to an ischemic injury, but the precise level of blood pressure that is likely to produce an insult is quite variable and partially dependent on synergistic factors such as nephrotoxic drugs, contrast media, or agents used to support cardiovascular function, such as epinephrine. In patients with sepsis, ATN may occur without systemic hypotension and is believed to be mediated by a variety of inflammatory factors such as vasoactive hormones, endotoxins, cytokines, and chemokines. The largest category of agents likely to produce an acute renal insult includes drugs, particularly those that may effect renal blood flow directly. Angiotensin-converting enzyme inhibitors (ACE-I) reduce the production of angiotensin II, which has a potent vasoconstrictive effect on the efferent arteriole, which in turn is fundamental for autoregulation of GFR (see Sec. 21.4 and Fig. 21-8). Because the autoregulation of GFR is more tenuously balanced in newborns (see Sec. 21.2), these drugs have been associated with precipitous and fulminant declines in GFR in full-term and premature infants. Similarly, if patients taking ACE-I become dehydrated, GFR will decline, and ATN can develop. In addition, nonsteroidal anti-inflammatory drugs (NSAIDs) inhibit prostaglandin production, which is a fundamental component of the dilatation of the afferent arteriole. Thus, patients who receive large doses of NSAIDs or these medications on a long-term basis are susceptible to the development of ATN. Because ibuprofen is frequently used in small children who are febrile and may become dehydrated, these children are at particular risk for developing ATN, and care should be taken to sustain hydration and prevent excess use of NSAIDs for the control of fever. Hospitalized children are exposed to a large variety of potentially nephrotoxic drugs, including aminoglycoside antibiotics, amphotericin, and immunosuppressive medications such as cyclosporine or chemotherapeutic agents. In most cases, any single insult alone would be unlikely to cause ATN and ARF. However, several insults (each below its individual threshold for injury), when occurring in combination, may have a devastating effect on renal tubule cells. For example, a patient may be on chemotherapeutic agents and an aminoglycoside antibiotic, each appropriately adjusted so that serum levels are nontoxic, but when these agents act in consort, a renal insult may occur.

Some patients will develop ARF without oliguria, termed nonoliguric ARF (see Fig. 21-18). In essence, these patients have sustained a state of glomerular tubular imbalance in which the GFR, although extremely low (usually <10 cc/min/1.73 m²), still exceeds the reabsorptive capacity of the damaged tubular epithelium. Patients with nonoliguric ARF are somewhat easier to manage because the restrictions on the volume of fluids that can be administered are much less stringent, but the overall outcome is not substantially different. Nonoliguric ARF is the classical presentation of aminoglycoside toxicity, contrast-medium-related renal injury, and asphyxia. Interestingly, patients with oliguric ATN actually have a phase of nonoliguric renal insufficiency during the early stages of recovery of renal function.

Tumor lysis syndrome (TLS) is a unique form of ARF that results from the lysis of tumor cells by antineoplastic agents. Patients with tumors with a high proliferative index, such as Burkitt lymphoma, B-cell acute lymphoblastic lymphoma, and acute lymphoblastic leukemia with a total white blood cell count greater than 10^{12}/L are at substantial risk for developing TLS (see Sec. 20.7). On rare occasions, TLS can occur spontaneously before induction of chemotherapy because of spontaneous involution of large tumors. In this clinical setting, the nephrotoxicity is caused by hyperuricemia and uricosuria that results in the precipitation of uric acid in concentrated, acidic tubular fluid, particularly in the distal portion of the nephron. Consequently, severe acidemia, nephrotoxic drugs, radiocontrast agents, and tumor infiltration of the kidney itself may increase the risk of developing TLS. The deposition of uric acid crystals is further compounded by hyperphosphatemia and the precipitation of calcium phosphate in the kidney.

Clinically, TLS presents with declining urine output in a patient undergoing chemotherapy for the treatment of a bulky tumor mass. These tumor cells are lysed, intracellular electrolytes and minerals are released into the plasma, and characteristic findings include an elevated serum uric acid, hyperkalemia, acidemia, hyperphosphatemia, and a reciprocal hypocalcemia. When renal function is concomitantly reduced, this pattern of abnormal electrolytes can become life threatening. The best therapeutic measures to prevent the development of TLS are (1) sustaining a high urine flow rate before the administration of the antineoplastic drugs and (2) inhibiting uric acid production by blocking the conversion of xanthine to uric acid with the drug allopurinol and attempting to maintain an alkaline urine. To substantially enhance the solubility of uric acid, the urine pH should be maintained at 7 or greater. However, the renal epithelium generally promotes an acid urine and tends to abhor an alkaline urine. Therefore, an overemphasis on alkalinizing the urine rather than sustaining a high urinary flow rate may produce substantial acid–base and electrolyte complications without significantly preventing acute urate nephropathy. A high tubular flow rate, regardless of the urine osmolality or pH, offers the best protection of the renal epithelium from TLS. Uric acid oxidase (uricase) converts uric acid to allantoin and represents the most effective means of preventing hyperuricemia and aborting the development of TLS. Once widely clinically available, this drug should essentially eliminate this form of acute renal failure.

For patients with established TLS, renal replacement therapy is almost always necessary, and because of the rate of production of the potentially toxic minerals and electrolytes, hemodialysis is the preferred mode of treatment. Recovery of renal function in children with TLS is excellent, and renal function frequently recovers completely, although in some instances, residual renal insufficiency may occur.

The prognosis for children and adolescents with ARF is more dependent on the associated medical problems and multiorgan failure than the severity of the renal insult per se. Over the past two decades, major advances in supportive care and dialysis therapy (see Sec. 21.14) have been developed, but the mortality for patients with ARF has not changed. Because of renal replacement therapy, patients die *with* but not *because of* ARF. For those patients who do recover, renal function may return to normal values, although concentrating ability may require several years to become maximal.

21.7.2   Therapy

For patients with ARF, therapy consists of prevention, supportive care, and renal replacement modalities. In clinical settings in which a renal insult may be anticipated, such as open heart surgery, administration of amphotericin or cisplatin, radiocontrast infusion, or severe hypotension, the prophylactic administration of mannitol or furosemide to create an osmotic diuresis appears to be effective. In patients who develop hemoglobinuria following severe hemolysis or myoglobinuria from rhabdomyolysis, sustaining a high urinary flow rate will prevent the development of tubular toxicity and ARF. Both in the experimental setting and clinically, achieving a urinary flow rate of 4 to 5 ml/kg/h will substantially reduce the incidence of hemoglobin- or myoglobin-induced ARF. In an accident in which massive crush injuries occurred, all victims who received an infusion of mannitol before the release of myoglobin from the injured muscles had renal function that was well sustained, and ARF did not develop. Once an acute renal insult is established and ATN has developed, diuretic agents have little or no role: mannitol may precipitate congestive heart failure, and furosemide may result in significant ototoxicity. Similarly, attempts to increase renal blood flow by the administration of low doses of dopamine are ineffective and, in fact, may worsen the degree of cellular necrosis.

Supportive care for patients with ARF must be directed toward appropriate fluid therapy to (1) maintain a normal intravascular volume and avoid volume overload with the development of congestive heart failure, (2) maintain physiological levels of S_{Na} and S_K as well as calcium and phosphorus, and most important, (3) provide adequate nutrition. The daily fluid requirement for children with ARF can be best estimated from insensible water losses (see Sec. 21.4) plus any urine output and nonrenal fluid losses. Daily assessment of intake and output, weight, and S_{Na} levels can be used to judge the adequacy of fluids being given. If an appropriate volume and composition of fluid is administered, the patient's weight will decrease by 0.5 to 1% per day, but the S_{Na} value will remain normal. A rapid decline in weight with an increase in S_{Na} suggests inadequate fluid replacement, whereas a fall in S_{Na} associated with a gain in weight suggests excessive fluid administration. During the early phase of recovery, polyuric patients may have substantial renal losses of salt and water that must be carefully monitored.

Patients with ARF are particularly susceptible to hyperkalemia (see Sec. 21.4), and potassium levels must be interpreted with respect to the other electrolytes and the acid-base status of the child (see Sec. 21.4). A mildly elevated serum potassium (S_K) is less troublesome in a patient with metabolic acidemia, because of the cellular shifts of potassium and hydrogen ion, than in patients with alkalemia. Severe hyperkalemia may be a life-threatening emergency and should be treated promptly and aggressively (see Sec. 21.4 and Table 21-8).

In patients with ARF, hyponatremia is usually iatrogenic either because of overzealous fluid administration in an attempt to prompt urine output or from an overestimation of free water requirements for patients with oligoanuria. Nonetheless, the hyponatremia should be carefully evaluated (see Sec. 21.4) and corrected to a value of 125 meq/L if the patient is symptomatic. Adjustment of fluids is usually sufficient to prevent severe hyponatremia. During the diuretic phase of recovery from ATN, hypernatremia may develop because of excessive free water losses in the urine.

The precipitous decrease in renal function that occurs in ARF results in hyperphosphatemia and hypocalcemia. Treatment for hyperphosphatemia consists of eliminating phosphorus from all parenteral fluids, reducing the phosphate content of any dietary products or medications (phosphate-containing enemas should never be used), and administration of oral phosphate-binding agents (see Sec. 21.14). In patients with TLS, hyperphosphatemia may be substantial and require hemodialysis for correction because of severe hypocalcemia. In ARF, hypocalcemia results from hyperphosphatemia, vitamin D deficiency, skeletal resistance to the action of PTH, and hypoalbuminemia. The latter will not affect ionized calcium levels that should be determined in this clinical setting. Hypocalcemia may potentiate the development of tetany, convulsions, or arrhythmias in critically ill patients with ARF and should be promptly addressed, particularly in patients with hyperkalemia. For patients who develop signs and symptoms consistent with hypocalcemia but who have no response to the intravenous infusion of calcium, hypomagnesemia should be considered (see Sec. 24.11).

Metabolic acidemia is inevitably a component of ARF because the renal epithelium is essential for the excretion of nonvolatile acids and reabsorption of bicarbonate. Because of the precarious and critical condition of many patients with ARF, the respiratory mechanisms that usually compensate for a metabolic acidosis may also be impaired, and a very severe acidemia develops. Severe acidemia will contribute to hyperkalemia, but caution must be taken in the administration of bicarbonate intravenously because these solutions are significantly hypertonic and can result in rapid shifts in serum pH, which, in the presence of a low ionized calcium, may result in tetany or seizures.

Nutritional support for children with ARF is essential, and the failure to provide adequate calories may perpetuate the renal injury and delay the recovery of renal function. Multiple attempts have been made to define the most ideal nutritional support for patients with ARF, but only general guidelines pertain. Specific adjustments must be made because of the highly variable clinical conditions associated with the development of ARF. Maintenance basal calories should be estimated from the patient's weight (see Table 21-4) and increased for temperature (12% per degree C above 37°), congestive heart failure, surgery (15–30% increase), or burns or sepsis (100% increase). If possible, enteral feedings are preferred, but, if not feasible, the parenteral administration of nutrition should be instituted early in the course of ARF. Protein intake should not be restricted, and a minimum of 0.6 g/kg/d with an optimal administration of 1.5 to 2 g/kg/d should be attempted. Additional protein will be needed if the patient is receiving renal replacement therapy (see Sec. 21.14). Lipids are an excellent source of calories and should provide not less than 30%, but no more than 50%, of the calories administered. Patients with concomitant hepatic failure or sepsis or respiratory distress syndrome may need to have lipid administration restricted. The primary source of calories is usually carbohydrate. In some cases, adequate delivery of carbohydrate calories may require insulin. Both inadequate and excessive nutritional support may be detrimental to recovery from ARF.

Renal replacement therapy is designed to remove endogenous and exogenous toxins and to maintain fluid, electrolyte, and acid-base status until renal function returns (see Sec. 21.14). No absolute criteria are available to determine initiation of acute dialysis, and strict criteria based on the level of S_{Cr} or BUN are not particularly helpful or relevant in all clinical situations. Overwhelmingly, the primary reason to initiate renal replacement therapy is to be able to provide adequate nutritional support, particularly for patients with oliguric ARF. In a minority of cases, acute dialysis is needed for the treatment of hyperkalemia, hyperphosphatemia, hypocalcemia, or hyperuricemia, particularly in patients with TLS. Renal replacement therapy may consist of peritoneal dialysis, hemodialysis, or continuous hemofiltration (see Sec. 21.14). Over the past many years, each of these techniques has been successfully adapted for the treatment of children of all ages, including premature and term newborns. Moreover, each modality has specific indications, contraindications, and risks. Thus, no single modality will be effective in every form of ARF, and in many cases, the best therapy for a given patient will be dependent on the expertise of the individuals responsible for initiating and sustaining renal replacement therapy.

References

Gouyon JB, Guignard J-P: Management of acute renal failure in newborns. Pediatr Nephrol 14:227–239, 2000

Norman UE, Asadi FK: A prospective study of acute renal failure in the newborn infant. Pediatrics 63:475–479, 1979

Stapleton FB: Renal complications of childhood cancer and chemotherapy. In: Holliday M, Barratt M, Avner E, eds: Pediatric Nephrology, 3rd ed. Philadelphia, Lippincott Williams & Wilkins, 1994:1204–1211

Van Why SK, Siegel NJ: Heat shock proteins in renal injury and recovery. Curr Opin Nephrol Hypertens 7:407–412, 1998

21.8 GLOMERULAR DISORDERS

Allison A. Eddy

Glomerular diseases may present clinically in several different ways depending on the nature and severity of the primary disease and the extent to which the normal physiological functions of the glomerulus are perturbed. Some children with glomerulonephritis are asymptomatic, found incidentally to have asymptomatic microscopic hematuria or proteinuria by a routine urinalysis. At the other extreme, children may become critically ill with oligoanuric rapidly progressive glomerulonephritis in need of urgent dialysis. A few glomerular diseases are inherited (see Sec. 21.9), but most forms of glomerulonephritis are acquired and are generally considered to be immunologically mediated. To present a practical approach to glomerulonephritis, focus will be placed on the three classical clinical syndromes that characterize glomerular injury: acute glomerulonephritis, defined by the triad of hematuria, hypertension, and azotemia; nephrotic syndrome, defined by proteinuria and hypoalbuminemia; and hemolytic uremic syndrome, defined by microangiopathic hemolytic anemia, thrombocytopenia, and renal insufficiency.

PRACTICAL APPROACH TO A PATIENT WITH GLOMERULONEPHRITIS

The patient with glomerular disease usually presents clinically with a constellation of features that may include hematuria, proteinuria, hypertension, edema, and renal insufficiency. The urinary sediment is characterized as active because of the presence of dysmorphic erythrocytes and cellular casts (see Fig. 21-12). A series of questions help to guide the initial plan of investigation and management.

1. **Does this patient have acute or chronic glomerulonephritis?** It is surprising how many patients with chronic glomerulonephritis appear relatively asymptomatic until the disease is fairly advanced. Clues of chronicity include significant anemia, evidence of renal osteodystrophy (abnormal bone radiographs or an elevated PTH level), or small echogenic kidneys by ultrasound examination. Left ventricular hypertrophy may reflect long-standing hypertension.

2. **Does this patient have isolated renal disease or involvement of extrarenal organ systems?** A careful systems review and physical examination should help to determine whether the investigation should move in the direction of primary (acquired) glomerulonephritis or toward multisystem disease associated with glomerulonephritis (Table 21-12). Extrarenal disease may be clinically silent. For example, in considering postinfectious glomerulonephritis, serology may be necessary (such as a streptozyme or anti–hepatitis B or anti–hepatitis C antibodies). When patients present with vasculitis caused by Wegener granulomatosis, involvement of the lung parenchyma or sinuses usually requires radiologic confirmation.

3. **Does this patient have hypocomplementemic glomerulonephritis?** A low serum C3 concentration generally indicates one of four diseases in children: acute postinfectious glomerulonephritis, lupus nephritis, membranoproliferative glomerulonephritis, and glomerulonephritis associated with chronic infections (subacute bacterial endocarditis and shunt nephritis).

4. **Does this patient have recurrent painless macroscopic hematuria?** If the answer is yes, the patient likely has IgA nephropathy, although this also is a fairly common presentation of Alport syndrome during the first decade of life.

5. **What is the age of the patient?** Although most forms of glomerulonephritis can occur in almost any age group, many diseases have a characteristic age range for onset of disease (Table 21-13). For example, glomerulonephritis in the newborn period is extremely rare and is often the result of a congenital infection.

6. **Does this patient have clinical evidence of rapidly progressive glomerulonephritis?** Such a course is usually caused by crescentic glomerulonephritis and, more rarely, may result from acute glomerulonephritis with superimposed acute tubular necrosis. Rapidly progressive glomerulonephritis should be considered an emergency in need of urgent histologic diagnosis. Most of these patients have aggressive diseases that can be treated adequately with immunosuppressive therapy only if therapy is initiated early and in high doses. In patients with anti-GBM nephritis, early plasmapheresis can also be extremely helpful.

7. **Does this patient have nephritic/nephrotic syndrome?** Although proteinuria is a hallmark of significant glomerular disease, frank nephrotic syndrome is a less common feature of the acute nephritic syndrome. In a patient presenting clinically with acute glomerulonephritis and a low serum C3 level, the presence of nephrotic syndrome should suggest membranoproliferative glomerulonephritis or lupus nephritis. Although the nephrotic syndrome can occur in association with acute poststreptococcal glomerulonephritis, it is not very common.

8. **Does this patient need a renal biopsy now?** The question of when to perform a renal biopsy is somewhat arbitrary. Renal biopsies are generally not necessary when the diagnosis is obvious and the disease is self-limited without specific therapy, ie, typical acute poststreptococcal glomerulonephritis and mild nephritis secondary to Henoch-Schönlein purpura. For most glomerular diseases, the only way to make a definitive diagnosis is by renal biopsy. For many of these patients, the only way to design a rational plan of therapy is by histologic determination of the diagnosis and the pattern and severity of renal damage (Table 21-14).

21.8.1 Glomerulonephritis

The pathophysiological sequence of events that leads to the development of the nephritic triad (hematuria, azotemia, and hypertension) is shown in Fig. 21-19. In each of the clinical entities with glomerular proliferation, the inflammation process leads to decreased glomerular perfusion, resulting in compromised renal function and retention of salt and water with potential development of hypertension and edema.

ACUTE POSTSTREPTOCOCCAL GLOMERULONEPHRITIS

Acute poststreptococcal glomerulonephritis (APSGN) is clearly the most frequent and best-characterized form of acute postinfectious glomerulonephritis. The clinical syndrome is often regarded as the prototype of the acute nephritic syndrome. However, numerous

TABLE 21-12

CLASSIFICATION OF COMMON PEDIATRIC GLOMERULAR DISEASES

CONGENITAL GLOMERULONEPHRITIS	GENETIC GLOMERULAR DISEASES	PRIMARY ACQUIRED GLOMERULAR DISEASES	MULTISYSTEM DISEASES WITH GLOMERULONEPHRITIS
Syphilis	Alport syndrome	Postinfectious glomerulonephritis	Goodpasture syndrome
Toxoplasmosis	Infantile nephrotic syndrome	IgA nephropathy	Lupus nephritis
Cytomegalovirus	Denys-Drash syndrome	Membranoproliferative glomerulonephritis	Henoch-Schönlein purpura nephritis
	Diffuse mesangial sclerosis	Idiopathic crescentic glomerulonephritis	Systemic vasculitis
	Nail-patella syndrome	Minimal change nephrotic syndrome	Hemolytic uremic syndrome
	Frasier syndrome	Focal segmental glomerulosclerosis	
		Membranous nephropathy	

infectious organisms, including many other bacteria, viruses, and parasites, may also induce postinfectious acute glomerulonephritis. Because the infection typically precedes nephritis by a few weeks, it may be difficult to identify the original causative agent. Group A β-hemolytic streptococcal disease has the advantage that the antecedent pharyngitis or pyoderma was often obvious clinically, and serologic testing is readily available to confirm recent infection. Without a good clinical history and a high index of suspicion, it is more challenging to prove the etiology of a nonspecific antecedent illness that is typically in the resolution phase when the patient presents acutely with glomerulonephritis. Nonetheless, if a patient appears to have acute postinfectious glomerulonephritis and a recent infection with group A β-hemolytic *Streptococcus* cannot be proven, the diagnosis of postinfectious glomerulonephritis may still be correct. APSGN accounts for 80 to 90% of such cases and is used as the prototype for this group of disorders.

EPIDEMIOLOGY AND PREDISPOSING FACTORS APSGN follows infection with specific "nephritogenic" strains of group A β-he-

TABLE 21-13

TYPICAL AGE AT PRESENTATION WITH GLOMERULAR DISEASE

DISEASE	PEAK INCIDENCE (YEARS)	YOUNGEST AGE REPORTED
Proliferative glomerulonephritis		
Primary		
Postinfectious glomerulonephritis	5–15	8 mo
IgA nephropathy	10–30	3 yr
Membranoproliferative glomerulonephritis	8–30	15 mo
Multisystem		
Goodpasture syndrome	20–30	2 yr
Lupus nephritis	15–45	6 wk
Henoch-Schönlein purpura nephritis	3–10	8 mo
Systemic vasculitis	Adults	? 7 yr
Nonproliferative glomerulopathies		
Minimal-change nephrotic syndrome	2–6	3 mo
Idiopathic focal segmental glomerulosclerosis	2–7	3 wk
Membranous nephropathy	Variable depending on etiology	5 mo

molytic *Streptococcus*. This organism has traditionally been characterized by two distinct outer cell wall proteins (M and T), leading to the recognition of more than 80 subtypes. APSGN was first linked to strain 12, and since that time, several other strains have been shown to be nephritogenic (1, 2, 3, 4, 18, 25, 49, 55, 57, 60) or are suspected of being nephritogenic (31, 52, 56, 59, 61). APSGN and acute rheumatic fever almost never occur simultaneously in the same patient. Antibiotic treatment of the prodromal disease does not appear to prevent acute glomerulonephritis, but treatment is important to prevent the spread of the nephritogenic bacteria. Although difficult to determine with certainty, the overall risk of developing APSGN after infection with a nephritogenic strain is in the range of 10 to 15%. Determining the true incidence is difficult because 50 to 85% of patients with APSGN may be asymptomatic.

APSGN is primarily a disease of school-age children (5–15 years; younger in epidemic forms) and is more common in boys. Although reported in an 8-month-old child, the disease is rare under 3 years of age (Table 21-13) and may occur as a sporadic or epidemic disease. The incidence of APSGN has decreased in the United States and Europe over the past two decades, largely as a result of the decline in the epidemic form of streptococcal skin infections. Some evidence suggests that the prevalence of certain nephritogenic stains is decreasing as well. A seasonal pattern exists for APSGN because in North America pharyngitis is more common in the winter and spring, and impetigo in the summer and fall.

CLINICAL MANIFESTATIONS The clinical manifestations of the classic form of APSGN begin abruptly. Patients are usually afebrile with a latency period following pharyngitis of 1 to 2 weeks and 3 to 6 weeks after a skin infection. The most common presenting features in symptomatic patients are edema (85%) and gross hematuria (30–50%). Essentially all the patients have microhematuria. The urine often has a unique color, described as smoky, cola-colored, or tea-colored (see Sec. 21.5 and Table 21-10). Hypertension is common (60–80%) but is usually mild to moderate; rarely, hypertensive encephalopathy has been reported. The pathogenesis of the hypertension is not entirely understood and results only in part from intracellular volume expansion. The degree of renal failure is usually mild. A form of rapidly progressive glomerulonephritis (associated histologically with crescent formation) is unusual and reported in less than 1% of children. Although many patients have significant proteinuria and a slightly depressed serum albumin level, fewer than 5% of symptomatic patients develop frank nephrotic syndrome. Severe complications including pulmonary hemorrhage and cerebral vasculitis have been reported. Spontane-

TABLE 21-14

CLASSICAL HISTOLOGIC FEATURES OF PEDIATRIC GLOMERULAR DISEASES[a]

DISEASE	LIGHT MICROSCOPY	IMMUNOFLUORESCENCE MICROSCOPY	ELECTRON MICROSCOPY
Postinfectious glomerulonephritis	• Hypercellularity (resident cells and infiltrating leukocytes) • Lobular accentuation of tufts	• Subepithelial deposits of IgG and C3 • May have "starry sky" appearance	• Large subepithelial electron-dense deposits (humps)
IgA nephropathy	• Focal segmental hypercellularity and mesangial matrix expansion	• Mesangial deposits of IgA essential; C3 and IgG often present as well	• Mesangial electron-dense deposits; 33% also have paramesangial or subendothelial deposits
Membranoproliferative glomerulo-nephritis type I	• Diffuse increase in mesangial matrix and cells giving a lobular appearance to tuft • GBM may appear split because of mesangial matrix interposition	• Subendothelial deposits of C3 and immunoglobulins • Mesangial deposits	• Subendothelial and mesangial electron-dense deposits • Interposition mesangial matrix into basement membrane
Membranoproliferative glomerulo-nephritis type II	• Glomerular hypercellularity and mesangial matrix increase causing lobular accentuation of tufts • Thickened segments of GBM	• C3 at periphery of mesangial and GBM intramembranous deposits (forming "rings")	• Electron-dense material within the GBM and often in the mesangium, along Bowman capsule
Anti-GBM nephritis	• Focal hypercellularity, often with necrotizing lesions • Crescents usually present • Interstitial inflammation common	• IgG usually with C3 in a linear pattern along the GBM; may also be present along some TBMs	• No electron-dense deposits • GBM may be widened with lucent subendothelial zones
Lupus nephritis	• Five patterns recognized by light microscopy: I. Normal; II. Mesangial, mild increase in mesangial matrix and cells; III. Focal proliferative, <50% glomeruli hypercellular with increased matrix; IV. Diffuse proliferative, >50% glomeruli have increased cells and matrix, may be thickened GBM segments ("wire-loops"); V. Membranous, thickened GBM, cellularity normal or mildly increased	• Complement and immunoglobulins (IgG>IgM>IgA); I, negative staining; II, mesangial deposits; III, mesangial deposits, GBM deposits; IV, mesangial and subendothelial deposits; V, subepithelial and mesangial deposits	• Electron-dense deposits, often in the location suggested by immunofluorescence microscopy • Fingerprint pattern in deposits • Tubuloreticular inclusions
Henoch-Schönlein purpura nephritis	• Variable from minimal abnormalities to focal or diffuse hypercellularity and mesangial matrix expansion • Crescents present in most severe cases • Rarely may have MPGN appearance	• IgA and C3 in mesangium; also along GBM in more severe cases • IgG present in 50% cases	• Electron-dense deposits in mesangial and paramesangial areas • Subendothelial and occasional subepithelial deposits seen in more severe cases
Renal vasculitis	• Focal and segmental proliferation with areas of fibrinoid necrosis • Crescents are common	• Typically negative for complement and immunoglobulins; fibrin present in necrotic areas	• No electron-dense deposits
Minimal-change lesion	• Typically no changes; in small subset mild hypercellularity present	• Usually negative • ~25% have mesangial IgM deposits	• Widening and effacement of epithelial foot processes (podocytes) during relapses
Focal segmental glomerulosclerosis	• Initially a few glomeruli (cortico-medullary junction) have segmental sclerosis • Lesion typically begins at the vascular pole	• Usually negative • IgM and/or C3 may be present in sclerotic regions	• Fusion of epithelial foot processes

(continued)

TABLE 21-14 Continued

DISEASE	LIGHT MICROSCOPY	IMMUNOFLUORESCENCE MICROSCOPY	ELECTRON MICROSCOPY
Membranous nephropathy	• Generalized thickening of GBM; by silver stain hallmark epithelial "spikes" may be seen • Cellularity usually normal in idiopathic variant; may be mildly increased in secondary variants	• Granular staining along the GBM for IgG and C3	• Subepithelial electron-dense deposits; size and position of deposit changes with stage (I to IV)
Hemolytic uremic syndrome	• Endothelial cell swelling, thickened capillary wall, and reduced capillary lumen • Glomeruli may be lobular and resemble MPGN • Thrombi may occlude extraglomerular arterioles	• Fibrin deposits • IgM and C3 may also be present along capillary loops	• Endothelial cell swelling; widening of glomerular capillary walls caused by an expanded subendothelial space filled with lucent granular material (fibrin)

[a] Terminology: (1) number of affected glomeruli focal (a subset, usually <50%) or diffuse (most glomeruli, at least 50%); (2) area affected within a single glomerulus segmental (only part is abnormal) or global (the entire glomerulus).

ous improvement typically begins within 1 week with resolution of the edema in 5 to 10 days and hypertension in 2 to 3 weeks, but the urinalysis may be abnormal for several years.

LABORATORY FINDINGS The critical initial diagnostic test in a child with acute nephritis is the serum C3 level that is usually below 50% of normal values in patients with APSGN. Up to 10% of patients may have a normal C3 level, and the percentage is even higher in patients with other forms of acute postinfectious glomerulonephritis. Although specialized testing may show in vitro evidence of activation of the classical pathway of complement, C4 levels are typically normal, and a significantly decreased C4 level should suggest an alternative diagnosis such as systemic lupus erythematosus, bacterial endocarditis, shunt nephritis, or idiopathic membranoproliferative glomerulonephritis (Fig. 21-20). The serum C3 level usually returns to normal within 6 to 12 weeks. Prolonged hypocomplementemia should point to alternative diagnoses, although it is occasionally reported in patients with APSGN. The urinalysis typically shows hematuria, proteinuria, and red cell casts, but on rare

occasions, patients may have a normal urinalysis. Evidence of a recent streptococcal infection makes the diagnosis of APSGN most likely, with a few caveats. A positive throat culture is insufficient to confirm the diagnosis, as 20% of normal school children are carriers and will have a positive throat culture. An antibody to the streptolysin O enzyme (ASO) is detected in 80% of children with antecedent pharyngitis, but the test is also positive in 16 to 18% of healthy children. After skin infections, a positive ASO is less frequent (50%), possibly because of the binding of the ASO enzyme to lipids in the skin. The streptozyme assay combines serologic testing to five different streptococcal antigens (streptolysin O, streptokinase, hyaluronidase, DNase B, and NADase) and increases the likelihood of positive testing to greater than 95% in patients with pharyngitis and to 80% in patients with skin infections. The DNase B test is quite reliable to establish a prior streptococcal infection. In the majority of patients, the clinical presentation and laboratory tests make the diagnosis of APSGN quite evident. There is no indication to perform a renal biopsy to confirm the diagnosis in such children.

SEQUENCE OF EVENTS IN ACUTE GLOMERULONEPHRITIS

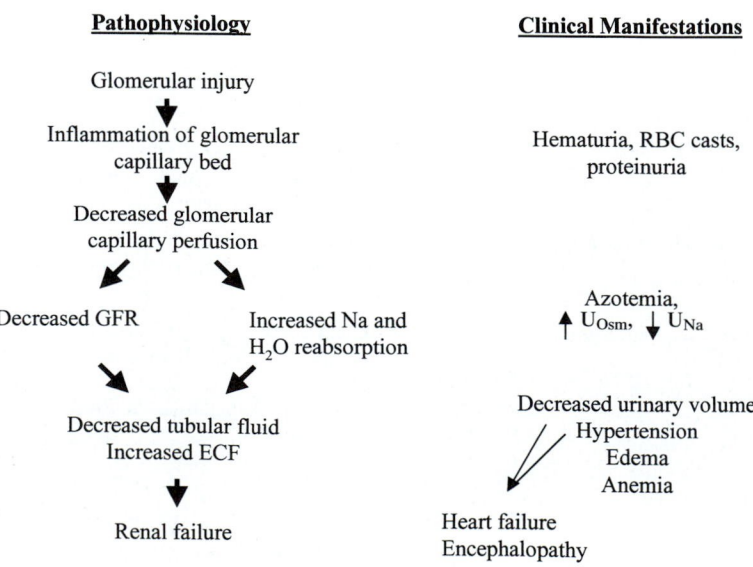

FIGURE 21-19 Sequence of pathophysiological events in acute glomerulonephritis and the associated clinical manifestations. RBC, red blood cell; U_{Osm}, urinary osmolarity, U_{Na}, urinary sodium concentration; ECF, extracellular fluid; GFR = glomerular filtration rate.

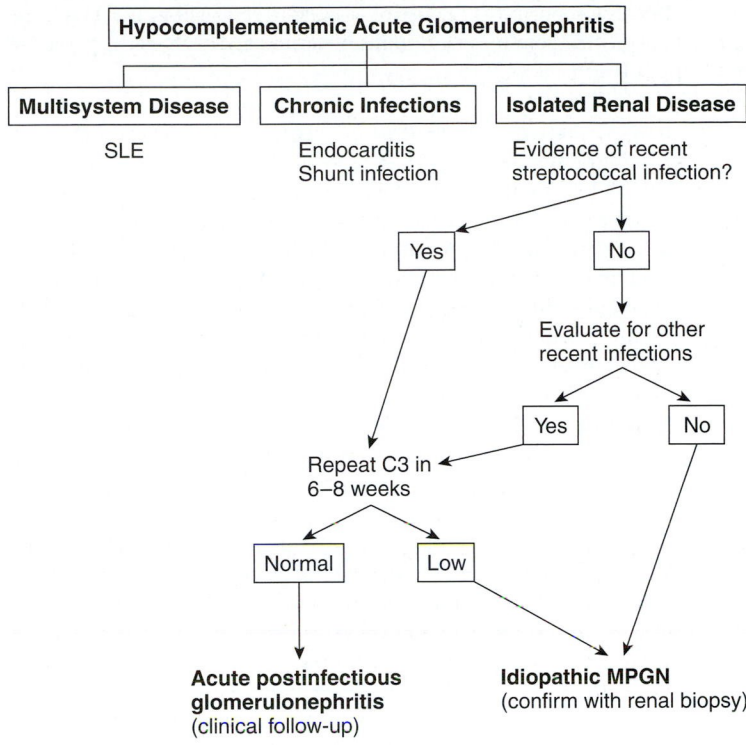

FIGURE 21-20 Causes of glomerulonephritis associated with hypocomplementemia. SLE, systemic lupus erythematosus; C3, third component of complement proteins; MPGN, membranoproliferative glomerulonephritis.

PATHOGENESIS Although APSGN is thought to be the prototype of immune complex–mediated glomerulonephritis, the precise nature of the antigen-antibody complex remains undefined. The latency period between the acute infection and the onset of nephritis is thought to represent the period required to generate sufficient IgG antistreptococcal antibodies to trigger immune complex formation. Although several streptococcal antigens have been identified in the glomerular immune deposits (eg, endostreptosins, nephritic strain-associated protein, nephritis plasma-binding protein), proving that these antigens are the target of immune attack that leads to the subsequent glomerular injury has not yet been possible. The traditional view that APSGN results from glomerular trapping of circulating immune complexes has fallen into disfavor. Current thinking is that the target antigen is initially trapped within the glomerulus with subsequent immune complex formation "in situ" within the kidney. This antigen may be derived from the streptococcal organism, or it may actually be a normal glomerular molecule that crossreacts with antibodies generated to the streptococcal antigens. IgG itself may become a planted antigen after it becomes desialated by streptococcal neuraminidase, with electrostatic IgG trapping related to the exposure of positive surface charges. Once glomerular immune deposits are formed, activation of the complement cascade and infiltration of circulating leukocytes appear to initiate the glomerular damage. APSGN is described as an "exudative" glomerulonephritis characterized in the acute phase by many intraglomerular neutrophils.

TREATMENT APSGN is an acute disease that resolves without specific therapy. Supportive care to manage the acute nephritis syndrome is essential, and occasionally patients succumb to complications. If not previously administered, antibiotics should be given to prevent the spread of the nephritogenic strain of *Streptococcus*. In the acute phase, most hospitalized patients are fluid-overloaded and may respond to loop diuretics. Fluids need to be balanced to prevent further intravascular volume overload, including appropri-

ate sodium and fluid restriction. Hypertension is typically not severe and can be managed with calcium channel blockers. In patients with more severe renal insufficiency, hyperkalemia, hyperphosphatemia, and acidosis are likely to occur and will require medical management. These patients rarely need dialysis. Despite the old wives' tale, bed rest is of no proven benefit once patients are well enough to ambulate. Spontaneous improvement should begin within 1 week. Corticosteroids and cytotoxic agents have no proven role and theoretically may be harmful. In the rare patient with rapidly progressive glomerulonephritis associated with crescentic nephritis (in greater than 30% glomeruli) on biopsy, anecdotal evidence suggests that immunosuppressive therapy may be beneficial. However, this is such a rare presentation that prospective clinical trials to evaluate the efficacy of therapy are impossible.

PROGNOSIS Gross hematuria and edema begin to resolve within a few days. Microscopic hematuria may persist for 1 year, occasionally exacerbated by intercurrent infections. Prolonged hematuria up to 5 years has been observed but is rare. Traditionally APSGN in children has been considered a completely reversible disease, and this is still generally true. In the exceptional patient with crescentic disease, prolonged oliguria, and massive proteinuria, recovery may not be complete. Currently no data are available on the evaluation of outcomes two to three decades after uncomplicated childhood APSGN. In the meantime, it seems reasonable to anticipate a good long-term outcome in children with APSGN, although those hospitalized with severe acute disease deserve long-term follow-up, as they may not have a completely benign long-term outcome.

GLOMERULONEPHRITIS WITH CHRONIC INFECTIONS

Immune responses may also induce glomerulonephritis in the face of certain persistent infections. In pediatric patients, the most important examples of this are congenital infections with cytomegalovirus or toxoplasmosis that may present clinically as infantile nephrotic syndrome (see Sec. 21.3), infective endocarditis, shunt nephritis, hepatitis B and C, and AIDS. In endemic tropical areas of the world, chronic infection with *Plasmodium malariae, Schistosoma mansoni,* and filariasis may cause more chronic forms of glomerulonephritis.

INFECTIVE ENDOCARDITIS With the decline in the incidence of acute rheumatic fever, subacute bacterial endocarditis (usually caused by *Streptococcus viridans*) has become a rare entity. Acute bacterial endocarditis is now more common, especially among intravenous drug abusers. *Staphylococcus aureus* is the most frequent pathogen, but several other organisms are occasionally implicated. The serum C3 and C4 levels are depressed in 90% of patients. The disease is considered to be immunologically mediated and resembles APSGN histologically. With appropriate antibiotic therapy, the glomerulopathy improves, but chronic renal failure may occur. Normalization of the serum complement levels is a good prognostic indicator.

SHUNT NEPHRITIS Shunt nephritis was first recognized in children with ventriculoatrial shunts used for the treatment of hydrocephalus. The risk of nephritis is reported to be 4% among patients with infected shunts. This complication is distinctly rare in patients with infected ventricluloperitoneal shunts. A similar form of nephritis has been reported in patients with infected vascular access grafts. Coagulase-negative *Staphylococcus* is the most common offending organism. Blood cultures may be negative, but the organism may be isolated from cultures of the graft itself. The renal disease often has an indolent presentation: Gross hematuria is common, and 25 to 30% may develop nephrotic syndrome. Serum C3 and C4 levels are usually depressed (90%). Histologically, the lesion is a diffuse proliferative glomerulonephritis that resembles idiopathic membranoproliferative glomerulonephritis type I. Treatment includes antibiotic therapy and removal of the infected shunt. The glomerular disease slowly resolves, but residual renal damage is fairly common.

CHRONIC HEPATITIS An association between hepatitis B (HB) and membranous nephropathy was first reported in 1969. Since the initial report, this association has been made worldwide but is particularly prevalent among children in Asia. Most children present with nephrotic syndrome or with nonnephrotic proteinuria during the chronic carrier stage of their disease. Most of the affected children do not have a history or clinical evidence of ongoing liver disease, although the serum transaminase levels are usually mildly elevated. Depressed serum C3 and C4 levels may be detected (15–64% of patients) but are not characteristic. In children the prognosis is excellent, with 95% having undergone a spontaneous remission within 5 to 7 years of diagnosis. Remission usually coincides with the disappearance of HBe antigenemia and the appearance of HB antibodies. Immunosuppressive therapy is contraindicated, especially in children, because of an increased risk of chronic active hepatitis. The prognosis is less favorable in adults. Interferon therapy has not been shown to be beneficial in children. Newer antiviral protocols are currently under investigation. Chronic infection with HB may also cause a serum-sickness-like syndrome and is less commonly associated with membranoproliferative glomerulonephritis (MPGN) and crescentic glomerulonephritis.

Hepatitis C was first identified as a cause of MPGN in a group of adults in 1993 and has since then been confirmed, but this association varies widely depending on the population tested. It has

also been reported as a cause of MPGN in renal allografts. Hepatitis C does not seem to be a significant cause of MPGN in the pediatric population.

HUMAN IMMUNODEFICIENCY VIRUS (HIV)-ASSOCIATED A proteinuric syndrome was first reported in association with HIV in 1984. The true incidence of HIV nephropathy is unknown but is thought to be in the range of 2 to 10% of infected patients. Most patients present with proteinuria, usually with nephrotic syndrome, which may be the first manifestation of HIV infection or may occur in patients with AIDS or AIDS-related complex. Although it was initially debated that renal disease in this setting may be heroin-induced nephropathy, it is now clear that it affects individuals, including infants, without a history of drug abuse. Although how is still unclear, evidence suggests that HIV itself plays a direct role in the pathogenesis of the glomerulopathy. When a renal biopsy is performed, a unique variant of focal segmental glomerulosclerosis (FSGS) is usually found. In addition to the typical FSGS lesion, "collapsed" glomeruli (also seen in a small subset of patients with idiopathic FSGS), degenerated and microcystic tubules, interstitial edema and inflammation, and glomerular endothelial tubuloreticular inclusions (reminiscent of those associated with SLE nephritis) are commonly observed features. The optimal treatment of HIV nephropathy is unknown. Many adults with HIV nephropathy progress rapidly to ESRD, whereas the lesion typically follows a more indolent course in children. Antiviral medication such as azidothymidine may slow the rate of progression. Anecdotal case reports suggest a benefical outcome in patients treated with steroids or cyclosporine. However, infectious complications were frequent, and the relative risks and merits of these more aggressive approaches to treatment need to be evaluated carefully. Angiotensin II inhibitors may have a protective role. In addition to the "collapsing" variant of FSGS, HIV-infected patients have an increased risk of developing other glomerulopathies including IgA nephropathy, a glomerular microangiopathy that resembles hemolytic uremic syndrome; mesangial hyperplasia; membranoproliferative glomerulonephritis; lupus-like glomerulonephritis; and minimal-change nephrotic syndrome.

IgA NEPHROPATHY

IgA nephropathy was first described by Berger and Hinglais in 1968 and is the most frequent glomerular disease throughout the world. Although it may occur at almost any age, it is much more common in children and young adults (in the second and third decades of life) but can occur in the first decade of life and has been diagnosed in children as young as 3 years of age. Even though the course of the disease is indolent in most patients, a significant number are at risk of ultimately developing ESRD.

EPIDEMIOLOGY/PREDISPOSING FACTORS The true incidence of IgA nephropathy is uncertain, as there are no serologic markers making renal biopsy the only way to confirm the diagnosis. Despite the fact that the indications for renal biopsy vary widely around the world, there is evidence that the disease is more common in some countries such as Japan and Australia, whereas prevalence rates are lower in North America. Genetic factors may play a role, although the basis for genetic predisposition is not yet clear. Although more common in Asians and whites, IgA nephropathy is rare in blacks and more common in Native Americans living in New Mexico. Even though familial clustering is rare, familial cases have been reported. The disease is more prevalent in male patients, with the male:female ratio ranging from 2:1 to 6:1.

IgA nephropathy might best be considered a syndrome. Although most cases appear to be idiopathic, several secondary forms of IgA nephropathy do exist. For many of the secondary forms, glomerular immune deposits containing predominately IgA are present, but the severity of renal injury is often mild. However, the awareness of these associations may ultimately shed light on the pathogenesis of idiopathic IgA nephropathy, an area of current uncertainty. IgA nephropathy has been reported in association with many systemic diseases: cirrhosis and other forms of severe liver disease; patients with portosystemic shunts; enteropathies such as celiac disease and Crohn disease; chronic lung diseases including obstructive bronchitis, cystic fibrosis, and idiopathic interstitial pneumonia; neoplasias such as IgA monoclonal gammopathy, various carcinomas, and mycosis fungoides; infections, including human immunodeficiency virus, *Mycoplasma*, toxoplasmosis, and leprosy; dermatitis herpetiformis; seronegative arthropathies; recurrent mastitis and episcleritis. Lupus nephritis is probably the only other renal disease that may be characterized by significant IgA deposits, but other unique features of this disease usually make the diagnosis obvious.

Most children with Henoch-Schönlein purpura (75%) have evidence of glomerulonephritis that resembles IgA nephropathy histopathologically. Many nephrologists consider these two entities to be different manifestations of the same disease, and a common pathogenesis may exist because both diseases share similar geographic distribution and both are rare in African-Americans; the two disorders have been reported to coexist in different individuals in the same family (including monozygotic twins), and rare patients with the idiopathic form of IgA nephropathy have been reported to develop Henoch-Schönlein purpura several years later. IgA nephropathy is best considered a syndrome of multiple causes: the idiopathic form is the most common; Henoch-Schönlein purpura is another relatively common cause but is usually a self-limited disease occurring in childhood.

CLINICAL MANIFESTATIONS Recurrent episodes of painless macroscopic hematuria represent the classic clinical presentation of IgA nephropathy. Very few other glomerular diseases have this clinical course. The first episode may mimic APSGN. In patients with Alport syndrome, recurrent episodes of macroscopic hematuria may occur mainly in the first decade of life (see Sec. 21.9). Gross hematuria may also be the initial presentation of children with membranoproliferative glomerulonephritis. The onset of macrohematuria is often preceded 24 to 48 hours earlier by an upper respiratory tract infection; associations with gastroenteritis, sinusitis, and strenuous exercise have also been reported but are much less common. This latency period between the onset of prodromal symptoms and macrohematuria is considerably shorter than that observed in patients with APSGN. Some of these children complain of flank or loin pain presumably because of swelling of the renal capsule; although dysuria has been reported, it is not a frequent symptom. The second most common presentation is the incidental finding of microhematuria usually associated with mild proteinuria. A subset of this group does develop future episodes of gross hematuria. Overall, gross hematuria is said to be much more common in children than adults, with up to 90% eventually experiencing at least one episode. For reasons that remain unclear, patients with recurrent gross hematuria have a better long-term prognosis. The gross hematuria typically resolves within a few days. The interval between

episodes is highly variable, ranging from a few months to many years. The frequency of the episodes decreases with age. Between these episodes, microscopic hematuria and variable degrees of proteinuria typically persist.

At least three rarer clinical presentations have been reported. Fewer than 10% of children present with an acute nephritic episode associated with edema, hematuria, hypertension, and renal insufficiency. In most patients, renal function returns to baseline levels without specific therapy, and the long-term prognosis remains relatively good. If a renal biopsy is performed during the acute nephrotic episode, the degree of glomerular disease does not account for the renal failure. Superimposed acute tubular necrosis is the likely explanation, with tubular toxicity from erythrocyte products such as hemoglobin and iron, possible contributory factors. Within this clinical subgroup, a very small number of patients may develop rapidly progressive glomerulonephritis caused by a severe crescentic form of IgA nephropathy, which is a serious presentation with a poor prognosis for long-term recovery of renal function. Fewer than 10% of children with IgA nephropathy may present with nephrotic syndrome. Within this group, a rare subset of children have minor glomerular histologic changes, and the nephrotic syndrome undergoes spontaneous remission or may respond to steroids. The remaining nephrotic patients have severe proliferative changes on renal biopsy and have a significant risk of developing chronic renal insufficiency.

LABORATORY FINDINGS There are currently no reliable serologic markers. With the first episode of gross hematuria, it is reasonable to rule out a diagnosis of APSGN with a serum C3 and ASO levels. Serum IgA levels may be elevated in 8 to 16% of children with IgA nephropathy. The percentage is higher in adults, but this test is not sufficiently specific to establish a diagnosis. Serum IgA-fibronectin aggregates, IgA immune complexes, and IgA rheumatoid factor may be detected, but these tests are not routinely performed and currently lack adequate sensitivity or specificity to be diagnostic. Likewise, IgA and C3 have been reported in the dermal capillaries of forearm skin biopsies in 20 to 50% of IgA nephropathy patients, but the usefulness of these findings needs further investigation. Most pediatric nephrologists would recommend a biopsy for IgA nephropathy patients with impaired renal function, hypertension, or significant proteinuria (greater than 1 g/24 h), as these patients are at increased risk of ultimately developing end-stage renal disease (see Sec. 21.5.3). Thus, it seems justified to treat this subset of patients with the most efficacious known therapy or to enter them into clinical studies designed to determine the best treatment.

PATHOGENESIS Despite an incredibly large number of studies, the pathogenesis of IgA nephropathy remains open to speculation. There is general agreement that it is an immune complex disease characterized by the predominance of immune complexes in the glomerular mesangial matrix. Whether these deposits represent immune complexes trapped from the circulation or complexes formed in situ in the kidney is debatable.

TREATMENT Therapy is controversial, and at present whether any therapy significantly alters the ultimate course of progressive IgA nephropathy is unclear. For many patients, the disease follows a benign course, and specific therapeutic intervention is unnecessary. However, a subset of patients is at risk of developing progressive renal insufficiency. Potential risk factors include male sex, older age, elevated serum creatinine, hypertension, persistent severe protein-

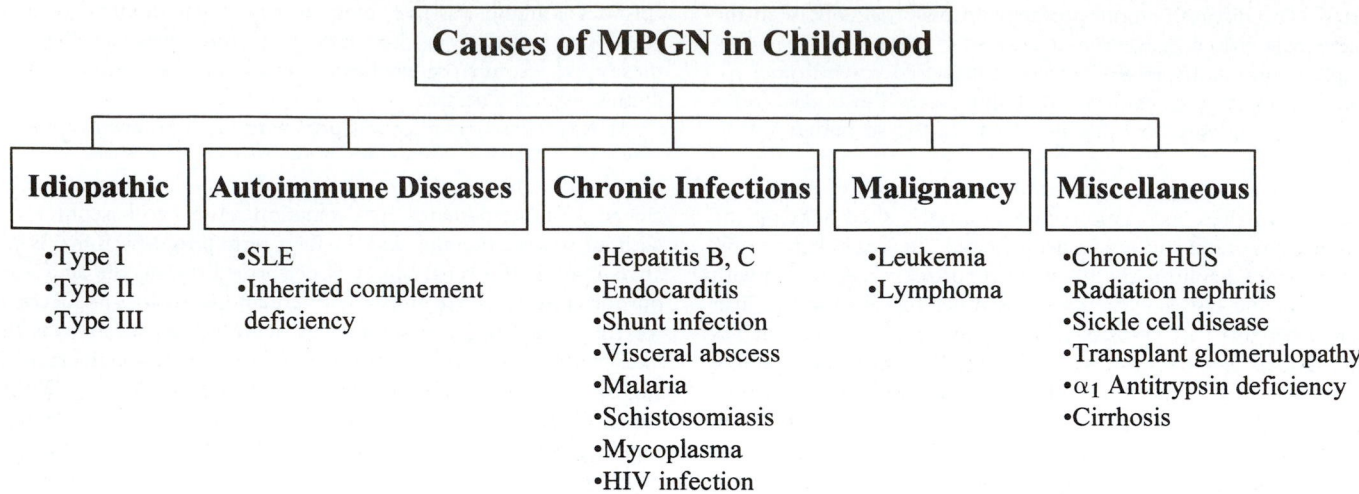

FIGURE 21-21 Causes of membranoproliferative glomerulonephritis (MPGN) in the pediatric population. SLE = systemic lupus erythematosus; HUS = hemolytic uremic syndrome.

uria, and the severity of the proliferative and sclerotic lesions on renal biopsy. Clear treatment guidelines will come only through prospective randomized double-blind studies, several of which are currently in progress. General recommendations include the following: (1) Hypertensive patients should be treated with angiotensin inhibitors that not only control the blood pressure but may slow the rate of decline in GFR. Theoretically normotensive patients excreting more than 1 g/24 h protein might benefit from treatment with an angiotensin-converting enzyme (ACE) inhibitor or an angiotensin II receptor antagonist, but definitive proof is currently lacking. (2) Treatment with ω-3 fatty acids in the form of fish oil (eicosapentaenoic acid and docosahexaenoic acid) has yielded conflicting results with two controlled studies showing no benefit, whereas a larger study demonstrated a slowing in the rate of progression of renal insufficiency. (3) Alternate-day steroids may be of benefit in patients with slowly progressive disease, although proof of efficacy has not been rigorously tested. If steroids are to be of benefit, it is likely that long-term therapy will be required. (4) There are very little data, mostly anecdotal, in the pediatric population about the use of more intensive immunosuppression, which should be considered only for patients with aggressive crescentic disease. Limited experience has reported beneficial outcomes with pulse steroids, plasmapheresis, intravenous immunoglobulin, and/or cytotoxic drugs.

PROGNOSIS/LONG-TERM OUTCOME IgA nephropathy is a disease with a highly variable outcome. For patients with self-limited episodes of recurring hematuria who do not develop significant proteinuria, the long-term outcome is quite good. The risk of developing ESRD has been better documented in adults than in children. In Japan, where diagnosis is usually made by screening urinalyses, 11% of children developed chronic renal insufficiency after 15 years of follow-up. Among 103 patients with clinical onset of IgA nephropathy before 18 years of age who were followed in Kentucky and Tennessee, 15% developed ESRD by 15 years, and 20% by 20 years. Risk factors for progressive disease appear to be similar in children and adults, although in general, patients with disease onset in childhood have a better prognosis. Genetic risk factors that might influence progression include black race and ACE gene polymorphisms.

MEMBRANOPROLIFERATIVE GLOMERULONEPHRITIS

Membranoproliferative glomerulonephritis (MPGN), less commonly referred to as mesangiocapillary glomerulonephritis, is a specific morphologic pattern of glomerulonephritis characterized by thickening of the GBM (from immune complex deposition and/or interposition of mesangial cell cytoplasm in the GBM) and hypercellularity (caused by proliferation of mesangial cells and the influx of leukocytes) that often produces a lobular appearance of the glomerular tuft. MPGN is not a distinct disease entity. This histologic pattern of glomerulonephritis is most often idiopathic in children, but numerous secondary causes are known, and these entities should be considered in all patients (Fig. 21-21). The idiopathic varieties are divided into two distinct and unrelated diseases. Type I appears to be an immune complex disease characterized by immune deposits along the subendothelial space of the GBM that contain C3 and immunoglobulins (IgG > IgM). Type III appears to be a histologic variant of type I except that prominent subepithelial deposits are also present. Splitting this latter group of patients into a subgroup distinct from type I is not universally accepted. Although subtle clinical and laboratory differences between patients with type I and type III exist, overall they are quite similar and are considered together. In contrast, type II MPGN, also known as dense intramembranous deposit disease, is clearly a distinct entity characterized ultrastructurally by the presence of dense ribbon-like deposits within that GBM. Similar deposits may be found in other kidney basement membranes and within the mesangium. The nature of this dense material remains unknown, but it appears to be biochemically similar to GBM itself, and this material does not appear to be composed of immune complexes but activates the alternative complement cascade with C3 characteristically lining the outer aspect of these deposits. Significant deposits of immunoglobulins are typically absent.

EPIDEMIOLOGY/PREDISPOSING FACTORS Idiopathic MPGN most commonly begins between the ages of 8 and 30 years, is distinctly rare under the age of 5 years (although cases as young as 15 months have been reported), and is mainly a disease of whites. Although uncommon, familial clusters are reported. Overall male and female patients are equally affected, but the condition is slightly more common in female adolescents. The disease appears to be decreasing in incidence over the past decade. Patients with type II MPGN are rarely seen anymore. There also appear to be fewer patients presenting with type I. In adults this may be because many patients previously thought to have idiopathic disease were found to be chronically infected with hepatitis C. However, the relationship between hepatitis C infection and MPGN in children is not strong, and the reason for the declining pediatric incidence of idiopathic MPGN is unclear.

CLINICAL MANIFESTATION Children with idiopathic MPGN may present clinically in one of several ways. Twenty to 30% develop an acute nephritic syndrome that mimics APSGN. In fact, many patients have had a preceding upper respiratory illness, and up to 40% have evidence of a recent streptococcal infection. The presence of nephrotic syndrome and a depressed serum C4 level are early clues to the diagnosis of MPGN rather than APSGN. In approximately 20 to 40% of the patients, the diagnosis is made after the incidental finding of proteinuria and hematuria. Nephrotic syndrome is a presenting feature in 30 to 50% of children, and even more children will develop the syndrome during the course of the disease. Much rarer presentations include recurrent episodes of gross hematuria mimicking IgA nephropathy and rapidly progressive glomerulonephritis. Subtle, but not substantial, differences exist between the clinical features at presentation of types I and II. Partial lipodystrophy (Barraquer-Simons disease) occurs in some patients with MPGN II.

LABORATORY FINDINGS A renal biopsy is required to establish the diagnosis, although a characteristic clinical presentation with persistent hypocomplementemia is highly suggestive. Type I patients have evidence of activation of the classical complement cascade with low serum C3 levels and borderline or low C4 levels. The complement profile in type II patients suggests alternative pathway activation with low C3 and normal C4 levels. The presence of C3 nephritic factor is characteristic of type II disease. This is an IgG autoantibody that binds to and stabilizes the C3 convertase of the alternative pathway (C3bBb), resulting in ongoing C3 breakdown. The serum C3 levels are depressed in 50% of patients with MPGN III; C4 may be normal or low. Overall, the serum C3 level is decreased in 75% of all patients at the time of initial presentation. The return of C3 levels to normal 6 to 8 weeks after presentation of acute nephritis will help differentiate MPGN from APSGN (Fig. 21-20). The levels are variable over time and do not have prognostic significance. A normocytic, normochromic Coombs-negative anemia is found in half of the patients and is not entirely explained by the degree of renal insufficiency.

PATHOGENESIS The pathogenesis of idiopathic MPGN remains enigmatic. Type I/III appears to be an immune-complex–mediated glomerular disease. The close association in some adult populations with hepatitis C infection and the declining overall incidence of this disease suggest that exogenous antigens trigger the disease. A small subset of patients with inherited complement deficiencies, especially of C2, are predisposed to develop MPGN. Whether complement directly contributes to the immunopathology or hypocomplementemia plays a role by predisposing to antecedent infections or by impairing the opsonization, solubilization, and clearance of immune complex is unknown. In type II MPGN, the nature of the renal electron-dense deposits remains unclear despite numerous attempts to isolate and characterize them. The only plausible explanation at present is that these deposits are biochemically modified renal basement membranes, perhaps because of the incorporation of sialic-acid-rich glycoproteins. Whether C3 nephritic factor plays a pathogenic role or is a disease marker or a secondary epiphenomenon remains unclear.

TREATMENT Responsiveness to treatment remains an unsettled issue, as the results of randomized clinical trials have not produced convincing evidence that any treatment, at least of relatively short duration, is beneficial. These studies have been criticized because MPGN is typically a chronic, slowly progressive disease, and effective treatment would need to be given for years. For many children without nephrotic syndrome, renal function may remain stable for many years without specific therapy. The consensus in North America is that children with idiopathic MPGN and significant proteinuria will do better if treated with a prolonged course (3–10 years) of alternate-day steroids. A variety of different protocols have been tried, but most involve a dose of 2 mg/kg every other day (maximum 60 mg) for at least 1 year with various tapering schedules thereafter. The role of antiplatelet therapy remains unclear. Limited and conflicting data on the use of cytotoxic drugs preclude reliable recommendations.

PROGNOSIS/LONG-TERM OUTCOME Limited data exist on the long-term outcome of children with MPGN. For many patients, the disease carries a poor prognosis, particularly if associated with nephrotic syndrome. In the follow-up of 50 children with MPGN, ESRD occurred in 53% at 10 years among patients presenting with nephrotic syndrome compared to 34% for the nonnephrotic group. Outcome is said to be worse for patients with type II MPGN. In other series of pediatric patients, the long-term prognosis is variable, with development of ESRD in 10 to 40% of patients at 10 to 20 years follow-up. The outcome may have improved in recent years, but because of the indolent course of this disease, long-term follow-up is necessary to confirm this impression. Spontaneous remissions have been reported in a very small subset of patients.

RAPIDLY PROGRESSIVE (CRESCENTIC) GLOMERULONEPHRITIS

Rapidly progressive glomerulonephritis (RPGN) is a clinical syndrome characterized by quick and progressive deterioration in renal function typically associated with oliguria. Without specific therapy, most patients progress to ESRD within a period of weeks to months. Histologically, this clinical syndrome is usually associated with crescents in more than 50% of the glomeruli. However, not all patients with crescentic nephritis present with RPGN, and, conversely, not all patients with a clinical syndrome of RPGN have crescentic glomerulonephritis. Nonetheless, RPGN is an important entity to recognize and understand and should be considered a nephrologic emergency because the overall prognosis is so poor in this group of patients. The only hope of renal recovery is early confirmation of the diagnosis by renal biopsy followed by immediate initiation of appropriate therapy.

EPIDEMIOLOGY/PREDISPOSING FACTORS RPGN is a rare disorder, particularly in childhood. On the basis of the immunopathologic features of this syndrome, crescentic glomerulonephritis is currently classified into three groups (Fig. 21-22): anti-GBM nephritis, immune complex nephritis, and pauci-immune disease. In

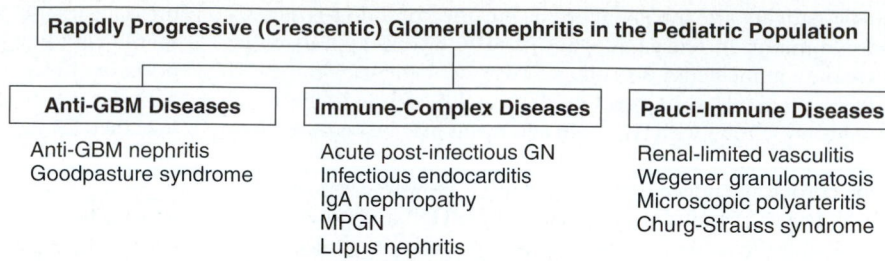

Rapidly Progressive (Crescentic) Glomerulonephritis in the Pediatric Population		
Anti-GBM Diseases	**Immune-Complex Diseases**	**Pauci-Immune Diseases**
Anti-GBM nephritis Goodpasture syndrome	Acute post-infectious GN Infectious endocarditis IgA nephropathy MPGN Lupus nephritis Henoch-Schönlein nephritis	Renal-limited vasculitis Wegener granulomatosis Microscopic polyarteritis Churg-Strauss syndrome

FIGURE 21-22   Causes of rapidly progressive glomerulonephritis in the pediatric population. GBM = glomerular basement membrane; GN = glomerulonephritis; MPGN = membrano-proliferative glomerulonephritis.

the pediatric population, 5 to 7% of the cases are caused by anti-GBM disease, 80 to 85% by immune complex nephritis, and 13 to 15% by pauci-immune disease. The last group may be more common than these figures indicate because its association with antineutrophil cytoplasmic antibodies (ANCA) was just made in the mid-1980s, providing an important serologic marker that was not previously available. There is a fourth entity, referred to as idiopathic crescentic glomerulonephritis, characterized as pauci-immune and ANCA-negative, that is very rare in children.

CLINICAL AND LABORATORY MANIFESTATIONS Patients with RPGN may present either with an acute nephritic syndrome (see Fig. 21-19) or in a more insidious manner with symptoms caused by chronic renal failure. Children with RPGN present with gross hematuria (50–85%), edema (13–80%), anemia (70%), and hypertension (63-85%). Nephrotic syndrome is uncommon, likely because of the rapid onset of renal insufficiency. The urinalysis typically reveals an active urine sediment with hematuria, proteinuria, and cellular casts. Serologic studies may be very helpful in establishing a tentative diagnosis, but biopsy confirmation is mandatory. Initial tests should include a C3, C4, antinuclear factor (ANF), anti-GBM antibody, and ANCA titer. Not only will the biopsy establish the diagnosis in most patients, but it will provide valuable information about the relative degree of acute (potentially treatable) and chronic histologic changes (see Table 21-14). In many patients, the kidney may be damaged beyond the point of repair, making immunosuppressive therapy, at least for the renal component of the disease, irrational.

TREATMENT Therapy is directed to specific disease entities, but a few general principles apply to all of these diseases (Fig. 21-22). Spontaneous resolution of RPGN is extremely unlikely. The prognosis is poor unless aggressive therapy is started early in the course of the disease. In contrast, if the outcome of ESRD is inevitable, patients should not be exposed to the risks of aggressive therapy. Virtually all diseases that cause crescentic nephritis are thought to be immunologically mediated, and the mainstay of therapy is immunosuppression. Because these disease are very rare and the prognosis is so poor, treatment guidelines based on randomized prospective clinical trials are not available. If immunosuppressive therapy is warranted, most centers would begin with high-dose intravenous methylprednisolone, followed by daily oral prednisone, often with the addition of cytotoxic therapy (usually cyclophosphamide). Plasmapheresis is clearly indicated in patients with anti-GBM disease, but other forms of crescentic glomerular diseases have not been shown to have a beneficial response. The long-term prognosis of children with crescentic nephritis is poorly delineated in the literature.

ANTI-GBM DISEASE

A rare and aggressive form of crescentic glomerulonephritis can be mediated by anti–glomerular basement membrane (anti-GBM) antibodies. These patients may have isolated renal disease or pulmonary involvement that typically causes pulmonary hemorrhage, Goodpasture syndrome.

EPIDEMIOLOGY/PREDISPOSING FACTORS Anti-GBM disease typically occurs in young adults and is most common in young men. Although rare in the first decade of life, it has been reported in children as young as 2 years. Although most cases are sporadic, miniepidemics have occurred, and evidence for a genetic predisposition in some patients has been suggested. Anti-GBM nephritis may occur as a rare complication of other renal diseases (after extracorporeal shock-wave lithotripsy or in association with staghorn calculi, membranous nephropathy, or minimal-change disease). Many patients have had an antecedent flu-like illness, and an association with influenza A_2 has been reported. Why some, but not all, patients develop pulmonary disease is unclear because the target antigen is present in all alveolar basement membranes. Experience with experimental models suggests that a second factor in addition to the anti-GBM antibody may be required before the lung becomes involved. Exposure to tobacco, hydrocarbons, cocaine, and viral pneumonitis, all of which may cause lung injury, has been associated with an enhanced likelihood of pulmonary hemorrhage. Another unique situation where anti-GBM nephritis may occur is in the small subset (3–4%) of patients with Alport syndrome who receive a normal kidney allograft (see Secs. 21.9 and 21.15).

CLINICAL MANIFESTATIONS Patients present with acute nephritis and, less commonly, with symptoms caused by chronic renal insufficiency. Progression to renal failure typically begins within weeks. Pulmonary hemorrhage presenting as hemoptysis usually precedes or accompanies the onset of nephritis. In 30% of patients, the pulmonary involvement may be clinically silent or follow the onset of glomerulonephritis. The episodes of hemoptysis may be life-threatening. A pulmonary-renal syndrome also occurs in systemic lupus erythematosus, systemic vasculitis, Henoch-Schönlein purpura, cardiovascular disease, and various infections.

LABORATORY FINDINGS More than 90% of patients have an anti-GBM antibody detected in the plasma at the time of clinical presentation, although the titer of the antibody does not correlate with disease severity. A subset of patients (up to 30%) may also have a positive ANCA. Some of these overlap patients have evidence of extrarenal disease caused by vasculitis, and, overall, this group seems to have a slightly better prognosis. Many patients have evidence of iron deficiency anemia as a complication of pulmonary hemorrhage. Because acute pulmonary hemorrhage can resolve quickly radiologically, other evidence of pulmonary hemorrhage would include the presence of hemosiderin-laden macrophages or an increased carbon monoxide diffusion capacity from the presence of hemoglobin in the alveoli. The diagnosis is confirmed by renal biopsy showing crescentic nephritis with linear deposits of IgG and C3 along the glomerular basement membrane (see Table 21-14).

PATHOGENESIS The Goodpasture target antigen is a normal structural component of renal and pulmonary basement membranes and consists of the last 36 amino acid residues of the carboxy-terminal region of the $\alpha3$ chain of type IV collagen. Basement membrane type IV collagen consists of six distinct polypeptide chains ($\alpha1$ to $\alpha6$) that combine to form triple helices. The relative abundance of the $\alpha3$ chain in glomeruli and alveoli likely explains the restriction of antibody-medicated disease to these organs. Most anti-GBM antibodies are IgG isotype, although a few patients with IgA antibodies have been reported.

TREATMENT If the patient has pulmonary disease and/or evidence of reversible renal disease, the mainstay of therapy is plasmapheresis to remove the circulating antibody. Immunosuppressive therapy (prednisone and cyclophosphamide) is particularly beneficial for patients with lung disease and is added to blunt further antibody production.

PROGNOSIS/LONG-TERM OUTCOME The potential to reverse the renal disease is poor unless treatment is started early. In most patients, anti-GBM antibody production is of limited duration, with the antibody disappearing from the circulation in 8 to 14 weeks, and is rarely detected after 6 months. Nonetheless, the capacity of this antibody to cause irreversible renal injury is remarkable. ESRD in adults is almost inevitable if the initial creatinine is greater than 6 mg/dL or 75% of the glomeruli have crescents on renal biopsy. The small group of patients who recover from the acute disease can do very well. Relapses have been reported but are extremely rare.

LUPUS NEPHRITIS

Systemic lupus erythematosus (SLE) is considered the prototype of multisystem diseases caused by immune complex–mediated tissue injury (see Chapter 12) to the kidney. In fact, in circumstances in which renal biopsies are performed routinely on all newly diagnosed patients, the finding of a completely normal kidney without IgG and C3 deposits is extremely rare. Renal biopsies are usually limited to patients with clinical or laboratory evidence of renal involvement and include 60 to 80% of children at the time of diagnosis. Another 10% subsequently develop renal disease, usually within 3 years of diagnosis.

EPIDEMIOLOGY/PREDISPOSING FACTORS Approximately 20% of SLE patients have childhood onset of the disease. Although it is less common in the first decade of life, it has been reported in a 6-week-old infant. The disease predominates in female patients, but the sex difference is somewhat less striking in childhood. The etiology of SLE is incompletely understood, but several factors are known to have an influence. Disease susceptibility is often an inherited trait. Familial cases are common, and the disease is more prevalent among individuals of African-American, Hispanic, and Asian decent. In some families, the disease is linked to the inheritance of specific HLA alleles. An increased risk of SLE occurs in patients with certain inherited defects of the immune system, in-

cluding deficiencies in early complement components (C2, C3, C4) and IgA. Several environmental factors have been implicated as triggers for onset of disease or exacerbation: viruses, sun exposure, and female sex hormones.

CLINICAL MANIFESTATIONS The clinical manifestations of lupus nephritis span the spectrum of glomerular diseases ranging from asymptomatic microscopic hematuria and/or proteinuria to rapidly progressive glomerulonephritis. Acute renal failure is a rare but recognized presentation (see Fig. 21-18). Usually other systemic manifestations of SLE are readily apparent, and a renal biopsy is almost never required to establish the diagnosis of SLE. The presence of 4 out of 11 American Rheumatism Association criteria for SLE confers a 96% sensitivity and specificity for the diagnosis of SLE (see Chapter 12). These criteria are malar rash, discoid rash, photosensitivity, oral ulcers, arthritis, serositis, renal disease, neurologic disease, hematologic disorders, immune serologic abnormalities, and a positive antinuclear antibody. Although most patients with lupus nephritis have nonrenal manifestations of SLE, AGN may rarely be the initial presentation, and a few patients may present with interstitial nephritis or renal disease associated with antiphospholipid antibodies that may cause renal infarction or thrombotic microangiopathy resembling hemolytic uremia syndrome (see Sec. 21.8.3).

A renal biopsy is not necessary to make the diagnosis of SLE, but it plays an important role in establishing the pattern of renal disease and guiding therapeutic options (see Table 21-14). The correlation between clinical manifestations and pathologic findings is not sufficiently strong to preclude renal biopsies. Of the several pathologic classifications of lupus nephritis, the modified World Health Organization (WHO) classification is most widely used. The distribution of the various forms of lupus nephritis does not vary significantly between childhood and adult-onset SLE. Class I is a normal biopsy on light microscopy. Class II (mesangial) occurs in 19 to 27% of patients and is characterized by mild mesangial matrix expansion, sometimes with mild mesangial hypercellularity, with immune complexes localized to the mesangium. Clinically these patients usually have mild hematuria with or without low-grade proteinuria. The proliferative forms of lupus nephritis are the most common and most serious. Class III is focal proliferative nephritis with involvement in less than 50% of the glomeruli, whereas class IV is generalized and referred to as diffuse proliferative lupus nephritis (DPLN). Many feel that class III and class IV represent a spectrum of quantitative differences in a similar pattern of glomerular injury. At the time of initial renal biopsy, 18 to 24% of patients have class III and 39 to 44% have class IV lupus nephritis. In addition to histologic features of glomerular inflammation, these proliferative diseases have immune deposits in the mesangium and along the capillary wall, mainly in a subendothelial position. There is considerable overlap of the clinical manifestations in patients with class III and class IV nephritis. Class V is a unique subtype of disease, membranous lupus nephritis, that is characterized by immune complexes in the subepithelial position. These patients are characterized clinically by significant proteinuria, often in the nephrotic range. Hematuria may be absent or microscopic, and cellular casts are typically absent in the urine sediment. Class V lupus nephritis may be increasing in frequency, with reported incidence ranging from 8 to 22%. Even though it may be easy to predict that patients with severe clinical disease have DPLN, this same histologic picture may be present in patients with relatively mild clinical manifestations. The presence of nephrotic syndrome is most likely to be associated with DPLN, but the syndrome is also present in more than 50% of patients with membranous lupus nephritis and, occasionally, in patients with focal proliferative and even mesangial lupus nephritis. The biopsy also provides important information about the acuity of the disease (indicating the potential for therapeutic responsiveness) and its chronicity, features that should be taken into consideration when therapeutic decisions are made.

LABORATORY FINDINGS In association with clinical manifestations of a multisystem disease, autoantibody production is a major feature of SLE (see Chapter 12). Multiple autoantigens may be targets, but the most frequent and best-characterized targets are DNA, ribonucleoprotein, and other nuclear and cytoplasmic proteins. Almost all patients have a positive antinuclear antibody (ANA), although this antibody can be detected in individuals who do not have SLE. True ANA-negative SLE is rare in childhood. The ANA titer bears no relationship to the severity of the renal disease. Antibodies to double-stranded DNA (dsDNA) and Smith antigen (Sm) are more specific but occur in only 70% and 25%, respectively, of untreated patients. A small subset of patients with SLE have antiphospholipid antibodies that are associated with a significant risk of thrombotic disease. Hypocomplementemia is another important finding in SLE patients with active disease. Anti-dsDNA titers and serum C3 levels are useful parameters for monitoring renal disease activity and response to therapy. No combination of these serologic studies will effectively predict the type (WHO class) or severity of renal involvement.

PATHOGENESIS The basic mechanism of tissue injury is the deposition of immune complexes. Most tissue deposits contain IgG and C3, but the presence of IgM and/or IgA is also common. The exact nature of the antigen within these deposits remains unclear. It has been difficult to verify the presence of DNA. Through the activation of complement, these deposits are thought to trigger an inflammatory response that causes tissue damage. No single genetic defect explains the polyclonal B-cell activation that leads to autoantibody production in these patients.

TREATMENT Although the best treatment of SLE patients remains debatable, several guidelines have been established. Even though SLE nephritis may be controlled with medical therapy, currently no known cure exists. For some patients, therapy will be determined by the severity of the extrarenal disease. However, for many patients, the severity of the renal disease guides the approach to immunosuppression (Fig. 21-23). The treatment of patients with mesangial lupus nephritis (Class II) should be determined by the extrarenal manifestations. This is a mild renal lesion that has an excellent prognosis. Patients with focal proliferative disease (class III) can generally be managed with prednisone alone. However, if patients have more aggressive histologic features such as focal necrotizing lesions or crescents, they are best treated as patients with DPLN.

Unfortunately, DPLN is an aggressive disease that will ultimately destroy the kidney if left uncontrolled. Several studies now indicate that the combined use of corticosteroids with immunosuppressive drugs results in a better long-term outcome than treatment with corticosteroids alone. Which immunosuppressive agent to use and for how long remains hotly debated. Although there are no compelling data that cyclophosphamide is superior to purine synthesis inhibitors, cyclophosphamide is commonly used. However, many of these patients, particularly those with good renal function, will have an excellent outcome if they are treated with prednisone and azathioprine. A new-generation inhibitor of purine metabolism, mycophenolate mofetil, is being evaluated to replace azathioprine as a first-line drug in the treatment of SLE. After an initial 6-month phase of aggressive treatment aimed at achieving disease remission, this group of patients needs long-term maintenance therapy to prevent relapses. Ideally this should include low-dose prednisone combined with a cytotoxic drug. To protect against significant gonadal toxicity and potential infertility, attempts should be made to limit exposure to cyclophosphamide to 3 to 6 months, particularly if patients have a brisk early response during the induction phase of therapy. Therefore, switching from a cytotoxic to purine metabolism inhibition is frequently attempted during maintenance therapy. Treatment must be individualized. Despite maintenance therapy, many patients experience renal flares. Rising anti-dsDNA titers and falling serum complement levels are warning signs of an impending flare, but alone, they are insufficient criteria to change therapy. It is also important to remember that aggressive cytotoxic therapy is not indicated in the treatment of DPLN characterized by advanced renal fibrosis because ESRD is inevitable in this patient group.

Good guidelines for the treatment of membranous lupus nephritis are not currently available. The group with pure membranous lesions (class Va) have a fairly good renal prognosis, and these patients are often managed as patients with idiopathic membranous nephropathy (see Sec. 21.8.2). Patients with superimposed proliferative lesions are probably best treated for the severity of the proliferative lesions because of a higher risk of developing renal insufficiency. There is some published experience with the use of methotrexate, cyclosporine, and intravenous IgG, but which patients with lupus nephritis are most likely to benefit from these therapies is currently unclear.

PROGNOSIS/LONG-TERM OUTCOME ESRD is still a significant problem in patients with DPLN, in part because of the subset of patients who have advanced renal scarring at the time of initial diagnosis and the subset of patients who are noncompliant with medication. Still other patients have aggressive disease that is difficult to control with current treatment protocols. The incidence of ESRD in SLE patients with DPLN has decreased from 50% in the 1950s to 20% in the 1990s. Whereas fewer than 10% of patients are currently receiving renal replacement therapy 5 years after diagnosis, a significant group with mild chronic renal insufficiency are likely to develop progressive renal insufficiency over several years. Patients with recurrent nephritic flares need to be treated appropriately and, overall, have a worse long-term outcome.

HENOCH-SCHÖNLEIN PURPURA NEPHRITIS

Henoch-Schönlein purpura (HSP) or anaphylactoid purpura is a syndrome characterized by a tetrad of clinical features that can occur in any order and at any time over several days to weeks: a purpuric rash, arthralgias, abdominal pain, and glomerulonephritis. Histologically the renal disease is indistinguishable from idiopathic IgA nephropathy. The incidence of renal disease is variably reported from 20 to 100%, depending on the diagnostic criteria used.

EPIDEMIOLOGY/PREDISPOSING FACTORS The peak incidence of HSP occurs in children between 4 and 5 years of age, with 75% of cases reported in children less than 7 years old, and is rare in children under 2 years but has been reported in an 8-month-old infant (see Table 21-13). HSP is more common in the winter and early

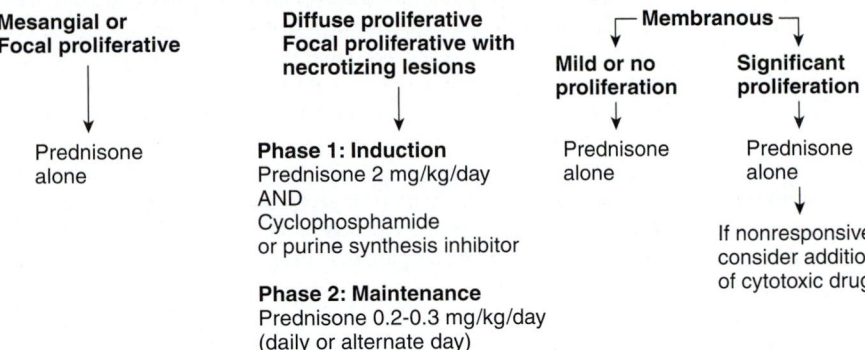

FIGURE 21-23 A suggested approach to the treatment of children with lupus nephritis based on WHO classification.

spring, and often, a history of an antecedent pharyngitis or upper respiratory infection is present, but only 20 to 30% of cases have serologic evidence of a recent infection with group A β-hemolytic *Streptococcus*. Both familial cases and small epidemics of HSP have been reported.

CLINICAL MANIFESTATIONS Most patients with HSP nephritis have asymptomatic hematuria and mild proteinuria. As many as 20% may have gross hematuria, and approximately 10% of the children with renal disease may present with an acute nephritic syndrome. Nephrotic syndrome and renal insufficiency are much less common. Almost all patients develop nephritis after the appearance of the rash, and in more then 90% of the patients, renal involvement is evident within 8 weeks of disease onset. Rare clinical presentations include hypertension with a normal urinalysis and microscopic hematuria caused by urethritis. Facial and/or scalp edema is common in children with HSP, unrelated to the severity of the renal disease. Children with significant renal disease are more likely to have severe abdominal pain than children without nephritis. Seventy percent of children with HSP are clinically well within 4 weeks, but recurrent episodes occur fairly commonly for the first 3 months and have been reported after an interval as long as 5 years. Renal disease is often more severe in the patients with recurrent attacks.

LABORATORY FINDINGS HSP is a clinical diagnosis based on the presence of palpable purpura, abdominal pain, and joint disease. There are no diagnostic tests. Rarely patients with ANCA-positive vasculitis, SLE, and even APSGN may present clinically with a syndrome that mimics HSP. Elevated serum IgA levels and IgA rheumatoid factor are detected in approximately 50% of patients. Serum complement levels are usually normal or elevated.

PATHOGENESIS The immunopathogenesis of HSP nephritis appears similar to idiopathic IgA nephropathy and is characterized by the deposition of IgA-containing immune complexes in the glomerular mesangium and, less commonly, along the glomerular capillary wall. The systemic disease is characterized as a hypersensitivity vasculitis afflicting small vessels. Although an antecedent respiratory illness is common, the role of infectious agents is unclear.

TREATMENT There is no definitive treatment for HSP nephritis, and most patients recover with supportive care. However, a subset of patients present with severe renal disease and are at risk of developing chronic and even end-stage renal disease. These severely

affected children should undergo renal biopsy to establish the extent of the glomerular injury, as clinical and pathologic findings do not always correlate. The histologic severity of HSP nephritis is usually graded on a scale of 1 to 6 based on criteria established by the International Study of Kidney Disease in Children. This grading system is weighted to the number of crescents, which is felt to be highly predictable of a poorer outcome: grade I, minor abnormalities; grade II, pure mesangial proliferation; grade III, focal or diffuse mesangial proliferation with crescents in fewer than 50% of glomeruli; grade IV, same as grade III except crescents in 50 to 75% of glomeruli; grade V, same as grade III but more than 75% of glomeruli have crescents. Grade VI is a rare variant resembling MPGN. Patients with grades III to VI have a less favorable prognosis and are generally treated with prednisone. Cytotoxic drugs (cyclophosphamide or azathioprine) may have some benefit. The optimal treatment protocol has not been established, and no controlled studies have established the benefit of immunosuppressive therapy.

PROGNOSIS/LONG-TERM OUTCOME Short-term follow-up indicates an excellent prognosis. More than 90% of patients recover, but the urinalysis is still abnormal in 50% of the children at 3 months and in 10 to 20% 2 years after symptoms have resolved. A few children (3–4%) have a catastrophic acute illness and develop a rapidly progressive clinical course with ESRD within months. Another group (~5%) have evidence of chronic renal damage, usually persistent proteinuria, with progression over a period of years. Poor prognostic features include an acute nephritic presentation, heavy proteinuria, and the presence of glomerular crescents (>75%) on biopsy. There are emerging data that all patients with severe acute renal involvement need to be followed up for many years. In a long-term follow-up study (averaging 23 years) of 78 patients with HSP, 44% of patients with nephrotic syndrome or acute nephritis at presentation had hypertension or a progressive decline in renal function, whereas 82% with hematuria alone were normal.

RENAL VASCULITIS (ANCA-POSITIVE FOCAL NECROTIZING GLOMERULONEPHRITIS)

Vasculitis occurs in many different diseases and syndromes in childhood. HSP is the most common form of systemic vasculitis in children. Vasculitis may also be a manifestation of connective tissue disorders such as SLE or of certain infections such as rickettsial disease (Rocky Mountain spotted fever), bacterial infections (gonococcal infections), viral infections (hepatitis B, parvovirus, HIV), and tuberculosis. The most widely used classification of vasculitis is based on the size of the vessels involved (Fig. 21-24).

Systemic vasculitis associated with antineutrophil cytoplasmic antibodies (ANCA) is discussed here. ANCA were first identified in the sera of patients with focal necrotizing glomerulonephritis in 1982, and the presence of these antibodies now appears to be a sensitive marker for three disorders associated with pauci-immune (minimal evidence of immune complex deposition) focal necrotizing glomerulonephritis. Two target ANCA antigens, both present in neutrophil lysosomes, have been identified: proteinase-3 produces a diffuse cytoplasmic staining pattern (cANCA), and myeloperoxidase provides a perinuclear staining pattern (pANCA). There are three small-vessel vasculitic syndromes associated with ANCA and focal necrotizing glomerulonephritis. Churg-Strauss syndrome is very uncommon in children. It is characterized by an initial phase of allergic asthma; followed by vasculitis associated with eosinophilic infiltrates and peripheral blood eosinophilia. Glomerulonephritis occurs in 30 to 40% of Churg-Strauss patients, but the degree of involvement is usually mild. This section focuses on microscopic polyarteritis and Wegener granulomatosis.

EPIDEMIOLOGY/PREDISPOSING FACTORS   Detailed pediatric epidemiologic studies are not available because these diseases are uncommon in the pediatric population and because the diagnosis was often unclear before a serologic marker became available in the mid-1980s. Wegener granulomatosis and microscopic polyarteritis are most common in adults in the fifth and sixth decades of life.

CLINICAL MANIFESTATIONS   There is tremendous overlap in the clinical manifestations of Wegener granulomatosis and microscopic polyarteritis except that necrotizing granulomatous vasculitis of the upper and lower airway is a diagnostic feature of Wegener granulomatosis and is absent in patients with microscopic polyarteritis. Both diseases typically present with a flu-like prodrome and systemic symptoms including myalgias, fever, anorexia, and weight loss. Skin involvement (purpura or urticaria) and arthritis or arthralgia are common. Lung disease is common in both syndromes, ranging from clinically silent involvement to life-threatening pulmonary hemorrhage. In microscopic polyarteritis, the lung disease results from alveolar capillaritis, whereas in Wegener disease, necrotizing granulomas, which may be microscopic or macroscopic, form pulmonary nodules or even cavitating lesions. Granulomatous involvement of the upper airway, sinuses, nasal passages, and ears is also present in many patients with Wegener. Renal involvement is very common in both diseases, approximately 90% with micro-

scopic polyarteritis and 80% with Wegener granulomatosis. There is a small subset of patients who present with renal-limited vasculitis. Histologically, the glomerular disease is similar in all three groups of patients, and the degree of involvement is usually severe. All patients with nephritis have hematuria, most have proteinuria, and more than 70% have a reduced glomerular filtration rate at presentation. Some patients present with rapidly progressive glomerulonephritis from severe glomerular damage caused by fibrinoid necrosis and crescents. Even though Wegener is classified as a granulomatous disease, granulomatous renal vasculitis is rare, detected in perhaps 5% of biopsied patients. Immune deposits are sparse or completely absent.

LABORATORY FINDINGS   In a patient with focal necrotizing glomerulonephritis often accompanied by extrarenal disease caused by vasculitis, antineutrophil cytoplasmic antibodies are positive in ~90% of patients with Wegener granulomatosis and microscopic polyarteritis. A small subset of patients with glomerulonephritis caused by anti-GBM antibodies or immune complex disease may also be ANCA-positive. Although there is some overlap, the type of ANCA may predict the nature of the disease. Proteinase-3 reactive antibody or cANCA is 90 to 98% sensitive and specific for Wegener granulomatosis, whereas patients with microscopic polyarteritis and renal-limited vasculitis are more likely to have antibodies to myeloperoxidase or pANCA. Monitoring the ANCA titer can be useful in evaluating disease activity. Relapses are unusual among patients with a persistently negative titer, whereas disease relapses are often accompanied by the reappearance of ANCA or a significant titer increase.

PATHOGENESIS   The pathogenesis of ANCA-positive vasculitis is unknown. Microscopic polyarteritis has been considered a hypersensitivity angiitis in some patients, possibly representing a reaction to a drug or an infectious agent. Although a flu-like prodrome is typical in many patients, suggesting an infectious trigger, candidate microorganisms have yet to be identified. Whether ANCA are pathogenetically important remains unclear.

TREATMENT   ANCA-associated systemic vasculitis is an aggressive disease. Before the current treatments, mean survival rates were less than 6 months. The introduction of cytotoxic drugs (cyclophosphamide in particular) has resulted in a dramatic improvement in outcomes, but significant morbidity and mortality remain. There is little role for corticosteroid therapy alone except to control the extrarenal localized disease. The first goal of therapy is to induce disease remission, and this generally involves the administration of high-dose corticosteroids and cyclophosphamide. The role of plas-

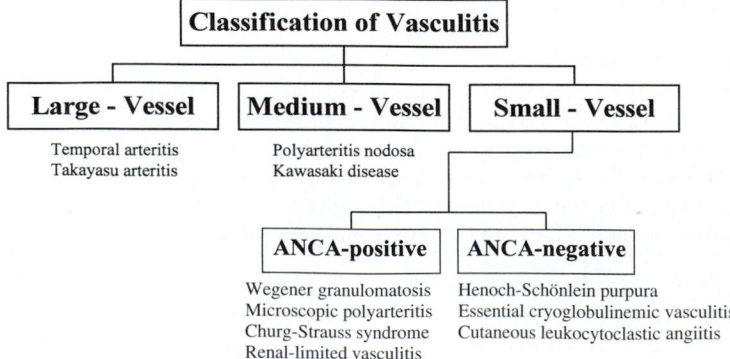

FIGURE 21-24   Classification of vasculitis taken from the Chapel Hill Consensus Conference on the nomenclature of systemic vasculitis. SOURCE: *Jennette JC, Falk RJ, Andrassy K, et al: Nomenclature of systemic vasculitides. Proposal of an international consensus conference. Arthritis Rheum 37:187–192, 1994, with copyright permission of the American College of Rheumatology.*

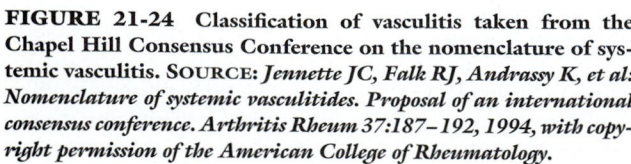

mapheresis is unclear, but it may be helpful in patients with severe dialysis-dependent acute glomerulonephritis. Once the disease is in remission (after an average of 6 months of therapy), low-dose maintenance immunosuppression may be indicated because of the high relapse rate, ~20 to 40% within 1 year of cessation of therapy. The ideal maintenance regimen has not been determined. Trimethoprim-sulfamethoxazole may be beneficial in the treatment of patients with Wegener granulomatosis.

PROGNOSIS/LONG-TERM OUTCOME Patient and kidney survival have improved dramatically with intensive immunosuppressive therapy. However, as many as 25% of patients with ANCA-associated vasculitis who are treated with prednisone and cyclophosphamide relapse after the initial treatment. Five-year survival in adults is now in the range of 70 to 85%. There are few long-term follow-up studies of children.

21.8.2   Nephrotic Syndrome

The pathophysiological sequence of events that lead to the classical clinical features in nephrotic syndrome, proteinuria, and hypoalbuminemias, are depicted in Fig. 21-25. Nephrotic syndrome (NS) is not a disease but a constellation of clinical findings common to a number of renal disorders. By definition, it comprises proteinuria greater than 50 mg/kg/24h (>40 mg/m²/h or a protein-to-creatinine ratio greater than 2.0), and hypoalbuminemia (serum albumin less than 3.0 g/dL); edema, and hypercholesterolemia are commonly present. The reason for the increased hepatic production of lipoproteins during the nephrotic state is not entirely understood but may be linked to the low plasma oncotic pressure or defects in lipoprotein catabolism. Nephrotic syndrome (NS) may be a manifestation of any of the glomerulonephropathies but more commonly occurs in children as an isolated entity without clinical evidence of nephritic features or evidence of significant glomerular inflammation on renal biopsy. The urinary sediment in patients with NS may show oval fat bodies and granular casts, but cellular casts are absent. In patients with both nephritic and nephrotic clinical findings, a diagnosis of systemic disorders (SLE, HSP, vasculitis) or MPGN is most likely.

The NS of childhood can be divided into three groups: infantile (see Sec. 21.3 and 21.9), secondary, and primary. Only 10 to 15%

of children have an identifiable secondary cause for their NS. Secondary causes are numerous, and new entities are described regularly. Four broad categories encompass the majority of secondary causes (only representative examples are given):

1. Infections: HIV, malaria.
2. Systemic diseases: Diabetes mellitus, SLE, HSP.
3. Drugs and toxins: NSAIDs, penicillin derivatives, ACE-I.
4. Mechanical factors: Renal vein thrombosis, pickwickian syndrome.
5. Tumors: Hodgkin disease, lymphoproliferative disorders.

The histologic lesions that are associated with secondary causes of NS are frequently indistinguishable from the idiopathic lesions, but the treatment and long-term outcome are more related to the specific underlying cause.

Primary (idiopathic) NS is the occurrence of the constellation of clinical findings that define NS (see Fig. 21-25) in the absence of an identifiable causative agent or disease and accounts for 85 to 90% of children with NS. Primary NS is classified into four histologic categories: minimal change, proliferative changes, focal segmental glomerulosclerosis, and membranous.

MINIMAL-CHANGE NEPHROTIC SYNDROME

Minimal-change nephrotic syndrome (MCNS), also known historically as "nil disease" or "lipoid nephrosis" to reflect the subtle changes present on light microscopic examination of the renal biopsy, is the most common cause of NS in childhood and accounts for 90% of patients presenting under 10 years of age and 80% of all pediatric patients with NS. In children, MCNS is usually idiopathic, although occasionally it occurs in association with malignancies (Hodgkin lymphoma and other T-cell malignancies), following exposure to nonsteroidal anti-inflammatory drugs, or in association with IgA nephropathy or immune-mediated diseases (SLE, Kimura disease). The incidence of MCNS is 2 to 7/100,000 children under the age of 16. The peak incidence is in preschool children with a median age of 2.5 years; 80% of patients present before their sixth birthday, and boys are slightly more affected. Familial cases have been reported but are not common (3% in some series). There appears to be a higher incidence in the Asian population. A history of atopy is reported in 30 to 60% of these children. MCNS is char-

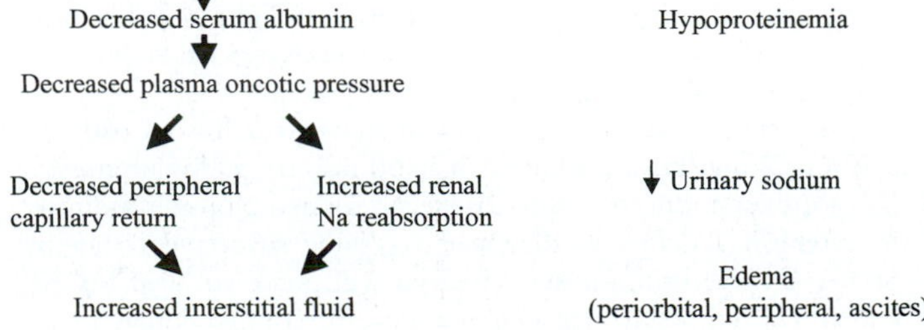

SEQUENCE OF EVENTS IN NEPHROTIC SYNDROME

FIGURE 21-25 Sequence of pathophysiological events in nephrotic syndrome and the associated clinical manifestations.

acterized by response to corticosteroids (>90%), a chronic relapsing course (60–80%), and an excellent long-term prognosis. The relationship between MCNS and the more severe disease, focal segmental glomerulosclerosis (FSGS), continues to be unclear, but these entities may represent different ends of a disease spectrum rather than disorders with different pathogenesis.

CLINICAL MANIFESTATIONS Most patients (95%) present with edema that is most striking in lax tissues and variable in severity because of gravity-dependent effects. Early morning swelling of the eyelids (periorbital edema) is common, and frequently, new patients are initially misdiagnosed as having an allergic reaction. Increasing abdominal girth from ascites is also common. Most episodes of NS, including relapses, are triggered by an antecedent infection. Less commonly, patients with MCNS initially present with symptoms secondary to complications of the nephrotic syndrome, especially infections (peritonitis, cellulitis) or thromboembolic complications. Hypertension is not typical, but a mildly elevated blood pressure has been reported in 13 to 21% of patients. Macroscopic hematuria is distinctly uncommon, and other causes of NS should be sought. Microscopic hematuria may be seen in 15 to 20% of patients.

LABORATORY FINDINGS In addition to proteinuria, the urinalysis may show oval fat bodies (maltese crosses) and waxy or hyaline casts. Granular casts are common when the patients are also volume-contracted. Cellular casts are not typical. At presentation, the serum creatinine is elevated in some patients, especially if intravascular volume contraction (frequently associated with an elevated hematocrit) is present. Hyponatremia is quite common (see Sec. 21.4). The serum C3 level is usually normal or elevated. Urinary protein losses may result in low serum levels of IgG, thyroxine-binding globulin (nephrotic infants are often picked up in neonatal thyroid screening), vitamin D–binding globulin, alternative complement pathway factor B, and antithrombin III. Serum fibrinogen levels are often elevated and may be used as a surrogate marker for the risk of thrombosis.

PATHOGENESIS In truth, little progress has been made in establishing the mechanism of disease. The most common hypothesis suggests that T cells release a soluble factor that damages the GBM, causing proteinuria. Although several candidate lymphokines have been proposed, the nature of the "nephrotic factor" remains elusive. Evidence for a circulating "nephrotic factor" is also supported by unique observations in renal transplant patients. When a patient received a kidney from a cadaveric donor with active MCNS, proteinuria decreased rapidly in the transplant recipient and remained persistently normal after 6 weeks. Conversely, MCNS was reported to recur in a renal allograft transplanted into a patient with a history of MCNS. Several subtle differences in the in vitro phenotype and function of lymphocytes (comparing cells harvested from nephrotic and nonnephrotic patients) can be ascribed to the nephrotic plasma milieu rather than to some intrinsic T-cell alteration.

Another potentially pathogenic mechanism in MCNS is the loss of charge selectivity of the glomerular capillary wall, which is caused by a decrease in the heparan sulfate proteoglycan content that constitutes many of the negatively charged sites along the GBM. However, the mechanisms responsible for this change remain unknown, and loss of charge selectivity is a feature in many other diseases associated with the nephrotic syndrome.

TREATMENT

SUPPORTIVE/SYMPTOMATIC TREATMENT Edema is mild in most patients and can be managed adequately with dietary salt restriction. Fluid intake is not usually restricted except in the face of severe hyponatremia. Diuretics are effective, but are rarely needed and must be used cautiously to avoid intravascular volume contraction. Intravenous albumin infusions may be hazardous but can be life-saving in patients with clinical signs and symptoms caused by severe hypovolemia. Intravenous albumin and furosemide can also be used, cautiously, in patients with symptomatic edema or anasarca. A low serum albumin level alone is not a reason to administer intravenous albumin, which is short-lived and can cause CHF or severe hypotension. Hypertension is relatively uncommon, even during corticosteroid therapy, but when present, it requires treatment with antihypertensive medications, which can usually be discontinued once the disease is in remission.

A major aspect of the initial management is parent education. The majority of patients will follow a chronic relapsing course, and the families need to be prepared in advance for this clinical course. All families should be taught to check the urine for protein using a dipstick. A diary of the urinary dipstick results along with drug doses and significant clinical events should be kept by the family. The importance of testing the urine during intercurrent illness needs emphasis. Whereas relapses are frequently triggered by an upper respiratory tract infection, transient low-grade proteinuria may also occur. Parents need to be encouraged to call for advice when proteinuria reappears so that true relapses can be treated before they become complicated, whereas transient episodes of low-grade proteinuria can be closely monitored but are not an indication to start corticosteroid therapy immediately.

Screening for tuberculosis should be done before high-dose corticosteroids are given. Children who have never had chickenpox should be treated with varicella immune globulin if exposed and should be vaccinated once they have been off prednisone for a few months. Administration of pneumococcal vaccine is also recommended. The use of nonsteroidal anti-inflammation drugs as antipyretics is best avoided in these patients.

CORTICOSTEROID THERAPY Treatment with corticosteroids was first introduced in 1956 and has proven to be a life-saving therapy. Because steroids will induce a remission in approximately 90% of children with MCNS, children with a clinical presentation that is typical of MCNS are generally treated without a renal biopsy. Some atypical features that would indicate the need for a renal biopsy before treatment might include age less than 1 year, macrohematuria along with hypertension, hypocomplementemia, or renal failure not caused by volume concentration. Although spontaneous remissions may occur, the current standard of care is to treat all full-blown relapses. The precipitating infection should be remitting when treatment begins. The optimal dose, schedule of administration, and total duration of steroid therapy have not been standardized and have undergone recent evaluation in light of rather compelling evidence that a longer initial course of steroids reduces the frequency of subsequent relapses.

Most children receive initial treatment with prednisone (60 mg/m²/d or 2 mg/kg/d, maximal dose 60 mg/d), and if a remission has not been induced in 8 to 10 weeks, a renal biopsy is indicated to establish a definitive diagnosis to guide subsequent therapy. Some of these unresponsive children will prove to have MCNS, which will ultimately respond to a more prolonged course of steroids or to an alkylating agent or cyclosporine.

The percentage of children who never relapse after this initial episode is unfortunately only 10 to 25%. There is no standard protocol for treatment of relapses, but reinduction of remission is usually necessary, followed by a gradual tapering off of the steroids. A common reason for nonresponsiveness to therapy during relapse is an insufficient dose of prednisone. Smaller reinduction doses simply prolong the duration of therapy, are often unsuccessful in inducing a sustained remission, and frequently result in the use of a higher cumulative dose of prednisone. Another cause for failure to respond during a relapse is an occult infection, commonly dental caries or sinusitis, the symptoms of which may be masked by treatment.

Unfortunately, almost 50% of children with MCNS experience multiple relapses: frequently relapsing nephrotic syndrome (FRNS) is defined as two or more relapses within 6 months of initial response or 4 or more relapses within any 12-month period, and steroid-dependent nephrotic syndrome (SDNS) is two consecutive relapses occurring during steroid therapy or within 14 days of its cessation. This group of patients is often managed after reinduction of remission with low-dose, alternate-day prednisone tapered to the patient's apparent "threshold dose" (the dose below which relapses occur) to reduce the number of relapses and the total cumulative dose of steroid therapy. Regular assessment of growth and monitoring for cataracts are imperative. The major challenge in treating children with MCNS is to balance carefully therapeutic intervention with potential side effects that may be permanent in a disease that, although recurrent, will eventually remit.

OTHER IMMUNOSUPPRESSIVE AGENTS Steroid toxicity, especially growth retardation, has led to the use of other potentially more toxic medications in children with SD- or FRNS or steroid-unresponsive MCNS. Before initiation of cytotoxic therapy, a biopsy is usually done in steroid-resistant patients but not in those with steroid-dependent or frequently relapsing disease. Although there is not a complete consensus on this topic, alkylating agents are often the next drug of choice. Cyclophosphamide for 8 to 12 weeks is generally well tolerated with minimal risk of gonadal toxicity. Chlorambucil is also effective but is less widely used, in part because of a reported risk of seizures as a side effect. The alkylating agent is ideally started after induction of remission (to minimize the risks of infections and hemorrhagic cystitis) and is used in combination with prednisone. Although a small proportion of patients have no discernible benefit with this therapy, approximately 50% remain in remission for 2 to 3 years. Cyclosporine is effective in inducing and sustaining remission in 85 to 90% of steroid-responsive nephrotics and has had a major impact in a small group of patients debilitated by the disease, steroid toxicity, and refractoriness to cyclophosphamide. Unfortunately, relapses commonly occur once cyclosporine is discontinued, and because of nephrotoxic side effects, cyclosporine levels must be carefully monitored, and serial renal biopsies may be required to evaluate the degree of interstitial fibrosis if therapy is continued for longer than 18 months.

PROGNOSIS/LONG-TERM OUTCOME Before the introduction of antibiotics and corticosteroids, 40% of these children died within 5 years of diagnosis. Deaths were most commonly caused by infectious complications. Although today more than 95% of these children are still alive at 20 to 25 years, mortality has not been completely eradicated. Deaths are usually secondary to infections, occasionally the result of thrombotic complications. Late-onset renal failure is very unusual, but a small number of patients develop acute tubular necrosis if a relapse occurs accompanied by sepsis and/or hypovolemia. Nonsteroidal anti-inflammatory drugs may also increase the risk of acute renal failure, especially during relapse. A young age at onset along with several relapses in the first year after diagnosis identifies a subgroup of patients most likely to have a protracted course.

Eight to 10 years after diagnosis, 80% of patients achieve a permanent remission. A small number continue to experience relapses even into adulthood. Although relapses after prolonged remission are very rare, cases have been reported to relapse 20 to 25 years later. Some patients who are initially steroid-responsive become steroid-resistant. Many of these patients have focal segmental glomerulosclerosis (which may have been missed on an early biopsy or may have evolved from MCNS) and have a significant risk of developing ESRD.

PROLIFERATIVE LESIONS

Many of the histologic lesions associated with glomerulonephritis may also present with NS, and clinical characteristics, treatment options, and outcome for these subgroups are discussed in Sec. 21.8.1. In some children with NS, mild, nonsclerotic widening of the mesangial matrix has been described and may include deposits in this area of the glomerulus (mesangial proliferative glomerulonephritis). Technically, such findings exclude the diagnosis of MCNS. However, this subgroup of children is frequently responsive to corticosteroids (75–80%) and, if refractory, most respond to alkylating agents. Although frequent relapses are common, the long-term outcome is quite good when sclerosing lesions are not present, and to a large extent these patients are considered to have a clinical course and outcome similar to children with MCNS.

FOCAL SEGMENTAL GLOMERULOSCLEROSIS (IDIOPATHIC)

Focal segmental glomerulosclerosis (FSGS) is an important cause of nephrotic syndrome. It is the most frequent glomerular disease to cause ESRD in childhood and is second only to congenital anomalies as a cause of pediatric ESRD. The histologic lesion is characterized by complete collapse of a segment of the glomerulus with mesangial sclerosis. Only some of the glomeruli are affected initially (ie, a focal rather than diffuse lesion), and the deep juxtamedullary glomeruli are involved first. Areas of tubular atrophy and interstitial fibrosis are frequently seen and may suggest the diagnosis even if glomerulosclerosis is not evident (see Table 21-14). Most children with FSGS present with nephrotic syndrome that is often resistant to steroids (75–80%). FSGS is idiopathic in most affected children, but secondary causes are well known. The secondary forms of FSGS may present with nonnephrotic range proteinuria and may be associated with a reduced nephron mass. In these patients, glomerular adaptive responses such as hyperfiltration and hypertrophy are thought ultimately to cause focal glomerular scarring. Examples include FSGS secondary to oligomeganephronia, unilateral renal agenesis, renal dysplasia, reflux nephropathy, or as a sequel to cortical necrosis or surgical ablation. Hyperfiltration may play a role in the genesis of FSGS in patients with sickle cell disease, morbid obesity, cyanotic congenital heart disease, and hypertension. Any progressive glomerular disease may produce renal scarring in a focal pattern resembling FSGS lesions, but in these cases, other histologic changes make the primary diagnosis evident. FSGS may be seen as a complication of HIV disease or heroin-associated nephropathy.

EPIDEMIOLOGY/PREDISPOSING FACTORS In the pediatric population, idiopathic FSGS typically begins between 2 and 7 years of age (Table 21-13). There is a slight predominance in boys, especially when present at a young age. There is also a higher incidence among African-Americans. The incidence of FSGS seems to be increased in both the pediatric and adult populations, an observation that is not simply explained by disease resulting from HIV nephropathy. In a small minority of patients, the disease appears to be inherited. One gene has recently been identified on chromosome 1 (*SRN1*, steroid-resistant idiopathic nephrotic syndrome gene 1) in a subgroup with autosomal recessive FSGS. In families with autosomal dominant inheritance, loci have been mapped to chromosomes 11q21-22 and 19q13.

CLINICAL MANIFESTATIONS   Most children (90%) with FSGS present with nephrotic syndrome that is initially indistinguishable from MCNS. Less commonly, patients may present with asymptomatic proteinuria with or without microhematuria. At the time of presentation, approximately 30% of children have mild hypertension, 55% have microscopic hematuria, and 20% have an elevated serum creatinine level. Macroscopic hematuria is rare.

LABORATORY FINDINGS   The diagnosis of FSGS can only be established with certainty by renal biopsy. A clue to the diagnosis is often the lack of responsiveness to corticosteroid therapy. Patients with FSGS have tubulointerstitial damage that may impair proximal tubular function, causing features of Fanconi syndrome such as glycosuria, phosphaturia, renal tubular acidosis, and low-molecular-weight proteinuria (see Sec. 21.11).

PATHOGENESIS   The etiology of FSGS is unclear. The high rate of recurrence of the disease in renal allografts, often within hours of the surgery, highlights the importance of a systemic factor(s). The nature of this factor and the reason for its production remain elusive. Further evidence is provided by reports of pregnant women with FSGS giving birth to infants with nephrotic syndrome that disappears spontaneously a few weeks after birth. A bioassay based on the ability of plasma from FSGS patients to increase albumin permeability of isolated rat glomeruli has been developed, and in some studies, the persistence of this factor correlates with a high risk for recurrent disease in a renal allograft, but this association has not been confirmed in all studies. MCNS and FSGS may be different manifestations of a single pathogenic process. The possibility also exists that the typical focal segmental scar is a consequence rather than a cause of proteinuria.

TREATMENT   No other glomerular disease is more challenging to treat. With a poor overall response rate to immunosuppressive therapy and a high rate of recurrence in renal allografts, this disease can be devastating. At best, 20 to 25% of patients achieve a remission after treatment with corticosteriods alone. Although steroid responsiveness bodes well for long-term prognosis, some of these children become steroid-unresponsive quickly with the first relapse of NS. The role of alkylating agents in treatment of FSCS is debated, but a subset of patients will respond, and these usually were those patients who had at least a partial response to prednisone therapy. Overall, approximately 50% of FSGS patients treated with alkylating agents experience some reduction in proteinuria. The best treatment results to date have been obtained with high-dose intravenous methylprednisone and oral prednisone, often in combination with an alkylating agent (The Tune-Mendoza protocol). After 6 years of follow-up, 66% of the initial group of patients were reported to be in remission, 9% had developed ESRD, and 16% had

chronic renal failure. Not all centers have had similar results, especially in African-American patients. In uncontrolled studies, treatment with cyclosporine plus corticosteroids has been reported to induce remission in 20 to 30% of patients. Cyclosporine needs to be continued for long periods of time because the NS frequently relapses once cyclosporine is discontinued. Pilot studies with plasmapheresis and protein A immunoabsorption have been disappointing.

PROGNOSIS/LONG-TERM OUTCOME   The single best prognostic indicator in FSGS patients is responsiveness to steroid therapy. Approximately 50% of the patients who do not achieve a remission of the NS develop ESRD within 5 years. The risks of progressive renal failure are higher among patients of Hispanic and African descent and children with disease onset under 1 year of age. The severity of the proteinuria and the degree of interstitial fibrosis on renal biopsy also correlate with the rate of progression to ESRD. Recurrance of proteinuria and NS after transplantation is well known (see Sec. 21.15).

MEMBRANOUS NEPHROPATHY (IDIOPATHIC)

Membranous nephropathy is a noninflammatory glomerular disease characterized by the presence of immune deposits (usually containing IgG and C3) within the basement membrane or along the subepithelial aspect of the glomerular capillary wall associated with proteinuria. Membranous nephropathy is a rare cause of nephrotic syndrome in childhood, accounting for approximately 1% of cases in North America. Unlike the disease in adults, which is often idiopathic, as many as 50% of the childhood cases are secondary to an underlying disorder (Table 21-15). Nephrotic syndrome secondary to membranous nephropathy does not usually respond to initial therapy with prednisone. When a renal biopsy establishes a diagnosis of membranous nephropathy, an exhaustive investigation is warranted to look for an underlying cause. Treatment is then based on the primary disorder, withdrawal of an incriminated medication, or specific treatment of the underlying autoimmune disease, infection, or malignancy.

TABLE 21-15

COMMON SECONDARY CAUSES OF MEMBRANOUS NEPHROPATHY IN CHILDREN

DISEASE CATEGORY	DISEASE EXAMPLES
Autoimmune diseases	Systemic lupus erythematosus
	Mixed connective tissue disease
	Autoimmune thyroiditis
Infections	Hepatitis B
	Congenital syphilis
	Malaria
Drugs	Penicillamine
	Gold
Neoplasia	Chronic lymphocytic leukemia
	Non-Hodgkin lymphoma
	Neuroblastoma
	Carcinoma
Miscellaneous	Sickle cell anemia
	De novo in renal allograft

EPIDEMIOLOGY/PREDISPOSING FACTORS Although this disease is rare in childhood, it occurs at any age including infants. Cases affecting identical twins and siblings have been reported. Detailed epidemiologic studies in childhood have not been conducted.

CLINICAL MANIFESTATIONS Proteinuria is the hallmark of membranous nephropathy. Among the features present at the time of diagnosis, 72% have nephrotic syndrome, 70% microhematuria, 2% macroscopic hematuria, and 22% are hypertensive. The disease is typically insidious in its onset and progression. Only 3% of children have renal failure at presentation. A rapid deterioration in renal function mandates a search for an additional cause. A small group of these patients develop a superimposed crescentic glomerulonephritis, sometimes from formation of anti-GBM antibodies. Although renal vein thrombosis is said to be a common complication among adult patients with membranous nephropathy, this complication is apparently rare in children.

LABORATORY FINDINGS As in most glomerular diseases a renal biopsy is required to establish a definitive diagnosis. Serologic tests including serum complement levels are typically normal. Where laboratory investigations are particularly helpful is in establishing a secondary cause. Hepatitis B serology, serum complement levels, and an ANA test should be done in all patients. The renal biopsy may point in the direction of a secondary cause if immune deposits are also found in the mesangium (SLE), if significant deposits of IgA are present (IgA nephropathy), or if there is evidence of cellular proliferation (postinfectious GM), all features that are atypical of the idiopathic disease. Rarely, patients with a secondary cause will present with NS and membranous nephropathy without clinical evidence of the primary disorder.

PATHOGENESIS Idiopathic membranous nephropathy appears to be an antibody-mediated disease even though the target antigen remains unknown. Most likely the immune complexes form "in situ" within the subepithelial space, where target antigens of either exogenous or endogenous origin come to reside. In a rat model of membranous nephropathy (Heymann nephritis), the antigen is a normal constituent of the glomerular epithelial cell that reacts with its antibody and is subsequently shed into coated pits adjacent to the GBM. Despite extensive investigation, the existence of a similar antigen in idiopathic human membranous nephropathy has yet to be established. In addition to the more common associations with autoimmune diseases listed in Table 21-15, membranous nephropathy has also been reported rarely in patients with insulin-dependent diabetes mellitus, Crohn disease, and primary biliary cirrhosis, suggesting that other candidate autoantigens will eventually be unveiled. Glomerular inflammation does not explain the proteinuria; rather, the terminal membrane attack complex of the complement cascade, C5b-9, appears to be the critical mediator.

TREATMENT Established treatment guidelines for children with idiopathic membranous nephropathy do not currently exist. Children who present with nonnephrotic proteinuria, a normal blood pressure, and normal renal function appear to have a good prognosis without specific therapy, but close observation is warranted. Immunosuppressive therapy should be reserved for patients with risk factors for progressive disease such as persistent nephrotic syndrome, hypertension, and/or an elevated serum creatinine level. Overall, children appear to have a better prognosis than do adults. In the adult population the best results to date have been achieved

with combined treatment with prednisone and an alkylating agent ("Ponticelli" regimen). In nephrotic children it may be reasonable to start with high-dose alternate-day prednisone first and to reserve alkylating agents (cyclophosphamide or chlorambucil) for nonresponsive patients. Such therapy appears to improve the short-term outcome of patients, but additional studies are still needed to confirm long-term efficacy. The place of cyclosporine in the treatment of this disease is unclear at present. There are also anecdotal case reports of clinical improvements after intravenous IgG and with mycophenolate mofetil therapy.

PROGNOSIS/LONG-TERM OUTCOME In a review of 163 pediatric membranous nephropathy patients from six published series, the following observations were made: 39% were in remission, 38% had active disease, and 19% had chronic renal insufficiency after a follow-up period ranging from 1 to 16 years. Membranous nephropathy is typically an indolent, slowly progressive disease with fewer than 5% of children developing ESRD 5 years after diagnosis. In adults, 14% have developed ESRD by 5 years. Good long-term follow-up studies are not yet available for patients who develop membranous nephropathy in childhood.

MEDICAL COMPLICATIONS OF NEPHROTIC SYNDROME

Persistence of nephrotic syndrome is associated with significant morbidity and even mortality. Short-term mortality is most frequently from infectious complications and less commonly from thromboembolic events. Long-term sequelae of hyperlipidemia are likely to be important, but the specific risks have not been clearly delineated, especially in children. Because nephrotic syndrome frequently follows a chronic relapsing course, children are at risk for several recognized complications. Not to be overlooked is the tremendous psychological stress that the patients and their families endure. The side effects of corticosteroids and cytotoxic drugs are also significant for many children.

INFECTIONS Even in the current medical era acute bacterial infections are relatively common and potentially fatal complications. The acute onset of fever in a child during relapse of NS needs urgent evaluation. Primary peritonitis still occurs in 2 to 6% of these children, and the infections include cellulitis, sinusitis, and pneumonia. Fever associated with abdominal pain must be considered as peritonitis until proven otherwise. Approximately 50% of cases are caused by *Streptococcus pneumoniae* while other encapsulated organisms are occasionally isolated, as well as gram-negative organisms (especially *Escherichia coli*). Patients with presumed peritonitis should be treated with antibiotics to cover both gram-positive and -negative organisms while culture results are awaited. Unfortunately, the peritoneal culture is negative in 15 to 50% of patients with a presumptive diagnosis of peritonitis. Prophylactic penicillin has not proven to be effective in the prevention of pneumococcal peritonitis. Once a nephrotic patient is in remission and off steroids for a few months, a pneumococcal vaccination should be given even though as many as 50% of vaccinated nephrotic patients will fail to maintain adequate antibody titers when tested 1 year later.

Several abnormalities associated with the nephrotic state appear to predispose patients to bacterial infections. Abnormalities of both cellular and humoral immunity, low serum IgG levels (only partly explained by urinary losses), decreased rates of immunoglobulin synthesis, and increased catabolism all contribute. Decreased serum

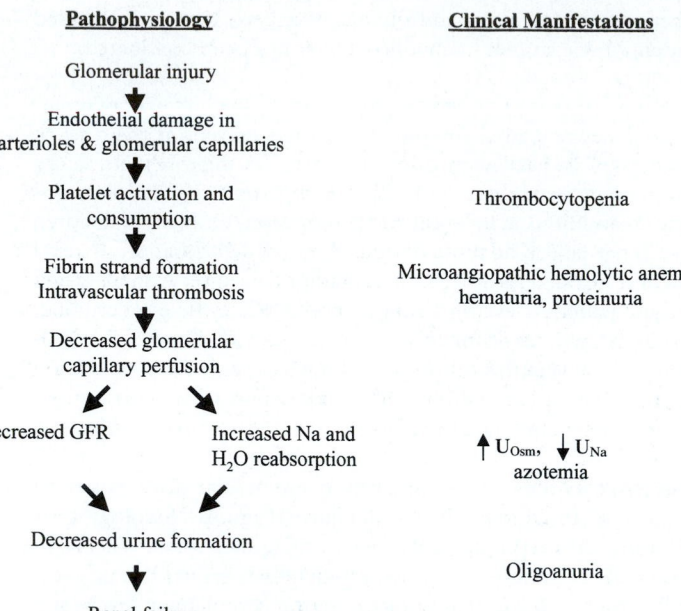

SEQUENCE OF EVENTS IN HEMOLYTIC UREMIC SYNDROME

FIGURE 21-26   Sequence of pathophysiological events in the hemolytic uremic syndrome and the associated clinical manifestations.

levels of complement proteins I and B of the alternative complement pathway impair plasma bacterial opsonic activity and may explain the predisposition to infections caused by encapsulated bacteria (see Sec. 19.6). Local factors related to tissue edema, breakdown of the skin barrier, and the presence of peritoneal fluid, which is a rich culture medium, might also facilitate infections. These factors are compounded by the use of immunosuppressive drugs.

THROMBOTIC DISEASE Thrombosis is one of the most serious potential complications of nephrotic syndrome. Virtually all nephrotic patients have a hypercoagulable state, and as many as 20% experience thrombotic events that are often clinically silent. The cause of the nephrotic syndrome may affect the absolute risk; thrombosis is relatively common in adults with membranous nephropathy and infrequent in children with MCNS. Which abnormalities of the clotting process best correlate with the risk of thrombosis is still unclear. Consequently, identifying the "at risk" population with a view to using prophylactic anticoagulant treatment is not feasible. Virtually every aspect of the hemostatic pathway (see Sec. 19.10) is perturbed in some way, but the changes that may be most important include increased serum levels of clotting factors (especially VIII, V, and fibrinogen), urinary loss of anticoagulants (antithrombin III, protein S), and increased platelet number and reactivity. Other contributing factors include hyperlipidemia and hyperviscosity. The risk of thrombotic disease is significantly enhanced in the presence of hypovolemia and during prolonged periods of immobilization. Indwelling venous catheters impose a major risk and should be avoided if at all possible.

The clinical presentation is highly variable and obviously dependent on the site of the clot. In children both arterial and venous clots occur. The renal vein and sagittal sinus are commonly involved as well as the pulmonary and femoral arteries. Many of these clots are clinically silent. Aspirin therapy may be recommended for patients with significant thrombocytosis. Guidelines for the duration of therapy once remission of the nephrotic syndrome has been achieved are not established.

Nephrotic patients may have low levels of clotting factor XII, which may cause a prolonged PTT on routine coagulation screening but is not associated with a risk of bleeding, so procedures such as renal biopsies can be safely performed.

CARDIOVASCULAR DISEASE An issue of significant concern is whether children with chronic relapsing nephrotic syndrome are at increased risk of developing premature atherosclerotic disease. Adequate data are currently not available, but this may be a valid concern. Children as young as 5 years dying with nephrotic syndrome have been found on autopsy to have atheromatous lesions. In adults with nephrotic syndrome, the relative risk of myocardial infarction is 5.5 compared with a control population after adjustment for other known risk factors. Several factors may contribute to the increased risk of cardiovascular disease and stroke, including hypertension and the use of steroids. However, the atherogenic plasma lipid profile that typifies nephrotic syndrome may add a significant risk. Plasma cholesterol and lipoprotein(a) levels are high. Whether hypercholesterolemia should be treated remains unclear. In the near future, data may be developed to better address this issue in children with nephrotic syndrome.

21.8.3   Hemolytic Uremic Syndrome

The pathophysiological sequence of events that results in the clinical manifestations of hemolytic uremic syndrome are depicted in Fig. 21-26. In these disorders, the initiating insult is damage to the endothelium with thrombosis, which results in the diagnostic triad of microangiopathic hemolytic anemia, thrombocytopenia, and renal insufficiency. Hemolytic uremic syndrome (HUS) is the most common cause of acute renal failure in a previously healthy child. Most children with HUS (90%) have an antecedent illness of diarrhea caused by a strain of *Escherichia coli* that produces a *Shigella*-like toxin. This group of patients has been classified as "typical" or "diarrhea-associated" (D+HUS) or *Shiga*-toxin–associated HUS. Approximately 10% of patients develop HUS for other reasons that may be broadly classified into secondary and idiopathic variants. HUS may occur in association with other infections (especially *Streptococcus pneumoniae* and rarely as a complication of HIV infection), following exposure to certain drugs (mitomycin C, cyclosporine, FK-506, cocaine, and quinine), or in association with other systemic diseases (cancer, SLE, cobalamin C disease, scleroderma). The idiopathic variants may be sporadic or genetic, with autosomal dominant and autosomal recessive patterns of inheritance reported. Some of these families have genetic deficiencies in complement proteins, especially factor H. A candidate gene is localized to chromosome 1q32, the location of genes encoding a family of complement regulatory proteins. The possibility of a genetic form of the disease should be considered in a child with an atypical presentation. HUS and thrombotic thrombocytopenic purpura (TTP) have overlapping clinical features caused by thrombotic microangiopathy. Although HUS and TTP may represent variable presentations of the same disease, different causes, pathogenesis, response rates to specific treatments, and clinical outcomes occur and are probably best considered separate syndromes. A syndrome resembling HUS can also be seen among patients with malignant hypertension.

EPIDEMIOLOGY/PREDISPOSING FACTORS More than 85% of children with HUS have been infected with *E. coli* 0157:H7, which is mainly a disease of infants and young children (9 months to 4 years of age). It occurs worldwide as both sporadic and epidemic cases. For unclear reasons HUS is uncommon in African-Americans. There is often a seasonal disease pattern, with greatest incidence in the summer and fall in North America. The primary reservoir for *E. coli* 0157:H7 is cattle, and in the United States approximately 1% of cattle harbor this bacteria. The bacteria can be killed by exposure to adequate heat; undercooked beef is frequently found to be the source of exposure. Contaminated lakes and swimming pools are occasionally identified as the source. Consumption of raw milk, fruits, fruit juices, or vegetables that have been contaminated with manure may also cause disease. Although less common, person-to-person spread has been documented. The risk of HUS in children under the age of 15 years with *E. coli* 0157:H7 colitis is in the range of 8 to 10%.

The best way to prevent infection with *E. coli* 0157:H7 is adequate cooking of ground beef and washing of fruits and vegetables. Good hand-washing practices will decrease the (low) risk of person-to-person spread. Routine irradiation of meat and vaccine development offer the best hope of disease control but are currently not available options. Studies are now in progress to determine if treatment of children with bloody diarrhea with Synsorb-Pk, a synthetic oligosaccharide receptor for *Shiga*-toxin bound to diatomaceous earth, can decrease the incidence of HUS.

CLINICAL MANIFESTATIONS The antecedent illness of *E. coli* 0157:H7–induced colitis is typically associated with abdominal pain and diarrhea that is often bloody (35–90%). Half of the patients have nausea and vomiting. Fever is typically low grade or absent. The colitis is usually self-limited, but complications may occur including rectal prolapse, toxic megacolon, bowel wall necrosis, and perforation. Strictures may develop as a late complication. The onset of HUS is usually abrupt, often occurring 2 to 14 days (median 6 days) after the onset of the diarrhea, as the colitis resolves. The presenting symptoms are often related to renal failure and depend on the volume status of the patient. Patients are noted to be pale and occasionally mildly icteric from the hemolytic anemia. The severity of the renal failure is highly variable, but close to

50% develop oligoanuria and require dialysis (see Sec. 21.7). Hypertension is variable, caused not only by fluid overload but also by activation of the renin-angiotensin system within the ischemic kidneys, and can be quite severe, which suggests a poorer prognosis. The mean duration of the renal failure is 2 weeks.

The microangiopathic hemolytic anemia causes sudden pallor and symptoms secondary to acute anemia. The degree of thrombocytopenia is variable, and patients may present with petechiae. Hemolysis may continue for several weeks. There is no correlation between the severity of the hemolysis and the degree of renal failure. During the recovery phase, the hemolytic process resolves more slowly than the other manifestations, and patients are often discharged with a persistent anemia from an inappropriately low reticulocyte count that cannot be explained by deficiency of folate, B_{12}, or iron. A recent study suggests that low serum erythropoietin levels may explain this phase of the anemia. The hemoglobin level eventually normalizes in most patients without specific intervention. Cholelithiasis has been reported as a late sequel to the hemolytic process.

Neurologic involvement is common. Most patients are very irritable and somnolent. However, more serious involvement is also seen and includes seizures in 20% and stupor or coma in 15% of children with HUS or cerebral infarcts. The neurologic manifestations may be the presenting feature and have an impact on acute mortality rates and long-term morbidity.

Although the bowel and the kidneys are always involved, virtually any organ can become damaged by microvascular thrombosis. Approximately 40% of patients have hepatomegaly and elevated serum transaminases. As many as 20% of patients have pancreatic involvement as indicated by an elevation of serum amylase and lipase levels. Less commonly, patients may develop hyperglycemia and even require insulin therapy. Although most of these patients ultimately are able to discontinue insulin when the acute illness resolves, some develop chronic insulin-dependent diabetes. Although primary cardiac involvement, not related to volume overload, is rare, myocarditis is a serious complication. Pericardial effusions may also occur. In patients with atypical forms of HUS, the clinical presentation is insidious in its onset and is not preceded by an enteric infection.

LABORATORY FINDINGS Biochemical evidence of renal insufficiency associated with microangiopathic hemolytic anemia and thrombocytopenia are the hallmark features of HUS (see Fig. 21-26). The PT and PTT are usually normal unless antibiotic therapy has caused vitamin K deficiency. Urinalysis typically shows hematuria and proteinuria. Although hypoalbuminemia is common at presentation, gastrointestinal losses are the most likely cause. Leukocytosis is common, and peripheral WBC counts greater than 20,000 correlate with a poorer prognosis.

When a patient presents with diarrhea-associated HUS, documentation of a *Shiga*-toxin–producing *E. coli* is important to identify the source of exposure and minimize the spread of the disease. Stool cultures should be obtained as soon as possible with special procedures to identify *E. coli* 0157:H7. Serum C3 and CH50 levels may be depressed, especially in familial cases.

PATHOGENESIS A major advance in our understanding of the pathogenesis of HUS was made in 1983 when Karmali and his associates discovered that more than 85% of HUS patients had been infected with a strain of *E. coli* that produced a *Shiga*-like toxin (SLT), a toxin that was first reported in association with *Shigella* *dysenteriae*. These toxins are also referred to as verotoxins because of their cytopathic effects on Vero cells, a cell line that is derived from African green monkey kidney cells. *E. coli* 0157:H7 can produce either one or two toxins, ST-1 and ST-2. These toxins bind to a glycolipid receptor (Gb3) that is abundantly expressed on human glomerular endothelial cells. *Shiga*-like toxins are also toxic to cultured renal tubular cells, an effect that likely contributes to renal injury in vivo. A few other bacterial strains have been shown to produce SLT, including *E. coli* 0103:H2, which was associated with HUS after causing a urinary tract infection. After the glomerular endothelial cells are injured by the toxin, a thrombotic microangiopathic reaction ensues that is characterized by fibrin deposition and damage to erythrocytes and platelets. A similar cascade of events may cause tissue injury in vascular beds in other organs. Serum levels of many prothrombotic substances are increased (tissue factor, platelet-activating factor, plasminogen activator inhibitor, von Willebrand factor, thromboxane A_2), whereas decreased levels have been reported for some antithrombotic systems (prostacyclin, thrombomodulin, plasminogen activator). *E. coli* also produce lipopolysaccharides that may stimulate the production of cytokines that may also contribute to endothelial injury. Although P1 blood group antigen (present in 75% of normal individuals) can bind SLT and could theoretically prevent individuals from developing HUS, convincing evidence for this hypothesis has not yet been documented.

A rare but important cause of secondary HUS may be as a complication of infection with *Streptococcus pneumoniae*. This organism produces neuraminidase, an enzyme that may cleave sialic acid residues on erythrocytes, platelets, and glomeruli to expose the cryptic Thomsen-Freidenreich antigen. Naturally occurring IgM antibodies to this antigen may induce hemolysis, thrombocytopenia, and glomerular capillary damage. These patients have a positive Coombs test, and difficulties are encountered with ABO crossmatching. Use of fresh-frozen plasma, an additional source of the pathogenic antibody, is contraindicated in these patients. Mortality in this variant of HUS is high, in the range of 50%.

TREATMENT   For typical diarrhea or SLT-associated HUS, supportive medical care is by far the most important aspect of treatment and is responsible for the drastic decline in mortality rates from >50% before 1970 (predialysis era) to current rates, which are less than 5%. Meticulous attention must be paid to fluid and electrolyte management. Volume loss from diarrhea and vomiting must be replaced, but care needs to be taken to avoid intravascular volume overload (see Secs. 21.4 and 21.7). Even with meticulous management, 40 to 50% of the patients develop oligoanuria and require acute dialysis. Packed red blood cell transfusions should be reserved for patients with clinical indications of severe anemia (Hct 15–18%) but are eventually required in ~75% of patients. Packed RBCs must be infused slowly with careful attention paid to the blood pressure. Platelet transfusions should be avoided unless the patients are actively bleeding or if they are needed in preparation for a significant surgical procedure. Careful attention should be paid to nutritional needs, as many of these patients are already catabolic and have had several days of poor calorie intake before presentation.

No specific therapeutic interventions have proven beneficial in the treatment of patients with HUS. Two limited randomized studies failed to show a beneficial effect of plasma infusions and plasmapheresis on acute mortality or long-term outcome. Antiplatelet drugs and fibrinolytic therapy are of no proven benefit but increase the risk of hemorrhagic complications and should be avoided. During the prodromal phase of colitis, antimotility drugs are contra-

indicated, and antibiotics actually increase the probability of developing HUS.

The optimal treatment of atypical forms of HUS is less clear. Because of the poorer overall prognosis of these patients, the higher relapse rates, and extrapolating from experience with the treatment of patients with TTP, most centers would recommend treatment with daily plasmapheresis until the condition of the patient stabilizes, and several anecdotal reports have suggested a good outcome, especially among patients with significant neurologic involvement.

PROGNOSIS/LONG-TERM OUTCOME   Acute mortality of diarrhea-associated HUS is now in the range of 3 to 5% and is often related to severe complications such as neurologic disease and cardiac failure or multiorgan involvement. Renal function spontaneously improves, and almost all patients are able to discontinue dialysis. Approximately 5% of survivors suffer severe sequelae to the kidney and/or brain. However, several recent long-term follow-up studies suggest that only 60% of patients fully recover normal renal function, and the rest have evidence of proteinuria, hypertension, and/or a reduced glomerular filtration rate of minimal clinical significance. Approximately 5 to 15% of patients will ultimately have slowly progressive renal insufficiency. Bad prognostic indicators include anuria for longer than 2 weeks, an initial neutrophil count greater than 20,000, coma on admission, and atypical forms of the disease. Although renal biopsies are not generally performed in these patients, late sequelae have been observed in 90% of patients with cortical necrosis and in 60% who had thrombi in more than 60% of the glomeruli. Involvement of extraglomerular renal vessels also portends a poorer prognosis. Recurrent disease in both native and transplant kidneys is extremely rare in diarrhea-associated HUS but occurs quite commonly in familial variants and in 18% of patients with atypical forms of the disease.

References

General

Couser WG: Glomerulonephritis. Lancet 353:1509–1515, 1999

Postinfectious Glomerulonephritis

D'Amico G: Renal involvement in hepatitis C infection: cryoglobulinemic glomerulonephritis. Kidney Int 54:650–671, 1998

Potter EV, Lipschultz SA, Abidh S, Poon-King T, Earle DP: Twelve- to seventeen-year follow-up of patients with poststreptococcal acute glomerulonephritis in Trinidad. N Engl J Med 307:725–729, 1982

IgA Nephropathy

Dillon JJ: Fish oil therapy for IgA nephropathy: efficacy and interstudy variability. J Am Soc Nephrol 8:1739–1744, 1997

Donadio JV Jr, Grande JP: Immunoglobulin A nephropathy: a clinical perspective. J Am Soc Nephrol 8:1324–1332, 1997

Galla JH: IgA nephropathy. Kidney Int 47:377–387, 1995

MPGN

McEnery P: Membranoproliferative glomerulonephritis: the Cincinnati experience—cumulative renal survival from 1957 to 1989. J Pediatr 116: S109–S114, 1990

Schwertz R, de Jong R, Gretz N, et al, and Arbeitsgemeinschaft Pädiatrische Nephrologie: Outcome of idiopathic membranoproliferative glomerulonephritis in children. Acta Pediatr 85:308–312, 1996

Tarshish P, Bernstein J, Tobin JN, Edelmann CM Jr: Treatment of mesangiocapillary glomerulonephritis with alternate-day prednisone—a report of the International Study of Kidney Disease in Children. Pediatr Nephrol 6:123–130, 1992

Crescentic Glomerulonephritis

Jardim HMPF, Leake J, Risdon RA, Barratt TM, Dillon MJ: Crescentic glomerulonephritis in children. Pediatr Nephrol 6:231–235, 1992

Goodpasture Syndrome

Bolton WK: Goodpasture's syndrome. Kidney Int 50:1753–1766, 1996

Lupus Nephritis

Bansal VK, Beto JA: Treatment of lupus nephritis: a meta-analysis of clinical trials. Am J Kidney Dis 29:193–199, 1997

Yang L-Y, Chen W-P, Lin C-Y: Lupus nephritis in children—a review of 167 patients. Pediatrics 94:335–340, 1994

HSP Nephritis

Goldstein AR, Akuse R, White RHR, Chantler C: Long-term follow-up of childhood Henoch-Schönlein nephritis. Lancet 339:280–282, 1992

Vasculitis

Jennette JC, Falk RJ: Small-vessel vasculitis. N Engl J Med 337:1512–1523, 1997

Rottem M, Fauci AS, Hallahan CW, et al: Wegener granulomatosis in children and adolescents: clinical presentation and outcome. J Pediatr 122:26–31, 1993

Minimal-Change Nephrotic Syndrome

Brodehl J: The treatment of minimal change nephrotic syndrome: lessons learned from multicentre co-operative studies. Eur J Pediatr 150:380–387, 1991

Tune BM, Mendoza SA: Treatment of the idiopathic nephrotic syndrome: regimens and outcomes in children and adults. J Am Soc Nephrol 8:824–832, 1997

Focal Segmental Glomerulosclerosis

Mendoza SA, Reznik VM, Griswold WR, Krensky AM, Yorgin PD, Tune BM: Treatment of steroid-resistant focal segmental glomerulosclerosis with pulse methylprednisolone and alkylating agents. Pediatr Nephrol 4:303–307, 1990

Sharma M, Sharma R, McCarthy ET, Savin VJ: "The FSGS factor": enrichment and in vivo effect of activity from focal segmental glomerulosclerosis plasma. J Am Soc Nephrol 10:552–561, 1999

Membranous Nephropathy

Cameron JS: Membranous nephropathy in childhood and its treatment. Pediatr Nephrol 4:193–198, 1990

Ponticelli C, Zucchelli P, Passerini P, et al: A 10-year follow-up of a randomized study with methylprednisolone and chlorambucil in membranous nephropathy. Kidney Int 48:1600–1604, 1995

Complications of Nephrotic Syndrome

Orth SR, Ritz E: The nephrotic syndrome. N Engl J Med 338:1202–1211, 1998

Hemolytic Uremic Syndrome

Kaplan BS, Meyers KE, Schulman SL: The pathogenesis and treatment of hemolytic uremic syndrome. J Am Soc Nephrol 9:1126–1133, 1998

Siegler RL, Milligan MK, Burningham TH, Christofferson RD, Chang S-Y, Jorde LB: Long-term outcome and prognostic indicators in the hemolytic-uremic syndrome. J Pediatr 118:195–200, 1991

Siegler RL, Pavia AT, Hansen FL, Christofferson RD, Cook JB: Atypical hemolytic-uremic syndrome: a comparison with postdiarrheal disease. J Pediatr 128:505–511, 1996

Wons CS, Jelacic S, Habeeb RC, Watkins SC, Tarr PI: The risk of hemolytic-uremic syndrome after antibiotic treatment of E. Coli 0157:47 infection. N Engl J Med 342(26):1930–1936, 2000

21.9 HEREDITARY GLOMERULOPATHIES

Clifford E. Kashtan

The hereditary glomerulopathies are a heterogenous group of disorders that present with either a nephritic or nephrotic pattern (see Figs. 21-19 and 21-25). A family history of renal disease is frequently present but may be vague or difficult to ascertain in many cases. The genetic and molecular abnormalities that lead to the development of these disorders are becoming well defined and provide considerable insight into the pathogenesis of a wide variety of renal diseases (Table 21-16).

ALPORT SYNDROME

Alport syndrome (AS) is a genetically heterogenous disease arising from mutations in genes coding for type IV collagen, the major collagenous constituent of basement membranes (BM). The features of AS reflect derangements of BM structure and function resulting from changes in type IV collagen expression. The cardinal finding in AS is persistent microhematuria. Affected boys and men inevitably develop proteinuria, hypertension, and renal failure, whereas renal failure is infrequent in affected girls and women. High-frequency sensorineural deafness and ocular defects such as perimacular pigmentary abnormalities and lenticonus are often associated with renal disease in AS.

About 80% of AS is X-linked, derived from mutations in *COL4A5*, the gene encoding the α5 chain of type IV collagen [α5(IV)]. A subtype of X-linked AS (XLAS) in which diffuse leiomyomatosis is an associated feature reflects deletion mutations involving the adjacent *COL4A5* and *COL4A6* genes. Most other patients have autosomal recessive AS (ARAS) as a result of mutations in *COL4A3* or *COL4A4*, which encode the α3(IV) and α4(IV) chains, respectively. The rare autosomal dominant form of AS has been mapped to chromosome 2 in the region of *COL4A3* and *COL4A4*.

Six isomers of type IV collagen, designated α1(IV) to α6(IV), have been identified. The α1(IV) and α2(IV) chains occur in all BM, while the α3(IV) to α6(IV) chains have restricted distributions. The distribution of α3(IV) to α5(IV) chains correspond to

TABLE 21-16
HEREDITARY GLOMERULOPATHIES

DISEASE	GENE	GENE PRODUCT	INHERITANCE
Alport syndrome	COL4A5	α5(IV)	X-linked
Alport syndrome	COL4A3 or COL4A4	α3(IV) or α4(IV)	Autosomal recessive
Benign familial hematuria (thin GBM disease)[a]	COL4A4 COL4A3?	α4(IV) α3(IV)?	Autosomal dominant
Finnish-type congenital nephrotic syndrome	NPHS1	Nephrin	Autosomal recessive
Denys-Drash syndrome	WT1	wt1	Autosomal recessive
Frasier syndrome	WT1	wt1	Autosomal recessive
Isolated diffuse mesangial sclerosis[a]	WT1	wt1	Autosomal recessive
Nail-patella syndrome	LMX1B	lmx1b	Autosomal recessive
Fabry disease	GLA	α-Galactosidase A	X-linked
Steroid-resistant nephrotic syndrome	NPHS2	Podocin	Autosomal recessive
Familial focal segmental glomerulosclerosis[a]	19q34	α-Actinin-4	Autosomal dominant
Collagen type III glomerulopathy	?	?	Autosomal recessive

[a] Mutations at other as yet unidentified genetic loci may result in this phenotype.

the major sites of dysfunction in AS: the kidney, eye, and ear. In the kidney, the α3(IV), α4(IV), and α5(IV) chains are normally expressed in glomerular BM (GBM), distal tubular and collecting tubule BM, and Bowman capsule. In most boys with XLAS, the α3(IV) to α6(IV) chains are completely lost from renal BM. Girls with XLAS usually exhibit mosaic expression of these chains, reflecting X-chromosome inactivation patterns (see Sec. 10.1). In ARAS, α3(IV) and α4(IV) chains are typically lost from all BM, and the α5(IV) chain is lost from GBM, but expression of α5(IV) and α6(IV) chains is preserved in Bowman capsule, distal and collecting tubule BM, and epidermal BM. Ocular BM expressing the α3(IV) to α5(IV) chains include the lens capsule, corneal BM, Descemet and Bruch membranes, and the internal limiting membrane of the retina. These chains are also found in several cochlear BM, including the basilar membrane and the BM of the inner and outer sulci, the spiral prominence, and the spiral limbus.

The diagnosis of AS still relies heavily on histologic studies, although molecular genetic analysis may eventually replace tissue diagnosis for many patients. Kidney biopsy diagnosis of AS has conventionally relied on electron microscopy, which reveals a characteristic reticulation and thickening of the GBM. Analysis of renal expression of α3(IV) to α5(IV) chains may be a useful adjunct to routine renal biopsy studies, especially when ultrastructural changes in the GBM are ambiguous. Absence of epidermal basement membrane expression of α5(IV) is diagnostic of XLAS, so in some cases kidney biopsy may not be necessary for diagnosis.

There are no specific therapies for AS. Naturally occurring canine models of XLAS are being used to study gene therapy and pharmacologic intervention. Renal transplantation in AS is usually very successful. Because AS patients who receive an intact kidney at transplantation are exposed to a previously absent antigen, occasional patients (5% or fewer) develop anti-GBM nephritis of the allograft, almost always resulting in graft loss (see Sec. 21.15).

BENIGN FAMILIAL HEMATURIA (THIN GLOMERULAR BASEMENT MEMBRANE DISEASE, THIN MEMBRANE NEPHROPATHY)

Isolated glomerular hematuria (including RBC casts) may occur as a familial or sporadic condition and is often associated with a renal biopsy finding of excessively thin GBM. When multiple family members are affected, and family history is negative for renal failure, the term *benign familial hematuria* (BFH) is appropriate. The sporadic form is designated *thin GBM disease* or *thin membrane nephropathy*. Several disorders that differ at the molecular level can be associated with GBM thinning. BFH and Alport syndrome (AS) are both inherited GBM disorders that are manifested by chronic hematuria but differ in several important respects: (1) extrarenal abnormalities are rare in BFH; (2) proteinuria, hypertension, and progression to ESRD are unusual in BFH; (3) gender differences in expression of BFH are not apparent; and (4) transmission of BFH is autosomal dominant. BFH and early AS may be difficult to distinguish histologically because diffuse GBM attenuation is characteristic of both. However, the GBM of BFH patients remains attenuated over time rather than undergoing the progressive thickening and multilamellation that are pathognomonic of AS. Some patients with supposed BFH who have developed proteinuria and hypertension may represent variants of AS in which the predominant abnormality of GBM is attenuation rather than thickening and multilamellation.

In a Dutch kindred, with BFH, affected individuals were found to be heterozygous for a missense mutation in COL4A4. However, linkage to the COL4A3 and COL4A4 genes has been excluded in other BFH families, indicating that BFH is a genetically heterogeneous condition. To date, immunohistologic studies of type IV collagen in GBM of patients with BFH or thin membrane disease have failed to uncover any abnormalities in the distribution of any of the six chains.

When a patient's family history indicates autosomal dominant transmission of hematuria with no history of chronic renal failure, and kidney and urinary tract imaging are normal, a presumptive diagnosis of BFH can often be made without kidney biopsy. When family history is negative or unknown, or there are atypical coexisting features such as proteinuria or deafness, renal biopsy may be extremely informative. A finding of thin GBM (<250 nm in adults, <200–250 nm in children, depending on age) may be further characterized by examining the distribution of type IV collagen α chains in the kidney. Normal distribution of these chains provides supportive, although not conclusive, evidence for a diagnosis of BFH.

Because BFH and thin membrane disease are nonprogressive, therapeutic interventions are not indicated.

FINNISH-TYPE CONGENITAL NEPHROTIC SYNDROME (NPHS1)

This autosomal recessive condition is the predominant cause of massive proteinuria in the first month of life (see Sec. 21.3). Although Finland has the world's highest incidence of NPHS1 (about 1.2 cases/10,000 pregnancies), many cases involving children of non-Finnish ancestry have been reported. Fetuses with NPHS1 exhibit proteinuria in utero, manifested by elevated levels of α-fetoprotein in the amniotic fluid. Edema frequently appears during the first week of life. Malnutrition, overwhelming infection, and thrombosis are important causes of severe morbidity and mortality. With aggressive therapy, these children can survive infancy and grow sufficiently to undergo renal transplantation, with excellent rates of patient and graft survival.

The *NPHS1* locus was recently identified by positional cloning, and the gene was first localized to the long arm of chromosome 19 (19q13.1) in both Finnish and non-Finnish kindreds. Sequencing in this chromosomal region revealed a previously unknown gene that exhibited specific expression in glomerular epithelial cells (podocytes). The product of the *NPHS1* gene has been given the name "nephrin." Nephrin belongs to the immunoglobulin (Ig) superfamily of cell adhesion molecules and has been localized specifically to the slit diaphragm, a specialized tight junction situated between podocyte foot processes. Kidneys of NPHS1 patients exhibit absence of podocyte foot processes and of slit diaphragms. These observations suggest that nephrin is a critical component of the slit diaphragm, which in turn plays a vital role in preventing the passage of protein across the glomerular capillary wall.

Two mutations in nephrin account for over 90% of Finnish *NPHS1* patients. The Fin_{major} mutation is a 2-bp deletion in exon 2 that generates a stop codon and is found in about 80% of Finnish patients. The Fin_{minor} mutation is a nonsense mutation in exon 26 and is found in about 17% of Finnish patients. A variety of deletion, insertion, nonsense, missense, and splicing mutations have been found in non-Finnish patients. *NPHS1* is the predominant, but not sole, cause of nephrotic syndrome in the first month of life (see Sec. 21.3).

FAMILIAL STEROID-RESISTANT NEPHROTIC SYNDROME

Both autosomal recessive and autosomal dominant forms of steroid-resistant nephrotic syndrome/focal segmental glomerulosclerosis (FSGS) have been described. Recently French investigators mapped recessive steroid-resistant nephrotic syndrome to the q25-31 region of chromosome 1 termed *NPHS2*. The protein product of this gene is termed podocin and functions as an integral membrane protein contributing to the filtration barrier of podocytes. A locus for autosomal dominant FSGS has been mapped to 19q34 and produces defective α-actinin-4, which renders the podocytes susceptible to damage resulting in sclerosis. In other families with autosomal dominant FSGS, 19q34 has been excluded as the site of the disease locus, demonstrating that this disease is genetically heterogeneous.

DIFFUSE MESANGIAL SCLEROSIS, DENYS-DRASH SYNDROME, AND FRASIER SYNDROME

These are rare disorders resulting from mutations in the *WT1* gene, which encodes a transcription factor known as the Wilms tumor suppressor. Progressive nephropathy and XY gonadal dysgenesis are features of both Denys-Drash syndrome (DDS) and Fraser syndrome, but these disorders exhibit important phenotypic differences that reflect differences in the underlying *WT1* mutations. Diffuse mesangial sclerosis (DMS), the characteristic renal lesion of DDS, can occur as an isolated entity; some patients with isolated DMS have *WT1* mutations.

The WT1 protein has the ability to repress or activate transcription of the genes to which it binds, depending on the target. Transcriptional repression by WT1 may be modulated by other proteins. WT1 is also capable of binding to RNA and may regulate gene expression by posttranscriptional as well as transcriptional mechanisms. WT1 mRNA is expressed during nephrogenesis in the condensed mesenchyme, renal vesicle, and podocytes, and expression persists in the podocytes of adult kidneys. The temporal and spatial patterns of WT1 mRNA expression suggest that WT1 participates in mediating differentiation of nephrogenic mesenchyme to glomerular epithelium and in maintaining the epithelial phenotype of the podocyte. Loss of WT1 function could then lead to uncontrolled growth of metanephric blastema cells, resulting in Wilms tumor, as well as aberrant podocyte differentiation. WT1 mRNA is also expressed in primordial tissue of the gonadal ridge, in ovarian follicular granulosa cells, and in Sertoli cells of the testis. Normal maturation of the gonads also appears to depend on the functional integrity of WT1.

DENYS-DRASH SYNDROME   DDS is a constellation of findings that includes Wilms tumor, XY gonadal dysgenesis with ambiguous genitalia, and a nephropathy that usually presents as an infantile-onset nephrotic syndrome and progresses to renal failure during the first 3 years of life. Children with DDS may exhibit the complete constellation of abnormalities or may exhibit nephropathy and genital abnormalities without Wilms tumor or nephropathy and Wilms tumor without genital abnormalities. As in other forms of XY gonadal dysgenesis, the risk of gonadoblastoma is high (see Sec. 20.15). If the diagnosis of DDS is established, bilateral nephrectomy should be considered because of the risk of Wilms tumor developing.

Patients with DDS consistently exhibit a specific glomerular lesion termed diffuse mesangial sclerosis (DMS). The characteristic lesion is observed in middle cortical glomeruli, which show mesangial expansion with obliteration of the capillaries, giving the tuft the appearance of a solid mass of matrix covered by a corona of hypertrophied podocytes.

The predominant defect is a missense mutation that converts ^{394}Arg to Trp in children with DDS. This mutation, and the less prevalent ^{396}Asp to Asn and ^{366}Arg to His mutations, abolish the DNA-binding activity of *WT1*. Almost all of these mutations appear to have arisen de novo, but inheritance of *WT1* mutations has been described.

Wilms tumors in patients with DDS are hemizygous for the mutant *WT1* allele, indicating that the tumors develop through a recessive mechanism. The persistence of nephrogenic rests (undifferentiated mesenchyme) in DDS kidneys likely results from the germline *WT1* mutation ("first hit"). A Wilms tumor will then result if a somatic mutation ("second hit") of the normal *WT1* allele occurs within a nephrogenic rest, resulting in unrestrained cell proliferation (see Sec. 20.2).

In contrast to Wilms tumor, DMS and gonadal dysgenesis in DDS do not occur by a recessive mechanism because patients with DDS are heterozygous for their *WT1* mutations. DDS mutations appear to behave in a dominant-negative fashion; ie, the mutant protein interferes with the function of the product of the wild-type allele. The association of mutant and wild-type proteins antagonizes *WT1*-mediated transcriptional repression. The dominant-negative effect of DDS *WT1* mutations helps explain why renal and genital abnormalities are more severe in DDS than in patients with

WAGR syndrome, who have one wild-type *WT1* allele, while the other is a null allele as a result of a deletion or frameshift mutation.

ISOLATED DMS DMS may occur as an isolated condition. *WT1* mutations have been described in four of 10 patients with isolated DMS. The absence of a *WT1* mutation in six of the patients indicates that isolated DMS is a genetically heterogeneous disease.

FRASIER SYNDROME Frasier syndrome is another rare disorder characterized by male pseudohermaphroditism and renal failure. These patients have normal female genitalia and an XY karyotype. Proteinuria appears during childhood, progressing to nephrotic syndrome and chronic renal failure by adolescence or early adulthood. Renal pathologic changes consist of focal and segmental glomerulosclerosis rather than DMS. Wilms tumor is extremely unusual in Fraser syndrome but may occur. Patients with Fraser syndrome may not be recognized until they undergo evaluation for primary amenorrhea. As in other forms of XY gonadal dysgenesis, gonadoblastoma is a frequent complication (see Sec. 20.15).

FABRY DISEASE

Fabry disease comprises the clinical and pathologic consequences of hereditary deficiency of α-galactosidase A (αGal A), which results in intracellular accumulation of neutral glycosphingolipids with terminal α-linked galactosyl moieties. A variety of mutations in the X-chromosomal αGal A gene have been identified in patients with Fabry disease. Most of these mutations are associated with the classic Fabry phenotype, in which there is multisystem involvement. Certain missense mutations have been identified in patients with a mild phenotype limited to left ventricular hypertrophy.

In boys with classic Fabry disease, the kidneys, heart, and peripheral and central nervous system exhibit the most serious structural and functional abnormalities (see Chapter 9). Clinical manifestations in heterozygous girls are typically mild. The nephropathy of Fabry disease typically manifests as mild to moderate proteinuria, at times associated with microhematuria, with onset in young adulthood. Nephrotic syndrome is unusual. Urinary oval fat bodies exhibiting a Maltese cross pattern when viewed under a polarizing microscope may be seen and reflect the large amounts of urinary glycosphingolipid. Deterioration of renal function is gradual, with hypertension and ESRD developing by the fourth or fifth decade. Heterozygous women typically display mild renal involvement but may develop ESRD. By light microscopy glomerular visceral epithelial cells appear to be enlarged and packed with small, clear vacuoles, which represent glycosphingolipid material extracted during processing. Segmental and global glomerulosclerosis develop over time. Electron microscopy reveals abundant lysosomal inclusions, particularly within visceral epithelial cells, consisting of layers of dense material separated by clear spaces, arranged concentrically ("myelin figures") or in parallel ("zebra bodies"). The progression of the Fabry nephropathy to ESRD probably reflects two parallel processes. Visceral epithelial cell dysfunction, which results in proteinuria, is followed by visceral epithelial cell detachment and necrosis, leading to capillary loop collapse and segmental sclerosis. Simultaneously, progressive impairment of arterial flow may develop as enlarging endothelial cells impinge on vascular lumina, resulting in ischemic glomerular damage. Renal transplantation is an effective treatment for advanced Fabry nephropathy but does not address extrarenal manifestations. Coronary artery and cerebrovascular disease are the major causes of death in transplanted patients with Fabry disease.

NAIL-PATELLA SYNDROME

Nail-patella syndrome (NPS) is an autosomal dominant disorder consisting of hypoplasia or absence of the patellae, dystrophic nails, dysplasia of the elbows, iliac horns, and renal disease. The NPS gene is localized to chromosome 9q34. Targeted disruption in mice of a transcription factor gene known as *LMX1B* was found to result in skeletal defects (hypoplastic nails and absent patellae) as well as renal dysplasia (see Sec. 10.3). The human homolog of *LMX1B* was found to map to chromosome 9q34, and mutations in *LMX1B* have been identified in patients with NPS. Although *LMX1B* appears to be important for normal limb and kidney development, the precise mechanisms for the renal effects of *LMX1B* mutations remain unclear.

Clinically apparent renal disease occurs in fewer than half of NPS patients. The nephropathy is usually benign, with about 10% of those with renal involvement eventually progressing to ESRD. The clinical signs of NPS nephropathy include microhematuria and mild proteinuria appearing in adolescence or young adulthood. Some patients develop nephrotic syndrome, and hypertension, if present, tends to be mild.

There are no specific light or immunofluorescence microscopic features of the NPS renal lesion, but characteristic abnormalities are observed by electron microscopy. In routinely-stained material, the GBM exhibits multiple irregular lucencies, which give a "moth-eaten" appearance. These lucent areas sometimes appear to contain cross-banded collagen fibrils. These fibrils may be observed in NPS kidneys in the absence of clinically evident renal disease but have not been found in extraglomerular basement membranes. No published studies have established the identity of the collagen fibrils found in the GBM of NPS patients.

Cross-banded fibrils identified as type III collagen have been seen in GBM of patients with glomerular disease but lacking nail or skeletal abnormalities, sometimes as a familial condition. Many of the patients with "collagen type III glomerulopathy" are children who have progressed rapidly to ESRD. In kindreds with collagen type III glomerulopathy, the disorder appears to be transmitted as an autosomal recessive trait. Thus, collagen type III glomerulopathy and NPS appear to be distinct diseases.

No specific therapy is available for the nephropathy of NPS. Renal transplantation has been performed successfully, without apparent recurrence of the disease in the transplanted kidney. Because NPS is an autosomal dominant disorder, careful evaluation of potential living related kidney donors for nonrenal features of the disease is essential.

References

Alport Syndrome

Barker DF, Hostikka SL, Zhou J, et al: Identification of mutations in the COL4A5 collagen gene in Alport syndrome. Science 248:1224–1227, 1990

Jefferson JA, Lemmink HH, Hughes AE, et al: Autosomal dominant Alport syndrome linked to the type IV collagen alpha 3 and alpha 4 genes (COL4A3 and COL4A4). Nephrol Dial Transplant 12:1595–1599, 1997

Kashtan CE, Michael AF: Perspectives in clinical nephrology: Alport syndrome. Kidney Int 50:1445–1463, 1996

Mochizuki T, Lemmink HH, Mariyama M, et al: Identification of mutations in the $\alpha3$(IV) and $\alpha4$(IV) collagen genes in autosomal recessive Alport syndrome. Nature Genet 8:77–82, 1994

Benign Familial Hematuria

Lang S, Stevenson B, Risdon RA: Thin basement membrane nephropathy as a cause of recurrent haematuria in childhood. Histopathology 16: 331–337, 1990

Lemmink HH, Nillesen WN, Mochizuki T, et al: Benign familial hematuria due to mutation of the type IV collagen α4 gene. J Clin Invest 98:1114–1118, 1996

Congenital Nephrotic Syndrome

Holmberg C, Antikainen M, Ronnholm K, Ala Houhala M, Jalanko H: Management of congenital nephrotic syndrome of the Finnish type. Pediatr Nephrol 9:87–93, 1995

Kestila M, Lenkkeri U, Mannikko M, et al: Positionally cloned gene for a novel glomerular protein—nephrin—is mutated in congenital nephrotic syndrome. Mol Cell 1:575–582, 1998

Mahan JD, Mauer SM, Sibley RK, Vernier RL: Congenital nephrotic syndrome: evolution of medical management and results of renal transplantation. J Pediatr 105:549–557, 1984

Somlo S, Munder P: Getting a foothold in nephrotic syndrome. Nature Genet 24:333–335, 2000

Familial Steroid-Resistant Nephrotic Syndrome

Fuchshuber A, Jean G, Gribouval O, et al: Mapping a gene (SRN1) to chromosome 1q25-q31 in idiopathic nephrotic syndrome confirms a distinct entity of autosomal recessive nephrosis. Hum Mol Genet 4: 2155–2158, 1995

Diffuse Mesangial Sclerosis, Denys-Drash Syndrome, and Frasier Syndrome

Barbosa AS, Hadjiathanasiou CG, Theodoridis C, et al: The same mutation affecting the splicing of WT1 gene is present on Frasier syndrome patients with or without Wilms' tumor. Hum Mutat 13:146–153, 1999

Coppes MJ, Huff V, Pelletier J: Denys-Drash syndrome: relating a clinical disorder to genetic alterations in the tumor suppressor WT1. J Pediatr 123:673–678, 1993

Habib R, Loirat C, Gubler MC, et al: The nephropathy associated with male pseudohermaphroditism and Wilms' tumor (Drash syndrome): a distinctive glomerular lesion—report of 10 cases. Clin Nephrol 24:269–278, 1985

Pelletier J, Bruening W, Kashtan CE, et al: Germline mutations in the Wilms' tumor suppressor are associated with abnormal urogenital development in Denys-Drash syndrome. Cell 67:437–447, 1991

Fabry Disease

Eng CM, Ashley GA, Burgert TS, Enriquez AL, D'Souza M, Desnick RJ: Fabry disease: thirty-five mutations in the alpha-galactosidase A gene in patients with classic and variant phenotypes. Mol Med 3:174–182, 1997

Nail-Patella Syndrome

Gubler MC, Dommergues JP, Foulard M, et al: Collagen type III glomerulopathy: a new type of hereditary nephropathy. Pediatr Nephrol 7: 354–360, 1993

McIntosh I, Clough MV, Schaffer AA, et al: Fine mapping of the nail-patella syndrome locus at 9q34. Am J Hum Genet 60:133–142, 1997

21.10 CYSTIC DISORDERS OF THE KIDNEY

Friedhelm Hildebrandt

DIAGNOSIS OF RENAL CYSTIC DISORDERS

HISTORY AND PEDIGREE ANALYSIS Cystic disorders of the kidney are among the most common causes for end-stage renal disease in children. Most renal cystic diseases (Table 21-17) are monogenic disorders, indicating that in an affected individual the disease is caused by a defect in a single gene (see Sec. 10.1). When the history is taken, emphasis should be placed on pedigree analysis to clarify whether the pattern of inheritance is compatible with a dominant or recessive mode. In *autosomal dominant* diseases, a genetic defect in only one allele of the disease gene (on one parental chromosome) leads to the disease phenotype. Typically, there are affected individuals in more than one generation, father-to-son transmission may be present (as opposed to X-linked diseases), and the disease course is usually milder than in recessive variants of the disease. In *autosomal recessive* diseases, defects in both alleles of a gene (on both parental chromosomes) are necessary for the disease to occur.

TABLE 21-17
CYSTIC RENAL DISORDERS[a]

	MODE OF INHERITANCE
Cystic dysplasia (multicystic dysplastic kidney)	
Polycystic kidney disease	
Autosomal recessive polycystic kidney disease (ARPKD) [263200]	AR
Autosomal dominant polycystic kidney disease (ADPKD1 and 2) [601313, 173910]	AD
Tuberous sclerosis type 2 (TSC2) [191092]	AD
Nephronophthisis/medullary cystic disease (NPH/MCKD) complex	
Juvenile nephronophthisis type 1 (NPH1) [256100]	AR
Infantile nephronophthisis type 2 (NPH2) [602088]	AR
Adolescent nephronophthisis type 3 (NPH3)	AR
Medullary cystic kidney disease type 1 (ADMCKD1) [704000]	AD
Medullary cystic kidney disease type 2 (ADMCKD2) [603860]	AD
Other renal cystic diseases	
Hypoplastic familial glomerulocystic disease [137920]	AD
Medullary sponge kidney	-
Oligomeganephronia	-
Renal cystic diseases in genetic syndromes	
Laurence-Moon-Bardet-Biedl syndrome [209901], [209900], [600151], [600374], [603650]	AR
Meckel-Gruber syndrome [249000]	AR

[a]OMIM numbering is given in brackets. Continuously updated information on the molecular genetics of these diseases can be retrieved from the World Wide Web: *http://www.ncbi.nlm.nih.gov/Omim/2000.*

Typically, there are affected individuals in only one generation, and the disease course is usually more severe than in a dominant variant of the disease. Knowledge of the mode of inheritance is an important guide for differential diagnosis, for genetic counseling, and for planning a molecular genetic diagnosis. In some diseases, defects in different genes localized in different chromosomal positions can give rise to identical or very similar disease phenotypes in different patients. This phenomenon is called "genetic locus heterogeneity" and is exemplified by autosomal dominant polycystic kidney disease (ADPKD) types 1 and 2.

MOLECULAR GENETIC DIAGNOSIS   In some renal cystic disorders the responsible gene has been identified, rendering *direct molecular genetic testing* possible. In these instances, the disease-causing mutation can be identified in affected patients. In principle, direct genetic testing can be performed in a single affected child of a family. However, because some rare mutations can be difficult to detect, exclusion of a genetic defect is possible only if the disease-causing mutation in a family is already known. If the disease-related gene has not yet been identified, but the chromosomal localization of a disease gene is known, only *indirect molecular genetic testing* by haplotype analysis is feasible (Fig. 21-27). Haplotype analysis, however, is possible only if an affected individual is already known to the family. Disadvantages of indirect genetic testing are that an affected individual already needs to be present in the kindred and that the diagnosis can be based on only an estimate of statistical likelihood, which depends on pedigree size. Updates on laboratories that perform molecular genetic diagnosis can be found at OMIM (*http://www.ncbi.nlm.nih.gov/Omim/2000*) or at the Gene Tests™ resource (*http://www.genetests.org/*). Molecular genetic diagnosis should as a rule be initiated only within the context of genetic counseling by an approved genetic counselor because there are many difficult ethical issues to consider (see Sec. 10.1).

TREATMENT   Most renal cystic disorders eventually lead to end-stage renal disease (ESRD). As yet, no treatment directed to the primary cause is available for these diseases. Therefore, therapy is symptomatic and is aimed at complications that might accelerate progression. For instance, unilateral nephrectomy may be indicated in a nonfunctional multicystic dysplastic kidney that has been the source of recurrent urinary tract infections. Another example is control of blood pressure in ADPKD to decelerate progression into renal failure. In the phase of compensated chronic renal insufficiency, symptomatic treatment for anemia, acidosis, growth retardation, and renal osteodystrophy is most important (see Sec. 21.13). Eventually, renal replacement therapy by dialysis and transplantation becomes necessary (see Secs. 21.14 and 21.15).

All renal cystic disorders lead to changes in renal ultrasonographic appearance within an age range specific for the disease. Therefore, an algorithm for differential diagnosis in cystic diseases of the kidney is based on results of renal ultrasound and stratified by certain age groups (Fig. 21-28).

21.10.1   Cystic Dysplasia

Cystic dysplasia, also termed *multicystic dysplastic kidney* (MCDK), results from a developmental defect in kidney organogenesis (see Sec. 21.3). In MCDK the abnormality can be unilateral, in contrast to other renal cystic disorders, where both kidneys are always affected. In cystic dysplasia the abnormal kidney involved is usually detected on ultrasound as a cluster of cysts with negligible renal parenchyma. In bilateral cystic dysplasia, ESRD may be present at birth or will develop at a variable rate postnatally (see Sec. 21.3).

21.10.2   Polycystic Kidney Disease

AUTOSOMAL RECESSIVE POLYCYSTIC KIDNEY DISEASE

Autosomal recessive polycystic kidney disease (ARPKD) leads to end-stage renal failure in the perinatal period, in childhood, or even later in adult life. Uniformly, there is bilateral kidney enlargement as a result of transformation of collecting ducts into fusiform cysts. ARPKD occurs in 1 in 6000 to 40,000 live births. ARPKD is always associated with hepatic fibrosis, which may not be clinically evident initially because renal failure develops earlier than clinical sequelae of hepatic fibrosis.

HISTORY AND CLINICAL FEATURES   In the neonate, oligohydramnios results from intrauterine renal failure. Oligohydramnios results in insufficient lung development and the typical "Potter facies," which is characterized by low-set ears, a flat nose, and a retracted chin. In these severe prenatal cases abnormal kidney growth can already be detected by ultrasound in the second half of pregnancy. Postnatally, prominent renal symptoms are palpable enlarged kidneys, the development of chronic renal insufficiency, and hypertension, starting at a median age of 6 months. Initial symptoms that lead to the diagnosis of ARPKD include (in decreasing order of frequency) palpable abdominal mass, hypertension, urinary tract infections, a positive family history or prenatal diagnosis, liver involvement, and growth failure.

ARPKD kidneys can be grossly enlarged so that palpable abdominal masses are common, as are hypertension and urinary tract infections. In a study of 66 boys and 49 girls with ARPKD, age at diagnosis was 11% prenatal, 41% neonatal, 23% infantile, and 25% juvenile. Glomerular filtration rate was reduced in 70% of patients with a medium onset of 0.6 years. Among extrarenal organ manifestations, congenital hepatic fibrosis is the most important, followed by the risk of GI bleeding from esophageal varices. The occurrence of portal hypertension is variable, but liver cell function is normal. However, there can be cerebral aneurysms and, rarely, cysts in the pancreas or spleen.

A few patients will not manifest the renal components of their disease and will have reasonably preserved renal function but will present with symptoms related to congenital hepatic fibrosis and portal hypertension.

COMPLICATIONS   Complications resulting from chronic renal failure are anemia, growth retardation, and osteodystrophy. There is a risk of cyst infection and urinary obstruction. Hypertension is frequent, and nephrolithiasis occurs in about 15% of cases. Hypersplenism can be present because of portal hypertension secondary to congenital hepatic fibrosis (see Chapter 18). Fertility- and pregnancy-related problems are also common.

DIAGNOSIS   Diagnosis in ARPKD rests on clinical signs and symptoms, renal and hepatic imaging, kidney and/or liver biopsy, and molecular genetic diagnosis (Fig. 21-28). Over time, cystic dilation of the bilary tree (Caroli disease) develops.

RENAL ULTRASOUND AND HISTOLOGY   Bilaterally enlarged hyperechogenic kidneys maintain a reniform shape even when grossly

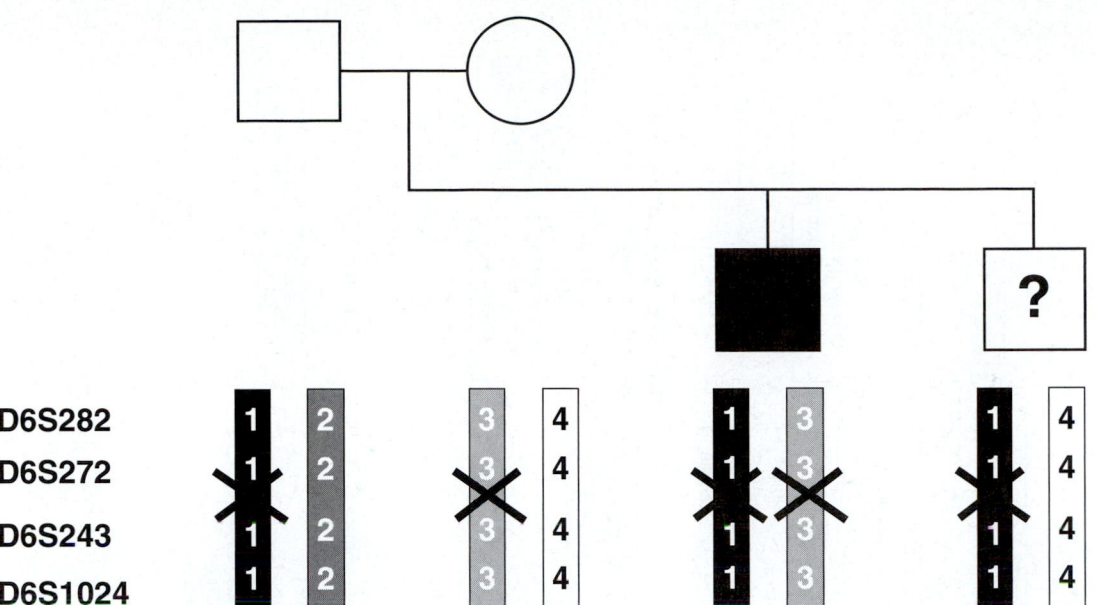

FIGURE 21-27 Principle of haplotype analysis for indirect molecular genetic diagnosis in an example of ARPKD. Polymorphic DNA markers from the genetic region for ARPKD on chromosome 6 are examined for their alleles by polymerase chain reaction. In this family with one boy affected by ARPKD *(black symbol)*, alleles of four markers from the ARPKD chromosomal region were examined and were assigned allele numbers. Consecutive alleles of neighboring markers are called a "haplotype" and allow identification of the paternal and maternal chromosomes in each individual. Chromosomes inherited from father and mother of an individual are coded in different shades of gray. The gene for ARPKD is positioned between flanking markers D6S272 and D6S243. In a recessive disease the affected child is carrying one defective gene from the father and one from the mother (indicated by Xs). The sibling who is to be diagnosed is carrying the paternal chromosome with the defective ARPKD allele; however, he inherited the healthy chromosome from the mother and can therefore be diagnosed as an unaffected heterozygous carrier of ARPKD.

enlarged. On ultrasound kidneys typically exhibit a "salt and pepper" appearance. In later stages distinct, rounded cysts appear. On hepatic ultrasound the liver is hyperechogenic, and later visible biliary cysts may develop. Renal and hepatic changes can be demonstrated by CT scan, MRI, or IVP. On MRI the radial arrangement of fusiformly dilated collecting ducts can be appreciated, but this is usually not required for diagnosis. In the kidney there are fusiform dilation and cyst development, involving 10 to 90% of collecting ducts, depending on severity and age of onset. Liver histology exhibits portal and interlobular fibrosis as well as biliary duct hyperplasia.

MOLECULAR GENETICS AND GENETIC COUNSELING A gene locus for ARPKD has been localized on chromosome 6p21.1-p12. There is no indication of genetic locus heterogeneity in ARPKD, even for early-onset perinatal cases. In ARPKD, a recessive disease, an a priori risk of 25% exists for a sibling of an affected individual. For prenatal diagnosis, ultrasound and the presence of oligohydramnios can be indicative. Unfortunately, diagnostic enlargement of fetal kidneys may not occur until after 24 to 28 weeks of gestation, making early diagnosis difficult, and a negative ultrasound early in gestation does not rule out ARPKD. For the diagnosis of ARPKD, a negative renal ultrasound in the parents is obligatory in order to distinguish the disease from early-onset autosomal dominant PKD. Because there is only one locus known for ARPKD, indirect molecular genetic diagnosis is possible by haplotype analysis in a family with at least one affected child (see Fig. 21-27).

Direct mutational analysis will be available only once the disease-related gene has been identified.

DIFFERENTIAL DIAGNOSIS For the differential diagnosis of ARPKD other cystic diseases that occur in infancy have to be considered (Fig. 21-28). Cystic dysplasia of the kidney can be distinguished from ARPKD by reduced kidney size, loss of reniform shape, and the presence of urinary tract malformations. Autosomal dominant polycystic kidney disease (ADPKD) may occur in infants if large deletions are present in the *PKD1* gene. Laurence-Moon-Bardet-Biedl syndrome can clearly be distinguished from ARPKD by the presence of retinitis pigmentosa and polydactyly together with obesity, mental retardation, and hypogonadism. Meckel-Gruber syndrome shows a wide variety of extrarenal organ involvement, including occipital encephalocele, renal dys-/agenesis, cleft palate, and ocular anomalies. Bilateral Wilms tumor is rare and can be distinguished from ARPKD by a highly irregular parenchymal pattern on imaging techniques.

TREATMENT Treatment of severe hypertension in young infants with ARPKD is difficult but essential to maximize preservation of renal function. Detection and treatment of UTI are also important. Management of portal hypertension frequently becomes a major problem. In end-stage renal disease, renal replacement therapy by dialysis and transplantation becomes necessary including combined kidney and liver transplantation or secondary liver transplantation after initial kidney transplantation if warranted.

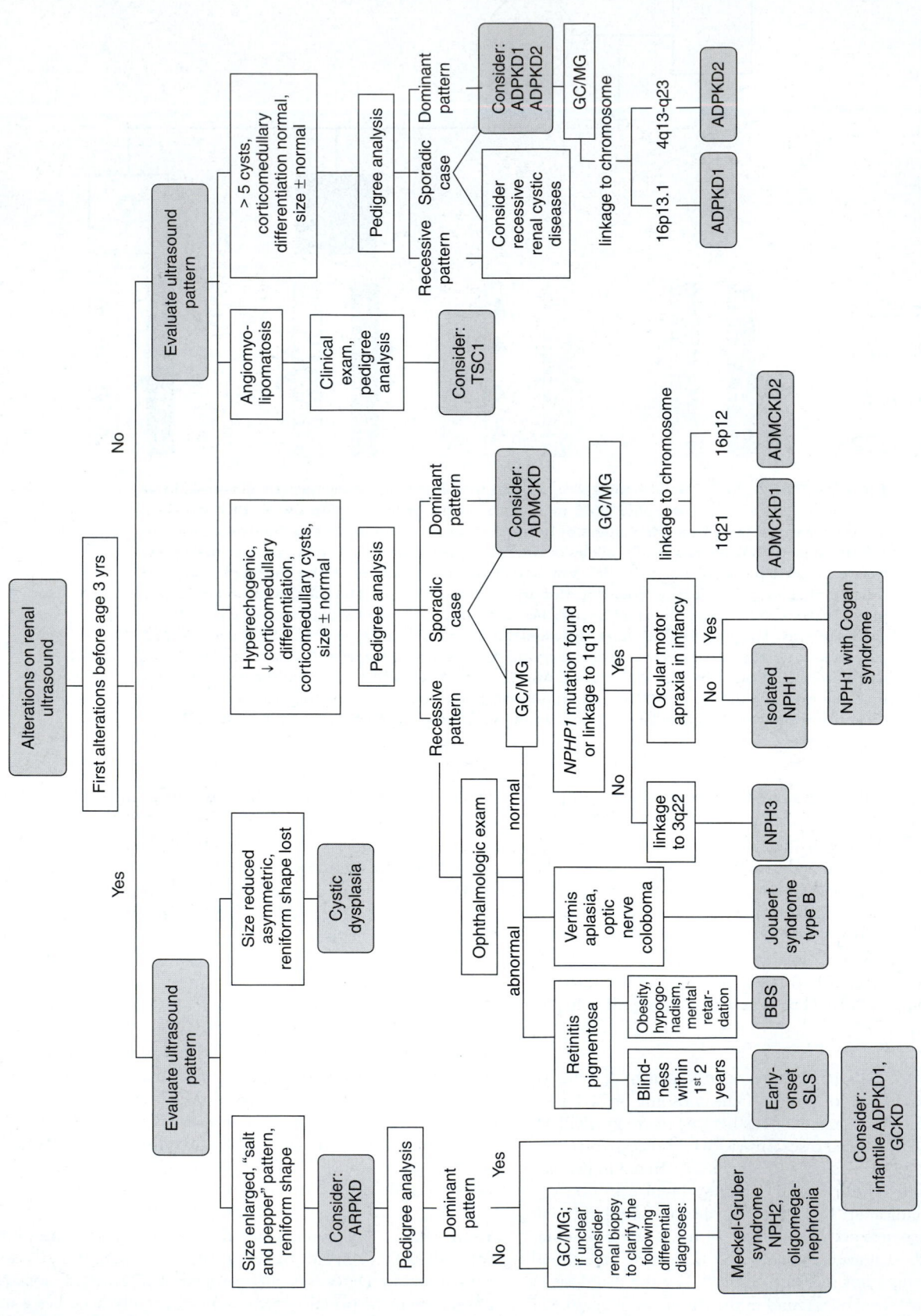

FIGURE 21-28 Algorithm for the evaluation of renal cystic disorders. GC/MG = initiate genetic counseling (GC) and potentially, as a consequence, molecular genetic diagnostic study (MG). ARPKD = autosomal recessive polycystic kidney disease; ADMCKD = autosomal dominant medullary cystic kidney disease; ADPKD = autosomal dominant polycystic kidney disease; BBS = Laurence-Moon-Bardet-Biedl syndrome; GCKD = glomerulocystic kidney disease; NPH1, 2, 3 = nephronophthisis type 1, 2, 3, respectively; SLS = Senior-Loken syndrome.

PROGNOSIS In ARPKD, survival at 1 year of age is 94% and 82% in male and female infants, respectively. Interestingly, among siblings a high concordance in the time course toward renal failure is observed.

AUTOSOMAL DOMINANT POLYCYSTIC KIDNEY DISEASE

AUTOSOMAL DOMINANT POLYCYSTIC KIDNEY DISEASE TYPE 1 Autosomal dominant polycystic kidney disease (ADPKD) is the most frequent disease of autosomal dominant inheritance in the United States and Europe. About 10 to 15% of all patients in adult chronic dialysis programs have ADPKD with a prevalence of 1:1000. End-stage renal disease usually develops between age 50 and 60 years. The gene *PKD1* is localized on chromosome 16p13.1 and codes for polycystin 1, a novel protein with a large transmembrane domain and a complex extracellular domain. Polycystin 1 is thought to bind to the gene product (polycystin 2) of the *PKD2* gene.

CLINICAL FEATURES Although ADPKD usually manifests in late adulthood, severe neonatal onset with Potter sequence occurs. Clinical symptoms in older children and adults include abdominal pain, palpable abdominal masses, hematuria, urinary tract infections, hypertension, and abdominal or inguinal hernias. Cerebral aneurysms and diverticulosis of the gut develop in adults with ADPKD.

RENAL ULTRASOUND In children who are known to be genetically at risk, the presence of even a single cyst in normal-sized kidneys is highly predictive for the development of ADPKD. Hepatic, pancreatic, or ovarian cysts are rarely detected before puberty.

MOLECULAR GENETICS Although a germline mutation segregates in affected families in an autosomal dominant fashion, the disease mechanism, by which renal cysts develop gradually over several decades, involves loss of heterozygosity (LOH) of the second allele in individual cysts, consistent with a "second hit mechanism" (see Sec. 20.2). Molecular genetic diagnosis of *PKD1* has now become available.

MANAGEMENT At-risk children should be followed annually for hematuria, hypertension, or palpable abdominal mass. Aggressive treatment of hypertension and/or urinary tract infection is indicated because both pose considerable risk for accelerated progression into ESRD. The presence of cerebral aneurysms should be evaluated by cranial CT or MRI in families with a history of this complication or if symptoms warrant, but routine screening is not usually undertaken.

INFANTILE-ONSET OF ADPKD1 ADPKD can in rare instances occur in infancy if patients carry large deletions, which affect the *PKD1* gene as well as the neighboring *TSC2* gene, a "contiguous gene deletion syndrome" (see Sec. 10.1). Among patients with tuberous sclerosis, apparently only individuals carrying such extensive deletions develop large bilateral renal cysts and exhibit infantile onset of ADPKD.

AUTOSOMAL DOMINANT POLYCYSTIC KIDNEY DISEASE TYPE 2 ADPKD2 is clinically highly similar to ADPKD1 but follows a somewhat milder course toward renal failure and does not present in childhood. Mutational analysis has been performed in patients with ADPKD2. In this way ADPKD1 and -2 can now be differentiated on a molecular genetic basis. This may be of particular interest if live-donor kidney transplantation is planned in a family with suspected or proven ADPKD1 or -2.

21.10.3 Nephronophthisis/Medullary Cystic Kidney Disease

Diseases of the so-called "nephronophthisis/medullary cystic kidney disease" (NPH/MCKD) complex are renal cystic diseases that share a virtually identical renal histology, which is characterized by thickening and disintegration of the tubular basement membrane, interstitial lymphocytic infiltrations, and distal tubular atrophy with ectasia. Over time, chronic sclerosing tubulointerstitial nephropathy develops, and cysts occur primarily at the corticomedullary junction of the kidneys. Although histology is similar in all forms of the disease, two different disease groups can be differentiated.

NEPHRONOPHTHISIS (NPH)

Autosomal recessive forms, termed nephronophthisis, have an infantile (NPH2), a juvenile (NPH1), and an adolescent-onset form (NPH3). Recessive juvenile nephronophthisis (NPH1) most frequently occurs with isolated renal involvement but may be associated with extrarenal involvement.

JUVENILE NEPHRONOPHTHISIS TYPE 1 In NPH1, a history of polyuria, polydipsia, anemia, and growth retardation is common. Because these children have a salt-losing nephropathy and, therefore, do not develop the usually expected symptoms of renal disease (hematuria, proteinuria, hypertension, or edema), the diagnosis is frequently unexpected, and renal insufficiency is found because of an evaluation for anemia, lethargy, or polyuria. NPH1 leads to end-stage renal failure at a median age of 13 years.

DIAGNOSIS Renal ultrasound is an important aid in diagnosis of NPH and demonstrates lack of corticomedullary differentiation, increased echogenicity, and, beyond the age of 9 years, cysts at the corticomedullary border of the kidneys. The characteristic concentrating defect of nephronophthisis has been studied using renal function scintigraphy.

JUVENILE NEPHRONOPHTHISIS TYPE 1 WITH EXTRARENAL ORGAN INVOLVEMENT Recessive juvenile nephronophthisis can be associated with extrarenal organ involvement. The inability to perform horizontal eye movements (ocular motor apraxia type Cogan) was found in infants and toddlers with NPH1 and homozygous deletions in the *NPHP1* gene. Retinitis pigmentosa is associated with NPH in Senior-Løken syndrome (SLS), and cerebellar vermis aplasia and coloboma of the eye in Joubert syndrome type B. An association of NPH with hepatic fibrosis or cone-shaped epiphyses has also been described. Finally, Jeune syndrome (asphyxiating thoracic dysplasia), Ellis-van Creveld syndrome, RHYNS syndrome, and Laurence-Moon-Bardet-Biedl syndrome have been found in combination with NPH.

INFANTILE NEPHRONOPHTHISIS TYPE 2 Recently, in a large Bedouin pedigree, a second gene locus (*NPH2*) for recessive NPH has been localized to chromosome 9q22-q31 by homozygosity mapping. This form of the disease is termed infantile nephronophthisis because of its prenatal, perinatal, or infantile onset. Because clinical course and histology in this disease are quite different from other forms of NPH, whether this disease should be classified within the NPH/MCKD complex is doubtful.

ADOLESCENT NEPHRONOPHTHISIS TYPE 3 A third locus for NPH was identified in a large Venezuelan kindred. This disease variant is termed "adolescent nephronophthisis" (NPH3). Onset of ESRD occurs 6 years later than in juvenile NPH1, with a median onset of terminal renal failure at age 19 years. Otherwise no significant difference was found regarding clinical symptoms or histology in comparison to NPH1.

MOLECULAR GENETICS Recent identification of the gene (*NPHP1*) responsible for juvenile nephronophthisis type 1 renders direct genetic diagnosis possible. The gene product nephrocystin codes for an SH3 ("*src* homology 3") domain, suggesting that this gene product may have a potential role in protein–protein interactions, eg, in signal transduction at focal adhesions, the contact points between cells and extracellular matrix. A defect in cell–matrix interaction would lend a potential explanation to the characteristic histologic picture of tubular basement membrane disruption in NPH. In about 85% of children, deletions of the *NPHP1* gene on both parental chromosomes are present. Therefore, molecular genetic diagnosis can be performed by demonstration of the presence of these deletions or of point mutations in the *NPHP1* gene (Fig. 21-28). Homozygous deletions of the *NPHP1* region have also been described in Cogan syndrome with oculomotor apraxia as well as in a late-onset form of retinitis pigmentosa. This disease is characterized by oculomotor apraxia in infancy and early childhood, where children compensate for lack of ocular mobility by jerking head movements.

AUTOSOMAL DOMINANT MEDULLARY CYSTIC KIDNEY DISEASE (ADMCKD)

Medullary cystic kidney disease, the second group of diseases of the NPH/MCKD complex, is characterized by autosomal dominant inheritance, adult-onset of end-stage renal failure, and lack of extrarenal involvement. These are termed "autosomal-dominant medullary cystic kidney disease" (ADMCKD). A gene locus (*MCKD1*) for ADMCKD1 has been localized to chromosome 1q21. A second locus (*MCKD2*) for a disease termed ADMCKD2 was localized to chromosome 16p12 by total genome linkage analysis. In many of the published ADMCKD pedigrees, the disease was associated with hyperuricemia and gouty arthritis in most of the affected individuals.

21.10.4 Glomerulocystic Kidney Disease

The term glomerulocystic kidney disease (GCKD) describes a heterogeneous group of diseases characterized by multiple small cortical cysts, resulting from cystic dilation of the Bowman space and the initial proximal convoluted tubule. The lack of further tubular involvement differentiates GCKD from other cystic diseases, in which cysts arise from tubular dilation. Although this histologic picture is found in families with ARPKD as well as in several rare diseases including orofacial-digital syndrome type I, a distinct disease entity, *familial hypoplastic glomerulocystic disease,* occurs and follows autosomal dominant inheritance.

CLINICAL FEATURES The typical presentation of non–autosomal dominant GCKD is an infant with abdominal masses and renal insufficiency. Hypertension is common at presentation. Hepatic cysts have been described. Some patients present only as adults with hypertension, flank pain, and hematuria. The degree of renal dysfunction is variable. Children with *familial hypoplastic GCKD* (autosomal dominant) have chronic renal failure early in life, but typically have stable courses without progression to ESRD.

RENAL ULTRASOUND In non–autosomal dominant GCKD, ultrasonography reveals bilateral renal enlargement without distortion of renal contour but with increased echogenicity of the cortex and renal medulla, loss of corticomedullary differentiation, and small cortical cysts. In contrast, in *familial hypoplastic GCKD* (autosomal dominant), kidneys are small, and an abnormality of medullary pyramids with abnormal collecting systems and absent papillae is present.

21.10.5 Other Renal Cystic Disorders

MECKEL-GRUBER SYNDROME

Meckel-Gruber syndrome in an autosomal recessive inherited disorder featuring developmental defects of different organs including the kidney (see Chapter 10). Diagnostic criteria include cystic dysplasia of the kidney, hepatic fibrosis, and occipital encephalocele. Postaxial polydactyly can also be present. Diagnosis is based on clinical criteria as well as on renal or liver biopsy. Prognosis is guarded in cases with onset of renal insufficiency in the neonatal period. In the differential diagnosis of Meckel-Gruber syndrome, ARPKD, Joubert syndrome type B, and carbohydrate-deficient glycoprotein disease have to be considered. Two gene loci have been mapped for the disease: *MKS1* is localized on 17q23-q23 and is most prevalent in Finland, whereas *MKS2* is localized on 11q13.

LAURENCE-MOON-BARDET-BIEDL SYNDROME

Laurence-Moon-Bardet-Biedl syndrome (BBS) is an autosomal recessive disease characterized by obesity, retinitis pigmentosa, hypogenitalism, polydactyly, mental retardation, and the occurrence of cystic dysplasia of the kidney (see Chapter 10). Renal histology is similar to nephronophthisis. There is genetic locus heterogeneity in BBS with four different chromosomal localizations (in parentheses): BBS1 (11q13), BBS2 (16q21), BBS3 (3p12), and BBS4 (15q22). Direct molecular genetic diagnosis of BBS is not possible at present.

MEDULLARY SPONGE KIDNEY

Medullary sponge kidney is a rare congenital cystic disorder in which there is ectasia of cortical ducts within the inner medulla of the kidney, resulting in a sponge-like appearance. Calcifications, which develop in these locations, are visible on plain x-ray films. There is a strong propensity to renal calculi and urinary tract infections. Recently, familial cases have been described within the familial ureteral abnormalities syndrome (FUAS), which raises the question of whether there might exist a monogenic form of this disorder. The characteristic pyelogram with linear striations from dilated collecting ducts and enlarged calices is usually diagnostic of the disease. Generally there is no role for sonography, CT, or arteriography. Prognosis is good because in the absence of complications, renal function is normal, and there is no increased morbidity or mortality resulting from the disease.

References

Guay-Woodford LM, Galliani CM, Musulman-Mroczek E, et al: Diffuse renal cystic disease in children: morphologic and genetic correlations. Pediatr Nephrol 12:173–182, 1998

Hildebrandt F: Renal cystic disease. Curr Opin Pediatr 11:141, 1999

Hildebrandt F, Otto E, Rensing C, et al: A novel gene encoding an SH3 domain protein is mutated in nephronophthisis type 1. Nature Genet 17:149–153, 1997

Zerres K, Rudnik-Schoneborn S, Steinkamm C, et al: Autosomal recessive polycystic kidney disease. J Mol Med 76:303–309, 1998

21.11 RENAL TUBULAR DISORDERS

Michel Baum

In adults, renal tubules reabsorb most of the glomerular ultrafiltrate and modify the composition of the tubular fluid to maintain salt and water balance. The kidney of the growing child maintains a positive balance for a number of filtered solutes that are necessary for growth (see Sec. 21.2). Disorders of tubular function can result from inherited primary defects in transporters responsible for the reabsorption of solutes and water or from inherited or acquired disorders that cause tubular injury. Renal transport disorders can be mild, with little or no clinical consequences, or can be life threatening, depending on which transporters are affected.

21.11.1   Fanconi Syndrome

The proximal tubule is responsible for the reabsorption of all of the filtered glucose, amino acids, and 80% of the filtered bicarbonate and phosphate (see Fig. 21-4). The luminal fluid entering the proximal tubule is an ultrafiltrate of plasma. Most solutes are transported across the apical membrane in conjunction with sodium. The driving force for solute transport is the low intracellular sodium generated by the basolateral Na,K ATPase. The preferential reabsorption of organic solutes, bicarbonate, and phosphate results in tubular fluid devoid of organic solutes and with a higher chloride and lower bicarbonate concentration than that in the peritubular plasma. Solutes can diffuse across the paracellular pathway down concentration gradients generated by active transport.

The Fanconi syndrome is a generalized proximal tubule transport disorder resulting in hypophosphatemia, hypokalemia, and a hyperchloremic metabolic acidosis. Evaluation of the urine reveals glucosuria, generalized aminoaciduria, and phosphaturia (fractional excretion of phosphate of at least 15%). A generalized decrease in proximal tubular transport could result from (1) primary injury to the Na,K ATPase pump, (2) a decrease in intracellular ATP that fuels the pump, or (3) an increase in the permeability of the proximal tubule paracellular pathway. Although the cellular basis for most causes of the Fanconi syndrome has not been determined, many studies have demonstrated that the proximal tubule transport defect is the result of a decrease in intracellular ATP.

TABLE 21-18

CAUSES OF THE FANCONI SYNDROME

Inherited disorders
  Primary
  Cystinosis
  Galactosemia
  Glycogen storage disease
  Tyrosinemia
  Hereditary fructose intolerance
  Wilson disease
  Lowe syndrome
  Dent disease
  Metachromatic leukodystrophy
  Pyruvate carboxylase deficiency
  Mitochondrial phosphoenolpyruvate carboxykinase deficiency
Toxins
  Ifosfamide
  Aminoglycosides
  Heavy metals
  Outdated tetracyclines
Acquired disorders
  Sjögren syndrome
  Dysproteinemias
  Vitamin D deficiency (can be inherited)
  Amyloidosis
  Multiple myeloma

The causes for the Fanconi syndrome are listed in Table 21-18. Cystinosis, the most common inherited cause of the Fanconi syndrome in children, is an autosomal recessive disorder in which cystine accumulates in lysosomes, where carrier-mediated transport of cystine from this compartment into the cytoplasm is impaired. Eventually the intracellular cystine burden increases to the point that there is impairment in cellular function. The diagnosis of cystinosis is made by finding elevated cystine levels in leukocytes or by finding corneal cystine crystals on slit lamp examination in children over 1 year of age (see Chapter 9).

Children with cystinosis usually are healthy for the first 6 months of life. Shortly thereafter, polydipsia, polyuria, constipation, unexplained fevers, and failure to thrive develop. Patients with cystinosis have hypophosphatemic rickets because of the loss of phosphate in the urine. These early signs and symptoms are the result of the electrolyte and mineral losses associated with the Fanconi syndrome. Patients with cystinosis develop progressive renal failure, and, without cysteamine therapy, end-stage renal disease (ESRD) occurs by 10 years of age. Endocrine disorders including hypothyroidism and diabetes mellitus can be seen in older children. Cystine can accumulate in the cornea, leading to photophobia and painful corneal ulcerations. Older patients with cystinosis can develop a retinopathy, cerebral atrophy, and central nervous system dysfunction. Gastrointestinal disturbances including swallowing difficulties are also common in older children and adults.

Two milder forms of cystinosis have been described. In the late-onset form of the disease, patients present in adolescence and have a slower rate of progression of renal disease. There is also a benign form of cystinosis, which presents with cystine crystals in the cornea seen on slit lamp exam but without other manifestations of cystinosis.

Cysteamine therapy has proven to be very effective in slowing or preventing the deterioration in renal function and improves the growth in patients with cystinosis. Cysteamine enters the lysosome, where it forms a mixed disulfide, and the cysteine-cysteamine complex exits across the lysosomal membrane via the lysine carrier. Cysteamine eye drops effectively dissolve corneal cystine crystals. However, cysteamine does not prevent or affect the severity of the Fanconi syndrome.

For patients with the Fanconi syndrome, treatment is focused on the primary disease (see Table 21-18). In patients with hereditary fructose intolerance, galactosemia, or tyrosinemia, removal of the nonmetabolized sugar or amino acid from the diet ameliorates the proximal tubular transport disorder (see Chapter 9). Patients with a toxin-induced form of the disease should avoid the offending agent. If the Fanconi syndrome is secondary to heavy metal toxicity or Wilson disease (see Chapter 18), chelation therapy should be initiated. If this approach is unsuccessful, therapy is centered on replacement of urinary solute losses. Hypophosphatemia and rickets can be successfully treated with oral phosphate supplements and 1,25-dihydroxycholecalciferol. Treatment of the proximal renal tubular acidosis is discussed below. The amount of solute replacement is dependent on the extent of the proximal tubular injury and the filtered load presented to the proximal tubule. In some patients with severe proximal tubule injury, reducing the filtered solute load by decreasing the glomerular filtration rate with either indomethacin or thiazide diuretics makes oral replacement more tolerable and feasible.

21.11.2   Renal Tubular Acidosis

PROXIMAL RENAL TUBULAR ACIDOSIS

The kidney serves two functions to maintain acid-base balance. The first is to reclaim the filtered load of bicarbonate, and the second is to excrete the acid that is generated from metabolism. In growing children, the kidney must also excrete the acid generated from new bone formation (see Sec. 21.2). Renal tubular acidosis is caused by impaired renal acidification and results in a hyperchloremic metabolic acidosis (see Sec. 21.4). With a normal kidney, acidemia is associated with increased urinary excretion of both titratable acid and ammonium to maintain serum pH. The amount of urinary ammonium excretion can be estimated by measuring the urinary cation gap: $U_{Cl} - (U_K + U_{Na})$. For example, in diarrhea both the acidosis and hypokalemia result in an increase in renal ammonia (NH_3) production. In the tubule fluid, NH_3 provides a buffer for the extra protons that must be excreted. As the distal tubule increases acid (H^+) secretion, an increase in urinary ammonium chloride results. Consequently, the urine chloride will be higher than the sum of the urine sodium and potassium because the ammonium of the ammonium chloride is not measured, resulting in a positive urinary cation gap. This approximation is frequently referred to as a negative anion gap because of the conventional use of the serum anion gap (see Sec. 21.4) to assess acid-base disorders. In renal tubular acidosis the urinary ammonium chloride concentration does not increase appreciably, and the urine cation gap is negative or zero. A blood gas should be obtained in the evaluation of a metabolic acidosis to insure that the low serum bicarbonate concentration is not the result of compensation for a respiratory alkalosis (see Sec. 21.4).

The proximal tubule reabsorbs most of the filtered load of bicarbonate (see Fig. 21-4). The serum bicarbonate concentration is maintained at a constant level, which is set by the bicarbonate reabsorptive capacity of the kidney. Ingestion or infusion of bicarbonate will increase the serum bicarbonate concentration above this threshold only transiently. The serum bicarbonate will quickly fall back to its original level as the excess bicarbonate is excreted in the urine. The proximal tubule is responsible for the reabsorption of 80% of the filtered bicarbonate and thus plays a major role in setting the bicarbonate threshold (ie, the serum bicarbonate level).

In proximal renal tubular acidosis, a decrease in proximal tubule bicarbonate reabsorptive capacity results in a low bicarbonate threshold. Because the serum bicarbonate concentration is lower than normal, the concentration of bicarbonate in the glomerular ultrafiltrate delivered to the tubules will also be lower. Thus, patients with proximal renal tubular acidosis can reabsorb all of their filtered bicarbonate, albeit at a lower serum bicarbonate level than normal. Patients with proximal renal tubular acidosis maintain a constant serum bicarbonate and do not have bicarbonaturia unless bicarbonate is administered. At their respective bicarbonate thresholds, both normal individuals and patients with proximal renal tubular acidosis have no bicarbonate in the tubular fluid delivered to the distal nephron. The distal tubule can excrete the metabolically generated acid in a urine with a pH less than 5.5. Hypokalemia is often seen with proximal renal tubular acidosis and results from the decrease in potassium reabsorption seen with metabolic acidosis.

Proximal renal tubular acidosis could be caused by a mutation in any of the genes of proximal tubule transporters or carbonic anhydrase. Although isolated proximal renal tubular acidosis has been described, it is almost always seen in conjunction with the Fanconi syndrome. As with the Fanconi syndrome, patients with isolated proximal renal tubular acidosis present with failure to thrive.

Therapy of proximal renal tubular acidosis is quite difficult. Over 10 to 15 meq/kg per day of alkali may need to be administered, which may result in only a modest improvement in the serum bicarbonate concentration. In addition, sodium bicarbonate or citrate will result in delivery of bicarbonate or citrate to the distal nephron, resulting in an increase in urinary potassium excretion. Bicarbonate or citrate should be administered as a mixture of sodium and potassium salts, and the serum potassium should be monitored closely. Reducing the glomerular filtration rate with either indomethacin or a thiazide diuretic will decrease the filtered load of bicarbonate delivered to the tubules and may make alkali therapy more successful.

CLASSICAL DISTAL RENAL TUBULAR ACIDOSIS

The distal nephron is responsible for secreting the acid generated from metabolism in adults. In growing children the formation of new bone liberates acid, which must also be secreted by the distal tubule. Luminal membrane proton secretion is via an $H^+ATPase$ and an H,K ATPase, which secretes a proton and simultaneously reabsorbs a potassium ion. The intracellular bicarbonate formed exits the cell via a Cl^-/HCO_3^- exchanger on the basolateral membrane. As in the proximal tubule, carbonic anhydrase aids in the conversion of CO_2 and H_2O to H_2CO_3 (see Fig. 21-6). Primary distal renal tubular acidosis can theoretically be caused by a defect in any of these transporters. Families with autosomal dominant distal renal tubular acidosis have been found to have a mutation in the gene for a basolateral membrane Cl^-/HCO_3^- exchanger that is responsible for bicarbonate exit from the cell. Distal renal tubular acidosis may also be inherited as a sex-linked or as an autosomal recessive disease. In children, distal renal tubular acidosis is usually sporadic, hereditary, or secondary to amphotericin B therapy (Table

TABLE 21-19

CAUSES OF DISTAL RENAL TUBULAR ACIDOSIS

Primary
   Hereditary (may be associated with deafness)
   Idiopathic
Hereditary, associated with other diseases
   Ehlers-Danlos syndrome
   Hereditary hypercalciuria
   Osteopetrosis with carbonic anhydrase II deficiency
   Hereditary elliptocytosis
   Sickle cell anemia
   Medullary cystic disease
   Fabry disease
   Wilson disease
Autoimmune diseases
   Sjögren syndrome
   Pulmonary fibrosis
   Chronic active hepatitis
   Biliary cirrhosis
   Systemic lupus erythematosus
   Thyroiditis
   Hypergammaglobulinemia
   Cryoglobulinemia
Diseases associated with nephrocalcinosis
   Hyperthyroidism
   Vitamin D intoxication
   Hypercalciuria
   Medullary sponge kidney
   Fabry disease
   Wilson disease
   Hyperparathyroidism
Drugs
   Amphotericin B
   Lithium
   Glue
   Analgesic nephropathy
   Cyclamate
   Cyclosporine
   Chronic furosemide therapy for treatment of bronchopulmonary dys-
      plasia
   Vanadate
Tubulointerstitial diseases
   Balkan nephropathy
   Chronic pyelonephritis
   Leprosy
   Obstructive uropathy
   Renal transplantation
   Hyperoxaluria

21-19). In renal tubular acidosis caused by amphotericin B therapy, proton secretion is intact, but the secreted protons diffuse back into cells through a channel created by the drug.

As with proximal renal tubular acidosis, patients with distal renal tubular acidosis present with failure to thrive. Laboratory evaluation reveals a hyperchloremic metabolic acidosis and hypokalemia. The hypokalemia can be severe enough to cause muscle weakness, cramps, and paralysis. The patient will have a negative urine cation gap. The chronic metabolic acidosis results in bone demineralization and hypercalciuria. Several features of distal renal tubular acidosis clearly distinguish it from a proximal disorder. Because the distal nephron is the segment responsible for final urinary acidification, patients with distal renal tubular acidosis are unable to excrete urine with a pH less than 5.5. Both acidosis and hypokalemia increase proximal tubule citrate reabsorption and cause hypoci-

traturia. Because citrate is the major factor that increases urinary calcium solubility, nephrocalcinosis and nephrolithiasis are frequently seen in patients with distal renal tubular acidosis. In proximal renal tubular acidosis, citrate reabsorption is usually impaired by tubular injury, and citrate excretion is normal or increased.

Distal renal tubular acidosis is treated by providing alkali in an amount equivalent to the protons normally secreted by the distal nephron. A combination of sodium and potassium citrate or bicarbonate of 3 to 5 meq/kg per day in three to four divided doses in children is sufficient to normalize the serum bicarbonate and prevent hypocitraturia. Children with primary distal renal tubular acidosis who are treated with alkali may not only grow normally but can have catch-up growth. Untreated patients or those with poor compliance also develop progressive nephrocalcinosis and renal insufficiency. In children who present with severe hypokalemia and acidosis, potassium must be corrected before initiation of alkali therapy to prevent a further decrease in the serum potassium (see Sec. 21.4).

RENAL TUBULAR ACIDOSIS WITH HYPERKALEMIA

Renal tubular acidosis associated with hyperkalemia has been designated type 4 renal tubular acidosis. The pathogenesis of this disorder is related to transporters in the cortical collecting tubule (see Fig. 21-6). The reabsorption of sodium and secretion of both potassium and protons are stimulated by mineralocorticoids. Deficiency or resistance to mineralocorticoids will thus result in hyperkalemia and hyperchloremic metabolic acidosis. Hyperkalemia results in lower ammonia production by the proximal tubule, which exacerbates the metabolic acidosis by limiting urinary buffer excretion.

A number of disorders are associated with either mineralocorticoid deficiency or a resistance to the action of mineralocorticoids (see Sec. 24.4). Addison disease is rare in children but can be the result of autoimmune disease, hemorrhage, tumors, tuberculosis, or severe infection. A decrease in mineralocorticoid production is seen in 21-hydroxylase deficiency, the most common form of adrenogenital syndrome. Boys with 21-hydroxylase deficiency do not have ambiguous genitalia and often present with dehydration resulting from renal salt wasting in the first 2 months of life. Converting enzyme inhibitors and chronic heparin administration can result in hypoaldosteronism. Hyporeninemic hypoaldosteronism in children is usually the result of drugs such as cyclosporine, nonsteroidal anti-inflammatory agents, and tubulointerstitial disease.

The most common causes for type 4 renal tubular acidosis are obstructive uropathy, interstitial renal disease, and multicystic dysplastic kidneys. In these disorders aldosterone secretion is normal, but damage to the cortical collecting tubule and resistance to the action of aldosterone occur. In these disorders the hyperkalemia is out of proportion to the severity of the renal insufficiency. Type 4 renal tubular acidosis is seen in patients with type 1 pseudohypoaldosteronism (see Sec. 24.4). There are two forms of type 1 pseudohypoaldosteronism. Both are characterized by unresponsiveness of the collecting tubule to aldosterone. In the more severe autosomal recessive form, there is a mutation of the amiloride-sensitive sodium channel in the cortical collecting tubule, causing loss of channel activity. The disease presents in neonates with salt wasting and volume depletion. Children with this disorder can fail to thrive and have numerous pulmonary infections. The sweat chloride levels are elevated, and this disorder has been mistaken for cystic fibrosis. The autosomal dominant or sporadic form results from a mutation in the mineralocorticoid receptor gene. The dominant form is milder, presents later in life, and tends to remit with age. In both types the serum aldosterone levels and plasma renin activities are elevated. Type 2 pseudohypoaldosteronism, or Gordon syndrome, is a rare autosomal dominant disorder characterized by hyperkalemia, renal tubular acidosis, and hypertension. The defect is thought to be caused by enhanced chloride permeability of the cortical collecting tubule, which results in volume expansion and suppression of renin and aldosterone. The latter causes type 4 renal tubular acidosis. Drugs can also cause type 4 renal tubular acidosis. Amiloride and triamterene block the apical sodium channel on the cortical collecting tubule, and spironolactone is an aldosterone receptor antagonist.

Treatment of type 4 renal tubular acidosis is focused at finding the cause and treating primary disease. Patients with glucocorticoid and mineralocorticoid deficiency must receive replacement therapy. Sodium bicarbonate therapy at 3 to 5 meq/kg in children and 1 meq/kg in adults corrects the acidosis and improves the hyperkalemia. Dietary potassium restriction is often required. Patients with type 1 pseudohypoaldosteronism should be treated with salt supplements in addition to treatment of hyperkalemia and metabolic acidosis. Gordon syndrome is treated with sodium restriction and thiazide diuretics.

21.11.3   Renal Glucosuria

Glucose is reabsorbed across the apical membrane of the proximal tubule via a Na^+-glucose cotransporter and exits across the basolateral membrane by facilitated diffusion through a Na^+-independent transporter. The Na^+-glucose cotransporter in the early proximal tubule is a low-affinity, high-capacity transporter that reabsorbs one sodium for every glucose molecule and has been designated SGLT2. In contrast, SGLT1 is a high-affinity, low-capacity transporter that transports two sodium ions for each glucose molecule and is located in the late proximal tubule and in the intestine, where both glucose and galactose are transferred.

If the serum glucose rises above the capacity of the tubules to reabsorb the filtered load, glucosuria results. The plasma concentration at which glucosuria appears is designated the threshold for glucose. Neonates born before 30 weeks of gestation often have glucosuria because of immaturity of the proximal tubule, which cannot reabsorb the filtered load of glucose. Infants born after 34 weeks of gestation reabsorb over 99% of the filtered glucose, and glucosuria is not detected (see Sec. 21.2).

Primary renal glucosuria is a benign condition, usually detected on a routine urinalysis, in which glucosuria occurs in the absence of hyperglycemia. No other renal abnormalities are present in primary renal glucosuria. Patients with this condition do not have polyuria, polydipsia, or hypoglycemia, and the HbA_{1c} is normal. Primary renal glucosuria is inherited in an autosomal recessive fashion and is caused by a mutation in SGLT2, the early proximal tubule Na-glucose transporter. No therapy is indicated, and no increased risk of developing diabetes mellitus exists.

Glucose-galactose malabsorption results from a mutation in SGLT1. In this autosomal recessive disorder, patients present with watery diarrhea because of an inability to transport dietary glucose and galactose. The stools are acidic and contain sugar. The patients may also have glucosuria because this transporter is in the late proximal tubule. The diarrhea disappears when the infants are fed a glucose- and galactose-free diet.

21.11.4   Renal Aminoacidurias

Amino acids are filtered by the glomerulus and reabsorbed by the proximal tubule. As with glucose, amino acid uptake across the apical membrane is sodium dependent, and amino acids exit the cell by facilitated diffusion. Aminoaciduria can result from an increase in the filtered load of amino acids presented to the proximal tubule, from an inherited metabolic defect that increases the serum concentration of specific amino acids, or from defects in renal transporters responsible for amino acid reabsorption.

CYSTINURIA

Cystinuria is an autosomal recessive disorder that is the most common inherited defect in renal tubular amino acid transport. In cystinuria, a defect in dibasic amino acid transport results in increased excretion of lysine, arginine ornithine, and cystine. The limited solubility of cystine in urine results in renal calculi (see Sec. 21.12). Stones can form at any age but are most prevalent in the second and third decades of life. Recurrent stones produce progressive renal damage. The gene for cystinuria has been cloned and designated *SLC3A1* (see Chapter 9).

Cystinuria should be suspected in any patient who has recurrent renal stones. The diagnosis is confirmed by a urinary cystine excretion greater than 250 mg per gram of creatinine. Urinalysis is very helpful because patients with cystinuria excrete hexagonal cystine crystals. Treatment of cystinuria is focused on preventing renal stone formation. Fluid intake to decrease the concentration of cystine in the urine is critical. Alkalinization of the urine (to a pH of 6.5–7.0) will increase urinary cystine solubility, but excessive alkalinization increases the risk of developing calcium phosphate stones. Some patients require chelation therapy with either penicillamine or α-mercaptopropionylglycine (Thiola).

IMINOGLYCINURIA

Iminoglycinuria is an autosomal recessive disorder of impaired renal tubular transport of proline, hydroxyproline, and glycine. In some patients there is also a defect in the intestinal transport of these amino acids. The serum levels of these amino acids are normal, which distinguishes iminoglycinuria from hyperhydroxyprolinemia, hyperprolinemia, and hyperglycinemia. Iminoglycinuria is a benign condition, and no therapy is indicated (see Chapter 9).

HARTNUP DISORDER

Hartnup disorder is an autosomal recessive disorder of neutral amino acid transport in both the intestine and kidney. Plasma levels of neutral amino acids are either normal or low. Most patients with Hartnup disorder are asymptomatic; however, some patients develop pellagra-like symptoms including a "sunburn-like" rash on exposed skin surfaces, ataxia, and behavioral disturbances. Patients who are symptomatic have niacin deficiency from impaired intestinal absorption and hyperexcretion of tryptophan. Symptomatic patients should be treated with nicotinamide (see Chapter 9).

21.11.5   Genetic Disorders of Electrolyte Transport

DENT DISEASE

Dent disease is an X-linked recessive disorder characterized by low-molecular-weight proteinuria, nephrocalcinosis, recurrent renal stones, and progressive renal insufficiency. This disorder is also known as X-linked hypercalciuric nephrolithiasis. Some patients with Dent disease have rickets, phosphaturia, glucosuria, and aminoaciduria. There is no defect in renal acidification in most patients.

Dent disease is caused by a defect in a renal chloride channel designated as CLC-5, but the mechanism by which this defect leads to the constellation of clinical features is not known. However, CLC-5 is expressed in endosomes, and a defect in CLC-5 would impair endosomal acidification, which could inhibit proximal tubule transport by affecting membrane trafficking and protein absorption. The diagnosis should be considered in male patients with hypercalciuria and proteinuria and in patients with recurrent renal stones who have low-molecular-weight proteinuria such as β_2-microglobulin, α_2-microglobulin, and retinol-binding protein. Treatment is directed at preventing renal calculi. Patients should have adequate fluid intake and eat a low-sodium diet. A thiazide diuretic should be prescribed to decrease calcium excretion.

BARTTER SYNDROME

Bartter syndrome is an autosomal recessive disorder that usually presents in the first year of life with failure to thrive. A history of polyhydramnios and prematurity is common. Infants and children have polydipsia and polyuria, which is caused by a renal concentrating defect. Older children can have a history of constipation, salt craving, and complain of muscle cramps that are the result of the chronic volume depletion resulting from renal salt losses.

Patients with Bartter syndrome have a hypokalemic metabolic alkalosis and may also have hyponatremia and hypomagnesemia (see Sec. 21.4). Blood pressure is usually normal, but orthostatic changes occur in their blood pressure and pulse. Plasma renin and aldosterone levels and urinary prostaglandin excretion are elevated as a result of volume depletion. Bartter found that affected patients had a blunted hypertensive response to intravenous infusion of angiotensin II that was also caused by chronic volume depletion, which contributed to the hypokalemic alkalosis by increasing serum aldosterone secretion.

This pathophysiological sequence is the same as would occur if a patient were chronically taking a diuretic that inhibits the Na/K/2Cl transporter in the thick ascending limb (see Fig. 21-6). In fact, many patients with Bartter syndrome have a mutation in the Na/K/2Cl cotransporter; however, mutations in the chloride and potassium channels, two other transporters necessary for NaCl transport in this segment, have also been described. This segment also reabsorbs potassium, calcium, and magnesium across the paracellular pathway because of a lumen-positive potential difference (see Sec. 21.2). Mutations in any of the transporters that cause Bartter syndrome result in a decrease in the lumen potential difference to zero. This contributes to the hypokalemia and can increase urinary magnesium and calcium excretion. Patients with Bartter syndrome usually have very high urinary calcium levels (U_{Ca}/U_{cr} is usually >0.40), which can cause nephrocalcinosis. However, some patients with chloride channel defects have normal rates of calcium excretion.

Treatment of patients with Bartter syndrome is centered on replacement of electrolytes lost in the urine. Neonates and infants require NaCl and KCl to increase the intravascular volume and correct the hypokalemia. Older children increase their salt intake themselves, and sodium supplements are usually not necessary. Magnesium supplementation should be provided in those patients with hypomagnesemia. An increase in renal prostaglandin production exacerbates urinary sodium losses. Indomethacin therapy can be very beneficial, but gastritis and gastrointestinal bleeding are a potential complication that must be monitored. Failure to thrive and hypotonia frequently persist in these children, and therapy is complex.

GITELMAN SYNDROME

Gitelman syndrome is an autosomal recessive disorder that is frequently confused with Bartter syndrome. Gitelman syndrome is also a renal salt-wasting disorder and results in volume contraction and a hypokalemic alkalosis (see Sec. 21.4). Unlike Bartter syndrome, patients with Gitelman are usually born at term, have no history of polyhydramnios, do not have failure to thrive, and usually present in late childhood. Many of these children will have a craving for pickles. Although hypomagnesemia is found in half of patients with Bartter syndrome, it is almost invariably present in Gitelman syndrome. The most profound difference is in the urinary calcium excretion, which is low in Gitelman syndrome (U_{Ca}/U_{cr} <0.1) but usually elevated in Bartter syndrome. Most patients with Gitelman syndrome have a history of tetany or weakness that is secondary to the hypomagnesemia.

The constellation of clinical features in Gitelman syndrome are comparable to a patient who is taking a thiazide diuretic, which inhibits the NaCl cotransporter in the distal convoluted tubule and decreases urinary calcium excretion (see Sec. 21.2). All patients studied with Gitelman syndrome characterized to date have an inactivating mutation in the gene for the NaCl cotransporter in the distal convoluted tubule (see Fig. 21-6). The pathophysiology of the hypomagnesemia is unclear.

The treatment of Gitelman syndrome is to provide magnesium and potassium supplements to replace that lost in the urine. Patients with this disorder have chronic volume depletion and will usually increase their salt intake to replete their urinary losses.

LIDDLE SYNDROME

Liddle syndrome is an autosomal dominant disorder characterized by hypertension, hypokalemia, and metabolic alkalosis (see Sec. 21.4). These are characteristic features of hyperaldosteronism. However, patients with Liddle syndrome have low plasma aldosterone levels. Liddle found that patients with this disorder normalized their blood pressure and the electrolyte disorder by treatment with a low-sodium diet and the sodium channel blocker, triamterene, but were unresponsive to spironolactone, an aldosterone receptor antagonist. The molecular basis for Liddle syndrome has been clarified with the cloning of the epithelial sodium channel (designated ENaC), which has three subunits. All the patients with this disorder have had a defect in one of the ENaC subunits. The number of sodium channels on the apical membrane is dependent on the rate of insertion and removal. In Liddle syndrome the mutations are in a portion of the channel that is necessary for sodium channel removal. Thus, a gain of function occurs, and augmented sodium transport and volume expansion result in the low plasma renin and aldosterone levels and the hypertension in these patients. As in hyperaldosteronism, the increased sodium reabsorption produces a more negative potential difference, which causes high rates of potassium and proton secretion, resulting in the hypokalemic alkalosis. Liddle syndrome can be effectively treated by decreasing dietary sodium intake and giving a sodium channel blocker such as amiloride or triamterene.

APPARENT MINERALOCORTICOID EXCESS

Patients with apparent mineralocorticoid excess have hypertension and hypokalemic metabolic alkalosis but have low plasma aldosterone levels (see Sec. 24.4). The pathophysiology of this disorder has recently been elucidated. Normally the concentration of cortisol is far greater than that of aldosterone. Both cortisol and aldosterone can bind to the mineralocorticoid receptor in the collecting tubule. Cortisol would have the same effect as aldosterone if it were not for 11β-hydroxysteroid dehydrogenase, which converts cortisol to cortisone and prevents cortisol binding to the mineralocorticoid receptor. Patients with 11β-hydroxysteroid dehydrogenase deficiency will have apparent hyperaldosteronism as a result of the mineralocorticoid effect of cortisol. The diagnosis is made by finding low levels of cortisone metabolites in the urine. 11β-Hydroxysteroid dehydrogenase can also be inhibited by glycyrrhizic acid, which is in black licorice and chewing tobacco.

GLUCOCORTICOID-REMEDIABLE ALDOSTERONISM

Glucocorticoid-remediable aldosteronism is a rare autosomal dominant disorder in which the patient appears to have primary hyperaldosteronism. These patients have hypertension and may or may not have hypokalemia and metabolic alkalosis. The serum aldosterone levels are high, and the renin levels are suppressed. In this disorder, ACTH regulates aldosterone production rather than the normal situation in which the renin-angiotensin system and serum potassium levels regulate aldosterone production. The genes for 11β-hydroxylase (which is regulated by ACTH) and aldosterone synthase are normally found in tandem on chromosome 8. Gene duplication and a crossover event result in a hybrid gene in which the regulatory portion of 11β-hydroxylase is fused to aldosterone synthase. Patients with this disorder have improvement in their hypertension and the associated electrolyte disturbances with the administration of glucocorticoids, which decrease ACTH secretion.

NEPHROGENIC DIABETES INSIPIDUS

The urine osmolality can range form 50 to 1200 mOsm/kg water in adults and from 50 to 500 mOsm/kg water in neonates (see Sec. 21.2). The urine osmolality is dependent on the formation of a hypertonic medullary interstitium and the secretion of arginine vasopressin (also called antidiuretic hormone, ADH). ADH is secreted by the neurohypophysis in response to hyperosmolality or volume depletion and acts on the collecting tubule to increase passive water transport. Vasopressin binds to the vasopressin 2 receptor, which triggers the insertion of water channels (designated aquaporin 2) into the luminal membrane; this increases collecting tubule water permeability. The hypertonic medullary interstitium is formed by the countercurrent system.

Nephrogenic diabetes insipidus is a disorder in which the collecting tubule is unresponsive to vasopressin. Congenital nephrogenic diabetes insipidus can present in the first week of life with irritability, vomiting, and unexplained fever. These infants may have repeated episodes of hypernatremic dehydration, which may be accompanied by seizures, until a diagnosis is reached and therapy is initiated. Repeated episodes of hypernatremia can result in mental retardation. Patients often fail to thrive because of their need to ingest water at the expense of food. Rarely the enormous urine

TABLE 21-20

CAUSES OF NEPHROGENIC DIABETES INSIPIDUS

Congenital
   Mutation in vasopressin 2 receptor (X-linked)
   Mutation in aquaporin 2 water channel (AR/AD)
Drugs
   Lithium
   Demeclocycline
Electrolyte disorders
   Hypokalemia
   Hypercalcemia
Renal and systemic diseases
   Sickle cell anemia
   Obstructive uropathy
   Medullary sponge kidney
   Polycystic kidney disease
   Sjögren syndrome
   Amyloidosis

volumes can result in urinary tract dilatation and cause diminished renal function.

Most patients with congenital nephrogenic diabetes insipidus have a mutation in the vasopressin 2 receptor. The gene for the vasopressin 2 receptor lies on the X chromosome. Although men with X-linked nephrogenic diabetes insipidus have severe disease, women with one mutant allele will have variable degrees of polydipsia and polyuria based on stochastic X chromosome inactivation (see Sec. 10.1). Nephrogenic diabetes insipidus can also result from a mutation in the aquaporin 2 water channel, which is usually inherited in an autosomal recessive fashion, although an autosomal dominant inherited defect of this water channel has been described in a few kindreds. Nephrogenic diabetes insipidus can also be secondary to drugs, electrolyte disorders, and a number of diseases Table 21-20). These secondary causes of nephrogenic diabetes insipidus result from an attenuated effect of antidiuretic hormone on the collecting tubule or a disruption of the medullary concentration gradient.

Congenital diabetes insipidus should be diagnosed early to prevent the manifestations of repeated hypernatremic dehydration. Treatment includes providing adequate water and decreasing the loss of free water. Thiazide diuretics and a low-salt diet promote volume depletion and decrease the filtered load of water, resulting in decreased urine water losses. Neonates should be fed a low-sodium formula. Thiazide diuretics can produce hypokalemia, and serum potassium levels must be monitored. Indomethacin can also be used to decrease the glomerular filtration rate, but gastrointestinal bleeding may occur.

References

Fanconi Syndrome

Baum M: The Fanconi syndrome of cystinosis: insights into the pathophysiology. Pediatr Nephrol 12:492–497, 1998
Bergeron M, Gougoux A, Vinay P: The renal Fanconi syndrome. In: Scriver CR, Beaudet AL, Sly WS, Valle D, eds: The Metabolic and Molecular Bases of Inherited Diseases, 7th ed. New York, McGraw-Hill, 1995: 3691–3704

Renal Tubular Acidosis

DuBose TD Jr, Alpern RJ: Renal tubular acidosis. In: Scriver CR, Beaudet AL, Sly WS, Valle D, eds: The Metabolic and Molecular Bases of Inherited Diseases, 7th ed. New York, McGraw-Hill, 1995:3655–3690

Glucosuria

Desjeuz J-F, Turk E, Wright E: Congenital selective Na+ D-glucose cotransport defects leading to renal glycosuria and congenital selective intestinal malabsorption of glucose and galactose. In: Scriver CR, Beaudet AL, Sly WS, Valle D, eds: The Metabolic and Molecular Bases of Inherited Diseases, 7th ed. New York, McGraw-Hill, 1995:3563–3580

Aminoacidurias

Levy HL: Hartnup disorder. In: Scriver CR, Beaudet AL, Sly WS, Valle D, eds: The Metabolic and Molecular Bases of Inherited Diseases, 7th ed. New York, McGraw-Hill, 1995:3629–3642

Segal S, Their SO: Cystinuria. In: Scriver CR, Beaudet AL, Sly WS, Valle D, eds: The Metabolic and Molecular Bases of Inherited Diseases, 7th ed. New York, McGraw-Hill, 1995:3581–3602

Genetic Disorders of Electrolyte Transport

Bartter FC, Pronove P, Gill JR Jr, MacCardle RC: Hyperplasia of the juxtaglomerular complex with hyperaldosteronism and hypokalemic alkalosis. Am J Med 33:811–828, 1962

Bichet DG, Oksche A, Rosenthal W: Congenital nephrogenic diabetes insipidus. J Am Soc Nephrol 8(12):1951–1958, 1997

Gitelman HJ, Graham JB, Welt LG: A new familial disorder characterized by hypokalemia and hypomagnesemia. Trans Assoc Am Physicians 79:221–235, 1966

Liddle GW, Bledsoe T, Coppage WS: A familial renal disorder simulating primary aldosteronism but with negligible aldosterone secretion. Trans Assoc Am Physicians 76:199–213, 1993

Scheinman SJ: X-linked hypercalciuric nephrolithiasis: clinical syndromes and chloride channel mutations. Kidney Int 53:3–17, 1998

Scheinman SJ, Guay-Woodford LM, Thakker RV, Warnock DG: Genetic disorders of renal electrolyte transport. N Engl J Med 340:1177–1187, 1999

Simon DB, Nelson-Williams C, Bia MJ, et al: Gitelman's variant of Bartter's syndrome, inherited hypokalemic alkalosis, is caused by mutations in the thiazide-sensitive Na-Cl cotransporter. Nature Genet 12:24–30, 1996

21.12 NEPHROLITHIASIS

Craig B. Langman

Nephrolithiasis is a general term, analogous to urolithiasis or kidney stone, that describes a process of stone formation or presence in the urinary tract, from kidney through the urethral meatus. Over 90% of urolithiasis are localized to the upper tracts and ureters, with a small minority residing in the bladder or urethra. The term is not specific as to type of stone, mechanism of stone formation, or likelihood of recurrence.

ETIOLOGY

Kidney stones most often occur as microcrystalline substances that arise as a consequence of an alteration in the multicomponent ionic environment of the urine related to a specific disease or clinical condition. The ionic homeostasis of the urine is termed metastable, which denotes that slight increases or decreases in the concentrations of critical substances or urinary pH may shift a series of equilibrium reactions to promote subsequent precipitation of components that form the nidus of a stone. An understanding of the clinical circumstances that maintain metastable urine environments is the science of stone formation and is directly translated into clinical disease pathogenesis and treatment.

The most direct means of determining the etiology of a kidney stone is to know the composition of the stone which is best delineated to by x-ray diffraction pattern, which is unique for a given stone type. The chemical composition of a stone may yield false impressions of etiology because minerals in urine may have been attracted to the stone surface without contributing substantially to its formation process. X-ray diffraction studies of a stone are readily available.

The overwhelming majority of kidney stones contain calcium as the major cation. Estimates of calcium-containing stones range from 60 to 80% of stone-forming adult patients who receive care at large stone-referral centers in the United States. This high prevalence has been validated in solo practice and community-based settings as well. Children who form stones have a similar, if not higher, incidence of calcium-containing stones. Calcium-containing stones may form in patients who are hypercalcemic or in those with a normal serum calcium level (Table 21-21). Hypercalcemia is quite rare in children, and kidney stones that form as a result of hypercalcemia are equally rare. Over 98% of kidney stones in children are formed in the presence of normocalcemia. However, over 70% of normocalcemic children with a calcium-containing kidney stone have at least one of several risk factors that predispose to stone formation (Table 21-22).

The most frequent urinary biochemical abnormality in children who form a kidney stone is the presence of excess calcium excretion, termed hypercalciuria. Of the many etiologies for hypercalciuria (Table 21-21), the most frequent is idiopathic. Idiopathic hyper-

TABLE 21-21

HYPERCALCIURIC CONDITIONS ASSOCIATED WITH KIDNEY STONE FORMATION

ASSOCIATED WITH HYPERCALCEMIA	ASSOCIATED WITH NORMAL SERUM CALCIUM LEVEL
Primary hyperparathyroidism	Idiopathic hypercalciuria
Sarcoid;	Mutations in kidney chloride gene *CLC-5*
Cat-scratch fever	
Idiopathic infantile hypercalcemia	Immobilization (common)
Immobilization (rare)	Prematurity and furosemide therapy
Neonatal Bartter syndrome	Renal distal tubular acidosis
Seyberth syndrome	Glycogen storage disease
Thyrotoxicosis	Hereditary hypophosphatemia with hypercalciuria
	Ketogenic diet
	Activating mutation of the extracellular calcium-sensor gene (hypocalcemia)
	Medullary sponge kidney
	Inflammatory diseases such as juvenile arthritis
	Corticosteroid therapy

TABLE 21-22

RISK FACTORS FOR RENAL STONES

Male gender
Higher dietary purine intake
Reduced urinary citrate
Reduced urinary glycosaminoglycans
Hydropenic life-style
Urinary infection
Reduced urinary magnesium
Lowered urinary pH

TABLE 21-24

CONDITIONS ASSOCIATED WITH CALCIUM PHOSPHATE KIDNEY STONES

Distal renal tubular acidosis
Alkaline urine
Calcium oxalate kidney stones
Hypocitraturia
Urine infection
Hereditary hypophosphatemia with hypercalciuria
Primary hyperparathyroidism

calciuria may produce asymptomatic, microscopic or gross, hematuria in addition to kidney stones (see Sec. 21.5), and a family history of kidney stone disease is not uncommon because the disease behaves as an autosomal dominant disease with incomplete penetrance (see Sec. 10.1). The exact cause is unknown but likely reflects an abnormality in vitamin D homeostasis. The active vitamin D metabolite, 1,25-dihydroxyvitamin D, is elevated in many patients with idiopathic hypercalciuria and renal stones. Whether the hypercalciuria may reflect increased bone turnover and subsequent loss of bone calcium that contributes to elevated urinary calcium is controversial. Determining bone mineral density in children with idiopathic hypercalciuria has been recommended by some.

The most frequent urinary anion that forms a crystal with calcium is oxalate, either as a mono- or a dihydrate form. The etiology of hyperoxaluria is diverse (Table 21-23). Urinary supersaturation of calcium oxalate, an index of likelihood of spontaneous kidney stone formation, is greatly increased by small increases in urine oxalate excretion. In comparison, larger fractional increases in urinary calcium excretion are required for equivalent changes in calcium-oxalate urinary supersaturation. Thus factors that may increase oxalate excretion, such as dietary intake, may precipitate stone formation (Table 21-23). The second most common anion associated with calcium in a kidney stone is phosphate. Whether increased urinary excretion of phosphate alone is sufficient to produce a kidney stone is unclear, but generally, calcium phosphate stones are seen with other pathologic conditions (Table 21-24).

Excess excretion of uric acid, another normal anionic component of urine, may predispose to either a uric acid stone or, interestingly, a calcium-containing kidney stone (Table 21-25). Rarely, increased urinary excretion of xanthine or hypoxanthine when patients are treated with xanthine oxidase inhibitors may predispose

to formation of stones containing those compounds, particularly in patients with Lesch-Nyhan syndrome (see Chapter 9).

Other constituents of normal urine may be excreted in excess and predispose to kidney stone formation. This includes the dibasic amino acid cystine (see Sec. 21.11), but conditions associated with diffuse aminoaciduria, such as Fanconi syndrome, are not associated with cystine kidney stones despite high urinary levels of the dibasic amino acids. Cystinuria consists of the abnormal excretion of cystine, ornithine, arginine, and lysine due to defect in tubule reabsorption of dibasic amino acids and is distinct from cystinosis, a metabolic disorder with multiorgan system involvement (see Chapter 9 and Sec. 21.11).

Rare metabolic defects (adenine phosphoribosyl transferase deficiency or hereditary xanthine oxidase deficiency) may produce kidney stones in children. Nephrolithiasis has been associated with use of protease inhibitors to treat HIV infection. Urinary tract infection with urea-splitting organisms, usually *Proteus mirabilis*, are associated with struvite stones. Other anionic constituents in normal urine may be protective for kidney stone formation, including citrate, which, when reduced in urine, is associated with a greater likelihood of calcium-containing kidney stone formation, particularly in patients with RTA (see Sec. 21.11).

PATHOPHYSIOLOGY OF KIDNEY STONE FORMATION

Kidney stones that begin as crystallites have unique free energies of formation, and reductions in the needed free energy of formation will increase the likelihood of stone formation, which may occur by a process termed heterotopic nucleation. In essence, a second substance promotes easier crystal formation, compared to monoionic, native crystal alone. An important clinical example of heterotopic nucleation occurs when a bacterial urinary pathogen is present and increases the likelihood of kidney stone formation of any type. Another example of heterotopic nucleation is the coexistence of hyperuricosuria in the urine of calcium-containing kidney stone patients.

TABLE 21-23

PRINCIPAL CAUSES OF HYPEROXALURIA

Primary overproduction of oxalate: Primary hyperoxaluria
   AGXT mutation: type I
   DGDH mutation: type II
   Unknown: type III

Secondary overproduction of oxalate
   Ethylene glycol poisoning
   Vitamin C excess
   Pyridoxine deficiency

Enteric overabsorption
   Increased serum bile acid levels
   Inflammatory bowel disease
   Dietary oxalate excess
   Dietary calcium deficiency
   Small bowel resection/disease

TABLE 21-25

PRINCIPAL CAUSES OF HYPERURICOSURIA

INCREASED PRODUCTION	INCREASED EXCRETION
Hemolytic anemia	Proximal tubular defect
Hematologic malignancy	Acidosis
Irradiation or treatment with cytotoxic agents	
Gout	
Lesch-Nyhan syndrome	

GENETICS OF KIDNEY STONES

Idiopathic hypercalciuria is an autosomal dominant disease with incomplete clinical penetrance. Most other inherited kidney stone disease is autosomal recessive. Most diseases in which kidney stone formation occurs as one aspect of the disease are also autosomal recessive.

CLINICAL PRESENTATIONS OF KIDNEY STONES

Infants, children, and adolescents present in two general ways with kidney stones: with acute colic or with urinary complaints of a seemingly minor nature.

Acute renal colic is a clinical emergency heralded by colicky abdominal or flank pain that radiates to the groin. Renal colic is excruciating pain, seldom forgotten by the patient, parent or physician. Often the patient has a mildly reduced blood pressure, abdominal distension, reduced intestinal peristalsis, and possibly a deep palpable abdominal pain over the area of the kidney stone. Nausea and vomiting are frequent accompaniments of children with renal colic, and urinary symptoms may include gross or microscopic hematuria, urgency, hesitancy, frequency, and dysuria. If urinary infection is coexistent, symptoms and signs of that process may be present also.

After pain relief, stabilization of intravascular volume status, and evaluation of kidney function and electrolytes, the patient should have an imaging study of the urinary tract performed. Renal ultrasonography is an adequate first approach to visualization of obstructing kidney stone but may miss a stone in the midureter. Plain abdominal radiography will reveal radiopaque stones but does not resolve issues of kidney obstruction or parenchymal characteristics that are seen easily with ultrasonography. Definitive studies usually require contrast computed tomography, although the radiation exposure is much higher than with conventional radiography. Lack of relief of acute renal colic in 12 to 24 hours generally, even with morphine or related drugs, and after an increased fluid intake administered parenterally, requires consideration of urologic intervention. Bilateral kidney stones with obstruction require immediate removal to protect renal function. Unilateral stones greater than 5 mm in diameter may not pass spontaneously in infants and children.

Minor signs and symptoms of kidney stones include urinary complaints of urgency, frequency, dysuria, hesitancy, incontinence in an otherwise continent child, and signs including microscopic hematuria, gross hematuria, and pyuria with or without urinary infection. Mild, chronic, recurrent abdominal pain may be present. Diseases in which kidney stone formation occurs will have other symptoms and signs referable to the specific disease process.

DIAGNOSIS OF KIDNEY STONES

Kidney stones are documented (1) by spontaneous passage of a stone and subsequent analysis that demonstrates a known stone composition or (2) by a radiologic imaging study that demonstrates kidney stones within the urinary tract. Factitious kidney stones will not have a true x-ray diffraction pattern consistent with known human kidney stones and may represent a sign of psychopathology.

A systematic diagnostic approach will yield a high likelihood of successfully determining the composition of kidney stones. The steps outlined in Table 21-26 can be carried out in the home environment with the patient eating his or her usual diet. This approach allows ascertainment of the metabolic cause of kidney stones

TABLE 21-26

STRATEGY FOR DIAGNOSIS OF KIDNEY STONE ETIOLOGY

- Obtain four 24-hour urine collections for determination of lithogenic substances while patient ingests usual diet
  - Under acid or thymol preservative, collect for calcium, citrate, oxalate, creatinine (two collections)
  - Without preservative, collect for phosphorus, uric acid, magnesium, creatinine, β_2-microglobulin (as a prototypic low-molecular-weight protein), albumin, dibasic amino acids
- Perform urine culture
- At end of urine collections, obtain blood for determination of kidney function, electrolytes with bicarbonate level, calcium, phosphorus, magnesium, uric acid; consider levels of intact parathyroid hormone, 25(OH)D, 1,25(OH)$_2$D; consider bone mineral density testing
- Compare urine excretions to normative data (Table 21-27)
- Obtain radiographic imaging studies, as needed

in over 93% of 250 children. Representative normative values for urinary constituents are shown in Table 21-27.

TREATMENT APPROACHES TO KIDNEY STONES

There is no medical therapy that can remove or dissolve existing kidney stones in the urinary tract of children, although limited data suggest that some urate stones in adults may undergo dissolution with parenteral bicarbonate-based fluid therapy. Medical therapy includes dietary alteration and liberal fluid intake as first principles. Medications designed to prevent new stone formation or to lessen the likelihood of increased size of existing stones should be considered. Medical therapies that normalize the abnormal urinary constituents associated with stone formation greatly reduce or eliminate the likelihood of new stone formation. Thiazide diuretics will markedly reduce hypercalciuria and are frequently used to treat idiopathic hypercalciuria and prevent excess calcium excretion and stone formation. For patients with metabolic stones, therapy must be related to the underlying defect or must compensate for the alterations in renal excretion of related compounds such as uric acid, xanthine, or cystine. Maintaining solubility of such compounds in the urine may be achieved by manipulating urine pH, osmolarity, or electrolyte content.

Stone removal may be needed with acute urinary obstruction, recurrent urinary infection, or other symptoms. Techniques include extracorporeal shock-wave lithotripsy (ESWL), percutaneous techniques for stone removal, or operative stone removal. The long-term safety of ESWL as related to kidney growth and development in infants and children is, as yet, undetermined.

TABLE 21-27

NORMATIVE DATA FOR EXCRETION OF SELECTED LITHOGENIC SUBSTANCES

SUBSTANCE	REFERENCE RANGE
Calcium	≤ 4 mg/kg/d for children ≥ 2 yr of age
Citrate	≥ 0.5 mg/mg creatinine/d
Oxalate	≤ 0.5 mmol/m^2/d
Uric acid	Varies with age, up to a maximum of 750 mg/d in adolescence

PROGNOSIS

Kidney stones represent a form of chronic disease that recurs with a high frequency if untreated. Prompt recognition of the causes of a kidney stone may allow institution of medical therapy that alters the natural history. Success at stone prevention requires a team of dedicated health professionals knowledgeable about the diseases that produce kidney stones and parents or guardians and children who are able to be compliant with life-long medical therapy.

References

Langman CB: L Genetics and the environment in pediatric urolithiasis. In: Rodgers AL, Hibbert BE, Hess B, Khan SR, Preminger GM (eds): Urolithiasis 2000, Book of Proceedings, Vol 2. 9th International Symposium on Urolithiasis, University of Cape Town, Cape Town, South Africa, 2000, pg 427–436

Neuhaus TJ, Belzer T, Blau N, Hoppe B, Sidhu H, Leumann E: Urinary oxalate excretion in urolithiasis and nephrocalcinosis. Arch Dis Child 82:322–326, 2000

Scheinman SJ, Cox JPD, Lloyd SE, et al: Isolated hypercalciuria with mutation in *CLCN5*: relevance to idiopathic hypercalciuria. Kidney Int 57(1):232–239, 2000

21.13 CHRONIC RENAL INSUFFICIENCY

Sandra L. Watkins

Recent interest in the outcomes of patients receiving dialysis and renal transplantation has heightened awareness of the importance of care for the pre–end-stage renal disease patient. This is especially true for pediatric patients, in whom growth and development may be impacted by chronic renal insufficiency long before end-stage renal disease (ESRD) is reached. Early intervention in the course of chronic renal failure may help to prevent progression to ESRD in addition to promoting improved outcomes of ESRD therapies.

The care of the young child with ESRD has changed dramatically in the last 30 years. By the early 1960s, both renal allotransplantation and chronic hemodialysis had been performed successfully. In the late 1970s and 1980s, the advent of home peritoneal dialysis greatly expanded the repertoire of care for children with ESRD. Today, renal replacement therapy is routinely available to infants and children of all ages with renal failure, and most are surviving well into adulthood. Thus, it becomes important to maximize the care of these patients during the years of progressive chronic renal insufficiency (CRI). The goal is to allow infants and children with chronic renal failure to reach their full developmental, intellectual, and physical potential while enhancing the quality of their lives.

ETIOLOGY

Approximately 60% of children with CRI have an underlying congenital structural abnormality as the etiology of their renal disease. This percentage approaches 80% in infants under 1 year of age. Glomerulonephritis accounts for 15% of chronic renal insufficiency cases, with the other 25% of underlying conditions being a potpourri of infections, malignancy, and other acquired diseases. Diabetic nephropathy rarely results in chronic renal insufficiency during childhood, but many adults who develop ESRD from diabetic nephropathy in their 20s and 30s presented with insulin-dependent diabetes during childhood.

EPIDEMIOLOGY

The point prevalence of ESRD in children in the United States is 66 per million, and the incidence is 13 per million. The prevalence and incidence of CRI are unknown because they are not tracked by the United States Renal Data System, but estimates are that CRI may be 5 to 10 times more common than ESRD. Children and adolescents account for only 3% of the total dialysis population of the United States.

PROGRESSION

Once CRI has become established, an inexorable progression to ESRD over time can be anticipated. This progression occurs even when the underlying process is inactive, such as in the case of renal dysplasia, treated glomerulonephritis, or resolved vesicoureteral reflux. End-stage kidneys demonstrate remarkably similar histologic patterns, suggesting that, regardless of initial disease, the response of the kidney at a cellular level represents a final common pathway. Unfortunately, the mechanisms responsible for the cellular response that leads to renal scarring are undetermined.

Experimental models, such as the remnant kidney model, provide evidence to suggest that (1) systemic hypertension and glomerular hypertension play a role in the progression of renal failure; (2) amelioration of increased glomerular pressures, eg, low-protein diets or the use of angiotensin–converting enzyme inhibitors (ACE I), protects against progressive glomerulosclerosis; (3) growth factors are increased and appear to play some role in the final common pathway of the end-stage kidney; (4) inhibition of transforming growth factor β demonstrates a slowing of progression of glomerulosclerosis. However, none of these models fully explains the progression to ESRD in humans, but these observations are the basis of some of the therapeutic interventions that are attempted with CRI patients.

Other factors have also been postulated to play a role in progressive renal scarring, including ongoing activity of the primary disease, other dietary factors in addition to protein, hyperlipidemia, altered coagulation, proteinuria, calcium/phosphate deposition, systemic hypertension, race, sex, and nephrotoxins.

21.13.1   Clinical Consequences and Pathophysiology

PROGRESSION OF RENAL INSUFFICIENCY

In the human, loss of renal tissue results in compensatory hypertrophy of the remaining renal mass and to increased glomerular filtration capacity so that initially no change in the serum creatinine concentration is evident. However, if the damage is extensive, the ultimate ongoing sclerosis will eventually translate into a rising creatinine and progression to ESRD. The level of GFR at which inexorable decline begins is not definitively known. Some studies suggest that patients with a GFR greater than 50% of normal may not progress to ESRD during their lifetime. A recent study in adult patients with GFR of 10 to 55 mL/min demonstrated that the average rate of loss of GFR, −4 mL/min/yr, was remarkably stable at all levels of initial GFR, although the progression of individual patients varied widely.

Changes in serum creatinine may be deceptive in following the course of CRI (see Sec. 21.5): (1) The S_{cr} will remain in the normal range until 50% of GFR is lost; (2) once S_{Cr} is elevated what appear to be rapid increases will occur because each halving of GFR results in doublings of S_{Cr}; and (3) as GFR declines, secretion of creatinine increases so that S_{Cr} underestimates GFR.

Tubular function is preserved until much later in the course of progression because hypertrophy of tubular mass allows more tubular reabsorption of various solutes such as phosphate. In fact, serum sodium concentration is maintained in the normal range until complete renal failure is reached.

MANIFESTATIONS OF UREMIA

As glomerular filtration rate falls, serum creatinine and blood urea nitrogen concentrations increase. These are surrogate markers for uremia but are not thought to be uremic toxins. Other compounds such as guanidines, amines that are products of metabolism of protein, homocysteine, and uncharacterized compounds of middle molecular weight (500–3000) have been implicated as the true uremic toxins. Regardless of the causative agents, uremia leads to a well-described constellation of symptoms affecting the neurologic, endocrine, gastrointestinal, dermatologic, hematologic, cardiovascular, and pulmonary systems (see Table 21-28). Many of these symptoms become evident early in the course of chronic renal insufficiency.

In children, the effects of uremia on development and neurologic function, nutritional needs, somatic growth, social adaptation, and the psychosocial functioning of the family and the relatively poor survival are unique. Many of these issues are particularly important during infancy. Other aspects of CRI are similar to those seen in adults, including renal bone disease, anemia, and electrolyte and acid-base disturbances.

GROWTH FAILURE Growth failure has long been recognized in children with chronic renal failure. Because recent advances in dialysis and transplantation offer the potential for the child with ESRD to live well into adulthood, the problem of growth failure is magnified, as these children are unlikely to reach normal adult stature.

Most children with renal insufficiency exhibit profound growth retardation. The average height of adults who suffered from chronic renal failure during childhood is 3 standard deviations below the mean. Further, 62% of boys and 41% of girls who experienced renal replacement therapy before the age of 15 have final adult heights less than the normal range. Because one-third of postnatal stature is attained in the first 2 years of life, infants with CRI demonstrate severe statural height failure. Older children parallel the growth pattern of the normal child but well below the median, and the adolescent has an attenuated pubertal growth spurt.

Growth failure can occur relatively early in the progression of CRI. In a large national registry of children with CRI, nearly 25% of those with a mild renal insufficiency (50–75% normal GFR) already had heights less than the fifth percentile for age, 60% of those with a GFR 20% of normal fell below the fifth percentile for height. Many factors are thought to contribute to the growth failure associated with chronic renal insufficiency, but the mechanisms responsible for their effects are poorly understood.

TABLE 21-28

SIGNS AND SYMPTOMS OF THE UREMIC SYNDROME

Neurologic
  Tiredness
  Weakness
  Inability to concentrate
  Poor memory
  Asterixis
  Seizures
  Peripheral neuropathy
  Restless leg syndrome
  Muscle cramping
Endocrine
  Poor statural growth
  2° hyperparathyroidism
  Hyperlipidemia
  Ovarian dysfunction
  Testicular dysfunction
  Altered thyroid function
Gastrointestinal
  Nausea/vomiting
  Anorexia
  Pancreatitis
Dermatologic
  Pruritus
  Calcifications
  Pigmentary changes
Hematologic
  Anemia
  Neutrophil dysfunction
  Platelet dysfunction
Cardiovascular
  Accelerated atherosclerosis
  Pericarditis
Pulmonary
  Atypical pulmonary edema
  Pleuritis

SOURCE: *Bailey JL, Mitch WE: Pathophysiology of uremia. In: Brenner BM, Rector FC, eds: The Kidney, 6th ed. Philadelphia, WB Saunders, 2000:2060.*

Poor nutritional intake can certainly influence growth in any setting, and chronic renal failure is no exception. Some modest improvement in height SD scores with nutritional intervention has been reported. Renal osteodystrophy, intercurrent infections, metabolic acidosis, and tubular defects have been correlated to poor growth, and specific therapy for these defects can be growth enhancing. Corticosteroids are well known to inhibit statural growth. Although chronic anemia was long thought to be a contributing factor to growth failure, early reports of correction of anemia with recombinant erythropoietin have been disappointing regarding improvement in nutrition or growth. Psychosocial factors have also been shown to affect the growth of children with impaired renal function.

Growth hormone levels and responses to provocative testing are elevated in children with renal failure. An inverse correlation between renal function and growth hormone levels and/or urinary growth hormone excretion has been demonstrated. However, increased serum concentrations of growth hormone may, in part, reflect diminished clearances, making interpretation of measurements difficult. Growth hormone functions by stimulating production and release of insulin-like growth factor I (IGF-I) as well as by more direct effects on target tissues. The status of IGF-I and binding proteins for growth hormone in uremic children is being investigated.

RENAL OSTEODYSTROPHY Renal failure has long been known to be associated with bone disease and major disturbances of mineral metabolism. The kidney plays an important role in the regulation of calcium, phosphorus, and magnesium homeostasis (see Sec. 24.11). The proximal tubule is the final site for the synthesis of 1,25-dihydroxyvitamin D through 1α-hydroxylation. The kidney is also one of the major target organs for parathyroid hormone. As with other aspects of uremia, the effects of bone disease can become more pronounced during periods of rapid growth, leading to prominent and long-lasting bony abnormalities in children with CRI.

As with growth failure, renal osteodystrophy can occur very early in the course of chronic renal insufficiency. Similarly, the severity can be quite variable. Elevated levels of parathyroid hormone can be seen in mild CRI. Changes in bone histology become apparent with moderate chronic renal insufficiency. With progression of the renal failure, renal osteodystrophy worsens, in some cases leading to severe muscle weakness and parathyroid gland enlargement.

The pathophysiology of renal osteodystrophy is complex and not completely understood. Certainly phosphate retention with progressive renal failure plays a major role. However, overt hyperphosphatemia does not generally occur until the GFR is 25 to 30% of normal and thus is a late sign of disordered mineral metabolism. Alterations in phosphate excretion lead to decreased levels of serum 1,25-dihydroxyvitamin D in early CRI, thus modifying parathyroid hormone secretion. Decreased levels of 1,25-dihydroxyvitamin D lead to impaired intestinal absorption of calcium from the diet, causing serum calcium levels to fall, which in turn triggers increased secretion of parathyroid hormone, thus perpetuating the problem. The primary histologic lesion seen in renal osteodystrophy is a high-turnover disorder leading to osteitis fibrosa. However, low-turnover lesions and impaired mineralization with osteomalacia can also occur.

Clinical manifestations of renal osteodystrophy include growth retardation, bone pain, slipped capital femoral epiphyses, muscle weakness, extraskeletal calcifications, and bony deformities, including bowing and rachitic changes such as rachitic rosary, frontal bossing, and widened metaphyses of the wrists and ankles.

ANEMIA Anemia of chronic renal insufficiency was recognized over 100 years ago and is characterized by a hypoproliferative, normocytic picture and, like other signs and symptoms of uremia, correlates somewhat with the degree of renal insufficiency. The primary problem is decreased production of red blood cells secondary to decreased synthesis of erythropoietin. Other less significant factors may include marrow fibrosis secondary to hyperparathyroidism, direct effects of uremic toxins on the marrow, aluminum accumulation, and dietary iron deficiency.

Erythropoietin, a glycoprotein, is synthesized by cells adjacent to proximal tubular cells in the inner cortex and outer medulla of the kidney. In response to an oxygen sensor in the kidney, erythropoietin is released and stimulates the hematopoietic stem cells to mature to erythroid cells. Erythropoietin further fosters the addition of iron to the heme moiety and may be effective in preventing apoptosis of erythroid progenitors.

As renal failure progresses, the synthesis of erythropoietin is decreased, leading to progressive anemia over time, which typically becomes a clinically significant problem when CRI reaches moderate proportions with GFR less than 50 mL/min/m². The anemia

of chronic renal failure contributes to many of the symptoms of uremia including poor appetite, tiredness, weakness, and poor school performance.

ELECTROLYTE AND ACID-BASE DISTURBANCES Tubular function is generally well preserved until late in the course of renal failure. However, in some situations electrolyte and acid-base homeostasis may be impaired when chronic renal insufficiency is still relatively mild. Infants and children with obstructive uropathy may have impaired sodium retention, which renders them prone to extracellular volume contraction, and this can be further exacerbated by an inability to adequately concentrate the urine. Thus, these children can become significantly volume depleted and require intervention.

The ability to excrete potassium is generally maintained until ESRD is reached. However, the balance is precarious and depends in part on the actions of aldosterone. If children with chronic renal insufficiency are given spironolactone, an agent that inhibits aldosterone activity, serious hyperkalemia can result. Similarly, these patients may be overly sensitive to angiotensin-converting enzyme inhibitors, which can cause hyperkalemia (see Sec. 21.4).

Metabolic acidosis can be related to CRI and is especially pronounced in conditions with tubular dysfunction such as obstructive uropathy or MCDK because of an inability to excrete acid in the distal tubule. Chronic acidosis can significantly impair growth and bone development.

Renal tubular disorders (see Sec. 21.11) such as Fanconi syndrome, renal tubular acidosis, hypophosphatemic rickets, Bartter syndrome, and others may require supplementation with potassium, phosphorus, and/or bicarbonate. If CRI develops, the renal wasting often improves with decreased filtered load and, paradoxically, the need for mineral and electrolyte supplementation decreases.

NEUROLOGIC DEVELOPMENT The developing central nervous system appears to be especially susceptible to injury leading to developmental delays and severe dysfunction. Although the intrauterine period is obviously a vulnerable time, rapid brain growth and myelination continue for the first 6 to 12 months of extrauterine life. Infants with chronic renal insufficiency appear to be especially susceptible to developmental delays and learning disabilities.

Suggested reasons for central nervous system and developmental abnormalities in this population have included aluminum toxicity, hyperparathyroidism and the resultant bone disease, deafness (may be as high as 40% in infants with congenital renal malformations), malnutrition, psychosocial and motor effects of frequent hospitalizations and physical restriction, anemia, and uremic toxins. Poor caloric intake has been demonstrated in infants with CRI because of anorexia, early satiety, gastroesophageal reflux, poor motility, vomiting, and abnormal gastrointestinal hormonal activity. Poor nutrition leads to abnormal cephalic growth and inevitably to developmental delay.

Recent practices of using non–aluminum-containing phosphate binders, 1,25-dihydroxyvitamin D, recognition of hearing defects, nasogastric and gastrostomy nutritional supplementation, home therapy, and recombinant erythropoietin have led to improvement in neurologic function and development in these infants. Studies of infants and toddlers followed longitudinally demonstrate reduced incidence of developmental delay, which is milder and more amenable to therapeutic intervention than that seen previously.

NUTRITION

Neurologic development, growth, renal osteodystrophy, and anemia are all impacted by the nutrition of the child. Poor nutritional intake in chronic renal insufficiency is probably multifactorial because of anorexia, vomiting, gastroesophageal reflux, and gastrointestinal hormonal imbalance. The anorexia is a major problem, leading to inadequate intake despite often heroic efforts by parents. Early placement of gastrostomy or nasogastric tube for supplemental feedings is often indicated and can lead to improvement in weight velocity, linear growth, and development.

21.13.2   Therapeutic Interventions

PROGRESSION OF RENAL INSUFFICIENCY

Early detection of anatomic abnormalities can often allow for surgical intervention before any permanent renal damage occurs. Fetal ultrasound that detects obstruction and vigorous early investigation of urinary tract infection are two maneuvers that may lead to early correction and prevention of renal injury. Screening programs for hematuria and urinary tract infections have generally been disappointing and not cost-effective.

Long-term clinical studies have clearly demonstrated that treatment of hypertension can slow the rate of renal progression. ACE Is and calcium channel blockers appear to have renal specific effects that may be beneficial in preserving renal function.

Moreover, ACE Is may have a protective effect on the kidney, even in nonhypertensive patients, related either to (1) effects on glomerular hemodynamics, (2) inhibition of transforming growth factor β, or (3) reduction in proteinuria. Progression of diabetic nephropathy has clearly been shown to be slowed with the use of an ACE I in combination with tight glucose control. Human studies in nondiabetic renal disease have been less convincing, and thus, use of ACE Is to prevent progression of chronic renal insufficiency in the nondiabetic remains largely theoretical at this time.

A number of other agents have been suggested for control of the progression of renal disease. These include β-blockers, calcium channel blockers, antihyperlipidemic agents, AT1 receptor blockers, nonsteroidals, and diuretics. None have yet been definitively shown to be useful in the clinical setting. Dietary protein restriction, despite encouraging animal studies, has not been shown in clinical trials to clearly alter the rate of renal failure progression. Because protein intake is so necessary for the growing child, protein restriction currently has no place in the treatment of pediatric renal disease.

CONSEQUENCES OF UREMIA

GROWTH FAILURE Multiple studies have confirmed the effect of recombinant growth hormone in overcoming the short stature associated with CRI in the prepubertal pediatric population. Although more difficult to assess, pubertal children with CRI are also believed to respond favorably to recombinant growth hormone treatment. A landmark randomized, double-blind placebo-controlled trial of recombinant growth hormone treatment of children with chronic renal insufficiency demonstrated doubling of the height velocity over the first year of therapy with an improvement of 1 standard deviation in score. To date concerns regarding potential long-term side effects on glomerulosclerosis and hyperlipidemia have not been borne out by experimental data.

The approach to the child with growth failure associated with CRI begins with a thorough search for contributing factors (Fig. 21-29). Nutrition must be maximized, with supplemental enteral feedings if necessary. Electrolyte abnormalities, acid-base disturbances, and renal osteodystrophy must be assessed and properly treated. If growth continues to be poor (height less than the fifth percentile for age and/or height velocity less than the 25th percentile for age), subcutaneous recombinant growth hormone should be initiated at a dose of 0.05 mg/kg/d (Fig. 21-29). Growth should be monitored at least quarterly. Bone age, hip and knee radiographs, and serum chemistries should be obtained at baseline and followed at regular intervals. Should a child reach predicted 50th percentile height, based on midparental heights, growth hormone therapy should be paused but resumed if growth velocity again falls.

RENAL OSTEODYSTROPHY Children with CRI should be monitored regularly for signs and symptoms of bone disease, including physical exam, serum calcium, phosphate, alkaline phosphatase, and intact parathyroid hormone level. The goal of therapy is to normalize growth and prevent the development of bony deformity, extraskeletal calcifications, and marked secondary hyperparathyroidism. Therapy with calcitriol should be instituted if parathyroid hormone levels are significantly elevated (see Sec. 21.14). Controversy exists regarding the optimal level of parathyroid hormone because concern has been raised that maintaining parathyroid hormone in the normal range may lead to adynamic bone disease or poor growth. Rising phosphorus levels require reduced-phosphate diets and phosphate binding with calcium carbonate or other phosphate binders (see Sec. 21.14). Serum phosphorus levels should be maintained in the 4 to 6 mg/dL range in children and adolescents. Infants should be kept at an age-appropriate level, which may be as high as 8 mg/dL for a premature infant. Some infants may actually require phosphorus supplementation. Aluminum-containing phosphate binders should be avoided because aluminum accumulates in CRI, leading to bone marrow and neurotoxicity. Calcium supplements are generally indicated and may be provided by calcium-containing phosphate binders. Target serum calcium level is the high-normal range.

ANEMIA As with growth failure, the first step in treating the anemia of chronic renal insufficiency is to exclude other causes of anemia, including blood loss, iron deficiency, folate and vitamin B_{12} deficiency, and other common causes of anemia (Fig. 21-30). Hypertension and renal osteodystrophy must be well controlled prior to initiation of recombinant erythropoietin. Once these entities are excluded and/or treated, therapy with recombinant erythropoietin should be initiated if the hemoglobin level is below 10 g/dL (Hct < 30%). A reticulocyte response is seen after two to three doses, which correlates with increased erythron transferrin uptake. Within several weeks of therapy the hemoglobin starts to rise.

Therapy should begin with 50 to 100 U/kg/dose subcutaneously, given two or three times weekly. Once the target hemoglobin of 11 to 13 g/dL (33–36% Hct) is reached, doses should be decreased to maintain a stable hemoglobin, generally a dose of 25 to 100 U/kg/dose one to three times per week.

Iron management is a crucial component to erythropoietin therapy. The major reason for the suboptimal erythropoietic response to recombinant erythropoietin is iron deficiency, which results, in part, from the increased rate of erythropoiesis and the associated demand for iron. Functional iron deficiency, a state in which transferrin-bound iron is rapidly depleted despite the presence of ade-

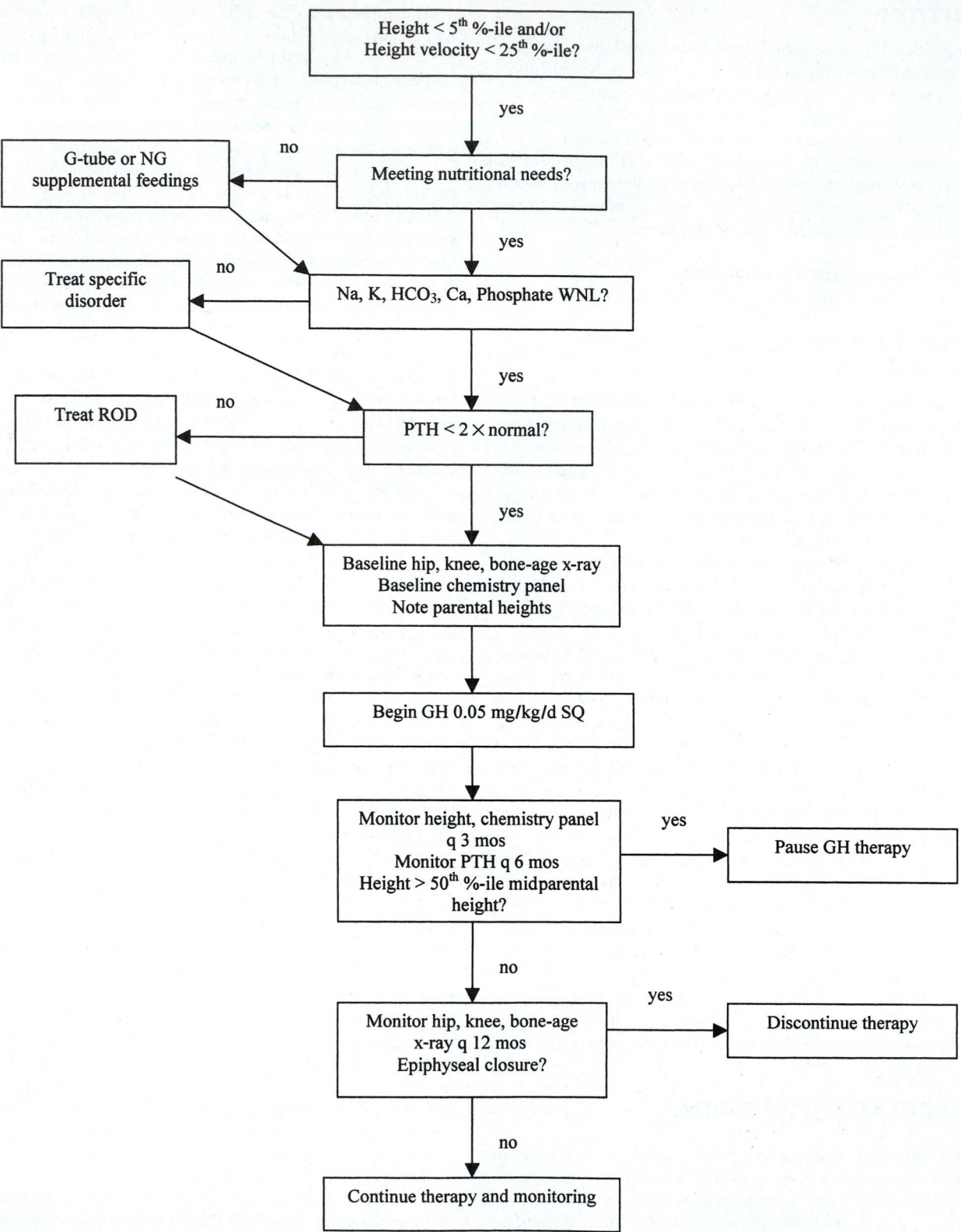

FIGURE 21-29 Management of growth failure in chronic renal insufficiency. G-tube = gastrostomy tube; NG = nasogastric; Na = sodium; K = potassium; HCO_3 = bicarbonate; Ca = calcium; WNL = within normal limits; PTH = parathyroid hormone; ROD = renal osteodystrophy; GH = recombinant growth hormone; SQ = subcutaneous.

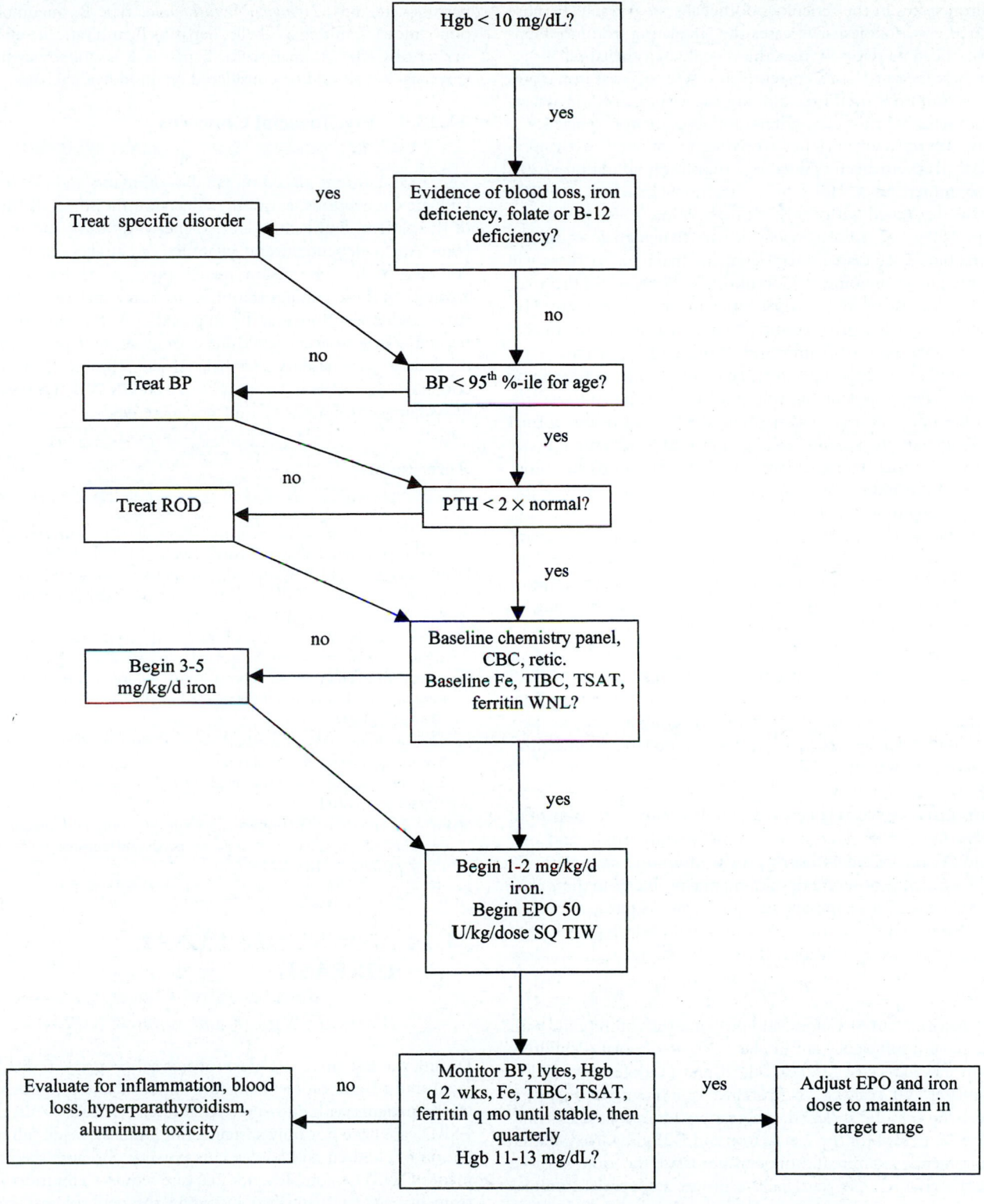

FIGURE 21-30 Management of the anemia of chronic renal failure. Hgb = hemoglobin; BP = blood pressure; PTH = parathyroid hormone; ROD = renal osteodystrophy; CBC = complete blood count; retic = reticulocyte count; Fe = iron; TIBC = total iron-binding capacity; TSAT = transferrin saturation; WNL = within normal limits; EPO = recombinant erythropoietin; SQ = subcutaneous; TIW = thrice weekly; lytes = electrolytes.

quate iron stores in the reticuloendothelial system results because stimulated erythropoiesis decreases the circulating iron more rapidly than it can be released from the reticuloendothelial cell.

The best measurements currently available to assess iron stores are the serum iron, total iron-binding capacity, transferrin saturation, and serum ferritin. The criteria for absolute iron deficiency in patients with renal insufficiency receiving recombinant erythropoietin have arbitrarily been defined as a transferrin saturation < 20% and a serum ferritin < 100 g/mL. Functional or relative iron deficiency is diagnosed with transferrin saturation >30% and serum ferritin >600 g/mL. Oral iron may be needed in high doses initially while red blood cell mass is increasing, and maintenance doses will be required in an ongoing fashion during erythropoietin therapy.

Adverse events related to erythropoietin therapy are rare. Hyperkalemia may occur in anephric patients as a result of markedly increased intake as appetite improves. Worsening hypertension was also encountered in 22% of patients, especially if patients are volume overloaded. Development of antibodies to recombinant erythropoietin has not been reported. Beneficial effects of nearly normal hemoglobin in these patients include improved patient survival, decreased left ventricular mass, decreased hospitalizations and other measures of morbidity, and improved quality of life, exercise tolerance, and cognitive function.

If resistance to the effects of erythropoietin appears to occur, underlying conditions such as aluminum toxicity, severe hyperparathyroidism with marrow fibrosis, inflammatory disease, true or functional iron deficiency, or occult gastrointestinal bleeding or other external blood loss should be assessed.

ELECTROLYTE AND ACID-BASE DISTURBANCES Infants with severe obstruction and dysplasia can have significant fluid and sodium needs that must be provided through nutritional intake (see Sec. 21.3). Tubular damage leads to polyuria secondary to concentration defects, salt wasting, and acidosis.

NEUROLOGIC ABNORMALITIES Careful attention to nutrition, avoidance of aluminum, control of renal osteodystrophy and anemia, and the use of recombinant growth hormone can greatly reduce the incidence of severe developmental problems in these children. Evaluation for deafness, visual problems, seizures, and delays should be pursued if indicated. Early testing for learning disabilities and referral for special education can be very helpful as the children mature.

NUTRITIONAL NEEDS Caloric and protein needs of the child with chronic renal insufficiency are similar to those of normal children. An infant should receive 115 kcal/kg/d, and an adolescent requires approximately 40 kcal/kg/d. Protein requirements of an infant may be as high as 2.2 g/kg/d, whereas an adolescent needs only 0.8 g/kg/d. Except for the special iron and 1,25-dihydroxyvitamin D requirements, vitamin and mineral needs are the same as those for healthy children. As renal failure progresses, special formulas with altered concentrations of sodium, potassium, phosphate, or protein may become necessary. A qualified pediatric renal dietitian is most helpful in the management of these patients.

21.13.3   General Health Maintenance

The ultimate goal for all children with renal failure is transplantation. Because after transplantation these children will be immunocompromised, immunizations should be complete for diphtheria,

pertussis, tetanus, *Hemophilus influenzae* type B, pneumococcus, polio, measles, mumps, rubella, hepatitis B, and varicella during the period of CRI. Vaccination for hepatitis A is still somewhat controversial but should be considered on an individual basis.

21.13.4   Psychosocial Concerns

The social burdens placed on families of infants and children with CRI are tremendous, as are the effects on the social development of the patient. Some children become withdrawn, and others become overly dependent and infantilized. Families express various emotions such as depression, denial, anger, hope, impatience, and anxiety. As these families transition to home dialysis, even greater stress and disruption may be imposed. Involvement of specially trained social workers, child-life therapists, and psychologists is needed to help patients and their families cope with this chronic condition. In addition, the impact of a child's CRI/ESRD on normal siblings should not be underestimated.

References

Brandt JR, Avner ED, Hickman RO, Watkins SL: Safety and efficacy of erythropoietin in children. Pediatr Nephrol 13(2):143–147, 1999

Fennell RS, Fennell EB, Carter RL, Mings EL, Klausner AB, Hurst JR: A longitudinal study of the cognitive function of children with renal failure. Pediatr Nephrol 4:11–15, 1990

Fine RN, Kohaut EC, Brown D, Perlman AJ, for the Genentech Cooperative Study Group: Growth after recombinant human growth hormone treatment in children with chronic renal failure: report of a multicenter randomized double-blind placebo-controlled study. J Pediatr 124(3): 374–382, 1994

Salusky IB, Ramirez JA, Goodman WG: Disorders of bone and mineral metabolism in chronic renal failure. In: Holliday MA, Barratt TM, Avner ED, eds: Pediatric Nephrology, 3rd ed. Baltimore, Williams & Wilkins, 1994:1287–1304

Sedman A, Griedman A, Boineau F, Strife FC, Fine R: Nutritional management of the child with mild to moderate chronic renal failure. J Pediatr 129:13s–18s, 1996

21.14 END-STAGE RENAL DISEASE

Beatriz D. Kuizon and Isidor B. Salusky

During the last three decades, substantial progress in dialysis and renal transplantation has markedly impacted the prognosis of pediatric patients with end-stage renal disease (ESRD). Advances in ESRD care have not only sustained life but also made full rehabilitation of children and adolescents possible. Because the management of ESRD is complex, optimal care requires a multidisciplinary team of pediatric specialists including the nephrologist, surgeon, urologist, psychologist or psychiatrist, dialysis nursing staff, occupational and physical therapist, play therapist, renal dietitian, social worker, and other personnel who are trained in pediatric ESRD care and who can contribute to improving the quality of life of the patient and the family while dialysis is utilized. Early referral to the pediatric ESRD centers should therefore be encouraged to facilitate coordination of these services.

Conservative management before dialysis is directed toward minimizing the progression of renal disease, preventing and treating the complications of renal failure, maximizing growth and development, as well as improving school attendance and academic performance (see Sec. 21.13). When progression of renal failure occurs, early counseling regarding the forms of renal replacement therapy (peritoneal dialysis, hemodialysis, renal transplantation) should be undertaken, allowing enough time for access placement and wound healing, patient/parent education, and initiation of dialysis before the patient becomes symptomatic. More importantly, efforts should be directed toward preparation for transplantation and evaluation of potential living donors because successful transplantation remains the optimal treatment of children and adolescents with ESRD.

21.14.1 Indications for Maintenance Dialysis

Although no predetermined threshold level of serum creatinine or blood urea nitrogen has been established above which dialysis should be started, regular dialysis is usually considered when the creatinine clearance has decreased below 10 mL/min/1.73 m^2. Children with advanced renal disease may present with nonspecific symptoms such as decreased appetite, nausea and vomiting, easy fatigability, reduced exercise tolerance, and poor school performance, which may prompt dialysis initiation (see Table 21-28). Poor growth may also suggest prompt dialysis, particularly in younger children. In addition, regular dialysis should be considered when nutritional requirements cannot be maintained because of severe fluid limitations. Stringent protein restriction in an attempt to maintain blood urea nitrogen levels within acceptable limits to delay dialysis therapy or attempt to prevent renal progression should be avoided because of the inherent risk of malnutrition. Other indications for initiation of dialysis are similar to those resulting from acute renal failure and include fluid overload associated with congestive heart failure or hypertension, uncontrolled hyperkalemia, metabolic acidosis, and hyperphosphatemia.

The need for dialysis should be anticipated in order to allow for proper patient and family education on treatment modalities, patient training, and for creation of a functioning vascular or peritoneal access even before dialysis is required. Whenever possible, dialysis should not be started as an emergency procedure because this usually necessitates placement of a temporary vascular access for hemodialysis. Precautions should be taken to preserve vessels for future vascular access.

CHOICE OF DIALYSIS MODALITY

Peritoneal dialysis (PD) and hemodialysis (HD) have both become standard treatments of ESRD in pediatric patients. Although neither modality has been shown to be more advantageous in this population, PD is the preferred treatment modality in pediatric patients in the United States, particularly in the youngest age group. In contrast, HD remains the predominant mode of dialysis in adult patients with ESRD. The advantages of PD include relatively stable serum biochemistries and blood pressure and fewer restrictions on dietary and fluid intake because dialysis is performed daily; simplicity of the procedure permits dialysis to be done at home, thus allowing greater flexibility of the dialysis regimen, infrequent interruptions of the school schedule, decreased reliance on the dialysis center, reduced requirements for erythropoietin and blood transfusions, and avoidance of venipunctures. Thus, PD is most suited for infants and young children, patients with severe cardiovascular disease or with vascular access difficulties, and those who live far from the dialysis center. Absolute contraindications for PD include

peritoneal membrane failure, presence of extensive abdominal adhesions that obstruct dialysate flow, surgically uncorrectable mechanical defects that prevent effective PD or increase the risk of infection (omphalocele, gastroschisis, diaphragmatic hernia, bladder extrophy), and inability to identify a person (usually a parent) who can be trained for PD if the patient is incapable of performing PD. Relative contraindications for PD include newly placed abdominal foreign bodies (ventriculoperitoneal shunt), peritoneal leaks, body size limitations, inability to tolerate exchange volumes required to achieve adequate clearance or fluid removal, inflammatory or ischemic bowel disease or frequent episodes of diverticulitis, morbid obesity, and severe malnutrition.

Hemodialysis is the preferred modality in a greater proportion of adolescent patients with ESRD. Reasons for choosing hemodialysis include shorter treatment time and freedom from dialysis responsibilities, and the main contraindication for hemodialysis is failure to maintain a vascular access. Cardiac failure and coagulopathy are relative contraindications to HD. Although hemodialysis can be offered in very young children, it is technically more challenging because of patient size, high rate of vascular access thrombosis or failure, and need for skilled and experienced dialysis personnel.

21.14.2 Dialytic Modalities

PERITONEAL DIALYSIS

Peritoneal dialysis is a process that facilitates transport of solutes and fluid between the capillary blood and the dialysate fluid through the peritoneal membrane, a serous membrane that lines the inner surface of the abdominal wall and reflects over the visceral organs. The procedure requires repeated instillation and drainage of dialysate solution into the abdominal cavity through a peritoneal dialysis catheter, which has been surgically placed through the abdominal wall. Because families are trained to perform peritoneal dialysis at home, in-center intermittent peritoneal dialysis is often reserved for the period of training for home care. Continuous dialysis can be delivered manually (continuous ambulatory peritoneal dialysis, CAPD) or through an automated cycler machine (continuous cycling peritoneal dialysis, CCPD, or automated peritoneal dialysis, APD), although the majority of patients in the United States prefer APD. In CAPD, the patient or the parent connects a bag of dialysate solution to the peritoneal dialysis catheter, and the dialysate solution is instilled into the peritoneal cavity using exchange volumes that range between 900 and 1100 mL/m^2 or 35 to 45 mL/kg. After 4 to 6 hours, the dialysate is drained into the same bag, which is disinfected, and a new bag is attached. Three or four such exchanges are done during the day, and an additional 6- to 8-hour exchange is carried out at night. The CCPD/APD technique, on the other hand, is performed using a cycler machine, generally involves five or six short-dwell exchanges over 10 to 12 hours at night, and may include a long exchange during the day. In infants, however, 8 to 12 hourly exchanges are usually needed for fluid removal. Both techniques are comparable in efficacy.

Peritoneal dialysis removes nitrogenous waste products such as urea and creatinine through the process of diffusion, whereby solutes move from a greater concentration to a lesser concentration (eg, from the blood compartment to the dialysate compartment) across the peritoneal membrane. Convection or solvent drag also contributes to solute transfer. High concentrations of glucose in the dialysate solution create an osmotic gradient that facilitates net movement of water into the peritoneal cavity (ultrafiltration). Additional fluid is absorbed by the subdiaphragmatic lymphatic system, however, so that the net fluid removal is the difference between ultrafiltration and lymphatic drainage. The glucose concentration of dialysate solution ranges from 1.5 to 4.25% (1.5 to 4.25 g/100 mL), and the concentration is adjusted to achieve the desired amount of ultrafiltration. Dialysate solutions also contain electrolytes in physiological concentrations to correct acid-base and electrolyte abnormalities. Dialysate sodium is lower (132 meq/L) than plasma levels because approximately half of the ultrafiltrate is composed of free water. Dialysate solutions do not contain potassium to facilitate its removal during dialysis. The buffer present in most commercially available peritoneal dialysate solutions is lactate (40 meq/L), which is rapidly converted to bicarbonate in patients with normal liver function. To avoid negative calcium balance, dialysate solutions also contain calcium (2.5–3.5 meq/L).

The main complications of PD are peritonitis and catheter-related infections. On average, one peritonitis episode occurs every patient year, and more frequently in younger children. Peritonitis is suspected when the patient presents with cloudy peritoneal fluid, abdominal pain and/or tenderness, and sometimes fever. Patients/parents are trained to obtain dialysate fluid for cell count, Gram stain, and culture before starting intraperitoneal antibiotics. A dialysate WBC count $\geq 100/\mu L$ with at least 50% polymorphonuclear cells is suggestive of peritonitis. Most patients are treated successfully with intraperitoneal antibiotics as outpatients except those with severe symptoms or persistent cloudy fluid, for whom hospitalization, administration of intravenous antibiotics, and/or catheter removal may be required. Most infections are caused by gram-positive organisms and to a lesser extent by gram-negative organisms. Fungal peritonitis occurs infrequently and is treated with antifungal medications and catheter removal. Multiple episodes of peritonitis may result in peritoneal membrane failure and eventual switch to HD. The other infectious complications of PD include infection at the catheter exit site, which presents as exudate and erythema of the skin, and tunnel infection, which manifests as erythema, tenderness, and swelling of the subcutaneous pathway of the catheter and may be associated with purulent discharge. Most common organisms are *Staphylococcus* species, followed by gram-negative organisms. Both infections are treated with oral or intraperitoneal antibiotics. A tunnel infection, however, may require catheter removal, especially when it results in peritonitis. Additional complications of PD include inflow/outflow catheter malfunction, catheter migration, subcutaneous leakage of dialysate fluid, hydrothorax, abdominal wall or inguinal hernia, and pain during inflow/outflow of dialysate fluid.

HEMODIALYSIS

Hemodialysis is a process whereby excess fluid and toxins are removed by the extracorporeal circulation of blood through a dialyzer. Blood is pumped from the patient to the dialyzer and then returned back to the patient via a central catheter or arteriovenous fistula. Diffusion occurs through a semipermeable membrane that separates the blood and the dialysate fluid. Because the direction of blood flow is opposite to that of the dialysate flow (countercurrent flow), the concentration gradient between the two compartments is maintained, thus maximizing diffusion of solutes. The pressure gradient across the membrane (transmembrane pressure) and the ultrafiltration coefficient (permeability of membrane to water) of the membrane regulate fluid removal from the blood to the dialysate compartment (ultrafiltration). As in PD, the dialysate solution used in HD contains electrolytes in physiological concentra-

tions to normalize the acid-base and electrolyte abnormalities. Dialysate sodium concentration is usually 140 meq/L to prevent hypotension and cramps from rapid fluid removal. Dialysate potassium concentration is adjusted based on the serum potassium level. Bicarbonate (35 meq/L) is the major buffer, which avoids blood pressure instability associated with acetate use. Similar to PD, HD solutions contain calcium (2.5–3.5 meq/L) to avoid negative calcium balance. Hemodialysis is required three to four times a week in most patients, with each procedure lasting 3 to 4 hours and preferably performed in a facility with experience caring for children and adolescents.

Hemodialysis requires vascular access that allows sufficient blood flow to support the extracorporeal circuit. Creation of an arteriovenous (AV) fistula between the radial artery and cephalic vein (Brescia-Cimino) has been standard practice in adult HD patients because of longer patency rate and lower rates of thrombosis and infection. In pediatric patients, however, this technique has been reserved for bigger children and adolescents because of vessel size. Ideally, placement of an AV fistula should be done a few months before the expected need for dialysis to allow maturation of the fistula and to avoid placement of a temporary HD catheter. In younger children, other options include placement of either an arteriovenous graft using synthetic material (polytetrafluoroethylene) or cuffed dual-lumen permanent catheter. Catheters should be placed in the internal jugular vein rather than in the subclavian vein, if possible, because of attendant risk of subclavian vein stenosis and/or thrombosis.

Access malfunction and infection are major complications of hemodialysis. Long maturation time and primary failure are problems associated with AV fistula placement in children. Stenosis at the venous anastomosis site is treated with angioplasty or surgical correction. Thrombosis of the HD catheter may be treated initially with intraluminal administration of thrombin plasminogen activator, but persistent dysfunction may require catheter stripping or replacement. Local infections are treated initially with antibiotics against gram-positive and gram-negative organisms, and the antibiotics are adjusted based on culture results. More extensive infection of the AV graft may require resection of the infected portion of the graft. Persistent bacteremia may require catheter removal. Other access complications include AV fistula aneurysm and arterial steal syndrome.

The other complications of hemodialysis are associated with the rapid rate of fluid and solute removal. Ultrafiltration of large volumes of fluid over a short period increases the likelihood of hypotension, especially in patients with poor cardiac function. Rapid solute shifts potentially precipitate cerebral edema and dialysis disequilibrium, which is characterized by headache, nausea, vomiting, or even seizures and coma and can be prevented by avoiding rapid solute removal and by administration of mannitol, particularly during the first few dialysis sessions, in patients with markedly elevated BUN levels.

HEMOFILTRATION/ HEMODIAFILTRATION

Continuous arteriovenous hemofiltration (CAVH), continuous venovenous hemofiltration (CVVH), or, with an additional dialysis component, continuous arteriovenous hemodiafiltration (CAVHD) and continuous venovenous hemodiafiltration (CVVHD) are alternative renal replacement therapies that may be offered in children with acute renal failure. The major advantage of continuous renal replacement therapies is the slow and gradual rate of fluid and solute removal; thus, these procedures are generally better tolerated than intermittent hemodialysis and are best suited for critically ill and hemodynamically unstable patients. In addition, continuous therapies may be considered in patients in whom peritoneal dialysis may be contraindicated (abdominal wall defects, diaphragmatic hernia, acute abdomen, respiratory failure). CAVH requires both arterial and venous catheters and adequate mean arterial pressures to provide blood flow through the extracorporeal circuit. CVVH, on the other hand, uses a double-lumen venous catheter and an external pump to provide blood flow through the filter. Although CAVH is a simpler setup, CVVH avoids the need for an arterial access, and the use of a pump ensures faster and more consistent blood flow rates. Both systems require anticoagulation to prevent clotting of the access, hemofilter, and tubings.

In continuous hemofiltration, fluid removal is achieved by the pressure gradient across a highly permeable membrane, and removal of small and medium-sized solutes occurs through convection or solvent drag. The composition of the fluid removed (ultrafiltrate) is similar to that of plasma. Continuous therapies require replacement fluid because large volumes of ultrafiltrate are removed. To improve solute clearance, dialysate fluid can be also added to the circuit (CAVHD or CVVHD). Most frequently, a 1.5% standard peritoneal dialysate solution is used as dialysate fluid. However, the high glucose content of the solution may lead to hyperglycemia, and the lactate content may result in worsening acidosis in patients with liver failure. In these instances, a bicarbonate-based solution with lower glucose concentration may be specially made by the pharmacy.

21.14.3   Clinical Consequences of ESRD

The clinical consequences of ESRD are similar to those encountered in patients with CRI (see Sec. 21.13). Although the pathophysiological mechanisms related to loss of renal function are the same, management of these clinical consequences must be modified in patients on dialysis.

GROWTH RETARDATION

Factors that have been thought to contribute to growth failure include protein and calorie malnutrition, metabolic acidosis, end-organ growth hormone (GH) resistance, anemia, and renal bone disease (see Sec. 21.13). In addition, linear growth is influenced by the age at onset of CRI and primary renal disease. Management of growth retardation includes provision of adequate nutrition; correction of acidosis, electrolyte abnormalities, and anemia; control of bone disease; and maximizing dialysis. Treatment with recombinant human growth hormone (rhGH) should be considered in patients with significant growth failure (Sec. 21.13 and Fig. 21-29). Although acceleration of growth velocity has been observed during administration of supraphysiological doses of rhGH in children with CRI on conservative management, less favorable responses have been demonstrated in patients undergoing regular dialysis and in transplant recipients. Although the reasons for the variable responses to rhGH administration have yet to be determined, differences in GH resistance, concomitant treatment with large doses of calcitriol, and steroid treatment in renal transplant recipients may be implicated.

ANEMIA

Clinical trials in adult and pediatric patients with ESRD established the efficacy of EPO therapy in increasing hematocrit levels and eliminating transfusion requirements in most patients. With correction of anemia, pediatric patients reported improvements in appetite, physical activity, exercise tolerance, and cognitive function, leading to a better quality of life overall. Erythropoietin therapy is usually initiated at 50 to 100 U/kg/dose one to three times a week when hematocrit levels fall below 30% or sooner if symptoms of anemia develop. Erythropoietin is administered subcutaneously in predialysis patients and in those treated with maintenance peritoneal dialysis (PD), but it is usually given intravenously in those undergoing HD. Intraperitoneal administration of erythropoietin may be considered for patients receiving PD who are unable to tolerate subcutaneous injections. The dose should be adjusted to maintain hematocrit levels between 33 and 36%. The most common cause of inadequate response to EPO therapy is iron deficiency; thus, iron studies (serum iron, total iron-binding capacity, serum ferritin) should be regularly performed, and supplemental iron therapy should be initiated either to replete or maintain adequate iron stores (see Sec. 21.13 and Fig. 21-30). Other reasons for EPO resistance include acute and chronic infection, severe osteitis fibrosa, aluminum toxicity, folate and vitamin B_{12} deficiency, and hemoglobinopathies.

ACIDOSIS

Although limited information regarding the effects of metabolic acidemia on skeletal growth in children with ESRD is available, recent data suggest that alterations in the GH–IGF-1 axis occur. Correction of the metabolic acidemia in most dialysis patients is achieved through lactate supplementation in the PD fluid and through the use of bicarbonate in the HD solution. Some patients, however, may require additional oral doses of sodium bicarbonate or sodium citrate or the use of higher sodium bicarbonate dialysate concentrations if serum bicarbonate levels remain below 22 meq/L. In patients treated with sodium citrate, concomitant use of aluminum-containing phosphate binders should be avoided because citrate increases intestinal aluminum absorption and, therefore, the risk of aluminum toxicity. Such binders are generally contraindicated because of CNS effects also (see Sec. 21.13).

RENAL OSTEODYSTROPHY

The management of children with renal osteodystrophy is aimed at achieving normal bone formation rates and turnover, which can generally be accomplished with dietary phosphorus restriction, phosphate-binding agents, and vitamin D analogs. Dietary phosphorus intake is generally restricted to 400 to 800 mg/d because the quantity removed by either PD (300–400 mg/day) or HD (800 mg/treatment) is often insufficient to prevent hyperphosphatemia. Phosphate-binding agents are often necessary because adherence to dietary restriction is difficult and because of protein requirements for growth. Serum phosphorus levels should be monitored regularly, and levels maintained within the range acceptable for age (see Sec. 21.13). Infants are particularly at risk for hypophosphatemia because of low dietary intake, use of large doses of phosphate binders, phosphate removal by dialysis, and possibly nutritional depletion. Severe and persistent hypophosphatemia can lead to bone disease such as osteomalacia and rickets, proximal myopathy, rhabdomyolysis, and congestive heart failure.

The phosphate-binding agents that are currently available include calcium salts, aluminum-containing compounds, and sevelamer hydrochloride (Renagel). Calcium salts (calcium carbonate, calcium acetate, calcium citrate) are widely prescribed phosphate binders and are also sources of supplemental calcium. Hypercalcemia is the most common side effect of calcium salts, particularly during vitamin D therapy, and can usually be reversed with reductions in the dose of binder or vitamin D or of dialysate calcium concentration. Aluminum-containing phosphate binders were frequently used in the past, but long-term treatment led to bone disease, encephalopathy, and anemia. This class of phosphate binders should be avoided. Sevelamer hydrochloride (Renagel) is a nonabsorbable calcium- and aluminum-free compound that has been reported to reduce serum phosphorus levels in adult patients treated with hemodialysis. Added benefits of lowering serum total serum cholesterol and low-density lipoprotein cholesterol levels and diminishing exogenous calcium load were also observed with Renagel treatment. However, further studies are warranted to evaluate the long-term effects of this new therapy on bone disease in children with ESRD.

Vitamin D analogs have been shown to suppress PTH secretion and reverse the biochemical, radiographic, and histologic changes of high-turnover bone disease. In pediatric patients receiving maintenance dialysis, calcitriol therapy may be started at a daily dose of 0.25 to 0.5 μg/d when serum PTH levels exceed 300 pg/mL. Alternatively, calcitriol may be given intermittently, at a starting dose of 0.5 to 1 μg three times per week administered orally or intravenously. Doses are gradually increased in 0.25- to 0.5-μg increments to achieve serum calcium levels between 10.0 and 10.5 mg/dL. Decreasing the dialysate calcium concentration may allow higher doses of calcitriol to be given. Calcitriol should be discontinued when PTH levels fall below 200 pg/mL in patients treated with dialysis. Long-term treatment with high pulse doses of calcitriol should be undertaken with caution because of the risk of adynamic bone and poor growth in prepubertal children with secondary hyperparathyroidism.

NUTRITION

Appropriate nutritional support and periodic nutritional assessment are important components of ESRD care. Calorie intake according to the recommended daily allowance (RDA) for chronological age should be prescribed initially and adjusted subsequently based on the patient's response (see Sec. 21.13). Because calorie supplementation above the RDA for age has not uniformly resulted in accelerated growth, this approach is not recommended at the present time. Additional calories (7–10 kcal/kg/d) from dialysate glucose absorption should be included in the total caloric intake in patients treated with PD. Because anorexia is common, nutritional supplements must be initiated, particularly in infants and young children, when voluntary intake does not consistently meet the RDA for energy and/or protein or when there is poor growth. Supplements can be given orally by adding carbohydrate, protein, or fat modules in the infant formula or using commercially available supplements for older children. Enteral tube feeding (nasogastric tube, gastrostomy tube) should be considered if oral supplementation alone does not meet the RDA or promote growth.

Patients treated with maintenance HD should initially be prescribed protein intake according to the RDA for chronological age (infants 1.6–2.2 g/kg/d, children aged 1–6 years 1.2 g/kg/d, 7–14 years 1 g/kg/d, and postpubertal patients 0.8 g/kg/d) plus an additional 0.4 g/kg/d. Children undergoing regular PD, on the other hand, require higher protein intake than those treated with HD because of daily protein and amino acid losses through the peritoneum. Initial recommendations should be based on the RDA for chronological age plus the expected peritoneal losses, taking into consideration that dialysate protein loss is greater in small

and young children. Nutritional assessment should be done regularly, and adjustments made as necessary.

Vitamin and mineral intake should also be monitored in patients with ESRD. Dietary intake should provide 100% dietary reference intake for water-soluble vitamins (B$_1$, B$_2$, B$_6$, B$_{12}$, folic acid) and 100% RDA for vitamins A, C, E, and K; copper; and zinc. Supplementation should be considered in patients who are unable to meet these goals.

References

Lerner GR, Warady BA, Sullivan EK, Alexander SR: Chronic dialysis in children and adolescents. The 1996 Annual Report of the North American Pediatric Renal Transplant Cooperative Study. Pediatr Nephrol 13: 404–417, 1999

National Kidney Foundation: NKF-DOQI clinical practice guidelines for peritoneal dialysis adequacy. Am J Kidney Dis 30:S67–S136, 1997

US Renal Data System, USRDS 2000 Annual Data Report. Bethesda: National Institutes of Health, National Institute of Diabetes and Digestive and Kidney Diseases, 2000

Warady BA, Alexander SR, Watkins S, Kohaut E, Harmon WE: Optimal care of the pediatric end-stage renal disease patient on dialysis. Am J Kidney Dis 33:567–583, 1999

21.15 PEDIATRIC RENAL TRANSPLANTATION

Samhar Al-Akash and Robert Ettenger

Kidney transplantation is the therapy of choice for children with end-stage renal disease (ESRD). Successful transplantation ameliorates clinical consequences of ESRD and also significantly improves, and often corrects, delayed skeletal growth, sexual maturation, cognitive performance, and psychosocial functioning. The child with a well-functioning kidney has a robust quality of life and can achieve at a high level.

21.15.1 Epidemiology Transplantation in Children

The most common primary diagnosis of ESRD in transplanted children is structural disease (49%), followed by various forms of glomerulonephritis (14%) and focal segmental glomerulosclerosis (12%) (Table 21-29). At the time of transplant, 46% of pediatric recipients of kidney transplants are >12 years of age, 34% are 6 to 12 years of age, 15% are between the ages of 2 and 5 years, and only 5% are <2 years of age. The mean age of pediatric patients receiving a kidney transplant is 10.9 years. Sixty percent are male, 62% are white, 16% are African-American, and 16% are Hispanic.

Over the last decade, the absolute numbers of pediatric kidney transplants have remained relatively constant and comprise 4 to 6% of all transplants in the United States. The rates for both living related and cadaver renal transplantation are more than double the corresponding rates for adults 20 to 44 years of age.

Virtually half of all pediatric kidney transplants come from living donors, and children continue to represent an ever-decreasing percentage of the waiting list for cadaver donors. Median waiting times continue to lengthen for potential pediatric recipients of cadaver donor transplants (from a minimum of 236 days for children 1–5 years of age to 561 days for adolescents).

TABLE 21-29

CAUSES OF ESRD IN TRANSPLANTED PEDIATRIC PATIENTS, 1987–1998

PRIMARY DISEASE	PERCENTAGE (%)
Structural disease	48.7
Glomerulonephritis	14.5
Focal segmental glomerulosclerosis	11.8
Hemolytic uremic syndrome	2.6
Congenital nephrotic syndrome	2.6
Familial nephritis (Alport)	2.4
Cystinosis	2.2
Renal infarct	1.8
Other	13.4

Transplantation should be considered when CRI is apparent (see Secs. 21.13 and 21.14) or once ESRD therapy is indicated. Most centers require a recipient to be at least 8 to 10 kg to minimize the risk of vascular thrombosis and to accommodate an adult-size kidney. However, transplantation has been successful in children <10 kg or <6 months of age at experienced centers.

Preemptive transplantation (ie, transplantation without prior dialysis) accounts for 24% of all pediatric renal transplants. The major reason cited by patients and families to undertake preemptive transplantation is the desire to avoid dialysis. No difference in graft outcome in pediatric recipients who have undergone preemptive transplantation is apparent when compared with those who have been dialyzed prior to transplantation. In fact, some studies demonstrate a small improvement in allograft outcome in pediatric patients who have received preemptive transplants, although the reasons for the improved graft survival are unknown. Because of the prolonged waiting time for cadaver donors, the vast majority of kidneys for preemptive transplants are from living donors.

21.15.2   Patient and Graft Survival

Survival rates for recipients of primary transplants are excellent for both cadaver and living donor groups: the 1-, 2-, and 5-year rates for recipients of living donor kidneys are 98, 97, and 95%; for those with cadaver donor kidneys 97, 96, and 93%. Patients <2 years old have the lowest survival: 91% and 80% at 3 years for recipients of living and cadaver donor kidneys, respectively. Bacterial infections account for approximately 15% of deaths; viral infections account for 10%, and other infections account for 9%. Other causes of death include cardiopulmonary disease, 16%; cancer/malignancy, 11%; and dialysis-related complications (after graft failure), 2.4%. Approximately 46% of patients who die do so with a functioning graft.

GRAFT SURVIVAL

Of the more than 6500 pediatric kidney transplants reported to the North American Pediatric Renal Transplant Cooperative Study (NAPRTCS) registry since 1987, slightly more than 24% have failed. Chronic rejection is the leading cause of graft failure, accounting for 31% of failures. Other causes include acute rejection (16%), vascular thrombosis (12%), recurrence of original disease (6%), patient noncompliance (3.6%), primary nonfunction (2.6%), infection (2.2%), malignancy (1.2%), and death from other causes (10%). Although some causes of failure, such as graft thrombosis and recurrence of the original disease, have remained constant over

the last 10 years, loss from acute rejection has fallen dramatically. On the other hand, loss from chronic rejection has increased and accounted for 41% of graft failures in the past year.

In recent years, there have been dramatic improvements in short- and long-term graft survival rates. Currently, graft survival is 92% at 1 year and 74% at 7 years in living-donor transplant recipients and 83% and 59% at the same time points in cadaver-donor graft recipients. A number of factors significantly influence allograft outcome in pediatric patients.

DONOR SOURCE   Graft and patient survival rates are better in recipients of living donor transplants in all pediatric age groups. Recipients of living donor kidneys have a 10 to 20% advantage in graft survival at 1, 3, and 5 years. The statistical improvement in transplant survival is greatest in younger transplant recipients. Shorter cold ischemia time, better HLA matching, lower acute rejection rates, and better preoperative preparation help account for the better outcome in recipients of living donor kidneys.

RECIPIENT AGE   Children <6 years, and especially those <2 years, have lower graft survival rates than older children, especially with cadaver donor kidneys. The 5-year graft survival in recipients <2 years of age is 80% and 52% for living and cadaver donor transplants, respectively. This is primarily because of early graft losses within the first 6 months after transplantation. Higher rates of vascular thrombosis and irreversible acute rejection help account for this early graft loss. Young renal transplant recipients have more severe outcomes from acute rejection. The 5-year graft survival rates for recipients >12 years of age are 5 to 10% lower than for those 2 to 12 years old. Higher rates of medication noncompliance have been cited as one cause for these outcomes.

DONOR AGE   Kidneys from donors aged 16 to 40 years provide optimal graft survival and function. Transplantation with cadaver kidneys from donors <6 years old is associated with markedly decreased graft survival, with a 22% increased risk for graft loss. Children <5 years old receiving a kidney from a donor <6 years old have a 100% increase in the rate of graft failure. Kidneys from cadaver donors >50 years of age are more likely to have a suboptimal renal function outcome. The older the donor, the greater is the decline of renal function with time, which is an important consideration in pediatric renal transplantation because optimal graft function is important for posttransplant growth.

RACE   In recipients of living-donor kidneys, African-American race is the most significant factor associated with poor outcome. In cadaver donor graft recipients, African-American race is second only to young recipient age as a predictor of graft failure.

HUMAN LEUKOCYTE ANTIGEN (HLA) MATCHING   Long-term graft survival is best when the donor is an HLA-identical sibling. Transplants from HLA haploidentical parental or sibling donors have a half-life (time to failure of 50% of grafts) of 12 to 14 years compared to 25 years in transplant recipients from HLA-identical siblings. Recently, it has been found that recipients of kidney transplants from haploidentical sibling donors bearing maternal antigens not inherited by the recipient have a significantly better long-term graft survival than transplant recipients of kidneys from sibling donors expressing paternal HLA antigens not inherited by the recipient. Cadaver donor transplants fully matched at the HLA-A, -B, and -DR loci have a 10 to 20% survival advantage at 5 years after transplantation compared to grafts that are fully mismatched. Surprisingly, graft survival with living unrelated donor transplants is comparable to that seen with living related donor transplants. The advantage of living unrelated donor transplantation over cadaveric transplantation appears mainly to result from shorter ischemia time.

Antibodies directed against the HLA antigens of the donor allograft produce immediate and irreversible "hyperacute" rejection. To guard against this, before transplantation, serum from the recipient is reacted against lymphocytes obtained from the donor in a test termed a "crossmatch." When donor-directed antibody is detected, the transplant is not performed.

Blood transfusions expose the recipient to a wide range of HLA antigens and may subsequently result in sensitization to these antigens leading to higher rates of rejection and graft failure. The NAPRTCS data base indicates that the graft failure rate is almost double in living-donor transplant recipients who received more than five blood transfusions before transplantation compared to those who had five or fewer transfusions. For cadaveric transplant recipients a similar pattern was noted, which is contradictory to older data that suggested that a large number of blood transfusions improved graft survival, especially for cadaveric transplants. Similarly, sensitization may result from rejection of a previous transplant, and graft survival for repeat cadaveric transplants is worse by approximately 20%.

IMMUNOLOGIC FACTORS Immunologic parameters in young children are different from those of older children and adults. Differences include higher numbers of T and B cells, higher $CD4^+$ to $CD8^+$ T-cell ratio, and increased spontaneous blastogenic responses. These differences may account for increased nonspecific immune responsiveness and may be in part responsible for the higher rates of irreversible rejection observed in young children.

TECHNICAL FACTORS/DELAYED GRAFT FUNCTION Small children present difficult operative challenges. The relatively large size of the graft may result in longer anastomosis times and ischemia times and, subsequently, high rates of early delayed graft function (DGF), which significantly reduces graft survival. In children who require dialysis within the first week after transplantation, the 3-year graft survival rates are reduced by approximately 20% and 30% in recipients of cadaver and living-donor kidneys, respectively.

The transplanted kidney is usually placed in an extraperitoneal location when possible to allow easier clinical monitoring and access to the graft. In smaller children, the aorta and inferior vena cava may be used for anastomosis to ensure adequate blood flow; in larger children and adolescents, the iliac vessels are used.

Establishing vascular anastomosis may be problematic in the child with previous hemodialysis accesses in the lower extremities. In such children, vessel patency must be evaluated by Doppler ultrasonography or magnetic resonance angiography before transplantation.

INDUCTION THERAPY WITH AN ANTILYMPHOCYTE BIOLOGICAL AGENT Antibody induction with either polyclonal or monoclonal antibodies is used in the immediate posttransplant period either for prophylaxis against rejection or in a sequential manner to avoid nephrotoxicity resulting from early use of calcineurin inhibitors. In the United States, polyclonal agents that are currently available include Atgam, an equine antithymocyte preparation, and thymoglobulin, a rabbit preparation; monoclonal agents include the mouse monoclonal OKT3, which targets the ϵ chain of the CD3 complex on the human T cell, and the humanized antibodies Daclizumab and Basiliximab, which target the α chain of the activated T cell's interleukin-2 receptor.

Registry data suggest that long-term graft survival in living-donor transplantation is improved only slightly by such therapy. In cadaver-donor transplantation, however, there is almost a 10% advantage in the 5-year graft survival rate when this form of therapy is used early posttransplantation.

RECURRENCE OF ORIGINAL DISEASE Recurrent disease in the renal graft accounts for graft loss in about 6% of primary transplants and 10% in repeat transplants. Both glomerular and metabolic diseases can recur after transplantation, with the majority of recurrences caused by glomerular disease. As a general rule, recurrence of glomerular disease is more likely after living-related-donor than cadaver-donor transplantation.

GLOMERULAR DISEASES

1. *Focal segmental glomerulosclerosis* (FSGS) is the most frequent cause of graft loss from recurrent disease and recurs in 30 to 40% of primary transplants and in 50 to 80% of subsequent transplants; it leads to graft failure in about half of these patients. Recurrence is usually characterized by massive proteinuria, hypoalbuminemia, and often the full-blown picture of nephrotic syndrome with edema or anasarca and hypercholesterolemia. It may present immediately or weeks to months after transplantation. Predictors of recurrence include rapid progression to ESRD at the time of initial diagnosis (less than 3 years), poor response to therapy, younger age at diagnosis (but more than 6 years of age), African-American race, and presence of mesangial proliferation in the native kidney. In recent years, a protein permeability factor has been isolated from sera of patients with FSGS, and its concentration has been found to correlate with recurrence of nephrotic syndrome in the transplanted kidney. The precise nature of this factor remains unclear, and there is no clinically approved assay. Living-donor transplants appear to have a higher rate of recurrence than cadaver-donor transplants. The potential for recurrence of FSGS is not generally regarded as a contraindication to living-donor transplantation, but if a first transplant has been lost to rapid recurrence, use of a living donor for a repeat transplant may not be indicated.

2. *Alport syndrome* itself does not recur, but anti–glomerular basement membrane (GBM) antibody-mediated glomerulonephritis may occur after transplantation and often leads to graft loss (see Sec. 21.9). Anti-GBM glomerulonephritis presents as rapidly progressive crescentic glomerulonephritis with linear deposits of IgG in the basement membrane and most commonly leads to graft loss. Asymptomatic cases with linear IgG deposits have also been reported. Fortunately, this complication is very rare and probably affects fewer than 5% of Alport recipients.

3. Histologic evidence of recurrence of *membranoproliferative glomerulonephritis I* (MPGN-I) varies widely, with reported rates from 20 to 70%. Graft loss occurs in up to 30% of cases wherein the disease recurs. Histologic recurrence of MPGN-II occurs in virtually all cases; however, most of these recurrences are benign and do not cause graft dysfunction or loss.

4. Histologic recurrence of *IgA nephropathy and Henoch-Schönlein purpura* with mesangial IgA deposits is common and occurs in about 50% of patients with IgA nephropathy and in 30% of patients with HSP. Most of the recurrences are asymptomatic, but graft loss may occur, often in association with crescent formation.

5. Recurrent *hemolytic uremic syndrome* (HUS) has been reported in up to 50% of cases in some series; however, rates as low as 1 to 4% have been observed in large series. The diarrhea-associated or "typical" form of HUS does not usually recur after transplantation.

Recurrence of the atypical form of HUS has been linked to the use of cyclosporine and more recently to tacrolimus.

6. In *anti-GBM disease,* a high level of circulating anti-GBM antibody before transplantation is felt to be associated with higher rate of recurrence. Therefore, waiting for 6 to 12 months after anti-GBM nephritis combined with an undetectable titer of anti-GBM antibody is recommended before transplantation. Reappearance of anti-GBM antibody in the serum may be associated with histologic recurrence, which has been reported in up to 50% of cases, with clinical manifestations of nephritis in only 25% of these cases. Graft loss is rare, and spontaneous resolution may occur.

7. *Congenital nephrotic syndrome* (CNS) of the Finnish type is an autosomal recessive disease that is caused by a mutation in the *NPHS1* gene located at chromosome 19q13.1 (see Sec. 21.9). CNS does not recur after transplantation; however, de novo steroid-resistant nephrotic syndrome has been reported in up to 24% of cases.

8. Recurrence of *membranous nephropathy* is characterized by development of posttransplant nephrotic syndrome. Such recurrence is relatively rare. De novo membranous nephropathy occurs more frequently, although it is still somewhat unusual, and manifests itself as posttransplant nephrotic syndrome in patients whose ESRD was caused by disorders other than membranous nephropathy.

9. Among other glomerular diseases, recurrence of *systemic lupus erythematosus* is rare, and recurrent disease does not cause significant clinical disease. *Wegener granulomatosis* (WG) recurs in a small number of patients, and although it rarely causes graft loss, pulmonary manifestations do occur.

METABOLIC DISEASES

1. *Primary hyperoxaluria type I (oxalosis)* results from deficiency of hepatic peroxisomal alanine glyoxylate aminotransferase (AGT; see Chapter 9). Deficiency of this enzyme leads to deposition of oxalate in all body tissues including the kidneys, myocardium, and bone. Renal transplantation alone does not correct the enzymatic deficiency, and therefore, graft loss is inevitable in these cases because of oxalate deposition in the graft. Combined or two-stage liver and kidney transplantation has led to higher rates of success. The transplanted liver corrects the enzymatic deficiency and helps to mobilize tissue oxalate, while the transplanted well-functioning kidney excretes the mobilized plasma oxalate.

2. Transplantation of children with *nephropathic cystinosis* corrects the transport defect in the kidney but not hypothyroidism, visual abnormalities, and central nervous system manifestations (see Chapter 9 and Sec. 21.11). After successful transplantation, ongoing therapy with cysteamine and thyroid hormone are usually required. Cystine crystals can be found in the renal graft interstitium within macrophages of host origin, but this does not result in recurrence of Fanconi syndrome or graft dysfunction.

3. The graft survival rate in patients with *sickle cell disease/ nephropathy* is very low with only about 25% functioning beyond 1 year after transplantation. The improvement in the hematocrit results in higher numbers of abnormal red blood cells, leading to sickling episodes in the graft.

21.15.3　Pretransplant Evaluation

LIVING DONOR

It is possible to consider an adult donor of almost any size for a child, no matter how young. Live donation from siblings is usually restricted to donors who have reached their 18th birthday, although the courts have given permission for younger children to donate under extraordinary circumstances (usually identical twins).

Transplants from HLA-identical sibling donors are optimal and enable the lowest amount of immunosuppression to be used. Usually, however, the first live donor for a child is a one-haplotype–matched parent. Theoretically, maternal live donor transplants should fare better than paternal ones, but differences in outcome, if any, are small. Second-degree relatives and zero-haplotype–matched siblings may also be considered as donors. Live unrelated donors who do not share HLA antigens are preferred to cadaver donors, even with better HLA matches.

The major ABO blood groups of renal transplant donors and recipients should be compatible in order to avoid antibody-mediated rejection from naturally occurring isohemagglutinins. One exception to this rule is the use of kidneys from donors with the A2 subtype for blood type O recipients.

RECIPIENT EVALUATION

The pediatric recipient of a renal allograft requires careful evaluation and preparation.

NEUROLOGIC DEVELOPMENT Infants with ESRD during the first year of life frequently suffer neurologic abnormalities. Some studies describe an improvement in psychomotor delay in some infants with successful transplantation, with a significant percentage of infants regaining normal developmental milestones. Tests of global intelligence show increased rates of improvement after successful transplantation.

A seizure disorder requiring anticonvulsant medication may be present in up to 10% of young pediatric transplant candidates. Whenever possible, seizures should be controlled with drugs that do not induce the CYP3A4 hepatic microsomal enzymes responsible for the metabolism of immunosuppressive agents, eg, cyclosporine (CsA), tacrolimus (Tac), sirolimus, and prednisone. Induction of these enzymes will result in marked reductions in the blood levels of these immunosuppressants.

PSYCHOEMOTIONAL STATUS Primary psychiatric problems may be amenable to therapy and should not exclude children from consideration for transplantation. Noncompliance is a particularly prevalent problem in adolescent transplant recipients. Patterns of medication and dialysis compliance should be established as part of the transplant evaluation. Psychiatric evaluation should be performed in high-risk cases. If noncompliance is identified or anticipated, behavioral modification programs or other interventions should be in place before transplantation.

CARDIOVASCULAR DISEASE Hypertension and chronic fluid overload during dialysis may predispose to left ventricular hypertrophy and/or dilatation, and severe hypertensive cardiomyopathy and congestive heart failure may supervene. The importance of control of hypertension in children with ESRD cannot be overemphasized.

INFECTION Urinary tract infections and infections related to peritoneal dialysis are the most common sources of bacterial infection in children with ESRD. Aggressive antibiotic therapy and prophylaxis of urinary tract infections in children may effectively suppress infection, although pretransplant nephrectomy is occasionally required for recalcitrant infections in children with reflux.

It is important to establish the cytomegalovirus (CMV) and Epstein-Barr virus (EBV) antibody status of the patient before transplantation. Both of these herpes viruses are important posttransplant pathogens, and knowledge of the antibody status helps to determine appropriate posttransplant prophylaxis.

IMMUNIZATION STATUS Before transplant, immunizations should be brought up to date (see Sec. 21.13). Live viral vaccines are contraindicated in the immunosuppressed patient. Every effort should be made to complete these vaccinations, including varicella vaccination, before transplantation. In addition, vaccination in the immunosuppressed host may fail to induce an adequate immune response, especially with the use of newer immunosuppressive agents.

UROLOGIC PROBLEMS Urologic problems are best addressed before transplantation. Intractable urinary tract infection, in the presence of hydronephrosis or severe reflux, may require nephrectomy before transplantation. The presence of an abnormal lower urinary tract is not a contraindication to transplantation. Malformations and voiding abnormalities (eg, neurogenic bladder, bladder dyssynergia, remnant posterior urethral valves, urethral strictures) should be identified and repaired if possible.

RENAL OSTEODYSTROPHY Aggressive diagnosis and treatment of hyperparathyroidism, osteomalacia, and adynamic bone disease are important in the pretransplant period. Control of hyperparathyroidism with vitamin D analogs, or even parathyroidectomy, may be required before transplantation (see Sec. 21.14). Posttransplant hypophosphatemia, hypercalcemia, and poor growth may be related to uncontrolled hyperparathyroidism.

NEPHROTIC SYNDROME In children with glomerular diseases, proteinuria usually diminishes as kidney function deteriorates. Occasionally, florid nephrotic syndrome may persist, particularly for patients with focal glomerulosclerosis. Control of heavy proteinuria before transplantation usually requires renal embolization or bilateral nephrectomy.

PORTAL HYPERTENSION In pediatric ESRD, portal hypertension is most common in autosomal recessive polycystic kidney disease (see Sec. 21.10). Esophageal varices require portal-systemic shunting. If neutropenia and thrombocytopenia are present, partial splenectomy or splenic embolization may be required before transplantation.

PRIOR MALIGNANCY Wilms tumor is the principal malignancy producing ESRD in children. A disease-free period of 1 year should be observed before transplantation is considered because earlier transplantation has been associated with development of recurrent or metastatic disease in nearly 50% of reported cases. Premature transplantation has also been associated with overwhelming sepsis, which may be related to chemotherapy for the tumor.

The presence of a primary nonrenal malignancy is not an absolute contraindication to transplantation, although an appropriate waiting time must be observed between tumor extirpation and transplantation.

21.15.4 Immunosuppressive Drugs

CORTICOSTEROIDS

The emergence of more powerful immunosuppressive agents has led to a dramatic improvement in acute rejection rates and has allowed the use of lower daily doses of steroids. Several steroid withdrawal trials have been conducted with variable degrees of success, and steroids continue to be used in most centers, with an increased tendency toward using lower daily maintenance doses or alternate-day dosing. However, even with reduced steroid doses, side effects such as hypertension, acne, obesity, hyperlipidemia, and retarded skeletal growth persist.

CALCINEURIN INHIBITORS

CYCLOSPORINE Both CsA and tacrolimus are "prodrugs" that exert their immunosuppressive action only after binding in the cell cytoplasm to a unique protein, termed an "immunophyllin." The CsA-immunophyllin complex blocks the action of a cytoplasmic phosphatase, calcineurin, which in turn inhibits the transcription of T-cell growth factors such as IL-2. More recent studies suggest that CsA induces the formation of the growth factor TGF-β, an immunosuppressive cytokine that also induces fibrosis. These actions explain, at least in part, both CsA's immunosuppressive activity and its propensity to foster chronic renal fibrosis.

CsA is currently used as the primary agent in about 75% of pediatric renal transplant recipients. The microemulsion formulation of CsA (Neoral) has more reliable absorption and a more consistent pharmacokinetic profile than that observed with the oil-based preparations (Sandimmune). Drugs that induce the hepatic P450 enzymes that metabolize CsA (and Tac) and are commonly used in pediatrics include phenobarbital, phenytoin (Dilantin), carbamazepine, and rifampin. Drugs that inhibit these enzymes and raise CsA (and Tac) levels include the antifungal azoles (eg, fluconazole), erythromycin, azithromycin, and calcium channel blockers such as verapamil and diltiazem. CsA appears to cause at least two forms of nephrotoxicity. The elaboration of thromboxane A_2 blocks the generation of the vasodilator prostaglandins and results in decreased renal blood flow and renal ischemia because of afferent arteriolar vasoconstriction. In the early postoperative period, this effect may cause or aggravate early graft dysfunction. CsA also has a chronic nephrotoxicity, the hallmark of which is interstitial fibrosis.

Other side effects of CsA include hypertension, electrolyte abnormalities, hyperlipidemia, hepatotoxicity, fine hand tremors, mild paresthesias, seizures, and cosmetic side effects including hypertrichosis, gingival hyperplasia, and coarsening of facial features. Hispanic and black children appear to be at higher risk of these complications. Calcium channel blockers worsen gingival hyperplasia. Because cosmetic side effects with Tac are far less pronounced, many centers have moved to using Tac in adolescent girls.

TACROLIMUS Tacrolimus is a potent immunosuppressive agent that acts in a similar fashion to CsA and is the primary immunosuppressive agent in approximately 25% of patients. It is being used with increased frequency because it yields results in graft survival that are similar to those seen with CsA at 1 and 4 years after transplant.

Hypertension, gingival hypertrophy, and hirsutism are significantly less prevalent and severe with Tac than with CsA. Posttransplant diabetes mellitus occurs with higher frequency with Tac in both adults (up to 20%) and children (about 10%) when compared to CsA (<5%). Tac is also associated with a higher rate of EBV-associated posttransplant lymphoproliferative disorder (PTLD).

The nephrotoxicity profiles with both tacrolimus and CsA are similar. Neurotoxicity with tacrolimus is more serious, with higher rates of seizures, insomnia, encephalopathy, and coma. Hypomagnesemia, tremors, and paresthesias are also more pronounced with tacrolimus. Other side effects seen with Tac include hair loss and nausea.

ANTIPROLIFERATIVE AGENTS

AZATHIOPRINE Azathioprine (Aza) is the nitroimidazole derivative of 6-mercaptopurine (6-MP) and is converted in the liver to 6-MP; it inhibits both DNA and RNA synthesis. Although it was the mainstay of immunosuppression in the 1960s, 1970s, and early 1980s, it is currently used in <20% of pediatric transplants. Megaloblastic anemia, bone marrow suppression (especially leukopenia), and hepatic toxicity are the most common side effects. The toxicity of Aza is potentiated by allopurinol and trimethoprim-sulfamethoxazole.

MYCOPHENOLATE MOFETIL (MMF) MMF is the 2-morpholino-ethyl ester of mycophenolic acid (MPA). MMF is hydrolyzed in the liver to MPA, the active metabolite. MPA selectively and reversibly inhibits inosine monophosphate dehydrogenase, thereby inhibiting de novo purine synthesis in T and B lymphocytes. MMF is used in 70% of pediatric renal transplants. When used in combination with CsA and prednisone, it reduces the rate of acute rejection to the range of 17 to 30% at 1 year.

Gastrointestinal and hematologic side effects are most commonly observed. Gastrointestinal complications include diarrhea, nausea, vomiting, and stomach upset. To ameliorate the upper gastrointestinal side effects, patients on MMF should always receive H_2 blockers or proton pump inhibitors. Hematologic side effects include leukopenia, thrombocytopenia and anemia. Because it is a potent immunosuppressive agent with some bone marrow toxicity, patients treated with MMF are at a moderately increased risk for viral and bacterial infections, and appropriate chemoprophylaxis should be employed. Prophylaxis against CMV is particularly important in pediatric patients receiving MMF.

BIOLOGICAL AGENTS: POLYCLONAL AND MONOCLONAL ANTIBODIES

Antibodies with specificity against surface antigens of T lymphocytes have proven useful to reverse acute rejection episodes, particularly those that have not responded to high-dose corticosteroid therapy. They can also be used in the immediate posttransplant period as induction therapy. This therapy is used for prophylaxis against rejection while calcineurin inhibitors are withheld to avoid early nephrotoxicity.

Currently, the only polyclonal antibodies widely available for clinical use in the United States are the equine antithymocyte globulin Atgam, and the rabbit antithymocyte globulin, thymoglobulin. Until recently, the only clinically available monoclonal antibody was OKT3, a murine monoclonal antibody with specificity for the ϵ chain of the CD3 antigen on T cells.

Early antibody therapy, whether for induction or rejection reversal, carries risks and inconveniences. Infections with CMV and EBV occur more frequently and with increased morbidity. PTLD also occurs with higher frequency, especially with repeated courses of therapy. "First-dose" reactions caused by cytokine release (fever, chills, diarrhea, headache, cerebral edema, and pulmonary edema) can occur with all of the agents and are especially frequent with OKT3. Other side effects include severe leukopenia and thrombocytopenia. Anti-idiotypic or anti-isotypic antibodies are formed against the murine OKT3 in over 40% of patients and can preclude the future use of OKT3. Finally, monitoring peripheral blood lymphocyte subsets to evaluate response to therapy and the need for further dosing is required with these agents, particularly OKT3, and daily administration is usually necessary for a minimum of 1 week, which prolongs the hospital stay and increases expenses.

NEW IMMUNOSUPPRESSIVE AGENTS

SIROLIMUS Sirolimus (Rapamune or Rapamycin) is a macrolide that structurally resembles Tac. Sirolimus, and another similar compound, everolimus, binds to the same immunophyllin as Tac but works through a different mechanism. The sirolimus/immunophyllin molecule inhibits the signal transduction protein mTOR (for mammalian target of Rapamycin). Studies in adult renal transplantation showed that sirolimus significantly reduced the rate of acute rejection episodes to 10 to 20% when used in combination with CsA and prednisone. Hyperlipidemia and thrombocytopenia are the major side effects. Data are similar for everolimus. There are no reported clinical studies on the safety and efficacy of sirolimus in children.

HUMANIZED MONOCLONAL ANTIBODIES THAT BLOCK THE IL-2 RECEPTOR

DACLIZUMAB (ZENAPAX) Daclizumab is a humanized monoclonal IgG1 antibody with specificity against the α subunit of the IL-2 receptor (CD25), expressed only on activated T cells. By targeting only T cells activated by the graft, this antibody reduces acute rejection episodes with no additional side effects.

BASILIXIMAB (SIMULECT) This is a chimeric humanized monoclonal antibody with high affinity for CD25. The mechanism of action is the same as for daclizumab. Data from pediatric clinical studies show that rates of acute rejection were improved with basiliximab, with no significant increase in adverse effects.

21.15.5 Posttransplant Medical Issues

ACUTE REJECTION

Acute rejection episodes (ARE) are characterized by elevated serum creatinine levels, sodium retention, hypertension, fever, and graft tenderness. With the newer immunosuppressive agents, most of these symptoms are absent or attenuated. Acute rejection accounts for 16% of pediatric renal graft failures in primary transplants and 15% in retransplants. An ARE occurs in about 25% of recipients of living-donor transplants and 30% of cadaveric transplant recipients. A first ARE occurs within the first 3 months after transplantation in about 50% of those who develop an ARE, with higher frequency and earlier recurrence in recipients of cadaveric transplants. The relative risk for ARE is higher in black patients, patients with one or two HLA-DR mismatches, those with early graft dysfunction, and in patients who did not receive induction therapy. An ARE is the single most important predictor of chronic rejection and precedes graft failure from chronic rejection in more than 90% of cases. Children under 6 years of age carry the highest risk for irreversible rejection.

In small recipients of large kidneys (eg, children receiving a parent's kidney), significant allograft dysfunction may be present despite little rise in the serum creatinine. Late diagnosis and treatment of an ARE is associated with higher incidence of resistant rejections and graft loss, especially in this clinical setting.

In addition to ARE, the differential diagnosis of acute allograft dysfunction includes acute tubular necrosis in the early posttransplant period, prerenal azotemia, CsA or Tac nephrotoxicity, urinary obstruction or leak, renal artery stenosis, bacterial or viral infections, and, rarely, thrombotic microangiopathy. Renal biopsy is the gold standard for diagnosis of an ARE.

CHRONIC REJECTION

Chronic rejection (CR) is the leading cause of graft failure in children. AREs, particularly late and/or multiple AREs, are the most common correlates of CR. The clinical picture of CR includes slowly increasing serum creatinine, hypertension, and moderate hyproteinuria. There is no treatment currently for CR. Prevention of AREs is the most important prevention strategy.

NONCOMPLIANCE

Noncompliance is the most important cause of late AREs. At least 50% of pediatric cadaveric transplant recipients (more than 60% in adolescents) demonstrate significant medication noncompliance, and this is the principal cause of graft loss in 10 to 15% of all pediatric kidney transplant recipients. Occasional medication noncompliance is virtually universal. Complete noncompliance is often the result of an underlying emotional or psychosocial stress or of health beliefs that are not in alignment with those of the medical team.

Accurately predicting who will be noncompliant is different. A disorganized family structure, female sex, adolescence, and a history of previous graft loss from noncompliance have been identified as significant risk factors. Personality problems related to low self-esteem and poor social adjustment are found with higher frequency in noncompliant patients. Studies indicate that compliance has no correlation with intelligence, memory, education, or number of drugs that a patient takes. The frequency of taking medications, on the other hand, does affect compliance rates, with decreasing compliance with increased frequency of medication dosing. Noncompliance must be suspected when diminished cushingoid features, unexplained weight loss, or unexplained swings in the patient's kidney function or CsA/Tac trough blood levels are observed.

POSTTRANSPLANT GROWTH

In spite of improvement in growth after transplantation, catch-up growth is usually not realized. The main factors influencing posttransplant growth include the following.

AGE AT TRANSPLANT Children under 6 years of age exhibit the best improvement in their height after transplantation. Older children grow, but at a lower rate. Children over 12 years of age tend to have minimal or no growth after transplantation, and the pubertal growth spurt is blunted or lost. The fact that youngest children benefit the most from early transplantation provides a strong argument for expedited transplantation in an attempt to optimize and perhaps normalize stature.

CORTICOSTEROID DOSE The exact mechanism by which steroids impair skeletal growth is unknown. Strategies to improve growth include the use of lower daily doses of steroids, the use of alternate-day steroid dosing, or dose tapering to complete withdrawal, each

of which has significant risks of rejection and/or diminished graft survival.

The use of recombinant growth hormone (rhGH) in pediatric renal transplant recipients significantly improves growth velocity, even in the presence of chronic graft dysfunction. AREs were not increased, and renal function did not differ between rhGH and control patients.

ALLOGRAFT FUNCTION A GFR of <60 mL/min/1.73 m² is associated with poor growth; optimal growth occurs with a GFR greater than 90 mL/min/1.73 m². Graft function is the most important factor after high corticosteroid dosage in the genesis of posttransplant growth failure.

SEXUAL MATURATION

Restoration of kidney function by transplantation improves pubertal development. Elevated gonadotropin levels and reduced gonadotropin pulsatility are found in patients with chronic renal failure; children with successful kidney transplants demonstrate a higher nocturnal rise and increased amplitude of gonadotropin pulsatility. In pubertal female patients, menses with ovulatory cycles usually return within 6 to 12 months after transplantation. Therefore, potentially sexually active adolescent patients should be given appropriate contraceptive information. Adolescent female transplant recipients have successfully borne children; the only consistently reported neonatal abnormality has been an increased incidence of prematurity. Adolescent boys can successfully father children. No consistent pattern of abnormalities has been reported in their offspring.

INFECTIONS

Infection remains the major cause of morbidity and mortality posttransplant (see Chapter 13).

BACTERIAL INFECTIONS Pneumonia and urinary tract infections (UTI) are the most common posttransplant bacterial infections. UTI can progress rapidly to urosepsis and may be confused with ARE.

VIRAL INFECTIONS The herpes group viruses (CMV, herpes virus, varicella-zoster, and Epstein-Barr virus) pose a special problem in view of their common occurrence in children. Many young children have not yet been exposed to these viruses, and because protective immunity is lacking, the predisposition for serious primary infection is high. The incidence of these infections is much higher in children who receive antilymphocyte antibody therapy as part of their induction therapy and following treatment of acute rejection with these agents or high-dose pulse steroids. Therefore, prophylactic therapy is advisable.

CYTOMEGALOVIRUS Cytomegalovirus can exist as a latent infection in lymphoid tissue. Moreover, the incidence of CMV seropositivity is approximately 30% in children over the age of 5 and rises to approximately 60% in teenagers. Thus, the younger the child, the greater the potential for primary infection when a CMV-positive donor kidney is transplanted. The manifestations of CMV infection include fever, leukopenia, thrombocytopenia, pneumonia, gastrointestinal ulcers, hepatitis, glomerular lesions and renal dysfunction, AREs, and immunodepression. CMV infection has been linked to CR in all transplanted organs. Agents to treat and/or prevent include CMV hyperimmune globulin, high-dose immune globulin, and the antiviral agents acyclovir, valacyclovir, ganciclovir, and valganciclovir. Prophylactic treatment with ganciclovir is indicated in CMV-negative recipients of a kidney from a CMV-positive donor.

VARICELLA-ZOSTER The most common manifestation of VZV in older pediatric recipients is a localized rash along a dermatomal distribution (shingles). In younger children, primary VZV infection can result in a rapidly progressive and overwhelming infection with encephalitis, pneumonitis, hepatic failure, pancreatitis, and disseminated intravascular coagulation. Seronegative children require varicella-zoster immune globulin (VZIG) within 72 hours of accidental exposure. VZIG is effective in favorably modifying the disease in 75% of cases. Children should be vaccinated with the varicella vaccine before transplantation (see Sec. 21.13). A child with a kidney transplant who develops chicken pox should begin receiving parenteral acyclovir without delay; with zoster infection there is less of a threat of dissemination, although acyclovir should also be used.

EPSTEIN-BARR VIRUS Approximately 50% of the pediatric population are seronegative for EBV, and infection will occur in approximately 75% of these patients. Even in immunosuppressed patients, most EBV infections are clinically silent.

PTLD (see Sec. 20.7) occurs in 0.5 to 2% of pediatric renal transplant recipients and is often related to EBV infection in the presence of vigorous immunosuppression. Signs and symptoms of PTLD include fever, weight loss, hepatosplenomegaly, diarrhea, lymphadenopathy, and, in the case of central nervous system (CNS) involvement, neurologic symptoms. Therapy consists of dramatically reducing the immunosuppression and, in the high-grade neoplastic lesions, appropriate chemotherapy or antilymphocyte therapy.

HERPES SIMPLEX The typical perioral herpetic ulcerations are common in immunosuppressed children and usually respond to oral acyclovir.

PNEUMOCYSTIS CARINII PNEUMONIA Trimethoprim-sulfamethoxazole prophylaxis is indicated during the first 3 to 6 months posttransplant.

HYPERTENSION AND CARDIOVASCULAR DISEASE

More than two-thirds of transplanted children treated with cyclosporine are hypertensive. The differential diagnosis includes acute and chronic rejection, obstruction, the effects of drugs such as CsA and corticosteroids, and renal artery stenosis. Calcium channel blockers are generally well tolerated and are the agents of choice for blood pressure management, as they appear to counteract the renal afferent arteriolar vasoconstrictive effects of CsA. However, gingival hypertrophy may be exacerbated by the combination of CsA and calcium channel blockers.

Concern regarding long-term posttransplant cardiovascular morbidity and mortality has generally been directed toward the adult posttransplant population. Risk factors should also be addressed in children who will presumably grow to adulthood with their transplants. Serum cholesterol levels are frequently higher than the "at risk" level for children (see Chapter 9). Dietary measures are appropriate to reduce hyperlipidemia. Currently insufficient data exist to recommend the use of lipid-lowering drugs in pediatric transplant recipients.

21.15.6 Quality of Life

Within a year of successful transplantation, the social and emotional functioning of the child and the child's family appear to return to preillness levels. Pretransplant personality disorders, however, continue to manifest themselves. Within 1 year after transplantation, more than 90% of children attend school, and fewer than 10% are not involved in any vocational or education programs. Three-year follow-up shows that nearly 90% of children are in appropriate school or job placement. Surveys of 10-year survivors of pediatric kidney transplants report that the overwhelming majority of patients consider their health to be good, engage in appropriate social, educational, and sexual activities, and experience a very good or excellent quality of life.

References

Al-Uzri A, Sullivan EK, Fine RN, Harmon WE: Living-unrelated renal transplantation in children: a report of the North American Pediatric Renal Transplantation Cooperative Study (NAPRTCS). Pediatr Transplant 2(2):139–114, 1998

Bartosh SM, Aronson AJ, Swanson-Pewitt EE, Thistlethwaite JR: OKT3 induction in pediatric renal transplantation. Pediatr Nephrol 7:45–49, 1993

Benfield MR, McDonald R, Sullivan EK, Stablein DM, Tejani A: The 1997 Annual Renal Transplantation in Children Report of The North American Pediatric Renal Transplant Cooperative Study (NAPRTCS). Pediatr Transplant 3(2):152–167, 1999

Cameron JS: Recurrent primary disease and de novo nephritis following renal transplantation. Pediatr Nephrol 5:412–442, 1991

Davis ID: Pediatric renal transplantation: back to school issues. Transplant Proc 31(Suppl 4A):61S–62S, 1999

Jabs K, Sullivan EK, Avner ED, Harmon WE: Alternate-day steroid dosing improves growth without adversely affecting graft survival or long-term graft function: a report of the North American Pediatric Renal Transplantation Cooperative Study (NAPRTCS). Transplantation 61(1):31–36, 1996

Matas AJ, Chavers BM, Nevins TE, et al: Recipient evaluation, preparation, and care in pediatric transplantation: the University of Minnesota protocols. Kidney Int 49(Suppl 53):S99–S102, 1996

Schurman SJ, McEnry PT: Factors influencing short-term and long-term pediatric renal transplant survival. J Pediatr 130(3):455–462, 1997

Shapiro R: Tacrolimus in pediatric renal transplantation: a review. Pediatr Transplant 2(4):270–276, 1998

21.16 UROLOGIC ABNORMALITIES OF THE GENITOURINARY TRACT

John W. Colberg

21.16.1   Anomalies of the Kidney and Ureter

URETEROPELVIC JUNCTION OBSTRUCTION

Obstruction of ureteropelvic junction (UPJ) is the most common cause of hydronephrosis in infancy and childhood. Most cases of UPJ obstruction are detected by prenatal ultrasonography. UPJ obstruction is suspected when only the renal pelvis is dilated without accompanying dilatation of the ureter. A voiding cystourethrogram may be required to exclude vesicoureteral reflux, which also can produce significant hydronephrosis. In cases of symptomatic UPJ obstruction, the clinical presentation is dependent on the age of the patient. Pain, hematuria, hypertension, and urinary tract infections are more common in older children. Initially, flank or abdominal pain may be attributed to gastrointestinal disease because the pain follows ingestion of liquids, which cause a diuresis and distention of the pelvis of the kidney. Hematuria associated with mild trauma reflects the increased susceptibility of dilated kidneys to injury (see Table 21-11). Clinical presentation in infants is usually associated with a palpable abdominal mass that must be differentiated from other causes of abdominal masses in the newborn (see Chapter 2 and Sec. 20.12).

UPJ obstruction is most often caused by an intrinsic narrowing or disarray of the musculature at the junction of the renal pelvis and ureter. Extrinsic compression by an aberrant crossing vessel or fibrous band is a less common etiology. The obstruction initially leads to an increased intrapelvic pressure and accumulation of urine proximal to the site of obstruction, which causes dilation of the renal pelvis and calyces. Long-standing obstruction leads to growth retardation of the affected kidney with compensatory growth of the contralateral unobstructed kidney.

The management of prenatally detected UPJ obstruction is controversial. Although a renal ultrasound is usually obtained shortly after delivery, the extent of dilatation of the renal pelvis may be underestimated because of the low urine flow rate in the newborn (see Sec. 21.2), and more definitive studies should be obtained when the infant is 4 to 6 months of age. Up to two-thirds of prenatally detected UPJ obstructions will have preserved renal function. Some systems will show improvement and even resolution of the obstruction. The degree of obstruction and the differential function of the affected kidney, as determined by diuretic renography, helps to determine management. Early pyeloplasty is indicated if the postnatal evaluation yields evidence of functional impairment (relative function of involved side <40% of total function) and/or massive dilation of renal pelvis (AP diameter >30 mm). Conservative management is indicated if the relative function of the affected kidney is greater than 40% of the total function. Indications to abandon conservative management in favor of pyeloplasty are deteriorating renal function, increasing hydronephrosis, development of pain, and persistence of obstruction with no improvement after 4 to 5 years of conservative management.

URETERAL DUPLICATION

Duplication is the most common structural anomaly of the upper urinary tract, affecting 1 in 160 individuals. Ureteral duplication can be complete or partial. When complete ureteral duplication exists, the medial and distal ureteral orifices drain from the ureter to the upper pole of the kidney (Meyer-Weigert law). The majority of complete and partial duplications remain asymptomatic and undetected. Symptoms occur as the result of vesicoureteral reflux (predominantly to the lower pole system), UPJ obstruction (usually involving the lower pole system), obstruction (resulting from the presence of a ureterocele usually involving the upper pole system), or ureteric ectopia (with associated obstruction or incontinence). Because the majority of uncomplicated duplications are not associated with dilatation, detection by ultrasonography is difficult. The basis of management is related to the degree of vesicoureteral reflux, the presence of a ureterocele, and the level of function of the affected systems.

URETERAL ECTOPIA

Ectopic ureters are rare in boys and usually present with urinary infection or epididymoorchitis. The ureter can drain into the vas deferens, seminal vesicles, prostatic urethra, or distal trigone. Because all of these locations are proximal to the external sphincter, continence is preserved. In girls, the possibility of an ectopic ureter must be considered when a lifelong history of urinary incontinence is present. The ureter can drain into the bladder neck, urethra, vagina, uterus, fallopian tubes, or vestibule. Because some of these locations are distal to the urinary sphincter, incontinence, both daytime and nighttime, can occur.

MEGAURETER

Wide and dilated (>7 mm) ureters are referred to as megaureters and are classified as refluxing or nonrefluxing, obstructive or nonobstructive, and are subdivided into primary and secondary types. Historically, obstructed megaureters presented with urinary tract infections, flank pain, or calculi. Presently, megaureters account for 10% of infants with prenatally detected uropathy.

A primary obstructed nonrefluxing megaureter is the result of a stenotic, aperistaltic segment of distal ureter at the level of the ureterovesical junction. Secondary obstructed nonrefluxing megaureters can result from neurogenic bladder, an obstructing ureterocele, or a tumor involving the bladder. A primary refluxing megaureter, which can be obstructed or nonobstructed, is a congenital anomaly associated with an inadequate ureteral tunnel length at the ureterovesical junction and is more likely to be bilateral than unilateral. Secondary refluxing megaureters occur as a result of abnormalities involving the bladder or urethra, such as neurogenic bladder, posterior urethral valves, or ureteroceles. At times, reflux and obstruction exist in the same ureter. The primary etiologic factor may need to be addressed in the management of secondary obstructed or refluxing megaureters. The diagnosis of a nonrefluxing nonobstructed megaureter is one of exclusion. The primary cause of this condition is unknown, and spontaneous resolution of the ureteral dilatation can occur.

The management of megaureters is based on the results of ultrasonography, a voiding cystourethrogram (VCUG), an IVP, and/or diuretic renography. Surgical management of megaureters is directed at either correction of the reflux or removal of the obstruction. With primary refluxing megaureters, intervention is required in patients with recurrent infections, with or without parenchymal loss, and in patients with a fixed ureteral orifice abnormality resulting in high-grade reflux. With primary obstructing nonrefluxing megaureters, indications for intervention include progressive hydronephrosis, parenchymal loss, and recurrent infections. The majority of infants with prenatally detected obstructed megaureters can be managed conservatively because they are asymptomatic, and their obstruction is often associated with preserved renal function. Close observation is required to detect any deterioration of renal function.

URETEROCELES

A ureterocele is a cystic dilation of the intravesical submucosal ureter and can be associated with a single system or, more commonly, with a duplex system. Ureteroceles that are associated with a duplex system (80% of cases) usually drain the upper pole of the kidney. Ureteroceles are classified as intravesical (contained entirely within the bladder) or ectopic (located at the bladder neck or in the urethra). Ureteroceles vary in size and may obstruct the collecting system that drains into them or the drainage of the ipsilateral or contralateral ureters, distort the trigone and result in vesicoureteral reflux, or obstruct the urethra, the last occurring more frequently in boys. The embryology of ureteroceles consists of incomplete dissolution of Chwalla membrane, resulting in an obstructed ureteral–meatal orifice. Girls are affected four to seven times more commonly than boys.

Many single-system ureteroceles are small and asymptomatic. The radiologic findings on IVP are pathognomonic, showing a "cobra head" deformity. In the absence of obstruction or recurrent infection, no treatment is necessary. Ureteroceles associated with a duplex system are commonly detected by prenatal ultrasonography or present clinically with a febrile urinary tract infection. A VCUG is necessary to evaluate the presence of vesicoureteral reflux, and nuclear renography is helpful in assessing the degree of function of the affected kidney.

The choice of strategy for the treatment of ureteroceles is based on the age of the patient, the amount of functioning renal parenchyma, whether the kidney is single or duplex, the location of the ureterocele, and the presence of vesicoureteral reflux. In the past, definitive surgical management included an upper pole partial nephrectomy with or without reimplantation of the ureter draining the lower segment. Endoscopic management with transurethral incision of ureteroceles has become a less invasive approach for selected patients with ureteroceles.

RETROCAVAL URETER

The retrocaval ureter is a congenital anomaly in which the upper one-third of the right ureter passes behind the vena cava with resultant obstruction. The anomaly results from an error in the development of the vena cava, specifically the persistence of the subcardinal vein ventral to the developing ureter. A retrocaval ureter is of clinical significance only when obstruction with resultant hydronephrosis result. This condition can be misdiagnosed as a simple ureteropelvic junction (UPJ) obstruction on ultrasonography, and further radiologic evaluation may be warranted.

21.16.2   Anomalies of the Bladder and Urethra

POSTERIOR URETHRAL VALVES

Posterior urethral valves are a congenital pair of obstructing leaflets in the region of the verumontanum in the prostatic urethra. The etiology is unclear, but they may form when the ventrolateral folds of the urogenital sinus fail to regress. Posterior urethral valves (PUV) are the most common cause of urinary obstruction in male infants and the most common type of obstructive uropathy leading to childhood renal failure. The incidence of PUV is 1 in 5000 to 8000 male infants.

Obstruction from urethral valves causes increased voiding pressures that result in dilatation of the prostatic urethra, hypertrophy of the bladder neck, bladder trabeculation, vesicoureteral reflux, renal dysplasia, and loss of renal function. The degree of obstruction creates a spectrum of damage. Massive unilateral vesicoureteral reflux is a unique entity in PUV patients and is described by the acronym VURD (valve, unilateral, reflux, and dysplasia) syndrome. Because of the pressure popoff afforded by the affected kidney, the contralateral kidney is protected, the ipsilateral side takes the brunt of the increased voiding pressure, and patients with VURD syndrome have a good prognosis for presentation of renal function.

Most infants with PUV are identified with bilateral hydroureteronephrosis in utero on prenatal ultrasonography. Other causes of bilateral hydroureteronephrosis include prune belly syndrome, vesicoureteral reflux, and bilateral ureterovesical junction (UVJ) obstruction. After birth the diagnosis is confirmed with a VCUG. If the diagnosis is not detected on prenatal ultrasonography, the infant may present with a wide range of signs and symptoms including delayed voiding, a distended bladder, palpable kidneys, a poor urinary stream with dribbling, and sepsis. Constitutional symptoms such as abdominal distension, failure to thrive, and vomiting may occur. An infant may present with a variable degree of renal failure with hyponatremia and hyperkalemia (see Sec. 21.4). Later in childhood, nonspecific voiding problems such as incontinence, nocturnal enuresis, frequency, recurrent urinary tract infections, and hematuria with mild trauma may be present.

Initial treatment in the infant is directed toward relief of the obstruction. Immediate stabilization of the baby with bladder drainage is mandatory. Sepsis, electrolyte abnormalities, acidemia, and fluid imbalance need aggressive management. After stabilization of the infant, primary transurethral valve ablation is performed when technically feasible. If the urethra is too small to accept an infant cystoscope, a temporary vesicostomy may be performed. High diversion with loop ureterostomies is reserved for infants whose renal function continues to deteriorate in spite of bladder drainage. Older boys can almost always undergo primary transurethral valve ablation because urethral size is not an issue, and overall renal function is usually better preserved.

Long-term complications from PUV include the development of bladder dysfunction and renal insufficiency. Bladder dysfunction may be manifest by detrusor instability and small noncompliant bladder. Some patients will develop the so-called "valve bladder" syndrome, which is characterized by persistent hydroureteronephrosis in the absence of an UVJ obstruction related to a small-capacity, high-pressure bladder. Some patients can be managed effectively with double voiding or anticholinergic medication and clean intermittent catheterization. If bladder capacity and hydroureteronephrosis does not improve, bladder augmentation may be required. The incidence of ESRD in PUV is approximately 25%. A useful predictor of renal failure is the nadir serum creatinine at 1 year of age. A serum creatinine <0.8 g/dL after the age of 1 makes renal failure less likely.

PRUNE BELLY SYNDROME

The prune belly syndrome is a complex consisting of congenital absence or deficiency of abdominal wall musculature, cryptorchidism, and anomalies of the urogenital tract, mainly dilation of the prostatic urethra, bladder, and ureters. The syndrome also is known as the triad syndrome, the Eagle-Barrett syndrome, and the urethral obstruction malformation complex. The incidence of this syndrome has been estimated to be 1 in 40,000 live births. Although cryptorchidism eliminates this syndrome in female patients, approximately 5% of cases occur in female patients with an incomplete form of the syndrome.

The severity of the disease varies widely. The most severe form or lethal variant results in death in the perinatal period because of complete urethral obstruction (without a patent urachus), renal insufficiency, and oligohydramnios with associated pulmonary hypoplasia. Advances in neonatal intensive care have improved the survival for some of these infants, but the prognosis is still poor.

Another group of newborns with prune belly syndrome lacks severe pulmonary hypoplasia but has significant involvement of the urinary tract and manifests moderate to severe renal insufficiency or failure and failure to thrive. The clinical course is one of either stabilization or progressive loss of renal function with an ultimate need for transplantation.

The last category of infants with prune belly syndrome have absence or deficiency of the musculature and undescended testes but normal renal function even though the urinary tract has a markedly abnormal radiographic appearance. These children comprise the majority of cases with prune belly syndrome and do not develop significant renal impairment.

Many theories have been proposed to explain the etiology and pathogenesis of prune belly syndrome. These include (1) in utero distal urinary obstruction resulting in dilatation of the entire urinary tract and subsequent pressure atrophy of the abdominal wall musculature; (2) embryologic aberrations of mesenchymal development resulting in defects in the genitourinary tract, the testes, and the abdominal wall; (3) an intrinsic defect in the urinary tract that causes bladder and ureteral dilatation; and (4) an error in the embryogenesis of the yolk sac and allantois. Unfortunately, none of these theories fully explains all aspects of this syndrome.

The most obvious defect in newborns with the syndrome is the shriveled, prune-like appearance of the abdominal wall. As the child begins to stand, a pear-shaped or pot-bellied appearance occurs. The weakness of the abdominal wall musculature may result in developmental delay in motor activities associated with axial balance. The lack of mechanical assistance from the abdominal wall contributes to respiratory infections and chronic constipation.

Abnormalities of the urinary tract are the major factors affecting the prognosis of children with prune belly syndrome. Typical radiologic features include elongated, tortuous, and dilated ureters that have poor or absent peristalsis and a large-capacity, smooth-walled bladder with a patent urachus. VUR is present in 70% of cases. The posterior urethra is dilated, and the prostate is absent or hypoplastic. Abnormalities in the epididymis, seminal vesicles, and vas deferens may be responsible for the infertility uniformly seen with this syndrome. The anterior urethra is usually normal; however, abnormalities range from urethral atresia to a fusiform or scaphoid megalourethra. Renal dysplasia and multicystic dysplastic kidney (MCDK) are common, and the extent of renal parenchymal involvement determines ultimate renal function. Bilateral cryptorchidism is a consistent finding of prune belly syndrome. The location of the testes is usually at the level of the iliac vessels in an apparent intraperitoneal position on a long mesorchium.

Varied approaches to the management of prune belly syndrome have been advocated. The goals of early management are to preserve renal function and prevent infection. Invasive procedures may complicate treatment of urinary tract infections and should be kept to the minimum.

Many infants require no early intervention. The dilatation of the urinary tract in prune belly syndrome is usually a low-pressure, nonobstructive system. However, if during the newborn period renal function deteriorates secondary to obstructive uropathy, intervention is warranted. Temporary urinary diversion with a vesicostomy or cutaneous pyelostomy may be required. More extensive reconstructive surgery (reduction cystoplasty and excision of distal ureters with tapering and reimplantation of the healthier upper portion of the ureters into the bladder) may be performed in an effort to reduce stasis and prevent urinary tract infections in older children. Early orchiopexy should be performed and may be performed in conjunction with reconstructive surgery or at the time of an abdominoplasty. Patients are usually placed on antibiotic prophylaxis to prevent UTI.

EPISPADIAS-EXSTROPHY COMPLEX

The epispadias-exstrophy complex is the result of a persistent cloacal membrane that does not retract normally toward the perineum. The persistent membrane prevents medial mesenchymal ingrowth, causing the future abdominal wall to remain laterally placed. With dehiscence of the cloacal membrane, the posterior wall of the bladder becomes exposed to the exterior on the surface of the abdominal wall. If dehiscence occurs after the urorectal septum has partitioned the cloaca, bladder exstrophy occurs. If dehiscence occurs before the division of the cloaca, a more severe defect occurs, cloacal exstrophy. Bladder exstrophy is almost always accompanied by epispadias. Epispadias alone results if persistence of the cloacal membrane occurs only inferiorly.

The most common anomaly in this complex is classic bladder exstrophy, occurring in 1 in 30,000 to 40,000 births with a male preponderance. The risk of recurrence in a given family is 1%. The typical features include a defect in the abdominal wall from the umbilicus inferiorly, with the bladder open and exposed to the exterior. The bony pelvis does not make a complete ring, resulting in a widely spaced, externally rotated symphysis pubis. In boys, the penis appears foreshortened and wider, with dorsal chordee and an open urethral plate. In girls, the mons and clitoris are bifid, and the entire urethra is open dorsally. In both sexes the reproductive organs are normal. Indirect hernias are common. The abnormal anatomy of the puborectalis muscle can result in rectal prolapse. The upper urinary tracts are usually normal; however, anomalies of renal development and fusion can occur (see Sec. 21.3). Bilateral vesicoureteral reflux is almost universal.

The goals of management of the exstrophy-epispadias complex include closure of the bony pelvis (with or without osteotomies), closure of the bladder and urethra, closure of the abdominal wall defect, preservation of renal function, and a functionally and cosmetically acceptable penis in boys. The surgical management is usually staged, with closure of the bladder performed in the first 48 hours. Epispadias reconstruction and penile lengthening are accomplished at 6 months to 1 year of age. The final stage of surgical reconstruction involves bladder neck reconstruction for urinary incontinence and ureteral reimplantation to correct vesicoureteral reflux, which is performed at approximately 4 to 5 years of age or when there is adequate bladder capacity. Recently, reconstruction of the epispadiac penis and closure of the bladder have been performed in a single stage, with good preliminary results. Despite successful bladder closure and epispadias repair, some bladders fail to grow. In these cases bladder augmentation with a bowel segment and clean intermittent catheterization are required. With a staged approach, success rates in terms of spontaneous voiding with urinary continence approach 75 to 85%.

ANTERIOR URETHRAL ANOMALIES

URETHRORRHAGIA Urethrorrhagia occurs only in boys and consists of terminal hematuria or spotting of blood on the underwear. It is occasionally associated with mild dysuria. The symptoms are usually intermittent but may last for up to a year or longer. The symptoms have a tendency to recur.

The diagnosis of urethrorrhagia is made by history and confirmed with a normal physical examination. The urinalysis may show microscopic hematuria but is often negative. Evaluation should include an ultrasound of the kidneys and bladder to exclude any structural anomalies if hematuria occurs. Cystoscopy is rarely indicated unless the symptoms persist beyond 6 months or the history is inconsistent with the diagnosis. Although this condition causes great concern and anxiety in parents, the process is self-limited, and reassurance and patience is the preferred treatment.

URETHRAL PROLAPSE   Urethral prolapse is the complete eversion of the urethral mucosa through the external meatus and is almost exclusively reported in African-American girls between the ages of 4 and 10. The etiology of the prolapse is unclear but may be related to an intrinsic anatomic defect involving the periurethral smooth muscle layers in association with episodic increases in intraabdominal pressure. Predisposing factors include coughing, constipation, trauma, and urinary and vaginal infections.

Vaginal bleeding or spotting on the child's underwear is often the presenting symptom, followed by mild dysuria. Physical examination often demonstrates a typical-appearing everted, hemorrhagic, donut-shaped periurethral mass. A prolapsed ureterocele or a vaginal rhabdomyosarcoma also must be considered with this presentation.

Management includes conservative medical treatment with reduction of the prolapse, sitz baths, and topical antibiotics. Surgical resection of the prolapsed portion of the urethra is frequently required after the acute inflammation has resolved.

21.16.3   Anomalies of the Penis

HYPOSPADIAS

Hypospadias is a congenital abnormality of the penis resulting from incomplete development of the anterior urethra, resulting in the abnormal positioning of the urethral meatus proximal to the tip of the glans. The urethral meatus may be located at any point along the ventral shaft of the penis or may open onto the scrotum or perineum. The more proximal the opening, the more likely the penis will demonstrate ventral shortening and curvature referred to as *chordee*. Typically, the prepuce is incompletely formed, with the skin on the ventral surface thin or absent and an abundance of dorsal skin that drapes over the glans as a dorsal hood.

Hypospadias is the most common congenital abnormality of the penis, occurring in 1 in every 300 male children. The diagnosis of all but minor forms of hypospadias is easily made on examination of newborn boys. The incomplete formation of the prepuce with the characteristic excess dorsal hood leads to the diagnosis of hypospadias. Because almost every hypospadias repair uses preputial skin, neonatal circumcision should *not* be performed. Bilateral cryptorchidism associated with hypospadias is a form of intersex, and appropriate evaluation should be performed (see Sec. 24.7). Isolated upper urinary tract abnormalities are uncommon, and no imaging is required in the evaluation of hypospadias. In severe cases of hypospadias, a utriculus masculinus may be present, which is usually uncomplicated except for occasional urinary tract infections and difficulty with catheter passage.

The objectives of surgical repair of hypospadias consist of providing a straight penis that is adequate for sexual intercourse, extending the urethral meatus to the tip of the glans, and making the appearance of the penis as normal as possible. Surgery should be performed before 2 years of age. A one-stage procedure for uncomplicated hypospadias is preferable, but for more severe forms of penoscrotal or perineal hypospadias with severe chordee, a two-stage repair may be required.

PENILE TORSION/CURVATURE

Penile torsion is the misalignment of the penile skin with respect to the shaft and glans of the penis and can occur in either a clock-wise or counterclockwise fashion with or without other associated abnormalities such as hypospadias or chordee. Most rotations are less than 90°, but occasionally the torsion can exceed 180°. Mild degrees of rotation are common and do not result in voiding or erectile dysfunction. Surgical correction of penile torsion involves degloving of the penis and realignment of the skin with shaft of the penis.

Penile curvature can occur in any direction. Ventral curvature is defined as chordee and is usually present with hypospadias but can occur in isolation. If associated with hypospadias, chordee is corrected at the time of the hypospadias repair. If the chordee is the result of skin tethering, degloving of the penis with ventral transposition of the dorsal foreskin will result in straightening of the penis. If the penis is still bent, the chordee may be related to urethral tethering or corporal disproportion. Dorsal plication of the tunica albuginea can be performed. Rarely, the urethra may need to be mobilized or divided and reconstructed to correct the chordee. Penile curvature occurring laterally, dorsally, or in other planes is most often the result of corporal disproportion. If significant enough to affect sexual intercourse, surgical intervention by plication of the tunica albuginea can be performed.

PHIMOSIS/PARAPHIMOSIS

Phimosis is a fibrotic contraction of the preputial opening that does not permit retraction of the foreskin. Iatrogenic injury from forcible retraction of the foreskin is a common cause of phimosis. Normal erections and manual retraction contribute to further scarring and infection. Most foreskins should easily be retracted by 4 years of age. Severe phimosis can impede the urinary flow with bulging of the foreskin during urination. Posthitis is preputial inflammation and cellulitis. If the infection progresses to involvement of the glans, it is referred to as balanitis. Treatment with topical and oral antibiotics and steroid creams as well as local hygiene is successful in most cases. Circumcision should be considered when the inflammation and swelling have resolved. Paraphimosis is the entrapment of a phimotic prepuce proximal to the coronal margin, causing edema and swelling of the glans and foreskin. Prompt reduction with sedation or local anesthesia is required. If unsuccessful, a dorsal slit or circumcision is indicated.

MEATAL STENOSIS

Meatal stenosis often is an overdiagnosed condition. Boys who have undergone circumcision are at risk for the development of meatal stenosis, usually secondary to trauma or meatitis. Accurate assessment of the size of the urethral meatus with visual inspection alone is almost impossible. One must observe the voiding process for evidence of straining and for the assessment of the caliber and deflection of the urinary stream. Intervention is indicated only if the child's urinary stream is thin and/or deflects in an abnormal direction, which is the most frequent indication for therapy. Meatal stenosis does not cause significant urinary obstruction or result in hydronephrosis; therefore, routine radiologic workup is not indicated. Treatment of meatal stenosis is ventral meatotomy.

MICROPHALLUS

Microphallus in the newborn is defined as a normally developed penis, without hypospadias or ambiguous genitalia, whose penile stretched length from the pubic symphysis to the tip of the penis is less than 2.5 cm (less than 2.5 SD below the mean). The etiology of microphallus is thought to be related either to a deficiency of gonadotropin secretion in the last two trimesters of gestation or to a local organ insensitivity to testosterone. The nature of the defect can be determined by the infant's response to gonadotropin stimulation. In most cases the the hypothalamic-pituitary–end organ axis distal to the hypothalamus is intact, indicating that the hypothalamus is the site of the primary defect. Central causes of microphallus are Kallman syndrome, Prader-Willi syndrome, and panhypopituitarism (see Secs. 10.1 and 24.2). Early treatment with local or systemic testosterone may prove beneficial in increasing phallic growth. For infants who fail to respond or have an androgen insensitivity syndrome, consideration should be given to gender reassignment at an early age.

PRIAPISM

Priapism is a painful, unremitting erection in which the corpora cavernosa are rigid, but the glans and corporus spongiosum remain flaccid. Prolonged erection will result in corporal fibrosis and impotence. Sickle cell disease is the most common cause of priapism in children (see Sec. 19.4). Nocturnal erections, dehydration, mild acidema related to hypoventilation, and masturbation are possible precipitating factors. In priapism associated with sickle cell disease, prompt treatment directed toward hydration, pain control, oxygen therapy, and transfusions to increase the level of hemoglobin A will usually result in detumescence. Other treatments include corporal aspiration and irrigation with α-adrenergic agonists (eg, phenylephrine) and caudal anesthesia. Recent data suggest that prompt irrigation with α-adrenergic agonists is efficacious in treatment of priapism in patients with sickle cell anemia. Priapism unresponsive to medical treatment in the first 24 to 48 hours indicates the need for surgical intervention with cavernoglandular shunting procedures. Impotence is not uncommon as the result of priapism, whether or not surgical intervention is performed.

Less common causes of priapism include leukemia, blunt perineal trauma, spinal cord injury, medications (trazodone, chloropromazine, clozapine, cocaine, and alcohol), and Fabry disease. Regardless of cause, principles of management include treatment of any underlying process, supportive measures, and shunt procedures when necessary.

21.16.4 Anomalies of the Testes and Scrotum

TESTICULAR TORSION

Torsion of the spermatic cord and testes is a true emergency. An accurate diagnosis and urgent surgical management are required for a favorable outcome. Time is a critical factor because viability of the testis relates directly to the duration of the torsion. Torsion of the testis must be differentiated from other causes of acute scrotal swelling (Fig. 21-31).

The frequency of spermatic cord torsion is 1 in 4000 boys and men younger than age 25. Most torsions occur in patients between 3 and 20 years of age, but testicular torsion can occur at any age. The peak incidence is in the preadolescent age group. Most testicular torsions in this age group occur within the tunica vaginalis and are referred to as intravaginal torsion, which is thought to result form the high insertion of the tunica vaginalis on the spermatic cord (bell clapper deformity), which allows for testicular mobility that predisposes the testis to twisting.

Acute onset of pain associated with nausea and vomiting is the prominent feature of testicular torsion. Scrotal edema and erythema and loss of the cremasteric reflex with a high-lying, horizontal testis frequently are found. A secondary hydrocele may be present. As the

acute scrotal inflammation continues, the intrascrotal contents become confluent, making the diagnosis of torsion more difficult to differentiate from other causes of acute scrotal pain and swelling (Fig. 21-31). If the diagnosis of testicular torsion is clinically apparent, no further investigation is warranted. If the involved testis is totally infarcted or necrotic, removal may be indicated. Immediate exploration and detorsion and contralateral testicular fixation are required because of the significant incidence of bilateral pathology with intravaginal torsion. Color-flow Doppler ultrasonography is the study of choice to try to differentiate testicular torsion from other causes of acute scrotal pain. With testicular torsion no flow will be seen in the affected testis. Imaging studies should not delay surgical intervention. Irreversible changes occur in testes within 4 to 6 hours, and after 24 hours of torsion, testicular infarction is the rule.

NEONATAL TESTICULAR TORSION Neonatal torsion is the torsion of the entire spermatic cord and testis outside the tunica vaginalis, referred to as extravaginal torsion, and occurs exclusively in neonates, often before birth. The etiology may be related to the lack of testicular fixation in the scrotum, allowing the testis, spermatic cord, and tunica vaginalis to twist. The finding of a painless, swollen, discolored hemiscrotum in the neonate is diagnostic of spermatic cord torsion. Although testicular salvage is rare when the condition is present at birth, some pediatric urologists recommend surgical exploration with orchiectomy and contralateral orchiopexy. The incidence of bilaterality with extravaginal torsion is significantly less than with intravaginal torsion, but the consequences are such that fixation of the contralateral gonad is recommended by some. Others advise observation because the incidence of torsion of the remaining testis is not significantly greater than what would be expected in the general population.

TORSION OF THE TESTICULAR APPENDAGES

Torsion of the appendix testes, a remnant of the cranial portion of the müllerian duct, and the appendix epididymis, a mesonephric tubule remnant, probably is the most common cause of acute scrotal pain in children and occurs in prepubertal boys between the ages of 3 and 13 years. Torsion of the appendix testes is the most common, comprising >90% of torsed appendages. Torsion of the testicular appendages can be clinically indistinguishable from testicular torsion. The pain, however, of a torsed testicular appendage tends to be less severe than that of testicular torsion, not associated with nausea or vomiting, and to resolve over several days. Examination in the early stages may reveal a palpable, tender nodule on the superior portion of the testicle with blue discoloration ("blue dot" sign). The testis usually is not enlarged or indurated early in the process. As the inflammatory response progresses, swelling and erythema of the scrotum may make differentiation between a torsed appendix testis and a torsed testis impossible. Color-flow Doppler ultrasonography can help distinguish torsion of the testicular appendages from torsion of the testis (Fig. 21-31). Almost all cases will resolve spontaneously with conservative measures. Surgical exploration is indicated only if the diagnosis is unclear or the pain is persistent or recurrent.

CRYPTORCHIDISM (UNDESCENDED TESTES)

Cryptorchidism or incomplete testicular descent occurs in up to 30% of premature infant boys. In boys born at term the incidence

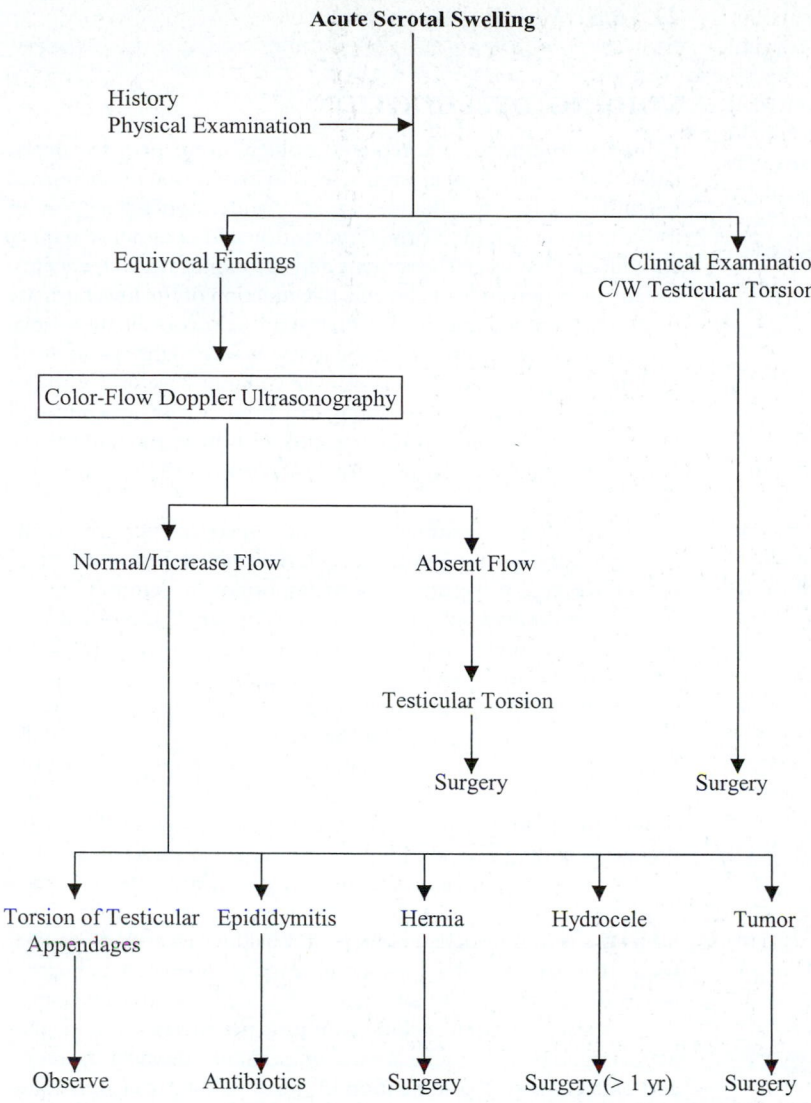

FIGURE 21-31   Evaluation and treatment of acute scrotal swelling in children. C/W = compatible with.

is 3 to 4%. By 1 year of life, testes have descended in all but 0.3% of boys. Cryptorchidism is the most common genital problem encountered in pediatric urology.

True undescended testes may be intraabdominal or in the inguinal canal. Ectopic testes are testes that are distal to the external inguinal ring but are not located in the scrotum. Although usually located just above the scrotum, ectopic testes can be located in the perineum or on the shaft of the penis. True undescended and ectopic testes must be distinguished from retractile testes. Retractile testes can be brought down to the bottom of the scrotum and are the result of a hyperactive cremasteric reflex. Retractile testes ultimately will reside in the scrotum spontaneously, although a small percentage can become entrapped in the inguinal region and require surgical correction. Undescended testes are usually associated with an inguinal hernia and, when intraabdominal, are at an increased risk for testicular torsion. Undescended testes have a 4 to 10 times higher risk for developing malignancy, seminoma being the most common tumor seen.

Testicular descent occurs late in fetal development and is regulated by many factors including shortening of the gubernaculum, intraabdominal pressure, and hormonal and neurologic influences. The function of the genitofemoral nerve has been implicated in testicular descent.

All general pediatric examinations should include documentation of testicular position. Repeated examinations with the patient in multiple positions are helpful. Usually treatment should be instituted between 1 and 2 years of age. Early treatment is predicated on preserving fertility because testes left in an undescended location past puberty will have decreased or absent spermatogenesis.

The goal of treatment is to relocate the undescended testis into the scrotum, which can be achieved by either hormonal or surgical treatment. Hormonal manipulation is based on the observation that increased testosterone may encourage testicular descent. Intramuscular human chorionic gonadotropin (hCG) is given in a series of injections. Success rates of approximately 30 to 40% have been reported but are not uniformly achieved. Surgical orchiopexy remains the treatment of choice in most patients. Palpable undescended testes are usually located within or emerging from the inguinal canal and are best managed through a standard inguinal incision. With bilateral nonpalpable testes, confirmation that testes are present is important before a series of invasive diagnostic or therapeutic modalities are begun. These patients should have measurement of serum follicle-stimulating hormone (FSH) (high values correlate with anorchia in prepubertal boys) and an hCG stimulation test (a testosterone spike in response to hCG stimulation indicates the presence of at least one functional testis). In approximately 60% of patients with a unilateral nonpalpable testis, the gonad is absent. Laparoscopy can be useful in this setting to help plan the surgical approach.

When the vas deferens and gonadal vessels are observed to end blindly proximal to the internal ring without a processus vaginalis (or hernia sac), the so-called intraabdominal vanishing testis syndrome, there is absence of the ipsilateral gonad, and a surgical exploration is obviated. When the testis is in a high intraabdominal position, division of the testicular artery or vein may be required so that the testis can reach the scrotum.

HERNIA/HYDROCELE

Inguinal bulges and scrotal masses in children are usually secondary to hernias or hydroceles. Hernias and hydroceles result from the failure of the fusion and obliteration of the processus vaginalis. The patency of the processus vaginalis allows peritoneal fluid, omentum, or viscera to enter the inguinal canal or the scrotum. Small defects allow only the passage of peritoneal fluid, resulting in a hydrocele. Larger defects may result in bowel within the hernia sac and potential ischemic injury to the testis. Noncommunicating hydroceles tend to resolve during the first year of life. Communicating hydroceles fluctuate in size, smaller when supine and larger when erect. Hydroceles transilluminate; hernias do not. Hydroceles that persist after 1 year of age should be repaired surgically. Inguinal hernias should be repaired when diagnosed. Incarcerated hernias should be manually reduced, and operative repair performed soon thereafter. Strangulated hernias require emergent surgical exploration to prevent necrosis of the bowel and testis.

Routine contralateral inguinal exploration is controversial. Approximately 29% of patients will eventually develop a contralateral inguinal hernia after previous unilateral repair. Indications for contralateral exploration include patients with peritoneal dialysis catheters or ventriculoperitoneal shunts and boys younger than 2 years of age with only one hernia that is clinically evident. Laparoscopy through the hernia sac at the time of exploration may aid in determining whether the contralateral side should be surgically explored.

VARICOCELES

A varicocele is an abnormal dilation and tortuosity of the testicular vein and pampinoform plexus of the spermatic cord and is present in approximately 15% of adolescent boys, but unusual prior to puberty. Varicoceles occur almost exclusively on the left side. Most varicoceles are asymptomatic and are discovered during routine physical examination. The etiology is related to the unique anatomy of the left testicular vein, which is longer than the right and enters the left renal vein instead of the vena cava. The lack of internal spermatic vein valves results in increased hydrostatic pressure and engorgement of the veins surrounding the testis. This causes an increase in scrotal temperature that can interfere with normal testicular development.

There is no consensus as to the indications for varicocele repair in adolescents. Although varicoceles in adults are the most common treatable cause of infertility, most men with varicoceles have normal fertility. These findings raise questions as to whether varicocele repair should be undertaken in adolescent boys who are too young to produce a semen specimen. Boys with atrophy or retarded growth of the left testis should undergo varicocele repair, whereas boys with a normal-sized left testis should be followed closely, and surgery performed at the first sign of decreased testicular growth. Semen analysis can be followed, and repair of the varicocele performed if the semen quality is abnormal.

21.16.5   Voiding Disorders

VOIDING DYSFUNCTION

Urinary incontinence is a frequent problem in the pediatric population, and the etiology is often a delay in maturation of the normal micturition pathways. Bladder capacity and emptying rely on an intact nervous system. Normal micturition and continence require coordination between the somatic and autonomic nervous systems, which are responsible for the effective function of the lower urinary tract. The cerebral cortex and brainstem help coordinate normal voiding. Daytime continence is achieved before nighttime control. By 4 to 5 years of age, the majority of children develop control of micturition. Dysfunctional voiding may present with a spectrum of findings including incontinence, recurrent urinary tract infections, frequency, urgency, dysuria, hydronephrosis, VUR, and renal failure.

Evaluation and treatment for urinary incontinence are usually not performed before 5 years of age. A complete history focusing on the pattern of wetting is most important in determining the etiology of the patient's incontinence (Fig. 21-32). Normal volitional voiding interspersed with continuous urinary leakage is suggestive of an ectopic ureter. Voiding without prior awareness suggests a sensory deficit, and bounding up and down on the soles of the feet before voiding suggests the presence of detrusor instability. Incontinence with stress (coughing, sneezing, lifting, and exercise) and with giggling can occur in children. The physical examination should focus on findings of an occult neuropathic bladder, suggested by finding a sacral dimple, café-au-lait spots, or a hairy tuft over the sacrum. Urinalysis and urine culture should be performed to rule out infection. All children with daytime incontinence should have an ultrasound of the kidneys and bladder to exclude an anatomic defect responsible for incontinence. Urodynamic evaluation is performed when there is a suspicion of a neuropathic abnormality. Treatment options include antibiotic prophylaxis, timed voiding, anticholinergic medications, imipramine, perineal exercises, and biofeedback. A combination of timed voiding and anticholinergics is the initial treatment for a sensory deficit and detrusor instability. Giggling incontinence is difficult to treat but may respond to anticholinergic medications. Perineal exercises and agents with α-adrenergic agonist properties, such as imipramine, are used to treat stress incontinence.

NOCTURNAL ENURESIS

Nocturnal enuresis is the involuntary loss of urine during sleep and may be either primary or secondary. Primary enuretics have never had a prolonged dry period. It affects 10% of children who are 5 years of age, with a spontaneous resolution rate of 15% per year. Boys are affected more frequently than girls. Forty percent of children with one parent who was affected will have nocturnal enuresis, and 70% will have nocturnal enuresis if both parents were affected. Although nocturnal enuresis does not cause physical harm to children, it can be emotionally disruptive to the child and family.

The etiologies of nocturnal enuresis include delayed maturational control of continence, emotional stress, the presence of a small bladder capacity, and poor sleep arousal. No one etiology can explain nocturnal enuresis, and the majority of children with enuresis do not have either organic or functional disease.

Appropriate evaluation requires only a complete history and physical examination (Fig. 21-32). Attention to daytime voiding patterns is important to exclude dysfunctional voiding. The physical

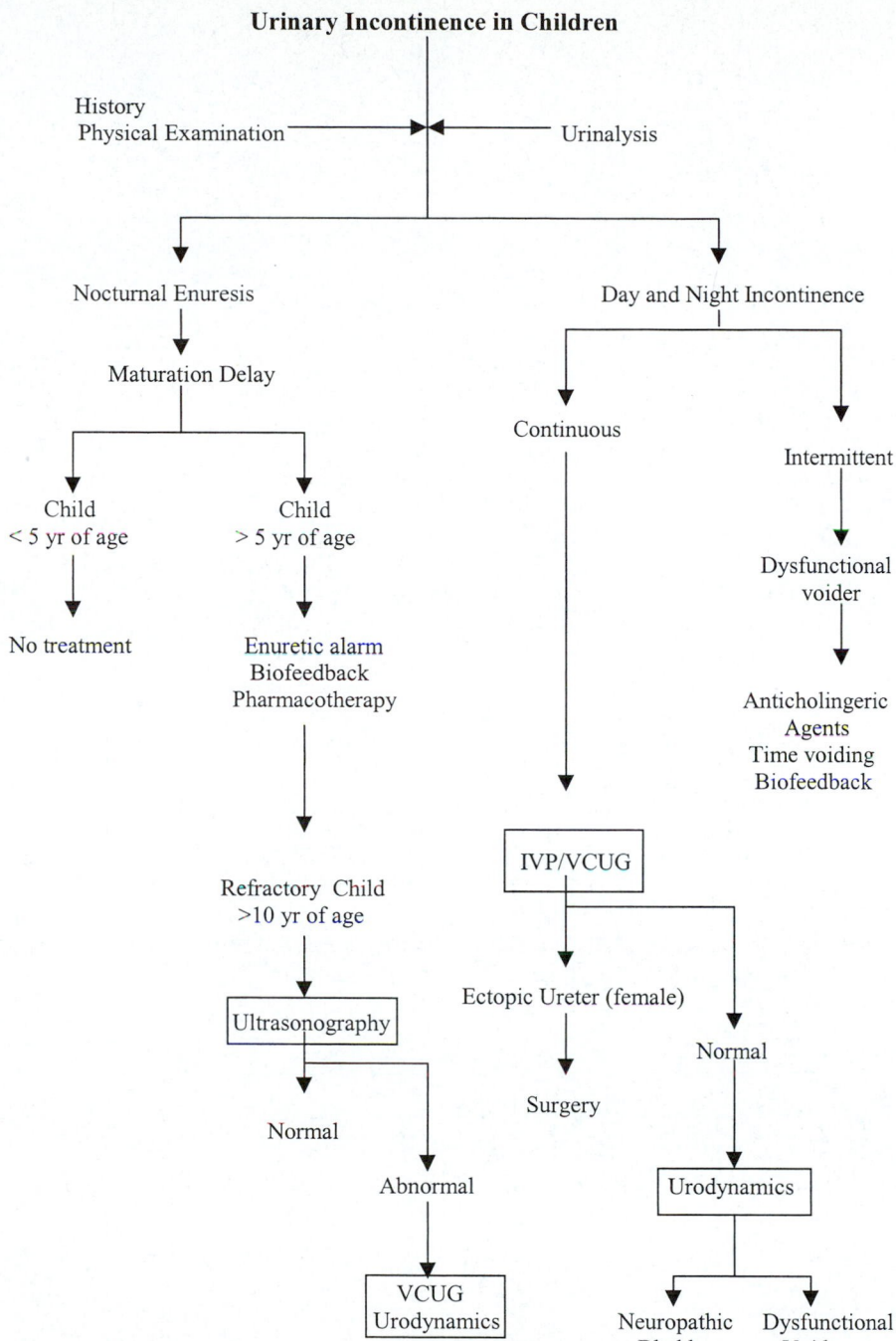

Urinary Incontinence in Children

FIGURE 21-32 Evaluation and treatment of urinary incontinence in children. IVP = intravenous pyelogram; VCUG = voiding cystourethrogram.

examination should include emphasis on the neurologic system to exclude an occult neuropathic bladder. A urinalysis and culture should be performed to look for infection. Imaging studies are not required for the evaluation of nocturnal enuresis if the history, physical examination, and urinalysis are normal. However, imaging studies in children older than 10 years of age with refractory nocturnal enuresis have been suggested.

Treatment includes the use of enuresis alarms, which are most effective in younger children. In older children, three medications are currently available: oxybutynin, imipramine, and desmopressin acetate (DDAVP). When, in addition to nocturnal enuresis, urgency or frequency is present, a combination of oxybutynin in the daytime and imipramine at night may be efficacious.

References

Gillenwater JY, Grayhack JT, Howards SS, Duckett JW, eds: Adult and Pediatric Urology, 3rd ed. St Louis, Mosby-Year Book, 1996

Gomella LG, ed: The 5-Minute Urology Consult, 1st ed. Philadelphia, Lippincott Williams & Wilkins, 2000

Kelalis PP, King LR, Belman AE, eds: Clinical Pediatric Urology, 3rd ed. Philadelphia, WB Saunders, 1992

Walsh PC, Retik AB, Vaughan ED Jr, Wein AJ, eds: Campbell's Urology, 7th ed, vol 2. Philadelphia, WB Saunders, 1998

Weiss RM, George N Jr, O'Reilly PH, eds: Comprehensive Urology, 1st ed. London, CV Mosby, 2001

THE CIRCULATORY SYSTEM

Julien I. E. Hoffman, Associate Editor

22.1 BASIC SCIENCE

22.1.1 Embryology

James D. Bristow

OVERVIEW OF CARDIAC DEVELOPMENT

During the first month of gestation, the primitive cardiac tube forms. It has four segments in series: the sinoatrium, primitive ventricle, bulbus cordis, and conotruncus (Fig. 22-1A). Blood enters the sinoatrium and leaves via the truncus. During the second month of gestation this simple tube changes to a heart with two systems in parallel, each system having an atrium, a ventricle, and a great artery. The increase from four to six components is accomplished by division of the proximal and distal segments into paired structures: the sinoatrium into right and left atria and the truncus into aorta and pulmonary artery. In contrast, the left and right ventricles form from the primitive ventricle and bulbus cordis, respectively. When the primitive heart tube loops to the right, the bulbus cordis and primitive ventricle come to lie side by side (Fig. 22-1B,C). While the two atria form, the atrioventricular (AV) canal is divided by the endocardial cushions into tricuspid and mitral inlets, both of which initially connect to the primitive ventricle. The transition to a double pumping system requires subsequent alignment of each ventricle with its respective AV valve proximally and the great arteries distally. The proximal alignment is achieved by rightward migration of the AV canal and leftward migration of the ventricular septum (Fig. 22-1D,E), so that the right atrium connects to the right ventricle. At the distal end of the cardiac tube, the transition is more complex. The distal end of the bulbus cordis divides into two muscular portions: the subaortic conus and the subpulmonic conus. The latter increases in length, but the subaortic conus resorbs as the aorta migrates posteriorly to connect with the left ventricle.

There are many places for error in this complex process, and as a result, congenital heart defects are the most common human malformations. Although the broad spectrum of congenital heart disease can be confusing, appreciation of the normal embryologic development of the heart provides a framework for understanding congenital heart disease. This is true because when normal development fails, the result is frequently the persistence of normal fetal structures or spatial relationships. This is true for each of the cardiac segments described above. For example, rightward migration of the AV canal normally aligns the tricuspid valve over the right ventricle. Failure of this process results in *double-inlet left ventricle* (a common form of single ventricle); both AV valves or a common AV valve connects to a large left ventricle, and there is a rudimentary right ventricular outflow chamber. This arrangement is identical to

that of the heart tube immediately after looping (Fig. 22-1C). Abnormalities of normal conal resorption also occur and lead to abnormal connections of the great arteries to the ventricles. For example, failure of resorption of the subaortic conus results in persistent connection of both great arteries to the right ventricle, a condition called *double-outlet right ventricle*. Similarly, failure of the truncus to divide into aorta and main pulmonary artery results in postnatal persistence of the *truncus arteriosus,* a normal fetal structure. In the sections that follow, normal development is described, followed by descriptions of perturbations that lead to common congenital heart defects.

CARDIAC LOOPING

During development, the heart is the first structure of the body to demonstrate left-right asymmetry, and the first sign of this asymmetry is looping of the primitive heart tube ventrally and to the right. This so-called *d*-loop places the bulbus cordis (the future right ventricle) to the right, leaving the primitive ventricle (the future left ventricle) to the left. The postlooped heart then rotates slightly to place the developing right ventricle in front of the left.

When the heart loops to the left rather than to the right (an *l*-loop), the normal positions of the ventricles are reversed within the thorax, with the morphologic right ventricle lying to the left and the morphologic left ventricle to the right. This left-right reversal can be accompanied by reversal of the left-right axis in all other organs, resulting in situs inversus. Remarkably, in most individuals with situs inversus, subsequent cardiac development is normal. However, patients with normal situs in whom an *l*-loop occurs may have severe congenital heart defects. It is not surprising that a defect occurring at such an early stage of heart formation might interfere with subsequent development. Frequently, an *l*-loop leads to failure of AV valve migration, resulting in *double-inlet left ventricle* (described above). If AV valve migration does occur, because the ventricles are reversed within the chest but the atria are not, the left ventricle becomes aligned with the right atrium and the left atrium with the right ventricle. In this circumstance, if development of the conus and truncus is normal (so that the right ventricle gives rise to the pulmonary artery and the left ventricle to the aorta), the result is *isolated ventricular inversion*. More commonly, an *l*-loop is also accompanied by misalignment of the ventriculoarterial connection so that the right ventricle gives rise to the aorta and the left ventricle to the pulmonary artery. The net result is interposition of the left ventricle between right atrium and pulmonary artery and right ventricle between left atrium and aorta. Because this arrangement allows a normal postnatal flow pattern, it is referred to as *congenitally corrected transposition of the great arteries* or simply *l-transposition*.

ATRIAL SEPTUM

The primitive common atrium is divided into two chambers by a septum formed from three structures: septum I, septum II, and a

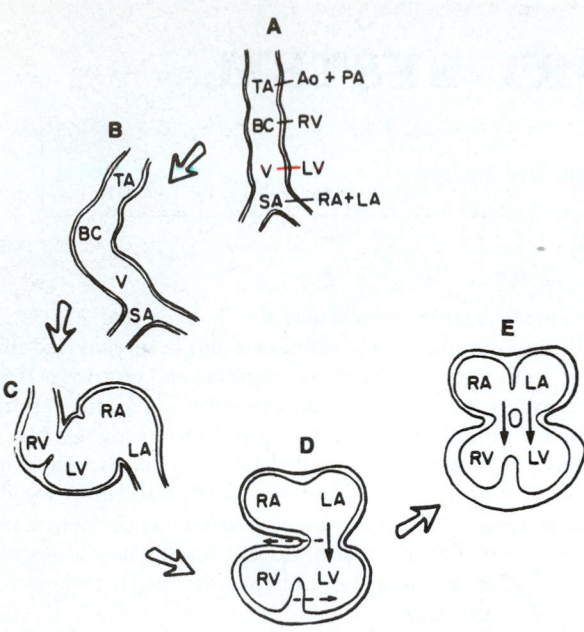

FIGURE 22-1 **Transition from straight cardiac tube to four-chamber heart. A: Straight cardiac tube stage with four segments in series. The sinoatrium (SA) is destined to become the right and left atria (RA, LA); the primitive ventricle (V) is precursor to the left ventricle (LV); the bulbus cordis (BC) becomes the right ventricle (RV); the truncus arteriosus (TA) divides into the aorta (Ao) and main pulmonary artery (PA). The proximal and distal ends of the tube are fixed. B: Differential growth results in the tube bending toward the right. C: The bulboventricular portion of the tube doubles over on itself, so that the right and left ventricles lie side by side. D: The right and left atria still connect to the left ventricle by the atrioventricular (AV) canal. The AV canal migrates toward the right, so that it lies over both ventricles. E: The anterior and posterior endocardial cushions meet and divide the AV canal into tricuspid and mitral orifices.**

small portion of endocardial cushion tissue (Fig. 22-2). Septum I arises as a crescent-shaped structure from the atrial roof and grows toward the AV canal to leave an interatrial opening (ostium primum) of decreasing size (Fig. 22-2A,B,C). Before the ostium primum closes, multiple perforations develop in the cephalad portion of septum I (Fig. 22-2C); they coalesce to form the ostium secundum and permit continued right-to-left flow when the ostium primum is obliterated (Fig. 22-2D,E). Septum II begins to form at the roof of the atrium just to the right of septum I. This septum grows along the atrial wall, but its free concave margin remains open centrally as the fossa ovalis (Fig. 22-2C,D,E). The thin tissue of septum I acts as a one-way valve, the valve of the foramen ovale, and permits passage of blood from right to left during fetal life (Fig. 22-2E).

Defects of the atrial septum may be of three types: foramen ovale or *secundum defects, primum defects,* and *sinus venosus defects.* Secundum defects occur if there is insufficient foramen ovale valve tissue to permit closure of the foramen. These defects are normal during development of septum II but should be closed by complete development of septum II. Sinus venosus defects are caused not by a deficiency of atrial tissue but by misalignment with straddling across the atrial septum of the structures derived from the right sinus horn (superior vena cava). Primum defects are best considered with endocardial cushion defects and are described below.

VENTRICULAR SEPTUM AND STRUCTURES DERIVED FROM THE ENDOCARDIAL CUSHIONS

The ventricular septum of the mature heart can be separated into three components with embryologically distinct origins: the muscular, outlet, and inlet septa. The first, the muscular septum, comprises the bulk of the ventricular septum; it arises from a flange of tissue lying at the junction of the primitive (left) ventricle and the bulbis cordis (right ventricle). Muscular *ventricular septal defects* result from incomplete extension of this tissue across the connection between these two chambers. Similarly, normal closure of the outlet ventricular septum occurs by inferior extension of the cono-

FIGURE 22-2 **Formation of the atrial septum and foramen ovale. A,B: Septum I begins to separate the chamber into right and left atria. C: Septum II forms a complete septum, with the exception of a central opening with a prominent muscular rim at its superior margin. This opening, the fossa ovalis, is covered by the tissue of septum I (the valve of the foramen ovale). Note that there is a small portion of atrial septum just above the AV valves that is formed by endocardial cushion tissue. The latter also forms the uppermost portion of the ventricular septum as well as portions of the tricuspid and mitral valves. D: Coalescence of perforations to form ostium secundum. E: Obliteration of ostium primum. RV and LV = right and left ventricles; TV and MV = tricuspid and mitral valves.**

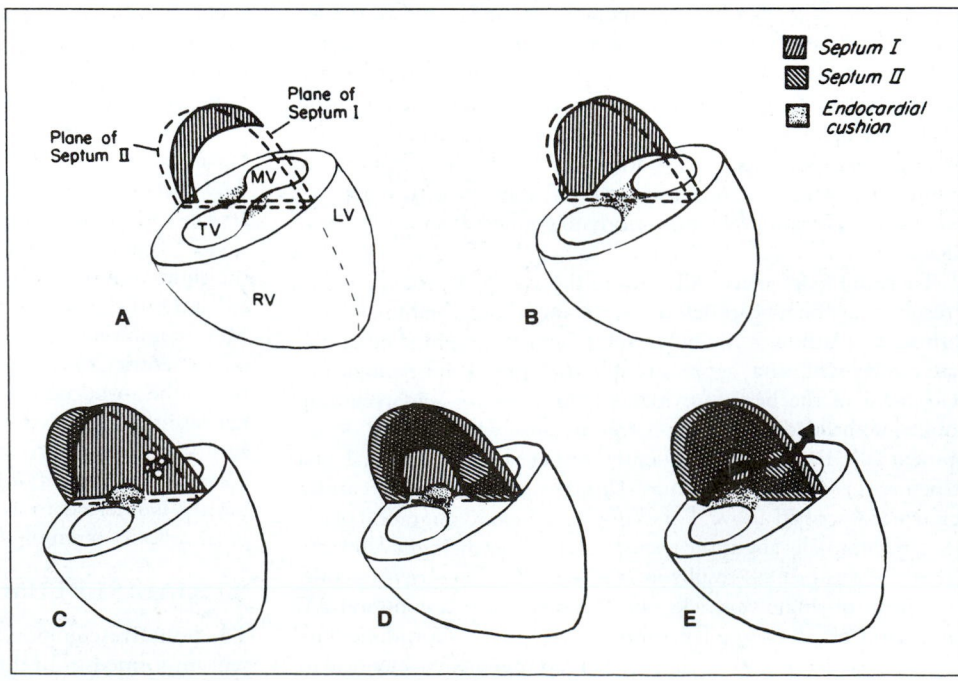

truncal septum that divides the aorta and pulmonary artery. Defects in this region are frequently called *supracristal ventricular septal defects* because they lie above the crista, a prominent muscle band within the right ventricle. *Inlet ventricular septal defects* are one type of endocardial cushion defect described below. The most common ventricular septal defects occur in the region where the muscular, inlet, and outlet portions of the septum meet. These defects are called *perimembranous ventricular septal defects*. Because relative deficiency of any of the three components of the ventricular septum can lead to a perimembranous defect, it is of little surprise that they are very common.

The inlet portion of the ventricular septum and the primum portion of the atrial septum are derived from the endocardial cushions and are thus considered along with morphogenesis of the AV canal. The AV canal initially connects the atria to the primitive ventricle but eventually overlies both ventricles because the AV canal shifts toward the right while the lower ventricular septum shifts toward the left (Fig. 22-1). Growth of the endocardial cushions ultimately divides the AV canal into the tricuspid and mitral channels while providing the lower portion of the atrial septum and the inlet portion of the ventricular septum. Deficiency of development in this region may result in various defects. The least severe is the ostium primum type of atrial septal defect, which usually has a large defect in the lowermost portion of the atrial septum, an anterior (septal) mitral leaflet cleft, and a displaced mitral valve as well as an insignificant ventricular septal defect below the AV valves. The most severe defect is the complete AV canal with large contiguous atrial and ventricular defects, a common AV valve straddling the ventricular septum, and deficiency of AV valve tissue. Less common types of endocardial cushion defects include isolated mitral clefts or isolated ventricular septal defects in the inlet region.

PULMONARY VEINS

The lung buds are outgrowths of the primitive foregut, and early in fetal life venous drainage is by the splanchnic plexus to the cardinal and umbilicovitelline veins (Fig. 22-3). The common pulmonary vein arises from the posterior left atrium as a small pouch that enlarges and connects with the splanchnic plexus. As pulmonary venous drainage via the common pulmonary vein increases, the anastomoses to the cardinal and umbilicovitelline venous systems disappear. The common pulmonary vein is incorporated into the posterior left atrial wall, and the pulmonary veins then connect directly to the left atrium (Fig. 22-3A). Should the common pulmonary vein fail to develop or connect to the splanchnic plexus, the primitive venous connections persist and result in *total anomalous pulmonary venous connection* to derivatives of the cardinal system (superior vena cava) or umbilicovitelline (portal) venous system (Fig. 22-3C). A closely related anomaly is *cor triatriatum*, in which the common pulmonary vein is poorly incorporated into the left atrium so that there is a stenotic membrane between the common pulmonary vein and the left atrium (Fig. 22-3B).

THE CONOTRUNCUS

The conotruncus is the most distal portion of the primitive heart tube, and its normal development is required for normal separation of the aorta and pulmonary outflow tracts and their normal alignment with the appropriate ventricles. Normal conotruncal development involves four distinct processes: proliferation of cells within the conotruncal cushions; migration of cells into the conotruncus from the cardiac neural crest; resorption of the subaortic conus; and leftward movement of the conotruncus. These processes and

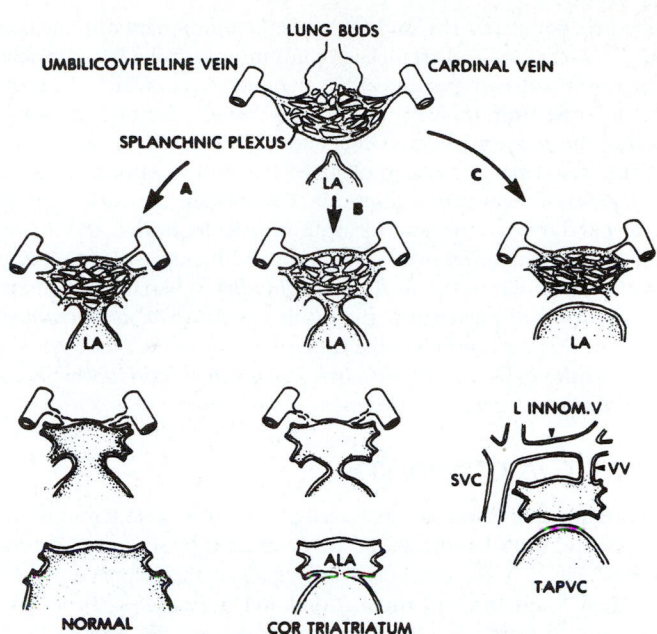

FIGURE 22-3   Embryology of normal pulmonary veins, cor triatriatum, and total anomalous pulmonary venous connection. A: Normal pulmonary venous development. B: Cor triatriatum. Narrowing of the common pulmonary vein/left atrial junction results in formation of a stenotic membrane that separates the left atrium from a chamber receiving the pulmonary veins, ie, the accessory left atrium (ALA). C: Total anomalous pulmonary venous connection (TAPVC). VV = vertical vein; L INNOM. V = left innominate vein; SVC = superior vena cava.

heart disease that results from their failed development are considered in turn.

The conotruncus contains endocardial swellings exactly analogous to the endocardial cushions in that they septate ventricular outflow tract just as the endocardial cushions septate ventricular inlet (the AV canal). The outflow cushions grow toward each other from ventral and dorsal positions to divide the conus into right and left ventricular outflows, and the truncus into the aortic and pulmonary valves. Meanwhile, the aortic sac above is septated by an invagination of the roof of the aortic sac that eventually fuses with the conus septum rising from below to complete the separation of the great arteries. Migration of neural crest cells into the expanding conotruncal septum is essential for its completion. It is not clear, however, whether the failure of separation that occurs in the absence of neural crest invasion results from a simple reduction in cell number or from the loss of essential patterning signals that are provided by the invading neural crest cells. In either event, when conotruncal septation fails, the result is *persistent truncus arteriosus*. In this lesion, the outlet septum is absent, and there is a single truncal valve rather than a pair of semilunar valves. There is a common aortic and pulmonary trunk, from which the branch pulmonary arteries arise in a variety of configurations.

Because the conotruncus is initially positioned over the future right ventricle, for appropriate separation of the aortic and pulmonary outflows to occur, the aortic portion of the conotruncus must move leftward so that the aorta is committed to the left ventricle. For this leftward migration to occur, muscle from the left portion of the conus must be resorbed. Failure of the subaortic conus to resorb prevents migration, and the result is double-outlet right ventricle. Sometimes the subpulmonary conus rather than the subaortic conus resorbs, and then it is the pulmonary outflow that migrates leftward and establishes continuity with the left ventricle. The result is d-*transposition of the great arteries* in which the great arteries arise from the wrong ventricles. Finally, even when resorption of the subaortic conus occurs normally, migration may be deficient, resulting in malalignment of the outlet septum with the remainder of the ventricular septum. Commonly, the outlet septum is deviated toward the anterior right ventricular outlet, and the result is an outlet VSD, overriding aorta and hypoplasia of the right ventricular outlet typical of *tetralogy of Fallot*. When the outlet septum is deviated posteriorly, the result is a *posterior malalignment VSD*. In this circumstance, the outlet septum frequently obstructs aortic outflow, producing *subaortic stenosis* and secondary hypoplasia of the aortic arch or *coarctation of the aorta*.

AORTIC ARCH SYSTEM

The ventral and dorsal aortas as well as their cervical extensions, the ventral and dorsal aortic roots, are connected by six pairs of aortic arches (Fig. 22-4). The aortic arches make their appearance sequentially, and three of these paired arches (arches I, II, and V) disappear without leaving permanent remnants, while another (arch III) connects the internal and external carotid arteries. The proximal portions of the sixth arches become the right and left pulmonary arteries, and the distal left sixth arch becomes the ductus arteriosus; rarely, the distal right sixth arch persists as a right ductus arteriosus. Normally, the left fourth arch forms the left aortic arch, and the proximal portion of the right fourth arch becomes the prox-

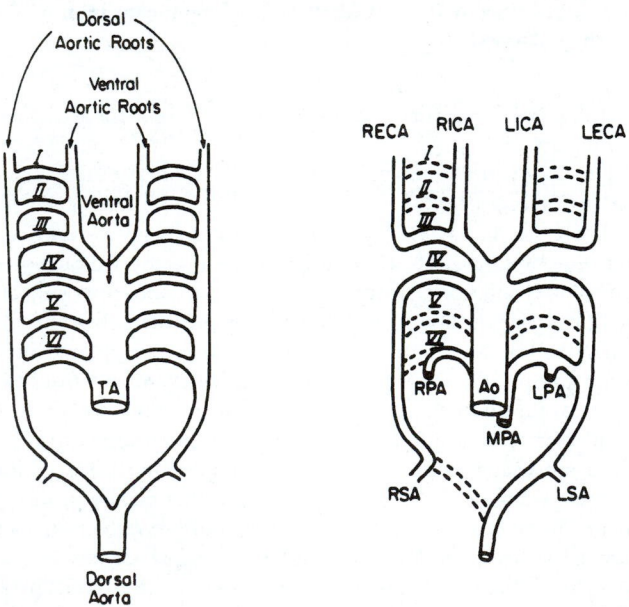

FIGURE 22-4 Schematic diagram of the embryonic aortic arch system. On the left the truncus arteriosus (TA) and the six arches that connect it to the dorsal aorta. The six arches appear sequentially, and those that regress do so at different times. Involution of the various aortic arches and portions of the dorsal aortic roots, as well as persistence of other segments, result in formation of the normal arterial pattern shown on the right. The structures are drawn to show their aortic arch derivations rather than their final anatomic positions. TA = truncus arteriosus; Ao = aorta; MPA = main pulmonary artery; RPA = right pulmonary artery; LPA = left pulmonary artery; RECA and RICA = right external and internal carotid arteries; LECA and LICA = left external and internal carotid arteries; RSA and LSA = right and left subclavian arteries.

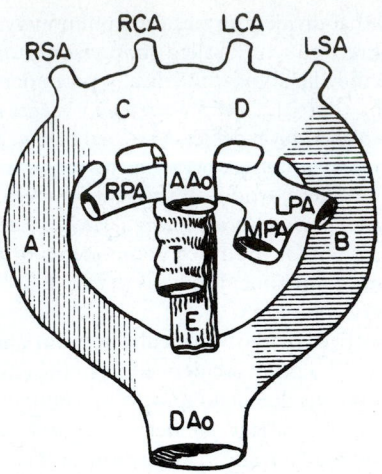

FIGURE 22-5 Schematic diagram of Edwards hypothetic double aortic arch and bilateral ductus arteriosi. Regression in shaded area *A* results in the normal left aortic arch; regression in shaded area *B* results in right aortic arch. Regression at location *C* results in left aortic arch and anomalous right subclavian artery, and regression at *D* results in right aortic arch and anomalous left subclavian artery. T = trachea; E = esophagus; MPA = main pulmonary artery; RPA and LPA = right and left pulmonary arteries; RSA and LSA = right and left subclavian arteries; RCA and LCA = right and left carotid arteries. These are the four most common types of arch anomalies; however, the number of possible arch anomalies is large because regression can occur almost anywhere. Lack of regression results in a double aortic arch.

imal portion of the right subclavian artery. The aortic arch system and the arterial structures that it subsequently forms are diagrammed in Fig. 22-4. Edwards and associates have devised a hypothetic double aortic arch system that simplifies the understanding of aortic arch anomalies (Fig. 22-5). The embryology of any aortic arch anomaly is apparent if one postulates regression of an aortic arch at an appropriate location; if there is no arch regression, then there will be a double aortic arch.

CONDUCTION SYSTEM

Before septation of the atria and ventricles, rings of specialized conducting cells form at the sinoatrial, ventriculobulbar, and bulbotruncal junctions. The conduction tissue appears to arise from cardiac myocytes in response to unknown signals. With looping of the cardiac tube, the AV ring is invaginated to lie at the base of the atrial septum so that some of its specialized cells contact the upper part of the ventriculobulbar ring, thereby providing continuity between the primitive AV node and the penetrating bundle of His. Failure of various portions of these specialized rings to make contact with each other causes congenital heart block. If the atrial septum and upper part of the ventricular septum are not normally aligned (as in *l*-transposition or in single ventricle), the normal posterior AV node cannot join the bundle of His. In this instance an anterior portion of the AV ring tissue may join the ventriculobulbar ring to produce an abnormally placed bundle of His.

References

Bristow J: Cardiac and myocardial structure and myocardial cellular and molecular function. In: Gluckman PD, Heymann MA, eds: Perinatal and Pediatric Pathophysiology. London, Edward Arnold, 1993:473

Clark EB: Morphogenesis, growth and biomechanics. In: Emmanouilides GC, Riemenschneider TA, Allen HD, Gutgesell HP, eds: Heart Disease in Infants, Children, and Adolescents, Including the Fetus and Young Adult. Baltimore, Williams & Wilkins, 1994:1

Epstein ML: Development of the cardiac conduction system. In: Moller JH, Neal WA, eds: Fetal, Neonatal, and Infant Cardiac Disease. Norwalk, CT, Appleton & Lange, 1990:25

Goor DA, Lillehei CW: Congenital Malformations of the Heart: Embryology, Anatomy, and Operative Considerations. New York, Grune & Stratton, 1975

Harvey RP, Rosenthal N: Heart Development. San Diego, Academic Press, 1999

Netter FH, Van Mierop LHS: Embryology. In: Netter FH, ed: The Ciba Collection of Medical Illustrations, Vol 5: Heart. Summit, NJ, Ciba, 1969

Stewart JR, Kincaid OW, Edwards JE: An Atlas of Vascular Rings and Related Malformations of the Aortic Arch System. Springfield, IL, Charles C Thomas, 1964

Wenink ACG: Embryology of the heart. In: Anderson RH, Macartney FJ, Shinebourne EA, Tynan M, eds: Paediatric Cardiology. Edinburgh, Churchill Livingstone, 1987:83

22.1.2   Fetal Circulation and Cardiovascular Adjustments After Birth

Abraham M. Rudolph

Although the most dramatic circulatory changes occur at birth, when gas exchange moves from the placenta to the lungs, cardiovascular function is changing both before and after birth. Most of our knowledge of the physiology and pathophysiology of the fetal circulation comes from studies in fetal lambs, but recent echocardiographic Doppler studies of the human fetus at various stages of gestational development have confirmed the similarity of the course of the circulation and its responses to stress in human and sheep fetuses.

COURSE AND DISTRIBUTION OF FETAL CIRCULATION

In adult mammals blood circulates serially through the right side of the heart to the lungs, then through the left side of the heart to the systemic circulation, and returns to the right side of the heart. Cardiac output is the volume of blood ejected by either ventricle per minute. In the fetus the series circulation does not occur because the right ventricle ejects only a small amount of blood to the lungs. Most of the right ventricular output passes directly into the systemic circulation through the ductus arteriosus (Figs. 22-6 and 22-7). We therefore consider fetal cardiac output to be the total output of both ventricles and term it the combined ventricular output (CVO). The CVO in fetal lambs from about halfway through gestation to term is 450 to 500 mL/kg fetal body weight per minute.

About 40% of the CVO or 200 mL/kg fetal weight per minute goes to the umbilical-placental circulation. Blood oxygenated in the placenta returns to the fetus through the umbilical veins; the main umbilical vein passes from the umbilicus to enter the portal venous system at the porta hepatis. After providing the portal branches to the left lobe of the liver, the umbilical vein gives rise to the ductus venosus and then arches to the right to join the portal vein. The portal veins entering the right lobe of the liver thus supply a mixture of well-oxygenated umbilical venous blood and poorly oxygenated portal venous blood. The venous supply to the left lobe of the liver comes exclusively from the umbilical veins. These blood flow pat-

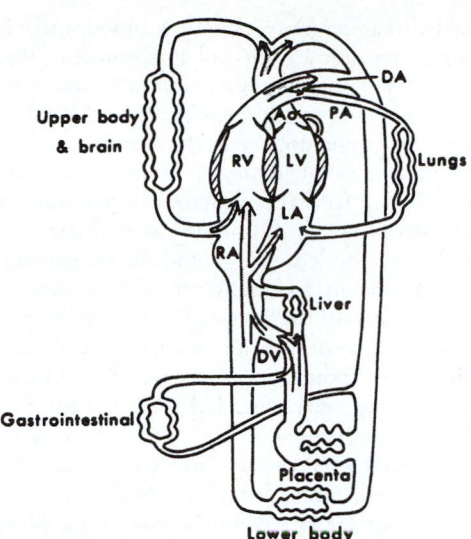

FIGURE 22-6   Course of fetal circulation. (For description see text.) DA = ductus arteriosus; Ao = aorta; PA = pulmonary artery; RV = right ventricle; LV = left ventricle; LA = left atrium; RA = right atrium; DV = ductus venosus. SOURCE: *Rudolph AM: Congenital Diseases of the Heart. Chicago, Year Book, 1974.*

terns account for the higher oxygen saturation in the left as compared with the right hepatic vein. The ductus venosus, passing from the umbilical vein directly to the inferior vena cava, allows about half the umbilical venous return to bypass the hepatic microcirculation; the other half reaches the inferior vena cava through the hepatic veins after first passing through the hepatic circulation.

Although the distal inferior vena caval, ductus venosus, and hepatic venous bloodstreams all enter the inferior vena cava just below the diaphragm, they do not mix completely in this vessel. Blood from the ductus venosus and the left hepatic vein, with higher oxygen saturations, passes into the right atrium and streams preferen-

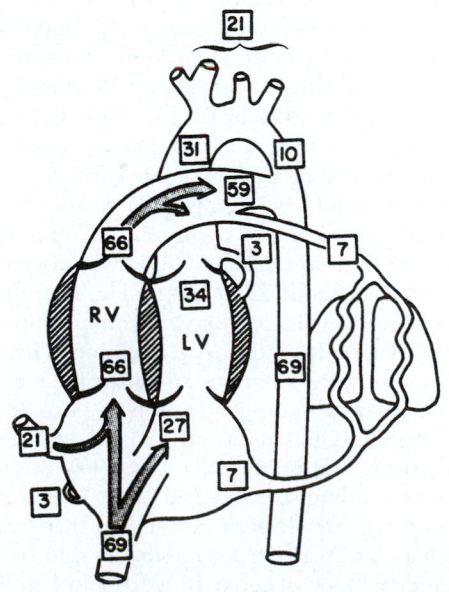

FIGURE 22-7   Percentages of CVO ejected by the left (LV) and right (RV) ventricles and passing through the major vascular channels are shown *(numbers in squares).* (For description, see text.) Measurements derived from studies in fetal lambs. SOURCE: *Rudolph AM: Congenital Diseases of the Heart. Chicago, Year Book, 1974.*

tially across the foramen ovale, providing blood with a higher oxygen content to the left atrium and left ventricle. Right hepatic venous blood, with a lower oxygen saturation, and most distal inferior vena caval blood passes preferentially to the right atrium and right ventricle, but some does cross the foramen.

In sheep, the blood flow returning in the inferior vena cava represents about 70% of total venous return to the heart. About one-third of the inferior vena caval blood passes directly through the foramen ovale into the left atrium, and the remaining two-thirds enters the right atrium and right ventricle. Superior vena caval blood is directed toward the tricuspid valve, and in normal fetuses an insignificant volume of superior vena caval blood passes through the foramen ovale. About 20% of the CVO returns to the heart through the superior vena cava, and thus, the right ventricle receives and ejects about 66% of the CVO. The major portion of blood ejected into the pulmonary trunk passes through the ductus arteriosus to the descending aorta (58% of CVO); only 7 to 8% of the CVO (or about 10 to 15% of the blood ejected by the right ventricle) enters the pulmonary circulation. The left atrium receives the blood returning to the heart from the lungs (7 to 8% of CVO) and the inferior vena caval blood that crosses the foramen ovale (25% of CVO). The left ventricle thus receives and ejects about 33% of the CVO. About 3% of the CVO perfuses the coronary arteries, and 20% of the CVO supplies the head, brain, neck, upper body, and arms. The remaining 10% of CVO ejected by the left ventricle flows across the aortic isthmus to the descending aorta. The proportions of CVO distributed to various fetal organs, as determined in near-term lambs, are: myocardium, 3 to 4%; lungs, 7 to 8%; gastrointestinal tract, 5 to 6%; brain, 3 to 4%; kidneys, 2 to 3%; and placenta, 40%.

In the human fetus, the brain is much larger relative to the body. If brain blood flow in relation to tissue weight is similar in humans and lambs, the output of the left ventricle, which supplies the brain, would be much higher in the human. I estimate that the human brain receives about 20 to 30% of CVO, so that the ratio of right to left ventricular output in the human fetus should be about 1.2:1 to 1.3:1, instead of the ratio of 2:1 found in the lamb fetus. Recent estimates from echocardiography and Doppler flow measurements have shown a ratio of right:left ventricular output of about 1.3:1 in human fetuses, with about 55% of the CVO ejected by the right ventricle and 45% by the left ventricle.

The oxygen tension of fetal arterial blood is much lower than that in the adult. Umbilical venous blood distributed to the ductus venosus and left liver lobe before any mixing with systemic venous blood has an oxygen tension of about 30 to 35 mm Hg. Blood in the distal inferior vena cava, superior vena cava, and portal vein has an oxygen tension of about 12 to 14 mm Hg. In the left atrium a small volume of blood with a low oxygen tension returning through the pulmonary veins reduces the oxygen tension of the blood passing into it from the ductus venosus across the foramen ovale. Left ventricular blood, with an oxygen tension of 24 to 28 mm Hg, is ejected into the ascending aorta and is largely distributed to the myocardium, brain, and upper body. Over 90% of superior vena caval blood passes through the tricuspid valve; mixture of this blood with the portion of inferior vena caval blood that passes into the right ventricle results in an oxygen tension in right ventricular and pulmonary arterial blood of about 18 to 19 mm Hg. Blood in the descending aorta comes predominantly from the main pulmonary artery through the ductus arteriosus, with a small proportion from ascending aortic flow across the aortic isthmus. The oxygen tension in descending aortic blood is about 20 to 23 mm Hg as compared with that in the ascending aorta of 24 to 28 mm Hg.

Because the fetus is surrounded by amniotic fluid, all fetal vascular pressures are recorded relative to amniotic cavity pressure. Vena caval and right atrial pressures are 3 to 5 mm Hg above, and left atrial pressure is 2 to 4 mm Hg above, amniotic cavity pressure. Right and left ventricular systolic pressures are usually equal, about 65 to 70 mm Hg in late gestation. Pulmonary arterial and aortic systolic and diastolic pressures are also usually equal, with systolic levels of 65 to 70 mm Hg and diastolic levels of 30 to 35 mm Hg. In late gestation right ventricular and pulmonary arterial systolic pressures are often 5 to 8 mm Hg higher than those in the left ventricle and aorta, probably as a result of mild constriction of the ductus arteriosus.

FETAL MYOCARDIAL PERFORMANCE

Fetal and adult myocyte diameters are, respectively, 5 to 7 and 20 to 25 micrometers. In contrast to the well-organized, parallel arrangement of the myofibrils within each cell in the adult myocardium, the fetal myocyte has fewer myofibrils with more random orientation. Friedman and associates have shown that isolated strips of myocardium from fetal lamb hearts develop less tension per unit mass of muscle than do adult myocardial strips. They ascribed this to a higher water content and fewer contractile elements than in the adult.

There has been controversy about the ability of the fetal heart to increase its output. Thornburg and co-workers and Gilbert showed that rapid fluid infusion into fetal lambs in utero caused left and right ventricular output to increase with filling pressure up to 2 to 3 mm Hg above the resting pressure of 2 to 3 mm Hg, but that no additional rise of output occurred with further increases of pressure. Reducing ventricular filling pressures resulted in a marked fall in ventricular output. They concluded that the fetal heart shows the Frank-Starling response of increasing stroke volume with increased diastolic volume or pressure, but only at low filling pressures. However, later studies by Hawkins and colleagues showed that the lack of increase in stroke volume at higher filling pressures resulted from the increased systemic arterial pressure resulting from infusion of fluid. When arterial pressure was fixed at specific levels, ventricular stroke volume increased with filling pressures of up to 10 to 12 mm Hg. Furthermore, when the afterload of the left ventricle is reduced in the fetal lamb in utero by ventilating the fetus, increasing filling pressure of the left ventricle will achieve left ventricular outputs noted after birth. In newborn lambs, the heart can eject the same stroke volume at filling pressures similar to those in the fetus, but at much higher arterial pressures, suggesting that myocardial performance has increased postnatally.

CIRCULATORY CHANGES AFTER BIRTH

Two dramatic events that occur immediately after birth are cessation of the umbilical-placental circulation and establishment of an adequate pulmonary circulation. The umbilical vessels are very reactive to mechanical stimulation, particularly stretch; in natural birth in animals the umbilical vessels constrict after being torn or bitten. The vessels also constrict when exposed to an increase in oxygen tension, and the rise in systemic arterial oxygen tension after birth probably maintains constriction; severe hypoxia could relax the vessels and cause hemorrhage. Removal of the placental circulation markedly reduces venous return through the inferior vena cava. The cessation of umbilical venous return also reduces flow through the ductus venosus, which closes within 3 to 7 days after birth, probably passively as a result of the reduced flow and pressure.

CHANGES IN PULMONARY CIRCULATION The low pulmonary blood flow in the fetus results from the high pulmonary vascular resistance. The small arteries in the fetal lungs have a thick medial smooth muscle layer, and maintained constriction of these vessels causes the high pulmonary vascular resistance. The total pulmonary vascular resistance markedly decreases with advancing gestation as a result of a great increase in the number of vessels during growth, resulting in an increase in cross-sectional area of the vascular bed. The pulmonary vessels are very reactive to several physiological and pharmacologic influences. A decrease in oxygen tension or in the pH of the blood perfusing the pulmonary vessels constricts them, and the vasoconstrictor responses to hypoxia and acidemia are additive. Studies in fetal lambs have shown a progressive increase in the magnitude of the vasoconstrictor response to hypoxia with advancing gestation. This cannot be explained by a morphologic change in the small pulmonary arteries that determine resistance because the ratios of the thickness of the smooth muscle layer to the diameter of the vessel do not change over the latter half of gestation.

Acetylcholine, histamine, tolazoline, and β-adrenergic catecholamines are potent vasodilators of the fetal pulmonary vessels, as are bradykinin, prostaglandins D_2, E_1, and E_2 (PGE_2), and prostacyclin (PGI_2). Leukotrienes, particularly LTD_4, are pulmonary vasoconstrictors. Recently, N Ω-nitro-L-arginine, a competitive inhibitor of the nitric oxide producer L-arginine, has been shown to cause pulmonary vasoconstriction in the fetus. This suggests that the pulmonary circulation is normally relaxed to some extent by release from endothelium of nitric oxide (NO).

The high fetal pulmonary vascular resistance has been attributed to hypoxic vasoconstriction because pulmonary vessels are subjected to the relatively low PO_2 of perfusing blood. Ventilating the lungs with air results in a four- to 10-fold increase in pulmonary blood flow by producing a marked fall in pulmonary vascular resistance. Before birth, the precapillary vessels are exposed to pulmonary arterial blood with an oxygen tension of about 18 mm Hg. Expansion of the alveoli with air subjects the vessels to a higher oxygen tension because oxygen diffuses into vessels proximal to the capillaries from adjacent alveoli.

The decrease in pulmonary vascular resistance associated with ventilation was long regarded as largely related to the effects of oxygenation, with physical expansion of the lung playing a minor role. Recent studies in fetal lambs in utero, however, have shown that expanding the lungs with a gas that does not change fetal blood gases markedly decreases pulmonary vascular resistance. Subsequent ventilation with oxygen produced further vasodilation. Gaseous expansion of the lung could influence pulmonary vessels either by altering surface forces by developing a gas-liquid interface in the alveoli or by releasing a vasodilator substance. Studies in fetal lambs have shown that prostaglandin I_2 (PGI_2) release in the lung is at least one factor responsible for pulmonary vasodilation associated with physical expansion of the lungs because this decrease is limited by the prostaglandin synthesis inhibitors indomethacin and meclofenamate.

Pulmonary vasodilation is associated with an increase in fetal PO_2 even when the lungs are not expanded with gas. Placing a ewe in a hyperbaric oxygen chamber, in the absence of ventilation, increases fetal arterial PO_2 and results in a marked fall of pulmonary vascular resistance. The effects of oxygen are exerted locally in the lung and are not related to reflexes arising from peripheral chemoreceptors. We do not know if the vasodilation is caused by release of chemical mediators or by a direct local effect of oxygen on the smooth muscle. Bradykinin, a potent pulmonary vasodilator, is released in the lung when oxygen tension is increased and has been thought to be responsible for postnatal pulmonary vasodilation; this does not completely explain the effects of oxygen because bradykinin levels are elevated for only a short time.

More recently, production of NO has been thought to be responsible for the vasodilator effect of oxygen because blockade of NO production markedly reduces, or may eliminate, the response to increased oxygenation.

The possibility that oxygen exerts a direct local dilator effect on pulmonary vascular smooth muscle has gained renewed interest because oxygen-sensitive potassium channels have been demonstrated in smooth muscle in lung vessels. Drugs that open these channels cause pulmonary vascular dilation, and those that close the channels cause constriction. Hypoxia closes these channels, and the rise in lung oxygen levels after birth could relax smooth muscle by opening potassium channels.

While the ductus arteriosus is widely patent, the pulmonary arterial pressure remains at systemic arterial levels, but constriction of the ductus separates the aorta and pulmonary artery, so that pulmonary arterial and right ventricular pressures fall when there is the normal fall in pulmonary vascular resistance.

The initial decrease in pulmonary vascular resistance results from release of vasoconstriction. In the 6 to 8 weeks after birth there is a further progressive fall caused by thinning of the smooth muscle layer in the media. The patterns of postnatal changes in pulmonary flow, vascular resistance, and pressure are shown in Fig. 22-8. The postnatal maturation of the pulmonary vessels is disturbed by conditions that interfere with normal oxygenation after birth, such as lung disease or exposure to high altitude, and also by congenital cardiac lesions, particularly those associated with pulmonary hypertension.

CLOSURE OF FORAMEN OVALE In the fetus, over half of inferior vena caval blood comes from umbilical venous return. Removal of the placental circulation markedly decreases the amount of inferior vena caval blood returning to the heart and causes a small drop in right atrial pressure, whereas the increase in pulmonary blood flow increases pulmonary venous return and elevates left atrial pressure. This combination of pressure changes closes the valve-like flap of the foramen ovale. In many infants the foramen ovale is incompletely closed, and a small opening with a small left-to-right shunt is present for several months. A small opening without left-to-right shunting persists throughout life in about 15 to 20% of people. In early infancy, and sometimes in later life, if right atrial pressure is raised above that in the left atrium, the foramen ovale may open, and right-to-left shunting of blood may occur.

CLOSURE OF DUCTUS ARTERIOSUS During fetal life the ductus arteriosus is a large channel with a diameter similar to that of the descending aorta. The ductus has a large amount of smooth muscle in the media, in contrast with the contiguous aorta and pulmonary artery, which have largely elastic tissue. The ductus was once thought to be kept open passively by the pressure within it. However, inhibiting prostaglandin synthesis with indomethacin or aspirin in pregnant animals or directly in the fetus constricts the ductus arteriosus; the pulmonary arterial pressure rises, and systemic arterial pressure is maintained or increases. This suggested that patency of the ductus in utero is maintained by prostaglandins. The ductus in vivo is relaxed by both prostacyclin (PGI_2) and prosta-

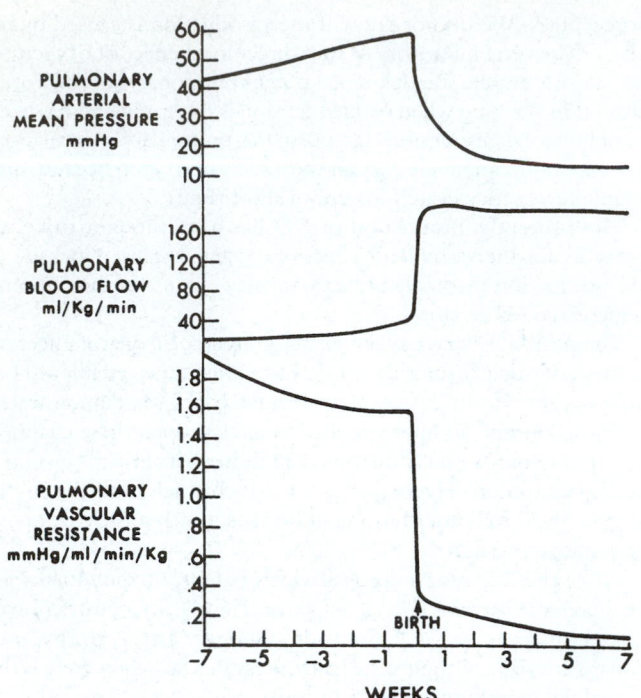

FIGURE 22-8 Changes in total pulmonary arterial pressure, pulmonary blood flow, and pulmonary vascular resistance (PVR) in the perinatal period. PVR decreases during the latter part of gestation, mainly because of an increase in the number of pulmonary vessels associated with growth. It falls dramatically at birth because of the vasodilator effect of ventilating the lungs with air; a further gradual decrease occurs as pulmonary vascular smooth muscle regresses. Pulmonary blood flow increases slightly during fetal growth, then increases dramatically after birth. Pulmonary arterial pressure falls rapidly immediately after birth and then more gradually, to reach adult levels after 6 to 8 weeks.

glandin E_2 (PGE_2), but it is much more sensitive to PGE_2. Isolated ductus tissue incubated with arachidonic acid, the fatty acid from which prostaglandins are synthesized, produces large quantities of PGI_2 but only small amounts of PGE_2. In the fetus, however, circulating levels of PGE_2 are high, approximately three to five times adult levels. We do not know whether ductus patency is caused by prostaglandins released locally or those that are circulating. The ductus arteriosus constricts rapidly after birth and in most mature infants is functionally closed within 10 to 15 hours. Permanent closure by thrombosis, intimal proliferation, and fibrosis is complete within 3 weeks.

The mechanisms responsible for closure of the ductus arteriosus after birth have not yet been fully delineated. During fetal life the ductus is exposed to a pulmonary arterial blood PO_2 of 18 to 20 mm Hg. An increase in the PO_2 to which the ductus is exposed is known to cause constriction. Postnatally, after pulmonary vascular resistance has fallen, blood flows through the ductus from the aorta to the pulmonary artery and exposes the ductus to the systemic arterial blood PO_2 of 80 to 90 mm Hg. Changes in prostaglandin metabolism are also involved; circulating blood levels of PGE_2 drop rapidly after birth, and the decrease in PGE_2 concentration may contribute to closure of the ductus.

There is a high incidence of persistent patency of the ductus arteriosus in preterm infants as compared with mature infants, perhaps because of the lower responsiveness of the ductus to oxygen-induced constriction in very immature fetuses. High circulating lev-

els of PGE_2 are maintained for a longer period after birth in premature as compared with mature infants. This could be related to increased production or decreased degradation of PGE_2 in the immature lungs. This could also account for the success in treating a patent ductus arteriosus in preterm infants with indomethacin to block synthesis of prostaglandins (see Sec. 2.16.2).

While the ductus arteriosus is still patent after birth, the reduction in pulmonary vascular resistance results in a left-to-right shunt through the ductus. If pulmonary vascular resistance is increased by hypoxia or other factors, right-to-left shunting of blood will occur through the ductus. If systemic arterial oxygen tension does not increase normally after birth, the ductus may remain patent; there is a high incidence of patent ductus arteriosus in individuals who are born at and continue to live at altitudes above 3000 m.

CHANGES IN CARDIAC OUTPUT AND DISTRIBUTION The CVO in the fetal lamb is 450 to 500 mL/kg fetal body weight per minute, with about 330 mL/kg/min being ejected by the right ventricle and 170 mL/kg/min by the left ventricle. After birth there is an increase in the total output of the heart during the first few days, with each ventricle ejecting about 350 mL/kg/min; there is thus a modest increase in right ventricular output but a considerable increase in left ventricular output. The cardiac output per kilogram of body weight falls fairly rapidly over the first 8 to 10 weeks after birth to about 150 mL/kg/min and then falls more slowly to the adult level of about 70 to 80 mL/kg/min. The increase in cardiac output after birth can be explained partly by the increased metabolism required to maintain body temperature; cardiac output parallels changes in oxygen consumption in the newborn lamb. Variations in metabolic activity, such as deviation from the neutral ambient temperature, increase oxygen consumption and cardiac output. In the human fetus, because left ventricular output is relatively higher than in the lamb, the increase in output after birth would be considerably less.

The high resting cardiac output in the early postnatal period and the rapid fall over the first 8 weeks are also related to replacement of fetal hemoglobin by adult hemoglobin in circulating erythrocytes. The oxygen equilibration curve of fetal blood is shifted to the left as compared with that for adult blood. Although this is advantageous during fetal life because it aids in uptake of oxygen by fetal blood in the placenta, it is disadvantageous postnatally because it interferes with release of oxygen in the tissues at the PO_2 levels prevailing after birth (see Sec. 19.1.4).

Because the resting cardiac output required to supply oxygen to the tissues is so high in relation to body weight in neonates, they have limited ability to raise cardiac output further as compared with adults. In the newborn lamb during the first postnatal week, cardiac output related to body weight can be increased by an average of only 35% during rapid intravenous infusion of fluids to raise left atrial pressure above 20 mm Hg. By 3 weeks, when resting output has fallen to about 300 mL/kg/min, output can be increased by about 50%, whereas by 8 weeks, when resting output has fallen to about 150 mL/kg/min, cardiac output can be increased by about 70% of resting levels. These findings indicate that the heart of the newborn animal can provide a large cardiac output but is limited in its reserve capabilities in view of the high cardiac output requirements necessary to meet oxygen needs at rest. Thus, the volume load of a left-to-right shunt imposed on the heart in the early postnatal period may not be well tolerated because it may interfere with blood flow to the body; later in infancy, however, a shunt of similar magnitude may be well tolerated.

CHANGES IN HEART RATE AND BLOOD PRESSURE Resting fetal heart rate averages 160 to 180 beats per minute. During the newborn period the heart rate averages about 120 beats per minute during sleep and increases to 140 to 160 beats per minute while the infant is awake. In premature infants the resting heart rate is higher, averaging 120 to 140 beats per minute. Heart rate gradually decreases with advancing age. Systemic arterial blood pressure in the fetus at term is about 60/35 mm Hg, as referred to amniotic cavity pressure. Arterial pressure in the mature infant averages 70/50 mm Hg, but it is lower in the premature infant. Arterial pressure gradually increases with age.

References

Clyman RI: Persistent patent ductus arteriosus. Int J Technol Assess Health Care 7(Suppl 1):70, 1991

Fineman JR, Soifer SJ, Heymann MA: Regulation of pulmonary vascular tone in the neonatal period. Annu Rev Physiol 57:115, 1995

Gilbert RD: Control of fetal cardiac output during changes in blood volume. Am J Physiol 238:H80, 1980

Hawkins J, Van Hare GF, Schmidt KG, et al: Effects of increasing afterload on left ventricular output in fetal lambs. Circ Res 65:127, 1989

Heymann MA, Rudolph AM: Effects of acetylsalicylic acid on the ductus arteriosus and circulation of fetal lambs in utero. Circ Res 38:418, 1976

Iwamoto HS, Teitel DF, Rudolph AM: Effects of lung distension and spontaneous fetal breathing on hemodynamics in sheep. Pediatr Res 33:639, 1993

Kinsella JP, Abman SH: Recent developments in inhaled nitric oxide therapy of the newborn. Curr Opin Pediatr 11:121, 1999

Klopfenstein HS, Rudolph AM: Postnatal changes in the circulation, and responses to volume loading in sheep. Circ Res 42:839, 1978

Lister G, Walter TK, Versmold HT, et al: Oxygen delivery in lambs: cardiovascular and hematologic development. Am J Physiol 237:H668, 1979

Rudolph AM: Distribution and regulation of blood flow in the fetal and neonatal lamb. Circ Res 57:811, 1985

Teitel D, Iwamoto HS, Rudolph AM: Effects of birth-related events on central blood flow patterns. Pediatr Res 22:557, 1987

Thornburg KL, Morton MJ: Filling and arterial pressures as determinants of RV stroke volume in the sheep fetus. Am J Physiol 244:H656, 1983

Thornburg KL, Morton MJ: Filling and arterial pressures as determinants of left ventricular stroke volume in the fetal lambs. Am J Physiol 251:H961, 1986

Van Hare GF, Hawkins JA, Schmidt KG, Rudolph AM: The effects of increasing mean arterial pressure on left ventricular output in newborn lambs. Circ Res 67:78, 1990

22.2   DIAGNOSTIC TOOLS

22.2.1   History and Physical Examination

Michael M. Brook

HISTORY

PREGNANCY A history of maternal illness or exposure to drugs and chemicals may disclose infectious agents or chemicals that are known teratogens. Maternal diabetes is associated with increased risk of both structural disease and cardiomyopathy.

FAMILY HISTORY See Table 22-1.

PERSONAL HISTORY Growth is often retarded with congestive heart failure or cyanotic heart disease. Edema is manifested by rapid weight gain, swelling of face or eyelids, and swelling of ankles or tightness of shoes. Exercise intolerance as a result of heart failure or inadequate oxygen supply to muscles may cause dyspnea or tachypnea at rest or exercise, orthopnea if there is pulmonary venous congestion, and muscle fatigue on effort. In infants, these symptoms show up as tachypnea on feeding or crying, abnormal sweating (on the entire torso) with crying or feeding, unusually slow feeding, and cool extremities; in school-age children, they may show up as inability to keep up with the child's peers. Questions about the volume and duration of feedings can be helpful in assessing fatigue in infants. A history of stridor or hoarseness, or dysphagia on eating solids, may indicate a vascular ring. Chest pain is seldom caused by heart disease but may rarely reflect myocardial ischemia (see Sec. 22.4.9). Syncope is seldom of cardiac origin (see Sec. 22.4.8) but can occur with severe aortic stenosis, hypertrophic cardiomyopathy or pulmonary hypertension, or very rapid or very slow heart rates. A history of squatting or cyanotic spells focuses attention on tetralogy of Fallot, but normal children also squat occasionally. Questions about heart rate and dropped or irregular heartbeats can be helpful in making decisions about further investigations for arrhythmias.

PHYSICAL EXAMINATION

It is important to decide if the child is ill or not, and to do a careful general examination with special attention to the features of the many genetic and malformation syndromes that can be associated with heart disease (see Sec. 10.3).

SKIN, HEAD AND NECK, AND EXTREMITIES

COLOR The color of the skin and mucous membranes should be noted. Severe anemia causes pallor, as does the vasoconstriction of congestive heart failure; the fingers are usually warm in the former but cool and moist in the latter from sympathetic stimulation. Cyanosis refers to a dusky purple-blue color caused by an excessive absolute amount of reduced hemoglobin. It is most readily apparent in superficial capillary-rich sites such as the lips, mucous membranes, and nail beds. Most physicians recognize definite cyanosis when arterial oxygen saturation is under 85%, but under optimal conditions of normal color vision, good ambient light, light skin

TABLE 22-1

IMPLICATIONS OF FAMILY HISTORY

POSITIVE FAMILY HISTORY	POSSIBLE IMPLICATIONS AND FOLLOW-UP
"Blue" babies, holes in heart, sudden death in infancy	Congenital heart disease
Recent viral illness in family	Viral myocarditis
"Heart attacks," especially under 50 years old	Measure cholesterol, prudent diet, avoid smoking
High blood pressure, strokes	Careful blood pressure measurement
Sudden death in children or adults	Congenital heart disease, cardiomyopathies, arrhythmias (especially long-QT syndrome)
Heart failure	Hypertension, atherosclerosis, cardiomyopathy
Murmurs	Too nonspecific to be of use

pigmentation, and normal hemoglobin concentration, minor degrees of cyanosis at arterial oxygen saturation levels of 90 to 92% can be detected. Children with mild desaturation can have a "ruddy" complexion with reddish discoloration of the cheeks. Cyanosis is less apparent clinically when there is severe anemia because the concentration of reduced hemoglobin is limited by the anemia. Conversely, cyanosis may occur with normal arterial oxygen saturation when the hematocrit is greatly increased (polycythemia).

It is essential to distinguish peripheral from central cyanosis. Peripheral cyanosis occurs with normal arterial saturation and is caused by slowed peripheral circulation with excessive oxygen extraction by the tissues, and thus an increased concentration of reduced hemoglobin at the venous end of the capillaries. This occurs in heart failure, a cold environment, polycythemia, or even in normal newborn infants (acrocyanosis); the extremities are cold and blue, but the tongue is pink. Central cyanosis, on the other hand, is caused by arterial desaturation and is best seen in the tongue and oral mucous membranes, which are always warm and have a high blood flow. Central cyanosis can be subtle; comparing the child's color to that of a family member can be helpful. Occasionally, there may be cyanosis in the toes and not the fingers because of right-to-left ductus shunting of desaturated blood with pulmonary hypertension or aortic arch obstruction. If the fingers but not the toes are blue, there is transposition of the great arteries with right-to-left shunting of saturated blood through the ductus.

Petechiae in the skin and nail beds may indicate infective endocarditis but also occur in other diseases and even with minor local trauma.

CAPILLARY REFILL   Capillary refill time is a crude test of skin circulation. If over 3 seconds, it indicates decreased skin flow from heart failure, shock, or sympathetic stimulation not caused by disease.

CLUBBING   Clubbing of the fingers and toes occurs in cyanotic heart disease, but seldom under 1 year of age. It also occurs in suppurative lung disease, infective endocarditis, and biliary cirrhosis; some clubbing is familial. The earliest sign of clubbing is filling in of the angle between the proximal nail bed and the soft tissue of the finger, just beneath the cuticle; this is best shown by apposing the dorsal parts of the terminal phalanges of the corresponding fingers of each hand and noting that the diamond-shaped space normally present has been reduced or filled in. The tissues in this region are shiny and tense. Pressing down on the proximal nail bed causes the nail to move toward the bone because with clubbing there is increased vascularity of the tissues in this area. More severe clubbing also has swelling of the terminal part of the finger (drumstick). Rounding and beaking of the distal nail bed in the absence of other signs of clubbing is familial and does not indicate disease. Some children with minimal arterial desaturation (88 to 92%) often have red, shiny fingertips, but so do normal children who suck their fingers.

EDEMA   Pitting edema of the ankles or sacrum occurs in congestive heart failure. It is rare in infants, who instead may have puffy eyelids; the parents should be asked if the eyelids look abnormally swollen because some people normally have this appearance. Recent rapid weight gain may be caused by increased fluid accumulation.

ARTERIAL PULSES   Radial, femoral, pedal, and carotid arteries should be felt on both sides because some anomalies or diseases can cause any of these to be weak or absent. The radial and femoral pulses, about equidistant from the heart, should be almost synchronous; a significant delay of the femoral pulse is typical of coarctation of the aorta. The pulse quality should be assessed: a *rapidly rising* pulse occurs with vasodilation (heat and marked anemia) or a runoff from the aorta, as in marked aortic incompetence, a large patent ductus arteriosus, or rapid ventricular ejection with a large ventricular septal defect or marked mitral incompetence; a slow-rising pulse indicates severe aortic stenosis or hypertension; a small and weak pulse occurs in shock from any cause. Finger and palmar pulses may be felt when there is marked vasodilation (eg, in a premature infant with a large left-to-right ductus shunt). Heart rate is best counted by auscultation of the heart rather than by feeling the pulse to avoid errors resulting from dropped beats. Measurement of blood pressure at each examination is essential (see Sec. 22.4.5).

VENOUS PULSES   Venous pulses are examined in the neck but may be difficult to see in infants. It is best to examine them while listening to the heart sounds to define systole and diastole. The mean jugular venous pressure assesses mean right atrial pressure. A venous wave seen just before the first heart sound is the *a* wave, caused by atrial contraction; an exaggerated *a* wave indicates right atrial hypertrophy and is most often caused by increased right ventricular diastolic pressure. The jugular venous pressure should then fall in systole (the *x* descent); if it remains high in systole and falls only after the second heart sound, then significant tricuspid incompetence is present. Intermittent giant *a* waves are cannon waves, caused by contraction of the right atrium against a closed tricuspid valve in heart block or other forms of atrioventricular dissociation. Exaggerated venous and arterial pulsations in the neck are typical of large intracranial arteriovenous malformations.

THE ABDOMEN   A spleen tip may be felt with deep inspiration in normal infants but is not normally palpable in older children. The liver edge can normally be as much as 3 cm below the costal margin in the right midclavicular line in infants and 1 to 2 cm below it in older children. The normal liver edge is soft, smooth, and nontender; a firm liver with a sharp edge or tenderness is abnormal. If the liver seems to be enlarged, make sure by percussion that the upper edge is in the fifth intercostal space and not pushed down; children with pulmonary disease, such as asthma, can appear to have an enlarged liver as a result of hyperinflation. A few normal children have an unusually large right hepatic lobe.

THE THORAX

INSPECTION   Look for the rate and depth of respiration and any retractions as well as asymmetries caused by precordial bulging from long-standing early cardiomegaly or unilateral lung hypoplasia. Pectus carinatum or excavatum may explain some murmurs and can occur in Marfan syndrome. The straight back syndrome also produces innocent murmurs. With marked overactivity of the ventricles, visible precordial pulsations may be seen. Infants with stridor may have tracheal compression from a vascular ring.

PALPATION   Palpation of the precordium with the patient supine assesses ventricular size and activity. The apical impulse should not be below the fifth intercostal space or lateral to the left midclavicular line; if it is beyond these limits, the left ventricle is enlarged or displaced. Try to define the quality of the impulse as normal, or as slowly rising and falling because of an obstructive lesion that causes a pressure load, or rapidly rising and falling ("slapping") with a large excursion because of a large volume load. Similarly, a pulsation felt at the left lower sternal border usually represents the right ventricle, which can be assessed for pressure or volume loads in the same way. Occasionally, pulsation in the left third intercostal space about an inch from the sternal edge denotes a hypertensive main pulmonary artery. Cardiac impulses in the right chest indicate dextrocardia or mediastinal shift. Thrills may be palpated with the flat of the hand and usually accompany loud murmurs.

PERCUSSION Percussion is valuable for lungs but inaccurate for estimating heart size in children. It is useful only for relating the left heart border to the apical impulse when a pericardial effusion is suspected, or in detecting a mediastinal shift.

AUSCULTATION Auscultation of the lungs for rales, rhonchi, and wheezing is discussed in Section 23.3.1. Auscultation of the heart should be done systematically at the apex, left lower sternal border, midleft sternal border, upper left and then upper right sternal borders, the axillae, and the back. First the bell and then the diaphragm should be used. The patient should be examined both sitting and supine, except in neonates. At each area, specifically listen for the first and second heart sounds and any other sounds or clicks and only then pay attention to systolic and diastolic murmurs. At the end of the examination, the physician should be able to describe each sound and each murmur at each area. In this way, even subtle signs will not be overpowered by a loud murmur that might not be the most important feature of the examination.

The first heart sound, heard best at the apex or lower left sternal edge, is usually single or narrowly split. Its intensity varies with the energy of atrioventricular valve closure. It is loud in mitral stenosis, increased ventricular contractility, or a short PR interval because the atrioventricular valves are deep in the ventricle and come together rapidly and forcefully at the onset of systole. The first heart sound is soft if the valves are nearly apposed when systole begins, as in aortic incompetence or a long PR interval; it is also soft with decreased contractility, especially in myocarditis. The first heart sound varies in intensity with complete atrioventricular block.

It is important to distinguish the first heart sound from systolic ejection or nonejection clicks. Ejection clicks arise early in systole at the base of the heart and may be confused with a first heart sound; however, the clicks are usually better heard at the base than at the apex and are high-pitched and clicking, rather than having the dull, lower-pitched quality of the first heart sound. First heart sounds are never heard better at the base than at the apex. Palpation of the pulse during auscultation also can help to distinguish these: first heart sounds precede the pulse, but an ejection click is generally synchronous with the pulse. Systolic ejection clicks occur with an enlarged great vessel at the base of the heart: an enlarged aorta in valvar aortic stenosis, bicuspid aortic valve, or tetralogy of Fallot; the large single vessel of a truncus arteriosus; and a large pulmonary artery as a result of valvar pulmonic stenosis, idiopathic dilatation of the pulmonary artery, or pulmonary hypertension, although they are uncommon with a large pulmonary artery caused by a large left-to-right shunt. They can be heard in normal infants from the first day after birth. These clicks are caused either by the opening snap of a semilunar valve or by sudden distension of the arterial wall in systole. Nonejection clicks are later in systole and are heard at the lower left sternal border or the apex. At the lower left sternal border, a click often represents the snap of a pseudoaneurysm associ-

ated with a closing ventricular septal defect. At the apex a click suggests mitral valve prolapse; there is an early or midsystolic click, often followed by a midsystolic or late systolic murmur of mitral incompetence.

In the newborn infant with moderately elevated pulmonary arterial pressure and a thin chest wall, pulmonic closure is often as loud as aortic closure and is heard at the lower as well as the upper left sternal border. Even in the first few years of life, normal pulmonary closure may be almost as loud at the upper left sternal border as is the aortic closure at the upper right sternal border. With severe pulmonary hypertension, however, the second sound may be louder than the aortic and is sometimes palpable.

If the first (aortic) component of the second heart sound is heard loudest at the upper left sternal border, then there is probably malposition of the aorta. In *l*-transposition of the great arteries (corrected transposition) and in *d*-transposition of the great arteries (classic transposition), the aortic valve is anterior and more superior than normal so that aortic closure is unusually loud and heard best at the upper left sternal border. In the tetralogy of Fallot, the aorta is wide and dextroposed, and the pulmonary artery that is anterior to it is smaller than usual; the second heart sound is usually single and heard loudest at the lower left sternal border. In aortic atresia there is a loud single (pulmonic) second sound heard best at the upper left sternal border.

Absence of splitting of the second heart sound may indicate atresia or severe stenosis of a semilunar valve but may be normal in the first 2 days after birth. In newborn infants with rapid heart and respiratory rates, the splitting may be too narrow to appreciate, even though it may be present on a phonocardiogram. An easily heard splitting of the second heart sound in an infant is generally abnormal and suggests a very large left-to-right atrial or venous level shunt, as in anomalous pulmonary venous drainage or arteriovenous fistula. In *d*-transposition of the great arteries, the pulmonary artery is posterior, and pulmonic closure may be too soft to be heard.

Wide splitting of the second heart sound suggests right bundle branch block, pulmonic stenosis, or atrial septal defect. Occasionally it occurs in normal children examined when supine; when they sit up, the width of the splitting decreases markedly, and the respiratory variation becomes more prominent, thus separating this from pathologic splitting of the second sound. Rarely infants and very young children with large atrial septal defects may have normal splitting and respiratory variation of the second heart sound for unknown reasons.

The second heart sound is usually soft when contractility is markedly decreased, as in myocarditis. The third heart sound ("gallop") occurs early in diastole and coincides with rapid ventricular filling. If it arises in the left ventricle, it usually does not change with respiration, but it may become prominent with ventricular hypertrophy. When there is also tachycardia, a protodiastolic gallop occurs and should be regarded as abnormal.

The fourth heart sound occurs in late diastole, when atrial contraction fills the ventricle. It is almost always abnormal and tends to be prominent with left or right atrial hypertrophy from any causes. With tachycardia it produces a presystolic gallop.

INNOCENT MURMURS Murmurs caused by normal turbulence and vibration that do not indicate present or future heart disease are termed *innocent* or *benign* murmurs. They are often called functional murmurs, but this term is ambiguous because all murmurs are related to cardiac function. Innocent murmurs are uncommon in infants (except for the PPPS murmur described below), but one or more of them can be heard in almost every child over 2 years of age provided that the child cooperates and the room is quiet. With age and increasing thickness of the chest wall, the murmurs become harder to hear and may be detected easily in only about 20% of adolescents and adults. Some people retain these murmurs throughout life. There are seven distinct types of innocent murmurs, all of which can and should be diagnosed by their specific features (Fig. 22-9) and not by failure to identify the murmur as being caused by a known organic lesion.

SYSTOLIC MURMURS Still's murmur is short, midsystolic, and musical, like a plucked string instrument or kazoo, with a low-pitched, regular fundamental frequency between 90 and 120 Hz (about one and one-half octaves below middle C) and some overtones. It is heard best in the lower precordium, is not heard in the back, and decreases in intensity during inspiration and with positional changes that decrease venous return. The mechanism of production is uncertain, but vibrations of the semilunar valves, ventricular wall, chordae tendinae, or false tendon have been suggested. The musical quality and timing easily distinguish this murmur from other murmurs in the lower precordium. Mitral incompetence murmurs are usually apical, with radiation to the axilla and back; they are high-pitched, blowing, and either pansystolic or late systolic. Ventricular septal defects have murmurs that are harsh, loud, and pansystolic, or, if the defect is very small, the murmurs may be very early in systole and have a high-pitched whistling or spray-can quality.

The *basal ejection systolic murmur,* heard at the base, is high-pitched and blowing, with no musical components. At the beginning of systole, blood just above the pulmonic valves is not moving and is sheared away from the wall when blood is ejected from the ventricles; eddies that occur produce the murmur. These murmurs can mimic pulmonic or aortic stenosis or a bicuspid aortic valve. The distinction may not be easy. If there is mild stenosis (severe stenosis can be diagnosed from other features), the murmur is usually harsher and longer, and there may be a systolic ejection click. If the murmur is short, soft, and blowing, and there is no other evidence of heart disease, it is wisest to regard it as innocent to avoid producing cardiac neurosis.

The *supraclavicular arterial bruit* is very short and early, ending within the first quarter or third of systole. It is caused by turbulence in the subclavian and carotid arteries as the blood is accelerated early in systole. Its extreme shortness and predominant supraclavicular site make it easy to diagnose; often the murmur decreases if the subclavian artery is compressed against the first rib or if the neck is hyperextended. The murmurs of aortic or pulmonic stenosis

may transmit to the neck, but they are heard best below the clavicles and are longer. Internal carotid arterial obstructive lesions are rare in children, and the bruits of thyrotoxicosis are accompanied by typical signs of that lesion.

The *physiological peripheral pulmonic stenosis murmur* (PPPS) is caused by the fetal anatomy. For some weeks after birth the right and left pulmonary arteries are much smaller than, and come off at a sharp angle from, the large main pulmonary artery. This creates turbulence and loss of pressure head as blood accelerates when passing from main to branch pulmonary arteries, and with this there is a soft stenotic murmur heard best in the axillae. As the child grows, the vessels remodel until the branch pulmonary arteries are similar in diameter to the main pulmonary artery and come off from it at a gentler curve. The turbulence and the murmur usually disappear by 6 to 9 months of age.

All of these systolic murmurs are short and usually soft (grade 2/6). They are all louder when supine than erect because stroke volume is greater when supine. They also get louder with exercise, anxiety, anemia, or fever because of greater stroke volume and acceleration of blood, but this phenomenon does not help to differentiate them from pathologic murmurs.

In addition, there is the *cardiorespiratory murmur,* which is rare, localized to the lower left sternal border, and squeaking or whiffing. It probably arises outside the heart when the lung is suddenly compressed by systolic cardiac movement. This murmur disappears during held expiration.

CONTINUOUS MURMURS The *venous hum* is caused by blood draining down the collapsed jugular veins into the dilated intrathoracic veins; the high velocity in the cervical veins makes the vein walls flutter and cause a low-pitched murmur. This explains the continuous nature of the murmur and accentuation in diastole or inspiration. It also explains why the murmur is often absent when supine, because the neck veins are distended, and there is no point of transition between collapsed and distended veins. The murmur can often be abolished by altering the position of the head (tilting, rotating), as this alters flow in the neck veins; it can also be abolished by occluding the veins in the neck with the thumb or by having the patient do a Valsalva maneuver. The murmur may be mistaken for a patent ductus arteriosus if it is on the left side or for other arteriovenous fistulas. Its characteristics and variability make it easily diagnosed.

A continuous murmur (the *mammary souffle*) may be heard over the breasts in pregnant or lactating women. It is usually soft. The setting makes the diagnosis easy, and it is important not to diagnose underlying heart disease.

Murmur	Position	Quality	Timing and duration		
			1		A2 P2
Still, vibratory	Medial to apex, LLSB	Musical, low pitch			
Basal	ULSB	Blowing, high pitch			
Supra-clavicular	Lower neck	Blowing, high pitch			
PPPS	Axillae, back, ULSB	Blowing, high pitch			
Cardio-respiratory	Apex, LLSB	Squeaking			

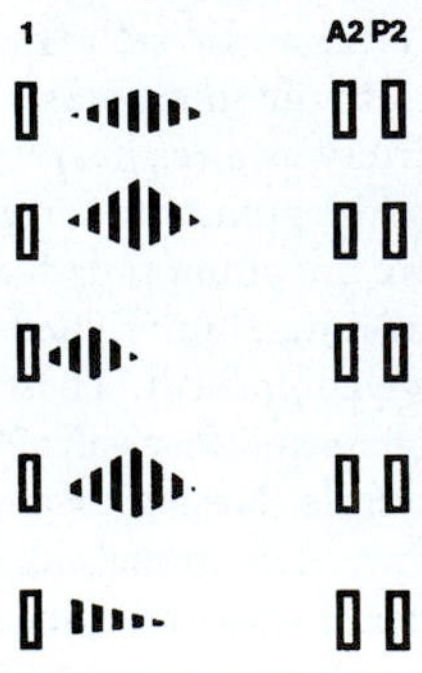

FIGURE 22-9 Description of innocent murmurs. LLSB = lower left sternal border; ULSB = upper left sternal border; 1 and 2 = first and second heart sounds; PPPS = physiological peripheral pulmonic stenosis; A = aortic; P = pulmonic.

SIGNIFICANCE These murmurs are important because of the marked anxiety that people have about heart disease. Many people equate murmurs with heart disease and death, and the physician can do great harm by transmitting uncertainty to the family. Therefore, the approach should be to assess the child's health and cardiac status by a thorough history and physical examination, with particular attention to the characteristics of the murmurs. Because it is possible to have an innocent murmur with a cardiac abnormality, such as a cardiomyopathy, cardiac normality must be assessed from all aspects of the cardiovascular examination, not only from the murmur.

Once an innocent murmur *and* a normal heart have been diagnosed, the parents should be told that the heart is normal and the murmur is a normal phenomenon ("He has an innocent murmur, and his heart is normal"). It may help to explain that normal turbulence causes murmurs, much as flowing water in a hose or pipe has a swishing sound or a river flowing around a bend ripples and splashes. It is essential to make sure that the parents realize that the murmur is not an indication of slight heart disease and that it is of no importance whether it goes away or stays. However, the physician must use judgment in discussing normal murmurs with parents because some people are overanxious and may misinterpret what is said. It is, of course, not always possible to be sure that a murmur is innocent, particularly in infants. It is reasonable to explain to the parents that the murmur either is normal or may indicate mild heart disease and that further assessment of the child or a cardiac consultation will probably make the definitive diagnosis.

PATHOLOGIC MURMURS Murmurs caused by heart disease differ from innocent murmurs in quality, intensity, position, and radiation and are often associated with other abnormal features of the cardiac examination. They are discussed in detail in sections dealing with specific cardiac lesions.

References

Bergman AB, Stamm SJ: The morbidity of cardiac nondisease in children. N Engl J Med 276:1008, 1967

Caceres CA, Perry LW: The Innocent Murmur. Boston, Little, Brown, 1967

Castle RF, Craige E: Auscultation of the heart in infants and children. Pediatrics 26:511, 1960

Fyler DC: Nadas' Pediatric Cardiology. Philadelphia, Hanley & Balfus, 1992

McKusick VA: Cardiovascular Sound in Health and Disease. Baltimore, Williams & Wilkins, 1972

Pelech AN: Evaluation of the pediatric patient with a cardiac murmur. Pediatr Clin North Am 46:167, 1999

22.2.2   Electrocardiography

George F. Van Hare

Normally, electrical depolarization begins in the sinoatrial (SA) node and spreads through the atria (Fig. 22-10). The wave of depolarization passes down, to the left and anteriorly, generating a potential detected on the body surface as the P wave. A force like this that has magnitude and direction is termed a *vector* and can be represented by an arrow with direction and magnitude proportional to the force. The impulse is delayed at the AV node, producing the P-R interval and allowing ventricular filling to be completed before

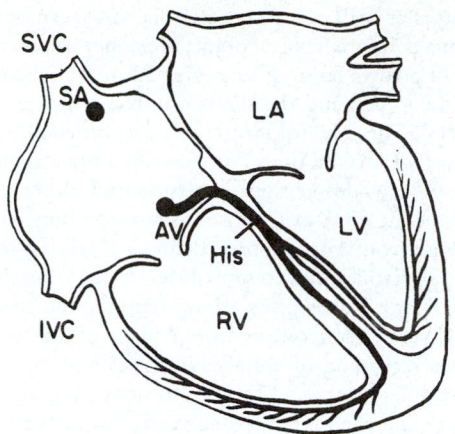

FIGURE 22-10   Diagram of conduction system. SA = sinoatrial node; AV = atrioventricular node; His = bundle of His, dividing into right and left bundles; RV and LV = right and left ventricles; SVC and IVC = superior and inferior venae cavae; LA = left atrium.

ventricular contraction begins. Beyond the AV node the impulse moves rapidly down the bundle of His into the right and left branches. As the impulses pass down the septum they activate septal muscle predominantly from the left side, so that the initial ventricular vector passes from left to right, anteriorly and superiorly (Fig. 22-11A), and begins the Q wave in lead V_6 or the first part of the R wave in lead V_1. After reaching the apex, the impulse invades the ventricular free walls from endocardium to epicardium and from apex toward the base, thus inscribing the R and S waves; the last part of the heart to be activated is the posterior ventricular muscle just under the AV ring. In adults and older children there is more left than right ventricular muscle, so that the major cardiac vectors point to the left and posteriorly and produce a tall R wave in V_6 and a deep S wave in V_1. In a newborn infant with a thick right ventricle, the major cardiac vectors pass to the right and anteriorly and produce a dominant R wave in V_1 and a large S wave in V_6. After depolarization has occurred, there is slower repolarization that produces the T wave.

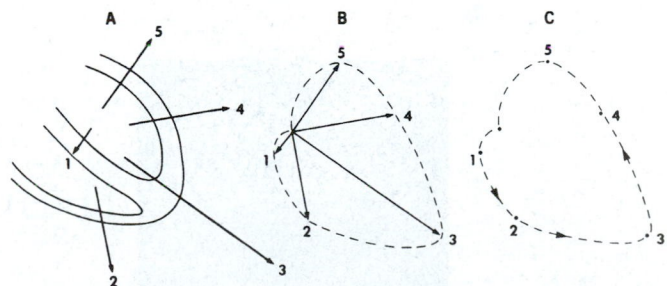

FIGURE 22-11   Normal ventricular depolarization, starting with 1 and ending with 5. A: Section through ventricles with thicker-walled left ventricle and thinner-walled right ventricle. *Arrows* are vectors, indicating direction and magnitude of electrical forces at each time. B: Vectors are superimposed on common center, and their tips are joined by a dashed line. C: The *dashed line* remains to give a vector loop. The vector at any moment would be a line joining the central point to the corresponding part of the loop. The *arrows* represent the direction of movement of the instantaneous vectors. In practice, direction is indicated by having each dash shaped like a teardrop with the blunt end leading, and the dashes occur each 0.0025 second of the cardiac cycle.

The vectors at each point in the cardiac cycle can be drawn as if arising from a common central point; thus, they can be represented by a series of arrows fanning out (Fig. 22-11B). The ends of the arrows can be joined and the shafts omitted to give a vector loop (Fig. 22-11C). These vector loops can be recorded directly by connecting electrodes to the body and recording the voltages between three sets of electrodes at right angles to each other. Leads from right to left define an X axis, those from top to bottom define a Y axis, and those from front to back define a Z axis. (A lead is a line joining two electrodes or two sets of electrodes.) Simultaneous recording of X and Y axes gives a loop representing the projection of the actual vector loop on the frontal plane of the body, whereas simultaneous recording of voltages in the X and Z axes gives the horizontal-plane projection of the vector loop (Fig. 22-12). The Y and Z axes define the sagittal-plane vector loop, but this adds no new information. Various lead systems give similar patterns but different values of various measurements, so that each needs its own standards. The beam is interrupted each 0.0025 second and usually has a blunt leading edge, so that it is possible to tell which way the vector is moving and at what speed.

The electrocardiogram is a recording of voltage against time, usually made at a paper speed of 25 mm/s, with 1 mV giving 10 mm of deflection. At any instant the mean vector present can be resolved into two components, one parallel to a lead and one at right angles to it. The latter affects both electrodes equally, so that there is no potential difference between them, whereas the former causes a voltage to appear between the two electrodes. This voltage is proportional to the projection made by the vector on the lead (Fig. 22-13A). The limb leads (I, II, III, aVR, aVL, aVF) represent the vector in the frontal plane, and the precordial leads essentially represent the vector in the horizontal plane (Fig. 22-13B); of these, the right chest leads (V_{4R}, V_{3R}, V_1, V_2) indicate anteroposterior forces, and the left chest leads (V_5, V_6) indicate left-to-right forces. Furthermore, certain parts of the left ventricle are reflected in certain groupings of leads: leads V_1 and V_2 show activity in the anteroseptal muscle, V_2 to V_5 in the anterior wall, V_5 and V_6 in the apex, I and aVL in the anterolateral wall, and II, III, and aVF in the inferior (diaphragmatic) wall. Remember that there is actually a three-dimensional vector in the heart and that the electrocardiogram and vectorcardiogram merely indicate the projection of that

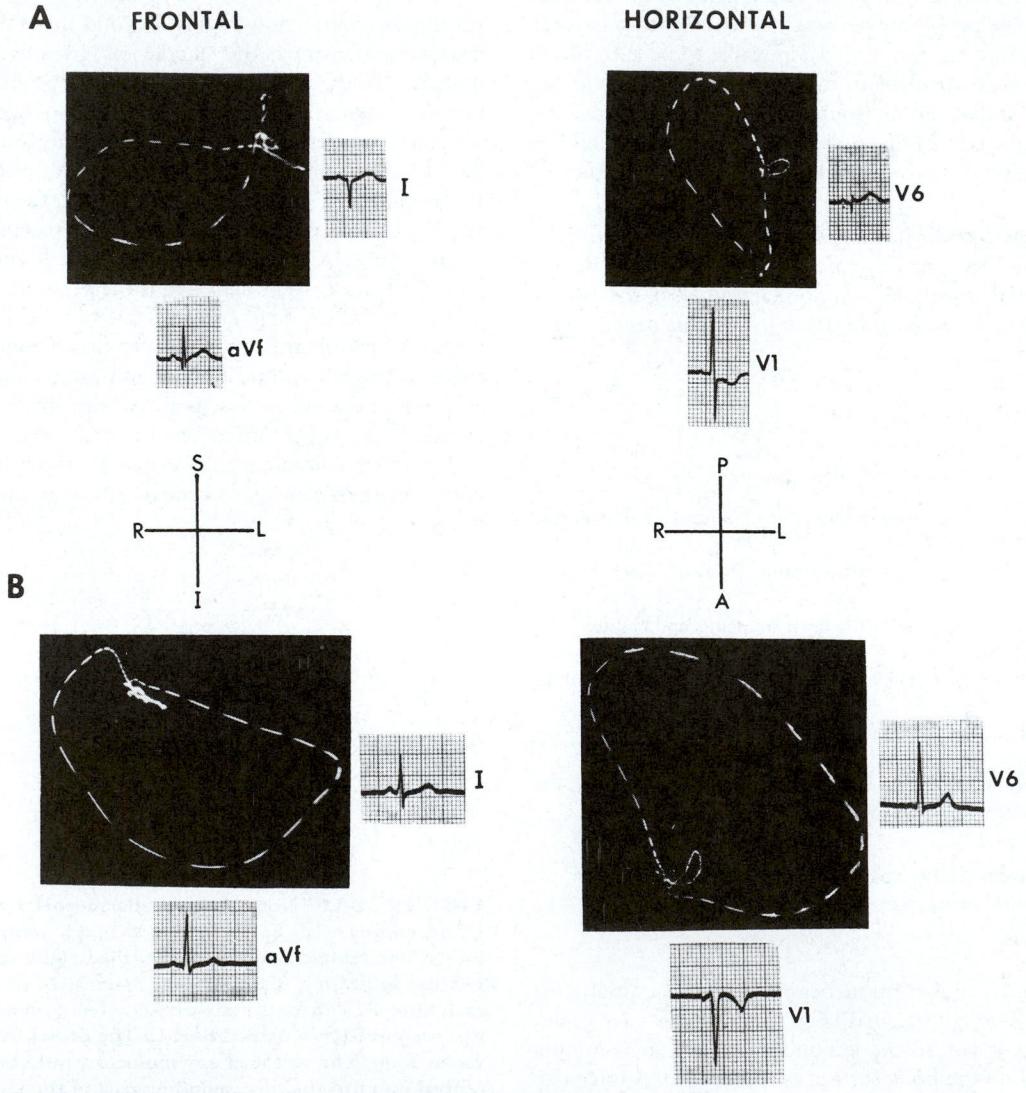

FIGURE 22-12   A: Frontal- and horizontal-plane vectors of a normal 3-week-old infant. B: Frontal and horizontal plane vectors of a normal 10-year-old child. Leads I and aVF from the corresponding electrocardiograms are shown in appropriate positions next to the frontal-plane loops; similarly, leads V_1 and V_2 are shown next to the horizontal loops.

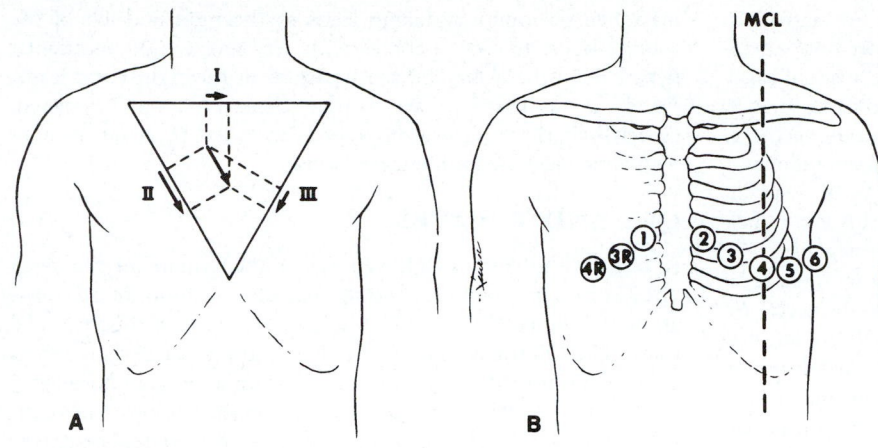

FIGURE 22-13 A: Einthoven equilateral triangle is superimposed on the frontal plane of the thorax. A mean QRS vector is shown in the triangle, and its projection on each of the limb leads is obtained by dropping perpendiculars (*dashed lines*) from the vector to each lead. Note that the angle the vector makes determines the magnitude of its projection in each lead and that the magnitude is greatest in the lead almost parallel to the vector. **B:** The conventional sites for electrode placement on the thorax (V leads). V_1 and V_2 are in the fourth intercostal space. V_4 is in the fifth space. V_3 is halfway between V_2 and V_4, and V_5 and V_6 are in the fifth space in the anterior and midaxillary lines, respectively. V_3R and V_4R are the right-sided counterparts of V_3 and V_4. These precordial leads lie roughly in the horizontal plane. MCL = midclavicular line.

vector on a particular lead or plane, respectively. The electrocardiogram is easier to take, and time intervals are more easily measured with it, whereas the vectorcardiogram gives more precise information about the vector at each moment in the cardiac cycle. Although vectorcardiograms are now rarely performed, the experienced electrocardiographer sees the electrocardiogram as a representation of the vectorcardiogram and visualizes the vector forces in interpreting the tracings.

APPROACH

The routine pediatric electrocardiogram involves the recording of 15 leads, the standard 12 plus leads to the right of V_1 (V_3R, V_4R), and at least one lead (V_7) to the left of V_6; if no Q wave is seen in V_7, then leads to the left of V_7 must be recorded. The electrocardiogram should be interpreted knowing the history, physical examination, drug therapy, and heart size, shape, and position as seen on the chest roentgenogram. It is best to read the electrocardiogram systematically. First measure atrial and ventricular rates and define the rhythm. Then record the P-R interval, QRS duration, and Q-T interval. Measure the frontal-plane mean axes of the P waves, QRS complex, and T waves. Finally, look for abnormalities of pattern in the waves and their interconnecting segments and note the voltages of P, Q, R, S, and T waves.

The electrocardiogram gives information about arrhythmias, hypertrophy of atria or ventricles, electrolyte changes, some myocardial or pericardial infections, and myocardial ischemia and infarction; and some specific patterns occur in certain congenital heart diseases. The electrocardiogram gives little information about myocardial function or ventricular cavity size.

MEASURING QRS AXIS To evaluate the mean frontal-plane QRS axis, the following features must be noted:

- Lead I runs from the left to the right arm; by agreement, a deflection passing toward the left arm is positive, and a deflection passing away from it is negative (Fig. 22-14A).
- Leads II and III are at 60° to each other and to lead I, and they can be superimposed on a common center (Fig. 22-14B). Note that the lower half of the frontal plane is assigned positive numbers and the upper half negative numbers.
- Lead aVF runs from the legs up to the heart and thus lies in the axis +90° to −90° (Fig. 22-14C). An impulse passing toward the leg thus gives a positive deflection.

- Leads aVR and aVL pass from the right and left shoulders, respectively, to the heart (Fig. 22-14D), and their axes are at 60° to each other and to lead aVF. Because they are unipolar leads, an impulse passing toward either shoulder will give a positive deflection despite the negative angles associated with the superior ends of the axes in the figure.
- All six leads may be superimposed on a central point (Fig. 22-14E) to give axes at 30° to each other.
- To use this hexaxial reference frame, first decide whether lead I is predominantly positive or negative. In general, this can be determined from the heights of the R and S waves. However,

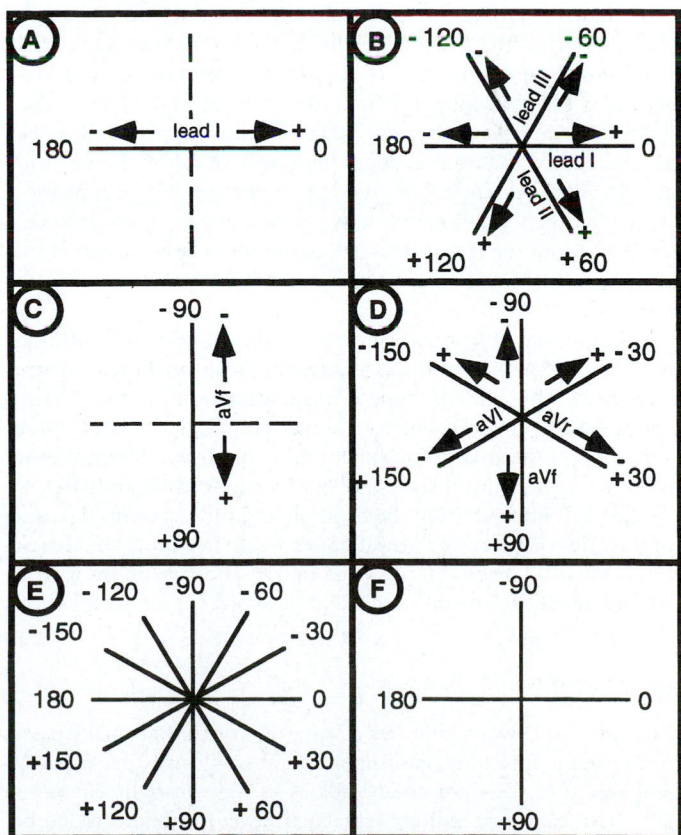

FIGURE 22-14 Measurement of mean frontal plane axes (see text).

because it is actually area that is assessed, a tall but narrow R wave might contribute less positivity than a short but wide S wave contributes negativity; if the Q wave is large, it should also be included in the assessment. If the result is positive, the net vector is passing to the left; if it is negative, the net vector is passing to the right. If the net voltage is zero (that is, equiphasic R and S complexes), the vector must be passing up at $-90°$ or down at $+90°$ (Fig. 22-14A). Next, examine aVF for its net voltage: if positive, the vector is passing down; if negative, it is passing up; if zero, it is passing directly right or left (Fig. 22-14C). These two leads can be integrated to assign the vector to one of four quadrants (Fig. 22-14F). Lead I+, aVF+ indicates the left lower quadrant; lead I+, aVF− indicates the left upper quadrant (left axis); lead I−, aVF+ indicates the right lower quadrant (right axis); lead I−, aVF− indicates the right upper quadrant, sometimes termed the "northwest" quadrant. The axis can be measured more closely by referring to the remaining leads; today this is done automatically by the computer in the electrocardiograph.

- Occasionally the R and S waves are almost equiphasic in several leads, perhaps in four or in all six. This implies that the QRS vector is mainly perpendicular to the frontal plane and in the frontal plane forms a rough circle, so that there is no true mean axis. This is sometimes termed an *indeterminate frontal-plane axis*. It has no clinical importance except insofar as it prevents the accurate determination of a mean QRS axis.
- The mean frontal axis of the P and T waves can be calculated in the same way.

P WAVE

Normally the right atrium is activated before the left atrium, so that the first part of the P wave is right atrial, the last part is left atrial, and forces from both atria make up the middle of the P wave. With right atrial hypertrophy, the duration of the P wave is not lengthened, but the P waves become taller and peaked, especially in lead II, and exceed the normal upper limit of 0.25 mV (2.5 mm at full standardization). In lead V_1 too, there may be a large biphasic P wave. With left atrial hypertrophy, the initial part of the P wave is unaltered, but the later part is larger and often lasts longer, so that the P waves are wider than normal and bifid with a large second component.

The normal P frontal-plane axis is about $+30°$ to $+60°$; any marked change from this axis suggests an abnormal focus of atrial activation. Thus, in true mirror-image dextrocardia, the P axis is about $+120°$, giving a negative P wave in lead I, whereas retrograde activation of the atria from a junctional focus gives a P axis of about $-30°$ to $-60°$; thus, P waves are negative in leads II and III.

The P-R interval, from the beginning of the P wave to the onset of the QRS complex, is about 0.13 second in newborns; it increases to about 0.16 second at 16 years of age and can be up to 0.21 second in adults. The interval is slightly shorter at more rapid heart rates at any age.

Q WAVE

Because the Q wave indicates a septal vector that normally passes to the right, anteriorly, and superiorly, it is normally present in V_6 and absent in the right chest leads. A Q wave in right but not in left chest leads may indicate septal activation from right to left because of left bundle branch block or ventricular inversion (corrected transposition of the great arteries). It can occur also if the heart is rotated so that the septum lies in the sagittal plane; the septal vector

may then be found by taking leads to the right and left of the routine leads. In some patients with very severe right ventricular hypertrophy there may be a qR pattern in the right chest leads. Finally, a tiny initial r wave in right chest leads may be missed, especially if the electrocardiogram is recorded by an instrument with an inadequate frequency response.

QRS AND T WAVES

At birth, with the thick right ventricle of the term infant, the mean QRS axis points anteriorly and to the right, giving right axis deviation (95% limits, 90° to 190°) and large R waves in right precordial leads. The QRS axis shifts to the left in the frontal plane and at about 3 months of age averages $+65°$, with a range in normal infants of 0° to $+105°$. It normally remains in the left lower quadrant throughout life. In the horizontal plane the axis rotates posteriorly until it is pointing leftward at 0° at about 3 months of age and posteriorly at about $-45°$ from age 3 years onward. This explains why with age the R wave decreases in V_1 and increases in V_6, whereas V_1 shows a large S wave after infancy. Although premature infants also show right ventricular dominance at birth, the QRS vector begins to swing posteriorly and to the left at about 1 month of age; this normal variant may cause overdiagnosis of left ventricular hypertrophy in preterm infants.

The mean T vector undergoes rapid and marked changes after birth. For the first 12 hours it points to the left and posteriorly and has a frontal-plane axis of about $+60°$; this gives a negative T wave in V_1. Then the T vector rotates anteriorly and to the right, giving a positive T wave in V_1 by 24 hours after birth. It remains anterior for 2 to 7 days and then moves posteriorly and to the left, so that the T wave again inverts in V_1. The reasons for these rapid changes are not clear. At about 12 years of age the T wave may become upright once again in V_1 in some children. T waves normally may be inverted in leads V_5 and V_6 during but not beyond the first day after birth; they may be inverted normally in V_4 until 5 years of age and in V_3 until 10 years of age. The frontal-plane T axis stays at about $+60°$ throughout childhood. Because the T and QRS vectors do not follow the same course in early childhood, the angle between them changes. At birth the frontal-plane mean QRS-T angle is about $+130°$, and it slowly falls until it reaches 30° to 60° by about 3 years of age; thereafter it remains under 60°, and any increase suggests some myocardial abnormality.

VENTRICULAR HYPERTROPHY

Ventricular hypertrophy is difficult to diagnose. Differences in heart position and chest shape affect how much of the cardiac potential is recorded from the body surface, and minor degrees of asynchrony of ventricular depolarization can alter the algebraic sum of the electrical forces at any moment. Because of the wide range of normality it is impossible to diagnose slight hypertrophy, especially as the voltages before the onset of hypertrophy are seldom known. Furthermore, no single sign on its own can be considered reliable; in particular, just an abnormal QRS axis or a single increased voltage should not lead to the diagnosis if there is no other supportive evidence.

LEFT VENTRICULAR HYPERTROPHY In infancy, with the increased mass of left ventricular muscle in left ventricular hypertrophy, the mean QRS axis moves to the left and posteriorly. Therefore, in the frontal plane the QRS axis moves to between 0° and 90°; an axis less than 30° is uncommon in infancy and suggests the possibility of left ventricular hypertrophy. This leftward shift of the

QRS axis increases the R wave and decreases the S wave in V_5 and V_6, and the posterior shift of the QRS axis decreases R waves and increases S waves in V_1. In older children and adults the QRS axis is normally to the left, posterior, and inferior, so that with left ventricular hypertrophy there is no further axis shift but only an increase in voltage. A left superior frontal axis ($0°$ to $-90°$) cannot be caused by increased inferiorly placed left ventricular muscle and is not the mark of left ventricular hypertrophy but of a conduction defect.

Without an axis shift to rely on, the diagnosis of left ventricular hypertrophy is based largely on voltage changes. Increased posterior forces are suggested by R waves below the fifth percentile or S waves above the 95th percentile in V_{3R} and V_1 (Fig. 22-15A). The increased left forces are suggested by R waves above the 95th percentile in V_5 and V_5 (Fig. 22-15B); smaller-than-normal S waves in V_5 and V_6 are not helpful because they can normally be very small. In addition, because the septum is usually involved in the hypertrophy, there is often an enlarged Q wave, which, when greater than 0.4 mV (4 mm at full standardization), suggests left ventricular hypertrophy. T-wave changes in the absence of voltage changes do not indicate left ventricular hypertrophy, but if the two changes are associated, they suggest either myocardial ischemia, as in severe aortic stenosis, or else what is termed left ventricular strain.

RIGHT VENTRICULAR HYPERTROPHY At birth the term infant has a right ventricular wall as thick as or slightly thicker than that of the left ventricle and thus, compared with the older child or adult, has physiological right ventricular hypertrophy. If there is pathologic excessive right ventricular hypertrophy, the mean QRS vector may move farther right and anteriorly, so that frontal-plane QRS axes more than $190°$ under 1 week of age or $105°$ over 1 month of age suggest right ventricular hypertrophy, provided that there is no conduction defect. The increased anterior and rightward forces produce taller R waves and smaller S waves in right chest leads and smaller R waves and larger S waves in left chest leads.

In addition, a pure R wave or a qR pattern in the right chest leads strongly suggests pathologic right ventricular hypertrophy, and so does an upright T wave in V_{4R} and V_1 between 7 days and about 8 years of age. Note that neither left nor right ventricular hypertrophy can be diagnosed confidently if there is an abnormally wide QRS complex, as occurs in bundle branch block or Wolff-Parkinson-White syndrome.

RIGHT BUNDLE BRANCH BLOCK If the right bundle is interrupted, septal activation from left to right is unchanged, and then the left ventricle is depolarized to give a force to the left and posteriorly; this force is more marked than usual because the counteracting right ventricular forces have not yet begun. As left ventricular depolarization is ending, the impulse eventually penetrates the right ventricular muscle and spreads slowly through it to give late-onset slow right and anterior forces. Therefore, in right chest leads there is a normal initial R wave followed by a deep narrow S wave and then a tall and wide R′ that brings the QRS duration to over 0.12 second in adults. (By convention, a deflection under 5 mm is written as a lowercase letter, eg, r, and a deflection over 5 mm is written as a capital letter, eg, R. Also, a second positive deflection is described as r′ or R′.) In left chest leads the pattern is of a qRS type, with a deep and wide terminal S wave. The terminal right and anterior forces, being unopposed by left ventricular forces, are large and serve to produce a marked right-axis shift in the frontal plane.

Because in the newborn infant the normal QRS duration is about 0.05 to 0.06 second, it is possible for complete right bundle branch block to widen the QRS but still be under the limit of 0.12 second that pertains to adults. If the child has had a right ventriculotomy, there may be a typical right bundle branch block pattern as a result of the cutting of many terminal conduction fibers in the free wall and not from damage to the main right bundle. Finally, many normal children have an rSr′ pattern that results from a delayed but otherwise normal terminal deflection caused by late depolarization of the posterior part of the right ventricle under the AV groove. This pattern has been termed *incomplete right bundle branch block,* but in children it usually has nothing to do with conduction changes in the right bundle and its major branches. Therefore, it is better to refer to this as a *minor right ventricular conduction delay,* and this pattern does not prevent one from reading the ECG as normal. A similar pattern is also seen in most children with atrial septal defects and in those with mild pulmonic stenosis, but the normal and abnormal causes for the pattern cannot be distinguished on the electrocardiogram.

In some newborn infants there may be a very tall and pure R wave in right chest leads that raises the suspicion of right ventricular hyperthrophy. Close inspection shows a slur or notch on the upstroke of the R wave; with time the slur becomes more marked, a deep notch develops to produce an rR′ pattern, and finally a typical rSr′ pattern develops. Therefore, a conduction defect in babies can

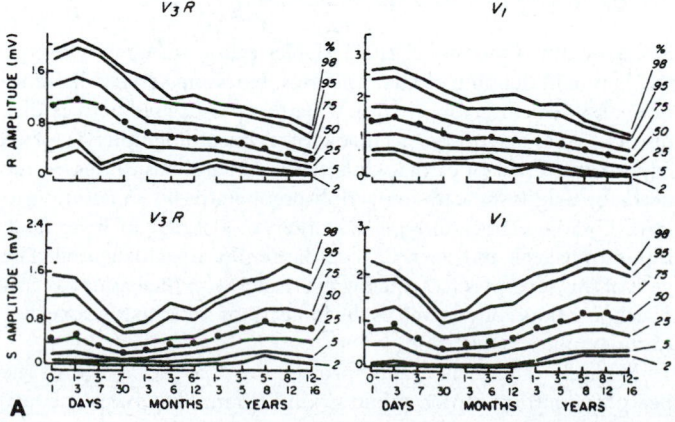
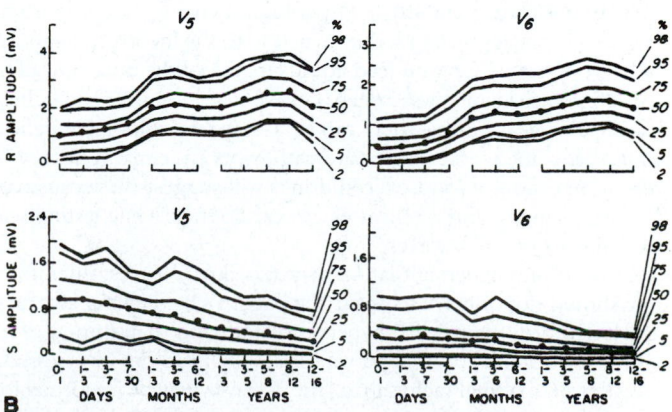

FIGURE 22-15 Normal values for R and S waves in (A) right and (B) left precordial leads at different ages. *Lines* represent percentiles, with dotted line the 50th percentile. SOURCE: *Davignon A, Rautaharju P, Boiselle E, et al: Normal ECG standards for infants and children. Pediatr Cardiol 1:123, 1979/1980.*

simulate right ventricular hypertrophy, but absence of other evidence of right ventricular pathologic changes and the evolution of the electrocardiogram lead to the correct diagnosis.

S-T SEGMENT AND T WAVES

S-T–segment and T-wave changes other than those related to maturation have similar causes in children and adults. Frequently they are secondary to changes in the QRS complex, such as widening of the QRS complex in conduction abnormalities or an increased QRS amplitude in hypertrophy. These secondary changes of T waves are usually associated with a normal QRS-T angle in the frontal plane. Primary T-wave changes are those occurring in the absence of QRS changes and may be classified as changes related to electrolyte disturbances; physiological changes (see below); or pathologic changes caused by drugs (especially digitalis glycosides), myocarditis or pericarditis, cardiomyopathy, degenerative neurologic diseases, and myocardial ischemia. The pathologic changes are discussed in their respective sections, but the other two groups are discussed briefly here.

ELECTROLYTE ABNORMALITIES *Hypocalcemia* lengthens, and *hypercalcemia* shortens, the QT interval. Because the QT interval normally varies with heart rate, a rate-independent corrected QT interval (QTc) is calculated as $QT/\sqrt{R\text{-}R}$. The normal value is 0.40, with a range of 0.36 to 0.44. A low magnesium level may intensify the effects of low calcium; clinically the long Q-T interval of hypocalcemia in infancy may remain after the calcium level has been restored to normal and improve only after magnesium is given. Other factors can also alter the Q-T interval: digitalis glycosides and pericarditis may shorten it slightly, and myocarditis and certain genetic syndromes may lengthen it.

A *high serum potassium* level gives high, peaked T waves that are clearly abnormal at concentrations above 7 meq/L. Higher potassium concentrations not only raise T waves further, but reduce QRS amplitude, widen QRS duration, and lengthen P-R interval. Above 9 meq/L there are usually atrial arrest and very wide QRS complexes that may lead to ventricular fibrillation. Preterm infants may be more resistant to these changes. *Low serum potassium* levels lower T waves, the effect being detectable below 3.5 meq/L. As potassium falls more, a U wave appears, and the S-T segment becomes depressed.

PHYSIOLOGICAL CHANGES Physiological changes are important because, if not appreciated, they may lead to the incorrect diagnosis of heart disease. Drinking iced liquids may cool the inferior wall of the left ventricle and cause deep T-wave inversion in the left chest leads. After heavy meals there can be T-wave inversion in left chest leads that some workers associate with hyperglycemia. A history of recent ingestion of food or iced drinks will suggest these causes of T-wave changes, and a repeat electrocardiogram while fasting will then show normal T waves.

Anxiety and hyperventilation may also alter T waves. Therefore, one should not only try to assess the patient's anxiety but also take an electrocardiogram with hyperventilation and then during exercise so that the effect of hyperventilation by itself can be assessed.

After paroxysmal tachycardia, the T waves may be abnormal for several hours or days, perhaps because of transient myocardial ischemia or potassium loss; the T waves usually return to normal, and there is probably no permanent damage.

Two other important normal variants should be considered. Some children and young adults have large upright T waves and elevated S-T segments in precordial or even limb leads, so that pericarditis might be suspected. This pattern is termed "early repolarization," although it is not clear that it represents any abnormality of the order of ventricular repolarization, and it should not be considered abnormal. What distinguishes this variant from pericarditis is that here the T waves are very large and do not evolve as they do in pericarditis. The second variant is that of isolated inversion of the T waves in leads over the left ventricular apex, although the T waves are upright in earlier and later leads. This change occurs most often in young men; it can vary from time to time and has no accepted explanation. Like other physiological T-wave changes, the T waves usually return to normal after oral potassium salts are ingested. Finally, athletes in peak training condition can have not only increased voltages diagnostic of left or right ventricular hypertrophy but also T-wave inversion in left ventricular leads. These are normal findings in this setting.

References

Davignon A, Rautaharju P, Boiselle E, et al: Normal ECG standards for infants and children. Pediatr Cardiol 1:123, 1979/1980

Fyler DC: Nadas' Pediatric Cardiology. Philadelphia, Hanley & Balfus, 1992

Garson A: Electrocardiography. In: Anderson RH, Macartney FJ, Shinebourne EA, Tynan M, eds: Paediatric Cardiology. Edinburgh, Churchill Livingstone, 1987:235

Grant RP: Grant's Clinical Electrocardiography: The Spatial Vector Approach. New York, McGraw-Hill, 1970

Guntheroth WA: Pediatric Electrocardiography. Philadelphia, WB Saunders, 1965

Liebman J, Plonsey R, Gillette PC: Pediatric electrocardiography. Baltimore, Williams & Wilkins, 1982

Liebman J, Plonsey R: Electrocardiography. In: Adams FH, Emmanouilides GC, Riemenschneider TA, eds: Heart Disease in Infants, Children, and Adolescents. Baltimore, Williams & Wilkins, 1989:35

Marriott HJL, Wagner G: Practical Electrocardiography. Baltimore, Williams & Wilkins, 1988

Schamroth L: An Introduction to Electrocardiography. Oxford, Blackwell, 1971

22.2.3 Echocardiography

Theresa A. Tacy and Norman H. Silverman

Standard two-dimensional and Doppler echocardiography plays a major role in defining cardiac anatomy, assessing ventricular function, and detecting abnormal flow patterns associated with cardiac disease. The diagnostic accuracy of echocardiography is often equivalent to that of cardiac catheterization and has decreased the need for diagnostic catheterization preoperatively. In addition to transthoracic echocardiography, other modalities such as fetal, transesophageal, and stress echocardiography are widely used. The goal of this section is to acquaint the reader with the basic concepts of echocardiography as well as the indications for each type of echocardiographic examination.

M-mode echocardiography provides an "ice-pick" view of the heart by emitting a narrow ultrasound beam. Structures encountered by the beam are reflected back and displayed as dots, and as the image scrolls through to display time, the motion of this site over the cardiac cycle is displayed (Fig. 22-16). The frame rate in M-mode echocardiography is 1000 to 4000 frames per second, yielding excellent time resolution. Thus M-mode provides the most

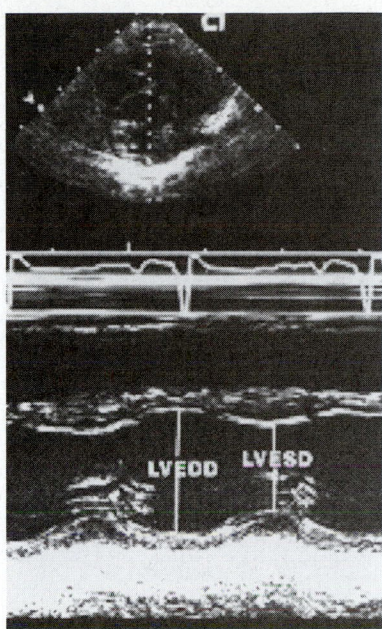

FIGURE 22-16 This M-mode from a normal subject is aligned properly for calculating fractional shortening, which is the percentage change between the left ventricular end-diastolic dimension (LVEDD) and the left ventricular end-systolic dimension (LVESD). In addition, this view is useful for measuring septal and posterior wall thickness and for confirming abnormal septal wall motion. Sweep speed 100 mm/s. *Calibrating marks* every 5 mm.

precise display of events that occur rapidly within the cardiac cycle, such as the opening and closing of valves, the motion of ventricular and atrial walls, and changes in cavity size during contraction and relaxation. However, because of the narrow area of interrogation, anatomic relationships are best left to other modalities such as the two-dimensional echocardiogram. To produce this, emitted beams of sound are steered, usually over 30 times a second, over an arc of approximately 90°, producing a fan-shaped or sector image. The sector is made up of many lines of information, and the ultrasound information represented on each line within this sector fan produces an image. The replay of this ultrasound image from the sector fan in time that is almost instantaneous with its generation has led to the technique being called "real-time imaging."

Two-dimensional echocardiography shows a slice of the heart that allows assessment of the spatial and anatomic relationships in the heart. Because each view is limited to one slice, multiple planes of the heart are investigated during a complete study to allow interrogation of all the heart. On a transthoracic study, these views are obtained from multiple sites on the chest, including parasternal position, cardiac apex, subcostal position in the midline below the subxiphoid process, and suprasternal position from the suprasternal notch. Only with complete display of the cardiac images from all of these positions can a reliable three-dimensional concept of cardiac anatomy be achieved (Figs. 22-17 to 22-20). Two-dimensional imaging is useful for anatomic information but does not assess flow patterns or hemodynamics. If performed alone, it may miss small or subtle lesions, valve leakage, or other subtle flow disturbances.

A second application of ultrasonography is to evaluate blood flow patterns in the heart and vessels by the Doppler principle. Johann Christian Doppler (1803–1853), an Austrian physicist, first showed that if the observer is moving relative to a sound source,

the detected and transmitted frequencies differ; an observer moving toward the sound source hears a higher-frequency tone than that heard by a stationary observer. This phenomenon, induced by the relative motion of the sound source and the observer, is referred to as the Doppler effect, and the resulting change in frequency of sound is called the Doppler shift.

The blood flow patterns within the heart and great vessels are evaluated by measuring blood velocity and displaying this information in various formats. Ultrasonic Doppler blood velocity measurement is performed by both spectral and color-flow Doppler. Spectral Doppler displays blood velocity vertically on a scale as a function of time (horizontal axis) (Fig. 22-21). If the direction of flow is toward the transducer, the flow velocity information is displayed above the baseline (as positive velocity values), and, if motion is away from the transducer, is displayed below the baseline. Spectral Doppler assessments of flow can be performed using one of two modes of ultrasound, either pulsed-wave (PW) or continuous-wave (CW) mode. In the PW mode, measurements can be performed within a small range, and at a precise site determined by the operator; however, the maximum velocity that can be measured is limited. Pulsed-wave Doppler velocimetry is used to define the origin of flow disturbances within the cardiovascular system, such as flow events through valve orifices, and the direction of blood flow. The CW mode has no limit to the maximum measurable velocity; however, the site of velocity measurement cannot be controlled, and blood flow at all depths along the axis of the Doppler beam is measured and displayed. Thus, in practice, the operator usually uses PW Doppler for precise determination of the site, direction, and pattern of flow and CW to measure higher velocities accurately.

Color Doppler flow mapping techniques have become important in the echocardiographic examination. In color Doppler echocardiography, information on blood flow velocity is computed, color encoded, and superimposed on the two-dimensional echocardiographic image. Flow moving toward the transducer has red hues, ranging from a deep red at low velocities to a yellow hue at higher velocities, whereas blood traveling away from the transducer is assigned a deep blue hue at lower velocities and a light blue at higher velocities. Disturbed flow is displayed as a mosaic color that includes green. The information is updated several times a second, producing a real-time map of flow during the cardiac cycle. Color Doppler provides information about direction, velocity, and flow disturbances so that normal and abnormal flow patterns can be easily identified (Fig. 22-22). Color flow mapping techniques are qualitative and not used for precise velocity measurements. Their main utility is for recognizing abnormal flow patterns and as an aid in aligning the spectral Doppler beam for accurate flow velocity measurement. Because M-mode echocardiography, two-dimensional echocardiography, and spectral and color Doppler velocity measurements each assess a different aspect of heart anatomy, function, or flow information, the complete echocardiogram includes all of them.

Echocardiography not only describes anatomy and flow aberrations but also is used to measure cardiac dimensions and function and to estimate pressure drop and shunt magnitude. Chamber and vessel dimensions measured by either M-mode or two-dimensional images are compared with normal data. This information aids in assessing the effects of a shunt lesion, such as finding left ventricular dilatation in a patient with aortic insufficiency. Normal plots of ventricular dimensions, valve sizes, or great vessel sizes related to patient body surface area, weight, or age and height exist for children and are useful for comparison.

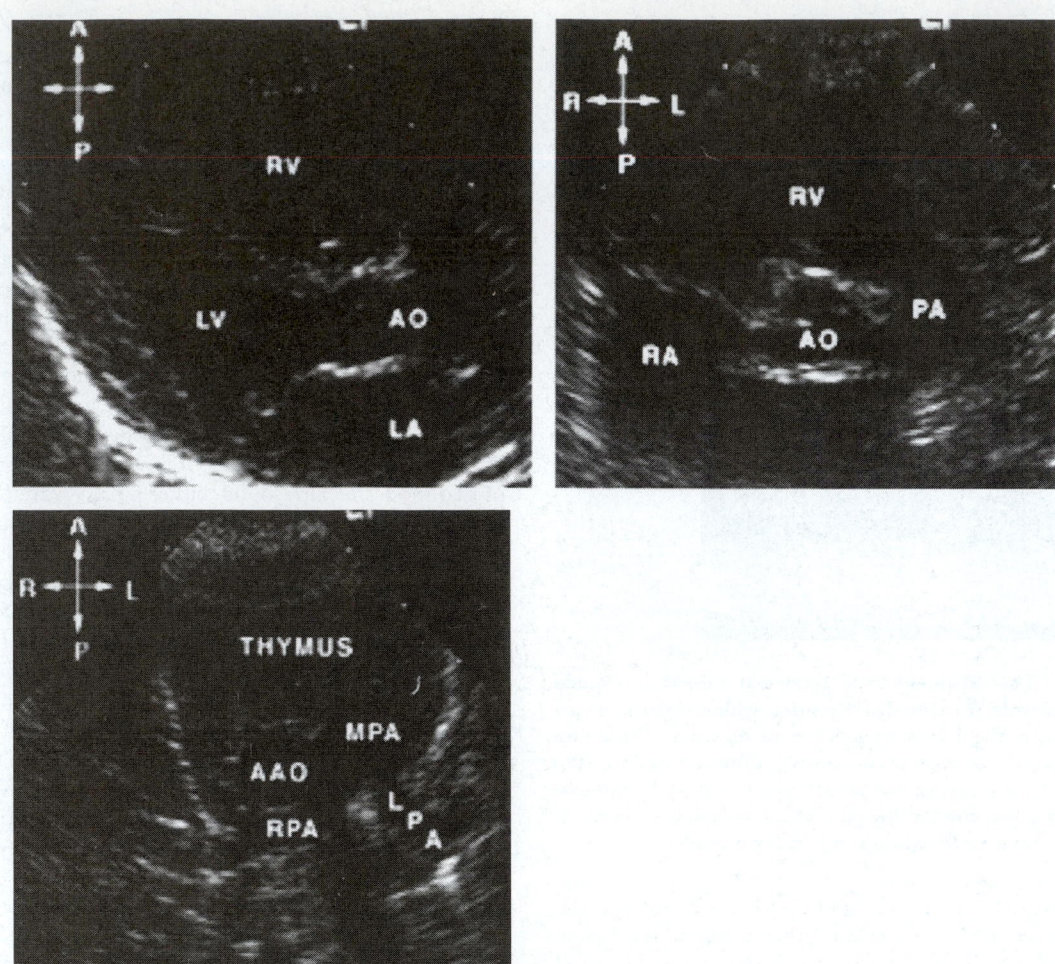

FIGURE 22-17 *Parasternal views.* **Upper left panel:** This frame, from a normal subject, is a parasternal long axis view taken slicing the heart from a parasternal location at the fourth left interspace, subtending a sector with the right ventricle (RV) anteriorly. The sound beams then pass through the ventricular septum and the aorta (AO), the left ventricular cavity (LV), and the left ventricular posterior wall. Behind the ascending aortic root is the left atrium (LA). A = anterior; P = posterior. **Lower left panel:** From the same normal subject in the parasternal short-axis view from the third intercostal space. The sector subtends the right side of the heart as it winds around the aortic root (AO) in the center of image. The right atrium (RA) is separated from the right ventricle (RV) by the tricuspid valve. The pulmonary artery (PA) is separated from the right ventricle by the pulmonary valve. The cusps of the aortic valve can also be identified in this figure. A = anterior; P = posterior; R = right; L = left. **Right panel:** A very high right parasternal view (in the right infraclavicular region) permits imaging of the main (MPA) and branch pulmonary arteries (RPA, LPA). The relationship of the RPA to the ascending aorta (AAO) is easily seen. The thymus is evident in this image. A = anterior; P = posterior; R = right; L = left.

Left ventricular function is commonly assessed during a routine examination by M-mode measurement of the left ventricular shortening fraction, the percentage change of the left ventricular chamber diameter during a cardiac cycle. Normal values for LV shortening fraction are constant throughout childhood and range from 28 to 44%. The LV shortening fraction is easily measured but does not take into account the loading conditions of the left ventricle and thus does not measure LV contractility alone. For example, a patient with severe systemic hypertension may have a depressed LV shortening fraction but normal contractility. Another limitation of the LV shortening fraction as a measure of ventricular function is its assumption of normal LV geometry. If flattened or paradoxic interventricular wall motion exists, shortening fraction will not reliably represent left ventricular function. With altered LV geometry,

change in volume or ejection fraction is measured from the two-dimensional image of the LV. One of the more common methods to determine the volume change is the Simpson rule method, based on the principle that the volume of any object, regardless of its shape, equals the sum of the volumes of multiple individual slices of known thickness that compose the object. On the two-dimensional image, the cavity of the ventricle is traced in systole and diastole, and the ultrasound machine assigns a series of discs of known thickness and a diameter determined by the LV dimensions. The volumes of these discs are then summed, and the change in volume between systole and diastole is computed and reported as an ejection fraction. Normal values for ejection fraction range from 56 to 78%. Although the Simpson rule method transcends most geometric assumptions, ejection fraction is load-dependent. De-

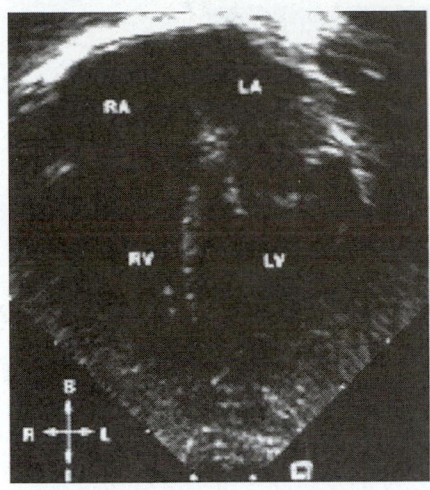
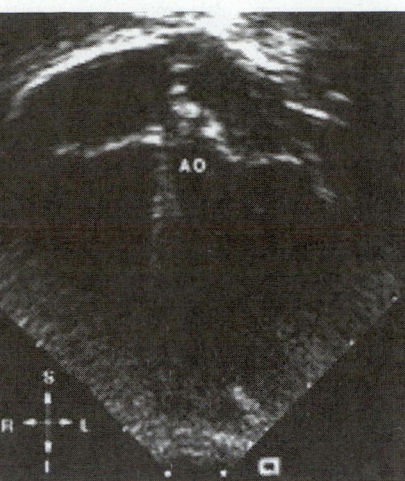

FIGURE 22-18 *Apical four-chamber views.* **Left panel:** A normal apical four-chamber view (A4 Ch), demonstrating the scan from the anterior to the posterior aspect of the heart (from the apex to base). The right atrium (RA) is separated from the left atrium (LA) by the faint echo of the interatrial septum, and the left and right ventricles (LV and RV) can be seen separated from their respective atria by the tricuspid and mitral valves in the open position and from each other by the ventricular septum. S = superior; I = inferior; R = right; L = left. **Right panel:** When the transducer is angulated anteriorly from the position shown above, the aortic root (AO) can be seen arising from the left ventricle. S = superior; I = inferior; R = right; L = left.

spite this limitation, it provides a useful index of ventricular function under many circumstances.

The quantitative assessment of flow events in the heart and great vessels is performed using spectral Doppler velocity measurement of flow velocities. The blood velocity can often be used to predict a pressure drop across the area of flow. The peak velocity is related to the pressure drop by the modified Bernoulli equation; ie, pressure drop = $4 \cdot$ (velocity in m/s)^2. Thus, a peak jet velocity of 3 m/s predicts a peak pressure drop of $4 \cdot (3)^2 = 36$ mm Hg. High-velocity jets can be measured arising from a ventricular septal defect, patent ductus arteriosus, valvar stenosis, valve regurgitation, or from a pulmonary artery band or aortic coarctation (Fig. 22-22). This gradient can be used to predict a chamber or vessel pressure or to assess stenosis severity. The flow volume across a region can also be estimated, such as the cardiac output. Volume per beat can be calculated by measuring the area under the curve of the velocity signal, and the cross-sectional area of the valve estimated using two-dimensional imaging. The volume of flow is determined as the product of flow cross-sectional area and the velocity-time integral of the Doppler signal. This product is the stroke volume across the area of interest, or volume per beat. The stroke volume across the aortic valve is converted to a cardiac output by multiplying the stroke volume by the heart rate.

Fetal echocardiography can reliably diagnose many heart defects as early as 16 weeks of gestation. Because of excellent resolution of the two-dimensional images along with improvements in color flow mapping techniques, most congenital heart defects can be diagnosed in utero except for minor abnormalities in heart valves or small septal defects. The most common indications for fetal echocardiography are a family history of congenital heart disease, an abnormal heart detected by obstetric fetal ultrasonography, maternal risk factors such as diabetes mellitus, and the suspicion of fetal arrhythmias. When severe heart disease not amenable to future therapy is diagnosed, treatment options currently include termination of the pregnancy, or delivery can be planned at a tertiary care facility so that immediate treatment can be given to the infant. Fetal arrhythmias can be diagnosed with fetal echocardiography, and in some instances treatment may be instituted. The fetus with complete heart block must be monitored for signs of hydrops, which may necessitate early delivery if detected. Cardiac compli-

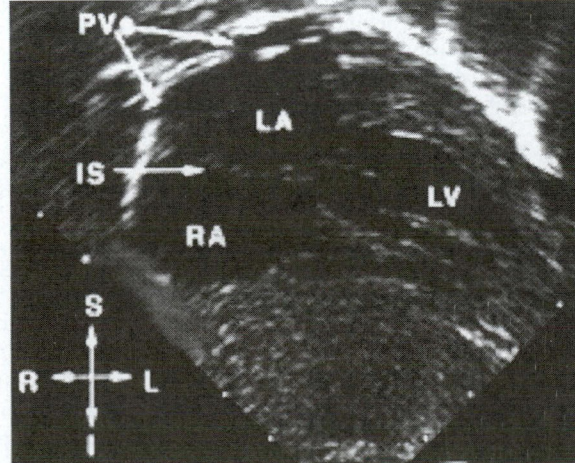
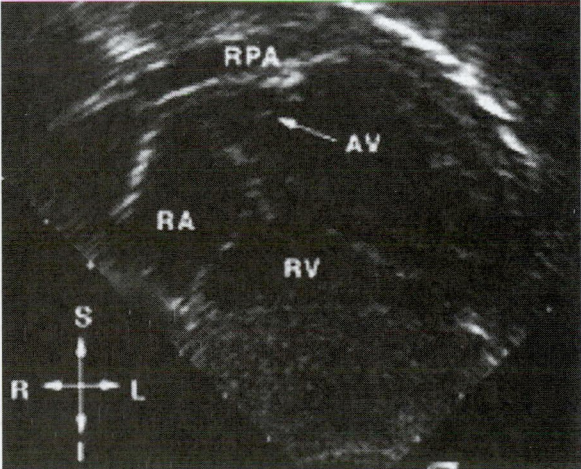

FIGURE 22-19 *Subcostal views.* **Left panel:** In the subcostal coronal plane with posterior angulation, the right atrium (RA), interatrial septum, and pulmonary veins (PV) entering the LA are seen well. S = superior; I = inferior; R = right; L = left. **Right panel:** When the transducer is swept anteriorly from position shown on the left, the plane of the beam goes through the left ventricular outflow tract. In this image, the tricuspid valve is seen between the RA and RV, as well as the aortic valve (AV). The right pulmonary artery (RPA), which courses underneath the ascending aorta, is also visible.

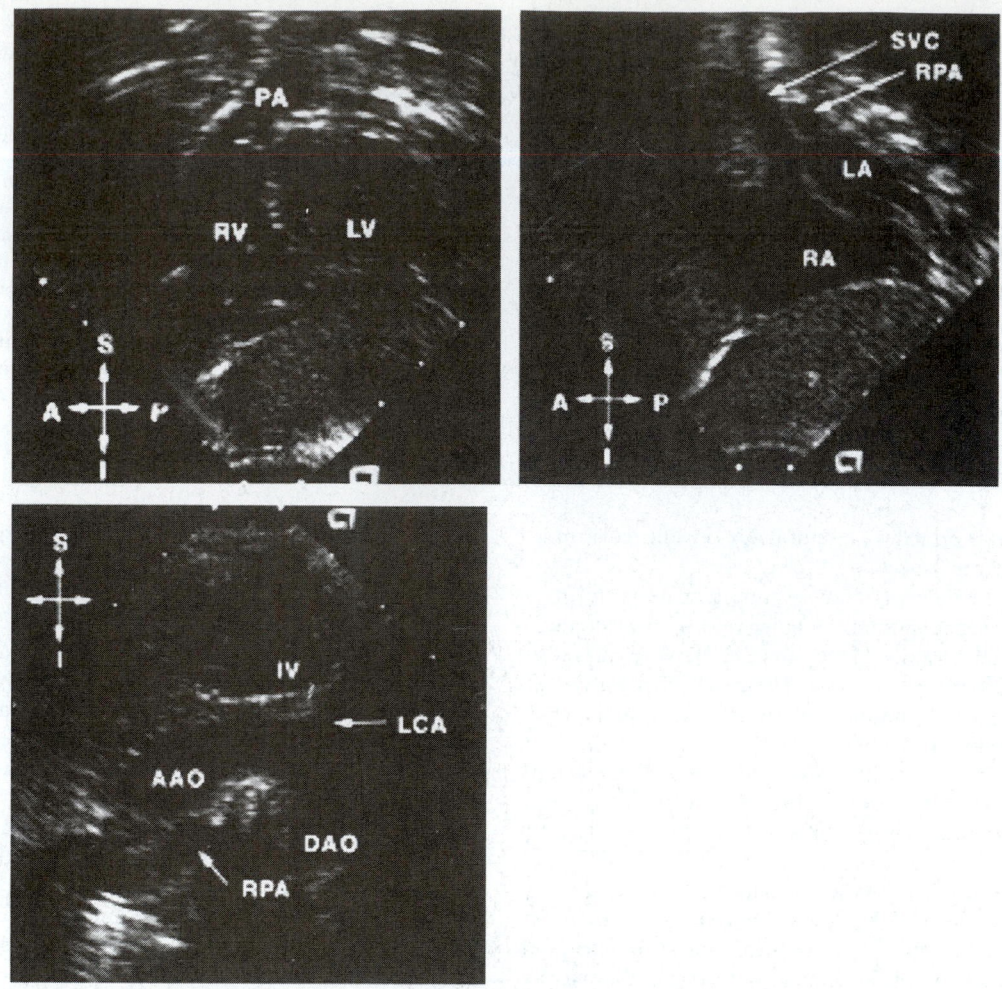

FIGURE 22-20 *Sagittal views.* **Upper left panel:** With the ultrasound beam oriented in the sagittal plane of the body and angulated leftward, the left ventricle (LV) is seen in cross section; the right ventricle (RV) and pulmonary artery (PA) can be seen wrapping around the left ventricle. S = superior; I = inferior; R = right; L = left. **Lower left panel:** With the ultrasound beam oriented in the sagittal plane of the body and angulated rightward, the superior vena cava is seen entering the RA, the LA is seen, as is the RPA in cross section passing behind the SVC. S = superior; I = inferior; R = right; L = left. **Right panel:** The aortic arch from the suprasternal notch sagittal view in a normal infant. The scan comes from the suprasternal notch area, and the sector subtends the innominate vein (IV) superiorly as it crosses in front of the ascending aorta (AAO). The whole arch is seen from the ascending aorta to the descending aorta (DAO). The left carotid artery (LCA) can be seen arising from the aortic arch. The circular right pulmonary artery (RPA) can be seen running under the arch. S = superior; I = inferior.

cations of twin pregnancies can be monitored and treatment initiated if fetal compromise is detected. Thus, monitoring and treatment of these fetuses and counseling of their parents requires a unified and informed team comprised of perinatologists, neonatologists, obstetricians, and pediatric cardiologists, which reviews each fetal malformation or compromise and establishes treatment plans, including the delivery of the patient.

Transesophageal echocardiography (TEE) has been used in children as small as 2.3 kg by inserting a phased-array ultrasound transducer mounted on the tip of a fiberoptic gastroscope as small as 6 mm in diameter. This device allows imaging of the heart from the esophagus and stomach when transthoracic images are of poor quality, when the chest is open, or when a transthoracic study is impractical because of extensive chest bandaging. The most common indication for TEE in children is during cardiac surgery. In-

traoperative TEE has had a great impact by providing additional information preoperatively that alters the planned surgical approach after the initial surgical procedure, identifying postoperative structural abnormalities that require additional surgical intervention while the patient is still in the operating room and identifying postoperative abnormalities that alter medical management immediately after separation from cardiopulmonary bypass support. Transesophageal echocardiography also can play an integral role during cardiac catheterization in placement of devices and stents and monitoring catheter placement during transseptal or ablation procedures.

Stress echocardiography is more common in adults but is increasing in children. Whereas standard echocardiographic studies are done at rest, stress echocardiography evaluates the patient during exercise or during an enhanced inotropic state (accomplished by

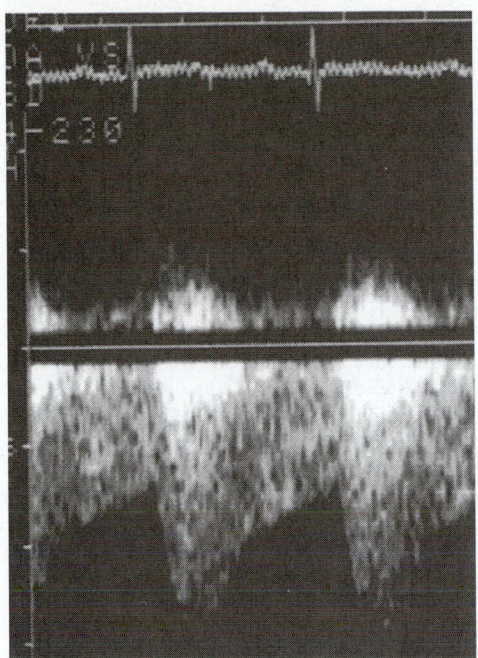

FIGURE 22-21 **Continuous-wave Doppler signal across an aortic coarctation taken from the suprasternal position, aiming inferiorly down the descending aorta. The velocity scale is in meters per second and identifies the scale of 0 to 6 m/s. The velocity of flow across the coarctation increases in systole, and because the direction of flow is away from the transducer, the signal is represented below the baseline. The signal increases to a velocity (V) of 2.6 m/s, which predicts a peak pressure gradient (PG) of 27 mm Hg.**

dobutamine infusion). Stress echocardiography may demonstrate abnormal ventricular function in asymptomatic patients with normal resting state assessments. It is useful in assessing exercise intolerance after surgical intervention and is helpful in evaluating the patient with Kawasaki disease.

Contrast echocardiography with cross-sectional or M-mode modalities is useful for detecting right-to-left intracardiac shunts as

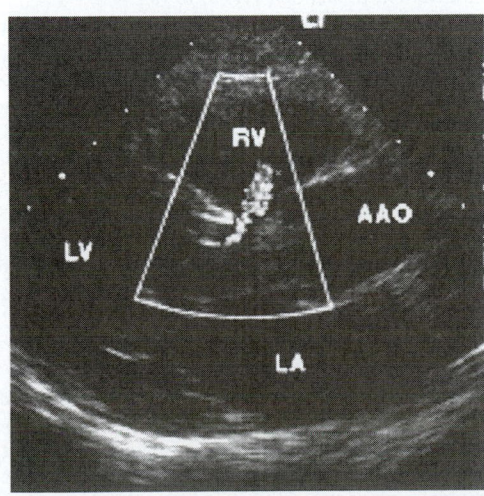

FIGURE 22-22 **This parasternal long-axis view with color Doppler demonstrates a small ventricular septal defect that permits shunting from the left ventricle (LV) to the right ventricle (RV) in systole. This flow is color encoded with red hues because in this view the direction of flow is toward the transducer.**

well as for validating cardiac structures. Microcavitations from agitated saline injected into a peripheral vessel or via catheter can be produced by injecting 1 to 2 mL of saline, dextrose, or other intravenous solution mixed with a small quantity of blood. As the capillary bed traps the microbubbles (less than 200 μm in diameter), they do not enter the systemic circulation when injected on the right side unless an intracardiac communication is present. The microbubbles, however, follow the blood flow patterns so that when right-to-left shunts occur, even in degrees not detectable by other techniques such as angiography or oximetry, these shunts can be detected by the microbubbles in the left heart. The technique is particularly valuable for defining intraatrial right-to-left shunting (Fig. 22-23).

Transtelephonic echocardiography is useful in areas where a pediatric echocardiographer is geographically distant but immediate review of studies is needed to determine patient management. This method uses one of a variety of means to transmit echocardiographic images by either videotransmission services or computer lines. The echocardiographic images are transferred to a regional tertiary care center, where a pediatric cardiologist can review the images while they are being performed or as soon as the study is completed. Often, real-time telephone connections between the sonographer doing the study and the pediatric cardiologist are established when the study begins, and the cardiologist assists the sonographer with verbal instructions. Thus far, transtelephonic echocardiography has been reliable and cost-effective for assessing

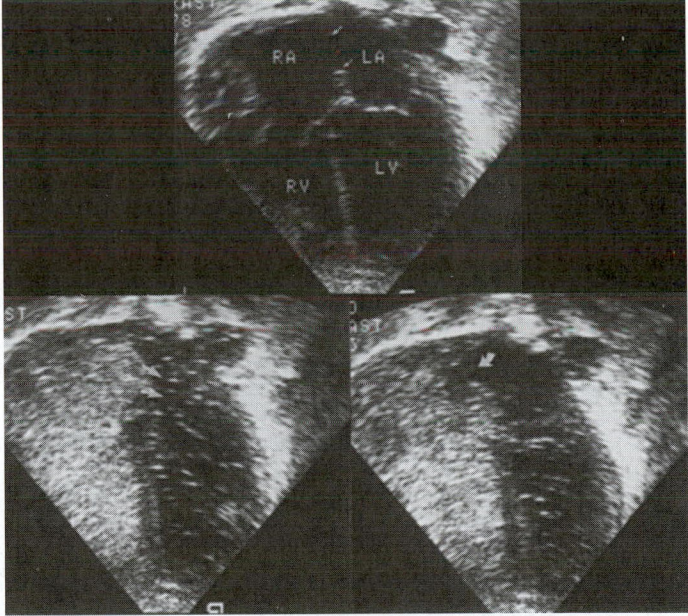

FIGURE 22-23 **These panels demonstrate the effect of an agitated saline contrast echocardiogram in a neonate with bidirectional atrial shunting. The top panel shows a control apical four-chamber view before injection. The four chambers of the heart are labeled as in the previous examples: the *small arrows* indicate the extent of the foramen ovale. The lower left panel demonstrates the arrival of saline contrast within the heart. Opacification appears dense in the right atrium and right ventricle, but the left atrium and left ventricle show opacification through the foramen ovale (arrow). This indicates a right-to-left atrial shunt. The lower right panel shows that the saline has been washed out of the left side. The right atrium remains filled with contrast material, and there is a silhouette effect of non–contrast-containing blood from the left atrium (arrow), which indicates the left-to-right atrial shunt.**

patients in remote locations and has been especially effective in avoiding unnecessary neonatal transports.

In today's managed care environment, cost-effective means for diagnosis is a major concern to the primary care physician, who must be a careful consumer of medical technology. However, the costs of and indications for echocardiography remain misunderstood by many primary care physicians. Patients are often referred for echocardiography alone instead of for a cardiology consultation to evaluate murmurs. Bensky et al studied potential causes of this practice and determined that the majority of referring physicians underestimated the cost of echocardiography drastically, believing it was cost-equivalent to cardiac consultation. Primary care physicians also believe a cardiologist will obtain an echocardiogram as part of their evaluation of a child with a murmur, despite ample published literature documenting that cardiology consultation alone is often sufficiently diagnostic and is a more cost-effective means for assessing a heart murmur. Despite these facts, the use of echocardiography among primary care physicians as a screening tool for heart disease is rising.

The impact of technician technical skill and experience when performing the echocardiogram is often underestimated. Echocardiography requires a multitude of decisions and actions by the performer: appropriate machine settings and transducers must be chosen, correct windows with full sweeps must be performed, and patient cooperation must often be coerced in the pediatric setting. Most often, cooperation is accomplished with reassurance, entertainment, and skill with children. In the hands of a skilled and patient technician, sedation is rarely required to complete a full echocardiogram. The operator-dependent nature of echocardiography has a profound impact on the accuracy of the test; one recent study demonstrated a high rate of clinically relevant diagnostic error in pediatric echocardiograms performed in adult laboratories. Because of the above comments, we believe that the echocardiogram is best utilized when ordered by a cardiologist and performed in a pediatric echocardiography laboratory.

References

Benheim A, Karr S, Sell J, et al: Routine use of transesophageal echocardiography and color flow imaging in the evaluation and treatment of children with congenital heart disease. Echocardiography 10:583, 1993

Bensky A, Covitz W, Durant R: Primary care physicians' use of screening echocardiography. Pediatrics 103:e40, 1999

Copel J, Pilu G, Kleinman C: Congenital heart disease and extracardiac anomalies: associations and indications for fetal echocardiography. Am J Obstet Gynecol 154:1121, 1986

Cortes R, Satomi G, Yoshigi M, Momma K: Maximal hemodynamic response after the Fontan procedure: Doppler evaluation during the treadmill test. Pediatr Cardiol 15:170, 1994

Danford D, Nasir A, Gumbiner C: Cost assessment of the evaluation of heart murmurs. Pediatrics 91:365, 1993

Finley J, Sharratt G, Nanton M, et al: Paediatric echocardiography by telemedicine—nine years' experience. J Telemed Telecare 34:200, 1997

Folland E, Parisi A, Moynihan P, et al: Assessment of left ventricular ejection fraction and volume by real-time two-dimensional echocardiography: a comparison of cineangiographic and radionucleide techniques. Circulation 60:760, 1979

Frommelt M, Frommelt P: Advances in echocardiographic diagnostic modalities for the pediatrician. Pediatr Clin North Am 46:427, 1999

Gardin J, Sung H, Yoganathan A, et al: Doppler flow velocity mapping in an in vitro model of the normal pulmonary artery. J Am Coll Cardiol 12:1366, 1988

Geva T, Hegesh J, Frand M: Reappraisal of the approach to the child with heart murmurs: is echocardiography mandatory? Int J Cardiol 19:107, 1988

Gutgesell H, Paquet M, Duff D, McNamara D: Evaluation of left ventricular size and function by echocardiography. Results in normal children. Circulation 56:457, 1977

Hahn K, Gal R, Sarnoski J, et al: Transesophageal echocardiographically guided atrial transseptal catheterization in patients with normal-sized atria: incidence of complications. Clin Cardiol 18:217, 1995

Jaffe C, Ellis K: Current Problems in Radiology: Angiocardiographic Quantitation of Ventricular Volume, Shape, and Mass. Chicago, Year Book Medical Publishers, 1974

Kantoch M, Frost G, Robertson M: Use of transesophageal echocardiography in radiofrequency catheter ablation in children and adolescents. Can J Cardiol 14:519, 1998

King D, Smith E, Huhta J, Gutgesell H: Mitral and tricuspid valve anular diameter in normal children determined by two-dimensional echocardiography. Am J Cardiol 55:787, 1985

Klewer S, Goldberg S, Donnerstein RL, et al: Dobutamine stress echocardiography: a sensitive indicator of diminished myocardial function in asymptomatic doxorubicin-treated long-term survivors of childhood cancer. J Am Coll Cardiol 19:394, 1992

Lai W, al-Khatib Y, Klitzner T, et al: Biplanar transesophageal echocardiographic direction of radiofrequency catheter ablation in children and adolescents with the Wolff-Parkinson-White syndrome. Am J Cardiol 71:872, 1993

Lam J, Neirotti R, Nijveld A, et al: Transesophageal echocardiography in pediatric patients: preliminary results. J Am Soc Echocardiogr 4:43, 1991

Levine R, Jamoh A, Cape E, et al: Pressure recovery distal to a stenosis: Potential cause of gradient "overstimulation" by Doppler echocardiography. J Am Coll Cardiol 13:706, 1989

Magni G, Hijazi ZM, Pandian NG, et al: Two- and three-dimensional transesophageal echocardiography in patient selection and assessment of atrial septal defect closure by the new DAS-Angel Wings device: initial clinical experience. Circulation 96(6):1722, 1997

Newburger J, Rosenthal A, Williams R, et al: Noninvasive tests in the initial evaluation of heart murmurs in children. N Engl J Med 308:61, 1983

Nidorf S, Picard M, Triulzi M, et al: New perspectives in the assessment of cardiac chamber dimensions during development and adulthood. J Am Coll Cardiol 19:983, 1992

Pahl E, Sehgal R, Chrystof D: Feasibility of exercise stress echocardiography for the follow-up of children with coronary involvement secondary to Kawasaki disease. Circulation 91:122, 1995

Porter K, Wagner P, Cabaniss M: Fetal board: a multidisciplinary approach to management of the abnormal fetus. Obstet Gynecol 72:275, 1988

Rice M, McDonald R, Reller MD, Sahn D. J Pediatr 128:1–14, 1996

Roge C, Silverman N, Hart P, Ray R: Cardiac structure growth pattern determined by echocardiography. Circulation 57:285, 1978

Rowland D, Gutgesell H: Noninvasive assessment of myocardial contractility, preload, and afterload in healthy newborn infants. Am J Cardiol 75:818, 1995

Seward J, Khandheria B, Oh J, et al: Transesophageal echocardiography: technique, anatomic correlations, implementation, and clinical applications. Mayo Clin Proc 63:649, 1988

Silverman N, Ports T, Snider A, et al: Determination of left ventricular volume in children: echocardiographic and angiographic determinations. Circulation 62:548, 1980

Simpson I, Valdez-Cruz L, Yoganathan A, et al: Spatial velocity distribution and acceleration in serial subvalve tunnel and valvular obstruction: an in vitro study using Doppler color flow mapping. J Am Coll Cardiol 13:241, 1989

Smythe J, Teixeira O, Vlad P, et al: Initial evaluation of heart murmurs: are laboratory tests necessary? Pediatrics 86:497, 1990

Snider A, Enderlein M, Teitel D, Juster R: Two-dimensional echocardiographic determination of aortic and pulmonary artery sizes from infancy to adulthood in normal subjects. Am J Cardiol 53:218, 1984

Stanger P, Silverman N, Foster E: Diagnostic accuracy of pediatric echo-cardiograms performed in adult laboratories. Am J Cardiol 83:908, 1999

St John Sutton M, Marier D, Oldershaw P, et al: Effect of age related changes in chamber size, wall thickness, and heart rate on left ventricular function in normal children. Br Heart J 48:342, 1982

Sutherland G, Fraser A: Colour flow mapping in cardiology: indications and limitations. Br Med Bull 45:1076, 1989

Sutherland G, Steumper O: Transthoracic versus transesophageal echocar-diography in the pediatric patient. Curr Opin Pediatr 5:598, 1993

Thomas J, Weyman A: Fluid dynamics model of mitral valve flow: descrip-tion with in vitro validation. J Am Coll Cardiol 13:221, 1989

22.2.4   Nuclear Medicine

Michael W. Dae

Radionuclide studies are used mainly to evaluate shunts, determine right and left ventricular function, and assess myocardial perfusion.

LEFT-TO-RIGHT SHUNTS

After rapid injection of a bolus of radionuclide into the circulation, its transit through the heart and lungs is monitored with a γ camera. For small infants, a butterfly needle can be used in a temporal scalp vein, and in older children and adults a butterfly needle or a small plastic catheter can be inserted into an external jugular or antecu-bital vein. Delivery of a compact, nonfragmented bolus of activity is critical to allow accurate determination of the size of the shunt. With good technique, the success rate should be over 90%. It may be necessary to sedate infants and some children because crying simulates a Valsalva maneuver and can impede bolus entry into the thorax and lead to fragmentation of the bolus. Tc-DTPA is the radionuclide most often used for shunt studies; doses are 200 μCi per kilogram of body weight, with a minimum dose of 2 mCi. The advantage of this over other Tc-based agents is its fairly rapid renal excretion, with prompt clearance of background activity so that, if needed, a second injection can be done. Generally, no more than two sequential injections are done because of dosimetry limitations.

The sequential flow study is reviewed for information about chamber orientation and vascular connections. With normal ana-tomic relationships, right heart structures appear, followed by the main pulmonary artery, lungs, and, subsequently, the left ventricle (levophase) and descending aorta. Persistent pulmonary activity re-sulting in the absence of a distinct levophase is consistent with a moderate to large left-to-right shunt and results from recirculation of activity from heart back to lungs across the shunt.

For quantification, time-versus-radioactivity curves are gener-ated from regions of interest over the superior vena cava, to assess the quality of the bolus and the periphery of the right lung, for shunt detection and magnitude (Fig. 22-24). A separate curve may be generated over the left lung if differential shunting is expected (as may occur with a patent ductus arteriosus). The normal pul-monary arterial curve has an ascending limb, reflecting the arrival of tracer in the pulmonary circulation, and a symmetric descending limb, reflecting the tracer exiting the lungs; a late peak reflects sys-temic recirculation. In a left-to-right shunt, a shoulder on the downslope indicates recirculation of activity back to the lungs across the shunt. For shunt quantification, the shape of the pul-monary portion of the curve is approximated by an algebraic ex-pression called a γ variate function. The area under this curve is proportional to pulmonary flow, Q_p. This fitted curve is then sub-tracted from the initial time-versus-radioactivity curve, and another γ variate fit is done on the remaining curve. The area under this second fitted curve is proportional to the shunt flow, Q_{sh}. The dif-ference between the two fitted curves is a measure of systemic flow, Q_s. The resultant calculation of pulmonary to systemic flow, $Q_p:Q_s$, is $Q_p:Q_s = Q_p/(Q_p - Q_{sh})$.

The $Q_p:Q_s$ calculation correlates very well with shunt size de-termined at cardiac catheterization over a clinically significant range of 1.2:1 to 3.0:1. Ratios under 1.2:1 are consistent with the absence of left-to-right shunts. Because the method depends on passage of all the injected radionuclide through the lungs, left-to-right shunts are overestimated in the presence of right-to-left shunts. Shunts with $Q_p:Q_s$ ratios over 3.0:1 are difficult to estimate, but this is not important, as any $Q_p:Q_s$ ratio over 3.0:1 is very large.

The radionuclide method has also been used to measure changes in shunt magnitude in response to oxygen therapy, to assess the

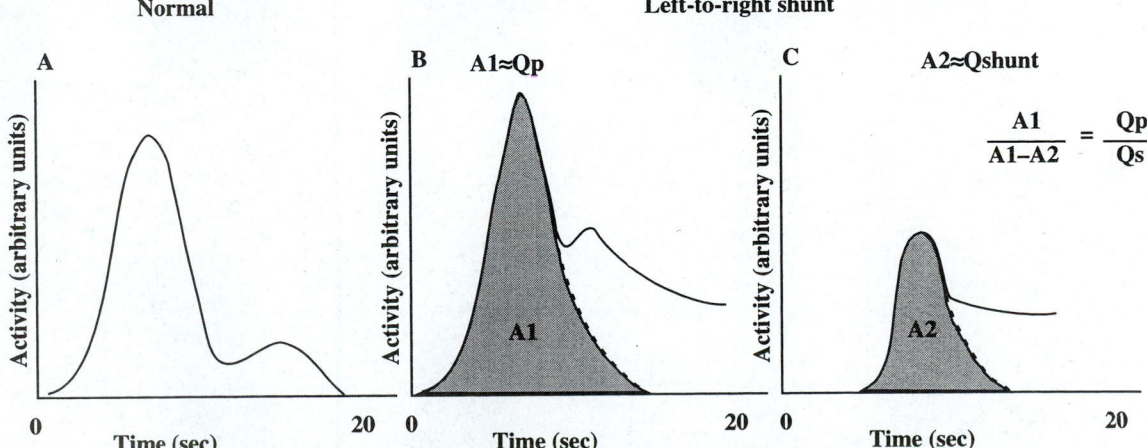

FIGURE 22-24   A: Normal pulmonary time-activity curves. B: Pulmonary time-activity curves with left-to-right shunt. Area under the first pass of tracer through the lungs as defined by a γ-variate extrapolation. Qp = pulmonary flow. C: Area under the portion of the curve corresponding to radiolabeled blood returning prematurely to the lung by the left-to-right shunt; Q_{SHUNT} = shunt flow; B − C = Q_s = systemic flow. SOURCE: *Treves ST: Pediatric Nuclear Medicine. New York, Springer-Verlag, 1985.*

reactivity of the pulmonary vascular bed in patients with large shunts and pulmonary hypertension, and in the postoperative assessment of residual shunt size in patients with murmurs and echo-Doppler evidence of persistent shunting after surgical correction of septal defects.

It is also possible to calculate the extent of left-to-right shunts using the equilibrium blood pool method. Stroke volume or amplitude images can be used to measure the difference in stroke volume between the ventricles, as is commonly done to evaluate regurgitant lesions. For each ventricle, the stroke volume is the difference between end diastolic and end systolic volumes determined from the radioactivity at each of these times. With a ventricular septal defect or a patent ductus arteriosus, the left ventricle handles the excess volume of the shunt flow, and its stroke volume is proportional to the pulmonary blood flow; the right ventricular stroke volume is proportional to the systemic blood flow. The pulmonary-to-systemic flow ratio can be calculated as: $Q_p:Q_s = $ LV stroke volume/RV stroke volume. For an atrial septal defect or anomalous pulmonary venous return, the right ventricle carries the excess shunt flow. The $Q_p:Q_s$ can be calculated as: $Q_p:Q_s = $ RV stroke volume/LV stroke volume. A good correlation ($r = .79$) has been noted between the shunt $Q_p:Q_s$ ratio calculated from stroke volume ratios and oximetry. This approach may be particularly useful when attempts at a good bolus injection were unsuccessful.

RIGHT-TO-LEFT SHUNT EVALUATION

Right-to-left shunts can be detected by inspecting the first-pass radionuclide angiogram for premature appearance of radioactivity in the left-sided chambers or aorta. Time-versus-radioactivity curves generated from regions of interest over the carotid artery can be analyzed by curve-fitting methods to quantify shunt size. Intravenous injections of an inert radioactive gas, such as ^{133}Xe or krypton-81m, can also be used to detect right-to-left shunts. Significant systemic activity of these agents, which should be totally extracted by the lungs and exhaled in the alveolar gas, indicates shunting.

The easiest and most commonly used method is the intravenous injection of ^{99m}Tc-labeled macroaggregated albumin (MAA) particles, similar to those used to assess pulmonary perfusion. In the absence of right-to-left shunting, all of the particles are trapped in the lungs. When right-to-left shunting occurs at any level, particles enter the systemic circulation in proportion to the shunt flow, lodging in the capillary and precapillary beds of systemic organs (Fig. 22-25). A series of whole-body images are taken to determine the percentage of right-to-left shunt as: whole-body counts − lung counts/whole-body counts. Pulmonary-to-systemic flow ratio can be calculated as: $Q_p:Q_s = $ lung counts/whole-body counts.

In spite of the general reluctance to administer particles to patients with known right-to-left shunts, the method has proven to be safe, accurate, and very easy to perform. The particle number should be kept below 50,000 in children.

ASSESSMENT OF VENTRICULAR FUNCTION

Radionuclide methods are well suited to assess ventricular size and function in congenital heart lesions. Both first-pass and gated equilibrium methods to determine ejection fraction have been validated in children. Quantitative assessment of absolute ventricular volumes and regurgitant fraction have also been reported in children. It is feasible to measure ejection fraction even in tiny premature infants

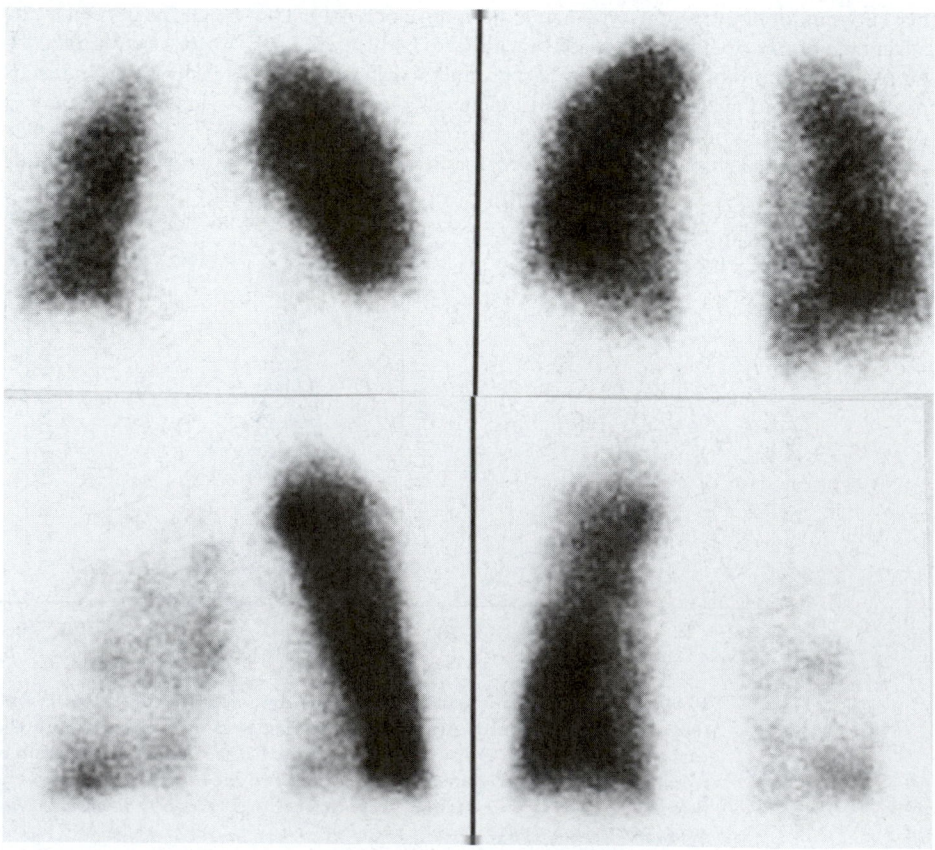

FIGURE 22-25 Shown is a posterior whole-body image. Technetium-labeled MAA particles were injected intravenously and show localization to lungs, kidneys, and brain, indicating a right-to-left shunt.

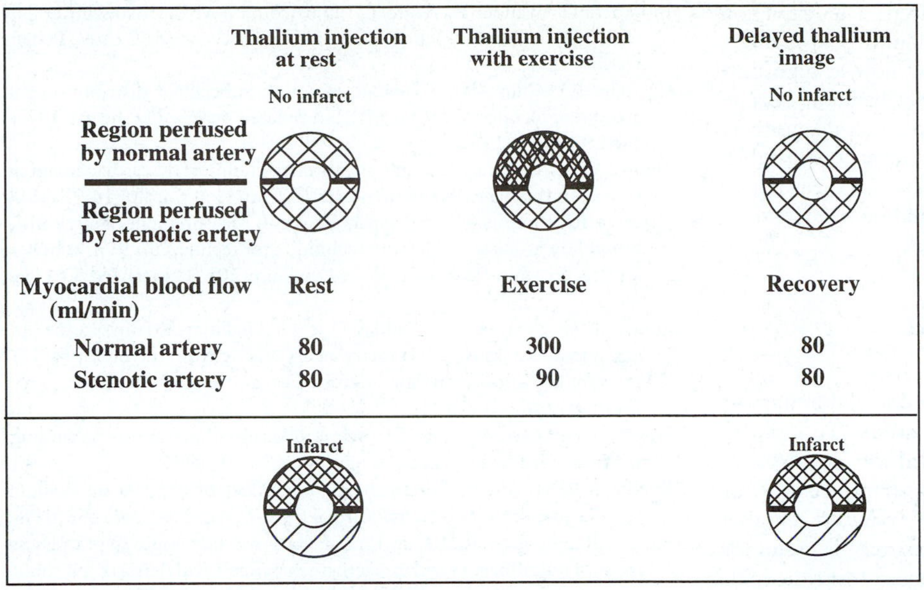

FIGURE 22-26 Diagrammatic illustration of the relationship between myocardial blood flow at rest and during exercise and regional myocardial ^{201}Tl uptake in zones perfused by normal and stenotic coronary arteries. (The darker shading represents higher blood flow.) When thallium is injected at rest, there is uniform distribution of the radionuclide throughout the myocardium (upper left). When thallium is injected during exercise, there is a relative diminution in thallium uptake in the zone perfused by the stenotic vessel (middle panel). Several hours following ^{201}Tl injection with exercise, there is "redistribution" and normalization of thallium uptake in normal and stenotic zones (upper right). SOURCE: *Beller GA: Radionuclide evaluation before and after medical or surgical myocardial revascularization. In: Gerson MC, ed: Cardiac Nuclear Medicine. New York, McGraw-Hill, 1987:349–369.*

with the use of the pinhole collimator. Ventricular size and function evaluations are useful at rest and with dynamic stress in a variety of congenital lesions, both before and after surgical correction.

ASSESSMENT OF MYOCARDIAL PERFUSION

Moderate coronary arterial narrowing or stenosis is tolerated during the resting state without reductions in coronary flow. As myocardial demands rise, eg, during exercise, the resulting increase in blood flow in a stenotic coronary artery is often not sufficient to maintain adequate function, and ischemic electrocardiographic changes and chest pain may occur. If normal blood flow is quickly restored, the chest pain resolves, electrocardiographic changes return to baseline, and contractile function returns. If there is some delay in restoration of flow, contractile function may remain depressed for up to weeks (stunned myocardium). If blood flow is chronically reduced at rest, resulting in chronic ischemia, contractile function may remain chronically depressed (hibernating myocardium). If blood flow is not restored, irreversible damage occurs, leading to myocardial necrosis and the eventual replacement of myocytes with scar.

THALLIUM-201

The most common agent for assessing myocardial perfusion is thallium-201. Thallium is a cyclotron-produced radionuclide with a 73-hour half-life and predominant emission energy of 80 keV. Physiologically, thallium behaves like potassium and is transported into cells largely by the sodium potassium ATPase pump. On the first exposure to the heart (first pass), over 85% of the thallium dose that reaches the myocardial cells is taken up. As a result, the initial distribution of thallium provides a static map of myocardial perfusion at the time of injection. Thallium extraction by the myocardium depends on the delivery of the tracer (perfusion) and on viable myocytes. Ischemic myocytes retain the ability to extract thallium (provided some perfusion is present). Only when ischemia is of sufficient severity and duration to lead to necrosis will thallium not be extracted.

Consider a coronary vascular territory supplied by a left anterior descending coronary artery with significant (>70%) stenosis. The two other major vessels (right coronary artery and left circumflex)

are normal. In all likelihood, an injection of thallium in such a patient at rest would lead to a homogeneous distribution, as in normals (Fig. 22-26). With increased coronary blood flow to maximal levels (generally up to four times baseline flow) either by maximal exercise or with a vasodilator such as dipyridamole, there will probably be less accumulation of thallium in the territory perfused by the stenotic LAD (septum and anterior wall), compared to the remaining myocardium perfused by the vessels without any stenosis (Fig. 22-26) because there will be less increase in flow in the LAD territory. This relative heterogeneity of blood flow is the most important finding on a thallium image. The underperfused area represents normal but transiently underperfused or ischemic myocardium. An identical pattern would appear in a patient who has suffered a myocardial infarction involving the LAD. How can we distinguish between the two situations?

Thallium in the heart will redistribute with time. After the initial accumulation in the heart, thallium slowly washes out into the blood. Regions with high blood flow and high concentrations of thallium wash out faster than regions with lower blood flow and low concentrations of thallium, so that intracellular concentration gradients of thallium in the heart tend to equalize. The resultant delayed thallium image shows a more homogeneous distribution (Fig. 22-26), if the initial region of reduced uptake represented ischemia in a region of viable myocytes. If the initial region of reduced uptake represented scar, a persistent defect will appear on the delayed images.

TECHNETIUM 99M-LABELED MYOCARDIAL PERFUSION TRACERS

Thallium-201 is a popular and useful myocardial perfusion agent, but it does have drawbacks. Its relatively long half-life (72 hours) limits the amount of activity that can be injected because of dosimetry concerns. The low energy (80 keV) of the major photon emission poses potential problems because of soft tissue attenuation. Also, ^{201}Tl is cyclotron produced, which limits its availability. Relative to ^{201}Tl, ^{99m}Tc has the advantage of higher energy (140 keV), leading to less attenuation; shorter half-life (6 hours), allowing the injection of larger doses; and ready availability because it is generator produced. ^{99m}Tc-Sestamibi, or Cardiolite, is a lipophilic cationic complex that has recently been introduced. The extraction fraction of sestamibi is lower than that of thallium (65% vs 85%), and so it may underestimate myocardial blood flow at high flow rates (>2 mL/min/g) to a greater degree than thallium. In spite of this diffusion limitation, clinical results comparing the sensitivity and specificity of thallium and sestamibi have been comparable. Another property shared by sestamibi and thallium is their dependence on viable myocytes for extraction. Sestamibi uptake is markedly diminished in irreversibly injured myocytes.

APPLICATIONS OF PERFUSION SCINTIGRAPHY IN CONGENITAL HEART DISEASE

Myocardial perfusion scintigraphy has been used in children, most often to identify an anomalous left coronary artery. To evaluate patients for this lesion, thallium-201 is injected intravenously, at rest, and images are acquired in multiple planar projections, or SPECT imaging is done. Thallium scintigraphy typically reveals a segmental perfusion abnormality at rest. This pattern is useful for identifying an anomalous left coronary as opposed to myocarditis or cardiomyopathy as the etiology for poor ventricular function in infants. The technique is also used to detect myocardial ischemia and infarction in Kawasaki syndrome.

Assessing myocardial perfusion is important in the follow-up of patients with transposition of the great vessels after the arterial switch procedure. Large perfusion abnormalities have occasionally been seen in the territories of occluded coronary arteries after the switch procedure.

RADIONUCLIDE ASSESSMENT OF INFLAMMATION

Gallium-67 accumulates in acute and chronic inflammatory lesions of bacterial as well as nonbacterial etiologies. Gallium uptake has been described in many instances of inflammatory heart disease, including bacterial endocarditis, myocardial abscess, and pericarditis. Animal studies have shown intense and uniform gallium accumulation in experimental myocarditis, and a high correlation between biopsy-proven myocarditis and gallium uptake has been found in patients. In nearly all reported instances of gallium uptake in myocarditis, the pattern of uptake is diffuse, even when there are characteristic ECG changes that mimic myocardial infarction.

Antimyosin antibody cardiac imaging has also shown success in detecting biopsy-proven myocarditis. Antimyosin localizes to regions of myocyte necrosis in myocarditis, as opposed to the localization of ^{67}Ga to the inflammatory component. Few studies have examined thallium uptake in myocarditis; however, focal perfusion defects have been reported. These defects, however, tend to be in nonvascular distributions.

References

Baker E, Ellam S, Lorber A, et al: Superiority of radionuclide over oximetric measurement of left to right shunts. Br Heart J 53:535, 1985

Baker E, Ellam S, Maisey M, Tynan M: Radionuclide measurement of left ventricular ejection fraction in infants and children. Br Heart J 51:275, 1984

Baker E, Ellam S, Tynan M, Maisey M: First-pass measurement of left ventricular function in infants and children. Eur J Nucl Med 10:422, 1985

Beanlands R, Dawood F, Wen W, et al: Are the kinetics of technetium-99m methoxyisobutyl isonitrile affected by cell metabolism and viability? Circulation 82:1802, 1990

Bjorkhem G, Evander E, White T, Lundstrom N: Myocardial scintigraphy with 201-thallium in pediatric cardiology: a review of 52 cases. Pediatr Cardiol 11:1, 1990

Carvalho PA, Chin MC, Kronauge JF, et al: Subcellular distribution and analysis of technetium-99m-MIBI in isolated perfused rat hearts. J Nucl Med 33:1516, 1992

Dec G, Palacios I, Yasuda T, et al: Antimyosin antibody cardiac imaging: its role in the diagnosis of myocarditis. J Am Coll Cardiol 16:97, 1990

DiRocco RJ, Rumsey WL, Kuczinski BL, et al: Measurement of myocardial blood flow using a coinjection technique for technetium-99m-teboroxime, technetium-96-sestamibi, and thallium-201. J Nucl Med 33:1152, 1992

Findley J, Howman-giles R, Gilday D, et al: Thallium-201 myocardial imaging in anomalous left coronary artery arising from the pulmonary artery: applications before and after medical and surgical treatment. Am J Cardiol 42:675, 1978

Folger G, Eltohami E, Hajar H: Acute myocardial-infarction-like findings with myocarditis in infancy. Angiology 45:737, 1994

Friedman BJ, Beihn R, Friedman JP: The effect of hypoxia on thallium kinetics in cultured chick myocardial cells. J Nucl Med 28:1453, 1987

Fujii A, Rabinovitch M, Keane J, et al: Radionuclide angiographic assessment of pulmonary vascular reactivity in patients with left to right shunts and pulmonary hypertension. Am J Cardiol 49:356, 1982

Hannon D, Gelfand M, Bailey W, Hall J, Kaplan S: Pinhole radionuclide ventriculography in small infants. Am Heart J 111:316, 1986

Hayes A, Baker E, Kakadeker A, et al: Influence of anatomical correction for transposition of the great arteries on myocardial perfusion: radionuclide imaging with Tc^{99m} methoxy isobutyl isonitrile. J Am Coll Cardiol 24:769, 1994

Hijazi Z, Udelson J, Snapper H, et al: Physiologic significance of chronic coronary aneurysms in patients with Kawasaki disease. J Am Coll Cardiol 24:1633, 1994

Hurwitz R, Papanicolaou N, Treves S, et al: Radionuclide angiography in evaluation of patients after surgical repair of transposition of the great arteries. Am J Cardiol 49:761, 1982

Hurwitz RA, Treves S, Freed M, et al: Quantitation of aortic and mitral regurgitation in the pediatric population: evaluation by radionuclide angiocardiography. Am J Cardiol 51:252, 1983

Kahn JK, McGhie I, Akers MJ, et al: Quantitative rotational tomography with 201-T1 and 99m-Tc 2-methoxy-isobutyl-isonitrile: a direct comparison in normal individuals and patients with coronary artery disease. Circulation 79:1282, 1989

Kramer R, Goldstein R, Hirshfeld J, et al: Accumulation of gallium-67 in regions of acute myocardial infarction. Am J Cardiol 33:861, 1974

Long R, Braunwald E, Morrow A: Intracardiac injection of radioactive krypton. Circulation 21:1126, 1963

Maltz OL, Treves S: Quantitative radionuclide angiocardiography. Determination of Q_p/Q_s in children. Circulation 47:1049, 1973

Moodie D, Cook S, Gill C, et al: Thallium-201 myocardial imaging in young adults with anomalous left coronary artery arising from the pulmonary artery. J Nucl Med 2:1076, 1980

Morguet A, Munz D, Emrich D: Scintigraphic detection of inflammatory heart disease. Eur J Nucl Med 21:666, 1994

Mullins LJ, Moor RD: The movement of thallium ions in muscle. J Gen Physiol 43:759, 1960

O'Connell J, Henkin R, Robinson J, et al: Gallium-67 imaging in patients with dilated cardiomyopathy and biopsy-proven myocarditis. Circulation 70:58, 1984

Parrish M, Graham T, Born M, et al: Radionuclide ventriculography for assessment of absolute right and left ventricular volumes in children. Circulation 66:811, 1982

Parrish M, Graham T, Born M, et al: Radionuclide stroke count ratios for assessment of right and left ventricular volume overload in children. Am J Cardiol 51:261, 1983

Peter C, Armstrong B, Jones R: Radionuclide quantitation of right-to-left shunts in children. Circulation 64:572, 1981

Pohost GM, Albert NM, Ingwall JS, Strauss HW: Thallium redistribution: mechanisms and clinical utility. Semin Nucl Med 10:70, 1980

Reduto L, Berger H, Johnstone D, et al: Radionuclide assessment of right and left ventricular exercise reserve after total correction of tetralogy of Fallot. Am J Cardiol 45:1013, 1980

Reeves W, Jackson G, Flickinger F, et al: Radionuclide imaging of experimental myocarditis. Circulation 63:640, 1981

Rigo P, Chevigne M: Measurement of left to right shunts by gated radionuclide angiography: Concise communication. J Nucl Med 23:1070, 1982

Schor R, Massie B, Botvinick E, Shames D: Gallium-67 uptake in silent myocardial infarction. Radiology 129:117, 1978

Sty J, Starshak R, Miller J: Particle body imaging in cardiopulmonary disorders. In: Wagner HN, ed: Pediatric Nuclear Medicine. New York, Appleton-Century-Crofts, 1983:46

Tamaki N, Yonekura Y, Kadota K, et al: Thallium-201 myocardial perfusion imaging in myocarditis. Clin Nucl Med 10:562, 1985

Treves S, Kuruc A: Radionuclide evaluation of circulatory shunts. Cardiol Clin 1:427, 1983

Tsan M: Mechanism of gallium-67 accumulation in inflammatory lesions. J Nucl Med 26:88, 1985

Wackers FJ, Berman DS, Maddahi J, et al: Technetium-99m hexakis 2-methoxyisobutyl isonitrile: human biodistribution, dosimetry, safety, and preliminary comparison to thallium-201 for myocardial perfusion imaging. J Nucl Med 30:301, 1989

Weindling S, Wernovsky G, Colan S, et al: Myocardial perfusion, function, and exercise tolerance after the arterial switch operation. J Am Coll Cardiol 23:424, 1994

22.2.5   Radiology

Charles B. Higgins

The diagnosis of the specific morphology of congenital heart disease (CHD) is established with imaging techniques. During the past two decades, noninvasive imaging has increasingly replaced cardiac catheterization and x-ray angiography for both preoperative diagnosis and postoperative monitoring of surgically corrected or palliated CHD. Echocardiography has assumed a dominant role, and its depiction of internal cardiac morphology has decreased dependence on the chest x-ray. The newer noninvasive imaging techniques, computed tomography (CT) and magnetic resonance imaging (MRI), have also been shown to be effective for depicting cardiovascular anatomy. Moreover, MRI can also provide quantification of ventricular function and blood flow. Here we focus upon the current role of the chest x-ray and the evolving role of MRI because CT has been used infrequently in CHD.

CHEST X-RAY

The chest x-ray gives reliable information about pulmonary edema, pulmonary vascularity, cardiac size, and the position and size of the thoracic aorta and pulmonary artery. It is usually not possible to assess specific chamber enlargement accurately, especially in the neonate. It is possible to classify CHD into five diagnostic groups (Table 22-2). Further refinement beyond these five groups of differential diagnoses may not be possible using the chest x-ray. The chest x-ray can also be useful for determining cardiac malposition and situs abnormalities. Postoperatively, the chest x-ray is employed to monitor pulmonary vascularity and heart size.

MRI

MRI provides a three-dimensional data set for depicting cardiovascular anatomy and quantifying ventricular volumes, mass, and function. There are four MR imaging sequences used for CHD: the spin-echo technique (black blood images) is used to demonstrate morphology; contrast (gadolinium chelate)-enhanced MR angiography (MRA) is used to depict morphology, especially for arteries and veins (Fig. 22-27); cine MRI is used to evaluate right and left ventricular function and volumes; velocity-encoded cine MRI enables quantification of blood flow.

MORPHOLOGIC DIAGNOSIS

The role of MRI in defining the morphology of CHD is supplementary to echocardiography; the most frequent applications at the current time are listed in Table 22-3.

MRI and contrast-enhanced MRA are the preferred techniques for imaging thoracic aortic anomalies. For example, they define the site and severity of coarctation and, important for surgical planning, the status of the aortic arch and isthmus (Fig. 22-28). Velocity-encoded cine MRI can estimate the gradient across the coarctation and the degree of collateral circulation. In arch anomalies, they define the specific anomaly as well as the site and severity of airway compression.

The presence and size of the main and central pulmonary arteries are effectively depicted by MR techniques. Consequently, they are used for preoperative evaluation of tetralogy of Fallot, pulmonary atresia, and other lesions in which hypoplasia or stenosis of the pulmonary arteries may be a component. A comparative study on the efficacy of MRI and echocardiography for assessing the pulmonary arteries postoperatively revealed greater effectiveness of MRI for evaluating the right and left pulmonary arteries (Fig. 22-29). MRI and especially contrast-enhanced MRA are the preferred imaging techniques for evaluating pulmonary venous anomalies, such as anomalous connections and stenosis.

The multiple imaging planes, wide field of view, and spatial resolution of MRI can be exploited for determining situs, atrioventricular and arteroventricular connection, valve atresias, and size of various cardiac chambers. Consequently, segmental analysis of MR images is effective for evaluating complex congenital heart disease such as univentricular hearts. The postoperative morphology of operative procedures for complex cyanotic congenital heart disease is displayed precisely by MRI. Cine MRI can be employed for the postoperative evaluation of volumes, mass, and function of the right as well as the left ventricle. Sequential studies in normal- and abnormal-shaped ventricles indicate that MRI is the most reproducible method available for quantifying ventricular volume and mass. Velocity-encoded cine MRI can be used to measure and monitor the volume of pulmonary regurgitation after surgery for right ventricular outlet obstruction.

MRI and electron-beam CT have been used in recent years to identify coronary artery anomalies. Contrast-enhanced coronary MRA has been proposed as the most effective technique for defining ectopic origin and anomalous course of coronary artery anomalies; however, this technique is still operator dependent for its reliability. Our experience has found electron-beam CT to be equally effective and image quality more reliable for this purpose.

MRI may be indicated for evaluating ventricular dysrhythmias in order to exclude right ventricular dysplasia, ventricular tumors, hypertropic cardiomyopathy, and ventricular dysfunction. MRI may be used to establish the diagnosis of right ventricular dysplasia by showing fatty deposition or focal thinning of the right ventricular free wall on spin-echo images and focal contraction abnormalities on cine MRI.

MRI is the preferred technique for the definitive diagnosis and staging of primary and secondary tumors of the heart. It effectively

TABLE 22-2

DIAGNOSTIC GROUPS OF CONGENITAL HEART DISEASE

ACYANOTIC	CYANOTIC			PULMONARY VENOUS CONGESTION, DISPROPORTIONATE CARDIOMEGALY	
1. PULMONARY OVERCIRCULATION	**2. ↓ PULMONARY VASCULARITY, NO CARDIOMEGALY**	**3. ↓ PULMONARY VASCULARITY, CARDIOMEGALY**	**4. ↑ PULMONARY VASCULARITY**	**5A. NON-STRUCTURAL HEART DISEASE (NEONATE)**	**5B. STRUCTURAL HEART DISEASE (NEONATE)**
Atrial septal defect	Tetralogy of Fallot	Ebstein anomaly	Transposition of great arteries	Asphyxia	Hypoplastic left heart syndrome
Partial anomalous pulmonary venous connection	*d*-TGA + PS + VSD	Pulmonary stenosis (critical) with ASD or patent foramen ovale	Truncus arteriosus	Hypervolemia, hyperviscosity	Total anomalous pulmonary venous connection below diaphragm
Atrioventricular septal defect (endocardial cushion defect)	Double-outlet right ventricle + PS + VSD	Some tricuspid atresia (restrictive ASD)	Total anomalous pulmonary venous connection	Overhydration	Coarctation of the aorta
Ventricular septal defect	Double-outlet left ventricle + PS + VSD	Pulmonary atresia with intact ventricular septum, type II	Tricuspid atresia	Asphyxia	Hypoplastic left heart syndrome
Patent ductus arteriosus	*l*-TGA + PS + VSD	Transient tricuspid regurgitation of the newborn	Single ventricle (univentricular atrioventricular connection)	Maternal–fetal transfusion	Endocardial fibroelastosis
Other aortic level shunts: ruptured sinus of Valsalva aneurysm, aorticopulmonary window, etc.	Single ventricle + PS		Double-outlet right ventricle	Excess stripping of cord	Anomalous origin of coronary artery from pulmonary artery
			Double-outlet left ventricle	Paroxysmal atrial tachycardia	Intrauterine myocarditis
			Atrioventricular septal defect (complete form)	Heart block	
			Hypoplastic left heart syndrome	Hypoglycemia	
			Pulmonary arteriovenous fistula(s)	Hypocalcemia	
				Hydrops fetalis Systemic hypertension	

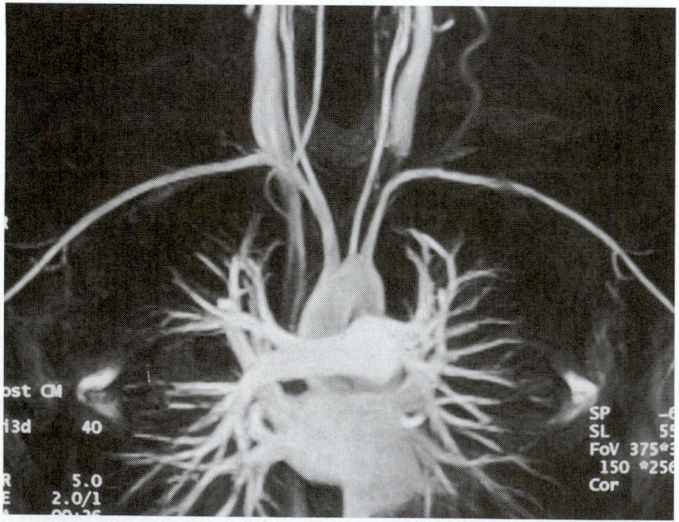

FIGURE 22-27 Contrast (gadolinium chelate)-enhanced three-dimensional MRA of the heart and great arteries displayed in the coronal plane.

demonstrates the extracardiac as well as intracardiac components of tumors (Fig. 22-30). It is the optimal procedure for evaluating suspected pericardial and paracardiac masses and possible extension of mediastinal tumors into the heart or pericardium.

MRI can also define pericardial abnormalities such as pericardial thickening in constrictive pericarditis or partial absence of the pericardium.

TABLE 22-3

MAJOR USES OF MRI FOR MORPHOLOGIC DIAGNOSIS OF CHD

1. Thoracic aortic anomalies (coarctation and arch anomalies)
2. Presence, size, stenosis of pulmonary arteries
3. Pulmonary venous connections
4. Complex cyanotic lesions (splenic syndromes; situs abnormalities; univentricular heart; atrioventricular valve atresia)
5. Coronary artery anomalies
6. Postoperative monitoring of complex CHD (tetralogy of Fallot; Fontan procedure; Rastelli procedure; Jatene procedure; Norwood procedure; etc)
7. Right ventricular dysplasia

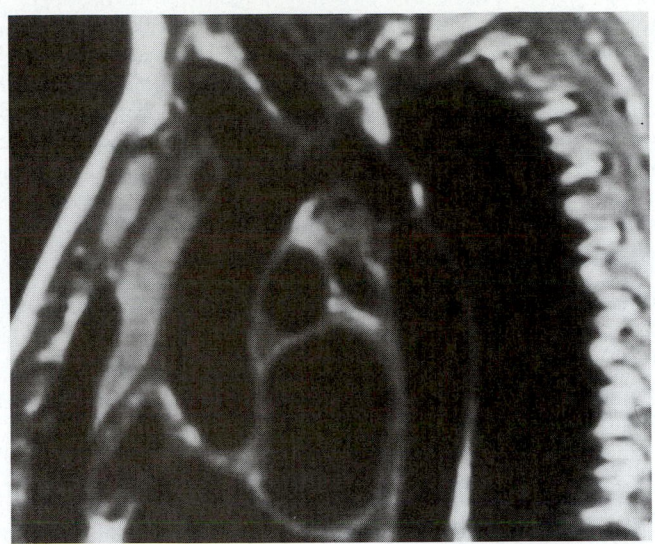

FIGURE 22-28   ECG-gated spin-echo image in the oblique sagittal plane demonstrates a discrete juxtaductal coarctation of the aorta.

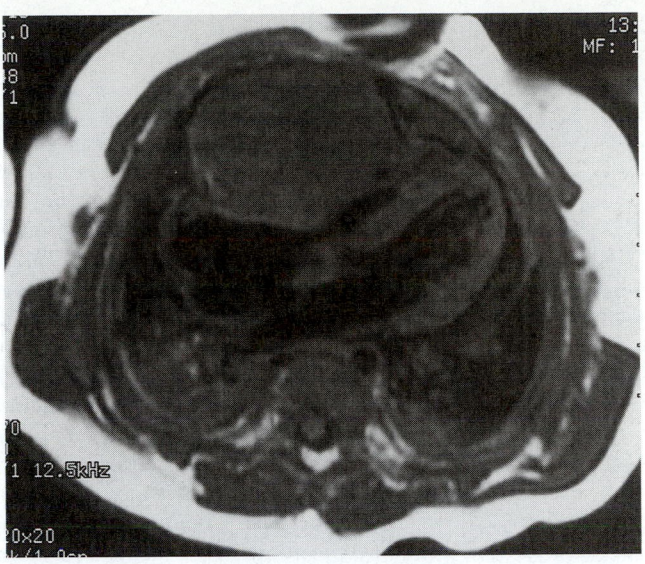

FIGURE 22-30   ECG-gated spin-echo image in an infant demonstrates a huge fibroma arising from the right ventricular wall and a pericardial effusion.

References

Blake L, Scheinman MM, Higgins CB: MR features of arrhythmogenic right ventricular dysplasia. Am J Roentgenol 162:809, 1994

Duerinckx AJ, Wexler L, Banerjee A, et al: Postoperative evaluation of pulmonary arteries in congenital heart surgery by MRI: comparison with echocardiography. Am Heart J 128:177, 1994

Higgins CB: Essentials of Cardiac Imaging. Philadelphia, Lippincott, 1992: 49

Higgins CB: MRI of congenital heart disease. In: Higgins CB, Hricak H, Helms CA, eds: Magnetic Resonance of the Body, 3rd ed. Philadelphia, Lippincott-Raven, 1997

Kersting-Sommerhoff BA, Diethelm L, Stanger P, et al: Evaluation of complex congenital ventricular anomalies with MRI. Am Heart J 120:133, 1990

McConnel MV, Ganz P, Selwyn AP, et al: Identification of anomalous coronary arteries and their anatomic course by MR coronary angiography. Circulation 92:3158, 1995

Oshinski JN, Parks J, Markou CP, et al. Improved measurement of pressure gradient in aortic coarctation by MRI. J Am Coll Cardiol 28:1818, 1996

Post JC, van Rossum AC, Bronzwaer JGF, et al: MRI of anomalous coronary arteries. Circulation 92:3163–3171, 1995

Rebergen SA, Chin JGJ, Ottenkamp J, et al: Pulmonary regurgitation in late postoperative follow-up of tetralogy of Fallot. Volumetric quantification by nuclear magnetic resonance velocity mapping. Circulation 88:2257–2266, 1993

Semelka RC, Tomei E, Wagner S, et al: Normal left ventricular dimensions and function: interstudy reproducibility of measurement with cine MRI. Radiology 174:763, 1990

Semelka RC, Tomei E, Wagner S, et al: Interstudy reproducibility of dimensional and functional measurements between cine MRI studies in abnormal left ventricle. Am Heart J 119:1367, 1990

Steffens JC, Bourne MW, Sakuma H, Higgins CB: Quantitation of collateral blood flow in coarctation of the aorta by velocity-encoded cine MRI. Circulation 90:937, 1994

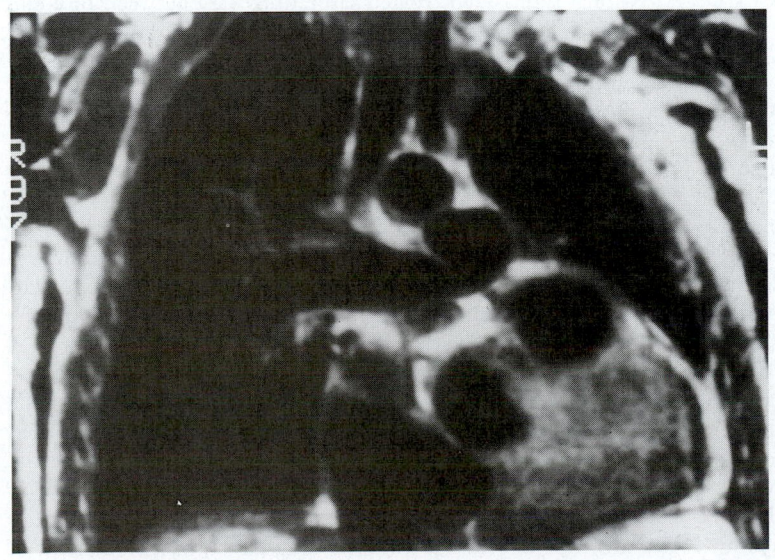

FIGURE 22-29   ECG-gated spin-echo image in the oblique coronal plane in a patient after Rastelli procedure shows a stenosis of the right pulmonary artery.

22.2.6   Cardiac Catherization

Jeffrey A. Feinstein and Phillip Moore

Today, most patients are diagnosed and sent to surgery after echocardiography without cardiac catheterization. Intraoperative transesophageal echocardiography supplements this information and draws attention to residual abnormalities that can be promptly corrected, reducing the need for postoperative cardiac catheterization. Cardiac catheterization is still needed to evaluate pulmonary vascular resistance and reactivity, to define lesions of peripheral pulmonary arteries that are not seen well with echocardiography, and to evaluate or confirm unusual or complex anatomic lesions. Patients may need cardiac catheterization to assess residual defects soon after surgery because surface echo-Doppler studies may be less accurate at this time. Infants and children need cardiac catheterization despite adequate noninvasive diagnosis if therapeutic procedures are to be done at the same time. Common interventional procedures include balloon septostomy in a neonate with transposition of the great arteries, balloon valvoplasty in pulmonic or aortic stenosis, balloon angioplasty of branch pulmonary artery stenosis or recoarctation, and coil occlusion of patent ductus arteriosus. Finally, the role of catheterization is expanding to become the primary treatment for some patients as new and improved tools and techniques are developed, such as device closure of atrial septal defects and stent correction of native coarctation.

Cardiac catheterization can rarely lead to serious complications, including arrhythmias, arterial obstruction, reactions to contrast medium, hemorrhage, cardiac perforation, hypoxemic episodes, infections, and death. The mortality rate is 0.2% with the highest risk associated with premature infants, critically ill neonates, and those undergoing complex interventional catheterization procedures. Older children at particular risk of death are those with a very high pulmonary vascular resistance and no means of shunting. In these children vagal episodes leading to decreased systemic output and death may occur during or soon after catheterization. In general, the risk of catheterization varies with the age and illness of the child, the type of lesion, and the experience of those doing the catheterization. Some desperately ill children undergoing emergency studies will die during or just after the study, but not because of it. About 3% of children may have significant but nonfatal complications.

TECHNIQUE

The most commonly used vessels for cardiac catheterization are the femoral, internal jugular, and subclavian veins and the femoral artery. The catheters are placed percutaneously by a modified Seldinger technique. Local infections and arterial complications are extremely rare, and the same vessels may be used repeatedly. In patients with congenital heart disease, the femoral approach often permits passage of a venous catheter into the left side of the heart through a patent foramen ovale or atrial septal defect, avoiding the use of the artery. Patients who have many repeat catheterizations may develop obstruction of the femoral or internal jugular veins, prohibiting their future use. If needed, vascular access can be safely obtained through percutaneous cannulation of the hepatic veins, called a "transhepatic approach."

Catheter manipulation is performed under fluoroscopy, with image intensification to reduce radiation exposure. Catheters, long thin plastic tubes with one or more holes at the end, come in many sizes, shapes, and materials. Angiographic catheters have multiple holes at their tip to allow rapid injection of contrast medium for angiography. Directional catheters come in many preformed shapes, have a single end hole, and are made out of stiff materials to provide excellent control (ie, "steerability") to facilitate manipulation into specific chambers and vessels. Balloon-tipped catheters have soft shafts and, with the balloon inflated, tend to follow the course of blood flow.

DIAGNOSTIC CATHETERIZATION

Measurements during the catheterization include oxygen saturations and pressures in the cardiac chambers and great vessels. This information is used to calculate blood flows, intracardiac shunts, and vascular resistances. Angiography in one or more chambers or vessels is then done to define the cardiac anatomy.

Oxygen Saturations

A small blood sample for oximetry is taken from each of the major vessels and cardiac chambers. Shunts are diagnosed by comparing oxygen saturations in great veins, chambers, and great vessels. This information must be interpreted with caution, as streaming may influence saturations, especially in the venae cavae and right atrium. For example, hepatic venous blood with medium saturation mixes poorly with highly saturated renal streams and less saturated femoral venous streams in the inferior vena cava. The lowest oxygen concentrations are found in coronary sinus blood, and because the coronary sinus enters just above the tricuspid valve, a sample in the right ventricle may be a little less saturated than one in the right atrium. An increase in oxygen saturation at a given level may be the result of a shunt at that level, a shunt at a more proximal level with streaming, or a shunt at a more distal level with regurgitation.

Although noninvasive methods, including echocardiography with color Doppler and nuclear medicine shunt studies, can be used to quantify cardiac shunts, oxygen saturation data remain the gold standard. Saturation data may be of limited use in quantifying multiple cardiac shunts. A patient with a large left-to-right atrial shunt has blood with very high oxygen saturation entering the right ventricle. A second shunt of equal magnitude at the ventricular level produces a relatively small additional increase in oxygen saturation. In view of these limitations, multiple cardiac shunts are best delineated by using both oxygen saturation data and angiography.

Normal right-sided oxygen saturations vary between 65% and 80%, depending on cardiac output and hemoglobin concentration. In patients breathing room air, left-sided saturations are usually 95% to 98%. This mild left-sided desaturation results from normal right-to-left shunting of desaturated pulmonary bronchial blood into the pulmonary veins.

Flows, Shunts, and Resistances

Flows and shunts may be calculated by the Fick (oxygen saturation) method, by angiographic volumes, or by indicator dilution techniques that today are done exclusively with cold saline and thermistor catheters. The Fick technique is by far the most widely used. It makes use of the fact that flow through an organ can be estimated by measuring the concentration of a substance (indicator) in arterial blood flowing to that organ, the amount of that substance added to or removed from blood as it passes through that organ, and the concentration of the substance in venous blood leaving that organ. For example, if blood entering the lung has an oxygen content of 150 mL/L, and blood leaving the lung has an oxygen content of 200 mL/L, then each liter of blood passing through the lungs picks up 50 mL of oxygen. If the oxygen consumption is 200 mL/min, then each minute 200 mL of oxygen is taken up by the lungs and carried away by $200/50 = 4$ L of blood. Hence the pulmonary flow (Q_p) is 4 L/min, calculated as:

$$\dot{Q}_p = \dot{V}O_2/(C_{pv} - C_{pa}),$$

where $\dot{Q}_p$ is pulmonary flow (L/min), $\dot{V}O_2$ is oxygen consumption (mL/min), C_{pv} is pulmonary venous oxygen content (mL/L of blood), and C_{pa} is pulmonary arterial oxygen content (mL/L of blood).

Note that the calculation uses oxygen content, not oxygen saturation. Oxygen *saturation* refers to the proportion of hemoglobin in blood that is combined with oxygen. It is expressed as a percentage and is independent of hemoglobin concentration. In contrast, oxygen *content* refers to the total amount of oxygen in a volume of blood and includes physically dissolved oxygen in addition to that bound to hemoglobin. It is expressed as either milliliters of oxygen per deciliter (100 mL) or liter of blood or as volume percent. Clearly, the oxygen content of blood with 50% oxygen saturation and a hemoglobin concentration of 20 g/dL is nearly twice that of blood with 50% oxygen saturation and a hemoglobin concentration of 10 g/dL. Oxygen *capacity* refers to the total content of oxygen that hemoglobin contains when 100% saturated.

In patients breathing room air, the physically dissolved oxygen (0.3 mL/L) is negligible in comparison with the oxygen bound to hemoglobin (13.6 mL/L at 100% saturation). A close approximation of the arterial-venous (AV) difference in oxygen content may be obtained by multiplying the arterial-venous difference in oxygen saturation by the oxygen capacity. Hence,

$$\dot{Q}_p = \dot{V}O_2/[(sat_{pv} - sat_{pa}) \times capacity]$$

where sat_{pv} is pulmonary venous oxygen saturation, and sat_{pa} is pulmonary arterial oxygen saturation.

With no right-to-left shunting, an aortic sample is preferable to a pulmonary venous sample because it is a mixture of blood from all four pulmonary veins. Similarly, with no left-to-right shunting, a pulmonary arterial sample is a representative mixture of systemic venous blood.

In a steady state, the amount of oxygen utilized in the tissues is equal to the amount taken into the lungs, and systemic flow is calculated with the same equation and oxygen consumption. Without shunts the systemic AV oxygen difference is the same as the pulmonary AV oxygen difference, and the calculated pulmonary flow ($\dot{Q}_p$) equals the systemic flow ($\dot{Q}_s$) or cardiac output. If there are shunts, then pulmonary and systemic flows must be calculated separately, the former from oxygen contents in pulmonary veins and pulmonary artery, the latter from aorta and mixed systemic venous blood.

Flow and shunt calculations are shown in examples 1 through 3. In each, the oxygen consumption ($\dot{V}O_2$) is assumed to be 150 mL/min/m², and the hemoglobin (Hb) concentration is assumed to be 14.7 g/dL blood or 147 g/L of blood. Because 1 g of Hb combines with 1.356 mL O_2, then

$$O_2 \text{ capacity} = 147 \text{ g Hb/L} \times 1.356 \text{ mL } O_2/\text{g Hb}$$
$$= 200 \text{ mL } O_2/\text{L}.$$

In the equations, saturations are given as fractions of unity. Thus 96% is given as 0.96.

Example 1: Left-to-Right Shunt

The most distal saturation that is proximal to the left-to-right shunt is used in the calculation, as it is usually the best-mixed venous sample available. Left-to-right shunt $= \dot{Q}_p - \dot{Q}_s = 3.75$ L/min/m².

Example 2: Right-to-Left Shunt

Right-to-left shunt $= \dot{Q}_s - \dot{Q}_p = 1.25$ L/min/m².

Example 3: Bidirectional Shunting

Calculation of bidirectional shunts requires the concept of effective pulmonary flow ($\dot{Q}_{EP}$), defined as the volume of systemic venous blood per minute that flows through the lungs. This volume does not include blood that is shunted in either direction because shunted blood is not effective; it neither picks up oxygen nor delivers it. In a patient with only a left-to-right shunt, effective flow equals systemic flow ($\dot{Q}_p - \dot{Q}_{EP}$ is the left-to-right shunt), and in a patient with only a right-to-left shunt, effective flow equals pulmonary flow ($\dot{Q}_s - \dot{Q}_{EP}$ is the right-to-left shunt). In patients with bidirectional shunting, the arteriovenous difference used to calculate effective pulmonary flow uses the mixed systemic venous and mixed pulmonary venous oxygen contents.

Left-to-right shunt $\dot{Q}_p - \dot{Q}_{EP} = 0.75$ L/min/m²; right-to-left shunt $= \dot{Q}_s - \dot{Q}_{EP} = 2.0$ L/min/m².

Pressures

Pressures are recorded in each chamber and vessel entered and are monitored continuously during catheter manipulation to assist in determining catheter position. Differences in pressure from site to site help to localize obstructions and are essential in assessing their severity. Pressure signals from the transducers are sent to a recording device that displays them on a monitor and prints them on paper or records them digitally for future reference.

Normal pressure measurements in children are shown in Table 22-4.

TABLE 22-4

AVERAGE NORMAL RANGES OF INTRACARDIAC AND INTRAVASCULAR PRESSURE

	INFANTS AND CHILDREN	NEWBORNS
Right atrium	$a = 5-8$	$M = 0-4$
	$v = 2-6$	
	$M = 2-6$	
Right ventricle	$15-25/2-5$	$35-80/1-5$
Pulmonary artery	$15-25/8-12$	$35-80/20-50$
	$(M = 10-16)$	$(M = 25-60)$
Pulmonary wedge	$a = 6-12$	
	$v = 8-15$	
	$M = 5-12$	
Left atrium	$a = 6-12$	$M = 3-6$
	$v = 8-15$	
	$M = 5-10$	
Left ventricle	$80-130/5-10$	
Systemic artery	$90-130/60-80$	$65-80/45-60$
	$(M = 70-95)$	$(M = 60-65)$

M = mean pressure.
SOURCE: *Rudolph AM: Congenital Diseases of the Heart. Chicago, Year Book, 1974.*

Vascular Resistance

The resistance to blood flow in the pulmonary and systemic circulations is calculated from the equations:

$$R_P = \frac{\text{mean PA pressure} - \text{mean PV or LA pressure}}{\dot{Q}_P}$$

$$R_S = \frac{\text{mean same pressure} - \text{mean RA pressure}}{\dot{Q}_S}$$

where PA and PV are pulmonary artery and vein, respectively, LA and RA are left and right atria, respectively, Ao is aorta, R_P is pulmonary vascular resistance (resistance units/mm²), $\dot{Q}_P$ is pulmonary flow (L/min/mm²), R_S is systemic vascular resistance (resistance units/mm²), and $\dot{Q}_S$ is systemic flow (L/min/mm²). When pressures are measured in millimeters of mercury, resistance units are equivalent to millimeters of mercury per liter per minute, commonly termed Wood units. Most of the resistance to flow is at the arteriolar level, and the calculated resistance is inversely related to the cross-sectional area of the arteriolar lumen. In the systemic circulation the calculated resistance is a mean value for several different vascular beds. The normal systemic vascular resistance varies between 15 and 30 units/m². Although high at birth, the pulmonary vascular resistance reaches values near low adult values after 2 to 4 weeks. So that these values can be compared at different ages, they are usually related to surface area. Normal values in children and adults are 1 to 3 units/m². Elevation to 10 units/m² suggests mild or moderate pulmonary vascular disease, often responsive to vasodilators. Marked elevation to >10 units/m² often suggests significant fixed pulmonary vascular disease.

Angiography

Positioning a catheter in a particular chamber and rapidly injecting iodinated contrast medium permits radiographic delineation of most cardiovascular structures. Multiple injection sites and angulation of the cameras are often necessary to obtain a complete anatomic diagnosis.

Angiograms may be recorded digitally or on film at 15, 30, or 60 frames per second. Biplane angiograms yield more information than single-plane angiograms while using the same volume of contrast material. This is important for patients with complicated abnormalities who require multiple angiograms and in newborns who may have a low tolerance to contrast medium. A video replay system permits immediate examination of angiograms. This not only ensures that the desired information has been recorded but also minimizes delays in treating critically ill newborns.

Additional Testing

Additional tests may be done during the procedure. Drug testing is done using isoproterenol or dobutamine infusion to simulate exercise, or with oxygen, nitric oxide, or prostacyclin to determine pulmonary vascular reactivity. Evaluating pulmonary vascular resistance and its responsiveness to pulmonary vasodilators is discussed in Sec. 22.3.9.

Endomyocardial biopsy is the gold standard for detecting rejection in cardiac transplant patients. Nearly all institutions screen their pediatric transplant patients with cardiac biopsies at regular intervals, although this is less common for neonates. Other, more controversial, indications for biopsy include new-onset cardiomyopathy and suspected myocarditis. Though in the past it was thought useful to biopsy both ventricles, right ventricular biopsy alone is now standard practice.

INTERVENTIONAL PEDIATRIC CARDIAC CATHETERIZATION

Interventional cardiac catheterization has become the standard of care for treating an increasing number of congenital heart lesions, but in others, it remains investigational (Table 22-5). These procedures are directed at avoiding, postponing, or complementing surgery with its attendant risks, scars, and lengthy hospitalization and recovery times. Occasionally there is no suitable surgical procedure. The therapeutic procedures performed in pediatric populations can be either dilations or closures. Dilations are performed using balloons alone or in combination with stents, whereas closures are accomplished using embolization coils or specially designed devices.

Enlarging or Creating Atrial Communications

An unrestrictive atrial septal defect may be necessary for patients with certain cardiac abnormalities. Adequate mixing through an atrial septal defect is essential for survival in neonates with *d*-transposition as well as in patients with a single ventricle with a small mitral valve, mitral, tricuspid, or aortic atresia, and total anomalous pulmonary venous connection. *Balloon atrial septostomy* (Rashkind procedure) involves passing a balloon-tipped catheter through the foramen ovale into the left atrium, inflating the balloon, and then pulling it back rapidly across the atrial septum. The resulting tear in the atrial septum usually permits improved mixing. Although balloon catheters successfully tear the thin valve of the foramen

TABLE 22-5

INTERVENTIONAL CARDIAC CATHETERIZATION

- **Treatment of dysrhythmias**
  - Intracardiac pacing for bradyarrhythmias
  - Overdrive pacing for tachyarrhythmias
  - Transcatheter electrical ablation of His bundle for uncontrollable supraventricular tachycardia
  - Transcatheter ablation of ectopic focus, AV nodal pathway, or bundle of Kent for tachycardia
- **Retrieval of embolized catheter fragments**
- **Enlarging or creating atrial septal defects**
  - Balloon atrial septostomy
  - Blade atrial septostomy
- **Occlusion of atrial septal defects**[a]
- **Occlusion of patent ductus arteriosus**[a]
- **Embolization of arteriovenous fistulas or bronchial collateral vessels**
- **Balloon angioplasty**
  - Coronary arteries (adults)
  - Branch pulmonary arteries
  - Aortic coarctation
  - Aortic recoarctation
  - Aortopulmonary shunts, eg, Blalock-Taussig or Waterston
- **Balloon valvuloplasty**
  - Pulmonic stenosis
  - Aortic stenosis
  - Mitral stenosis

[a] Still experimental.

ovale of neonates, the thicker septum of older infants is not usually amenable to balloon septostomy. Techniques used to open the septum in older infants and children include *blade atrial septostomy* (Park procedure), *static balloon septoplasty,* and *atrial septal stenting.*

Valvoplasty

Balloon pulmonary valvoplasty is safe and highly successful in reducing the transvalvar gradient while producing little pulmonary insufficiency. With large balloons that exceed the size of the pulmonary valve annulus by 20 to 40%, pulmonary valve gradients are typically reduced to <15 mm Hg with little or no resulting pulmonary insufficiency. The residual obstruction may be minimally greater than that seen after surgery; however, the insufficiency appears to be less. The low mortality and morbidity associated with balloon pulmonary valvoplasty, now done as an outpatient procedure, as well as the lack of thoracotomy, cardiopulmonary bypass, transfusions, general anesthetic, and scars make it the procedure of choice. Thick dysplastic valves, as occur in Noonan syndrome, and stenosis in the main pulmonary artery just above the valve may respond poorly to balloon dilatation and require surgery.

For similar reasons *balloon aortic valvoplasty* is the treatment of choice in patients with valvar aortic stenosis and can be performed with low mortality, good relief of aortic obstruction, and variable but usually mild aortic insufficiency. Patients with calcific aortic stenosis, moderate to severe aortic insufficiency, or annular hypoplasia are not good candidates for valvoplasty. Early and medium-length follow-up studies show acute results comparable to primary surgery; usually there is less aortic regurgitation, but occasionally severe aortic regurgitation necessitates valve replacement. The risks of valvoplasty include arrhythmias, emboli, neurologic events, and injury to access vessels. In contrast, surgical risks include mortality, risks of anesthesia, cardiopulmonary bypass, and blood products, and the disadvantages of a long hospitalization, an undesirable scar, and greater cost. Both balloon valvoplasty and surgical valvotomy are palliative, and a repeat procedure will usually be needed in the future. Longer-term follow-up suggests that repeat treatment for either recurrent stenosis or worsening insufficiency is needed in 50% of patients within 8 years of valvoplasty. In some patients who develop restenosis after surgical or balloon procedures, balloon valvoplasty has been used as a means of deferring valve replacement; such delays are particularly important in small children who would otherwise require multiple valve replacements.

Balloon *mitral valvoplasty* has been performed via a transseptal approach in a few children in the United States, and a larger number in Asia and the Middle East. Preliminary results indicate very good relief of obstruction with minimal resulting mitral insufficiency in children with rheumatic mitral stenosis. Results for congenital stenosis are quite variable, with a greater propensity for developing mitral insufficiency.

Balloon Angioplasty

Angioplasty of obstructed vessels in children has been performed since 1982. Relief of obstruction is achieved by tearing the intimal and medial layers. The most commonly involved vessels are arteries, specifically the pulmonary arteries and aorta, though some postoperative venous obstructions are amenable to dilatation as well. Recent advances in balloon catheter technology, allowing for smaller balloon catheters that can be inflated to extremely high

pressures (20 atm), has made these procedures safer and more effective. For some lesions, such as distal pulmonary artery stenosis, direct surgical relief is not possible, and angioplasty is the only available treatment.

Stenosis of the branch pulmonary arteries may be congenital, acquired, or postsurgical (ie, at shunt insertion sites, bands, or conduits). Examples of congenital pulmonary artery branch stenosis (PABS) include tetralogy of Fallot with pulmonary atresia, Williams syndrome, Alagille syndrome, and congenital rubella.

Stenoses caused by scarring from previous Blalock-Taussig or other aortopulmonary shunts are usually amenable to balloon palliation. This is not always so for native stenoses or hypoplastic pulmonary arteries, with a success rate of 75%. In some patients there may be modest initial improvement in the size of the pulmonary arteries, which then show significant growth thereafter.

A combined surgical-transcatheter approach to patients with complex pulmonary artery stenosis has now become commonplace. Surgical attention to proximal stenoses and any intracardiac defects plus transcatheter therapy of distal pulmonary stenosis and recurrent obstruction improve short- and long-term outcomes.

Balloon dilatation of native *aortic coarctation* in neonates and children is successful in 80% of patients but has been associated with significant complications, including aortic rupture and death (<1%) as well as late aneurysm formation at the site of the previously torn vessel (5%). Recurrence of coarctation following dilatation in neonates occurs in up to 75%, and for this reason most cardiac centers recommend surgical treatment of neonatal coarctation. The role of this procedure for native coarctation in older children is unsettled, though most centers offer dilatation as an alternative treatment to surgery. On the other hand, recoarctation angioplasty has achieved wide acceptance because the surrounding scar from the previous surgery may act as a protective barrier to minimize the risk of aneurysm formation, and surgical repair may be difficult. The early results of recoarctation balloon angioplasty appear to be at least as good as reoperation, although there have been some deaths and morbidity.

Endovascular Stents

Balloon-expandable stents (metallic mesh tubes) are now used to treat many lesions that are not amenable to balloon dilatation alone. Lesions with significant elastic recoil that resist tearing can often be treated with endovascular stents.

The largest experience in pediatrics is with stenting for branch pulmonary artery stenosis. Results have shown an increase in vessel diameter, a fall in peak systolic gradient across the obstruction, an increase in flow to the stented lung, and a decrease in right ventricular pressure. Restenosis is rare, occurring in only 3% of patients, and redilatation has been effective. Similar success has been reported with stents in postoperative right ventricular to pulmonary artery conduit stenosis, and stent placement has become the treatment of choice for systemic venous obstruction. Stent placement as primary treatment of coarctation of the aorta, both native and recurrent, has become a preferred therapy for adolescent patients at many centers. Procedural success is excellent in over 95%; however, mid- and late-term follow-up are not yet available.

Coil Embolization

Aortopulmonary collaterals, arteriovenous malformations, Blalock-Taussig shunts, venous collaterals, coronary artery fistulas, and patent ductus arteriosus have all been successfully occluded by coil embolization. The embolization coils consist of a straight metal wire, either stainless steel or platinum, with or without Dacron strands, available in multiple sizes, lengths, and shapes, that coil into a helix when extruded from the catheter. Although PDA or coronary artery fistula embolization may obviate the need for surgery, most embolizations serve either to reduce the cardiac workload by decreasing the amount of shunting or simplify a planned surgical procedure.

PDA coil occlusion has become standard therapy for most older infants and nearly all children and adults. Recent reports have demonstrated closure rates of nearly 100% with PDAs measuring 3.5 mm or less and have been successful in PDAs as large as 6 mm. The coil is deployed with one loop of coil in the pulmonary artery and the rest in the ductal ampulla. Because the ductus is often funnel shaped, this arrangement anchors the coil in the ductus and prevents embolization to the pulmonary bed or lower body. If, in a large PDA, a single coil does not completely close it, multiple coils can be placed until no residual shunting exists. Complications are exceedingly rare and most often consist of coil embolization to the pulmonary artery; the coil can be retrieved and removed from the patient in the catheterization laboratory with minimal effort. Pulse loss is a risk for small infants but can be minimized by a venous approach. Rarely recanalization, documented by color flow Doppler, has been reported.

The technique for *coil closure of collaterals* or other communications is straightforward. A catheter is placed in the vessel to be occluded, and a selective angiogram is done to delineate the anatomy and diameter of the vessel to be closed. Coils are chosen that are slightly larger than the diameter of the vessel, as the vessel will distend when the coil is deployed. With a long "pusher" wire, the coil is advanced through the catheter and deployed in the vessel. Repeat angiography is performed to confirm complete closure. If residual flow remains, additional coils are placed.

Device Closure of Septal Defects

Surgical closure is the standard treatment of choice for atrial and ventricular septal defects but requires cardiopulmonary bypass and its inherent risks. In addition, the resultant scar, a relatively long recovery, and some morbidity have led to the development of nonsurgical alternatives. Transcatheter closure of atrial septal defects, currently under multicenter investigation in the United States, has been shown to be safe and effective in >96% of patients, with zero mortality and complications in <3%. Approximately 60% of patients currently undergoing surgical closure may be device candidates. Device closure of ventricular septal defects has been performed successfully but remains in the early phase of clinical trials.

Current device designs can be classified as single- or double-sided systems. In the single-sided system, the Sideris button device, the large square foam occluder is placed against the left atrial side of the septum, and a counteroccluder, comprised of a stiff wire, is secured on the right atrial side of the septum, holding the device in place. Double-sided devices can be either double umbrella or double disk devices. In the first system, two Dacron-covered umbrellas each with four flexible metal arms are connected by a single post. When implanted, the umbrellas open toward each other and hold the septal tissue between them. The second system is comprised of a self-expanding shape memory wire mesh made from Nitinol (nickel-titanium alloy). The two disks are linked together by a short connecting waist and, when deployed, have a shape similar to a chocolate sandwich cookie. To increase its thrombogenicity, the device's discs and waist are filled with polyester patches that are sewn to the wire frame.

These devices are currently approved and available for use in Europe. In the United States, only a single device (the CardioSEAL double umbrella) has been FDA approved, but only for compassionate use in children with complex heart problems. Clinical trials of these devices are ongoing in the United States, with approval expected in the year 2001.

References

Bridges ND, Freed MD: Cardiac catheterization. In: Emmanouilides GC, Riemenschneider TA, Allen HD, Gutgesell HP, eds: Heart Disease in Infants, Children, and Adolescents, Including the Fetus and Young Adult. Baltimore, Williams & Wilkins, 1995:310

Freedom RM, Mawon JB, Yoo SJ, Benson LN, eds: Congenital Heart Disease Textbook of Angiocardiography. Armonk, NY, Futura Publishing, 1997

Ing FF, Grifka RG, Nihill MR, Mullins CE: Repeat dilation of intravascular stents in congenital heart defects. Circulation 92:893, 1995

Lloyd TR, Fedderly R, Mendelsohn AM, et al: Transcatheter occlusion of patent ductus arteriosus with Gianturco coils. Circulation 88(part 1): 1412, 1993

Lock JE, Keane JF, Perry SB: Diagnostic and Interventional Catheterization in Congenital Heart Disease, 2nd ed. Norwell, MA, Kluwer Academic Publishers, 2000

Moore P, Egito E, Mowrey H, et al: Mid-term results of balloon dilation of congenital aortic stenosis: Predictors of success. J Am Coll Cardiol 27:1257–1263, 1996

Mullins CE, O'Laughlin MP: Therapeutic cardiac catheterization. In: Emmanouilides GC, Riemenschneider TA, Allen HD, Gutgesell HP, eds: Heart Disease in Infants, Children, and Adolescents. Baltimore, Williams & Wilkins, 1995:439

O'Laughlin MP, Slack MC, Grifka RG, et al: Implantation and intermediate-term follow-up of stents in congenital heart disease. Circulation 88:605, 1993

Rudolph AM: Congenital Diseases of the Heart. Chicago, Year Book, 1974

Stanger P, Cassidy SC, Girod DA, et al: Balloon pulmonary valvuloplasty: results of the valvuloplasty and angioplasty of congenital anomalies registry. Am J Cardiol 65:75, 1990

Vitiello R, McCrindle BW, Nykanen D, et al: Complications associated with pediatric cardiac catheterization. J Am Coll Cardiol 32:1433, 1998

22.3   CONGENITAL HEART DISEASE

22.3.1   Incidence and Recurrence

Julien I. E. Hoffman

Congenital heart diseases occur in at least 10 per 1000 live-born children; the incidence is much higher in stillborn infants and in spontaneous abortuses. This figure excludes bicuspid aortic valves, patent ductus arteriosus in premature infants, and tiny muscular ventricular septal defects with respective incidences of 10 to 20, 4 to 5, and 30 to 40 per 1000 live-born children. The distributions of various common types of congenital heart diseases at birth are given in Table 22-6.

TABLE 22-6

RELATIVE AND ABSOLUTE INCIDENCE OF MAJOR CONGENITAL HEART LESIONS AND THEIR RECURRENCE RATES

LESION[f]	PERCENTAGE OF ALL CHD 25–75% (MEDIAN)	PER MILLION LIVE BORN CHILDREN 25–75% (MEDIAN)	% RECURRENCE SIBLINGS	% RECURRENCE OFFSPRING
Ventricular septal defect	27.1–42.0 (32.4)	1667–3142 (2267)	4–6	2–22
Atrial septal defect	6.8–11.7 (7.5)	403–910 (563)	3	2–14
Patent ductus arteriosus[a]	5.3–11.0 (7.1)	350–774 (471)	2.5–3	2–11
Pulmonic stenosis	5.0–8.6 (7.0)	280–641 (404)	3	3–18
Coarctation of the aorta	3.8–5.8 (5.0)	289–419 (332)	2–7	2–8
Transposition of the great arteries	3.5–5.3 (4.5)	275–380 (327)	2	0[e]–5
Tetralogy of Fallot	3.9–6.8 (5.2)	261–500 (311)	2–3	1–4
Atrioventricular septal defect[d]	2.6–5.1 (3.8)	213–346 (284)	2–3	5–15
Aortic stenosis	3.3–5.9 (4.0)	155–339 (283)	3	3–18
Hypoplastic left heart[b]	1.6–3.4 (2.9)	151–255 (230)	1–4	—
Hypoplastic right heart[c]	1.4–3.2 (2.3)	105–197 (171)	1	5
Double-inlet left ventricle	0.7–1.7 (1.4)	54–126 (87)	3	5
Persistent truncus arteriosus	0.7–1.7 (1.4)	61–145 (86)	1–14	8
Double-outlet right ventricle	1.0–3.9 (1.2)	69–238 (79)	2	4
Total anomalous pulmonary venous connection	0.6–1.7 (1.0)	47–93 (53)	3	5
Miscellaneous	8.0–14.8 (11.4)	536–1058 (804)		

[a] Excluding preterm infants.
[b] Mainly aortic and mitral atresia.
[c] Mainly tricuspid atresia and pulmonary atresia with an intact ventricular septum.
[d] Excluding trisomy 21.
[e] Close to zero for simple transposition of the great arteries.
[f] The lesions are arranged in order of absolute incidence rates.

ETIOLOGY

Congenital heart diseases result from interaction between genetic and environmental factors.

GENETIC FACTORS Single classic mendelian mutant genes account for 3% of congenital heart diseases; 5% are caused by gross chromosomal aberrations, 3% by known environmental factors (eg, rubella, fetal alcohol syndrome), and the rest by multifactorial gene effects or single gene effects modulated by random events.

Single mutant genes (autosomal dominant or recessive or X-linked) usually cause congenital heart disease as part of a complex of abnormalities. The most common of these is Noonan syndrome, with pulmonic stenosis and hypertrophic cardiomyopathy as the most frequent cardiac lesions; other syndromes with their most common cardiac lesions include Apert syndrome (ventricular septal defects, coarctation of the aorta), Holt-Oram syndrome (atrial and ventricular septal defects), and Ellis-van Creveld syndrome (single atrium).

Chromosomal abnormalities also cause congenital heart diseases as part of a complex of lesions. Many of these syndromes have a high incidence of congenital heart diseases: cri-du-chat syndrome (20%), XO (Turner) syndrome (50%), trisomy 21 (Down) syndrome (50%), trisomy 13 (90%), and trisomy 18 (99%). Ventricular septal defects are the most common cardiac lesions in all except Turner syndrome, which predominantly has bicuspid aortic valves and coarctation of the aorta.

Multifactorial gene factors are believed to be the basis for patent ductus arteriosus. They were thought to be the basis for other congenital heart diseases as well, but some evidence now suggests other

possible factors, such as single gene effects modulated by random events.

ENVIRONMENTAL FACTORS

FETAL ENVIRONMENT Women taking lithium salts during pregnancy may have children with congenital heart diseases, with a high incidence of mitral and tricuspid valve lesions, especially Ebstein syndrome. Diabetic women or those taking progesterone in pregnancy have an increased risk of having children with congenital heart diseases. About half the children of alcoholic mothers have congenital heart diseases (usually left-to-right shunts). Retinoic acid used to treat acne may cause several types of congenital heart lesions.

VIRAL LESIONS Rubella embryopathy is often associated with peripheral pulmonic stenosis, patent ductus arteriosus, and valvar pulmonic stenosis. Other viruses, notably coxsackieviruses, have been thought to cause congenital heart diseases because of an increased frequency of rising serum titers to this virus in mothers whose infants have congenital heart disease. Mumps virus is responsible for endocardial fibroelastosis.

COUNSELING FAMILIES

When a child is found to have congenital heart disease, the parents frequently have severe guilt feelings and are almost always worried about the risk of occurrence of congenital heart disease in future children. These issues should be discussed openly with the parents, who are often reticent about mentioning them. An explanation of what is known of the causes of congenital heart diseases and reassurance that the parents did not cause it by acts of omission or commission are arguments that can be used to help allay guilt feelings. This approach must be correlated with all the other aspects of giving continued support to parents with chronically ill children.

RECURRENCE

The risk of occurrence of cardiac lesions in future children concerns parents. If the cardiac lesion is part of a syndrome caused by a single gene mutation, then in general autosomal dominant genes will appear in 50% of offspring, whereas autosomal recessive genes produce disease in 25% of offspring. Chromosomal abnormalities have risks of recurrence that vary with the specific chromosomal change involved. Other forms of inheritance produce a much lower risk of recurrence (Table 22-6). Furthermore, if two first-degree relatives have congenital heart disease, then the risk of heart disease in the next infant is about three times as high as the figures just cited. The risk of transmission of congenital heart disease to children if the parent, especially the mother, has congenital heart disease averages about 5 to 10%.

If another child has congenital heart disease, it is most often similar in type (concordant) to that in the parent or sibling.

References

Burn J: The aetiology of congenital heart disease. In: Anderson RH, Macartney FJ, Shinebourne EA, Tynan M, eds: Paediatric Cardiology. Edinburgh, Churchill Livingstone, 1987:15

Hoffman JIE: The incidence of congenital heart disease. I. Postnatal incidence. Pediatr Cardiol 16:103, 1995

Kitchen LW: Psychological factors in congenital heart disease in children. J Fam Pract 6:777, 1978

Mitchell SC, Korones SB, Berendes HW: Congenital heart disease in 56,109 births. Incidence and natural history. Circulation 43:323, 1971

Mitchell SC, Sellmann AH, Westphal MC, et al: Etiologic correlates in a study of congenital heart disease in 56,109 births. Am J Cardiol 28:653, 1971

Newman TB: Ventricular septal defects. Pediatrics 76:741, 1985

Nora JJ, Nora AH: Update on counseling the family with a first-degree relative with a congenital heart defect. Am J Med Genet 29:137, 1988

Rose V, Gold RJM, Lindsay G, et al: A possible increase in the incidence of congenital heart defects among the offspring of affected parents. J Am Coll Cardiol 6:376, 1985

Ursell PC, Byrne JM, Strobing RA: Significance of cardiac defects in the developing fetus: a study of spontaneous abortuses. Circulation 72:1232, 1985

Whittemore R, Hobbins JC, Engle MA: Pregnancy and its outcome in women with and without surgical treatment of congenital heart disease. Am J Cardiol 50:641, 1982

22.3.2   Left-to-Right Shunts

Julien I. E. Hoffman

GENERAL FEATURES

A shunt from systemic to pulmonary circulation through an abnormal communication, termed a *left-to-right shunt,* lets oxygenated blood recirculate through the lungs without entering the peripheral arterial circulation. This shunt is wasted flow that adds to cardiac work without improving delivery of oxygenated blood. A left-to-right shunt may be present alone or associated with right-to-left shunting (bidirectional shunting) or obstructive lesions.

Anatomic Classification

Left-to-right shunts are classified anatomically by the level at which the systemic and pulmonary circulations communicate (Table 22-7).

Effects in Fetus

With defects that produce left-to-right shunts after birth, fetal somatic development is unaltered, and blood flow to the fetal organs and placenta is probably normal. However, alterations of flow patterns in the fetal heart and great vessels may affect their development. When some left ventricular output is shunted away from the ascending aorta, as may occur in endocardial cushion defects, a large ventricular septal defect, or double-outlet right ventricle, particularly with aortic or subaortic obstruction, then decreased aortic isthmus flow may cause hypoplasia or even interruption of the aortic isthmus. Altered streaming patterns may change the composition of blood leaving the heart. Thus, with an endocardial cushion defect or large ventricular septal defect, the oxygen tension of blood leaving the right ventricle and perfusing the lungs may be higher than that in the normal fetus. This higher oxygen tension may alter the development of pulmonary resistance vessels, thereby affecting postnatal clinical features.

Factors Influencing Left-to-Right Shunts

Three major interrelated factors control the amount of left-to-right shunting postnatally: the size of and therefore the resistance to flow offered by the communication, the difference in pressures between the chambers or vessels, and the total outflow resistances (including peripheral resistances) of the chambers or vessels.

TABLE 22-7
LEFT-TO-RIGHT SHUNTS

Pretricuspid
  Left atrium or pulmonary veins to right atrium (partially dependent)
    Atrial septal defects: incompetent foramen ovale, primum, secundum, sinus venosus
    Partial anomalous pulmonary venous connection
Posttricuspid
  Aorta to pulmonary artery (dependent)
    Patent ductus arteriosus
    Aortopulmonary fenestration
    Hemitruncus arteriosus
    Lobar sequestration
    Coronary-pulmonary fistula
    Anomalous origin of left coronary artery from pulmonary artery
  Aorta to right ventricle (dependent)
    Sinus of Valsalva fistula
    Coronary arteriovenous fistula
  Aorta to right atrium or systemic vein (obligatory)
    Systemic arteriovenous fistula
    Sinus of Valsalva fistula
    Coronary arteriovenous fistula
  Left ventricle to right ventricle (dependent)
    Ventricular septal defect
    Endocardial cushion defect
  Left ventricle to right atrium (obligatory)
    Left ventricular to right atrial communication
    Endocardial cushion defect

If the communication at any level is small, it offers a high resistance to flow through it so that the left-to-right shunt will be small, no matter what the pressures or resistances are (Fig. 22-31A). The latter two factors come into play only with medium-sized or big communications. In pretricuspid (atrial level) communications, atrial pressures are low and almost equal, and the amount and direction of shunting depends only on the resistance to emptying of the left and right atria into their respective ventricles. Before and immediately after birth, systemic and pulmonary vascular resistances and pressures are high and equal, and both ventricles have similar wall thicknesses and distensibility. Therefore, diastolic inflow into each ventricle is similar, and even with a large atrial septal communication, there will be little left-to-right atrial shunting. Over the next few weeks, systemic pressures and vascular resistances increase while pulmonary vascular resistances and pressures decrease, and the ventricular wall becomes thinner and the diastolic distensibility greater in the right than the left ventricle. Therefore, more blood flows from right atrium to right ventricle than from left atrium to left ventricle, so that a larger left-to-right shunt develops. (Think of the atria as a single chamber with two exits. More blood will enter the more distensible receiving chamber.). Note that the large left-to-right shunt can develop only after pulmonary arterial resistance and pressure have decreased greatly.

In a posttricuspid shunt such as a ventricular septal defect or patent ductus arteriosus, when the communication is large, systolic pressures in the ventricles or great arteries are equal (Fig. 22-31B,C), and the magnitude and direction of shunting will be determined by the relative outflow resistance of each ventricle or great artery. If left-sided outflow resistance is much higher than that of the right side, there will be a large left-to-right shunt (Fig. 22-31B). If right-sided outflow resistance increases and approximates that of the left side, or if systemic resistance falls, the left-to-right shunt will be small (Fig. 22-31C). If the outflow resistance is higher for the right than the left side, there will be a shunt from right to left. The outflow resistance may be at a semilunar valve orifice, in a great

vessel, in peripheral resistance vessels, or any combination of these. In the absence of aortic or pulmonic stenosis, the relationship between pulmonary and systemic vascular resistances determines the magnitude of shunting. Because systemic vascular resistance is normally high and changes little after birth, alteration in pulmonary vascular resistance is a major regulator of shunting through an aortopulmonary or interventricular defect, particularly in the first months after birth, when the normal progressive fall in pulmonary vascular resistance occurs. This type of shunting, in which the ratio of pulmonary vascular resistance to systemic vascular resistance determines the shunt, is termed *dependent* shunting, and it applies to both pre- and posttricuspid shunts.

Another group of left-to-right shunts has a communication between a high-pressure ventricle and a low-pressure chamber or vessel, such as a direct left ventricular to right atrial communication or a systemic arteriovenous fistula (Fig. 22-31D). The magnitude of the shunt depends on the size of the communication and the pressure difference between the chambers or vessels involved and not on the pulmonary vascular resistance; the shunt is therefore termed *obligatory*.

General Pathophysiology and Clinical Correlates

The site of the defect determines some of its specific features; however, many features associated with left-to-right shunting are common to several defects. A small left-to-right shunt has little hemodynamic effect on the heart and presents only with specific murmurs related to turbulent flow across the defect. Larger shunts, however, have prominent effects that depend on the level at which shunting occurs because this determines which part of the circulation receives the additional blood flow.

In an aortopulmonary left-to-right shunt, some of the left ventricular output leaves the systemic circulation and increases pulmonary blood flow by that amount. The resultant greater pulmonary venous return to the left atrium and left ventricle increases left ventricular diastolic volume and thus increases left ventricular stroke volume and stroke work by the Frank-Starling mechanism. The left ventricle is enlarged and hyperactive, with a forceful and hyperactive apical impulse. Because of the increased left ventricular output, there may be a third heart sound caused by rapid left ventricular filling in early diastole and a fourth heart sound from left atrial hypertrophy. Also, when pulmonary venous return to the left atrium approximately doubles, there may be a low-frequency apical middiastolic rumbling murmur from increased and turbulent diastolic flow across a normal mitral valve. Dilatation of the left ventricle elevates left ventricular end-diastolic and left atrial pressures and, if marked, causes left heart failure and pulmonary venous congestion (Fig. 22-32). Left atrial dilatation may stretch the atrial septum, causing incompetence of the valve of the foramen ovale and a left-to-right atrial shunt that may be clinically significant. The right ventricle does not handle an extra volume load (unless there is an atrial shunt) but will have an increased pressure load if there is pulmonary hypertension. This produces a forceful heave felt at the lower left sternal border enlargement and a loud pulmonic valve closure sound (P_2).

Similar hemodynamic effects may follow a left-to-right shunt at the ventricular level, but the right ventricle will also have some volume overload, so that the right ventricular impulse also is hyperactive. Left-to-right shunts at the atrial level increase volume load only on the right atrium and ventricle, and if there is some

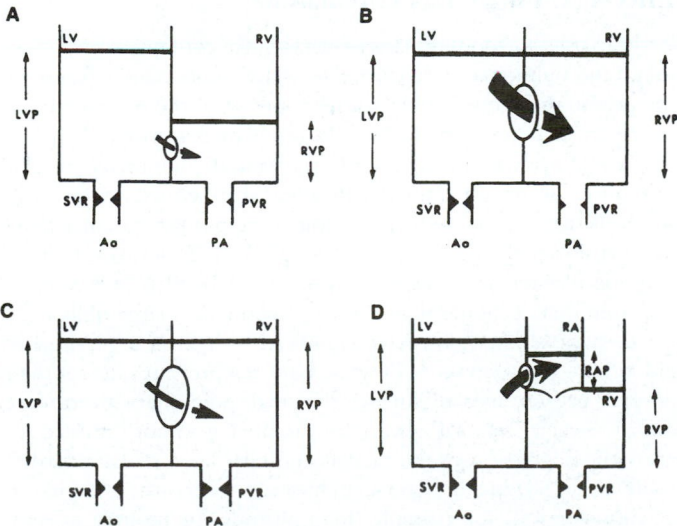

FIGURE 22-31 Diagrammatic representations of the major factors that regulate the magnitude of left-to-right shunting in congenital heart disease. LV = left ventricle; RV = right ventricle; RA = right atrium; Ao = aorta; PA = pulmonary artery; LVP = left ventricular systolic pressure; RVP = right ventricular systolic pressure; RAP = right atrial mean pressure; SVR = systemic vascular resistance; PVR = pulmonary vascular resistance.

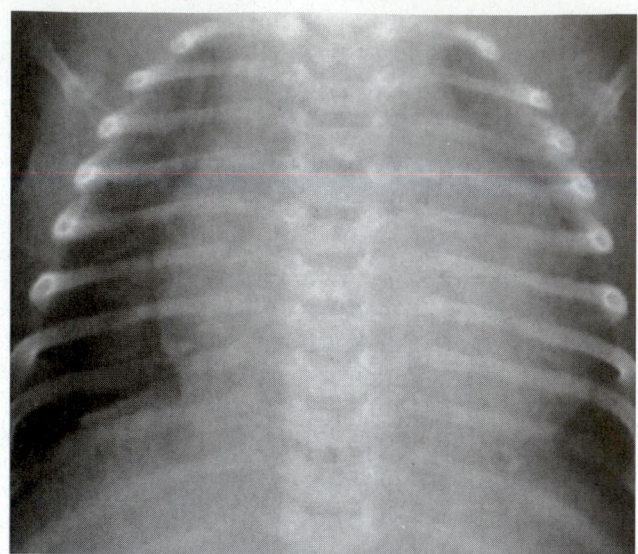

FIGURE 22-32   Chest roentgenogram in newborn infant with left ventricular failure demonstrating marked cardiomegaly and pulmonary venous congestion, the latter suggested by haziness of the lung fields.

outflow obstruction, a moderately increased right ventricular systolic pressure load may also occur. Therefore, a hyperactive impulse is felt over the right but not the left ventricle. An increase in right ventricular end-diastolic pressure with a subsequent increase in right atrial and systemic venous pressures is not usual. With obligatory shunts, volume overloading of both ventricles occurs, and both right and left ventricular impulses are hyperactive. Persistently increased precordial activity with cardiac enlargement in infants and young children often produces anterior bulging of the left hemithorax.

The sympathetic-adrenal system and myocardial hypertrophy help to maintain adequate myocardial performance, normal systemic output, and adequate tissue oxygenation in the face of a large left-to-right shunt. There is increased catecholamine release from the adrenal glands and sympathetic nerve fibers within the myocardium, so that heart rate and the force of myocardial contraction increase. This increased sympathetic-adrenal activity also accounts for the excessive sweating seen in left ventricular failure, particularly in infants. These compensatory mechanisms are well developed in older children and adults but not fully developed in newborn, particularly premature, infants. In addition, because myocardial structure matures during fetal and neonatal development, premature infants are less capable of handling a volume overload than are mature or older infants. If the increased volume or pressure load on the ventricles persists, the muscle fibers hypertrophy, and the increased amount of contractile protein helps to handle the load without excessive ventricular dilatation or sympathetic stimulation.

The increased work load and mass of the left ventricle increase myocardial oxygen requirements. Delivery of oxygen to the myocardium depends on coronary blood flow and the oxygen content of arterial blood. Coronary perfusion to the left ventricle occurs during diastole and depends on the systemic arterial–intramyocardial diastolic pressure difference as well as the duration of diastole. Therefore, a reduction in arterial diastolic pressure (as in an aortopulmonary communication with a large left-to-right shunt), an

increase in left ventricular end-diastolic pressure and therefore subendocardial intramyocardial pressure (as with left ventricular failure), and a reduction in diastolic period (as with tachycardia) are all detrimental to myocardial perfusion and oxygen delivery. In the right ventricle, myocardial blood flow is unlikely to be compromised unless the right ventricle has a systemic systolic pressure and is hypertrophied.

A low hemoglobin content, as occurs with physiological anemia in early infancy or after repeated blood sampling during intensive nursery care, also jeopardizes oxygen delivery to the myocardium and may precipitate left ventricular failure. A shift of P_{50} to the left (alkalosis, some abnormal hemoglobins, fetal hemoglobin) also makes it more difficult to supply oxygen to the myocardium. In addition, anemia or a left shift of P_{50} places a further demand on the left ventricle to increase systemic output to supply adequate oxygen to the entire body. Similarly, infections may further stress the left ventricle by increasing tissue oxygen demands and thereby requirements for cardiac output.

Chest roentgenograms of posttricuspid shunts show left ventricular and left atrial enlargement, and in aortopulmonary communications, the ascending aorta, which carries the increased flow, may be dilated. Increased pulmonary blood flow is manifested by prominent dilated main and branch pulmonary arteries extending into the lung fields (Fig. 22-33). If there is left ventricular failure, the roentgenogram shows the features described in Sec. 22.4.4. In pretricuspid shunts, the right ventricle and atrium are enlarged, and increased pulmonary blood flow is evident.

Electrocardiographic evidence of atrial and ventricular hypertrophy depends on the duration and magnitude of the shunt. Electrocardiographic features vary with the different types of atrial communication and are discussed later.

Echocardiographic findings also depend on the magnitude of left-to-right shunting and the degree of heart failure as well as on the specific lesion.

Effects on Pulmonary Circulation

With a large aortopulmonary or ventricular communication, systemic and pulmonary arterial pressures are similar, and because of the persistent high pulmonary arterial pressure, the medial muscle of the small pulmonary arteries does not regress as rapidly or as much as in normal individuals. Thus, although pulmonary vascular resistance falls rapidly immediately after birth because of the onset of ventilation, the subsequent decline in pulmonary vascular resistance is slower than normal (see Sec. 22.3.9). The lowest pulmonary vascular resistance reached is usually delayed 2 to 3 months and even then is higher than normal. Infants with large obligatory left-to-right shunts also have significantly increased pulmonary blood flow and therefore pulmonary arterial pressures higher than normal, because in early infancy the small pulmonary arteries are not distensible; this will also delay the medial smooth muscle regression. Regression of the medial muscular layer is also retarded by anything producing hypoxic pulmonary vasoconstriction in the newborn period, for example, high altitude, pulmonary disease, chronic upper airway obstruction, or obstruction of the major airways by dilated pulmonary arteries produced by a large left-to-right shunt. In patients with atrial communications, the pulmonary arterial pressure and pulmonary vascular resistance fall normally in the postnatal period, and small pulmonary arteries undergo the normal regression of medial smooth muscle.

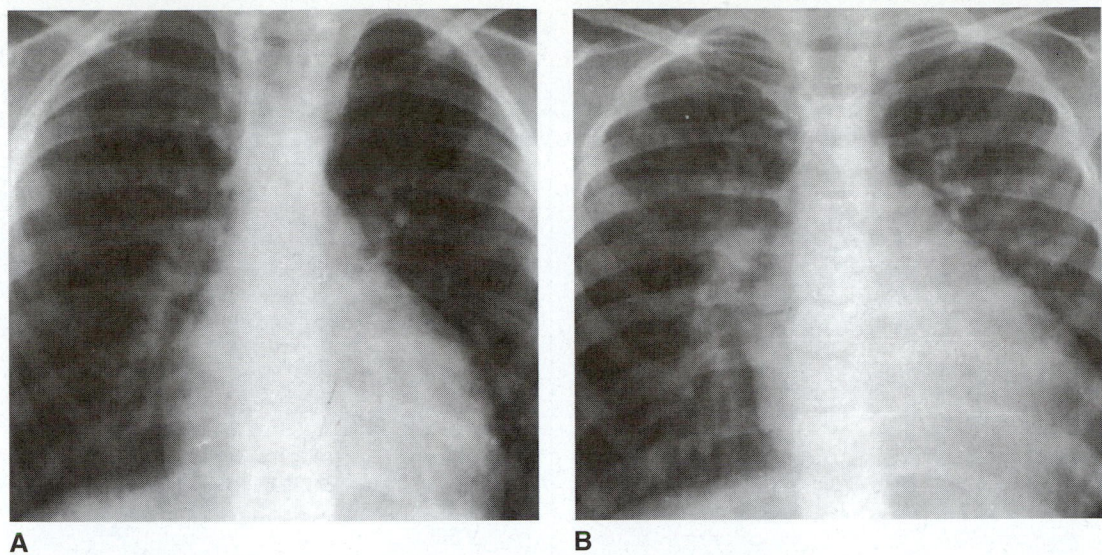

FIGURE 22-33 Chest roentgenograms in (A) a child with a small ventricular septal defect with a moderate left-to-right shunt and (B) a child with a large ventricular septal defect with a large left-to-right shunt and pulmonary arterial hypertension.

PATENT DUCTUS ARTERIOSUS

Postnatal closure of the ductus arteriosus is effected by constriction of smooth muscle in its wall. In full-term infants, this functional closure normally occurs within 10 to 15 hours after birth; however, complete anatomic obliteration of the ductus arteriosus is slower and may not be complete until the third postnatal week. Because pulmonary vascular resistance falls as soon as the lungs expand, in the first 10 to 15 hours when the ductus arteriosus is still open, a left-to-right shunt through the ductus arteriosus may occur, and a murmur may be heard.

Causes of Persistent Patency

A clinically apparent patent ductus arteriosus occurs in 30 to 40% of premature infants with birth weights under 1750 g. The mechanisms responsible for continued patency are related to the inability of the ductus arteriosus in immature infants to respond normally to an increased oxygen tension and to changes in prostaglandin concentrations. The incidence of persistent patency of the ductus arteriosus in full-term infants born at high altitude is significantly higher than in those born at sea level, probably because of the lower atmospheric oxygen tension. Persistent patency of the ductus arteriosus in full-term and occasional preterm infants at lower altitudes is generally related to a structural abnormality of the ductus arteriosus itself. No cause has been established in most patients, but a genetic basis has been inferred because this lesion fits the classic model of polygenic inheritance. Maternal rubella in the first trimester of pregnancy, however, is associated with a high incidence of persistent patency of the ductus arteriosus, and rubella virus has been cultured from ductus arteriosus tissue.

Clinical Manifestations in Mature Infants

The diagnosis of patent ductus arteriosus is easier in full-term infants or older children than in immature infants. Because of continuous runoff of blood from the aorta to the pulmonary artery through the ductus arteriosus, the murmur in older infants and children is continuous (Fig. 22-34) and has a rumbling, machinery-like quality, usually with late systolic accentuation of the murmur. It is heard best below the left clavicle. If the ductus arteriosus is small, this may be the only abnormal finding. If it is larger, the increase in left ventricular output is associated with an increase in stroke volume that causes a rapid rise in the aortic pulse pressure as a result of rapid left ventricular ejection and also causes left ventricular hyperactivity. The diastolic runoff through the aortopulmonary communication plus the peripheral vasodilatation that usually occurs account for the low diastolic pressure and the collapsing pulse. The increased volume load enlarges the left atrium and ventricle, with roentgenographic evidence of dilatation and electrocardiographic evidence of hypertrophy. Because the ascending aorta receives the increased left ventricular output, it is dilated. On x-ray, the pulmonary vascular markings indicate increased pulmonary blood flow. If there is pulmonary hypertension, there may be signs of right ventricular pressure overload.

Differential Diagnosis

In premature infants, particularly those under 1000 g birth weight, there is little chance that clinical findings suggestive of a patent ductus arteriosus are caused by some other congenital heart defect. However, in larger premature and full-term infants, sometimes a patent ductus arteriosus cannot be differentiated clinically from aortopulmonary window, truncus arteriosus, ventricular septal defect with aortic regurgitation, or arteriovenous fistula. A major problem may occur when there is severe heart failure with a markedly reduced cardiac output; the peripheral pulses may not be bounding, the murmur may be soft and not continuous, and the precordium may not be hyperactive. After appropriate therapy for left ventricular failure, the classic physical findings usually reappear. Echocardiography is diagnostic.

Outcome

In the full-term infant with a patent ductus arteriosus, spontaneous closure may occur, but much less commonly than in the premature

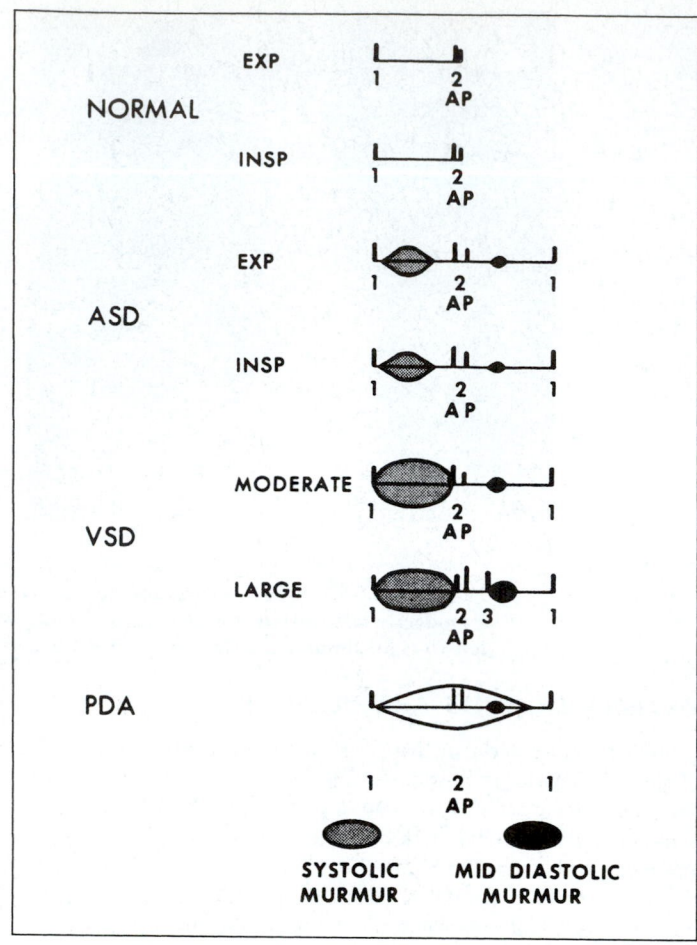

FIGURE 22-34 Diagrammatic representation of the auscultatory findings in normal children and children with atrial septal defect (ASD), ventricular septal defect (VSD), and patent ductus arteriosus (PDA). EXP = at end-expiration; INSP = at end-inspiration; 1 = first heart sound; 2 = second heart sound; A = aortic component of second heart sound; P = pulmonic component of second heart sound; 3 = third heart sound. The continuous murmur of the PDA is indicated by the two curved lines that enclose a clear area. The murmur begins just after S1, reaches a maximal intensity near S2, and dies away in diastole. To qualify as continuous, a murmur must continue from systole into diastole; it need not occupy all of diastole.

infant. Medical management, if needed, should be instituted, and at a convenient time surgical closure should be done. Even if there is no heart failure, there are two reasons to close a patent ductus arteriosus. If there is marked pulmonary hypertension as a result of a large communication, the danger of the development of pulmonary vascular disease necessitates closure, preferably before 6 to 8 months of age. In the older child with a small patent ductus arteriosus, closure should still be advised in view of the risk of infective endocarditis. Transcatheter closure with a coil is satisfactory if the diameter of the ductus is below 5 mm, but larger ductuses need surgery, which can be done safely by open thoracotomy. Recently ductus closure by thoracoscopy has been introduced.

AORTOPULMONARY FENESTRATION

Aortopulmonary fenestration, caused by failure of formation of the base of the spiral septum, generally produces a large aortopulmonary communication just above the semilunar valves. The pulses are typically bounding or collapsing, like those of a large patent ductus arteriosus. However, the murmur more closely resembles that of a high ventricular septal defect in that it is generally not continuous, has a rough, often crescendo-decrescendo character, and is heard maximally along the left sternal border in the third and fourth intercostal spaces. The diagnosis can be made by two-dimensional echocardiography and confirmed by cardiac catheterization and angiocardiography. Surgical closure during cardiopulmonary bypass is corrective.

ANOMALOUS ORIGIN OF LEFT CORONARY ARTERY

See Sec. 22.3.8 for a detailed discussion.

HEMITRUNCUS ARTERIOSUS AND LOBAR SEQUESTRATION

In hemitruncus arteriosus, either the left or more often the right pulmonary artery arises from the aorta. In lobar sequestration a portion of the lung, usually a lobe or part of a lobe, gets its arterial blood supply from an abnormal artery arising from the aorta. The involved pulmonary artery does not communicate with the main pulmonary artery. The flow into the lung or portion of lung is controlled by the pulmonary vascular resistance and the resistance offered by the communicating vessel itself. The clinical presentation in children with these lesions also depends on the magnitude of the shunt and will be very similar to that found with a patent ductus arteriosus. However, the murmur, often continuous, may be better heard more laterally or even in the back.

One important feature of a hemitruncus is that the normally arising pulmonary artery carries the total right ventricular output, which is the total systemic venous return. Normally this flow is distributed between the two pulmonary arteries. Pressure in the normally arising pulmonary artery is generally normal, and therefore the risks of subsequent pulmonary vascular disease are similar to those in children with atrial septal defects and a pulmonary blood flow about twice normal. However, with an associated left-to-right shunt, blood flow to the normal lung is more than doubled; thus, there may be pulmonary hypertension and subsequent pulmonary vascular disease. The lung supplied by the abnormally arising vessel is at risk not only from increased flow but also from increased pressure because this lung is perfused at systemic pressure less the pressure fall offered by the channel itself. If the abnormally arising pulmonary artery is adequately developed, implantation into the main pulmonary artery can be done. If a significant portion of lung is involved in lobar sequestration, a lobectomy is indicated.

Unilateral Absence of Pulmonary Artery

Although this is not a lesion with a left-to-right shunt, it resembles a hemitruncus. The right or the left pulmonary artery may be congenitally absent, either isolated or with other congenital cardiac defects. Absence of the left and right pulmonary arteries has the same incidence when these are isolated lesions and when they are associated with most cardiac defects; however, if there is a patent ductus arteriosus, then it is usually the right pulmonary artery that is absent, and in the tetralogy of Fallot it is almost always the left artery that is missing. The lung on the affected side is usually hypoplastic and supplied by bronchial arteries, so that the chest roentgenogram shows a small hemithorax, no hilar pulmonary artery, and often a diffuse reticular pattern of bronchial collaterals. Because ventilation can still take place on that side, there is wasted ventilation and usually dyspnea on effort.

The chief importance of the lesion is its tendency to produce pulmonary hypertension and pulmonary vascular disease in all except those with the tetralogy of Fallot. Because there is only one pulmonary artery, it receives the total right ventricular output. Therefore, even if there are no other lesions, that lung receives twice its normal blood flow; if there are left-to-right shunts in addition, it gets more than this. In infancy, before pulmonary arterial muscle has regressed, this increased flow leads to hypertension and can eventually cause severe pulmonary vascular disease, which has been reported in 18% of patients with no other lesions and 88% of those with cardiac lesions.

Diagnosis is made by angiography or magnetic resonance imaging. Treatment is directed at repairing the associated defects and avoiding anything that might affect the pulmonary vessels of the normal lung (eg, living at high altitude or taking contraceptive pills).

SINUS OF VALSALVA FISTULA

Rupture of a sinus of Valsalva into one of the cardiac chambers is secondary to a structural abnormality in the sinus. Most commonly these changes involve the anterior (right coronary) aortic valve sinus, and subsequent rupture produces a communication from the right coronary sinus into the right ventricle or right atrium. Less commonly, rupture involves the noncoronary or the left coronary sinus; rupture into the left atrium or ventricle is discussed in Sec. 22.3.3. The aneurysmal dilatation of the sinus that precedes rupture is often related to a ventricular septal defect. Connective-tissue disorders such as Marfan syndrome may also have associated aneurysmal dilatation of the aortic sinuses, but these do not rupture. Small fistulas may occur after infective endocarditis, but more extensive rupture usually occurs after trauma or spontaneously with progressive weakening of the sinus. Acute rupture, although more common in young adults, does occur in children. At the time of rupture there frequently is an episode of acute chest pain and dyspnea, with sudden onset of a murmur and congestive heart failure; however,

a more insidious onset has been described. With rupture into the right ventricle, the physical signs resemble those of a patent ductus arteriosus, with a loud continuous superficial murmur along the left sternal border, but with the addition of an increased right ventricular volume load. With rupture into the right atrium, this lesion will behave as an obligatory shunt, and the features are those of a patent ductus arteriosus and an atrial shunt combined. The diagnosis can be made by two-dimensional echocardiography, including Doppler and contrast echocardiography. Accurate differentiation from other lesions may require cardiac catheterization and angiocardiography. Surgical closure of the fistula can be done with cardiopulmonary bypass.

CONGENITAL CORONARY ARTERIOVENOUS FISTULA

In this lesion a fistula usually passes from one of the coronary arteries directly into the right ventricle (the most common site) or into the right atrium (either directly or through the coronary sinus). Communications with the left ventricle, left atrium, or pulmonary artery are much less common, except for small coronary-pulmonary fistulas that are of little importance.

The most striking clinical feature is a continuous murmur superficial in character and heard best along the lower left sternal border. The murmur is generally maximal in diastole and has very high-pitched components. Ventricular hyperactivity and a middiastolic rumble depend on the magnitude of shunting, which is not usually great. A continuous thrill may be palpable. The diagnosis can be made by two-dimensional echocardiography with Doppler and contrast echocardiography, but the specific diagnosis may require cardiac catheterization and angiocardiography. Treatment involves either ligation of the fistulous communication with the coronary sinus, right atrium, or pulmonary artery or specific surgical repair when the communication is with the right ventricular cavity. Occasionally occlusion can be done by a coil introduced through a catheter.

SYSTEMIC ARTERIOVENOUS FISTULA

Placental arteriovenous fistulas may produce a large increase in fetal cardiac output, particularly in descending aortic blood flow. Although the fistula is no longer present after birth, residual signs may remain in the neonate. These include peripheral edema, cardiomegaly, and a dilated descending aorta.

The most common sites for large arteriovenous communications in children are intracranial, hepatic, or in the extremities. However, fistulas have been described between internal mammary vessels or other major systemic arteries and their related veins, and with more frequent use of two-dimensional echocardiography and color Doppler, these are being encountered more frequently. They may be seen as part of Rendu-Osler-Weber syndrome. They can also be traumatic in origin, most commonly between renal vessels after needle biopsy of the kidney and in the femoral triangle after needling of the femoral vessels.

Because these lesions are obligatory left-to-right shunts, the hemodynamic and clinical features depend on the size of the communication and thus its resistance to flow. The majority of systemic arteriovenous fistulas are small and so do not produce major hemodynamic changes. The exceptions to this are hepatic or intracranial arteriovenous fistulas, particularly those that involve the great vein of Galen or its tributaries.

Certain clinical features are common to all types of arteriovenous fistulas: a systolic or continuous murmur over the site of the fistula, occasionally a pulsatile mass, and distended and sometimes pulsatile veins draining the region of the fistula. Increased limb size and swelling may occur with peripheral arteriovenous fistulas. Hepatic arteriovenous fistulas generally do not involve one feeder vessel but are usually hemangiomatous.

Intracranial arteriovenous fistulas usually produce the most severe hemodynamic changes because they involve vessels of large caliber and the left-to-right shunt is often large. In early infancy they may produce severe congestive heart failure, and they are among the few cardiovascular lesions that produce hydrops fetalis or severe congestive failure in the first days after birth. Clinically they generally present with continuous murmurs over either side of the skull and with bounding carotid pulses and distended jugular veins. The superior vena cava is generally markedly dilated on chest radiograph, and there is significant right and left ventricular volume overload. Peripheral pulses are bounding and even collapsing, unless heart failure is so marked that all pulses except the carotids are feeble. If the shunt is not large, cardiovascular manifestations may be mild, and neurologic sequelae dominate the clinical picture (see Sec. 25.8.9). Contrast two-dimensional echocardiography with Doppler is helpful in diagnosis, but the definitive diagnosis of these lesions may require cardiac catheterization and angiocardiography. Surgical ligation or excision of the fistula is generally effective, although intracranial fistulas, particularly those involving the great vein of Galen, may also have multiple feeding arteries, have a poorer outcome, and may not be operable. Newer arterial embolization methods show promise for treating some of these lesions.

VENTRICULAR SEPTAL DEFECT

Congenital defects of the interventricular septum are the most common of all congenital heart lesions, accounting for approximately 30 to 60% of all full-term patients with congenital heart malformations; this percentage is equivalent to three to six of every 1000 live births. This excludes the 3 to 5% of neonates with tiny muscular ventricular septal defects that usually close within the first year. A ventricular septal defect usually occurs as an isolated abnormality but may be associated with other congenital cardiac malformations. In view of the pattern of blood flow in the heart and great vessels of a fetus with a ventricular septal defect, with diversion of blood from the aortic isthmus, narrowing of the aortic isthmus or true coarctation should always be considered when an infant with a ventricular septal defect has severe heart failure. Ventricular septal defects are also associated with other forms of congenital cardiac malformations. They are common in corrected transposition of the great arteries, in which systemic atrioventricular valve regurgitation and complete heart block are also frequent. They are always present in a truncus arteriosus communis and in a double-outlet right ventricle that, in the absence of pulmonic stenosis, has the clinical features of an isolated ventricular septal defect.

An isolated ventricular septal defect may occur anywhere in the interventricular septum. At birth, about 90% of these defects occur in the muscular septum, but because these usually close spontaneously within 6 to 12 months of birth, the membranous septum becomes the most common site after infancy. Defects vary in size from minute openings to almost complete absence of the interventricular septum (a common ventricle). Most muscular (except multiple, so-called "Swiss cheese") and perimembranous defects have a high chance of spontaneous closure, unlike large inlet subtricuspid defects, subarterial outlet defects (subaortic as in tetralogy of Fallot

or large subpulmonic as in "supracristal" defects), or doubly committed subarterial ventricular septal defects. Spontaneous partial closure of subpulmonic or doubly committed subarterial defects often involves prolapse of the aortic valve cusp into the defect with development of aortic regurgitation; this form of defect occurs in 5% of whites but in about 35% of Japanese and Chinese. Spontaneous closure of perimembranous defects often is associated with ventricular septal pseudoaneurysm formation; early detection of such an aneurysm indicates a high likelihood of closure.

Clinical Manifestations

The pathophysiology of left-to-right shunting through a ventricular septal defect involves left and right ventricular volume overloads because the extra volume of the left-to-right shunt passes into the right ventricle before passing into the pulmonary artery.

The systolic murmur of a ventricular septal defect is generally harsh and of the plateau type (Fig. 22-35). With a small shunt the murmur may be heard only in early systole; as the shunt increases, however, the murmur becomes holosystolic and ends at the aortic component of the second sound. The intensity of the murmur is not necessarily related to the size of the defect, and loud murmurs may be heard with hemodynamically insignificant defects (maladie de Roger). Loud murmurs are usually associated with systolic thrills. The murmur is generally heard best at the lower left sternal border, and it radiates throughout the precordium, but maximally toward the subxiphoid area. However, with a high subpulmonic ventricular septal defect, the maximal intensity may be at the middle to upper left sternal border, with radiation to the right of the sternum. Occasionally the murmur of a very small defect has a crescendo-decrescendo high-pitched quality and must be distinguished from an innocent murmur. When the left-to-right shunt is large enough to produce a ratio of pulmonary flow to systemic flow higher than 2:1, a middiastolic rumbling murmur may be audible at and inside the apex, and a third sound may appear. As the shunt increases, so does precordial activity.

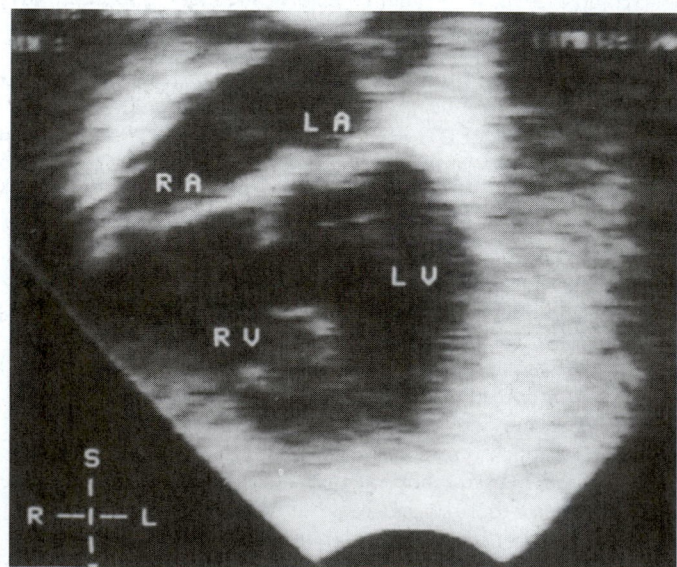

FIGURE 22-35   Posterior muscular ventricular septal defect demonstrated in the apical four-chamber view; the defect is about 1 cm in diameter. I = inferior; L = left; LA = left atrium; LV = left ventricle; R = right; RA = right atrium; RV = right ventricle; S = superior.

If the defect is small or medium in size, marked pulmonary hypertension is absent, and the pulmonic component of the second sound is either of normal or minimally increased intensity. If there is pulmonary hypertension, the pulmonic component of the second sound is accentuated. With a small or moderate-sized shunt, the chest roentgenogram shows no or slight increase in left ventricular and left atrial size and pulmonary vascular markings (Fig. 22-33A). As the volume of shunting increases, cardiac enlargement and pulmonary vascularity also increase (Fig. 22-33B), and pulmonary edema may be seen. Because the shunt is at the ventricular level, the ascending aorta is not dilated. The electrocardiogram is normal if the defect is small; it shows increasing left ventricular hypertrophy as the left-to-right shunt increases, and when there is much right ventricular hypertension, right ventricular hypertrophy is added. A two-dimensional echocardiogram can be used to show the size and position of the ventricular septal defect (Fig. 22-35). Doppler with imaging techniques can localize the defect by detecting disturbed flow in the right ventricle, and color Doppler flow mapping can demonstrate single or even multiple defects. In the most severe form of ventricular septal defect, single ventricle complex, magnetic resonance imaging may help to delineate the anatomy.

If there is a large left-to-right shunt, there are clinical signs and symptoms of volume overload and cardiac failure. In full-term infants this occurs most commonly between 2 and 6 months of age, but it may occur earlier in premature infants. Although the left-to-right shunt should generally be greatest between 2 and 3 months of age, when pulmonary vascular resistance has dropped to its lowest level, congestive heart failure occasionally occurs in term infants under 1 month of age. It is in these infants that the ventricular septal defect is often associated with anemia, significant left-to-right shunt at the atrial or ductus arteriosus levels, or coarctation of the aorta. In addition, infants who have double-outlet right ventricle with ventricular septal defect are at risk of developing congestive failure earlier than expected. This is probably because in fetal life the pulmonary vasculature is perfused with blood that has a higher oxygen tension than normal, and thus, there may be unusually low pulmonary vascular resistance after birth.

Management

Isolated ventricular septal defects are the most common types of congenital heart disease, so that all pediatricians need to know how they can be managed. The decision tree is shown in Table 22-8 and the circled numbers in the table are discussed below.

1. About 3 to 5% of all liveborn babies have small muscular ventricular septal defects, most of which close spontaneously within the next 6 to 12 months. It is neither practical nor reasonable to obtain echocardiograms in all of them, provided there appears to be nothing more than a small ventricular septal defect. Note that a neonate with a large ventricular septal defect usually has no murmur in the newborn nursery; a large defect with a small shunt across it because of a high pulmonary vascular resistance produces little turbulence. In fact, a typical ventricular septal defect murmur heard in the newborn nursery is almost certainly caused by a small defect.
2. Because defects in the perimembranous or muscular portions of the septum have a high incidence of spontaneous closure, it is appropriate to treat them medically for up to 1 year in the hope that surgery can be averted. Several different mechanisms may be responsible for spontaneous closure of a ventricular septal defect. These include growth and hypertrophy of the muscular portion of the defect, formation of a membranous diaphragm (from intimal proliferation), apposition of the septal leaflet of the tricuspid valve

against the defect, or prolapse of the aortic valve cusp, which can lead to aortic regurgitation. When the defect is getting smaller, the systolic murmur may first increase in intensity, but with progressive decrease in size, the murmur becomes softer, and when the defect is extremely small, the murmur becomes shorter and acquires a crescendo-decrescendo high-pitched whistling quality that often portends complete closure. Spontaneous closure may eventually occur in up to 70% of patients, and many of these closures occur by 3 years of age. In a further 25% the defect becomes smaller but may not close completely; however, the hemodynamic effects are significantly reduced. Because of these statistics, if the defect seems to be becoming smaller, surgical correction should be delayed in the hope of spontaneous closure.

Table 22-8 also shows reasons for considering early surgery without waiting for the defect to close spontaneously.

3. Children with trisomy 21 appear to get early pulmonary vascular disease, so that surgery should not be deferred if the defect remains large.
4. Severe social problems are rare reasons for early surgery. These include inability of the parents to bring the child for frequent medical supervision because of distance from the doctor or negligence. In addition, some of these infants are very difficult to manage. They require 2-hourly feeds and consume so much attention that other children in the family are neglected; marriages may even be threatened.
5. Although all infants with large ventricular septal defects grow poorly, with weights usually below the fifth percentile and heights below the 10th percentile, catch-up growth usually occurs once the defect is closed (spontaneously or after surgery). In most of these infants the growth of head circumference is normal, but in a few head growth falls off rapidly by 3 or 4 months of age. Head growth will return to normal if the defect is closed at this time but fails to catch up if surgery is delayed more than 1 to 2 years.
6. If the patient does not need early surgery for one of the reasons mentioned above, it is appropriate to wait for about 12 months in the hope that the defect will close or become smaller.
7. If the shunt remains large after 1 year of age, there has to be a reason for *not* closing a large ventricular septal defect because of the increasing risk of irreversible pulmonary vascular disease. By 2 years of age, about 33% of these children have irreversible pulmonary vascular disease.
8. If the left-to-right shunt becomes smaller, there will be clinical improvement, manifested by decreasing cardiac hyperactivity and heart size, diminishing intensity and eventual disappearance of the middiastolic murmur, decreasing intensity and changing character of the systolic murmur, lessening and then disappearance of tachypnea, improved appetite and growth, and lessening demand for drug therapy. It is crucial not to be misled into thinking that this improvement necessarily indicates a smaller VSD because it might also reflect the development of pulmonary vascular disease or, less often, infundibular stenosis. Echocardiography and perhaps cardiac catheterization are mandatory to make decisions about future management at this stage.
9. In most patients with a ventricular septal defect, severe pulmonary vascular disease does not occur until after 1 year of age. However, it can occur earlier, and this will be indicated by a decrease in the left-to-right shunt, a finding that indicates the need for further studies. With obstructive pulmonary vascular disease there is often little or no left-to-right shunting and no significant right-to-left shunting for several years. However, generally by 5 to 6 years of age, there is increasing cyanosis, particularly during ex-

TABLE 22-8
DECISION TREE FOR MANAGEMENT OF VSD

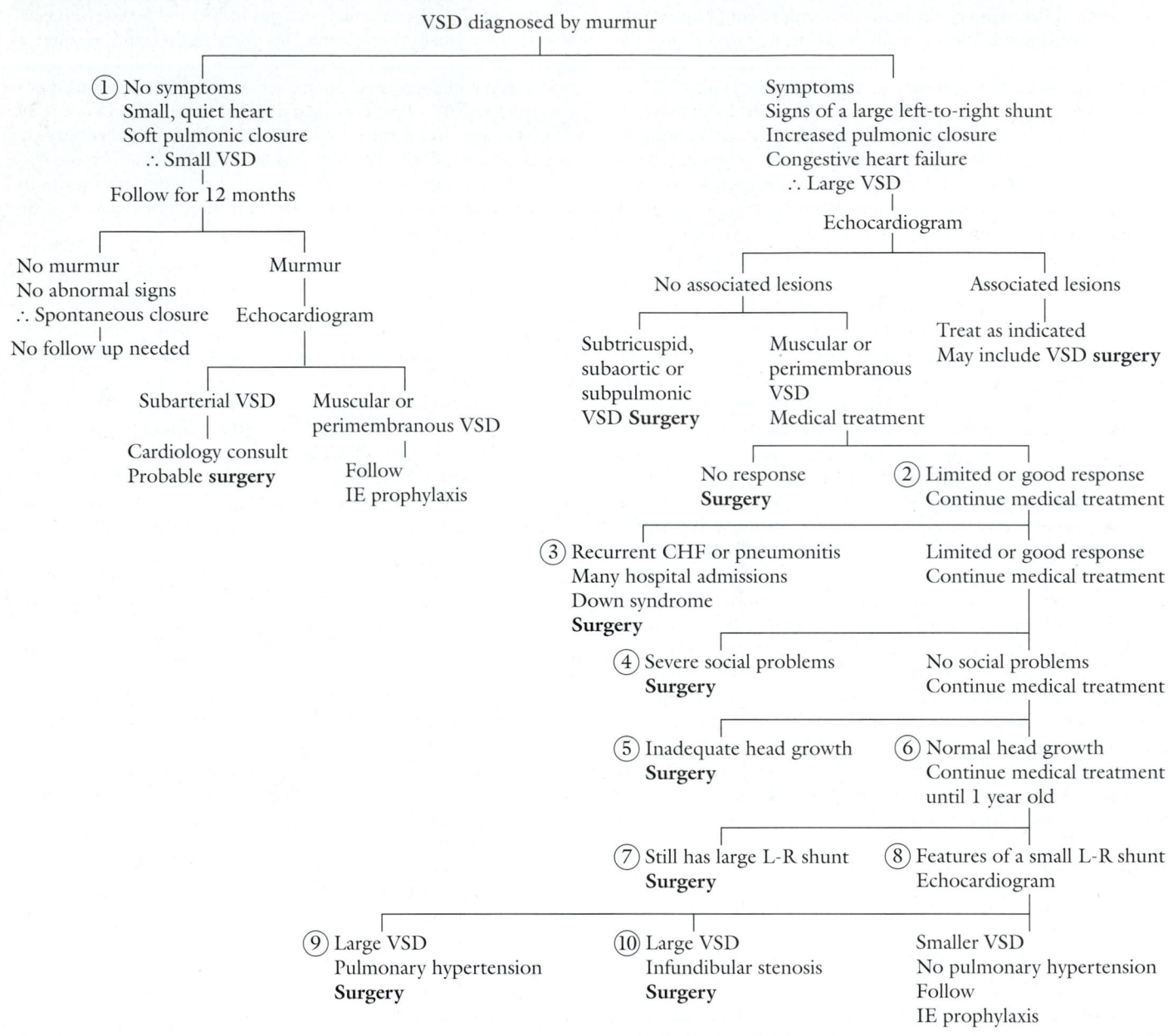

ercise (Eisenmenger syndrome). As severe pulmonary hypertension develops, the main pulmonary artery segment becomes markedly dilated, and the peripheral pulmonary vascular markings on the chest roentgenogram decrease (Fig. 22-36). Obstructive pulmonary vascular disease may progress rapidly in some infants and become irreversible by the age of 12 to 18 months; this should never be allowed to occur. Any doubt as to the cause of any change in clinical status should be investigated by two-dimensional echocardiography with Doppler or if necessary by cardiac catheterization, and there is good reason to consider routinely recatheterizing children with large ventricular septal defects at 9 to 12 months of age to detect early pulmonary vascular disease that is not clinically apparent.

10. Infundibular hypertrophy generally develops fairly rapidly,

and there may be only a short period in which the left-to-right shunting is present. Soon thereafter there will be cyanosis, initially on exercise only but then persistently, and the features of the tetralogy of Fallot can develop. In those infants who develop right ventricular outflow obstruction, the incidence of spontaneous closure of a ventricular septal defect is low; a right-to-left shunt can be further complicated by cerebral thrombosis, embolism, or abscess, and the development of infundibular hypertrophy leads to more difficult surgical repair, so that closure of the defect and infundibular resection, if necessary, should be considered early.

Primary surgical closure of the defects can be done with very low mortality. If primary closure is not feasible because of multiple muscular defects or other complicating factors, then banding the

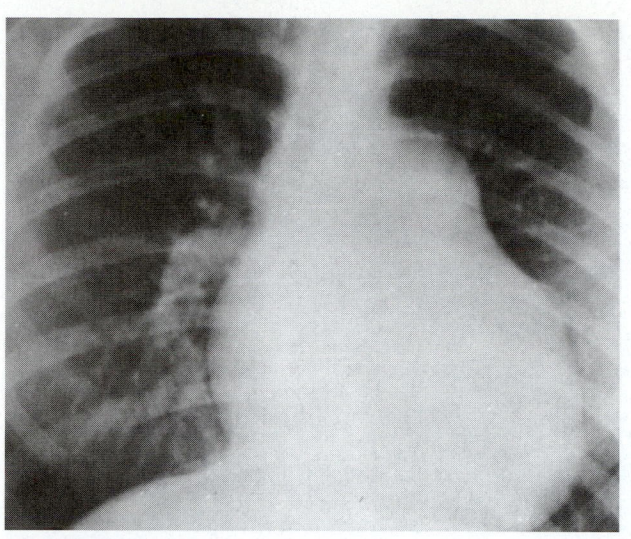

FIGURE 22-36   Chest roentgenogram in a young girl with a ventricular septal defect and pulmonary vascular disease (Eisenmenger syndrome). Marked dilatation of the main pulmonary artery and decreased peripheral vascular markings are shown.

pulmonary artery will decrease the left-to-right shunt, reduce pulmonary arterial blood flow and pressure, and relieve congestive heart failure. Banding has its own complications, and removal of the band when the defect is closed later adds to the mortality of the procedure.

Consequence and Complications

In several infants with significant reductions in left-to-right shunts caused by spontaneous closing of the ventricular septal defects, mid- to late systolic clicks have become audible. In these children, aneurysmal dilatation of the thin membranous septum or tricuspid valve tissue that has grown to close the defect has occurred, with bulging of pseudoaneurysm into the right ventricle. A small opening often present at the apex of the pseudoaneurysm allows a small left-to-right shunt. Normally the defect closes, and the pseudoaneurysm slowly shrinks, but rarely it may enlarge progressively. These pseudoaneurysms can be demonstrated by echocardiography.

A number of infants have developed progressive aortic insufficiency associated with ventricular septal defect, particularly if it is subarterial. There is prolapse of an aortic valve leaflet with dilatation of the aortic valve sinus, and rupture of the aortic sinus or cusp may occur. The development of insufficiency has been attributed to stress on the unsupported aortic valve cusp and perhaps suction on it by the jet of the shunt passing through the defect. Even with a small ventricular septal defect, or one showing evidence of closure, aortic insufficiency requires surgical closure of the defect to prevent further prolapse. It may in fact be prudent to close subarterial ventricular septal defects even before evidence of aortic valve cusp involvement is apparent.

Infective endocarditis is an additional problem; rarely, it can occur even after spontaneous closure of the defect. If infective endocarditis involves the tricuspid leaflet sealing the ventricular septal defect, rupture may occur and produce a direct left-ventricular-to-right-atrial communication. Antibiotic prophylaxis should therefore be continued in those children with small defects; most pediatric cardiologists do not advocate prophylaxis once complete spontaneous closure has been demonstrated.

LEVOTRANSPOSITION OF THE GREAT ARTERIES

Levotransposition (*l*-transposition) occurs when the primitive cardiac tube loops to the left instead of to the right during early development. The anatomic left ventricle is on the right side and connects the right atrium with its tricuspid valve to the pulmonary artery. The anatomic right ventricle on the left side receives oxygenated blood from the left atrium through a mitral valve and ejects into an anteriorly placed left-sided aorta. There is thus *l*-transposition of the great arteries and inversion of the ventricles, but the combination of discordant atrioventricular and discordant ventriculoarterial connections allows normal flow of venous blood to the lungs and arterial blood to the body; hence, the designation (physiologically) corrected transposition.

If there are no other lesions, people with this anomaly may live normal lives, but almost all have ventricular septal defects, many have pulmonic stenosis, some have an Ebstein-like malformation of the left-sided systemic tricuspid valve that produces left-sided atrioventricular regurgitation, and many have defects of atrioventricular conduction (particularly complete atrioventricular block). Those with normal conduction at birth develop complete heart block at a rate of 1 to 2% per year. The symptoms and signs depend on the severity and nature of these associated lesions.

In addition to the murmurs of ventricular septal defects or pulmonic stenosis, these patients characteristically have a loud second heart sound, often single, best heard at the upper left sternal border because of the high left anterior position of the aortic valve. The electrocardiogram may show atrioventricular conduction defects and will show right- or left-sided hypertrophy as appropriate for associated lesions. In about 80% of these patients the electrocardiogram shows Q waves in right chest leads and no Q waves on the left, the pattern reflecting the activation of the septum from right to left.

Frequently the chest roentgenogram indicates the diagnosis because the levoposed aorta produces a straight shoulder on the left heart border (Fig. 22-37). Echocardiograms disclose the abnormal position of the great arteries, the morphology of the right- and left-sided ventricles, as well as another typical anatomic feature, the anteroposterior orientation of the ventricular septum.

Surgical correction of these lesions is more hazardous than correction of similar lesions without ventricular inversion. The abnormal conduction system increases the risk of surgically produced complete atrioventricular block when a ventricular septal defect is closed. Large coronary arteries often run across the outflow tract of the pulmonic ventricle, where an incision would have to be made. The pulmonary artery is very posterior, so that correcting pulmonic stenosis is difficult, particularly because the obstruction is seldom a valvar stenosis but more often a subpulmonic fibromuscular narrowing or else a mass of accessory tissue from the adjacent mitral valve. For these reasons, surgery is not advised if patients are doing well. If they deteriorate, then the pulmonary artery may be banded for a large left-to-right shunt, or else an aortopulmonary shunt is done to palliate severe cyanosis. Complete correction should be attempted only by a skilled surgeon and only after the risks have been fully assessed.

ATRIAL SEPTAL DEFECTS

The development of the atrial septum is discussed in Sec. 22.1.1. Interference with the development of the septum primum at its lower margin, associated with abnormal development of the en-

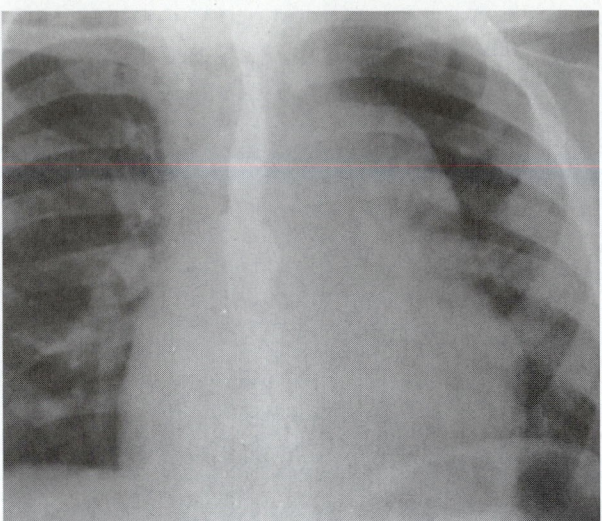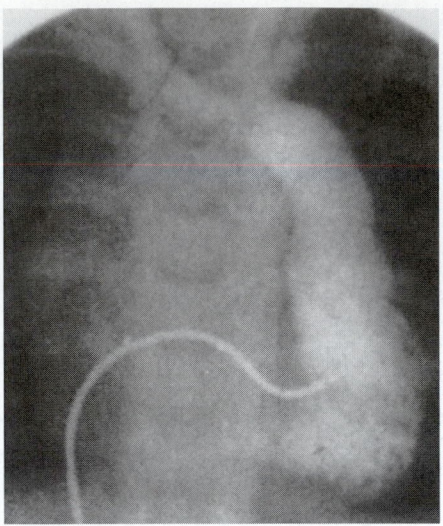

FIGURE 22-37 On the **left** is the typical chest roentgenogram in corrected transposition, with the filled-in upper left heart border resulting from the levoposed aorta, as shown in the angiogram on the **right**.

docardial cushions, produces an ostium primum atrial septal defect with no inferior rim of atrial septal tissue. This lesion is generally associated with abnormalities of the mitral and tricuspid valves (which form from the endocardial cushions) as well as defective formation of the upper portion of the interventricular septum.

A second type of atrial septal defect is the so-called ostium secundum defect. This is a defect in the central portion of the septum in relation to the foramen ovale; it results from inadequate closure of the central hole in the septum primum by the septum secundum and is more appropriately termed a fossa ovalis defect.

A third type of atrial septal defect is the sinus venosus defect, that is, in the superior portion of the atrial septum, and generally extends into the superior vena cava.

INCOMPETENT (PATENT) FORAMEN OVALE With the onset of ventilation after birth, pulmonary venous return increases markedly, and left atrial pressure rises. The foramen ovale is therefore normally functionally closed by the membranous valve of the foramen ovale, apposed to the crista dividens and the lower portion of the septum secundum. Although normally functionally closed shortly after birth, the foramen ovale often remains probe-patent. When pulmonary vascular resistance does not fall normally after birth, the resultant pulmonary hypertension and increased right ventricular end-diastolic pressure and right atrial pressure often cause right-to-left shunting across the foramen ovale and systemic hypoxemia.

In some infants, although the normal atrial pressure relationships occur after birth, the valve of the foramen ovale does not completely cover the foramen, either because the valve is too short or because the foramen ovale has become enlarged and stretched in infants in whom left atrial pressure and volume are increased, as with patent ductus arteriosus, ventricular septal defect, or left ventricular outflow obstruction secondary to aortic stenosis or coarctation. Significant left-to-right shunting may occur through an incompetent foramen ovale when left atrial pressure is high. If the cause of the increased left atrial pressure is relieved, atrial shunting generally decreases or disappears. In some congenital heart defects, survival after birth depends on persistent patency of the foramen ovale. These defects include tricuspid and mitral atresia and total anomalous pulmonary venous connection. In aortopulmonary

transposition a patent foramen ovale may be the only communication between the systemic and pulmonary circulations. Right-to-left shunting across the foramen ovale is also associated with right ventricular obstructive lesions such as pulmonic stenosis and with pulmonary hypertension, particularly in newborns.

OSTIUM SECUNDUM ATRIAL SEPTAL DEFECT Ostium secundum defects vary in size from a small defect to one in which only a rim of atrial tissue separates the defect from the AV valves. Usually ostium secundum defects are isolated lesions, but some may be associated with partial anomalous pulmonary venous connection (usually draining the right lung) or pulmonic stenosis.

The magnitude of left-to-right shunting depends on the size of the defect, the relationship of inflow resistances of the left and right ventricles, and the outflow resistance of each ventricle. Small atrial communications are therefore associated with small shunts. Large defects are associated with large left-to-right shunts if there is a low inflow resistance of the right ventricle and a low pulmonary resistance. The effect of a large shunt at the atrial level is a marked increase in flow through the right atrium and right ventricle. This extra volume load is tolerated well by the right ventricle because it is handling the increased volume at a low pressure. Therefore, cardiac failure is unusual in infancy and, when it occurs, is generally precipitated by either a combination of defects or some other complication.

Children with large atrial septal defects are generally asymptomatic. However, when there is pulmonary hypertension because of congenital or acquired lung disease, especially in preterm infants, the atrial septal defect may contribute to the symptoms as well as to right-to-left intracardiac shunting. The increased right ventricular volume load causes precordial hyperactivity along the left sternal border. The first heart sound is normal, and the second heart sound is characteristically widely split, with absence of the normal respiratory variation in the width of splitting (Fig. 22-34). Both components of the second sound are of normal intensity. Although fixed splitting of the second sound is characteristic in older children, this sign is occasionally absent, especially in infants or when the communication is not large. Several mechanisms have been invoked to explain the wide splitting; increased right ventricular stroke volume, prolongation of the systolic ejection period, and a low pulmonary vascular impedance are those most generally accepted. If there is pulmonary hypertension, the second sound may be less widely split; this may account for the lack of splitting in early infancy, when pulmonary vascular resistance has not fallen to its normal low level.

Flow across the atrial septal defect is not associated with a murmur; however, a long systolic ejection murmur that is crescendo-decrescendo in type is generally heard at the upper left sternal border as a result of increased flow across the right ventricular outflow tract and pulmonic valve. The murmur associated with atrial septal defects can usually be differentiated from an innocent pulmonary flow murmur, which is usually shorter, by the response to the Valsalva maneuver. When intrathoracic pressure is increased, systemic venous return is immediately reduced, right ventricular stroke volume decreases immediately, and the intensity of an innocent pulmonary flow murmur suddenly decreases. However, with a large atrial septal defect, the left-to-right shunt across the atrial communication maintains right ventricular stroke volume for several beats despite the decrease of systemic venous return; thus, there is little, if any, change in the intensity of the murmur in the first three to four beats. If the left-to-right shunt is fairly large, there is often a low-frequency, rumbling, early or middiastolic murmur caused by increased flow across the tricuspid valve that is heard best at the lower left sternal border. Also, a prominent third heart sound is often heard at the lower left sternal border.

The chest roentgenogram shows enlargement of the right atrium and ventricle and sometimes the outflow region of the right ventricle. The main pulmonary artery is dilated, and pulmonary vascular markings are increased. However, the relationship between prominence of the pulmonary vascularity and the magnitude of the left-to-right shunt is unreliable. The electrocardiogram generally shows right axis deviation with normal atrial complexes and normal conduction. There is right ventricular hypertrophy with a typical rsR′ or rSR′ pattern in the right precordial leads, and the S wave in the inferior leads is usually notched.

Two-dimensional echocardiography shows an increase in diastolic size of the right ventricle together with paradoxic motion of the interventricular septum. Other similar hemodynamic disturbances, such as partial anomalous pulmonary venous return and pulmonary or tricuspid regurgitation, may give similar findings. Septal dropout is often seen, indicating the site of the atrial septal defect, and color Doppler clearly demonstrates the flow patterns and often the defect itself. A negative shadow in the right atrium during contrast echocardiography can delineate the defect (Fig. 22-23).

Diagnostic cardiac catheterization and angiocardiography have been replaced by echocardiography.

Persistent right-to-left shunting is unusual in ostium secundum defects, but transient right-to-left shunting is common after any Valsalva-like maneuver. However, with sinus venosus defects there may be right-to-left shunting from the superior vena cava into the left atrium, and slight arterial oxygen desaturation may be found. Infective endocarditis is rare in uncomplicated secundum atrial septal defects. Obstructive pulmonary vascular disease may occur, but not usually before the late second decade or third decade. This becomes evident by a decrease in the physical findings associated with the left-to-right shunt and later by right-to-left shunting. It is concern about the possible development of pulmonary vascular disease that generally leads to surgical closure of the communication. Atrial arrhythmias, especially atrial fibrillation or flutter (probably caused by atrial enlargement), congestive heart failure, mitral in-

competence, and strokes from paradoxic embolization may occur in adult life, and these are added reasons for considering closure of atrial defects in children. However, several years after simple surgical closure, atrial arrhythmias still can develop. Nonsurgical closure using an umbrella- or clamshell-like device manipulated into the defect by means of a large catheter is being investigated as an alternative for surgical closure of small or medium-sized defects (see Sec. 22.2.6).

OSTIUM PRIMUM DEFECTS AND ATRIOVENTRICULAR SEPTAL (ENDOCARDIAL CUSHION) DEFECTS   Ostrium primum and atrioventricular septal defects result from arrested or abnormal development of the endocardial cushions in the primitive atrioventricular (AV) canal; they range in severity from a small ostium primum atrial septal defect to a complete AV canal. The severity and type of anatomic defect depend on which endocardial cushions are involved and the stage of developmental failure. Because the cushions are involved in the development of both atrial and ventricular septa, as well as mitral and tricuspid valves, many different combinations of abnormalities in this region are found. They may occur as isolated lesions in otherwise normal infants; however, they are often seen with other congenital abnormalities in trisomy 21 (Down), asplenia or polysplenia, and Ellis-van Creveld syndromes.

Fetal somatic development is essentially normal; however, there is a high incidence of secondary hemodynamic alterations in the aorta in this group of lesions. Subaortic outflow obstruction, although often of only minor severity, is common; when associated with the potential obligatory shunt in utero, it may result in significant alterations in the patterns of blood flow during fetal life. Therefore, aortic isthmus narrowing and juxtaductal coarctation are found in many infants with this defect.

OSTIUM PRIMUM DEFECT   Ostium primum defect is the most benign form of endocardial cushion defect; it is also termed partial AV canal defect. The central portion of the atrial septum in the region of the mitral and tricuspid valve rings is absent, and the defect is usually large. The anterior (or septal) mitral valve leaflet is displaced and usually cleft. The tricuspid valve is generally not involved but may also have a small cleft in the septal leaflet. The magnitude of the atrial left-to-right shunt is controlled by the same mechanisms in ostium primum as in secundum atrial septal defects. The clinical features are similar and include right ventricular hyperactivity, increased pulmonary blood flow, and a widely split second sound. In addition to the right ventricular outflow murmur and the tricuspid middiastolic flow murmur, murmurs of mitral or tricuspid regurgitation, or both, may be present if significant clefts in these valves are present. However, marked regurgitation is unusual, particularly in infancy and early childhood. The electrocardiogram characteristically shows left axis deviation, generally in the $-20°$ to $-60°$ range, and right ventricular hypertrophy with an rsR′ pattern in right precordial leads. Chest roentgenographic findings depend on the magnitude of left-to-right shunting. Two-dimensional echocardiography and color Doppler flow mapping usually clearly delineate the anatomy. Congestive heart failure and arrhythmias occur, usually in late teenage or early adult life.

COMPLETE AV CANAL DEFECT   Complete AV canal defects involve failure of development of separate tricuspid and mitral valve rings. In addition to the ostium primum defect, there is a ventricular septal defect in the posterior portion of the interventricular septum and clefts in the septal leaflets of both the tricuspid and mitral valves. The anterior and posterior segments of each septal leaflet are not separated (as in normal development) but join each other through the defect, so that in the most severe form there is a large common anterior mitral-tricuspid valve leaflet as well as a smaller common posterior mitral-tricuspid valve leaflet. The earlier the stage of arrested development of the endocardial cushions has occurred, the larger the ventricular septal defect and the more primitive the development of the AV valves. Although the most severe form may occur as an isolated defect, it may be associated with other complex anomalies such as asplenia or polysplenia syndromes and single ventricle.

In general, the more severe or primitive the defect, the more marked the clinical manifestations. The ventricular septal defect behaves like any other ventricular septal defect in producing a left ventricular volume load and, if it is large, pulmonary hypertension and a right ventricular pressure load. The characteristic murmur of a ventricular septal defect will be present, as will a middiastolic rumble caused by increased pulmonary venous return with increased diastolic flow across the mitral valve. If the cleft in the mitral valve is significant, mitral regurgitation may be present, and an apical pansystolic blowing murmur may be heard. The middiastolic rumble will then be further accentuated by the even larger flow across the mitral valve, and left ventricular enlargement will be more prominent. The ostium primum defect portion of the complete canal will present with physical findings similar to those in an isolated atrial septal defect; these include right ventricular volume overload, a tricuspid diastolic flow rumble, and a right ventricular outflow murmur. Should tricuspid regurgitation be present, a pansystolic blowing murmur in the tricuspid area and systolic pulsation of the jugular veins may be evident, and the increased flow across the tricuspid valve will accentuate the middiastolic murmur. Both the atrial and ventricular shunts are dependent. However, often the cleft in the misplaced mitral valve allows ventricular blood to pass through it and the ostium primum defect to enter the right atrium, so that there is an obligatory shunt from left ventricle to right atrium. There may at times be minor right-to-left shunting and mild cyanosis.

Heart failure often occurs by 2 months after birth. However, symptoms may develop very early in infancy if there is an obligatory large left-ventricle-to-right-atrium shunt or with significant AV valve dysfunction; an additional defect, such as a patent ductus arteriosus, may also lead to early symptoms. These symptoms are primarily related to severe congestive heart failure and include tachypnea, sweating, and difficulty with feeding. Systemic cardiac output is generally low, and the infant then has poor pulses, tachycardia, hepatomegaly, and peripheral pallor. Marked cardiomegaly is common.

As with ostium primum defects, the electrocardiogram shows left axis deviation (superior axis), but in most complete AV canal defects it is even more negative, in the range $-60°$ to $-150°$. The frontal-plane vector loop is counterclockwise. The P-R interval is often prolonged. Ventricular and atrial hypertrophy depend on the level of maximal shunting and the amount of AV valve regurgitation. The left axis deviation is not pathognomonic of an atrioventricular septal defect; it may also be found with double-outlet right ventricle, with tricuspid or pulmonary atresia, or even in normal children. The absence of left axis deviation does not exclude the diagnosis of an atrioventricular septal defect but is strongly against it. Chest roentgenographic findings depend on the level of shunting and the amount of AV valve regurgitation. Two-dimensional echocardiography and Doppler color flow mapping yield specific anatomic information and permit detecting differences between in-

complete and complete forms of this defect. Magnetic resonance imaging may contribute to anatomic detail.

Infants with this defect are at high risk of developing obstructive pulmonary vascular disease from severe pulmonary hypertension and a large left-to-right shunt, so that early surgery is advisable. Many infants have poor responses to vigorous medical management, although this may buy a little time. Complete surgical repair of these lesions can be done in infancy with a mortality rate of about 5 to 10% providing the two ventricles are about of equal size. Infants with Down syndrome tend to have a more favorable anatomy for correction. The availability of transesophageal echocardiography during surgery adds to the effectiveness of surgery, particularly when mitral regurgitation is a major component. If the ventricles are unbalanced, then some form of single ventricle repair can be done. If for some reason complete correction is not appropriate, intractable cardiac failure may be improved by pulmonary artery banding, which will increase the outflow resistance of the right ventricle and so decrease the amount of dependent shunting. However, in most infants with complete AV canal defects the large left-ventricle-to-right-atrium shunt or AV valve regurgitation will be unaffected by pulmonary artery banding.

PARTIAL ANOMALOUS PULMONARY VENOUS CONNECTION

Partial anomalous pulmonary venous connection without an associated atrial septal defect is rare. The anomalous pulmonary veins almost always drain either the complete right lung or a portion of it, and they may connect with the superior vena cava or directly with the right atrium. In addition, there is a specific entity (scimitar syndrome) in which the pulmonary veins from the lower lobe and sometimes the middle lobe of the right lung drain by a common channel into the inferior vena cava. Associated with this is underdevelopment as well as lobar sequestration of that portion of the lung. The chest roentgenogram in scimitar syndrome is typical, and the anomalous vessel is generally seen easily. The clinical presentation of these lesions resembles that of secundum atrial septal defects, except that the second heart sound is generally normally split. Partial anomalous pulmonary venous connection, when associated with an atrial septal defect, does not generally contribute any specific clinical features.

References

Alzamora-Castro V, Battilana G, Abugattas R, et al: Patent ductus arteriosus and high altitude. Am J Cardiol 5:761, 1960

Campbell M: Natural history of persistent ductus arteriosus. Br Heart J 30:4, 1968

Campbell M: Natural history of atrial septal defect. Br Heart J 32:820, 1970

Chin AJ, Keane JF, Norwood WI, et al: Repair of common atrioventricular canal in infancy. J Thorac Cardiovasc Surg 84:437, 1982

Clyman RI, Heymann MA: Pharmacology of the ductus arteriosus. Pediatr Clin North Am 28:77, 1981

Dickinson DF, Arnold R, Wilkinson JL: Ventricular septal defect in children born in Liverpool 1960 to 1969. Br Heart J 46:47, 1981

Feldt RH, Porter CJ, Edwards WD, et al: AVSDs. In: Emmanoulides GC, Allen HD, Riemenschneider TA, et al, eds: Heart Disease in Infants, Children, and Adolescents. Baltimore, Williams & Wilkins, 1995:704

Fournier A, Young ML, Garcia OL, et al: Electrophysiologic cardiac function before and after surgery in children with atrioventricular canal. Am J Cardiol 57:1137, 1986

Freedom RM, White RD, Pieroni DR, et al: The natural history of the so-called aneurysm of the membranous ventricular septum in childhood. Circulation 49:375, 1974

Frontera-Izquierdo P, Cabezuelo-Huerta G: Natural and modified history of isolated ventricular septal defect: a 17-year study. Pediatr Cardiol 13:193, 1992

Godart F, Rey C, Francart C, et al: Two-dimensional echocardiographic and color Doppler measurements of atrial septal defect, and comparison with the balloon-stretched diameter. Am J Cardiol 72:1095, 1993

Gray DT, Fyler DC, Walker AM, et al: Clinical outcomes and costs of trans-catheter as compared with surgical closure of patent ductus arteriosus. The Patent Ductus Arteriosus Closure Comparative Study Group. N Engl J Med 329:1517, 1993

Henze A, Huttunen H, Björk VO: Ruptured sinus of Valsalva aneurysms. Scand J Thorac Cardiovasc Surg 17:249, 1983

Hiraishi S, Agata Y, Nowatari M, et al: Incidence and natural course of trabecular ventricular septal defects: two-dimensional echocardiography and color Doppler flow imaging study. J Pediatr 120:409, 1992

Hobbs RE, Millit HD, Raghavan PV, et al: Coronary artery fistulae: a 10-year review. Cleve Clin Q 49:191, 1982

Hoffman HJ, Chuang S, Hendrick EB, Humphreys RP: Aneurysm of the vein of Galen. Experience at The Hospital for Sick Children, Toronto. J Neurosurg 57:316, 1982

Hoffman JIE: Ventricular septal defect: indications for therapy in infants. Pediatr Clin North Am 18:1091, 1971

Hoffman JIE, Heymann MA: Normal pulmonary circulation. In: Scarpelli EM, ed: Pulmonary Physiology: Fetus, Newborn, Child, Adolescent. Philadelphia, Lea & Febiger, 1990:233

Hoffman JIE, Rudolph AM, Heymann MA: Pulmonary vascular disease with congenital heart lesions: pathologic features and causes. Circulation 64:873, 1981

Hornberger LK, Sahn DJ, Krabill KA, et al: Elucidation of the natural history of ventricular septal defects by serial Doppler color flow mapping studies. J Am Coll Cardiol 13:1111, 1989

Kano Y, Abe T, Tanaka M, et al: Electrophysiological abnormalities before and after surgery for atrial septal defect. J Electrocardiol 26:225, 1993

Kidd L, Driscoll DJ, Gersony WM, et al: Second natural history study of congenital heart defects. Results of treatment of patients with ventricular septal defects. Circulation 87:38, 1993

King RM, Puga FJ, Danielson GK, et al: Prognostic features and surgical treatment of partial atrioventricular canal. Circulation 74:142, 1986

Kirklin JW, Barratt-Boyes BG: Congenital aneurysm of the sinus of Valsalva. In: Kirklin JW, Barratt-Boyes BG, eds: Cardiac Surgery. New York, Wiley, 1993:825

Konstantinides S, Kasper W, Geibel A, et al: Detection of left-to-right shunt in atrial septal defect by negative contrast echocardiography: a comparison of transthoracic and transesophageal approach. Am Heart J 126:909, 1993

Mahoney LT, Truesdell SC, Krzmarzick TR, et al: Atrial septal defects that present in infancy. Am J Dis Child 140:1115, 1986

Mehta AV, Chidambaram B: Ventricular septal defect in the first year of life. Am J Cardiol 70:364, 1992

Meyer RA, Korfhagen JC, Covitz W, et al: Long-term follow-up study after closure of secundum atrial septal defect in children: an echocardiographic study. Am J Cardiol 50:143, 1982

Moller JH, Patton C, Varco RL, Lillehei CW: Late results (30 to 35 years) after operative closure of isolated ventricular septal defect from 1954 to 1960. Am J Cardiol 68:1491, 1991

Morris CD, Menashe VD: 25-year mortality after surgical repair of congenital heart defect in childhood. A population-based cohort study. JAMA 266:3447, 1991

Murphy JG, Gersh BJ, McGoon MD, et al: Long-term outcome after surgical repair of isolated atrial septal defect. Follow-up at 27 to 32 years. N Engl J Med 323:1645, 1990

Musewe NM, Smallhorn JF, Burrows PE, et al: Echocardiographic and Doppler evaluation of the aortic arch and brachiocephalic vessels in cerebral and systemic arteriovenous fistulas. Pediatr Cardiol 12:1529, 1988

Pool PE, Vogel JHK, Blount SG Jr: Congenital unilateral absence of a pulmonary artery. Am J Cardiol 9:706, 1962

Ramaciotti C, Keren A, Silverman NH: Importance of pseudoaneurysms of the ventricular septum in the natural history of isolated perimembranous ventricular septal defects. Am J Cardiol 57:268, 1986

Roguin N, Du Z-D, Barak M, et al: High prevalence of muscular ventricular septal defect in neonates. J Am Coll Cardiol 26:1545, 1995

Samánek M: Children with congenital heart disease: probability of natural survival. Pediatr Cardiol 13:152, 1992

Schmidt KG, Cassidy SC, Silverman NH, et al: Doubly committed subarterial ventricular septal defects: echocardiographic features and surgical implications. J Am Coll Cardiol 12:1538, 1988

Silverman NH, Zuberbuhler JR, Anderson RH: AVSDs: cross-sectional echocardiographic and morphologic comparisons. Int J Cardiol 13:309, 1986

Smallhorn JF: Patent ductus arteriosus—evaluation by echocardiography. Echocardiography 4:101, 1987

Soto B, Ceballos R, Kirklin JW: Ventricular septal defect: a surgical viewpoint. Pediatr Cardiol 14:1291, 1989

Williams RG: Doppler color flow mapping and prediction of ventricular septal defect outcome. J Am Coll Cardiol 13:1119, 1989

Winslow TM, Redberg RF, Foster E, et al: Transesophageal echocardiographic detection of abnormalities of the tricuspid valve in adults associated with spontaneous closure of perimembranous ventricular septal defect. Am J Cardiol 70:967, 1992

22.3.3   Regurgitant Lesions

James H. Moller

Each of the cardiac valves may be affected pathologically so that the valve orifice is unguarded, and blood regurgitates across it from the higher-pressure to the lower-pressure region. Because of retrograde blood flow across the valve, there is increased anterograde blood flow as well that reflects not only the normal flow (the cardiac output) but also the returning regurgitant volume. The anatomic consequence of regurgitation is dilatation of the cardiac chamber or great vessel on either side of the insufficient valve. In each condition associated with regurgitation of the left or right side of the heart, the left or right ventricle is dilated proportionally to the degree of regurgitation. Because of the normally higher pressures in and the conical shape of the left ventricle, it tolerates regurgitant lesions less well than does the crescent-shaped right ventricle, which functions normally at a low systolic pressure. Thus, congestive cardiac failure is more common in the former than the latter.

The diagnostic process with a regurgitant lesion has three steps. The first is recognition that the patient has a regurgitant lesion, the major diagnostic clue being the typical murmur. All regurgitant murmurs include an isovolumetric period. In mitral and tricuspid insufficiency, the murmur typically begins with the first heart sound, thus encompassing the isovolumetric contraction period and extending into the ejection phase of systole. The murmurs of aortic and pulmonary insufficiency begin with the second heart sound, thus encompassing the isovolumetric relaxation period, and extend further into diastole. The specific valve involved can usually be identified by the location on the thorax where it is heard maximally and by the pitch. The four major sites of cardiac auscultation are the aortic (upper right sternal border), pulmonic (upper left sternal border), mitral (cardiac apex), and tricuspid (lower left sternal border) areas. The murmurs of regurgitation of the various valves are heard best in these respective areas. In most patients, the murmurs of aortic and mitral regurgitation are high pitched, from the large pressure difference across the valve, and thus are heard better with a diaphragm. The murmurs of pulmonary and tricuspid regurgitation are low pitched because of the low pressure difference ordinarily present across these valves and thus are heard better with a bell. The murmurs are usually characteristic enough to allow a correct clinical diagnosis.

The second step is assessing the severity of the condition by evaluating the effect of the regurgitant volume on the cardiac chamber or great artery on either side of the regurgitant valve. This can be done simply by the history, physical examination, electrocardiogram, and chest x-ray.

Third, the possible etiologic factors and anatomic cause of the particular valvar abnormality leading to regurgitation must be sought. It is not enough to be satisfied with a diagnosis of aortic insufficiency, for example, without efforts to determine its etiology. Etiologic factors often determine natural history, methods of treatment, and prognosis.

With the availability of echocardiography, more precise assessment of hemodynamics and anatomy can be obtained. This diagnostic technique, however, is often unnecessary at the initial evaluation or at each subsequent visit if the physician can apply basic clinical skills and diagnostic techniques, which are often less expensive.

AORTIC REGURGITATION

The primary finding of aortic regurgitation is a high-pitched, early diastolic murmur that starts at the aortic component of the second heart sound. The length and loudness of the murmur increase with the severity of regurgitation.

Most children with this condition are asymptomatic, but if it is at least moderately severe, they have fatigue on exercise. Those with either significant chronic regurgitation or acutely developing regurgitation may develop congestive heart failure. With acute onset of aortic regurgitation, as from ruptured sinus of Valsalva (discussed below), symptoms develop abruptly.

With moderate or severe aortic regurgitation, the pulse pressure is widened, the systolic pressure being elevated by the augmented left ventricular stroke volume (cardiac output plus regurgitant volume), and the diastolic pressure is lowered because of "runoff" into the left ventricle as well as baroceptor-induced peripheral vascular vasodilatation. On auscultation, an aortic systolic ejection murmur is frequently present from the augmented forward flow across the aortic valve and/or structural abnormality of the valve itself. There may be at the apex a low-pitched, middiastolic murmur (Austin Flint murmur) attributed to the regurgitant aortic jet striking the anterior leaflet of the mitral valve, making it vibrate.

An electrocardiogram may show tall R waves in the left precordial leads from left ventricular dilatation. T waves become flat or inverted in these leads if coronary perfusion is impaired by low aortic diastolic pressure.

Chest x-rays are normal if regurgitation is mild but show cardiac enlargement with a left ventricular contour when moderate or severe regurgitation is present. The ascending aorta may appear prominent along the upper right side of the mediastinum from either the large stroke volume or anatomic features secondary to the condition causing the regurgitation, such as Marfan syndrome or aortic stenosis.

The echocardiogram is very helpful in assessing the hemodynamics and anatomic causes of this regurgitation. The regurgitant jet can be identified and assessed by color echo Doppler; the breadth and extent of the jet correlate with the degree of regurgitation. In addition, measurement of left ventricular dimensions can

assess the regurgitant volume, and the ejection or shortening fraction the ventricular response to the volume overload. The appearance of the aortic valve, surrounding structures, and ascending aorta is critical to determine the underlying cardiac abnormality or etiologic factor.

Regurgitation from the aorta into the left ventricle results from a variety of congenital or acquired cardiac conditions, which occasionally coexist (Table 22-9).

Congenital aortic stenosis usually occurs secondary to a bicuspid valve that during childhood may develop minimal aortic regurgitation, recognizable only as a soft murmur and minimal regurgitation on echo Doppler. The usual treatment of moderate or severe aortic stenosis is by valvotomy or valvuloplasty. After either procedure, the degree of regurgitation increases, but rarely enough to result in symptoms or more than minimal hemodynamic disturbance, except in an occasional patient following balloon valvuloplasty.

TABLE 22-9

IMPORTANT ANATOMIC CAUSES OF VALVAR REGURGITATION

Aortic regurgitation
  Bicuspid aortic valve
  Aortic stenosis following valvotomy or valvuloplasty
  Membranous subaortic stenosis
  Infective endocarditis
  Sinus of Valsalva aneurysm
  Aortico–left ventricular tunnel
  Ventricular septal defect with prolapsed aortic cusp
  Marfan syndrome
  Rheumatic fever
  Infective endocarditis
Mitral regurgitation
  Mitral valve prolapse
    Idiopathic
    Marfan syndrome and other connective tissue disorders
    Mucopolysaccharidosis
    Atrial septal defect
  Rheumatic fever
  Infective endocarditis
  Primary abnormalities of valve
    Cleft in anterior leaflet
    Double orifice
  Secondary to myocardial ischemia
    Anomalous left coronary
    Kawasaki disease
    Neonatal myocardial ischemia
  Secondary to other cardiac anomalies
    Endocardiac cushion defect
    Severe aortic stenosis
    Hypertrophic cardiomyopathy
Pulmonary regurgitation
  Postoperative valvotomy, valvuloplasty, or outflow patch placement
  Absent pulmonary valve with/without associated ventricular septal defect
Tricuspid regurgitation
  Transient tricuspid insufficiency of the neonate
  Ebstein malformation
  Secondary to right ventricular dysfunction
    Postoperative atrial baffle
    Postoperative right ventriculotomy
    Severe pulmonary stenosis
  Infective endocarditis

In *membranous subaortic stenosis,* the jet through the membrane, which is located slightly below the aortic valve, strikes one of the aortic valve cusps, distorting and thickening it, so it may become mildly incompetent.

Sinus of Valsalva aneurysm results from separation between the aortic media and the heart at the level of the annulus fibrosis, as the aneurysm is below the level of the valve. The aneurysm can occur in any of the three aortic sinuses and may rupture into the adjacent cardiac chamber. With progressive prolapse, aortic regurgitation develops. If the aneurysm ruptures, congestive cardiac failure and a murmur of aortic regurgitation develop abruptly.

Aortico–left ventricular tunnel is a rare condition in which a vascular-like structure arises above the aortic valve and passes through the ventricular septum to the left ventricle. This results in findings resembling significant aortic valve regurgitation.

With a *ventricular septal defect* adjacent to the aortic annulus, usually a *subpulmonary ventricular septal defect,* the support of the adjacent aortic cusp is weakened. The cusp tends to sag into the left ventricle, and the left-to-right shunt through the ventricular septal defect exerts force on the cusp through the defect. The presence of the cusp in the ventricular septal defect tends to narrow it, while the aortic regurgitation worsens. The findings are those of a ventricular septal defect plus aortic insufficiency. Repair of the defect may buttress the aortic cusp sufficiently to reduce the aortic regurgitation and obviate surgery on the aortic valve.

Marfan syndrome is associated with dilated sinuses of Valsalva and ascending aorta. Aortic regurgitation that may be severe can result. The echocardiographic findings are diagnostic, showing greatly dilated aortic sinuses, symmetric enlargement of the ascending aorta, and often mitral valve prolapse. The diagnosis is made by characteristic features involving a number of organ systems because of abnormalities in connective tissue caused by defective fibrillin. Establishing a diagnosis of Marfan syndrome is critical because of the potential danger of aortic dissection when the ascending aorta becomes excessively dilated (>5 cm in diameter in adults). Serial echocardiograms are used to monitor progression of ascending aortic aneurysm formation.

Rheumatic fever is a major cause of aortic incompetence worldwide, although today this is uncommon in the United States.

Finally, *infective endocarditis* can occur on a malformed aortic valve. Staphylococcal endocarditis in particular can destroy the valve, leading to significant aortic regurgitation.

MANAGEMENT Most patients can be followed routinely. In those with more significant regurgitation, periodic echocardiograms to assess left ventricular function should be performed to help guide decisions about operation. Afterload reduction is used with moderate or severe aortic regurgitation to lessen the regurgitant volume. Operations that involve valve replacement are reserved for those patients with chronic regurgitation who are symptomatic and have developed left ventricular dysfunction, often indicated by progressive dilatation of the left ventricle, or those patients who have developed aortic regurgitation acutely and are in failure.

MITRAL REGURGITATION

The primary feature of mitral insufficiency is an apical high-pitched murmur that, if moderately severe, radiates to the left axilla and left posterior thorax. Typically, it begins with the first heart sound and may continue throughout systole (pansystolic) and so occupies both the isovolumetric contraction and ejection phases of systole.

In mitral valve prolapse (discussed below), the murmur begins later in systole because of the anatomic features of the valve.

Once the regurgitant volume equals or exceeds the cardiac output, several findings develop. The first heart sound becomes loud, and a third heart sound is heard at the apex. A low-pitched, mid-diastolic murmur is heard at the cardiac apex. Large R waves are found in the left precordial leads. On chest x-ray, there may be cardiac enlargement from left ventricular dilatation and left atrial enlargement, evident as elevation of the left mainstem bronchus or, if severe, as an enlarged left atrial appendage along the upper left cardiac border.

Once the regurgitant volume is twice the cardiac output, so that left ventricular volume is three times normal, the degree of left ventricular dilatation is excessive. Then cardiac failure with its associated symptoms and signs appears.

The echocardiogram allows assessment of hemodynamics and anatomic features of the mitral valve. Mitral regurgitation can develop secondary to both acquired and congenital anomalies of the mitral valve that are reviewed below and in Table 22-9. Internationally, the most common cause is rheumatic fever, whereas in the United States, it is usually secondary to mitral valve prolapse (up to 5% of the population).

MITRAL VALVE PROLAPSE In this condition, the posterior leaflet of the mitral valve, and occasionally the anterior leaflet as well, prolapses into the left atrium. The reasons for prolapse are unknown. Mitral valve prolapse occurs in increased frequency in patients with connective tissue disorders of Marfan or Ehlers-Danlos syndromes and also with mucopolysaccharidoses, ruptured chordae (perhaps from subacute bacterial endocarditis), and certain cardiac anomalies (such as atrial septal defect) associated with reduced left ventricular volume. Because the leaflets of the mitral valve are tethered by the chordae tendineae to the left ventricular papillary muscles, the extent and duration of the prolapse depend on the left ventricular volume. Left ventricular volume is larger when the patient reclines and is smaller when the patient sits or stands. Thus, in the former state, the mitral valve prolapses less and for a shorter period of time than in the latter positions.

Mitral valve prolapse can be recognized by typical auscultatory findings that are usually diagnostic. At the apex, a late systolic crescendo murmur is heard, often initiated by a click. When the patient sits or stands, the murmur is louder and longer, and when the patient squats or reclines, it becomes softer, shorter, and later in systole. Most patients are asymptomatic, but some have chest pain or palpitations, and the causal relationship is unknown. There are no typical electrocardiographic or radiographic findings, but the echocardiogram, if performed, demonstrates the anatomic and hemodynamic features. There is an association with thoracic anomalies, such as pectus excavatum, scoliosis, or straight back syndrome.

Mitral valve prolapse is common in Marfan syndrome because of the elongated chordae tendineae. The resultant mitral regurgitation can become significant, causing major left atrial enlargement to such a degree that atrial fibrillation may develop. The physical findings in a patient with Marfan syndrome are generally typical and diagnostic (see Sec. 10.3.6 and Table 10-14).

Mitral regurgitation can occur secondary to primary anomalies of the mitral valve, which include *cleft in the anterior leaflet* and *double orifice.* Only the echocardiogram is diagnostic of these conditions. *Papillary muscle dysfunction* from anomalous left coronary artery (Sec. 22.3.8) or conditions with left ventricular hypertrophy can result in mitral regurgitation. In the former, the electrocardiogram is typical (Sec. 22.3.8), and in the latter, generally the cause of left ventricular hypertrophy can be found on clinical examination, electrocardiograms, or echocardiograms.

In some patients, mitral regurgitation improves following medical or surgical treatment of the underlying condition (eg, left atrial myxoma, endocardial cushion defect, anomalous left coronary artery, severe aortic stenosis, idiopathic hypertrophic subaortic stenosis). In these, improvement occurs without direct treatment of the mitral valve. Mitral regurgitation secondary to neonatal asphyxia or hypoglycemia generally improves spontaneously during the first year of life, as the ischemic left ventricular myocardium recovers. Many patients require no treatment, but in those who become symptomatic or have moderate regurgitation, afterload reduction may lessen the regurgitant volume and delay valve replacement.

A cleft mitral valve may be repaired directly, but other forms of mitral regurgitation generally require valvuloplasty or valve replacement. Replacement is reserved for those with symptoms and/or deteriorating left ventricular function when a conservative operation is not possible.

PULMONARY REGURGITATION

The primary finding of pulmonary regurgitation is an early decrescendo diastolic murmur beginning with the pulmonary component of the second heart sound. The murmur is usually low pitched, unlike a murmur of aortic regurgitation, because of the low pulmonary artery diastolic pressure. The murmur is high pitched when pulmonary hypertension is present, as in a neonate or a patient with pulmonary vascular disease in whom pulmonary regurgitation develops.

Pulmonary regurgitation is usually well tolerated because of the low pulmonary artery diastolic pressure and shape of the right ventricle. Thus, children are asymptomatic with this condition and have a near-normal exercise tolerance. Congestive cardiac failure is uncommon unless there is pulmonary hypertension or abnormal right ventricular function.

If the regurgitant volume exceeds twice normal, a soft pulmonary systolic ejection murmur may be heard, accompanied by widened, but variable, splitting of the second heart sound. Because of the increased anterograde flow into the pulmonary trunk and proximal pulmonary arteries, the pulmonary arterial pulse pressure is increased, and the pulmonary arteries are pulsatile, as shown by imaging techniques. On a chest x-ray, the pulmonary trunk and proximal pulmonary arteries may be dilated. With increasing volumes of blood in the right ventricle, the right ventricle dilates, leading to cardiomegaly on a chest x-ray and an rSr' in the right precordial electrocardiographic leads.

The most common cause of pulmonary regurgitation is postoperatively after relief of pulmonary stenosis, either isolated or combined with a ventricular communication (most frequently tetralogy of Fallot). After either a valvotomy or a balloon valvoplasty for valvar pulmonary stenosis, the degree of regurgitation and the hemodynamic alterations are usually minimal. In patients in whom pulmonary stenosis has been relieved by a transannular patch or in whom a ventriculotomy is done for an intracardiac repair, fatigue or cardiac failure may develop, cardiomegaly is found, and the electrocardiogram shows complete right bundle-branch block. In these instances, probably the combination of the degree of pulmonary regurgitation and the altered right ventricular function results in hemodynamic dysfunction that might not have been present with a normally functioning right ventricle. These patients may develop

exercise fatigue from inability of the right ventricle to increase cardiac output during exercise and eventually right heart failure.

Congenital pulmonary regurgitation is rare and may be associated with either an intact ventricular septum or a ventricular septal defect. Isolated pulmonary insufficiency with intact ventricular septum can cause cardiac failure in the immediate neonatal period because of the elevated pulmonary artery pressure normally present at this age. This elevation greatly augments regurgitation and leads to profound and sometimes fatal cardiac failure.

In those with a coexistent ventricular septal defect (tetralogy of Fallot with absent pulmonary valve), although there may be symptoms and signs of cardiac failure, these usually develop later in infancy and usually are overshadowed by marked respiratory symptoms secondary to bronchial compression from enlarged pulsatile central pulmonary arteries. Because of pulmonary hypertension in both of the previous scenarios, the diastolic murmur is higher pitched.

MANAGEMENT

Most patients with pulmonary regurgitation after valvuloplasty, valvotomy, or transannular patch do not require treatment but should be followed periodically. If symptoms or evidence of significant decreased right ventricular function is determined by echocardiography, valve replacement should be performed.

In infants with coexistent ventricular septal defect and absent pulmonary valve, an operation to close the ventricular septal defect and plicate the main pulmonary arteries should be done.

For a neonate with absent pulmonary valve and intact ventricular septum, giving nitric oxide via a ventilator may relax pulmonary arterioles and lower pulmonary vascular resistance. Once pulmonary artery pressure reaches normal levels, the symptoms disappear.

TRICUSPID REGURGITATION

In tricuspid regurgitation, the primary finding is a pansystolic murmur along the lower left sternal border; the murmur may radiate towards the right. The murmur is usually low pitched because of the low right ventricular systolic pressures but is higher pitched if associated with a high right ventricular systolic pressure.

Because of the increased right arterial volume, the right lower cardiac border of the chest x-ray may be rounded and prominent, and the electrocardiogram shows tall and slightly broadened P waves of right atrial enlargement. If significant, jugular veins are distended, and the liver is enlarged.

Because of the increased anterograde flow, a low-pitched middiastolic murmur is present in the tricuspid area. Once the right ventricular volume exceeds twice normal, cardiomegaly and an rSR' (lead V_1) may be found.

Because of the low right ventricular systolic pressure, compliant right ventricle, and right ventricular shape, this condition is usually well tolerated and unassociated with congestive cardiac failure unless right ventricular dysfunction coexists.

Tricuspid regurgitation is common, secondary to congenital or acquired conditions associated with right ventricular dilatation, although the degree is often mild and detectable only by color Doppler interrogation of the tricuspid valve. Two particularly critical conditions causing tricuspid regurgitation can present in the neonatal period.

TRANSIENT TRICUSPID INSUFFICIENCY OF THE NEONATE In some neonates with severe perinatal stress, marked tricuspid regurgitation may develop secondary to right ventricular myocardial ischemia. Affected neonates often have acidosis and hypoglycemia. Myocardial enzyme levels (creatine kinase MB band) are elevated. Pulmonary hypertension frequently coexists and accentuates the degree of regurgitation.

Cardiac failure may be present, accentuated by the elevated pulmonary vascular resistance and myocardial dysfunction. There are no distinguishing clinical findings other than the perinatal history and frequently ST segment and T-wave changes on an electrocardiogram. Treatment is supportive with inotropes to improve myocardial function, ventilator support to reduce oxygen consumption, and nitric oxide.

The tricuspid regurgitation generally resolves during infancy as pulmonary resistance declines and the right ventricular myocardium recovers. Usually by 6 months of age, there are no abnormal findings.

EBSTEIN MALFORMATION This congenital cardiac anomaly must be considered in the differential diagnosis of tricuspid insufficiency and is discussed in Sec. 22.3.5.

SECONDARY TO RIGHT VENTRICULAR DYSFUNCTION Tricuspid regurgitation may develop secondary to right ventricular dysfunction. The two common situations in which this occurs in childhood are right ventricular failure and severe pulmonary stenosis. The former is found late in the postoperative course of children following atrial baffle procedures for complete transposition or right ventriculotomy (plus conduit placement), as in tetralogy of Fallot.

In those patients following atrial baffle procedures, because the right ventricle is connected to the aorta, systemic afterload reduction reduces the degree of regurgitation. Among those following repair of tetralogy of Fallot who have significant postoperative pulmonary regurgitation, repair of this problem often reduces right ventricular volume and lessens the tricuspid regurgitation. In children with severe pulmonary stenosis, tricuspid regurgitation may develop from either coexistent structural anomalies of the tricuspid valve or right ventricular dysfunction. In these patients, the regurgitation is accentuated by the elevated right ventricular systolic pressure. Relief of the pulmonary stenosis is generally sufficient to diminish the tricuspid regurgitation.

Rare causes of tricuspid regurgitation include *endocarditis,* which occurs on a normal valve in addicts following intravenous injection of contaminated drugs. *Carcinoid* disease is another very rare cause. Other primary congenital anomalies of the tricuspid valve are also rare and include isolated cleft of the septal leaflet, abnormal chordae tendineae, or structural abnormalities of the leaflets.

References

Aortic Regurgitation

Bonow RO, Lakatos E, McIntosh BJ, et al: Serial long-term assessment of the natural history of asymptomatic patients with chronic aortic regurgitation and normal left ventricular systolic function. Circulation 84: 1625, 1991

Bouchard A, Yock P, Schiller NB, et al: Value of color Doppler estimation of regurgitant volume in patients with chronic aortic insufficiency. Am Heart J 117:1099, 1989

Child JS, Perloff JK, Kaplan S: The heart of the matter: cardiovascular involvement in Marfan's syndrome. J Am Coll Cardiol 14:429, 1989

Flint A: On cardiac murmurs. Am J Med Sci 44:29, 1862

Grayburn PA, Smith MD, Handshoe R, et al: Detection of aortic insufficiency by standard echocardiography, pulsed Doppler echocardiography, and auscultation. Ann Intern Med 104:599, 1986

Henry WL, Bonow RO, Borer JS, et al: Observations on the optimum time for operative intervention for aortic regurgitation. Circulation 61:471, 1980

Lemon DK, White CW: Annuloaortic ectasia: angiographic, hemodynamic and clinical comparison with aortic valve insufficiency. Am J Cardiol 41: 482, 1978

Marsalese DL, Moodie DS, Vacante M, et al: Marfan's syndrome: natural history and long-term follow-up of cardiovascular involvement. J Am Coll Cardiol 14:422, 1989

Scognamiglio R, Fasoli G, Ponchia A, et al: Long-term nifedipine unloading therapy in asymptomatic patients with chronic severe aortic regurgitation. J Am Coll Cardiol 16:424, 1990

Mitral Regurgitation

Blieden LC, Moller JH: Cardiac involvement in inherited disorders of metabolism. Prog Cardiovasc Dis 16:615, 1974

Boudoulas H, Kolibash AJ, Baker P, et al: Mitral valve prolapse and the mitral valve prolapse syndrome: a diagnostic classification and pathogenesis of symptoms. Am Heart J 118:796, 1989

Braunwald E: Mitral regurgitation: physiological, clinical and surgical considerations. N Engl J Med 282:425, 1969

Davachi R, Moller JH, Edwards JE: Diseases of the mitral valve in infancy: anatomic analysis of 55 cases. Circulation 43:565, 1971

Galve E, Candell-Riera J, Pigrau C, et al: Prevalence, morphologic types, and evolution of cardiac valvular disease in systemic lupus erythematosus. N Engl J Med 319:817, 1988

Gidding SS, Shulman ST, Ilbawi M, et al: Mucocutaneous lymph node syndrome (Kawasaki disease): delayed aortic and mitral insufficiency secondary to active valvulitis. J Am Coll Cardiol 7:894, 1986

Glesby MJ, Pyeritz RE: Association of mitral valve prolapse and systemic abnormalities of connective tissue: a phenotype continuum. JAMA 262: 523, 1989

Hirata K, Triposkiadis F, Sparks E, et al: The Marfan syndrome: cardiovascular physical findings and diagnostic correlates. Am Heart J 123:743, 1992

Leier CV, Call TD, Fulkerson PK, et al: The spectrum of cardiac defects in the Ehlers-Danlos syndrome, types I & III. Ann Intern Med 92:171, 1980

Marcus RH, Sareli P, Pocock WA, et al: Functional anatomy of severe mitral regurgitation in active rheumatic carditis. Am J Cardiol 63:577, 1989

Maron BJ, Bonow RO, Cannon RO, et al: Hypertrophic cardiomyopathy: interrelation of clinical manifestations, pathophysiology and therapy. N Engl J Med 316:780, 884, 1987

Petrone RK, Klues HG, Panza JA, et al: Coexistence of mitral valve prolapse in a consecutive group of 528 patients with hypertrophic cardiomyopathy assessed with echocardiography. J Am Coll Cardiol 20:55, 1992

Sanyal SK, Leung RKF, Tierney RC, et al: Mitral valve prolapse syndrome in children with Duchenne's muscular dystrophy. Pediatrics 63:116, 1979

Smallhorn J, de Leval M, Stark J, et al: Isolated anterior mitral cleft: two-dimensional echocardiographic assessment and differentiation from "clefts" associated with atrioventricular septal defect. Br Heart J 48:109, 1982

Pulmonary Regurgitation

Berman W Jr, Fripp RR, Rowe SA, et al: Congenital isolated pulmonary valve incompetence: neonatal presentation and early natural history. Am Heart J 124:248, 1992

Ito T, Engle MA, Holswade GR: Congenital insufficiency of the pulmonic valve: a rare cause of neonatal heart failure. Pediatrics 28:712, 1961

Rabinovitch M, Grady S, David J, et al: Compression of intrapulmonary bronchi by abnormally branching pulmonary arteries associated with absent pulmonary valves. Am J Cardiol 50:804, 1982

Snir E, de Leval MR, Elliott MJ, et al: Current surgical technique to repair Fallot's tetralogy with absent pulmonary valve syndrome. Ann Thorac Surg 51:979, 1991

Tricuspid Regurgitation

Bucciarelli RL, Nelson EM, Egan EA, et al: Transient tricuspid insufficiency of the newborn: a form of myocardial dysfunction in stressed newborns. Pediatrics 59:330, 1977

Giuliani ER, Fuster V, Brandenburg RO, et al: Ebstein's anomaly. The clinical features and natural history of Ebstein's anomaly of the tricuspid valve. Mayo Clin Proc 54:163, 1979

Ilbawi MN, Idriss FS, DeLeon SY, et al: Factors that exaggerate the deleterious effects of pulmonary insufficiency on the right ventricle after tetralogy repair. J Thorac Cardiovasc Surg 93:36, 1987

Newfeld EA, Cole RB, Paul MH: Ebstein's malformation of the tricuspid valve in the neonate: functional and anatomic pulmonary outflow tract obstruction. Am J Cardiol 19:727, 1967

Pinsky WW, Nihill MR, Mullins CE, et al: The absent pulmonary valve syndrome: considerations of management. Circulation 54:159, 1978

Shimazaki Y, Blackstone EH, Kirklin JW: The natural history of isolated congenital pulmonary valve incompetence: surgical implications. J Thorac Cardiovasc Surg 32:257, 1984

22.3.4   Obstructive Lesions

Phillip Moore

Obstructive congenital cardiac lesions are conveniently classified as obstructions on the left or right sides of the heart in Tables 22-10 and 22-11, respectively.

GENERAL FEATURES

Obstruction of flow because of a congenital abnormality may occur in any part of the pulmonary and systemic vascular systems, but the outflow tracts of each ventricle are most often affected. The obstruction may be so mild as to produce no significant hemodynamic effects or so severe as to cause total obstruction of flow. Mild or moderate obstruction is called *stenosis,* whereas complete obstruction is termed *atresia.* Atresia may occur at an atrioventricular valve, at a semilunar valve, or in the aortic arch. With atresia, blood is diverted from its normal pattern of flow and is directed through abnormal pathways to maintain systemic or pulmonary blood flow. Most of these complex lesions involve complete admixture of pulmonary and systemic venous returns and thus produce both right-to-left and left-to-right shunting; they are considered in Sec. 22.3.5. When the obstruction is incomplete, blood flow is largely maintained through normal pathways, and the basic anatomy is unaltered. However, to maintain a normal output through the stenosis, an unusually high pressure proximal to the obstruction is required, causing an increased pressure load proximal to the obstruction. For example, narrowing of the aorta increases left ventricular systolic pressure; with severe obstruction, left ventricular end-diastolic pressure rises. Left atrial and pulmonary venous pressures then increase, and pulmonary edema may occur. This causes pulmonary hypertension and eventually right ventricular failure, with an increase in systemic venous pressure. In association with the increased pressure, the chamber of the heart involved dilates and eventually hypertrophies in order to maintain the pressure load.

TABLE 22-10

LEFT-SIDED OBSTRUCTIVE LESIONS

Pulmonary venous obstruction
Obstruction within the left atrium
  Cor triatriatum
  Tumor (myxoma)
  Supravalvar stenosing ring
Mitral valve obstruction
  Atresia
  Stenosis
  Parachute mitral valve
Hypoplastic left ventricle
Left ventricular outflow tract obstruction
  Subaortic stenosis
    Diffuse (idiopathic hypertrophic)
    Discrete
  Valve obstruction
  Valvar aortic stenosis
Supravalvar aortic stenosis
Aortic arch obstruction
  Interruption
  Hypoplasia
  Coarctation
Abdominal coarctation
Peripheral systemic arterial stenosis

If this cannot be accomplished, cardiac failure occurs, and cardiac output and arterial blood pressure fall. It is important to remember that although the foramen ovale is functionally closed soon after birth, it may allow shunting between the two circulations in either direction if there is an obstruction distal to it.

LEFT HEART OBSTRUCTION

Left heart obstruction can occur in the pulmonary veins, left atrium, mitral valve, left ventricular outflow tract, aortic valve, and aorta.

PULMONARY VENOUS OBSTRUCTION Obstruction to pulmonary venous return is generally associated with abnormal connection of the pulmonary veins, either below the diaphragm to the

TABLE 22-11

RIGHT-SIDED OBSTRUCTIVE LESIONS

Systemic venous obstruction
Right atrium
  Tumor (myxoma)
  Thrombus
Tricuspid valve
  Atresia
  Stenosis
Hypoplastic right ventricle
Right ventricular outflow tract obstruction
  Right ventricular muscle bands
  Subvalvar stenosis: diffuse infundibular, discrete
  Valvar pulmonic stenosis
  Pulmonary atresia
Supravalvar pulmonary stenosis
Peripheral pulmonic stenosis
  Central
  Peripheral
Pulmonary vascular (arterial) obstruction

IVC or above, to the SVC (see Sec. 22.3.5). Although surgical repair can be done, obstruction may recur early because of scar tissue formation. Obstruction of normally connected pulmonary veins does occur occasionally as a result of external compression by a posterior mediastinal mass, fibrosis, or an intrinsic abnormality in the pulmonary veins; single or multiple pulmonary veins may be involved. Intrinsic narrowing may be caused by diffuse hypoplasia, a localized diaphragm, or narrowing of the pulmonary veins as they enter the left atrium.

Pulmonary venous pressure increases with an anatomic obstruction to pulmonary venous return. The rise in pulmonary venous pressure causes increased transudation of fluid through the capillary walls into the interstitial lung spaces, from where it passes into alveoli or lymphatics. Should lymphatic drainage be unable to remove the increased fluid volume, fluid accumulates in the interstitial spaces and the alveoli, commonly known as pulmonary edema. Capillary permeability determines the amount of fluid leaving the vascular system when venous pressure is raised. It has been suggested that capillary permeability is greater in infants than in adults and is even greater in prematures. If this is so, premature infants may get severe pulmonary edema at lower pulmonary venous pressures. The fluid accumulation in the alveoli is clinically apparent as respiratory distress and rales and by interfering with gas exchange, particularly of carbon dioxide, and increasing arterial blood carbon dioxide tension. As fluid accumulates, there is lymphatic engorgement that on chest roentgenogram is associated with Kerley B lines, fluid in the major fissures, and eventually pleural effusion. In some infants in whom congenital lymphangiectasis has been diagnosed, subsequent autopsy examination has revealed pulmonary venous obstruction, usually associated with total anomalous pulmonary venous connection.

Frequently an increased pulmonary venous pressure is associated with an increased pulmonary vascular resistance. The suggested mechanisms that produce this effect include a decrease in oxygen tension to which the resistance vessels are exposed, with resultant pulmonary vascular constriction, and compression of the resistance vessels by edema fluid. With the increase in pulmonary vascular resistance, pulmonary arterial pressure rises, causing a pressure overload on the right ventricle.

The clinical presentation includes the signs and symptoms of pulmonary edema and pulmonary hypertension. It can be difficult, particularly in young infants, to differentiate certain forms of chronic pulmonary disease from pulmonary venous obstruction, which should therefore always be considered if chronic lung disease and pulmonary edema are present.

Treatment of pulmonary venous obstruction is surgical repair. Anomalous veins are attached to the left atrium; intrinsically stenotic veins are enlarged with a patch. Recurrence of stenosis with the need for multiple surgeries is common. Nonsurgical catheter-based treatment, including balloon dilatation, alone or with stent placement, has been used. Although immediate improvement is common, recurrence of stenosis is frequent, and therefore this therapy has limited use. Lung transplantation remains an option for those patients who have failed repeated conventional surgeries.

OBSTRUCTION WITHIN THE LEFT ATRIUM *Cor triatriatum* is a membrane in the midportion of the left atrium; the membrane obstructs flow from the pulmonary veins to the mitral valve. It occurs when failure of resorption of the common pulmonary vein results in division of the left atrium into upper and lower chambers (Fig. 22-3) during development. The pulmonary veins drain into the proximal chamber that communicates through an obstructive opening with the distal portion of the atrium, which in turn is connected to the atrial appendage and the mitral valve. The physiological effects and clinical presentation are the same as in pulmonary venous obstruction. The diagnosis is made by echocardiography, which may show a membrane in the left atrial cavity; it may be confirmed by cardiac catheterization with angiocardiography or magnetic reasonance imaging. Treatment consists of surgical excision of the obstructing membrane and is curative.

An equally uncommon lesion producing obstruction within the left atrium is a *supravalvar mitral ring,* often associated with a parachute mitral valve, subaortic stenosis, and coarctation of the aorta (Shone syndrome). The supravalvar mitral ring is a membrane that develops in the left atrium adjacent to the mitral valve and restricts leaflet motion, causing obstruction. A tumor within the left atrium, usually a *myxoma,* can also produce obstruction within the left atrial chamber, and it generally mimics mitral stenosis; however, because such a tumor is often on a pedicle, the obstruction to the mitral valve orifice (and hence the clinical features) may be intermittent. Treatment of supravalvar mitral ring and myoma is by surgical resection, which is curative.

MITRAL VALVE OBSTRUCTION Obstruction to outflow from the left atrium either by abnormalities of the mitral valve apparatus or by left ventricular failure increases atrial pressure. The left atrium dilates and hypertrophies. Left atrial pressure loading may be inferred clinically on hearing a well-marked fourth heart sound that suggests more forceful contraction by the hypertrophied atrium. Electrocardiographically there may be a widely notched P wave in lead II and in leads V_5 and V_6, and the P wave in V_1 may be enlarged with a prominant negative or biphasic component suggesting left atrial enlargement. On a chest roentgenogram the typical signs of left atrial dilatation, prominent left upper heart silhouette and superiorly deviated left bronchus, may be seen. An increased pulmonary venous pressure is manifested by tachypnea, the cardinal sign of left ventricular failure.

The most severe form of mitral valve obstruction is mitral atresia, discussed in Sec. 22.3.5. Congenital mitral stenosis may be an isolated defect or may be associated with other abnormalities such as an atrial or ventricular septal defect, aortic stenosis, coarctation of the aorta, or endocardial fibroelastosis. Congenital malformations of the mitral valve may produce grossly abnormal valve cusps or a valve that appears normal but has fused commissures or else fusion of chordae tendineae below the valve ring. Parachute mitral valve, in which the chordae tendineae are all attached to a single papillary muscle, also obstructs flow at the mitral valve level. This may occur as an isolated lesion, but it is more commonly part of a complex group of left heart obstructions, know as Shone syndrome.

The congenital forms of mitral stenosis are generally severe and present in early infancy with symptoms and physical findings of pulmonary edema; if pulmonary hypertension occurs, severe congestive cardiac failure may supervene. The pulmonic component of the second sound is accentuated, its intensity depending on the severity of pulmonary hypertension. A rumbling apical diastolic murmur with presystolic accentuation is usually present; however, with severe cardiac failure the murmur may not be heard but may appear when cardiac failure is controlled. Various degrees of mitral incompetence may be associated with the stenosis, and there may be an apical blowing murmur of mitral insufficiency. An opening snap of the mitral valve may be heard, but this is not common because the valve is very thick and immobile. Tricuspid regurgitation may occur if there is severe pulmonary hypertension with right ventricular dilatation. On the electrocardiogram the P waves are broad and notched, suggesting left atrial enlargement, and right ventricular hypertrophy may be present. The chest roentgenogram shows only moderate enlargement of the cardiac silhouette caused by left atrial and possibly right ventricular enlargement. The pulmonary vascular markings depend on the severity of obstruction. The specific diagnosis may be made by echocardiography and rarely needs confirmation by cardiac catheterization and angiocardiography. Two-dimensional echocardiography and color Doppler flow mapping are valuable in assessing the anatomy and function of the valve and its chordal attachments, the anatomy of the valve ring and the supravalvar region, the size of the left ventricle, and any additional or associated abnormalities. Doppler evaluation can also estimate the flow and the pressure difference across the valve. In older children, a transesophageal echocardiogram may be needed to define the mitral valve abnormalities.

Medical treatment of severe congenital mitral stenosis with intractable heart failure in infancy and early childhood is usually unsuccessful. Surgical management, because of the marked thickening and deformity of the mitral valve, generally involves inserting a prosthetic valve; however, in older patients valve repair may be tried. The prosthetic valve has a limited effective life, and surgical replacement with a larger prosthetic valve is needed to accommodate growth. In addition, children with a prosthetic mitral valve must be given anticoagulants to prevent thrombosis of the valve. Recently dilatation of the stenotic valve with a balloon catheter has shown promise, particularly in older patients (see Sec. 22.2.6). If the left ventricle is hypoplastic, then repair of the mitral valve may not be appropriate, and a Fontan or single ventricle type surgical repair may be needed.

LEFT VENTRICULAR OUTFLOW OBSTRUCTION Most left ventricular obstructive lesions do not occur rapidly, and compensatory myocardial hypertrophy therefore occurs in response to the increased systolic pressure in the chamber. The increased muscle mass allows increased cardiac work to be performed with little ventricular dilatation and without greatly increased end-diastolic pressures. As an additional response to stress, increased sympathetic activity occurs and produces greater contractile force and rate of ejection, thus shortening systole and lowering end-diastolic pressure. However, with severe obstruction, even these compensatory mechanisms may fail, and the left ventricle dilates and end-diastolic pressure increases.

A further important consideration in the response of the myocardium to an increased pressure load is the ability to provide an adequate oxygen supply. The oxygen requirements of the left ventricular myocardium are related to the systolic pressure generated within the ventricle, the thickness of the wall, the diameter of the cavity, and the degree of sympathetic stimulation. The amount of oxygen supplied to the myocardium is related to the aortic diastolic pressure, the left ventricular diastolic pressure, the duration of diastole, and the oxygen-carrying capacity of blood perfusing the myocardium. Therefore, with severe obstruction oxygen requirements are significantly increased, but the supply of oxygen may be compromised if there is left ventricular failure with an increase in ventricular end-diastolic pressure and a shortened diastolic duration because of the compensatory tachycardia.

The left ventricular response to obstruction is manifested by left ventricular hypertrophy, inferred from a slow forceful heave of the left ventricular apex. Hypertrophy by itself does not significantly enlarge the external heart dimensions, for the increased wall thick-

ness may be only a few millimeters, but if there is associated dilatation, the left ventricular apex is displaced downward and to the left. The heart may or may not show enlargement on a roentgenogram; even if it is not enlarged there may be a slightly more rounded left ventricular contour than seen normally. There are no specific changes in the first or second heart sounds, but a third heart sound may appear; if there is systemic hypertension, aortic closure is loud. Electrocardiography shows increased left inferior and posterior forces. The mean frontal-plane QRS axis is normal with pure left ventricular hypertrophy because an inferiorly placed ventricle with a normal sequence of depolarization does not produce the left superior axis termed left axis deviation.

Several congenital cardiovascular malformations obstruct ejection of blood from the left ventricle. The most common of these is obstruction of the aortic valve cusps themselves; however, the left ventricular outflow tract may be obstructed by an abnormally situated mitral valve leaflet or papillary muscle, by muscular hypertrophy of the ventricular septum, by a subvalvar fibrous ring, by a thin subvalvar membrane with a small orifice, or by supravalvar aortic narrowing. Because valvar aortic stenosis is the most common form of aortic stenosis, it is described in detail, and differences associated with other forms of left ventricular outflow tract obstruction are identified.

VALVAR AORTIC STENOSIS About 85% of congenitally stenotic aortic valves are bicuspid, with one small and one large cusp and an eccentric fish-mouth orifice between them. Another 14% have no obvious separation into leaflets, so that there is a thick monocusp with an eccentric orifice shaped like a teardrop. The obstruction results in part from the small orifice left by commissural fusion and in part from thickening and lack of mobility of the valve.

Somatic development is usually normal at the time of birth. If the stenosis was severe in utero, then blood will have been diverted from the left ventricle, so that it and the ascending aorta are hypoplastic. Because of the high left ventricular pressure, there may be marked endocardial thickening (secondary endocardial fibroelastosis) that further impairs left ventricular performance.

PATHOPHYSIOLOGY If there is a high systolic pressure and left ventricular hypertrophy, and if aortic diastolic pressure is low and diastole is short, subendocardial blood flow may be inadequate, and subendocardial ischemia may result. This explains the subendocardial necrosis and fibrosis often noted with severe aortic stenosis. It also explains why exercise in moderately severe aortic stenosis may cause anginal pain and S-T depression or T-wave inversion in the left ventricular electrocardiographic leads. Ischemia or ischemic damage may also be responsible for the occasional sudden death, almost certainly because of ventricular fibrillation. One other symptom of aortic stenosis is syncope, usually following exertion of prolonged standing. Lesser degrees of stenosis cause left ventricular hypertrophy with no evidence of ischemia at rest or exercise, and the mildest stenotic lesions produce only a murmur with no left ventricular hypertrophy.

After birth, in an infant with severe aortic stenosis, if the foramen ovale is competent, left atrial pressure rises, and left ventricular output is well maintained, but at the expense of pulmonary edema. If, however, the foramen ovale is incompetent and allows a large left-to-right shunt, left atrial pressure may not rise as much, so there may be less pulmonary edema but at the expense of a lower cardiac output. In either circumstance left ventricular dilatation may be marked, and left ventricular failure occurs. Infants with less severe aortic stenosis are generally capable of maintaining cardiac output and of developing adequate hypertrophy to overcome the obstruction.

Congenital aortic stenosis is usually progressive. As the child grows and cardiac output increases, the valve orifice may not grow to keep pace with increased cardiac output requirements; thus, the obstruction becomes more severe, and the pressure difference between the aorta and left ventricle increases. Rapid changes in the severity of aortic stenosis may occur with rapid growth spurts.

CLINICAL FEATURES Severe aortic stenosis generally presents in the immediate postnatal period. The physical findings are those of a systolic murmur of variable intensity, depending on the left ventricular output. This systolic murmur is often best heard at the middle left sternal border in infants; it can be confused with the murmur of ventricular septal defect. If cardiac output is greatly reduced, the murmur may be very soft or even absent. An early systolic ejection click is common. Peripheral perfusion and pulses depend on the degree of failure, but they are generally decreased; these infants can be misdiagnosed as having septic shock. Evidence of significant atrial left-to-right shunting with right ventricular hyperactivity is often present. Chest roentgenograms show marked cardiomegaly with severe pulmonary venous congestion. The electrocardiogram often shows increased right ventricular forces; increased left ventricular forces are rarely present in the neonate. An echocardiogram may show the abnormal aortic valve and usually demonstrates a dilated, poorly contractile left ventricle, sometimes with bright subendocardial echos that indicate secondary fibroelastosis.

In older children with aortic stenosis, the murmur usually draws attention to the defect. Chest or epigastric pain or syncopal episodes are generally associated with severe stenosis and are uncommon presenting symptoms. They may, however, develop in a child known to have aortic stenosis, where they indicate progression in severity of the stenosis. Many of the physical findings of aortic stenosis correlate roughly with the severity of the stenosis. Left ventricular hypertrophy causes an increased apical impulse. If there has been long-standing severe obstruction from infancy, a left precordial bulge and an apical impulse in the left anterior axillary line may be evident. In children with moderately severe stenosis, the systemic arterial pulse is usually normal. In adults, as the stenosis becomes more severe, the upstroke of the pulse is slowed, and pulse volume is decreased; this sign is uncommon in children, even those with moderately severe stenosis. The first heart sound may be normal or soft in severe stenosis. Commonly, an early systolic ejection click is heard along the left sternal border and is usually transmitted toward the apex of the heart.

Because of prolonged left ventricular ejection, the aortic component of the second heart sound can be delayed, and the splitting of the second sound therefore narrows. The aortic component may be softer than normal. In more severe stenosis, left ventricular ejection is prolonged even more, and the splitting of the second sound may disappear because of superimposition of the aortic and pulmonic components. Rarely the aortic component may even follow the pulmonic component, so that the second sound narrows with inspiration and widens with expiration (paradoxic splitting). A prominent apical third sound is frequently heard, and in severe stenosis a fourth sound may also be present. A loud crescendo-decrescendo systolic murmur, often grade 4 to 5 in intensity and associated with a suprasternal notch thrill, is characteristic of aortic stenosis. The murmur starts with the first sound and reaches peak intensity early in systole in mild stenosis and later in systole in more severe stenosis. A more reliable sign of severity is the frequency of

the murmur; the smaller the orifice the greater the velocity of blood being ejected, and therefore the higher the pitch of the murmur. The murmur is usually best heard at the upper right sternal border and radiates well into the suprasternal notch and into the neck. In infants and young children it is often better heard at the upper left sternal border or even over the upper sternum. A short grade 2 to 3/6 decrescendo blowing regurgitant murmur may occasionally be heard at the middle left sternal border.

The electrocardiogram may show left ventricular hypertrophy, but this is a poor index of the severity of the stenosis. T-wave flattening or inversion and S-T segment depression in left ventricular precordial leads indicate left ventricular strain from severe aortic outflow obstruction and indicate the need for treatment. These changes may not be present at rest but may be brought out by graded exercise. The chest roentgenogram occasionally shows left ventricular enlargement, but more often the only abnormal finding is poststenotic dilatation of the ascending aorta. Two-dimensional echocardiography can define the anatomy of the aortic valve area (Fig. 22-38). A Doppler examination gives a relatively accurate indication of severity by estimating the pressure difference across the valve from the velocity signal.

It is important to realize that symptoms, physical findings, chest roentgenograms, and electrocardiograms are not reliable in predicting the severity of aortic stenosis. Children with severe stenosis and large pressure differences between aorta and left ventricle may have a benign course and no evidence or minimal evidence of left ventricular stress, whereas some children with only moderately large pressure differences may have more significant physical findings. It is for this reason, and because sudden death may occur in children with moderate stenosis and relatively minor physical findings, that the pressure difference between aorta and left ventricle and the hemodynamic status should be evaluated carefully by Doppler examination or cardiac catheterization.

Echocardiography with Doppler examination is essential for any child with aortic stenosis with or without symptoms, congestive heart failure, or electrocardiographic changes of left ventricular hypertrophy. If there is no evidence of myocardial ischemia at rest, an exercise test may help to determine the adequacy of myocardial perfusion. Any suggestion that the stenosis is severe should lead to referral for treatment. In most centers cardiac catheterization is performed when there are doubts about the echocardiographic findings or the stenosis is severe enough to warrant treatment. If valvotomy is not needed, these patients should be followed at least yearly with electrocardiograms at rest and during exercise and by echocardiogram-Doppler study because of the tendency of this lesion to become more severe.

TREATMENT Symptoms such as chest pain or syncope warrant immediate evaluation and treatment, as does evidence of ischemia on ECG. A pressure gradient of greater than 70 mm Hg measured with echo Doppler velocity generally correlates with a direct catheterization measurement of greater than 50 mm Hg and indicates the need for treatment in an asymptomatic patient. This most often correlates with a valve area of less than 0.65 cm^2/m^2 body surface area, normal being greater than 2.0 cm^2/m^2. Treatment historically has been surgical valvotomy, but balloon valvoplasty has become the treatment of choice (see Sec. 22.2.6). Both forms of valvotomy are only palliative; the valve commissure can be opened to reduce the obstruction, but the valve orifice is usually not opened maximally because that causes massive aortic incompetence. In fact, the average gradient reduction with balloon dilation is 65% with a 15% chance of developing mild incompetence. Palliation is lifesaving

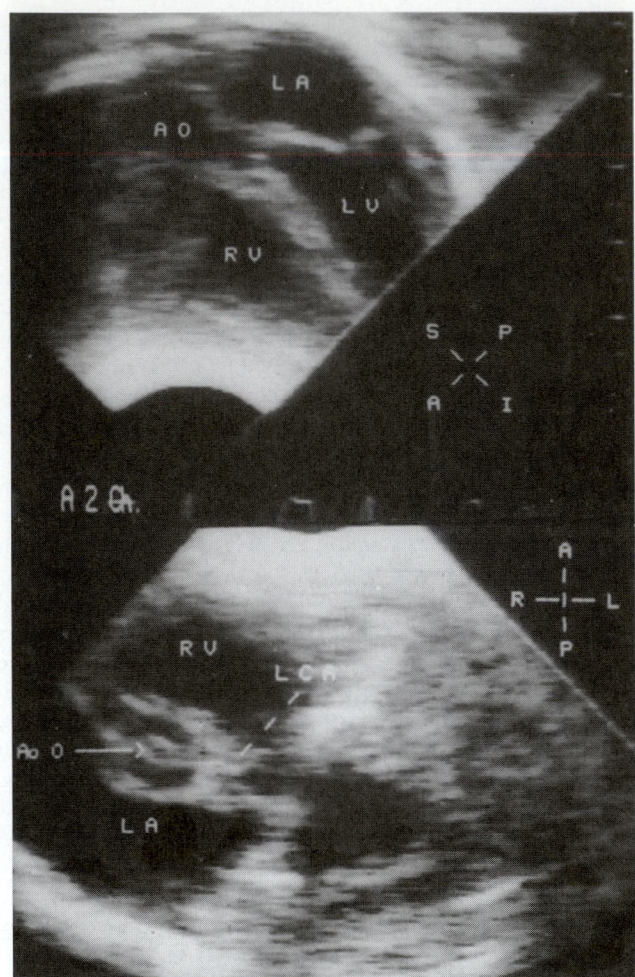

FIGURE 22-38   Apical four-chamber view *(top)* **and parasternal short-axis view** *(bottom)* **in a patient with critical aortic stenosis.** *Top:* **In the apical four-chamber view, all chambers of the heart are observed. The thickened aortic valve leaflets are seen in the systolic projection to be barely separating, and ascending aorta (Ao) is dilated. A = anterior; I = inferior; LA = left atrium; LV = left ventricle; RV = right ventricle.** *Bottom:* **A parasternal short-axis view through the aortic root shows the pinhole orifice of a pseudounicuspid aortic valve (AoO). The left coronary artery (LCA) is identified. A = anterior; L = left; LA = left atrium; P = posterior; RV = right ventricle.**

and may produce a good functional result that lasts for many years. However, there is a high incidence of recurrence of stenosis, often associated with calcification, and 40% of patients require repeat treatment within 10 years. Although repeat balloon dilatation is successful, eventually most patients with severe aortic valve stenosis may require surgical treatment, either the Ross procedure or mechanical valve replacement. The Ross procedure consists of moving the pulmonary valve ring with the valve intact into the aortic annulus and placing a homograft aortic valve into the right ventricular outflow tract. By having the patient's own valve in the aortic position, there is no need for anticoagulation and an excellent hemodynamic result with an extremely low incidence of restenosis. However, the aortic homograft (new pulmonary valve) does not grow and becomes insufficient over time, necessitating surgical replacement every 10 to 15 years. Surgical repair, either mechanical valve replacement or the Ross procedure, should be deferred until

the patient is fully grown if possible, in order to avoid the need for repeat surgical procedures.

BICUSPID AORTIC VALVE   Bicuspid aortic valve is present in 1 to 3% of the population. There is an asymmetric orifice, and the valve may not open fully in systole, but there need not be any obstruction to left ventricular ejection. Bicuspid valves are found in 50% of patients with coarctation of the aorta but more often are isolated anomalies. Sometimes they are associated with a grade 1–2/6 systolic ejection murmur and click at the right upper sternal border, but often they are not clinically apparent. The diagnosis is best made by two-dimensional echocardiography.

The importance of bicuspid aortic valves is that they may produce aortic stenosis in later life; middle-aged adults with calcific aortic stenosis usually have congenitally bicuspid aortic valves. The likelihood of late development of calcific aortic stenosis is uncertain but may be high. Occasionally, bicuspid aortic valves are the seat of infective endocarditis; thus, if bicuspid aortic valves are diagnosed, prophylaxis against infective endocarditis should be given.

DISCRETE SUBVALVAR AORTIC STENOSIS   Subvalvar aortic stenosis may be caused by either a thin membranous diaphragm or a thick fibromuscular obstruction. The aortic valve itself may be thickened and distorted by the high-velocity jet stream passing through the subaortic obstruction and may be insufficient. The clinical features are similar to those observed with valvar aortic stenosis, and there are no reliable clinical criteria to differentiate valvar from subvalvar obstruction. However, in the discrete form of subvalvar stenosis a systolic ejection click is unusual, a diastolic regurgitant murmur is heard often, suprasternal notch thrills are uncommon, and aortic dilatation (although present in some patients with subaortic stenosis) is less marked than in patients with valvar aortic stenosis. The two-dimensional echocardiogram may be used to define more accurately the type, thickness, and site of obstruction present. In addition to the subaortic obstruction, there may be hypoplasia of the aortic annulus itself. Aortic valve motion may be compromised by altered flow patterns, and the echocardiogram may show normal valve opening with abrupt partial closure in midsystole. Differentiation between valvar and subvalvar aortic stenosis by echocardiography or occasionally by cardiac catheterization and angiocardiography is important because a subvalvar diaphragm is readily removed at surgery with good results and because even mild subvalvar obstruction may cause progressive aortic valve damage and regurgitation. Some children may have subvalvar obstruction from an abnormally placed papillary muscle and displaced mitral valve. This is much more difficult to alleviate surgically, and it may be complicated by mitral regurgitation.

DIFFUSE SUBAORTIC STENOSIS   Diffuse subaortic left ventricular outflow stenosis may be associated with any cause of diffuse hypertrophy of the left ventricle. It occurs with valvar aortic stenosis and with certain types of cardiomyopathy such as glycogen storage disease. Infants born to diabetic mothers have a high incidence of a mild form of diffuse cardiomyopathy, although a few may have severe asymmetric septal hypertrophy. In both, the abnormality is temporary and generally resolves within several months. Some children with Noonan syndrome have a specific form of eccentric subaortic stenosis. Tumors, such as rhabdomyomas, may also cause outflow obstruction. In premature infants with chronic lung disease treated with steroids, a diffuse symmetric hypertrophy may develop.

This regresses spontaneously once steroid treatment is discontinued.

The most common form of diffuse subaortic stenosis is idiopathic. This entity has been called idiopathic hypertrophic subaortic stenosis (IHSS), hypertrophic obstructive cardiomyopathy (HOCM), hypertrophic cardiomyopathy (HCM), or asymmetric septal hypertrophy (ASH). The disease is transmitted as a mendelian dominant with variable expression and is usually seen in more than one member of a family. In some families there is a tendency to ventricular arrhythmias and less severe outflow tract obstruction, whereas in others there is severe obstruction. About 50% of patients have mutations that map to the myosin heavy chain on chromosome 14; many different mutations are now known. Other mutations affect cardiac troponin T and α-tropomyosin. Linkage studies have also suggested mutations on chromosomes 1, 11, and 15 as well.

Many of the physical findings are similar to those in valvar aortic stenosis, but certain features usually distinguish them. A double or triple apical impulse, described as a *precordial ripple*, is often seen or palpated. The first heart sound may be normal or soft; systolic clicks are rarely heard. The suprasternal notch thrill is absent. A delayed-onset crescendo-decrescendo systolic murmur, usually of grade 2–4/6 intensity, may be heard best at the middle left to upper right sternal border, and a systolic thrill may be palpable over the precordium. In some children there is moderate to marked mitral incompetence as well. The second heart sound may be narrow or even paradoxically split. Third and fourth heart sounds are common; diastolic murmurs are unusual. The pulses are unusual in that there is a fast rise, and a bifid carotid pulse may be palpable. Maneuvers that reduce venous return, such as the Valsalva maneuver or assuming an erect posture, are often associated with an increase in the intensity of the systolic murmur because of a decrease in left ventricular size with exaggeration of the obstruction. If the patient squats, thereby increasing venous return and peripheral vascular resistance, the murmur decreases in intensity as a result of left ventricular dilatation. All these maneuvers tend to produce opposite effects in valvar aortic stenosis. The chest roentgenogram shows left ventricular enlargement without dilatation of the ascending aorta. The electrocardiogram is variable, but with severe or moderately severe hypertrophy, there are markedly increased left ventricular forces often associated with S-T segment depression and T-wave flattening or inversion in the left precordial leads. Deep Q waves in the left precordial leads indicative of septal hypertrophy are more evident than in valvar aortic stenosis.

The two-dimensional echocardiogram has been of great help in diagnosing this lesion. It demonstrates the asymmetric septal hypertrophy (Fig. 22-39), and during systole it usually shows anterior movement of the mitral valve (SAM), which touches the septum and in part causes the outflow tract obstruction. SAM is not always demonstrated but usually can be provoked by maneuvers that precipitate outflow obstruction, such as amyl nitrite inhalation or the Valsalva maneuver.

Children with this disease are more likely to die from arrhythmias than from obstruction and heart failure. The results of treatment of this lesion are variable. Some children respond fairly well to β-adrenergic-receptor blockers; however, this is generally of only temporary benefit. Calcium antagonists are useful, particularly when the major problem is decreased diastolic ventricular distensibility. Surgical excision of the hypertrophied muscle has produced marked improvement in some children. Atrioventricular sequential pacing in conjunction with β-adrenergic blocker therapy has been

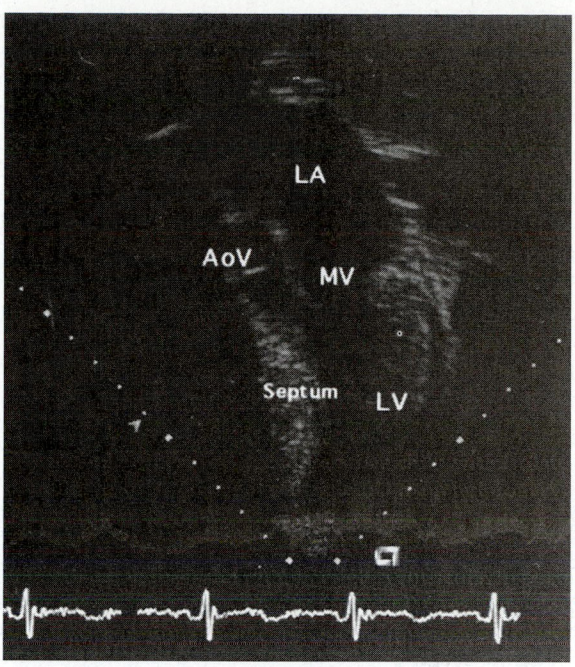

FIGURE 22-39 Two-dimensional echocardiogram of the left ventricule (LV) in a child with hypertrophic cardiomyopathy. The excessive and asymmetric bulging of the septum is characteristic of this disease. The anterior leaflet of the mitral valve (MV) is close to the septum, and if the two come in contact during systole, they obstruct the left ventricular outflow tract, a phenomenon termed systolic anterior motion of the mitral valve.

used successfully. Because the ventricle is stimulated from the right side of the septum, there is asynchronous contraction of the left ventricle, the septum relaxes before the rest of the ventricle contracts, and outflow tract obstruction is reduced. Controlled comparisons in adult patients suggest that surgical resection may be more effective than pacing at gradient reduction. In the late 1990s a catheter-based treatment was developed consisting of intentional infarction of the hypertrophied septum by instilling alcohol solution into a septal perforating coronary artery. This has been used successfully in adults to reduce the outflow obstruction; however, long-term follow-up is not available, and the technique has not been applied to children.

SUPRAVALVAR AORTIC STENOSIS Supravalvar aortic stenosis is a localized or diffuse narrowing just above the level of the coronary arteries and the superior annular margin of the sinuses of Valsalva. The coronary arteries usually arise proximal to the obstruction and are often tortuous, with thickened medial and intimal layers. Coronary perfusion may be compromised by involvement of the coronary ostia in fibrous tissue. Although supravalvar aortic stenosis may occur as an isolated lesion, it is often associated with Williams syndrome, also known as idiopathic infantile hypercalcemia. This disorder features mental retardation, cocktail personality, peculiar facies, and narrowings of peripheral systemic and pulmonary arteries (see Table 10-10). On auscultation the aortic closure sound is frequently accentuated; an ejection click is unusual, and the systolic murmur is best heard at the base and toward the neck. If peripheral pulmonic stenosis is associated, a continuous murmur may be heard laterally in the chest. Characteristically, blood pressure is about 15 mm Hg higher in the right than the left arm. The chest roentgenogram does not show poststenotic dilatation of the ascending aorta. The electrocardiogram shows left ventricular hypertrophy as well as T-wave inversion in left chest leads if there is severe stenosis. Magnetic resonance imaging and echocardiography demonstrate the supravalvar narrowing, and Doppler study can assess the pressure gradient. Cardiac catheterization and angiography are done to confirm the severity of the supravalvar obstruction and associated peripheral pulmonic stenosis. If obstruction is severe, the diffuse supravalvar narrowing can be relieved surgically with excellent long-term results. If severe peripheral pulmonary artery stenosis is associated with the supravalvar obstruction, cardiac catheterization with balloon dilatation of the branch pulmonary stenoses is often performed before surgical repair.

AORTIC OBSTRUCTIONS

Obstructive lesions of the aorta may be subdivided into diffuse narrowing (hypoplasia) or interruption of a portion of the aortic arch, discrete narrowing (thoracic coarctation) closely related to the attachment of the ductus arteriosus with the aorta, pseudocoarctation, and abdominal coarctation. The discrete thoracic coarctation is the most common lesion and is usually associated with a normally developed aortic arch.

HYPOPLASIA OR INTERRUPTION In normal fetal life the aortic isthmus (the portion of aorta between the origin of the left subclavian artery and the ductus attachment) conducts only about 10 to 12% of the combined output of both the left and right ventricles. This probably explains why in normal full-term infants the diameter of the aortic isthmus is about three-fourths that of the descending aorta; this difference usually disappears by about 6 months of age.

Pathologic hypoplasia of the aortic arch is noted most commonly in the aortic isthmus but may occur in other parts of the aortic arch. The most severe form of this lesion is complete interruption of the aortic arch. With rare exceptions, infants with aortic arch interruption or hypoplasia have associated major congenital cardiac defects, such as a large ventricular septal defect, double-outlet right ventricle, Taussig-Bing anomaly, tricuspid atresia with aortopulmonary transposition, or endocardial cushion defect. During the newborn period the ductus arteriosus is invariably patent. The reason for these associations is that aortic outflow obstruction associated with these intracardiac lesions may divert flow during fetal life, with a consequent reduction in the growth of the aortic arch. The clinical course of infants with these lesions will be dictated by the intracardiac lesions (usually a ventricular septal defect with or without other complicating defects), by the magnitude of right-to-left flow across the ductus arteriosus, and by the degree of obstruction of the aorta.

With complete interruption, descending aortic blood flow is provided only by right-to-left flow through the ductus arteriosus. In hypoplasia of the arch, some of the descending aortic blood flow will pass through the aortic arch, the amount depending on the severity of the obstruction and the ability of the left ventricle to overcome the increased afterload. Because there is generally a significant left-to-right shunt across a ventricular septal defect, the increased pulmonary blood flow usually delays the normal postnatal fall in pulmonary vascular resistance. This elevated pulmonary vascular resistance promotes right-to-left shunting into the descending aorta through the patent ductus arteriosus and maintains lower body blood flow. Initially, while the ductus arteriosus is dilated, there may be no arterial blood pressure difference between the upper and lower body. There may be cyanosis of the toes and feet

with normal color of the fingers and hands because of the right-to-left shunt at the ductus arteriosus level. However, with progressive constriction of the ductus arteriosus, the lower body arterial blood pressure falls, and its pulse pressure narrows. The progressive fall in pulmonary vascular resistance after birth further interferes with the flow of blood across the ductus arteriosus because flow will preferentially go through the pulmonary circulation rather than to the lower body. Left ventricular myocardial performance, already affected by the increased afterload, is further stressed by this volume load so that there may be severe left ventricular failure. The time course of these changes varies. As perfusion to the lower body further decreases, metabolic acidemia develops, and there may be oliguria or anuria related to inadequate renal blood flow.

In many infants the clinical presentation of these lesions is that of a large left-to-right intracardiac shunt with left-sided failure. In some of these the hypoplasia is not severe, and the arch anomaly is only of secondary importance, but in others the arch may be severely hypoplastic or even interrupted. Two-dimensional echocardiography defines clearly the intracardiac abnormalities associated with aortic arch interruption. Clear definition of the arch itself, however, is not always possible with echocardiography alone and may require cardiac catheterization with angiography.

Infants with aortic arch narrowing and an associated intracardiac lesion may respond to medical management, including digitalis and particularly diuretics. Prostaglandin E_1 infusions have been extremely beneficial in many of these infants. After dilatation of the ductus arteriosus, lower body perfusion is often restored, renal function returns, and the infants clear acidemia. This temporizing measure then allows stabilization before surgery. Surgical repair should be done, even in premature infants, if the narrowing is severe or the arch is interrupted. At the time of correction of the aortic arch anomaly, surgical measures to correct or palliate the intracardiac lesion may be necessary.

LOCALIZED JUXTADUCTAL COARCTATION OF AORTA Several terms, such as postductal or adult-type coarctation, have been applied to this lesion. However, localized narrowing of the aorta (coarctation of the aorta) is always closely related to the insertion of the ductus arteriosus into the aorta; in fact, the posterolateral shelf that forms the localized narrowing is generally directly opposite the ductus arteriosus. For this reason the term *juxtaductal aortic coarctation* seems more appropriate. With closure of the ductus arteriosus and growth of the child, the usual concentric obstruction seen in older children and young adults will develop. Unlike hypoplastic aortic arches, major intracardiac anomalies are not commonly found with isolated coarctation of the aorta; however, there is a high association of this lesion with Turner syndrome and with bicuspid aortic valve. Other associated abnormalities include aberrant origins of the subclavian arteries, ventricular septal defect, persistent patency of ductus arteriosus, and the group of defects associated with parachute mitral valve.

Because the ductus arteriosus is wide during fetal life, localized juxtaductal coarctation is unlikely to produce significant alteration in the distribution of blood flow during fetal life, and fetal development is normal. Normally after birth the ductus arteriosus constricts at its pulmonary artery end first, so that although it is functionally closed, an aortic ampulla of the ductus arteriosus persists for several days to several months. There is generally a progressive reduction in the size of the ampulla as the ductus arteriosus constricts progressive toward its aortic end. If there is a juxtaductal aortic coarctation directly opposite the aortic end of the ductus arteriosus, and the aortic ampulla remains moderately large, flow from the ascending aorta to the descending aorta is not impeded by the posterolateral shelf, so there will be no clinical evidence of the coarctation. However, as the aortic end of the ductus arteriosus constricts, blood flow becomes obstructed; obstruction is facilitated by constriction of an extension of ductus smooth muscle that forms a sling around the posterior shelf. If the posterolateral shelf is large, and obstruction develops rapidly, a sudden increase in afterload to the left ventricle causes left ventricular failure.

The clinical presentation is often similar to that of severe aortic stenosis in the neonatal period and mimics the circulatory collapse associated with overwhelming sepsis. Significant left-to-right atrial shunting may occur through a stretched foramen ovale, and when there is severe left ventricular failure, all pulses may be weak. However, with improvement in left ventricular function, a significant pressure difference develops between the arms and the legs. Because there has been no obstruction during fetal life and failure has occurred rapidly, collateral circulation is not usually well developed in the newborn. Specific murmurs are not a feature of this lesion in infancy; however, if the ductus arteriosus is still patent, a continuous murmur may be heard at the upper left sternal border. As with aortic stenosis in infancy, the electrocardiogram typically shows right axis deviation and right ventricular hypertrophy. The chest roentgenogram shows marked generalized cardiomegaly with pulmonary venous congestion secondary to left ventricular failure. Two-dimensional echocardiography can often define the anatomy of the coarctation and, together with evaluation of the Doppler velocity signals in both the ascending and descending aorta, can give a good idea of the severity of the obstruction. If the anatomy is not clarified by echocardiography, then aortography should be done in an infant and MRI in the older child. In general, infants who have rapidly developed severe congestive failure from a coarctation in the neonatal period respond poorly to medical treatment, and surgical excision of the coarctation should be performed as soon as the patient is stable. If left ventricular function is severely depressed, inotropic support should be given. Infusion of PGE_1 has been of great benefit in many of these infants in preparation for surgery, as it may dilate the ductus arteriosus, permitting blood to flow around the constricting shelf and relieve the acute aortic obstruction.

If the aortic shelf is not very prominent, or the ampulla of the ductus arteriosus occludes gradually, aortic obstruction develops slowly over several weeks or months. Rapid left ventricular failure is less likely because compensatory mechanisms such as myocardial hypertrophy and development of collateral circulation have time to occur. Collateral anastomoses generally involve the periscapular, intercostal, transverse cervical, and internal mammary arteries. If there are large collateral vessels, only minor pressure differences may be apparent between the ascending and descending aorta at rest; larger differences may be brought out by exercise. Cardiac failure may appear at 3 to 6 months as the coarctation becomes more severe. However, if failure does not occur by 6 months of age, it is rare until adult life. In older children the presenting symptoms may be related to hypertension in the ascending aorta or to decreased blood flow to the legs during exercise, with intermittent claudication. Cerebrovascular accidents associated with hypertension are rare before the age of 7 years and may be associated with rupture of berry aneurysms. Hypertension above and below the coarctation has been described, but the mechanism is unclear. Intimal thickening of the coronary arteries may occur. Infective endocarditis is also common with coarctation and usually involves the aortic wall in the dilated poststenotic segment, but it may occur on the bicuspid aortic valve.

The clinical findings in a child with coarctation of the aorta include easily palpable collateral arteries above the clavicle and over the lateral and inferior scapular margins. The arm pulses are strong, but femoral pulses are decreased and delayed relative to the arm pulses. Because there is a high association of abnormality of one of the subclavian arteries, palpation of both subclavian arteries as well as carotid arteries should be routine. An aberrant right subclavian artery arising below the coarctation gives a low blood pressure in the right arm; the left subclavian artery arises normally but may be hypoplastic, so that left arm pressures also may be low. Blood pressure measurements in the arm and leg confirm the palpated differences. Depending on the severity of the coarctation, the heart may or may not be enlarged, and an increased left ventricular impulse palpable. The heart sounds are generally normal; however, with hypertension or an associated bicuspid aortic valve, an ejection systolic click and a third heart sound may be heard. Soft high-frequency continuous murmurs are often audible over the large collateral vessels. A short, soft ejection systolic murmur may be heard at the upper sternal area or posteriorly to the left of the spine.

The chest roentgenogram (Fig. 22-40) has several classic features. Cardiac enlargement and left ventricular enlargement depend on the severity of the stenosis. The ascending aorta is often dilated and displaces the superior vena cava to the right. On the left border of the aortic arch and descending aortic shadow, the area of poststenotic dilatation below the coarctation and the dilated aortic segment just above the coarctation may be seen as the "3" sign. Notching of the lower margin of the ribs at about the junction of the middle and medial thirds, caused by erosion of the bone by large intercostal arteries, may be seen after 1 year of age in half the patients. The electrocardiogram demonstrates left ventricular hypertrophy from the obstruction. Older children may have S-T depression and T-wave flattening or inversion in left chest leads, but these changes are uncommon. Two-dimensional echocardiography and color Doppler flow mapping are valuable in assessing the anatomy of the coarctation and the adjacent aorta and vessels; Doppler eval-

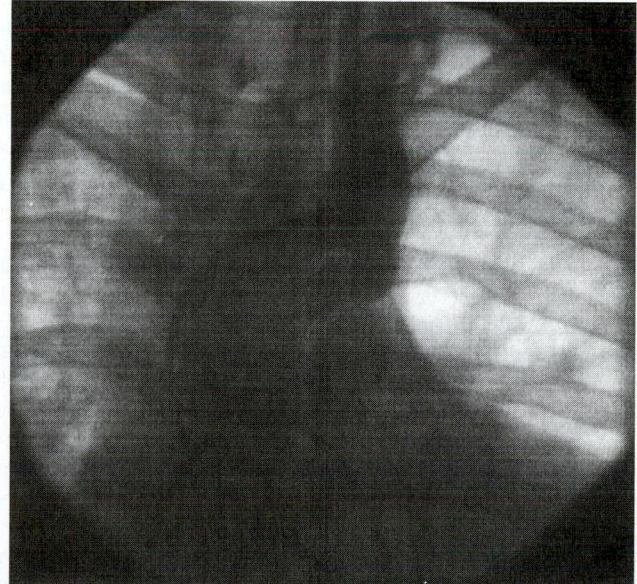

FIGURE 22-40 Posteroanterior roentgenogram of upper thorax. There is a catheter in the transverse aortic arch through which contrast material has been injected to show the coarctation. Opposite the coarctation, the left fourth rib shows prominent notching due to erosion by an enlarged collateral intercostal artery.

uation can estimate the pressure difference across the coarctation but usually exaggerates the severity as compared to upper to lower extremity blood pressure measurements. Magnetic resonance imaging can accurately define the anatomy and should be performed if the echocardiogram is unclear.

If the coarctation is not treated, there may be persistent hypertension, rupture of a berry aneurysm of the circle of Willis, congestive heart failure, infective endocarditis, hypertensive encephalopathy, or rupture of the aorta; the latter has been reported only in adults. For these reasons, treatment is recommended at the time of diagnosis. Surgery remains the treatment of choice in infants and young children. Excision with direct anastomosis is the surgical technique of choice whenever possible; however, widening of the aorta with a patch or part of the subclavian artery to reduce the chances of recoarctation is sometimes necessary. Surgery has become very safe and effective, even for neonates. Recoarctation is more common if surgery is done before 2 years of age; however, its incidence is decreasing with improved surgical techniques. In addition, there is evidence that the earlier the repair, the less likely there is to be persistent "essential" hypertension, which sometimes follows coarctation surgery. Balloon angioplasty for older children and angioplasty with stent placement for adolescents and adults are excellent less invasive therapeutic alternatives to surgery. This treatment requires minimal hospitalization with return to full activities within 2 days. Balloon angioplasty of both native (unoperated) coarctation and postoperative recoarctation is effective in 80% of patients and has become the treatment of choice for all recoarctation patients. Angioplasty with stent placement is effective in over 95% of patients but has been reserved for older children and adults because of the limitations of stent size on vessel growth (Fig. 22-41).

POSTCOARCTECTOMY SYNDROME   Fever, abdominal pain of varying degree, abdominal distension, nausea, and vomiting may commence 1 to 3 days after surgical repair of aortic coarctation and last for several days. Systemic hypertension is always present. In the most severe forms, infarction of segments of bowel has occurred, but in most children the syndrome is mild. This complication may be secondary to arteritis in thin mesenteric and renal arteries suddenly perfused with pulsatile flow at pressures higher than those to which they have previously been exposed. The mainstay of treatment is to lower blood pressure with antihypertensive agents. Other therapy includes fluid and electrolyte maintenance and, if necessary, abdominal decompression by nasogastric suction. Rarely, resection of an infarcted area of bowel becomes necessary.

PSEUDOCOARCTATION   Increased length of the aortic arch occurs occasionally and causes kinking of the descending thoracic aorta. Murmurs caused by turbulent flow across the arch, as well as minor pressure differences between the arms and the legs, may lead one to suspect a true coarctation of the aorta. The diagnosis is made by either cardiac catheterization with angiocardiography or magnetic resonance imaging; the distal portion of the aortic arch is generally angled anteriorly. Usually, no specific treatment is required, although rarely aortic dissection has been reported in adults.

ABDOMINAL COARCTATION   Obstruction of the lower thoracic or abdominal aorta by an intrinsic narrowing is considerably less common than the usual form of coarctation of the aorta. Rather than the short segment of constriction seen in juxtaductal coarctation, a long narrow segment is usually present, and one or several major branch arteries of the abdominal aorta are usually involved. The diagnosis is generally suspected when there is a difference between

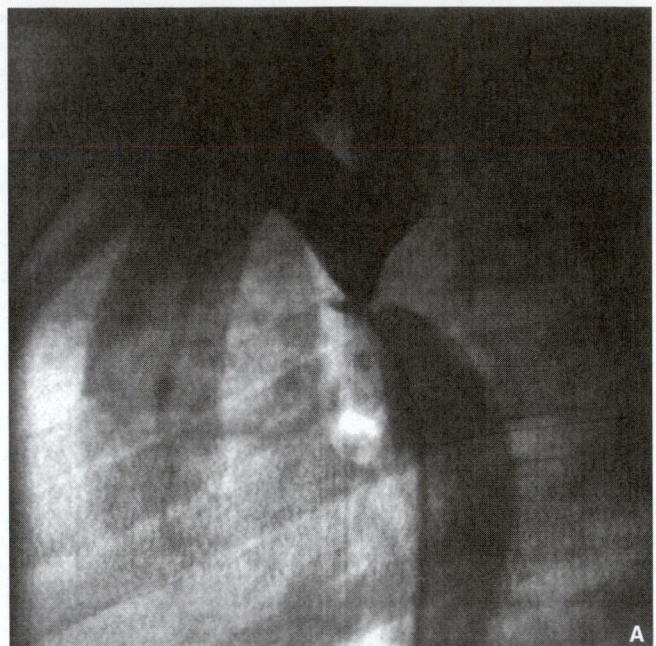

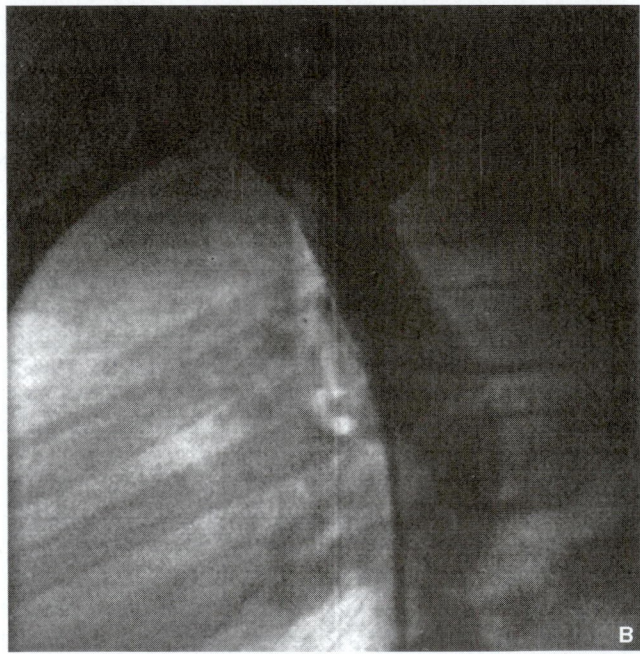

FIGURE 22-41   A: Aortogram of a tight coarctation of the aorta just below the left subclavian artery. The contrast medium is injected into the ascending aorta, and the image below the coarctation is less dense because little of the material reaches the descending aorta. B: An aortogram in the same patient after balloon dilatation of the coarctation and placement of a stent to keep the aorta wide. The stent can be seen faintly as a wire mesh where the previous obstruction was.

the upper- and lower-limb pulse volumes and arterial blood pressures without any indication of thoracic collateral arterial circulation or a murmur in the chest. A systolic or continuous murmur is frequently heard over the abdomen and is best heard posteriorly. The diagnosis is confirmed by two-dimensional echocardiography with Doppler or cardiac catheterization and angiocardiography. Treatment involves surgical removal of the obstructed segment, which may be difficult because arterial branches to vital organs may be involved in the coarcted segment. If the area is not adjacent to major abdominal aortic branches, angioplasty with stent placement can be effective in the older patient.

PERIPHERAL SYSTEMIC ARTERIAL STENOSIS Peripheral systemic arterial stenoses may occur in any systemic artery; however, renal artery stenosis is the most common. In rubella syndrome, peripheral pulmonic stenosis is commonly accompanied by multiple peripheral systemic arterial stenoses, often involving the renal arteries and causing renovascular systemic hypertension. Takayasu arteritis causes stenosis of the origins of medium-sized systemic or pulmonary arteries (see Sec. 12.6.6).

RIGHT HEART OBSTRUCTION

Right heart obstruction can occur in the pulmonary capillary bed, pulmonary arteries, pulmonary valve, RVOT, tricuspid valve, and systemic veins.

GENERAL FEATURES The responses of the right ventricle to an increased afterload are similar to those described for the left ventricle. Right ventricular hypertrophy produces a forceful slow lift felt best along the left sternal border and behind the sternum. If there is pulmonary hypertension, the pulmonary artery may be felt in systole in the third interspace at the left sternal border, the pulmonic component of the second heart sound is accentuated, and there may be an ejection systolic click at the base. The ventricle will appear enlarged on roentgenogram only if dilated; even if the heart is not enlarged, the apex may be tipped up. If there is pulmonary hypertension, the main pulmonary artery may be enlarged. The ECG shows right axis deviation, tall R waves, or a qR complex in the right precordial leads, and there may be upright T waves at an age when they should be inverted or deep inversion of the right precordial T waves, described as a strain pattern.

When right atrial pressure rises, systemic venous return is obstructed, and systemic venous pressure rises. Right atrial pressure loading may be reflected in a fourth heart sound, some dilatation of the right atrium on roentgenogram, and tall peaked P waves in leads II and V_1 of the electrocardiogram. Should the systemic venous pressure be elevated, then characteristic enlargement of liver, spleen, and distention of the jugular veins occurs. Peripheral edema of the soft tissues is a late finding, very uncommon in younger children.

Right atrial pressure elevation is usually the result of right ventricular failure. Right ventricular pressure elevation is frequently the result of pulmonary hypertension caused by a raised pulmonary venous pressure, which in turn follows left ventricular failure. Because left ventricular pressure overload, as in coarctation of the aorta, can cause a right ventricular pressure overload via a raised pulmonary venous pressure and vascular resistance, it is possible for the clinical picture of left heart obstruction to be dominated by the right ventricular signs.

SYSTEMIC VENOUS OBSTRUCTION Obstruction to superior or inferior vena caval return may result from an extrinsic lesion such as a mediastinal mass or an intrinsic lesion such as thrombosis, or it may occur secondarily to intracardiac surgical procedures such as an atrial baffle procedure for aortopulmonary transposition. Acute obstruction may present with venous distension and edema of that portion of the body drained by the obstructed vein. Peripheral organs, particularly the liver and spleen, become congested and enlarged, and peripheral edema may result. Increased systemic venous

pressure in the intestine may result in bowel edema and eventually ascites leading to poor food absorption, nausea, vomiting, and abdominal pain. However, collateral venous channels generally form rapidly, and these signs soon diminish. Venous collateral channels may be evident superficially. If symptoms persist, treatment by either surgical patch or balloon angioplasty with stent placement can be very effective. Congenital interruption of the inferior vena cava occurs commonly with cardiac and visceral malposition; polysplenia is commonly associated. Venous drainage is effected through an enlarged azygous system, and there is usually no venous obstruction.

OBSTRUCTION IN THE RIGHT ATRIUM A tumor in the right atrium, generally a myxoma but occasionally an extension of a Wilms tumor or a hepatic tumor, may obstruct venous return. The clinical presentation usually mimics that of tricuspid stenosis, with intermittent obstruction when there is a myxoma. Right atrial myxomas are far less common than those in the left atrium. Thrombus formation in the right atrium may also produce venous obstruction; this is rare in children but may complicate indwelling caval or atrial catheters.

TRICUSPID VALVE OBSTRUCTION The most severe form of tricuspid valve obstruction is tricuspid atresia (discussed in Sec. 22.3.5). Isolated congenital tricuspid stenosis is rare, and more often underdevelopment of the tricuspid valve and its annulus is associated with underdevelopment of the whole right ventricle. Underdevelopment of the right ventricle (hypoplastic right ventricle) is usually associated with either severe pulmonic stenosis or pulmonary atresia. Whether or not the ventricular septum is intact, a hypoplastic right ventricle generally presents in infancy with severe cyanosis as a result of right-to-left shunting at the atrial level.

If the interatrial septum is intact, the physical findings of tricuspid stenosis include those of venous obstruction. On auscultation there is usually a middiastolic rumbling murmur at the lower left sternal border as well as a prominent third sound, and in severe stenosis an audible fourth sound. The electrocardiogram may show tall peaked P waves indicative of right atrial enlargement, and the latter may be seen also on the chest roentgenogram.

Treatment of tricuspid stenosis often depends on the associated right heart abnormalities. Isolated valve stenosis can be repaired surgically with an annuloplasty. Associated right ventricular hypoplasia may require a palliative approach with placement of a Glenn shunt (SVC to RPA), thereby requiring the small RV to pump only the lower body blood flow.

RIGHT VENTRICULAR OUTFLOW OBSTRUCTION As with left ventricular outflow obstruction, right ventricular outflow obstruction may occur at the level of the pulmonic valve or above or below the valve leaflets. Valvar pulmonic stenosis is the most common form of right ventricular outflow obstruction. Complete obstruction, pulmonary atresia, is discussed in Sec. 22.3.5.

VALVAR PULMONIC STENOSIS In valvar pulmonic stenosis the valve annulus is usually normally formed, but there are abnormalities of the valve leaflets. In less severe forms there are three normally formed cusps, but the raphae are partly fused, so that the leaflet movement is restricted. In more severe forms there is less clear separation of the cusps, which are thickened to varying degrees and form a dome. Right ventricular hypertrophy occurs in response to the valve obstruction, with significant infundibular (subvalvar) stenosis developing in more severe forms of valvar pulmonic stenosis; this tends to be progressive, producing a secondary outflow obstruction. With the more severe forms of valvar pulmonic stenosis, the valve annulus and even the entire main and major branch pulmonary arteries may be underdeveloped (hypoplastic). In children with Noonan syndrome, there is a high incidence of valvar pulmonic stenosis with thick and myxomatous cusps.

Somatic development is usually normal at the time of birth in infants with pulmonic stenosis. Although the right ventricle is normally the dominant ventricle in the fetus and ejects about two-thirds of the combined ventricular output, total fetal cardiac output is probably normal in the face of right ventricular outflow obstruction. Systemic venous return is probably diverted across the foramen ovale and ejected by the left ventricle, which assumes dominance. The wider-than-normal ascending aorta and aortic isthmus found in infants with severe pulmonic stenosis or pulmonary atresia supports this thesis.

With valvar pulmonic stenosis, development of the right ventricle and tricuspid valve in the fetus probably depends on the stage of gestation at which the stenosis occurs. If stenosis develops early in gestation, venous return is likely to be diverted across the foramen ovale, with subsequent underdevelopment of the right ventricle and the tricuspid valve and even eventual development of pulmonary atresia. However, if the stenosis occurs later, right ventricular development is more likely to be normal.

PATHOPHYSIOLOGY In pulmonic stenosis the right ventricle requires increased amounts of oxygen and therefore coronary blood flow. Currently no information is available as to the exact pressure levels at which right ventricular myocardial ischemia occurs; however, severe pulmonic stenosis is required for some time before this becomes a major factor. Even infants with RV pressures 150% above systemic pressures do not show evidence of ischemia on ECG if treated early.

After birth, the course of the circulation and the clinical presentation depend on the severity of the pulmonic stenosis and the degree of development of the right ventricular chamber and outflow tract, the tricuspid valve, and the main and branch pulmonary arteries. In severe pulmonic stenosis the right ventricle is incapable of ejecting the total systemic venous return, and therefore, pulmonary blood flow derived from the right ventricle is limited. Infants with this form of severe pulmonic stenosis, also termed "critical pulmonic stenosis," behave as if complete pulmonic atresia were present, and most of the pulmonary blood flow will then have to be provided through a patent ductus arteriosus.

Right ventricular hypertension caused by severe valvar obstruction leads to tricuspid regurgitation and elevated right atrial pressures. Most of the systemic venous return is directed across the interatrial septum to the left atrium, causing cyanosis. The degree of cyanosis is determined by the amount of atrial shunt and pulmonary blood flow through the patent ductus. The atrial shunt is generally through a patent foramen ovale, although true atrial septal defects do occur with pulmonic stenosis. In early infancy, obstruction to flow across the interatrial septum is unusual because the foramen ovale has carried a significant volume of blood in fetal life. However, if the interatrial communication becomes inadequate, systemic output may not be maintained, and systemic venous obstruction may occur.

In moderately severe pulmonic stenosis adequate anterograde pulmonary blood flow is present when the ductus arteriosus closes. The right ventricle hypertrophies in response to the increased pressure load, and it can usually maintain an adequate output with mod-

erately severe obstructions. Infants with this degree of obstruction are therefore able to maintain normal pulmonary blood flow; even if they have interatrial communication, they have neither right-sided failure nor right-to-left atrial shunting. With more severe pulmonic stenosis, the right ventricle may be incapable of maintaining the high pressure required to overcome the obstruction and provide a normal output, and right-sided cardiac failure may therefore develop within a few months after birth. If there is an interatrial communication, right-to-left atrial shunting of moderate to mild degree may occur and cause cyanosis. Most infants and children with mild or moderate pulmonic stenosis develop and grow normally. Systemic and pulmonary blood flows therefore increase with age, and if the orifice of the obstructed pulmonic valve does not grow, the right ventricular systolic pressure increases gradually to maintain output. Furthermore, because the normal resting heart rate of an infant is higher than that of an older child, the decrease in heart rate causes stroke volume to increase significantly, and systolic flow across the stenotic valve increases commensurately.

CLINICAL FEATURES Severe pulmonic stenosis presents in the immediate postnatal period and resembles pulmonary atresia with severe cyanosis and cardiac collapse as the ductus closes. In moderately severe pulmonic stenosis during infancy, mild cyanosis may be present if the foramen ovale remains patent. However, if the foramen ovale becomes sealed, the cyanosis disappears. Right ventricular failure may become evident after about 6 months, but if it does not occur at that time it is generally delayed until early adulthood. Right ventricular failure will be evidenced by rapid onset of hepatomegaly, prominent pulsatile neck veins (large *a* waves), and a low-output state.

The majority of children have moderately severe pulmonic stenosis, are asymptomatic, and are detected because of a murmur. Many of the physical findings of pulmonic stenosis correlate roughly with the severity of the stenosis. When right ventricular enlargement is produced, a fairly diffuse forceful parasternal impulse along the lower left border of the sternum may be palpable. A systolic thrill is generally palpable at the upper left sternal border. The auscultatory findings are summarized diagrammatically in Fig. 22-42. The first heart sound is usually normal but may be accentuated. A systolic ejection click is often heard along the entire left sternal border and is softer in patients with severe stenosis. With

VALVAR PULMONIC STENOSIS

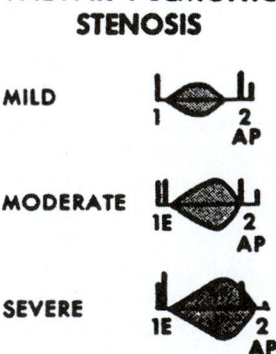

FIGURE 22-42 Diagrammatic representation of the auscultatory findings in valvar pulmonic stenosis. 1 = first heart sound; E = systolic ejection click; 2 = second heart sound; A = aortic component of second heart sound; P = pulmonic component of second heart sound.

progressive development of secondary right ventricular outflow obstruction from infundibular hypertrophy, an ejection click previously heard may disappear. The time interval between the q wave of the electrocardiogram or the first heart sound and the ejection systolic click shortens as the stenosis becomes more severe. The second heart sound is usually moderately soft, and as the stenosis becomes more severe, the pulmonic component of the second sound becomes softer and more delayed. Eventually in the most severe forms of pulmonic stenosis, the pulmonic component of the second sound may completely disappear. With marked hypertrophy a fourth heart sound is often heard, and with right ventricular failure a third heart sound may be present.

The murmur of pulmonic stenosis is an ejection systolic murmur of the crescendo-decrescendo type best heard at the upper left sternal border, with radiation to the left infraclavicular area. The intensity of the murmur does not correlate well with the severity of the stenosis, although it is generally louder in severe stenosis than in very mild stenosis. However, as pulmonic stenosis becomes more severe, right ventricular ejection is prolonged; thus, with more severe obstruction the peak intensity will be later in systole, and the murmur will become longer, until eventually the aortic component of the second sound becomes obscured. The frequency of the murmur correlates with the severity of stenosis, with higher frequencies heard with severe stenosis and low to medium frequencies heard with mild stenosis. During the Valsalva maneuver, as intrathoracic pressure is increased and systemic venous return and right ventricular stroke volume are reduced, the murmur of pulmonic stenosis decreases immediately unless there is congestive heart failure or severe infundibular hypertrophy.

The electrocardiogram shows right atrial hypertrophy with peaked P waves. There will also be right ventricular hypertrophy and right axis deviation, the degree depending on the severity of the stenosis. The right precordial leads show tall R waves, and with severe stenosis, they may also show T-wave inversion and S-T segment depression.

The chest roentgenogram shows right ventricular prominence with an upturned apex. The magnitude of enlargement depends on the severity of the stenosis and subsequent development of right ventricular hypertrophy. The main and left pulmonary arteries are prominent because of poststenotic dilatation (Fig. 22-43). The pulmonary vascular markings are generally within normal limits, or they may appear slightly diminished. Valve cusp thickening, annular narrowing, right ventricular free wall thickening, and pulmonary arterial enlargement are seen on two-dimensional echocardiography (Fig. 22-44). Doppler examination reliably indicates the severity of the obstruction.

NATURAL HISTORY Some children with moderate stenosis show little or no change in right ventricular systolic pressure over many years, indicating that the valve orifice has probably enlarged with growth. However, other children have a marked increase in right ventricular systolic pressure, suggesting either inadequate growth of the pulmonic valve orifice, development of infundibular stenosis, or both. If this should occur, right ventricular end-diastolic pressure eventually rises, and right heart failure may develop. An additional factor causing right ventricular failure may be inadequate myocardial perfusion.

Mild valvar pulmonic stenosis with a small increase in right ventricular systolic pressure may not affect right ventricular output or the right ventricular myocardium significantly. In many instances, with growth of the child there is little or no increase in right ven-

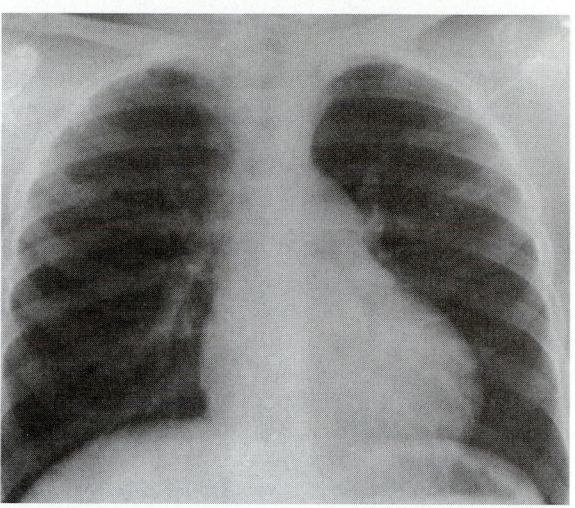

FIGURE 22-43 Chest roentgenogram in a child with isolated valvar pulmonic stenosis. The right ventricle and main pulmonary artery are enlarged; the pulmonary vessels are normal.

tricular systolic pressure, and minimal right ventricular hypertrophy may occur. The long-term outcome for mild RV pressure elevation is excellent, with minimal impact on cardiac function until late adult years.

TREATMENT Those children with severe stenosis (right ventricular systolic pressure greater than systemic) should undergo immediate pulmonary balloon valvoplasty or, if this cannot be done, surgical valvotomy. The majority of children with severe valvar pulmonic stenosis also have infundibular hypertrophy; however, this regresses once the valvar stenosis is relieved. All symptomatic patients with exercise intolerance or fatigue and those with significant right ventricular hypertrophy should be treated, even if the measured gradient is relatively mild. Without symptoms or hypertrophy, a right ventricular systolic pressure of over 50 mm Hg in children warrants

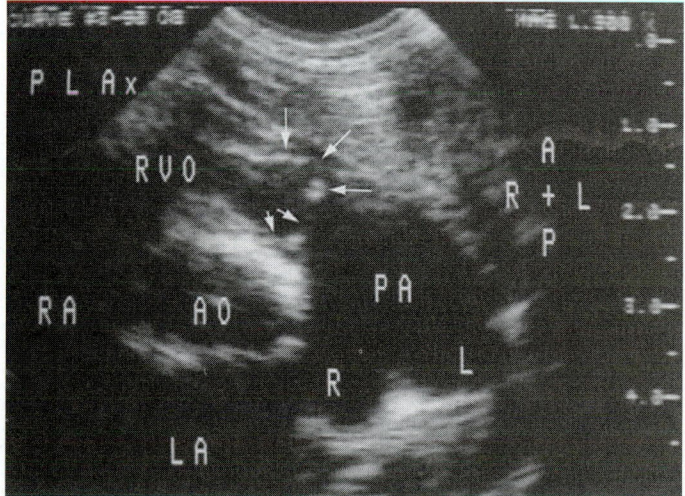

FIGURE 22-44 Thickened, domed pulmonary valve and marked poststenotic dilatation of the main and main branch pulmonary arteries are shown. PA = pulmonary artery; L = left; R = right; LA = left atrium; Ao = aorta; RA = right atrium; RVO = right ventricular outflow.

treatment because over a prolonged period such pressure elevation may lead to myocardial fibrosis. Balloon valvoplasty done at cardiac catheterization is the treatment of choice in most patients, even infants; it can be performed as an outpatient procedure using sedation alone. The relief of obstruction is excellent, on average 60%, with minimal short- or long-term complications (see Sec. 22.2.6).

SUBVALVAR PULMONIC STENOSIS Isolated diffuse infundibular pulmonic stenosis with a normal pulmonic valve is rare. It is more likely to be associated with a ventricular septal defect. The most common type is tetralogy of Fallot, where the aorta overides a large outlet VSD and the right ventricular outflow tract is displaced medially, causing subvalvar pulmonic obstruction (see Sec. 22.3.5). Double-chambered right ventricle, also quite common, is caused by large aberrant muscular bands that divide the right ventricular cavity into two separate chambers and obstruct flow through the subpulmonic infundibular area. This anomaly is usually but not always associated with a ventricular septal defect, is often progressive, and should be treated if significant obstruction is present or there is evidence of RVH. Treatment by surgical resection of the aberrant muscle bundles with closure of the VSD is usually curative.

Diffuse interventricular septal hypertrophy secondary to marked left ventricular hypertrophy may bulge into the right ventricle or outflow tract and thereby produce obstruction (Bernheim effect). Myocardial tumors, particularly those involving the interventricular septum, may also produce right ventricular outflow obstruction.

The clinical features of these lesions are similar to those of valvar pulmonic stenosis. An ejection click is less commonly heard, however, and poststenotic dilatation of the pulmonary artery is less prominent or absent. The systolic murmur is usually maximal at the third or fourth interspace along the left sternal border. These findings lead one to suspect subvalvar stenosis, and the diagnosis can be confirmed by echocardiography. If the anatomy or the degree of obstruction is not well defined by echocardiography, then cardiac catheterization or MRI is needed before surgical repair can be done.

SUPRAVALVAR PULMONIC STENOSIS Stenosis of the major pulmonary arteries may occur anywhere along the entire length of the pulmonary arterial tree. Obstruction may be single or multiple and may be by a diaphragm, localized narrowing, or more diffuse constrictions. Often there are long hypoplastic segments as well as multiple areas of discrete stenosis. There is often an association with intrahepatic cholestasis (Alagille syndrome).

STENOSIS OF MAIN PULMONARY ARTERY In stenosis of the main pulmonary artery a constricting ring is usually present in the main pulmonary artery, either at or shortly beyond the tips of the pulmonic valve leaflets. This type of stenosis is commonly associated with rubella syndrome, where it is produced by a thick fibrous ring. In addition, children with peculiar facies and associated supravalvar stenosis without a history of rubella have been reported, and in them a thin supravalvar diaphragm is present. The clinical findings in this lesion are similar to those of valvar pulmonic stenosis, but the second heart sound is usually normal. The diagnosis can be made at cardiac catheterization or by echocardiography. Although balloon dilatation has been tried, results are poor. Optimal treatment is surgical patch repair. Immediate results are excellent, although there is a small incidence of restenosis at the patch site because of poor growth or scar tissue formation.

PERIPHERAL BRANCH STENOSIS In the newborn period a physiological branch pulmonary arterial stenosis is present, and it ac-

counts for innocent murmurs in many infants up to 6 to 12 months of age. True peripheral pulmonary arterial branch stenosis or hypoplasia may occur as an isolated defect or may be associated with underdevelopment of part or all of one lung or with underdevelopment of the right heart. Peripheral pulmonary arterial stenosis is frequently noted in infants with rubella syndrome, often in association with patent ductus arteriosus. Peripheral branch pulmonary arterial stenosis may also be found with other intracardiac congenital heart diseases, especially tetralogy of Fallot.

The clinical features vary and may mimic either valvar pulmonic stenosis or a patent ductus arteriosus. The murmur is generally harsh and systolic and suggestive of pulmonic stenosis, but it usually has wider radiation into the infraclavicular regions (particularly toward the right) and the axillae; occasionally the murmur is continuous. The second heart sound is not consistently altered, and an ejection click is unusual. The electrocardiogram shows right ventricular hypertrophy in the more severe lesions; in rubella syndrome, left axis deviation is common. The chest roentgenogram may show right ventricular enlargement and occasionally shows multiple dilated pulmonary artery segments caused by poststenotic dilatation. If the peripheral stenosis involves only one lung or one segment of lung, undervascularization of that segment may be evident. Central stenoses may be shown by two-dimensional echocardiography, but peripheral stenoses are not. Echocardiography is useful at assessing the significance of peripheral stenoses by estimating the right ventricular pressure. In addition, radionuclide pulmonary flow scans can demonstrate the presence and physiological significance of peripheral pulmonary artery stenoses. To define the location and anatomy of these defects, cardiac catheterization with angiography is necessary. Treatment depends on the severity and the number of stenoses; multiple peripheral lesions in the parenchyma of the lung are best treated with interventional catheterization techniques (see Sec. 22.2.6) whereas more central lesions may be relieved surgically. Transvascular placement of stents has markedly improved the ability to dilate branch pulmonary arteries and to maintain dilatation even of tortuous or kinked vessels; multiple as well as more peripheral stenoses are also manageable by this new approach.

PERSISTENT PULMONARY HYPERTENSION IN THE NEWBORN This syndrome, characterized by a high pulmonary vascular resistance and diminished pulmonary blood flow, is discussed in Sec. 22.3.9 and 2.17.11.

References

Amaral FT, Ribeiro PJ, Salgado HC: Congenital coarctation of the lower thoracic aorta. A rare surgically correctable cause of hypertension in the young—case report. Int J Cardiol 39:109, 1993

Arensman FW, Francis PD, Helmsworth JA, et al: Early medical and surgical intervention for tetralogy of Fallot with absence of pulmonary valve. J Thorac Cardiovasc Surg 84:430, 1982

Asherson RA, Oakley CM: Pulmonary hypertension and systemic lupus erythematosus. J Rheumatol 13:1, 1986 (erratum J Rheumatol 13:840, 1986)

Beekman RH, Rocchini AP, Behrendt DM, et al: Long-term outcome after repair of coarctation in infancy: subclavian angioplasty does not reduce the need for reoperation. J Am Coll Cardiol 8:1406, 1986

Berman LB, Neches WH, Patrode RE, et al: Coarctation of the aorta in children: late results after surgery. Am J Dis Child 134:464, 1980

Berner M, Beghetti M, Ricou B, et al: Relief of severe pulmonary hypertension after closure of a large ventricular septal defect using low dose inhaled nitric oxide. Intensive Care Med 19:75, 1993

Bove EL, Minich LL, Pridjian AK, et al: The management of severe subaortic stenosis, ventricular septal defect, and aortic arch obstruction in the neonate. J Thorac Cardiovasc Surg 105:289, 1993

Carpentier A: Congenital malformations of the mitral valve. In: Stark J, de Leval M, eds: Surgery for Congenital Heart Disease. New York, WB Saunders, 1993

Cohen M, Fuster V, Steele PM, et al: Coarctation of the aorta: long-term follow-up and prediction of outcome after surgical correction. Circulation 80:840, 1989

Danilowicz D, Hoffman JIE, Rudolph AM: Serial studies of pulmonary stenosis in infancy and childhood. Br Heart J 37:808, 1975

DeBoer DA, Robbins RC, Maron BJ, et al: Late results of aortic valvotomy for congenital valvar aortic stenosis. Ann Thorac Surg 50:69, 1990

Elkins RC, Knott-Craig CJ, Razook JD, et al: Pulmonary autograft replacement of the aortic valve. J Card Surg 9:198, 1994

Fletcher SE, Nihill MR, Grifka RG, et al: Balloon angioplasty of native coarctation of the aorta: midterm follow up and prognostic factors. J Am Coll Cardiol 25:730–734, 1995

Friedman WF: The intrinsic physiologic properties of the developing heart. In: Friedman WF, Lesch M, Sonnenblick EM, eds: Neonatal Heart Disease. New York, Grune & Stratton, 1973

Greenwood RD, Rosenthal A, Crocker AC, et al: Syndrome of intra-hepatic biliary dysgenesis and cardiovascular malformations. Pediatrics 58:243, 1976

Grifka RG, O'Laughlin MP, Nihill MR, et al: Double-transseptal, double-balloon valvoplasty for congenital mitral stenosis. Circulation 85:123, 1992

Hausdorf G, Schneider M, Schirmer KR, et al: Anterograde balloon valvoplasty of aortic stenosis in children. Am J Cardiol 71:460, 1993

Haworth SG: Pulmonary vasculature. In: Anderson RH, Macartney FJ, Shinebourne EA, Tynan M, eds: Paediatric Cardiology. Edinburgh, Churchill Livingstone, 1987:123

Hayes CJ, Gersony WM, Driscoll DJ, et al: Second natural history study of congenital heart defects. Results of treatment of patients with pulmonary valvar stenosis . Circulation 87(2)(Suppl 1):I28, 1993

Heymann MA, Rudolph AM: Effects of congenital heart disease on the fetal and neonatal circulations. Prog Cardiovasc Dis 15:115, 1972

Ho SY, Anderson RH: Coarctation, tubular hypoplasia and the ductus arteriosus. Br Heart J 41:268, 1979

Hoffman JIE: Aortic stenosis. In: Moller JH, Neall WA, eds: Fetal, Neonatal and Infant Cardiac Disease. East Norwalk, CT, Appleton & Lange, 1990:451

Hoffman JIE, Heymann MA: Normal pulmonary circulation. In: Scarpelli EM, ed: Pulmonary Physiology: Fetus, Newborn, Child, Adolescent. Philadelphia, Lea & Febiger, 1990:233

Hoffman JIE, Rudolph AM, Heymann MA: Pulmonary vascular disease with congenital heart lesions: pathologic features and causes. Circulation 64:873, 1981

Hughes GRV: The antiphospholipid syndrome: ten years on. Lancet 342:341, 1993

Johnson MC, Canter CE, Strauss AW, et al: Repair of coarctation of the aorta in infancy: comparison of surgical and balloon angioplasty. Am Heart J 125:464, 1993

Jonas RA, Quaegebeur JM, Kirklin JW, et al: Outcomes in patients with interrupted aortic arch and ventricular septal defect: a multi-institutional study. J Thorac Cardiovasc Surg 107:1099–1113, 1994

Keane JF, Driscoll DJ, Gersony WM, et al: Second natural history study of congenital heart defects. Results of treatment of patients with aortic valvar stenosis. Circulation 87:I-16, 1993

Kelly DP, Strauss AW: Inherited cardiomyopathies. N Engl J Med 330:913, 1994

Kitchiner DJ, Jackson M, Walsh K, et al: Incidence and prognosis of congenital aortic valve stenosis in Liverpool (1960–1990). Br Heart J 69:71, 1993

Knott-Craig CJ, Elkins RC, Ward KE: Neonatal coarctation repair: influence of technique on late results. Circulation 88(Suppl 2):198–204, 1993

Lakier JB, Lewis AB, Heymann MA, et al: Isolated aortic stenosis in the neonate: natural history and hemodynamic considerations. Circulation 50:801, 1974

Levin DL, Heymann MA, Kitterman JA, et al: Persistent pulmonary hypertension of the newborn infant. J Pediatr 89:626, 1976

Levin PL, Mills LJ, Weinberg AG: Hemodynamic, pulmonary vascular and myocardial abnormalities secondary to pharmacologic constriction of the fetal ductus arteriosus. Circulation 60:360, 1979

Lewis AB, Heymann MA, Stanger P, et al: Evaluation of the subendocardial ischemia of valvar aortic stenosis in children. Circulation 49:978, 1974

Li MD, Coles JC, McDonald AC: Anomalous muscle bundle of the right ventricle. Br Heart J 40:1040, 1978

Marian AM, Roberts R: Molecular basis of hypertrophic and dilated cardiomyopathy. Texas Heart Inst J 21:6, 1994

Maron BJ, Roberts WC: Cardiomyopathies in the first two decades of life. In: Engle MA, ed: Pediatric Cardiovascular Disease. Philadelphia, FA Davis, 1981:35

Maron BJ, Tajik AJ, Ruttenberg HD, et al: Hypertrophic cardiomyopathy in infants: clinical features and natural history. Circulation 65:7, 1982

Masura J, Burch M, Deanfield JE, et al: Five-year follow-up after balloon pulmonary valvoplasty. J Am Coll Cardiol 21:13, 1993

Mendelsohn AM, Bove EL, Lupinetti FM, et al: Intraoperative and percutaneous stenting of congenital pulmonary artery and vein stenosis. Circulation 88:II-210, 1993

Moore P, Adatia I, Spevak PJ, et al: Severe congenital mitral stenosis in infants. Circulation 89:2099–2106, 1994

Muhler EG, Neuerburg JM, Ruben A, et al: Evaluation of aortic coarctation after surgical repair: role of magnetic resonance imaging and Doppler ultrasound. Br Heart J 70:285, 1993

Mullins CE, Nihill MR, Vick GW III, et al: Double balloon technique for dilation of valvular or vessel stenosis in congenital and acquired heart disease. J Am Coll Cardiol 10:107, 1987

Nishimura RA, Pieroni DR, Bierman FZ, et al: Second natural history study of congenital heart defects. Aortic stenosis: echocardiography. Circulation 87:I-66, 1993

O'Connor BK, Beekman RH, Lindauer A, et al: Intermediate-term outcome after pulmonary balloon valvoplasty: comparison with a matched surgical control group. J Am Coll Cardiol 20:169, 1992

O'Connor BK, Beekman RH, Rocchini AP, et al: Intermediate-term effectiveness of balloon valvoplasty for congenital aortic stenosis. A prospective follow-up study. Circulation 84:73, 1991

O'Laughlin MP, Slack MC, Grifka RG, et al: Implantation and intermediate-term follow-up of stents in congenital heart disease. Circulation 88:605, 1993

Ostman-Smith I, Silverman NH, Oldershaw P, et al: Cor triatriatum sinistrum. Diagnostic features on cross sectional echocardiography. Br Heart J 51:211, 1984

Palevsky HI, Fishman AP: Vasodilator therapy for primary pulmonary hypertension. Annu Rev Med 36:563, 1985

Rabinovitch M, Grady S, David I, et al: Compression of intrapulmonary bronchi by abnormally branching pulmonary arteries associated with absent pulmonary valves. Am J Cardiol 50:804, 1982

Ramaciotti C, Chin AJ: Noninvasive diagnosis of coarctation of the aorta in the presence of a patent ductus arteriosus. Am Heart J 125:179, 1993

Rao PS: Transcatheter treatment of pulmonary outflow tract obstruction: a review. Prog Cardiovasc Dis 35:119, 1992

Redington AN, Hayes AM, Ho SY: Transcatheter stent implantation to treat aortic coarctation in infancy. Br Heart J 69:80, 1993

Reid LM: Structure and function in pulmonary hypertension. New perceptions. Chest 89:279, 1986

Rich S: Primary pulmonary hypertension. Prog Cardiovasc Dis 31:205, 1988

Roberts N, Moes CAF: Supravalvar pulmonary stenosis. J Pediatr 82:838, 1973

Rowe RD: Maternal rubella and pulmonary artery stenosis. Am J Cardiol 24:318, 1969

Rudolph AM, Heymann MA, Spitznas U: Hemodynamic considerations in the development of narrowing of the aorta. Am J Cardiol 30:514, 1972

Sade RM, Crawford FA, Hohn AR, et al: Growth of the aorta after prosthetic patch aortoplasty for coarctation in infants. Ann Thorac Surg 38: 21, 1984

Shaddy RE, Boucek MM, Sturtevant JE, et al: Comparison of angioplasty and surgery for unoperated coarctation of the aorta. Circulation 87:793, 1993

Sime F, Banchero N, Peñaloza D, et al: Pulmonary hypertension in children born and living at high altitudes. Am J Cardiol 11:150, 1963

Strafford MA, Griffiths SP, Gersony WM: Coarctation of the aorta: a study in delayed detection. Pediatrics 69:159, 1982

Suarez de Lezo J, Pan M, Romero M, et al: Immediate and follow-up findings after stent treatment for severe coarctation of the aorta. Am J Cardiol 83:400–406, 1999

Sullivan ID, Robinson PJ, Leval M, et al: Membranous supravalvar mitral stenosis: a treatable form of congenital heart disease. J Am Coll Cardiol 8:159, 1986

Talsma M, Witsenburg M, Rohmer J, et al: Determinants for outcome of balloon valvoplasty for severe pulmonary stenosis in neonates and infants up to six months of age. Am J Cardiol 71:1246, 1993

Teien DE, Wendel H, Bjornebrink J, et al: Evaluation of anatomical obstruction by Doppler echocardiography and magnetic resonance imaging in patients with coarctation of the aorta. Br Heart J 69:352, 1993

Van der Hauwaert LG, Fryus JP, Doumoulin M, et al: Cardiovascular malformations in Turner's and Noonan's syndrome. Br Heart J 40:500, 1978

Van Son AM, Schaff HV, Danielson GK, et al: Surgical treatment of discrete and tunnel subaortic stenosis: late survival and risk of reoperation. Circulation 88:II-159, 1993

Vogelpoel L, Schrire V: Auscultatory and phonocardiographic assessment of pulmonary stenosis with intact ventricular septum. Circulation 22: 55, 1960

Watkins H, McKenna WJ, Thierfelder L, et al: Mutations in the genes for cardiac troponin T and α-tropomyosin in hypertrophic cardiomyopathy. N Engl J Med 332:1058, 1995

Watkins H, Rosenzweig A, Hwang D-S, et al: Characteristics and prognostic implications of myosin missense mutations in familial hypertrophic cardiomyopathy. N Engl J Med 326:1108, 1992

Wennevold A, Jacobsen JR: Natural history of valvular pulmonic stenosis in children below the age of two years. Long-term follow-up with serial heart catheterizations. Eur J Cardiol 8:371, 1978

Wessel DL: Inhaled nitric oxide for the treatment of pulmonary hypertension before and after cardiopulmonary bypass. Crit Care Med 21:S-344, 1993

Zeevi B, Keane JF, Castaneda AR, et al: Neonatal critical valvar aortic stenosis: a comparison of surgical and balloon dilation therapy. Circulation 80:831, 1989

Zeevi B, Keane JF, Fellows KE, et al: Balloon dilation of critical pulmonary stenosis in the first week of life. J Am Coll Cardiol 11:821, 1988

22.3.5   Right-To-Left Shunts

David F. Teitel

GENERAL FEATURES

In the normal circulation, all the systemic venous return of desaturated or right-sided blood is directed via the right atrium and ventricle to the pulmonary arteries for oxygenation, and the fully saturated pulmonary venous blood is returned via the left atrium and ventricle to the aorta to provide oxygen for the body. Many congenital heart lesions are associated with redirection of some of the right-sided blood to the aorta, thus causing systemic arterial

hypoxemia that leads to cyanosis. This pathophysiological process is called a right-to-left shunt. (Diversion of some of the oxygenated blood back into the lungs is termed a left-to-right shunt.)

PATHOPHYSIOLOGICAL CLASSIFICATION

Three pathophysiological groups are associated with right-to-left shunts (Fig. 22-45). Each group has fairly reproducible pathophysiological processes that dictate the clinical presentation. The first group has a right-to-left shunt only (Fig. 22-45B,C,D). Because systemic blood flow is normal in these patients, the right-to-left shunt must necessarily decrease pulmonary blood flow; the less the pulmonary blood flow, the more the cyanosis. The second group has normal to increased pulmonary blood flow but is associated with cyanosis because the aorta is transposed over the ventricular septum (Fig. 22-45E). Thus, the aorta primarily receives systemic venous return, and the patient usually presents with severe cyanosis. The third group of defects not only has a right-to-left shunt and thus some systemic arterial desaturation but also has a left-to-right shunt (Fig. 22-45F). Frequently the blood is fully mixed in the heart, and the degree of cyanosis depends on the relative pulmonary and systemic blood flows. If neither circulation is obstructed, much more blood tends to be delivered to the lungs because, even at birth, pulmonary vascular resistance is less than systemic. The elevated pulmonary blood flow in these patients limits the degree of cyanosis, and their symptoms usually are related to the elevated pulmonary blood flow, which frequently causes respiratory symptoms and failure to thrive.

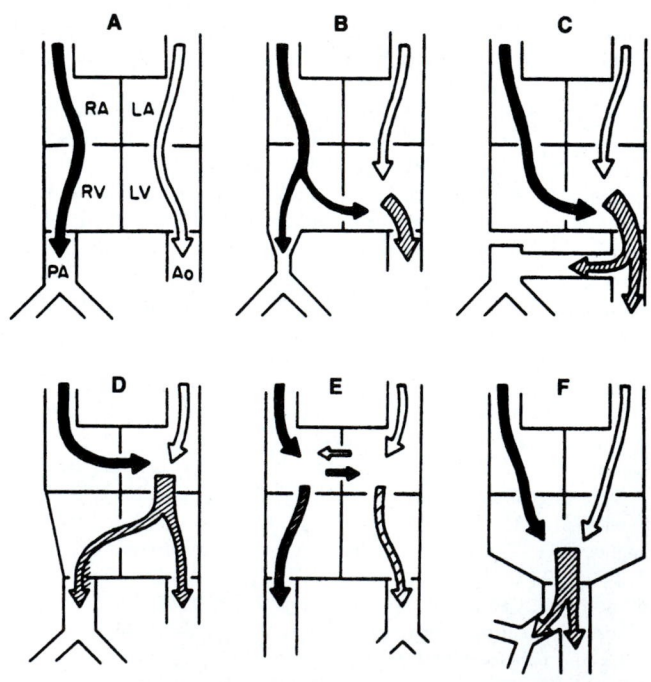

FIGURE 22-45 Diagrams of normal heart (**A**), tetralogy of Fallot (**B**), pulmonary atresia (**C**), tricuspid atresia (**D**), aortopulmonary transposition (**E**), and truncus arteriosus (**F**). *White arrows* indicate fully saturated pulmonary venous return in all diagrams, and also a small left-to-right shunt in diagram E. *Black arrows* indicate desaturated systemic venous return in all diagrams as well as a right-to-left shunt in all diagrams except A. *Cross-hatched arrows* indicate blood of intermediate saturation because of mixing of fully saturated and desaturated bloodstreams.

PURE RIGHT-TO-LEFT SHUNT (DECREASED PULMONARY BLOOD FLOW)

GENERAL Pure right-to-left shunts occur when the inflow or outflow of the right side of the heart is redirected or obstructed or when one of the right-sided valves is insufficient. It is best to think of this group of lesions along lines of blood flow (Table 22-12). For example, the first level of redirection of flow is at the level of the systemic veins, some of which can flow directly into the left atrium, as occurs in an unroofed coronary sinus. The first level of obstruction or insufficiency within the heart is at the tricuspid valve. Obstruction may be caused either by complete absence of the valve (tricuspid atresia) or stenosis (hypoplastic right heart syndrome). Insufficiency of the valve may be secondary to perinatal asphyxia, causing transient papillary muscle dysfunction, or may be secondary to a primary valve abnormality, as in Ebstein anomaly. Whatever the cause, right atrial pressure is elevated, and thus systemic venous blood is directed across the atrial septum to the left side of the heart and causes cyanosis. Obstruction of the outflow of the right ventricle can occur with a ventricular septal defect (tetralogy of Fallot) or without it (critical pulmonary stenosis or pulmonary atresia with intact ventricular septum). Pulmonary arterial stenoses usually occur in association with tetralogy of Fallot but can be isolated, as in Williams syndrome. Last, pulmonary arterial blood flow can be redirected just before it is about to reach the capillary bed for oxygenation, as occurs in pulmonary arteriovenous malformations.

INITIAL PRESENTATION The degree of cyanosis is determined by the amount of pulmonary blood flow in these patients. In neonates with critical obstruction or insufficiency, systemic arterial oxygen tension falls rapidly over the first hours or days of life, and prostaglandin E_1 (PGE_1) infusion is essential to maintain adequate pulmonary blood flow via the ductus arteriosus. In any newborn with significant cyanosis in the first hours of birth, infusion of PGE_1 should be started immediately on the assumption that pulmonary blood flow is compromised. The primary complications of PGE_1 are systemic vasodilatation and respiratory depression. As long as blood pressure is kept normal with volume infusion and vasoconstrictor support as necessary, and as long as ventilatory support is available in the event of respiratory depression, PGE_1 is never absolutely contraindicated and may be life-saving in patients with decreased pulmonary blood flow. Oxygen therapy is of very limited value because pulmonary blood flow is decreased and pulmonary venous blood is nearly fully saturated, but it may increase oxygen content in the blood slightly by adding oxygen dissolved in the blood. If hemoglobin concentrations are relatively low, blood transfusions can increase oxygen uptake in the lung by increasing the amount of hemoglobin to which the oxygen can bind.

Metabolic acidemia is rarely present unless the cyanosis is extremely severe. Prostaglandin E_1 will usually rapidly increase pulmonary blood flow and lead to resolution of the acidosis, but if acidosis is moderately severe, intravenous infusions of sodium bicarbonate can be given. Undiluted molar sodium bicarbonate (1 meq/mL) is generally given to the neonate intravenously in 5-mL amounts. After each injection, arterial or mixed venous pH should be reassessed so that the time and amount of subsequent injections can be based on the response. The infant should also be kept at an optimal temperature (skin temperature about 36.5°C) to minimize oxygen needs. In the very sick infant, tracheal intubation, muscle paralysis with neuromuscular blocking agents, and mechanical ventilation may conserve energy and ensure the best possible ventilation. These very sick infants often have acute gastric dilatation, and removal of stomach contents and limitation of oral intake may be necessary to prevent aspiration.

Hypoglycemia is common because anaerobic metabolism accelerates glycolysis. Blood glucose levels should be checked early, and glucose infusions should be given if the levels are low. Hypocalcemia may occur and also should be treated.

Definitive diagnosis is usually made by echocardiography. Cardiac catheterization is rarely indicated except for those in whom the catheterization may be therapeutic (such as balloon pulmonary valvuloplasty in infants with critical pulmonary stenosis or coil embolization of pulmonary arteriovenous malformations). Unlike those patients with transposition of the great vessels, the atrial communication is usually large, and thus balloon atrial septostomy is rarely indicated. This is because the obstruction is present in utero, and thus a much larger amount of blood than the normal 35 to 45% of combined venous return crosses the foramen ovale to the left atrium and ventricle. This increased blood flow across the foramen ovale is thought to increase the size of the foramen ovale and lead to true secundum atrial septal defects in many infants. Diagnostic catheterization is generally reserved for patients with pulmonary arterial abnormalities (for example, patients with pulmonary atresia, ventricular septal defect, and major aortopulmonary

TABLE 22-12
PURE RIGHT-TO-LEFT SHUNT LESIONS

LEVEL	PATHOPHYSIOLOGY	LESION
Systemic veins	Redirection of flow	Systemic vein to left atrium (usually left superior vena cava)
		Unroofed coronary sinus
Tricuspid valve	Obstruction	Tricuspid atresia
		Tricuspid stenosis (usually hypoplastic right ventricle with pulmonary atresia)
	Insufficiency	Ebstein anomaly
		Papillary muscle dysfunction (perinatal asphyxia)
Right ventricle	Obstruction	Double-chamber right ventricle
		Infundibular stenosis (usually with tetralogy of Fallot)
Pulmonary valve	Obstruction	Tetralogy of Fallot (either pulmonary valve stenosis or atresia)
		Pulmonary stenosis with intact septum
		Pulmonary atresia with intact septum
	Insufficiency	Absent pulmonary valve syndrome
Pulmonary arteries	Obstruction	Supravalvar pulmonary stenosis (usually Williams syndrome)
		Branch pulmonary artery stenosis (usually Alagille or rubella syndrome)
	Redirection	Pulmonary arteriovenous malformation

collaterals) because echocardiography does not afford a good view of the peripheral pulmonary vascular bed.

LONG-TERM MEDICAL THERAPY Although most patients now undergo definitive or at least palliative procedures at a very early age to increase pulmonary blood flow and systemic arterial oxygen saturation to acceptable levels, some patients either do not present to medical care or are not amenable to corrective procedures. These patients have sequelae of chronic cyanosis. The most common group of patients with chronic, persistent cyanosis are those with severe tetralogy of Fallot (with or without pulmonary valve atresia) who have extremely abnormal pulmonary vascular beds that are unable to accept normal amounts of blood flow, so that the ventricular septal defect cannot be closed. Patients with inflow obstruction to the right side of the heart tend to progress to Fontan procedures at an early age so that cyanosis is resolved.

Polycythemia with increased hemoglobin and hematocrit is an important consequence of arterial oxygen desaturation; it is a hematopoietic adaptation to the hypoxic stimulus. The increased oxygen content achieved by this compensatory mechanism is advantageous until the hematocrit exceeds about 55%, when the effects of the high blood viscosity begin to outweigh the advantages of the increased circulating oxyhemoglobin. It is important that hypochromic microcytic anemia be recognized in the severely cyanotic patient with high erythrocyte counts but relatively normal hemoglobin and hematocrit levels; this anemia can easily be corrected by oral iron administration.

The increased blood viscosity in severe cyanotic polycythemia may cause cerebral, mesenteric, renal, or pulmonary thromboses. Dehydration increases the danger of thrombosis, and adequate fluid intake should be maintained, particularly during febrile illnesses and hot weather. Anemia (hypochromic microcytic) in association with hypoxemia has also been implicated, particularly in infants, as one mechanism for cerebrovascular accidents (see Sec. 22.4.11).

Brain abscesses may occur in patients with right-to-left shunts because bacteria normally filtered out in the pulmonary circulation may be shunted directly into the systemic circulation.

Cyanotic patients with long-standing severe polycythemia may have *thrombocytopenia* and abnormalities of the soluble coagulation system, particularly in the older patient; caution is advised in regard to excessive postoperative bleeding.

The prolonged and severe hypoxemia of cyanotic congenital heart disease often results in retarded physical growth that is most striking in the musculature. Preschool children with cyanotic heart disease, as a group, may have slightly lower IQ scores and may perform less well with perceptual motor tasks than do children with acyanotic heart disease.

SPECIFIC LESIONS Although there are a large number of congenital heart defects associated with decreased pulmonary blood flow, the most prevalent and representative of specific groups of lesions are presented below, along lines of blood flow.

Abnormal Systemic Venous Drainage Although abnormal systemic venous connections are sometimes associated with complex cyanotic malformations, isolated abnormal systemic venous connections to the heart are rare and relatively occult causes of cyanotic congenital heart disease without any other abnormal clinical signs or findings. These abnormal connections include termination of the right or left superior vena cava, the inferior vena cava, or hepatic vein in the left atrium. A left superior vena cava usually drains into

the heart via the coronary sinus, so that the drainage of left superior vena caval blood into the left atrium is often referred to as "unroofed coronary sinus." Rarely, a large persistent eustachian valve directs blood from a normally connected inferior vena cava through the foramen ovale. Diagnosis may at times be suspected with careful two-dimensional Doppler and color echocardiographic examination and two-dimensional echocardiographic contrast studies, but appropriate venous angiography should be used to define operative possibilities.

Tricuspid Atresia Tricuspid atresia constitutes 1% of all congenital heart disease in the first year of life. There is agenesis of the tricuspid orifice with no opening from the right atrium to the right ventricle, and the only outlet from the right atrium for systemic venous return is an interatrial communication, usually a widely patent foramen ovale (Fig. 22-45D). Mixing of the entire pulmonary venous return and systemic venous return occurs in the left atrium, and consequently, systemic arterial oxygen desaturation depends on pulmonary blood flow. Left ventricular output is then distributed directly to the aorta and indirectly through a ventricular septal defect or patent ductus arteriosus to the pulmonary vascular bed. Pulmonary blood flow is usually severely diminished in tricuspid atresia because of the small, restrictive ventricular septal defect and the underdeveloped stenotic right ventricular outflow tract. Less often, if there is no ventricular septal defect, pulmonary atresia and an extremely hypoplastic right ventricle may be present; pulmonary blood flow must then come from the aorta via a patent ductus arteriosus or aortopulmonary collateral vessels. Increased pulmonary blood flow is uncommon in tricuspid atresia but may occur when the ventricular septal defect is large and the pulmonary outflow tract from the right ventricle is well developed, or when transposition of the great arteries is present and the pulmonary artery arises directly from the left ventricle.

Clinical Manifestations Intense cyanosis usually occurs within hours to days after birth as the ductus arteriosus begins to close, unless the ventricular septal defect and right ventricular outflow tract are widely patent. Right heart failure, manifested by hepatomegaly and occasionally by presystolic hepatic pulsations, is rarely present but will occur if right-to-left shunting is obstructed at the patent foramen ovale. The precordium is quiet. This is an important clinical finding and distinguishes tricuspid atresia from almost all other common forms of cyanotic congenital heart disease except for hypoplastic right heart syndrome. Neonates within this group with outflow obstruction, or neonates with transposition of the great arteries or bidirectional shunts, have either pressure or volume loading of the right ventricle and thus present with either normal or increased right ventricular impulses. There is usually a harsh systolic murmur along the left sternal border caused by flow through the ventricular septal defect and right ventricular infundibular stenosis. The second heart sound is narrowly split, with a soft pulmonary component. If the ventricular septum is intact, there may be no significant murmur or only the very faint continuous bruit of a small patent ductus arteriosus, and the second heart sound is single. Few infants survive beyond 6 months of age without surgical palliation, but for those who do, clubbing, polycythemia, and poor physical development may be apparent.

In contrast, infants with tricuspid atresia and large ventricular septal defect (often with transposition of the great arteries) present with increased pulmonary blood flow and show only minimal cyanosis after the newborn period. Congestive heart failure, with tachypnea, dyspnea, excessive perspiration, hepatomegaly, and pulmonary rales, appears by 3 to 6 weeks of age. The findings in these infants are those of a large left-to-right shunt: precordial hyperactivity, a long harsh pansystolic murmur along the left sternal border, and a prominent middiastolic rumbling murmur at the apex.

Roentgenography The roentgenographic findings in the *usual* infant with tricuspid atresia and small ventricular septal defect include diminished pulmonary vasculature and a small heart with a distinctive rounded or apple configuration resulting from deficiency of the right ventricular and pulmonary artery segments. In contrast, the infant with a large ventricular septal defect or transposition has increased pulmonary markings and a large cardiac silhouette because of left ventricular enlargement.

Electrocardiography The electrocardiographic findings of left superior axis deviation and left ventricular hypertrophy are helpful clues because the two most prevalent cyanotic heart lesions, tetralogy with diminished pulmonary blood flow and complete transposition of the great arteries with increased pulmonary blood flow, usually manifest right axis deviation and prominent right ventricular forces (both normal for a newborn). Right atrial hypertrophy with prominent peaked P waves in limb lead II is also common, and the P-R interval is often abnormally short. In tricuspid atresia with transposition of the great arteries, the QRS axis is usually in the left lower quadrant, but this is still relatively leftward as compared to a normal newborn.

Echocardiography The two-dimensional echocardiogram readily establishes the absence of a tricuspid orifice and valve leaflet apparatus (Fig. 22-46). There is an enlarged left ventricle and usually a hypoplastic right ventricular outflow tract. Tricuspid atresia variants

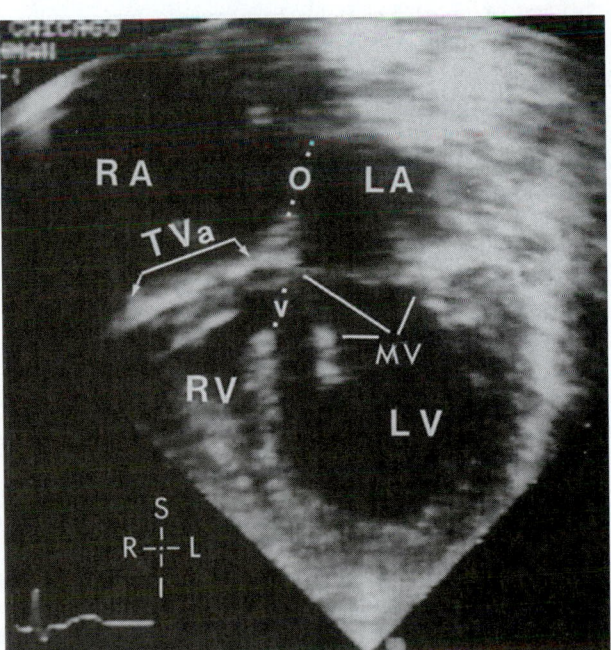

FIGURE 22-46 Tricuspid atresia. Two-dimensional echocardiogram, apical view, showing absence of any tricuspid valve or orifice (TVa) entering the right ventricle (RV). Note large patent interatrial foramen (O), enlarged left ventricle (LV), hypoplastic right ventricle, and ventricular septal defect (V). MV = mitral valve.

with large ventricular septal defect or with transposition of the great arteries can easily be distinguished, as can more complex tricuspid (right- or left-sided AV valve) atresia malformations with ventricular and great artery inversion.

Cardiac catheterization is rarely indicated in the newborn period because the pulmonary arteries are normally developed and the foramen ovale is usually widely patent. Catheterization is generally reserved for the patient following palliative surgical procedures in anticipation of further surgery.

Treatment Treatment of infants with tricuspid atresia and diminished pulmonary blood flow is surgical and often urgent. After the initial presentation of cyanosis and the subsequent institution of PGE_1, the patient usually undergoes a palliative systemic-pulmonary shunt, a modified Blalock–Taussig anastomosis (with Gore-Tex conduit interposition). The operative survival is excellent (~95%) and with stable and prolonged augmentation of the pulmonary blood flow. In the older infant or young child, the shunt is replaced by a cavopulmonary connection that decreases the amount of blood returning to the left ventricle and thus its work. The typical procedure connects the superior vena cava directly to the main pulmonary artery, which is either banded or completely disconnected from the right ventricle (bidirectional Glenn procedure). A late complication reported with the Glenn shunt has been the occurrence of intrapulmonary arteriovenous shunts in dependent portions of the lungs or large superior-to-inferior vena caval collaterals, both with a resultant increase in cyanosis.

The modified Fontan-Kreuzer operation is the final palliative procedure in these children. It diverts the inferior vena caval return directly to the pulmonary arteries, either using an external conduit or a lateral tunnel within the right atrium. After this procedure, all systemic venous blood (except the relatively small coronary circulation, which returns directly to the heart via the coronary sinus) goes directly to the lungs so that the patients are no longer cyanotic. Success of the Fontan operation depends on appropriate selection of patients with adequate sized pulmonary arteries, low pulmonary artery pressure and vascular resistance, and good left ventricular function without significant mitral regurgitation. The results can be very satisfactory, although there is concern about deterioration 15 years or more after the surgery. Heart failure and atrial arrhythmias are the most common late complications, and there is a significant late mortality secondary to these developments. Because the systemic venous pressure is always higher than normal, some patients develop protein-losing enteropathy that is also very difficult to manage.

Neonates with tricuspid atresia, large ventricular defects, with or without transposition of the great arteries, present with markedly increased pulmonary blood flow and usually have early surgical palliation with pulmonary artery banding to restrict the pulmonary blood flow in order to prevent pulmonary vascular disease. Subsequent medical and surgical approaches to these patients are similar to those for the usual patient with tricuspid atresia.

Ebstein Anomaly This is a rare malformation in which the posterior and septal leaflets of the tricuspid valve are displaced downward and attached anomalously to the right ventricular wall. The abnormally placed tricuspid valve divides the right ventricle into a proximal "atrialized" segment and a distal functional ventricle. The atrialized ventricular segment and the right atrium together are usually enormously dilated, and there is severe tricuspid incompetence (Fig. 22-47). Hemodynamic abnormalities are related to the

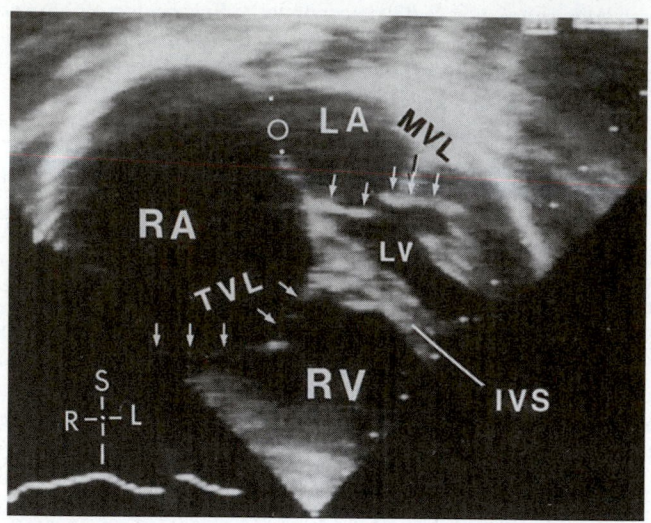

FIGURE 22-47 Ebstein anomaly. Two-dimensional echocardiogram, subcostal view, showing grossly dilated right atrium (RA), prominent downward (apical) displacement of tricuspid valve leaflets (TVL) into right ventricular cavity (RV). IVS = interventricular septum; MVL = mitral valve leaflets; LA = left atrium; LV = left ventricle; O = patent foramen ovale.

extent of the tricuspid regurgitation, to the small size of the remaining functional right ventricle and its outflow (which may be severely obstructed), and to the subsequent degree of right-to-left shunting through a patent foramen ovale.

Clinical Manifestations Wide variations in hemodynamic derangements cause the clinical symptoms to vary widely. In the most extreme lesions, severe tricuspid insufficiency presents in utero, and death occurs secondary to hydrops fetalis. Many neonates present with severe cyanosis. Although this decreases dramatically in the first few days of life because of the rapid perinatal decrease in the pulmonary vascular resistance, some have persistent severe cyanosis requiring placement of a systemic-pulmonary shunt. Those infants usually have severely hypoplastic ventricles and obstructed outflow tracts. The long-term approach is similar to that of tricuspid insufficiency, with a modified Fontan circulation being the final palliative procedure. In most patients, cyanosis resolves in the first few days of life and does not recur, if at all, until later childhood or young adulthood. Although there frequently is little limitation to activities during childhood, exercise tolerance eventually deteriorates. Episodes of paroxysmal supraventricular tachycardia occur in 20 to 25% of patients.

On auscultation a characteristic triple or quadruple heart sound rhythm overrides a soft high-pitched systolic murmur of tricuspid regurgitation. There is also a characteristic soft scratchy middiastolic murmur at the left sternal border and apex. The second heart sound is usually widely split with little respiratory variation.

Roentgenography The roentgenographic findings include moderate or marked cardiomegaly with striking enlargement of the right atrium and usually diminished pulmonary vascular markings. The heart is often globular.

Electrocardiography The electrocardiogram may also be characteristic, usually showing right atrial hypertrophy, prolonged P-R interval, and incomplete or complete right bundle branch block

patterns. Preexcitation patterns (Wolff-Parkinson-White syndrome) occur in about 10 to 15%.

Echocardiography The two-dimensional echocardiogram is diagnostic and shows a large tricuspid orifice with apical displacement of the septal leaflet of the tricuspid valve (Fig. 22-47). The valve displacement is often dramatic, but the extent of displacement and the size of the right atrium correlate poorly with clinical severity. Of more importance are Doppler studies of the extent of tricuspid regurgitation and the right ventricular outflow tract blood flow. Cardiac catheterization is often complicated by induced tachyarrhythmias and is seldom indicated, even for preoperative evaluation.

Treatment Moderate congestive heart failure can be effectively treated with digitalis and diuretics, and disturbing dysrhythmias can usually be controlled pharmacologically. Surgical treatment is seldom necessary in infancy or childhood. When major tricuspid incompetence is associated with progressive congestive heart failure, surgical maneuvers directed at realigning the tricuspid valve leaflets to their true annulus, resecting redundant atrialized tissue, or placing a prosthetic tricuspid valve have been done with reasonably satisfactory functional results.

The life expectancy of the patient with Ebstein anomaly varies widely, depending on the severity. Because the pathologic substratum is so variable, management of these patients must be individualized. The usual cause of death is congestive heart failure in the second or third decade of life. In the child or young adult, the more severe the cyanosis the poorer the prognosis; the onset of florid congestive heart failure is usually followed by death within a few years.

Pulmonary Atresia with Intact Ventricular Septum Two percent of infants who present with severe congenital heart disease in the first year after birth have pulmonary atresia or critical pulmonary valve stenosis with intact ventricular septum. The majority have a hypoplastic but thick-walled right ventricle with a markedly hypoplastic tricuspid orifice and valve (Fig. 22-48). About 15% have a right ventricle of normal or large volume, with tricuspid valve incompetence, and these often have critical stenosis rather than atresia. Intermediate forms occur. In all of the patients there is little or no blood flow across the pulmonary valve; rather, systemic venous return crosses the atrial septum to the left heart and the aorta. The pulmonary circulation is sustained primarily through a patent ductus arteriosus (Fig. 22-49).

Clinical Manifestations Cyanosis occurs early in the neonatal period, and these infants usually deteriorate rapidly and die unless PGE₁ is started. Gross cardiac failure occurs rarely, and only if there is severe tricuspid incompetence. Similar to tricuspid atresia, the precordium is quiet unless there is marked tricuspid incompetence.

If murmurs are heard they are usually faint. A soft systolic blowing murmur, representing insufficiency of the hypoplastic tricuspid valve, may be heard along the lower left and right sternal borders; a soft continuous bruit of a small patent ductus arteriosus may be heard at the upper left sternal border. The second heart sound at the pulmonary area is single, reflecting only aortic valve closure.

Roentgenography On chest roentgenogram the infant with a markedly hypoplastic tricuspid orifice shows a small heart; diminished pulmonary vascular markings are the rule, except rarely with a large persistent patent ductus arteriosus or with an infusion of

PGE$_1$. Even with high pulmonary blood flow, however, the central arteries are not large, so the pulmonary vascular markings may appear diminished. Infants with marked tricuspid insufficiency and large right ventricular and atrial volumes have gross cardiomegaly.

Electrocardiography   On the electrocardiogram left ventricular hypertrophy is common in the first days or weeks of life, but right ventricular hypertrophy becomes evident as the right ventricular muscle hypertrophies further. In contrast to tricuspid atresia, where there is continuing left ventricular hypertrophy and usually a superior left QRS axis deviation, the infant with pulmonary atresia shows an inferior QRS axis and right ventricular hypertrophy.

Echocardiography   A two-dimensional echocardiogram shows the small right ventricle, hypoplastic tricuspid valve, pulmonary valve atresia, and intact ventricular septum. Doppler interrogation sometimes documents retrograde right ventricular coronary sinusoid-to-coronary artery blood flow in systole and may demonstrate flow across the pulmonary valve if there is critical pulmonary stenosis rather than atresia.

Cardiac Catheterization   In contrast to many other lesions, cardiac catheterization is indicated in all patients with pulmonary atresia/critical pulmonary stenosis for both diagnosis and therapeutic reasons. Catheterization shows right atrial hypertension, a massive right-to-left interatrial shunt, and right ventricular hypertension, often with peak systolic pressures far greater than systemic. A right ventricular selective angiogram establishes the diagnosis by demonstrating the obstruction between the right ventricle and the pulmonary artery, and the extent of hypoplasia of the ventricular cavity and tricuspid orifices. In ventricular systole, intramyocardial sinusoids may fill from the dead-end right ventricular cavity and drain retrograde into the coronary arterial system (Fig. 22-48A).

Occasionally, there is no connection between some of these coronary arteries and the aorta; this is called a right ventricular dependent coronary circulation. Although the prognosis for pulmonary atresia in general is poor, with midterm survival in the 60 to 80% range, the prognosis for infants with a dependent coronary circulation is particularly poor, so it should be sought out in every patient. The pulmonary artery will be seen to fill through a tortuous ductus arteriosus (Fig. 22-49). Pulmonary valvuloplasty is attempted in most of these patients, even with atretic valves, as discussed below.

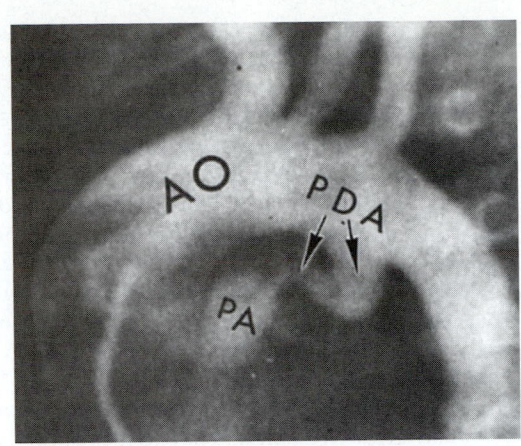

FIGURE 22-49   Angiocardiogram (lateral view) showing long, tortuous, persistent patent ductus arteriosus (PDA) providing tenuous pulmonary blood flow in neonate with pulmonary atresia and intact ventricular septum. PA = pulmonary artery; AO = aorta.

Treatment   Immediate intravenous infusion of PGE$_1$ on diagnosis has greatly improved outcome in these patients. At catheterization an attempt at pulmonary valvuloplasty is made, even if the valve is atretic, except when the tricuspid valve and right ventricle are so diminutive that they cannot contribute significantly to the circulation. If a valvuloplasty is successful, PGE$_1$ is continued for several days because the severe right ventricular hypertrophy prevents adequate filling and the patient remains ductus dependent for adequate pulmonary blood flow. However, the ventricle remodels rapidly if the obstruction is relieved, and the PGE$_1$ usually can be discontinued within a week.

If the valvuloplasty is unsuccessful or considered inadequate after 7 to 10 days, surgery is indicated. Patients in whom a right ventricular outflow tract is identified angiographically should have a pulmonary valvotomy performed. A small right ventricular cavity alone does not preclude executing a valvotomy. However, if the coronary arterial supply is mainly from sinusoids, decompression of the right ventricle must be avoided. In infants with an adequate right ventricular size, pulmonary valvotomy alone is advised, but PGE$_1$ infusion is continued for a few days postoperatively as in pulmonary valvuloplasty. If the right ventricle is considered inadequate initially or after several days, a systemic-pulmonary shunt is also performed. The valvotomy permits the right ventricle to eject some blood and promotes progressive chamber enlargement,

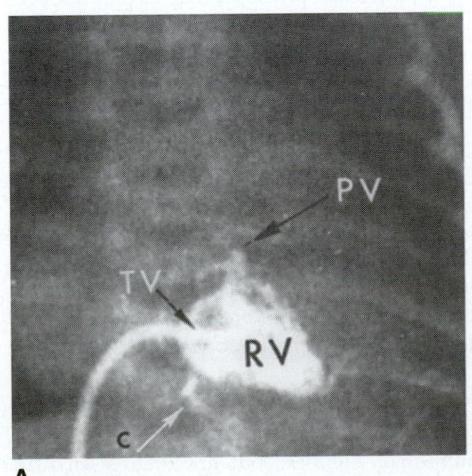

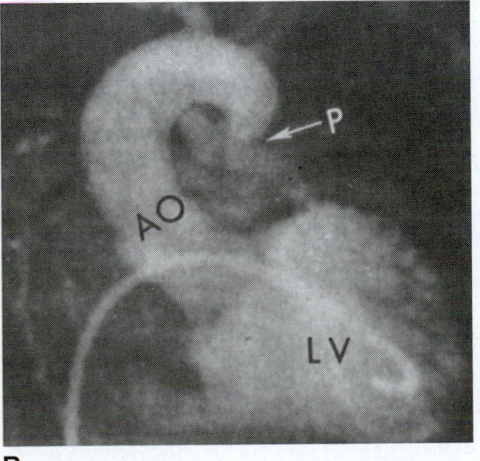

A   B

FIGURE 22-48 Angiocardiogram (anteroposterior view) in neonate with pulmonary valve (PV) atresia and intact ventricular septum. A: Right ventricular injection showing hypoplastic right ventricular cavity (RV), tricuspid valve (TV), and retrograde filling of coronary arteries (c). B: Left ventricular injection showing larger left ventricle (LV), wide aorta (AO), and aortic isthmus, and small pulmonary blood flow derived through patent ductus arteriosus (P).

whereas the anastomosis initially provides the bulk of increased pulmonary blood flow that is essential for survival. The pulmonary valvotomy and shunt performed in the neonatal period for this malformation usually do not provide optimal long-term results. Reoperation 3 to 5 years later usually becomes necessary because of persistent or recurrent right ventricular outflow tract obstruction. The second-stage operation involves right ventricular outflow tract reconstruction and placement of an outflow patch graft with ligation of the shunt. If the right ventricle remains inadequate, either a bidirectional Glenn procedure is performed so that the right ventricle handles only inferior vena caval blood or, in the worst patients, a modified Fontan-Kreuzer procedure is done.

Tetralogy of Fallot Tetralogy of Fallot is the most common cyanotic heart lesion encountered in untreated patients with cyanotic congenital heart disease who survive beyond infancy. Four structural abnormalities constitute the tetralogy: right ventricular outflow tract stenosis, ventricular septal defect, dextroposition of the aorta, and right ventricular hypertrophy (Figs. 22-50 and 22-51). There is wide anatomic variation, with resultant physiological and clinical variations.

Embryology and Morphology The basic lesion is anterocephalad malalignment of the outlet septum relative to the muscular septum. This is associated with unequal division of the truncus arteriosus into small pulmonary and large aortic components. The malalignment together with secondary hypertrophy of the muscle form the primary site of obstruction to blood flow in the infundibulum or outflow tract of the right ventricle (Fig. 22-50). In addition, the pulmonary valve is often stenotic, and the pulmonary valve annulus and pulmonary arteries are often hypoplastic. In the most severe form (tetralogy of Fallot with pulmonary atresia), the distal infundibular outflow tract and pulmonary valve are atretic (Fig. 22-51), and the pulmonary artery and main pulmonary arterial branches may be severely hypoplastic or atretic. Often most of the lung is supplied by large aortopulmonary collaterals. The ventricular septal defect is usually large, perimembranous with outlet extension, and near the tricuspid and aortic valves. The aorta arises directly over the ventricular septal defect; the degree of overriding varies greatly. An important diagnostic feature is the frequent occurrence (~25%)

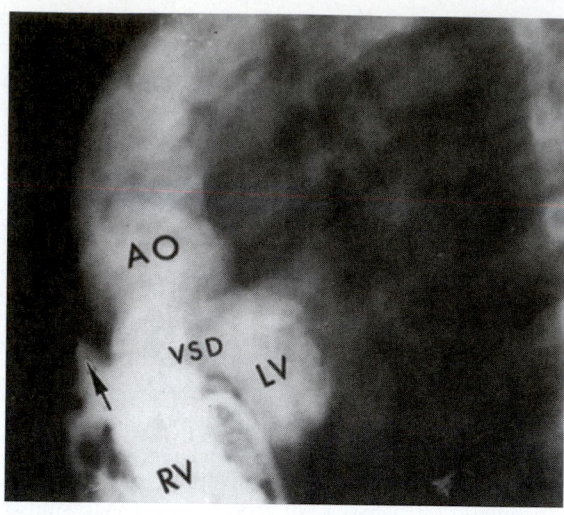

FIGURE 22-51 Angiocardiogram in tetralogy of Fallot with pulmonary atresia. Lateral oblique view showing large ventricular septal defect (VSD) confluent with large overriding aortic orifice. *Arrow* indicates atretic right ventricular outflow tract.

of a right-sided aortic arch. Particularly with a right-sided aortic arch, partial deletion of chromosome 22 occurs. This is diagnosed by FISH analysis and is associated with thymic and parathyroid hypoplasia (DiGeorge or CATCH 22 syndrome) and facial hypoplasia with soft palate insufficiency (velocardiofacial or Shprintzen syndrome).

Hemodynamics Because of the pulmonary outflow tract obstruction, varying amounts of systemic venous blood are shunted across the ventricular septal defect into the aorta, resulting in cyanosis. Pulmonary artery pressure and pulmonary blood flow are reduced. The clinical features reflect the magnitude of the pulmonary blood flow, which in turn depends on the severity of right ventricular outflow tract obstruction, the relative resistances to ventricular outflow imposed by the systemic and pulmonary circulations, and on any systemic-to-pulmonary collateral blood supply via bronchial arteries or, rarely, a persistent patent ductus arteriosus.

Because the ventricular septal defect in the tetralogy of Fallot is usually large, right ventricular peak systolic pressure equals that in the left ventricle and aorta, and right and left ventricular pressure contours are similar. Rarely, the ventricular septal defect is anatomically or functionally small because of apposition of a tricuspid valve leaflet to the defect; right ventricular pressures then exceed left ventricular pressures.

The acute severe episodes of dyspnea and hypoxemia, termed *blue spells* or *hypercyanotic episodes*, in some infants with the tetralogy reflect a further acute reduction in the pulmonary blood flow. These spells may occur even if the infant is not cyanotic at rest. The precipitating mechanisms are probably multiple: prolonged crying may decrease pulmonary blood flow because of prolonged expirations; decreases in right ventricular preload and systemic vascular resistance because of sleeping, fever, or spontaneous vasomotor changes decrease pulmonary blood flow and increase the right-to-left shunt; and constriction of the right ventricular infundibulum may occur, further decreasing pulmonary blood flow, although it is uncertain whether this truly occurs.

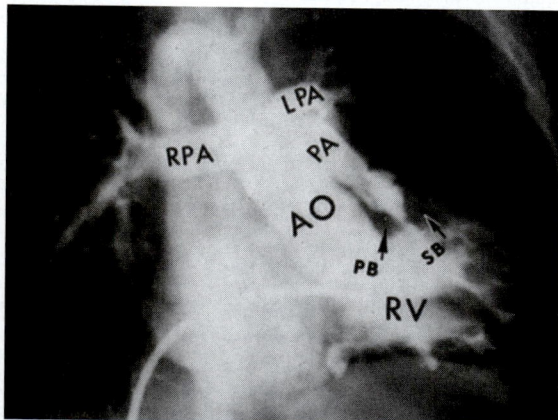

FIGURE 22-50 Angiocardiogram in tetralogy of Fallot; right ventricular (RV) selective injection showing severe infundibular obstruction *(arrows)* and early filling of aorta (AO); PA, LPA, and RPA = main, left, and right pulmonary arteries; PB = parietal band; SB = septal band.

Clinical Manifestations The clinical findings at birth vary with the severity of the pulmonary stenosis, but few infants with the tetralogy of Fallot remain asymptomatic or acyanotic. Cyanosis may not be present at birth; as long as the ductus arteriosus remains patent there may be adequate pulmonary blood flow, or the outflow tract obstruction may not be severe at birth. When right ventricular outflow tract obstruction and ventricular septal defect of the general morphology of the tetralogy of Fallot are present without significant right-to-left shunt, the anomaly is termed *acyanotic Fallot.* Hypercyanotic episodes with paroxysmal hyperpnea may occur spontaneously or after early morning feedings or prolonged crying. The attacks may last only a few moments and have no sequelae; they may cause obtundation, limpness, deep exhaustion, or sleep; rarely, they may end in unconsciousness, convulsions, or even death. Because approximately one-third of patients with the tetralogy of Fallot begin to have hypoxic spells by 4 or 5 months of age, corrective surgery is usually done electively within a few months of birth. Thus, the pediatrician rarely sees these episodes any more. In the very rare instance in which an infant does not undergo correction, exercise tolerance in the child varies in proportion to the severity of the cyanosis. Young children with the tetralogy of Fallot and severe cyanosis often adopt a characteristic squatting position after exertion. This maneuver results in an increased arterial oxygen saturation, probably by increasing systemic arterial resistance. A final group of patients shows little or no evidence of cyanosis in infancy or early childhood (acyanotic Fallot); cyanosis on exertion gradually becomes more manifest as they grow older. Occasionally, even in this group, very rapid clinical change toward the classic severely cyanotic tetralogy can occur.

In the rare, untreated patient, major late complications include brain abscess, cerebral thrombosis with hemiplegia, and infective endocarditis. Growth and development are generally delayed in proportion to the degree of cyanosis. Infective endocarditis is particularly common in children who have palliative systemic-pulmonary shunts rather than correction. Prophylactic antibiotic therapy should be given when surgical procedures involving teeth, throat, ear, nasal, bronchial, gastrointestinal, and genitourinary tracts are undertaken.

Physical examination shows a right ventricular systolic heave along the lower left sternal border. A systolic thrill is usually not appreciated because the ventricular shunt is usually right to left. The first heart sound is usually accentuated at the lower left sternal border, and in some patients an early systolic ejection click, aortic in origin, may be heard maximally at the left sternal border and apex. A single loud second heart sound corresponding to aortic valve closure is generally heard best at the lower left sternal border. When closure of the pulmonary valve is audible at the upper left sternal border, it is delayed and diminished in intensity. In patients with moderate right ventricular outflow tract obstruction, the systolic murmur is loud and harsh, stenotic or pansystolic in quality, and best heard at the middle or lower left sternal border. The systolic murmur begins early in systole and stops short of the second heart sound because the murmur is caused by outflow of blood across the right ventricular outflow tract; in general, the more severe the obstruction to pulmonary blood flow, the shorter the murmur. In extreme pulmonary outflow tract stenosis or pulmonary atresia, and at the height of a paroxysmal hypoxemic spell, the murmur may be absent or very short and faint. A faint continuous murmur may be heard over the anterior or posterior chest, particularly in children with pulmonary atresia; this bruit represents flow through enlarged bronchial collateral vessels. Rarely, a continuous murmur of persistent ductus arteriosus is heard at the upper left sternal border.

Roentgenography The heart is of normal size, and lung fields are poorly vascularized, signifying diminished pulmonary blood flow (Fig. 22-52). The right ventricular outflow tract and main pulmonary artery segments are usually hypoplastic, resulting in a concavity of the upper left margin of the cardiac silhouette instead of the normal convexity. A characteristic "coeur en sabot" or boot-shaped heart may be present, particularly with pulmonary atresia. The ascending aorta is generally large. In about 25% of the patients a right-sided aortic arch is present and is recognized by observing a right-sided rather than left-sided indentation on the trachea. The superior vena caval shadow may be displaced to the right. When bronchial collateral circulation is well developed, diffuse fine vascular markings are noted throughout the lung. Rarely, markedly decreased left lung vascular markings indicate absence or stenosis of the left pulmonary artery.

Electrocardiography The electrocardiogram shows right axis deviation and right ventricular hypertrophy, although in the newborn infant the diagnosis of pathologic right ventricular hypertrophy by electrocardiogram is more difficult because of the normal right ventricular dominance at this age. In the acyanotic tetralogy patient, combined ventricular hypertrophy may be noted at first, with progression into pure right ventricular hypertrophy as cyanosis develops.

Echocardiography In tetralogy of Fallot, the dilated aortic root overrides a large adjacent ventricular septal defect (Fig. 22-53), and varying degrees of right ventricular infundibular obstruction, pulmonary valve stenosis, and hypoplasia or narrowing of the main pulmonary artery and left pulmonary artery are revealed. Doppler examination confirms the severity of the obstruction and demonstrates systolic turbulence in the main pulmonary artery. With pulmonary atresia, no flow can be detected immediately beyond the right ventricular outflow tract, but in the pulmonary artery there will be systolic and diastolic turbulence because of flow through the ductus arteriosus or aortopulmonary collateral vessels into the central pulmonary arteries. Last, abnormal courses of the coronary

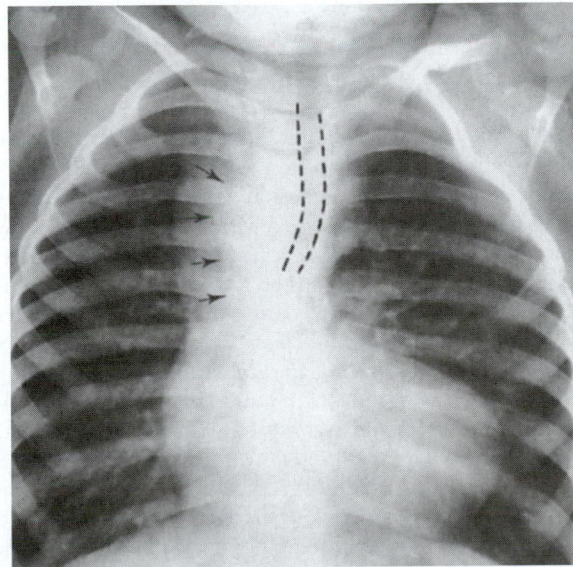

FIGURE 22-52   **Chest roentgenogram in tetralogy of Fallot. *Arrows* indicate right-sided aortic arch and upper thoracic aorta. *Dashed lines* indicate right-sided aortic indentation on the air tracheogram.**

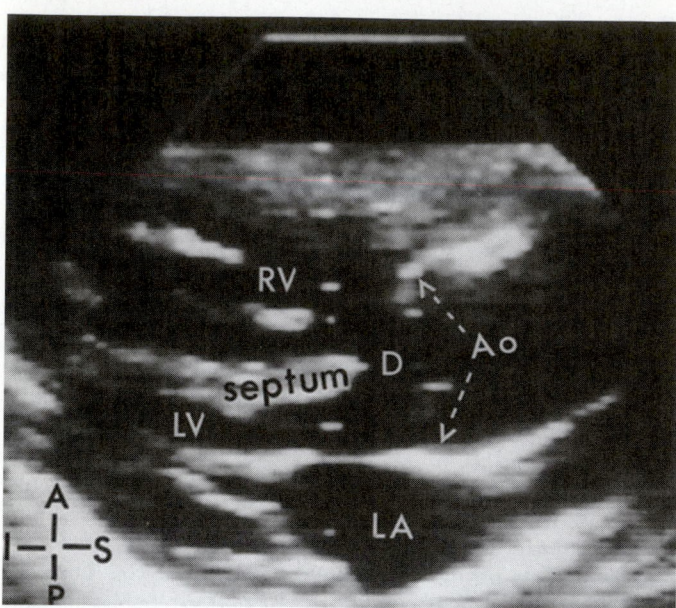

FIGURE 22-53 Long-axis view showing the aorta (Ao) entering the right (RV) and left (LV) ventricles. LA = left atrium; D = ventricular septal defect.

arteries are frequent in tetralogy of Fallot and can be defined by echocardiography. Of particular importance is the left anterior descending artery arising from the right coronary artery and coursing across the right ventricular outflow tract. This is particularly important to recognize in the infant with severe right ventricular outflow tract obstruction, in whom a right ventricular outflow patch is contemplated.

Cardiac Catheterization In most patients, careful evaluation and correlation of the clinical findings, roentgenogram, electrocardiogram, and two-dimensional echocardiogram establish the diagnosis. Cardiac catheterization with selective arteriography provides more detailed morphologic and physiological information if required. It is usually reserved for the patient with pulmonary atresia and is done to define the source and distribution of blood flow to the lungs (Fig. 22-54).

Treatment As with many significant congenital heart abnormalities, the treatment is ultimately surgical. For the neonate with prominent cyanosis, prompt infusion of PGE_1 is important. Corrective surgery is usually performed within 2 to 4 months of birth, but in the rare patient who has not had palliative or corrective surgery, medical therapy is primarily directed toward acute relief of hypercyanotic episodes and preventing the complications of right-to-left shunts. A hypercyanotic episode may be treated by placing the infant on the abdomen in a knee-chest position or holding the infant with the legs flexed on the abdomen. Oxygen should be given to lessen dyspnea and cyanosis but is not very helpful because of the very low pulmonary blood flow. Morphine sulfate (0.2 mg/kg body weight subcutaneously) is especially effective in terminating a prolonged or severe attack. If the spell is protracted and severe and does not respond to the foregoing therapy, metabolic acidemia ensues, and correction with intravenous sodium bicarbonate is essential. Vasopressors can be given either early in the attack or if other therapy fails; phenylephrine, 0.02 mg/kg IV or 0.1 mg/kg IM, will raise systemic resistance and thus increase pulmonary blood flow. If possible, it should be given by continuous intravenous in-

fusion, generally at a dose of 2 to 5 μg/kg/min. In infancy these attacks may be precipitated by a relative iron-deficiency anemia (hypochromic microcytic), and such patients should have iron therapy until the hematocrit reaches levels of 50 to 55%. Further increase in the hematocrit results in a marked rise in blood viscosity, with progressive impediment to blood flow and risk of cerebral thrombosis. Any hypercyanotic episode is an absolute indication for surgery, so it is now rare to need to treat anemia except in the immediate preoperative period. If surgery is contraindicated for some reason, oral propranolol has been given at a dosage of 0.5 to 1.0 mg/kg orally every 6 hours to prevent or reduce the frequency of paroxysmal dyspneic attacks.

Early elective surgery is indicated for infants with tetralogy of Fallot or tetralogy with pulmonary atresia, even in the absence of symptoms. Patients with the tetralogy of Fallot and patent right ventricular outflow tracts can have intracardiac surgical repair of the malformation by skilled congenital heart surgeons in the first months of life with an operative mortality under 5%. The ventricular septal defect is closed, the infundibular muscle is resected, and sometimes right ventricular outflow and main pulmonary artery patches are placed to augment the outflow tract. Pulmonary valvotomy is also performed in most patients, but enlargement of the pulmonary valve annulus with a transannular patch is avoided unless the annulus is critically small. This is because a patch is associated with a greater degree of pulmonary valve insufficiency, often requiring homograft interposition between the right ventricle and pulmonary artery at a later age. Rarely, an infant cannot be repaired because of marked pulmonary artery hypoplasia, and a systemic-pulmonary anastomosis or a right ventricular outflow patch is performed without closure of the ventricular septal defect. Balloon dilatation of the pulmonary arteries can then be performed in the catheterization laboratory in anticipation of later correction.

Although repair of tetralogy of Fallot with pulmonary atresia has in recent years become increasingly successful, the operative risk and late complications and death are higher than for uncomplicated tetralogy. Unifocalization of the often discontinuous sources of pulmonary blood flow to a central system is required before the standard repair. This may be done in one or multiple stages. The 10- and 20-year survival rates *excluding operative and early hospital deaths* are approximately 80 and 65%, respectively, as against 95% for simple tetralogy over the same intervals.

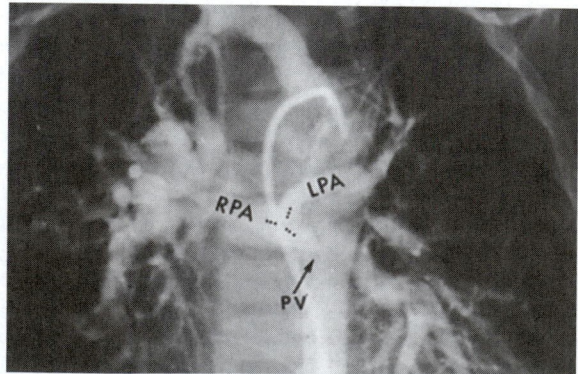

FIGURE 22-54 Angiocardiogram (anteroposterior view) in tetralogy of Fallot with pulmonary atresia and injection into aorta. Multiple large aortopulmonary collateral vessels and patent ductus arteriosus providing blood flow to distal pulmonary artery branches; retrograde filling of small proximal pulmonary artery branches (RPA and LPA) and main pulmonary artery terminating in atretic pulmonary valve (PV).

Surgical correction for most patients with uncomplicated tetralogy of Fallot results in excellent, long-lived functional results with over 90% freedom from reoperation. Residual or recurrent small left-to-right shunts are uncommon, but residual mild or moderate right ventricular-pulmonary outflow tract obstruction and incompetence are common. A few patients have surgically induced complete atrioventricular block and require an implanted pacemaker. About 1 to 3% have serious late dysrhythmias, particularly ventricular tachycardia, probably related to reentry mechanisms at the site of right ventricular tissue excisions, and about 1 to 2% die suddenly, presumably from dysrhythmias. Dysrhythmias should be suspected if these patients after surgery complain of dizzy spells, syncope, or palpitations, and appropriate diagnostic studies and therapy applied.

Tetralogy-like Lesions The clinical findings in patients with double-outlet right ventricle, single ventricle, or *d*- or *l*-transposition of the great arteries with a ventricular septal defect, when associated with severe pulmonic or subpulmonic stenosis, may closely resemble the findings in tetralogy of Fallot. These other malformations can be diagnosed with ease by two-dimensional and Doppler echocardiography.

Pulmonary Arteriovenous Malformation Occasionally fistulas connect pulmonary artery and vein so that some pulmonary blood flow bypasses the alveoli. The fistulas may be large and discrete, single or multiple, or there may be numerous small fistulas scattered throughout the lungs. Coil embolization of the fistulas can be performed in the catheterization laboratory to improve arterial oxygen saturation, although they are frequently multiple and may recur in the same or other lung segments.

AORTIC MALPOSITION

GENERAL The second major group of congenital heart defects that present with severe cyanosis in the newborn period has the common finding that the aorta is malposed across the ventricular septum to arise from the right ventricle (Table 22-13). This malposition occurs in such a manner (anterior and to the right with situs solitus) that the aorta is committed to receiving systemic venous return. Thus, even with a very large pulmonary blood flow, the patient can be very cyanotic. The most common heart lesion with aortic malposition is complete *d*-transposition of the great arteries. In this defect, the pulmonary artery is also malposed, arising from the left ventricle. In most patients, the ventricular septum is intact (Fig. 22-55). Because the great vessels arise from the inappropriate ventricles, these are discordant ventriculoarterial connections. The atrioventricular connections, however, are normal (concordant).

Although associated defects occur in fewer than half of patients with complete *d*-transposition of the great arteries, a wide variety may occur (Table 22-13). Defects in the ventricular septum or aortic arch are the most common. In association with a ventricular septal defect, pulmonary stenosis often occurs. If the ventricular septal defect lies below the pulmonary valve, the pulmonary artery frequently arises from the right ventricle as well, a form of double-outlet right ventricle called the Taussig-Bing anomaly. This defect is very often associated with subaortic stenosis and aortic arch abnormalities, as the pulmonary outflow tract compresses the aortic outflow tract anteriorly (much the same way that an overriding aorta is associated with subpulmonic stenosis in tetralogy of Fallot).

TABLE 22-13
AORTIC MALPOSITIONS[a]

LEVEL	ASSOCIATED LESION
Atrial septum	Atrial septal defect
Atrioventricular valve	Tricuspid atresia
	Atrioventricular canal defect
Ventricles	Ventricular septal defect
	Double-outlet right ventricle (Taussig-Bing anomaly)
	Subvalvar aortic stenosis (usually with Taussig-Bing anomaly)
	Subvalvar pulmonary stenosis
Pulmonary valve	Pulmonary valve stenosis or atresia
	Pulmonary stenosis with intact septum
	Pulmonary atresia with intact septum
Aortic arch	Aortic interruption (usually with Taussig-Bing anomaly)
	Aortic coarctation (often with ventricular septal defect)
	Patent ductus arteriosus

[a] Aorta is malposed over the venous ventricle as isolated lesion associated with other lesions.

INITIAL PRESENTATION In the absence of a ventricular septal defect, the aorta receives all of the desaturated systemic venous return and can receive pulmonary venous blood only via an interatrial communication. However, these infants often do not have atrial septal defects. Thus, as occurs normally, pulmonary blood flow increases dramatically at birth, and the increase in pulmonary venous return tends to close the foramen ovale. If this occurs, the neonate with transposition may become critically cyanotic soon after birth,

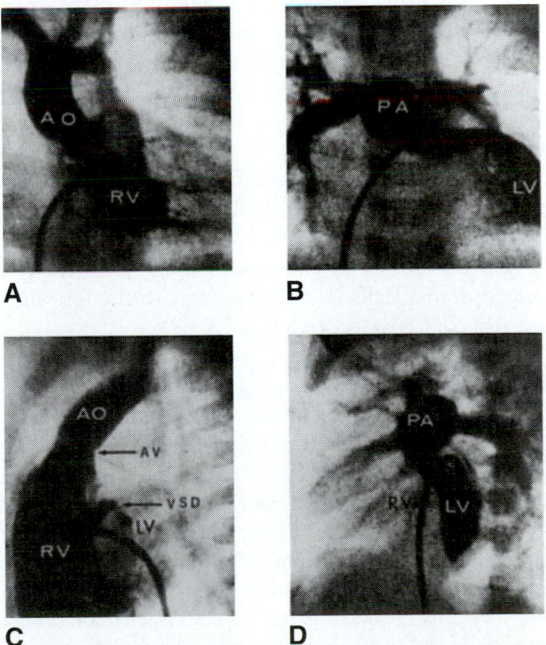

FIGURE 22-55 Selective right (A,C) and left (B,D) ventricular angiograms in infant with transposition of the great arteries and small ventricular septal defect. A,B: Anteroposterior views. C,D: Lateral views. RV = right ventricle; LV = left ventricle; AO = aorta; PA = pulmonary artery; VSD = ventricular septal defect; AV = aortic valve level.

a problem intensified by closure of the ductus arteriosus. If this occurs, an emergency atrial septostomy to establish an atrial left-to-right shunt should be performed. In the interim, particularly if the infant is not at a major medical center with a neonatal cardiology program, PGE_1 can be very beneficial by increasing pulmonary blood flow, which in turn increases pulmonary venous return and left atrial pressure and thus forces pulmonary venous blood to cross to the right atrium. This may be life saving but may occur at the expense of very high left atrial pressures. Thus, the neonate should be intubated if there are signs of any respiratory compromise. In addition, immediate supportive therapy for metabolic acidemia and maintenance of body temperature should be instituted.

The balloon atrial septostomy is performed via the femoral or umbilical vein during neonatal cardiac catheterization or even under echocardiographic visualization in the intensive care nursery. A transvenously introduced catheter bearing a balloon is advanced through the foramen ovale into the left atrium, where the balloon is inflated to a diameter of 8 to 10 mm. The catheter and inflated balloon are then abruptly withdrawn into the right atrium, thus rupturing the septum primum valve of the fossa ovalis, enlarging the interatrial communication, and providing for more adequate mixing of blood. The systemic arterial oxygen tension often rises initially, but if it remains low despite PGE_1 and an adequate balloon septostomy, a transfusion of blood is often helpful. By increasing circulating volume and atrial pressures, a transfusion can dramatically increase the left-to-right atrial shunt. After a few days of stabilization, almost all infants with simple transposition today undergo surgical repair.

SPECIFIC LESIONS In order to consider this group of lesions along lines of blood flow, one has to make the initial assumption that the aorta is committed to the systemic venous (right) ventricle and then consider blood flow from the right atrium onward. Defects in the atrial, atrioventricular, and ventricular septa may occur, the latter of which is frequently associated with either pulmonic stenosis or with double-outlet right ventricle (Taussig-Bing anomaly), which itself is associated with aortic outflow obstruction.

COMPLETE (d-)TRANSPOSITION OF GREAT ARTERIES Complete transposition of the great arteries is the most common cardiac cause of cyanosis in the neonate, and until recently it accounted for the majority of deaths in infants with cyanotic congenital heart disease under 1 year of age. Once almost universally fatal, the prognosis has changed dramatically in recent years with the introduction of palliative and corrective procedures.

Morphology and Physiology In complete transposition of the great arteries, the systemic venous return traverses the right atrium and right ventricle and is ejected into the transposed aorta arising from the right ventricle; the pulmonary venous return traverses the left atrium and left ventricle and is ejected back into the lungs via the transposed pulmonary artery. There are thus two separate circulations in parallel instead of in series. This arrangement is incompatible with life without some communications to permit oxygenated pulmonary venous blood to enter the systemic circulation and systemic venous blood to enter the pulmonary circulation. In over half the patients with complete transposition the ventricular septum is intact, and intracardiac shunting occurs only through a stretched foramen ovale or, rarely, a secundum atrial defect; consequently, cyanosis is extreme. Infants with an associated large ventricular septal defect have better mixing between the two circulations and so have higher systemic oxygen saturations. Although a patent ductus

arteriosus may be demonstrated in about half of the newborn infants with transposition, it closes functionally and anatomically soon after birth in most patients. A persistent large patent ductus arteriosus is uncommon, particularly malignant, and requires prompt recognition and therapy. Left ventricular outflow tract stenosis of varying degrees also may be present; it most often results from a fibrous ridge or collar in the outflow tract of the left ventricle. Common AV canal, AV valve atresia, severe pulmonary valve stenosis or atresia, coarctation of the aorta, or right aortic arch is rare in complete transposition of the great arteries.

The major consequences of transposition of the great arteries are severe hypoxemia, metabolic acidemia, and congestive heart failure. The level of systemic arterial oxygen saturation depends on the transfer of oxygenated pulmonary venous blood to the systemic circuit as well as the reciprocal transfer of systemic venous return to the pulmonary circuit. These transfers are a function of the size of the shunting sites: foramen ovale, ostium secundum defect, ventricular septal defect, patent ductus arteriosus, and bronchial collateral circulation. Other important factors, particularly in patients with large ventricular septal defect, are the hemodynamic consequences of pulmonary outflow tract stenosis and increased pulmonary vascular resistance; if outflow resistance is high, it will restrict the pulmonary blood flow and the volume of the oxygenated pulmonary venous return and reduce the systemic arterial oxygen saturation. The existence of the systemic and pulmonary circulatory pathways in parallel instead of in series usually results in high cardiac outputs for both the right and left ventricles, with consequent cardiac dilatation and myocardial failure. Myocardial function can be further compromised by the markedly desaturated aortic blood flow entering the coronary circulation.

Pulmonary vascular obstructive disease has been observed both by microscopy and by cardiac catheterization to be more common and to progress at an unusually rapid rate in infants with transposition of the great arteries and large ventricular septal defect, as contrasted to infants with large ventricular septal defect and normally related great arteries. About 75% of all infants with transposition of the great arteries and large ventricular septal defect older than 1 year of age have advanced pulmonary vascular obstructive disease. Associated pulmonic stenosis, intracardiac correction with closure of the ventricular septal defect, or early surgical pulmonary artery banding protects against the development of pulmonary vascular obstructive disease in this lesion. Histologic studies demonstrate moderate pulmonary vascular disease lesions in many infants with large ventricular septal defect by 3 to 4 months of age. Accordingly, palliative pulmonary artery banding or intracardiac repair should be considered before this age. Significant pulmonary vascular obstructive disease has even been seen in about 5% of the transposition patients with intact ventricular septum who survive early infancy.

Clinical Manifestations Most infants with an intact ventricular septum become critically ill the first few hours after birth, but if there is a large ventricular septal defect, cyanosis may be slight, and congestive heart failure may not become evident until a few weeks after birth. Characteristically, attention is first directed to the infant with inadequate intracardiac mixing by nursery personnel who observe cyanosis in an otherwise apparently healthy infant. A high index of suspicion is needed for early diagnosis; except for persistent cyanosis and progressive hyperpnea in the first hours after birth, the infant may appear well developed and minimally distressed, and the findings on chest roentgenogram and electrocardiogram may be deceptively normal.

On auscultation the second heart sound is usually interpreted as loud and single and is heard best usually at the upper left sternal border, but careful auscultation often reveals narrow splitting with a soft pulmonary valve closure. The murmurs are usually unimpressive in the newborn with an intact ventricular septum, but there may be a short grade 2–3/6 ejection systolic murmur at the middle of the left sternal border. A loud harsh systolic murmur in a slightly older infant usually indicates a ventricular septal defect or left ventricular outflow tract stenosis. In the former the murmur is pansystolic and maximal along the middle and lower left sternal border; in the latter the murmur is more stenotic and is maximal at the middle left sternal border, but with transmission toward the upper right sternal border.

Infants with transposition of the great arteries and large ventricular septal defect develop prominent cardiac failure and modest cyanosis by 3 to 4 weeks of age. Increasing tachypnea, dyspnea, and excessive perspiration are noted. Cyanosis may increase, but often it remains relatively mild because of good circulatory mixing. Pulmonary rales and hepatomegaly may be striking.

Electrocardiogram The electrocardiogram may not be helpful in the newborn infant because it shows right axis deviation and right ventricular hypertrophy of a degree that may be normal for a neonate. After 5 days of age, however, persistence of a positive T wave over the right precordium suggests abnormal right ventricular hypertrophy. In the older infant with an intact ventricular septum, right atrial hypertrophy and overt right ventricular hypertrophy are present. If there is a large ventricular septal defect, left ventricular hypertrophy may also develop in the first few months of life.

Roentgenography The roentgenographic findings can vary from near normal to grossly abnormal. In the neonate the heart is small, but it enlarges over the first 1 to 2 weeks after birth. The pulmonary vascular markings may appear normal or minimally increased initially (Fig. 22-56A), and only later do the characteristic findings of increased pulmonary vascularity appear. The classic transposition cardiac silhouette, an egg-shaped or oval heart with a narrow superior mediastinum and small thymic shadow, is diagnostic, but it is present early in only about one-third of the newborn infants (Fig. 22-56B).

The chest roentgenogram in infants with large ventricular septal defect, after the initial newborn period, characteristically shows a larger, more globular heart with very prominent pulmonary vascular markings.

Echocardiography Two-dimensional and Doppler echocardiography constitute the major tools for morphologic diagnosis and functional assessment, showing the transposed great arteries, with the aorta arising anterior and to the right from the morphologic right ventricle, and the pulmonary artery arising posterior and to the left from the morphologic left ventricle. The sites, direction, and magnitude of shunts can be seen, and assessments of ventricular pressures can be made.

Cardiac Catheterization Cardiac catheterization in the neonate plays an important therapeutic role in effecting hemodynamic and clinical improvement by doing a balloon atrial septostomy. Often the procedure is performed under echocardiographic guidance at the bedside, and limited diagnostic data are obtained. If it is performed in a catheterization laboratory, hemodynamic data show that oxygen saturation of the blood in the pulmonary artery is higher than that in the aorta. In the immediate newborn period, if the ventricular septum is intact, the left ventricular systolic pressure may equal right ventricular systolic pressure; however, after a few days left ventricular pressure usually falls to one-half or less of right ventricular pressure unless some left ventricular outflow tract obstruction is present. A pressure difference across the atrial septum is common, with left atrial pressures exceeding those on the right, before the balloon septostomy.

Selective right ventricular angiography demonstrates the high anterior position of the aorta arising from the right ventricle, the status of the ventricular septum, and the ductus arteriosus. Selective left ventricular angiography demonstrates a pulmonary artery arising from the posterior ventricle, the status of the ventricular septum, and any left ventricular outflow tract stenosis (Fig. 22-55).

Treatment After initial stabilization with balloon atrial septostomy, PGE$_1$ infusion, intubation and ventilation, and correction of any metabolic derangements, the patient is allowed to stabilize for a few days. During that time, full evaluation of associated lesions and coronary arterial anatomy is made. In the absence of lesions such as subpulmonary or pulmonary valve stenosis, arterial switch surgery is performed. It is now the treatment of choice, primarily because it returns systemic ventricular function to the left ventricle and because midterm follow-up studies indicate preservation of normal ventricular function and no significant incidence of postoperative arrhythmias. The operation involves transecting the great arteries, switching their attachments above the semilunar valves, and transplanting the coronary arteries from the preoperative an-

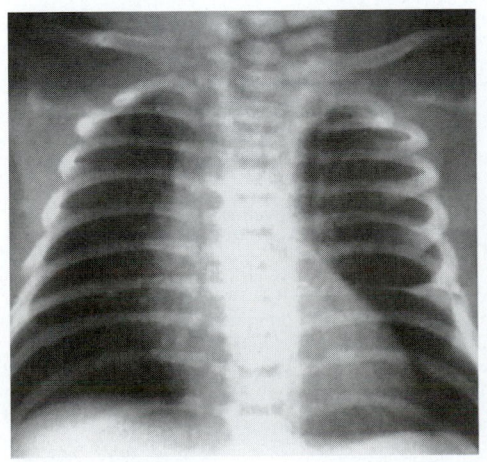
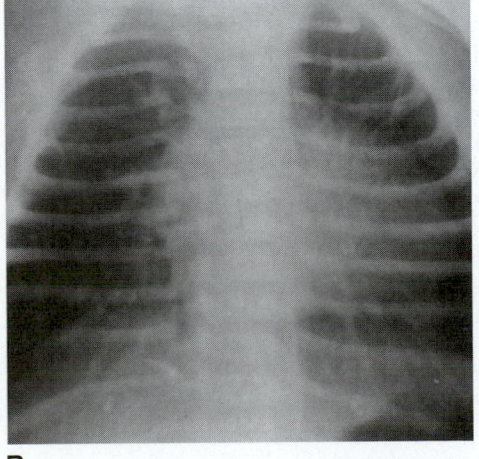

A   **B**

FIGURE 22-56 Chest roentgenogram in *d*-transposition of the great arteries. A: Infant 1 day old with deceptively normal-appearing heart size and pulmonary vascular markings. B: Infant 1 day old with more classic oval-shaped and enlarged heart with slightly increased vascular markings.

terior aortic root (new pulmonary root) to the preoperative posterior pulmonary arterial root (new aortic root). For infants with intact ventricular septum or an insignificant ventricular septal defect, it is critical to perform this operation under 8 weeks of age while the left ventricular pressure and muscle mass have not yet regressed to those of a low pressure, thin-walled pulmonary ventricle dictated by the transposition physiology. Current experience for the one-stage arterial switch repair in neonates in centers with neonatal cardiac surgical proficiency indicates early operative survival of 95% or more. Freedom from reoperation (most often done to relieve surgically induced supravalvar pulmonic stenosis) is also 90 to 95%.

For the infant with complete transposition and a large ventricular septal defect, the primary management problems are left ventricular failure and pulmonary hypertension with the early onset of pulmonary vascular disease. Occasionally there may be myocardial ischemia caused by coronary arterial problems associated with the switch. Currently, neonatal arterial switch repair with closure of the ventricular septal defect has significantly improved the prognosis for this subset of transposition patients to about 90% survival over 5 years.

TRANSPOSITION OF THE GREAT ARTERIES WITH PULMONARY STENOSIS In the infant with transposition of the great arteries and intact ventricular septum, slight or moderate left ventricular outflow tract stenosis may be present or develop in the subpulmonary region. This obstruction may be predominantly muscular and dynamic or predominantly fibromuscular and fixed. A distinct fibrous ridge often develops where the septal mitral leaflet is apposed to a prominent septal muscular bulge. The bulge is convex to the left ventricle and caused by the higher right than left ventricular pressure. The degree of obstruction is usually modest and only severe degrees of anatomic obstruction should be relieved by resection or conduit bypass at the time of the open-heart procedure.

When a ventricular septal defect is present with severe subvalvar left ventricular outflow tract stenosis, the clinical picture may mimic the tetralogy of Fallot. Symptoms may begin at birth, with severe cyanosis and paroxysmal hypoxemic spells; the pulmonary vascular markings on the roentgenogram are decreased. If the pulmonary stenosis is not severe, cyanosis and clinical symptoms are not extreme initially, but they may become so as the infant matures. Two-dimensional echocardiography and selective left ventriculography can define the extent and site of the pulmonary stenosis.

In the extremely cyanotic newborn infant with transposition and severe subpulmonary or pulmonary stenosis or atresia, the safest treatment is to perform a systemic-pulmonary shunt. Intracardiac repair is difficult and should be postponed until past the age of 1 to 2 years. Surgical repair (Rastelli procedure) consists of repair of the ventricular septal defect with an intracardiac ventricular baffle so as to connect the left ventricle to the aorta. Then an extracardiac valve-bearing conduit is placed between the right ventricle and the distal stump of the pulmonary artery, to bypass completely the severely stenosed left ventricular outflow tract.

TAUSSIG-BING ANOMALY Double-outlet right ventricle (DORV) is a rare group of lesions that is one of the types of malposition of the great arteries. Both the aortic and pulmonary valves are positioned over the right ventricle, there is often conal (outlet septum) tissue below both orifices, and the only outflow from the left ventricle is through the ventricular septal defect, which may be either subpulmonary or subaortic, or rarely uncommitted. When the pulmonary artery is committed to the right ventricle and the aorta

overrides the ventricular septal defect, there is usually subpulmonic stenosis, and the physiology and treatment are similar to tetralogy of Fallot. When the aorta is committed to the right ventricle and the pulmonary orifice is related to and overriding the ventricular septal defect (Taussig-Bing anomaly), the hemodynamics and clinical findings are similar to those of transposition of the great arteries with large ventricular septal defect and pulmonary hypertension. An associated coarctation of the aorta is present in about 25% of these patients.

Corrective surgical procedures are increasingly successful for Taussig-Bing anomaly. Arterial switch repair as for complete transposition is the operation of choice, providing the great arteries are not too different in diameter, with early and midterm outcomes similar to that of transposition with a large ventricular septal defect. Often aortic arch abnormalities are present. If so, they are corrected surgically either before or at the same time as the intracardiac repair. When the arterial size discrepancy is severe or intracardiac anatomy makes correction problematic, a pulmonary artery band is often performed at the same time as the aortic arch repair, and definitive surgery is delayed until a later date.

BIDIRECTIONAL (RIGHT-TO-LEFT AND LEFT-TO-RIGHT) SHUNTS

GENERAL In this group of lesions systemic arterial desaturation is present because some of the systemic venous blood is directed out the aorta. However, pulmonary venous blood also is directed back to the pulmonary arterial circulation (Table 22-14). When there is no obstruction to either circulation, usually far more blood passes into the pulmonary circulation. This occurs whether the shunt occurs at the level of the veins, atria, ventricles, or great arteries. At the venous/atrial level (for example, total anomalous pulmonary venous return without obstruction), pulmonary blood flow exceeds systemic because the compliance of the right ventricle is greater than that of the left ventricle. At the ventricular/great vessel level (for example, truncus arteriosus), pulmonary blood flow exceeds systemic because pulmonary vascular resistance falls to well below systemic levels soon after birth.

INITIAL PRESENTATION The presentation of this group of lesions varies over time, as pulmonary vascular resistance decreases rapidly in the first hours and days, and right ventricular compliance in-

TABLE 22-14
BIDIRECTIONAL SHUNTS

LEVEL	LESION
Veins	Total anomalous pulmonary venous connection
Atrial septum	Absent atrial septum (usually in heterotaxy syndromes)
Atrioventricular valves	Complete atrioventricular septal defect with minimal septa (often with heterotaxy syndromes)
Ventricles	Single ventricle (usually double-inlet left ventricle, sometimes atresia of one atrioventricular valve)
	Hypoplastic left ventricle (with a ductus arteriosus)
Truncal/aortopulmonary septum	Truncus arteriosus

creases over the first few weeks. It also depends on whether there is obstruction to the inflow or outflow of the left side of the heart and whether the ductus arteriosus is patent.

In the absence of obstruction, the infant may present transiently with systemic hypoxemia that is rarely severe enough to cause symptoms and often is not appreciated clinically. Over time, pulmonary blood flow increases, causing increasing rate and effort of breathing. This is associated with diaphoresis and poor feeding. The poor feeding is associated with increased caloric demands associated with increased cardiorespiratory work, so that poor growth is nearly universal. If no murmurs are present, as occurs in total anomalous pulmonary venous connection without obstruction, and if the respiratory symptoms are not appreciated, the presentation may be that of failure to thrive, and diagnosis of cardiac disease may be greatly delayed.

With inflow obstruction (for example, total anomalous pulmonary venous connection with obstruction), the infant presents with severe respiratory distress and hypoxemia. The absence of murmurs and a small heart on chest radiograph often suggest the diagnosis of pulmonary hypertension, so that echocardiography with color Doppler studies must be performed on all neonates with this presentation. In the infant with mitral hypoplasia or atresia (hypoplastic left heart syndrome), all pulmonary venous return crosses the atrial septum to the right atrium and joins the systemic venous return across the right ventricle to the pulmonary artery. Pulmonary blood flow is high, causing respiratory distress, and systemic blood flow depends entirely on the patency of the ductus arteriosus. As the ductus arteriosus begins to close, the infant then presents in cardiovascular collapse, with severe metabolic acidosis. Therapy includes intubation and ventilation because of pulmonary edema and PGE_1 if the lesion is associated with ductal-dependent systemic blood flow.

SPECIFIC LESIONS There are a wide variety of lesions with a wide variety of presentations.

TOTAL ANOMALOUS PULMONARY VENOUS CONNECTION Total anomalous pulmonary venous connection accounts for about 2% of all congenital heart malformations seen in the first year of life and is characterized by absence of any direct connection between the pulmonary veins and the left atrium. The pulmonary veins are connected either directly to the right atrium or to various systemic veins draining toward the right atrium, such as right superior vena cava, azygous vein, left innominate vein, coronary sinus, ductus venosus, or various combinations of these connections. The pulmonary veins almost always come together to form a common channel that lies behind but is separate from the left atrium. This proximity provides the key to successful corrective surgery. The embryologic basis for the malformation is a failure of development of the connection of the common pulmonary vein with the left atrium, and consequently an anomalous union occurs between the pulmonary vein plexus of the developing lung buds and one of several systemic venous structures. Three main anatomic types of connection have been described: supracardiac, cardiac, and infracardiac (also called infradiaphragmatic). In about 25% of the patients, pulmonary venous return to the heart proceeds from the confluence immediately posterior to the left atrium via a left vertical venous trunk that joins the left innominate vein, which joins the right superior vena cava in normal fashion. In about 25% the anomalous drainage pathway descends below the diaphragm, usually to connect with the ductus venosus, and the pulmonary venous drainage eventually returns to the heart via the inferior vena cava. In the cardiac type the pul-

monary veins may be connected directly to the right atrium or the coronary sinus.

The physiological and clinical features of one important subgroup of infants with total anomalous pulmonary venous connection are dictated by pulmonary venous obstruction at some level in the pulmonary venous drainage pathway. In the infradiaphragmatic type, severe obstruction to pulmonary venous return is invariable. Obstruction may result from the length and narrowness of the common trunk itself, compression in the esophageal hiatus of the diaphragm, or more often from the constriction that normally occurs in the ductus venosus and the resistance that the total pulmonary venous return faces when it must pass through the portal-hepatic circulation (Fig. 22-57). Supracardiac drainage pathways also may manifest pulmonary venous obstruction, but this occurs much less frequently. The site of obstruction may be a localized intrinsic constriction, but more frequently it occurs where the left vertical vein is compressed at it passes between the left pulmonary artery anteriorly and the left bronchus posteriorly, rather than passing anterior to the pulmonary artery. Obstruction may also occur with other types of anomalous connection.

Associated intracardiac anomalies have been described in up to 30% of patients with total anomalous pulmonary venous connection. These anomalies are usually complex lesions such as common AV canal or transposition or single-ventricle complexes and are most often associated with heterotaxy syndrome (right or left atrial isomerism).

Hemodynamics All pulmonary venous blood returns to the right atrium, where it mixes with the systemic venous return. A variable proportion then passes to the systemic circulation through a stretched patent foramen ovale into the left atrium, ventricle, and aorta; the remainder passes to the pulmonary circulation through the tricuspid valve into the right ventricle and pulmonary artery. Systemic arterial desaturation is present as a result of the obligatory right-to-left shunting of blood at the atrial level, although rarely streaming of pulmonary venous blood into the left atrium gives near-normal aortic saturations. The arterial oxygen saturation varies

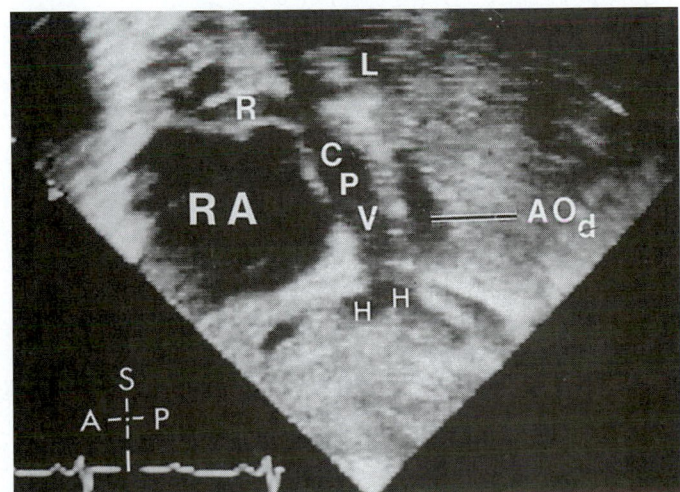

FIGURE 22-57 Total anomalous pulmonary venous connection—intradiaphragmatic type. Two-dimensional echocardiogram, subcostal view, showing drainage pathway from right and left pulmonary veins (R,L) to vertical common pulmonary vein (CPV) and descending pulmonary venous channel entering the hepatic-portal (H) system and eventually the inferior vena cava and right atrium. AO_d = descending aorta.

widely but is rarely decreased significantly enough to impair oxygen delivery and depends on the ratio of pulmonary to systemic blood flow. Because the pulmonary venous blood joins with systemic venous blood at or before the right atrium, the oxygen saturations tend to be similar in all four chambers of the heart and in the two great arteries.

The majority of infants with supracardiac and cardiac types have little or no pulmonary venous obstruction and consequently have high pulmonary blood flow, various degrees of pulmonary hypertension, and relatively low pulmonary vascular resistance. These infants generally survive the first few weeks and months of life but may succumb to severe congestive heart failure during the first year of life unless surgically corrected. All infants with the infradiaphragmatic type and about one-third of the infants with the supracardiac type manifest severe pulmonary venous obstruction and so have severe pulmonary hypertension, restricted pulmonary blood flow, pulmonary venous engorgement, and interstitial pulmonary edema. Pulmonary artery pressures often exceed systemic pressures, and death is common in the first weeks of life if the disorder is not corrected. In all types of total anomalous pulmonary venous connection, the pressures in the right atrium are invariably higher than those in the left atrium, and occasionally pulmonary venous obstruction may result from restriction of flow across the foramen ovale.

Clinical Features   About 80 to 90% of all patients manifest tachypnea, congestive heart failure, and failure to thrive early in infancy. In the group without pulmonary obstruction, cyanosis may be minimal, but cyanosis becomes more significant as congestive heart failure progresses. In the newborn period the heart is hyperdynamic, but heart sounds are normal; murmurs are only rarely heard. If diagnosis is delayed, the auscultatory findings change. A quadruple gallop rhythm frequently develops. A soft ejection systolic murmur is present along the left sternal border, and a middiastolic inflow rumble is usually heard at the lower left sternal border and apex. At times a continuous murmur or venous hum may be heard originating from some point in the venous channels.

In infants with the obstructed form of total anomalous pulmonary venous drainage, there is very early onset of severe dyspnea. The clinical picture is that of rapidly progressive dyspnea, pulmonary edema, cyanosis, and right heart failure. The second heart sound is loud and narrowly split, and a gallop rhythm may be heard. Murmurs are not prominent, but a soft blowing systolic murmur of tricuspid regurgitation may be heard at the lower left sternal border.

Roentgenography   In the unobstructed group the roentgenographic examination shows marked cardiac enlargement with pulmonary vascular engorgement. A pathognomonic configuration termed "figure of eight" or "snowman" may be recognized beyond infancy; this silhouette is formed by the dilated left vertical vein, innominate vein, and right superior vena cava sitting astride the dilated heart.

A characteristic chest roentgenogram is present in those infants with pulmonary venous obstruction. The heart is normal or slightly enlarged, and the lung fields show a diffuse, hazy reticulated pattern superficially resembling the ground-glass appearance seen in the respiratory distress syndrome (Fig. 22-58). Because of this and the lack of diagnostic murmurs, one is likely to misdiagnose these patients as having some form of diffuse interstitial pneumonitis if one relies on the roentgenogram alone. Early two-dimensional echo-

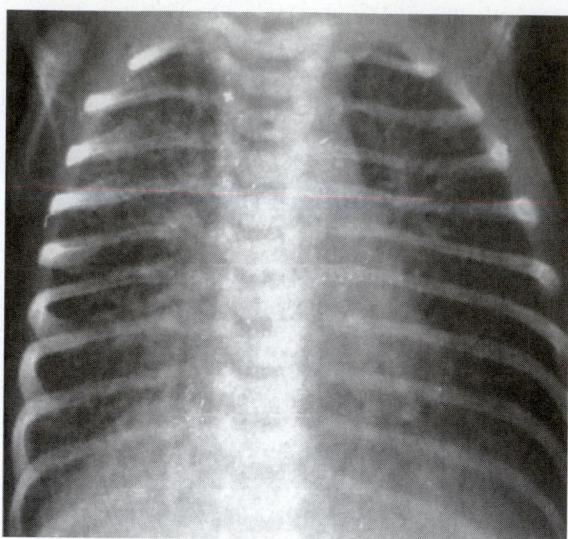

FIGURE 22-58   Chest roentgenogram in neonate with obstructed subdiaphragmatic type of total anomalous pulmonary venous drainage showing slight cardiac enlargement and characteristic reticulated peripheral lung markings.

cardiographic diagnosis of a normal versus an abnormal heart is critical, especially if the apparent lung disease is not improving.

Electrocardiography   The electrocardiogram shows right ventricular hypertrophy and commonly also right atrial hypertrophy. The hypertrophy is often in excess of the normal right ventricular dominance at birth, as demonstrated by a qR complex in the right precordial leads, poor left forces, and the lack of inversion of the T waves over the first few days of life.

Echocardiography   Two-dimensional echocardiography can establish the diagnosis and anatomy subtype of pulmonary venous connection with a high degree of sensitivity and specificity particularly in infants who have atrial situs solitus, unifocal rather than mixed pulmonary venous connections, and no evidence of other major congenital defects (Fig. 22-57). It is thus critical that all infants with severe respiratory distress and cyanosis at birth undergo echocardiography early in their course, particularly if extra corporeal membrane oxygenation (ECMO) is being considered. Cardiac catheterization with angiography in these critically ill infants, no matter how carefully executed, may make them even more ill and is of little diagnostic value. It should be considered only in infants with complex intracardiac anatomy in whom pulmonary venous connections are likely to be mixed and cannot be clearly delineated by echocardiography.

Treatment   For the severely obstructed group rapid clinical deterioration and early death are invariable without surgical treatment. Aggressive treatment of hypoxemia and metabolic acidemia should be instituted, diuretics given, and continuous positive airway pressure with oxygen supplementation should be provided while preparations are made for surgical correction with cardiopulmonary bypass.

With all types of single connections, the aim of surgical correction is to reincorporate the common pulmonary vein into the left atrium. Because this chamber may be small, correction is carried out with a wide parallel incision between the posterior aspect of the atria and the anterior wall of the common pulmonary vein as the heart is lifted out of the pericardium. The interatrial septum may be replaced to the right of the anastomosis to enlarge the functional left atrium. The anomalous connection is simply ligated and divided.

In the unobstructed type, corrective surgery dramatically restores the normal circulatory pathways with a modest surgical risk of 5% or less under the best circumstances. When severe pulmonary venous obstruction is present, particularly for the infradiaphragmatic type, the surgical mortality has been higher, but prompt referral, aggressive management of metabolic acidemia, and early emergency surgery have had increasing success, with excellent long-term results. However, it is important to note that early (2 to 4 months) postoperative pulmonary venous obstructions have been observed in about 10% of these patients. These obstructions result either from an anastomotic stricture or from a particularly malignant form of diffuse pulmonary venous fibrosis at the venous ostia or within the lobar veins. The prognosis in the latter group of patients is very poor.

HYPOPLASTIC LEFT HEART SYNDROME The term *hypoplastic left heart syndrome* describes a group of malformations characterized by marked underdevelopment of the entire left side of the heart. The right side of the heart is dilated and hypertrophied and supports both pulmonary and systemic circulations through a patent ductus arteriosus (Fig. 22-59). The specific anatomic abnormalities include underdevelopment of the left atrium and ventricle, stenosis or atresia of the aortic or mitral orifices, and marked hypoplasia of the ascending aorta (Fig. 22-60). Most commonly, aortic and mitral atresia coexist, and the left ventricular cavity is minute or completely obliterated. Rarely, mitral atresia is present associated with a ventricular septal defect. Hypoplastic left heart syndrome accounted for nearly 25% of cardiac deaths in the first year of life (New England Regional Infant Cardiac Registry).

Hemodynamics The essential hemodynamic abnormality is the absence or gross inadequacy of left ventricular function. Pulmonary venous blood passes from left to right atrium via the patent foramen

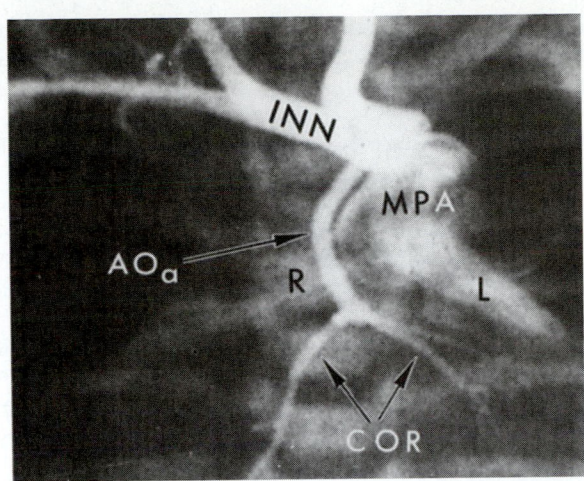

FIGURE 22-60 Angiocardiogram (anteroposterior view) in hypoplastic left heart complex (age 2 days). Injection into region of innominate artery (INN) and aortic arch shows markedly hypoplastic ascending aorta (AO$_a$) with flow to coronary arteries (COR). MPA, R, and L indicate retrograde filling of large pulmonary arteries.

ovale, and this interatrial communication is often small and restrictive to blood flow, causing severe left atrial and pulmonary venous hypertension. The ventricular septum is almost always intact. The right ventricle functions as the systemic ventricle as well as the pulmonary ventricle by delivering blood into the aorta through the widely patent ductus arteriosus. The pulmonary vascular resistance must be high to provide for this systemic function of the right ventricle. Furthermore, as the ductus arteriosus constricts intermittently, there is intermittent restriction to systemic blood flow.

In the rare condition of mitral atresia with ventricular septal defect, all the pulmonary venous blood passes through a foramen ovale to mix with systemic venous return. Blood then enters the enlarged right ventricle from which it passes into the pulmonary artery and, through a ventricular septal defect, into the hypoplastic left ventricle and the aorta. If the foramen ovale permits a large left-to-right shunt, these infants initially do quite well but then go into congestive heart failure because of a torrential pulmonary blood flow.

Clinical Features Most infants with hypoplastic left heart complex are acutely ill, with signs of congestive heart failure within the first days or weeks after birth; those with aortic atresia succumb usually within the first few days after birth.

There are signs and symptoms of severe right-sided and left-sided heart failure: cyanosis of varying degree, and often a characteristic grayish pallor and poor peripheral pulses, which contrast with hyperdynamic cardiac pulsations. Characteristically the peripheral pulses may diminish from time to time and then reappear, presumably related to episodes of constriction of the ductus arteriosus. The major hemodynamic abnormalities are pulmonary venous hypertension and inadequate maintenance of the systemic circulation. Murmurs are not prominent, but a short soft midsystolic murmur and middiastolic rumble may be present. The second heart sound is single, heard loudest at the upper left sternal border, and is accentuated until clinical deterioration with gross right heart failure is advanced. A systolic ejection click may be heard.

Roentgenography The roentgenogram shortly after birth may show only slight cardiac enlargement, but with clinical deteriora-

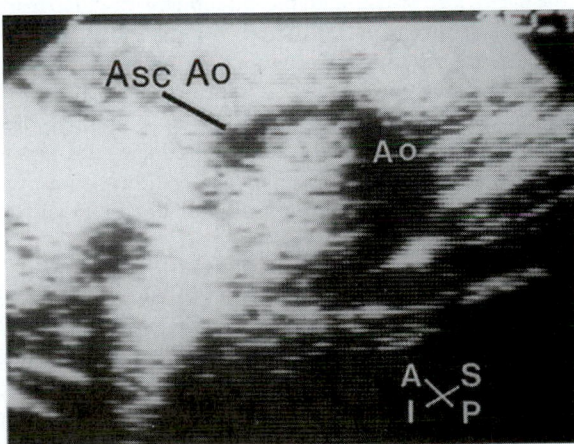

FIGURE 22-59 Hypoplastic left heart complex (aortic atresia). Two-dimensional echocardiogram, suprasternal notch sagittal plane, showing an image of the hypoplastic ascending aorta (Asc Ao) in a patient with aortic atresia. The transverse aorta (Ao) is of normal caliber, and the vessels to the head and neck can be seen to arise from it. As the arch descends into the thorax toward the coronary arteries, it becomes hypoplastic where the innominate artery arises. Orientation: A = anterior; I = inferior; P = posterior; S = superior.

tion, striking generalized cardiac enlargement and moderately prominent pulmonary vascular markings appear. Pulmonary venous obstruction may be indicated by hazy lung markings.

Electrocardiography The electrocardiogram at birth may show normal right ventricular dominance, but if the infant survives a few days, right atrial and right ventricular hypertrophy are usual. Left-sided forces are often decreased, as evidenced by the absence of a septal q wave even out to V_7 and V_8 and only a small r wave in V_5 and V_6.

Echocardiography The two-dimensional echocardiogram is diagnostic by imaging a hypoplastic ascending aorta, atresia or marked stenosis of the mitral and aortic orifices, and an obliterated or minute posterior left ventricle in conjunction with a dilated, large anterior right ventricle and large patent ductus arteriosus (Fig. 22-59). These findings together with the clinical picture obviate the need for any additional invasive diagnostic studies. The patients who present difficult therapeutic decisions have transitional ventricles, with moderately hypoplastic mitral and aortic valves. The decision about whether to attempt a one- or two-ventricle repair is often difficult.

Treatment Supportive therapy directed at congestive heart failure, hypoxemia, and metabolic acidemia is of only limited benefit, and survival beyond the first week or 10 days of life is rare in the absence of maintenance of ductus patency with PGE_1. Although the anatomic and functional abnormalities in hypoplastic left heart syndrome are formidable, two different management programs are being pursued in some centers. First, an innovative surgical intervention (Norwood procedure) has been applied to the available structures to salvage a physiologically effective circulation by a three-stage operative approach. Ductus closure, the immediate cause of rapid circulatory collapse and death in these neonates, is modified by a PGE_1 infusion to maintain a widely patent ductus arteriosus. In the first surgical stage, the main pulmonary artery is transected, and the patent ductus arteriosus is ligated. Output from the right ventricle to the aorta is established by using the proximal main pulmonary artery to reconstruct the diminutive ascending aorta and aortic arch. Pulmonary blood flow is reestablished with a systemic-pulmonary shunt such as a modified right Blalock-Taussig shunt. If the foramen ovale is small, as often occurs, an atrial septectomy is performed to enable the pulmonary venous blood to return to the right atrium and ventricle without restriction. After survival for about 4 to 6 months, a bidirectional Glenn procedure is done (see above), followed later in childhood by completion of the inferior vena caval–pulmonary artery connection (modified Fontan operation). There is a fairly high surgical mortality with the first stage. Experience with the subsequent stages of "corrective" surgery is limited, and present results are disappointing.

In the rare patients with mitral atresia and ventricular septal defect, the ascending aorta may be large enough so that augmentation with the main pulmonary artery is not necessary. They may require pulmonary arterial banding to decrease pulmonary blood flow and pressure and protect the pulmonary vessels until a subsequent caval–pulmonary arterial connection can be done. If the foramen ovale is restrictive, the atrial septum must be opened. Thereafter, these infants are managed like the previous group while they await a caval–pulmonary connection.

The second approach consists of neonatal orthotopic cardiac transplantation. Although there are major difficulties related to shortage of donor hearts and the uncertainty about the long-term

effects of immunosuppression therapy, excellent short-term results have been obtained with a low operative mortality (under 10%) in a few institutions. While the child is awaiting transplantation, the ductus arteriosus may be kept open by a stent.

SINGLE VENTRICLE A single-ventricle (or univentricular) malformation is diagnosed when there is one ventricular chamber that receives both the mitral and tricuspid orifices or a common AV orifice. About 70 to 80% of single-ventricle malformations are derived from an *l*-bulboventricular loop (as opposed to the normal *d*-looping) and manifest bulboventricular inversion. These hearts have a single right-sided, morphologically left, ventricle with absence of the inflow portion of the right ventricle. There is persistence of a rudimentary anterior and left-sided right ventricular outflow chamber that communicates proximally with the single ventricle through a ventricular septal defect (persistent bulboventricular orifice) and distally with an *l*-transposed aorta. The pulmonary artery is posterior and arises from the single ventricle. Stenosis or atresia of the pulmonary outflow tract is also common, as is coarctation of the aorta, although they do not coexist—as in all congenital heart lesions, one or the other outflow tract may be obstructed, but almost never both. Subaortic stenosis as a result of a decrease in size of the bulboventricular orifice is relatively common and may occur after the pulmonary artery has been banded. Complex associated anomalies are usual, and they include dextrocardia, right atrial isomerism, common atrioventricular canal, and total anomalous pulmonary venous connection.

The term *common ventricle* has been used to distinguish a rare type of single-ventricle heart that has a well-developed right as well as left ventricular inflow tract; in such a heart the univentricular chamber represents essentially a huge ventricular septal defect.

Hemodynamics The hemodynamics and clinical picture vary, depending on the pulmonary blood flow and the associated intracardiac malformations. Some degree of systemic arterial desaturation is always present because of mixing of the pulmonary and systemic venous blood in the single ventricle or, in some, a common atrium. With significant pulmonary stenosis or atresia, cyanosis may be severe, the heart size small, and the pulmonary vascular markings diminished. In contrast, when there is no pulmonary stenosis the clinical and hemodynamic findings are dictated by the relationship between pulmonary and systemic vascular resistances and blood flows. In the infant, and in the older child when pulmonary vascular resistance is low, there will be torrential pulmonary blood flow with marked cardiomegaly and severe congestive heart failure. In the surviving child, increasing pulmonary vascular disease may moderate the excessive flow to the lungs.

Clinical Features With severe pulmonary stenosis the systolic ejection murmur is usually loud; with pulmonary atresia no murmurs may be heard except in the presence of atrioventricular valve insufficiency. An aortic ejection click may be heard; the second heart sound is usually single and loud. With markedly increased pulmonary blood flow, cyanosis may be quite mild, the systolic ejection murmur pansystolic, the second heart sound loud and narrowly split, and a third heart sound and short middiastolic rumble are often present.

Roentgenography The chest roentgenogram establishes the extent of cardiomegaly and pulmonary blood flow and the shape of the heart silhouette—straightened left heart border is often characteristic (Fig. 22-37) and should suggest the diagnosis of a single left

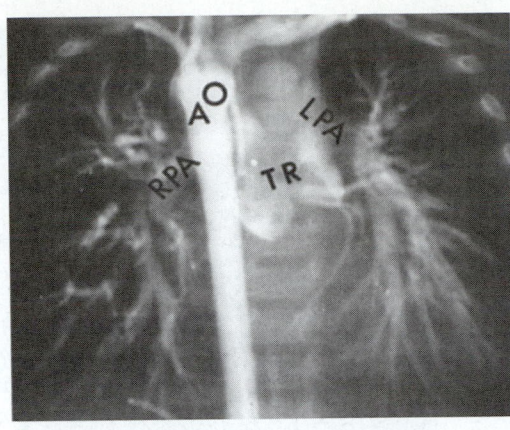 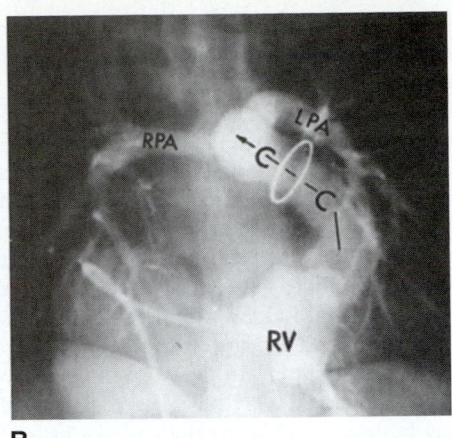

A   B

FIGURE 22-61 A: Angiocardiogram (anteroposterior view) in truncus arteriosus showing origin of the pulmonary arteries (RPA, LPA) and aorta (AO) from the truncus (TR). **B:** Angiocardiogram (anteroposterior view) in truncus arteriosus following corrective surgery with placement of valved conduit (C-C) from right ventricle (RV) to main pulmonary artery and closure of ventricular septal defect.

ventricle with small rudimentary right ventricular outflow tract associated with *l*-malposition of the great arteries.

Electrocardiography The electrocardiogram is nonspecific, presenting either right or left axis deviation and a precordial QRS pattern suggesting either right, combined ventricular, or left ventricular dominance. Large unchanging equiphasic or negative complexes across the entire precordium should raise a suspicion of single-ventricle malformation.

Echocardiography Two-dimensional echocardiography can establish the diagnosis of single-ventricle complex and provide additional anatomic details such as the presence of two AV orifices or one large common orifice, the orientation of the rudimentary outflow chamber, pulmonary outflow tract stenosis, and possibly anomalous pulmonary venous connections.

Cardiac Catheterization Cardiac catheterization and angiography may be helpful in differentiating certain particularly complex malformations such as "criss-cross" or "upstairs-downstairs" hearts and for identifying pulmonary or subpulmonary stenosis, measuring the pulmonary vascular resistance, establishing the anatomic course of the rudimentary small outlet chamber and the spatial relationships and connections of the cardiac chambers and great vessels, and the details of abnormal pulmonary or systemic venous connections. Magnetic resonance imaging is also helpful for assessing complex anatomic details.

Treatment The clinical course and prognosis are often grave, but palliation and long-term salvage have been effected for infants with decreased pulmonary blood flow by surgically creating either systemic-pulmonary or cavopulmonary anastomoses and for infants with increased pulmonary blood flow by pulmonary artery banding, with subsequent progression to the modified Fontan circulation. If there is subaortic stenosis, the proximal pulmonary arterial trunk can be anastomosed to the aorta (Damus-Stansel-Kaye procedure). Occasionally, surgical procedures have successfully placed a prosthetic septum in some forms of single-ventricle hearts. These formidable procedures have been significantly aided by the recent recognition in such hearts of abnormal disposition of the cardiac

specialized conduction tissue arising from an anterior rather than a normal posterior atrioventricular node and coursing as the bundle of His astride the anterior (conal) septum.

TRUNCUS ARTERIOSUS Truncus arteriosus, constituting 2% of all congenital heart lesions, is characterized by the emergence of only a single arterial trunk from the ventricular chambers, and this vessel supplies the coronary, pulmonary, and systemic circulations proximal to the aortic arch. A truncal valve, usually with three or four leaflets, overrides a ventricular septal defect, which is always present. The pulmonary arteries generally arise as a single vessel or as two separate vessels from the posterior or lateral wall of the truncus (Fig. 22-61A). Truncus arteriosus must not be confused with the relatively common lesion tetralogy of Fallot with pulmonary atresia, also characterized by a single large vessel, the aorta, that arises from the heart. In tetralogy of Fallot with pulmonary atresia, however, there is a hypoplastic or atretic pulmonary artery attached to the right ventricular outflow region, and the lungs are supplied with blood by pulmonary arteries arising from a ductus arteriosus or from major aortopulmonary collateral vessels usually arising from the thoracic descending aorta. Similar to these patients, though, a large percentage of infants with truncus arteriosus have partial deletion of chromosome 22. Rarely, interrupted aortic arch is present with the descending aorta being supplied from the main pulmonary artery via the ductus arteriosus.

Hemodynamics The right and left ventricles eject blood at systemic pressure into the common arterial trunk; thus, the coronary arteries, pulmonary arteries, and aorta receive a mixture of venous and oxygenated blood at systemic pressure. The pulmonary blood flow is markedly increased in infancy because there are usually primary pulmonary artery branches of adequate size and the pulmonary vascular resistance is initially not greatly increased. Consequently, cyanosis is minimal, and the hemodynamics as well as the clinical picture are those of a large left-to-right shunt. The pulmonary circulation may be restricted in a few patients by the development of pulmonary vascular obstructive disease or rarely by hypoplastic or stenotic pulmonary arteries arising from the truncus; in 16% of patients, one pulmonary artery is absent.

Clinical Features Symptoms usually appear in the first weeks or months of life and are consistent with a large left-to-right shunt: left heart failure, dyspnea, wheezing, frequent respiratory infections, and poor physical development. Failure to thrive is universal. In the infant, cyanosis is often not apparent or is minimal at rest because the pulmonary blood flow is so high. The heart is hyperdynamic, and peripheral pulses are prominent or bounding. The second heart sound is loud and single because of the single set of semilunar valves. A prominent systolic ejection click is heard very commonly at the lower and middle left sternal border. A harsh systolic murmur may best be heard along the middle left sternal border, and a continuous murmur is heard at the base or lateral chest wall in older infants and children. In newborn or young infants, particularly those with marked congestive heart failure, only a systolic murmur may be heard, similar to the findings in some newborn infants with a large patent ductus arteriosus. Severe truncal valve incompetence may be suspected from a prominent to-and-fro quality in the murmur. Truncal valve stenosis occurs rarely.

If pulmonary blood flow is restricted, either by high pulmonary vascular resistance or by stenotic or hypoplastic pulmonary arteries, cyanosis is more severe, congestive heart failure is unusual, only a minimal systolic murmur of short duration and low intensity is heard, and there may be a faint continuous bruit representing bronchial pulmonary collateral flow.

Roentgenography Roentgenographic findings also depend on the size of the pulmonary arteries and the pulmonary blood flow pattern. In most infants there is considerable cardiac enlargement, with increased pulmonary vascular markings. When pulmonary blood flow is decreased, both heart size and pulmonary vascular markings are less prominent. A right aortic arch is common (30 to 50%), and the hilar origin of the pulmonary artery may appear superiorly displaced.

Electrocardiography The electrocardiogram demonstrates right ventricular or combined ventricular hypertrophy.

Echocardiography Two-dimensional echocardiography establishes the diagnosis by demonstrating a large, single arterial vessel overriding the ventricular septum and identifying a main or primary branch pulmonary artery arising directly from this common trunk (Fig. 22-62). The ductus arteriosus is often absent except with an interrupted aortic arch. Cardiac catheterization is rarely indicated in the young infant, but, if performed, selective angiography reveals the common trunk arising from the heart and the origin of the pulmonary arteries from the truncus (Fig. 22-61A).

Treatment The prognosis is variable, depending to a considerable degree on the pulmonary blood flow pattern; most infants (about 75%) if unoperated die within the first 3 to 12 months from heart failure. Corrective surgery has been developed and widely applied, provided the patient is free from significant pulmonary vascular disease, which often develops by 3 to 4 months of age. The ventricular septal defect is closed to leave the aorta arising from the left ventricle, the pulmonary arteries are removed from their common truncus origin, and a valved conduit is placed from the free right ventricular wall to the pulmonary arteries (Fig. 22-61B) to form a new right ventricular outflow tract (Rastelli procedure). At present, the lowest operative mortality (under 10%) and the highest long-term yield of good results are achieved by corrective surgery done under 3 months of age. The child will have the initial small conduit changed to a larger size after 3 to 7 years and will have to have the

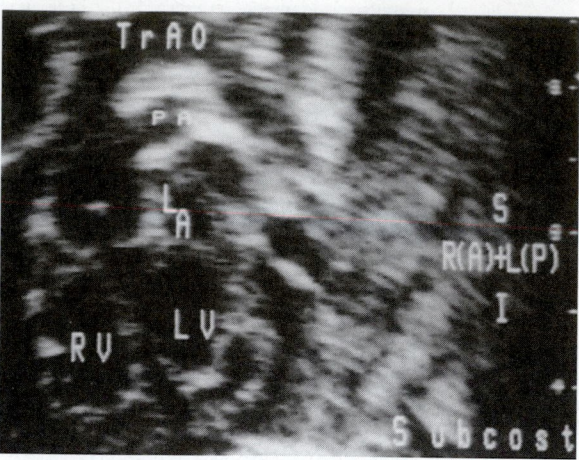

FIGURE 22-62 **Truncus arteriosus. This frame, taken from the subcostal coronal plane, demonstrates the origin of the truncus above and overriding both the left (LV) and right (RV) ventricles. The truncus gives origin to the pulmonary artery (PA) and then continues as the aorta. The transverse aorta (TrAO) can be seen coursing to the left side. LA = left atrium. Orientation: I = inferior; R(A) = right, anterior; S = superior; L(P) = left, posterior.**

second conduit changed to a larger size after 5 to 10 years. Truncal valve insufficiency, modest in about 25% but severe in about 5 to 10%, remains an important factor in late mortality; sometimes truncal valve replacement is needed.

References

General References

Freedom RM, Culham JAG, Moes CAF: Angiography of Congenital Heart Disease. New York, Macmillan, 1984

Fyler DC, Buckley LP, Hellebrand WE, et al: Report of the New England Regional Infant Cardiac Program. Pediatrics 65(Suppl):375, 1980

Gutgesell HP: Echocardiograph as an alternative to cardiac catheterization prior to surgery for congenital heart disease. In: Kron KL, Mavroudis C, eds: Innovations in Congenital Heart Surgery. Philadelphia, Hanley and Belfus, 1989

Hallidie-Smith KA: Prostaglandin E$_1$ in suspected ductus dependent cardiac malformations. Arch Dis Child 59:1020, 1984

Kirklin JW, Barratt-Boyes BG: Cardiac Surgery. New York, Wiley, 1993

Moller JH, Anderson RC: 1,000 consecutive children with a cardiac malformation with 26- to 37-year follow-up. Am J Cardiol 70:661, 1992

Morris CD, Menashe VD: 25-year mortality after surgical repair of congenital heart defect in childhood. JAMA 266:3447, 1991

Stark J: Do we really correct congenital heart defects? J Thorac Cardiovasc Surg 97:1, 1989

Tetralogy of Fallot

Boncheck LI, Staff A, Sunderland CO, et al: Natural history of tetralogy of Fallot in infancy. Clinical classification and therapeutic implications. Circulation 48:392, 1973

Ilbawi MN, Greico J, Deleon SY, et al: Modified Blalock-Taussig shunt in newborn infants. J Thorac Cardiovasc Surg 88:770, 1984

Joffe H, Georgapolous D, Celermajer DS, et al: Late ventricular arrhythmia is rare after early repair of tetralogy of Fallot. J Am Coll Cardiol 23:1146, 1994

Karl TR, Sano S, Pornviliwan S, Mee RB: Tetralogy of Fallot: favorable outcome of nonneonatal transatrial, transpulmonary repair. Ann Thorac Surg 54:903, 1992

Kreutzer J, Perry SB, Jonas RA, et al: Tetralogy of Fallot with diminuitive pulmonary arteries: preoperative pulmonary valve dilatation and transcatheter rehabilitation of pulmonary arteries. J Am Coll Cardiol 27:1741, 1996

Lillehi CW, Varco RL, Cohen M, et al: The first open heart corrections of tetralogy of Fallot: a 26–31-year follow-up of 106 patients. Ann Surg 204:490, 1986

Murphy JG, Gersh BJ, Mair DD, et al: Long-term outcome in patients undergoing surgical repair of tetralogy of Fallot. N Engl J Med 329:593–599, 1993

Reddy VM, Liddicoat JR, McElhinney DB, et al: Routine primary repair of tetralogy of Fallot in neonates and infants less than three months of age. Ann Thorac Surg 60:S592, 1995

Reddy VM, Petrossian E, McElhinney DB, et al: One stage complete unifocalization in infants. When should the ventricular septal defect be closed? J Thorac Cardiovasc Surg 113:858, 1997

Sreeram N, Saleem M, Jackson M, et al: Results of balloon pulmonary valvuloplasty as a palliative procedure in tetralogy of Fallot. J Am Coll Cardiol 18:159, 1991

Tricuspid Atresia

Dick M, Rosenthal A: The clinical profile of tricuspid atresia. In: Rao PS, ed: Tricuspid Atresia. Mount Kisco, NY, Futura Publishing, 1982:83

Franklin RC, Spiegelhalter DJ, Sullivan ID, et al: Tricuspid atresia presenting in infancy. Survival and suitability for the Fontan operation. Circulation 87:427, 1993

Mair DD, Puga FJ, Danielson GK: Late functional status of survivors of the Fontan procedure performed during the 1970s. Circulation 86(Suppl II):106, 1992

Pulmonary Atresia with Intact Ventricular Septum

Bull C, Kostelka M, Sorensen K, de Leval M: Outcome measures for the neonatal management of pulmonary atresia with intact ventricular septum. J Thorac Cardiovasc Surg 107:359, 1994

Freedom RM: Pulmonary Atresia and Intact Ventricular Septum. Mount Kisco, NY, Futura Publishers, 1989

Giglia TM, Jenkins KJ, Matitiau A, et al: Influence of right heart size on outcome in pulmonary atresia with intact ventricular septum. Circulation 88:2248, 1993

Hanley FL, Sade RM, Freedom RM, et al: Outcomes in critically ill neonates with pulmonary stenosis and intact ventricular septum: a multiinstitutional study. J Am Coll Cardiol 22:183, 1993

Kasznica J, Ursell PC, Blanc WA, et al: Abnormalities of the coronary circulation in pulmonary atresia and intact ventricular septum. Am Heart J 114:1415, 1987

Rabinovitch M, Herreva-DeLeon V, Castaneda AR, et al: Growth and development of the pulmonary vascular bed in patients with tetralogy of Fallot with or without pulmonary atresia. Circulation 64:1234, 1981

Rosenthal E, Qureshi SA, Kakadekar AP, et al: Technique of percutaneous laser-assisted valve dilatation for valvar atresia in congenital heart disease. Br Heart J 69:556, 1993

Ebstein Anomaly

Celermajer DS, Bull C, Till JA, et al: Ebstein's anomaly: presentation and outcome from fetus to adult. J Am Coll Cardiol 23:170, 1994

Danielson GK, Driscoll DJ, Mair DD, et al: Operative treatment of Ebstein's anomaly. J Thorac Cardiovasc Surg 104:1195, 1992

Hing YM, Moller JH: Ebstein's anomaly: a long-term study of survival. Am Heart J 125:1419, 1993

Leung MP, Baker EJ, Anderson RH, et al: Angiographic spectrum of Ebstein's malformation: its relevance to clinical presentation and outcome. J Am Coll Cardiol 11:154, 1988

Rusconi PG, Zuberbuhler JR, Anderson RH, Rigby ML: Morphologic-echocardiographic correlates of Ebstein's malformation. Eur Heart J 12:784, 1991

Transposition of the Great Arteries

Bonhoeffer P, Bonnet D, Piechaud JF, et al: Coronary artery obstruction after the arterial swich operation for transposition of the great arteries in the newborn. J Am Coll Cardiol 29:202, 1997

Martin RP, Qureshi SA, Ettedgui JA, et al: An evaluation of right and left ventricular function after anatomical correction and intra-atrial repair operations for complete transposition of the great arteries. Circulation 82:808, 1990

Paul MH: Complete transposition of the great arteries. In: Adams FH, Emmanouilides GC, Riemenschneider TA, eds: Heart Disease in Infants, Children, and Adolescents. Baltimore, Williams & Wilkins, 1989

Serraf A, Lacour-Gayet F, Bruniaux J, et al: Anatomic correction of transposition of the great arteries in neonates. J Am Coll Cardiol 22:193, 1993

von Segesser LK, Fry M, Senning A, Turina MI: Atrial repair for transposition of the great arteries: current approach in Zurich based on 24 years of follow-up. Thorac Cardiovasc Surg 39(Suppl 2):185, 1991

Williams WG, Trusler GA, Kirklin JW, et al: Early and late results of a protocol for simple transposition leading to an atrial switch (Mustard) repair. J Thorac Cardiovasc Surg 95:717, 1988

Double-Outlet Right Ventricle

Aoki M, Forbess JM, Jonas RA, et al: Result of biventricular repair for double-outlet right ventricle. J Thorac Cardiovasc Surg 10:338, 1994

Hagler DJ, Tajik AJ, Seward JB, et al: Double outlet right ventricle: wide angle two-dimensional echocardiographic observations. Circulation 63:419, 1981

Sidi D, Lecompte Y: Transposition and malposition of the great arteries with ventricular septal defects. In: Moller JH, Hoffman JIE, eds: Pediatric Cardiovascular Medicine. New York, Churchill Livingstone, 2000:363

Single Ventricle

Driscoll DJ, Offord KP, Feldt RH, et al: Five-to-fifteen year follow-up after Fontan operation. Circulation 85:469, 1992

Huhta JC, Seward JB, Tajik AJ, et al: Two-dimensional echocardiographic spectrum of univentricular atrioventricular connection. J Am Coll Cardiol 5:149, 1985

Kreuzer EA, Kreutzer J, Kreutzer GO: Univentricular heart. In: Moller JH, Hoffman JIE, eds: Pediatric Cardiovascular Medicine. New York, Churchill Livingstone, 2000:469

Lui RC, Williams WG, Trusler GA, et al: Experience with the Damus-Stansel-Kaye procedure for children with Taussig-Bing hearts or univentricular hearts with subaortic stenosis. Circulation 88(Suppl II):170, 1993

Malm T, Pawade A, Karl TR, Mee RB: Recent results with the modified Fontan operation. Scand J Thorac Cardiovasc Surg 27:65, 1993

Pridjian AK, Mendelsohn AM, Lupinetti FM, et al: Usefulness of the bidirectional Glenn procedure as staged reconstruction for the functional single ventricle. Am J Cardiol 71:959, 1993

Total Anomalous Pulmonary Venous Drainage

Cobanoglu A, Menashe VD: Total anomalous venous connection in neonates and young infants: repair in the current era. J Thorac Cardiovasc Surg 104:728, 1992

Jenkins KJ, Sanders SP, Orav EJ, et al: Individual pulmonary vein size and survival in infants with total anomalous pulmonary venous connection. J Am Coll Cardiol 22:201, 1993

Lucas RV Jr Lock JE, Tanlon R, et al: Gross and histologic anatomy of total anomalous pulmonary venous connections. Am J Cardiol 62:292, 1988

Wang JK, Lue HC, Wu MH, et al: Obstructed total anomalous pulmonary venous connection. Pediatr Cardiol 14:28, 1993

Truncus Arteriosus

Bove EL, Lupinetti FM, Pridjian AK, et al: Results of a policy of primary repair of truncus arteriosus in the neonate. J Thorac Cardiovasc Surg 105:1057, 1993

Calder L, van Praagh R, van Praagh S, et al: Truncus arteriosus communis: clinical, angiographic, and pathologic findings in 100 patients. Am Heart J 92:23, 1976

Ceballos R, Soto B, Kirklin JW, et al: Truncus arteriosus: an anatomical-angiographic study. Br Heart J 49:589, 1983

Hanley FL, Heinemann MK, Jonas RA, et al: Repair of truncus arteriosus in the neonate. J Thorac Cardiovasc Surg 105:1047, 1993

Stanger P: Truncus arteriosus. In: Moller JH, Neal WA, eds: Fetal, Neo-natal, and Infant Cardiac Disease. Norwalk, CT, Appleton & Lange, 1990:587

Hypoplastic Left Heart

Bove EL, Mosca RS: Surgical repair of the hypoplastic left heart syndrome. Prog Pediatr Cardiol 5:23, 1996

Chiavarelli M, Gundry SR, Razzouk AJ, Bailey LL: Cardiac transplantation for infants with hypoplastic left-heart syndrome. JAMA 270:2944, 1993

Farrell PE Jr, Chang AC, Murdison KA, et al: Outcome and assessment after the modified Fontan procedure for hypoplastic left heart syndrome. Circulation 85:116, 1992

Pulmonary Arteriovenous Fistula

Hodgson CH, Burchell HB, Good CA, Clagett OT: Hereditary hemor-rhagic telangiectasia and pulmonary arteriovenous fistula. N Engl J Med 261:625, 1959

Jeffrey GP, Prince RL, Van der Schaaf A: Fatal intrapulmonary arteriove-nous shunting in cirrhosis—diagnosis by radionuclide lung perfusion scan. Med J Aust 152:549, 552, 1990

Kravath RE, Scarpelli EM, Bernstein J: Hepatogenic cyanosis: arteriovenous shunts in chronic active hepatitis. J Pediatr 78:238, 1971

LeRoux BT: Pulmonary arteriovenous fistulae. Q J Med 28:1, 1959

LeRoux BT: Pulmonary "hamartomata." Thorax 19:236, 1964

22.3.6 Malpositions

Paul Stanger

A heart abnormally situated in the thorax is said to show malposi-tion. Such hearts often have abnormalities of chamber localization and great artery attachments as well as septal defects, valve anom-alies, and outflow obstructions. Describing the basic structure of such a complex heart requires description of three cardiac segments (atria, ventricles, and great arteries) and should include not only positional interrelationships but also connections of ventricles to atria and great arteries.

SITUS AND ATRIA

The right and left atria may be regarded as extensions of the sys-temic and pulmonary veins, respectively, so that the body situs in-dicates the positions of the atria. Body situs is determined by certain organs that are normally asymmetric. The normal body configu-ration, *situs solitus* (Fig. 22-63), is characterized by a right lung with three lobes and an eparterial bronchus, a left lung with two lobes and a hyparterial bronchus, asymmetric tracheobronchial branching, a liver with a major lobe on the right, a left-sided stom-ach and spleen, right-sided venae cavae, morphologically distinct atria, and a specific orderly arrangement of the gastrointestinal tract. *Situs inversus* is characterized by a mirror-image configuration of the asymmetric organs, including the gastrointestinal tract. In addition to these two asymmetric forms of situs, two roughly sym-metric body configurations have been found with *right* and *left atrial isomerism*. Right atrial isomerism is characterized by bilateral right-sidedness, with bilateral three-lobed lungs, each with a typical right bronchial branching pattern, a horizontal liver with equal-sized lobes, and bilateral morphologic right atria, each with a si-noatrial node. The spleen is usually absent (asplenia), and this may also be regarded as a feature of bilateral right-sidedness. In contrast, left atrial isomerism is characterized by bilateral left-sidedness in-volving lungs, bronchi, and the atria. There are usually multiple (2 to 30), roughly equal-sized spleens with a total mass equal to that of a normal sized spleen clustered together on both sides of the dorsal mesogastrium (polysplenia). This is in contrast to accessory spleens, which are small isolated splenic masses in addition to a normal spleen. Malrotations of the bowel are common in both as-plenia and polysplenia. Right and left atrial isomerism replace the terms asplenia and polysplenia, respectively, because splenic mor-phology and isomerism do not always match. In general, organ symmetry is more variable with left than with right isomerism.

VENTRICLES

The primitive cardiac tube normally bends to the right and forms a *d*-loop, so that the anatomic right ventricle lies to the right of the anatomic left ventricle. Such a loop is appropriate or *concordant* for a situs solitus individual; that is, the right atrium connects to the right ventricle and the left atrium to the left ventricle. Conversely, an *l*-loop is concordant for a situs inversus individual (Fig. 22-63). Occasionally a discordant loop forms (*l*-loop in situs solitus or *d*-loop in situs inversus); the anatomic right atrium connects to the anatomic left ventricle and anatomic left atrium to anatomic right ventricle.

GREAT ARTERIES

Great arteries may be described by their ventricular connections and positional interrelationships. Ventricular connections may be nor-mal (pulmonary artery from right ventricle, aorta from left ventri-cle), double-outlet right or left ventricle (DORV or DOLV, re-spectively), or transposition (aorta from right ventricle, pulmonary artery from left ventricle). The positional interrelationships may be described as *d* (dextro), where the aortic valve is to the right of the pulmonary artery, *l* (levo), where the aortic valve is to the left, or *o* (ortho), where the aorta is directly in front of the pulmonary artery; these terms are not to be confused with *d*-loops and *l*-loops. Usually great-artery interrelationships reflect ventricular interrelationships; however, there are enough exceptions that description of both seg-ments is preferable.

The right ventricular infundibulum (or conus) is usually the most anterior cardiac structure and connects with the anterior great artery. Accordingly, normally related great arteries usually have an anterior pulmonary artery, transpositions have an anterior aorta,

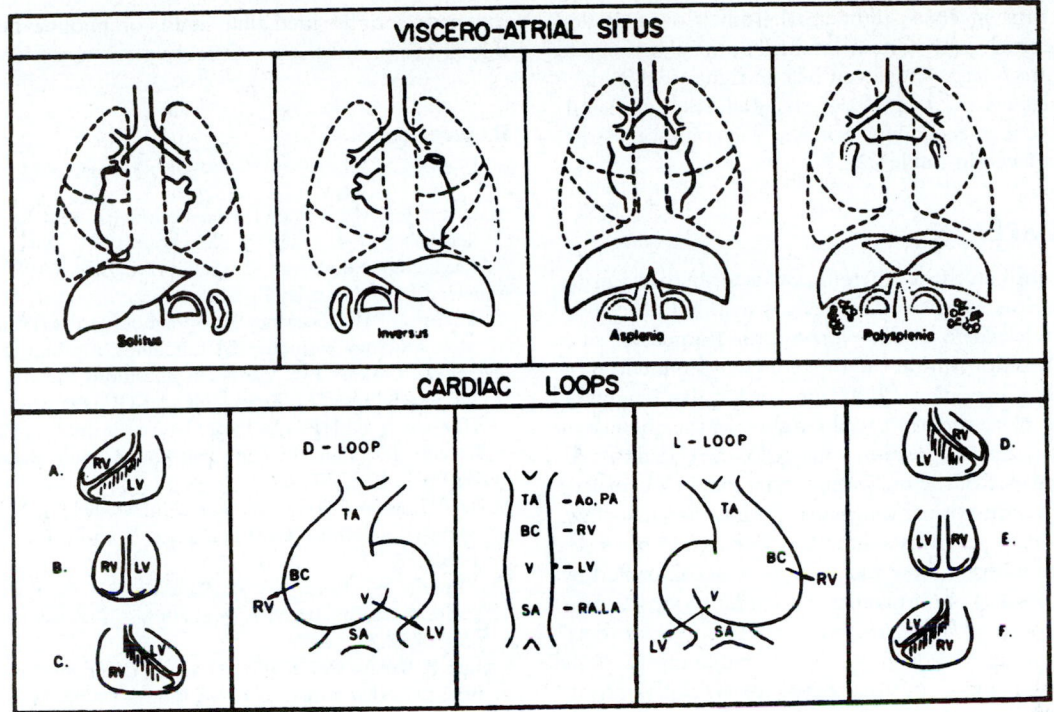

FIGURE 22-63   Anatomic factors in cardiac malpositions. **Top:** Diagrams of the four basic body configurations or situses: solitus, inversus, asplenia (right atrial isomerism), and polysplenia (left atrial isomerism). For asplenia and polysplenia, the outlines indicate abdominal organs (liver, spleen, stomach) with variable lateralization. **Bottom:** The central diagram is of the straight cardiac tube and its four segments. The truncus arteriosus (TA), at the cephalad end, divides coronally into an anterior portion that becomes the aorta and a posterior portion that becomes the pulmonary artery. The sinoatrium (SA) is at the caudal end and divides sagitally into the right- and left-side atria. The morphology of the atria depends on the situs. The bulbus cordis (BC) becomes the morphologic right ventricle, and the primitive ventricle (V) becomes the morphologic left ventricle. The lateral interrelationships of the ventricles depend on the direction of bulboventricular looping. Rightward looping (*d*-looping) places the morphologic right ventricle (RV) to the right of the morphologic left ventricle (LV). This interrelationship is reversed with *l*-looping. Although looping determines the interrelationship of the ventricles, the cardiac position is determined by the degree of pivoting of the ventricles (A–F).

and double-outlets tend to have side-by-side vessels. Vessels arising from the left ventricle almost always lack a conus, and so their valves are more caudad than are those arising from the right ventricle.

Discordant loops (solitus/*l*-loop or inversus/*d*-loop) are almost always associated with transposition of the great arteries. The sequential arrangement of chambers and great arteries in these patients is such that the flow is potentially normal, and so these lesions have been called (physiologically) corrected transposition of the great arteries. Any abnormal circulation in these hearts is the result of associated abnormalities such as septal defects or AV valve stenoses or regurgitation, one or more of which occur in nearly all. The conduction pathways are also abnormal and may produce various degrees of AV block.

A simplified nomenclature for describing complex hearts (after van Praagh and colleagues) follows:

Situs

- Solitus
- Inversus
- Right atrial isomerism
- Left atrial isomerism

Ventricles

- *d*-Loop: morphologic RV to right of morphologic LV
- *l*-Loop: morphologic LV to right of morphologic RV
- *d*- or *l*-single-ventricle: outlets of both atria to a large primitive ventricle with small outlet chamber that has no AV valve; as the outflow chamber is the RV outflow, its position determines *d* or *l* designation

Great arteries

- *d*: Aortic valve to right of pulmonic
- *l*: Aortic valve to left of pulmonic
- *o*: Aortic valve directly anterior
- Normal: PA from RV, Ao from LV
- DORV: PA and Ao from RV
- DOLV: PA and Ao from LV
- Trans: Ao from RV, PA from LV
- Malposition: unusual arrangement of vessels not conforming to above

Hence, segmental sets may be described as follows: solitus/*d*-loop/*d*-trans is the usual transposition of the great arteries in situs solitus; inversus/*d*-loop/*d*-trans is corrected transposition of the great arteries in situs inversus; right atrial isomerism/*d*-single/ *d*-trans is single ventricle with aorta from small outlet chamber and pulmonary artery from large single ventricle in right atrial isomerism. Additional defects (eg, septal defects, stenoses, anomalous veins) must be described separately. Some of the common associated anomalies are listed in Table 22-15.

CARDIAC POSITION

A heart predominantly in the left hemithorax is termed *levocardia* and is normal for situs solitus. If the heart is mainly in the right hemithorax, it is referred to as *dextrocardia,* the normal for situs inversus. Cardiac position within the thorax may be influenced by external forces (eg, a hypoplastic right lung or left diaphragmatic eventration may displace the heart to the right). In the absence of such external factors, cardiac position is most closely related to concordance or discordance of the bulboventricular loop. Concordant loops nearly always have normal ventricular position for that situs, that is, left-sided heart for situs solitus and right-sided heart for situs inversus. Exceptions are few and tend to be accompanied by less severe, if any, cardiac abnormalities. Discordant loops in situs solitus or situs inversus and (because atrial symmetry precludes concordance) all loops in atrial isomerisms have variable cardiac positions; for example, an *l*-loop in situs solitus (or atrial isomerism)

can have a right-sided, left-sided, or midline heart. Similarly, a *d*-loop in situs inversus or atrial isomerism can have any position.

References

Anderson RH, Macartney FJ, Shinebourne EA, et al: Terminology. In: Anderson RH, Macartney FJ, Shinebourne EA, Tynan M, eds: Paediatric Cardiology. Edinburgh, Churchill Livingstone, 1987:65

Anderson RH, Macartney FJ, Shinebourne EA, et al: Atrial isomerism. In: Anderson RH, Macartney FJ, Shinebourne EA, Tynan M, eds: Paediatric Cardiology. Edinburgh, Churchill Livingstone, 1987:473

Hagler DJ, O'Leary PW: Cardiac malpositions and abnormalities of atrial and visceral situs. In: Emmanouilides GC, Riemenschneider TA, Allen HD, Gutgesell HP, eds: Heart Disease in Infants, Children, and Adolescents, Including the Fetus and Young Adult. Baltimore, Williams & Wilkins, 1994:1307

Moller JH: Malposition of the heart. In: Moller JH, Neal WA, eds: Fetal, Neonatal, and Infant Cardiac Disease. Norwalk, CT, Appleton & Lange, 1990:755

Shinebourne EA, Macartney FJ, Anderson RH: Sequential chamber localization—logical approach to diagnosis in congenital heart disease. Br Heart J 38:327, 1976

Stanger P, Benassi RC, Korns ME, et al: Diagrammatic portrayal of variations in cardiac structure. Circulation 37(Suppl IV):1, 1968

TABLE 22-15

MOST COMMON CARDIAC ANOMALIES FOUND IN EACH TYPE OF BODY CONFIGURATION

SEGMENTAL SET	COMMON NAME	ASSOCIATED CARDIAC ANOMALIES	MISCELLANEOUS
Solitus/*d*-loop/ *d*-normal	Normal heart of situs solitus; may have abnormal cardiac position because of dextroposition (cardiac displacement from extracardiac forces) or dextrorotation (rightward pivoting of the ventricular portion of the heart)	Variable, but usually atrial septal defects, ventricular septal defects, or patent ductus arteriosus	
Inversus/*l*-loop/ *l*-normal	Normal heart of situs inversus	Usually normal, but may have associated lesions including transposition	Often have nonmotile cilia and tendency to have sinusitis and bronchiectasis (Kartagener syndrome)
Solitus-/*l*-loop/ *l*-trans	Corrected transposition of situs solitus	High incidence of ventricular septal defect or pulmonic stenosis, Ebstein malformation of the systemic ventricle, and AV block	
Inversus/*d*-loop/*d*-trans	Corrected transposition of situs inversus		
Right atrial isomerism/*d*-or *l*-loop		Almost all have transposition of the great arteries, severe pulmonic stenosis or atresia, and AV canal with large ventricular septal defect or single ventricle; two-thirds have anomalous pulmonary venous connection to vena cava or portal system	Severe cyanosis from birth on; symmetric liver and bronchi; malrotation of bowel common; Heinz or Howell-Jolly bodies or pitted red cells on peripheral blood smear; 80% have asplenia
Left atrial isomerism/*d*- or *l*-loop		Most commonly have left-to-right shunts through atrial septal defects, ventricular septal defects, endocardial cushion defects, or double-outlet right ventricle; may also have left-sided obstructive lesions like aortic stenosis or coarctation; transposition and pulmonic stenosis are unusual; pulmonary veins may connect to either or both atria; two-thirds have interruption of the inferior vena cava	Cyanosis usually mild or absent; congestive heart failure common; malrotation of bowel common; symmetric liver, but less so than in right atrial isomerism; superior P axis in ECG common; occasional biliary atresia; usually have polysplenia

Van Mierop LHS, Gessner IH, Schiebler GL: Asplenia and polysplenia syndrome. Birth Defects 8:74, 1972

Van Praagh R: Nomenclature and classification: morphologic and segmental approach to diagnosis. In: Moller JH, Hoffman JIE, eds: Pediatric Cardiovascular Medicine. New York, Churchill Livingstone, 2000: 275

22.3.7   Vascular Rings and Slings

Julien I. E. Hoffman

These anomalies arise from abnormal persistence and dissolution of all or some of the paired embryonic aortic arches that connect the embryonic truncus arteriosus to the paired dorsal aortas (Figs. 22-4 and 22-5). Abnormal development of these arteries may produce no symptoms (aberrant right subclavian artery, right aortic arch) or may press on the esophagus or trachea and cause dysphagia and airway obstruction. Therefore, diagnosis can usually be made by examining the characteristic indentations that the abnormal arteries make on the barium-filled esophagus or the trachea. Confirmation by echocardiography, computed tomography, or magnetic resonance imaging has replaced aortography. Physical examination of the heart and the electrocardiogram are usually normal.

Infants with severe obstructions are very ill with vomiting, choking, and often dysphagia, so that feeding and weight gain are poor. Wheezing and stridor, usually inspiratory, are often prominent and made worse by feeding. Frequently these infants hyperextend their heads to reduce tracheal compression. Episodes of cyanosis, apnea, or unconsciousness occur. Most of these infants develop symptoms below 3 months of age. Less severe obstruction may present with recurrent respiratory infections.

The most common anomaly is an aberrant right subclavian artery. When the proximal rather than the distal part of the right fourth arch is absorbed, the right subclavian artery runs posteriorly from the descending thoracic aorta to reach the right arm, passing obliquely up and to the right behind the esophagus and indenting it posteriorly (Fig. 22-64). This anomaly so rarely causes symptoms that even if it is found, some other cause of esophageal or respiratory symptoms should be sought.

If the distal fourth arch disappears on the left rather than on the right, there will be a right aortic arch and a mirror-image arrangement of arteries to the arms and head. This is not a cause of symptoms, but the prominent roentgenographic shadow that the arch casts on the right side of the mediastinum may be mistaken for enlarged nodes or a tumor. A right aortic arch is found in about 25% of patients with the tetralogy of Fallot and about 50% with truncus arteriosus.

Most anomalies that cause serious symptoms encircle the esophagus and trachea to form a vascular ring (Fig. 22-65). The most common of these is the double aortic arch, which can result from failure of absorption of any part of the embryonic fourth arches. The right and left arches indent the right and left sides of the trachea and the esophagus, and the right arch indents the esophagus posteriorly as it passes to the left behind the esophagus to join the left arch, usually the smaller arch, and form the descending aorta. Sometimes the descending aorta is right-sided, and the left arch is retroesophageal. Division of one of the arches, usually the smaller posterior one, opens the constricting ring and is curative; this can be done by open or thoracoscopic surgery. However, deformity of the tracheobronchial tree may cause residual postoperative airway problems.

Almost as common is the right aortic arch that becomes a con-

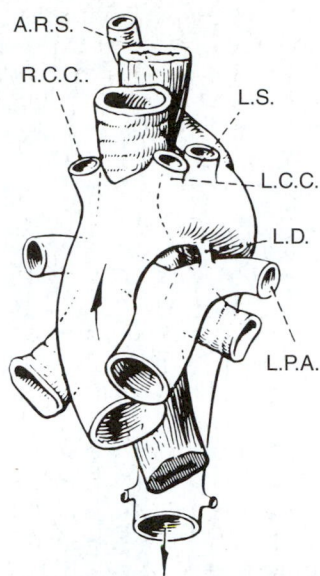

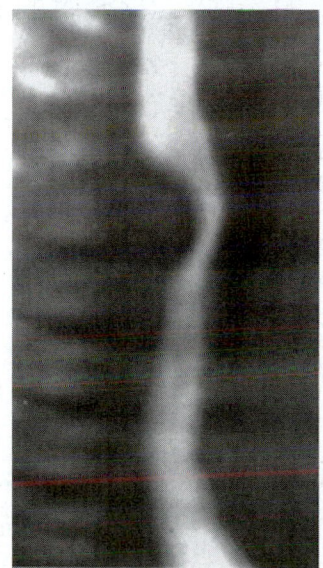 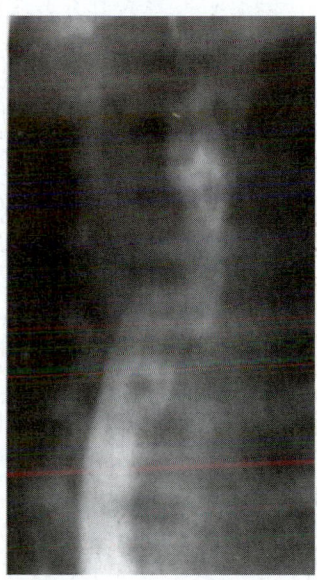

FIGURE 22-64   **Upper panel: Diagram of aberrant right subclavian artery (A.R.S.) arising distal to the left subclavian artery (L.S.). R.C.C. and L.C.C. = right and left common carotid arteries; L.D. = ductus arteriosus or ligamentum arteriosum; L.P.A. = left pulmonary artery. SOURCE: *Stewart JR, Kincaid OW, Edwards JE: An Atlas of Vascular Rings and Related Malformations of the Aortic Arch. Springfield, IL, Charles C Thomas, 1964, by permission of the authors and the publishers.* Lower panels: Lateral *(left)* and frontal *(right)* barium esophagrams in patient with aberrant right subclavian artery. SOURCE: *Courtesy of Dr. H. Taybi.***

stricting ring because of a retroesophageal left-sided patent ductus arteriosus or ligamentum arteriosum. The combination produces indentations on the esophagus and trachea similar to those that occur with a double arch. Division of the ductus or ligamentum is curative. Note that infants with any of these aortic arch anomalies may have a complete or partial DiGeorge syndrome, associated with a deletion in chromosome 22q11.

Occasionally a carotid or innominate artery compresses the anterior margin of the trachea. This may show up on roentgenograms of the tracheal air column or on a tracheogram, but the esophagram

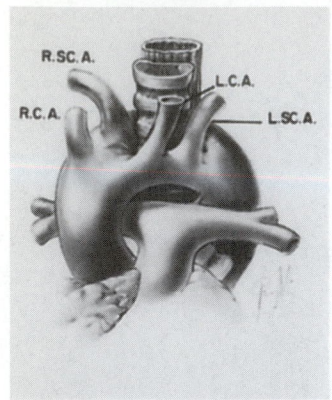
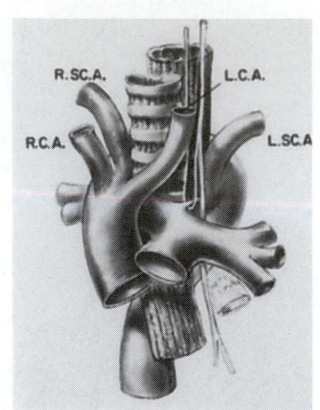

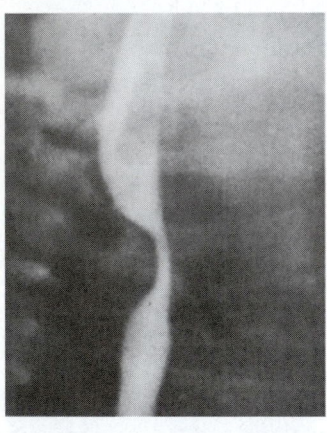
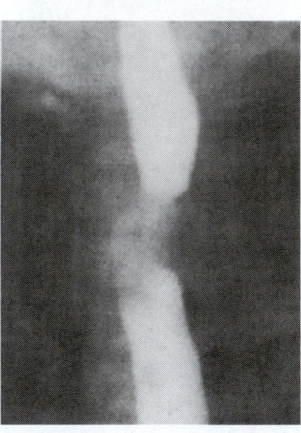

FIGURE 22-65 **Upper left panel: Diagram of double aortic arch. R.C.A. and L.C.A. = right and left common carotid arteries; R.SC.A. and L.SC.A. = right and left subclavian arteries. Upper right panel: Diagram of vascular ring from ligamentum arteriosum, identified by the recurrent laryngeal nerve that loops around it. The ligamentum arteriosum completes the ring. Abbreviations as in left panel.** SOURCE: *Arcinieges A, Hakimi M, Hertzler IH, et al. Surgical management of congenital vascular rings. J Thorac Cardiovasc Surg 77:721, 1979, by permission of the authors and the publishers.* **Lower panels: Lateral** *(left)* **and frontal** *(right)* **barium esophagrams in patient with double aortic arch. The esophagus is narrowed in the frontal view, and the right arch is higher than the left arch.** SOURCE: *Courtesy of Dr. H. Taybi.*

is normal. If needed, the compressing artery can be displaced anteriorly at surgery.

Although not a vascular ring, the anomalous left pulmonary artery also causes airway obstruction. The left pulmonary artery arises from the right pulmonary artery and passes between the esophagus and trachea, compressing the trachea and the right main bronchus. It is the only important vascular anomaly to indent only the anterior edge of the esophagus (Fig. 22-66). The infants may have cough, wheezing, stridor, and episodes of choking, cyanosis, or apnea, but dysphagia is rare. There may be collapse or hyperinflation of part of the right lung. Associated cardiovascular anomalies are common. Diagnosis is made by a combination of esophagrams, bronchoscopy, and angiography. Surgical reattachment of the left pulmonary artery to the main pulmonary artery relieves the obstruction, but tracheal stenosis often leads to suboptimal results.

References

Arciniegas A, Hakimi M, Hertzler JH, et al: Surgical management of congenital vascular rings. J Thorac Cardiovasc Surg 77:721, 1979

Backer CL, Idriss FS, Holinger LD, Mavroudis C: Pulmonary artery sling: results of surgical repair in infancy. J Thorac Cardiovasc Surg 103:683, 1992

Backer CL, Ilbawi MN, Idriss FS, Deleon SY: Vascular anomalies causing tracheoesophageal compression: review of experience in children. J Thorac Cardiovasc Surg 97:725, 1989

Berdon WE, Baker DH: Vascular anomalies and the infant lung: rings, slings and other things. Semin Roentgenol 7:39, 1972

Blake HA, Manion WC: Thoracic arterial arch anomalies. Circulation 26: 251, 1962

Conley ME, Beckwith JB, Mancer JFK, et al: The spectrum of DiGeorge syndrome. J Pediatr 94:883, 1979

Edwards JE: Vascular rings and slings. In: Moller JH, Neal WA, eds: Fetal, Neonatal, and Infant Cardiac Disease. Norwalk, CT, Appleton & Lange, 1990:745

Jonas RA, Spevack PJ, McGill T, Castaneda A: Pulmonary artery sling: primary repair by tracheal resection in infancy. J Thorac Cardiovasc Surg 97:548, 1989

Klinkhamer AC: Esophagography in Anomalies of the Aortic Arch System. Baltimore, Williams & Wilkins, 1969

Marmon LM, Haas JM, Balsara RK, Dunn JM: Vascular rings and slings: long-term follow-up of pulmonary function. J Pediatr Surg 19:683, 1984

Ruckman RN: Anomalies of the aortic arch complex. In: Adams FH, Emmanouilides GC, Riemenschneider TA, eds: Heart Disease in Infants, Children and Adolescents. Baltimore, Williams & Wilkins, 1989:255

FIGURE 22-66 **Left panel: Diagram of anomalous left pulmonary artery showing its passage between esophagus and trachea and compression of the right main bronchus.** SOURCE: *Clarkson, Ritter, Rahimtoola, et al: Am J Dis Child 113:373, 1967, by permission of the authors and the publishers.* **Right panel: Barium esophagram to show indentation of the anterior wall of the esophagus and the posterior wall of the trachea.** SOURCE: *Dupuis et al: Am J Cardiol 61:177, 1988, by permission of the authors and the publishers.*

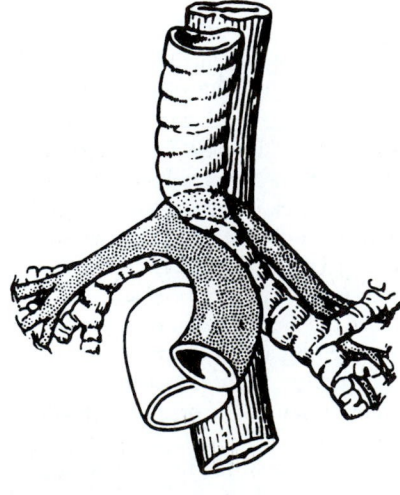
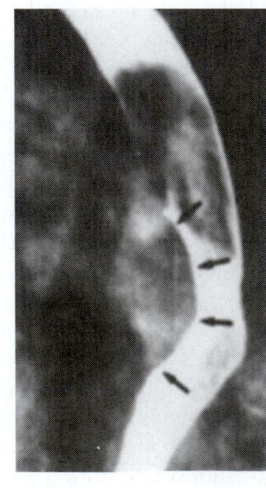

Stewart JR, Kincaid OW, Edwards JE: An Atlas of Vascular Rings and Related Malformations of the Aortic Arch. Springfield, IL, Charles C Thomas, 1964

Wilson DI, Goodship JA, Burn J, et al: Deletions within chromosome 22q11 in familial congenital heart disease. Lancet 340:573, 1992

22.3.8   Coronary Arterial Anomalies

Julien I. E. Hoffman

ANOMALOUS ORIGIN OF LEFT CORONARY ARTERY

The left coronary artery arises from the pulmonary artery, and the right coronary artery arises normally from the anterior aortic sinus. During fetal life, with similar pulmonary arterial and aortic pressures and saturations, myocardial perfusion and oxygenation are normal. However, after birth, pulmonary arterial pressure decreases, and blood flows from the right coronary artery through collateral vessels into the left coronary artery and then into the pulmonary artery. Thus a small left-to-right shunt is produced, and blood destined for the myocardium is diverted to the pulmonary artery through these channels. Usually the anterolateral wall of the left ventricle is involved.

Generally patients present with myocardial failure from ischemia or even a myocardial infarct between 2 weeks and 6 months of age. Episodes of restlessness and crying, as if in pain, associated with pallor and sweating have been described in infants with this anomaly, but poor feeding, tachypnea, and respiratory symptoms related to left ventricular failure are more usual. Severe cardiomegaly is the rule, and mitral insufficiency murmurs often result from dilatation of the mitral valve ring or papillary muscle infarction. Prominent third and fourth heart sounds are common. The electrocardiogram shows an anterolateral infarct pattern, with broad, deep Q waves in leads I, aVL, and the left precordium, often associated with persistent S-T segment and T-wave changes in these leads. Increased left ventricular forces are usual. The chest x-ray shows cardiomegaly and usually pulmonary venous congestion. Other lesions that present with similar findings include endocardial fibroelastosis, myocarditis, and glycogen storage disease involving the heart. Because anomalous origin of the left coronary artery is treatable, this diagnosis must be considered when there is unexplained left ventricular failure in infancy; it can be suspected on two-dimensional echocardiography but often must be confirmed by cardiac catheterization and angiocardiography. Treatment consists of reimplanting the coronary artery into the aorta or by aortocoronary bypass grafting. If these are not feasible, ligating the anomalous left coronary artery, if there is a left-to-right shunt from the coronary artery into the pulmonary artery, prevents runoff and thereby permits better perfusion of the surviving myocardium through the collateral vessels.

ANOMALOUS AORTIC ORIGIN OF CORONARY ARTERIES

Occasionally the left coronary artery arises from the right aortic sinus of Valsalva, or the right coronary artery arises from the left aortic sinus of Valsalva. The anomalously arising artery may reach its territory of supply by passing between the aorta and the pulmonary artery. Patients with this anomaly have episodes of chest pain, syncope, or even sudden death, which unfortunately may be the first abnormal event. Almost invariably these symptoms occur during or just after strenuous exercise. The anomaly is almost never familial.

The anomaly cannot be diagnosed clinically. However, unexplained chest pain or syncope on exercise require screening by echocardiography and, even if this is normal, by coronary angiography, computed tomography, or magnetic resonance imaging. The anomalous artery can be implanted surgically into its correct sinus to prevent further danger.

CORONARY ARTERIOVENOUS FISTULAS

See Section 22.3.2.

MISCELLANEOUS ANOMALIES

Some coronary arteries come off a single trunk from the aorta. Other than an increased risk if there is coronary atheroma, these patients occasionally die suddenly, most often when the single trunk passes between the aorta and pulmonary artery. The clinical presentation and diagnosis are the same as for anomalous aortic origin of the coronary arteries.

Rarely the whole coronary arterial system is hypoplastic. There may be ischemic symptoms or sudden death. Diagnosis is made by angiography. There is no specific treatment.

Sudden death has also occurred in patients with normally attached coronary arteries who, at autopsy, have had slitlike orifices of a coronary artery and in whom the first part of the coronary artery emerges tangentially rather than being perpendicular to the aortic wall.

References

Askenazi J, Nadas AS: Anomalous left coronary artery originating from the pulmonary artery: report on 15 cases. Circulation 51:976, 1975

Cheitlin MD, Decastro CM, McAllister HA: Sudden death as a complication of anomalous left coronary origin from the anterior sinus of Valsalva: a not-so-minor congenital anomaly. Circulation 50:780, 1974

Hoffman JIE: Congenital anomalies of the coronary vessels and the aortic root. In: Emmanouilides GC, Riemenschneider TA, Allen HD, Gutgesell HP, eds: Heart Disease in Infants, Children, and Adolescents, Including the Fetus and Young Adult. Baltimore, Williams & Wilkins, 1994:769

Kragel AH, Roberts WC: Anomalous origin of either the right or the left main coronary artery from the aorta with subsequent coursing between aorta and pulmonary trunk: analysis of 32 necropsy cases. Am J Cardiol 62:771, 1988

Liberthson RR, Dinsmore RE, Fallon JT: Aberrant coronary artery origin from the aorta. Report of 18 patients, review of literature and delineation of natural history and management. Circulation 59:748, 1979

Moodie DS, Fyfe D, Gill GC, et al: Anomalous origin of the left coronary artery from the pulmonary artery (Bland-White-Garland syndrome) in adult patients. Long-term follow-up after surgery. Am Heart J 106:381, 1983

Roberts WC: Major anomalies of coronary arterial origin seen in adulthood. Am Heart J 111:941, 1986

Shirani J, Roberts WC: Solitary coronary ostium in the aorta in the absence of other major congenital cardiovascular anomalies. J Am Coll Cardiol 21:137, 1993

Virmani R, Chun PKC, Goldstein RE, et al: Acute takeoffs of the coronary arteries along the aortic wall and congenital ostial valve-like ridges: association with sudden death. J Am Coll Cardiol 3:766, 1984

Wesselhoeft H, Fawcett JS, Johnson AL: Anomalous origin of the left coronary artery from the pulmonary trunk. Its clinical spectrum, pathology, and pathophysiology, based on a review of 140 cases with seven further cases. Circulation 38:403, 1968

22.3.9 Pulmonary Hypertension and Increased Pulmonary Vascular Resistance

Jeffrey R. Fineman

After about 1 week of age, pulmonary arterial blood pressure is normally under 25/12 mm Hg. Any higher pressure is regarded as pulmonary arterial hypertension, although slight increases are usually not clinically important. To evaluate the causes of pulmonary arterial hypertension, consider the concept of vascular resistance (R), which is, by definition, the ratio of the pressure drop across a vascular bed to the blood flow through it. For the pulmonary circulation the pressure drop is from the pulmonary artery (P_a) to the pulmonary veins (P_V) and is normally 4 to 10 mm Hg at rest. The flow is the pulmonary blood flow (Q_P), which at all ages is about 3.5 L/min for each square meter of body surface area. Thus, resting pulmonary vascular resistance is about 1 to 3 mm Hg/L/min/m². On exercise in the normal subject, pulmonary blood flow can increase three- to fourfold with little rise in pulmonary arterial pressure; the resistance falls to one-third or one-quarter of its resting value because the small resistance vessels dilate and new vessels are recruited.

The resistance equation $R = (P_a - P_V)/Q_P$ can be rearranged as $P_a = RQ_P + P_V$, an expression that gives the simplest classification of the causes of pulmonary arterial hypertension. Pulmonary arterial pressure (P_a) rises with an increase in pulmonary vascular resistance, pulmonary blood flow, or pulmonary venous pressure, provided that a rise in one variable does not alter the others; an increase in flow normally causes a fall in pulmonary vascular resistance that tends to prevent a rise in pulmonary arterial pressure. Thus, pulmonary arterial pressures are usually normal or only minimally elevated with exercise or with the large pulmonary flows found with large atrial septal defects. Conversely, the high pulmonary arterial pressures seen with large ventricular septal defects (which equalize pressures between the two ventricles) indicate the failure of pulmonary vascular resistance to fall when pulmonary blood flow increases, so that increases in both Q_p and R are responsible for the pulmonary arterial hypertension.

If pulmonary venous pressure rises (eg, because of total anomalous pulmonary venous connection with obstruction, mitral stenosis, or left ventricular failure), then pulmonary arterial pressure rises by about the same amount. Sometimes these patients also have an increased pulmonary vascular resistance secondary to vascular narrowing, and the pulmonary arterial pressure rises more than pulmonary venous pressure.

To analyze pulmonary vascular resistance in more detail, consider the relationship found by Poiseuille for the resistance offered by a glass tube to the steady flow of liquid through it: Resistance equals pressure drop across the tube divided by the flow through it, and the value of this ratio (the resistance) = $(8/\pi)\,(l/r^4)\,(\eta)$. That is, resistance depends on a constant $(8/\pi)$, the geometric factor of tube length (l) divided by the fourth power of the radius (r), and the viscosity (η). Although pulsatile blood flow through a vascular bed is not the same as steady flow of water through a glass tube, the factors determining resistance are similar in both, with one major difference: In the lung, resistance is inversely related to kr^4, where k is the number of resistance vessels.

The main causes of an increased pulmonary vascular resistance are an increase in blood viscosity or a decrease in total cross-sectional area of the resistance vessels; this decreased area may result from fewer vessels or else a normal number of vessels but with some or all of them narrowed. The most common cause of increased blood viscosity is a raised hematocrit, as occurs with cyanotic heart disease. As a rough approximation, a rise in hematocrit from 40 to 70% doubles viscosity and hence doubles pulmonary vascular resistance.

A decreased total number of resistance vessels occurs at times with congenital heart diseases, such as ventricular septal defects, or with congenital lung lesions such as lung hypoplasia, emphysema, or cystic changes. If there is a single pulmonary artery, so that all right ventricular output goes to one lung, then in effect the number of vessels available for receiving that output has fallen by about half. The number of vessels can also be reduced postnatally if they are occluded by tumor or blood emboli. The antiphospholipid syndrome and other rheumatologic diseases may be associated with embolic and thrombotic pulmonary arterial lesions in adolescents and young adults.

Most often the number of vessels is normal, but their luminal diameters are decreased, either by acute vasoconstriction or by organic changes of the arterial wall that may be permanent. Vasoconstriction can be caused by many biologically active agents (eg, serotonin, norepinephrine, endothelin-1), but by far the most important cause is alveolar hypoxia, especially potentiated by metabolic acidemia. Some of the major causes of hypoxia in children are upper airway obstruction; sleep apnea; central nervous system depression from many causes, including prematurity; thoracic cage impairment by obesity (Pickwickian syndrome); neuromuscular diseases; kyphoscoliosis; congenitally small thoracic cage (achondroplasia, Jeune syndrome); large diaphragmatic hernia; extensive parenchymal or small airway disease (meconium aspiration, severe bronchiolitis, cystic fibrosis, infections); and high altitude. Most of these factors cause multiple changes of acid-base balance and blood gases, but the likelihood of pulmonary arterial hypertension and even right-sided congestive heart failure must be considered too. Hypoxic pulmonary vasoconstriction can be reversed by raising alveolar oxygen tension (if possible) or by giving a pulmonary vasodilator. It is important to note that pulmonary arterial hypertension causes muscular hypertrophy of the pulmonary arterial wall, thereby making it thicker and the lumen narrower. Relief of hypoxic vasoconstriction may not return pulmonary vascular resistance to normal at once because of the residual organic change. However, if pulmonary arterial pressure remains low, the hypertrophied smooth muscle of the media returns to normal over several weeks.

Organic changes in the walls, other than muscular hypertrophy, have many causes. The most common of these are secondary to congenital heart disease with high pulmonary blood flows secondary to large left-to-right shunts. The initial high pulmonary vascular resistance in infants with large left-to-right shunts results only from an increased amount of medial smooth muscle that extends more distally than expected for age. Subsequently, however, true pulmonary vascular disease may occur: proliferation of the intimal cells, with intimal thickening and hyalinization, narrowing of the lumen, fibrosis, and eventually thrombosis. The mechanisms producing these intimal changes are probably related to high shear stresses that damage endothelial cells. Pulmonary vascular endothelial cells regulate pulmonary vascular tone and vascular smooth muscle remodeling by producing several vasoactive substances such as nitric oxide (NO), prostacyclin (PGI_2), and endothelin-1 (ET-1). The endothelial damage reduces local formation of NO and PGI_2, both pulmonary vasodilators, inhibitors of smooth muscle mitogenesis, and inhibitors of platelet aggregation. In addition, there is increased production of ET-1, a potent pulmonary vasoconstrictor and promoter of smooth muscle mitogenesis. Therefore, this disturbance in endothelial cell function causes active vasoconstriction and promotes both vascular smooth muscle growth and platelet aggregation. Once platelets aggregate on damaged endothelium, they degranulate and release substances that not only encourage more platelet aggregation but also stimulate mitosis and migration of subintimal cells via a platelet-derived growth factor (PGDF). Penetration of these large molecules into the media is encouraged by disintegration of the internal elastic lamina, mediated by production of a local elastase.

Although early organic changes are reversible by repair of the cardiac defect, the intimal proliferative changes of hyalinization and fibrosis are not reversible. As more and more small pulmonary arteries become involved, there is a progressive increase in pulmonary vascular resistance, so that left-to-right shunting decreases, as does evidence of left ventricular failure. Eventually no left-to-right shunt remains, and later right-to-left shunting may occur. Children with pulmonary vascular disease also have decreased numbers of acinar small pulmonary arteries, the decrease being proportional to the severity of the increased resistance. In severe pulmonary vascular obstructive disease, arteriovenous malformations may also develop, and hemoptysis may occur.

The risk and age of developing advanced pulmonary vascular disease depends on the physiology of the underlying cardiac defect. For example, atrial septal defects produce increased pulmonary blood flow with normal pulmonary arterial pressures. These patients have the normal muscular regression, and their small pulmonary arteries are thin-walled and easily distensible. Therefore, advanced intimal vascular changes occur in only about 10 to 20% of patients and are delayed generally until after the second decade. In contrast, defects that produce increased pulmonary blood flow and increased pulmonary arterial pressures (ie, large ventricular septal defects) have a higher risk of developing advanced pulmonary vascular disease within the first decade of life. Blood viscosity also plays a significant role in producing this damage because shear stresses increase as viscosity rises; therefore, infants who have not only left-to-right shunts with increased pulmonary blood flow and pressure but also chronic hypoxemia with a high hematocrit are at even greater risk of developing pulmonary vascular disease (ie, truncus arteriosus and transposition of the great vessels). With current noninvasive techniques and more widespread awareness of the problem, the incidence of irreversible pulmonary vascular disease secondary to congenital heart disease has decreased significantly. Children with trisomy 21 seem to be at increased risk of developing pulmonary vascular disease.

Organic changes in the walls can occur in many other systemic and pulmonary diseases such as collagen diseases and schistosomiasis; the granulomatous lesions caused by schistosomal ova are common causes of severe childhood pulmonary arterial hypertension in endemic regions such as Puerto Rico, Egypt, and southern Africa.

These considerations usually allow the cause of the pulmonary arterial hypertension to be diagnosed, but occasionally no known cause can be found; the disease is termed primary or idiopathic pulmonary arterial hypertension. One form of this is a progressive disease, often familial, that eventually causes right heart failure and death; the disease may begin in early childhood or as late as early adult life.

CLINICAL MANIFESTATIONS

In children with secondary increases in pulmonary vascular resistance, the underlying pathologic condition may be evident during the cardiac examination. The pulmonary hypertension produced by the increased pulmonary vascular resistance produces a narrowly split second heart sound with the pulmonic component accentuated. In severe pulmonary hypertension, the pulmonic component of the second sound is markedly accentuated; a systolic ejection click is common, and an early diastolic decrescendo murmur of pulmonary regurgitation may be heard. In addition, right ventricular failure (cor pulmonale) may occur with dilatation of the right ventricular cavity and subsequent tricuspid regurgitation, especially in newborn infants. Tricuspid regurgitation may cause a systolic murmur best heard at the lower left sternal border; if the regurgitation is severe, a middiastolic flow rumble may be heard, although this is unusual. Right ventricular enlargement may be evident on the chest roentgenogram or electrocardiogram, depending on the duration of the increased pulmonary vascular resistance.

Children with primary pulmonary vascular disease present with a very loud pulmonic component of the second sound that is often palpable at the upper left sternal border. A diastolic regurgitant pulmonic insufficiency murmur is often heard, and in severe pulmonary hypertension, right heart failure may occur. Syncope and chest pain are common. On the chest roentgenogram the pulmonary artery is markedly dilated, and right atrial and ventricular enlargement are observed. The electrocardiogram may also show right ventricular and right atrial hypertrophy.

TREATMENT

In those lesions that produce secondary increases in pulmonary vascular resistance, the underlying disease state should be treated whenever possible. For example, infants and children with enlarged tonsils and upper airway obstruction may develop subsequent right heart failure that is generally cured by a tonsillectomy and adenoidectomy. Likewise, removal of a retropharyngeal or retrolaryngeal mass relieves the hypoxia caused by these lesions. During sleep, the rate and depth of respiration normally decrease, so that an elevation in pulmonary vascular resistance associated with hypoxia increases further during sleeping hours; thus, the delivery of positive airway pressure via mask can be helpful at night. Underlying pulmonary abnormalities cannot always be treated, and in diseases such as cystic fibrosis, transplantation may be ultimately needed. In older children with primary pulmonary hypertension, chronic intravenous PGI_2 infusions may provide long-term reductions in pulmonary vascular resistance and beneficial effects on symptoms. However, mortality in this disease remains high, and prostaglandin therapy is often used as a bridge to transplantation. Reactive pulmonary hypertension, particularly associated with correction of congenital heart defects following cardiopulmonary bypass, may respond to vasodilators such as inhaled nitric oxide or PGI_2 in addition to O_2.

PERSISTENT PULMONARY HYPERTENSION IN THE NEWBORN

This syndrome, characterized by a high pulmonary vascular resistance and diminished pulmonary blood flow, is discussed in Sec. 22.17.11.

References

Alzamora-Castro V, Battilana G, Abugattas R, et al: Patent ductus arteriosus and high altitude. Am J Cardiol 5:761, 1960

Asherson RA, Oakley CM: Pulmonary hypertension and systemic lupus erythematosus. J Rheumatol 13:1, 1986 (erratum J Rheumatol 13:840, 1986)

Atz AM, Wessel DL: Inhaled nitric oxide in the neonate with cardiac disease. Semin Perinatol 21:441, 1997

Barst RJ: Recent advances in the treatment of pulmonary artery hypertension. Pediatr Clin North Am 46:331, 1999

Campbell M: Natural history of persistent ductus arteriosus. Br Heart J 30:4, 1968

Campbell M: Natural history of atrial septal defect. Br Heart J 32:820, 1970

Fineman JR, Soifer SJ: Pulmonary vascular regulation in newborns, infants and children after surgery for congenital heart disease. Prog Pediatr Cardiol 4:125, 1995

Frontera-Izquierdo P, Cabezuelo-Huerta G: Natural and modified history of isolated ventricular septal defect: a 17-year study. Pediatr Cardiol 13:193, 1992

Giaid A, Yanagisawa M, Langleben D, et al: Expression of endothelin-1 in the lungs of patients with pulmonary hypertension. N Engl J Med 328:1732, 1993

Giaid A, Saleh D: Reduced expression of endothelial nitric oxide synthase in the lungs of patients with pulmonary hypertension. N Engl J Med 333:214, 1995

Haworth SG: Pulmonary hypertension. In: Moller J, Hoffman JIE, eds: Pediatric Cardiovascular Medicine. New York, Churchill Livingstone, 2000:709

Heymann MA, Rudolph AM: Effects of congenital heart disease on the fetal and neonatal circulations. Prog Cardiovasc Dis 15:115, 1972

Hoffman JIE, Heymann MA: Normal pulmonary circulation. In: Scarpelli EM, ed: Pulmonary Physiology: Fetus, Newborn, Child, Adolescent. Philadelphia, Lea & Febiger, 1990:233

Hoffman JIE, Rudolph AM, Heymann MA: Pulmonary vascular disease with congenital heart lesions: pathologic features and causes. Circulation 64:873, 1981

Hughes GRV: The antiphospholipid syndrome: ten years on. Lancet 342:341, 1993

McLaughlin VV, Genthner DE, Panella MM, Rich SR: Reduction in pulmonary vascular resistance with long-term epoprostenol (prostacyclin) therapy in primary pulmonary hypertension. N Engl J Med 338:273, 1998.

Pool PE, Vogel JHK, Blount SG Jr: Congenital unilateral absence of a pulmonary artery. Am J Cardiol 9:706, 1962

Rabinovitch M: Elastase and cell matrix interactions in the pathobiology of vascular disease. Acta Paediatr Jpn 37:657, 1995

Rabinovitch M: It all begins with EVE (endogenous vascular elastase). Isr J Med Sci 32:803, 1996

Rabinovitch M, Bothwell T, Hayakawa BN, et al: Pulmonary artery endothelial abnormalities in patients with congenital heart defects and pulmonary hypertension. Lab Invest 6:632, 1986

Reid LM: Structure and function in pulmonary hypertension. New perceptions. Chest 89:279, 1986

Rich S, Kaufmann E, Levy PS: The effect of high doses of calcium-channel blockers on survival in primary pulmonary hypertension. N Engl J Med 327:76, 1992

Roos A: Poiseuille's law and its limitations in vascular systems. Med Thorac 19:224, 1962

Rubin LJ: Primary pulmonary hypertension. N Engl J Med 336:111, 1997

Rudolph AM: The changes in the circulation after birth: their importance in congenital heart disease. Circulation 41:343, 1970

Rudolph AM, Yuan S: Response of the pulmonary vasculature to hypoxia and H+ ion concentration changes. J Clin Invest 45:399, 1966

Sime F, Banchero N, Peñaloza D, et al: Pulmonary hypertension in children born and living at high altitudes. Am J Cardiol 11:150, 1963

22.3.10   Arrhythmias

George F. Van Hare and Paul Stanger

GENERAL PRINCIPLES

ANATOMY AND PHYSIOLOGY The heart has specialized cells collected into nodes and tracts (Fig. 22-10). The sinoatrial (SA) node, near the junction of the superior vena cava and right atrium, has a rich vagal and sympathetic nerve supply and normally controls heart rate. Conduction of impulses from the SA node to the atrioventricular (AV) node occurs without a specialized conducting system. The slow cell-to-cell conduction through atrial myocardium explains the relatively long duration of the P wave.

The AV node is in the interatrial septum just anterior and superior to the mouth of the coronary sinus; it is also innervated by vagal and sympathetic fibers and consists of a mesh of very thin fibers that conduct impulses very slowly. As a result, the AV node delays conduction, giving time for ventricular filling; in atrial fibrillation the AV node limits the number of impulses reaching the ventricles. From the AV node the bundle of His passes through the central fibrous body into the ventricular septum just behind and below its membranous portion. The bundle of His has large, rapidly conducting fibers and has vagal nerves only proximally; more distally, there is only sympathetic innervation of conduction tissues. Near the summit of the muscular ventricular septum the bundle of His gives off the compact right bundle branch, which has wide fibers, and then the left branch bundle, which is a diffuse fan of thinner fibers. The bundle is insulated from surrounding myocardium and normally does not activate the ventricular myocardium until it branches and ramifies into the Purkinje fibers. These peripheral conducting fibers ramify just beneath the endocardium so that the ventricular walls are depolarized from subendocardium to subepicardium. Rapid conduction down the His-Purkinje system allows the entire ventricular myocardium to contract nearly simultaneously, explaining the narrow QRS complex in normals.

Some people have accessory pathways connecting atrial and ventricular myocardium. One type, the *bundle of Kent*, is a muscular bridge spanning the AV groove. With some Kent bundles, conduction is possible in both anterograde and retrograde directions; in others, it is exclusively retrograde. Anterograde conduction causes early depolarization of the ventricles (*preexcitation*); retrograde conduction causes rapid reentry between the atria and the ventricles, causing sustained tachyarrhythmias. A second type of accessory pathway, the *Mahaim fiber*, is thought to be made up of specialized conducting fibers and to connect directly to the specialized conducting system. The most common type, called the atriofascicular connection, connects atrial myocardium with elements of the right bundle branch. In general, with Mahaim pathways only anterograde conduction is possible, and tachycardia occurs as a result of anterograde conduction from the atrium to the distal conducting system and then retrograde conduction to the bundle of His, AV node, and back to the atrium.

Finally, some people have *dual AV node pathways*. These pathways are functionally and anatomically distinct, with the atrial approaches to the slow pathway being posterior and inferior to the compact AV node and the approaches to the fast pathway being anterior and superior to the node. The effective refractory period is usually shorter in the slow than the fast pathway. Dual pathways may lead to *atrioventricular node reentry tachycardia*, when, after a premature atrial contraction blocks in the fast pathway and con-

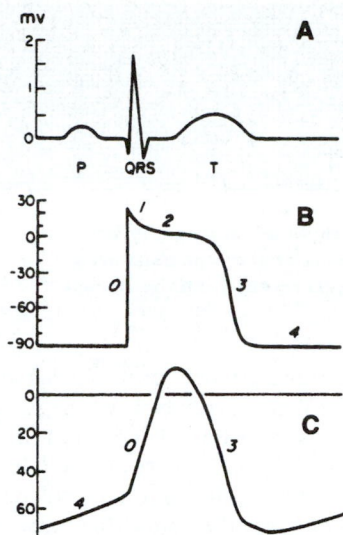

FIGURE 22-67 **A: Typical electrocardiogram lead II. B: Transmembrane potential of cardiac muscle cell. C: Transmembrane potential of pacemaker cell.**

ducts down the slow, the impulse may reenter the fast pathway retrograde, setting up sustained reentrant tachycardia.

CELLULAR ELECTROPHYSIOLOGY If a microelectrode is placed in a cardiac muscle cell, the potential between it and an electrode outside the cell is the transmembrane potential. In diastole this potential (the resting potential) is −80 to −90 mV. When the cell is stimulated, an action potential results (Fig. 22-67B). Rapid depolarization (phase 0) results from rapid sodium influx; the rapid return to near zero potential (phase 1) results from chloride influx. The less negative the transmembrane potential at the onset of depolarization, the slower the rate of depolarization (V_{max}) in phase 0; in turn, reduced V_{max} slows the velocity of propagation of the impulse through the fibers. Antiarrhythmic agents with class I activity (eg, procainamide, flecainide) block sodium influx, reduce V_{max}, and therefore slow conduction. Phase 1 is followed by a plateau (phase 2) during which slow inward calcium and sodium currents are nearly balanced by potassium leaking out of the cell. Potassium conductance then increases, and potassium efflux causes the potential to become more negative rapidly (phase 3) until the resting membrane potential is reached. During phase 4, sodium is actively pumped out of the cell in exchange for potassium.

Once the action potential has begun, the cell is completely refractory to stimulation until it attains a transmembrane potential of about −55 mV in phase 3, and from this value until it reaches a resting potential of −85 mV in phase 4 the cell gradually regains excitability. Between absolute refractoriness and complete responsiveness is the relative refractory period; in keeping with the relationship between V_{max} and transmembrane potential, a stimulus early in the refractory period produces a slow and poorly conducted action potential. Prolongation of action potential duration and absolute and relative refractory periods occurs with slowing of the rate of depolarization, a long R-R interval thus giving a longer refractory period of the next beat. Refractory periods are also prolonged by disease (myocarditis, ischemia) and by some antiarrhythmic drugs (ibutalide, sotalol).

Certain cells have a different pattern (Fig. 22-67C). The resting potential starts at about −80 mV but then automatically becomes more positive. When the potential reaches a threshold of about −50 mV, the action potential begins spontaneously; thus, these cells are called *automatic cells* and are said to have *automaticity*. Normally, most cardiac muscle cells do not have automaticity; those that do may be found anywhere in the heart but are mainly in the SA node, the lower part of the AV node, muscle in the mitral and tricuspid valves, and the conduction system. The repetition rate at which groups of automatic cells depolarize depends mainly on the slope of spontaneous depolarization; the more rapid it is, the sooner the threshold is reached. Diastolic depolarization rate is accelerated by catecholamines, vagal blockade, a raised temperature, lowered extracellular potassium or calcium, or a fall in tissue pH or oxygen tension; these changes thus tend to increase heart rate.

Diastolic depolarization rate and thus automaticity are reduced by vagal stimulation, β-adrenergic blockade, increased extracellular potassium, and drugs such as quinidine, procainamide, lidocaine, and phenytoin. The effect of these drugs in reducing automaticity makes them useful in treating many arrhythmias. It is important to note that different automatic cells have different sensitivities for changes induced by these agents. Thus, phenytoin increases atrial diastolic depolarization but decreases ventricular diastolic depolarization, and lidocaine has a marked effect on ventricular automaticity but not on atrial automaticity. Normally the discharge rate is highest for automatic cells in the SA node, which is thus the usual pacemaker for the heart. Collections of automatic cells (latent pacemakers) lower in the conducting system have slower diastolic depolarization, the slowest being those in the ventricles. Normally these lower (or ectopic) pacemakers are discharged by impulses from the SA node before they can discharge spontaneously, and thus, they are usually suppressed by impulses from above. The typical discharge rate of each pacemaker varies with age (Table 22-16).

Most normal cardiac muscle and automatic cells show rapid depolarization and also conduct rapidly; thus they are known as *fast-responding cells*. However, some cells show a slow response. Their transmembrane resting potential is only about −60 mV, depolarization is slow, as is conduction, and in phase 4 there is an after-depolarization that normally does not reach the threshold for initiating another action potential. Slow-responding cells are found normally in the SA and AV nodes and the AV valves. Fast-responding cells can be converted into slow-responding cells by ischemia, digitalis toxicity, excess potassium or catecholamines, or chronic

TABLE 22-16

NORMAL PACEMAKER RATES AT VARIOUS AGES

	AGE				
PACEMAKER	**0–1 MO**	**1 YR**	**5 YR**	**10 YR**	**ADULT**
SA node	100–180	110–180	60–120	55–110	50–100
AV node	80–90				50–70
Ventricles	50–70				35–50

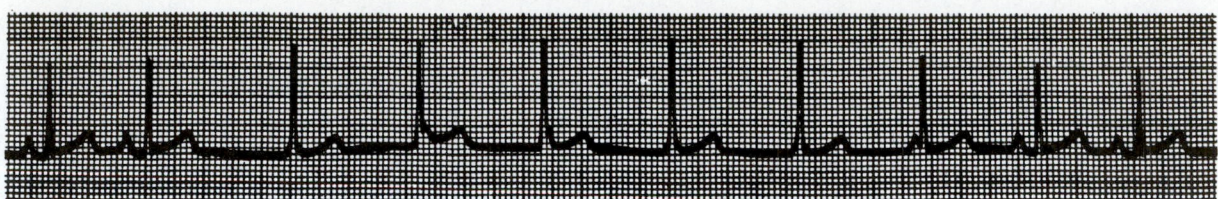

FIGURE 22-68 Junctional escape beats in a healthy boy. The basic rhythm is sinus arrhythmia; the first two and last two impulses are conducted to the ventricles. Junctional escape beats occur when the sinus rate slows. The notched QRS complex in the escape beats results from the normal P wave coinciding with the junctional escape beat.

dilatation. In all these cells the rapid sodium influx of phase 1 is absent, and depolarization is achieved mainly by the slow inward calcium current and can be blocked by calcium channel blockers (verapamil, diltiazem).

BASIC FEATURES OF ARRHYTHMIAS

There are three major types of disorders: abnormal automaticity (impulse formation), abnormal conduction, and fibrillation.

DISORDERS OF AUTOMATICITY If the SA node discharges abnormally slowly or the impulse from it is not conducted, an ectopic lower pacemaker, either atrial or more commonly junctional (a term used in lieu of "AV nodal" because it is uncertain if the AV node has pacemaker potential), takes over. If the block is in the AV node or bundle of His, a ventricular pacemaker may take over. In this way, lower pacemakers escape from suppression by higher pacemakers. Escape may occur for a single beat, for a few beats, or may result in a permanent lower pacemaker rhythm if the higher pacemaker does not regain control. Escape beats or rhythms indicate abnormality of the higher pacemaker or abnormal conduction from it, and the escape is a normal response. An escape beat is recognized by its late appearance (R-R interval longer than normal) and evidence of an ectopic focus (abnormal P wave axis and morphology for an atrial ectopic focus; no P wave, very short P-R, or retrograde P wave for junctional focus). An escape rhythm is characterized by an ectopic rhythm that is slower than a normal sinus rhythm (Fig. 22-68).

The other disorder of automaticity is premature discharge of a lower pacemaker. One or two of these beats are termed *premature beats* or *extrasystoles,* but three or more in a row constitute *ectopic tachycardia.* If the ectopic focus is in the atrium or is junctional, the descending impulse reaches the ventricles through the His-Purkinje system, and a normal QRS complex usually occurs (but see Aberrant Conduction, below). If the ectopic focus is ventricular, the impulse spreads slowly through muscle cells and produces a wide, bizarre QRS-T complex with the polarities of the QRS complex and the T wave opposite to each other. If the premature beat begins in the right ventricle, then this ventricle is depolarized before the left ventricle, and the QRS pattern resembles a left bundle branch block. Conversely, a left ventricular ectopic beat resembles a right bundle branch block. The basic difference between bundle branch block and ectopic patterns is that in the former only the terminal part of depolarization is slow, whereas in the latter the whole QRS complex is slowed and distorted. It may be difficult to make this differentiation in practice. However, in children, most aberrantly conducted beats with bundle branch block follow a premature atrial beat. Therefore, a wide QRS complex without a premature P wave is likely to be ventricular in origin.

With a ventricular premature beat, the retrograde impulse is often blocked at the AV node, and the basic rhythm of the SA node is usually unaltered, so that the first sinus beat after a ventricular extrasystole follows a full compensatory pause. That is, the interval between the sinus beat preceding the extrasystole and the sinus beat following it is at least twice the normal R-R interval (Fig. 22-69). However, with atrial or junctional premature beats, the SA node is usually discharged; thus, the next sinus beat usually occurs after an incomplete compensatory pause (less than twice the normal R-R interval).

Ectopic tachycardias have QRS complexes like those of the corresponding ectopic beats: usually normal if the focus is supraventricular, almost always widened if it is ventricular, but widened if there is a supraventricular focus with aberrant conduction. These are differentiated below.

The effect of premature atrial beats on P-wave morphology depends on the site of the atrial focus. If it is near the SA node, an almost normal P wave occurs (Fig. 22-70); if it is near the AV node, then the atrial axis is directed superiorly, leading to inverted P waves in leads II, III, and aVF (Fig. 22-69B). Therefore, low atrial and high His-bundle premature beats give similar P waves, although, because of the time taken for retrograde conduction through the AV node to the atria, an infranodal pacemaker is more likely to give P waves buried in the QRS complex or following it. If the ectopic focus is ventricular, there can be a retrograde P wave after the QRS

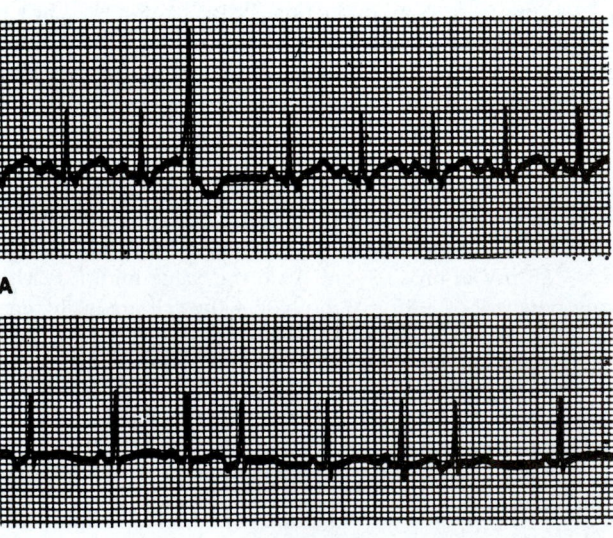

A

B

FIGURE 22-69 Compensatory pauses following ectopic beats. **A:** Premature ventricular ectopic beat followed by a full compensatory pause. **B:** Premature atrial contractions with incomplete and full compensatory pauses. Both strips are lead II.

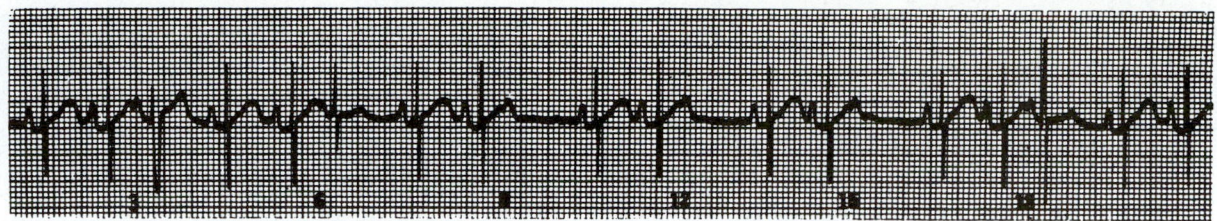

FIGURE 22-70   Premature atrial contractions with varying coupling intervals and the different types of ventricular responses. Every third P wave is a premature atrial ectopic beat; however, the interval between the atrial ectopic beat and the preceding QRS complex varies. The sixth and 18th beats are atrial ectopic beats that occur relatively late and reach the ventricles when they have almost completely repolarized; the resulting QRS complex is similar to the normal ventricular complexes. The ninth, 12th, and 15th atrial beats occur early and are not conducted because the impulses reach the AV node or ventricles while they are still refractory (interference). The third beat is a premature atrial contraction that is intermediate in timing and shows aberrant conduction from refractoriness of one of the bundle branches.

complex, but often the retrograde impulse is blocked in the AV node, and the atrium is activated normally from the SA node at a different rate.

Premature beats may be caused by increased automaticity of an ectopic focus; they have many causes, including endogenous catecholamines, drugs, and disease. Frequently the mechanism of ectopic tachycardias relates to the slow response that can occur in damaged fibers. Unlike fast-response fibers, which can be inhibited by rapid impulses from higher pacemakers, the slow-response fibers react to rapid stimuli with increasing amplitude of afterdepolarizations that may reach threshold and initiate the repetitive action potentials characteristic of an ectopic tachycardia.

Tachycardias may also result from reentry, a circular form of depolarization that occurs when there are two parallel pathways with unidirectional block and often a protected zone of slow conduction. For example, consider a strip of damaged ventricular muscle that does not conduct anterograde but does conduct slowly retrograde. The normal sinus impulse descends and depolarizes the normal but not the abnormal muscle. The wave of depolarization eventually passes slowly retrograde up the abnormal strip that has not been depolarized; by the time the impulse emerges from the abnormal muscle, the rest of the muscle is responsive and is depolarized prematurely—a ventricular premature beat. Usually the wave of depolarization does not continue to circulate because the abnormal muscle, having been depolarized, is then refractory to impulses from any direction. The sequence may be repeated to produce ventricular bigeminy. Because normally there is slow conduction through the AV node, reentry through it is believed to explain many types of extrasystoles. If the recirculating wave of depolarization is itself slowed in some other portion of muscle, then the wave may return to the original abnormal muscle strip when it has regained excitability, and a rapid repetitive depolarization (reentry tachycardia) will occur. Reentry is the cause of tachycardia in Wolff-Parkinson-White syndrome, in which a premature impulse blocks in the accessory pathway but descends through the slowly conducting AV node, returns to the atrium through the rapidly conducting bundle of Kent, and continues around the circuit.

DISORDERS OF CONDUCTION   Conduction may be impaired either by an abnormal increase in the refractory period (pathologic or primary) or by interference from another impulse that alters the refractory period (physiological or secondary). Physiological factors that affect conduction include *concealed conduction* and *physiological interference*. When conduction through tissue cannot be de-

tected on the electrocardiogram but is inferred by its effect on conduction of a subsequent impulse, then it is termed concealed conduction. This may well be shown, for example, if there is an interpolated (very early) ventricular premature beat (Fig. 22-71). The retrograde impulse from the ventricular focus enters the AV node and prolongs the AV nodal refractory period but does not capture the atrium, which is still refractory from the last beat. The next impulse from the SA node is conducted more slowly than normal through the AV node because it is still partially refractory. The resulting long P-R interval is the evidence for concealed retrograde conduction.

Interference is shown most simply if there is a very early isolated atrial premature beat. In Fig. 22-70, the ninth P wave is seen on the T wave of the preceding QRS complex, but because the AV node or ventricle is still refractory, the impulse is not conducted. This is physiological, not pathologic, failure of conduction. A more prolonged episode of physiological interference may occur if the sinus pacemaker slows or a junctional pacemaker speeds up so that the atria and ventricles beat at roughly similar rates but are controlled by different pacemakers (see Figs. 22-67 and 22-72). This is one form of *atrioventricular dissociation* (the other main form being complete atrioventricular block). Despite a normal AV conduction system, the descending impulse from the SA node does not pass the AV node, which has been made refractory by the retrograde impulse from the ventricle or bundle of His. In turn, this retrograde impulse does not capture the atrium, which has been made refractory by the sinus beat. Failure of the SA node to capture the ventricle is thus not because of an abnormality of conduction but of physiological effects on refractory periods. An electrocardiogram with this type of interference shows unrelated P waves and

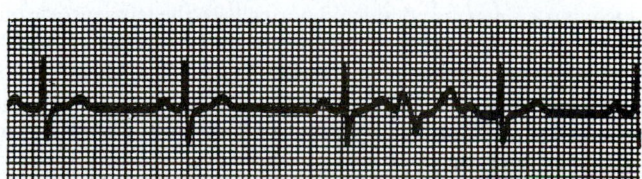

FIGURE 22-71   Interpolated ventricular ectopic beats and concealed conduction. The basic rhythm is sinus and is not altered by the ventricular ectopic beats. Impulses from the ventricular ectopic beats pass retrograde to the AV node. The next sinus beat reaches the AV node before it has fully recovered, and the P-R interval is therefore prolonged after each ectopic beat.

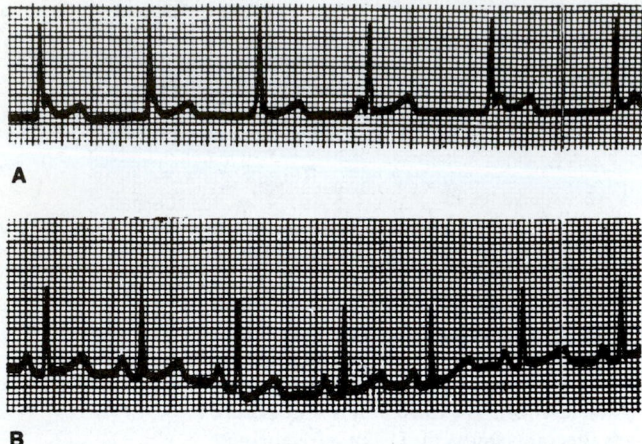

A

B

FIGURE 22-72 **AV dissociation. A: Independent atrial and ventricular contractions, with neither depolarizing the other. The atrial rate is slower than the ventricular; consequently, the dissociation may be the result of an accelerated junctional pacemaker whose rate exceeds that of the sinus pacemaker. B: Mild exercise speeds up the sinus pacemaker, resulting in conduction to the ventricles and suppression of the junctional pacemaker.**

QRS complexes with the ventricular rate faster than the atrial rate. Occasionally ventricular and atrial rates are the same, but the P-R interval is too short to diagnose a sinus rhythm; this is termed *isorhythmic dissociation*. Sometimes the interference occurs in the atrium or the ventricle rather than in the AV node, and then it produces atrial or ventricular *fusion beats*, the latter being more important. Typically a ventricular premature beat has a wide QRS complex. However, if the ventricular premature beat begins while the normal sinus impulse is descending the His-Purkinje system, then some of the ventricle will be depolarized normally and the rest slowly; the resulting QRS complex (the fusion beat) will usually be intermediate in form between the normal complex and that associated with the ventricular ectopic beat (Fig. 22-73; see also Fig. 22-85). A fusion beat strongly implies that other wider beats are ventricular in origin.

ABERRANT CONDUCTION Whenever a supraventricular impulse reaches the AV node or bundle of His in the relative refractory period, the impulse may be transmitted aberrantly because of uneven loss of refractoriness in the AV node or bundle branches. The impulse may arrive at the AV node or bundle at this time because of a premature supraventricular beat, supraventricular tachycardia, or a prolonged Q-T interval of the preceding beat. In most people, the right bundle branch normally has a longer refractory period than the left bundle. Therefore, premature supraventricular beats or tachycardias may be conducted normally to the left ventricle but slowly to the right ventricle, giving the pattern of right bundle branch block and a wide QRS complex (Fig. 22-70). However, left bundle aberration occurs occasionally. Bundle branch aberration after single premature supraventricular beats is quite common, particularly if the beat follows a long pause (Ashman phenomenon). However, sustained bundle branch aberration with supraventricular tachycardia is less common in children than adults, and *most sustained wide QRS tachycardias in children are caused by ventricular tachycardia.*

An important form of aberration occurs when the ventricle during tachycardia is activated entirely or in part from an accessory AV connection. Activation from a Kent bundle does not use the His-

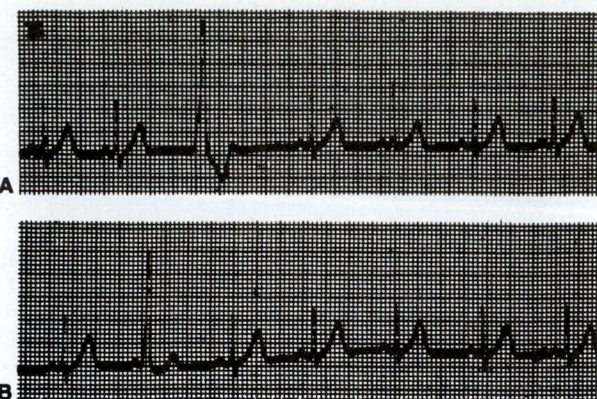

A

B

FIGURE 22-73 **Ventricular fusion beat. A: Premature ventricular ectopic beat. B: Fusion beat resulting from a premature ventricular ectopic beat occurring just after the P wave, so that part of the myocardium is depolarized slowly by the ectopic beat and the remainder by the sinus impulse reaching the ventricles via the His-Purkinje system.**

Purkinje system, so that conduction through the ventricle is slow, as with a ventricular ectopic focus. This phenomenon is seen in Wolff-Parkinson-White syndrome with atrial tachycardia or fibrillation or in antidromic reentry with conduction anterograde in the pathway and retrograde in the AV node. It is also seen during reentry involving a Mahaim atriofascicular connection, in which conduction is down the pathway to the right bundle branch with retrograde activation to the atrium via the bundle of His and AV node.

ATRIOVENTRICULAR BLOCK If conduction is delayed through the AV node or the bundle of His, then various degrees of AV block occur. If there is merely a long P-R interval but all beats are conducted, it is a *first-degree AV block* (Fig. 22-74). If no atrial beats are conducted, so that the ventricles are driven by a junctional or ventricular focus, then there are normal P waves at one rate and QRS complexes at a slower rate, usually with no fixed relationship between P waves and QRS complexes. This is *complete* or *third-degree AV block* (Fig. 22-75).

Whenever atria and ventricles are controlled by independent pacemakers, there is AV dissociation. This may result either from complete AV block or from junctional or ventricular tachycardia or accelerated rhythm without retrograde conduction. The former has faster atrial than ventricular rates; the descending impulse cannot reach the lower pacemaker because a conduction block exists. The latter has faster ventricular than atrial rates, *but coexistent anterograde conduction block is not excluded*. The absence of anterograde conduction block is demonstrated when a critically timed atrial impulse conducts to the ventricles and suddenly shortens the R-R interval. In ventricular tachycardia, this shortened R-R interval is associated with shortening of, or normalization of, the QRS com-

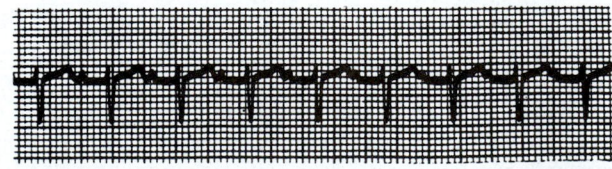

FIGURE 22-74 **First-degree AV block in a newborn infant. The P-R interval is 0.18 seconds, which is prolonged for the patient's age and heart rate.**

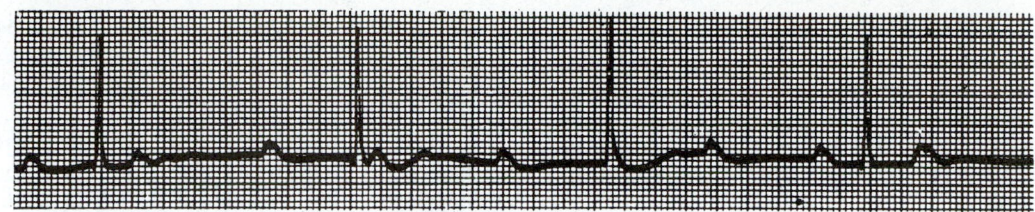

FIGURE 22-75   Third-degree AV block. The P waves and QRS complexes have no consistent temporal relationship. The atrial rate is 90 beats per minute, and the ventricular 38 beats per minute.

plex. In junctional tachycardia, the QRS remains relatively unchanged in capture beats. If there is doubt about AV conduction, one can determine if block is present by increasing atrial rate with exercise or hyperventilation and noting whether or not ventricular capture occurs (Fig. 22-72).

If some sinus beats are conducted to the ventricle but others do not reach it, there is *second-degree AV block*. Type I second-degree AV block is characterized by Wenckebach conduction, which usually occurs in the AV node. The first atrial impulse of a group of beats is conducted normally, but the next atrial impulse reaches the AV node while it is still partly refractory and thus is conducted more slowly, giving a longer P-R interval. The next atrial impulse arrives even earlier in the AV nodal refractory period, with an even longer P-R interval as a result. Eventually the atrial impulse reaches the AV node in its absolute refractory period and is blocked, so that no QRS complex follows (Fig. 22-76). The effect of this on the QRS complexes is to make them occur with progressively shorter R-R intervals until an unusually long R-R interval indicates that one ventricular complex has dropped out. Two other features are typical of this arrhythmia. The largest increment in P-R intervals is in the second beat after the dropped beat; the first has the shortest P-R interval because the long pause has allowed the AV node to recover. Furthermore, the duration of the longest R-R interval is always less than twice the short R-R intervals because these cycles contain the longest P-R intervals. This feature of progressive shortening of the R-R intervals until a long R-R interval that is less than two of the shorter R-R intervals occurs is the hallmark that allows Wenckebach phenomenon to be diagnosed even when P waves are not easily seen. Finally, the phenomenon of *group beating* provides a clue to Wenckebach conduction. Atrioventricular block occurs with a repetitive pattern, often 3:2 or 4:3, so that there are repetitive groups of 2 or 3 QRS complexes followed by pauses.

Type II (Mobitz) second-degree AV block occurs when a QRS complex drops out without prior lengthening of the P-R intervals and usually occurs distal to the AV node. It is less common but more serious than type I second-degree AV block and is more likely to lead to complete AV block.

Second-degree AV block does not imply a fixed relationship between atrial and ventricular complexes. There may be 2:1 second-degree AV block, in which only alternate atrial impulses are conducted to the ventricle; 3:1 second-degree AV block indicates that every third atrial impulse is conducted to the ventricles. There may be higher grades of second-degree block, such as 4:1, 5:1, or block may vary, with no consistent relationship between the numbers of conducted and blocked atrial impulses. This lack of group beating helps to differentiate type II from type I block. In addition, there is no shortening of P-R interval after a blocked beat in type II second-degree AV block.

MYOCARDIAL FIBRILLATION   Sometimes a stimulus to a region that has repolarized is conducted at different rates in some directions and blocked in others. As a result, an irregular wavefront of depolarization takes a tortuous path through the muscle and leaves behind it an irregular path of refractory cells. Portions of the wavefront return to regions that were formerly refractory but are now excitable. The wave of depolarization becomes more irregular, and eventually there is chaotic fragmented contraction that is termed *fibrillation*.

To produce fibrillation two conditions are needed. First, there must be asymmetric slowing of conduction or asymmetric shortening of refractoriness, which can result from hypoxemia, ischemia, electrolyte abnormalities, or many drugs. Second, there must be a premature stimulus such as an external electric shock, a premature beat, or tachycardia that occurs very early before all the muscle has repolarized. The fact that an extrasystole can occur so early is itself evidence of decreased refractoriness of some muscle.

If the chaotic rhythm occurs in the atria, there is *atrial fibrillation*, which is easily provoked by rapid atrial pacing. However, in children, atrial fibrillation is usually not sustained and reverts to sinus rhythm unless the atria are enlarged. If the chaotic rhythm occurs in the ventricles, there is *ventricular fibrillation:* the vulnerable period in which a shock (or rarely, an ectopic beat) can cause fibrillation is at the apex of the T wave.

DIAGNOSIS

Arrhythmias are best diagnosed with knowledge of the history and physical findings and with all previous electrocardiograms from that

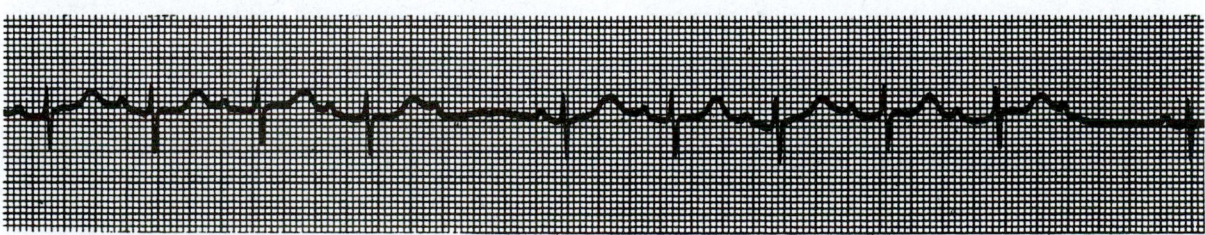

FIGURE 22-76   Second-degree AV block. The tracing shows two Wenckebach cycles with progressive lengthening of the P-R interval until the atrial beat is not conducted to the ventricles.

patient. The electrocardiogram of the arrhythmia under study should be a routine full electrocardiogram plus some very long strips, lasting about 1 minute or more. In sinus rhythm, leads II and V_1 are most likely to show good P waves, but with ectopic atrial foci, other leads may be better. Sometimes special maneuvers are needed to bring out P waves, such as using modified chest, esophageal, or intracardiac leads.

The electrocardiogram should be examined carefully for P waves. These should be inspected for variations in rate, morphology, and mean axis, for P-R intervals and their possible variation, and to find out if the P waves are likely to be the source of the impulse causing the QRS complex. Then the QRS complex should be examined for its rate, rhythm, and morphology.

Maneuvers that increase AV block (eg, vagal stimuli) may slow ventricular rate and allow better definition of atrial and ventricular complexes. They should be performed only while the electrocardiogram is running, for safety as well as for future analysis.

Most arrhythmias can be diagnosed by careful diagnosis of the electrocardiogram during tachycardia and in the baseline state. Often, however, additional methods are helpful. Recordings of paroxysmal tachycardias are often difficult to obtain, particularly at their onset or offset, which are the most important features for analysis. If episodes occur daily, a 24-hour ambulatory electrocardiogram (Holter monitor) may capture the episode. If they are less frequent, transtelephonic event recorders or memory loops that are activated by the patient when symptoms occur may capture an episode. Sometimes tachycardias are precipitated by exercise, and an exercise test may elicit the arrhythmia. Invasive electrophysiological study is the definitive method of diagnosing cardiac arrhythmias. As many as four electrode catheters are inserted by veins into the heart for pacing and recording the intracardiac electrograms. Both SA and AV node function are assessed, and arrhythmias may be induced, diagnosed, and mapped to determine their origin and route of conduction by programmed electrical stimulation.

ARRHYTHMIAS WITH REGULAR RHYTHM AT NORMAL RATE
A regular rhythm at normal rate is most likely to be sinus rhythm, but the electrocardiogram should be inspected carefully to exclude atrial tachycardia with 2:1 AV block, atrial flutter with 4:1 AV block, accelerated junctional or idioventricular rhythms, or atrial fibrillation with an independent idioventricular rhythm caused by a coexistent atrioventricular block.

PAUSES   Occasional pauses are most commonly caused by nonconducted very early atrial extrasystoles; these may not always be readily apparent, as the P waves may be superimposed on the preceding T wave. They can also result from marked sinus arrhythmia, second-degree AV block, or SA exit block as well as concealed conduction of junctional extrasystoles that has made the AV node refractory.

GROUPS OF BEATS   *Bigeminy* means that beats occur in pairs. Most commonly this is because of extrasystole coupled to the previous normal beat, but it can also indicate a 3:2 AV block (every third atrial beat not conducted) or an escape beat paired with the next normal beat. Similarly, *trigeminy* means groups of three beats. These could be two normal beats and one premature beat, one normal and two premature beats, 4:3 AV block, and so on. Wenckebach periods often produce beats that are grouped in pairs, triplets, or larger groups.

IRREGULAR RHYTHMS   Occasional irregularities result from premature beats or escape beats, the latter occurring with sinus pauses,

blocked atrial premature beats, or second-degree AV block. These are usually easy to differentiate. At times it is difficult to distinguish atrial fibrillation from a second-degree AV block with Wenckebach periods occurring in a tachycardia where P waves are not easy to find. The diagnosis is made by the characteristic features of Wenckebach periods: progressive shortening of the R-R interval before a long pause, with the longest R-R interval being less than two of the shortest intervals.

TACHYCARDIAS   A rapid heart rate with normal P waves and P-R intervals, and with variations in rate from moment to moment, is a sinus tachycardia. A rapid fixed rate with complete regularity, normal QRS complexes, and either P waves on the T waves or else no clear P waves is probably a supraventricular tachycardia; vagal stimulation causes either no change or an abrupt reversion to sinus rhythm. A rapid rate, usually fixed and regular, with a wide QRS complex is either a ventricular tachycardia or a supraventricular tachycardia with ventricular aberration or preceding bundle branch block. A ventricular tachycardia can be diagnosed by examining the QRS patterns (see above), by finding fusion beats, or by noting that the QRS complexes are similar to ventricular ectopic beats found in other electrocardiograms. Vagal stimulation usually does not affect this arrhythmia. If a slower atrial rhythm is noted from P waves usually deforming the T waves variously from beat to beat, then ventricular tachycardia is likely. However, retrograde P waves at the same rate as the ventricles can occur with junctional or ventricular tachycardias. A rapid supraventricular tachycardia can also be caused by atrial flutter with a regular block; this is differentiated from a plain supraventricular tachycardia by the typical sawtooth flutter waves, although these waves may be seen in only one or two leads. It could also result from atrial fibrillation, detected by slight variations in the R-R intervals. In both these arrhythmias the rate is slowed and the variability is increased by increasing AV nodal block with vagal stimulation or digitalis.

TREATMENT

PRINCIPLES OF TREATMENT   In addition to correctly identifying the arrhythmia, proper management of arrhythmias requires attention to four questions.

1. *Does the arrhythmia need treatment?* In many children no treatment is needed. Many of the most effective antiarrhythmic agents may cause new, or worsen existing, arrhythmias or even cause sudden death. Arrhythmias that require treatment are those that threaten to cause ventricular fibrillation or asystole (eg, ventricular tachycardia, multiform ventricular ectopic beats) and those in which ventricular rate is too slow or too fast for effective cardiac output. In general, the effects of abnormal ventricular rates depend not only on the rates but also on how much they differ from the patient's usual rate. Thus, a chronically slow ventricular rate of 50 beats per minute is accompanied by ventricular dilatation and hypertrophy and well-maintained cardiac output. On the other hand, a sudden drop from 100 to 50 beats per minute may be poorly tolerated.

2. *Can underlying causes be removed?* In children, particularly neonates, most clinically significant arrhythmias are caused by apnea, hypoxemia, acidemia, electrolyte disturbances, or drugs such as digitalis or catecholamines. If the arrhythmia is treated without attention to the underlying cause, the patient may deteriorate.

3. *Do secondary effects need treatment?* Arrhythmias that reduce cardiac output may cause hypotension and acidemia, with subse-

quent increase in sympathetic tone, which helps to maintain the arrhythmia.

4.   *What specific therapeutic strategy is needed for the arrhythmia?* Consider two patients with 2:1 AV block, one with an atrial rate of 260 beats per minute, the other with an atrial rate of 100 beats per minute. The first patient has an adequate ventricular rate of 130 beats per minute, and therapy should be directed at slowing the atrial rate; the AV block should not be treated because it is useful in preventing too many impulses from reaching the ventricles and causing a harmful rapid ventricular rate. In the second patient, therapy should be directed to increasing the ventricular rate of 50 beats per minute by improving AV conduction or by pacing the ventricles.

PHARMACOLOGIC MANAGEMENT Methods of controlling arrhythmias are chosen with the mechanism of the specific arrhythmia in mind. However, caution is needed when extrapolating pharmacologic effects observed in normal cardiac muscle to diseased muscle. For example, in ischemic heart muscle, lidocaine prolongs conduction and refractoriness, whereas it increases conduction velocity in normal fibers; in fact, its effectiveness against some ventricular arrhythmias may depend on this action (blocking reentry) rather than on its depression of excitability. For this reason, selection of the appropriate antiarrhythmic agent should be based on experience as well as theory.

BRADYCARDIAS A slow ventricular rate may be caused by severe sinus bradycardia or arrest or second- or third-degree AV block. The slowing either causes a cardiac output that is too low or allows breakthrough of potentially dangerous ventricular escape beats or tachycardia. Treatment is aimed at increasing the ventricular rate. *Atropine* (0.01 mg/kg subcutaneously or intravenously) may increase SA nodal discharge rate or accelerate AV conduction, but it does not speed up low ventricular pacemakers because the vagus does not supply conduction tissue below the bundle of His. *Isoproterenol* (0.05 to 0.5 µg/kg/min) may increase pacemaker discharge rates and conduction at any level but should be used with care if there are ventricular arrhythmias as well. Slowed conduction through the AV node, especially if induced by digitalis, may be improved by phenytoin. If drug therapy is ineffective or contraindicated, then temporary or permanent artificial cardiac pacing may be needed.

ECTOPIC BEATS AND ECTOPIC TACHYCARDIAS Arrhythmias with premature beats or tachycardias have abnormalities related to increased automaticity of cardiac cells, to increased afterdepolarizations of slow-response fibers, or to uneven conduction times that result in reentry. Proposed mechanisms of antiarrhythmic action include raising the threshold at which cells depolarize, decreasing sodium conductance so that phase 0 depolarization is slowed and conduction velocity along the fiber is reduced, thereby converting unidirectional block to bidirectional block and stopping reentry; decreasing the slow calcium current and preventing afterdepolarization; prolonging the effective refractory period relative to the action potential duration so that at any heart rate there is less time for a reentrant or ectopic impulse to depolarize the cell; and decreasing phase 4 depolarization so that it takes longer to reach the threshold for depolarization. Many drugs act in more than one way but often have one major action, so that it is possible to avoid using two drugs with the same basic mode of action.

Vagal stimulation (carotid sinus massage, Valsalva maneuver, baroreceptor reflex to hypertension, anticholinesterase drugs) re-

duces automaticity and shortens the action potential duration and the effective refractory period of atrial muscle; it also slows atrial and AV nodal conduction and lengthens the refractory period of the AV node. These actions may abolish paroxysmal supraventricular tachycardia, and they decrease ventricular response in atrial flutter or fibrillation. Because of sparse ventricular innervation, vagal stimulation has little effect on ventricular arrhythmias.

Should vagal stimulation fail, the drug of choice for treating atrial arrhythmias is *digoxin*. This increases ventricular automaticity and so increases the chances of getting ventricular premature beats and tachycardias, which explains in part why digoxin is not the drug of choice for treating ventricular arrhythmias. At therapeutic doses, both excitability and conduction velocity are depressed in the atrium. At all doses, AV nodal conduction is slowed, so that first the P-R interval lengthens; with larger doses second- or third-degree AV nodal block occurs. Digoxin shortens the action potential duration and the refractory period in atria and ventricles, thus shortening the QT interval. To abolish paroxysmal supraventricular tachycardias that rely on the AV node as part of the reentrant circuit, *adenosine* is now the drug of choice. Many experts use *propranolol* or *verapamil* to slow the ventricular response in atrial flutter or fibrillation; verapamil is ineffective in this regard when Wolff-Parkinson-White syndrome is present.

Antiarrhythmic drugs are classified by their major electrophysiological properties; the major groups are described in Table 22-17, as are their main indications and contraindications.

NONPHARMACOLOGIC MANAGEMENT

ACUTE MANAGEMENT Drug therapy is not always successful in abolishing arrhythmias. *Electrical cardioversion* by a depolarizing shock is mandatory in ventricular fibrillation and is the method of first or second choice in treating acute tachycardias (paroxysmal atrial or ventricular tachycardias, atrial flutter, or fibrillation), especially if they cause serious cardiovascular difficulties. Rapid overdrive pacing, using temporary electrodes inserted by a transvenous or esophageal route, may be used to drive the heart fast enough to prevent the emergence of ventricular ectopic beats, to abolish reentrant tachycardias, or to prevent the recurrence of tachycardias.

PERMANENT ANTIBRADYCARDIA PACING Permanent pacemaker implantation is often needed to manage bradyarrhythmias. Implantation may be transvenous, by the subclavian or cephalic vein, with the pulse generator placed infraclavicularly. Implantation may, alternatively, be epicardial, with a subxiphoid generator. The epicardial route is reserved for the smallest children and those in whom transvenous pacing is contraindicated because of the risk of thromboembolism (eg, those with an intracardiac shunt and those with no venous access to the ventricle, such as those with the Fontan procedure).

Pacemakers are classified by a three-letter code (V = ventricle; A = atrium; D = dual; I = inhibit; T = triggered) that describes the chamber paced, the chamber sensed, and the response to a sensed event. For example, VVI means that the ventricle is both paced and sensed, and generator output is inhibited when intrinsic ventricular activity is sensed. With the advent of the fully automatic DDD pacemaker, only three configurations are now commonly implanted: VVI, AAI, and DDD. An extra letter, R, is added for those pulse generators with a variable rate response to physical demands. These demands are sensed by sensing either the body's motion, thoracic impedance, body temperature, or minute ventilation.

TABLE 22-17

MAJOR GROUPS OF ANTIARRHYTHMIC DRUGS*

	CLASS 1A		CLASS 1B		CLASS 1C		CLASS 2:	CLASS 3			CLASS 4:	CLASS 5: BRETYL-IUM TOSY-LATE
	QUINI-DINE	PROCAIN-AMIDE	LIDO-CAINE	MEXILE-TINE	FLECAI-NIDE	PROPAFE-NONE	PROPRAN-OLOL	AMIODA-RONE	SOTALOL	IBUTILIDE	VERAPA-MIL	
Major indications	Serious ventricular arrhythmias, recurrent PAT with WPW, atrial flutter, or fibrillation	Serious ventricular arrhythmias, PAT	Serious ventricular arrhythmias, digitalis-induced arrhythmias; may decrease AV block	Oral treatment of serious recurrent ventricular arrhythmias	Refractory ventricular arrhythmias, slow conduction in accessory pathways	Automatic junctional or atrial tachycardia, SVT with accessory pathways	Serious supra- or ventricular arrhythmias; prevention of SVT in WPW; slowing ventricular rate in atrial fibrillation	Any serious arrhythmia refractory to other therapies	Atrial and ventricular arrhythmias, particularly in patients with structural heart disease	Conversion of atrial flutter or atrial fibrillation	SVT, but not with WPW; slowing ventricular rate in atrial fibrillation	*Main:* reversion to VF after defibrillation *Other:* Serious ventricular arrhythmias
Major contraindications	Known hypersensitivity to quinidine, myocardial depression, sick sinus syndrome, impaired conduction, including complete AV block, long QT	Myocardial depression, sick sinus syndrome, impaired conduction, including complete AV block, long QT			Myocardial depression, serious structural heart disease	Myocardial depression	Asthma, hypoglycemia, AV block	Severe pulmonary disease	↓ K^+ and Mg^{2+} concentrations	Previously documented hypersensitivity	β-Adrenergic blockade; infants <1 year old; myocardial depression	Postural hypotension
Dose Oral	Sulfate: 30–60 mg/kg/d children, 10 mg/kg/d adults divided 6h Gluconate: 20% higher dose, every 8–12 h, 6 mg/kg every 2–4 h, 3–5 times daily	50–100 mg/kg/d divided q4h; if slow-release form, q6h		Children: 1.4–5.1 mg/kg/dose q8h Adults: 450–1200 mg/d divided 8h	50–200 mg/m²/d div 12h or 6.7–9.5 mg/kg/d div q12h	300–400 mg/m²/d div q6h	2 mg/kg/d div q6h to start, then up to 6 mg/kg/d	Loading 5–10 mg/kg/d for 5–10 d, then 5 mg/kg/d qd	2–8 mg/kg/d div TID	NA	4–7 mg/kg/d div, TID or QD or BID with slow-release forms	

(continued)

TABLE 22-17 Continued

| | CLASS 1A | | CLASS 1B | | CLASS 1C | | CLASS 2: | CLASS 3 | | | CLASS 4: | CLASS 5: |
	QUINI-DINE	PROCAIN-AMIDE	LIDO-CAINE	MEXILE-TINE	FLECAI-NIDE	PROPAFE-NONE	PROPRAN-OLOL	AMIODA-RONE	SOTALOL	IBUTILIDE	VERAPA-MIL	BRETYL-IUM TOSY-LATE
IV	Not recommended	10–15 mg/kg over 30–45 min, then 30–80 μg/kg/min	1–2 mg/kg slowly, then 10–50 μg/kg/min infusion		NA		0.01 mg/kg every 2 min to 0.1 mg/kg total	5 mg/kg by central line over 30–60 min (diluted in 5% DW); maintenance 10 mg/kg/d by continuous infusion		0.01 mg/kg over 1 min, maximal dose 1 mg; can repeat 10 min after end of first infusion	0.15 mg/kg over 1 min; can repeat in 30 min	5 mg/kg, can repeat every 10–20 min to total of 30 mg/kg
Pharmacokinetics Therapeutic plasma levels (μg/mL)	2–5	4–10	1.5–5	0.5–2	0.2–1	<1	0.05–0.10	0.5–2	?<5	Unknown	0.1–0.3	
Side effects Cardiovascular	Myocardial depression, hypotension, prolonged AV conduction and PR, QRS and QT durations (but may increase AV conduction by vagolytic action), asystole, ventricular flutter or fibrillation	Hypotension, prolonged AV conduction and PR, QRS, and QT durations, AV block, asystole	Conduction abnormalities		Myocardial depression, AV block (rare), makes ventricular arrhythmias worse, prolong PR, QRS	Proarrhythmic in 2% of patients, myocardial depression, prolonged PR, QRS; bradycardia	Myocardial depression, AV block	Severe bradycardia AV block; ventricular arrhythmias; makes heart refractory to pacing	Torsades de pointes, bradycardia, myocardial depression	QT interval prolongation, proarrhythmia, esp. PVCs (5%), VT (5%), Torsades de pointes and polymorphous VT (4%). Risk higher with congestive heart failure, ↓ K$^+$, ↓ Mg^{2+}, or history of torsades. Clinician must be prepared to perform DC cardioversion.	Myocardial depression; AV block; bradycardia	Postural hypotension

1851

(continued)

TABLE 22-17 Continued

	CLASS 1A		CLASS 1B		CLASS 1C		CLASS 2: PROPRAN-OLOL	CLASS 3			CLASS 4: VERAPA-MIL	CLASS 5: BRETYL-IUM TOSY-LATE
	QUINI-DINE	PROCAIN-AMIDE	LIDO-CAINE	MEXILE-TINE	FLECAI-NIDE	PROPAFE-NONE		AMIODA-RONE	SOTALOL	IBUTILIDE		
Central nervous system	Tinnitus, confusion, seizures	Hallucina-tions, con-fusion	Seizures, ataxia, coma	Ataxia, tremor	Dizziness, headache, blurred vi-sion	Dizziness, headache, tremor, taste dis-turbance	Lethargy, fa-tigue	Dizziness, ataxia	Lethargy, fa-tigue, diz-ziness	Headache (4%)	Dizziness	
Gastro-intestinal	Nausea, vom-iting, diar-rhea	Anorexia, nausea, vomiting		GI upset, hepatitis		Anorexia, nausea, vomiting, constipa-tion		GI upset, hepatitis	Nausea	Nausea (2%)	Nausea	Nausea, vom-iting, pa-rotid pain
Hema-tologic Hyper-sensitiv-ity	Thrombo-cytopenia Fever, col-lapse, rash, respiratory arrest	Agranulo-cytosis SLE syn-drome, fe-ver, joint pains, rash		Blood dyscra-sias								
Other							Broncho-spasm, hy-poglycemia	Skin discolor-ation and photosensi-tivity; cor-neal depos-its; altered thyroid function; pulmonary fibrosis				

*Note that there are often complex drug interactions that should be considered when these medications are used. For some of the drugs there is limited experience in children. And, many patients in whom these drugs are used may also be receiving other medications, e.g. digoxin or coumadin, whose metabolism is affected by the antiarrhythmics.

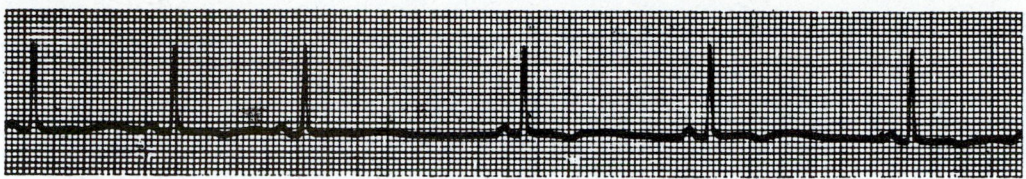

FIGURE 22-77   Sinus arrhythmia. A normal variant in which the sinus rate varies with respiration.

As a pulse generator nears the end of its battery life (typically 5 to 10 years), it exhibits a characteristic behavior, depending on the manufacturer and model. This is commonly a prolongation of pulse width, slowing of the rate, or the onset of asynchronous pacing. Another common cause of unusual behavior is lead fracture, when the pulse generator may oversense and fail to fire, fail to capture, or revert to asynchronous pacing. All children with implanted pacemakers should have regular follow-up, including transtelephonic monitoring, so that such problems can be detected promptly.

ANTITACHYCARDIA PACING   For selected patients who can be easily converted from a reentrant supraventricular tachycardia by rapid pacing, permanent antitachycardia pacing may be used. In terms of classification, the letter T is added for those pulse generators that have antitachycardia pacing capability. For example, an AAI-T device provides atrial demand pacing but also is capable of converting sensed episodes of paroxysmal tachycardia back into sinus rhythm by burst pacing or programmed stimulation; the modalities used are programmed by the clinician.

IMPLANTABLE CARDIOVERTER-DEFIBRILLATOR (ICD)   Children with life-threatening ventricular arrhythmias unresponsive to medical management may need implantation of a device that senses the onset of ventricular fibrillation and delivers one or more direct current defibrillation shocks directly to the heart via large epicardial patches. These devices all have the capability of antibradycardia pacing, antitachycardia pacing, and cardioversion or defibrillation. With the development of smaller generators and transvenous coils, most systems currently implanted are transvenous. Recently, "dual-chamber systems" have become available in which leads are placed in both the atrium and ventricle. These provide dual-chamber pacing and ventricular antitachycardia, cardioversion, and defibrillation capabilities.

RADIOFREQUENCY ABLATION   The development of techniques to map and ablate abnormal foci or pathways in the heart using radiofrequency (RF) energy revolutionized the management of patients with abnormal tachycardia. The RF ablation procedure is performed in the cardiac catheterization laboratory as part of an electrophysiology study. Once the diagnosis is made and the abnormal pathway or focus is located precisely, a special electrode catheter is placed at that site, and RF energy is delivered between the electrode of the catheter and a large chest patch, creating a tiny region of thermal injury. If properly placed, such a lesion may interrupt conduction in an accessory pathway, modify the AV node, or eliminate an automatic focus. All forms of abnormal tachycardia are amenable to RF ablation at relatively low risk, although risks are higher in infants. Success rates are over 90% for the common forms of supraventricular tachycardia but are lower for other forms of abnormal tachycardia.

SURGERY   Although RF ablation has replaced cardiac surgery for definitive cure of the mechanism of abnormal tachycardia in most patients, surgery may be recommended for patients who have failed RF ablation and in infants with incessant ventricular tachycardia secondary to cardiac hamartomas.

SINUS RHYTHM AND ITS VARIANTS

SINUS TACHYCARDIA   Sinus tachycardia is most often caused by anxiety or exercise but may result from fever, anemia, hypovolemia, shock, congestive heart failure, hyperthyroidism, and many medications. It is often confused with abnormal tachycardias, particularly in sick patients, and differentiation may be difficult. The rate seldom exceeds 200 beats per minute, even in newborns, and varies with time or activity. The electrocardiogram usually shows normal P waves, but at fast rates the P wave may be superimposed on the previous T wave. Vagal stimulation gradually slows the heart rate, in contrast to the abrupt slowing that it may cause with a paroxysmal supraventricular tachycardia. The best diagnostic modality is to treat the likely underlying cause of sinus tachycardia and observe slow resolution.

SINUS BRADYCARDIA   Sinus bradycardia is physiological in well-trained athletes as well as with vagal stimulation; it is also seen in pathologic states, including increased intracranial pressure, hyperkalemia, hypothermia, hypothalamic seizures, hypothyroidism, hypoxemia, obstructive jaundice, muscarinic poisoning, vagal effects of digitalis intoxication, and surgical damage to the SA node. It is occasionally seen for no known reason. Note that a slow sinus rhythm implies that the lower pacemakers have an even lower discharge rate than the SA node.

SINUS ARRHYTHMIA   Sinus arrhythmia (Figs. 22-77 and 22-78) is a normal variant in which the sinus rate varies; usually but not always the rate increases with inspiration and slows with expiration. This arrhythmia usually occurs when there is good vagal tone with a slow or normal heart rate; it is rare in newborns. During expiration the sinus rate may be sufficiently slowed to allow escape beats from an atrial or junctional pacemaker. Sinus arrhythmia with atrial escape beats has also been called *wandering atrial pacemaker*. The variants of sinus arrhythmia are important only in that they should not be mistaken for serious arrhythmias.

SINUS ARREST   *Sinus arrest* is a prolonged cessation of SA nodal pacemaker activity for more than two cycles (Fig. 22-79). With no sinus beats there may be escape beats from a lower pacemaker, but if there are long pauses with no atrial or ventricular activity, then there is failure of the lower pacemakers as well as the SA node.

In *sinoatrial block* (SA exit block), the SA pacemaker is discharging, but occasionally an impulse does not depolarize the atria. This

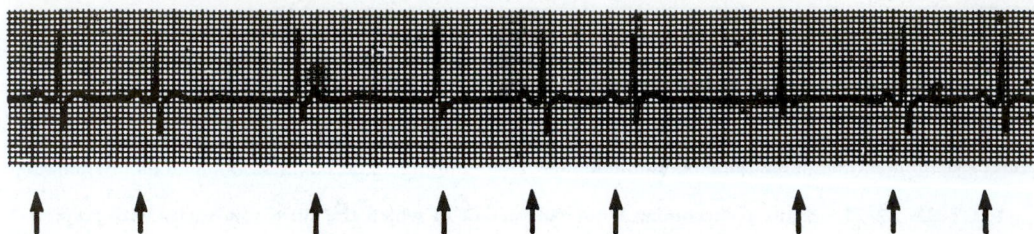

FIGURE 22-78 Sinus arrhythmia with escape beats. During sinus slowing, the sinus rate is less than that of a lower pacemaker. QRS complexes 3, 4, and 7 are probably junctional escape beats. The *arrows* indicate the sinus P waves.

is recognized by pauses that approximate multiples of a normal P-P interval.

Some children have *sick sinus syndrome* or *bradycardia-tachycardia syndrome*. They have episodes of marked sinus slowing or prolonged sinus arrest in which the lower pacemakers do not take over appropriately. As a result, there may be profound slowing of the heart rate or even asystole for several seconds. At other times there may be episodes of tachycardia. This syndrome is seen most often after atrial surgery (eg, repair of atrial septal defects, atrial baffles in transposition of the great arteries, or the Fontan procedure), but it may rarely arise spontaneously. Attempts to suppress the tachycardias with drugs may lead to unacceptable episodes of slowing or asystole, and artificial pacemakers may be required.

ECTOPIC SUPRAVENTRICULAR RHYTHMS

Because atrial and junctional ectopic pacemakers can produce similar QRS complexes and either similarly abnormal P waves or else no visible P waves, they are usually discussed together.

Ectopic atrial rhythm, also called coronary sinus rhythm, is similar to a normal sinus rhythm except for a superior P vector that gives P waves in leads II, III, and aVF. This is a normal variant, and heart rates are normal and may show respiratory variation. It is common in sinus venosus atrial septal defects and polysplenia syndromes.

ATRIAL PREMATURE BEATS *Atrial premature beats* (extrasystoles) are characterized by P waves that occur prematurely, usually differ in shape from normal P waves, and are followed by a near-normal P-R interval and either a normal or sometimes an aberrant QRS complex (Figs. 22-69 and 22-70). In older children there is usually an incomplete compensatory pause, but in infants the pause is occasionally complete. Very premature atrial extrasystoles may not be conducted because the impulse reaches the AV node or ventricles while these are still refractory (Fig. 22-70). Very early, blocked atrial extrasystoles are the most common causes of occasional pauses in rhythm. Isolated infrequent atrial extrasystoles are

unimportant. They are often seen in newborns and usually disappear by 2 to 6 weeks of age; even if they remain, they are usually of no concern. Multiple atrial premature beats may indicate an underlying mechanism for supraventricular tachycardia, such as an accessory pathway, or can cause transient atrial fibrillation that will not be sustained if the atrium is of normal size. Atrial bigeminy in which the premature atrial beats are blocked may cause a persistently low ventricular rate.

PAROXYSMAL SUPRAVENTRICULAR TACHYCARDIA *Paroxysmal supraventricular tachycardia (PSVT)* includes several mechanisms of tachycardia. It is characterized by rapid atrial rates, generally 180 to 300 beats per minute, and usually each beat is conducted to the ventricles (Fig. 22-80). Initial episodes are most frequent in early infancy, but they can occur at any age and even in utero. Brief episodes may cause no symptoms, although the parents may note mild pallor and a dynamic precordium. Older children may be aware of rapid heartbeats or fluttering in the chest. The episodes usually start and end abruptly. Short episodes of tachycardia usually do not harm the patient, but episodes of several hours or more may cause congestive heart failure, particularly in infants. Infants may even present with shock and heart failure, and the tachycardia may not be recognized as the cause of illness.

Specific causes of the tachycardia usually are not found, although many infants have their paroxysm during a respiratory illness. In adolescents and adults, emotional stress, fatigue, excess caffeine ingestion, tobacco, and drugs such as amphetamines may precipitate attacks. Underlying congenital heart disease is uncommon. About 5 to 10% of patients with paroxysmal supraventricular tachycardias show ventricular preexcitation between the attacks: Wolff-Parkinson-White syndrome (Fig. 22-80).

Patients with Wolff-Parkinson-White (WPW) syndrome have one or more bridges of muscle (bundle of Kent) between the atria and ventricles, so that impulses from the atrium can reach the ventricles through two pathways. While the impulse is delayed in the AV node there is rapid transmission to the ventricles via the bundle

FIGURE 22-79 Sinus arrest. There is cessation of SA nodal activity for more than two cycles. The long pause is terminated by an atrial escape beat with a P wave that is slightly different from those of sinus node origin. The second beat after the long pauses has an abnormal QRS complex because of aberrancy.

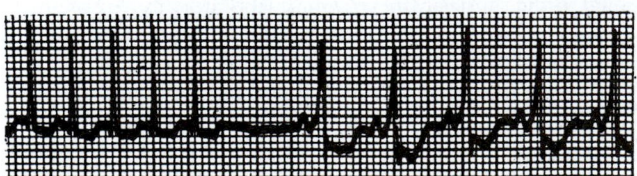

FIGURE 22-80 Supraventricular tachycardia ending abruptly and converting to sinus rhythm with preexcitation of the Wolff-Parkinson-White type. Note the short P-R interval and the δ wave at the beginning of the QRS complexes when there is sinus rhythm but not during the tachycardia.

of Kent. There is early but slow depolarization of the ventricle adjacent to the bundle of Kent, which produces a short P-R interval and then a slow initial part of the QRS complex—the δ wave. During this slow spread through part of the ventricular muscle the normal activation by the conduction system occurs, and the rest of the ventricles depolarize normally. The two waves of ventricular depolarization meet to produce one form of fusion beat. During the tachycardia the impulse descends through the AV node and reenters by the abnormal connection; thus, the QRS complex is normal. Approximately 50% of patients with preexcitation have tachyarrhythmias.

Other patients, without preexcitation, may have a *concealed accessory pathway,* in which the bundle of Kent is capable only of retrograde conduction. The tachycardia circuit is identical to that in WPW syndrome. One important form of concealed accessory pathway is the *permanent form of junctional reciprocating tachycardia (PJRT).* There is a concealed slowly conducting accessory pathway near the mouth of the coronary sinus, and slow retrograde conduction in this pathway leads to incessant tachycardia, which may in turn lead to cardiomyopathy. Patients without preexcitation may alternatively have *atrioventricular node reentry tachycardia,* in which there are two AV node pathways, one fast and one slow. Reentry occurs within the AV node, with conduction down the slow and up the fast pathway. Such patients may have relatively short PR intervals in sinus rhythm as a result of conduction down the fast pathway.

The harmful cardiac effects of supraventricular tachycardias are caused by inadequate ventricular filling because of the short diastole and also loss of atrial contraction at the right time in the cycle. In addition, there can be myocardial ischemia from impaired coronary flow; ischemia probably causes the S-T depression and T-wave inversion that are common in the attack. Finally, incessant tachycardias such as atrial ectopic tachycardia, junctional ectopic tachycardia (below), and PJRT, if allowed to continue for weeks or months, may lead to cardiomyopathy. Sometimes atrial tachycardia is seen with 2:1 AV block. Although this may represent atrial flutter or tachycardia with a very rapid atrial rate, in children taking digoxin digitalis intoxication must be considered (Fig. 22-81). Digoxin causes the ectopic tachycardia and, by its effect on the AV node, allows only every second impulse to reach the ventricles. As a result, these patients have ventricular rates of about 100 to 150 beats per minute; they may easily be thought to have sinus tachycardia if the alternating blocked P waves are not seen or if the lack of variation of the ventricular rate is not noted. This arrhythmia is important because it may be a prelude to more serious digitalis-induced arrhythmias, including ventricular fibrillation.

Treatment of paroxysmal supraventricular tachycardia is aimed at stopping the attack and preventing future attacks. Treatment of the acute episode depends on the clinical severity. If the child is not very ill, begin by stimulating the vagus nerve. The electrocardiogram should always be recorded before and during vagal stimulation so that there will be a record of the arrhythmia and of vagal effects on it. The vagus nerve can be stimulated mechanically by massaging *one* carotid sinus at a time, by causing gagging with posterior pharyngeal stimulation, by inserting a finger into the anus, by placing a damp cold cloth wrapped around crushed ice on the face and nose for 30 to 40 seconds (diving reflex), or by placing ice water in the stomach with a nasogastric tube. Although stimulating the diving reflex has a high success rate, it should be done with caution in young infants in whom ventricular fibrillation has, rarely, followed its use. Eyeball pressure should be avoided. If these simple measures are ineffective, then the vagus can be stimulated by raising the blood pressure suddenly and producing a baroreceptor reflex. To do this, inject *phenylephrine* (Neo-Synephrine), 0.02 mg/kg intravenously, slowly. The vagus may also be stimulated by giving *edrophonium chloride* (Tensilon), an anticholinesterase. If this is given rapidly intravenously and undiluted at a dose of 2 mg for infants, 5 mg for those 1 to 5 years old, and 10 mg for older children, there will be a sudden but temporary vagal stimulation that may stop the attack. Atropine should be available to treat any bronchospasm that might occur, and edrophonium must not be used if there is a history of asthma. In practice, the use of such drugs to elicit a vagal response has become rare because of the availability of adenosine.

Adenosine is valuable in acute management of supraventricular tachycardias that involve the atrioventricular node as part of the reentrant circuit, such as atrioventricular node reentrant tachycardia and atrioventricular reciprocating tachycardia of Wolff-Parkinson-White syndrome, concealed accessory pathways, and PJRT. When given rapidly by intravenous injection, adenosine induces a very brief episode of complete atrioventricular block, thereby interrupting the reentrant circuit. The onset of effect is usually less than 15 seconds, the half-life in blood is under 10 seconds, and the resulting atrioventricular blockade is, therefore, brief and self-limited. Other forms of abnormal tachycardia such as atrial tachycardia and ventricular tachycardia may also be sensitive to adenosine, independent of the effect on the AV node, but the effect is not as reliable as in the tachycardias listed above. Successful conversion of supraventricular tachycardia with adenosine may provide evidence against other forms of tachycardia, such as atrial tachycardia, that do not involve the atrioventricular node as part of the reentrant circuit.

Digoxin is a well-tested drug for treating supraventricular tachycardias in children. It is often successful in stopping the attack even if no other therapy is given, but because it may take some time to act, there is no reason not to try vagal stimulation while digoxin is being absorbed. Furthermore, because digoxin sensitizes the heart to vagal stimulation, repeating the vagal stimulation after digitalization is often successful in stopping a persistent attack.

If the infant is severely ill with shock and heart failure, simple maneuvers like an ice pack on the face or carotid sinus massage can be tried, for a very brief period. If there is no response, the arrhythmia may be stopped by an electric shock synchronized so that it does not fall in the vulnerable period (cardioversion). It is then essential to insert an intravenous line for administration of drugs, including sodium bicarbonate to combat acidemia, and to attempt to raise blood pressure with phenylephrine.

Infants with supraventricular tachycardias may have recurrences for the next 6 months but often lose their propensity for tachycardia by 1 year of age. Children whose tachycardias begin later are more likely to have recurrent attacks for many years, and many of those

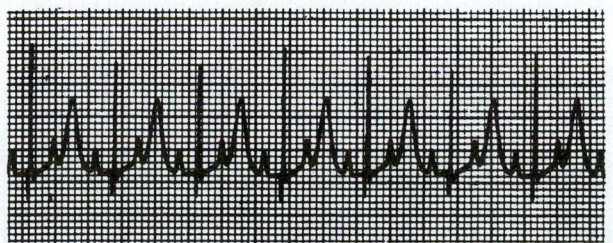

FIGURE 22-81 Paroxysmal atrial tachycardia with 2:1 AV block in a neonate with digitalis toxicity. Although the atrial rate was 240 beats per minute, the ventricular rate was 120 beats per minute, and the patient tolerated the arrhythmia well.

who lose their tachycardia in the first year experience recurrences later, often around 4 to 6 years of age. Digoxin is usually the most useful agent for preventing recurrences in the first year, but if it is ineffective, then propranolol may be added. If the patient has ventricular preexcitation, digoxin should be avoided. Occasionally other drugs such as sotalol, flecainide, or even amiodarone may be needed. Some older children have recurrent attacks of supraventricular tachycardia with several months between attacks. If the attacks do not cause heart failure, and if the patient and family can be reassured, it may be better for them to tolerate the attacks rather than take daily medications to prevent a rare event. These patients can often be taught how to stop an attack with a Valsalva maneuver or some other form of vagal stimulation. They can also be given a prescription for propranolol to be used if an attack persists.

On the other hand, patients occasionally have frequent, disabling attacks that do not respond to any form of medical therapy; they may need electrophysiological investigation and radiofrequency ablation for interruption of anomalous pathways, or other forms of nonpharmacologic management.

Supraventricular tachycardia in the fetus requires treatment because of the high incidence of fetal death and nonimmune hydrops fetalis. If the infant is near term, consideration should be given to immediate delivery, after which conventional treatment can be given. If the infant is very premature, a trial of antiarrhythmic agents that cross the placenta is warranted. Digitalizing the mother rapidly (0.25 mg intravenously 2-hourly for three doses) is the first choice, but if it fails to restore sinus rhythm, other agents may be needed. In particular, flecainide has been used with success in fetuses who have already developed hydrops fetalis. Recent reports suggest that potent antiarrhythmic agents that do not cross the placenta in adequate concentrations, such as amiodarone, may be given to the fetus by direct fetal cordocentesis.

JUNCTIONAL TACHYCARDIA An accelerated junctional pacemaker produces a ventricular rate that may be normal for a sinus pacemaker but is high for a junctional pacemaker. This rhythm is seen most often after surgery near the AV node (such as closure of ventricular septal defect) or with digitalis intoxication or myocarditis. Often it needs no specific treatment. When an accelerated junctional focus is very fast, it is termed *junctional ectopic tachycardia* (JET). It may be postoperative or congenital, has a high mortality rate, and is difficult to control with antiarrhythmic agents. This rhythm always requires cardiac consultation.

ATRIAL FLUTTER *Atrial flutter* is characterized by rapid atrial rates of about 300 per minute in older children and adolescents and as high as 450 to 500 beats per minute in newborns. In the typical form, there is a sawtooth configuration of atrial waves (F waves) best seen in leads II, III, and V_1, with variable AV block (Fig. 22-82). However, after extensive atrial surgery, atrial flutter may be atypical, and the typical sawtooth F waves may not be present. The ventricular rate may be regular or irregular; if regular, the ratio of atrial rate to ventricular rate can range from 2:1 (most frequent) to 8:1. With a reasonable ventricular rate, the arrhythmia may be tolerated well for a long time, but with rapid ventricular responses, severe symptoms can occur. Treatment should initially be with digoxin to increase the AV block and slow ventricular rate; if this does not suffice, then propranolol can be added. Sometimes this treatment will cause sinus rhythm to return, but if it does not, then the addition of quinidine may abolish the arrhythmia, or else electrical cardioversion may be successful. Atrial flutter is rare in infants and children and is usually associated with structural heart disease,

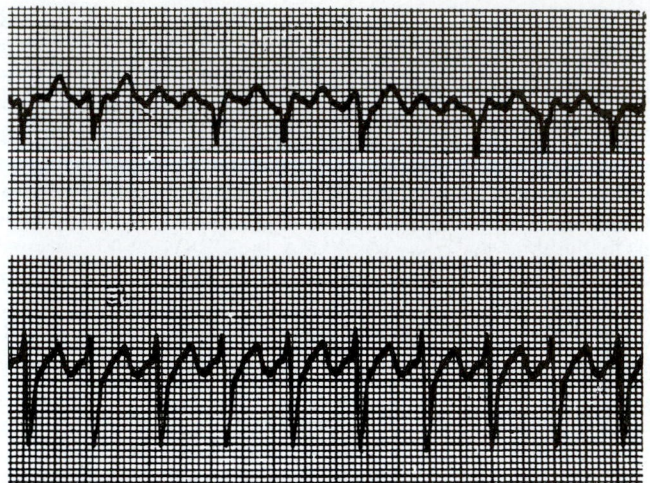

FIGURE 22-82 Atrial flutter. **A: Atrial flutter with varying conduction to the ventricles. Note the rapid atrial rate (270 beats per minute) and the sawtooth configuration of the atrial complexes (F waves). B: Tracing obtained from the same patient a few minutes later shows atrial flutter with 2:1 AV block. Every other F wave is buried in a T wave; consequently, this arrhythmia might be misinterpreted as a sinus tachycardia.**

particularly with dilated atria. It sometimes occurs transiently in otherwise normal newborn infants. Because atrial flutter has been implicated in sudden death after the Mustard or Senning repair of transposition of the great arteries, an aggressive approach to abolishing the arrhythmia has been recommended. Interruption of the flutter circuit by RF ablation or surgery has been successful.

ATRIAL FIBRILLATION Atrial fibrillation is rare in children. It is characterized by disordered atrial activity, and the electrocardiogram shows no P waves but instead has fine or coarse fibrillatory or f waves (Fig. 22-83). The ventricular response is very irregular and usually rapid; generally it is hard to find two exactly equal R-R intervals. Treatment is initially with digoxin or other agents such as diltiazem infusion to decrease ventricular rate. If the atrium is enlarged, then atrial fibrillation may be sustained. To restore sinus rhythm, antiarrhythmic agents such as quinidine or sotalol may be added, but cardioversion is generally more effective. After sinus rhythm is restored, quinidine or sotalol may be used to maintain it. If the atrial fibrillation keeps recurring, it is usually better to aim only for control of the ventricular rate with digoxin; if ventricular rates still rise unduly with exercise, then propranolol or verapamil may be added. When atrial fibrillation occurs in the presence of an accessory pathway (Wolff-Parkinson-White syndrome), conduction to the ventricle over the pathway may be dangerously rapid with

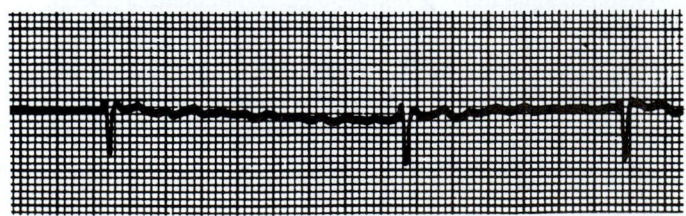

FIGURE 22-83 Atrial fibrillation. The undulating baseline indicates disordered atrial activity. The ventricular response is slow because of digoxin therapy.

wide QRS complexes and is thought to be the mechanism of sudden death in this syndrome. Because digoxin may shorten the anterograde effective refractory period of the accessory pathway, allowing even faster ventricular rates, it is contraindicated for the acute and chronic treatment of patients of any age with the Wolff-Parkinson-White syndrome except when an electrophysiological study has documented that digoxin may be used safely.

ECTOPIC VENTRICULAR ARRHYTHMIAS

VENTRICULAR EXTRASYSTOLES Ventricular extrasystoles may occur infrequently or in a fixed ratio with normal beats: bigeminy, trigeminy, quadrigeminy, and so on (Figs. 22-69, 22-73, and 22-84). If there is a single ectopic focus, then the coupling interval (the interval between the normal QRS complex and the ectopic one that follows it) is constant or almost constant, and the wide QRS complex is uniform in configuration. These *uniform ventricular extrasystoles* are common in normal adolescents. When the heart rate increases with exercise or anxiety, the extrasystoles usually disappear because the faster sinus rate discharges the ectopic focus before it can produce the premature beats. With mild exercise the sympathetic stimulation may actually increase the frequency of these ectopic beats, and it is only when heart rates exceed 150 to 160 beats per minute that these benign ectopic beats may disappear. Alcohol, caffeine, tobacco, fatigue, amphetamines, or other sympathomimetic drugs may increase the frequency of ventricular extrasystoles. In clinically healthy people, uniform ventricular ectopic beats are usually benign. However, if there is evident underlying heart disease, more attention should be paid to these extrasystoles, especially if they are of recent onset. If the extrasystoles appear in a patient receiving catecholamines or digoxin, they should be regarded as possible signs of toxicity, and the dosage should be reduced, or the drug should be stopped. Should there be frequent ventricular extrasystoles, particularly if they are known to be of recent onset, cardiac consultation should be obtained in order to exclude underlying heart disease such as mitral valve prolapse, myocarditis, or cardiomyopathy.

More importance should be attached to *multiform ventricular extrasystoles* (ie, those with different coupling intervals and varying QRS complexes and axes); these are particularly common in digitalis intoxication in adults, but are unusual in children. They cause concern for two reasons. First, they are often a sign of significant underlying cardiac disease, especially with poor myocardial function. Second, multiform ventricular ectopy is more likely to be associated with unstable ventricular tachycardia or ventricular fibrillation.

Couplets in which two extrasystoles follow a normal beat may be serious and require cardiac consultation. Ventricular premature beats sometimes occur early after cardiac surgery, particularly ventriculotomy. Unless they are very frequent, multiform, or repetitive, they need no treatment. They usually disappear with time. If they appear later, or if exercise testing brings out frequent or multiform ventricular ectopic beats, then cardiac consultation should be sought.

VENTRICULAR TACHYCARDIA Ventricular tachycardia is defined as a series of three or more ventricular ectopic beats, often manifesting as a rapid tachycardia with wide QRS complexes (Fig. 22-85A). Although in children the QRS complex can be relatively narrow (Fig. 22-85B), it always differs from the QRS in sinus rhythm. Often there is AV dissociation, with the P waves occurring less often

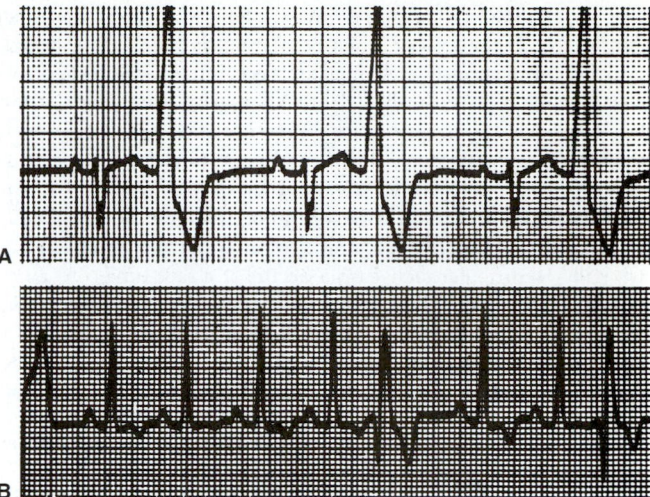

FIGURE 22-84 Ventricular extrasystoles. A: Ventricular bigeminy in which every other beat is a premature ventricular ectopic. The coupling interval is constant, and the ectopic complexes are uniform in configuration. B: Multiform ventricular ectopic beats. There are at least three different ectopic foci, each having its own coupling interval and QRS pattern.

than QRS complexes; this may be seen by slight variations of the T waves caused by varying superimposition of P waves on them. However, in about one-half the patients, there may be retrograde capture of the atria, particularly at slower ventricular rates, so that there is a 1:1 relationship between atrial and ventricular contractions. The major differential diagnosis is from supraventricular tachycardia with aberrant conduction. Proof of the ventricular origin of the arrhythmia can be obtained if the QRS complexes resemble typical ventricular extrasystoles in previous electrocardiograms or if ventricular fusion beats are seen (Figs. 22-73 and 22-85).

Ventricular tachycardia may cause severe symptoms and often leads to ventricular fibrillation. It should usually be treated as an emergency. Because most wide QRS tachycardias in children represent ventricular tachycardia, they should nearly always be treated as ventricular tachycardia unless one is certain of a supraventricular origin. Inappropriate treatment of ventricular tachycardia (with di-

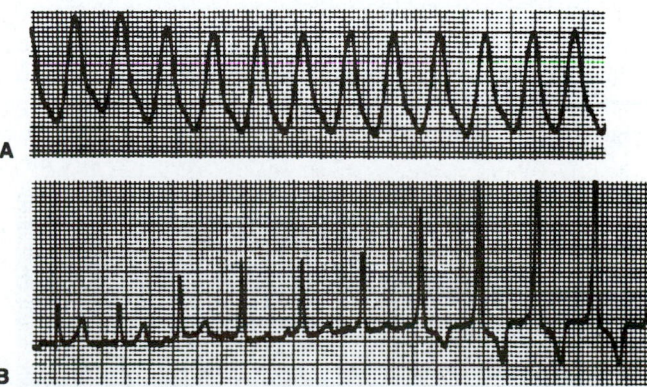

FIGURE 22-85 Ventricular tachycardia. A: Common form of ventricular tachycardia with rapid rate (160 beats per minute) and broad bizarre QRS complexes. B: Ventricular tachycardia with moderately rapid rate (120 beats per minute) and relatively narrow complexes. The sequence of fusion beats at the onset of the arrhythmia clearly identifies it as being ventricular in origin.

goxin or verapamil, for example) may be fatal. Cardioversion is usually effective. If the patient is hemodynamically stable, lidocaine can be given intravenously at 1 mg/kg over 1 to 2 minutes, or else procainamide intravenously at 10 to 15 mg/kg over 30 to 45 minutes, taking care to monitor blood pressure and to slow or stop the infusion should hypotension occur. Phenytoin can also be used, especially if the arrhythmia is caused by digoxin toxicity. Future attacks may be prevented with quinidine, propranolol, or mexiletine; occasionally sotalol, flecainide, or amiodarone is needed. Occasionally, ventricular tachycardia occurs at a rate similar to a normal sinus rate and with a relatively narrow QRS complex (Fig. 22-85) and is called *ventricular accelerated rhythm*. If it causes no circulatory difficulties, it may be fairly benign. It will usually not require treatment, and, when seen in the newborn, episodes usually disappear within several weeks or months.

VENTRICULAR FIBRILLATION Ventricular fibrillation produces a recording with no QRS complexes on it; there is just a wavy line (Fig. 22-86). P waves can be present. There is no cardiac output, and cardiopulmonary resuscitation should be commenced while preparations are made for electrical defibrillation.

Ventricular fibrillation is often the terminal event in many illnesses. It may follow hypoxemia, hyperkalemia, digitalis or quinidine intoxication, myocarditis, myocardial infarction, catecholamine infusions, anesthetics, and many drugs. It may be seen in patients with dilated cardiomyopathy. It is also a consequence of other arrhythmias, particularly ventricular tachycardia or multiple multiform ventricular ectopic beats.

Ventricular fibrillation may occur in two other settings. People with complete (third-degree) AV block have episodes of transient ventricular fibrillation that cause syncope (Adams-Stokes attacks) and indicate the need for artificial pacemakers. Occasionally these attacks occur when the complete heart block is intermittent and is brought on by vagal or other stimuli. Ventricular fibrillation is also the cause of the syncope and death that occur in Jervell-Lange-Nielsen and Romano-Ward syndromes. In both of these there is hereditary prolongation of the Q-T interval, and in the first there is congenital deafness. The arrhythmia starts with an unusual form of ventricular tachycardia called *torsades de pointes,* in which there are polymorphous complexes that seem to rotate around an imaginary isoelectric line. Several of these patients have died suddenly of fright or on hearing an unexpected loud noise. The prolonged Q-T interval is related to specific heritable abnormalities in cardiac potassium or sodium channels. To date, at least four specific genes coding for channels have been identified that may be abnormal because of mutations or deletion, but many patients with prolonged QT syndrome have none of these known mutations. Treat-

ment of these syndromes always requires chronic β-adrenergic blockade. In addition, permanent overdrive pacing is recommended to suppress ventricular ectopy and eliminate sudden pauses that are thought to be important in the onset of torsades. Finally, some patients with recurrent attacks not responding to the above measures may benefit from an implantable cardioverter-defibrillator.

ABNORMALITIES OF CONDUCTION

FIRST-DEGREE AV BLOCK First-degree AV block (Fig. 22-74) may occasionally occur without any evidence of heart disease, or with congenital heart disease such as endocardial cushion defect or corrected transposition of the great arteries. It may also occur with acute infections such as in acute rheumatic fever, diphtheria, and other infections, and its appearance does not necessarily mean that there is myocarditis. It also occurs with strong vagal stimulation and with digoxin administration. The mechanism may be delay of conduction through the atrium, AV node, or His-Purkinje system. It needs no treatment but should be considered carefully to determine if there is an underlying problem and followed to find out if the conduction defect will get worse and produce higher degrees of heart block.

SECOND-DEGREE AV BLOCK Type I second-degree AV block (Fig. 22-76) may occur in normals, particularly athletes with slow sinus rates. In this setting it occurs at night and is probably caused by increased vagal tone. If it is asymptomatic in someone with no structural or functional heart disease, it does not require aggressive evaluation or treatment. If it causes symptoms, it usually responds to atropine. This type of AV block can also be caused by drugs such as digoxin. Type II second-degree AV block usually results from disease of the His-Purkinje system and always requires careful evaluation. There is a significant risk of progression to third-degree AV block or syncope, with the chance of sudden death, and permanent pacemaker implantation is often recommended.

THIRD-DEGREE AV BLOCK Third-degree (complete) AV block is often congenital or occurs early in childhood. In two-thirds of these children there is no underlying heart disease, but the others may have a variety of congenital lesions, the most common being corrected transposition of the great arteries. The block often occurs in utero, and at times cesarean section has been done because of fetal distress inferred from the slow heart rate. There is a strong association with systemic lupus erythematosus or mixed connective tissue disease in the mother, who may even develop overt disease later, after the child's birth. Complete heart block may also follow surgery when patches are placed in the region of the AV node and the bundle of His. Occasionally, drugs may cause complete heart block, and it has been seen in digitalis intoxication.

Although some infants with congenital heart block develop congestive heart failure, most remain asymptomatic for several decades. These patients adjust to the slow rate by increasing stroke volume and by cardiac hypertrophy; they often have systolic flow murmurs over the base and middiastolic flow murmurs over the mitral and tricuspid valves because of the increased stroke volume. The first heart sound varies in intensity because of varying P-R interval, and there are cannon waves in the jugular veins. Occasionally, atrial sounds may be heard. On the electrocardiogram there are regular P waves at a normal rate, but these will be completely unrelated to the less-frequent QRS complexes (Figs. 22-75 and 22-87). The QRS complexes are usually narrow and normal, indicating that the

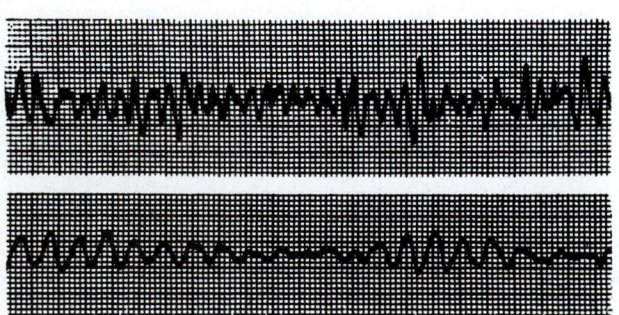

FIGURE 22-86 Ventricular fibrillation may be coarse (top) or undulating (bottom).

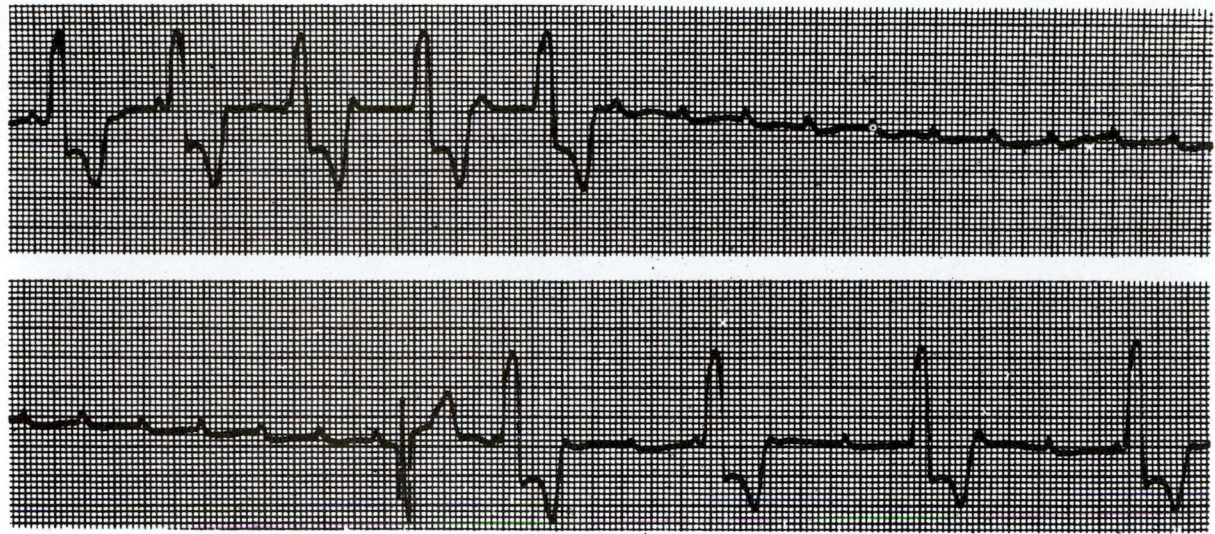

FIGURE 22-87   Adams-Stokes attack in a patient with postoperative third-degree AV block. There was a sudden asystole lasting 6 seconds, during which the patient fainted.

pacemaker is high in the bundle of His. Sometimes the QRS complexes are wide because the pacemaker is in the ventricles.

Artificial pacemakers are needed when the ventricular rate is too slow to sustain an adequate cardiac output or if these patients have syncope that may be from Adams-Stokes attacks (episodes of syncope from sudden asystole, ventricular tachycardia, or ventricular fibrillation—see Fig. 22-87). Usually these episodes last between 6 and 60 seconds, and then the ventricles resume their slow beat spontaneously, but sometimes the episodes are fatal. The attacks are more common after surgical block than with congenital block and more common with a wide than a narrow QRS complex. Should they occur, a ventricular pacemaker should be inserted promptly. Isoproterenol at 0.05 to 0.5 μg/kg/min may be infused to speed the ventricles before inserting the artificial pacemaker. All drugs that are potentially cardiac depressants should be avoided, as they can depress the idioventricular pacemaker. Another group that should be considered for permanent pacing is that of asymptomatic patients whose mean daytime ventricular rates are below 50 beats per minute, or who have long pauses with R-R intervals greater than 3 seconds, because of their tendency to have syncope or sudden death. By adulthood most if not all patients with complete congenital AV block will have pacemakers implanted because of the development of symptoms or to prevent them.

In fetuses with isolated complete atrioventricular block, a favorable outcome has usually been found at heart rates over 55 beats per minute. If the fetal heart rate is lower, perinatologists have attempted to increase it either with tocolytic agents that are also β-sympathomimetic agents (Ritodrine or Terbutaline) or by fetal placement of a pacemaker. These treatments are still undergoing clinical trials at this time.

SURGICAL BUNDLE BRANCH BLOCK   After closure of a ventricular septal defect, either isolated or in a tetralogy of Fallot, there may be damage to the right bundle branch and the anterior fibers of the left bundle. There will then be a right bundle branch block and a left anterior hemiblock manifested by a left superior QRS axis deviation of about -30 to $-90°$. These patients have only the posterior fibers of the left bundle for AV conduction and so are at risk of developing complete AV block should these remaining fibers be injured (eg, by slow fibrosis). No treatment is indicated, but care

must be paid to any symptoms that might suggest episodes of complete AV block. Electrophysiological study to determine if the residual fibers can conduct normally may be indicated.

References

Benson DW Jr, Dunnigan A: Disturbances of cardiac rhythm. In: Moller JH, Neal WA, eds: Fetal, Neonatal, and Infant Cardiac Disease. Norwalk, CT, Appleton & Lange, 1990:835

Deal BJ, Keane JF, Gillette PC, et al: Wolff-Parkinson-White syndrome and supraventricular tachycardia during infancy: management and follow-up. J Am Coll Cardiol 5:130, 1985

Garratt C, Linker N, Griffith M, Ward D, Camm AJ: Comparison of adenosine and verapamil for termination of paroxysmal junctional tachycardia. Am J Cardiol 64:1310, 1989

Garson A Jr, Gillette PC, McVey P, et al: Amiodarone treatment of critical arrhythmias in children and young adults. J Am Coll Cardiol 4:749, 1984

Garson A Jr, Randall DC, Gillette PC, et al: Prevention of sudden death after repair of tetralogy of Fallot: treatment of ventricular arrhythmias. J Am Coll Cardiol 6:221, 1985

Hohnloser SH, Woosley RL: Drug therapy: sotalol. N Engl J Med 331:31, 1994

Jackman WM, Wang XZ, Friday KJ, et al: Catheter ablation of accessory atrioventricular pathways (Wolff-Parkinson-White syndrome) by radiofrequency current. N Engl J Med 324:1605–1611, 1991

Kalman JM, Van Hare GF, Olgin GE, et al: Ablation of "incisional" reentrant atrial tachycardia complicating surgery for congenital heart disease: use of entrainment to define a critical isthmus of slow conduction. Circulation 93:502, 1996

Kleinman CS, Copel JA, Weinstein EM, et al: In utero diagnosis and treatment of fetal supraventricular tachycardia. Semin Perinatol 9:113, 1985

Kugler JD, Danford DA: Pacemakers in children: an update. Am Heart J 117:665, 1989

Kugler JD, Danford DA, Deal BJ, et al: Radiofrequency catheter ablation for tachyarrhythmias in children and adolescents. N Engl J Med 330: 1481, 1994

Lambert EC, Menon R, Wagner HR, et al: Sudden unexpected death from cardiovascular disease in children. Am J Cardiol 34:89, 1974

Michaelsson M, Jonzon A, Riesenfeld T: Isolated congenital complete atrioventricular block in adult life. A prospective study. Circulation 92:442, 1995

Moak JP, Smith RT, Garson A Jr: Newer antiarrhythmic drugs in children. Am J Cardiol 113:180, 1987

Perry JC, McQuinn RL, Smith RT, et al: Flecainide acetate for resistant arrhythmias in the young: efficacy and pharmacokinetics. J Am Coll Cardiol 14:185, 1989

Perry JC, Garson A: Supraventricular tachycardia due to Wolff-Parkinson-White syndrome in children: early disappearance and late recurrence. J Am Coll Cardiol 16:1215–1220, 1990

Saul JP, Hulse JE, De W, et al: Catheter ablation of accessory atrioventricular pathways in young patients: use of long vascular sheaths, the transseptal approach and a retrograde left posterior parallel approach. J Am Coll Cardiol 21:571–583, 1993

Simpson JM, Sharland GK. Fetal tachycardias: management and outcome of 127 consecutive cases. Heart 79:576, 1998

Van Hare GF, Lesh MD, Stanger P: Radiofrequency catheter ablation of supraventricular arrhythmias in patients with congenital heart disease: results and technical considerations. J Am Coll Cardiol 22:883–890, 1993

Vetter VL, Tanner CS, Horowitz LN: Electrophysiologic consequences of the Mustard operation for complete transposition of the great arteries. J Am Coll Cardiol 10:1265, 1987

22.4   ACQUIRED CARDIOVASCULAR DISEASE

22.4.1   Diseases of Myocardium

James D. Bristow

The myocardium can be affected by disease processes unrelated to abnormal pressure or volume loads; these processes may be inflammatory, metabolic, infiltrative, ischemic, or primary, with significant overlap. Myocardial diseases may present acutely, with signs of congestive heart failure: tachypnea often with rales, tachycardia, an enlarged but quiet heart, soft heart sounds that may have a tic-tac rhythm, cardiac gallops, and either no murmurs or systolic murmurs of mitral or tricuspid incompetence. Alternatively, they may present chronically with failure to thrive, decreased exercise tolerance, and more subtle findings of heart failure. Occasionally, the predominant process may be an arrhythmia, either atrial or ventricular tachycardia/fibrillation or heart block. These present clinically with palpitations, syncope, or sudden death.

The electrocardiogram and chest x-ray are useful in suggesting heart disease but are rarely diagnostic. In acute presentations, the chest x-ray usually shows diffuse cardiac enlargement, passive pulmonary congestion, and interstitial edema; the electrocardiogram shows normal or reduced QRS voltages (because hypertrophy has not yet had time to develop), and S-T segment depressions with T-wave inversion in the anterolateral precordial leads. The echocardiogram often shows diffuse cardiac dilatation, decreased contractions, and atrioventricular valve regurgitation.

Chronic myocardial diseases (cardiomyopathies) present in one of three configurations, as defined in the World Health Organization classification, that are useful in diagnosis and therapy. Most commonly, the ventricle is *dilated* and shows decreased contractility; systolic function is impaired. Less often, the ventricular wall is thickened or *hypertrophic* and can cause obstruction to systolic outflow or impair diastolic filling. Least often there is a *restrictive* cardiomyopathy with grossly impaired filling that produces a small heart; systolic function is normal, but diastolic function is impaired.

Dilated cardiomyopathy is considered most often to be primary or a sequel of viral myocarditis; nutritional and toxic factors may be involved in some patients, and chronic tachycardias are uncommon but important causes. Several kindreds in which dilated cardiomyopathy is inherited have been reported; as additional families are found and studied, the importance of genetic causes will grow. Hypertrophic cardiomyopathy is frequently genetic, resulting from mutations in genes encoding sarcomeric proteins, genes involved in energy metabolism, or as part of several neuromuscular disorders. Restrictive cardiomyopathy is often associated with infiltration of the myocardium by cells or unusual chemicals.

In chronic cardiomyopathies, the chest x-ray may show profound cardiomegaly (dilated type) or a heart of normal size. The lung fields are usually clear. The electrocardiogram often shows left ventricular hypertrophy, frequently with left axis deviation, increased left precordial and inferior forces, and S-T segment flattening with T-wave inversion. The clinical, ECG, and chest x-ray findings are frequently nonspecific, but the echocardiogram distinguishes the three cardiomyopathic configurations. In dilated cardiomyopathy there is marked cardiac enlargement, ventricular wall thinning, and reduced systolic function. In hypertrophic cardiomyopathy there is thickening of the ventricles that may affect the septum more than the ventricular free walls or may be uniform. Hypertrophy is frequently massive at the time of diagnosis, and systolic function may be hyperdynamic or normal. Finally, in restrictive cardiomyopathy, ventricular appearance and systolic function are near normal, but there are markedly dilated atria and restricted ventricular filling. Specific tests for diagnosis depend on the likely etiology of the disease process, but cardiac biopsy is only occasionally useful for making a specific diagnosis.

INFLAMMATORY DISEASES

Inflammatory diseases of the myocardium may be infectious or autoimmune mediated, acute or chronic. Acute infection is the most common inflammatory process that directly affects the heart. Acute myocarditis can occur at any age, including the fetus, and its course ranges from very mild to fulminant, with death in a few days or weeks. Often there is a history of a recent upper respiratory tract infection, and viruses are usually the causative agents. Historically, the enteroviruses (coxsackie and echoviruses) have been considered most common, but specific diagnosis is hampered by the difficulty in isolating the virus from affected patients. Recently, polymerase chain reaction (PCR) of myocardial biopsy specimens has detected viral genomes in many patients with acute and chronic myocarditis; adenovirus is the most common virus associated with myocarditis and dilated cardiomyopathy. Interestingly, adenovirus and coxsackievirus share a cellular receptor that is important for viral entry into the cell, which may explain their particular prevalence. Many other viruses including parvovirus, HIV, mumps, cytomegalovirus, and varicella can cause myocarditis, as can other pathogens (*Rickettsiae, Toxoplasma gondii, Mycoplasma pneumoniae, Chlamydia trachomatis, Borrelia burgdorferi*). Diphtheria exotoxin causes profound myocardial damage by interfering with mitochondrial energy metabolism and is often associated with heart block, ventricular tachycardia, and fibrillation; mortality is high. *Trypanosoma cruzi* (Chagas disease) is a common cause of myocarditis in South and Central America; the acute myocarditis can be severe and is the primary cause of death in the acute phase of the illness, although chronic myocardial dysfunction, occurring after a long latent period, is a far more common result of *T. cruzi* infection.

Immune-mediated myocarditis can also occur acutely. Rheumatic myocarditis may occur early in acute rheumatic fever and is almost always accompanied by endocardial (mitral or aortic valve insufficiency) involvement and sometimes by pericarditis. Kawasaki syndrome causes myocardial and pericardial inflammation, although myocardial dysfunction is rarely severe in the absence of significant obstructive coronary arterial lesions. Many other autoimmune diseases may affect the myocardium, including systemic lupus erythematosus, which may cause acute myocardial or pericardial inflammation, or chronic endocardial disease (Libman-Sachs endocarditis). Maternal systemic lupus erythematosus is also associated with conduction system damage and heart block in the fetus.

Treatment of acute myocarditis is supportive; bedrest, diuretics, inotropic agents, afterload reduction, and occasionally ventilatory support may all be necessary. Viral myocarditis is associated with ventricular dysrhythmias and conduction abnormalities that may be potentiated by digoxin; if used, it should be given in low dose, and with careful cardiac monitoring. Specific therapies include steroids in acute rheumatic (but not viral) myocarditis, γ-globulin and salicylates in Kawasaki syndrome, γ-globulin in viral myocarditis, antitoxin in diphtheria, and antimicrobials in bacterial, parasitic, mycoplasma, or rickettsial myocarditis. The diagnosis of myocarditis can be inferred by documenting a specific clinical pattern (as in rheumatic myocarditis, Kawasaki syndrome, or diphtheria), documenting myocardial inflammation by nuclear isotope scans, or by isolating a potentially causative virus in the throat or feces in association with an appropriate antibody response. *Proof* of a specific virus as the cause requires its isolation from the myocardium or localization by other techniques such as PCR, although this is rarely necessary in the clinical setting.

Chronic inflammation of the myocardium also occurs. Occasionally viral myocarditis presents with chronic congestive heart failure, dysrhythmias, and cardiomegaly with hypertrophy. Finding inflammatory infiltrates on myocardial biopsy suggests ongoing inflammation and perhaps separates this disease from idiopathic dilated cardiomyopathy. However, many authors now suggest that the latter is a later manifestation of viral infection. Indeed, viral genomes can be isolated from the myocardium of many patients with dilated cardiomyopathy, even when an inflammatory infiltrate is not found on biopsy. This may reflect the patchy nature of the inflammatory process. Viral genomes have not been amplified from the myocardium of control patients with structural heart disease, suggesting that this test is specific for persistent viral infection. Cardiomyopathy is believed to result from ongoing inflammation and release of inflammatory cytokines that may lead to myocyte death. Steroids or azathioprine have been used with only occasional success, probably because symptoms occur late in the process, when cardiac reserve is exhausted.

Myocarditis causing a dilated cardiomyopathy is a common finding in HIV infection. Although the HIV virus has been isolated from the myocardium at autopsy or localized by polymerase chain reaction, other viral genomes are recovered at least as frequently in HIV-infected children, suggesting that HIV infection may predispose patients to persistent myocardial infection with other viruses.

METABOLIC DISORDERS

Myocardial function may be impaired by dietary deficiencies or excesses of various substances, or primarily by enzymatic defects that impair energy utilization. Low calcium or magnesium levels may occasionally cause cardiac dilatation and heart failure, particularly in premature infants. Clinically, there may be hyperreflexia; electro-

cardiographically there usually is a prolonged Q-T interval and occasionally atrioventricular block. Severe hypophosphatemia may also cause reversible heart failure. Hypokalemia and hyperkalemia are discussed in Secs. 21.4.4 and 22.2.2. Severe hypoglycemia can cause cardiac dilatation and heart failure in newborns, particularly in infants born prematurely, with intrauterine growth retardation, with severe cyanotic heart disease, or in infants of diabetic mothers. Infants of diabetic mothers can also have an obstructive cardiomyopathy that resembles hypertrophic cardiomyopathy with asymmetric septal hypertrophy. The heart usually returns to normal over several months (see Sec. 22.3.4).

Deficiencies of vitamins (thiamine, causing beriberi), trace metals (selenium, causing Keshan disease), amino acids (taurine), or cofactors (carnitine) can cause cardiac dilatation and heart failure. These deficiencies can be either nutritional or, rarely, caused by an inborn error of metabolism. For example, carnitine deficiency may be secondary to a variety of chronic illnesses including mitochondrial myopathies or may be a primary process. Treatment in all is toward redressing the specific deficiency. Hormonal abnormalities can also cause myocardial dysfunction. Hypothyroidism not only causes bradycardia, low cardiac output, and pericardial effusion but also can cause myocardial degeneration with S-T and T-wave changes. Pheochromocytoma may produce left ventricular hypertrophy and heart failure from sustained or paroxysmal hypertension; in addition, high catecholamine blood levels can cause subendocardial hemorrhages and myocardial degeneration that further impair cardiac function.

Other causes of myocardial dysfunction include toxic effects of drugs (chloroquine, ipecac, cocaine, and adriamycin, the last of which may cause severe, long-lasting myocardial damage), radiation (particularly mediastinal radiotherapy for lymphoma), metabolic by-products (uremic cardiomyopathy, which is rapidly reversible with hemodialysis), and severe anemia.

Genetic metabolic disorders are increasingly recognized as causes of severe myocardial disease in early infancy. These disorders generally produce cardiomyopathy by interfering with energy metabolism. Specific defects may affect transport of substrate or cofactors into mitochondria (eg, carnitine-palmitoyl transferase-1 deficiency), or directly affect mitochondrial enzymes involved in β-oxidation of fatty acids (eg, long-chain and medium-chain acyl dehydrogenase deficiency) or electron transport. These defects can be associated with dilated or hypertrophic cardiomyopathy and produce profound but episodic cardiac failure. Although rare, diagnosis of these disorders is important because familial incidence is frequent.

INFILTRATIVE DISEASES

Many substances can infiltrate the myocytes or interstitium and impair cardiac function. Abnormal deposition of glycogen (especially type II glycogen storage or Pompe disease) or glycolipid (Fabry disease) in the myocytes causes massive ventricular hypertrophy and obstruction. Hemosiderin may be deposited in the interstitium, causing myocardial fibrosis and subsequent systolic and diastolic dysfunction. This may be primary but is more commonly secondary to repeated blood transfusions in thalassemia, sickle cell anemia, and aplastic anemia. Mucopolysaccharidoses can produce myocardial degeneration. Hurler and Hunter syndromes also cause intimal thickening of the coronary arteries and, with Morquio and Scheie syndromes, can cause valvar regurgitation. Other syndromes associated with myocardial infiltration and fibrosis include cystinosis, amyloidosis, and sarcoidosis.

Infiltration may also be caused by neoplastic processes. The infiltration may be generalized, as in leukemia and lymphoma, or may be localized. Localized tumors are described in Sec. 22.4.2.

ISCHEMIA

Myocardial ischemia is rare in childhood. It may be caused by embolism, particularly in the perinatal period when venous thrombi easily cross the foramen ovale, but is more commonly caused by coronary artery abnormalities. Most frequent among these are congenital defects in which the coronary arteries communicate with another vascular bed, producing ischemia through a vascular steal syndrome. Examples include anomalous origin of the left or right coronary artery from the pulmonary artery, arteriovenous fistula, and arteriocameral fistula. Coronary insufficiency also results from inborn errors of metabolism (homozygous type 2 hyperlipidemia, homocystinuria), idiopathic calcification of the coronary arteries, and vasculitides. The most common vasculitis affecting the coronary arteries occurs in Kawasaki syndrome; coronary arterial aneurysms occur in up to 20% of patients, although this incidence can be greatly reduced by early administration of γ-globulin (see Sec. 12.6.2). Prolonged administration of low-dose aspirin, other antiplatelet agents, or coumadin may decrease the incidence of thrombosis once aneurysms have occurred. Other vasculitides, including juvenile rheumatoid arthritis, polyarteritis nodosa, and systemic lupus erythematosus, may also affect coronary arteries. Obliterative coronary arteritis has been associated with transplant rejection. All of these diseases can produce myocardial ischemia, its extent varying with the size and number of arteries involved and the amount of collateral formation. There may be cardiac dilatation, arrhythmias, and often mitral incompetence from damage to the papillary muscles.

Chronic atrial or ventricular tachycardias are associated with a dilated cardiomyopathy that can be cured if the arrhythmia is controlled. Myocardial ischemia is the likely but unproven mechanism.

PRIMARY

Diseases that primarily alter the structure of the myocyte can be separated into known neuromuscular disorders and unknown (or idiopathic) disorders. The most common neuromuscular disorders affecting myocytes include Friedreich ataxia, which causes cardiac dilatation or hypertrophy and heart failure in older children and adolescents, and progressive (Duchenne or Becker) muscular dystrophy, which may cause left ventricular hypertrophy and S-T and T-wave changes. There are many less common diseases, often with abnormalities in mitochondrial structure or function, that affect cardiac as well as skeletal myocytes.

Familial examples of isolated dilated cardiomyopathy have also been reported. One kindred with X-linked inheritance and isolated dilated cardiomyopathy has been mapped to the dystrophin locus, the gene responsible for Duchenne muscular dystrophy. Mutations in cardiac actin were recently described as a cause of dilated cardiomyopathy with autosomal dominant inheritance. Five other families have been studied and mapped to a chromosomal interval, but specific mutations have not yet been identified.

Idiopathic dilated cardiomyopathy occurs in children of all ages. Treatment is supportive and includes nutritional supplementation, diuretics, inotropic agents, and vasodilators; β-adrenergic blockade may be of value. Many children are candidates for cardiac transplantation. An unusual and perhaps genetically determined cardiomyopathy affects the right ventricle (arrhythmogenic right ventric-

ular dysplasia), which is dilated and hypokinetic and generates severe arrhythmias.

One specific pathologic type of cardiomyopathy is *endocardial fibroelastosis*, in which the ventricles or atria are lined with thick white tissue that on microscopy shows marked endocardial and subendocardial fibroelastic proliferation. These changes may be secondary to severe obstructive lesions; they may occur in the left ventricle and atrium with severe aortic stenosis or coarctation of the aorta, in the left atrium with mitral atresia and a small foramen ovale, or in the right ventricle with severe pulmonary stenosis or atresia. More often they are primary. *Primary (idiopathic) endocardial fibroelastosis*, a disease of unknown origin, usually occurs before 1 year of age. The disease may appear in clusters, suggesting an infective origin. Many of these infants have had positive skin reactions to inactivated mumps antigen, and in a recent report, mumps virus was recovered by PCR from the myocardium of patients with endocardial fibroelastosis but not others. The endocardial thickening is accompanied by myocardial hypertrophy, impaired myocardial function, and mitral and tricuspid regurgitation. The clinical features are those of any chronic myocardial disorder with congestive heart failure, as are the radiologic and electrocardiographic features. Because the clinical findings are nonspecific, the diagnosis can be proved only by biopsy or autopsy. However, the echocardiogram often shows bright endocardial echoes. Treatment is symptomatic. Most children get worse and die months or years after the onset, but spontaneous remissions have been described.

Hypertrophic cardiomyopathy may affect the left and right ventricular free walls but most commonly causes massive septal hypertrophy. It is generally transmitted in an autosomal dominant pattern, with nearly complete penetrance if patients are followed lifelong. Genetic hypertrophic cardiomyopathy is a disease of the sarcomere. Mutations have been identified in seven different sarcomeric proteins (β-myosin heavy chain, troponin I, troponin T, α-tropomyosin, myosin binding protein-C, and the regulatory and essential myosin light chains). Although clinical outcomes may be correlated with specific mutations, routine molecular diagnosis is not yet available. It is discussed in detail in Sec. 22.3.4. Similar hypertrophic cardiomyopathies have been noted in Pompe disease, Friedreich ataxia, some rare mitochondrial disorders, and Noonan syndrome.

Restrictive cardiomyopathy is extremely rare in childhood and is characterized by severe biatrial dilatation in the presence of normal ventricular dimensions. It is generally sporadic and idiopathic, and the prognosis is poor, with a median survival of less than 2 years.

References

Inflammatory Diseases

Acute

Acierno LJ: Cardiac complications in acquired immunodeficiency syndrome (AIDS): a review. J Am Coll Cardiol 13:1144, 1989

Bowles NE, Richardson PJ, Olsen EGJ, et al: Detection of coxsackie-B-virus–specific RNA sequences in myocardial biopsy samples from patients with myocarditis and dilated cardiomyopathy. Lancet 2:1120, 1986

Dec GW Jr, Palacios IF, Fallon JT, et al: Active myocarditis in the spectrum of acute dilated cardiomyopathies. N Engl J Med 312:885, 1985

Drucker NA, Colan SD, Lewis AB, et al: γ-Globulin treatment of acute myocarditis in the pediatric population. Circulation 89:252, 1994

Hicks RV, Mellish ME: Kawasaki syndrome. Pediatr Clin North Am 3: 1151, 1986

Kao CH, Hsieh KS, Wang YL, et al: Tc-99m HMPAO labeled WBC scan for the detection of myocarditis in different phases of Kawasaki disease. Clin Nucl Med 17:185, 1992

Marcin-Garcia J, Sheridan R, Hanissian AS: Echocardiographic detection of early cardiac involvement in juvenile rheumatoid arthritis. Pediatrics 73:394, 1984

Martin AB, Webber S, Fricker FJ, et al: Acute myocarditis in children. Circulation 90:330, 1994

Morgan BC: Cardiac complications of diphtheria. Pediatrics 32:549, 1963

Ni J, Bowles NE, Kim YH, et al: Viral infection of the myocardium in endocardial fibroelastosis. Molecular evidence for the role of mumps virus as an etiologic agent. Circulation 95:133, 1997

Rosenberg HS, McNamara DG: Acute myocarditis in infancy and childhood. Prog Cardiovasc Dis 7:179, 1964

Woodruff JF: Viral myocarditis. A review. Am J Pathol 101:25, 1980

Chronic

Ansari A, Larson PH: Heart disease in systemic lupus erythematosus: diagnosis and management. Texas Heart Inst J 12:9, 1985

Bowles NE, Rose ML, Taylor P, et al: End-stage dilated cardiomyopathy: persistence of enterovirus-RNA in myocardium at cardiac transplantation and lack of immune response. Circulation 80:1128, 1989

Calabrese LH, Profitt MR, Yen-Lieberman B, et al: Congestive cardiomyopathy and illness related to the acquired immunodeficiency syndrome (AIDS) associated with isolation of retrovirus from myocardium. Ann Intern Med 107:691, 1987

Diitrich H, Chow L, Denaro F, et al: Human immunodeficiency virus, coxsackievirus and cardiomyopathy. Ann Intern Med 108:108, 1988

Galve E, Candell-Riera J, Pigrau C, et al: Prevalence, morphologic types, and evolution of cardiac valvular disease in systemic lupus erythematosus. N Engl J Med 319:817, 1988

Giacca M, Severini GM, Mestroni L, et al: Low frequency of detection by nested polymerase chain reaction of enterovirus ribonucleic acid in endomyocardial tissue of patients with idiopathic dilated cardiomyopathy. J Am Coll Cardiol 24:1033, 1994

Matsumori A, Kawai C: An animal model of congestive (dilated) cardiomyopathy: dilatation and hypertrophy of the heart in the chronic stage in DBA/2 mice with myocarditis caused by encephalomyocarditis virus. Circulation 66:355, 1982

Svantesson H, Bjorkhem G, Elborgh R: Cardiac involvement in juvenile rheumatoid arthritis. A follow up study. Acta Paediatr Scand 72:345, 1983

Towbin JA: Pediatric myocardial disease. Pediatr Clin North Am 46:289, 1999

Waterson AP: Virological investigations in congestive cardiomyopathy. Postgrad Med J 54:505, 1978

Metabolic Disorders

Secondary

Gottdiener JS, Katin MJ, Borer JS, et al: Late cardiac effects of therapeutic mediastinal irradiation. N Engl J Med 308:569, 1983

Hung J, Harris PJ, Uren RF, et al: Uremic cardiomyopathy—effect of hemodialysis on left ventricular function in end-stage renal failure. N Engl J Med 302:547, 1980

Krug SE: Cocaine abuse: historical, epidemiologic, and clinical perspectives for pediatricians. Adv Pediatr 36:369, 1989

Riggs JE, Klingberg WG, Flink EB, et al: Cardioskeletal mitochondrial myopathy associated with chronic magnesium deficiency. Neurology 42: 128, 1992

Tang S-C, Liu Y-X, Jin Z-H, et al: M-mode echocardiographic features of children with Keshan disease: a preliminary observation of 106 cases. Chin Med J 97:795, 1984

Tenaglia A, Cody R: Evidence for a taurine-deficiency cardiomyopathy. Am J Cardiol 62:136, 1988

Primary

Ino T, Sherwood WG, Benson LN, et al: Cardiac manifestations in disorders of fat and carnitine metabolism in infancy. J Am Coll Cardiol 11:1301, 1988

Kelly DP, Hale DE, Rutledge SL, et al: Molecular basis of inherited medium-chain acyl-CoA dehydrogenase deficiency causing sudden child death. J Inher Metab Dis 15:171, 1992

Mathur A, Sims HF, Gopalakrishnan D, et al: Molecular heterogeneity in very-long-chain acyl-CoA dehydrogenase deficiency causing pediatric cardiomyopathy and sudden death. Circulation 99:1337, 1999

Nagai T, Tuchiya Y, Taguchi Y, et al: Fatal infantile mitochondrial encephalomyopathy with complex I and IV deficiencies. Pediatr Neurol 9: 151, 1993

Servidei S, Bertini E, Dimauro S: Hereditary metabolic cardiomyopathies. Adv Pediatr 41:1, 1994

Shoffner JM, Wallace DC: Heart disease and mitochondrial DNA mutations. Heart Dis Stroke 1:235, 1992

Tripp ME, Katcher ML, Peters HA, et al: Systemic carnitine deficiency presenting as familial endocardial fibroelastosis: a treatable cardiomyopathy. N Engl J Med 305:385, 1981

Waber LJ, Valle D, Meill C, et al: Carnitine deficiency presenting as familial cardiomyopathy: a treatable defect in carnitine transport. J Pediatr 101: 700, 1982

Infiltrative Diseases

Hayflick S, Rowe S, Kavanaugh-McHugh A, et al: Acute infantile cardiomyopathy as a presenting feature of mucopolysaccharidosis VI. J Pediatr 120:269, 1992

Krovetz LJ, Lorincz AE, Schiebler GL: Cardiovascular manifestations of the Hurler syndrome. Hemodynamic and angiographic observations in 15 patients. Circulation 31:132, 1965

Nordvag BY, Ranlov I, Riise HM, et al: Retrospective molecular detection of transthyretin Met-111 mutation in a Danish kindred with familial amyloid cardiomyopathy, using DNA from formalin-fixed and paraffin-embedded tissues. Hum Genet 92:265, 1993

Schieken RM, Kerber RE, Ionasescu VV, et al: Cardiac manifestations of mucopolysaccharidoses. Circulation 52:700, 1975

Ischemia

Askenazi J, Nadas AS: Anomalous left coronary artery originating from a pulmonary artery. Circulation 51:976, 1975

Bernstein D, Finkbeiner WE, Soifer S, et al: Perinatal myocardial infarction: a case report and review of the literature. Pediatr Cardiol 6:313–317, 1986

Cheitlin MD: Coronary arterial anomalies: Clinical and angiographic aspects. In: Virmani R, Forman MB, eds: Nonatherosclerotic Ischemic Heart Disease. New York, Raven Press, 1989:125

Dardir M, Ferrans VJ, Roberts WC: Coronary artery disease in familial and metabolic disorders. In: Virmani R, Forman MB, eds: Nonatherosclerotic Ischemic Heart Disease. New York, Raven Press, 1989:185

Hamsten A, Norberg R, Björkholm M, et al: Antibodies to cardiolipin in young survivors of myocardial infarction: an association with recurrent cardiovascular events. Lancet 1:113, 1986

Kato H, Ichinose E, Kawasaki T: Myocardial infarctions in Kawasaki disease: clinical analysis in 195 cases. J Pediatr 108:923, 1986

Newburger JW, Takahashi M, Burns JC, et al: The treatment of Kawasaki syndrome with intravenous gamma globulin. N Engl J Med 315:341, 1986

Takahashi M, Mason W, Lewis A: Regression of coronary artery aneurysms in patients with Kawasaki syndrome. Circulation 75:387, 1987

Virmani R, Rogan K, Cheitlin MD: Congenital coronary artery anomalies. In: Virmani R, Forman MB, eds: Nonatherosclerotic Ischemic Heart Disease. New York, Raven Press, 1989:153

Wesselhoeft H, Fawcett JS, Johnson AL: Anomalous origin of the left coronary artery from the pulmonary trunk: its clinical spectrum, pathology and pathophysiology based on a review of 140 cases with 7 further cases. Circulation 38:403, 1968

Primary

Berko BA, Swift M: X-linked dilated cardiomyopathy. N Engl J Med 316:1186, 1987

Burch M, Mann JM, Sharland M, et al: Myocardial disarray in Noonan syndrome. Br Heart J 68:586, 1992

Chan DP, Allen HD: Dilated congestive cardiomyopathy. In: Emmanouilides GC, Riemenschneider TA, Allen HD, Gutgesell HP, eds: Heart Disease in Infants, Children, and Adolescents, Including the Fetus and Young Adult. Baltimore, Williams & Wilkins, 1994:1365

Clark CE, Henry WL, Epstein SE: Familial prevalence and genetic transmission of idiopathic hypertrophic subaortic stenosis. N Engl J Med 289:709, 1973

Ehlers KH, Engle MA, Levin AR, et al: Eccentric ventricular hypertrophy in familial and sporadic instances of 46XX,XY Turner phenotype. Circulation 45:639, 1972

Factor SM, Sonnenblick EH: The pathogenesis of clinical and experimental congestive cardiomyopathies: recent concepts. Prog Cardiovasc Dis 27:395, 1985

Fananapazir L, Dalakas MC, Cyran F, et al: Missense mutations in the beta-myosin heavy-chain gene cause central core disease in hypertrophic cardiomyopathy. Proc Natl Acad Sci USA 90:3993, 1993

Ferencz C, Neill CA: Cardiomyopathy in infancy: observations in an epidemiologic study. Pediatr Cardiol 13:65, 1992

Geisterfer-Lowrance AA, Kass S, Tanigawa G, et al: A molecular basis for familial hypertrophic cardiomyopathy: a beta cardiac myosin heavy chain gene missense mutation. Cell 62:999, 1990

Griffin ML, Hernandez A, Martin TC, et al: Dilated cardiomyopathy in infants and children. J Am Coll Cardiol 11:139, 1988

Kelly DP, Strauss AW: Inherited cardiomyopathies. N Engl J Med 330:913, 1994

Lewis AB: Clinical profile and outcome of restrictive cardiomyopathy in children. Am Heart J 123:1589, 1992

Magliocco AM, Mitchell LB, Brownell AKW, et al: Dilated cardiomyopathy in multicore myopathy. Am J Cardiol 63:150, 1989

Manning JA, Keith JD: Fibro-elastosis in children. Prog Cardiovasc Dis 7:172, 1964

Marian AM, Roberts R: Molecular basis of hypertrophic and dilated cardiomyopathy. Texas Heart Inst J 21:6, 1994

Maron BJ: Hypertrophic cardiomyopathy. In: Emmanouilides GC, Riemenschneider TA, Allen HD, Gutgesell HP, eds: Heart Disease in Infants, Children, and Adolescents, Including the Fetus and Young Adult. Baltimore, Williams & Wilkins, 1994:1337

Maron BJ, Tajik AJ, Ruttenberg HD, et al: Hypertrophic cardiomyopathy in infants: clinical features and natural history. Circulation 65:7, 1982

Michels VV, Moll PP, Miller FA, et al: The frequency of familial dilated cardiomyopathy in a series of patients with idiopathic dilated cardiomyopathy. N Engl J Med 326:77, 1992

Moller JH, Lucas RV, Adams P Jr, et al: Endocardial fibroelastosis: a clinical and anatomic study of 47 patients with emphasis on the relationship to mitral insufficiency. Circulation 30:759, 1964

Rosenzweig A, Watkins H, Hwang DS, et al: Preclinical diagnosis of familial hypertrophic cardiomyopathy by genetic analysis of blood lymphocytes. N Engl J Med 325:1753, 1991

Spivak P: Myocardial disease. In: Moller JH, Neal WA, eds: Fetal, Neonatal, and Infant Cardiac Disease. Norwalk, CT, Appleton & Lange, 1990:809

Taliercio CP, Seward JP, Driscoll DJ, et al: Idiopathic dilated cardiomyopathy in the young: clinical profile and natural history. J Am Coll Cardiol 6:1126, 1985

Thiene G, Nava A, Corrado D, et al: Right ventricular cardiomyopathy and sudden death in young people. N Engl J Med 318:129, 1988

Thierfelder L, Watkins H, MacRae C, et al: Alpha-tropomyosin and cardiac troponin T mutations cause familial hypertrophic cardiomyopathy: a disease of the sarcomere. Cell 77:701, 1994

Towbin JA, Hejtmancik JF, Brink P, et al: X-linked dilated cardiomyopathy. Molecular genetic evidence of linkage to the Duchenne muscular dystrophy (dystrophin) gene at the Xp21 locus. Circulation 87:1854, 1993

Watkins H, Rosenzweig A, Hwang DS, et al: Characteristics and prognostic implications of myosin missense mutations in familial hypertrophic cardiomyopathy. N Engl J Med 326:1108, 1992

Neuromuscular

Ades LC, Gedeon AK, Wilson MJ, et al: Barth syndrome: clinical features and confirmation of gene localisation to distal Xq28. Am J Med Genet 45:327, 1993

Child JS, Perloff JK, Bach PM, et al: Cardiac involvement in Friedreich's ataxia: a clinical study of 75 patients. J Am Coll Cardiol 7:1370, 1986

Goldberg SJ, Stern LZ, Feldman L, et al: Serial left ventricular wall measurements in Duchenne's muscular dystrophy. J Am Coll Cardiol 2:136, 1983

Muller-Felber W, Rossmanith T, Spes C, et al: The clinical spectrum of Friedreich's ataxia in German families showing linkage to the FRDA locus on chromosome 9. Clin Invest 71:109, 1993

Neustein HB, Lurie PR, Dahms B, et al: An X-linked recessive cardiomyopathy with abnormal mitochondria. Pediatrics 64:24, 1979

22.4.2 Cardiac Tumors

Julien I. E. Hoffman

Cardiac tumors, especially primary tumors, are rare at any age. Most primary tumors have no systemic symptoms. They present with pericardial involvement (pain, effusion, tamponade), features of obstruction to blood flow (congestive heart failure, syncope, murmurs, chest pain), conduction defects, arrhythmias (including sudden death), or peripheral embolization. Occasionally they are found incidentally during cardiac imaging done for some other reason, including in fetuses. Some tumors, especially myxomas, may present with fever, malaise, weight loss, and increases in erythrocyte sedimentation rate, globulin, or interleukin-6 concentrations; these systemic features often simulate collagen vascular diseases or infective endocarditis.

Diagnosis of suspected tumors is usually by an imaging technique, usually transthoracic echocardiography. It can be supplemented by transesophageal echocardiography, magnetic resonance imaging, and cardiac catheterization and angiography.

PRIMARY NONMALIGNANT TUMORS (IN ORDER OF FREQUENCY)

Rhabdomyomas are the most common tumors. They are single or multiple, in the ventricles or ventricular septum, and distinguishable from the surrounding compressed myocardium. They usually cause death under 5 years of age by obstructing blood flow but often regress. They may also cause arrhythmias or heart block. About half of them are associated with the syndrome of tuberous sclerosis, and about half the patients with tuberous sclerosis have cardiac rhabdomyomas. Surgery can be done for isolated tumors.

Fibromas are usually solitary and in the ventricular walls; they are probably hamartomas. They may cause obstruction but more often cause heart block or ventricular arrhythmias. Surgical excision has been successful.

Myxomas are benign, usually pedunculated tumors that usually arise from the atrial septum near the foramen ovale; occasionally they attach elsewhere in the atria or the ventricles. They are more common in left than right atrium. Atrial myxomas may simulate mitral or tricuspid valve disease because they often prolapse into the valve ring to produce obstruction or incompetence; chest pain, dyspnea, or syncope may result. They can embolize to systemic or pulmonary arteries or obstruct pulmonary veins. They may be associated with fever, weight loss, anorexia, Raynaud syndrome, and increases in sedimentation rate, γ-globulins, and serum antihyaluronidase titers. These systemic symptoms result from release of cytokines, especially interleukin-6. The diagnosis may be suspected clinically, especially if the mitral or tricuspid murmurs change from time to time or with differences of position. Surgical removal is usually successful, except that recurrences often occur in the familial types. Myxomas may occur rarely with some familial cutaneous or endocrine syndromes.

Teratomas are rare and usually occur in infants. They arise at the base of the heart or within the pericardium and may cause obstruction or arrhythmias. Surgical excision is possible.

Hemangiomas are usually in the atrial walls and may cure themselves by thrombosis and fibrosis.

Atrioventricular nodal tumors are vascular lesions of the atrioventricular node. Most of the patients have complete heart block. Some present with sudden death. Because the tumors are small and confined to the AV node, they are easily missed at routine autopsy.

MALIGNANT TUMORS

The rare *primary malignant tumors* are usually sarcomas. They are often anaplastic and invasive and spread beyond the heart. Cure by surgery or chemotherapy is rare. Kaposi sarcoma, now seen more often because of its association with AIDS, is more often epicardial than myocardial and usually does not affect cardiac function.

Secondary metastatic malignant tumors can occur with non-Hodgkin lymphoma, neuroblastoma, Wilms tumor, and a variety of sarcomas. They may produce obstruction, usually right-sided.

References

Balian AA, Hogan TF: Cardiac tumors. In: Moller JH, Neal WA, eds: Fetal, Neonatal, and Infant Cardiac Disease. Norwalk, CT, Appleton & Lange, 1990:869

Burke B, Edwards JE, Titus JL: Tumors and tumor-like lesions of the heart and great vessels in the young. Advances in Pathology and Laboratory Medicine 5:357, 1992

Burke AP, Virmani R: Cardiac myxoma. A clinicopathologic study. Am J Clin Pathol 100:671, 1993

Carney JA, Gordon H, Carpenter PC, et al: The complex of myxomas, and endocrine overactivity. Medicine 64:270, 1985

Castells E, Ferran V, Octavio de Toledo MC, et al: Cardiac myxomas: surgical treatment, long-term results and recurrence. J Cardiovasc Surg 34: 49, 1993

Chan HS, Sonley MJ, Moes CA, et al: Primary and secondary tumors of childhood involving the heart, pericardium, and great vessels. A report of 75 cases and a review of the literature. Cancer 56:825, 1985

Colucci WS, Braunwald E: Primary tumors of the heart. In: Braunwald E, ed: Heart Disease: A Textbook of Cardiovascular Medicine, 4th ed. Philadelphia, WB Saunders, 1992:1451

Garson A Jr, Gillette PC, Titus JL, et al: Surgical treatment of ventricular tachycardia in infants. N Engl J Med 310:1443, 1984

Jourdan M, Bataille R, Seguin J, et al: Constitutive production of interleukin-6 and immunologic features in cardiac myxomas. Arthritis Rheum 33:398, 1990

Markel ML, Waller BF, Armstrong WF: Cardiac myxoma. A review. Medicine 66:114, 1987

Marx GR: Cardiac tumors. In: Emmanouilides GC, Riemenschneider TA, Allen HD, Gutgesell HP, eds: Heart Disease in Infants, Children, and Adolescents, Including the Fetus and Young Adult. Baltimore, Williams & Wilkins, 1994:1773

Molina JE, Edwards JE, Ward HB: Primary cardiac tumors: experience at the University of Minnesota. Thorac Cardiovasc Surg 38(Suppl 2):183, 1990

Rhodes AR, Silverman RA, Harrist TJ, et al: Mucocutaneous lentigines, cardiomucocutaneous myxomas and multiple blue nevi: the LAMB syndrome. J Am Acad Dermatol 10:72, 1984

Salcedo EE, Cohen GI, White RD, Davison MB: Cardiac tumors: diagnosis and management. Curr Prob Cardiol 17:73, 1992

Van Gelder HM, O'Brien DJ, Staples ED, Alexander JA: Familial cardiac myxoma. Ann Thorac Surg 53:419, 1992

Wiedermann CJ, Reinisch N, Fischer-Colbrie R, et al: Proinflammatory cytokines in cardiac myxomas. J Intern Med 232:263, 1992

22.4.3 Diseases of Pericardium

Julien I. E. Hoffman and Paul Stanger

Pericardial diseases cause pericarditis, pericardial effusion, or both; if the effusion makes the pericardium tense and impairs cardiac filling, then there is cardiac tamponade.

ACUTE PERICARDITIS

Acute pericarditis is an acute inflammation of the parietal pericardium and superficial myocardium. It is manifested by pain, a friction rub, electrocardiographic changes, and sometimes fever. The pain is precordial or referred to epigastrium, neck, shoulder, or left arm; it may be relieved by leaning forward and made worse by deep inspiration or coughing. Pain is not always present. The friction rub, heard most often along the left sternal border, has a grating sound like that produced by sandpaper on wood or may resemble creaking leather. Often the rub is brought out by firm pressure of the stethoscope on the chest or by having the patient lean forward, and it may vary with respiration or posture. It may be soft or loud, is often to-and-fro or with three components, and is always in phase with the heart sounds. The examiner must make sure that the stethoscope does not slip over the skin, particularly over bony prominences, because this may produce a sound like a friction rub. The electrocardiogram initially shows elevation of the S-T segments in most leads; after about 1 week the S-T segments return to normal and are associated with T-wave flattening and then inversion in the same leads. These changes may persist for months after the acute lesion has gone.

PERICARDIAL EFFUSION

Pericardial effusion may be serous, purulent, or bloody. It distends the pericardium and moves the parietal pericardium away from the heart. With a large effusion, the heart is quiet to palpation, all heart sounds are muffled, and on percussion the left border of cardiac dullness extends to the left of the apex beat. If there is pericarditis there may be a friction rub and the typical S-T and T-wave changes, but effusions may cause low QRS voltages or electrical alternans as well. Radiographically the cardiac silhouette is large and cannot be distinguished with certainty from cardiac dilatation, although the latter often shows associated pulmonary venous congestion. The diagnosis of pericardial effusion is best confirmed by echocardiography.

CARDIAC TAMPONADE Cardiac tamponade may occur with relatively little fluid if the pericardium is indistensible or if the fluid accumulates very rapidly. In contrast, a large effusion can form in a lax pericardium without causing tamponade. Once the pericardium becomes tense, pressure in the pericardial cavity rises and impairs cardiac relaxation and filling. Ventricular end-diastolic, atrial, and venous pressures rise on both sides of the heart by about equal amounts, and the liver enlarges. With reduced cardiac filling, cardiac output and stroke volume fall, giving tachycardia, low blood pressure, a narrow pulse pressure, and peripheral vasoconstriction with clammy, cold extremities and reduced skin perfusion.

Normally, with inspiration, intrathoracic pressure falls, and abdominal pressure rises, so that systemic venous return increases. With tamponade this increment in venous return cannot be accommodated in the heart; thus, the jugular venous pressure rises with inspiration (Kussmaul sign), although this sign is seen less frequently in tamponade than in constrictive pericarditis. Furthermore, with inspiration the pulmonary venous return and left ventricular output fall for two reasons. The increased systemic venous return distends the right atrium and ventricle, which, because of the tense pericardium, compress the left atrium and ventricle and reduce their input and thus their output. Second, the tense pericardium acts as a rigid box around the heart, so that when intrathoracic pressure falls on inspiration the pressure gradient from pulmonary veins to left atrium is reduced, and again left-sided filling is reduced. As a result of these mechanisms, inspiration causes aortic blood pressure to fall more than usual—the *pulsus paradoxus.* Normally, deep inspiration may drop aortic blood pressure 4 to 10 mm Hg; any greater fall is abnormal. To detect this change, place a sphygmomanometer cuff on the arm and determine the blood pressure in the usual way. Then inflate the cuff to just above systolic pressure, and deflate the cuff slowly until the first Korotkoff sounds appear. Maintain pressure and determine if the sounds disappear with inspiration. If they do, lower cuff pressure in steps of 2 mm Hg and note when the sounds first persist throughout the respiratory cycle. The difference between the two levels is the amount of pulsus paradoxus. The difference is also noted in diastole but is easier to measure in systole. Pulsus paradoxus also occurs with airway obstruction, as in asthma, but the pulmonary findings identify this cause. It has also been noted with a big pulmonary embolus or tense ascites. Pulsus paradoxus may be absent in tamponade if there is preexisting severe left ventricular failure, hypovolemia, an atrial septal defect, or severe aortic incompetence.

Although the diagnosis of pericardial effusion may be verified by echocardiography, cardiac tamponade is best diagnosed by physical examination; Kussmaul sign in the jugular veins and the pulsus paradoxus are the crucial criteria. Recently Doppler echocardiography has shown that in tamponade there is an inspiratory increase in early diastolic flow across the tricuspid valve but a decrease in early diastolic mitral flow. It is important to note that tamponade can occur with a relatively small effusion if the effusion forms rapidly

or the pericardium is indistensible, so that the size of the cardiac shadow may not be significant in diagnosis. Furthermore, patients with enlarged hearts can get an effusion and tamponade that might be interpreted as worsening of heart failure; here, too, pulsus paradoxus will lead to the right diagnosis.

PERICARDIOCENTESIS Pericardiocentesis may be used to remove pericardial fluid for diagnostic study or to decompress the pericardial cavity if there is severe tamponade. Lesser degrees of tamponade may be managed conservatively, provided that the patient can be observed closely during treatment; vital signs should be taken frequently. If tamponade gets worse or is severe when the patient is first seen, then fluid should be removed.

Have the patient, sedated if necessary, lying at about 45° to the horizontal with the head raised. Clean and sterilize the precordium and apply sterile drapes with full aseptic technique. Infiltrate the skin and subcutaneous tissue with local anesthetic just below the xiphoid process. Connect the patient to the limb leads of an electrocardiograph and attach the V lead by a sterile connector to a 20-gauge needle on a syringe. (Make sure that the electrocardiograph has been checked to exclude any significant current leakage.) Start the paper of the electrocardiograph running, insert the needle through the skin just below the xiphoid process, and push it slowly toward the midthoracic spine; the needle should be at an angle of about 20° below the perpendicular to the body wall. Attempt to remove fluid with the syringe after each 1 or 2 mm of penetration; as soon as fluid enters the syringe, clamp a hemostat to the needle at the point of entry into the skin to avoid further penetration. If the needle touches the heart, the V lead will show marked S-T elevation because of an injury current; this current is too local to be seen on the usual limb leads. When this injury current is seen, withdraw the needle until the S-T segment returns to normal. Remove the fluid until it ceases to come out easily, and do not try to get more out by moving the needle, as this may injure the heart. A safer method of removing pericardial fluid is to place a 22-gauge lumbar puncture needle with a stylet into a 20-gauge flexible plastic tube, such as Angiocath. Once fluid comes out through the needle, advance the plastic tube over the needle, which can then be withdrawn; the soft plastic tube is less likely to cause myocardial damage. If the fluid does not come out or is thick, refer to a surgeon, who can then remove fluid through a small opening in the pericardium. Pericardiocentesis can be lifesaving but can also cause dysrhythmias or serious bleeding into the pericardium. Therefore, except in emergencies, it should be done only when adequate help is available and when facilities for resuscitation are present. If available, guidance by two-dimensional echocardiography reduces risks and is particularly helpful if the effusion is loculated.

CHRONIC CONSTRICTIVE PERICARDITIS

Chronic constrictive pericarditis is an uncommon sequel to acute pericarditis. It is seen most often after tuberculous or suppurative pericarditis or mediastinal radiation and is very rare after acute rheumatic pericarditis. There is massive fibrous proliferation that obliterates the pericardial cavity and often calcifies. This produces chronic tamponade, so that there is gradual development of marked hepatomegaly, ascites, and pleural effusion, but peripheral edema is not marked, and pulmonary edema is rare. Intestinal venous congestion may cause protein-losing enteropathy and hypoalbuminemia, leading to the misdiagnosis of liver disease or nephrosis.

The heart is quiet to palpation and often not much enlarged. A prominent early third sound (pericardial knock) is common and coincides with the rapid fall in jugular venous pressure (steep descent) when the tricuspid valve opens and blood rushes from the high-pressure right atrium to the relatively indistensible right ventricle. A raised jugular venous pressure with Kussmaul sign and pulsus paradoxus are more frequent than with acute tamponade. The electrocardiogram may show low-voltage and nonspecific T-wave changes. The echocardiogram is also nonspecific but often shows a flattened posterior left ventricular wall with little motion. With inspiration, early diastolic flow increases at the tricuspid valve but decreases at the mitral valve. These changes help to distinguish constrictive pericarditis from restrictive cardiomyopathy. The thick pericardium is best shown by computerized axial tomography or magnetic resonance imaging. The diagnosis can be confirmed at cardiac catheterization. Treatment consists of surgical removal of the restricting fibrous tissue. The results are not always good, either because the fibrous tissue was not completely removed, coronary arteries were damaged, or diffuse fibrosis extended into the myocardium from the surface. To decrease the risk of occurrence of constrictive pericarditis, patients with purulent or tuberculous pericarditis should be referred early for surgical treatment.

SPECIFIC DISEASES

The causes of pericarditis are given in Table 22-18, and some of them are discussed in more detail below.

INFECTION

RHEUMATIC FEVER Acute rheumatic fever with extensive pancarditis is now uncommon in the United States. Pericarditis usually occurs after or with valvulitis and myocarditis, but the friction rub and effusion may mask the other features. Tamponade and constrictive pericarditis are very rare. Treatment is discussed above.

ACUTE NONSPECIFIC PERICARDITIS Acute nonspecific pericarditis, thought to be viral, often follows a respiratory infection. Sometimes the causative agent can be identified in pericardial fluid by serologic tests or PCR. The pericarditic phase is manifested by fever, malaise, anorexia, and pericardial pain; in infants there are also tachycardia and tachypnea. There is a polymorphonuclear leukocytosis. A pericardial friction rub and effusions are common, and typical electrocardiographic changes are seen. The patients are not usually very ill, and tamponade and constrictive pericarditis are rare. Recovery occurs spontaneously in 2 to 4 weeks. Treatment is usually symptomatic with or without nonsteroidal antiinflammatory agents, but steroids may be needed occasionally for recurrent or unusually severe or long-lasting disease.

About 25 to 50% of children with HIV have an effusion, but tamponade is rare.

PURULENT PERICARDITIS Purulent pericarditis usually occurs by extension from a septic focus in the lung (pneumonia or empyema) but may occur with septicemia or, rarely, after cardiac surgery. The common organisms are staphylococci, pneumococci, streptococci, *Haemophilus influenzae,* and meningococci; these organisms can usually be isolated from blood and pericardial fluid. The incidence of *H. influenzae* infections has, however, been declining with early immunization practices. The illness has an acute onset, with a high swinging fever, marked polymorphonuclear leukocytosis, and severe toxicity. Often symptoms are modified if the patient has been

TABLE 22-18

ETIOLOGY[a] OF PERICARDITIS

A. **Idiopathic, presumed viral**
B. Acute infections:
  (1) **Viral-coxsackie A and B,** echovirus, adenovirus, mumps virus, influenza virus, varicella zoster and vaccinia viruses, infectious mononucleosis, psittacosis-lymphogranuloma venereum group, cytomegalovirus, rubella, herpes simplex, **human immunodeficiency virus**
  (2) **Bacterial-staphylococci, pneumococci, *Haemophilus influenzae,*** meningococci, streptococci, *Salmonella,* mycobacteria with HIV infection
  (3) Mycoplasma
  (4) Protozoa—amebae, toxoplasmosis
  (5) Rickettsia— *Coxiella burnetii*
C. Physical causes:
  (1) **Hemopericardium and pericarditis after chest trauma or cardiac surgery**
  (2) **Serous or serosanguineous effusions after cardiac trauma, cardiac surgery, or myocardial infarction; all may result from autoimmune mechanisms**
  (3) Perforation of right atrium by indwelling lines, even soft silastic catheters
  (4) Chest wall radiation
D. Chronic infections:
  (1) **Tuberculosis,** actinomycosis, nocardiasis
  (2) Fungi—histoplasmosis, coccidiomycosis, *Candida* sp, aspergillosis, blastomycosis
  (3) Hydatid disease
E. Associated with anasarca in congestive heart failure, nephrosis, or cirrhosis of the liver
F. Vasculitis syndromes, especially systemic lupus erythematosus, rheumatoid arthritis, and rheumatic fever, but also scleroderma, polyarteritis, Wegener granulomatosis, Behçet syndrome, Reiter syndrome, Whipple disease
G. Metabolic disorders—uremia, **myxedema,** gout
H. Hemodialysis
I. Congenital heart disease, cardiomyopathy
J. Benign and malignant tumors
K. Foreign bodies in the pericardial cavity
L. Drugs—hydralazine, procainamide, phenytoin, isoniazid, phenylbutazone, methysergide, penicillin, anticoagulants, practolol, minoxidil
M. Certain anemias—sickle cell disease, thalassemia, congenital aplastic anemia
N. Miscellaneous—dissecting aneurysm, acute pancreatitis, sarcoidosis, multiple myeloma, amyloidosis, Kawasaki syndrome, ulcerative colitis

[a] The most common causes are printed in **bold** type.

treated with antibiotics for the primary illness. In these patients in particular, tamponade is common. Intensive treatment with appropriate antibiotics alone has a high mortality. Addition of surgical drainage of the pericardial cavity reduces mortality and decreases the risk of later constrictive pericarditis. Close observation for tamponade is essential. Constrictive pericarditis may follow cure, so that an extended follow-up is necessary.

TUBERCULOUS PERICARDITIS Tuberculous pericarditis usually complicates tuberculosis elsewhere. It starts insidiously with malaise, anorexia, low-grade fever, and night sweats, and then the typical features of pericarditis develop; there may be an effusion. Diagnosis is by a positive tuberculin test, isolation of tubercle bacilli from pericardial fluid, sputum, or gastric washings, and histologic examination of the pericardium. Adenosine deaminase concentrations in the pericardial fluid usually exceed 50 U/L. PCR may help to identify the organism. Antituberculous therapy is effective, but because constrictive pericarditis is a common sequel, some experts advocate early pericardiectomy to avoid having to remove dense fibrous tissue later. Other causes of chronic infectious pericarditis are various fungi as well as actinomycosis or nocardiosis.

NONINFECTIOUS CAUSES

TRAUMA Hemopericardium occurs after blunt or penetrating trauma, including cardiac massage, and tamponade may occur rapidly, so that emergency pericardiocentesis may be needed while preparations are made for surgery. Constrictive pericarditis is a rare sequel. Tamponade may also occur with bleeding after cardiac surgery and must be considered whenever there is a low-cardiac-output syndrome in the postoperative period.

COLLAGEN DISEASES In rheumatoid arthritis, pericarditis and high fevers may precede joint involvement. Treatment should be by salicylates first, with steroids reserved for refractory lesions. Systemic lupus erythematosus may have associated pericarditis with effusions and occasionally cardiac tamponade. The effusion may persist after other symptoms disappear with steroid therapy. Other collagen vascular diseases may also cause pericarditis.

UREMIA Pericarditis and effusions, even tamponade, may occur with chronic uremia. The disorder may be difficult to diagnose because of cardiomegaly and heart failure in some patients. With longer survival as a result of hemodialysis or transplantation, constrictive pericarditis has occasionally developed.

MISCELLANEOUS Pericarditis and effusions may occur after radiation of the chest, with foreign bodies in or near the pericardium, and with the rare tumors that occur there. If effusions after radiation persist beyond 2 to 3 months, a pericardial window may be created surgically to permit drainage. Dissecting aneurysm, hypothyroidism, sarcoidosis, multiple myeloma, and acute pancreatitis are rare causes. Pericardial effusions are seen with fetal hydrops.

POSTPERICARDIOTOMY SYNDROME The postpericardiotomy syndrome may follow any operation in which the pericardium is opened. The syndrome is not common in infants. Up to 30% of these patients have attacks of acute pericarditis and fever beginning about 1 to 4 weeks (range 3 days to 6 months) after surgery. There is often a pericardial effusion and sometimes a pleural effusion that need not be on the side of the thoracotomy. Although echocardiography is the mainstay of diagnosis, an effusion per se does not make the diagnosis because about 50% of children after a cardiac operation with a pericardiotomy have a small effusion at the time of discharge from hospital. There are a mild polymorphonuclear leukocytosis and an increased sedimentation rate. Patients with the syndrome have high titers of a heart-reactive antibody, and 70% show an acute rise of antibodies to adenoviruses, coxsackie B, or cytomegalovirus. The current belief is that an immune response is triggered by viral invasion of traumatized myocardial tissue. A similar syndrome can occur after pulmonary infarction.

Treatment by bed rest and acetylsalicylic acid (120 mg/kg/d) is usually effective. Once the acute attack is under control, the acetylsalicylic acid can be slowly withdrawn over 6 weeks; more rapid withdrawal may lead to recurrences, which may occur in 10 to 15% of patients in any event. Occasionally steroids may be needed if there is no response to this treatment.

CONGENITAL LESIONS Congenital pericardial lesions are rare. Localized *pericardial defects* occur most often on the left side. The left atrium can herniate through the defect, and this may cause chest pain, syncope, or dysrhythmias. If the defect is larger, so that the left ventricle herniates through, the coronary artery could be compressed; death from this cause has been reported. The pulmonary artery may herniate and give the appearance of a dilated pulmonary artery. Congenital pericardial cysts or diverticula usually occur on the right side. They are seldom large but cause problems of diagnosis. Echocardiography, computerized tomography, magnetic resonance imaging, and angiography are helpful in diagnosis.

References

Congenital Lesions

Gehlmann HR, Van Ingen GJ: Symptomatic congenital complete absence of the left pericardium. Eur Heart J 10:670, 1989

Nasser WK: Congenital defects of the pericardium. In: Fowler NO, ed: The Pericardium in Health and Disease. Mt Kisco, NY, Futura, 1985

Nasser WK, Helman C, Tavel ME, et al: Congenital absence of the left pericardium: clinical, electrocardiographic, radiographic, hemodynamic, and angiographic findings in 6 cases. Circulation 41:469, 1970

Van Son JAM, Danielson GK, Schaff HV, et al: Congenital partial and complete absence of the pericardium. Mayo Clin Proc 68:743, 1993

Pericarditis

Dupuis C, Gronnier P, Kachaner J, et al: Bacterial pericarditis in infancy and childhood. Am J Cardiol 74:807, 1994

Engle MA, Ehlers KM, O'Loughlin JE, et al: The post-pericardiotomy syndrome: iatrogenic illness and immunologic and virologic components. Cardiovasc Clin 11:381, 1981

Engle MA, Gay WA Jr, Kaminsky ME, et al: The postpericardiotomy syndrome then and now. Curr Probl Cardiol 3:1–40, 1978

Fowler, NO: Cardiac tamponade. A clinical or an echocardiographic diagnosis? Circulation 87:1738, 1993

Golinko RJ, Kaplan N, Rudolph AM: The mechanism of pulsus paradoxus during acute pericardial tamponade. J Clin Invest 42:249, 1963

Hier-Madsenk K, Sauamäki KI, Wulff J, et al: Purulent pericarditis in children. Scand J Thorac Cardiovasc Surg 19:185, 1985

Hoit BD: Imaging the pericardium. Cardiol Clin 8:587, 1990

Huggo-Hamman CT, Scher H, De Moor MM: Tuberculous pericarditis in children: a review of 44 cases. Pediatr Infect Dis 13:13, 1994

Klein AL, Cohen GI: Doppler echocardiographic assessment of constrictive pericarditis, cardiac amyloidosis, and cardiac tamponade. Cleve Clin J Med 59:278, 1992

Komsuoglu B, Goldeli O, Kulan K, Komsuoglu SS: The diagnostic and prognostic value of adenosine deaminase in tuberculous pericarditis. Eur Heart J 16:1126, 1995

Maisch B: Immunologic regulator and effector functions in perimyocarditis, postmyocarditis heart muscle disease and dilated cardiomyopathy. Basic Res Cardiol 81:217, 1986

Masui T, Finck S, Higgins CB: Constrictive pericarditis and restrictive cardiomyopathy: evaluation with MR imaging. Radiology 182:369, 1992

Pandian NG, Brockway B, Simonetti J, et al: Pericardiocentesis under two dimensional echocardiographic guidance in located pericardial effusion. Ann Thorac Surg 45:99, 1988

Permanyer-Miralda G, Sagrista-Sauleda J, Soler-Soler J: Primary acute pericardial disease: a prospective study of 231 consecutive patients. Am J Cardiol 56:623, 1985

Reddy PS, Leon DF, Shaver JA: Pericardial Diseases. New York, Raven Press, 1982

Reeder GS: Pericardial disease: echocardiographic and hemodynamic aspects. Curr Opin Cardiol 4:417, 1989

Shabetai R: The Pericardium. New York, Grune & Stratton, 1981

Shabetai R: Pericardial and cardiac pressure. Circulation 77:1, 1988

Spodick DH: Advances in the diagnosis and management of clinical pericardial disease. Curr Opin Cardiol 4:412, 1989

Spodick DH: Acute clinically noneffusive ("dry") pericarditis. In: Spodick DH, ed: The Pericardium: A Comprehensive Textbook, vol 1. Amsterdam, Marcel Dekker, 1997

Vaitkus PT, Kussmaul WG: Constrictive pericarditis versus restrictive cardiomyopathy: a reappraisal and update of diagnostic criteria. Am Heart J 122:1431, 1991.

22.4.4   Congestive Heart Failure

Norman S. Talner and Michael P. Carboni

The clinical syndrome of congestive heart failure as seen in infants and children represents the inability of the heart and circulation to meet the metabolic demands of the body despite various compensatory hemodynamic and neurohumoral mechanisms. This clinical picture may emerge when the myocardium is subjected to excessive loading conditions (volume and/or pressure), primary alterations in contractile function, marked changes in chronotropic state (tachy- or bradydysrhythmias), or various combinations of these factors. As a result, signs develop of pulmonary and systemic venous congestion, impaired systemic perfusion, and findings that indicate such adaptive mechanisms as changes in heart rate, vasoconstrictor tone, renal function, and ventricular hypertrophy. Over time, these changes may become maladaptive.

Congestive heart failure in a child represents an extremely high-risk situation that demands prompt recognition, stabilization of the patient, and safe transport to a pediatric cardiovascular center for management that in many instances may include surgical intervention.

ETIOLOGIC BASIS FOR HEART FAILURE

The specific etiology for heart failure in the pediatric age group tends to vary with the patient's age at presentation, eg, fetus, newborn, young infant, older child, or adolescent. The following discussion presents the leading causes of heart failure in each of these groups.

In the fetus, nonimmune hydrops fetalis, the clinical expression of heart failure in utero, is usually associated with tachyarrhythmias, blood group incompatibilities (Rh), or inflammatory disorders (parvovirus) and is only rarely associated with an underlying cardiac malformation. This is primarily because of the presence of the placenta for gas exchange, the fetal flow pathways that permit a bypass for obstructive lesions, and the high pulmonary vascular resistance that limits pulmonary blood flow. A large systemic arteriovenous fistula or massive tricuspid regurgitation as with the Ebstein malformation are exceptions, producing severe heart failure in utero.

Heart failure that presents during the first week of life is primarily from congenital cardiac malformations with usually a component of ductus arteriosus–dependent systemic perfusion (hypoplastic left heart syndrome, interruption of aortic arch, and coarctation of the aorta). Non–ductus-dependent systemic blood flow compromise may also be seen with critical aortic stenosis as well as myocardial ischemia secondary to birth asphyxia. Other causes include inflammatory diseases of the myocardium, adrenal

disease, hyper- and hypothyroidism, renal artery hypertension, tachyarrhythmias, and the high-output state of a large arteriovenous malformation. Total anomalous venous return with pulmonary venous obstruction in this age group may have satisfactory systemic perfusion because of a right-to-left shunt via the foramen ovale, so that severe hypoxemia in association with pulmonary venous congestion dominates the clinical picture, one that is often confused with a primary pulmonary disorder.

In the preterm infant a patent ductus arteriosus is the most common cause of heart failure, usually as a complication of respiratory distress syndrome. The early presentation with left-to-right shunting with a PDA is probably related to the limited ability of the small pulmonary arteries of the premature infant to constrict, coupled with the limited distensibility of immature myocardium that diminishes its ability to tolerate a volume load.

Congestive heart failure after the first 2 weeks of life may still arise from coarctation of the aorta or aortic stenosis, so that the clinician must be alert to this possibility as well as entertaining the diagnosis of a septic process when an infant presents with the acute onset of impaired systemic perfusion. Beyond 2 weeks and up to 3 months of age, large-volume left-to-right shunt lesions with increased pulmonary blood flow predominate. This type of lesion requires a postnatal fall in pulmonary vascular resistance before clinical manifestations become evident. Examples include the large ventricular septal defect, patent ductus arteriosus, and atrioventricular canal defect as well as the less common mixing lesions such as single ventricle, truncus arteriosus, and transposition of the great arteries with a large ventricular communication. The common mixing group may present earlier because of a hypoxemic component in addition to the increase in pulmonary blood flow, or in certain instances one ventricle doing the work of two. Another lesion that depends on the postnatal decrease in pulmonary vascular resistance is that of the anomalous origin of the left coronary artery from the pulmonary trunk.

Heart failure that presents initially in the older child and adolescent may be caused by an acquired disease or be a complication of an existing cardiac malformation (bacterial endocarditis, residual defects, arrhythmias, myocardial dysfunction), particularly if the child has had prior palliative cardiac surgery or repair. The acquired diseases include myopericarditis, acute rheumatic carditis and heart disease, other vasculitides, dilated and hypertrophic cardiomyopathies, metabolic derangements, neuromuscular diseases, cardiotoxic drugs (anthracyclines), immune deficiency diseases, Kawasaki syndrome, severe anemias, Lyme disease, substance abuse, and chronic airway obstructive disease (enlarged tonsils and adenoids, cystic fibrosis).

The etiology of congestive heart failure based on age at presentation is listed in Table 22-19.

FUNDAMENTAL MECHANISMS

Heart failure from any cause represents the inability of the heart to meet the demands for blood flow without excessive use of physiological compensatory mechanisms. Of these causes, the most prominent is an increase in stroke volume associated with an increase in ventricular volume—the Frank-Starling effect. When symptoms arise, they represent the effect of increased filling volumes and pressure on the pulmonary and systemic circulations. The Frank-Starling mechanism operates irrespective of the cause of the clinical syndrome. With volume loading (valvar regurgitation, left to right shunts, A-V fistulas, severe anemia), there is a need for

TABLE 22-19

ETIOLOGY OF HEART FAILURE BASED ON TIME OF PRESENTATION

Fetus
  Tachyarrhythmia
  Anemia
    Hemolytic diseases
    Parvovirus
  Arteriovenous malformation
  Tricuspid regurgitation (Ebstein malformation)
  Premature closure of foramen ovale
  Complete heart block
At birth
  Structural malformations
    Tricuspid regurgitation
    Pulmonary regurgitation
    Arteriovenous malformation
  Perinatal asphyxia
    Global dysfunction
    Tricuspid regurgitation
  Tachyarrhythmia
  Complete heart block
Age 1–7 days
  Structural abnormalities
    Hypoplastic left heart syndrome
    Aortic stenosis
    Anomalous pulmonary venous return with obstruction
    PDA (preterm infants)
  Common mixing lesions
    Truncus arteriosus
    Single ventricle with TPBF
  Pulmonary disorders
    Persistent pulmonary hypertension
    Airway obstruction
  Renal disease
    Failure
    Hypertension
  Endocrine disease
    Hyperthyroid
    Adrenal
    Infant of diabetic mother with left heart obstruction
Infancy (1–6 weeks)
  Structural abnormalities
    Coarctation

  Left-to-right shunt lesions
    VSD, AV canal, PDA, etc
  Common mixing lesions
  Anomalous left coronary artery
Disorders of cardiac muscle
  Glycogen storage disease
  Dilated cardiomyopathies
Renal disease (as above)
Endocrine (as above) and hypothyroidism
Airway obstructive disease
Older child and adolescent
  Preexisting structural heart disease (with or without preceding surgery)
    AV or semilunar valve regurgitation
    Decreased inotropic state
    Infectious endocarditis
    Pulmonary vascular obstructive disease
    Chronic tachyarrhythmia
  Cardiomyopathies
    Dilated
    Hypertrophic
    Restrictive
    Postmyocarditis
  Inflammatory disorders
    Myocarditis
    Collagen vascular disease
    Rheumatic fever and RHD
    Kawasaki syndrome
    HIV
    Sepsis (meningococcal, staphylococcal, etc)
  Endocrine disease (as previous)
  Renal disease (as previous)
  Systemic hypertension
  Primary pulmonary hypertension
  Chronic tachyarrhythmia
  Heart block
Miscellaneous
  Neuromuscular diseases
  Marfan syndrome
  Noonan syndrome
  Hunter-Hurler syndrome

higher stroke volumes, which the circulatory system provides by increasing ventricular filling volumes and pressures until symptoms occur. If the heart has an increase in afterload (impedance to ejection), such as in aortic or pulmonary stenosis and systemic or pulmonary hypertension, a primary decrease in myocardial contractility, or diastolic dysfunction, stroke volume is decreased for any given end-diastolic pressure. To maintain stroke volume, end-diastolic pressure and volume are increased, and the patient becomes symptomatic.

Disorders in the chronotropic function of the heart (tachyarrhythmias) or associated with pericardial disease may acutely impede cardiac filling and cardiac output. In their chronic stages, tachyarrhythmias may also be associated with depressed systolic function. Chronic pericardial disease with constriction leads to elevated filling pressures, particularly left ventricular, and venous congestion ensues. With acute tamponade, however, the primary response is that of poor forward cardiac output and less pulmonary vascular congestion.

MATURATIONAL ASPECTS OF CARDIOVASCULAR PERFORMANCE

There are important developmental aspects of cardiac performance that influence the appearance of the clinical signs of heart failure. The normal maturing cardiovascular system operates at a high diastolic volume, and thus diastolic reserve in the infant may be less than in the adult. The myocardial response to an acute increase in afterload in the young also appears to be impaired, a factor that relates to a diminished ability to develop tension as impedance to ejection is raised. Although the developing myocardium appears to respond appropriately to sympathetic stimulation, contractile reserve appears to be limited as norepinephrine stores are diminished. An increase in heart rate via the sympathetic nervous system and the ability to vasoconstrict and modify regional organ perfusion, however, occur at all postnatal ages.

The mechanical properties of the developing myocardium differ from those of the adult. Ventricular compliance is diminished, and the heart exhibits a greater resting tension for any increment in diastolic stretch. Excitation-contraction coupling studies in the developing mammal also indicate that the movement of calcium ion from extracellular sites to the contractile elements occupies a greater role in the excitatory process than the release of calcium from the sarcoplasmic reticulum.

ADAPTIVE MECHANISMS

The clinician must understand not only the fundamental alterations in myocardial performance that may result in heart failure but also the important contributions of the major neurohumoral mechanisms that play a key role in the pathophysiology of heart failure, particularly in its the later stages. The Frank-Starling mechanism increases ventricular wall stress and myocardial oxygen demands. An early adaptive mechanism that occurs during the clinical course of heart failure is myocardial hypertrophy in which wall stress moves closer to normal. This occurs as a response to a variety of hemodynamic, neurohumoral, hormonal, and pathologic stimuli as the heart attempts to adapt to the increased demands for cardiac work by increasing muscle mass. At the cellular level, the cardiac myocyte responds to mechanical stress by initiating a number of processes that lead to hypertrophy. The induction of natriuretic peptides and fetal contractile proteins characterizes the hypertrophic response along with recent evidence that myocyte loss may occur as a result of programmed cell death (apoptosis). The signaling pathways for cardiac hypertrophy and heart failure are now potential therapeutic and molecular targets. Although the hypertrophic response is important in attempting to maintain systolic function, there are maladaptive consequences as well. These include increased metabolic demands for the coronary circulation and increased production of fibrous tissue as well as muscle mass, which may interfere with ventricular filling by altering ventricular compliance.

Considerable attention has been focused on neurohumoral elements that are activated in response to the hemodynamic stresses that cause heart failure. An increase in sympathoadrenal activity combining catecholamines released from synaptic nerve terminals and from the adrenal gland occupies an important role in the adaptation to heart failure. The major effects of adrenergic stimulation include sinus tachycardia, an increase in vasomotor tone, which permits a redistribution of cardiac output to vital organ systems (heart and brain) while limiting blood flow to other areas (skin, kidneys, gastrointestinal tract), and an initial increase in myocardial contractility. Chronic activation of the adrenergic systems may have deleterious consequences as well. These include an increase in metabolic rate that raises oxygen demands, sweating, and eventually desensitization of the myocardial adrenergic pathway. The latter has been associated with a decrease in density of β-adrenergic receptors on the surface of myocardial cells and functional loss of the catecholamine-mediated positive inotropic response. These observations have led to the therapeutic use of β-adrenoreceptor blockade in chronic congestive heart failure secondary to a dilated cardiomyopathy in order to modulate many of these adverse effects.

Similarly, the circulating humoral agent angiotensin II, a potent vasoconstrictor, participates in key adaptive responses that are initially useful but become maladaptive. Mechanical stress on cardiac myocytes, as might be induced by cardiac dilatation, causes the myocardium to release local angiotensin II secretory granules, which then act to initiate the hypertrophic response (protooncogene expression). At the same time, however, angiotensin II acts on cardiac fibroblasts to promote fibrosis. Thus, although the hypertrophic response is adaptive by restoring wall stress to normal,

by initiating fibrosis and thereby altering ventricular compliance, it is maladaptive as well. These observations on the function of angiotensin II have led to the development of angiotensin-converting enzyme inhibitors and angiotensin-receptor blockade in order to provide vasodilatation and thereby decrease afterload on the myocardium and, in addition, to modulate the ventricular remodeling process.

Although the adrenergic system and angiotensin II appear to be the principal neurohumoral mechanisms in congestive heart failure, other mechanisms have been implicated, although their precise roles remain to be clearly defined. These include atrial natriuretic factor, neuropeptide Y, endothelin, and nitric oxide as well as a number of growth factors, particularly tissue necrosis factor.

There is now evidence at the cellular level that points to a key role of the sarcolemmal sodium-calcium exchanger in the adaptive response to the various stresses induced by a dilated cardiomyopathic process. This exchanger functions as a regulator of cytosolic and stored calcium in cardiac myocytes and thus serves as a major determinant of systolic and diastolic function.

The regulation of body fluid volume (sodium and water excretion) in heart failure patients is controlled by cardiac output and the peripheral circulation. Thus, either a fall in cardiac output or arterial vasodilatation causes arterial underfilling, which activates the various neurohumoral mechanisms that stimulate sodium and water retention. This explains why a volume increase occurs with either a low- or high-cardiac-output form of heart failure. The decrease in relative filling of the arterial circulation results in an increase in sympathetic nervous system activity, nonosmotic release of arginine vasopressin, and activation of the renin-angiotensin-aldosterone system. Each of these serves to decrease renal perfusion and provide the basis for decreased sodium and water excretion and the increase of blood volume that contributes to the hemodynamic alterations observed in heart failure patients.

An additional compensatory mechanism that permits improved oxygen delivery to the tissues by facilitating oxygen unloading resides in the red blood cell. A rightward shift in the oxyhemoglobin dissociation curve via increased 2,3-diphosphoglycerate results in an increase in P50 (oxygen tension at 50% oxygen saturation), thus favoring oxygen release to the tissues. Increased levels of 2,3-DPG have been found in certain infants in heart failure but not in newborns or preterm infants who have a high proportion of fetal hemoglobin.

THE CLINICAL EXPRESSION OF HEART FAILURE

PULMONARY VENOUS CONGESTION Elevation of left-sided filling pressures (atrial and pulmonary venous) causes transudation of fluid into the pulmonary interstitial space and, if massive, into alveolar spaces as well. Increased water in the pulmonary interstitial space stimulates receptors that produce rapid shallow breathing (60–80/min) or tachypnea. If the alveolar spaces are invaded, then and only then may rales be heard. Thus, interstitial pulmonary edema may exist without auscultatory evidence of alveolar involvement. Lung water is cleared via peribronchial and perivascular spaces into lymphatics. As this takes place, there may be peribronchiolar edema that increases airway resistance and may become manifest as wheezing. This can easily be confused with the findings observed in bronchiolitis or acute asthma. The important point is that wheezing may arise from several causes, one of which is an elevated pulmonary venous pressure. The increase in respiratory rate and effort increases oxygen demands by the increased work of breathing and makes the infant tire easily while feeding.

SYSTEMIC VENOUS CONGESTION The elevation of right-sided filling pressures that may occur with heart failure produces systemic venous congestion. In the infant this is most commonly manifest as hepatomegaly. In the older child distended neck veins and edema, particularly of the eyelids, may be observed; peripheral edema and ascites are relatively rare.

SYSTEMIC PERFUSION When heart failure is dominated by impaired systemic perfusion, as with coarctation and cardiomyopathies, the clinical picture is dominated by signs of diminished arterial pulsations and impaired capillary refill. Therefore, a careful appraisal of pulse volume including the brachial, femoral, and carotid pulses are in order together with blood pressure determinations in both arms and leg. It should be emphasized that a 20 mm Hg difference between arm and leg is a significant difference when perfusion is impaired by the marked curtailment in systemic blood flow.

Pulse volume may be increased in heart failure when there is a low systemic resistance (anemia, arteriovenous malformation) or aortic or truncal runoff lesions such as patent ductus arteriosus, aorticopulmonary window, truncus arteriosus, or severe aortic regurgitation (all of which also dilate peripheral arterioles).

CARDIAC FINDINGS Precordial activity may be exaggerated with volume loading, whereas activity is diminished with impaired ventricular contractility or accumulation of fluid in the pericardial space. A gallop rhythm may be appreciated in patients with myocardial or pericardial disease and suggests diminished filling of a stiff, poorly compliant ventricle. In many of the cardiac malformations that may be associated with heart failure, the classical murmur of the defect may be present but may be modified by respiratory complications or diminished cardiac output.

In the newborn, in severe heart failure, always listen over the anterior fontanelle for a bruit that might indicate a systemic arteriovenous fistula.

The adaptive mechanisms that operate as heart failure develops are responsible for many of the clinical findings. Evidence for enhanced sympathoadrenal activity includes tachycardia, pallor (vasoconstriction), decreased urine output (decreased renal blood flow), and sweating. The major chronic effect of impaired cardiac performance, particularly in the infant, is that of growth failure, whereas in the older child diminished exercise tolerance tends to predominate.

The principal clinical-physiological correlates are listed in Table 22-20.

LABORATORY AIDS IN DIAGNOSIS

CHEST ROENTGENOGRAM A chest x-ray that shows an enlarged cardiac silhouette strongly supports the clinical observations. In addition, the film may document increased pulmonary vascular markings with increased pulmonary blood flow lesions or pulmonary venous congestion compatible with pulmonary venous obstruction or a left-sided obstructive defect. Pulmonary venous congestion may also be seen with a normal-sized heart shadow in the cyanotic infant with anomalous pulmonary venous connection with obstruction to pulmonary venous return. There may also be lobar emphysema or collapse secondary to compression by a dilated pulmonary

TABLE 22-20

THE CARDINAL SIGNS AND SYMPTOMS OF CONGESTIVE HEART FAILURE AND THEIR PATHOPHYSIOLOGICAL MECHANISMS

SIGNS AND SYMPTOMS	MECHANISMS
Pulmonary venous congestion	↑ Left-sided filling pressure
Tachypnea	Interstitial pulmonary edema
Wheezing	Bronchiolar edema
Crepitant rales	Alveolar edema
Feeding difficulties	↑ Work of breathing
Systemic venous congestion	↑ Right-sided filling pressure
Hepatomegaly	Hepatic venous congestion
Peripheral edema (may only be facial)	↑ Fluid transudation, ↑ aldosterone
↑ Antidiuretic hormone	↓ Renal blood flow
↓ Cardiac output	↓ Inotropic state
↓ Precordial activity	↓ Inotropic function or pericardial effusion
↓ Arterial pulsations	↓ Systemic perfusion
↓ Capillary refill	↓ Systemic perfusion
Irritability	↓ O_2 transport
Volume loading	Chamber dilatation
↑ Precordial activity	Preserved inotropic state
Gallop sounds	↑ Ventricular filling
Murmurs	Valvar regurgitation, left-to-right shunt
Bruits	Possible AVMs
Pressure loading	↑ Afterload
Gallop sounds	↓ Compliance, ↑ wall stress
Murmurs (ejection)	Poststenotic turbulence
Adaptive changes	↑ Neurohumoral responses
Tachycardia	↑ β_1-Adrenergic activity
Pallor (vasoconstriction)	↑ α_1 and angiotensin II response
Low urine output	↓ Renal perfusion
Growth failure	↑ Metabolic demands, ↓ systemic blood flow
Sweating	↑ Sympathetic and cholinergic stimulation

artery and an enlarged left atrium and left ventricle. The heart may be only minimally enlarged early in the presentation of acute myocardial inflammatory disease, although the lung markings will usually show pulmonary venous congestion. Lung vascular markings may be diminished with severe pulmonary valve stenosis with intact ventricular septum or the Ebstein malformation, together with clinical signs of systemic venous congestion and cyanosis from right-to-left shunting via the foramen ovale.

ELECTROCARDIOGRAM An electrocardiogram may provide useful data as to chamber enlargement, or S-T and T-wave alterations that indicate myocardial ischemia as seen with myopericarditis or neonatal asphyxial states and severe obstruction to systemic or pulmonary blood flow. Low voltages suggest myopericardial inflammation. A true myocardial infarction pattern can be seen with the anomalous left coronary artery malformation. The electrocardiogram can also document a significant cardiac dysrhythmia that might have caused cardiac failure, particularly tachyarrhythmias such as supraventricular tachycardia or atrial fibrillation.

ECHOCARDIOGRAPHY An ultrasound study of the heart with Doppler interrogation is a vital part of the evaluation, but it should be stressed that heart failure is a clinical diagnosis with the echocardiogram providing valuable supportive information relative to basic cardiac structure and function once the diagnosis is suspected.

MYOCARDIAL ENZYME CHANGES When perinatal asphyxia, a coronary artery abnormality, or myopericardial disease is suspected with electrocardiographic evidence of S-T and T-wave alterations, blood should be drawn for myocardial enzyme determination, specifically myocardial creatine kinase (CK) and troponin T. Elevation of these factors provides supporting evidence for an acute myocardial ischemic insult.

BLOOD GAS AND ACID-BASE DETERMINATION The blood gas tensions, pH, and acid-base studies provide valuable indicators of the severity of the compromise in systemic perfusion (metabolic acidosis with lactic acid accumulation) or indicate compromise of ventilatory function if $PaCO_2$ is elevated, as with large left-to-right shunt lesions. Furthermore, a significantly decreased arterial PO_2 level may go along with impaired ventilatory function or a lesion that, in addition to producing pulmonary and systemic venous congestion, has a significant right-to-left shunt component.

OTHER LABORATORY STUDIES Blood glucose levels should be obtained in the infant with heart failure, as the newborn myocardium preferentially uses carbohydrates for its metabolic requirements. Serum calcium determination is important, particularly when lesions associated with the DiGeorge syndrome are present (truncus arteriosus, interrupted aortic arch, tetralogy of Fallot, or double-outlet right ventricle). Significant anemia can be detected by hemoglobin and red blood cell counts. Anemia in a 2- to 3-month-old contributes to the postnatal fall in pulmonary vascular resistance by decreasing blood viscosity and favors an increase in left-to-right shunting in patients with a large ventricular communication or ductus arteriosus.

MANAGEMENT

Although treatment of the pediatric patient with cardiac failure is usually under the supervision of a pediatric cardiologist, the pediatrician should know about, and be updated on, current treatment strategies, particularly the specific pharmacologic agents being utilized. This includes the mode of action of the various therapeutic agents, desired clinical response, potential side effects, possible deleterious drug interactions, and important changes in the patient's clinical status that warrant reevaluation.

INOTROPIC AGENTS

The inotropic state of the myocardium may be improved by pharmacologic agents given intravenously in treatment of acute congestive heart failure or orally when given chronically.

INOTROPIC AGENTS FOR ACUTE LOW-OUTPUT HEART FAILURE

DOPAMINE This is a catecholamine-like inotropic drug widely used to manage acute low-output states, particularly those after open heart surgery. Its principal mode of action is to increase myocardial contractility by stimulating norepinephrine release from cardiac adrenergic receptor sites. In addition to its myocardial effect, it dilates peripheral vascular beds via its action on dopamine receptors to inhibit norepinephrine release. These effects are achieved at relatively low doses and are associated with augmented coronary and renal perfusion. At high doses, α-adrenoreceptor stimulation induces vasoconstriction and a decrease in renal blood flow.

DOBUTAMINE This is a synthetic analog of dopamine that has β_1-adrenergic stimulating effects that enhance myocardial contractility. In addition to its myocardial effect, this drug is a mild vasodilator. When given by infusion pump, with appropriate patient monitoring, cardiac output increases as systemic vascular resistance falls, with usually only minimal changes in heart rate and blood pressure.

EPINEPHRINE This produces mixed α- and β-adrenoreceptor stimulation. In postoperative, low-output states, with intense vasoconstriction present, epinephrine may actually dilate these beds, and this together with its very potent inotropic effects justifies its use when responses to dopamine or dobutamine are unsatisfactory.

AMRINONE AND MILRINONE These drugs belong to the class of nonglycosidal, noncatecholamine agents that exert positive inotropic and vasodilator effects by inhibiting phosphodiesterase. As with the other titratable medications, they must be given by infusion pump with close patient monitoring. These drugs may have a special role in those patients with chronic congestive heart failure who, when treated with repeated dopamine infusions, have had desensitization of β_1-adrenoreceptors and a diminished inotropic response. Because these agents act beyond the receptor site, a positive inotropic response may still be achieved. Milrinone has an additional therapeutic advantage in that it can be given orally.

INOTROPIC AGENTS FOR CHRONIC USAGE

DIGITALIS GLYCOSIDES Digitalis glycosides, notably digoxin, continue to be the most widely used inotropic agents in the treatment of congestive heart failure, although their use acutely and for specific lesions such as large-volume left-to-right shunts has been questioned. Their principal mode of action is to inhibit the sodium pump at its receptor site (Na,K ATPase). As a consequence, intracellular sodium increases, with subsequent calcium entry from activation of the Na^+-Ca^{2+} exchange mechanism. This increase in intracellular calcium then produces a positive inotropic response. Another important effect of the glycoside is to inhibit sympathetic nerve traffic and so decrease metabolic demands while preserving contractility enhancement—certainly a desirable effect in chronic CHF.

The cardiac glycoside digoxin is now given primarily by mouth. Although loading doses have been recommended in the past, many patients are now started on a maintenance dose and achieve full digitalization over approximately 1 week. Parents must be instructed on how to measure out the medication, the proper timing of administration, safe storage of the drug out of reach of the patient or siblings, and potential toxic effects. All calculated doses should be carefully checked to avoid potential lethal ingestions.

Serum digoxin levels are being determined less frequently today, with more dependence on clinical response and electrocardiographic changes to indicate the possibility of digitalis toxicity. If, however, there may be potential harmful drug interactions, hepatic or renal dysfunction, or serum electrolyte disorders, serum digoxin levels may be helpful. Drug interactions that increase serum digoxin level concentration include quinidine, verapamil, amiodorone, β-adrenoreceptor blockers, tetracycline, and erythromycin. Low serum digoxin levels may be observed with rifampin, kaolin-pectin, neomycin, and cholestyramine.

Acute Digoxin Intoxication The primary care physician must be alert to clinical signs of digitalis intoxication. The major features of toxicity include gastrointestinal symptoms such as nausea, vomiting, and diarrhea, neurologic manifestations such as colored vision, confusion, and vertigo, and cardiac symptoms such as palpitations and arrhythmias, some potentially lethal. Treatment depends on the clinical severity, varying from merely withholding the medication and then altering the dosage to using digoxin-specific antibodies for effective therapy of life-threatening toxicity.

TREATMENT OF PULMONARY AND SYSTEMIC VENOUS CONGESTION

DIURETICS Diuretics remain the principal agents used to control pulmonary and systemic venous congestion. The kidneys respond to the apparent volume deficit in cardiac failure by increasing sodium reabsorption, which leads to volume expansion and exacerbates congestion of the pulmonary and systemic circulations. The fundamental aim of therapy is to increase renal perfusion using the agents described in the previous section and increase sodium transport in the kidney to distal diluting sites. Diuretic agents are designed to maximize sodium loss by increasing renal excretion of sodium and other ions by inhibiting tubular reabsorption of sodium at various sites along the nephron.

LOOP DIURETICS These include furosemide, bumetamide, and ethacrynic acid, which inhibit the sodium-potassium-chloride cotransporter in the ascending limb of the loop of Henle to block sodium and chloride reabsorption. This causes increased tubular luminal concentrations of sodium, potassium, chloride, and hydrogen ions, which are then lost in the urine. There is thus the potential for such electrolyte abnormalities as hyponatremia, hypokalemia, hypochloremia, and metabolic alkalosis. There also may be accompanying hypercalciuria.

DIURETIC AGENTS AFFECTING THE CORTICAL DILUTING SEGMENT These include the thiazides and metolazone, which block sodium and chloride reabsorption in the region of renal tubule concerned with the generation of free water—the cortical diluting segment of the ascending limb and the proximal portion of the distal convoluted tubule. As a result, more sodium reaches the distal tubules, where it can be exchanged with potassium. In addition, thiazides increase the active excretion of potassium ion. By acting at different sites than the loop diuretics, these drugs may produce additive effects on electrolyte losses.

Metalozone, when given as a single daily dose, may produce profound diuresis and carries the risk of excessive volume depletion. Therefore, it should be given only in hospital under close medical observation.

POTASSIUM-SPARING DIURETIC AGENTS Spironolactone is the main potassium-sparing agent used in infants and children with congestive heart failure. It acts on the distal tubule at the site of aldosterone activity to inhibit sodium-potassium exchange. This impairs the reabsorption of sodium and the excretion of potassium and hydrogen ions, thus sparing potassium loss. The principal use of spironolactone is in conjunction with loop diuretics to minimize potassium losses. Recent evidence has shown that concurrent use of spironolactone and angiotensin-converting enzyme inhibitors re-

duces mortality in severe congestive heart failure. Potassium levels should be followed closely in these patients to avoid hyperkalemia.

COMPLICATIONS OF PROLONGED DIURETIC TREATMENT

HYPONATREMIA Hyponatremia reflects increased renal sodium losses in the face of an inability to excrete free water. There also may be an increase in arginine vasopressin antidiuretic hormone activity and increased activity of angiotensin II. Management of this complication includes restricting water intake in combination with furosemide and an ACE inhibitor.

METABOLIC ALKALOSIS This abnormality is observed frequently when loop diuretics are given over a prolonged time.

HYPOKALEMIA The risk of hypokalemia is present when loop diuretics are given intravenously in high doses; the low serum potassium may precipitate cardiac arrhythmias and digitalis intoxication. This complication can usually be avoided by providing potassium supplements or using potassium-sparing diuretics or ACE inhibitors.

VOLUME CONTRACTION Significant depletion of intravascular volume may occur, particularly when the more potent diuretics such as furosemide or metolazone are given. When these agents are used, frequent checks of perfusion status, serum electrolytes, creatinine, and urea nitrogen are required if this serious complication is to be avoided.

VASODILATORS

Pharmacologic interventions to manipulate ventricular loading conditions are major advances in the treatment of congestive heart failure. Vasodilator drugs now occupy prominent roles in the treatment of infants with cardiac failure secondary to a large left-to-right shunt, postoperative low-output states, severe AV valve and semilunar valve regurgitation, and dilated cardiomyopathies. These medications are used with inotropic agents to improve pump function and diuretics to decrease pulmonary and systemic congestion, with the focus being to augment function by lowering resistances in the pre- and postcapillary vascular beds and improving cardiovascular performance.

ACE INHIBITORS In treating chronic severe congestive heart failure such as that encountered with dilated cardiomyopathies, the ACE inhibitors are now favored; their principal role is to inhibit the maladaptive neurohumoral responses initiated by the renin-angiotensin-aldosterone axis. Several well-controlled studies in adults have shown that the outcome in dilated cardiomyopathy has been markedly improved by adding angiotensin-converting enzyme inhibition to cardiac glycosides and diuretics. In addition to their vasodilating effect, there is now evidence that inhibiting angiotensin alters ventricular remodeling. Increased production of bradykinin may also be important in the decrease in afterload. When ACE inhibitors are given, blood pressure must be carefully monitored, particularly during the initial phases of therapy. Neutropenia may occur so that blood counts should be obtained as part of the monitoring process. These inhibitors occasionally cause a rise in creatinine and rarely cause angioneurotic edema. Potassium supplements and potassium-sparing diuretics should be used with caution in conjunction with ACE inhibition.

Captopril and *enalapril,* the commonly used ACE inhibitors, have been shown to decrease the left-to-right shunt in infants with large communications at the ventricular level as well as to improve the hemodynamic status of patients with severe congestive but not restrictive cardiomyopathies.

SODIUM NITROPRUSSIDE This is the most widely used acute vasodilator in acute situations such as after cardiopulmonary bypass, when manipulation of afterload is required. Nitroprusside is a smooth muscle dilator of both arterioles and venules and acts to decrease filling pressures and systemic and pulmonary vascular resistances. The mode of action is probably by the formation of the relaxing factor nitric oxide. When it is used, attention must be directed to intravascular volume and to the possibility of the development of cyanide toxicity if the medication is given for more than 48 hours.

β-ADRENORECEPTOR BLOCKADE

Low-dose β-adrenoreceptor blockade has been added to the treatment of dilated cardiomyopathy with encouraging results, based on well-controlled studies in adult populations. The basis for this approach is the potential for these agents to interfere with the deleterious effects of increased sympathoadrenal activity. Workload and ventricular relaxation improve without an increase in myocardial oxygen consumption. Exercise capacity has also been enhanced. Obviously, these drugs must be used with caution, as myocardial performance may deteriorate initially before improvement is noted. Some of the newer selective β_1-adrenoreceptor blockers such as metoprolol appear to produce the most encouraging therapeutic effects. Up-regulation of β-adrenoreceptors has been described in patients with dilated cardiomyopathy undergoing treatment with these blocking agents, thereby restoring responsiveness to inotropic interventions. Another advantage of the newer selective β blockers is possible avoidance of bronchospasm as a complication.

SUPPORTIVE MEASURES

NUTRITION An important adjunct to the management of the infant or child in congestive failure is providing an adequate caloric and fluid intake to permit at least weight stabilization or, ideally, to allow for weight gain. One important criterion for successful treatment of the infant, in particular, is its ability to grow. Growth limitation represents an adaptive mechanism to limit metabolic demands and preserve vital organ function. Frequent small feedings appear to be tolerated in infants reasonably well. If not, either intermittent or continuous gavage feedings are recommended. The increased metabolic rate of infants in congestive heart failure requires a higher than normal intake of calories if growth is to take place. The required caloric intake may be as high as 150 cal/kg/day for infants, with progressively lower caloric requirements for those over a year of age. Direct measurement of oxygen consumption offers a way of calculating caloric requirements.

Infant formulas should be concentrated up to 24 to 28 cal/ounce (or more) in order to provide an adequate caloric intake while limiting fluid intake. Severe fluid restriction is not indicated, nor should diets very low in sodium be given. Instructing parents in proper feeding techniques requires a supportive nursing staff, as feeding of the infant or child in cardiac failure can be very frustrating. Before discharge from the hospital, care solely by parents should be started in order to build up the parents' knowledge and confidence when management takes place at home.

POSITIONING Positioning the infant or child in a semiupright position may lessen pulmonary congestion and decrease the work of breathing. Attention should be directed to pulmonary toilet with measures such as suctioning, chest physiotherapy, and postural drainage.

SUPPLEMENTAL OXYGEN Oxygenation is required for certain patients if pulse oximetry indicates compromise of blood oxygenation. A few words of caution, however, are indicated. In a large-volume left-to-right shunt, oxygen decreases pulmonary vascular resistance and raises systemic vascular resistance. These changes increase left-to-right shunting. In an infant with a lesion that has ductus-dependent systemic blood flow, oxygen may further constrict the ductus arteriosus while increasing pulmonary blood flow and thus further compromise systemic perfusion.

VENTILATION On occasion, respiratory failure accompanies cardiac failure, particularly in the infant with pulmonary overcirculation. A superimposed pulmonary infection, such as RSV, may precipitate this complication. Intubation and positive-pressure ventilation usually normalize the blood gas tensions and pH and lessen metabolic demands. Respiratory failure usually signifies that surgical intervention will be needed once stabilization has been attained.

BED REST In an older patient with acute congestive heart failure, bed rest initially remains an important component of management, particularly during the acute phase of heart failure or when an exacerbation occurs. This is of special importance in myocarditis. There must be adequate time for sleep, some limitation of disturbing interventions, and the availability of a television screen and computer games for entertainment. Parental support is needed, and arrangements for home schooling should be made for the older child and adolescent. As the patient improves, rehabilitation programs are in order to maximize the activity level in concert with the cardiovascular status.

MECHANICAL CIRCULATORY SUPPORT DEVICES Mechanical circulatory support has been used, particularly postoperatively in high-risk infants and older patients as well as as a bridge toward heart transplantation. Support may take a number of forms: these include intraaortic balloon pump counterpulsation, extracorporeal membrane oxygenation, ventricular assist devices, and abdominal compression devices.

PARENT-STAFF CONFERENCES It is imperative that the pediatrician, cardiologist, and nursing staff discuss with parents the nature of the underlying condition and what the term heart failure really means for that particular infant, child, or adolescent. We tend to avoid this term if possible and use such other terms as lung congestion, liver congestion, and impaired pumping ability, as the connotation of failure is very depressing to a concerned parent. The staff should stress that although the heart may be functioning well, the underlying defect such as a hole in the heart has caused overcirculation to the lungs with lung congestion and liver congestion as well. A definitive plan of action should be elaborated with alternatives offered depending on the clinical response of the patient.

ROLE OF PEDIATRICIAN IN PATIENT FOLLOW-UP

After initial hospitalization for management of congestive heart failure, almost all patients require close medical supervision to monitor clinical progress. Here the pediatrician occupies a central role in evaluating the infant or child to confirm signs of heart failure, ability to grow, intercurrent infections that can affect heart function, and possible signs of drug toxicity. Communication between the primary care physician and pediatric cardiologist must be close, and the cardiologist should keep the primary care physician updated on management plans and changes. The patient and family should be kept informed regarding limits of exercise, sports participation, antibiotic prophylaxis for dental and surgical procedures, and clinical signs and symptoms that require reevaluation (fever, chest pain, rhythm disturbances, syncope, decrease in exercise tolerance).

SPECIFIC MANAGEMENT SCHEMATA

Three typical clinical problems associated with heart failure are outlined, and their management discussed.

THE ACUTE LOW-CARDIAC-OUTPUT PICTURE DEVELOPING WITH COARCTATION OF THE AORTA The clinical picture in a neonate less than 2 weeks of age with critical coarctation of the aorta demands prompt recognition and stabilization before surgical repair or balloon dilatation. The sudden development of tachypnea, pallor, and decreased arterial pulsations should immediately raise the suspicion of a lesion such as coarctation (or critical aortic stenosis) with ductus-dependent systemic perfusion, although septic shock can produce a similar picture. The acute onset of these symptoms with coarctation develops when the aortic end of the ductus arteriosus constricts. The left ventricle is then subjected to an abrupt increase in afterload that quickly produces ventricular dilatation and impaired contractility. Cardiac output is severely compromised, as shown by a metabolic acidosis. Once this diagnosis is suspected, these infants require a venous access route so that prostaglandin E_1 can be given to dilate the ductus arteriosus as well as to provide for volume expansion if necessary. To improve contractility, an infusion of dopamine should be begun, and the acidemia corrected with sodium bicarbonate. Because prostaglandin E_1 may induce respiratory arrest, the infant should be intubated and ventilated, with the added benefit that metabolic demands are decreased. A satisfactory response is indicated by an improvement in the quality of the upper arm pulses (the leg pulses may still be decreased); capillary refill improves, the skin is warmer, and the pH is close to normal. When the infant has stabilized, transfer to a pediatric cardiovascular center for balloon dilatation or surgical repair is done. The approach, as outlined above, has resulted in marked improvement in morbidity and mortality outcomes in the critically ill infant with coarctation.

A LARGE-VOLUME LEFT-TO-RIGHT SHUNT (VSD) Typically a 3-week- to 2-month-old irritable, tachypneic infant has a history of poor feeding with a rapid heart rate and a hyperdynamic precordium, usually with a loud holosystolic murmur along the left sternal border. A chest x-ray reveals an enlarged heart with prominent pulmonary vascular markings. Echocardiography shows a large communication at the ventricular level with dilated cardiac chambers and normal ventricular contractility. The therapeutic challenge is to manage the pulmonary edema, limit the left-to-right shunting, provide nutrition, and allow the infant to grow in the hope that the defect may get smaller over time. To accomplish this, diuretic therapy with intravenous furosemide is initiated, and attempts are made to provide adequate caloric intake by concentrating the formula and offering frequent small-volume feedings, possibly by nasogastric tube. The use of digoxin in this situation is controversial

because ventricular contractility is normal. However, we believe that digoxin is indicated, not primarily for its inotropic effect but because of its ability to produce sympathoadrenal withdrawal and thereby lessen metabolic demands while preserving myocardial pumping function.

Two additional approaches have been used, both aimed at reducing the left-to-right shunt. The first uses the ACE inhibitor captopril, which, by decreasing afterload, augments systemic blood flow while reducing pulmonary blood flow. A second approach is to correct any relative anemia by blood transfusion to raise hemoglobin levels to 13 to 14 g/dL, which will raise pulmonary vascular resistance and reduce the left-to-right shunt while preserving oxygen delivery to the tissues.

If there is respiratory failure ($PaCO_2 > 50$ mm Hg), mechanical ventilation with PEEP may be required. This decreases metabolic requirements, lessens pulmonary edema, and aids in stabilizing the infant before surgical intervention.

These interventions make the patient a better candidate for surgical repair. If control of heart failure with resumption of normal growth cannot be achieved, then surgery is certainly indicated, sooner rather than later.

MANAGEMENT OF DILATED CARDIOMYOPATHY Congestive heart failure resulting from a dilated cardiomyopathy presents the clinician with a challenging problem. The patient may be of any age with a myopathy arising from any of a number of etiologies. One has to use measures aimed at improving ventricular contractility, decreasing filling pressures and volumes, lessening pulmonary and systemic venous congestion, and preventing thromboembolic and arrhythmic complications. The endpoint of all of this may in some instances be a mechanical assist device as a bridge to transplantation unless there is a dramatic improvement in cardiovascular performance. The current therapeutic approach to the patient with a dilated cardiomyopathy is based on large group control studies in primarily adult populations. This includes digoxin for inotropic support, furosemide to provide control of pulmonary edema and systemic venous congestion, and ACE inhibition to induce vasodilatation and modulate the ventricular remodeling process. Patients treated in this fashion have shown improved exercise performance and lessened morbidity and mortality. Nevertheless, return of normal function is the exception.

β-Adrenoreceptor blockade has been introduced into the above drug regimens, and relatively large controlled studies in adults indicate substantial benefits from this approach. The aim with β-blockade is to minimize the maladaptive alterations on cardiovascular performance induced by excessive sympathoadrenal stimulation. The demonstration that β-adrenergic blocking agents as well as ACE inhibitors can improve symptoms, morbidity, and survival and also appear to slow the progression of myocardial dysfunction is related to their effects in the myocardial remodeling process. As a result, new strategies for inhibiting the sympathetic nervous system and renin-angiotensin system (angiotensin receptor blockers) are being evaluated in adult heart failure patients. Additional factors that may contribute to the remodeling process include endothelin, inflammatory cytokines, and reactive oxygen species. New therapeutic strategies may, therefore, include inhibition of endothelin receptors, and agents that reduce inflammatory cytokines and oxidative stresses.

The pediatric experience with β-adrenergic blockade, however, has been limited, but based on the adult experience and anecdotal pediatric reports, this treatment warrants cautious introduction into the pediatric armamentarium for the patient in congestive heart failure with a dilated cardiomyopathy who is refractory to the standard drug regimens.

OTHER SPECIFIC INTERVENTIONS

There are a few therapeutic interventions that are aimed at specific disease processes that warrant citation. These include (1) giving digoxin or other antiarrhythmics to the mother to control a supraventricular tachyarrhythmia in the fetus, (2) pacing for heart block associated with compromised cardiac output, (3) immune globulin for acute myocarditis, (4) transfusions for heart failure associated with anemia, and (5) carnitine replacement for documented disorders of fatty acid metabolism.

In addition, there is experimental evidence that probucol, a lipid-lowering drug with strong antioxidant properties, may protect against adriamycin-induced cardiomyopathy without interfering with the antitumor actions of the drug.

MANAGEMENT OF DIASTOLIC HEART FAILURE Diastolic heart failure rarely occurs in the isolated form but may certainly accompany systolic failure. Pure diastolic heart failure is defined hemodynamically as an elevated end-diastolic pressure in the presence of a normal ventricular volume. The ejection fraction is also normal. Unfortunately, therapy for this functional impairment is rarely successful. β-Adrenoreceptor and calcium channel-blocking agents have been tried with limited success. ACE inhibitors have also been used to try to minimize myocardial fibrosis. All of these agents have been most effective in the treatment of systemic hypertension, where they appear to inhibit the maladaptive components of the ventricular hypertrophic response. Paramount in any consideration of impairment of diastolic function, however, is the importance of ruling out constrictive pericarditis as the causative factor producing clinical signs of systemic venous congestion.

References

General

Artman M, Graham TP Jr: Congestive heart failure in infancy: recognition and management. Am Heart J 103:1040, 1982

Artman H, Parrish MD, Graham TP Jr: Congestive heart failure in childhood and adolescence: recognition and management. Am Heart J 105: 471, 1983

Friedman WF, George BL: New concepts and drugs in the treatment of congestive heart failure. Pediatr Clin North Am 31:1197, 1984

Gessner IH, Victorica BE: Pediatric Cardiology: A Problem Oriented Approach. Philadelphia, WB Saunders, 1993:117–129

Talner NS, Carboni M, McGovern J: Congestive heart failure. In: Moller JH, Hoffman JIE, eds: Pediatric Cardiovascular Medicine. New York, Churchill Livingstone, 2000:817

Pathophysiology

Anderson PAW, Kleinman CS, Lister G, Talner NS: Cardiovascular function during normal fetal and neonatal development and with hypoxic stress. In: Polin RA, Fox WW, eds: Fetal and Neonatal Physiology. Philadelphia, WB Saunders 1998:837–890

Hunter JJ, Chien KR: Signaling pathways for cardiac hypertrophy and failure. N Engl J Med 341:1276, 1999

Katz AM: Heart failure in 2001. Am J Cardiol 70:126c, 1992

Klitzner TS, Friedman WF: A diminished role for the sarcoplasmic reticulum in newborn myocardial contraction. Pediatr Res 26:98, 1989

Lakatta EG, Houser SR: Myocyte dysfunction in heart failure. Sci Med 6: 8, 1999

Lister G, Talner NS: Oxygen transport in congenital heart disease. Cardiovasc Clin 2:129, 1980

Opie LH: The heart: physiology from cell to circulation. In: Heart Failure and Neurohumoral Responses. Philadelphia, Lippincott-Raven, 1998: 475–511

Sagawa K, Maughan L, Suga H, Sunagawa K: Cardiac Contraction and the Pressure-Volume Relationship. New York, Oxford Press, 1988:299–339

Schrier RW, Abraham WT: Hormones and hemodynamics in heart failure. N Engl J Med 341:577, 1999

Staub NC: Pulmonary edema. Physiol Rev 54:360, 1974

Teitel D, Sidi D, Chin T, et al: Developmental changes in myocardial contractile reserve in the lamb. Pediatr Res 6:887, 1972

Therapy

Artman M, Graham TR Jr: Guidelines for vasodilator therapy in infants and children. Am Heart J 113:994, 1987

George BL, Friedman WF: Treatment of heart failure in infants. Compr Ther 12:8, 1986

Givertz MM, Colucci WS: Treatment of heart failure—new approaches. In: Colucci WS, ed: Atlas of Heart Failure. Philadelphia, Current Medicine, 1999:11.2–11.19

Thier SO. Diuretic mechanisms as a guide to therapy. Hosp Pract 22:61, 1987

22.4.5   Systemic Hypertension

Donald E. Potter and Julien I. E. Hoffman

Hypertension is defined as systolic or diastolic systemic arterial blood pressure above normal for age (Fig. 22-88). Moderate or severe arterial hypertension in children is uncommon and usually secondary to a detectable lesion. In adults, most arterial hypertension has no detectable cause and is termed essential or primary. Essential hypertension is common; there are about 60 million people with arterial pressures above 140/90 mm Hg in the United States. Milder forms of hypertension may be common at all ages.

STANDARDS

Normal values are 5 to 10 mm Hg higher for those above the 95th percentile for weight or height than for those in the 50th percentiles. Systolic pressures are slightly higher, and diastolic pressures slightly lower, with the patient supine rather than erect. Different sets of standards may therefore differ from each other by as much as 10 mm Hg, and minor departures from normal standards should not be overemphasized, particularly because blood pressures (especially diastolic) can vary markedly from week to week.

MEASUREMENT OF BLOOD PRESSURE

The first time a patient is seen, measure blood pressure in at least one arm. If it is high, then measure pressures in the other arm and at least one leg. At subsequent visits, measurement in one arm is adequate as long as all pulses feel equal and the patient is over 2 months old. When pressure is measured in the arm, the patient should be resting and relaxed, in a quiet room, and either sitting or supine. Place the arm at heart level and apply a cuff firmly to the upper arm so that the center of the rubber bag within the cuff is over the brachial artery. The rubber bag must be wide enough to cover two thirds of the length of the upper arm and long enough to cover at least three fourths of the arm circumference. ***One of the***

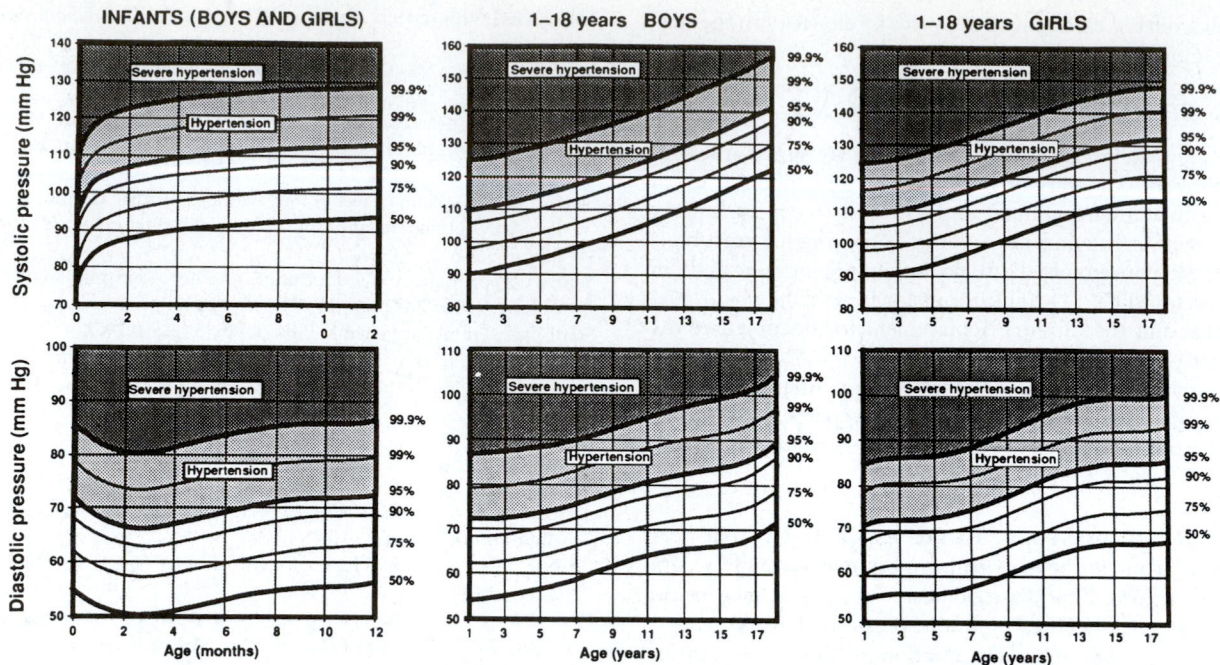

FIGURE 22-88 Normal values for systolic and diastolic (fourth phase) blood pressures adapted from the data provided by the Task Force. There are some minor differences less than 5 mm Hg between some of the values depicted in this figure and in the figures produced by the Task Force. These differences are less than those observed in different sets of normal values. Severe hypertension, based on clinical experience, and described by the Task Force, is approximately at the 99.9th percentile.

most common causes of apparent hypertension is erroneous measurement from using too small a blood pressure cuff. Feel the brachial or radial pulse and inflate the cuff until the pulse disappears, then deflate the cuff and note the pressure at which the pulse reappears. After about 15 seconds, reinflate the cuff to about 30 mm Hg above the palpatory systolic pressure, place the stethoscope on the brachial artery, and deflate the cuff by 2 to 3 mm Hg per second. The first Korotkoff sounds indicate the systolic pressure. The sounds become louder, then suddenly become muffled, and finally disappear. The point of muffling (fourth phase) may be a better estimate of diastolic pressure than is the point of disappearance (fifth phase), which occasionally gives a false low reading. Repeat the measurements twice; often the third pressure is the lowest because the patient is more relaxed. Record the pulse rate with each measurement because tachycardia may denote anxiety that increases blood pressure. Leg pressures are measured with the patient prone so that the stethoscope can be placed on the popliteal artery. The rubber bag should cover two thirds of the thigh length and at least three fourths of its circumference; thus, a larger cuff is needed for the leg than for the arm.

In infants, blood pressure may be difficult to obtain by this method but can be measured by ultrasound (Doppler) devices.

EFFECTS OF HYPERTENSION

Long-standing hypertension causes congestive heart failure or degenerative vascular diseases of the brain, kidneys, or heart. In adults it is the most common cause of congestive heart failure and is the precursor of most cerebral vascular accidents. By causing renal arteriolar damage, it contributes to renal failure. It is also a major risk factor in coronary artery disease, especially in women.

There is no particular level of blood pressure at which complications occur; each increment of pressure above the normal pres-

sures adds to the risk of developing cardiovascular disease. A raised systolic pressure is as harmful as a raised diastolic pressure; the complications of hypertension depend on the average blood pressure load throughout the day. All these cardiovascular complications are uncommon in children unless pressures are extremely high. Nevertheless, because mild hypertension can progress to severe hypertension and eventually lead to these complications, recording and assessing blood pressures are important parts of any pediatric examination.

BASIC MECHANISMS

Arterial hypertension is caused by a decreased compliance of the large arteries, an increased resistance of the systemic arterioles, or an increased cardiac output.

Isolated systolic hypertension occurs with normal arterial compliance and a large stroke volume, as occurs in marked bradycardia, severe aortic incompetence, a large patent ductus arteriosus or arteriovenous fistula, or peripheral vasodilatation from heat, anemia, or thyrotoxicosis. It also occurs beyond middle age, when the compliance of large arteries may decrease. In both of these situations, ejection leads to excessively high systolic pressures, but diastolic pressures are normal or reduced, and the pulse pressure is wide.

For other forms of hypertension, increased diastolic and systolic pressures can be understood by realizing that blood pressure is the product of cardiac output and peripheral resistance. An increase in either of these will raise blood pressure as long as the other variable does not decrease. Thus, a high cardiac output in anemia does not cause hypertension because peripheral resistance falls, but it does raise blood pressure with anxiety, in which peripheral resistance is high.

Mechanisms of increased cardiac output and peripheral resistance are given in Table 22-21.

TABLE 22-21

MECHANISMS PRODUCING HYPERTENSION

Increased cardiac output
Sympathetic stimulation (anxiety)
Increased blood volume
Infused blood or saline
Excess salt intake
Renal failure (decreased GFR)
Mineralocorticoid excess
Increased peripheral resistance
α-Adrenergic receptor stimulation
Stimulation of certain cortical and hypothalamic centers
Effect of angiotensin on area postrema
Decreased baroreceptor inhibition
Increased circulating catecholamines
Pheochromocytoma
Neuroblastoma
Increased sensitivity to local catecholamines
Glucocorticoids
Inhibit catechol-*ortho*-methyltransferase
Angiotensin
Stimulates norepinephrine formation and release
Inhibits neuronal reuptake of norepinephrine
? Vasopressin
Increased renin-angiotensin activity
Renal parenchymal disease
Renal artery obstruction: thrombosis, stenosis
Renal vein thrombosis (late)
Renin-secreting tumor of juxtamedullary cells
Wilms tumor
Mechanical factors
Coarctation of the aorta
Thickened arteriolar medial muscle, often secondary to hypertension
Increased sodium content of arteriolar walls
Polycythemia
Decreased production of vasodilators (all but the first are putative)
Renal prostaglandins, possible cause of preeclampsia
Dopamine
Kallikrein
Bradykinin
Atrial natriopeptide

CAUSES OF HYPERTENSION

The common causes of hypertension at different ages are given in Table 22-22. A more comprehensive list of the causes of hypertension is given in Tables 22-23 and 22-24. For convenience these have been divided into hypertension that is associated with another,

TABLE 22-22

AGE-RELATED COMMON CAUSES OF HYPERTENSION

AGE GROUP	LESIONS
Neonate	Renal artery thrombosis or stenosis, renal malformations, coarctation of the aorta, bronchopulmonary dysplasia
Infants to 6 years	Renal parenchymal diseases, coarctation of the aorta, renal artery stenosis
6–10 years	Renal parenchymal diseases, renal artery stenosis, essential hypertension
Adolescence	Essential hypertension, obesity, renal parenchymal diseases

TABLE 22-23

CAUSES OF HYPERTENSION (OFTEN ACUTE) ASSOCIATED WITH OTHER DISORDERS

Nervous system disorders
Encephalitis, meningitis
Raised intracranial pressure
After intracranial surgery or cranial trauma
Poliomyelitis; Guillain-Barré syndrome
Familial dysautonomia
Severe emotional stress
Acute renal disease
Acute glomerulonephritis
Hemolytic-uremic syndrome
Acute pyelonephritis
Renal vein thrombosis
Vasculitides
Transplant rejection
Metabolic disorders
Hypernatremia
Hypercalcemia
Acute intermittent porphyria
Steroid ingestion (contraceptive pills with estrogen, anabolic steroids, therapeutic)
Drug abuse
Cocaine, amphetamines, phencyclidine
Hypervolemia
Miscellaneous
Bronchopulmonary dysplasia
Preeclampsia
Stevens-Johnson syndrome
Leukemia
Mercury or lead poisoning
Burns
Prolonged bed rest and traction
Hypervitaminosis A or D
Congenital rubella
Pseudoxanthoma elasticum
Genitourinary tract surgery
Closure of abdominal wall defects
Familial chloride-losing enteropathy
Cyclic vomiting
Extracorporeal membrane oxygenation
Syndromes
Turner syndrome
Williams syndrome
Cushing syndrome

usually obvious disease (Table 22-23), is often acute, and subsides when the associated disease is cured, and sustained hypertension that often cannot be diagnosed by a preliminary history and examination and is usually secondary to renal or endocrine disorders (Table 22-24).

APPROACH TO DIAGNOSIS

It is important to diagnose the cause of hypertension and treat it if it is significant, but equally important to avoid diagnosing or labeling a patient as hypertensive when pressures are normal or transiently elevated. Overdiagnosis leads to unnecessary and expensive tests, and false labeling may adversely affect the subject's application for work or life insurance.

A diagnostic evaluation is undertaken in children whose blood pressures are repeatedly above the 95th percentile. Diagnosis is approached by knowing the causes of hypertension (Tables 22-22,

TABLE 22-24
CAUSES OF SUSTAINED HYPERTENSION

Miscellaneous
  Obesity
  Coarctation of the aorta
  Takayasu syndrome
  Lead poisoning
Renal disease
  Parenchymal diseases
    Glomerulonephritis
    Pyelonephritis
    Collagen vascular diseases
    Liddle syndrome
  Renin-secreting tumors
  Congenital malformations: cystic, dysplastic, and hypoplastic kidneys
  Obstructive uropathy
  Renal vascular disease
    Renal artery thrombosis (NB: Umbilical artery catheterization)
    Renal artery stenosis: fibromuscular, atheromatous
  Extrinsic vascular compression
	Endocrine disease
	  A. Catecholamine-induced
	    Catecholamine-secreting tumors: pheochromocytoma, neuroblastoma
	    Sudden catecholamine release; large intravenous doses of reserpine or α-methyldopa
	    Supersensitivity to circulating catecholamines; eating foods with a high tyramine content (aged cheeses, pickled herring, beer, red wine) while taking monamine oxidase inhibitors
	    Taking sympathomimetic amines (decongestants, eye drops), especially if taking reserpine or α-methyldopa
	  B. Excess mineralocorticoids
	    Aldosterone-producing adenomas
	    Adrenal hyperplasia $\pm$ dexamethasone-suppressible aldosteronism
	    Adrenal carcinoma
	    Congenital adrenal hyperplasia
	    11β- or 17α-hydroxylase deficiency
	    Apparent mineralocorticoid excess
	    Excess licorice ingestion
	    Ketaconozole administration
	  C. Excess glucocortioids
	    Cushing syndrome
	    Iatrogenic
	  D. Sex hormones
	    Contraceptive pills with estrogen
	    Testosterone
	    Anabolic steroids

22-23, and 22-24) and relating these to findings ascertained from a complete history and physical examination (Tables 22-25 and 22-26) and from basic laboratory tests (Table 22-27). Most of the common causes of hypertension will usually be evident after this

TABLE 22-25
HISTORY

HISTORY	RELEVANCE
Family history of hypertension	Essential hypertension
	Dexamethasone-suppressible hypertension
Family history of renal disease	Many congenital renal diseases
Urinary tract infections	Chronic pyelonephritis
Medications	Sympathomimetic drugs, contraceptive pills
Substance abuse	Cocaine, amphetamines, phencyclidine, anabolic steroids
Prescribed medications	Contraceptive pills, steroids, sympathomimetics
Exposure to lead	Renal hypertension from lead
Heat intolerance, sweating, weight loss	Hyperthyroidism
Headaches, pallor, sweating, palpitations	Pheochromocytoma

TABLE 22-26
FINDINGS ON PHYSICAL EXAMINATION

PHYSICAL FINDINGS	RELEVANCE
General features	
Obesity	Obesity-related hypertension
Moonface, buffalo hump, striae	Cushing syndrome
Webbed neck, low hairline, widely spaced nipples	Turner syndrome
Elfin facies, mental retardation	Williams syndrome
Virilization, hypogonadism, pseudohermaphroditism	Congenital adrenal hyperplasia
Café-au-lait spots	Neurofibromatosis + renal artery stenosis or pheochromocytoma
Warm, moist skin; tachycardia, hyperactive reflexes, thyromegaly	Thyrotoxicosis
Regional features	
Papilledema, slow heart rate	Increased intracranial pressure
Retinal arterial changes	Severe or chronic hypertension
Forceful or displaced LV apex beat	Left ventricular hypertrophy
Decreased blood pressure and pulses in legs	Coarctation of the aorta
Abdominal masses	Wilms tumor, neuroblastoma, cystic kidney, hydronephrosis
Bruits in epigastrium or renal angles	Renal artery stenosis

evaluation and can be addressed as appropriate. If no cause is discovered, and if blood pressure remains near the 95th percentile, the child is observed at 3- to 6-month intervals. Mild hypertension in children does not require treatment, and elaborate studies to identify its cause are not warranted. A schema for diagnosis is given in Fig. 22-89.

In children with more severe hypertension, the decision to proceed with further testing is influenced by several factors. The younger the child with significant hypertension or the higher the blood pressure, the more likely there is to be a correctable cause, and thus, further investigations should be pursued. If the child is markedly overweight, obesity is the likely cause. If there is a strong family history of essential hypertension, particularly in an adolescent patient, there is less need to look for another cause.

The more intensive investigations listed in Table 22-28 are used to diagnose renal and endocrine abnormalities, including tumors.

MINERALOCORTICOIDS Patients with aldosterone-secreting tumors or hyperplasia of the adrenals may develop hypertension. This

TABLE 22-27
BASIC INVESTIGATIONS

INVESTIGATION	RELEVANCE
Urinalysis	Pyelonephritis, glomerulonephritis, some renal anomalies
Urine culture (girls)	Pyelonephritis
Serum blood urea nitrogen, creatinine	Renal insufficiency
Serum electrolytes	Hypokalemia and alkalosis (hyperaldosteronism), hypernatremia, hypercalcemia

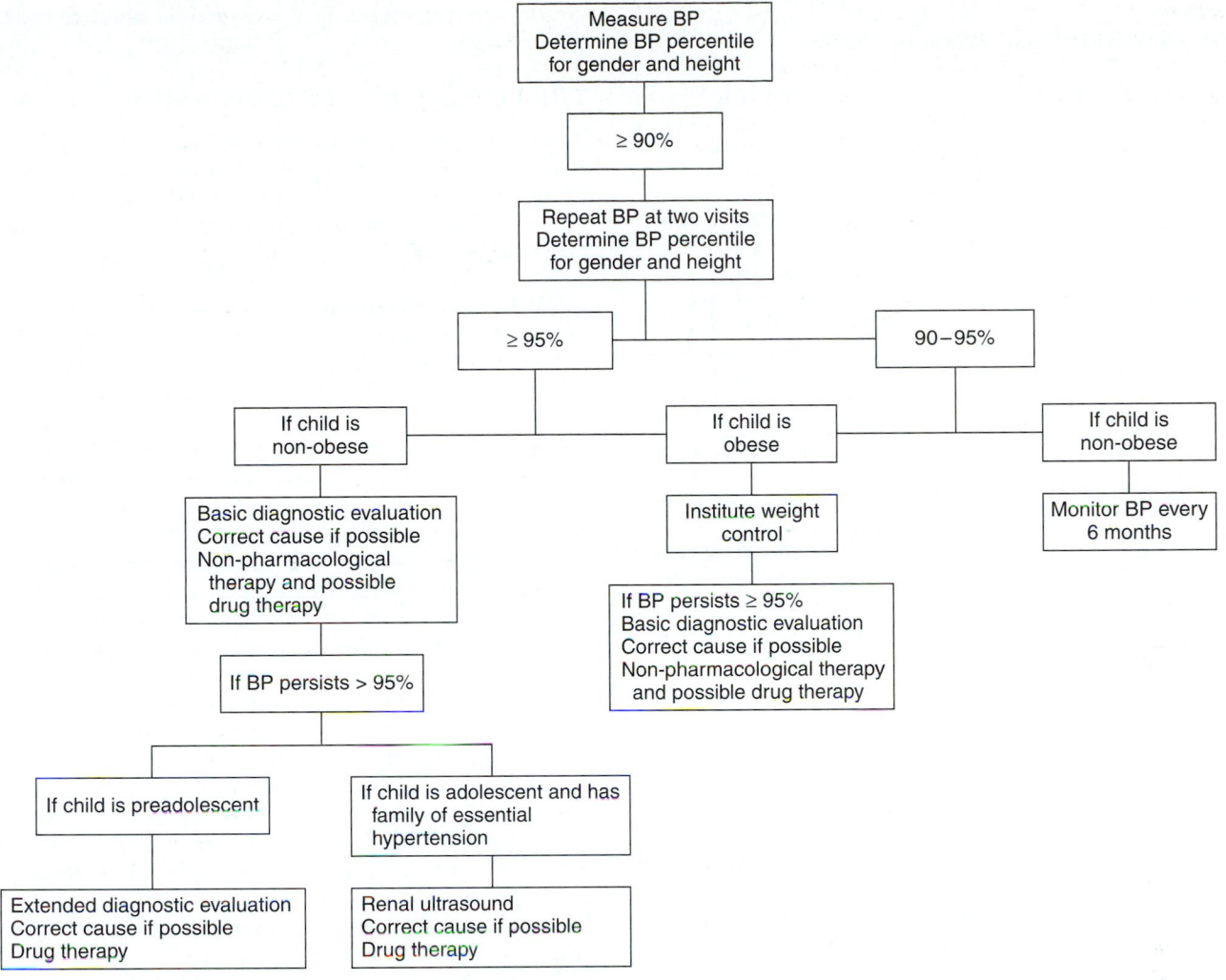

FIGURE 22-89   **Flow chart to show how to manage a child with arterial hypertension. The boxes that indicate the need for basic and extended evaluation refer to Tables 22-27 and 22-28 in conjunction with Tables 22-23 to 22-26.**

is usually associated with hypernatremia, hypokalemia, metabolic alkalosis, increased plasma volume, a low and fixed plasma renin level, and increased aldosterone secretion rates. Serum electrolytes provide a fairly good screening test for this disorder, and they can be followed by measuring peripheral renin levels after 2 hours in the erect position. Persistently low renin levels then indicate the need for the more time-consuming and expensive measurements of aldosterone concentrations or secretion rates as well as tests to determine if aldosterone can be suppressed by giving a high salt intake and dexamethasone. Low renin activity does not prove mineralocorticoid excess because renin is low in about 20% of patients with essential hypertension.

There may be hypertension in adrenogenital syndromes because of 11β- and 17α-hydroxylase deficiencies. The former tend to have virilization and hyperkalemia with hyponatremia; the latter often have hypokalemic alkalosis. The hypertension is associated with increased fluid and sodium retention caused by overproduction of desoxycorticosterone. There are also hypertensive patients with overproduction of 18-hydroxydesoxycorticosterone.

GLUCOCORTICOIDS Blood pressure should be checked frequently in those taking high dosages of steroids. Hypertension occurs in

Cushing syndrome. These patients usually have the typical cushingoid facies, buffalo hump, obesity, striae, hyperglycemia, and polycythemia; thus, routine measurements of 17-hydroxycorticosteroids or urinary free cortisol in an otherwise asymptomatic hypertensive patient without cushingoid features are not justified.

SEX HORMONES Girls taking oral contraceptives can develop hypertension, but if the agent is stopped, the pressure usually falls in 2 to 3 months. Testosterone administration may also cause blood pressure to rise. Preeclampsia should always be considered in girls of childbearing age.

RENAL DISORDERS Any type of renal parenchymal or vascular disease can cause hypertension. About 80% of secondary hypertension is caused by renal disease, four-fifths of which is related to renal anomalies and renal parenchymal disease and the rest to renal vascular abnormalities. Renal anomalies and parenchymal disease are diagnosed by renal ultrasound and DMSA scan. Renovascular disease may be detected by renal Doppler ultrasound, by magnetic resonance imaging, or by renal isotope scans with labeled MAG3 to show the relative distribution of blood flow to each kidney. The greatest sensitivity and specificity appear if these scans are done

TABLE 22-28
MORE INTENSIVE INVESTIGATIONS

INVESTIGATION	RELEVANCE
Electrocardiogram, echocardiogram	Left ventricular hypertrophy
Renal ultrasound	Renal anomalies, hydronephrosis, renal scars, Wilms tumor, neuroblastoma
Renal Doppler ultrasound, MRI	Renal artery stenosis
Plasma renin concentration	Increased in renal artery stenosis; decreased in primary hyperaldosteronism, dexamethasone-suppressible hypertension
Plasma aldosterone concentration	Increased in renal artery stenosis, primary hyperaldosteronism, dexamethasone-suppressible hypertension
Plasma deoxycorticosterone	Increased in congenital adrenal hyperplasia
Urinary steroids	Apparent mineralocorticoid excess, congenital adrenal hyperplasia
Urinary catecholamines, metanephrines, VMA	Pheochromocytoma, neuroblastoma
Dimercaptosuccinic acid (DMSA) scan	Chronic pyelonephritis
Captopril renal scan	Renal artery stenosis
Renal arteriogram	Renal artery stenosis

after giving captopril. These tests depend on differences between the two sides and so are of less value if there is bilateral renal artery stenosis. All these tests are 90 to 95% sensitive and 95% specific in detecting renal artery stenosis in adults, but there are few studies in children. In children, unlike adults, arterial lesions are more common in branch arteries than in the renal artery and are thus more difficult to detect.

Plasma renin may be measured before the patient gets out of bed in the morning, again after he or she has been erect for 2 hours, and perhaps again after institution of a low-sodium diet; each institution has its own method of doing these tests and its own standard. The captopril test is useful for evaluating renovascular disease. The patient, on a normal salt intake and on no antihypertensive drugs, has blood pressure and blood for plasma renin activity (PRA) measured after sitting quietly for 30 minutes and then 1 hour after being given captopril 0.3 mg/kg. Renovascular disease is indicated by stimulated PRA of 12 ng/mL/h plus an absolute increase in PRA of 10 ng/mL/h or more plus a percentage increase in PRA over 150%. Aldosterone may also be measured. Finally, renal vein renin may be measured at catheterization, and renal arteriography might be done; intraarterial digital subtraction angiography gives excellent images with low amounts of contrast material. Because these are the most invasive and the most expensive steps, they should not be done without good cause or before consultation with experts in the field.

MODERATE AND SEVERE HYPERTENSION

Moderate and severe hypertension includes those with pressures above the 99th percentile. Severity is defined by the features listed in Table 22-29, and those with severe hypertension should be admitted to hospital. They may even need to have their blood pres-

sures lowered before investigations to prevent serious complications (Table 22-30).

TREATMENT OF HYPERTENSION

If the cause cannot be removed, or while awaiting definitive treatment, it may be necessary to lower the blood pressure. The aims of treatment are to lower blood pressure and reverse organ damage without inducing significant side effects. If there is renal disease, then renal function can deteriorate as pressures are lowered.

EMERGENCY TREATMENT Hypertensive emergencies are those with very high blood pressures or with any of the features discussed earlier. If the blood pressure needs to be lowered rapidly, then the agents listed in Table 20-30 should be considered.

LONG-TERM THERAPY Because therapy for chronic hypertension may need to go on for years, even for life, it is essential to be sure that therapy is needed and then to commence with simpler forms before using more powerful and more complex drug treatment. It may be prudent to obtain 24-hour blood pressure measurements, which often show that the highest pressure is that in the doctor's office ("white coat hypertension"). Attempts to restore that atypical pressure to normal may lead to unacceptable hypotension.

Reduction of weight is important because obesity is an independent cause of left ventricular hypertrophy. Regular exercise should be encouraged. The patient should avoid smoking and a diet high in saturated animal fats because these factors add to the risk of later atherosclerosis. The diet should be high in potassium, which may help to lower pressures. Salt should be restricted, but because not all hypertensives are salt sensitive, the restriction can be relaxed if it is found not to lower pressure. Recent studies suggest that the chloride in salt causes the pressure elevation.

Psychotherapy to help the patient deal with stresses may be of value.

Sedative drugs such as barbiturates or benzodiazepines (Valium) can be very helpful, provided that they are used with precautions about excessive sedation and the risk of addiction.

PRINCIPLES OF DRUG THERAPY Hypotensive drugs may work at one or more levels in the body to lower cardiac output or cause systemic arterial vasodilatation (Table 22-31). Often the primary action is partly or completely counteracted by compensatory changes. For example, vasodilatation may cause a rise in heart rate and cardiac output that returns pressure to its former level, and this may also happen if a fall in cardiac output causes reflex vasoconstriction. Furthermore, reducing blood volume with a diuretic usually increases renin secretion. On the other hand, lowering blood pressure may increase renin production and lead to sodium reten-

TABLE 22-29
FEATURES OF SEVERE HYPERTENSION

Blood pressure	Above the 99.9th percentile or increasing rapidly
Neurologic	Focal or generalized seizures, localizing signs, isolated facial nerve palsy, headaches
Visual	Blurred vision, papilledema, retinal hemorrhages and exudates, constriction of retinal arteries
Cardiac	Left ventricular hypertrophy, pulmonary edema
Renal	Severe back or abdominal pain, abdominal or renal masses or bruits, decreasing renal function

tion and an increase in blood volume, thus restoring blood pressure to its former level. Therefore, if blood pressure is not effectively lowered by moderate doses of a drug, it is best to add another drug with a different mode of action. Not only does this lower blood pressure more effectively, but unwanted side effects are minimized by keeping the dose of each drug relatively low. When treating for the long term, it is important to start on low doses of drugs and increase the dose only after 3 to 7 days. This reduces the chances of incurring severe hypotension or severe side effects. Pressures should be measured with the patient supine and erect to detect excessive postural hypotension. If hypertension has been chronic, do not attempt to lower blood pressure to normal too rapidly. Hypertension thickens arteriolar walls, so that the minimal vascular resistance is higher than normal. Under these circumstances the only way to reduce blood pressure to normal is to decrease cardiac output below normal. It is better to reduce blood pressure moderately at first, wait some weeks until the vessels are presumably less thick, and then attempt to return blood pressures to normal in stages.

Not all agents that lower blood pressure reverse left ventricular hypertrophy. Those that do include adrenergic blocking agents, calcium blockers, and angiotensin-converting enzyme inhibitors, whereas diuretics and smooth muscle vasodilators on their own are less effective, probably because they do not interfere with sympathetic reflexes and so lead to tachycardia and increase of cardiac output. Therefore, sometimes with severe hypertension one or more of the first group of agents are used first, but a diuretic is added if there is fluid retention, or a smooth muscle vasodilator is

TABLE 22-31

SITES OF ACTION OF HYPOTENSIVE AGENTS

MAIN SITE AND BASIC MECHANISM OF ACTION	DRUG
Hypothalamus	Reserpine
Medulla	Methyldopa, clonidine, barbiturates
Sympathetic ganglia (blockade)	Trimethaphan camsylate (Arfonad)
Postganglionic adrenergic nerves (depression)	Guanethidine, bethanidine, debrisoquin
Adrenergic nerve endings (catecholamine depletion)	Reserpine
α-Adrenergic receptors (blockade)	Phentolamine, phenoxybenzamine, prazosin labetalol
β-Adrenergic receptors (blockade)	Propranolol, esmolol, labetalol, metoprolol
Arteriolar smooth muscle (relaxation)	Hydralazine, minoxidil, diazoxide, diuretics, nitroprusside, angiotensin-converting enzyme inhibitor, angiotensin receptor blockade, calcium channel blockade
Decrease in body sodium and blood volume	Thiazides, furosemide, spironolactone, triamterene

TABLE 22-30

DRUGS FOR HYPERTENSIVE EMERGENCIES

DRUG	DOSE	MAXIMAL DOSE	ROUTE	COMMENTS
Sodium nitroprusside (Nipride)	0.5 μg/kg/min initially	10 μg/kg/min	IV	Marked postural effect; monitor pressure frequently; check arterial pH for metabolic acidemia; if used over 48 hours may be toxic if thiocyanate concentrations exceed 12 mg/dL blood
Phentolamine (Regitine)	0.02 mg/kg; if no response, 0.1 mg/kg	—	IV	Only if pheochromocytoma is suspected
Diazoxide (Hyperstat)	2 mg/kg; if no response, 1 mg/kg every 10 minutes	5 mg/kg	IV	Give rapidly without dilution; may cause tachycardia
Hydralazine (Apresoline)	0.15–0.6 mg/kg	6 mg/kg/d	IV	Give 4–6 hourly; action starts in 20–30 minutes; peak at 2 hours; may cause tachycardia
Minoxidil	0.1–0.2 mg/kg	1 mg/kg	PO	
Nifedipine (Adalat)	0.2–0.5 mg/kg	20 mg/dose	PO or sublingual	Capsules contain 10 mg in 0.34 mL or 20 mg in 0.45 mL; chew and swallow or use a tuberculin syringe; do not expose to light; may give headaches
Esmolol	500 μg/kg loading dose, then 200 μg/kg/min; can increase by 50–100 μg/kg every 5–10 min	1 mg/kg	IV	Avoid in asthmatics, heart failure, heart block
Labetalol (Normodyne, Trandate)	0.3 mg/kg/dose every 20 minutes until pressure is controlled, or 1 mg/kg/h	300 mg/day or 3 mg/kg/h	IV	Avoid in asthmatics, heart failure, heart block
α-Methyldopa (Aldomet)	10 mg/kg	50 mg/kg/d	IV	Takes 1–2 hours to act; somnolence
Enalaprilat (Vasotec IV)	25–100 μg/kg every 6 hours	—	IV	Precipitous fall of BP in high-renin states

added if pressures need to be lowered more. Furthermore, although β-adrenergic blockers have been used successfully for many years, they often produce unacceptable lethargy, weakness, and tiredness; therefore, they are less favored for monotherapy than they were.

SPECIFIC FEATURES OF DRUGS USED IN AMBULATORY TREATMENT   The doses in common use are listed in Table 22-32. Many of these doses are based on adult doses corrected for weight because there have not been enough careful studies of all of these agents in children; consequently, different authorities recommend different doses of some of these drugs.

Angiotensin-converting enzyme inhibitors decrease angiotensin concentrations and so reduce vasoconstriction and aldosterone concentrations and cause increased excretion of salt and water despite the increase in plasma renin. They also increase bradykinin concentrations, which may cause coughing. To avoid severe hy-

TABLE 22-32
AMBULATORY TREATMENT OF HYPERTENSION

DRUGS	DOSE (MG/KG/DAY)		INTERVAL BETWEEN DOSES (HOURS)
	INITIAL	MAXIMAL	
Diuretics			
Chlorothiazide	10	20	12–24
Hydrochlorothiazide	0.5	2	12–24
Furosemide	1	6	12–24
Vasodilators			
Hydralazine	0.75	7.5	6–12
Minoxidil	0.1	1	24
Central α_2-adrenergic antagonists			
Clonidine	0.005	0.025	12
α-Methyldopa	10	60	8–12
β-Adrenergic blocking agents			
Propranolol	1	8	8–12
Metoprolol	1	5	12
Atenolol	1	8	24
Nadolol	0.5	4	24
Labetalol	2	10	8–12
α-Adrenergic blocking agents			
Prazosin	0.02	0.4	8–12
Phentolamine	0.2[a]	1.0[a]	
Phenoxybenzamine	1	5	24
Calcium channel blockers			
Verapamil	4	8	12–24
Nifedipine (long acting)	30[b]	120[b]	12–24
Diltiazem	1.5	3.5	12–24
Amlodipine	0.1	0.3	24
Converting enzyme inhibitors or receptor blockade			
Captopril	1	6	8–12
Enalapril	0.1	0.75	12–24
Lisinopril	0.1	0.75	24
Losartan	1	2	12–24

[a] Given as single doses; see text.
[b] Total daily dose (mg).

potension, these drugs should be started in low dosage, particularly if the patient is dehydrated. Angiotensin receptor blockers block AT-1 receptors and do not affect bradykinin, and so may avoid the irritating cough. All these agents can rarely cause angioneurotic edema and renal failure.

Calcium blockers can now be given once or twice daily with slow release (SR) preparations. Nifedipine and amlodipine are among the most popular and effective drugs for children with hypertension and renal disease. Side effects of reflex tachycardia and headache occasionally limit their use.

No β-*adrenergic receptor blocker* is markedly superior to the others in lowering blood pressure, but they differ in side effects and frequency of dosage. These agents decrease renin secretion but may cause salt and water retention, so that diuretics may be needed as well. Decreased sympathetic β-adrenergic receptor stimulation of the airways and intestines leaves unopposed vagal action, which can cause bronchospasm and, rarely, diarrhea; cardioselective agents such as metoprolol or atenolol are less likely to cause bronchospasm than is propranolol. Because these drugs cross the blood-brain barrier, they may cause changes of mood or behavior.

α-*Adrenergic receptor blockers* such as prazosin act on presynaptic α-adrenergic receptors. Prazosin differs from the others in this group in not causing significant hypotension with exercise and not causing much postural hypotension and tachycardia. This is believed to result from blockade of the reuptake of norepinephrine by presynaptic nerve endings. Prazosin may cause profound postural hypotension after the first dose; thus, patients should take the first dose at night and be warned not to stand up suddenly. Other α-adrenergic blockers have limited usefulness. Phentolamine is used to test for increased circulating catecholamines as the cause of the hypertension, and phenoxybenzamine, given once daily and so better for long-term administration, is used to prepare patients with pheochromocytomas for surgery. Its dose can be increased at 7- to 14-day intervals. These agents, too, are used in treating the rebound hypertension caused by α-methyldopa or clonidine withdrawal.

CNS sympathetic inhibitors such as α-methyldopa and clonidine act predominantly in the central nervous system to reduce sympathetic outflow. In addition, α-methyldopa replaces norepinephrine in the storage granules of the vesicles and acts as an inefficient neurotransmitter. If the drugs are stopped suddenly, there may be sympathetic overactivity and severe rebound hypertension, which may limit their use in unreliable patients. A transdermal patch that releases clonidine at a fixed rate and is changed every 7 days has been used effectively in children, especially in those who dislike taking pills. The patch may cause contact dermatitis.

Peripheral adrenergic blocking agents such as reserpine and guanethidine affect the formation, storage, and release of norepinephrine in the storage granules of the postganglionic sympathetic nerve endings. They are used little today because of unacceptable side effects.

Diuretics reduce salt and water retention and so reduce blood volume but may also have some direct vasodilator effect. They may be all that is needed in mild hypertension. They are given once daily each morning. Doses (Table 22-32) are lower than those used in treating congestive heart failure. Doses can be increased after 1 to 2 weeks if there is an inadequate therapeutic effect. Thiazides are most often used, but better diuresis, if needed, may be obtained with oral furosemide. The hypotensive effects of these diuretics can be overcome if salt intake is high, and people tend to increase their salt intake when they take these diuretics. Therefore, patients should avoid salty foods and not add salt when food is brought to the table. A salt substitute may be helpful. Salt restriction is particularly important in renal hypertension, in which sodium excretion is often markedly impaired and in which an increased blood volume is often a major factor in the hypertension. Thiazides may increase blood glucose and lipoprotein concentrations.

Direct arteriolar vasodilators such as hydralazine usually increase renal blood flow and do not alter glomerular filtration rate. By lowering blood pressure, however, they may increase renin secretion as well as salt and water retention, so that they should be combined with diuretics. At high dosages, hydralazine causes a syndrome that resembles systemic lupus erythematosus and is reversible on withholding the drug. Minoxidil is a powerful vasodilator that is used in hypertension refractory to other forms of therapy.

RENOVASCULAR DISEASE

Renovascular disease causing hypertension is uncommon but should be considered seriously in investigating significant hypertension; it is proportionately more common in children than in adults.

ESSENTIAL HYPERTENSION

Typically, essential hypertension is recognized in the third decade of life and progresses slowly over many years. Studies emphasize not only the strong familial incidence of essential hypertension but also that young children of hypertensive parents tend to have pressures at the upper limits of normal. In some children these pressures remain at the upper limits of normal and rise with age, and it might be these who in the third decade have pressures recognized as being above an arbitrary level and thus are diagnosed as having essential hypertension.

Whether the cause of essential hypertension is genetic, environmental, or a mixture of both is unknown, and we do not know if this is a single disease or a syndrome common to many different diseases. Adults with essential hypertension have various combinations of high, normal, and low renin and aldosterone concentrations, so that they are different physiologically. Similar studies have not yet been reported in children. Recently, abnormal fluxes of sodium and potassium across the red cell membranes have been found in essential hypertension. Hypercalcemia (mild) and failure of the kidneys to produce dopamine in response to a salt load have also been suggested as causal mechanisms. The role of renal antihypertensive factors has been supported by the finding that patients with renal failure secondary to essential hypertension lose their hypertension after renal transplantation. Central nervous system factors and resetting of baroreceptors are also important, and an imbalance of endothelial dilator and constrictor factors has been invoked. Recently there has been interest in the association between hypertension and increased concentrations of angiotensinogen, and investigators have found linkage between the angiotensinogen gene locus and essential hypertension.

Essential hypertension is diagnosed from a family history and by excluding other causes of hypertension. In adults, lowering blood pressure by various means can reduce the cardiovascular complications of hypertension, even if it is fairly mild. However, no one has yet used medications to treat children with mild essential hypertension, because the long-term effects of the available drugs are unknown. Probably the wisest course would be use of preventive measures such as eliminating causes of stress, avoiding obesity and smoking, taking regular exercise, and eating a prudent diet. Salt intake should be reduced. Medications should, however, be used if blood pressure is high or if there are signs that it is causing damage.

Before hypertensive children are allowed to do strenuous exercise, formal exercise testing may be valuable. Maximal pressures over 230 mm Hg systolic or 130 mm Hg diastolic are taken by some authorities as reason to bar strenuous exercise because of concern about the cumulative effects of stressing the vascular system.

References

General

Avar MY, Hogg, RJ, Arant BS JR, Seikaly MG: Etiology of sustained hypertension in children in the southwestern United States. Pediatr Nephrol 8:186, 1994

Balfe JW, Levin L, Tsuru N, et al: Hypertension in childhood. Adv Pediatr 36:201, 1989

Bao W, Threefoot SA, Srinivasan SR, Berenson GS: Essential hypertension predicted by tracking of elevated blood pressure from childhood to adulthood: the Bogalusa Heart Study. Am J Hypertens 8:657, 1995

Caulfield M, Lavender P, Farrall M, et al: Linkage of the angiotensinogen gene to essential hypertension. N Engl J Med 330:1629, 1994

Deal JE, Snell ME, Barratt TM, Dillon MJ: Renovascular disease in childhood. J Pediatr 25:55, 1992

Hediger ML, Schall JI, Katz SH, et al: Resting blood pressure and pulse rate distributions in black adolescents. The Philadelphia blood pressure project. Pediatrics 74:1016, 1984

Hilton PJ: Cellular sodium transport in essential hypertension. N Engl J Med 221, 1986

Horan MJ, Lenfant C: Epidemiology of blood pressure and predictors of hypertension. Hypertension 15(Suppl I):1, 1990

Ingelfinger JR: Pediatric Hypertension. Philadelphia, WB Saunders, 1982

Jorgensen RS, Houston BK: Family history of hypertension, personality patterns, and cardiovascular reactivity to stress. Psychosom Med 48:102, 1986

Kaas IK: Blood pressure in offspring of hypertensive parents. Acta Paediatr Scand 73:842, 1984

Kurtz TW, Al-Bander HA, Morris RC Jr: "Salt-sensitive" essential hypertension in man. N Engl J Med 317:1043, 1987

Lauer RM, Burns TL, Clarke WR: Assessing children's blood pressure: considerations of age and body size. The Muscatine study. Pediatrics 75:1081, 1985

Lauer RM, Clarke WR, Beaglehole R: Level, trend, and variability of blood pressure during childhood. The Muscatine study. Circulation 69:242, 1984

Lifton, RP: Molecular genetics of human blood pressure variation. Science 272:676, 1996

Loggie JMH: Hypertension in children and adolescents. I. Causes and diagnostic studies. J Pediatr 74:331, 1966

Mahoney LT, Clark WR, Burns TL, Lauer RM: Childhood predictors of high blood pressure. Am J Hypertens 8:6085, 1991

Pickering TG, Laragh JH: Renovascular hypertension. In: Brenner BM, Rector FC, eds: The Kidney. Philadelphia, WB Saunders, 1991

Report of the Second Task Force on Blood Pressure Control in Children—1987. Pediatrics 79:1, 1987

Rosner B, Cook NR, Evans DA, et al: Reproducibility and predictive values of routine blood pressure measurements in children. Am J Epidemiol 126:1115, 1987

Sinaiko AR: Hypertension in children. N Engl J Med 335:1968, 1996

Sokolow M, Perloff D, Cowan R: Contribution of ambulatory blood pressure to the assessment of patients with mild to moderate elevation of office blood pressure. Cardiovasc Rev Rep 1:295, 1980

Strauer BE, Bayer F, Brecht HM, Motz W: The influence of sympathetic nervous activity on regression of cardiac hypertrophy. J Hypertens 3(Suppl 4):39, 1985

Update on the 1987 Task Force on High Blood Pressure in Children and Adolescents: A Working Group Report from the National High Blood Pressure Education Program. Pediatrics 98:649, 1996

Voors AW, Webbe LS, Berenson G: Relationship of blood pressure levels to height and weight in children. Cardiovasc Med 3:911, 1978

Weinberger MH, Miller JZ, Luft FC, et al: Definitions and characteristics of sodium sensitivity and blood pressure resistance. Hypertension 8(Suppl II):127, 1986

Williams RR, Hung SC, Hasstedt SJ, et al: Multigenic human hypertension: evidence for subtypes and hope for haplo-types. J Hypertens 8(Suppl 7):S39, 1990

Zachariah PK, Sheps SG, Ilstrup DM, et al: Blood pressure load—a better determinant of hypertension. Mayo Clin Proc 63:1085, 1988

Treatment

De Quattro V: Treating hypertensive crises: which drugs for which patient? J Crit Illness 2:24, 1987

Freis ED: Should mild hypertension be treated? N Engl J Med 307:306, 1982

Garcia JY, Vidt DG: Current management of hypertensive emergencies. Drugs 34:263, 1987

MacMahon SW, Wilcken DE, MacDonald GJ: The effect of weight reduction on left ventricular mass. A randomized controlled trial in young, overweight hypertensive patients. N Engl J Med 314:334, 1986

Sinaiko AR: Treatment of hypertension in children. Pediatr Nephrol 8:603, 1994

Wollam GL, Hall WD, Porter VD, et al: Time course of regression of left ventricular hypertrophy in treated hypertensive patients. Am J Med 75(Suppl):100, 1983

Wood AJJ: Pharmacologic differences between beta blockers. Am Heart J 108:1070, 1984

Exercise

Kaplan NM, Deveraux RB, Miller HS Jr: Task Force 4: systemic hypertension. J Am Coll Cardiol 24:885, 1994

Maron BJ, Mitchell JH: Revised eligibility criteria for competitive athletes with cardiovascular abnormalities. J Am Coll Cardiol 24:848, 1994

Nudel DB, Gootman N, Brunson SC, et al: Exercise performance of hypertensive adolescents. Pediatrics 65:1073, 1980

Strong WB: Hypertension and sports. Pediatrics 64:693, 1979

22.4.6 Pediatric Heart Transplantation

Daniel Bernstein and Clifford Chin

The first human heart transplant was done by Barnard in 1966. Poor initial survival dampened enthusiasm for heart transplantation, but after cyclosporine was introduced in 1980, widespread interest in the procedure was renewed.

Initially, most pediatric transplants were done on adolescents, but by 1984 heart transplantation was extended to infants below 1 year of age. Over the last 5 years, between 350 and 400 pediatric heart transplants were done annually worldwide. Survival for all patients under 18 years of age listed in the registry of the International Society for Heart Transplantation is 75% at 1 year and 65% at 5 years (Fig. 22-90), comparing favorably to survival rates in adults. Early posttransplant survival is slightly lower in patients under 1 year of age, but this difference disappears after 7 years posttransplant. The long-term outlook for pediatric heart transplant

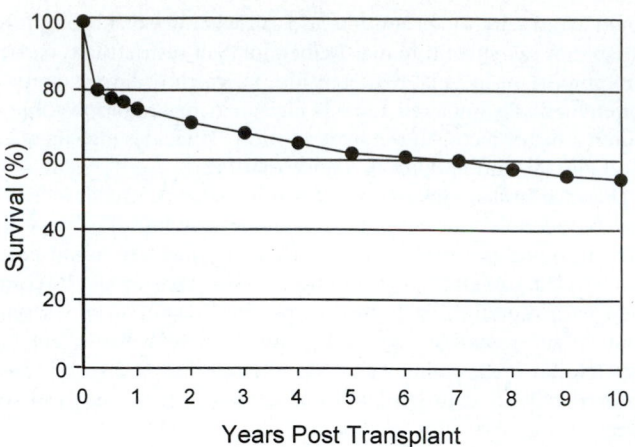

FIGURE 22-90 Actuarial survival after pediatric heart transplantation. Data are from 3493 patients under 18 years of age transplanted between 1982 and 1997 and entered into the Registry of the International Society for Heart and Lung Transplantation. SOURCE: *Boucek et al: J Heart Lung Transplant 17:1141, 1998.*

recipients is improving; a growing number of children are approaching 10 and even 20 years of survival. At present, cardiac transplantation is accepted as therapy for infants and children with cardiomyopathies for which no standard surgical alternative exists and for some forms of complex congenital heart disease for which surgical procedures are extremely high risk or ineffective.

INDICATIONS FOR PEDIATRIC HEART TRANSPLANTATION

Over 1 year of age, cardiomyopathies are the most common indication, accounting for about 60% of the combined worldwide experience in heart transplantation. Although transplantation is not considered the primary therapy for most patients with congenital heart disease, many patients with complex congenital heart disease who have had conventional surgery for congenital heart lesions (eg, the Mustard, Fontan, or Norwood procedures) present with late myocardial dysfunction; these patients now account for nearly 40% of transplants between 1 and 10 years of age. The one group of patients with congenital heart disease in whom primary cardiac transplantation is considered is those neonates with hypoplastic left heart syndrome. However, donor scarcity still limits the availability of this option. Because of this, and the increased success rate of the Norwood operation, many pediatric transplant centers do not recommend primary heart transplantation for these patients.

RECIPIENT AND DONOR SELECTION

Potential heart transplant recipients are screened for other serious medical problems, such as systemic infection, severe hepatic or renal dysfunction, or severe malnutrition, that may disqualify them. Pulmonary vascular resistance is measured, and patients with pulmonary vascular resistance above 5 to 8 mm Hg/L/min nonresponsive to pulmonary vasodilators may be candidates for combined heart-lung allografts. The family support system is evaluated to ensure compliance with the complicated posttransplant medical regimen. While awaiting transplantation, patients with poor left ventricular function are placed on maximal anticongestive therapy, often parenterally. Oral β-adrenergic blocking agents (eg, metoprolol, carvedilol) and high-dose angiotensin-converting enzyme (ACE) inhibitors (eg, captopril and enalapril) have significantly improved the survival of adult patients with cardiomyopathy while awaiting transplantation. The safety and efficacy of these agents are currently being investigated in children. In patients with poor ventricular function, anticoagulants are added to reduce the risk of mural thrombosis and thromboembolism. Patients should be routinely screened for arrhythmias, and antiarrhythmic drugs and/or implantable cardioverter-defibrillators may be used to manage potential life-threatening arrhythmias.

Donor availability is a serious problem for children. Potential recipients are listed on a computerized registry, and allografts are selected by matching ABO blood groups and approximate body weight and heart size. Specific HLA matching is not currently feasible in heart transplantation, and in the cyclosporine era the advantage offered by such matching is controversial. Contraindications for organ donation include preexisting severe cardiac disease, prolonged cardiac arrest, evidence of systemic illness or infection, and cardiac dysfunction. Because of the scarcity of pediatric-age donors, a history of resuscitation or easily repairable congenital heart disease (eg, atrial or ventricular septal defect) is not an automatic exclusion.

OPERATIVE AND POSTOPERATIVE MANAGEMENT

Both donor and recipient hearts are excised, leaving the posterior atrial walls containing the venae cavae and pulmonary veins. The great vessels are divided distal to the semilunar valves. The donor atria are then sutured to the remaining posterior portion of the recipient's atria, and the great vessels are anastomosed. Most pediatric heart transplant recipients can be extubated within the first 48 hours posttransplant. Without complications, patients can usually be discharged within 1 to 2 weeks.

Immediate postoperative immunosuppression is achieved at most centers with a combination of cyclosporine (10 mg/kg/d), azathioprine (1 to 2 mg/kg/d), and prednisone started at 0.6 mg/kg/d and tapered to 0.2 mg/kg/d over the first 6 weeks. Many centers also use induction therapy with either murine antihuman T lymphocyte antibody (OKT3) or antilymphocyte globulin (ATG). Newly developed antibodies directed against the IL-2 receptor on activated T cells have the advantage of increased selectivity for activated lymphocytes. Through genetic engineering, a "humanized" form of this antibody has been developed in which side effects have been significantly reduced. In children without graft rejection, steroids are tapered to an alternate-day regimen after the first 6 to 12 months and can sometimes be totally eliminated. In some centers, steroids are not routinely included for maintenance immunosuppression but are added later if rejection becomes uncontrollable. Some centers now use tacrolimus (FK-506) instead of cyclosporine as the primary immunosuppressive agent. Pediatric patients treated with tacrolimus have similar rates of survival and rejection as those treated with cyclosporine; however, they have a reduced need for steroids and less hypertension. Tacrolimus does not cause hirsutism or ginigival hyperplasia, often a problem with cyclosporine, although it may cause a higher incidence of diabetes. Newer immunosuppressive agents such as mycophenolate mofetil are currently being used in selected children in lieu of azathioprine and may offer some advantage, especially in those patients with resistant rejection.

DIAGNOSIS AND TREATMENT OF REJECTION

Posttransplant management centers on preventing acute graft rejection, the second leading cause of death in both adult and pedi-

atric heart transplant recipients. The incidence of acute graft rejection is greatest within the first 3 to 6 months after transplantation, and most children have at least one episode of rejection within the first year after transplantation. Evidence of acute rejection may include fatigue, fluid retention, fever, diaphoresis, a gallop rhythm, reduced voltage on the electrocardiogram, atrial or ventricular arrhythmia or heart block, and radiologic changes of an enlarged heart or pulmonary edema. However, the routine use of cyclosporine has resulted in loss of sensitivity of these markers of rejection, and most rejection episodes occur without any detectable clinical symptoms. Echocardiographic indices of systolic and diastolic left ventricular function are currently being evaluated as predictors of early rejection. However, most transplant centers do not rely on noninvasive methods alone in rejection surveillance.

Currently, right ventricular myocardial biopsy remains the most reliable method of rejection surveillance and can be performed safely in infants and children. In adolescents, myocardial biopsies may be performed as often as every 1 to 4 weeks during the first 6 months. If the patient remains rejection-free, the frequency is reduced to three or four biopsies per year. In infants and toddlers, surveillance biopsies are usually performed less often and can be as infrequent as once or twice yearly.

Cardiac rejection is graded according to a system developed by the International Society for Heart and Lung Transplantation (ISHLT) based on the amount of cellular infiltration and myocyte necrosis. Grade 1 or 2 rejection does not lead to a change in treatment, but a repeat biopsy specimen is usually obtained within 1 to 2 weeks; 21 to 43% of these episodes progress to grade 3 or greater rejection, and the rest resolve spontaneously. For grade 3 or 4 rejection, intravenous methylprednisolone or an increase in oral prednisone is given for one or two short courses. If rejection persists, several additional therapeutic regimens are available, including switching to another primary immunosuppressant (tacrolimus, mycophenolate), a repeat course of OKT3, antithymocyte globulin, or total lymphoid irradiation. The ultimate treatment for refractory rejection is retransplantation.

LONG-TERM COMPLICATIONS

INFECTION Infection is the most serious complication of chronic immunosuppression and is the major cause of morbidity in these patients. Between one-quarter and one-third of all deaths are from infection. The incidence of infection is greatest in the first 3 to 6 months posttransplant when immunosuppressive doses are highest. Fortunately, cyclosporine, by allowing a reduction in steroid dose, has reduced the mortality from serious infectious episodes in children from 26% to 11%. Viruses are the most common agents of infection, and although most normal childhood viral illnesses are well tolerated, herpes simplex and cytomegalovirus often lead to serious disease. Cytomegalovirus infections account for as many as 25% of infectious episodes and may occur either as a primary infection or as a reactivation. Severe cytomegalovirus infection is disseminated, associated with pneumonitis, and often associated with graft rejection. Ganciclovir prophylaxis has reduced the incidence of this serious infection. Bacterial infections are the next most frequent, with the lung being the most common site (35%), followed by the blood, urinary tract, and, less commonly, the sternotomy site. Fungi (14%) and protozoa (6%) also cause posttransplant infections. Those children treated without steroids have less infection.

RENAL FUNCTION AND HYPERTENSION Cyclosporine may cause chronic tubulointerstitial nephropathy in adult heart transplant recipients. Although most children develop a gradual increase in serum creatinine during the first posttransplant year, renal dysfunction resolves in most of them when cyclosporine dosage is reduced; severe nephrotoxicity is less common. Hypertension is more common, being reported in as many as 90% of pediatric heart transplant recipients, although it is less common with tacrolimus. It results from a defect in renal sodium excretion and from plasma volume expansion rather than from activation of the renin-angiotensin or sympathetic nervous system. Corticosteroids may thus potentiate cyclosporine-induced hypertension.

HEMATOLOGIC   Mild generalized bone marrow suppression is common with azathioprine and less common with mycophenolate. Moderate to severe anemia has occasionally been associated with tacrolimus.

METABOLIC   Elevations in hepatic transaminases can occur with azathioprine and are usually reversible. New-onset diabetes mellitus has been associated with tacrolimus and may be associated with higher doses and with concomitant pulse steroid therapy. Hyperlipidemia is common and may play a role in the development of graft coronary artery disease (see below).

GROWTH RETARDATION   The growth-inhibiting effects of chronic steroid administration are significant. Fortunately, with careful monitoring, most children can be tapered to alternate-day steroid regimens associated with improved linear growth, and some can be weaned off steroids entirely. In long-term studies, 75% of pediatric heart transplant recipients achieve normal growth by 5 years posttransplant.

NEUROLOGIC SEQUELAE   The most common neurologic problems are side effects of cyclosporine and include tremor, seizures, myalgias, and paresthesias. Intracranial infections, such as meningitis, brain abscess, and encephalitis, are less common; the most common organisms are *Aspergillus*, *Cryptococcus neoformans*, and *Listeria monocytogenes*. Many of the expected clinical findings, such as nuchal rigidity, may be absent in immunosuppressed patients, so that early diagnosis requires a heightened index of suspicion.

ORTHOPEDIC SEQUELAE   Bone disease, such as osteoporosis and aseptic necrosis, has been described only rarely in pediatric heart transplant recipients but is an added reason for reducing the corticosteroid dosage as soon as tolerated

LYMPHOPROLIFERATIVE DISEASE   A serious complication of immunosuppressive therapy for transplantation has been the appearance of neoplasms, the most common being lymphoma. Many of these posttransplant lymphomas are associated with infection by Epstein-Barr virus and are now classified as "lymphoproliferative disorders" because of their more favorable prognosis and often dramatic response to reduction of immunosuppression.

GRAFT CORONARY ARTERY DISEASE   Accelerated graft coronary vascular disease occurs in 33 to 50% of adult heart transplant recipients. In children, graft atherosclerosis is more variable, ranging in different series from 10 to 30%. Unlike typical coronary atherosclerosis, graft coronary artery disease is diffuse with distal vessel involvement and is presumed to result from immunologically mediated vessel injury. Because the graft lacks innervation, angina pectoris is absent, and thus, routine coronary angiography is done annually to detect this disorder. Standard medical and surgical therapies are usually not useful, and repeat heart transplantation has been the only effective treatment. Calcium channel blockers have recently been shown to reduce the occurrence of graft coronary disease. Careful control of hyperlipidemia with the "statin" drugs (atorvastatin, pravastatin) may also be protective.

COSMETIC ISSUES   Corticosteroid therapy may result in a cushingoid facial appearance and steroid acne. Cyclosporine has also been implicated in the development of a change in facial features, hypertrichosis, and gingival hyperplasia. Many of these complications are dose related and improve with adjustments in immunosuppressive medications.

REHABILITATION

The ultimate goal of heart transplantation is return to normal activity and life style, which must be sufficiently likely to outweigh the complications listed above. For heart transplantation in children, the prospect for rehabilitation is excellent; at most centers 90 to 100% of patients discharged from hospital are in New York Heart Association functional class I. In the Stanford experience, one-quarter of pediatric heart transplant recipients have never been hospitalized for illness after their initial operation.

Pediatric transplant recipients can return to school and obtain regular employment on graduation. They participate in both noncompetitive and competitive sports and other age-appropriate activities with almost no limitations; contact sports should be avoided. Major adjustments occur in the family, as the child who was formerly severely limited begins to experience the newfound freedom associated with a return to full physical activity. Psychological adjustment to the transplant experience, as assessed by standardized personality/behavior inventories, is usually good in children. There is, however, a disturbing incidence of noncompliance in patients once they reach adolescence, similar to that encountered in other chronic illnesses. Early counseling interventions may be able to prevent the life-threatening consequences if these teenagers discontinue their immunosuppressive medications.

Both invasive and noninvasive tests of ventricular function show excellent long-term results. Myocardial growth is excellent, although persistent mild hypertrophy is common. The pulmonary arterial and aortic anastomotic sites grow adequately in all but patients operated on for the hypoplastic left heart syndrome, in whom aortic coarctation may recur. Because the transplanted heart is denervated, cardiac function depends on the release of circulating catecholamines. Thus, the increase in heart rate and cardiac output during exercise is slower than normal, and maximal heart rate and cardiac output responses are attenuated. However, rarely are these abnormalities associated with overt symptoms.

CONTROVERSIES AND NEW FRONTIERS

HYPOPLASTIC LEFT HEART SYNDROME   There is still controversy regarding the best surgical management of neonates with hypoplastic left heart syndrome, ie, transplantation versus palliation with the Norwood procedure. Early survival is now similar for both options; however, the problem of donor availability may limit the number of neonates who will benefit from this procedure. One approach to this problem is to perform the first stage of the Norwood procedure as a bridge to transplantation in later infancy.

NEW IMMUNOSUPPRESSIVE AGENTS The development of new, more specifically targeted immunosuppressive drugs should help to reduce posttransplant morbidity and mortality. Mycophenolate mofetil is associated with less generalized bone marrow suppression than azathioprine; however, randomized controlled studies have been performed only in adults, and there is still controversy as to whether this agent should be routinely substituted for azathioprine. Tacrolimus (FK-506) has gained favor in many pediatric centers as a substitute for cyclosporine because of the absence of gingival hyperplasia and hirsutism. Many centers still use cyclosporine-azathioprine-prednisone as their primary immunosuppressive regimen but switch to mycophenolate or tacrolimus when a patient develops excessive or resistant rejection episodes. "Humanized" antilymphocyte preparations that are more specific for activated T cells may eventually replace antilymphocyte globulin or OKT3. Total lymphoid irradiation has now been used successfully to treat refractory rejection in several children and holds the theoretical advantage of conferring long-term graft tolerance.

HEART-LUNG AND UNILATERAL LUNG TRANSPLANTATION The experience with heart-lung transplantation in children is growing. Indications include pulmonary hypoplasia associated with congenital heart disease, Eisenmenger syndrome, primary pulmonary hypertension, and cystic fibrosis. Initial results in both adults and children demonstrate 65% 1-year and 54% 3-year survival rates; however, improved patient selection and postoperative management are improving survival statistic. Postoperative indices of cardiopulmonary function and exercise capacity show significant improvement. Obliterative bronchiolitis, a form of chronic rejection, remains a major limitation to long-term survival. Problems of donor availability are even more severe with lung transplantation. The selected use of living-related lung transplantation, in which a lobe from a parent is transplanted into a child, may partially alleviate this problem.

NONINVASIVE METHODS OF REJECTION SURVEILLANCE Despite recent advances, there is still no universally accepted noninvasive method to detect cardiac rejection in children. Computerized electrocardiographic analysis and echocardiographic indices of systolic and diastolic ventricular function appear promising in early studies.

References

Addonizio LJ, Gersony WM, Robbins RC, et al: Elevated pulmonary vascular resistance and cardiac transplantation. Circulation 76(Suppl V): 52, 1987

Asante-Korang A, Boyle GJ, Webber SA, et al: Experience of FK506 immune suppression in pediatric heart transplantation: a study of long-term adverse effects. J Heart Lung Transplant 15:415, 1996.

Bailey NA, Lay P: New horizons: infant cardiac transplantation. Heart Lung 18:172, 1989

Baum D, Bernstein D, Starnes VA, et al: Pediatric heart transplantation at Stanford: results of a 15 year experience. Pediatrics 88:203, 1991

Baum D, Miller WW, eds: Pediatric Heart, Heart-Lung, and Lung Transplantation. Prog Pediatr Cardiol 4(2), 1993; 3(1), 1994

Bernstein D, Baum D, Berry G, et al: Neoplastic disorders after pediatric heart transplantation. Circulation 88(Part 2):230, 1993

Bernstein D, Kolla S, Miner M, et al: Cardiac growth after pediatric heart transplantation. Circulation 85:1433, 1992

Bernstein D, Starnes VA, Baum D: Pediatric heart transplantation. In: Barness L, ed: Advances in Pediatrics, vol 37. Chicago, Year-Book, 1990: 413

Billingham M, Cary N, Hammond M, et al: A working formulation for the standardization of nomenclature in the diagnosis of heart and lung rejection: heart rejection study group. J Heart Transplant 9:587, 1990

Boucek MM, Novick RJ, Bennett LE, et al: The registry of the International Society of Heart and Lung Transplantation: second official pediatric report—1998. J Heart Lung Transplant 17:1141, 1999

Fricker FJ, Griffith BP, Hardesty RL, et al: Experience with heart transplantation in children. Pediatrics 79:138, 1987

Gao SZ, Schroeder JS, Alderman EL, et al: Clinical and laboratory correlates of accelerated coronary artery disease in the cardiac transplant patient. Circulation 76(Suppl 5):56, 1987

Grattan MT, Moreno-Cabral CE, Starnes VA, et al: Cytomegalovirus infection is associated with cardiac allograft rejection and atherosclerosis. JAMA 261:3561, 1989

Green M, Wald ER, Fricker FJ, et al: Infections in pediatric orthotopic heart transplant recipients. Pediatr Infect Dis 8:87, 1989

Hotson JR, Enzmann DR: Neurologic complications of cardiac transplantation. Neurol Clin 6:346, 1988

Kirklin JK, Bourge RC, McGiffin DC: Recurrent or persistent cardiac allograft rejection: therapeutic options and recommendations. Transplant Proc 29(Suppl 8A):40S, 1997

Kobashigawa JA: Controversies in heart and lung transplantation immunosuppression: tacrolimus versus cyclosporine. Transplant Proc 30: 1095, 1998

Kobashigawa J, Miller L, Renlund D, et al: A randomized active-controlled trial of mycophenolate mofetil in heart transplant recipients. Transplantation 66:507, 1998

Lawrence KS, Fricker FJ: Pediatric heart transplantation: quality of life. J Heart Transplant 6:329, 1987

Pope SE, Stinson EB, Daughters GT, et al: Exercise response of the denervated heart in long-term cardiac transplantation recipients. Am J Cardiol 46:213, 1980

Schroeder JS, Gao SZ, Alderman EL: A preliminary study of diltiazem in the prevention of coronary artery disease in heart transplant recipients. N Engl J Med 3:164, 1993

Uzark K, Crowley D, Behrendt D, et al: Effects of pediatric heart transplantation on the family. Circulation 76(Suppl IV):145, 1987

Vincenti F, Kirkman R, Light S, et al: Interleukin-2-receptor blockade with daclizumab to prevent acute rejection in renal transplantation. N Engl J Med 338:161, 1998

Wagner K, Webber SA, Kurland G, et al: New-onset diabetes mellitus in pediatric thoracic organ recipients receiving tacrolimus-based immunosuppression. J Heart Lung Transplant 16:275, 1997

Wood AJ, Maurer G, Niederberger W, et al: Cyclosporine: pharamacokinetics, metabolism, and drug interactions. Transplant Proc 15(Suppl 1): 2409, 1983

22.4.7   Atherosclerosis

Julien I. E. Hoffman

INCIDENCE

In the Western world, coronary atherosclerosis causes about 30 to 40% of all deaths and is a major cause of disability and death in middle-aged and even young adults. Advanced atheroma was found at autopsy in a large percentage of US soldiers killed in Korea and Vietnam. In the West, deaths from coronary atherosclerosis are decreasing, but in former Eastern bloc countries, this disease process is increasing at an alarming rate. Although complications of atherosclerosis are rare before middle age, the atherosclerotic process begins in childhood. Furthermore, habits acquired in childhood predispose to the development and progression of atherosclerosis in later life.

PATHOLOGY

Atherosclerosis affects all large arteries, sparing only upper limb arteries. The earliest lesions are (inflammatory) focal intimal fatty streaks: thin yellow, raised streaks caused by accumulation of T cells and fatty droplets inside macrophages (foam cells). These lesions may regress, but populations with a high incidence of fatty streaks have a high incidence of advanced coronary atheromata. Then lesions appear that include foam cells formed from macrophages and transformed smooth muscle cells, T lymphocytes, and a few extracellular lipid droplets. More advanced lesions include fibrous plaques—raised white lesions caused by focal intimal accumulations of foam cells with a collagen cap over a deeper and larger deposit of extracellular lipids, cellular debris, and T lymphocytes. The plaques initially are eccentric and do not compromise arterial blood flow, but later they bulge into the lumen and restrict blood flow. Advanced plaques may calcify and/or rupture, leading to platelet-rich thrombi on these plaques that partially or completely occlude the artery. Thrombi or plaque fragments may embolize to distal coronary arteries, abdominal organs, lower limbs, or brain. Atherosclerotic arteries have reduced ability to dilate and are prone to vasospasm so that there can be myocardial ischemia without physical occlusion.

PATHOGENESIS

The arterial endothelium normally limits intimal penetration by large molecules like very low-density (VLDL) or low-density (LDL) lipoproteins. However, smaller particles such as high-density lipoproteins (HDL) move freely across the endothelium, thus explaining how HDL participates in removing cholesterol from cells in general and foam cells in particular. HDL is also associated with an enzyme, paraoxonase, which hydrolyzes lipid peroxides and limits LDL oxidation. Endothelial cells produce prostacyclin (PGI_2) and nitric oxide, which inhibit platelet aggregation and prevent vasospasm.

The first pathologic change in atherosclerosis might be increased endothelial permeability to large molecules like lipoproteins—a nonspecific response to viruses, toxins, immune complexes, products of activated white blood cells, or platelets. It can also result from a raised apolipoprotein B–containing lipoprotein concentration in the blood. When lipoproteins enter the intima, the main protein moiety of LDL and VLDL (apolipoprotein B) binds to negatively charged glycosoaminoglycans and elastin in the intima, causing lipoproteins to accumulate there. The LDL may be modified (oxidized and acetylated) by 15-lipoxygenase and only then is taken up by macrophages (scavenger cells) via the acetyl-LDL receptors, creating foam cells. Oxidized LDL is immunogenic.

Further chemical modifications of LDL occur. Modified LDL produces a chemotactic factor and is cytotoxic to endothelial cells. Blood monocytes become attracted to the endothelium, adhere to it, enter the subendothelial space, and become macrophages. As they fill with lipid droplets of cholesteryl esters that they cannot metabolize, they raise the endothelium into an irregular surface; endothelial permeability increases, and the lumen is compromised. T lymphocytes are also found. (Monocyte chemotaxis and intimal penetration may also initiate atherogenesis.) Endothelial damage induces platelets to aggregate on their luminal surface, degranulate, and produce ADP and thromboxane A_2, which lead to more platelet aggregation. Platelets, endothelial cells, macrophages, and T lymphocytes produce cytokines such as colony-stimulating factors, insulin-like growth factor 1, TGF-β, interleukin-1, and TNF-α, all of which have many inflammatory actions stimulating the growth of the atheroma. One of these factors is platelet-derived growth factor (PDGF), which causes smooth muscle cells to divide, migrate into the intima, and take up lipoproteins to become foam cells, produce elastin and collagen, and form fibrous plaques. Other cytokines have similar actions.

The atheromas appear in low-shear regions except for the coronary arterial atheroma that occurs in transplant recipients.

ETIOLOGY

Many factors that promote coronary atherosclerosis are either familial, promote endothelial injury, or both. Others are common to affluent industrial societies, such as more sedentary work and mental stress, excessive fat and carbohydrate intake, cigarette smoking, obesity, and less heavy exercise. There may be different factors responsible for the underlying atheroma and the subsequent thrombosis.

One major risk factor is a family history of coronary arterial disease under 55 years of age. There are many mechanisms for this relationship.

1. Not only are there many genetically determined lipoprotein and apolipoprotein abnormalities (see Sec. 9.14), but more recently various restriction-fragment length polymorphisms of apolipoproteins have been associated with coronary atherosclerosis. Small LDL particles and some isoforms of lipoprotein(a) are also independent risk factors.
2. Abnormal clotting factors are associated with an increased risk of myocardial infarction. These include a high plasma fibrinogen concentration and mutations of factor V (Leiden), factor VII, tissue plasminogen activator, plasminogen-activator inhibitor, and platelet glycoprotein IIb/IIA receptor.
3. Obesity, diabetes mellitus, hyperinsulinemia.
4. Hypertension.

Low-estrogen states are associated with an increased risk of coronary atheroma and myocardial infarction; these are male gender and the postmenopausal state in women. Estrogen lowers LDL and raises HDL concentrations, protecting the premenopausal woman.

Endothelial dysfunction is prominent in atheromatous subjects. Some important causes are:

1. Smoking (also increases platelet adhesiveness and lowers HDL concentrations).
2. Sedentary life style.
3. High homocysteine concentration. This is thought to facilitate atherosclerosis, an important issue because the concentrations can be lowered by an adequate folic acid intake.
4. Hypercholesterolemia, independent of HDL concentrations.

Many infections damage the endothelium, and people with coronary heart disease have an increased incidence of antibodies to *Chlamydia pneumoniae*. This may be why an increased C-reactive protein concentration is associated with an increased risk of myocardial infarction.

Reactive oxygen free radicals have also been implicated in atheroma.

The importance of cholesterol is clear. It forms a large part of the atheromatous lesion. Atheromata are more frequent in those with hypercholesterolemia associated with apolipoprotein B–containing lipoproteins, whether genetic or not, and strict reduction of blood cholesterol concentration can cause regression of atheroma. (Raising HDL concentrations independently can also cause regression of atheromata.) How much excess dietary cholesterol is responsible for causing atheroma is less clear, although the role of excess intake of saturated fats is more certain. It is difficult to distinguish between the role of diet and the many other factors described above.

PREVENTION

Because of the strong familial association, a pediatric history should ask about diabetes mellitus, hypertension, premature coronary disease, sudden death, xanthomata, clotting disorders, and raised blood cholesterol levels in close relatives. Positive responses should lead to careful assessment of factors that could promote coronary atherosclerosis and to screening of blood lipids. It is as important to determine the relative LDL/HDL cholesterol concentrations as to measure total serum cholesterol. There are no current recommendations for lipid screening of all children, although there are proponents of this approach.

The Surgeon General and the National Research Council have recommended a decreased intake of saturated fat and cholesterol in everyone over 2 years of age. The American Heart Association recommends a prudent diet in which less than 30% of calories come from fat and less than 10% of calories come from saturated fats; cholesterol intake should be under 200 mg/day. Some authorities question the importance of this last requirement. Not only is it very restrictive, the amount being that in one egg, but there is no clear evidence that dietary cholesterol intake, per se, affects blood lipoprotein concentrations. A reduction in saturated fatty acids is beneficial, but the role of polyunsaturated fatty acids is unclear. Some studies show that monounsaturated fatty acids such as oleic acid help to lower blood cholesterol concentrations without the lowering of HDL concentrations that occurs when the diet is high in polyunsaturated fatty acids. On the other hand, *trans*-unsaturated fatty acids probably promote atheromatosis. One recent study showed that replacing saturated and *trans*-unsaturated fatty acids with mono- and polyunsaturated fatty acids had a greater effect than did reducing total fat intake in decreasing coronary arterial disease in women. By adopting these prudent measures, we can avoid recommending some arbitrary cutoff point of serum cholesterol concentration for implementing a diet in healthy children. The total caloric intake should allow normal but not excessive weight gain, and parents should be made aware that an overweight child is not healthy. Organ meats and fatty meats should be limited. Skim or low-fat milk should be substituted for whole milk and butter, and intake of whole-milk cheeses should be minimized. Cottage cheese made from skim or low fat milk is a good source of protein with little fat or cholesterol. It is important for growing children to avoid as much as possible the products of fast food stores, which promote meals consisting largely of deep fat fried french fries, a high-fat-content hamburger with cheese, mayonnaise, and a fat-based dressing, not to mention the milk shake made with cream. These meals are inexpensive, so that children with minimal money to spend on food can take in as much fat and calories at one of these meals as they should in a week.

Physical exercise, isotonic and not isometric, should be encouraged. Thirty minutes of strenuous exercise three times weekly may be as protective as more intensive exercise regimens. One effect of exercise is to increase HDL concentrations that protect against coronary heart disease.

Smoking cigarettes should be absolutely discouraged.

Hypertension should be controlled.

Add fish to the diet. Cold water fatty fish have little arachidonic acid but much eicosapentaenoic acid, an ω-3 fatty acid. Eicosapentaenoic acid competes with arachidonic acid for the same enzyme system, so that instead of thromboxane A_2, thromboxane A_3 with negligible platelet-aggregating and vasoconstrictive effects is produced. This may be in part why Greenland Eskimos who have high total blood cholesterol concentrations and high intake of fats from seal and whale meat have little coronary heart disease.

Fruits and vegetables contain flavonoids (eg, quercetin and reveritrol in grape juice), antioxidants (eg, α-tocopherol and lycopene found in tomatoes and pink grapefruit), vitamins, and folic acid (which lowers homocysteine concentrations in serum). These dietary elements may play an important role in preventing atheromata, although the definitive clinical trials remain to be done. Eating these foods also helps to replace some of the mass of the diet, thus reducing the quantity of fat and carbohydrates in the meal.

Giving estrogen to women with low estrogen concentrations (ovarian failure, postmenopausal) reduces the risk of coronary heart disease.

References

Ascherio A, Katan MB, Zock PL, et al: Trans fatty acids and coronary heart disease. N Engl J Med 340:1994, 1999

Berenson GS, Srinivasan S, Bao W, et al: Association between multiple cardiovascular risk factors and atherosclerosis in children and young adults. N Engl J Med 338:1650, 1998

Breslow JL, Deeb S, Lalouel JM: AHA conference report on cholesterol. Workshop II. Genetic susceptibility to atherosclerosis. Circulation 80: 724, 1989

Burke AP, Farb A, Malcolm JT, et al: Coronary risk factors and plaque morphology in men with coronary disease who died suddenly. N Engl J Med 336:1276, 1997

Chait A, Brazg RL, Tribble DL, Krauss RM: Susceptibility of small, low density lipoproteins to oxidative modification in subjects with atherogenic lipoprotein phenotype, pattern B. Am J Med 94:350, 1993

Clarke R, Daly L, Robinson K, et al: Hyperhomocysteinemia: an independent risk factor for vascular disease. N Engl J Med 324:1149, 1991

Constant J: Alcohol, ischemic heart disease, and the French paradox. Clin Cardiol 20:420, 1997

Davidson M, Kuo C-C, Middaugh JP, et al: Confirmed previous infection with *Chlamydia pneumoniae* (YWAR) and its presence in early coronary atherosclerosis. Circulation 98:628, 1998

Daviglus ML, Stamler J, Orencia AJ, et al: Fish consumption and the 30-year risk of fatal myocardial infarction. N Engl J Med 336:1046, 1997

Després J-P, Lamarche B, Mauriège P, et al: Hyperinsulinemia as an independent risk factor for ischemic heart disease. N Engl J Med 334:952, 1996

Diaz MN, Frei B, Vita JA, Keaney JF Jr: Antioxidants and atherosclerotic heart disease. N Engl J Med 337:40, 1997

Freedman DS, Srinivasan SR, Shear CL: The relation of apolipoproteins A_1 and B in children to parental myocardial infarction. N Engl J Med 315: 721, 1986

Fuster V, Badimon L, Badimon JJ, Chesebro JH: The pathogenesis of coronary artery disease and the acute coronary syndromes. N Engl J Med 326:242 and 310, 1992

Goodman DS, Bradford RH, Brewer HB Jr. AHA conference report on cholesterol. Workshop IV. Diagnosis, evaluation and treatment: current status and issues. Circulation 80:735, 1989

Grodstein F, Stampfer MJ, Manson JE, et al: Postmenopausal estrogen and progestin use and the risk of cardiovascular disease. N Engl J Med 335: 453, 1996

Grundy SM, Broen WV, Dietschy JM. AHA conference report on cholesterol. Workshop III. Basis for dietary treatment. Circulation 80:729, 1989

Hajjar DP: Viral pathogenesis of atherosclerosis. Impact of molecular mimicry and viral genes. Am J Pathol 139:1195, 1991

Hansson GK, Jonasson L, Seifert P, Stemme S: Immune mechanisms in atherosclerosis. Atherosclerosis 9:567, 1989

Havel RJ, Goldstein JL, Brown MS: Lipoproteins and lipid transport. In: Bondy PK, Rosenberg LE, eds: Metabolic Control and Disease. Philadelphia, WB Saunders, 1980

Hegele RA, Huang L-S, Herbert PN: Apolipoprotein B-gene DNA polymorphisms associated with myocardial infarction. N Engl J Med 315: 1509, 1986

Hu FB, Stampfer MJ, Manson JE, et al: Dietary fat intake and the risk of coronary heart disease in women. N Engl J Med 337:1491, 1997

Iacoviello L, Di Castelnuevo A, De Kniff P, et al: Polymorphisms in the coagulation factor VII gene and the risk of myocardial infarction. N Engl J Med 338:79, 1998

Klag MJ, Ford DE, Mead LA, et al: Serum cholesterol in young men and subsequent cardiovascular disease. N Engl J Med 328:313, 1993

Koenig W, Resch KL, Ernst E: Fibrinogen and cardiovascular risk. Primary Cardiol 20:39, 1994

Kromhout D, Bosschieter EB, Coulander CL: The inverse relation between fish consumption and 20-year mortality from coronary heart disease. N Engl J Med 312:1205, 1985

Kwiterovich PO Jr: Biochemical, clinical, genetic, and pathologic data in the pediatric age group relevant to the cholesterol hypothesis. Pediatrics 78:349, 1986

Lauer RM: National Cholesterol Education Program. Report of the Expert Panel on Blood Cholesterol Levels in Children and Adolescents. Pediatrics 89(Suppl):525, 1992

Lawn RM: Lipoprotein(a) in heart disease. Sci Am 266:54, 1992

Leaf A, Weber PC: Cardiovascular effects of n-3 fatty acids. N Engl J Med 318:549, 1988

Lee J, Lauer RM, Clarke WR: Lipoproteins in the progeny of young men with coronary artery disease: children with increased risk. Pediatrics 78: 330, 1986

Malinow MR, Duell PB, Hess DL, et al: Reduction of plasma homocyt(e)ine levels by breakfast cereal fortified with folic acid in patients with coronary heart disease. N Engl J Med 338:1009, 1998

Marmot M, Elliott P: Coronary Heart Disease Epidemiology. Oxford, Oxford University Press, 1992

McGill HC Jr: Questions about the natural history of human atherosclerosis. In: Glagov S, Newman WP III, eds: Pathobiology of the Atherosclerotic Plaque. New York, Springer Verlag, 1990:1

Nygård O, Nordrehaug JE, Refsum H, et al: Plasma homocysteine levels and mortality on patients with coronary artery disease. N Engl J Med 337:230, 1997

Ridker PM, Cushman M, Stampfer MJ, et al: Inflammation, aspirin, and the risk of cardiovascular disease in apparently healthy men. N Engl J Med 336:973, 1997

Rimm EB, Stampfer MJ, Ascherio A, et al: Vitamin E consumption and the risk of coronary heart disease in men. N Engl J Med 328:1450, 1993

Ross R: The pathogenesis of atherosclerosis: a perspective for the 1990s. Nature 362:801, 1993

Ross R: Atherosclerosis—an inflammatory disease. N Engl J Med 340:115, 1999

Saikku P, Leinonen M, Tenkanen L, et al: Chronic *Chlamydia pneumoniae* infection as a risk factor for coronary heart disease in the Helsinki Heart Study. Ann Intern Med 116:273, 1992

Scanu AM: Lipoprotein(a). A genetic risk factor for premature coronary heart disease. JAMA 267:3326, 1992

Stampfer MJ, Hennekens CH, Manson JE, et al: Vitamin E consumption and the risk of coronary disease in women. N Engl J Med 328:1444, 1993

Stampfer MJ, Sacks FM, Salvini S, et al: A prospective study of cholesterol, apolipoproteins, and the risk of myocardial infarction. N Engl J Med 325:373, 1991

Stary HC: The sequence of cell and matrix changes in atherosclerotic lesions of coronary arteries in the first forty years of life. Eur Heart J 11:3, 1990

Stary HC: The Evolution of Human Atherosclerotic Lesions. West Point, PA, Merck & Co, 1993

Stary HC, Blankenhorn DH, Chandler AB, et al: A definition of the intima of human arteries and of its atherosclerosis-prone regions. Circulation 85:391, 1992

Steinberg D: Antioxidants in the prevention of human atherosclerosis. Circulation 85:2338, 1992

Steinberg D, Carew TE, Fielding C, et al: AHA conference report on cholesterol. Workshop I. Lipoproteins and the pathogenesis of atherosclerosis. Circulation 80:719, 1989

Steinberg D, Parthasarathy S, Carew TE, et al: Beyond cholesterol. Modifications of low-density lipoprotein that increase its atherogenicity. N Engl J Med 320:915, 1989

Strong JP: Atherosclerotic lesions: natural history, risk factors, and topography. Arch Pathol Lab Med 116:1268, 1992

Strong JP, McGill HC Jr: The pediatric aspects of atherosclerosis. J Atherosclerosis Res 9:251, 1969

Sytkowski PA, Kannel WB, D'Agostino RB: Changes in risk factors and the decline of mortality from cardiovascular disease. N Engl J Med 322: 1635, 1990

Tybjaerg-Hansen A, Steffensen R, Meinertz H, et al: Association of mutations in the apolipoprotein B gene with hypercholesterolemia and the risk of ischemic heart disease. N Engl J Med 338:1577, 1998

Wang XL, Wilcken DEL, Dudman NPB: Neonatal apo A-1, apo B, and apo(a) levels in dried blood spots in an Australian population. Pediatr Res 28:496, 1990

Welch GN, Loscalzo J: Homocysteine and atherothrombosis. N Engl J Med 338:1042, 1998

Yater WM, Traum AH, Brown WG, et al: Coronary artery disease in men eighteen to thirty-nine years of age. Am Heart J 36:334, 481, 683, 1948

Young SG, Parthsarathy S: Why are low-density lipoproteins atherogenic? West J Med 160:153, 1994

22.4.8 Syncope

Julien I. E. Hoffman

Syncope is defined as transient complete loss of consciousness and postural tone. About 15% of children experience syncope, and syncope accounts for 1% of pediatric emergency room admissions.

PATHOPHYSIOLOGY

The basic mechanism of syncope is transient cerebral ischemia. Normally, there are potent defenses that maintain cerebral blood flow. For example, standing up or relaxing after strenuous exercise causes blood to pool in the legs, thus reducing venous return and ventricular filling. Ventricular stretch receptors fire less often, and the decreased brainstem afferent input increases sympathetic output, causing tachycardia and peripheral vasoconstriction. In some people, for unknown reasons, this defense mechanism is followed by paradoxical activation of ventricular mechanoreceptors, increase of afferent traffic to the brainstem, sympathetic inhibition, peripheral arteriolar and venous dilatation, and profound hypotension. There is often bradycardia from increased vagal stimulation. Other mechanisms must occur, however, because syncope can occur with a transplanted denervated heart. Occasionally, cerebral ischemia occurs from a profound decrease in cardiac output from cardiac disease. Rarely, cerebral ischemia occurs in the absence of changes in peripheral blood flow or pressure.

ETIOLOGY AND CLINICAL FEATURES

The most common cause is *vasodepressor or neurocardiogenic syncope,* the simple fainting attack, that is more frequent in adolescents and is triggered by injury or fear of injury, pain, anger, disgust, or the sight of blood. The subject feels weak, dizzy (not true vertigo), nauseated, and has blurred vision (starting in the periphery) and a rushing sound in the ears. Blood pressure falls, and the subject becomes pale and sweaty and develops profound bradycardia and loss of consciousness. Myoclonic movements may occur, but true tonic-clonic seizures are rare. Because of the warning symptoms, injury is rare. The attack is aborted or terminated by lying down but may recur if the subject stands up too soon.

In *orthostatic hypotension* there is an abrupt fall in blood pressure on standing, with little change in heart rate at first. This is common in those standing still for a long time in warm surroundings, for example, on parade or in church services. It is more likely in subjects with a decreased central blood volume, in those with impaired autonomic nervous system responses, and after certain drugs (Table 22-33).

Cardiac causes include obstructive lesions and arrhythmias (Table 22-33). Obstructive lesions can usually be diagnosed clinically

TABLE 22-33
CAUSES OF SYNCOPE

Neurocardiogenic syncope
Orthostatic hypotension
  Decreased central blood volume
    Acute hemorrhage, acute diarrhea, excessive diuresis, adrenal insufficiency, pregnancy, prolonged standing, poor muscle tone, eg, after prolonged recumbency
  Autonomic insufficiency
    Peripheral neuritis
      Diabetes mellitus, alcoholic neuritis, familial dysautonomia (Riley-Day syndrome), amyloidosis, porphyria
    Central autonomic failure (Shy-Drager syndrome)
    Idiopathic (Bradbury-Eggleston syndrome)
    Spinal cord lesions
  Medications and intoxications
    Vasodilators, antiarrhythmics, antidepressants, anticonvulsants, nitrates, symptholytics, narcotics, cocaine, alcohol
Cardiac diseases
  Obstructive lesions
    Severe aortic or pulmonic stenosis, hypertrophic cardiomyopathy, left atrial myxoma, malfunctioning prosthetic mitral or aortic valve, tetralogy of Fallot, severe pulmonary hypertension without shunts, abnormal origin or course of coronary arteries, cardiac tamponade, acute pulmonary embolism
  Arrhythmias
    Tachycardias: supraventricular, ventricular
    Bradycardias: sinus node dysfunction, atrioventricular block
    Pacemaker malfunction
    Long-QT syndrome
Vagal syncope
  Micturition, deglutition, glossopharyngeal neuralgia, postgastrectomy (dumping syndrome)
Other vascular causes
  Cerebral vascular diseases, including transient ischemic attacks; subclavian steal; basilar artery migraine; carotid sinus hypersensitivity (all but the last of these do not affect peripheral blood flow and pressure)
Noncardiovascular
  Atypical seizures; cough syncope; hyperventilation; hysteria; sudden increase in intracranial pressure

and by echocardiogram, but coronary artery anomalies may need imaging techniques (angiography, MRI) for their diagnosis. Arrhythmias can cause syncope. If there has been an incision in the atria (eg, atrial baffle for transposition of the great arteries, Fontan procedure, closure of atrial septal defect), the possibility of a sick sinus syndrome (bradycardia-tachycardia syndrome) must be considered, as well as the possibility of conduction defects caused by injury to the atrioventricular node. If a ventricular septal defect has been closed, there are two causes of syncope. Suturing of the patch causes overt or concealed damage to the atrioventricular node or His bundle, with permanent or intermittent complete heart block. Alternatively, especially after a ventriculotomy, the scar may cause episodes of ventricular tachycardia. If the history suggests an arrhythmia, an electrocardiogram and a Holter monitor may help to make the diagnosis; however, sometimes exercise testing or electrophysiological testing may be required. Everyone with syncope deserves an electrocardiogram, which is the only way to diagnose the long-QT syndrome.

True *vagal syncope* produces severe bradycardia when the vagus is stimulated, for example, by swallowing cold foods or liquids or sudden decompression of a full bladder. It is uncommon. *Carotid sinus hypersensitivity* is a variant of this in which there is a fall in blood pressure when the carotid sinus is stimulated by pressure or a tight collar.

Local decreases in cerebral blood flow include a *subclavian steal,* often when use of an arm diverts blood from the head. Cerebral vascular obstructive lesions may present in this way. Finally, *basilar artery migraine* may cause syncope by causing vascular spasm in brainstem arteries.

Nonvascular causes include atypical seizures, hyperventilation, cough syncope, prolonged Valsalva maneuver, sudden rise in intracranial pressure, and hysterical syncope. Typical seizures and breath-holding spells do not present as syncope.

DIAGNOSIS

Initially this is based on the history and physical examination. Emphasis should be placed on any recent acute illness, use of licit or illicit drugs, psychosocial factors, previous illnesses (including migraine), and a family history of syncope or heart disease. Blood pressure should be measured with the patient supine and then immediately after standing up. In the absence of findings of heart disease or gross autonomic dysfunction, vasodepressor syncope is the most common cause. Any suggestion of an arrhythmia warrants an electrocardiogram and a 24-hour Holter monitor. Findings consistent with heart disease warrant echocardiographic examination.

Confirmation of vasodepressor syncope may be obtained by the tilt table test. After control blood pressure and heart rate are recorded, the patient is tilted head up to 60 to 80° for 10 to 45 minutes (there is variation from one institution to the other). Hypotension and bradycardia indicate a positive test, and the patient may lose consciousness. If these changes do not develop, the patient is placed flat again, and the test is repeated with an intravenous infusion of isoproterenol; this often provokes a positive response. The sensitivity and specificity of this test are not good; however, if syncope occurs, the patient can verify if it resembles the original syncopal event, which was usually not observed by a physician.

Referral to a cardiologist is indicated if there is evidence of structural heart disease or a long QT interval, if there is chest pain or palpitations, an abnormal electrocardiogram, or if syncope is related to exercise, causes injury, or is recurrent.

THERAPY

No one treatment works for all patients. Any cause found, including causes of postural hypotension, must be dealt with. Vasodepressor syncope should first be treated by increasing blood volume by increasing fluid intake (3 to 4 liters daily for an adolescent) and salt intake (250 to 1000 mg thrice daily); if necessary, fludrocortisone can be added. Caffeine should be eliminated from the diet. If these measures fail, β-adrenergic blocking agents often help; pindolol, 10 mg two to three times daily for adolescents, is popular. α-Adrenergic agonists such as pseudoephedrine (15 to 30 mg TID) have been successful. Scopolamine patches and disopyramide have been effective, as have serotonin blockers (fluoxetine or sertraline hydrochloride). Tight support stockings may be needed. Those who are sedentary may be helped by aerobic fitness training. Occasionally pacemakers are needed, but because they do not affect the hypotension, they are of limited use in classical vasodepressor syncope.

Cardiac syncope in most countries and states must be reported to the motor vehicle licensing authorities, who will probably withdraw or refuse to issue a driver's license. Permission to drive may be reinstated after successful medical or pacemaker therapy.

References

Cox MM, Perlman BA, Mayor MR, et al: Acute and long-term beta-adrenergic blockade for patients with neurocardiogenic syncope. J Am Coll Cardiol 26:1293, 1995

Dambrink JHA, Imholz BPM, Karemaker JM, Wieling W: Circulatory adaptation to orthostatic stress in health 10–14-year old children investigated in a general practice. Clin Sci 81:51, 1991

Driscoll DJ, Jacobsen SJ, Porter CJ, Wollan PC: Syncope in children and adolescents. J Am Coll Cardiol 29:1039, 1997

Fish FA, Strasburger JF, Benson DW Jr: Reproducibility of a symptomatic response to upright tilt in young patients with unexplained syncope. Am J Cardiol 70:605, 1992

Grubb BP, Kosinski D: Tilt table testing; concepts and limitations. PACE 20(Pt II):781, 1987

Grubb BP, Temesy-Armos P, Moore J, et al: The use of head upright tilt table testing in the evaluation and management of syncope in children and adolescents. PACE 15:742, 1992

Grubb BP, Samoil D, Kosinski D, et al: Use of sertraline hydrochloride in the treatment of refractory neurocardiogenic syncope in children and adolescents. J Am Coll Cardiol 24:490, 1994

Natale A, Sra J, Dhala A, et al: Efficacy of different treatment strategies for neurocardiogenic syncope. PACE 18:655, 1995

Perna GP, Ficola V, Salvatori MP, et al. Increase of plasma beta endorphins in vasodepressor syncope. Am J Cardiol 65:929, 1990

Perry JC, Garson A Jr: The child with recurrent syncope: autonomic function testing and beta-adrenergic sensitivity. J Am Coll Cardiol 17:1168, 1991

Pratt JL, Fleisher GR: Syncope in children and adolescents. Pediatr Energ Care 5:80, 1989

Scott WA, Pongiglione G, Bromberg BJ, et al: Randomized comparison of atenolol and fludrocortisone acetate in the treatment of pediatric neurally mediated syncope. Am J Cardiol 76:400, 1995

Strieper MJ, Campbell RM: Efficacy of alpha-adrenergic agonist therapy for prevention of pediatric neurocardiogenic syncope. J Am Coll Cardiol 22:594, 1993

22.4.9   Chest Pain

John Fahey

Chest pain is a very common pediatric complaint, resulting in visits to pediatricians, emergency departments, cardiologists, and pul-

monologists. Media attention has, rightfully, focused on the importance of chest pain in adults as the initial symptom of a "heart attack" and severe underlying cardiac disease. These implications frequently spill over to the pediatric patient, and chest pain usually is associated with anxiety and urgency for both patients and their families. Most often the child and the parents want to know if the pain is related to the heart, if it is life threatening, and what are the long-term implications. Chest pain is best approached by separation into acute onset of severe, unremitting chest pain or chronic and recurrent episodes of less severe chest pain because the focus of the history and physical examination, as well as the need and usefulness of ancillary laboratory studies, are quite different for these two presentations.

ACUTE-ONSET SEVERE CHEST PAIN

These children are usually distressed, seek urgent medical attention, and are more likely to have the chest pain at the time of the visit. The history and physical examination should be brief and focused to quickly categorize the pain as cardiac or noncardiac. The history should focus on two areas: the pain and associated symptoms, and underlying and predisposing medical conditions. The history should define the onset and duration of the pain, its quality, intensity, location, and radiation, as well as factors that provoke or relieve the pain. Associated symptoms, such as fever, coughing, vomiting, lightheadedness, syncope, palpitations, breathlessness, or diaphoresis, should be noted. Significant underlying medical conditions include congenital and acquired heart disease, diseases of the lung and chest wall, and diseases of the upper abdomen. Ancillary testing with electrocardiogram, echocardiogram, and chest x-ray are more likely to be useful in this group.

CARDIAC CAUSES

PERICARDIAL PAIN Inflammation and irritation of the pericardium (pericarditis) causes severe substernal chest pain that may be described as squeezing or tightening and therefore closely mimics cardiac angina. The pain is worse with movement, including breathing. The patients are uncomfortable, preferring to lean forward and refusing to lie down. The pain may be reproduced by sternal pressure. There is usually a friction rub. If a significant effusion has developed, there may not be a rub, and the heart sounds may be distant. The patient must be evaluated for signs of tamponade. The differential diagnosis of pericarditis is discussed in Sec. 22.4.3.

ANGINA AND ACUTE MYOCARDIAL INFARCTION Although the most feared, this is one of the rarest causes of acute chest pain in children. The pain is severe and substernal, described as pressure, burning, or gripping. The radiation may be to the neck or left arm. The pain usually follows effort and is relieved by rest. The cardiac examination may be normal. The electrocardiogram should show signs of ischemia (S-T segment elevation and T-wave changes over the involved myocardium, with reciprocal S-T segment depression in the opposite leads). Specific questions should be asked about a history of hypertrophic cardiomyopathy or Kawasaki disease. In addition, a history of illicit drug use, especially cocaine or crack, should be obtained, especially if there is no underlying cardiac disease. Cocaine causes adrenergic stimulation and coronary vasospasm, leading to myocardial ischemia and infarction. This pain will be nonexertional. An echocardiogram will detect anomalies or aneurysms of the coronary arteries as well as hypertrophic cardiomyopathy.

ARRHYTHMIA Tachyarrhythmias, especially supraventricular tachycardia, may cause acute chest pain. Although usually described as chest discomfort, especially in the younger child, very fast rates may compromise myocardial blood flow and produce myocardial ischemia. The pain is usually not associated with exercise but is frequently associated with lightheadedness, syncope, or palpitations. The pain should resolve immediately on termination of the arrhythmia. An electrocardiogram during the arrhythmia is diagnostic. In addition, there may be signs of myocardial ischemia after termination of the arrhythmia.

AORTIC DISSECTION The pain is usually acute and sharp (or tearing) in nature. Referral of the pain is related to the area of the aorta in question: ascending dissections with anterior chest pain, arch dissection with superior radiation (to the neck), and descending aortic dissection with posterior radiation (usually to the back). A history or typical stigmata of Marfan or Elhers-Danlos syndrome are most common. The dissection may be spontaneous or follow seemingly minimal trauma. Dissection should be suspected in any patient with severe chest trauma or hemopericardium. In experienced hands, transesophageal echocardiography aids in rapid diagnosis. This is a surgical emergency.

NONCARDIAC CAUSES

PULMONARY Spontaneous pneumothorax causes severe unilateral chest pain, which may be difficult for the patient to localize. This is usually followed by dyspnea. Unilaterally decreased breath sounds should be diagnostic, as is a shift of the trachea from the midline. A history of asthma, cystic fibrosis, Marfan syndrome, or trauma should be sought. Pleural irritation may cause acute onset of chest pain, which is classically inspiratory pain (pleuritic pain). Viral etiologies are most common and may be epidemic (pleurodynia) and associated with fever and a pleural rub on examination. Bacterial pneumonia with empyema should be considered in the highly febrile or toxic-appearing child. Obviously, this is an emergency in the child with sickle cell disease. Pulmonary embolism is rare in pediatric patients but should be considered if there is cough, dyspnea, or hemoptysis associated with acute pleuritic pain, especially if there is a history of leg trauma or an adolescent female on oral contraceptives.

ESOPHAGEAL/GASTRIC Although the pain of gastroesophageal reflux and resultant esophagitis is usually retrosternal, burning, and not severe, it may occasionally be gripping and angina-like. The relation of the pain to food and the complaint that the pain is worse when supine may be helpful clues. An esophageal foreign body may cause severe retrosternal pain. Esophageal spasm and esophageal tear from vomiting are rare in childhood but can cause this type of pain.

Diaphragmatic irritation classically radiates to the shoulder or lower chest, and a subphrenic or hepatic abscess should be considered in the febrile patient with a normal chest wall, lung, and heart examination. Splenic flexure syndrome, splenic infarct, or splenic sequestration syndrome may present as left shoulder pain. Pancreatitis causes epigastric pain, which may radiate to the back. It may also cause pleural effusions, which may complicate the diagnosis.

CHRONIC AND RECURRENT CHEST PAIN

These patients are more likely to be seen in an office setting on a nonemergency basis. The patient is unlikely to have the pain at the time of the visit. The physical examination is likely to be normal, and the history is the most important part of the visit. As for acute severe chest pain, the characteristics of the pain as well as associated symptoms and underlying medical conditions should be delineated. Because the pain may have been occurring intermittently over weeks, months, or even years, the history may be extensive. Important issues will involve events occurring at the onset of the pain (including family stresses, illnesses, or deaths), the level of concern of the child and the parents, the extent to which the pain interferes with the child's activities, school work and attendance, as well as any prior workup or tentative diagnoses that may have been made. Occasionally, the child may sense that the adults around him doubt the existence of the pain, its severity, or the motivation behind the complaints.

It is important to impart information to the patient during the interview and the examination. Acknowledge that no one doubts the presence or effects of the pain. Inform them that most often, but not always, the etiology of the pain can be determined. Ensure them that cardiac causes, the only ones potentially life-threatening, will be ruled out in a logical and sequential fashion. Following this, the differential diagnosis will then focus on other real, but benign causes (Table 22-34). A practical explanation for the patient would be that the structures that can cause pain are, logically, only the ones present in or on the chest: the chest wall and overlying structures, the lungs, the esophageal-gastric unit, and the heart, with the heart being the least common cause. Although psychogenic chest pain is an important cause, discussion of this is best approached after the history and physical examination.

THE CHEST WALL Musculoskeletal pain involving the chest wall is probably the most common cause of chest pain when an etiology can be determined. The pain is usually localized, nonradiating, and reproducible. The pain is usually worse with exercise because of the increase in ventilatory rate and effort, leading the patient to suspect that the pain is cardiac in origin. The entire surface of the thorax should be examined for bruising or skin lesions (ie, zoster). The breasts should be examined in both boys and girls for nodules, mastitis, bruising, or fat necrosis. Muscle pain from injury or overuse is common, especially when athletes participate in new events, change training intensity, or change sports. Palpation along the ribs and sternum may reproduce the pain.

There are a variety of syndromes, frequently confused or used interchangeably, describing rib and sternal pain. *Costochondritis* is characterized by pain and tenderness of the anterior chest at the costochondral or costosternal articulations. There is no swelling involved. The pain may be mild to severe, is most often unilateral, with the left fourth to sixth costochondral junctions being most frequently involved. This syndrome is slightly more common in girls and may follow a viral illness or intense exercise. It is diagnosed by reproducing the pain by palpating at the site.

Tietze syndrome describes pain and nonsuppurative swelling of the anterior chest wall, usually of the second or third costochondral junction unilaterally, without involvement of the overlying skin. The pain and swelling are usually intermittent but may last months to years, and there is no sex predilection. *Precordial catch* is characterized by the sudden onset of severe, sharp, or shooting chest pain that is very localized, most often at the cardiac apex, and lasts between 30 seconds and a few minutes. The pain occurs at rest or during mild activity and may occur several times a day. The pain is worse with deep inspiration, causing one to hesitate and then resume breathing at a shallow level. The etiology is unknown. *Slipping rib syndrome* involves the eighth, ninth, or tenth ribs at their

TABLE 22-34

CHRONIC, RECURRING CHEST PAIN

CAUSE	CHARACTERISTICS OF PAIN	EVALUATION
Chest wall	Localized, sharp, stabbing Reproducible by palpation Not brought on by exertion but may be worse with exertion	History, examination with attempts to reproduce by palpation
Lungs (EIA)	Midsternal pain, deep chest tightness during inspiration, after exercise	Pediatric exercise stress testing, with pulmonary function
Gastroesophageal	Low retrosternal or left precordial burning; worse at bedtime or lying down or with meals	Trial of antacid before referral
Cardiac (angina)	Pressure or gripping deep in chest, may radiate to neck or arm; brought on by exertion, relieved by rest	Referral to pediatric cardiology if angina suspected
Psychogenic	Vague, poorly localized, difficult to describe, varying in location; related to stressful events	History to determine stressful events at onset of pain Examination

anterior tip. These ribs do not attach directly to the sternum, but the tips are united by fibrous tissue. Fibrous tissue damage may allow one of these ribs to override the one above it, causing the pain. The pain is of sudden onset, may be sharp and stabbing or dull, may last for hours, and the area may remain tender for days. The pain may be reproduced by the "hooking maneuver," that is, hooking the fingers under the inferior rib margin and pulling anteriorly. *Hypersensitive xiphoid* causes low substernal or epigastric pain associated with a tender xiphoid cartilage. The pain may occur at rest or with exertion. In children, this pain may occur at the xiphoid insertion of the abdominal muscles as a result of overuse of these muscles with prolonged running or calisthenics.

With chest wall pain, reproducing the pain is diagnostic, and no further workup or testing is needed. The treatment begins with assuring the patient and parents that the pain is noncardiac and benign. Combinations of rest and mild analgesics (acetaminophen or nonsteroidal antiinflammatory agents) until the pain subsides are usually all that is necessary. The patient should be reminded that such pains often recur. Specific therapies (mastitis, zoster, etc) are instituted as necessary.

THE LUNGS

Exercise-induced asthma (EIA) has become an increasingly important cause of chest pain in pediatrics. During bronchospasm, these children may experience a deep and sharp substernal pain associated with chest "tightness." It is important to remember that EIA is worst during the 5 to 10 minutes during recovery from exercise and then slowly improves over the subsequent 20 to 30 minutes. The associated chest pain may be exertional or immediately post-exertional. Using a specially designed rapidly increasing ramp exercise protocol, Weins et al. diagnosed EIA in 72% of children referred to a pediatric cardiology clinic for evaluation of chronic chest pain, most of whom developed chest pain during the study. Thus, EIA should be considered in the differential diagnosis of exertional chest pain.

Children with chronic asthma are at risk for recurrent chest pain because of the bronchospasm as just noted, as well as muscle strain associated with chronic coughing. In addition, over 40% of children with asthma will have exercise-induced asthma.

The association of pneumothorax and chest pain in this population has been mentioned.

As more children participate in organized athletic activities requiring training, a "stitch" has become a common complaint. The pain is felt in the right upper quadrant and under the right costal margin, with occasional radiation to the right shoulder or xiphoid. The pain is a sharp, cramping sensation occurring while running or walking and always relieved by rest.

THE GASTROINTESTINAL TRACT

Gastroesophageal reflux with esophagitis is diagnosed with increasing frequency in children, especially in those with chronic chest pain of unknown etiology. The pain is most often retrosternal or left precordial, or combinations of these two. Worsening of the pain with meals, increased abdominal pressure, or lying down are suggestive but not always present. Manometry and esophagoscopy are diagnostic, but a trial of antacids or H_2 blockers may be warranted if the history is highly suggestive. Esophageal foreign body, achalasia, and diffuse esophageal spasm are other less common causes of similar pain in children.

THE HEART

Except for the acute pericardial syndromes outlined above, most cardiac chest pain in children is anginal in etiology, related to a mismatch between myocardial oxygen supply and demand. This is caused by either coronary artery obstruction by congenital malformations or acquired disease, or ventricular hypertrophy and excessive myocardial oxygen demands with normal coronary arteries. Chronic anginal pain is intermittent, brought on by exercise, and eases with rest. It is most often described as a pressure or gripping sensation and only rarely described as sharp or burning in nature. Association of the pain with palpitations, lightheadedness, or syncope is worrisome.

Congenital coronary artery malformations may be associated with ischemic heart disease in young children or be delayed to adolescence and adulthood (see section 22.3.8). The most common anomaly is *anomalous origin of the left coronary artery from the pulmonary artery*. These patients usually become symptomatic in infancy, but rarely, a patient may remain asymptomatic until adolescence and present with angina. In some children, the *left coronary arises anomalously from the right sinus of Valsalva or the right coronary artery arises from the left sinus of Valsalva*. In these, the orifice of the coronary artery may be slit-like and stenotic, or the artery may course between the aorta and pulmonary artery and be compressed during exercise by distension of the aorta and pulmonary artery. As a result, exercise-related angina develops. *Coronary*

TABLE 22-35

CAUSES OF SUDDEN UNEXPECTED DEATH

DISEASE

Hypertrophic cardiomyopathy
Anomalous origin of a coronary artery
Myocarditis
Right ventricular dysplasia
Mitral valve prolapse
Long-QT syndrome
Idiopathic left ventricular concentric hypertrophy
Miscellaneous coronary arterial disease
   Premature atherosclerosis
   After Kawasaki syndrome
Mechanical factors
   Ruptured aorta (Marfan syndrome)

arterial fistulas may steal flow from the normal coronary artery, resulting in ischemia.

Kawasaki disease is the most common acquired coronary disease. Resultant coronary aneurysms may heal with narrowing, or thrombosis of the aneurysms may lead to coronary stenosis and insufficiency. A history of Kawasaki disease should be obtained, but the diagnosis might have been missed. Disorders of lipoprotein metabolism, such as familial hypercholesterolemia, may result in premature atherosclerotic coronary artery disease and insufficiency. Skin lesions of planar xanthomas may be present at birth and lead to the diagnosis. Other metabolic disorders such as mucopolysaccharidoses and homocystinuria may have coronary artery involvement with narrowing and thrombosis.

With marked ventricular hypertrophy, the subendocardial layers of the heart may be inadequately perfused at times of increased myocardial demands, as with exercise, leading to myocardial ischemia and exertional angina. Severe ventricular hypertrophy may result from marked pulmonary or aortic valve stenosis, hypertrophic cardiomyopathy, or severe systemic or pulmonary hypertension. These patients are at risk for anginal chest pain and sudden death.

Mitral valve prolapse has been associated with atypical chest pain, but this association has recently been questioned. Arfken found no difference in the incidence of chest pain between children with and without mitral valve prolapse. Also, mitral valve prolapse is not more common in children with chest pain than in the general population. There is a greatly increased incidence of gastroesophageal causes of chest pain in children with prolapse.

Tachyarrhythmias, especially supraventricular tachycardia, may cause angina-like chest pain and should always be considered in the differential diagnosis of chest pain. A history of palpitation associated with the chest pain is highly suggestive.

PSYCHOGENIC CAUSES

Psychogenic factors may be responsible for a large percentage of chronic chest pain in children and adolescents. A history of a specific stressful situation around the onset of the chest pain can frequently be obtained, such as death, coronary artery disease in family or friends, divorce, separation from friends, school failure, or a physical disability. Other family members may have similar complaints. The pain may be very vague and difficult for the child to localize or describe. The pain may vary in location and intensity. Chest pain has been associated with hyperventilation syndrome, depression, and somatization. Frequently there is tenderness over the left ventricular apex.

References

Leung AK, Robson WL, Cho SH: Chest pain in children. Can Fam Physician 42:1156 and 1163, 1996

Rowe BH, Dulberg CS, Peterson RG, et al: Characteristics of children presenting with chest pain to a pediatric emergency department. Can Med Assoc J 143:388, 1990

Selbst SM: Consultation with the specialist. Chest pain in children. Pediatr Rev 18:169, 1997

Selbst SM, Ruddy R, Clark BJ: Chest pain in children. Follow-up of patients previously reported. Clin Pediatr 29:374, 1990

Taubman B, Vetter VL: Slipping rib syndrome as a cause of chest pain in children. Clin Pediatr 35:403, 1996

Tunaoglu FS, Olgüntürk R, Akcabay S, et al: Chest pain in children referred to a cardiology clinic. Pediatr Cardiol 16:69, 1995

Wiens L, Sabath R, Ewing L, et al: Chest pain in otherwise healthy children and adolescents is frequently caused by exercise-induced asthma. Pediatrics 90:350, 1992

Woolf PK, Gewitz MH, Berezin S, et al: Noncardiac chest pain in adolescents and children with mitral valve prolapse. J Adolesc Health 12:247, 1991

Zavaras-Angelidou KA, Weinhouse E, Nelson DB: Review of 180 episodes of chest pain in 134 children. Pediatr Emerg Care 8:189, 1992

22.4.10   Sudden Death

Julien I. E Hoffman

The pediatrician often is responsible for verifying that a child can play competitive sports, and there will be concern about the occasional child who drops dead during or just after strenuous exercise. The following guidelines may be helpful.

Sudden unexpected death, probably caused by an arrhythmia but occasionally from mechanical factors, has been observed in subjects with various conditions (Table 22-35); hypertrophic cardiomyopathy accounts for about half of all these deaths, and coronary arterial anomalies for 10 to 20%.

DIAGNOSTIC SCREENING

A *positive family history* includes sudden death, syncope, chest pain, arrhythmias, or "heart disease." It is particularly likely in hypertrophic cardiomyopathy, right ventricular dysplasia, mitral valve prolapse, long-QT syndrome, premature atherosclerosis, and Marfan syndrome.

A *positive personal history* includes syncope, chest pain, arrhythmias, murmurs, or "heart disease." It may be present in any of the lesions in Table 22-35.

Positive signs include left ventricular enlargement or hypertrophy, specific murmurs, and Marfanoid body habitus. There are no abnormal signs with anomalous aortic origin of a coronary artery, coronary arterial aneurysms after Kawasaki syndrome, or the long-QT syndrome.

Electrocardiography and echocardiography may be diagnostic, but some patients may need electrophysiological testing or coronary arterial imaging.

Reference

Maron BJ: Sudden cardiac death in the young athlete and the preparticipation cardiovascular examination. In: Moller J, Hoffman JIE, eds: Pediatric Cardiovascular Medicine. New York, Churchill Livingstone, 2000:891

22.4.11 Common Management Problems

Paul Stanger and Julien I. E. Hoffman

Once heart disease has been diagnosed, day-to-day management is needed for the many minor problems and questions that arise. This is true not only of the common minor heart lesions but also of those major lesions that have had surgery or will need surgery in the future.

EFFECTS OF ALTITUDE

With increasing height above sea level, atmospheric oxygen tension falls, and so do alveolar oxygen tension and oxygen tension and saturation of pulmonary venous blood (Table 22-36). Up to 3000 feet there is no noticeable effect on oxygenation of blood in the lungs; at 5000 feet saturation falls slightly; and above 8000 feet pulmonary venous oxygen saturation decreases substantially. Therefore, patients with cyanotic heart disease should live at altitudes below 5000 feet so that there will be no further compromise of oxygen delivery to the body. Whether they should be allowed to go to high altitudes temporarily (eg, when the family goes skiing) depends mainly on the severity of their disease. Those who are tolerating their lesions well should be allowed to try the higher altitudes but should be warned to return to lower altitudes quickly if they become at all distressed. Oximetry while breathing mixtures with reduced oxygen concentrations may help to assess which patients might have difficulty. An exception to this is children with tetralogy of Fallot, who are at risk of having hypoxemic spells; they should avoid high altitudes until after surgery to increase pulmonary blood flow. Any patient with significant pulmonary hypertension from pulmonary vascular disease should avoid altitudes over 3000 feet, especially if actively exercising, because the reduced alveolar oxygen tension may increase pulmonary vasoconstriction. Patients with only one pulmonary artery are at risk of developing pulmonary edema at altitude and should remain below an altitude of 5000 feet. However, patients with large left-to-right shunts usually have no difficulty at high altitudes, and in fact, any pulmonary vasoconstriction that altitude causes will reduce the left-to-right shunt and produce some mild improvement while they are at high altitude.

Similar considerations apply to flying in commercial aircraft. These are pressurized to the equivalent of 7000 to 8000 feet above sea level, which could be hazardous for children who are deeply cyanotic. All commercial aircraft are required to have a supply of oxygen, and this can be made available to the patient; however, the airlines prefer prior arrangements to be made for a special oxygen supply for patients. They are often reluctant to take responsibility and may request that the patient's physician approve the flight. It is important to note that signs of distress during flight may not be cardiac in origin. Distress, especially during descent, may be the result of aerotitis; this can be avoided by having the infant feed and swallow during ascent and descent and also by not flying during or just after an upper respiratory tract infection.

CEREBRAL COMPLICATIONS

Patients with cyanotic heart disease may develop cerebral vascular accidents or brain abscesses; the former are most common under 2 years of age, the latter are rare under 18 months of age. Each of these complications occurs more often with greater arterial desaturation and more cyanosis. Thrombosis usually presents rapidly, with seizures or paralysis, usually a hemiparesis; brain abscess has a more insidious onset marked by headaches, low-grade fever, personality changes, vomiting, and occasionally seizures or paralysis.

Cerebral thrombosis may occur with either very high or relatively low hematocrits. When the hematocrit is over 65% the blood becomes very viscous and is more likely to clot. However, cerebral thromboses are also frequent in very cyanotic children with relatively low hematocrits. These children have marked arterial desaturation but, because of iron deficiency, have an inappropriately low hematocrit that may be only about 40 to 50%. Their tendency to have cerebral vascular accidents may be ascribed to iron deficiency damaging endothelial cells, hypoxemia damaging brain tissue, causing edema and thus slowing flow, or increased rigidity of the red cells. It is therefore important in any cyanotic infant or young child to check repeatedly at least the hematocrit and hemoglobin. If their ratio is greater than 3:1, then the red cell count and the appearance of the red cells on a smear should be checked so that iron deficiency can be detected and treated. Should the hematocrit rise to very high levels (this often follows iron therapy), then that is itself an indication for surgery. If this cannot be done, the hematocrit should be reduced by periodic removal of whole blood; if the volume removed is large, it should be replaced with an equal amount of albumin solution. Reducing the hematocrit to about 55% not only

TABLE 22-36
EFFECTS OF ALTITUDE

| ALTITUDE (FT) | ATMOSPHERE | | ALVEOLAR OXYGEN TENSION (MM HG)[a] | | PULMONARY VENOUS OXYGEN SATURATION(%) | |
	TOTAL PRESSURE (MM HG)	OXYGEN TENSION (MM HG)	ACUTE	ACCLIMATIZED	ACUTE	ACCLIMATIZED
0	760	159	110	110	98	98
3,000	681	143	92	95	94	95
5,000	632	132	78	82	93	94
8,000	565	118	66	68	89	90
11,000	503	105	54	60	80	86
14,000	446	93	44	52	70	80

[a] The alveolar values are approximate because they depend on metabolism, ventilation, and the alveolar–arterial oxygen difference. With acclimatization and chronic hyperventilation, the alveolar oxygen rises.

reduces the risk of thrombosis but also increases oxygen delivery to tissues by lowering blood viscosity. Before removing red cells, however, it is essential to exclude relative iron deficiency.

Cerebral vascular accidents can occur spontaneously but are more likely if oxygen requirements are raised by fever or if blood viscosity is increased further by dehydration from vomiting or diarrhea. Therefore, in cyanotic patients, these ailments need prompt treatment. Another precaution required in the adolescent cyanotic girl is to avoid the use of oral steroid contraceptives because these have been associated with an increased incidence of cerebral thromboses.

FEBRILE ILLNESSES

It is a rare child who does not have febrile illnesses. However, if the child has heart disease, there are more than the usual number of things to think about. If the child has cyanotic heart disease, then the possibility of a high fever causing cerebral thrombosis must be considered, as well as the possibility that fever is caused by a brain abscess or endocarditis. In a child with a large left-to-right shunt, the chest should be carefully examined both clinically and by roentgenography because these children have an increased incidence of pneumonitis. Furthermore, congestive heart failure may be precipitated or made worse by a fever of any origin because of the increased oxygen requirements that ensue. If the child has had recent cardiac surgery, the postpericardiotomy syndrome and the postpump syndrome caused by infection with cytomegalovirus must be considered, as should hepatitis and urinary tract infection.

All febrile children known to have heart disease must be assessed carefully to exclude infective endocarditis. However, it is important not to start treatment for infective endocarditis without good cause; otherwise, almost all children with heart disease will be treated unnecessarily for what is usually an intercurrent infection. In general, infective endocarditis does not present with sudden onset of high fever. Therefore, a child who has heart disease and is seen at the onset of an acute febrile illness is likely to have one of the common causes of fever and should be investigated and treated like any child of the same age. The use of antibiotics without a specific diagnosis, just because the child has a heart lesion, is unwarranted.

Not all these children need blood cultures during febrile illnesses unless clinical features suggest infective endocarditis. However, if the fever persists without obvious cause for more than 1 to 3 days, it is then advisable to obtain blood cultures to exclude infective endocarditis. Under some circumstances, however, blood cultures should be taken at the onset of fever. Stenotic or bicuspid aortic valves are common sites of infective endocarditis; valve destruction by infection may be early and devastating, and systemic embolization from an infected aortic valve is common. Therefore, blood cultures should be taken early if a patient with a known aortic valve lesion becomes febrile. Prompt action is also needed if a patient has had a valve replaced with a prosthetic, heterograft, or homograft valve because once an infection becomes established on foreign material, it may be impossible to cure it with antibiotics.

ANTIBIOTIC PROPHYLAXIS

Prophylaxis should always be given against infective endocarditis, especially at times of dental treatment (see Sec. 13.1.10). The dental treatment to be covered includes extractions, scaling and cleaning of the teeth by a dental hygienist, and most drilling to prepare cavities for filling. In addition, fitting of braces and major readjustments to braces require prophylaxis. However, the frequent minor readjustments that are made should probably not be accompanied by prophylaxis because then there would be the risk of colonizing the mouth with antibiotic-resistant organisms. For these reasons, too, the decision to start orthodontic treatment in children with heart disease should be made carefully, and minor unimportant orthodontic procedures should probably be avoided. However, corrective procedures in children may reduce the amount of dental care needed later and thus reduce the risk of infective endocarditis then. Decisions must be individualized; a child may be more handicapped by having buckteeth than by having mild pulmonic stenosis. Other oral procedures, such as tonsillectomy or oral trauma, also require prophylaxis, as does gastrointestinal or urinary tract surgery.

Children who have had rheumatic fever should take penicillin prophylaxis for many years to prevent recurrences and cardiac damage (see Sec. 13.2.32).

EXERCISE RESTRICTIONS

Exercise increases oxygen consumption, cardiac output, heart rate, and systemic blood pressure and thus increases cardiac work. This by itself is no reason to restrict children with most types of heart disease. Most children with cyanotic heart disease or left-to-right shunts restrict themselves because they become dyspneic or fatigued on effort, and there is no evidence that this causes any harm. The decision to restrict exercise is more difficult when patients have obstructive lesions: aortic or pulmonic stenosis, coarctation of the aorta, or systemic or pulmonic hypertension. If the stenosis is severe, it will probably come to early valvotomy and may no longer be a problem; however, the vascular lesions or moderate stenotic lesions are more difficult to manage because with exercise there may be no symptoms despite potentially dangerous and damaging levels of pressure. Management is difficult and is best left to the cardiologist. The following are some of the considerations.

In all but the mildest of obstructive lesions, exhausting exercise should be avoided. This includes competitive sports and team sports, in which the children may feel obliged to play as hard as possible and may forget their restrictions. In patients with mild or moderate obstructive lesions, examining the effects of different levels of exercise on the circulation may prove useful. If there is no excessive hypertension or hypotension, and no ischemic S-T changes with exercise, then normal exercise can probably be allowed safely; competitive sports should still be avoided. With aortic stenosis the electrocardiogram is a useful but not infallible guide to how much can be done. If there are any ischemic S-T changes at any exercise level, that patient should probably undergo surgery; however, normal electrocardiographic patterns do not completely exclude subtle ischemic damage. Estimating the left ventricular systolic pressure by Doppler methods provides more useful information.

If pulmonic stenosis is mild, there will be no electrocardiographic changes with exercise. The only guide is to measure the right ventricular pressures during exercise by Doppler methods or by cardiac catheterization; if after this there is no indication for valvotomy, then strenuous, noncompetitive exercise can be permitted.

If there is severe pulmonary hypertension without a communication between the two circulations (primary pulmonary hypertension or residual severe pulmonary vascular disease after closure of a ventricular septal defect or a ductus arteriosus), then all levels of exercise should be avoided. An increase in cardiac output will produce severe right ventricular hypertension and can cause acute right ventricular failure and death.

Exercise restriction may be needed in some children who have had their lesions repaired surgically. Those with obstructive lesions have already been discussed. Some of those who have had ventriculotomies, especially for repair of a tetralogy of Fallot, have been shown to have bursts of ventricular tachycardia with exercise, and because these could give rise to ventricular fibrillation, it is advisable to evaluate the electrocardiographic responses to exercise before deciding how much exercise can be allowed.

Clearance for competitive sports and the risk of sudden death in these children are discussed in Sec. 22.4.10.

PSYCHOLOGICAL SUPPORT

Any child with heart disease is probably worried about it, as are the parents and possibly the siblings. Insofar as is possible, the anxieties of these people should be elicited, and support should be given. Fear of sudden death is common, but sudden death is rare in most forms of childhood heart disease; reassurance can validly be given. If there is a very sick infant who requires a great deal of care, it is common for the siblings to be neglected, and even for marriages to break up. Although the pediatrician is not necessarily the best person to counsel the family on these issues, the pediatrician should certainly be aware of the problems and attempt to ease them.

Older children are apt to be concerned about differences that set them apart from their peers; clearly this is accentuated if they are restricted. Thus, it is important to look for these problems, attempt to discuss them with the child and the parents, and avoid unnecessary restrictions.

In adolescents, marriageability and the ability to have children are often matters of great concern. Reassurance can usually be given to patients with mild or treated heart disease. It should be noted, however, that their children are at greater-than-normal risk of also having congenital heart disease (see Sec. 22.3.1). Most girls with severe cyanotic heart disease are infertile; if one does become pregnant, her health will usually not be compromised. Obstructive lesions, especially mitral stenosis, increase risks of pregnancy because of the increase in cardiac output and blood volume that occur during pregnancy. Patients with atrial septal defects may go into congestive heart failure at term. The one group for whom pregnancy is contraindicated is the group with severe pulmonary hypertension without a ventricular septal defect or a ductus arteriosus. To allow pregnancy to continue to term often results in maternal death; thus, contraception (other than oral steroids) or sterilization is mandatory.

POSTOPERATIVE PROBLEMS

When a child leaves the hospital after cardiac surgery, the referring physician needs to be familiar with certain common problems.

CARDIAC MEDICATIONS The child may still need cardiac medications to manage congestive heart failure, especially if surgery has been to correct a ventricular septal defect, atrioventricular canal, tetralogy of Fallot, truncus arteriosus, or transposition of the great arteries. Even if the defects have been completely repaired, it may take weeks or months before the ventricles function normally. Once signs of congestive heart failure disappear, the anticongestive medications can gradually be decreased every 3 to 7 days until they have

all been discontinued, as long as congestive heart failure does not recur.

ANEMIA Some children are moderately anemic after open heart surgery and usually need only iron and careful follow-up of hemoglobin and hematocrit. Rarely, an intravascular hemolytic syndrome occurs in children after repair of an atrioventricular canal defect; residual high-velocity jets of blood striking the patch cause mechanical red cell destruction. Sometimes these children present as if they had infective endocarditis, but evidence of hemolysis makes the diagnosis. Often, only treatment with iron is needed until the hemolysis disappears, but occasionally reoperation is needed.

FEVER Any child can become febrile, with or without preceding cardiac surgery, but certain postoperative problems need to be considered:

1. Pneumonitis or lung collapse related to postoperative lung problems.
2. Urinary tract infections caused by the indwelling bladder catheter that many of these children have had for a few days.
3. Blood-transmitted infections such as hepatitis or cytomegalovirus disease, even though blood-banking methods have markedly reduced the incidence of these infections.
4. Infective endocarditis, particularly with staphylococci or gramnegative organisms.
5. Wound infection or mediastinitis.
6. Postpericardiotomy syndrome (see Sec. 22.4.3). Sometimes this syndrome may begin a few weeks after leaving the hospital. It may be characterized by chest pain or a pericardial friction rub, but these signs are not always present. Rarely, this syndrome may cause pericardial tamponade. Echocardiography proves the diagnosis.
7. Rarely there may be a drug fever.
8. There is an ill-defined entity termed *conduit fever* that occurs in children with conduits. Because there is no specific test for this cause, it is a diagnosis of exclusion.

CARE OF THE WOUNDS By the time of discharge from hospital, the wounds in the heart, blood vessels, and soft tissues will have begun to heal. It takes about 4 weeks for incisions in the heart to form firm fibrous tissue; therefore, excessive activity should be avoided for this period. The sternum, like most broken bones, takes about 6 weeks for firm union and is the last tissue to heal completely. Therefore, for the first 6 weeks, activities that might injure the chest wall should be avoided (swinging the child by the hands, picking the child up under the arms, bicycle or horse riding, rough play with friends).

The sternal incision should be kept clean and dry until the edges are united or covered by a firm crust; tub baths where the incision could become wet should be avoided until the steristrips or dressings fall off or the sutures are removed. Most sutures will be removed before the child leaves hospital, but sometimes they need to be left in for longer periods and should not be removed without consulting the surgeon or cardiologist. Finally, the scar on the chest will initially be red, raised, very sensitive to sunlight, and susceptible to sunburn; it should be kept covered when the child is outdoors. This sensitivity is lost after about 6 months, when the scar has become flatter and paler.

EXERCISE The child should be restricted to normal activities around the house for 3 weeks and can then return to school as long as no stressful activity is undertaken for another 3 weeks. Then, if all is well, the child may be allowed to increase activity gradually and participate in noncompetitive sports and physical education. Preferably, participation in this activity should be approved by the pediatric cardiologist.

INSURANCE PROBLEMS

Insurability of children with heart disease is of concern to parents. Many forms of mild or completely repaired congenital heart lesions can often be insured at standard rates. Other lesions may be insurable at increased rates, but some are still uninsurable (Table 22-37). However, because there is no unanimity among insurance companies, several may need to be approached to obtain the best rates for a given lesion.

References

Allen HD, Franklin WW, Fontana ME: Employability and insurability. In: Emmanouilides GC, Riemenschneider TA, Allen HD, Gutgesell HP, eds: Heart Disease in Infants, Children, and Adolescents, Including the Fetus and Young Adult. Baltimore, Williams & Wilkins, 1994:683

Beekman RH: Exercise recommendations for adolescents after surgery for congenital heart disease. Pediatrician 13:210, 1986

Hollister AS: Orthostatic hypotension. Causes, evaluation, and management. West J Med 157:652, 1992

Manolis AS, Linzer M, Salem D, Estes NAM III: Syncope: current diagnostic evaluation and management. Ann Intern Med 112:850, 1990

Maron BJ, Roberts WC, McAllister HA, et al: Sudden death in young athletes. Circulation 62:218, 1980

Samoil D, Grubb BP, Kip K, Kosinski DJ: Head-upright tilt table testing in children with unexplained syncope. Pediatrics 92:426, 1993

Selbst SWM: Chest pain in children. Pediatrics 75:1068, 1985

Truesdell SC, Skorton DJ, Lauer RM: Life insurance for children with cardiovascular disease. Pediatrics 77:687, 1986

22.4.12   Rheumatic Fever

Julien I. E. Hoffman

Rheumatic fever is an inflammatory disease that follows infection with certain strains of group A streptococci. The disease affects the heart, joints, central nervous system, and subcutaneous tissue. In the United States, after a decline in incidence for many years, new outbreaks of this disease have been reported.

ETIOLOGY AND PATHOLOGY

Epidemiologic studies suggest an individual propensity to develop rheumatic fever, a nonsuppurative complication of group A streptococcal infection of the upper respiratory tract, which occurs most commonly in children 5 to 15 years of age (Sec. 13.2.32). Rheumatic fever occurs in 3% of patients who carry an infecting strain for more than 3 weeks after convalescence, whereas persons carrying the organism for less than 3 weeks have an incidence of only 0.3%. Individuals with increases in antistreptolysin O titers greater than 250 U/mL after streptococcal infection have a 5% incidence of rheumatic fever; whereas less than 1% of those with increases of less than 100 U/mL develop the disease. Patients with streptococcal infections and a history of previous rheumatic fever have a 5 to 50% greater incidence of rheumatic fever than do patients with no prior history of the disease; this tendency declines with age. Environmental factors (latitude, altitude, humidity), nutrition, crowding, and age appear to influence the incidence of rheumatic fever, probably because the same factors influence the incidence of streptococcal infection.

Pathologic changes are found throughout the body in connective tissue and around small blood vessels. The pathognomonic lesion of rheumatic fever is the Aschoff body, an inflammatory lesion associated with swelling and fragmentation of collagen fibers and alterations in the staining characteristics of connective tissue. Endocarditis produces a verrucous valvitis that may heal with fibrous thickening and adhesions of valve commissures and chordae tendineae, resulting in variable degrees of valve stenosis and insufficiency. The mitral and aortic valves are affected most commonly, the tricuspid less frequently, and the pulmonary valve rarely.

Pathologic changes in the joints consist of exudation with edema of synovial membranes, focal necrosis in the joint capsule, edema and inflammation in periarticular tissue, and joint effusion. These changes are completely reversible. Subcutaneous nodules seen during the acute phase of the disease resemble Aschoff bodies and are granulomas with localized areas of fibrinoid swelling of collagen and perivascular infiltration with large cells, pale nuclei, and prominent nucleoli. "Rheumatic pneumonia" consists of exudative and

TABLE 22-37
INSURABILITY OF HEART DISEASE

STANDARD RATES	INCREASED RATES	USUALLY UNINSURABLE
Mild pulmonic stenosis	Mild or moderate aortic or mitral insufficiency	Severe aortic insufficiency
Mitral valve prolapse, no regurgitation	Some arrhythmias	Large atrial septal defect
Rheumatic fever, no carditis	Mild or moderate aortic stenosis	Moderate/severe coarctation of the aorta
Postoperative with no residual defect:	Mild coarctation of the aorta	Ebstein anomaly
Atrial septal defect	Small atrial or ventricular septal defect	Complete transposition of the great arteries
Ventricular septal defect	Postoperative with no or mild residua:	Endocardial cushion defect
Patent ductus arteriosus	Coarctation of the aorta	Hypertrophic subaortic stenosis
	Endocardial cushion defect	Patent ductus arteriosus
	Complete transposition of the great arteries	Mitral valve prolapse with arrythmias
	Total anomalous pulmonary venous return	Moderate/severe pulmonic stenosis
	Ventricular septal defect with small shunt	Tricuspid atresia
	Tetralogy of Fallot	Tetralogy of Fallot
		Truncus arteriosus
		Lesions with pulmonary vascular disease
		Operated lesions with severe residua

inflammatory changes without Aschoff bodies. Pathologic changes in patients with chorea are not consistent, and little postmortem information is available because patients with active chorea rarely die.

CLINICAL FEATURES

Many of the clinical manifestations of rheumatic fever occur in other collagen vascular disorders. A patient presenting with cardiac, joint, and dermatologic abnormalities whould be evaluated for rheumatic fever, rheumatoid arthritis, and SLE (see Sec. 12.4 and Sec. 12.7). Any one of these disorders can be diagnosed only by a complete clinical and laboratory evaluation of all three.

The major clinical manifestations of rheumatic fever include: polyarthritis, carditis, chorea, subcutaneous nodules, and erythema marginatum (Table 22-38). A patient with two major or one major and two minor manifestations probably has rheumatic fever (Jones criteria). Frequently, however, the patient does not meet the Jones criteria and may still have rheumatic fever, but with less certainty of diagnosis.

In classic rheumatic fever there is *acute migratory polyarthritis* associated with fever. The joints are red, hot, swollen, exquisitely tender, and painful if moved. In general the larger joints of the extremities are affected, but arthritis may occur in the spine and other joints such as the temporomandibular and sternoclavicular joints; arthritis of fingers and toes is commoner in older than younger patients. Usually, as pain and effusion subside in one joint, another becomes involved, but several joints may be involved simultaneously. The arthritis lasts less than 1 month, even if untreated.

Most patients with *rheumatic carditis* do not have cardiac symptoms. Carditis may affect the endocardium (valves), myocardium, or pericardium. *Endocarditis* is manifested by organic murmurs. The most frequent murmur is an apical systolic murmur of mitral regurgitation; the third heart sound is frequently accentuated. With severe mitral regurgitation, the third heart sound may be followed or replaced by a low-pitched mid-diastolic rumble. (This murmur may occur in other forms of acute carditis as well as in severe anemias.) Some patients have a soft middiastolic murmur heard only at the apex (Carey Coombs murmur); the murmur is due to the mitral vegetations. The murmur of aortic regurgitation is the second most common murmur heard in patients with rheumatic fever. Patients without murmurs may have mild valve incompetence by color Doppler flow studies, but this finding by itself should not be used to diagnose acute rheumatic fever.

Myocarditis may be manifested by tachycardia disproportionate to the fever, a gallop rhythm, heart sounds with a "tic-tac" quality, or arrhythmias. Sometimes there may be only cardiomegaly on x-ray. If severe, there may be congestive heart failure. There may be conduction abnormalities: prolongation of the P-R interval occurs in over 20%, but is non-specific and alone does not constitute an acceptable criterion for diagnosing rheumatic carditis; dropped beats may occur with second degree atrioventricular block, but complete heart block is very rare. *Pericarditis* may appear suddenly and may be associated with precordial pain, a friction rub, or a striking increase in heart size. More often, however, patients with pericarditis are asymptomatic, an an increase in heart size is detected on routine roentgenograms. Pericarditis seldom appears without endocarditis and myocarditis, the combination being termed *pancarditis*. Death may occur during the acute phase of carditis or after clinical recovery; permanent cardiac damage may result in long-

TABLE 22-38

MODIFIED JONES CRITERIA FOR THE DIAGNOSIS OF ACUTE RHEUMATIC FEVER

Major manifestations
  Carditis
  Polyarthritis
  Chorea
  Erythema marginatum
  Subcutaneous nodules
Minor manifestations
  Clinical
    Arthralgia
    Fever
  Laboratory findings
    Increased acute phase reactants:
      Increased erythrocyte sedimentation rate
      Increased C-reactive protein
  Prolonged P-R interval

term disability, usually because of mitral or aortic valvular insufficiency or stenosis.

Sydenham's chorea is characterized by sudden, aimless, irregular movements of the extremities frequently associated with emotional instability and muscle weakness. The onset may be gradual, with complaints that the child is nervous. The patient may become clumsy and may stumble, fall, or drop objects. Often there are complaints from the school of poor attention and deteriorating handwriting. Facial grimacing and various speech disorders occur. As the chorea becomes more severe, the irregular jerking movements can be sufficiently violent to cause injuries. Muscle weakness may be profound. Most of the choreiform movements subside during sleep and are exaggerated by emotions. Characteristically, if the patient is asked to extend the arms, hands, and fingers, flexion of the wrists and hyperextension of the metacarpo-phalangeal joints are observed. The pronator sign may be elicited: after the arms are raised above the head there is gradual pronation of the hands (apposition of the dorsal aspects of the hands). Other signs are an inability to hold the tongue still when it is protruded and spasmodic contractions of the hands when the patient intentionally grips objects or the examiner's hand. Chorea is not often associated with other features of rheumatic fever except perhaps mild carditis. It can also be caused by diseases other than rheumatic fever.

Subcutaneous nodules are painless small (0.5 to 1 cm) swellings over bony prominences, primarily over the extensor tendons of the hands, feet, elbows, scalp, scapulae, and vertebrae. Nodules tend to occur in crops and may persist for days to months after the onset of acute rheumatic fever. Subcutaneous nodules are not specific for rheumatic fever and may occur in rheumatoid arthritis as well as SLE.

Erythema marginatum occurs in only 10% of patients. The characteristic rash associated with rheumatic fever consists of an evanescent, pink, erythematous macule, often with a clear center and serpiginous outline. The rash is transient, migratory, and nonpruritic; it blanches with pressure and is found primarily on the trunk and proximal extremities.

Other clinical features of rheumatic fever, the so-called minor Jones criteria, are of little value in diagnosis. Fever may be variable and may persist for weeks. Arthralgia is frequently present, but in the absence of objective migratory polyarthritis does not assume major diagnostic importance.

LABORATORY EVALUATION

The erythrocyte sedimentation rate and C-reactive protein are almost always elevated in acute rheumatic fever, the degree of elevation being influenced by previous salicylate or steroid therapy, anemia, and congestive heart failure. Because these studies may be abnormal in virtually any other inflammatory state, they are of little value for the specific diagnosis of acute rheumatic fever. Leukopenia or urinalysis abnormalities probably do not occur in rheumatic fever, and if found in a patient with joint cardiac abnormalities suggest SLE.

Isolation of group A streptococci from a patient suspected of having acute rheumatic fever provides strong evidence for the diagnosis. Caution is needed, however, as many normal children may be carriers of streptococci. Failure to isolate streptococci from patients with known rheumatic fever may be related to prior antibiotic therapy, to only small numbers of organisms, or to inadequate cultures.

Probably the most specific and most reliable proof of a previous streptococcal infection can be obtained from studies of serum antibody titers against the organism. A rising antibody titer to specific streptococcal antigens is more significant than a single elevated value. However, if the physician sees the patient more than 2 months after acute streptococcal infection, antibody titers may be declining or low. This occurs most frequently in patients whose initial or only manifestation of rheumatic fever is carditis or chorea. The most widely used serologic test is antibody formation against streptolysin O (AS)). Titers of at least 333 U in children and 250 U in adults are considered elevated. Other available antibody tests are antideoxyribonuclease B (anti-DNase B), antihyaluronidase (AH), antistreptokinase (ASK), and antinicotinamide-adenine dinucleotidase (anti-NADase). A twofold rise in titer to one or more of the above antigens can be demonstrated in virtually all cases of acute or recurrent rheumatic fever is serum samples are obtained within 2 months of the streptococcal infection. Patients who present with fever, rash, arthritis, or carditis should have studies to exclude abnormalities associated with SLE and rheumatoid arthritis. These include antinuclear antibodies, anti-DNA titers, and rheumatoid factor.

TREATMENT

In acute rheumatic fever, a course of penicillin should be given even if cultures for group A streptococci are negative. Either 1.2 million U of benzathine penicillin G as a single intramuscular injection or 600,000 U of procaine penicillin G given as a daily injection for 10 days is effective therapy. Erythromycin, 1 g orally for 10 days, may be substituted for penicillin in patients allergic to penicillin. Prophylaxis against recurrent rheumatic fever should be instituted immediately after acute therapy. The most effective prophylaxis consists of 1.2 million U of benzathine penicillin G intramuscularly given every three weeks; the injection is painful and may lead to reactions. Alternative therapy consists of either 200,000 U of penicillin given orally twice to three times each day (depending on size) or 1 g of sulfadiazine given orally once each day; compliance may be a problem. The optimal duration of prophylaxis is uncertain, and the safest recommendation is to continue therapy indefinitely. An alternative is to stop after adolescence, but start again when patients become re-exposed to streptococcal infections (eg, living in barracks or dormitories, or having small children who have streptococcal disease).

If a child has acute rheumatic fever but no clinical carditis, normal activity can be resumed once the pain and fever have disappeared, usually after 5 to 7 days. If there is mild carditis, then at least 10 to 15 days of bed rest are needed to ensure that there is no progressive deterioration. It is pointless to wait for the murmur to disappear, because it may never do so. In both these groups, too, the erythrocyte sedimentation rate is not a good guide to the course of the illness; sometimes the rate will remain high until after the patient ambulates. On the other hand, if there is severe carditis, as shown by marked cardiomegaly or congestive heart failure, the patient should be kept at rest for several weeks, until the heart size either returns to normal or is at least stable.

Salicylates and steroids are of value in controlling the acute clinical manifestations. Arthritis and fever respond dramatically to salicylate therapy, often within hours of initiation of treatment. Acetylsalicylic acid is usually used, in a dose of 80 to 100 mg/kg/d. The duration of treatment is related to the course and severity of the disease; the minimum period is usually 6 weeks. When steroids or salicylates are discontinued, the dose should be reduced gradually over 2 to 4 weeks. If rebound occurs, full therapy may have to be reinstituted for an additional 4 to 6 weeks. Some physicians do not use such large doses and give salicylates only as needed for pain and fever.

Studies of patients with moderate to severe carditis treated with salicylates or steroids do not demonstrate any superiority of either drug in modifying the duration of acute disease or residual heart damage after 5 years of follow-up. On the other hand, patients who develop congestive heart failure should be treated with steroids (prednisone in a dose of 2 mg/kg/d). Although digitalis may fail to benefit the patient with severe myocarditis, it is often successful in controlling congestive heart failure in patients with valvular insufficiency. Digitalis should be started cautiously, because toxic manifestations occur with relatively small doses when acute myocarditis is present. Occasionally surgical implantation of a prosthetic valve is needed if severe incompetence of aortic or mitral valves leads to refractory heart failure; this can be done in the face of high fever.

Specific treatment for chorea is not available. Physical and mental stress should be reduced, and adequate protective measures instituted to prevent injury during severe episodes. Occasionally, in very severe disease, steroids have been helpful. Phenobarbital and valproic acid may give symptomatic relief.

PROGNOSIS

Approximately 75% of patients with acute rheumatic fever are well after 6 weeks, and beyond 6 months less than 5% are symptomatic with chorea or intractable carditis. Rheumatic fever does not recur in the absence of recurrent infection when more than 8 weeks has elapsed after stopping treatment. Up to 70% of patients who develop carditis during the initial episode of acute rheumatic fever recover without any residual heart disease. Approximately 70% of the patients with congestive heart failure and pericarditis during acute rheumatic fever develop permanent heart disease, versus 20% of patients with only mild carditis during the acute disease. In individual patients the clinical course during recurrent episodes of rheumatic fever tends to be similar to that seen during the initial episode. Patients with recurrent rheumatic fever have a greater incidence of permanent heart damage after carditis than do patients having only a single episode. Patients who have had chorea without clinical carditis may present years later with mitral stenosis.

Patients with a well-documents history of acute rheumatic fever and those with documented evidence of rheumatic heart disease should receive continuous antibiotic prophylaxis to prevent recurrent episodes triggered by group A streptococcal pharyngitis. Although patients without rheumatic heart disease are at lower risk of recurrence than are patients with carditis or valvular disease, prophylaxis for all patients with rheumatic fever should be continued for 5 years or until the age of 21 years, whichever is longer. Prophylactic regimens include 1.2 million units of benzathine penicillin G intramuscularly every 4 weeks or 250 mg of penicillin V orally twice a day. Oral sulfadiazine of sulfisoxazole in a single daily dose of 0.5 gram for patients weighing less than 27 kg (60 lb) or 1.0 gram for patients weighing more than 27 kg may be substituted. Erythromycin 250 mg twice a day is an alternative regimen for patients allergic to penicillin or sulfonamide drugs.

References

Aron AM, Freeman JM, Carter S: The natural history of Sydenham's chorea: review of the literature and long-term evaluation with emphasis on cardiac sequelae. Am J Med 38:83, 1965

Berrios X, del Campo E, Guzman B, Bisno AL: Discontinuing rheumatic fever prophylaxis in selected adolescents and young adults. Ann Int Med 118:401, 1993

Bisno AL: Acute rheumatic fever: a present-day perspective. Medicine 72: 278, 1993

Burge DJ, DeHoratius RJ: Acute rheumatic fever. Cardiovasc Clin 23:3, 1993

Dajani AS, Bisno AL, Chung KJ, et al: Prevention of rheumatic fever. Circulation 78:1082, 1988

Feinstein AR, Spagnulo M, Wood H, et al: Rheumatic fever in childhood and adolescence. Long-term epidemiologic study of subsequent prophylaxis: Streptococcal infections and clinical sequelae. Ann Intern Med 60:86, 1964

Folger GM Jr, Hajar R, Robida A, Hajar HA: Occurrence of valvar heart disease in acute rheumatic fever without evident carditis: colour-flow Doppler identification. Br Heart J 67:434, 1992

Kaplan EL: Global assessment of rheumatic fever and rheumatic heart disease at the close of the century. Influences and dynamics of populations and pathogens: a failure to realize prevention? Circulation 88:1964, 1993

Spagnulo M, Pasternack B, Taranta A: Risk of rheumatic fever recurrences after streptococcal infections: prospective study of clinical and social factors. N Engl J Med 285:641, 1971

Special Writing Group of the Committee on Rheumatic Fever, Endocarditis, and Kawasaki Disease of the Council of Cardiovascular Disease in the Young of the American Heart Association: guidelines for the diagnosis of rheumatic fever. Jones criteria, 1992 update. JAMA 268:2069, 1992

Veasey LG, Weidermeyer SE, Ormond SG: Resurgence of acute rheumatic fever in the intermountain area of the United States. N Engl J Med 316: 421, 1987

THE RESPIRATORY SYSTEM

Thomas A. Hazinski, Associate Editor

23.1 LUNG GROWTH IN INFANCY AND CHILDHOOD

Elizabeth A. Perkett

The lung of the term infant is fully capable of meeting the respiratory needs of the newborn infant, but anatomically it is not a miniature adult lung. Detailed morphometric studies of lungs at autopsy, plus correlation with animal studies, have provided insight into the postnatal development of the lung.

FIVE PHASES OF LUNG DEVELOPMENT

Lung development is divided into five stages, four of which are completed before birth at term. The *embryonic* phase of lung development involves the growth of the major airways and is complete at 6 weeks of gestation. From 6 to 16 weeks, the *pseudoglandular* phase, the airways branch, and the acinus (the future gas-exchanging region) begins to develop. Branching of the airways is complete by 16 weeks; as a result, even the most premature infant has fully developed its conducting airways. The *canalicular* phase, from 16 to 28 weeks of gestation, encompasses the vascularization of the distal mesenchyme and development of the acinus. Initially a double capillary bed grows into the developing walls of the air spaces; postnatally the capillaries fuse and become single. During the canalicular phase, capillaries come into close proximity to airway epithelium, resulting in the potential for gas exchange. Thus, an extremely premature newborn infant may be viable even though there are no true alveoli. The *saccular* phase, of lung development, 26 to 36 weeks of gestation, involves the further development of the gas exchange surface, with secondary crests that subdivide the saccules to form alveoli. The increased air-blood interface makes adequate gas exchange much more likely if the infant is born prematurely. The *alveolar* phase of lung development begins at 36 weeks of gestation and continues in the postnatal period.

AIRWAYS

The basic pattern of a newborn infant's airways is the same as that found in an adult lung because airway branching is complete by 16 weeks of gestation. Once branching is complete, it is estimated that there are 25,000 terminal bronchioles. After birth, further airway growth occurs by an increase in length and diameter. The trachea and main bronchi grow more rapidly than the small airways, with the trachea ultimately increasing threefold in diameter and the bronchioles twofold in diameter (Fig. 23-1). Airway smooth muscle is present in the large airways by 8 weeks of gestation and continues to develop as more distal airways appear. At birth, bronchial smooth muscle is mature and is responsive to factors that influence muscle tone. In the larger airways the proportion of the bronchial wall occupied by smooth muscle is about 3% in both the child and adult. In small airways, smooth muscle comprises 10% of the airway wall in children but 20% in adults.

MAJOR BLOOD VESSELS

Pulmonary arterial development closely follows the development of the large airways in utero. Pulmonary arteries run together with bronchi and have a similar branching pattern. As a result, when lung tissue is hypoplastic or absent, airway and artery are both absent or proportionally reduced. The total number of preacinar arteries is present by 20 weeks of fetal life. Intraacinar vessels develop during fetal life and grow rapidly during the first few years of life with the postnatal increase in alveoli. The intrapulmonary bronchial arteries develop and are supplied by the aorta. The bronchial arteries normally supply only preacinar airways; they end before terminal bronchioles and do not participate in gas exchange.

ALVEOLI

True alveoli first appear at about 36 weeks of gestation, but most alveolar development occurs postnatally. Alveoli increase in number by the growth of secondary septa from the walls of saccules. Further increases come from segmentation of the primitive alveoli and development of respiratory bronchioles from terminal bronchioles. With the development of new alveoli there is accompanying growth of capillaries to allow gas exchange. Recent evidence indicates that vascular endothelial growth factor (VEGF) and its receptors are necessary for acinar development. Fusion of the double capillary network can be seen by 1 month postnatally and is complete by 18 months of age. In the newborn the alveolar–arterial ratio is 20:1; it is 12:1 by age 2 and further decreases to 8:1 in childhood. Throughout postnatal lung growth, the internal surface area of the lung closely follows body growth and remains about 1 m²/kg body weight.

Following birth there is very rapid alveolar multiplication, with estimates of 20 million alveoli at birth, which increase to 200 million by 3 years of age. Although there is no agreement on the age at which alveolar multiplication ceases, it markedly decreases in rate after age 2 to 3 years. Estimates of the number of alveoli in adult lungs vary from 200 million to 600 million. The reason for the marked variability in number of alveoli in adults is not known; perhaps genetic, environmental, or metabolic factors are involved. In a normal adult the surface area of the air–blood interface is approximately 70-fold greater than the surface area of the skin.

The alveolar surface is lined with type I and type II epithelial cells, which are well developed at birth. The flat type I cells cover 93% of the distal airway surface, whereas the type II cells are more numerous but, because of their cuboidal shape, cover only 7% of the surface area. Type II cells produce surfactant and molecules involved in host defense against infection and inflammation. Type II cells are also the progenitor cells of the type I cells and thus are

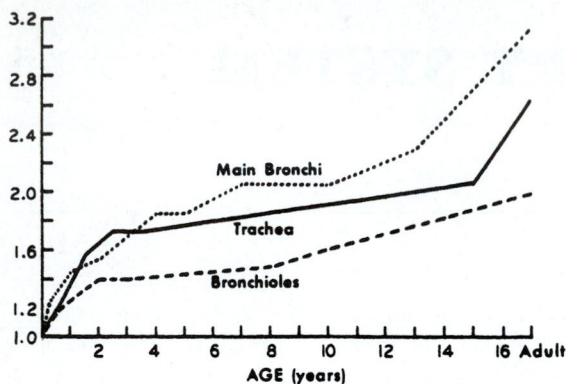

FIGURE 23-1 The relative change in diameters of large airways as a function of age. Note the rapid growth during the first two years of life. SOURCE: *From Engel S: Lung Structure. Springfield, IL, Charles C. Thomas, 1962.*

critical in the maintenance of the distal airway epithelium throughout life.

AIRWAY LINING CELLS

Perhaps a dozen or more cell types have been identified by morphologic or histochemical methods on or just below the airway surface, but the function of these cells is unknown. Ciliated epithelial cells are found lining large airways by 16 weeks of gestation. Mucus-producing cells are also found in the early fetal lung and account for 30% of the lining cells in midgestation. However, their number then decreases so that the newborn lung has fewer mucus-producing cells than the adult lung. Following birth there is an increase in the number of mucous cells. Nonciliated bronchial epithelial cells, termed Clara cells, appear late in gestation at about 36 weeks. Submucosal glands develop in early fetal life, and there does not appear to be any new gland formation postnatally. After birth, apparent increases in gland area with growth and with conditions that stimulate secretions are the result of hypertrophy and increased activity of existing glands.

COLLATERAL VENTILATION CHANNELS

Collateral ventilatory channels are reduced or absent in the newborn lung. In the adult lung gas can pass through pores of Kohn (holes between alveoli) and through canals of Lambert (channels between terminal bronchioles and adjacent alveoli). Although lack of collateral airflow is not important for ventilation, airflow via collateral channels may prevent gas absorption in lung units distal to obstructed airways. It is possible that the lack of collateral ventilation contributes to the common finding of patchy atelectasis in airway diseases in young children.

CONNECTIVE TISSUE SPACE

At birth there is some cartilage in the trachea, main bronchi, and segmental bronchi, but airways are very compliant and easily compressed by extrinsic masses or even by forced exhalation. A loose connective sheath surrounds airways by the 16th week of gestation. This sheath contains lymphatic channels near the acinus and lymphatic vessels adjacent to larger airways and are essential to maintain a dry air–blood barrier for gas exchange. The sheath grows with the airways and extends to a few generations of bronchioles proximal to the terminal bronchioles. There is further development of

cartilage in more distal bronchi for about 2 months postnatally. After that time the existing cartilage increases in mass as the airway dimensions grow, and airway walls become rigid.

The interstitial space contains little collagen and elastin at birth, which may make the air space more vulnerable to injury from high pressure (barotrauma) or lung stretch. Elastin is linked with alveolar growth and increases with the rapid alveolarization in the postnatal period.

CONTROL OF LUNG GROWTH

Intrauterine lung growth has been extensively studied in animal models and is complex with multiple mechanisms including growth factors, hormones, mechanical factors, mesenchymal-epithelial cell interactions, matrix deposition, and nutritional status. Factors that have been implicated in postnatal growth inhibition include absent fetal breathing movements, corticosteroids, hyperoxia, space limitation (kyphoscoliosis, abdominal masses, diaphragm defects, etc), malnutrition, and decreased pulmonary blood flow. Stimulation of lung growth has been seen with high-altitude exposure, acromegaly, exercise, and postpneumonectomy. In animal models, vitamin A (retinol) and its metabolite retinoic acid appear to be essential for the proper maturation and maintenance of airway epithelium and the acinar space. Studies suggest that premature infants may have low vitamin A stores, resulting in poor healing following newborn respiratory diseases and making them more vulnerable to the development of chronic lung disease. Hyperoxia and dexamethasone have been shown to disrupt alveolar development in rats and in larger animals. Although this response has not been proven to occur in humans, these are common therapies in premature infants, and thus, there is concern whether alveolar development could be impaired. Studies in rats suggest that retinoic acid can counteract the deleterious effects of hyperoxia and steroids and can stimulate the development of new alveoli in mature lungs; however, a similar response to retinoic acid has not yet been demonstrated in humans. For premature infants, the maintenance of adequate nutrition, including vitamin A, is likely important for optimizing postnatal lung growth.

Metabolic needs can influence lung growth as reflected in finding that the lungs of high-altitude natives are slightly larger than those from sea-level inhabitants. More striking is the diffusing capacity, which is 20 to 30% greater in high-altitude residents. This is partially explained by increased numbers and size of alveoli. Trained athletes tend to have larger lungs, which could be secondary to the metabolic needs as well as the stimulation of stretching with deep breathing.

SUMMARY

The first 3 years of life are a critical time for lung growth, particularly for the formation of alveoli. Prospects for normal lung growth are enhanced by proper nutrition and adequate oxygenation. However, neonatal lung injury, intercurrent respiratory infections, and exposure to environmental inhalant hazards such as tobacco smoke may adversely influence lung growth.

References

Burri PH: Fetal and postnatal development of the lung. Annu Rev Physiol 46:617, 1984

Chytil F: The lungs and vitamin A. Am J Physiol 262:L517, 1992

Jeffery PK: The development of large and small airways. Am J Respir Crit Care Med 157:S174, 1998

Massaro GD, Massaro D: Postnatal treatment with retinoic acid increases the number of pulmonary alveoli in rats. Am J Physiol 270:L305, 1996

Merkus PJFM, ten Have-Opbroek AAW, Quanjer PH: Human lung growth: a review. Pediatr Pulmonol 21:383–397, 1996

Shenai JP, Chytil F, Jhaveri A, et al: Plasma vitamin A and retinol binding protein in premature and term neonates. J Pediatr 99:302–305, 1981

Thurlbeck WM: Pre- and postnatal organ development. In: Chernick V, Mellins RB, eds: Basic Mechanisms of Pediatric Respiratory Disease. Philadelphia, BC Decker, 1991:23

23.2 PHYSIOLOGICAL BASIS OF PULMONARY FUNCTION

Greg Omlor and John McBride

Like all mammals, humans take up oxygen and eliminate carbon dioxide by allowing respiratory gases to diffuse across a large and permeable interface. The success of this strategy depends on developing and maintaining a complex gas exchange system involving the brain, airways, alveoli, heart and great vessels, and respiratory muscles. From late fetal life to the end of adolescence, the respiratory system changes in structure, size, and functional capacity. Just before birth the lung holds just a few hundred milliliters of fluid and has little blood flow and a low level of liquid ventilation to and from its relatively few and large air spaces. By adolescence it has increased 30- to 40-fold in volume, developed many new alveoli and capillaries, and is contained in a much stiffer and stronger chest wall. Of these and other changes, the most extensive occur in the first few weeks and months of life. Survival and normal development depend on the lung's ability to maintain adequate gas exchange through this transformation. It is not surprising that, under certain circumstances, the function of the developing lung is vulnerable, particularly in the face of lower respiratory diseases. This section reviews the basics of pulmonary function and how these functions are affected by changes in lung structure with age.

AIR SPACES (ALVEOLI)

The gas-exchanging portion of the lung resembles a sponge made up of millions of individual alveoli, each of which might be considered to resemble a tiny balloon. Like balloons, the individual alveoli (and the lung as a whole) will collapse unless supported by the chest wall. The force with which the unsupported lung deflates is called the recoil pressure of the lung. It is important that lung recoil be low enough that the lung can be easily stretched with breathing but, at the same time, adequately high to keep the airways and alveoli throughout the lung evenly expanded. If the lung is too stiff, the work of breathing is too high; if it is too compliant, airways will become compressed, leading to airflow obstruction. Only about one-third of lung recoil is supplied by the elastin and collagen fibers of the lung tissue. The other two-thirds of this force results from the surface tension of the microscopic layer of fluid lining the alveoli. The low recoil pressure of the healthy lung and the even distribution of lung recoil throughout the millions of alveoli would not be possible without pulmonary surfactant to decrease the surface tension of the alveolar lining fluid and to allow it to fluctuate with changes in lung volume. High lung recoil in immature infants with surfactant deficiency grossly increases the work of breathing and disrupts normal alveolar function.

THE RESPIRATORY PUMP

The tendency for the unsupported lung to collapse is counterbalanced by the stiffness of the rib cage and its tendency to spring outward. The balance of these forces is adequate to keep the lung inflated even when the respiratory muscles are totally relaxed. In older children the volume of air remaining in the lung when the respiratory muscles are completely relaxed, which is termed the functional residual capacity (FRC) or equilibrium volume, is about 50% of the total lung capacity (TLC, the volume of air in the lung with a maximal inspiration). In the first few months of life, the relaxed lung volume is much lower, usually only 20 to 30% of TLC, because the bones and cartilage of the rib cage have not stiffened adequately to hold the lung as far open as later in childhood. This has important implications for infant lung function.

The most important muscle of inspiration is the diaphragm. Its contraction expands the volume of the chest cavity and thus the volume of the lungs by two mechanisms. Shortening of the diaphragmatic fibers increases the cephalocaudal dimension of the rib cage. In addition, the descent of the diaphragmatic dome pushes the abdominal contents caudally and thereby increases the abdominal pressure. The increased abdominal pressure is applied not only to the abdominal wall but also to the bottom of the rib cage, causing both to move outward, which expands the thorax in the ventral and lateral directions. Diaphragmatic paralysis or weakness is serious at any age but is particularly problematic in infancy, when the relaxation lung volume is lowest. An often overlooked but essential respiratory muscle is the genioglossus, the muscle that moves the tongue forward just before every diaphragm contraction. If this muscle is weak, or if the tongue is large or posteriorly placed, diaphragm contraction can pull the tongue into the airway and create upper airway obstruction. Other muscles of respiration, such as the sternocleidomastoids and trapezius, expand the chest by lifting the upper ribs. These muscles can support ventilation by themselves if the lung is normal but are usually not active during quiet breathing at rest. They are not as efficient in infancy because the rib cage itself is unstable and does not move as a unit when the upper ribs are lifted. The intercostal muscles primarily act to stiffen the rib cage, a particularly important function in the neonate, when the rib cage is most flexible. When the lung is stiff or airways are narrowed, contractions of these accessory respiratory muscles become visible and are signs of respiratory distress at any age. Despite the relative weakness and mechanical inefficiency of the respiratory muscles early in life, most clinical problems of these muscles in infancy and childhood are related to neuromuscular diseases (eg, spinal muscular atrophy) or to damage to nerves within the brachial plexus from injury at birth.

LUNG VOLUMES

Total lung capacity (TLC) is limited primarily by the stiffness of the lung. With inflation, the lung becomes stiffer and stiffer until it can not be further expanded by the respiratory muscles. Residual volume (RV), the amount of air contained in the lung at the end of a maximal expiration, is determined in healthy individuals primarily by the chest wall and is usually 20% of TLC. At RV the diaphragm is maximally stretched, and the ribs can be pushed together no further. In children with airway obstruction, RV may be increased if airway "closure" traps gas within the alveoli. The volume of an average breath or tidal volume (TV) is usually about

10% of TLC at rest and can increase to 50% of TLC with maximal effort.

One of the most important lung volumes is the functional residual capacity (FRC), the volume of air in the lung at the end of a normal tidal breath. If the FRC is too low during tidal breathing, the small volume of gas in the lung and the effect of low lung volumes on airway function (see below) can compromise gas exchange. In older children and adults, the respiratory muscles are totally relaxed at the end of a normal breath, and so FRC is equal to the equilibrium volume or about 50% of total lung capacity. This is an efficient breathing strategy because no energy is required to maintain lung volume between breaths. If FRC were equal to the equilibrium volume during infancy (only 20–30% of TLC), breathing at this low lung volume would lead to atelectasis and compromised gas exchange. Infants maintain FRC above this volume (but still below 50% of TLC) because of their rapid respiratory rate: the lung never has time to return to the equilibrium volume between breaths. On the other hand, infants have a greater tendency than older children to develop hypoxemia during sleep when respiratory rate decreases and the end-expiratory volume falls toward the equilibrium volume.

AIRWAY FUNCTION

The airways must move gas to and from millions of alveoli with a minimum of energy expenditure. The upper extrathoracic and lower intrathoracic airways behave fundamentally differently in that the upper airways tend to narrow during inspiration, whereas the lower airways tend to narrow during expiration.

Upper airway obstruction normally causes difficulty on inspiration and presents as inspiratory stridor. Severe upper airway obstruction dramatically increases the work of breathing. Inspiratory narrowing of the nasal and pharyngeal airways is normally minimized by the tonic and phasic contraction of the muscles of the upper airway such as the alar nasae, genioglossus, and pharyngeal muscles. Excessive relaxation of the genioglossus and pharyngeal muscles during sleep is a fundamental cause of obstructive sleep apnea in both children and adults. Laryngeal narrowing is inhibited primarily by the intrinsic stiffness of the laryngeal cartilage. In the first year of life a lack of stiffness of the laryngeal cartilages may cause stridor that usually resolves with age (laryngomalacia). The relatively small diameter of the cricoid cartilage just below the larynx in the first years of life may explain the tendency of young children to develop stridor with mucosal edema associated with respiratory viral infections (croup).

Obstruction of the intrathoracic airways usually causes expiratory obstruction and wheezing. Narrowing of the central intrapulmonary airways during expiration is normally resisted by the cartilage rings (trachea) and plates (bronchi) in the walls of these airways. Peripheral airway narrowing is counteracted by the attachments between the airway walls and the connective tissue skeleton of the lung parenchyma. At high lung volumes such as those seen in patients with severe asthma or bronchiolitis, the lung is stiffest, and the intrapulmonary airways receive the greatest support from the surrounding parenchyma attachments. In this situation, wheezing may actually disappear or decrease, only to return as lung volumes return toward normal. Intrathoracic airway obstruction increases the work of breathing and leads to an uneven distribution of inspired air to the alveoli, leading in turn to hypoxemia and the need to increase total alveolar ventilation to achieve adequate carbon dioxide elimination. Infants and young children are prone to

expiratory airway obstruction because of the relatively poor support provided to the intrapulmonary airways by the developing lung parenchyma.

An increase in expiratory effort can eventually narrow the intrathoracic airways so severely that a point is reached at which increasing effort does not result in greater flow. This point of flow limitation can be reached in individual pulmonary airways at very modest flows, even in healthy lungs. The maximum flow achievable decreases with decreasing lung volume because airway diameters and lung recoil decrease as lung volume falls. In intrathoracic airway obstruction, flow limitation at low lung volumes can lead to local gas trapping. This in turn results in a very unequal distribution of ventilation and disruption of gas exchange. Flow limitation and gas exchange are exacerbated in infancy by the normally narrow airways and by further narrowing when there is inflammation, edema, or secretions.

Flow limitation is the basis of some of the most useful tests of airway function in both children and adults. Everyone can achieve flow limitation even at high lung volumes by exhaling as rapidly as possible after a maximal inspiration. An individual's level of flow limitation during maximal expiration (as measured by spirometric parameters or a flow–volume curve) reflects lung recoil, airway narrowing, and the floppiness of airways, all of which are important components of airway dysfunction in individuals with asthma or obstructive lung diseases. In contrast, airway resistance reflects only physical airway narrowing and is therefore a less useful measure of airway dysfunction in children with common airway diseases.

WORK OF BREATHING

The work of breathing, the energy required to accomplish ventilation includes the energy required to move air through the airways, to stretch the lung, and to expand the rib cage. In the healthy lung, the energy required to move air through the airways is relatively small compared to the energy required to stretch the lung. During quiet breathing, exhalation is passive, and the overall work of breathing is usually less than 1% of the total resting energy expenditure. Airway obstruction and parenchymal disease will increase the work of breathing by tenfold or more, especially when exhalation requires the use of intercostal and abdominal muscles.

PULMONARY CIRCULATION

The pulmonary vessels deliver systemic venous blood into pulmonary capillaries and independently adjust the muscular tone in the thousands of small pulmonary arteries to match perfusion to local alveolar ventilation. If perfusion of any lung unit is excessive relative to ventilation, Po_2 falls. This local change in oxygen tension in the perivascular space leads to constriction of the local pulmonary vessels and a decrease in blood flow to that area of lung until the balance of perfusion and ventilation is restored. The pulmonary vessels at birth have a large amount of muscle that disappears over the first few months of life. Persistence of this musculature can lead to high pulmonary vascular resistance throughout the lung, pulmonary hypertension, and an impaired ability to match perfusion to ventilation, particularly during episodes of lower airway infection. This is particularly common in children with high pulmonary blood flow, usually associated with left-to-right cardiac shunts.

GAS EXCHANGE

Gas exchange across the alveolar capillary membrane depends on (1) breathing inspired air with an adequate oxygen concentration,

(2) maintaining an appropriate level of alveolar ventilation, (3) exposure of the entire output of the right ventricle to the gas-exchanging membrane, (4) even matching of the air and blood across the entire lung, and (5) the appropriate size and permeability of the alveolar surface area.

The corresponding causes of hypoxemia are (1) breathing air with a low oxygen concentration such as at high altitude, (2) hypoventilation, (3) anatomic shunt, (4) ventilation–perfusion mismatching, and (5) diffusion block. Hypoventilation can occur in children with muscle weakness or with central respiratory depression caused by sedation or CNS disorders. Anatomic right-to-left intracardiac and intrapulmonary shunts can occur in patients with congenital heart disease, pulmonary hypertension, pulmonary hypoplasia, or chronic liver failure. However, the most common cause of hypoxemia in patients of all ages with pulmonary disorders is the mismatching of ventilation and perfusion. When ventilation and perfusion are mismatched, both CO_2 elimination and O_2 uptake are affected. Carbon dioxide elimination is usually easily enhanced by increasing the rate or depth of respiration; the resultant overventilation of well-perfused lung units will reduce the PCO_2 in this pulmonary venous blood to low levels. Increasing the level of ventilation, however, has little effect on oxygen uptake and PO_2 because hemoglobin is almost completely saturated. Therefore, the hallmark of mild to moderate ventilation–perfusion mismatch is a low PO_2 when the patient is breathing room air. The low PO_2 can usually be increased by breathing gas with an increased oxygen concentration. By contrast, an increased PCO_2 signals that a severe ventilation–perfusion mismatching is present and that respiratory failure is imminent. For the many reasons noted earlier (low lung volumes, small airways, low lung recoil, etc), young children are particularly prone to the development of hypoxemia related to ventilation–perfusion mismatching with a respiratory infection, upper airway obstruction, asthma, pulmonary edema, or respiratory muscle weakness.

23.3   TOOLS FOR DIAGNOSIS AND MANAGEMENT OF RESPIRATORY DISORDERS

Thomas A. Hazinski

This section reviews the signs and symptoms, diagnostic procedures, and therapy that are common to all respiratory diseases.

23.3.1   Signs and Symptoms

ANXIETY AND RESTLESSNESS

Inability to breathe with ease produces anxiety. A decrease in oxygen (ie, hypoxemia) and accumulation of carbon dioxide (ie, hypercarbia) in arterial blood accentuate this feeling. Restlessness, agitation, diaphoresis, and vigorous respiratory efforts are the first signs of hypoxemia. The infant with respiratory muscle fatigue who suddenly becomes more active may not actually be improving; paradoxically, increased activity may indicate a general worsening of the condition and be a sign of respiratory failure.

BREATHING PATTERN

The breathing pattern provides important clues to the degree of respiratory distress (see Sec. 4.1.1). At rest in patients with normal lungs, there usually is a pause between breaths at end-exhalation, corresponding to the functional residual capacity or FRC. Pulmonary diseases may cause either a rapid breathing rate (tachypnea) or slow respiratory rate (with prolonged expiratory or inspiratory time because of airway obstruction during expiration or inspiration, respectively), but generally causes a *disappearance of the respiratory pause at FRC*. In addition, the patient with respiratory distress will often initiate another inhalation before exhalation to FRC, resulting in hyperinflation and an increase in the anterior-posterior diameter of the chest.

RETRACTIONS

The nonrigid parts of the chest wall tend to retract when intrathoracic pressure is negative with respect to the atmospheric pressure. Retraction of the lower sternum and the suprasternal and intercostal spaces occurs even during normal respiration of the very young infant, in whom these structures are very compliant. In the older infant and child who has a more rigid chest wall, retractions during inspiration indicate that intrapleural pressure is markedly below atmospheric pressure because of increased effort to overcome either airway obstruction or reduced lung compliance.

CYANOSIS

When airway or parenchymal disease is severe, even maximal respiratory efforts cannot provide sufficient ventilation to deliver oxygen to the alveoli to saturate the arterial blood fully. When the amount of unoxygenated hemoglobin exceeds 5 g/dL, the child will appear cyanotic. If a child is anemic, however, significant hypoxemia may be present without cyanosis. The degree of cyanosis is difficult to estimate when there is peripheral vasoconstriction, as in shock. Under this circumstance, the child will be pale, and oxygen tension in arterial blood must be estimated by oximetry or measured directly to determine the adequacy of oxygenation.

RESPIRATORY SOUNDS

Breath sounds are influenced by the depth of breathing, velocity of the air flow, position of the patient, and the presence of fluid in the air spaces. The pitch of breath sounds depends on the size of the orifices or the diameter of the airways: the smaller the orifice or airway, the higher the pitch. The intensity of breath sounds varies directly with the velocity and rate of the airflow. Extrathoracic airways tend to narrow during inspiration, whereas intrathoracic airways narrow during exhalation. Therefore, the quality of breath sounds varies with the phase of respiration. Young infants may have intermittently sonorous breathing that often is misinterpreted by caretakers as wheezing or "rattling in the chest." These infants may have a mild form of laryngomalacia or micrognathia. It is a self-limiting problem that resolves with age, and it does not require further evaluation unless there are additional signs and symptoms of respiratory distress or growth failure.

Nasopharyngeal obstruction causes a gargling or snoring sound. Obstruction of the larynx and extrathoracic trachea produces a relatively high-pitched, harsh noise during inspiration called *stridor*. Because laryngeal obstruction is worsened during inspiration and reduced during expiration, laryngeal stridor is predominantly inspiratory. Masses at the base of the tongue and in the anterior phar-

TABLE 23-1

DIFFERENTIAL DIAGNOSIS OF COUGH

DIAGNOSIS	CLUES TO DIAGNOSIS
Sinusitis	Cough occurs after lying down; face pain, morning post-tussive emesis, transient relief by antibiotic therapy
Foreign body	Acute onset of choking, asymmetric breath sounds or wheezing
Cystic fibrosis	Frequent or severe respiratory illnesses; chronic sinusitis, growth failure, clubbing, steatorrhea
Asthma	Cough elicited by exercise, occurs at night, chest radiograph shows thickened bronchial walls with or without hyperexpansion
Gastroesophageal reflux	Frequent wet burps, dirty lung appearance, cough associated with meals, failure to thrive, postprandial cough
Habit cough, psychogenic cough	Distinctive sound, disappears while asleep
Vocal cord dysfunction	Wheeze-like sound, intermittent hoarse voice, disappears when asleep
Tracheoesophageal fistula, laryngeal cleft, discoordinated swallow	Choking and cough associated with drinking liquids; poor response to asthma or reflux therapy; patchy infiltrates on chest radiograph
Hypersensitivity pneumonitis	Dyspnea, exposure to potential inhalant hazard, dry cough; normal lung sounds
Tobacco smoke exposure	Heavy tobacco smoke exposure
Immune deficiency (including AIDS)	Frequent, prolonged infections; growth failure, lymphadenopathy
Cilia dysmotility syndrome	Sinusitis, chronic otitis, situs inversus
Allergic bronchopulmonary aspergillosis	Eosinophilia, high IgE levels, patchy infiltrates on chest radiograph
Tuberculosis	Tuberculosis exposure, positive skin test, abnormal chest radiograph
Pertussis/pertussis syndrome	Paroxysmal severe cough clusters following an upper respiratory infection
Tourette syndrome	Verbal tics, cough disappears when asleep

ynx are more likely to obstruct the larynx and cause stridor when the patient is supine. Vocal cord abnormalities, either subglottic or masses just beneath them, can cause hoarseness or a weak cry. (The differential diagnosis of stridor is discussed in Secs. 15.4.2 and 23.6) An obstruction of the extrathoracic trachea creates noises of somewhat higher pitch during inspiration than obstruction of the larynx does. The sounds of obstruction of the intrathoracic trachea and bronchi are predominantly expiratory. Partial blockage of the smaller airways hinders both the inflow and outflow of gas, creating wheezing. Wheezes are most prominent during expiration, but the clinician should recognize that a forceful exhalation can create high-pitched sounds in a normal person through glottic closure or voluntary vocal cord adduction. A diagnostic approach to wheezing is presented in Table 23-9 (Sec. 23.7). With atelectasis and consolidation, and also in thin people, breath sounds have an auditory quality as if they were emanating from a tube (ie, tubular breathing). Mucus or edema in distal respiratory units creates crackling sounds or rales. Patients with interstitial edema and inflammation usually have normal breath sounds. Patients with focal bronchiectasis may have very musical inspiratory sounds, which change after coughing.

COUGH

A cough is a voluntary or involuntary explosive expiration. After a deep inspiration, the glottis is closed and the expiratory muscles contract, compressing the lung and raising intrapulmonary pressure above the atmospheric pressure. The glottis then opens, and gas is expelled at a rapid rate. The cough reflex is initiated by the stimulation of subepithelial mechanoreceptors in the trachea, bronchi, and interstitium. Cough receptors may be activated by dust, chemicals, inflammation, mucus, airway distortion, or rapid changes in airway volume. A series of coughs that is difficult to stop is called a *paroxysm* and is common in pertussis, viral infections, cystic fibrosis, gastroesophageal reflux, and asthma. During paroxysms of coughing, central venous blood pressure rises, cerebral venous blood flow falls, and intracranial pressure increases. This may pro-

duce signs of cerebral hypertension such as headache, vomiting, conjunctival hemorrhage, or blurred vision. When foreign bodies or excess mucus is present, coughing is essential to eliminate the obstruction or facilitate mucociliary clearance. The high intrathoracic pressures that are created during active expiration, however, can collapse and obstruct the unstable airways of young infants or patients with bronchiectasis. A chronic cough may be uncomfortable or even harmful, causing chest pain, musculoskeletal pain, pulmonary air leaks, or rib fracture. A diagnostic approach to chronic cough is presented in Table 23-1.

HEMOPTYSIS

Hemoptysis is defined as bleeding that originates from the airway or the lung parenchyma but is observed in the upper airway or in expectorated secretions. Acute hemoptysis results from inflammation or trauma to the nasopharynx, larynx, or esophagus. Epistaxis and hematemesis also may be confused with hemoptysis, and these sites must be considered in the evaluation of a patient suspected to have hemoptysis. Intermittent hemoptysis is common in chronic conditions such as cystic fibrosis and bronchiectasis in which there is chronic infection. Significant bleeding into lung parenchyma (eg, that seen in pulmonary hemosiderosis or pulmonary vasculitis syndromes) may not cause obvious hemoptysis because much of the blood is swallowed or retained in the interstitial space or alveoli. Pulmonary arteriovenous malformations anywhere in the respiratory tract may also cause hemoptysis.

Flexible fiberoptic bronchoscopy can be useful in evaluating patients with unexplained hemoptysis. Either the site of bleeding may be directly visualized, or analysis of lavage may reveal hemosiderin-laden macrophages, thus establishing the diagnosis of pulmonary hemorrhage when the bleeding site cannot be seen. A diagnostic approach to hemoptysis is presented in Fig. 23-2.

CHEST PAIN

Chest pain is a frequent complaint, but it rarely indicates serious organic disease such as pulmonary embolus, pneumothorax, or car-

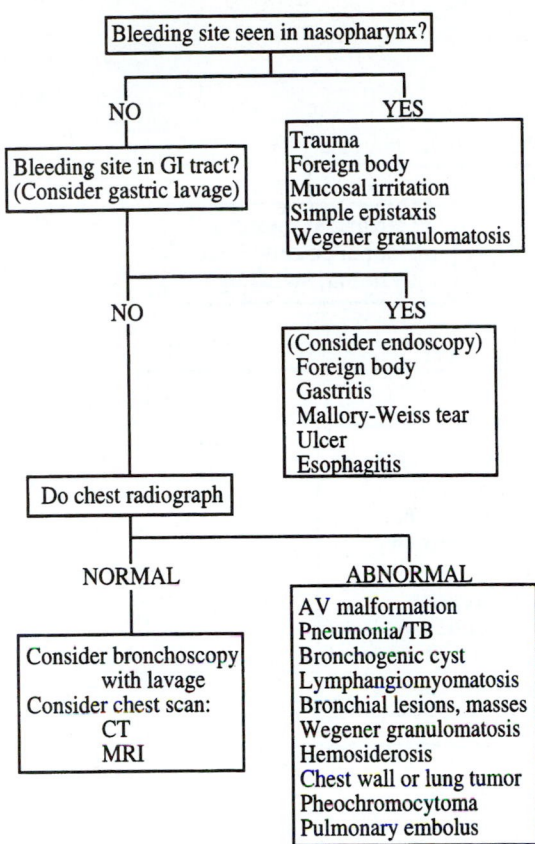

FIGURE 23-2 Diagnostic approach to hemoptysis.

diac diseases. The trachea and major bronchi have sensory innervation, and children with asthma may complain of vague substernal discomfort at rest or exercise. The pleural and periostial surfaces also are innervated so that inflammation at these sites can cause chest pain augmented by posture or breathing. Most chest pain is either functional or of musculoskeletal origin. A diagnostic approach to chest pain is presented in Fig. 23-3 and also discussed in detail in Sec. 22.4.9.

PLEURAL EFFUSIONS

In each hemithorax, there is always 0.25 mL/kg of fluid between the visceral and parietal pleura. Under pathologic conditions, the amount of fluid increases, and its chemical composition changes. Pleural effusions are traditionally classified as either transudates or exudates, based on a variety of criteria. In contrast to a transudate, an exudate has the following characteristics: protein concentration in pleural fluid greater than 50% of the protein concentration in plasma, a lactate dehydrogenase (LDH) concentration in pleural fluid greater than 60% of the LDH concentration in serum, and an absolute LDH concentration in pleural fluid > 200 IU/mL. A differential diagnosis of transudates and exudates is shown in Table 23-2.

Pleural effusions can be suspected clinically in the presence of decreased breath sounds, but most often pleural effusions are detected by routine chest radiography as a blunting of one or both costophrenic angles. Lateral decubitus radiographs can also demonstrate the mobility of the fluid, thereby differentiating fluid from an intrathoracic mass or pulmonary consolidation. Chest ultraso-

nography can be used to identify fluid and some use it to estimate the viscosity of the fluid.

In practice, pleural effusions can be classified as either infectious or noninfectious, and when pleural fluid is obtained, it should always be stained and examined microscopically and cultured for likely pathogens. Infected pleural effusions tend to be transudates and to have high concentration of neutrophils and neutrophil-derived proteins such as elastase and lysozyme. Other laboratory tests should be obtained as guided by the clinical situation. For example, if malignancy is suspected, the fluid sample should be examined cytologically. If pancreatic disease is suspected, the amylase and lipase concentrations in pleural fluid should be obtained.

References

Heffner JE, Brown LK, Barbieri CA: Diagnostic value of tests that discriminate between exudative and transudative pleural effusions. Chest 111: 970–980, 1997

Noppen M, DeWalel M, Li R, et al: Volume and cellular content of normal pleural fluid in humans. Am J Respir Crit Care Med 162:1023–1026, 2000

23.3.2 Imaging Modalities

CONVENTIONAL RADIOLOGIC IMAGING

In patients with suspected upper airway obstruction, it often is useful to obtain both anteroposterior and lateral films of the neck while the arms are down, the back of the head is up, and the neck is slightly extended. A high-quality plain neck or chest radiograph often can show the size and shape of the air-filled larynx, trachea, or major bronchi; can indicate the side of the aortic arch; and may reveal sites of airway obstruction or distortion. Airway compression, exaggerated dilatation, diaphragm dysfunction, or airway instability (tracheomalacia) can be determined with fluoroscopy. Video cinefluoroscopy is useful to examine swallowing function in children with chronic pulmonary symptoms. In patients with stridor, wheezing, or chronic cough, a barium esophagram is essential to detect foregut malformations, constricting vascular rings, H-type tracheoesophageal fistulas, and clefts. An esophagram can also be used to support the diagnosis of gastroesophageal reflux.

COMPUTED AXIAL TOMOGRAPHY

Computed tomography (CT) is a powerful diagnostic tool for examining the airway, lung parenchyma, and mediastinal structures. Chest CT exposes the patient to ionizing radiation and usually requires intravenous injection of a contrast agent. The procedure generally requires sedation, but newer high-speed devices permit the examination of unsedated patients. High-resolution, thin-cut scanning devices produce excellent images even in patients with tachypnea or who are uncooperative. Chest CT can also be used to guide transthoracic needle biopsy and aspiration of peripheral chest masses. Recent experience suggests that CT also may be useful in the diagnosis and management of interstitial lung diseases. To optimize the value of this imaging modality, prior consultation with an experienced pediatric radiologist is strongly advised so that the most appropriate scanning protocol and contrast agent can be employed.

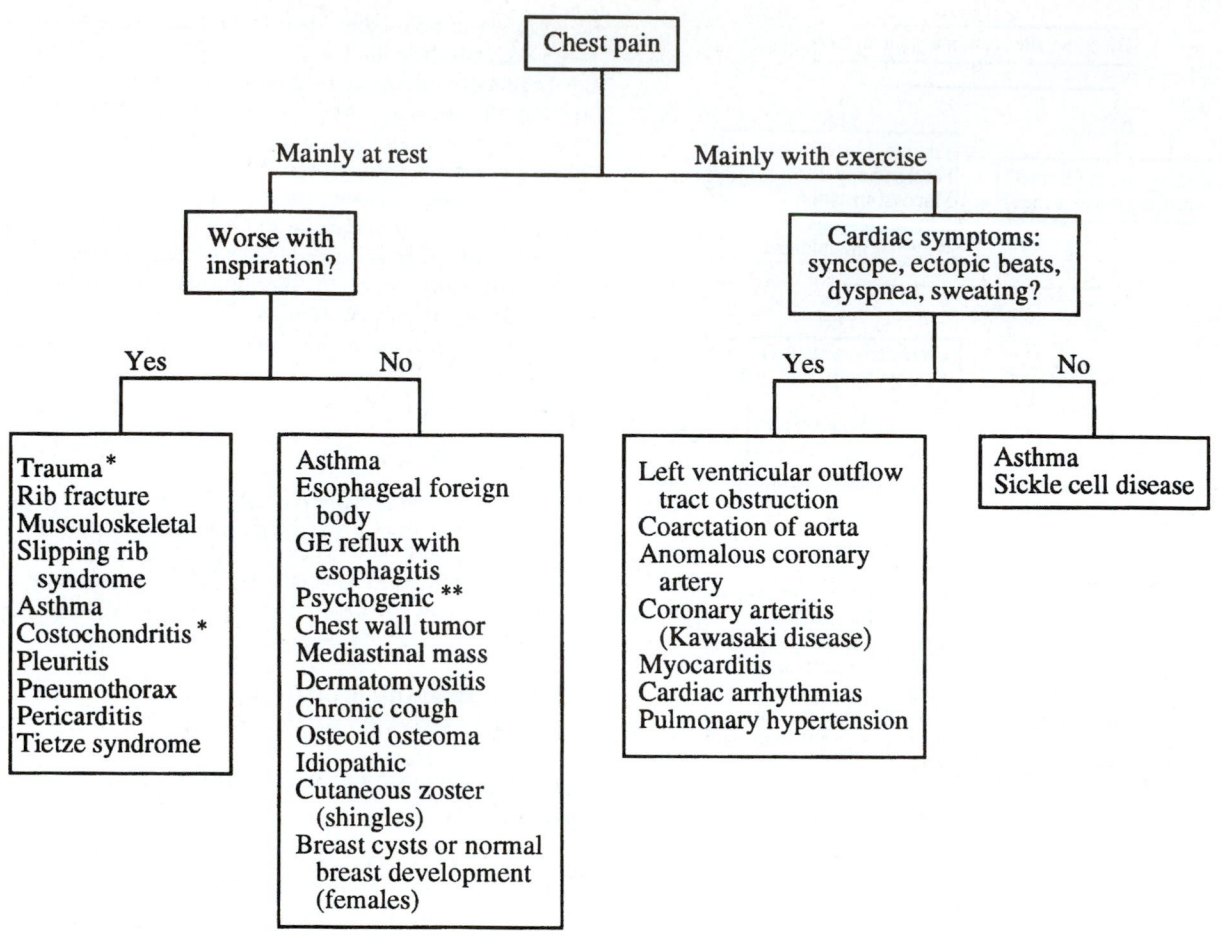

FIGURE 23-3   **Diagnostic approach to chest-pain. *Associated with chest-wall tenderness. **Disappears with sleep.**

MAGNETIC RESONANCE IMAGING

Magnetic resonance imaging (MRI) is not used often to examine the respiratory system, but it is useful when anomalous blood ves-

TABLE 23-2
CAUSES OF PLEURAL EFFUSIONS

Transudates
  Congestive heart failure
  Nephrotic syndrome
  Cirrhosis
  Hypoalbuminemia
  Pulmonary edema
Exudates
  Bacterial pneumonia
  Tuberculosis
  Trauma
  Pleuropericarditis
  Collagen vascular diseases
  Pancreatitis (pancreaticopleural fistula)
  Pulmonary embolus
  Postpericardiotomy syndrome
  Malignancy
Miscellaneous
  Thoracic duct injury or malformation
  Complications of central venous catheterization

sels or lesions that are within or adjacent to bone are suspected. MRI does not require ionizing radiation, and it cannot ordinarily be used in patients with implanted metallic devices such as wire sutures, pacemakers, or surgical staples. Recently, velocity-encoded cine MRI has been used to measure pulmonary blood flow and pressure and to identify abnormal vessels in the chest.

ULTRASONOGRAPHY

Chest ultrasonography rarely is employed beyond the newborn period because air distorts the ultrasound signal. However, there are some circumstances where ultrasonography and Doppler velocimetry are useful. These include determining the size and viscosity of pleural effusions, estimating diaphragm motion, detecting anomalous blood vessels within infected pulmonary sequestrations, and confirming that a displaced but normal thymus is present in infants with apparent cardiomegaly or mediastinal mass.

VENTILATION/PERFUSION LUNG SCANNING

The inhalation and injection of radioactive nuclides can yield semiquantitative information about the absolute and relative amounts of ventilation and blood flow in lung segments. It is less frequently employed in children than in adults but can be useful in assessing the functional importance of focal lung or pulmonary vascular disorders.

References

Knisely VL, Broderick LS, Kuhlman JE: MR imaging of the pleural and chest wall. MRI Clin North Am 8:125–141, 2000

23.3.3   Respiratory Monitoring Devices

Routine pediatric pulmonary function testing usually includes some estimate of arterial blood gas tensions from measurements of arterial oxygen saturation (SaO_2) that are made using a pulse oximeter, a skin-surface monitor of PO_2 or PCO_2 (PsO_2 and $PsCO_2$, respectively), or an end-tidal PCO_2 monitor. Devices that are designed to make these measurements are commercially available, safe, and relatively easy to use. However, a thorough understanding of how they operate is essential if the data they provide are to be interpreted properly (see Sec. 4.2.1 for more detail).

PULSE OXIMETRY

Continuous estimates of SaO_2 by pulse oximetry represent the most important innovation in noninvasive monitoring. The pulse oximeter uses light-emitting diodes (LED) to send light pulses of two different wavelengths through tissues such as fingers or toes. As it passes through the tissues, the light is absorbed by venous blood, tissue pigments, and arterial blood. Absorption by arterial blood is pulsatile and can be differentiated from the constant absorption by tissue pigments and venous blood. In the red region of the spectrum, reduced hemoglobin absorbs more light than does oxyhemoglobin, whereas in the infrared region, oxyhemoglobin absorbs more light than does reduced hemoglobin. By rapidly switching between red and infrared LEDs, the pulse oximeter can estimate the oxygen saturation, but *not* the partial pressure of oxygen (PaO_2), of arterial blood. To use oximetry correctly, it is important to remember that the relationship between PaO_2 and saturation is not linear; rather, it is described by the sigmoid hemoglobin–oxygen dissociation curve. For example, at normal pH, a PaO_2 of 60 mm Hg results in a saturation of 90%.

TRANSCUTANEOUS (SKIN SURFACE) OXYGEN AND CARBON DIOXIDE RECORDING

Skin-surface (ie, transcutaneous) blood gas monitoring uses skin-surface PaO_2 electrodes that are standard Clark PaO_2 electrodes modified so that they can be heated and mounted on the skin. On the skin, the electrode measures the flow of oxygen from the skin surface into the sensor and, using the in vitro calibration data, expresses this flow as PsO_2. Oxygen flow from the blood vessels beneath the skin, and therefore the PsO_2, is affected by several factors, only one of which is PaO_2.

Fortunately, at a skin temperature in infants of 44°C, the PsO_2 is approximately equal to the PaO_2. In older children and adults, however, skin thickness increases, skin resistance relative to electrode membrane resistance increases, and PsO_2 usually is lower than PaO_2, especially if the skin perfusion is compromised or edema is present. In older individuals, heating the skin surface to 45°C may be sufficient to adjust the PsO_2 so that it is closer to the PaO_2. Because of delays that are imposed by the circulation, the skin, membrane, and electrode itself, changes in PaO_2 are detected by the PsO_2 electrode after a lag time of as much as 45 seconds.

TABLE 23-3

FACTORS AFFECTING SKIN SURFACE PCO_2 ($PsCO_2$)

Acting to increase $PsCO_2$
  Increased $PaCO_2$
  Increased electrode temperature
  Increased skin carbon dioxide production
  Decreased skin blood flow
Acting to decrease $PsCO_2$
  Decreased $PaCO_2$
  Decreased electrode temperature

The skin-surface PCO_2 electrode is a conventional glass pH electrode that is immersed in a buffer, covered with a semipermeable membrane, and surrounded by a silver ring that acts as both a reference electrode and a heater. Carbon dioxide diffuses across the membrane, dissolves in the buffer, and produces a change in pH that can be related to the PCO_2 by calibration with a standard gas. The electrode differs from the PO_2 electrode in that it measures carbon dioxide concentration, not flow, and therefore is relatively unaffected by changes in skin resistance. It is, however, affected by changes in skin perfusion, so like the PsO_2 electrode, it should be heated to 43 to 44°C to produce vasodilatation of skin blood vessels. Because this heating increases both local $PaCO_2$ and skin carbon dioxide production, the $PsCO_2$ of heated skin always is higher than arterial PCO_2. The ratio between $PsCO_2$ and $PaCO_2$ at any given temperature, however, is constant, and adjustment factors have been derived so that it is easy to predict accurately the $PaCO_2$ from the $PsCO_2$. These adjustments can be built into the preamplifier so that the readout of $PsCO_2$ can closely approximate $PaCO_2$ (Table 23-3).

Transcutaneous blood gas recording has been valuable in controlling oxygen administration to premature infants. It has documented previously unrecognized causes of hypoxemia and hypercarbia such as excessive handling, suctioning, and feeding. Other uses include exercise testing and evaluation of gas exchange during sleep.

END-TIDAL PCO_2 MONITORING (CAPNOGRAPHY)

The carbon dioxide concentration in expired gas can be measured continuously using an infrared technique. Because exhaled alveolar air contains carbon dioxide but inhaled air does not, the continuous measurement of carbon dioxide in respiratory gas has been used to estimate arterial PCO_2 in many clinical settings including the home.

References

Hansen TN, Tooley WH: Skin surface carbon dioxide tension in sick infants. Pediatrics 64:942, 1979

Jennis MS, Peabody JL: Pulse oximetry: an alternative method for the assessment of oxygenation in newborn infants. Pediatrics 79:524, 1987

Landers S, Hansen TN: Skin surface oxygen monitoring. Perinatol Neonatol 8:39, 1984

Meredith KS, Monaco FJ: Evaluation of a mainstream capnometer and end-tidal carbon dioxide monitoring in mechanically ventilated infants. Pediatr Pulmonol 9:254, 1990

Peabody JL, Gregory GA, Willis MM, Tooley WH: Transcutaneous oxygen tension in sick infants. Am Rev Respir Dis 118:83, 1978

Poets CF, Southall DP: Noninvasive monitoring of oxygenation in infants and children: practical considerations and areas of concern. Pediatrics 93:737, 1994

Ramanathan R, Durand M, Larrazabal C: Pulse oximetry in very low birth weight infants with acute and chronic lung disease. Pediatrics 79:612, 1987

23.3.4 Diagnostic Procedures

AIRWAY ENDOSCOPY: LARYNGOSCOPY, RIGID BRONCHOSCOPY, AND FLEXIBLE BRONCHOSCOPY

Visualization of the airway by direct laryngoscopy is useful in the diagnosis of airway obstruction and structural or functional abnormalities of the upper airway. Rigid bronchoscopy is useful for examining the upper airway and trachea, but it may cause distortion of the upper airway and larynx that can obscure dynamic lesions such as laryngomalacia. Examination with a rigid bronchoscope in infants and children requires general anesthesia. The rigid bronchoscope has excellent optics, can be used to ventilate the patient, and permits the use of laser therapy, foreign-body removal, and biopsy of bronchial lesions. However, because of its size and rigidity, it is difficult to visualize the larynx and smaller distal airways.

The flexible fiberoptic bronchoscope avoids much of the difficulty that is associated with rigid bronchoscopes. Instruments less than 3 mm in diameter can be used to examine the airways of small infants and to obtain lung secretions for analysis. The nasopharynx, glottis, trachea, and bronchi can be easily visualized while the subject breathes around the scope. In older patients, direct biopsy of an endobronchial mass or a transbronchial biopsy can be performed. Often only light sedation is needed, but the requirements for anesthesia should be individualized. Fiberoptic bronchoscopes have been most useful in evaluating patients with unexplained pulmonary infiltrates, focal bronchial obstruction, stridor, atelectasis, or persistent wheezing. Fiberoptic bronchoscopy also may be used to obtain bronchoalveolar lavage specimens from specific regions of the lung, particularly in patients suspected to have unusual infections or in patients with immunodeficiency syndromes. Critically ill patients can be examined in intensive care units, thus facilitating diagnosis and therapy without the need for more invasive procedures or transport.

BRONCHOALVEOLAR LAVAGE

The cellular, microbiological, and biochemical composition of the airway and alveolar spaces can be estimated from distal airway secretions using bronchoalveolar lavage (BAL) during either flexible or rigid bronchoscopy. The technique is safe and simple to perform, but it requires both an experienced endoscopist and careful planning to ensure that the lavage sample can be obtained and processed appropriately to yield interpretable results. Bronchoalveolar lavage through a fiberoptic bronchoscope is useful in patients with unexplained pulmonary infiltrates in whom aspiration or pulmonary hemosiderosis is considered. In these cases, analysis of lavage fluid for lipid-laden or hemosiderin-laden macrophages will strongly support the diagnosis. BAL may also be useful in three groups of children with suspected pulmonary infection: (1) critically ill children in whom a specific etiologic diagnosis must be made to guide antimicrobial therapy; (2) children who have deteriorated while receiving conventional antimicrobial therapy; and (3) children with pneumonia who have either a congenital or acquired immunodeficiency. Although contamination of the bronchoalveolar lavage fluid by upper airway flora may sometimes yield inconclusive data, precise identification of some organisms (*Mycobacterium tuberculosis, Pneumocystis carinii, Legionella,* and so on) is diagnostic of infection and may eliminate the need for lung biopsy.

THORACOSCOPY

Once used exclusively to examine pleural disease, the thoracoscope and other related endoscopic instruments have been found to be useful in performing lung and node biopsies, nerve blocks, pericardial windows, and mediastinal evaluation. Ventilation of the contralateral lung usually is necessary during thoracoscopy, and the capacity to perform a conventional thoracotomy should be available. A classification of mediastinal masses based on anatomic localization is presented in Table 23-4.

LUNG BIOPSY

Biopsies of lung tissue or regional lymph nodes often are necessary to diagnose localized or diffuse parenchymal disease, diagnose malignancy, or detect pathogens in situ. The most common indication for open lung biopsy, however, is the suspicion of an unusual pulmonary pathogen in a patient who is immunodeficient or immunosuppressed and who has failed to improve after conventional antibiotic treatment.

As with bronchoalveolar lavage, clinical judgment must be applied when organisms such as cytomegalovirus, atypical mycobacteria, and *Candida* are isolated. Techniques other than thoracot-

TABLE 23-4
CLASSIFICATION OF MEDIASTINAL MASSES

Anterior mediastinum and paratracheal area
  Normal thymus
  Substernal thyroid
  Thymoma/thymic cyst
  Teratoma
  Lymphoma/lymphosarcoma
  Fibrosing mediastinitis
  Hilar adenopathy
    Tuberculosis
    Histoplasmosis
    Sarcoidosis
    Malignancy
    Chronic infection/AIDS
  Inflammatory pseudotumor (plasma cell granuloma)
Middle mediastinum
  Granulomatous disease (tuberculosis, histoplasmosis)
  Sarcoidosis
  Lymphoma
  Bronchogenic cyst
  Esophageal duplication cyst
  Extralobar sequestration
  Fibrosing mediastinitis
Posterior mediastinum/paravertebral sulcus
  Neuroblastoma
  Anterior neural tube defect
  Sarcoma
  Ganglioneuroblastoma
  Neurofibroma

omy may be employed to obtain tissue for histologic examination. These include percutaneous needle biopsy, high-speed drill trephine biopsy, transbronchial biopsy, and thoracoscopy. These methods often are used in conjunction with CT or ultrasonographic localization.

CARDIAC ECHOCARDIOGRAPHY

Echocardiography, with or without contrast enhancement, is often useful in excluding the possibility of heart disease in patients with chronic respiratory complaints. It is also useful to determine the presence and degree of pulmonary hypertension and in determining whether pulmonary disease has affected right ventricular function. Contrast-enhanced echocardiography is used to detect the presence of pulmonary arteriovenous malformations.

BLOOD GASES, PH, ELECTROLYTES

Assessment of gas exchange and acid-base regulation often requires the analysis of arterial blood. Depending on the age of the child, several sampling sites usually are available. In the young infant with a small amount of scalp tissue, the temporal artery is easily palpated and entered with a small-gauge needle. Radial, dorsalis pedis, and posterior tibial arteries also are easily cannulated. When a sample directly from an artery is unobtainable, arterialized capillary blood can be used. Warming a heel of an infant or a finger of an older child accelerates local blood flow so that the pH and $PaCO_2$ of capillary and arterial samples are similar. Arterialized capillary PaO_2 almost always is lower than that of arterial blood. Capillary pH, PaO_2, and $PaCO_2$ therefore must be interpreted with caution. Sluggish skin blood flow makes arterialized capillary blood gas measurements particularly unreliable. In any child with peripheral vasoconstriction or shock, arterial samples are required to evaluate ventilatory status. Transcutaneous PaO_2 and $PaCO_2$ monitoring also may be used to assess gas exchange noninvasively, but these techniques have largely been supplanted by pulse oximetry and end-tidal carbon dioxide monitoring (see Sec. 4.2.1).

In patients suspected to have chronic hypoventilation, the analysis of venous blood may be useful because sustained hypercapnia causes pH to decrease and bicarbonate concentration to increase. Similarly, patients with chronic lung or heart disorders requiring chronic diuretic therapy may be monitored for evidence of metabolic alkalosis.

PULMONARY FUNCTION TESTS

Numerous methods are available to assess lung volumes, distribution of ventilation and perfusion, and airflow (see Sec. 23.3.5).

INSPIRATORY AND EXPIRATORY PRESSURE (FORCE) MEASUREMENT

When respiratory muscle or chest wall disorders are suspected, estimation of the inspiratory or expiratory muscle strength is quite useful. To measure these variables, the patient is asked to perform a maximal inspiration or expiration against a complete obstruction while the airway pressure is measured. The pressure that is generated during these maximal maneuvers is proportional to the respiratory muscle strength. Serial measurement of inspiratory force is useful in the care of patients with Guillain-Barré syndrome, muscular dystrophy, or other neuromuscular and skeletal disorders that may impair respiratory muscle tone, power, or coordination.

23.3.5 Pulmonary Function Testing

Greg Omlor and John McBride

Pulmonary function tests are objective measures of lung function that can be used to identify the underlying cause of respiratory symptoms in children and adolescents and to monitor the status of those with chronic lung diseases. Some tests can be performed reliably and safely in the home. More sophisticated and technically difficult tests must be carried out in a pulmonary function laboratory. It is imperative that these tests be performed with satisfactory technique and interpreted appropriately. This is particularly true for tests that require the cooperation and maximum effort of the patient. Although reliable measurements in adolescents can often be obtained in a general medical pulmonary laboratory, tests in younger children should be performed in a pediatric pulmonary laboratory if at all possible. Inaccurate results can be misleading at best and dangerous at worst.

Pulmonary function tests include measurements of gas exchange (blood gases, diffusing capacity), of the mechanical function of the lung (peak expiratory flow, spirometry, lung volumes, and changes in these parameters in response to medication or stimuli), of respiratory muscle strength, and of the ability to exercise. In laboratories with particular expertise, measurements that were previously possible only in cooperative older subjects can now be done in infants and young children.

TESTS OF GAS EXCHANGE

The most direct tests of gas exchange are measurements of oxygen and carbon dioxide in samples of arterial blood (see Secs. 4.2.1, 23.3.3, and 23.3.4). These tests usually identify that gas exchange is normal or abnormal but do not usually reveal the cause of an abnormality. Another measure of gas exchange, the diffusing capacity of the lung for carbon monoxide, is available only in pediatric pulmonary function laboratories and is useful in a relatively small number of specific situations.

ASSESSING THE ETIOLOGY OF ABNORMAL GAS EXCHANGE

The physiological causes of disordered gas exchange include (1) breathing gas with an abnormally low oxygen level, (2) acute or chronic hypoventilation, (3) anatomic shunt of pulmonary arterial blood through unventilated lung units, arterial-venous malformations in the lung, or across septal defects, (4) mismatching of ventilation and perfusion within the lung, and (5) block to diffusion of gas across the alveolar–capillary interface.

The mismatching of ventilation and perfusion is the most common cause of hypoxemia. Diffusion block is almost never the primary mechanism of hypoxemia. Effective management of children and adolescents with respiratory disorders depends on the accurate recognition of the mechanism of disordered gas exchange. This can usually be accomplished by appropriate measurements of oxygenation and carbon dioxide and consideration of the clinical context (Table 23-5) (see Sec. 4.1.1).

DIFFUSING CAPACITY

The diffusing capacity of the lung is usually measured by having a child take a deep breath of a gas mixture containing small amounts of carbon monoxide and helium and measuring the exhaled con-

TABLE 23-5

ASSESSING THE CAUSE OF ABNORMALITIES OF GAS EXCHANGE

CAUSE	P_{O_2}	P_{CO_2}	RESPONSE TO OXYGEN	COMMENT
Low inspired O_2	↓	nl or ↓	Normalization of P_{O_2}	High altitude most common setting
Hypoventilation	↓	↑	P_{O_2} improves; P_{CO_2} may worsen	P_{CO_2} and P_{O_2} inversely and approximately equally abnormal
Shunt	↓↓	nl or ↓	Only modest improvement in P_{O_2} with 100% oxygen	
Diffusion block	↓	nl or ↓	Improved P_{O_2}	Extremely rare
Ventilation–perfusion mismatch	↓ or ↓↓	nl or ↓	Improved P_{O_2}	Elevated P_{CO_2} is late finding relative to low P_{O_2}
				Most common cause of hypoxemia in patients with lung disease

nl = normal.

centrations of these gases after a 10-second breath hold. The diffusing capacity is a reflection of the size and function of the alveolar–capillary surface for gas exchange. Its interpretation, however, is complicated by the complex effects of circulating hemoglobin concentration, lung volume, and cardiac output. Diffusing capacity is frequently used to detect or monitor interstitial lung diseases such as that associated with cancer chemotherapy (decreased diffusing capacity) or to recognize acute alveolar hemorrhage (increased diffusing capacity). The fact that the diffusing capacity is increased in many individuals with asthma can also be helpful in confusing situations.

LUNG MECHANICS (LUNG VOLUMES AND AIRWAY FUNCTION)

Among the most useful PFTs in pediatric practice are those that measure the size of the lungs as reflected by their volume (spirometry and measurement of absolute lung volumes) and airway function (maximal flows and resistance/conductance). Because these measurements usually require the patient's cooperation, adequate values can often be obtained only in children over 5 years of age. The devices used to measure lung mechanics range from simple and inexpensive to sophisticated and expensive. Several can be used in any office. The simplest is a peak flow meter. A computer-based office spirometer can provide more helpful information but requires staff training, regular calibration, and equipment maintenance to prevent transmission of infectious agents. More sophisticated measurements, such as airway challenge tests, tests of absolute lung volumes by body plethysmography, and measurements of lung function during exercise, are best accomplished in a pediatric pulmonary function laboratory.

LUNG VOLUMES

The vital capacity, the deepest breath that can be taken from full expiration to full inspiration, is easily measured by spirometry. Vital capacity is reduced in patients with restrictive lung disease, and it can be an easily measured and useful parameter for following such children. An accurate assessment of lung size, however, requires a technique that measures all of the air in the lung, including the air remaining in the lung at full expiration (the residual volume) that is not included in the vital capacity. In individuals with airway obstruction, the vital capacity is low because the residual volume is very large (gas trapping) rather than because overall lung size is small. In this situation, a small vital capacity reflects airway obstruction rather than lung restriction.

The total volume of gas in the lung can be measured in a fully equipped pulmonary laboratory. The most commonly used method involves a body plethysmograph, a large rigid cabinet in which the subject is enclosed. As the child breathes in and out through a mouthpiece, measurements of pressures in the cabinet and at the subject's mouth allow calculation of lung volume using the Boyle law, a mathematical description of the relationship between gas volume and pressure. Body plethysmography permits estimation of residual volume, functional residual capacity (the volume of air in the lung at the end of a relaxed breath), and the total lung capacity (the volume of air in the lung at full inspiration).

Restrictive lung disease is present when the total lung capacity is decreased, but obstruction can also reduce vital capacity (see Pulmonary Function Test Interpretation). In the absence of airway obstruction and gas trapping, the serial measurement of vital capacity can be used to monitor restrictive processes such as interstitial pneumonitis, scoliosis, and chest wall disorders. Respiratory muscle weakness is one cause of restrictive lung disease; muscle strength should be measured in any child found to have low lung volumes.

AIRWAY FUNCTION Airway obstruction, the most common respiratory problem of children and adolescents, is most reliably assessed by analyzing flows during a maximal forced expiration. This requires that the child understand the maneuver and be willing and able to cooperate. Measurements of airway or pulmonary resistance or conductance that do not involve a forced expiration can also be helpful but require more complicated techniques and are not as easily interpreted.

SPIROMETRY (TESTS OF MAXIMAL EXPIRATION) Spirometry involves the measurement of expired volume and/or flow while the subject exhales as rapidly as possible from full lung inflation to residual volume. Most children over 5 or 6 years of age are able to perform this maneuver with careful coaching, but it is effort-dependent. Interpretation of a suboptimal maneuver can result in misleading information; therefore, both the individual coaching the child during the test and the physician interpreting the results must be able to recognize and reject an inadequate effort. Criteria for an acceptable maneuver are a maximal effort and an exhalation of at least 6 seconds (or, for children, an exhalation that continues for at least one second beyond the end of expiratory flow). At least three maneuvers with values for FEV_1 and vital capacity that agree among tests within 200 mL should be recorded.

The most useful numerical parameters derived from forced expiration include forced vital capacity (FVC), peak flow (PF), forced expiratory volume in 1 second (FEV_1), and forced expiratory flow between 25% and 75% of vital capacity (FEF_{25-75}). Additional information is obtained from examining the maximal expiratory flow–volume curve, a plot of flow rate on the vertical axis against lung volume on the horizontal axis. FVC, the volume exhaled from the deepest inspiration possible to the end of exhalation, is usually nearly identical to vital capacity measured during a slow exhalation but may be slightly smaller in individuals with airway obstruction. FEV_1, the volume exhaled during the first 1 second of exhalation, is the most dependable indicator of airway obstruction. In children who have a small vital capacity because of restrictive lung disease, the absolute value of FEV_1 is often lower than predicted even in the absence of airway obstruction. In this situation, the FEV_1/FVC ratio, the fraction of the vital capacity exhaled in the first second, is a more reliable indicator of obstruction. An FEV_1/FVC ratio greater than 80% indicates normal airway function. The FEF_{25-75} is usually considered an indication of peripheral airway obstruction and is, therefore, abnormal earlier in the evolution of obstructive disorders such as asthma. However, it is more variable than the FEV_1, so an isolated abnormal FEF_{25-75} should be considered pathologic only after careful consideration.

PEAK EXPIRATORY FLOW   Peak expiratory flow rate (PEFR), the highest flow achieved during exhalation, is derived from spirometry but can also be measured easily with a hand-held peak flow meter. Peak expiratory flow rate is determined predominantly by the patient's effort, muscle strength, and by the caliber of the larger airways. The peak flow is very effort-dependent, and an adequate value may not be measured if the child either purposefully or inadvertently does not provide full effort.

Even when used properly, however, PEFR varies dramatically among normal children of the same size and also among different peak flow devices. Therefore, comparing a child's peak flow to predicted normal values is often not useful. Peak flow values are most helpful when a particular child has mastered the technique and can regularly achieve reproducible values. The child's "personal best" value can then be estimated confidently from serial measurements over weeks or months so long as the child continues to use the same device. Reliable peak flow measurements can be a useful adjunct to the management of children with asthma. Although peak flow may be relatively normal when asthma symptoms are triggered, expiratory flow rates at lower lung volumes are markedly decreased. Therefore, it must be recognized that inadequate measurements can be confusing and can result in inappropriate treatment decisions unless corroborated by symptom assessment, physical examination, or other pulmonary function measurements.

INSPIRATORY/EXPIRATORY FLOW–VOLUME CURVES   The shape of the flow–volume loop can be helpful in identifying the site and potential cause of a child's lung problem, particularly when a maximum inspiration is also recorded. The shape of the curve is remarkably reproducible for each individual; failure to record identical curves from repeated maneuvers or to achieve a smooth expiratory limb without coughing or interruptions is an indication of inadequate effort or poor cooperation. The shape of a normal flow–volume loop and variations typical of various pathologic situations are illustrated in Fig. 23-4. The "scooped out" pattern of intrapulmonary airway obstruction in which the expiratory flow limb sags toward the x (volume) axis is particularly characteristic.

AIRWAY RESISTANCE/CONDUCTANCE   Airway resistance, the pressure required to move air through the airways divided by the flow rate, is increased in children with obstructive lung diseases. This measurement, usually made in the pulmonary function lab using the body plethysmograph, requires more sophisticated equipment but less patient cooperation than spirometry. Resistance can sometimes be measured in young children unable to perform an adequate forced expiration. It is particularly useful for assessing children who develop bronchospasm with maximal expiratory efforts, in whom spirometry is not reliable. The interpretation of this measurement is less straightforward than spirometry. It is sometimes expressed as the inverse of resistance, or conductance. This is attractive because conductance divided by lung volume, called specific conductance, is the same value for normal children and adults regardless of size and is decreased in individuals with airway obstruction.

AIRWAYS REACTIVITY   One of the most useful indications for pulmonary function testing is the measurement of airway reactivity in patients suspected to have asthma but who have atypical symptoms or who have normal spirometry at rest. The majority of children with asthma have airway hyperreactivity that can be demonstrated either by an increase in expiratory flow rates after treatment with a bronchodilator or by a decrease in expiratory flow rates after inhalation of agents that elicit bronchoconstriction. The absence of hyperreactivity does not rule out asthma because an asthmatic child in good control may have normal reactivity. The easiest of these tests is spirometry before and after the administration of an inhaled dose of a bronchodilator such as albuterol. Hyperreactivity is usually defined as a 12% improvement in FEV_1 after a standard bronchodilator treatment. Some pulmonologists consider a 25 to 30% improvement in FEF_{25-75} or airway conductance to be evidence of reversible airflow limitation even with a smaller change in FEV_1.

The diagnosis of asthma can be challenging in children who are maximally bronchodilated at the time of testing and therefore have normal pre- and postbronchodilator spirometry. In this situation, hyperreactivity can be confirmed by demonstrating an exaggerated bronchoconstrictor response to any of several stimuli: exercise, hyperventilation of cold air, or by breathing increasing concentrations of methacholine, histamine, or, rarely, by inhalation of an antigen to which the individual is sensitive. Each of these provocative tests, however, involves the risk of inducing severe bronchospasm, so the patient must be closely monitored and a strict protocol followed. A physician and equipment for emergency treatment must be available. A common bronchoconstrictor protocol is the exercise challenge test. The subject exercises for 4 to 6 minutes at 80% of the predicted maximal heart rate. Spirometry is then recorded at 5-minute intervals for 20 to 30 minutes. A 10 to 15% fall in FEV_1 is considered evidence of airway hyperreactivity.

RESPIRATORY MUSCLE STRENGTH

Respiratory muscle strength is tested by measuring the maximal positive pressure created by forceful exhalation after full inspiration and the maximal negative pressure that can be developed breathing in after a maximal expiration. The maximal inspiratory pressure (NIP or NIF) estimates the strength of the diaphragm and accessory inspiratory muscles. NIFs more negative than -60 cm H_2O can be generated by individuals with normal respiratory muscle function; values less negative than -40 cm H_2O are considered abnormal. The maximal expiratory pressure estimates the strength of the abdominal and thoracic musculature.

Respiratory muscle strength should be evaluated in every child with restricted lung volumes to rule out muscle weakness as a cause for this problem. It is also useful to measure muscle strength serially

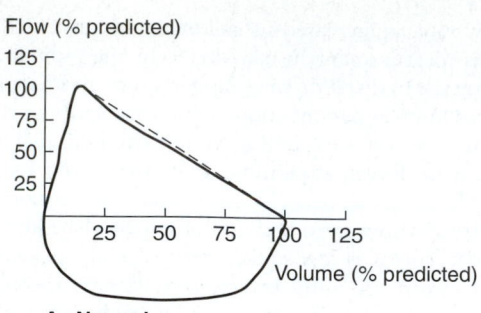

A. Normal

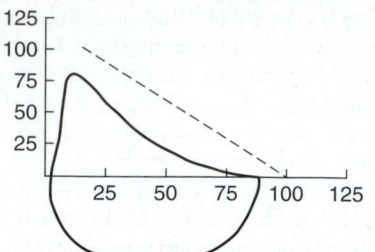

B. Obstructed Intrapulmonary Airways

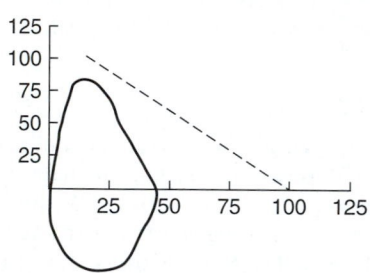

C. Restrictive Lung Disease

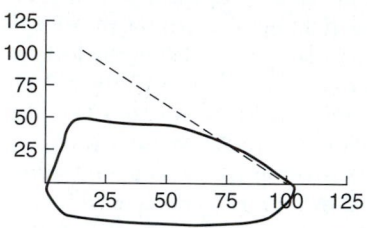

D. Fixed Central or Upper Airways Obstruction

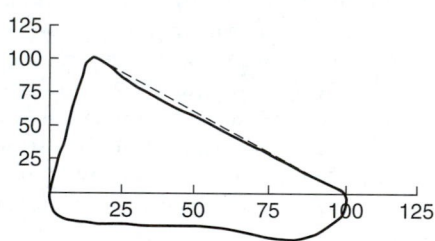

E. Variable Upper Airway Obstruction

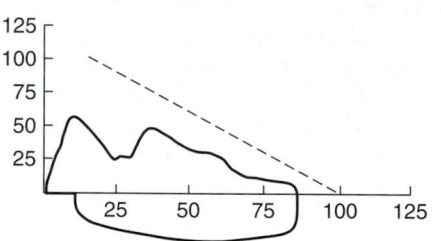

F. Inadequate Effort

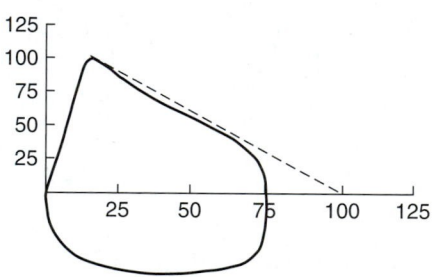

G. Incomplete Exhalation

FIGURE 23-4   Maximum inspiratory and expiratory flow-volume loops that represent normal, disease states and unacceptable recordings. Flow (*y* axis) and volume (*x* axis) are both shown as percent predicted. **A.** Normal curve. Peak flow occurs in the first 20% of exhalation (shown as positive flow). Once peak flow is reached, flow decreases smoothly and nearly linearly as the lung empties. The dashed line indicates predicted normal curve. The inspiratory curve (below *x* axis) has a different shape because inspiratory flow is not dependent on lung volume as is expiratory flow. Flows on expiration and inspiration at 50% of the FVC are approximately equal. **B.** Obstructed intrapulmonary airways. Maximal flows are lower than predicted and the curve is convex toward the volume (*x*) axis. This scooping of the expiratory limb is typical for asthma and cystic fibrosis. **C.** Restrictive lung disease. Vital capacity is reduced, but maximal flows at higher lung volumes are close to normal. There is no scooping. **D.** Fixed central or upper airways obstruction. The expiratory curve is truncated, there is no scooped pattern, and inspiratory flows are approximately equally reduced. **E.** Variable upper airway obstruction. Inspiratory flow loop is truncated. Expiratory flow/inspiratory flow ratio at 50% of the FVC is >2. **F.** Inadequate effort. Loop is not smooth. Flows are submaximal over much of lung volume. **G.** Incomplete exhalation. Premature termination of exhalation causes an abrupt drop in flow at low lung volumes. Curves F and G are not acceptable and should not be interpreted.

in patients with scoliosis, chronic neuromuscular disorders, and acute demyelinating disorders such as Guillain-Barré syndrome to follow their progress.

PULMONARY FUNCTION TEST INTERPRETATION

To interpret pulmonary function tests, compare a child's values to those of children of the same height, sex, and age. It is therefore critical that the subject's height is measured accurately. Interpretation can be difficult for children whose height is abnormal, as in children with scoliosis or meningomyelocele. In such situations, arm span can be used as the height. Vital capacity and total lung capacity should be greater than 80% of the predicted value, and the residual volume less than 30% of the total lung capacity. Restrictive lung disease cannot be definitively diagnosed from measurement of vital capacity alone because airway obstruction with gas trapping can result in a small vital capacity despite a normal total lung capacity. The most dependable indication of airway obstruction is an FEV_1 less than 80% of the predicted value in a subject with normal lung volumes or an FEV_1/FVC ratio less than 80% regardless of lung volume. In individuals with a normal FEV_1 mild or early airway obstruction can be suggested by an FEF_{25-75} less than 60% of predicted, an elevated residual volume, or an abnormal configuration of the flow–volume curve (see Fig. 23-4).

Pulmonary function tests are particularly useful in monitoring the status of children and adolescents with known respiratory disease. In addition to diagnosing and monitoring restrictive and obstructive lung diseases, pulmonary function tests can provide objective measures of such diverse respiratory problems as diaphragmatic weakness, upper airway obstruction, vocal cord dysfunction, interstitial fibrosis, and pulmonary hemorrhage. Many primary care physicians are comfortable interpreting common measurements such as those of lung volume and spirometry. The assistance of an experienced pediatric respiratory specialist can be helpful in considering the implications of more complex tests such as diffusing capacity and tests of airway reactivity.

23.3.6   Exercise Testing

Dan Michael Cooper

Participation in physical activity by both healthy children and those with chronic diseases and disabilities has dramatically changed in recent years as a result of social, cultural, and nutritional factors as well as advances in clinical care. Great progress has also been made in using exercise as a diagnostic and therapeutic tool in both healthy children and those with chronic disease and disability (Table 23-6).

In healthy children, inappropriately low levels of physical activity are associated with obesity, early onset of type 2 diabetes, reduced bone mineralization (and osteoporosis later in life), and increased cardiovascular risk factors. Excessive exercise is associated with eating disorders, impaired growth, and exercise- or sports-related musculoskeletal injuries. Unfortunately, formalized training in evaluation of physical activity or the use of exercise either diagnostically or therapeutically is lacking among most pediatricians and child health-care professionals. This section presents a brief overview of the role played by physical activity in healthy children and in those with chronic disease or disability and reviews the elements of exercise testing and its role as a diagnostic tool in child and adolescent health.

TABLE 23-6

EXAMPLES OF CURRENT CLINICAL USES OF EXERCISE IN CHILDREN AND ADOLESCENTS

Diagnostic
  Elucidation of bronchial reactivity
  Growth hormone deficiency
  Preparticipation sports physical in children
  Establishing reduced physical activity as an etiology for obesity
  Evaluating fitness and the efficacy of therapy in patients with a variety of congenital heart diseases
  Evaluating long-term outcomes of surgical repair of single-ventricle congenital heart lesions
  Determination of optimal hematocrit in patients with congenital anemia
  Quantifying the functional disability caused by chronic diseases of childhood and developing an exercise prescription
  Predicting outcomes in cystic fibrosis
  Establishing the diagnosis of the long-QT syndrome

Therapeutic and rehabilitation
  Training respiratory muscles in patients with chronic lung disease
  An adjunct to chest physiotherapy in patients with cystic fibrosis
  Stabilization of glycemia in insulin-dependent diabetes
  An adjunct to diet in the treatment of childhood obesity
  Nonpharmacologic treatment of juvenile hypertension
  Increasing school and social participation in children with osteogenesis imperfecta
  Amelioration of exercise-induced asthma
  Pediatric cardiac rehabilitation
  Improving functional performance in children with cerebral palsy

There is mounting research identifying physiological, molecular, and structural mechanisms that link exercise with processes of growth and development in health and disease. Natural patterns of exercise in healthy children are characterized by many brief episodes (about 85 per hour, mean of 20-sec duration) that vary greatly in intensity. The majority of these pulses of exercise are relatively low-intensity, but in about 20%, the exercise intensity is likely to be above the anaerobic or lactate threshold. During these high-intensity exercise periods, increases in circulating levels of growth hormone, insulin-like growth factor-I (IGF-I), and inflammatory mediators (eg, interleukin-6) can occur. Current research suggests that physical activity influences growth and development through these anabolic and catabolic mediators.

In many countries, there appears to be an epidemic of childhood obesity. Although the mechanisms are complex and multifactorial, reduced levels of physical activity seem to be a playing a role in the pathophysiology of this condition. The increased cardiovascular morbidity and insulin resistance associated with obesity later in life is profound, costly, and well documented. Because not all obese children are unfit, exercise testing in obese children is useful because it can identify those individuals in whom fitness is truly low and guide the clinician in developing an appropriately structured exercise intervention. The ability of exercise to enhance peak bone mass is substantial but may be limited to childhood and adolescence. On the other hand, physical inactivity during childhood may also contribute to osteoporosis later in life. Excessive physical activity can have adverse health consequences in children as well. Impaired growth, delayed puberty, bone demineralization, and stress or overuse fractures can occur in children who participate in sports at a highly competitive and intense level. In addition, the long-term psychosocial consequences to young children of participating in overly competitive and inappropriately stressful training are not yet known.

The pediatrician can play an important role in identifying and managing the wide variety of conditions that are associated with both insufficient and excessive physical activity. Studies in adults have demonstrated that relatively simple counseling and educational programs in the primary care setting can alter patterns of physical activity. Pediatricians can become more proactive in quantifying physical activity levels in routine health assessments of children. In cases where subjective or clinical evidence exists for abnormal physical activity (eg, obesity), formal exercise testing may be useful to prescribe an exercise intervention appropriate for the child's current level of physical activity. Finally, primary care pediatricians ought to be aware of the fact that the "preparticipation physical," often a requirement for child and adolescent sports participation, is not yet a standardized procedure. Substantial controversy still exists regarding what the focus of the examination should be and to what extent it can actually work to assess the suitability of a particular child for a specific sport.

THE ROLE OF EXERCISE TESTING AND TRAINING IN CHILDREN WITH DISEASE AND DISABILITY

Exercise testing can give the pediatrician insight into cardiorespiratory and metabolic disease mechanisms and provide the basis for effective exercise "prescriptions." With specialized groups of patients, exercise testing can provide minimally invasive ways of gaining potentially useful information about cardiorespiratory and metabolic function. In the following, I highlight three conditions (congenital heart disease, asthma, and cystic fibrosis) in which exercise testing or therapy has proved to be clinically useful.

EXERCISE TESTING IN CONGENITAL HEART DISEASE   Exercise testing and training programs have been used extensively in many children, adolescents, and adults with a variety of congenital heart lesions. Particularly illustrative have been studies on patients with complex congenital heart defects or single ventricular lesions. The Fontan procedure, in which the systemic and pulmonary circulations are separated, has become the surgical therapy of choice for selected patients.

Although the Fontan intervention has resulted in improvements in cardiorespiratory function, the long-term outlook remains guarded, and additional surgical or medical interventions are often necessary. Cardiorespiratory function under resting conditions is of limited value in determining physiological impairment; however, exercise testing in patients who have undergone the Fontan procedure has come to be an important tool for making clinical decisions and for evaluating outcomes in these patients. An example of how a relatively simple, minimally invasive exercise test can highlight pathophysiology in patients with single ventricle lesions following the Fontan-type repair is illustrated in Fig. 23-5.

EXERCISE TESTING IN ASTHMA   Currently, the most common use of diagnostic exercise testing is in the evaluation of exercise-induced asthma (EIA) (see Fig. 23-6). EIA, a common feature of asthma, especially in children, is characterized by a short and sometimes severe asthmatic attack following exercise. As EIA occurs in about 60 to 80% of asthmatic children, it can be used as one of the diagnostic tests to establish the disease. An exercise challenge is a more specific indicator of asthma than either histamine or methacholine challenges and probably has a wider margin of safety. In

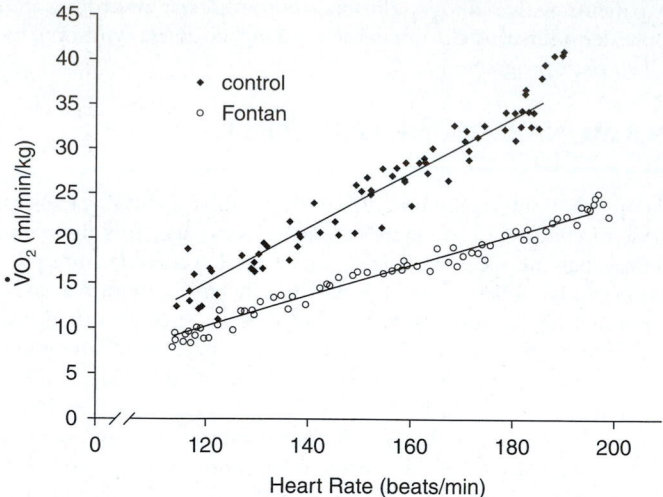

FIGURE 23-5   Relationship between oxygen uptake ($\dot{V}O_2$) and heart rate (HR) during progressive exercise in individual 12-year-old control and Fontan subjects. In both cases, there was a characteristic largely linear relationship between the two variables (solid lines indicate best-fit lines by linear regression). As demonstrated in these individuals, the slope of the relationship ($\dot{V}O_2$/HR) was lower in the Fontan subjects, consistent with an impaired stroke volume response to exercise. SOURCE: *Figure from Troutman et al. JACC 31:668, 1998.*

addition, patients without asthma may have exercise-associated signs and symptoms as a result of deconditioning, cardiac disorders, or emotional or psychological factors. The successful completion of a formal exercise protocol may give reassurance to both the patient and the family that exercise can be safely performed.

During the first few minutes of exercise in a subject with asthma, lung function changes little or may even improve. Toward the end of exercise or few minutes after, FEV_1 begins to fall. The maximum fall in lung function occurs 5 to 10 minutes after the end of exercise, after which recovery in lung function will take place in about 30 to 45 minutes. In a small proportion of asthmatic subjects, a so-called late-phase reaction may develop from exercise-induced airway inflammation.

The upper limit of postexercise fall in FEV_1 in normal children is 6 to 8%, so that a decrease of more than 10% suggests airway

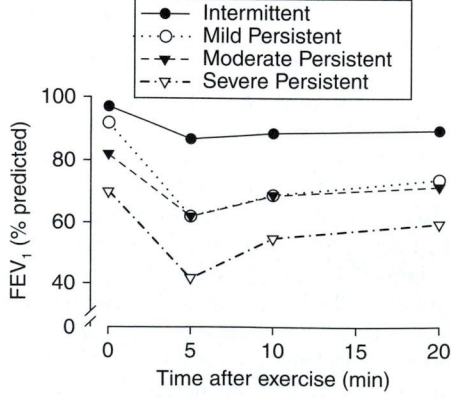

FIGURE 23-6   Time course of forced expiratory volume in 1 second as percent predicted (FEV_1 % predicted) after exercise in children with varying degrees of asthma severity. SOURCE: *Redrawn from Cabral et al. AJRCCM 159:1819, 1999.*

hyperreactivity. In asthmatic children the severity of EIA may be influenced by the severity of asthma and by preexposure to allergens. Practical guidelines for the performance of exercise challenge testing for the diagnosis of asthma are reviewed elsewhere.

EXERCISE TESTING IN CYSTIC FIBROSIS   Recently, it was demonstrated that there is a positive relationship between physical fitness and longevity in patients with cystic fibrosis (CF). The research extended a series of previous investigations that had shown the feasibility and possible benefits of exercise as therapy in CF. The idea that a potentially modifiable behavior such as exercise could contribute to patient health and quality of life in CF remains compelling. There clearly are several mechanisms responsible for the health benefits of exercise in CF. Specific disease-related effects, such as improved mucociliary clearance, likely play a role. In addition, the ability of exercise to stimulate a metabolic state that promotes anabolism contributes to improved health in CF. Recent data demonstrate that anabolic effects of exercise are caused by exercise stimulation of the growth hormone–insulin-like growth factor-I axis (GH–IGF-I) and other growth mediators, receptors, and binding proteins that control somatic and tissue growth. Intriguing new data demonstrate that exercise can also stimulate inflammatory cytokines, leading to a neuroendocrine "catabolic state" even in healthy children. The current idea that exercise stimulates both anabolic and catabolic mediators is particularly relevant to children and adolescents with CF. Chronic hypoxia, pulmonary inflammation, increased basal energy expenditure, and malnutrition lead to a catabolic state in many patients with CF. The feasibility of medically supervised exercise interventions has been demonstrated in recent studies and suggest that cardiorespiratory exercise testing in children, adolescents, and adults provides the clinician with valuable information both to gauge the degree of impairment and to prescribe an effective, trackable exercise intervention. An example of a typical ventilatory response to exercise in a child with cystic fibrosis is shown in Fig. 23-7.

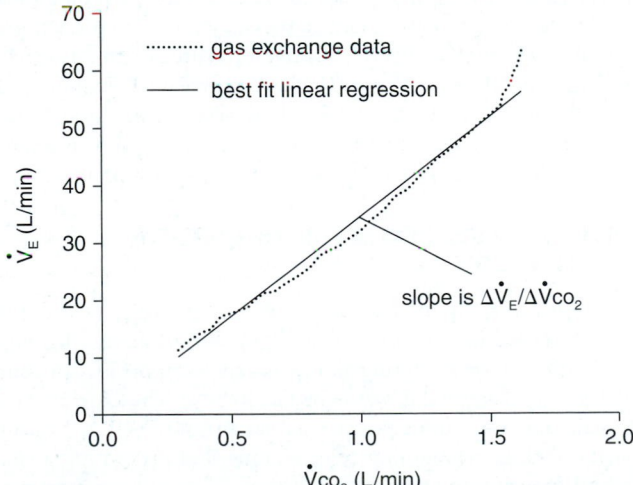

FIGURE 23-7   The relationship between ventilation ($\dot{V}_E$) and carbon dioxide output ($\dot{V}CO_2$) during a progressive exercise test in a 9-year-old girl with CF. Since $\dot{V}_E$ is driven by $\dot{V}CO_2$, these data tend to have a high signal-to-noise ratio and can be used to assess cardiorespiratory responses to exercise without the need for a maximal effort. The slope of the $\dot{V}_E$-$\dot{V}CO_2$ relationship is easily calculated using standard linear regression techniques.

THE FUTURE OF EXERCISE TESTING AND TRAINING IN CHILDREN

Exercise is a major and necessary biological task of children, and identifying reliable molecular, biochemical, structural, and functional markers of optimal physical activity remains a challenge for clinical research in the years to come. For healthy children, devising strategies to encourage exercise in the physically inactive child and to define both upper and lower limits of physical activity that produce optimum growth and development will require additional research. For the child with chronic disease or disability, the challenge is to determine how best to use physical activity that will lead to improvements in long-term health and quality of life. Increasingly, pediatricians and child health-care professionals will be called on to guide and prescribe levels of physical activity for their patients as well as to utilize the remarkable diagnostic tools that exercise testing can offer.

References

Adams GR: Role of insulin-like growth factor-I in the regulation of skeletal muscle adaptation to increased loading. In: Holloszy JH, ed: Exercise and Sports Science Reviews. Baltimore, Williams & Wilkins, 1998:31–60

Berman N, Bailey RC, Barstow TJ, Cooper DM: Spectral and bout detection analysis of physical activity patterns in healthy, perpubertal boys and girls. Am J Hum Biol 10:289–297, 1998

Boas SR, Joswiak ML, Nixon PA, Fulton JA, Orenstein DM: Factors limiting anaerobic performance in adolescent males with cystic fibrosis. Med Sci Sports Exer 28:291–298, 1996

Cabral AL, Conceiecaao GM, Fonseca-Guedes CH, Martins MA: Exercise-induced bronchospasm in children: effects of asthma severity. Am J Respir Crit Care Med 159:1819–1823, 1999

Calfas KJ, Long BJ, Sallis JF, Wooten WJ, Prat M, Patrick K: A controlled trial of physician counseling to promote the adoption of physical activity. Prev Med 25:225–233, 1996

Cantwell JD: Preparticipation physical evaluation: getting to the heart of the matter. Med Sci Sports Exer 30:S341–S344, 1998

Cooper DM: Exercise and cystic fibrosis: the search for a therapeutic optimum. Pediatr Pulmonol 25:143–144, 1998

Cooper DM, Poage J, Barstow TJ, Springer C: Are obese children truly unfit? Minimizing the confounding effect of body size on the exercise response. J Pediatr 116:223–230, 1990

Cooper DM, Springer C: Pulmonary function assessment in the laboratory during exercise. In: Chernick V, Boat TF, eds: Kendig's Disorders of the Respiratory Tract in Children. Philadelphia, WB Saunders, 1998: 214–237

Cooper DM, Weiler-Ravell D, Whipp BJ, Wasserman K: Aerobic parameters of exercise as a function of body size during growth in children. J Appl Physiol 56:628–634, 1984

Danielson GK: Cardiorespiratory response to exercise after modified Fontan operation: determinants of performance. JACC 29:785–790, 1997

Eliakim A, Brasel JA, Mohan S, Cooper DM: Increased physical activity and the growth hormone insulin-like growth factor-I axis in adolescent males. Am J Physiol 275:R308–R314, 1998

Luepker RV: How physically active are American children and what can we do about it? Int J Obes Rel Metab Dis 23(Suppl 2):S12–S17, 1999

Nixon PA, Orenstein DM, Kelsey SF, Doershuk CF: The prognostic value of exercise testing in patients with cystic fibrosis. N Engl J Med 327: 1785–1788, 1992

Reybrouck T, Mertens L, Schepers D, Vinckx J, Gewillig M: Assessment of cardiorespiratory exercise function in obese children and adolescents by body mass-independent parameters. Eur J Appl Physiol Occup Physiol 75:478–483, 1997

Rowland T, Potts J, Potts T, Son-Hing J, Harbison G, Sandor G: Cardiovascular responses to exercise in children and adolescents with myocardial dysfunction. Am Heart J 137:126–133, 1999

Scheett TP, Milles PJ, Ziegler MG, Stoppani J, Cooper DM: Effect of exercise on cytokines and growth mediators in prepubertal children. Pediatr Res 46:429–434, 1999

Troutman WB, Barstow TJ, Galindo AJ, Cooper DM: Abnormal dynamic cardiorespiratory responses to exercise in pediatric patients after Fontan procedure. J Am Col Cardiol 31:668–673, 1998

Weinsier RL, Hunter GR, Heini AF, Goran MI, Sell SM: The etiology of obesity: relative contribution of metabolic factors, diet, and physical activity. Am J Med 105:145–150, 1998

23.3.7 General Therapies

Thomas A. Hazinski

OXYGEN

When hypoxemia is present, increasing the oxygen concentration of inspired gas will reduce anxiety, decrease the respiratory rate and depth of breathing, decrease the work of breathing, decrease pulmonary vascular resistance, and improve cardiovascular function. Inspired oxygen concentrations as high as 100% may be necessary to bring PaO_2 to normal levels, but most commonly low-flow oxygen therapy is used.

There are several methods for delivering oxygen to children, with the method of choice depending on the amount of oxygen that is needed. A tent has a large volume and many leaks, and even at high flow rates, an oxygen concentration greater than 35 to 40% is difficult to maintain. Oxygen flowing at 4 to 5 L/min through a 4- to 5-L plastic hood over the infant's head will produce a concentration of close to 100%; oxygen flowing through nasal cannulas into the nasopharynx at 4 L/min will provide a concentration of up to 45 to 50%. The inspired oxygen concentration may approach 100% if a tightly fitting oxygen mask with a reservoir bag is used.

In infants and children with chronic lung disease, arterial desaturation may always be present or occur during sleep. Oxygen breathing rarely depresses respiration or causes hypercarbia as in adults. Indeed, oxygen therapy alone may improve ventilation. Frequent arterial blood gas measurements and continuous measurement of oxygenation by pulse oximetry and ventilation by end-tidal carbon dioxide will permit adjustment of the oxygen dose and identify the patient who responds to oxygen breathing with hypoventilation. Improved oxygenation decreases pulmonary vasoconstriction and increases pulmonary blood flow to units that have been ventilated but not perfused. This increases elimination of carbon dioxide, even though the total ventilation may be unaffected.

HELIOX

A mixture of 30 to 40% oxygen and 60 to 70% helium may be used to treat postextubation stridor, infectious croup, and other causes of transient upper airway obstruction. Helium is a low-density gas that decreases resistance to airflow in areas with turbulence. Patients receiving heliox should be carefully monitored, but its use may prevent intubation or reintubation of some patients.

INHALED NITRIC OXIDE (NO)

The administration of NO is used to increase pulmonary blood flow and PO_2 in critically ill patients with a variety of acute pulmonary and cardiac diseases. NO causes vascular smooth muscle relaxation by interacting with the enzyme guanylate cyclase to increase cyclic GMP. NO is a specific pulmonary vasodilator that owes its specificity to the fact that it is rapidly inactivated by hemoglobin when it enters the circulation and is dissolved in blood. NO may also have antioxidant and anti-inflammatory effects. Clinical studies are under way to establish optimal timing and dosages. In addition, drugs to indirectly increase NO levels in pulmonary vascular smooth muscle are being developed. Adverse effects are methemoglobinemia and interference with hemostasis.

INHALATION-BASED THERAPIES

The number of drugs that can be delivered to the lung by the aerosol route continues to increase. For disorders such as asthma, it has become the preferred treatment route. Inhalation-based drug-delivery methods employ aerosol-driven canisters with volume spacers, compressed air nebulizers, and patient-driven powder inhalers. Nebulizers also have been used to administer recombinant DNase and antibiotics to patients with cystic fibrosis and other patients at risk for chronic airway infections. The rationales for inhaled drug delivery are to confine the therapeutic effect to specific lung sites, to deliver high doses of drug that might be toxic if given parenterally, and to limit systemic side effects. Although drug delivery is difficult to measure, these goals usually can be achieved with careful choice of the drug dose and delivery device and thorough training and retraining of the family and patient about their proper use.

AIRWAY CLEARANCE METHODS AND DEVICES

If a patient cannot cough effectively or has a chronic suppurative lung disease, mucociliary clearance is impaired and increases the patient's susceptibility to atelectasis, complicated respiratory infections, and progressive respiratory failure. Such patients include those with cerebral palsy, scoliosis, neuromuscular disorders, cystic fibrosis, bronchiectasis, COPD, lung or chest wall malformations, and tracheostomies. A variety of physical methods and devices have been developed to augment mucociliary clearance, including those that vibrate airway walls (manual percussion techniques, flutter valve, vibrating pneumatic vest, positive-pressure breathing devices) or inflate and deflate the lung (IPPB, Coughalater®, manual bagging with chest compression). The early and routine use of these devices and techniques in patients with these conditions is important in improving quality of life and in avoiding hospitalization.

NONINVASIVE POSITIVE-PRESSURE VENTILATION

Developed originally to treat nocturnal upper airway obstruction in adults, several devices are now available for home use that augment ventilation by delivering air or oxygen under positive pressure to the airway using nasal masks or face masks. These devices can also maintain continuous positive airway pressure (CPAP) during exhalation, thus maintaining lung volume and preventing atelectasis and reducing the work of breathing. Bilevel positive-pressure ventilation (BiPAP®) has been used extensively in patients with neuromuscular disorders, severe scoliosis, and other chronic lung disorders. It has also been used to treat severe pulmonary exacerbations of patients with advanced lung disease who are awaiting lung transplantation. In some cases, conventional mechanical ventilators can be configured to deliver positive-pressure ventilation via a snug-fitting mask, avoiding the morbidity associated with endotracheal intubation.

CARE OF THE PATIENT WITH CHRONIC PULMONARY DISEASES

A variety of congenital and acquired conditions can lead to chronic respiratory insufficiency that requires treatment with a wide variety of devices. Settings for ongoing care of these children include the acute-care hospital, extended-care facility, and home. The first two options provide skilled care in a traditional setting, but they separate children from their families. The third option, home care, provides an alternative to prolonged hospital care for infants and children with such problems. Under appropriate circumstances, home care is safe and provides the best environment for these patients. Children with severe bronchopulmonary dysplasia, neuromuscular disorders, congenital sleep hypoventilation syndrome, severe tracheobronchomalacia, and many other chronic respiratory problems are now routinely mechanically ventilated at home.

To provide technologically sophisticated care at home, the chronically ill child and family must fulfill specific criteria. First, the child's condition must be stable. The definition of stability will vary with the diagnosis, but in the ventilator-dependent child, ventilator settings should be unchanged for 3 to 8 weeks, with no adjustments in drug regimen for at least 5 days. Ideally, the child's ventilatory requirements should be able to be maintained by manual ventilation with oxygen and a bag-valve-tube system for at least 2 hours. This latter criterion allows a margin of safety should equipment fail, and it permits safe transport of the child to medical facilities for emergency care. Second, the family must commit themselves to learn about all home-care devices and methods without undue pressure from medical personnel, insurance companies, or others, and they must have the financial means of providing home care. Finally, appropriate resources such as skilled nurses, respiratory therapists, medical equipment suppliers, and an appropriately skilled physician must be available in their community. If the family and child meet these criteria, home care can be a viable option for most children.

Follow-up care must provide careful surveillance of oxygen requirements, reactive airways disease, fluid balance abnormalities, medical equipment needs, and complications such as equipment malfunction, tracheostomy-related problems, respiratory infections, nutrition and gastrostomy tube–related concerns. Doses of medications such as diuretics, potassium chloride, and bronchodilators must be adjusted to compensate for growth, side effects, and natural history of the chronic lung disease. Diuretic therapy can cause hypokalemia, metabolic alkalosis, nephrocalcinosis, ototoxicity, and dehydration. During episodes of gastroenteritis and low fluid intake, the effects of diuretics can become life-threatening; for these reasons, diuretic therapy should be used with caution and monitored closely, especially when digitalis is also used. In spite of these risks, however, diuretics should be given to those patients who demonstrate improved lung function and clinical stability with their use. Bronchodilator and inhaled corticosteroid therapy is given by aerosol if reversible airway obstruction is documented and there is a beneficial clinical response. Inhaled antibiotic therapy may be useful to treat or prevent chronic tracheobronchial infections. Growth and development are important indicators of patient progress, and these should be documented carefully. Routine immunizations and all other well-child care should be provided. Caloric intake should be adjusted and monitored to permit normal growth, but in immobile patients, conventional caloric intake can cause obesity. Caretakers also should be familiar with the purpose and side effects of all prescribed drugs and devices.

For the ventilator-dependent child, close contact and periodic evaluation by a physician and health care team who are knowledgeable about chronic ventilator management are essential for appropriate adjustments and occasional temporary increases in ventilator support. Although some families are able to provide total care for such a child, the majority require additional assistance in the form of skilled nursing. Some families require 24-hour-a-day skilled nursing at home for a few months before being able to provide the majority of care. Skilled home nursing care also may be needed for patients who require supplemental oxygen, tracheostomy care, or other complex therapies but who are not ventilator-dependent because skilled assessment permits the early treatment of illness that otherwise might require hospitalization or mechanical ventilation. Periodic pulse oximetry and end-tidal PCO_2 monitoring also can be performed at home or in the office to assess the adequacy of gas exchange.

Of all therapies for the treatment of chronic respiratory insufficiency, none is more important than supplemental oxygen. The most common method for delivering oxygen at home is a nasal cannula that is connected to an oxygen source. It should be fixed securely so that the oxygen flow is maintained continuously. In infants, this usually is accomplished by securing the cannula with an adhesive dressing extending across the upper lip to the middle of the zygomatic arch or beyond. A number of nonocclusive, hypoallergenic dressings with excellent adhesion are available.

The source of oxygen depends on the flow that is required. For 0.5 L/min or less, large tanks of compressed oxygen may suffice. These heavy tanks must be secured properly. At 1 L/min or higher, an oxygen concentrator or a liquid oxygen system is used. Small cylinders or a portable liquid oxygen system can be used for short trips and for emergencies. Oxygen flow rates should be measured with flowmeters that are accurate in the ranges required. At high flow rates, humidification of oxygen may be necessary to avoid excessive dehydration of the upper airways.

The goal of oxygen therapy is to maintain a normal level of oxyhemoglobin saturation most of the time. Feeding, sleep state, crying, and activity level all may cause arterial oxygen desaturation, which sometimes is marked. Transient episodes of slight desaturation such as occur in normal infants and children are acceptable. Consequently, the oxygen need should be evaluated for each of these states with a goal to maintain oxygen saturation at 92% or greater as judged by pulse oximetry. In patients with pulmonary hypertension or in patients with widely fluctuating oxygen requirements, saturations in the 94 to 96% range may be necessary. If an oximeter is available in the home, it should be used properly, and movement artifact should be recognized as a frequent cause for abnormal results. Oximetry results should not be used as a substitute for clinical assessment.

If a patient on a ventilator becomes severely hypoxemic or develops significant apnea with bradycardia, cardiorespiratory monitoring at home will alert parents to the presence of changes in heart and respiratory rates and prevent prolonged hypoxemia and its consequences. The monitor should be simple to use and reliable. The supplier also must provide initial training and continuous on-call service for monitor malfunctions and maintenance, and health-care providers must provide support for the emotional difficulties that surface with such technical problems and home monitoring in general.

Caretakers must be skilled at cardiopulmonary resuscitation (CPR). Resuscitative techniques must be practiced under the supervision of an experienced instructor who is trained in the resuscitation of chronically ill infants and children. In addition to CPR, parents must learn to evaluate respiratory distress, including counting respiratory rate, evaluating retractions, and, in some children, listening for rales (crackles) and wheezes. If the child requires tube feedings, gastrostomy care, or other special treatment, parents must learn these as well. Just before discharge, a few days of "rooming in" for the parents is a valuable, confidence-building experience.

References

Signs and Symptoms, Diagnosis, and Treatment of Lung Disease

Cohn RC, Kercsmar C, Dearborn D: Safety and efficacy of flexible endoscopy in children with bronchopulmonary dysplasia. Am J Dis Child 142: 1225, 1988

Comroe JH Jr, Forester RE II, Dubois AB, et al: The Lung, 2nd ed. Chicago, Year Book, 1962

Criner G, Brennan K, Travaline JM, Kreimer D: Efficacy and compliance with noninvasive positive pressure ventilation in patients with chronic respiratory failure. Chest 116:667–675, 1999

Flaherty KR, Kazerooni EA, Martinez FJ: Differential diagnosis of chronic airflow obstruction. J Asthma 37:201–223, 2000

Green CG, Eisenberg J, Leong A, et al: Flexible bronchoscopy of the pediatric airway. Am Rev Respir Dis 145:233, 1992

Hunt CE, Corwin JM, Lister G, et al: Longitudinal assessment of hemoglobin oxygen saturation in healthy infants during the first six months of age. J pediatrics 135:580–586, 1999

Irwin RS, Madison JM: The diagnosis and treatment of cough. N Engl J Med 343:1715–1721, 2000

Kemper KJ, Ritz RH, Benson MS, Bishop MS: Helium-oxygen mixture in the treatment of postextubation stridor in pediatric trauma patients. Crit Care Med 19:356, 1991

Patteshall EN, Noyes BE, Orenstein DM: Use of bronchoalveolar lavage in immunocompromised children with pneumonia. Pediatr Pulmonol 5:1, 1988

Polgar G, Promadhat V: Pulmonary Function Testing in Children: Techniques and Standards. Philadelphia, WB Saunders, 1971

Ramsey BW, Dorkin HL, Eisenberg JD, et al: Efficacy of aerosolized tobramycin in patients with cystic fibrosis. N Engl J Med 328:1740, 1993

Care of the Child with Chronic Pulmonary Diseases

Campbell AN, Zarfin Y, Groenveld M, Bryan MH: Low flow oxygen therapy in infants. Arch Dis Child 58:795, 1983

Criner G, Brennan K, Tavaline JM, Kreimer D: Efficacy and compliance with noninvasive positive pressure ventilation in patients with chronic respiratory failure. Chest 116:667–675, 1999

Hazinski TA, Rush MG: Current therapy for bronchopulmonary dysplasia. Semin Perinatol 19:563, 1992

Lucas J, Golesi J, Sleeper G, Ryan JA: Home Respiratory Care. Norwalk, CT, Appleton & Lange, 1988

Plant PK, Elliott MW: Non-invasive positive pressure ventilation. J Col Physicians 33:521–525, 1999

23.4 CONGENITAL DISORDERS OF THE LOWER RESPIRATORY TRACT

Thomas A. Hazinski

TRACHEAL LESIONS

TRACHEAL AGENESIS This rare condition (also referred to as *aplasia* or *atresia of the trachea*) has three anatomic types described by Landing and Dixon. In type I, the proximal trachea is atretic, and the distal part communicates with the esophagus through a fistula. In type II, the bronchi meet in the midline and communicate with the esophagus through a fistula. In type III, both bronchi independently communicate with the esophagus. Associated anomalies are common and include abnormalities of the cardiovascular, gastrointestinal, genitourinary, and central nervous systems as well as agenesis of the lungs and chromosomal abnormalities. At birth, there is immediate respiratory distress, and affected infants die shortly after birth from respiratory failure. The diagnosis should be suspected when the trachea cannot be intubated despite adequate visualization of the larynx, which is hypoplastic. Establishing ventilation through the esophageal communication to the airways may allow the patient to survive long enough for diagnostic procedures and attempts at correction.

TRACHEAL STENOSIS Most commonly, tracheal stenosis presents as segmental stenosis anywhere along the trachea. Clinical signs are severe retractions (especially with agitation or a respiratory infection), dyspnea, inspiratory and expiratory stridor, hypercarbia, and hypoxemia. Tracheal stenosis also should be considered in the differential diagnosis of recurrent, severe, or prolonged croup. The diagnosis can be suspected by demonstrating a fixed intrathoracic obstruction pattern on inspiratory-expiratory flow–volume curves and confirmed by bronchoscopy, CT scan, or magnetic resonance imaging (MRI) scanning (Fig. 23-8). Because of the risk for complete obstruction of the trachea, endoscopy and imaging studies should be performed by experienced personnel. If symptoms are severe, the stenotic segment should be either resected or, in some instances, stented. Extracorporeal membrane oxygenation may be used to ensure there is adequate gas exchange during surgery. Successful resection of even a long stenotic segment has been reported. With hypoplasia of the entire trachea because of a generalized abnormality of cartilage formation (eg, chondrodysplasia punctata), the prognosis is poor.

TRACHEOMALACIA AND BRONCHOMALACIA The terms *tracheomalacia* and *bronchomalacia* denote instability of the trachea or bronchi resulting from abnormally soft or pliable tracheal cartilages.

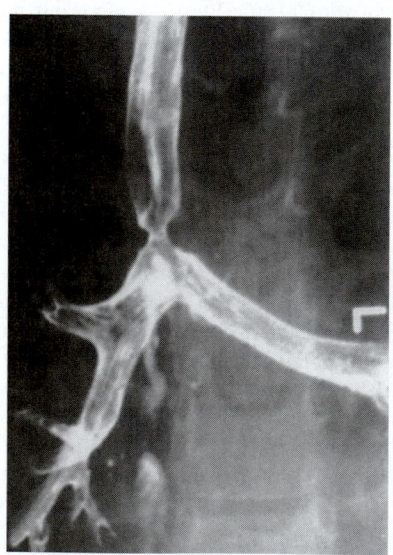

FIGURE 23-8 Tracheal stenosis. Tantalum tracheogram showing marked tracheal stenosis just above the carina.

Normally, intrathoracic airways widen during inhalation and narrow slightly during exhalation. The degree of narrowing is limited by cartilage, by tonic airway muscle contraction, and by traction forces exerted by lung parenchyma. With a delay in development of the supportive structures of large airways, excessive narrowing may occur during exhalation, and airway obstruction may be severe, especially if the infant becomes agitated and makes forceful respiratory maneuvers. Classification of the condition is based on the anatomic area that is involved (eg, tracheomalacia, tracheobronchomalacia, bronchomalacia).

Clinical signs include stridor, wheezing, respiratory distress, and hyperinflation, either diffuse or localized. Cough is usually absent, and growth is not impaired. Signs and symptoms usually disappear during sleep but become evident during agitation or respiratory infections. The diagnosis is established by airway fluoroscopy or flexible fiberoptic bronchoscopy. When wheezing results from tracheomalacia, inhalation of bronchodilator drugs may worsen airway instability and increase wheezing. Malacia may be caused by a delay in development of the supporting structures of the airways or by other abnormalities such as tracheoesophageal fistula and compression by anomalous vascular rings, bronchogenic cysts, or tumors. Symptoms usually lessen with time, and in most patients, no specific therapy is indicated. In the most severe instances, supplemental oxygen, continuous positive airway pressure, tracheoplasty, or tracheostomy may be necessary. Recently, expandable stents have been inserted with some success.

LARYNGOTRACHEOESOPHAGEAL CLEFTS Laryngotracheoesophageal clefts are rare and divided into three types: (1) posterior laryngeal cleft, (2) cleft of larynx and upper trachea, and (3) complete cleft of larynx and trachea to the level of the carina. Symptoms are similar to those for tracheoesophageal fistula, with which clefts may be mistaken, and may include difficulty with oral secretions, recurrent pneumonia, respiratory distress with feedings, aspiration pneumonitis, and weak or absent cry (see Sec. 13.4.1). Polyhydramnios is common, probably because of the inability of the fetus to swallow. The diagnosis should be suspected when, on laryngoscopy, the larynx appears large and the vocal cords long. Anatomic findings are often subtle and may require multiple imaging modalities for assessment.

There often are associated anomalies, including the G syndrome (ie, abnormal facies, prominent occiput and forehead, short lingual frenulum, stridor, hoarse cry, hypospadias, cryptorchidism, and laryngotracheoesophageal cleft). For infants with large clefts, the prognosis for survival is guarded.

VASCULAR RINGS AND SLINGS After repair of a vascular ring or sling, residual tracheomalacia or tracheal stenosis may persist postoperatively and may require arteriopexy, tracheoplasty, or airway stenting for relief of symptoms (see Sec. 22.3.7).

TRACHEOBRONCHIAL OBSTRUCTION CAUSED BY HEART DISEASE Bronchial obstruction may occur because of cardiomegaly, cardiomyopathy or congenital heart disease, enlarged left atrium or mispositioned great vessels, or from a persistent patent ductus arteriosus or ductus remnant. Primary or secondary pulmonary hypertension is associated with dilated pulmonary arteries, which can compress one or both mainstem bronchi. If airway obstruction is complete, there is atelectasis. If it is partial, there may be focal hyperinflation. Pulmonary symptoms usually resolve with correction of the cardiovascular abnormalities. With absence of the pulmonary valve, the pulmonary arteries become massively dilated, and bilateral airway obstruction usually is severe (see Sec. 22.3.3); because of severe distortion of the airways, infants may have persistence of respiratory distress for months after corrective cardial surgery.

OTHER TRACHEAL LESIONS Tracheal obstruction also may be caused by a hemangioma, papillomas, cystic hygroma, congenital goiter, or ectopic thyroid tissue. Intrathoracic tumors rarely cause tracheal obstruction; when they do, therapy and prognosis depend on the specific type of tumor. Tracheal obstruction may occur from necrotizing tracheobronchitis, which is an idiopathic disorder associated with mechanical ventilation. Severe obstruction is associated with frequent cyanotic spells and may require endoscopic removal of the abnormal tissue.

A rare cause of neonatal respiratory distress is tracheobiliary (or bronchobiliary) fistula. Symptoms are those of aspiration pneumonia. Diagnosis is by bronchoscopic observation of bilious fluid entering the airway via the fistulous tract, and treatment is surgical excision.

BRONCHIAL OBSTRUCTION AND LOBAR EMPHYSEMA

Overdistension of a lung lobe (usually an upper lobe) with fluid or air can cause respiratory distress during the neonatal period. Fluid in the distended lobe may be slowly absorbed after birth; therefore, the distended lobe may give the initial impression of a tumor on chest radiography. Whether filled with air or fluid, the distended, emphysematous lobe pushes the mediastinum to the opposite side and compresses the rest of the lung on both sides of the thorax, often resulting in respiratory distress (Fig. 23-9). The subsequent hyperinflation and adjacent atelectasis seen on the chest radiograph can be misinterpreted as congenital pneumonia, but mediastinal shift is rare in simple neonatal pneumonia and should alert the clinician to the diagnosis of lobar emphysema, especially when an upper lobe is hyperlucent. Abnormalities of bronchial cartilage or compression of the bronchial vessels by cysts in the affected lobe are found in about one-half of patients with congenital lobar emphysema (Fig. 23-10). In these patients, the alveolar histology usually is normal. In the remaining patients, alveoli, alveolar ducts, and respiratory bronchioles are cystic in appearance. Tachypnea, grunting, and retractions often begin shortly after birth or within the first

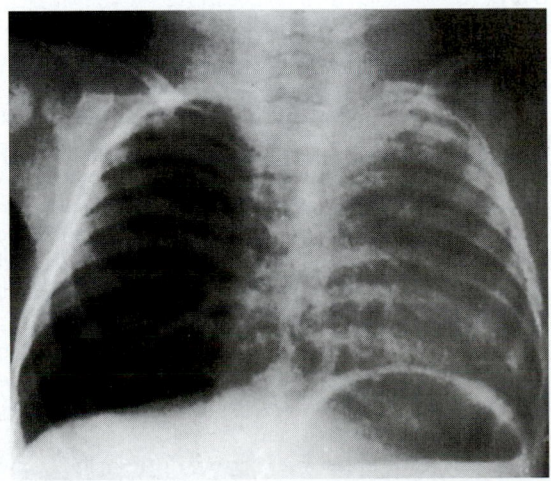

FIGURE 23-9   Chest radiograph showing hyperinflation (flat hemidiaphragm) of the right lung with mediastinal shift to the left.

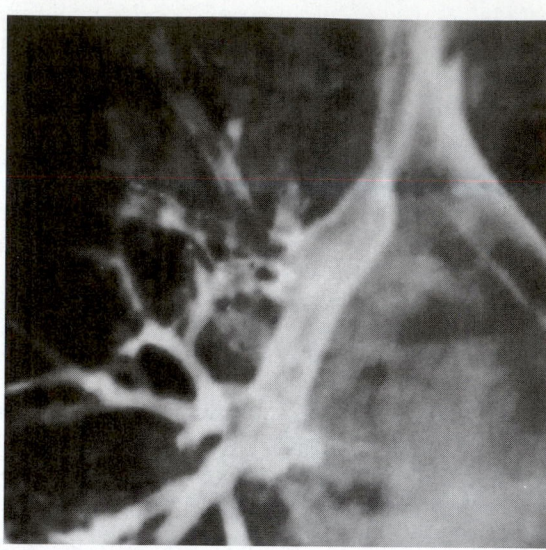

FIGURE 23-10   Cinebrochiogram of the same patient shown in Fig. 23–9. A small segment of the right mainstem bronchus, just below the carina, is narrow on forced expiration.

6 months of life. Occasionally, the defect is discovered during the evaluation of a respiratory infection.

Lobar emphysema is not always congenital. It also can be caused by extrinsic airway compression resulting from cardiovascular defects, intrinsic lobar obstruction, or bronchial injury during positive-pressure ventilation.

Increased resonance, decreased breath sounds, expiratory wheeze, and a shift in the location of heart sounds and trachea are the signs found on physical examination. High-resolution computed axial tomography can provide important clues to the underlying anatomic abnormality.

Medical management of lobar emphysema with supplemental oxygen and transient mechanical ventilation has been successful in mildly ill patients with single-lobe involvement. Surgery should be avoided if possible because long-term studies have found no differences in pulmonary function between surgically treated and medically treated patients.

PARENCHYMAL AND VASCULAR LESIONS

PULMONARY HYPOPLASIA As the mortality rates from other neonatal respiratory diseases, especially the respiratory distress syndrome, have decreased in the past several years, pulmonary hypoplasia has become an increasingly common cause of neonatal mortality. It is present in up to 20% of all neonatal autopsies. Certain physical factors are necessary for normal fetal lung growth, including adequate intrathoracic space, adequate amounts of amniotic fluid, and fetal breathing movements. Interference with any of these factors can result in pulmonary hypoplasia, which can be associated with a variety of clinical conditions (Table 23-7). With premature rupture of the membranes, the risk of pulmonary hypoplasia is relative to the degree of prematurity at the time of the membrane rupture and to the severity and duration of oligohydramnios.

With pulmonary hypoplasia, respiratory distress almost always is present at birth. Assisted ventilation often leads to pneumothorax because of decreased compliance and small lung volumes. Severe

hypoxemia and hypercarbia are common. Other clinical findings depend on the condition causing the pulmonary hypoplasia. In the case of lesions within the thorax, the chest has a normal shape and size. With oligohydramnios, the chest may appear to be small; associated findings include Potter facies and limb contractures. Chest radiographs may show a specific abnormality (eg, congenital diaphragmatic hernia) or merely small lung volumes, high diaphragms, and an apparently large heart. The diagnosis of pulmonary hypoplasia can be inferred from the clinical findings and associated conditions, but it can be made with certainty only with postmortem measurements of lung size, lung DNA content, and lung morphometry.

The prognosis depends on the severity of both the pulmonary hypoplasia and the associated anomalies. In the most severe lesions, the lungs are too small to permit survival. In less severe hypoplasia, lung growth may occur if the infant is maintained with prolonged mechanical ventilation or extracorporeal membrane oxygenation (ECMO). In infants who survive, prolonged oxygen administration may be necessary. Some infants with historical factors and clinical presentation that are consistent with marked pulmonary hypoplasia show unexplained, rapid improvement over a period of hours to days in response to assisted ventilation. Because of this, vigorous resuscitative efforts should be used even for those infants with apparently severe pulmonary hypoplasia.

CONGENITAL MISALIGNMENT OF PULMONARY VESSELS (ALVEOLAR CAPILLARY DYSPLASIA) This is a rare condition consisting of a decreased number of pulmonary capillaries, anomalous veins in bronchovascular bundles, and hypertrophy of pulmonary arteriolar muscle. In contrast to pulmonary hypoplasia, lung size is normal. These infants present in the perinatal period with severe pulmonary hypertension that is refractory to treatment. It may be associated with left-sided congenital heart disease but is usually an isolated abnormality. Survival to a few weeks or months of life has been reported with the use in ECMO or inhaled nitric oxide, but the disorder is fatal. The diagnosis is confirmed by lung biopsy.

SCIMITAR SYNDROME The scimitar syndrome is a rare vascular malformation in which pulmonary venous blood from all or part of

TABLE 23-7

CONDITIONS ASSOCIATED WITH PULMONARY HYPOPLASIA

Space-occupying lesions of the thorax
  Congenital diaphragmatic hernia
  Intrathoracic tumors (eg, cystic adenomatoid malformation)
  Pleural effusions (eg, hydrops fetalis, Pena-Shokier syndrome)
Oligohydramnios
  Prolonged rupture of membranes
  Renal lesions (renal agenesis, obstructive uropathy, infantile polycystic disease)
  Abdominal pregnancy
Thoracic abnormalities
  Asphyxiating thoracic dystrophy
  Thanatophoric dwarfism
  Giant omphalocele
Absent or deficient fetal breathing movements
  Werdnig-Hoffmann disease (with intrauterine onset)
  Congenital muscular dystrophy
  Anencephaly
  Agenesis of phrenic nerves

the right lung returns to the inferior vena cava just above or below the diaphragm. There often is hypoplasia of the right lung. Some instances of the scimitar syndrome are associated with the "horseshoe lung" (ie, hypoplasia of the right lung and fusion of the posteroinferior segments of both lungs behind the heart and anterior to the esophagus and spine). Two types of scimitar syndrome have been described. The *adult* form has a small shunt between the right pulmonary veins and the inferior vena cava, which usually is well tolerated. Symptoms typically do not appear until after infancy, and there is a good prognosis. The *infantile* form has a large shunt between the anomalous arteries to the right lower lung (sometimes called the *vascular sequestration*) and the inferior vena cava. This form is severe, with early onset of respiratory distress, pulmonary hypertension, and heart failure, and has a poor prognosis for survival. Recent reports suggest that the most effective treatment is ligation of the aberrant systemic arteries to the right lung. Ligation of the associated patent ductus arteriosus is associated with a high mortality rate, and excision of the "sequestered" region of lung may aggravate the already present pulmonary hypoplasia.

PULMONARY ARTERIOVENOUS FISTULAS *Congenital* pulmonary arteriovenous (AV) fistula is one manifestation of several disorders that affect many organ systems. Hereditary hemorrhagic telangiectasia (HHT or Rendu-Osler-Weber syndrome), an autosomal dominant disorder, is the most common cause. Bleeding from the respiratory tract can occur at any age (see Sec. 12.8). Pulmonary arteriovenous malformations develop in up to 20% of HHT patients. The diagnosis is made during infancy in approximately 15% of patients with congenital pulmonary AV fistula. HHT accounts for more than 70% of all patients with congenital AV malformations. Therefore, if a pulmonary arteriovenous malformation is discovered at an early age, the possibility of HHT should be considered strongly.

Acquired pulmonary AV fistulas occur with pulmonary hypertension that is associated with mitral stenosis, cystic fibrosis, and chest trauma. Microscopic pulmonary AV fistulas can occur in children with chronic liver disease and cause hypoxemia (hepatopulmonary syndrome). Systemic-to-pulmonary vascular connections may also develop in patients with cyanotic congenital heart disease.

Clinical findings in pulmonary AV fistulas are caused by right-to-left shunting of systemic venous blood directly into pulmonary veins and the left heart. Signs include dyspnea, hemoptysis, epistaxis, and exercise intolerance. Cyanosis and clubbing are less common. A systolic or continuous bruit is occasionally found. Because the blood flows under low pressure, congestive heart failure is very uncommon. Pneumothorax and hemothorax rarely occur. There is an increased risk for septicemia and brain abscess. Polycythemia with hematocrits of 60 to 80% may occur and lead to thrombosis and embolism. Oxygen saturation is low, decreases further with exercise, and increases (but not to normal levels) with supplemental oxygen. In patients with HHT, chest radiographs show noncalcified nodular densities. CT lung scanning reveals that the densities are enhanced by contrast agents. In patients with the hepatopulmonary syndrome, both chest radiograph and CT scans may be normal. The diagnosis is confirmed by excluding cyanotic congenital heart disease and by demonstrating the fistulas by pulmonary angiography or by contrast echocardiography or by lung perfusion scanning with technetium-labeled macroaggregated albumin.

In symptomatic patients, the fistula(s) can be ablated by the administration of embolizing agents during pulmonary angiography. If the fistulas are large, or if embolization is unsuccessful, sur-

gical excision may be necessary. In patients with the hepatopulmonary syndrome, liver transplantation usually causes regression of the fistulas.

PULMONARY SEQUESTRATIONS Pulmonary sequestrations result from disturbed embryogenesis, which leads to a mass of lung-like tissue that does not function and receives its blood supply from anomalous systemic arteries. Intralobar sequestrations are contained within the normal visceral pleura, and their venous drainage is into pulmonary veins. Extralobar sequestrations have their own separate pleura and venous drainage into systemic or portal veins.

Intralobar sequestrations usually occur in the lower lobe of either lung, but they may occur in other lobes or below the diaphragm. Arterial supply is from the thoracic or abdominal aorta, usually through a large vessel; drainage usually is through the pulmonary veins. Communications with the esophagus are uncommon, but such a connection is suggested when infection or air-filled cysts are present. Intralobar sequestrations generally are isolated anomalies, and most are recognized before 20 years of age (Fig. 23-11).

Extralobar sequestrations occur just above or below the diaphragm; 90% are on the left side. Arterial supply usually is from small anomalous branches of a pulmonary or systemic artery, and venous drainage is via a systemic vein. Communication with the foregut is common, as are associated anomalies such as bronchial agenesis, duplication of the colon, vertebral anomalies, and diaphragmatic defects. Boys are affected three to four times as often as girls. Signs may be present in the neonatal period, and most instances are diagnosed before 2 years of age.

Respiratory distress is the most common presenting symptom. Others include recurrent pneumonia, hemoptysis, fever, and other signs of pulmonary infection. Pleuritic chest pain out of proportion to clinical or radiographic findings is often present.

Occasionally, presenting signs are those of a very large left-to-right shunt through the sequestration, with congestive heart failure and low systemic blood flow. The physical examination may be normal, or there may be rales, dullness to percussion, and a continuous murmur that is heard over the posterior lung base. Pectus excavatum also may be present. Differential diagnosis includes pneumonia, empyema, lung abscess, bronchiectasis, neoplasms, cystic adenomatoid malformation, bronchogenic or enterogenic cysts, diaphragm hernia, and intrathoracic kidney.

The chest radiograph is usually abnormal, but the findings may be subtle or obscured by the cardiac silhouette. CT is helpful, and ultrasonography with Doppler flow studies is useful in diagnosis if an anomalous systemic artery can be identified. Bronchoscopy and bronchography usually are not helpful because there is no connection between the sequestration and the normal airway. Because of the risk of recurrent infection, treatment of a pulmonary sequestration is surgical resection.

SPONTANEOUS PNEUMOTHORAX

A spontaneous pneumothorax may occur in pediatric patients who have no apparent history of pulmonary or chest wall disease, chest trauma, or other obvious precipitating factor. The pathogenesis is somewhat speculative, but in most cases, air from distended lung bullae enters the lung interstitium and causes rupture of mediastinal parietal pleura. This produces a pneumomediastinum and then a pneumothorax. It is not clear if the bullae are congenital or acquired. Tall and thin individuals are at increased risk for sponta-

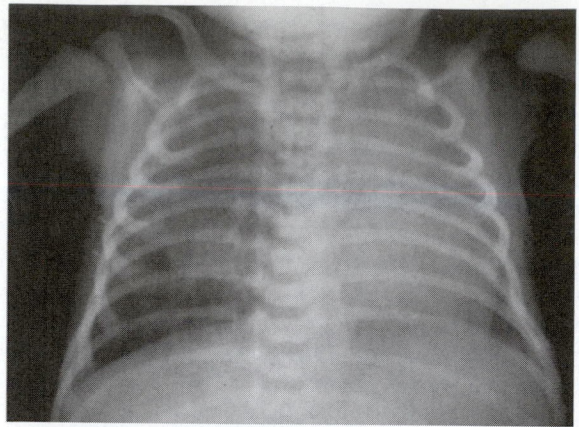

A

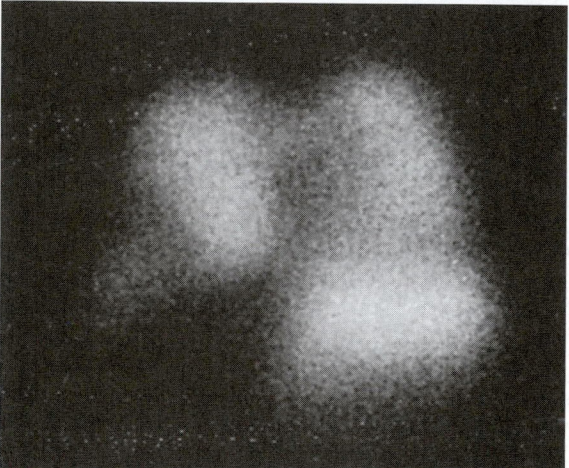

B

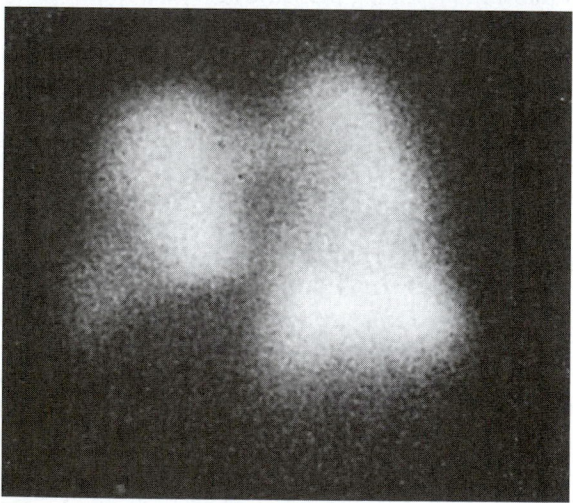

C

FIGURE 23-11 Pulmonary sequestration in a newborn infant who presented with respiratory distress and congestive heart failure. **A.** Chest radiograph on the day of birth showing a relatively lucent area in the right lower lung field with shift of the mediastinum to the left. **B.** Ventilation scan of the lungs (age, 7 days) showing a filling defect in the right lower lung field. **C.** Perfusion scan of the lungs showing a filling defect in the same area. The next day, the infant underwent operative removal of an intralobar sequestration of the right lower lobe. The sequestered tissue was supplied by a large anomalous artery that arose from the abdominal aorta.

neous pneumothorax. Most episodes occur at rest and are not associated with vigorous activity or coughing. Pleuritic chest pain is present, but shoulder or upper quadrant abdominal pain on the affected side may be present. The pain is described as sharp or steady, and often the patient can recall similar episodes that were less severe. Physical examination may be normal if the pneumothorax is small, but breath sounds may be diminished on the affected side. Dyspnea and hypoxemia may be severe if the pneumothorax is large or displaces the mediastinum to the contralateral side. The diagnosis is confirmed by chest radiography, but the findings may be subtle. Radiographs taken after exhalation to residual volume may be necessary to visualize the air leak. Initial treatment depends on the patient's symptoms and on the size and duration of the air leak and range from simple needle aspiration to chest tube drainage, thoracoscopic stapling, and pleurodesis.

The risk of recurrence is difficult to estimate in pediatric populations. In adults, the risk of a second spontaneous pneumothorax ranges from 20 to 50%. Risk factors for recurrence include a thin body habitus, young age, and smoking. Most recurrences seem to occur within 2 years. The presence of pleural bullae can be confirmed by chest CT scan, but their presence does not appear to correlate with recurrences. After a second recurrence, the risk of a third increases by as much as twofold.

CONGENITAL PULMONARY LYMPHANGIECTASIS

See Sec. 23.3.4.

CYSTIC LESIONS

Congenital cystic lesions in the thorax can be classified into three categories.

BRONCHOGENIC CYSTS AND DERMOID CYSTS Dermoid cysts are rare lesions that differ from bronchogenic cysts only in their histologic appearance. They are lined by keratinized, stratified, squamous epithelium, and they may contain sweat glands and ducts; some of these cysts communicate with a bronchus. Clinical and radiologic findings are similar to those caused by bronchogenic cysts.

Bronchogenic cysts result from abnormal budding or branching of the tracheobronchial tree. They may be an incidental finding on chest radiography but can cause respiratory signs, including dyspnea, because of the compression of adjacent tissue, recurrent infections, and atelectasis resulting from airway compression. Bronchogenic cysts have been classified according to their location. *Paratracheal cysts* attach to the trachea above the carina. *Carinal cysts* attach at the carina and also may attach to the anterior esophageal wall. *Hilar cysts* attach to one of the main lobar bronchi. *Paraesophageal cysts* have no communication with the tracheobronchial tree but may attach to or communicate with the esophagus. Bronchogenic cysts also have been found below the diaphragm. Histologically, bronchogenic cysts are lined by ciliated columnar epithelium and have cartilage and smooth muscle within the wall.

Most bronchogenic cysts are unilocular and filled with mucoid material. Mediastinal shift is rare unless there is extensive lobar obstruction and atelectasis. These cysts appear on radiography as round or oval homogenous masses with a density similar to that of water. Cysts that communicate with the airways or esophagus may be fluid-filled, air-filled, or have an air–fluid level; some cysts may have each of these appearances at different times (Fig. 23-12). Pneumothorax or hemoptysis may occur if the cyst ruptures. Di-

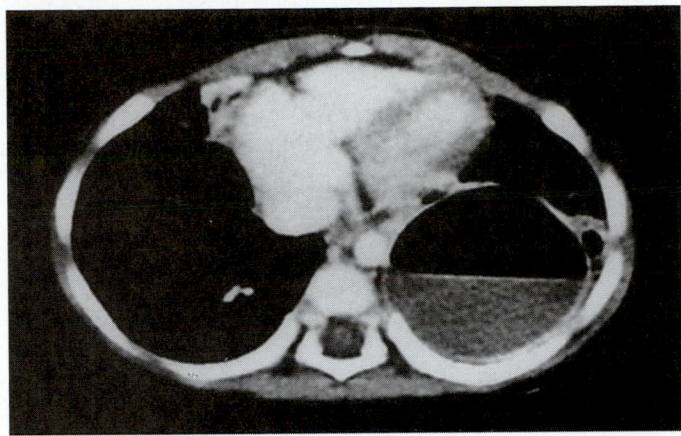

A

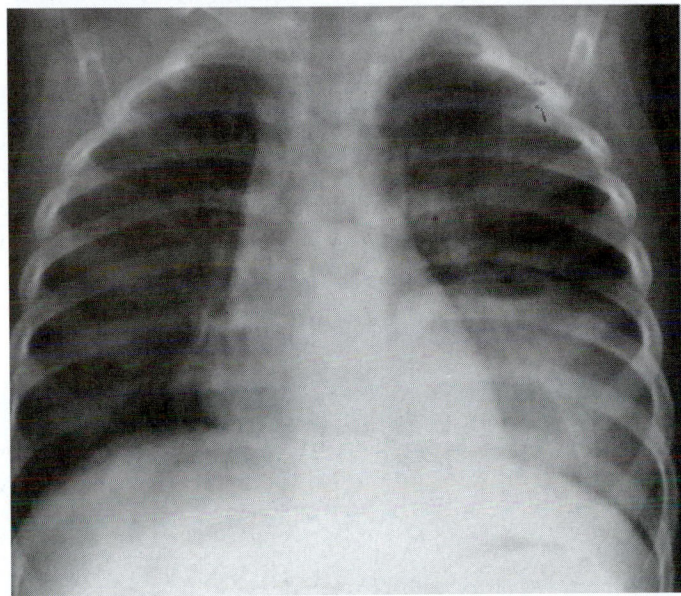

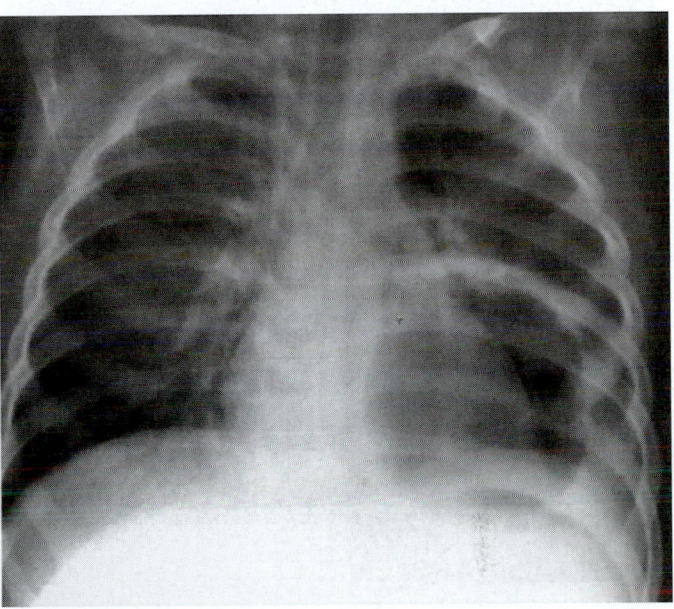

B

FIGURE 23-12   Bronchogenic cyst in an infant at 11 months of age who presented with respiratory distress. **A.** Computed tomographic scan of the chest with the infant recumbent showed the mass to be half-filled with fluid. **B.** Two weeks later, a chest radiograph (infant upright) showed a round lesion on the left lower lung field. Except for a small amount of air at the upper edge of the mass, the mass appeared to be solid, homogeneous, and almost completely filled with fluid. **C.** Three weeks later, the mass was completely filled with air. The mass was resected, with resolution of the respiratory distress. Pathologic examination showed the mass to be a bronchogenic cyst.

agnosis is assisted by CT or MRI. Some cysts may become infected or are discovered incidentally during the evaluation of an acute respiratory infection. The differential diagnosis includes lung abscess or a foreign body. Treatment of bronchogenic cysts is excision. Transthoracic CT-guided needle aspiration of the cyst has been described, but cyst rupture and spillage into unaffected lung may occur.

CONGENITAL CYSTIC ADENOMATOID MALFORMATION Congenital cystic adenomatoid malformation (CCAM) is an uncommon anomaly of the lung with a broad spectrum of clinical presentations. It may present before or after birth. Lesions are characterized by an increase in structures resembling bronchioles that are lined by columnar epithelium; cartilage usually is absent. Based on whether the predominant component of the lesion is cystic or solid, CCAM can be categorized into three types: (1) type I, consisting of a few very large cysts; (2) type II, macrocystic tumors that have single or multiple cysts with a diameter of 1 cm; and (3) type III, solid tumors with cysts less than 5 mm in diameter. A few reports of hyperplastic cells in excised specimens have raised the possibility that CAMs may have an increased risk of malignant transformation.

With prenatal diagnosis of CCAM by ultrasonography, a variety of outcomes have been recognized. Some lesions show little change during fetal life and can be resected postnatally. In a few, the lesions seem to regress and even disappear. Large lesions with mediastinal shift and fetal hydrops have a poor prognosis and a high likelihood of fetal death or severe postnatal respiratory failure because of an inadequate amount of normal pulmonary tissue. In some instances of fetal CCAM with large cysts, in utero drainage or removal of the cysts has led to improvement in the fetus and expansion of the normal lung tissue.

Postnatally, an infant with a CCAM presents with respiratory distress, the severity of which depends on the size of the lesion. Very small lesions cause few, if any, symptoms. There may be mediastinal shift and overdistension resulting from trapped air and replacement of much of the lung with the cystic mass (Fig. 23-13). Treatment of CCAM is resection of the affected lung tissue. Subsequent outcome depends on the amount of lung tissue remaining and the degree of distortion of the remaining airways, which also may be hypoplastic because of compression in utero. If a large volume of abnormal tissue is removed in the neonatal period, the pos-

sibility of secondary scoliosis and its complications should be anticipated.

References

Tracheobronchial Lesions

Altman KW, Wetmore RF, Marsh RR: Congenital airway abnormalities in patients requiring hospitalization. Arch Otolaryngol 125:525–528, 1999

Benjamin B: Tracheomalacia in infants and children. Ann Otol Rhinol Laryngol 93:438, 1984

De Lorimier AA, Harrison MR, Hardy K, et al: Tracheobronchial obstructions in infants and children. Experience with 45 cases. Ann Surg 212: 277, 1990

Filler RM, Messineo A, Vinograd I: Severe tracheomalacia associated with esophageal atresia: results of surgical treatment. J Pediatr Surg 27:1136, 1992

Furman RH, Backer CL, Dunham ME, Donaldson J, Mavroudis C, Hollinger L: The use of balloon-expandable metallic stents in the treatment of pediatric tracheomalacia and bronchomalacia. Arch Otolaryngol 125: 203–207, 1999

Han MT, Hall DG, Manche A, Rittenhouse EA: Double aortic arch causing tracheo-esophageal compression. Am J Surg 165:628, 1993

Howell L, Smith JD: G syndrome and its otolaryngologic manifestations. Ann Otol Rhinol Laryngol 98:185, 1989

McLaughlin RB, Wetmore RF, Tavill MA, Gaynor JW, Spray TL: Vascular anomalies causing symptomatic tracheobronchial compression. Laryngoscope 109:312–319, 1999

Ogawa T, Yamataka A, Miyano T, et al: Treatment of laryngotracheoesophageal cleft. J Pediatr Surg 24:341, 1989

Panitch HB, Keklikian EN, Motley RA, et al: Effect of altering smooth muscle tone on maximal expiratory flows in patients with tracheomalacia. Pediatr Pulmonol 9:170, 1990

Stanger P, Lucas RV Jr, Edwards JE: Anatomic factors causing respiratory distress in acyanotic congenital cardiac disease. Pediatrics 43:760, 1969

Van Son JA, Julsrud PR, Hagler DJ, et al: Surgical treatment of vascular rings: The Mayo Clinic experience. Mayo Clin Proc 68:1056, 1993

Parenchymal and Vascular Lesions

Al-Hathlol K, Phillips S, Seshia MK, Casiro O, Alvaro RE, Rigatto H: Alveolar capillary dysplasia. Report of a case of prolonged life without ECMO and review of the literature. Early Hum Dev 57:85–94, 2000

Baumann MH, Strange C, Heffner JE, et al: Management of spontaneous pneumothorax. Chest 119:590–602, 2001

Burke CM, Safai C, Nelson DP, Raffin TA: Pulmonary arteriovenous malformations: a critical update. Am Rev Respir Dis 134:334, 1986

Coran AG, Drongowski R: Congenital cystic disease of the tracheobronchial tree in infants and children. Arch Surg 129:521, 1994

Dupuis C, Charaf LAC, Breviere GM, Abou P: "Infantile" form of the scimitar syndrome with pulmonary hypertension. Am J Cardiol 71: 1326, 1993

Dupuis C, Remy J, Remy-Jardin M, et al: The "horseshoe" lung: six new cases. Pediatr Pulmonol 17:124, 1994

Gao YA, Burrows PE, Benson LN, et al: Scimitar syndrome in infancy. J Am Coll Cardiol 22:873, 1993

Huber A, Schranz D, Blaha I, et al: Congenital pulmonary lymphangiectasis. Pediatr Pulmonol 10:310, 1991

Karnack I, Senocak ME, Ciftci AO, Buyukpaukcu N: Congenital lobar emphysema: diagnostic and therapeutic considerations. J Pediatr Surg 34: 1347–1351, 1999

Krowka MJ: Hepatopulmonary syndromes. Gut 46:1–4, 2000

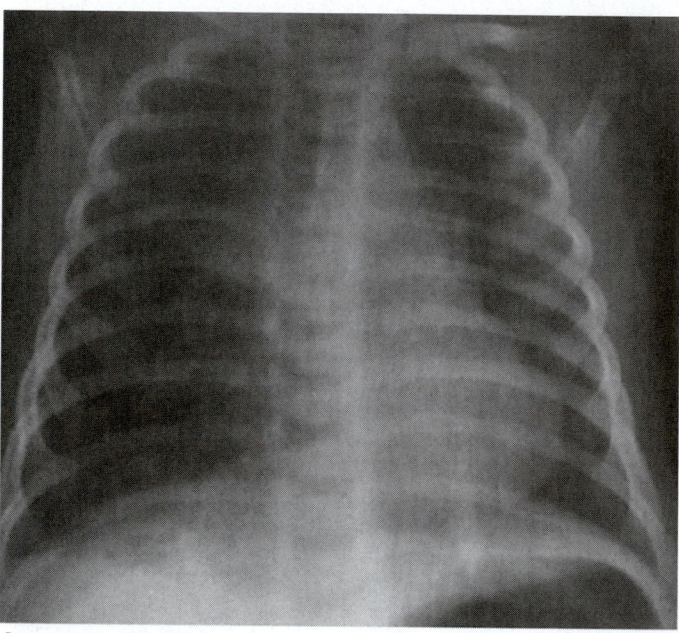

A

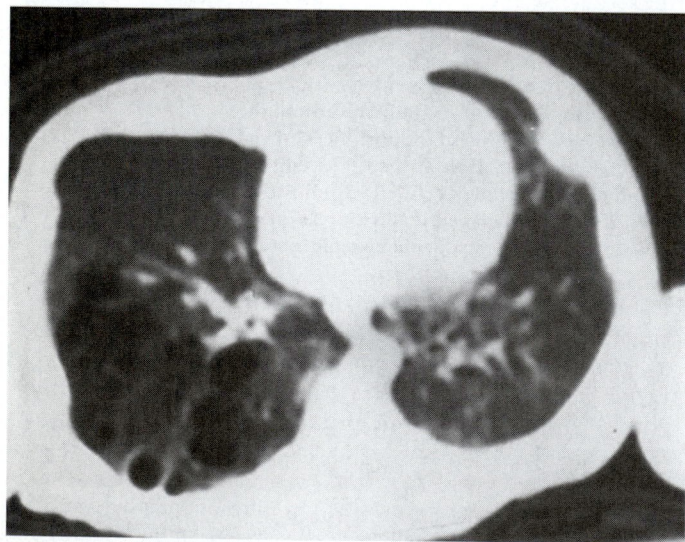

B

FIGURE 23-13 Cystic adenomatoid malformation of the right lower lobe in a newborn infant who presented shortly after birth with tachypnea. A. Chest radiograph showing abnormal lung tissue in the right lower lung field. B. Computed tomographic scan of the thorax showing several small cystic areas in the right lower lobe.

Noonan JA, Walters LR, Reeves JT: Congenital pulmonary lymphangiectasis. Am J Dis Child 120:314, 1970

Page DV, Stocker JT: Anomalies associated with pulmonary hypoplasia. Am Rev Respir Dis 125:216, 1982

Rodgers BM, Harman PK, Johnson AM: Bronchopulmonary foregut malformations: the spectrum of anomalies. Ann Surg 203:517, 1986

Sahn SA, Heffner JE: Spontaneous pneumothorax. N Engl J Med 342:868–874, 2000

Schwartz DS, Reyes-Mugica M, Keller MS: Imaging of surgical disease of the newborn chest. Radiol Clin North Am 37:1067–1078, 1999

Shovlin CL, Letarte M: Hereditary hemorrhagic telangiectasia and pulmonary arteriovenous malformations: Issues in clinical management and review of pathogenic mechanisms. Thorax 54:714–729, 1999

Vergani P, Ghindini A, Locatelli A, et al: Risk factors for pulmonary hypoplasia in second-trimester premature rupture of membranes. Am J Obstetr Gynecol 170:1359, 1994

Weissberg D, Raefaely Y: Pneumothorax: experience with 1,199 patients. Chest 117:1279–1285, 2000

Werner HA, Pirie GE, Nadel HR, et al: Lung volumes, mechanics and perfusion after pulmonary resection in infancy. J Thorac Cardiovasc Surg 105:737, 1993

Wigglesworth JS, Desai R: Use of DNA estimation for growth assessment in normal and hypoplastic fetal lungs. Arch Dis Child 56:601, 1981

23.5   DISORDERS OF RESPIRATORY CONTROL

It is well recognized that respiratory control requires complicated machinery to sense blood gas tensions and H[+], generate rhythmic breathing, tense and relax the muscles of the upper airway and the respiratory pump, and integrate these processes in a coordinated fashion. Sometimes these processes can be dissected to identify the precise mechanism for a disturbance of breathing, and other times our understanding is more descriptive than mechanistic. Accordingly, the following section groups important disorders where control of respiratory function is disturbed at one or more of the levels described above.

23.5.1   Chronic Alveolar Hypoventilation

Debra E. Weese-Mayer and Jean M. Silvestri

Most chronic respiratory control disorders in infants and children are manifested primarily by alveolar hypoventilation both awake and asleep. However, others are manifest during sleep only. This section reviews the diagnosis and management of the infant or child with chronic alveolar hypoventilation. For the purpose of this discussion, alveolar hypoventilation is described as inadequate ventilation resulting in increased carbon dioxide levels and decreased oxyhemoglobin saturation.

GENERAL CONSIDERATIONS

Alveolar hypoventilation may be *congenital* (present at birth) or *acquired*. Alveolar hypoventilation may be subdivided further into *idiopathic* or *secondary* to an anatomic, physiologic, or metabolic disorder. For example, congenital central hypoventilation syndrome (CCHS), a cause of congenital alveolar hypoventilation, is considered idiopathic because its etiology is unknown and it is a diagnosis of exclusion. However, alveolar hypoventilation associated with Chiari II malformation and Mobius syndrome are congenital and thought to be secondary to hypoplasia of brainstem nuclei. Alveolar hypoventilation in the infant with a congenital myopathy is secondary to neuromuscular weakness. Likewise, alveolar hypoventilation associated with Leigh disease is thought to be caused by spongiform degeneration of the brainstem. Finally, alveolar hypoventilation associated with pyruvate dehydrogenase deficiency and carnitine deficiency results from metabolic abnormalities. Disorders causing obstructive sleep apnea are discussed in Sec. 23.5.3.

DISORDERS CAUSING CONGENITAL ALVEOLAR HYPOVENTILATION

IDIOPATHIC CONGENITAL CENTRAL HYPOVENTILATION SYNDROME   CCHS is a rare disorder with approximately 100 published cases and fewer than 200 patients worldwide. Children with CCHS typically present in the newborn period. CCHS is characterized by generally adequate ventilation while the patient is awake but alveolar hypoventilation (*not* apnea) during sleep. When apnea is present, it occurs after discontinuation of mechanical ventilation and before initiation of spontaneous breathing. Typically during sleep, infants with CCHS will have normal respiratory rates but diminished tidal volume, leading to progressive hypoxemia and hypercapnia. Gas exchange is impaired regardless of sleep state, although ventilation is better in rapid eye movement (REM) sleep than in non-REM sleep. More severely affected children hypoventilate both when awake and asleep. During sleep, they also have absent or negligible ventilatory sensitivity to either hypercarbia or hypoxemia. When asleep, patients with CCHS do not awaken in response to hypercarbia, to hypoxemia, or to the combined stimulus of both. When awake, ventilatory responsiveness to hypercarbia and hypoxemia is generally absent, and they have a markedly impaired perception of asphyxia (ie, behavioral awareness of hypercarbia and hypoxemia), even when awake minute ventilation is adequate. Interestingly, the heart rate response to exercise is normal, but these children do not accelerate their heart rate in response to hypoxia.

Conditions associated with CCHS include Hirschsprung disease, ganglioneuroma, neuroblastoma, ganglioneuroblastoma, lack of heart rate variability, and eye abnormalities including diminished pupillary light response and visual perceptual deficits. Feeding difficulty with esophageal dysmotility in infancy, breath-holding spells, poor temperature regulation with the basal body temperature typically <37°C, and sporadic profuse sweating episodes with cool extremities have also been described. Children with CCHS lack a perception of dyspnea but maintain voluntary control of breathing; for example, when asked to take a deep breath, they do so. During exercise these children may be at risk for hypercarbia and hypoxemia, though the degree of exercise and the severity of the CCHS likely affect the response for each child. Perception of anxiety is also decreased among children with CCHS.

CCHS is a lifelong condition. Patients continue to demonstrate abnormalities in control of breathing, and some patients eventually require daytime/awake ventilatory support as well. Because of its rarity, the diagnosis of CCHS may be delayed. Delayed diagnosis after varying degrees of hypoxia probably explains much of the observed variation in neurodevelopmental outcome. Further, practitioners often provide ongoing care to a chronically ventilated child without attention to the unique needs of the child with CCHS. For these reasons, strong consideration should be given to referral of these patients to health centers with expertise in the diagnosis and management of CCHS.

ALVEOLAR HYPOVENTILATION DUE TO CHIARI II MALFORMATION The brainstem abnormality in patients with Chiari II malformation results in a variable degree of alveolar hypoventilation. These patients have mild alterations in breathing patterns that are clinically insignificant, but approximately 30% of these patients will have variable degrees of alveolar hypoventilation and bradypnea in the presence of normal or even increased tidal volume. The most severely affected Chiari II patients lack ventilatory responsiveness to hypoxemia and hypercarbia both awake and asleep. These patients typically lack an arousal response from sleep regardless of the extent of asphyxia. During wakefulness there is typically no perception of asphyxia.

The brainstem abnormalities in patients with Chiari II malformation include "beaking" of the midbrain, caudal elongation of the fourth ventricle and cerebellar vermis to the cervical level, and hydromyelia. Possible mechanisms for the associated alveolar hypoventilation include hypoplasia of brainstem nuclei or stretching of arteries that results in either dysfunction of respiratory control centers or compression of the brainstem, leading to dysfunction on the basis of mechanical damage.

OTHER CAUSES OF CONGENITAL HYPOVENTILATION *Mobius syndrome* is a complex congenital disorder involving hypoplasia/dysfunction of several brainstem nuclei. Affected infants may present with alveolar hypoventilation indistinguishable from CCHS but without the associated autonomic findings. *Leigh encephalomyelopathy* is an autosomal recessive disorder that represents an inborn error of metabolism. Alveolar hypoventilation with Leigh disease may precede the progressive neurologic deterioration and can be initially confused with CCHS. Infants with *congenital myopathies* may demonstrate alveolar hypoventilation on the basis of neuromuscular weakness, though reduced respiratory drive has also been proposed. *Pyruvate dehydrogenase deficiency* and *carnitine deficiency* represent inborn errors of metabolism that are associated with alveolar hypoventilation in infants, although the mechanism is not understood.

DISORDERS CAUSING ACQUIRED ALVEOLAR HYPOVENTILATION

Acquired causes of chronic alveolar hypoventilation include structural lesions in the brainstem, high cervical spinal cord, or lower motor neuron. These include patients with severe birth asphyxia, with profound hypoventilation as part of a severe and typically global insult to the central nervous system. Infectious processes such as encephalitis may result in acquired hypoventilation secondary to impaired chemoreceptor drive and also related to discoordinated control of inspiratory and expiratory muscles. Wild-type and vaccine-associated poliomyelitis can affect the brainstem and spinal cord, causing chronic alveolar hypoventilation. Posttraumatic hypoventilation has been reported and is the cause of hypoventilation in children with high cervical injuries that involve the phrenic nerves (cervical nerves 3, 4, and 5). Although the brainstem respiratory centers in these patients may be normal, the respiratory efferent output cannot be transmitted peripherally because of more peripheral defects. The resultant paralysis of diaphragm and accessory muscles of respiration thus causes alveolar hypoventilation. Infarction, emboli, and tumors in and around the brainstem may also cause hypoventilation.

DIAGNOSIS AND MANAGEMENT OF CHRONIC ALVEOLAR HYPOVENTILATION

Children with CCHS typically present in the newborn period. Presenting symptoms include lethargy and duskiness or cyanosis on falling asleep. In these infants, noninvasive gas exchange monitoring during sleep reveals decreasing oxyhemoglobin saturation with increasing carbon dioxide levels with little or no increase in breathing frequency, heart rate, or awakening. Most infants with CCHS have some degree of chest wall movement, but some will appear apneic both awake and asleep. In infants with CCHS, even alarming degrees of hypoxemia and hypercarbia will become normal shortly after the infant awakens. Generalized weakness is absent, and muscle tone and reflexes are normal. Because CCHS is a diagnosis of exclusion, myasthenia gravis, airway obstructive lesions, diaphragm dysfunction, structural CNS abnormalities, and Mobius syndrome should be considered. Studies should be performed to rule out primary neuromuscular, lung, or cardiac disease or an identifiable brainstem lesion. Specific metabolic diseases such as Leigh disease, pyruvate dehydrogenase deficiency, and carnitine deficiency should also be considered. The initial evaluation should include a detailed neurologic evaluation that may require a muscle biopsy, a chest x-ray, fluoroscopy of the diaphragm, bronchoscopy, an electromyogram with nerve conduction velocities, echocardiogram, and an MRI of the brain/brainstem. Serum and urinary carnitine levels to rule out an inborn error in fatty acid metabolism should be obtained from a laboratory with known expertise in their assessment. The infant with carnitine deficiency may require a muscle biopsy for confirmation of the diagnosis. A detailed ophthalmologic evaluation should be performed to assess for pupillary reactivity and optic disc anatomy. A rectal biopsy should be considered in the event of abdominal distension and delayed defecation to assess for Hischsprung disease. Each infant should have gas exchange monitoring both awake and asleep. The recording montage should include at a minimum tidal volume (pneumotachograph), movement of the chest and abdomen, hemoglobin saturation with oximetry, end-tidal carbon dioxide measurement, and electrocardiogram. Careful observation should be made of the infant's tidal volume and respiratory frequency response to the endogenous challenges of hypercarbia and hypoxemia both awake and asleep. The distinction of need for artificial ventilatory support asleep only or awake and asleep should be made after several detailed evaluations in a controlled laboratory setting.

If other causes of alveolar hypoventilation are excluded, and the diagnosis of CCHS is made, a tracheostomy should be performed, and mechanical ventilation should be provided while the infant is asleep. If the diagnosis is uncertain and the degree of hypoventilation is mild, a trial of noninvasive ventilatory support devices can be attempted (see below). A transition to a home mechanical ventilator should be made to allow ample time for parental training before discharge. Arrangement for discharge to home with the primary mechanical ventilator and a back-up ventilator should be completed and requests for adequate home nursing care made. Often 24-hour per day care with highly trained registered nurses is required to optimize patient management. At home, monitoring of hemoglobin saturation is useful and reassuring; end-tidal carbon dioxide monitoring is also occasionally necessary to provide objective evidence of clinical deterioration or of "outgrowing" initial ventilator settings. The goals of management of this infant is the prevention of hypoxemia and cor pulmonale. Because the child with CCHS does not demonstrate dyspnea in response to chronic hypoventilation or acute pulmonary infection, objective measures of physiological compromise are necessary to ensure early clinical intervention.

Rarely a child will present with seemingly classic symptoms of CCHS later in infancy. In these cases, it is essential that an acquired abnormality resulting in prior apparent life-threatening events that resulted in damage to their control of breathing be considered. All available medical records should be reviewed to seek an etiology for the alveolar hypoventilation. It is remotely possible that an infant will have such subtle disease that the child's condition will go undetected until later in infancy.

VENTILATORY SUPPORT OPTIONS Several ventilatory support options are available for the infant and child with chronic alveolar hypoventilation. Typically the infant who requires ventilatory support 24 h/d will have a tracheostomy and use a mechanical ventilator that delivers positive-pressure ventilation. As the infant becomes ambulatory, the possibility of diaphragm pacing by phrenic nerve stimulation should be considered to allow for increased daytime mobility and improved quality of life, particularly in the child with CCHS. Although pacing has been used successfully in children with CCHS, Chiari II malformation, and others, it would not be successful in the child with progressive neuromuscular or neurodegenerative diseases. Older infants and toddlers may use a Passy-Muir one-way speaking valve while awake, allowing for vocalization and use of the upper airway on exhalation. The child with CCHS will likely have success with training of the upper airway, but this would not be successful in the child with altered pharyngeal tone (Chiari II malformation) or neuromuscular weakness. The paced child with CCHS may also be assessed for capping of the tracheostomy tube during pacing while awake, thereby allowing for inspiration and exhalation via the upper airway. Nonetheless, these 24-h/d supported CCHS patients will still require a tracheostomy for the nighttime mechanical ventilation. It might also be feasible in the older child with an entirely normal airway to provide diaphragm pacing while awake and positive-pressure mask ventilation while asleep, thereby eliminating the need for a tracheostomy. However, because respiratory infections commonly increase the need for ventilatory support, such a child would require interim endotracheal intubation to allow for adequate ventilation.

Those children with CCHS or other disorders who consistently require ventilatory support during sleep only and who are able to cooperate can be considered as candidates for noninvasive support with either positive-pressure mask ventilation or negative-pressure ventilation. If successful, a tracheal decannulation can be considered, but with the recognition that in the event of a significant respiratory infection, endotracheal intubation will be necessary. Conversely, the child who usually requires ventilatory support only during sleep may require ventilatory assistance awake and asleep during an intercurrent illness. Regardless of the method of ventilatory support, the goal is to normalize oxygenation and ventilation for each child. Typically the recommendation is for hemoglobin saturation values $\geq$ 95%. The end-tidal carbon dioxide range may be broad with limits of 30 to 45 mm Hg, allowing for variation with sleep position.

For each of the above-described modalities, the goal is to match the patient with the optimal technology for her or his life-style needs. Although diaphragm pacing is not typically recommended in the young child who requires therapy only at night, in the older child with CCHS this might be an appropriate consideration.

LONG-TERM MANAGEMENT Long-term care requires the coordinated efforts of a devoted family and a primary care physician in conjunction with a subspecialist and team with recognized expertise in disorders of respiratory control. Routine evaluations should include assessment of growth, speech, and neurologic development. Periodically, evaluation should include an in-hospital evaluation with detailed recording during sleep and wakefulness in a respiratory physiology laboratory to monitor the adequacy of ventilation. Because many infants with CCHS appear to acquire awake hypoventilation at 2 to 3 years of age, when the natural decrease in respiratory frequency occurs, toddlers in this age group must be closely monitored to assure adequate ventilatory support. With advancing age, physiological assessment of oxygenation and ventilation during exercise and recovery from exercise should be performed on a routine basis. An echocardiogram should be performed every 6 months to evaluate for right ventricular hypertrophy and pulmonary hypertension, which, if present, indicate that ventilatory support is not optimal. A Holter recording should be considered annually to assess for transient arrhythmias, especially in the event of dizziness or syncope. Bronchoscopy should be performed if there is a suspicion of tracheostomy-related complications or if there is difficulty in phonation when the child is breathing spontaneously. Detailed developmental and ophthalmologic assessments should be performed every 12 months to verify that the child is on track and to provide guidance for intervention.

LONG-TERM OUTCOME

Although little is known about the long-term outcome of all patients with chronic alveolar hypoventilation, published data show prolonged survival of children with CCHS as well as overall good quality of life. Because patients with CCHS have unique physiological responses to exercise and infections, they are not like other children who require chronic mechanical ventilation. It is difficult to determine whether adverse neurodevelopmental outcome is related to a diffuse central nervous system process specific to the underlying disorder or if it is secondary to intermittent or previously undetected hypoxemia. These studies of neurodevelopmental follow-up serve to emphasize the importance of early diagnosis, ongoing vigilant care in the day-to-day management, with appropriate ongoing involvement of professionals with experience with disorders of respiratory control.

References

Mellins RB, Balfour HH Jr, Turino GM, Winters RW: Failure of automatic control of ventilation (Ondine's curse). Medicine 49(6):487–504, 1970

Weese-Mayer DE, Brouillette RT, Naidich TP, McClone DG, Hunt CE: Magnetic resonance imaging and computerized tomography in central hypoventilation. Am Rev Respir Dis 137:393–398, 1988

Weese-Mayer DE, Hunt CE, Brouillette RT, Silvestri JM: Diaphragm pacing in infants and children. J Pediatr 120(1):1–8, 1992

Weese-Mayer DE, Shannon DC, Keens TG, Silvestri JM: American Thoracic Society statement on idiopathic congenital central hypoventilation syndrome: diagnosis and management. Am J Respir Crit Care Med 160: 368–373, 1999

Weese-Mayer DE, Silvestri JM, Kenny AS, et al: Diaphragm pacing with a quadripolar phrenic nerve electrode: an international study. Pace 19: 1311–1319, 1996

Weese-Mayer DE, Silvestri JM, Menzies LJ, Morrow-Kenny AS, Hunt CE, Hauptman SA: Congenital central hypoventilation syndrome: diagnosis, management, and long-term outcome in thirty-two children. J Pediatr 120:381–387, 1992

23.5.2 Apnea and SIDS

Jean M. Silvestri and Debra E. Weese-Mayer

APNEA

Apnea is a common problem in premature infants. The incidence is inversely related to gestational age, with >50% of infants <32 weeks of gestation having significant apnea. Apnea in a term infant is always considered abnormal and requires a thorough evaluation.

DEFINITIONS Apnea must be distinguished from periodic breathing. Apnea is the absence of respiratory airflow and is classified as *central* (no respiratory effort, no airflow), *obstructive* (respiratory effort, usually with paradoxic inward movement of the chest and outward movement of the abdomen, absent airflow), or *mixed* (both central and obstructive components). Apnea may be pathologic if there is cessation of airflow for ≥20 seconds or shorter, associated with significant bradycardia or cyanosis. Periodic breathing, defined as three or more respiratory pauses of ≥3 seconds with less than 20 seconds of respiration between pauses, is a normal and common pattern for preterm infants. In the laboratory, it can be induced by mild hypoxia and can be abolished by increasing inspired oxygen or carbon dioxide.

Apnea of prematurity is periodic breathing with apnea in a preterm infant that usually resolves by 37 weeks of gestation but may persist for several weeks past term. The terms *apnea of prematurity*, or *apnea of infancy* (AOI) in term infants, should be used only after all other underlying causes for apnea have been ruled out or treated. If apnea or prematurity is associated with hypoxemia or bradycardia, then intervention with monitoring and supplemental oxygen may be indicated.

It is important to note that normal and appropriate infant behavior can be misinterpreted as serious apnea. For example, the newborn infant who is fed by an anxious or inexperienced person may choke and stop breathing for a few seconds as an airway protection reflex. Similarly, an overzealous caretaker may observe normal 5- to 6-second episodes of respiratory pauses and report them as being of longer duration. Breath-holding spells may also cause breathing irregularities, but their relationship to disciplinary or painful stimuli in awake infants provides clues to this diagnosis.

ETIOLOGY In the preterm infant, recurrent apnea may be multifactorial and related to delayed maturation of cardiorespiratory control. Indeed, in areas where premature infants are routinely discharged from hospital with heart rate/impedance monitors, the monitoring devices themselves may erroneously signal the presence of apnea where none is actually present (see Sec. 4.2.1). However, in infants with recurrent apnea, specific pathophysiological disorders must be considered. These include:

- Hypoxia with decreased oxygen delivery (pulmonary and cardiac disease, patent ductus arteriosus, anemia)
- Infection (pneumonia, bronchiolitis, sepsis, meningitis, necrotizing enterocolitis, pertussis, botulism)
- Central nervous system pathology (asphyxia, seizures, hydrocephalus, IVH, CNS malformations, intentional and unintentional trauma)
- Metabolic disorders (hypoglycemia, hypocalcemia, hypo/hypernatremia, hypermagnesemia, hyperammonemia)

- Perinatal and postnatal drugs (maternal drug abuse, magnesium sulfate, morphine, sedatives, antihistamines, anesthetics)
- Cardiac arrhythmias
- Environmental factors (high or low ambient temperature, NG tubes, suctioning, bilirubin mask)
- Anatomic factors (upper airway malformation, vascular rings, diaphragm dysfunction)
- Gastroesophageal reflux or oropharyngeal aspiration

Of the etiologic factors listed above, the most frequent causes of recurrent apnea are sleep-associated hypoxemia and gastroesophageal reflux.

The differential diagnosis and evaluation of the infant with apnea is determined by consideration of several factors. Age of onset of apnea may provide a clue to the diagnosis. A thorough history and physical examination, directed at associated symptoms and signs of the potential etiologies listed above, is essential. Laboratory testing and imaging procedures should be directed by the history and physical examination.

MANAGEMENT The management of recurrent apnea depends on the etiology. Infants are typically monitored with heart rate/impedance monitors, and it should be noted that impedance-based monitors detect chest wall motion and thus will not detect obstructive apnea unless the episode produces significant bradycardia. Therefore, it is important to monitor heart rate and hemoglobin saturation in those infants with apnea to determine the frequency and severity of episodes as well as careful observation and appropriate diagnostic tests to detect any associated conditions.

If treatable causes are excluded, treatment options from least invasive to most invasive include tactile stimulation, low-flow oxygen, oscillating/rocking water beds, methylxanthines, nasal CPAP, nasal ventilation, and intubation with mechanical ventilation. Methylxanthines may be effective in the treatment of apnea of prematurity by stimulating central respiratory drive. Theophylline and caffeine reduce the severity and incidence of apnea; dosing regimens vary, and serum levels should be monitored periodically. However, side effects of increased metabolic rate and feeding intolerance may pose further problems for the VLBW infant and for those infants with gastroesophageal reflux. Methylxanthines can cause tachycardia, jitteriness, GI distress, and seizures.

FOLLOW-UP Apnea of prematurity typically resolves at term, but in some infants, particularly those of VLBW (24–27 weeks of gestation), apnea may persist postterm. Rarely, term infants will be diagnosed with apnea of infancy as well. Regional practices vary as to the period of time an infant needs to be observed for the absence of apnea to be discharged without a home monitor. Twelve- and 24-hour recordings of chest wall impedance and ECG (pneumograms) are not recommended before discharge because they are not predictive of subsequent apnea or SIDS. If monitoring is chosen at nursery discharge, basic cardiopulmonary resuscitation should be taught to all caregivers. Should subsequent apneic/bradycardia episodes be suggested either by caregiver report or by frequent monitor alarms, a memory monitor (also known as event recording or documented monitoring, which are recordings of impedance and electrocardiogram to distinguish true from false alarms) is recommended because of the high incidence of false alarms.

It is important to recognize that neither apnea of infancy nor apnea of prematurity is a risk factor for SIDS. However, prematurity itself is a risk factor for SIDS. A review of factors that reduce the risk for SIDS (supine sleep position, smoke-free environment, firm sleeping surface, avoidance of overbundling or overheating of the infant) is recommended at the time of discharge for all caregivers.

APPARENT LIFE-THREATENING EVENTS

An apparent life-threatening event (ALTE) is defined as an acute unexpected episode that is frightening to the observer and is characterized by some combination of apnea (central and occasionally obstructive), color change (usually cyanotic or pallid but occasionally erythematous or plethoric), marked change in muscle tone (usually marked limpness, rarely stiffness), and choking or gagging that requires significant intervention (vigorous stimulation, mouth-to-mouth breathing, or full cardiopulmonary resuscitation) to revive the infant and restore normal breathing. Typically, infants with ALTE are less than 18 months of age, and the acute episode often resolves by the time the infant is examined by a health-care provider. Note that the definition of ALTE may include apnea, but ALTE can also occur without apparent apnea as well. The definition of an ALTE is often confounded by the subjective nature of eyewitness accounts and by the unknown efficacy of any resuscitative efforts initiated. In those infants who have experienced an ALTE for whom no specific cause can be found, the diagnosis of idiopathic ALTE is given. The term ALTE should not be applied to infants who present with stupor or coma or to those infants with known underlying disorders known to cause severe symptoms. Etiology and management are discussed in Sec. 4.3.2.

SUDDEN INFANT DEATH SYNDROME

Sudden unexpected infant death has been described for centuries, even referenced in biblical times. However, it was not accepted as a death certificate diagnosis until the late 1960s. In the 1970s the US Congress legislated the need to increase public awareness of SIDS. A definition and an ICD-9 code, vital to insure uniformity in the diagnosis of SIDS, was not established until 1979.

DEFINITION SIDS is defined as the sudden death of an infant under 1 year of age that remains unexplained after thorough case investigation, including performance of a complete autopsy, examination of the death scene, and review of the clinical history. In the United States SIDS is the third leading cause of death in infants after congenital anomalies and conditions related to prematurity. Through decades of research, the pathology and epidemiology of SIDS are better understood, and intriguing clues to its etiology have come from the identification of pre- and postnatal risk factors. Despite these advances, the causes of SIDS remain unknown.

INCIDENCE Through identification of modifiable risk factors, especially the recommendation that infants sleep on their backs or sides, the incidence of SIDS has decreased dramatically. In the United States, slow declines in SIDS were observed in the 1980s (SIDS rate 1.51/1000 live births in 1979, 1.46/1000 live births in 1983, and 1.40/1000 live births in 1988). However, from 1995 to 2000, SIDS rates fell over 40% after campaigns by the American Academy of Pediatrics endorsed nonprone sleeping in 1992 and "back to sleep" in 1996. In 1998, the SIDS death rate was 0.64/1000.

PATHOLOGY In the 1970s Naeye described tissue markers of hypoxia associated with SIDS deaths. These included abnormal thickening of the smooth muscle in the small pulmonary arteries, hypertrophy of the right ventricle, increased periadrenal brown fat, increased hepatic erythropoiesis, increased chromaffin in the adrenal medulla, gliosis in the brainstem, and carotid body abnormalities. However, no markers have been consistently identified in subsequent studies. Abnormalities of the CNS found in victims of SIDS include delayed myelination, increased brain weight, periventricular and subcortical leukomalacia, and increased density of brainstem dendritic spines. These are nonspecific findings, and hence, more detailed studies examining neuropathology and neurotransmitters in the brain and brainstem associated with cardiorespiratory function and arousal are being performed to further understand pathologic mechanisms. For example, the recent finding of more neuronal apoptosis in the hippocampus and brainstem of SIDS victims as compared to controls lends more weight to the argument that SIDS is triggered by an acute hypoxemic event.

The diagnosis of SIDS is one of exclusion. All aspects of any sudden unexpected infant death must be thoroughly reviewed, emphasizing the importance of a complete anatomic and biochemical autopsy, review of infant and family history, and examination of the death scene. Recent reports suggest that rare inborn errors of metabolism, such as medium-chain acyl-CoA dehydrogenase (MCAD) deficiency, should be excluded by postmortem genetic analysis. In addition, national guidelines are published for death scene investigation. Death scene investigations can help to rule out accidental, environmental, and intentional causes of sudden unexplained infant deaths and provide information to researchers on risk factors for SIDS.

EPIDEMIOLOGY SIDS is rare in the first month of life, with the peak incidence occurring between 2 and 4 months of age, and with ~90% of all SIDS deaths occurring before 6 months of age. Although deaths attributable to SIDS have been reported in the second year of life, the diagnosis of SIDS is not recommended for infants who die beyond 1 year of age.

SIDS occurs more often in boys than girls. The incidence of SIDS increases with decreasing gestational age and is increased in infants with intrauterine growth retardation. A seasonal incidence is also observed, with higher rates in cold-weather months irrespective of the hemisphere one lives in. Deaths typically occur after midnight and before 8 a.m. The incidence is higher among African-American and Native American infants as compared to white, Asian, and Hispanic infants. Although the vast majority of infants with SIDS are thought to have been asleep when they died, compelling and reliable accounts describe the syndrome as occurring in awake infants.

ENVIRONMENTAL RISK FACTORS FOR SIDS In examining risk factors associated with SIDS it is striking that sociodemographic factors often play more of a role than medical factors. The following are characteristic maternal and antenatal risk factors associated with an increased SIDS risk: low socioeconomic status, young maternal age, higher parity, shorter interpregnancy interval, late or absent prenatal care, maternal infections (UTI and STD), prenatal cocaine and opiate exposure, and smoking, both during pregnancy and passive exposure after birth. Smoking remains a highly significant and modifiable risk factor in the "back to sleep" era.

Although past data have suggested that SIDS risk is increased in an infant whose sibling has died of SIDS, more recent data cast doubt on this possibility. Interpretation of the SIDS sibling data is often confounded by the lack of a consistent definition for SIDS, the age range of SIDS victims, and absence of a death scene investigation. Also, it is unclear how these data have been influenced by the "back to sleep" recommendation. Nonetheless, overall there appears to be a slightly higher risk of SIDS and other infant mortality among SIDS siblings. There are also other distinguishing infant risk factors. Although the risk of SIDS is increased among preterm infants, apnea of prematurity is *not* a risk factor for SIDS. Infants who are breast-fed have a decreased incidence of SIDS; however, breast-feeding appears to have less of a protective effect in the "back to sleep" era. Infants who have had a prior ALTE have an increased risk of SIDS. There is no statistical association of SIDS and immunizations; recent studies even suggest that receiving immunizations (DTP and OPV) appears to have a protective effect.

SLEEPING POSITION AND SIDS RISK The risk of SIDS is decreased in those infants who are positioned on their backs to sleep, on a firm sleeping surface, without loose bedcovers, and who are not overbundled or overheated. Although cosleeping (infant and mother in the same bed) can alter sleep patterns of the mother and infant, there are no data to support the proposition that cosleeping decreases SIDS. However, cosleeping under certain conditions such as maternal alcohol use and cigarette smoking may actually increase the risk of SIDS.

The single risk factor that has had the greatest impact on reduction of SIDS rates has been placing infants on their backs to sleep. Data emerged in the early 1990s from New Zealand demonstrating that infant sleep position, cigarette smoking, and lack of breast-feeding accounted for a high proportion of SIDS deaths. Fortunately, these are behaviors that are amenable to intervention, with the simplest being altering infant sleep position from prone to supine. After intervention campaigns in New Zealand and other countries, SIDS rates dramatically fell. Even though worldwide SIDS rates fell, it took longer for the acceptance of the "back to sleep" message in the United States. The prevalence of prone sleeping in the United States has finally decreased at the end of the century, and this has been associated with a decreased incidence of SIDS in the United States as well. In conjunction with intervention campaigns, there have been attempts to guide infant caretakers to avoid certain SIDS risk factors, that is, those factors that one can modify.

Although one cannot predict the infant who will die of SIDS, one can identify and modify environmental risk factors that may reduce the risk. These modifiable risk factors include smoking cessation or at a minimum decreasing the number of cigarettes smoked during pregnancy because this is a dose-dependent effect, maintaining a smoke-free environment for the infant, placing an infant on the back to sleep, using a firm sleeping surface without loose bedding, and not overheating or overbundling the infant. In addition, those infants who are "secondary" prone sleepers (infants not placed prone but who turn to prone) or inexperienced prone sleepers (infants not usually placed prone and then placed prone) are also at increased risk for SIDS. Thus, it is of particular importance that this education and practice of avoidance of SIDS risk factors should extend to all caregivers of infants under 12 months of age including babysitters and daycare providers.

PATHOPHYSIOLOGY The strong association of prone sleeping and SIDS has led to a number of studies examining the mechanisms that may account for this association. Studies have demonstrated increased quiet sleep and sleep efficiency when prone, thus suggesting an inability to respond to potentially adverse stimuli. The prone position has also been associated with airway obstruction and possible airway occlusion, thermal imbalance with potential hyperthermia, altered arousal responses to auditory stimuli, and decreased cardiac responses to auditory stimuli. Prone sleeping

on a soft sleeping surface with loose bedding can result in the rebreathing of exhaled air and subsequent hypercapnia.

Although the causes of SIDS remain unknown, numerous hypotheses exist. For many years much research was driven by the "apnea hypothesis," ie, that sleep-associated apnea was the main mechanism and the terminal event in SIDS. This led to the use of home cardiorespiratory monitoring to detect prolonged apnea and bradycardia. However, subsequent studies and use of memory monitors did not show a strong association of apnea in SIDS victims before death. Moreover, no study has demonstrated that home cardiorespiratory monitoring saves lives. Although there is decreased enthusiasm for the apnea hypothesis, home memory monitoring has revealed episodes of terminal bradycardia before death. These latter episodes could be interpreted as a secondary event before death.

Autonomic nervous system dysfunction has been implicated in SIDS. Some investigators have found evidence of brainstem dysfunction with respiratory pattern abnormalities, altered cardiac control, prolonged Q-T interval, abnormal chemoreceptor sensitivity, deficient arousal responses, inability to self-resuscitate, and abnormal thermoregulation.

As a result, current evidence supports the following speculation: It is likely that multiple risk factors can act through different mechanisms on a vulnerable infant at a vulnerable point during gestation or infancy and result in a sudden terminal cardiorespiratory event. This concept was characterized and proposed by Filiano and Kinney as the "triple risk model" and emphasizes that for SIDS to occur there must be an interaction among three critical conditions: (1) a vulnerable infant who is exposed to (2) an exogenous stressor during a (3) critical developmental period of rapid growth and development.

Research continues to improve understanding of the pathophysiological processes occurring in SIDS so efforts can be made to identify at-risk infants, provide intervention, and avert these tragic deaths. However, all of these data rely on studying large populations of infants and retrospectively examining the responses of infants who have died of SIDS, studies of infants with severe ALTEs that survive, or autopsy studies. As SIDS incidence continues to decrease, all of these studies will be more difficult to perform.

SIDS, like many other medical disorders, may have more than one explanation and thus more than one means of prevention. This may also account for the varied characteristics of SIDS infants. Avoidance of SIDS risk factors may be increasing the survival of infants who may otherwise have died; however, it is unknown whether vulnerable infants will go on to mature and pass on an as yet unidentified and potentially inheritable risk factor.

References

Apnea

Miller MJ, Martin RJ: Apnea of prematurity. Clin Perinatol 19(4):789–808, 1992

Weese-Mayer DE, Brouillette RT, Morrow AS, Conway LP, Klemka-Walden LM, Hunt CE: Assessing validity of infant monitor alarms with event recording. J Pediatr 115:702–708, 1989

Weese-Mayer DE, Morrow AS, Conway LP, Brouillette RT, Silvestri JM: Assessing clinical significance of apnea exceeding fifteen seconds with event recording. J Pediatr 117(4):568–574, 1990

ALTE

Brooks JG: Apparent life-threatening events and apnea of infancy. Clin Perinatol 19(4):809–838, 1992

Samuels MP, Poets CF, Noyes JP, Hartmann H, Hewertson J, Southall DP: Diagnosis and management after life threatening events in infants and young children who received cardiopulmonary resuscitation. Br Med J 306:489–492, 1993

SIDS

Dwyer T, Ponsonby AB, Newman NM, Gibbons LE: Prospective cohort study of prone sleeping position in sudden infant death syndrome. Lancet 337:1244–1247, 1991

Filiano J, Kinney HC: A perspective on neuropathologic findings in victims of the sudden infant death syndrome: the triple risk model. Biol Neonate 15:194–197, 1990

Fleming PJ, Blair PS, Bacon C, et al: Environment of infants during sleep and risk of the sudden infant death syndrome: results of 1993–5 case-control study for confidential inquiry into stillbirths and deaths in infancy. Br Med J 313:191–195, 1996

Hoffman HJ, Hoffman LS: Epidemiology of the sudden infant death syndrome: maternal, neonatal, and postneonatal risk factors. Clin Perinatol 19(4):717–738, 1992.

Kinney HC, Filiano JJ, Sleeper LA, Mandell F, Valdes-Dapena M, Frost W: Decreased muscarinic receptor binding in the arcuate nucleus in sudden infant death syndrome. Science 269:1446–1450, 1995

Malloy MH, Hoffman HJ: Prematurity, sudden infant death syndrome, and age of death. Pediatrics 96:464–471, 1995

Mitchell EA, Ford RP, Stewart AW, et al: Smoking and the sudden infant death syndrome. Pediatrics 91:893–896, 1993

Mitchell EA, Scragg R, Stewart AW, et al: Results from the first year of the New Zealand cot death study. NZ Med 104:71–76, 1991

Panigraphy A, Filiano JJ, Sleeper LA, et al: Decreased kainate receptor binding in the arcuate nucleus of sudden infant death syndrome. J Neuropathol Exp Neurol 56:1253–1261, 1997

Ponsonby AL, Dwyer T, Gibbon LE, Cochrane JA, Wang Y-G: Factors potentiating the risk of sudden infant death syndrome associated with the prone position. N Engl J Med 329:377–382, 1993

Ramanathan R, Corwin MJ, Hunt CE, et al and CHIME: Cardiorespiratory events recorded on home monitors: comparison of healthy infants with those at increased risk for SIDS. JAMA 285:2199–2207, 2001

Schoendorf KC, Kiely JL: Relationship of sudden infant death syndrome to maternal smoking during and after pregnancy. Pediatrics 90:905–908, 1992

Valdes-Dalpena M: The sudden infant death syndrome: pathologic findings. Clin Perinatol 19(4):701–716, 1992

Waters KA, Meehan B, Huang JQ, Gravel RA, Michaud J, Cote A: Neuronal apoptosis in sudden infant death syndrome. Pediatr Res 45:166–172, 1999

Willinger M, James LS, Catz C: Defining the sudden infant death syndrome (SIDS): deliberations of an expert panel convened by the National Institute of Child Health and Human Development. Pediatr Pathol 11:677–684, 1991

Useful Website

www.sidsalliance.org

23.5.3   Obstructive Sleep Apnea and Other Sleep-Related Disorders

Sally L. Davidson Ward

Perhaps the most enduring description of the impact of obstructive sleep apnea in childhood was penned by Charles Dickens in 1837 in his classic *The Pickwick Papers.* Joe, the "fat boy," undoubtedly suffered from obesity-hypoventilation syndrome, also known as Pickwickian syndrome. Throughout the novel Joe snores loudly, falls asleep during his daytime activities, and eats voraciously. Sir William Osler wrote the first medical description of pediatric obstructive sleep apnea in 1892: "Chronic enlargement of the tonsillar tissues is an affectation of great importance, and may influence in an extraordinary way the mental and bodily development of children.... At night the child's sleep is greatly disturbed; the respirations are loud and snoring, and there are sometimes prolonged pauses, followed by deep, noisy inspirations. The child may wake up in a paroxysm of shortness of breath." However, it was not until nearly a century had passed that the first series of eight children with obstructive sleep apnea confirmed by polysomnography was reported by Guilleminault in 1976.

Obstructive sleep apnea syndrome (OSAS) in children is very different from that in adults. These differences must be kept in mind, as they limit the value of applying the principles used to diagnose and treat adults to children. Pediatric OSAS is a disorder characterized by loud, habitual snoring, episodes of complete or partial upper airway obstruction, hypoventilation, hypoxemia, and abnormal sleep patterns.

Obstructive apnea is the result of complete upper airway obstruction during sleep with cessation of airflow at the nose and mouth despite respiratory efforts. This is distinct from central apnea, in which cessation of airflow is caused by a lack of respiratory efforts. Many children with OSAS actually exhibit partial airway obstruction associated with hypoxemia and hypoventilation rather than complete airway obstruction; this can be termed obstructive hypoventilation. Discrete episodes of partial airway obstruction identified by a reduction in airflow, especially with associated paradoxic breathing, hypoxemia, and arousal from sleep, are termed obstructive hypopneas.

EPIDEMIOLOGY

OSAS occurs in children of all ages, including neonates. Craniofacial anomalies are responsible for most OSAS in infancy. Beyond infancy, the peak incidence is between 3 and 6 years of age, which is the age when the tonsils and adenoids are the largest in relation to the oropharyngeal size. OSAS has been estimated to occur in nearly 1% of 4- to 5-year-old children, whereas habitual snoring occurs in about 10%. In the prepubertal age range, it occurs equally among boys and girls. This is in contrast to adult OSAS, where there is a distinct male predominance.

NORMAL RESPIRATION DURING SLEEP

Sleep is a period of vulnerability for the respiratory system. Ventilation during sleep is decreased compared to the awake state and varies with the stage of sleep. During non–rapid eye movement (NREM) sleep, breathing is regular, but tidal volume and respiratory rate are decreased. This results in a decrease in minute ventilation, a decrease in lung volume, and a marked increase in upper airway resistance. During wakefulness, breathing is under the dual control of involuntary (or chemical control of breathing) and voluntary drives (behavioral control of breathing). This allows for coordination between the need to adjust breathing for voluntary activities of respiration, such as speaking and swallowing, with the need to maintain normal oxygen and carbon dioxide levels as metabolic demands change. However, during NREM sleep, neurologic control of breathing is completely dependent on chemoreceptor responses, and voluntary control of breathing is absent.

During rapid eye movement (REM) sleep, voluntary control of breathing predominates, and the breathing pattern is more irregular, with a variable respiratory rate and tidal volume and frequent pauses in respiration. Another characteristic of REM sleep is the active inhibition of skeletal muscle tone, which spares only the diaphragm and the extraocular muscles. Inhibition of the activity of the muscles of the chest wall during REM sleep results in a further decrease in lung volume. Hypotonia of the upper airway muscles increases the risk of obstructive apnea during REM sleep. In addition, both hypoxic and hypercapnic ventilatory drives decrease during sleep. During wakefulness, there is a continuous barrage of sensory input to the central nervous system, which serves as a nonspecific stimulus to ventilation. The withdrawal of this so-called "wakefulness stimulus" is another important reason for the relative depression of ventilation during sleep. Thus, during sleep, there is an increase in $PaCO_2$ and a decrease in PaO_2 and S_aO_2 as compared to wakefulness. Other important respiratory reflexes, such as coughing and swallowing, are depressed or absent during sleep. This leads to an accumulation of respiratory secretions during sleep. It is not surprising, therefore, that the effects of these normal changes in the respiratory system that occur with sleep are magnified in patients with underlying pulmonary or upper airway disease.

In infants, the changes that occur during sleep in pulmonary and chest wall mechanics, upper airway resistance, ventilatory muscle function, and ventilatory pattern are even more pronounced. This is an important consideration because infants spend more time sleeping than older children and adults, and a greater percentage of sleep time is spent in REM sleep, when upper airway function is most compromised. In REM sleep in infants, functional residual capacity (FRC) is decreased from the loss of chest wall muscle tone and the more compliant chest wall. The upper airway is also more compliant, predisposing to airway obstruction. In neonates, hypoxia results in respiratory depression rather than stimulating ventilation. In the first few months of life, infants are preferential nose breathers. Thus, upper airway obstruction with OSAS can occur with isolated nasal obstruction. Nasal congestion secondary to an otherwise mild viral upper respiratory tract infection can result in significant respiratory distress in young infants, especially during sleep and feeding.

Airway obstruction is observed frequently during periodic breathing in preterm infants. Periodic breathing is a respiratory pattern characterized by repetitive short apneas separated by bursts of normal breathing. Periodic breathing is a normal feature of the respiratory pattern during sleep in infancy. Obstructed breaths are commonly identified at the resumption of respiratory efforts following periodic apnea. An imbalance between central drive to the diaphragm and the upper airway dilating muscles may exist in premature infants. It should be appreciated, then, that when OSAS occurs in infancy, it is superimposed on these preexisting features of normal infant sleep and breathing.

PATHOPHYSIOLOGY OF OSAS

The pathophysiology of OSAS is multifactorial and not fully understood. OSAS occurs when the balance between the factors maintaining upper airway patency and those promoting airway collapse is disturbed. This balance is determined by the interactions among central ventilatory responses to hypoxia, hypercapnia and airway occlusion, upper airway neuromuscular tone, the effects of sleep state and arousal, and the anatomic size and resistance of the upper airway.

Because the normal upper airway is a single structure burdened with multiple functions, it is necessarily a complex area and involves the coordinated activity of more than 30 pairs of muscles. The pharynx must be mobile and compliant in order to facilitate speaking and swallowing. However, the respiratory function of the pharynx would be best served by a rigid tube, and muscles of the upper airway are also called on to maintain the upper airway patent. The need to serve these dual, and in many ways opposing, functions underlies the complexity and instability of the upper airway.

One of the pharyngeal dilators, the genioglossus muscle, forms the base of the tongue and receives innervation from the hypoglossal nerve (cranial nerve IX). The nucleus of the hypoglossal nerve receives central respiratory control input. In adults, a decrease in phasic genioglossus activity is associated with the onset of obstructive sleep apnea, whereas an increase in activity accompanies termination of the obstructive event. However, genioglossus hypotonia is not felt to play a role in childhood OSA, but, similar to adults, an increase in genioglossus tone terminates airway obstruction. In premature infants, sustained genioglossus activity was not present during normal breathing, but an increase in genioglossus activity occurred at the termination of obstructive apnea.

Recent evidence demonstrates that the upper airway in both children and adults behaves as predicted by the Starling resistor model. This model has been well described in a number of biological systems such as blood vessels and the lower airways. It predicts that in the upper airway, under conditions of flow limitation, maximal inspiratory airflow is determined by the pressure changes upstream (toward the nose) from a collapsible site of the upper airway. This occurs independent of the downstream (toward the trachea) pressures generated by the diaphragm. The pressure at which the upper airway collapses has been termed the critical closing pressure. This value can be used to quantify the tendency of the upper airway to collapse. Studies of the critical closing pressure demonstrate that adults and children with OSAS have more collapsible upper airways than either normal subjects or snorers without OSAS. These studies also show that children have a less collapsible upper airway than adults.

This may partially explain why OSAS in adults is generally more severe than in children. Normal infants, as compared to older children, have intermediate critical closing pressures consistent with the increased tendency of the infant airway to collapse.

Patients with OSAS tend to have either a narrow upper airway (eg, from adenotonsillar hypertrophy, craniofacial anomalies, or obesity) or abnormal upper airway neuromotor tone (eg, from muscular dystrophy, myopathy, or cerebral palsy). Even patients with severe OSAS usually maintain upper airway patency during wakefulness through the tonic activity of upper airway muscles. When children with OSAS fall asleep, the wakefulness stimulus is withdrawn, and the upper airway collapses, with resultant complete or partial airway obstruction. Upper airway obstruction is associated with increasingly vigorous, often paradoxic, respiratory efforts. Eventually, obstructive apneas are terminated by a gasp. In most adults with OSAS, the increased upper airway tone terminating an apnea is secondary to arousal from sleep. Arousals are usually manifested as transient changes in sleep state and body movements. Arousals may occur hundreds of times each night, causing sleep fragmentation and deprivation with excessive daytime somnolence as the result. In children with OSAS, arousals occur less frequently, and repeated complete or partial airway obstruction (obstructive apneas, hypopneas, or hypoventilation) may continue without arousal. For this reason, the overall sleep pattern (termed sleep architecture) in children with OSAS may be normal, with normal proportions of REM and NREM sleep. This may explain why children with OSAS are less likely than adults to present with a complaint of excessive daytime sleepiness. Abnormal ventilatory control has been proposed to play a role in adult OSAS. But children with OSAS secondary to adenotonsillar hypertrophy have normal ventilatory responses to hypercapnia and hypoxia during wakefulness. This suggests that, unlike the case in adults, abnormal central ventilatory drive plays little role in childhood OSAS.

CONDITIONS THAT PREDISPOSE TO OSAS

In children, decreased airway size secondary to adenotonsillar hypertrophy is the leading cause of OSAS. However, the severity of OSAS cannot be predicted simply by the size of the tonsils and adenoids. In most children, OSAS resolves completely following adenotonsillectomy. Children with sickle cell disease have a high incidence of OSAS because of lymphoid hyperplasia involving the tonsils and adenoids. This may also develop from significant hypoxemia during sleep as a result of underlying lung disease.

Infants and children with craniofacial anomalies are at high risk for OSAS. Any anomaly associated with midfacial hypoplasia, micrognathia, macroglossia, hypotonia, malformations of cranial base, or obesity may cause OSAS. Children with Down syndrome are at especially high risk for OSAS because they have midfacial hypoplasia, hypotonia, macroglossia, and are frequently overweight. Unrecognized or undertreated hypothyroidism can exacerbate OSAS in Down syndrome by depressing ventilatory responses.

Obesity is associated with severe OSAS. The incidence of OSAS in childhood obesity is not known, but many overweight children do not have OSAS, suggesting that obesity alone does not cause sleep-disordered breathing. Fat deposition in the pharynx and increased work of breathing because of the mechanical load imposed on the chest and abdomen may contribute to the severity of OSAS in obese children. Because the incidence of obesity in childhood is on the rise in the United States, obesity-related OSAS will be of increasing importance in the future.

Neuromuscular disease increases the risk of developing OSAS. Children with cerebral palsy have an increased incidence of OSAS because of incoordination or spasticity of their upper airway muscles. They may also have upper airway obstruction during wakefulness. Frequently, these children have associated problems with swallowing and upper airway reflexes that can cause chronic lung disease as a result of recurrent aspiration. Thus, in addition to OSAS, children with cerebral palsy may have hypoxemia during sleep. Patients with muscular dystrophy are at risk for OSAS because of weakness of the upper airway muscles. Obesity may also be present in these patients, further increasing the risk of OSAS. OSAS may precede the onset of respiratory failure caused by ventilatory muscle weakness.

Laryngomalacia is the most common cause of congenital stridor in infancy. It is usually a self-limited problem that improves with growth and maturation over the first year of life. However, severe laryngomalacia may also result in OSAS in infants. Frequently, infants with laryngomalacia sufficiently severe to cause OSAS also suffer from feeding difficulties and failure to thrive.

EVALUATION OF THE CHILD SUSPECTED OF OSAS

HISTORY   Most children with OSAS present with a history of loud, habitual snoring and difficulty breathing during sleep. Parents can

usually describe restlessness, retractions, paradoxic breathing, and episodes of increased respiratory effort associated with decreased or absent airflow. These episodes may be followed by gasping, choking, movement, or arousal. Cyanosis is only rarely noted. Enuresis is commonly reported in children with OSAS. Diaphoresis may be present. Children may assume an unusual sleep posture such as sleeping with their neck hyperextended in order to promote airway patency. For this reason they may sleep in an unusual location such as on the floor, couch, or in a chair. Many parents of children with OSAS are so concerned about their child's breathing that they sleep with their child and reposition them or shake them awake throughout the night to terminate apneas. Some children will come to medical attention after they have been excluded from daycare because of frightening respiratory behavior observed during daytime naps.

Even with dramatic breathing difficulties during sleep, breathing during wakefulness is usually relatively normal. Daytime symptoms related to adenotonsillar hypertrophy, such as mouth breathing, frequent upper respiratory tract infections, and dysphagia, may occur. Hyponasal or muffled speech may be present. Excessive daytime sleepiness is possible but is seen much less commonly than in adults with OSAS. In children presenting with excessive daytime sleepiness, narcolepsy and poor sleep habits are part of the differential diagnosis. Children with OSAS and obesity may have hypoventilation when awake and are prone to excessive daytime sleepiness.

OSAS in young infants is more subtle and therefore difficult to recognize because respiratory efforts are less forceful during obstructed breaths. Infant feeding can be compromised in OSAS because successful feeding requires unlabored and well-coordinated breathing. Upper airway obstruction causes infants to struggle and choke during feedings. A combination of increased effort to feed with decreased caloric intake may add to failure to thrive.

PHYSICAL EXAMINATION   Usually, physical examination during wakefulness is unremarkable (unless speech is abnormal and the tonsils are extremely large). This commonly leads to a delay in diagnosis, as the physician rarely has the opportunity to see the child asleep. The presence of mouth breathing, adenoidal facies, or craniofacial anomalies should be noted. The patency of the nasal passages should be assessed, and the pharynx should be evaluated for the size of the tongue, tonsils, and uvula. Palatal integrity should be inspected. Pectus excavatum may be present. The lungs are usually clear to auscultation. Cardiac examination may reveal signs of pulmonary hypertension. Muscle tone, developmental status, and growth parameters should be assessed.

During sleep, the child will usually snore loudly. Breathing is labored, and tachypnea, retractions (particularly suprasternal), and paradoxic inward motion of the chest during inspiration are present. During periods of complete obstruction, the patient will be noted to be making respiratory efforts, but no snoring is heard, airflow is absent, and breath sounds cannot be heard. Apneic episodes may be terminated by body movements or awakening. In infants the apneic episodes may be short, and the obstructed breaths difficult to appreciate because they often occur simultaneously with movement and awakening.

COMPLICATIONS OF OSAS

The complications of OSAS result from chronic nocturnal hypoxemia, increased work of breathing, and sleep disruption. A significant decrease in sleeping energy expenditure following adenotonsillectomy has been reported, and body weight percentiles often improve significantly following therapy. This suggests that growth failure may be related to increased energy expenditure during sleep. Elevated energy expenditure during sleep in OSAS may be secondary to increased work of breathing. Chronic hypoxemia and hypoventilation may lead to pulmonary hypertension or cor pulmonale. Systemic hypertension is common in adults with OSAS but is not seen with OSAS in children.

Severe neurobehavioral complications are infrequent. However, children may have developmental delay, poor school performance, hyperactivity, aggressive behavior, and social withdrawal. Rare cases of severe asphyxial brain damage, seizures, and coma have been reported. The frequency and significance of more subtle manifestations of cognitive impairment are yet to be determined. Excessive daytime sleepiness can occur in children with OSAS, especially if they are obese. Children with obesity-related OSAS may be unable to participate in school, family life, or other normal childhood activities because of their extreme sleepiness. Children with craniofacial anomalies and cerebral palsy may have underlying syndromes that include neurodevelopmental disabilities.

LABORATORY EVALUATION

POLYSOMNOGRAPHY Polysomnography is usually required to establish the diagnosis of OSAS, as history is often misleading. In addition, polysomnography can exclude other causes of sleep-related symptoms, such as nocturnal seizures or narcolepsy. It provides objective measures of severity, which are important in scheduling surgery and in planning the postoperative management. Polysomnography provides a baseline for those children whose condition does not resolve postoperatively.

With the use of appropriate facility, equipment, and personnel, polysomnography can be performed successfully in all infants and children. Technicians skilled in working with children are essential. It is preferable to study children during natural, nocturnal sleep rather than during sleep induced by sleep deprivation, sedation, or daytime nap. Nap polysomnography may have some value in children with uncomplicated OSAS secondary to adenotonsillar hypertrophy because it has been shown that an abnormal polysomnogram predicts an abnormal overnight polysomnographic study. However, a normal nap study does not rule out the possibility of significant OSAS.

During polysomnography, a wide variety of physiological variables are serially recorded. Sleep state, nasal and oral airflow, chest and abdominal wall motion, arterial oxygen saturation (SaO_2), oximeter pulse waveform, end-tidal (exhaled) PCO_2, and electrocardiogram are usually monitored. Because children with OSAS frequently demonstrate prolonged obstructive hypoventilation rather than discrete obstructive apneas, assessment of end-tidal CO_2 is essential. An audiovisual system to record snoring and sleep behavior is helpful. Sleep state is monitored by electroencephalogram (EEG), electrooculogram, and electromyogram. If a neurologic condition, such as nocturnal seizures, is suspected, additional EEG leads are used. The technician's observations are also important and are documented throughout the study. Physiological data can be recorded on a paper strip chart recorder or by a computerized acquisition system. Computerized systems allow for viewing the data in expanded or compressed time scales, can tabulate the number and severity of abnormal variables, and greatly decrease the space required to store patient records. Complete reliance on automated scoring systems is discouraged because currently available systems are not sufficiently accurate to separate artifacts from true events.

The accuracy of home studies has not yet been evaluated in the pediatric population.

The study should be scored for total sleep time, sleep efficiency, distribution of sleep stages, body movements and position, arousals, and sleep behaviors. The presence or absence of snoring, stridor, retractions, and gasping should be noted. Abnormalities in respiratory or cardiac rate should be reported. Respiratory events should be scored as central, obstructive, or as containing elements of both (mixed apnea) along with their number, length, and associated sequelae such as hypoxemia or arousal. Discrete episodes of partial airway obstruction may occur (hypopneas). Hypopneas are usually defined as a reduction in airflow of more than 50% from baseline. When accompanied by desaturation or arousal, a hypopnea may be more significant. The presence of hypoventilation, hypoxemia, and paradoxic breathing should be reported. Because breathing during sleep changes with age, age-appropriate normative values should be used. Table 23-8 outlines normal values for polysomnography in children. Brief periods of desaturation are common in normal infants less than 6 months of age, especially in the first weeks of life and with apnea or periodic breathing. These events appear to be part of normal respiratory behavior in young infants, although baseline arterial oxygen saturation is generally greater than 95%.

Some children have snoring, labored breathing, diaphoresis, paradoxic breathing, and disrupted sleep yet do not have discrete obstructive apneas or hypopneas. This has been termed the upper airway resistance syndrome (UARS). Adults with UARS present with excessive daytime sleepiness as a result of multiple arousals from sleep triggered by increased respiratory efforts. UARS is associated with large negative pressures in the thorax documented by intraesophageal pressure catheters. However, monitoring intraesophageal pressures is not practical for routine polysomnography in children, and the diagnostic criteria for UARS in children have not been defined. For example, it is not known if hypoxemia occurs frequently in UARS, and presence or absence of hypoventilation documented by end-tidal carbon dioxide measurements has not been reported. There may be overlap between UARS and obstructive hypoventilation in the pediatric population.

The timing of polysomnography in infants and children with craniofacial anomalies is important. The severity of OSAS may

TABLE 23-8

SUGGESTED NORMAL POLYSOMNOGRAPHY VALUES FOR CHILDREN AGE 1 TO 18 YEARS

TST (hours)	≥ 6
Sleep efficiency (%)	≥ 85
REM sleep (% TST)	15–30
NREM sleep (% TST)	55–80
Spontaneous arousals (N/h)	6–10 in children <10 years
	10–18 in children 10 to 18 years
Obstructive apnea index (N/h)	≤ 1
Peak $P_{ET}CO_2$ (mm Hg)	≤ 53
Duration of hypoventilation ($P_{ET}CO_2$ > 50 mm Hg) (%TST)	≤ 8
Lowest SaO_2 (%)	≥ 92
Desaturation events > 4% (N/h TST)	≤ 1.4

Sleep efficiency: TST as percentage of total recording time. TST = total sleep time; REM = rapid eye movement; NREM = non-REM; N/h = number of events per hour; $P_{ET}CO_2$ = end-tidal carbon dioxide tension; SaO_2 = arterial oxygen saturation. SOURCE: *Marcus CL, Omlin KJ, Basinski DJ, et al: Normal polysomnographic values for children and adolescents. Am Rev Respir Dis 146:1235–1239, 1992.*

change with growth, maturation, or after surgical procedures such as cleft palate or velopharyngeal incompetence repair. It is important to obtain a baseline study in infants and children with syndromes commonly associated with OSAS. This can then be used for comparison with subsequent studies if symptoms change, to document improvement following therapy, or to predict safety of general anesthesia. If a tracheotomy has been performed to maintain an unobstructed airway, repeat polysomnography with a small, occluded tracheostomy can be performed in the future to confirm resolution of OSAS after adequate facial growth or reconstructive surgery.

OTHER STUDIES Multiple sleep latency testing (MSLT) can be used to quantify excessive daytime sleepiness and to diagnose narcolepsy. In most children, extensive radiologic evaluation of the upper airway is unnecessary. A single lateral neck film for soft tissues of the nasopharynx will suffice for documenting hypertrophy of the adenoids or tonsils. In patients with craniofacial abnormalities, airway CT, MRI, fluoroscopy, or cephalometry can aid the planning of the surgical approach. However, there are few normative data for such studies in children. Patients with severe OSAS should have an electrocardiogram and echocardiogram to assess for pulmonary hypertension. Arterial blood gas measurement may be indicated for patients with severe obesity-related OSAS who are at risk for hypoventilation during wakefulness. The finding of an elevated bicarbonate or total CO_2 content in a sample of venous blood suggests that hypercarbia has been severe and chronic enough to provoke renal compensation for a chronic respiratory acidosis.

In the appropriate clinical setting, polysomnography may not always be necessary. For example, the obese child with snoring, a convincing history of periodic obstructed breathing when asleep, enlarged tonsils and adenoids, and mild right ventricular hypertrophy can be referred for otolaryngologic evaluation.

TREATMENT

The standard treatment of childhood OSAS is adenotonsillectomy. OSAS results from the function and relative size of the upper airway structures rather than the absolute size of the tonsils and adenoids. Therefore, both tonsils and adenoids should be removed, even if only one appears to be the primary abnormality. Adenotonsillectomy should be the initial treatment of OSAS in children with other predisposing factors (eg, obesity, Down syndrome), although further treatment may be necessary. Children with OSAS (especially very young children or those with underlying conditions) are at increased risk for postoperative complications and require careful monitoring postoperatively. OSAS can be temporarily treated with supplemental oxygen, continuous or bilevel positive airway pressure, or with nasopharyngeal tubes. Systemic or nasal steroids may decrease the size of airway lymphoid tissue. Supplemental oxygen in moderately severe OSAS may improve sleep architecture and respiratory pattern without increasing hypoventilation or central apneas. However, patients with severe OSAS, especially those with Down syndrome or obesity, may be subject to respiratory depression and hypoventilation if hypoxic drive is inhibited by supplemental oxygen. Thus, supplemental oxygen should not be used until simultaneous monitoring of arterial or end-tidal PCO_2 has confirmed that respiratory depression has not been induced.

Continuous positive airway pressure (CPAP) is used in those children who are not candidates for, or are not cured by, adenotonsillectomy. It is effective and well tolerated by most children but requires training and appropriately sized equipment. A significant number of children with OSAS in association with obesity or craniofacial anomalies continue to have symptoms postadenotonsillectomy and will benefit greatly from CPAP. CPAP is delivered via a nasal mask or prongs and acts as a pneumatic splint to maintain airway patency during sleep. The pressures necessary to overcome airway obstruction must be titrated during overnight polysomnography. Adequate preparation and training of the parents and child are essential to insure acceptance of the device. Skilled nurses, therapists, and technicians are required to select the correct equipment, monitor skin integrity at the mask site, and assess oxygenation. Patients who do not feel comfortable with CPAP may be successfully treated with bilevel positive airway pressure (BiPAP), which allows selection of different pressures during inspiration and exhalation.

Weight loss is recommended for all obese patients with OSAS but may be difficult to achieve. However, even modest weight loss can improve OSAS. Uvulopharyngopalatoplasty (UPPP) is frequently used to treat adults with OSAS. UPPP involves resection of the uvula, tonsils, and redundant palatal and pharyngeal mucosa. It has not been extensively evaluated in children but has been reported to be successful in the treatment of children with Down syndrome and cerebral palsy. Craniofacial surgery such as midface advancement with intermaxillary fixation for patients with midface hypoplasia can be helpful. Some infants with Pierre Robin sequence and mandibular hypoplasia or retrognathia will improve with a tongue-lip adhesion (glossopexy). This may enhance feeding as well as breathing. Prone positioning during sleep, supplemental oxygen, and home apnea and bradycardia monitoring are also useful supportive therapies in these infants because they will improve during the first year of life with growth and maturation. Epiglottoplasty will improve obstructive apnea in infancy caused by laryngomalacia. Tracheotomy may still be required if other measures are ineffective.

PROGNOSIS AND NATURAL HISTORY

The natural course and long-term prognosis of pediatric OSAS are unknown. Recurrence of OSAS in adolescents who had been successfully treated by adenotonsillectomy during childhood has been reported. This suggests that children with OSAS may be at risk for a recurrence of their disease in adulthood if they acquire additional risk factors such as obesity or alcohol ingestion. A genetic predisposition is being explored. In addition, little is known about the outcome of children who snore, yet have normal laboratory studies, although small series report a low risk for development of OSAS. The answer to the questions of when and if such children need to be reevaluated will need to be addressed by population-based longitudinal studies.

References

Betancourt D, Beckerman RC: Craniofacial syndromes. In: Beckerman RC, Brouillette RT, Hunt CE, eds: Respiratory Control Disorders in Infants and Children. Baltimore, Williams & Wilkins, 1992:294–305

Carroll JL, Loughlin GM: Obstructive sleep apnea syndrome in infants and children: diagnosis and management. In: Ferber R, Kryger M, eds: Principles and Practice of Sleep Medicine in the Child. Philadelphia, WB Saunders, 1995:193–216

Guilleminault C, Korobkin R, Winkle R: A review of 50 children with obstructive sleep apnea syndrome. Lung 159:275–287, 1981

Loughlin GM, Brouillette RT: Standards and indications for cardiopulmonary sleep studies in children. Am J Respir Crit Care Med 153:886–878, 1996

Mallory GB, Beckerman RC: Relationship between obesity and respiratory control abnormalities. In: Beckerman RC, Brouillette RT, Hunt CE, eds: Respiratory Control Disorders in Infants and Children. Baltimore, Williams & Wilkins, 1992:294–305

Marcus CL, Omlin KJ, Basinski DJ, et al: Normal polysomnographic values for children and adolescents. Am Rev Respir Dis 146:1235–1239, 1992

Osler W: Chronic tonsillitis. In: The Principles and Practice of Medicine. New York, Appleton and Co, 1892:335–339

Roloff DW, Aldrich MS: Sleep disorders and airway obstruction in newborns and infants. Otolaryngol Clin North Am 23:639–649, 1990

Ward SLD, Marcus CL: Obstructive sleep apnea in infants and young children. J Clin Neurophysiol 13:198–207, 1996

23.6   DISORDERS CAUSING INSPIRATORY OBSTRUCTION

Thomas A. Hazinski

The extrathoracic airways narrow during inspiration and widen during expiration. Obstruction of the extrathoracic airway causes intraluminal pressure distal to the obstruction to fall during inspiration, which adds to the obstruction. Inspiratory stridor, hoarseness, and both suprasternal and intercostal retractions are signs of a partial obstruction of the larynx and extrathoracic trachea. If the obstruction is severe, then agitation, cyanosis, acidosis, and respiratory failure occur. Although acute stridor usually is caused by acute airway infections, other disorders may be present and should be considered when symptoms are severe, prolonged, or recurrent. In these patients, imaging studies and endoscopy may be necessary. The differential diagnosis of stridor is discussed in Sec. 15.4.2.

NONINFECTIOUS CAUSES OF UPPER AIRWAY OBSTRUCTION

Laryngomalacia is the most common noninfectious cause of persistent stridor (see Sec. 15.4.2). However, teratoma of the tonsil, nasopharyngeal angiofibromas, fibroleiomyomas, and adenocarcinomas also cause stridor. These are rare in childhood, but when they do occur, they can cause severe airway obstruction. Neurofibromas of the upper airway may be associated with café-au-lait spots. Hemangiomas of the upper airway may be associated with superficial hemangiomas. Signs and symptoms that hemangiomas produce are intermittent and depend on the degree of vascular engorgement. Corticosteroid therapy may cause shrinkage of the hemangioma with a striking decrease in symptoms.

Papillomas that are caused by human papilloma virus can occur from the pharynx to the bronchi. The virus may be transmitted from mother to infant during the perinatal period. Excision by laser may be required, but papillomas recur and can easily be seeded into the lower airway. Surgical removal should be undertaken only when there are signs and symptoms of obstruction.

SUBGLOTTIC FOREIGN BODIES

Foreign bodies may lodge just below the vocal cords or in the upper esophagus and produce signs and symptoms similar to croup or asthma. As with bronchial foreign bodies, the episode frequently is not observed, so the possibility of a foreign body must be considered in any patient with acute onset of respiratory distress. If the inhaled object differs in density from the surrounding soft tissue, it can be detected on neck radiography. Upper airway and chest radiography is recommended when there is an abrupt onset of symptoms of upper airway obstruction. Endoscopic inspection of the upper airway may be necessary when the onset of stridor is abrupt.

GASTROESOPHAGEAL REFLUX–ASSOCIATED STRIDOR

Gastroesophageal reflux and aspiration have been linked to upper respiratory symptoms, including apnea, choking spells, laryngospasm, noisy breathing, chronic cough, and stridor. Acid-induced laryngospasm may be severe enough to cause hypoxia and seizures. Respiratory symptoms from reflux can occur without vomiting or growth failure. In addition, the possibility of reflux should be considered in an infant with laryngomalacia whose stridor increases. Further complicating the picture, reflux is more common in children and infants with acute and chronic respiratory illnesses, and it often is impossible to know with certainty whether there is a connection between the two.

Infants with reflux-associated stridor present with a history of intermittent or waxing and waning stridor. At laryngoscopy, the larynx often appears to be inflamed, but it otherwise is normal. An esophageal pH recording in conjunction with careful concurrent documentation of respiratory status will demonstrate a chronologic relationship between the episodes of reflux and increased stridor. Reflux treatment usually provides effective relief within days to weeks, thus confirming the relationship between reflux and airway obstruction (see Sec. 17.10.4).

BURNS

Caustic chemicals and heat can injure the upper airway and cause severe stridor and obstruction. The etiology of such injuries usually is known, and the intervention that is required will depend on the severity of the impairment. Endotracheal intubation or emergency tracheotomy in the acute setting may be necessary. Impairment of the lower respiratory tract also is very common in heat injury. Steroids and nebulized antibiotics have not proven to be effective in burns (see Sec. 4.3.6).

ANGIOEDEMA AND ANGIONEUROTIC EDEMA

Angioedema, which sometimes is referred to as "giant urticaria," consists of localized edema of rapid onset in response to a number of triggers, including infection, drugs (especially angiotensin-converting enzyme inhibitors and aspirin), exercise, allergens, insect bites, serum sickness, collagen vascular diseases, and malignancies. It commonly affects the upper airway, causing life-threatening obstruction. Subcutaneous epinephrine, 0.01 mL/kg of 1:1000 concentration, provides rapid relief. A variety of antihistamines (eg, diphenhydramine) provide longer-term control. Occasionally, systemic steroids are required to control the problem.

Hereditary angioneurotic edema is a rare autosomal dominant disorder that produces low or defective C1 esterase inhibitor. Rare acquired forms are associated with lymphoproliferative disorders and autoantibody disease. The upper airway is a frequent site of involvement that can require tracheotomy; other acute-care measures include antihistamines and steroids. Long-term treatment is evolving and includes attenuated androgens, antifibrinolytics, and supplementation of C1 esterase inhibitor, but use of these agents is considered to be experimental (see Sec. 11.5.1).

INFECTIOUS CAUSES OF UPPER AIRWAY OBSTRUCTION

CROUP SYNDROME Croup refers to the acute or subacute onset of inspiratory stridor, barking or brassy cough, and hoarseness. The course of the disease varies from a mild viral illness that lasts 3 to 4 days to a severe acute periepiglottitis, usually caused by grampositive bacteria or, in unimmunized populations, *Hemophilus influenzae* type b.

ACUTE EPIGLOTTITIS Acute epiglottitis is an infection of the larynx, with rapid swelling of the epiglottis and increasing inspiratory difficulty. It usually is caused by *H. influenzae* type b and requires early and aggressive treatment. The widespread use of *Hemophilus* b vaccine has reduced the incidence of this disease, but it still must be considered in any child with acute, croup-like symptoms. The child with acute epiglottitis usually is older than 3 years of age. Onset is acute, with inspiratory stridor, drooling, and increasing agitation. The disease progresses over 4 to 12 hours to almost total airway obstruction. There usually are fever and other signs of systemic toxicity. In contrast to a child with viral laryngotracheobronchitis, there is rarely any history of an antecedent upper respiratory infection, and there is absence of spontaneous cough.

When obstruction is severe, breath sounds are diminished over the lung fields. The child tends to remain in a sitting position with chin extended and may complain of pain in his or her throat on swallowing. Secretions are not swallowed. As the obstruction progresses, stridor may decrease as breathing becomes shallow and rapid.

In patients with good air exchange, a cautious examination of the posterior pharynx (being careful not to touch the wall of the pharynx with the tongue blade) will reveal a grossly edematous epiglottis. This swollen epiglottis has been described as resembling a bright red raspberry. Once the tip of the swollen epiglottis is visualized, examination of the pharynx should stop—any further manipulation of the inflamed epiglottis may cause complete laryngeal obstruction. It is essential that appropriate equipment and personnel who are trained to perform endotracheal intubation or tracheostomy be present when a child with possible epiglottitis is examined. The examination should be performed only in an emergency room, intensive care unit, operating room, or similar setting, where a surgical airway can be established if necessary. The diagnosis of epiglottitis also may be suggested by identifying a plump, swollen epiglottis on a lateral neck radiograph.

A child with confirmed epiglottitis should be intubated. A tube that is 0.5 to 1.0 mm smaller than usually is appropriate for the child's size should be selected. Endotracheal intubation may be difficult; tracheotomy may be necessary. The average duration of endotracheal intubation after starting antibiotics is 2 to 4 days. The incidence of postintubation complications is low. Pulmonary edema can complicate both acute epiglottitis and viral croup, and it may cause hypoxemia and pulmonary infiltrates that are seen on chest radiographs.

After blood for culture is obtained (which are often positive with epiglottitis), immediate treatment with intravenous cefuroxime, 75 mg/kg/d, should begin. The child should be monitored in an intensive care unit.

ACUTE LARYNGOTRACHEITIS (VIRAL CROUP)

Acute laryngotracheitis is the most common cause of acute stridor that is encountered in pediatric practice. It usually occurs in the late fall and winter months, when viral respiratory infections reach their peak incidence. It is more common in boys than in girls, and occurs more often in children between 6 months and 6 years of age who have had an upper respiratory infection for 2 to 3 days before inspiratory stridor develops. Many children have a "barking seal" cough and wheezing. Fever usually is present, but the child generally does not appear to be very ill. On cautious examination of the posterior pharynx, the epiglottis may be slightly red and mildly edematous, which is quite different from the gross swelling of acute epiglottitis. The obstruction in acute laryngotracheobronchitis is primarily subglottic in location and produces the so-called "steeple sign" on posteroanterior neck radiographs because the airway appears to taper gradually to a very narrow segment. Parainfluenza type 1 viruses are the most common cause of viral croups, accounting for up to 65% of the incidents, and parainfluenza type 3, influenza A and B viruses, adenoviruses, respiratory syncytial virus, and echovirus cause most of the rest. *Mycoplasma pneumoniae* also can produce croup symptoms in older children.

Most children with croup do not require hospitalization. Treatment at home consists of air humidification, avoidance of agitation, and reduction of fever. An oral electrolyte solution may be offered to mildly affected infants, but those with respiratory distress or cough-induced vomiting should be fed with caution. Oropharyngeal suctioning should be avoided because stimulating the posterior pharynx may cause reflex laryngeal and bronchial constriction. If signs of severe obstruction develop, treatment with an aerosol of racemic epinephrine (2.25%), nebulized with 100% oxygen, frequently provides relief. Frequent aerosol treatments may be needed for the first few hours. A single parenteral dose of dexamethasone, 0.6 mg/kg, is effective in decreasing the length and severity of respiratory symptoms that are associated with viral croup. Inhaled corticosteroid therapy has also been used with some success, but parenteral dexamethasone is somewhat easier. Intubation or tracheostomy rarely is necessary. Sedation should be either avoided or used in a monitored environment. Arterial pH and blood gas measurements may help in guiding treatment, but they are not a substitute for good clinical judgment. Arterial blood gas values may not be representative of the child's overall condition, and arterial puncture may cause further agitation. Heliox has been used successfully to maintain gas exchange in critically ill patients who might otherwise have required intubation. Estimation of arterial saturation by pulse oximetry can be used to monitor oxygenation. Intubation rarely is necessary, but if required, the presence of an underlying congenital lesion such as subglottic stenosis or a vascular ring should be considered.

The differential diagnosis of viral croup includes epiglottitis, foreign body, and angioneurotic edema. Careful history taking usually can distinguish viral croup from these other disorders. Some children have recurrent croup, usually as a result of recurrent infection with viruses that are known to cause the disease. In these patients, however, other congenital and acquired causes of stridor should be considered, especially with infants. In patients with frequent episodes or the inability to sustain long symptom-free intervals, barium esophagram and bronchoscopy should be performed to exclude structural disorders (see Sec. 15.4).

SPASMODIC CROUP

Spasmodic croup (ie, acute spasmodic laryngitis) is characterized by acute attacks of inspiratory stridor that tend to occur suddenly during the evening or at night, last several hours, and then subside, only to recur during the next several days. It usually is seen in children between 6 months and 3 years of age. Its etiology is uncertain, but it may represent recurrent viral laryngotracheitis. The child with spasmodic croup usually awakens with a barking, metallic cough and marked inspiratory stridor. The degree of inspiratory obstruction can be striking, with retractions of the supraclavicular and substernal areas. Fever is absent, and although the child may have had a mild upper respiratory infection preceding the attack, examination of the posterior pharynx reveals only minimal, if any, signs of inflammation. Acute adductor spasm of the vocal cords also may be a cause, possibly triggered by a mild viral illness or allergy.

Placing the child in a closed bathroom in which a hot shower is running may bring relief in a few minutes. Paradoxically, exposure to the cool night air while en route to a hospital frequently breaks the attack before the hospital is reached. Aerosol treatment with racemic epinephrine usually terminates the attack. If symptoms are atypical or frequent, structural causes of recurrent stridor should be considered. Occurrence in later childhood and adolescence suggests psychogenic illness, especially if symptoms do not occur during sleep.

DIPHTHERITIC CROUP

Diphtheria must be considered in the differential diagnosis with acute infectious croup; a history of completed immunizations for diphtheria makes the diagnosis very unlikely. Typically, a child with diphtheritic croup has been ill for 1 to 2 days, looks sick, and has a serous or serosanguineous nasal discharge. Cutaneous lesions and cervical lymphadenopathy also may be present. Examination of the posterior pharynx may reveal a gray-white membrane over the tonsils, with possible extension to the uvula. Occasionally, this membrane is limited to the larynx, making it difficult to visualize and the diagnosis difficult to make. Treatment requires immediate administration of diphtheria equine antitoxin and either penicillin or erythromycin (see Sec. 13.2.13).

BACTERIAL TRACHEITIS (PSEUDOMEMBRANOUS CROUP)

Bacterial tracheitis is a rare but important cause of severe upper airway obstruction and should be considered in older patients with stridor or in infants who do not respond to racemic epinephrine inhalation. Children with this condition initially have symptoms that are similar to epiglottitis or severe viral laryngotracheitis. Lateral neck radiographs show subglottic narrowing and foreign material in the tracheal lumen. Endoscopy reveals extensive sloughing of the respiratory epithelium and large amounts of mucopurulent secretions and debris blocking the trachea. These secretions may be difficult to remove and progressively occlude the airway. *Staphylococcus aureus* is the most common organism that is associated with this condition; nontypable *H. influenzae, Branhamella catarrhalis,* and *Streptococcus pneumoniae* are less often the cause. Treatment includes culture of secretions, appropriate intravenous antibiotics, oxygen, avoidance of fluid overload, and endotracheal intubation if there are signs of progressive respiratory failure.

RETROPHARYNGEAL AND PERITONSILLAR ABSCESS

Abscess formation in the retropharyngeal space rarely follows a viral infection of the nasopharynx or a penetrating pharyngeal injury. In this age of frequent antibiotics use, this is a rare but urgent problem. These abscesses form in children who are under 5 years of age and who present with sudden onset of fever, dysphagia, drooling, neck

rigidity, and noisy and labored breathing. Examination of the pharynx can reveal bulging of the posterior wall. Widening of the retropharynx is easily seen on a lateral neck radiograph. Surgical drainage and broad-spectrum parenteral antibiotics are required. Group A *Streptococcus* is the most common cause, but anaerobes (eg, *Bacteroides* sp.) also can cause this infection. Intubation may be needed to protect the airway during the acute phase of the illness.

Abscess of the peritonsillar space generally occurs in older children, who present with severe throat pain and a muffled voice. Examination of the pharynx reveals medial displacement of the soft palate, tonsil, and uvula. The abscess must be drained surgically with an endotracheal tube in place to protect the airway. Antibiotics are given as for a retropharyngeal abscess.

References

Flom LL: Upper airway obstruction in the pediatric patient. Emerg Med Clin North Am 9:757, 1991

Zalzal GH: Stridor and airway compromise. Pediatr Clin North Am 36: 1389, 1989

Inspiratory Obstruction (Stridor)

Barsum WJ, Miller MA, Marcon MJ, et al: Cefuroxime therapy for bacteremic soft tissue infections in children. Am J Dis Child 139:1141, 1985

Friedberg J: An approach to stridor in infants and children. J Otolaryngol 16:203, 1987

Friedman EM, Vastola AP, McGill TJI, Healy BG: Chronic pediatric stridor: etiology and outcome. Laryngoscope 100:277, 1990

Gay BB Jr, Atkinson GO, Vanderzalm T, et al: Subglottic foreign bodies in pediatric patients. Am J Dis Child 140:165, 1986

John SD, Swischuk LE: Stridor and upper airway obstruction in infants and children. Radiographics 12:625, 1992

Klassen TP, Feldman ME, Watters LK, et al: Nebulized budesonide for children with mild-to-moderate croup. N Engl J Med 331:285, 1994

Kuusela AL, Vesikari T: A randomized double-blind, placebo-controlled trial of dexamethasone and racemic epinephrine in the treatment of croup. Acta Paediatr Scand 77:99, 1988

McClurg FLD, Davans DA: Laser laryngoplasty for laryngomalacia. Laryngoscope 104:247, 1994

Moulin D, Bertrand JM, Buts JP, et al: Upper airway lesions in children after accidental ingestion of caustic substances. J Pediatr 106:408, 1985

Poole SR, Mauro RD, Fan LL, Brooks J: The child with simultaneous stridor and wheezing. Pediatr Emerg Care 6:33, 1990

Skinner DW, Bradley PJ: Psychogenic stridor. J Laryngol Otol 103:383, 1989

Skolnik NS: Treatment of croup. A critical review. Am J Dis Child 143: 1045, 1989

Trunkel DE, Zalzal GH: Stridor in infants and children: ambulatory evaluation and operative diagnosis. Clin Pediatr 31:48, 1992

Winter PH, Koopmann CF Jr: Juvenile myasthenia gravis: an unusual presentation. Int J Pediatr Otorhinol 19:273, 1990

Zach MS, Schnall RA, Landow LI: Upper and lower airway hyperreactivity in recurrent croup. Am Rev Respir Dis 121:979, 1980

Zeitouni A, Manoukian J: Epiglottoplasty in the treatment of laryngomalacia. J Otolaryngol 22:29, 1993

Croup

Ausejo M, Saenz A, Kellner JD, Johnson DW, Moher D, Klassen TP: The effectiveness of glucocorticoids in treating croup: meta-analysis. Br Med J 319:595–600, 1999

Johnson DW, Jacobson S, Edney PC, Hadfield P, Mundy ME, Schuh S: A comparison of nebulized budesonide, intramuscular dexamethasone, and placebo for moderately severe croup. N Engl J Med 339:498–503, 1998

Tumors

Guarisco JL: Congenital head and neck masses in infants and children. Ear Nose Throat J 70:75, 1991

Hawkins DB, Crocket DM, Kahlstron EJ, MacLaughlin EF: Corticosteroid management of airway hemangiomas: long term follow up. Laryngoscope 94:633, 1984

Sie KC, McGill T, Healy GB: Subglottic hemangioma: ten years' experience with the carbon dioxide laser. Ann Otol Rhinol Laryngol 103:167, 1994

Gastroesophageal Reflux

Colombo JL, Hallberg TK: Recurrent aspiration in children: lipid-laden macrophage quantitation. Pediatr Pulmonol 3:86, 1987

Irwin RS, Zawacki JK, Curley FJ, et al: Chronic cough as the sole presenting manifestation of gastroesophageal reflux. Am Rev Respir Dis 140:1294, 1989

Nielson DW, Heldt GP, Tooley WH: Stridor and gastroesophageal reflux in infants. Pediatrics 85:1034, 1990

Orenstein SR, Orenstein DM: Gastroesophageal reflux and respiratory diseases in children. J Pediatr 112:847, 1988

Burns

Harjacek M, Konberg AE, Yates EW, Montgomery P: Thermal epiglottitis after swallowing hot tea. Pediatr Emerg Care 8:342, 1992

Herndon DN, Langner F, Thompson P, et al: Pulmonary injury in burned patients. Surg Clin North Am 67:31, 1987

Angioedema and Angioneurotic Edema

Sim TC, Grant JA: Hereditary angioneurotic edema: its diagnostic and management perspectives. Am J Med 88:656, 1990

Thompson T, Frable MA: Drug-induced, life-threatening angioedema revisited. Laryngoscope 103:10, 1993

Epiglottitis

Beck RA, Kambiss S, Bass JW: The retreat of *Hemophilus influenza* type B invasive disease: analysis and immunization program and implications for OTO-HNS. Otolaryngol Head Neck Surg 109:712, 1993

Cressman WR, Myer CM: Diagnosis and management of croup and epiglottitis. Pediatr Clin North Am 41:265, 1994

Viral Croup

Skolnik NS: Treatment of croup. A critical review. Am J Dis Child 143:1045, 1989

Wagener JS, Landau LI, Olinsky A, et al: Management of children hospitalized for laryngotracheobronchitis. Pediatr Pulmonol 2:159, 1986

Bacterial Tracheitis

Donaldson JD, Maltby CC: Bacterial tracheitis in children. J Otolaryngol 18:101, 1989

Kasian GF, Bingham WT, Steinberg J, et al: Bacterial tracheitis in children. Can Med Assoc J 140:46, 1989

Retropharyngeal Abscess

Coulthard M, Isaacs D: Retropharyngeal abscess. Arch Dis Child 66:1227, 1991

Glasier CM, Stark JE, Jacob RF, et al: CT and ultrasound imaging of retropharyngeal abscess in children. Am J Neuroradiol 13:1191, 1992

23.7   DISORDERS CAUSING EXPIRATORY OBSTRUCTION

Thomas A. Hazinski

Foreign bodies, inflammation, edema, intrinsic airway lesions, mucus, or mediastinal masses may occlude the lower airway. In addition, the child's poorly supported large airways collapse during expiration (see Sec. 4.1.1), and this is exaggerated with crying or agitation. In narrowed airways, gas flow accelerates, pressure differences across the walls of the large bronchi increase, and the force tending to distort their walls increases. Thus, obstruction or instability of the lower airway causes wheezing or noisy exhalation. A differential diagnosis of wheezing is presented in Table 23-9.

After complete obstruction of an airway, gas is absorbed distal to the blockage, producing an atelectatic lung segment. Pulmonary blood flow to the atelectatic unit decreases immediately, so cyanosis usually is absent even when an entire lobe is involved. The atelectatic area may enlarge as it fills with mucus. In the absence of blood flow as well as the cleansing action of the cilia and mucous lining, the likelihood of secondary infection increases. Abscesses may form, or chronic inflammation may slowly erode and destroy the wall of the airway, causing focal bronchiectasis.

TABLE 23-9

DIFFERENTIAL DIAGNOSIS OF RECURRENT WHEEZING

Generalized
  Foreign body
  Asthma
  Cystic fibrosis
  Aspiration
    Neurologic
    Structural abnormality of trachea or esophagus
  Gastroesophageal reflux
  Fictitious asthma (vocal cord dysfunction)
  Pulmonary edema (cardiogenic, noncardiogenic)
  Hemosiderosis
  Tracheomalacia
  Vascular ring
Focal
  Foreign body
  Bronchial obstruction
    Intrinsic
      Papilloma
      Granuloma
      Hemangioma
    Extrinsic
      Adenopathy (tuberculosis, histoplasmosis, malignancy, AIDS)
      Congenital malformation
      Mediastinal mass
      Dilated pulmonary arteries

After partial obstruction of an airway, air trapping and segmental hyperinflation may develop. If the obstruction is generalized, as in asthma or bronchiolitis, there will be relatively uniform hyperinflation. If the obstruction is localized, the lung adjacent to the obstruction will expand. Occasionally, cystic lesions form and may become infected.

BRONCHIAL ADENOMAS, PAPILLOMATA, AND BRONCHOGENIC CYSTS

Bronchial adenomas are rare in childhood, and they may arise from the cells of the mucous glands and ducts of the bronchus. There are two histologic types. Ninety percent are the carcinoid type, which resemble the carcinoid tumors of the small bowel but without symptoms of the carcinoid syndrome; 10% are the cylindromatous type, which are made of cuboidal or flattened epithelial cells closely resembling the mixed tumors of the salivary gland. Of these, 40% are malignant.

Papillomatosis of the trachea and bronchi has been reported in children and is caused by the human papilloma virus. Papillomas frequently are multiple and pedunculated, and they may move during inspiration and expiration. Dyspnea and stridor are common. Secondary obstructive changes with obstructive emphysema, atelectasis, pneumonia, bronchiectasis, and multiple cystic lesions (Fig. 23-14) may occur when papillomata are in the distal parts of the tracheobronchial tree. Occasionally, they have given rise to squamous carcinomas, usually after radiation therapy. When they obstruct a major airway, they must be removed. This must be done with care because a dislodged fragment can seed other areas of the lung. Unfortunately, however, they almost always return, so children with this condition usually undergo many bronchoscopic procedures. Immunomodulatory and antiviral therapies have been disappointing.

Bronchogenic cysts arising in bronchial walls or lymphatic tissue are common. These may occur in any part of the lung but most often are found in the subcarinal area and mediastinum. Adenomas and cysts cause wheezing, repeated episodes of infection, and hemoptysis. If they obstruct a large airway, they cause dyspnea, retractions, and cyanosis. Adenomas usually obstruct bronchi, but they may occlude the trachea. Respiratory symptoms that are associated with tracheal adenomas typically are relieved by flexing the neck and are aggravated by hyperextension. Because of their posterior placement, cysts ordinarily cause anterior displacement and compression of the major bronchi or trachea. Bronchial adenomas and cysts usually should be removed because of the risk of obstruction, infection, and rupture.

ASPIRATION OF FOREIGN BODIES

Most young children place a wide variety of dangerous objects into their mouths, but fortunately, aspiration is infrequent. Seeds, nuts, and peanuts are the most frequently aspirated items. However, hot dogs, small toys, coins, jewelry, and firm vegetables are common culprits as well. Aspirated material tends to lodge in the lower lobe of the right lung, but any lobe (or lobes) can be involved. Foreign bodies in the esophagus also can cause severe respiratory distress, especially in infants, where the posterior membranous portion of the trachea is large. Pathogenesis and management of foreign body aspiration are discussed in detail in Sec. 4.3.5.

GASTROESOPHAGEAL REFLUX AND ASPIRATION

Gastric contents occasionally reflux into the esophagus in everyone. It is especially common in the first year after birth and rarely causes any symptoms. However, reflux of acidic gastric fluid causes respiratory symptoms even when pulmonary aspiration is absent. The most convincing data to date have shown a temporal relationship between gastroesophageal reflux and certain respiratory symptoms that improve with effective management of the reflux. Gastroesophageal reflux is discussed in detail in Sec. 17.10.4.

BRONCHIOLITIS OBLITERANS

Bronchiolitis obliterans is a chronic lung disease in which small bronchi and bronchioles are obstructed by intraluminal masses of fibrous tissue. Although there have been a number of reported causes of bronchiolitis obliterans (Table 23-10) in children, the majority have followed lower respiratory tract infection with adenovirus, particularly types 3, 7, and 21. Infections with these agents have occurred both in utero and at all ages throughout childhood. The incidence of bronchiolitis obliterans is highest when the initial infection occurs between 6 months and 2 years of age. The incidence of chronic lung disease following an episode of adenovirus pneumonitis during childhood is approximately 30%, but it has approached 60% in certain populations of Native Americans in North America and New Zealand Maoris.

Bronchiolitis obliterans also has been described following the inhalation of acids and sulfur dioxide. However, its clinical importance is the result of its emergence as the major long-term complication of lung transplantation. In addition, lesions resembling bronchiolitis obliterans have been identified in bone marrow transplant patients, where it usually is associated with graft-versus-host disease.

Bronchiolitis obliterans begins as a severe necrotizing pneumonitis with destruction of the bronchiolar epithelium. The bronchiolar lumen is filled with cellular debris. As healing occurs, large polypoid masses of granulation tissue obstruct the lumen of the

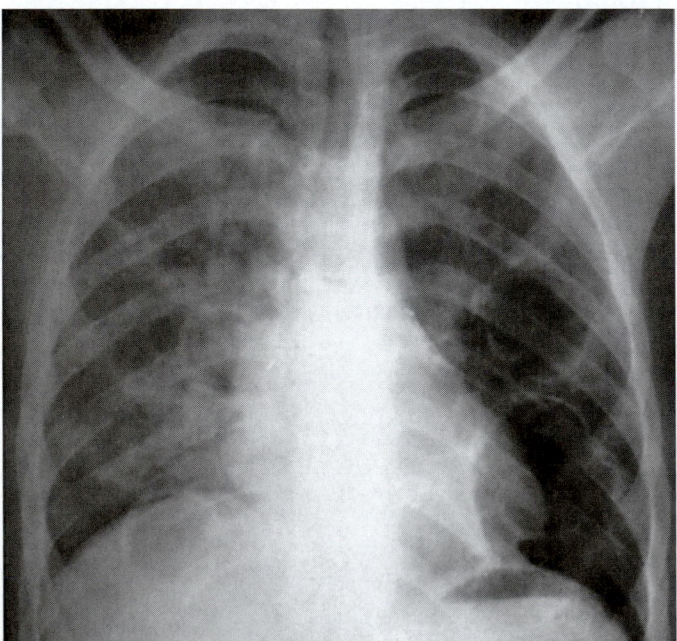

FIGURE 23-14   Chest radiograph of a 13-year-old boy with papillomatosis. Note the large bilateral cysts.

TABLE 23-10
CAUSES OF BRONCHIOLITIS OBLITERANS

Inhalation of irritant substances
  Fumes
    Concentrated ammonia
    Nitric, hydrochloric, and sulfuric acids
    War gases (chlorine, phosgene, chloropicrine)
    Burning radiographic film
  Talcum powder
  Zinc stearate
Infections
  Adenovirus
  Influenza viruses
  Pertussis
  Measles
  Tuberculosis
Aspiration
  Amniotic fluid
  Lipids
  Foreign bodies
  Stomach acid (gastroesophageal reflux)
Immunologic
  Lung transplantation
  Bone marrow transplantation (graft-vs-host disease)

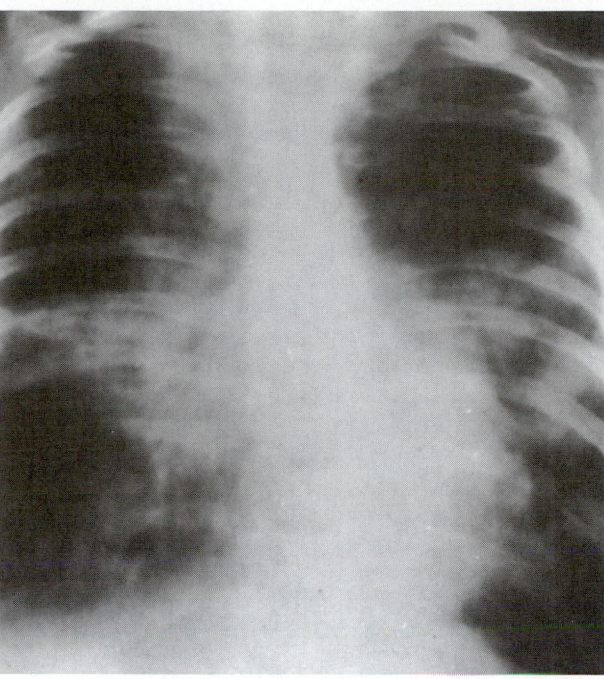

FIGURE 23-16 Chest radiograph obtained in a patient with bronchiolitis obliterans, demonstrating marked bilateral hyperaeration and pulmonary edema.

bronchioles and small bronchi. Later, these masses of tissue become fibrotic, causing partial or total obliteration of the airway (Fig. 23-15). There is a decrease in the size of the pulmonary capillary bed, and airway resistance and the work of breathing increase. Perfusion of poorly ventilated lung units causes hypoxemia, and a fall in effective ventilation causes hypercarbia. The chronic hypoxia, airway obstruction, and reduction in the size of the pulmonary vascular bed often lead to pulmonary edema that further compromises gas exchange.

In the acute phase, the disease is indistinguishable from acute bronchiolitis or an interstitial pneumonia. After a brief period of partial or even total apparent recovery, however, there is a gradual return to the symptoms of obstructive lung disease with dyspnea, tachypnea, and chronic cough. Chest examination reveals rales and

wheezing. On the chest radiograph, the lungs are overaerated and have increased interstitial markings. Pulmonary edema is common, but focal pulmonary infiltrates are rare (Fig. 23-16). The diagnosis is suggested by the clinical course, chest radiograph, and CT, but it is confirmed by lung biopsy and pathologic examination.

Treatment is supportive and includes oxygen, good nutrition, and the avoidance of secondary lung injury from aspiration, reflux, or secondary infection. Chronic oxygen administration usually is necessary to prevent pulmonary hypertension and congestive heart failure. Diuretics are valuable in treating obvious pulmonary edema, and a trial of bronchodilators may be warranted. It is possible that

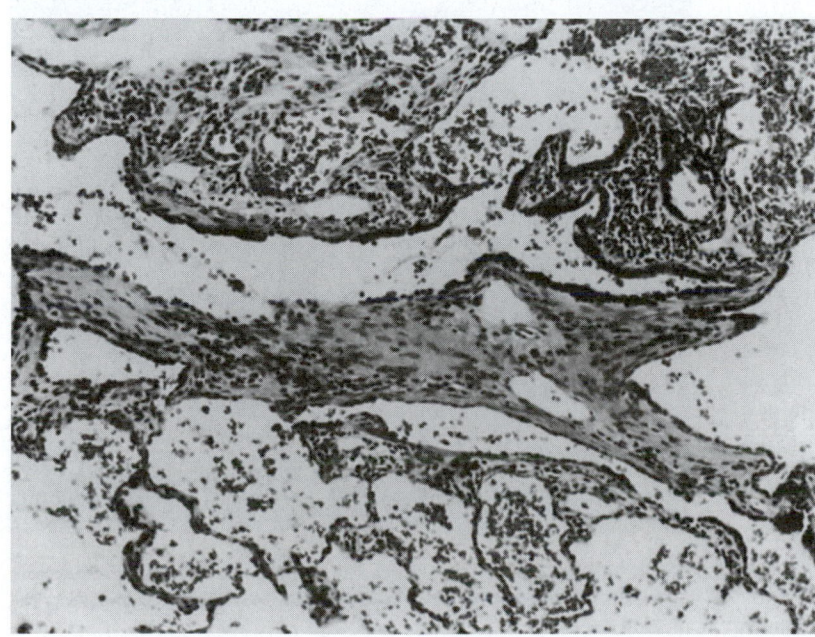

FIGURE 23-15 A lung biopsy specimen from the same patient as in Figure 23-16, revealing fibrous plugging of a bronchiole and marked interstitial round cell infiltration.

glucocorticoids may limit disease progression by slowing cellular and matrix proliferation. There have been several reports of clinical improvement in adults with bronchiolitis obliterans following treatment with high-dose corticosteroids as well as with immunomodulatory agents if the disease is associated with graft-versus-host disease.

Occasionally, the obliterative process is predominantly unilateral, resulting in the unilateral hyperlucent lung or Swyer-James syndrome. In this condition, the affected lung is hyperinflated, but its total size is normal. This unilateral overinflation and impairment of ventilation often are readily detectable on careful examination of the chest. Chest radiographs show increased lucency on the involved side, and fluoroscopy may demonstrate a shift of the mediastinum toward the less affected side during expiration. Bronchoscopy reveals no obstruction of the major airways. Treatment is supportive, but surgical removal of a severely affected lobe occasionally may be indicated.

The prognosis of children with bronchiolitis obliterans varies. Some children seem to improve gradually, especially after 8 to 10 years of age. Others, however, continue to have significant pulmonary disability, with chronic obstruction, bronchiectasis, and recurrent infections. Some progress to respiratory failure and die shortly after the onset of symptoms. In a few instances, lung transplantation has been employed.

Recently a distinct pathologic entity termed bronchiolitis obliterans–organizing pneumonia (BOOP) has been described. It has been associated with a wide variety of lung diseases, including infectious pneumonias, toxic inhalants, and collagen vascular disease (see Sec. 23.13.1). The pathologic appearance is similar to bronchiolitis obliterans except that the alveolar septa are thickened by a chronic inflammatory cell infiltrate and type II cell hyperplasia. Corticosteroid therapy is often effective.

POSTTRANSPLANT LUNG

Acute noninfectious interstitial pneumonitis and bronchiolitis have been described in patients who have undergone solid organ or bone marrow transplantation. In these patients, the pneumonitis is thought to be related to graft-versus-host disease or a chemotherapy-induced pneumonitis and responds to immunomodulatory therapy once pulmonary infection has been excluded.

In lung transplant recipients, one or more episodes of acute rejection are common, with one-half of these episodes occurring within 3 months. These episodes are characterized by the onset of new pulmonary symptoms, confirmed by excluding infection by lavage or lung biopsy, and effectively treated with high-dose, short-term corticosteroid therapy.

An ominous late complication of lung transplantation is bronchiolitis obliterans, which develops in up to 50% of long-term survivors. The etiology of this complication is unknown. Chronic viral infection, especially with cytomegalovirus, has been implicated, but recent evidence suggests that it is a unique form of organ rejection. An immunologic mechanism is suspected because lung biopsies reveal perivascular lymphocytic cuffing and interstitial fibrosis. These findings are consistent with pulmonary rejection or drug-induced pneumonitis. Post–lung transplant bronchiolitis obliterans is unresponsive to current therapy and may be irreversible.

BRONCHIECTASIS

Bronchiectasis, or dilatation of the bronchi, occurs when the bronchial wall is so damaged by infection and chronic inflammation that it becomes susceptible to distension and distortion during

breathing. Radiographically, bronchiectasis is seen as failure of the bronchi to taper in distal lung segments. Focal bronchiectasis may be reversible, but in most instances, bronchiectasis implies irreversible airway damage. Bronchiectasis usually develops after months or years, but a congenital form of bronchiectasis also has been described.

Bronchiectasis may be focal (ie, associated with a discrete infection, intrinsic or extrinsic mass, foreign body, inflammatory reaction) or generalized (ie, secondary to cystic fibrosis, chronic aspiration, ciliary dysmotility syndromes, immune deficiencies, or allergic bronchopulmonary aspergillosis). Bronchiectasis usually is accompanied by chronic inflammation that produces a chronic productive cough and often is complicated by recurrent infection. The chest is enlarged, and musical rales and rhonchi always are present throughout the lungs even during symptom-free intervals. Clubbing of the fingers is common. Children with extensive bronchiectasis fatigue easily and have reduced exercise capacity and slow growth. Bronchography and CT demonstrate dilated bronchi (Fig. 23-17) that do not taper peripherally. Atelectasis and abscess formation may occur when the obstruction is complete; when obstruction is partial, there is regional hyperinflation. Bronchial hyperreactivity may be present, and the patient may benefit from treatment with inhaled bronchodilators.

Children with advanced bronchiectasis frequently have a large total lung capacity, large FRC, and a small vital capacity. There are increased airway resistance and decreased expiratory flow rates. Ventilation and pulmonary perfusion are unevenly distributed. Some areas of the lung may have little ventilation and a large blood flow, which causes a decreased PaO_2. Other areas of the lung receive little blood flow and may be relatively well ventilated; this tends to increase the respiratory dead space, decrease ventilatory efficiency, and increase the work of breathing. In some patients with severe bronchiectasis, bronchodilator inhalation may increase airway instability, thus leading to further airway obstruction.

Children with severe asthma and excessive production of airway mucus probably constitute the largest group of patients who tend to develop localized dilation of the airways. This type of bronchi-

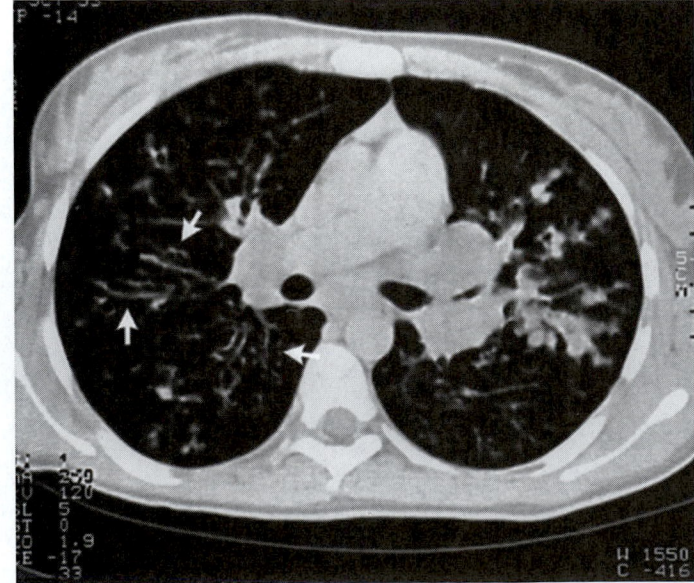

FIGURE 23-17   Chest CT scan showing multilobar bronchiectasis in a child with hypogammaglobulinemia. Note the lack of airway tapering *(arrows)*.

ectasis usually is reversible, and surgery for bronchiectasis in children with asthma is very rarely needed. Atelectasis of the right middle lobe may occur in children with severe or undertreated asthma; this focal bronchiectasis usually is reversible with improved asthma therapy. A persistent right middle lobe infiltrate or atelectasis generally is associated with asthma, cystic fibrosis, bronchial stenosis, or a foreign body. Surgical removal of the right middle lobe rarely is necessary unless it is associated with active clinical symptoms, hypoxemia, or clinical deterioration despite optimal medical management.

Treatment of chronic bronchiectasis includes daily bronchodilator inhalation (if clinical assessment and spirometry indicate no ill effects) followed by vigorous postural drainage or the use of airway clearance devices. If bronchiectasis results from allergic bronchopulmonary aspergillosis, systemic corticosteroid therapy is indicated. Specific infections are treated with short courses of conventional antibiotics. Recently, inhaled antibiotic therapy has been used to treat patients with intractable symptoms. Prolonged antibiotic prophylaxis may be necessary to suppress chronic infection and control clinical symptoms. As noted earlier, when bronchiectasis is localized, removal of the segment or lobe may be necessary if the patient remains symptomatic despite maximum medical therapy. Surgical resection also is indicated for patients with generalized bronchiectasis if there is massive or recurrent hemoptysis that can be localized.

DYSMOTILE CILIA SYNDROMES

Normal ciliary motility is necessary for adequate clearance of fluid and foreign materials from both the upper and lower respiratory tracts (Fig. 23-18). Cilia normally beat synchronously 7 to 22 times per second. Impairment of ciliary beat or synchrony results in reduced mucociliary clearance and recurrent episodes of upper and lower respiratory infections. Chronic ciliary dysfunction is one cause of bronchiectasis in children.

Several rare abnormalities of cilia morphology are associated with immotility. Absence of one or both dynein arms, which is an autosomal recessive disorder, is the most common structural abnormality associated with ciliary immotility and is the defect found in most patients with Kartagener syndrome. This syndrome is a sporadic or familial condition consisting of sinusitis, bronchiectasis, situs inversus, and reduced male fertility. Less common structural abnormalities affecting ciliary function include defects in the radial spoke linkages, with disorientation of the central microtubular doublets and absence of the central microtubular doublet with replacement by a doublet from the outer ring. In addition, there are rare individuals with abnormal ciliary function in whom no structural abnormality can be identified. It also is known that structurally abnormal cilia can be identified in normal individuals and that cilia morphology can be transiently altered by acute infection or inflammation.

Patients with respiratory cilia dysfunction have recurrent or chronic otitis media, sinusitis, rhinitis, nasal polyposis, and bronchiectasis. Male patients also may have immotile spermatozoa. In approximately 50% of patients, embryonic ciliary immotility is associated with situs inversus.

The diagnosis should be suspected in any child with bronchiectasis and sinusitis, chronic otitis media, or situs inversus. Cystic fibrosis, immunodeficiency syndromes, and chronic aspiration should be excluded by appropriate testing. The diagnosis is made by electron-microscopic examination of cilia that are obtained by nasal scrapings or mucosal biopsy. These samples should be ob-

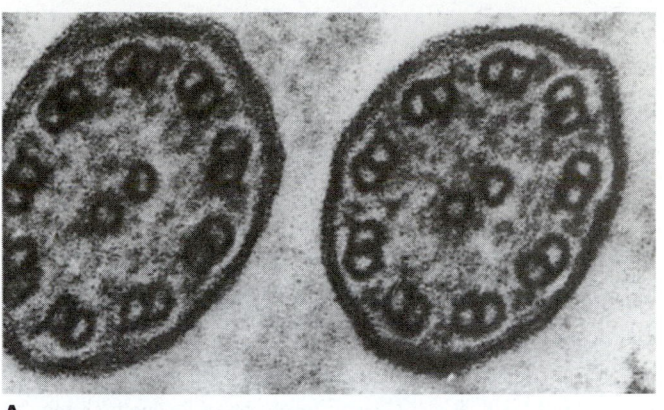

A

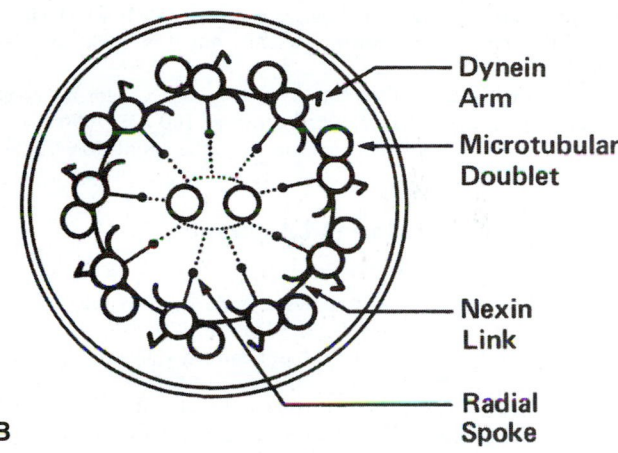

B

FIGURE 23-18   A. Electron micrograph of normal cilia. B. Diagram of normal cilium. Ciliary beating results from sliding of adjacent microtubular doublets. The radial spokes and nexin links convert this sliding into a bending motion. Energy for ciliary beating is provided by ATP and ATPase activity in the dynein arms.

tained when the patient is free of acute infection. Some physicians obtain ciliated cells by gently scraping the nasal mucosa and then examining a wet-mount preparation of these cells microscopically. The finding of rhythmically beating cilia is reassuring, but the accuracy of this qualitative technique is unknown, and a negative result is inconclusive. In older patients, mucociliary clearance also can be assessed by measuring the clearance rate of inhaled technetium-labeled albumin microspheres. In some centers, cilia beat frequency and synchrony can be quantified.

Treatment is the same as for bronchiectasis. Prognosis is good, with substantial remission of symptoms occurring after adolescence.

References

Disorders Causing Lower Airway Obstruction

Brodsky L, Siddiqui SY, Stanievich JF: Massive oropharyngeal papillomatosis causing obstructive sleep apnea in a child. Arch Otolaryngol Head Neck Surg 113:882, 1987

Brünner S, Poulsen PT, Vesterdal J: Cysts of the lung in infants and children. Acta Paediatr Scand 49:39, 1960

Chun K, Colombani PM, Dudgeon DL, Haller JA: Diagnosis and management of congenital vascular rings: A 22-year experience. Ann Thorac Surg 53:597, 1992

Leventhal BG, Kashima HK, Mounts P, et al: Long-term response of recurrent respiratory papillomatosis to treatment with lymphoblastoid interferon alfa-N1. Papilloma Study Group. N Eng J Med 325:613, 1991

Schnadig VJ, Clark WO, Clegg TJ, Yao CS: Invasive papillomatosis and squamous carcinoma complicating juvenile laryngeal papillomatosis. Arch Otolaryngol Head Neck Surg 112:966, 1986

Verska JJ, Connolly JE: Bronchial adenomas in children. J Thorac Cardiovasc Surg 55:411, 1968

Foreign Bodies

Aytac A, Yurdakul Y, Ikizler C, et al: Inhalation of foreign bodies in children. Report of 500 cases. J Thorac Cardiovasc Surg 74:145, 1977

Mantel K, Butenandt I: Tracheobronchial foreign body aspiration in childhood. A report of 224 cases. Eur J Pediatr 145:211, 1986

Puhakka H, Svedström E, Kero P, et al: Tracheobronchial foreign bodies—a persistent problem in pediatric patients. Am J Dis Child 143:543, 1989

Steen KH, Zimmerman T: Tracheobronchial aspiration of foreign bodies in children: A study of 94 cases. Laryngoscope 100:525, 1990

Weissberg D, Schwartz I: Foreign bodies in the tracheobronchial tree. Chest 91:730, 1987

Gastroesophageal Reflux and Aspiration

Bauer ML, Figueroa-Colon R, Georgeson K, Young DW: Chronic pulmonary aspiration in children. South Med J 86:789, 1993

Colombo JL, Hallberg TK: Recurrent aspiration in children: Lipid-laden macrophage quantitation. Pediatr Pulmonol 3:86, 1987

Irwin RS, Zawacki JK, Curley FJ, et al: Chronic cough as the sole presenting manifestation of gastroesophageal reflux. Am Rev Respir Dis 140:1294, 1989

Mansfield LE: Gastroesophageal reflux and respiratory disorders: a review. Ann Allergy 62:158, 1989

McVeagh P, Howman-Giles R, Kemp A: Pulmonary aspiration studied by radionuclide milk scanning and barium swallow roentgenography. Am J Dis Child 141:917, 1987

Nielson DW, Heldt GP, Tooley WH: Stridor and gastroesophageal reflux in infants. Pediatrics 8:6, 1990

Orenstein SR, Orenstein DM: Gastroesophageal reflux and respiratory diseases in children. J Pediatr 112:847, 1988

Bronchiolitis Obliterans

Azizirad H, Polgar G, Borns PF, Chatten J: Bronchiolitis obliterans. Clin Pediatr 14:572, 1975

Becroft DMO: Bronchiolitis obliterans, bronchiectasis, and other sequelae of adenovirus type 21 infection in young children. J Clin Pathol 24:72, 1971

Cumming GR, MacPherson RI, Chernick V: Unilateral hyperlucent lung syndrome in children. J Pediatr 78:250, 1971

Hardy KA, Schidlow DV, Zaeri N: Obliterative bronchiolitis in children. Chest 93:460, 1988

Swyer PR, James GCW: A case of unilateral pulmonary emphysema. Thorax 8:133, 1953

Posttransplant Lung

Gaynor JW, Bridges ND, Clark BJ, Spray TL: Update on lung transplantation in children. Curr Opin Pediatr 10:256–261, 1998

Noyes BE, Kurland G, Orenstein DM, et al: Experience with pediatric lung transplantation. J Pediatr 124:261, 1994

Stillwell PC, Mallory GB: Pediatric lung transplantation. Clin Chest Med 18:405–414, 1997

Bronchiectasis

Lewiston NJ: Bronchiectasis in childhood. Pediatr Clin North Am 31:865, 1984

Similä S, Linna O, Lanning P, et al: Chronic lung damage caused by adenovirus type 7: a 10-year follow-up study. Chest 80:127, 1981

Dysmotile Cilia Syndromes

Eliasson R, Mossberg B, Camner P, Afzelius BA: The immotile-cilia syndrome: a congenital ciliary abnormality as an etiologic factor in chronic airway infections and male sterility. N Engl J Med 297:1, 1977

Engesaeth VG, Warner JO, Bush A: New associations of primary ciliary dyskinesia syndrome. Pediatr Pulmonol 16:9, 1993

Rooklin AR, McGeady SJ, Mikaelian DO, et al: The immotile cilia syndrome: a cause of recurrent pulmonary disease in children. Pediatrics 66:526, 1980

Steinkamp G, Van der Hardt H, Simmermann HJ: Pulmonary resection for localized bronchiectasis in cystic fibrosis. Report of three cases and review of the literature. Acta Pediatr Scand 77:569, 1988

Turner JAP, Corkey CWB, Lee JYC, et al: Clinical expressions of immotile cilia syndrome. Pediatrics 67:805, 1981

23.8   ASTHMA

Mark H. Ross, Christopher M. Mjaanes, and Robert Lemanske, Jr.

Asthma is the most common and best understood chronic disease in childhood, but the diagnosis and management of this disorder is a challenge for pediatricians and for the entire health-care system. Cardinal pathophysiological features of asthma include airway obstruction, airway inflammation, and hyperresponsiveness. No single test can unequivocally diagnose asthma. Instead, clinicians must base the diagnosis on several factors including family history, risk factors, symptom patterns, diagnostic tests, and responses to therapy. Occasionally, the diagnosis of asthma is established by the exclusion of diseases or anatomic abnormalities of the respiratory tract that mimic asthma (Table 23-11). Multiple patterns of disease activity suggest that numerous genetic, microbiological, environmental, and age-related factors contribute significantly to the initiation, propagation, and, in many cases, resolution of the syndrome that has been termed asthma.

EPIDEMIOLOGY

From data available from the National Heart, Lung, and Blood Institute (*www.nhlbi.nih.gov*), asthma ranks among the common chronic conditions in the United States, affecting an estimated 14.9 million persons in 1995 and causing over 1.5 million emergency department visits, 500,000 hospitalizations, and over 5500 deaths. The prevalence of asthma has been increasing since the early 1980s for all age, sex, and racial groups. The overall age-adjusted prevalence of asthma increased 75% from 1980 to 1994; among children up to 4 years of age, asthma prevalence increased 160%. Asthma disproportionately affects children and blacks. Within the general population, asthma affects women more than men; however, among children, it affects boys more. From a more global perspective, asthma is more prevalent in some countries than others. For

TABLE 23-11

DISEASES OR ABNORMALITIES THAT CAN MIMIC ASTHMA

UPPER RESPIRATORY TRACT	MIDDLE RESPIRATORY TRACT	LOWER RESPIRATORY TRACT
Allergic rhinitis	Laryngeal webs	Viral bronchiolitis
Infectious rhinitis	Laryngomalacia	Cystic fibrosis
Sinusitis	Tracheomalacia	Bronchopulmonary dysplasia
Adenoidal/tonsillar hypertrophy	Tracheoesophageal fistula	Foreign body
Foreign body	Tracheal stenosis	Gastroesophageal reflux
	Bronchial stenosis	Chronic aspiration
	Vascular rings	Bronchiectasis
	Enlarged lymph nodes	Pulmonary hemosiderosis
	Tumor	*Chlamydia trachomatis*
	Foreign body	Bronchiolitis obliterans
	Pertussis	Toxic inhalation
	Epiglottitis	Tumor
	Laryngotracheobronchitis	Hyperventilation syndrome
	Toxic inhalation	
	Vocal cord dysfunction	

example, it is infrequent in Eastern Europe and Asia but much more common in the United Kingdom, Australia, New Zealand, Ireland, and North America. An affluent life-style is associated with a higher prevalence, but serious asthma clusters in disadvantaged populations.

PATHOPHYSIOLOGY

AIRFLOW OBSTRUCTION In asthma, *airflow obstruction* is produced by several pathogenic abnormalities. The precise contribution of each of these abnormalities varies among asthmatic patients and no doubt contributes to the diversity and severity of clinical manifestations. Airflow obstruction in asthma is largely reversible, although current evidence suggests some patients may develop an irreversible component of obstruction termed *remodeling*.

BRONCHIAL SMOOTH MUSCLE SPASM Bronchial smooth muscle spasm contributes significantly to airway obstruction. Evidence suggests that either the quantity or the function of bronchial smooth muscle in asthma is abnormal. Autopsy specimens obtained from asthmatic patients dying of their disease have demonstrated hypertrophy of the smooth muscle lining the airways. Some investigators have demonstrated a greater maximal response to contractile agonists and an impaired relaxation to β-agonists and theophylline in vitro. The airway contains a number of resident cells (mast cells, alveolar macrophages, airway epithelium, and endothelium) as well as immigrating inflammatory cells (eosinophils, lymphocytes, neutrophils, basophils, and platelets) that are capable of generating a wide variety of mediators and signaling molecules that can induce bronchospasm. These include histamine, platelet-activating factor, and a number of derivatives of arachidonic acid including prostaglandin D_2 and the cysteinyl leukotrienes (LTC_4, LTD_4, LTE_4). Thus, it is likely that infiltration of inflammatory cells into the airway walls contributes to bronchial smooth muscle tone through the local effects of these various mediators.

EDEMA OF AIRWAY MUCOSA *Edema* of the airway mucosa results from increased capillary permeability with leakage of serum proteins into interstitial areas. A number of cell-derived mediators are capable of inducing edema formation, including histamine, prostaglandin E, LTC_4, LTD_4, LTE_4, platelet-activating factor, and bradykinin. Resulting edema and cellular inflammation cause increased airway wall thickness in patients, which contributes to the mechanics of airway narrowing.

MUCOUS IMPACTION OF BRONCHI *Mucous impaction of bronchi* is another characteristic pathologic feature seen in untreated or undertreated asthma. Mucus production results from hyperplasia and metaplasia of goblet cells lining the airway. Impacted mucus leads to hyperinflation, focal atelectasis, and a productive cough.

AIRWAY INFLAMMATION *Airway inflammation* has long been recognized to be a major feature of the histopathologic findings in many patients with fatal status asthmaticus. More recently, transbronchial biopsies of patients with even mild intermittent asthma have demonstrated significant inflammation that extends to the most distal airways. Significant findings include denudation of the airway epithelium, mucous plugging of segment bronchi and bronchioles, collagen deposition beneath the epithelial basement membrane, edema of the submucosa, infiltration by polymorphonuclear leukocytes (predominantly eosinophils), and smooth muscle hypertrophy. Eosinophil infiltration is more predominant in children who will develop allergic asthma, whereas it is less prominent in children with nonallergic wheezing. This pattern of inflammation is consistent with a helper T-cell type 2 (T_H2) paradigm. The recognition of the key role of chronic inflammation in the pathogenesis of asthma provides the scientific rationale for the prophylactic use of drugs with anti-inflammatory properties.

AIRWAY HYPERRESPONSIVENESS Airway hyperresponsiveness, defined as an exaggerated bronchoconstrictor response to many stimuli, is an important physiological characteristic of asthma, but it is not a unique diagnostic feature of the disease. Many factors contribute to hyperresponsiveness seen in asthma, including genetic factors, preexisting lung disease, airway architecture (related to the patient's age and to edema, smooth muscle hypertrophy, and collagen deposition), and time of the day (nighttime vs daytime). At present, airway inflammation is thought to be the principal mechanism defining the degree of bronchial hyperresponsiveness in asthma. This principle provides the rationale for the daily administration of drugs with anti-inflammatory properties in order to reduce the magnitude of bronchial hyperresponsiveness. However, although airway inflammation contributes to the level of bronchial hyperresponsiveness in asthma, bronchial hyperresponsiveness can be demonstrated in asthmatics who have not wheezed for years or in subjects without asthma.

GENETICS

The inheritance pattern of asthma demonstrates that it is a complex genetic disorder with environmental influences as with hypertension, atherosclerosis, arthritis, and diabetes mellitus. One of the greatest challenges faced by investigators in this area is the marked heterogeneity of the asthmatic phenotype. Although wheezing, coughing, and shortness of breath are common clinical endpoints for the asthmatic disease process, any individual with asthma will respond differently to triggering factors (eg, allergens, viruses, cold air, tobacco smoke, exercise). The variability in the patterns and severity of the disease, its close clinical association with various atopic diseases, and the manner in which the symptoms change in relationship to age or in response to therapeutic intervention have made finding a single genetic "marker" elusive. Because asthma is frequently associated with atopy and is characterized by marked increases in airway responsiveness and inflammation, it should come as no surprise that various gene candidates related to smooth muscle contractile mechanisms and to the immune system have been sought. Thus, linkage to 11q13 (the high-affinity IgE receptor), 5q (the cytokine gene cluster), 12q (IFN-γ), 14q (T-cell antigen receptor), as well as others have been considered as possible candidate loci. Polymorphisms in genes such as the α subunit of the IL-4 receptor, the β_2-adrenergic receptor, and the major cell surface receptor for endotoxin (CD14) may further influence disease expression and the response to therapy. The importance of environmental factors that may be necessary for complete expression of the disease phenotype needs to be more precisely defined.

DIAGNOSIS

Diagnosing asthma in infants and children begins with a review of the patient's history and physical exam. Symptoms include recurrent wheezing, shortness of breath, chest tightness, exercise limitation, mucoid vomiting, and chronic day and night cough. Associated conditions include rhinitis and atopy. Precipitating factors that trigger these symptoms include viral infections, tobacco smoke, vigorous exercise, allergen or irritant exposures, breathing cold dry air, aspirin, aspiration, or acid reflux. The history may also indicate that these symptoms were improved with the use of inhaled or oral asthma medications but did not improve with antibiotics or antihistamine therapy. On physical examination during a symptom-free interval, asthmatic signs are minimal and may include only a prolonged expiratory time and a wet-sounding voluntary cough. During acute exacerbations, however, there may be wheezing with reduced airflow throughout the lung fields, chest hyperinflation, tachypnea, and the use of accessory muscles. However, wheezing in children, particularly in infancy, does not mean that chronic asthma will develop. At least 20% of children less than 2 years of age experience transient episodes of wheezing during viral respiratory infections related, at least in part, to an age-related disproportionate relationship between airway diameter relative to lung volume. As these infants grow, this relationship becomes more normal, and it is thought that these are the children who "outgrow" their asthma. However, at least 15% of children who wheeze during infancy continue to wheeze beyond 6 years of age. Finally, at least 15% of children develop late-onset wheezing patterns characterized by the initial development of symptoms beyond 6 years of age.

The Global Initiative for Asthma (GINA) report has proposed a classification to define asthma severity (Table 23-12). This scale is based on symptoms and, where possible, pulmonary function data that are present before introduction of treatment. Asthma can be subdivided by severity into intermittent or persistent disease. Persistent disease can further be divided into mild, moderate, or severe. With an asthma exacerbation, the severity of disease can change abruptly and dramatically. Classifying asthma in this manner can be helpful in choosing the appropriate medications to initiate treatment or to adjust treatment in patients whose disease remains persistent.

PULMONARY FUNCTION STUDIES Abnormalities in pulmonary function are a measure of the degree of airflow obstruction and reflect the consequence of asthma on airway mechanics. Typical spirometric abnormalities seen in the child whose asthma is active include reductions in FEV_1 and the FEV_1/FVC ratio and an increase in the FEV_1 ($>12-15\%$) in response to a bronchodilator. However, failure to demonstrate an improvement with bronchodilator therapy should not be interpreted as absolute evidence of irreversible disease of the airways, but rather that the major component of obstruction is inflammation, not bronchospasm. Peak expiratory flow rate (PEFR) is often decreased only as a late manifestation of worsening airway obstruction because it does not measure airflow in small airways and may be normal in patients with active disease.

In children less than 5 years of age, pulmonary function testing is usually not feasible because of the patient's inability to cooperate and generate maximal expiratory maneuvers. In this age group, history and response to bronchodilator or anti-inflammatory therapy become essential to making the diagnosis. In some research hospitals, infant pulmonary function testing may be performed to assess the degree of airway obstruction or response to therapeutic intervention, but even when these latter tests are negative, a trial of asthma therapy is probably warranted.

In older children and adolescents, spirometry can document baseline airflow obstruction and the extent to which this obstruction is reversible after a single dose of inhaled bronchodilator therapy. Spirometry is also useful to assess the response to chronic therapy. It is important to remember that expiratory flow rates are effort-dependent and can be influenced by a number of factors including age (inability to comprehend or cooperate with the procedure), technical malfunction (broken peak flow meter), or symptom formation or amplification in patients with psychosocial disorders.

When baseline spirometry is normal, but the diagnosis of asthma is highly suspect, *bronchoprovocation* can be performed using methacholine (or histamine) or exercise. A positive methacholine test (decrease of $FEV_1 > 15\%$ from baseline) is indicative of airway hyperresponsiveness but is not a diagnostic test for asthma. Many individuals with acute (viral infections or irritant exposures) and chronic respiratory tract conditions (allergic rhinitis, cystic fibrosis, bronchitis) will demonstrate an enhanced bronchial response to methacholine inhalation. As a group, asthmatic patients may be the most sensitive, but the threshold of reactivity may fluctuate over time based on exposure to recent triggering factors or concurrent medication use. Because a positive response to methacholine is almost always demonstrable in asthmatic patients, a negative methacholine challenge test can be useful in potentially eliminating asthma from further diagnostic or therapeutic consideration. Exercise bronchoprovocation may be less sensitive than methacholine in demonstrating airway hyperresponsiveness, but a positive re-

TABLE 23-12

STEPWISE APPROACH FOR MANAGING ASTHMA IN TEENAGERS/ADULTS AND IN CHILDREN OVER 5 YEARS OLD: CLASSIFY SEVERITY ON BASIS OF CLINICAL FEATURES BEFORE TREATMENT[a]

	SYMPTOMS[b]	NIGHTTIME SYMPTOMS	LUNG FUNCTION
Step 4 Severe persistent	Continual symptoms Limited physical activity Frequent exacerbations	Frequent	•FEV_1/PEF ≤60% predicted •PEF variability >30%
Step 3 Moderate persistent	Daily symptoms Daily use of inhaled short-acting β_2-agonist Exacerbations affect activity Exacerbations >2 times a week: may last days	>1 time a week	•FEV_1/PEF >60% to <80% predicted •PEF variability >30%
Step 2 Mild persistent	Symptoms >2 times a week but <1 time a day Exacerbations may affect activity	>2 times a month	•FEV_1/PEF ≥80% predicted •PEF variability 20%–30%
Step 1 Mild intermittent	Symptoms ≤2 times a week Asymptomatic and normal PEF between exacerbations Exacerbations brief (from a few hours to a few days); intensity may vary	≤2 times a month	•FEV_1/PEF ≥80% predicted •PEF variability <20%

SOURCE: *National Asthma Education and Prevention Program: Clinical Practice Guidelines. Expert Panel Report 2. Guidelines for the diagnosis and management of asthma. NIH publication No. 97–4051, July 1997.*

[a] The presence of one of the features of severity is sufficient to place a patient in that category. An individual should be assigned to the most severe grade in which any feature occurs. The characteristics noted in this table are general and may overlap because asthma is highly variable. Furthermore, an individual's classification may change over time.

[b] Patients at any level of severity can have mild, moderate, or severe exacerbations. Some patients with intermittent asthma experience severe and life-threatening exacerbations separated by long periods of normal lung function and no symptoms.

sponse is more specific for asthma. This type of challenge can be very helpful because it re-creates the conditions associated with induction of respiratory symptoms. An FEV_1 decrease of greater than 10% is suspicious, and one of 15% or more is diagnostic of EIB (see Sec. 23.3.6).

CHEST RADIOGRAPHS In contrast to pulmonary function testing, which facilitates both diagnostic and therapeutic decision making, routine chest radiographs for patients suspected of having asthma are often useful in excluding disorders that mimic asthma. In infants and young children, the finding of peribronchial thickening, heavy lung markings, or hyperinflation on a chest radiograph taken when the child seems clinically well is another indication that chronic lung inflammation and asthma are present.

LABORATORY STUDIES *Peripheral white blood cell counts* add little to the short- and long-term management of asthma. Because adrenergic agents and corticosteroids cause demargination of polymorphonuclear leukocytes and corticosteroids increase bone marrow output of neutrophils, interpretation of differential white blood cell determinations is confounded following the introduction of these medications. Eosinophilia is a general marker for atopy, which coexists with asthma, allergic rhinitis, atopic dermatitis, and food allergy. It is useful to help identify atopic individuals who are at risk of having asthma but is not necessarily as a marker for asthma per se.

Arterial blood gas (ABG) measurements provide important information about the efficiency of gas exchange in patients with a severe exacerbation but are not routinely used because they are invasive. Pulse oximetry is used as a surrogate indicator of disease severity in patients with mild to moderate exacerbations. Although some have concluded that oxygen saturations greater than 92% are associated with a low risk for respiratory failure, others have argued

that the sensitivity and specificity of saturations in this range are inadequate to predict the potential for eventual hospital admission.

DIFFERENTIAL DIAGNOSIS

INFANTS AND CHILDREN The differential diagnosis for the two most common symptoms of asthma, coughing and wheezing, is extensive in children. Patients and their parents can describe the same sound in many different ways, and, on physical examination, the transmission of upper airway noise to the lower airway can also pose challenges in locating the source of the abnormality. The clinician should also be aware that individuals with normal lung function can generate a wheezing sound during forced exhalation; this sound emanates from the larynx and is often seen in patients with fictitious asthma. Proper location of the problem within the airway is a useful starting point in developing the differential diagnosis (see Table 23-11).

In the *upper respiratory tract,* allergic rhinitis, infectious rhinitis, sinusitis, choanal atresia, adenoidal or tonsillar hypertrophy, micrognathia, and other structural abnormalities can produce sonorous breathing sounds that parents may describe as "wheezing," "whistling," or "rattling." Because antigen-specific IgE antibody responses do not develop to aeroallergens (eg, house dust mites, pollens, molds, animal danders) until after the first 2 to 3 years of life, allergic disease would be an unusual etiologic factor for any airway problem in this age group. Rarely, foods may induce attacks of asthma, but airway symptoms are almost always accompanied by cutaneous or gastrointestinal manifestations.

Middle respiratory tract problems that may occasionally mimic asthma include structural abnormalities that produce turbulent airflow in the large airways, such as foreign body, laryngeal webs, laryngomalacia, tracheomalacia, tracheoesophageal fistula, vocal cord paralysis, tracheostenosis, bronchostenosis, and vascular rings.

Cervical or intrathoracic masses that cause either internal or external compromise or compression of the airway (eg, tumors or enlarged lymph nodes caused by granulomatous diseases) also produce adventitious sounds that may be mistaken for asthma. Other confounding problems may arise from infectious causes (epiglottitis, laryngotracheobronchitis, pertussis), toxic causes (inhalation of dust, gas, or talc), or dysfunction of the vocal cords or larynx from neurologic or psychological factors.

Lower respiratory tract causes of wheezing and coughing are the most difficult to differentiate from asthma because asthma initially affects small airways. Children with a history of prematurity and mechanical ventilation are at risk for the development of bronchopulmonary dysplasia or pulmonary interstitial emphysema. Many of these children eventually develop severe chronic obstructive lung disease, which is indistinguishable from asthma in many instances. Cystic fibrosis (CF) may also present with recurrent asthma-like symptoms (and many children with CF can also have asthma and/or allergic rhinitis), but digital clubbing is rarely seen in asthma, whereas it is often present in patients with CF.

Viral bronchiolitis is one of the most difficult entities to differentiate from asthma in very young children because wheezing and abnormalities of gas exchange are important alterations found in both, and viruses are a major contributing factor to asthma in this age group. Viruses, such as respiratory syncytial virus, may provoke isolated episodes of wheezing in children, but when wheezing occurs repetitively with colds, asthma should be considered as the underlying cause producing the symptoms. Foreign body aspiration can produce both acute and chronic wheezing (both unilateral and bilateral) and coughing typically in children younger than 2 years of age. Gastroesophageal reflux can cause wheezing and cough by itself or can exacerbate symptoms in the patient with asthma. In physically impaired children with dysfunctional swallowing mechanisms, chronic aspiration may contribute to airway abnormalities that can either mimic or exacerbate asthma. Finally, less common causes such as α_1-antitrypsin deficiency, bronchiectasis, hypersensitivity lung diseases (molds, birds, fibers), pulmonary eosinophilia (Loeffler syndrome), pulmonary hemosiderosis, *Chlamydia trachomatis* infection, obliterative bronchiolitis, and pulmonary edema from heart diseases have occasionally produced diagnostic challenges to clinicians evaluating children and young adults for asthma.

TEENAGERS AND YOUNG ADULTS   Many of the same factors that can cause wheezing in younger children and masquerade for asthma are found in teenagers. These include upper airway obstruction, foreign bodies, tracheal compression, intramural tracheal disease, and ultraluminal tracheal disease. Of these, the most frequent confounding problem is vocal cord dysfunction. Other causes of wheezing to consider include pulmonary embolus, foreign body aspiration, gastroesophageal reflux disease, and carcinoid. Although eosinophilia is a characteristic feature of asthma, a number of other pulmonary diseases have wheezing, pulmonary infiltration, and eosinophilia. These include allergic bronchopulmonary aspergillosis (ABPA), chronic eosinophilic pneumonia, and Churg-Strauss syndrome. Findings of recurrent, persistent, or focal infiltrates on chest radiographs are indications that the patient does not have uncomplicated asthma.

COEXISTING ISSUES IN CHILDHOOD ASTHMA

SINUSITIS AND ASTHMA   The association between asthma and sinusitis in children has been the subject of debate for many years.

Much of the difficulty in defining this relationship results from the uncertainties in making the clinical diagnosis of sinusitis. There is little debate that children with asthma have a high rate of upper respiratory signs and symptoms and an increased frequency of abnormal sinus radiographs. However, there is relatively little information regarding the positive and negative predictive values of sinus radiographs in patients with asthma. Abnormal sinus radiographs can be observed in 33 to 65% of children with asthma, especially if computerized tomography (CT) is used to screen for sinus abnormalities. The interpretation of these radiologic images can be misleading in children, whose sinus development is variable and asymmetric. Moreover, patients with simple acute nasopharyngitis can have abnormal sinus CT scans. Further, children with asthma often have clinical signs and symptoms compatible with sinusitis during acute exacerbations of asthma, raising the possibility that bacterial sinusitis causes increased lower respiratory symptoms. Aggressive treatment of sinus disease may decrease medication requirements to control concomitant asthmatic symptoms.

GASTROESOPHAGEAL REFLUX AND ASTHMA   Gastroesophageal reflux disease (GERD) is an important consideration in two clinical presentations of the wheezing child: first, in the wheezing infant without asthma who has postprandial vomiting, coughing, or wheezing; and second, in the child with asthma who is poorly responsive to therapy. Some of these children may complain of dysphagia, regurgitation, or vague substernal chest discomfort, presumably from acid esophagitis. Although it is clear that reflux can trigger wheezing and cough, GERD with or without aspiration may cause bronchospasm. Conversely, airway obstruction in asthma increases transdiaphragmatic pressure swings that can promote reflux by decreasing lower esophageal sphincter (LES) pressure. Agents used to treat asthma, such as theophylline, may also lower the LES pressure and predispose to GERD.

EXERCISE AND ASTHMA   In both asthmatic and nonasthmatic individuals, the initiation of exercise causes bronchodilation and an increase in expiratory flow rates. However, more vigorous or prolonged exercise can trigger asthma symptoms. Exercise-induced asthma (EIA) is occasionally seen in adolescents who have no other signs or symptoms of asthma at rest, sleep, or during respiratory infections. These patients typically develop cough or dyspnea after 6 to 10 minutes of strenuous exercise, especially exercise in cold dry air. In these children with only exercise-related symptoms, pretreatment with cromolyn sodium or a short-acting β-adrenergic agent will prevent symptom formation. In other patients with persistent asthma, exercise may be one of several triggers of asthma symptoms.

Asthma is often considered in the differential diagnosis of children who have reduced exercise tolerance or who develop pulmonary symptoms after brief periods of exercise. In these patients, deconditioning (lack of fitness), unreasonable amounts of stress associated with athletic competition, or other psychological factors should be explored.

VOCAL CORD DYSFUNCTION AND ASTHMA (FICTITIOUS WHEEZING)   Both glottic closure and vocal cord adduction during exhalation can produce a high-pitched wheezing sound that can be misdiagnosed as asthma. This can occur in patients without asthma and has an epidemiology and risk factors similar to patients with tics or habit cough. Like other tics, the symptom disappears during sleep. The formation of this symptom requires concentrated effort and cannot usually be sustained for long periods. In contrast to patients with asthma, cough and hypoxemia are absent, and these patients will often stop wheezing when they believe they are unobserved or if they are distracted. Treatment of these patients may be difficult. In some patients, flexible fiberoptic endoscopy has been used to illustrate the symptom to the patient, and symptom formation may be reduced by stress reduction techniques.

Fictitious wheezing can also occur in patients with asthma who amplify their symptoms for secondary gain or for psychological reasons. This is an extremely challenging situation, and acute wheezing episodes in these patients require a thorough assessment of every exacerbation to determine whether fictitious or authentic wheezing is present.

REFRACTORY ASTHMA With proper education and medication, most patients with asthma can achieve long symptom-free intervals and engage in all age-appropriate activities. When asthma symptoms become difficult to control, three possibilities should be considered: (1) another disorder, such as cystic fibrosis, ABPA, vocal cord dysfunction, hypersensitivity pneumonitis, or obstructive sleep apnea, may be present; (2) exacerbating factors, such as environmental tobacco smoke exposure, reflux, or sinusitis, may be present; or (3) poor understanding and adherence to the recommended asthma treatment program. Even when these factors have been excluded or treated, up to 5% of pediatric patients may have severe asthma and are characterized clinically by persistently abnormal lung function, rapid onset of severe symptoms, and the need for high doses or prolonged courses of oral corticosteroids to maintain symptom-free intervals. Whether these patients constitute a distinct physiological or pathologic group is unclear. The economic cost of the treatment of this small subgroup is enormous.

GROWTH OF ASTHMATIC CHILDREN Children with chronic perennial asthma frequently exhibit linear growth retardation in part because of chronic respiratory symptoms and the adoption of a sedentary life-style. Thus, cross-sectional comparison of asthmatic children with their pubertal peers often reveals a temporary relative slowing of growth velocity even though growth potential and eventual adult height attained are likely to be normal. Delays in height attainment correlate well with delays in skeletal maturation and pubertal development and seem to be independent of the severity of asthma. Based on a number of short-term term studies evaluating linear growth in asthmatic children receiving inhaled corticosteroids (ICS), the US Food and Drug Administration now mandates that manufacturers of all ICS medications include a warning in their product labeling indicating that treatment with this class of compounds has the potential of affecting linear growth. More recent studies suggest that low- and moderate-dose ICS therapy does not adversely effect either linear growth or skeletal mineralization. Because ICS are extremely effective long-term controller medications, this warning should not deter physicians from prescribing them when indicated. Careful monitoring of growth and growth velocity is obviously indicated, and clinicians should attempt various strategies to minimize ICS doses while maintaining acceptable asthma control.

TREATMENT

The treatment of asthma is one of the greatest challenges in pediatrics today. The National Heart, Lung, and Blood Institute has published a clinician's guide, both for general asthma management and specifically for managing pediatric asthma, containing many valuable educational materials, including asthma treatment plan work sheets that are designed for office use. The overall goals of therapy include maintaining age-appropriate activity levels at home and school, maintaining optimal pulmonary function, preventing chronic symptoms (eg, coughing or breathlessness in the night, early morning, and after exertion), preventing recurrent exacerbations of asthma, and avoiding adverse effects of asthma medications. These goals should be formulated in regard to the cognitive and social development of the child and the social situation at home and school. Specific areas to be addressed include asthma education, mediations, and asthma treatment plans including environmental control of allergens and emergency care plans. The child and family must be educated (and periodically reeducated) about asthma, dedicated to the therapeutic goals, have all asthma medications available at home, and have telephone access to an asthma expert.

When pharmacotherapy is considered for patients with asthma, special consideration must be given to potential side effects of medications and also to the method of drug delivery. Adverse effects on either growth or behavior are particularly undesirable during this period of rapid physical and intellectual development. However, it should be recognized that untreated or undertreated asthma results in days lost from school or work, exercise limitation, sleep disruption, and adoption of a sedentary life-style, all of which can adversely affect development.

Inhaled medications are usually administered by either nebulizer or pressurized metered-dose inhaler (MDI) attached to a volume spacer device. Volume spacer devices improve the delivery of inhaled medications to the lung surface and reduce systemic absorption of the drug by trapping most of the large aerosol droplets, while the smaller particles are held in a reservoir until they are inhaled. Some brands of spacers, such as the Aerochamber, may be equipped with either mouthpieces or variable-size masks, which are suitable for use by children under 3 years of age. The use of a spacer with inhaled corticosteroids may also reduce the incidence of oral candidiasis and hoarse voice. Dry powder inhalers have been developed in response to a demand for chlorofluorocarbon-free alternatives to propellant-driven MDIs. Although compressed air nebulizers have traditionally been used in medical facilities for treatment of acute asthma, MDIs provide bronchodilation that is faster and equal or greater in magnitude but require meticulous attention to the technical aspects of administration. It is of primary importance to understand the various delivery systems and to teach patients to use them correctly. Unfortunately, children and adolescents may not be able to use MDIs/spacer or dry powder inhalers correctly and thus may not derive full benefit from the medications delivered in these ways.

LONG-TERM TREATMENT OF PERSISTENT ASTHMA In patients with mild intermittent asthma, the avoidance of symptom triggers and the occasional use of a short-acting β_2 agonist agent such as albuterol may be effective when used before exercise or for a few days during viral respiratory infections. These patients can sustain long symptom-free intervals and usually have no nocturnal symptoms. However, if the frequency of bronchodilator therapy increases, or if the patient develops chronic symptoms, the use of daily preventive therapy should be considered. Therapy for persistent asthma must be directed at suppression of inflammation, elimination of asthma symptoms, and the early identification and treatment of acute exacerbations (Table 23-13). Control of asthma with the smallest amount of medication and minimal risk for adverse effects is the aim of asthma therapy.

TABLE 23-13

USUAL DOSAGES FOR LONG-TERM CONTROL MEDICATIONS

MEDICATION	DOSAGE FORM	ADULT DOSE	CHILD DOSE	COMMENTS
Inhaled corticosteroids	See Table 23-14		See Table 23-14	
Systemic corticosteroids				
Methylprednisolone	2-, 4-, 8-, 16-, 32-mg tablets	8–64 mg daily in a single dose or qid as needed for control	0.25–2 mg/kg daily in single dose or qid as needed for control	For long-term treatment of severe persistent asthma, administer single dose in AM either daily or on alternate days (alternate-day therapy may produce less adrenal suppression)
Prednisolone	5-mg tabs, 5 mg/5.0 mL, 15 mg/5.0 mL	Short-course "burst" 40–60 mg per day as single or 2 divided doses for 3–10 days	Short-course "burst:" 1–2 mg/kg/day, maximum 60 mg/day, for 3–10 days	Short courses or "bursts" are effective for establishing control when initiating therapy or during a period of gradual deterioration
Prednisone	1-, 2.5-, 5-, 10-, 20-, 25-mg tabs, 5 mg/ml solution			The burst should be continued until patient achieves 80% PEF personal best or symptoms resolve. This usually requires 3–10 days but may require longer. There is no evidence that tapering the dose following improvement prevents relapse
Cromolyn and nedocromil				
Cromolyn	MD [1 mg/puff] Nebulizer solution 20 mg/ampule	2–4 puffs tid-qid 1 ampule tid-qid	1–2 puffs tid-qid 1 ampule tid-qid	One dose before exercise or allergen exposure provides effective prophylaxis for 1–2 hours
Nedocromil	MD [1.75 mg/puff]	2–4 puffs bid-qid	1–2 puffs bid-qid	See cromolyn above
Long-acting inhaled β_2 agonists	**Inhaled**			
Salmeterol	MD [21 μg/puff, 60 or 120 puffs] DP [50 μg/blister]	2 puffs q 12 hr 1 blister q 12 hr	1–2 puffs q 12 hr 1 blister q 12 hr	May use one dose nightly for symptoms Should not be used as rescue inhaler for symptom relief or exacerbations
Methylxanthines				
Theophylline (numerous manufacturers)	Liquids Sustained-release tablets and capsules	Starting dose 10 mg/kg/day up to 300 mg max; usual max 800 mg/day	Starting dose 10 mg/kg/day; usual max: $\geq$1 year of age: 16 mg/kg/day <1 year: 0.2 (age in weeks) +5 = mg/kg/day	Adjust dosage to achieve peak serum concentration of 5–15 μg/mL at steady-state (at least 48 hours on same dosage) Due to wide interpatient variability in theophylline metabolic clearance, routine serum theophylline level monitoring is important
Leukotriene modifiers				
Zileuton	300-mg tablet 600-mg tablet	2400 mg daily (2 300-mg tablets or 1 600-mg tablet, qid)		Monitor hepatic enzymes (alanine aminotransferase [ALT]
Zafirlukast	20-mg tablet	40-mg tablet (1 tablet bid)		Administration with meals decreases bioavailability; take at least 1 hour before or 2 hours after meals
Montelukast	5-mg chewable tablet 10-mg tablet	10 mg QHS	5–10 mg QHS 5 mg dose for children <40 kg and 10 mg dose for >40 kg	

MD = metered dose.

SOURCE: *National Asthma Education and Prevention Program: Clinical practice guidelines. Expert Panel Report 2. Guidelines for the diagnosis and management of asthma. NIH publication No. 97–4051, July 1997. http://www.nhlbi.nih.gov/guidelines/asthma/asthgdln.htm*

Asthma medications are categorized into two general classes: *long-term control medications,* which are taken daily on a long-term basis to achieve and maintain control of persistent asthma, and *quick-relief medications,* which provide prompt reversal of acute airflow obstruction and bronchoconstriction. The National Asthma Education Program has developed algorithms to aid in the management of children with mild, moderate, and severe asthma (Figs. 23-19 and 23-20). Of the controller medications, cromolyn and

	Long-Term Control	Quick-Relief

Step 4
Severe Persistent
	Daily anti-inflammatory medications:
	• High-dose inhaled corticosteroid with spacer/holding chamber and face mask.
	    AND
	• If needed, add systemic corticosteroids 0.25-2 mg/kg/day and reduce to lowest daily or alternate-day dose that stabilizes symptoms.
		• Short-acting bronchodilator as needed for symptoms. Intensity of treatment depends on severity of exacerbation.
		• Either:
		  → Inhaled short-acting beta$_2$-agonist by nebulizer or spacer/holding chamber and face mask.
		    OR
		  → Oral beta$_2$-agonist.
		
		Daily or increasing use of short-acting, inhaled beta$_2$-agonists may indicate need for additional long-term control therapy.*

Step 3
Moderate Persistent
	Daily anti-inflammatory medications. Either:
	• Medium-dose inhaled corticosteroid with spacer/holding chamber and face mask.
	  OR, once control is established,
	• Low-to-medium-dose inhaled corticosteroid and nedocromil.
	    OR
	• Low-to-medium-dose inhaled corticosteroid and long-acting bronchoditator (theophylline).
		• Short-acting bronchodilator as needed for symptoms. Intensity of treatment depends on severity of exacerbation.
		• Either:
		  → Inhaled short-acting beta$_2$-agonist by nebulizer or spacer/holding chamber and face mask.
		    OR
		  → Oral beta$_2$-agonist.
		
		Daily or increasing use of short-acting, inhaled beta$_2$-agonists may indicate need for additional long-term control therapy.*

Step 2
Mild Persistent
	Daily anti-inflammatory medication. Either:
	• Cromolyn (nebulizer preferred, or MDI) or nedocromil (MDI) tid-qid. Infants and young children usually begin with a trial of cromolyn or nedocromil.
	    OR
	• Low-dose inhaled corticosteroid with spacer/holding chamber and face mask.
		• Short-acting bronchodilator as needed for symptoms. Intensity of treatment depends on severity of exacerbation.
		• Either:
		  → Inhaled short-acting beta$_2$-agonist by nebulizer or spacer/holding chamber and face mask.
		    OR
		  → Oral beta$_2$-agonist.
		
		Daily or increasing use of short-acting, inhaled beta$_2$-agonists may indicate need for additional long-term control therapy.*

Step 1
Mild Intermittent
	• No daily medication	• Short-acting bronchodilator as needed for symptoms <2×/wk. Intensity of treatment depends on severity of exacerbation.
		• Either:
		  → Inhaled short-acting beta$_2$-agonist by nebulizer or spacer/holding chamber and face mask.
		    OR
		  → Oral beta$_2$-agonist.
		
		Daily or increasing use of short-acting, inhaled beta$_2$-agonists may indicate need for additional long-term control therapy.*

Step Down		***Step Up**
Review treatment every 1 to 6 months; a gradual stepwise reduction in treatment may be possible.		If control is not maintained, consider stepping up. First, review patient medication technique, adherence, and environmental control (avoidance of allergens and/or other factors that contribute to asthma severity).

Courtesy of: American Academy of Allergy, Asthma, and Immunology. Pediatric Asthma, Promoting Best Practice: Guide for Managing Asthma in Children. 1999.

FIGURE 23-19 Stepwise approach to managing asthma in infants and young children (≤5 years of age) with acute or chronic asthma symptoms.

---

nedocromil are considered first-line anti-inflammatory medications in children with moderate asthma because of proven efficacy and a paucity of side effects. The drugs are extremely safe and must be given by inhalation at least three or four times per day. More recently, the development and testing of leukotriene receptor antagonist drugs in children 4 years of age or older has been completed. These studies suggest that this class of compounds, which are given orally, may be very effective in certain children as a single agent or

	Long-Term Control	Quick-Relief

Step 4
Severe Persistent
	Daily medications:
	• Anti-inflammatory: high-dose inhaled corticosteroid.
	    AND
	• Long-acting bronchoditator (e.g., either long-acting, inhaled beta$_2$-agonist or sustained-release theophylline).
	    AND
	• Corticosteroid tablets or syrup long-term (2 mg/kg/day, generally not to exceed 60 mg per day); make repeated attempts to reduce systemic corticosteroids and maintain control with high-dose inhaled corticosteroids
		• Short-acting bronchodilator inhaled beta$_2$-agonist as needed for symptoms. Intensity of treatment depends on severity of exacerbation.
		
		Daily or increasing use of short-acting, inhaled beta$_2$-agonists may indicate need for additional long-term control therapy.*

Step 3 Moderate Persistent	Daily medication: • Anti-inflammatory: either medium-dose inhaled corticosteroid. OR • Low-to medium-dose inhaled corticosteroid and add a long-acting bronchodilator, especially for nighttime symptoms (e.g., either long-acting, inhaled beta$_2$-agonist or sustained-release theophylline). • If needed, medium-to high-dose inhaled corticosteroid and long-acting bronchodilator, especially for nighttime symptoms.	• Short-acting bronchodilator: inhaled beta$_2$-agonist as needed for symptoms. Intensity of treatment depends on severity of exacerbation. **Daily or increasing use of short-acting, inhaled beta$_2$-agonists may indicate need for additional long-term control therapy.***

Step 2
Mild Persistent
	One daily medication:
	• Anti-inflammatory: EITHER
	  → Low-dose inhaled corticosteroid
	    OR
	  → Cromolyn or nedocromil (children usually begin with a trial of cromolyn or nedocromil).
	• Sustained-release theophylline (to serum concentration of 5-15 mcg/mL) is an alternative, but not preferred, therapy.
	• A leukotriene modifier may be considered although their position in therapy is not fully established.
		• Short-acting bronchodilator: inhaled beta$_2$-agonist as needed for symptoms. Intensity of treatment depends on severity of exacerbation.
		
		Daily or increasing use of short-acting, inhaled beta$_2$-agonists may indicate need for additional long-term control therapy.*

Step 1 Mild Intermittent	• No daily medication needed.	• Short-acting bronchodilator: inhaled beta$_2$-agonist as needed for symptoms. Intensity of treatment depends on severity of exacerbation. **Daily or increasing use of short-acting, inhaled beta$_2$-agonists may indicate need for additional long-term control therapy.***
Step Down		***Step Up**
Review treatment every 1 to 6 months; a gradual stepwise reduction in treatment may be possible.		If control is not maintained, consider stepping up. First, review patient medication technique, adherence, and environmental control (avoidance of allergens and/or other factors that contribute to asthma severity).

Courtesy of: American Academy of Allergy, Asthma, and Immunology. Pediatric Asthma, Promoting Best Practice: Guide for Managing Asthma in Children. 1999.

FIGURE 23-20 Stepwise approach for managing asthma in children >5 years of age with acute or chronic asthma symptoms.

combined with inhaled corticosteroids to control persistent asthma. If the response to these medications is not satisfactory, a long-acting β-adrenergic agent is added to the regimen. In rare cases, daily oral corticosteroid therapy is necessary.

Once stability is achieved, periodic reductions in dosages should be attempted to establish the minimum amount of medications needed to maintain acceptable symptom control. Unresponsiveness to the regimens described should prompt a review of exposure to triggers (allergens, tobacco smoke, sinusitis), inhaler technique, adherence to medication regimen, and other possible diagnoses, such as cystic fibrosis, allergic bronchopulmonary aspergillosis, GERD, or vocal cord dysfunction.

Corticosteroids, both inhaled and oral, are the most effective anti-inflammatory agents available for the treatment of asthma and the only agents shown to reverse the histologic manifestations of asthma. Their efficacy is related to many factors, including a diminution in inflammatory cell function and activation, stabilization of vascular permeability, a decrease in mucus production, and an increase in β-adrenergic responsiveness. Chronic administration of oral corticosteroids can result in several adverse effects, including hypothalamic-pituitary-adrenal (HPA) axis suppression, osteoporosis, cataracts, hyperglycemia, hypertension, weight gain, dermal thinning and striae, and growth retardation. To minimize these effects, inhaled corticosteroid therapy has been developed. Five preparations of inhaled corticosteroids (ICS) are currently available in the United States (Table 23-14). The choice of ICS depends on a number of factors including potency, systemic absorption, taste, delivery system, and cost. The potencies of these preparations are quite variable, and the clinician should understand that "not all puffs are created equal." Systemic bioavailability of ICS result from a combination of oral, gastrointestinal, and transpulmonary absorbtion and can be reduced by the use of a volume spacer. Fortunately, because ICS are efficacious in children and young adults, the need for chronic oral corticosteroid regimens has diminished substantially. ICS therapy has an increasingly large body of evidence documenting its safety and efficacy in reducing exacerbations and hospitalizations and the need for oral corticosteroid therapy. Early reports of growth retardation related to ICS use have not been substantiated with larger long-term studies.

One additional complication of corticosteroid therapy deserves mentioning. Although single case reports of fatal varicella infection in children with asthma receiving systemic steroids suggest a potential danger, there is no clear evidence that treatment with inhaled corticosteroids places patients at an increased risk of serious infectious complications.

Cromolyn sodium and *nedocromil sodium* are anti-inflammatory medications for the treatment of chronic asthma with impressive safety records. They are effective in attenuating exercise-induced bronchospasm if given before exercise. The mechanism of action is not well understood. They do not have direct bronchodilating effects and have no efficacy in the treatment of acute exacerbations. Cromolyn sodium is available in both an MDI form and a form for nebulization. In some children and adolescents, nebulized cromolyn sodium may be comparable to ICS in controlling symptoms. Comparative studies of nedocromil sodium (MDI preparation only) and cromolyn sodium suggest that nedocromil sodium may be more effective in treating reversible airway obstruction and at lower doses than cromolyn sodium. Reported adverse effects for cromolyn sodium are rare but include increased cough and wheeze, dermatitis, myositis, and gastroenteritis. The adverse effects reported for nedocromil sodium include nausea, vomiting, sore throat, cough, and headache.

TABLE 23-14

ESTIMATED COMPARATIVE DAILY DOSAGES OF INHALED CORTICOSTEROIDS FOR CHILDREN

DRUG	LOW DOSE	MEDIUM DOSE	HIGH DOSE
Beclomethasone	84–336 μg	336–672 μg	>672 μg
42 μg/puff	(2–8 puffs)	(8–16 puffs)	(>16 puffs)
84 μg/puff	(1–4 puffs)	(4–8 puffs)	(>8 puffs)
Budesonide Turbuhaler 200 μg/dose	100–200 μg	200–400 μg (1–2 inhalations—200 μg)	>400 μg (>2 inhalations—200 μg)
Flunisolide, 250 μg/puff	500–750 μg (2–3 puffs)	1000–1250 μg (4–5 puffs)	>1250 μg (>5 puffs)
Fluticasone MDI, 44, 110, 220 μg/puff	88–176 μg (2–4 puffs—44 μg)	176–440 μg (4–10 puffs—44 μg) or	>440 μg (>4 puffs—110 μg)
DPI: 50, 100, 250 μg/dose	(2–4 inhalations—50 μg)	(2–4 puffs—110 μg) (2–4 inhalations—100 μg)	(>4 inhalations—100 μg)
Triamcinolone acetonide 100 μg/puff	400–800 μg (4–8 puffs)	800–1200 μg (8–12 puffs)	>1200 μg (>12 puffs)

NOTE:
- The most important determinant of appropriate dosing is the clinician's judgment of the patient's response to therapy. The clinician must monitor the patient's response on several clinical parameters and adjust the dose accordingly. The stepwise approach to therapy emphasizes that once control of asthma is achieved, the dose of medication should be carefully titrated to the minimum dose required to maintain control, thus reducing the potential for adverse effect.
- See National Asthma Education and Prevention Program: Clinical Practice Guidelines. Expert Panel Report 2. Figure 3-5c, Estimated Clinical Comparability of Doses for Inhaled Corticosteroids, for an explanation of the rationale used for the comparative dosages. The reference point for the range in the dosages for children is data on the safety of inhaled corticosteroids in children, which, in general, suggest that the dose ranges are equivalent to beclomethasone dipropionate 200–400 μg/day (low dose), 400–800 μg/day (medium dose), and >800 μg/day (high dose).
- Some dosages may be outside package labeling.
- Metered-dose inhaler dosages are expressed as the actuator dose (the amount of drug leaving the actuator and delivered to the patient), which is the labeling required in the United States. This is different from the dosage expressed as the valve dose (the amount of drug leaving the valve, not all of which is available to the patient), which is used in many European countries and in some of the scientific literature. Dry powder inhaler doses (eg., Turbuhaler) are expressed as the amount of drug in the inhaler after activation.

MDI = metered-dose inhaler; DPI = dry powder inhalers.

SOURCE: *National Asthma Education and Prevention Program: Clinical practice guidelines. Expert Panel Report 2. Guidelines for the diagnosis and management of asthma. NIH publication No. 97-4051, July 1997. http://www.nhlbi.nih.gov/guidelines/asthma/asthgdln.htm*

Long-acting β_2-agonists, which bind with high affinity to β_2 receptors, provide bronchodilation up to 12 hours in duration. Salmeterol is the first such medication approved for use in the United States. It is added to the treatment regimen of patients with chronic persistent asthma as an adjunct to inhaled corticosteroids. Addition of salmeterol to an existing steroid regimen may provide greater benefit than increasing the current steroid dose. The patient should be cautioned that, unlike short-acting β_2-agonists such as albuterol or terbutaline, salmeterol has a much slower onset of action and therefore should not be used to treat acute bronchospasm.

Leukotriene modifiers are the newest oral agents for the treatment of asthma. Leukotrienes are biologically active fatty acids derived from the oxidative metabolism of arachidonic acid. A role for leukotrienes in the pathogenesis of asthma has been suggested by their presence in the lungs of asthmatics and on the findings that leukotrienes exhibit both proinflammatory and bronchoconstrictor properties. This class of drugs includes agents that either inhibit leukotriene production (5-lipoxygenase inhibitors) or inhibit leukotriene binding to receptors (LTD_4 antagonists). The first of these approved for use in the United States, zafirlukast, is an orally active LTD_4 receptor antagonist. This compound has been demonstrated to attenuate the acute airway obstructive response to allergen and exercise challenge and to improve chronic asthma control. Montelukast, a once-daily dosed LTD_4 receptor antagonist, has been approved for use in children as young as 4 years of age. It can improve exercise-induced bronchospasm, improve chronic objective and subjective signs and symptoms, and allows for reduction of ICS therapy in some patients. Zileuton, a 5-lipoxygenase inhibitor, has also demonstrated efficacy in exercise-induced and aspirin-induced bronchospasm and also exerts an ICS-sparing effect. Zileuton can be hepatotoxic and should be used only in conjunction with strict monitoring of hepatic function. Safety issues with the use of leukotriene modifiers remain to be fully addressed. In clinical trials, most adverse events have been mild. Reported adverse effects include headache, dyspepsia, macular rashes, and reversible liver enzyme elevations. The appropriate positioning of these compounds in the management of asthma awaits more extensive clinical experience with their use both as prophylactic agents and in the management of chronic disease activity.

Theophylline is a methylxanthine bronchodilator with extrapulmonary effects, including enhancement of respiratory muscle contractility. Theophylline is an old medication that is being replaced by newer treatment modalities that require less acute monitoring and have wider margins of safety. Serum levels of theophylline, which is extensively metabolized by the liver, are markedly affected by a number of variables including age, diet, disease states, tobacco smoke, and drug interactions, all of which contribute to the complexity of using this medication. Because of the variability of theophylline metabolism, as well as a narrow therapeutic index, children using theophylline must have serum levels monitored periodically with the goal of a serum concentration of 5 to 20 μg/mL. When compared with β_2-agonists, theophylline has a slower onset of action and a lower peak effect, making it less suitable for acute therapy. Unfortunately, theophylline may produce a number of dose-related side effects including gastrointestinal symptoms and possible adverse behavioral effects. Its use as a first-line drug for persistent asthma has all but disappeared, although it may have a role in the treatment of severe respiratory failure in status asthmaticus.

Inhaled *anticholinergic agents* (eg, ipratropium bromide) are available and may produce bronchodilation by reducing intrinsic cholinergic tone of the airway. In clinical trials of asthma, there has been little evidence to support their use in long-term management. In general, anticholinergics are less potent than β_2-agonists and have a slow onset of action to maximal effect (ie, 30 to 60 minutes). In some, but not all, patients with acute exacerbations, ipratropium bromide has shown additive effects with inhaled short-acting β_2-agonists. Anticholinergics have also been effective in treating asthma exacerbations in patients who are taking β-adrenergic antagonist drugs such as propranolol and related compounds.

The role of monoantigen *immunotherapy* in the treatment of asthma remains controversial. Immunotherapy is effective in the treatment of allergic rhinitis that coexists in many children with asthma. Immunotherapy can attenuate the late response after allergen challenge in children, suggesting that it may play an immunomodulatory role in the pathogenesis of allergic airway inflammation. However, randomized controlled clinical trials have not shown strong or consistent beneficial effects. It is possible that immunotherapy can be beneficial in situations in which patients or their parents have difficulty following asthma medication treatment plans or environmental control measures. Poorly controlled labile asthma remains a contraindication to immunotherapy use.

Immunomodulation using newer forms of therapy, eg, a parenterally administered monoclonal antibody to IgE, also show promise in asthma clinical trials in both children and adults. This agent substantially reduces plasma IgE concentrations and can significantly reduce both inhaled and oral corticosteroid use in many patients. Unlike conventional allergen immunotherapy, treatment with anti-IgE antibody is associated with little to no risk of systemic reactions.

ACUTE ASTHMA TREATMENT Inhaled rapid-onset β_2-agonists (albuterol, terbutaline, pirbuterol, and a newer nonracemic form of albuterol) are first-line drugs for rescue treatment of acute asthmatic symptoms in patients of all ages (Table 23-15). Because of the potential for the development of progressive life-threatening symptoms if treatment of acute exacerbations of asthma is delayed, it is recommended that children with asthma who attend daycare centers or school have these drugs available. Children who have sufficient maturity to control the use of inhaled medications should be permitted to carry their β_2-agonist inhalers with them at school and use them as needed.

As in other age groups, the treatment of acute exacerbations of asthma in children and adolescents will depend on the severity of airflow obstruction, as assessed by objective measurements (physical findings, spirometry, pulse oximetry, and, where appropriate, peak flow rates) and the initial response to bronchodilator therapy. Additional algorithms based on the same principles have been established for managing acute asthma at home (Fig. 23-21) and in the hospital (Fig. 23-22). Several studies have demonstrated conclusively that oral or parenteral corticosteroid therapy is essential for the treatment of acute exacerbations of asthma that respond poorly to bronchodilator therapy. When given early in the course of an asthma exacerbation, they can reduce the need for hospitalization. The development of an acute episode of asthma should prompt the clinician to reevaluate the current asthma prevention program and make appropriate modifications.

β_2-Adrenergic drugs are the most potent and rapidly acting bronchodilators in clinical use. Their availability in multiple formulations (short- and long-acting, nonracemic form) and delivery systems (MDIs, nebulizer solutions, and respirable powders) gives them wide clinical versatility. Paradoxically, the rapid onset of action and potent bronchodilator activity may lead to deterioration of asthma disease control if the patient uses β-agonists to the ex-

TABLE 23-15

USUAL DOSAGES FOR QUICK-RELIEF MEDICATIONS

MEDICATION	DOSAGE FORM	ADULT DOSE	CHILD DOSE	COMMENTS
Short-acting inhaled β_2-agonists				
	MDI			
Albuterol	90 μg/puff, 200 puffs	2 puffs q4h as needed and q5 min before exercise	1–2 puffs q4h as needed and q5 min before exercise	An increasing use or lack of expected effect indicates diminished control of asthma
Albuterol HFA	90 μg/puff, 200 puffs			
Pirbuterol	200 μg/puff, 400 puffs			Not generally recommended for long-term treatment
				Three to four doses in 1 day or regular use on a daily basis indicates the need for additional therapy
				Differences in potency exist so that all products are essentially equipotent on a per puff basis
				May double usual dose for mild exacerbations
				Nonselective agents (ie, epinephrine, isoproterenol, metaproterenol) are not recommended
	DPI			
Albuterol Rotahaler	200 μg/capsule	1–2 capsules q4-6h as needed and before exercise	1 capsule q4-6h as needed and before exercise	
	Nebulizer solution			
Albuterol	5 mg/mL (0.5%)	1.25–5 mg (0.25–1 mL) in 2–3 mL of saline q4-8h	0.05 mg/kg (min 1.25 mg, max 2.5 mg) in 2–3 mL of saline q4-6h	May mix with cromolyn or ipratropium nebulizer solutions
				May double dose for mild exacerbations
Anticholinergics				
	MDI			
Ipratropium	18 μg/puff	2–3 puffs q6h	1–2 puffs q6h	Evidence is lacking for producing added benefit to β_2-agonists in long-term asthma therapy
	Nebulizer solution			
	0.2 mg/mL (.02%)	0.25–0.5 mg q6h	0.25 mg q6h	
Systemic corticosteroids				
Methylprednisolone	2-, 4-, 8-, 16-, 32-mg tablets	Short-course "burst;" 40–60 mg/day as single or 2 divided doses for 3–10 days	Short-course "burst;" 1–2 mg/kg/day, maximum 60 mg/day, for 3–10 days	Short courses or "bursts" are effective for establishing control when initiating therapy or during a period of gradual deterioration
Prednisolone	5-mg tabs, 5 mg/5.0 mL, 15 mg/5.0 mL			The burst should be continued until patient achieves 80% PEF personal best or symptoms resolve. This usually requires 3–10 days but may require longer. There is no evidence that tapering the dose after improvement prevents relapse
Prednisone	1-, 2.5-, 5-, 10-, 20-, 25-mg tabs; 5 mg/mL solution			

HFA = hydrofluoroalkane; MDI = metered-dose inhaler; DPI = dry powder inhaler; PEF = peak expiratory flow.

SOURCE: *National Asthma Education and Prevention Program: Clinical practice guidelines. Expert Panel Report 2. Guidelines for the diagnosis and management of asthma. NIH publication No. 97-4051, July 1997. http://www.nhlbi.nih.gov/guidelines/asthma/asthgdln.htm*

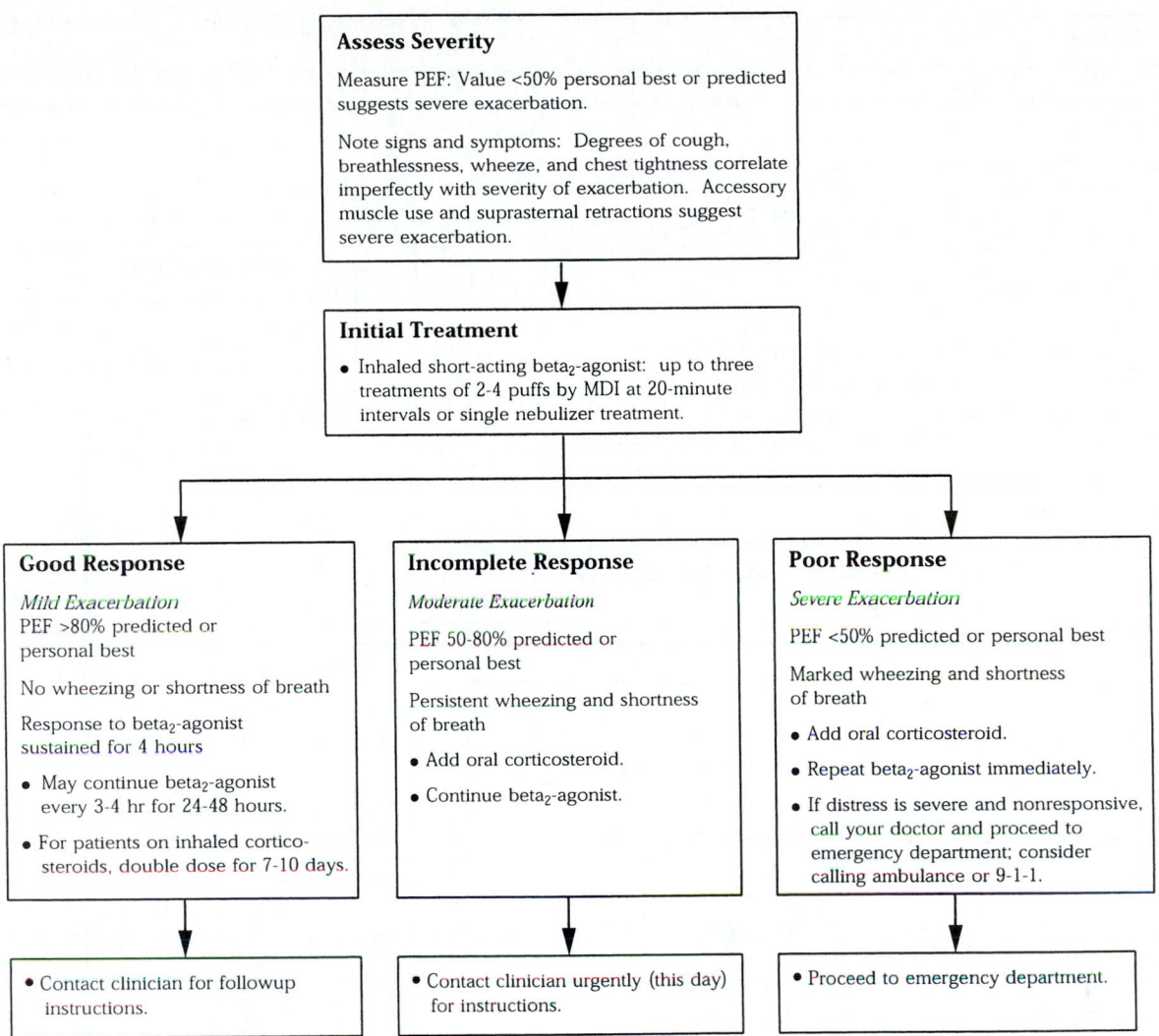

Assess Severity

Measure PEF: Value <50% personal best or predicted suggests severe exacerbation.

Note signs and symptoms: Degrees of cough, breathlessness, wheeze, and chest tightness correlate imperfectly with severity of exacerbation. Accessory muscle use and suprasternal retractions suggest severe exacerbation.

Initial Treatment

- Inhaled short-acting beta$_2$-agonist: up to three treatments of 2-4 puffs by MDI at 20-minute intervals or single nebulizer treatment.

Good Response

Mild Exacerbation
PEF >80% predicted or personal best

No wheezing or shortness of breath

Response to beta$_2$-agonist sustained for 4 hours

- May continue beta$_2$-agonist every 3-4 hr for 24-48 hours.
- For patients on inhaled corticosteroids, double dose for 7-10 days.

- Contact clinician for followup instructions.

Incomplete Response

Moderate Exacerbation
PEF 50-80% predicted or personal best

Persistent wheezing and shortness of breath

- Add oral corticosteroid.
- Continue beta$_2$-agonist.

- Contact clinician urgently (this day) for instructions.

Poor Response

Severe Exacerbation
PEF <50% predicted or personal best

Marked wheezing and shortness of breath

- Add oral corticosteroid.
- Repeat beta$_2$-agonist immediately.
- If distress is severe and nonresponsive, call your doctor and proceed to emergency department; consider calling ambulance or 9-1-1.

- Proceed to emergency department.

FIGURE 23-21   Note: Patients at high risk of asthma-related death should receive immediate clinical attention after initial treatment. Additional therapy may be required. PEF = peak expiratory flow.

clusion of anti-inflammatory medications. Therefore, increasing frequency of β-agonist use should be considered as an indicator of inadequate disease control and as signaling the need for a medical evaluation. Side effects of selective β$_2$-agonists include tremor, tachycardia, and increased anxiety, but these effects are minimal when β-agonists are administered via inhalation. Oral β-agonist therapy, like theophylline therapy, is rarely used for either acute or chronic therapy.

For acute rescue management of asthma exacerbations, albuterol or related agents may be delivered continuously via nebulizer or intermittently every 3 to 6 hours by either nebulizer or MDI. A need for more frequent administration than every 4 hours, more than eight inhalations from a metered-dose inhaler per day, or the use of more than one inhaler per month should alert the treating physician that the child needs more aggressive anti-inflammatory therapy. Short-acting β-agonists are also very effective for prophylaxis of allergen- or exercise-induced asthma. The long-acting β-agonist salmeterol is also effective for these types of exposures.

MONITORING ASTHMA Some children with asthma may have a limited ability to perceive the degree of obstruction in their own airways. Spirometry is the most accurate and preferred method of monitoring airway obstruction when used in a setting that provides maximal patient cooperation and effort. Unfortunately, spirometry is not always available in offices, urgent care centers, and emergency rooms. Therefore, alternative measurement tools must be used. Peak flow meters provide a reasonably accurate and portable means of obtaining objective pulmonary function measurements. These devices measure the peak expiratory flow rate (PEFR), which is the greatest flow velocity (liters per second) that is generated during forced expiration. In motivated patients using good technique, this measurement correlates with FEV$_1$ and provides a measurement of airway obstruction. However, peak flow is an effort-dependent test, and erroneously high or low values can be obtained. Thus, PEFR values may be manipulated by some children in order to avoid school or participation in physical education classes. Properly performed, peak flow measurements can be used by the patient, parent, and physician to make decisions about asthma therapy. Use of a peak flow meter may also allow patients to effectively manage most asthmatic exacerbations, providing positive feedback for the asthma treatment plan and increasing feelings of self-control over their chronic disease. Peak flow meters may also be useful in evaluating

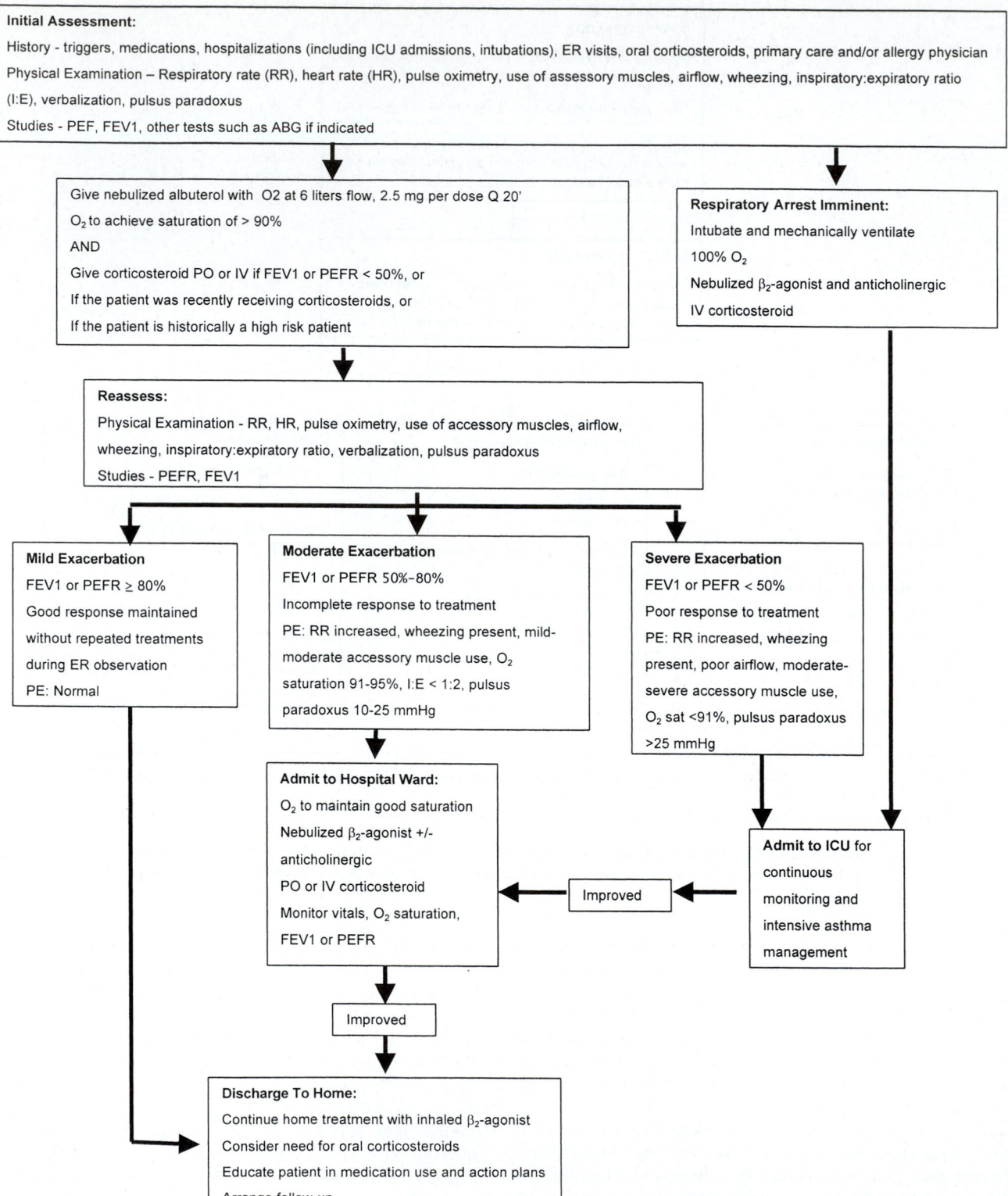

FIGURE 23-22 Emergency management of asthma exacerbations in children. PEF = peak expiratory flow.

the possibility of asthma in a patient who has suggestive symptoms at night or after exercise yet has normal pulmonary function in the clinic. It should be emphasized that neither peak flow monitoring nor spirometry is a substitute for a comprehensive asthma management and education program.

A useful protocol for using peak flow meters in managing asthma is outlined in the *Guidelines for the Diagnosis and Management of Asthma* published by the US Department of Health and Human Services (Fig. 4-5 at *www.nhlbi.nih.gov/guidelines/asthma/asthgdln.htm*). The first goal is to ascertain the patient's personal best peak flow rate, which requires the appropriate use of medications to maximize pulmonary function. Once this value has been established, the calculation of green (80–100% of personal best), yellow (50–80% of personal best), and red (<50% of personal best) zones can be accomplished. Peak flow rates in the green zone indicate stable disease activity, provided that no other warning signs are present (nocturnal awakenings caused by asthma, exercise intolerance, etc). If the patient's peak flow rate is in the yellow zone and the administration of a β-agonist does not result in bringing the peak flow value back into the green zone, many asthma specialists would recommend doubling the maintenance dose of anti-inflammatory therapy until peak flow rates are consistently back in the green zone. If peak flow rates continue to deteriorate while in the yellow zone, or if they are in the red zone, oral corticosteroid therapy should be initiated, and the patient should contact a physician as soon as possible.

CONTROL OF ENVIRONMENTAL ALLERGENS AND IRRITANTS

Respiratory allergies are a major factor in the pathogenesis of asthma in children. Furthermore, limiting exposure to relevant indoor allergens may lead to reductions in asthma symptoms, bronchial hyperresponsiveness, and use of asthma medications. Relevant indoor allergens include dust mite, cockroach, and cat and dog dander. One seemingly easily avoided irritant is environmental tobacco smoke. However, despite increased public awareness of the detrimental effect of smoking, it is often difficult to avoid secondhand smoke.

PREVENTION

Asthma prevention continues to be an important area of current study. Potential contributing factors in the development of asthma currently under investigation can be divided into prenatal and postnatal factors. Prenatal factors can further be subdivided into fixed and variable factors. Fixed factors include a family history of allergy or asthma, male gender, and the in utero cytokine environment. Variable factors include perinatal tobacco smoke exposure resulting in low birth weight and smaller airways relative to lung volume at birth and early life. Postnatal factors include exposure to tobacco smoke, indoor allergens, the development of allergy, and possibly exposure to certain viral respiratory infections. Overall, there remain large gaps in the current understanding of the pathogenesis of allergic diseases in children that have hindered the development of truly effective preventative strategies. The greatest preventative strategy at present is avoidance of tobacco smoke.

EDUCATION

Asthma education is the cornerstone of asthma therapy. Understanding the nature of asthma, recognizing and responding to asthma symptoms, and reducing triggers can help recognize and prevent exacerbations. The importance and proper administration of medications should be reviewed periodically during office visits when the patient is well. Asthma education conveyed to patients and families during the stress of an ED visit or hospitalization is rarely effective unless reinforced by later educational sessions. The correct use of a peak flow meter and implementation of an action plan should be rehearsed. Finally, compliance with the prescribed plan and periodic communication with the health-care team should be encouraged. The education team can be of a variety of backgrounds including physicians, nurses, respiratory therapists, and pharmacists.

PROGNOSIS

The prognosis of asthma in childhood is excellent. Approximately 20% of children who wheeze with lower respiratory illnesses in the first year of life will no longer wheeze by the age of 3; follow-up of these children at 6 years of age indicates a persistence of diminished lung function that probably was responsible for their symptom pattern in the first few years of life, but these children do not have clinical asthma. In contrast, 15% of wheezing infants will go on to develop persistent wheezing beyond the age of 3 years and should be given a diagnosis of asthma. Risk factors that predict persistent symptoms beyond infancy into childhood include male gender, presence of atopy (especially atopic dermatitis), environmental tobacco smoke exposure, and maternal history of asthma.

When evaluations are done of the relationship of childhood asthmatic symptoms at age 7 years with the presence of similar symptoms at age 25 years, a slightly different risk profile emerges. Risk factors measured at age 7 years that independently predicted current asthma as an adult included female gender, history of atopic dermatitis, presence of low midexpiratory flow rates, maternal or paternal history of asthma, presence of childhood asthma with the first episode after the age of 2, or having more than 10 attacks.

Most children with asthma tended to improve during adolescence. In an Australian study more than half of the subjects whose wheezing began before 7 years of age and then ceased before adolescence remained free of wheezing. Of the subjects who ceased wheezing at 14 years, 45% had minor occurrences between ages 14 and 21 years. Fewer than 20% of those children who wheezed persistently during childhood became totally free of wheezing during adolescence. Thus, persistent wheezing during the childhood years is a marker of unfavorable prognosis.

Although these findings are somewhat reassuring, it must be recognized that the prognosis of any single individual cannot be accurately predicted, so the objective of asthma treatment is to do whatever is necessary to produce long symptom-free intervals and allow the child and family to engage in all age-appropriate activities.

SPECIALIST REFERRAL

Primary care physicians can manage the majority of patients with asthma. Referral to an asthma specialist should be considered when the diagnosis is uncertain or when the therapeutic response is suboptimal. Consultation with an asthma specialist should also be considered in patients with serious asthma, as evidenced by admission to the pediatric intensive care unit, numerous admissions to the hospital, frequent utilization of the emergency room, or use of oral steroid therapy more than two or three times per year.

References

American Academy of Allergy, Asthma, and Immunology: Pediatric Asthma, Promoting Best Practice: Guide for Managing Asthma in Children, 1999. Published and authored by American Academy of Allergy, Asthma, and Immunology, Milwaukee, WI. See also *www.aaaai.org/professional/pediatricasthmaguidelines*

American Thoracic Society Workshop Report: refractory asthma. Am J Respir Crit Care Med 162:2341–2351, 2000

Gern JE, Lemanske RF, Busse WW: Early life origins of asthma. J Clin Invest 104:837–843, 1999

Global Initiative for Asthma. In: Global Strategy for Asthma Management and Prevention. Bethesda/Geneva, NHLBI/WHO Workshop Report, 1993

Lemanske RF Jr, Busse WW: Asthma. JAMA 278:1855–1873, 1997

Mannino DM, Homa DM, Pertowski CA, et al: Surveillance for asthma—United States, 1960–1995. MMWR 47:SS-1, 1998

Martinez FD, Helms PJ: Types of asthma and wheezing. Eur Respir J 27:3–8s, 1998

National Institutes of Health: Guidelines for the Diagnosis and Management of Asthma. Bethesda, NIH, Pub No. 97–4051, 1997 (*http://www.nhlbi.nih.gov/guidelines/asthma/asthgdln.htm*)

Stein RT, Holberg CJ, Sherrill D, et al: Influence of parental smoking on respiratory symptoms during the first decade of life: the Tucson Children's Respiratory Study. Am J Epidemiol 149:1030–1037, 1999

23.9 BRONCHOPULMONARY DYSPLASIA

Thomas A. Hazinski

Bronchopulmonary dysplasia (BPD) is the term applied to a set of persistent respiratory signs and symptoms in infants who had developed respiratory failure after birth. Its pathogenesis is related to the treatment of neonatal respiratory failure, which interacts with other factors in the immature developing lung to cause further injury and to delay repair. These factors include the oxidant stress of oxygen therapy, lung stretch from mechanical ventilation, and perinatal infection. There is also preliminary evidence that genetic factors are involved, but because BPD is a syndrome, its genetic antecedents are likely to be complex and polygenic. More than 80% of infants who develop BPD are less than 30 weeks of gestation, indicating that lung immaturity is the most important risk factor for its development. Other pre- and postnatal risk factors are discussed below.

The definition of BPD is based on clinical criteria applied at certain intervals after birth. The classic definition of BPD proposed by Northway in 1967 consisted of oxygen dependency, persistent signs of respiratory distress, and an abnormal chest radiograph at 28 days of life. This definition was based on clinical and autopsy findings in infants greater than 1500 g at birth, a cohort that rarely if ever develops BPD today. The definition has been challenged by those who note that the definition fails to consider the effect of gestational age (ie, not all 28-day-old infants are at the same stage of lung development). As a result, some prefer to define BPD at 36 weeks postconceptional age. Epidemiologic and intervention studies have employed both definitions. From a functional point of view, approximately 30 to 40% of infants who require supplemental oxygen therapy at 28 days of age will require supplemental oxygen at discharge from the NICU. Each year in the United States, approximately 10,000 infants develop BPD severe enough to require oxygen therapy at home, and the treatment of these infants is the subject of this section.

PREVENTION OF BPD

Prenatal corticosteroid therapy and delay of premature birth to beyond 30 weeks of gestation are the only two prenatal strategies that might reduce the incidence of BPD. Postnatally, only one intervention, parenteral vitamin A (retinol palmitate) given in doses to normalize the retinol concentration in serum, has been shown to reduce the incidence of BPD. Other postnatal therapies, such as dexamethasone, high-frequency or patient-triggered ventilation, antiproteases and antioxidant therapy, have been found to be ineffective or, in the case of dexamethasone, harmful. Surfactant ther-

apy, which improves the survival rate of premature infants with neonatal respiratory failure, may actually increase the number of infants with BPD. Clinical trials of inhaled nitric oxide (NO) are currently under way to test the hypothesis that NO exerts anti-inflammatory or antioxidant effects and reduces the incidence or severity of BPD.

RISK FACTORS FOR BPD

Although premature birth and severe neonatal respiratory failure are the most important risk factors for the development of BPD, recent studies have identified other factors that have led experts to propose that a new form of BPD now exists. This "new BPD" is no longer related to the severity of respiratory failure at birth because, at least in the United States, at least two-thirds of infants who develop BPD have either mild or delayed onset of respiratory insufficiency. In these infants, postnatal factors such as infection, altered innate immunity, patent ductus arteriosus, protein-calorie malnutrition, regulation of lung fluid balance, and micronutrient deficiency may play amplifying and interactive roles in the evolution of BPD. In addition, the recent finding that infants destined to develop BPD have increased levels of cytokines in their amniotic fluid suggests that prenatal infection or dysregulated innate immunity may be of etiologic importance. Center-to-center differences in BPD incidence have been observed even after adjustment for known risk factors, suggesting that other factors such as nursing care practices, infection control, or fluid management may influence the risk of BPD.

PATHOLOGY OF BPD

Surprisingly, little is known about the pathology of BPD beyond the immediate neonatal period, and even within the neonatal period, pathologic data have been obtained from autopsy specimens. These latter studies, often performed in less immature or more atypical cases, described airway and interstitial abnormalities, including squamous metaplasia of airway epithelium, airway muscle and mucous gland hypertrophy, interstitial edema, and fibrosis. Newer observations in humans who survive and in highly plausible animal models indicate that airway damage and fibrosis are less severe, but there is evidence of more distal and functionally important abnormalities in the acinus. These studies indicate that *arrested acinar development with abnormal alveolar capillary growth* is the hallmark of the "new BPD." This failure of lung septation and capillary development explains why oxygen therapy is still necessary in infants with BPD who have few or no respiratory symptoms or radiographic abnormalities. Current studies are needed to determine whether these abnormalities persist or whether postnatal alveolarization can be accelerated. It is also possible that lung development can be enhanced by therapies that enhance lung growth.

PATHOPHYSIOLOGY OF BPD

Infants with BPD have increased airway resistance, reduced lung compliance, and probably a reduced capillary surface area, leading to the development of wheezing, rales (crackles), tachypnea, hypoxemia, and increased work of breathing. Resting energy expenditure is increased in BPD infants, which may explain why some infants with BPD grow slowly and have increased caloric requirements. Some infants with BPD have pulmonary hypertension, but its incidence is unknown. Systemic hypertension may also be present, but its relationship to BPD is unknown, and not all centers have detected it.

TREATMENT OF BPD

The treatment of BPD has been derived empirically from consideration of the observed physiological abnormalities and, to a lesser degree, from short-term randomized clinical trials.

LOW-FLOW OXYGEN Of all the treatments for BPD, oxygen has the strongest rationale and the widest margin of safety. Chronic or intermittent hypoxemia can cause cor pulmonale and pulmonary hypertension and can slow growth and development. Low-flow oxygen therapy via nasal cannula does not produce inspired oxygen concentrations that can cause oxygen toxicity or respiratory depression. Oxygen therapy is guided by pulse oximetry obtained during precisely defined clinical conditions, usually when the infant is awake and quiet. The goal of oxygen therapy is to maintain oxyhemoglobin saturation between 92 and 96% when the infant is awake and asleep. The need for supplemental oxygen can usually be adjusted downward in the first few months after discharge; oxygen therapy is rarely needed beyond 8 to 10 months of age, but this cannot be predicted. Intercurrent respiratory infections may require a transient increase in oxygen therapy, but a persistent or increasing oxygen requirement or new pulmonary symptoms should prompt an investigation for comorbidities such as aspiration, congestive heart failure, asthma, pulmonary hypertension, subglottic stenosis, or tracheoesophageal malformations.

DIURETICS WITH KCl The rationale for diuretic therapy is derived from short-term clinical studies and the clinical finding of rales and pulmonary infiltrates on chest radiograph that disappear after diuretic administration. Short-term studies of daily and alternate-day furosemide therapy suggest improvement in lung mechanics and gas exchange in most infants. The mechanisms by which furosemide improves lung function is uncertain. Because electrolyte and calcium loss in urine is inevitable with daily furosemide therapy and can lead to a primary metabolic alkalosis and other side effects, additional KCl should be provided. Diuretic therapy should be reserved for infants with severe disease as evidenced by hypercarbia and a primary respiratory acidosis with renal compensation. In these infants, the adequacy of KCl supplementation must be assessed by measuring the pH of venous blood and not by measurements of electrolyte concentrations in serum. In hypercarbic infants, venous pH should be in the 7.30 to 7.35 range. If the venous pH is normal or in the alkaline range, additional KCl should be administered because this indicates that furosemide is causing a primary metabolic alkalosis. Thiazide-type diuretics cause a diuresis, but it is not clear that lung function is improved. Diuretic therapy is usually discontinued before oxygen therapy is reduced.

Acute fluid overload may also accompany infectious exacerbations, and short-term furosemide therapy may be effective in infants with infectious exacerbations who have clinical or radiologic evidence of acute pulmonary edema.

BRONCHODILATOR THERAPY The rationale for bronchodilator therapy is based on the finding of wheezing and hyperinflation in some infants with chronic BPD. On the other hand, up to 30% of infants with BPD have some degree of tracheomalacia. In these infants, bronchodilator therapy may cause more airway instability during exhalation. The use of inhaled bronchodilator drugs should

be based on objective evidence of clinical improvement. Short-term bronchodilator therapy may also be useful in those who develop acute wheezing during infectious exacerbations.

CORTICOSTEROID THERAPY The rationale for corticosteroid therapy is based on the finding of high levels of proinflammatory signaling factors and cytokines in bronchoalveolar lavage fluid in infants with BPD. Single-center clinical studies also suggested that 7 to 21 days of parenteral dexamethasone therapy hastened extubation in ventilator-dependent infants. Unfortunately, at least three recent large multicenter trials of parenteral dexamethasone could identify no evidence of clinical or economic benefits but did find evidence of adverse gastrointestinal and neurologic effects. As a result of these observations, the use of dexamethasone therapy for the treatment of BPD cannot be recommended. Inhaled corticosteroid therapy is not effective to prevent the evolution of BPD but may be useful in older infants with signs and symptoms of asthma. Short-term treatment with oral corticosteroids may be useful in older infants with BPD who have evidence of recurrent episodes of bronchial hyperreactivity and asthma.

NUTRITION If oxygenation and caloric intake are adequate, infants with BPD should gain 20 to 40 g per day (averaged over 14- to 30-day periods). Weight gain below this level requires investigation, starting with the possibility that oxygen therapy is inadequate. If oxygenation is adequate, the infant's nutrition should be adjusted either by increasing total fluid intake or by increasing the caloric density of the formula. If weight gain is still slow, comorbidities such as gastroesophageal reflux, gastric outlet obstruction, swallowing dysfunction, oral aversive behavior, or maternal–child interaction problems should be considered. In some infants with severe disease in whom comorbidities have been excluded, slow growth may be an adaptive response to slow lung repair. In these infants, growth will not accelerate until lung repair occurs.

PULMONARY HYPERTENSION Indirect clinical evidence and the autopsy finding of right ventricular hypertrophy suggest that some infants with BPD have pulmonary hypertension. Oxygen therapy can reduce pulmonary artery pressure in some infants. Captopril and other ACE inhibitors have also been used, but there is little evidence to support their effectiveness. Low-dose nitric oxide (NO) has also been employed, but its use is considered experimental at this time.

PROPHYLAXIS AGAINST RSV BRONCHIOLITIS Infants with BPD have an increased incidence of both RSV and non-RSV bronchiolitis, which can be severe. An effective vaccine against RSV is not yet available, but passive immunization with monthly doses of an anti-RSV antibody has been shown to reduce the risk of hospitalization. It should be emphasized that good hand-washing, influenza vaccination of family members, avoidance of people with respiratory infections, and avoidance of environmental tobacco smoke are also highly effective ways to prevent respiratory complications in these infants.

TREATMENT OF PULMONARY EXACERBATIONS Pulmonary exacerbations are usually caused by respiratory infections but occasionally can be caused by the premature discontinuation of oxygen or diuretic therapies. Even an upper respiratory infection can prompt respiratory distress and hypoxemia if nasal obstruction reduces the efficacy of oxygen delivery via nasal cannula. Viral infections can trigger wheezing, especially in an infant with a family history of asthma. In general, an increase in rales suggests pulmonary edema, and an increase in wheezing suggests airway infection or inflammation, but any infant with BPD must be assessed individually. Diuretic and inhaled bronchodilator therapy are begun or increased, and the effectiveness of these interventions is assessed by their effect on oxygenation and on clinical signs. If wheezing is recurrent or severe, a short course of corticosteroid therapy is warranted.

Antibiotic therapy is usually begun with drugs that are suitable for respiratory infections in non-BPD infants because there is no evidence that infants with BPD are at risk for infections with unusual pathogens. However, if oropharyngeal aspiration is suspected on clinical grounds, penicillin or clindamycin may be used.

The infant with BPD who has a tracheostomy is a special situation that must be managed properly. Tracheostomies are commonly colonized with *Pseudomonas* or other gram-negative bacteria, but these bacteria rarely cause serious pulmonary symptoms. Antibiotics directed at these commensal organisms should not be employed unless there is evidence of an extremely serious infection or if a course of conventional antibiotic therapy has not eliminated the symptoms. For these reasons, cultures of tracheostomy tube secretions should not be obtained except perhaps if the infant fails to respond to a 7- to 14-day course of conventional antibiotic therapy. Likewise, repetitive tracheostomy cultures should not be used to direct the duration of antibiotic therapy because eradication of commensal organisms is extremely unlikely. In selected infants, a 10- to 21-day course of inhaled tobramycin (80–160 mg BID) may be employed to treat clinically symptomatic tracheal infections that have not responded to conventional antibiotic therapy.

Prophylactic antibiotic therapy has not been shown to reduce the incidence of pulmonary exacerbations and should probably be avoided. In infants in whom asthma is suspected, prophylaxis with inhaled budesonide or cromolyn sodium should be considered. In infants in whom recurrent aspiration is suspected, an evaluation of swallowing function and the temporary placement of a gastrostomy should be considered. The possibility of gastroesophageal reflux should be considered in infants with persistent wheezing, cough, or failure to thrive. All infants with BPD should be immunized with all recommended age-appropriate immunizations.

LONG-TERM OUTCOME

Because BPD is most frequent and severe in the most immature surviving infants, it has been difficult to determine precisely which outcomes are unique to BPD and which outcomes are related to the effects of extreme prematurity. Ultimate height may be lower than that of gestational age–matched premature infants without BPD. Neurodevelopmental outcome may also be less than expected, but it is likely that these findings are also attributable to neurologic complications observed in very low-birth-weight infants, to frequent rehospitalization, and to the overall quality of the postnatal environment rather than to BPD per se.

The majority of older children and adolescents with BPD do not have significant respiratory symptoms that interfere with participation with all age-appropriate activities. Some infants with BPD can have pectus excavatum or other chest wall deformities that do not usually impair lung function. Young children who had BPD have slightly reduced expiratory flow rates and increased RV/TLC ratios that are clinically insignificant, but up to 30% of infants may

develop persistent asthma requiring daily prophylactic medications. Older children and young adults have slightly reduced lung volumes, airway hyperreactivity, and mild obstructive ventilatory defects, but exercise performance is usually normal.

References

Abman SH, Groothuis JR: Pathophysiology and treatment of bronchopulmonary dysplasia. Current issues. Pediatr Clin North Am 41:277, 1994

Avery ME, Tooley WH, Keller JB: Is chronic lung disease in low birth weight infants preventable? A survey of eight centers. Pediatrics 79:26, 1987

Bland RD, Coalson JJ: Chronic lung disease in early infancy. In: Lenfant C, ed: Lung Biology in Health and Disease, Vol 137. New York, Marcel Dekker, 2000.

Bonikos DS, Bensch KG, Northway WH Jr, Edwards DK: Bronchopulmonary dysplasia: the pulmonary pathologic sequel of necrotizing bronchiolitis and pulmonary fibrosis. Hum Pathol 7:643, 1976

Bruce MC, Schuryler M, Martin RJ, et al: Risk factors for the degradation of lung elastic fibers in the ventilated neonate. Implications for impaired lung development in bronchopulmonary dysplasia. Am Rev Respir Dis 146:204, 1992

Cabal LA, Larrazabal C, Ramanathan R, et al: Effects of metaproterenol on pulmonary mechanics, oxygenation, and ventilation in infants with chronic lung disease. J Pediatr 110:116, 1987

Carlton DP, Cummings JJ, Scheerer RG, et al: Lung overexpansion increases pulmonary microvascular protein permeability in young lambs. J Appl Physiol 69:577, 1990

Coalson JJ: Experimental models of BPD. Biol Neonate 71(1): 35–38, 1997

Collaborative Dexamethasone Trial Group: Dexamethasone therapy in neonatal chronic lung disease: an international placebo-controlled trial. Pediatrics 88:421, 1991

Engelhardt B, Elliott S, Hazinski TA: Short- and long-term effects of furosemide on lung function in infants with bronchopulmonary dysplasia. J Pediatr 109:1034, 1986

Frank L: Antioxidants, nutrition and bronchopulmonary dysplasia. Clin Perinatol 19:541, 1992

Goodman G, Perkin RM, Anas NG, et al: Pulmonary hypertension in infants with bronchopulmonary dysplasia. J Pediatr 112:67, 1988

Greenough A: Bronchopulmonary dysplasia: early diagnosis, prophylaxis and treatment. Arch Dis Child 65:1082, 1990

Groneck P, Götze-Speer B, Oppermann M, et al: Association of pulmonary inflammation and increased microvascular permeability during the development of bronchopulmonary dysplasia: a sequential analysis of inflammatory mediators in respiratory fluids of high-risk preterm neonates. Pediatrics 93:712, 1994

Impact-RSV Study Group: Palivizumab, a humanized RSV monoclonal antibody, reduces hospitalization from RSV infection in high-risk infants. Pediatrics 102:531–537, 1998

Jobe AJ: The new BPD: an arrest of lung development. Pediatri Res 46: 641–643, 1999

Kao LC, Durand DJ, Phillips BL, Nickerson BG: Oral theophylline and diuretics improve pulmonary mechanics in infants with bronchopulmonary dysplasia. J Pediatr 111:439, 1987

Kao LC, Durand DJ, McCrea RC, et al: Randomized trial of long-term diuretic therapy for infants with oxygen-dependent bronchopulmonary dysplasia. J Pediatr 124:772, 1994

Kao LC, Warburton D, Platzker ACG, Keens TG: Effect of isoproterenol inhalation on airway resistance in chronic bronchopulmonary dysplasia. Pediatrics 73:509, 1984

Kazzi NJ, Brans YW, Poland RL: Effect of dexamethasone therapy on fibronectin and albumin levels in lung secretions of infants with bronchopulmonary dysplasia. J Pediatr 121:597, 1992

Kennedy JD: Lung function outcome in children of premature birth. J Paediatr Child Health 35:516–521, 1999

Mammel MC, Green TP, Johnston DE, Thompson TR: Controlled trial of dexamethasone therapy in infants with bronchopulmonary dysplasia. Lancet 1:1356, 1983

Margraf LR, Tomashefski JF Jr, Bruce MC, Dahms BB: Morphometric analysis of the lung in bronchopulmonary dysplasia. Am Rev Respir Dis 143:391, 1991

Meredith KS, de Lemos RA, Coalson JJ, et al: Role of lung injury in the pathogenesis of hyaline membrane disease of premature baboons. J Appl Physiol 66:2150, 1989

Merritt TA, Cochrane CH, Holcomb K, et al: Elastase and α-proteinase inhibitor activity in tracheal aspirates during respiratory distress syndrome. Role of inflammation in the pathogenesis of bronchopulmonary dysplasia. J Clin Invest 72:656, 1983

Morray JP, Fox WW, Kettrick RG, Downes JJ: Improvement in lung mechanics as a function of age in the infant with severe bronchopulmonary dysplasia. Pediatr Res 16:290, 1982

Northway WH, Rosan RC, Porter DY: Pulmonary disease following respiratory therapy of hyaline membrane disease. Bronchopulmonary dysplasia. N Engl J Med 276:357, 1967

Northway WH Jr, Moss RB, Carlisle KB, et al: Late pulmonary sequelae of bronchopulmonary dysplasia. N Engl J Med 323:1793, 1990

Panitch HB, Keklikian EN, Motley RA, Wolfson MR, Schidlow DV: Effect of altering smooth muscle tone on maximal expiratory flows in patients with tracheomalacia. Pediatr Pulmonol 9:170–176, 1990

Rotschild A, Solimano A, Puterman M, et al: Increased compliance in response to salbutamol in premature infants with developing bronchopulmonary dysplasia. J Pediatr 115:984, 1989

Rush MG, Engelhardt B, Parker RA, Hazinski TA: Double-blind, placebo-controlled trial of alternate-day furosemide therapy in infants with chronic bronchopulmonary dysplasia. J Pediatr 117:112, 1990

Rush MG, Hazinski TA: Current therapy of bronchopulmonary dysplasia. Clin Perinatol 19:563, 1992

Sluis KB, Darlow BA, Vissers MCM, Winterbourn CC: Proteinase-antiproteinase balance in tracheal aspirates from neonates. Eur Respir J 7:251, 1994

Southall DC, Samuels MP: Bronchopulmonary dysplasia: a new look at management. Arch Dis Child 65:1089, 1990

Speer CP: Inflammatory mechanisms in neonatal chronic lung disease. Eur J Pediatr 158:S18–S22, 1999

Taghizadeh A, Reynolds EOR: Pathogenesis of bronchopulmonary dysplasia following hyaline membrane disease. Am J Pathol 82:241, 1976

Tammela OKT: First-year infections after initial hospitalization in low birth weight infants with and without bronchopulmonary dysplasia. Scand J Infect Dis 24:515, 1992

Tammela OKT, Koivisto ME: Fluid restriction for preventing bronchopulmonary dysplasia? Reduced fluid intake during the first weeks of life improves the outcome of low-birth-weight infants. Acta Paediatr 81:207, 1992

Tyson JE, Wright LL, Oh W, et al: Vitamin A supplementation for extremely-low-birth weight infants. N Engl J Med 340:1962–1968, 1999

Walti H, Tordet C, Gerbaut L, et al: Persistent elastase/proteinase inhibitor imbalance during prolonged ventilation of infants with bronchopulmonary dysplasia: evidence for the role of nosocomial infections. Pediatr Res 26:351, 1989

Watts CL, Bruce MC: Effect of dexamethasone therapy on fibronectin and albumin levels in lung secretions of infants with bronchopulmonary dysplasia. J Pediatr 121:597, 1992

Wilkie RA, Bryan MH: Effect of bronchodilators on airway resistance in ventilator-dependent neonates with chronic lung disease. J Pediatr 111:278, 1987

Yoder MC Jr, Chua R, Tepper R: Effect of dexamethasone on pulmonary inflammation and pulmonary function of ventilator-dependent infants with bronchopulmonary dysplasia. Am Rev Respir Dis 143:1044, 1991

Yoon BH, Romero R, Jun JK, et al: Amniotic fluid cytokines and the risk for the development of BPD. Am J Obstet Gynecol 177:825–830, 1997

23.10 CYSTIC FIBROSIS

David M. Orenstein

Cystic fibrosis (CF) is the most common life-shortening inherited disease in North America. In 1938, Dr Dorothy Andersen first described the complex of respiratory and digestive signs and symptoms that make up this syndrome, but references to a childhood disorder characterized by salty sweat and early death date at least to the middle ages. The cellular and molecular bases for the disorder have recently been elucidated. CF affects virtually every organ system with epithelial surfaces—most importantly, the lungs, pancreas, intestinal mucous glands, liver, the reproductive tracts, and sweat glands. A common pathogenetic mechanism in major target systems is abnormal ion transport across epithelial surfaces. Impermeable chloride channels and overactive sodium pumps of these epithelial cells lead to biochemical and bioelectric abnormalities within organ lumina, leading in turn to viscid intralumenal secretions in the affected organs. These abnormally viscous secretions cause the blockage of ducts and air passages.

GENETICS, PREVALENCE, AND MOLECULAR AND CELLULAR PATHOPHYSIOLOGY

Cystic fibrosis is inherited as an autosomal recessive disorder. It is most common in those of northern European extraction, with an incidence of approximately 1 in every 3200 live births. It is seen in about 1 in every 15,000 births in African-Americans and is much less common in Asian populations. It has been found in virtually every ethnic and racial group. Some 4% of whites are heterozygous for CF (ie, carry one CF allele); heterozygotes have no evidence of clinical disease. The most common mutation in the CF gene is a three-base-pair deletion that leads to the loss of a single phenylalanine at position 508 of the protein product ("$\Delta F508$"). The $\Delta F508$ mutation accounts for 70 to 80% of CF chromosomes; about 50% of CF patients in North America are homozygous for this mutation. More than 850 other mutations at the CF locus have been discovered, but these account for only a small additional proportion of CF cases. In a few ethnic groups, a small number of mutations account for a large proportion of cases of CF (Table 23-16). Prenatal testing and carrier testing can be accomplished in virtually every family having a family member with CF whose genotype is known, using direct mutation analysis or a combination of mutation analysis and marker testing employing restriction fragment length polymorphisms. Testing for CF mutations in utero or newborn screening in the absence of a family history is being discussed but is not yet thought to be appropriate. Population screening for heterozygotes is not yet practical.

The gene for CF is on the long arm of chromosome 7 and spans 250 kb. Its product is a 1480–amino acid protein that regulates transmembrane ion transport. It serves as the most important apical membrane chloride channel and also influences sodium and water transport across epithelial cells of many organs and glands. Because of this functional role, both the protein product and the gene itself are called CFTR (cystic fibrosis transmembrane conductance regulator). The gene is transcribed into mRNA, which is translated into protein in the endoplasmic reticulum (Fig. 23-23). Then, the CFTR protein is glycosylated in the Golgi apparatus and folded into a configuration that allows it to travel through the cytoplasm to the apical surface of airway and mucus gland epithelium. Once

TABLE 23-16

CHARACTERISTICS OF VARIOUS CFTR MUTATIONS

MUTATION	GEOGRAPHIC/ ETHNIC INCIDENCE	OTHER	CLASS
ΔF508	70–75% in North America	Pancreatic insufficiency	II
W1282X	50–60% in Ashkenzai Jews; 2% worldwide	Pancreatic insufficiency	I
G542X	3.4% worldwide	Pancreatic insufficiency	I
G551D	2.4% worldwide	Pancreatic insufficiency	III
3905insT	2.1% worldwide	Pancreatic insufficiency	I
N1303K	1.8% worldwide	Pancreatic insufficiency	II
R553X	1.3% worldwide	Pancreatic insufficiency	I
621 + 1G → T	1.3% worldwide	Pancreatic insufficiency	
1717 − 1G → T	1.3% worldwide	Pancreatic insufficiency	
A455E[a]	3–7% in Netherlands; 0–0.2% in North America	Pancreatic sufficiency; mild lung disease	
3849 + 10kb C → T[a]	1.4% worldwide; 4% in Israel	Normal sweat chloride; most males not sterile; lung disease varies from mild to severe	I
R1162X	20% of non-ΔF508 CF chromosomes in NE Italy; rare in rest of world	Pancreatic insufficiency	I
R117H[a]	0.8% worldwide	Pancreatic sufficiency	IV
R334W[a]		Pancreatic sufficiency	IV
P574H[a]		Pancreatic sufficiency	
Y563N[a]		Pancreatic sufficiency	

[a] Compound heterozygotes in most cases have one copy of the mutation noted and one other CF mutation (usually ΔF508).

resident in the apical membrane, it must have appropriate regulation, in that it must be able to respond to regulatory molecules. Finally, normal conductance of chloride and other ions depends on the channel's remaining open for the appropriate time.

CFTR mutations can be classified according to which step in this sequence of events is defective (Fig. 23-23). As in vitro studies have shown restored chloride conductance with various interventions in each of these classes, there is hope that clinically useful class-specific treatment might someday be possible.

Although much is known about the physiological consequences of many CF mutations, it is not yet clear how the ion transport abnormality leads to the characteristic clinical abnormalities in the lungs and pancreas of CF patients. Regardless of the mechanism by which the abnormal gene and protein lead to the luminal abnormalities, virtually all organs with epithelial lining cells are affected. In addition, it is not yet clear how the different mutations affect clinical disease. Most CF genotypes, such as those patients who are homozygous for the ΔF508 mutation, are associated with pancreatic insufficiency, but a few alleles appear to confer pancreatic sufficiency. Other CF alleles appear to be associated with a delayed onset and slower progression of pulmonary disease. Characteristics of some of the most common CFTR mutations are listed in Table 23-16. Because within the population of ΔF508 homozygotes there is substantial phenotypic variation, it is thought that there are genes other than CFTR that can modify the phenotypic expression of CF.

CLINICAL MANIFESTATIONS

Gastrointestinal Tract

The typical CF patient has exocrine pancreatic insufficiency, with maldigestion of fats and protein, and consequent malabsorption, steatorrhea, and failure to thrive. Pancreatic insufficiency is present at birth in only 50% of CF patients, and develops by age 9 years in another 35 to 40%. This is important to keep in mind, since the diagnosis of CF is often delayed or missed in patients without typ-

ical GI involvement. Pancreatic insufficiency is determined in large part by genetic factors, as certain genotypes (for eg, ΔF508) are nearly always associated with pancreatic insufficiency, while others confer pancreatic sufficiency (Table 23-17).

Bowel obstruction, a result of thickened intestinal mucus and pancreatic insufficiency, is present at birth (meconium ileus) in 10 to 20% of patients, especially those who are ΔF508 homozygotes. Later in life distal intestinal obstruction syndrome, DIOS (previously termed meconium ileus equivalent), occurs in 20 to 25%. Rectal prolapse, caused by the same factors and by malnutrition with loss of anal sling musculature, is seen in 20% of CF patients in the first years of life. Intussusception is much less common, but CF patients account for a substantial portion of the patients with intussusception after 1 year of age. Gastroesophageal reflux, which may complicate the pulmonary disease, interfere with nutrition, or both, occurs with increased frequency in infants (and older children) with CF. Reflux may be worsened, especially in infants, by head-down positioning for chest physical therapy. Acid peptic disease can result from gastric acid hypersecretion and deficient pancreatic bicarbonate secretion. Cholelithiasis is more common in CF than healthy control populations. Liver pathology, including non-specific steatosis, cholestasis, and the specific lesion, focal biliary cirrhosis, occur in up to 10% of infants and children with CF. However, the clinical manifestation of cirrhosis with hepatic failure or portal hypertension with hypersplenism, bleeding esophageal varices, or both, is much less common. These hepatic complications will probably increase as life span increases. Children or adults, particularly those with normal exocrine pancreatic function, may develop recurrent episodes of acute pancreatitis. Endocrine pancreas dysfunction also can occur, leading to carbohydrate intolerance and diabetes mellitus that is unassociated with ketoacidosis.

SWEAT GLANDS The epithelial ion transport defect is expressed in the sweat glands, leading to the high salt content of CF sweat, long recognized as a hallmark of this disorder. In patients without CF, sweat precursor fluid is isotonic to plasma, and as the fluid moves

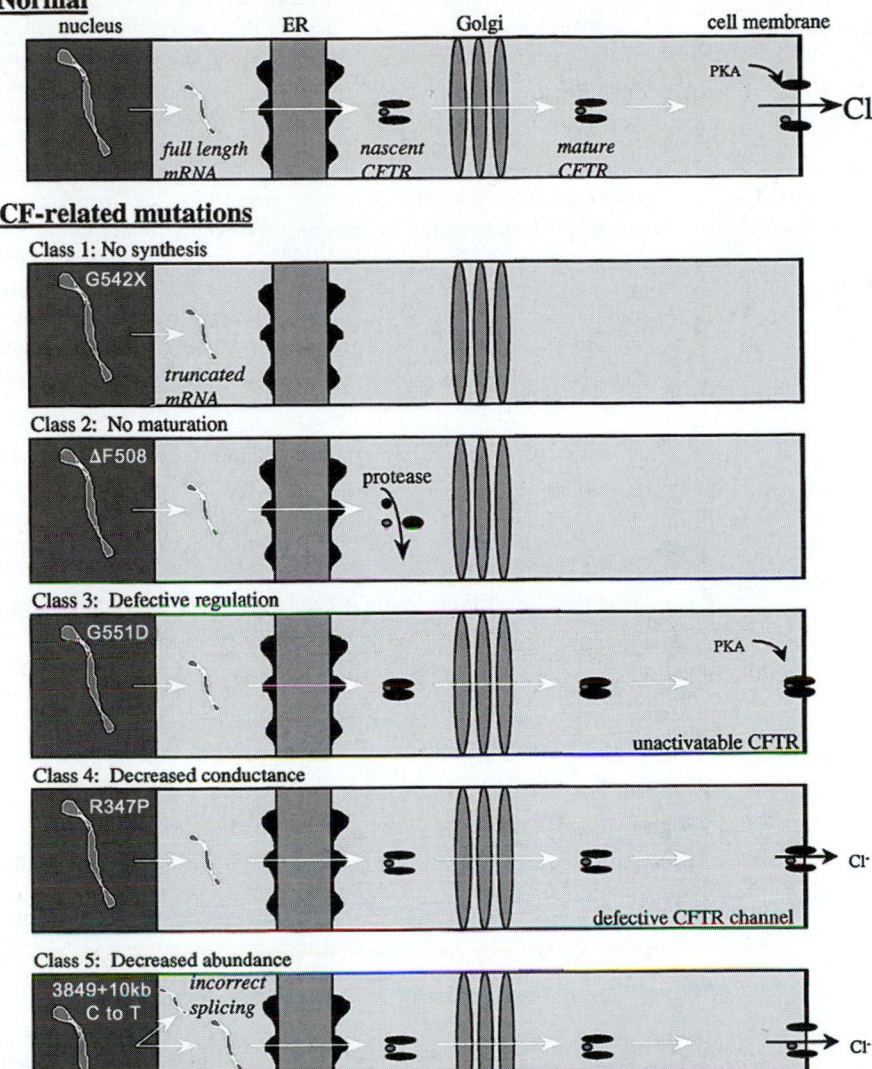

FIGURE 23-23 Steps in the production, delivery, and functioning of normal CFTR (cystic fibrosis transmembrane conductance regulator protein) in epithelial cells, and the corresponding classes of abnormalities encoded by different CFTR gene mutations. In normal epithelia (top), the CF gene is transcribed into mRNA, which is translated in the endoplasmic reticulum (ER) to CFTR protein. Next, the nascent CFTR is glycosylated in the Golgi apparatus before insertion in the cell membrane. In class 1 CF mutations, there is failure of CFTR translation, typically due to stop mutations (e.g., G542X). In class 2 mutations, including ΔF508, the most common mutation, CFTR fails to mature and is degraded by proteases in the ER. Class 3 mutations are fully processed and protein inserted in the membrane, but the protein is not properly responsive to activation (e.g., with the G551D mutation, CFTR fails to conduct chloride in response to protein kinase A). In class 4 mutations, the mature protein is activated normally, but the chloride conductance of the channel is reduced. Class 5 mutations result in decreased abundance of full-length mRNA, and therefore a decrease in the amount of fully functional CFTR at the cell membrane. SOURCE: *(From Pilewski JM, Frizzell RA. Role of CFTR in airway disease. Physiol Rev 70 [Suppl 1]:S215–S255, 1999.)*

through the sweat apparatus toward the skin, chloride is reabsorbed, with sodium following to maintain electrical neutrality. This results in sweat on the skin surface that is hypotonic to plasma and usually has a sodium and chloride concentration below 40 meq/L. In CF, the absent or poorly functioning CFTR chloride channel makes chloride reabsorption substantially below normal. The resultant fluid that emerges as sweat at the skin surface has sodium and chloride concentrations greater than 60 meq/L. This ion transport defect in the sweat apparatus provides the basis for the sweat test (discussed later). CF patients lose more salt during exercise in the heat than do persons without CF, and they may experience dehydration or heat prostration. Infants may develop hyponatremia and hypochloremia. For unknown reasons, African-American infants with CF seem to be at greater risk than white infants for this complication.

RESPIRATORY TRACT The upper respiratory tract is involved in virtually all CF patients, with radiographic evidence of pansinusitis. This is much more evident radiographically than symptomatically. It occasionally is helpful diagnostically because (particularly in childhood) persistent pansinusitis is uncommon except in CF, and CF is extremely uncommon without pansinusitis. Nasal polyps may

be found in as many as 25% of CF patients and may be recurrent. Indeed, the finding of large nasal polyps in children less than 12 years of age should prompt the clinician to consider CF.

The lower respiratory tract involvement in CF accounts for over 90% of the morbidity and mortality. Although the lungs are his-

TABLE 23-17

ETHNIC GROUPS WHERE A FEW MUTATIONS ACCOUNT FOR MOST OF THE CYSTIC FIBROSIS CHROMOSOMES

GROUP	NUMBER OF MUTATIONS	% OF CF CHROMOSOMES
Alberta (Canada) Hutterites	2	100
Welsh	29	99.5
Brittany Celts	19	98
Ashkenazi Jews	5	97
Belgian	17	94.3

SOURCE: *Orenstein DM: Cystic Fibrosis: A Guide for Patient and Family, 2nd ed. Philadelphia, Lippincott-Raven, 1997:211, courtesy of Dr. Gary Cutting.*

tologically and radiographically normal at birth, the respiratory epithelium is abnormal electrophysiologically, leading to obstruction of small airways by viscid mucus, by airway inflammation, and by recurrent endobronchial infection, which typifies the disease. Invading organisms and inflammatory cells release inflammatory mediators and leave behind large amounts of DNA when the cells lyse, adding further to the viscosity of lung mucus. Because of these factors, obstructive pulmonary disease, beginning in the small airways, eventually is present in almost all patients with CF. Recurrent cough, wheeze, or both, which may be diagnosed initially as recurrent bronchiolitis, asthma, or pneumonia, are often the first indications of pulmonary involvement. As the disease progresses, hyperinflation and crackles become apparent, and diffuse bronchiectasis eventually develops.

Pulmonary function tests reveal a pattern of obstructive airways disease: decreased forced expiratory volume in 1 second, decreased peak expiratory flow, and increased residual volume, indicative of air trapping. These obstructive changes show varying responses to bronchodilator inhalation: some patients improve, whereas many do not change, and a few actually worsen because bronchiectatic airways may require bronchoconstrictor tone to remain stable. The response to bronchodilators is not consistent over time. Exercise testing typically shows reduced exercise tolerance and fitness, with comparatively large minute ventilation for the oxygen consumed, presumably because of greater than normal dead-space ventilation. Often, a higher than normal proportion of the ventilatory capacity is required at peak workloads. Male patients have greater exercise tolerance and cardiopulmonary fitness than female subjects. The pulmonary function and exercise tests are relatively sensitive tools for following progression of disease in the older, cooperative child (see Sec. 23.3.6).

Chronic pulmonary infection and inflammation, with episodes of acute exacerbation, are typical of CF patients. The chronic and acute condition is most accurately thought of as purulent bronchiolitis and bronchitis. Exacerbations are characterized by increased cough, often productive of purulent sputum, particularly in the morning on arising and with exertion; decreased exercise tolerance; lethargy, malaise, and weight loss. Fever is often absent. In the early stages of the disease, the bacterial organisms most commonly colonizing the lower respiratory tract of patients with CF include *Staphylococcus aureus*. *Hemophilus influenzae,* and a variety of gram-negative organisms. Eventually most patients permanently acquire *Pseudomonas aeruginosa* and related gram-negative organisms, many of which become resistant to conventional antibiotic therapy. Increasing numbers of patients have *Pseudomonas* species at diagnosis; whether this represents a true increase in prevalence or represents better microbiology laboratory performance is uncertain. There seems to be a unique relationship between CF patients and *Pseudomonas;* at least half of all CF patients are colonized with a peculiar mucoid strain of this organism that is seldom seen in other human disease states. Some studies have suggested that early colonization of the respiratory tract with *Pseudomonas* is an independent risk factor for progressive pulmonary disease. Recently, other organisms, such as *Aspergillus fumigatus, Burkholderia* (formerly *Pseudomonas*) *cepacia, Alcaligenes xylosoxidans* and *Stenotrophomonas maltophilia,* have become increasingly important as pulmonary pathogens

Despite the universal finding of chronic pulmonary colonization and infection, extrapulmonary infection is unusual, indicating that any defect in innate immunity is limited to the lungs. Pulmonary defenses are almost certainly inhibited by viscid mucus, and mu-

cociliary transport rates are dramatically reduced. It is not yet clear whether the ion transport abnormalities affect microbial adherence. The abnormal salt concentration in the thin aqueous layer on the airway surface may inhibit the function of naturally occurring antimicrobial peptides. Alternatively, airway surface liquid may be normal in tonicity yet deficient in volume, rendering cilia ineffective in clearing secretions and microbes. In addition, there appear to be circulating or locally secreted toxins, some from neutrophils and some from *Pseudomonas* organisms themselves, that inhibit the phagocytosis and killing of *Pseudomonas* by pulmonary alveolar macrophages and neutrophils. Whatever the bacterial burden, there is also an overabundance of neutrophil-derived inflammatory mediators that add to airways inflammation and obstruction. Current research is focused on a better understanding of the mechanisms of lung inflammation in CF.

PROGRESSION OF CF LUNG DISEASE The rate of progression of the lung disease varies widely among individuals, influenced in part by environmental factors, with second-hand cigarette smoke and recurrent viral infection being two proven factors associated with worse pulmonary prognosis.

The initial histologic lesion is bronchiolitis, reflected physiologically as small airways obstruction and radiographically as overinflation and prominent bronchial markings (Fig. 23-24). Further worsening of the lung disease includes extension from bronchiolitis to bronchitis, with thickened bronchial walls demonstrable on radiographs as circular lesions if the bronchi are projected in cross section, or characteristic parallel linear opacities ("tram tracks") if the bronchi are projected longitudinally. With further progression and the development of bronchiectasis and small cysts, rounded densities become evident on radiographs. The right upper lobe is commonly affected earlier and more severely than other lobes (Fig. 23-25). With more advanced disease, small abnormal areas coalesce to form larger cysts (which may be dense when filled with mucopurulent secretions or lucent when relatively empty) and regions of

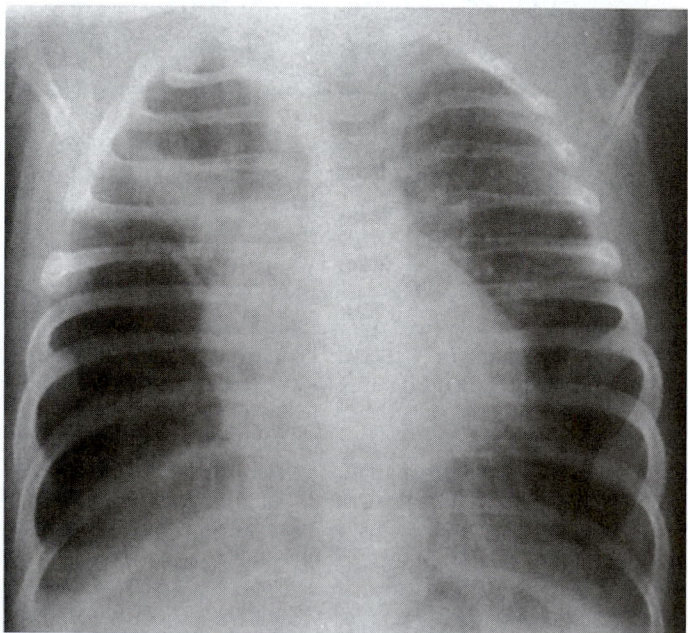

FIGURE 23-24 **Two-month-old infant with cystic fibrosis. Chest radiograph shows markedly overinflated lungs and atelectasis in the right upper lobe.**

fibrosis. Enlarged tortuous bronchial arteries may contribute to the opacities visible on chest radiographs and may also lead to hemoptysis. Large apical blebs may form and rupture, leading to pneumothorax (Fig. 23-26).

Pulmonary complications include chest pain, pneumothorax, hemoptysis, segmental and lobar atelectasis, pulmonary hyperten-

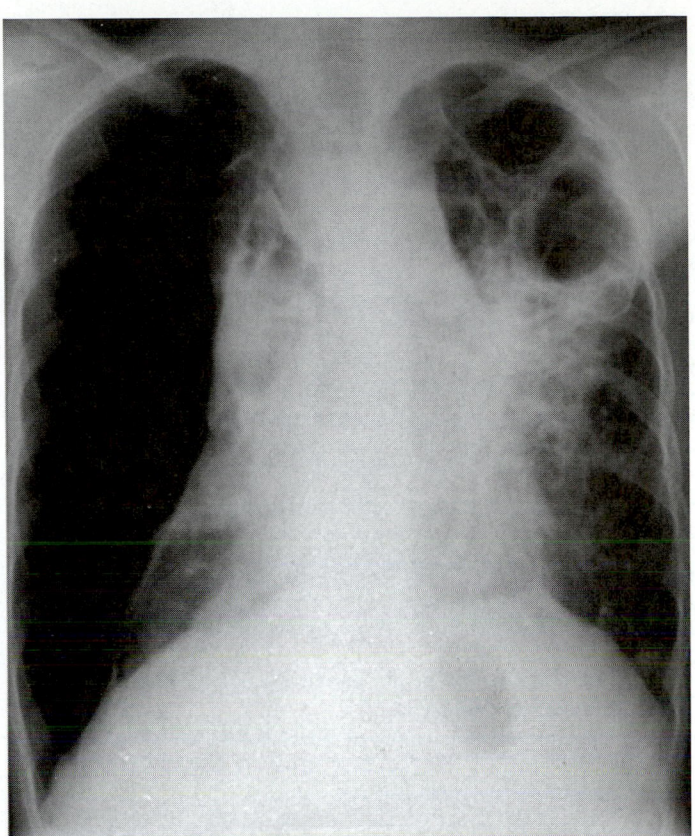

FIGURE 23-26 Fifteen-year-old boy with a right tension pneumothorax, probably resulting from rupture of an apical subpleural bleb. The left upper lobe exhibits extensive atelectasis and several large bullae. Such a large pneumothorax is unusual in patients with cystic fibrosis. Although the lungs tend to be noncompliant, they may also adhere to the inside of the chest wall because of pleural inflammation, which limits the amount of alveolar collapse when there is extra-alveolar air. Therefore, a tension pneumothorax can be present with a relatively small amount of extrapulmonary air apparent on radiographs.

sion leading to cor pulmonale, and respiratory failure (see Treatment of Pulmonary Complications). Digital clubbing is a nearly universal finding in patients with even mildly abnormal lung function.

OTHER ORGAN SYSTEMS The reproductive tract is involved in most male patients, with atresia of the vas deferens and consequent obstructive azoospermia and sterility. However, male CF patients can produce children through in vitro methods. In female patients, thick cervical mucus often results in decreased fertility. Delayed puberty may be seen in either sex as a consequence of chronic illness and poor nutrition. Some adolescents and adults display a unique pattern of hyperglycemia and abnormal glucose tolerance tests, but diabetic ketoacidosis is rare, and microvascular complications of diabetes are less frequent. With improved survival, there may be more microvascular diabetic complications. Occasional patients, particularly those with severe lung disease, have hypertrophic pulmonary osteoarthropathy involving the long bones and adjacent joints. This complication is characterized clinically by joint (especially knee) pain and radiographically by periostial thickening. A systemic vasculitis syndrome with arthritis and a vasculitic skin rash has also been described in CF patients.

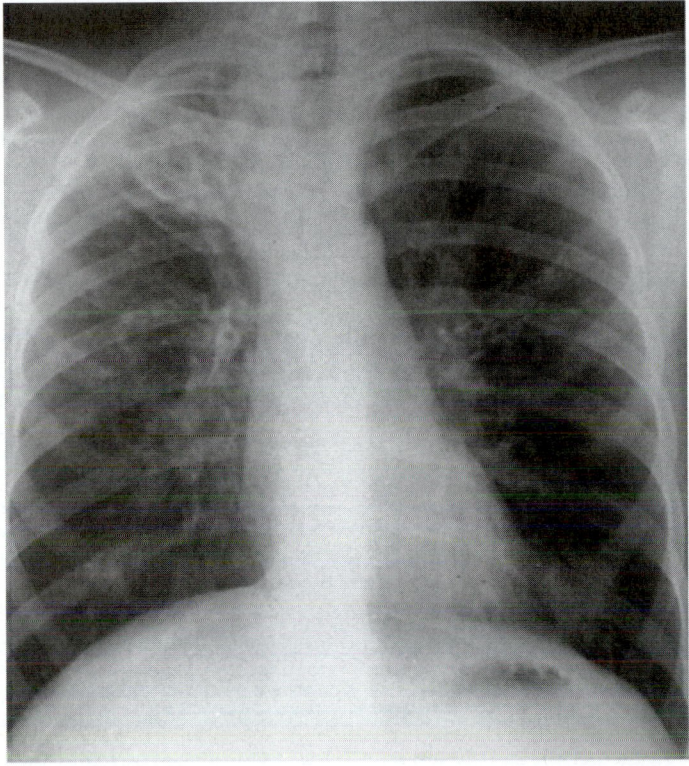

A

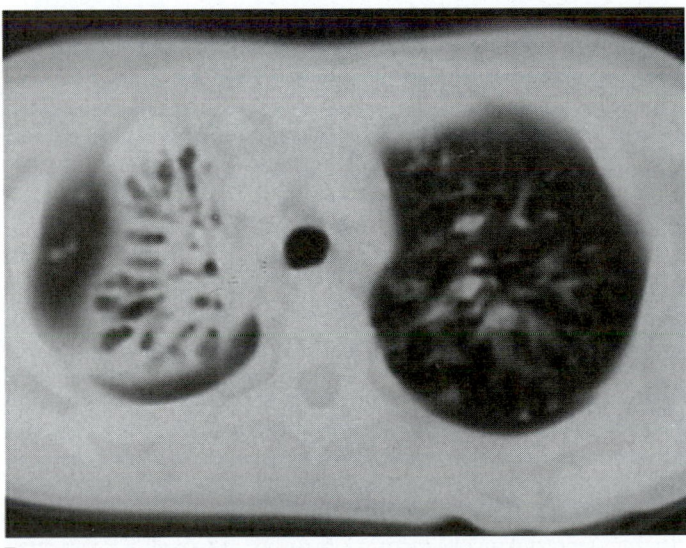

B

FIGURE 23-25 Thirteen-year-old girl with disease most severely involving right upper lobe. **A.** Chest radiograph shows inhomogeneous opacification and volume loss in right upper lobe. **B.** Computed tomographic section shows extensive bronchiectasis in partially collapsed lobe.

DIAGNOSIS

As shown in Table 23-18, the accepted criteria for diagnosis of CF are (1) one or more characteristic phenotypic features (chronic obstructive pulmonary disease, exocrine pancreatic insufficiency, sweat salt loss syndrome, pansinusitis, male infertility), (2) CF in a full sibling or a positive newborn screen, and (3) laboratory confirmation, via (a) a positive sweat test (a sweat chloride concentration greater than 60 meq/L on a sample of at least 100 mg, obtained after maximal stimulation by pilocarpine iontophoresis), (b) identification of two CFTR mutations known to cause CF, or (c) an abnormal nasal potential difference (see below). Even today, in the era of molecular diagnostics, the diagnosis is almost never made without a positive sweat test because it is not yet feasible to test for over 600 mutations. Theoretically, the sweat test is simple, but false positives and false negatives are extremely common in tests performed outside established CF centers. Contrary to widespread belief, sweat tests can be accomplished in young infants, although some young infants might not produce a large enough volume of sweat for analysis. Concentrations of sodium and chloride in sweat are below 40 meq/L in normals, whereas nearly all patients with CF demonstrate values greater than 60 meq/L. Very few patients fall in the intermediate or borderline range (40–60 meq/L), and in these patients, genotype analysis and nasal potential difference measurements may be required for definitive diagnosis. Patients with intact exocrine pancreatic function have somewhat lower sweat chloride concentrations than those with pancreatic insufficiency, but their values are still well outside the normal range. Table 23-19 lists conditions giving false-positive and false-negative sweat test results.

Although the sweat test remains the gold standard for the confirmation of the diagnosis of CF, DNA analysis is increasingly used for CF diagnosis. Demonstration of two of the known CFTR mutations in DNA in the appropriate clinical setting is considered definitive for the diagnosis. Until more CF gene mutations can be detected inexpensively, there will be some patients with CF with one or both unidentified alleles. Therefore, DNA analysis cannot yet definitively rule out CF, nor can it positively identify all CF patients. DNA analysis should be performed in those patients for whom sweat testing is logistically difficult (live far from a CF center) or has yielded equivocal results. DNA analysis for CF is relatively easy for the referring physician: blood, buccal brushings, or chori-

TABLE 23-18
DIAGNOSTIC CRITERIA FOR CYSTIC FIBROSIS[a]

CLINICAL/HISTORY	LABORATORY EVIDENCE OF ABNORMAL CFTR/CFTR FUNCTION
• One or more characteristic phenotypic features (chronic obstructive pulmonary disease, exocrine pancreatic insufficiency, sweat salt loss syndrome, male infertility)	• A positive sweat test (a sweat chloride concentration >60 meq/L on a sample of at least 100 mg, obtained after maximal stimulation by pilocarpine iontophoresis
• CF in a sibling or a positive newborn screen	• Identification of two CFTR mutations known to cause CF
	• Diagnostic nasal potential difference

[a] Diagnosis requires at least one from each column.

TABLE 23-19
CONDITIONS GIVING FALSE-POSITIVE AND FALSE-NEGATIVE SWEAT TEST RESULTS

False positive (> 60 meq/L)
  Laboratory error
  Adrenal insufficiency syndromes
  Anorexia nervosa
  Ectodermal dysplasia
  Familial cholestasis (Byler syndrome)
  Fucosidosis
  Glycogen storage disease (type I)
  Hypoparathyroidism
  Hypothyroidism
  Malnutrition
  Mauriac syndrome
  Mucopolysaccharidoses
  Munchausen by proxy syndrome (addition of table salt to sweat sample)
  Nephrogenic diabetes insipidus
False negative (< 40 meq/L)
  Laboratory error
  Edema, hypoproteinemia
  Rare cystic fibrosis mutations

onic villous samples can be sent by overnight courier to any of a number of commercial laboratories, with results often available within a week. The commercial laboratories examine DNA for 25 to 100 of the most common mutations, which together account for >95% of all CF patients. Therefore, results must be interpreted with caution. For example, an individual may be found to have one abnormal cystic fibrosis allele and one unknown allele. This second allele may be normal, and the person is a CF carrier, or it may be one of the mutations that is not included in the laboratory's panel, and the person has the disease. In the event of such a result (one CF allele and one "negative"), advice should be sought from individuals who are experienced in the genetics of cystic fibrosis.

The function of the CFTR protein in respiratory epithelium can be assessed directly in vivo with measurement of the bioelectric voltage difference across nasal epithelium, the "nasal potential difference," or nasal PD. The nasal PD can be measured in a few specialized cystic fibrosis centers. Three abnormalities characterize the CF nasal PD (Fig. 23-27): (1) more negative than normal PD (reflecting abnormally high Na$^+$ transport across a Cl$^-$-impermeable barrier), (2) greater-than-normal inhibition of PD with perfusion with amiloride, a Na$^+$ channel blocker (reflecting inhibition of greater-than-normal Na$^+$ transport), and (3) little or no change in PD with perfusion with isoproterenol and a Cl$^-$-free solution (reflecting the absence of Cl$^-$ secretion).

The key to making the diagnosis is a high index of suspicion in the presence of any of the manifestations. Table 23-20 lists the indications for a sweat test. Most physicians are sufficiently aware of the disease that few children with the triad of growth failure, steatorrhea, and chronic pulmonary disease escape diagnosis. However, atypical patients, especially those who have no clinically apparent pancreatic involvement (as many as 15% of all CF patients, and as many as 50% of young infants with CF) or who have normal growth may escape diagnosis for years. There is no such thing as a child who "looks too good" to have CF.

NEWBORN SCREENING Most newborns with CF have an elevation of blood immunoreactive trypsinogen (IRT). The assay for IRT can be carried out on the dried blood spots obtained from

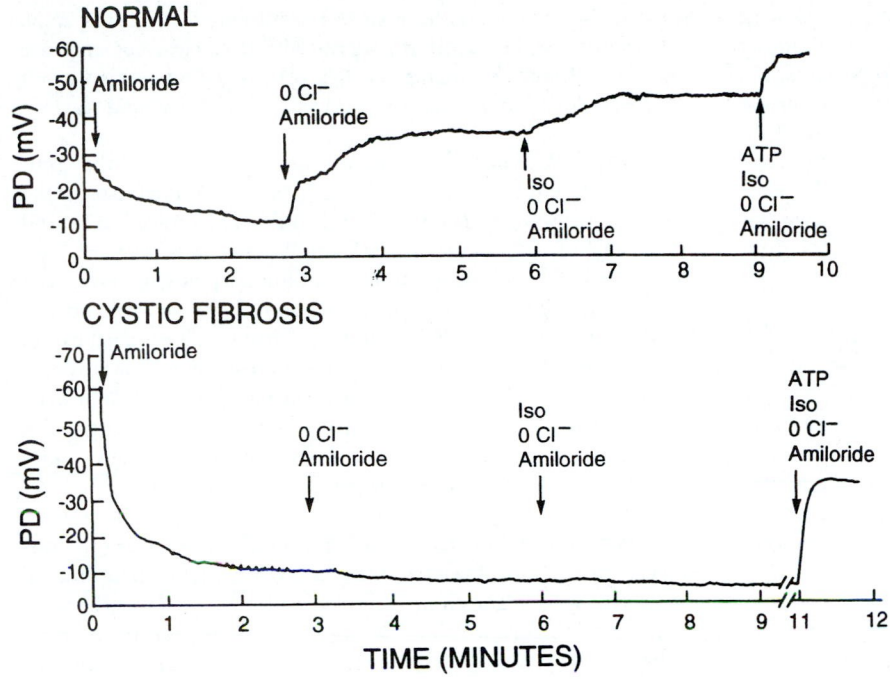

FIGURE 23-27 Nasal potential (PD) tracings in a normal subject (upper panel) and one with cystic fibrosis (lower). Note the (1) more negative than normal PD, (2) greater-than-normal inhibition of PD with perfusion with amiloride, and (3) little or no change in PD with perfusion with isoproterenol and a C-free solution. SOURCE: *(From Orenstein DM, Rosenstein BJ, Stern RC. Cystic Fibrosis Medical Care. Lippincott Williams & Wilkins, Philadelphia, 2000. Original adapted from Knowles MR, Paradiso AM, Boucher RC. In vivo nasal potential difference: Techniques and protocols for assessing efficacy of gene transfer in cystic fibrosis. Human Gene Therapy 1995;6:445, with permission.)*

newborns for routine screening for other genetic and metabolic diseases. The IRT test has been used in a number of states and countries, and its use is likely to continue. There appear to be very

TABLE 23-20
INDICATIONS FOR SWEAT TESTING

Gastrointestinal tract
　Chronic diarrhea
　Steatorrhea
　Meconium ileus
　Meconium plug syndrome
　Rectal prolapse
　Cirrhosis/portal hypertension
　Prolonged neonatal jaundice
　Pancreatitis
　Deficiency of fat-soluble vitamins (especially A, E, K)
Respiratory tract
　Upper
　　Nasal polyps
　　Pansinusitis on radiographs
　Lower
　　Chronic cough
　　Recurrent bronchiolitis
　　Recurrent wheezing
　　Intractable "asthma"
　　Recurrent or persistent atelectasis
　　Obstructive pulmonary disease
　　Staphylococcal pneumonia
　　Pseudomonas aeruginosa (especially mucoid colony types) recovered from throat, sputum, or bronchoscopic cultures
Other
　Digital clubbing
　Family history of cystic fibrosis
　Failure to thrive
　Hyponatremic, hypochloremic alkalosis
　Severe dehydration incompatible with clinical history
　Heat prostration
　"Tastes salty"
　Male infertility

few false negatives with this screen, but the false-positive rate is as high as 90%. This high false-positive rate requires repeating the analysis for IRT after one positive test. If the second test (usually at several weeks of age) still shows elevated IRT, definitive genetic or sweat testing must be carried out as soon as possible. Some laboratories are using polymerase chain reaction (PCR) technology on blood spots found to have elevated IRT levels to look for the most common CF mutations (ΔF508 and several others).

Recent studies suggest that the early diagnosis of CF and the institution of an aggressive treatment program can improve the quality and length of life. Efforts at pursuing the diagnosis quickly and aggressively will be rewarded by the family's peace of mind in the case of a negative result and the knowledge of an improved outlook for the child in the event of a positive result.

TREATMENT

Cystic fibrosis is a complex disease, and patients require a comprehensive evidence-based approach. This is usually best carried out in, or at least coordinated by, a specialized CF diagnosis and treatment center where different specialists focusing on cystic fibrosis are available. Survival is greater for patients followed in CF centers than for those followed outside centers. Therapy has three primary components: pulmonary, gastrointestinal, and psychological.

PULMONARY THERAPY The goal of pulmonary therapy is to prevent or delay progression of the pulmonary involvement. This is accomplished through the relief of airway obstruction and inflammation, and the control of infection.

THERAPY TO IMPROVE MUCOCILIARY CLEARANCE Chest physical therapy (CPT) with percussion and postural drainage is the mainstay of all treatment programs in CF patients with evidence of pulmonary disease. Most patients undergo CPT to all pulmonary segments one to four times daily, with increased frequency at the time of clinical pulmonary exacerbations. Many patients have found that mechanical percussors ease this arduous task. Newer methods of airway clearance, including the "flutter valve," forced expiratory technique (FET), use of forced expiratory efforts into a mask with positive expiratory pressure (PEP masks), or the use of a vibrating vest, have all been introduced, each with its own proponents. No definitive studies indicate the ideal time for instituting the airway clearance therapy or the benefits of various techniques. Bronchoscopy and airway lavage have demonstrated mucus plugs in the airways of even asymptomatic infants, implying that airway-clearance procedures should be instituted very early in life. Head-down positions should probably be avoided during chest physical therapy in infants, as they increase gastroesophageal reflux.

EXERCISE Aerobic exercise (jogging and swimming) are beneficial for CF patients in terms of increased cardiopulmonary fitness (oxygen consumption, VO_2) and work capacity. Further, high aerobic fitness is correlated with prolonged survival. There is some suggestion that various kinds of exercise may be as effective as traditional CPT in relief of pulmonary obstruction, but studies examining this question have had conflicting results. Therefore, until a definitive study is available, most experts advise the use of both exercise and CPT.

INHALATION-BASED THERAPY Various kinds of aerosols have been employed for patients with CF in order to dilate bronchi, reduce mucus viscosity, reduce mucosal edema and inflammation, suppress microbial growth, and, in rare cases, even to correct the cellular abnormality in functioning CFTR. Bronchodilators increase airflow acutely in some patients, make no difference in many, and actually reduce airflow in a few patients with severe disease where smooth muscle relaxation causes airway instability during exhalation. There have been few studies of the effects of long-term bronchodilator aerosol use. Mucolytic agents (eg, N-acetylcysteine) are effective in vitro, but they may cause irritation, bronchoconstriction, and bronchorrhea in vivo. Recombinant human DNase, which can degrade neutrophil-derived DNA and decrease the viscosity of airway secretions, has been shown to reduce the rate of pulmonary function decline and has been helpful for many patients. Vasoconstrictors (eg, phenylephrine) are sometimes used to reduce mucosal edema, although their efficacy has yet to be established. Antibiotics, especially aminoglycosides and semisynthetic penicillin derivatives, can be delivered by aerosols, with favorable results.

Several experimental aerosol therapies have been introduced and await definitive study to assess their safety and efficacy. Amiloride may make airway luminal contents less viscous by blocking the absorption of sodium and water from airway secretions. Uridine triphosphate, UTP, appears to open auxiliary chloride channels in CF epithelial cells and therefore may also improve the hydration of airway secretions. α_1-Antitrypsin and other inhibitors of neutrophil and bacterial-derived proteases may diminish the damaging effects of chronic airway infection and inflammation. Several other anti-inflammatory agents are undergoing clinical trials, as are some new agents thought to increase delivery of CFTR protein to the airway epithelial cell surface or to improve its function. Airway delivery of healthy genes via various viral and nonviral vectors is also being studied.

ANTI-INFLAMMATORY THERAPY FOR CF Several approaches have been proposed to reduce airway inflammation in cystic fibrosis, including the use of oral corticosteroids and ibuprofen. Clinical trials of corticosteroid therapy suggest some benefits (improved pulmonary function over a 4-year period) and some drawbacks (decreased growth velocity and possible glucose intolerance). Cromolyn sodium has been shown in a small study to be ineffective.

Inhaled topical steroids have shown small benefits in a few small studies but may be useful in patients who have clear-cut evidence of asthma. Ibuprofen therapy seems to benefit some patients, but the therapeutic index is narrow, and side effects may limit its use.

THERAPY FOR INFECTION There is general agreement that antibiotic treatment has been the single most important factor in the greatly improved prognosis in CF. Chronic airway colonization and infection with *Staphylococcus* and later *Pseudomonas* are nearly universal, and clinical exacerbations of pulmonary disease have been convincingly linked to worsened infection. *Staphylococcus* and *Hemophilus* may occasionally be eliminated from the bronchial tree in CF, but once *Pseudomonas* colonization is established, it is almost never eradicated. Its emergence as a chronic airway resident may, in some cases, be delayed for a prolonged period with aggressive treatment (eg, with an oral quinolone and aerosol aminoglycoside) after the initial positive throat or sputum culture.

ANTIBIOTIC STRATEGIES Some CF centers advocate continuous inhaled or oral prophylactic antibiotic treatment, with additional treatment with intravenous antibiotics for acute exacerbations. There is some concern that this approach might lead to the early emergence of drug-resistant pathogens in the airways. Another approach is to restrict the use of antibiotics to times of exacerbation of pulmonary disease, as evidenced by increased symptoms or signs (such as cough or sputum production) or worsening objective data, such as chest radiograph or pulmonary function test results. Some patients, especially those with advanced disease, suffer exacerbations whenever they are not being treated with antibiotics; in such patients, virtually continuous treatment is indicated. A third approach is to treat with an aggressive course of antibiotics (oral, aerosol, or IV), based on culture results, for 2 to 3 weeks every 1 or 2 months in patients with any evidence of pulmonary disease (morning cough, abnormal x-ray, etc). For example, CF patients in some European countries whose cultures grow *Pseudomonas aeruginosa* are hospitalized for 2 weeks of intravenous antibiotics and aggressive chest physiotherapy every 3 months, regardless of their clinical condition. Survival has increased dramatically since the institution of this approach. An algorithm for the approach to CF lung infection used in one American center is shown in Fig. 23-28. Because of the extremely large variation in CF from patient to patient, most centers employ an individualized approach to this issue, which includes a thorough discussion of the risks and benefits of any proposed therapeutic approach.

A cornerstone of most successful treatment programs is frequent comprehensive clinical evaluation of patients, including microbiological examination of respiratory tract flora by a laboratory that is experienced in the detection of potential cystic fibrosis pathogens. Oral antibiotics (amoxicillin/clavulanate, cephalexin, trimethoprim-sulfamethoxazole, erythromycin, clarithromycin, or azithromycin) at the first sign of worsening respiratory symptoms may successfully treat a pulmonary exacerbation. Some of these drugs (eg, the macrolides, including erythromycin) have anti-inflammatory effects unrelated to their bactericidal effects.

The quinolones (eg, ciprofloxacin, ofloxacin, levofloxacin) are a class of oral antibiotics with impressive in vitro activity against *Pseudomonas* and good penetration into the lung. Simultaneous treatment with rifampin may prevent the rapid emergence of resistant organisms, which is otherwise common during treatment with quinolones. The quinolones have been useful and apparently safe in children as young as 4 years, although the possibility of quinolone-associated arthropathy must be considered.

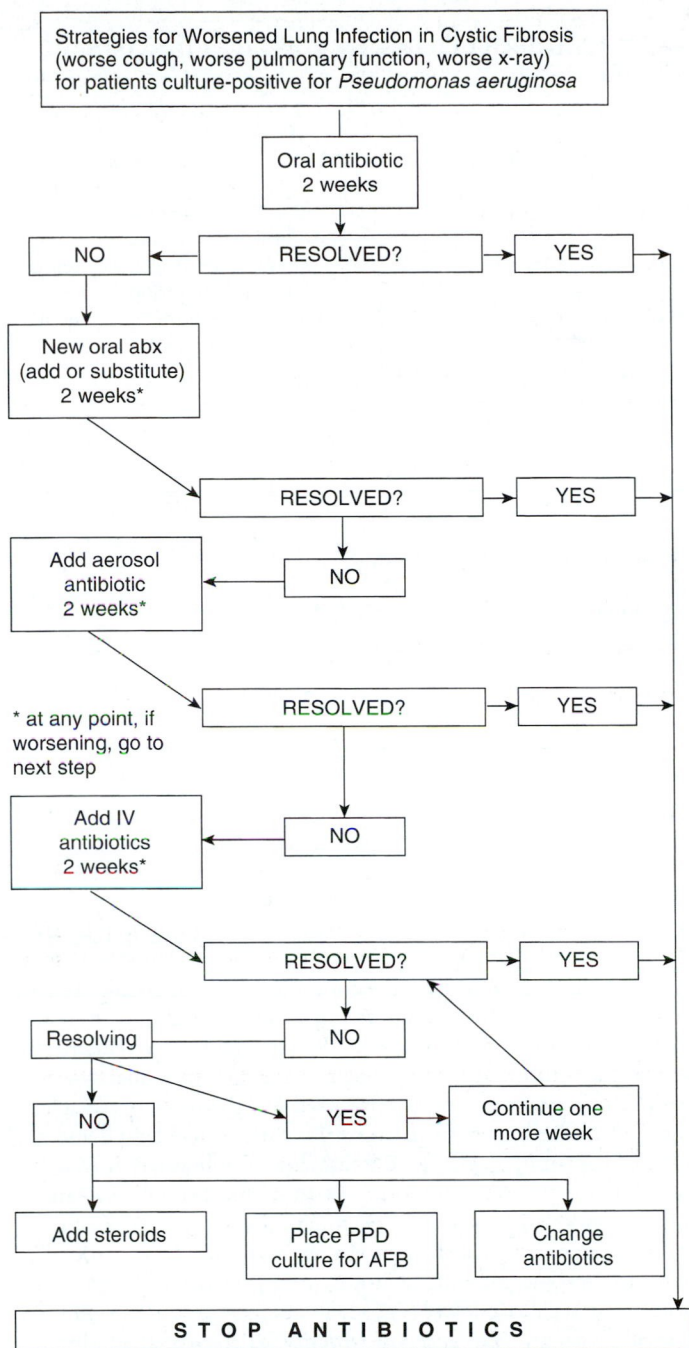

FIGURE 23-28 Approach to lung infection at one cystic fibrosis center. In each instance of antibiotic use, the choice of antibiotics will be based in part on recent cultures of respiratory tract secretions. If recent cultures are unhelpful, consider adding empiric treatment for *Pseudomonas aeruginosa* or *Staphylococcus aureus*, even if these organisms have not been recovered. Also consider performing bronchoscopy and bronchoalveolar lavage to obtain better cultures and to examine the cells recovered for evidence of aspiration (large numbers of lipid-filled macrophages). Also consider evaluating or treating empirically for gastroesophageal reflux. Abx = antibiotic; AFB = acid-fast bacillus; PPD = tuberculin skin test.

Aerosolized antibiotics, especially tobramycin, may be effective in many patients colonized with *Pseudomonas*. High endobronchial concentrations of tobramycin can be achieved via the inhaled route that would be impossible to achieve with intravenous dosage. Pa-

tients who cannot tolerate certain drugs (eg, colistin) intravenously may do well with the same drugs delivered by aerosol. In patients with severe airways obstruction, aerosol penetration into the lung may be limited and render this form of treatment less valuable. The sequential use of inhaled bronchodilators or DNase may increase antibiotic deposition.

Intravenous antibiotics are indicated when the patient does not respond to outpatient oral or aerosol antibiotic therapy. The important consideration in the decision to begin parenteral therapy is whether the child is sicker than his or her own baseline and not whether the child seems dreadfully ill. It is clear that a significant amount of lung can be lost irreversibly while a child still looks reasonably well. Because *Pseudomonas aeruginosa* is usually the offending organism, intravenous therapy is commonly carried out with an aminoglycoside and a semisynthetic anti-*Pseudomonas* penicillin or a third-generation cephalosporin. Intravenous antibiotics are usually administered during hospitalization, but in carefully selected cases they may successfully be administered at home, either initially or for 1 or 2 weeks following hospitalization. Response to treatment is often slower or absent at home, and the burden on a family of administering two or three different antibiotics on different schedules around the clock should not be underestimated. The most commonly used intravenous antibiotics, dosing schedules, and toxicities are listed in Table 23-21. Intravenous antibiotic treatment should be continued until the patient's pulmonary status has reached a plateau, as assessed by physical examination, oximetry, and spirometry. The time to reach this plateau is most commonly 2 to 3 weeks but can be longer in sicker patients. On occasion the new plateau may be better than the previous level of functioning. On other occasions, because cystic fibrosis remains a progressive disease, the patient may not regain his or her previous level of functioning. Most patients will be able to maintain levels they achieve during hospitalization for at least a few weeks after discharge, but most will not continue to improve after intravenous antibiotics have been discontinued.

Intravenous antibiotics are most often administered during a hospitalization. Studies have shown that the benefits of hospitalization cannot be explained completely by the use of intravenous antibiotics alone. Some patients improve in the hospital even if intravenous antibiotics are not given. Possible benefits of hospitalization include effective and frequent chest physical therapy and aerosol treatments, improved nutritional support, relatively clean air, absence of inhalant hazards and aeroallergens, enforcement of a strict therapeutic regimen, and opportunities for continuing patient education.

TREATMENT OF PULMONARY COMPLICATIONS

CHEST PAIN Chest pain is reasonably common in CF, particularly in patients with advanced lung disease. If the onset of the pain is abrupt, unilateral, pleuritic, and associated with shortness of breath, the most likely and the most ominous cause is pneumothorax (see below). Other causes of chest pain include pleural inflammation and musculoskeletal strains, especially from prolonged paroxysmal coughing episodes. The musculoskeletal strains usually respond to rest, anti-inflammatory treatment, or both. Pleural inflammation is usually secondary to underlying parenchymal infection and is treated with antibiotics. The occasional patient reports chest pain that is relieved when a hard coughing spell produces a large mucus plug. Esophageal pain from gastroesophageal reflux or "pill esophagitis" should be treated with antiacid therapy (antacids, H_2-block-

TABLE 23-21

INTRAVENOUS ANTIBIOTICS FOR TREATING PULMONARY EXACERBATIONS IN CYSTIC FIBROSIS

DRUG	24-H DOSE (mg/kg)	DOSES PER 24 h	LEVEL	TOXICITY	MONITOR
Gentamicin	7.5–10[a]	1–3	Peak = 10 mg/L[b] Trough <2 mg/L	Nephrotoxicity; ototoxicity	Blood urea nitrogen, creatinine, urinalysis; hearing
Tobramycin	7.5–10[a]	1–3	Peak = 10 mg/L[b] Trough <2 mg/L	Nephrotoxicity; ototoxicity	Blood urea nitrogen, creatinine, urinalysis; hearing
Amikacin	15–30	2–3	Peak = 30 mg/L Trough <5 mg/L	Nephrotoxicity; ototoxicity	Blood urea nitrogen, creatinine, urinalysis; hearing
Carbenicillin	250–450	4–6		Platelet aggregation, allergy, salt load, vein irritation	
Ticarcillin	200–300	4–6			
Ticarcillin/ clavulanate	200–300	4–6			
[d]Piperacillin/ tazobactam	240[c]	4		Platelet aggregation	
[d]Imipenem	50–100	3–4		Nausea during infusion, vein irritation, seizures	
[d]Meropenem	60	3		Vein irritation	
Ceftazidime	250	3–4		Allergy	
Aztreonam	150	3–4			
Colistin	5–10	3		Headache, nephrotoxicity	Blood urea nitrogen, urinalysis, creatinine

[a] Starting dose; adjust upward to achieve appropriate serum levels.
[b] Peak will be much higher with once-a-day dosing.
[c] Refers to amount of piperacillin.
[d] Not approved for children.

ers, etc) and adequate fluids for swallowing the large numbers of pills and capsules required for CF treatment.

PNEUMOTHORAX Many patients with advanced pulmonary disease have apical blebs. In 10% of CF patients, these blebs can rupture, leading to the accumulation of air in the pleural space. Many pneumothoraces eventually resolve with bed rest and oxygen therapy or with simple chest tube drainage, but recurrence rates of 50 to 100% are likely. Therefore, therapy to prevent recurrence is advisable. The instillation of chemical sclerosing agents has been used with some success but is painful and may not reduce the risk of recurrences. The most successful treatment for early resolution of the pneumothorax, prevention of subsequent episodes, and least morbidity has been open thoracotomy through a small subaxillary incision, identification and excision of any apical blebs, stripping of the apical pleura, and manual abrasion of the remainder of the accessible pleura. Thoracoscopic surgery has also been employed for excising apical blebs and stripping the pleura.

In some centers, surgical or chemical ablation of the pleural space is considered a contraindication to lung transplantation. A stepwise approach to the first episode of pneumothorax has been advocated, whereby simple chest tube drainage is undertaken first. If the air leak does not resolve within the next few days, or if an episode recurs, an attempt should be made to identify and seal apical blebs via the thoracoscope or a small thoracotomy. If these steps fail, formal open thoracotomy with pleurectomy should be performed.

HEMOPTYSIS Minor hemoptysis (blood-streaked sputum) is a common complication. Massive hemoptysis, defined as more than 300 mL in 24 hours, is much less common, occurring in 5 to 10% of patients, and, although terrifying to patient and family, rarely is severe enough to interfere with gas exchange or to require transfusion. Deaths have been reported but are exceedingly rare. Massive hemoptysis is thought to be the result of local infection that erodes one of the tortuous bronchial vessels adjacent to bronchiectatic airways. The appropriate treatment for all but the most overwhelmingly brisk bleeding is to reassure the patient and family and to initiate or continue aggressive treatment of pulmonary infection, including intravenous antibiotics. Because infection plays a causative role and blood reduces ciliary function and is a fertile bacterial medium, aggressive chest physical therapy should be continued if possible. In some patients, hemoptysis may be associated with the platelet-aggregation defect (eg, seen with aspirin, carbenicillin, or ticarcillin therapy). Because CF patients malabsorb fat-soluble vitamins, treatment of hemoptysis includes supplementing with vitamin K. With brisk bleeding, intravenous pitressin can be effective. In the rare recalcitrant case of hemoptysis, embolization of the offending bronchial artery under radiologic guidance may bring resolution of the bleeding. Lobectomy is seldom necessary.

ATELECTASIS Even early in the course of the disease, lobar or segmental atelectasis, particularly in the upper lobes, can develop (Fig. 23-25). Segmental or lobar atelectasis is best treated with antibiotics, bronchodilators, and vigorous chest physical therapy. It may take weeks or months for atelectasis to resolve. Bronchoscopy is unlikely to speed the resolution but should be considered when the atelectasis is associated with an otherwise unexplained deterioration; in these cases, culture of bronchoscopically obtained specimens may yield an unexpected organism that can be used to guide antimicrobial therapy.

COR PULMONALE Pulmonary hypertension, with enlargement of the right ventricle, is common in end-stage CF. Overt heart failure with enlarged liver and peripheral edema is much less common but more ominous. One study has suggested that survival is less than 8 months after the onset of heart failure, although more recent results have been better. Diuretics are usually helpful, but digitalis is not used unless there is also left ventricular dysfunction. Salt intake should be restricted. Treatment of the underlying suppurative lung disease and administration of supplemental oxygen are the approaches most likely to be of benefit. In CF patients with advanced pulmonary disease and cor pulmonale, simultaneous heart and lung transplantation may be employed.

RESPIRATORY FAILURE Respiratory failure in CF is almost always the end result of a long devastating course. Occasionally, it can be seen acutely in a previously stable patient who had been doing well and abruptly worsens due to a severe viral infection, trauma, or following surgery for nonpulmonary problems. For acute respiratory failure in a previously relatively healthy patient, there should be extremely aggressive treatment, with oxygen, antibiotics, aerosols, and airway clearance. Mechanical ventilation may be indicated for those individuals with good lung function before an acute deterioration. The prognosis for regaining the previous status is good.

With chronic respiratory failure, the prognosis is much different, and therefore the approach to the patient is different. Oxygen therapy is indicated to keep oxygen saturation above 90%. If the patient has carbon dioxide retention (a very late finding in CF), oxygen should be administered with caution in order to avoid suppression of the hypoxic drive to breathe. This is much more a theoretical problem than a real one, however, because the majority of patients with cystic fibrosis will either not change or actually improve their ventilation with supplemental oxygen. In these patients, supplemental oxygen may improve gas exchange by reducing anxiety and improving respiratory muscle function. Emphasis should be on patient comfort. Terminally ill CF patients may have CO_2 narcosis and be comfortable, whereas in others, air hunger from hypoxemia may dominate the clinical picture. Morphine may be helpful in these latter patients, in decreasing anxiety and promoting comfort. Morphine must be used carefully in this setting, as some terminal CF patients appear to be exquisitely sensitive to the drug, perhaps because of acidosis. Some centers use a starting dose as low as 0.1 mg (not 0.1 mg/kg) and double the dose until the desired result is achieved.

A number of options are available to support ventilation in CF patients with respiratory failure. These include conventional invasive approaches using endotracheal intubation or tracheotomy and mechanical ventilation, to less invasive devices such as intermittent positive-pressure breathing or mask BiPAP. The choice of techniques may be different in those patients who are lung transplant candidates and those who are not. Without transplantation, once patients begin these therapies, they have little chance of being able to stop them. Long-term mechanical ventilation is unlikely to enhance the quality of life of CF patients with respiratory failure and is not recommended. At some centers, some patients accepted for lung transplantation have been supported for weeks or months with mask BiPAP or conventional mechanical ventilation as a "bridge" to transplantation. Some patients have died on ventilators awaiting the availability of suitable donor lungs. Some centers view mechanical ventilation as a contraindication to transplantation and feel that initiating such treatment unconscionably complicates the letting-go, dying, and grieving process. These issues are best addressed with patients and families on multiple occasions when the patient is not in impending respiratory failure.

LUNG TRANSPLANTATION Heart-lung or double-lung transplantation has been successful in a limited number of CF patients with end-stage disease. One-year survival ranges from 50 to 85%. Donor-organ availability is a limiting factor for most North American lung transplant programs, and pretransplant mortality is high among those on transplant waiting lists. After transplantation, medical care is even more complex than that for cystic fibrosis before transplantation. Postoperative problems with immunosuppression, infection, acute and chronic organ rejection, finances, and psychological adjustment require constant attention. Nonetheless, some patients have had excellent results, with return to full-time work or school. Because waiting lists for donor lungs are as long as 2 years, most centers begin discussing transplantation with patients before they have respiratory failure, perhaps when pulmonary status begins to decline rapidly and oxygen therapy is required.

GASTROINTESTINAL THERAPY

NUTRITION AND ENZYME REPLACEMENT THERAPY Longitudinal surveys of growth patterns in CF patients indicate that maintaining a normal weight-to-height ratio is associated with a slower pace of lung function deterioration. For this reason, the main goal of gastrointestinal therapy is to provide good nutrition and to teach and reinforce age-appropriate nutritional habits. Since pancreatic enzyme replacement preparations and especially enteric-coated preparations became available, this once insurmountable problem has become quite manageable. The correct dose of enzyme is determined by trial and error, titrating against the symptoms and signs of maldigestion and malabsorption (steatorrhea, abdominal discomfort, excessive hunger, and poor weight gain). Enzyme doses greater than 2500 units/kg/meal of the lipase component are rarely necessary. Some patients who seem to require very large numbers of enzyme capsules may do better if they are treated with H_2 blockers, which enhance the bioavailability of ingested enzymes. In these patients, it is likely that gastric acid hypersecretion, along with the usual absence of pancreatic bicarbonate, has rendered their duodenum and jejunum sufficiently acidic to prevent the complete dissolution of the enteric coating of the enzyme supplements.

Supplemental vitamins, especially the fat-soluble vitamins A and E, should be administered at twice their recommended daily doses. Diet need not be specially tailored for the CF patient as long as adequate balanced calories are supplied at 100 to 150% RDA. For those who have difficulty gaining or maintaining weight, a high-calorie (usually high-fat) diet is recommended. In many patients, oral high-calorie nutritional supplements may be indicated to maintain adequate nutrition. Even these supplements may prove inadequate in an important subset of CF patients who simply cannot eat enough to offset caloric losses. These patients may have the anorexia of chronic illness or may have greater than normal caloric expenditure because of chronic infection or increased ventilatory muscle energy expenditure. Many of these patients do well with nocturnal enteral feeds provided through a gastrostomy or jejunostomy tube. Formula can be provided continuously overnight to provide much of the patient's caloric needs, including "catch-up" needs. Elemental formulas can be used and may reduce the need for pancreatic enzyme supplements, but many patients have thrived on much more standard, less expensive, formulas with enzyme replacement at bedtime and in the morning.

GASTROINTESTINAL COMPLICATIONS Abdominal pain is relatively common in patients with CF and can be caused by a large number of problems, not all of which are CF-related (Table 23-22).

Meconium ileus and distal intestinal obstruction (DIOS) can usually be treated with careful administration of hyperosmolar enemas, such as meglumine diatrizoate (Gastrografin). DIOS in its early stages (ie, abdominal distension and constipation without complete obstruction) may respond to large volumes of oral or nasogastric GoLytely, eliminating the need for enemas. Chronic constipation can often be prevented from leading to DIOS by adjusting pancreatic enzyme dosing or by the use of lactulose or newer agents such as Miralax. Fibrosing colonopathy is a recently recognized serious complication of very high doses of pancreatic enzymes. Patients may have abdominal pain, bloody diarrhea, or signs of obstruction. Surgery is usually required. The problem has not been seen in patients taking less than 5000 units of lipase per kilogram of body weight per meal.

As in any patient, appendicitis, cholecystitis, *C. difficile* colitis, hepatitis, trauma, and other causes must be considered in the differential diagnosis of acute abdominal pain.

Rectal prolapse is treated by gentle manual pressure on the protruding rectum and is prevented by adjustment of diet and enzymes to reduce bulky stools.

Gastroesophageal reflux in infants should be treated conservatively, with use of the prone position and avoidance of the seated position, as that position is provocative for reflux. The head-down chest physical therapy position should be avoided in infants. Reflux manifest in infants as regurgitation with loss of calories is treated by thickening formula feedings with one tablespoon of rice cereal per ounce of formula. Reflux manifest at any age as esophagitis with heartburn or feeding refusal is treated with H_2 blockers. Reflux manifest as reflex bronchospasm is also treated with H_2 blockers and bronchodilators. In any of these manifestations of reflux, the administration of a prokinetic agent may increase lower esophageal sphincter tone and promote gastric emptying.

In patients with reflux symptoms who do not respond to medical management, the possibility of gastric outlet obstruction should be excluded with gastric emptying studies.

LIVER DISEASE IN CF PATIENTS There is no proven treatment for advanced cirrhosis except liver transplantation. In a few uncontrolled studies bile salts, in the form of ursodeoxycholic acid, have appeared to reduce or stabilize hepatic enzyme levels in CF patients with milder forms of cholestasis. In the rare cases of symptomatic esophageal varices, endoscopic sclerotherapy or variceal banding may be life saving and may eliminate the need for portocaval shunting. Where sclerotherapy or banding fails, transjugular intrahepatic portosystemic shunting (TIPS) has been successful in reducing portal hypertension. The TIPS procedure avoids more invasive shunting procedures, and has left liver transplantation as a future option. Liver transplantation has been carried out in a few patients with CF, with results similar to those recipients without cystic fibrosis. Surprisingly, pulmonary function has not worsened and may even have improved in these CF patients after transplantation, raising the possibility that the immunosuppressive drugs may have beneficial effects on chronic pulmonary infection.

OTHER CF-RELATED COMPLICATIONS Hyperglycemia, termed CF-associated carbohydrate intolerance, occurs in a small but important group of CF patients, who may require insulin therapy. In some patients, dietary manipulations, including use of high-calorie, low-carbohydrate supplements, may help. In others, oral hypoglycemic agents have eliminated or delayed the need for insulin injections. However, reluctance to begin insulin therapy may be misguided, as institution of insulin therapy can improve growth and pulmonary function.

Salt loss may be excessive, especially during exertion in warm weather, but can be prevented if the infants are well hydrated. Older children and adults will generally regulate their salt intake quite adequately if given free access to salt and water. CF patients underestimate their fluid needs during exercise in the heat and need to be encouraged to drink more than they think they need at such times. Salt tablets are not necessary and may be harmful.

PSYCHOLOGICAL CONSIDERATIONS The emotional burdens of a genetic, incurable, progressive, life-shortening, financially draining, and activity-limiting disease on patient and family are substantial. It is remarkable how well the large majority of patients and families

TABLE 23-22

ABDOMINAL PAIN IN CYSTIC FIBROSIS

CAUSE	CHARACTERISTICS	TREATMENT
Constipation	Difficult stooling	Oral lactulose; prune juice; fiber
DIOS (distal intestinal obstruction syndrome)	Crampy pain, feel well between waves of pain; no stools; with or without emesis	Oral or nasogastric GoLytely; Gastrografin enema
Fibrosing colonopathy	Abdominal pain; bloody diarrhea; signs of obstruction	Surgery
Gastroenteritis	Vomiting and diarrhea	Supportive
Pancreatitis	Largely restricted to those with intact pancreatic function	No oral intake; pain control; then low-fat diet; pancreatic enzymes may help
Intussusception	Intermittent; crampy; with or without currant jelly stools	Contrast enema; surgery
Gallstones	Epigastric right upper quadrant, crampy; may be worse after fatty meal	Surgery
Peptic ulcer disease	Epigastric pain; with or without vomiting	Antacids; H_2 blockers; proton pump inhibitors
Appendicitis	Fever, anorexia, right lower quadrant abdominal pain; can also be chronic	Surgery
Abdominal wall (from coughing)	Tender to palpation	Supportive

adjust, with a very low incidence of depression. Issues that patients must face include education and vocation, marriage, reproduction, medical expenses, independent living, and anticipation of disability and death. Establishing and maintaining a positive, optimistic, yet realistic attitude are extremely important. These goals are attainable, especially if the primary physician shares this attitude and maintains a close, supportive relationship with the patient and family. Knowledge of the tremendously improved prognosis over the past decades facilitates such an attitude.

PROGNOSIS

Institution of specialized CF centers and comprehensive aggressive treatment programs beginning in the 1950s has improved the prognosis tremendously. National median survival was 10.6 years in 1966, 20 years in 1981, and 32 years in 1998. It is important to note that these advances in survival have not resulted entirely from major conceptual breakthroughs or new classes of antibiotics but mostly from the adoption of aggressive treatment programs that emphasize daily attention to the complex details of CF care. There are currently many patients in their 20s and 30s with excellent lung function, and, at the end of 1998, 37% of CF patients in the United States were 18 years old or older. Survival probably depends on several factors, including inherent severity of the disease, determined in part by genotype; aggressiveness of the treatment program as prescribed by the physician and carried out by the patient and family; and some degree of chance, especially concerning contact with various bacterial and viral pathogens. Exposure to cigarette smoke speeds pulmonary decline. In general, the survival of male patients is better than that of girls. Survival has recently been shown to been closely correlated with physical fitness, as measured during an exercise test, with fitness being a stronger correlate of survival than even pulmonary function. Perhaps most importantly, long-term prognosis may depend on the timing of diagnosis and institution of treatment. Several studies indicate that those CF patients who are diagnosed early and who begin an aggressive treatment program before the onset of significant pulmonary damage have significantly better pulmonary function and survival than those discovered and treated only after considerable pulmonary tissue has been lost.

What does the future hold for patients with CF? The recent discovery of the CF gene, the improved understanding of the basic cellular and molecular defects, and the success of gene-transfer and protein-repair techniques to reverse the basic defect in CF cells in vitro have all raised hopes for improved treatments and even the possibility of a cure within the foreseeable future. Current research efforts are directed at the further understanding of the molecular pathogenesis of CF and screening of drugs that show beneficial effects in animal models and CF cells. The next wave of therapeutic modalities based on this research is likely to improve survival even further.

References

Andersen D: Cystic fibrosis of the pancreas and its relation to celiac disease: a clinical and pathological study. Am J Dis Child 56:344–399, 1938

Anonymous: Gene therapy for cystic fibrosis utilizing a replication-deficient recombinant adenovirus vector to deliver the human cystic fibrosis transmembrane conductance regulator cDNA to the airways. A phase I study. Hum Gene Ther 5(8):1019–1057, 1994

Anonymous: Correlation between genotype and phenotype in patients with cystic fibrosis. The Cystic Fibrosis Genotype-Phenotype Consortium. N Engl J Med 329:1308–1313, 1993

Collins F: Cystic fibrosis: molecular biology and therapeutic implications. Science 256:774–779, 1992

Davis PB, Drumm M, Konstan MW: Cystic fibrosis. State of the art. Am J Respir Crit Care Med 154:1229–1256, 1996

Drumm M, Pope H, Cliff W, et al: Correction of the cystic fibrosis defect in vitro by retrovirus-mediated gene transfer. Cell 62:1227–1233, 1990

Eigen H, Rosenstein BJ, FitzSimmons S, Schidlow DV: A multicenter study of alternate-day prednisone therapy I patients with cystic fibrosis. J Pediatr 126:515–523, 1995

Fredericksen B, Koch C, Hoiby N: Antibiotic treatment of initial colonization with *Pseudomonas aeruginosa* postpones chronic infection and prevents deterioration of pulmonary function in cystic fibrosis. Pediatr Pulmonol 23:330–335, 1997

Harms HK, Matouk E, Tournier G, et al, on behalf of DNase International Study Group: Multicenter, open-label study of recombinant human DNase in cystic fibrosis patients with moderate lung disease. Pediatr Pulmonol 26:155–161, 1998

Hodson ME, Geddes DM, eds: Cystic Fibrosis. London, Chapman & Hall Medical, 1995

Knowles M, Church N, Waltner W, et al: A pilot study of aerosolized amiloride for the treatment of lung disease in cystic fibrosis. N Engl J Med 322:1189–1194, 1990

Knowles M, Gatzy J, Boucher R: Increased bioelectric potential difference across respiratory epithelia in cystic fibrosis. N Engl J Med 305:1498–1495, 1981

Koletzko S, Stringer D, Cleghorn G, et al: Lavage treatment of distal intestinal obstruction syndrome in children with cystic fibrosis. Pediatrics 83:737–733, 1989

Konstan MW, Byard PJ, Hoppel CL, Davis PB: Effect of high-dose ibuprofen in patients with cystic fibrosis. N Engl J Med 332:848–854, 1995

LeGrys VA: Sweat testing for the diagnosis of cystic fibrosis: practical considerations. J Pediatr 129:892–897, 1996

Madden B, Hodson M, Tsang V, et al: Intermediate-term results of heart-lung transplantation for cystic fibrosis. Lancet 339:1583–1587, 1992

McElvaney N, Hubbard R, Birrer P, et al: Aerosol alpha-1 antitrypsin treatment for cystic fibrosis. Lancet 1:392–394, 1991

Mendeloff EN, Huddleston CB, Mallory GB, et al: Pediatric and adult lung transplantation for cystic fibrosis. J Thorac Cardiovasc Surg 115:404–413, 1998

Nixon PA, Orenstein DM, Kelsey SF, Doershuk CF. The prognostic value of exercise testing in patients with cystic fibrosis. N Engl J Med 327:1785–1788, 1992

Orenstein DM: Cystic Fibrosis: A Guide for Patient and Family. Philadelphia, Lippincott-Raven, 1997

Orenstein DM, Rosenstein BJ, Stern RC: Cystic Fibrosis Medical Care. Philadelphia, Lippincott Williams & Wilkins, 2000

Orenstein DM, Stern RC, eds: Treatment of the hospitalized cystic fibrosis patient. In: Lenfant C, ed: Lung Biology in Health and Disease, vol 109. New York, Marcel Dekker, 1998

Ramsey BW, Pepe MS, Quan JM, et al: Intermittent administration of inhaled tobramycin in patients with cystic fibrosis. N Engl J Med 340:23–30, 1999

Riordan J, Rommens J, Kerem B-S, et al: Identification of the cystic fibrosis gene: cloning and characterization of complementary DNA. Science 245:1066–1073, 1989

Rosenstein BJ, Zeitlin PL: Cystic fibrosis (seminar). Lancet 851:277–282, 1998

Spector M, Stern R: Pneumothorax in cystic fibrosis: a 26-year experience. Ann Thorac Surg 47:204–207, 1989

Zabner J, Couture LA, Gregory RJ et al: Adenovirus-mediated gene transfer transiently corrects the chloride transport defect in nasal epithelia of patients with cystic fibrosis. Cell 75:207–216, 1993

Useful Websites

Cystic Fibrosis Foundation: *www.cff.org*
Cystic Fibrosis Handbook: *www.cystic-I.org/handbook*

23.11 TYPICAL AND ATYPICAL PNEUMONIAS

Thomas A. Hazinski

23.11.1   Bacterial Pneumonias

GENERAL CONSIDERATIONS

Bacterial pneumonias continue to be an important cause of severe illness, particularly in the winter months. Moreover, pathogen resistance to conventional antimicrobial therapy is becoming a problem of worldwide importance and concern.

Because the surface of the lung is exposed continuously to many infectious agents, respiratory infections would be common if the defense mechanisms of the respiratory tract were not so efficient. The lung's defenses include (1) upper airway reflexes that prevent aspiration of infected pharyngeal secretions; (2) a mucociliary clearance system that serves to clear the respiratory epithelium of aspirated microorganisms; (3) a cough reflex that propels foreign material out of the lower tract; (4) a mucous blanket of the respiratory tract to which airborne organisms adhere; (5) antibodies and immune effector cells residing in the airway lining fluid that interact with pathogens; and (6) cells of the pulmonary immune system that process and present microorganisms to focal lymphatic tissue.

Acute primary bacterial pneumonias have many common features, and they can affect any of the lung's lobes or segments. As lobes or segments become consolidated and airless, lung compliance and vital capacity decrease, and the work of breathing increases. This is reflected in young infants and children by expiratory grunting, *retractions, tachypnea,* and *flaring* of the alae nasae. Crackles (rales) or tubular breath sounds are often heard, but a lobar pneumonia may produce no adventitious sounds at all. Vital capacity and lung compliance usually are lower than would be predicted from the extent of consolidation. These changes probably reflect the involvement of inflamed areas of the lung that appear to be normal radiographically. Arterial oxygen tension falls and carbon dioxide tension rises when the lung is extremely stiff or inspiration is limited by pain or fatigue. Whether the child is hospitalized or treated at home depends on the age of the child, severity of the illness, suspected organism, and adequacy of the caretakers. Although many older children can be treated at home, there should be a low threshold for admitting the young infant to the hospital. Indications for hospitalization include severe respiratory distress, dehydration, hypoxia, apnea, poor feeding, deterioration of clinical status after starting therapy, or an associated complication such as empyema. If admitted, the child should be given maintenance fluids and started on an appropriate antibiotic for the suspected bacteria. Potential culture sites to identify the offending bacteria include blood, pleural fluid, and, in selected patients, bronchoalveolar lavage fluid. The culture of sputum does not usually provide accurate information. Because a specific diagnosis in children with pneumonia often cannot be made rapidly, it is prudent initially to use an antibiotic that is effective against the most common bacterial causes of pneumonia, including *Streptococcus pneumoniae,* group A streptococci, nontypable *Hemophilus influenzae,* and *Staphylococcus aureus.* A second-generation cephalosporin such as cefuroxime is effective initial therapy in children with disease caused by an unknown bacteria, although it should be recognized that pneumonia caused by *Mycoplasma pneumoniae* is not adequately treated with this antibiotic. Pulse oximetry measurements should be done on all hospitalized patients, and supplemental oxygen given if needed to maintain an oxygen saturation of 92% or greater. Intravenous antibiotic therapy should be continued until the patient is afebrile, has significant reduction in the work of breathing, and no longer requires supplemental oxygen. At that time, oral antibiotics can be given for a total antibiotic course of 10 to 21 days. Radiographs may remain abnormal for 6 to 8 weeks.

For unknown reasons, patients with parapneumonic effusions and patients with prolonged fever are being seen with increasing frequency in most pediatric centers. The effusions are usually sterile. Antibiotic therapy should be reevaluated if the patient develops prolonged or recurrent fever, but prolonged fever is usually not attributable to persistent infection; it is usually caused by either a prolonged production of fever-producing cytokines or a secondary infection.

PNEUMOCOCCAL PNEUMONIA

Streptococcus pneumoniae rarely causes a primary infection, usually invading the lung after the respiratory tract has been damaged by a viral or chemical agent. Pneumococcal pneumonia is characterized by a rapid onset of inflammatory edema and exudation of serum and red blood cells into the alveoli. Within 24 to 48 hours, the alveoli become filled with pneumococci and fibrin, leukocytes, and serosanguineous fluid. The onset is abrupt, with fever, chills, chest pain, and dyspnea. Mild cough, which may produce blood-tinged sputum, is present early but may disappear as the lobes consolidate. The child appears to be acutely ill, has tachycardia, and breathes rapidly and shallowly. There is dullness to percussion over the affected segment of the lung, breath sounds are diminished, and bronchial breathing and pleural friction rubs may be heard. Crackles may not be heard until later in the course of the disease. Small, sterile, pleural effusions are common, and empyema may be a late complication. Thoracentesis may be necessary to distinguish between these two complications, and pleural fluid should be obtained to guide therapy if possible. When pneumonia is complicated by bacteremia, leukopenia and shock may occur. The combination of leukopenia, shock, and pneumonia has a poor prognosis; mortality rates of up to 50% have been reported.

Children with sickle-cell disease are particularly likely to develop pneumococcal pneumonia because of impaired splenic function. These children usually are given prophylactic oral penicillin, and they should be immunized with polyvalent pneumococcal vaccine.

Although penicillin is still effective against the majority of *S. pneumoniae* isolates, second-generation cephalosporin therapy has become the standard of care for most patients. However, strains resistant to one or more cephalosporins are reported frequently. For critically ill children with pneumonia, additional antimicrobial therapy for possible penicillin or β-lactam resistance should be considered at the outset and then modified as needed after susceptibilities are known. For hospitalized children with severe hypersensitivity to the β-lactam agents, clindamycin or vancomycin is acceptable. All children with meningitis in addition to pneumonia will require vancomycin. Clindamycin is a useful alternative for penicillin-allergic children treated as outpatients. Most children respond rapidly and require only 10 days of antibiotics. No specific isolation procedures are required for hospitalized patients with pneumococcal pneumonia. Of concern are recent reports describing an increase in the number of penicillin-resistant *S. pneumoniae* isolates in the United States, approaching 40% in some regions. When a penicillin-resistant organism is isolated, antibiotic selection and dosage is best guided by serum mean inhibitory concentration values.

Although sterile pleural effusions may persist for several weeks, these usually resolve without treatment. Clinically significant empyemas may require closed-suction drainage or decortication. Occasionally, pneumatoceles may develop. These almost always are asymptomatic, disappear in days to weeks, and do not require surgical excision.

STREPTOCOCCAL PNEUMONIA

Pneumonia caused by group A β-hemolytic streptococci usually follows childhood exanthemata, particularly rubeola, varicella, and scarlet fever, but it also occurs in children without previous illness. In the early stage, most of the inflammatory reaction is interstitial, but eventually, the inflammatory response also involves the airways. Widespread edema develops, and shedding of the alveolar epithelium occurs. Pneumatoceles or abscess formation can occur as well.

Streptococcal infections have a sudden onset, with sore throat, hoarseness, fever, chest pain, cough, marked respiratory distress, and leukocytosis. When pneumonia develops, there is dullness to percussion over the affected lung, and rales and decreased breath sounds are heard during auscultation. If an effusion is present, crepitant rales and pleural friction rubs usually are heard. A chest radiograph may show segmental involvement, diffuse peribronchiolar densities, or effusion; findings rarely may resemble an interstitial pneumonia caused by viruses. Pneumatoceles are common and similar to those occurring with staphylococcal lung infections. These always disappear spontaneously. The most common complications are abscesses and empyema. Less common complications are pericarditis and peritonitis. Uncomplicated illness may be treated with oral penicillin for 10 to 14 days. Large doses of intravenous penicillin G for longer periods are required in more seriously ill children.

Clinical response, decrease in the white blood cell count, and disappearance of *Streptococcus* may proceed slowly after penicillin therapy is initiated. Three to four weeks of treatment may be required, and empyema usually requires closed-suction drainage. *Streptococcus* causes a necrotizing pneumonia, and residual focal bronchiectasis and fibrosis may occur.

STAPHYLOCOCCAL PNEUMONIA

Although less common than pneumococcal, β-hemolytic *Streptococcus,* or viral pneumonias, staphylococcal pneumonia is still a serious disease. Unless it is treated early and vigorously, infants with staphylococcal pneumonia may develop pneumatoceles, pneumothoraces, and empyema. The organisms first produce a diffuse inflammation in one or more segments of the lung that may resemble a viral pneumonitis. The right lung more often is affected than the left. Inflamed bronchi become partially occluded, and pneumatoceles form beyond the obstruction. The bacteria multiply rapidly, producing a necrotizing toxin that causes tissue destruction. Microabscesses form around small bronchi and in pneumatoceles. Pneumatoceles and abscesses extend toward the pleural space and frequently rupture into it, causing empyema and pneumothorax.

Staphylococcal pneumonias have a rapid onset, with fever, tachypnea, dyspnea, tachycardia, and cyanosis. They often are preceded by an upper respiratory infection for which antibiotics have

been given. The child with staphylococcal pneumonia may be lethargic or irritable. Ileus and abdominal distension can occur. Physical signs reflect the progress of the disease. The chest radiograph may show a lobar distribution of radiodensities, effusion, or pneumothorax; most characteristic are discrete areas of overinflation and distinct pneumatoceles. Staphylococci often can be grown from the blood. Bilateral or multilobe involvement or a white blood cell count of less than 10,000 cells/μL are poor prognostic signs.

Because staphylococcal pneumonia may be fulminant, every patient in whom this condition is suspected should be hospitalized, and therapy begun after appropriate cultures are obtained. A penicillinase-resistant penicillin should be given for at least 2 weeks, or longer for severe illnesses with complications. Approximately 11% of staphylococcal isolates in the United States are methicillin resistant, and vancomycin should be given when these organisms are isolated, when the patient has risk factors for MRSA (eg, recent contact with known carrier, recent hospitalization, presence of intravascular catheter or tracheostomy), or when the patient is not responding to initial therapy. The patient with *Staph. aureus* pneumonia requires contact isolation.

If the course is complicated by a pneumothorax, it should be decompressed. Large pneumatoceles may resemble a pneumothorax, however, so careful radiographic examination must be done to distinguish them. Pneumatoceles are part of the healing process, are seen 3 to 4 days after treatment has begun, and usually disappear. If empyema is present and the patient is recovering slowly, it must be treated promptly by closed-suction drainage.

Follow-up studies of patients who had staphylococcal pneumonia with empyema in early childhood indicate no clinical or radiologic abnormalities.

HEMOPHILUS INFLUENZAE PNEUMONIA

With the widespread use of the *Hemophilus* vaccine, pneumonias caused by encapsulated *H. influenzae* type b organisms are now rare. Clinical presentation with lobar distribution may be indistinguishable from pneumococcal pneumonia, although the onset usually is more insidious. The bronchopneumonic variety may mimic acute bronchiolitis during the early stages, but increasing interstitial edema, producing a "shaggy" appearance on radiographs, should alert the physician to the presence of a bacterial infection.

Ampicillin is the drug of choice for children with mild pulmonary disease. Children with moderate pulmonary disease should be treated with an oral antibiotic resistant to β-lactamase such as ampicillin/clavulanic acid (Augmentin). A second-generation cephalosporin (eg, ceftriaxone, cefotaxime, ceftazidime) given intravenously usually is effective for severe disease.

KLEBSIELLA PNEUMONIAE PNEUMONIA

Klebsiella pneumoniae are found in the respiratory and gastrointestinal tracts of many healthy children, but they rarely cause pneumonia in children. Occasional epidemics of *K. pneumoniae* infection occur in newborn nurseries. However, when *K. pneumoniae* pneumonia occurs in older children, they usually are immunocompromised or have had prolonged endotracheal intubation. The clinical picture is indistinguishable from other varieties of pneumonia, but copious, thick, purulent secretions should suggest the diagnosis. Older children are prone to develop pulmonary abscesses and cavitation (ie, pneumatoceles). Bacteremia and empyema are common.

Klebsiella pneumonia may not respond to antibiotics that are used to treat usual pulmonary infections in childhood (ie, ampicillin and penicillinase-resistant penicillins). However, cefotaxime and an aminoglycoside usually are effective.

Klebsiella and other gram-negative bacteria may also colonize tracheostomy tubes but rarely cause clinical symptoms. If this organism is cultured from the tracheostomy tube of a patient with indolent symptoms who does not respond to conventional therapy, a trial of inhaled aminoglycoside therapy is warranted.

ANAEROBIC BACTERIAL PNEUMONIA

Children who are prone to aspirate oropharyngeal secretions typically have some form of neurologic impairment or structural abnormality of the airway and esophagus. Like gram-negative enteric bacteria, *S. aureus* and *S. pyogenes,* anaerobic bacteria cause tissue necrosis and abscess formation. Sputum with a putrid smell strongly suggests anaerobic infection. Most of the anaerobic bacteria causing pneumonia are highly susceptible to penicillin. Some strains of *Bacteroides fragilis* produce β-lactamase and therefore are resistant to penicillin. Therefore, in severely ill patients with suspected anaerobic infection, it is reasonable to begin therapy with clindamycin or ticarcillin/clavulanic acid with an aminoglycoside if concomitant gram-negative infection is suspected (see Sec. 13.2.2).

COMPLICATIONS OF BACTERIAL PNEUMONIAS

LUNG ABSCESS There has been a sharp drop in the incidence of lung abscess during the past 20 years, probably because of better respiratory therapy of abscess-prone patients. Abscesses without pneumonia (ie, *primary abscesses*) may follow aspiration of an infected foreign body or oropharyngeal secretions. Children with gingival disease, particularly those with swallowing dysfunction, also may develop a lung abscess. An abscess that complicates a bacterial pneumonia is called a *secondary abscess* because it forms in an area of lung consolidation that reestablishes a connection with an airway. A third form of lung abscess occurs in patients with a pre-existing cystic lesion, cavity, or lung malformation that becomes secondarily infected (eg, patients with a bronchogenic cyst, sequestration, or adenomatoid malformation).

The most common organisms found in primary abscesses in childhood are staphylococci and β-hemolytic streptococci. Anaerobes may be the causal agent in children with gingivitis and discoordinated swallowing. Most lung abscesses can be treated with antibiotics alone. If fever persists, or the abscess does not decrease in size despite an adequate course of antibiotics for the infecting organism, surgical intervention may be required. Because of the possibility of retained foreign body or congenital malformation, patients with lung abscess should be followed closely, and both clinical and radiologic resolution of the abscess should be documented.

PLEURAL EFFUSION AND EMPYEMA If a pulmonary infection disrupts the normal pathways of pleural fluid production and elimination, pleural fluid can accumulate, sometimes rapidly, and be detected clinically or radiographically as a pleural effusion. Ultrasonography and lateral decubitus radiographs of the chest may be necessary to differentiate pleural fluid from lung consolidation. Sterile, low-viscosity, alkaline, and relatively acellular fluid is termed a *parapneumonic effusion.* If pulmonary inflammation extends beyond the pleural surface, the pleural effusion will be purulent,

acidic, and contain high concentrations of inflammatory cells; occasionally, the pathogen will be seen or cultured from this fluid. This latter fluid is termed an *empyema.* Empyemas may be a complication of any bacterial pneumonia, but it most commonly is caused by *S. aureus* or *S. pneumoniae.*

The management of pleural effusion and empyema is controversial. If the patient is seriously ill, a small amount of fluid should be obtained for appropriate culture and miscoscopic examination [Gram stain, KOH preparation, and stain for acid-fast bacilli (AFB)]. If respiratory distress or hypoxemia is severe, thoracostomy tube drainage may be necessary. An empyema may cause prolonged fever and leukocytosis as well as a protracted hospitalization. Almost all cases of empyema can be successfully treated with appropriate antibiotics. If the pleural effusion is increasing in size, or the patient has respiratory distress, hypoxemia, or prolonged fever, thoracotomy with decortication and chest-tube drainage may be necessary. Long-term follow-up indicates that the majority of children who have recovered from empyema have normal lung function and chest radiographs.

HILAR ADENOPATHY The finding of possible hilar adenopathy during the evaluation of a child with pneumonia should prompt the consideration that a granulomatous disease is present, such as tuberculosis, histoplasmosis, rare fungal infections, sarcoidosis, and malignancies. A chest CT scan with intravenous contrast is helpful in establishing the degree and functional importance of hilar nodes and may yield additional information about the presence of parenchymal or node calcification.

RECURRENT PNEUMONIA During the evaluation of a patient with acute pneumonia, the medical history may reveal that the current illness is one of many episodes of pneumonia. In these patients, previous chest radiographs should be reviewed and correlated with the patient's history to determine if the symptoms and infiltrates are persistent or recurrent. In all of these patients, a sweat test should be performed to exclude the possibility of cystic fibrosis. In patients whose evaluation suggests that recurrent pneumonias have occurred in *different* lobes each time and the patient has no chronic respiratory symptoms, recurrent aspiration, ciliary dysmotility syndrome, and disorders of immune function should be considered. If chest radiographs indicate that the *same* lung segment is involved each time, a congenital malformation or foreign body should be suspected. In patients with a history of recurrent pneumonia, it is often discovered that the patient has recurrent atelectasis and mucoid bronchial impaction secondary to undetected asthma triggered by viral infections. These children may have chronic pulmonary symptoms such as chronic night cough or exercise-induced cough, even when they are not acutely ill. Review of previous chest radiographs indicates that the same areas of atelectasis are repeatedly imaged and misinterpreted as acute pulmonary infections. For these reasons, patients with a history of recurrent pneumonia should be reevaluated periodically until they have both clinical and radiologic resolution of their signs and symptoms. Failure to reestablish a symptom-free and a normal chest radiograph should prompt a search for other disorders.

References

Asher MI, Spier S, Beland M, et al: Primary lung abscess in childhood: the long-term outcome of conservative management. Am J Dis Child 136: 491, 1982

Brook I: Lung abscesses and pleural empyema in children. Adv Pediatr Infect Dis 8:159, 1993

Brook I, Finegold SM: Bacteriology of aspiration pneumonia in children. Pediatrics 65:1115, 1980

Centers for Disease Control and Prevention: Drug-resistant *S. pneumoniae*—Kentucky and Tennessee, 1993. JAMA 271:421, 1994

Chartrand SA, McCracken GH Jr: Staphylococcal pneumonia in infants and children. Pediatr Infect Dis 1:19, 1982

Mason EO, Kaplan SL, Lamberth LB, Tillman J: Increased rate of isolation of penicillin-resistant *Streptococcus pneumoniae* in a children's hospital and in vitro susceptibilities to antibiotics of potential therapeutic use. Antimicrob Agents Chemother 36:1703, 1992

McLaughlin FJ, Goldman DA, Rosenbaum DM, et al: Empyema in children: clinical course and long-term follow-up. Pediatrics 73:587, 1984

Murphy D, Lockhart CH, Todd JK: Pneumococcal empyema: outcome of medical management. Am J Dis Child 134:659, 1980

Parker LA, Melton JW, Delany DJ, Yankaskas BC: Percutaneous small bore catheter drainage of lung abscesses. Chest 92:213, 1987

Peter G: The child with pneumonia: diagnostic and therapeutic considerations. Pediatr Infect Dis 7:453, 1988

Pollak JS, Passik CS: Intrapleural urokinase in the treatment of pleural effusions. Chest 105:868, 1994

Sahn SA: Management of complicated parapneumonic effusion. Am Rev Respir Dis 148:813, 1993

Shann F, Barker J, Poore P: Clinical signs that predict death in children with severe pneumonia. Pediatr Infect Dis 8:852, 1989

Soto M, Demis T, Landau LI: Pulmonary function following staphylococcal pneumonia in children. Aust Paediatr J 19:172, 1983

Stark JM: Lung infections in children. Curr Opin Pediatr 5:273, 1993

23.11.2   Mycotic and Fungal Infections

Symptoms that are produced by most mycotic infections are mild, often diagnosed as a flu-like illness, rarely require treatment, and resolve without sequelae. Histoplasmosis and coccidioidomycosis are examples. However, mycotic infections can be severe in children with diminished immunologic competence because of malnutrition, congenital or acquired immunodeficiency disorder, and in children who are receiving immunosuppressive therapy for leukemia, malignancy, or organ transplantation.

HISTOPLASMOSIS

Primary infection of the lung with *Histoplasma capsulatum* is common in endemic areas such as the Southeast and Mississippi valley in the United States. There is a wide spectrum of pulmonary disease that can result from infection with *H. capsulatum* (Table 23-23). Most primary histoplasmosis infections are asymptomatic and are diagnosed in retrospect because of the development of pulmonary calcifications and calcified hilar adenopathy observed on a chest radiograph that was obtained for other reasons. Rarely, a heavier inoculum can result in acute pulmonary histoplasmosis manifested by fever, anorexia, malaise, chest pain, tachypnea, uncalcified hilar adenopathy, and cough. Histoplasmosis can also cause miliary pneumonia and disseminated disease. See Sec. 13.5.7 for clinical findings, diagnosis, and treatment.

Histoplasmosis also can present as asymptomatic mediastinal masses resulting from enlarged hilar lymph nodes detected by chest radiography (ie, mediastinal granuloma). Before calcifications develop within the enlarged nodes, the possibility of lymphoma or other malignancy should be considered in the differential diagnosis. Tuberculosis should be excluded by skin testing and appropriate cultures. Occasionally, enlarged nodes can erode or obstruct a bronchus and cause hemoptysis or a secondary postobstructive

TABLE 23-23

CONSEQUENCES OF INHALATION OF *HISTOPLASMA CAPSULATUM* SPORES INTO ALVEOLI

Asymptomatic
  Self-limited infection
Symptomatic
  Dissemination
  Regional lymphadenopathy
    Nonsegmental pneumonitis
      Resolution
      Histoplasmoma
    Resolution
    Residual nodes with or without calcification
    Mediastinal granuloma
    Mediastinal fibrosis with obstruction of:
      Superior vena cava and azygous vein
      Pulmonary arteries and veins
      Bronchi
      Esophagus
      Coronary arteries
    Pericarditis

pneumonia. Surgical removal of enlarged nodes sometimes is necessary.

Another complication of histoplasmosis is fibrosing mediastinitis. In this condition, a diffuse fibroproliferative reaction causes distortion or obliteration of mediastinal structures, which can result in obstruction of the pulmonary artery, pulmonary veins, coronary arteries, esophagus, trachea, and superior vena cava (see Sec. 13.5.7). Histologically, the tissue is not calcified and resembles keloid. No specific treatment is available. Surgical resection usually is impossible because of the extensive fibrous tissue, which obliterates fascial planes. The disease may occasionally regress in children, but it is usually slowly progressive. Signs and symptoms are related to the mediastinal structure obliterated by the fibroproliferation.

COCCIDIOIDOMYCOSIS

Primary infection of the lungs with *Coccidioides immitis* is very common in arid regions of the southwestern United States, Mexico, and Central America. Children with primary coccidioidomycosis have a low-grade fever, minimal lung involvement, and erythema nodosum. Almost all instances of primary coccidioidomycosis heal without treatment, leaving small, calcified pulmonary scars. In the San Joaquin Valley of California, it is called *valley fever*. Occasionally, there is progressive, primary lung inflammation or dissemination that must be treated vigorously. Treatment then consists of intravenous amphotericin B until there is a decrease in serum antibodies; this may take several months. Children treated with amphotericin B should have frequent measurements of renal function. Serologic testing for coccidioidal precipitins and complement-fixing antibodies are the most sensitive methods of following the response to treatment (see Sec. 13.5.5).

ASPERGILLOSIS

Aspergillus sp. are widely distributed in soil, decaying vegetable matter, and bird droppings. Aspergilli, particularly *A. fumigatus,* commonly are found in the sputum of patients with chronic pulmonary disease, notably in those with cystic fibrosis. These usually are saprophytic commensals, but they can cause pulmonary disease, ranging from hypersensitivity reactions to invasion of the parenchyma with formation of fungus balls (see Secs. 13.5.2 and 23.13.2). Patients with neutropenia and with chronic granulomatous disease are particularly susceptible to developing invasive aspergillosis.

BLASTOMYCOSIS

When inhaled, *Blastomyces dermatitis* spores can cause lung disease. Blastomycosis pneumonia most often is seen in the United States in the midwestern river basins and in the southeastern states. Symptoms include fever, malaise, productive cough, chest pain, vomiting, and occasional pulmonary hemorrhage. Chest radiographs can resemble the myriad of findings seen with tuberculosis; a pleural effusion also may be present. Cutaneous ulcerated lesions are seen with this infection as well. Diagnosis usually can be made by sputum culture. Complement-fixation and skin tests often are negative. Treatment with amphotericin B is indicated for patients with severe disease; either ketoconazole or itraconozole has been recommended for patients with mild indolent symptoms (see Sec. 13.5.3).

CRYPTOCOCCOSIS, CANDIDIASIS, AND SPOROTRICHOSIS

Cryptococcus and *Candida* sp. often cause pulmonary inflammation in immunologically incompetent children. Diagnosis must be made by lung biopsy. Treatment is amphotericin B or 5-fluorocytosine. *Sporotrichum* occasionally has been identified as an organism that is responsible for chronic pulmonary inflammation. This infection responds to some extent to therapy with potassium iodide, but amphotericin B probably is the drug of choice (see Secs. 13.5.4, 13.5.6, and 13.5.9).

MUCORMYCOSIS

Mucormycosis is a rare infection during childhood, and it usually occurs in immunocompromised individuals. Up to one-half of patients present with pneumonia or lung abscess. Treatment consists of antifungal chemotherapy, usually with amphotericin B, and surgical debridement (see Sec. 13.5.10).

ACTINOMYCOSIS

Actinomycosis is a chronic suppurative infection that is characterized by abscess and sinus tract formation in the cervicofacial area. This disease can occur in children who are immunologically competent, and pulmonary infection should alert the physician to possible cervicofacial spread, foreign-body aspiration, poor dental hygiene, or chronic aspiration. The clinical picture of a chronic pulmonary infection is cough, sputum, fever, dyspnea, and weight loss. Pulmonary hemorrhage also may occur. Multiple abscesses may be present. Extension into the pleural cavity or pericardium or involvement of the ribs and subcutaneous tissues with sinus formation is common. The differential diagnosis includes chest wall sarcoma and skin tumor. Anaerobic cultures are necessary to grow the organism, but the diagnosis can be strongly suspected by finding sulfur granules in the pus from a draining cutaneous sinus. The treatment of choice is high doses of penicillin, 10 million IU/d intravenously, for several weeks, followed by oral penicillin for a minimum of 6 months (see Sec. 13.2.1).

NOCARDIOSIS

This chronic suppurative disease resembles actinomycosis. Abscesses and sinuses are less common, however, and in children, the lung often is involved. It may occur as a complication of immunodeficiency diseases such as chronic granulomatous disease. There are a persistent cough, intermittent septic fever, hepatosplenomegaly, and progressive pulmonary insufficiency. Treatment with sulfadiazine or a combination of trimethoprim-sulfamethoxazole has been effective in the early stages of this disease (see Sec. 13.2.1).

References

Causey WA, Sieger B: Systemic nocardiosis caused by *Nocardia brasiliensis*. Am Rev Respir Dis 109:134, 1974

Heffner JE: Pleuropulmonary manifestations of actinomycosis in nocardiosis. Semin Respir Infect 3:352, 1988

Kirchner SG, Hernanz-Schulman M, Stein S, et al: Imaging of pediatric mediastinal histoplasmosis. Radiographics 11:365, 1991

Kline MW: Mucormycosis in children: review of the literature and report of cases. Pediatr Infect Dis 4:672, 1985

Loyd JE, Tillman BF, Adkinson JB, Des Pres RM: Mediastinal fibrosis complicating histoplasmosis. Medicine 67:295, 1988

Newson BD, Hardy JD: Pulmonary fungal infection: survey of 159 cases with surgical implications. J Thorac Cardiovasc Surg 83:218, 1982

Powell DA, Schuit KE: Acute pulmonary blastomycosis in children: clinical course and follow-up. Pediatrics 63:736, 1979

Schoumacher RA, Berkow RL: Invasive pulmonary aspergillosis in an infant: an unusual presentation of chronic granulomatous disease. Pediatr Infect Dis J 6:215, 1987

23.11.3   Viral Respiratory Infections

INFECTIOUS BRONCHIOLITIS

Infectious bronchiolitis is a common disease of infancy and childhood, and it most often occurs in the winter and spring months. It often is preceded by symptoms of nasopharyngitis, poor feeding, and low-grade fever but proceeds to cause cough, wheezing, and tachypnea. These symptoms are associated with intercostal and subcostal retractions and progressive hyperinflation of the lungs. The course of the disease is relatively mild in older infants and children, and recovery occurs in 4 to 5 days. Infants who are under 1 year of age or who have chronic cardiopulmonary disease usually have more severe respiratory distress, and death can occur in these groups (see also Sec. 13.4.19).

ETIOLOGY   Bronchiolitis was first described as a complication of measles and mumps, but it now is associated with many respiratory viruses. Most commonly, bronchiolitis is caused by the respiratory syncytial virus (RSV). RSV can be detected in nasopharyngeal washings at the onset of symptoms. The virus usually disappears within 7 days, but it can persist for a month or longer in very young infants. Infants under 6 months of age with an RSV infection produce less RSV-specific antibodies than do older children, which may explain why the virus can be recovered for a longer period of time and why the disease is more severe and occasionally recurrent in younger infants. Risk factors for severe RSV bronchiolitis include tobacco smoke exposure, crowded living conditions, a family history of asthma, and low birth weight. Spread of RSV is by large particles and self-inoculation after contact with contaminated surfaces. Hospital and day-care outbreaks can be reduced by handwashing before and after patient contact.

The respiratory viruses cause inflammation and necrosis of the airway mucosa. The walls of the small bronchi and bronchioles become edematous, and the mucosa is disrupted and infiltrated with inflammatory cells. Lumina of the airways often are completely occluded with leukocytes, mucus, and cell debris. Medium-sized bronchi may be similarly affected. Adenoviruses cause a more severe disruption of the mucosa than RSV and also produce a necrotizing bronchiolitis with residual bronchiectasis. Mortality is rare, but morbidity from RSV and other viruses can be quite high. Some infants develop chronic inflammatory changes that can cause chronic peribronchiolar inflammation and bronchiolitis obliterans.

CLINICAL FEATURES   The inflammation and necrosis of the airways exposes the irritant receptors, which, when stimulated by deep breaths, cause coughing. To prevent coughing and reduce the work of breathing, infants and children breathe rapidly and shallowly. Along with partial obstruction of small airways, this breathing pattern tends to trap a portion of each breath and leads to hyperinflation. Deep breaths are accompanied by rales and expiratory wheezing and usually are followed by a paroxysm of coughing. Cyanosis may occur and be most marked during sleep when the drive to respiration is blunted. Hypercapnia is common in infants who are less than 1 year of age, particularly when they are agitated or coughing. In addition to cough, stimulation of the irritant receptors also causes reflex constriction of the larynx. Increased nasopharyngeal secretions can cause further upper airway obstruction and increase the work of breathing. Both central and obstructive apnea can occur in infants who are less than 2 to 3 months of age, presumably related to prematurity and nasopharyngitis. Suprasternal, sternal, and intercostal retractions become marked. As the intrapleural pressure falls, venous return to the heart increases, thereby increasing lung microvascular pressure just as the pericapillary interstitial pressure is falling. The hydrostatic pressure changes favor the development of pulmonary edema. In addition, edema is further enhanced by increased levels of antidiuretic hormone. As edema fluid accumulates between alveoli and around small airways, peribronchial receptors are stimulated, causing tachypnea. Pulmonary edema decreases lung compliance, which, along with the bronchoconstriction, increases the work of breathing.

The radiologic appearance of bronchiolitis is nonspecific and includes both hyperinflation and diffuse pulmonary infiltrates. Pleural effusions are rare.

TREATMENT   The treatment of bronchiolitis is supportive. The most important treatment is oxygen if the infant is hypoxemic. Oxygen should be delivered by head hood, tent, or nasal cannula and guided by the results of accurately performed pulse oximetry. Fluids should be given to treat or prevent dehydration, but overhydration should be avoided to reduce the risk of pulmonary edema. A therapeutic trial of inhaled β-agonist therapy should be strongly considered. Some studies suggest that inhaled racemic epinephrine improves clinical status better than do agents with only β-adrenergic effects. Small infants tend to permit their carbon dioxide tension to rise, and many infants will tolerate PCO_2 values of 60 mm Hg without difficulty during the acute phase of the disease. Secondary bacterial infection is rare but should be considered in critically ill patients or in patients who appear to improve and then worsen. If the patient has a history of recurrent episodes of wheezing, corticosteroid therapy (as for the treatment of status asthmat-

icus) should be considered as well. Extracorporeal membrane oxygenation has been used to treat refractory respiratory failure with good results.

Ribavirin, which is a nucleoside analog that inhibits viral replication, has been used to treat RSV infections of the lower respiratory tract in both infants and children. Ribavirin is given in an aerosol that is produced by a specially designed device; a variety of protocols have been proposed. In many institutions, ribavirin is delivered via a double hood or endotracheal tube in a closed system to reduce the exposure of caretakers. The use of ribavirin is controversial because some clinical trials have yielded small clinical benefits relative to expense and complexity of the protocol for inhalation. Its use should be considered in patients with immunodeficiency or in infants with extremely severe disease.

Infants who have had bronchiolitis are more likely to have wheezing with subsequent respiratory tract infections, and they also are more likely to develop chronic asthma. The association between asthma and RSV probably is indirect. RSV is an easily identifiable pathogen causing bronchiolitis, and infants with asthma are more likely to wheeze with any viral infection (see Sec. 23.8).

Prospects for the prevention of RSV bronchiolitis remain poor, and no vaccine is yet available. In preterm infants and in infants with BPD, the requirement for hospitalization can be reduced substantially by monthly administration of anti-RSV-enriched IVIG or a monoclonal anti-RSV antibody, but either treatment is expensive, does not prevent infection, and is not life saving.

VIRAL PNEUMONIAS

Many viruses can cause pneumonia in infants and children. These include RSV, parainfluenza viruses, adenoviruses, rhinoviruses, influenza viruses, and both varicella and rubeola viruses. The latter can cause particularly severe disease in immunocompromised patients. After several days of upper respiratory tract symptoms or rash, lower respiratory tract involvement is heralded by the sudden onset of tachypnea, nonproductive and often paroxysmal cough, substernal discomfort, low-grade fever, and malaise. There may be dullness over the lung, diminished breath sounds, as well as fine and crepitant rales. Often, however, there are no physical signs of lung disease. This is in stark contrast to the radiographic picture, which often has marked perihilar and parenchymal infiltrates.

Most viral pneumonias respond to nonspecific treatment, including rest and adequate fluid intake. If signs of airway obstruction are present, bronchodilators and other previously outlined measures for diseases of the airway should be considered based on clinical response, but they are not routinely warranted. If there is significant hypoxemia, oxygen should be given. The mortality rate is low, but convalescence often is prolonged. Some infections, particularly in young infants, may cause extensive damage and require 1 year or more to resolve completely; chronic interstitial lung disease also may develop and require both oxygen and anti-inflammatory therapy (see Sec. 23.7).

Specific antiviral therapy is available for some viral pneumonias. Ribavirin appears to be safe and effective in populations who are at high risk for significant RSV bronchiolitis and pneumonia, including those with complicated heart disease, bronchopulmonary dysplasia, immunodeficiency (both primary and acquired, such as AIDS, and patients undergoing chemotherapy or bone marrow transplantation), and cystic fibrosis. Varicella-zoster virus pneumonia can be reduced in susceptible individuals by administration of varicella-zoster immune globulin on exposure, and treatment with acyclovir usually is effective in preventing severe pneumonia. The combination of ganciclovir and cytomegalovirus immune globulin has been reported to be effective in bone marrow transplant patients with cytomegalovirus pneumonitis. Recently, an outbreak of hantavirus pneumonia occurred in the southwestern United States. This rodent-borne virus, unlike other viruses, was not associated with an upper respiratory infection–type syndrome. Mortality was high, and intravenous ribavirin, although experimental for this indication, was thought to be beneficial.

Residual lung disease, particularly hyperreactive airways, is common. Some infants with severe adenovirus bronchiolitis and pneumonia develop bronchiolitis obliterans (see Sec. 23.7).

References

Gozal D, Colin AA, Jaffe M, Hochberg Z: Water, electrolyte, and endocrine homeostasis in infants with bronchiolitis. Pediatr Res 27:204, 1990

Groothuis JR, Salbenblatt CK, Lauer BA: Severe respiratory syncytial virus infection in older children. Am J Dis Child 144:346, 1990

Henderson FW, Clyde WA, Collier AM, Denny FW: The etiologic and epidemiologic spectrum of bronchiolitis in pediatric practice. J Pediatr 95:183, 1979

Howard TS, Hoffman LH, Stang PE, Simoes EA: RSV pneumonia in the hospital setting: Length of stay, charges, and mortality . J Pediatrics 137:227–232, 2000

Klassen TP: Recent advances in the treatment of bronchiolitis and lyaryngitis. Pediatr Clin North Am 44:249–261, 1997

Koppi M, Reijonen T, Poysa L, Juntunen-Backman K: A 2 to 3 year outcome after bronchiolitis. Am J Dis Child 147:628, 1993

Mallory GB Jr, Motoyama EK, Koumbourlis AC, et al: Bronchial reactivity in infants in acute respiratory failure with viral bronchiolitis. Pediatr Pulmonol 6:253, 1989

Menon KI, Sutcliffe T, Klassen TP: A randomized trial comparing the efficacy of epinephrine with salbutamol in the treatment of acute bronchiolitis. J Pediatr 126:1004–1007, 1995

Perlstein PH, Kotagal U, Schoettker PJ, et al: Sustaining the implementation of an evidence-based guideline for bronchiolitis. Arch Pediatr Adolesc Med 154:1001–1007, 2000

Reese AC, James IR, Landau LT, Lesouef PN: Relationship between urinary cotine level and diagnosis in children admitted to hospital. Am Rev Respir Dis 146:66, 1992

Sanchez I, DeKoster J, Powell RE, et al: Effect of racemic epinephrine and salbutamol on clinical score and pulmonary mechanics in infants with bronchiolitis. J Pediatr 122:145, 1993

Simoes EA: Respiratory syncytial virus infection. Lancet 354:847–852, 1999

Welliver RC, Wong DT, Sun M, McCarthy N: Parainfluenza virus bronchiolitis. Am J Dis Child 140:34, 1986

Wohl MEB, Chernick V: Bronchiolitis: state of the art. Am Rev Respir Dis 118:759, 1978

23.11.4 Infectious Interstitial Pneumonias

MYCOPLASMA PNEUMONIA

Mycoplasma pneumoniae and the related species *M. hominis, M. genitalium,* and *Ureaplasma urealyticum* cause an acute interstitial pneumonitis. It is the most common treatable cause of lower respiratory infection in children over 5 years of age. *Mycoplasma* pneumonia can be severe and cause pleural effusions, myocarditis, encephalopathy, and ARDS. A characteristic prodrome of headache, fever, malaise, and pharyngitis may precede the onset of non-

productive cough and dyspnea. Crackles may be heard bilaterally, and chest radiography often reveals an interstitial infiltrate, although lobar involvement is possible. Pleural effusions are present in up to 30% of cases. The diagnosis can be confirmed serologically with rapid ELISA-based methods; 50% of patients will have a positive cold agglutinin titer, and the diagnosis can be suspected if the patient's blood is shown to reversibly agglutinate when chilled. A course of macrolide or tetracycline therapy will shorten the course of the illness.

The clinical course, diagnosis, and treatment are detailed in Sec. 13.2.22.

CHLAMYDIAL INFECTIONS

CHLAMYDIA **PNEUMONITIS** *Chlamydia trachomatis* causes trachoma, inclusion conjunctivitis, urethritis, and pneumonia. It commonly is found in the female genital tract, and infants who are born to infected mothers have approximately a 50% chance of having conjunctivitis and a 10 to 20% chance of developing pneumonia. Pulmonary infection usually develops gradually over the first weeks of life. Often, it is preceded by a nasal or eye discharge. In some patients, the incubation period may be 2 to 3 months. Signs of pneumonia start with a nonproductive cough and tachypnea, usually between 3 and 19 weeks of age. Fever is absent. Chest radiographs show hyperinflated lungs and diffuse interstitial infiltrate. As the disease progresses, respiratory distress becomes more marked, with rales, intercostal retractions, and occasionally wheezing. The cough often is marked and paroxysmal, and the respiratory rate may be at or near 100 breaths per minute for many weeks. This may interfere with feeding. Occasionally, *C. trachomatis* can cause myocarditis. Serum IgM and IgG levels usually are high, and there may be eosinophilia. The diagnosis is made by culture of *C. trachomatis,* presence of specific serum antibodies, or rapid antigen-detection methods (eg, direct fluorescent antibodies, enzyme immunoassay, DNA probe) of respiratory or conjunctival secretions. Erythromycin, 40–50 mg/kg/d, in divided doses for 14 days, is the treatment of choice for chlamydial conjunctivitis or pneumonia. An alternate therapy is sulfisoxazole, 150 mg/kg/d for 14 days, for infants beyond the immediate neonatal period. Oral erythromycin has been associated with idiopathic hypertrophic pyloric stenosis in infants less than 6 weeks of age, but the risk with other macrolides (e.g. azithromycin) is unknown. A causal link has not been established (see Sec. 13.2.11).

Other *Chlamydia* organisms, formerly termed *Chlamydia TWAR* and now designated *Chlamydia pneumoniae,* have been isolated from older patients with mild febrile pneumonia syndromes. Bronchospasm is common. Occasionally, these agents also may cause myocarditis as well. The treatment for *Chlamydia pneumoniae* infection is erythromycin or tetracycline.

PSITTACOSIS-ORNITHOSIS PNEUMONIA The responsible organism, which previously was regarded as a large virus, is now classified with the chlamydial group, *Chlamydia psittaci* and *Chlamydia pecorum.* The signs and symptoms of infection are indistinguishable from those that are associated with viral infections of the lung, although chest pain, hemoptysis, and headache may be more frequent. A history of contact with birds, particularly caged birds who are not necessarily ill, should suggest the diagnosis. Treatment with erythromycin, azithromycin, or tetracycline will shorten the duration of the illness (see Sec. 13.2.11).

Q FEVER

Coxiella burnetii, which is a rickettsial organism, causes an acute pneumonitis that is characterized by the infiltration of the peribronchiolar and perivascular spaces with plasma cells and lymphocytes. The disease is endemic in sheep, and it frequently is transmitted to sheep handlers. The clinical features, diagnosis, and treatment are detailed in Sec. 13.3. A recent report of this illness in 18 children under 3 years of age suggested that Q fever may be more common than previously thought.

PNEUMOCYSTIS CARINII PNEUMONIA

Pneumocystis carinii occurs as an asymptomatic infection in most young children. *P. carinii* pneumonia occurs in immunosuppressed infants and children as well as debilitated infants. Originally described as an infection in premature infants occurring sporadically and occasionally in epidemics, it now is primarily diagnosed in children of all ages with either congenital and acquired immune deficiency disorders and in patients receiving immunosuppressive drugs for malignancies or organ transplantation. *P. carinii* pneumonia is the most common pulmonary infection in patients with human immunodeficiency virus (HIV) infection, including infants and young children with perinatally acquired HIV infection.

The first symptom in infants is a low-grade fever, followed by nonproductive cough in the absence of upper respiratory tract symptoms. Vomiting and diarrhea are common. Older children may complain of pain in the anterior part of the chest or substernal region, and the onset in them may be more rapid. Over a period of 1 to 4 weeks, the child develops increasing tachypnea and cyanosis and appears to be acutely ill. Rapidly progressive pneumonia can occur. Auscultatory findings may be surprisingly few, but areas of fine crepitant rales may be present, particularly after coughing. A chest radiograph in the early stages of the disease shows a bilateral perihilar interstitial haziness, progressing to diffuse linear shadows that radiate toward the periphery. In moderately advanced pneumonia, there are generalized, irregular patches of consolidation that are surrounded by areas of increased translucency. Bilateral diffuse consolidation occurs in advanced pneumonia. Patients with AIDS often have atypical radiographic patterns, including unilateral disease, cystic disease, and effusions. Diagnosis and treatment are discussed in Sec. 13.6.5.

FILARIA PNEUMONITIS (TROPICAL EOSINOPHILIA)

Tropical eosinophilia is a common cause of pneumonitis in India and some areas of Central America and Southeast Asia. Most disease occurs in children who are under 10 years of age. The disease is characterized by diffuse, interstitial pulmonary edema and interalveolar infiltration of eosinophils. The onset is insidious, with low-grade fever, hacking dry cough, wheezing, and nocturnal respiratory distress. Rales may be heard at the bases of the lungs. Chest radiographs show diminished translucency with an increase in hilar markings. The eosinophil count is always elevated to at least 2500 cells/mL. Treatment with diethylcarbamazine, 6 mg/kg TID for 14 days, usually is successful (see Sec. 13.6.2).

LEGIONELLA PNEUMOPHILA (LEGIONNAIRES DISEASE)

Legionella pneumophila was first described after an outbreak of rapidly progressive hemorrhagic pneumonia in Philadelphia in 1977.

In infants and children, there is nothing characteristic about the signs and symptoms that are associated with *L. pneumophila*. The disease is less severe in children than in adults. The infection usually is heralded by fever followed by cough and respiratory distress. Gastrointestinal symptoms and diarrhea are common, and neurologic signs, notably ataxia, may occur. *L. pneumophila* is most severe in immunosuppressed children. The diagnosis may be made by isolation of *L. pneumophila* from the airway or blood, specific immunofluorescence, or a rise in antibody titer of at least fourfold. The organism is sensitive to erythromycin, but a 3- to 4-week course may be required. The combination of rifampin and erythromycin is additive and perhaps synergistic, and this should be used in immunosuppressed patients and others who are critically ill.

References

Carlson NC, Kuskie MR, Dobyns EL, et al: Legionellosis in children: an expanding spectrum. Pediatr Infect Dis J 9:133, 1990

Grayston JT: *Chlamydia pneumoniae,* strain TWAR pneumonia. Annu Rev Med 43:317, 1992

Grayston JT: *Chlamydia pneumoniae* (TWAR) infections in children. Pediatr Infect Dis J 13:675, 1994

Harrison HR, English MG, Lee CK, Alexander ER: *Chlamydia trachomatis* infant pneumonitis: comparison with matched controls and other infant pneumonitis. N Engl J Med 298:702, 1978

Hauger SB: Guidelines for the care of children and adolescents with HIV infection: Approach to the pediatric patient with HIV infection and pulmonary symptoms. J Pediatr 119:S25, 1991

Levy H, Simpson SG: Hantavirus pulmonary syndrome. Am Rev Respir Crit Care Med 149:1710, 1994

Martin RE, Bates JH: Atypical pneumonia. Infect Dis Clin North Am 5: 585, 1991

Mok JYQ, Waugn PR, Simpson H: *Mycoplasma pneumoniae* infection: A follow-up study of 50 children with respiratory illness. Arch Dis Child 54:506, 1979

Pui CH, Hughes WT, Evans WE, Crist WM: Prevention of *Pneumocystis carinii* in children with cancer. J Clin Oncol 12:1522, 1994

Richardus JH, Dumas AM, Huisman J, Schaap GJ: Q fever in infancy: a review of 18 cases. Pediatr Infect Dis 4:369, 1985

Sabato AR, Martin AJ, Marmion BP, et al: *Mycoplasma* pneumonias: acute illness, antibiotics, and subsequent pulmonary function. Arch Dis Child 59:1034, 1984

Schonwald S, Gunjaca M, Kolacny-Babic L, et al: Comparison of azithromycin and erythromycin in the treatment of atypical pneumonias. J Antimicrob Chemother 25(Suppl A):123, 1990

Simonds RJ, Oxtoby MJ, Caldwell MB, et al: *Pneumocystis carinii* pneumonia among US children with perinatally acquired HIV infection. JAMA 270:470, 1993

Stagno S, Brasfield DM, Brown MB, et al: Infant pneumonitis associated with cytomegalovirus, *Chlamydia, Pneumocystis,* and *Ureaplasma:* a prospective study. Pediatrics 68:322, 1981

Starke JM: Lung infections in children. Curr Opin Pediatr 5:273, 1993

23.11.5   Aspiration Syndromes

Thomas A. Hazinski

In theory, aspiration syndromes can be divided into two types: The aspiration of oropharyngeal flora or infected secretions leading to *aspiration pneumonia,* and the aspiration of gastric contents leading to *aspiration pneumonitis.* In practice it is often difficult to distinguish between the two conditions. In both cases, the aspiration event may be unwitnessed or accompanied by few if any acute symptoms.

ASPIRATION PNEUMONIA

Patients with normal neuromuscular function, immune function, and airway protective reflexes probably experience frequent episodes of microaspiration of colonized oropharyngeal secretions with no ill effects. However, aspiration pneumonia most often occurs in patients with chronic neuromuscular disorders which cause dysphagia, impaired gastroesophageal motility, poor oral hygiene, diminished gag reflex, and a weak cough. In these patients, aspiration pneumonia may follow an upper respiratory infection and aspiration of infected secretions, which contain not only bacteria but cytokines and pro-inflammatory molecules. The presence of a tracheostomy does not eliminate the possibility of aspiration pneumonia.

The diagnosis of acute aspiration pneumonia should be considered when a patient with impaired neurologic function develops fever, tachypnea, cough, and respiratory distress, especially following a few days of upper respiratory symptoms. Chest radiography may demonstrate a focal infiltrate in independent lung segments; ie, the posterior segments of upper lobes and apical segments of lower lobes.

The treatment of acute aspiration pneumonia should be logically based on the bacteriology of the disorder, but modern studies have not systemically addressed this issue. Older studies emphasized the importance of anaerobic organisms, and penicillin, its derivatives, and clindamycin have been recommended most often. In adults, more recent studies suggest that the bacteriology of aspiration pneumonia more closely resembles that of community-acquired pneumonia in general. In these patients, treatment with a second-generation cephalosporin with or without penicillin may be sufficient. If aspiration pneumonia is suspected in critically ill or chronically hospitalized patients, the risk of gram-negative organisms increases, and more broad-spectrum antibiotic regimens have been suggested (eg, either ciprofloxacin, piperacillin-tazobactam, ceftazadime, or cefipime along with an aminoglycoside or metronidazole).

ASPIRATION PNEUMONITIS

The acute and chronic aspiration of gastric acid or food can cause acute airway and parenchymal inflammation in the absence of bacteria. Aspiration can occur during swallowing or indirectly following episodes of reflux or vomiting. Acute aspiration pneumonitis can occur in patients with chronic neuromuscular disorders, in otherwise normal patients with a depressed level of consciousness (seizures, general anesthesia, drug overdose, etc) or in infants who are force-fed, fed inappropriate foods, or fed by inexperienced individuals. The clinical presentation of acute aspiration pneumonitis varies from a single witnessed severe choking or aspiration episode with the immediate onset of cough, cyanosis, wheezing, and diffuse rales. Respiratory failure and ARDS may also develop. Because the clinical presentation overlaps so much with aspiration pneumonia, the treatment of acutely ill patients usually includes the administration of antibiotics appropriate for aspiration pneumonia.

Chronic microaspiration occurs in patients with chronic neuromuscular disorders. In these patients, the onset of symptoms is much slower, with chronic nonproductive cough, oxyhemoglobin saturation in the low normal range, or wheezing which does not respond completely to inhaled bronchodilator therapy. In these patients, chest radiography demonstrates streaky infiltrates typically in the lower lobes with peribronchial thickening. The evaluation of these patients includes an assessment of their swallowing function, the integrity of their gastroesophageal junction, and gastric emptying capability. Flexible fiberoptic bronchoscopic examination will reveal increased numbers of lipid-laden macrophages in lavage fluid; this finding supports the suspicion of aspiration, but lipid-laden macrophages may be seen in other pulmonary conditions as well. Late complications include bronchiectasis and chronic oxygen dependency.

References

Knauer-Fischer S, Ratjen F: Lipid-laden macrophages in bronchoalveolar lavage fluid as a marker for pulmonary aspiration. Pediatr Pulmonol 27: 419–422, 1999

Marik PE: Aspiration pneumonitis and aspiration pneumonia. New Engl J Med 344:665–671, 2001

Morton RE, Wheatley R, Derby UK: Respiratory tract infections due to direct and reflux aspiration in children with severe neurodisability. Dev Med Child Neur 41:320–334, 1999

Warner MA, Warner ME, Warner DO, Warner LO, Warner EJ: Perioperative pulmonary aspiration in infants and children. Anesthesiology 90: 66–71, 1999

23.12 CHEMICAL PNEUMONITIS

Thomas A. Hazinski

HYDROCARBON PNEUMONITIS

The inhalation or aspiration of aliphatic hydrocarbons into the lungs causes a widespread inflammatory reaction that is characterized by patchy bilateral pulmonary infiltrates, fever, shortness of breath, and hypoxemia (see Sec. 4.3.3). Hydrocarbons are widely present in the vicinity of curious toddlers, although the exact products change with time. Kerosene and furniture polish were frequent causes in the past, but recently gasoline, scented lamp oil, and charcoal lighter fluid have been causative agents. Cardiac and central nervous system dysfunction also have been reported, but these symptoms are probably secondary to hypoxemia and not a result of absorption into the circulation. The aspiration of aromatic hydrocarbons such as benzene and toluene produces similar pulmonary toxicity but also may produce extrapulmonary effects.

Because of their low viscosity, hydrocarbon aspiration is inevitable either during swallowing or after vomiting unless the volume is very small. Respiratory symptoms begin with aspiration; the larger the aspirated volume, the more marked the symptoms. It frequently is written that the onset of pulmonary symptoms may not be evident for 12 to 24 hours, but this "asymptomatic interval" is not well documented.

Treatment mainly is supportive. The induction of emesis or gastric lavage may result in increased aspiration and should be avoided. Children with respiratory symptoms or an abnormal chest radiograph should be observed in a medical facility. If there are no symptoms, and the chest radiograph is normal 3 to 4 hours after the ingestion of simple hydrocarbons, however, the child can be observed at home.

Fever and dyspnea may last for up to 2 weeks in severe disease, but with oxygen, respiratory physiotherapy to help clear secretions, adequate fluid and caloric intake, and antibiotics for secondary bacterial infection, most children will recover completely. After the first week, it is not uncommon for pneumatoceles to develop in areas of extensive consolidation. These cysts rarely, if ever, rupture. Corticosteroid therapy has been recommended, but there is no convincing evidence that it alters the course of disease. Counseling parents on the potential dangers of common household substances must be a regular part of follow-up care. If kept in the house, volatile hydrocarbons should be kept out of the reach of children, preferably in locked cupboards.

SILO-FILLER DISEASE

Acute pneumonitis can develop in patients following exposure to freshly filled silos. The disease is caused by inhaling nitrogen dioxide, which is a dense gas that accumulates just above freshly-cut grain. The intraalveolar septa become edematous and filled with an accumulation of mononuclear cells and fibroblasts. Diffuse alveolar damage with hemorrhagic edema and hyaline membrane formation is characteristic. At the time of exposure, cough and dyspnea occur, followed by several days of apparent improvement. Then comes an abrupt onset of chills, fever, dyspnea, cyanosis, and cough, with rales throughout the lungs. Radiologically, there is diffuse pulmonary infiltration. Corticosteroids may help to prevent progression to severe bronchiolitis obliterans. However, the course may be fulminating, and the mortality rate is as high as 20%. The disease may be prevented by using proper silo ventilation.

PARAQUAT LUNG

Paraquat, which is a dipyridilium compound, is a potent herbicide that, if ingested, is highly toxic in humans. Respiratory failure develops a few days to 2 weeks after ingestion. The mortality rate is very high. Paraquat is corrosive and, if ingested, results in immediate painful lesions of the mouth and esophagus. Renal excretion causes tubular damage with azotemia and hematuria.

Pulmonary symptoms can occur after cutaneous absorption, although the mouth is the usual route. Storing paraquat in spray bottles or other containers that children find attractive has often led to oral ingestion. The basic lung lesion is a proliferative bronchiolitis and alveolitis, with pulmonary hemorrhage causing intraalveolar hyaline membranes and fibrosis. Gas exchange is impaired early, and progression to acute respiratory distress syndrome is common. No effective treatment is known. General supportive measures and forced osmotic diuresis to increase excretion have been recommended. Experimental data in animals suggest that breathing high concentrations of oxygen may increase the pulmonary toxicity.

PNEUMONITIS FROM OTHER CHEMICALS

Many industrial and agricultural chemicals, if inhaled in high concentrations, may cause acute interalveolar edema and mononuclear infiltration, with sudden onset of cough, substernal pain, and cyanosis. Prolonged exposure to lower concentrations of the same agent may cause chronic interstitial pneumonitis, which is characterized by interalveolar granuloma formation similar to that seen in sarcoidosis. Organic compounds such as shellac, seed oil, tobacco juice, gum arabic, and polyvinylpyrrolidone (a substance found in hair spray) and inorganic substances such as beryllium, mercury vapors, and chlorine may cause this reaction. If a child is exposed to these agents and develops respiratory symptoms, treatment

should be guided by information from a regional poison control center or by on-line search of toxicology data bases.

References

Anas N, Namasonthi V, Ginsburg CM: Criteria for hospitalizing children who have ingested products containing hydrocarbons. JAMA 246:840, 1981

Anene O, Castello FU: Myocardial dysfunction after hydrocarbon ingestion. Crit Care Med 22:528, 1994

Bergeson PS, Hales SW, Lustgarten MD, et al: Pneumatoceles following hydrocarbon ingestion. Am J Dis Child 129:49, 1975

Brook MP, McCarren MM, Mueller JA: Pine oil cleaner ingestion. Ann Emerg Med 18:391, 1989

Zwemer FL, Pratt DS, May JJ: Silo filler's disease in New York State. Am Rev Respir Dis 146:650, 1992

23.13 INFLAMMATORY DISEASES OF THE LUNG PARENCHYMA

Cynthia Epstein and Leland Fan

23.13.1   Interstitial Lung Diseases of Childhood

Interstitial lung disease (ILD) in children comprises a large, heterogeneous group of chronic pulmonary conditions characterized by restrictive lung disease and disordered gas exchange. Our knowledge of pediatric ILD is based largely on what has been described in small case series and anecdotal case reports. Although more is known about ILD in adults, the spectrum and distribution of disease as well as the prognosis and response to therapy are somewhat different in children.

CLASSIFICATION

ILD in the pediatric population can be categorized according to known and unknown etiology, as shown in Tables 23-24 and 23-25. The idiopathic forms of ILD can be further classified by histologic criteria. The Liebow classification of interstitial pneumonias was recently updated by Katzenstein and Meyers to include four entities: usual interstitial pneumonitis (UIP), desquamative interstitial pneumonitis (DIP), acute interstitial pneumonitis (AIP), and nonspecific interstitial pneumonitis (NSIP). In the past, the term idiopathic pulmonary fibrosis (IPF) was used interchangeably with

TABLE 23-24

PEDIATRIC INTERSTITIAL LUNG DISEASES OF KNOWN ETIOLOGY

Aspiration syndromes
Chronic infection (viral, bacterial, fungal, parasitic)
  Immunocompetent host
  Immunocompromised host
Bronchopulmonary dysplasia
Hypersensitivity pneumonitis (and other environmental exposures)
Lipid storage diseases

TABLE 23-25

PEDIATRIC INTERSTITIAL LUNG DISEASES OF UNKNOWN ETIOLOGY

Primary pulmonary disorders
  Usual interstitial pneumonitis (UIP)
  Desquamative interstitial pneumonitis (DIP)
  Lymphocytic interstitial pneumonitis (LIP) and related disorders
  Nonspecific interstitial pneumonitis
  Pulmonary hemosiderosis
  Pulmonary infiltrates with eosinophilia
  Bronchiolitis obliterans
  Bronchiolitis obliterans with organizing pneumonia (BOOP)
  Alveolar proteinosis
  Pulmonary vascular disorders (proliferative and congenital)
  Pulmonary lymphatic disorders
  Pulmonary microlithiasis
Systemic disorders with pulmonary involvement
  Connective tissue disease
  Malignancies
  Histiocytosis
  Sarcoidosis
  Neurocutaneous syndromes

ILD, but it should now be restricted to characterize only classical UIP.

The remainder of this section focuses on the description of idiopathic forms of ILD and summarizes the current understanding of ILD with regard to clinical presentation, evaluation, treatment, and outcome.

USUAL INTERSTITIAL PNEUMONITIS UIP is a progressive process with variable distribution of interstitial changes within the lung. The heterogeneity of the lesions results from the recruitment of initially normal lung tissue by an inflammatory and later fibrotic process. Therefore, areas of interstitial fibrosis, inflammation, honeycomb change, and normal lung exist together within the lung tissue. Honeycomb change is a result of lung scarring and remodeling that is irreversible and is not specific to UIP. It is commonly referred to as "end-stage lung."

There have been a number of case reports of children with UIP and related disorders. However, in one study, the diagnosis was established without a lung biopsy in 40 of 65 patients, and others have combined DIP and UIP for their evaluation. Case series that are restricted to patients who have undergone lung biopsy suggest that true UIP in children is extremely rare and carries a poor prognosis as it does in adults.

DESQUAMATIVE INTERSTITIAL PNEUMONITIS In contrast to the heterogeneity seen in UIP, DIP is characterized by a uniform and monotonous histologic process with hyperplasia of alveolar epithelial cells and increased number of macrophages within the air spaces. Fibrosis is not a notable feature of this process, but widening of alveolar septa by connective tissue is seen. In adults, DIP is linked to smoking, and its incidence is decreasing. DIP in childhood is probably a different process because it is not decreasing in incidence and it is not linked to smoking. There is a wide distribution of age of onset for DIP, with a review reporting 15 cases having an age of onset of less than 1 year and 10 cases older than 1 year of age. Familial cases of DIP are reported to carry a very poor prognosis.

ACUTE INTERSTITIAL PNEUMONITIS AIP, also known as Hamman-Rich syndrome, is an acute, severe, and rapidly progressive process with a high fatality rate. It is characterized by an active diffuse interstitial process consisting of proliferating fibroblasts and myofibroblasts within thickened alveolar septa. The appearance of this injury is similar to what is observed in UIP except that the process is diffuse rather than focal. Honeycomb changes are the final result of this progressive process.

NONSPECIFIC INTERSTITIAL PNEUMONITIS NSIP does not represent a single specific disease entity but rather is a designation for a heterogeneous group of interstitial pneumonias that fit specific histologic parameters. The histologic changes in NSIP appear to have occurred over a single time period. This temporal uniformity distinguishes NSIP from UIP. Overall, a nonspecific pattern of inflammation and fibrosis within the alveolar wall is observed, with either inflammation with minimal fibrosis (50%) or a mixture of inflammation and fibrosis (40%) in the majority of cases. However, fibrosis with minimal inflammation is present in about 10% of cases. These changes can be either patchy or diffuse. NSIP has been found to occur in children, although the incidence is unknown. A recent study of ILD in children documented 8 of 25 cases as NSIP by lung biopsy.

LYMPHOCYTIC INTERSTITIAL PNEUMONITIS LIP remains in the differential diagnosis for ILD in childhood, although it is a form of pulmonary lymphoproliferative disease. LIP is characterized by a diffuse infiltrate of mature and immature lymphocytes, plasma cells, and histiocytes in the alveolar septa and pulmonary interstitium. Nodular formation of lymphocytes is commonly seen, occasionally with germinal centers. The blood vessels and airways are not involved in this process, and fibrosis is not a typical feature. However, if there is a significant nodular component, it may distort the pulmonary architecture.

LIP is the most common form of classically described ILD. It most often occurs with underlying conditions, such as autoimmune disease (juvenile rheumatoid arthritis and Sjögren syndrome), and immunodeficiency states (AIDS and congenital immunodeficiency syndromes). However, LIP also exists in idiopathic and familial forms. LIP is a CDC class B disease in HIV-infected patients, indicative of a better prognosis then other AIDS-defining illnesses. It occurs in 25 to 40% of children affected perinatally with HIV and usually presents in the second or third year of life. This differs dramatically from the adult incidence of only 3%.

BRONCHIOLITIS OBLITERANS ORGANIZING PNEUMONIA BOOP is a rare type of pediatric ILD characterized by patchy areas of inflammation and organizing pneumonia with obstruction of airways by intraluminal polyps of fibrous tissue. Extensive fibrosis or honeycombing is not a notable feature of BOOP. It can be idiopathic, AIDS-related, or a complication of chemotherapeutic regimens or bone marrow transplantation with graft-versus-host disease.

CLINICAL PRESENTATION

A thorough history is crucial to the evaluation of a patient with suspected ILD. There are specific topics in the history that may help establish the diagnosis or focus the diagnostic evaluation. A careful feeding history may elicit a potential cause for aspiration. A detailed environmental history may uncover potential exposures such as birds or molds. Previous or frequent respiratory infections or other illnesses are important clues to underlying immunodeficiency states such as AIDS, congenital immunodeficiency syndromes, or Wegener granulomatosis. A systemic process, such as collagen vascular disorders or the vasculitis syndromes, may be suspected with a history of joint disease, rash, or renal involvement. A family history of a similar disorder may be found in DIP or LIP. The onset of symptoms for ILD is usually insidious, with many patients having symptoms for years before their diagnosis.

The typical symptoms of ILD include tachypnea, cough, dyspnea, exercise intolerance, and frequent respiratory infections. Although wheezing is elicited from history in 50% of patients, it is found on physical exam in only 20% of patients. Some patients have been misdiagnosed as having asthma and are treated with bronchodilators, but without appreciable benefit. A factor that can be useful to differentiate between these two conditions is that symptoms of ILD tend to be more continuous compared with the episodic symptoms of asthma.

On physical exam, the most common findings include retractions, tachypnea, and basilar crackles. Evidence of growth failure, cyanosis, digital clubbing, and increased second heart sound are present in the more severe cases. Salivary gland enlargement and generalized lymphadenopathy are commonly detected in patients with LIP.

LABORATORY DIAGNOSTIC EVALUATION

Because the differential diagnosis for ILD is large, it is essential to approach the evaluation of pediatric patients with ILD in a systematic fashion. Diagnostic studies can be differentiated into those used to (1) assess extent and severity of disease, (2) identify disorders that predispose to ILD, and (3) identify the primary ILD (see Tables 23-24 and 23-25). A diagnostic process that begins with a complete history and physical exam, continues with noninvasive tests, and finally involves invasive tests has been demonstrated to be beneficial (Table 23-26). This approach was used in 51 patients with ILD and provided a specific diagnosis in 35 patients, with 9 not requiring a lung biopsy for diagnosis.

Although most laboratory tests are not helpful in identifying specific etiologies in ILD, they can provide supportive evidence for

TABLE 23-26
DIAGNOSTIC STUDIES

To assess extent and severity of disease
   Chest films, high-resolution computed tomography
   Pulmonary function studies: spirometry, pulse oximetry and arterial
      blood gases (resting, sleeping, and with exercise), diffusion, pressure-
      volume curve, infant studies
   Electrocardiogram, echocardiogram
To identify primary disorders that predispose to ILD
   HIV ELISA
   Immune studies: immunoglobulins including IgE, skin tests for delayed
      hypersensitivity, response to immunizations, T and B subsets, com-
      plement, others as indicated
   Barium swallow, pH probe
To identify primary ILD
   Antinuclear antibody
   Angiotensin converting enzyme
   Antineutrophil cytoplasmic antibody
   Anti-glomerular basement membrane antibody
   Hypersensitivity screen
   Infectious disease evaluation: cultures, titers, skin tests
   Cardiac catheterization (in selected cases)
   Bronchoalveolar lavage and transbronchial biopsy
   Transthoracic biopsy

ILD = interstitial lung disease.

a disorder. Microcytic anemia unresponsive to iron may indicate pulmonary hemosiderosis. Other tests described in Table 23-26 are utilized to facilitate diagnosis in particular collagen vascular disorders, sarcoidosis, congenital immunodeficiencies, and AIDS.

PULMONARY FUNCTION TESTING   Pulmonary function testing in ILD demonstrates a pattern of restrictive lung disease with reduced forced vital capacity (FVC) and forced vital capacity in one second (FEV_1) as well as a normal FEV_1/FVC ratio. Although total lung capacity (TLC) may be reduced, functional residual capacity and residual volume (RV) are variable. FVC/TLC and RV/TLC ratios are usually elevated, which may indicate either a relative decrease in TLC or true hyperinflation.

Pulse oximetry may indicate hypoxemia at rest or exercise and has been shown to correlate with severity of illness and may have prognostic significance. Chronic hypoxia can lead to pulmonary hypertension, which is often indicative of a poor prognosis.

RADIOLOGIC EVALUATION   A chest radiograph (CXR) is abnormal most often in pediatric ILD. There are particular terms used to describe the patterns seen on plain films that are not disease specific, such as reticular, nodular, ground glass, and honeycombing. Although a CXR can be useful to detect abnormalities, high-resolution computed tomography (HRCT) scans provide more precise information about the extent and distribution of the parenchymal disease. With this enhanced detail, favorable biopsy sites can be selected. In a recent study of 20 children with biopsy-proven ILD, the correct histologic diagnosis was accurately predicted from HRCT findings in 56% of the cases.

BRONCHOALVEOLAR LAVAGE   The analysis of bronchoalveolar lavage (BAL) fluid has been used to diagnose pulmonary disorders and is especially useful for diagnosis of infection in an immunocompromised host. The diagnostic yield of BAL for a specific infectious agent in eight studies of immunocompromised children without HIV was 47%. In five studies of children with AIDS the yield improved to 77%. BAL is also useful in immunocompetent children with suspected ILD. A prospective study of 29 patients with ILD revealed that BAL was diagnostic for the primary disorder in 5 patients, narrowed the differential diagnosis in 15 patients, and uncovered a secondary disorder in 8 patients.

In addition to infection, other disorders that can be diagnosed with BAL include aspiration, pulmonary hemorrhage, alveolar proteinosis, lysosomal storage diseases, and histiocytosis. The diagnosis of aspiration by lipid-laden macrophages in BAL is a sensitive but not specific test. A novel diagnostic method utilizing immunohistochemistry to detect specific milk proteins in a murine model of milk aspiration shows promise as a more specific test.

LUNG BIOPSY   Lung biopsy remains the gold standard for the diagnosis of pediatric ILD. Transbronchial lung biopsy has limited use in pediatric ILD, especially in young children, where adequate and representative tissue samples are difficult or impossible to obtain. Either open lung biopsy (OLB) or video-assisted thoracoscopy (VAT) is the preferred method to obtain lung tissue for diagnosis. VAT was shown to have less morbidity with respect to duration of surgery, chest tube, and hospitalization while demonstrating a similar diagnostic yield as OLB. Thus, VAT is becoming the method of choice for lung biopsy in children. Whatever method is used, the lung biopsy specimen must be processed in a consistent manner and should be analyzed by an experienced pediatric pathologist. However, even a properly obtained and processed biopsy does not guarantee a diagnosis. In a prospective study of 30 children with a lung biopsy for suspected ILD, a specific diagnosis was made in 56% of cases. The cause for this low yield was largely an extremely low yield in children less than 2 years of age.

TREATMENT

The treatment for patients with pediatric ILD involves both supportive care and pharmacologic therapy. It is very important to assure adequate nutrition, aggressive therapy of intercurrent infections, avoidance of tobacco smoke and other inhaled irritants including causative environmental agents, oxygen therapy for chronic hypoxia, selective use of bronchodilators, and an annual influenza vaccine. A carefully supervised exercise and fitness program can be beneficial as long as the patients are adequately oxygenated during exercise.

The pharmacologic therapy of choice for pediatric ILD remains corticosteroids, based on the theory that suppression of ongoing inflammation and fibrosis is beneficial. Unfortunately, because of the rarity of these conditions, there are no controlled clinical trials to provide conclusive evidence to substantiate this assumption. However, experience gained from case reports and retrospective studies have demonstrated that treatment with steroids leads to clinical improvement in 40% of the children with ILD. An alternative to treatment with daily oral steroids is pulse intravenous steroid therapy, given in very high doses (30 mg/kg/d of methylprednisolone for 3 days each month). This therapy may be equally effective and cause fewer systemic side effects. Other treatment regimens include immunosuppressive agents such as hydoxychloroquine, azathioprine, cyclophosphamide, methotrexate, and cyclosporine as well as intravenous immunoglobulin. Of these alternative methods, hydroxychloroquine is used most frequently and has been found to be effective in a number of case reports for the treatment of LIP, DIP, and pulmonary hemosiderosis, with a steroid-sparing effect. The recommended dose for therapy for children with ILD is 10 mg/kg/d. The ultimate treatment option for pediatric ILD is lung transplantation, which is becoming more common and carries a comparable survival rate to other conditions requiring transplantation.

OUTCOME/PROGNOSIS

The prognosis for children with ILD remains variable, although the overall mortality rate is high. A study of children with DIP revealed a 50% mortality rate overall, with survival of only 1 out of 10 patients with a positive family history for DIP. Fan and colleagues reviewed the outcome of 99 children with ILD over a 15-year period. A severity-of-illness score based on the need for supplemental oxygen and the presence of pulmonary hypertension was predictive of a negative outcome, with a high score associated with a higher probability of decreased survival.

References

Andiman WA, Shearer WT: Lymphoid interstitial pneumonitis. In: Pizzo PA, Wilfert CM, eds: Pediatric AIDS: The Challenge of HIV Infection in Infants, Children, and Adolescents, 3rd ed. Baltimore, Lippincott Williams & Wilkins, 1999:323–334

Avital A, Godfrey S, Maayan CH, et al: Chloroquine treatment of interstitial lung disease in children. Pediatr Pulmonol 18:356–360, 1994

Balasubramanyan N, Murphy A, O'Sullivan J, et al: Familial interstitial lung disease in children: response to chloroquine treatment in one sibling with desquamative interstitial pneumonitis. Pediatr Pulmonol 23:55–61, 1997

Battistini E, Dini G, Savioli C, et al: Bronchiolitis obliterans organizing pneumonia in three children with acute leukemia treated with cytosine arabinoside and anthracyclines. Eur Respir J 10:1187–1190, 1997

Bridges ND, Mallory GB, Huddleston CB, et al: Lung transplantation in infancy and early childhood. J Heart Lung Transplant 15:895–902, 1996

Buchino J, Keenen WJ, Alegren JJ, et al: Familial desquamative interstitial pneumonitis occurring in infants. Am J Med Genet [Suppl]3:283–291, 1987

Bush A, Sheppard MN, Warner JO: Chloroquine in idiopathic pulmonary hemosiderosis. Arch Dis Child 67:625–627, 1992

Campos JMS, Simonetti JP: Treatment of lymphoid interstitial pneumonia with chloroquine. J Pediatr 122(3):503, 1993

Church JA, Isaacs H, Saxon A, et al: Lymphoid interstitial pneumonitis and hypogammaglobulinemia in children. Am Rev Respir Dis 124:491–496, 1981

Colombo JL, Halberg JK: Recurrent aspiration in children: lipid laden alveolar macrophage quantitation. Pediatr Pulmonol 3:86–89, 1987

Desmarquest P, Tamalet A, Fauroux B, et al: Chronic interstitial lung disease in children: response to high-dose intravenous methylprednisolone pulses. Pediatr Pulmonol 26:332–338, 1998

Elidemir O, Fan LL, Colasurdo GN: A novel diagnostic method for pulmonary aspiration in a murine model: immunohistochemical staining of milk proteins in alveolar macrophages. Am J Respir Crit Care Med 161:622–626, 2000

Fan LL: Pediatric interstitial lung disease. In: Schwarz MI, King TE, eds: Interstitial Lung Disease. Hamilton, BC, Decker, 1998:103–118

Fan LL, Kozinetz CA: Factors influencing survival in children with chronic interstitial lung disease. Am J Respir Crit Care Med 156:939–942, 1997

Fan LL, Kozinetz CA, Deterding RR, et al: Evaluation of a diagnostic approach to pediatric interstitial lung disease. Pediatrics 101(1):82–85, 1998

Fan LL, Kozinetz CA, Wojczak HA, et al: Diagnostic value of transbronchial, thoracoscopic, and open lung biopsy in immunocompetent children with chronic interstitial lung disease. J Pediatr 131:565–569, 1997

Fan LL, Langston C: Interstitial lung disease. In: Chernick V, Boat TF, eds: Kendig's Disorders of the Respiratory Tract in Children, 6th ed. Philadelphia, WB Saunders, 1998:607–616

Fan LL, Lum Lung MC, Wagener JS: The diagnostic value of brochoalveolar lavage in immunocompetent children with chronic diffuse pulmonary infiltrates. Pediatr Pulmonol 23:8–13, 1997

Fan LL, Mullen ALN, Brugman JM, et al: Clinical spectrum of chronic interstitial lung disease in children. J Pediatr 121:867–872, 1992

Farrell PM, Gilbert EF, Zimmerman JJ, et al: Familial lung disease associated with proliferation and desquamation of type II pneumocytes. Am J Dis Child 140:262–266, 1986

Hepburn B: Interstitial lung disease in childhood rheumatic disorders. In: Laraya-Cuasay LR, Hughes WT, eds: Interstitial Lung Disease in Children, vol III. Boca Raton, CRC Press, 1988:114–115

Inove T, Toyoshima K, Kikui M: Idiopathic bronchiolitis obliterans organizing pneumonia in childhood. Pediatr Pulmonol 22:67–72, 1996

Katzenstein AA, Fiorelli RF: Nonspecific interstitial pneumonitis/fibrosis. Am J Surg Pathol 28(2):136–147, 1994

Katzenstein AA, Myers JL: Idiopathic pulmonary fibrosis. Am J Respir Crit Care Med 157:1301–1315, 1998

Kleinau I, Perez-Carto A, Schmid HJ, et al: Bronchiolitis obliterans, organizing pneumonia, and chronic graft-versus-host disease in a child after allogeneic bone marrow transplantation. Bone Marrow Transplant 19(8):841–844, 1997

Kurland G, Noyes BE, Jaffe R, et al: Bronchoalveolar lavage and transbronchial biopsy in children following heart-lung and lung transplantation. Chest 104(4):1043–1048, 1993

Lamberts SW, Bruining HA, DeJong FH: Corticosteroid therapy in severe illness. N Engl J Med 337:1285–1292, 1997

Leahy F, Pasterkamp H, Tal A: Desquamative interstitial pneumonia responsive to chloroquine. Clin Pediatr 24(4):230–232, 1984

Liebow AA: Definition and clarification of interstitial pneumonias in human pathology. Prog Respir Res 8:1–33, 1975

Lovell D, Lindsley C, Langston C: Lymphoid interstitial pneumonia in juvenile rheumatoid arthritis. J Pediatr 105(6):947–950, 1984

Lynch DA, Hay T, Newell JD, et al: Pediatric diffuse lung disease: diagnosis and classification using high-resolution CT. Am J Roentgenol 173:713–718, 1999

Myers JL: NSIP, UIP and the ABC's of idiopathic interstitial pneumonias. Eur Respir J 12:1003–1004, 1998

Nicholson AG, Kem H, Corrin B, et al: The value of classifying interstitial pneumonias in childhood according to defined histological parameters. Histopathology 33:203–211, 1998

Noyes BE, Kurland G, Orenstein DM: Lung and heart-lung transplantation in children. Pediatr Pulmonol 23:39–48, 1997

Rogers BB, Browning I, Rosenblatt H, et al: A familial lymphoproliferative disorder presenting with primary pulmonary manifestations. Am Rev Respir Dis 145:203–208, 1992

Schneider RF: Lymphocytic interstitial pneumonitis and nonspecific interstitial pneumonitis. Clin Chest Med 17(4):763–766, 1996

Sharief N, Crawford OF, Dinwiddie R: Fibrosing alveolitis and desquamative interstitial pneumonitis. Pediatr Pulmonol 17:359–365, 1994

Springer C, Maayan C, Katzir Z, et al: Chloroquine treatment in desquamative interstitial pneumonia. Arch Dis Child 62:76–77, 1987

Waters KA, Bale P, Isaacs D, et al: Successful chloroquine therapy in a child with lymphoid interstitial pneumonitis. J Pediatr 119(6):989–991, 1991

Zahran J, Herold B, Abrahams C, et al: Bronchiolitis obliterans organizing pneumonia in a child with acquired immunodeficiency syndrome. Pediatr Infect Dis J 15:448–451, 1996

Zapetal A, Houstek M, Samarek M, Copora M, Paul T: Lung function in children and adolescents with idiopathic interstitial pulmonary fibrosis. Pediatr Pulmonol 1(3):154–167, 1985

23.13.2 Allergic Bronchopulmonary Aspergillosis

The fungi *Aspergillus fumigatus, bipolaris,* and *currulasia* have been isolated from the sputum of immunocompetent persons, the lungs of persons with other primary pulmonary diseases, and the lungs of patients with invasive pulmonary aspergillosis. In 1952, Hinson and colleagues isolated *Aspergillus* from the sputum or intrabronchial mucus of eight adults with wheezing and proximal bronchiectasis; three had chronic bronchial asthma. Since that initial report of bronchopulmonary aspergillosis, many examples have been reported, and in 1970, the first well-documented pediatric patient was described. Allergic bronchopulmonary aspergillosis (ABPA) occurs predominantly in patients with asthma and cystic fibrosis.

Bronchopulmonary aspergillosis is a chronic pulmonary disease whose clinical course is characterized by recurrent exacerbations of wheezing and respiratory distress that are separated by symptom-free intervals of variable duration. Although the diagnosis has been confirmed in children without cystic fibrosis or asthma, these patients typically have asthma of variable severity. Wheezing episodes are accompanied by productive cough, dyspnea, and low-grade fever. Chest pain and hemoptysis may be present if central bronchial involvement is extensive. Sputum examination or culture reveals *A. fumigatus* organisms or other *Aspergillus* species, and the patient may expectorate "brown stones" (ie, masses of *Aspergillus* hyphae). Patchy peribronchial pulmonary infiltrates are seen on the chest radiograph, and if advanced disease is present, proximal bronchial walls are thickened, and the airways are dilated. Pulmonary function tests indicate large airway obstruction. The most distinctive laboratory abnormality is a marked elevation of serum IgE that persists for several months after an acute exacerbation. Precipitating IgG and IgE antibodies to *Aspergillus* antigens are present in serum and are rarely present in patients with asthma. This latter finding helps to separate asthmatic patients with high IgE levels from patients with ABPA. Intradermal skin testing with *Aspergillus* antigens demonstrates positive immediate and late reactions. Recent systemic corticosteroid therapy may suppress the skin test and IgE responses.

Allergic bronchopulmonary aspergillosis is characterized histologically by bronchocentric granulomatosis, mucoid impaction of bronchi, and eosinophilic infiltration. *Aspergillus* organisms are confined to bronchial surfaces or mucous plugs, which differentiates this disease from invasive aspergillosis.

The most serious complication of ABPA is progressive saccular bronchiectasis, which usually begins centrally. Central bronchiectasis may be diagnosed by CT or bronchoscopy, but it also may be discovered at thoracotomy, as the initial presentation suggests a focal disease, foreign body, lung abscess, lymphoid malignancy, or lung metastasis.

The pathogenesis of bronchopulmonary aspergillosis is not understood. *Aspergillus* spores are probably inhaled and grow in endobronchial fluid as hyphae. Most patients have no history of unusually intense or prolonged exposure to molds. Although the disease has been termed *allergic bronchopulmonary aspergillosis,* most of the circulating IgE in these patients is not specific for any known *Aspergillus* antigen, and other signs of atopy may be absent. All other tests of humoral and cell-mediated immunity are normal. Parenteral or inhaled antifungal therapy does not eradicate the fungus or improve symptoms. Recently, fungi other than *Aspergillus* have been reported to cause an allergic bronchopulmonary aspergillosis-like illness.

There is no specific therapy, but treatment goals are the control of asthmatic symptoms, if present, and prevention of recurrent episodes that can lead to progressive bronchiectasis and pulmonary fibrosis. Asthmatic symptoms usually are easily controlled with combined bronchodilator and anti-inflammatory therapy. Serial immunoglobulin E determinations may be helpful in differentiating acute exacerbations of this disease from either acute asthma or pneumonia because the clinical and radiographic signs are similar. In some patients, a rise in the IgE level occurs immediately before or during an exacerbation of bronchopulmonary aspergillosis, whereas a stable or falling IgE level suggests other causes. Symptomatic or radiographic recurrences are treated with corticosteroids daily for 2 to 4 weeks; some children have required alternate-day corticosteroid therapy for months. The serum IgE level can be used in conjunction with clinical status to guide the dose and duration of steroid therapy. This regimen is associated with a decrease in the number and severity of recurrences. If bronchiectasis is present, bronchodilator therapy, prophylactic antibiotics, and daily chest physiotherapy may be indicated.

The prognosis in children is not clear. The subsequent clinical course cannot be predicted by the severity of asthma or of the bronchial involvement that is present at diagnosis. Either interstitial fibrosis or bronchiolitis obliterans may occur. Case clustering of bronchopulmonary aspergillosis has been reported from cystic fibrosis treatment centers; the clinical and therapeutic implications of this interaction are unknown.

Recent reports indicate that up to 10% of patients with cystic fibrosis have ABPA or a clinical syndrome resembling it.

References

Cockrill BA, Hales CA: Allergic bronchopulmonary aspergillosis. Annu Rev Med 50:303–316, 1999

Greenberger PA: Immunologic aspects of lung diseases and cystic fibrosis. JAMA 278:1924–1930, 1997

Imbeau SA, Cohen M, Reed CE: Allergic bronchopulmonary aspergillosis in infants. Am J Dis Child 131:1127, 1977

Kaltzenstein AL, Leibow AA, Friedman PJ: Bronchocentric granulomatosis, mucoid impaction and hypersensitivity reaction to fungi. Am Rev Respir Dis 111:497, 1975

Knutsen AP, Slavin RG: Allergic bronchopulmonary aspergillosis in patients with cystic fibrosis. Semin Respir Infect 7:179, 1992

Lake FR, Froudist JH, McAleer R, et al: Allergic bronchopulmonary aspergillosis caused by *Bipolaris* and *Curvularia*. Aust NZ J Med 21:871, 1991

Slavin RG, Bedrossian CW, Hutcheson PS, et al: A pathologic study of allergic bronchopulmonary aspergillosis. J Allergy Clin Immunol 81: 718, 1988

23.13.3   Hypersensitivity Pneumonitis

In this past decade, many previously "idiopathic" chronic interstitial lung diseases have been linked to a patient's exposure to specific organic materials. Resourceful detective work often reveals unusual environmental sources of these antigens. Bird fancier's lung, farmer's lung, and humidifier/forced-air system lung probably are the most common alveolar hypersensitivity lung diseases described in children, although the list is continually increasing (Table 23-27). In addition, chemotherapeutic agents such as methotrexate, bleomycin, chlorambucil, and cyclophosphamide have been linked to the development of hypersensitivity pneumonitis.

The clinical features of hypersensitivity pneumonitis include nonproductive cough, dyspnea, exercise intolerance, clear lung sounds or crackles, diffuse pulmonary infiltrates, digital clubbing, and pulmonary function tests that are consistent with restrictive lung disease. The diffusing capacity for carbon monoxide is reduced. High-resolution CT often reveals extensive interstitial disease when chest radiography indicates only scant infiltrates. Hypoxemia may be present at rest or may occur during exercise or travel to high altitude. Obstructive pulmonary disease and wheezing usually are not present, and expiratory flow rates (corrected for vital capacity) often exceed predicted values. Histologically, mononuclear, proliferative, and granulomatous changes are present in the interstitium, along with variable amounts of interstitial fibrosis; vasculitis and bronchiolar inflammation usually are absent.

Exposure to putative antigens may elicit the acute onset of symptoms. Equally important, symptoms may disappear during some seasons or with lengthy absences from the offending agent or environment; either of these should raise the suspicion that an environmental factor may be of etiologic importance. The clinical course is characterized by slowly progressive pulmonary disability. Occasionally, the associated constitutional symptoms may be so extensive that the clinical presentation resembles anorexia nervosa, inflammatory bowel disease, or cystic fibrosis.

The pathogenesis of hypersensitivity pneumonitis is unknown. Lung biopsy and analysis of lavage fluid that is obtained after antigen challenge show evidence of inflammation in the absence of the abnormalities of commonly performed immunologic tests of

TABLE 23-27

POSSIBLE ETIOLOGIC AGENTS IN HYPERSENSITIVITY PNEUMONITIS

MAJOR ANTIGENS	EXPOSURE OR SOURCE	DISEASE
Thermophilic bacteria		
Micropolyspora faeni	Moldy hay	Farmer's lung
Thermoactinomyces vulgaris	Moldy grain	Grain handler's lung
M. faeni, T. vulgaris	Mushroom compost	Mushroom worker's lung
T. sacchari	Moldy sugar cane (bagasse)	Bagassosis
T. vulgaris, T. candidus, M. faeni	Heated water reservoirs	Humidifier or air conditioner lung
Other bacteria		
Bacillus subtilis	Water	Detergent worker's lung
B. sereus	Water reservoir	Humidifier lung
True fungi		
Cryptostroma corticale	Moldy bark	Maple bark stripper's lung
Aspergillus clavatus	Moldy malt, barley	Malt worker's lung
Aureobasidium pullulans and *Graphium* sp.	Moldy redwood dust	Sequoiosis
Mucor stolonifer	Moldy paprika pods	Paprika splitter's lung
Sitophilus granarius	Infested wheat flour	Wheat weevil's disease
Penicillium caseii	Cheese mold	Cheese worker's lung
P. frequentans	Moldy cork dust	Suberosis
Aspergillus spores	Water reservoir	Aspergillosis
Animal proteins		
Avian proteins (serum and excreta)	Pigeons, parakeets	Bird breeder's lung
Chicken feathers (serum)	Chickens	Chicken handler's lung
Turkey feathers (serum)	Turkeys	Turkey handler's lung
Duck feathers	Ducks	Duck fever
Rat urine (serum)	Rats	Rodent handler's disease
Porcine and bovine pituitary protein	Pituitary snuff	Pituitary snuff-taker's lung
Amoeba		
Acanthamoeba	Water	Humidifier lung
Bacterial products		
Endotoxin (?)	Cotton brac	Byssinosis
Streptomyces verticillus glycopeptides	Bleomycin	Bleomycin hypersensitivity lung

serum or skin. This indicates that the lung can respond to antigen stimulation in a specific and isolated fashion. In animal models, the lesions of hypersensitivity pneumonitis can be induced by inhaled antigens only if there is preexisting lung inflammation. Clinically, parents often are able to associate the onset of the symptoms of hypersensitivity pneumonitis with a family or classroom outbreak of a viral respiratory infection. Recent reports have emphasized the importance of genetic and acquired factors that appear to alter the susceptibility of the lung to this type of injury.

The diagnosis of hypersensitivity pneumonitis should be considered in a patient with interstitial lung disease and a history of prolonged or recurrent exposure to inhaled organic dusts. Questions concerning exposure to birds and other sources of antigen must be specific. Some patients who ultimately prove to have bird fancier's lung initially deny any exposure to pets or birds because they regard these animals as intimate family members, as belonging to other people in the home, or as a home-based business or hobby.

The diagnosis is supported by demonstrating circulating antibody to antigens that are prepared from the suspected source, although these antibodies may be present in asymptomatic persons. For example, 40% of pigeon breeders have precipitins to pigeon serum, but fewer than 5% of this group have demonstrable pulmonary disease. Total serum IgG and IgA levels also may be elevated in these patients. Intradermal injections or inhalation of suspected antigens often yields nonspecific results. In severely affected patients, lung biopsy should be performed before therapy is initiated if an unusual pulmonary infection is suspected but cannot be ruled out by serologic testing or bronchoalveolar lavage. Care must be taken to obtain representative tissue samples for histologic and microbiological examination.

Avoidance of the offending antigen is the most important treatment. If extensive pulmonary disease is present with oxygen desaturation, either at rest or during exercise, the response to glucocorticoid administration can be dramatic, and a 3- to 6-month course of treatment should be tried. Glucocorticoids can be used to abort acute attacks, but they should not replace removal of the antigen from the patient's environment. Antihistamines and bronchodilators usually have no effect. Pulmonary function tests, including oximetry, should be used to objectively assess the effects of steroid therapy.

Prognosis usually is good if antigen avoidance and a short course of steroids are begun. If extensive pulmonary fibrosis is present in multiple biopsy samples, a poor response to steroid therapy may be expected, and progressive respiratory insufficiency may occur. In these individuals, other immunosuppressive drugs such as azathioprine or chloroquine have been used. It probably is best to recommend that children permanently avoid the antigen source. However, long-term follow-up of adults with farmer's lung indicates that some patients can return to farming with no further deterioration in pulmonary function.

References

Braun SR, doPico GA, Tsiatis A, et al: Farmer's lung disease: long-term clinical and physiologic outcome. Am Rev Respir Dis 119:1985, 1979

Cunningham AS, Fink JN, Schlueter DP: Childhood hypersensitivity pneumonitis due to dove antigens. Pediatrics 58:436, 1976

Reynolds HY: Hypersensitivity pneumonitis. Clin Chest Med 3:503, 1982

Roberts RC, Moore VL: Immunopathogenesis of hypersensitivity pneumonitis. Am Rev Respir Dis 116:1075, 1977

Stiehm ER, Reed CE, Tooley WH: Pigeon breeder's lung in children. Pediatrics 39:904, 1967

23.13.4   Sarcoidosis

Sarcoidosis is a rare granulomatous disease of unknown cause that is characterized by involvement of many organs, including the lung, joints, lymph nodes, skin, eyes, liver, spleen, muscle, and brain. The multisystem nature of this disease along with its unpredictable course, pathologic appearance of involved tissue, and analysis of lung lavage fluid all strongly indicate an immunologically mediated disorder. Recent data from bronchoalveolar lavage analyses suggest that activated T lymphocytes play an important role in the pathogenesis of this disease.

The incidence of sarcoidosis in children is difficult to ascertain. Cases seem to cluster in discrete regions of the United States. In countries that have comprehensive health screening with chest radiography (eg, Sweden and Japan), the incidence is close to 1 in 5000, but most of these patients are asymptomatic. The majority of affected patients are adults in their fourth decade of life. Although the diagnosis has been made in infants, the usual age at presentation of symptomatic sarcoidosis in pediatric patients is in the second decade. Boys and girls are equally susceptible, but black and Hispanic children seem to have a two- to 10-fold risk relative to whites. The etiology of sarcoidosis is unknown, but case clustering suggests that an infectious or toxic agent may be responsible.

CLINICAL PRESENTATION

Children and young adults most often present with symptoms of fatigue and weight loss. Cough and dyspnea usually indicate pulmonary involvement, but even extensive pulmonary involvement may be clinically undetectable. When hilar adenopathy is present, it is usually bilateral and somewhat symmetric, in contrast to most other granulomatous pulmonary diseases. Laryngeal involvement may cause hoarseness, dyspnea, and dysphagia. Cardiac involvement may be present initially and cause an arrhythmia or dyspnea with congestive heart failure. Bone and joint pain, parotid gland swelling, visual symptoms (eg, eye pain, blurry vision, ocular swelling), headache, and unexplained fevers may be present. The most frequent physical finding is generalized lymph node enlargement. Lymph nodes are firm, nontender, and movable. A skin rash resembling erythema nodosum may be present. Joint effusions and hepatosplenomegaly also are observed.

Laboratory abnormalities are nonspecific and include hyperproteinemia with a low albumin : globulin ratio, elevated erythrocyte sedimentation rate, eosinophilia, hypercalciuria, and, rarely, hypercalcemia. The serum concentration of angiotensin-converting enzyme may be elevated. Chest radiography may be the first test that suggests this diagnosis. Radiographic staging of pulmonary sarcoidosis has been described, although its prognostic value is uncertain. Between 40 and 60% of symptomatic children will have hilar adenopathy alone or in combination with parenchymal infiltrates. Chest tomography may reveal hilar adenopathy that cannot be demonstrated by plain-film radiography. Static and dynamic tests of pulmonary function usually reveal restrictive lung disease, although hilar lymph node enlargement, bronchial compression, or bronchiectasis may cause obstructive ventilatory defects.

DIAGNOSIS

The diagnosis of sarcoidosis should be considered when a patient presents with multisystem complaints, even when respiratory complaints are absent. Evidence of pulmonary disease that is associated with rash, uveitis, or arthritis strongly suggests the diagnosis. The diagnosis can be more securely established by histologic evidence of noncaseating granulomas in an organ or tissue. When pulmonary disease is prominent, open-lung or transbronchial biopsy may be performed. Bronchoalveolar lavage reveals an abnormally high percentage of lymphocytes (especially T lymphocytes) in lavage fluid relative to blood, even when lung disease is minimal or absent.

Biopsy of extrathoracic tissue also can support or suggest the diagnosis in a patient who is being evaluated for some other disease. Granulomas have been identified in lymph node, skin, conjunctiva, salivary gland, liver, spleen, epiglottis, and epididymis. Recently, scintigraphic scanning of the lung after infusion of gallium-67 has been shown to identify areas of active thoracic and extrathoracic involvement.

The differential diagnosis includes malignancy, connective tissue disorders, hepatitis, and opportunistic pulmonary infections.

PROGNOSIS AND TREATMENT

In some children, sarcoidosis behaves as a subacute infectious disease, with gradual improvement in a few months. Approximately 30 to 40% remain symptomatic, although radiographic evidence of lung injury may persist for many years, even if the symptoms disappear. Some patients will develop progressive cystic emphysema or bronchiectasis. Severe restrictive pulmonary disease results in exercise-induced hypoxemia. Bronchial hyperactivity may be present and may respond to bronchodilator therapy. In patients with multisystem involvement, systemic corticosteroid therapy usually is tried. Controlled trials in adults suggest that steroids are of little benefit in the management of chronic lung disease, but beneficial responses to acute therapy have been observed. Increases in angiotensin-converting enzyme levels and changes in the gallium lung scan may accompany or predict exacerbations. As with any chronic lung disease, the hazards of smoking and heavy dust or inhalant exposure should be avoided. Periodic ophthalmologic examinations can identify eye disease that appears to respond to corticosteroid therapy.

References

Hunninghake GW, Garrett KC, Richerson GH, et al: Pathogenesis of the granulomatous lung diseases. Am Rev Respir Dis 130:476, 1984

Pattishall EN, Strope GL, Spinola SM, Denny FW: Childhood sarcoidosis. J Pediatr 108:169, 1986

Poe RH, Levy PC: Diagnosis and treatment of sarcoidosis. Compr Ther 19:209, 1993

Valeyre D, Saumon G, Bladier D, et al: The relationships between noninvasive explorations in pulmonary sarcoidosis of recent origin, as shown in bronchoalveolar lavage, serum, and pulmonary function tests. Am Rev Respir Dis 126:41, 1982

23.14 α_1-ANTITRYPSIN DEFICIENCY (α_1-PROTEASE INHIBITOR DEFICIENCY)

Thomas A. Hazinski

A genetic deficiency of plasma glycoprotein, called α_1-*antitrypsin* or α_1-*protease inhibitor* (α_1-PI), was described over 25 years ago in adults with cirrhosis, pulmonary emphysema, or both. α_1-PI is pre-dominantly produced in the liver and normally accounts for approximately 10% of the total protein in plasma. The function of α_1-PI is to inhibit serine proteases such as elastase, which are released from activated neutrophils and macrophages. If these proteases are unopposed by a sufficient amount of α_1-PI, lung tissue is destroyed, and emphysema will occur. Protease-induced lung injury also may occur if α_1-PI is present but inactivated by tobacco smoke, high oxygen concentrations, and gram-negative bacteria.

α-PI deficiency is inherited as an autosomal recessive condition. Its incidence is approximately 1 in 4000 births, and it occurs almost exclusively in whites, especially those of northern European descent. Over 75 molecular variants of α_1-PI have been identified, but the majority do not result in a major reduction of serum α_1-PI levels. Clinical manifestations of α_1-PI deficiency occur predominantly in persons who are homozygous for the PI Z variant and have α_1-PI levels less than 11 μmol/L. A rare *null-null* variant also has been described that results in no α_1-PI synthesis. The Z allele is caused by a single amino acid substitution (ie, Glu to Lys at position 342) because of a G-A mutation in the fifth exon of the gene, which is located on the long arm of chromosome 14. This substitution results in the synthesis and accumulation of an α_1-PI molecule that cannot be secreted by the liver into the circulation.

Lung disease is uncommon in the pediatric age group. Cirrhosis may develop during infancy in 10 to 15% of patients with the ZZ genotype. Prenatal diagnosis and accurate genetic counseling are now possible for this condition (see Sec. 18.4).

PULMONARY MANIFESTATIONS

Pulmonary symptoms of α_1-PI deficiency are rare in pediatric patients, and α_1-PI deficiency accounts for fewer than 4% of all adult patients with emphysema. In a cohort of US patients who were diagnosed by newborn screening, all 22 patients had normal pulmonary function tests and clinical examinations at a mean age of 15 years. Dyspnea, chronic cough, and spirometric evidence of obstructive disease eventually occur in 80% of patients, but usually not until the fifth decade of life. There is good evidence that either tobacco smoking or heavy inhalant exposure hastens this process. On the chest radiograph, there is evidence of hyperinflation and bullae formation, particularly in the lower lung fields. Rarely, symptoms resembling bronchial asthma are present as well, but screening of childhood asthma populations has only rarely detected a patient with α_1-PI deficiency.

Rapidly progressive pulmonary disease may develop suddenly in adolescents with α_1-PI deficiency who have had long-standing hepatic involvement. In addition, recent reports have described the formation of pulmonary cysts following acute pulmonary infections in infants and young children with α_1-PI deficiency and cirrhosis. An example of this is shown in Fig. 23-29, which is a chest radiograph of a 4-month-old infant who presented with fever, jaundice, and a history of a pulmonary infiltrate and initially responded to the usual antibiotic therapy. The serum α_1-PI concentration was 15% of normal values, and the PI phenotype was ZZ. Over the next month, the lung cyst increased in size, hepatic function rapidly worsened, and the infant died of multiorgan failure. Autopsy revealed massive cirrhosis and panacinar emphysema that was confined to the left lower lobe. Anecdotal instances such as this suggest that early emphysema can be initiated by an acute infection that activates granulocytes and leads to increased protease activity. Pulmonary cysts also have been described following pneumonia in a

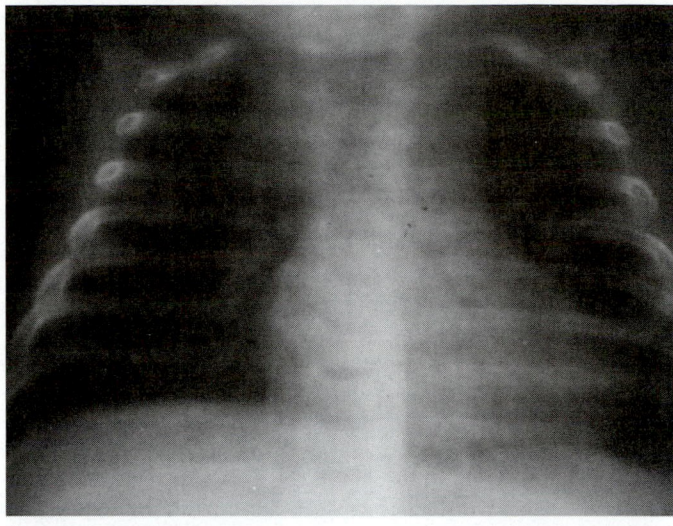

A

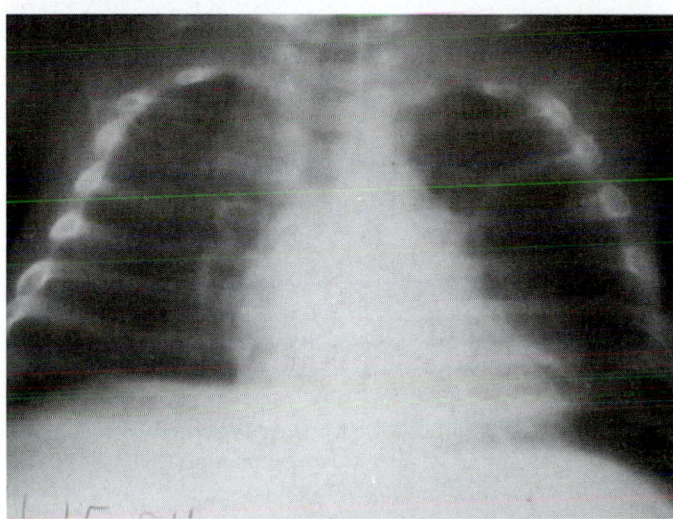

B

FIGURE 23-29   A. Chest radiograph of a 4-month-old child with α_1-protease inhibitor deficiency. Note the cyst in the left midlung field. B. Chest radiograph of the same infant taken 1 month later. Note that the cyst has greatly increased in size.

child with the PI MZ phenotype, which is a subgroup with intermediate levels of α_1-PI and no increased risk of emphysema. A high risk of emphysema is present only for those patients with the *null-null* genotype; the risk of emphysema in these patients is 20 to 50%.

DIAGNOSIS

The diagnosis of α_1-PI deficiency should be considered in children with severe asthma or an otherwise unexplained chronic obstructive pulmonary disease. The diagnosis is made by demonstrating a low level of α_1-PI in serum. In ZZ homozygotes, α_1-PI levels are less than 15% of normal (ie, MM) subjects. The precise variant can be determined from blood by protein electrophoresis with isoelectric focusing. Recombinant DNA methods may be used to isolate and amplify specific α_1-PI genes from genomic DNA that is obtained from the patient's blood or from fetal cells obtained for prenatal diagnosis.

TREATMENT

Liver transplantation can prevent progressive pulmonary disease, and corticosteroid therapy can reduce protease activity. Protease activity also can be reduced by avoiding tobacco smoke and other lung irritants. Because emphysema develops as a result of reduced serum α_1-PI levels, weekly or monthly infusions of plasma-derived or recombinant α_1-PI can be administered to maintain serum levels in the normal range. In addition, the potential value of aerosolized α_1-PI protein or the α_1-PI gene is being explored.

References

Brantley M, Nukiwa T, Crystal RG: Molecular basis of alpha₁-antitrypsin deficiency. Am J Med 84:13, 1988

Edmonds BK, Hodge JA, Reitschel RL: Alpha-1-antitrypsin deficiency-associated panniculitis: care report and review of literature. J Pediatr Dermatol 8:296, 1991

Guidelines for the approach to the patient with severe hereditary alpha-1-antitrypsin deficiency. Am Rev Respir Dis 140:1494, 1989

Newman SL, Sexson W, Courtney S, Goodwin C: Cystic degeneration of the lung in an infant with alpha₁-antitrypsin deficiency. Clin Pediatr 22: 830, 1983

Rovner MS, Stoller JK: Therapy for alpha-1-antitrypsin deficiency: rationale and strategic approach. Clin Pulm Med 1:135, 1994

Specks U, Homburger HA: Anti-neutrophil cytoplasmic antibodies. Mayo Clin Proc 69:1197, 1994.

Stoller JK: Clinical features and natural history of severe alpha₁-anti-protease deficiency. Chest 111:123S–128S, 1997

Sveger T: Prospective study of children with alpha₁-antitrypsin deficiency: eight-year-old follow-up. J Pediatr 104:91, 1984

Wall M, Moe E, Eisenburg J, et al: Long-term follow-up of a cohort of children with alpha-1-antitrypsin deficiency. J Pediatr 116:248, 1990

23.15 PULMONARY VASCULITIS SYNDROMES

Thomas A. Hazinski

IDIOPATHIC PULMONARY HEMOSIDEROSIS

Idiopathic pulmonary hemosiderosis (IPH) is a rare disease of uncertain etiology. It has been proposed that the development of IPH requires an immunologic response to antigens that reach antibody-producing cells via already damaged lung or gut epithelium. Both sexes are equally affected, and the disease has been described in several family members. It may be classified as *primary* when no extrapulmonary disorder is present or as *secondary* when a cardiac, systemic vasculitis, or collagen vascular disease is present. In either one, recurrent bleeding into the lung interstitium results in the deposition of iron (ie, hemosiderin), which is unavailable for hematopoiesis. Patients with IPH have migratory, patchy infiltrates on chest radiographs that may be interpreted as recurrent pneumonia. Myocardial disease and cardiac arrhythmias also have been associated with primary IPH. A microcytic, hypochromic anemia that is characteristic of iron deficiency may be present, and the reticulocyte count varies. Iron therapy may not improve the anemia. Clinical manifestations include pallor, nonproductive cough, fatigue, low-grade fever, and wheezing. Hemoptysis is present in approximately 50% of patients and may be life-threatening. Hemosiderin-laden macrophages may be detected in lung lavage fluid, laryngeal swab specimens, or serial morning samples of gastric aspirate. Demonstrating hemosiderin in these macrophages establishes that the bleeding is of pulmonary origin, and it may eliminate the need for lung biopsy if other clinical features are present. Melena and hematemesis are infrequent, but gastrointestinal bleeding occasionally is so severe that gastrointestinal disease is initially suspected. The presence of significant hematuria, rash, or arthralgia suggests that a multisystem disease is present.

Intrapulmonary hemorrhage also may occur in pulmonary vasculitis syndromes, cocaine intoxication, pulmonary embolism, venoocclusive diseases, heart failure, and in pulmonary AV malformations. The histologic appearance of the lung in IPH is not specific. Areas of focal hemorrhage that are associated with hemosiderin-laden macrophages, interstitial fibrosis, and chronic interstitial pneumonitis may be present. In some patients, pulmonary vasculitis is extensive. Fluorescent staining with antibodies to immunoglobulin and complement is nonspecific, and the capillary basement membrane ultrastructure is normal.

Pulmonary function studies reveal a restrictive ventilatory defect. Vital capacity and other lung volumes and lung compliance are low; flow rates (corrected for vital capacity) are normal or high. An obstructive ventilatory defect may be detected during acute peribronchiolar bleeding. Hypoxemia may be present or detected during mild exercise. Pulmonary hypertension may be present because of either vascular obliteration or chronic hypoxemia, and some patients may require continuous or nocturnal oxygen therapy.

For unknown reasons, some patients with IPH improve when cow's milk products are eliminated from their diet. Although the clinical response to milk and the presence of milk precipitins strongly suggest that immune mechanisms are involved, unique immunologic abnormalities have not yet been demonstrated. Milk precipitins have been found in the sera of 5 to 10% of normal children and in 50% of patients with IgA deficiency; IPH rarely, if ever, occurs in this latter group. In addition, some children with milk precipitins and chronic interstitial lung disease do not show hemosiderosis on lung biopsies. Nevertheless, some patients with IPH appear to improve when a milk-free diet is begun, whether or not milk precipitins are present in their sera. Hemosiderosis has been described in patients with gluten enteropathy, and in these patients, a gluten-elimination diet has improved the pulmonary symptoms.

There is no specific therapy for IPH; however, a 4- to 6-week trial of cow's milk avoidance is warranted whether or not milk precipitins are demonstrable. Iron therapy or blood transfusion may be necessary if severe anemia is present, although some experts believe that iron deposition in the lungs may be accelerated by this therapy. Corticosteroids, azathioprine, and cyclophosphamide have been used for both short- and long-term management of IPH, and these appear to be valuable in many patients. A few children originally thought to have primary IPH have developed glomerulonephritis or signs of collagen vascular diseases months to years after their initial onset of symptoms; for this reason, blood pressure determination and urine examination should be performed routinely in these patients. The natural history of this disease is characterized by remissions and exacerbations. Progressive pulmonary fibrosis, pulmonary hypertension, or massive hemoptysis may be fatal, but the course of any individual patient cannot be predicted.

GOODPASTURE SYNDROME AND ITS VARIANTS

The clinical association of pulmonary hemosiderosis and severe glomerulonephritis was described in 1958 and termed *Goodpasture syndrome*. In the past, this syndrome probably has included several diseases. It currently is used to designate a group of patients with renal and pulmonary disease in whom antibodies to specific glomerular basement-membrane antigens can be demonstrated. Goodpasture syndrome rarely has been diagnosed during childhood. There have been several recent reports, however, of children with immunopathologic evidence of immune complex–mediated glomerulonephritis, hemosiderosis, and pulmonary hemorrhage. These children resembled patients with Goodpasture syndrome, but basement-membrane antibody could not be identified in their sera. These patients may represent variants of Goodpasture syndrome.

Renal or pulmonary involvement in classical Goodpasture syndrome or its variants may be subtle and precede one another by months or years. Other disorders that may present with kidney and lung involvement are systemic lupus erythematosus, polyarteritis, uremic pneumonitis, and other collagen vascular diseases. These diseases usually can be differentiated by other clinical and laboratory findings.

Long-term corticosteroid or immunosuppressive therapy has been used in these patients. Bilateral nephrectomy or plasmapheresis has been reported to improve pulmonary function in young adults with classical Goodpasture syndrome. Kidney transplantation and subsequent immunosuppressive therapy may improve pulmonary symptoms.

COLLAGEN VASCULAR DISEASES

Juvenile rheumatoid arthritis, systemic lupus erythematosus, dermatomyositis, mixed connective tissue disease, scleroderma, and ankylosing spondylitis represent the most common collagen vascular diseases in pediatric patients; these are discussed in detail in Chapter 12. Pulmonary manifestations have been found in all of these disorders, and in some patients, drugs used to treat the disease (eg, gold salts, methotrexate) have been associated with development of a drug-induced interstitial pneumonitis. The chest wall, diaphragm, and extrathoracic airways also may be involved in these diseases, even when the lung parenchyma is only minimally affected. The most common cause of acute pulmonary disease in patients with collagen vascular diseases is infection, especially infection with opportunistic organisms. Therefore, appropriate cultures, serologic tests, and histopathologic examination of lavage fluid and, perhaps, biopsy material should be performed before pulmonary findings are attributed to the underlying disease.

Parenchymal involvement is suggested by cough, chest pain, exercise intolerance, and dyspnea. Rales and wheezing may be present, and there is diffuse interstitial disease on chest radiography. Vital capacity and other lung volumes and lung compliance are low, and the diffusing capacity for carbon monoxide may be reduced. Histologic examination reveals lymphocytic proliferation, interstitial pneumonitis, vasculitis, and pulmonary fibrosis.

Involvement of the pleura is suggested by pleuritic pain or pleural effusions. Distinctive immunologic abnormalities of the pleural fluid have not been demonstrated, but when an effusion is present, a pleural fluid culture should be strongly considered because of the risk of coexisting opportunistic infection. Complete removal of pleural fluid may be necessary if there is respiratory distress; decortication of the pleura rarely is necessary.

Diaphragm and chest wall involvement may occur in all collagen vascular diseases, and this may explain why respiratory symptoms develop in patients with normal chest radiographs. Pulmonary function tests both at rest and during exercise may be useful in objectively assessing these symptoms. This is particularly true in patients with dermatomyositis, where occlusive vasculitis and degeneration of striated muscle fibers occur; this can result in progressive alveolar hypoventilation and respiratory insufficiency. Patients with ankylosing spondylitis may develop fusion of multiple costovertebral joints, resulting in chest wall restriction.

Vasculitis, intimal proliferation, and sclerosis of pulmonary capillaries may result in hemoptysis. Even when hemoptysis is absent, however, pulmonary hypertension and pulmonary heart failure can occur. If there is hemorrhage around small airways, obstructive pulmonary symptoms may be present, and bronchodilator therapy may be beneficial. In those patients with arthritis, involvement of the cricoarytenoid joint can cause stridor and, occasionally, life-threatening upper airway obstruction. Noninfectious inflammation of the epiglottis with airway obstruction has been reported to occur in adults with systemic lupus erythematosus. Abnormal esophageal motility, which is prominent in several collagen vascular diseases, may predispose patients to repeated aspiration pneumonitis.

Corticosteroids and immunosuppressive therapy rarely are necessary to control the pulmonary manifestations of these diseases. When these drugs are used for other indications, however, improvement in pulmonary function may occur.

SYSTEMIC VASCULITIDES (SYSTEMIC VASCULITIS SYNDROME)

There is a group of multisystem diseases that are predominantly characterized by inflammation and necrosis of blood vessels, especially medium-sized arteries. Despite widespread vessel involvement, clinical pulmonary involvement is rare, but pulmonary infiltrates and hemoptysis can occur (see Sec. 12.6). Most of these disorders have been associated with immunologic abnormalities, most notably the presence of non–organ-specific autoantibodies in patients' sera. Polyarteritis nodosa, Kawasaki disease, and Henoch-Schönlein purpura are the most common examples of these disorders in pediatric patients.

By contrast, upper and lower respiratory tract involvement frequently is seen in patients with Wegener granulomatosis. Sinusitis, chronic otitis media, mastoiditis, and nasal ulceration may precede lower respiratory involvement. Hemoptysis and nodular pulmonary infiltrates usually are present and represent necrotizing granulomatous vasculitis. Diffuse pulmonary infiltrates are probably secondary to hemorrhage. Granulomatous lesions may cause subglottic stenosis or obstruct lobar bronchi. Glomerulonephritis may be present. The diagnosis is supported by finding antineutrophil cytoplasmic (cANCA) and anti-protein-3 antibodies in serum. Daily corticosteroid therapy combined with either cyclophosphamide or methotrexate has been of value in these patients. Recurrences after years of apparent quiescence are not uncommon.

Pulmonary vasculitis may also occur in the Churg-Strauss syndrome (allergic granulomatous angiitis), a rare disorder that is even rarer in children. Clinical findings include dyspnea, cough, hemoptysis, pulmonary infiltrates, blood and lung tissue eosinophilia, and vasculitic skin lesions.

References

Idiopathic Pulmonary Hemosiderosis

Beckerman RC, Taussig LM, Pinneas JL: Familial idiopathic pulmonary hemosiderosis. Am J Dis Child 133:609, 1979

Colombo JL, Stolz SM: Treatment of life-threatening primary pulmonary hemosiderosis with cyclophosphamide. Chest 102:959, 1992

Gaum WE, Aterman K: Complete left bundle branch block in idiopathic pulmonary hemosiderosis. J Pediatr 85:633, 1974

Levy J, Wilmott RW: Pulmonary hemosiderosis. Pediatr Pulmonol 2:384, 1986

Reading R, Watson JG, Platt JW, Bird AG: Pulmonary hemosiderosis and gluten. Arch Dis Child 62:513, 1986

Stafford HA, Palmar SH, Boat TF: Immunologic studies in cow's milk induced pulmonary hemosiderosis. Pediatr Res 11:898, 1977

Goodpasture Syndrome and Its Variants

Bergram H, Jervall J, Broadwell EJ, et al: Goodpasture's syndrome: A report of seven patients including long-term follow-up of three who received a kidney transplant. Am J Med 68:54, 1980

Care Records of the Massachusetts General Hospital: Case 16, 1993. N Engl J Med 328:1183, 1993

Loughlin JM, Taussig LM, Murphy SA, et al: Immune complex mediated granulonephritis and pulmonary hemorrhage simulating Goodpasture's syndrome. J Pediatr 93:181, 1979

Collagen Vascular Diseases

Dabich L, Sullivan DB, Cassidy JT: Scleroderma in the child. J Pediatr 85:770, 1974

Gelfand EW: The use of intravenous immune globulin in collagen vascular disorders: A potentially new modality of therapy. J Allergy Clin Immunol 84:613, 1989

Hunninghake GW, Fauci AS: Pulmonary involvement in the collagen vascular diseases. Am Rev Respir Dis 119:471, 1979

Jacobs JC, Hui RN: Cricoarytenoid arthritis and airway obstruction in juvenile rheumatoid arthritis. Pediatrics 59:292, 1977

Miller RW, Salcedo JR, Fink RJ, et al: Pulmonary hemorrhage in pediatric patients with systemic lupus erythematosus. J Pediatr 108:576, 1986

Pachman LM, Cook N: Juvenile dermatomyositis: A clinical and immunologic study. J Pediatr 96:226, 1980

Singsen BH, Bernstein GH, Cornreich HK, et al: Mixed connective tissue disease in childhood. J Pediatr 90:893, 1977

Walravens PA, Chase HP: The prognosis of childhood systemic lupus erythematosus. Am J Dis Child 130:929, 1976

Systemic Vasculitides

Rottem M, Fauci AS, Hallahan CW, et al: Wegener granulomatosis in children and adolescents: Clinical presentation and outcome. J Pediatr 122:26, 1993

Wright WK, Krous HF, Griswold WR, et al: Pulmonary vasculitis with hemorrhage in anaphylactoid purpura. Pediatr Pulmonol 17:269, 1994

23.16 PULMONARY ALVEOLAR PROTEINOSIS (ALVEOLAR PHOSPHOLIPOPROTEINOSIS)

Thomas A. Hazinski

Pulmonary alveolar proteinosis is a rare chronic disease of the lung in which there is intraalveolar deposition of periodic acid–Schiff-positive proteinaceous material rich in phospholipids and resembling tubular myelin. Despite this alveolar filling, alveolar architecture is maintained. An abnormality of type II cell phospholipid production or defective phospholipid clearance by lung macrophages has been implicated in the pathogenesis of this disorder. Some severe instances of alveolar proteinosis in neonates are associated with surfactant protein B deficiency. The condition is characterized by dyspnea that is associated with a persistent dry cough, fatigue, and weight loss. Physical examination may reveal a few scattered rales and, rarely, digital clubbing. Chest radiographs show fine, diffuse perihilar, radiating, feathery, or nodular densities that are similar to those seen in pulmonary edema.

Diagnosis requires lung biopsy. Immunodeficiency disorders have been found in some patients with pulmonary alveolar proteinosis, which may explain the coincidence of bacterial and fungal infections that occur with this disease.

The clinical picture and histologic appearance of the lung in some patients are similar to those of desquamative interstitial pneumonitis. Corticosteroids and repeated pulmonary lavage have been recommended, and there is suggestive evidence that they improve the restrictive ventilatory defect. Lengthy remission periods have been observed in more than one-half of all affected adults, but anecdotal reports suggest that the disease is more progressive in children.

References

De Mello DE, Nogee LM, Heyman S, et al: Molecular and phenotypic variability in the congenital alveolar proteinosis syndrome associated with inherited surfactant protein B deficiency. J Pediatr 125:43, 1994

Gilmore LB, Talley FA, Hook GER: Classification and morphometric quantitation of insoluble materials from the lungs of patients with alveolar proteinosis. Am J Pathol 133:252, 1988

Prakash UBS, Barham SS, Carpenter HA, et al: Pulmonary alveolar phospholipoproteinosis: Experience with 34 cases and a review. Mayo Clin Proc 62:499, 1987

23.17 CHEST WALL AND RESPIRATORY MUSCLE DISEASES

Mary K. Schroth and Christopher G. Green

PHYSIOLOGY

Chest wall and neuromuscular diseases can impair the efficiency of ventilation by adversely affecting the respiratory pump. An understanding of the respiratory pump is important in planning treatment for patients with these disorders.

Inspiration is achieved by the contraction of respiratory muscles, which stiffen the chest and lower intrathoracic pressure, causing air to flow into the airway and lungs. Expiration is generally passive and depends on the elastic properties of the lungs and the chest wall. Active expiration occurs during coughing, exercise, and during episodes of respiratory distress.

The chest wall includes the rib cage, the associated intercostal and accessory muscles, and the diaphragm. The diaphragm is the main muscle of inspiration. It is innervated by cervical segments 3, 4, and 5. Contraction of the diaphragm flattens the dome of the diaphragm and moves the diaphragm caudally. This flattening and the accompanying increase in intraabdominal pressure moves the lower ribs outward and increases the intrathoracic volume.

Contraction of the external intercostal muscles lifts the ribs in a bucket handle fashion during inspiration and increases the volume of the thorax. The internal intercostal muscles lower the ribs and thereby aid in expiration and expiratory maneuvers such as coughing, sneezing, and speech.

The accessory or extrathoracic muscles of respiration (abdominal and pelvic wall muscles, scalenes, sternocleidomastoids, shoulder girdle muscles, and serratus anterior) are important during respiratory distress such as in patients with significant obstructive lung disease. The scalenes, sternocleidomastoids, shoulder girdle muscles, and serratus anterior aid inspiration. The abdominal and pelvic muscles are important in aiding exhalation and of particular importance during the expiratory phase of coughing.

Upper airway patency is maintained by the alae nasi, pharyngeal wall muscles, genioglossus, posterior cricoarytenoid, and thyroarytenoid muscles. The action of these muscles may be impaired by neuromuscular weakness, which results in an increase in upper airway resistance and, if severe, to upper airway obstruction. These changes are particularly prominent during sleep, especially rapid eye movement (REM) sleep.

Physiological assessment of the respiratory system in chest wall and neuromuscular diseases is an important aspect of clinical management. Spirometry is a key tool in children and teenagers with these disorders. Exhaled volumes and expiratory flows are decreased when neuromuscular weakness is significant or in the presence of severe chest wall deformities. The FEV_1/FVC is typically elevated in contrast to the fall in FEV_1/FVC seen in obstructive airway disease.

Maximal inspiratory and expiratory pressures provide assessment of respiratory muscle strength (see Sec. 23.3.4). These measurements may be obtained periodically in patients to assess disease progression and response to treatment. Noninvasive measurements of gas exchange, hemoglobin oxygen saturation (SpO_2), and end-tidal carbon dioxide ($ETCO_2$) can be obtained during wakefulness and during sleep.

CHEST WALL MALFORMATIONS

KYPHOSCOLIOSIS Kyphoscoliosis results in varying degrees of chest wall malformation and deformity. Kyphosis refers to the angulation of the spine in the anterior-posterior direction. Scoliosis refers to the angulation of the spine in the lateral direction. Etiologies for kyphoscoliosis include idiopathic, which accounts for 80 to 85% of diagnosed scoliosis; congenital vertebral or rib abnormalities; and neuromuscular disease. The spine curvature causes vertebral body rotation and distortion of all attached structures. As a result of the rib rotation, the rib cage is prominent over the posterior chest on the convex side of the curve, with anterior flattening and widening of the interspaces. The concave side of the scoliosis has the opposite deformity. The resulting anatomic deformity results in functional pulmonary disability, most commonly restrictive lung disease. When scoliosis is severe, large airways and pulmonary vessels may be distorted as well. Because of the functional limitations and the natural history of untreated scoliosis resulting in reduced life expectancy, screening programs for scoliosis in school-age children have been developed. The goal of screening is to identify children with scoliosis before their adolescent growth spurt, which has the potential to cause significant curve progression. The degree of curvature is determined by the Cobb method, which is the angle of the intersection of perpendiculars from the end plates of the most tilted superior and inferior vertebrae. In general, cardiorespiratory compromise occurs when scoliosis exceeds 90° or more.

Idiopathic scoliosis is divided into three categories based on the age of presentation. Infantile scoliosis occurs between ages 0 and 3 years, juvenile scoliosis occurs between 3 and 10 years, and adolescent scoliosis occurs after age 10 years. Infantile scoliosis occurs more frequently in boys than girls. Juvenile and adolescent idiopathic scoliosis occurs more frequently in girls than boys. The prevalence of a scoliotic curve of 10° or more is about 3% in the general population. A curve of 20° or more has a prevalence of 0.5%.

In the majority of patients, scoliosis is not life-threatening. However, the natural history of untreated idiopathic scoliosis in adolescents demonstrates a death rate 2.2 times greater than in a cohort of adolescents without scoliosis. Deaths occur in the fourth and fifth decades of life and are from cardiopulmonary insufficiency. Survivors had dyspnea, back pain, and exercise limitation. Death may occur earlier in congenital scoliosis.

Mild scoliosis is typically painless and causes no symptoms at rest or during exercise. The convex side of the lung reveals normal vesicular sounds. In contrast, on the concave side breath sounds are decreased, and inspiratory crackles may be present. A chest radiograph may demonstrate volume loss on the concave side and recurrent or chronic atelectasis. Evaluation of pulmonary function includes spirometry and lung volumes, using arm span to estimate height. When the thoracic curve exceeds 50°, pulmonary function abnormalities are detectable. Scoliosis causes altered chest wall mechanics and diaphragm dysfunction, which result in decreased chest wall compliance. These changes cause individuals with scoliosis to breathe with a smaller than normal tidal volume, and as a result, the amount of dead space is increased relative to their tidal volume. If individuals are unable to compensate by increasing their respiratory rate in order to maintain adequate minute ventilation, alveolar hypoventilation will occur. Furthermore, ventilation–perfusion mismatch has been documented in severe scoliosis, contributing to alveolar hypoventilation. In moderate to severe scoliosis, the degree of restrictive lung disease is related to the severity of the curves. In mild scoliosis, although a reduction of lung volume has been reported, there is little correlation between the degree of curvature and lung volume.

Management depends on the patient's age and the severity of the scoliosis. Respiratory function should be monitored periodically for evidence of compromise, and respiratory infections treated aggressively. Ideally, progression of the curve can be prevented by bracing. Nonprogressive curves are followed clinically. However, for congenital and infantile scoliosis that is symptomatic or progressive, options for treatment include serial body casting and orthoses.

Surgery is often required in an effort to either straighten the spine or to prevent further progression of the curve. The majority of children with neuromuscular weakness will require surgical correction of their scoliosis because of weak muscle support of the spine. Results following scoliosis surgery have been inconsistent. In individuals with neuromuscular disorders who use a wheelchair for mobility or who have pain when sitting, spine stabilization often results in improved quality of life with decreased pain and improved wheelchair positioning. If surgery is planned, the patient should begin a preoperative program of incentive spirometry and chest physiotherapy; familiarity with these techniques may help to speed recovery postoperatively.

PECTUS EXCAVATUM   Also called funnel chest, pectus excavatum is the depression of the midsternum. This chest wall malformation may be congenital, familial, or acquired. The etiology of congenital pectus excavatum is not well understood. In Marfan syndrome, the suspected etiology is a defect in osteogenesis and chondrogenesis resulting in the midportion of the sternum becoming misaligned. Acquired pectus excavatum can occur in infants with bronchopulmonary dysplasia and in young children with chronic and severe airway obstruction.

Pectus excavatum alone generally does not cause significant cardiac or respiratory dysfunction either at rest or during exercise. Mitral valve prolapse may be present. Moderately severe pectus excavatum shifts the heart leftward and narrows the anterior-posterior diameter of the chest; when this occurs, a chest radiograph will depict the normal right hila of the lung, and the patient may be misdiagnosed as having an acute pneumonia. Cardiac function is usually normal at rest. Alterations in cardiac function have been reported in adults with pectus excavatum, but only during strenuous exercise. Spirometry is usually normal unless there is underlying lung disease.

Surgical candidates include individuals with pectus excavatum who have an associated thoracic scoliosis. Correction of the sternum will result in correction of the scoliosis. However, the most common reason for repair is to improve the appearance of the chest wall. Published data generally do not demonstrate physiological improvement in lung function after repair, but a few studies suggest that pectus repair may result in a modest improvement in cardiac output or exercise tolerance.

PECTUS CARINATUM   Also called pigeon breast, pectus carinatum is the protrusion of the sternum accentuated by lateral depression of the costal cartilages. The deformity is usually symmetric but can be unilateral. Pectus carinatum is rarely symptomatic. Typically, it results from an overgrowth of rib cartilage. Surgical repair is performed for cosmetic reasons.

ASPHYXIATING THORACIC DYSTROPHY (JEUNE SYNDROME)   Asphyxiating thoracic dystrophy is an autosomal recessive disorder characterized by skeletal malformations including a small, narrow rib cage with shortened ribs and renal disease. Short-limb dwarfism, pelvic and phalangeal abnormalities, polydactyly, and hepatic disorders are possible associated manifestations. Typically, the diagnosis is made shortly after birth from the characteristic findings of a narrow and bell-shaped thoracic cage with short horizontal ribs and flaring of the costochondral junctions. These findings are associated with a fixed chest wall and result in restrictive lung disease because of the mechanical limitations of the chest. These children are at risk for recurrent atelectasis, pneumonia, and impaired lung growth. Many patients die soon after birth as a result of respiratory failure, but milder cases may be managed by long-term mechanical ventilation. Thoracoplasty to enlarge the chest is not usually effective.

NEUROMUSCULAR DISEASES

Neuromuscular diseases are divided into neurologic disorders and myopathies. Neurologic disorders include spinal muscular atrophy, spinal cord injuries, and neuropathies such as Guillain-Barré syndrome. The myopathies include Duchenne, Becker, and limb-girdle muscular dystrophies. In general, children with neuromuscular disease who must use a wheelchair for ambulation also have significant respiratory muscle weakness and are at risk for respiratory failure, especially during intercurrent respiratory infections.

SPINAL MUSCULAR ATROPHY   Spinal muscular atrophy (SMA) is the second most common lethal autosomal recessive inherited disorder after cystic fibrosis. Clinical features of SMA include hypotonia, muscle weakness including extensive involvement of the intercostal muscles, muscle atrophy, and fasciculations. The neuropathologic lesion is degeneration of the anterior horn cells and, variably, the bulbar nuclei. Muscle weakness is symmetric, greater proximally, and typically more profound in the legs than the arms. There are no sensory deficits and no intellectual impairment associated with SMA. The gene defect for SMA is localized to chromosome 5q and was discovered in 1990. The gene and its protein product, survivor motor neuron (SMN), were identified in 1995.

SMA is divided into three classifications, which are best distinguished by their age of onset of disease and clinical course. SMA type I (Werdnig-Hoffmann disease or severe infantile SMA) is the most severe disorder and generally presents before 6 months of age with profound hypotonia and weakness, swallowing dysfunction, and tongue fasciculations; the disease generally results in respiratory insufficiency and death by 2 years of age unless long-term mechanical ventilation is employed.

SMA type II (intermediate or chronic infantile SMA) has an estimated incidence of 1/15,000 to 1/25,000 live births. Children with SMA type II may initially achieve normal motor milestones, but these are lost during the first 2 years of life. Median age of death is 12 years unless long-term mechanical ventilation is employed. Children with SMA type II may not be able to sit independently. Weakness may be static for long periods, with progression of weakness during intercurrent illness or immobilization. Bulbar musculature is generally intact. The onset of SMA type III (Kugelberg-Welander or mild SMA) may be between 2 and 17 years of life, and children are usually able to stand and walk unaided.

Clinical examination, laboratory evaluation (including normal serum creatine kinase), EMG, and muscle biopsy were used in the diagnosis of SMA. The discovery of the gene in 1995 resulted in diagnosis by gene mutation screening alone in 95% of cases. Laboratory data demonstrate subtle differences in the SMA types. Therefore, Dubowitz uses functional status to distinguish the types; ie, in severe SMA, children are unable to sit; in intermediate SMA, children are able to sit unsupported but cannot stand or walk unaided; with mild SMA, children are able to stand and walk unaided.

Management of children with SMA includes aggressive respiratory, nutritional, and orthopedic management. Children with SMA who use a wheelchair for ambulation are at risk for nocturnal hypoventilation. Evaluation includes assessment of lung function with spirometry, lung volumes, respiratory muscle strength measurements, and pulse oximetry. Hypoventilation is best evaluated by polysomnography with multiple channel measurements including end-tidal CO_2 and pulse oximetry. Hypoventilation is managed using respiratory support such as noninvasive positive-pressure ventilation while sleeping. During viral respiratory infections, aggressive airway clearance of increased secretions is critical to the child's survival, as outlined below. Annual influenza and pneumococcal vaccinations are recommended.

Nutritional evaluation and counseling are frequently needed because of poor weight gain secondary to diffuse motor weakness contributing to swallowing dysfunction and malnutrition. High-calorie diets and supplements are recommended, and gastrostomy tube placement is sometimes required, although obesity should be avoided. Orthopedic concerns must be actively managed including bracing of the extremities to promote optimal function and to limit pain. Progressive scoliosis is managed initially with bracing to fa-

cilitate sitting, although improper bracing can actually impair ventilation. Scoliosis may require surgical correction. These interventions contribute significantly to quality of life.

The option of tracheostomy and long-term mechanical ventilation should be discussed with patients and family members well before the onset of respiratory failure.

GUILLAIN-BARRÉ SYNDROME Guillain-Barré syndrome is an acute inflammatory ascending demyelinating disease of the peripheral nervous system. The vast majority of affected individuals have a history of recent nonspecific illness, but Guillain-Barré is also associated with cytomegalovirus and Epstein-Barr virus infection. The ascending paralysis and weakness progresses, typically over hours to several days. Involvement of the diaphragm and intercostal muscles results in hypoventilation, and tidal breathing may occur well below the patient's usual functional residual capacity. Progressive weakness involving the cranial nerves may result in laryngeal and vocal cord dysfunction with resulting upper airway obstruction. Respiratory support is required when hypoventilation occurs or when the individual cannot clear lower airway secretions. Serial monitoring of vital capacity and respiratory muscle function is critical. Treatment includes intravenous immunoglobulin, corticosteroids, and aggressive respiratory support. Recovery ranges from days to months and is usually complete.

DUCHENNE MUSCULAR DYSTROPHY Duchenne muscular dystrophy is the most common childhood form of muscular dystrophy. Duchenne muscular dystrophy occurs in 1:3000 male births and is an X-linked recessive progressive neuromuscular disease caused by mutations in the dystrophin gene resulting in deficiency of normal dystrophin protein. The gene was localized to the short arm of the X chromosome (Xp21) in 1986. Boys typically present between 2 and 6 years old with frequent falling, a waddling gait, and toe walking. Classic features of Duchenne muscular dystrophy include calf muscle pseuodohypertrophy and the Gower sign (climbing up the legs using the hands when rising from a seated position on the floor). Serum creatine kinase is elevated. The diagnosis is made by muscle biopsy, which reveals missing or significantly deficient dystrophin. A milder form of muscular dystrophy called Becker muscular dystrophy also affects the dystrophin gene and protein. Individuals present at a later age and walk until midteens to early 20s. Muscle biopsy reveals a decreased dystrophin concentration. Genetic testing identifies 60 to 65% of affected individuals with Duchenne or Becker muscular dystrophy.

Progression of motor weakness in Duchenne muscular dystrophy results in loss of ambulation by a mean age of 11 years. Respiratory muscle function parallels gross motor weakness and is complicated by progressive scoliosis. In the late teens and early 20s, disease progression results in further respiratory muscle weakness and increasing difficulty handling respiratory infections because of poor airway clearance of secretions and, ultimately, fatal respiratory failure. In addition, individuals with Duchenne and Becker muscular dystrophy develop cardiomyopathy, which contributes to their early death.

Management is supportive and directed at maintaining respiratory function and muscle strength. Corticosteroids slow muscle destruction in Duchenne muscular dystrophy, but the side effects of current preparations limit their use. Supporting ambulation for as long as possible facilitates airway clearance and maintains quality of life. Interventions include supportive bracing and surgical muscle releases. Scoliosis typically begins before the loss of ambulation and progresses rapidly after individuals require a wheelchair for ambulation Surgical correction of scoliosis is usually necessary to maintain comfort in positioning and may also slow the loss of vital capacity.

Lung function should be monitored, especially after loss of ambulation, with spirometry, lung volumes, and respiratory muscle strength measurements. The usual pattern is restrictive lung disease with increased residual volume secondary to weaker respiratory muscles of expiration compared to inspiration that are unable to actively expire to lung volumes below the functional residual capacity.

An additional feature of reduced expiratory muscle strength is an ineffective cough. During respiratory infections, aggressive airway clearance is critical and includes using manual cough assist and mechanical cough assist devices. In addition, respiratory support may be required, and noninvasive ventilation is the preferred route. Long-term invasive ventilation with tracheostomy is controversial and should be discussed with family members before a critical event. In addition, obesity contributes to increased work of breathing and worsening restrictive lung disease, and weight control may be necessary.

MYASTHENIA GRAVIS Myasthenia gravis is a rare disease in pediatric patients but is the most common primary disorder of neuromuscular transmission. The postsynaptic receptors for acetylcholine are functionally reduced in number by autoimmune mechanisms or by abnormal protein formation, and thus, the postjunctional membrane is less sensitive to released acetylcholine. Neonatal myasthenia gravis results from the transplacental transmission of maternal acetylcholine receptor antibodies to the neonate. Symptoms are usually present within the first day of life. Clinical presentation includes hypotonia, a weak cry, difficulty feeding, facial weakness, and palpebral ptosis. Respiratory compromise is caused by aspiration secondary to dysphagia and progressive respiratory muscle weakness, and respiratory failure is possible. Neonatal myasthenia resolves within 2 to 6 weeks as the antibodies are cleared and the receptors are regenerated.

Congenital myasthenia gravis is an autosomal recessive inherited disorder with variable age of onset. These individuals do not have circulating antibodies to the acetylcholine receptor. Juvenile myasthenia gravis is an acquired autoimmune disorder of neuromuscular transmission and affects girls more commonly than boys. Circulating acetylcholine receptor autoantibodies are present in 80 to 90% of affected individuals. Juvenile myasthenia gravis accounts for approximately 10% of all cases of myasthenia gravis, and onset is typically over 10 years of age. The course of juvenile myasthenia gravis is generalized progressive muscle weakness including the muscles of respiration. Muscle weakness is exacerbated by repetitive muscle use. Ocular muscles are involved in the majority of cases.

Diagnosis of myasthenia gravis is based on transient clinical improvement following administration of anticholinesterase medication such as intravenous edrophonium chloride or intramuscular neostigmine methylsulfate. In addition, electromyography (EMG) studies and the presence or absence of circulating acetylcholine receptor antibodies aid in the diagnosis and classification of myasthenia gravis.

Management includes using oral anticholinesterase medications, which increase the concentration of acetylcholine at the receptor site. Supportive care may also be required, eg, in the case of respiratory failure. Immunosuppression may induce remission within

3 years in up to 70% of patients but may not be sustained. Thymectomy may induce remission in up to 60% of patients. Plasmapheresis may be useful as a short-term intervention for acute symptomatic deterioration. The administration of intravenous immunoglobulins has demonstrated promising results in high doses.

DIAPHRAGMATIC PARALYSIS Unilateral and bilateral paralysis of the diaphragm is rare in pediatric patients. However, it may be overlooked during the evaluation of infants with unexplained hypoxemia, atelectasis, or tachypnea. In the neonatal period, diaphragm paralysis is most frequently caused by complications during delivery or following thoracic or neck surgery. The phrenic nerve fibers arise from C3, C4, and C5. The superficial location of the phrenic nerve in the neck and within the thorax contributes to the risk of injury during delivery. During cardiovascular surgery, the phrenic nerve may be injured by cooling, stretching, or accidental direct injury. In addition, high cervical spine trauma or tumors can result in diaphragm paralysis, and neuromuscular disease may be complicated by diaphragm paralysis.

The neonate is at much greater risk of respiratory compromise from diaphragm paralysis. Older children and adults tolerate unilateral diaphragm paralysis well. Diaphragm paralysis should be considered in any infant with unexplained respiratory distress with tachypnea and hypoxemia, especially after a difficult delivery, or in a child following thoracotomy who fails to wean from mechanical ventilation. Chest radiographs demonstrating an elevated hemidiaphragm or elevation of both diaphragms are suspect for diaphragm paralysis. Diagnosis is made by ultrasound or fluoroscopy, which shows very little movement with breathing, or paradoxic (upward) movement of the diaphragm with inspiration. Transcervical nerve stimulation may be helpful in determining whether the phrenic nerve is intact.

Management options include respiratory support until the diaphragm(s) recover and surgical plication if recovery is incomplete. Following thoracic or neck surgery, recovery may occur up to 6 months later in up to 90% of affected individuals if the phrenic nerve is intact. Infants may require positive-pressure ventilation, either invasively or noninvasively, until the diaphragm recovers. In individuals with permanent unilateral diaphragm paralysis, diaphragm plication may be helpful. In individuals with irreversible bilateral diaphragm paralysis, eg, spinal cord injury or neuromuscular disease, respiratory support with mechanical ventilation will be required. Older children and adult patients tolerate the diaphragm limitation relatively well, although they may require nocturnal respiratory support only.

MALFORMATION OF THE DIAPHRAGM

EVENTRATION Eventration of the diaphragm is a marked elevation of the diaphragm. This is usually congenital but may be acquired after phrenic nerve injury from surgery or birth trauma. The diaphragm is thin and fibrous rather than muscular. This defect is more common on the left than on the right and more common in boys than in girls. Symptoms in some cases are similar to those of a diaphragmatic hernia (tachypnea, dyspnea, retractions, and cyanosis). In other cases the symptoms are less severe. Some cases are asymptomatic or are recognized because of recurrent pneumonia in the poorly ventilated ipsilateral lung. Diagnosis is made by noting unilateral decreased ventilation on physical examination, by chest radiograph demonstrating the eventration, and by fluoroscopy, which shows paradoxic movement of the affected portion of the diaphragm. Persistently symptomatic cases are treated initially with intubation and ventilator support. Definitive treatment is plication of the affected diaphragm. Asymptomatic cases are treated conservatively.

ACCESSORY DIAPHRAGM Accessory diaphragm is a rare anomaly in which a fibromuscular band divides the hemithorax (usually the right) into two parts. Occasionally, the lesion may be an incidental finding on chest radiography. More commonly, there are associated symptoms that may include neonatal respiratory distress or later onset of dyspnea, recurrent infections, and hemoptysis. In most, there is hypoplasia of the ipsilateral lung with the mediastinum shifted to that side. Diagnosis usually is made by lateral radiography. When symptomatic, the accessory diaphragm should be removed.

CONNECTIVE TISSUES DISEASES/ COLLAGEN VASCULAR DISORDERS

Chronic inflammatory musculoskeletal disease is frequently associated with pulmonary complications. Systemic lupus erythematosus (SLE), polymyositis-dermatomyositis, ankylosing spondylitis, and rheumatoid arthritis are connective tissue diseases that involve the respiratory system. SLE is a disease of immune dysregulation characterized by arthritis, serositis, renal disease, neurologic disease, hematologic disease, cutaneous manifestations, and the presence of antinuclear antibodies (ANA). Children typically present with fever, malaise, arthritis and arthralgias, and rash. The most common respiratory complications of SLE is pleuritis with chest pain, with or without pleural effusion. Pleural effusions may be unilateral or bilateral and occur in 40 to 50% of individuals with SLE. Costovertebral joint involvement may result in restrictive lung disease even without SLE-associated lung parenchymal involvement. Additional complications include acute lupus pneumonitis, which is similar to adult respiratory distress syndrome. Pulmonary alveolar hemorrhage may complicate lupus pneumonitis. Interstitial lung disease can occur but is less common. Complications of SLE are treated with immunosuppressive therapy including corticosteroids.

Dermatomyositis is an inflammatory myopathy with associated cutaneous lesions of unknown etiology. The disease is characterized by proximal muscle weakness and tenderness, elevation of serum muscle enzymes, muscle necrosis, and cellular inflammation. Childhood dermatomyositis is associated with HLA-B8/DR3. In children, respiratory muscle weakness in combination with dysphagia may lead to aspiration. These individuals are also at risk for hypoventilation and death. In addition to muscle weakness, interstitial lung disease can occur. The prognosis for patients with dermatomyositis with interstitial fibrosis is poor. Treatment is with corticosteroids.

Ankylosing spondylitis is a disorder of the axial skeleton associated with HLA-B27. The sacral spine and sacroiliac-iliac joints are affected, and boys are affected more commonly than girls. Uveitis is a common associated symptom. Diagnosis includes serology with negative rheumatoid factor and ANA titers. Pleuropulmonary disease occurred in 1.3% of individuals at one center. As the disease progresses, the chest wall compliance decreases dramatically secondary to progressive immobilization of the costovertebral joints, resulting in a significant decrease in chest wall compliance. However, the chest wall becomes fixed in a more expanded position, resulting in mildly reduced vital capacity and normal functional re-

sidual capacity and residual volumes. Interstitial lung disease does not occur. The goal of therapy is to relieve pain and maintain function.

Juvenile rheumatoid arthritis (JRA) is a disease of chronic synovitis of unknown etiology. The disease is characterized by a symmetric deforming inflammatory polyarthritis. Systemic JRA is characterized by extraarticular manifestations including erythematous rash, fever, hepatosplenomegaly, lymphadenopathy, and cardiopulmonary disease. The prevalence of pulmonary disease associated with JRA has been estimated to be 4 to 8% with more pleural involvement than parenchymal. Reported pleural disease includes pleuritis, effusions, and pleural thickening. Parenchymal disease includes interstitial pneumonitis, rheumatoid nodules, lymphoid hyperplasia, and obliterative bronchiolitis. In addition, drug therapy has induced pulmonary side effects. JRA is not life-threatening.

MANAGEMENT OF CHRONIC RESPIRATORY FAILURE

Respiratory muscle weakness, thoracic deformities including scoliosis, and compromised nutritional status are contributing factors to respiratory insufficiency and early death in at-risk children. In children with SMA type I or II, marked atrophy of the intercostal muscles causes paradoxic breathing. Instead of the ribs rising and lifting the chest wall upward during inspiration, the chest wall is pulled downward as the diaphragm descends, which leads to development of a bell-shaped chest. These factors result in decreased chest wall compliance, lung underdevelopment, and decreased ability to cough. Three stages are seen in the decline of respiratory function in neuromuscular disorders (NMD): difficulty clearing secretions and atelectasis; nocturnal hypoventilation; and daytime hypoxemia. Over time, respiratory failure develops, followed by death. With the development of nocturnal hypoventilation, patients with neuromuscular weakness require respiratory support while they sleep. This respiratory deterioration occurs in the first 2 years in children with SMA type I. In contrast, individuals with Duchenne muscular dystrophy do not develop respiratory compromise until the middle of or late in the second decade of life.

Objective assessment of pulmonary function should be performed periodically in these patients when they are free of intercurrent infections. Evaluation of pulmonary function includes spirometry, lung volumes, respiratory muscle strength measurements, and pulse oximetry while awake every 6 to 12 months for individuals who require wheelchairs for ambulation. Assessment of hypoventilation and sleep quality may be assessed by overnight polysomnography.

During respiratory infections, individuals with chest wall malformations and neuromuscular diseases are placed at a further mechanical disadvantage. Secretion-filled airways and inflamed lung tissue increase the load on respiratory muscles and on the muscles that are used to generate forceful coughs. Atelectasis and hypoxemia can progress to respiratory failure and death.

Respiratory support includes both assisted ventilation and airway clearance techniques (see Sec. 23.3.7). Airway expansion is necessary to promote lung growth and facilitate airway clearance. Assisted ventilation techniques include inspiratory muscle aids such as using a resuscitator bag with mask to provide intermittent positive-pressure breaths, intermittent positive-pressure breathing (IPPB), which delivers synchronized breath support to a preset inspiratory pressure, and the In-exsufflator cough machine (JH Emerson Co, Cambridge, MA). Incentive spirometers are readily available, but these rely on the patient's inspiratory effort and are therefore not as effective as those that actively inflate the lung. Airway clearance techniques include chest physiotherapy using a manual or electric percussor, postural drainage, and intrapulmonary percussive ventilation (IPV, Percussionaire® Corp, Sandpoint, ID). These techniques loosen secretions in the lower airways. However, to facilitate removal of the loosened secretions from the airways in children with spinal muscular atrophy, a manual cough assist technique or the In-exsufflator cough machine should be used. The In-exsufflator cough machine provides airway expansion through a mouthpiece or face mask followed by a negative pressure that results in coughing and improved airway clearance of lower airway secretions. The In-exsufflator cough machine significantly increases peak cough expiratory flow rates in patients with neuromuscular disease compared to their spontaneous cough. Furthermore, compared to manually assisted coughing, mechanical insufflation is significantly more effective in producing more normal and effective peak cough expiratory flows (see Table 23-28).

The options for ventilatory support include invasive and noninvasive forms of ventilation. Invasive ventilation refers to using positive-pressure mechanical ventilation through a tracheostomy tube. Because of advancing technology with improved face-mask design, noninvasive ventilation is a reasonable option for individuals with neuromuscular weakness and progressive chest wall deformities. The categories of noninvasive ventilation include positive-pressure and negative-pressure ventilation. Positive-pressure ventilation is accomplished using a nasal mask, face mask, or mouthpiece connected to a mechanical ventilator. The ventilator is adjusted and designed to compensate for the large anticipated air leak. The same face masks and mouthpieces can also be attached to devices that produce bilevel positive airway pressure or BiPAP®, which augments the patient's spontaneous breaths. BiPAP refers to a type of ventilation that senses airway pressure changes at the mouth and provides a higher inspiratory positive airway pressure (IPAP) during inspiration, alternating with a lower expiratory positive airway pressure (EPAP). BiPAP provides more comfortable and more effective respiratory support than CPAP. BiPAP levels should be high enough to support adequate gas exchange.

TABLE 23-28

DEVICES USEFUL FOR PATIENTS WITH CHRONIC RESPIRATORY FAILURE

Airway expansion
  Resuscitator bag and mask
  Intermittent positive-pressure breathing (IPPB)
  In-exsufflator cough machine
Airway clearance
  Chest physiotherapy
  Postural drainage
  Intrapulmonary percussive ventilation (IPV)
  Manual cough assist
  In-exsufflator cough machine
Airway support
  Positive pressure with nasal mask
    CPAP
    BiPAP®
    Mechanical ventilator
  Negative pressure with NEV®-100 ventilator
    Pulmowrap®
    Soft seal chest shell
    Porta-lung™

Negative-pressure ventilation (NPV) requires that a patient reside in a rigid chamber in which cycles of subatmospheric pressure are generated around the chest to produce inspiratory airflow (the patient's head is outside the chamber). The chamber encircles the thorax and upper abdomen. Negative-pressure ventilation is accomplished using chambers such as the Pulmowrap®, the soft seal chest shell, or the Porta-lung™ with a pump called the NEV®-100 extrathoracic ventilator (see Table 23-28).

The key to management of chronic respiratory failure is anticipation of a patient who is at risk for respiratory failure, preparation of the physician and the patient for the possibility, recognition of developing respiratory failure, and appropriate intervention in a timely fashion.

References

Physiology

Allen JL, Wohl MEB: Neuromuscular and chest-wall disorders. In: Taussig LM, Landau LI, eds: Pediatric Respiratory Medicine. St Louis, CV Mosby, 1999:1154–1171

Chest Wall Malformations

Kyphoscoliosis

Canet E, Praud J-P, Bureau MA: Chest wall diseases and dysfunction in children. In: Chernick V, Boat TF, eds: Kendig's Disorders of the Respiratory Tract in Children, 6th ed. Philadelphia, WB Saunders, 1998: 787–815

Kearon C, Viviani GR, Kirkley A, Killian KJ: Factors determining pulmonary function in adolescent idiopathic thoracic scoliosis. Am Rev Respir Dis 148:288–294, 1993

Kennedy JD, Staples AJ, Brook PD, et al: Effect of spinal surgery on lung function in Duchenne muscular dystrophy. Thorax 50:1173–1178, 1995

Pectus Excavatum and Pectus Carinatum

Besier GD, Epstein SE, Stampfer M, Goldstein RE, Noland SP, Levitsky S: Impairment of cardiac function in patients with pectus excavatum, with improvement after operative correction. N Engl J Med 287:267–272, 1972

Karrer FM, Hall RJ, Lilly JR: Noncardiac thoracic surgery in children: an overview. Surg Ann 25(Pt 2):117–149, 1993

Asphyxiating Thoracic Dystrophy (Jeune Syndrome)

Barnes ND, Hull D, Sumons JS: Thoracic dystrophy. Arch Dis Child 44: 11–17, 1969

Finegold MJ, Katzew H, Genieser NB, Becker MH: Lung structure in thoracic dystrophy. Am J Dis Child 122:153–159, 1971

Todd DW, Tinguely SJ, Norberg WJ: A thoracic expansion technique for Jeune's asphyxiating thoracic dystrophy. J Pediatr Surg 21:161–163, 1986

Neuromuscular Diseases

Spinal Muscular Atrophy

Dubowitz V: Color Atlas of Muscle Disorders in Childhood. Chicago, Year-Book Medical Publishers, 66, 1989

Russman BS, Iannaccone ST, Buncher CR, et al: Spinal muscular atrophy: new thoughts on the pathogenesis and classification schema. J Child Neurol 7:347–353, 1992

Families of SMA website: *www.fsma.org*

Duchenne Muscular Dystrophy

Iannaccone ST: Current status of Duchenne muscular dystrophy. Pediatr Clin North Am 39:879–894, 1992

Muscular Dystrophy Association website: *www.mdausa.org*

Myasthenia Gravis

Boonyapisit K, Kaminski HJ, Ruff RL: Disorders of neuromuscular junction ion channels. Am J Med 106:97–113, 1999

Myasthenia Gravis Foundation of America (MGFA) website: *www.myasthenia.org*

Diaphragmatic Paralysis

Commare MC, Kurstjens SP, Barois A: Diaphragmatic paralysis in children: a review of 11 cases. Pediatr Pulmonol 18:187–193, 1994

Eventration of the Diaphragm

Deslauriers J: Eventration of the diaphragm. Chest Surg Clin North Am 8: 315–330, 1998

Connective Tissues Diseases/Collagen Vascular Disorders

Athreya BH, Doughty RA, Bookspan M, Schumacher HR, Sewell EM, Chatten J: Pulmonary manifestations of juvenile rheumatoid arthritis. A report of eight cases and review. Clin Chest Med 1:361–374, 1980

Todd NW, Wise RA: Respiratory complications in the collagen vascular diseases. Clin Pulm Med 3:101–112, 1996

Management of Chronic Respiratory Failure

Bach JR: Mechanical insufflation-exsufflation: comparison of peak expiratory flows with manually assisted and unassisted coughing techniques. Chest 104:1553–1562, 1993

Bach JR: Update and perspective on noninvasive respiratory muscle aids, part 2: the expiratory aids. Chest 105:1538–1544, 1994

Lyager S, Steffensen B, Juhl B: Indicators of need for mechanical ventilation in Duchenne muscular dystrophy and spinal muscular atrophy. Chest 108:779–785, 1995

Robert D, Willig TN, Paulus J: Long-term nasal ventilation in neuromuscular disorders: report of a consensus conference. Eur Respir J 6:599–606, 1993

THE ENDOCRINE SYSTEM

Walter L. Miller, Associate Editor

24.1 MECHANISMS OF HORMONE ACTION

Pinchas Cohen and Philip L. Ballard

Hormones are molecules that are involved in signaling within an organism. Hormones act as endocrine factors when they are secreted from a gland or tissue, and they act at distal sites. For example, insulin is secreted from pancreatic β cells and acts on skeletal muscle. When a hormone or growth factor is secreted from a cell and acts on a nearby cell, it is said to act in a *paracrine* manner, for example, glucagon stimulates insulin release within pancreatic islet cells. When a hormone acts on the cell that secreted it, as when insulin inhibits its own secretion, it operates in an *autocrine* manner. Some growth factors act in an *intracrine* manner, signaling within the cell that produced them without being secreted. Hormones represent a variety of structural classes of compounds, including relatively small molecules (eg, the neurotransmitter acetylcholine); larger molecules, such as iodinated amino acids, steroids, fatty acids, and oligopeptides; and very large molecules, such as glycoproteins with molecular masses of tens of thousands of daltons.

A large proportion of circulating steroid and thyroid hormones and some growth factors are associated with specific binding proteins in plasma, whereas most catecholamine and polypeptide hormones travel in a free state. In general, only unbound hormones are active (available to cells), whereas bound hormones apparently serve as reservoirs. The insulin-like growth factors (IGFs), however, are bound to binding proteins (IGFBPs), which appear to have an essential role in distribution to target cells and binding receptors. Some of these binding proteins can themselves act as growth factors independently of IGFs. Most hormones are secreted and transported in their active form. Exceptions include testosterone, which is converted to dihydrotestosterone in most target tissues, and thyroxine (T_4), which is deiodinated to the more active triiodothyronine (T_3) in target cells.

Despite the diversity of structure and amount, most hormones exert their effects through interaction with specific receptors at target cells. Hormone receptors are specific proteins that contain molecular sites where hormones are initially bound by cells. The receptors transduce and often amplify the extracellular hormonal signals through secondary messengers. Subsequent modulation of specific gene expression or protein function leads to the observed changes in cellular function.

Hormones and growth factors have three general biologic roles in developing and adult organisms. First, during embryogenesis, they influence the commitment of multipotential cells to specific cell lineages. For example, it is likely that a variety of growth factors acting in a paracrine manner (ie, on neighboring cells) are important in early organogenesis. Second, hormones influence cell proliferation and the timing of terminal differentiation of determined cells. For example, IGFs in conjunction with other hormones, such as T_4, control proliferation of chondrocytes throughout growth. Third, hormones modulate cellular metabolism and mediate the stress response in postnatal organisms. Examples include hormonal action of insulin, glucagon, and catecholamines on glycogen metabolism. The diversity of hormonal effects results from modulation of specific proteins (eg, by phosphorylation) or activation of different networks of genes in the various target cells. The availability of specific genes for activation by hormones appears to be determined by differential tissue expression of DNA binding proteins, also called *transcription factors*, which influence the responsiveness to activating signals.

RECEPTOR PROPERTIES

Many different cellular and plasma proteins are capable of binding hormones. Receptor proteins are differentiated from these (nonspecific) binding proteins by a number of properties that indicate physiologic importance for hormone action. Criteria for receptor function are as follows: binding to a receptor occurs at physiological concentrations of free hormone; there are relatively few receptor molecules per cell; the binding affinity of a hormone and its analogs (agonists, partial agonists, or antagonists) correlates with biologic potency; biologically inactive analogs do not bind to the receptor; the kinetics of binding are sufficiently rapid to account for the hormonal response; receptors are present in responsive tissues; and loss of receptor from a cell is associated with loss of hormone response. Thus receptors are characterized by high affinity and specificity of binding, tissue distribution, and indispensability for hormone effects.

The binding reaction is governed by the law of mass action, and the extent of hormone effect is determined by the concentration of receptor-hormone complex. The interaction between hormone and receptor is strong but reversible, involving noncovalent binding. The chemical nature of binding involves interaction of specific portions of the hormone molecule with a specific region of the receptor (binding site) through hydrophobic, electrostatic, and van de Walls bonding.

In systems responsive to catecholamine and polypeptide hormones, a maximal biologic response often is achieved when only a relatively small proportion of the total receptors on a cell are occupied. The circumstance in which more receptors are present than are needed to elicit a maximal response has been called *spareness*. Such receptors are not truly spare or extra, because their presence influences, through mass action, both the dose-response relation (increased sensitivity to hormone) and the kinetics of hormone binding (faster binding and slower dissociation). Figure 24-1 shows the effects of changes in receptor number and affinity on a theoretical system (eg, the response to insulin) in which a reduced response to hormone stimulation can occur with or without a change in the equilibrium constant of the hormone to the receptor (K_d).

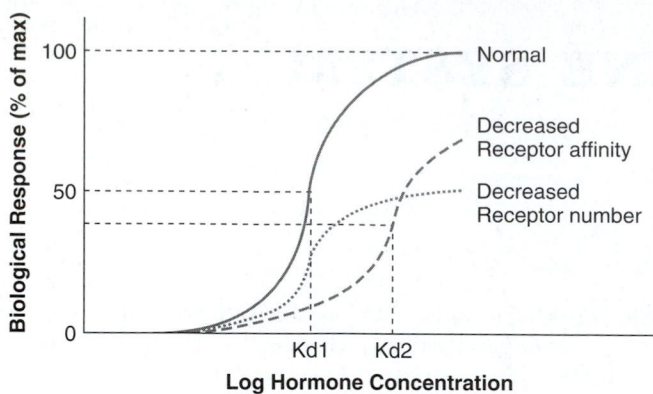

FIGURE 24-1   **Effects of decrease in hormone receptor number or affinity on response to stimulation. A dramatic decrease in receptor number to overcome the spare receptor effect decreases the response to a hormonal stimulus without changing the equilibrium constant (K_d). Mutation of a receptor can decrease affinity and response with a higher K_d.**

Receptors for steroids, such as sex steroids and cortisol, are present in both the cytoplasm and nucleus of cells; no intermediary messengers are involved. Membrane receptors have been identified for most other hormones, and the effects of these hormones often are mediated through secondary messengers. These receptors are characterized by an extracellular domain that contains the ligand binding sites, a hydrophobic transmembrane portion (often several membrane-spanning regions), and a cytoplasmic domain that couples receptor to other proteins (eg, G proteins or kinases of various sorts). Some hormonal systems can activate several different signal transduction pathways. For example, the various β-adrenergic receptors can activate adenylate cyclase, cyclic adenosine monophosphate (cAMP), or mobilization of calcium ion (Ca^{2+}). The insulin receptor can activate several insulin response elements and phosphorylates a number of other substrates, which explains the diverse effects of insulin on metabolism and gene transcription.

NUCLEAR RECEPTORS

STEROID RECEPTORS   Steroids enter target cells by means of passive diffusion, although facilitated entrance through membrane binding sites also can occur. Steroid receptors have a ligand binding domain and a DNA binding domain. These receptors bind their respective ligands in the cytoplasm and diffuse into the nucleus, where they dimerize and bind gene promotors at specific response elements. A multiprotein transcriptional complex forms around the receptor dimer, and new synthesis of messenger RNA (mRNA) and protein eventually leads to the observed hormonal effects (Fig. 24-2).

The rate of formation of receptor-steroid complexes is proportional to the concentration of both hormone and receptor. In general, receptor occupancy is closely correlated with hormonal response. Thus decreased hormonal effect can be caused by a deficiency of either hormone or its receptor. Changes in receptor concentration also can affect the dose-response kinetics of hormone action.

Whereas receptors for androgens, estrogens, progesterone, and aldosterone are restricted to respective target tissues, glucocorticoids affect most, if not all, tissues. The particular effects of glucocorticoids on enzymes of metabolic pathways in different tissues depend on the specific genes, which are under hormonal regulation.

The anti-inflammatory effects of glucocorticoids occur at the level of transcription but primarily involve antagonism of the inductive effects of cytokines and other proinflammatory agents. Evidence has accumulated that many of these glucocorticoid responses involve an inhibitory effect on the transactivation activity of nuclear factor-$\kappa\beta$, which increases the expression of many genes involved in immune and inflammatory responses, including cytokines, complement-related factors, cell adhesion molecules, and various immunoreceptors of both resident tissue cells and inflammatory cells from the circulation.

OTHER NUCLEAR RECEPTORS   A family of nuclear receptors, which also function as transcription factors, has been identified that act through heterodimerization with a common partner called the *retinoid-X receptor* (RXR). These receptors include the thyroid hormone receptor, the retinoid receptor, the vitamin D receptor, and the peroxisome proliferator activating receptor-γ (PPARγ). These receptors form dimers with RXR and signal through specific response elements, influencing different gene groups. The RXR can also form homodimers and signal through a specific element. This receptor system is critical to growth and development and to the differentiation of various tissues. Vitamin D is critical for the regulation of calcium homeostasis. Thyroid receptors regulate energy metabolism through the control of the expression of other genes, primarily β-adrenergic receptors. In most tissues there is considerable conversion of T_4 to T_3, which binds to the receptor with much higher affinity. Retinoid receptors are important in the processes of organogenesis and other developmental events. PPARγ receptors are necessary for adipogenesis, and they mediate insulin sensitivity. The natural ligands for PPAR are fatty acids; however, a new class of drugs that act as potent agonists of PPAR are emerging as important therapies for diabetes (by reversing insulin resistance). Additional receptors, related to known nuclear receptors, have been identified. Because the endogenous ligand and function of these putative receptors are currently unknown, they have been designated *orphan receptors*. The functions of these receptors in cell metabolism and differentiation are being unraveled and may hold the key to understanding and controlling a variety of diseases. The amino acid sequence of the DNA binding regions of the various nuclear receptors is highly conserved. There also is homology in the ligand-binding domains that in general parallels the structural

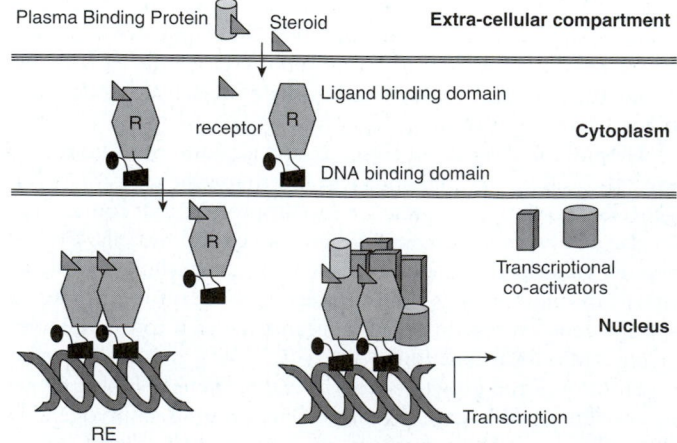

FIGURE 24-2   **A model of steroid receptor action. Signaling of the steroid receptor–dimer complex through binding to its response element (*RE*).**

relatedness of the hormones. The DNA binding domain of nuclear receptors is composed of two zinc-binding fingers. It is proposed that these loops of amino acids bind to DNA and associate with other DNA binding proteins. In this action, the hormone receptor complex acts as an enhancer or inhibitor of specific gene expression.

PLASMA MEMBRANE RECEPTORS

Most hormones and growth factors exert their effects through binding to receptors in the plasma membrane of target cells. Stimulation of a receptor by its agonist initiates a cascade of biochemical events that produce a change in cellular function. Transduction of the hormonal signal involves phosphorylation and generation of secondary and often tertiary messenger molecules in both membrane and cytoplasm. Membrane receptors can mediate rapid events such as glucose transport in response to insulin, which occurs within seconds, or protein production in response to growth factors, which can take days.

There is a continuous turnover of most membrane receptors. In many cases, the binding of hormone to receptors is followed by aggregation of receptors at sites on the cell surface. The receptor–hormone complexes then undergo pinocytosis followed by fusion with liposomes and either degradation of the proteins or recycling of the receptor back to the cell surface. In the case of low-density lipoproteins, internalization leads to hydrolysis and release of cholesterol, which acts by a feedback mechanism to inhibit cholesterol biosynthesis. Membrane receptors signal through a number of second messengers.

CYCLIC AMP Catecholamines and many polypeptide hormones exert their effects through cell membrane receptors and activation of the adenylate cyclase–cAMP system. Interactions of these hormones with membrane receptors activate adenylate cyclase, a membrane enzyme linked to guanine nucleotide regulatory protein (G protein). This enzyme catalyzes conversion of adenosine triphosphate (ATP) to cAMP, which acts as a second messenger of hormone action. In most systems, cAMP binds to the regulatory subunits of cAMP-dependent protein kinase (protein kinase A), releasing the catalytic subunits to catalyze phosphorylation of proteins that contain the amino acid sequence Arg-Arg-X-Ser. The particular proteins or enzymes phosphorylated that thereby become altered in function are unique for different hormones in different tissues, thus providing specificity to the hormone effect. Cyclic AMP is degraded to $5'$AMP by cAMP phosphodiesterase. This enzyme is inhibited by a number of drugs, such as methylxanthines. Hormones that activate adenylate cyclase increase cAMP levels within a few minutes, and changes in enzyme activity occur soon thereafter. Responses that involve phosphorylation of nuclear proteins, with subsequent alterations in RNA or DNA synthesis, can take several hours to reach maximal effect.

Cyclic AMP also modifies the content of specific cellular proteins by regulating gene expression. This effect is mediated by protein kinase A phosphorylation of nuclear proteins that bind at cAMP response elements (CRE) in the target genes. A family of CRE-binding proteins contain phosphorylation sites for protein kinase A and other kinases, positively charged domains for DNA binding, and domains rich in the amino acid leucine that facilitate protein–protein interaction. Phosphorylation of CRE-binding protein appears to induce conformational changes in the protein that facilitate interaction with other transcriptional proteins. The result is an increase in the rate of gene transcription.

GUANINE NUCLEOTIDE REGULATORY PROTEINS The guanosine triphosphate–binding, or G, proteins are involved in regulation of a variety of intracellular pathways. Alterations in G protein function are involved in acquired and in genetic diseases. In cholera, the toxin catalyzes ADP ribosylation of the subunit and causes sustained synthesis of cAMP in intestinal mucosal cells. This produces excessive secretion of fluid into the intestine, which is characteristic of cholera. In pertussis, toxin-induced ADP ribosylation inactivates subunit α_1, which is coupled with the β_2-adrenergic receptor. This system normally modulates the effects of β_2-adrenergic agonists, which stimulate production of cAMP. Inactivation of α_1 by pertussis toxin causes unrestrained synthesis of cAMP and clinical symptoms.

McCune-Albright syndrome, originally described as a triad of bone, skin, and endocrine abnormalities, is associated with a mutation in the G_s-α subunit. The mutations occur in variable abundance in different tissues in a manner consistent with somatic mutation and mosaicism. The affected tissues have constitutively active glandular function, which causes sexual precocity and other features of the condition.

HYDROLYSIS OF PHOSPHATIDYLINOSITOL Inositol triphosphate (IP_3) is generated from phosphatidylinositol, a cell membrane phospholipid, through hormone activation of a phosphodiesterase (phospholipase C) and lipid kinase enzymes in the cell membrane. Inositol triphosphate binds to its receptor on intracellular membranes and promotes mobilization of intracellular Ca^{2+} (a "tertiary" messenger), resulting in activation of Ca^{2+} calmodulin-dependent protein kinases and phosphorylation of specific proteins. Inositol triphosphate is recycled into phosphatidylinositol. A rapidly reversible effect occurs when the hormone is removed.

The other product of phosphodiesterase action is diacylglycerol. This compound directly stimulates protein kinase C, a phospholipid- and Ca^{2+}-dependent enzyme. The result is phosphorylation of specific proteins that are, in general, distinct from the substrates for the Ca^{2+}-dependent protein kinases. Protein kinase C proteins transduce extracellular signals (hormones and neurotransmitters) into the target cell. An extracellular signal triggers migration of protein kinase C from the cytosol, where it is relatively inactive, to the plasma membrane or nuclear membrane, where it is activated by phospholipids and calcium phosphorylates other protein kinases that in turn phosphorylate and activate other enzymes or target proteins to elicit the biologic response.

CALCIUM Calcium functions as an ionic second messenger in many cells. It conveys signals across the cell membrane and propagates intracellular signaling. The concentration of intracellular calcium is maintained at low levels relative to extracellular fluid as a result of the low permeability of the plasma membrane to calcium and the presence of membrane-bound calcium pumps, which transport calcium out of the cell. In response to various extracellular signals, calcium channels open in the plasma membrane. The result is a transient increase in intracellular calcium concentration. Intracellular calcium is bound by the protein calmodulin, which interacts with the calcium pump to increase its efficiency and sensitivity to calcium ions. An initial response is mobilization of intracellular calcium from the endoplasmic reticulum. In smooth muscle the calcium-calmodulin complex increases the activity of myosin light-chain kinase as an early step in muscle contraction. In liver it mediates glycogen degradation through activation of glycogen phosphorylase and inactivation of glycogen synthetase. Cytosolic free calcium also acts through binding to other proteins that mediate responses such as exocytosis and ion flux.

ACTIVATION OF SIGNAL TRANSDUCTION THROUGH KINASES
Phosphorylation of a receptor after hormone binding is a critical early event in many membrane receptor systems. In the case of insulin, for example, the various biological effects are mediated through specific high-affinity cell surface receptors without involvement of cAMP or phosphatidylinositol hydrolysis. Insulin receptors are integral membrane glycoproteins composed of two α subunits (M_r 130,000), which contain the insulin binding sites, and two β subunits (M_r 90,000), which have intrinsic tyrosine kinase activity. One of the earliest responses to the binding of insulin is autophosphorylation of tyrosine residues on the β subunit. This event increases the kinase activity of the insulin receptor and renders it independent of insulin. The biological effects of insulin are caused by phosphorylation of various cellular proteins by the tyrosine kinase activity of the insulin receptor. The insulin receptor also is susceptible to phosphorylation on serine and threonine residues by action of protein kinase A, protein kinase C, and possibly other kinases. Phosphorylation of these residues in general decreases both the autophosphorylation and tyrosine kinase activity of the insulin receptor, thus downregulating its activity. Receptor is inactivated by dephosphorylation of tyrosine residues by phosphatase enzymes.

The phosphorylation mechanism of receptor activation has been demonstrated for the receptors of epidermal growth factor, platelet-derived growth factor, and IGF-I. In the case of insulin, IGF-I, and other growth factors, the initial phophorylation event leads to a cascade of events orchestrated through insulin-responsive substrates (IRS). Whereas insulin and IGFs both can phosphorylate IRS-I and IRS-II, IRS-I is mainly involved in insulin action and IRS-II primarily in IGF action. These IRS molecules cause activation of two major pathways of signal transduction—the mitogen-activated kinase (MAP-K) pathway and the PI3-Akt pathway. Both of these signaling cascades rely on serial phosphorylation events.

Phosphatidylinositol 3-kinase (PI3K) has a central role in a broad range of biological effects. The PI3K-Akt pathway is a potent mediator of cell survival signals. On binding of growth factors and autophosphorylation of receptor kinases, binding sites for PI3K are produced in their cytoplasmic domains, thus recruiting active PI3K to the inner surface of the plasma membrane. There PI3K acts on membrane phosphoinositides to generate phosphatidylinositol-3,4-bisphosphate and phosphatidylinositol-3,4,5-triphosphate. These phospholipids are foci for recruiting and activating a number of signaling proteins to the membrane. Among these proteins are the serine-threonine kinases of the *Akt* family (*Akt*-1, *Akt*-2 and *Akt*-3, collectively called *Akt*), which are critical regulators of apoptosis. The tumor-suppressor gene *PTEN* functions as a lipid phosphatase and specifically antagonizes the action of PI3K. Loss of *PTEN* in tumors leads to deregulation of the PI3K pathway and unregulated activation of *Akt*. As a result, PTEN-deficient tumor cells may be protected from apoptosis. Therefore it is likely that deregulated PI3K *Akt* contributes to tumorigenesis in a large number of tumors among humans.

Another unique signaling cascade is the JAK-STAT pathway. Typical of GH and cytokine signaling, the janus-activated kinases (JAK) phosphorylate a corresponding family member of the signal transducers and activators of transcription (STAT), which migrates to the nucleus and influences gene transcription. The TGF-β receptor superfamily activates a family of second messengers called Smads, which modulate transcription by migrating into the nucleus and acting directly as part of the transcriptional machinery.

A unique signaling mechanism activated by the tumor necrosis factor (TNF) receptor family is conversion of sphingomyelin into ceramide. Ceramide is an essential molecule in the activation of caspases, which cause apoptosis. Ceramide activates ceramide-activated protein phosphatase, which is key to TNF-induced apoptosis.

REGULATION OF RECEPTOR PROPERTIES

The binding activity of many receptors is subject to regulation by homologous hormone, other hormones, or metabolic influences. The most common pattern is negative ("down") regulation of the concentration of receptor by the homologous hormone. This occurs for insulin, growth hormone (GH), thyrotropin-releasing hormone (TRH), catecholamines, gonadotropins, glucagon, ACTH, and the steroid hormones. Positive ("up") regulation of receptor number also occurs in some instances. Angiotensin II increases its own receptors in adrenal glomerulosa cells, and prolactin may increase its receptors in liver cells.

For membrane receptors, the mechanism of negative regulation by homologous ligands appears to involve both phosphorylation and internalization of a receptor. Binding of hormone enhances the mobility of a receptor within cell membranes and the formation of receptor clusters that then undergo endocytosis. Thus continued occupancy of receptors by ligand causes receptor inactivation (uncoupling) or degradation with subsequent desensitization of the cell to hormone. This process is reversed on removal of the hormone as newly synthesized receptor reaches the plasma membrane. Negative regulation of receptors as a mechanism for reducing responsiveness in the presence of high hormone concentration may be biologically advantageous. In hyperinsulinemia, for example, reduced sensitivity of peripheral tissues to insulin would blunt the hypoglycemic effect.

The secretion of many hormones is pulsatile rather than continuous. In the case of hypothalamic releasing hormones, for example, episodic secretion under the influence of pulse generator neurons is a potent stimulus for secretion of pituitary hormones. In contrast, continuous infusion of releasing hormones inhibits secretion of pituitary hormones by down-regulating receptors in the pituitary gland. This regulatory event provides the basis for management of true precocious puberty. Injection of a potent, long-acting agonist of luteinizing hormone-releasing factor suppresses gonadotropin secretion and controls the physical manifestations of precocious puberty among children.

Negative regulation of receptor function through reduced binding affinity apparently occurs with insulin. Binding in this system displays negative cooperativity, meaning that binding of insulin to receptor decreases the affinity of other binding sites for subsequent insulin molecules. Metabolic influences can affect either binding affinity or receptor number. For example, low pH decreases the affinity of insulin receptors, and sodium depletion increases angiotensin-II receptors in the adrenal glands.

Receptors can be affected by heterologous hormones. β-Adrenergic receptor concentration is increased by thyroid hormone in the heart and by glucocorticoids in the lung. Muscarinic receptor agonists promote desensitization of β-adrenergic receptors in the heart, acting through stimulation of protein kinase C, which phosphorylates β-adrenergic receptors and impairs interaction with G proteins. Estrogen regulates adrenergic receptors, angiotensin II, and progesterone receptors in the uterus; receptors for progesterone and prolactin in the mammary glands; and androgen receptors

TABLE 24-1

DISEASES INVOLVING ALTERATIONS OF HORMONE RECEPTORS

DISEASE	RECEPTOR ABNORMALITY
Nuclear Receptors	
Some cases of type 2 diabetes mellitus	PPAR mutations leading to insulin resistance
Vitamin D–resistant rickets	Vitamin D receptor
Testicular feminization	Androgen receptor
Generalized resistance to thyroid hormone	Thyroid receptor
Primary cortisol resistance	Glucocorticoid receptor
Membrane Receptors	
Laron dwarfism	Growth hormone receptor
Pseudohypoparathyroidism	Parathyroid hormone receptor and associated G protein
Leprechaunism	Insulin receptor
Growth hormone deficiency	GHRH receptor
Nephrogenic diabetes insipidus	Vasopressin receptor
Obesity	Leptin receptor
Familial glucocorticoid deficiency	ACTH receptor
Activating Mutations	
Hyperinsulinism	Sulfonylurea receptor
McCune-Albright syndrome	G protein mutations affecting gonadotropin and other hormone signaling
Testotoxicosis	Constitutively activated luteinizing hormone receptor
Familial benign hypocalciuric hypercalcemia and hyperparathyroidism	Mutations in the calcium-sensing receptor
Congenital nonautoimmune hyperthyroidism	Thyroid-stimulating hormone receptor activating mutations

PPAR = peroxisome proliferator activating receptor; GHRH = growth hormone-releasing hormone; ACTH = adrenocorticotropin hormone.

in the oviducts of chicks. Glucocorticoids decrease receptors for $1,25(OH)_2$ vitamin D in bone cells, which is perhaps in part responsible for the osteopenia of long-term glucocorticoid therapy. Hormones can cross-react with other receptors. This occurs in particular with protein hormones that have a high degree of structural homology. Examples include ACTH binding to melanocyte-stimulating hormone receptors (causing skin darkening), chorionic gonadotropin binding to the same receptor as luteinizing hormone (LH), chorionic somatomammotropin interaction with both GH and prolactin receptors, insulin binding to IGF receptors (and causing acanthosis nigricans), and cross-binding of vasopressin and oxytocin to their receptors. Cross-reactivity also can occur with steroid hormones, but this is generally limited to pharmacologic concentrations of hormone. Antihormonal compounds have been synthesized that bind to receptor and act as an antagonist by preventing DNA binding. Examples include tamoxifen (anti-estrogen) and RU-486 (anti-progesterone and anti-glucocorticoid).

RECEPTORS AND DISEASE

Resistance to hormones, defined as a defect in responsiveness of target tissues to a hormone, occurs at several levels. Endocrine abnormalities at the prereceptor level usually involve abnormal hormones. Because of the critical role of receptors in hormone action, it is not surprising that a number of diseases involve a defect in the

receptor mechanism that can be either inherited or acquired. Table 24-1 lists some of those diseases caused by receptor mutations.

The most common alterations involve diminished receptor affinity for the hormonal ligand. Examples are mutations in the androgen receptor causing testicular feminization or in the GH receptor causing Laron syndrome, which is indistinguishable from GH deficiency. Some patients with severe insulin resistance have various point mutations in the insulin receptor, which account for loss of function and development of diabetes. Mutation in PPARγ can also cause insulin resistance and diabetes. Other diseases are caused by activating mutations in receptors. Examples of this include testotoxicosis, which involves the LH receptor and congenital hyperinsulinism caused by activating mutations in the sulfonylurea receptor. Another type of alteration involves the presence of antibodies to receptors. In the case of Graves disease, anti-TSH receptor antibodies (LATS) mimic the action of thyroid stimulating hormone (TSH) and increase production of thyroid hormones. Antibodies to receptor block neuromuscular transmission in myasthenia gravis and prevent insulin binding in a form of insulin-resistant diabetes. It is likely that additional diseases will be shown to involve alteration in receptor number or function caused by mutations, protein modification, or antibodies.

References

Bazzoni F, Beutler B: The tumor necrosis factor ligand and receptor families. N Engl J Med 334:1717, 1996

Brown EM, Pollak M, Seidman JG, Chou YH, Riccardi D, Hebert SC: Calcium-ion sensing cell-surface receptors. N Engl J Med 333:234, 1995

Ihle JN: Cytokine receptor signalling. Nature 377:591, 1995

Ji TH, Grossmann M, Ji I: G protein-coupled receptors: I. diversity of receptor-ligand interactions. J Biol Chem 273:17299, 1998

Lowell BB: PPARγ: an essential regulator of adipogenesis and modulator of fat cell function. Cell 99:239, 1999

Schillace RV, Scott JD: Organization of kinases, phosphatases, and receptor complexes. J Clin Invest 103:761, 1999

Virkamaki A, Ueki K, Kahn CR: Protein-protein interaction in insulin signaling and the molecular mechanisms of insulin resistance. J Clin Invest 103:931, 1999

24.2 DISORDERS OF THE ANTERIOR PITUITARY GLAND, HYPOTHALAMUS, AND GROWTH

Edward O. Reiter and A. Joseph D'Ercole

24.2.1. Physiology of the Anterior Pituitary Gland and Hypothalamus

The anterior pituitary is crucial for normal growth, sexual maturation, and endocrine function. The pituitary integrates, mediates, and modulates the influence of the brain and the hypothalamus on the endocrine system (Fig. 24-3). The hypothalamus regulates anterior pituitary function by synthesizing small peptides that either promote or inhibit pituitary hormone secretion (Table 24-2). Release of these factors is controlled in part by central nervous system neurotransmitters, such as dopamine, norepinephrine, serotonin,

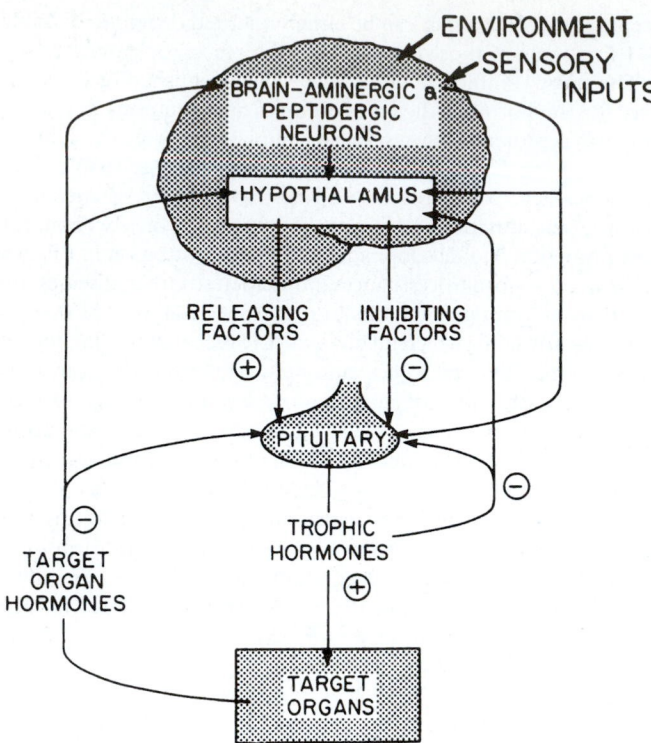

FIGURE 24-3 Brain-hypothalamic-pituitary-target organ axis. This schema depicts the complex regulatory interrelations among brain neurotransmitters and peptides, hypothalamic releasing and inhibiting factors, pituitary trophic hormones, and target organ hormones. *Arrows* indicate the avenues of regulation. Signs (+ or −) indicate whether the effect is stimulatory or inhibitory, respectively. Negative feedback of target gland hormones is illustrated by the *arrows on the left*. The short and ultra-short-loop negative feedback mechanism is illustrated on the *right* by the inhibitory effects of trophic hormones on secretions from the hypothalamus.

and endogenous opioids. They are then carried by the hypothalamic-hypophyseal portal circulation to anterior pituitary cells, where they act. Pituitary hormones can modulate their own secretion by affecting secretion of hypothalamic peptides or by acting directly on the pituitary glands. These phenomena are called *short* and *ultra-short* feedback loops, respectively (see Fig. 24-3). The peripheral endocrine glands, whose secretion of hormones is stimulated by pituitary trophic hormones, also exert negative feedback on anterior pituitary function at the level of the hypothalamus, the pituitary gland, or both. Through these exquisitely sensitive and complex interactions, the anterior pituitary gland regulates much of the endocrine milieu of the body.

EMBRYOLOGY AND DEVELOPMENT

The anterior pituitary gland is derived from evagination of ectodermal cells in the roof of the primitive oral cavity, whereas the posterior pituitary gland (neurohypophysis) is derived from neural cells in the floor of the third ventricle. A complex cascade of homeobox genes encode multiple transcription factors that direct temporal and anatomic development of the gland. The pituitary gland is housed at the base of the brain in the sella turcica, a cavity of the sphenoid bone. It is connected by a stalk to the hypothalamus and separated from the brain by a reflection of the dura mater. The hypothalamic-releasing and -inhibiting factors reach the anterior pituitary gland through the hypothalamic-hypophyseal portal cir-

culation. At its source in the floor of the hypothalamus, this vascular system is a dense network of arterioles and capillaries. In the pituitary stalk it is composed of portal veins that drain into sinusoidal capillaries in the anterior pituitary gland. Arterial blood derived from branches of the internal carotid artery brings to the pituitary gland the modulating signals from distant endocrine organs as well as the nutrient and oxygen supply.

ANTERIOR PITUITARY HORMONES: SYNTHESIS, STRUCTURE, AND REGULATION

The anterior pituitary gland is composed of five major classes of secretory cells defined by the hormone that they predominantly synthesize. Traditional staining methods do not define reliably the hormone product of individual cells. In general, however, somatotropins (cells that secrete growth hormone) and mammotropins (cells that secrete prolactin) are the more numerous acidophilic staining cells. Corticotropins, thyrotropins, and gonadotropins exhibit basophilic staining. Somatotropins and lactotropins arise from

TABLE 24-2

HYPOTHALAMIC PEPTIDES INVOLVED IN REGULATION OF ANTERIOR PITUITARY HORMONE SECRETION

Growth hormone-releasing hormone, growth hormone-releasing factor (GHRH, GRF)	Three molecular forms containing 44, 40, or 37 amino acids; IV injection causes serum growth hormone (GH) level to increase within minutes; poor GH response among elderly persons
Somatostatin, somatotropin release-inhibiting factor	Inhibits GH secretion; 14 amino acid residues; member of a family of somatostatin-like peptides that are widely distributed in the body and have varied effects. These include inhibition of thyroid-stimulating hormone (TSH) and insulin secretion, inhibition of secretion of a variety of gastrointestinal hormones, and direct effects on the digestive tract
Thyrotropin-releasing hormone (TRH, TRF)	A tripeptide; stimulates release of TSH and prolactin secretion, although the physiological importance of the latter is not known. Present in tissues other than the hypothalamus and has a variety of effects on central nervous system function
Corticotropin-releasing hormone (CRH, CRF)	41 Amino acids; glucocorticoids inhibit CRH secretion by the hypothalamus and response of pituitary gland to CRH
Gonadotropin-releasing hormone (GnRH), luteinizing hormone-releasing hormone (LHRH)	A decapeptide; stimulates secretion of both LH and follicle-stimulating hormone (FSH); the FSH response to GnRH is selectively inhibited by inhibin, a gonadal hormone; LH responses to GnRH are absent or poor before puberty but increase with the onset of puberty

the same precursor cell. Differentiation requires expression of at least two specific transcription factors, PIT-1 (also called GH factor I, or GHF-1) and PROP-1. Defects in the regulation of somatotropin differentiation also cause TSH deficiency, indicating that thyrotropin differentiation and function are regulated in part by the same transcription factors. Gonadotropins and corticotropins differentiate by independent mechanisms, although children with PROP-1 gene abnormalities may have hypogonadotropic hypogonadism that is evident at puberty.

The pituitary hormones are synthesized as precursor molecules. Preprohormones, the products of mRNA translation, contain an amino terminal amino acid sequence called a *leader* or *signal sequence,* which directs the protein to its intracellular site of storage. The hormone is usually stored as a prohormone. During transport through the secretory pathway, precursor molecules are processed by various proteolytic cleavages into smaller proteins that usually are the biologically active substances. For example, pro-opiomelanocortin is an mRNA translation product cleaved in corticotropins to ACTH and β-lipotropin. ACTH can be further cleaved to β-melanotropin, and β-lipotropin can be processed to β-endorphin and γ-lipotropin, although the latter is present only to a limited degree in corticotropins. The latter processing steps, however, are the norm in the intermediate lobes of lower animals, where α-melanocyte-stimulating hormone and β-endorphin are the major gene products. Processing of the same precursor molecules, therefore, can be different in different cells.

Thyrotropin, LH, and follicle-stimulating hormone are glycoproteins (contain carbohydrate moieties) and share a common α-chain subunit (Table 24-3). The β-subunit of each hormone is distinct and confers biological and immunologic specificity. The

TABLE 24-3
HUMAN ANTERIOR PITUITARY HORMONES

Peptides

Growth hormone (GH)	191 Amino acids, single chain
Prolactin	198 Amino acids (homologous with GH)
Proopiomelanocortin is cleaved to:	
ACTH	39 Amino acids
Secondarily cleaved to:	13 Amino acids (ACTH 1–13)
α-Melanotropin	
CLIP peptide	
Lipotropin (LPH)	22 Amino acids (ACTH 18–39)
Secondarily cleaved to:	
β-Endorphin	31 Amino acids (β LPH 61–91)
γ-Lipotropin	58 Amino acids (β LPH 1–58)
β-Melanotropin	18 Amino acids (β LPH 41–58)
Glycoproteins	
α Subunit is common to each hormone and has 96 amino acids plus carbohydrate moieties; β subunit confers specificity	
Follicle-stimulating hormone	α Subunit and a 115-amino-acid β subunit; 32% carbohydrate by weight
Luteinizing hormone	α Subunit and a 115-amino-acid β subunit; 16% carbohydrate
Thyroid-stimulating hormone (thyrotropin)	α Subunit and a 112-amino-acid β subunit; 16% carbohydrate

CLIP = corticotropin-like intermediate lobe peptide; ACTH = adrenocorticotropin hormone.

hypothalamic-pituitary gonadol hormones are discussed in Sec. 24.8.2.

GROWTH HORMONE AND INSULIN-LIKE GROWTH FACTOR AXIS

Growth hormone, a major promoter of anabolism, is a single-chain peptide with three intrachain disulfide bonds that contain 191 amino acids. Growth hormone stimulates RNA and protein synthesis in the liver and in many other tissues. Among the proteins synthesis of which is stimulated by GH are IGF-I and IGF-II, or somatomedins that mediate many of the growth-promoting effects of GH. The name *somatomedin* was coined to describe peptides induced by GH that promote cellular proliferation in cartilage and other peripheral tissues. Two somatomedin (IGF) peptides circulate in serum, and each has structural homology (~40%) with proinsulin. Similarities with insulin in structure and function led to the use of the name *insulin-like growth factor.* Somatomedin-C (IGF-I) is a 7650-Da basic peptide that is markedly GH dependent. Growth hormone regulates synthesis of IGF-I at the transcriptional level, with the result that blood levels of IGF-I vary depending on GH secretory status. They are low in hypopituitarism and high in acromegaly. Insulin-like growth factor II, a neutral 7471-Da peptide, is only partially dependent on GH. Its serum concentrations are decreased modestly in states of GH deficiency, but they are not elevated in acromegaly. The influence of GH on IGF-II is at least partly at the level of mRNA abundance.

The insulin-like actions of each IGF include stimulation of glucose uptake and oxidation (actions opposite to those stimulated by GH). These actions are caused partly by the insulin-like structure of these substances, which allows interaction with the cell surface receptor for insulin. Both IGFs primarily interact with another receptor called the type 1 IGF receptor. This receptor is structurally similar to the insulin receptor and can mediate insulin-like actions in addition to signaling the events involved in cell proliferation. Insulin-like growth factor II also binds to a distinct receptor that is identical to the cation-independent mannose-6-phosphate receptor. This receptor does not appear to mediate the growth promoting actions of IGF-I but facilitates the uptake of IGF-II and its transport to lysosomes for degradation.

Because IGFs are synthesized in almost all tissues and their receptors are ubiquitous, it is believed that they may act on target tissues by autocrine or paracrine mechanisms, as well as by classic endocrine mechanisms. The liver appears to be the primary source of the IGFs that circulate in the blood.

In serum, IGFs are bound to several high-molecular-weight carrier or binding proteins (IGFBPs). Most IGF circulates in a complex of 150,000-Da that contains a 53,000-Da binding protein, called IGFBP-3, and a separate, acid-labile protein. Three low-molecular-weight IGF-binding proteins, IGFBP-1, IGFBP-2, and IGFBP-4, also appear in the blood. IGFBPs increase the concentrations of IGF in the blood and prevent rapid fluctuations. These IGFBPs also affect the action of IGF, by means of inhibiting it to make the IGF unavailable for interaction with the type 1 receptor or by augmenting the action, possibly by delivering IGFs to the type 1 receptor. In some circumstances, IGFBPs alter cell function through direct action on their own distinct membrane receptors.

Plasma IGF-I concentrations are relatively low early in life and increase through childhood to values at puberty that are two to three times those of healthy adults. Values decline through adult life. There is minimal diurnal variation in IGF-I level, and values do not fluctuate dramatically in response to eating or other daily activities. Some IGFBPs are regulated by nutritional changes and insulin secretion (eg, IGFBP-1 and IGFBP-2). The result is modest diurnal changes in concentration of circulating IGF-I.

The two major known regulators of IGF-I are GH and nutritional status. Values of IGF-I are low among patients with GH deficiency and elevated among persons with GH excess. Although helpful in the diagnosis of GH deficiency, low serum IGF-I concentration cannot be used to confirm a diagnosis, because levels also are decreased in malnutrition, hypothyroidism, prolonged fasting, and a variety of chronic illnesses, many of which can cause growth failure. Measurement of IGF-I is useful for detecting GH excess caused by GH-secreting pituitary tumors and for monitoring the response of such patients to therapy. Results of studies with human subjects suggest that both dietary energy and proteins are important in the maintenance of IGF-I level and in restoring this peptide among persons with malnutrition. IGFBP-3 also is regulated by GH and can be measured to give an indirect indication of GH secretion and action.

Regulation of GH secretion is extraordinarily complex and includes a variety of endogenous diurnal rhythms, as well as external influences, presumed to be mediated by the central nervous system and integrated by the hypothalamus. Growth hormone, like other pituitary hormones, has a relatively short half-life in serum (20 to 25 minutes). Therefore blood must be sampled frequently to detect secretory surges. Large amounts of GH are released normally within 1 hour of the onset of deep sleep. Other surges occur 2 to 3 hours after eating and in response to vigorous exercise and physical and emotional stress. Each of these secretory bursts is probably mediated by hypothalamic release of GH-releasing hormone (GHRH), which is regulated by neurotransmitters emanating from higher central nervous system centers. The predominant influence of the hypothalamus on the pituitary gland is stimulatory. Somatostatin (somatotropin-release inhibitory factor) is produced by the hypothalamus in response to influences such as hyperglycemia and elevation of free fatty acids and inhibits GH secretion by the pituitary gland. Negative feedback is important in inhibiting GH release. Specifically, GH and IGF-I stimulate the release of somatostatin by the hypothalamus and thereby inhibit GH release. Insulin-like growth factor I also appears to inhibit stimulation of GH release by GHRH at the level of the pituitary gland. A putative hypothalamic peptide, GH-releasing peptide may also act on specific pituitary or hypothalamic receptors to enhance GH secretion. The hormonal milieu of the pituitary gland also modulates many of the aforementioned regulatory influences. For example, estrogens, testosterone, or thyroid hormone enhances the magnitude of GH release, whereas glucocorticoids may have the opposite effect.

PROLACTIN

Human prolactin is a 198-amino-acid protein homologous with GH. It is stored in the pituitary gland in about 50-fold lower quantities than is GH. Prolactin is needed for milk production, but prolactin alone is not sufficient for this purpose. Estrogen, progesterone, and insulin, and perhaps other substances, are needed for the breast to respond to prolactin. Prolactin also may have other physiological roles, such as salt retention and inhibition of gonadal function.

Like GH, prolactin is released in surges and has a short half-life in the blood (15 to 20 minutes). Blood concentrations increase progressively during pregnancy (approximately tenfold) and decline after delivery. Suckling is an important stimulus to prolactin release.

It causes an immediate, dramatic increase in prolactin in the blood. Stress also stimulates prolactin secretion. Among nonpregnant, nonlactating persons, the level of prolactin in the blood increases during sleep. This surge of prolactin occurs later and is more prolonged than that of GH.

Unlike other pituitary hormones, which are secreted under the influence of releasing factors, the main regulatory mode of prolactin is tonic inhibition of secretion. Dopamine appears to be the main factor responsible for inhibiting prolactin secretion, although γ-aminobutyric acid also produces this effect. Although TRH injected intravenously stimulates prolactin secretion, the physiological importance of TRH in regulating prolactin secretion in humans is uncertain.

24.2.2 Overview of Normal Growth

Growth is a complex process that involves the interaction of multiple, diverse factors and represents the sum of these influences on cell replication and programmed cell death, called *apoptosis*, as well as on cell differentiation. Growth is ultimately governed by the genome of a person and its interactions with external factors, such as nutrition and psychosocial well-being. Despite the complexity, healthy children grow linearly in a remarkably predictable manner. Change from a normal growth pattern often is the first manifestation of a disease, either an endocrine or a nonendocrine disorder that can involve almost any organ system. Frequent and accurate assessment of growth therefore is of primary importance in the care of children.

CHARACTER OF NORMAL GROWTH

Growth rates differ during intrauterine life, early and middle childhood, and adolescence. Growth ceases after fusion of long bone and vertebral epiphyses. During gestation, growth averages 1.2 to 1.5 cm per week but increases dramatically to a midgestational peak of 2.5 cm per week with a decline to 0.5 cm per week immediately before birth. Growth velocity during the first 2 years of life averages about 15 cm per year and slows to approximately 6 cm per year during middle childhood. Pubertal growth begins earlier among girls than among boys but is 3 to 5 cm greater in magnitude among boys than among girls. The peak height velocity during the pubertal growth spurt is similar to the rate of growth during the second year of life (7 to 11 cm/yr). The time of onset of puberty and consequently the age at the pubertal growth spurt varies among healthy children. On average girls complete puberty earlier than do boys and thus stop growing earlier (at 14 to 15 years of age compared with 16 to 17 years for boys). This accounts for the approximately 13-cm difference in the adult heights of women and men. A delay in the onset of puberty appears to be more common among boys than among girls. Early onset of puberty is more common among girls. Nonetheless, among most healthy children, final height is not influenced by the chronologic time of onset of the pubertal growth spurt.

Because heredity is an important determinant of growth, it is important to relate a patient's height to that of siblings and parents. Tanner and associates developed a method by which stature of children can be assessed relative to midparental height. Mean parental height is calculated, and 6.5 cm is added for boys or subtracted for girls. The 2-SD range for this calculated parental target height is approximately 10 cm. Although this is a rough approximation, the possibility of an underlying pathologic condition is considered when a child's growth pattern clearly deviates from that of the parents.

MEASUREMENTS

Accurate height measurements are necessary for the evaluation of growth. Measurement of supine length should be used for children younger than 2 years and erect height for older children. Supine length can be readily determined in a box constructed with an inflexible board against which the head is placed and a movable footboard on which the feet are placed perpendicular to the plane of the supine length of the infant. Under ideal conditions, the child is relaxed, the legs are fully extended, and the head is positioned so that a perpendicular plane to the long axis of the trunk is made by a line connecting the outer canthus of the eyes and the external auditory meatus. This is called the *Frankfurt plane.*

For older children who are physically capable, standing or erect height is measured with a wall-mounted device. The traditional measuring device with a flexible arm mounted to a weight balance is notoriously unreliable and should be avoided. As with supine length, the position of the child is crucial to accuracy and reproducibility. The child should be fully erect with heels together, with the head in the Frankfurt plane, and the back of the head, thoracic spine, buttocks, and heels should touch the measuring device. An effort should be made to correct discrepancies related to lordosis or scoliosis. Because erect height undergoes day-time lowering, serial measurements ideally should be made at the same time of day.

Length and height are measured in triplicate by a trained person. The variation should be no more than 0.3 cm, and the mean of the measurements should be recorded. To estimate height velocity, two measurements (preferably made by the same person) no less than 4 months apart should be used. Even when every effort is made to obtain accurate height measurements, measurement every 9 to 12 months is preferable to minimize error.

ASSESSMENT OF MEASUREMENTS (USE OF GROWTH CHARTS)

Once obtained, growth data must be evaluated against normal standards. Most US pediatric clinics use charts that are derived from cross-sectional data; that is, data from a large population in which each person is measured once. These charts allow comparison of an individual child's growth with that of a normal US population graphically displayed in percentiles. When applied to an individual child, however, these charts have the following limitations: (1) children below the third or above the 97th percentiles, for whom there is the most concern, are not well defined, and (2) because differences in the timing and tempo of the onset and progression of puberty influence normal growth rates, evaluation of growth during adolescence can be misleading. Such data are most useful in computing standard deviation scores (SDSs), because a short child can be quantitatively described as, for example −4.2 or −2.5 SDS from normal. Height SDS for age is calculated as follows: SDS equals height minus mean height for healthy children at this age and sex divided by the SD of height for healthy children at this age and sex. Because these values are defined by cross-sectional data, however, childhood SDSs are not directly comparable with SDS during adolescence, when variation in growth rate and maturational tempo can be large. To address this issue, Tanner and colleagues developed growth charts combining longitudinal data to construct the curve shapes with percentile widths obtained in a large cross-sectional survey, thus accounting for variability in the timing of puberty.

The data from cross-sectional and longitudinal growth studies have been used to develop height velocity standards. It is important to emphasize that carefully documented height velocity data are invaluable in assessing a child for abnormalities of growth. Although there is considerable variability in normal height velocity among children of different ages, between the age of 2 years and the onset of puberty, children normally grow with remarkable fidelity relative to the normal growth curves. Any crossing of height percentiles during this age period warrant further evaluation.

Standardized US growth charts for clinical use can be downloaded from the Centers for Disease Control and Prevention at (www.cdc.gov/growthcharts). Syndrome-specific growth curves have been developed for a number of clinical conditions associated with growth failure, such as Turner syndrome, achondroplasia, and Down syndrome. These growth profiles are invaluable for tracking the growth of children with these disorders. Deviation of growth from the appropriate growth curve suggests a second underlying cause.

24.2.3   Approach to the Evaluation of Aberrant Growth

When disorders of linear growth appear to be caused by abnormalities intrinsic to the growth plate, they are called *primary growth abnormalities. Secondary growth disorders* refer to growth failure caused by chronic disease or endocrine disorders. The approach to evaluation of the child with poor growth is also discussed in Sec. 1.1.2, and the approach to the child with failure to gain weight is discussed in Sec. 17.5.1. Deficiency of growth hormone is discussed in Sec. 24.2.4 and other endocrine causes of growth retardation in Sec. 24.2.5. The term *idiopathic short stature* usually refers to variants of normal growth, such as constitutional delay of growth and maturation and genetic short stature. Evaluation of a child with growth failure requires consideration of all of these potential etiologic factors. Clues to causes are provided by the growth pattern, medical history, and physical examination. There are no universally accepted criteria to evaluate children for growth failure, but evaluation is considered for the following patients:

- Any child whose height is more than 3 SD below the mean height for age. Three SD below the mean value for age can be approximated by means of measuring the vertical distance on a growth chart from the mean to the third percentile (−2SD) and multiplying this value by 1.5.
- Any child, regardless of absolute height, with a subnormal growth rate that is falling away from the normal growth channel.
- Any child whose height percentile clearly differs from that of midparental height.

If a child meets these criteria, the evaluation includes a complete medical history with a genetic pedigree and documentation of the stature of ancestors and a search for evidence of perinatal insult. Adequacy of diet; stooling and urination patterns; presence of symptoms of respiratory, gastrointestinal, and infectious disease; and headaches and other symptoms suggestive of an intracranial lesion are determined. Specific attention is focused on the medical and social history during periods in which growth failure occurred.

In the physical examination the child's weight and height are compared. Among children who are underweight for height, a chronic systemic disease is more likely than is hypopituitarism or an endocrine abnormality. An endocrine disorder is more likely among short children whose weight percentile is greater than height percentile. Evidence of disproportionate body segments suggests a disorder such as a chondrodysplasia. In this regard other measurements of the body are useful. They include occipitofrontal head circumference, lower body segment or distance from top of pubic symphysis to the floor, upper body segment or sitting height (height of stool is subtracted from standing height), and arm span. Published standards for these body proportion measurements show the age-related changes. For example, the upper to lower segment ratio drops from 1.7 for neonates to slightly less than 1.0 for adults.

If no diagnostic clues are forthcoming from the history and physical examination, selected laboratory tests are performed to screen for some of the silent causes of growth failure (Table 24-4). Although it has no specific diagnostic value, radiography of the hand and wrist to assess "bone age" is useful because it provides a reflection of somatic maturity. It is useful in determining the potential for growth and can help in assessing the time when growth retardation began. The ossification centers of the left hand and wrist appear and progress in a predictable sequence in healthy children, thus they can be compared with the normal age and sex standards of Greulich and Pyle. Skeletal age in hypopituitarism usually is delayed in conformity with height age.

Plasma levels of IGF-I and IGFBP-3, which are GH-dependent, are measured before complete pituitary function testing is undertaken (Fig. 24-4). A normal IGF-I concentration renders GH deficiency unlikely. A low value does not prove GH deficiency, because such values occur in malnutrition, hypothyroidism, and other chronic illnesses. In general, the same holds for IGFBP-3. Nonetheless, abnormal values of these GH-dependent peptides strongly suggest either GH deficiency or resistance to GH action. Children who fulfill growth criteria and for whom history, physical examination, and laboratory screening tests yield no clues other than low

TABLE 24-4
SCREENING TESTS FOR CHILDREN WITH GROWTH FAILURE

TEST	PURPOSE
Complete blood cell count with erythrocyte sedimentation rate (ESR)	Screening test for inflammatory bowel disease with anemia and elevated ESR
Renal function tests (urine, pH, and specific gravity, urea nitrogen, serum creatinine, carbon dioxide, and electrolytes)	Exclude chronic renal failure with acidosis; exclude renal tubular disease
Serum calcium, phosphorus, and alkaline phosphatase	Screening tests for rickets
Serum free thyroxine and thyroid-stimulating hormone	Exclude hypothyroidism not apparent at physical examination
IGF-I and IGFBP-3	Growth hormone deficiency unlikely if normal
Anti-endomysial antibody, serum IgA or anti-*trans*-glutaminase antibody	Exclude celiac disease
Karyotype (girls only)	Exclude Turner syndrome not apparent at physical examination
Radiographs of hand and wrist	Determine bone age, which is delayed in hypopituitarism and most other causes of growth failure; sometimes not delayed in bone dysplasia

IGF = insulin-like growth factor; IGFBP = IGF-binding protein.

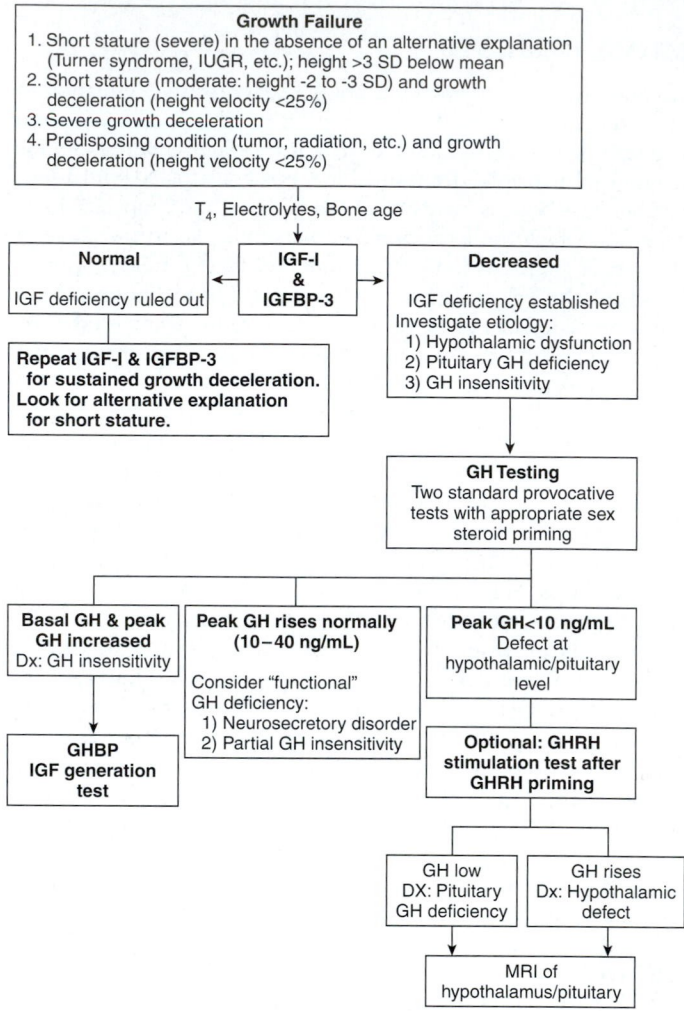

BIOCHEMICAL EVALUATION OF GROWTH FAILURE

FIGURE 24-4 Biochemical assessment of a child with growth failure. Primary screening evaluation is to establish IGF deficiency. Subsequent studies localize causation at hypothalamic or pituitary dysfunction or GH resistance. SOURCE: (*Reiter EO, Rosenfeld RG: In: Wilson DW, Foster JD, Kronenberg HN, Larsen PR, eds.: Textbook of Endocrinology, 9th ed. Philadelphia, Saunders, 1998:1474.*)

or borderline levels of the GH-dependent peptides can undergo pituitary function testing. Figure 24-4 outlines the approach to further evaluation.

Because GH is secreted episodically, adequacy of GH production cannot be determined with random blood samples. It is necessary to measure GH frequently over many hours or to assess the GH response to provocative stimuli.

To assess GH secretion, most physicians perform two or more pharmacologic provocative tests (Table 24-5), because failure to respond to a single stimulus is not sufficient evidence to confirm the diagnosis of GH deficiency. Determining which short children have GH deficiency and which children are to be treated with GH is difficult, because the severity of GH deficiency forms a continuum between complete and modest partial deficiency. Furthermore, values obtained with any single test may not reflect true GH secretory capacity. Although maximal poststimulus serum GH values of 7 to 10 ng/mL or less have generally been accepted as evidence of impaired GH secretion, most physicians accept that these

TABLE 24-5

CLINICAL TESTS OF GROWTH HORMONE SECRETION

TEST	TEST CONDITIONS	TIME OF GROWTH HORMONE RESPONSE
Screening tests		
Exercise	Patient should be fasting; 15 min moderate exercise, then 5 min vigorous exercise	20–40 min after exercise is begun
Sleep	Increase in GH level occurs with deep sleep (EEG stages 3,4); with EEG monitoring and frequent sampling, can be used as a more definitive test	Initial peak within 1 h after onset of deep sleep; awaken patient for sample
Formal tests		
Insulin	Regular cyrstalline insulin, 0.05–0.1 U/kg IV; 50% decrease in blood sugar is necessary for adequate test; lowest blood sugar occurs 20–30 min after insulin is given	45–75 min
Arginine	L-Arginine monohydrochloride, 5–10% solution, 0.5 g/kg (30 g for adults) infused over 30 min	60–120 min
L-Dopa	0.5 g/1.73 m² by mouth. Growth hormone responses often are improved by administering priming doses of 0.25 g/1.73 m² of L-dopa for 1 or more days before test dose	45–120 min
Glucagon	0.03 mg/kg IM or SC (maximum of 1 mg)	120–180 min
Clonidine	4 μg/kg by mouth	60–120 min
Propranolol (used to augment responses to primary stimuli)	30–40 mg (children 0.75 mg/kg) by mouth 30-60 min before glucagon, insulin, arginine, L-dopa, or exercise tests	As with primary stimuli
Estrogen	Used to "prime" the patient to improve the GH response	As with primary stimuli

GH = growth hormone; EEG = electroencephalogram.
SOURCE: *Modified from Underwood LE, Van Wyk JJ: In Wilson JD, Foster DW, eds: Williams Textbook of Endocrinology, 8th ed. Philadelphia, Saunders, 1992, p 1120.*

cutoff values are arbitrary. Strict adherence to these values can lead to inappropriate treatment of some patients. Contrary to earlier opinions, it appears that measurement of GH with round-the-clock blood sampling is not a definitive diagnostic procedure.

Measurement of GH secretion in response to the injection of GRF has some diagnostic value. If the GH response is absent or minimal, GH deficiency is likely. The underlying lesion, however, could be pituitary or hypothalamic in origin, the latter occurring among patients who have not secreted enough endogenous GH to "prime" the GH-secreting cells of the pituitary gland. If, however, the GH response to GRF is normal in the presence of a deficient response to provocative stimuli, hypothalamic hypopituitarism caused by GRF deficiency is responsible for the GH deficiency. It is becoming increasingly apparent that tests for GH secretion are of modest value in diagnosing or excluding GH deficiency. Children who secrete GH normally may not secrete GH during testing, and children with deficiency may muster what appear to be good responses during testing. More emphasis therefore is being placed on auxologic data (height and growth rate) and measurements of indices of GH action, such as IGF-I and IGFBP-3. At this time, integrity of the GH-IGF axis usually is screened by means of measurement of IGF-I and IGFBP-3 with GH provocative tests to confirm secretory adequacy.

Table 24-6 lists tests useful in the complete evaluation of pituitary function. Children with isolated GH deficiency have normal serum thyroxine levels, and their TSH level does not differ from normal. ACTH deficiency can be evaluated by means of measuring cortisol in the serum and cortisol after injection of synthetic ACTH or by means of measuring 11-desoxycortisol response after administration of metyrapone. Abnormalities of gonadotropin secretion are difficult to detect before puberty. For most children proved to

have GH deficiency, it is almost impossible to predict whether they will enter puberty spontaneously.

Radiographs of the sella turcica can show enlargement of the sella, erosion of the sphenoid bone, or calcification from a craniopharyngioma. Approximately one-third of patients with idiopathic hypopituitarism have an abnormally small sella turcica, suggesting that the pituitary gland is small and hypofunctioning. Magnetic resonance (MR) imaging studies have shown characteristic developmental abnormalities in the hypothalamic-pituitary area.

24.2.4   Abnormalities of the Anterior Pituitary Gland and Hypothalamus

HYPOPITUITARISM WITH DEFICIENCY OF GROWTH HORMONE

Most children with deficient pituitary function secrete inadequate amounts of GH, therefore the term *hypopituitarism* is used interchangeably with GH deficiency. Children who have diabetes insipidus caused by isolated deficiency of antidiuretic hormone and those uncommon children who have isolated gonadotropin deficiency (Kallmann syndrome) are exceptions. They have normal GH secretion but have pituitary dysfunction. Deficiency of GH can occur alone (isolated GH deficiency) or in conjuction with overt deficiency of one or more other pituitary hormones (some physicians use the term *panhypopituitarism* to refer to multiple pituitary hormone deficiencies). Deficiency of GH is severe when no increase in GH level is measured in the serum after exposure to provocative stimuli and partial when modest GH responses can be elicited. Although there are exceptions, patients with multiple pituitary hor-

TABLE 24-6

TESTS OF PITUITARY FUNCTION USEFUL IN DETERMINING WHETHER A CHILD HAS HYPOPITUITARISM

PROCEDURE	INFORMATION OBTAINED
Magnetic resonance imaging	Presence of abnormalities of the hypothalamus and pituitary, associated brain anomalies
Serum level of IGF-I and IGFBP-3	GH secretion and action
Tests of GH secretion (eg, insulin-induced hypoglycemia, arginine, clonidine, L-dopa, sleep)	Direct measurement of GH secretory capacity (see Table 24-5); insulin-induced hypoglycemia for cortisol response to stress
GH response to GRF	Localization to hypothalamus or pituitary gland of a lesion causing impaired GH secretion
Basal serum concentration of cortisol and cortisol 45 min after injection of 0.25 mg cosyntropin	Assessment of basal adrenal function; response to ACTH is modulated by previous exposure of adrenal gland to endogenous ACTH
Serum 11-desoxycortisol response to metyrapone given orally	Integrity of hypothalamic-pituitary-adrenal axis
Serum total or free thyroxine	Presence of chemical hypothyroidism
TSH response to TRH given intravenously	Localization of lesion to hypothalamus or pituitary gland

IGF = insulin-like growth factor; IGFBP = IGF = binding protein; GH = growth hormone; GRF = growth hormone-releasing factor; ACTH = adrenocorticotropin hormone; TSH = thyroid-stimulating hormone; TRH = thyrotropin-releasing hormone.

monal deficiencies tend to have more severe GH deficiency. The incidence of GH deficiency is not known; the most accurate estimate is that it affects 1 in every 4000 school-age children. The congenital forms of multiple pituitary hormone deficiency occur three or four times more often among boys than among girls.

The causes of hypopituitarism with GH deficiency include hypothalamic disorders that impair secretion of GHRH, and lesions of the pituitary gland or pituitary stalk that cause GH deficiency directly (Table 24-7). The precise location of the offending lesion sometimes is difficult to determine. The cause of hypopituitarism usually is not found; thus the term *idiopathic hypopituitarism* is used. Growth failure typically is diagnosed among such children by the end of the first year after birth. Because as many as 70% of children with idiopathic hypopituitarism have histories of some form of perinatal insult, it has been postulated that hypoxia from maternal bleeding, breech delivery, or asphyxia during the birth process may cause hypothalamic dysfunction. However, MR imaging studies have shown abnormality of the pituitary stalk, ectopic posterior pituitary gland, and anterior pituitary hypoplasia in at least 30% of these patients. It is now widely believed that some children with so-called idiopathic hypopituitarism actually have developmental defects of the pituitary gland and hypothalamus. The inference that hypothalamic dysfunction causes hypopituitarism among these infants comes from the observation that these children with GH deficiency often are able to secrete GH after injection of GHRH as well as from studies of TSH release in response to TRH. Deficiency of GH also may be associated with a variety of midline central nervous system and facial developmental defects, which are presumably mediated by defects in an array of genes regulating brain development. Such defects range from severe abnormalities of brain development, as in holoprosencephaly, to cleft lip and cleft palate. Hypopituitarism also can occur in association with hypotelorism or single upper central incisor. *Septooptic dysplasia* is a form of midfacial central nervous system hypoplasia in which GH deficiency and other pituitary hormone deficiencies are associated with small optic disc, nystagmus, blindness, and often absence or underdevelopment of the septum pellucidum.

Inherited genetic defects with autosomal recessive transmission have been shown to cause hypopituitarism. A variety of coding defects for transcription factors, for example, PIT-1 or PROP-1, cause failure of development of somatotropins, lactotropins, and thyrotropins. Patients with such defects have hypopituitarism with GH, prolactin, and usually TSH deficiency. Gonadotropin deficiency can occur with PROP-1 errors. Specific mutations, especially deletions, in the gene encoding GH have been described.

The incidence of hypopituitarism caused by central nervous system irradiation has increased with the improved survival of children with leukemia or middle-ear or nasopharyngeal tumors after radiation therapy. Deficiency of GH has been estimated to occur among more than 65% of these children if irradiation exceeds 250 cGy. Growth failure caused by GH deficiency has been described among children with emotional disturbances caused by living in hostile and inadequate environments. These so-called psy-

TABLE 24-7

CAUSES OF PITUITARY DWARFISM AND IGF-I DEFICIENCY SYNDROME

Disorders of the pituitary gland
Aplasia, hypoplasia
Genetic syndromes: deletion of the GH gene, familial panhypopituitarism and familial isolated GH deficiency
Intrasellar tumor: craniopharyngioma, adenoma
Nontumorous destruction: Infarction associated with trauma, infection, or irradiation of the head
Hypothalamic disorders: growth hormone-releasing hormone deficiency
Developmental abnormalities
    Infundibular dysgenesis (anterior pituitary hypoplasia, stalk attenuation or absence, ectopic posterior pituitary); often associated with birth trauma and other forms of perinatal insult
    Midline central nervous system and facial developmental defects: septooptic dysplasia, holoprosencephaly, cleft lip or palate, single upper central incisor
Infection
Histiocytosis
Hypothalamic tumor
    Craniopharyngioma
    Hamartoma
    Neurofibroma
    Glioma
    Germinoma
Psychosocial dwarfism
Idiopathic disorder
Disorders of GH responsiveness (GH high, IGF-I low)
Primary GH receptor abnormalities
    Laron syndrome
Secondary conditions
    Protein-calorie malnutrition
    Chronic illness and inflammatory disease
    IGF-I gene defects

IGF = insulin-like growth factor; GH = growth hormone.

chosocial dwarfs are withdrawn and have bizarre eating habits, polydipsia, and tendencies to ingest contaminated food and drink. They also gorge and vomit. If tested immediately after they enter the hospital, they often show evidence of GH deficiency, and sometimes of ACTH deficiency. After the children spend a brief period in a supportive environment, pituitary function, mental status, and dietary habits improve remarkably, and linear growth is accelerated. Hypothalamic dysfunction, therefore, seems to be mediated through higher cortical centers.

CLINICAL PRESENTATION AND MANAGEMENT OF HYPOPITUITARISM

The clinical presentation of hypopituitarism with GH deficiency varies depending on the age at presentation. Infants with intrauterine hypopituitarism at birth can have hypoglycemic seizures and prolonged jaundice; boys have micropenis and undescended testes. Because most affected patients have idiopathic hypopituitarism, growth failure often is apparent by the end of the first year. Growth rates are slow during childhood, rates of less than 4 to 5 cm/yr being common. The onset of growth failure after a period of normal growth suggests the presence of an intrasellar or suprasellar tumor.

Among patients with early-onset disease, there is a 10% incidence of hypoglycemic seizures and a 20% incidence of chemical hypoglycemia. Attacks of hypoglycemia are limited primarily to young children and occur typically after periods of fasting, such as before breakfast and during illnesses when dietary intake is reduced. Hypoglycemia among these patients is caused by deficiencies of the hormones that antagonize the action of insulin. It is corrected by means of treatment with both GH and cortisol. Children with hypopituitarism are normally proportioned for age, have a prominent calvarium, tend to be overweight for height, and have prominent subcutaneous deposits of abdominal fat (Fig. 24-5). Many affected patients do not undergo puberty at the appropriate age because of concurrent gonadotropin deficiency. Because adrenal secretion of mineralocorticoids is not dependent on pituitary ACTH, children with hypopituitarism rarely have an electrolyte imbalance. Most children show no clinical signs of thyroid hormone deficiency, although serum thyroxine concentrations may be less than normal. Diabetes insipidus is rare among patients with idiopathic hypopituitarism. When present, it suggests the presence of a tumor or another structural hypothalamic lesion (eg, septooptic dysplasia).

Therapy for hypopituitarism necessitates replacement of all deficient hormones. The growth response to GH of children with hypopituitarism is a function of the logarithm of the GH dose. The recommended starting dose is 0.03 to 0.05 mg/kg/d given subcutaneously. Children with GH deficiency typically have an increase in growth rate of 3.5 to 4 cm/yr before treatment to a mean of 8.0 to 11.0 cm/yr during the first year of therapy. As treatment continues, growth rate declines somewhat, so that after 3 to 4 years of therapy, it may be average for age and developmental status. The advent of GH prepared by means of recombinant DNA methods has made it possible to increase the doses of GH administered to achieve optimal growth over prolonged periods, an alternative not available when only limited amounts of pituitary-extracted GH were available. In general, children with the most profound GH deficiency respond best to GH. The success of GH treatment depends to a considerable extent on early diagnosis and treatment, the best results being achieved by children who never have the psychological consequences of short stature. In one recent study, the mean final adult height was at −0.7 SD, or very close to the middle of the normal range of heights. Children treated appropriately with GH can expect to reach genetically expected adult heights. The attainment of such adult stature can be facilitated in some situations if the onset of puberty is delayed by treating children with GH deficiency with potent agonists of gonadotropin-releasing factor (GnRH). The beneficial effects of obtaining a greater adult height must be balanced against the adverse effects of delaying puberty.

If a child does not respond to GH therapy, the diagnosis of GH deficiency is reconsidered, and the possibility of a problem that impairs the GH response is considered. The possibilities include failure to administer the hormone properly, development of hypothyroidism, or formation of growth-attenuating antibodies to GH. Such growth-attenuating antibodies are uncommon, present in fewer than 1% of patients. However, they are particularly likely to be present in children with abnormalities of the GH gene. Growth hormone resistance syndromes (see Sec. 24.2.5) involving abnormalities of structure or function of the GH receptor exist on an inherited or acquired basis and cause failure of IGF generation with consequent growth impairment. Growth hormone treatment of children has few side effects. Glucose intolerance among treated

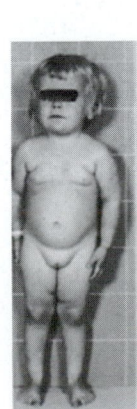 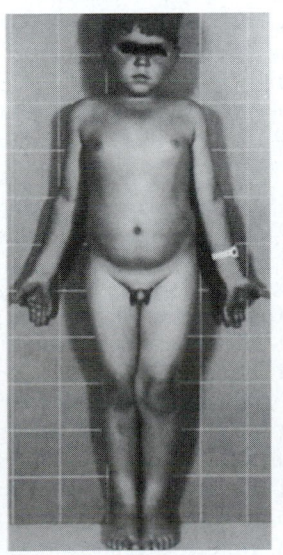 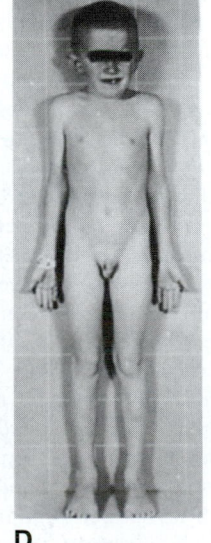

A   B   C   D

FIGURE 24-5   Children with GH deficiency have an immature appearance in addition to short stature. Patient A and B are typical of most GH deficient patients, being overweight for height with folds of ripply fat, particularly on the trunk. Because growth of the cranium is determined primarily by the growth of the brain, whereas growth of the face is dependent on GH, the calvarium often is large relative to the face. *Patient C* had a small penis and impaired response to exogenous gonadotropins, suggesting gonadotropin deficiency. *Patient D* is quite thin.

patients is extremely rare. Concern had been raised that GH treatment may predispose patients to leukemia, but no relation between GH and leukemia has been established. Slipped capital femoral epiphysis, pseudotumor cerebri, gynecomastia, and pancreatitis are possible adverse effects of GH treatment.

Many children do not have the classic criteria of GH deficiency but may benefit from GH therapy. Some of these children have constitutional growth delay (idiopathic short stature), a frequently diagnosed disorder characterized by growth failure for a finite period early in life (6–26 months), a normal or near-normal growth rate for most of childhood, pubertal development delayed 2 or more years, and eventual attainment of normal adult stature and hormonal function. At least 50% of boys with this disorder have accelerated linear growth in response to GH. Results of GH treatment of a group of such children suggest a mean adult height gain of about 2 inches (5 cm), but there are a wide range of growth responses. Evaluation of the use of GH to treat girls with delayed puberty and transiently diminished GH secretion is important, because even low-dose estrogen therapy can cause undue skeletal maturation and diminished final height. The possible side effects of GH therapy among those children are not known but appear minimal. Nonetheless, therapy with GH for any condition other than the US Food and Drug Administration approved uses, which include hypopituitarism, Turner syndrome, and chronic renal insufficiency, is considered experimental.

Craniopharyngioma is the most common tumor causing hypopituitarism among children. A remnant of the Rathke pouch, an outpouching of the roof of the embryonic pharynx, craniopharyngioma is composed of epithelial cells that proliferate and occupy space inside and above the sella, encroaching on adjacent pituitary and hypothalamic tissue. These rests of embryonic cells usually proliferate and become manifest in the first few years of life but may not be apparent clinically for decades. Craniopharyngioma can be solid or contain cysts filled with a thick fluid the consistency and color of motor oil. Many such tumors calcify, particularly among older children.

Although this tumor usually impinges on both the hypothalamus and the pituitary gland, it can manifest as an intrasellar or a suprasellar mass. Most often the symptoms are caused by central nervous system involvement by the tumor. They include headaches, vomiting, visual disturbances, symptoms of diabetes insipidus, and change in sensorium. Some patients have no signs of endocrine deficiency. Others have obvious growth arrest and pubertal delay. If the tumor invades the hypothalamus, signs of impaired vegetative function, including poikilothermia, hypersomnia, and obesity, can occur. Because nearly 90% of patients have suprasellar or intrasellar calcification, plain radiographs of the skull can be useful in diagnosis. Magnetic resonance imaging, however, usually is performed for the diagnosis and evaluation of these lesions. Even when calcification is not present, there often is ballooning of the sella or erosion of the sella walls and posterior clinoid processes. Surgical excision, when possible, is the preferred treatment. When complete excision of the tumor is not possible, drainage of the cyst followed by radiation therapy is recommended. Transsphenoidal decompression of the cyst combined with radiation therapy is most efficacious in the management of large craniopharyngioma.

Microadenoma of the pituitary can occur with Cushing syndrome (see Sec. 24.4.8). Hypothalamic glioma, often associated with neurofibromatosis, and germinoma can cause pituitary insufficiency and many of the neurologic signs of craniopharyngioma. Although therapy for the tumor is based on its nature, location, and size, radiation usually is the primary mode of therapy after a histologic diagnosis is made. Parenchymal cell tumor of the pituitary gland is rare among children. Such tumors can secrete pituitary hormones, as they do among adults. Whether functional or not, these tumors can cause hypopituitarism by compressing adjacent normal pituitary tissue. They can produce neurologic signs by impinging on the optic nerves and adjacent brain. When possible, the tumor is excised by the transsphenoidal route. Enough pituitary tissue is left for return of normal pituitary function.

Empty sella syndrome is an uncommon disorder among children. It occurs when the diaphragma sellae does not surround the pituitary stalk tightly. The result is herniation of the arachnoid into the pituitary fossa and compression of normal pituitary tissue onto the walls of the sella turcica. The sella turcica can be expanded, and intrasellar hypodensity may be apparent at computed tomography (CT). Many patients with empty sella syndrome have no symptoms or signs of pituitary dysfunction. As many as 30%, however, have pituitary hypofunction. The prevalence of empty sella syndrome increases among patients with pituitary adenoma.

Most children with hypopituitarism do not have clinical hypothyroidism. Some, however, may have serum T_4 concentrations less than normal. Others may have a decline in serum T_4 level once GH therapy is started. This may attenuate the growth response. In either instance, replacement doses of levothyroxine are indicated.

Because signs of hypoadrenalism are uncommon among children with hypopituitarism, administration of glucocorticoids is not indicated unless the patient has syncope, postural hypotension, attacks of hypoglycemia, or laboratory evidence of pituitary-adrenal axis hypofunction. Because glucocorticoid excess attenuates growth, the dose usually is limited to 5 to 10 mg cortisol per square meter of body surface area per day by mouth. Four to 10 times this dosage is needed during periods of stress.

Diabetes insipidus often occurs after operations on the region of the pituitary gland and hypothalamus. It is uncommon with idiopathic hypopituitarism. Diabetes is managed effectively with desmopressin, a synthetic analog of vasopressin. This agent is administered intranasally in a dosage of 5 to 15 μg one to two times a day.

Long-acting testosterone enanthate is administered intramuscularly to boys with hypopituitarism who have no signs of puberty by 14 years of age. Beginning with a dosage of 50 mg a month, the dosage is gradually increased over several years to 200 mg every 2 weeks. This androgen often markedly enhances the growth response to GH. Girls who need estrogen replacement are given conjugated estrogen (0.3–0.6 mg daily) or ethinyl estradiol (5–10 μg a day initially). After 9 to 12 months of continuous estrogen therapy, cycling with a synthetic progestin is begun; the dosage of ethinyl estradiol is gradually increased.

ISOLATED DEFICIENCIES OF PITUITARY HORMONES OTHER THAN GROWTH HORMONE

Isolated deficiency of gonadotropins occurs sporadically or in families, as in *Kallmann syndrome*, which is associated with anosmia (see Sec. 24.8.5). Intrauterine gonadotropin deficiency causes cryptorchidism or microphallus among some boys. The most common symptom among both boys and girls is lack of pubertal development. The syndrome is caused by failure of the hypothalamus to secrete GnRH. After repeated pulsatile administration of GnRH, these children can secrete follicle-stimulating hormone (FSH) and LH. Treatment of boys includes producing pubertal changes by means of administration of testosterone. Because such therapy does not produce testicular growth and spermatogenesis, the usual practice is to administer recombinant human gonadotropins when the patient desires fertility. Girls are given estrogen and progesterone to achieve pubertal development. They also need gonadotropins to stimulate ovulation when pregnancy is being considered. Administration of GnRH can induce both pubertal development and fertility among patients with hypothalamic GnRH deficiency. Gonadotropin-releasing factor has a short half-life and must be given parenterally in a pulsatile manner to achieve the desired effect. These factors have limited the use of this approach. Isolated deficiencies of TSH and ACTH are rare.

EXCESS OF PITUITARY GROWTH HORMONE

Excess of pituitary GH is a rare condition among children. *Gigantism* is the predominant feature of GH excess among children whose bony epiphyses have not yet fused. Many affected children have features found among adults with *acromegaly*. These include overgrowth of the mandible, enlargement of the hands and feet, thickening of the skin, and excessive sweating. Pituitary tumors that cause GH excess can occur spontaneously or possibly as a consequence of prolonged stimulation by hypothalamic GHRH. Extrahypothalamic tumors that secrete GHRH and stimulate the pituitary gland to produce excessive GH also can cause gigantism. In rare instances, tumors that secrete GHRH can cause acromegaly among adults.

Screening for GH excess can be accomplished by means of measuring the concentration of IGF-I in the plasma. This value is consistently elevated among patients with active acromegaly and provides a better index of disease severity than does level of GH itself. The diagnosis is confirmed by means of administering an oral glucose load and determining whether serum level of GH is suppressed. Among patients with pituitary GH excess, complete suppression of GH does not occur. The tallness of children with GH excess may be caused by compression on normal pituitary tissue by a pituitary tumor. This delays the onset and progression of puberty and allows a longer period of growth. Treatment consists of removal of the growth-hormone-secreting tumor. This is best attempted by the transsphenoidal route. During the operation, efforts are made to preserve normal pituitary tissue. If surgery is unsuccessful, irradiation of the pituitary gland is appropriate. Administration of bromocriptine or an analog of somatostatin is useful for suppressing secretion of GH in some patients. An antagonist of GH action at its receptor is being extensively tested.

24.2.5   Other Endocrine Causes of Growth Retardation

HYPOTHYROIDISM

Growth usually is retarded among children with hypothyroidism. Although growth failure depends on the age at onset, the duration, and the severity of disease, it often is profound and frequently is the most prominent manifestation of acquired hypothyroidism. Linear growth can nearly cease and is invariably more affected than weight gain, so children usually are overweight for height. Because the symptoms of hypothyroidism are subtle, diagnosis often is delayed. One study showed a 4.2-year delay between the onset of decrease in linear growth rate and the diagnosis. At the time of diagnosis, girls were 4.0 SD below and boys 3.2 SD below mean height for age. In diagnosis, it is helpful to look for immaturity in facial appearance and in body proportion with an increased upper to lower body segment ratio. These findings are caused by delayed skeletal maturation, which can be judged by delay in bone age. Although chronic hypothyroidism usually is associated with delayed puberty, precocious puberty and premature menarche can occur. The development of newborn screening programs for congenital hypothyroidism has resulted in prompt diagnosis and treatment of affected newborns (approximately 1/4,000 live births), almost eliminating congenital hypothyroidism as a cause of poor growth.

In general the diagnosis of primary hypothyroidism is straightforward with low serum T_4 concentrations and elevated TSH levels. The diagnosis of *Hashimoto thyroiditis,* the most common cause of acquired childhood hypothyroidism, is assumed when antithyroid antibodies are detected. Secondary or tertiary hypothyroidism, because of TSH or TRH deficiency, respectively, is a rare cause of hypothyroidism (see Sec. 24.6).

Replacement treatment of infants and children with congenital hypothyroidism maintains normal growth. Treatment of children with acquired hypothyroidism results in rapid catch-up growth. Not infrequently, however, the accelerated growth may not allow full growth potential, especially among children with long-standing disease, because rapid skeletal maturation often occurs during the first 18 months of treatment. Catch-up growth can be particularly compromised when therapy is initiated near puberty.

GLUCOCORTICOID EXCESS

Regardless of the source (endogenous adrenal production, as in Cushing syndrome, adrenal tumor, or exogenous administration), glucocorticoid excess interferes with bone metabolism by inhibiting osteoblastic activity and enhancing bone resorption. The result is retarded skeletal growth. Because children exposed to glucocorticoid excess frequently do not attain target heights, it appears that some of the deleterious effects of glucocorticoids on the epiphysis persist after correction of chronic glucocorticoid excess. Treatment with glucocorticoids should be limited to the minimum that the underlying condition allows, frequently by the use of alternate-day therapy or carefully monitored inhalants.

GROWTH HORMONE RESISTANCE

Children with characteristics of GH deficiency accompanied by normal or elevated serum GH levels and decreased IGF-I level are said to have *GH resistance.* Primary GH resistance can be caused by abnormalities of the GH receptor, postreceptor defects of GH signal mechanisms, or primary errors of IGF-I biosynthesis. Growth hormone resistance can be acquired and appears to be a component of the pathophysiological mechanism of malnutrition and a variety of hepatic, renal, and other chronic diseases. It can also be caused by acquisition of antibodies to GH or to the GH receptor.

Children with genetic defects in the GH receptor have clinical features identical to those of children with IGF deficiency caused by GH deficiency. Basal levels of GH in the serum are elevated, and serum levels of IGF-I, IGF-II, and IGFBP-3 are profoundly reduced. The hallmark of the diagnosis, however, is lack of response to GH treatment. A variety of mutations in the GH receptor gene have been described, including deletions and a number of point mutations (missense, nonsense, and abnormal splicing) that result in absence of the receptor or in receptors with reduced function. Most of the point mutations are in the extracellular or GH binding domain of the GH receptor. Measurement of serum GH binding protein (GHBP) can be helpful in making the diagnosis, because GHBP is a cleavage product of the extracellular portion of the GH receptor. Inability to detect GHBP in the serum thus suggests an absence of GH receptor. The presence of GHBP, however, does not exclude a disorder of the GH receptor, because mutations in the GH receptor gene that affect function often have normal GHBP levels.

Only one person with a defect in the gene for IGF-I has been described. He had a partial gene deletion that yields a truncated IGF-I molecule. At diagnosis the patient was 15 years of age. He had both prenatal and postnatal (−6.7 SDS) growth retardation and resistance to exogenous GH. He also had sensorineural deafness, mental retardation, and microcephaly, indicating the importance of IGF-I to central nervous system development. He had undetectable serum levels of IGF-I, as expected, but normal serum IGFBP-3 and GHBP levels.

24.2.6 Primary Disorders of Growth Retardation

OSTEOCHONDRODYSPLASIA

Achondroplasia and hypochondroplasia are among the more common forms of osteochondrodysplasia, which now encompasses more than 100 inherited disorders characterized by abnormalities in size and structure of cartilage and bone. The unique radiologic features of each of this heterogeneous group of disorders usually provide a specific diagnosis. As the genetics of each disorder is elucidated, genomic analysis often can establish the diagnosis. For example, both achondroplasia and hypochondroplasia are caused by activating mutations in the gene for fibroblast growth factor receptor 3 on chromosome 4p16.3. Diminished growth velocity is present from infancy in achondroplasia, such that average adult height among men is 130 cm and among women is 120 cm. The phenotypic features and short stature are less pronounced in hypochondroplasia; adult height usually is 120 to 150 cm. Growth curves for children with achondroplasia are useful in evaluating the growth of these children. These disorders are discussed in more detail in Secs. 10.3.5 and 10.3.6.

CHROMOSOMAL ABNORMALITIES

Growth failure, which occurs both in utero and postnatally, is a frequent manifestation of chromosomal defects. It often is associated with a variety of somatic abnormalities and mental retardation.

DOWN SYNDROME (TRISOMY 21) This syndrome always is accompanied by growth retardation. Birth weight and length are low and the low growth velocity continues postnatally. Typically the pubertal growth spurt is delayed and incomplete, as is skeletal maturation. Adult height ranges from 135 to 170 cm among men and 127 to 158 cm among women. Although the mechanisms for growth failure in Down syndrome are not clear, there is evidence of borderline normal GH secretion accompanied by low serum concentration of IGF-I. These children also have a high incidence of hypothyroidism, usually caused by Hashimoto thyroiditis, and celiac disease which further slows growth rate if the patient is not treated. All children with Down syndrome are routinely screened for hypothyroidism and celiac disease (see also Sec. 10.2).

TURNER SYNDROME (GONADAL DYSGENESIS) The diagnosis of Turner syndrome is considered whenever a girl has unexplained growth failure. Short stature is the single most common feature of

Turner syndrome. Growth of these girls has a distinct pattern characterized by (1) mild intrauterine growth retardation (IUGR) with mean birth weights and lengths of 2800 g and 48.3 cm, respectively, (2) subnormal height velocity between birth and 3 years of age, (3) a further gradual decline in height velocity from 3 years of age until approximately 14 years of age that results in a progressive deviation from normal height percentiles, and (4) a prolonged adolescent growth phase with a partial return toward normal height as the result of delayed epiphyseal fusion. In the United States and Europe, mean adult height ranges from 142 to 147 cm, among women with Turner syndrome, approximately 20 cm less than the mean among healthy women. Individual genetic factors, however, influence adult height in Turner syndrome, because parental height correlates well with final patient height. In other words, patients with this syndrome tend to be taller if their parents are tall. The allelic absence of the *SHOX* gene (in the pseudoautosomal region of the X chromosome) appears to be involved in the growth failure that occurs in Turner syndrome. Although there is little evidence of abnormalities in the GH–IGF-I axis in Turner syndrome, GH therapy is effective in both accelerating short-term growth and increasing adult height.

PRADER-WILLI SYNDROME In the neonate this syndrome comprises low birth weight, hypotonia, feeding difficulty, and among boys cryptorchidism and microphallus caused by hypogonadotropic hypogonadism. After birth growth failure often becomes more marked and is accompanied by hyperphagia and obesity. Deletions in the short arm of the paternally derived chromosome 15 at q11-13 or maternal uniparental disomy of chromosome 15 have been found in some patients. The mechanisms of growth failure, however, are not known. Although GH responses to provocative tests can be low, as can serum concentration of IGF-I, these abnormalities may be caused by obesity rather than being the cause of growth failure. When growth velocity is low and IGF-I levels are below the normal range, the possibility of GH deficiency is greater. Nonetheless, results of some studies suggest that GH treatment is beneficial in that it may improve exercise tolerance and body composition.

INTRAUTERINE GROWTH RETARDATION

Growth failure in utero has numerous causes and is broadly defined to include all infants with birth lengths or weights below the tenth percentile for gestational age, that is, small for gestational age (SGA). Intrauterine growth retardation (IUGR) often is associated with alterations in the intrauterine environment imposed by maternal undernutrition or hypertension or by abnormalities of the placenta. In most cases the reason for abnormal fetal growth is unclear. Deficits in IGF-I expression may mediate IUGR in many cases, because the concentration of IGF-I in cord or fetal blood usually is low in SGA regardless of the apparent cause of growth failure. The importance of IGF-I to fetal growth is suggested by results of many studies that show serum IGF-I levels correlate with birth size.

After birth, some SGA infants continue to have attenuated growth with persistent height deficits throughout childhood and adolescence. This failure to catch up may reflect an abnormality intrinsic to the infant or an irreversible effect imposed by an altered intrauterine milieu. The earlier in gestation that fetal growth is impaired, the less likely is catch-up growth. Intrauterine growth retardation can have implications that extend to adult life, because there is an increased risk of hypertension, adult-onset diabetes, and cardiovascular disease among adults who are born SGA. A number of syndromes involve marked IUGR. They include the Russell-Silver, Cockayne, and Noonan syndromes. Results of several studies suggest that treatment with GH may accelerate growth rate in children with a history of IUGR.

24.2.7 Secondary Causes of Growth Retardation

MALNUTRITION Undernutrition or malnutrition is the most common cause of growth failure. It usually represents deficits in intake of protein and other nutrients as well as dietary components, such as zinc, iron, and vitamins necessary for normal growth and development (see also Sec. 17.5). Undernutrition manifests as a decrease in weight gain followed by a deceleration in linear growth. Depending on severity, progression to linear growth failure occurs within weeks or months among neonates. Among older children, this may not occur for years. As discussed later, undernutrition likely causes the growth failure that accompanies many chronic diseases. Alterations in the GH/IGF system probably mediate the growth failure in undernutrition. Serum levels of IGF-I are decreased despite normal or elevated GH levels.

GASTROINTESTINAL DISEASE Growth failure can be the predominant or the only manifestation of intestinal disease among children. Therefore it is considered in the evaluation of any child with growth retardation. Children with celiac disease and Crohn disease often have decreased serum IGF-I levels. The growth failure undoubtedly accrues from the effects of undernutrition (caused by malabsorption or anorexia) and chronic inflammation, both of which can decrease IGF-I expression. Among children with Crohn disease, glucocorticoid therapy also contributes to growth failure. Even with appropriate therapy, impaired linear growth results in deficits of final height among approximately 30% of children with Crohn disease. Most children with celiac disease, however, achieve a normal final height with appropriate dietary management.

CHRONIC LIVER DISEASE Decreased food intake, malabsorption of fat and fat-soluble vitamins, and deficiency of trace elements result in poor linear growth and short stature among children with chronic liver disease. Alteration of the GH-IGF system with evidence of GH resistance appears to mediate the growth failure. After liver transplantation, linear growth accelerates but may be delayed by drug therapy or complications of transplantation.

CARDIOVASCULAR DISEASE Growth failure can accompany cyanotic congenital heart disease and chronic congestive failure. Among children with the former, the degree of cyanosis correlates with the degree of growth impairment. It is likely related to the increase in basal metabolic rate caused by increases in cardiac and respiratory work and to caloric intake insufficient to compensate for the increased work. Chronic congestive heart failure, however, also is associated with malabsorption that includes protein-losing enteropathy, intestinal lymphangiectasia, and steatorrhea. Corrective surgery often restores normal growth among these children.

RENAL DISEASE Impaired growth almost invariably occurs among children with altered renal function. As with gastrointestinal disorders, growth failure can be the first clinical sign of uremia or renal tubular acidosis. Among children with chronic renal failure, decreased caloric intake, metabolic acidosis, protein wasting, chronic anemia, compromised cardiac function, altered vitamin metabolism, and other factors contribute to the growth failure. Although GH secretion and serum IGF-I and IGF-II levels usually are normal among these children, serum level of IGFBPs often is increased. It seems likely that IGFBPs inhibit the action of IGF and, in turn, growth. In nephrotic syndrome, however, serum levels of IGF-I and IGFBP-3 are low because of urinary losses. Chronic glucocorticoid therapy for some renal disorders can exacerbate growth retardation by diminishing GH release and blunting the action of IGF-I at growth plates. Growth hormone treatment of children with renal failure is effective in accelerating linear growth, likely by increasing the molar ratio of IGF peptides to IGFBPs and thereby overcoming the inhibitory action of IGFBPs. Before the use of GH in the care of these children, about two-thirds of children had final adult heights more than 2 SD below the mean. Despite successful renal transplantation, height often is either not restored to normal, or no catch-up growth occurs. In these situations, GH administration may be useful.

HEMATOLOGIC DISORDERS Children with chronic anemia, such as thalassemia and sickle cell disease, often have growth failure, especially as teenagers. They also often have delayed onset of puberty and late menarche. Impaired oxygen delivery, increased cardiovascular work, and inadequate nutrition likely contribute to the growth alteration. Therapy with repeated transfusions, and the hemosiderosis that can result, can cause endocrine deficiencies, such as hypothyroidism, gonadal failure, hypogonadotropic hypogonadism, and possibly GH resistance, as in other chronic diseases. Each of the latter factors can contribute to growth failure. Nonetheless, the final adult height of patients with sickle cell disease and other forms of chronic anemia, depending on severity and therapy, can be normal.

DIABETES MELLITUS Most children with insulin-dependent (type 1) diabetes mellitus grow normally, even if glycemic control is marginal. However, deceleration of growth velocity is not unusual immediately before or during puberty among children who do not maintain reasonable glycemic status. With long-standing poor control, severe growth retardation can occur. Accompanied by hepatomegaly, this condition is called *Mauriac syndrome*. Glycemic control is inversely correlated with serum IGF-I concentration and positively with IGFBP-1 concentrations, but neither value corresponds well with growth velocity.

INBORN ERRORS OF METABOLISM Children with many of the inborn errors of metabolism, such as glycogen storage disease, mucopolysaccharidosis, glycoproteinosis, and mucolipidosis, have growth retardation that can be severe. The association of marked skeletal dysplasia with these disorders suggests that intrinsic abnormalities of bone growth are a component of the growth failure. In contrast, children with organic acidosis, such as methylmalonic or propionic aciduria, have features of GH resistance in that they have low serum level of IGF-I with apparently normal GH secretion. The latter may be caused by altered nutritional and acid-base status.

PULMONARY DISEASE Among children with asthma, height velocity is related to disease severity. With chronic stress accompanied by increased production of endogenous glucocorticoids, impaired nutrition and increased energy requirements appear to be the mechanisms of growth failure. Systemic glucocorticoid therapy further impairs growth among these children, especially because the synthetic glucocorticoids most commonly used, such as prednisone or dexamethasone, appear to have greater growth-suppressive effects than do their putative equivalent cortisol doses (see Sec. 24.4.9). Nonetheless, normal adult height usually is achieved by all but the most severely affected children. Use of alternate-day or aerosolized glucocorticoids appears to minimize the growth retarding effects of glucocorticoid therapy, but systemic absorption can still effect growth, depending on the specific drug and dose used.

Infants with bronchopulmonary dysplasia usually have poor growth exacerbated by treatment with high doses of glucocorticoids, which can transiently halt linear growth. Growth of surviving infants is poor through early childhood but can be normal in late childhood when the lung disease resolves. Chronic hypoxemia, poor nutrition, chronic pulmonary infection, and reactive airway disease contribute to the poor early growth.

Children with cystic fibrosis usually have retarded growth and delay in sexual maturation. This is caused by many factors, including chronic pulmonary infection with bronchiectasis, pancreatic insufficiency with both exocrine and endocrine inadequacy, malabsorption, and undernutrition. The degree of growth retardation, however, is best related to the severity of the pulmonary disease rather than to pancreatic dysfunction, possibly because of the attention paid to nutritional supplementation for these children. On average, children with cystic fibrosis have heights at about the twentieth percentile and weights at the tenth percentile, but adult heights approach normal range.

CHRONIC INFECTION Growth failure can accompany any chronic infection or inflammatory disease during childhood. For example, among children with acquired immunodeficiency syndrome (AIDS), length and weight during early childhood are approximately 1 SD below the mean. Delayed bone age and late onset and progression of puberty have been found among boys with hemophilia and human immunodeficiency virus infection. The diminished growth resulting from chronic infectious and inflammatory diseases may be mediated by cytokines, because these substances are known to influence the endocrine system at many levels. They also impair mineral and nutrient metabolism, growth and remodeling of bone, and the production and action of IGFs.

24.2.8 Tall Stature

Most tall children are normal, and their stature is linked to genetic background and an optimal environment for growth. Tall stature is concerning only if a child's tallness is inappropriate for parental height or when linear growth velocity accelerates inappropriately. A number of endocrine and nonendocrine disorders cause excessive linear growth during childhood and adolescence. Endocrine causes of accelerated growth include GH excess or acromegaly (see Sec 24.2.4); thyrotoxicosis; excess androgenic hormones, as in congenital adrenal hyperplasia and virilizing tumors; and sexual precocity. The latter disorders are readily apparent on physical examination because of accompanying signs of androgen excess or sexual maturation. Adolescents with hypogonadotropic hypogonadism also can be tall and have a eunuchoid habitus. Other clinical entities that can cause an increase in absolute height or accelerated height velocity include obesity, Marfan syndrome, homocystinuria, total lipodystrophy, neurofibromatosis, and chromosomal abnormalities such as Klinefelter syndrome, and 48XXYY and 47XYY syndromes.

CONSTITUTIONAL TALL STATURE

When the prediction of adult height for a girl exceeds 180 cm, height is considered excessive by some families. Concern about the final adult height of boys is rarely about overgrowth but rather about short stature and delayed adolescent maturation. In general, tall children have tall parents, their body proportions are normal, their height has been greater than the 97th percentile since early childhood, and height velocity is within the normal range. Children with constitutional tall stature may have augmented GH responses to some stimuli and increased levels of IGF-I.

Treatment of excessively tall girls is a therapeutic dilemma for pediatricians and endocrinologists. Considerable data suggest that high-dose estrogen therapy markedly restricts final height to less than predicted. The vagaries of height prediction and the ever-present risk of dangerous long-term side effects of hormonal therapy dictate careful consideration of each patient's clinical state, self-image, and desire for treatment. Height restriction is a cosmetic alteration, so the final decision must be made by well-informed parents and the child, not the physician. In recent years, hormonal therapy rarely has been used to diminish final height. Societal acceptance of tall women has markedly lowered the unease previously felt by tall women. In the rare instances in which treatment is desired, a conjugated estrogen preparation such as Premarin is given cyclically: 10 mg/d for 21 days, followed by no treatment for 8 to 10 days. A progestational agent (5 mg) can be added for the last 5 to 10 days of the treatment period. Therapy is initiated when skeletal age is 10 to 12 years. Hormonal treatment is continued until growth ceases, usually when the bone age is 15 to 16 years. Postmenarchal girls do not usually need exogenous estrogen therapy; as maximum growth after menarche is not more than 5 to 10 cm. The average diminution of final adult height as a result of high-dose estrogen administration appears to be about 4 cm (range 0 to 9 cm).

OTHER OVERGROWTH DISORDERS

Several disorders are considered in the differential diagnosis of tall stature. *Cerebral gigantism* (Sotos syndrome) is associated with large size at birth, macrocrania, large ears, a prominent mandible, subnormal intelligence, and poor coordination. Growth velocity is increased during the first years of life, but later it decelerates and follows a channel above but parallel to the 97th percentile. No endocrine abnormalities have yet been uncovered among these children. *Beckwith-Wiedemann syndrome* manifests among newborns as macrosomia, macroglossia, omphalocele, and hypoglycemia. The mechanism of overgrowth is not certain in this disorder, but evidence of abnormal IGF-II gene regulation has been found among some affected children, suggesting that IGF-II stimulates overgrowth in this syndrome.

References

Boersma B, Otten BJ, Stoelings GBA, Wit JM: Catch-up growth after prolonged hypothyroidism. Eur J Pediatr 155:362–367, 1996

Cohen MMJ: A comprehensive and critical assessment of overgrowth and overgrowth syndromes. Adv Hum Genet 18:181–303, 1989

Drop SL, De Waal WJ, de Muinck Keizer-Schrama SM: Sex steroid treatment of constitutionally tall staure. Endocr Rev 19:540–558, 1998

Du Caju MVL, Rooman RP, Op De Beeck L: Longitudinal data on growth and final height in diabetic children. Pediatr Res 38:607–611, 1995

Jones JI, Clemmons DR: Insulin-like growth factors and their binding proteins: biologic actions. Endocr Rev 16:3–34, 1995

Kohaut EC: Chronic renal disease and growth in childhood. Curr Opin Pediatr 7:171–175, 1995

Laron Z, Blum W, Chatelain P, et al: Classification of growth hormone insensitivity syndrome. J Pediatr 122:241, 1993

Magiakou MA, Mastorakos G, Oldfield EH, et al: Cushing's syndrome in children and adolescents. Presentation, diagnosis, and therapy. N Engl J Med 331:629–636, 1994

Moye J, Rich KC, Kalish LA, et al: Natural history of somatic growth in infants born to women infected by human immunodeficiency virus. J Pediatr 128:58–69, 1996

Procter AM, Phillips JA, Cooper DN: The molecular genetics of growth hormone deficiency. Hum Genet 103:255–272, 1998

Rivkees SA, Bode HH, Crawford JD: Long-term growth in juvenile acquired hypothyroidism. N Engl J Med 318:599–602, 1988

Rosenfeld RG, Attie KM, Frane J, et al: 1998. Growth hormone therapy of Turner's syndrome: beneficial effect on adult height. J Pediatr 132:319–324, 1998

Rosenfeld RG, Rosenbloom AL, Guevara-Aguirre J: Growth hormone (GH) insensitivity due to primary GH receptor deficiency. Endocr Rev 15:369–390, 1994

Schuurmans FM, Pulles-Heintzberger CF, Gerver WJ, Kester AD, Forget PP: Long-term growth of children with congenital heart disease: a retrospective study. Acta Pediatr 87:1250–1255, 1998

Tanner JM: Normal growth and techniques of growth assessment. Clin Endocrinol Metab 15:411–451, 1986

Veznedaroglu E, Armonda RA, Andrews DW: Diagnosis and therapy for pituitary tumors. Curr Opin Oncol 11:27–31, 1999

Woods KA, Camacho-Hubner C, Savage MO, Clark AJL: Intrauterine growth retardation and postnatal growth failure associated with deletion of the insulin-like growth factor I gene. N Engl J Med 335:1342–1349, 1996

Zeitler PS, Travers S, Kappy MS: Advances in the recognition and treatment of endocrine complications in children with chronic disease. Adv Pediatr 46:101–150, 1999

24.3 PRIMARY DISTURBANCES OF WATER HOMEOSTASIS

Joseph A. Majzoub

24.3.1 Physiology of Water Homeostasis

Maintenance of the tonicity of extracellular fluids within a very narrow range is crucial for proper cell function because extracellular osmolality regulates cell shape and intracellular concentrations of ions and other osmolytes. Proper extracellular ionic concentrations are necessary for the correct function of ion channels, generation of neural action potentials, and other modes of intercellular communication. Normal blood tonicity is maintained over a 10-fold variation in water intake. Control of plasma osmolality involves a complex integration of endocrine, neural, and paracrine pathways. Plasma osmolality is regulated principally through vasopressin release from the posterior pituitary gland. Volume homeostasis is determined largely through the action of the renin-angiotensin-aldosterone system with contributions from both vasopressin and the natriuretic peptide family. Dysfunction in any of these systems can result in abnormal regulation of blood osmolality. If not properly recognized and controlled, the abnormality can cause life-threatening hypersosmolality or hypoosmolality. The evaluation and approach to the child with polyuria, polydipsia, and abnormalities of serum electrolytes and a osmolality are discussed in Sec. 21.4.

VASOPRESSIN SYNTHESIS, METABOLISM, AND ACTION

The nine-amino-acid peptide vasopressin consists of a six-amino-acid disulfide ring and a three-amino-acid tail with amidation of the carboxy teminus. It is synthesized in hypothalamic paraventricular and supraoptic magnocellular neurons. The axons of these neurons transport the hormone to the posterior pituitary gland, the site of storage and release into the systemic circulation. The bilaterally paired hypothalamic paraventricular and supraoptic nuclei are separated from one another by relatively large distances (~1 cm). The axons course caudally, converge at the infundibulum, and terminate at different levels within the pituitary stalk and posterior pituitary gland. Vasopressin also is synthesized in the parvocellular neurons of the paraventricular nucleus, where it may help regulate the hypothalamic-pituitary-adrenal axis, and in the hypothalamic suprachiasmatic nucleus, where it may participate in generation of circadian rhythms.

During synthesis and perhaps after secretion into the bloodstream, vasopressin is bound to neurophysin, a 10,000-Da protein. Neurophysin may function to protect vasopressin against degradation during intracellular storage or to promote more efficient packaging or posttranslational processing of vasopressin with secretory granules. A single gene consisting of three exons encodes both vasopressin and neurophysin. Exon 1 encodes the signal and vasopressin peptides and the amino-terminal 9 amino acids of neurophysin. Exon 2 encodes most neurophysin. Exon 3 codes for the carboxy-terminal end of neurophysin followed by an additional 39 amino acid–long glycopeptide. A synthetic analog of vasopressin, desamino-D-arginine vasopressin (desmopressin) has twice the antidiuretic potency and 100 times the duration of action of vasopressin.

Once in the circulation, vasopressin has a half-life of only 5 to 10 minutes, because of its rapid degradation by a cysteine amino-terminal peptidase called *vasopressinase*. Desmopressin is insensitive to amino-terminal degradation and thus has a much longer half-life, 8 to 24 hours. During pregnancy, the placenta secretes large amounts of vasopressinase, resulting in a fourfold increase in the rate of metabolic clearance of vasopressin. Healthy pregnant women compensate for this increased rate of degradation with an increase in vasopressin secretion. If there is a preexisting deficit in vasopressin secretion or action, diabetes insipidus can develop in the last trimester. This disorder resolves in the immediately postpartum period. This form of diabetes insipidus responds to treatment with desmopressin, which is resistant to degradation by vasopressinase, but not vasopressin.

Vasopressin binds to three different G protein–coupled cell surface receptors, designated V1, V2, and V3. The major sites of V1 receptor expression are on vascular smooth muscle and hepatocytes, where receptor activation causes vasoconstriction and glycogenolysis, respectively. The serum concentration of vasopressin required to increase blood pressure significantly is severalfold higher than that required for maximal antidiuresis. The V3 receptor is present on corticotrophs in the anterior pituitary gland, and vasopressin binding increases ACTH secretion. Modulation of water balance is mediated by the action of vasopressin on V2 receptors, which are located primarily on the blood (basolateral) side of the renal collecting tubule (Fig. 24-6). Activation of cAMP-dependent protein kinase causes insertion of aggregates of a water channel, called *aquaporin 2,* into the luminal membrane. This activity causes up to a 100-fold increase in water permeability and allows water movement from the tubular lumen along its osmotic gradient into the hypertonic inner medullary interstitium and excretion of concentrated urine.

REGULATION OF WATER BALANCE

Water balance is controlled by a balance of water ingestion and loss. Thirst stimulates water ingestion, which restores past water losses, and vasopressin secretion, which stimulates water reabsorption by the kidney, thereby reducing water losses. Ideally, these two systems work in concert to regulate extracellular fluid tonicity efficiently. However, each system can maintain plasma osmolality in the nearly normal range by itself. For example, in the complete absence of vasopressin secretion, urine output increases to as much as 5 to 10 L/m², but with free access to water, thirst increases ingestion of water to compensate. Conversely, an intact vasopressin secretory system can compensate for some degree of disordered thirst regulation. However, when both vasopressin secretion and thirst are compromised, either by disease or iatrogenic means, life-threatening abnormalities in plasma osmolality can occur.

Vasopressin secretion is stimulated by an increase in the plasma concentration of osmotically active substances (those not freely permeable across cell membranes, principally sodium chloride) and by nonosmotic mechanisms. Normal blood osmolality ranges between 280 and 290 milliosmoles per kilogram of water (mOsm/kg), the threshold for vasopressin release being approximately 283 mOsm/kg. Above this threshold, an osmosensor outside the blood-brain barrier near the anterior hypothalamus that can detect as little as a 1 to 2% change in blood osmolality, signals the posterior pituitary

gland to secrete vasopressin. Vasopressin level increases in proportion to plasma osmolality, up to a maximum concentration of about 20 pg/mL at a blood osmolality of about 320 mOsm/kg. The sensation of thirst is determined by hypothalamic neurons anatomically distinct from those that make vasopressin. The threshold for thirst is slightly higher (~293 mOsm/kg) than that for vasopressin release. During the development of hyperosmolality, vasopressin is released first. The increase in water intake follows when water reabsorption by the kidney is activated. This prevents a persistent diuretic state.

Vasopressin is also secreted in response to nonosmotic stimuli, such as a decrease in intravascular volume and pressure. Afferent baroreceptor pathways arising from the right and left atria and the aortic arch (carotid sinus) are stimulated by increasing intravascular volume and stretch of vessel walls, which send signals to the hypothalamic paraventricular and supraoptic nuclei that inhibit vasopressin secretion. Although minor changes in plasma osmolality evoke linear increases in plasma vasopressin level, no change in vasopressin secretion occurs until there are large reductions in blood volume, at least 8%. Vasopressin concentration then increases exponentially with further reductions in blood volume. When blood volume decreases approximately 25%, vasopressin concentration increases 20- to 30-fold above normal, vastly exceeding the levels required for maximal antidiuresis and high enough to cause vasoconstriction through the V1 vascular receptors.

Other triggers of vasopressin secretion include nausea, pain, hypoglycemia, psychological stress, and exposure to ethanol or chlorpropamide. Vasopressin secretion is inhibited by glucocorticoids. Regulation of vasopressin by glucocorticoids is lost with primary or secondary glucocorticoid deficiency, which enhances both hypothalamic vasopressin production and directly impairs free water excretion, which can cause hyponatremia.

24.3.2   Central Diabetes Insipidus

CAUSES OF CENTRAL DIABETES INSIPIDUS

Among children, central diabetes insipidus, also known as *hypothalamic, neurogenic,* or *vasopressin-sensitive diabetes insipidus,* is most often the result of congenital anatomic defects of the hypothalamic-pituitary axis, neoplasm, or neurosurgery or trauma that damages vasopressin-secreting neurons. It also can be caused by infiltrative, autoimmune, and infectious disease that affects vasopressin neurons or fiber tracts. The least common cause is disorders of vasopressin gene structure. Among approximately 10% of children with central diabetes insipidus, the cause cannot be determined. Nephrogenic causes of diabetes insipidus are discussed in Sec. 21.4.3.

HYPOTHALAMIC-PITUITARY SURGERY The most common cause of central diabetes insipidus is neurosurgical destruction of vasopressin neurons after hypothalamic-pituitary surgery. It is important to differentiate polyuria associated with the onset of acute postsurgical central diabetes insipidus from that caused by normal diuresis of fluids given during surgery. In both cases, the urine can be dilute and of high volume, exceeding 200 mL/m²/h. In postsurgical central diabetes insipidus, however, serum osmolality is high. With excess hydration it is normal. The axons of vasopressin-containing magnocellular neurons extend uninterrupted to the posterior pituitary gland over a distance of approximately 10 mm. These axons terminate at various levels within the stalk and gland.

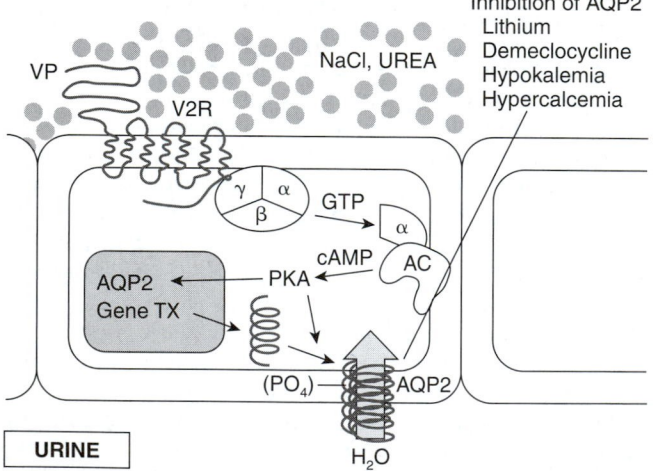

FIGURE 24-6 Action of vasopressin in the kidney. Vasopressin (*VP*) binds to the V2 receptor (*V2R*) to cause dissociation of the trimeric G protein (α, β, γ) and allowing $G_s\alpha$ to activate adenylate cyclase (*AC*). The result is an increase in cyclic adenosine monophosphate and activation of protein kinase A (*PKA*). The catalytic subunit of PKA phosphorylates the aquaporin 2 (*AQP2*) water channel, causing it to aggregate as a homotetramer in the luminal membrane of the collecting duct. The result is in an increase in water flow down its osmotic gradient from the urine into the hypertonic renal medullary interstitium containing sodium chloride and urea (*closed circles*). Demeclocycline, lithium, high calcium and low potassium levels interfere with these processes.

Because surgical interruption of these axons can cause retrograde degeneration of hypothalamic neurons, lesions closer to the hypothalamus affect more neurons and cause greater permanent loss of hormone secretion. Not infrequently, a triple-phase response follows hypothalamic pituitary surgery. During the initial phase, transient diabetes insipidus lasts $\frac{1}{2}$ to 2 days, possibly owing to edema that interferes with normal vasopressin secretion. If there is substantial destruction of vasopressin-secreting neurons, a second phase of inappropriate vasopressin secretion lasts as long as 10 days because of unregulated release of vasopressin by dying neurons. This is followed by a third phase of permanent diabetes insipidus if more than 90% of vasopressin cells are destroyed. A marked degree of inappropriate vasopressin secretion in the second phase usually portends permanent diabetes insipidus. It is important to recognize that in some patients with coexisting defects in vasopressin secretion and ACTH secretion (for example, after resection of anterior and posterior pituitary gland for craniopharyngioma), symptoms of diabetes insipidus can be masked because cortisol deficiency (resulting from ACTH deficiency) impairs renal free water clearance. In such cases, diabetes insipidus manifests with initiation of glucocorticoid replacement therapy.

BENIGN AND MALIGNANT TUMORS   Because hypothalamic vasopressin neurons are distributed over a large area within the hypothalamus, tumors that cause diabetes insipidus must be extremely large, be infiltrative, or be strategically located at the point of convergence of the hypothalamoneurohypophyseal axonal tract in the infundibulum. Germinoma and pinealoma typically arise near the base of the hypothalamus where vasopressin axons converge before entering the posterior pituitary gland. For this reason these lesions are among the most common primary brain tumors associated with diabetes insipidus. Germinoma causing the disorder can be small and undetectable at MR imaging for several years after the onset of polyuria. For this reason, quantitative measurement of the β subunit of human chorionic gonadotropin, which is often secreted by germinoma and pinealoma, and repeated MR imaging of the brain are performed for children with unexplained diabetes insipidus.

INFILTRATIVE DISORDERS   Langerhans cell histiocytosis and lymphocytic hypophysitis are the most common types of infiltrative disorders causing diabetes insipidus. Approximately 10% of patients with histiocytosis have diabetes insipidus, usually those with more prolonged, multisystem disease. Anterior pituitary deficits often accompany posterior pituitary deficits. Magnetic resonance imaging characteristically shows thickening of the pituitary stalk. Radiation to the pituitary region within 14 days of the onset of symptoms of diabetes insipidus may result in return of vasopressin secretion. Diabetes insipidus never is caused by irradiation of the hypothalamic-pituitary region. Lymphocytic infundibuloneurohypophysitis, which can be associated with other autoimmune diseases, may account for more than one-half of cases of "idiopathic" central diabetes insipidus. Image analysis shows an enlarged pituitary gland and thickened stalk and magnocellular hypothalamic nuclei. A necrotizing form of this entity has been described that also causes anterior pituitary failure and responds to glucocorticoid treatment.

TRAUMA OR SHOCK   Permanent diabetes insipidus can be caused by seemingly minor trauma to the base of the brain. Swelling around or severance of the vasopressin-containing axons can cause transient or permanent defects in vasopressin secretion. Approximately one-half of patients with fractures of the sella turcica have permanent diabetes insipidus. Diabetes may not manifest for as long as 1 month after the trauma. During this time, the neurons of the severed axons undergo retrograde degeneration. Septic shock and postpartum hemorrhage also are associated with pituitary infarction (Sheehan syndrome) and cause varying degrees of diabetes insipidus. *Empty sella syndrome,* possibly caused by unrecognized pituitary infarction, can be associated with diabetes insipidus among children.

INHERITED AND DEVELOPMENTAL DEFECTS   Midline anatomic abnormalities of the brain such as septooptic dysplasia with agenesis of the corpus callosum, holoprosencephaly, and familial pituitary hypoplasia with absent stalk can be associated with central diabetes insipidus that usually manifests within the first month of life. These disorders often are associated with signs of anterior pituitary dysfunction, jaundice, and among boys, microphallus. Central diabetes insipidus and midline brain abnormalities can be accompanied by defects in thirst perception. Vasopressin deficiency occurs in the DIDMOAD syndrome, which consists of diabetes insipidus, diabetes mellitus, optic atrophy, and deafness. This syndrome, also know as *Wolfram syndrome,* is caused by recessive mutations in the recently identified gene *wolframin* on chromosome 4p16. The normal function of this gene, which is expressed in several tissues including brain and pancreas, is unknown.

Familial, autosomal dominant central diabetes insipidus manifests by about 5 years of age. Vasopressin secretion, initially normal, gradually declines until diabetes insipidus of variable severity ensues. Patients respond well to vasopressin replacement therapy. The disease has a high degree of penetrance but can be of variable severity within a family. Several different single nucleotide mutations in the vasopressin gene cause the disease, most occurring in the neurophysin region.

OTHERS   Infections involving the base of the brain, such as meningococcal, cryptococcal, *Listeria,* and toxoplasmosis meningitis; congenital cytomegalovirus infection; and nonspecific inflammatory disease of the brain, can cause central diabetes insipidus. The disease often is transient, suggesting that it is caused by inflammation rather than destruction of vasopressin-containing neurons. Diabetes insipidus can be associated with pulmony granulomatous disease, including sarcoidosis. It has been suggested that children with enuresis have a primary central deficiency in vasopressin secretion because children with enuresis often lack a nocturnal increase in plasma level of vasopressin, although the same findings can be caused solely by excessive water intake by these children. The use of desmopressin has been highly effective in abolishing bed wetting (see Sec. 21.5.9).

MANAGEMENT OF CENTRAL DIABETES INSIPIDUS

A person with an intact thirst mechanism and free access to fluids can maintain plasma osmolality and sodium in the high normal range, although at great inconvenience. An adult with uncontrolled diabetes insipidus with a maximum urine concentrating ability of about 100 mOsm/kg needs to ingest about 5 L of fluid per day. For children, long-standing intake of these high fluid volumes can cause hydroureter or hyperfluorosis in communities that fluoridate the water.

The management of central diabetes insipidus generally rests on replacement with vasopressin or desmopressin. There are two situations in which central diabetes insipidus often is best managed solely with high levels of fluid intake—treatment of neonates and young infants and during immediately postoperative management of central diabetes insipidus caused by neurosurgery. Because neonates and young infants receive all of their nutrition in liquid form, the obligatory high oral fluid requirements ($3 \text{ L/m}^2/\text{d}$) combined with vasopressin treatment are likely to cause complications of hyponatremia. In difficult cases, thiazide or amiloride diuretics can be added to facilitate renal proximal tubular sodium and water reabsorption, and decrease oral fluid requirements. When a child begins to eat solid foods, obligate fluid intake decreases and desmopressin therapy can be initiated more safely.

After neurosurgical procedures, immediate management of central diabetes insipidus is complicated by the variable timing of emergence of the inappropriate vasopressin secretion phase of the triple-phase response to neurosurgical injury discussed earlier. For these reasons, it is often best to treat young children who have acute postoperative diabetes insipidus with fluids alone, avoiding the use of vasopressin. This method consists of matching input and output once an hour using 1 to $3 \text{ L/m}^2/\text{d}$ (40 to $120 \text{ mL/m}^2/\text{h}$). If intravenous therapy is used, a basal $40\text{-mL/m}^2/\text{h}$ infusion of 5% dextrose in $\frac{1}{4}$ normal-saline solution is administered. Potassium chloride can be added to the basal solution if oral intake is to be delayed for several days. No additional fluid is administered for hourly urine outputs less than $40 \text{ mL/m}^2/\text{h}$, and then any additional urine volume is replaced with 5% dextrose in water (D_5W) up to a total of $120 \text{ mL/m}^2/\text{h}$. For example, for a child with a surface area of 1 m^2 (approximately 30 kg), the basal infusion rate is 40 mL/h of $D5_{1/4}NS$. If hourly urine output is 60 mL, an additional 20 mL/h, for a total infusion rate of 60 mL/h, is administered. For urine outputs greater than 120 mL/h, the maximum infusion rate is 120 mL/h. This type of therapy should maintain serum level of sodium at approximately 150 Eq/L. The patient is in a mildly volume contracted state, which allows assessment of both thirst sensation and return of either normal vasopressin secretion or the emergence of inappropriate secretion of vasopressin. Mild hypoglycemia can occur during this therapy, especially among patients receiving postoperative glucocorticoids. This fluid management protocol, however, because it does not entail use of vasopressin, eliminates any risk of hyponatremia.

Intravenous therapy with synthetic aqueous vasopressin (Pitressin) is useful in the management of central diabetes insipidus of acute onset. If vasopressin is administered in continuous infusion, fluid intake must be limited to $1 \text{ L/m}^2/\text{d}$ (assuming normal solute intake and nonrenal water losses). The potency of synthetic vasopressin is measured by means of bioassay and is expressed in bioactive units, 1 mU being equivalent to approximately 2.5 ng of vasopressin. For intravenous vasopressin therapy, a dose of 1.5 mU/kg per hour results in blood vasopressin concentrations of approximately 10 pg/mL, twice that needed for full antidiuretic activity. The effect of vasopressin is maximal within 2 hours of the start of infusion. In the care of patients treated with vasopressin for postneurosurgical diabetes insipidus, intravenous administration is changed to oral fluid intake at the earliest opportunity. Thirst sensation, if intact, helps regulate blood osmolality. Intravenous desmopressin is not used in the immediate management of postoperative central diabetes insipidus. It offers no advantage over vasopressin, and its long half-life compared with that of vasopressin is a distinct disadvantage, because it can increase the risk of water intoxication.

Outpatient treatment of children with central diabetes insipidus beyond infancy begins with oral desmopressin tablets. Young children may respond to 25 or 50 μg at bedtime. If the dose is effective

but has too short a duration of action, it can be increased further, or a second, morning dose can be added. Patients need to escape the antidiuretic effect of treatment for at least 1 hour before the next dose to ensure that any excessive water is excreted. Otherwise, water intoxication can occur. Desmopressin is available for intranasal administration (10 μg/0.1 mL). The initial dose is 0.025 mL (2.5 μg) given by means of rhinal tube at bedtime. Desmopressin is available as a nasal spray in the same concentration, each spray delivering 10 μg (0.1 mL). This is the standard preparation used to manage primary enuresis. When switching from nasal to oral desmopressin, the equivalent oral dose is 10- to 20-fold greater than the nasal dose.

A special problem arises when a patient undergoing long-term treatment of central diabetes insipidus is to undergo an elective surgical procedure necessitating general anesthesia. Two options can be considered. The patient can receive the usual regimen of desmopressin the morning of the operation. The alternative is to hold desmopressin the evening before and the morning of the operation. In either case, intra- and postoperative intravenous fluids are limited to 1 to $3 \text{ L/m}^2/\text{d}$ until the antidiuretic effect of desmopressin wanes. Therapy then is switched to oral fluid intake as soon as possible to allow thirst to guide replacement. Another special situation arises when a patient with central diabetes insipidus needs high volumes of fluid for therapeutic reasons, such as for cancer chemotherapy. These patients can be treated by means of discontinuation of antidiuretic therapy and an increase in fluid intake or with a low dose of intravenous vasopressin (0.1 mU/kg/h, approximately one-eighth the full antidiuretic dose), with which the partial antidiuretic effect allows administration of higher amounts of fluid without causing hyponatremia.

References

Boulgourdjian EM, Martinez AS, Ropelato MG, Heinrich JJ, Bergada C: Oral desmopressin treatment of central diabetes insipidus in children. Acta Paediatr 86:1261–1262, 1997

Miller WL: Molecular genetics of familial central diabetes insipidus. J Clin Endocrinol Metab 77:592–595, 1993

24.4 THE ADRENAL CORTEX

Walter L. Miller

24.4.1 Embryology and Anatomy

The adrenal cortex produces three principal categories of steroid hormones that regulate a wide variety of physiological processes. Mineralocorticoids, principally aldosterone, regulate renal retention of sodium and thus profoundly influence electrolyte balance, intravascular volume, and blood pressure. Glucocorticoids, principally cortisol, are named for their carbohydrate-mobilizing activity but are ubiquitous physiological regulators that influence a wide variety of bodily functions. Adrenal androgens serve no known physiological role but do mediate some secondary sexual characteristics among women, and overproduction may result in virilism.

EMBRYOLOGY

The cells of the adrenal cortex are mesodermal, unlike the ectodermal adrenal medulla. Between the fifth and sixth week of fetal development, the gonadal ridge develops near the rostral end of the mesonephros. These cells give rise to the steroidogenic cells of the gonads and to the adrenal cortex. The adrenal and gonadal cells separate, the adrenal cells migrating retroperitoneally and the gonadal cells migrating caudally. Between the seventh and eighth weeks of gestation, the adrenal cells are invaded by sympathetic neural cells that give rise to the adrenal medulla. By the end of the eighth week, the adrenal gland has become encapsulated and is clearly associated with the upper pole of the kidney, which at this time is much smaller than the adrenal gland.

The fetal adrenal cortex consists of an outer, *definitive* zone, the principal site of glucocorticoid and mineralocorticoid synthesis, and a much larger, *fetal* zone that makes androgenic precursors for the placental synthesis of estriol. The fetal adrenal gland is huge in proportion to other structures. At birth, the adrenal glands weigh 8 to 9 g, roughly twice the size of adult adrenal glands, and represent 0.5% of total body weight, compared with 0.0175% in adults.

ANATOMY

Unlike most other organs, the arteries and veins serving the adrenal glands do not run in parallel. Arterial blood is provided by several small arteries arising from the renal and phrenic arteries, the aorta, and sometimes the ovarian and left spermatic arteries. The veins are more conventional, the left adrenal vein draining into the left renal vein and the right adrenal vein draining directly into the vena cava. Arterial blood enters the sinusoidal circulation of the cortex and drains toward the medulla, so that medullary chromaffin cells are bathed in high concentrations of steroid hormones.

The adult adrenal cortex consists of three histologically recognizable zones: the glomerulosa is immediately below the capsule, the fasciculata is in the middle, and the reticularis lies next to the medulla. The glomerulosa, fasciculata, and reticularis, respectively, constitute about 15%, 75%, and 10% of the adrenal cortex of older children and adults. These zones appear to be distinct functionally as well as histologically, but considerable overlap exists. Immunocytochemical data show that the zones interdigitate physically. After birth, the large fetal zone begins to involute and disappears by 1 year of age. The definitive zone simultaneously enlarges, but two of the adult zones—glomerulosa and fasciculata—are not fully differentiated until about 3 years of age. The reticularis may not be fully differentiated until about 15 years of age.

24.4.2   Steroid Hormone Synthesis

EARLY STEPS: CHOLESTEROL UPTAKE, STORAGE, AND TRANSPORT

The human adrenal gland may synthesize cholesterol de novo from acetate, but most of its supply of cholesterol comes from plasma low-density lipoproteins (LDLs) derived from dietary cholesterol. Adequate concentrations of LDL suppress 3-hydroxy-3-methylglutaryl coenzyme A (HMG-CoA) reductase, the rate-limiting enzyme in cholesterol synthesis. ACTH, which stimulates adrenal steroidogenesis, also stimulates the activity of HMG-CoA reductase, LDL receptors, and uptake of LDL cholesterol. Esters of LDL cholesterol are taken up by means of receptor-mediated endocytosis and are stored directly or converted to free cholesterol and used for steroid hormone synthesis. Storage of cholesterol esters in lipid droplets is controlled by the action of two opposing enzymes, cholesterol esterase (cholesterol ester hydrolase) and cholesterol ester synthetase. ACTH stimulates the esterase and inhibits the synthe-

tase, increasing the availability of free cholesterol for steroid hormone synthesis.

STEROIDOGENIC ENZYMES

The principal pathways of human adrenal steroid hormone synthesis are shown in Fig. 24-7. Most steroidogenic enzymes are members of the cytochrome P450 group of oxidases. *Cytochrome P450* is a generic term for a large number of oxidative enzymes, all of which have about 500 amino acids and contain a single heme group. They are termed *P450 (pigment 450)* because all absorb light at 450 nm in their reduced states. Five distinct P450 enzymes are involved in adrenal steroidogenesis. P450scc, present in adrenal mitochondria, is the cholesterol side-chain cleavage enzyme that mediates the series of reactions formerly called *20,22 desmolase*. Two distinct isozymes of P450c11, also present in mitochondria, mediate 11-hydroxylase, 18-hydroxylase, and 18-methyl oxidase activities. P450c17, present in the endoplasmic reticulum, mediates the activity of both 17α-hydroxylase and 17,20 lyase. P450c21 mediates 21-hydroxylation of both glucocorticoids and mineralocorticoids. In the gonads, and elsewhere, P450aro in the endoplasmic reticulum mediates aromatization of androgens to estrogens.

In addition to the cytochrome P450 enzymes, a second class of enzymes termed *hydroxysteroid dehydrogenases* is involved in steroidogenesis. These enzymes do not have heme groups, and they require the oxidized form of nicotinamide adenine dinucleotide (NAD^+) or the oxidized form of NAD phosphate ($NADP^+$) as cofactors. Whereas most steroidogenic reactions catalyzed by P450 enzymes are caused by the action of a single form of P450, each of the reactions catalyzed by hydroxysteroid dehydrogenases can be catalyzed by at least two isozymes. Members of this family include the 3β-, 11β-, and 17β-hydroxysteroid dehydrogenases.

P450scc   Conversion of cholesterol to pregnenolone in mitochondria is the first, rate-limiting, and hormonally regulated step in the synthesis of all steroid hormones. This involves three distinct reactions, 20α-hydroxylation, 22-hydroxylation, and scission of the cholesterol side chain to yield pregnenolone and isocaproic acid. However, a single protein, termed *P450scc* (where *scc* refers to the side-chain cleavage of cholesterol) encoded by a single gene on chromosome 15, catalyzes all the steps between cholesterol and pregnenolone. These three reactions occur on a single active site that is in contact with the hydrophobic bilayer membrane.

StAR   Acute and chronic regulation of steroidogenesis occur at different levels. Chronic regulation, meaning the net steroidogenic capacity of the gland, is determined by transcriptional regulation of the gene for P450cc. Acute regulation, such as rapid synthesis and release of steroids in response to acute stress, is at the level of movement of cytoplasmic cholesterol into the mitochondria, where it can then be converted to pregnenolone by P450scc. The essential factor in this cholesterol flux is the steroidogenic acute regulatory protein (StAR). This short-lived protein acts on the mitochondria to move cholesterol from the outer to inner mitochondrial membrane. The action of StAR in the adrenal glands and gonads is essential, but other steroidogenic tissues that do not need to increase steroidogenesis rapidly, such as the placenta and brain, lack StAR.

3β-HYDROXYSTEROID   **DEHYDROGENASE/$\Delta^5 \rightarrow \Delta^4$**   **ISOMERASE**   Once pregnenolone is produced from cholesterol, it can undergo 17α-hydroxylation by P450c17 to yield 17-hydroxypregnenolone,

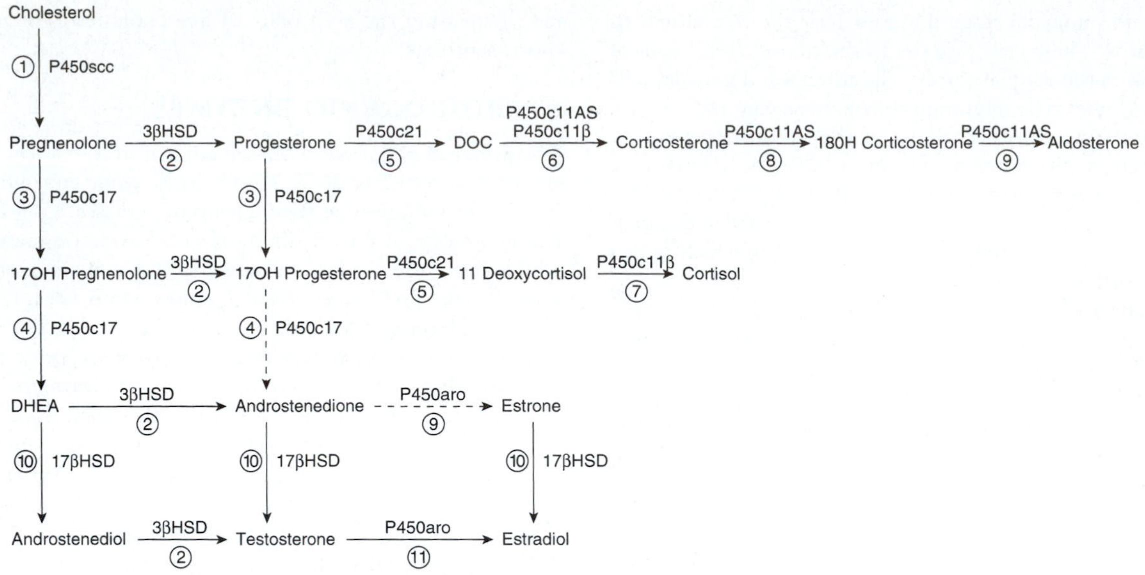

FIGURE 24-7   Principal pathways of human adrenal steroid hormone synthesis. Other quantitatively and physiologically minor steroids also are produced. The chemical identities of the enzymes are shown by each reaction. Reaction 1: Mitochondrial cytochrome P450scc mediates 20α-hydroxylation, 22-hydroxylation, and scission of the C20-22 carbon bond to convert cholesterol to pregnenolone. Reaction 2: 3β-HSD, a non-P450 enzyme bound to the endoplasmic reticulum, mediates 3β-hydroxysteroid dehydrogenase and isomerase activities. Reaction 3: P450c17 catalyzes the 17α-hydroxylation of pregnenolone to 17α-hydroxypregnenolone and of progesterone to 17α-hydroxyprogesterone (17OHP). Reaction 4: The 17,20-lyase activity of the 21-hydroxylation of both progesterone and 17OH pregnenolone to dihydroepiandrostenedione (DHEA), but very little 17OHP is converted to Δ^4 androstenedione. Reaction 5: P450c21 catalyzes the 21-hydroxylation of both progesterone and 17OHP. Reaction 7: P450c11β converts 11-deoxycortisol to cortisol. Reactions 6, 8, and 9: In the adrenal zona glomerulosa, deoxycorticosterone (DOC) is converted to corticosterone and then to 18OH-corticosterone and finally to aldosterone by a single enzyme, P450c11AS. DOC also can be converted to corticosterone by P450c11β in the zona fasciculata. Reactions 10 and 11 occur principally in the testes and ovaries. Reaction 10: Several isozymes of 17βHSD, a reversible non-P450 enzyme of the endoplasmic reticulum, mediate both 17-ketosteroid reductase and 17β-hydroxysteroid dehydrogenase activities, converting DHEA to androstenediol, androstenedione to testosterone, and estrone to estradiol. Reaction 11: Testosterone is converted to estradiol by P450aro. (SOURCE: *Modified from Miller WL: The molecular biology of steroid hormone synthesis. Endocr Rev 9:295, 1988.*)

or it can be converted to progesterone, the first biologically important steroid in the pathway. A single enzyme, 3β-hydroxysteroid dehydrogenase (3βHSD) catalyzes both conversion of the hydroxyl group to a keto group on carbon 3 and isomerization of the double bond from the B ring (Δ^5 steroids) to the A ring (Δ^4 steroids). This single enzyme converts pregnenolone to progesterone, 17α-hydroxypregnenolone to 17α-hydroxyprogesterone, dehydroepiandrosterone (DHEA) to androstenedione, and androstenediol to testosterone.

P450c17   Both pregnenolone and progesterone may undergo 17α-hydroxylation to 17α-hydroxypregnenolone and 17α-hydroxyprogesterone (17OHP). These latter 17-hydroxylated steroids then can undergo scission of the C17,20 carbon bond to yield DHEA, but 17OHP is not effectively converted to androstenedione by the adrenal glands or gonads of humans. All of these reactions are mediated by a single enzyme, P450c17, which is bound to smooth endoplasmic reticulum. Because P450c17 has both 17α-hydroxylase activity and C17,20 lyase activity, it is the key branch point in steroid hormone synthesis. If neither activity of P450c17 is present, pregnenolone is converted to mineralocorticoids; if 17α-hydroxylase activity is present but 17,20 lyase activity is not, pregnenolone

is converted to the glucocorticoid cortisol; if both activities are present, pregnenolone is converted to sex steroids. P450c17 is encoded by a single gene on chromosome 10 that is structurally related to the genes for P450c21 (21-hydroxylase).

P450c21   After synthesis of progesterone and 17OHP, these steroids are hydroxylated at the 21 position to yield deoxycorticosterone (DOC) and 11-deoxycortisol, respectively. The nature of the 21 hydroxylating step has been of great clinical interest because disordered 21-hydroxylation causes more than 90% of all congenital adrenal hyperplasia. Congenital adrenal hyperplasia has been extensively studied clinically. Adrenal 21-hydroxylase activity is catalyzed by P450c21, which is encoded by a single functional gene on chromosome 6p21. Because this gene lies in the middle of the major histocompatibility locus, disorders of adrenal 21-hydroxylation are closely linked to specific HLA types (see Sec. 24.4.6).

P450c11β AND P450c11AS   Two closely related enzymes, P450c11β and P450c11AS, catalyze the final steps in the synthesis of both glucocorticoids and mineralocorticoids. These two isozymes have 93% amino acid sequence identity and are encoded by duplicated genes on chromosome 8. Like P450scc, the two forms of P450c11 are present in the inner mitochondrial membrane and use adrenodoxin and adrenodoxin reductase to receive electrons from NADPH. By far the more abundant of the two isozymes is P450c11β, which is the classic 11β-hydroxylase that converts 11-deoxycortisol to cortisol and 11-DOC to corticosterone. The less abundant isozyme, P450c11AS, is present only in the zona glomerulosa, where it has 11β-hydroxylase, 18-hydroxylase, and 18-methyl oxidase (aldosterone synthase) activity; thus P450c11AS can catalyze all the reactions needed to convert DOC to aldosterone. P450c11β is primarily induced by ACTH through cAMP and is suppressed by glucocorticoids such as dexamethasone. Patients with disorders in P450c11β have classic 11β-hydroxylase deficiency but can still produce aldosterone. Patients with disorders in P450c11AS have rare forms of aldosterone deficiency (so-called corticosterone methyl oxidase deficiency) and retain the ability to produce cortisol.

17β-HYDROXYSTEROID DEHYDROGENASES Dehydroepiandrosterone is converted to androstenediol, androstenedione is converted to testosterone, and estrone is converted to estradiol by a series of enzymes called *17-ketosteroid reductase* or *17β-hydroxysteroid dehydrogenase* (17βHSD). At least four forms of 17βHSD are important in human steroidogenesis, although it is clear that other forms exist. Type I (17βHSD-I) is a purely estrogenic enzyme (produces estradiol and estriol) present in the placenta and ovary. Type III (17βHSD-III) is a purely androgenic enzyme (produces androstenedione and testosterone) present in the testes. These two enzymes can each inactivate estrogens or androgens, thus reversing the reactions catalyzed by 17βHSD-I and 17βHSD-III.

STEROID SULFOTRANSFERASE AND SULFATASE Steroid sulfates can be synthesized directly from cholesterol sulfate or be formed by sulfation of steroids by cytosolic sulfotransferases. Steroid sulfates also can be hydrolyzed to the native steroid by steroid sulfatase. Because of the association between steroid sulfatase deficiency and X-linked ichthyosis, much is known about this enzyme. In fetal adrenal glands and placenta, sulfatase deficiency decreases the pool of free DHEA available for placental conversion to estrogen, resulting in low concentrations of estriol in the maternal blood and urine, prolonged gestation, and prolonged, delayed labor. Accumulation of steroid sulfates in the stratum corneum of the skin causes ichthyosis. Study of genomic DNA from persons with this syndrome indicates deletions in this gene on chromosome Xp22.3 are a common cause of X-linked ichthyosis.

AROMATASE: P450aro Although not adrenal enzymes, aromatase and other steroidogenic enzymes are considered with adrenal steroidogenic enzymes. Estrogens are produced by aromatization of androgens, including adrenal androgens, by means of a complex series of reactions catalyzed by a single microsomal enzyme, P450aro. This typical cytochrome P450 is encoded by a single, large gene on chromosome 15q21.1. Expression of P450aro in extraglandular tissues, especially fat, can convert adrenal androgens to estrogens. Expression of aromatase in the epiphyses is responsible for local conversion of testosterone to estradiol, accelerating epiphyseal fusion and terminating growth.

5α-REDUCTASE Testosterone, a potent androgen, is converted to dihydrotestosterone, an even more potent androgen, by 5α-reductase, an enzyme present in some cells where testosterone acts. There are two distinct forms of 5α-reductase. The type I enzyme, present

in the scalp and other peripheral tissues, is encoded by a gene on chromosome 5. The type II enzyme, the predominant form in male reproductive tissues, is encoded by a structurally related gene on chromosome 2p23. The syndrome of 5α-reductase deficiency, a disorder of male sexual differentiation, is caused by a wide variety of mutations in the gene that encodes the type II enzyme.

11β-HYDROXYSTEROID DEHYDROGENASE Although certain steroids are categorized as glucocorticoids or mineralocorticoids, cloning and expression of the "mineralocorticoid" (glucocorticoid type II) receptor shows it has equal affinity for both aldosterone and cortisol. However, cortisol does not act as a mineralocorticoid in vivo. In tissues sensitive to mineralocorticoids, including liver and kidney, cortisol is enzymatically converted to cortisone, a metabolically inactive steroid. The interconversion of cortisol and cortisone is mediated by two isozymes of 11β-dehydrogenase (11βHSD). The type I enzyme (11βHSD-I) is expressed mainly in glucocorticoid-responsive tissues such as the liver, testis, lung, and proximal convoluted tubule. 11βHSD-I can catalyze both the oxidation of cortisol to cortisone with NADP$^+$ as the cofactor and reduction of cortisone to cortisol with NADPH as the cofactor. The reaction catalyzed depends on which cofactor is available, but the enzyme can only function with a high concentration of steroid (K_m = 1mmol/L). 11βHSD-II catalyzes only the oxidation of cortisol to cortisone with NADH and can function with low concentrations of steroid (K_m = 10–100nmol/L). 11βHSD-II is expressed in mineralocorticoid-responsive tissues and thus serves to defend the mineralocorticoid receptor by inactivating cortisol to cortisone, so that only true mineralocorticoids, such as aldosterone or DOC, can exert a mineralocorticoid effect.

FETAL ADRENAL STEROIDOGENESIS

Fetal adrenocortical steroidogenesis begins quite early, approximately the sixth week of gestation. Fetuses with genetic lesions of adrenal steroidogenesis can produce sufficient adrenal androgen to virilize a female fetus to a nearly male appearance (see Sec. 24.4.6). This masculinization of the genitalia is complete by the 12th week of gestation. The definitive zone of the fetal adrenal gland produces steroid hormones according to the pathways in Fig. 24-7. In contrast, the large fetal zone of the adrenal gland is relatively deficient in 3βHSD and has relatively abundant 17,20 lyase activity of P450c17. Thus it produces a huge amount of DHEA and its sulfate (DHEAS). The fetal adrenal gland also has considerable sulfotransferase activity but little steroid sulfatase activity, also favoring conversion of DHEA to DHEAS. The resulting DHEAS cannot be a substrate for adrenal 3βHSD; instead, it is secreted, 16α-hydroxylated in the fetal liver, and then acted on by placental 3βHSD-I, 17βHSD-I, and P450aro to produce estriol, or the substrates can bypass the liver to yield estrone and estradiol. Placental estrogens inhibit adrenal 3βHSD activity and provide a feedback system to promote production of DHEAS. Fetal adrenal steroids account for 50% of the estrone and estradiol and 90% of the estriol in the maternal circulation.

Although the fetoplacental unit produces huge amounts of DHEA, DHEAS and estriol, as well as other steroids, these substances do not appear to have an essential role. Successful pregnancy depends on placental synthesis of progesterone, which suppresses uterine contractility and prevents spontaneous abortion; however, fetuses with genetic disorders of adrenal and gonadal steroidogenesis develop normally, reach term, and are delivered normally. Mineralocorticoid and glucocorticoid production is needed postnatally but not prenatally, estrogens are not needed, and androgens are needed only for male sexual differentiation.

Regulation of steroidogenesis and growth of the fetal adrenal gland are not fully understood, although excess ACTH is clearly involved in adrenal growth and overproduction of androgens among fetuses with congenital adrenal hyperplasia. Prenatal suppression of ACTH can greatly decrease production of fetal adrenal androgens and thus decrease virilization of female fetuses. The hypothalamic-pituitary-adrenal axis functions early in fetal life. In contrast, anencephalic fetuses lacking pituitary ACTH have adrenal glands that retain the capability of steroidogenesis. Fetal adrenal steroidogenesis is regulated by both ACTH-dependent and ACTH-independent mechanisms.

24.4.3 Regulation of Steroidogenesis

GLUCOCORTICOID SECRETION: THE HYPOTHALAMIC-PITUITARY-ADRENAL AXIS

Hypothalamus: Corticotropin-Releasing Factor and Arginine Vasopressin

The principal steroidal product of the human adrenal gland is cortisol, which is mainly secreted in response to ACTH produced in the pituitary gland. Secretion of ACTH is stimulated primarily by corticotropin-releasing factor (CRF) from the hypothalamus. These are the major, but by no means the sole, components of the hypothalamic-pituitary-adrenal axis. Hypothalamic CRF is a 41-amino-acid peptide synthesized mainly by neurons in the paraventricular nucleus. These same hypothalamic neurons also produce the decapeptide arginine vasopressin (AVP, also known as antidiuretic hormone). Corticotropin-releasing factor and AVP travel through axons to the median eminence, which releases them into the pituitary portal circulation, although most AVP axons terminate in the posterior pituitary gland. Corticotropin-releasing factor and AVP stimulate synthesis and release of ACTH through different cellular mechanisms. Corticotropin-releasing factor is the more important physiological stimulator of ACTH release, although maximal doses of AVP can elicit a maximal ACTH response. When given together, CRF and AVP act synergistically, as is expected from the independent mechanisms of action.

Pituitary Gland: ACTH and Proopiomelanocortin

Pituitary ACTH is a 39-amino-acid peptide derived from proopiomelanocortin (POMC), a 241-amino-acid protein. This protein undergoes a series of proteolytic cleavages to yield several biologically active peptides (Fig. 24-8). The N-terminal glycopeptide (POM C1–75) can stimulate steroidogenesis and may function as an adrenal mitogen. POMC 112–150 is ACTH 1–39, POMC 112–126 and POMC 191–207 constitute α and β melanocyte stimulating hormone, respectively, and POMC 210–241 is β-endorphin. POMC also is produced in small amounts by the brain, testes, and placenta, but this extrapituitary POMC does not contribute greatly to circulating ACTH. Malignant tumors commonly produce "ectopic ACTH" in adults and rarely in children. This ACTH also is derived from POMC. Only the first 20 to 24 amino acids of ACTH are needed for its full biological activity, and synthetic ACTH 1–24 is widely used in diagnostic tests of adrenal

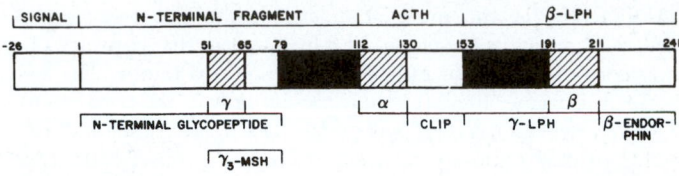

HUMAN PRE-PRO-OPIOMELANOCORTIN

FIGURE 24-8 Structure of human preproopiomelanocortin (POMC). The *numbers* are amino acid positions. Number 1 is assigned to the first amino acid of POMC after the 26-amino-acid signal peptide, which directs the protein to be secreted from the cell. The α, β, and γ melanocyte-stimulating hormone (MSH) regions, which characterize the three constant regions, are indicated by *diagonal lines*. The variable regions are *solid*. The amino acid numbers shown refer to the N-terminal amino acid of each cleavage site. Because these amino acids are removed, the numbers do not correspond exactly with the amino acid numbers of the peptides used in the text. LPH = lipotrophin. (SOURCE: *Miller WL, Baxter JD, Eberhardt NL: In: Krieger DT, Brownstein MJ, Martin JB eds Brain Peptides. New York, Wiley, 1983.*)

function. However, these shorter forms of ACTH have a shorter half-life than does native ACTH 1–39.

Actions of ACTH

ACTH stimulates steroidogenesis by interacting with receptors that stimulate production of cAMP. This elicits short- and long-term effects. ACTH through cAMP stimulates production of LDL receptors and uptake of LDL cholesterol, stimulates cholesterol esterase while inhibiting cholesterol ester synthase to increase intracellular free cholesterol, and stimulates synthesis and phosphorylation of StAR to increase cholesterol flux into mitochondria to deliver cholesterol substrate to P450scc. All of these actions occur within minutes and constitute the "acute" effect of ACTH on steroidogenesis. The adrenal glands contain relatively modest amounts of steroid hormones; thus release of preformed cortisol does not contribute a great deal to the acute response to ACTH. The long-term ("chronic") effects of ACTH are mediated primarily by increasing the transcription of the genes for the steroidogenic enzymes, thus increasing the net steroidogenic capacity of the adrenal glands.

The role of ACTH and other peptides derived from POMC in stimulating growth of the adult adrenal glands remain uncertain. In fetal adrenal glands, however, ACTH stimulates local production of IGF-II and of basic fibroblast growth factor. These two factors, possibly in conjunction with epidermal growth factor, are mediators of ACTH-induced growth of fetal adrenal glands.

Diurnal Rhythms of ACTH and Cortisol

Plasma concentrations of ACTH and cortisol tend to be high in the morning and low in the evening. Peak ACTH concentration usually occurs at 4 to 6 a.m. and peak cortisol value at about 8 a.m. Both ACTH and cortisol are released episodically in pulses every 30 to 120 minutes throughout the day, but the frequency and amplitude of these pulses is much greater in the morning. At least four related factors appear to play a role in the rhythm of ACTH and cortisol: intrinsic rhythmicity of synthesis and secretion of CRF by the hypothalamus; light-dark cycles; feeding cycles; and inherent rhythmicity in the adrenal glands, possibly mediated by adrenal innervation. In healthy persons, cortisol is released before lunch and supper, but not at these times in persons who eat continuously during the day. Thus glucocorticoids, which increase blood glucose level, appear to be released at times of fasting and are inhibited by feeding.

As most parents know, infants do not have a diurnal rhythm of sleep or feeding. Infants acquire such behavioral rhythms in response to their environment long before they acquire a rhythm of ACTH and cortisol. The diurnal rhythm of ACTH and cortisol begins to be established by 6 months of age but may not be well established until after 3 years of age. Once established, this rhythm is changed only with difficulty. When persons move to different parts of the world, their ACTH-cortisol rhythms generally take 15 to 20 days to adjust appropriately.

Physical stress, such as blood loss or high fever, can increase secretion of both ACTH and cortisol, but minor surgery and minor illnesses, such as upper respiratory infections, have little effect on ACTH and cortisol secretion. Most psychoactive drugs, such as anticonvulsants, neurotransmitters, and antidepressants, do not affect the diurnal rhythm of ACTH and cortisol, although cyproheptadine (a serotonin antagonist) effectively suppresses ACTH release.

Adrenal Glands: Glucocorticoid Feedback

The hypothalamic-pituitary-adrenal axis is a classic example of an endocrine feedback system. ACTH increases production of cortisol, and cortisol decreases production of ACTH. Cortisol and other glucocorticoids exert feedback inhibition of both CRF and ACTH. Like the acute and chronic phases of the action of ACTH on the adrenal glands, there are acute and chronic phases of the feedback inhibition of ACTH and presumably of CRF. The acute phase, which occurs within minutes, inhibits release of ACTH and CRF from secretory granules. With prolonged exposure, glucocorticoids inhibit ACTH synthesis by directly inhibiting transcription of the gene for POMC.

MINERALOCORTICOID SECRETION: THE RENIN-ANGIOTENSIN SYSTEM

Renin is a serine protease enzyme synthesized largely by the juxtaglomerular cells of the kidney. Decreased blood pressure, upright posture, sodium depletion, vasodilatory drugs, kallikrein, opiates, and β-adrenergic stimulation all promote release of renin. In the circulation, renin enzymatically attacks angiotensinogen, the renin substrate, to release the amino-terminal 10 amino acids of angiotensinogen, referred to as *angiotensin I*. This decapeptide is biologically inactive until converting enzyme, present primarily in the lungs and blood vessels, cleaves off its two carboxy-terminal amino acids to produce the octapeptide angiotensin II. Inhibition of the action of converting enzyme by agents such as captopril is useful in both the diagnosis and management of hyperreninemic hypertension.

Angiotensin II has two principal actions, both of which increase blood pressure. It directly stimulates arteriolar vasoconstriction within a few seconds and stimulates synthesis and secretion of aldosterone within minutes. An increased plasma level of potassium is also a powerful and direct stimulator of aldosterone synthesis and release. Aldosterone, secreted by the glomerulosa cells of the adrenal cortex, has the greatest mineralocorticoid activity of all naturally occurring steroids. Aldosterone causes renal sodium retention and potassium loss with a consequent increase in intravascular volume and blood pressure. Angiotensin II functions through receptors that stimulate production of phosphatidylinositol, mobilize intracellular and extracellular Ca^{2+}, and activate protein kinase C.

Although the renin-angiotensin system is clearly the main regulator of mineralocorticoid secretion, ACTH and possibly other POMC-derived peptides can promote secretion of aldosterone. Ammonium ion, hyponatremia, and dopamine antagonists can stimulate secretion of aldosterone, and atrial natriuretic factor is a potent physiological inhibitor of aldosterone secretion.

ADRENAL ANDROGEN SECRETION: REGULATION OF ADRENARCHE

Dehydroepiandrosterone, DHEAS, and androstenedione, which are almost exclusively secreted by the adrenal zona reticularis, are generally called *adrenal androgens* because they can be peripherally converted to testosterone. However, these steroids have little capability of binding to and activating androgen receptors, hence are really androgen precursors. The adrenal glands of young children secrete small amounts of DHEA, DHEAS, and androstenedione until the onset of adrenarche, usually approximately 8 years of age. Adrenarche is independent of puberty, the gonads, or gonadotropins, and the mechanism by which the onset of adrenarche is triggered remains unknown. Secretion of DHEA and DHEAS continues to increase during and after puberty and reaches maximal value in young adulthood, after which there is a gradual decrease in secretion of these steroids into the eight and ninth decades of life ("adrenopause") (Fig. 24-9). Despite the huge increases in adrenal secretion of DHEA and DHEAS during adrenarche, circulating concentrations of ACTH and cortisol do not change with age. Thus ACTH plays a permissive role in adrenarche but does not trigger it. Searches for hypothetical polypeptide hormones that might specifically stimulate the zona reticularis have been unsuccessful. Studies of adrenarche have focused on the roles of $3\beta HSD$ and P450c17. The abundance of $3\beta HSD$ protein in the zona reticularis appears to decrease with the onset of adrenarche, and the adrenal expression of cytochrome b_5, which fosters the 17,20 lyase activity of P450c17, is almost exclusively confined to the zona reticularis. Both of these factors strongly favor production of DHEA. Premature and exaggerated adrenarche has been found in association with insulin resistance. Girls with premature exaggerated adrenarche appear to be at much higher risk of polycystic ovary syndrome as adults (characterized by hyperandrogenism, fewer ovulatory cycles, insulin resistance, and hypertriglyceridemia). Evidence is accumulating to suggest that replacing DHEA lost during adrenopause may improve memory and a sense of well-being among the elderly. Results of studies of the physiological, biochemical, and clinical correlates of adrenarche point to premature adrenarche as an early sign of a metabolic disorder.

24.4.4   Plasma Steroids and their Disposal

All steroid hormones are derivatives of pregnenolone (Fig. 24-10). Because pregnenolone and its derivatives contain 21 carbon atoms, they are often called *C21 steroids*. Each carbon atom is numbered to indicate the location at which the various steroidogenic reactions occur (eg, 21-hydroxylation, 11-hydroxylation). The 17,20 lyase activity of P450c17 cleaves the bond between carbon atoms 17 and

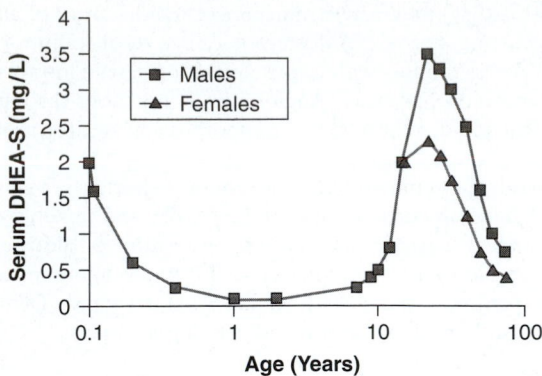

FIGURE 24-9   Concentrations of DHEAS as a function of age. The x-axis is a log scale.

20 to yield C19 sex steroids. Steroids that have a double bond between carbon atoms 4 and 5 are called Δ^4 *steroids*. Their precursors that have a double bond between carbon atoms 5 and 6 are called Δ^5 *steroids;* 3βHSD converts Δ^5 to Δ^4 steroids.

More than 50 different steroids have been isolated from adrenocortical tissue, but only a few are secreted in sizable quantities. Adult secretion of cortisol is approximately 15 mg per 24 hours. Secretion of corticosterone, a weak glucocorticoid, is approximately 2 mg per 24 hours. However, the adult secretion rate of aldosterone is only approximately 0.1 mg per 24 hours. This 200-fold molar difference in secretory rates of cortisol and aldosterone must be remembered when the effects of plasma steroid binding proteins are being considered and when the consequences of incomplete defects in steroidogenesis are being conceptualized.

Most circulating steroids are bound to plasma proteins, including corticosteroid-binding globulin (CBG, also called *transcortin*), albumin, and α_1-acid glycoprotein. Transcortin has a high affinity for cortisol but a relatively low binding capacity. Albumin has a low affinity and high capacity. α_1-Acid glycoprotein is intermediate for the two variables. The result is that approximately 90% of circulating cortisol is bound to transcortin and a small amount more is bound to other proteins. These steroid-binding proteins are not transport proteins. The biologically important steroids are water soluble in physiologically effective concentrations, and persons without transcortin have no obvious untoward effects. However, these plasma proteins do act as a reservoir for steroids. This ensures

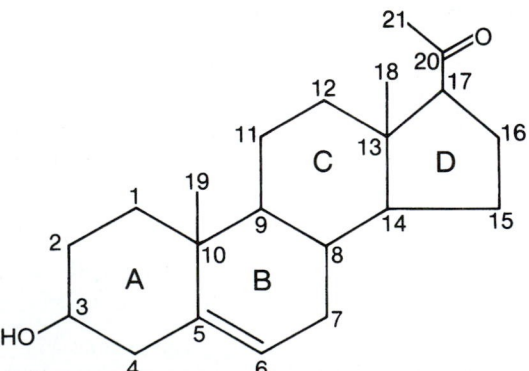

FIGURE 24-10   Structure of pregnenolone. The carbon atoms are *numbered.* **These indicate the sites of action of the various enzymes. The isomerase activity of 3β-hydroxysteroid dehydrogenase moves the double bond between carbons 5 and 6 in the B ring (Δ^5 compounds) to between carbons 4 and 5 in the A ring (Δ^4 compounds).**

that peripheral tissues are bathed in roughly equal concentrations of cortisol and greatly diminishes the physiological effect of the diurnal variation in cortisol secretion. The synthetic glucocorticoids used in therapy do not bind to a great extent to transcortin and bind poorly to albumin, partially accounting for increased potency and increased receptor-binding affinity. Aldosterone is not bound well by any plasma protein. Changes in plasma protein concentration therefore do not affect plasma aldosterone concentration but greatly influence plasma cortisol concentration. Estradiol and testosterone bind strongly to another plasma protein, called *sex steroid–binding globulin* and also bind weakly to albumin.

It is often thought that the concentration of "free" (unbound) circulating steroids determines biological activity. However, the target tissues for many steroid hormones contain enzymes that modify those steroids. Thus many actions of testosterone are actually caused by dihydrotestosterone produced by local 5α-reductase. Cortisol has differential actions on various tissues because of the presence or absence of 11βHSD, which inactivates cortisol to cortisone. Similar peripheral metabolism occurs through "extraglandular" 21-hydroxylase, P450aro, 3βHSD, and 17-ketosteroid reductase. Thus circulating steroids are both classic hormones and precursors of locally acting paracrine factors.

Only about 1% of circulating plasma cortisol and aldosterone are excreted unchanged in the urine. The rest is metabolized by the liver. There are many hepatic metabolites of each steroid. Most carry additional hydroxyl groups or are linked to a glucuronide moiety, rendering them more soluble and readily excreted by the kidney.

24.4.5   Clinical and Laboratory Evaluation of Adrenal Function

CLINICAL EVALUATION

Astute clinical evaluation usually discloses the presence of primary adrenal deficiency or hypersecretion before laboratory tests are performed. Most patients with chronic adrenal insufficiency have weakness, fatigue, anorexia, weight loss, hypotension, and hyperpigmentation. Patients with acute adrenal insufficiency can have hypotension, shock, weakness, apathy, confusion, anorexia, nausea, vomiting, dehydration, abdominal or flank pain, hyperthermia, and hypoglycemia. Girls with deficient adrenal androgen secretion have decreased virilizing secondary sexual characteristics (pubic and axillary hair, comedomes, axillary odor). Early signs of glucocorticoid excess include increased appetite, weight gain, and growth arrest without concomitant delay in bone age. Chronic glucocorticoid excess among children causes typical cushingoid facies, but the buffalo hump and centripetal distribution of body fat characteristic of adult Cushing disease occur only with long-standing undiagnosed disease. Mineralocorticoid excess is characterized principally by hypertension, but this condition can be masked if the patient is consuming a very low sodium diet (eg, is a newborn). Hypersecretion of adrenal androgens is characterized by accelerated growth with a disproportionate increase in bone age, increased muscle mass, acne, hirsutism, deepening of the voice, and virilism. An important feature of any physical examination of a virilized boy is careful examination and measurement of the testes. Bilateral enlargement of the testes suggests central (true) precocious puberty. Unilateral testicular enlargement suggests testicular tumor. Prepubertal testes in a virilized boy indicate an extratesticular source of androgen, such as the adrenal glands.

TABLE 24-8

MEAN SEX STEROID CONCENTRATION AMONG INFANTS AND CHILDREN

	PROG	17OHP	DHEA	DHEA-S (μg/dL)	Δ^4-A	E_1	E_2	T M	T F	DHT M	DHT F
Cord blood	36,000	1900	600	235	90	1400	810	30	25	6	6
Premature infants	350	250	800	400	200			120	10	30	4
Term newborns		35	570	160	150			200	40	25	10
Infants	30	30	110	30	20	<1.5	<1.5	190	<10	40	<3
Children 1–6 yr			30	10	25	<1.5	<1.5		5		<3
6–8 yr			90	20	25	<1.5	<1.5		5		<3
8–10 yr			160	50	25	<1.5	<1.5		5		<3
Male											
Pubertal stage I	20	40	160	35	25	1.1	0.8		5		<3
II	20	50	300	95	45	1.6	1.1		40		8
III	25	60	390	120	70	2.1	1.6		190		20
IV	35	80	400	200	80	3.3	2.2		370		35
V	40	100	500	230	100	3.2	2.1		550		45
Adult	35	100	450	270	115	3.0	2.0		620		50
Female											
Pubertal stage I	20	30	160	40	25	1.3	0.8		5		<3
II	30	50	330	70	65	2.1	1.6		20		8
III	40	70	390	90	120	3.0	2.5		25		10
IV	290	90	430	120	130	3.6	4.7		25		10
V	160	110	540	150	160	6.1	11.0		30		10
Adult											
Follicular	30	45	450	150	165	6.0	5.0		30		10
Luteal	750	165	450	150	165	11.0	13.0		30		10

All values except DHEAS are ng/dL of plasma.
PROG = progesterone; 17OHP = 17 hydroxyprogesterone; DHEA = dehydroepiandrosterone; DHEAS = DHEA sulfate; Δ^4A = androstenedione; E_1 = estrone; E_2 = estradiol; T = testosterone; DHT = dihydrotestosterone; M = male; F = female.
SOURCE: *Data adapted from Endocrine Sciences, Tarzana, CA.*

Imaging studies are of limited usefulness in the diagnosis of adrenal disease. Computed tomography and MR imaging only rarely depict pituitary tumors hypersecreting ACTH. More than 90% of such tumors are invisible to current imaging techniques, although preliminary results with MR imaging with gadolinium enhancement suggest better results. Small size, odd shape, and location of the glands near other structures compromise use of imaging of the adrenal glands. Patients with Cushing disease or congenital adrenal hyperplasia have modest enlargement of the adrenal glands, but this is not consistently detectable with imaging. The gross enlargement of the adrenal glands in congenital lipoid adrenal hyperplasia, hypoplasia in hereditary ACTH unresponsiveness syndrome, and many malignant tumors, however, can be diagnosed with imaging studies. Many adrenal adenomas are too small to be detected.

LABORATORY EVALUATION

The diagnostic evaluation of adrenal function is essentially chemical. The nonspecificity of many of the clinical signs and the disappointing results of imaging studies remind us that any proper evaluation of hypothalamic-pituitary-adrenal function must rely on a series of carefully performed physiological tests and biochemical assays. Highly specific, sensitive immunoassays can be performed on small volumes of plasma to allow direct examination of most adrenal steroids.

PLASMA CONCENTRATIONS OF CORTISOL AND OTHER STEROIDS Plasma cortisol is measured routinely with a variety of techniques, including radioimmunoassay and high-pressure liquid chromatography (HPLC). It is important to know which procedure one's hospital or commercial laboratory is using and precisely what it is measuring. All immunoassays have some degree of cross-reactivity with other steroids. Most cortisol immunoassays detect both cortisol and cortisone; these substances are readily differentiated with HPLC. Because the plasma of a newborn contains mainly cortisone rather than cortisol during the first few days of life, comparison of newborn data obtained with HPLC to published standards obtained by means of immunoassay may incorrectly suggest adrenal insufficiency. Tables 24-8 and 24-9 summarize normal plasma concentrations of a variety of steroids in infancy and childhood. With the notable exception of DHEAS, most adrenal steroids have diurnal variation based on the diurnal rhythm of ACTH. Because the stress of illness or hospitalization can increase adrenal steroid secretion and because diurnal rhythms may not be well established among children younger than 3 years, it is best to obtain two or more samples for measurement of any steroid. Not all endocrine laboratories can assay all steroids, and depending on the assay procedures used, various laboratories can have different normal values. Most central hospital and commercial laboratories are designed primarily to serve adult rather than pediatric patients. It is important to know whether the available assays are sufficiently sensitive with small volumes of blood to be useful in measuring pediatric values. This is especially true for measurement of sex steroids and gonadotropins, which can have pathological elevations among children and still be below the limit of detection of most "adult" assays.

PLASMA RENIN Renin usually is not measured directly but is assayed according to its enzymatic activity. Plasma renin activity

TABLE 24-9
MEAN GLUCOCORTICOID AND MINERALOCORTICOID CONCENTRATIONS

	CORTISOL	DOC	CORTICOSTERONE	18-OH CORTICOSTERONE	ALDOSTERONE	PLASMA RENIN ACTIVITY
Cord blood	13	180	650	—	85	1800
Premature infants	6.5	—	—	200	100	8000
Newborns	5	—	230	350	95	2100
Infants	9	20	545	80	30	1200
Children (8 a.m.)						
1–2 yr	4–20	—	—	65	2→8[a]	535
2–10 yr	As adults	10	—	45	10→30[a]	300
10–15 yr	As adults	—	—	25	5→20[a]	120
Adults (8 a.m.)	10–20	7	425	20	7→13[a]	100→145[a]
(4 p.m.)	5–10	—	130	—		

All values in ng/dL plasma except cortisol (μg/dL) and plasma renin activity (ng/dL/h).
[a] Two values separated by an arrow indicate those in supine and upright posture.
DOC = deoxycorticosterone.

(PRA) is simply an immunoassay of the amount of angiotensin I generated per milliliter of serum per hour at 37°C. In normal serum, the concentration of both renin and angiotensinogen, the renin substrate, is limiting. Another test, plasma renin content, is performed to measure the amount of angiotensin I generated in 1 hour at 37°C in the presence of excess concentration of angiotensinogen.

Plasma renin activity is sensitive to dietary sodium intake, posture, diuretic therapy, activity, and sex steroids. Because PRA values can vary widely with these variables, it is best to measure renin twice, once in the morning after overnight supine posture and then again after maintenance of upright posture for 4 hours. A simultaneous 24-hour collection of urine for measurement of total sodium excretion usually is needed to interpret PRA results. Low levels of dietary and urinary sodium, low intravascular volume, and presence of diuretics and estrogens increase PRA. Sodium loading, hyperaldosteronemia, and increased intravascular volume decrease PRA.

Renin measurements are used in the evaluation of hypertension and in the management of congenital adrenal hyperplasia. Children with simple virilizing adrenal hyperplasia who do not have clinical evidence of urinary salt wasting (hyponatremia, hyperkalemia, acidosis, hypotension, shock) can nevertheless have increased PRA, especially when dietary sodium is restricted. Therapy for simple virilizing 21-hydroxylase deficiency with sufficient mineralocorticoid to suppress PRA into the normal range reduces the child's requirement for glucocorticoids and maximizes final adult height. Children with congenital adrenal hyperplasia need to have mineralocorticoid replacement therapy monitored routinely with measurement of PRA.

URINARY STEROID EXCRETION Measurement of 24-hour urinary excretion of steroid metabolites is one of the oldest procedures for assessing adrenal function and is one of the most useful. Examination of total 24-hour excretion of steroids eliminates fluctuation in serum samples caused by time of day, episodic bursts of ACTH and steroid secretion, and transient stress, such as a visit to the clinic or difficult venipuncture. Collection of a complete 24-hour urinary sample can be difficult for infants or small children. It is strongly recommended that two consecutive 24-hour collections

be obtained and that each be assayed for creatinine to monitor the completeness of the collection. Because of the diurnal and episodic nature of steroid secretion, one should never obtain 8- or 12-hour collections and attempt to infer the 24-hour excretory rate from such partial collections.

Urinary 17-hydroxycorticosteroids (17OHCS), assayed with the colorimetric Porter-Silber reaction, are used to measure the major urinary metabolites of cortisol and cortisone. It is also used to measure metabolites of 11-deoxycortisol, which are increased in 11-hydroxylase deficiency or after treatment with metyrapone, a commonly used diagnostic agent (see later). Urinary secretion of 17OHCS increases in obesity, hyperthyroidism, and anorexia nervosa. It decreases in starvation, hypothyroidism, renal failure, liver disease, and pregnancy. Drugs that induce hepatic enzymes, such as phenobarbital, can cause low urinary 17OHCS values by stimulating hepatic metabolism of circulating steroids to excreted compounds not detected with the Porter-Silber reaction. Phenothiazines, spironolactone, hydroxyzine, and some antibiotics can interfere with the colorimetric assay directly, giving falsely elevated values.

Measurement of urinary free cortisol avoids the nonspecificity and drug interference problems inherent with 17OHCS. This test is highly reliable in the diagnosis of Cushing syndrome among adults, but there is less experience in the care of children with Cushing syndrome. Excretion of urinary free cortisol is 15 to 20 μg/g of creatinine among healthy children and as much as 40 μg/g of creatinine among obese children. Values in Cushing syndrome exceed these. These values emphasize the need to measure creatinine to monitor the completeness of the collection and to allow a simple means of adjusting for body size.

Urinary 17-ketosteroids, assayed with the Zimmerman reaction, are used to measure 17-ketosteroids by means of generation of a colored compound. The reaction is used principally to measure metabolites of DHEA and DHEAS and thus correlates with adrenal androgen production, but androstenedione, testosterone, and dihydrotestosterone are not measured. Penicillin, nalidixic acid, spironolactone, phenothiazines, and nonspecific urinary chromagens can spuriously increase values of 17-ketosteroids. Measurement of plasma DHEAS has largely replaced the use of urinary 17-ketosteroids.

TABLE 24-10

RESPONSES OF ADRENAL STEROIDS TO A 60-MINUTE ACTH TEST

STEROID	INFANT		PREPUBERTAL		PUBERTAL	
	BASAL	STIMULATED	BASAL	STIMULATED	BASAL	STIMULATED
17OH-Pregnenolone	225	—	55	320	120	800
17-Hydroxyprogesterone	25	190	50	190	60	160
Dehydroepiandrosterone	40	—	70	125	260	560
11-Deoxycortisol	80	—	60	200	60	170
Cortisol (μg/dL)	10	30	13	30	10	25
Deoxycorticosterone	20	80	8	55	8	55
Progesterone	35	100	35	125	60	150

All values are mean values in ng/dL of plasma, except cortisol, which is μg/dL.
SOURCE: *Data adapted from Endocrine Sciences, Tarzana, CA.*

PLASMA ACTH Accurate routine immunoassay of plasma ACTH is now available from several commercial laboratories. The samples must be handled with care. Samples are drawn into a plastic syringe containing heparin or ethylenediamine tetraacetic acid (EDTA) and quickly transported in plastic tubes on ice, because ACTH adheres to glass and is quickly inactivated. Elevated plasma ACTH concentrations can be highly informative, but most tests cannot detect low or low-normal values, and such values can be spurious if the samples are handled badly. For adults and older children who have well-established diurnal rhythms of ACTH, normal 8 a.m. values rarely exceed 50 pg/mL, whereas values between 8 p.m. and midnight usually are undetectable. Patients with Cushing disease often have normal morning values, but the diagnosis can be suggested by increased evening values.

SECRETORY RATES The secretory rates of cortisol, aldosterone, and other steroids can be measured by means of administering a small dose of tritiated cortisol or aldosterone and measuring the specific activity of one or more known metabolites in a 24-hour urine collection. Results with this and other procedures show that children and adults secrete about 6 to 9 mg cortisol per square meter of body surface area per day. This number is of considerable importance in estimating physiologic replacement doses of glucocorticoids (see Sec. 24.4.9).

DEXAMETHASONE SUPPRESSION TEST Administration of small doses of dexamethasone, a potent synthetic glucocorticoid, suppresses secretion of pituitary ACTH and of adrenal cortisol and allows one to determine whether glucocorticoid excess is caused primarily by pituitary disease or by adrenal disease. Because dexamethasone also suppresses adrenal androgen secretion, this test is useful for differentiating adrenal and gonadal sources of sex steroids. A complete, formal dexamethasone suppression test necessitates measurement of basal values and those obtained in response to both low and high doses of dexamethasone. This is described in the evaluation of Cushing syndrome in Sec. 24.4.8. Variations of this test are commonly used in the care of adults, notably the single-dose 1.0-mg overnight suppression test. This is a useful outpatient screening procedure for differentiating Cushing syndrome from exogenous obesity. It can be useful for the same purpose in the care of adolescents and older children but is otherwise of limited usefulness in pediatrics. An overnight high-dose dexamethasone suppression test is probably more reliable than the conventional 2-day, high-dose test in differentiating adults with Cushing disease from

those with ectopic ACTH syndrome. However, the usefulness of this test in the care of pediatric patients has not been established.

STIMULATION TESTS Direct stimulation of the adrenal glands with ACTH is a rapid, safe, and easy way to evaluate adrenocortical function. A single bolus of synthetic ACTH (1-24) (cosyntropin) is administered intravenously, and cortisol values are measured at 0 and 60 minutes. Normative data for this test are shown in Table 24-10. The usual dose is 0.1 mg for newborns, 0.15 mg for children up to 2 years of age, and 0.25 mg for children older than 2 years and adults. All of these doses are pharmacologic. A very-low-dose (1 μg) test may be useful in assessing adrenal recovery from glucocorticoid suppression. One of the widest uses of intravenous ACTH tests in pediatrics is diagnosis of congenital adrenal hyperplasia. Stimulating the adrenal glands with ACTH increases steroidogenesis, resulting in accumulation of steroids proximal to the disordered enzyme. For example, impaired activity of P450c21 (21-hydroxylase) leads to accumulation of 17OHP. Measuring the response of 17OHP to a 60-minute ACTH test is the single most powerful and reliable means of diagnosing 21-hydroxylase deficiency. Comparing the patient's basal to ACTH-stimulated values of 17OHP against those from large numbers of well-studied patients usually allows differentiation from healthy persons, heterozygotes, patients with nonclassic congenital adrenal hyperplasia, and patients with classic congenital adrenal hyperplasia, although there inevitably is some overlap between groups (Fig. 24-11).

Insulin-induced hypoglycemia is no longer widely used to test adrenal function. It must be remembered, however, that hypoglycemia stimulates release of "counterregulatory" hormones that act to increase plasma glucose concentrations: ACTH and cortisol, growth hormone, epinephrine, and glucagon. Thus, a blood sample for measurement of these hormones should be obtained while the patient is hypoglycemic when one is evaluating hypoglycemia of unknown causation, especially if a newborn appears otherwise healthy.

METYRAPONE TEST Metyrapone blocks the action of P450c11β and, to a much lesser extent, P450scc. It is a chemical means of inducing transient deficiency of 11-hydroxylase activity, which results in decreased cortisol secretion and subsequent increase in ACTH secretion. Metyrapone testing is done to assess the capability of the pituitary gland to produce ACTH in response to a physiological stimulus. This test has largely been replaced by direct measurement of ACTH.

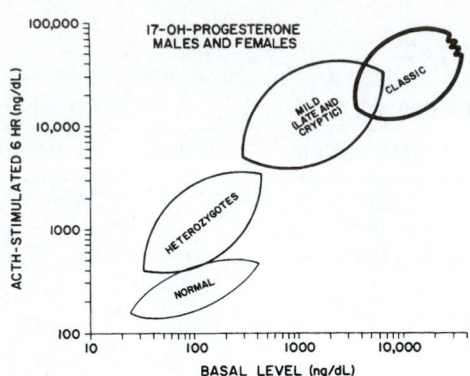

FIGURE 24-11 Correlation between basal and ACTH-stimulated plasma concentration of 17-hydroxyprogesterone in normal persons, heterozygotes, and homozygotes for 21-hydroxylase deficiency. (SOURCE: *Rosenfeld S, Miller WL: In: Mahesh JB, Greenblatt RB, eds: Hirsutism and Virilism. Wright-PSG, 1983.*)

CRF TESTING Corticotropin-releasing factor is now generally available as a test of pituitary ACTH reserve, but there is relatively little experience in the care of children. Testing with CRF may be useful for differentiating hypothalamic from pituitary causes of ACTH deficiency and may be a useful adjunct in establishing the diagnosis of Cushing disease.

24.4.6 Genetic Lesions in Steroidogenesis

One or more autosomal recessive genetic disorders disrupts each of the steps in the pathway shown in Fig. 24-7. Most of these diminish synthesis of cortisol. In response to adrenal insufficiency, the pituitary gland synthesizes increased amounts of POMC, the large protein precursor of adrenocorticotropin hormone (ACTH). ACTH promotes increased steroidogenesis (see Sec. 24.4.3) and stimulates adrenal hypertrophy and hyperplasia. The term *congenital adrenal hyperplasia* refers to a group of diseases traditionally grouped together on the basis of the most prominent finding at autopsy.

In theory, congenital adrenal hyperplasia is easy to understand. A genetic lesion in one of the steroidogenic enzymes interferes with normal steroidogenesis. The signs and symptoms of the disease are caused by deficiency of the steroidal end product and the effects of accumulated steroidal precursors proximal to the blocked step. Thus reference to the pathways in Fig. 24-7 and a knowledge of the biological effects of each steroid should allow one to deduce the manifestations of the disease.

In practice, congenital adrenal hyperplasia can be confusing, both clinically and scientifically. The clinical, laboratory, and therapeutic features of each form of congenital adrenal hyperplasia are summarized in Table 24-11. As discussed in Sec. 24.4.2, each steroidogenic enzyme has multiple activity, and many extraadrenal tissues contain other enzymes that have similar steroidogenic activities. Elimination of an adrenal enzyme may not result in elimination of certain steroids from the circulation. Cloning of the genes for the steroidogenic enzymes allows direct study of these diseases.

CONGENITAL LIPOID ADRENAL HYPERPLASIA

Congenital lipoid adrenal hyperplasia, which is the most severe form of CAH, is caused by mutations in StAR, which facilitates movement of cholesterol into mitochondria, where it is converted

to pregnenolone. Mutations in StAR disrupt steroidogenesis in the adrenal glands and gonads but not in the placenta or brain, hence affected fetuses reach term and are normally developed. In the absence of testicular testosterone, however, XY genetic boys have normal female genitalia at birth. The disease usually becomes clinically apparent in the first month of life with symptoms of glucocorticoid and mineralocorticoid insufficiency, including poor feeding, lethargy, diarrhea, vomiting, hypotension, dehydration, hyponatremia, hyperkalemia, and acidosis. Early treatment with appropriate replacement doses of cortisol or cortisone acetate and with 9α-fluorocortisol is essential and effective. Genetic boys with this disorder are reared as girls and undergo orchiectomy in early childhood. Lipoid congenital adrenal hyperplasia is common among Japanese, Korean, and Palestinian populations but is rare among other groups. The phenotype results from both the loss of the StAR-mediated acute steroidogenic response and from subsequent accumulation of intracellular cholesterol esters and cell death. Because the ovary makes little or no steroid before puberty, these cells remain relatively intact, so affected 46XX girls undergo fairly normal puberty.

3β-HYDROXYSTEROID DEHYDROGENASE DEFICIENCY

Nearly complete absence of 3βHSD activity is rare. It presents signs and symptoms of glucocorticoid and mineralocorticoid deficiency and is fatal if not diagnosed early. In the most severe, classic form of this disorder, genetic girls are mildly virilized because the fetal adrenal glands overproduce large amounts of DHEA, a small portion of which is converted to testosterone by extraadrenal pathways. Patients with 3βHSD deficiency have mutations in the 3βHSD-II gene, which is expressed in the adrenal glands and gonads. The 3βHSD-I gene, which is expressed in the liver, placenta, brain, and other tissues never is affected; mutation of 3βHSD-I interrupts placental synthesis of progesterone, which causes spontaneous abortion. Activity of 3βHSD-I in extraglandular tissues can obfuscate the diagnosis of 3βHSD deficiency, because the large amounts of 17OH-pregnenolone produced by the disordered adrenal glands can be converted to 17OHP by the liver and other tissues so that the concentration of 17OHP can be nearly as high as in patients with 21-hydroxylase deficiency. The diagnosis can be established by means of examining the ratios of 17OHP to 17OH-pregnenolone and of androstenedione to DHEA after acute stimulation with an intravenous ACTH test.

Mild or partial defects of adrenal 3βHSD activity not associated with salt loss have been described in several large studies. Typical patients are young women or teenagers with hirsutism and virilism, but they also come to medical attention for premature adrenarche. Genetic studies have shown that few of these patients have 3βHSD mutations. The basis of increased secretion of Δ^5 steroids in these individuals is unknown. Among adults, the hirsutism can be ameliorated and regular menses restored by suppressing ACTH with 0.5 mg dexamethasone given orally each day. However, treatment of children with premature adrenarche is more conservative and must be considered carefully after a complete endocrine evaluation. Unnecessary administration of glucocorticoids has an adverse effect on normal growth.

P450c17 (17α-HYDROXYLASE/17,20 LYASE) DEFICIENCY

P450c17, a single enzyme present in both the adrenal glands and gonads, has both 17α-hydroxylase and 17,20 lyase activities. De-

TABLE 24-11

CLINICAL AND LABORATORY FINDINGS IN CONGENITAL ADRENAL HYPERPLASIA

ENZYME DEFICIENCY	PRESENTATION	LABORATORY FINDINGS	THERAPEUTIC MEASURES
Lipoid CAH (StAR)	Salt-wasting crisis Male pseudohermaphroditism	Low levels of all steroid hormones, with decreased/absent response to ACTH Decreased/absent response to hCG in male pseudohermaphroditism ↑ ACTH ↑ PRA	Glucocorticoid and mineralocorticoid replacement Salt supplementation Sex hormone replacement consonant with sex of rearing Gonadectomy of male pseudohermaphrodite
3βHSD	Salt-wasting crisis Male and female pseudohermaphroditism Precocious adrenarche	↑ Baseline and ACTH-stimulated Δ^5 steroids (pregnenolone, 17OH pregnenolone, DHEA) ↑ Δ^5/Δ^4 serum steroids Suppression of elevated adrenal steroids after glucocorticoid administration ↑ ACTH ↑ PRA	Glucocorticoid and mineralocorticoid replacement Salt supplementation Surgical correction of genitalia and sex hormone replacement as necessary consonant with sex of rearing

P450c21	Classic form:
	  Salt-wasting crisis
	  Female pseudohermaphroditism
	  Pre- and postnatal virilization
	Nonclassic form:
	  Precocious pseudoadrenarche, disordered puberty, menstrual irregularity, hirsutism, acne, infertility
		↑ Baseline and ACTH-stimulated 17OHP
		↑ Serum androgens and urine 17-ketosteroids
		Suppression of elevated adrenal steroids after glucocorticoid administration
		↑ ACTH ↑ PRA
			Glucocorticoid and mineralocorticoid replacement
			Salt supplementation
			Vaginoplasty and clitoroplasty in female pseudohermaphroditism

P450c11β	Female pseudohermaphroditism Postnatal virilization in males and females	↑ Baseline and ACTH-stimulated 11-deoxycortisol and DOC ↑ Serum androgens and urine 17-ketosteroids Suppression of elevated steroids after glucocorticoid administration ↑ ACTH ↓ PRA Hypokalemia	Glucocorticoid administration Vaginoplasty and clitoral recession in female pseudohermaphroditism
P450c11AS	Failure to thrive Weakness Salt loss	Hyponatremia, hyperkalemia ↑ Corticosterone ↓ Aldosterone, ↑ PRA	Mineralocorticoid replacement Salt supplementation
P450c17	Male pseudohermaphroditism Sexual infantilism Hypertension	↑ DOC, 18-OHDOC, corticosterone, 18-hydroxycorticosterone Low 17α-hydroxylated steroids and poor response to ACTH Poor response to hCG in male pseudohermaphroditism Suppression of elevated adrenal steroids after glucocorticoid administration ↓ PRA ↑ ACTH Hypokalemia	Glucocorticoid administration Surgical correction of genitalia and sex steroid replacement in male pseudohermaphroditism consonant with sex of rearing Sex hormone replacement in female

ACTH = adrenocorticotropin hormone; hCG = human chorionic gonadotropin; PRA = plasma renin activity; 3βHSD = 3β-hydroxysteroid dehydrogenase; DHEA = dehydroepiandrosterone; 17OHP = 17α-hydroxyprogesterone; DOC = deoxycorticosterone; ↑ = increased; ↓ = decreased.
SOURCE: *Miller WL, Levine LS: Molecular and clinical advances in congenital adrenal hyperplasia. J Pediatr 111:1–17, 1987.*

ficient 17α-hydroxylase activity and deficient 17,20 lyase activity are not truly separate genetic diseases. They represent the clinical manifestations of different lesions in the same gene.

Deficiency of P450c17 is rare. Deficient 17α-hydroxylase activity decreases cortisol synthesis with consequent overproduction of ACTH and stimulation of the steps proximal to P450c17. These patients may have mild symptoms of glucocorticoid deficiency, but this is not life threatening, because the lack of P450c17 causes overproduction of corticosterone, a weak glucocorticoid. These patients typically overproduce DOC in the zona fasciculata, resulting in sodium retention and hypertension but also suppressing aldosterone secretion from the zona glomerulosa. Absence of 17α-hydroxylase and 17,20 lyase activity also means that adrenal and gonadal sex steroids are not produced. As a result, genetic boys can have completely female external genitalia or have incomplete development (male pseudohermaphroditism) (see Sec. 24.7.4). Affected girls are phenotypically normal but do not undergo adrenarche and puberty. The classic presentation is that a teenage girl has sexual infantilism and hypertension. The diagnosis is readily made by means of finding low or absent 17-hydroxylated C21 and C19 plasma steroids and low urinary 17OHCS and 17-ketosteroids, which respond poorly to stimulation with ACTH. Serum levels of DOC, corticosterone, and 18OH-corticosterone are not routinely measured in most laboratories, but if they are, the value is elevated and shows hyperresponsiveness to ACTH and suppression after treatment with glucocorticoids. Isolated 17,20 lyase deficiency, in which 17α-hydroxylase activity remains nearly normal, has been found in a few patients. It is caused by P450c17 mutations that compromise electron transfer from P450 reductase.

P450c21 (21-HYDROXYLASE) DEFICIENCY

Deficiency of 21-hydroxylase accounts for approximately 95% of the genetic disorders of steroidogenesis. The severe forms occur among approximately 1 in 14,000 persons, but the mild, nonclassic form is much more common, probably affecting more than 1 in 1000 persons. Patients having complete deficiency of P450c21 are unable to convert progesterone to DOC, causing aldosterone deficiency. In the absence of aldosterone, the kidney cannot retain sodium normally. Serum sodium concentration decreases to 100 to 110 mmoL/L, and the kidney inappropriately retains K^+ and H^+, resulting in hypotension, shock, cardiovascular collapse, and death. Once the diagnosis is made, children with this disorder can continue to be highly resistant to mineralocorticoid therapy. They have the clinical signs and symptoms of type IV renal tubular acidosis. Because control of fluids and electrolytes in the fetus can be maintained by the placenta and the mother's kidneys, this salt-losing crisis develops only after birth, usually during the second week of life.

Inability to convert 17OHP to 11-deoxycortisol (and hence, to cortisol) results in glucocorticoid deficiency. In addition to impairing postnatal carbohydrate metabolism and other processes, cortisol deficiency manifests prenatally. It is believed that low concentration of fetal cortisol increases production and secretion of ACTH from the fetal pituitary gland. In addition to stimulating adrenal hyperplasia, ACTH stimulates transcription of the genes for all of the steroidogenic enzymes, especially P450scc, the rate-limiting enzyme in steroidogenesis. This increased gene transcription increases enzyme production and activity, and non-21-hydroxylated steroids, especially 17OHP, accumulate. As the pathways in Fig. 24-7 indicate, these steroids are converted to androstenedione and testosterone.

In the male fetus, the testes produce high concentrations of testosterone in early to middle gestation. This testosterone differentiates external male genitalia from the pluripotent embryonic precursor structures. In the female fetus, the ovaries are steroidogenically quiescent. No sex steroids or other factors are needed for differentiation of the female external genitalia; that is, the default phenotype of the human fetus is female. In a male fetus with 21-hydroxylase deficiency, the additional androstenedione and testosterone produced in the adrenal glands has little if any demonstrable phenotypic effect. In a female fetus with 21-hydroxylase deficiency, the testosterone inappropriately produced by the adrenal glands causes varying degrees of virilization of the external genitalia. This can range from mild clitoromegaly with or without posterior fusion of the labioscrotal folds to complete labioscrotal fusion, including a urethra that traverses the enlarged clitoris (Fig. 24-12). At birth, these female infants, who retain normal ovaries, fallopian tubes, and a uterus, can have "ambiguous" genitalia or can be sufficiently virilized to appear male. The result is errors of sex assignment at birth.

The diagnosis of 21-hydroxylase deficiency is suggested by genital ambiguity among girls, a salt-losing episode for either sex, or rapid growth and virilization among boys. Plasma 17OHP level is markedly elevated (>2000 ng/dL after 24 hours of age) and hyperresponsive to stimulation with ACTH (see Fig. 24-11). Measurement of other steroids, such as 11-deoxycortisol, 17-hydroxypregnenolone, DHEA, and androstenedione, is important because some adrenal and testicular tumors can produce abundant 17OHP. High 17OHP values that increase further after administration of ACTH also occurs in 3βHSD and P450c11 deficiencies. It is important to remember that 17OHP level is normally high in cord blood but decreases to "normal" levels in healthy newborns after 12 to 24 hours. Endocrinologically normal premature infants and

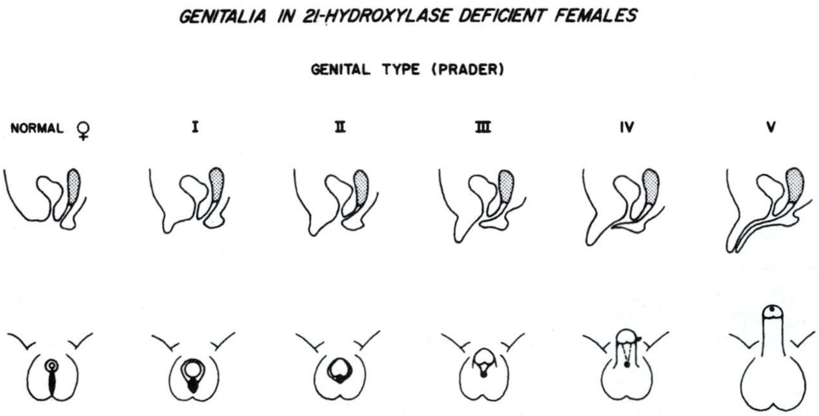

GENITALIA IN 21-HYDROXYLASE DEFICIENT FEMALES

GENITAL TYPE (PRADER)

	NORMAL ♀	I	II	III	IV	V

PERCENTAGE OF TYPE ,W/WO SALT LOSS

	I	II	III	IV	V
SL:	11	28	53	88	100
NSL:	89	72	47	12	0

PERCENTAGE OF SL'S & NLS'S WITH TYPE

	I	II	III	IV	V
SL:	1	11	51	31	5
NSL:	13	31	50	5	0

FIGURE 24-12 Virilization of the external genitalia. Continuous spectrum from normal female to normal male in both sagittal section (*top*) and perineal views (*bottom*). Disorders of external genitalia (*I-V*) can occur either through virilization of a normal female, as in congenital adrenal hyperplasia, or through an error in testosterone synthesis in the male. Among girls with congenital adrenal hyperplasia due to 21-hydroxylase deficiency, the degree of virilization correlates poorly with the presence of absence of clinical signs of salt loss.

term infants under severe stress (eg, cardiac or pulmonary disease) can have persistently elevated concentrations of 17OHP with normal 21-hydroxylase levels.

Clinical Forms of 21-Hydroxylase Deficiency

There is a wide range of clinical variants of congenital adrenal hyperplasia. These are often described as different diseases but should be considered part of a continuous spectrum of manifestations of this disease. These range from the severe salt-losing form to clinically inapparent forms that can be normal variants.

Salt-Losing Congenital Adrenal Hyperplasia

The clinical situation described earlier is that of a patient with salt-losing 21-hydroxylase deficiency. This disorder frequently is diagnosed at birth among girls because of the virilized external genitalia. When this happens, the mineralocorticoid and glucocorticoid deficiencies can be replaced orally, and the ambiguous genitalia can be corrected with plastic surgical procedures. Replacement steroid management is difficult, especially in the case of a rapidly growing child. These patients can have decreased fertility, short stature, and other problems as adults. This disorder generally is undiagnosed at birth among boys. The infant comes to medical attention during the salt-losing crisis that follows 5 to 15 days after birth, or he dies.

Simple Virilizing Congenital Adrenal Hyperplasia

Girls with virilized, ambiguous genitalia and increased concentrations of 17OHP but who do not have a salt-losing crisis have the simple virilizing form of congenital adrenal hyperplasia. Boys with this disorder often escape diagnosis until 4 to 7 years of age, when they come to medical attention because of inappropriate virilization (phallic enlargement; pubic, axillary, and facial hair; deepening of the voice). Although these children grow rapidly and are tall for age when the diagnosis is made, bone age advances at a disproportionately rapid rate; therefore, ultimate adult height is invariably compromised. Untreated or poorly treated children with congenital adrenal hyperplasia do not undergo normal puberty. Boys may have small testes and azoospermia caused by the feedback effects of the adrenally produced testosterone on hypothalamic-pituitary production of gonadotropins. Because the adrenal glands normally produce 100 to 200 times as much cortisol as aldosterone, mild defects (point mutations) in P450c21 are much less likely to affect mineralocorticoid secretion than they are cortisol secretion. Patients with simple virilizing congenital adrenal hyperplasia simply have a less severe disorder of P450c21, usually a mutation that changes isoleucine 172 to asparagine. Although they do not have clinically significant salt loss, these patients have disordered aldosterone synthesis. This is reflected physiologically by increased PRA after moderate salt restriction, which reflects hyperstimulation of the mineralocorticoid pathway.

Nonclassic Congenital Adrenal Hyperplasia

Many persons have mild forms of 21-hydroxylase deficiency. These may be evidenced by mild to moderate hirsutism, virilism, menstrual irregularities, and decreased fertility among women (so-called late-onset congenital adrenal hyperplasia), or there may be no phenotypic manifestations other than an elevated response of plasma 17OHP in response to administration of ACTH (so-called cryptic congenital adrenal hyperplasia). Despite the minimal manifestations of this disorder, these persons also have hormonal evidence of mild

subclinical impairment in mineralocorticoid secretion, as predicted from the existence of a single adrenal 21-hydroxylase.

Genetics of 21-Hydroxylase Deficiency

Two P450c21 genes are tandemly duplicated with the C4 genes that encode the fourth component of serum complement. This gene cluster lies in the middle of the class III region of the major histocompatibility locus (HLA locus) on the short arm of chromosome 6. Both human C4 genes are functional, but only the human P450c21B gene encodes adrenal 21-hydroxylase. Although P450c21A carries several mutations so that it cannot encode 21-hydroxylase, it has a great effect on the genetics of the locus. Over many generations, the P450c21A and B loci have exchanged DNA back and forth (gene conversion) so that the P450c21A and B genes are similar — 98% of their DNA bases are identical.

Congenital adrenal hyperplasia can be caused by three types of mutations—gene deletions, large gene conversions, and gene microconversions (Table 24-12). Microconversions, which resemble point mutations, account for about 75% of cases of congenital adrenal hyperplasia. Gene deletions in congenital adrenal hyperplasia extend from the middle of the P450c21A gene to a precisely homologous point in the P450c21B gene, producing a single hybrid, nonfunctional A/B gene. In gene conversion, part or all of the B gene acquires A sequences, so that there are two A genes or an A gene and an A/B hybrid. All deletions and large gene conversions in the homozygous state cause salt-losing congenital adrenal hyperplasia. Many point mutations also cause salt-losing congenital adrenal hyperplasia. Because a great number of genetic lesions cause the same clinical syndrome, most such patients are compound heterozygotes.

The location of the P450c21 genes in the HLA locus means that congenital adrenal hyperplasia is tightly linked to HLA mark-

TABLE 24-12

FREQUENCY OF GENETIC LESIONS CAUSING 21-HYDROXYLASE DEFICIENCY

LESION	PERCENTAGE IN CAH	PERCENTAGE AMONG HEALTHY PERSONS
Both genes grossly intact (includes normal, point mutations, and small intragenic gene conversions)	65.6	84.5
Deletion of P450c21A pseudogene	3.4	14.3
Duplication of P450c21 pseudogene	6.9	1.2
Large gene conversion	11.2	0
Large gene deletion	11.2	0
Other lesions	1.7	0

As revealed by Southern blotting studies of DNA from 116 affected and 84 normal haplotypes. Numbers percentage of P450c21B genes having a given structure and not the percentage of patients. Most patients are compound heterozygotes, that is, have different lesions affecting their maternal and paternal P450c21 genes.

SOURCE: *Data from Morel Y, Andre J, Urings-Lambert B, et al: Rearrangements and point mutations of P450c21 genes are distinguished by 5 restriction endonuclease haplotypes identified by a new probing strategy in 57 families with congenital adrenal hyperplasia. J Clin Invest 83:527, 1989.*

ers, especially HLA-B, HLA-C, and HLA-D. Knowledge of the HLA types of both parents and of one affected child can establish which unaffected children are carriers and whether a fetus will or will not be affected. Certain characteristic HLA markers are strongly linked to specific clinical forms of congenital adrenal hyperplasia. Approximately 40% of haplotypes for nonclassic congenital adrenal hyperplasia bear HLA-B14, and most, but not all, haplotypes bearing HLA-Bw47 have P450c21B gene deletions.

HLA typing can be done on cells obtained at amniocentesis. In conjunction with measuring amniotic fluid 17OHP, a highly accurate prenatal diagnosis can be made at 14 to 20 weeks of gestation. Use of chorionic villus sampling and analysis of the 21-hydroxylase gene can provide an accurate diagnosis as early as 8 weeks of gestation. Because this is approximately the time when the genital anomaly (labioscrotal fusion) begins, some physicians have attempted prenatal therapy for congenital adrenal hyperplasia by giving the mother synthetic glucocorticoid hormones that cross the placenta. This is experimental treatment, and authorization is required for human experimentation.

LESIONS IN THE ISOZYMES OF P450c11: 11β-HYDROXYLASE DEFICIENCY AND DISORDERS OF ALDOSTERONE SYNTHESIS

Two isozymes of P450c11, called *P450c11β* and *P450c11AS,* are encoded by a tandemly duplicated pair of genes on chromosome 8. P450c11β is abundantly expressed in the zona fasciculata and appears only to catalyze 11β-hydroxylation, converting 11-deoxycortisol to cortisol and DOC to corticosterone. P450c11AS is expressed only in the zona glomerulosa and is present in rather small quantities. P450c11AS catalyzes 11β-hydroxylase and 18 methyl oxidase (aldosterone synthetase) activity and thus converts DOC to corticosterone, 18OH-DOC, 18OH corticosterone, and aldosterone.

Disorders of P450c11β are rare except in the Middle East, where it accounts for about 15% of cases of congenital adrenal hyperplasia among both Arab and Sephardic Jewish populations. Severe deficiency of P450c11β decreases secretion of cortisol and causes congenital adrenal hyperplasia and virilization of affected girls as described earlier for P450c21 deficiency. The diagnosis usually is made when there are high basal concentrations of 11-deoxycortisol (the substrate for P450c11) and hyperresponsiveness to ACTH. Unlike those with the typical salt-losing syndrome of 21-hydroxylase deficiency, patients with 11-hydroxylase deficiency retain sodium normally because the substrate for 11-hydroxylation in the mineralocorticoid pathway, DOC, is itself a mineralocorticoid. Although DOC has much less potent mineralocorticoid activity than aldosterone, it is secreted at higher levels in 11-hydroxylase deficiency, so salt is retained, and serum level of sodium remains normal. Newborns occasionally have mild, transient salt loss, whereas older children often produce enough DOC to have hypertension. Therapy for 11β-hydroxylase deficiency consists of glucocorticoid replacement therapy, as in 21-hydroxylase deficiency. Some newborns may need treatment with mineralocorticoids and salt for 1 to 2 years as indicated by PRA.

Disorders of P450c11AS are rare. Complete absence of this enzyme causes so-called corticosterone methyl oxidase I deficiency, in which activity of both 18-hydroxylase and 18 methyl oxidase is absent. In such patients synthesis of cortisol and corticosterone, catalyzed by P450c11β, remains intact. Mutations in P450c11AS

that disrupt 18 methyl oxidase activity while preserving 18-hydroxylase activity cause corticosterone methyl oxidase II deficiency, better called *aldosterone synthetase deficiency.* Both groups of patients have failure to gain weight as infants and have mild to moderate hyponatremia and hyperkalemia, profound hyperreninemia, extremely low concentrations of aldosterone, and possibly hypotension, dehydration, and acidosis. Type I patients, who lack 18-hydroxylase activity, are characterized by extremely low concentrations of 18OH-DOC and 18OH-corticosterone. Type II patients have high concentrations of these steroids. Aldosterone synthetase deficiency is common among Jews of Iranian ancestry. Patients with any of these forms of hypoaldosteronism need treatment with salt and mineralocorticoids. Doses are adjusted according to blood pressure, electrolyte concentrations, and PRA rather than size, age, or body surface area, as is done for glucocorticoid therapy.

Defects in aldosterone biosynthesis have to be differentiated from other heritable forms of salt loss, including the autosomal dominant and recessive forms of *pseudohypoaldosteronism* in which aldosterone resistance is caused by in the genes for the α and β subunits of the amiloride-sensitive sodium channel.

A third disorder of the P450c11 genes is glucocorticoid-suppressible hyperaldosteronism. This rare disorder is caused by a gene duplication event that produces a hybrid P450c11 gene. The functional, hybrid gene has 5'-flanking (regulatory) sequences and the first two or three exons of P450c11β and the remainder of its sequences from P450c11AS. As a result, transcription of this hybrid is induced by ACTH, as would normally occur with P450c11β, but the encoded protein has aldosterone synthetase activity, so that the zonae fasciculata and reticularis contain a form of P450c11AS. This results in oversecretion of aldosterone and hypertension. Treatment is to suppress pituitary ACTH with glucocorticoids, thus suppressing production of the abnormal P450c11AS.

24.4.7 Adrenal Insufficiency

Adrenal insufficiency can be caused by hypopituitarism and ACTH deficiency, or it can be caused by a primary adrenal disorder. Primary adrenal insufficiency is commonly called *Addison disease.* Before 1950, most patients with Addison disease had tuberculosis of the adrenal glands, but more than 80% of adult patients today have autoimmune adrenalitis; therefore the term *Addison disease* is widely used to indicate an autoimmune or idiopathic cause. The various causes of adrenal insufficiency are listed in Table 24-13. Signs and symptoms of adrenal insufficiency are shown in Table 24-14.

CHRONIC PRIMARY ADRENAL INSUFFICIENCY

Autoimmune Adrenalitis

Autoimmune adrenalitis is most common among adults 25 to 45 years of age, about 70% of whom are women. The incidence among adults is about 1 in 25,000, but is much lower among children. Among young children, boys constitute about 75% of patients. Early in the course of autoimmune adrenalitis one may see signs of glucocorticoid deficiency (weakness, fatigue, weight loss, hypoglycemia, anorexia) without signs of mineralocorticoid deficiency (hyponatremia, hyperkalemia, acidosis, tachycardia, hypotension, low voltage on electrocardiogram, small heart on chest radiograph) or

TABLE 24-13

CAUSES OF ADRENAL INSUFFICIENCY

Primary adrenal insufficiency
   Autoimmune adrenalitis
   Autoimmune polyglandular syndrome (types I and II)
   Tuberculosis, fungal infection
   Sepsis
   AIDS
   Congenital adrenal hyperplasia
   Adrenal hemorrhage or infarction
   Congenital adrenal hypoplasia
   Adrenoleukodystrophy
   Primary xanthomatosis
   Unresponsiveness to ACTH
Secondary adrenal insufficiency
   Withdrawal from glucocorticoid therapy
   Hypopituitarism
   Hypothalamic tumors
   Irradiation of the central nervous system

evidence of mineralocorticoid deficiency without glucocorticoid deficiency. In primary chronic adrenal insufficiency, low concentrations of plasma cortisol stimulate hypersecretion of ACTH and other POMC peptides, including melanocyte stimulating hormone. Consequently, chronic primary adrenal insufficiency also is characterized by hyperpigmentation of the skin and mucous membranes. Such hyperpigmentation is most prominent in skin exposed to sun and in flexor surfaces such as the knees, elbows, and knuckles. The diagnosis is suggested by the aforementioned signs and symptoms, verified with a low morning cortisol level with a high ACTH level and confirmed with a minimal response of cortisol to a 60-minute intravenous ACTH test. Associated findings often include the appearance of a small heart on chest radiograph, anemia, azotemia, eosinophilia, lymphocytosis, and hypoglycemia. Therapy for chronic primary adrenal insufficiency consists of glucocorticoid and mineralocorticoid replacement in physiologic doses (see Sec. 24.4.9).

The diagnosis of an autoimmune mechanism for chronic adrenal insufficiency is based largely on the finding of circulating anti-adrenal antibodies. Autopsy studies of children and adults show lymphocytic infiltration of the adrenal cortex. Autoimmune dysfunction of other endocrine tissues frequently is associated with autoimmune adrenalitis. Approximately one-half of adult patients with lymphocytic adrenalitis also have disease of another endocrine system and high titers of antibodies specific to the affected tissues. The term *Schmidt syndrome* refers to the relatively common association of thyroiditis or diabetes mellitus with autoimmune adrenal insufficiency. This disease triad, which occurs mainly among adults, sometimes is called *type 2 autoimmune polyglandular syndrome* and is linked to HLA-DR3 and HLA-DR4. Among older children and adults, primary ovarian failure but not primary testicular failure occurs among approximately one-fourth of patients with primary lymphocytic autoimmune adrenalitis.

Hypoparathyroidism, pernicious anemia, and chronic mucocutaneous infection with *Candida albicans* (moniliasis) often occur together without associated adrenalitis among girls. When adrenalitis is present, boys and girls are affected equally. This associated group of disorders is more common among children than among adults and sometimes is called *type 1 autoimmune polyglandular syndrome*. It can include atrophic gastritis, hypergonadotrophic hy-

pogonadism, chronic active hepatitis, alopecia, or vitiligo. Unlike type 2 autoimmune polyglandular syndrome, a specific HLA association has not been found for this disorder.

Metabolic Causes

Rare metabolic disorders that cause chronic primary adrenal insufficiency include adrenoleukodystrophy (Schilder disease), primary xanthomatosis (Wolman disease), cholesterol ester storage disease, and hereditary unresponsiveness to ACTH.

Adrenoleukodystrophy is caused by mutations in a specific, very-long-chain fatty acid acyl-coenzyme A synthase encoded by a peroxisomal membrane transporter gene. The mechanism by which mutations in the encoded ALDP protein cause disease is unclear. The gene is on chromosome Xq28, and hence only boys are affected, although a rare severe infantile autosomal recessive form also occurs among girls. The disease is characterized by high ratios of C26 to C22 very-long-chain fatty acids in plasma and tissues, allowing diagnosis of the carrier state as well as detection among affected fetuses and individual patients. Symptoms commonly develop in mid-childhood, but a variant of the disorder, called *adrenomyeloneuropathy*, manifests in early adulthood. Both adrenoleukodystrophy and adrenomyeloneuropathy are caused by mutations in the same gene. The same mutation can cause either form of the disease; hence it is likely that other genetic loci also are involved. Earliest findings are associated with central nervous system leukodystrophy and include behavioral changes, poor school performance, dysarthria, and poor memory that progresses to severe dementia. Symptoms of adrenal insufficiency usually appear after symptoms of white matter disease. In contrast, in adrenomyeloneuropathy the disorder begins with adrenal insufficiency in childhood and adolescence, and signs of neurologic disease follow 10 to 15 years later.

Wolman disease and *cholesterol ester storage disease* appear to be two allelic variants in the secreted form of lysosomal acid lipase

TABLE 24-14

SIGNS AND SYMPTOMS OF ADRENAL INSUFFICIENCY

Features shared by acute and chronic insufficiency
   Anorexia
   Apathy and confusion
   Dehydration
   Fatigue
   Hyperkalemia
   Hypoglycemia
   Hyponatremia
   Hypovolemia and tachycardia
   Nausea and vomiting
   Postural hypotension
   Salt craving
   Weakness
Features of acute insufficiency (adrenal crisis)
   Abdominal pain
   Fever
Features of chronic insufficiency (Addison disease)
   Sparse pubic and axillary hair
   Diarrhea
   Hyperpigmentation
   Low-voltage electrocardiogram
   Small heart on radiograph
   Weight loss

(cholesterol esterase) that mobilizes cholesterol esters from adrenal lipid droplets. The gene for this enzyme on chromosome 10q has been cloned, and the mutations in it that caused one case of Wolman disease have been identified. Because insufficient free cholesterol is available to P450scc, there is adrenal insufficiency. The disease is less severe than congenital lipoid adrenal hyperplasia (see Sec. 24.4.6) with respect to steroidogenesis, and patients may survive for several months after birth. However, the disease affects all cells, not only steroidogenic cells, because all cells must store and use cholesterol; hence, the disorder is relentless and fatal. Vomiting, steatorrhea, failure to thrive, hepatosplenomegaly, and adrenal calcification are the usual findings. The diagnosis is established when bone marrow aspiration yields foam cells containing large lysosomal vacuoles engorged with cholesterol esters. The diagnosis is confirmed when there is no cholesterol esterase activity in fibroblasts, leukocytes, or marrow cells. Cholesterol ester storage disease appears to be a milder defect of the same enzyme, generally presenting in childhood or adolescence among the 10 reported cases.

Hereditary unresponsiveness to ACTH (familial glucocorticoid deficiency) can manifest as an acute adrenal crisis precipitated by an intercurrent illness in infancy or with the signs and symptoms of chronic adrenal insufficiency in childhood. Unlike patients with autoimmune adrenalitis or other forms of destruction of adrenal tissue, patients with hereditary unresponsiveness to ACTH continue to produce mineralocorticoids normally, because production of aldosterone by the adrenal zona glomerulosa is regulated principally by the renin-angiotensin system. Thus the presenting features are failure to thrive, lethargy, pallor, hyperpigmentation, delayed milestones, and hypoglycemia, often associated with seizures. Serum electrolyte values are normal, and dehydration occurs only as part of the precipitating intercurrent illness. The disorder is transmitted as an autosomal recessive trait. Some but not all patients have mutations of the gene that encodes the ACTH receptor on chromosome 18p11, indicating the heterogeneous nature of the defect. Another autosomal recessive form of familial glucocorticoid deficiency is associated with achalasia, alacrima, a complex neurologic disorder, and intellectual impairment; rare patients also have mineralocorticoid deficiency.

Adrenal hypoplasia congenita (congenital adrenal hypoplasia) is caused by mutations of the *DAX-1* gene on chromosome Xp21. This gene encodes a nuclear transcription factor that participates at various steps in the differentiation of adrenal and gonadal tissues, as well as in gonadotropin expression, so that successfully treated children may not enter puberty. In this disorder the definitive zone of the fetal adrenal glands does not develop, and the fetal zone is vacuolated and cytomegalic. Poor function of the fetal zone causes low concentration of maternal estriol during pregnancy, but parturition is normal. Neonatal glucocorticoid and mineralocorticoid deficiencies manifest as a typical salt-wasting crisis and respond well to replacement therapy. Deletions of the *DAX-1* gene can encompass adjacent genes, causing glycerol kinase deficiency, Duchenne muscular dystrophy, and mental retardation.

Other Causes

Some cases of chronic adrenal insufficiency have causes other than autoimmunity. Adrenal hypoplasia, hemorrhage, and infections, all discussed later as causes of acute primary adrenal insufficiency, may spare some adrenal tissue, leaving severely compromised rather than totally absent adrenal function. The result, as with autoimmune adrenalitis, is a chronic disorder with insidious onset of the broad range of nonspecific findings described earlier. Tuberculosis, fungal infection, and amyloidosis can cause similar clinical features.

ACUTE PRIMARY ADRENAL INSUFFICIENCY

Acute adrenal crisis occurs most commonly among children with undiagnosed chronic adrenal insufficiency who undergo additional severe stress, such as major illness, trauma, or surgery. The symptoms and signs include abdominal pain, fever, hypoglycemia with seizures, weakness, apathy, nausea, vomiting, anorexia, hyponatremia, hypochloremia, acidemia, hyperkalemia, hypotension, shock, cardiovascular collapse, and death. Treatment consists of fluid and electrolyte resuscitation, ample doses of glucocorticoids, chronic glucocorticoid and mineralocorticoid replacement, and control of the precipitating illness.

Acute adrenal crisis can manifest in the second week of life among infants with congenital adrenal hyperplasia, especially boys with salt-losing 21-hydroxylase deficiency. These infants escape earlier diagnosis prompted by observation of a genital anomaly. A similar presentation in infancy occurs with congenital adrenal hypoplasia and with congenital lipoid adrenal hyperplasia. In both diseases absence of fetal adrenal synthesis of DHEA results in very low maternal estriol concentrations, which appear to have no influence on the outcome of the pregnancy. These two causes of low maternal estriol levels are readily differentiated from a more common cause, anencephaly, by means of ultrasonographic examination of the fetus.

Massive adrenal hemorrhage with shock caused by blood loss can occur among large infants who have undergone traumatic delivery. A flank mass is usually palpable and can be differentiated from renal venous thrombosis by microscopic rather than gross hematuria. The diagnosis is confirmed with intravenous pyelography or ultrasonography. Massive adrenal hemorrhage is more commonly associated with meningococcemia (Waterhouse-Friderichsen syndrome). Meningitis is often but not always present. The characteristic petechial rash of meningococcemia can progress rapidly to large ecchymosis. Blood pressure decreases and respiration becomes labored, frequently leading rapidly to coma and death. Immediate intervention with intravenous fluids, antibiotics, and glucocorticoids is not always successful. A similar adrenal crisis can occur in rare instances with septicemia from *Streptococcus* sp., *Pneumococcus* sp., or diphtheria.

SECONDARY ADRENAL INSUFFICIENCY

Chronic adrenal insufficiency is caused by extraadrenal disorders of two general types—insufficient tropic stimulation of the adrenal glands and tissue insensitivity to adrenal steroids. Insufficient tropic stimulation of the adrenal glands can be caused by idiopathic hypopituitarism, central nervous system tumors that damage the cells producing CRF or POMC, or chronic suppression of these cells by long-term glucocorticoid therapy.

Idiopathic hypopituitarism, or deficient secretion of multiple anterior pituitary hormones, is principally a hypothalamic rather than a pituitary disorder. The deficient secretion of growth hormone, gonadotropins, TSH, and ACTH is caused by insufficient stimulation of the pituitary gland by the corresponding hypothalamic hormones. Isolated growth hormone deficiency, a common disorder, and isolated ACTH deficiency, a rare disorder, are simply variants. In hypopituitarism of most causes, secretion of GH is generally lost first, followed in order by gonadotropins, TSH, and ACTH. Combined deficiency of GH and ACTH strongly predisposes the patient to hypoglycemia, because both hormones raise plasma level of glucose. Patients with ACTH deficiency, with or without deficiency of other anterior pituitary hormones, have a relatively mild form of adrenal insufficiency. Mineralocorticoid secretion is normal; cortisol secretion is decreased but not absent. Adrenal reserve is severely compromised by chronic understimulation of biosynthesis of the steroidogenic enzymes. Because some cortisol continues to be made, the diagnosis may not be apparent unless a CRF or metyrapone test of pituitary ACTH production and an intravenous ACTH test of adrenal reserve are performed. This can be especially true when TSH deficiency is a component of hypopituitarism. Hypothyroidism caused by TSH deficiency slows metabolism of the small amount of cortisol produced and therefore protects the patient from the symptoms of adrenal insufficiency. Management of such hypothyroidism with T_4 accelerates metabolism of these small amounts of cortisol and unmasks adrenal insufficiency caused by ACTH deficiency. On occasion it precipitates acute adrenal crisis. Careful evaluation of the pituitary-adrenal axis is needed in the management of hypopituitarism with secondary hypothyroidism. Many clinicians choose to "cover" a patient with small doses of glucocorticoids (one-fourth to one-half of physiological replacement) during initial therapy for such secondary hypothyroidism.

Hypothalamic tumors, such as craniopharyngioma, are associated with ACTH deficiency in about 25% of cases, perhaps more if the patient has a tumor such as germinoma or astrocytoma. Adrenal insufficiency is rarely the presenting problem, but it can contribute to the clinical features. Surgery and radiation therapy usually cause secondary ACTH deficiency. All such patients receive glucocorticoid coverage during treatment regardless of the status of the hypothalamic-pituitary-adrenal axis when the tumor is identified. Cortisol is needed for the kidney to excrete free water. Therapy for secondary adrenal insufficiency in some central nervous system tumors can unmask a previously inapparent deficiency of vasopressin and thus precipitate diabetes insipidus.

Long-term glucocorticoid therapy can suppress POMC gene transcription and the synthesis and storage of ACTH. Long-term therapy apparently decreases the synthesis and storage of CRF and diminishes the number of CRF receptors in the pituitary gland. Therefore recovery of the hypothalamic-pituitary axis from long-term glucocorticoid therapy entails recovery of general components in a sequence and hence often requires considerable time. Patients successfully withdrawn from glucocorticoid therapy or successfully treated for Cushing disease may have fairly rapid normalization of plasma cortisol values while continuing to have diminished adrenal reserve for more than 6 months.

Glucocorticoid treatment of pregnant women can suppress the fetal adrenal glands. Treatment of pregnant women with cortisone or prednisone causes minimal suppression of the fetal adrenal glands because placental $11\beta HSD$ converts the biologically active form of these steroids, cortisol and prednisolone, back to their biologically inactive parent compounds. When radiolabeled cortisol or prednisolone is administered to a pregnant woman, the equilibrium concentrations in maternal plasma are 10 times higher than those in cord plasma. However, dexamethasone is not subject to a cycle of activation and inactivation by 11-oxidoreductase/$11\beta HSD$. Administration of even relatively low doses of dexamethasone (0.5 mg/d) to a pregnant woman can affect fetal adrenal steroidogenesis. This has led to experimental therapy for congenital adrenal hyperplasia in fetal life by means of maternal administration of dexamethasone. Early results suggest there may be a role for such an

approach, but the safety and efficacy of such therapy are not established.

24.4.8   Adrenal Excess

Aside from the congenital adrenal hyperplasia, causes of excess adrenal steroid production are rare, falling into three categories—glucocorticoid excess (Cushing syndrome), mineralocorticoid excess (Conn syndrome), and virilizing and feminizing adrenal tumors.

CUSHING SYNDROME

The term *Cushing syndrome* often is used to describe any form of glucocorticoid excess. Following general practice, we reserve the term *Cushing disease* for hypercortisolism caused by pituitary overproduction of ACTH. The related disorder caused by ACTH of nonpituitary origin is called *ectopic ACTH syndrome.* The term *Cushing syndrome* sometimes is used to refer specifically to hypersecretion of cortisol from adrenal tumors, but this use is ambiguous and should be avoided. Other causes of Cushing syndrome include adrenal adenoma, adrenal carcinoma, and multinodular adrenal hyperplasia. All of these disorders are distinct from *iatrogenic Cushing syndrome,* which is the clinical constellation caused by administration of supraphysiologic quantities of ACTH or glucocorticoids.

Although generally described in great detail and illustrated with striking photographs in endocrinology textbooks, Cushing disease is fairly rare among adults. It is widely believed that Cushing syndrome is extremely rare among children. Although the true incidence of Cushing syndrome is unknown, it is clear that this disorder is more common than previously recognized, especially among children. Many patients first seen as adults actually experience the onset of symptoms in childhood or adolescence. Harvey Cushing's original patient was a woman of only 23 years whose history and clinical features indicated long-standing disease. Hence many cases of Cushing syndrome can be detected while the patient is in the pediatric age group. Among adults and children older than 7 years, the most common cause of Cushing syndrome is true Cushing disease (adrenal hyperplasia caused by hypersecretion of pituitary ACTH). Among infants and children younger than 7 years, adrenal tumors predominate. Among 60 infants younger than 1 year with Cushing syndrome, 48 had adrenal tumors.

Clinical Findings

The physical features of Cushing syndrome are familiar to almost all physicians. Central obesity, moon facies, hirsutism, and facial flushing occur among more than 80% of adults with Cushing syndrome. Striae, hypertension, muscular weakness, back pain, buffalo hump fat distribution, psychological disturbances, acne, and easy bruising also are common (35% to 80%) (Table 24-15). However, these are the signs and features of advanced Cushing disease. When annual photographs of such patients are available, it is usually evident that these features can take 5 years or longer to develop (Fig. 24-13). Thus, the classic cushingoid appearance usually is not the initial picture seen in the child with Cushing syndrome. The earliest, most reliable indicators of hypercortisolism in children are weight gain and growth arrest. Any overweight child who stops growing should be evaluated for Cushing syndrome. By contrast, children with simple dietary obesity often grow more rapidly and are tall for their age (presumably due to chronic secondary hyper-

TABLE 24-15

FINDINGS AMONG 39 CHILDREN WITH CUSHING DISEASE

FINDING	PERCENTAGE OF PATIENTS
Symptoms	
Weight gain	92
Poor growth	84
Fatigue	67
Delayed puberty	60
Compulsive behavior	44
Bruising	28
Headache	26
Nocturia	8
Signs	
Osteopenia	74
Hypertension	63
Plethora	46
Acne	46
Hirsutism	46
Striae	36
Buffalo hump	28
Delayed bone age	13
Laboratory Studies	
Absent diurnal rhythm	100
High urinary level of 17-hydroxycorticosteroid	100
High urinary cortisol	86
Unresponsive to low-dose dexamethasone	86
Suppression by high-dose dexamethasone	86

SOURCE: *Data from: Devoe DJ, Miller WL, Conte FA, et al: Long-term outcome in children and adolescents after transsphenoidal surgery for Cushing's disease. J Clin Endocrinol Metab 82:3196-3202, 1997.*

insulinism). The obesity of Cushing disease in children is initially generalized rather than centripetal, and a buffalo hump is evidence of long-standing disease. Psychological disturbances, especially compulsive over-achieving behavior, are distinct from the depression often seen in adults with Cushing disease. It is likely that Cushing syndrome is generally regarded as a disease of young adults because the diagnosis was missed, rather than absent, during adolescence. In rare instances, Cushing syndrome caused by adrenal carcinoma or the ectopic ACTH syndrome can produce a rapid fulminant course.

Cushing Disease

More than 90% of adults with Cushing disease have identifiable pituitary microadenomas. These tumors are generally 2 to 10 mm in diameter, are not encapsulated, have ill-defined boundaries, and frequently can be detected with contrast-enhanced pituitary MR imaging. These tumors often can be identified only from minor differences in appearance and texture from surrounding tissue. The frequency of surgical cure correlates with the technical skill of the surgeon. Although histologic techniques may not help differentiate the tumor from normal tissue, molecular biological techniques confirm increased synthesis of POMC in these tissues. Among children and adolescents, approximately 80% to 85% of those with Cushing disease have surgically identifiable microadenoma. Although removal of the tumor usually appears curative, about 25% of such "cured" patients have a relapse and manifest Cushing disease within about 6 years.

For most patients, the circadian rhythms of ACTH and cortisol return to normal postoperatively, ACTH and cortisol respond appropriately to hypoglycemia, cortisol is easily suppressed by low doses of dexamethasone, and the other hypothalamic-pituitary systems return to normal, indicating that hypothalamic function has recovered. However, some patients with Cushing disease have no

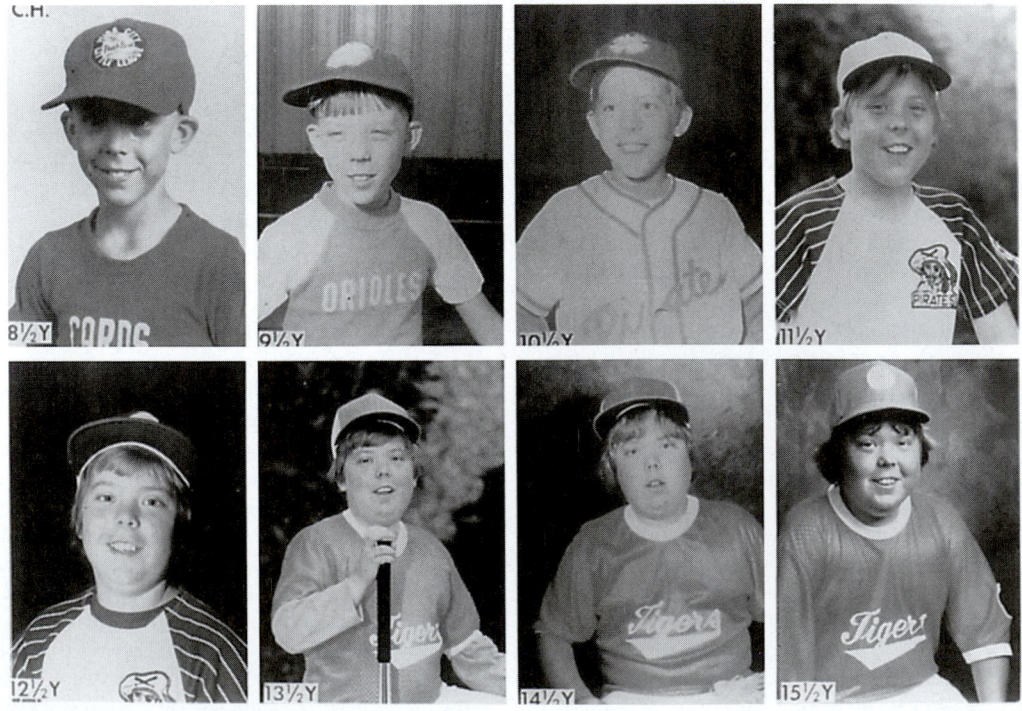

FIGURE 24-13 Development of Cushing disease. Serial photographs show a boy referred for evaluation of short stature at 16 years of age. Onset of Cushing disease was between $10\frac{1}{2}$ and $11\frac{1}{2}$ years of age.

identifiable microadenoma, and some "cured" patients have relapses. This suggests that this smaller population of patients may have a primary hypothalamic disorder. Effective therapy for Cushing disease with cyproheptadine, a serotonin antagonist, has been reported among adults, further suggesting a hypothalamic disturbance. Results of current clinical investigation suggest that Cushing disease usually is caused by primary pituitary adenoma but that it sometimes is caused by hypothalamic dysfunction. Microsurgery can be curative of the former but not of the latter. No diagnostic maneuver is available to differentiate the two possibilities. Transsphenoidal exploration remains the preferred initial therapeutic approach to Cushing disease.

Other therapeutic approaches include hypophysectomy, pituitary irradiation, cyproheptadine, adrenalectomy, and drugs that inhibit adrenal function. All have disadvantages, especially in the care of children. Hypophysectomy and pituitary irradiation eliminate pituitary secretion of GH, TSH, and gonadotropins, causing growth failure, hypothyroidism, and failure to progress in puberty. Deficiency of various pituitary hormones can be delayed after pituitary irradiation, and the delayed onset in elimination of the hypersecretion of ACTH further compromises the final adult height of the child with Cushing disease. Large doses of radiation increase the risk of cerebral arteritis, leukoencephalopathy, leukemia, glial neoplasms, bone tumors involving the skull, and of congenital defects in subsequent offspring. Cyproheptadine has met with virtually no success in therapy for pediatric Cushing disease, in part because of the unacceptable side effects (weight gain, irritability, hallucinations) that often occur with the needed doses. Adrenalectomy is performed if transsphenoidal surgery fails. In addition to eliminating normal production of glucocorticoids and mineralocorticoids, removal of the adrenal glands eliminates the physiological feedback inhibition of the pituitary gland. This causes development of pituitary macroadenoma in some patients, and the tumor produces large quantities of ACTH. The tumor can expand and impinge on the optic nerves and can produce sufficient POMC to yield enough melanocyte-stimulating hormone to produce profound darkening of the skin (Nelson syndrome). Children may be more prone to Nelson syndrome than are adults; as many as 25% of children have this complication. Drugs that inhibit steroidogenesis, such as ketoconazole, are useful treatment for selected patients. Metyrapone is not useful for long-term therapy. Mitotane, an adrenolytic agent, can be used to effect chemical adrenalectomy, but the side effects of nausea, anorexia, and vomiting are severe.

Other Causes of Cushing Syndrome

Ectopic ACTH syndrome is common among adults with oat cell carcinoma of the lung, carcinoid tumors, pancreatic islet cell carcinoma, and thymoma. Although it is rare among children, ectopic ACTH syndrome has been found among infants younger than 1 year. Associated tumors have included neuroblastoma, pheochromocytoma, and islet cell carcinoma of the pancreas. Because the malignant tissues producing the ectopic ACTH tend to be unresponsive to feedback by cortisol, ectopic ACTH syndrome is typically associated with ACTH concentrations 10 to 100 times higher than those of Cushing disease. However, both adults and children with this disorder may have little or no clinical evidence of hypercortisolism, probably because of the typically rapid onset of the disease and the general catabolism associated with malignant disease. Unlike patients with Cushing disease, adults and children with ectopic ACTH syndrome frequently have hypokalemic alkalosis, presumably because the extremely high levels of ACTH stimulate

production of DOC by the adrenal fasciculata and may also stimulate the adrenal glomerulosa in the absence of hyperreninemia.

Adrenal tumors, especially adrenal carcinoma, are the more typical cause of Cushing syndrome among infants and small children. These tumors tend to occur with much greater frequency among girls; the reason for this is unknown. Adrenal adenoma almost always secretes cortisol with minimal secretion of mineralocorticoids or sex steroids. In contrast, adrenal carcinoma tends to secrete both cortisol and androgens. Congenital bodily asymmetry (hemihypertrophy) can be associated with adrenal adenoma or carcinoma, with or without association with the Beckwith-Wiedemann syndrome. Computed tomography and MR imaging are useful in the diagnosis of adrenal tumors. Management of both adenoma and carcinoma is surgical, although the prognosis for adrenal carcinoma is poor. A few patients have done well with adjunctive therapy with mitotane, but the side effects of nausea and anorexia can be quite severe.

ACTH-independent multinodular adrenal hyperplasia is a rare entity characterized by secretion of both cortisol and adrenal androgens. It occurs among infants, children, and young adults; girls are affected more frequently. Somatic cell mutations of a G-protein that activates the ACTH receptor have been found in a few patients, and a similar form of multinodular adrenal hyperplasia occasionally occurs in McCune-Albright syndrome. Complete adrenalectomy usually is indicated, although in some instances, success has been reported with subtotal resection.

Differential Diagnosis

Suspicion of Cushing syndrome among children usually is raised when the child has weight gain, growth arrest, mood change, and change in facial appearance (plethora, acne, hirsutism). Because the diagnosis often is being sought at a relatively early point in the cause of disease, diagnosis can be subtle and difficult. Absolute elevations in a concentration of ACTH and cortisol in the plasma often are absent. Rather than finding morning concentrations of cortisol greater than 20 $\mu g/dL$ or of ACTH greater than 50 pg/mL, it is more typical to find mild, often equivocal elevations in afternoon and evening values. This loss of the diurnal rhythm evidenced by continued secretion of ACTH and cortisol throughout the afternoon, evening, and night usually is the earliest reliable laboratory index of Cushing disease. In contrast, the values for ACTH and cortisol typically are extremely high in ectopic ACTH syndrome, whereas cortisol level is elevated but ACTH is suppressed in the presence of adrenal tumors and in multinodular adrenal hyperplasia (Table 24-16).

Low- and high-dose dexamethasone suppression tests can be useful when performed with care. Children are admitted to the hospital, preferably to a "metabolic" service or pediatric clinical research department. Two days of baseline (control) data are obtained. Low-dose dexamethasone (20 $\mu g/kg/d$) is given, divided into equal doses given every 6 hours for 2 days followed by high-dose dexamethasone (80 $\mu g/kg/d$) given in the same manner. Eight a.m. and 8 p.m. values for ACTH and cortisol and 24-hour urine collections for 17OHS, 17-ketosteroid, free cortisol, and creatinine (to monitor the completeness of the collection) are obtained on each of the 6 days of the test. Because of variations caused by episodic secretion of ACTH, the 8 a.m. and 8 p.m. blood values are drawn in triplicate at 8:00, 8:15, and 8:30. In tests of patients with exogenous obesity or other non-Cushing disorders, levels of cortisol, ACTH, and urinary steroids are suppressed readily by low doses of dexamethasone. Plasma level of cortisol should be less than 5 $\mu g/100$ mL, ACTH less than 20 pg/mL, and 24-hour urinary

TABLE 24-16

DIAGNOSTIC VALUES IN VARIOUS CAUSES OF CUSHING SYNDROME

TEST		NORMAL VALUE	ADRENAL CARCINOMA	ADRENAL ADENOMA	NODULAR ADRENAL HYPERPLASIA	CUSHING DISEASE	ECTOPIC ACTH SYNDROME
Plasma cortisol concentration	a.m.	>14	↑	↑	↑	±	↑↑
	p.m.	<8	↑	↑	↑	↑	↑↑
Plasma ACTH concentration	a.m.	<100	↓	↓	↓	↑	↑↑
	p.m.	<50	↓	↓	↓	↑	↑↑
Low-dose dex suppression	Cortisol	<3	No Δ	No Δ	No Δ	±	No Δ
	ACTH	<30	No Δ	No Δ	No Δ	±	No Δ
	17OHCS	<2	No Δ	No Δ	No Δ	±	No Δ
High-dose dex suppression	Cortisol	↓↓	No Δ	No Δ	Usually no Δ	↓	No Δ
	ACTH	↓↓	No Δ	No Δ	Usually no Δ	↓	No Δ
	17OHCS	↓↓	No Δ	No Δ	Usually no Δ	↓	No Δ
IV ACTH test	Cortisol	>20	No Δ	± or ↑	± or ↑	↑	No Δ
Metyrapone test	Cortisol	↓	± or ↓	No Δ	± or ↓	↓	± or ↓
	11 Deoxycortisol	↑	± or ↑	No Δ	± or ↑	↑	± or ↑
	ACTH	↑	No Δ	No Δ	± or ↑	↑	No Δ
	17OHCS	↑	No Δ	No Δ	±	↑	No Δ
24-Hour urinary excretion (basal)	17OHCS		↑↑	↑	↑	↑	↑
	17KS		↑↑	± or ↑	↑	↑	↑
Plasma concentration	DHEA or DHEAS		↑↑	↓	± or ↑	↑	↑

Cortisol concentration in mg/dL; ACTH concentration in pg/mL; 17OHCS in mg/24h. ↑ = increase; ↑↑ = large increase; ↓ = decrease; ↓↓ = large decrease; ± = incomplete response; Δ = change; ACTH = adrenocorticotropin hormone; dex = dexamethasone; 17OHCS = 17-hydroxycorticosteroid; 17KS = 17-ketosteroid; DHEA = dehydroepiandrosterone; DHEAS = DHEA sulfate.

17OHS less than 1 mg/g of creatinine. Patients with adrenal adenoma, adrenal carcinoma, or ectopic ACTH syndrome have values relatively insensitive to both low- and high-dose dexamethasone, although some patients with multinodular adrenal hyperplasia may respond to high-dose suppression. Patients with Cushing disease classically respond with suppression of ACTH, cortisol, and urinary steroids during the high-dose treatment but not during the low-dose treatment. Some children, however, especially early in the course of illness, may have partial suppression in response to low-dose dexamethasone. If the low dose given exceeds 20 $\mu g/kg/d$ or if the assays used are insufficiently sensitive to differentiate partial from complete suppression, test results may be falsely negative. In general, the diagnosis of Cushing disease is considerably more difficult to establish for children than it is for adults.

VIRILIZING AND FEMINIZING ADRENAL TUMORS

Most virilizing adrenal tumors are adrenal carcinoma that produces a mixed array of androgens and glucocorticoids. Virilizing tumors in boys manifest in a manner similar to that of simple virilizing congenital adrenal hyperplasia. There is phallic enlargement, erections, pubic and axillary hair, increased muscle mass, deepening of the voice, acne, and scrotal thinning, but testicular size is prepubertal. Elevated concentration of testosterone among young boys alters behavior. The boy has increased irritability, rambunctiousness, and hyperactivity and plays roughly but has no evidence of libido. Diagnosis is based on the presence of hyperandrogenemia that cannot be suppressed with glucocorticoids. Treatment is surgical. All such tumors are handled as if they are malignant. Care is exerted not to cut the capsule and seed cells onto the peritoneum. The pathologic distinction between adrenal adenoma and carcinoma can be difficult.

Feminizing adrenal tumors are extremely rare among either sex. Feminizing adrenal (or extraadrenal) tumors can be differentiated from true (central) precocious puberty among girls because of absence of increased circulating concentrations of gonadotropins and a prepubertal response of LH to an intravenous challenge of GnRH. Among boys, such tumors cause gynecomastia, which resembles the benign gynecomastia that often accompanies puberty. However, as with virilizing adrenal tumors, testicular size and the gonadotropin response to GnRH testing are prepubertal. The diagnosis of a feminizing tumor in a pubertal boy can be extremely difficult, but it usually is suggested by an arrest in pubertal progression and can be proved by the persistence of circulating plasma estrogens after administration of testosterone.

CONN SYNDROME

Conn syndrome, characterized by hypertension, polyuria, hypokalemic alkalosis, and low plasma renin activity caused by aldosterone-producing adrenal adenoma is exquisitely rare among children. The diagnostic task is to differentiate primary aldosteronism from physiological secondary hyperaldosteronism occurring in response to another physiological disturbance. Any loss of sodium, retention of potassium, or decrease in blood volume causes hyperreninemic secondary hyperaldosteronism. Renal tubular acidosis, treatment with diuretics, salt-wasting nephritis, or hypovolemia caused by nephrosis, ascites, or blood loss is typical of physiological secondary hyperaldosteronism. Primary aldosteronism is characterized by hypertension and hypokalemic alkalosis. The cause is a small adrenal adenoma, usually confined to one adrenal gland. Both adrenal

glands need to be explored surgically because adrenal vein catheterization is not possible for children and is difficult for adults.

24.4.9 Glucocorticoid Therapy and Withdrawal

Since they were introduced into clinical medicine in the early 1950s, glucocorticoids have been used to manage almost every known disease. At present, rational use falls into two broad categories—replacement in adrenal insufficiency and pharmacotherapeutic use. The latter category is largely related to the anti-inflammatory properties of glucocorticoids but also includes lysis of leukemic leukocytes, decreasing plasma calcium concentration, and decreasing high intracranial pressure. Almost all of these actions are mediated through glucocorticoid receptors, which are present in most cells. Because there appears to be only one major type of glucocorticoid receptor, all glucocorticoids affect all tissues that contain such receptors. The only differences among the various glucocorticoid preparations are the ratio of glucocorticoid to mineralocorticoid activity, capacity to bind to various binding proteins, molar potency, and biological half-life. A common use of dexamethasone, a synthetic glucocorticoid, is decreasing high intracranial pressure and brain edema. Neurosurgical experience indicates that the optimal doses are 10 to 100 times those that would thoroughly saturate all available receptors, suggesting that this action of dexamethasone may not be mediated through the glucocorticoid receptor.

Glucocorticoids are so called because of their major actions to increase plasma concentrations of glucose. This occurs through induction of the transcription of many genes, including most of the enzymes of the Embden-Meyerhof glycolytic pathway and other hepatic enzymes that divert amino acids, such as alanine, to the production of glucose. The coordinated action to increase transcription of these genes can increase plasma concentrations of glucose and cause obesity and muscle wasting. The other features of Cushing syndrome are similarly attributable to the increased transcriptional activity of specific glucocorticoid-sensitive genes.

REPLACEMENT THERAPY

The goal of all forms of replacement therapy is to return to the body that which it cannot produce. With glucocorticoids, replacement therapy is complicated by undesirable side effects with even minor degrees of overtreatment or undertreatment. Overtreatment can cause the signs and symptoms of Cushing syndrome. Even minimal overtreatment can impair the growth of children. Undertreatment causes the signs and symptoms of adrenal insufficiency only if the extent of undertreatment (dose and duration) is considerable. However, undertreatment can impair capability to respond to stress. Among children, glucocorticoid replacement therapy is most commonly used to manage congenital adrenal hyperplasia. In this setting, undertreatment causes overproduction of adrenal androgens. The result is hastening of epiphyseal maturation and closure and compromise of ultimate adult height. In the formulation of a program of adrenal replacement therapy for a growing child, it is much more crucial to mimic normal endogenous production of glucocorticoids than it is in treatment of adults, who have already achieved maximal growth potential. To optimize pediatric glucocorticoid replacement therapy, doses approximate the endogenous secretory rate of cortisol, approximately 8 $mg/m^2/d$, although there is considerable individual variation. Several additional factors must be considered in tailoring a specific child's glucocorticoid replacement regimen.

The *specific form of adrenal insufficiency* for which the patient is being treated influences therapy. In the management of autoimmune adrenalitis or any other form of Addison disease, it is prudent to err slightly on the side of undertreatment. This eliminates the possibility of glucocorticoid-induced iatrogenic growth retardation and allows the pituitary gland to continue to produce normal to slightly elevated concentrations of ACTH. This ACTH continues to stimulate the remaining functional adrenal steroidogenic machinery and is a fairly convenient means of monitoring the effects of therapy. In contrast, in the management of severe virilizing congenital adrenal hyperplasia, adrenal function is suppressed more completely. Essentially all adrenal steroidogenesis produces unwanted androgens with consequent virilization and rate of advancement of bony maturation more rapid than the rate of advancement of height. As stated earlier, however, overtreatment also compromises growth.

The *presence or absence of associated mineralocorticoid deficiency* is an important variable. Children with mild degrees of mineralocorticoid insufficiency, such as those with simple virilizing congenital adrenal hyperplasia, may continue to have mildly elevated ACTH values, suggesting insufficient glucocorticoid replacement in association with elevated PRA. Some children have an ACTH level elevated in response to chronic, compromised hypovolemia. The excess secretion is an attempt to stimulate the adrenal glands to produce more mineralocorticoid. For these children, who do not have overt signs and symptoms of mineralocorticoid insufficiency, treatment with mineralocorticoid replacement may allow a decrease in the amount of glucocorticoid replacement needed to suppress plasma ACTH and urinary 17-ketosteroid levels. This decrease in glucocorticoid therapy reduces the likelihood of compromise of adult height.

The *specific formulation of glucocorticoid used* is of great importance. Extremely potent, long-acting glucocorticoids, such as dexamethasone or prednisone, are preferred in the treatment of adults but are rarely appropriate for replacement therapy among children. Because children are continually growing and changing in weight and body surface area, it is necessary to adjust doses frequently. Small, incremental changes are more easily made with relatively weaker glucocorticoids. The efficacy of attempting to mimic the physiological diurnal variation in steroid hormone secretion is controversial. Because ACTH and cortisol concentrations are high in the morning and low in the evening, it is appealing to attempt to duplicate this circadian rhythm in replacement therapy. However, the results do not clearly indicate that better growth is achieved by giving relatively larger doses in the morning and lower doses at night. This probably reflects the fact that ACTH and cortisol secretion are episodic throughout the day and that this well-established circadian variation is not smooth. The pattern of high in the morning and low in the evening is only an averaged result. Furthermore, the adrenal glands release cortisol episodically throughout the day in response to various physiological demands, such as hypoglycemia, exercise, and stress. Under normal circumstances plasma concentration is high when the clearance and disposal rates also are high. A planned program of replacement therapy cannot possibly anticipate these day-to-day variations.

Dosage equivalents among various glucocorticoids can be misleading. Because most preparations of glucocorticoids are intended for pharmacotherapeutic use rather than replacement therapy, and because the most common indication for pharmacologic dosage of glucocorticoids is for their anti-inflammatory properties, almost all tables of glucocorticoid equivalencies are based on anti-inflammatory, immunosuppressive equivalencies. However, the differences in plasma half-life and ability to bind to plasma proteins cause different biological equivalencies. Thus dexamethasone is widely reported as being 25 to 30 times more potent than cortisol when its anti-inflammatory capabilities are measured, but the growth-suppressant activity of dexamethasone is about 80 times that of cortisol (Table 24-17). Thus there is no unanimity in recommendations for designing a glucocorticoid replacement regimen. However, understanding these variables allows appropriate monitoring and encourages the physician to vary treatment according to the responses and needs of the child.

GLUCOCORTICOIDS

Commonly Used Glucocorticoid Preparations

Numerous chemical derivatives and variants of naturally occurring steroids are commercially available in a huge array of dosage forms, vehicles, and concentrations, all carrying confusing and uninformative brand names. Choosing the appropriate product can be simplified by considering only the most widely used steroids (Table 24-17). As indicated in the table, there are four relevant considerations in the choice of which drug to use.

First, the glucocorticoid potency of the various drugs is generally calculated and described according to anti-inflammatory potency. Second, the growth-suppressant effect of a glucocorticoid preparation can differ greatly from its anti-inflammatory effect. This difference is caused by differences in half-life, metabolism, protein binding, and receptor affinity (potency). It is not caused by receptor specificity, because all known receptor-mediated effects of glucocorticoids are mediated through a single type of receptor. Third, the mineralocorticoid activity of various glucocorticoid preparations varies widely. As discussed in Sec. 24.4.2, both glucocorticoid and mineralocorticoid hormones can bind to both glucocorticoid (type I) and mineralocorticoid (type II) receptors. Mineralocorticoid activity is intimately related to the activity of the enzyme 11β-dehydrogenase, which metabolizes glucocorticoids to a form that cannot bind the receptor but cannot metabolize mineralocorticoids. The relative mineralocorticoid potency of various steroids is determined by both their affinity for the type II receptor and their resistance to the activity of 11β-dehydrogenase. Some commonly used glucocorticoids, especially cortisol and cortisone, have marked mineralocorticoid activity, so "stress doses" provide sufficient mineralocorticoid activity to meet physiological needs. Mineralocorticoid supplementation may not be needed in those cases. Fourth, the plasma half-life and biological half-life of the various preparations vary widely and may not be coordinated. This is mainly related to binding to plasma proteins, hepatic metabolism, and hepatic activation. For example, cortisone and prednisone are biologically inactive (and even have mild steroid antagonist actions) until they are metabolized by hepatic 11β-dehydrogenase to their active forms, cortisol and prednisolone. The relative glucocorticoid potency of these preparations also is affected by liver function. Cortisone and prednisone are cleared more rapidly by patients taking drugs such as phenobarbital or phenytoin that induce hepatic enzymes and are cleared more slowly by patients with liver failure.

Route of administration is important. Glucocorticoids are available for oral, intramuscular, intravenous, intrathecal, intraarticular, inhalant, and topical use. Topical preparations include those designed for use on skin, mucous membranes, and conjunctiva. Each preparation is designed to deliver the maximal concentration of

TABLE 24-17

POTENCY OF VARIOUS THERAPEUTIC STEROIDS RELATIVE TO THE POTENCY OF CORTISOL

STEROID	ANTI-INFLAMMATORY GLUCOCORTICOID EFFECT	GROWTH-RETARDING GLUCOCORTICOID EFFECT	SALT-RETAINING MINERALOCORTICOID EFFECT	PLASMA HALF-LIFE (min)	BIOLOGICAL HALF-LIFE (h)
Cortisol (hydrocortisone)	1.0	1.0	1.0	80–120	8
Cortisone acetate (oral)	0.8	0.8	0.8	80–120	8
Cortisone acetate (IM)	0.8	1.3	0.8	—	18
Prednisone	3.5–4	5	0.8	200	16–36
Prednisolone	4	—	0.8	120–300	16–36
Methylprednisolone	5	7.5	0.5	—	—
Betamethasone	25–30	—	0	130–330	—
Triamcinolone	5	—	0	—	—
Dexamethasone	30	80	0	150–>300	36–54
9α-Fluorocortisol	15	—	200	—	—
Deoxycorticosterone acetate[a]	0	—	20	—	—
Aldosterone[b]	0.3	—	200-1000	—	—

[a] No longer commercially available.

[b] Not commercially available; shown for comparison.

SOURCE: *Data compiled from various sources, primarily Tyrrell JB: Glucocorticoid therapy. In: Felig P, Baxter JD, Frohman LA, eds: Endocrinology and Metabolism, 3rd ed. New York, McGraw-Hill, 1995:855, and Styne DM, Richards GE, Bell JJ, et al: Growth patterns in congenital adrenal hyperplasia: correlation of glucocorticoid therapy with stature. In: Lee PA, Plotnick LP, Kowarski AA, Migeon CJ, eds: Congenital Adrenal Hyperplasia. Baltimore, University Park Press, 1977:247.*

steroid to the desired tissue while delivering less steroid systemically. However, all such preparations are absorbed to varying extents, so even topically administered steroids used to treat eczema or inhaled steroids for asthma can cause growth retardation and other signs of Cushing syndrome. In general, and in contradistinction to many other drugs, orally administered steroids are absorbed rapidly but incompletely, whereas intramuscularly administered steroids are absorbed slowly but completely. If the secretory rate of cortisol is 8 mg/m^2 of body surface area, the intramuscular or intravenous replacement dose of cortisol (hydrocortisone) is 8 mg/m^2, but the oral equivalent is about 20 mg of hydrocortisone. The efficiency of absorption of glucocorticoids can vary considerably depending on diet, gastric acidity, intestinal transit time, and other individual factors. This emphasizes that the dosage equivalents listed in Table 24-17 and similar tables are only general approximations. The equivalencies shown are estimated biological equivalencies with a broad range of variability and are not physical chemical equivalents.

ACTH can be used for glucocorticoid therapy because of its action to stimulate endogenous adrenal steroidogenesis. Although ACTH is extremely useful in diagnostic tests of adrenal function (see Sec. 24.4.5), its use as a therapeutic agent is no longer favored, principally because it stimulates synthesis of mineralocorticoids and adrenal androgens as well as glucocorticoids and because it must be administered parenterally. At present, intramuscular ACTH 1–39 in a gel form is recommended for and is the best therapy for infantile spasms and possibly also for other forms of epilepsy among infants resistant to conventional anticonvulsants. Whether this action is mediated by ACTH itself, by other peptides in the biological preparation, by adrenal steroids, or by ACTH-responsive synthesis of novel neurosteroids in the brain has not been determined. The risk of complications of such therapy, mineralocorticoid-induced hypertension, can be avoided by use of a low-sodium diet (eg, baby food). Treatment with daily injections of ACTH results in less hypothalamic-pituitary suppression than does treatment with equivalent doses of oral glucocorticoids, presumably because the effect on the adrenal glands is transient. Adrenal suppression does not occur in ACTH therapy. Because the effects of ACTH on adrenal steroidogenesis are highly variable, it is even more difficult to determine dosage equivalencies for ACTH and oral steroid preparations than it is among the various steroids. A rough guide from studies with adults is that 40 units of ACTH (1–39) gel is approximately equivalent to 100 mg of cortisol.

Pharmacologic Steroid Therapy

Pharmacologic (supraphysiological) doses of glucocorticoids are used in a variety of clinical situations. Immune suppression in organ transplantation, tumor chemotherapy, management of autoimmune collagen vascular and nephrotic syndromes, and inflammatory bowel disease are the most common indications for protracted high-dose glucocorticoid therapy. Asthma, pseudotumor cerebri, dermatitis, certain infections, neuritis, and certain forms of anemia are often managed with glucocorticoids. The decision to use glucocorticoid treatment in these situations is left to the appropriate specialist, but risks, especially growth suppression, must be balanced with benefits. The choice of glucocorticoid preparation to be used is guided by the pharmacologic parameters described earlier and in Table 24-17 and by custom. For example, dexamethasone and betamethasone are equally effective in escaping the effects of placental 11β-dehydrogenase because they enter the fetal circula-

tion after maternal administration. Betamethasone, however, is used almost universally to induce fetal lung maturation.

Pharmacologic doses of glucocorticoids administered for more than 1 or 2 weeks cause the signs and symptoms of iatrogenic Cushing syndrome. These are similar to the glucocorticoid-induced findings of Cushing disease but may be more severe because of the high doses involved (Table 24-18). Other differences in the clinical and laboratory findings of iatrogenic Cushing syndrome as opposed to Cushing disease are related to the absence of adrenal androgen effects and the usual absence of mineralocorticoid effects in iatrogenic Cushing syndrome. To ensure that such undesired mineralocorticoid effects are held to a minimum, steroids with high ratios of glucocorticoid to mineralocorticoid activity usually are chosen.

The use of alternate-day therapy can decrease the glucocorticoid-induced features of iatrogenic Cushing syndrome. This seems to be especially true of suppression of the hypothalamic-pituitary-adrenal axis and suppression of growth. The basic premises of alternate-day therapy are that the disease can be suppressed with intermittent therapy and that there is marked recovery of the unwanted glucocorticoid effects during the off day. It is crucial to choose a relatively short-acting glucocorticoid and administer it only once in the morning of each therapeutic day to ensure that the off day is truly off. Long-acting glucocorticoids, such as dexamethasone, triamcinolone, and betamethasone, are not used for alternate-day therapy. Results are best with oral prednisone or methylprednisolone.

Withdrawal of Glucocorticoid Therapy

Withdrawal of glucocorticoid therapy can be difficult and can cause symptoms of glucocorticoid insufficiency. When glucocorticoid therapy has been used for only 1 week or 10 days, therapy can be discontinued abruptly, even if high doses have been used. Although only one or two doses of glucocorticoid are needed to suppress the hypothalamic-pituitary-adrenal axis, this axis recovers rapidly from short-term suppression. When therapy has persisted for 2 weeks or longer, recovery of hypothalamic-pituitary-adrenal function is slower, and tapering of dosage of glucocorticoids is indicated. Abrupt discontinuation of treatment of such patients causes symptoms of glucocorticoid insufficiency, the so-called steroid withdrawal syndrome. This symptom complex does not include salt loss; adrenal glomerulosa function, regulated principally by the renin-angiotensin system, remains normal. However, blood pressure can decrease abruptly, because glucocorticoids are needed for

TABLE 24-18

COMPLICATIONS OF HIGH-DOSE GLUCOCORTICOID THERAPY

SHORT-TERM THERAPY	LONG-TERM THERAPY
Gastritis	Gastric ulcer
Growth arrest	Short stature
Increased appetite	Weight gain
Hypercalciuria	Osteoporosis, fractures
Glycosuria	Slipped epiphysis
Immune suppression	Ischemic bone necrosis
Masked symptoms of infection, especially fever and inflammation	Poor wound healing
	Catabolism
	Cataracts
Toxic psychosis	Bruising (capillary fragility)
	Adrenal and pituitary suppression
	Toxic psychosis

the action of catecholamines in maintaining vascular tone. Steroid withdrawal syndrome can entail all the signs of glucocorticoid insufficiency (see Sec. 24.4.7), but the most prominent symptoms are malaise, anorexia, headache, lethargy, nausea, and fever. In reducing the doses of glucocorticoids of children receiving pharmacologic, supraphysiological doses, it might appear logical to reduce the dosage precipitously to "physiological" replacement doses. However, this is rarely successful and occasionally disastrous. Even when given "physiological" replacement, patients who have been receiving pharmacologic doses of glucocorticoids have steroid withdrawal. Although the mechanism is not known with certainty, it is most likely that long-term pharmacologic glucocorticoid therapy inhibits transcription of the genes for glucocorticoid receptors, reducing the number of receptors per cell. If this is so, physiological concentrations of glucocorticoids elicit a subphysiological cellular response. The result is steroid withdrawal syndrome. For this reason, it is necessary to taper from the outset. The duration of glucocorticoid therapy is a critical consideration in designing a glucocorticoid withdrawal program. Therapy for 2 months completely suppresses the hypothalamic-pituitary-adrenal axis but does not cause adrenal atrophy. Therapy of years' duration can cause almost-total atrophy of the adrenal fasciculata and reticularis. It may necessitate a withdrawal regimen that takes months.

Procedures for tapering steroids are empirical. Success is greatly determined by the length and mode of therapy and by individual patient responses. Patients who have been taking alternate-day therapy can be withdrawn more easily than those receiving daily therapy, especially daily therapy with a long-acting glucocorticoid such as dexamethasone. Among patients undergoing long-standing therapy, 25% reduction in the previous level of therapy per week is generally recommended. A patient with a body surface area of 1 m^2 has a secretory rate of cortisol of approximately 9 mg/d, equivalent to 20 mg/d of orally administered cortisone acetate. If the patient has been taking daily therapy equivalent to 100 mg of cortisone acetate for many months, a tapering protocol over 8 to 10 weeks may be needed. A protocol of 75% of the previous week's dose would thus be 75 mg/d for the first week, 56 mg/d for the second, then 42, 31.5, 24, 18, 13.5, 10, 7.5, 5.5 mg/d, then off treatment. A more practical regimen based on the sizes of tablets available is 75, 50, 37.5, 25, 17.5, 12.5, 10, 7.5, and 5 mg/d. Tapering can be more rapid for most patients, but all patients need to be observed closely. When withdrawal is done with steroids other than cortisone or cortisol, measurement of morning cortisol values can be useful. A morning cortisol value of 10 μg/dL or more indicates the dose can be reduced safely.

Even after successful discontinuation of therapy, the hypothalamic-pituitary-adrenal axis is not entirely normal. As in the care of a patient successfully treated for Cushing disease (see Sec. 24.4.8), the hypothalamic-pituitary-adrenal axis may be incapable of responding to severe stress for 6 to 12 months after successful withdrawal from long-term, high-dose glucocorticoid therapy. Evaluation of the hypothalamus and pituitary gland with a CRF or metyrapone test and evaluation of adrenal responsiveness to pituitary stimulation with an intravenous ACTH test are performed at the conclusion of a withdrawal program and 6 months thereafter. The results of these tests indicate whether steroid coverage is needed for acute surgical stress or illness.

Stress Doses of Glucocorticoids

Cortisol secretory rate increases markedly during physiological stress such as trauma, surgery, or severe illness. Patients receiving glucocorticoid replacement therapy or those recently withdrawn from pharmacologic therapy need coverage with stress doses of steroids in such situations. The specific indications for this coverage and the appropriate dosage are controversial and difficult to establish. Most practitioners prefer to err on the side of steroid overdosage. This is the safest tactic in the short term, but overdosage and increased dosage when it is not needed can, over a period of years, have a profound effect on growth.

It is generally said that doses 3 to 10 times physiological replacement are needed for "the stress of surgery." The stress accompanying a surgical procedure can vary greatly. Modern techniques of anesthesiology; better anesthetic, analgesic, and muscle-relaxing drugs; and increased awareness of the particular needs of children in managing intraoperative fluids and electrolytes have greatly reduced the stress of surgery. In the past, a considerable amount of such stress had to do with pain and hypovolemia, but these problems are less important in contemporary children's hospitals and inpatient services. Similarly, part of the stress of acute illness is fever and fluid loss, factors now familiar to all pediatricians. Although it remains appropriate and necessary to give about three times the physiological requirements during such periods of stress, it probably is not necessary to give much higher doses. It also is not necessary to triple a child's physiological replacement regimen during simple colds, upper respiratory infection, otitis media, or after immunizations, unless the patient becomes dehydrated or febrile.

Preoperative preparation of a patient with adrenal hypoplasia and receiving replacement therapy is simple if it is well planned. Although it is true that stress doses of steroids can be administered intravenously by the anesthesiologist during an operation, the results have been suboptimal. Doses administered as an intravenous bolus are short acting and may not provide coverage throughout the procedure. The transition from hospital ward to surgical theater to recovery room usually involves a transition among three or more teams of personnel, increasing the risk of error. Because intramuscularly administered cortisone acetate has a biological half-life of approximately 18 hours, we recommend intramuscular administration of twice the day's physiological requirement 18 hours before the operation and again 8 hours before the operation. This provides the patient with a body reservoir of glucocorticoid throughout the operation and the immediately postoperative period. Regular therapy at two to three times physiological requirements can be reinstituted the day after the surgical procedure.

MINERALOCORTICOID REPLACEMENT

Replacement therapy with mineralocorticoids is indicated for salt-losing congenital adrenal hyperplasia (see Sec. 24.4.6) and in syndromes of adrenal insufficiency that affect the zona glomerulosa (see Sec. 24.4.7). A variety of mineralocorticoid preparations have been used over the years. However, only one mineralocorticoid, 9α-fluorocortisol (Florinef) is currently available. This is unfortunate because 9α-fluorocortisol can be administered only orally; no parenteral mineralocorticoid preparation is available.

Mineralocorticoids are perhaps unique among pharmacotherapeutic agents in that the doses used are essentially the same irrespective of the size and age of the patient. Newborns are quite insensitive to mineralocorticoids and may need larger doses than do adults. This is reflected in the substantial age-dependent decrease in circulating aldosterone concentrations (Fig. 24-14). In general, the replacement dose of 9α-fluorocortisol is 0.05 to 0.10 mg daily. It is important to realize that a mineralocorticoid by itself is nearly useless; sodium must be available to the nephrons for min-

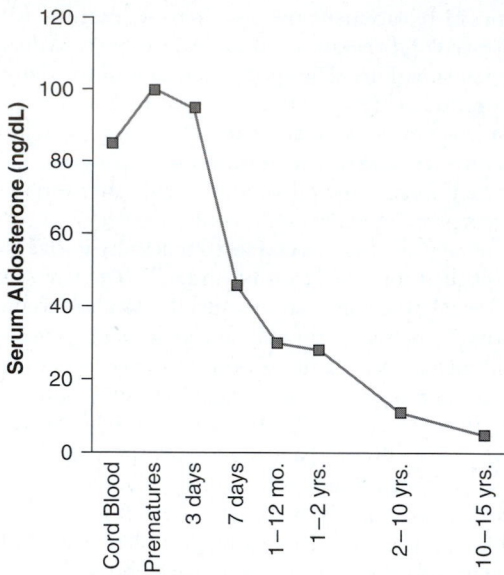

FIGURE 24-14 **Concentrations of aldosterone as a function of age.**

eralocorticoids to promote reabsorption of sodium. A newborn with salt-losing congenital adrenal hyperplasia must be treated with both mineralocorticoids and sodium chloride. Mineralocorticoids also cause hypertension only by retaining sodium. When long-acting parenteral mineralocorticoid preparations were available, they could be administered without fear of causing hypertension, hypernatremia, or hyponatremia, because the biological effects could be titrated by varying the amount of salt given daily.

Although 9α-fluorocortisol is the only mineralocorticoid per se available, it is not the only steroid that has mineralocorticoid activity. Cortisol has marked mineralocorticoid activity; approximately 20 mg cortisol or cortisone administered intravenously has a mineralocorticoid action equivalent to 0.1 mg of 9α-fluorocortisol (Table 24-17). When cortisol or cortisone is given in stress doses as described earlier, it provides adequate mineralocorticoid activity, and mineralocorticoid replacement can be interrupted. This situation occurs frequently when patients with salt-losing congenital adrenal hyperplasia undergo surgical treatment. The stress doses of intramuscular cortisone acetate and the intravenous saline solutions administered during and after the operation suffice for the mineralocorticoid requirements. Additional 9α-fluorocortisol is not needed until the supraphysiological stress doses of cortisol are decreased. Because 9α-fluorocortisol can be administered only orally and because this may not be possible in the postoperative period, the appropriate drug for glucocorticoid replacement is cortisol or cortisone. These drugs have mineralocorticoid activity, unlike synthetic steroids such as prednisone or dexamethasone, which have little mineralocorticoid activity.

References

General

Auchus RJ, Geller DH, Lee TC, Miller WL: The regulation of human P450c17 activity: relationship to premature adrenarche, insulin resistance, and the polycystic ovary syndrome. Trends Endocrinol Metab 83: 1399, 1998

Bamberger CM, Schulte HM, Chrousos GP: Molecular determinants of glucocorticoid receptor function and tissue sensitivity to gluococorticoids. Endocr Rev 17:245, 1996

Bose HS, Sugawara T, Strauss JF III, Miller WL: The pathophysiology and genetics of congenital lipoid adrenal hyperplasia. N Engl J Med 335: 1870, 1996

Clark AJL, Weber A: Adrenocorticotropin insensitivity syndromes. Endocr Rev 19:828, 1998

Fardella CE, Miller WL: Molecular biology of mineralocorticoid metabolism. Annu Rev Nutr 16:433, 1996

Forest MG, Morel Y, David M: Prenatal treatment of congenital adrenal hyperplasia. Trends Endocrinol Metab 9:284, 1998

Gonzalez FJ: The molecular biology of cytochrome P450s. Pharmacol Rev 40:243, 1989

Joehrer K, Geley S, Strasser-Wozak EMC, et al: CYP11B1 mutations causing non-classic adrenal hyperplasia due to 11β-hydroxylase deficiency. Hum Mol Genet 6:1829, 1997

Lajic S, Wedell A, Bui TH, Ritzen EM, Holst M: Long-term somatic follow-up of prenatally treated children with congenital adrenal hyperplasia. J Clin Endocrinol Metab 83:3872, 1998

Lashansky G, Saenger P, Dimartino-Nardi J, et al: Normative data for steroidogenic response of mineralocorticoids and their precursors to ACTH in a healthy pediatric population. J Clin Endocrinol Metab 75: 1491, 1992

Lashansky G, Saenger P, Fishman K, et al: Normative data for adrenal steroidogenesis in a healthy pediatric population: age and sex-related changes after ACTH stimulation. J Clin Endocrinol Metab 73:674, 1991

Mellon SH: Neurosteroids: biochemistry, modes of action and clinical relevance. J Clin Endocrinol Metab 78:1003–1008, 1994

Miller WL: Congenital adrenal hyperplasia in the adult patient. Adv Intern Med 44:155, 1999

Miller WL: Congenital lipoid adrenal hyperplasia: the human gene knockout of the steroidogenic acute regulatory protein. J Mol Endocrinol 19: 227, 1997

Miller WL: Genetics, diagnosis, and management of 21-hydroxylase deficiency. J Clin Endocrinol Metab 78:241, 1994

Miller WL: Prenatal treatment of congenital adrenal hyperplasia: a promising experimental therapy of unproven safety. Trends Endocrinol Metab 9:290, 1998

Miller WL: Steroid hormone biosynthesis in the materno-feto-placental unit. Clin Perinatol 25:799, 1998

Moser HW: Adrenoleukodystrophy. Curr Opin Neurol 8:221, 1995

New MI, White PC: Genetic disorders of steroid hormone synthesis and metabolism. Baillieres Clin Endocrinol Metab 9:525, 1995

New MI, Wilson RC: Steroid disorders in children: congenital adrenal hyperplasia and apparent mineralocorticoid excess. Proc Natl Acad Sci USA 96:12790, 1999

Pang S: The molecular and clinical spectrum of 3β-hydroxysteroid dehydrogenase deficiency disorder. Trends Endocrinol Metab 9:82, 1998

Rosner W: The functions of corticosteroid binding globulin and sex hormone binding globulin: recent advances. Endocr Rev 11:80, 1990

Sklar CA, Kaplan SL, Grumbach MM: Evidence for dissociation between adrenarche and gonadarche: studies in patients with idiopathic precocious puberty, gonadal dysgenesis, isolated gonadotropin deficiency, and constitutionally delayed growth and adolescence. J Clin Endocrinol Metab 51:548, 1980

Streck WS, Lockwood DH: Pituitary-adrenal recovery following short-term suppression with corticosteroids. Am J Med 66:910, 1979

Watkins PA, Gould SJ, Smith MA, et al: Altered expression of ALDP in X-linked adrenoleukodystrophy. Am J Hum Genet 57:292–301, 1995

White PC: Disorders of aldosterone biosynthesis and action. N Engl J Med 331:250, 1994

White PC, Mune T, Agarwal AK: 11β-Hydroxysteroid dehydrogenase and the syndrome of apparent mineralocorticoid excess. Endocr Rev 18:135, 1997

Yanase T, Simpson ER, Waterman MR: 17α-Hydroxylase/17,20 lyase deficiency: from clinical investigation to molecular definition. Endocr Rev 12:91, 1991

24.5 ADRENAL MEDULLA, PHEOCHROMOCYTOMA, AND MULTIPLE ENDOCRINE NEOPLASIA SYNDROMES

Steven D. Chernausek

The adrenal medulla and the sympathetic nerves and ganglia are derived from neural crest ectoderm. During embryogenesis, primitive sympathetic cells (sympathogonia) migrate ventrally from the neural tube and differentiate into neuroblasts that give rise to ganglion cells. Aggregations of these cells form sympathetic ganglia that become linked together to make the sympathetic trunks. Other primitive cells are transformed into pheochromoblasts and then to chromaffin cells that move to the anlagen of the adrenal cortex, penetrate its substance, and compose the primordial adrenal medulla. Chromaffin cells are widely distributed among the sympathetic ganglia. A large mass of them, composing the organ of Zuckerkandl, is adjacent to the origin of the inferior mesenteric artery. The extraadrenal chromaffin tissues dominate during fetal life and early infancy but subsequently degenerate as chromaffin cells of the adrenal medulla mature. In rare instances ectopic rests of chromaffin tissue persist and are present in various sites in the neck, chest, and abdomen.

The sympathetic nerves and the adrenal medullae both release catecholamines and are commonly called the *sympathoadrenal-neuroendocrine system*. Neural and hormonal communication takes place within this system, which controls many physiological processes in the body. The catecholamine norepinephrine functions primarily as a neurotransmitter. It is released from the sympathetic postganglionic axon terminals directly at the effector cell on blood vessels and viscera. Noradrenergic fibers are widely distributed in the body to form an intricate network within the innervated tissues. They have an important role in direct and indirect metabolic regulation of many cell types.

24.5.1 Biochemistry and Physiology of Catecholamines

Catecholamine biosynthesis is illustrated in Fig. 24-15. Enzymatic conversion of tyrosine to dihydroxyphenylalanine by tyrosine hydroxylase is the rate-limiting step in catecholamine biosynthesis. High concentrations of glucocorticoids, which are present in the adrenal medulla because of the enveloping adrenal cortex, enhance conversion of norepinephrine to epinephrine by inducing the enzyme phenylethanolamine N-methyl transferase. The adrenal medulla is the only location in the sympathetic nervous system where this conversion takes place. Metabolism of primary adrenal medullary products is shown in Fig. 24-16. Measurement of epinephrine, norepinephrine, or their metabolic products is the principal means of diagnosing pheochromocytoma.

Catecholamines are products of the sympathetic nervous system that exert effects both in the circulation as hormones and within the nervous system as neurotransmitters. Catecholamines have important effects on the cardiovascular system. They regulate vascular tone and stimulate cardiac output by means of increases in heart rate and contractility. They are involved in fuel homeostasis, constituting an important defense against hypoglycemia by rapidly stimulating hepatic glucose output. They contribute to energy mobilization in times of stress by stimulating lipolysis. Almost every organ and physiological system are influenced, directly or indirectly, by catecholamine status. Their widespread effects are mediated by specific cell-surface receptors classified as either α-adrenergic (generally excitatory for smooth muscle) or β-adrenergic (generally inhibitory of smooth muscle). Each major class of receptor has been subdivided further. For example, the α_1 receptor subtype mediates arteriolar constriction in vascular smooth muscle. Activation of the

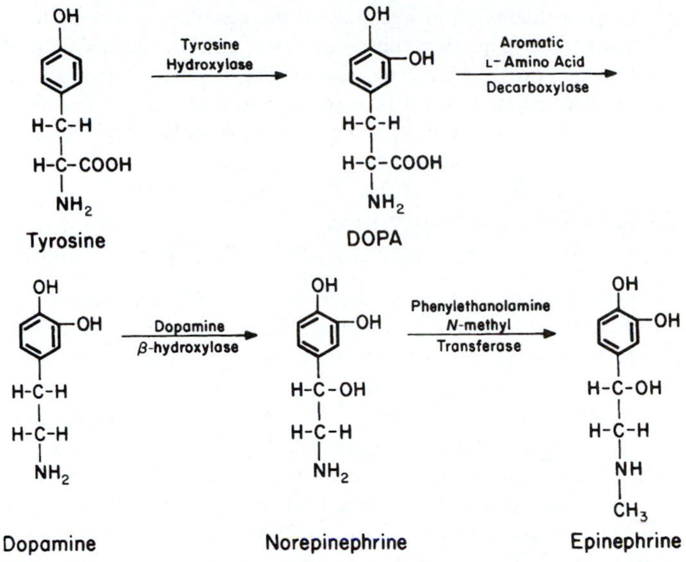

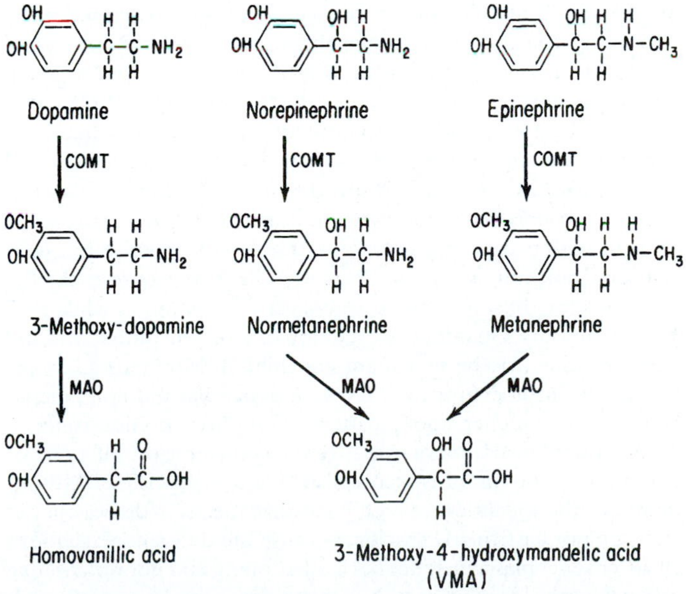

FIGURE 24-15 The principal pathways for synthesis of catecholamines.

FIGURE 24-16 Schematic shows formation of principal catecholamine metabolites. COMT = catechol-*O*-methyl transferase; MAO = monoamine oxidase.

β_2 receptor dilates smooth muscle of the vasculature and tracheo-bronchial tree. The β_3 receptor mediates catecholamine-induced lipolysis and brown fat thermogenesis. Pharmacologic agents have different interactions with these receptor subclasses. For example, propranolol blocks both β_1 and β_2 receptors, whereas atenolol is specific for the β_1 (cardiac) receptor subtype.

24.5.2   Pheochromocytoma

Pheochromocytoma is a rare, catecholamine-producing tumor usually found in the adrenal medulla, although it can occur in any sympathetic ganglion. They are usually benign, unilateral, and sporadic. Although most pheochromocytomas appear to be sporadic, 10 to 20% occur in the context of a genetic syndrome, von Hippel-Lindau disease (VHL), multiple endocrine neoplasia type 2 (MEN2), and neurofibromatosis being the most common. Von Hippel-Lindau disease is characterized by angiomata of the retina and hemangioblastoma of the cerebellum and is caused by mutations in the *VHL* gene. Missense mutations of the *VHL* gene are typically associated with pheochromocytoma. Mutations of the *RET* oncogene cause MEN 2 (see Sec. 24.5.3).

CLINICAL FEATURES The classic presentation of pheochromocytoma is paroxysmal headache, tachycardia, and diaphoresis. However, clinical manifestations can be quite variable; headache is common. Some reports suggest that most children with pheochromocytoma have sustained hypertension. Patients with tumors detected because of screening for genetic syndromes may have no symptoms but simply have elevated urinary catecholamine secretion. Indications for evaluation for pheochromocytoma include presence of the classic symptom complex, a family history of pheochromocytoma or MEN, unidentified adrenal tumor, severe hypertension and tachycardia in response to general anesthesia or surgery, and hypertension that is unexplained and poorly responsive to standard therapy.

DIAGNOSIS Quantitation of urinary catecholamine excretion by measuring epinephrine, norepinephrine, metanephrine, or homovanillic acid in a 24-hour collection is the most important step toward diagnosis. These values are highly sensitive (>90%). It is probably best to avoid medications during collection, but most common antihypertensive agents (eg, diuretics, calcium channel blockers) usually do not obscure the diagnosis. Measurement of plasma catecholamine concentration usually is not necessary. Some patients with paroxysmal symptoms may show only episodic excessive catecholamine secretion. Probably the best way to make the diagnosis for those patients is to collect urine samples while they have symptoms. Quantitative excretion of vanillylmandelic acid and metanephrine may be similar among children with neuroblastoma and pheochromocytoma, but levels of dopamine and norepinephrine are much higher among patients with pheochromocytoma.

After demonstration of excessive catecholamine production, localization of the tumor is accomplished with either CT or MR imaging. Both modalities are highly sensitive means of detection, but they are not particularly specific, because the differential diagnosis of adrenal neoplasia includes both functioning and nonfunctioning adrenal cortical tumors as well as those arising in the medulla. It is appropriate to begin the radiographic search for the adrenal tumor only after excessive secretion of catecholamines has been documented. Metaiodobenzyl guanidine (MIBG) scanning is specific for pheochromocytoma. Localized increased uptake is found among approximately 90% of patients. Because CT and MR imaging are so useful, MIBG scanning usually is considered a second-line test. Its role may be principally for determining the extent of metastasis in malignant pheochromocytoma or for localizing nonadrenal tumors.

TREATMENT Once the diagnosis of pheochromocytoma is established, surgical extirpation is the best treatment. Patients are at high risk of perioperative complications, such as hypertensive crisis, myocardial dysfunction, and shock. The preoperative and intraoperative treatment of patients undergoing surgical removal of pheochromocytoma necessitates careful attention. Preoperative α-adrenergic blockade with phenoxybenzamine is the most commonly used approach. Patients initially receive 5 to 10 mg twice a day (0.25–2 mg/kg/d), which is gradually increased until the symptoms of hypertension resolve. This generally takes 1 to 2 weeks. A β-blocker such as propranolol or atenolol can be added to the regimen in the event that tachycardia or arrhythmia develops during phenoxybenzamine therapy, but only after α-adrenergic blockade has been accomplished. This is because the hypertension can worsen if the vasodilating effects of the β-blocker are allowed at a time when the α-adrenergic receptors remain stimulated. Even with adequate preoperative preparation, careful monitoring is needed during the procedure and in the postoperative period. Pulmonary edema and impaired myocardial function can occur in the postoperative period.

PROGNOSIS Most patients with a single adrenal pheochromocytoma are cured because 90% of the tumors are benign. It is not possible to determine malignant potential on the basis of microscopic cellular features. Malignant disease is diagnosed only when there is evidence of invasion or metastasis. Recurrence rates in the contralateral adrenal gland are low except among patients with genetic syndromes predisposing them to pheochromocytoma. Because pheochromocytoma is so rare among children, the possibility of an underlying genetic syndrome always is considered when pheochromocytoma is diagnosed at a young age.

24.5.3   Multiple Endocrine Neoplasia Syndromes

The MEN syndromes are rare genetic diseases characterized by multicentric endocrine hyperplasia and neoplasia in specific tissues. They are inherited in a mendelian autosomal dominant manner with the clinical manifestations developing over several decades of life. Long disease-free periods in early life are typical, but penetrance of disease is ultimately very high (>90%). Even though clinical manifestations are uncommon in childhood, knowledge of these conditions is important for the pediatrician because the diagnosis of MEN in a relative affects the subsequent care of a pediatric patient. The diseases occasionally manifest in childhood, so that monitoring for endocrine disease and prophylactic treatment during childhood is indicated. The advent of modern molecular genetic diagnostics facilitates the identification of patients at risk and allows for a focus on those truly at high risk of disease.

Two well-defined genetic disorders constitute the MEN syndromes (Table 24-19). Multiple endocrine neoplasia type 1 is caused by mutations of the *MEN1* gene and characteristically produces hyperfunction of the parathyroid gland, pituitary gland, and islet cells of the pancreas. Multiple endocrine neoplasia type 2 is produced by mutations in the *RET* oncogene. The principal en-

TABLE 24-19

CLASSIFICATION AND FEATURES OF THE MULTIPLE ENDOCRINE NEOPLASIA SYNDROMES

SYNDROME	PRINCIPAL CLINICAL FEATURES	GENETIC ABNORMALITY	PROBABLE DISEASE MECHANISM
MEN 1	Hyperplasia or neoplasia of the pituitary gland, parathyroid glands, and endocrine pancreas (3Ps)	*MEN1* mutation	Loss of tumor suppressor function
MEN 2A	Medullary thyroid cancer, parathyroid hyperplasia, pheochromocytoma	*RET* oncogene mutation	Persistent activation (gain of function) of growth factor receptor (RET protein)
MEN 2B	Medullary thyroid cancer, pheochromocytoma with marfanoid body habitus, and multiple mucosal neuromas	Single, specific *RET* oncogene mutation (codon 918) found in nearly all patients	Enhance function of intracellular tyrosine kinase domain of growth factor receptor (RET protein)
Familial medullary carcinoma of the thyroid	Medullary thyroid cancer	*RET* oncogene mutation	Similar to MEN 2A. Persistent activation of growth factor receptor (RET protein)

docrine abnormality of MEN 2 is medullary carcinoma of the thyroid. In some families, medullary carcinoma of the thyroid is the only manifestation; in others it is associated with pheochromocytoma and hyperparathyroidism (MEN 2A) or with multiple mucosal neuromas. The distinct clinical syndromes of MEN 2 are determined by the specific nature of the mutation in the *RET* oncogene.

The strategy for clinical management of MEN is to remove the diseased gland or organ before malignant growth occurs or hormone hypersecretion causes illness. To do that, one must first establish the diagnosis in the proband, determine which family members are at risk, and screen those at risk with periodic testing so that timely intervention takes place. The methods used to identify those at risk have evolved over the last several years and now incorporate molecular genetic testing. Nonetheless, the basic strategic principles remain the same.

MULTIPLE ENDOCRINE NEOPLASIA TYPE 1

ETIOLOGY Multiple endocrine neoplasia type 1 is caused by mutations in the *MEN1* gene, which is located on chromosome 11 and encodes the protein menin. Mutations in *MEN1* that produce the syndrome are those that typically would cause loss of function, including nonsense mutations, large deletions, or frameshift mutations distributed widely over the coding sequence. The mechanism by which this inherited defect in menin produces disease in an autosomal dominant manner is unknown, as is the exact function of menin. It is postulated that menin acts as a tumor suppressor much like the Wilms tumor gene product. Loss of function caused by mutation of the *MEN1* gene is not sufficient to induce cell overgrowth of endocrine tissue because the remaining allele functions normally. If a specific cell loses a small segment of chromosome 11 that includes the remaining normal *MEN1* gene, a clone of cells deficient in the tumor suppressor initially exhibits abnormal growth regulation and eventually becomes neoplastic. This is called *loss of heterozygosity*.

CLINICAL FEATURES Presentation of MEN 1 before age 10 years is rare; it is unusual before 20 years of age. Patients with MEN 1 typically do not have symptomatic disease until the fourth to the sixth decades of life. However, when patients at risk are screened

regularly with biochemical measures, clinical disease is detected about 10 years earlier.

The most common manifestation of MEN 1 is hyperparathyroidism, which is present in 95% of cases. Demonstrating hypercalcemia with a circulating concentration of parathyroid hormone (PTH) that is either elevated or inappropriately normal (for the elevated calcium level) establishes the diagnosis. Mild hypercalcemia with a normal PTH level also occurs in familial hypocalcuric hypercalcemia, but this condition usually is easy to differentiate from parathyroid hyperplasia on the basis of the family history and assessment of calcium excretion.

Pancreatic islet cell tumors are next in prevalence, found among as many as 75 to 80% of patients with MEN 1 over their lifetimes. Gastrinoma is the most common tumor and produces Zollinger-Ellison syndrome (severe peptic ulcer disease and gastric acid hypersecretion caused by a gastrin-producing islet cell tumor). Malignant gastrinoma is the principal cause of death attributable to MEN 1. About one-third of pancreatic tumors are insulinoma. Less common are tumors producing pancreatic polypeptide or vasoactive intestinal peptide. The latter can manifest as diarrhea.

Tumors of the pituitary gland are third in overall frequency in MEN 1 but may be a more frequent presentation among adolescents. Clinical manifestations of pituitary tumors are caused by the mass effect (eg, headache or abnormalities of vision) or hormone excess. Prolactinoma is the most common pituitary tumor in MEN 1. Hyperprolactinemia can produce galactorrhea and delayed or interrupted puberty. The latter occurs because high circulating concentrations of prolactin block release of LH and FSH, resulting in hypogonadism. Growth hormone–secreting tumors also are relatively common. It takes several years of excess GH secretion to produce clinical features of acromegaly or gigantism.

TREATMENT The main mode of treatment is surgical removal of the diseased glandular tissues once the abnormalities are identified. In the case of hyperparathyroidism, hyperplasia, not adenoma formation, is the main pathologic feature. Thus removal of several glands is needed, with retention of a small amount of parathyroid gland for maintenance of calcium homeostasis. Removal of all parathyroid glands with autotransplantation of a portion of one of the glands to the forearm also can be performed. Surgery is needed for islet cell tumors. The disease of the pancreas can be multicentric and thus necessitate more extensive surgery than does removal of a solitary adenoma. Surgery also is indicated for GH-secreting tumors. Initial therapy for prolactinoma typically is a dopamine agonist (bromocriptine or cabergoline).

MULTIPLE ENDOCRINE NEOPLASIA TYPE 2

ETIOLOGY   Multiple endocrine neoplasia types 2A and 2B and familial medullary carcinoma of the thyroid are caused by specific mutations in *RET,* an oncogene. The RET protein is a cell-surface growth factor receptor, the normal function of which appears to be to mediate action of nervous system growth regulatory peptides such as glial cell–derived neurotrophic factor and neuroturin. The *RET* gene is expressed in tissues derived from the neural crest tissues and parathyroid gland, that is, tissues that eventually become diseased in patients with MEN 2. Unlike the wide variety of mutations that produce MEN 1, a limited number of mutations cause MEN 2. In the case of MEN 2A and familial medullary carcinoma of the thyroid, mutations almost always involve replacement of one of the cysteine residues located near the transmembrane domain of *RET*. A single amino acid substitution in the intracellular tyrosine kinase domain (threonine for methionine at codon 918) produces MEN 2B, the disorder associated with multiple mucosal neuroma. These mutations appear to be gain-of-function mutations that lead to constitutive activation of the RET protein. Therefore, one can consider the receptor for glial cell–derived neurotrophic factor and neuroturin to be persistently in the switched-on position. It is believed that this unabated stimulation of the cells causes cellular hyperplasia and produces predisposition to neoplasia. In contrast, loss-of-function *RET* mutations produce Hirschsprung disease, and on occasion, intestinal neuronal dysplasia occurs in families with MEN 2B (see Sec. 17.27.3).

CLINICAL FEATURES   Multiple endocrine neoplasia type 2 is subdivided into three clinical syndromes: MEN 2A, 2B, and familial medullary carcinoma of the thyroid only. Medullary carcinoma of the thyroid is the predominant lesion of all MEN 2 syndromes. More than 90% of patients with one of the characteristic *RET* mutations eventually have medullary carcinoma of the thyroid, which is cancer of the parafollicular, or C, cells that are of neural crest origin. C cells secrete calcitonin, a hormone that has calcium-regulating properties but the function in humans is unclear. Measurement of serum concentration of calcitonin is extremely helpful in identifying patients with C-cell hyperplasia or medullary carcinoma of the thyroid.

Patients with MEN 2A have familial medullary carcinoma of the thyroid in association with either pheochromocytoma or hyperparathyroidism. The risk of pheochromocytoma appears to be 50% among patients with MEN 2A. It usually develops after the diagnosis of medullary carcinoma of the thyroid is made. Hyperparathyroidism occurs among fewer then 20% of patients.

An unusual somatic appearance and abnormal development of neural ganglia distinguish patients with MEN 2B. Thick lips and slender limbs with long fingers (marfanoid body habitus) occur in association with multiple mucosal neuromas and hypertrophy of the corneal nerves. The neuromas can occur throughout the gastrointestinal tract and usually are visible on the tongue as small, pearly nodules. Dysplasia of the neural ganglia appears to produce motility dysfunction and frequently causes gastrointestinal symptoms such as constipation, bloating, and failure to thrive. The gastrointestinal abnormalities may be the dominant presenting features among children with MEN 2B. The risk of medullary carcinoma of the thyroid

and pheochromocytoma appears to be similar to that of MEN 2A, but hyperparathyroidism is uncommon.

Patients with familial medullary carcinoma of the thyroid have medullary carcinoma of the thyroid only. That is, there is no pheochromocytoma or hyperparathyroidism in the pedigree, and the person has a normal external appearance. It was not clear initially that this condition was related to MEN 2 until *RET* mutations were identified among families with medullary carcinoma of the thyroid only.

TREATMENT   Medullary carcinoma of the thyroid typically has local metastasis and gradual but continued growth of the tumor. Tumor growth can be slow, but does pose real risks. Surgical treatment is the only therapy proven effective and can be curative if performed early in the course of disease. Most patients with a neck mass already have local spread of medullary carcinoma of the thyroid and are not cured with surgical treatment. Therefore (also see Sec. 24.6.10) identification of patients at risk and screening either biochemically through calcitonin measurements or with molecular genetic methods that identify the *RET* gene mutation are the best way to manage MEN 2. The goal is to perform total thyroidectomy before the spread of tumor beyond the thyroid gland. Patients with *RET* mutations need annual assessment of urinary catecholamine excretion to detect occult pheochromocytoma and need abdominal CT or MR imaging when values are elevated.

PREVENTION AND SCREENING   The value of identifying patients at high risk of medullary carcinoma of the thyroid who need prophylactic thyroid surgery is clearly established. Before the use of molecular genetic diagnostic methods, relatives of patients with heritable medullary carcinoma of the thyroid were screened with measurement of calcitonin in the plasma after stimulation, usually with intravenous pentagastrin with or without calcium. Because this test was designed to identify early C-cell hyperplasia, a negative test result at a young age did not mean the patient was free of risk. Therefore multiple testing at intervals was needed. The ability to identify family members carrying *RET* oncogene mutations has greatly simplified the approach to care of families with MEN 2A and familial medullary carcinoma of the thyroid. Because relatively few mutations are known to produce MEN 2, genetic screening is relatively straightforward and offered at several commercial sites.

When evaluating relatives of a patient with MEN 2, most experts recommend total thyroidectomy for all patients with *RET* oncogene mutations, irrespective of calcitonin status. This is because of the high risk of development of medullary carcinoma of the thyroid over the patient's life span, the proven efficacy of prophylactic thyroidectomy, the relative ease of managing athyrotic patients, and the fact that medullary carcinoma of the thyroid in situ has been found among some patients with *RET* mutations who have normal results of calcitonin stimulation tests. Thyroidectomy can be performed safely by an experienced pediatric surgeon on patients 2 to 4 years of age. This therapy prevents almost all medullary carcinoma of the thyroid among patients with MEN 2A and familial medullary carcinoma of the thyroid. Patients with MEN 2B generally do not need genetic screening because they are recognized by their phenotypic features. Earlier thyroidectomy may be indicated for MEN 2B because of the allegedly more aggressive nature of medullary carcinoma of the thyroid among these patients.

The usefulness of genetic screening for MEN 1 is less clear than it is for MEN 2. Screening has not yet proved to alter the course of disease, and no specific intervention is considered solely on the basis of carrying a mutation for MEN 1. Furthermore, the wide variety of potential mutations make screening for MEN 1 more complex and expensive than screening for MEN 2. However, ascertainment of MEN 1 carrier status allows biochemical screening to be focused on patients at risk and allows family members with normal MEN 1 gene status to escape repetitive clinical testing. Once a patient is identified as at risk, regular biochemical screening is indicated. The optimal age at which to begin screening has yet to be established. Annual screening that incorporates the medical history and physical examination with measurements of ionized calcium, prolactin, and gastrin beginning at 5 to 10 years of age is reasonable.

References

Carlson KM, Dou S, Chi D, et al: Single missense mutation in the tyrosine kinase catalytic domain of the RET protooncogene is associated with multiple endocrine neoplasia type 2B. Proc Natl Acad Sci USA 91: 1579–1583, 1994

Evans DB, Fleming JB, Lee JE, Cote G, Gagel RF: The surgical treatment of medullary thyroid carcinoma. Semin Surg Oncol 16:50–63, 1999

Friedrich CA: Von Hippel-Lindau syndrome: a pleomorphic condition. Cancer 86:2478–2482, 1999

Iler MA, King DR, Ginn-Pease ME, O'Dorisio TM, Sotos JF: Multiple endocrine neoplasia type 2A: a 25-year review. J Pediatr Surg 34:92–96, 1999

Krausz Y, Rosler A, Guttmann H, Ish-Shalom S, Shibley N, Chisin R, Glaser B: Somatostatin receptor scintigraphy for early detection of regional and distant metastases of medullary carcinoma of the thyroid. Clin Nucl Med 24:256–260, 1999

Marx SJ, Agarwal SK, Kester MB, et al: Multiple endocrine neoplasia type 1: clinical and genetic features of the hereditary endocrine neoplasias. Recent Prog Horm Res 54:397–438, 1999

Ponder BA: The phenotypes associated with ret mutations in the multiple endocrine neoplasia type 2 syndrome. Cancer Res 59:1736s–1741s, 1999

Ponder BAJ: The gene causing multiple endocrine neoplasia type 2 (MEN2). Ann Med 26:199–203, 1994

van Heurn LW, Schaap C, Sie G, et al: Predictive DNA testing for multiple endocrine neoplasia 2: a therapeutic challenge of prophylactic thyroidectomy in very young children. J Pediatr Surg 34:568–571, 1999

24.6　THE THYROID

Delbert A. Fisher

24.6.1　Normal Thyroid Function

METABOLISM OF DIETARY IODINE

The thyroid gland concentrates iodide from the blood and returns it to peripheral tissues in a hormonally active form. The major substrates for thyroid hormone synthesis are iodide and tyrosine. Iodine is absorbed from the upper gastrointestinal tract into the blood, where it is distributed within the extrathyroidal iodide pool. This pool has the approximate dimensions of the extracellular space and is constantly cleared of iodide through renal excretion. The proportion of dietary iodide accumulated by the thyroid gland in organic form is directly related to the rate of iodide trapping and the rate of conversion of iodide into organic compounds. The rate of thyroid iodide trapping is inversely related to the rate of renal

iodide excretion. Iodide is excreted largely in urine through glomerular filtration; 1 to 2% may be excreted in sweat under basal conditions and as much as 10% with severe sweating. There is continuous secretion of iodide by the salivary and digestive glands, but this is reabsorbed; there is no substantial fecal excretion.

BIOSYNTHESIS OF THYROID HORMONES

The steps in synthesis and release of thyroid hormones are summarized in Figure 24-17. They are as follows:

1. Iodide trapping by the thyroid gland
2. Synthesis of tyrosine-containing thyroglobulin as iodine acceptor
3. Organification of trapped iodide as iodotyrosine
4. Coupling of the iodotyrosines monoiodotyrosine (MIT) and diiodotyrosine (DIT) to form the iodothyronines thyroxine (T_4) and triiodothyronine (T_3) and storage in follicular colloid
5. Endocytosis of colloid droplets and hydrolysis of colloid thyroglobulin to release MIT, DIT, T_4, and T_3
6. Deiodination of MIT and DIT with intrathyroidal recycling of the iodotyrosine iodine

IODIDE-CONCENTRATING MECHANISM Iodide is transported across the cell membrane into the thyroid follicular cell by a sodium-iodide symporter. This is the first and rate-limiting step in biosynthesis of thyroid hormone. The symporter normally gener-

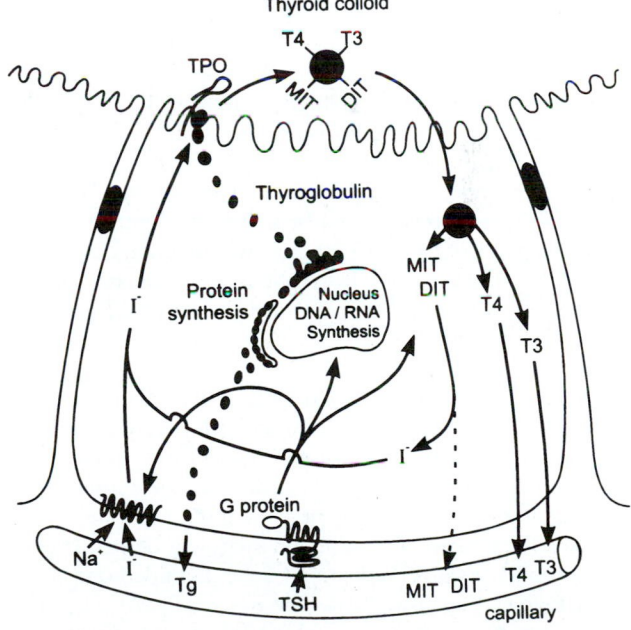

FIGURE 24-17　Steps in the biosynthesis, storage (as follicular colloid), and secretion of thyroid hormones. The synthesis, organification, and degradation of thyroglobulin, the iodothyronine prohormone, occur within the same thyroid follicular cell. Through the G-protein couple, the thyroid-stimulating hormone (TSH) receptor stimulates iodide trapping through the sodium-iodide symporter, thyroglobulin synthesis, and thyroglobulin endocytosis and degradation. Iodide, derived from iodotyrosine deiodinase–mediated deiodination of mono- and diiodotyrosine (MIT, DIT), is recycled within the gland. Secretion products include thyroxine (T_4), triiodothyronine (T_3), MIT, and DIT. Thyroglobulin also reaches the circulation, probably largely through the thyroid lymphatic vessels.

ates a thyroid to serum ratio concentration gradient of 30- to 40-fold. This gradient can reach several hundredfold when the thyroid gland is stimulated by a low-iodine diet, by thyroid-stimulating hormone (TSH), by thyroid-stimulating immunoglobulins in Graves disease, or by drugs that impair the efficiency of hormone synthesis. Other tissues, including the salivary glands, gastric mucosa, and placenta, are capable of transporting inorganic iodide. Certain anions are capable of competitively inhibiting iodide transport. Several of these, in order of increasing potency, include bromide (Br^-), nitrite (NO_2^-), thiocyanate (SCN^-), perchlorate (ClO_4^-), and technetium (TcO_4^-).

ORGANIFICATION OF TRAPPED IODIDE Biosynthesis of thyroid hormone begins with oxidation of iodide to an active intermediate followed by iodination of thyroglobulin-bound tyrosyl residues to form the iodotyrosines MIT and DIT. The half-time of incorporation of iodide into protein approximates 2 minutes. Both iodide oxidation and organification are catalyzed by thyroid peroxidase, a membrane-bound enzyme located at the cell colloid-lumen interface. Iodide reacts with the peroxidase, forming an oxidized iodine species that is incorporated into the tyrosyl residues of thyroglobulin. Thyroglobulin is an iodinated glycoprotein with a molecular weight approximating 660,000. It is composed of two subunits, each comprising two to four peptide chains. A normal thyroid gland contains 50 to 100 mg thyroglobulin for every 1 g of gland. Monoiodotyrosine, DIT, T_3, and T_4 are present within thyroglobulin as iodoaminoacyl residues that can be cleaved by proteolytic enzymes. The tyrosyl residues, the iodine acceptors of thyroglobulin, constitute about 3% of the weight of the protein.

In addition to catalyzing the formation of iodotyrosines, thyroid peroxidase catalyzes the coupling of iodotyrosines within the thyroglobulin molecule to form T_3 and T_4. Diiodotyrosine and MIT couple, with loss of an alanine side chain, to form T_3; DIT and DIT couple to form T_4. The relative proportions of T_3 and T_4 formed depend on the amount of available iodide and the extent of thyroglobulin iodination. With adequate iodine intake, 70% of the iodoprotein is iodotyrosine, the rest is iodothyronine with a T_4 to T_3 ratio ranging from 10:1 to 20:1. Low-iodine diets increase the MIT to DIT ratio, increase T_3 synthesis, and increase the thyroglobulin T_3 to T_4 ratio. High-iodine diets increase DIT production and favor T_4 synthesis.

SECRETION OF THYROID HORMONES Thyroglobulin is stored in colloid, and before thyroid hormones are released, the colloid must be ingested by the follicular cell. This process of endocytosis is under control of TSH. Ingested colloid droplets fuse with apically streaming proteolytic enzyme-containing lysosomes to form phagolysosomes, where thyroglobulin hydrolysis occurs. Digestion of thyroglobulin involves reduction of the disulfide bonds by glutathione followed by proteolysis. The free MIT, DIT, T_3, and T_4 within the phagolysosomes are released into the cytoplasm and diffuse into blood (see Fig. 24-17). An outer-ring iodothyronine deiodinase catalyzes monodeiodination of T_4 to T_3. The enzyme activity is stimulated by TSH with the result that the ratio of T_3 to T_4 secreted from the thyroid gland increases with increasing TSH stimulation. Thyroid-stimulating immunoglobulins in Graves disease probably produce a similar effect, accounting at least in part, for the increased T_3 to T_4 secretion ratio in Graves hyperthyroidism.

DEIODINATION OF IODOTYROSINES The MIT and DIT released during hydrolysis of thyroglobulin are largely deiodinated under the influence of an iodotyrosine deiodinase. The released iodide

enters the intracellular iodide pool and is reused for new hormone synthesis. Nonthyroidal tissues also are capable of deiodinating iodotyrosines and presumably contain a similar iodotyrosine deiodinating system. A defect in thyroidal or nonthyroidal iodotyrosine deiodinase causes release of iodotyrosines into the circulation and increased excretion in urine. The loss from the thyroid gland of this normally recycled iodine, amounting to 70% to 80% of the daily thyroidal iodine supply, can cause serious iodine deficiency and variable degrees of hypothyroidism.

REGULATION OF THYROID GROWTH AND FUNCTION

Thyroid follicular cell function is regulated by TSH, which stimulates most aspects of thyroid metabolism within minutes. Thyroid-stimulating hormone activates adenylate cyclase and stimulates production of intracellular cAMP, which mediates most of the effects of TSH on thyroid metabolism (iodide trapping, iodothyronine synthesis, thyroglobulin synthesis, glucose oxidation, pinocytosis, hormone release, and thyroid growth). Human chorionic gonadotropin (hCG) competes with TSH for receptors on thyroid follicular cells, as do TSH receptor-stimulating antibodies (TSA) in patients with choriocarcinoma and Graves disease, respectively. Thyroid-stimulating hormone increases mRNA levels for thyroid peroxidase and thyroglobulin in thyroid follicular cells. Thyroid cell DNA synthesis and growth are separately stimulated by TSH, TSA, IGF-1, and epidermal growth factor, and these stimuli may act synergistically to augment thyroid growth.

The average level of plasma iodide also influences thyroid follicular cell function. Variation in iodine intake in the physiological range modulates thyroid membrane iodide trapping. In pharmacologic doses, iodide blocks organification (Wolff-Chaikoff effect), thyroglobulin synthesis, hormone release, and thyroid growth. At least one important mechanism for these effects is the inhibitory action of iodide on the stimulation of cAMP by TSH.

The hypothalamus controls the secretion of TSH by the pituitary gland. Removal of the pituitary gland causes thyroid atrophy, but thyroid cell integrity and function are maintained at a basal level. Thus TSH functions as a tropic hormone. Secretion of TSH is modulated by thyrotropin-releasing hormone (TRH), a tripeptide synthesized in the hypothalamus and secreted into the pituitary portal vascular system for transport to the anterior pituitary thyrotrope cell. One important factor regulating TRH production is environmental temperature. Both peripheral thermal receptors and neuronal thermal receptors in the anterior hypothalamus monitor environmental and central temperature. These receptors modulate neuronal output to the hypothalamic centers that regulate TRH secretion. Decreasing environmental and body temperatures increase TRH release and increase the tonic level of TSH release. Somatostatin and dopamine can inhibit TSH release by actions at the pituitary level, and these inhibitory transmitters contribute to central nervous system modulation of TSH release. Norepinephrine and serotonin can inhibit TSH release, but the importance is not clear. Glucocorticoids inhibit TSH release at the pituitary level, but the mechanism is unknown. There is diurnal variation of TSH secretion with peak values at 2 a.m. to 4 a.m. and nadir levels at 4 p.m. to 6 p.m.

THYROID HORMONE METABOLISM

METABOLISM OF THYROGLOBULIN Some thyroglobulin escapes into the circulation from the endoplasmic reticulum in the process of synthesis and intracellular transport. Circulating thyroglobulin

TABLE 24-20

SERUM THYROGLOBULIN CONCENTRATIONS FOR HEALTHY PERSONS

	SERUM THYROGLOBULIN (ng/mL)
Cord blood (term)	15–101
Birth to 35 mo	11–92
3–11 yr	5.6–42
12–16 yr	2.3–40
Adults	3.5–56
Athyroid infants	<1.0

SOURCE: *Data from Quest Diagnostics, Nichols Institute Clinical Correlations Division. Values are 2SD range.*

concentration in healthy adults ranges from less than 1 to 30 ng/mL (1 to 30 μg/L). Thus thyroglobulin is a normal secretory product of the thyroid gland and is under TSH control. Values increase after administration of TSH and decrease during administration of thyroid hormone. Among persons who live in an area where goiter is endemic, there is a high correlation between serum TSH and serum thyroglobulin levels. There is evidence that thyroglobulin reaches the general circulation through thyroidal lymphatic vessels.

The average half-life of circulating thyroglobulin in humans varies from 13.8 hours to 4.3 days. The half-time of the low-molecular-weight species is only a few hours. Clearance presumably occurs by means of hepatic uptake. In rats asialothyroglobulin is cleared four times more rapidly than is the intact protein. Receptors for thyroglobulin have been found on splenic and thymic cells in rats and on peripheral and thyroidal lymphocytes in humans.

Changes in mean concentration of thyroglobulin in the serum that occur with age are summarized in Table 24-20. The progressive decrease with age presumably reflects a decrease in the rate of production of thyroid hormone (normalized for body or thyroid weight). As among adults, thyroid ablation among infants results in unmeasurable blood levels of thyroglobulin. The absence of measurable thyroglobulin in the serum of infants with congenital hypothyroidism supports a diagnosis of thyroid agenesis or defective thyroglobulin synthesis.

Circulating levels of thyroglobulin can be high among patients with a variety of thyroid disorders, reflecting thyroidal hyperactivity. These include endemic goiter, subacute thyroiditis, Graves disease, and toxic multinodular goiter. There is little information regarding the serum levels of thyroglobulin of patients with Hashimoto thyroiditis because the presence of serum antithyroglobulin antibody precludes reliable measurement of thyroglobulin by means of immunoassay. Serum concentration of thyroglobulin also increases, often markedly, among patients with thyroid adenoma and papillary-follicular carcinoma, although not among those with anaplastic or medullary carcinoma. Thus measurement of thyroglobulin is useful in differentiating medullary from papillary-follicular carcinoma. Measurement of thyroglobulin also is useful in the follow-up evaluation of patients who have been treated for papillary-follicular carcinoma.

DISTRIBUTION OF THYROID HORMONES Both T_3 and T_4 are present in blood in association with plasma proteins. The thyroid gland is the sole source of T_4, but most of the T_3 in blood is derived from nonglandular sources through monodeiodination of T_4 in peripheral tissues. The concentration of T_4 in human blood is 50 to 100 times greater than that of T_3. The concentrations of both are relatively constant in the steady state. Average values for children relative to age are shown in Table 24-21.

The circulating thyroid hormone-binding proteins include thyroxine-binding interalphaglobulin (TBG), thyroxine-binding prealbumin (transthryretin), and albumin. The binding reactions are such that the euthyroid steady-state concentrations of free T_4 and free T_3 approximate 0.03% and 0.30%, respectively, of the total hormone concentrations. Absolute mean free T_4 and T_3 concentrations approximate 2.0 and 0.40 ng/dL, respectively (25.7 and 5.2 pmol/L). Thyroxine-binding interalphaglobulin, which has the lowest plasma concentration of the several binding proteins (10 to 40 mg/L), binds about half of the total T_3 and 70% of T_4. Transthyretin, with a plasma concentration of 100 to 200 mg/L, binds only about 1% of T_3 and 20% of T_4. Albumin, with a concentration several thousandfold greater (20 to 50 g/L), binds about half of T_3 and only about 10% of T_4.

METABOLISM OF THYROID HORMONES Deiodination is the main pathway of thyroid hormone metabolism mediated by iodothyronine monodeiodinase enzymes. The first step in T_4 metabolism is deiodination either to T_3 or to reverse T_3 (rT_3). Monodeiodination of the β or outer ring (relative to the alanine side chain) produces T_3, which has three to four times the metabolic potency of T_4. Monodeiodination of the α or inner ring produces rT_3, which is largely inactive metabolically. Under normal circumstances T_3 and rT_3 are produced at approximately similar rates (Fig. 24-18).

TABLE 24-21

NORMAL VALUES FOR SERUM THYROID HORMONE CONCENTRATION

AGE	T_4 (μg/dL)	FT_4 (ng/dL)	T_3 (ng/dL)	TSH (mU/L)	TBG (mg/dL)
1–4 d	11–21.5	2.2–5.3	97–740	1.0–39	2.2–4.2
1–4 wk	8.2–17.2	0.9–2.3	104–344	1.7–9.1	—
1–12 mo	5.9–16.3	0.8–1.8	104–247	0.8–8.2	1.6–3.6
1–5 yr	7.3–15.0	0.8–2.1	104–266	0.7–5.7	1.2–2.8
6–10 yr	6.4–13.3	1.0–2.1	91–240	0.7–5.7	1.2–2.8
11–15 yr	5.5–11.7	0.8–2.0	84–214	0.7–5.7	1.4–3.0
16–20 yr	4.2–11.8	0.8–2.0	78–208	0.7–5.7	1.4–3.0
21–50 yr	4.3–12.5	0.9–2.5	71–201	0.4–4.2	1.7–3.6

Values are 2SD range.
T_4 = thyroxine; FT_4 = free T_4; T_3 = triiodothyronine; TSH = thyroid-stimulating hormone; TBG = thyroxine-binding globulin.
SOURCE: *Data from Quest Diagnostics Nichols Institute Clinical Correlations Division.*

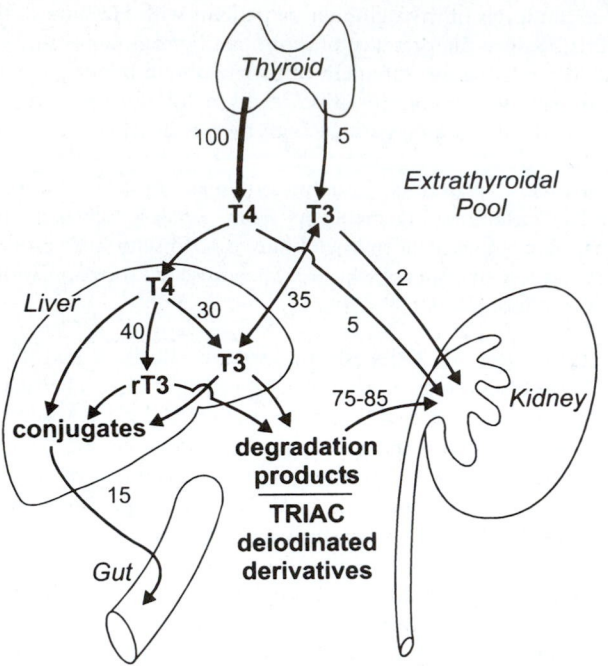

FIGURE 24-18   Routes of metabolism, clearance, and excretion of thyroid hormones. The numbers show approximate pathway flows. One hundred micrograms of thyroxine (T_4) secretion daily would be metabolized in peripheral tissues, largely liver, to triiodothyronine (T_3, 30%) or reverse T_3 (rT_3, 40%), which diffuse into extracellular fluid. For every 100 μg of T_4, approximately 5 μg of T_3 is secreted. Although small amounts of T_4 and T_3 are excreted intact in urine, most of both iodothyronines are metabolized through deiodination, side-chain alteration (to analogs including tetraiodothyroacetic and triiodothyroacetic acid, _TRIAC_), and glucuronide or sulfate conjugation (largely in liver for excretion in bile). The products are excreted through the intestine (15%) or kidney 75 to 85%.

In most tissues, particularly liver, and excluding brain and brown adipose tissue, T_3 and rT_3 generated through T_4 monodeiodination diffuse rapidly from tissue to interstitial fluid to plasma. Large amounts of T_3 and small amounts of rT_3 are synthesized and released by the thyroid gland. Thus circulating levels of T_3 and rT_3 reflect both secretion and peripheral production. From 70% to 90% of circulating T_3 is derived from peripheral conversion and 10 to 25% from the thyroid gland; respective values for rT_3 are 96 to 98% and 2 to 4%. Progressive tissue monodeiodination reactions degrade T_3 and rT_3 to diiodo, monoiodo, and noniodinated thyronine.

The alanine side chain of the inner ring of the iodothyronines is subject to degradative reactions, including transamination, deamination, and decarboxylation. Pyruvic acid analogs and small amounts of lactic acid analogs have been observed in urine and bile. These have minimal biological activity. The acetic acid analogs in tissue, bile, and urine have some activity.

Thyroid hormones are excreted in urine and stool in both free and conjugated forms. The conjugation reactions involve both glucuronide conjugation and sulfoconjugation. Glucuronide conjugation occurs mainly in liver through microsomal glycuronyl transferase. Sulfoconjugation also is prominent in the liver and may be an obligatory step for hepatic monodeiodination reactions. Iodothyronine sulfation markedly augments outer-ring deiodination in the liver. In the fetus, where outer-ring deiodinase activity is de-

velopmentally low, the major thyroid hormone metabolites are sulfate conjugates, which are biologically inactive.

ACTIONS OF THYROID HORMONES

Thyroid hormones influence growth and development, oxygen consumption and heat production, nerve function, and metabolism of lipids, carbohydrates, proteins, nucleic acids, vitamins, and inorganic ions. They also have important effects on other hormone actions. The free hormones penetrate the cell membranes and bind to specific nuclear receptors. Triiodothyronine is the active hormone and binds to the nuclear receptors with approximately 10 times the affinity of T_4. Triiodothyronine also binds to plasma membrane and mitochondrial inner-membrane receptors. The major effects of thyroid hormones are probably mediated by the nuclear T_3 receptors; T_3 receptor binding stimulates gene transcription and modulates synthesis of mRNA and proteins that mediate thyroid hormone effects in various tissues. The importance of the plasma membrane and mitochondrial receptors is not clear.

The thyroid hormone nuclear receptors are members of the steroid hormone–retinoic acid receptor superfamily and function as DNA transcription factors. In humans two genes code for thyroid hormone nuclear receptors: one on chromosome 3, designated β, and one on chromosome 17, designated α. Each gene is translated to several mRNA species, the importance of which is not yet clear. The effects of thyroid hormones as related to known thyroid actions at the molecular level are summarized in Table 24-22.

FETAL AND NEWBORN THYROID FUNCTION

FETAL THYROID FUNCTION The fetal thyroid and pituitary glands are well formed by 10 to 12 weeks of gestation. The thyroid gland can accumulate iodide and synthesize hormone, and the pituitary gland contains TSH by this time. Fetal serum TSH, T_4, and T_3 concentrations are either undetectable or very low before midgestation. The placenta is relatively impermeable to thyroid hormones. Most of the thyroid hormone that crosses the placenta is deiodinated, but there is limited transfer of T_4 from mother to fetus, and there are low levels of T_4 in the cord blood of an athyroid fetus (ranging from 30 to 70 nmol/L; 2.3 to 5.4 μg/dL). The placenta contains an active inner-ring iodothyronine deiodinase that converts T_4 to rT_3 and T_3 to T_2 (also an inactive metabolite). The high levels of rT_3 in amniotic fluid and, in part, those in fetal blood are probably the result of placental monodeiodination activity.

The placenta is impermeable to TSH. Between 18 and 24 weeks of gestation there is a progressive increase in pituitary TSH content and concentration and a progressive increase in fetal serum concentration of TSH. By 24 weeks fetal serum levels of TSH exceed paired maternal values. There is a parallel increase in fetal thyroid uptake of radioiodine. This abrupt stimulation of TSH synthesis and secretion at midgestation correlates with maturation of the hypothalamic-pituitary portal blood vascular system and an increase in hypothalamic production of TRH (Fig. 24-19).

Between midgestation and term, fetal serum TSH concentrations remain relatively high and stimulate a progressive increase in fetal serum T_4 concentration. There also is a progressive increase in serum TBG concentration between midgestation and 30 to 35 weeks of gestation, but the progressive increase in free T_4 indicates a progressive saturation of protein binding sites. Taken together,

TABLE 24-22
EFFECTS OF THYROID HORMONES

Central nervous system development
General
  Stimulation of cell migration and neuronal cell maturation
  Stimulation of dendritic arborization and synaptic density
  Increases myelinogenesis
Specific gene regulated by triiodothyronine
  Major myelin proteins
  Nerve growth factor and its receptors
  Neurotropin 3
  Mitochondrial genes
  Neural cell adhesion molecules
  Cerebellar Purkinje cell protein 2
  Prostaglandin D_2 synthase
Effects on growth and development
Stimulation of pituitary growth hormone (GH) synthesis and
  secretion
Potentiation of GH stimulation of insulin-like growth factor (IGF) syn-
  thesis and action
Stimulation of growth factor production
  Epidermal growth factor
  Nerve growth factor
  Erythropoietin
Stimulation of bone metabolism and growth
  Cartilage response to IGF-I
  Osteoblastic and osteoclastic bone remodeling
Thermogenic effects
Stimulation of mitochondrial enzyme synthesis
Stimulation of thermogenin
Stimulation of membrane Na/K ATPase synthesis
Metabolic effects
Hepatic protein
  Induction of hepatic lipogenic enzymes
  Stimulation of hepatic glutamine synthetase and α-amino-
    levulinic acid synthetase
  Potentiation of prolactin stimulation of lactalbumin synthesis
  Potentiation of GH stimulation of B_2 englobulin synthesis
Plasma membrane effects
  Stimulation of glucose transport
  Stimulation of adrenergic receptor binding

these data suggest a progressive increase in fetal T_4 secretion during the last trimester of pregnancy. The fetal thyroid gland can concentrate iodide during the second trimester, but the iodide transport mechanism is immature and is not suppressed by exposure to high plasma iodide levels. Thus the fetus is susceptible to iodide-induced hypothyroidism (Wolff-Chaikoff effect).

FETAL TRIIODOTHYRONINE DEFICIENCY Thyroxine in the fetus is metabolized largely to inactive iodothyronines. The iodothyronine deiodinase, type III, in fetal liver and skin and in placenta degrades T_4 to rT_3 and T_3 to T_2. The low fetal T_3 production rate results from low levels of hepatic outer-ring iodothyronine deiodinase activity in fetal liver. Fetal blood rT_3 and rT_3S levels are high by 20 to 24 weeks of gestation because of increased rT_3 production. Fetal pituitary, brain, and brown adipose tissues contain an active outer-ring iodothyronine deiodinase isoenzyme (type II), capable of local T_3 production from T_4. This type II iodothyronine deiodinase in brain and brown adipose tissue is inhibited by thyroid hormone, and activity increases in the hypothyroxinemic fetus. The liver enzyme is stimulated by thyroid hormone, and activity is re-

duced in the T_4-deficient fetus. Both effects tend to augment availability of T_3 to brain tissue in the event of fetal T_4 deficiency.

NEWBORN THYROID FUNCTION With parturition, a newborn infant is transformed from a state of chemical T_3 deficiency to chemical T_3 thyrotoxicosis (see Fig. 24-19). The increase in serum T_3 level at term occurs in two phases. During the first phase, beginning at about 30 weeks of gestation, there is a progressive decrease in fetal type III iodothyronine monodeiodinase activity and increasing type I activity, the latter caused at least in part by increased fetal cortisol production. During the second phase, at parturition, placental T_3 monodeiodination ceases. With extrauterine exposure, serum concentration of TSH increases rapidly to a mean peak level of 80 to 90 μU/mL (80 to 90 U/L) by 30 minutes, probably stimulated by cooling of the neonate in the extrauterine environment. In response, serum T_3, T_4, free T_4, and free T_3 levels increase briskly. Serum concentration of TBG, in contrast, remains un-

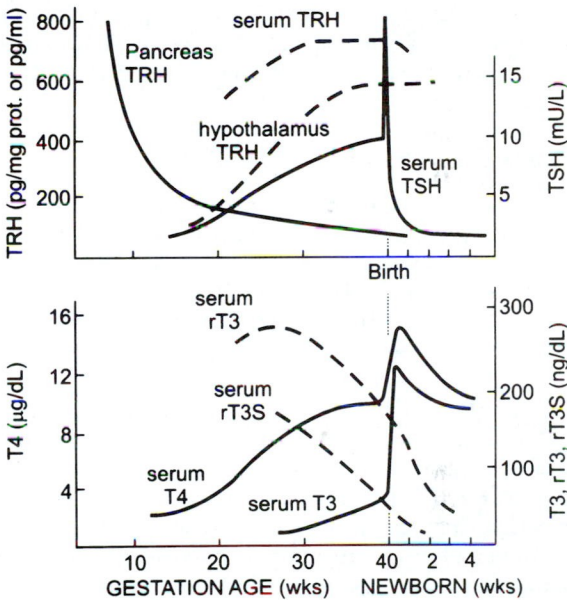

FIGURE 24-19 Maturation of thyroid function in the fetal and neonatal periods. Thyrotropin-releasing hormone (*TRH*) is produced in the fetal and neonatal periods. It is produced in the fetal environment from placenta and fetal gastrointestinal tissues, largely pancreas. Serum levels are relatively high because of this extrahypothalamic production and lack of degrading enzymes in fetal plasma. There is a progressive increase in fetal hypothalamic TRH concentration beginning at midgestation associated with a progressive increase in fetal serum thyroid-stimulating hormone (*TSH*). Fetal serum thyroxine (*T_4*) levels increase progressively during the latter half of gestation largely because of increased fetal hepatic production of thyroid hormone-binding globulin (*TBG*). Fetal serum T_4 concentration also increases progressively in response to increasing TSH secretion and progressive maturation of fetal thyroid TSH responsiveness. Most fetal T_4 is converted in peripheral tissues to inactive reverse triiodothyronine (*rT_3*) and inactive sulfated iodothyronines (represented by rT_3 sulfate, rT_3S). At 28–32 weeks of gestation decreasing production of rT_3 and sulfated analogs and increased production or decreased degradation of T_3 cause decreases in serum rT_3 and rT_3S levels and increases in T_3 concentration. At parturition, a cold-stimulated TSH surge peaks at 30 minutes followed by increased T_4 and T_3 secretion and serum concentration of T_4 and T_3. Serum T_3 levels after birth remain elevated because of increased T_4 to T_3 conversion and decreased placental deiodination.

changed, and the high levels of serum T_3 decrease only gradually to adult values during the first 2 to 3 weeks after birth. The levels of iodothyronine sulfate conjugates decrease rapidly after birth because of the increased activity of the tissue outer-ring iodothyronine monodeiodinase. Local T_3 production from T_4 in brown adipose tissue augments production of thermogenin, the mitochondrial protein that uncouples oxidative phosphorylation and potentiates norepinephrine-stimulated brown fat thermogenesis. Brown fat and thyroxine are essential for thermogenesis and extrauterine survival.

24.6.2   Transient Thyroid Dysfunction in the Premature Infant

The complexity of ontogenesis of the thyroid system provides opportunities for a variety of potential defects or immaturities of thyroid function of the newborn. As a rule, defects in the early phases of ontogenesis cause permanent thyroid dysfunction. Transient disorders of thyroid function among premature infants are related to the late maturing events of thyroid ontogenesis. These disorders are summarized in Table 24-23.

TRANSIENT HYPOTHYROXINEMIA

Serum T_4 concentration increases progressively with gestational age. All premature infants have some degree of hypothyroxinemia. Ninety-seven to 98% of term infants have serum T_4 concentrations greater than 6.5 μg/dL (84 nmol/L). The prevalence of serum T_4 values less than 6.5 μg/dL approximates 50% among infants delivered before 30 weeks of gestation. The prevalence among all premature infants approximates 25%. Infants with hypothyroxinemia (T_4 less than 6.5 μg/dL, or 84 nmol/L) also have low levels of free T_4. The relatively low levels of free T_4 are associated with normal or even low basal serum TSH values and normal TSH and T_4 responses to TRH, which indicate responsive pituitary and thyroid glands. Such infants appear to have a state of hypothalamic, or tertiary, hypothyroidism or immaturity that represents a normal stage of development of the thyroid system. The hypothyroxinemia is transient, correcting spontaneously over 4 to 8 weeks with progressive maturation. Postnatal growth and development of such infants are normal. These infants do not need treatment, unless serum TSH concentration increases to more than 20 mU/L.

TRANSIENT PRIMARY HYPOTHYROIDISM

Transient primary hypothyroidism, which is characterized by low serum T_4 and high TSH concentrations, is more common in Europe than in North America. In Belgium, approximately 20% of premature infants have transient hypothyroidism, the incidence increasing with decreasing gestational age. In North America the incidence approximates 0.2% among low birth weight and 0.4% among very low birth weight premature infants. Such infants have hypothyroxinemia associated with the decrease in free T_4 levels to values observed among infants with congenital hypothyroidism. Serum concentration of TSH increases into the primary hypothyroid range (>40 mU/L). The cord blood T_4 and TSH levels of these infants usually are in the normal range for premature infants. The primary hypothyroid state develops during the first 1 to 2 weeks of extrauterine life and is superimposed on the usual state of transient hypothyroxinemia characteristic of prematurity. Urinary iodine excretion and thyroid iodine content are reduced among these infants, suggesting that the acquired primary hypothyroidism is the result of limited iodine substrate relative to the increased thyroid hormone needs of early infancy.

The hypothyroidism is transient but may persist for several weeks; thus treatment is recommended. In a series of such infants treated with T_3 (5 μg/kg/d in three divided doses), serum T_4 levels increased spontaneously during the period of T_3 treatment, indicating spontaneous recovery of thyroid functional capacity. The average time to recovery of function and discontinuation of treatment was 50 days. The prevalence of transient hypothyroidism among premature neonates depends on the extent of iodine deficiency in the environment. Term infants can have transient neonatal hypothyroidism in areas of low iodine intake (endemic goiter). Iodine supplementation of neonates in areas of iodine deficiency prevents transient hypothyroidism.

Premature infants are particularly susceptible to transient, *iodine-induced hypothyroidism*. Either in utero or in the postnatal period, administration of iodine-containing drugs to the mother or amniotic injection of radiographic contrast agents for amniofetography can induce hypothyroidism. The hypothyroidism, with or without goiter, is characterized by low serum total T_4 and free T_4 concentrations and high levels of TSH. These infants are treated at birth, and treatment should continue for 2 to 3 months or until the goiter disappears. Transient hypothyroidism also has occurred among term infants exposed to iodine in utero.

In iodine-sufficient areas, including North America and Japan, the mechanism of acquired neonatal hypothyroidism is likely to be iodine overload, exposure to antithyroid medications, or placental transfer from mother to fetus of TSH-receptor blocking antibodies, the latter producing a hypothyroid state that lasts until maternal immunoglobulin is degraded. The prevalence of maternal TSH receptor antibody–induced transient hypothyroidism among neonates is low, approximately 1 in 40,000 to 80,000 newborns. The neonatal hypothyroid state induced by TSH receptor antibody can be severe, and the maternal blocking antibody can be detected for many months in newborn serum. Such infants must be treated.

TABLE 24-23

TRANSIENT THYROID DYSFUNCTION AMONG PREMATURE INFANTS

TRANSIENT DISORDER	T_4	FT_4	T_3	TSH	TSH RESPONSE TO TRH
Hypothyroxinemia	↓	↓	↓	N	N
Primary hypothyroidism	↓	↓	↓	↑	↑
Hypothalamic-pituitary hypothyroidism	↓	↓	↓	N	N or prolonged
Low T_3 syndrome (nonthyroidal illness)	N or ↓	N or ↑	↓ ↓	N	N or ↓

TRH = thyrotropin-releasing hormone. See Table 24-21 for key to other abbreviations. ↓ = decrease; ↑ = increase; ↓ ↓ = large decrease; N = normal.

TRANSIENT HYPOTHALAMIC-PITUITARY HYPOTHYROIDISM

In very low birth weight premature infants, T_4 and free T_4 concentrations decrease to nadir values at 1 to 2 weeks of postnatal age, usually without an increase in serum TSH concentration. In perhaps 10% of very low birth weight infants, serum free T_4 levels decrease to less than 0.5 ng/dL (7 pmol/L). The mechanism appears to be thyroid glandular immaturity and relative iodine deficiency, but hypothalamic-pituitary immaturity also is postulated because serum TSH values remain low. Thyroxine therapy prevents transient hypothyroxinemia. Preliminary data suggest that such therapy improves intelligence later. However, further controlled studies are necessary to better define the need and indications for treatment of such infants.

LOW T_3 SYNDROME (NONTHYROIDAL ILLNESS)

Premature infants have an increased susceptibility to neonatal morbidity of several varieties. Infants born at less than 34 weeks of gestation have a high incidence of respiratory distress, and premature infants in general have great increased risk of birth trauma, vascular accidents, hypoxia, hypoglycemia, hypocalcemia, infection, and relative malnutrition. All of these factors tend to inhibit further conversion of T_4 to T_3 in the neonatal period and to aggravate the extent of the low T_3 state. Serum T_3 values may remain low in these infants (below 80 ng/dL, or 1.23 nmol/L) for 1 to 2 months; T_4 given to such infants increases concentrations of rT_3 but not of T_3.

Features of low T_3 syndrome among premature infants are similar to those among older children or adults. These include low serum T_3 concentration caused by low rate of conversion of T_4 to T_3 in nonthyroidal tissue, variable serum rT_3 levels with values equal to or lower than concentrations among otherwise healthy premature infants, and normal or low total serum T_4 concentrations with free T_4 levels usually in the range of values for healthy premature infants of matched gestational age and weight. Some of these infants have low serum levels of TBG; others have an inhibitor of T_4 binding to TBG as described for adults with low T_3 syndrome. Serum TSH concentrations are normal. The mechanism(s) for these changes is unclear, but cytokines, including tumor necrosis factor, have been implicated.

24.6.3   Thyroid Hormone Carrier Protein Abnormalities

THYROID-BINDING GLOBULIN DEFICIENCY   Deficiency of TBG is transmitted as an X-linked trait and the prevalence approximates 1 in 5000. Serum TBG levels measured by means of either immunoassay or T_4-binding capacity are low among affected men and boys and approximately half-normal among female carriers. In about one-half of affected families, TBG level at radioimmunoassay is low. In the other half, the defect is partial. Serum T_4 levels vary similarly, but affected persons are euthyroid with normal serum free T_4 concentrations and normal serum TSH responses to exogenous TRH. A variety of structural defects in the TBG molecule account for the variably decreased T_4 binding. In some patients, non-T_4-binding (denatured) TBG can be detected with a radioimmunoassay, and a defective TBG molecule with reduced stability and decreased binding capacity can be characterized.

HIGH TBG LEVEL   Persons with increased levels of TBG have increased total serum T_4 concentrations with normal free T_4 and TSH levels; thus they are euthyroid. The prevalence varies from 1 in 40,000 persons in North America to 1 in 6000 in England. Studies similar to those among persons with low TBG concentrations have shown a correlation between TBG production rates and serum levels, suggesting that the mechanism for high TBG concentration is increased production, presumably by the liver. Levels of TBG increase as much as 4.5 times normal among affected boys and men, and females carriers have serum concentrations intermediate between normal value and the high levels among affected men and boys. Early reports suggested a dominant mode of inheritance, but results of subsequent studies are more compatible with an X-linked mode of inheritance.

HIGH (TBPA) TRANSTHYRETIN   In 1982 Moses et al. reported the case of a 53-year-old euthyroid man with an elevated serum level of T_4 not corrected by use of a free T_4 index but with normal free T_4, total serum T_3, and TSH concentrations and normal TSH and T_3 responses to TRH. Serum TBG and albumin levels were normal, but the serum TBPA concentration measured by means of radioimmunoelectrophoresis was 2.5 to 3.0 times above the level in a normal human serum pool. Moreover, 70% of serum T_4 was selectively removed by an anti-TBPA immunoglobulin affinity column. One of the man's three children had a similar abnormality, but the mode of inheritance was not clearly defined. Since this report, variant forms of TBPA associated with familial amyloidotic polyneuropathy and rare families with TBPA of high affinity or with increased TBPA concentrations have been reported.

FAMILIAL DYSALBUMINEMIC HYPERTHYROXINEMIA   Several groups of investigators have described euthyroid patients with increased serum T_4 concentrations not corrected by use of the free T_4 index correction and with normal free T_4, total serum T_3, and TSH levels. There is increased binding of T_4 to albumin, and the albumin in these patients has an affinity for T_4 binding intermediate between TBG and TBPA. Triiodothyronine is less avidly bound, accounting for the preferential increase in serum concentration of T_4. Patients with the disorder are euthyroid with normal thyroid hormone production rates. The abnormal albumin seems to be transmitted as an autosomal dominant trait. There is male to male transmission, and an affected-to-unaffected ratio of one or greater among first-degree relatives. The diagnosis of abnormalities of thyroid hormone binding can be confirmed with combined protein electrophoresis and radioimmunoassay of T_4 and of the binding protein species. These methods are available in reference laboratories.

24.6.4   Congenital Hypothyroidism

Cretinism is an ancient term that has long been used in Europe to describe a form of imbecility and dwarfism common in areas of endemic goiter. The implications of this term are vague. The term is still applied to characterize endemic congenital goiter, but the term *congenital hypothyroidism* is now preferable in nonendemic areas. Nonendemic congenital hypothyroidism can be caused by defective thyroid embryogenesis, hypothalamic-pituitary defects, inborn defects in thyroid hormone synthesis or action, or intrauterine exposure to goitrogenic agents. These abnormalities are summarized in Table 24-24.

TABLE 24-24
THYROID DISORDERS OF CHILDREN

Fetal thyroid dysfunction	**Iodine deficiency syndromes**
Goiter	Goiter
Hypothyroidism	Mental impairment
Maternal TSH receptor-blocking antibody	Cretinism
Goitrogenic drugs	**Thyroid hormone resistance syndromes**
Dyshormonogenesis	Thyroid hormone β receptor (TRβ) mutations
Hyperthyroidism	Peripheral tissue resistance syndrome
Maternal TSH receptor-stimulating antibody	Pituitary resistance syndrome
Thyroid dysfunction among premature infants	**TSH receptor mutations**
Transient hypothyroxinemia	Loss of function, hypothyroidism
Transient primary hypothyroidism	Gain of function, hyperthyroidism
Transient hypothalamic-pituitary hypothyroidism	**Autoimmune thyroid disease**
Nonthyroidal illness	Hashimoto thyroiditis
Sporadic congenital hypothyroidism	TSH receptor autoantibody disease
Thyroid dysgenesis	Stimulating antibody, Graves disease
Idiopathic (95%)	Blocking antibody, hypothyroidism
Athyrosis	**Infectious thyroiditis**
Hypoplasia	Suppurative thyroiditis
Ectopia	Subacute thyroiditis
Genetic (5%)	**Adolescent goiter**
Athyrosis	Nonthyroidal illness (low T$_3$ syndrome)
TTF-1 mutations	**Thyroid neoplasia**
TTF-2 mutations	Adenoma
Hypoplasia	Nonfunctional
PAX-8 mutations	Functional
TSH receptor mutations	Cystic
Thyroid dyshormonogenesis	Papillary-follicular carcinoma
Sodium-iodide symporter defect	Medullary carcinoma
Organification defects	MEN 2A, 2B, *RET* mutations
Abnormal thyroglobulin	Sporadic
Pendrin defect (Pendred syndrome)	Undifferentiated
Iodotyrosine deiodinase defect	Metastatic
Hypothalamic-pituitary hypothyroidism	**Miscellaneous**
Anencephaly	G protein mutations (nonautoimmune hyperthyroidism)
Holoprosencephaly	Cystinosis
Septooptic dysplasia	Chromosomal disorders
Median facial syndromes	
TSHβ mutations	
Pit-1 mutations	
PROP-1 mutations	
Idiopathic	
Transient hypothyroidism	
Maternal TSH receptor-blocking antibody	
Goitrogenic drugs	
Iodine excess or deficiency	

TSH = thyroid-stimulating hormone; T$_3$ = triiodothyronine; MEN = multiple endocrine neoplasia.

DEFECTIVE THYROID EMBRYOGENESIS (THYROID DYSGENESIS)

Thyroid dysgenesis causes decreased thyroid function among most infants with permanent congenital hypothyroidism detected in screening programs. The prevalence approximates 1 in 4000 newborns. The term *thyroid dysgenesis* describes ectopia or hypoplasia of the thyroid glands (or both) or total thyroid agenesis among infants. Some thyroid tissue is probably present among 40 to 60%

of these infants and represents a spectrum of severity of thyroid deficiency. Thyroid isotope scanning, ultrasonography, and uptake tests may not be sensitive enough to detect small amounts of residual functioning thyroid tissue. In such infants, normal or near-normal circulating levels of T$_3$ in the face of a low T$_4$ value suggest residual thyroid tissue, as do measurable levels of serum thyroglobulin.

The pathogenesis in most patients is unclear. Thyroid dysgenesis is more prevalent among girls than among boys; the girl to boy ratio approximates 2:1. Although the disorder usually is sporadic, familial examples have been described. These presumably are caused by mutations of the homeobox genes, *TTF-1*, *TTF-2*, and *PAX-8*, which are involved in thyroid gland embryogenesis (see Table 24-24). The disorder is less prevalent among black infants (1 in 11,000 births), and more prevalent among Hispanics relative to white infants. The prevalence also is high among infants with Down syndrome. A seasonal incidence, peaking during summer, has been reported in Japan and Australia. In rare instances, thyroid dysgenesis occurs in association with maternal autoimmune thyroiditis. In those instances the disorder is attributed to transplacentally acquired antithyroid factors. However, there usually is no correlation between thyroid dysgenesis and the presence of maternal autoimmune thyroiditis or circulating thyroid autoantibodies.

Most infants with thyroid dysgenesis have no symptoms, and few have signs of hypothyroidism during the early weeks of life. Consequently, fewer than 5% of cases of hypothyroidism among infants are detected according to clinical criteria before the chemical screening diagnosis. Most affected infants have low serum T$_4$ and high TSH concentrations in cord blood or in filter paper blood spots collected at 1 to 5 days of age. An additional group of infants has T$_4$ levels in the low-normal or normal range and increased TSH values. These infants usually have ectopic thyroid tissue on scans and may constitute 10 to 15% of infants with congenital thyroid dysgenesis. One percent to 5% of infants with congenital hypothyroidism have a low serum TSH level at birth and an increase to primary hypothyroid levels during the first 2 to 3 months of life. These infants may be missed with newborn screening.

TRANSIENT CONGENITAL HYPOTHYROIDISM

Ingestion of goitrogenic substances by a mother can cause fetal goiter and neonatal hypothyroidism. The most frequently ingested drug is iodide, usually prescribed in expectorants or as therapy for maternal thyrotoxicosis. Common goitrogenic agents are listed in Table 24-25. The mothers of these children often have taken iodide for many years without having large goiters and have been euthyroid during pregnancy. The fetus is unusually sensitive to iodide-induced hypothyroidism, probably because the mechanisms for decreasing thyroid iodide uptake to compensate for high plasma iodide levels are immature. Other goitrogens that have caused neonatal goiter include the thioureas, sulfonamides, and hematinic preparations containing cobalt. Neonatal goiters caused by propylthiouracil are uncommon unless large doses (more than 150 mg/d near term) of propylthiouracil or other drugs are given to the mother. Transient hypothyroidism also is caused by transplacentally acquired maternal TSA. These can be measured as TSH binding inhibiting immunoglobulin (TBII) or as cAMP (TSH) blocking antibodies (TBA). These mothers usually have atrophic thyroiditis. The antibody half-life in the neonate approximates 2 weeks, and hypothyroidism can persist for 2 to 4 months.

TABLE 24-25
GOITROGENIC AGENTS

Anions
Iodine (in large amounts)
Perchlorate
Thiocyanate
Cations
Cobalt (in certain hematinic preparations)
Arsenic salts
Lithium salts
Drugs
Propylthiouracil
Methimazole
Aminosalicyclic acid
Aminoglutethimide
Phenylbutazone
Amiodarone
Naturally occurring substances
Goitrin (1,5-vinyl-2-thiooxazolidone) (present in cabbage and other members of the genus *Brassica*)
Soybeans (not soybean milk as currently prepared)
Linamarin (a glycoside in cassava)

HYPOTHALAMIC PITUITARY DEFECTS

Permanent congenital hypothyroidism caused by a decrease in effective TSH stimulation of thyroid hormone secretion can be caused by various abnormalities in TSH synthesis and metabolism (see Table 24-24). Affected infants can have anomalous hypothalamic or pituitary development or a sporadic or familial deficiency in TRH or TSH secretion, either alone or in association with other pituitary hormone deficiencies. Syndromes that have been described and reviewed include hypothalamic hypothyroidism with TRH deficiency or resistance, or both, isolated TSH deficiency, familial panhypopituitarism, congenital absence of the pituitary gland, and panhypopituitarism with absence of the sella turcica. Hypopituitarism can be associated with major and minor midline defects, including holoprosencephaly, cleft lip and palate, and septooptic dysplasia, or genetic defects, including *Pit-1, PROP-1,* and other autosomal-recessive gene defects. The combined prevalence of these abnormalities associated with congenital hypothyroidism probably approximates 1 in 60,000 to 100,000 births. Hypothalamic (tertiary) hypothyroidism caused by TRH deficiency is suspected because of the presence of persistently low serum T_4, T_3, and free T_4 values with low or normal-range serum concentrations of TSH.

INBORN DEFECTS OF THYROID HORMONE SYNTHESIS OR EFFECT

Patients with inborn defects in thyroid metabolism represent the second most common cause of congenital nonendemic hypothyroidism. These defects often are called *goitrous hypothyroidism* or *familial goiter.*

CONGENITAL ISOLATED TSH DEFICIENCY Thyroid-stimulating hormone is one of several closely related pituitary glycoprotein hormones composed of a common α and specific β subunits. Several cases of congenital hypothyroidism have been reported with low T_4 and T_3 levels and unmeasurable TSH in the presence of normal levels of the other pituitary hormones LH and FSH. Several mutations of the TSHβ subunit gene have been described in these patients. Most are single base substitutions in the CAGYC region

of the β-subunit gene associated with a conformational change that prevented α and β subunit binding.

DECREASED TSH RESPONSIVENESS Resistance to TSH is caused by mutations of the TSH receptor gene. The TSH receptor belongs to the superfamily of seven transmembrane domain receptors coupled to the G-protein cellular signaling system. Reported mutations have involved the extracellular, transmembrane, and intracellular domains of the protein with graded effects on receptor function. The clinical phenotype ranges from mild TSH receptor resistance with euthyroid hyperthyrotropinemia to rare congenital hypothyroidism. The disorder usually is transmitted as a recessive trait, most resistant patients being compound heterozygotes. Non–TSH receptor, non-TSHβ, and non-G-protein-mediated TSH resistance has been reported in three families with dominant rather than recessive inheritance.

THYROID IODIDE TRANSPORT DEFECTS Several patients have been described who had hyperplastic thyroid glands but only minimal uptake of radioactive iodide 24 hours after administration of the iodide. The thyroid glands of these patients are enlarged two to four times, and the patients have been hypothyroid. Other iodine-concentrating tissues (salivary glands, gastric mucosa) also did not concentrate iodide from the circulation. The thyroid follicular cell membrane iodide transport protein has been cloned and characterized as a sodium-iodide symporter, a member of a family of sodium-dependent cotransporters. The sodium-iodide symporter is predicted to have 12 transmembrane domains and sequence homology with the sodium-glucose cotransporter. The gene is expressed in thyroid follicular cells, salivary glands, mammary glands, and gastric mucosa. The rare patients with sodium-iodide symporter mutations reported to date have had homozygosity for a defect from consanguineous parents or compound heterozygosity from a nonconsanguineous union.

IODIDE ORGANIFICATION DEFECTS Absence or deficiency of the peroxidase enzymes necessary to oxidize thyroidal iodide to reactive iodine has been described in more than 200 patients. Patients with the defect usually have goitrous cretinism. Giving thiocyanate or perchlorate to such patients 2 hours after a test dose of radioiodine causes a precipitous decrease in thyroid radioactivity. This perchlorate (or thiocyanate) discharge indicates an organification defect, assuming the patient has no other reason for defective iodination (eg, antithyroid drugs, high iodine intake, or Hashimoto thyroiditis). Diagnosis of the specific defect is confirmed by means of measuring low or absent levels of thyroid peroxidase activity in thyroid tissue obtained by means of biopsy. More than 90% of the patients described have had deficient thyroid peroxidase activity. The thyroid peroxidase gene has been cloned and resides on chromosome 2. The gene mutations in affected patients have produced variable functional impairment of enzyme activity, usually because of homozygosity of a single mutation or compound heterozygosity.

In 1896, Pendred described two deaf sisters with goiter who lived in a nonendemic goiter area. Many such patients have been described since and are referred to as having *Pendred syndrome.* The prevalence is estimated to be 1.5 to 3 per 100,000 schoolchildren. The syndrome includes high-tone or complete congenital neural deafness, goiter of variable degree appearing in middle or late childhood, and euthyroidism or mild hypothyroidism. Approximately one-third of patients have the complete syndrome; others have no hearing loss or only mild goiter. The Pendred gene (*pendrin*) has been cloned and found to encode a chloride-iodide cotransport protein. The gene was mapped to chromosome 7 whether *pendrin* functions as a chloride or an iodide transporter is unclear, as is its role in the deafness associated with the syndrome.

IODOTYROSINE DEIODINASE DEFECT Deficiency of the iodotyrosine dehalogenase enzyme can produce a hereditary defect that causes either congenital hypothyroidism or a less severe form of familial goiter. Failure to deiodinate thyroid MIT and DIT as they are released from thyroglobulin leads to severe iodine wastage, because these nondeiodinated iodotyrosines diffuse out of the thyroid and are excreted in urine. The iodine is thus lost rather than being recycled within the thyroid gland. Iodotyrosine deiodinases are present in thyroid cells and in peripheral tissues, and abnormalities involving both deiodinase systems have been described. Several patients have been reported with euthyroid goiter and partial defects in deiodination of iodotyrosine in both thyroid and peripheral tissues, in peripheral tissues only, or in thyroid tissue only. Such patients may remain compensated without or with a small goiter if they are in areas of high iodine intake.

DEFECTS IN THYROGLOBULIN SYNTHESIS OR TRANSPORT Abnormalities of thyroglobulin structure can produce a variety of functional abnormalities including decreased iodination, reduced MIT and DIT coupling efficiency, and increased iodination of alternative substrates (iodoalbumin). The large thyroglobulin gene has been cloned and contains a large number of exons and the large introns that predispose this gene to mutation-induced transcriptional errors. Both quantitative and qualitative defects have been described in animals and in humans. Patients with quantitative defects have low levels of thyroglobulin in blood and thyroid tissue. Patients with a qualitative defect produce an abnormal form of thyroglobulin. The result is defective iodothyronine synthesis or defective transport of the molecule to the follicular lumen. Thyroglobulin defects occur with an incidence of 1:80,000 to 100,000 newborns.

DECREASED PERIPHERAL RESPONSIVENESS TO THYROID HORMONES: THYROID HORMONE RESISTANCE Refetoff and associates in 1967 first described a familial syndrome among three deaf-mute siblings with stippled epiphyses, retarded skeletal age, goiter, greatly elevated levels of serum free T_4 and free T_3, and normal plasma TSH concentrations. Growth rate, metabolic rate, and intelligence were normal. Kinetic studies indicated that the thyroid glands were secreting about five times the normal amount of T_4 daily. Administration of 1000 μg/d of T_4 or 375 μg/d of T_3 produced little or no metabolic effects. As the patients matured, plasma level of T_4 tended to return to normal, the epiphyses closed, and the goiters disappeared. Recent studies of the youngest affected sibling showed a normal TSH response to TRH despite threefold elevated serum free T_4 and free T_3 levels. Administration of T_3 produced a suppression of the TSH and prolactin responses to TRH. These results indicate that the pituitary gland shares TSH resistance.

The syndromes of thyroid resistance are characterized by increased levels of total and free T_4 and T_3, normal TSH values, and reduced clinical and biochemical manifestations of thyroid hormone actions relative to the increased hormone levels. There are two varieties, *generalized tissue resistance* and *pituitary resistance*. The prevalence of each remains unclear. More than 400 cases have been reported. Two genes code for the nuclear T_3 receptor proteins—an α receptor gene on chromosome 17 and a β receptor

gene on chromosome 3. Together these genes program production of two major thyroid (T_3) receptors, β_1 and α_1, distributed among the body tissues in varying proportions relative to age. A third receptor, β_2, is present in pituitary tissue. To date, the defects characterized in more than 50 families have involved the β-receptor gene. Most defects have involved minor alterations at the DNA level or single nucleotide substitutions that alter single amino acids in the hormone-binding domain of the receptor.

Clinical features of generalized tissue resistance often are subtle. The disorder is not detected with newborn screening because T_4 levels are high and TSH level is normal or slightly elevated. Some tissues are more involved than others, probably reflecting the individual molecular defect and the distribution of the α receptors. Short stature, failure to thrive, or delayed mental development can occur but are uncommon. Goiter, hyperactivity, restlessness, nervousness, and tachycardia are common features among children, and a hyperactivity syndrome or hyperthyroidism may be the suspect diagnosis. The presumed cause is a variable tissue responsiveness to thyroid hormone related to the functional status of the α and β receptor interaction. Treatment is difficult and must be individualized.

Isolated pituitary resistance results in peripheral tissue hyperthyroidism. This disorder can be misdiagnosed as Graves disease if the level of TSH in the serum is not measured. Recent data suggest that selective pituitary resistance and generalized resistance to thyroid hormone are not qualitatively different syndromes in that a β-receptor defect similar to others reported in children with generalized resistance has been described in a patient with apparent pituitary resistance.

MATERNAL INGESTION OF GOITROGENIC DRUGS Ingestion of goitrogenic substances by a pregnant woman can cause fetal goiter and neonatal hypothyroidism. These disorders are discussed earlier in the section on transient congenital hypothyroidism.

CLINICAL AND LABORATORY FEATURES OF CONGENITAL HYPOTHYROIDISM

Infants with congenital hypothyroidism are born with little or no clinical evidence of thyroid hormone deficiency. Detection on the basis of signs and symptoms usually is delayed 6 to 12 weeks or longer. Table 24-26 shows the frequencies of some of the common symptoms and signs of hypothyroidism at certain ages. The classic signs, including the characteristic facies, enlarged protruding tongue, and growth and developmental retardation, evolve progressively during the first few months of life. Early clinical diagnosis therefore must be based on a high index of suspicion regarding nonspecific symptoms and signs. Although many of the signs of hypothyroidism are absent or subtle among newborns, the diagnosis should be considered when any infant has prolonged jaundice, transient hypothermia, an enlarged (greater than 1 cm) posterior fontanelle, failure to nurse properly, or respiratory distress with feeding.

The classic facies among older infants represent myxedema of the subcutaneous tissues and in the tongue. The thickened tongue becomes protuberant, and the infant has increasing difficulty nursing and handling salivary secretions. The cry is hoarse because of myxedema of the vocal cords. Prolonged hypothyroidism causes marked muscular hypotonia and mental torpor, hypothermia, umbilical hernia, potbelly, constipation, bradycardia, and diminished pulse pressure. The cardiac silhouette can be enlarged. An electro-

TABLE 24-26

SIGNS AND SYMPTOMS AMONG 182 INFANTS WITH CONGENITAL HYPOTHYROIDISM BEFORE TREATMENT

SIGN OR SYMPTOM	AGE 5 WK (N = 163)	AGE 10 WK (N = 19)
Prolonged jaundice (>7 d)	31	20
Umbilical hernia	23	27
Constipation	21	27
Macroglossia	21	7
Feeding problems	19	13
Distended abdomen	16	23
Hypotonia	16	13
Hoarse cry	16	7
Large posterior fontanelle (>1 cm)	13	7
Dry skin	10	13
Hypothermia	5	7
Goiter (palpable)	2	7
Retarded bone age	40	5

Two groups of infants with congenital hypothyroidism detected by means of screening at birth and again at 4–6 weeks of age. Average age at diagnosis for the two groups was 36 and 69 days. Values are percentage of infants.

SOURCE: *Data collated from LaFranchi SH, Hanna CE, Krainz PL, et al: Screening for congenital hypothyroidism with specimen collection at two time periods: results of the northwest regional screening. Pediatrics 76:734, 1985*

cardiogram shows low voltage and a prolonged conduction time. The extremities are cool and can have extreme pallor and circulatory mottling.

Thyroid hormone deficiency present from birth leads to marked delay in central nervous system development. Growth and arborization of nerve cells are delayed, axodendritic interaction and connectivity are reduced, vascularization and myelination proceed at subnormal rates, and irreversible mental retardation occurs if treatment is delayed. The period of central nervous system thyroid hormone dependency extends to 2 to 3 years of age among human infants. The onset of hypothyroidism after this time does not produce mental deficiency. Replacement therapy with thyroid hormone minimizes mental retardation among infants with cretinism when begun in the early neonatal period.

NEWBORN SCREENING FOR CONGENITAL HYPOTHYROIDISM

Newborn screening is routine in most industrialized areas of the world. Filter paper blood spots are used in conjunction with phenylketonuria and other newborn genetic screening tests. Screening for congenital hypothyroidism is conducted either with combined T_4 and TSH testing or with TSH testing alone. Approximately 1 in 4000 newborns has congenital hypothyroidism. Screening and follow-up evaluation are accomplished within 2 to 3 weeks, at which time hypothyroidism is suspected clinically in fewer than 5% of cases. Screening data confirm that serum T_4 value is low and TSH concentration high among newborns with primary hypothyroidism. Most screening programs report only infants with elevated filter-paper blood-spot TSH concentrations. Because 10 to 15% of infants with congenital hypothyroidism have T_4 values in the normal range (7 to 10 μg/dL, or 90 to 127 nmol/L), it is desirable, in programs in which T_4 is followed by TSH screening, to maintain the T_4 cutoff (for TSH testing) at the 10 percentile level (or at 10 to 11 μg/dL, or 127 to 140 nmol/L if an absolute cutoff is used).

In both T_4-TSH and TSH screening programs, 8 to 10% of infants with congenital hypothyroidism have a screening TSH value less than 50 μU/ml (50 mU/L). One in 20 to 30 infants with hypothyroidism (about 1 in 100,000 to 1 in 150,000 newborns) has a screening TSH level less than 20 μU/ml (20 mU/L), and the abnormality may not be detected. Infants with TSH deficiency probably will be missed in any screening program. Clinicians need to remember that 5 to 7% of infants with congenital hypothyroidism escape detection in newborn screening programs and that the diagnosis must be made on clinical grounds.

The diagnosis of congenital hypothyroidism must be confirmed with measurement of serum T_4 and TSH concentrations for any infant with suspicious screening results. Usually the T_4 level is less than 6 μg/dL and the TSH level is greater than 50 μU/mL (77 nmol/L and 50 mU/L). However, a serum level of T_4 less than 10 μg/dL with a TSH level greater than 20 μU/mL (130 nmol/L and 20 mU/L) suggests the presence of the disorder. Repetition of the test is desirable for infants with T_4 values between 6 and 10 μg/dL (77 and 130 nmol/L) and TSH levels of 20 to 40 μU/ml (20 to 40 mU/L).

Secondary hypothyroidism is more difficult to diagnose. A low serum T_4 and a low T_3 resin uptake (with a low corrected T_4 result) or a low free T_4 concentration indicates hypothyroidism rather than low TBG concentration. A normal or low serum level of TSH in these circumstances suggests secondary or tertiary hypothyroidism rather than primary hypothyroidism. If there is a subnormal TSH response to TRH, a diagnosis of pituitary hypothyroidism is in order. If the peak level of TSH after administration of TRH is normal (not increased), *hypothalamic TRH deficiency* can be inferred. The TSH deficiency can be isolated or associated with other pituitary hormone deficiencies. Thus tests of GH and ACTH secretory capacity are in order.

MANAGEMENT OF CONGENITAL HYPOTHYROIDISM

Therapy for hypothyroidism requires exogenous thyroid hormone (Table 24-27). Sodium-L-thyroxine is the drug of choice because of its uniform potency and reliable absorption. Moreover, synthetic T_4 produces normal serum levels of both T_4 and T_3, the latter because of peripheral conversion. The best guide to adequacy of therapy is periodic measurement of circulating levels of T_4 and TSH. During the initial stages of treatment, T_3 determination also may be of value. The history and physical examination are important in follow-up evaluation, but mild hypothyroidism or hyperthyroidism cannot always be excluded on clinical grounds. Using Na-L-thyroxine for treatment, the physician adjusts serum T_4 to the upper normal range (10 to 14 μg/dL, or 130 to 180 nmol/L), at which

TABLE 24-27

REPLACEMENT DOSE OF SODIUM-L-THYROXINE IN INFANCY AND CHILDHOOD

AGE	RANGE OF DOSE	
	(μg/kg/d)	(μg)
1–12 mo	15–7	25–50
1–5 yr	7–5	50–100
5–10 yr	5–3	100–150
10–20 yr	4–2	100–200

time serum T_3 levels should be normal (70 to 220 ng/dL, or 1.07 to 3.38 nmol/L). Serum TSH levels can be normal or modestly elevated if the patient is adequately treated during the first year of life. The thyroid hormone feedback set point seems to be altered among many infants with congenital hypothyroidism. Serum concentration of TSH thus remains mildly elevated in the face of adequate T_4 replacement with normal or even elevated serum T_4 levels. Inappropriately elevated levels of TSH after 1 year are uncommon. The usual starting dose of Na-L-thyroxine for hypothyroid infants is 10 to 15 μg/kg/d. For infants with more severe hypothyroidism at birth (low T_4 and retarded bone age), this dose results in a 5 to 10 point increase in intelligence relative to infants treated with lesser T_4 dosages.

Infants with presumably transient hypothyroidism caused by maternal use of goitrogenic drugs need not be treated unless the low serum T_4 and elevated TSH levels persist for longer than 2 weeks. Therapy usually can be discontinued after 8 to 12 weeks. Mothers with hyperthyroidism who are taking propylthiouracil can breast-feed their infants, because the concentration of drug in breast milk is low. Infants with hypothyroidism born of a mother with autoimmune thyroiditis need measurement of TSH receptor blocking autoantibodies (TBII or TBA) in maternal, cord, or newborn blood. These infants are treated, but therapy can be discontinued if the autoantibody titer has dissipated by 3 to 4 months of age.

Adequate dosage of Na-L-thyroxine in the first year ordinarily ranges between 25 to 50 μg daily. The growth rate should accelerate after therapy is initiated, and any growth deficit usually is restored within a few months. Bone age is a sensitive index of thyroid deficiency; delayed bone maturation suggests inadequate dosage when other signs of hypothyroidism have been obliterated.

24.6.5   Acquired Juvenile Hypothyroidism

Hypothyroidism can develop at any age among previously healthy children; it is more common among girls. The onset usually is insidious. A high proportion of patients have circulating antithyroid antibodies. Among these children, the hypothyroidism probably is the result of an autoimmune process (Hashimoto thyroiditis). Among others, acquired juvenile hypothyroidism can be caused by exposure to goitrogenic agents, thyroid dysgenesis, late onset of hypothyroidism caused by an inborn error of thyroidal biosynthesis, acquired hypothalamic or pituitary hypothyroidism, or endemic factors (see Table 24-24).

EXPOSURE TO GOITROGENIC AGENTS

Any food or drug that interferes with synthesis of thyroid hormone is a potential cause of goiter and hypothyroidism. A partial list of such agents is given in Table 24-25. Dietary goitrogens can be difficult to identify, because they can reach the person through devious routes. The prevalence of goiter among schoolchildren in selected areas of the Appalachian Mountains approached 30%, particularly in Kentucky and northern Virginia, in the 1980s. There is no iodine deficiency in these areas, but bacterial contamination of groundwater has been repeatedly demonstrated, and the presence of unidentified goitrogens in groundwater has been postulated. Reevaluation has shown a high prevalence of antithyroid antibodies in the general population. It seems likely that both environmental (region-specific) and immunologic (genetic) factors have a role.

COMPENSATED OR PARTIALLY COMPENSATED THYROID DYSGENESIS

Ectopic thyroid glands in children first come to attention during childhood because of the presence of an enlarging mass at the base of the tongue or along the course of the thyroglossal duct. Usually only one sibling is affected, but rare familial instances have been reported. The enlargement can occur at any age; it usually accelerates a short time before adolescence. Degrees of hypothyroidism range from barely detectable to severe. The term *cryptothyroidism*, by analogy with *cryptorchidism*, has been applied to such ectopically located thyroid tissue. Children with unilateral thyroid aplasia have a functional *hemithyroid gland*. Such patients usually do not have hypothyroidism. They may be given the mistaken diagnosis of functioning thyroid nodule. Most instances of thyroid dysgenesis and ectopic thyroid gland are detected in newborn screening programs, but an occasional patient with a normal T_4 level or minimal TSH elevation at birth can be missed in the screening program. Complete substitution treatment usually reduces the thyroid tissue enlargement, so surgery can be avoided. Full substitution must be continued for life. Severe hypothyroidism occasionally follows surgical removal of what has been presumed to be a *thyroglossal duct cyst*. As with lingual thyroid, masses high in the neck may prove to be the only functional thyroid tissue present. In some patients, enlargement of the mass is correlated with failing thyroid function before surgery.

AUTOIMMUNE THYROIDITIS

Hashimoto thyroiditis (chronic thyroiditis, lymphadenoid goiter, autoimmune thyroiditis) was defined in 1912 when Hashimoto reported on four patients with goiter characterized by diffuse infiltration of plasma cells and lymphocytes, fibrosis, parenchymal atrophy, and eosinophilic degeneration in some of the acini. The disease occurs in a genetically predisposed population. Thirty percent to 40% of patients have a family history of thyroid disease. The disease also has a marked predilection for girls and women. Chronic thyroiditis is the most common cause of goiter and hypothyroidism among children older than 6 years in North America.

The onset of the disorder usually is insidious. Approximately 5% to 10% of patients, particularly adolescents, have tachycardia, nervousness, and other signs of thyrotoxicosis, but most have a euthyroid goiter or a goiter with mild hypothyroidism. The thyroid gland usually is irregularly enlarged and firm with accentuation of the normal lobular architecture (bosselated). The goiter occasionally gives rise to the sensation of local pressure and difficulty in swallowing.

If the patient is not treated, the course of Hashimoto thyroiditis is variable. The gland usually undergoes progressive atrophy, and the patient has acquired hypothyroidism without a recognized period of compensatory hypertrophy. The yearly incidence of hypothyroidism among adult patients with Hashimoto thyroiditis is 5 to 7%. Spontaneous remission can occur among 30% of adolescent patients.

The spectrum of autoimmune thyroid disease in children includes euthyroid goiter, hypothyroid goiter, Graves disease, hashitoxicosis, nodular goiter, thyroid antigen-antibody nephritis, and multiple endocrine deficiency disease. The last includes diabetes mellitus, adrenal insufficiency, hypoparathyroidism, moniliasis, and, less commonly, pernicious anemia and thrombocytopenia. The most common clinical association is Hashimoto thyroiditis and diabetes mellitus with or without adrenal cortical insufficiency

(Schmidt syndrome). Studies have shown that 30% of children with diabetes mellitus have thyroid autoantibodies and approximately 10% have elevated serum TSH levels. All children with diabetes mellitus need screening for autoimmune thyroid disease. Autoimmune thyroid disease among pregnant women can be associated with transient neonatal hypothyroidism caused by transplacental passage of TSH receptor-blocking antibodies (Fig. 24-20).

Most patients have detectable levels of circulating antithyroid antibodies. Types of antibodies described include antibodies against thyroglobulin, against a colloid component other than thyroglobulin, against the peroxidase enzyme, against the sodium-iodide symporter protein, against thyroid nuclei, and against thyroid TSH receptors. Antithyroglobulin and antimicrosomal antibodies are most prevalent, and these are the antibodies that have been most useful in diagnosis. The peroxidase enzyme is a microsomal enzyme, and there is a high correlation between antimicrosomal and antiperoxidase antibody levels among affected patients. These antithyroid antibodies are not pathognomonic of Hashimoto thyroiditis. Among 15 to 20% of adults without thyroiditis, significant antibody titers occur, but at least some of these persons are genetically predisposed and have not yet developed thyroiditis. Antithyroid antibodies also are present in patients with untreated Graves

disease. The familial prevalence of antithyroid antibody helps identify the familial predisposition to autoimmune thyroid disease.

Blood from almost all patients with Hashimoto thyroiditis and Graves disease can be shown to contain a population of thymus-dependent (T) lymphocytes sensitized against the particulate portion of thyroid cells (microsomes and cell membranes). A genetically determined defect in the immune surveillance system has been postulated. Both T lymphocytes sensitized against thyroidal components and humoral antibodies directed at various thyroidal components produce the thyroid abnormality. The latter antibodies are produced by B rather than T lymphocytes. It is known that the interaction of T and B lymphocytes plays a crucial role in the elaboration of immunoglobulins by B lymphocytes.

COMPENSATED OR PARTIALLY COMPENSATED DEFECT IN THYROID HORMONE BIOSYNTHESIS

Most patients with hypothyroidism caused by defective hormone synthesis have congenital hypothyroidism. Infants with a compensated defect and normal T_4 values can escape detection, however, in a neonatal T_4 screening program even though serum concentration of TSH is elevated. Moreover, the appearance of goiter among these patients can be delayed, as can detection. Thus some patients have a goiter and compensated hypothyroidism and have apparent acquired hypothyroidism after infancy. The goiter in these patients, including those with peripheral resistance to T_3, is diffuse, soft, and variable in size. The Hashimoto glands, however, tend to be firm and bosselated and only moderately enlarged.

ACQUIRED HYPOTHALAMIC-PITUITARY HYPOTHYROIDISM

Hypothalamic or pituitary disorders can be acquired after head trauma, tumors such as craniopharyngioma, granulomatous disease, meningitis, head irradiation, or rare vascular accidents including Sheehan syndrome (postpartum hemorrhage). Growth failure caused by GH or TSH deficiency usually is the earliest manifestation of pituitary hypofunction, but other features related to the primary disease, neurologic disorder, or hypothalamic dysfunction can be prominent.

ENDEMIC GOITER AND HYPOTHYROIDISM

Endemic goiter is the most common thyroid disease worldwide—300 million persons are affected. Iodine deficiency is the most important etiologic factor, but other environmental agents and genetic factors have a role. Endemic goiter occurs in regions with no iodine deficiency, such as Tasmania, Italy, Finland, Japan, Sri Lanka, China, and some areas of the United States. Both dietary goitrogens, the most important of which is thiocyanate derived from cassava, and goitrogenic factors in groundwater (bacterial contamination, disulfides of aliphatic hydrocarbons from sedimentary rocks) have been implicated in endemic goiter. In many areas of the world, vegetables of the Brassicae family, particularly cassava, have been shown to potentiate the effects of iodine deficiency. The goitrogenic action of cassava is caused by release of cyanide from linamarin, a glycoside present in large amounts in cassava, and conversion of cyanide to thiocyanate by a human after ingestion.

Iodide deficiency, with or without the additive effect of a goitrogen, causes production of deficient thyroid hormone, increased

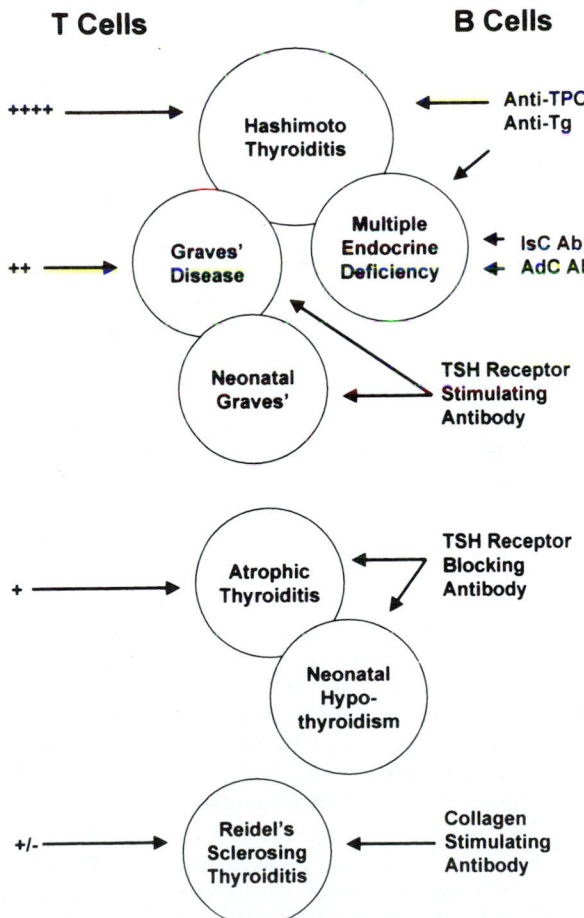

FIGURE 24-20 Relation of T-cell infiltrate of thyroid tissue and B-cell antibody production to clinical autoimmune thyroid disease phenotypes. Extent of lymphoid infiltration shown as ++++ to ±. Anti-TPO = antiperoxidase antibody; Anti-Tg = antithyroglobulin antibody; IsCA and AdCA are islet cell and adrenal antibodies. The correlations are only approximate.

TSH secretion, increased iodide trapping, goiter, and an increased T_3 to T_4 ratio of secreted thyroid hormone. These adaptive responses compensate to a variable extent for the deficient iodine substrate or impaired hormone biosynthesis. Thus clinical manifestations range from euthyroidism with variable goiter to goitrous hypothyroidism among adults and cretinism among children. The prevalence of endemic cretinism may be as high as 5 to 8% because of combined maternal and fetal hypothyroidism in areas of severe iodine deficiency. Two extreme types of neurologic and myxedematous cretinism have been described. *Neurologic cretinism* includes mental retardation and various neurologic defects, such as deafness and aphonia, pyramidal tract syndrome of the lower limbs, and extrapyramidal signs such as ataxia and strabismus. Thyroid function is characteristic of compensated hypothyroidism, but the patients usually are clinically euthyroid. *Myxedematous cretinism* includes the signs and symptoms of longstanding hypothyroidism, such as dwarfism, myxedema, and mental retardation. The goiters usually are small.

MISCELLANEOUS CAUSES OF ACQUIRED HYPOTHYROIDISM

Hypothyroidism appears to occur with increased frequency in association with several *chromosomal disorders,* including Turner syndrome, Down syndrome, and Klinefelter syndrome. Autoimmune thyroiditis is more prevalent with all of these disorders. With Down syndrome there is also an increased prevalence of thyroid dysgenesis. Compensated hypothyroidism occurs frequently and early among children with nephropathic *cystinosis.* Some children with the disorder have overt hypothyroidism. The thyroid gland has extensive destruction and infiltration of the epithelium with cystine crystals.

DIAGNOSIS OF ACQUIRED HYPOTHYROIDISM

The most useful aid in recognizing acquired hypothyroidism among children is a serial record of growth. Considerable time usually elapses between the onset of hypothyroidism and the emergence of classic signs of myxedema. If growth records are available, however, the onset of hypothyroidism can be readily documented with a progressive downward deviation from previously normal growth. Weight tends to increase. For most patients, weight for age is proportionately greater than height for age (Fig. 24-21).

The possibility of thyroid deficiency is considered when any child is not growing normally. Retardation of bone age in hypothyroidism almost always equals or exceeds the retardation in linear growth, but delayed bone age also is present in other forms of dwarfism and is not pathognomonic of hypothyroidism. A patient with thyroid deficiency usually has slowing of the deep tendon reflexes with a delayed relaxation phase. Varying clinical manifestations of myxedema related to organ hypofunction (eg, cardiac intestinal, skin, renal) occur with prolonged or severe hypothyroidism.

Sexual development of most children with hypothyroidism is delayed in approximate proportion to the retardation of skeletal maturation. However, some children with severe hypothyroidism are sexually precocious. Girls have precocious menstruation, breast development, and galactorrhea. Among boys this syndrome is associated with excessive enlargement of the penis and testes. Most of these patients lack sexual hair, and bone age is retarded in keeping with the duration of the hypothyroid state. Many have an en-

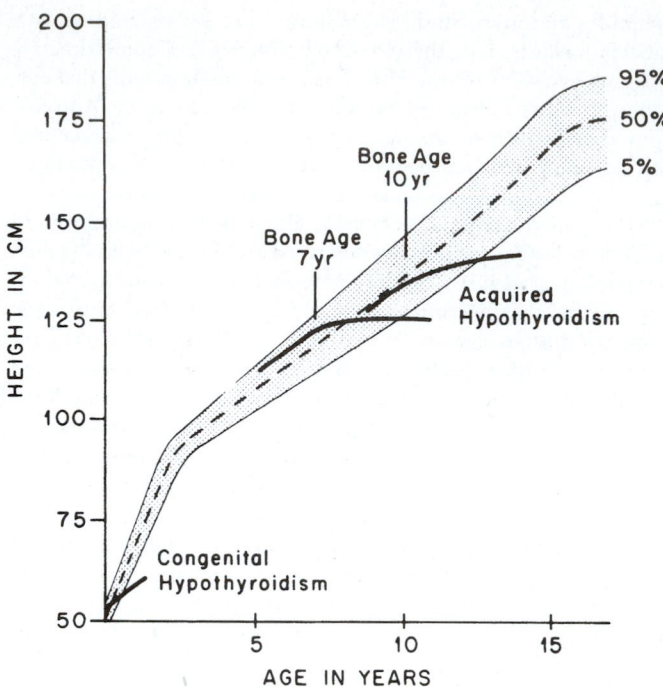

FIGURE 24-21   **The evolution of clinical hypothyroidism in childhood and adolescence usually is slow, and the early manifestations are subtle. The earliest sign is a slowing of linear growth as indicated for two children with thyroid failure at 7 and 10 years, respectively. The rate of bone age maturation also slows markedly. Bone age can be used to estimate the time of onset of thyroid failure. Growth failure also is an early manifestation of congenital hypothyroidism.**

larged sella turcica. Serum levels of prolactin and FSH are elevated among some children, but the mechanism is not clear. The increase in serum prolactin level can be explained by the fact that TRH stimulates both TSH and prolactin release from the pituitary gland. A paracrine action on gonadotropes may explain the increased gonadotropin secretion. When the hypothyroid state is alleviated, the manifestations of sexual precocity regress, and normal puberty occurs when the general level of maturity has progressed appropriately (see Sec. 24.8).

The diagnosis of *Hashimoto thyroiditis* is based on a series of characteristic findings. The thyroid gland is moderately enlarged, firm, and bosselated in 80 to 90% of patients. Increased titers of antithyroglobulin, antimicrosomal, or antiperoxidase antibody occur in 90 to 95% of patients. Serum concentration of TSH is elevated in 30 to 40% of patients, who may have an associated low serum T_4 concentration, a normal or near-normal serum T_3 concentration, and an elevated T_3 to T_4 concentration ratio.

Hypothyroidism usually is a lifelong disease. The diagnosis always must be supported with tests of thyroid function before treatment is instituted. Minimal documentation includes plasma levels of T_4 and TSH. If a goiter exists, antithyroid antibodies are measured. If not, a thyroid scan is useful to exclude thyroid dysgenesis. An elevated TSH level establishes that the disease originates in the thyroid rather than the pituitary gland. A low T_4 (and free T_4) level with a low serum TSH level indicates hypothalamic or pituitary hypothyroidism. Whenever the latter is suspected, it is mandatory that other pituitary deficiencies be sought with a complete set of pituitary function studies, including provocative tests of ACTH and growth hormone secretion, and the response of TSH to administration of TRH. Computed tomography or MR imaging of the brain and visual field examination are performed to exclude a pituitary or hypothalamic tumor.

THERAPY FOR ACQUIRED HYPOTHYROIDISM

Substitution treatment of older children with hypothyroidism follows the guidelines for the management of congenital hypothyroidism (see earlier). Most children respond well to an initial dose of L-thyroxine equivalent to about 100 $\mu g/m^2$ of body surface. After treatment begins, a child with hypothyroidism resumes growth at a rate greater than normal, the period of so-called catch-up growth. Accurate serial height measurements provide assurance that the dosage provided is adequate. Excessive dosage is marked by disproportionate advancement in skeletal age. This must be avoided because it hastens closure of epiphyses and can shorten adult stature. Among patients with pituitary TSH deficiency or deficiency of other anterior pituitary hormones, treatment with adrenal glucocorticoids or GH is provided as necessary.

24.6.6   Nonthyroidal Illness (Low T₃ Syndrome)

A selective deficiency of tissue and serum T_3 has been described among patients dying of severe prolonged illness, termed "euthyroid sick" or *low T_3 syndrome* or *nonthyroidal illness*. This syndrome of low total and free serum T_3, normal or low total serum T_4, normal or high free T_4, and normal serum TSH concentrations has now been reported among fetuses, patients with protein-calorie malnutrition or anorexia nervosa, fasting patients, postoperative patients, and patients with various severe acute and chronic illnesses. The last include patients with diabetic ketoacidosis, severe trauma, burns, febrile states, hepatic cirrhosis, renal failure, and toxemia of pregnancy. The following drugs have been found to produce a similar syndrome of selective T_3 deficiency: dexamethasone, selected radiocontrast agents, propylthiouracil, propranolol, and amiodarone.

The low serum T_3 levels in this syndrome occur as a result of inhibition of iodothyronine β or outer-ring monodeiodinase activity and a decreased rate of T_3 production from T_4 in body tissues. Alpha or inner-ring monodeiodination is not impaired; thus, rT_3 production is not reduced. Moreover, rT_3 degradation is decreased because the conversion of rT_3 to DIT is mediated by the same deiodinase that mediates T_4 to T_3 conversion. Thus serum T_3 levels decrease while rT_3 levels remain normal or increase. The three patterns of change in serum T_4 levels are low, normal, and elevated T_4. Among patients with low T_4 concentrations, TBG levels can be reduced; an inhibitor of T_4 binding to TBG has been described. Serum free T_4 levels, however, usually are normal or even increased, and serum TSH levels are normal. Patients with high T_4 concentrations appear to have an abnormality in T_4 disposal or clearance, usually induced by a drug such as amiodarone.

The importance of the T_3 deficiency in this syndrome is unclear. Treatment is directed at the primary systemic illness. There is no convincing evidence that treatment with thyroid hormone, either T_4 or T_3, is indicated. The T_3 deficiency has been interpreted as a compensatory mechanism to reduce metabolic rate and tissue catabolism among sick patients with reduced substrate intake. Treatment increases tissue metabolism.

24.6.7   Diffuse Nontoxic Goiter (Simple Colloid Goiter, Adolescent Goiter)

The term *adolescent goiter* is useless for diagnostic purposes, because the incidence of most types of goiter increases in the years before the onset of puberty, particularly among girls. Simple, or idiopathic, goiter is a common disorder in Europe and Scandinavia, where the prevalence is approximately 2% among school children and the female to male ratio is 7:1 to 8:1. The prevalence in North America appears to be lower. A common finding in the disorder is a family history of goiter. Among many children with a strong family history of thyroid disease, detailed tests of thyroid function do not reveal identifiable defects. The genetic pattern in such families suggests an autosomal dominant mode of transmission, with greater expression among female family members. Results of thyroid function tests are normal. Thyroid biopsy reveals only colloid goiter. Simple enlargement of the thyroid usually regresses spontaneously. Many patients with nodular goiters in the third, fourth, and fifth decades of life have a history of a mild diffuse thyroid enlargement during childhood or adolescence. Nodular goiters in such patients may have developed from recurring episodes of hyperplasia and involution. Whether subtle genetic defects in thyroid hormone biosynthesis exist among such patients is not known.

24.6.8   Infectious Thyroiditis

SUBACUTE THYROIDITIS This is self-limited inflammation of the thyroid that usually follows or is associated with an upper respiratory illness. A few patients have had evidence of associated mumps virus infection and others have had cat-scratch fever. Several viral agents may be responsible. Unlike that of other thyroid disease, the incidence of subacute thyroiditis is the same for the two sexes. Onset is accompanied by fever and pain that may occur locally or may be referred to the angles of the jaw. The thyroid gland can be exquisitely sensitive to palpation or only mildly tender.

During the acute phase, a characteristic increase in serum T_4 and T_3 levels presumably is caused by release of stored hormone by the damaged thyroid follicular cells; signs and symptoms of hyperthyroidism may develop. Thyroidal radioiodine uptake at this time is low or absent, also indicating thyroid cell damage. Signs and symptoms of hyperthyroidism, including tachycardia, are present and persist for 1 to 4 weeks. After this time there is a period of transient hypothyroidism as the thyroid gland recovers. The total course runs 2 to 9 months, depending on severity, but essentially all patients recover spontaneously.

Symptoms usually can be controlled with large doses of acetylsalicylic acid or, in severe disease, glucocorticoids. Antithyroid antibodies usually do not develop, and most patients recover with no residual defect in thyroid function. Subacute thyroiditis can be difficult to differentiate from acute purulent thyroiditis, but the latter condition is now rare.

SUPPURATIVE THYROIDITIS Bacterial infection of the thyroid gland is rare among children. It usually is associated with an embryologic remnant or left pyriform sinus tract. The left lobe is most often involved. Suppurative thyroiditis can be associated with other head and neck infections. Among older children and adolescents, bacterial thyroiditis can be associated with bacteremic spread from distant infection. Children usually have acute pain, often with dysphagia, and unilateral or bilateral thyroid enlargement, fever, and local tenderness. The gland is firm initially, and an abscess may develop later. Leukocytosis is common, and results of thyroid function tests usually are normal. Early differentiation from subacute thyroiditis can be difficult, but signs and symptoms of hyperthyroidism are uncommon, and the course usually is limited to 2 to 4 weeks. The common organisms are *Staphylococcus aureus, Streptococcus pyogenes,* and *Streptococcus pneumoniae.* Fine-needle aspiration biopsy and culture are helpful in the selection of an antimicrobial agent.

24.6.9 Hyperthyroidism

JUVENILE GRAVES DISEASE

Pathogenesis

Thyrotoxicosis in childhood and adolescence most commonly occurs as a consequence of diffuse thyroid hyperplasia (Graves disease). Graves disease is a multisystem disease involving hyperthyroidism, eye manifestations, and dermopathy. Among children, unlike adults, the latter manifestations are absent or mild. The disease occurs among preschool children. In rare instances it begins in infancy. However, the incidence increases sharply as children approach adolescence. Girls are affected 6 to 8 times more often than are boys. Graves disease, like Hashimoto thyroiditis, has a genetic basis. A high proportion of patients have a family history of goiter, hyperthyroidism, or hypothyroidism. It is believed that both Graves disease and Hashimoto thyroiditis arise randomly in a genetically predisposed population. The concordance rate for Graves disease among monozygotic twins has been reported to be 30 to 60%. Among dizygotic twins it is only 3 to 9%. Family studies have disclosed a high percentage of circulating antithyroid antibodies in close relatives. Certain HLA haplotypes, such as HLA B8 and Dr3 in whites, are prevalent in Graves disease.

The three principal autoantigens of Graves disease (the TSH receptor, thyroid peroxidase, and thyroglobulin) have been cloned. The TSH receptor autoantibodies have a major pathogenetic role in Graves disease. Thyroid-stimulating hormone receptor-stimulating antibodies can be identified by means of bioassay and receptor assay techniques. These antibodies displace TSH from membrane TSH receptors and stimulate adenylate cyclase and cAMP production in thyroid follicular cell lines in culture. Autoantibodies measured only by displacement of radiolabeled TSH from thyroid cell membrane TSH receptor are called *TSH binding-inhibiting immunoglobulin* (TBII) or TBIA.

The production of TSA by B lymphocytes probably is a secondary response to a cell-mediated immune reaction that requires involvement of T lymphocytes in a manner similar to that postulated for Hashimoto thyroiditis (see Fig. 24-20). Cell cultures of lymphocytes from patients with Graves disease produce immunoglobulins only after stimulation with phytohemagglutinin. Because the latter substance stimulates only T cells, which are incapable of secreting immunoglobulins, it can be inferred that cell-mediated as well as humoral immune mechanisms are involved in the genesis of the thyrotoxic state.

Clinical Features

The onset of thyrotoxicosis usually is insidious, with a period of increasing nervousness, palpitation, increased appetite, and muscle weakness. Some patients have marked weight loss, usually in association with a voracious appetite. Some children and, especially,

adolescents have a weight increase with the onset of the disease. There is a tendency for children with thyrotoxicosis to be in the upper percentile channels for height. Except for exophthalmos and other eye signs, the symptoms of thyrotoxicosis are nonspecific and for prolonged periods can be mistaken for another condition. Behavior abnormalities, declining school performance, and emotional instability are common. Some patients have prominent cardiovascular signs, and attention is focused on a cardiac murmur or decreased exercise tolerance. Fatigability and objective muscle weakness occur among 60 to 70% of patients with juvenile thyrotoxicosis. Myopathy varies in severity from fatigability to periodic paralysis and, as for adults, can be the most prominent manifestation of the disease. In rare instances, juvenile Graves disease occurs in association with myasthenia gravis, another autoimmune disorder.

Most of the signs and symptoms of Graves disease are similar to those produced by a hyperactive sympathetic nervous system and can be stimulated by anxiety, fright, or acute illness. Even among patients with unimpressive tachycardia, the pulse pressure is widened and the precordium is overactive. Underlying heart disease is difficult to exclude in the presence of cardiomegaly, ejection murmurs, precordial thrill, and gallop rhythms. Other signs of sympathetic overactivity are tremor, excessive perspiration, rapid tendon reflex relaxation times, and emotional lability. The size of the thyroid gland is highly variable, and the goiter can escape notice if the gland is only slightly enlarged.

A better appreciation of thyroidal size and consistency can be gained if the patient is examined in the supine position with the neck thrust forward by hyperextension. Bimanual palpation during swallowing and during digital displacement of each lobe delineates the thyroid from other structures. Tracings of the two-dimensional projection of the gland, outlined with a skin pencil, provide a valuable method of recording serial changes. The characteristics of the thyroid to be assessed at physical examination are size, uniformity, and consistency. A bruit or thrill provides some indication of the degree of hyperplasia but has no specific diagnostic value. During phases of active hyperplasia, the thyroid typically has a resilient bulging that is lost as recovery takes place.

Severe Graves ophthalmyopathy is much less common among children than among adults, and malignant exophthalmos is almost unknown. The eye findings in this disease are grouped as those caused by sympathetic hyperactivity and those caused by specific pathologic changes in the orbit. Those caused by sympathetic hyperactivity give the appearance of stare owing to retraction of the upper lid and a wide palpebral aperture. There also is a lag in descent of the upper lid on looking downward (lid lag) as well as infrequent blinking and absence of forehead wrinkling on upward gaze. The eyes frequently present a glazed appearance. These findings, to a large extent, parallel the severity of the disease and disappear as the patient is rendered euthyroid.

Changes in the orbit are caused by infiltration of mucopolysaccharides, lymphocytes, and edema fluid within the ocular muscles, lacrimal glands, and retroorbital fat. These changes cause exophthalmos, ophthalmoplegia, chemosis of the conjunctiva, pain, swelling, and irritation. Although the inflammatory changes usually improve with control of the hyperthyroid state, the course of the thyroid and eye manifestations can differ. Some degree of exophthalmos tends to remain after recovery from thyrotoxicosis.

Accumulation of mucopolysaccharides in skin and subcutaneous tissues, *Graves dermopathy* or *pretibial myxedema,* is rare among children. Graves disease and Hashimoto thyroiditis occasionally are encountered in the same patient. These children have clinical and laboratory features of Hashimoto thyroiditis and have thyrotoxicosis and resistance to thyroidal suppression by T_3. The somewhat whimsical term *hashitoxicosis* has been applied to these patients.

Laboratory Diagnosis

The initial laboratory tests should include serum TSH, serum T_4, free T_4 (with T_3 resin uptake), and serum T_3 measurement. The serum TSH level is suppressed below the limit of detection of second-generation TSH assays, and usually below 0.04 mU/L in the third-generation ultrasensitive assays. A serum TSH level above 1.0 μU/mL suggests TSH-dependent hyperthyroidism. Measurement of serum levels of TSH receptor autoantibody (TSA and TBII) confirm the diagnosis.

Treatment Options

Therapy for thyrotoxicosis must be directed at decreasing the secretory rate of thyroid hormones and, if possible, blunting the toxic effects produced by high circulating levels. Three principal methods are available for reducing thyroid hormone secretion: subtotal or total ablation of the thyroid gland with radioactive iodine, subtotal surgical thyroidectomy, and blocking thyroid hormone biosynthesis with drugs.

Treatment with Radioactive Iodine   In terms of ease, cost, efficacy, and short-term safety, treatment with iodine-131 is undoubtedly superior. This approach, however, has been used relatively infrequently to treat children and adolescents because of the high prevalence of posttreatment hypothyroidism and the potential risks of leukemia, thyroid cancer, and genetic damage. Late development of primary hypothyroidism after ^{131}I therapy has occurred in every series of patients studied, regardless of the dosage of radioiodine used. Approximately 10 to 20% of patients treated with radioiodine are hypothyroid within 1 year, and the incidence of hypothyroidism thereafter approximates 3% per year. Prolonged medical follow-up care and lifelong medication cannot be avoided with this mode of treatment.

Radioactive iodine has been used to treat adults for a sufficient time to alleviate fears of inducing leukemia and thyroid carcinoma. There is no evidence of reproductive dysfunction or increased prevalence of anomalies among offspring of treated patients. However, thyroid glands of young animals are much more susceptible to induction of thyroid carcinoma by ionizing radiation than are those of older animals. Radiation to the neck in infancy has been incriminated as an important cause of thyroid cancer among children, whereas this is infrequent among adults. Several children treated with radioiodine have been reported to have thyroid adenoma. Reports of treatment of more than 500 children and adolescents have appeared since 1950. There have been no recent reports of thyroid neoplasia in this population.

Most clinics reserve the use of radioiodine for management of thyrotoxicosis in the care of older adolescents who do not follow a medical regimen and who cannot be adequately prepared for surgical thyroidectomy. However, a number of recent reports of the successful treatment of children and adolescents with radioiodine suggest that this approach may be safe enough to consider as initial treatment of selected patients, particularly those 10 years or older.

Surgical Treatment   With proper preparation of the patient for surgical thyroidectomy, the immediate operative mortality approximates that of other major surgical procedures. With proper surgical treatment, most patients achieve satisfactory remission, and requirements for intensive medical follow-up care are less rigorous

than those for patients treated exclusively with drugs. The availability of an experienced thyroid surgeon is an important criterion for successful surgical treatment. The incidence of permanent hypoparathyroidism and recurrent laryngeal nerve damage after subtotal thyroidectomy is appreciable, and these serious complications will persist and may necessitate lifelong treatment. The surgeon attempts to leave enough thyroid tissue that the patient is euthyroid postoperatively. The patient may, however, have recurrence of thyrotoxicosis or may have late hypothyroidism after many years.

Medical Management   Management of Graves disease with antithyroid drugs requires a prolonged period of drug therapy (usually 2 to 5 years) and close supervision by a physician for years. Even among patients treated successfully, not more than 60 to 70% have permanent remission with drug therapy alone. Combined therapy with an antithyroid drug plus Na-L-thyroxine in replacement dosage has been used to suppress increased serum TSH levels and minimize the need for frequent adjustment of antithyroid drug dosage. A small percentage of patients are hypersensitive to propylthiouracil or methimazole. These reactions usually are mild and disappear when the drug is withdrawn, but severe reactions can occur (see later).

Approach to Therapy

The choice of therapy for thyrotoxicosis must be individualized. Other illnesses, the quality of thyroid surgery available, and the socioeconomic factors involved in determining the success of a prolonged medical regimen must be considered. Patients with weight loss and decreases in body mass index and a large goiter are more resistant to drug therapy. In most instances, however, treatment is begun with antithyroid drugs, and a decision regarding surgery or radioiodine therapy is made when the patient becomes euthyroid. Most pediatric endocrinologists prefer a drug therapy regimen, but there is an increasing trend to use of radioiodine as definitive therapy.

For patients with severe toxicosis, the β-adrenergic blocking agent propranolol is of value in controlling many of the manifestations of Graves disease. The drug is useful for initial treatment in the time before specific antithyroid drugs become effective. It has proved effective in preoperative preparation for subtotal thyroidectomy.

In the United States, propylthiouracil and methimazole are the antithyroid drugs most commonly used. Both inhibit the coupling of iodotyrosines and oxidation and organic binding of iodide and thereby block synthesis of thyroid hormones. Propylthiouracil reduces conversion of T_4 to T_3 in nonthyroid tissue. Methimazole has a longer half-time of degradation than does propylthiouracil. Propylthiouracil must be given every 6 to 8 hours. On occasion, maintenance therapy with methimazole can be accomplished with a single daily dose. The rapidity of response to therapy correlates best with the initial size of the thyroid gland, rather than with the degree of thyrotoxicity. Patients with a small gland and rapid thyroidal turnover usually improve in a few weeks, whereas those with very large glands may not achieve a satisfactory euthyroid state for 2 to 3 months.

The initial dosage of propylthiouracil varies from 300 to 600 mg daily (175 mg/m^2, or 5 to 7 mg/kg) in doses spaced at 6- or 8-hour intervals. The dosage of methimazole is about one-tenth that of propylthiouracil. Toxic reactions to propylthiouracil or methimazole are relatively common. Skin rashes occur among approximately 5% of patients treated with propylthiouracil or methimazole early in the course of therapy, but disappear when the drug is withheld. Often these rashes are mild and can be controlled with antihistamines. Persistent granulocytopenia can occur, usually after 4 to 8 weeks of therapy. Recovery usually occurs with drug withdrawal. With severe agranulocytosis, recovery usually follows protective isolation and glucocorticoid and antibiotic treatment. Severe reactions are rare but can be life threatening. These include lupus-like syndromes, drug fever, hepatitis, nephritis, and splenomegaly.

After the manifestations of thyrotoxicosis have disappeared, the best clinical prognostic guide in judging when to discontinue therapy is the size of the thyroid gland. Most patients with continued thyroid enlargement will have a relapse if antithyroid drugs are discontinued. It is also possible to monitor the level of circulating TSA. When circulating TSA disappears in a patient in clinical remission during drug treatment, remission outside treatment is more likely. Combined therapy with an antithyroid drug and T_4 offers advantages of a smoother course and avoids TSH-induced goiter. Administration of T_4 in the usual replacement dosage is begun after the euthyroid state is well established (3 to 6 months). The T_4 dosage is adjusted to maintain normal blood levels.

Sodium ipodate and iopanoate are iodinated radiographic contrast agents shown to be effective antithyroid drugs. They inhibit T_4 to T_3 conversion and reduce thyroid hormone production from the thyroid gland. Treatment over 6 to 12 months has been successful for 50 to 90% of adult patients with Graves disease. The effect of the drugs is transient, however, so they serve as useful adjuncts to other antithyroid regimens and for preoperative management. The dosage is 5 to 10 mg/kg daily.

Iodide in large doses blocks synthesis of thyroid hormone, inhibits the release of preformed thyroid hormone, and renders the gland less vascular. Iodine blockade can be maintained for only a limited time (4 to 16 weeks) before escape occurs, and a fully euthyroid state may not be achieved. The use of inorganic iodine is reserved for patients with severe toxicosis and impending thyroid storm and occasionally for the immediately preoperative preparation of patients who are about to undergo subtotal thyroidectomy.

NEONATAL THYROTOXICOSIS

Neonatal thyrotoxicosis usually is caused by TSA acquired from the mother through placental transport (neonatal Graves disease). Rare cases of neonatal hyperthyroidism caused by activating mutations of the TSH receptor have been reported. A familial history of absence of TSA should arouse suspicion.

Neonatal Graves disease is uncommon, accounting for about 1% of cases of Graves disease among children and adolescents. The rarity is presumed to be caused by the low incidence of thyrotoxicosis in pregnancy (1 to 2 cases per 1000 pregnancies) and because the neonatal disease occurs in only about 1 in 70 thyrotoxic pregnancies. In most instances, the disease is caused by transplacental passage of TSA from a mother with active or inactive Graves disease or Hashimoto thyroiditis (see Fig. 24-20). Thus neonatal Graves disease cannot be predicted from the maternal clinical status alone. However, one can predict neonatal disease among offspring of women with high TSA or TBII titers. One report described six neonates with overt thyrotoxicosis and four with chemical thyrotoxicosis among 104 mothers with Graves disease during pregnancy. All had suppressed levels of TSH and positive TBII titers in cord blood with variable T_4 concentrations.

Graves disease among newborns manifests as irritability, flushing, tachycardia, hypertension, poor weight gain or excessive

weight loss, thyroid enlargement, and exophthalmos. Thrombocytopenia with hepatosplenomegaly, jaundice, and hypoprothrombinemia also has been observed. Arrhythmia, cardiac failure, and death can occur if the thyrotoxicity is severe and treatment is inadequate. Mortality approaches 25% if disease is severe enough to be diagnosed.

Although neonatal Graves disease can manifest at birth, among some infants the onset of symptoms and signs usually is delayed as long as 8 to 9 days. This is the result of postnatal depletion of transplacentally acquired blocking doses of antithyroid drugs and the dramatic increase in newborn T_3 concentration normally associated with birth.

The diagnosis of neonatal Graves disease is confirmed with high levels of T_4, free T_4, and T_3 in postnatal blood. Cord blood values can be normal or near-normal, whereas levels 2 to 5 days after birth can be markedly high. Serum level of TSH is low. Neonatal Graves disease usually resolves spontaneously as maternal TSA in the newborn are degraded; the half-life approximates 12 days. The usual clinical course of neonatal Graves disease extends 3 to 12 weeks.

Management of hyperthyroidism among newborns includes sedatives and digitalization as necessary. Iodide or thionamide drugs are administered to decrease secretion of thyroid hormone. These drugs have additive effects with regard to inhibition of hormone synthesis; iodide also rapidly inhibits hormone release. Lugol solution (5% iodine and 10% potassium iodide; 126 mg of iodine per milliliter) is given in doses of 1 drop (about 8 mg) three times a day. Methimazole is administered in a dosage of 0.5 to 1 mg/kg/d in divided doses at 8-hour intervals. The dosage of propylthiouracil is 5 to 10 mg/kg/d in divided doses every 8 hours. A therapeutic response should be observed within 24 to 36 hours. If the response is not satisfactory, the dose of antithyroid drug and iodide can be increased by 50%. Adrenal glucocorticoids in antiinflammatory dosage and propranolol (1 to 2 mg/kg/d) also can be helpful. Radiographic contrast agents can be useful because the disease is transient. Sodium ipodate, 100 mg daily, or 0.3 to 0.5 g every 2 to 3 days, either alone or in conjunction with antithyroid drugs, has been effective.

THYROTROPIN-DEPENDENT HYPERTHYROIDISM

PITUITARY TUMORS TSH-secreting pituitary tumors associated with clinical hyperthyroidism have been reported among adults and in children. Among children, the local manifestations of the tumor are prominent. These included visual changes, optic atrophy, hydrocephalus, and amaurosis. Children with hyperthyroidism and measurable serum TSH concentrations need to be examined for neurologic dysfunction and visual abnormalities; brain MRI imaging for careful evaluation of the sella turcica is indicated if this evaluation arouses suspicion or if the serum concentration of TSH is normal or elevated.

SELECTIVE PITUITARY T_3 RESISTANCE Hyperthyroidism with diffuse goiter and elevated serum levels of TSH has been reported among several patients without enlargement of the pituitary gland. These patients have resistance to the feedback effect of T_3 on TSH release because of thyroid hormone receptor β gene mutation (see Sec. 24.6.4). Many cases have been misdiagnosed as Graves disease. Pituitary resistance to thyroid hormone is suspected when any patient has elevated thyroid hormone levels in the presence of normal or elevated TSH concentrations. If symptoms are of concern, therapy may be indicated. Dopaminergic drugs, triidothyroacetic acid, and single morning doses of T_3 have been tried. Thyroid ablative therapy may be necessary.

HYPERTHYROIDISM DUE TO AUTONOMOUS THYROID NODULE

The thyroid function of patients with thyroid nodules is variable. Most patients are euthyroid. Most functioning thyroid nodules occur in association with multinodular goiter. Somatic gain-of-function mutations of the TSH receptor have been found to be a major cause of benign toxic thyroid adenoma. Activating germline TSH receptor mutations, in contrast, produce congenital or childhood onset of thyroid hyperplasia and hyperthyroidism. Autonomously functioning thyroid nodules are rare among children. Most authors report that the incidence of thyroid carcinoma in functioning nodules is less than 1%. Functioning thyroid carcinoma is unusual enough that a number of examples have been reported; in most of these, malignancy criteria (see Sec. 24.6.10) were present.

Functional nodules do not usually produce clinical thyrotoxicosis; large nodules (more than 3-cm diameter) are most likely to do this. Autonomous nodules, however, suppress normal thyroid tissue if they secrete large amounts of hormone. Autonomy can be diagnosed by means of measurement of serum concentration of TSH. Suppressed levels, found with a highly sensitive assay, in the presence of euthyroid levels of thyroid hormones indicates a non-TSH thyroid stimulator or thyroid autonomy.

Functioning nodules that produce clinical and chemical thyrotoxicosis necessitate treatment. Radioiodine treatment tends to be reserved for patients older than 40 years. Antithyroid drug therapy is considered only for short-term management. Surgery is the most common therapy. Complete lobectomy with removal of pericapsular lymph nodes and preservation of the recurrent laryngeal nerve is the most desirable procedure. The course of functioning thyroid nodules in euthyroid patients is variable. Most likely, however, such patients remain euthyroid. The nodule often degenerates, presumably through recurrent hemorrhage. Follow-up care is essential because thyrotoxicosis can develop.

HYPERTHYROIDISM CAUSED BY ACTIVATING THYROID-STIMULATING HORMONE RECEPTOR MUTATIONS

Several families have been reported to have hyperthyroidism segregating as an autosomal dominant trait in the absence of autoimmune disease of the thyroid. The affected persons have goiter, increased total and free levels of T_4, and suppressed TSH concentration. Among patients treated surgically, the thyroid glands have diffuse hyperplasia without lymphocytic infiltration. Gain-of-function germline mutations of the TSH receptor have been found among these patients. Functionally, the transfected mutated receptors had abnormally increased constitutive cAMP stimulating activity.

This form of hyperthyroidism usually is detected during childhood or adolescence, but a few diagnoses have been made before the patient was 2 years of age or in the neonatal period. The abnormality is congenital, and it is possible that some of the earlier reported cases of familial persistent neonatal Graves disease have instead manifested unrecognized activating TSH-receptor mutations. Treatment of such infants is difficult because the disorder is not transient. Antithyroid drugs for short-term management and partial thyroidectomy seem the best therapies at present.

HYPERTHYROIDISM CAUSED BY ACTIVATING G-PROTEIN MUTATIONS

The guanine nucleotides (G proteins) are a family of signal transducing molecules that couple the seven-transmembrane-helix family of cell membrane receptors, including the TSH receptor, to activating cellular effector systems such as adenylcyclase. Activating mutations of the α-subunit of the stimulatory G protein, G_s, increase formation of cAMP and the associated endocrinopathies of McCune-Albright syndrome. It is postulated that the mutation occurs during embryonic development with a mosaic tissue distribution. The clinical manifestations are related to the tissues involved. They include polyostotic fibrosis dysplasia of bone and hyperfunction of one or more endocrine glands. The latter include ovarian cysts, gonadal hyperfunction and precocious puberty, pituitary adenoma causing adrenal hyperplasia or hypersecretion of GH, and hyperthyroidism. The thyroid hyperplasia and hyperthyroidism resemble those of Graves disease but without ophthalmologic features and without autoantibodies. Treatment options include antithyroid drugs, surgery, and radioiodine.

24.6.10　Thyroid Neoplasia

Classification

A thyroid neoplasm is suspected whenever a child is found to have a solitary thyroid mass with a consistency differing from that of the rest of the thyroid gland. A solitary nodule during the first two decades of life has a much greater likelihood of being malignant than those at older ages. The prevalence of cancer among children with thyroid nodules approximates 30%. The ratio of girls to boys among children with thyroid cancer is 2:1, in contrast to the much higher predominance of girls with thyroid enlargement from other causes. Nodular enlargement among boys is somewhat more likely to be cancerous than it is among girls. Thyroid cancer accounts for 0.5% of all cases of cancer for all ages and 1 to 1.5% of all childhood cancer.

Fifty percent or more of solitary thyroid nodules during childhood prove to be a *cystic lesion* or *benign adenoma*. Hyperfunctioning adenoma is exceedingly uncommon during the first two decades of life. Well-differentiated follicular carcinoma accounts for more than 90% of malignant lesions in this age group. Characterization of the histopathologic type as follicular, papillary, or papillary-follicular does not alter therapy. However, papillary and papillary-follicular carcinomas have higher recurrence rates than does follicular disease.

Other malignant tumors of the thyroid gland during childhood include *medullary carcinoma* arising in the parafollicular cells, *poorly differentiated thyroid carcinoma,* and tumors such as *lymphoma* and *metastatic carcinoma* arising in other tissues. The prognosis for these tumors is much worse than that for well-differentiated adenocarcinoma of the thyroid. It is important to establish a tissue diagnosis as early as possible and design treatment accordingly. Well-differentiated carcinoma has little tendency to become an undifferentiated neoplasm.

Etiology

A frequent predisposing cause of development of carcinoma of the thyroid gland during infancy and childhood is radiation exposure of the neck. In series of children described in the 1950s with thyroid cancer, 80% had a history of radiation therapy. Radiotherapy usually had been administered during early infancy to the upper mediastinum and neck for control of an "enlarged" thymus gland. Cancer also occurred after irradiation of hypertrophied tonsils and adenoids or acne among older children and adolescents. The average time between irradiation and recognition of cancer approximates 10 years. The estimated absolute risk of cancer is 4.4 per million children per rad of radiation dose (1 rad = 0.01 Gy). The most recent epidemic of radiation-induced thyroid cancer among children followed the Chernobyl nuclear accident in Russia in 1986. The radiation dose to exposed children ranged from 0.5 to 600 rad (0.005–6 Gy) in a group of 107 children detected by 1992 with a mean of 20 rad (0.2 Gy). The age at exposure ranged from 0 to 11 years, and the age at diagnosis 4 to 16 years. Thus cancer, predominantly papillary adenocarcinoma, developed in most cases within 3 to 5 years. However, the number of cases has continued to increase.

Hormonal Manifestations of Medullary Carcinoma

Medullary thyroid carcinoma arises from the parafollicular or C cells of the thyroid gland. It is said to be 4% to 10% of thyroid carcinoma. There are distinctive histologic characteristics—large deposits of amyloid situated among sheets of pleomorphic epithelial cells. Although many sporadic examples of medullary carcinoma of the thyroid have been described, at least one-half occur in kindreds and are apparently inherited as an autosomal dominant trait. Many of these familial instances are associated with MEN, which includes pheochromocytoma and parathyroid adenoma (see Sec. 24.5.3).

The distinctive feature of medullary carcinoma of the thyroid is excessive secretion of calcitonin. Other substances, including ACTH, melanocyte-stimulating hormone, histaminase, serotonin, prostaglandins, somatostatin, and β-endorphin may be produced. Although calcitonin levels are invariably high among patients with palpable tumors, the tumor can be detected in children before development of a palpable mass by means of measurement of calcitonin in the serum before or after stimulation tests with intravenous calcium or pentagastrin. Management in MEN 2A is discussed in Sec. 24.5.3.

Diagnosis and Management

Most children with papillary follicular carcinoma of the thyroid have a midneck or lateral neck mass. Most (60 to 80%) have one or more palpable neck lymph nodes that contain metastatic thyroid cells found at histologic examination. One-third to one-half of patients have extracapsular extension and 10% have distant metastasis, usually to the lungs. Fine-needle aspiration biopsy is the diagnostic approach of choice with analysis by an experienced cytopathologist. Fine-needle aspiration biopsy can be omitted if *malignancy criteria* are present. These include a history of radiation to the head or neck, a rapidly growing nodule that is very firm or hard, satellite lymph nodes, hoarseness or dysphagia, or evidence of distant metastasis.

The initial approach to therapy for a thyroid nodule is surgical with simple removal of the affected lobe. No further surgery is necessary if the mass proves to be a cystic lesion or benign adenoma. If a frozen section examination shows carcinoma, total lobectomy is performed on the side of origin, and as much of the contralateral lobe is excised as is compatible with preservation of the parathyroid glands and recurrent laryngeal nerve. Well-differentiated carcinoma is likely to involve multifocal sites in the thyroid gland.

Although accessible regional nodes are removed, mutilating neck dissection is not warranted. Routine use of therapeutic dosages of radioiodine after surgery is controversial in the care of patients with well-differentiated carcinoma of the thyroid and no evidence of metastasis. However, in the care of patients with lymph node involvement or other evidence of metastasis, radioiodine is administered postoperatively to ablate any residual functioning thyroid tissue. Patients are observed after surgery and radioiodine treatment by means of measurement of serum thyroglobulin concentration as a reliable tumor marker. A concentration of thyroglobulin in the serum less than 1 ng/mL (1 μg/L) while the patient is undergoing T_4 suppression treatment, or less than 10 ng/mL (10 μg/L) outside T_4 suppression, indicates remission. Higher values suggest metastasis. Metastatic disease usually is managed with high-dose radioiodine. After surgery or surgery with radioiodine, the patient maintenance therapy is provided with full substitution dosages of exogenous thyroid hormone to protect the gland from further stimulation by TSH.

Prognosis

The prognosis among children with well-differentiated follicular cell cancer of the thyroid is far better than that of most other types of childhood cancer. The course usually is indolent with long periods in which there is little progression. In a review only 13 of 540 patients had died of the disease 12 to 33 years postoperatively. However, as many as 35% of patients have local or distant recurrence, and constant surveillance is needed. Because spread to the lymph nodes occurs before surgical treatment of some patients, the excellent prognosis may be related more to the biological nature of this form of cancer than to total removal of all cancerous cells at the initial operation. Thyroid hormone suppression cannot be overemphasized and is prescribed in doses adequate to suppress TSH in the serum (assessed with a high-sensitivity TSH assay) but to avoid evidence of toxicity. Mortality from thyroid carcinoma during childhood and adolescence is primarily accounted for by the relatively uncommon instances of medullary carcinoma and undifferentiated carcinoma. In these lesions radical surgery combined with radiation or cancer chemotherapy is fully justified.

References

General

Apriletti JW, Ribeiro RCJ, Wagner RL, et al: Molecular and structural biology of thyroid hormone receptors. Clin Exp Pharmacol Physiol 25: S2–S11, 1998

Hsu JH, Brent GA: Thyroid hormone receptor gene knockouts. Trends Endocrinol Metab 9:103–112, 1998

Oppenheimer JH, Schwartz HL, Strait KA: An integrated view of thyroid hormone action in vivo. In: Weintraub BD, ed: Molecular Endocrinology. New York, Raven Press, 1995:249–268

Fetal and Newborn Thyroid Function

Burrow GN, Fisher DA, Larsen PR: Maternal and fetal thyroid function. N Engl J Med 331:1072–1078, 1994

Fisher DA: Fetal thyroid function: diagnosis and management of fetal thyroid disorders. Clin Obstet Gynecol 40:16–31, 1997

Fisher DA: Thyroid function in premature infants: the hypothyroxinemia of prematurity. Clin Perinatol 25:999–1014, 1998

La Franchi S: Thyroid function in preterm infants. Thyroid 9:71–78, 1999

Congenital Hypothyroidism

Abramwicz MJ, Duprez L, Parma J, Vassart G, Heinrichs C: Familial congenital hypothyroidism due to inactivating mutation of the thyrotropin receptor causing profound hypoplasia of the thyroid gland. J Clin Invest 99:3018–3024, 1997

Asteria C, Rajanayagam O, Collingwood TN, et al: Prenatal diagnosis of thyroid hormone resistance. J Clin Endocrinol Metab 84:405–410, 1999

Delange F: Neonatal screening for congenital hypothyroidism: results and perspectives. Horm Res 48:51–61, 1997

Derksen-Lubsen G, Verkerk PH: Neuropsychologic development in early treated congenital hypothyroidism: analysis of literature data. Pediatr Res 39:51–566, 1996

de Vijlder JJ, Ris-Stalpkers C, Vulsma T: Inborn errors of thyroid hormone biosynthesis. Exp Clin Endocrinol Diabetes 105 (Suppl 14):32–37, 1997

Devreiendt K, Vanhole C, Mattijs G, Dezegher F: Deletion of thyroid transcription factor-1 gene in an infant with neonatal thyroid dysfunction and respiratory failure. N Engl J Med 338:1317–1318, 1998

DiLauro R, Damante G, DeFelice M, et al: Molecular events in the differentiation of the thyroid gland. J Endocrinol Invest 18:117–119, 1995

Doeker BM, Pfaffle RW, Pohlenz J, Andler W: Congenital central hypothyroidism due to a homozygous mutation in the thyrotropin β subunit gene follows an autosomal recessive inheritance. J Clin Endocrinol Metab 84:129–133, 1998

Rosenbloom AL, Almonte AS, Brown MR, Fisher DA, Baumbach L, Parks JS: Clinical and biochemical phenotype of familial anterior hypopituitarism from mutation of the PROP-1 gene. J Clin Endocrinol Metab 84:50–57, 1999

Scott DA, Wang R, Kreman TM, Sheffield VC, Karniski LP: The Pendred syndrome gene encodes a chloride-iodide transport protein. Nature Genet 21:440–443, 1999

Juvenile Hypothyroidism and Goiter

Goldsmith JR, Grossman CM, Morton WE, et al: Juvenile hypothyroidism among two populations exposed to radioiodine. Environ Health Perspect 107:303–308, 1999

Grimeorp-Papendieck L, Chiesa A, Martinez A, Heinrich JJ, Bergado C: Nocturnal TSH surge and TRH test response in the evaluation of thyroid axis in hypothalamic pituitary disorders in childhood. Horm Res 50:252–257, 1998

Surks MI, Sievert R: Drugs and thyroid function. N Engl J Med 333:1688–1694, 1995

Weetman AP: Autoimmune thyroid disease and other autoimmune endocrinopathies. Curr Opin Endocrinol Diabetes 1:140–144, 1995

Hyperthyroidism

Akamizu T, Mori T, Nakao K: Pathogenesis of Graves' disease: molecular analysis of anti-thryotropin receptor antibodies. Endocr J 44:633–646, 1997

Glaser NS, Styne DM: Predictors of early remission of hyperthyroidism in children. J Clin Endocrinol Metab 82:1719–1726, 1997

Gruters A, Schoneberg T, Bieberman H, et al: Severe congenital hyperthyroidims caused by a germline neomutation in the extracellular portion of the thyrotropin receptor. J Clin Endocrinol Metab 83:1431–1436, 1998

Kopp P, Muirhead S, Jourdain N, Gu WX, Jameson JL, Rodd C: Congenital hyperthyroidism caused by a solitary toxic adenoma harboring a novel somatic mutation (serine 282-isoleucine) in the extracellular domain of the thyrotropin receptor. J Clin Invest 100:1634–1639, 1997

Polak M: Hyperthyroidism in early infancy: pathogenesis, clinical features and diagnosis, with a focus on neonatal hyperthyroidism. Thyroid 8:1171–1177, 1998

Rivkees SA, Sklar C, Freemark M: The management of Graves' disease in children with special emphasis on radioiodine treatment. J Clin Endocrinol Metab 83:3767–3776, 1998

Thyroid Neoplasia

Feinmesser R, Lubin E, Segal K, Noyek A: Carcinoma of the thyroid in children: a review. J Pediatr Endocrinol Metab 10:561–568, 1997

Heshmati HM, Gharib H, Van Heerden JA, Sizemore GW: Advances and controversies in the diagnosis and management of medullary thyroid carcinoma. Am J Med 103:60–69, 1997

Khurana KK, Labrador E, Izquierdo R, Mesonero CE, Pisharodi LR: The role of fine needle aspiration biopsy in the management of thyroid nodules in children and adolescents and young adults: a multi-institutional study. Thyroid 4:383–386, 1999

Learoyd DL, Twigg SM, Zedenius JV, Robinson BG: The molecular genetics of endocrine tumors. J Pediatr Endocrinol Metab 11:195–228, 1998

Schlumberger MJ: Papillary and follicular tyroid carcinoma. N Engl J Med 338:297–306, 1998

24.7 ABNORMALITIES OF SEX DETERMINATION AND DIFFERENTIATION

Melvin M. Grumbach

The terms *hermaphroditism* and *intersexuality* are generally used to describe the condition in which a person has gonads of one or both sexes and some degree of ambisexual differentiation of the accessory sexual structures. Depending on the morphologic features of the gonad, persons with these congenital abnormalities have been described as having *male pseudohermaphroditism* when testes are present, *female pseudohermaphroditism* when ovaries are present, or *true hermaphroditism* when both testicular and ovarian tissue can be identified. This definition does not include postnatal virilization or feminization or transsexualism.

24.7.1 Human Sex Differentiation

The human embryo is potentially a bisexual organism equipped with gonadal and genital primordia capable of differentiating as either male or female phenotypes. Sex determination and differentiation are conveniently divided into three ordered phases: genetic sex (sex determination); gonadal sex, differentiation of the gonad as a testis or ovary; and phenotypic sex (sex determination), sex-specific differentiation of the paired genital ducts, the urogenital sinus, and external genitalia determined by the action of two fetal testicular hormones. Each of these processes depends on and is governed by the action of specific genes. The genetic sex of the zygote is established by fertilization of a normal ovum by an X- or Y-bearing sperm. In humans the heterogametic sex (XY) is male and the homogametic sex (XX) is female. The Y chromosome functions as a dominant male determiner. The mechanisms involved in translating genetic sex into the dimorphic phenotypic sex of male and female newborn infants are incompletely understood.

The sex chromosomes and the autosomes contain genes that effect sex determination and, as a consequence, gonadogenesis. The male-determining region located on the short arm of the Y chromosome, the testis-determining factor, leads to differentiation of the paired bipotential indifferent gonads of the embryo as testes. Although the presence of only a single X chromosome (as in 45,X gonadal dysgenesis) can lead to the beginning of ovarian organogenesis, with rare exceptions two X chromosomes are needed for survival of oocytes in utero and the development of a normal ovary at birth. X chromosomes (in the absence of a Y chromosome or translocation of its testis-determining factor region to an X chromosome) are needed for ovarian organogenesis of the bipotential gonad. Studies involving patients with disorders of gonadogenesis, including 46,XY females patients with gonadal dysgenesis and 46,XX male patients, indicate that a small segment of the distal short arm of the Y chromosome just proximal to the pseudoautosomal (pairing) region contains the testis-determining factor and is essential for testicular organogenesis. The Y-linked testis-determining factor gene, named *SRY* (sex-determining region on Y), is located in the smallest region of the Y chromosome that can cause sex reversal. The corresponding *Sry* gene in the mouse is expressed in the genital ridge during a 2-day critical period just before and during the time when testis differentiation of the previously indifferent primordial gonad begins. It may be expressed even earlier, because *Sry* expression is detectable in the preimplantation mouse embryo. *SRY* encodes a member of the high-mobility group DNA-binding proteins, which contain a conserved high-mobility group box domain. The SRY protein does not function as a traditional transcription factor but instead bends DNA in a sequence-specific manner to bring together more distant DNA sequences that affect the transcription of downstream genes. Deletions or point mutations of the high-mobility group box domain of the *SRY* gene occur among about 15 to 20% of XY girls with complete gonadal dysgenesis.

Even though *SRY* is the master testis-determining switch, control of gonadogenesis is a much more complicated process. Several other autosomal and X-linked genes are involved in this transcription cascade. WT1, the Wilms tumor suppressor locus at chromosome 11p13 affects development not only of the kidney but differentiation of the urogenital ridge into the bipotential primordial gonad and acts before the *SRY* gene and ovarian-determining genes. Mutations in this gene occur in the Denys-Drash, Fraser, and WAGR syndromes (see Sec. 24.7.3). Moreover, duplication of the *DAX-1* gene on the short arm of the X chromosome (Xp21) in XY persons causes XY gonadal dysgenesis and sex reversal despite the presence of the *SRY* gene. Deletion of this locus does not affect testis differentiation but causes X-linked congenital adrenal hypoplasia and hypogonadotropic hypogonadism. Steroidogenic factor-1, an orphan nuclear receptor coded by an autosomal gene, is a major regulator of adrenal and gonadal steroidogenic enzymes. It is expressed in the indifferent bipotential gonad. Disruption of the gene encoding steroidogenic factor-1 in mice leads to programmed cell death (apoptosis) of the fetal gonads and adrenal glands. In a single case report a heterozygote mutation caused XY gonadal dysgenesis and adrenal insufficiency. A mutation in a single allele of the autosomal *SOX9* gene can cause both XY gonadal dysgenesis and camptomelic dysplasia; 9p- and 10q- deletions also can cause defective testicular organogenesis and male intersex.

Among approximately 80% of XX boys, an X-Y interchange occurred during paternal meiosis, and they express *SRY*. However, among 20% of XX boys and in all but a small proportion of XX true hermaphrodites, the *SRY* gene is not present. In these instances,

mutations in either autosomal or X-linked genes affecting gonadogenesis are quite likely involved.

The embryonic gonad is the first structure to emerge from the indifferent stage. During the seventh week of gestation, testicular differentiation occurs. Ovarian differentiation does not begin until about 11 or 12 weeks, when oogonia are first transformed into oocytes. The bipotential primordial germ cells, progenitors of oogonia and spermatogonia, arise from an extragonadal site, migrate to the urogenital ridge, and implant themselves in the primitive undifferentiated gonad. This earliest sex differentiation is followed by sex-specific development of the genital ducts and subsequently the urogenital sinus and external genitalia. Although the embryo possesses a male and a female set of duct primordia, normally only the homologous pair develops completely; the opposite set retrogresses, persisting as vestigial structures. In boys, the wolffian ducts form the vas deferens, epididymis, and seminal vesicles. In girls, the müllerian ducts differentiate into the fallopian tubes, the uterus, and the upper portion of the vagina. The urogenital sinus and the anlage of the external genitalia are neutral primordia that give rise to homologous structures in boys and girls. These homologous structures include the clitoris and penis, the labia majora and scrotum, the labia minora and corpus spongiosum that encloses the penile urethra, and the paraurethral glands and prostate.

The role of the gonad in embryogenesis of the accessory sex structures has been clarified in fetal castration experiments and through analysis of abnormalities of human sex differentiation. In the absence of testes and their hormones, the fetus has an inherent tendency to develop along female lines irrespective of chromosomal sex. The fetal testicular hormones are essential for differentiation of male sex structures and for retrogression of the female ducts. The fetal testis secretes two hormones critical to male sex differentiation—a glycoprotein, müllerian duct inhibitory factor (anti-müllerian hormone or müllerian inhibitory substance) secreted by Sertoli cells, and testosterone secreted by fetal Leydig cells. The müllerian duct inhibitory factor gene is regulated, in part, by the orphan nuclear receptor steroidogenic factor-1. The local action of müllerian duct factor on its receptor causes ipsilateral regression of the paired müllerian (female) ducts. Testosterone stimulates growth of the wolffian (male) ducts and male development of the urogenital sinus and external genitalia. Testosterone promotes male differentiation of the somatic sex structures by two mechanisms. It acts directly and probably ipsilaterally on the wolffian duct to bring about differentiation of the epididymis, vas deferens, and seminal vesicle. It is also the prohormone for dihydrotestosterone, which is formed by means of enzymatic reduction by 5 α-reductase type 2 in the target tissue, the urogenital sinus, and external genitalia. Dihydrotestosterone is the hormone that induces masculinization of the urogenital sinus, with formation of the prostate and male-type urethra, and masculinization of the primordia of the external genitalia to cause differentiation of the penis, penile urethra, and scrotum. Whereas a functioning fetal gonad is not a prerequisite for development of a female genital system, exposure of the female fetus to androgenic hormones can arrest female differentiation of the urogenital sinus and external genitalia and induce masculinization of the lower genital tract.

Abnormalities of sex differentiation can be divided into two broad categories: (1) errors in (primary) sex determination, such as sex chromosome anomalies, which lead to abnormalities of gonadogenesis, and (2) errors in sex differentiation that cause abnormal development of the somatic sex structures—the genital ducts, urogenital sinus, and external genitalia. Intrinsic or extrinsic factors that adversely affect any of the stages of these mechanisms can cause anomalies of sexual structure. These factors include a sex chromosome abnormality arising in the ovum or sperm of the parent or in the zygote after fertilization that affects gonadogenesis, as in the syndrome of gonadal dysgenesis (Turner syndrome) and seminiferous tubule dysgenesis (Klinefelter syndrome); translocation of sex-determining genes involving too minute an amount of chromosomal material to be visible at light microscopic examination (eg, between the *SRY* gene on the Y chromosome and an X chromosome), which can lead to an XX phenotype in a boy; a mutant gene, as in the feminizing testis form of male pseudohermaphroditism, which causes end-organ resistance to testosterone and other androgens in fetal and postnatal life; exposure of the fetus at a critical stage to inappropriate sex hormones that modify sex-specific differentiation of the derivatives of the urogenital sinus and the primordia of the external genitalia, as in the form of female pseudohermaphroditism caused by congenital virilizing adrenal hyperplasia; and undefined genetic or environmentally determined abnormalities in differentiation of the primordial genital tract.

SEX CHROMATIN PATTERN: X- AND Y-CHROMATIN The two X chromosomes in female diploid somatic cells exhibit striking morphologic and functional differences. One X chromosome is in a highly condensed (heteropyknotic) state in interphase and is visible as sex chromatin (Barr body). It completes DNA synthesis later than any other chromosome, and the action of genes located on the precociously condensed segments is suppressed (silent X) by transcriptional inactivation. The other X chromosome, the single X chromosome in male somatic cells, is in a highly extended (isopyknotic) state during interphase. It completes DNA replication with most of the complement and is genetically active. This discordant behavior of the two homologous X chromosomes in female somatic cells serves as a mechanism of dosage compensation. Inactivation of much of the genic activity of all but one X chromosome in persons with X polysomy minimizes phenotypic expression of the extra X chromosome or chromosomes in somatic cells.

24.7.2 Female Pseudohermaphroditism

Table 24-28 provides a convenient classification of anomalous sexual development for clinical use. Persons with *female pseudohermaphroditism* have a 46,XX karyotype, ovaries, female ducts, and variable degrees of masculine differentiation of the urogenital sinus and external genitalia. The sex chromatin pattern is positive (female). The syndrome illustrates well the complexity of pathogenetic factors that can cause similar malformations.

ANDROGEN-INDUCED

CONGENITAL VIRILIZING ADRENAL HYPERPLASIA This is the most common cause of female pseudohermaphroditism, accounting for approximately one-half of all cases of ambiguous external genitalia. This disorder is caused by an inborn error of adrenocortical biosynthesis that results in relative deficiency of hydrocortisone production, increased secretion of ACTH, and relative excess of androgenic hormones and other steroids. There are six types, all of which have in common an inborn error in the biosynthesis of cortisol. The defect in 21-hydroxylation is by far the most common, accounting for about 95% of the heritable disorders of steroid biosynthesis. The mode of inheritance is autosomal recessive. The functional B gene for 21α-hydroxylase (cytochrome P450c21) is on the short arm of chromosome 6, within the class III region of

the histocompatibility locus adjacent to C4b (a fourth component of complement) between HLA-B and HLA-D. The genetics and resulting abnormal physiological characteristics of 21α-hydroxylase deficiency are described in Sec. 24.4.6.

At birth the external genitalia of affected girls are, as a rule, conspicuously abnormal, whereas the genitalia of affected boys are normally differentiated. The degree of masculinization can be judged by the size of the clitoris and the completeness of labioscrotal fusion, which determines the size of the urogenital sinus (Fig. 24-22). The phallus is invariably enlarged, often approximating the size of a penis (Figs. 24-23). It is generally bound in chordee, behind which a perineal hypospadias is situated. In rare instances, the urethra extends to the tip of the phallus. The labia majora commonly look like a bifid scrotum. Within the perineal opening of the urogenital sinus lie the orifices of the vagina and the urethra. Greater or lesser degrees of fusion of the labioscrotal folds produce a perineal opening that varies in size from that of a small urethra-like opening to a relatively normal female introitus with a separate urethra and vagina (see Fig. 24-22).

The appearance of the external genitalia is not specific, and the genital abnormality can be indistinguishable from that in other forms of hermaphroditism with bilateral cryptorchidism. The feature that sets 21-hydroxylase deficiency apart from all other varieties of hermaphroditism is secretion of excessive quantities of adrenal androgen precursors. The urine contains 17-ketosteroids and, in patients with defective 21-hydroxylation, pregnanetriol in greater amounts than in any of the other forms of abnormal sex differentiation. (Normal excretion of 17-ketosteroids during the first 2 weeks can be as high as 2.5 mg/d, later diminishing to less than 1 mg/d.) The concentration of 17OHP in the plasma is strikingly elevated in patients with 21-hydroxylase deficiency (both salt losers and non-salt-losers). Measurement of this hormone is the most useful diagnostic test (see Sec. 24.4.6). Concentration of 17OHP in the plasma is high in affected newborn infants, for whom this determination can lead to rapid and early detection. In healthy newborns, the 17OHP concentration, high at birth, decreases rapidly during the first 24 hours; however, some stressed infants have values as high as 1000 mg/dL from the third to the seventh days of age. Infants with the life-threatening salt-losing form of 21-hydroxylase deficiency, which occurs among approximately 80% of patients with classic 21-hydroxylase deficiency rarely have clinical evidence of adrenal insufficiency before 4 days of age. It is essential to monitor serum electrolyte concentrations for infants at risk of this disorder. When the pattern of serum electrolyte values is not clearly abnormal, determination of plasma renin activity is useful. Older children have signs of virilization, rapid growth, and accelerated skeletal development. In addition to 21-hydroxylase deficiency, 11β-hydroxylase (P450c11β) deficiency causes virilization of female fetuses. Other forms of congenital adrenal hyperplasia not accompanied by virilization or with minimal virilization of the female fetus have been described (see Sec. 24.4.6).

AROMATASE DEFICIENCY Placental aromatase has a critical role in protecting the female fetus and the mother from exposure to large amounts of testosterone synthesized mainly by the placenta. When placental aromatase is deficient because of mutation in the P450arom gene, the concentration of androgen or androgen precursors exceeds the capacity for aromatization. As a consequence, the fetal placenta is unable to convert fetal adrenal androgen precursor to estrogen. This autosomal recessive disorder results in hypergonadotropic hypogonadism, multicystic ovaries, and the potential for tall stature after the age of puberty.

TABLE 24-28

CLASSIFICATION OF ANOMALOUS SEXUAL DEVELOPMENT

I. Disorders of gonadal differentiation
   A. Seminiferous tubule dysgenesis (Klinefelter syndrome)
   B. Syndrome of gonadal dysgenesis and its variants (Turner syndrome)
   C. Complete and incomplete forms of XX and XY gonadal dysgenesis
   D. True hermaphroditism

II. Female pseudohermaphroditism
   A. Androgen-induced
      1. Congenital virilizing adrenal hyperplasia
      2. CYP19 (P450arom) aromatase deficiency
      3. Androgens and synthetic progestagens transferred from maternal circulation
   B. Other teratologic factors (non-androgen-induced) associated with malformations of intestine and urinary tract

III. Male pseudohermaphroditism
   A. Testicular unresponsiveness to human chorionic gonadotropin (hCG) and luteinizing hormone (LH) (Leydig cell agenesis or hypoplasia caused by hCG/LH receptor defect)
   B. Inborn errors of testosterone biosynthesis
      1. Enzyme deficits affecting synthesis of both corticosteroids and testosterone (variants of congenital adrenal hyperplasia)
         a. Δ^7-Sterol reductase deficiency (Smith-Lemli-Opitz syndrome)
         b. Deficiency of steroidogenic acute regulatory protein (congenital lipoid adrenal hyperplasia)
         c. 3β-Hydroxysteroid dehydrogenase/ Δ^5 isomerase type II (3βHSD-II) deficiency
         d. CYP17 (P450c17[17α-hydroxylase/17,20 lyase]) deficiency
      2. Enzyme defects primarily affecting testosterone biosynthesis by the testes
         a. CYP17(P450c17[17,20 lyase]) deficiency
         b. 17β-Hydroxysteroid dehydrogenase type III (17βHSD-III) deficiency
   C. Defects in androgen-dependent target tissues
      1. End-organ resistance to androgenic hormones
         a. Syndrome of complete androgen resistance and its variants
         b. Syndrome of incomplete androgen resistance and its variants (Reifenstein syndrome)
         c. Androgen resistance in phenotypically normal boys
      2. Defects in testosterone metabolism by peripheral tissues; 5α-reductase-2 (SRD5A2) deficiency (pseudovaginal perineoscrotal hypospadias)
   D. Dysgenetic male pseudohermaphroditism
      1. XY gonadal dysgenesis (incomplete)
      2. XO/XY mosaicism, structurally abnormal Y chromosome, XP+, 9p−, 10q−
      3. Denys-Drash syndrome (*WT1* mutation)
      4. WAGR syndrome (*WT1* deletion)
      5. Camptomelic dysplasia (*SOX9* mutation)
      6. *SF1* mutation
      7. Testicular regression syndrome
   E. Defects in synthesis, secretion, or response to antimüllerian hormone: persistent müllerian duct syndrome (female genital ducts in otherwise normal men; herniae uteri inguinale)
   F. Maternal ingestion of progestagens
   G. Environmental chemicals

IV. Unclassified forms of abnormal sexual development
   A. Boys
      1. Hypospadias
      2. Ambiguous external genitalia in XY boys with multiple congenital anomalies
   B. Girls: absence or anomalous development of the vagina, uterus, and uterine tubes (Rokitansky-Küster-Hauser syndrome)

PLACENTAL TRANSFER OF ANDROGENS FROM THE MOTHER
In some instances, androgen-induced female pseudohermaphroditism is caused by placental transfer of androgens from the mother. In rare instances, a virilizing ovarian or adrenal tumor in the mother during pregnancy or in the female fetus autosomal recessive mutations in the gene that encodes aromatase partially masculinize the external genitalia of the female fetus. More frequently the maternal source has been therapeutic administration of steroids with androgenic activity during pregnancy. In several instances, testosterone or a testosterone analog has been administered during pregnancy. Comparable examples have been associated with certain oral semisynthetic progestins, such as 17α-ethynyltestosterone (Lutocylol, Pranone, Nugestoral), 17α-ethynyl-19-nortestosterone(Norlutin), norethynodrel (Enovid), and medroxyprogesterone acetate, given

to pregnant women in an effort to control habitual or threatened abortion. This practice is no longer in favor. In rare instances, female pseudohermaphroditism occurs as a consequence of maternal ingestion of danazol, usually for endometriosis. Fusion of the labioscrotal folds and formation of a urogenital sinus occur when androgen has been given before the 13th week of gestation, but enlargement of the clitoris can follow androgen treatment of the mother at any time during pregnancy. In rare instances, diethylstilbestrol, an estrogen, has been suggested as a possible fetal masculinizing agent. Maternal ingestion of stilbestrol and related synthetic estrogens during pregnancy has been associated, among adolescents and young women, with increased risk of clear cell adenocarcinoma of the vagina and cervix and vaginal adenosis. This risk is much lower than initially believed.

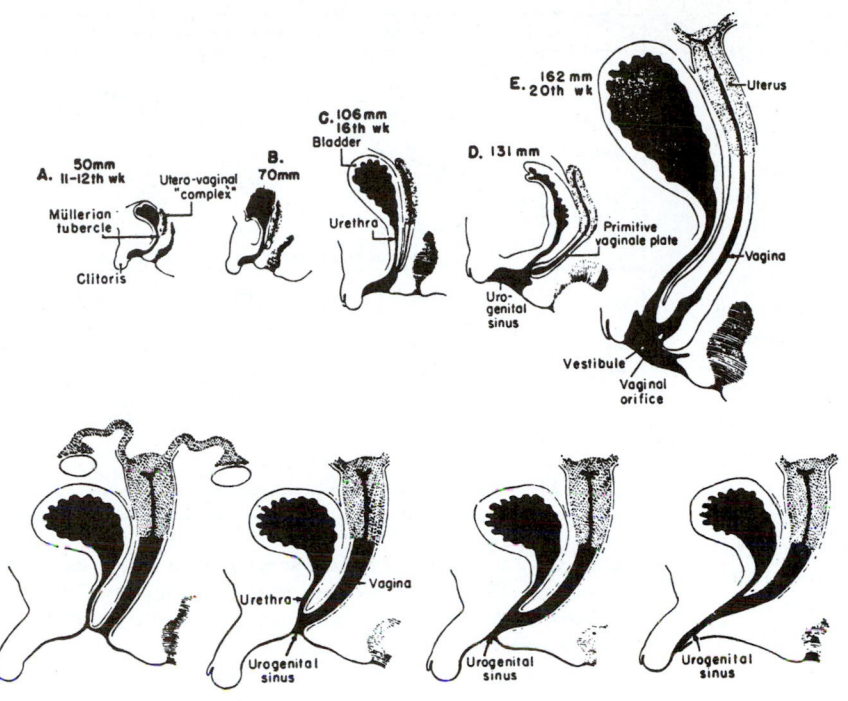

FIGURE 24-22 Development of female pseudohermaphroditism. **Top:** Sequence of differentiation of female accessory sex structures. Gradual descent of uterovaginal complex is evident (adapted from Koff). To modify differentiation of the urogenital sinus, especially the urethral groove, it seems that androgens must act on the female fetus before the 13th week of gestation, although enlargement of the clitoris can be induced at later stages. **Bottom:** Variations in degree of masculinization of urogenital sinus and external genitalia in androgen-induced female pseudohermaphroditism. (SOURCE: *From Grumbach MM, Ducharme JR: The effects of androgens on fetal development: androgen-induced female pseudohermaphrodism. Fertil Steril 11:157, 1960.*)

NON-ANDROGEN-INDUCED

In rare instances, female pseudohermaphroditism is not caused by androgen excess. In these instances, there are usually also developmental anomalies of the urinary tract and cloaca, including atresia of the rectum or rectovaginal fistula. There also may be absence of a fallopian tube or an ovary, and the uterus may be poorly developed. Stenosis of the urethra can cause urinary retention in early infancy.

24.7.3 Male Pseudohermaphroditism

Persons with *male pseudohermaphroditism* have testes, variable degrees of ambisexual development of the genital ducts or the urogenital sinus and external genitalia, or both, and chromatin-negative nuclei (Fig. 24-24). The karyotype is 46,XY, except in some patients with dysgenetic male pseudohermaphroditism. The appearance of the external genitalia varies from that of a normal girl to that of a boy with a penile urethra and either bilateral or unilateral cryptorchidism. Perineal hypospadias is common. The testes may be inside the abdomen, sometimes in the position of ovaries, in the inguinal region, or in the labioscrotal folds.

Male pseudohermaphroditism occurs in a heterogeneous group of disorders that have in common failure of the fetal testis to bring about complete masculinization of the somatic sex structures or impaired end-organ responsiveness to fetal testicular secretions. The classification of disorders in this group of intersexes is shown in Table 24-28. It is convenient to categorize male pseudohermaphroditism with incomplete masculinization because of a defect in testicular differentiation as dysgenetic male pseudohermaphroditism. The gonadal defect usually is caused by an anomaly of the sex chromosomes (eg, XO/XY mosaicism or a structural abnormality of the Y chromosome) or, less frequently, to an X-linked, autosomal or *SRY* mutant gene that causes defective gonadogenesis (XY gonadal dysgenesis). It is in these forms that a variable degree of differentiation of the müllerian ducts occurs. Among

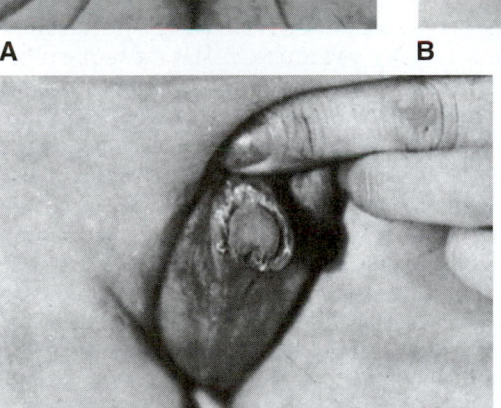

A   **B**

C

FIGURE 24-23   A: External genitalia of a 2-week-old infant with female pseudohermaphroditism and congenital adrenal hyperplasia. Enlarged phallus, bound in chordee, overlies funnel-shaped orifice of urogenital sinus. Labioscrotal folds look like bifid scrotum. B: Enlargement of clitoris without fusion of labioscrotal folds in 4-year-old girl with congenital adrenal hyperplasia. Hypertrophy of clitoris was found at birth. Separate vaginal and urethral orifices were identified by means of inspection. Sparse pubic hair also was present. C: Penile urethra in child with female pseudohermaphroditism at 45 months of age. Child has congenital adrenal hyperplasia.

these and other patients with dysgenetic testes, failure of the internal and external genitalia to undergo full male differentiation correlates well with incomplete testicular differentiation.

Many infants with male pseudohermaphroditism have an XY sex chromosome constitution and normal embryonic differentiation of the testes. Among such patients, defective male development of the somatic sex structures is a consequence of failure of the normally differentiated fetal testis to overcome the inherent tendency to feminize the derivatives of the urogenital sinus and external genitalia. This failure can be caused by insensitivity of the fetal testis to hCG and fetal pituitary LH, by inborn errors in testosterone biosynthesis by the fetal testis, or by failure of the target tissues to respond normally to testosterone stimulation. All of these categories are hereditary disorders caused by a single mutant gene. None involves development of müllerian derivatives (fallopian tubes, uterus). A rare form is caused by mutation of the gene that encodes the müllerian duct inhibitory factor that causes defective synthesis of the müllerian duct inhibitory factor or of its receptor, rendering the müllerian duct unresponsive. Both müllerian duct derivatives (fallopian tubes and uterus) as well as wolffian duct development are found, whereas the external genitalia usually are male. The classification of male pseudohermaphroditism in Table 24-28 is according to this scheme.

RESISTANCE TO HUMAN CHORIONIC GONADOTROPIN AND LUTEINIZING HORMONE (LEYDIG CELL HYPOPLASIA)

Mutations in the gene that encodes the hCG-LH receptor, a G protein–coupled seven-transmembrane α-helical receptor, cause fetal and postnatal testosterone deficiency. The external genitalia vary from female to ambiguous to hypoplastic male. Müllerian derivatives are absent. Plasma levels of 17OHP, androstenedione, and testosterone are low, and stimulation with hCG evokes little or no increase. Basal FSH and LH levels are elevated in infancy and at puberty.

INBORN ERRORS OF TESTOSTERONE BIOSYNTHESIS

Figure 24-7 shows the major pathways in testosterone biosynthesis. Each step is associated with an enzymatic defect inherited as an autosomal recessive trait that causes incomplete masculinization of the urogenital sinus or external genitalia but not differentiation of müllerian duct structures (see Sec. 24.4.2).

Δ^7-STEROL REDUCTASE DEFICIENCY (SMITH-LEMLI-OPITZ SYNDROME) This syndrome of multiple congenital anomalies, including male pseudohermaphroditism, is an inborn error of metabolism caused by autosomal recessive mutation of the gene encoding Δ^7-sterol reductase, a membrane-bound protein involved in cholesterol synthesis. The prevalence is estimated to be 1 in 20,000 to 30,000 persons of northern or central European ancestry. The phenotype is variable and related to the severity of the defect. The defects include growth and mental retardation; hypotonia; ptosis; microcephaly with a high forehead, short nose, and anteverted nostrils; cleft palate; micrognathia; central nervous system, cardiac, and renal malformations; and commonly syndactyly of the second and third toes. Among affected XY persons, the external geintalia vary from female to ambiguous (more than 70% of cases) to isolated hypospadias to normal. Less commonly, evidence of adrenal insufficiency is present with low concentration of sodium in the serum and high concentration of potassium and increased plasma renin

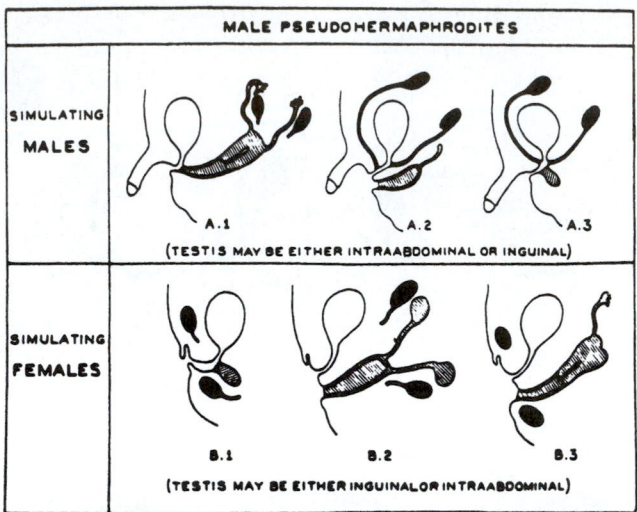

FIGURE 24-24 Common anatomic findings in male pseudohermaphroditism. *Black* structures are testes, derivatives of wolffian ducts. *Cross-hatched* areas include derivatives of müllerian ducts and female urogenital structures.

activity with an inappropriately low level of plasma aldosterone, which may not appear during the first 6 months of life. Cortisol production may be impaired.

The level of cholesterol in the serum is low in more than 90% of patients. The concentration of 7-dehydrocholesterol in the serum is invariably elevated. The diagnosis can be made prenatally with detection of 7-dehydrocholesterol in amniotic fluid or a chorionic villus sample. The concentration of estriol in maternal serum usually is low. Administration of cholesterol by mouth with bile salts can improve growth and behavior but not mental development.

CONGENITAL LIPOID ADRENAL HYPERPLASIA (STEROIDOGENIC ACUTE REGULATORY DEFICIENCY, MALE PSEUDOHERMAPHRODITISM, SEXUAL INFANTILISM, ADRENAL INSUFFICIENCY) This defect in the conversion of cholesterol to pregnenolone is discussed in Sec. 24.4.6. The patients have enormous accumulations of lipid in the cells of the adrenal cortex but surprisingly not in the gonads, severe adrenal insufficiency, and death in early infancy if not treated. Boys have pseudohermaphroditism, including a blind vaginal pouch, undescended testes, and with a severe defect, female external genitalia. The enlarged adrenal glands displace the kidneys caudally. Girls have a normal phenotype but also have life-threatening salt loss and cortisol deficiency. Girls feminize normally at puberty because lipids have not accumulated and destroyed the cells before pubertal secretion of gonadotropins.

3β-HYDROXYSTEROID DEHYDROGENASE TYPE II DEFICIENCY (MALE PSEUDOHERMAPHRODITISM AND ADRENAL INSUFFICIENCY) This is a rare form of adrenal hyperplasia in which salt loss is caused by aldosterone deficiency and there is a defect in cortisol and sex steroid secretion as a consequence of mutations in the gene encoding 3βHSD-II on chromosome 9. It is transmitted as an autosomal recessive trait. Boys are incompletely masculinized. High levels of 17-ketosteroids in the urine associated with elevated urinary and plasma levels of DHEA, 17-hydroxy-Δ^5-pregnenolone, and other 3β-hydroxysteroids confirm the diagnosis. In the less severe form, salt loss is not manifested clinically.

17α-HYDROXYLASE (P450c17) DEFICIENCY (MALE PSEUDOHER-MAPHRODITISM, SEXUAL INFANTILISM, HYPERTENSION, AND HYPOKALEMIC ALKALOSIS) Patients with this disorder have impaired synthesis of 17OHP and 17α-hydroxypregnenolone and their products (androgens, estrogens, and cortisol) caused by an autosomal-recessive mutant gene. A single gene, P450c17, located on chromosome 10, encodes both the adrenal and testicular enzyme that catalyzes 17-hydroxylation of pregnenolone and progesterone and removal of the C21 side chain of 17-hydroxypregnenolone (C17-20-lyase) to form C19 steroid DHEA. Increased secretion of corticosterone and deoxycorticosterone causes hypokalemic alkalosis and low-renin hypertension. Plasma concentration of gonadal steroids and excretion of urinary 17-ketosteroids are low. Affected boys are incompletely masculinized and may appear to be phenotypic girls.

ERRORS PRIMARILY AFFECTING TESTOSTERONE SYNTHESIS

17,20-LYASE (P450c17) DEFICIENCY These patients have ambiguous external genitalia and inguinal or intraabdominal testes because of mutations in the P450c17 gene that cause deficient 17,20 lyase function of the single P450c17 enzyme with little involvement of the 17α-hydroxylase reaction. At puberty, incomplete masculinization can occur. Gynecomastia has not been described. If the disorder is diagnosed in infancy, these patients can be reared as boys and treated with testosterone to induce male secondary characteristics and phallic growth. Plasma levels of testosterone, androstenedione, estradiol, and DHEA are low. After stimulation with hCG, the ratio of C21 steroids (cortisol, 17OHP) to C19 steroids increases. Among prepubertal children with male pseudohermaphroditism, 17,20 lyase deficiency must be differentiated from 5α-reductase-2 deficiency and from 17βHSD-III deficiency.

17β-HYDROXYSTEROID OXIDOREDUCTASE TYPE 3 (17β-HYDROXYSTEROID DEHYDROGENASE 17-KETOREDUCTASE) DEFECT This autosomal recessive genetic defect in testosterone biosynthesis is caused by mutations in the gene encoding 17β-hydroxysteroid oxidoreductase type 3. Patients have female or ambiguous external genitalia, inguinal testes, male genital duct development, and progressive virilization at puberty, usually with concomitant breast development. The type 3 isozyme, the last enzyme in the biosynthetic pathway for testosterone, is expressed primarily in the testis. Levels of androstenedione and estrone are strikingly elevated because their conversion to testosterone and estradiol is impaired. The usual testosterone to androstenedione ratio is reversed in peripheral and spermatic vein blood at puberty and among prepubertal patients stimulated with hCG gonadotropin. These patients must be differentiated from those with incomplete androgen resistance syndrome or 5α-reductase 2 deficiency, who have a similar phenotype but not a similar sex steroid pattern.

DEFECTS IN ANDROGEN-DEPENDENT TARGET TISSUES

Abnormalities in the action of testosterone are caused by various degrees of resistance to the action of testosterone in fetal and postnatal life. The resistance is caused by a heritable defect in the androgen receptor or its activation of intracellular events or by a familial deficiency of 5α-reductase that causes defective conversion of testosterone to dihydrotestosterone in peripheral tissues.

SYNDROME OF COMPLETE ANDROGEN RESISTANCE AND ITS VARIANTS (TESTICULAR FEMINIZATION) This syndrome is a common and well-defined form of male pseudohermaphroditism. These patients are genetically male. Their sex chromosome constitution is XY. They have testes that usually are in the inguinal canal or in the labial folds. Because these patients have a normal female appearance, the diagnosis often is not suspected. The occurrence of multiple examples within a family is frequent, and family pedigrees show X-linked inheritance consistent with the location of the gene on Xq11-12. The external genitalia are female in configuration. In some instances the clitoris is slightly enlarged and the labioscrotal folds are partially fused. There is a characteristic blind vaginal pouch, absent müllerian duct derivatives, and absent or hypoplastic wolffian ducts. Development of the genital ducts is variable, but the uterus is absent. At puberty, estrogenic steroids secreted by the testes bring about feminization of body habitus, development of breasts, and estrogenization of the vaginal mucosa despite elevated testosterone levels, but menstruation does not occur. The testes secrete testosterone, and at puberty the concentration of plasma testosterone usually is within the normal range for boys. However, both genital and somatic end organs do not respond to androgens in the fetus or at puberty, which leads to female differentiation of the urogenital sinus and external genitalia and to feminization at puberty. The hypothalamic feedback mechanism lacks normal sensitivity to testosterone, which elevates serum levels of LH but concentration of FSH in the serum usually is normal. Castration causes a decrease in plasma levels of estradiol and testosterone, an increase in both FSH and LH levels, and menopausal symptoms. Among most patients, pubic and axillary hair are absent or sparse, a manifestation of the impaired response to androgen of the hair follicles that give rise to sexual hair. In the classic form of the syndrome, large amounts of testosterone or dihydrotestosterone do not induce either masculinization or an appropriate degree of protein anabolism.

The underlying defect is a mutation in the androgen receptor, a ligand-regulated transcription factor that binds both dihydrotestosterone and testosterone (Fig. 24-25). The androgen receptor is a typical zinc-finger DNA-activating protein similar to the receptors for other steroids, vitamin D, thyroid hormone, and retinoic acid (see Sec. 24.1). The androgen receptor, like other members of this family, has three major, highly conserved regions: (1) the amino terminal end of the receptor is essential for transcriptional activation; (2) the cysteine-rich DNA-binding domain with two zinc fingers (transcriptional enhancer nucleotide sequences); and (3) the androgen (or ligand) binding domain is in the carboxyterminal portion of the protein. A wide range of mutations of the androgen receptor gene affect the steroid-binding, transcription-activating, and DNA-binding functions of the androgen receptor.

The discovery of a testis in an inguinal or labial hernia usually is the only clue to the diagnosis in the absence of a familial history. Affected infants have a high-normal to modestly elevated concentration of testosterone in the plasma for age and male genetic sex. The diagnosis is considered when an adolescent girl has primary amenorrhea (it is the third most common cause after gonadal dysgenesis and congenital absence of the vagina) in the presence of otherwise female secondary sexual characteristics (including breast development), especially when associated with absent or sparse sexual hair and unilateral or bilateral hernial masses. There is a propensity for the testes to undergo neoplastic transformation. Orchiectomy is recommended by late adolescence, and it is followed by estrogen replacement therapy.

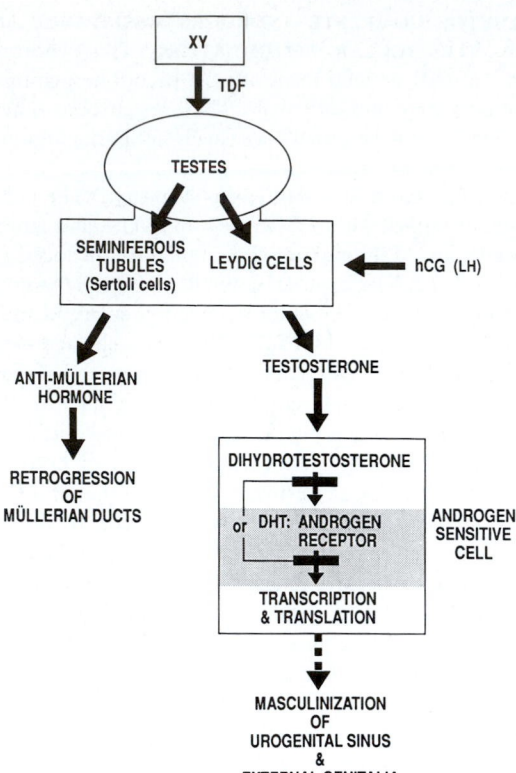

FIGURE 24-25 Pathogenesis of male pseudohermaphroditism caused by end-organ resistance to androgen (mutations in the gene encoding the androgen receptor). TDF = testis determining factor (*SRY*).

INCOMPLETE VARIANTS Some patients with androgen resistance and a pattern of X-linked inheritance have distinct clinical findings. These patients, although they have breast development at puberty, undergo variable degrees of masculinization. There is clitoral enlargement at birth, and some patients have ambiguous external genitalia. They usually show partial resistance to testosterone. The gene mutation encodes a defective but partially functional androgen receptor. Phenotypic boys with infertility as the sole manifestation of a deficiency of androgen receptors have been described. They represent one extreme of the highly variable phenotype of androgen resistance.

MALE PSEUDOHERMAPHRODITISM WITH NORMAL VIRILIZATION AT PUBERTY The preceding categories of male pseudohermaphroditism can be attributed to defective androgen biosynthesis or defective end-organ response, but there are other familial forms of male pseudohermaphroditism in which virilization occurs at puberty. In these patients, secretion of testosterone is normal or elevated. The karyotype is uniformly XY, and only male genital ducts are present. As with other forms of male pseudohermaphroditism, these forms encompass the full spectrum of external sexual ambiguity, extending from persons with only mild hypospadias and a normal-sized phallus to persons more closely resembling girls. They have minimal clitoral enlargement and incomplete masculinization of the urogenital sinus. One form has been well defined—a target cell defect in 5α-reductase type 2. Other forms may be related to differences in site and degree of an end-organ defect in the action of androgen.

5α-REDUCTASE TYPE 2 DEFICIENCY (PSEUDOVAGINAL PERINEOSCROTAL HYPOSPADIAS) Patients with this syndrome have an XY karyotype, normally differentiated testes, male internal genital ducts, and ambiguous external genitalia. At birth, the phallus usually is small and hypospadiac. There is persistence of the urogenital sinus with a blind vaginal pouch. In severe disease, separate vaginal and urethral orifices are present. These patients have a deficiency of 5α-reductase 2 at the target cell and impaired enzymatic transformation of testosterone to its active hormone (dihydrotestosterone) at these end organs. The disorder is autosomal recessive and caused by mutations in the 5α-reductase type 2 gene on chromosome 2. At puberty, these patients masculinize, and the phallus enlarges. There also is growth of axillary and pubic hair, and many children have male sex identity. The striking masculinization at puberty is attributable, at least in part, to the expression of the type 1 enzyme expressed at puberty but not in the fetus. Acne, facial hair, and temporal recession of the hairline are minimal or absent. Unlike patients with androgen receptor defects, these patients do not have gynecomastia. The findings suggest that male differentiation of the urogenital sinus and external genitalia requires the more potent androgen dihydrotestosterone and not testosterone, whereas differentiation of male genital ducts is mediated primarily by its precursor, testosterone. The diagnosis is suggested by the finding of an abnormally high plasma testosterone to dihydrotestosterone ratio after administration of hCG (1000 IU every other day twice). It is confirmed with an assay of 5α-reductase in cultures of skin fibroblasts, detection of an increased 5β/5α ratio of urinary C19 and C21 steroid metabolites, and with molecular genetic studies of the 5α-reductase type 2 gene. Early diagnosis is critical because selection of male gender assignment necessitates testosterone or dihydrotestosterone therapy to induce growth of the phallus. Repair of hypospadias is performed in early childhood.

DYSGENETIC MALE PSEUDOHERMAPHRODITISM

Defective testicular organogenesis results in ambiguous development of the genital ducts, urogenital sinus, and external genitalia. A heterogeneous group of disorders, including 45,X/46,XY mosaicism, structural abnormalities of the Y chromosome, and the sporadic and heritable forms of XY gonadal dysgenesis manifest defective gonadogenesis and masculinization.

MALE PSEUDOHERMAPHRODITISM AS VARIANT OF GONADAL DYSGENESIS A highly diverse phenotype has been described among patients with XO/XY mosaicism or structural abnormality of the Y chromosome. The appearance can range from a sexually infantile female phenotype with or without the somatic anomalies of Turner syndrome and with bilateral streak gonads, through variable degrees of masculine differentiation of the external genitalia, urogenital sinus, and genital ducts, to almost normal male differentiation of the genital tract. Some patients have a dysgenetic testis on one side and a streak gonad on the other. Short stature and the somatic anomalies of Turner syndrome are inconstant features. The dysgenetic testes must be removed because of the increased tendency toward development of malignant tumors.

INCOMPLETE FORM OF FAMILIAL XY GONADAL DYSGENESIS These XY patients are of normal stature and do not have the components of Turner syndrome. The testes are dysgenetic, and there are usually both müllerian and wolffian duct derivatives. The external genitalia are ambiguous. The gonads have variable degrees of dysgenetic testicular differentiation, and some virilization occurs at puberty. Gonadotropin levels are elevated. The defective testes are removed because of the risk of neoplastic transformation. These patients have variants of familial XY gonadal dysgenesis, which is transmitted as an X-linked recessive or sex-limited autosomal dominant trait, or they harbor a mutant *SRY* gene. Both the complete form, which has a female phenotype, and the incomplete form can occur in the same pedigree.

ASSOCIATED WITH DEGENERATIVE RENAL DISEASE   One form of dysgenetic male pseudohermaphroditism, *Denys-Drash syndrome,* is associated with degenerative renal disease (nephrotic syndrome, interstitial nephritis, or end-stage failure) and hypertension and commonly with Wilms tumor at a median age of 18 months. Both the testes and the kidneys are dysgenetic and predisposed to malignant transformation. A second form, *Fraser syndrome,* in addition to female or ambiguous external genitalia manifests as later-onset nephropathy (focal segmental glomerulosclerosis) and a predisposition for gonadoblastoma but not Wilms tumor. In Wilms tumor–aniridia–gonadoblastoma–mental retardation (WAGR) contiguous gene deletion (WT1) syndrome, affected boys often have ambiguous or hypoplastic male genitalia. All three syndromes are caused by mutations of the Wilms tumor suppressor gene (WT1).

ASSOCIATED AUTOSOMAL MUTATIONS IN THE SOX-9 OR STEROIDOGENIC FACTOR-1 (SF1) GENE   Heterozygous mutations in the *SOX*-9 (*SRY*-related high-mobility group box) gene are associated with a severe bone dysmorphology syndrome, camptomelic dysplasia, and frequently dysgenetic male pseudohermaphroditism. A heterozygous mutation is present in the gene encoding steroidogenic factor-1, an orphan nuclear receptor involved in regulation of gonadal and adrenal organogenesis and genes encoding StAR and steroidogenic enzymes. An XY phenotypic female patient has had primary adrenal insufficiency in the first weeks of life. At laparotomy bilateral dysgenetic testes with normal development of the uterus and fallopian tubes were present without woffian derivatives.

PERSISTENT MÜLLERIAN DUCT SYNDROME   Patients with this syndrome have normal male development of the external genitalia, testes, normal male ducts, and müllerian duct derivatives. The diagnosis often is made by the finding of a fallopian tube and uterus in a patient undergoing inguinal hernia repair, orchiopexy, or abdominal surgery. The disorder is inherited as a sex-limited autosomal-recessive trait and is caused by mutations in the gene encoding the antimüllerian hormone or its receptor.

UNCLASSIFIED FORMS OF ABNORMAL SEX DIFFERENTIATION

Some abnormalities of sex differentiation have not been well defined. For example, ambiguous external genitalia are associated with malformation syndromes such as Aarskog-Scott, Opitz, CHARGE, and VATER syndromes (see Sec. 10.3). Finasteride, an inhibitor of 5α-reductase type 2, used cosmetically as therapy for hair loss, causes male pseudohermaphroditism when given to pregnant rodents and monkeys in high doses.

24.7.4   True Hermaphroditism

Persons who have both an ovary and a testis or, more commonly, in whom one or both gonads are ovotestes have *true hermaphro-*

ditism. More than 350 patients have been described, including several affected sets of siblings, in which a single gene mutation may be the cause. The sex chromatin pattern can be negative or positive; the chromatin-positive pattern predominates. Development of the accessory sexual structures is highly variable. Three-fourths of these patients have been reared as boys, but they have variable degrees of hypospadias. Cryptorchidism and inguinal hernia that contains a gonad or vestigial uterus and fallopian tube are present in 50% of patients. Predominantly masculine or feminine maturation occurs at puberty. Most patients do not have a sex chromosome abnormality. In about 70% of patients, an XX sex chromosome constitution is found. About 20% are sex chromosome mosaics or chimerics, such as XX/XY, and about 10% are XY. Only a small proportion of children with XX true hermaphroditism, including some in pedigrees with XX boys, are *SRY* positive. The pathogenesis of most cases of XX true hemaphroditism cannot be explained with a Y to X or Y to autosome translocation or with hidden sex chromosome mosaicism or chimerism. The XX/XY chimerism is caused by double fertilization of a binucleate ovum or by fusion of two independently fertilized zygotes. Some of these patients are potentially fertile. When possible, the sex of rearing is chosen, and an attempt is made to preserve the appropriate gonad or gonadal segment, especially if an ovary is present in the mesosalpinx or a testis is attached to its exocrine ducts in the scrotum. There is, however, an increased risk of gonadal neoplasia.

24.7.5   Syndrome of Gonadal Dysgenesis and Variants

TURNER SYNDROME

The syndrome of gonadal dysgenesis (*Turner syndrome, gonadal dysplasia, ovarian agenesis, Bonnevie-Ullrich syndrome*) is characterized by female phenotype, short stature, sexual infantilism, streak gonads, and a diversity of associated somatic anomalies (Fig. 24-26). These features are caused by haploinsufficiency of the X chromosome (45,X karyotype). The most common associated congenital malformations include atypical facies, broad shield-like chest, low hairline over the nape of the neck, webbed neck (in about 30%), congenital lymphedema of the extremities, especially the hands and feet (30%), coarctation of the aorta (20%), hypertension, bicuspid aortic valve (unassociated with coarctation), short fourth metacarpal (50%), high arched palate, a variety of skeletal anomalies including cubitus valgus and Madelung (or bayonet) deformity of the wrist, hypoplastic and malformed nails, microthelia, and cutaneous (pigmented nevi and predisposition to keloid formation), ocular, otitic (tendency for recurrent otitis media, perceptible hearing loss), and renal (most commonly horseshoe kidney) abnormalities (50%). Renal ultrasonography is performed to detect a surgically correctable renal anomaly. Deficits of space-form recognition and directional sense are common despite a normal intelligence quotient. Skeletal maturation is normal or mildly delayed before puberty. Diminished mineralization of the hands, feet, and elbows is common.

The habitus is typical. It consists of a short stocky build; shield-like chest; short neck; prominent, low-set ears; and small mandible. Increased numbers of pigmented nevi are common. No true gonad is present. In each mesosalpinx is a ridge of connective tissue devoid of any germinal elements. Persons with Turner syndrome have none of the secondary sexual characteristics caused by secretion of estro-

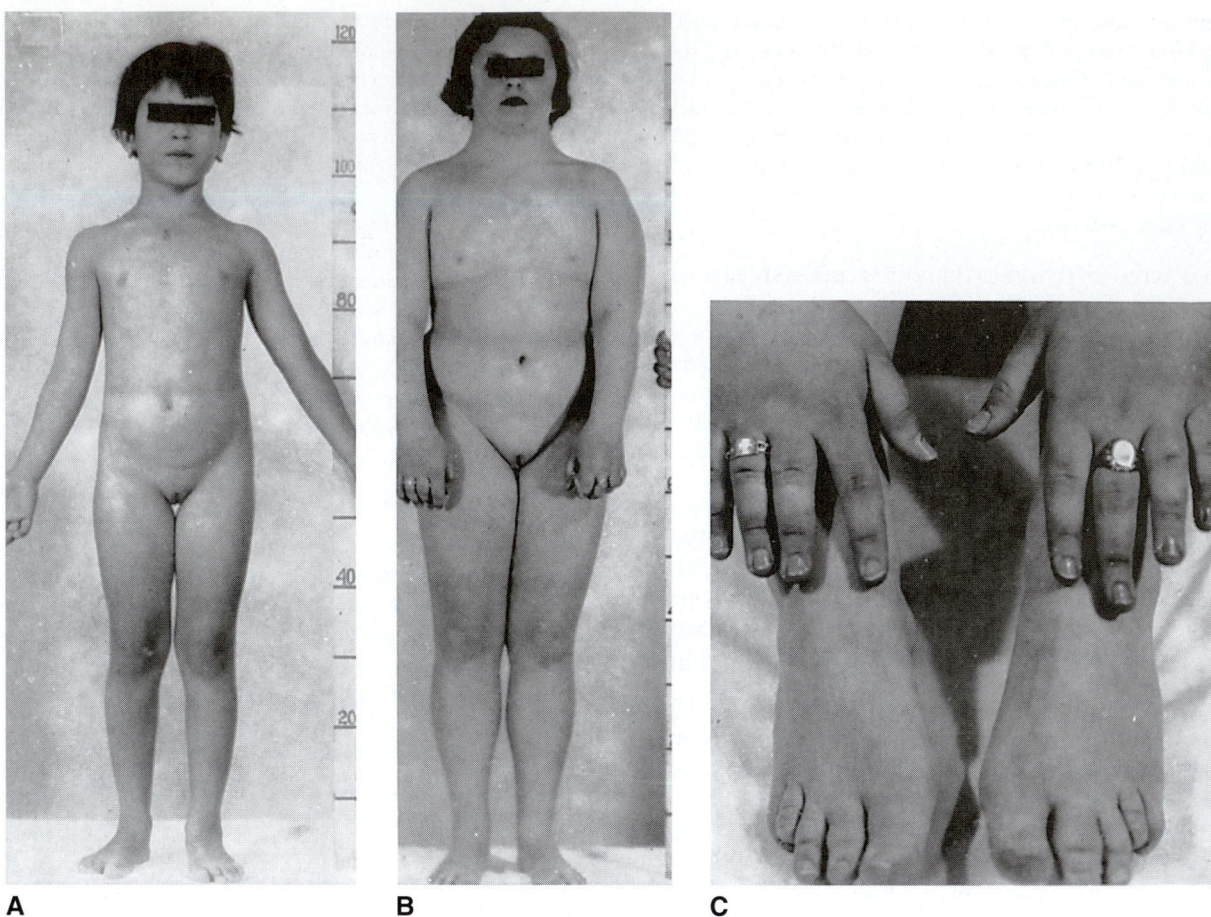

A   **B**   **C**

FIGURE 24-26 Two patients with syndrome of gonadal dysgenesis (Turner syndrome), chromatin-negative somatic nuclei, and 45,XX karyotype. **A.** Age 9 years. Short stature was presenting problem. **B.** Age 15 years. Classic aspect of Turner syndrome. **C.** Hands and feet of patient in **B** show useful clinical signs of conspicuous shortening of fourth digits caused by underdevelopment of metacarpals and metatarsals, puffiness over dorsum of digits between interphalangeal joints, convexity of nails, and prominence of pulp of finger beyond tip of fingernail.

gen at puberty, but unlike hypopituitary dwarfs, they do have sexual hair. In rare instances, some degree of feminization occurs at puberty, and some patients have been fertile. The mean mature height is 143 cm (range 133 to 153 cm). Associated disorders include Hashimoto thyroiditis, aortic rupture, osteopenia, obesity, inflammatory bowel disease, and rheumatoid arthritis. During adolescence serum concentrations of FSH and LH and excretion of urinary gonadotropins increase to castrated levels. Elevated levels of FSH in the serum frequently are detected in infancy and early childhood but not between approximately 4 and 10 years of age (see Sec. 24.8). In 45,X patients, ovaries are absent, and streak gonads can be detected with pelvic sonography or coronal MR imaging. The characteristics of the syndrome, especially lymphedema and loose folds of skin around the nape of the neck (Bonnevie-Ullrich syndrome), suggest the diagnosis as early as the neonatal period (Fig. 24-27). Pleural effusion can occur among newborns.

Intrauterine growth retardation is common; the mean birth weight and lenth are 1 SD below the value for healthy infants of comparable gestational age. Maternal age is not advanced. There is increased prevalence of twinning, but familial instances are exceedingly rare. About 7% of spontaneous abortions have a 45,X karyotype. It is estimated that about 2% of all zygotes are XO, but less

than 0.2% of 45,X fetuses survive to term. The infant mortality rate is high. The frequency of 45,X phenotypic gonadal dysgenesis among girls in surveys of newborn nurseries is 0.1 to 0.6 per 1000.

Other sex chromosome abnormalities have been described, all of which represent a less than complete absence of a second sex chromosome. The variable deficiency of the sex chromosome is associated with a highly diverse modification of the classic 45,X phenotype. These clinical variants of the syndrome of gonadal dysgenesis occur among patients with sex chromosome mosaicism involving an XO cell line (such as XO/XX, XO/XX/XXX, and XO/XY mosaicism) or a structural abnormality of an X or Y chromosome such as a long arm isochromosome X (XXqi), an X or Y chromosome deletion, or a ring X or Y chromosome. Structural abnormalities of the sex chromosomes are commonly associated with XO mosaicism owing to loss of the heteromorphic chromosome from some cells, such as XO/XXqi, XO/X ring X.

Sex chromosome mosaicism involving an XO cell line and structural abnormalities of the X or Y chromosome usually modify phenotypic expression of the classic form of the syndrome of gonadal dysgenesis associated with an XO karyotype. The modifications of the typical Turner phenotype in the variant forms of the syndrome are toward a more normal phenotype, and that can involve all or

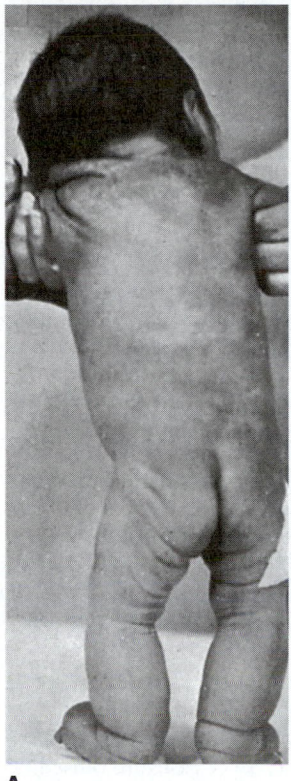
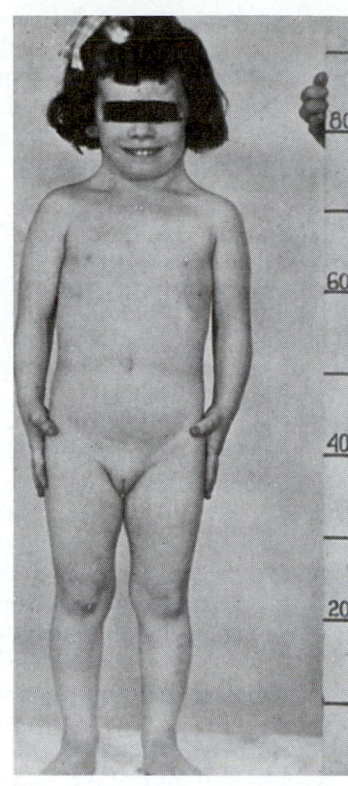

A   **B**

FIGURE 24-27   Patient with syndrome of 45,X gonadal dysgenesis and features of Bonnevie-Ullrich syndrome. A. Appearance at 7 days of age is massive edema of distal parts of lower extremities, webbed neck, puffiness of hands, and loose folds of skin over nape of neck. Dressing covers site of skin biopsy. B. At 4 years of age, patient has webbed neck, broad chest and microthelia. (SOURCE: *From Grumbach MM, Barr: Recent Prog Horm Res 14:255, 1958.*)

any of the following aspects of the disorder: gonadal differentiation and function, stature, and associated somatic stigmata. Patients with XO/XX or XO/XX/XXX mosaicism can achieve normal stature and a variable degree of ovarian function, including ovulation and fertility. The associated somatic anomalies can be absent or minimal. Among other persons with the same type of mosaicism, the phenotype cannot be differentiated from that of a 45,X person.

XO/XY mosaicism is associated with a diverse phenotype (see earlier). The karyotype can be associated with a variable degree of testicular differentiation, in some cases causing ambisexual development of the external genitalia and in others almost normal male phenotype.

Therapy is directed at maximizing final height and correcting remediable congenital anomalies and sexual infantilism. Preliminary results of treatment with subcutaneous daily injections of human GH suggest a mean gain in final height of 9 cm after 3 to 7 years of therapy. Among phenotypic girls with elevated urinary levels of gonadotropin, treatment with low-dosage estrogen (eg, 0.3 mg conjugated estrogen or less or 5 μg ethinyl estradiol daily) is initiated at approximately 13 years of age, continues for 6 months, and then is administered cyclically for 3 of 4 weeks to bring about the development of feminine secondary sexual characteristics and estrogen-withdrawal bleeding. The dose of estrogen should be increased gradually with the aim of administering the minimum dose to maintain secondary sex characteristics and menses and hinder development of involutional osteoporosis. It is useful to administer

an oral progestin (eg, medroxyprogesterone acetate, 5 mg daily) during the last 10 days of estrogen therapy. Gonadectomy is recommended in XO/XY and related forms of mosaicism because of the increased risk of gonadal neoplasm in the presence of a Y chromosome. Counseling of the patient throughout childhood and adolescence, and of the parents, is a vital part of treatment. Advances in in vitro fertilization and embryo transplantation have made childbearing a possibility.

XY GONADAL DYSGENESIS

The term *XY gonadal dysgenesis* has been used to describe a female phenotype with an XY karyotype, streak gonads, sexual infantilism, normal or tall stature, and lack of the somatic components of Turner syndrome. The prevalence of gonadal neoplasms such as seminoma and gonadoblastoma is greatly increased. Familial occurrence is common. In some sets of siblings, an affected sibling has had male pseudohermaphroditism with dysgenetic testes and ambiguous external genitalia. The reported pedigrees suggest X-linked recessive or sex-limited autosomal-dominant inheritance. A duplication of the *DAX1* gene in chromosome Xp21 is suspected in some familial cases. About 10 to 15% of patients have a deletion or mutation in the *SRY* gene on the short arm of the Y chromosome.

FAMILIAL XX GONADAL DYSGENESIS

These are children with a female phenotype who have normal stature, sexual infantilism, bilateral streak gonads, normal female external and internal genitalia, primary amenorrhea, elevated levels of gonadotropins, low values of serum and urinary estrogens, and XX karyotypes. The habitus often is eunuchoid, and the somatic anomalies associated with XO gonadal dysgenesis are absent or minimal. Families in which multiple siblings are affected are not uncommon, and the transmission is consistent with autosomal-recessive inheritance. In some families, the gonadal defect is associated with sensorineural deafness. The disorder rarely is recognized before puberty.

XX AND XY TURNER PHENOTYPE (NOONAN SYNDROME)

Among the group of children with a male phenotype and features of so-called *male Turner syndrome,* a distinctive entity with a prevalence of about 1 in 2000 live births has been described. This has led to recognition of its counterpart among girls and its differentiation from the syndrome of gonadal dysgenesis. These patients often have characteristic facies—ptosis; antimongoloid palpebral slant; broad, flat nose; webbed neck; short stature; high arched palate; and malformed ears (Fig. 24-28). Congenital heart disease (most commonly atrial septal defect or pulmonic stenosis but rarely coarctation of the aorta) is a cardinal but not invariable feature. An electrocardiogram frequently shows left axis deviation. Hypertrophic cardiomyopathy, sometimes with subaortic or subpulmonic stenosis, is common. Pectus excavatum, cubitus valgus, and impaired mental development are frequent associated findings. In boys, one or both testes may be undescended. Some boys have germinal cell aplasia, hypoplasia of the testis, and evidence of androgen deficiency. Girls have functioning ovaries. In both sexes the karyotype is normal, and gonadal differentiation is consistent with the chromosomal and phenotypic sex. Familial examples of autosomal-dominant transmission have been described.

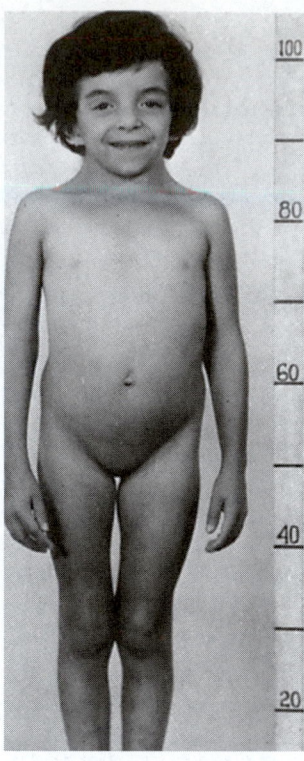

FIGURE 24-28   Phenotypic 8-year-old girl with syndrome of webbed neck, ptosis, congenital heart disease (pulmonary stenosis and atrial septal defect), short stature, triangular facies, prominent brow, hypertelorism, antimongoloid slant of palpebral fissures, broad apex nasi, low-set ears, and pectus excavatum (Noonan syndrome); 46,XX karyotype. (SOURCE: *From Grumbach MM, Barr: Recent Prog Horm Res 14:255, 1958.*)

24.7.6   Dysgenesis of the Seminiferous Tubules (Klinefelter Syndrome)

The most common human sex chromosomal aberration, a 47,XXY karyotype, is associated with dysgenesis of the seminiferous tubules (*Klinefelter syndrome*). This disorder, a common cause of primary hypogonadism and infertility among men, is characterized by male phenotype, by small, firm, defective testes (less than 3.0 cm long), and among adults by azoospermia and sterility. During or after puberty the variable features of gynecomastia and androgen deficiency with signs of eunuchoidism are present among about one-half of patients. The concentration of FSH and LH in the serum is elevated after 12 to 13 years of age. Testosterone concentrations are normal or low, whereas the concentration of plasma estradiol is normal or high. Cryptorchidism is infrequent. These patients tend to grow tall (mean adult height at the 75th percentile). The characteristic feature is disproportionately long legs, which may be detected before puberty. Epiphyseal fusion usually is not delayed, and osseous development follows the male pattern. The diagnosis is suspected when a long-legged adolescent boy has small, firm testes, gynecomastia, and poorly developed male secondary sex characteristics. Most XXY boys need help in reading and spelling. Mean IQ is between 85 and 99, but there is wide variation. Severe mental retardation is rare. Poor motor skills and delayed emotional development are common, but most patients do not have behavioral disorders. As a group, men with Klinefelter syndrome are little different from other men with hypogonadism in terms of education,

employment, socioeconomic status, social adjustment, and criminal behavior. The prevalence of germ cell neoplasms, especially in the mediastinum, is high. These tumors can secrete hCG and cause sexual precocity with prepubertal-sized testes. About 20% of male patients with primary mediastinal germ cell tumors have Klinefelter syndrome. Down syndrome and, among adults, chronic pulmonary disease, varicose veins, and mild diabetes mellitus also occur with increased frequency in this disorder. Carcinoma of the breast is 20 times more frequent than among other men.

In surveys of newborn infants, the 47,XXY abnormality has a frequency of 0.9 in 1000, and 0.15 in 1000 are XY/XXY mosaics. About 50% of XXY fetuses die in utero. Because the XY cell line can have a beneficial effect, some persons with XY/XXY mosaicism are potentially fertile.

The histopathologic features of the testis vary. Among XXY infants, testicular structure can be normal, but the prepubertal testis has a diminished number of germ cells. With the onset of puberty, and associated with the action of pituitary gonadotropins, the characteristic testicular defect is evident: hyalinization and atrophy of seminiferous tubules, absence of peritubular elastic tissue, aggregation and pseudoadenomatous groupings of Leydig cells, and occasional tubules lined by Sertoli cells. In rare instances, spermatogenesis occurs in isolated tubules.

The typical sex chromosome aberration is 47,XXY. Forty-two percent of male XXY arise from meiotic nondisjunction during oogenesis. In 53% of cases the nondisjunction occurs during spermatogenesis at the first meiotic division; 5% of cases are caused by mitotic nondisjunction in an early division of the fertilized zygote.

Other sex chromosome anomalies are less common in this disorder. These include XX/XXY and XY/XXY mosaicism, XX karyotype, and XXXY sex chromosome complex. In the last form, radioulnar synostosis is a useful clinical sign. The XY cell line can have an ameliorating effect, and some patients with this form of mosaicism have been fertile. About 90% of 46,XX boys have a Y to X translocation, which includes the gene on the short arm of the Y critical for testis determination; 10% have hypospadias or ambiguous external genitalia. Additional clinical features are characteristic of certain variants of the XXY karyotype. For example, XXYY persons, as a group, are taller and more long-legged than XXY patients, and quite consistent dermatoglyphic patterns have been described. Most of these patients have severe mental retardation.

The testicular lesion in Klinefelter syndrome is irreversible. Androgen deficiency can be managed at adolescence to enhance secondary sex characteristics and potential and to improve general well-being. Therapy is initiated with a long-acting repository preparation such as testosterone enanthate in oil, 50 to 100 mg intramuscularly every 4 weeks and gradually increased to the adult dose of 200 mg every 2 weeks. Testosterone therapy can decrease gynecomastia. Once gynecomastia is advanced, it is rarely affected by hormonal treatment, and reduction mammoplasty may be necessary for psychological and cosmetic reasons. Early diagnosis and appropriate counseling improve the prognosis.

24.7.7   Diagnosis and Management of Abnormalities of Sex Differentiation

DIAGNOSIS

Among infants with ambisexual development, it is of greatest importance to establish a diagnosis as soon after birth as possible, not only for psychological and social reasons but also because of the dangers inherent in failure to recognize the salt-losing form of congenital adrenal hyperplasia. Table 24-29 lists the features that should alert the physician to consider an anomaly of sex.

Ambiguous or incomplete masculinization of the external genitalia is a cardinal feature of intersexuality, and this diagnosis must be excluded before such an infant is considered to have male cryptorchidism and hypospadias. The appearance of the external genitalia can be highly variable; in some instances the phallus resembles a large clitoris. Usually, however, there is some fusion of the labioscrotal folds and only a single perineal orifice. The presence of a palpable gonad in a labioscrotal fold or in the groin is a strong point against the diagnosis of female pseudohermaphroditism. As indicated in Table 24-28, the appearance of the external genitalia in some forms of intersexuality is not ambiguous. Among children with male pseudohermaphroditism and complete androgen resistance syndrome, the external genital structures are female (see Fig. 24-24). Children with female pseudohermaphroditism in which the orifice of the urogenital sinus is located at or close to the tip of the phallus (see Fig. 24-23), have the appearance of boys with cryptorchidism. Klinefelter syndrome, XXY syndrome, and Turner syndrome are not associated with anomalous development of the external genitalia. The diagnosis of the syndrome of complete androgen resistance or insensitivity is suspected when an infant has the female phenotype and a firm mass in the inguinal region or labium majus. If a previous sibling or a relative has an abnormality of sex differentiation, the external genitalia of a newborn infant are examined with special care. Additional tests are performed even if the external genitalia are normal, depending on the nature of the disorder in the affected person. Phenotypic female infants with prominent edema of the hands and feet and loose folds of skin over the nape of the neck may have the syndrome of gonadal dysgenesis (Bonnevie-Ullrich syndrome). Figure 24-29 summarizes the diagnostic procedures of value in the differential diagnosis of ambiguous external genitalia or other causes of abnormality of sex.

Female pseudohermaphroditism must be differentiated from other forms of intersexuality in which there is bilateral cryptorchidism. The configuration of the external genitalia is not distinctive. The history may reveal other siblings with congenital virilizing adrenal hyperplasia, signs of progressive virilization, or dehydration, vomiting, collapse suggestive of an addisonian-like electrolyte disorder, or perinatal death. The mother and obstetrician are asked about hormones administered during pregnancy.

Detection of a 46,XX karyotype quickly limits the diagnostic possibilities to female pseudohermaphroditism or to true hermaphroditism with undescended gonads. In virilizing adrenal hyperpla-

sia, in which there is a defect in 21-hydroxylation, concentration of 17OHP in the plasma is strikingly elevated (see Sec. 24.4.6). Laparotomy is a superfluous diagnostic procedure in the evaluation of this disorder. Serum concentrations of electrolytes are measured whenever an infant is believed to have adrenal hyperplasia.

Patients who are 46,XX and have normal values for steroids in the plasma may have either true hermaphroditism or nonadrenal female pseudohermaphroditism, a distinction that can be based on the clinical features or for the former after laparotomy and gonadal biopsy. Patients whose mothers received potential masculinizing agents during pregnancy or who have evidence of a virilizing tumor or fetal aromatase deficiency do not need surgical exploration. Sonography and MR imaging of the pelvis and perineum are performed to identify the urogenital sinus when separate urethral and vaginal orifices cannot be identified with inspection and to search for a uterus and gonads in the abdomen. Müllerian duct derivatives are absent in testicular biosynthetic defects and androgen insensitivity and 5α-reductase-2 deficiency. A renal sonogram is of value for detecting anomalies of the urinary tract.

Persons who are XY and have abnormal external genitalia may have either male pseudohermaphroditism (including a variant of the syndrome of gonadal dysgenesis) or true hermaphroditism. Studies of plasma levels of sex steroids before and after administration of hCG and ACTH, karyotyping, and assessing the activity of the androgen receptor, especially DNA studies, usually clarifies the issue. Exploratory laparotomy and bilateral gonadal biopsy are necessary in selected instances for a definitive diagnosis. Before operation, the anatomic findings are defined with imaging studies. Urethroscopic examination is performed at surgery.

MANAGEMENT

The responsibility of the physician lies in recognition of ambisexual development, especially among infants. Early diagnosis and skillful management obviate many of the serious psychological and social problems of the patients and their parents, as well as the difficult decisions that may face the physician when the diagnosis is incorrect or the selection of sex is indecisive or delayed until childhood. The first problem in the care of a newborn infant with ambiguous genitalia is how to discuss it with the parents. The parents need to be told that the "true sex" of the infant is uncertain, and the ambiguity of the genitalia must be explained to them. They need to be reassured that, with modern diagnostic tests, a definitive diagnosis can be made expeditiously but that naming the baby, sending out birth announcements, and filing the birth certificate should be delayed. The parents need support, reassurance, and advice on how to deal with relatives and others. A simple explanation of the normal mechanism of sex differentiation presented with illustrative materials is useful. Introducing the parents to parents of children with a similar disorder and providing educational material can help to assuage some of their concerns. The parents need to know that they will be supported by a group experienced in dealing with these clinical problems. It must be clearly stated that the anatomic abnormalities can be surgically repaired, that hormone replacement can be given at an appropriate time, and that psychosocial support is available.

The physician and consultants recommend assignment of gender, but the ultimate decision is that of well-informed parents. These discussions must take into account the parental concerns, religious views, cultural factors, social mores, and the parents' level of understanding. It is critical to discuss with the parents what is known and what is not known about the long-term follow-up care of patients with intersex and the results of reconstructive genital surgery in terms of genital sensitivity and sexual gratification and

TABLE 24-29

FEATURES SUGGESTING AN ANOMALY OF SEX

During infancy
　Ambiguous appearance of external genitalia
　Male phenotype with cryptorchidism, especially if phallus is small
　Female phenotype with mass in groin or labium majus
　Affected sibling with sexual anomaly
　Female phenotype with prominent edema of distal parts of extremities
　　and loose folds of skin over nape of neck

After infancy
　Short girl, especially with features of syndrome of gonadal dysgenesis
　Girl with clitoral enlargement
　Adolescent boy with small testes, especially if associated with gynecomastia and eunuchoidism
　Primary amenorrhea in adolescent girl associated with breast development and sparse or absent pubic and axillary hair

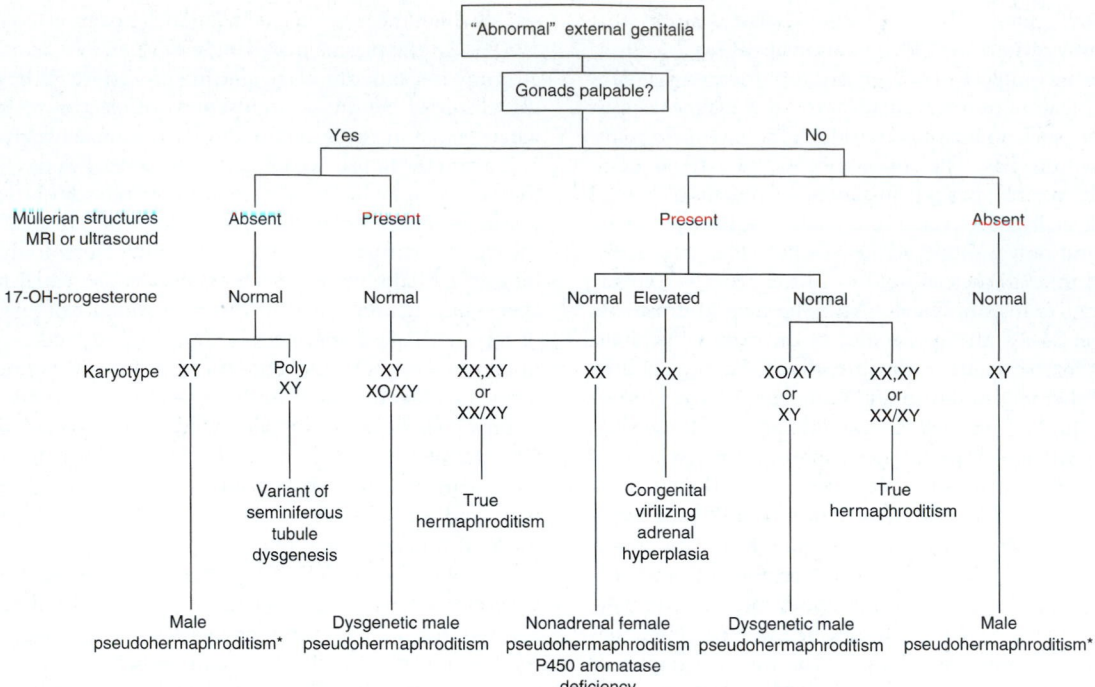

1. History: family history, pregnancy (hormones, virilization inspection). Palpation of inguinal region and labioscrotal folds; rectal examination. Karyotype analysis.
   Initial studies: plasma 17-hydroxyprogesterone and 17-hydroxypregnenolone, androstenedione, dehydroepiandrosterone, testosterone, and dihydrotestosterone.
   Serum electrolytes.
   Sonogram or MRI of kidneys, ureters, and pelvic contents.
   Provisional diagnosis.

2. "Vaginogram" (urogenital sonogram): selected cases.
   Endoscopy, laparotomy, gonadal biopsy: restricted to male pseudohermaphrodites, true hermaphrodites, and selected instances of nonadrenal female pseudohermaphroditism.

3. Molecular genetic studies (see specific disorders and Table 24-28).

* Plasma 17-hydroxyprogesterone levels may be modestly elevated in patients with P450c11β and 3β-hydroxysteroid dehydrogenase deficiency-2, and are "low" in patients with P450c17 and P450scc deficiency.

FIGURE 24-29   Steps in the diagnosis of intersexuality in infancy and childhood. *Step 1* involves evaluation and provisional diagnosis. *Step 2* is used in selected cases, and *Step 3* can be used for specific disorders. (SOURCE: *Adapted from Grumbach MM, Conte FA: Disorders of sex differentiation. In: Wilson JD, Foster DW, eds: Williams Textbook of Endocrinology, 8th ed. Philadelphia, Saunders, 1992.*)

of reproductive potential. The physician needs to be aware of the variable masculinizing effect of fetal androgens on postnatal gender behavior and our lack of knowledge of the effects of sex-linked and autosomal genes on gender orientation.

There has been a vigorous challenge to the previous model of "modified psychosexual neutrality" at birth as one issue in the decision to assign the sex of rearing and the timing and type of surgical treatment. This reexamination has been highlighted by great advances in diagnosis and understanding of the pathogenesis of disorders of sex differentiation and by the voice of nonprofessional support groups, psychologists, ethicists, and social scientists. Societal changes in attitudes toward sexual differences and increased access to information through the World Wide Web also has had an effect.

Assignment of infants with female pseudohermaphroditism as girls and repair of the external genitalia at 6 to 8 weeks of age to reinforce gender identity is recommended. Genital reconstruction of the urogenital sinus and vagina are deferred until adolescence or until requested by the patient or parents. Because these patients have ovaries, fallopian tubes, and uterus, they are potentially fertile.

Among infants with male pseudohermaphroditism, the basis for deciding on the sex of rearing is more complex, and many aspects remain controversial. Male gender assignment for patients with a phallus that can respond to testosterone therapy is most often cho-

sen. This includes infants with LH/hCG unresponsiveness, biosynthetic errors in testosterone biosynthesis, or 5α-reductase 2 deficiency and dysgenetic male pseudohermaphroditism. The care of patients with partial androgen resistance is more complex. For some patients with ambiguous external genitalia, high-dose testosterone therapy can increase phallus size to allow for sexual function. Because these patients are sterile, fertility usually is not a consideration.

The recommendation for gender assignment in true hermaphroditism is based on the morphologic features of the external genitalia and gonads. When the ambiguity of the genital structures is such that the child can be reared as a male or female, consideration of the selection of sex depends on whether the ovarian or testicular elements are better developed, the risk of malignant disease in dysgenetic-appearing testicular elements, and on the potential for fertility in the ovarian constituent. The gonad contrary to the selected sex is removed before puberty.

Previous tendencies by some physicians and many parents to withhold the diagnosis of ambiguous genitalia from the patient in an attempt to avoid any "doubt" about the assigned sex had dire psychosocial consequences. These patients have free access to their medical records in adolescence and adulthood, and the discovery of the deception in later life can be distressing. It is prudent for parents and physician to fully disclose, in stages keeping with the emotional maturity of the patient, all aspects of the diagnosis, pathophysiological mechanism, and management of the patient's "ambiguous genitalia."

The decision to remove the gonads is based on the type of secondary sexual development expected at puberty and the risk of malignant changes in later life. The latter consideration is not important in childhood or adolescence; the gonads can be monitored with sonography or MR imaging. In rare instances, a malignant tumor of the gonad has been detected before the age of puberty among patients with intersex, especially patients with dysgenetic testes (dysgenetic male pseudohermaphroditism), including XY persons with streak gonads. Gonadal tissue can be removed with laparoscopy.

References

Ahmed SF, Cheng A, Dovey L, et al: Phenotypic features, androgen receptor binding, and mutational analysis in 278 clinical cases reported as androgen insensitivity syndrome. J Clin Endocrinol Metab 85:658–665, 2000

Bender BG, Harmon RJ, Linden MG, et al: Psychological competence of unselected young adults with sex chromosome abnormalities. Am J Med Genet 88:200–206, 1999

Bin-Abbas B, Conte FA, Grumbach MM, Kaplan SL: Congenital hypogonadotropic hypogonadism and micropenis: effect of testosterone treatment on adult penile size—why sex reversal is not indicated. J Pediatr 134:579–583, 1999

Diamond M, Sigmundson HK: Sex reassignment at birth. Arch Pediatr Adolesc Med 151:248–304, 1997

Grumbach MM, Auchus RJ: Estrogen: Consequences and implications of human mutations in synthesis and action. J Clin Endocrinol Metab 84:4677–4694, 1999

Hadjiathanasious CG, Grauner R, Lortat-Jacob S, et al: True hemaphroditism: genetic variants and clinical management. J Pediatr 125:738–744, 1994

Imbeaud S, Carre-Eusebe D, Rey R, et al: Molecular genetics of the persistent müllerian duct syndrome: a study of 19 families. Hum Mol Genet 3:125–131, 1994

Imbeaud S, Faure E, Lamarre I, et al: Insensitivity to anti-müllerian hormone due to a mutation in the human anti-müllerian hormone receptor. Nature Genet 11:382–388, 1995

Koziell A, Gurndy R: Fraser and Denys-Drash syndromes: different disorders or part of a spectrum? Arch Dis Child 81:365–369, 1999

Kuhnle U, Bullinger M, Schwarz HP: The quality of life in adult female patients with congenital adrenal hyperplasia: a comprehensive study of the impact of genital malformations and chronic disease on female patient's life. Eur J Pediatr 154:708–716, 1995

Latronico AC, Anasti J, Arnhold IJP, et al: Brief report: testicular and ovarian resistance to luteinizing hormone caused by homozygous inactivating mutation of the luteinizing hormone receptor gene. N Engl J Med 334:507–512, 1996

Meyer-Bahlburg HFL: Gender assignment and reassignment in 46,XY pseudohermaphroditism and related conditions. J Clin Endocrinol Metab 84:3455–3458, 1999

Parker KL, Schedl A, Schimmer BP: Gene interactions in gonadal development. Ann Rev Physiol 61:417–433, 1999

Rao E, Weiss B, Takami M, et al: Pseudoautosomal deletions encompassing a novel homeobox gene cause growth failure in idiopathic short stature and Turner syndrome. Nature Genet 16:54–62, 1997

Saenger P: Turner syndrome. N Engl J Med 323:1749–1754, 1996

Slijpar FME, Drop SLS, Molenar JC, et al. Long-term psychological evaluation of intersex children. Arch Sex Behav 27:125–144, 1998

Swain A, Lovell-Badge R: Mammalian sex determination: a molecular drama. Genes Dev 13:755–767, 1999

Wilson JD: The role of androgens in male gender role behavior. Endocr Rev 20:726–737, 1999

24.8 NORMAL PUBERTAL DEVELOPMENT

Dennis M. Styne and Leonna Cuttler

The striking changes of secondary sexual development during puberty are caused by changes in hypothalamic-pituitary-gonadal endocrine function. The endocrine changes of puberty are divided into (1) gonadarche, or the awakening of gonadal action during which pituitary gonadotropins cause the secretion of gonadal steroids, and (2) adrenarche, or the awakening of adrenal androgen secretion caused by undefined factors.

Age at onset of menarche (as a reflection of the age of puberty) has decreased 2 to 3 months per decade in the developed world over the last two centuries. This trend has ceased in the United States since about 1940. Mothers and daughters now have a similar age of menarche. Children of a parent who entered puberty at an earlier or later age tend to follow familial patterns rather than following an ever earlier age at onset of puberty.

24.8.1 Secondary Sexual Development

The method to describe the stages of pubertal development popularized by Tanner is widely accepted. Sometimes called *sexual maturity ratings*, it provides an objective, consistent description of physical development (Fig. 24-30). Separately describing breast development (caused by ovarian estrogens) and pubic hair development (caused by adrenal androgens) is important because they are usually, but not always, coordinated (eg, premature adrenarche). Separately describing testicular and penile development from pubic hair development among boys likewise is useful because the adrenal gland can produce its own androgens out of sequence with testicular androgen secretion and cause disparate development. Prepuberty is stage 1 for any of the ratings, and there is no stage 0.

The onset of normal male puberty is heralded by an increase in diameter of the testes to more than 2.5 cm, excluding the epididymis. Volume measurements of the testes are accomplished by means of comparison with the standard ellipsoids of a Prader orchidometer. The onset of puberty corresponds to an increase in testicular volume to more than 4 mL. If other signs of pubertal development occur without an increase in testicular volume, an adrenal or exogenous source of androgen production is the cause. Stage 2a is proposed as a stage when testicular volume reaches 3 mL because 82% of boys progress through puberty within 5 months after this milestone.

Breast development among girls can start unilaterally. Asymmetric breast development of an early pubertal girl is not abnormal, and surgery is not indicated, although sadly such surgery has been performed.

Other physical changes occur during puberty that are not described with Tanner staging. The presence and prominence of axillary hair are used to describe this progression of puberty. For girls, the prepubertal reddish color of the vaginal lining becomes pink and dull because of cornification of the vaginal mucosa and secretion of a whitish discharge stimulated by estrogen. The labia minora and majora thicken under estrogen stimulation, and fat develops in the mons pubis. Percentage of body fat increases during puberty among girls, and subcutaneous fat deposition accounts for the change in body shape. The brow, nose, and chin develop more among boys, and the larynx changes shape to cause the change in voice of puberty.

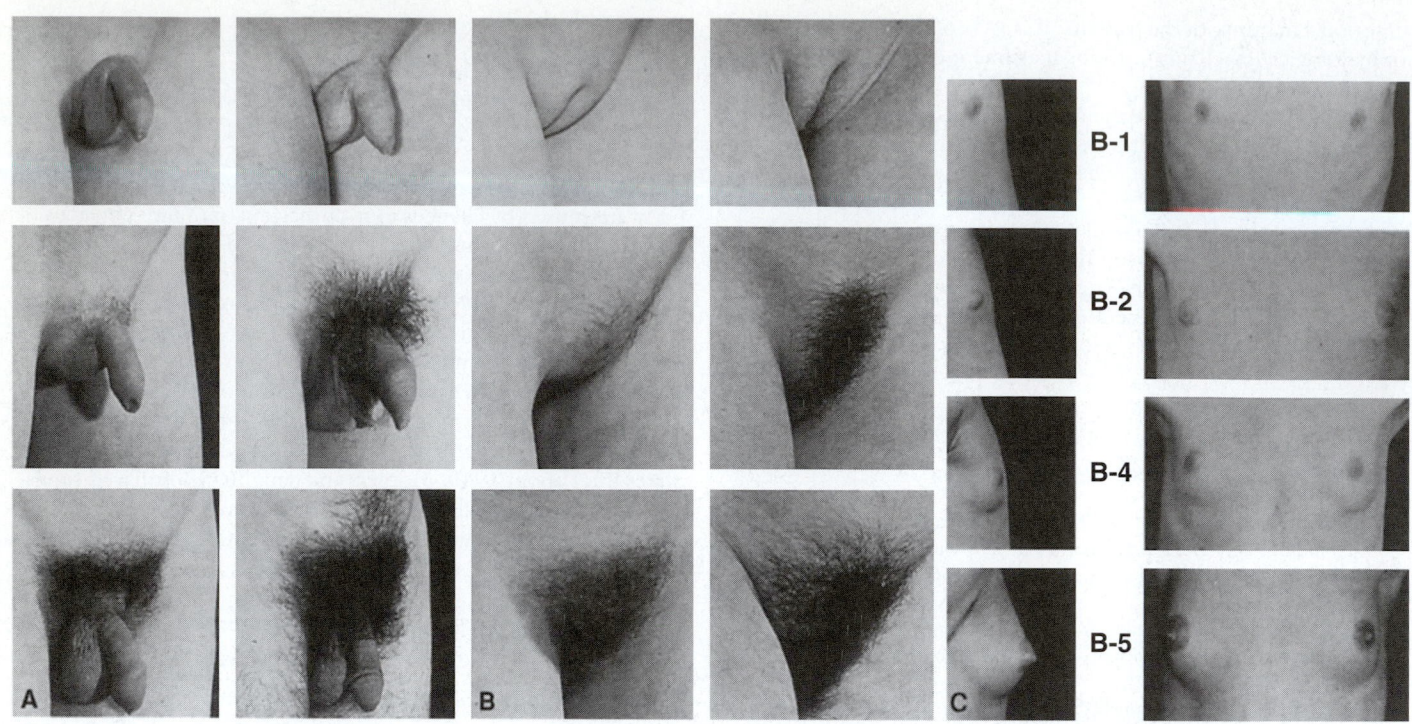

FIGURE 24-30   A. Genital development and pubic hair growth among boys. Stage G1 (*upper left*), prepubertal. Stage G2 (*upper right*), enlargement of testis to more than 2.5 cm, appearance of scrotal reddening, and increase in rugations. Stage G3, increase in length and to a lesser extent breadth of penis with further growth of testis. Stage G4, further increase in size of penis and testes and darkening of scrotal skin. Stages G5 and G6 (*lower panels*) adult genitalia. Stage P1 (*upper panels*) preadolescent, no pubic hair. Stage P2 (*middle left*), sparse growth of slightly pigmented, slightly curved pubic hair mainly at the base of the penis. Stage P3 (*middle right*), thicker curlier hair spread laterally. Stage P4 (*lower left*), adult-type hair that does not yet spread to medial thighs. Stage P5 (*lower right*), adult-type hair spread to medial thighs. B. Appearance of pubic and labial hair among girls. Stage PH1 (*upper left*), prepubertal, no pubic hair. Stage PH2 (*upper right, middle left*), sparse growth of long, straight, or slightly curly minimally pigmented hair, mainly on labia. Stage PH3 (*middle right*), considerably darker and coarser hair spreading over mons pubis. Stage PH4 (*lower left*), thick adult-type hair that does not yet spread to the medial surface of the thighs. Stage PH5 (*lower right*), hair is adult type and is distributed in the classic inverse triangle. C. Breast development. Stage B1 (*upper panels*), prepubertal, elevation of the papilla only. Stage B2, breast buds visible or palpable with enlargement of the areola. Stage B3, further enlargement of the breast and areola with no separation of their contours (not shown). Stage B4, projection of areola and papilla to form a secondary mound over the rest of the breast. Stage B5 (*lower panel*), mature breast with projection of papilla only.

PUBERTAL GROWTH SPURT

The pubertal growth spurt is the most rapid period of growth after the fetal and neonatal periods. The mean 5-inch (12.5 cm) difference in adult height between men and women is partially related to the fact that, on average, the male pubertal growth spurt occurs 2 years later than the pubertal growth spurt of girls and partially to the difference in height gained during the growth spurt. The pubertal growth spurt is thus an early pubertal event for girls and occurs before menses. For boys, it is a late pubertal event.

The endocrine factors that produce the pubertal growth spurt are complex. Insulin-like growth factors and GH exert important effects. Concentration of IGF-I in the serum is low at birth but increases throughout childhood until puberty, when a severalfold increase in serum concentration of IGF-I occurs. Serum values of IGF-I then decrease to the adult range. Serum IGF-I concentrations are best correlated with bone age rather than chronologic age. Children with delayed puberty who have serum concentrations of IGF-I appropriate for their delayed bone age but not their chro-

nologic age do not have GH deficiency, as often is mistakenly assumed.

The increase in serum concentrations of IGF-I at puberty is multifactorial. Secretion of GH increases at puberty because of increased secretion of sex steroids. Children with delayed puberty do not have this increase and may even have the concentrations of GH that occur in GH deficiency. Thus the diagnosis of GH deficiency on the basis of peak serum level of GH becomes even more problematic in the care of children with delayed puberty than in the care of younger children. Increased secretion of GH stimulates production of IGF-I. Thus sex steroids indirectly stimulate IGF-I production. Secretion of sex steroids increases production of IGF-I directly from effects on the cartilage independent of changes in secretion of GH.

SKELETAL DEVELOPMENT

Growth in stature is accompanied by advancement of skeletal development, which can be evaluated by means of comparison of a radiograph of the left hand of a subject with an image in a bone-age atlas. Determination of bone age does not in itself confirm the diagnosis of a disorder but can assist in differential diagnosis. Determination of bone age can, however, allow prediction of adult height. The farther bone age is from the age of epiphyseal fusion (15 years for girls and 17 years for boys), the more growth remains. Knowledge of a patient's age and bone age can be predictive of adult height for children older than 6 years if Bailey–Pinneau tables are used. If age and weight and parental heights are available, the Roche–Wainer–Thissen method provides increased accuracy. Bone age can be delayed by many conditions, including diseases such as hypothyroidism and constitutional delay in growth, which is a benign, self-limited variation of normal. A bone age of 13 years correlates with the onset of menarche, after which most girls achieve 2 to 7 cm of growth. Bone age is advanced in sexual precocity and accounts for the paradox of a child with early puberty having tall stature but ultimately having short adult stature. Epiphyseal fusion requires estrogen in both boys and girls. In persons with estrogen receptor defects who cannot respond to estrogen and others with aromatase deficiency who cannot produce estrogen, the epiphyses remain open after the age of 20 years, allowing continued and excessive growth into the third decade of life and resulting in tall adult stature.

Bone density increases during puberty, which along with infancy is the time of maximal accretion of bone. The peak of calcium deposition is 2 years later for boys than for girls, but both sexes achieve maximal bone density after the pubertal growth spurt. Delayed puberty, especially caused by permanent gonadal failure, decreases ultimate bone mass and in the most severe cases causes osteoporosis later in life.

THE AGE OF NORMAL PUBERTAL DEVELOPMENT

A cross-sectional survey of more than 17,000 girls in the United States showed that 2.4% of African-American girls had breast development by 5 years, 3.4% had pubic hair by 5 years, 15.4% had breast development at 7 years, and 17.7% had pubic hair by 7 years. Among white girls, 1.5% had breast development by 5 years, 0.4% had pubic hair by 5 years, 5% had breast development by 7 years, and 2.8% had pubic hair by 7 years. Thus African-American girls who enter puberty after their sixth birthday and white girls who enter puberty after their seventh birthday can be considered normal, not precocious. These data do not indicate that puberty today is earlier than it was 20 or 30 years ago because no comparable data have been available. These ages may have been the norm for the last several decades. Boys normally enter puberty after 9 years of age. Recent data suggest a trend that may decrease this lower limit of male puberty by 6 to 12 months.

If a boy does not enter puberty by 14 years of age and girls by 13 years, puberty is considered delayed. Any state of chronic disease or malnutrition can delay the onset of menses and puberty. These are the most common causes of delayed puberty worldwide. Obesity tends to advance skeletal maturation, increase growth rate, and decrease age at menarche. However, pathologic obesity can delay puberty and menarche.

24.8.2   The Endocrine Changes of Puberty

THE HYPOTHALAMIC-PITUITARY-GONADAL HORMONES

The hormones that cause pubertal development and reproduction emanate from the hypothalamus, the pituitary gland, the gonads, and the adrenal glands. Hypothalamic gonadotropin-releasing hormone (GnRH) is a 10-amino-acid peptide (coded by a gene on chromosome 8) secreted from the median eminence into the hypophyseal portal system in a pulsatile manner to reach the pituitary gland. The GnRH pulse generator is affected by biogenic amine neurotransmitters, peptidergic neuromodulators, neuroexcitatory amino acids, and neural pathways. Aminobutyric acid exerts a suppressive effect on GnRH secretion and can be an important factor in the relative quiescence of gonadotropin secretion that characterizes the "juvenile pause" that occurs after infancy and ends before the endocrine activity of puberty resumes. Sex steroids, mainly testosterone, estrogen, and progesterone, also inhibit GnRH pulse frequency in a negative feedback inhibition, whereas estrogen has the additional ability to exert positive feedback on gonadotropin secretion at midpuberty.

Gonadotropin-releasing hormone acts on the gonadotropes of the pituitary gland to increase intracellular calcium concentration and cause phosphorylation of protein kinase, which stimulates secretion of luteinizing hormone (LH) and follicle-stimulating hormone (FSH), in a pulsatile manner owing to the pulsatile nature of GnRH secretion. Gonadotropes exposed to continuous rather than episodic LH and FSH decrease the number of GnRH receptors, decrease the action of the occupied receptors, and decrease gonadotropin secretion (down-regulation).

Follicle-stimulating hormone and LH are glycoprotein hormones composed of two subunits, an α subunit, which is identical for all the pituitary glycoproteins, and distinct β subunits, which confer specificity. Human chorionic gonadotropin (hCG), produced by the placenta, is similar in structure to LH and causes the same biological effects as LH. The LH β-subunit gene is on chromosome 19q13.32, close to the gene for β-hCG, while the β-FSH gene is on 11p13. The half-life of injected LH is much shorter than that of FSH, although the metabolic clearance rate for LH is much faster than that of FSH. Such metabolic differences may explain the differing serum concentrations of LH and FSH achieved in response to a single hypothalamic peptide, GnRH. A variation in pulse frequency of GnRH changes the ratio of LH to FSH in the serum.

In boys, circulating LH activates membrane-bound receptors on testicular Leydig cells to stimulate testosterone secretion. After exposure to LH, the number of receptors for LH and the postreceptor pathway decrease their responsiveness to LH for at least 24 hours. This explains the clinical finding of resistance to LH after daily injections of LH compared with every-other-day injections of LH. Follicle-stimulating hormone supports spermatogenesis by attaching to its receptor on the cellular membrane of the seminiferous tubules. The main component responsible for growth of the testes is enlargement of the seminiferous tubules, not Leydig cell development. Thus patients with excess hCG have only minimal enlargement of the testes but secrete exceptional amounts of testosterone from the Leydig cells.

In girls, FSH binds to cell-surface receptors on ovarian follicular cells to stimulate secretion of estrogen. Luteinizing hormone becomes important later in pubertal development in completing the menstrual cycle of girls when it affects the theca cell after the onset of ovulation. Luteinizing hormone binds to membrane receptors and stimulates the activity of adenyl cyclase to produce cAMP, which stimulates production of the low-density lipoprotein (LDL) receptor to increase binding and uptake of LDL cholesterol and the formation of cholesterol esters. As in boys, LH stimulates P450scc, initiating steroidogenesis.

Less than 3% of circulating sex steroid is free and active. The rest is bound to sex hormone–binding globulin. Androgen decreases and estrogen stimulates formation of sex hormone–binding globulin. Thus testosterone secretion increases the fraction of free testosterone and magnifies the androgen effect. At the target cell, testosterone dissociates from the binding protein, diffuses into the cell, and can be converted by 5α-reductase to dihydrotestosterone or be converted to estrogen by aromatase, depending on the target cell. Testosterone and dihydrotestosterone bind to androgen receptors, which are encoded by a gene on the long arm of the X chromosome, but dihydrotestosterone is a substantially more potent androgen. The action of testosterone is sufficient to achieve some aspects of male sexual differentiation, whereas others require dihydrotestosterone (see Sec. 24.7.1). Testosterone suppresses LH secretion and maintains wolffian ducts, whereas dihydrotestosterone is needed for virilization of the external genitalia and for much of the secondary sexual characteristics of puberty. Androgens exert other effects in the body: testosterone stimulates muscle development, enzymatic activity in the liver, and hemoglobin synthesis and decreases the level of high-density lipoprotein cholesterol. Androgens susceptible to aromatization stimulate bone maturation at the epiphyseal plate only after conversion to estrogen. The main active estrogen in humans is estradiol. Estradiol produced at puberty affects the breast and uterus and the distribution of adipose tissue and bone, but estradiol has no role in normal female fetal development.

OTHER HORMONAL CHANGES AT PUBERTY

Pituitary lactotrophs produce prolactin, but unlike the other pituitary hormones stimulated by hypothalamic hormones, prolactin is suppressed by dopamine in the basal state. Serum concentration of prolactin increases in normal female puberty but is not affected by male puberty. Serum concentration of prolactin is valuable in diagnosis. Hypothalamic disease can decrease dopamine production and increase prolactin secretion. Pituitary disease can destroy lactotrophs and decrease prolactin secretion.

Inhibin is a heterodimeric glycoprotein that suppresses FSH secretion. Inhibin is produced by testicular Sertoli cells, ovarian granulosa cells, and the placenta. The suppressive effect of inhibin on FSH allows GnRH to achieve varying serum concentrations of LH and FSH throughout development and throughout the menstrual cycle. The reason for the remarkable elevations of serum concentration of FSH over LH in gonadal failure is the lack of inhibin production. Activin is a subunit of inhibin and has the opposite effect of inhibin; activin stimulates secretion of FSH.

Leptin is a polypeptide hormone produced and secreted by adipose cells and which attaches to receptors in the hypothalamus. Leptin suppresses appetite and has effects on physical activity. The absence of leptin or its receptors has been associated with an absence of gonadotropin secretion, and leptin treatment of a girl with leptin deficiency and hypogonadotropic hypogonadism led to gonadotropin secretion and progression of pubertal development. However, the role of leptin in normal puberty is uncertain. At present, leptin appears to be necessary but not sufficient for pubertal development.

ONSET OF PUBERTAL GONADAL ACTIVITY (GONARCHE)

The hormone levels characteristic of puberty are similar to those in the fetus. Gonadotropin secretion from the fetal pituitary gland increases during fetal life through midgestation under the stimu-

lation of hypothalamic GnRH. Central nervous system inhibition of GnRH secretion increases toward term with a resultant decrease in LH and FSH secretion. The fetal testes secrete testosterone under stimulation by LH and hCG. After birth and release from inhibition by placental estrogen, neonatal pituitary secretion of serum LH and FSH peaks. Gonadotropin secretion is followed by peaks of estrogen up to the fourth year of postnatal age in girls and peaks of testosterone up to the second year in boys. Infant boys may have transient elevations of serum testosterone concentration equal to those found in the midpubertal period. After infancy, concentrations of serum gonadotropins and sex steroids decline for a period of time labeled the *juvenile pause*. In the normal situation, the juvenile pause continues until the time of pubertal development, being caused by central suppression of hypothalamic function. If a tumor or other cause of increased intracranial pressure, such as hydrocephalus, or disordered central nervous system function occurs, central precocious puberty may develop.

Endocrine activity of the hypothalamic-pituitary-ovarian axis increases in the peripubertal period, before the physical changes of secondary sexual development become apparent. Increased GnRH secretion causes gonadotropin levels to increase, first during the night, causing a pattern of diurnal variation, and later during the entire day and night with an absence of diurnal variation. An increase in LH is the best indicator of gonadarche. In the past, a 2- or 4-hour GnRH stimulation test was necessary to determine whether the pubertal increase in gonadotropin secretion had occurred. Development of ultrasensitive gonadotropin assays (third-generation assays) now allow evaluation of gonadarche with a single measurement of LH. The serum concentration of estradiol in girls is extremely variable throughout the day. Most commercial assays are so insensitive that a single low value of estradiol is not helpful in ruling out pubertal endocrine activity, but elevations in estradiol level can confirm the appearance of pubertal endocrine activity. In contrast, serum level of testosterone remains more stable throughout the day. For boys, a single measurement of testosterone is useful for indicating pubertal activity. After the initial period of slightly elevated testosterone concentrations of early puberty, there is a steep increase in secretion during gonadal stage 3 (from approximately 40 ng/mL to more than 100 ng/mL). Standard laboratories may not be able to detect the low levels of estradiol and testosterone early in puberty, so samples must be sent to one of the few laboratories that specialize in pediatric endocrine analysis. An ultrasensitive bioassay for estradiol has been developed for research but is not yet available commercially.

ONSET OF MENSES (MENARCHE)

The advent of positive feedback of estrogen on GnRH secretion is the hallmark of regulation of the menstrual cycle in midpuberty and is an indication of reproductive maturity. As the pattern of gonadotropin secretion changes from diurnal variation to a more constant pattern, a progression of changes brings about this mature state. Secretion of FSH always is greater in girls than in boys, and FSH stimulates follicle formation in the early pubertal ovary. The follicle produces estrogen, which increases GnRH secretion, increases pituitary sensitivity to GnRH, and increases gonadotropin secretion. Each subsequent pulse of GnRH primes the gonadotropes to increase gonadotropin secretion further. Finally the sequence is in place to allow a critical mass of estrogen to cause a sharp release of LH. This same peak of estrogen suppresses FSH to allow the follicular cells to luteinize, increasing progesterone production, which increases LH secretion. The LH peak also stimulates prostaglandin, which causes an inflammatory response in the follicle, which leads to ovulation.

The increased endocrine activity of the midcycle ovary stimulates growth of the endometrium, but the decrease in endocrine activity toward the end of the cycle leaves the hyperplastic endometrium with no endocrine support. This and the local action of prostaglandins and constriction of arterioles leads to necrosis of the endometrium, and the menstrual flow begins.

A follicle must be of adequate size to produce sufficient estrogen to exert the positive feedback effect, the pituitary gland must have sufficient readily releasable LH to effect a surge of LH release, and the hypothalamus must be able to secrete adequate GnRH to cause stimulation of the pituitary gland to cause a pulse of LH to be released. These conditions do not develop until well into puberty, and ovulation is a middle to late pubertal event. The first 2 years of menses are anovulatory in 55 to 90% of cycles, but by 5 years after menarche only 20% of periods are anovulatory. Nonetheless, girls may be fertile before physical sexual maturity, and pregnancy has preceded the first documented menstrual period in many cases (see Sec. 3.4.1).

ONSET OF PUBERTAL ADRENAL GLAND ACTIVITY (ADRENARCHE)

An increase in level of adrenal androgens occurs several years before the onset of increasing gonadotropin secretion. This elevation in the level of the androgen precursor dehydroepiandrosterone (DHEA) and its sulfate (DHEAS) occurs at 6 to 7 years of age in girls and 7 to 8 years in boys, but it takes about 2 more years for pubic hair to appear. Serum concentration of DHEAS continues to increase through midpuberty and reaches maximal values in the mid-20s. Control of adrenarche is unknown but is separate from the mechanisms of gonadotropin stimulation. ACTH is necessary but not sufficient for adrenarche to occur. Premature adrenarche occurs when the increase in DHEAS level occurs at a younger than average age, and growth of pubic hair soon follows.

24.8.3   Early Puberty, Sexual Precocity

Onset of puberty among white girls as early as 7 years of age or among African-American girls as early as 6 years of age can be considered normal in the absence of neurologic symptoms or signs of increased intracranial pressure, in the absence of rapid advancement in pubertal development or bone age, or extremely early onset of menses. If there is a family history of a pattern of early pubertal development, the child is even more likely to have a variant of normal rather than a pathologic condition causing sexual precocity. Among boys the earliest limit of normal puberty is 9 years of age. Onset earlier than these limits is considered sexual precocity.

Sexual precocity is the general term for early puberty. *Isosexual precocity* refers to a girl who feminizes or a boy who virilizes early. *Central precocious puberty* or *true precocious puberty* is a term reserved for children with GnRH-dependent early puberty that follows the normal pubertal pattern with the normal control mechanisms triggered by GnRH. The only difference from normal puberty is the earlier age at onset. Central precocious puberty can be idiopathic or caused by organic conditions such as a brain tumor or hamartoma of the tuber cinereum. *GnRH-independent isosexual precocity* is caused by excessive estrogen secretion in girls or androgen secretion in boys from the gonads or the adrenal glands. Gonadotropins are suppressed because sex steroid secretion is autonomous. *Contrasexual precocity* refers to girls who virilize and boys

who feminize. Investigation of the causes of all types of sexual precocity are directed at determining whether the cause is endogenous or exogenous. The classification schema and causes of precocious puberty are outlined in Table 24-30.

TRUE CENTRAL PRECOCIOUS PUBERTY (GnRH DEPENDENT)

All children with sexual precocity have the effects of increased sex steroids such that growth is faster than appropriate for chronologic age, and bone age advances too quickly. Among boys, muscle development and deepening of the voice occur along with erections and increased aggressiveness. Boys with central precocious puberty have a testicular diameter greater than 2.5 cm or a volume greater than 4 mL. Girls have an increased growth rate even before development of the breasts, but the breast development is more easily detected. Breast development is noticed among girls with all types of isosexual precocity, but usually menarche occurs only in GnRH-dependent precocious puberty. There is an increased risk of development of carcinoma of the breast in adulthood with early menses, and this presumably also is true after central precocious puberty.

Although some children progress rapidly through precocious puberty, some follow a waxing and waning course. The more severely affected children have a bone age that advances faster than height velocity. If untreated, these patients achieve a severely decreased adult height because of premature epiphyseal closure. Older data indicated that girls not treated for sexual precocity reached a mean final height of 151 to 152 cm compared with a mean final height in the United States of 164 cm. These data mixed girls with severe sexual precocity with those who today might be considered to have a variant of normal and probably represent an overestimation. Boys not treated for sexual precocity reached a final height of 161 cm compared with an average final height in the United States of 178 cm.

Some children start puberty somewhat early compared with current standards but not strikingly so and may be manifesting a family tendency or *familial constitutional precocious puberty*. The milder cases with no marked advancement of bone age, no marked elevation of serum level of IGF-I, and among girls, no marked elevation of serum level of estrogen may not need treatment and still achieve acceptable final height. Others with unsustained precocious puberty can likewise be observed rather than treated, but their condition should be followed closely.

The psychological stress of early sexual development and menarche among girls can influence a decision toward therapy. Fertility can be achieved early by both boys and girls with central precocious puberty. One 6-year-old bore a child because of a combination of precocious puberty and sexual abuse.

CENTRAL NERVOUS SYSTEM CAUSES The most common cause of central precocious puberty is *hamartoma of the tuber cinereum*. These congenital masses of heterotopic tissue are derived from the embryonic hypothalamus but are not normally suppressed by the central nervous system during childhood and hence cause pulsatile secretion of gonadotropins and stimulation of the gonads. These hamartomas are not neoplasms because they do not grow or cause progressive problems. They can be associated with gelastic or laughing seizures, petit mal or grand mal seizures. Hamartoma of the tuber cinereum has the characteristic appearance on MR images of a sessile or pedunculated mass attached to the posterior hypothalamus between the tuber cinereum and the mamillary bodies projecting into the suprasellar cistern. Biopsy is not needed for di-

TABLE 24-30

CAUSES AND CLASSIFICATION OF SEXUAL PRECOCITY

Complete isosexual precocious puberty (GnRH-Dependent sexual precocity or premature activation of the hypothalamic pulse generator)

Familial or constitutional central precocious puberty
Idiopathic true precocious puberty
CNS tumors
   Hamartoma of the tuber cinereum
   Craniooptic glioma associated with neurofibromatosis type 1
   Hypothalamic astrocytoma
   Ependymoma
Other CNS disorders
   Encephalitis
   Static encephalopathy
   Brain abscess
   Sarcoid or tubercular granuloma
   Head trauma
   Hydrocephalus
   Pharyngioma
   Arachnoid cyst
   Myelomeningocele
   Vascular lesion
   Cranial irradiation
True precocious puberty after late therapy for congenital virilizing adrenal hyperplasia or other previous chronic exposure to sex steroids
Incomplete isosexual precocity (hypothalamic GnRH-independent)
Boys
   Gonadotropin-secreting tumors
      hCG-secreting CNS tumor (eg, chorioepithelioma, germinoma, teratoma)
      hCG-secreting tumors outside the CNS (hepatoma, teratoma, choriocarcinoma)
   Increased androgen secretion by adrenal gland or testis
      Congenital adrenal hyperplasia (CYP21 and CYP11B1 deficiencies)
      Virilizing adrenal neoplasm
      Leydig cell adenoma
      Familial testotoxicosis (sex-limited autosomal-dominant pituitary gonadotropin-independent precocious Leydig cell and germ cell maturation)
      Cortisol resistance syndrome
Girls
   Ovarian cyst
   Estrogen-secreting ovarian or adrenal neoplasm
   Peutz-Jeghers syndrome
Both sexes
   McCune-Albright syndrome
   Hypothyroidism
   Iatrogenic or exogenous sexual precocity (including unintentional exposure to estrogens in food, drugs, or cosmetics)
Variations of pubertal development
   Premature thelarche
   Premature isolated menarche
   Premature adrenarche
   Adolescent gynecomastia of boys

CNS = central nervous sytem; hCG = human chorionic gonadotropin.

agnosis or surgical management of central precocious puberty, because the lesion is responsive to GnRH agonists (see later). Many children previously thought to have idiopathic precocious puberty before the advent of CT and MR imaging were subsequently shown to have hamartoma of the tuber cinereum with the use of these noninvasive, benign techniques. Those who have no hamartoma or other definable cause of central precocious puberty have idiopathic precocious puberty.

Almost any manner of central nervous system disease can, depending on the location and severity of the lesion, advance the age of puberty or delay puberty. The most ominous causes of central precocious puberty are brain tumors in the posterior hypothalamic-pituitary region. The tumors can cause other symptoms, such as headache, abnormalities of vision, optic atrophy, and diabetes insipidus. Although precocious puberty occurs more frequently among girls than among boys, central nervous system tumor as a cause of precocious puberty is more common among boys than among girls. Craniopharyngioma, astrocytoma, ependymoma, and optic or hypothalamic glioma and ependymoma all interfere with the normal juvenile pause and cause central precocious puberty, as can optic glioma or neurofibroma in the hypothalamic area associated with neurofibromatosis type 1 or von Recklinghausen disease. Radiation to the central nervous system for cancer has become a more common cause as the long-term survival of patients with central nervous system cancer improves. The combination of GH deficiency and central precocious puberty occurs with central nervous system irradiation for brain tumors but can be missed clinically because the precocious puberty increases growth rate and masks the decreased growth rate caused by GH deficiency. These patients must be treated with both GH and GnRH agonist to improve final height.

High intracranial pressure caused by hydrocephalus or a subarachnoid cyst can cause precocious puberty, which is reversed solely by means of release of intracranial pressure. Fetal or childhood central nervous system infections of any type, such as tuberculosis and brain abscess, can cause precocious puberty, as can cerebral vascular accidents and central nervous system trauma. Developmental delay of various causes, including static cerebral encephalopathy, can cause precocious adrenarche (see later) or full central precocious puberty. Congenital defects of the central nervous system such as septooptic dysplasia may cause central precocious puberty.

ANDROGEN EXPOSURE Children exposed to high serum concentrations of androgens, such as those treated at a late age with glucocorticoids for virilizing congenital adrenal hyperplasia, have advanced bone age and advanced maturation of the hypothalamus, which frequently causes central precocious puberty. Thus a child with poorly or late controlled congenital adrenal hyperplasia may need a GnRH agonist in addition to the standard treatment with a glucocorticoid and mineralocorticoid. Likewise, children with androgen-secreting tumors removed after years of virilization can subsequently have central true precocious puberty.

CHILDREN ADOPTED FROM DEVELOPING COUNTRIES Girls adopted into Western families after an infancy in the Third World are reported to have central precocious puberty. This is postulated to be linked to early malnutrition followed by normal or excessive nutrition.

GnRH-INDEPENDENT SEXUAL PRECOCITY (INCOMPLETE ISOSEXUAL PRECOCITY)

Sexual precocity occurring in the absence of an increase in GnRH is caused by either autonomous secretion of sex steroids in both sexes or, among boys, to production of hCG, which stimulates testicular testosterone secretion. Thus FSH and LH are suppressed to nondetectable concentrations in the face of often extremely elevated sex steroid concentrations. Agonists of GnRH have no effect on those conditions in the initial phases, although it is possible that after therapy for an initially virilizing condition, exposure to sex steroids may stimulate early hypothalamic maturation, causing central precocious puberty that necessitates treatment with a GnRH agonist.

Causes among Boys

Germ cell tumors secrete hCG, which in high concentrations stimulates the Leydig cells to produce testosterone. Human chorionic gonadotropin does not stimulate the seminiferous tubules, so these boys have only slight enlargement of the testes (to a degree far less than occurs in central precocious or normal puberty). The penis enlarges, serum level of hCG is elevated, and levels of FSH and LH are not. For this evaluation to be meaningful, it is essential to use assays that can differentiate hCG from LH. The lesion responsible can be teratoma, chorioepithelioma, dysgerminoma, or a mixed germ cell tumor, which can be in the hypothalamus, the mediastinum, the lungs, the gonads, or the retroperitoneal cavity. Hepatoblastoma also can be causative. The tumors may secrete α-feto protein as well as hCG. Boys with 47,XXY Klinefelter syndrome have an increased incidence of hCG-secreting mediastinal germ cell neoplasms.

Virilizing congenital adrenal hyperplasia can be caused by 21-hydroxylase deficiency, which can be associated with the salt-loss of mineralocorticoid deficiency, or can be caused by 11β-hydroxylase deficiency, which can be accompanied by hypertension because of excess mineralocorticoid secretion. These conditions cause virilization without testicular enlargement, because the androgen comes from the adrenal glands. Because gonadotropins are suppressed, the testes can be small for age. The classical form manifests during infancy as salt loss and a normal genital appearance. Without salt loss, the condition can manifest as sexual precocity at 3 to 7 years of age (see Sec. 24.4.6). *Virilizing adenoma and carcinoma of the adrenal gland* secrete large amounts of DHEA and DHEAS, which are peripherally converted to androgens. When the adrenal gland is the cause of the virilization, the testes remain prepubertal in size. Leydig cell tumors are rare among boys but manifest as asymmetrically enlarged testis or testes.

Familial gonadotropin-independent sexual precocity with premature Leydig and germ cell maturation (or testotoxicosis) is a rare, sex-limited dominant condition that manifests only among boys. The boy grows rapidly but achieves a decreased adult height; affected girls are normal. Affected boys have enlargement of the penis and virilization but only minimal enlargement of the testes because there is predominant stimulation of Leydig cells and relatively less enlargement of the seminiferous tubules. These patients have elevated testosterone levels with low gonadotropin concentrations. The cause of the disorder is a mutation in the LH receptor, which renders it constitutionally activated, so that it constantly stimulates testosterone production. These children have a remarkably limited decrease in final height and normal fertility when they reach adulthood. Later in life, these patients become responsive to GnRH, although they were not responsive in childhood, and central precocious puberty occurs. This phenomenon appears similar to hypothalamic pituitary gonadal maturation as occurs among patients with premature puberty after therapy for virilizing disorders. Affected patients do not initially respond to GnRH agonists. Spironolactone, an antimineralocorticoid and antiandrogen agent used to limit androgen effect, has been combined with testolactone, an

inhibitor of aromatase that limits bone age advancement, as treatment of these boys. An alternative is cyproterone acetate, a powerful antiandrogen that blocks the androgen receptor, which can be used alone. Later, with the maturation of the hypothalamic-pituitary-gonadal axis and development of central precocious puberty, additional therapy with GnRH agonists is effective.

Causes among Girls

Gonadotropin-independent isosexual precocity among girls can be caused by ovarian cysts or neoplasms, exposure to exogenous estrogens, or abnormalities of the adrenal glands. Prepubertal girls normally have small ovarian cysts, but some cysts enlarge and secrete sufficient estrogen to cause breast development and even withdrawal bleeding. Most cysts do not recur, but repetitive cyst formation has been described. Affected girls secreted more FSH than normal prepubertal girls, and this may be the cause of the condition. A cyst can cause serum concentration of estrogen to reach the high level characteristic of tumors, but usually only pubertal values are encountered.

Several neoplasms can cause gonadotropin-independent isosexual precocity among girls. Granulosa cell tumors of the ovary are rare but are discovered at bimanual examination in 80% of cases. Antimüllerian hormone and inhibin are useful tumor markers for postoperative follow-up evaluation of these tumors. Gonadoblastoma can arise in streak gonads and secrete estrogen or even testosterone. It is benign but can harbor malignant ovarian tumors. Estrogen-secreting adrenal neoplasms are infrequent compared with those that secrete androgens. Tumors that secrete hCG cause no physical pubertal changes in girls. Girls and boys can be exposed to estrogens through ingestion of their mothers' oral contraceptives or contact with estrogen-containing ointment. Feminization also has been attributed to estrogen contamination of milk, meat, or even vitamins prepared on machinery previously used to package estrogen.

Causes among Girls and Boys

McCune-Albright syndrome is a common disorder comprising irregular café-au-lait spots, polyostotic fibrous dysplasia (cysts in the long bones and thickening of the skull), and autonomous endocrine function, usually GnRH-independent sexual precocity. The skin and skeletal manifestations develop after birth. This syndrome is most common among girls but can affect boys. Patients may have autonomous hyperactivity of the somatotropes (acromegaly or gigantism), thyroid cells (thyrotoxicosis), parathyroid glands, or adrenal glands (Cushing syndrome). The cause of such widespread endocrine activity was obscure until the discovery of mutations of the stimulatory G-protein subunit of the adenyl cyclase system attached to the membrane receptor of the affected cells. Because these are somatic cell mutations and are not in the germline, the disease is genetic but not heritable and affects some organs while skipping others, leading to the variable manifestations.

The sexual precocity of the McCune-Albright syndrome is initially autonomous, but exposure to estrogens or androgens eventually can mature the hypothalamic-pituitary-gonadal axis and cause GnRH-dependent precocious puberty. Testolactone, medroxyprogesterone acetate, and cyproterone acetate have been effective as initial treatment of girls with McCune-Albright syndrome. Agonists of GnRH have been effective later in childhood in managing secondary central precocious puberty, which occurs after maturation of the hypothalamic-pituitary-gonadal axis.

Severe, uncontrolled *hypothyroidism* can be associated with in-

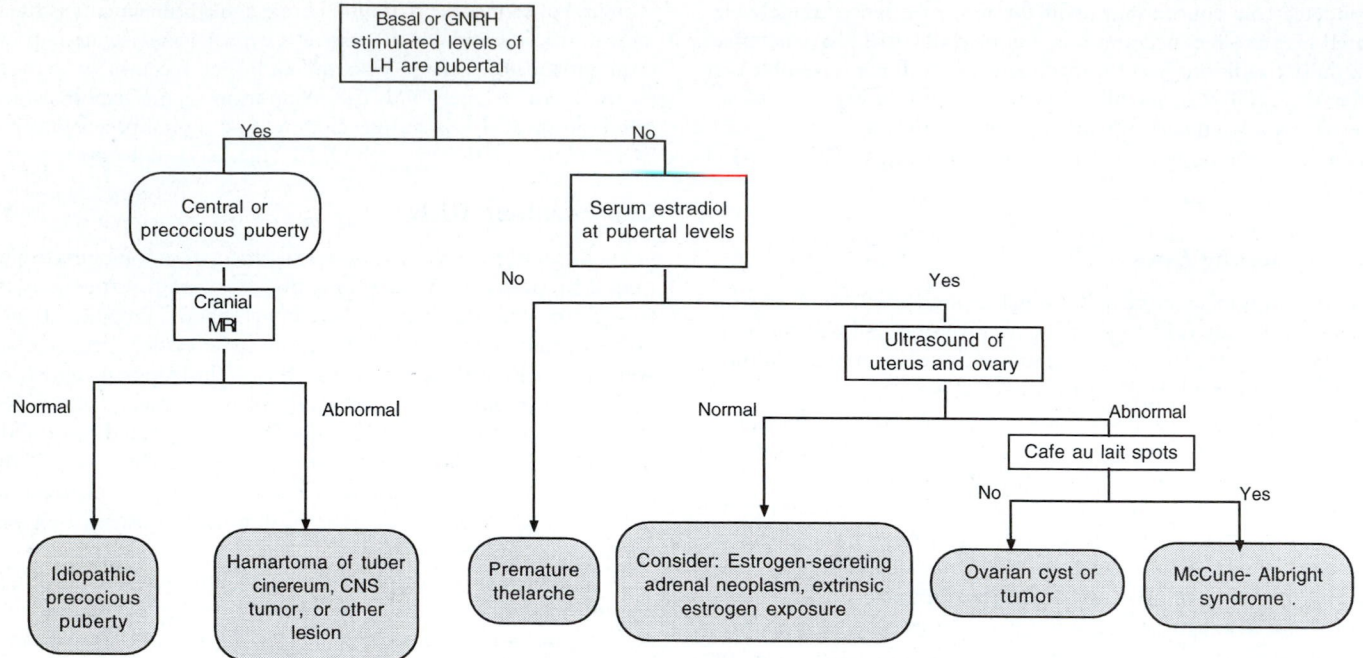

FIGURE 24-31   Diagnostic algorithm for breast development before 7 years among white girls and 6 years among African-American girls. GnRH = gonadotropin-releasing hormone.

complete sexual precocity of both boys and girls. The extremely high levels of TSH caused by hypothyroidism can stimulate LH and FSH receptors (hormonal overlap syndrome). Plasma level of prolactin is elevated, and galactorrhea can occur, especially among girls. Growth is impaired as for any child with hypothyroidism, so there is no pubertal growth spurt. Girls may have breast development, menstrual flow, and estrogen effects on the vaginal mucosa. The size of the testes may increase because of enlargement of the seminiferous tubules. The pituitary gland may enlarge and erode the sella turcica in a manner incorrectly suggesting a tumor because of increased TSH secretion and thyrotroph hyperplasia. Once hypothyroidism is controlled, sexual precocity reverts and the sella turcica becomes smaller.

DIAGNOSIS AND MANAGEMENT OF SEXUAL PRECOCITY

The approach to diagnosis of the cause of sexual precocity is shown in Figs. 24-31, 24-32, and 24-33. The goal in diagnosis of sexual precocity is first to eliminate the possibility of life-threatening tumors or other central nervous system conditions and second to determine optimal therapy to suppress pubertal development and bone age advancement. If the possibility of a central nervous system tumor has not been eliminated by establishing another diagnosis, patients with central precocious puberty need an MR imaging evaluation of the brain that is concentrated on the hypothalamic region.

FIGURE 24-32   Diagnostic algorithm for pubic hair before 7 years among white girls and 6 years among African-American girls. DHEAS = dehydroepiandrostenedione sulfate; 17OHP = 17α-hydroxyprogesterone.

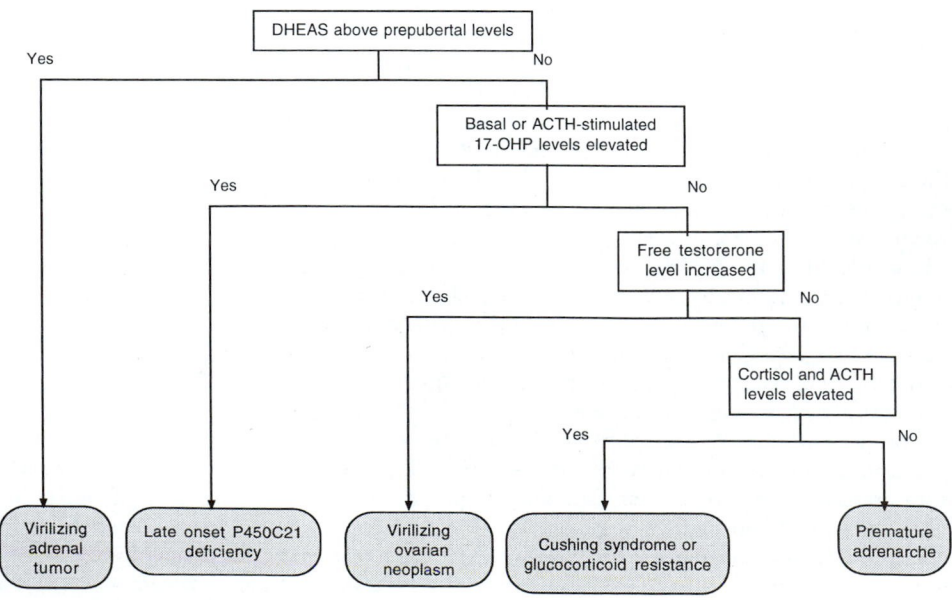

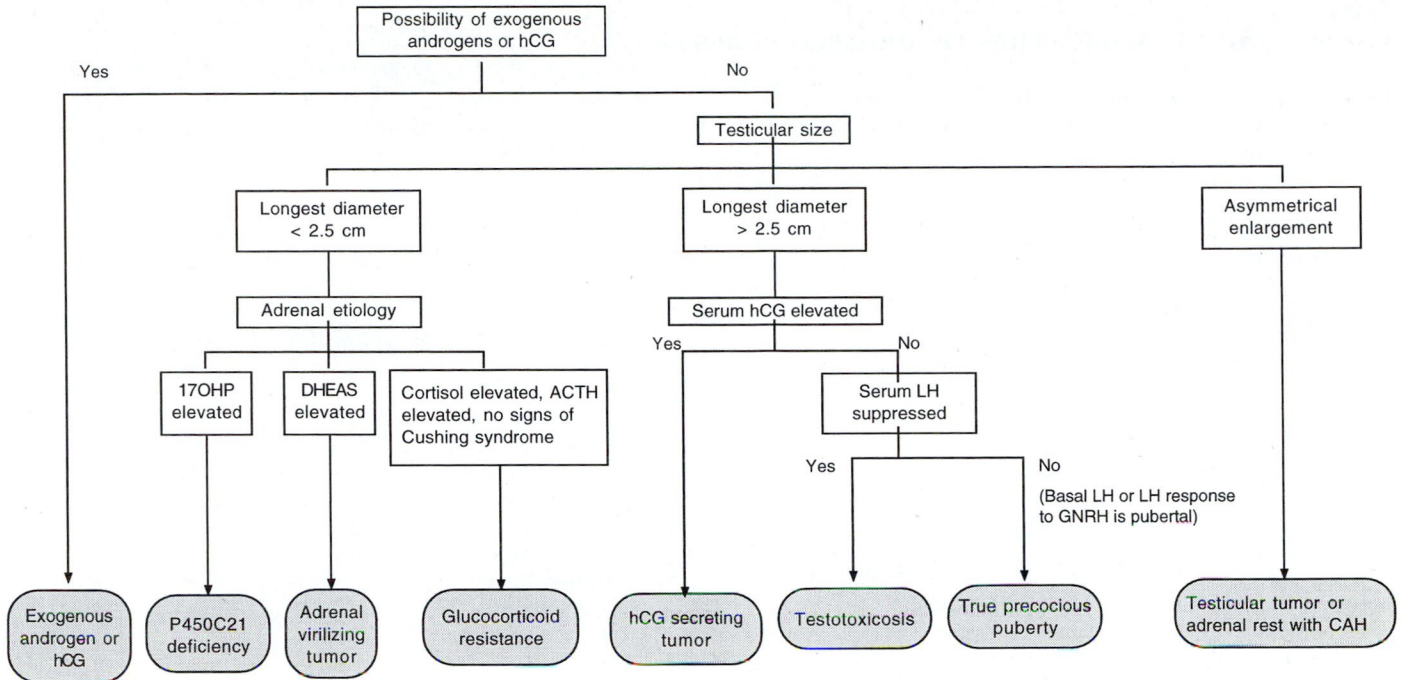

FIGURE 24-33 Diagnostic algorithm for precocious puberty among boys before 9 years of age. DHEAS = dehydroepiandrostenedione sulfate; 17OHP = 17α-hydroxyprogesterone

Patients with true precocious puberty have many laboratory findings similar to the results obtained in normal puberty. Alkaline phosphatase is elevated for chronologic age but not for bone age. Resting concentrations of gonadotropin are elevated to the pubertal range when measured with sensitive third-generation assays. Nocturnal episodic gonadotropin secretion increases, as does gonadotropin response to administration of GnRH. Laboratories have their own guidelines, but in general, if LH level increases more than 10 IU/mL after 100 μg GnRH is administered, the response is considered pubertal.

Idiopathic central precocious puberty is a diagnosis of exclusion. All aspects of the pubertal process mirror the normal condition, albeit at an early age. Children can enter puberty before their first birthday without a sign of an organic condition as the cause. These patients are treated with a GnRH agonist to allow the child to reach a final height that is close to normal.

Central precocious puberty is best managed with administration of GnRH agonists that have a strong binding affinity for the GnRH receptor and resist enzymatic degradation. After brief stimulation of LH and FSH secretion, binding to the receptor down-regulates the GnRH receptor, which almost eliminates further LH and FSH secretion. Levels of sex steroids decrease, bone age advancement decreases, and growth rate decreases. If therapy is started early enough, adult height equals or approximates the genetic potential. Menses ceases in girls. The most widely used preparation, leuprolide acetate, is available in a once-per-month injection or a daily preparation. Side effects include a decrease in bone density and bone accretion, so calcium supplementation is needed. Allergic reactions or sterile abscesses are rare. Agonists of GnRH are used to manage most types of central precocious puberty, including hematoma of the tuber cinereum (these congenital lesions do not necessitate surgery). Agonists of GnRH are not indicated for children with borderline early onset of puberty who are progressing slowly, have not had menarche, and have no central nervous system signs or symptoms.

24.8.4 Variations of Early Pubertal Development

PREMATURE THELARCHE

Premature thelarche most frequently occurs among girls by 2 years of age and almost always before 4 years. In most cases, breast development regresses within 6 months of onset, but in some cases it remains for years after diagnosis. Results of long-term follow-up studies suggest no untoward effects on later health or development. The cause of premature thelarche may be development of a small ovarian cyst, but usually by the time the outward physical manifestations occur, the cyst has regressed and no cause can be found. An elevated FSH level can cause premature thelarche, but patients do not have a pubertal result of a GnRH test. New supersensitive estrogen bioassays indicate a small increase in estrogen secretion is associated with premature thelarche, but such assays are not yet commercially available. Some girls with apparently classic premature thelarche later have central precocious puberty, so continued follow-up care of girls is essential, even if therapy is not initially indicated. In most cases, premature thelarche is a benign, self-limited disorder that is managed with reassurance.

PREMATURE ISOLATED MENARCHE

There are rare reports of girls who have menarche at an early age with no breast development. This can occur as an isolated incident or over a period of years. These girls then have normal pubertal development later in childhood. They must be differentiated from girls who have vaginal bleeding due to a foreign body, a local tumor, or vaginal trauma possibly caused by child abuse. The cause of premature isolated menarche is unknown.

PREMATURE ADRENARCHE

Some children have elevated levels of adrenal androgens years before the normal age of onset of adrenarche and have pubic and

TABLE 24-31

CAUSES AND CLASSIFICATION OF DELAYED PUBERTY

Idiopathic (constitutional) delay in growth and puberty
Hypogonadotropic hypogonadism: delayed puberty related to gonadotropin deficiency
CNS disorders
  Tumor
    Craniopharyngioma
    Germinoma
    Other germ cell tumors
      Hypothalamic and optic glioma
    Astrocytoma
    Pituitary tumor
  Other causes
    Langerhans histiocytosis
    Granulomatous and postinfectious lesions of the CNS
    Vascular abnormalities of the CNS
    Radiation therapy
    Congenital malformations especially associated with
      craniofacial anomalies
    Head trauma
Isolated gonadotropin deficiency
  With hyposmia or anosmia: Kallmann syndrome
  Without anosmia
  Congenital adrenal hypoplasia (*DAX1* mutation)
  Isolated LH deficiency
  Isolated FSH deficiency
Idiopathic and genetic forms of multiple pituitary hormone deficiencies
  Miscellaneous disorders
    Prader-Willi syndrome
    Laurence-Moon and Bardet-Biedl syndromes
Functional gonadotropin deficiency
Chronic systemic disease and malnutrition
  Sickle-cell disease
  Cystic fibrosis
  Acquired immune deficiency syndrome
  Chronic gastroenteric disease
  Chronic renal disease
  Malnutrition
  Anorexia nervosa
  Bulimia

Psychogenic amenorrhea
Impaired puberty and delayed menarche in female athletes and ballet
  dancers (exercise amenorrhea)
Hypothyroidism
Diabetes mellitus
Cushing disease
Hyperprolactinemia
Marijuana use
Gaucher disease
Hypergonadotropic hypogonadism: delayed puberty related to gonadal failure
Girls
  Syndrome of gonadal dysgenesis (Turner syndrome) and its variants
  XX and XY gonadal dysgenesis
    Familial and sporadic XX gonadal dysgenesis and its variants
    Familial and sporadic XY gonadal dysgenesis and its variants
  Other forms of primary ovarian failure
    Premature menopause
    Radiation therapy
    Chemotherapy
    Autoimmune oophoritis
    Resistant ovary
    Galactosemia
    Glycoprotein syndrome type 1
    FSH receptor gene mutators
    LH-hCG resistance
    Polycystic ovarian disease
    Noonan or pseudo-Turner syndrome
Boys
  Syndrome of seminiferous tubular dysgenesis and its variants (Klinefelter syndrome)
  Other forms of primary testicular failure
    Chemotherapy
    Radiation therapy
    Testicular biosynthetic defects
    Sertoli only syndrome
    LH resistance
    Anorchism and cryptorchidism

CNS = central nervous systems; LH = luteinizing hormone; FSH = follicle-stimulating hormone; hCG = human chorionic gonadotropin.

---

axillary hair development and acne years before the normal age of onset of normal puberty. Premature adrenarche must be differentiated from nonclassic 21-hydroxylase deficiency. In premature adrenarche, serum level of DHEAS is elevated to early midpubertal levels, whereas in nonclassic adrenal hyperplasia, serum levels of 17OHP and DHEAS may be elevated in the basal state, but 17OHP hyperresponds after ACTH stimulation to concentrations higher than normal in puberty. Bone age in premature adrenarche usually is not advanced over chronologic age, and growth velocity is similarly minimally increased or normal for age. Some girls with premature adrenarche have mild insulin resistance and are at increased risk of polycystic ovary syndrome in adulthood. Premature adrenarche necessitates careful follow-up evaluation because it is not a benign condition.

ADOLESCENT GYNECOMASTIA

More than 75% of healthy boys in the first and second stages of puberty have unilateral or bilateral breast development as a self-

limited and transient condition that rarely lasts more than 2 years. It is intensified by obesity and minimized to some degree by weight loss. Gynecomastia can cause much psychological distress during adolescence. Plastic surgery is indicated in only the most severe and persistent cases of gynecomastia and in the absence of an organic cause such as Klinefelter syndrome or a variant of androgen resistance syndrome. Such pathologic conditions must be ruled out before the diagnosis of adolescent gynecomastia is made. No medical therapy is available, but nonaromatizable androgen therapy is under study.

24.8.5 Delayed Puberty

Causes of delayed puberty are shown in Table 24-31. A boy who has not initiated spontaneous secondary sexual development by 14 years of age or a girl who has not done so by 13 years of age has delayed puberty. This can be caused by constitutional delay in adolescence or by a pathologic condition as serious as a brain tumor.

Evaluation of children for delays in pubertal development before these age guidelines would result in unnecessary testing of large numbers of children. Because 0.6% of the healthy population enters puberty spontaneously at an age later than these guidelines, even these age cutoffs include normal children with late spontaneous puberty. In some pathologic conditions, abnormalities of the hypothalamic-pituitary-gonadal axis allow a normal age at onset of puberty followed by cessation of progression. Thus patients who do not progress in secondary sexual development also should be considered for evaluation.

CONSTITUTIONAL DELAY IN GROWTH AND ADOLESCENCE: TEMPORARILY DELAYED PUBERTY

Patients who are healthy but have a slower rate of physical development than average have constitutional delay in growth and adolescence. These patients have a history of stature shorter than their age-matched peers throughout childhood, but their height is appropriate for bone age, and skeletal development is delayed more than 2.5 SD. They usually are thin and often have a family history of delayed puberty. Patients with a combination of a family tendency toward short stature and constitutional delay are the most likely to seek evaluation. They quite often seek evaluation when classmates or friends undergo pubertal development and growth, thereby accentuating their delay. Although mental development is appropriate for age, social development can lag if the patient, because of immature appearance, has been treated as younger than actual age by family, teachers, and peers. A family history of delay is common, so mothers should be asked their age at onset of menarche or other aspects of puberty, and fathers their age at shaving or at reaching adult height. Secondary sexual development generally occurs when a bone age of 12 years is reached for boys and 11 years for girls. Permanent gonadotropin deficiency is most likely if a patient does not start puberty spontaneously by 18 years of age. Cases of spontaneous pubertal development are rarely reported after 18 years of age. Before that age, in the absence of a classic presentation of constitutional delay in puberty, central nervous system disease, or other diagnostic characteristics, it is difficult to differentiate the temporary condition, constitutional delay in puberty, from permanent hypogonadotropic hypogonadism.

PERMANENT CONDITIONS OF SEXUAL INFANTILISM

HYPOGONADOTROPIC HYPOGONADISM Abnormalities of the hypothalamus or pituitary gland cause absence of onset of pubertal development associated with low serum levels of gonadotropins. If only gonadotropins are affected, the patient is of normal height but may have eunuchoid proportions of long legs and arms and an upper-to-lower-segment ratio well below the normal adult values. If GH also is deficient, the patient's growth rate also is decreased, often to a severe degree. Unlike patients with constitutional delay in puberty and those with GH deficiency, patients with *isolated gonadotropin deficiency* are of normal height until the adolescent age range, when, because of an absent pubertal growth spurt, they fall behind healthy persons. Because of delayed epiphyseal closure, they may continue to grow and reach a normal adult height albeit with characteristic eunuchoid proportions.

KALLMANN SYNDROME This disorder consists of hyposmia or anosmia and gonadotropin deficiency. Within a family, patients may have disorders of smell with normal gonadal function, and others may have abnormal gonadal function and a normal sense of smell. Some kindreds have members with Kallmann syndrome and others that appear to have constitutional delay in adolescence that suggests an etiologic relation between the two. In some cases, the disorder is caused by a mutation in a gene on Xp22.3 for an adhesion molecule that participates in normal migration of hypothalamic GnRH-secreting cells from the fetal volmeronasal organ (primitive nose) to the mediobasal hypothalamus. More than 80% of patients have absence of the olfactory sulci or olfactory bulbs on MR images, demonstrating the associated disordered development of the olfactory system.

ABNORMALITIES OF THE CENTRAL NERVOUS SYSTEM: GONADOTROPIN DEFICIENCY WITH OTHER PITUITARY HORMONE DEFICIENCIES

IDIOPATHIC HYPOPITUITARISM Congenital absence of any of the pituitary hormones can be found in idiopathic hypopituitarism. Because GH deficiency itself can delay the onset of puberty in an untreated patient, it can be difficult to determine which patient also has gonadotropin deficiency until the teenage years. Most cases are sporadic, but familial hypopituitarism can follow an X-linked or an autosomal recessive pattern in some kindreds. Hypopituitarism is discussed in Sec. 24.2.4.

DISORDERS OF THE CNS Patients with congenital midline defects may have gonadotropin deficiency as well as other types of hypothalamic-pituitary disorders. These conditions usually manifest in the neonatal period (see Sec. 24.2.4). Central nervous system tumors, particularly those involving the hypothalamic-pituitary region can cause precocious or delayed puberty (see Sec. 24.8.3). The same type of tumor can either delay or precipitate puberty, depending on the specific location. Prolactin-secreting tumors can delay puberty because of an inhibitory effect of prolactin on gonadotropin release or because of a mass effect of the tumor. Dopaminergic agents suppress progression of the tumor and prolactin secretion in some cases, but larger tumors necessitate surgical removal. Langerhans histiocytosis can cause isolated diabetes insipidus and can affect other hypothalamic-pituitary hormones. Granuloma of tuberculosis or sarcoid, postinfectious inflammation, and vascular lesions of the central nervous system all can impair hypothalamic-pituitary function, as can hydrocephalus, trauma caused by accidents, child abuse, or surgery. Radiation treatment can affect hypothalamic-pituitary function long after therapy is completed; this can include gonadotropin deficiency that delays puberty.

OTHER DISORDERS WITH DELAYED PUBERTY

Prader-Willi syndrome (see Sec. 24.2.6), Laurence-Moon or Bardet-Biedl syndromes of polydactyly, obesity, short stature, mental retardation, and retinitis pigmentosa can be associated with hypogonadotropic hypogonadism or hypergonadotropic hypogonadism, as can Turner syndrome and Klinefelter syndrome (see Sec. 24.7.5). Hypothyroidism inhibits the onset of puberty and menses, and hypothyroidism that occurs after the onset of puberty stops the progression of puberty.

Weight loss caused by chronic disease, malnutrition, and even dieting to less than 80% of ideal weight without definable psychiatric disease can cause hypogonadotropic hypogonadism. Weight loss of this degree is common in anorexia nervosa and causes a reversion of gonadotropin secretion patterns to prepubertal, low-amplitude pulsatile secretion that converts to the normal pubertal pattern months after weight regain. Increased physical activity in the presence of weight loss, as among ballerinas, or even in the maintenance of normal body weight, such as among swimmers or ice skaters, can cause cessation of menses. When increased activity ceases, as after an injury, menses recurs. Extreme exercise and weight control programs, such as those of young girls in competitive gymnastics, have been linked with a decrease in adult height and a decrease in bone density if puberty is delayed.

EVALUATION

The approach to the evaluation of delayed development of secondary sexual characteristics is outlined in Figs. 24-34 and 24-35. The first step in laboratory diagnosis of delayed puberty is differentiating primary gonadal disease (and hypergonadotropic hypogonadism) from hypothalamic-pituitary disease (and hypogonadotropic hypogonadism). If gonadotropin levels are high for age, a karyotype is obtained to evaluate the possibility of Turner syndrome or Klinefelter syndrome or their variants. Chronic disease, malnutrition, and excessive voluntary weight loss can delay puberty. Hypothyroidism must be ruled out by measurement of free T_4 and TSH. Prolactin is measured, although prolactin level can be elevated in cases of severe primary hypothyroidism.

If a patient has a low serum concentration of gonadotropin, differentiation between constitutional delay in puberty and permanent hypogonadotropic hypogonadism is challenging. A complete neurologic evaluation is performed to uncover any indication of a central nervous system tumor. If a tumor is being considered, MR imaging is performed. If midline abnormalities or anosmia are present, the diagnosis is likely to involve permanent impairment. If there is a compelling family history of delayed but ultimately spontaneous puberty, the diagnosis is likely to be constitutional delay in puberty. If the diagnosis still is in doubt, the patient is observed for

signs of spontaneous pubertal development or an increase in sex steroid concentrations. If a patient has not gone through the changes of puberty spontaneously by the age of 18 or 19 years, it is unlikely that he or she will do so. Several diagnostic methods have been suggested to differentiate constitutional delay in puberty from gonadotropin deficiency, but none has achieved wide acceptance. One promising method measures gonadotropin response after administration of GnRH agonist.

TREATMENT

A patient's immature appearance causes stress. In the worst case, it can lead to depression and suicidal ideation or attempts. In general, delayed puberty among boys is said to cause more distress than this condition among girls. Psychological support is offered as needed. Sex steroids are given to bring on pubertal development in permanent hypogonadism and also can be useful in constitutional delay. In the frequent situation in which the difference between the two cannot be established, short-term low-dose sex steroid therapy can be used to treat patients feeling the pressure of appearing immature, who are not comforted by the thought of "waiting for nature to take its course." The goal is to cause progression of secondary sexual development without advancing bone age and decreasing final height.

Boys

After the age of 14 years (the upper age of onset of normal pubertal development), boys can be given 50 to 100 mg of testosterone enanthate or cypionate intramuscularly every month for 3 months. If no sign of spontaneous puberty occurs in the 3 months after treatment, another course of testosterone can be offered. Patients with known hypogonadotropic hypogonadism need continuous testosterone therapy in increasing doses until the final dose of 250 to 300 mg per month is reached over 6 to 12 months. A dermal patch can be used to administer testosterone. Some teenagers prefer this to injections, but the patches must be changed daily. Some

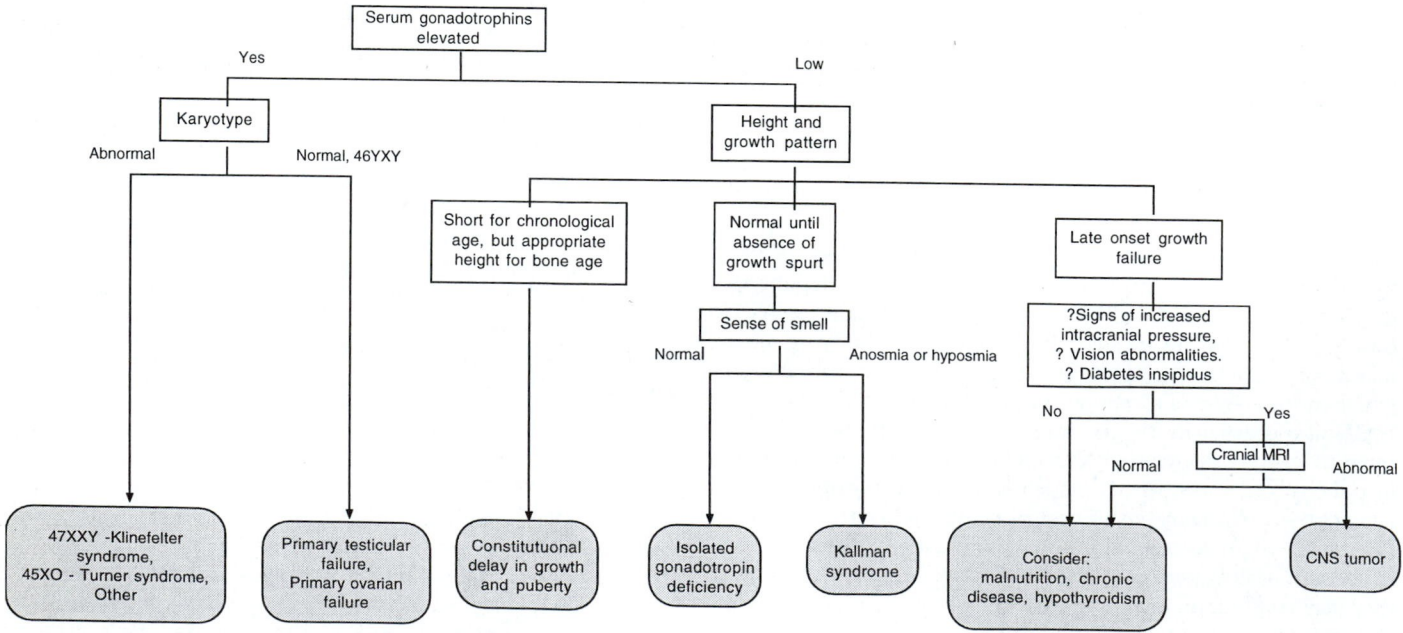

FIGURE 24-34   Evaluation of absence of secondary sexual development among boys at 14 years and girls at 13 years.

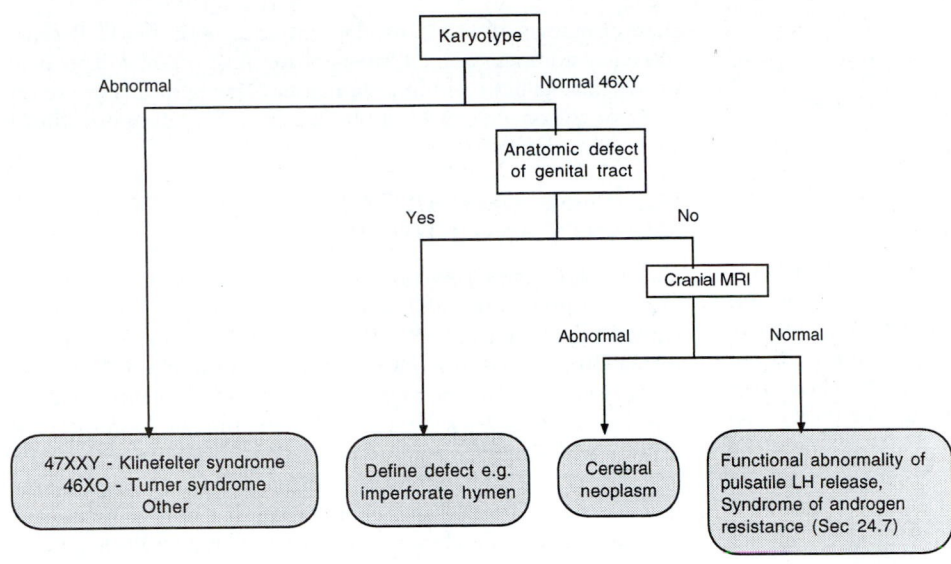

FIGURE 24-35 Evaluation of primary amenorrhea with normal secondary sexual development.

men need hCG injections in addition to testosterone to further pubic hair development and to achieve a more normal adult appearance. Patients with delayed puberty and growth hormone deficiency who have been treated regularly since an early age usually can receive this sex steroid treatment regimen. If the patient remains quite short or has not been treated before the teenage years, testosterone therapy can be withheld for a while or used at a lower dosage to ensure that maximal growth is reached before epiphyseal fusion eliminates the ability to respond to growth hormone.

Girls

Girls with delayed puberty can be treated with low-dose estrogen therapy. Ethinyl estradiol can be made into capsules and administered at 5 μg/d for 3 months. If hypogonadotropic hypogonadism is proved, or if the patient has hypergonadotropic hypogonadism, 10 to 15 μg/d of ethinyl estradiol is given after feminizing effects appear. After several months, estradiol is given only on the first to 21st days of the month. Withdrawal bleeding usually occurs each month after the end of estradiol administration. After several more months, a progestational agent such as medroxyprogesterone acetate (5 to 10 mg) is given on the 12th to 21st day of the cycle. Because of the suspected increase in risk of uterine carcinoma with exogenous estrogen treatment, it is recommended that a girl taking estrogen therapy undergo yearly pelvic examinations. Breast examinations also are needed because of the relation between estrogen and breast cancer. Patients with a family history of breast cancer need even closer observation. Girls with GH deficiency should not receive long-term or high-dose estrogen therapy until growth rate is normalized by administration of GH.

All Patients

All patients with hypogonadism, even those with temporarily delayed puberty, need at least the recommended 1500 mg elemental calcium per day to diminish the likelihood of osteoporosis in the future. All children and teenagers need the recommended daily allowance of calcium, but it is more important for those with disorders of puberty. Sex steroid therapy for the permanent conditions also can decrease the risk of osteopenia or osteoporosis later in life.

MENSTRUAL DISORDERS

Menstrual disorders and dysmenorrhea are discussed in Sec. 3.5.3.

References

Ahmed ML, Ong KK, Morrell DJ, et al: Longitudinal study of leptin concentrations during puberty: sex differences and relationship to changes in body composition. J Clin Endocrinol Metab 84:899–905, 1999

Dacou-Voutetakis C, Dracopoulo M: High incidence of molecular defects of the CYP21 gene in patients with premature adrenarche. J Clin Endocrinol Metab 84:1570–1574, 1999

Herman-Giddens ME, Slora EJ, Wasserman RC, et al: Secondary sex characteristics and menses in young girls seen in office practices: a study from the Pediatric Research in Office Settings Network. Pediatrics 99:505–512, 1997

Ibañez L, de Zegher F, Potau N: Anovulation after precocious pubarche: early markers and time course in adolescence. J Clin Endocrinol Metab 84:2691–2695, 1999

Kaplowitz PB, Oberfield SE: Reexamination of the age limit for defining puberty is precocious in girls in the United States: implications for evaluation and treatment. Drug and Therapeutics and Executive Committees of the Lawson Wilkins Pediatric Endocrine Society. Pediatrics 104:936–941, 1999

Kornreich L, Horev G, Blaser S, Daneman D, Kauli R, Grunebaum M: Central precocious puberty: evaluation by neuroimaging. Pediatr Radiol 25:7, 1995

Manasco PK, Umbach DM, Muly SM, et al: Ontogeny of gonadotropin, testosterone, and inhibin secretion in normal boys through puberty based on overnight serial sampling. J Clin Endocrinol Metab 80:2046–2052, 1995

Mitamura R, Yano K, Suzuki N, et al: Diurnal rhythms of luteinizing hormone, follicle-stimulating hormone, and testosterone secretion before the onset of male puberty. J Clin Endocrinol Metab 85:1074–1080, 2000

Palmert MR, Malin HV, Boepple PA: Unsustained or slowly progressive puberty in young girls: initial presentation and long-term follow-up of 20 untreated patients. J Clin Endocrinol Metab 84:415–423, 1999

Styne DM: New aspects in the diagnosis and treatment of pubertal disorders. Pediatr Clin North Am 44:505–529, 1997

Styne DM, Harris DA, Egli CA, et al: Treatment of true precocious puberty with a potent luteinizing hormone-releasing factor agonist: effect on growth, sexual maturation, pelvic sonography, and the hypothalamic-pituitary-gonadal axis. J Clin Endocrinol Metab 61:142–151, 1985

24.9 HYPOGLYCEMIA

Morey W. Haymond and Agneta L. Sunehag

Concentration of glucose in the plasma is maintained in a relatively narrow range in most persons but requires a delicate balance between glucose production and use. Euglycemia is maintained if the rate of appearance of glucose into the plasma space equals the rate of disappearance. If the rate of appearance of glucose exceeds the rate of disappearance, the plasma concentration of glucose increases. If the rate of appearance of glucose is lower than the rate of disappearance, plasma concentration decreases. Abnormalities in hormone secretion, substrate interconversion, and mobilization of metabolic fuels contribute to abnormalities in glucose production and use, which can result in hypoglycemia. Understanding the physiological mechanism of normal glucose metabolism is necessary to determine the pathophysiological mechanism of hypoglycemia and hyperglycemia.

24.9.1 Normal Glucose Homeostasis

The factors that regulate glucose homeostasis in adults and children are similar, but two aspects of glucose homeostasis are unique to the newborn infant and young child. The first concerns the transition from the intrauterine life to the first fast after delivery. The second is the high rate of glucose use in infants and children compared with that in adults.

TRANSITION TO EXTRAUTERINE LIFE

Glucose is rapidly transported across the placenta by means of facilitated diffusion. The result is a constant supply of glucose to the fetus. Thus the fetus is not dependent on its own glycogenolytic or gluconeogenic capability. Maternal glucose is the only source of glucose for a term infant at birth. Little is known about the time of induction of the hepatic gluconeogenic enzymes in the human fetus. Animal experiments show the activity of rate-limiting gluconeogenic enzymes (pyruvate carboxylase, phosphoenol pyruvate carboxykinase, glucose-6-phosphatase, and fructose-1,6-bisphosphatase) is low at birth but increases rapidly during the first hours of life. However, studies with fetal sheep suggest that hepatic glucose production can be hormonally modulated to some extent in utero.

Over the last trimester of gestation, the fetus accumulates body stores of fat and glycogen, and the activity of a number of enzymes necessary for mobilization of glucose, free fatty acids, and amino acids increases. This prepares the infant for its first fast after delivery and for cessation of continuous intravenous feeding with the clamping of the umbilical cord.

At delivery, a healthy newborn infant has adequate stores of fat and glycogen to sustain a short period of caloric deprivation and is capable of mobilizing these substrates as energy sources. The postnatal decrease in respiratory quotient and increase in plasma concentrations of glycerol and free fatty acids indicate that the newborn infant is mobilizing and oxidizing fat soon after birth. During the first 2 hours after birth, the plasma concentration of glucose decreases to reach a nadir approximately 1 to 2 hours postnatally. However, the decrease in insulin and increase in plasma concentrations of glucagon, epinephrine, and GH that occurs after birth stimulate glycogenolysis, gluconeogenesis, and lipolysis. The increase in fatty acid oxidation reduces use of glucose. Collectively these changes increase glucose concentration in the blood. Because glycogen stores are limited, the neonate must become dependent on gluconeogenesis within a short time. Newborn infants are capable of gluconeogenesis from both alanine and glycerol within 4 to 8 hours of delivery.

GLUCOSE REQUIREMENTS OF INFANTS AND CHILDREN

The absolute rate of glucose production and use (μmol $\cdot$ min^{-1}) increases throughout childhood with the increase in body and brain mass. Up to an age of 6 to 8 years and a body weight of approximately 20 kg, there is a linear relation between absolute glucose use and body weight that extends to premature infants weighing less than 1000 g. After the age of 8 years, the rate of glucose use decreases, achieving an adult value of 11 to 13 μmol $\cdot$ kg^{-1} $\cdot$ min^{-1} ($\sim$2 mg $\cdot$ kg^{-1} $\cdot$ min^{-1}) by late adolescence. Glucose use by the brain is as much as 20 times greater than that of nonbrain tissue. The larger brain to body weight ratio of children results in glucose flux rates (production and use) on a body weight basis that are three times higher in a young child than in an adult. In the postabsorptive state (4 to 14 hours of fast), the flux rate of glucose in children (younger than 8 years) is approximately 35 μmol $\cdot$ kg^{-1} $\cdot$ min^{-1} (6 mg $\cdot$ kg^{-1} $\cdot$ min^{-1}) compared with 13 μmol $\cdot$ kg^{-1} $\cdot$ min^{-1} (2 mg $\cdot$ kg^{-1} $\cdot$ min^{-1}) for adults. After a 30-hour fast, glucose flux decreases to 9 to 10 μmol $\cdot$ kg^{-1} $\cdot$ min^{-1} (1.8 mg $\cdot$ kg^{-1} $\cdot$ min^{-1}) and 23 μmol $\cdot$ kg^{-1} $\cdot$ min^{-1} (4.1 mg $\cdot$ kg^{-1} $\cdot$ min^{-1}) for adults and children, respectively (Table 24-32).

REQUIREMENTS FOR MAINTENANCE OF GLUCOSE HOMEOSTASIS

Maintenance of plasma concentration of glucose in the normal range regardless of age depends on (1) a normal endocrine system for integrating and modulating substrate mobilization, interconversion, and use, (2) functionally intact enzymes for glycogenolysis, gluconeogenesis, and use of other metabolic fuels, and (3) an adequate supply of endogenous fat, glycogen, and potential gluconeogenic substrates (amino acids, glycerol, and lactate). Although differences between men and women in glucose response to fasting have been identified (Fig. 24-36), adults can maintain a nearly normal blood concentration of glucose, even when totally deprived of calories for days or, in the case of obese persons, weeks. In contrast, healthy neonates and young children are less able to meet the obligatory demands for glucose and have a progressive decrease in plasma glucose concentration to hypoglycemic values after even short fasts (24 to 48 hours).

During overnight fasting, 50 to 60% of plasma glucose is derived from hepatic glycogen, whereas with prolonged fasting, gluconeogenesis becomes the main source of glucose production. Little is known about the dynamic and quantitative aspects of glucose production from glycogenolysis or gluconeogenesis or the factors affecting use of glucose by normal infants or children who have fasted. It is clear, however, that there is a more precarious balance between obligatory glucose requirements and ability to maintain an adequate supply of glucose during caloric deprivation. If glycogenolysis were the only source of glucose production, the hepatic glycogen content of healthy children would be sufficient to meet the glucose demands for no more than 5 to 10 hours. During a fast, the contribution from glycogenolysis decreases gradually and that from gluconeogenesis increases. For healthy children who have fasted overnight, gluconeogenesis accounts for about 50% of glucose production. After 24 to 36 hours of fasting, a young child is most likely totally dependent on gluconeogenesis as the primary source of endogenous plasma glucose. This is reflected clinically by a blunted or absent glycemic response to exogenous glucagon under these fasting conditions. A substantial percentage of the carbon for de novo glucose production after prolonged fasting in adults is derived from amino acids (glutamine and alanine) as a result of muscle proteolysis and from glycerol as a result of lipolysis. Because the mass of muscle relative to that of the entire body is smaller in newborns, infants, and young children than in adults, the ability to mobilize sufficient endogenous gluconeogenic substrate to maintain the higher rates of glucose production for a prolonged period of fast may be compromised.

The availability of endogenous stores of fatty acids for oxidative metabolism is of substantial importance in the maintenance of glucose homeostasis in infants and children. Free fatty acids are used by nearly every tissue of the body except brain. Although free fatty acids cannot be used, ketone bodies cross the blood-brain barrier and can supplant more than half of the glucose requirements of the brain in the fetus and neonate, as well as in adult animals. Conversely, defective oxidation of fatty acids by body tissues can result in a relative increase in the rates of glucose use.

The metabolic response to brief periods of fasting results in greater decreases in plasma concentration of glucose and increases in concentration of ketone bodies in children than in adults. This suggests that the relative increase in glucose requirements among children accelerates the adaptive mechanisms of fasting. As a result, abnormalities in modulation of mobilization, interconversion, and use of substrates among children frequently are accompanied by hypoglycemia.

HEPATIC GLYCOGENOLYSIS AND GLUCONEOGENESIS

Regulation of hepatic glucose production is basic to the maintenance of glucose homeostasis. Although the kidney is capable of glycogen synthesis, glycogenolysis, and gluconeogenesis, it does not contribute a great deal to net glucose production in adults except during prolonged fasting or metabolic acidosis. No information is available to determine the quantitative contribution of renal glucose production to glucose homeostasis in children. The enzymes responsible for storage and release of hepatic glycogen are discussed in Sec. 9.6.

Four enzymes are important in gluconeogenesis from three-carbon substrates such as lactate and pyruvate. Glucose-6-phosphatase hydrolyzes glucose-6-phosphate to glucose and is the final enzy-

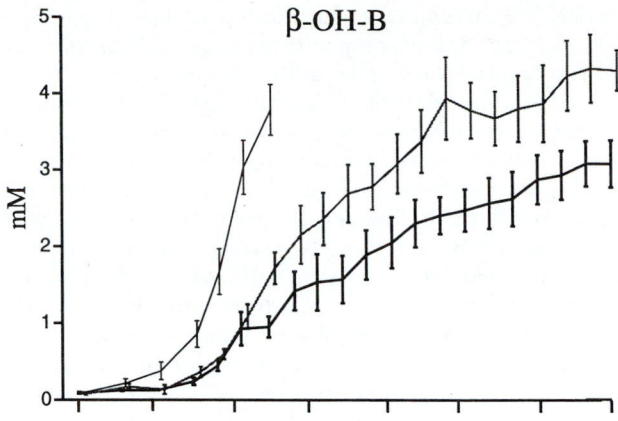

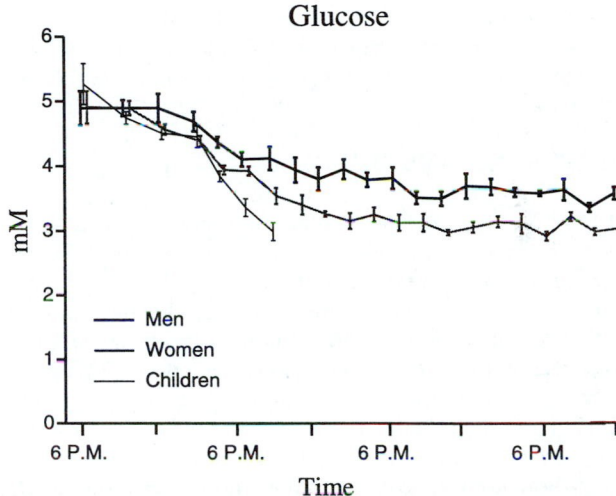

FIGURE 24-36   Plasma concentrations of glucose and β-hydroxybutyrate for men and women during 84 hours of fasting and for prepubertal children during a 30-hour fast. Zero time of the fast was 1800 hours, 1 hour after the last meal. All data are expressed as mean $\pm$ SE. (SOURCE: *Haymond MW: Hypoglycemia in infants and children. Endocrinol Metab Clin North Am 18:211–252, 1989, with permission.*)

matic step by which the liver and kidney release free glucose derived from either glycogenolysis or gluconeogenesis except for a small fraction, which theoretically can be derived from debrancher enzyme activity. Fructose-1,6-bisphosphatase catalyzes hydrolysis of

TABLE 24-32

EFFECTS OF FASTING ON GLUCOSE FLUX IN CHILDREN AND ADULTS

CONDITION	μmol/kg/min	μmol/100 g BRAIN/min	μmol/m²/min
Adults			
Postabsorptive[a]	12.8 ± 0.5	64 ± 3	483 ± 19
30-hour fast	9.8 ± 0.5	49 ± 3	370 ± 19
Healthy children			
Postabsorptive[a]	35 ± 2	70 ± 4	907 ± 52
30-hour fast	23 ± 3	43 ± 6	596 ± 78
Children with epilepsy			
Postabsorptive[a]	35 ± 2	59 ± 5	977 ± 56
30-hour fast	19 ± 1	31 ± 4	536 ± 11

[a] 14-hour fast.

SOURCE: *Haymond MW, Howard C, Ben-Galim E, et al: Effects of ketosis on glucose flux in children and adults. Am J Physiol 1983; 245:E373–E378.*

fructose-1,6-bisphosphate to fructose-6-phosphate, bypassing the energy-yielding enzyme phosphofructokinase. This enzyme has an important regulatory role in hepatic gluconeogenesis.

A second and perhaps more important regulatory site for hepatic gluconeogenesis exists between pyruvate and phosphoenolpyruvate and involves two enzymes of gluconeogenesis (pyruvate carboxylase and phosphoenolpyruvate carboxykinase) and one enzyme of glycolysis, pyruvate kinase. Pyruvate carboxylase is a mitochondrial enzyme that catalyzes conversion of pyruvate to oxaloacetate by the addition of carbon dioxide. Pyruvate carboxylase is biotin and manganese dependent and has very low activity in the absence of acetyl-coenzyme A, its positive modulator. Thus, only when the availability of acetyl-coenzyme A is increased (fasting or poorly controlled diabetes), can increased amounts of pyruvate be converted to oxaloacetate, the first step in gluconeogenesis. Phosphoenolpyruvate carboxykinase is present in both the cytosol and mitochondria. Although these two enzymes are the first steps in hepatic gluconeogenesis, hormonal regulation of hepatic glucose production is thought to occur at the level of pyruvate kinase and phosphofructokinase.

ENDOCRINE SYSTEM

INSULIN Insulin is the predominant hormone regulating blood glucose, because it is the only hormone which acts to decrease endogenous glucose production and accelerate glucose use. Insulin stimulates (1) transmembrane movement of glucose into skeletal and cardiac muscle and adipose tissue as a result of the GLUT4 glucose transporter and (2) conversion of glucose to glycogen and triglyceride. At even low concentrations, insulin is a potent inhibitor of adipose tissue lipolysis and decreases the rate of proteolysis. The net effect of these actions on peripheral tissues is to accelerate glucose disappearance from the blood and decrease the supply of gluconeogenic substrates (glycerol and amino acids) presented to the liver. In concert with these peripheral actions, insulin stimulates hepatic glycogen synthesis, decreases glycogenolysis, and decreases release of glucose from hepatic gluconeogenesis. Insulin appears to activate glycogen synthetase and inhibit the phosphorylase system.

Pancreatic arterial glucose concentration is the primary but not sole determinant of insulin release. A number of substrates, including free fatty acids, ketone bodies, and some amino acids, can either directly stimulate insulin release from the β cell or potentiate the effect of glucose on hormone secretion. Oral ingestion of fat and glucose provokes secretion of enteric factors that themselves augment or facilitate insulin release. During fasting, plasma concentration of insulin decreases to less than 5 $\mu U \cdot mL^{-1}$ in children. Concentrations greater than this in association with blood glucose concentrations less than 2.8 mmol/L (50 mg $\cdot$ dL^{-1}) are distinctly abnormal. Systemic insulin concentrations are substantially lower than the concentration in the portal vein, reflecting both transhepatic removal (approximately 50% is removed in one transhepatic passage) and dilution in the total vascular space.

COUNTERREGULATORY HORMONES The actions of cortisol, glucagon, epinephrine, and growth hormone oppose the hypoglycemic effects of insulin. These hormones increase the ambient blood glucose concentration by (1) inhibiting glucose uptake by muscle (epinephrine, cortisol, and growth hormone), (2) increasing the availability of endogenous gluconeogenic amino acids by increasing muscle proteolysis (cortisol), (3) activating lipolysis and providing increased free fatty acids as a source of energy and glycerol for glu-

coneogenesis (epinephrine, glucagon, growth hormone, and cortisol), (4) inhibiting insulin secretion from the pancreas (epinephrine), (5) acutely activating glycogenolytic and gluconeogenic enzymes (epinephrine and glucagon), and (6) chronically inducing gluconeogenic enzyme synthesis (glucagon and cortisol).

24.9.2 Hypoglycemic Syndromes

Hypoglycemia among infants and children has traditionally been divided into *transient neonatal hypoglycemia* and *hypoglycemia of infancy and childhood*. The definition of hypoglycemia is somewhat arbitrary, depending on the age of the patient and the conditions under which the samples are obtained. For example, a plasma glucose concentration of 3.3 mmol/L (60 mg $\cdot$ dL^{-1}) can be distinctly abnormal 1 hour after a carbohydrate load for any child or adolescent, whereas healthy women who fast for 4 days can have plasma glucose values less than 2.2 mmol/L (40 mg $\cdot$ dL^{-1}) without symptoms. Children usually have symptoms of hypoglycemia when plasma glucose concentrations decreases to approximately 2.2 mmol/L (40 mg $\cdot$ dL^{-1}). Any child or infant who has a plasma glucose concentration less than 2.8 mmol/L (<50 mg $\cdot$ dL^{-1}) during an elective fast should be observed carefully. At concentration less than 2.2 mmol/L (<40 mg $\cdot$ dL^{-1}), the patient is considered to have hypoglycemia, and diagnostic and therapeutic intervention is initiated. The definition of hypoglycemia among newborns continues to be a source of controversy, particularly in the first hours of life. Plasma concentration of glucose decreases over the first hours of life, a time of physiological hypoglycemia. After these first hours, plasma level of glucose less than 2.2 mmol/L (40 mg $\cdot$ dL^{-1}) is considered hypoglycemia, and appropriate treatment is initiated (feeding or intravenous glucose, depending on the patient's maturity, clinical status, and glucose concentration).

The symptoms associated with a rapid decrease in plasma concentration of glucose reflect increased adrenergic activity (tachycardia, shaking) and cholinergic activity (sweating, weakness, and hunger). If the hypoglycemia is not relieved, manifestations of progressive symptoms of cerebral dysfunction, such as headache, irritability, mental confusion, psychotic behavior, seizures, and coma, can develop. With frequent or prolonged episodes of hypoglycemia, permanent central nervous system damage or even death can occur. Symptoms of hypoglycemia are less obvious among neonates than they are among adults and may be overlooked. Careful, prospective monitoring of plasma concentration of glucose is indicated in the early hours of life and for longer periods in the care of infants at high risk of hypoglycemia.

NEONATAL HYPOGLYCEMIA

Hypoglycemia is caused by either decreased rates of glucose production or increased rates of use. Small-for-gestational-age infants have low glycogen, muscle, and fat stores, making them prone to hypoglycemia caused by inadequate glucose production from glycogen and by gluconeogenesis (see Sec. 2.7.4). Infants whose mothers have diabetes frequently have severe hypoglycemia after birth, presumably caused by chronic exposure to high ambient glucose concentrations during gestation with resultant β-cell hyperplasia. After birth, excessive insulin is secreted with resultant hypoglycemia (see Sec. 2.15). Other disorders that can cause hypoglycemia in the newborn include glucagon deficiency and disorders that increase the rates of glucose utilization such as neonatal sepsis. The differential diagnosis and management of hypoglycemia in the newborn infants are discussed in Sec. 2.17.4.

HYPOGLYCEMIA OF INFANCY AND CHILDHOOD

As in the newborn period, hypoglycemia in infancy and childhood is caused by either decreased rates of glucose production or increased use. Decreased glucose production can be caused by increased insulin secretion, as in hyperinsulinemia with persistent hyperinsulinemic hypoglycemia of infancy, islet cell dysplasia, or adenoma. Other causes of hypoglycemia not discussed herein include accidental or intentional, as in Munchausen syndrome by proxy, administration of oral hypoglycemic agents or insulin. Ingestion of salicylates or ethyl alcohol also causes hypoglycemia. Hepatic enzyme deficiencies, including disorders of glycogen metabolism, fructose-1,6-bisphosphatase deficiency, galactosemia, and hereditary fructose metabolism, also cause severe hypoglycemia (see Sec. 9.5.3). Other metabolic disorders, especially fatty acid oxidation defects and ketotic hypoglycemia, are discussed in Sec. 9.1.5. Hepatic failure can be complicated by hypoglycemia (see Sec. 18.12). Endocrine disorders, especially adrenal insufficiency or panhypopituitarism, can manifest as severe hypoglycemia.

PERSISTENT HYPERINSULINEMIC HYPOGLYCEMIA OF INFANCY This disorder most commonly appears during the first year of life. Early recognition and management of persistent hyperinsulinemic hypoglycemia of infancy (PHHI) are of utmost importance to avoid or minimize permanent neurologic damage. A sigmoid relationship normally exits between plasma level of glucose and insulin concentration. Only small amounts of insulin are secreted when the plasma level of glucose falls to less than 3.3 mmol/L (60 mg · dL^{-1}). Among children with β-cell dysplasia, this relation is disturbed or disrupted. Although insulin increases the transport and metabolic clearance of glucose, the primary effect of insulin on glucose metabolism is a decrease in hepatic glucose production. The incidence of PHHI is approximately 1:50,000 in northern Europe. It is much higher in countries with a high prevalence of consanguinity (1:2675 in Saudi Arabia). The following four gene defects on chromosome 11 have been identified: (1) sulfonylurea receptor defects (*SUR1*); (2) defects on the inward rectifying potassium channel *KIR6.2* gene; (3) regulatory mutations on the glutamate dehydrogenase gene, and (4) an activating glucokinase mutation. At least 13 different mutations of the sulfonylurea receptor gene on chromosome 11p15 have been described, but only a few patients have been found to have lesions in the *KIR6.2* gene. The *SUR1* and *KIR6.2* mutations result in absence of KATP activity in the β cells, which leads to closure of the potassium channel, depolarization of the cell membrane, influx of calcium ions, and increased insulin release. A form of congenital hyperinsulinemia characterized by hypoglycemia and hyperammonemia is caused by defects on the glutamate dehydrogenase gene.

Glucokinase controls glucose metabolism in the β cells and is responsible for glucose-mediated regulation of insulin secretion. Loss-of-function mutation of this gene is associated with maturity-onset diabetes of the young (see Sec. 24.10). However, the mutation Val455Met in the glucokinase gene causes autosomal-dominant familial hyperinsulinism by lowering the K_m for glucose 65%. The long-term effects of this mutation are not clear, but the oldest affected patient had diabetes later in life. The Val203Ala and Val455Met mutations cause disease among both heterozygotes and homozygotes. The disease in homozygotes is more severe and difficult to manage. Among heterozygotes the disease is milder, manifests later, and responds well to pharmacologic treatment.

Both focal and diffuse histopathologic abnormalities are associated with PHHI. Focal abnormalities occur among 30 to 50% of patients treated surgically. Some patients with the focal form have lost the maternal allele of chromosome 11p15 in the hyperplastic lesion. Some of these patients have a mutant *SUR1* gene inherited from the father. Loss of the maternal allele caused hemizygosity or homozygosity of the paternal defective allele of the *SUR1* gene and caused a recessive endocrine disorder associated with focal β-cell hyperplasia and hyperinsulinemia.

The primary aim of therapy for childhood hyperinsulinemic hypoglycemia is to prevent neurologic symptoms and sequelae, including seizures and mental retardation. The therapeutic approaches to PHHI are directed at decreasing insulin secretion pharmacologically or surgically. It is important to differentiate the focal and diffuse forms as early as possible, because the focal form responds well to partial pancreatectomy.

Medical management of hyperinsulinemia includes diazoxide, which blocks the sulfonylurea receptors on the β cells. The result is opening of the potassium channels and decreased insulin release. Doses of 5 to 20 mg/kg/d are administered. Side effects arc hypertrichosis, advanced bone age, mild hyperuricemia, decreased IgG concentration and neutrophil counts, and sodium and water retention. Water retention can be reduced with concomitant administration of hydrochlorothiazides, which further reduce insulin secretion. Life-threatening complications such as ketoacidosis, congestive heart failure, and nonketotic hyperosmolar coma can be avoided with appropriate monitoring of plasma level of glucose, urinary levels of ketones, and fluid balance. If treatment with diazoxide is not successful, somatostatin analogs and Ca^{2+}-channel blockers can be tried. However, long-term follow-up studies of the potential side effects of these drugs are not available. Glucagon may be useful during the initial stabilization period and before surgery. Insulin-like growth factor I has been reported to inhibit insulin secretion among persons with hyperinsulinemia.

When hyperinsulinemia is proved and medical therapy does not control hypoglycemia, surgical exploration is indicated for any child past the first weeks of life. Selective resection of focal anomalies often is curative. The diffuse form necessitates subtotal pancreatectomy, in which 95% of the pancreas is removed while leaving the spleen intact. The variable results of surgery reflect differences in the pathophysiological mechanism and the extent of pancreatectomy. After subtotal pancreatectomy, exogenous insulin may be needed for several months to control hyperglycemia. Conversely, recurrence of hypoglycemia within days of surgery portends future problems in the establishment of reasonable control of glucose homeostasis. Sufficient exocrine pancreas usually is preserved to avoid fat malabsorption. Careful follow-up care of each patient is needed to evaluate the long-term effects of subtotal pancreatectomy on endocrine and exocrine pancreatic function. When surgical results are poor, medical management must be continued.

ISLET CELL DYSPLASIA OR ADENOMA These rare disorders can manifest as hypoglycemia. In the care of older children and adolescents, other endocrine abnormalities (hyperparathyroidism, hypergastrinemia, and pituitary tumors) must be sought in the patient and his or her family to exclude MEN 1. The plasma insulin response to fasting or insulin secretagogues does not differentiate

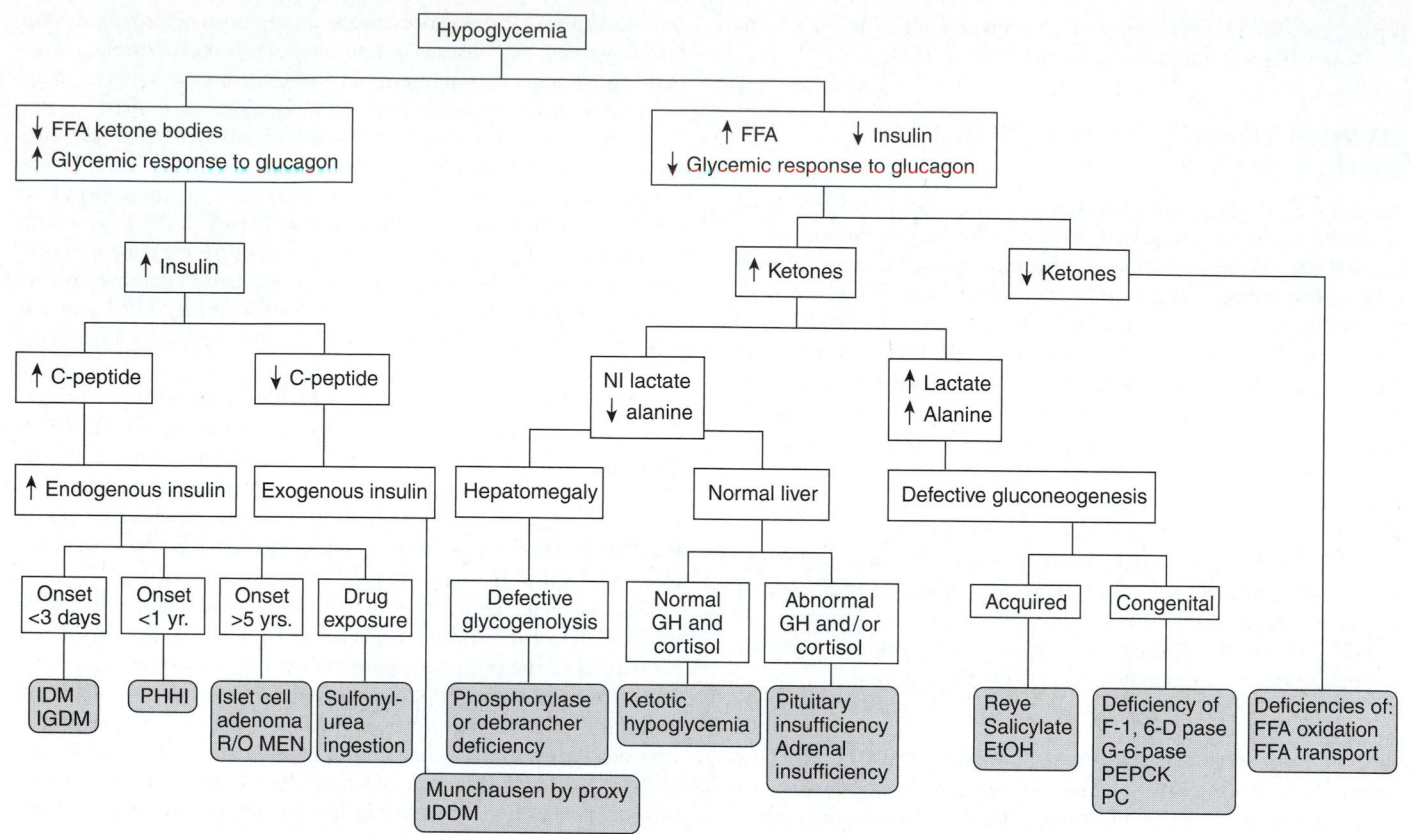

FIGURE 24-37   Diagnostic approach to hypoglycemia among children. *IDM* **and** *IGDM* **= infants of mothers with insulin-dependent or gestational-onset diabetes, respectively;** *PHHI* **= persistent hyperinsulinemic hypoglycemia of infancy;** *MEN* **= multiple endocrine neoplasia syndrome;** *FFA* **= free fatty acid;** *EtOH* **= Alcohol;** *F-1,6-Dpase* **= fructose 1,6 diphosphatase;** *G-6-pase* **= glucose-6-phosphatase;** *PEPCK* **= phosphoenolpyruvate carboxykinase;** *PC* **= pyruvate carboxylase;** *IDDM* **= insulin dependent diabetes mellitus.**

these various disorders. Because adenomas are generally less than 1 cm in diameter and are rare among infants and young children, celiac arteriography, MR imaging, and CT are of little diagnostic value. Percutaneous and intraoperative ultrasonography are highly sensitive techniques in identifying some insulin-producing tumors of the pancreas.

DIAGNOSTIC EVALUATION OF HYPOGLYCEMIA

The diagnostic evaluation of the newborn with hypoglycemia is discussed in Sec. 2.17.4. The approach to the evaluation of a child with hypoglycemia and suspected metabolic disease is discussed in Sec. 9.1.5. When any child is believed to have hypoglycemia, a low blood glucose value is quickly confirmed with a test strip. Sufficient blood *always* should be obtained before therapeutic intervention to confirm the diagnosis. Semiquantitative methods for estimating the concentration of glucose in the blood are useful for monitoring the condition of patients with suspected hypoglycemia. Because these methods are not reliable when glucose concentration is less than 2.8 mmol/L (50 mg · dL⁻¹), the diagnosis of hypoglycemia must rest on samples obtained in a quantitative analysis of plasma derived from blood placed in a tube containing NaFl (to inhibit erythrocyte glycolysis) and a method specific for glucose (most commonly, glucose oxidase).

If possible, adequate blood should be obtained to allow initial

evaluation of plasma concentrations of hormones (insulin, C-peptide, cortisol, GH, IGF-I, IGF-II, and IGFBP-1) and substrates (β-hydroxybutyrate, lactate, ammonium, free fatty acids, amino acids, and free and total carnitine). This single sample is the most valuable guide for further evaluation of a child with hypoglycemia as outlined in Fig. 24-37.

Historical factors helpful in defining the cause of hypoglycemia include the presence or absence of hypoglycemic symptoms at birth, age at onset, growth and development, frequency of hypoglycemic episodes, specific food intolerance or aversions, temporal relation to meals, family history, potential drug exposure, and unexplained infant death.

The findings from the history, physical examination, initial plasma sample (if available), and a provocative fast guide further testing. However, no elective fast is undertaken until the patient is shown to have normal plasma free and total carnitine concentrations because under most circumstances, fasting is contraindicated if carnitine level is low. Hypoglycemia in the face of relatively low plasma concentrations of ketone bodies, free fatty acids, or IGFBP-1 immediately focuses attention on abnormalities of insulin secretion. Hyperinsulinism is best documented with simultaneous measurement of plasma levels of glucose and insulin at times of hypoglycemia. Levels greater than 3 to 5 μU/mL when plasma level of glucose is less than 2.2 mmol/L (40 mg/dL) whether or not the patient is fed or fasted indicate the need for further studies to document hyperinsulinism. Intravenous glucagon (0.03 mg ·

kg^{-1}, maximum 1 mg) at the time of hypoglycemia can be both therapeutic and diagnostic. A clear glycemic response (increase greater than 1 mmol/L or 15 to 20 mg/dL) over the first 10 to 20 minutes after administration of glucagon reflects inappropriate sequestration of hepatic glycogen and strongly suggests hyperinsulinemia or glucagon deficiency. When hyperinsulinemia is strongly suspected or proved, blood is obtained for DNA analysis to identify (1) any of the sulfonylurea receptor or potassium channel defects, (2) increased expression of IGF-II gene on chromosome 11p15.5 (Beckwith-Wiedemann syndrome), and (3) mutations of the glutamate dehydrogenase gene (suspected when hypoglycemia is associated with hyperammonemia). Levels of IGFBP-1 can be of diagnostic value in differentiating hyperinsulinism from other hypoglycemic disorders. During fast-induced hypoglycemia, IGFBP-1 concentration does not increase or increases minimally in children with hyperinsulinism. In healthy children and children with ketotic hypoglycemia, IGFBP-1 concentration increases severalfold.

When a child has hypoglycemia as a part of multiorgan symptoms such as enteropathy, coagulopathy, and neuropathy, carbohydrate-deficient glycoprotein syndrome is suspected. Hypoglycemia in association with hypoketonemia but high plasma concentrations of free fatty acids directs the investigation toward fatty acid oxidation disorders. Symptomatic fasting hypoglycemia associated with ketonuria and ketonemia without hepatomegaly and with an onset after 18 months of age strongly suggests the diagnosis of ketotic hypoglycemia. The diagnosis of galactosemia or hereditary fructose intolerance is considered when an infant has hypoglycemia in the immediately postprandial period, particularly with hepatomegaly and failure to thrive. Fasting hypoglycemia, hepatomegaly, and metabolic acidosis associated with episodic hyperventilation are highly suggestive of glucose-6-phosphatase or fructose-1,6-bisphosphatase deficiency.

References

Haymond MW: Hypoglycemia in infants and children. Endocrinol Metab Clin North Am 18:211–252, 1989

Haymond MW, Sunehag A: Controlling the sugar bowl: regulation of glucose homeostasis in children. Endocrinol Metab Clin North Am 28: 663–694, 1999

Katz LE, Ferry RJ Jr, Stanley CA, Collett-Solberg PF, Baker L, Cohen P: Suppression of insulin oversecretion by subcutaneous recombinant human insulin-like growth factor I in children with congenital hyperinsulinism due to defective beta-cell sulfonylurea receptor. J Clin Endocrinol Metab 84:3117–24, 1999

Schwitzgebel VM, Gitelman SE: Neonatal hyperinsulinism. Clin Perinatol, 25:1015–1038, 1998

Stanley CA, Lieu YK, Hsu BY, et al: Hyperinsulinism and hyperammonemia in infants with regulatory mutations of the glutamate dehydrogenase gene. N Engl J Med 338:1352–1357, 1998

24.10 DIABETES MELLITUS

Stephen E. Gitelman

Diabetes mellitus encompasses a heterogeneous group of disorders defined by a derangement in carbohydrate metabolism caused by a defect in either insulin secretion or insulin action. The effects can be acute and life threatening, such as diabetic ketoacidosis, or chronic, resulting from long-term end-organ damage caused by chronic hyperglycemia. Aside from asthma, diabetes mellitus is the most common chronic illness of childhood, affecting more than 125,000 children in the United States, with approximately 13,000 new cases per year. Currently, 15% of the US health care budget is spent on diabetes and its complications. Maintenance of the glucose concentration of blood in a nearly normal range can prevent or minimize long-term damage. Assuring optimal management of this disorder over the patient's lifetime places a tremendous amount of responsibility on the patient, family, and health care team.

24.10.1   Diagnostic Criteria and Screening

The diagnostic criteria for diabetes mellitus are summarized in Table 24-33. The diagnosis is established when any one of the criteria are met. An elevated blood glucose level must be confirmed with any one of these methods on a subsequent day to confirm the diagnosis, unless there is unequivocal hyperglycemia with acute metabolic decompensation. The cutoff for fasting glucose result that establishes the diagnosis has been decreased from 140 to 126 mg/dL, more closely approximating an abnormal response in an oral glucose tolerance test (OGTT). Epidemiologic studies have shown that a fasting glucose level greater than 125 mg/dL corresponds to the point of increased risk of later vascular disease from chronic hyperglycemia.

A fasting glucose level has largely supplanted the OGTT for screening because it is quicker, less expensive, and more convenient and acceptable to patients. The OGTT is subject to greater intraindividual variation than is fasting glucose level. Levels of glycohemoglobin, or subfractions such as hemoglobin A_{1C} (HbA_{1C}), are used to measure the nonenzymatic covalent bonding of glucose to hemoglobin, and represents a 3-month average of blood glucose values. Although these tests are valuable for monitoring glycemic control and response to therapy and do not require a fasting sample, they are not as sensitive as a fasting glucose level for screening. Another problem is that many different glycosylated hemoglobin assays are used, making it impossible to derive a consistent standard. Thus routine use of such assays for diagnosis is not currently recommended. These studies also can be altered by factors that affect erythrocyte survival, such as an underlying hemoglobinopathy. In such cases, a fructosamine assay is used, which represents noncovalent glycation of serum proteins over a 2-week period.

Derangement in carbohydrate metabolism proceeds along a

TABLE 24-33

CRITERIA FOR THE DIAGNOSIS OF DIABETES MELLITUS

1. Randomly measured plasma concentration of glucose of 200 mg/dL or greater with classic signs and symptoms of diabetes (polyuria, polydipsia, weight loss, fatigue)
   or
2. Fasting plasma concentration of glucose 126 mg/dL or greater with no caloric intake for at least 8 hours previously
   or
3. Abnormal result of an oral glucose tolerance test [1.75 g/kg by mouth of anhydrous glucose dissolved in water (to a maximum of 75 g)] and plasma concentration of glucose after glucose load of 200 mg/dL or greater

Any one of these criteria must be repeated on a subsequent day to confirm the diagnosis, unless there is unequivocal hyperglycemia with acute metabolic decompensation (diabetic ketoacidosis).

continuum, and a given person can have a slow evolution from euglycemia toward diabetes mellitus (Table 24-34). Persons with fasting glucose level less than 110 mg/dL, or less than 140 mg/dL after an OGTT are euglycemic. Those with a fasting glucose level greater than 110 but less than 126 mg/dL or OGTT values more than 140 but less than 200 mg/dL are considered to have impaired glucose tolerance. These persons are at high risk of progression to overt diabetes over time; 1.5 to 7.3% of cases of impaired glucose tolerance advance to diabetes mellitus per year.

Although diabetes is common, routine screening is recommended only for persons considered at risk. Children who have had hyperglycemia during acute stress usually do not have diabetes mellitus. Nearly 4% of children without diabetes treated in emergency departments have a glucose level greater than 150 mg/dL. These children usually have serious illness (fever, need for hospital admission, or need for intravenous fluids), but only 2.3% of such children with hyperglycemia eventually have diabetes mellitus. However, children with incidental hyperglycemia in the absence of serious illness have a much greater risk of diabetes mellitus. As many as one-third have type 1 diabetes mellitus within 18 months. The presence of autoantibodies to islet β cells can help identify a subset of patients at risk of progression to type 1 diabetes mellitus. There are now investigational protocols to screen persons at risk of type 1 diabetes mellitus well before they have the disorder, but such studies are not yet recommended in routine practice. The rapidly increasing incidence of type 2 diabetes mellitus among children suggests that some of the risk factors considered for adult screening may be applicable to the younger population. Current recommendations are to screen those who are overweight (body mass index more than 85th percentile, weight for height more than 85th percentile, or weight greater than 120% ideal weight) and who have two or more of the following: (1) family history of type 2 diabetes mellitus in a first- or second-degree relative, (2) non-European ancestry, and (3) signs of insulin resistance or a condition associated with insulin resistance (eg, acanthosis nigricans, syndrome X, polycystic ovary syndrome). For these patients, the level of glucose in the blood while the patient is fasting is measured at 10 years of age, or earlier if puberty has started, and every 2 years thereafter.

CLASSIFICATION OF DIABETES MELLITUS

The types of diabetes mellitus can be classified by the underlying cause (Table 24-35). This is more useful than the traditional treatment-based classification of insulin-dependent diabetes mellitus versus non-insulin-dependent diabetes mellitus. Type 1 and type 2 diabetes mellitus are by far the most common disorders, but there are several rarer disorders that do not fall within the two primary groupings. Characterization of some of these disorders at the molecular and cellular level has provided important insights into normal physiologic mechanisms. Awareness of these disorders is important because of their association with other pathologic conditions.

TYPE 1 DIABETES MELLITUS Type 1 diabetes mellitus entails destruction of β cells. This is most often caused by a cell-mediated autoimmune process with linkage to particular HLA types. It can be marked by the presence of autoantibodies directed against β cells (Table 24-36). This form of diabetes mellitus was previously considered *juvenile onset,* but it can occur at any age. Insulin deficiency causes catabolism, weight loss, and a tendency toward diabetic ketoacidosis. Persons with type 1 diabetes mellitus rarely are obese when the disease manifests, although obesity is not inconsistent with the diagnosis. Some persons with type 1 diabetes mellitus have a variant form, sometimes called atypical diabetes mellitus. Among these persons the disease manifests during acute stress with diabetic ketoacidosis and necessitates insulin therapy. Between acute events the person has reduced insulin needs, and his or her condition may stabilize with oral medication. This type of diabetes mellitus occurs most often among African-Americans and Asians, usually with an autosomal-dominant pattern of transmission. Unlike the usual form of type 1 diabetes mellitus, atypical diabetes mellitus lacks an association with specific HLA types, and autoantibodies are absent.

TYPE 2 DIABETES MELLITUS Type 2 diabetes mellitus is approximately 10 times more common than type 1 (Table 24-36). It once was called *adult-onset diabetes mellitus,* but children and adolescents have type 2 diabetes mellitus with increasing frequency. There is a strong genetic predisposition toward type 2 diabetes mellitus which probably represents a heterogeneous group of conditions caused by defects in several genes. As these defects are characterized, further subdivision of this category will be possible. Type 2 diabetes mellitus is marked by a combination of insulin resistance, often associated with obesity, coupled with a defect in insulin secretion. A common physical finding associated with insulin resistance is acanthosis nigricans, a hyperpigmented, velvety overgrowth of skin around the neck and intertriginous areas. Insulin levels are readily measurable and can be quite high in type 2 diabetes mellitus. Persons with type 2 diabetes mellitus may have only hyperglycemia or mild diabetic ketoacidosis during acute stress. However, diabetic ketoacidosis at presentation does not exclude the diagnosis of type 2 diabetes mellitus. Because of the insidious onset, approximately 50% of persons with type 2 diabetes mellitus are unaware of their condition. Among adults the diagnosis is made an average of 7 years after the onset of disease. Except during diabetic ketoacidosis, these patients need not be treated with insulin, instead responding to oral agents.

GENETIC DEFECTS OF β-CELL FUNCTION Of the known genetic defects of β-cell function, the best characterized forms are *maturity-onset diabetes of the young* (MODY), which account for 2 to 5% of all cases of diabetes. These are autosomal-dominant single gene mutations that cause derangements in insulin secretion. Age at onset usually is younger than 25 years, and the person often is not obese. At least five MODY loci have been identified. The first MODY defect to be characterized was an inactivating mutation of glucokinase. This enzyme is the first and rate-limiting step in glu-

TABLE 24-34

SPECTRUM OF DERANGEMENT IN CARBOHYDRATE METABOLISM

TEST	NORMAL VALUE	IMPAIRED GLUCOSE TOLERANCE	DIABETES MELLITUS
Fasting glucose level	<110 mg/dL	≥110 to 125 mg/dL	≥126 mg/dL
Oral glucose tolerance test	<140 mg/dL	≥140 to 199 mg/dL	≥200 mg/dL

TABLE 24-35

ETIOLOGIC CLASSIFICATION OF DIABETES MELLITUS

I.   Type 1 diabetes (β-cell destruction, leading to insulin deficiency)
   A.   Immune mediated
   B.   Idiopathic
II. Type 2 diabetes (insulin resistance, coupled with insulin secretory defect)
III. Other specific types
   A.   Genetic defects of β-cell function, including
      1.   Maturity-onset diabetes of the young
      2.   Mitochondrial defects
      3.   Wolfram syndrome
   B.   Genetic defects in insulin action
      1.   Kahn type A insulin resistance syndrome
      2.   Hypoandrogenism, insulin resistance, acanthosis nigrans (HAIRAN)
      3.   Polycystic ovary syndrome
      4.   Leprechaunism
      5.   Rabson-Mendenhall syndrome
      6.   Lipoatrophic syndromes
   C.   Disease of the exocrine pancreas
      1.   Pancreatitis
      2.   Trauma, pancreatectomy
      3.   Neoplasia
      4.   Cystic fibrosis
      5.   Hemochromatosis
      6.   Fibrocalculous pancreatopathy
   D.   Endocrinopathy
      1.   Acromegaly
      2.   Cushing syndrome
      3.   Glucagonoma
      4.   Pheochromocytoma
      5.   Hyperthyroidism
      6.   Somatostatinoma
      7.   Aldosteronoma
   E.   Drug or chemical-induced disorder
      1.   Nitrosourea, including pentamidine
      2.   Other (see Table 24-37)
   F.   Infection
      1.   Congenital rubella
      2.   Coxsackie virus B
      3.   Adenovirus
      4.   Cytomegalovirus
      5.   Mumps
   G.   Uncommon forms of immune-mediated diabetes
      1.   Anti-insulin receptor antibodies (Kahn type B syndrome)
      2.   Stiff man syndrome
   H.   Other genetic syndromes sometimes associated with diabetes
      1.   Down syndrome
      2.   Klinefelter syndrome
      3.   Turner syndrome
      4.   Friedreich ataxia
      5.   Huntington chorea
      6.   Laurence-Moon-Biedl syndrome
      7.   Myotonic dystrophy
      8.   Porphyria
      9.   Prader-Willi syndrome
   I.   Neonatal diabetes
IV. Gestational diabetes mellitus

cose metabolism, in which glucose is converted to glucose-6-phosphate (Fig. 24-38). Glycolysis within β cells increases the ratio of ATP to ADP, which in turn is coupled to insulin secretion by an ATP-sensitive K^+ channel. Glucokinase acts as the glucose sensor

for β cells. Glucokinase abnormalities increase the threshold for insulin release, so insulin concentration is low for the degree of hyperglycemia present. MODY defects have also been linked to four different transcription factors, all of which seem to influence insulin gene transcription, as well as overall β-cell mass. Hepatocyte nuclear factors (HNF)-1α and -1β are members of the homeobox superfamily, and their expression is regulated in turn by HNF-4α, a member of the steroid hormone receptor superfamily. Heterozygous mutations in insulin promoter factor-1 (IPF-1) (also known as PAX-1 or IDX-1) are associated with MODY, and homozygous mutations cause agenesis of the pancreas. Of these defects, glucokinase mutations appear to be the most common, at least among the French population, in which it has been most thoroughly evaluated. Approximately 25% of Europeans and most non-Europeans with MODY have no known gene defect, suggesting the existence of additional loci yet to be characterized.

Diabetes is associated with *mitochondrial DNA defects*, most commonly in base pair 3243, affecting leucine transfer RNA. Patients commonly have sensorineural hearing loss. This mutation has also been observed in the MELAS syndrome (mitochondrial myopathy, encephalopathy, lactic acidosis, and stroke-like episodes), but diabetes mellitus has not been observed with this syndrome. *Kearns-Sayre syndrome*, which includes progressive ophthalmoplegia, pigmentary retinopathy, and cardiac conduction defects, also is associated with diabetes mellitus. The mechanism by which these disorders cause diabetes mellitus may be similar to that implicated for glucokinase deficiency, in which diminished generation of ATP causes a shift in the insulin secretion curve of the β cell.

Wolfram syndrome, also known as DIDMOAD (diabetes insipidus, diabetes mellitus, optic atrophy, and deafness), had been considered to be caused by a mitochondrial defect. However, this neurodegenerative disorder has been linked to a novel transmembrane protein on chromosome 4p that apparently affects β-cell survival. This syndrome is associated with nonautoimmune, insulin-deficient diabetes mellitus; has a mean age at onset at 6 years; and accounts for as many as 1 in 150 cases of diabetes mellitus among children.

GENETIC DEFECTS IN INSULIN ACTION Structural abnormalities of the insulin molecule are a rare autosomal-dominant cause of diabetes mellitus. Defects in the enzyme that converts proinsulin to insulin also have been described. More commonly, these insulin resistance syndromes are caused by defects in either the insulin receptor or the postreceptor signaling cascade. Diabetes mellitus can range from mild hyperglycemia in the face of hyperinsulinemia to severe diabetes mellitus, depending on the nature of the defect. These disorders often are associated with acanthosis nigricans and hyperandrogenism. *Leprechaunism* is the most severe form of insulin resistance. Documented defects in the insulin receptor cause severe intrauterine and postnatal growth retardation, lipoatrophy, hypertrichosis, dysmorphic features, and acanthosis nigricans. Most patients die within the first year of life. These patients have hyperinsulinemia with postprandial hyperglycemia but paradoxical fasting hypoglycemia. *Rabson-Mendenhall syndrome* is a related syndrome of severe insulin resistance with persisting hyperglycemia associated with acanthosis nigricans, dysmorphic facies, abnormal nails and dentition, hyperandrogenism, abdominal distension, and pineal gland hyperplasia. *Kahn type A syndrome* is suspected when a women has a lean, muscular body habitus and coarse facial features, acanthosis, hirsutism, and irregular menses. A milder form of this syndrome occurs among adolescent girls; it consists of hyperandrogenism, insulin resistance, and acanthosis nigricans (*HAIRAN syndrome*) and often is associated with obesity. *Polycystic*

TABLE 24-36

FEATURES OF TYPE 1 AND TYPE 2 DIABETES MELLITUS

FEATURE	TYPE 1	TYPE 2

Pathophysiological mechanism	Insulin deficient
	    autoantibody-positive
	    insulin level and C-peptide decreased
		Insulin resistant
		    autoantibody-negative
		    insulin, C-peptide increased

Presentation	Ketosis prone	Usually mild or no ketosis
Onset	Frequently younger than 18 yrs	Usually adults older than 40 yr
Body habitus	Thin	Obese, often acanthosis nigricans
Family history	Negative in 90% of cases	Often positive
Prevalence in United States	1.7 million	15 million

ovary syndrome shares the features of hyperandrogenism and insulin resistance, but affected women have irregular menses and do not necessarily have acanthosis nigricans. The *lipodystrophy syndromes* are associated with severe insulin resistance and either complete absence of subcutaneous fat or partial absence localized to distinct body areas. The clinical course is marked by severe hypertriglyceridemia, which leads to pancreatitis, and fatty infiltration of the liver with consequent cirrhosis. These disorders appear to be caused primarily by defects downstream from the insulin receptor in the signal transduction cascade.

DISEASE OF THE EXOCRINE PANCREAS Any process that causes diffuse injury to the exocrine pancreas can cause diabetes. Islets are distributed throughout the pancreas, so there must be substantial destruction before diabetes mellitus occurs. Examples include pancreatitis, trauma, infection, pancreatectomy, and neoplasia. Diabetes mellitus also can be caused by chronic obstruction of ductal flow, as by calculi or inspissated secretions in cystic fibrosis. Diabetes mellitus is encountered more among persons with cystic fibrosis, because life span has increased. As many as 40% of adults with cystic fibrosis have diabetes mellitus, and aggressive glucose control may improve their overall outcome. Iron overload syndromes, such as those that occur with hemochromatosis or with repeated transfusions (eg, thalessemia) also destroy β cells. Aggressive iron chelation therapy can minimize the risk of diabetes mellitus.

ENDOCRINOPATHY Several forms of endocrinopathy are associated with diabetes mellitus. Growth hormone, cortisol, glucagon, and epinephrine are counterregulatory hormones that antagonize a number of the effects of insulin. Overproduction of such hormones can unmask diabetes mellitus, especially among children who already have underlying risk. Somatostatinoma and aldosterone-secreting tumors also cause diabetes mellitus, at least in part through inhibition of insulin secretion. In all these cases, diabetes mellitus resolves when the underlying endocrinopathy is controlled.

DRUGS OR CHEMICAL INDUCERS Exposure to some drugs is associated with the development of diabetes mellitus. The nitrosoureas, such as the rat poison Vacor, streptozocin, and pentamidine, cause β-cell destruction. Many other medications either impair insulin secretion or inhibit insulin action (Table 24-37). Exposure to

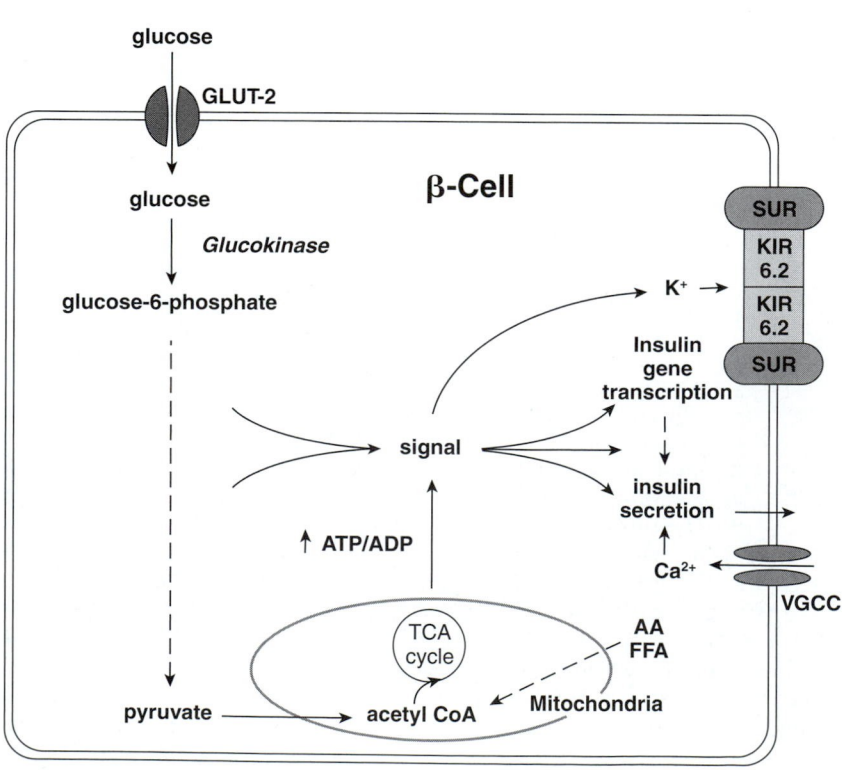

FIGURE 24-38   Signals in the β cell leading to insulin secretion. Glucose enters the cell through a glucose transporter (GLUT2). Glycolysis begins with glucokinase, which converts glucose to glucose-6-phosphate. This step is rate limiting, and defects in this enzyme are associated with one form of maturity-onset diabetes of the young. Gain-of-function mutations have been associated with neonatal hyperinsulinism. Production of ATP results from further glycolysis and processing in the tricarboxylic acid (TCA) cycle. Amino acids (AA) and free fatty acids (FFA) also contribute to ATP production. The net result of these metabolic pathways is an increase in insulin production. The increase in intracellular ATP/ADP ratio activates the sulfonylurea receptor (SUR), and closes the inward-rectifying potassium channel (KIR6.2). The cell membrane then depolarizes, and calcium influx through voltage-gated calcium channels (VGCC) triggers insulin secretion. Sulfonylureas enhance insulin secretion by binding to the SUR and closing the KIR6.2 channel, causing membrane depolarization. Diazoxide functions in the opposite manner to inhibit insulin secretion. Dashed lines represent pathways with intermediate steps not shown.

TABLE 24-37

DRUGS THAT INDUCE DIABETES MELLITUS

DRUG	DECREASES INSULIN SECRETION	IMPAIRS INSULIN ACTION
Diuretics	+	±
Diazoxide	+	+
β-Adrenergic antagonists	+	+
Diphenylhydantoin	+	−
Glucocorticoids	−	+
Oral contraceptives	−	+
Pentamidine	+	
Cyclosporine	+	+
FK506	+	−
Opiates	+	±
Asparaginase	+	−

+ = Effect present; − effect absent; ± effect may or may not be present.
SOURCE: *Modified from National Diabetes Group: Diabetes in America, 2nd ed. NIH publication no. 95-1468, 1995:76.*

one or more of these agents, in combination with stress or an underlying predisposition to diabetes mellitus, can cause diabetes mellitus. Such patients often are encountered after organ transplantation or during therapy for illnesses such as cancer or asthma. The diabetes mellitus may resolve quickly when these agents are discontinued.

OTHER MISCELLANEOUS CAUSES Infection can have a role in β-cell destruction, although a direct association has been difficult to prove. Commonly implicated infections and organisms include congenital rubella, coxsackievirus B, adenovirus, cytomegalovirus, and mumps. An increased incidence of diabetes mellitus also occurs among children with the genetic syndromes listed in Table 24-35, although diabetes usually is not the primary manifestation. Two uncommon forms of immune-mediated diabetes mellitus are classified separately from type 1 diabetes mellitus. *Kahn type B syndrome* is caused by autoantibodies directed against the insulin receptor. The severe insulin resistance and clinical manifestations are similar to those that occur with insulin receptor defects. This disorder can be associated with other systemic autoimmune diseases, such as lupus erythematosus. *Stiff man syndrome* occurs among adults. It is caused by antibodies directed against glutamate decarboxylase, an enzyme that produces glutamate in neural tissue and in β cells. The patients have stiffness and spasms of the axial muscles; as many as one-third have diabetes mellitus.

NEONATAL DIABETES Hyperglycemia occurring within the first month of life and lasting for more than 2 weeks occurs among approximately 1 in 500,000 newborns. It is more common among infants with intrauterine growth retardation. Approximately one-half of such children have permanent diabetes, one-fourth have transient diabetes, and one-fourth enter a remission phase but have a recurrence years later. The HLA haplotypes may or may not be those associated with type 1 diabetes mellitus, and there is no evidence of autoimmune destruction of β cells. Paternal uniparental disomy of chromosome 6q22-23 has been found in a few cases of transient neonatal diabetes mellitus. Neonatal diabetes mellitus probably represents a heterogeneous group of conditions and may include disorders in β-cell development or pancreatic agenesis, such as Wolcott-Rallison syndrome.

GESTATIONAL DIABETES Approximately 4% of all pregnancies are complicated by gestational diabetes. The problem often is found in the third trimester, when insulin resistance is most marked. Diagnosis and aggressive control of gestational diabetes are important in reducing perinatal morbidity and mortality, especially with regard to fetal overgrowth. Although gestational diabetes resolves spontaneously after delivery, as many as 60% of these women may later have impaired glucose tolerance of frank diabetes mellitus, often type 2. Maternal management of diabetes mellitus affects the offspring's later risk of diabetes mellitus.

24.10.2   Type 1 Diabetes Mellitus

EPIDEMIOLOGY

The prevalence of type 1 diabetes mellitus in the United States is approximately 1 in 2500 by 5 years of age. It increases to 1 in 300 by 20 years of age. There is an equal distribution between the sexes and across socioeconomic status. Whites of northern European descent are much more likely to have type 1 diabetes mellitus than are blacks, Asians, or Native Americans, suggesting a role for underlying genetic susceptibility. There are two peaks of onset, at 5 to 7 years of age and at puberty. However, type 1 diabetes mellitus can manifest at any age, approximately 50% of cases occurring among those older than 18 years. As many as 27% of lean Scandinavian adults previously considered to have type 2 diabetes mellitus actually may have a slowly progressive form of type 1 diabetes mellitus, called *latent autoimmune diabetes of adulthood.*

Results of epidemiologic studies suggest a possible infectious cause of type 1 diabetes mellitus. The onset of type 1 diabetes mellitus is seasonal, presenting more frequently in the fall and winter. Small epidemics of diabetes mellitus, with clusters of disease outbreak in various locales also suggest an infectious cause. However, in most cases diabetes mellitus appears to be caused not by acute infection but by the stress of an acute illness, which unmasks β-cell destruction that has occurred over months to years (Fig. 24-39). Type 1 diabetes mellitus is rare among those who live near the equator. The incidence increases in the more temperate regions of the world. The incidence is as low as 0.7/100,000 in Shanghai, China, and is highest among the Finns, at approximately 40/100,000, with an intermediate incidence in the United States of 12 to 14/100,000. The incidence of type 1 diabetes mellitus has doubled over the past 20 years in Finland and is increasing at 3.6% per year in northern Europe. The greatest risk is among those younger than 5 years. This distinct increase has not been consistently found in other parts of the world. In populations that migrate from a region of relatively low risk to a region of high risk, the immigrants assume a higher overall risk of type 1 diabetes mellitus that approaches the indigenous rate. Japanese children who have emigrated from Tokyo, a region of extremely low risk, to Honolulu have a twofold to threefold higher incidence of type 1 diabetes mellitus. Aside from infectious considerations, changes in diet and life-style must be entertained as causative factors. The higher incidences of type 1 diabetes mellitus correlate with societies in which atherosclerosis is most prevalent, which have greater consumption of dairy products, fat, and red meat.

PATHOPHYSIOLOGY

Type 1 diabetes mellitus is caused by autoimmune destruction of β cells. Histopathologic examination of the pancreas soon after diagnosis shows distinctive insulitis with infiltration of the islets with lymphocytes and macrophages. Activation of the immune system against islet cell antigens also is detected at diagnosis. Autoantibodies are found in as many as 90% of patients, and cellular autoimmunity to islet cell antigens is detected as well. The β-cell destruction is probably caused by cell-mediated immunity, rather than autoantibodies. Diabetes recurs among persons who have undergone pancreatic transplantation, even from an identical twin, suggesting that β cells are the targets of immune destruction. Treatment of persons with newly diagnosed diabetes with immunosuppressive agents such as cyclosporine and azathioprine induces transient remissions in as many as 50% of patients. A subset of persons with type 1 diabetes mellitus have other autoimmune diseases, especially thyroiditis, suggesting that, at least among these persons, disordered regulation of the immune system is responsible for the diabetes. Results with animal models lend further support to this notion. Diabetes can be adoptively transferred with infusion of lymphocytes from an animal with diabetes to an unaffected animal, and modulation of the immune system can be used to prevent diabetes.

Genetics

Family studies have demonstrated that susceptibility to type 1 diabetes mellitus is inherited by means of nonmendelian genetics. Most cases are sporadic. Only 10 to 15% of persons with type 1 diabetes have an affected family member. The risk of acquiring diabetes mellitus increases from 1 in 300 to 1 in 20 if a first-degree relative has the disease. The risk among siblings increases fourfold if the proband had diabetes mellitus before 9 years of age (Table 24-38). Identical twins have a concordance rate for diabetes mellitus as high as 70%, although there may be a wide discrepancy in the age at which the disease develops. Identical twins have identical genotypes, but their immunoregulatory genes (T-cell receptors, immunoglobulins) undergo random recombination events, which may account for the differences in susceptibility to diabetes mellitus. A twofold to threefold higher risk of diabetes mellitus exists if one's father rather than one's mother has the disease. This suggests imprinting has a role in this process or that maternal (perhaps transplacental) factors modify the risk.

As many as 20 genetic loci have been reported to increase susceptibility to type 1 diabetes mellitus, but approximately 50% of genetic risk is associated with the HLA locus on chromosome 6p21. An HLA-identical sibling has a 15% risk of developing type 1 diabetes mellitus, whereas a sibling with no shared alleles has only a

TABLE 24-38

INCREASED LIFETIME RISK OF TYPE 1 DIABETES MELLITUS WITH AN AFFECTED FAMILY MEMBER

RELATIONSHIP TO PROBAND	PERCENTAGE RISK OF DIABETES MELLITUS
Parent	3
Offspring	6
Of diabetic father	8
Of diabetic mother	3
Sibling	5
Share no HLA alleles	1
Share one HLA allele	5
HLA-identical	15
Identical twin	33 (up to 70 with long-term follow-up evaluation)
General population	0.3–0.4

SOURCE: *Modified from Atkinson MA, Maclaren NK: The pathogenesis of insulin-dependent diabetes mellitus. N Engl J Med 331:1428–1436, 1994.*

1% risk (see Table 24-38). Specific haplotypes of the class II HLA locus are most strongly associated with future risk of diabetes mellitus. This region encodes three dimeric molecules, DP, DQ, and DR, each composed of an α and a β chain. These molecules are expressed on the surface of antigen-presenting cells, and they present peptides to the T-cell receptor of T lymphocytes. With proper recognition, the T cell is then activated, and the strength of the interaction affects the robustness of that response. A risk of diabetes as high as tenfold is associated with the class II DR3 and DR4 antigens, and 95% of whites with type 1 diabetes mellitus bear these haplotypes. However, 45% of the general population also has these haplotypes. These particular haplotypes are in linkage disequilibrium with specific DQ alleles, which confer disease susceptibility. Because this is such a diverse locus containing so many possible allelic variants, a complex nomenclature has been adopted to categorize the chain (A for α, B for β) and specific allele (numeric designation). The highest risk of diabetes mellitus is associated with DQA1*0301/DQB1*0302 with DR4 and DQA1*0501/DQB1*0201 with DR3.

Specific amino acid changes within the DQ A and B chains are important in diabetes susceptibility. The presence of aspartic acid (Asp) at position 57 in one or both alleles in DQ B confers pro-

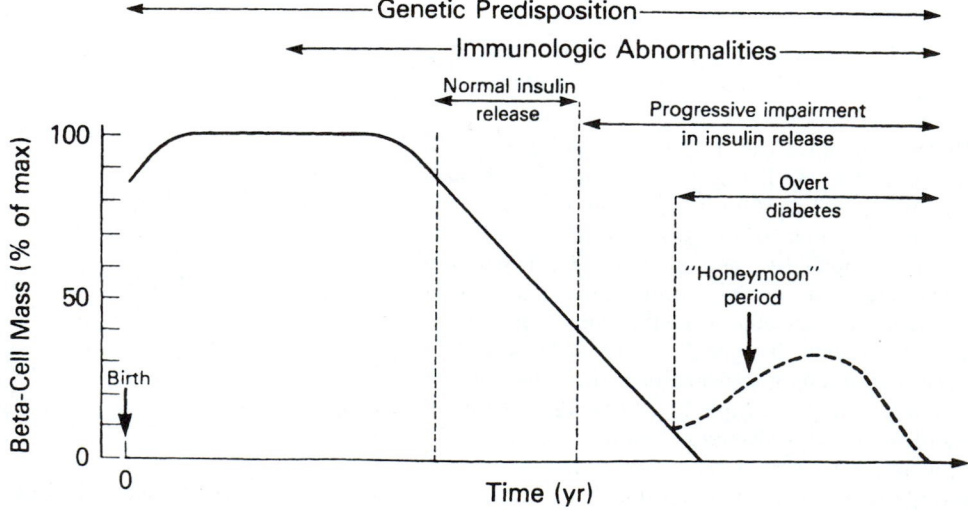

FIGURE 24-39 The proposed natural history of β-cell destruction leading to type 1 diabetes mellitus. Clinical presentation does not occur until 80 to 90% of β-cell mass has been destroyed. (SOURCE: *Medical management of Type 1 Diabetes, 3rd ed. Alexandria, VA, American Diabetes Association; 14, 1998.*)

tection against diabetes mellitus, whereas homozygous absence of Asp at this location confers approximately a 100-fold risk of the disorder, even if the amino acid change is conservative. Yet approximately 20% of Americans are homozygous for the absence of the Asp 57 allele, but only 5% of these persons have diabetes mellitus. Additional factors must be considered, such as other amino acid changes in these high-risk alleles. The presence of arginine (Arg) at position 52 in DQ A coupled with the absence of Asp 57 in DQ B confers additive risk of DM. Forty percent of those with type 1 diabetes mellitus are homozygous for both the absence of Asp 57 in DQ B and the presence of Arg 52 in DQ A. Both residues lie within the binding pocket for antigens that are being presented to the T-cell receptor. These sequence variants, along with other possible amino acid changes, can alter the shape of this pocket and modulate the immune response to a specific antigen. The net result may be a more vigorous response to a specific β-cell autoantigen, with resultant β-cell destruction or failure to induce normal tolerance.

To complicate matters further, some haplotypes appear to protect the person from diabetes, such as DR11 and DR15 and DQA1* 0102/DQB1*0602 in association with DR2. Although the DQB1*0602 allele is present in more than 20% of the general population, it occurs in less than 1% of patients with type 1 diabetes mellitus. In the presence of one haplotype conferring risk and one conferring protection, the effect from the protective allele dominates. Regional and ethnic differences in susceptibility to diabetes mellitus may be related to differences in the HLA types expressed in these populations. The HLA locus contains many other genes, and there certainly may be additional genes in linkage disequilibrium with the class II haplotypes that affect risk of diabetes.

Other, non-HLA loci also contribute to disease susceptibility. The IDDM 2 locus is mapped to a variable number of tandem repeat sequences lying upstream from the insulin gene on chromosome 11p15. The number of repeats may influence ectopic expression of insulin in the thymus, during development, thereby affecting tolerance to insulin. Expression of some genes in this locus is affected by parental imprinting, possibly explaining the difference in risk of diabetes mellitus conferred to offspring from mothers as opposed to fathers with diabetes mellitus. Costimulatory molecules that facilitate the interaction between antigen-presenting cells and T cells also are logical candidates for diabetes susceptibility. One such molecule, cytotoxic T-lymphocyte-associated-4 (CTLA-4) (in the IDDM 12 locus), has attracted interest for its possible role in diabetes risk and as a target for disease prevention.

Environment

Genetic risk alone does not appear to account fully for the development of type 1 diabetes mellitus. Environmental insults must synergize with underlying genetic risk. Characterization of environmental risk factors is difficult. We all are exposed to similar surroundings, and yet only a small number have diabetes. Viruses may play an important role, as is implied by epidemiologic observations. The strongest case is for congenital rubella: 20% of exposed fetuses eventually have diabetes. In a few cases, coxsackievirus has been cultured directly from the β cells of affected persons soon after diagnosis. Although diabetes mellitus can be caused by direct viral injury, coxsackievirus may induce an indirect immune response. The viral antigen P2-C shares homology with a portion of a β-cell antigen, glutamate decarboxylase. Thus immune response to P2-C may cause molecular mimicry, in which there is cross-reactivity with

the β-cell antigen. Mumps, cytomegalovirus, and other viruses have been implicated as potential pathogens.

Exposure to enviromental toxins also may increase risk of progression to diabetes. In addition to nitrosoureas and other drugs, much attention has centered on dietary risk. Nitrosamines from cooked meats promote β-cell injury, and repeated exposure may predispose to diabetes. Epidemiologic findings suggest that exposure to whole cow's milk in the first 3 months of life increases risk of diabetes and that breast milk may be protective. Societies in which breast-feeding is more common have lower risk of diabetes. Retrospective studies have shown that the incidence of diabetes mellitus changes in parallel with changes in the infant feeding practices in a given society. It remains unclear whether breast milk contains a protective factor or cow's milk harbors a sensitizing factor for diabetes mellitus. Autoantibodies directed against a 17-amino-acid peptide in bovine serum albumin are present in persons with new-onset diabetes mellitus, and this antibody cross-reacts with β-cell antigen p69. However, the importance of this antibody remains uncertain. It is present in those with unrelated chronic illnesses, and there is no comparable cell-mediated immune response against this antigen. Further studies are needed to determine whether cow's milk does indeed pose a risk of diabetes mellitus. In the meantime, the recommendation is to encourage breast-feeding through the first year of life, particularly for children with a strong family history of type 1 diabetes mellitus, and to avoid exposure to whole cow's milk during that time. There is no evidence linking diabetes mellitus with the use of commercial infant formula that contains cow's milk protein. These formulas are an appropriate alternative to breast-feeding. Ingestion of soy protein is associated with an increased risk of diabetes mellitus in animal models, and thus routine infant feeding with soy-based formulas is not recommended. Studies are underway to evaluate future risk of diabetes mellitus among infants fed elemental formulas.

Emotional and physical stress is a possible environmental trigger that may cause diabetes. Many new diagnoses of diabetes are preceded by traumatic family events, such as an accident, the death of a parent, or divorce. The underlying mechanism is unclear, but activation of the glucocorticoid axis may directly affect immunologic responses, and the counterregulatory effects of cortisol may unmask diabetes in person with limited β-cell mass. Difficulty quantifying and documenting stress continue to limit our understanding of how it intersects with diabetes.

Integrated View of the Destructive Process

A person at risk of type 1 diabetes mellitus has one or more genetic susceptibility alleles and lacks protective alleles. With this genetic risk, the person must be exposed to one or more environmental triggers that initiate and promote β-cell destruction. These early effector mechanisms are not yet delineated. β-Cell injury may be mediated directly, through β-cell-tropic viruses or specific toxins or through interaction between cytotoxic CD8+ T cells and class I antigens on the β-cell surface. The latter response may occur through molecular mimicry, in which activation of immune responses against a viral protein or a factor in cow's milk causes cross-reaction with a β-cell antigen. The β cell may then be destroyed by the Fas ligand, perforin, or other cytotoxic molecules. An essential component in this cascade may be the specific subpopulation of helper T (T_H) cells that are activated. T_H1 cells elaborate factors such as interleukin-2 (IL-2), interferon-α (IFN-α), and tumor necrosis factor-β (TNF-β); T_H2 cells secrete IL-4, IL-5, IL-10, and other cytokines. The importance of these subtypes is that T_H1 cells stimulate cell-mediated immune responses, whereas T_H2 cells mediate humoral responses. Type 1 diabetes mellitus may result from predominance of the T_H1 subtype. Type 1 diabetes mellitus often manifests soon after a viral infection. However, diabetes mellitus often does not result from an acute process but from slow destruction that may wax and wane over months to years (see Fig. 24-39). The person does not come to medical attention until 80 to 90% of β-cell mass is destroyed and seeks evaluation of hyperglycemia or diabetic ketoacidosis. Two markers provide a view of this process: autoantibodies against β cells are immunologic markers, and the intravenous glucose tolerance test is a metabolic marker. Islet cell autoantibody is an indirect immunofluorescence assay of the patient's serum against a section of normal pancreas. As many as 60 to 80% of patients with new-onset type 1 diabetes mellitus react, but only 0.5% of the general population and 3 to 4% of first-degree relatives have islet cell antibodies. The subset of specific autoantigens has been characterized further and includes a number of cell surface or cytoplasmic components of islets. The insulin autoantibody is the only one specific to β cells. It is often the first antibody detected, usually precedes diabetes mellitus in younger children, and is present in 30 to 50% of those with new-onset type 1 diabetes mellitus. Antibodies against glutamate decarboxylase are found in up to 80 to 90% of persons at diagnosis. These three antibody tests are available commercially, and additional autoantibodies to antigens such as ICA512 (also known as IA-2, a membrane-associated intracellular tyrosine phosphatase) will be available soon. Increased risk of diabetes mellitus correlates with a greater number of antibodies present in a given person and with higher titers of the antibodies. Whether the antibodies actually play a role in the destructive process remains unclear. They may represent epiphenomena related to destruction of the β cell and presentation of autoantigens to the immune system but may not themselves be primary initiators of the destructive process.

CLINICAL PRESENTATION

Insulin is an anabolic hormone. Secretion of insulin in response to feeding governs use of glucose in peripheral tissues, such as muscle, through enhanced glucose uptake and glycolysis. Insulin facilitates energy storage in the forms of glycogen, fat, and protein. Adipogenesis is approximately 10 times more sensitive to the effects of insulin than are the carbohydrate effects. The effects on carbohydrate metabolism are the first manifestation of relative insulin de-

ficiency (Fig. 24-40). Hyperglycemia is caused by limited glucose uptake into cells and by diminished insulin effects on the liver with increased hepatic glucose production from both breakdown of glycogen stores and increased gluconeogenesis.

As serum level of glucose exceeds the renal threshold for glucose reabsorption at approximately 180 mg/dL, osmotic diuresis occurs, and the classic symptoms of polyuria and compensatory polydipsia ensue. The urinary symptoms may prompt evaluation for secondary enuresis or for associated candidal diaper dermatitis or vaginitis. Fatigue and weakness are common from nocturia, disturbed sleep, and breakdown of protein from muscle to provide amino acids as substrate for gluconeogenesis. Polyphagia and weight loss also are common. Visual disturbance can be caused by diffusion of glucose into the lens and subsequent swelling. Further elevation in serum level of glucose, and hence osmolality, can cause lethargy. Many patients become stuporous and comatose at more than 340 mOsm. Slowly progressive, insidious symptoms can persist for days to weeks before diagnosis, although for more than two-thirds of patients, a diagnosis is made before the patient progresses to the more severe metabolic decompensation of both carbohydrate and fat metabolism known as diabetic ketoacidosis.

With more profound insulin deficiency, the patient's condition progresses to derangements in both carbohydrate and fat metabolism and development of diabetic ketoacidosis (see Fig. 24-40). Secretion of counterregulatory hormones (epinephrine, glucagon, cortisol, and GH) accelerates the rate and extent of lipolysis and conversion of free fatty acids to ketone bodies, β-hydroxybutyrate, acetoacetate, and acetone. As the rate of ketone production exceeds utilization or renal clearance, net accumulation results in metabolic acidosis, and serum pH decreases to less than 7.3 and bicarbonate concentration to less than 15 meq/L, and anion gap increases. Respirations are often deep and labored (Kussmaul), reflecting reflexive attempts to correct metabolic acidosis with compensatory respiratory alkalosis. The fruity odor of acetone can be discerned on the patient's breath, indicating underlying ketoacidosis. Ketone excretion in urine further exacerbates the osmotic diuresis from glucose loss, and ketosis often causes nausea and vomiting, which limits oral intake and exacerbates dehydration.

Patients also may present with a markedly elevated serum level of glucose (>600 mg/dL) and increase in serum osmolality, causing lethargy or obtundation. Yet they may have absent or minimal ketoacidosis. This presentation, referred to as *nonketotic hyperosmolar coma* (NKHC), is most frequent among debilitated elderly

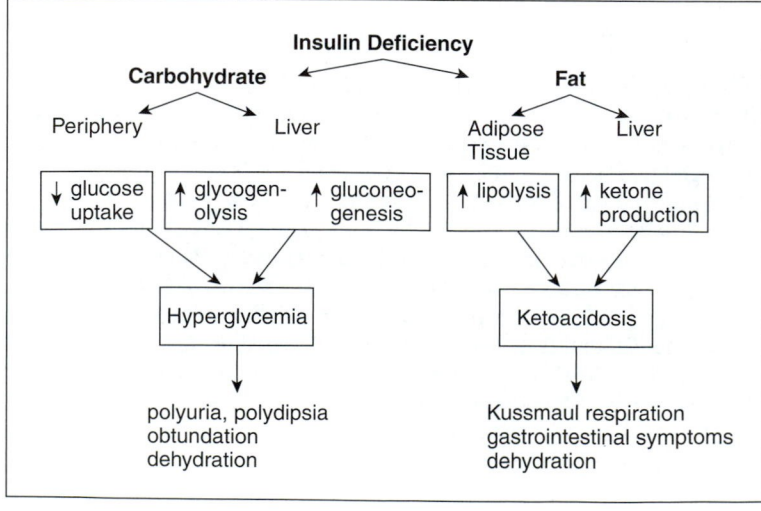

FIGURE 24-40 Pathophysiological mechanism underlying diabetic ketoacidosis with the consequent clinical signs and symptoms. Insulin effects on fat are approximately 10 times more potent than those on carbohydrate metabolism. Patients with both type 1 and type 2 diabetes mellitus have derangements in carbohydrate metabolism, but it is primarily those with type 1 diabetes mellitus with more severe insulin deficiency who have lipolysis and diabetic ketoacidosis. (**SOURCE:** *Siperstein MD: Diabetic ketoacidosis and hyperosmolar coma. Endocrinol Metab Clin North Am 21:415–432, 1992.*)

patients with type 2 diabetes mellitus but occurs infrequently among children with type 1 diabetes mellitus. Hyperglycemia can develop insidiously and more often occurs among patients with limited access to fluid, such as in those with preexisting neurologic damage. These patients may be profoundly dehydrated by the time they come to medical attention. The absence of ketones has been explained by the presence of enough residual insulin to spare lipolysis, as may be the case of persons with type 2 or early type 1 diabetes mellitus. In some instances, NKHC may not be associated with marked elevation of counterregulatory hormones, or hyperosmolality may blunt lipolysis. Nonketotic hyperosmolar coma is one end of the spectrum for manifestations of acute diabetes. Most patients do not have a pure picture of diabetic ketoacidosis or NKHC but are on a continuum between the two extremes.

For patients with established diabetes mellitus, the most common causes of diabetic ketoacidosis are failure to take insulin (the most common cause of recurrent diabetic ketoacidosis among adolescents), acute stress caused by trauma or illness, and poor sick-day management, which typically consists of not giving insulin because the child is not eating or failing to increase insulin for the illness as dictated by blood glucose monitoring (see Sec. 24.10.4).

24.10.3   Immediate Treatment

DIABETIC KETOACIDOSIS

Diabetic ketoacidosis is a life-threatening medical emergency that necessitates prompt and aggressive intervention. The mortality has decreased, but 0.1 to 3% of patients die, mainly of cerebral edema. Specific treatment protocols are useful (Table 24-39), but the keys to successful therapy consistently include the following:

1. Stabilization of the airway, respiration, restoration of circulatory volume
2. Institution of insulin therapy to correct hyperglycemia and clear ketoacidosis
3. Correction of fluid and metabolic abnormalities
4. Determination of the cause of diabetic ketoacidosis; rule out infection
5. Avoidance of complications of therapy, including cerebral edema, hypokalemia, and hypoglycemia

Initial Evaluation and Fluid Management

As in any medical emergency, protection of the airway and maintenance of respiration and circulation are of paramount and immediate concern. Patients with diabetic ketoacidosis rarely need intubation and ventilation. Comatose patients may need a nasogastric tube to prevent emesis and aspiration. Some patients have 10 to 15% dehydration, although many do not have profound fluid loss, and the degree of dehydration is often overestimated. The initial goal of fluid resuscitation is to restore circulation, usually with a 10- to 20-mL/kg bolus of isotonic saline solution or Ringer lactate over 30 to 60 minutes. As resuscitation is being initiated, emergency laboratory studies are performed to confirm the diagnosis and guide further therapy. These include serum glucose, electrolytes, venous blood gas, blood urea nitrogen, creatinine, calcium, phosphorus, magnesium, complete blood cell count with differential, urine glucose and ketones, and any cultures or radiologic studies that may be warranted to assess for infection. A complete history and physical examination may reveal the precipitating factors for the episode of diabetic ketoacidosis. In most instances, hospitalization in a facility equipped to treat acutely ill children where vital signs, neurologic status, and blood chemistries can be frequently monitored is necessary. This is particularly important for new-onset in the care of a child younger than 5 years, or if there is recurrent vomiting, an associated illness, or concerns about the level of family function. Patients with an initial pH less than 7.25 or serum bicarbonate concentration less than 12 meq/L always need hospitalization. Those brought to attention earlier with only mild metabolic abnormalities can sometimes be treated during an extended stay in the emergency department, particularly if this is a recurrence in an established patient with a reliable family, and if close follow-up care can be maintained by telephone and in the outpatient clinic.

Rehydration

Unlike standard recommendations for fluid replacement during dehydration from illnesses such as gastroenteritis, rehydration for diabetic ketoacidosis occurs slowly and evenly over the first 48 hours in a manner similar to that used for hypernatremic dehydration (see Sec. 21.4.4). Gradual correction of hyperosmolality minimizes the risk of cerebral edema. The daily rate of fluid replacement is calculated as follows: Deficit replacement, administered evenly over the first 48 hours (include the initial fluid bolus replacement as part of deficit correction) plus (maintenance fluids at the rate of 1500 mL/m^2/d) plus (ongoing losses including emesis, nasogastric drainage, or diarrhea). Urinary losses usually are not included because maintenance fluid replacement already accounts for some urinary loss, and further replacement often causes overrhydration. Once insulin therapy is initiated and serum level of glucose decreases, urinary losses should decrease rapidly.

Half-normal saline solution usually is an appropriate choice of fluid for this phase of therapy. If there is substantial hyperosmolality, use of isotonic saline solution (0.9% saline solution) is considered. Formal calculation of the sodium deficit with correction of 50% over the first 12 hours of therapy and the rest over the following 36 hours is useful. The patient's fluid status is reassessed frequently and readjusted as deemed necessary by the clinical course. Poor perfusion with prolonged capillary refill time can necessitate additional boluses of normal saline solution. Urinary output is not necessarily a reliable indicator of hydration status; glycosuria can lead to continued polyuria. Fluid replacement continues intravenously until the patient is not vomiting and has a clear sensorium, which is often 12 to 24 hours into therapy. Thereafter, intravenous fluids can be decreased or discontinued, and the patient can proceed with oral rehydration. Fluid replacement in excess of 4 L/m^2/d can be associated with cerebral edema. It is advised that no more than this amount be infused unless necessary to maintain perfusion.

Insulin Therapy

Diabetic ketoacidosis is caused by insulin deficiency, thus insulin therapy must begin as soon as possible to reverse the condition. Most patients need a 0.1-U/kg bolus of regular insulin intravenously, followed by a continuous infusion of regular insulin of 0.1 U/kg/h. Younger children, or those with less severe ketoacidosis, may be more sensitive to insulin, and an insulin bolus and hourly infusion of 0.05 U/kg/h may be adequate. Intravenous insulin has a plasma half-life of only 5 minutes and a biological half-life of 20 minutes, so continuous infusion must follow soon after the bolus. In preparation of an insulin drip, the tubing must first be flushed with the insulin solution to saturate any nonspecific binding sites. Insulin is infused through a separate line so that it

TABLE 24-39

MANAGEMENT OF DIABETIC KETOACIDOSIS

START OF TREATMENT	PHASE 1	PHASE 2	PHASE 3	PHASE 4 (48 HOURS)
	Patient with decreased peripheral circulation, coma **Short phase of rapid rehydration** Hour 1 to 2 When peripheral circulation restored or if initially well hydrated, proceed to phase 2	pH <7.30; glucose >15 mmol/L (270 mg/dL) **Slow rehydration** Blood glucose should decrease at no more than 4–5 mmol/L/h (75–100 mg/dL)	pH <7.30; glucose <15 mmol/L (270 mg/dL) **Slow rehydration** Keep blood glucose at 9–14 mmol/L (150–250 mg/dL)	pH >7.30 **Slow rehydration** Blood glucose can be lowered to 6–10 mmol/L (should fall by not more than 4–5 mmol/L/h; 75–100 mg/dL)
Fluid type	**NaCl (0.9%)** 10–20 mL/kg over 30–60 min If shock, give 5% albumin first (20–25 mL/kg over 30 min)	**NaCl (0.45 or 0.9%)** Replace Na deficit over 48 hours If blood glucose falls at greater than 8 mmol/L/h (140 mg/dL/h) or to value of 8–14 mmol/L (150–250 mg/dL) add 5% glucose to infusion	**5% Dextrose/NaCl (0.45%)** Increase glucose infusion further if falls below 8 mmol/L (150 mg/dL)	**5% Dextrose/NaCl (0.45%)**
Fluid rate	12.5 mL/kg/h, max 500 mL/h	Maintenance plus deficit over 48 hours (include initial fluid bolus in calculation of deficit volume) plus losses of emesis or diarrhea (not urine)	As for phase 2	As for phase 2 Decrease IV fluid immediately when patient begins to drink. IV and oral should equal 4 mL/kg/h.
Potassium	None	Add K 20 mmol/L when serum K <5 mmol/L; increase to 40 mmol/L if serum K <4 mmol/L; may use KPO$_4$ or K acetate to replace deficiencies.		Add K per laboratory results
Insulin	0.1 U/kg IV followed by infusion of 0.1 U/kg/h (for children younger than 5 yr begin with infusion of 0.05 U/kg/h) Prime tubing to absorb insulin and give through separate line from hydration			Blood glucose U/kg/h >10 mmol/L 0.1 5–10 mmol/L 0.075 3–5 mmol/L 0.05 <3 mmol/L 0.025 Then convert to subcutaneous, home-like regimen
Monitoring and laboratory tests	Initially and every 20 to 30 min obtain: pulse rate, respiratory rate, blood pressure, neurologic observations for signs of cerebral edema (headache, agitation, disorientation, combativeness, papillary changes, posturing)	*Tests initially and 2 hours:* Blood glucose (laboratory method) for calculation of corrected serum Na Serum Na, K, BUN, Osm, pH *Tests initially, then every 12 to 24 hours:* Serum Ca, PO$_4$, Mg *Test to assess other contributing factors to diabetic ketoacidosis* Complete blood cell count with differential Chest radiograph	*Tests every hour:* Blood glucose (bedside method) Serum Na (if measured value does not increase) Serum K (if <3 or >6 mmol/L)	Additional precautions: Keep mannitol at bedside for initiation of cerebral edema treatment (1g/kg over 15 min IV, repeat every 2 to 4 hours) Give insulin only after initial fluid therapy is started IV and oral fluids must not exceed 4 mL/kg/h (check this every hour) Decrease serum osmolarity by no more than 4–5 mOsm/h

SOURCE: *Adapted from Ragnar Hanas, MD.* http://www.ispad.org/dka/dka-swe2.htm

can be adjusted independently of the rehydration fluids. An insulin drip provides insulin in a controlled manner, gradually reversing the associated metabolic derangements. Subcutaneous insulin is much less effective in this setting, with slower onset of action from dehydration and poor peripheral perfusion. However, subcutaneous Lispro insulin (see later) or intramuscular regular insulin (which is absorbed more rapidly than subcutaneous regular insulin) is appropriate for treatment of those with mild diabetic ketoacidosis or as a temporizing measure if intravenous therapy cannot be initiated.

The goal of insulin therapy is to reduce the serum concentration of glucose by 75 to 100 mg/dL/h and minimize dramatic shifts in serum osmolality. Serum concentration of glucose often decreases rapidly in the first 1 to 2 hours of therapy because of initial hydration. The result is dilution from volume expansion and improvement in glomerular filtration rate with consequent increased glycosuria. However, concern over this decrease should not delay initiation of insulin therapy. If serum glucose is decreasing too rapidly, 5% dextrose can be added to the intravenous fluids to blunt the rate of decrease. As glucose level approaches 250 mg/dL, 5% dextrose is added to maintain the blood level of glucose in the 150 to 250 mg/dL range. The insulin infusion must be continued until ketoacidosis resolves, which is often longer than it takes for the serum concentration of glucose to normalize. Thus if serum level of glucose continues to decrease to less than 150 mg/dL, increasing the dextrose infusion is preferable to decreasing the insulin infusion rate. If serum concentration of glucose does not decrease steadily with the insulin drip, the infusion rate should be increased to achieve the desired effect. Insulin requirements of up to 0.2 to 0.3 U/kg/h can indicate severe insulin resistance (eg, with serious infection), or a problem with the insulin solution (eg, admixture error or inactive insulin).

The insulin infusion can be discontinued when diabetic ketoacidosis has been successfully controlled such that pH is greater than 7.3, bicarbonate level is greater than 15 meq/L, glucose less than 300 mg/dL, and the patient is ready to resume enteral intake. This transition ideally occurs during the day and before a meal. The insulin infusion must be continued for 30 to 60 minutes after the first subcutaneous dose is administered to allow for delayed onset of action of the injected insulin. Calculation of an appropriate subcutaneous dose is empiric, and various approaches are successful. Some clinicians prefer to administer 0.2 to 0.4 U/kg per dose of regular insulin subcutaneously at 6-hour intervals, on a sliding scale, and then devise a regimen based on the observed insulin needs. However, a patient with diabetic ketoacidosis is insulin resistant, needing up to 2.4 U/kg/d, and insulin requirements often vary over the ensuing days. It usually is more effective to initiate therapy with an outpatient regimen (see Sec. 24.10.4). Established patients may simply resume their previous insulin regimen, unless problems have been identified with its efficacy. A day in the hospital does not mimic a patient's life at home, with differences in food intake, stress, and activity. The patient need not stay in the hospital for an extended period to fine-tune the insulin regimen. This is better done in the outpatient setting when the child has resumed a usual life-style.

Electrolyte Abnormalities and Metabolic Acidosis

Sodium

Hyponatremia is common among patients with diabetic ketoacidosis. Urinary or gastrointestinal losses can cause sodium deficits of 5 to 25 meq/kg. Hyponatremia also reflects an influx of water from the intracellular space to the extracellular compartment to balance hyperglycemia and the resultant hyperosmolality. Spuriously low sodium levels are caused partially by osmolar dilution by glucose and the sodium-free lipid fraction of plasma. The corrected serum concentration of sodium is estimated with the following formula:

$$\frac{Na + (Glucose\ in\ mmol/L - 5.6)}{2}$$

To convert the glucose value from milligrams per deciliter to millimoles per liter, divide by 18. Serum concentration of sodium should increase slowly as the deficit is replaced with intravenous fluids containing sodium and as ongoing insulin therapy decreases serum levels of glucose and inhibits lipolysis. Failure of serum level of sodium to increase suggests excessive free water administration or the syndrome of inappropriate antidiuretic hormone (SIADH) and is a harbinger of cerebral edema.

Potassium

Total body potassium stores are depleted in diabetic ketoacidosis with deficits of 4 to 10 meq/kg, yet when the patient is first seen, serum concentration of potassium often is in the normal range or mildly elevated. Potassium is primarily an intracellular cation, and thus levels in the serum do not reflect total body stores. Diabetic ketoacidosis shifts potassium from the intracellular space to the extracellular space, partly from an exchange with hydrogen ions as a buffering mechanism and partly from insulin deficiency that decreases glucose-mediated intracellular potassium transport. Marked potassium loss occurs from vomiting and renal excretion. During therapy for diabetic ketoacidosis, serum level of potassium can decrease precipitously as insulin therapy facilitates intracellular glucose uptake and with potassium shift back into the intracellular compartment as acidosis resolves. In anticipation of these shifts, one must begin potassium replacement early in the course of therapy for diabetic ketoacidosis. If the patient is urinating and potassium level is 5 meq/L or less, potassium replacement is initiated with up to 40 meq/L added to the maintenance fluids. The goal is to provide 2 to 5 meq/kg/d. Patients with more marked deficits may need potassium replacement at up to 0.5 meq/kg/h. Supplementation can be achieved solely with KCl, or in part with K-acetate, which is converted to bicarbonate, or with K-phosphate, which can aid in phosphate repletion. Hypokalemia and hyperkalemia can be associated with life-threatening cardiac arrhythmias. All patients with diabetic ketoacidosis need cardiac monitoring.

Phosphate and Calcium

Patients with diabetic ketoacidosis often have a modest phosphate deficiency of approximately 0.5 to 4 mmol/kg. Like potassium, phosphate is primarily an intracellular ion but shifts to the extracellular compartment in diabetic ketoacidosis and is lost with urinary excretion of ketoacids. In theory, phosphate replacement leads to increased production of 2,3-bisphosphoglycerate, which improves oxygen availability in peripheral tissues and reduces lactic acidosis. However, randomized, prospective trials of phosphate replacement have not shown benefit in management of diabetic ketoacidosis. Because phosphate replacement can precipitate hypocalcemia and ectopic calcification, routine phosphate replacement is not currently recommended. However, severe phosphate deficiency (<1 mg/dL) can cause muscle weakness with respiratory and cardiac dysfunction and can even progress to rhabdomyolysis, hemolytic anemia, and neuroencephalopathy. Phosphate replacement with potassium phosphate (usually use as one half of the potassium supplement) is warranted if serum levels of phosphate are low, especially when less than 1.5 mg/dL. Serum levels of calcium and phosphate must be monitored carefully if replacement is pursued, and calcium supplementation may be needed to manage hypocalcemia.

Metabolic Acidosis

Metabolic acidosis in diabetic ketoacidosis is of paramount concern. It is caused by both ketoacidosis from insulin deficiency and lactic acidosis from osmotic diuresis and dehydration. Both components should improve steadily during the course of rehydration and insulin therapy. Persistent acidosis may reflect a need for more insulin or increased fluid replacement. To differentiate these two possibilities, one must frequently reexamine the patient to assess hydration. The acid-base status is readily evaluated with serial blood gas determinations or inspection of both the serum bicarbonate and anion gap from an electrolyte panel. Urinary or plasma ketone measurements are helpful in the initial diagnosis of diabetic ketoacidosis but are not useful to evaluate response to therapy. Most ketone measurements are based on a nitroprusside reaction, which detects acetoacetate but not β-hydroxybutyrate. These ketones are normally present in a 3:1 ratio (β-hydroxybutyrate to acetoacetate), but the ratio can be 8:1 or higher in diabetic ketoacidosis. As the patient's condition improves, the ratio decreases, and the ketone measurement may show a paradoxical rise, suggesting that the patient's condition has worsened when it actually is improving. Sodium bicarbonate rarely is indicated for the management of diabetic ketoacidosis. Prospective, randomized trials have shown it has not improved the outcome for patients with diabetic ketoacidosis, and it may even increase hepatic ketogenesis. Therapy with $NaHCO_3$ can induce paradoxical acidosis in the central nervous system because it does not freely cross the blood-brain barrier, but it can be converted to CO_2, which can diffuse into the brain, worsen cerebral acidosis, and exacerbate obtundation. Rapid alkalinization with $NaHCO_3$ also is detrimental because it can (1) cause potassium to shift intracellularly and precipitate hypokalemia with consequent cardiac arrhythmia, (2) decrease the level of ionized calcium and induce symptoms of hypocalcemia; and (3) shift the oxyhemoglobin dissociation curve to the left, which diminishes oxygen delivery to peripheral tissues and exacerbates lactic acidosis. Bicarbonate is usually not necessary if adequate fluid replacement and insulin therapy are provided. However, if the patient has severe, persistent acidosis with a pH less than 7.1 and there is concern that the metabolic acidosis is compromising cardiovascular function, bicarbonate can be used judiciously. The recommended dose is 1 to 2 meq/kg intravenously over 2 hours. Therapy is discontinued as pH increases to more than 7.1 or serum level of bicarbonate is more than 10 meq/L.

Complications of Therapy for Diabetic Ketoacidosis

Complications can arise during therapy for diabetic ketoacidosis. In addition to electrolyte abnormalities, adult respiratory distress syndrome occurs among some children after aggressive fluid resuscitation. Pneumomediastinum also has been described. It is presumed to be caused by pressure gradients between alveolus and interstitium that develop with hyperventilation or retching.

The most feared complication of diabetic ketoacidosis is cerebral edema. It occurs among fewer than 3% of children with diabetic ketoacidosis and is rarely encountered among those older than 20 years. Fifty percent of patients with diabetic ketoacidosis and cerebral edema die or suffer from permanent neurologic deficits. The cause of cerebral edema remains unknown. The most likely explanation is disequilibrium in osmolality between the intracellular compartment in the central nervous system and extracellular spaces that develops during diabetic ketoacidosis. To maintain cellular volume, intracellular osmolality increases through production of idiogenic osmols, which include taurine, glutamate, and polyols (eg, sorbitol). During therapy for diabetic ketoacidosis, fluid resuscitation and insulin can cause a dramatic decrease in serum osmolality before the cells in the brain dissipate the solutes responsible for increased intracellular osmolality. As a result, water shifts rapidly from the extracellular space to the intracellular compartment with consequent expansion of the brain tissue within a confined space and resultant cerebral edema. Support for this hypothesis includes observations that cerebrospinal fluid pressure increases among adults with diabetic ketoacidosis during treatment. In children subclinical brain swelling has been observed on cranial CT scans during therapy for diabetic ketoacidosis. However, one study of children with diabetic ketoacidosis showed decreased ventricular size on CT scans before initiation of therapy. Rare cases of cerebral edema have been described even before initiation of therapy. Thus it remains unclear whether cerebral edema is caused by the underlying disease or is a complication of therapy. Although hydration rate and tonicity of administered fluids, rapid decrease in serum level of glucose and osmolality, and the use of sodium bicarbonate and insulin all have been considered, none has been linked definitively to cerebral edema in retrospective analyses. The cause of cerebral edema remains unknown.

Patients at highest risk of cerebral edema are young, usually younger than 5 years, and those with diabetic ketoacidosis as the initial manifestation of disease. The symptoms often develop in the first 5 to 12 hours of treatment as the patient is otherwise improving. Approximately one-half of the patients with cerebral edema have neurologic changes before respiratory arrest. These changes include headache; behavioral change, often with lethargy progressing to decreased arousal but sometimes with delirious outbursts; incontinence; polyuria from diabetes insipidus rather than diabetes mellitus; temperature dysregulation; seizure; pupillary changes, such as asymmetry or fixed, dilated pupils; and hypertension with bradycardia. The patient should be examined at least once an hour for changes in neurologic findings during therapy for diabetic ketoacidosis. If cerebral edema is suspected, quick action must be taken to prevent herniation. Mannitol should be available at the bedside; 0.25 to 1 g/kg intravenously can be administered every 2 to 4 hours. Additional treatment measures include fluid restriction, elevation of the head of the bed, intubation with hyperventilation, and immediate consultation with a neurosurgeon. Neuroimaging helps differentiate cerebral edema from other possible causes of coma, such as central nervous system infection, hematoma, or thrombosis.

As many as one-half of patients with cerebral edema do not appear to have a prodromal phase to herald incipient herniation. These patients may die suddenly or have severe morbidity. Among those with warning signs, approximately one-half still have adverse outcomes. Limited understanding of the pathogenesis of cerebral edema and high risk of a poor outcome necessitate a focus on prevention of diabetic ketoacidosis.

Family Issues and Discharge Planning

Families of children newly diagnosed with diabetes need substantial emotional support and education during the hospitalization. Most families are in a state of disbelief and grief regarding the diagnosis, and this must be acknowledged by the health-care team. A social worker or counselor is helpful in assessing the family structure and support systems and helping to facilitate the grief process and devise appropriate coping strategies. These initial interactions with the family make lasting impressions that cement a working relationship for the years ahead. A large amount of medical information can be imparted to the family at this time, but many families are overwhelmed and may not be ready for a scholarly lecture on diabetes mellitus. Simple, basic principles of daily diabetes management must be emphasized, ideally taught by physicians, nurses, and dietitians who are certified diabetes educators. Before hospital discharge, the family and child must show competence in glucose monitoring; insulin administration; various aspects of nutrition, especially related to carbohydrate intake; recognition and management of hypoglycemia and hyperglycemia; when and how to check for urinary ketones; and what to do during intercurrent illnesses (see Sec. 24.10.5). The child must be given close follow-up care in the outpatient clinic and by telephone and be given 24-hour access to a physician in the event of an emergency. Families need clear guidelines on when and how to call for help. In the early stages, many families need daily telephone calls for reassurance, to assess glucose control, and to adjust the insulin regimen. A visiting home health nurse can help assess the family's management skills and facilitate the transition to outpatient therapy.

MANAGEMENT OF NONKETOTIC HYPEROSMOLAR COMA

Management of NKHC is similar to that of diabetic ketoacidosis with some important additional considerations. The onset of NKHC often is insidious. Patients may have even more profound fluid deficits and hyperosmolality at initial presentation than do those with diabetic ketoacidosis. The hyperosmolar state must be corrected slowly. Normal saline solution is an appropriate choice for initial fluid resuscitation and deficit replacement. In the absence of ketoacidosis, these patients often are more sensitive to insulin, so beginning the insulin drip at 0.05 U/kg/h is prudent. Fluid shifts during therapy can be substantial. As insulin enhances glucose uptake, water follows passively into the cell to maintain osmolality, and an acute decrease in vascular volume may ensue. Fluid requirements must be reassessed frequently during therapy. Repeated small boluses of saline solution may be needed to maintain vascular volume. Some patients need more than $4 \text{ L/m}^2/\text{d}$. Monitoring and management during therapy are otherwise similar to those described for diabetic ketoacidosis in Table 24-39.

HYPERGLYCEMIA WITHOUT KETOACIDOSIS

Patients with hyperglycemia without ketoacidosis and who appear otherwise well may not need intensive treatment with an insulin drip and may not even need hospitalization. These patients may have an early presentation of type 1 or type 2 diabetes mellitus. Such patients can be treated as outpatients, especially if a diabetes team is readily available to provide the necessary training and education. At the outset of outpatient therapy, insulin is dosed con-

servatively to avoid hypoglycemia. The care provider must maintain accessibility both in the clinic and by telephone.

24.10.4   Outpatient Management in Type 1 Diabetes Mellitus

GOALS

The goals of treatment of children with type 1 diabetes mellitus are as follows:

1. Stabilize blood level of glucose within a target range
2. Avoid metabolic decompensation (diabetic ketoacidosis, severe hypoglycemia)
3. Ensure normal growth and development at both a physical and emotional level
4. Prevent long-term complications of both hyperglycemia and hypoglycemia

The best means to achieve these goals have been established through several long-term studies involving adolescents and adults, most notably the Diabetes Control and Complications Trial (DCCT). This 9-year prospective multicenter trial compared outcomes among patients who underwent intensive treatment in an attempt to maintain euglycemia with outcomes among those treated in the conventional manner, in which the goal was clinical well-being. Patients in the intensive therapy group received three or more insulin injections per day or used an insulin pump; measured blood glucose several times a day; had monthly clinic visits with the health-care team and weekly follow-up telephone calls; and were encouraged to use a dynamic regimen with adjustments for variation in daily food intake and activities. Those in the conventional treatment group received one or two insulin injections per day, were seen in the clinic every several months, and followed a static daily insulin regimen. This study showed definitively that tighter glucose control reduces the risk of long-term complications of type 1 diabetes mellitus, decreases risk of development of microvascular complications, and slows progression of preexisting lesions 35 to 75%. The average blood concentration of glucose achieved by this carefully selected, highly motivated, intensive treatment group was 155 mg/dL. Fewer than 5% of the participants were able to maintain an average glucose value in the euglycemic range throughout the study. Thus this lofty goal may not be attainable in most populations. The intensively treated adolescents in the DCCT had even greater difficulty achieving the target ranges; they had an average glucose level of 171 mg/dL. Nonetheless, the American Diabetes Association has adopted these target ranges for adolescents and adults. The goals are as follows:

1. Preprandial glucose concentration 80 to 120 mg/dL
2. Two-hour postprandial glucose concentration less than 180 mg/dL
3. Bedtime glucose concentration 100 to 140 mg/dL
4. HbA_{1C} within 1 percentage point of high normal for the assay used

The DCCT showed that any improvement in glucose control lowers the risk of long-term complications. Every 10% decrease in HbA_{1C} is associated with a 40 to 45% lower risk of progression of retinopathy. Therefore, even if the stated target range is not achieved, any incremental decrease in blood glucose value decreases the risk of future microvascular disease. The relation between glucose level and long-term risk is exponential, such that severe hyperglycemia conveys greater risk of complications than does mild hyperglycemia. Some experts have suggested that there may even be a threshold effect, such that tighter glucose control below a certain range (at an average glucose level of approximately 180 mg/dL and HbA_{1C} of 8 for diabetic nephropathy) may not significantly reduce the risk of future complications. However, the United Kingdom Prospective Diabetes Study, a long-term study of outcomes among patients with type 2 diabetes mellitus and several smaller studies of patients with type 1 diabetes mellitus do not support the notion of a threshold phenomenon.

The major risks associated with intensive glucose control in the DCCT were weight gain and hypoglycemia. With tighter control of blood levels of glucose, ingested nutrients were stored more efficiently, and intensively treated patients gained an average of 4.5 kg. With aggressive attempts to achieve euglycemia, these same patients had a threefold higher incidence of severe hypoglycemic events than the conventional treatment group. The current challenge is to balance the benefit of tighter blood glucose control with the risk of excessive treatment.

Application of the DCCT criteria to the care of prepubertal children is controversial because the balance of benefits and risks with intensive therapy can differ between children and adults. Microvascular changes are rarely detected in prepubertal children, regardless of the duration of diabetes, so the benefit of intensive glucose control is uncertain. However, results of some studies with young adults suggest that the time to onset of microvascular complications after puberty is related to glucose control before puberty. Prepubertal children with diabetes mellitus may accrue subtle microvascular changes, albeit at a slower rate than before puberty. The benefits of tight glucose control for children are not as clearly defined as for adults. Further studies are needed to clarify this issue. The risk of intensive therapy is greater among children because they usually have more fluctuation in daily activities, less predictable intake, and increased insulin sensitivity. Hypoglycemic episodes are more common, and recognition of these episodes can be difficult. Several studies have shown that children with onset of diabetes mellitus before 6 years of age have an increased risk of neurocognitive deficits from recurrent hypoglycemia. The long-term risks for recurrent hypoglycemia among children older than 6 years and among adults is less clear.

There is no consensus among pediatric diabetologists on specific target ranges for glucose control during childhood, but the foregoing considerations suggest that goals should be adjusted by age. For the child younger than 6 years, the long-term risks of recurrent hypoglycemia appear to outweigh the possible benefits of tight control. Thus a looser target range is warranted, avoidance of hypoglycemia being the primary goal. Some experts have suggested target ranges of 100 to 200 mg/dL or even looser, especially for toddlers to provide a margin of safety for the inevitable wider excursions in glucose control. For prepubertal school-age children, one can assume a tighter target range than for toddlers, although the benefit of tight control in this age group has not been fully defined, and the risk of recurrent hypoglycemia appears to be greater than among adults. For adolescents in puberty, the benefits of tight control have been established by the DCCT. These patients need tighter target ranges, similar to those used by adults. Ideally, the HbA_{1C} for children older than 6 years should be within 1 to 2 percentage points of high normal for the assay used. The goals are somewhat looser for preschoolers. An HbA_{1C} in the normal or nearly normal range is not always reassuring; recurrent hypoglycemia depresses the overall average.

The family must appreciate the need to balance the risks of excessive treatment with the benefits of tight control. Their perceptions of the relative risks and benefits color their approach to management. Therapeutic goals must be individualized for each family. Some organized, highly functional families and children can maintain glucose level in a near euglycemic range without incurring recurrent hypoglycemia. They should be encouraged in their ongoing efforts. Pediatricians need to foster healthy habits in daily diabetes management that will remain with the child for life. Even if the target ranges are somewhat looser than for adults, the daily process of diabetes management is the same.

Although the goals are controversial, the means by which tighter glucose control was achieved in the DCCT have become the standard of care of all persons with diabetes (Table 24-40). Children are cared for by a pediatric diabetes team consisting of a nurse practitioner or certified diabetes educator, social worker or other mental health professional, registered dietitian, and a pediatric endocrinologist. The family receives ongoing diabetes education, so that they are empowered with self-management skills. Visits with a health-care professional are ideally scheduled at 3- to 4-month intervals but are more frequent for patients with new-onset disease, or unable to achieve goals, or those with other problems related to diabetes mellitus. After the honeymoon phase, the insulin regimen consists of three or more injections per day with adjustment for exercise or variation in diet. Blood level of glucose is measured routinely before each meal and at bedtime, occasionally in the middle of the night, and whenever the child has symptoms. The family maintains a written record of glucose levels, insulin doses, and variation in daily routine. These records are reviewed by the diabetes team at regular intervals between clinic visits to reassess and adjust the daily regimen as needed.

THE HONEYMOON PHASE

The insulin needs of a child with new-onset diabetes mellitus can change considerably in the days after hospital discharge. Activity level may increase, decreasing insulin requirements. A ravenous appetite during recovery from the catabolic state may precipitate a need for more insulin. Nonetheless, as many as two-thirds of patients enter a "honeymoon" or remission phase within days to sev-

TABLE 24-40
OUTPATIENT MANAGEMENT OF DIABETES

Family and patient expectations
Measure glucose before each meal, at bedtime, occasionally during the night, and when symptoms occur
Maintain written glucose logs
Follow meal plan with attention to carbohydrate intake
Outside the honeymoon period, administer three or more insulin injections per day; make adjustments for exercise and variation in intake
Provider expectations
Health care visit at least every 3–4 months with HbA_{1C}
  More frequent visits if not meeting goals
Regular access to a diabetes team, with ongoing education
  Diabetologist, nurse educator, dietitian, counselor
Frequent telephone contact with family between visits
  Review of glucose logs, adjustment of regimen as needed
  Availability for sick-day management
Screening for long-term complications
  Begin when patient has had diabetes for 5 years *and* is in puberty
  Assess with yearly retinal examination and measurement of microalbumin in urine

eral weeks of therapy. This phase consists of decreasing insulin needs and an increasing tendency toward hypoglycemia. The family needs to be forewarned about this phenomenon, and insulin doses must be decreased accordingly. The remission phase is caused by resumption of endogenous insulin secretion from the remaining 10 to 20% of β cells present at initial diagnosis (see Fig. 24-39). Chronic hyperglycemia is toxic to the β cell and inhibits the usual coupling between elevated blood level of glucose and insulin secretion. Yet when glucose level is consistently maintained closer to normal range with exogenous insulin, the toxicity is reversible, allowing the remaining β cells to resume normal function. As a result, blood level of glucose often is maintained in a nearly euglycemic range during the honeymoon phase despite simple insulin regimens (Fig. 24-41A). The nadir in insulin requirements usually occurs approximately 3 months after diagnosis, doses less than 0.5 U/kg/d being typical. Some patients (<5%) may have no need for exogenous insulin, but continuing a minimal twice-daily injection schedule is recommended to impress upon the family that diabetes mellitus has not been cured and because results of preliminary studies suggest that more aggressive insulin therapy at this time may help prolong the honeymoon phase. It often is quite traumatic for a child and family to reinitiate injections once they have been discontinued. Nonetheless, with ongoing autoimmune destruction of β cells, the honeymoon phase invariably ends, sometimes after only a month, but it can last for as long as 2 years. Dwindling endogenous insulin secretion manifests as a gradual increase in insulin needs with more erratic glycemic control. In general, younger children have no or a limited honeymoon, whereas older children and adolescents have longer honeymoon phases, probably reflecting the more virulent autoimmune destruction of β cells at younger ages.

INSULIN THERAPY

The goal of insulin replacement therapy in type 1 diabetes mellitus is to mimic the function of the β cell. However, exogenous insulin cannot be delivered in a closed-loop feedback system, that is, with a glucose sensor to regulate the appropriate amount of insulin secreted into the portal circulation. Current therapy for diabetes mellitus entails an open-loop system with intermittent glucose sensing by means of monitoring blood concentrations of glucose and clinical symptoms. A person who does not have diabetes has continuous secretion of insulin from the β cells at a basal level and pulsatile secretion in response to food, modulation by various gastrointestinal hormones, absorbed nutrients and neural controllers, and secretion into the portal circulation so that concentrations reaching the liver exceed peripheral levels. Thus exogenous insulin delivery remains crude compared with endogenous regulated insulin delivery.

INSULIN PREPARATIONS AND PHARMACOKINETICS

Most children are now treated only with recombinant human insulin, which is less antigenic than bovine or porcine insulins. Some diabetologists, however, still use animal insulins, especially when they want a more prolonged insulin effect. Several human insulin preparations are now available with varying durations of action (Table 24-41). The different properties of these insulin preparations are related to their variable tendencies to aggregate into larger complexes. To be absorbed from the injection site, insulin must dissociate from hexamers into a monomeric form. In each hexamer, six insulin molecules aggregate around a zinc ion. As the injected insulin is diluted by interstitial fluid, the hexamers dissociate into di-

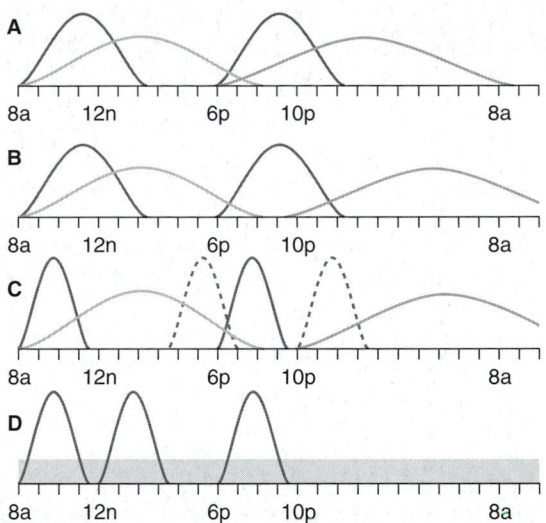

FIGURE 24-41 **Examples of commonly used insulin regimens for patients with type 1 diabetes mellitus. A. Standard split-mixed regimen with short-acting and intermediate-acting insulins (in this case regular and NPH) given before breakfast and dinner. B. Three-shot regimen with the NPH moved to bedtime to prevent nocturnal hypoglycemia, provide better coverage through to breakfast, and minimize effects from the dawn phenomenon. C. Four-shot regimen commonly used by school-age children with no injections during school. Lispro has been substituted for regular insulin at breakfast and dinner. An extra injection of Lispro is offered in the midafternoon if needed to cover snacks and to minimize hyperglycemia before dinner. It also may be needed with bedtime NPH to cover that snack (dashed lines). D. Insulin regimen called "the poor man's pump" in which Ultralente administered at breakfast and dinner covers basal insulin needs (shaded areas), and Lispro at meals provides bolus coverage for carbohydrate intake and correction of glucose levels above target range.**

mers and then monomers, at which point the insulin molecules traverse the endothelium and enter the circulation. The protamine in neutral protamine Hagedorn (NPH) and higher zinc concentration in Lente and Ultralente retard the dissociation, delay formation of monomeric insulin, and delay the insulin effect. In contrast, the biological activity of intravenous regular insulin is rapid because when diluted in solution, this form of insulin rapidly dissociates into monomers.

Until recently, regular insulin had been the fastest-acting insulin preparation. However, its pharmacokinetics are too slow to match food intake. Peak postprandial carbohydrate absorption often occurs 1 hour after a meal, whereas the peak effect of regular insulin occurs 2 to 4 hours after an injection. As a result, blood level of glucose may increase dramatically in the 1 to 2 hours after a meal,

TABLE 24-41

PHARMACOKINETICS OF HUMAN INSULIN PREPARATIONS

INSULIN	ONSET	PEAK	DURATION
Lispro	5–15 min	30–90 min	3–4 h
Regular	30–60 min	2–4 h	5–8 h
NPH	1–2 h	4–8 h	10–18 h
Lente	1–3 h	4–10 h	12–20 h
Ultralente	2–6 h	8–14 h	18–30 h

before the peak of action of regular insulin is realized. Thereafter, blood level of glucose may drop precipitously, coincident with the delayed peak insulin effect. This decrease often necessitates a snack to blunt the subsequent decrease in serum level glucose and to prevent hypoglycemia. To compensate for these pharmacokinetics, patients are instructed to take their regular insulin injection 15 to 30 minutes before a meal (even longer if blood level of glucose is elevated) and to avoid foods that are absorbed rapidly, such as juice or soda. Patients may not be able to adhere consistently to these recommendations. In practice many inject their regular insulin immediately before a meal.

Lispro insulin (Humalog) is an advance in subcutaneous therapy. It circumvents many of the problems of regular insulin (see Table 24-41). The name refers to the reversal of the proline and lysine residues at positions 28 and 29 in the insulin β chain. This novel molecule dissociates rapidly from the hexameric configuration into a monomeric state and has a rapid onset and shorter duration of action. As a result, Lispro insulin can be taken immediately before eating. If intake is uncertain, as with toddlers, one can administer a dose after a meal without causing serious postprandial hyperglycemia. Lispro insulin also allows rapid correction of hyperglycemia. It also can reduce hypoglycemia, because its peak action occurs coincident with peak carbohydrate absorption. This feature may be of particular benefit for those who exercise after meals, for insulin coverage in the evening or night, or for those who do not want to snack between meals. However, caution must be exercised with the use of Lispro insulin for coverage of fatty foods, which are digested and absorbed slowly. The patient may have hypoglycemia 1 to 2 hours after a fatty meal. With foods such as pizza, regular insulin may be needed or Lispro insulin can be injected after the meal. The benefit of Lispro insulin is also its disadvantage: The discrete, rapid onset of action is ideally suited for several well-spaced meals per day. With larger snacks between meals or grazing, several injections of Lispro insulin may be needed, or more practically, longer-acting insulins such as regular insulin may have to be used. Mixtures of Lispro and regular insulin can be considered to cover both meals and snacks.

A number of factors influence the insulin pharmacokinetics shown in Table 24-41. Smaller insulin doses tend to have a shorter duration of action, and larger doses extend the duration of action. The exception is Lispro insulin because larger doses only minimally extend the duration of action. Insulin tends to have a faster onset and shorter duration of action in younger children. The vials of insulin used should be kept at room temperature, where they remain stable for at least 30 days. Refrigerated insulin has a slower onset of action and stings on injection. The site of insulin injection influences action, except for Lispro insulin which has similar absorption from all sites. Insulin tends to be absorbed fastest and most reliably from the abdomen, with arm, leg, and buttocks progressively slower sites of absorption. The injection sites should remain consistent within a general area for a given time of day. For example, if the arm is the injection site of choice for dinner, it should be used at dinner every day. Toddlers may benefit from injections in the buttocks, because insulin tends to act more rapidly in younger children, and this will serve to slow insulin absorption and prolong its action. Injection into a site that will be used soon afterward for exercise accelerates insulin action, such as injection into the leg before running. Rubbing of the injection site and heat also accelerate absorption. One must be careful that insulin is injected subcutaneously and not intramuscularly. Deeper injection accelerates the action of insulin. Insulin syringes with short needles are available to avoid such problems.

Injection sites and technique should be reviewed with children and families at regular intervals. Frequent reinjection into the same site can cause lipohypertrophy, an overgrowth of adipose tissue readily detected at physical examination. Such sites become favored because they are relatively anesthetic, but use of these areas can cause delayed or erratic insulin absorption. Children should rotate their injection sites within a given area to avoid development of such areas. Lipohypertrophy often is resorbed within 3 to 6 months of disuse of the site. Lipoatrophy, the loss of subcutaneous fat at the injection site, occurs with use of animal but not human insulin, presumably because of allergic reactions.

After all these variables are taken into account, one still finds that subcutaneous insulin has intrinsic variation in action; intrasubject variation is 10 to 50%. Lispro insulin has the most reproducible pharmacokinetics; longer-acting forms of insulin have the least predictable actions. Patients using insulin regimens with frequent injections of short-acting insulin may have more reliable responses than do those relying more heavily on intermediate- or longer-acting insulin.

Insulin Regimens

In designing an insulin regimen, one can use any combination of insulin preparations. Sample regimens are shown in Fig. 24-41. Total daily insulin needs vary with age and pubertal status; many children need approximately 1 U/kg/d, but toddlers may need as little as 0.25 to 0.5 U/kg/d, and adolescents may need more than 1.5 U/kg/d. The simplest insulin regimen, often prescribed soon after diagnosis, is a *split-mixed regimen*, in which a combination of short- and intermediate-acting insulin (traditionally regular and NPH) is administered before breakfast and dinner. As a rough guide, two-thirds of the total insulin is given before breakfast and one-third before dinner. The higher morning dose is needed to cover carbohydrate absorption during the daytime meals. Of the morning injection, one-third consists of regular and two-thirds of NPH insulin. The evening injection is split evenly between regular and NPH. With this regimen, breakfast intake theoretically is covered by the morning regular insulin, lunch by the morning NPH, dinner by the evening regular, and overnight insulin needs by the evening NPH. However, this is a gross oversimplification. The timing and nature of food intake, exercise, and insulin pharmacokinetics all must be considered in adjusting the regimen. Two common problems with this regimen are hyperglycemia before dinner and hypoglycemia before lunch. The former problem often stems from a large afternoon snack. One can attempt to increase the morning NPH dose to cover this interval, but the insulin may still not have enough peak effect to cover the snack effectively. Further increases in the morning NPH dose may skew its pharmacokinetics so that the peak is broader and the action extends over a longer time. It may even overlap with the evening insulin dose and precipitate nocturnal hypoglycemia and yet still not adequately cover the midafternoon snack. The most appropriate intervention may be to restrict carbohydrate intake in the midafternoon or to administer another injection of short-acting insulin to cover carbohydrate intake at the time (Fig. 24-41C). An additional problem with this regimen is hypoglycemia in the mid- to late morning. The morning regular insulin dose may be too strong and may overlap with the onset of NPH action. Either the regular dose has to be reduced or an earlier or larger mid-morning snack has to be eaten. An alternative is to switch from regular to Lispro insulin. Many children no longer use regular insulin, but the more discrete action of Lispro insulin often necessitates an increase in NPH doses and additional Lispro insulin injections (Fig. 24-41C).

Patients may awaken with elevated fasting glucose levels as a result of the *Somogyi reaction,* in which counterregulatory hormones have been secreted to compensate for a hypoglycemic event earlier in the morning. The patient may or may not awaken during the night with nightmares, a restless sleep pattern, or headaches. Other patients, particularly adolescents, may need more insulin coverage from 4 a.m. to 8 a.m. because of the *dawn phenomenon,* in which resistance tends to increase from nocturnal peaks in GH secretion. To differentiate the dawn phenomenon and a Somogyi reaction, blood level of glucose must be measured during the night, especially at 2 to 3 a.m., when glucose values less than 100 mg/dL suggest a Somogyi reaction. Higher blood levels of glucose that continue to increase into breakfast are indicative of the dawn phenomenon. Regardless, the evening NPH dose often has to be moved from dinner to bedtime, so that the insulin lasts until breakfast and the peak effect more closely matches the dawn phenomenon, without placing the patient at risk of nocturnal hypoglycemia (Fig. 24-41B).

The success of these two- or three-shot regimens requires that the patient be restricted to a specific routine of activity and meals. One can achieve increased flexibility and improved metabolic control through frequent short-acting insulin injections, which mimic endogenous insulin secretion. For a child reluctant to take a lunch injection, the regimen can incorporate a fourth injection with Lispro insulin after school to cover the midafternoon snack. Lispro also may be needed with bedtime NPH to cover that snack as well (Fig 24-41C). In an even more sophisticated regimen, sometimes called the *poor man's pump,* Lispro injections are used before each meal and are coupled with a longer-acting or basal insulin (Fig. 24-41D).

No matter which insulin regimen is selected, the treatment plan must match the daily life-style of the child and family, so that the family does not have to dramatically alter its schedule to meet the demands of the insulin. No single regimen can be applied to every family. The intensity of the regimen must be balanced with the energy and interest that the family can mount for daily diabetes care. It is vital that the child have direct, ongoing supervision from an adult each day to ensure that injections are taken as directed. Especially with the more complicated regimens, children may begin to miss injections and at times may benefit from return to a simpler regimen.

One increasingly popular option for insulin delivery is an *insulin pump,* which is worn by more than 60,000 persons with diabetes in the United States. This external device is about the size of a beeper. It continuously infuses insulin through silicone tubing into the subcutaneous tissue (often called *continuous subcutaneous insulin infusion*). As with traditional injection therapy, this is an open-loop system; that is, the operator determines the amount of insulin to be delivered through the pump. The pump is programmed to deliver preset amounts of basal insulin during the day that should maintain one's blood glucose in a steady range if there is no carbohydrate intake. Bolus doses of insulin are delivered through the pump to cover ingested carbohydrate and to correct high blood sugar levels according to formulas derived for each patient. The pump delivers only short-acting insulin, most commonly Lispro. Without long-acting insulin, blood glucose control usually is tighter and insulin responses more predictable with fewer erratic swings in glucose level. Additional advantages of the pump include minimizing hypoglycemic events; the ability to deliver insulin at specific times and places, such as increased basal coverage during a

particular part of the night to cover the dawn phenomenon; and ease of insulin administration for persons already taking several injections per day. Life-style considerations are important. For example, the patient can sleep late and eat meals or snacks as desired, rather than according to a schedule. The pump can be detached easily for showers or exercise. Although once reserved for adults and adolescents, pumps are now being used more liberally by younger children.

A potential complication of use of a pump is the risk of diabetic ketoacidosis if insulin infusion is disrupted. The pump wearer must be committed to frequent glucose measurement, must be carefully trained on how to troubleshoot possible pump malfunctions, and must know how to revert to injected insulin if necessary to avoid diabetic ketoacidosis. Although the machine itself can malfunction, most problems are related to dislodgment of the tubing from its site of placement or to related technical problems. Pump wearers are at risk of development of infection at the site of set placement, but adequate skin cleansing when the catheter is introduced and regular set changes minimize this risk. Finally, children must accept having a device attached to their body, which may be a hurdle, particularly for those overly concerned with body image. Trial placement of an infusion set and wearing a pump with saline infusion for several days can help allay these fears. The ideal pump candidate is a highly motivated child with strong family support and supervision, who has consistently shown an ability to measure blood glucose frequently, to keep an organized glucose log, and to use an algorithm to determine insulin dosing.

Glucose Monitoring and Regimen Changes

To evaluate any regimen, the concentration of glucose in the blood must be measured before each meal, at bedtime, whenever a child has symptoms, and occasionally at 2 to 3 a.m. (see Table 24-40). Urine glucose monitoring is a far less accurate means of assessing response to therapy and has no place in current diabetes management. A myriad of glucometers are available for home glucose monitoring. These measure either whole blood or plasma glucose, the latter reading 10 to 15% higher than the former. These meters are accurate to within 10 to 15% with greater deviation at more extreme glucose concentrations. Most machines store several hundred data points, with time and date of the testing, which facilitates record keeping. Families should be instructed to keep a daily diary of these readings, along with insulin doses and variation in daily activities. Software applications allow direct downloading of stored information from the glucometer to a computer, for sophisticated data analysis. Although helpful, these analyses often cannot capture the nuances of each day and do not substitute for traditional logbook entries. Preparation of these diaries becomes tedious for parents and children, but it remains necessary for assessment of the insulin regimen.

Families must be trained to look for patterns in the glucose logs, such as consistent deviations at a particular time of day. In general, changes are considered if a particular pattern is evident for 2 to 3 consecutive days. Then a 10% change in the insulin covering that period of the day is instituted. In the most efficacious regimens, the insulin doses are not static but vary with changes in meal plan or for exercise. Families need an algorithm to correct high blood sugar values with extra-short-acting insulin. The amount needed for such sliding scales varies according to the age of the child and the time of day and must be derived empirically. Most children need 0.5 to 1 U for each 50 mg/dL that blood level of glucose is elevated above target range. Toddlers may need as little as 0.25 units for each

50 mg/dL that the blood level of glucose is elevated, whereas adolescents may need more than 2 U for each 50-mg/dL elevation in blood level of glucose. Because of the dawn phenomenon, some children need more insulin to correct a high blood level of glucose in the morning than they do in the evening. The dose of supplemental insulin also has to be adjusted for the presence of overlapping long-acting insulin, as in correction of hyperglycemia at lunch for a child who received morning NPH.

Some patients present factitious glucose logbooks. It may be helpful to download the glucometer to verify that written entries correspond with recorded data. Measurement of HbA_{1C} helps corroborate the logbook entries. Reasons behind data fabrication include frustration with the daily grind of management of diabetes mellitus, inability to maintain glucose levels within expected target range, or lack of compliance with cessation of actual glucose monitoring. The family or health-care team may attach a value judgment to the glucose values themselves, such that a number within target range translates into "goodness," even though swings in glucose values may be entirely beyond the child's control. Every effort should be made to handle glucose levels solely as information on which to base future decisions. In other words, praise the child for the behavior (glucose monitoring) but not the outcome (actual glucose value). The child and family must be reassured that no one is perfect. Empathy should be offered regarding the demanding daily schedule and imperfect nature of diabetes management. The physician's nonjudgmental view of glucose levels fosters open interaction with the family.

Devices to Facilitate Diabetes Management

A number of devices have been developed to facilitate daily diabetes management. Lancet devices for sampling blood glucose have fine needles and adjustable tips to minimize the depth of penetration. Laser devices are in limited use to obtain blood samples without a needle. Insulin syringes have evolved so that the needles are finer and as short as 1/3 inch (0.8 cm) to minimize the risk of intramuscular injection. Insulin "pens" eliminate the need to carry both insulin syringe and vial outside the home. These devices hold an insulin cartridge, and the insulin dose to be delivered can be dialed into the pen in increments as small as 0.5 U. Such devices facilitate insulin administration in school and are convenient for an active child who needs supplemental insulin during the course of a busy day. Air-powered injectors have been developed as an alternative to traditional needle injections. Insulin is delivered subcutaneously in an aerosolized burst. These devices are expensive, the discomfort may be similar to that of injection, and insulin delivery may be more erratic than that achieved with traditional injections.

DIETARY AND NUTRITIONAL GUIDELINES

Blood concentration of glucose is affected not only by insulin therapy but also by food intake. Thus one of the cornerstones of diabetes management is nutritional therapy. A registered dietitian with specialized training in pediatric diabetes should work within the framework of the family's dietary preferences to develop an individualized daily meal plan that provides adequate energy intake to promote normal growth and development. Actual caloric needs are calculated by age and weight, but careful monitoring of weight gain and linear growth is needed to modify the meal plan. The food types from which caloric intake is derived are the same for children with diabetes mellitus as they are for the general population. Carbohydrates should constitute 45 to 60% of the total daily calories.

Because of long-term concerns about atherosclerosis, 30% or less of total calories should come from fat, less than 10% from saturated fat. Protein should constitute 10 to 20% of daily caloric intake.

Patients traditionally were taught to use a complex system for meal planning to monitor protein, fat, and carbohydrate intake. However, carbohydrate is the primary nutrient affecting postprandial glycemic response, and thus attention is now focused primarily on carbohydrate intake. One system, called *carbohydrate counting,* focuses solely on carbohydrate intake. It is a simpler and less structured approach to meal planning. In the past, complex carbohydrates were most of the carbohydrate in the daily meal plan, and simple carbohydrates were minimized because of concern that the latter would cause greater glycemic excursion. In particular, concentrated sweets such as sucrose were excluded from the diet of persons with diabetes mellitus. However, many studies have shown that the total amount of carbohydrate ingested, not the source, determines blood glucose levels. Treats such as cookies and candy can be incorporated into a meal plan to provide a more flexible diet without resentment of food restrictions. If such foods are forbidden, a child often consumes them anyway and feels guilty about sneaking foods. Sanctioning such treats allows the child to learn how to incorporate such foods into the meal plan with appropriate insulin coverage. As with any child, one must provide limits for such treats and offer them within the context of a healthful meal plan. Lispro insulin provides an efficient means of blunting surges in postprandial glucose after ingestion of simple carbohydrates and allows liberalization of previous restrictions. Ingestion of simple carbohydrates such as juice has different effects on blood levels of glucose depending on the rate of absorption. If consumed when the stomach is empty, the carbohydrate is rapidly absorbed. If consumed with a meal, the juice carbohydrate empties from the stomach more slowly as a component of the mixed meal, and serum values of glucose do not increase dramatically.

In the early stages of diabetes mellitus, families must familiarize themselves with the foods that contain carbohydrate and the amount present in a given portion. Food models, food lists (such as the exchange lists prepared by the American Diabetes Association and the American Dietetics Association), and packaged food with detailed food labels all serve to assist the family in this process. Many food choices can be considered in convenient 15-g units, called *exchanges* or *carbos,* as shown in Table 24-42. The child does not need to eat a specific food at a given meal but can interchange foods such that the total amount of carbohydrate ingested adds to a specified amount at a given meal. The family is initially offered a fixed meal plan (with a corresponding insulin dose) based on usual eating patterns. The plan indicates a prescribed amount of carbohydrate for each meal, and for snacks between meals and at bedtime. Insulin doses may have to be decreased if a child does not want a snack at a particular time of day. The use of Lispro insulin can obviate snacks.

TABLE 24-42

COMMON FOODS THAT CONTAIN 15 GRAMS OF CARBOHYDRATE

4 ounces (120 mL) of juice
1 slice of bread
1/2 cup of beans (127 g), potatoes (133 g), or pasta (133 g)
1/3 cup of rice (80 g)
1 small piece of fruit
8 ounces (240 mL) of milk

Some families are content to continue with a fixed meal plan and accept daily regimentation. Consistency in blood sugar readings is related to a reproducible pattern of food intake each day. However, many families find such a plan limiting and prefer to adjust food intake according to appetite and food availability. These patients are best served by a formula for calculating insulin dose on the basis of a given amount of carbohydrate ingested known as an *insulin to carbohydrate ratio*. This ratio varies according to age, most children needing 0.5 to 1 U of short-acting insulin for every 15 g of carbohydrate ingested. Toddlers may need only 0.5 U for 30 g of carbohydrate ingested, and adolescents frequently need 2 to 3 U per 15 g ingested. As with high sugar corrections, this formula can vary at different times of the day. The dawn phenomenon necessitates use of more insulin per unit of carbohydrate at breakfast, especially for adolescents. These ratios must be derived for each patient. They can be calculated from inspection of past records, in which the patient has eaten a known amount of carbohydrate while simultaneously recording blood glucose and insulin doses. An alternative is to assign an empiric ratio and adjust as necessary from subsequent records. With such a ratio, the patient has increased flexibility and control over food intake and can eat according to appetite, rather than being forced to ingest the prescribed carbohydrate. The family gains confidence for handling special occasions such as Halloween and birthday parties, and the child with diabetes mellitus does not have to be restricted from participation. Such an approach can be particularly useful for toddlers because their food intake often is erratic. The family can count carbohydrates ingested at a meal and then offer the matching dose of Lispro insulin immediately after the meal, avoiding food battles and forced feeding.

EXERCISE

Exercise is an important part of a child's daily life and should be encouraged for those with diabetes mellitus. Benefits of sports participation include improved self-esteem and sense of well being, increased fitness with associated cardiovascular benefits, and decreased concentration of lipids in the serum. Unlike the situation for type 2 diabetes mellitus, exercise should not be prescribed as a means of blood sugar control for patients with type 1 diabetes mellitus. Although exercise improves insulin sensitivity, there is no evidence that it directly improves overall metabolic control. During exercise, a complex shift in fuel substrates must occur to meet the energy needs of the working muscle, while maintaining glucose homeostasis. This adaptation is mediated by an intricate balance between insulin and counterregulatory hormones. Among persons without diabetes, insulin secretion is spontaneously decreased to maintain euglycemia. Such a balance is not achieved as readily in children with type 1 diabetes mellitus. If the child exercises with too little insulin in circulation, the associated increase in counterregulatory hormones increases serum level of glucose, and ketones may be produced. On the other hand, an excess of insulin can block mobilization of fuel substrates, and hypoglycemia occurs. Hypoglycemia is an especially difficult problem for active children because it can occur during the event, soon afterward, or even hours later as depleted glycogen stores are being replenished. Thus insulin and carbohydrate intake must be modified in anticipation of and after exercise.

Specific exercise guidelines must be developed for each child and for each activity. The family must gather information on each activity and measure glucose before, during, and after the event. The insulin regimen must be adjusted so that exercise does not coincide with peak insulin effect. The insulin dose may have to be decreased from 10 to 20% up to 50% for more strenuous exercises. The child may need a snack before and during the event to avoid hypoglycemia, ingesting up to 15 to 30 g of carbohydrate for every 30 minutes during the exercise period. Diluted juice in a water bottle is an inconspicuous way to supply simple carbohydrate and maintain hydration status. The nighttime insulin dose may have to be decreased or the bedtime snack liberalized to avoid nocturnal hypoglycemia.

SICK DAYS

Families must receive anticipatory guidance for diabetes management during acute illnesses. With frequent glucose measurement, adherence to the guidelines outlined later, and ready telephone access to a health-care provider, most hospital readmissions for diabetes mellitus can be averted. Illness, even a mild upper respiratory tract infection, or stress can greatly alter the daily insulin needs of a patient, increasing insulin resistance and the tendency toward diabetic ketoacidosis. Insulin doses may have to be increased 10 to 20% or more to compensate for the increased production of counterregulatory hormones. If blood level of glucose remains greater than 250 mg/dL over 4 to 6 hours or if there are gastrointestinal symptoms, the child should be evaluated for urinary ketones. Urinary ketones may be detected well before the development of severe systemic acidosis from diabetic ketoacidosis. However, if ketone levels are moderate or high, the family should speak to the physician for further guidance on insulin dosing. Ketones increase insulin resistance considerably. The child may need as much as 10 to 20% of the total daily insulin dose given as a single supplemental injection of short-acting insulin to manage the underlying insulin deficiency. The family needs to measure blood glucose and urinary ketone levels every 2 to 4 hours. Doses of short-acting insulin may have to be repeated every 2 to 4 hours to manage hyperglycemia and curtail further ketoacidosis. Clear fluids should be encouraged to maintain hydration status and help clear ketones. When glucose level is more than 250 mg/dL, sugar-free solutions are used. As glucose level decreases, sugar-containing solutions are introduced in much the same way that intravenous fluids are selected for management of diabetic ketoacidosis in the hospital. The presence of Kussmaul respirations indicates severe diabetic ketoacidosis and prompt an immediate physician evaluation.

If the patient is vomiting, diabetic ketoacidosis must be differentiated from a primary gastrointestinal process, most often gastroenteritis. One common mistake is to omit insulin in the absence of enteral intake, but even if glucose values are not elevated, patients must continue to take insulin to cover their basal needs and to avoid diabetic ketoacidosis. The insulin dose can be adjusted by giving small doses of short-acting insulin at 2- to 4-hour intervals according to a sliding scale to adjust for variation in intake and glucose level. An alternative is to give one-half to two-thirds of the usual intermediate- or long-acting insulin to provide basal needs and give additional doses of short-acting insulin as needed. Hydration status is monitored closely, and oral intake of electrolyte-containing solutions is encouraged. Promethazine hydrochloric suppositories or another antiemetic agent can be particularly helpful to those with recurrent vomiting and enable continued outpatient management. The principal disadvantage to use of antiemetics is the risk of sedation and, more rarely, extrapyramidal symptoms. Nonetheless, in the care of a diabetic patient the benefits of such agents greatly outweigh the risks, and can save unnecessary emergency department visits and hospitalizations. In exploring the cause of vomiting, one must always consider the possibilities that the current insulin has lost its potency, and the family may need to use a new bottle; that preceding insulin injections may have been omitted; or that the child has a serious underlying problem unrelated to diabetes mellitus, such as appendicitis.

SURGERY

Some of the considerations for illness apply to diabetes management during surgery. Surgery with general anesthesia can cause great stress, and insulin resistance for patient with diabetes can increase considerably. Minor procedures with local anesthesia have minimal effects on carbohydrate metabolism. For minor, elective surgery, the procedure should be scheduled as the first operation of the day. The patient takes the usual nighttime insulin and the following morning omits short-acting insulin but takes one-half to two-thirds of the usual intermediate-acting insulin before the procedure. An alternative for limited, short procedures is that the nighttime insulin dose may last through the morning operation; the patient can hold the morning insulin dose until resuming enteral intake in the mid- to late morning. The anesthesiologist must help counsel the family on how to manage possible hypoglycemia before surgery. A clear, sugar-containing fluid usually poses no risk of aspiration if ingested several hours before the procedure. Hospitalization may be needed the day before the procedure to coordinate diabetes management with the surgical team. Subcutaneous short-acting insulin can be used perioperatively for immediate correction of hyperglycemia. Selection of dextrose concentration in the intravenous fluids can be gauged according to serum level of glucose. The goal is to avoid hypoglycemia and prevent blood glucose values from increasing to more than 200 mg/dL, thereby minimizing osmotic diuresis.

With more extensive procedures, or if the child is acutely ill, greater control of serum level of glucose can be gained through discontinuation of subcutaneous insulin and reliance on an intravenous insulin drip. In the absence of diabetic ketoacidosis, one can approximate the dose by adding the total injected insulin dose over a 24-hour interval and then dividing to calculate an hourly infusion rate. Usually only about 50% of this dose is needed, because the patient does not have substantial enteral intake in the perioperative period, and the 5% dextrose often used in intravenous fluids does not constitute a substantial carbohydrate load. The insulin dose has to be increased for the insulin resistance of an ill child; 0.1 U/kg/h or more is needed if there is concomitant diabetic ketoacidosis. While the drip is being administered, serum level of glucose should be measured hourly, and the insulin infusion rate adjusted accordingly. It can be difficult to predict enteral intake during the recovery phase. Thus the insulin infusion should be continued until solid food intake has been reestablished.

HYPOGLYCEMIA

One of the most important limitations in diabetes therapy is the risk of hypoglycemia. Because exogenous insulin is not delivered in a closed-loop feedback system, the inevitable mismatches between administered insulin, carbohydrate availability, and exercise cause hypoglycemia. The brain depends on a continuous glucose supply from the circulation, and as glucose levels decrease, a series of counterregulatory mechanisms are activated. Among persons without diabetes, insulin secretion is curtailed as glucose levels decrease into the lower range of normal. With further decrements, signals from the central nervous system activate the autonomic nervous system, stimulating first glucagon release and then epinephrine secretion. Growth hormone and cortisol also are involved in the counterreg-

ulatory response, but they are slower and less critical as initial defenses against acute hypoglycemia.

The signs and symptoms of hypoglycemia assume a hierarchy, depending on severity. Mild to moderate episodes of hypoglycemia are associated with autonomic nervous system activation. They include shakiness, palpitations, irritability, anxiety, diaphoresis, hunger, and tingling. Awareness of hypoglycemia is largely the result of recognition of this constellation of symptoms. More profound decreases in serum level of glucose result in a lack of glucose delivery to the brain with symptoms that include weakness, difficulty thinking, headache, slurred speech, blurred vision, and personality changes with irrational or combative behavior. These symptoms are more difficult for the affected child to recognize but are often reported by friends and family members. Further decreases in glucose level can cause extreme lethargy that progresses to loss of consciousness, coma, and death. Generalized tonic-clonic or focal seizures can occur, and the patient may have transient focal postictal deficits. Neuroimaging studies may be necessary to rule out structural lesions, but usually there are no focal findings, and deficits resolve spontaneously.

More than 50% of hypoglycemic events occur at night. Although some patients awaken with symptoms, or later report nightmares or restless sleep, many have no symptoms and sleep through these events, which can last for several hours. Sympathetic responses to hypoglycemia can be blunted during sleep. Therefore one must be careful to avoid overly aggressive glucose control during the night. Glucose monitoring during the night, at 2 to 3 a.m. or at additional time points, may be necessary to detect such events. Nocturnal hypoglycemia may have occurred if the fasting glucose level is low or normal or if there is severe hyperglycemia (possible Somogyi effect).

The first line of management of hypoglycemia is oral ingestion of a rapidly absorbed carbohydrate (Table 24-43). Families should be cautioned to use a pure simple carbohydrate, because mixed foods containing protein and fat, such as chocolate, are absorbed more slowly. Small boxes of juice or glucose tablets are convenient

---

TABLE 24-43

MANAGEMENT OF HYPOGLYCEMIA IN DIABETES MELLITUS

Have simple carbohydrates available at all times
Verify signs and symptoms with a glucometer reading
Follow the "rule of 15s":
    take 15 g of simple carbohydrate orally
    recheck glucose in 15 minutes
    repeat cycle if not above 100 mg/dL
For severe hypoglycemia:
    consider use of oral glucose if conscious
    may require intramuscular glucagon injection if combative or unconscious
        0.3 mg if < 6 years of age (<30 kg)
        0.5 mg if > 6 years of age
Anticipatory guidance to prevent recurrent hypoglycemia, hypoglycemic unawareness
    may need more frequent glucose monitoring
    consider loosening target ranges
    retrain to recognize subtle signs and symptoms of hypoglycemia
    make sure simple carbohydrates are always readily available
    review the use of glucagon, and stock it at home and school
    introduce a dynamic regimen, with adjustments for changes in daily schedule, eg, for exercise, decrease insulin and/or increase carbohydrate intake

and acceptable choices. Many parents offer candy, but the child needs to be made aware that hypoglycemia is a serious medical problem, so that he or she does not incur hypoglycemic episodes in anticipation of a treat. These items must be readily available for the child throughout the day. The child also should carry a source of carbohydrate outside the home, and the school classroom should be stocked with supplies. The amount of carbohydrate ingested to control hypoglycemia varies and must be individualized. As a rough guide, 15 g ingested raises the blood level of glucose of an adult approximately 50 mg/dL. Families should follow the rule of 15s, whereby the symptoms of hypoglycemia are first confirmed with a glucometer, and then the child ingests 15 g of carbohydrate with repeat glucose monitoring in 15 minutes. If the glucose value remains less than 100 mg/dL, the cycle is repeated until the glucose level is greater than 100 mg/dL. Smaller children may need less simple carbohydrate for hypoglycemia correction (0.3 g/kg). Those with more profound hypoglycemia may need more carbohydrate for recovery. Depending on the time of day, relation to meals, and activity level, additional food may have to be offered in the form of a complex carbohydrate with protein and fat to avoid another episode of hypoglycemia. After a hypoglycemic event, glucose level can be elevated from overingestion of carbohydrate (related to the child's hunger or anxiety in response to the hypoglycemia) or from rebound hyperglycemia related to counterregulatory hormonal secretion.

With moderate or severe hypoglycemia, a child may need assistance to appropriately manage hypoglycemia, especially because irrational behavior may result from the hypoglycemia. Forceful administration of carbohydrate to the patient may be necessary. Juice can be given through a syringe, or a more viscous form of simple carbohydrate, such as a glucose gel or cake frosting, can be applied to the buccal mucosa. If the patient is combative, or is not fully alert or conscious, initial therapy consists of an intramuscular glucagon injection. Although larger doses often are used, children younger than 6 years (<30 kg) have a brisk response to 0.3 mg, and 0.5 mg suffices for older children and adults. The glycemic response is transient, and glucose levels begin to decline again after about 90 minutes, so the patient should be encouraged to eat when alert. Recovery usually is uneventful, but the family must speak to the health-care team to reevaluate the current regimen and make necessary changes to prevent future episodes of severe hypoglycemia. Glucagon can cause vomiting, which complicates recovery. If the patient does not respond to the treatment, or if hypoglycemia recurs, transfer to a hospital for intravenous dextrose administration is indicated. Glucagon is the first line of treatment for severe hypoglycemia outside the hospital. All children with diabetes should have a glucagon emergency injection kit, and the family and school personnel must be well trained in administration.

Persons with tighter blood glucose control are at greater risk of severe hypoglycemia. In the short term, a person who has had a brief episode of moderate hypoglycemia has blunted symptoms and hormonal responses to hypoglycemia the following day. This phenomenon is caused by an adaptive response in which glucose is transported more efficiently from serum to the central nervous system, thereby preserving substrate availability to the brain but also impairing the central sympathetic response to hypoglycemia. These persons subsequently have neurogenic symptoms of hypoglycemia at a lower glucose threshold and are therefore unable to recognize and manage evolving hypoglycemia. They may suddenly have only neuroglycopenic symptoms in the face of severe hypoglycemia, a condition called *hypoglycemic unawareness.* The net result is that the person may not become aware of hypoglycemia until reaching

a more profoundly depressed level, at which there is greater risk of seizure and loss of consciousness. This scenario can become a vicious circle, in which hypoglycemia becomes a risk factor for further hypoglycemic events.

The mechanism of hypoglycemic unawareness is reversible. However, after several years with diabetes, patients may lose their glucagon secretory response to hypoglycemia and may later have a diminished response to epinephrine. At this point, the patient is at even higher risk of hypoglycemia, because of both the defective counterregulatory response and the depressed threshold for hypoglycemic symptoms.

Practical measures can be instituted to minimize recurrent hypoglycemia, especially for those with hypoglycemic unawareness or who have had a severe adverse event (see Table 24-43). More frequent glucose monitoring helps patients identify mild hypoglycemic events early in the course. Less stringent glucose control with looser target ranges may be necessary for a time to eliminate even mild hypoglycemia and help reset the threshold for hypoglycemic symptoms. The child and family need to be retrained to recognize the more subtle signs and symptoms of neuroglycopenia. They need to review the management of hypoglycemia and make sure that simple carbohydrates are readily available at all times, that the appropriate treatment protocol is being followed, and that glucagon is accessible. The physician should review the glucose log carefully to determine when and why such events are occurring. A more dynamic insulin regimen often is needed with the use of insulin to carbohydrate ratios and specific adjustments for exercise. The physician must be particularly attentive to the risk of nocturnal hypoglycemia. Periodic glucose measurements should be obtained at 2 to 3 a.m.. Additional carbohydrate may have to be consumed or insulin dose decreased at bedtime on more active days. A bedtime snack that contains carbohydrate, protein, and fat or a snack bar containing uncooked cornstarch can prolong carbohydrate absorption and minimize the risk of nocturnal hypoglycemia. Providers must remember that hypoglycemia can cause not only acute problems but also chronic neurologic sequelae.

24.10.5　Conditions Associated with Type 1 Diabetes Mellitus

POOR GROWTH Growth can be poor if food intake is restricted as a means to control blood level of glucose or because of poor glycemic control. An extreme form of such poor control is *Mauriac syndrome,* in which chronic inadequate insulin administration results in short stature, hepatomegaly from a fatty liver, osteopenia, and delayed adolescence. Celiac disease must also be considered as a cause of poor weight or linear growth. Hypothyroidism usually causes only poor linear growth.

JOINT AND SKIN DISORDERS Some persons with poor glycemic control also have limited joint mobility, which may be first identified in the interphalangeal joints with inability to approximate the palms and fingers (called the *prayer sign*). This condition often is associated with tight, waxy overlying skin similar to scleroderma. It may be caused by cross-linking of glycosylated collagen and is frequently associated with microvascular complications. *Necrobiosis lipoidica diabeticorum* is a rare skin manifestation that occurs primarily among girls and women with diabetes mellitus. It consists of shiny atrophic areas of breakdown and ulceration on the shins. The cause is unknown, but it appears to be independent of glucose control.

CELIAC DISEASE   Celiac disease occurs among 1 to 8% of persons with type 1 diabetes mellitus. The underlying cause is unknown, but both type 1 diabetes mellitus and celiac disease are associated with the HLA-DR3 genotype. All children with poor weight gain or linear growth should be screened for celiac disease with anti-endomysial or anti-transglutaminase antibody tests. Both are serum IgA antibodies, so IgA level must be measured to assure that a false-negative result is not obtained because of IgA deficiency. Intestinal biopsy is the standard for the diagnosis of celiac disease (see Sec. 17.18.2). Celiac screening of all persons with type 1 diabetes mellitus should be considered because many have minimal or no symptoms. Delays in diagnosis can result in dental abnormalities, osteoporosis, constitutional delay in growth and development, and possibly later development of lymphoma of the small intestine. Treatment consists of intake of a gluten-free diet, which requires careful instruction from a dietitian.

THYROIDITIS   As many as 40% of persons with diabetes have detectable thyroid autoantibodies. A smaller subpopulation (6% of children and a higher percentage of adults) eventually have overt primary hypothyroidism caused by Hashimoto thyroiditis. There is also an increased risk of Graves disease with type 1 diabetes mellitus. Thyroid-stimulating hormone should be measured after diagnosis of diabetes mellitus. If the linear growth rate is normal and there are no clinical symptoms, screening studies usually are not necessary, but a careful thyroid examination should be performed at routine intervals. Any suggestion of goiter warrants evaluation of thyroid function. Some experts advocate routine yearly thyroid hormone testing. In rare cases, type 1 diabetes mellitus can constitute part of a larger *polyglandular autoimmune syndrome*. Type II syndrome is associated with HLA-DR3 and -DR4 haplotypes; 50% of patients have diabetes mellitus with hypothyroidism or Graves disease and Addison disease (see Sec. 24.4.7).

LONG-TERM COMPLICATIONS OF TYPE 1 DIABETES MELLITUS

Persons with diabetes eventually may have complications of vascular compromise. These problems manifest as microvascular changes, which result in nephropathy, retinopathy, and neuropathy, or macrovascular changes with atherosclerosis and attendant problems such as coronary artery or cerebrovascular disease. The underlying mechanisms precipitating these complications are unclear. Current hypotheses include (1) accelerated nonenzymatic glycosylation of proteins that forms so-called advanced glycosylated end products, which interfere with protein function, (2) activation of the aldose-reductase pathway with accumulation of the toxic end-product sorbitol, and (3) activation of the intracellular protein kinase C pathway, which affects downstream events such as extracellular matrix production. Microvascular complications rarely are encountered among children with diabetes before puberty and are uncommon among adults within the first 5 years of diagnosis. An increasing incidence thereafter reaches a plateau after 25 years. Current recommendations are to begin screening for end-organ damage when the person has had diabetes for at least 5 years and is in puberty. Screening for complications includes yearly ophthalmologic and detailed neurologic examinations and measurement of urinary microalbumin.

RETINOPATHY   Almost every patient with diabetes mellitus has retinal changes (see Sec. 26.11.5). Initial alterations include background nonproliferative changes in the retinal capillaries with dot and blot hemorrhages, microaneurysms, and hard exudates. None of these changes threatens vision or necessitates treatment. However, leaky blood vessels near the macula cause macular edema, which can impair vision. Forty percent to 60% of cases of leakage never progress beyond this stage, but after 10 to 15 years of diabetes mellitus the others may begin to advance on to proliferative retinopathy with infarcts in the nerve layer (cotton-wool exudates) and resultant neovascularization into the vitreous and near the disc or retinal periphery. These fragile vessels can hemorrhage into the vitreous (preretinal hemorrhages). Subsequent healing produces scarring and retinal detachment. Macular edema, vitreous hemorrhage, and retinal detachment all compromise vision, and laser photocoagulopathy may be needed to preserve vision. Vision also can be compromised by changes in the lens caused by hyperglycemia. The problem resolves with improved glycemic control. In rare instances, patients have cataracts with persisting white opacity from sorbitol accumulation; these must be removed surgically.

NEPHROPATHY   The earliest renal changes are detected within 2 to 5 years of diagnosis with thickening of the glomerular basement membrane. In the first decade, increasing matrix is found within the mesangium. Some patients have progression to sclerosis of the glomerular capillaries in a diffuse or nodular pattern. Loss of renal function ensues as the glomerulus becomes a fibrous scar (see Sec. 21.8). An increase in albumin excretion often is found at diagnosis but reverts to normal with intensive glucose control. Some persons have gradually developing microalbuminuria, the earliest sign of diabetic nephropathy. Without treatment, 9% of these patients per year have macroalbuminuria, and almost all of these have end-stage renal disease within 7 to 10 years.

Screening for microalbuminuria begins 5 years after the onset of disease. It begins at puberty if the disease is diagnosed during early childhood. In the past, 24-hour or timed urine collections were used for screening, but these are cumbersome for patients and are subject to timing errors and collection inaccuracies. Studies indicate that a spot urine collection for the ratio of urinary albumin to creatinine is comparable with timed collections. Values less than 30 μg albumin per milligram creatinine are normal. Values of 30 to 300 or more than 300 μg correspond to micro- and macroalbuminuria, respectively. Typical urine dipsticks detect total protein rather than albumin and are much less sensitive and thus inadequate for screening. Sensitive semiquantitative commercial urine dipsticks for microalbumin detection are now available. If an abnormal screening collection is obtained, the study should be verified on one or more occasions to determine accuracy. Other causes of proteinuria must be considered (see Sec. 21.5.5).

The clinical course of diabetic nephropathy can be modified by a number of factors. Tighter metabolic control prevents progression of renal disease, and this must be pursued aggressively with each patient. Treatment with an agent to lower blood pressure, even if the patient does not have hypertension helps protect the kidney. Angiotensin-converting enzyme inhibitors have been shown to reduce the amount of proteinuria and slow progression of nephropathy. The drug should be initiated for those with microalbuminuria detected in two of three urine collections over a 6-month period. For those with overt diabetic nephropathy, restriction of dietary protein retards disease progression. Exposure to nonsteroidal anti-inflammatory agents should be minimized. Smoking is a risk factor for progression of renal disease and should be eliminated.

NEUROPATHY Diabetic neuropathy affects both the peripheral and the autonomic nervous system. Peripheral disease most commonly manifests as bilateral symmetric sensory polyneuropathy with paresthesia, pain, numbness, and loss of deep tendon reflexes. It often begins in the lower extremities at the tips of the toes and progresses in a stocking-glove distribution proximally. Such neurologic dysfunction is a risk factor for the development of ulcerations and the need for lower extremity amputation. Autonomic dysfunction includes gastroparesis with delayed gastric emptying, diarrhea, orthostatic hypotension, resting tachycardia with reduced heart rate variability during respiration, neurogenic bladder, and erectile dysfunction. These problems rarely are encountered among pediatric patients.

MACROVASCULAR DISEASE Macrovascular disease is rarely encountered in the pediatric population, but healthy habits in childhood can help prevent the development of atherosclerosis later in life. In addition to tight glucose control, regular exercise and healthy eating habits should be encouraged with appropriate moderation of fat intake. Screening lipid panels should be obtained, especially if there is a strong family history of lipid disorders or vascular disease manifesting at an early age. If the results are normal, the measurements can be repeated every 5 years. As with nephropathy, hypertension is a risk factor for macrovascular disease. Blood pressure should be monitored routinely, and early pharmacologic intervention is warranted for hypertension. Smoking accelerates the risk of any form of vascular disease among persons with diabetes mellitus and should be strongly discouraged.

PSYCHOSOCIAL ISSUES

Diabetes is a unique chronic illness. It differs from conditions such as cancer and asthma in that it is unrelenting and remains pervasive in everyday life. The specter of long-term complications raises a host of issues for the patient and family, including fear, guilt, and frustration. The child and family need ongoing care by a team that is sensitive to these issues. They often benefit from regular visits with a professional trained in individual and family therapy and with experience in the management of diabetes.

Families often request age-specific guidelines for when a child should be able to perform particular diabetes tasks, that is, when can the parents relinquish certain daily tasks and have the child assume more direct responsibility. There are no age-specific norms by which certain skills should be mastered. These decisions are based on the child's emotional and cognitive maturity, temperament, and external stresses and particular family situation. Daily activities can help dictate how and when a child assumes more direct management of the diabetes. For example, a child who wants to spend the night at a friend's house is motivated to learn glucose monitoring and injection therapy (although adult supervision still may be necessary). In the past, families and health-care providers took great pride in the ability of a child to assume independence in diabetes management. We now know that most children are not able to maintain such independence. They need structure and supervision from an adult. By the time they reach young adulthood, children with diabetes have become exhausted and frustrated by years of struggling alone with diabetes management. It is more beneficial for the family to share the task of management of diabetes mellitus with the child, but this interdependence requires a delicate balance between the parents and child with continual renegotiation over specific responsibilities and obligations. For many families, it helps to approach the daily diabetes tasks as routine household

chores, whereby the expectations of the child are clearly delineated, and failure to perform the tasks is associated with an agreed-on consequence (such as loss of a privilege). Vivid descriptions of long-term complications usually are counterproductive. The resultant fear and negative imagery leave some children with the sense that complications are inevitable and that efforts to prevent them are useless.

Type 1 diabetes mellitus places a child at risk of emotional and psychiatric disorders. The prevalence of low self-esteem and clinical depression increases among persons with diabetes, and anxiety disorders occur with greater frequency. Although erratic glucose control accounts for some symptoms, one must not dismiss a possible underlying psychiatric disorder. Such disorders can interfere with the ability to obtain intensive glucose control. Some children with diabetes mellitus have recurrent diabetic ketoacidosis and hospital readmissions, presumed the result of insulin omission. This behavior may be a manifestation of a child's anger and rebellion and denial of the diabetes. Some children use such situations for secondary gain, such as lashing out at their families or avoiding school. Such patients need an insulin regimen that is as simple as possible— a fixed insulin dose administered twice a day. Their parents must remain actively involved in daily management and directly observe each insulin injection.

Repeated episodes of diabetic ketoacidosis indicate a family is poorly equipped to supervise their child. Referral to children's protective services and placement into foster care may be necessary. Children can manipulate diabetes management in other ways for secondary gain. A small percentage purposefully induce hypoglycemia, either by missing meals or by administering excessive insulin. The diabetes team must carefully assess whether this behavior represents a suicidal gesture. Some children feign a hypoglycemic seizure to gain attention.

As many as one-third of women with type 1 diabetes mellitus have eating disorders, manifested as underdosing of insulin or insulin omission in an attempt to promote glycosuria and subsequent weight loss. In effect, this behavior is similar to the binging and purging of bulimia. Reinstitution of insulin therapy may be associated with acute fluid retention and edema, as in refeeding syndromes, and can prompt further insulin omission for fear of weight gain. This behavior may account, at least in part, for the greater number of hospital readmissions for diabetic ketoacidosis among female as opposed to male adolescents.

These issues are complex and usually are beyond the scope of most busy general practitioners. Community diabetes support groups can help in dealing with some of the more common concerns that arise in diabetes management. Diabetes summer camps are an invaluable resource. They provide peer support and role models for children with diabetes mellitus. In such settings, many children often are relieved to find that they are not alone with this disease and that diabetes mellitus need not pose limitations on their life if they have greater understanding of the disease and plan accordingly. In more difficult cases, trained mental health care professionals should be consulted.

ADOLESCENT ISSUES

Adolescence can be a particularly difficult time for intensive diabetes management. Aside from the psychosocial issues discussed earlier, teenagers often have an increasingly varied and busy daily life and consequently devote less time and energy to management of diabetes mellitus. Increased insulin resistance must be countered with increased insulin doses, and yet tight glucose control can remain elusive. Some young women may notice that insulin needs increase several days before menses, and insulin doses have to be adjusted accordingly at this time in the cycle. Contraception is vital for sexually active girls with diabetes mellitus, because hyperglycemia early in gestation can function as a teratogen. The adolescent needs to be reassured that she will be capable of having her own children, but ideally this is planned, with optimal metabolic control before conception. Boys may wonder about their risk of erectile dysfunction caused by autonomic dysfunction and should be reassured that tight glucose control minimizes their risk of any complication. Adolescents should be counseled regarding the risks of hypoglycemia while driving and the need for increased vigilance in glucose monitoring and carbohydrate availability.

Risk-taking behavior can pose particular problems for adolescents with diabetes mellitus. Experimentation with drugs impairs the person's decision making about diabetes. Recreational drugs can mask hypoglycemia and alter appetite, which results in missed meals and insulin injections. Ethanol ingestion can be especially dangerous because severe hypoglycemia can develop in the fasting state as gluconeogenesis is blocked. Adolescents must be advised of the need to stay in control of diabetes mellitus at all times, preferably avoiding drugs altogether. If one is to consume alcohol, it should only be taken in moderation and never on an empty stomach. Glucose levels should be measured more frequently. Cigarette smoking synergizes with chronic hyperglycemia to further increase risk of long-term complications and should be avoided altogether.

OTHER POTENTIAL TREATMENT APPROACHES

ALTERNATIVE INSULINS AND DELIVERY METHODS Investigators are developing new insulin analogs as well as alternative means of insulin delivery. One current gap in therapy is an insulin preparation that acts as a true basal insulin to provide continuous coverage over an extended time without a peaking effect. Glargine insulin (HOE 901) is a novel recombinant insulin that is soluble at an acidic pH but precipitates in the interstitial space at neutral pH and is then slowly absorbed. Results of clinical trials suggest that this may be a good alternative to Ultralente insulin. Many alternative routes for insulin delivery have been considered over the years in an attempt to circumvent daily injections. Trials are now underway with inhaled insulin, which has similar pharmacokinetics to injected Lispro insulin. In addition to external insulin pumps, intraperitoneal insulin pumps have been used in the care of a small number of adults. This surgically implanted device delivers insulin directly into the peritoneal cavity, where it is rapidly absorbed into the portal circulation. Basal and bolus rates are programmed with a handheld transmitter, and a large insulin reservoir is periodically refilled with a concentrated insulin preparation.

PANCREAS OR ISLET TRANSPLANTATION Whole pancreas or islet transplantation is possible but requires ongoing immunosuppression to inhibit graft rejection by the recipient. The well-known risks of such therapy render routine transplantation inappropriate, except for patients who need an additional organ transplant (as in the case of concomitant renal failure). Pancreas transplantation in this setting is now quite successful. The 5-year graft survival is as high as 75%. Current research efforts are directed at means to bypass the immune system to make immunosuppression unnecessary.

ARTIFICIAL PANCREAS Although the technology exists for insulin delivery through insulin pumps, construction of a reliable glu-

cose sensor has proved to be a formidable hurdle. The ideal sensor would be noninvasive, and efforts have been made to use radiation technology, similar to infrared pulse oximetry for measuring oxygen saturation. These devices have not proved reliable. Invasive glucose monitors are closer to clinical applicability, with development of sensors that reside within a blood vessel or that sample interstitial fluid from subcutaneous sites. By linking a glucose sensor to an insulin pump, one will have a closed-loop feedback system that approximates the β cell. These systems are experimental.

SCREENING AND PREVENTION AMONG HIGH-RISK POPULATIONS By the time of diagnosis, only 10 to 20% of β-cell mass remains. Thus interventions at this stage may be too late in effecting lasting remission. A number of different agents have been used at this stage, including immunosuppression with cyclosporine, azathioprine, and glucocorticoids, but all have limited efficacy. Remission has been induced in some patients, but has been sustained for only 2 years in a minority. With discontinuation of the drugs all patients need exogenous insulin. As with transplantation, the risk of use of these drugs currently outweighs the benefits, and such broad-spectrum immunosuppression is not warranted at the time of diagnosis. A variety of prevention strategies, including use of free radical scavengers, insulin therapy before disease becomes apparent, and exclusion of cow's milk from the diet, are being evaluated.

24.10.6 Type 2 Diabetes Mellitus

EPIDEMIOLOGY, RISK FACTORS, AND PATHOGENESIS

Type 2 diabetes mellitus used to be considered rare among children, constituting 2 to 3% of cases of diabetes mellitus. However, the incidence is increasing rapidly, from 0.7 to 7.2/100,000 over a 14-year period in one midwestern city in the United States, with 33% of new-onset cases among 10- to 19-year-olds caused by type 2 diabetes mellitus. It is now estimated that 10 to 20% of children with diabetes mellitus have type 2. The mean age at diagnosis is 12 to 14 years, which probably relates to the increased insulin resistance found during puberty. Most studies note a female to male predominance of type 2 diabetes mellitus. As is type 1, type 2 diabetes mellitus is caused by synergy between an underlying genetic risk and environmental exposures (Table 24-44). Type 2 diabetes mellitus is a polygenic disorder, but unlike type 1 diabetes mellitus, it has a strong family history. Ethnicity also influences one's risk of type 2 diabetes mellitus, fewer than 10% of whites have this disease, but 10 to 20% of hispanics, blacks, and Asians and as many as 50% of Pima Indians have this disorder. The thrifty gene hypothesis

TABLE 24-44

RISK FACTORS FOR TYPE 2 DIABETES MELLITUS IN CHILDREN

Family history of type 2 diabetes mellitus
Ethnicity
Obesity, with acanthosis nigricans
Puberty
History of impaired glucose tolerance
Pattern of evolving syndrome X (hypertension, hyperlipidemia, insulin resistance, atherosclerosis) or polycystic ovarian syndrome
History of being large-for-gestational-age or of intrauterine growth retardation at birth

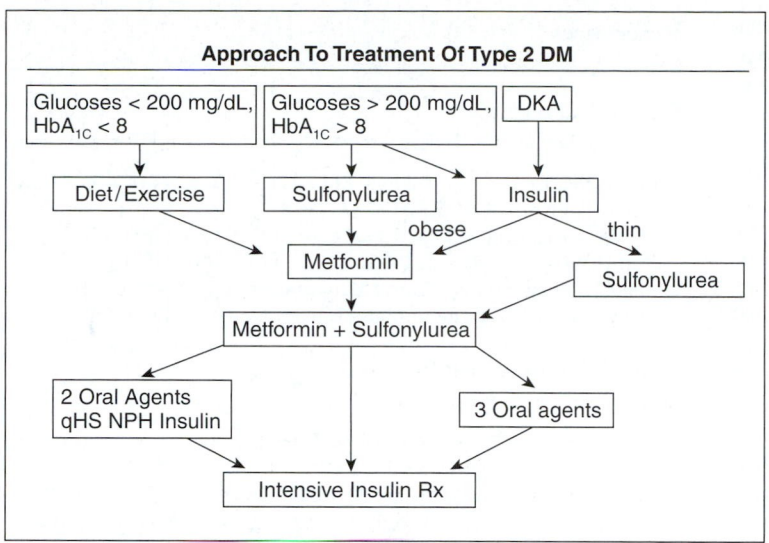

Approach To Treatment Of Type 2 DM

- Glucoses < 200 mg/dL, HbA$_{1C}$ < 8 → Diet/Exercise
- Glucoses > 200 mg/dL, HbA$_{1C}$ > 8 → Sulfonylurea
- DKA → Insulin

Sulfonylurea → Metformin (obese)
Insulin → Sulfonylurea (thin)

Metformin + Sulfonylurea
→ 2 Oral Agents qHS NPH Insulin
→ 3 Oral agents
→ Intensive Insulin Rx

FIGURE 24-42 Approach to the treatment of a child with type 2 diabetes mellitus. With only mild hyperglycemia, dietary and life-style interventions can be performed first. Persisting or worsening hyperglycemia necessitates pharmacologic intervention. Marked hyperglycemia necessitates initial therapy with a sulfonylurea or insulin with later transition to metformin, especially for obese patients. Persistent hyperglycemia necessitates use of additional agents. DKA = diabetic ketoacidosis, Hb = hemoglobin, NPH = NPH insulin.

suggests that our current genotype evolved from times of limited food availability, when efficient energy storage in times of famine represented a selective advantage. Such efficiency no longer matches the current life-style in much of the world. We have changed from a hunter-gatherer society to a more sedentary urban life-style, with less daily exercise and with ready access to an abundance of food. The result has been a dramatic increase in obesity, which is a risk factor for type 2 diabetes mellitus. The intrauterine milieu also influences the fetus's later risk of type 2 diabetes mellitus. Many children with a history of intrauterine growth retardation or those who are infants of mothers with diabetes later have increased insulin resistance and are thus at increased risk of type 2 diabetes mellitus as they age.

The primary lesion causing type 2 diabetes mellitus is not clear, although many consider it to be increased insulin resistance rather than an insulin secretory defect. Postulated causes of the resistance include down regulation of the insulin receptor, a decrease in receptor kinase activity, a decrease in phosphorylation of receptor substrates or defects in other aspects of the downstream signaling cascade, or defects in the glucose transporter system. The β cell is initially able to overcome such resistance with hypersecretion of insulin, but over time is not able to maintain this output, and impaired glucose tolerance and later type 2 diabetes mellitus ensue. Impending β-cell failure is preceded by a diminished response to a glucose load, a change in the normal oscillatory pattern of insulin secretion, and an increase in the secretion of proinsulin relative to processed insulin.

The challenge for the clinician is how to determine which child has type 2 rather than type 1 diabetes mellitus (see Table 24-36). In general, one expects a person with type 2 diabetes mellitus to be obese, often with acanthosis nigricans, to have a strong family history of diabetes, and to be of an ethnic background strongly associated with the disorder. Persons with type 2 diabetes mellitus frequently have hyperglycemia but without ketoacidosis, but diabetic ketoacidosis does not necessarily exclude the diagnosis. A lean person without ketoacidosis may have an early stage of type 1 diabetes mellitus, or a form of maturity-onset diabetes of the young (MODY) if the family history suggests an autosomal-dominant pattern of inheritance. Autoantibodies and insulin or C-peptide levels may be helpful in differentiating the types of diabetes. The clinical course clarifies this issue. Demonstration of endogenous insulin secretion more than 2 years after the initial diagnosis suggests type 2

diabetes mellitus. Diabetes among black youths can be especially difficult to categorize.

MANAGEMENT OF TYPE 2 DIABETES MELLITUS

A number of new options are available for the management of type 2 diabetes mellitus (Fig. 24-42). The cornerstone of therapy remains modification of diet and increased daily exercise. For some patients, loss of as little as 5 to 10 kg can reverse the hyperglycemia. Elimination of simple carbohydrates, especially soda and juice, with reduction of fat intake is a necessary life-style change. Moderate daily exercise can influence underlying insulin resistance. Most persons can not implement and maintain such interventions and need to move on to pharmacologic approaches.

If glucose level is frequently more than 200 mg/dL and HbA$_{1C}$ is greater than 8%, life-style modifications and pharmacologic intervention are begun. Options for pharmacologic therapy are described below, and a treatment selection algorithm is shown in Fig. 24-42. For the child with diabetic ketoacidosis who is presumed to have type 2 diabetes mellitus, the approach is similar to that to type 1 diabetes mellitus. An insulin drip may be needed for severe acidosis (pH <7.25) or with severe hyperglycemia (>600 mg/dL).

SULFONYLUREAS These agents increase the secretion of insulin from β cells. With modestly elevated glucose values but without severe ketoacidosis, sulfonylurea therapy alone often is effective within 3 to 7 days. Although inexpensive and conveniently dosed (1 or 2 times per day), there are several disadvantages to use of sulfonylureas, as follows: (1) insulin is secreted in an unregulated manner, and hypoglycemia can occur, (2) enhanced insulin secretion helps overcome insulin resistance but often leads to further weight gain, and (3) many patients eventually become refractory to such agents, presumably because of β-cell exhaustion, which necessitates addition of another medication.

INSULIN Because type 2 diabetes mellitus is not a condition of absolute insulin deficiency, the regimens may be much simpler than those for type 1 diabetes mellitus. Many patients benefit from initial treatment with bedtime NPH insulin to help minimize fasting hyperglycemia while continuing daytime sulfonylurea therapy. Insulin eventually may be needed during the day as well. Premixed insulin, such as 70/30 (70% NPH, 30% regular), can be dosed before breakfast and dinner. The disadvantage of premixed insulin is that the short-acting component cannot be increased for acute hyperglycemia or change in diet. Large insulin doses may be needed to overcome the insulin resistance of type 2 diabetes mellitus. As with sulfonylureas, the disadvantage of insulin is the risk of hypoglycemia and tendency to weight gain. A more sophisticated insulin regimen with Lispro insulin before meals and NPH insulin at bedtime may allow tighter glucose control with less insulin and may minimize the risks of weight gain and hypoglycemia.

METFORMIN (GLUCOPHAGE^R) This agent is a biguanide and has become the first-line drug for management of type 2 diabetes mellitus. The mechanism of action has not been fully delineated, but the primary function is to decrease hepatic glucose production. It also lowers insulin resistance in muscle and fat. Metformin decreases hyperlipidemia, and it induces modest weight loss. It may cause nonspecific gastrointestinal symptoms. Therapy should be initiated at a low dose and slowly titrated up to therapeutic levels. For a patient with severe hyperglycemia, therapy may have to be initiated with insulin or sulfonylurea. Then the transition is made to treatment with metformin. In rare cases, metformin has been associated with lactic acidosis. Its use is contraindicated in the treatment of patients with renal or liver failure or underlying metabolic acidosis. Metformin must be discontinued in any acute disorder in which renal clearance may be compromised, including major surgery, severe infection, or use of intravenous iodinated contrast media.

THIAZOLIDINEDIONES This novel class of drugs is thought to function primarily by decreasing peripheral insulin resistance within muscle and fat. The drugs serve as a ligand for the peripheral peroxisomal activator γ-receptor, a transcription factor that activates adipocyte differentiation and insulin-responsive genes. The first of this class of drug, troglitazone was effective in glucose control but has been withdrawn from the market because of liver toxicity. Pioglitazone and rosiglitazone are related compounds that have been approved and that may have no associated liver toxicity.

α-GLUCOSIDASE INHIBITORS Acarbose and related agents serve as competitive inhibitors of the enzymes on the small-intestinal brush border. They limit carbohydrate absorption and minimize postprandial hyperglycemia. Complications of carbohydrate malabsorption include bloating, flatulence, and diarrhea. Many children and adolescents do not consider these side effects tolerable, and thus this medication may have only a limited role for this population.

If blood levels of glucose are not tightly regulated with one of the aforedescribed medications, a different class of drug has to be added to the regimen in much the same manner as the management of hypertension or asthma (see Fig. 24-42). In the United Kingdom Prospective Diabetes Study, adults with type 2 diabetes mellitus often became refractory to the initial medication after 4 years, and the effect of a new medication appeared to be additive. Persons with type 2 diabetes mellitus are at the same risk as those with type 1 of long-term complications of hyperglycemia. The UK study showed definitively that tighter glucose control of type 2 diabetes mellitus among adults is associated with reduced risk of such complications. Unlike the situation with type 1 diabetes mellitus, euglycemia can be achieved by children with type 2 diabetes mellitus without high risk of hypoglycemia. These patients often have coexisting problems with hypertension and hyperlipidemia, and appropriate therapy for these conditions further reduces the risk of long-term complications.

References

General Overview

Kaufman FR: Diabetes in children and adolescents: areas of controversy. Med Clin North Am 82:721–738, 1998

Medical Management of Type 1 Diabetes, 3rd ed. Alexandria, VA, American Diabetes Association, 1998

Plotnick L, Henderson R: Clinical Management of the Child and Teenager with Diabetes. Baltimore, Johns Hopkins University Press, 1998

Type 1 Diabetes Mellitus

American Diabetes Association: Clinical practice recommendations. Diabetes Care 22(Suppl 1): S5-23, 1999

Bhisitkul DM, Morrow AL, Vinik AI, Shults J, Layland JC, Rohn R: Prevalence of stress hyperglycemia among patients attending a pediatric emergency department. J Pediatr 124:547–551, 1994

Froguel P, Vaxillaire M, Velho G: Genetic and metabolic heterogeneity of maturity-onset diabetes of the young. Diabetes Rev 5:123–130, 1997

Herskowitz-Dumont R, Wolfsdorf JI, Jackson RA Eisenbarth GS: Distinction between transient hyperglycemia and early insulin-dependent diabetes mellitus in childhood: a prospective study of incidence and prognostic factors. J Pediatr 123:347–354, 1993

Manske CL: Risks and benefits of kidney and pancreas transplantation for diabetic patients. Diabetes Care 22(Suppl 2): B114–120, 1999

Rabinovitch A, Skyler JS: Prevention of type 1 diabetes. Med Clin North Am 82:739–755, 1998

Slover RH, Eisenbarth GS: Prevention of type 1 diabetes and recurrent beta cell destruction of transplanted islets. Endocr Rev 18:241–258, 1997

Type 2 Diabetes Mellitus

American Diabetes Association Consensus Statement: Type 2 diabetes in children and adolescents. Diabetes Care 23:381–389, 2000

Glaser NS: Non-insulin dependent diabetes mellitus in childhood and adolescence. Pediatr Clin North Am 44:307–337, 1997

Kruszynska Y, Olefsky JM: Cellular and molecular mechanisms of non-insulin dependent diabetes mellitus. J Invest Med 44:413–428, 1996

Pinhas-Hamiel O, Dolan LM, Daniels SR, Standiford D, Khoury PR, Zeitler P: Increased incidence of non-insulin-dependent diabetes mellitus among adolescents. J Pediatr 128:608–615, 1996

Rosenbloom RL, Joe JR, Young RS, Winter WE: Emerging epidemic of type 2 diabetes in youth. Diabetes Care 22:345–354, 1999

United Kingdom Prospective Diabetes Study Group: Intensive blood-glucose control with sulphonylureas or insulin compared with conventional treatment and risk of complications in patients with type 2 diabetes (UKPDS 33). Lancet 352:837–853, 1998

United Kingdom Prospective Diabetes Study Group: Effect of intensive blood-glucose control with metformin on complications in overweight patients with type 2 diabetes (UKPDS 34). Lancet 352:854–865, 1998

24.11 OBESITY

Dennis M. Styne and Nancy Schoenfeld-Warden

24.11.1 Definition and Incidence of Obesity

Obesity among children and adolescents is an increasing problem in the United States and the rest of the world, even in locations previously prone to malnutrition. *Obesity* refers to excess body fat, not excess body weight. Previous indicators of obesity, such as the weight for age and weight to height ratio did not adequately adjust for height or were prone to false-positive descriptions of obesity, respectively. Obesity is now defined with a measure that provides a better reflection of the amount of body fat than previous measures. The new measure is age-specific value of *body mass index* (BMI), which is calculated as follows: Weight in kilograms/Height^2 in meters. Body mass index for age is shown in Table 24-45, and new height and weight charts composed by the United States National Center for Health Statistics are available at: (http://www.cdc.gov/nchs/about/major/nhanes/growthcharts/charts.htm). More accurate measurements of body composition than BMI are used in clinical research and epidemiologic studies. Dual-energy x-ray absorptiometry (DEXA) is used to determine bone mineral content and full body fat. Computed tomography or MR imaging best shows the distribution of body fat, especially the amount of intra-abdominal adipose tissue or visceral fat. Visceral fat is considered to be the most metabolically active fat depot and to be responsible for many of the comorbidities of obesity among adults. This relation has not been proved among children. Densitometry through underwater weighing, determining the displacement of air by the body (BodPod), determination of skinfold thickness, and bioelectric impedance analysis indicate amounts of body fat and body water.

Body fat percentages change normally with age. Infants have a relatively high BMI followed by a decrease at 5 to 6 years of age, the adiposity rebound. An early adiposity rebound is predictive of persistent overweight status with an odds ratio of 6. In childhood the values approximate 12% for boys and 15% for girls, with a temporary increase among boys until values at puberty return to childhood levels. Among girls the amount of body fat increases to 22 to 24% in late puberty. When BMI in children exceeds the 95th percentile, body fat percentage by DEXA or bioelectric impedance exceeds 40%.

Between the second National Health Examination Survey (NHANES II) in 1984 and NHANES III in 1993, the prevalence of BMI greater than the 95th percentile (defined as obesity by some and overweight by others) in the 6- to 11-year-old population increased from 6.5% to 11.4% for boys and 5.5 to 9.9% for girls. Among 12- to 17-year-olds it increased from 4.7% to 11.4% among boys and from 4.9% to 9.9% among girls. The prevalence of BMI in the 85th to 95th percentile (classified as at risk of obesity) increased to 22% during the same period. Hispanic and African-American children have a higher BMI, are more prone to obesity, and are at higher risk of type 2 diabetes mellitus than are white and Asian Americans at most ages.

The explanation for this dramatic increase in the incidence of obesity is multifactorial. Energy intake comes from food, and energy expenditure occurs as the result of a combination of basal metabolism, activity, and growth. If these factors are equal, weight stays stable along a growth or BMI percentile. When energy intake exceeds energy expenditure in a positive balance, weight gain with fat deposition occurs. Genetic factors modify the efficiency of conversion of energy intake to tissue as well as the energy expended for a given amount of activity in each person. Specific alleles of the mitochondrial uncoupling protein-2 are associated with obesity among children. Obese children and adults may be more efficient in their use of consumed calories. Thus with the same caloric intake and energy expenditure, one child may gain excess weight while another does not. Because the genetic factors relating to energy use have not changed, environmental influences that affect energy intake and expenditure are primarily responsible for the increased trend toward obesity among children. In most cases, obesity is caused by a subtle positive increase in caloric balance in a genetically susceptible person over a prolonged time. There is a 50% likelihood that obesity will persist into adulthood if the BMI in adolescence is greater than the 95th percentile. Parental fatness, low socioeconomic status, high birth weight, earlier and rapid secondary sexual maturation, and inactivity are predictive of persistence of obesity into adulthood.

The risk of morbidity from being overweight is unclear for children. Adults have an increased rate of complications as BMI increases to more than 25, which is approximately the 90th percentile BMI for the adult population. A BMI of 30 is approximately the 99th percentile. The BMI linked to complications in childhood has not been established, but a BMI above the 85th percentile is considered worrisome. Counseling is needed to prevent further weight gain. If risk factors such as a personal or family history of hypertension or dyslipidemia are present, weight loss is recommended. Hypertension and dyslipidemia also are more common when BMI is greater than the 85th percentile. Therefore it is reasonable to consider obese any child or adolescent with a BMI above the 95th percentile. The goal of prevention and management of obesity is improvement of metabolic function, not emulation of thin body types.

24.11.2   Consequences of Childhood Obesity

Medical or Health Consequences of Obesity

Complications of childhood obesity are shown in Table 24-46. These include hyperlipidemia, hypertension, increased incidence of type 2 diabetes mellitus (see Sec. 24.10), acanthosis nigricans, slipped capital femoral epiphysis, and obstructive sleep apnea. Advanced skeletal development also occurs, although with this complication children usually are short as adults because puberty occurs at an earlier age. The relatively early time of menarche is associated with an increased incidence of breast cancer later in life, and obesity is associated with development of hirsutism and irregular menses (ovarian hyperandrogensism). Hepatic steatosis, sometime associated with fibrosis (see Sec. 18.11) is increasingly recognized among obese children, as is cholelithiasis. Orthopedic disorders, including slipped capital femoral epiphysis and Blount disease of the tibia also have been associated with obesity.

Thirty percent of obese adults were obese as children, and 50% were obese as adolescents. Obesity starting at a young age causes more serious consequences among adults than does obesity that starts in adulthood. A 50-year follow-up survey as part of the Har-

TABLE 24-45
BODY MASS INDEX* IN CHILDREN

AGE (YRS)	BOYS 50%	BOYS 95%	GIRLS 50%
5	15.6	18.3	15.1
8	16.2	21.5	15.8
11	17.8	25.7	17.9
14	19.8	27.8	20.2
17	21.8	30.1	21.2

* Body mass index (BMI) = weight (kg)/height^2 (m)
(See:*http://www.cdc.gov/nchs/about/major/nhanes/growthcharts/charts.htm* for complete data charts)

TABLE 24-46

MEDICAL CONSEQUENCES OF CHILDHOOD AND ADOLESCENT OBESITY

Metabolic
  Insulin resistance (type 2 diabetes mellitus)
  Hyperlipidemia
Cardiopulmonary
  Hypertension
  Obstructive sleep apnea
  Obesity hypoventilation syndrome (pickwickian syndrome): CO_2 retention, hypoxia, polycythemia, right ventricular hypertrophy
  Increased incidence asthma
Dermatologic
  Acanthosis nigricans
  Heat rash
  Intertrigo
  Monilial dermatitis
Orthopedic
  Slipped capital femoral epiphysis
  Blount disease of the tibia
Gastrointestinal
  Hepatic steatosis and fibrosis
  Cholelithiasis
  Gastroesophageal reflux
Other
  Early puberty and menarche
  Advanced skeletal development: tall child, short adult
  Ovarian hyperandrogenism
  Idiopathic intracranial hypertension
  Lower extremity venous stasis disease
  Urinary stress incontinence

vard Growth Study of 1922–1935 showed increased risk of mortality from all causes (1.8 times) and morbidity from coronary heart disease (2.3 times), atherosclerotic cerebrovascular disease (13.2 times), and colorectal cancer (9.1 times) among men but not among women who had a BMI greater than the 75th percentile during adolescence. Overweight in adolescence was a more powerful predictor of mortality than weight in adulthood. A British study also showed a twofold increase in all causes of death after 57 years of follow-up study (1.9 times for ischemic heart disease and 1.6 times for generalized cardiovascular disease) among persons with a BMI above the 97th percentile compared with those between the 25th and 29th percentiles, at 7 years of age. Mean levels of fasting glucose, systolic and diastolic blood pressure, type 2 diabetes mellitus, and cardiovascular disease were greatest among adults who were classified in the highest childhood weight category at 9 to 13 years of age. In the Bogalusa Heart Study, being overweight during adolescence was associated with a statistically significant increase in prevalence of elevated cholesterol, LDL, and HDL levels in adulthood.

Psychological and Social Consequences of Obesity

From an early age, society stigmatizes obese persons as lazy, stupid, slow, and self-indulgent. Children express negative attitudes toward their obese peers as early as kindergarten and even prefer a playmate who uses a wheelchair or has a major physical disability to one who is obese. Adults, including physicians, inappropriately ascribe personal failings such as poor self-control and hedonism as the main cause of obesity. Because of these societal attitudes, almost all obese children are teased at some point. Obese children and adolescents have lower levels of self-esteem than do their nonobese counter-

parts. This likely explains their increased risk of smoking and drinking alcohol. A school-age child is at a critical period for the development of body image and self-esteem. Initiation of weight management at 6 to 9 years of age can improve the chance of overall sucess. Socioeconomic complications of obesity among teenage girls include persistent and severe disturbances in body image, lower likelihood of marriage, fewer years of education, low income, and a high incidence of poverty. Overweight men are less affected in these ways.

24.11.3   The Biology of Obesity

Adipocyte Development

The adipocyte is derived from preadipocytes in the pericapillary endothelium. Differentiation factors, including peroxisome proliferator–activated nuclear hormone receptor (PPARα2), CCAAT enhancer–binding protein (C/EBPα), and adipocyte determination and differentiation–dependent factor 1 (ADD1/SREPB1), control the expression of adipocyte-specific genes and the differentiation of adipocytes. Insulin, glucocorticoids, some prostaglandins, and various medications all can affect this process. Adipocytes increase in size during infancy, but this hypertrophy ceases in nonobese children at about 2 years of age. Among obese children, hypertrophy continues until adolescence. Hyperplasia of fat cells occurs at a greater rate among obese than among nonobese children. Although there appears to be a genetic basis for these differences, weight loss among obese children may decrease the rate of adipocyte hyperplasia.

Control of Appetite

Control of appetite is discussed in Sec. 17.8. Many central nervous system factors affect dietary intake in mammals in a redundant and complex manner to provide a failure-proof mechanism to ensure adequate energy intake. The ventromedial hypothalamus is one of the hypothalamic centers that regulates appetite and feeding behavior. Destruction by trauma or a brain tumor greatly increases intake and decreases metabolic rate, leading to massive obesity. Agents that stimulate appetite include drugs such as α-adrenergic agents, cyproheptadine, glucocorticoids, orexins, and neuropeptide Y. Agents that suppress appetite include β-adrenergic agents, ACTH-releasing factor, dopamine, serotonin, glucagon-like peptide-1, and leptin.

Leptin is a highly conserved protein hormone produced by adipocytes. It interacts with its hypothalamic receptor to regulate feeding through a leptin-melanocortin pathway in the hypothalamus. Serum leptin concentrations are mainly determined by white fat mass (as opposed to brown fat), but other factors such as sex hormones and nutritional factors also modulate levels. Abnormalities in five of the genes found in the leptin-melanocortin pathway are known to cause obesity among humans (Fig. 24-43). A few consanguineous kindreds have autosomal-recessive genetic defects in the production of leptin or in the receptor for leptin: affected children have exceptional weight gain starting in infancy. One 9-year-old child with leptin deficiency had 50% body fat, an insatiable appetite, and low gonadotropin secretion despite an advanced bone age of 13 years. Recombinant human leptin treatment decreased weight and appetite and increased pulsatile gonadotropin secretion, indicating the onset of pubertal activity. The average obese human has increased leptin secretion because of increased fat mass, but

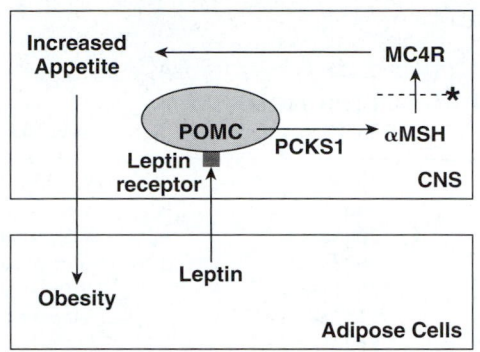

FIGURE 24-43   The leptin-melanocortin pathway in humans. Leptin is secreted by the adipose cell into the circulation. It binds with a membrane receptor in the hypothalamus to stimulate production of proopiomelanocortin (*POMC*), a prohormone cleaved into α-melanocyte-stimulating hormone (*αMSH*) (as well as ACTH and other molecules) by prohormoneconvertase-2 (*PC2*) or proportion converters subtilisin/kexin type 1 (*PCSK*1) enzymes. αMSH interacts with αMSH receptor 4 (*MC4R*) to stimulate appetite, which increases food ingestion. Mutations of the POMC gene cause early-onset obesity and red hair because of elimination of αMSH effects through MCR4 on appetite and on pigmentation. A more common mutation in a POMC locus associated with obesity is found in the Mexican American population. Mutations in MC4R cause obesity among 3 to 7% of morbidly obese children in an autosomal-dominant mendelian pattern. The agouti protein of mice (----*) is a paracrine factor that antagonizes the binding of αMSH to MCR1 in the skin (causing yellow color) and to MC4R in the central nervous system, causing obesity. A similar factor has not yet been described for humans.

appetite is not reduced, suggesting a degree of resistance to leptin. Leptin treatment does not promote weight loss in common forms of obesity among humans.

Genetics of Obesity

The obesity gene map (http://www.obesity.chair.ulaval.ca/genemap.html) lists at least 98 chromosomal loci for body weight, body fat, fat-pad weight (white adipose tissue), and other obesity-related traits in animal models and 59 traits in humans. Twenty-six mendelian disorders include obesity as a phenotype, including Prader-Willi and Bardet-Biedl syndromes, among others. Thirty-nine genes have associations with BMI, body fat, or other obesity-related phenotypes (Table 24-47).

A genetic tendency toward obesity is strongly suggested by epidemiologic observations. If either parent is obese, the likelihood that the child will be an obese adult increases fivefold. The BMIs of monozygotic twins are closer than those of dizygotic twins. The weights of monozygotic twins reared apart are similar, again indicating that genetic factors have a major effect on weight. The BMIs of adopted children are closer to those of their biological parents than to those of their adoptive parents. There is little effect of environment. Combining the results of studies leads to an estimate that at least 40% of obesity is heritable.

Environment

Several observations suggest that the intrauterine environment can affect ultimate weight control. Infants of mothers with diabetes have a higher prevalence of obesity by 10 years of age, but because diabetes is more common among obese mothers, it is possible that this can be explained as a genetic trend. Mothers who starve during the first and second trimesters but have adequate nutrition thereafter have had infants of normal weight who had an increased tendency to obesity 20 years later. The effect of the intrauterine environment on weight remains uncertain.

There is little doubt that the extrauterine environment can alter ultimate weight. Learned habits in regard to diet and activity affect the weight achieved. This likely explains the increased tendency toward obesity in the United States. An excess of only 50 kcal/d (eg, an additional pat of butter), all other thing being equal, leads to a gain of 5 pounds (2.25 kg) per year. For a person with a genetic susceptibility to obesity, an alteration in dietary habits can lead to obesity. A good example is provided by the Pima Indians of Mexico and Arizona, who have the same genetic background. The Arizona Pima once had a higher incidence of obesity than did the Mexican Pima, likely because of the high caloric density they ingested and reduced activity. As the diet and activity of the Mexican Pima change so that they are more similar to those of the Arizona Pima, the incidence of obesity is approaching that of the Arizona Pima.

Childhood activity is decreased in many developed nations, and television watching is increased. A relation between the prevalence of obesity and the amount of time watching television has been demonstrated in numerous studies. An average US child watches 20 hours of television per week and by the end of high school has watched 3 years of television. This decreases the time engaged in other physical activities and exposes them to numerous commercials that encourage the intake of high-calorie, low-fiber foods. Activity decreases with increasing age among children, more among girls than boys. Social factors further decrease activity in childhood; examples are concerns over safety of parks, limited family activity time, and after-school jobs. Participation in physical education decreases with advancing grade; by 11th and 12th grade, fewer than half of students have gym class.

Possibly because of lack of adequately sensitive techniques, there is no proof that overweight children expend less energy than do average-weight children. A 4-year longitudinal study of children showed that sex, initial adiposity, and parental adiposity were related to weight gain in childhood but found no evidence that reduced energy expenditure had a role. However, one study in which recording pedometers were used showed that nonobese children had a higher intensity of activity than did obese children, although total time spent in activity was the same.

Differences in activity level may affect overall energy expenditure, basal energy expenditure (basal metabolic rate) being altered by activity. Increased activity may increase resting energy expenditure as well. Resting energy expenditure decreases during weight loss; thus it becomes more difficult to lose weight as weight decreases.

Endocrine Changes and Obesity

Secretion of GH decreases in obesity, so an incorrect diagnosis of GH deficiency might be entertained. Paradoxically, the level of IGF-I in the serum is normal in obesity. This is the reverse of starvation or anorexia nervosa, in which the level of GH increases and that of IGF-I is low. Serum values of GH-binding protein are directly proportional to BMI and are high in obesity. Increased binding sites for GH may explain the normal serum level of IGF-I and excellent growth among obese children despite low GH secretion. IGFBP1 is suppressed by insulin, and serum values are low in obesity because of increased insulin secretion.

Hypothyroidism often is thought to be a cause of obesity. However, even among untreated children with hypothyroidism, weight

TABLE 24-47

OBESITY-RELATED SYNDROMES WITH KNOWN MAP LOCATIONS

SYNDROME	CANDIDATE GENE	CHROMOSOMAL LOCUS	INHERITANCE
Achondroplasia (ACH)	*FGFR3*	4p16.3	Autosomal dominant
Albright hereditary osteodystrophy 2 (AHO2)	None	15q	Autosomal dominant
Albright hereditary osteodystrophy (AHO)	*GNAS1*	20q13.2	Autosomal dominant
Alstrom syndrome	None	2p13-p12	Autosomal recessive
Angelman syndrome with obesity	None	15q11-q13	Autosomal dominant
Bardet-Biedl syndrome 1 (BBS1)	None	11q13	Autosomal recessive
Bardet-Biedl syndrome 2 (BBS2)	None	16q21	Autosomal recessive
Bardet-Biedl syndrome 3 (BBS3)	None	3p13-p12	Autosomal recessive
Bardet-Biedl syndrome 4 (BBS4)	*MYO9A*	15q22.3-23	Autosomal recessive
Bardet-Biedl syndrome 5 (BBS5)	None	2q21	Autosomal recessive
Berardinelli-Scip congenital lipodystrophy (BSCL)	None	9q34	Autosomal recessive
Börjeson-Forssman-Lehmann syndrome (BFLS)	*FGF13*	Xq26.3	X-linked
Carbohydrate-deficient glycoprotein syndrome type 1a (CDGS1A)	*PMM2*	16p13	Autosomal recessive
Choroideremia with deafness (CHOD)	None	Xq21.1-21.2	X-linked
Cohen syndrome (COH)	None	8q22-q23	Autosomal recessive
Familial partial lipodystrophy Dunnigan (FPLD)	*Lamin A/C*	1q21-q31	Autosomal dominant
Fanconi-Bickel syndrome (FBS)	*SLC2A2*	3q26.1-26.3	Autosomal recessive
Insulin resistance syndromes (IRS)	*INSR*	19p13.3	Autosomal dominant
Mehmo syndrome (MEHMO)	None	Xp22.13-21.1	X-linked
Posterior polymorphous corneal dystrophy (PPCD)	None	20q11	Autosomal dominant
Prader-Willi Syndrome (PWS)	*SNRPN*	15q11-q13	Autosomal dominant
Simpson-Golabi-Behmel 1 (SGBS1)	*GPC3, GPC4*	Xq26	X-linked
Simpson-Golabi-Behmel 2 (SGBS2)	None	Xp22	X-linked
Thyroid hormone resistance syndrome (THRS)	*THRB*	3p24.3	Autosomal dominant
Ulnar-mammary syndrome (UMS) or Schinzel syndrome	*TBX3*	12q23-24.1	Autosomal dominant
Wilson Turner	None	Xp21.1-q22	X-linked

SOURCE: Derived from Chagnon YC, Perusse L, Weisnegal SJ, et al. The human obesity gene map: the 1999 update. *Obes Res* 2000, 8:89–117

gain is modest, and massive obesity rarely is explained by hypothyroidism. Treatment does produce modest weight loss. Most obese children are euthyroid. Adrenal function is normal in most cases of obesity, although cortisol secretion rate and urinary levels of 17OHCs may be elevated, incorrectly suggesting Cushing disease as a cause of obesity. Cushing disease can be differentiated from uncomplicated obesity because obese patients have normal urinary levels of free cortisol and normal diurnal rhythms of serum levels of cortisol. An overnight or low-dose dexamethasone suppression test can be useful for the differential diagnosis of obesity and Cushing disease if a question remains (see Sec. 24.4.8).

24.11.4   Evaluation and Management of Obesity

EVALUATION

All children with a BMI greater than the 85th percentile and severely obese children younger than 2 years and those of any age rapidly gaining excessive weight need evaluation. The history focuses on family weight tendencies, obesity-related complications (see Table 24-46 and Fig. 24-44), and exclusion of other diseases or syndromes that may be associated with obesity. A history of headaches or neurologic symptoms, evidence of polyuria and polydipsia, or evidence of a psychopathologic condition may indicate a central nervous system tumor. Constipation, cold intolerance, and dry skin may suggest hypothyroidism. Linear growth failure is uncommon among obese children, who usually are tall for age. Cush-

ing syndrome, pseudohypoparathyroidism, and hypothalamic lesions must be considered if the child is short and obese. Developmental delay should lead to consideration of the many syndromes associated with obesity (see Table 24-47). The child's activity level, television watching, and dietary history are reviewed. The physical examination is focused on blood pressure, BMI, distribution of fat, optic disc contour, and the presence of acanthosis nigricans. Laboratory evaluation may be needed to exclude the causes of obesity discussed earlier. If none of these causes is suspected, the appropriate laboratory evaluation is directed at screening for complications of obesity. For a child with a BMI in the 85th to 94th percentile, only a fasting lipid profile is recommended unless the risk factors include cigarette smoking, the presence of diabetes mellitus, low physical activity, high blood pressure, a family history of early cardiovascular disease, or a family history that suggests diabetes or hyperlipidemia. In such cases, and for all children with a BMI greater than 95th percentile, laboratory evaluation includes a fasting lipid profile; fasting insulin and glucose; measurement of liver transaminases, calcium, and phosphorus; and an electrocardiogram. Depending on the history and physical findings, a Holter monitor study, extremity radiographs for orthopedic complications, thyroid function tests (free T_4 and TSH), morning cortisol or dexamethasone suppression test, or a sleep study to assess respiratory complications may be indicated.

TREATMENT

Obese children and their families need counseling regarding the risks of obesity. It is important that the health-care professional

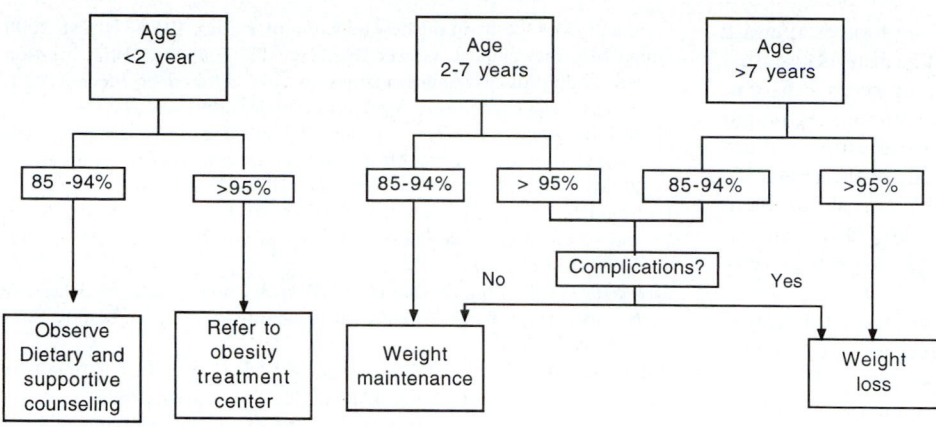

FIGURE 24-44 Weight loss and weight gain in pediatric obesity therapy. Percentage values refer to body mass index (BMI). (SOURCE: Modified from Barlow SE, Dietz WH: *Obesity evaluation and treatment: expert committee recommendations. Maternal and Child Health Bureau, Health Resources and Services Administration and the Department of Health and Human Services. Pediatrics 102:E29, 1998.*)

candidly discuss the effects of being overweight on the child's self-image and social interactions. It is useful to discuss the genetic predisposition to obesity and to recognize the challenges of a weight loss regimen. The following discussion is directed specifically at management of obesity. Therapy for comorbid conditions are not addressed.

Mild, uncomplicated cases of obesity usually can be approached in the primary physician's office. Severe or complicated cases necessitate a comprehensive approach, which is available in relatively few centers. The goals of a weight management program are improvement of medical and psychological health and prevention of comorbidities of obesity. Modification of diet and activity and behavior therapy are the essential components of a program aimed at a lasting effect. Weight management programs are less successful if there are delayed recognition of the weight problem, unrealistic expectations, lack of specific recommendations, lack of follow-up and maintenance programs, negative counseling techniques, and lack of readiness of the child and family. Adult weight control programs are not appropriate for children. A group program, such as the Shapedown Pediatric Obesity Program (http://www.shapedown.com), a structured weight loss and weight management program for children between the ages of 6 and 20 years, is aimed at children and adolescents. Obesity is best considered a chronic disease requiring constant awareness of food choices and activity levels. Treatment is aimed at acquiring healthful daily habits. A practitioner who is frustrated by the problem or prejudiced against obese persons and family or who has inadequate time to attend to the problem should not attempt treatment.

NUTRITION EDUCATION A change in diet that maintains weight stability or promotes slow weight loss is the most reasonable approach for most children. Weight loss goals should be obtainable and should allow for normal growth. Goals initially are small, so that the child does not become overwhelmed or discouraged. Two kilograms to 4 kg is a reasonable first goal; if preferred, a rate of 0.5 to 2 kg a month can be established. Lessons on healthful eating, portion control, choosing appropriate foods, label reading, and modification of recipes are essential to help the family and child achieve successful weight management. Limitation of fat intake is beneficial above and beyond the effect on calories. Keeping a dietary log helps the person concentrate on desired changes. It is necessary to provide parents with a specific calorie-per-day recommendation that follows guidelines for percentages of fat, protein, and carbohydrates. Tobacco use must be discouraged; some teenagers smoke in a misguided attempt to control weight.

In the most severe cases (usually among adolescents with apparent comorbidities such as sleep apnea and pseudotumor cerebri)

weight loss with a protein-sparing modified fast may be invoked. The protein-sparing modified fast is a severely caloric restricted diet of, for example, 600 to 900 kcal/d containing 1.5 to 2 g of high-biological-quality protein per kilogram per day with vitamin and mineral supplementation and considerable water (>1.5 L/d). Regular observation by a physician is essential to avoid severe complications. Carbohydrate is eliminated, so ketosis develops, which helps decrease appetite and fosters adherence to the diet. Arrhythmias are documented, so rhythm recording with a Holter monitor is performed before the fast. This program usually is limited to less than 5 months and aims for rapid weight loss, which should be maintained thereafter. Protein-sparing modified fasting rarely is indicated.

PHYSICAL ACTIVITY A child cannot exercise enough to burn off a high-calorie diet. A children's meal of cheeseburger, french fries, and a milk shake in a fast-food restaurants exceeds 750 calories; large-size children's meals that exceed 1000 calories have appeared. It would take more than 1.5 to 2 hours on a ski machine or stationary bicycle to work off such a single meal. The goal is to avoid such high-calorie loads and to reduce sedentary activity rather than to encourage a regimen of exercise to which no one can adhere. Fostering activities that can be carried through life is best. Some centers suggest the use of hip-hop or other popular dances as exercise. Self-monitoring with an activity log (or inactivity log) is helpful for child and parent to understand the behaviors and make changes. Setting weekly activity goals assists a gradual increase in activity. A benefit of increased activity is limitation of the loss of fat-free mass during decreased caloric intake. The most important change a family can make is to turn off the television or electronic games or limit these activities to no more than 1 hour per day.

BEHAVIOR MODIFICATION The essence of behavioral therapy is (1) functional analysis of the association between eating and activity behaviors and environmental events and (2) systematic modification of eating, activity, or other behaviors thought to contribute to or maintain obesity. Cognitive behavioral strategies for weight management should provide concrete skills for children and families to change the behavior and achieve a healthier lifestyle. Behavioral therapy sessions usually are conducted in small groups. A team approach to weight management is optimal; various combinations of a social worker, psychologist, dietitian, nurse, and physician participate.

The programs focus on a variety of skills that aid in altering eating and activity patterns. Enhancement of parenting skills is important so that parents do not tell children they are "bad" but rather praise healthy food choices, set consistent limits, and provide appropriate meal times without television. Using food as a reward is discouraged, and instruction on provision of healthy foods rather than junk foods is provided. The child or family keeps a diary to monitor activity and patterns of food intake. Children are taught to identify environmental cues associated with overeating and underactivity. These issues are addressed. Children are encouraged to become aware of their negative thoughts and beliefs about themselves and their weight. Stress management skills (other than eating) are taught and the child and family are taught to problem solve to facilitate healthful eating.

Family participation is essential for the program to succeed among children younger than 10 years. For teenagers, the degree of parental involvement needs to be individually assessed. In some instances, it may be counterproductive. It is also important that the treating health-care professionals be empathetic and compassionate. Physicians and others often communicate their own prejudice and poor understanding of obesity by oversimplifying the problem. Many physicians continue to believe that obesity is caused solely by gluttony or slothlike behavior that can be easily remedied if willpower is adequate.

SURGERY Gastric bypass or banding has benefits among morbidly obese adults with sustained weight loss. Monitoring for nutritional complications of protein deficiency, malnutrition, vitamins A, D, and B_{12}, and folic acid is important. Other complications include dumping syndrome and surgical adhesion. There is a little experience with this therapy in childhood and young adolescence. This approach therefore cannot be recommended.

MEDICATIONS No medications have been approved as therapy for obesity among persons younger than 16 years. They are being tested on children 12 to 16 years of age. Sibutramine, a serotonin reuptake inhibitor, can be used by older adolescents to increase the feeling of satiety and decrease intake. A side effect is a slight increase in blood pressure. Orlistat is an intestinal lipase inhibitor that decreases absorption of fat. Side effects such as bloating, flatulence, and diarrhea occur if fat intake is not reduced. As the biological mechanism of appetite control and obesity is elucidated, it is expected that better targeted, safer agents will become available.

References

Barlow SE, Dietz WH: Obesity evaluation and treatment: expert committee recommendations. Maternal and Child Health Bureau, Health Resources and Services Administration and the Department of Health and Human Services. Pediatrics 102:E29, 1998

Barsh GS, Farooqi IS, O'Rahilly S: Genetics of body-weight regulation. Nature 404:644–651, 2000

Bray GA, Tartaglia LA: Medicinal strategies in the treatment of obesity. Nature 404:672–677, 2000

Chagnon YC, Chen WJ, Perusse L, et al: Linkage and association studies between the melanocortin receptors 4 and 5 genes and obesity-related phenotypes in the Quebec Family Study. Mol Med 3:663–673, 1997

Claement K, Vaisse C, Lahlou N, et al: A mutation in the human leptin receptor gene causes obesity and pituitary dysfunction. Nature 392: 398–401, 1998

Dietz DW: Childhood weight affects adult morbidity and mortality. J Nutr 128(2 Suppl):411S–414S, 1998

Dietz WH, Robinson TN: Use of the body mass index (BMI) as a measure of overweight in children and adolescents. J Pediatr 132:191–193, 1998

Epstein LH: Family-based behavioural intervention for obese children. Int J Obes Relat Metab Disord 20:S14–S21, 1996

Friedman JM: Obesity in the new millennium. Nature 404:632–634, 2000

Goran MI, Shewchuk R, Gower BA, Nagy TR, Carpenter WH, Johnson RK: Longitudinal changes in fatness in white children: no effect of childhood energy expenditure Am J Clin Nutr 67:309–316, 1998

Hixson JE, Almasy L, Cole S, et al: Normal variation in leptin levels is associated with polymorphisms in the proopiomelanocortin gene, POMC. J Clin Endocrinol Metab 84:3187–3191, 1999

Ludwig DS, Pereira MA, Kroenke CH, et al: Dietary fiber, weight gain, and cardiovascular disease risk factors in young adults. JAMA 282: 1539–1546, 1999

Montague CT, Farooqi IS, Whitehead JP, et al: Congenital leptin deficiency is associated with severe early-onset obesity in humans. Nature 387: 903–908, 1997

Robinson TN: Reducing children's television viewing to prevent obesity: a randomized controlled trial. JAMA 282:1561–1567, 1999

Rosenbaum M, Leibel RL: The role of leptin in human physiology. N Engl J Med 341:913–915, 1999

Schonfeld-Warden N, Warden CH: Pediatric obesity: an overview of etiology and treatment. Pediatr Clin North Am 44:339–361, 1997

Schwartz MW, Woods SC, Porte DJ, Seely RJ, Baskin DG: Central nervous system control of food intake. Nature 404:661–671, 2000

Whitaker RC, Dietz WH: Role of the prenatal environment in the development of obesity. J Pediatr 132:768–776, 1998

24.12 DISORDERS OF CALCIUM AND PHOSPHORUS METABOLISM

Allen W. Root

24.12.1   Regulation of Mineral Homeostasis

CALCIUM, PHOSPHORUS, ALKALINE PHOSPHATASE

Calcium is the most abundant body cation. It is present largely (99%) in the skeleton as calcium phosphate in the mineral hydroxyapatite. The 1% of body calcium in cells, the circulation, and the extracellular fluid serves as an intercellular and intracellular messenger and is important for neuronal and neuromuscular communication, muscular contraction, enzyme function, clotting, protein synthesis and secretion, and cellular proliferation. In serum, 40 to 50% of calcium is present in the biologically active ionized state (Ca^{2+}); 40 to 50% is bound to albumin and globulins, where it is inert; and 10% is complexed to citrate, lactate, bicarbonate, phosphate (PO_4^{2-}), and sulfate. Systemic acidosis decreases calcium binding to albumin and increases serum levels of Ca^{2+}, whereas alkalosis increases calcium binding to albumin and lowers Ca^{2+} values. The Ca^{2+} concentration is regulated within narrow limits by the plasma membrane Ca^{2+} receptor, parathyroid hormone (PTH) and its receptor (PTHR1), calcitonin and its receptor, and the vitamin D hormone system acting on the intestines, bone, and kidney (Fig. 24-45). Calcium ion moves across cell membranes through selective Ca^{2+} channels and through paracellular transport channels. The skeleton contains 85% of the phosphate in the body complexed to Ca^{2+} in hydroxyapatite. Phosphorus is present in the serum as the anions HPO_4^{2-} or $H_2PO_4^-$; 12% is bound to proteins. Phosphate is filtered in the renal glomerulus and reabsorbed in the proximal and distal tubules. It is transported across cell membranes by sodium-phosphate cotransporter proteins. This ion is an integral component of nucleic acids, phospholipids, energy generating, and

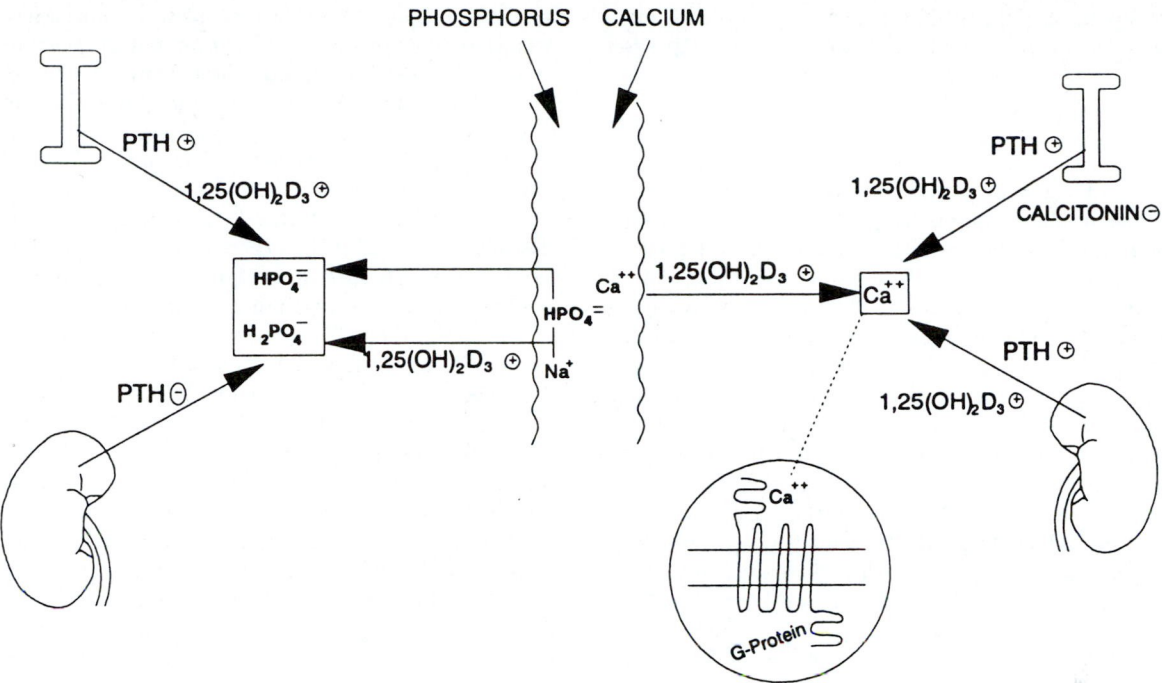

FIGURE 24-45 Maintenance of calcium homeostasis. Dietary calcium is absorbed in the proximal small intestine under the influence of calcitriol. Bone calcium is resorbed by PTH and calcitriol-dependent osteoclastic bone resorption, PTH-dependent short-term osteocyte-mediated calcium exchange, and long-term exchange of calcium between blood and bone; 98 to 99% of filtered calcium is reabsorbed in the renal tubules, a process partly regulated by PTH and calcitriol. Calcitonin inhibits resorption of calcium from bone. The Ca^{2+}-sensing receptor modulates secretion of PTH and renal tubular handling of calcium. CT = calcitonin; PTH = parathyroid hormone; $1,25(OH)_2D_3$ = calcitriol. (SOURCE: *From Root AW: Recent advances in the genetics of disorders of calcium homeostasis. Adv Pediatr 43:77–125, 1996, with permission.*)

intracellular signal transduction systems. It is essential for normal development and function of every cell.

Concentration of total calcium in the serum peaks in utero, decreases during the first 1 to 2 days after birth, stabilizes, and then decreases slightly over the first 18 months of life. Serum levels of calcium are slightly higher among children and adolescents than they are among adults. Because of both decreased glomerular filtration and increased tubular reabsorption of phosphate, calcium concentration is maximum in neonates and infants, decreases during childhood and adolescence, and achieves adult values by 17 years of age. The recommended daily adequate intakes and allowances of calcium, phosphorus, and vitamin D are shown in Table 17-1. Optimal bone mineralization during childhood and adolescence requires larger calcium intakes (ages 2 through 8 years, 1000 mg/d; ages 9 through 17 years, 1600 mg/d; ages 18 through 30 years, 1100 mg/d).

The effect of the serum Ca^{2+} on cellular function is mediated by the Ca^{2+}-sensing receptor (CASR), a cell wall protein that binds Ca^{2+} and magnesium. The CASR establishes the set point for release of PTH, the serum concentration of Ca^{2+} at which secretion of PTH is half-suppressed. The CASR is present on the plasma membranes of parathyroid chief cells, renal tubular cells of the thick ascending limb of the loop of Henle and the collecting ducts, thyroid parafollicular cells, bone, lung, adrenal, breast, intestinal, and nervous tissue. The CASR interacts through its intracellular carboxyl terminal with a guanosine triphosphate–linked heterotrimeric protein (G protein). On binding of Ca^{2+} to CASR the α subunit of the G protein ($G_s\alpha$) dissociates from the $\beta\gamma$ subunit

complex and activates membrane-bound phospholipase C-β1, initiating the reactions that follow cleavage of membrane phosphatidylinositol-4,5-bisphosphate into diacylglycerol and inositide trisphosphate and increases in cytosolic concentrations of Ca^{2+}. In the parathyroid glands, increasing cytosolic Ca^{2+} levels suppress release of PTH. In the kidney, binding of Ca^{2+} to the CASR depresses renal tubular reabsorption of Ca^{2+}, increasing urinary calcium excretion, and lowers the number of apical water channels in the inner medullary collecting ducts, thereby opposing vasopressin-induced tubular water permeability and causing polyuria. The CASR also regulates urinary excretion of magnesium in a manner similar to that of Ca^{2+}. Both loss-of-function (familial hypocalciuric hypercalcemia [FHH]) and gain-of-function (autosomal dominant hypoparathyroidism) mutations in the CASR have been described.

Three tissue-specific—intestinal, placental, germ cell—isoforms of alkaline phosphatase have genes clustered at chromosome 2q34-q37, and one tissue-nonspecific—bone, liver, kidney—form of alkaline phosphatase is on chromosome 1p36.1-p34. By alternative processing during translation, the osteoblast secretes a unique bone-specific form of alkaline phosphatase. In bone, alkaline phosphatase (1) binds to collagen type I to prepare skeletal matrix for mineralization, (2) hydrolyzes organically bound phosphate to increase its local concentration and exceed the $Ca^{2+} \times PO_4^{2-}$ product, resulting in deposition of calcium phosphate as hydroxyapatite, (3) transports phosphate and Ca^{2+} into the cell, and (4) hydrolyzes pyrophosphate and other inhibitors of mineralization. Tissue-nonspecific alkaline phosphatase activity is high in infants, somewhat lower during childhood, and high during adolescence to peak values at 10 to 12 years for girls and 12 to 14 years for boys coincident with peak growth velocities. Activity declines thereafter to adult values.

BONE

Eighty percent of the mineralized skeleton consists of cortical (compact) bone in the cranium, scapula, mandible, ileum, and shafts of the long bones. Twenty percent is cancellous (trabecular or spongy) bone in the vertebrae, basal skull, pelvis, and ends of the long bones. Eighty percent to 90% of cortical bone volume is calcified, but only 15 to 25% of trabecular bone is calcified. Because of its greater surface area, trabecular bone has a high turnover rate and is more metabolically active than compact bone, making it more susceptible to disorders that affect bone mineralization. Intramembranous bone formation of the skull occurs by means of local condensation of mesenchymal cells that differentiate into preosteoblasts and osteoblasts. Growth hormone enhances membranous bone formation. In bone of cartilaginous origin (long bones, vertebrae), chondrogenesis begins with mesenchymal cell differentiation into prechondroblasts and chondroblasts that evolve into a layer of resting chondrocytes. At the ends of the long bones, secondary ossification centers (epiphyses) are separated from the metaphysis by the cartilaginous epiphyseal growth plate. Chondrocyte proliferation within the growth plate allows linear growth of the long bone until it is completely ossified. Growth hormone supports differentiation of resting chondrocytes from the reserve zone of the epiphyseal cartilage plate and stimulates local synthesis of IGF-I, which increases proliferation of chondrocytes. Parathyroid hormone–related protein (PTHrP) slows the rate of chondrocyte maturation to allow greater chondrocyte proliferation. Endochondral bone formation, the process by which bone replaces cartilage, begins with differentiation of resting chondrocytes into proliferating chondrocytes that secrete organic matrix. As chondrocytes divide and mature, they become hypertrophic and eventually apoptotic. Vascular endothelial growth factor secreted by the terminal hypertrophic chondrocyte stimulates vascular invasion of cartilage by metaphyseal blood vessels. Accompanying these invading blood vessels are chondroclasts (monocyte-derived cells that resorb apoptotic chondrocytes and remodel cartilage) and osteoblasts that bring about development of mature bone.

Osteoblasts are bone-forming cells that secrete organic matrix (osteoid) into which calcium and phosphate are deposited as hydroxyapatite. They are derived from mesenchymal precursor cells under the direction of core binding factor α_1, a transcription factor that promotes synthesis of osteoblast-specific proteins including collagen type I(α_1) and noncollagenous matrix proteins—bone alkaline phosphatase, osteocalcin, fibronectin, bone sialoprotein, osteopontin—that bind to hydroxyapatite, influence mineralization and cell attachment, and assist osteoclast binding to bone matrix, respectively. Osteoblasts express receptors for PTH and calcitriol. Although primarily characterized as a bone resorptive agent, PTH also enhances bone formation through its effects on osteoblast function. Osteoblast function is stimulated by PTH, calcitriol, GH, and IGF-I, among other factors. After completing matrix synthesis, mature osteoblasts become embedded in bone as osteocytes.

Osteoclasts are multinucleated giant cells that can resorb bone mineral. They are derived from mononuclear hematopoietic stem cells (the colony-forming units from which macrophages also evolve) under the influence of osteoblast–stromal cell–secreted macrophage colony-stimulating factor and an osteoclast differentiation factor expressed on the osteoblast–stromal cell plasma

membrane (Fig. 24-46). The osteoblast–stromal cell is essential for osteoclast differentiation and function. Under the influence of macrophage colony-stimulating factor, hematopoietic stem cells differentiate into osteoclast precursors that express a transmembrane protein called *receptor activator of nuclear factor-κB* (NF-κB) (RANK), a protein that signals cellular action through NF-κB and c-Jun N-terminal kinase. RANK expressed on the surface of a prefusion osteoclast binds to the RANK-ligand (RANKL), an osteoclast-differentiating factor expressed on the membrane of the osteoblast–stromal cells to induce osteoclast fusion, osteoclast activation, and bone resorption. Parathyroid hormone, calcitriol, IL-11, and other cytokines stimulate expression of RANKL, whereas IL-1 enhances osteoclast fusion and function.

Other cytokines involved in osteoclast differentiation and function include IL-6, TGF-α, TNF, lymphotoxin, osteoclastopoietic factor, and prostaglandins of the E series. Osteoclast differentiation is antagonized by TGF-β and osteoprotegerin, a secreted member of the TNF receptor superfamily that acts as a soluble decoy receptor and binds RANKL and inhibits its effects on osteoclast differentiation and function. Osteoclastic bone resorption is stimulated by PTH and PTHrP (acting through osteoblastic RANKL) and by thyroid hormone. It is depressed by calcitonin, estrogen, IFN-γ, glucocorticoids, bisphosphonates, and other drugs. Osteoclasts express receptors for calcitonin and to a limited extent for PTH. Activated multinuclear osteoclasts reabsorb bone by adhering to endosteal and periosteal bone surfaces. There they generate (carbonic anhydrase II) and secrete protons (H^+) that dissolve the adjacent mineral phase and lysosomal proteolytic enzymes, such as cathepsin K, a cysteine protease, and metalloproteinases, that reabsorb osteoid matrix. Bone remodeling is a continuous process in which old bone is reabsorbed and replaced by new bone. It takes place in the four following stages: (1) *activation,* in which a resting bone surface is converted into a remodeling unit by the invasion of osteoclasts leading to (2) *bone resorption* followed by (3) *reversal,* in which osteoblasts enter the area of resorbed bone, and (4) renewed *bone formation,* when osteoblasts secrete osteoid into which hydroxyapatite is deposited.

About 35% of bone is composed of organic matrix proteins, 85 to 90% of which is type I collagen, a coiled triple helix of two polypeptide chains of collagen $\alpha_1(I)$ and one of $\alpha_2(I)$. They are cross-linked intramolecularly by disulfide bonds and intermolecularly at the amino (N) and carboxyl (C) telopeptides by pyridinium compounds that allow gathering of collagen molecules into fibrils and fiber bundles (Fig. 24-47). Every third amino acid of the collagen chain is glycine, which allows the collagen molecule to coil. Proline, hydroxyproline, and glycosylated hydroxylysine also are present in large quantities. N- and C-terminal extensions of the propeptides of collagen are proteolytically removed during formation of the mature collagen molecule and partially secreted into extracellular space and serum. Pyridinoline (PYR, hydroxylysyl-pyridinoline) and deoxypyridinoline (D-PYR, lysyl-pyridinoline) form nonreducible pyridinium cross-links between mature collagen fibers, rendering them insoluble. Type I collagen (composed of two procollagen α_1 and one procollagen α_2 polypeptide chains) predominates in bone but also is present in ligaments, tendons, fascia, and skin. Cartilage is primarily composed of type II collagen (three procollagen α_1 chains). Type III collagen is present in bone, tendons, arteries, and intestine. Serum concentrations of the procollagen I extension peptides, such as the C-terminal extension of procollagen type I and the N-terminal extension of procollagen type III, reflect bone and collagen formation and are highest among infants. Concentration decreases during childhood and adolescence

MODULATION OF OSTEOCLASTOGENESIS

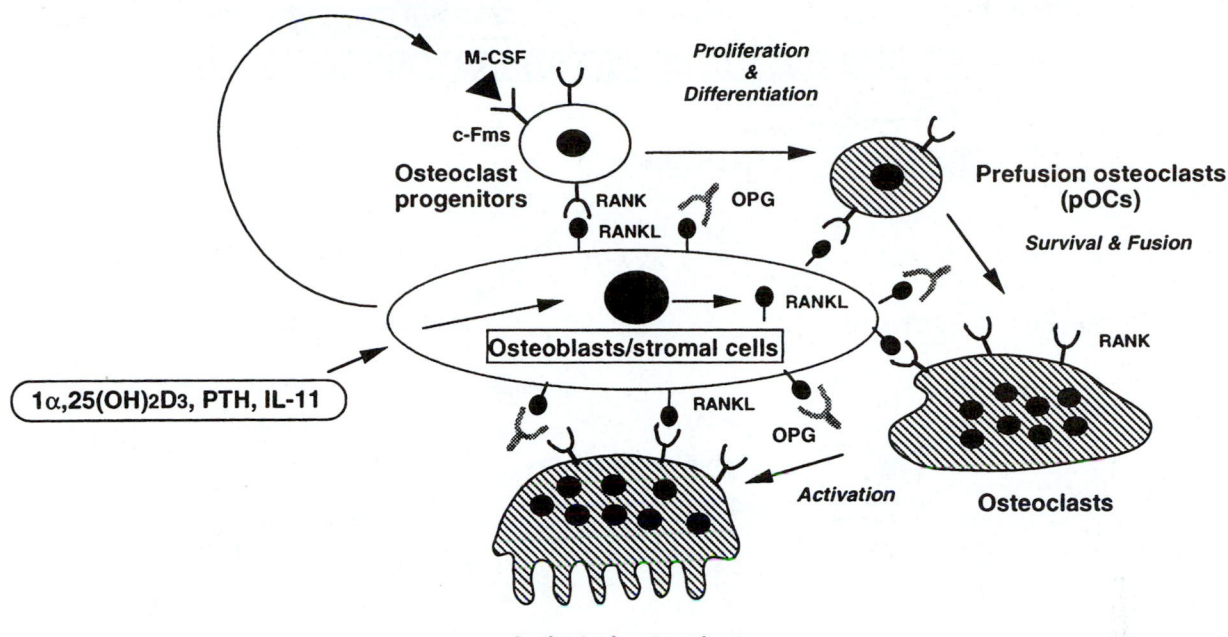

FIGURE 24-46   Osteoclastogenesis. OPG = osteoprotegerin; RANK = receptor activator of nuclear factor-*κ*B; (NF-*κ*B); RANKL = RANK ligand; M-CSF = macrophage colony-stimulating factor. (SOURCE: *From Suda T, Takahashi N, Udagawa N, et al: Modulation of osteoclast differentiation and function by the new members of the tumor necrosis factor receptor and ligand families. Endocrine Rev 20:345–357, 1999, with permission.*)

to adult levels. When mature bone matrix is degraded by osteoclasts, PYR, D-PYR, and the C- and N-telopeptides are released in both free and peptide-bound form. Urinary excretion of hydroxyproline, hydroxylysine, PYR, D-PYR, and N-telopeptides thus reflect collagen type I breakdown and bone resorption. In addition to collagen, 10 to 15% of bone matrix is composed of noncollagenous peptides, for the most part products of the osteoblast, including proteoglycans (chondroitin sulfate, heparan sulfate), growth-stimulating proteins, cell attachment peptides, and *γ*-carboxylated proteins. Bone morphogenetic protein, TGF-*β*, IGF-I, and IGF-II also are present in collagen matrix.

BONE MINERAL DENSITY   Calcium accretion begins in utero and continues throughout childhood and adolescence. Skeletal calcium content increases from 25 g at birth to 1200 g in adulthood. Sixty percent of adult bone calcium is accumulated during adolescence, when approximately 1600 mg of elemental calcium must be ingested daily to retain the 220 mg/d of calcium necessary to achieve optimal adult skeletal mass. Calcium supplementation can increase radial and femoral bone calcium levels substantially, particularly when spontaneous calcium intake is less than 900 mg/d. Peak adult bone mass is determined to a large extent (80%) by genetic factors such as race, sex, and body size. Bone mass also is influenced by nutrition, exercise, hormonal status, and timing of onset of puberty. It is essential that peak bone mass be maximized to avoid osteopenia and osteoporosis in later life. During childhood and adolescence peripheral (radial) and axial (vertebral) areal (surface area) bone mineral density (BMD) correlates with age, height, weight, body mass index, pubertal status, calcium intake, and exercise. Estrogens play a major role in bone mineralization in both girls and boys.

Boys with aromatase deficiency or with mutations of the estrogen receptor have marked osteopenia. Growth hormone is essential for normal bone calcium accretion. Children and adults with GH deficiency have marked osteopenia, which is reversible with GH therapy. Black persons of both sexes have greater lumbar BMD than do white persons.

Areal BMD is measured by single and dual photon absorptiometry and with dual-energy x-ray absorptiometry (DEXA). In DEXA minimal radiation is used to provide data about the peripheral and axial skeleton and body composition. Bone mineral density also can be assessed with quantitative ultrasonography of the calcaneus, tibia, patella, and digits. This method is attractive because it involves no radiation exposure, but experience in examinations of children is limited. DEXA demonstrates a doubling of lumbar vertebral (L2-L4) BMD between 4 and 15 years of age among boys (0.565 to 1.050 g/cm²) and girls (0.565 to 1.090 g/cm²) with maximal rates of increase in BMD between birth and 5 years of age among both sexes, 13 to 15 years among boys, and 12 to 14 years among girls. Because of the larger skeletal size of boys, total bone mineral content is greater. Peak bone mineral content and BMD are reached at 18 to 20 years in both sexes. For young adults, mean lumbar and femoral BMD approximates 1.1 to 1.2 g/cm². Girls with earlier menarche (before 12 years) have greater peak BMD (at age 18 to 19 years) than do those with later menarche (after 14 years). Men with constitutional delay in linear growth and sexual maturation have lower vertebral BMD than do those with pubertal onset at the usual age (11–12 years). Measurement of volumetric BMD (vBMD) by means of quantitative CT or calculation from DEXA data has been recommended to correct for variations in bone size. The goal is to lessen the dependent relations between vBMD

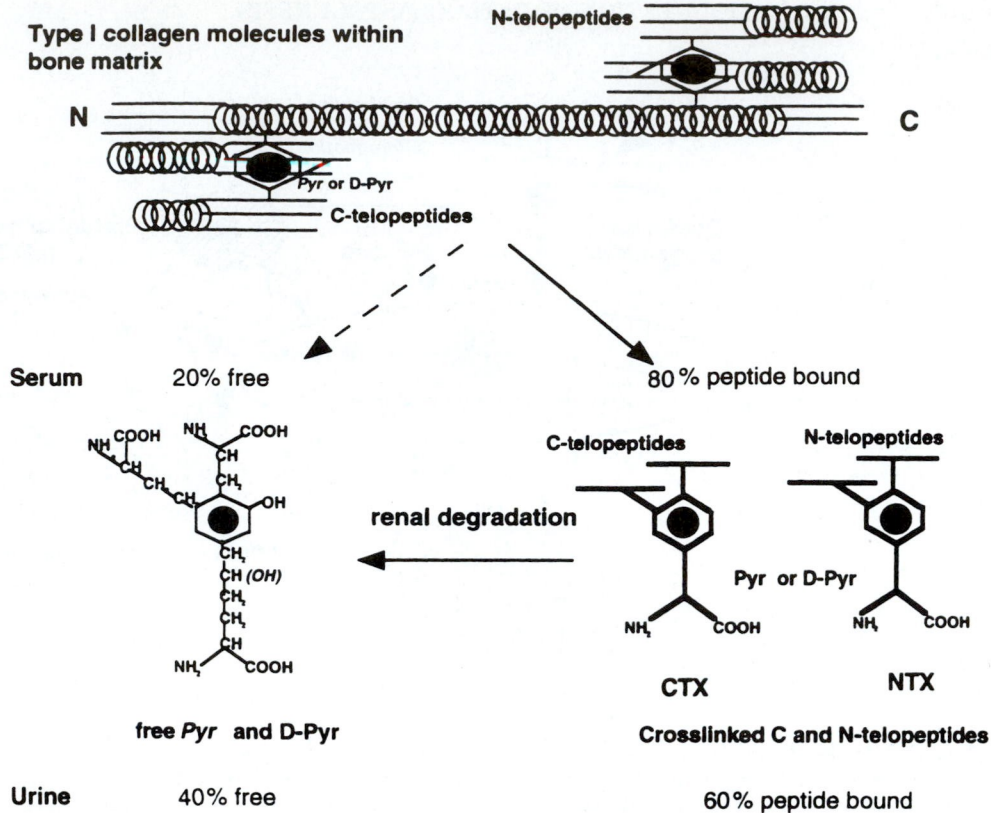

FIGURE 24-47   Pyridinium and telopeptides of collagen. N- and C-terminal extensions (*NTx*, *CTx*) of the propeptides of collagen are proteolytically removed during formation of mature collagen and secreted into extracellular space and serum. Pyridinoline (*PYR*, hydroxylysyl-pyridinoline) and deoxypyridinoline (*D-PYR*, lysyl-pyridinoline) form nonreducible pyridinium crosslinks between mature collagen fibers, rendering them insoluble. (SOURCE: *From Garnero P, Delmas PD: Biochemical markers of bone turnover: applications for osteoporosis. Endocrinol Metab Clin North Am 27:303–323, 1998, with permission.*)

and age, size, sex, and race. However, the usefulness and validity of this measurement have not yet been fully verified. Vertebral vBMD is similar and increases in both boys and girls during puberty. During childhood, lumbar vBMD is similar for blacks and whites. During puberty black boys and girls gain twice the vBMD recorded for whites with no sex difference.

VITAMIN D

Cholecalciferol, the principal D_3 vitamin of the body, is synthesized in the skin from cholesterol (Fig. 24-48). Cholecalciferol is transported in serum bound to the 58-kDa vitamin D binding protein, an α-globulin, to the liver where it is hydroxylated at carbon-25 by vitamin D_3-25-hydroxylase, a mitochondrial cytochrome P450 enzyme (P450c27), to form 25-hydroxycholecalciferol (25OHD$_3$, or calcidiol). The activity of vitamin D_3-25-hydroxylase is inhibited to a limited extent by calcidiol. Bound to vitamin D binding protein, calcidiol is transported to the kidney, where it is hydroxylated by cells in the proximal convoluted and straight renal tubules at carbon-1 to yield the active metabolite 1,25-dihydroxyvitamin D_3 [1,25(OH)$_2$D$_3$, or calcitriol] or carbon-24 to yield inactive 24R,25-dihydroxyvitamin D_3 [24R,25(OH)$_2$D$_3$] by means of the mitochondrial cytochrome P450 enzymes 25OHD$_3$-1α-hydroxylase (P450clα) or 25OHD$_3$-24-hydroxylase (P450c24), respectively. The gene for P450clα is located on chromosome 12q13.3.

P450clα is a 56-kDa protein that, like other mitochondrial cytochrome P450 class I enzymes, requires electrons from NADPH and the electron transport proteins—ferredoxin and ferredoxin reductase—for catalytic function. It is expressed in proximal renal tubular cells, keratinocytes, brain, testes, and activated mononuclear cells. 25OHD$_3$-1α-hydroxylase activity is increased by low levels of Ca^{2+}, phosphate, PTH, PTHrP, 24R,25(OH)$_2$D$_3$, GH, IGF-I, prolactin, cAMP, and protein kinase A in the serum and tissues. Its activity is suppressed by increased levels of Ca^{2+}, phosphate, and calcitriol in the serum and tissues. Calcitriol circulates primarily bound to vitamin D binding protein, although only the free fraction is biologically active. Calcitriol is catabolized by glucuronidation, sulfation, multisite (carbons-24-26) hydroxylation, and lactone formation to biologically inert, water-soluble compounds and is excreted in the urine and bile.

Serum concentrations of calcidiol reflect body stores of vitamin D. Values are higher among white than among black persons, in sunny than in cloudy climates, and in summer than in winter. In cord blood, calcidiol values are related to maternal levels. After infancy, the calcidiol levels of persons with normal intake of vitamin D reflect exposure to sunlight. Serum concentrations of calcitriol, the main biologically active metabolite of vitamin D_3, are high in infancy, somewhat lower during childhood, increase transiently during puberty, and then decline to adult values. The recommended supplemental daily intake of vitamin D is 100 IU (2.5 μg)

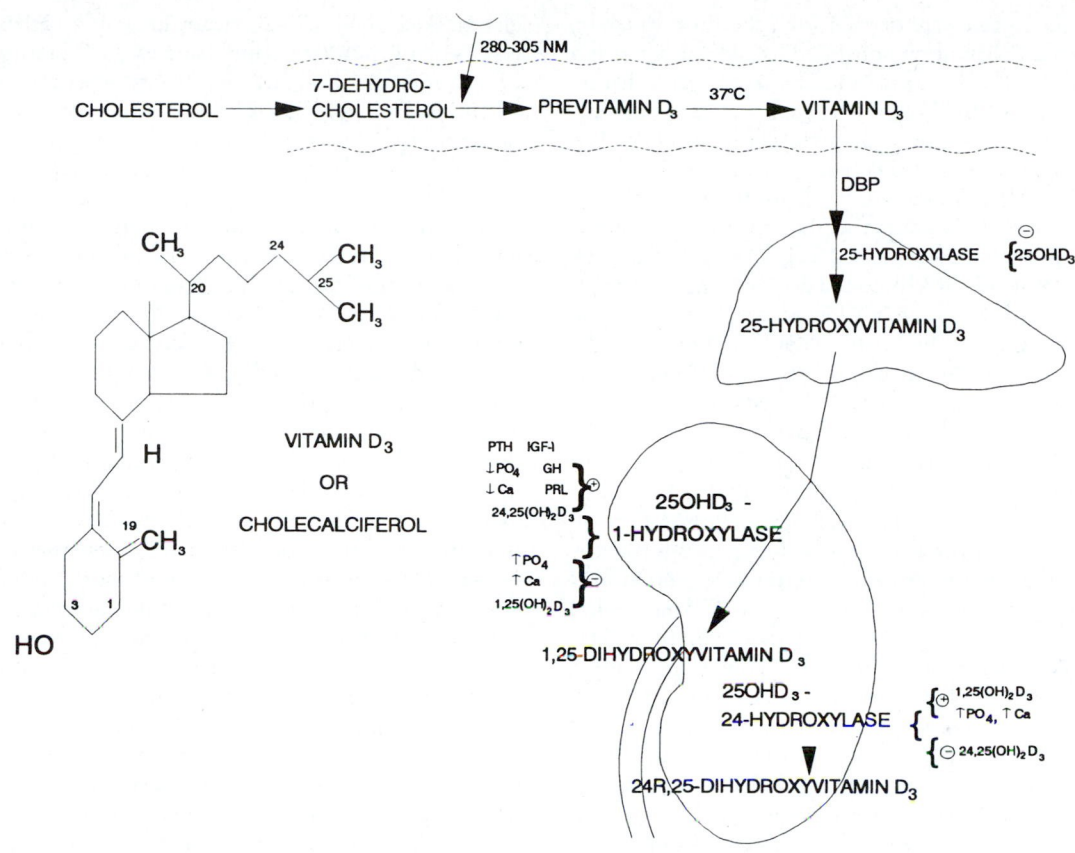

**FIGURE 24-48   Metabolism of vitamin D. Cholecalciferol is synthesized in skin from choles-
terol, metabolized to calcidiol in the liver, and to calcitriol in the kidney. Factors that regulate
these processes are depicted. (SOURCE: *From Mimouni FB, Root AW: Disorders of calcium metabolism in the newborn. In: Sperling MA, ed: Pediatric Endocrinology. Philadelphia, Saunders, 1996:95–
115, with permission.*)**

per 100 kcal of formula intake for neonates and infants and up to
400 IU (10 μg) for children and adolescents.

The vitamin D receptor, encoded by a gene on chromosome
12q13-14, is a member of the steroid-thyroid receptor gene superfamily of nuclear transcription activating factors. The vitamin D
receptor has a 24-amino-acid, amino-terminal segment, a DNA
binding domain with two zinc fingers, a hinge region, and a ligand
(calcitriol) binding domain at the carboxyl terminus. The three *vitamin D receptor* mRNA isoforms result from alternative splicing,
and there are polymorphisms in the 5′ and 3′ untranslated regions
of the vitamin D receptor gene that may account in part for individual differences in intestinal calcium absorption, growth in infancy, BMD, and the synthesis of vitamin D–regulated products.
Such polymorphisms have been linked to development of hyperparathyroidism and parathyroid tumors. The stimulatory or inhibitory effects of the vitamin D receptor on gene expression follow
the interaction of its DNA binding domain with DNA acceptor
segments in the promoter regions of genes regulated by calcitriol,
such as those for osteocalcin, 25OHD$_3$-24 hydroxylase, and osteopontin. The vitamin D receptor binds to DNA primarily as a heterodimer combined with the retinoid-X-receptor bound by 9-*cis*-
retinoic acid. The vitamin D receptor is expressed in the intestine,
distal renal tubules, osteoblast, keratinocyte, hair follicle, fibroblast,
smooth and cardiac muscle, lung, bladder, thyroid, parathyroid
glands, pancreas, adrenal cortex and medulla, pituitary gland, placenta, uterus, ovary, testis, prostate, activated T and B cells, mac-

rophages, monocytes, spleen, thymus and tonsil, brain, spinal cord,
and sensory ganglia. Although the primary role of calcitriol is to
enhance intestinal absorption of Ca^{2+} and phosphate, it also mobilizes Ca^{2+} from bone and increases its reabsorption from the distal
renal tubule, thereby enhancing bone mineralization and maintaining serum levels of calcium within a narrowly defined range. Calcitriol stimulates osteoblast differentiation and secretion of osteocalcin, alkaline phosphatase, and osteopontin, among other
substances. Calcitriol indirectly enhances osteoclast differentiation
from monocytic progenitor cells by stimulating osteoblast/stromal
cell production of osteoclast differentiating factors (macrophage
colony-stimulating factor, RANKL). Calcitriol also enhances bone
resorption by stimulating osteoblast production of osteopontin,
which is recognized by osteoclast surface integrin receptors. By
stimulating synthesis of osteocalcin, it suppresses osteoblast production of collagen and further supports bone resorption. Calcitriol
inhibits secretion of PTH by increasing serum concentration of
Ca^{2+} and by suppressing expression of PTH. Calcitriol both suppresses (decreased IL-2 production) and enhances (cell differentiation) immune function.

PARATHYROID HORMONE AND
PARATHYROID HORMONE–LIKE
HORMONE

Parathyroid hormone is synthesized and secreted by the chief cells
of the parathyroid glands at the superior and inferior poles of the

thyroid gland. These glands are derived from the third (inferior) and fourth (superior) pharyngeal pouches. Occasionally there is a fifth parathyroid gland, or a gland is located within the thyroid parenchyma or in the mediastinum. The gene for PTH on chromosome 11p15.3-p15.1 encodes a prepro-PTH molecule of 115 amino acids that is processed by a convertase (furin) to pro-PTH (90 amino acids) and then to mature PTH (84 amino acids). Full biological activity of PTH is present in the first 34 amino acids. Packaged in secretory granules, intact PTH is released from the parathyroid gland primarily in response to decreases in plasma concentration of Ca^{2+}. Once secreted PTH is rapidly metabolized (half-life less than 4 minutes) by hepatic Kupffer and renal tubular cells. Circulating PTH is heterogeneous with 5 to 30% intact 84-amino-acid PTH and the rest a variety of C- and N-terminal fragments resulting from proteolysis between amino acids 33 and 34 or 36 and 37 by Kupffer cells. Degradation of PTH can occur within the parathyroid cell. The half-life (20 minutes) of the carboxyl terminal fragments of PTH is prolonged, because they are cleared by means of glomerular filtration and degraded further by the kidney. Parathyroid hormone increases serum concentration of Ca^{2+} by stimulating resorption of Ca^{2+}, primarily from cortical bone by enhancing osteoblast synthesis of RANKL and by increasing its renal tubular and gastrointestinal absorption by augmenting synthesis of calcitriol. Parathyroid hormone increases urinary excretion of phosphate by decreasing renal tubular reabsorption. Hypocalcemia increases PTH mRNA, but hypercalcemia does not depress it. Hypocalemia increases PTH mRNA by means of posttranscriptional binding of PTH mRNA to cytosolic proteins that decrease its degradation rather than to increased transcription. Phosphate also influences PTH mRNA levels; hypophosphatemia suppresses and hyperphosphatemia enhances PTH secretion. Calcitriol directly inhibits transcription of the PTH gene by binding of vitamin D receptor to its promoter. Parathyroid hormone stimulates calcitriol synthesis through a direct effect on renal expression of P450c1α.

Secretion of PTH is stimulated by β-adrenergic agents, dopamine, and prostaglandin E acting through stimulatory G proteins, potassium by decreasing cytosolic Ca^{2+} levels, and prolactin and lithium, the latter by altering the set point for PTH release. Glucocorticoids, estrogens, and progestins enhance PTH release. Prostaglandin $F_{2\alpha}$ and α-adrenergic agonists depress PTH secretion through inhibitory G proteins. Fluoride suppresses PTH release by increasing cytosolic Ca^{2+}. Both low and high serum levels of magnesium inhibit secretion but not synthesis of PTH. Within its secretory granule, PTH is colocalized with chromogranin A, a 439-amino-acid protein that is a precursor to several peptides, including pancreastatin, a peptide that inhibits secretion of both PTH and pancreatic insulin. Chromogranin A and PTH are cosecreted, suggesting that pancreastatin released from chromogranin A can have an autocrine paracrine role in modifying further PTH release.

Parathyroid hormone–related protein, a protein structurally related to PTH, is the principal cause of hypercalcemia of malignant disease. Parathyroid hormone and PTHrP have evolved from a common ancestral protein, share partial structure, and use a common PTH/PTHrP receptor (PTHR1). Parathyroid hormone–related protein has somewhat greater effects than PTH on bone resorption and is less active than PTH on intestinal and renal function. The gene for PTHrP encodes isoforms of PTHrP with identical sequences through the first 139 amino acids. Eight of the first 13 amino acids of PTHrP are shared with PTH. Thereafter, the two proteins are dissimilar. Parathyroid hormone–related protein is expressed by the parathyroid glands, placenta, mammary glands, skin, brain, kidney, heart, lung, and perichondrial cells as well as by the pituitary gland, pancreas, and uterine myometrium. It acts primarily in a paracrine manner. Serum concentration of PTHrP is low except when PTHrP is secreted by tumors, in which case it causes humoral hypercalcemia of cancer. The effects of PTHrP on calcium, phosphate, and vitamin D metabolism are similar to those of PTH, but PTHrP also affects development of the teeth, cartilage, and endochondral bone. Parathyroid hormone–related protein is the main hypercalcemic agent synthesized by the fetal parathyroid glands. It may modulate placental trophoblast transport of Ca^{2+} and magnesium, thus maintaining the high fetal serum concentrations of calcium necessary for normal fetal homeostasis and skeletal mineralization. Large amounts of PTHrP in amniotic fluid are produced by the amnion and may affect fetal gastrointestinal, pulmonary, and epithelial function. Released by the prehypertrophic chondrocytes, perichondrial PTHrP acts on the chondrocyte to delay its differentiation into a hypertrophic chondrocyte, increase metaphyseal chondrocyte proliferation, and slow cartilage ossification. Parathyroid hormone–related protein is produced by mammary tissue and is abundant in human milk, suggesting that PTHrP may be important for calcium transport into milk and perhaps absorption of calcium by breast-fed infants. Serum concentrations of PTHrP are higher among lactating than among nonlactating women. The implication is that it can mobilize Ca^{2+} from the maternal skeleton. Parathyroid hormone–related protein also may act as a growth, transforming, and differentiation factor, particularly in human skin keratinocytes and lymphocytes. It also relaxes smooth muscle in the uterus, urinary bladder, intestinal tract, and vascular tissue. Secretion of PTHrP is inhibited by a peptide released from chromogranin A (amino acid residues 1–40).

Parathyroid hormone and PTHrP have a common receptor (PTHR1), which mediates most of their physiological processes. A gene on chromosome 3p22-p21.1 encodes this transmembrane G protein–coupled receptor. The PTHR1 is structurally similar to receptors for calcitonin, GHRH, secretin, and a number of other peptide hormones. A distinct receptor (PTHR2) selectively recognizes $^{1-34}$PTH but also binds $^{7-34}$PTHrP. The PTHR2 is 70% homologous to the PTHR1. The PTHR2 is expressed predominantly in brain, testis, placenta, and pancreas; its physiological role is unknown. Clinical disorders associated with either loss-of-function (Blomstrand chondrodysplasia) or gain-of-function (Murk Jansen syndrome) mutations in PTHR1 have been reported.

CALCITONIN

Calcitonin is a 32-amino-acid hypocalcemic peptide encoded by a gene that is alternatively transcribed and translated into two groups of products: (1) a 141-amino-acid precursor of calcitonin and katacalcin, a 21-amino-acid hypocalcemic peptide adjacent to calcitonin at its carboxyl terminal, and (2) a 128-amino-acid precursor of the 37-amino-acid calcitonin gene–related peptide. Calcitonin is secreted primarily by neural crest–derived thyroid parafollicular or C cells. In avian species, parafollicular cells form the ultimobranchial bodies. Although also secreted in small amounts by C cells, calcitonin gene–related peptide is primarily of neuronal origin and functions as a neurotransmitter and vasodilating agent. Calcitonin also is expressed in the anterior pituitary gland and by neuroendocrine cells in the lung and elsewhere where it can exert paracrine effects. The primary stimulus to calcitonin secretion is increasing serum concentrations of Ca^{2+}. Members of the gastrin-cholecystokinin intestinal peptide hormone family also stimulate calcitonin secretion. This principle is used in diagnostic testing for the hypercalcitonemia that accompanies medullary carcinoma of the thyroid. [1-40]Chromogranin A inhibits and [403-428]chromogranin A stimulates calcitonin secretion. Calcitonin secretion decreases when Ca^{2+} values decrease. Calcitonin has a brief half-life and is metabolized primarily by the kidney. Serum concentrations of calcitonin are high in the fetus and newborn, decrease quickly after birth, and decrease slowly until 3 years of age. Values change little thereafter. After 10 years of age, calcitonin levels are lower among girls than among boys. Calcitonin values are low among patients with primary congenital or acquired hypothyroidism. The most important function of calcitonin is to inhibit osteoclastic bone resorption and decrease concentration of serum Ca^{2+}. Salmon calcitonin is used therapeutically, because it is less rapidly degraded than human calcitonin and thus more biologically effective.

The biological effects of calcitonin are mediated through its G protein–coupled receptor, CALCR. There are two sequences for CALCR, one of which contains an insert of 16 amino acids in the first intracellular domain. The structure of CALCR is similar to that of the receptors for PTH and secretin.

OTHER BONE REGULATORY FACTORS

Growth hormone decreases urinary phosphate excretion and increases serum levels of phosphate and alkaline phosphatase. It directly stimulates colony formation of chondrocyte progenitor cells and their proliferation and differentiation. Through GH-mediated local and distal synthesis, IGF-I supports clonal expansion of differentiated chondrocytes in individual columns. Growth hormone stimulates proliferation and functional differentiation of osteoblasts, acting in part through osteoblast synthesis of IGF-I and IGF-BP3. Growth hormone also increases osteoclast differentiation and function. GH and IGF-I augment cortical bone mineralization in experimental animals and patients with acromegaly. Children and adults with low levels of somatotropin often have osteopenia, a situation reversible with GH treatment. Sex hormones, especially estrogens, directly stimulate cartilage proliferation, maturation, epiphyseal calcification, and bone formation. They increase bone mass. Estrogen inhibits production of the osteoclast activating factor IL-6 by bone and marrow stromal cells. Thyroid hormone stimulates cartilage growth and maturation as well as osteoclast activity and bone resorption.

24.12.2 Hypocalcemia

CAUSES OF HYPOCALCEMIA

Causes of hypocalcemia are listed Table 24-48. In a healthy term infant, concentration of total calcium in umbilical cord serum is approximately 12 to 13 mg/dL. Immediately after delivery the serum concentration of calcium begins to decrease, reaching a nadir 24 to 48 hours after birth coincident with a decline in secretion of PTHrP by the fetal parathyroid glands. Serum levels of calcium stabilize as calcitonin secretion declines and that of PTH increases, rising to normal adult levels by 14 days of age. Neonates with hypocalcemia may have no symptoms or may be irritable. They may have hyperacusis, laryngospasm, tetany, or seizures. Neonatal hypocalcemia can be of early (before 72 hours of age) or late (after 96–120 hours of age) onset. Early neonatal hypocalcemia (total calcium <7.5 mg/dL) often is associated with antenatal maternal illness, such as diabetes mellitus, toxemia, hyperparathyroidism, or familial hypocalciuric hypercalcemia (FHH), or with perinatal asphyxia, respiratory distress, or sepsis in infants. Low birth weight

infants, whether premature or with growth retardation caused by an intrauterine insult, are at increased risk of hypocalcemia (<7.0 mg/dL), perhaps because of an exaggerated increase in calcitonin secretion or delayed secretion of or decreased renal responsiveness to PTH. Infants with late-onset neonatal tetany characteristically are born of multiparous women of marginal socioeconomic status and vitamin D intake and are born during the winter months. Among infants with late-onset hypocalcemia, ingestion of large amounts of phosphate in proprietary formulas may exceed the renal excretory capacity of the neonate and cause hyperphosphatemia. Transient and permanent forms of hypoparathyroidism can occur in the newborn period. Transient congenital hypoparathyroidism (persistent neonatal hypocalcemia necessitating treatment for several months after birth before resolution) can be followed by a period of eucalcemia of several years' duration with later onset of hypocalcemia as residual parathyroid function is exhausted. Neonatal hypocalcemia often is caused by hypomagnesemia. For these infants, administration of magnesium alone restores the eucalcemic state.

Hypocalcemia among children or adolescents can manifest as episodes of muscle cramps, tetany, or paresthesias or can be asymptomatic and unrecognized until detected at chemical screening performed for another purpose or until a seizure occurs. Among these patients, hypocalcemia can be caused by hypoparathyroidism, which can result from a late-manifesting congenital anomaly of parathyroid gland formation, parathyroid destruction by autoimmune disease or surgery, synthesis of abnormal PTH, or impaired cellular responsiveness to PTH. Hypocalcemia is present in patients with restricted exposure to sunlight and decreased vitamin D intake, abnormal metabolism of vitamin D, or impaired cellular responsiveness to calcitriol. Inadequate calcium intake or excessive urinary excretion of calcium also causes hypocalcemia. Hypomagnesemia impairs the secretion but not the synthesis of PTH and impedes tissue responsiveness to PTH.

Hypoparathyroidism

Hypoparathyroidism can be sporadic or familial, transmitted as an autosomal-dominant, autosomal-recessive, or X-linked trait. Both autosomal-dominant and autosomal-recessive hypoparathyroidism have been associated with mutations of the gene for PTH, which cause errors in transcription, translation, or posttranslational processing or synthesis of an inactive protein. *Autosomal-dominant hypoparathyroidism* can be caused by gain-of-function mutations in the CASR. The mutant receptor has extreme sensitivity to very low levels of Ca^{2+}. The sensitivity causes suppression of PTH secretion and often symptomatic hypocalcemia, even seizures. In the kidney, decreased Ca^{2+} resorption results in hypercalciuria and decreased urinary concentrating ability. Persons with this disorder are sensitive to vitamin D. Administration of vitamin D can lead to further hypercalciuria, nephrocalcinosis, and impaired renal function. An autosomal-dominant form of familial hypoparathyroidism caused by aplasia or hypoplasia of the parathyroid glands has been associated with sensorineural deafness and renal dysplasia (*Barakat syndrome*) and linked to chromosome 10pter-p13. A probable autosomal-recessive familial association of congenital hypoparathyroidism, intrauterine and postnatal growth failure, and dysmorphic facial features has been described, but no genetic abnormality has been identified. The X-linked form of familial hypoparathyroidism on Xq26-27 is caused by an isolated defect in formation of the parathyroid glands. *Kearns-Sayre syndrome* is a mitochondrial disorder of ocular, cardiac, and peripheral myopathy associated with

TABLE 24-48

CAUSES OF HYPOCALCEMIA

I. Neonatal hypocalcemia
  A. Early onset
    1. Maternal illness
      a. Diabetes mellitus
      b. Toxemia of pregnancy
      c. Hyperparathyroidism
    2. Respiratory distress, sepsis
    3. Low birth weight
    4. Hypomagnesemia
  B. Late onset
    1. High phosphorus load
    2. Hypoparathyroidism
      a. Transient
      b. Permanent
II. Hypoparathyroidism
  A. Congenital
    1. Transient neonatal
    2. Familial
      a. Autosomal recessive
      b. Autosomal dominant
        (1) gain-of-function mutation of *CASR*
        (2) with sensorineural deafness and renal dysplasia
      c. Sex-linked recessive
    3. Dyshormonogenesis
    4. DiGeorge syndrome
    5. Kenny-Caffey syndrome
    6. Kearns-Sayre syndrome
  B. Resistance to parathyroid hormone
    1. Blomstrand chondrodysplasia (loss-of-function mutation *PTHR1*)
    2. Pseudohypoparathyroidism types Ia, Ib
    3. Pseudohypoparathyroidism type II
    4. Pseudopseudohypoparathyroidism
  C. Acquired
    1. Autoimmune
      a. Sporadic
      b. Familial—polyglandular syndrome type I
    2. Postsurgical, radiation insult
    3. Infiltrative (excessive iron or copper deposition, amyloidosis, sarcoidosis)
    4. Hypomagnesemia
    5. Idiopathic

III. Vitamin D deficiency (see disorders of mineralization)
IV. Others
  A. Deficiency of calcium
    1. Nutritional deprivation
    2. Hypercalciuria
  B. Hypomagnesemia
    1. Congenital
      a. Malabsorption
      b. Hypermagnesuria
        (1) Primary
        (2) Bartter syndrome
        (3) Renal tubular acidosis
    2. Acquired
      a. Acute renal failure
      b. Diuretics
  C. Hyperphosphatemia
    1. Renal failure
    2. Phosphate administration (IV, oral, rectal)
    3. Tumor cell lysis
    4. Muscle injuries (crush, rhabdomyolysis)
    5. Bisphosphonate administration
  D. Hypoproteinemia
  E. Drugs
    1. Furosemide
    2. Calcitonin
    3. Antineoplastic agents (plicamycin, asparaginase, cisplatin, cytosine arabinoside, doxorubicin)
    4. Citrated blood products
  F. Hungry bone syndrome
  G. Critical illness
    1. Rhabdomyolysis, toxic shock syndrome, acute pancreatitis, chronic renal failure

hypoparathyroidism and other endocrinopathies (hypogonadism, diabetes mellitus, GH deficiency). Mutations of mitochondrial DNA produce a mosaic pattern of tissue loss because of locally impaired energy generation. *Kenny-Caffey syndrome* type 2 is an autosomal dominant disorder that manifests as extreme short stature, dense tubular bones with narrow marrow cavities (medullary stenosis), hypocalcemia, hypophosphatemia, low serum levels of PTH, and absence of parathyroid tissue. *Blomstrand chondrodysplasia* is an autosomal recessive, lethal disorder caused by mutations of the PTH receptor, characterized by short-limbed dwarfism, accelerated skeletal maturation, increased bone mineralization, decreased numbers of resting and proliferating chondrocytes in the cartilage growth plates, hypocalcemia, hyperphosphatemia, and elevated serum concentrations of PTH.

DiGeorge syndrome is caused by anomalous development of the derivatives of the third and fourth pharyngeal pouches caused by abnormal migration of neural crest cells from the neural fold. It manifests as variable deficiencies of thymic and parathyroid gland function and anomalies of the face and cardiovascular system (Table 24-49). It can occur sporadically or be inherited as an autosomal-dominant characteristic with variable penetrance. DiGeorge syndrome has been associated primarily with deletions and translocations of chromosome 22q11.2, although other chromosomal anomalies and malformations (holoprosencephaly; CHARGE anomaly; and fetal alcohol, Kallman, and Zellweger syndromes) have occurred among these patients. DiGeorge syndrome shares anomalies with other syndromes (velocardiofacial, Shprintzen, Takao) associated with deletions of chromosome 22q11.2 collectively called *CATCH22* (cardiac abnormality, abnormal face, T-cell deficit caused by thymic hypoplasia, cleft palate, and hypocalcemia caused by hypoparathyroidism resulting from 22q11 deletion). The incidence of del-22q11 is 13 per 100,000 live births. Within the DiGeorge critical region on chromosome 22q11, mutation of *UFD1L* (ubiquitin fusion degradation) has been specifically associated with DiGeorge syndrome. This gene encodes a protease involved in degradation of ubiquitinated proteins by the 26S protea-

TABLE 24-49

CLINICAL CHARACTERISTICS OF THE DIGEORGE SYNDROME

Hypoparathyroidism
   Severe and permanent *or* mild and transient
Thymic dysfunction
   Mild or severe deficiency of T lymphocytes (CD4, CD4/CD8)
Facial malformations
   Mandibular hypoplasia
   Hypertelorism
   Short philtrum
   Small mouth
   Malformed/low-set ears
Cardiovascular anomalies
   Right aortic arch
   Interrupted aortic arch type B
   Ventricular/atrial septal defects
   Pulmonic stenosis
   Tetrology of Fallot
   Truncus/pseudotruncus arteriosus
Other
   Short stature
   Cleft palate
   Developmental delay

some. The protein substrate for this proteolytic pathway has not been identified, but its accumulation interferes with normal migration of neural crest cells. Haploinsufficiency of the *UFD1L* protein appears sufficient to cause DiGeorge syndrome, although the variable clinical manifestations of DiGeorge syndrome suggest that additional gene products may be involved. Neonates with DiGeorge syndrome may have transient or persistent hypocalcemia and variable deficits in thymus-mediated immune function. Restoration of the eucalcemic state can be accomplished with calcitriol and calcium supplementation. When there is no T-cell proliferative response to mitogens, DiGeorge syndrome can be fatal. Bone marrow transplantation is performed if possible.

Isolated autoimmune destruction of the parathyroid glands can be difficult to identify because antibodies to parathyroid tissue are detected in few patients. When hypoparathyroidism is part of autosomal-recessive autoimmune polyglandular disease type I (autoimmune polyendocrinopathy, candidiasis, ectodermal dysplasia), it is associated with hypoadrenocorticism, hypogonadism, insulin-dependent diabetes mellitus, pernicious anemia, chronic mucocutaneous candidiasis, vitiligo, enamel hypoplasia, alopecia, keratopathy, intestinal malabsorption, and chronic active hepatitis. Candidiasis usually develops by the time the child is 5 years of age. Hypoparathyroidism is the most common and frequently the first of the associated endocrinopathies and most often appears before 10 years of age. Autoimmune polyglandular syndrome type I has been linked to chromosome 21q22.3 and mutations in *AIRE* (autoimmune regulator), a gene that probably encodes a transcription factor the target genes of which are being sought.

The parathyroid glands can be excised or the blood supply compromised during thyroid surgery. They may be injured by radiation or destroyed by deposition of iron (hemochromatosis) or copper (Wilson disease) or by infiltrative processes (sarcoidosis).

Parathyroid Hormone Resistance

Through its carboxyl terminal, the PTH receptor PTHR1 is coupled to a stimulatory G protein the α subunit of which binds GTP

($G_s\alpha$). PTHR1 is coupled through $G_s\alpha$ to adenylyl cyclase and cAMP and further to protein kinase phosphorylation of serine and tyrosine residues of specific proteins. PTHR1 also is coupled to phospholipase C and metabolism of membrane phospholipids to increase intracellular Ca^{2+} leading to the physiological response to PTH. After binding of PTH or PTHrP to PTHR1, GTP displaces guanosine diphosphate (GDP) from the α subunit; $G_s\alpha$ dissociates from its $\beta\gamma$ subunit complex and activates adenylyl cyclase and phospholipase C. Intracellular concentrations of cAMP and Ca^{2+} increase and initiate the signal transduction pathways that lead to cell action. The gene for $G_s\alpha$ is located on chromosome 20q13.2.

In *Albright hereditary osteodystrophy,* loss-of-function mutations of $G_s\alpha$, either partial or complete gene deletion of one allele or point mutations that reduce $G_s\alpha$ activation by its hormone ligand or that impede binding of GTP, decrease signal intensity. Albright hereditary osteodystrophy is characterized by short stature, brachydactyly (usually shortening of the third through fifth metacarpal bones and the distal phalanx of the thumb), round face, obesity, ectopic subcutaneous calcifications, developmental delay, hypocalcemia, hyperphosphatemia, and elevated PTH concentrations (pseudohypoparathyroidism type Ia). Exogenous PTH does not increase serum level of calcium or urinary excretion of nephrogenous cAMP or phosphate. The gene for $G_s\alpha$ is imprinted (gene expression in some tissues is determined by the parent of origin) such that the paternal allele is expressed only weakly in the renal cortex. Therefore the clinical manifestations of a loss-of-function mutation of $G_s\alpha$ depend on whether the mutated gene is transmitted by the mother or father. When the mutated gene is transmitted from mother to child, the child expresses both the Albright hereditary osteodystrophy phenotype and *pseudohypoparathyroidism type Ia.* When the mutated gene is transmitted from father to child, the offspring usually expresses only Albright hereditary osteodystrophy (pseudopseudohypoparathyroidism) and may not be resistant to the biological activity of PTH. An as yet unidentified maternal factor is needed for the full clinical and hormonal expression of a loss-of-function mutation of $G_s\alpha$. Patients with Albright hereditary osteodystrophy and pseudohypoparathyroidism type Ia are resistant not only to PTH but also often to other hormones that signal through $G_s\alpha$-protein (thyrotropin, vasopressin, GHRH).

In *pseudohypoparathyroidism type Ib,* patients have hypocalcemia and hyperphosphatemia. They are fully resistant to the biological effects of PTH but have a normal phenotype. The cause of pseudohypoparathyroidism type Ib has not been identified. Mutations have not been found in the genes for $G_s\alpha$, PTH, or PTHR1, although some patients have had reduced expression of PTHR1. Pseudohypoparathyroidism type Ib and $G_s\alpha$ both map to chromosome 20q13.3. Because $G_s\alpha$ is paternally imprinted, a mutation in the $G_s\alpha$ promoter that specifically inactivates only its renal expression may be responsible for pseudohypoparathyroidism type Ib. In *pseudohypoparathyroidism type II,* the phenotype is normal, but the patient has hypocalcemia and hyperphosphatemia. In response to PTH, urinary cAMP excretion increases but that of phosphate does not.

Other Causes of Hypocalcemia

Deficiency of vitamin D intake, metabolism, or bioactivity can cause hypocalcemia (see Sec. 24.12.1). When administering vitamin D to a patient with vitamin D deficiency or one who has undergone parathyroidectomy for hyperparathyroidism and has skeletal demineralization, it is important to monitor serum levels of calcium closely and to prescribe supplemental calcium. Rapid deposition of

Ca^{2+} and phosphate can occur once mineralization of bone matrix is initiated and can cause hypocalcemia (hungry bone syndrome). Drugs that inhibit osteoclast resorption of bone or renal reabsorption of Ca^{2+} cause hypocalcemia. Hyperphosphatemia induced by intravenous infusion or by oral or rectal administration of phosphate-containing solutions for intestinal cleansing, acute cellular destruction, or renal failure can be accompanied by hypocalcemia. Hypocalcemia often occurs among acutely ill children and adolescents because of functional hypoparathyroidism, hypercalcitonemia, decreased calcitriol synthesis, alkalosis, and increased free fatty acids, which increase binding of Ca^{2+} to albumin.

EVALUATION OF HYPOCALCEMIA

When an infant has hypocalcemia, the maternal history and that of the pregnancy, labor, and postpartum period are important in identifying the cause (Fig. 24-49). A history of maternal hypercalcemia is helpful, but when an infant is the product of an uncomplicated, term pregnancy, delivery, and postpartum course, maternal calcium concentration should be measured to identify asymptomatic hyperparathyroidism or familial hypocalciuric hypercalcemia (FHH). A family history of hypocalcemia or associated immunodeficiency or autoimmune disorders may be helpful. The physical examination may reveal unusual facial features, cardiovascular or ectodermal defects, or osteochondrodystrophy. After it is confirmed that hypocalcemia is not caused by hypoproteinemia by means of measuring total calcium and ionized Ca^{2+} values, an increased concentration of calcium in the urine may suggest an abnormality in the CASR. If the concentration of calcium in the urine is low, as it is most commonly, the serum level of PTH is measured usually with values for phosphate, magnesium, creatinine, and alkaline phosphatase. Low PTH concentration suggests a primary abnormality of PTH synthesis or secretion. Among patients with hypoparathyroidism, calcium and PTH concentrations are low, phosphate values high, and magnesium levels normal. Among those with hypomagnesemia, magnesium concentrations are quite low. A critically ill patient with hypocalcemia also has an inappropriately low PTH level. A chest radiograph to measure the thymus can help identify DiGeorge syndrome. Because neonatal hypocalcemia from diverse causes in a nondysmorphic newborn often resolves after 14 to 21 days of age, definitive investigation of parathyroid gland function usually is reserved for infants with hypocalcemia that persists into the second month of life.

Patients with hypocalcemia and increased serum concentrations of PTH may be secreting an abnormal PTH molecule, have a loss-of-function mutation of PTHR1 or its associated G protein (pseudohypoparathyroidism), or a secondary PTH hypersecretory response to hypocalcemia. Renal responsiveness to PTH can be assessed by means of administering biosynthetic $^{1-34}$PTH and measuring the changes in serum concentrations of Ca^{2+}, phosphate, cAMP, and calcitriol and urinary level of cAMP and phosphate excretion. Infants with pseudohypoparathyroidism may be recognized initially in neonatal screening programs for congenital hypothyroidism because they often have elevated serum levels of thyrotropin without an anatomic or functional abnormality of the thyroid. The serum level of calcidiol is low among patients with deficiency of vitamin D. Children with P450c1α deficiency have low serum levels of calcitriol. Those with vitamin D receptor mutations have calcitriol concentrations that are increased manyfold and normal calcidiol concentrations. Patients with renal failure have high serum values of creatinine.

MANAGEMENT OF HYPOCALCEMIA

Neonates with hypocalcemia are treated if serum levels of calcium decrease to less than 6 mg/dL (Ca^{2+} <0.72 mmol/L). In an emergency, eucalcemia can be restored rapidly by means of cautious, monitored intravenous administration of calcium (10% calcium gluconate; 9 mg Ca^{2+}/dL, 2 mg/kg over 10 minutes; repeated every 4 hour if necessary). For many infants with neonatal hypocalcemia, a low-phosphate formula and oral calcium (calcium glubionate; 115 mg Ca^{2+}/5 mL) adjusted to maintain the calcium to phosphate intake ratio at 4:1 is sufficient to increase and maintain calcium levels. A patient with hypomagnesemia is best treated with magnesium while the cause of magnesium deficiency is sought (magnesium sulfate 50% solution; 0.1–0.2 mL/kg intramuscularly; repeated after 12–24 hours if needed). Patients with vitamin D deficiency improve after exposure to sunlight or ingestion of vitamin D (1000–2000 IU/d for several weeks) with supplemental calcium (40 mg/kg/d). Physiologic doses (10 ng/kg/d) of calcitriol usually restore Ca^{2+} and phosphate levels to normal in patients with renal $25OHD_3$-1α-hydroxylase deficiency. Patients with loss-of-function mutations of the vitamin D receptor need extraordinarily large amounts of calcitriol (up to 1000 μg/d) or parenteral calcium for even partial normalization of serum levels of calcium and phosphate. Calcitriol (20–60 ng/kg/d) and supplemental calcium (calcium glubionate or calcium citrate 30 to 75 mg Ca^{2+}/kg/d) restore eucalcemia in patients with hypoparathyroidism or pseudohypoparathyroidism. Because transient hypoparathyroidism among infants can be the initial manifestation of late-onset hypoparathyroidism, it is important to assess calcium homeostasis for such patients throughout childhood. Reevaluation of patients with isolated hypoparathyroidism periodically enables identification of autoimmune disorders in the patient or family. Assessment of thymic function is important in the care of patients with findings suggestive of DiGeorge syndrome. Because pseudohypoparathyroidism is associated with resistance to a number of hormones that act through stimulation of $G_s\alpha$, it is important to assess pituitary thyroid, pituitary gonadal, and vasopressin function periodically. In the care of children receiving calcium or calcitriol, serum and urine values of calcium and creatinine should be measured and renal sonography performed frequently to avoid hypercalcemia, hypercalciuria, and nephrocalcinosis.

24.12.3 Hypercalcemia

CAUSES OF HYPERCALCEMIA

Causes of hypercalcemia in infants, children, and adolescents are listed in Table 24-50. When serum concentrations of protein are normal, hypercalcemia is caused by increased resorption of bone mineral or enhanced intestinal absorption of calcium that exceeds renal excretory capacity for calcium. Neonatal hypercalcemia sometimes is associated with maternal hypoparathyroidism or excessive vitamin D intake. Infant formula and various brands of milk occasionally contain severalfold more vitamin D than the stated amounts, raising the possibility of hypervitaminosis D among infants who drink large volumes of these products. Long-term ingestion of formula for premature infants that is fortified with excess vitamin D has caused hypercalcemia. Hypophosphatemia is accompanied by hypercalcemia in a compensatory effort to maintain a constant calcium X phosphorus product. It can develop during provision of parenteral nutrition. Subcutaneous fat necrosis occurs

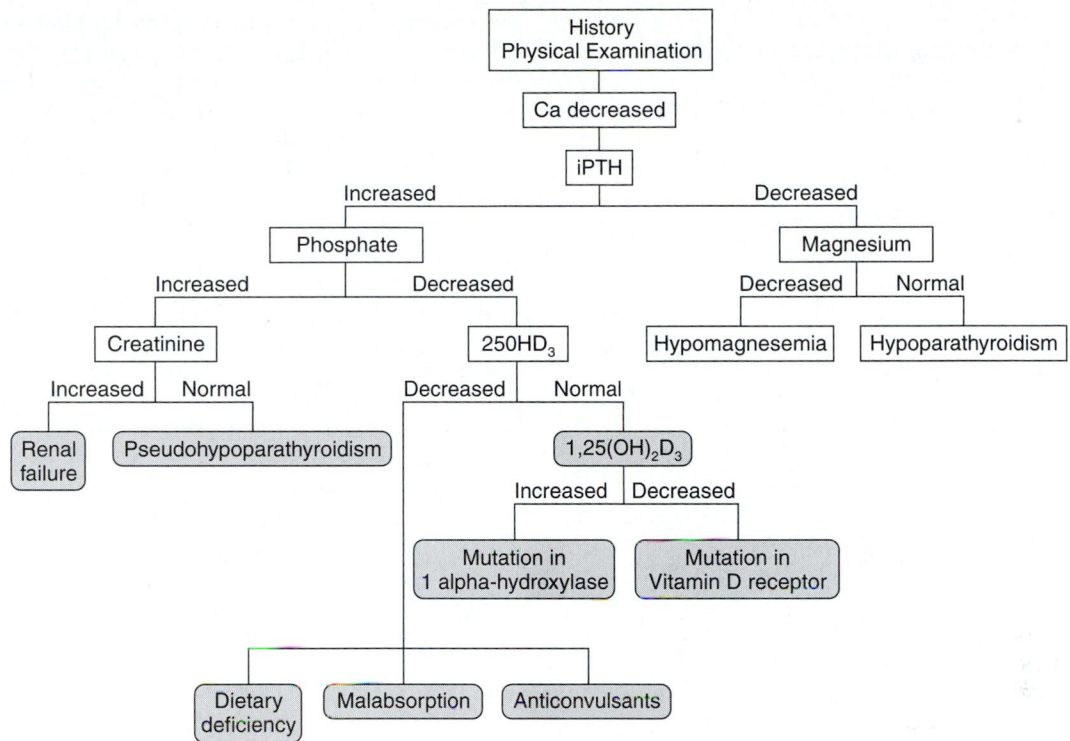

FIGURE 24-49   **Evaluation of hypocalcemia. iPTH = immunoreactive parathyroid hormone; Mg = serum magnesium; Phos = serum phosphorus; 25OHD₃ and 1,25(OH)₂D₃ = 25 and 1,25 hydroxyvitamin D.**

among severely asphyxiated infants. The associated hypercalcemia is caused by both reabsorption of the dystrophic calcification of these lesions and by the attendant inflammatory process and monocytic expression of $25OHD_3$-1α-hydroxylase activity with increased production of calcitriol. Hypercalcemia occurs among patients with the infantile form of hypophosphatasia. Idiopathic infantile hypercalcemia has been described and attributed to excessive vitamin D intake, although similar infants with increased levels of PTHrP also have been described. Congenital hyperparathyroidism can occur as an isolated or familial disorder. The latter may be a manifestation of FHH.

WILLIAMS-BEUREN SYNDROME   This autosomal-dominant disorder manifests as hypercalcemia in infancy, elfin face (epicanthal folds, full nasal tip, prominent lips, long philtrum, malocclusion), supravalvular aortic stenosis, stenotic pulmonary arteries, short stature, renal anomalies, developmental delay (except for adroit verbal skills with a large vocabulary and enhanced auditory memory, particularly for names), and unusual musical aptitude (including the ability to memorize, play, and sing many musical compositions). The pathophysiological mechanism of the hypercalcemia, which in rare instances persists into adulthood, is unknown. Hemizygotic microdeletions of either maternal or paternal chromosome 7q11.23 with loss of several contiguous genes in this region have been associated with this syndrome. Deletions of elastin have been found in most patients with Williams-Beuren syndrome. However, deletions and loss-of-function mutations of elastin cause isolated supravalvular aortic stenosis without the other features of this syndrome. It is likely that there are other genes at chromosome 7q11.2 the loss of which may be responsible for certain aspects of the phenotype.

FAMILIAL HYPOCALCIURIC HYPERCALCEMIA   This disorder is most often a benign autosomal-dominant trait in which there is asymptomatic hypercalcemia. Nevertheless, the clinical spectrum of FHH ranges widely. It includes severe life-threatening hypercalcemia and parathyroid gland hyperplasia in infancy. Familial hypocalciuric hypercalcemia is caused by an inactivating (loss-of-function) mutation of the gene for the CASR. The syndrome is associated most commonly with asymptomatic hypercalcemia, hypermagnesemia, hypocalciuria, and hypophosphatemia. Serum levels of calcitonin, calcidiol, and calcitriol are normal. Many heterozygous loss-of-function mutations in the CASR have been identified, primarily in the extracellular Ca^{2+}-binding domain of the receptor, that lower its affinity for Ca^{2+}. Because of decreased parathyroid chief cell membrane CASR number and function, the set point for Ca^{2+} suppression of PTH secretion is increased. Thus concentrations of total calcium (11–12 mg/dL) and Ca^{2+} are elevated, whereas serum levels of PTH usually are normal. In the renal tubule, decreases in CASR number and function result in hypocalciuria (calcium clearance/creatinine clearance <0.01) but nearly normal urinary concentrating ability. In other forms of hypercalcemia, urinary calcium excretion is increased and concentrating power depressed. Usually, FHH is a benign condition that requires no therapy, but it must be differentiated from mild primary hyperparathyroidism.

Neonates with homozygous loss-of-function mutations of the CASR (neonatal severe hyperparathyroidism), may have life-threatening hypercalcemia (total calcium levels 14–20 mg/dL), hypotonia, skeletal demineralization, and failure-to-thrive. Neonatal severe hyperparathyroidism also can occur among infants who are heterozygous for loss-of-function mutations in the CASR, probably because the mutated CASR exerts a strong dominant-negative ef-

TABLE 24-50

CAUSES OF HYPERCALCEMIA IN INFANCY, CHILDHOOD, AND ADOLESCENCE

I. Neonatal
   A. Maternal factors
      1. Hypocalcemia
      2. Excessive intake of vitamin D
   B. Hyperparathyroidism
      1. Sporadic, isolated
      2. Familial
         a. Neonatal severe hyperparathyroidism (familial hypocalciuric hypercalcemia—loss-of-function mutation of *CASR*)
         b. Murk Jansen syndrome (gain-of-function mutation of *PTHR1*)
   C. Williams syndrome
   D. Other causes
      1. Excessive vitamin D intake
      2. Hypophosphatemia
      3. Subcutaneous fat necrosis
      4. Hypophosphatasia
II. Childhood/adolescence
   A. Hyperparathyroidism
      1. Sporadic
      2. Familial
         a. Isolated
         b. Multiple endocrine neoplasia types I, IIa
   B. Familial hypocalciuric hypercalcemia
   C. Hypervitaminosis D
      1. Nutritional
      2. Associated with inflammatory/granulomatous diseases
         a. Sarcoidosis, tuberculosis, histoplasmosis, coccidioidomycosis, leprosy
         b. Chronic inflammatory disorders
         c. Neoplasms—lymphomas
   D. Immobilization
   E. Neoplasia
      1. Osseous metastases
      2. Production of PTH-related protein
      3. Production of cytokines/osteoclast-activating factors
   F. Other causes
      1. Hypophosphatemia
      2. Drugs
         a. Thiazides, lithium, vitamin A analogs, calcium, alkali
      3. Hyperthyroidism
      4. Hypoadrenalism
      5. Pheochromocytoma
      6. Vasoactive intestinal polypeptide-secreting tumor
      7. Acute or chronic renal failure/administration of aluminum

fect. Some infants with heterozygous mutations in the CASR have eucalcemic mothers. This suggests that the normally increased fetal serum concentration of calcium must be even higher in a fetus with a loss-of-function mutation in the CASR that causes severe in utero and postnatal secondary hyperparathyroidism and hypercalcemia.

PRIMARY HYPERPARATHYROIDISM Either adenoma or hyperplasia of the chief cells of the parathyroid glands causes primary hyperthyroidism. It most often occurs sporadically but can be transmitted as an isolated autosomal-dominant disorder or as part of the autosomal-dominant complex of MEN 1 and MEN 2. Primary hyperparathyroidism is relatively rare among children and adolescents,

who account for 2% of patients with this disorder. Girls are more commonly affected than are boys. Patients with primary hyperparathyroidism have both a set-point abnormality in the relation between serum concentrations of calcium and PTH and variable calcium-independent PTH secretion, possibly related to the mass of the tumor. The MEN syndromes are autosomal-dominant disorders characterized by the development of tumors of two or more endocrine glands within the same person (see Sec. 24.5.3). Multiple endocrine neoplasia type 1 is associated with hyperplasia or adenoma of the parathyroid glands and tumors of the anterior pituitary gland (nonfunctional or secreting prolactin, GH, or adrenocorticotropin), pancreas (secreting gastrin, insulin, glucagon, pancreatic polypeptide, or vasoactive intestinal polypeptide), and occasionally of the adrenal and thyroid glands. Hyperparathyroidism is the most common endocrinopathy of MEN 1, occurring in 95% of patients with this disorder. Boys and girls are affected with equal frequency. Multiple endocrine neoplasia type 2A (pheochromocytoma, medullary carcinoma of the thyroid, parathyroid hyperplasia or tumors), MEN 2B (medullary carcinoma of the thyroid, pheochromocytoma, marfanoid habitus, mucosal neuromas), and familial isolated medullary carcinoma of the thyroid are caused by germline gain-of-function mutations in the *RET* protooncogene.

MURK JANSEN SYNDROME This syndrome of autosomal dominant metaphyseal chondrodysplasia consists of short-limbed dwarfism; abnormal long bones, digits, spine, and pelvis; choanal atresia; highly arched palate; micrognathia; widely open cranial sutures (in infancy); sclerosis of the basal cranial bones; disorganization of the metaphyses (delayed chondrocyte differentiation, abnormal mineralization); and excessive loss of cortical bone despite the existence of normal trabecular bone. Patients have hypercalcemia and hypophosphatemia and have increased calcitriol and elevated urinary excretion of cAMP in the presence of low or undetectable levels of PTH and PTHrP in the serum. This hyperparathyroid-like state without hyperparathyroidism has been linked to constitutively activating mutations of PTHR1.

HYPERVITAMINOSIS D Ingestion of excessive amounts of vitamin D or calcitriol for therapeutic reasons (therapy for rickets, hypoparathyroidism, or other forms of hypocalcemia), megavitamin intake, or excessive fortification of milk causes hypervitaminosis D. Many granulomatous (sarcoidosis, tuberculosis, histoplasmosis, coccidioidomycosis, candidiasis), chronic inflammatory (collagen-vascular), and neoplastic disorders (primarily Hodgkin and non-Hodgkin B-cell lymphoma) are associated with hypercalcemia caused by monocytic (macrophage and other cells) expression of $25OHD_3$-1α-hydroxylase activity and excessive production of calcitriol. Unlike renal tubular cells, 1α-hydroxylase activity in monocytes is easily suppressed with glucocorticoids and it is not regulated by PTH, calcitriol, calcium, or phosphate. It may be stimulated by interferon-γ, nitric oxide, and leukotriene C_4. Among some children with hypercalcemia, excessive prostaglandin production can be of pathogenetic importance.

OTHER CAUSES OF HYPERCALCEMIA *Acute immobilization* of a growing child, particularly a male adolescent, decreases bone mineral accretion and uncouples the integrated action of osteoblasts and osteoclasts (acute disuse osteoporosis). Skeletal resorption of calcium continues and causes hypercalcemia, hypercalciuria, and, at times, acute renal insufficiency and hypertension. Hypercalciuria occurs soon after immobilization, and hypercalcemia develops several days to 2 to 3 weeks later. This condition can occur among

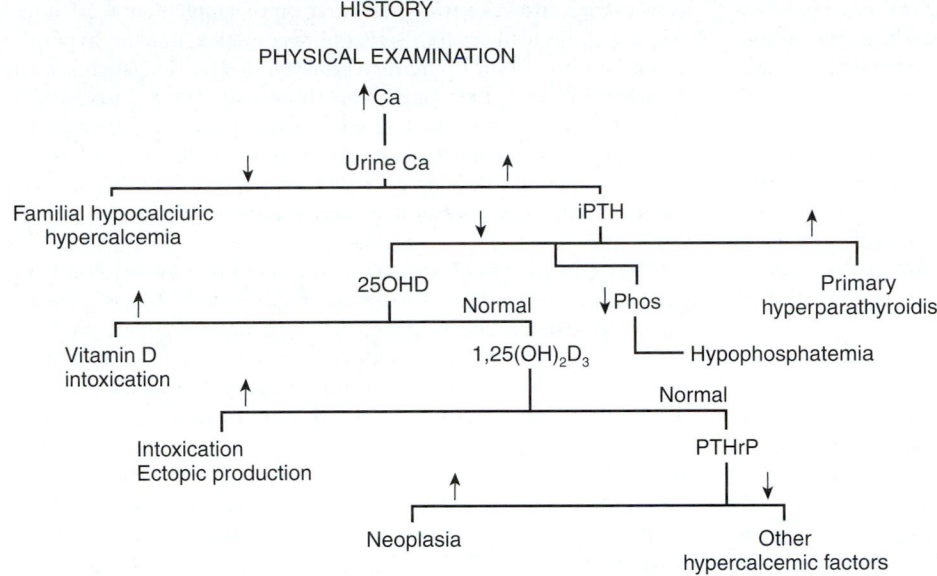

FIGURE 24-50 Evaluation of hypercalcemia. Ca = calcium; iPTH = immunoreactive parathyroid hormone; PTHrP = parathyroid-related hormone; 25OHD and $1,25(OH)_2D_3$ = 25 and 1,25 hydroxyvitamin D.

persons with hypoparathyroidism or vitamin D depletion. *Tumor-associated hypercalcemia* can be the consequence of neoplastic secretion of PTHrP, synthesis of calcitriol caused by expression of $25OHD_3$-1α-hydroxylase, or direct invasion and destruction of bone. Hypercalcemia occurs among fewer than 1% of children with cancer; being most common among children with leukemia, Hodgkin and non-Hodgkin lymphoma, rhabdomyosarcoma, hepatoblastoma, neuroblastoma, and Ewing sarcoma. Excessive ingestion of calcium (milk or calcium-containing antacids) and alkali can lead to absorptive hypercalcemia. A number of drugs cause hypercalcemia: thiazide diuretics enhance renal tubular resorption of calcium and decrease plasma volume; vitamin A and its retinoic acid analogs increase bone resorption; lithium alters the set point of PTH secretion. Hypercalcemia among patients with thyrotoxicosis is caused by the stimulatory effect of thyroid hormone on osteoclast function. Among patients with hypoadrenocorticism, the pathophysiological mechanism of hypercalcemia is uncertain. Hypercalcemia occurs in patients with acute and chronic renal failure, particularly those receiving large amounts of aluminum, and after renal transplantation, the latter related to secondary hyperparathyroidism. Prolonged, uncontrolled secondary hyperparathyroidism can cause relatively autonomous parathyroid hyperfunction (tertiary hyperparathyroidism) in patients with chronic renal failure or hypophosphatemic rickets receiving large amounts of phosphate. Parenteral nutrition with excessive calcium or aluminum or too little phosphate also causes hypercalcemia.

EVALUATION OF HYPERCALCEMIA

Patients with mild hypercalcemia (<12 mg/dL) usually have no symptoms. The disorder is detected during routine chemical screening for another purpose or during evaluation for renal calculi, osteopenia, pathologic fractures, or family screening. Marked hypercalcemia (>14 mg/dL) often is associated with weakness, anorexia, nausea, vomiting, peptic ulceration, acute pancreatitis, constipation, polydipsia, and polyuria (calcium acts as an osmotic diuretic; hypercalcemia impairs distal renal tubular concentrating ability). Hypercalcemia also is associated with neurologic dysfunction, such as impaired concentration, disturbed sleep, and altered consciousness, varying from confusion and lethargy to irritability, depression, stupor and coma. Among infants and young children,

hypercalcemia usually manifests as poor weight gain and growth (failure to thrive), anorexia, and polydipsia.

Evaluation (Fig. 24-50) begins with the history, during which the family and patient are asked about excessive intake of vitamin D, vitamin A (for management of acne), calcium (perhaps to "prevent" osteoporosis), or drugs that affect calcium metabolism (thiazide diuretics can unmask the presence of hyperparathyroidism by increasing borderline high calcium concentrations into the persistently hypercalcemic range). A family history of disordered calcium homeostasis (FHH, renal calculi) or familial neoplasms (prolactinoma, gastrinoma) is sought. Except in the extreme instance in which hypertension (if normally hydrated), dehydration, and an altered state of consciousness are present, physical examination of a patient with hypercalcemia is unremarkable. Rarely is a parathyroid mass palpable. In neonates with subcutaneous fat necrosis, hard masses usually are palpable. The diagnosis of Williams-Beuren syndrome is suggested by the presence of an elfin face, supravalvular aortic stenosis, and the marker chromosomal deletion (7q11.2). A child with Murk Jansen syndrome is extremely short and has a characteristic face (prominent eyes, micrognathia). Laboratory data show hyperparathyroidism except that the serum concentration of PTH is low or undetectable. Analysis of the gene for PTHR1 is needed for specific diagnosis of this disorder.

After the presence of hypercalcemia is confirmed, urinary excretion of calcium is measured. If it is low, the probability of FHH is high; if urine excretion of calcium is high, other possibilities are explored. Use of sensitive and specific immunochemiluminometric assays for intact [1–84]PTH in comparison with calcium values allows differentiation of patients with hyperparathyroidism from those with other causes of hypercalcemia who have low PTH values. In the absence of secondary hyperparathyroidism (chronic renal insufficiency, ingestion of thiazide diuretics or lithium), consistently elevated PTH concentration in a person with hypercalcemia, hypophosphatemia, and hypercalciuria suggests primary hyperparathyroidism. Although hyperparathyroidism is usually quite dramatic among children and adolescents, for an occasional patient repeated measurements of calcium and PTH may be necessary to establish the diagnosis. Among newborns with severe neonatal hyperparathyroidism, asymptomatic hypercalcemia from FHH, in one or both parents, is common. Radiographic examination of the bones of a child or adolescent with hyperparathyroidism may reveal osteitis fibrosa cystica or subperiosteal and endosteal bone resorption; BMD is likely to be decreased. Preoperatively, a parathyroid adenoma may be localized with high-resolution ultrasonography, CT, MR imaging, or radionuclide scanning with the isonitrile drug, ^{99m}Tc-sestamibi. Selective venous catheterization with sampling of local PTH levels or arteriography to identify the site of a parathyroid adenoma are only occasionally necessary. Evaluation for associated endocrine tumors is indicated if the family history suggests the possibility of MEN or there are clinical findings to suggest pheochromocytoma. When pheochromocytoma is identified, it should be removed before parathyroidectomy.

Patients with hypercalcemia and hypervitaminosis D have high serum concentrations of calcidiol (unless they are receiving calcitriol). Patients with granulomatous, chronic inflammatory, and lymphomatous diseases have high serum levels of calcitriol. A few children with humoral hypercalcemia of malignant disease have high serum concentrations of PTHrP. In the care of patients with hypercalcemia and hypocalciuria, the diagnosis of FHH is established through the family history, the asymptomatic state of the patient, normal PTH values, hypermagnesemia, and inappropriately low urinary calcium excretion. The diagnosis is confirmed by means of identification of a loss-of-function mutation in the gene for the CASR.

MANAGEMENT OF HYPERCALCEMIA

Patients with hypercalcemia (total calcium concentration >12 mg/dL) need vigorous hydration with isotonic saline solution (twice maintenance volume over 24–48 hours). This results in increased glomerular filtration of calcium, decreased reabsorption of calcium in the proximal and distal renal tubules, and calciuresis. Furosemide, 1 mg/kg slowly by means of intravenous infusion administered after restoration of extracellular fluid volume with saline solution, inhibits renal tubular calcium absorption and increases calciuresis. Serum concentration of Ca^{2+} can be monitored by means of measure of the length of the QT interval on an electrocardiogram; the QT interval is shortened by hypercalcemia. When hypercalcemia does not respond to the foregoing measures or serum concentration of calcium is quite high (>14 mg/dL), more specific antihypercalcemic agents such as calcitonin or bisphosphonates are used. Bisphosphonates (etidronate, pamidronate, alendronate) are phosphatase-resistant analogs of pyrophosphate, a naturally occurring inhibitor of osteoclast function. Bisphosphonates interfere with osteoclast differentiation, attachment to hydroxyapatite, and function. Intravenous administration of pamidronate (0.5–1.0 mg/kg per dose over 4–6 hours) repeated as indicated has been effective in decreasing serum concentration of calcium in children with hypercalcemia. Salmon calcitonin acts quickly but transiently to lower serum concentration of calcium. It is administered in several daily subcutaneous injections (2–4 U/kg per injection every 6–12 hours). Glucocorticoids usually are ineffective in the management of hyperparathyroidism. In rare instances it may be necessary to perform hemodialysis (with low- or zero-calcium dialysate) if a patient has severe hypercalcemia resistant to conventional therapy.

For infants with neonatal severe hypercalcemia, medical treatment can be useful, but most patients have needed parathyroidectomy. The effectiveness of bisphosphonates in the treatment of these neonates requires evaluation. In the care of children and adolescents with parathyroid adenoma, preoperative localization followed by operative removal by an experienced surgeon usually is required. Postoperatively many patients have transient hypocal-

cemia that improves with administration of supplemental calcium. Among those with severe osteitis fibrosa cystica, marked hypocalcemia can be caused by hungry bone syndrome. In patients with parathyroid hyperplasia (including those with MEN), total parathyroidectomy with implantation of slices of parathyroid tissue into a forearm pocket of muscle can prevent development of permanent hypoparathyroidism. When hypoparathyroidism develops, it is managed with administration of calcitriol and supplemental calcium as needed.

Hypervitaminosis D or excessive production of calcitriol and hypercalcemia associated with granulomatous and chronic inflammatory disease can be managed with glucocorticoids to suppress expression of 25OHD$_3$-1α-hydroxylase. Ketoconazole (3–9 mg/kg/d in three divided doses), an antifungal agent that also inhibits 25OHD$_3$-1α-hydroxylase activity, promptly decreases calcitriol and calcium values among children and adults with these disorders. Patients treated with ketoconazole may have nausea, vomiting, or abdominal pain, depressed secretion of gonadal steroids, or adrenal production of cortisol. Therefore careful observation of patients receiving ketoconazole is essential.

The hypercalcemia of immobilization is most appropriately managed by preventing its development. For acutely immobilized children and adolescents, as much active movement as possible should be prescribed, and a low-calcium diet and adequate hydration should be provided. Serum and urine levels of calcium should be measured frequently and increased fluids supplied if hypercalciuria develops. Once present, hypercalcemia is best managed with movement. Additional methods such as saline diuresis and furosemide therapy may be necessary until eucalcemia is restored. Antiprostaglandins may be useful in the treatment of some children with hypercalcemia caused by excessive prostaglandin production. Specific therapy for diseases accompanied by hypercalcemia (thyrotoxicosis, hypoadrenocorticism) often restores the eucalcemic state.

24.12.4 Disorders of Bone Mineralization

RICKETS AND OSTEOMALACIA

Rickets, a deformative disease that occurs among children, and osteomalacia, an adult disorder associated with increased fractures, are characterized by deficient mineralization of the bone matrix as a result of deficiencies of calcium or phosphorus or both. Rickets is caused by defective mineralization at the growth plate and osteomalacia at the corticoendosteal level. Rickets and osteomalacia are characterized histologically by excessive amounts and impaired mineralization of osteoid, evidenced by wide osteoid seams. Among persons with chronic hypophosphatemia, primarily the trabeculae are undermineralized. These illnesses can be caused by nutritional deficiencies of vitamin D, calcium, or phosphate; inability to absorb vitamin D or retain these ions; impaired synthesis of active vitamin D metabolites or insensitive tissue response to calcitriol; subnormal activity of alkaline phosphatase, chronic renal disease; or inhibitors of mineralization (Table 24-51).

Among very low birth weight infants or infants who need prolonged parenteral alimentation, osteopenia and fractures are common. In older infants and children, rickets is manifested by widening (flaring) of the metaphyses of the long bones, prominence of the costochondral junctions (rachitic rosary), flaring of the lower anterior thoracic wall, frontal bossing, and occasionally craniotabes. After the child begins to walk and bear weight, genu valgum or genu varum develops. Systemic manifestations of rickets include muscular weakness, anorexia, and increased susceptibility to infec-

TABLE 24-51

DISORDERS OF BONE MINERALIZATION

I. Abnormalities of vitamin D
  A. Nutritional deprivation
    1. Low birth weight infants
    2. Socioeconomic factors
    3. Malabsorption/hepatobiliary dysfunction/short gut syndrome
    4. Anticonvulsant drugs (phenytoin)
  B. Metabolic errors
    1. Deficiency of 25-hydroxylase
      a. Loss-of-function mutation of *CYP27*
      b. Severe liver disease
    2. Deficiency of 25-OH-vitamin D_3-1-hydroxylase
      a. Loss-of-function mutation of *CYP1α*
      b. Chronic renal disease
    3. Loss-of-function mutation of vitamin D receptor (*VDR*)
    4. Mucolipidosis 2
II. Deficiency of calcium
  A. Nutritional deprivation
  B. Hypercalciuria
III. Deficiency of phosphorus
  A. Nutritional deprivation
    1. Low birth weight infant
    2. With antacid intake
  B. Hyperphosphaturia
    1. X-linked familial hypophosphatemic rickets (*PHEX*)
      a. with hypercalciuria
    2. Oncogenic hypophosphatemic osteomalacia
    3. X-linked recessive hypophosphatemic rickets (*CLCN5*)
    4. Autosomal recessive hypophosphatemic rickets with hypercalciuria
    5. Renal tubular acidosis
      a. Fanconi syndrome
      b. Primary
      c. Tyrosinemia type 1
IV. Hypophosphatasia
  A. Perinatal, infantile, childhood, adult forms
  B. Pseudohypophosphatasia

V. Inhibitors of mineralization
  A. Aluminum
VI. Osteoporosis/osteopenia
  A. Hypogonadism
    1. Primary
      a. Gonadal dysgenesis
      b. Aromatase deficiency
      c. Estrogen receptor deficiency
    2. Hypogonadotropism
      a. Kallmann syndrome
      b. Excessive physical activity
      c. Hyperprolactinemia
  B. Malnutrition
    1. Cystic fibrosis
    2. Anorexia nervosa
  C. Cranial radiation
  D. Diabetes mellitus
  E. Drugs—glucocorticoids, aluminum
  F. Hyperparathyroidism
VII. Osteogenesis imperfecta
  A. Types I, II, III, IV
VIII. Osteosclerosis*
  A. Osteoporosis
    1. Infantile, intermediate, adult forms
    2. Deficiency of carbonic anhydrase II
  B. Other forms of osteosclerosis
    1. Dysosteosclerosis
    2. Endosteal hyperostosis
    3. Infantile cortical hyperostosis
    4. Metaphyseal dysplasia
    5. Pyknodysostosis
    6. Progressive diaphyseal dysplasia
    7. Fluorosis
    8. Hypervitaminosis A, D
    9. Ionizing radiation

SOURCE: Modified from Whyte MP: Sclerosing bone dysplasias. In: Favus MJ (ed): *Primer on the Metabolic Bone Diseases and Disorders of Mineral Metabolism,* 3rd ed. Lippincott-Raven, Philadelphia, 1996, 363–379.

tion among patients with vitamin D deficiency (a manifestation) of the effect of vitamin D on the immune system). Radiographic evaluation reveals osteopenia, pseudofracture lines, cupping of the distal metaphyses of the long bones, and widening of the epiphyseal cartilage (Fig. 24-51). Most children with rickets have normal or low serum levels of total calcium, low phosphate level and increased alkaline phosphatase and PTH concentrations (Table 24-52).

NUTRITIONAL DEFICIENCY CAUSING OSTEOPENIA OR RICKETS Among very low birth weight infants or newborns who need prolonged parenteral nutrition, osteopenia is primarily the result of calcium or phosphate deficiency and, to a limited extent, vitamin D deficiency. Sufficient elemental calcium (approximately 150 mg/kg/d) and phosphorus (approximately 100 mg/kg/d) and vitamin D (200 U/d) must be provided to the very low birth weight infants to prevent osteopenia of prematurity. Among older children, isolated dietary calcium deficiency or hypercalciuria has resulted in rickets.

Vitamin D deficiency still occurs in otherwise normal populations, particularly among dark-skinned infants and children who

stay indoors with little exposure to daylight, who wear clothing that shields the entire body from sunlight, and who ingest a diet low in vitamin D (breast milk from a vegetarian or poorly nourished mother or little or no milk, meat, eggs, or fish). Among patients with celiac disease, biliary obstruction, gastric resection, pancreatic insufficiency, or other malabsorption syndromes, vitamin D is poorly absorbed. Anticonvulsant drugs (eg, phenytoin) accelerate the catabolism of vitamin D to water-soluble metabolites, hastening their urinary loss. Serum concentrations of calcidiol are low in patients deprived of vitamin D_3, whereas calcitriol values can be high, normal, or low (Table 24-52). The optimal management of vitamin D deficiency is prevention by means of administration of 200 to 400 units of vitamin D daily to infants and children. When vitamin D deficiency rickets occurs, administration of vitamin D_3 1000 to 2000 U daily for several weeks or intramuscular injection of 600,000 U vitamin D_3 heal the rachitic process. A child with vitamin D deficiency who is receiving this agent must consume elemental calcium 40 mg/kg/d to avoid the hypocalcemia that accompanies remineralization of bone matrix (hungry bone syndrome).

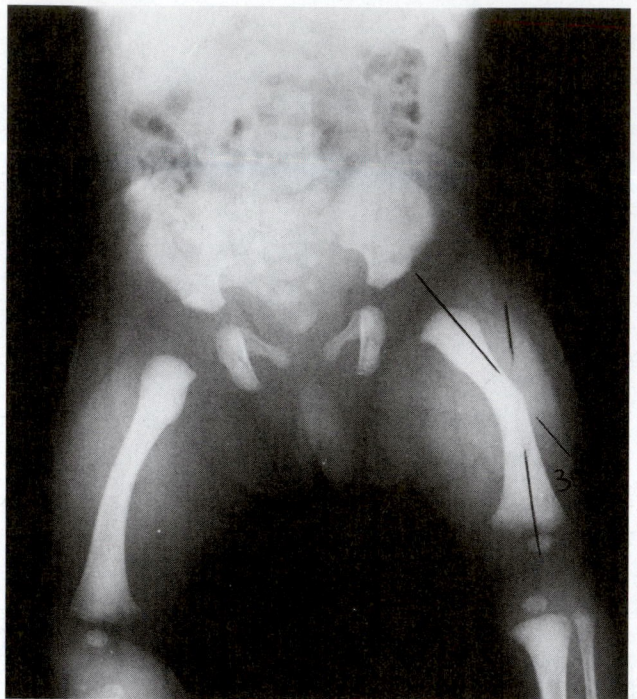
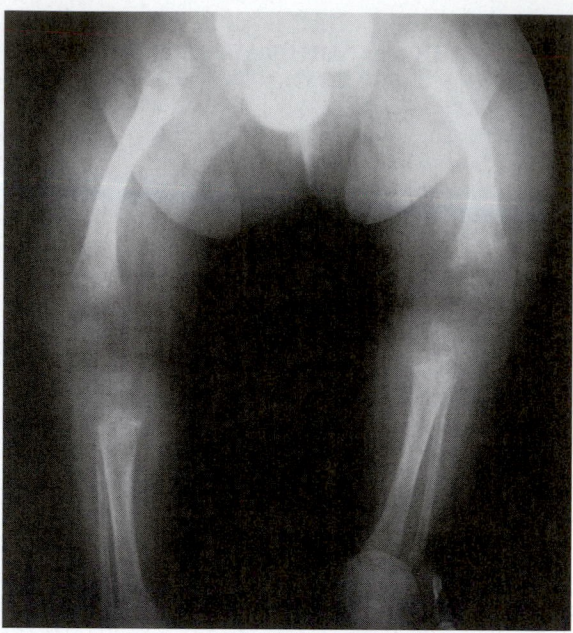
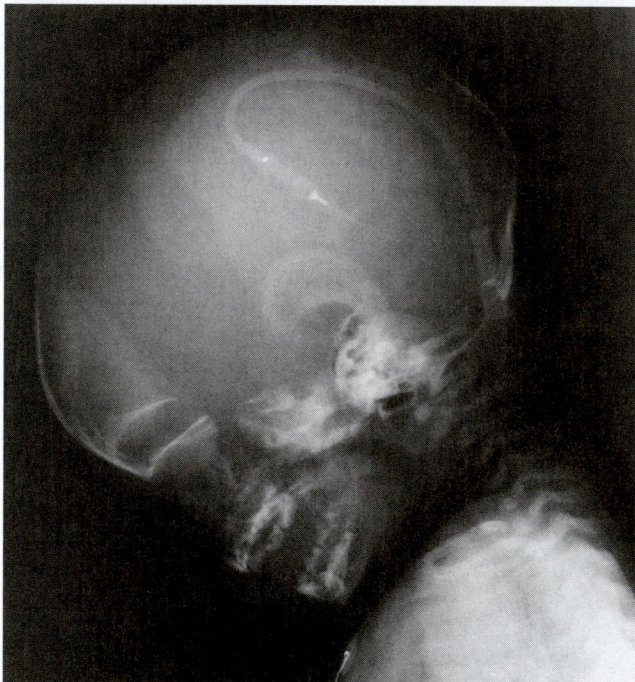

FIGURE 24-51 **A.** At birth, this infant with the infantile form of hypophosphatasia had normal radiographs of the hips and femur with physiologic bowing of the left femur. **B.** Hypercalcemia was found when the patient was evaluated for failure to thrive at 5 months of age, at which point radiographs showed rickets of the long bones and **C.** decreased mineralization of the skull. Hypercalcemia decreased after administration of calcitonin and pamidronate.

X-LINKED HYPOPHOSPHATEMIC RICKETS This is the most common form of rickets in developed countries (1:20,000 births). X-linked hypophosphatemic rickets (XHR) is expressed in both affected hemizygous males and heterozygous females, but there is substantial intrafamilial and inter- and intrafamilial variation in the clinical extent of the disease. Children and adults with XHR have short stature with deformities of the lower limbs (genu varum or genu valgum) that develop when the infant begins to walk, flaring of the metaphyses, rachitic rosary, frontal bossing, increased frequency of dental abscesses caused by abnormalities of dentin, bone pain, and joint stiffness. They usually do not have craniotabes, and muscle strength is normal. Adults with XHR have osteomalacia and a high fracture rate, dental abscesses, and bone pain. Serum concentrations of total calcium and Ca^{2+} are normal; hypophospha-

TABLE 24-52

LABORATORY DATA IN RICKETS

	CALCIUM	PHOSPHATE	ALKALINE PHOSPHATASE	CALCIDIOL	CALCITRIOL	PTH
Vitamin D deficiency						
Mild	N, ↓	N, ↓	↑	↓	N	N
Moderate	N, ↓	↓	↑↑	↓	↓, N, ↑	↑
Severe	↓	↓	↑↑	↓↓	↓	↑↑
Loss-of-function *PHEX* (X-linked hypophosphatemic rickets)	N	↓↓	↑	N	N, ↓	N
Loss-of-function *CYP27* (25-hydroxylase)	↓	↓	↑	N	N, ↓	N
Loss-of-function *CYP1α* (1α-hydroxylase)	↓↓	↓↓	↑↑↑	N	↓↓↓	↑↑↑
Loss-of-function *VDR* (resistance to calcitriol)	↓↓	↓↓	↑↑↑	N	↑↑↑	↑↑↑

PTH = parathyroid hormone; N = normal; ↑ = increased; ↓ = decreased.

temia and hyperphosphaturia are marked because of decreased renal tubular reabsorption of filtered phosphate and limited intestinal absorption of phosphate. Levels of PTH and calcidiol are normal, and calcitriol values are inappropriately low for the degree of hypophosphatemia. Alkaline phosphatase activity is increased. This disorder probably is related to the lack of an unidentified, humoral phosphaturic substance that augments renal tubular reabsorption of phosphate, although an intrinsic defect in the osteoblasts of these patients may be present. Among most patients, XHR is linked to mutations in the *PHEX* gene on chromosome Xp22.1 (phosphate regulating gene with homologies to endopeptidases on the X-chromosome), which encodes an endopeptidase that acts on a precursor form of an unidentified substance called *preprophosphotonin,* translating it into an active product (phosphotonin) that enhances renal tubular phosphate reabsorption and inhibits renal $25OHD_3$-24-hydroxylase activity. Among patients with inactivating mutations of *PHEX,* preprophosphotonin is not cleaved to phosphotonin, but the precursor is able to block the physiologic effects of its product, thereby depressing renal tubular reabsorption of phosphate, increasing phosphaturia and leading to hypophosphatemia, and increasing production of 24,25-dihydroxyvitamin D, thus depressing calcitriol synthesis. Some mesenchymal tumors associated with hypophosphatemic rickets and osteomalacia are thought to secrete unprocessed preprophosphotonin.

The diagnosis of XHR is established through the family history (when the patient is not the initial mutant) and radiographic and laboratory data in the absence of other causes of hypophosphatemia and hyperphosphaturia (Table 24-52). The mainstays of therapy are calcitriol (20–60 ng/kg/d) and elemental phosphorus 2 to 4 g daily in 5 or 6 divided doses (beginning at a dose of 30 mg/kg/d in divided doses and increasing in amount as tolerated). If hypercalciuria develops, the dose of calcitriol must be lowered. If that leads to renewal of the rachitic process, amiloride, a diuretic that increases renal tubular reabsorption of calcium, can be added cautiously to the therapeutic regimen. It is essential to assess radiographic changes; measure serum and urine levels of calcium, phosphate, and creatinine frequently; and to measure PTH periodically. High doses of phosphate can cause counterproductive secondary (and rarely tertiary) hyperparathyroidism. Yearly renal sonograms to find evidence of nephrocalcinosis are recommended. The development of nephrocalcinosis is related to the amount of phosphate

the patient has received. Hyperoxaluria also has been found in such patients and implicated in the pathogenesis of nephrocalcinosis. Complications of therapy include failure to heal the rickets, nephrocalcinosis (which occurs in as many as 80% of patients), renal failure, and tertiary hyperparathyroidism. Cooperative management with an experienced orthopedist is important. The orthopedist may prescribe braces or perform corrective osteotomies for patients with extreme deformities.

By 5 years of age, the heights of many children with XHR are considerably below the norm, but patients with minimal involvement may grow more normally. In many instances, treatment of a child with XHR with calcitriol and phosphate improves growth rate, in part because of correction of the deformities of the lower extremities. Height gain during puberty is normal among boys (+28.2 cm) and girls (+24.2 cm) with XHR, indicating that the compromised adult stature in XHR is related to impaired prepubertal growth. Administration of GH increases serum levels of phosphate and accelerates the rate of growth of children with XHR, but whether therapy improves adult stature is unknown. The clinical status of an adult with XHR varies. Most untreated adults have hypophosphatemia, elevated alkaline phosphatase activity, and osteomalacia, but they have no symptoms except frequent dental abscesses and degenerative hip disease caused by deformities of the lower limbs. Bone mineral density tends to be normal among adults with XHR (despite the histomorphologic abnormalities), suggesting that these persons are not at increased risk of osteoporotic fractures. However, approximately 25% of adults with XHR have clinical evidence of osteomalacia, such as progressive lower limb deformities, bone pain, fractures, and pseudofractures. Treatment with calcitriol and phosphate can be beneficial.

DEFECTS IN VITAMIN D METABOLISM AND FUNCTION Mutations in $25OHD_3$-1α-hydroxylase (P450c1α) have been described in patients with *pseudovitamin D deficiency rickets,* also called *vitamin D–dependent rickets type 1.* Onset in early infancy consists of hypocalcemia, hypophosphatemia, weakness, growth retardation, and rachitic deformities of the long bones. Serum concentration of calcidiol is normal, but calcitriol level is low, particularly in the presence of marked hypocalcemia and hypophosphatemia and elevated serum concentrations of PTH. Calcitriol concentrations do not increase after administration of vitamin D or calcidiol. Small amounts of calcitriol (10 ng/kg/d) completely reverse the clinical, hormonal, and radiographic abnormalities of this disorder. This form of rickets is quite frequent in a segment of the French-Canadian population of Quebec but occurs in all races and diverse geographic regions.

Inactivating mutations of the vitamin D receptor are transmitted in an autosomal-recessive manner and cause resistance to the biological effects of calcitriol. Depending on the site of mutation, the mutant receptors may be unable to dimerize, bind calcitriol, translocate to the appropriate DNA region, bind to the DNA, or initiate gene transcription after DNA binding. Calcitriol insensitivity is marked by severe rickets, hypocalcemia and hypophosphatemia, and extraordinarily elevated levels of calcitriol (as high as 1000 pg/mL) and PTH. Many of these patients also have alopecia, indicative of the essential role of vitamin D in the epithelium. Although spontaneous remission of the rachitic process occurs in rare instances, therapy for this disorder is difficult. High doses of calcitriol have been effective for a few patients. Continuous administration of large amounts of calcium into a central vein (elemental calcium 0.4–1.4 g/m²/d) has been reported to normalize calcium, phosphate, alkaline phosphatase, and PTH values; to heal the rickets; and to increase growth rate. Complications of this mode of therapy include catheter sepsis, cardiac arrhythmia, hypercalciuria, and nephrocalcinosis. After healing of the rickets with parenteral calcium, some patients can take large maintenance doses of oral calcium (elemental calcium 3.5–9 g/m²/d). For younger infants who do not yet have florid rickets, high doses of oral calcium can ameliorate but not completely heal the rickets.

HYPOPHOSPHATASIA Mutations of the gene for the bone-specific isoenzyme of tissue-nonspecific alkaline phosphatase are transmitted in an autosomal-recessive manner. The severity of clinical manifestations reflects the extent of loss of function of the mutant protein. Accumulation of inhibitors of mineralization such as pyrophosphate and inability to increase phosphate levels at the site of calcium-phosphate deposition limit matrix calcification. There are four clinical presentations of hypophosphatasia: (1) Perinatal—a lethal disorder with deformities of the thoracic rib cage limiting respiration; short, bowed, fractured extremities; rachitic rosary; metaphyseal flaring; softened skull; and marked osteopenia on radiographic examination, (2) Infantile—developing within the first 6 months after birth and manifesting as growth retardation, deformities of the long bones, functional craniosynostosis, hypotonia, constipation, hypercalcemia, and radiographic evidence of rickets; approximately 50% of these infants die of respiratory insufficiency, (3) Childhood—variable manifestations ranging from isolated premature shedding of deciduous teeth to clinical and radiographic evidence of osteopenia and rickets, (4) Adult—either subclinical, identified during an evaluation of the family of a child with hypophosphatasia or associated with premature loss of teeth, increased susceptibility to fracture, or pseudogout. Odontohypophosphatasia manifests only as dental disease such as periodontitis.

Hypophosphatasia is diagnosed from laboratory values, including absolutely or inappropriately low serum alkaline phosphatase activity, increased serum levels of pyrophosphate and pyridoxal-5'-phosphate, and increased urinary excretion of phosphoethanolamine and pyrophosphate. Patients with pseudohypophosphatasia are similar phenotypically and biochemically to those with the classic forms of hypophosphatasia except that their serum alkaline phosphatase activity is normal with artificial substrate in vitro but abnormal with natural substrates in vivo. No specific or effective therapy for hypophosphatasia is available; enzyme replacement has

been of only occasional benefit. Administration of even small doses of vitamin D or its metabolites usually is avoided because these patients experience hypercalcemia easily. Hypercalcemia among infants with hypophosphatasia responds to bisphosphonates and transiently to calcitonin. Phosphate can ameliorate the symptoms of mild hypophosphatasia for some children.

RENAL OSTEODYSTROPHY Compromised renal function causes excessive secretion of PTH (high-turnover lesions) or accumulation of metabolites that inhibit bone formation (eg, aluminum) (low-turnover lesions). When glomerular filtration rate decreases to less than 30% of normal, urinary phosphate excretion is impeded. The result is intracellular and extracellular phosphate accumulation, hyperphosphatemia and mild hypocalcemia, secondary hyperparathyroidism, osteoclast activation, and increased resorption of bone. Depressed calcitriol synthesis caused by both hyperphosphatemia and impaired proximal renal tubular function and partial skeletal resistance to PTH raises the set point for PTH release and parathyroid hyperplasia and increases PTH secretion. Bone biopsy shows histologic changes of secondary hyperparathyroidism among most children undergoing dialysis with renal osteodystrophy and some with osteomalacia. Therapy for renal osteodystrophy is to decrease phosphate intake and to administer calcitriol to inhibit phosphate absorption and suppress PTH production. Preparation of dialysis fluids with aluminum-free water, avoidance of aluminum-containing antacids, and use of phosphate binders have decreased the frequency of aluminum-induced bone disease among patients with chronic renal failure. Hypercalcemia can follow renal transplantation if there has been long-term dialysis and parathyroid hyperplasia and may necessitate parathyroidectomy.

OTHER CAUSES OF RICKETS *Autosomal-recessive hypophosphatemic rickets with hypercalciuria* occurs among patients of Middle Eastern origin. It is associated with high serum levels of calcitriol. Complete remission occurs with administration of phosphate alone. *Autosomal-dominant hypophosphatemic bone disease* has distinct radiographic features and normal calcitriol levels. Administration of calcitriol alone helps these patients. *Aluminum toxicity,* most commonly caused by administration of antacids to low birth weight infants or larger infants for management of gastroesophageal reflux and of aluminum in parenteral nutrition, can cause hypophosphatemia and decrease bone mineralization. Aluminum impairs osteoblast differentiation, proliferation, and function. This results in decreased collagen formation and bone mineralization. *X-linked recessive hypophosphatemic rickets* has been attributed to a mutation in a chloride channel.

OSTEOPENIA

Prevention of osteoporosis in adulthood necessitates that children and adolescents maintain adequate calcium intake, vitamin D stores, and activity to assure maximal bone development. However, because of ingestion of fruit juices and soft drinks, most U.S. women consume only 55 to 70% of the recommended daily calcium intake, which requires four to five 8-ounce (240 mL) glasses of milk (300 mg of calcium per glass) to be ingested to approximate the recommended intake. Sufficient protein, vitamins C and K, and copper also must be consumed for optimal bone matrix synthesis. Nutritional deprivation and diseases that prevent normal bone mineralization during childhood and adolescence predispose the affected person to later development of osteoporosis and its complications.

Osteoporosis is a metabolic bone disease of reduced bone mass and abnormal microarchitecture that results in decreased skeletal strength and increased risk of fracture. Osteoporotic bone is characterized by decreased width of bone cortex, decreased number of and increased distance between trabeculae, decreased osteoid, and depressed mineralization activity, which suggests decreased synthesis of bone matrix by osteoblasts.

Decreased cortical and trabecular bone formation and osteopenia are present in children and adolescents with gonadal dysgenesis (Turner syndrome), primary hypogonadism (Klinefelter syndrome, galactosemia, aftermath of radiation therapy), or secondary hypogonadism (anorexia nervosa, excessive physical training, hypogonadotropism). Among children with central precocious puberty, 1 to 2 years of treatment with an analog of gonadotropin-releasing hormone that suppresses pituitary-gonadal function causes a decline or halt in accumulation of bone mineral in the peripheral and the axial skeleton, a process that can be prevented or reversed by the coprovision of 1 g calcium per day during therapy. Among men with constitutional delay in growth and sexual maturation during adolescence, BMD is less than that among men with normal timing of pubertal maturation. Children with GH deficiency have a decrease in bone mineral content. Adults with congenital hypothyroidism have a 10% decrease in radial bone mass, perhaps the result of chronic hypocalcitonemia. Children and adolescents who have been treated with thyroxine ($120\ \mu g/m^2/d$ for 1–8 years) have less radial BMD than those who have not, emphasizing the necessity not to totally suppress serum thyrotropin in such patients.

Patients with anorexia nervosa have decreased BMD caused by poor nutrition, chronic acidemia, and functional hypogonadism. Bone mineral density also is decreased in severely burned patients and those with Marfan syndrome, homocystinuria, diabetes mellitus, lysinuric protein intolerance, or propionic and methylmalonic aciduria. Glucocorticoids impair bone mineralization by inhibiting protein and matrix synthesis and intestinal calcium absorption and by increasing urinary calcium excretion and bone resorption. The incidence of osteopenia among long-term survivors of childhood-onset acute lymphoblastic leukemia approaches 80% with a fracture rate of 40%, likely being caused by multiple factors, including the effects of glucocorticoid and antimetabolite drugs, suboptimal nutrition, delayed or arrested adolescent development, abnormalities of vitamin D intake or metabolism, possible GH deficiency among those who have received cranial radiation, and direct effects of radiation on bone itself. Patients with low BMD need therapy with adequate calcium and vitamin D to improve bone mass and possibly with bisphosphonates. However, the usefulness and safety of bisphosphonates in the treatment of children with osteopenia is a subject of investigation.

Juvenile osteoporosis is characterized by generalized osteopenia, vertebral collapse, and metaphyseal fractures that begin in middle to late childhood and resolve during puberty. Calcitriol has been of benefit in the care of some patients. However, some patients given the diagnosis of juvenile osteoporosis in the past may actually have osteogenesis imperfecta.

Osteogenesis imperfecta or brittle bone disease is a disorder of formation of type I collagen caused by loss-of-function deletions, insertions, frameshift or point mutations within the genes encoding procollagen (α_1)I and procollagen (α_2)I chains that reduce the amount of collagen produced or alter the structure and properties of the collagen molecule. There are four forms of osteogenesis imperfecta, and they typically present at different ages. Their features include blue sclerae, scoliosis, joint laxity, conductive hearing loss, abnormal dentition, and short stature (see Sec. 10.3.5). Children and adolescents with severe osteogenesis imperfecta have responded to the intermittent (2–3 times a year) intravenous administration of the bisphosphonate pamidronate with marked increase in BMD and decline in fracture rate as well as symptomatic improvement.

OSTEOSCLEROSIS

Osteosclerosis, increased bone density, occurs among patients with hypercalcemia caused by hypervitaminosis D and milk-alkali syndrome and among those with fluorosis, hypoparathyroidism, and a number of metabolic and genetic abnormalities of bone formation (craniodiaphyseal-craniometaphyseal dysplasia, infantile cortical hyperostosis, metaphyseal dysplasia, pyknodysostosis, and osteopetrosis). Osteopetrosis (marble bone disease) is caused by failure of osteoclast-mediated bone resorption. Clinical forms vary widely. *Autosomal-recessive infantile osteopetrosis* manifests as poor growth and delayed development; impaired function of cranial nerves II, III, VII, and VIII as bone overgrowth narrows the cranial foramina; leukopenia leading to increased susceptibility to infection and hepatosplenomegaly caused by decrease in bone marrow space; increased frequency of fractures; failure of tooth eruption from the sclerotic jaw, which leads to mandibular osteomyelitis; and death, often within the first several years of life, caused by sepsis, anemia, or hemorrhage. *Intermediate osteopetrosis* is associated with recurrent fractures, short stature, compromise of cranial nerve function, and anemia. *Autosomal-dominant adult osteopetrosis* is typified by an enlarged, sclerotic cranial vault and diffuse vertebral sclerosis (type I) or thickening of the vertebral endplates (rugger jersey spine) and sclerotic bands of bone in the pelvis (type II). In all of these disorders, radiographs of the bones show extreme density. Osteopetrotic bone contains many quiescent osteoclasts and an accumulation of calcified cartilage within bone that ordinarily would have been removed during remodeling. Osteoclast dysfunction has been attributed to an intrinsic functional abnormality of the osteoclast or to an extrinsically mediated abnormality, although mutations in macrophage colony-stimulating factor, RANK, and RANKL have not yet been identified among patients with osteopetrosis. Serum levels of acid phosphatase and the brain isoform of creatine kinase are increased. Therapeutic efforts that decrease calcium intake may lead to hypocalcemia, rickets, and secondary hyperparathyroidism. Some osteopetrotic children have responded to therapy with interferon-γ and high doses of calcitriol. Other children have improved after bone marrow transplantation with replacement of defective osteoclasts by new monocytic precursors. With improved treatment, life span has been prolonged and developmental progress has been fair.

Osteopetrosis caused by deficiency of carbonic anhydrase II and renal tubular acidosis is an autosomal-recessive disorder associated with mutations in the corresponding gene (chromosome 8q). The disorder manifests in late infancy or early childhood as retardation of growth and development, hypotonia, and fractures. Cerebral calcifications often are present after 5 years of age. These patients have metabolic acidosis associated with proximal or distal renal tubular acidosis, or both, and decreased or absent activity of carbonic anhydrase II in erythrocytes and urine. Carbonic anhydrase enhances the reaction of carbon dioxide and water to form carbonic acid ($CO_2 + H_2O \rightarrow H_2CO_3$), which then dissociates to form hydrogen ions (H^+) and bicarbonate (HCO_3^-). Cytosolic carbonic anhydrase II is the most active isoform of this enzyme and is present in normal osteoclasts. This enzyme is the primary stimulus to acid (H^+) formation by the osteoclasts. Absence of carbonic anhydrase II impairs resorption of hydroxyapatite despite the presence of systemic acidosis. Correction of metabolic acidosis does not necessarily improve osteoclast function.

References

Antoniazzi F, Bertoldo F, Lauriola S, et al: Prevention of bone demineralization by calcium supplementation in precocious puberty during gonadotropin releasing hormone agonist treatment. J Clin Endocrinol Metab 84:1992–1996, 1999

Bonjour JP, Carrie AL, Ferrari S, et al: Calcium-enriched foods and bone mass growth in prepubertal girls: a randomized, double-blind, placebo-controlled trial. J Clin Invest 99:1287–1294, 1997

Boot AM, de Ridder MAJ, Pols HAP, et al: Bone mineral density in children and adolescents: relation to puberty, calcium intake, and physical activity. J Clin Endocrinol Metab 82:57–62, 1997

Byers PH, Wallis GA, Willing MC: Osteogenesis imperfecta: translation of mutation to phenotype. J Med Genet 28:433–442, 1991

Carpenter TO: New perspectives on the biology and treatment of X-linked hypophosphatemic rickets. Pediatr Clin North Am 44:443–446, 1997

Charles JM, Key LL: Developmental spectrum of children with congenital osteopetrosis. J Pediatr 132:371–374, 1998

Chattopadhay N, Mithal A, Brown EM: The calcium-sensing receptor: a window into the physiology and pathophysiology of mineral ion metabolism. Endocr Rev 17:289–307, 1996

De Luca F, Baron J: Molecular biology and clinical importance of the Ca^{2+} sensing receptor. Curr Opin Pediatr 10:435–440, 1998

Dixon PH, Christie PT, Wooding C, et al: Mutational analysis of the PHEX gene in X-linked hypophosphatemia. J Clin Endocrinol Metab 83:3615–3623, 1998

Findlay DM, Martin TJ: Receptors of calciotropic hormones. Horm Metab Res 29:128–134, 1997

Fu GK, Lin D, Zhang MYH, et al: Cloning of human 25-hydroxyvitamin D-1α-hydroxylase and mutations causing vitamin D-dependent rickets type I. Mol Endocrinol 11:1961–1970, 1997

Garnero P, Delmas PD: Biochemical markers of bone turnover: applications for osteoporosis. Endocrinol Metab Clin North Am 27:303–323, 1998

Gerber H-P, Vu TH, Ryan AM, et al: VEGF couples hypertrophic cartilage remodeling, ossification and angiogenesis during endochondral bone formation. Nature Med 6:623–628, 1999

Glorieux FH, Bishop NJ, Plotkin H, et al: Cyclic administration of pamidronate in children with severe osteogenesis imperfecta. N Engl J Med 339:947–952, 1998

Haussler MR, Haussler CA, Jurutka PW, et al: The vitamin D hormone and its nuclear receptor: molecular actions and disease states. J Endocrinol 154:S57–S73, 1997

Juppner H, Schipani E, Bastepe M, et al: The gene responsible for psuedohypoparathyroidism type Ib is paternally imprinted and maps in four unrelated kindreds to chromosome 20q13.3. Proc Natl Acad Sci USA 95:11798–11803, 1998

Key LL Jr: Nutritional rickets. Trends Endocrinol Metab 2:81–85, 1991

Lteif A, Zimmerman D: Bisphosphonates for treatment of childhood hypercalcemia. Pediatrics 102:990–993, 1998

Malloy PJ, Pike JW, Feldman D: The vitamin D receptor and the syndrome of hereditary 1,25-dihydroxyvitamin D–resistant rickets. Endocr Rev 20:156–188, 1999

Markert ML, Hummell DS, Rosenblatt HM, et al: Complete DiGeorge syndrome: persistence of profound immunodeficiency. J Pediatr 132:15–21, 1998

Root AW: Recent advances in the genetics of disorders of calcium homeostasis. Adv Pediatr 43:77–125, 1996

Rubin K: Turner syndrome and osteoporosis: mechanisms and prognosis. Pediatrics 102:481–485, 1998

Simonet WS, Lacey DL, Dunstan CR, et al: Osteoprotegerin: a novel secreted protein involved in regulation of bone density. Cell 89:309–319, 1997

Steendijk R, Hauspie RC: The pattern of growth and growth retardation of patients with hypophosphatemic vitamin D-resistant rickets: a longitudinal study. Eur J Pediatr 151:422–427, 1992

Suda T, Takahashi N, Udagawa N, et al: Modulation of osteoclast differentiation and function by the new members of the tumor necrosis factor receptor and ligand families. Endocr Rev 20:345–357, 1999

Wang JT, Lin CJ, Burridge SM, et al: Genetics of vitamin D 1α-hydroxylase deficiency in 17 families. Am J Hum Genet 63:1694–1702, 1998

Weaver CM, Peacock M, Johnston CC Jr: Adolescent nutrition in the prevention of postmenopausal osteoporosis. J Clin Endocrinol Metab 84:1839–1843, 1999

Weisinger JR, Bellorin-Font E: Magnesium and phosphorus. Lancet 352:391–396, 1998

Whyte MP: Hypophosphatasia and the role of alkaline phosphatase. Endocr Rev 15:439–461, 1999

24.13 DISORDERS OF MAGNESIUM METABOLISM

Colin D. Rudolph

24.13.1   REGULATION OF MAGNESIUM

Magnesium (Mg^{2+}) is the second most common cation in the intracellular fluid. It is important for normal bone formation and is an essential component of critical enzymatic reactions including many kinases, ATPase and GTPase. Body magnesium is distributed such that 54% is in the skeleton as a component of bone, 45% is in the intracellular fluid, and only 1% is in the extracellular space. Approximately 0.3% Mg^{2+} is distributed in plasma; about 30% is bound to protein. Normal serum concentrations of Mg^{2+} range from 1.5 to 2.3 mg/dL (0.7–1.0 mmol/L). Serum concentrations of magnesium in neonates have been reported to be somewhat lower, with total serum magnesium levels of 1.4 to 2.0 mg/dL (0.58–0.83 mmol/L) and ionized Mg^{2+} levels of 0.97 to 1.26 mg/dL (0.40–0.56 mmol/L).

Magnesium is ubiquitous in foods, but it is particularly abundant in dairy products, bread, cereals, leafy vegetables, and meat. Intake varies between 200 and 600 mg per day in normal adults. Thirty to 50% is absorbed, predominantly in the distal small bowel. The mechanism of absorption is unclear (either a saturable carrier-mediated mechanism or a paracellular route), but rare genetic isolated defects in intestinal magnesium absorption suggest a specific magnesium transport mechanism exists. Vitamin D enhances intestinal Mg^{2+} absorption but to a much lesser extent than for Ca^{2+} absorption. The efficiency of Mg^{2+} absorption decreases with increasing intake. Absorption increases following magnesium depletion, during periods of rapid growth, and with ingestion of large quantities of phosphate.

Magnesium is primarily excreted by the kidney. In the adult, the proximal tubule reabsorbs only 10% of the filtered magnesium (fractional reabsorption of sodium and calcium is in excess of 70%), but in the neonate, the proximal tubule reabsorbs about 70% of the filtered magnesium. The permeability of the proximal tubule changes during development so that less Mg^{2+} is reabsorbed in the proximal tubule. In the adult, about 70% of filtered magnesium is reabsorbed in the thick ascending limb of the loop of Henle by a passive mechanism through a paracellular pathway. The remaining

5 to 10% of filtered Mg^{2+} is absorbed in the distal convoluted tubule by active transcellular transport through selective channels on the apical membrane. Magnesium entry across the apical membrane is the rate-limiting step in transepithelial reabsorption. Cellular Mg^{2+} is extruded at the basolateral membrane by a sodium-dependent exchange mechanism. Changes in distal tubular absorption of Mg^{2+} provide for selective magnesium conservation when intake decreases or if there are increased losses due to intestinal malabsorption. Increased serum Mg^{2+} or Ca^{2+} inhibits Mg^{2+} uptake through activation of the extracellular Ca^{2+}/Mg^{2+}-sensing receptor (CASR).

24.13.2   HYPOMAGNESEMIA

ymptoms of hypomagnesemia include neuromuscular, cardiovascular, and metabolic complications. Most occur in association with hypocalcemia, which results from reduced parathyroid hormone secretion and target-tissue resistance to the actions of parathyroid hormone due to hypomagnesemia. Neuromuscular symptoms include lethargy, nausea, muscle cramps, paresthesia, and mental abnormalities such as irritability and disorientation. Esophageal spasm leading to dysphagia, tremor, fasciculations, tetany, and seizure may occur. Cardiovascular complications include prolongation of the PR and QT intervals and flattening of the T waves with ventricular dysrhythmias. Hypomagnesemia, like hypokalemia, predisposes patients to digitalis toxicity. Because magnesium is required for Na,K ATPase activity, Mg^{2+} deficiency can cause potassium deficiency by inhibiting K^+ reabsorption in the proximal tubule.

A variety of inherited or acquired conditions can lead to hypomagnesemia (Table 24-53). Decreased intake rarely causes hypomagnesemia since magnesium is present in many foods; if intake is reduced, the kidney compensates by increasing absorption. Administration of parenteral nutrition without added magnesium or prolonged protein-calorie malnutrition may result in hypomagnesemia. Endocrine disorders including hyperparathyroidism, hypothyroidism, and diabetes mellitus may cause hypomagnesemia. Most alterations in magnesium balance are due to congenital or acquired disorders that decrease gastrointestinal absorption or increase renal losses of magnesium.

GASTROINTESTINAL CAUSES OF HYPOMAGNESEMIA

MALABSORPTION   Disorders such as short bowel syndrome, celiac disease, and chronic pancreatitis are all associated with hypomagnesemia. Biliary or small bowel fistulas may also result in increased losses of magnesium since the secreted Mg^{2+} is not reabsorbed in the distal small intestine.

FAMILIAL HYPOMAGNESEMIA   This rare inherited disorder, also known as familial hypomagnesemia with secondary hypocalcemia (HSH), is characterized by extremely low levels of serum concentrations of magnesium and by hypocalcemia. The usual age of presentation is within the first months of life, when severe hypomagnesemia results in hypocalcemia, and symptoms include restlessness, tremor, tetany, and seizures. The specific cause of the disorder is unknown, but it is thought to result from a defect in intestinal magnesium absorption. Urinary magnesium absorption is normal. Genetic linkage mapping has identified a mutation of chromosome 9 (9q12-9q22.2) associated with this disorder in three Bedouin kindreds. Patients treated with oral supplementation

TABLE 24-53
CAUSES OF HYPOMAGNESEMIA

Decreased intake
  Starvation
  Prolonged parenteral nutrition without magnesium supplementation
  Alcoholism
Impaired absorption
  Inherited
    Familial hypomagnesemia with secondary hypocalcemia
  Generalized malabsorptive disorders
    Short bowel syndrome
    Celiac disease
    Fistulas (small bowel, biliary)
    Chronic diarrhea
    Laxative abuse
    Chronic pancreatitis
    Cholestatic liver disease
Renal losses
  Inherited
    Gitelman syndrome
    Bartter syndrome
    Hypomagnesemia with secondary hypocalcemia
    Infantile primary hypomagnesemia with autosomal dominant inheritance
    Infantile primary hypomagnesemia with recessive inheritance
    Idiopathic hypermagnesuria
    Hypomagnesemia with hypercalciuria and nephrocalcinosis
    Autosomal dominant hypoparathyroidism
    Familial hypocalciuric hypercalcemia
  Drug-induced
    Diuretics (except potassium-sparing agents)
    Aminoglycosides
    Carbenicillin, ticarcillin
    Amphotericin B
    Cisplatin
    Pentamidine
    Cyclosporine, tacrolimus
    Fluoride poisoning
  Other
    Renal tubular acidosis
    Postobstructive diuresis
    Interstitial nephritis
    Diabetes mellitus with glucosuria
Endocrine/Metabolic
  Hypoparathyroidism
  Hyperthyroidism
  Vitamin D overdose
  Primary hyperaldosteronism
  Hungry bone syndrome
Other
  Burns
  Sepsis

of magnesium sulfate in doses of 0.5 to 0.75 mmol/kg/day have had normal growth and development but have a life-long requirement for Mg^{2+} supplementation.

RENAL CAUSES OF HYPOMAGNESEMIA

INHERITED DISORDERS   *Gitelman syndrome* often presents in late childhood with hypokalemic metabolic alkalosis and low serum concentration of magnesium. Patients may be asymptomatic, or symptoms may be of such severity as to cause hypomagnesemic tetany. Patients have hypocalciuria and renal magnesium wasting but do not have nephrocalcinosis. Some children present with growth retardation resulting from rickets. A variant of Gitelman syndrome has been described that is characterized by intermittent electrolyte abnormalities but severe growth failure associated with growth hormone deficiency, partial vasopressin insufficiency, and empty sella syndrome. Gitelman syndrome is genetically linked to a locus at 16q13, with causative mutations demonstrated in the chlorothiazide-sensitive NaCl cotranporter in the distal convoluted tubule. The reason for renal magnesium wasting with this defect is not totally understood. Treatment with oral magnesium corrects the magnesium deficit but not the metabolic alkalosis.

Infantile isolated renal magnesium wasting is an autosomal-dominant condition associated with few symptoms other than chondrocalcinosis. Patients always have hypocalciuria and mild hypomagnesemia. The disorder maps to chromosome 11q23 in two large Dutch families. An autosomal-recessive variant of this disorder has also been described.

Hypomagnesemia with hypercalciuria and nephrocalcinosis is a distinct autosomal-recessive syndrome characterized by persistent hypomagnesemia, marked hypercalciuria, and unlike Gitelman syndrome, early nephrocalcinosis. It is distinguished from other conditions by the absence of infantile hypocalcemic tetany and normal plasma potassium. Other distinctive features include ocular abnormalities, including myopia, nystagmus, and chorioretinitis; hearing impairment; tetany; seizures; chondrocalcinosis; rickets; and hypertension. The disorder has been associated with mutations in the gene that codes for a tight junctional protein located in the paracellular pathway of the thin ascending loop of Henle, *claudin 16*. The hypomagnesemia does not improve with oral magnesium administration. Early renal transplantation is often required due to the nephrocalcinosis; calcium and magnesium handling is normal following transplantation.

Inherited disorders of the extracellular CASR are also associated with hypomagnesemia (see Sec. 24.12). Up to 30% of patients with Bartter syndrome (see Sec. 21.11.5) may have hypomagnesemia as a result of renal magnesium wasting.

OTHER DISORDERS WITH RENAL MAGNESIUM LOSSES Drugs that commonly cause hypomagnesemia are listed in Table 24.53. Disorders associated with abnormalities of renal tubular function may also result in magnesium wasting.

TREATMENT OF HYPOMAGNESEMIA

Identification of the underlying cause of hypomagnesemia is often obvious following recognition of the disorder. Secondary causes are far more common than primary defects in magnesium metabolism.

Routine monitoring of serum concentrations of magnesium during administration of parenteral nutrition in patients with malabsorptive disorders, who require refeeding following severe malnutrition, or who are at risk for hungry bone syndrome allows therapy before patients are symptomatic (usually at serum levels below 0.65 mmol/L or 1.5 mg/dL). Mild or asymptomatic cases of hypomagnesemia can be treated with oral supplementation using magnesium oxide, magnesium chloride, or magnesium hydroxide. Overly aggressive oral supplementation will lead to diarrhea. Severe symptomatic hypomagnesemia may be treated with magnesium sulfate given intravenously. Adult doses of 2 to 4 g of 50% magnesium sulfate (16.6–33 meq) diluted in dextrose can be safely administered over 30 to 60 min. With life-threatening arrhythmias the same dose may be given by intravenous push. Pediatric doses of 1 meq/kg are effective. Subsequent doses of 0.5 meq/kg/d should be given over the following 3 to 5 days to replete body stores (1.0 mL/kg/d of 50% magnesium sulfate [USP]). In neonatal hypomagnesemia, intravenous administration of 6 mg elemental magnesium sulfate over 1 hour has been shown to be effective.

24.13.3   HYPERMAGNESEMIA

Symptomatic hypermagnesemia is infrequent and usually iatrogenic. Manifesting with neuromuscular blockade and respiratory depression, hypermagnesemia is most common in patients with renal impairment but can occur with administration of magnesium-containing antacids, purgatives, or rectal administration of magnesium-containing solutions. Hypermagnesemia can also occur in Addison disease, hypothroidism, lithium therapy, and with the milk-alkali syndrome.

Symptoms can be transiently reversed by the intravenous administration of calcium chloride. Insulin and dextrose can be administered to promote influx of magnesium into the intracellular space, similar to therapy for hyperkalemia. In severe cases, dialysis may be necessary.

References

Caddell JL: Magnesium in perinatal care and infant health. Magnes Trace Elem 10:229–250, 1991

Cole DEC, Quamme GA: Inherited disorders of renal magnesium handling. J Am Soc Nephrol 11:1937–1947, 2000

Walder RY, Shalev H, Brennan TMH, et al: Familial hypomagnesemia maps to chromosome 9q, not to the X chromosome: genetic linkage mapping and analysis of a balanced translocation breakpoint. Hum Mole Genet 6:1491–1497

THE NERVOUS SYSTEM

David Pleasure and Darryl C. De Vivo, Associate Editors

25.1 A CLINICAL APPROACH TO NEUROLOGIC DISEASE

Darryl C. De Vivo and David Pleasure

We have just exited the "decade of the brain." The advances in neuroscience achieved during the past 10 years have been stunning, particularly in molecular neurogenetics and developmental neurobiology. Our society will be the beneficiary of these successes because the social and economic burdens of potentially chronic and devastating neurological afflictions are enormous. Approximately one-third to one-half of infants and children admitted to tertiary pediatric care facilities exhibit evidence of nervous system dysfunction. This statistic underscores the relatively high incidence of neurologic disturbances in this selected patient population.

To some extent, this statistic reflects our progress in other areas of pediatrics. For example, the successes in salvaging infants born very prematurely and infants with complex congenital heart lesions has produced a new population of patients at risk of developing cerebral palsy, mental retardation, epilepsy, and learning disabilities. The value of the newer brain imaging techniques in detecting clinically silent intracranial hemorrhages in these premature infants is noteworthy. The child with leukemia or with a primary brain tumor is another example of a patient at risk for developing neurologic complications either from the disease process itself or from the vigorous treatment that must be directed at the nervous system. In addition, we are now recognizing abnormalities of the nervous system before patients become symptomatic. The development of sophisticated brain imaging techniques that includes computed tomography (CT); magnetic resonance (MR) imaging, angiography (MRA), and spectroscopy (MRS); positron emission tomography (PET); single-photon emission tomography (SPECT); and near-infrared spectroscopy (NIRS) has enabled physicians to recognize and diagnose intracranial and intraspinal abnormalities safely and early. Similarly, clinical applications of neurophysiologic techniques, event-mediated potentials in particular, have uncovered other abnormalities within the brain. In contrast to the use of the electroencephalogram (EEG), which reveals the integrated activities of neuronal populations within cortical regions having complex and multipurpose functions, evoked potentials can be used to assess the conduction and the processing of information within specific sensory pathways. Consequently, it is now possible to evaluate the integrity of the visual, auditory, and somatosensory pathways selectively and to uncover single and multiple lesions within the nervous system.

The sections that follow in this chapter are organized to present a comprehensive overview of neurologic diseases as they evolve developmentally in a static or progressive manner or as they are acquired during early infancy or childhood. The starting point in each section is the neurologic history and examination. The neurologist then selects from the array of sophisticated techniques available to substantiate the clinical diagnosis and to prepare the patient for therapeutic intervention.

Eliciting a careful history and performing a neurologic examination remain the cornerstones for initial evaluation of children suspected of having neurologic disease. The skillful physician will frequently narrow down the diagnostic considerations as the older patient participates in the interview or the younger patient wanders about the office. The physician's approach to the child with neurologic disease must be tailored to fit the circumstances. The physician must sort out the factors contributing to the neurologic complaint and make the necessary observations during the examination before deciding whether to wait or to proceed rapidly with various ancillary diagnostic procedures. Unfortunately, the development of CT and MR imaging has dulled our clinical senses and diminished our diagnostic acumen. Not every patient needs a diagnostic procedure; rather, these procedures should be considered only after a detailed history has been collected and a careful examination performed. In fact, one should view the advent of these brain-imaging techniques as an opportunity to refine further the clinicoradiologic correlation and to obviate the need for the more invasive procedures frequently needed in the past, which were associated with a higher risk to the patient.

NEUROLOGIC HISTORY

The purpose of the history is to define the nature and temporal profile of the neurologic complaint. One needs to determine whether the problem is congenital or acquired, chronic or episodic, static or progressive. Recognition of similar complaints in other family members or relatives is relevant because many neurologic disorders are genetically determined. As much history as possible should be obtained from the child. However, a hyperactive child may need to be excused from the room so that the distracted and harassed parents can give the physician their full attention. When possible, children should describe the symptoms in their own words, because the patient's perception of the complaints is the basis for the physician's interpretation. If the complaints are paroxysmal and stereotyped, it is frequently useful to ask the patient to describe the most recent episode in detail. The symptoms must be defined clearly because some commonly used terms have different meanings to different people. It is necessary, for example, to explore whether the "dizzy" child is experiencing vertigo or faintness. The history should be obtained from the patient and parents, but observations of teachers or others are also often of importance. This is particularly relevant when episodic disturbances are associated with altered consciousness. Noting the time when the ictus occurred may provide clues to the disorder. Typically, for example, a young child with ketotic hypoglycemia may present with a convulsive disorder that often occurs on Sunday about midmorning. The circumstances surrounding head trauma may be most important. Thus, a child who was noted to slump to the ground before striking his or her head may well have had a convulsion or an intracranial catastrophe leading to the fall and secondary head trauma. Also, a history of antecedent diseases may explain why a child is presenting in coma; these include metabolic disorders (especially diabetes mellitus), hematologic disorders, congenital heart disease, recent viral illness, and acute otitis media.

Children presenting with headaches, abdominal pain, or reluctance to attend school may well have associated neurologic disturbances. Contributing factors may include previously unrecognized mental retardation, specific learning disabilities, and depression. Less frequently, such complaints may be the harbingers of more serious neurologic illness such as hydrocephalus or subacute sclerosing panencephalitis. In addition, systemic diseases such as acute glomerulonephritis with hypertension may appear initially with neurologic disturbances.

Certain complaints commonly encountered by pediatricians immediately bring to mind specific diagnostic considerations. *Delayed development* during the first months or years of life may imply a static or a progressive process. Information concerning the prenatal, perinatal, and early neonatal period is often helpful in identifying an etiologic factor. Recognition of mental retardation may first appear as a delay in language and speech development. Other considerations include deafness and, less frequently, a seizure disorder or autism. Loss of previously acquired psychomotor skills implies a progressive disorder of the nervous system and requires further testing.

Large or small head size often implies intracranial abnormalities, although this predisposition may be familial. It is necessary, therefore, to evaluate the head sizes of other family members. Macrocephaly and microcephaly are generally accompanied by deficits in psychosocial development, but there are many exceptions. *Swallowing difficulties* may be associated with brainstem abnormalities or with neuromuscular dysfunction. *Disturbances in vision or ocular motility* can develop abruptly or gradually. Sudden loss of vision suggests optic neuritis, whereas gradual diminution suggests a slowly progressive process such as optic glioma or a degenerative disease. Diplopia implies an imbalance between the movements of the two eyes and is often associated with increased intracranial pressure (cranial nerve VI palsy). Head tilt may result from involvement of the trochlear nerve or the superior oblique muscle. More often, head tilt implies a disturbance in the vestibulocerebellar connections in association with a posterior fossa tumor.

Disorders of movement must be clearly defined. Such disorders may include tics, developmental clumsiness, ataxia, chorea, myoclonus, or dystonia. A tic represents a stereotyped behavior or mannerism that can be suppressed voluntarily by the patient. When this is accompanied by vocalizations and obscene utterances, one should consider Gilles de la Tourette syndrome. Developmental clumsiness often accompanies minimal cerebral dysfunction. Ataxia may involve the limbs (appendicular) or the trunk (axial) and represents involvement of cerebellar pathways. Unilateral appendicular ataxia suggests a lesion of the ipsilateral cerebellar hemisphere, and isolated axial ataxia is compatible with a midline cerebellar lesion. Generalized ataxia can occur as a consequence of loss of sensory input to the cerebellum (eg, in the Guillain-Barré syndrome), or as a consequence of the toxicity of antiepileptic drugs. Intermittent ataxia suggests a metabolic disease; acute onset, an infectious-inflammatory process involving the brain; and gradual development, a neoplastic or heredodegenerative process. Both chorea and myoclonus involve sudden jerky movements of selected muscle groups. Chorea is asynchronous, whereas myoclonus is often symmetric. Athetosis is characterized by a slow writhing movement. Dystonia

is manifested by sustained spasms of the neck, trunk, or limb muscles resulting in a fixed postural deformity; it may be a manifestation of idiopathic torsion dystonia, hepatolenticular degeneration (Wilson disease), or a static encephalopathy associated with perinatal trauma. Choreoathetosis and dystonia may represent toxic manifestations of medications, including phenytoin and phenothiazines.

Certain neurologic complaints may be *paroxysmal* in nature, such as recurrent unresponsiveness or headaches. The differential diagnosis includes seizure states, vascular or tension headaches, and, rarely, certain metabolic disorders.

Children who demonstrate *poor performance at school* may have specific learning disabilities, previously unrecognized mental retardation, or depression. With gradual deterioration in school performance accompanied by changes in personality and behavior, one should consider an intracranial neoplasm or a degenerative process that is biochemical or infectious in origin.

NEUROLOGIC EXAMINATION

GENERAL PRINCIPLES Accurate observation provides the basis for correct interpretation. The clinician must learn to document observations accurately and to be careful in the use of terminology, because not all persons necessarily use precisely the same definitions (various neurologic terms are defined later in this chapter).

The general physical examination frequently provides clues to the neurologic disease. Vital signs and anthropometric measurements must be recorded accurately. The head circumference of all infants and young children and, where appropriate, the head circumferences of other family members should be recorded. Inspection of the hair, nails, and skin may allow an immediate diagnosis (eg, neurocutaneous syndrome or steely hair disease [Menkes syndrome]). The Wood's lamp is useful in bringing out depigmented skin lesions characteristic of tuberous sclerosis; this test should be performed on all infants presenting with infantile spasms. Examination of the lungs and the breathing pattern may uncover disturbances in respiration that reflect brainstem disease or neuromuscular abnormalities. Similarly, the presence of a mass in the abdomen or hepatosplenomegaly may provide clues to the nature of a focal or diffuse process within the central nervous system. Asymmetries of the limbs may suggest atrophy or hemihypertrophy and provide clues to the underlying disease.

The neurologic examination is traditionally compartmentalized: mental status, craniospinal examination, cranial nerve examination, motor and sensory examinations, evaluation of coordination, and assessment of autonomic function. With a young infant or child, a complete neurologic examination is best conducted without following a rigid format. The variables of age and cooperation can tax the skills of the examiner in this regard, but with some imagination, sensitivity, patience, and increasing experience one can expect to complete the examination satisfactorily in every instance.

MENTAL STATUS Orientation, memory, intellect, judgment, and affect are the elements of mentation that are assessed in children. Many observations relating to these cognitive elements can be made while taking the history. For example, the child's ability to converse can be a measure of vocabulary, ability to use language, and general fund of knowledge. Also, one develops a general impression of the child's intelligence and judgment. The child's ability to recall personal historical information reflects memory capacity. Responses to stress and frustration may also provide insight into mood and adaptive behavior. Specific pencil-and-paper tasks can augment these observations. One should note the child's hand preference. Handedness frequently appears by 3 years of age and is well established by 5 years of age. The appearance of handedness at a younger age often implies a deficit affecting the contralateral limb. The expectations of a child's performance are predicted on the physician's awareness of the ages at which children usually achieve certain major developmental milestones (see Sec. 1.2). Older children should be asked to write their names and the alphabet or, if possible, a sentence. The drawing of various geometric figures such as circle, square, triangle, and diamond should be mastered at the ages 3, 4, 5, and 6 to 7 years, respectively. Similarly, one should assess the ability of older children to read and retain material. Often it is useful to ask a child to draw a person or to draw some other familiar object such as a house, clock, or flower; the quality of the performance will provide the experienced examiner with a reasonable assessment of the child's intelligence. These impressions can be buttressed by formal psychometric testing when necessary. Sequential observations will also provide valuable information as to whether the child is developing normally or is regressing.

CRANIOSPINAL EXAMINATION The basic principles of inspection, palpation, percussion, and auscultation are used to evaluate the cranium and the spine. The contour of the skull may be long and narrow in the anteroposterior diameter (scaphocephaly), suggesting premature closure of the sagittal suture, or the contour may be broad in the biparietal diameter (brachycephaly), as seen with premature closure of the coronal sutures or with bilateral subdural effusions in infancy. Midline defects over the nasion, occipital area, or lumbosacral area suggest an underlying abnormality such as a lipoma, dermoid, meningocele, or encephalocele. The fontanelles may be normal, large, or small, bulging or concave, and the venous pattern over the scalp may be prominent, suggesting cerebral venous sinus occlusion or hydrocephalus. Percussion of the skull may produce a sound reminiscent of that from a cracked pot (Macewen sign), indicating split cranial sutures and increased intracranial pressure. Points of tenderness over the spine suggest paraspinal abnormality or infection of the epidural or intervertebral disc spaces. Auscultation over the cranium, carotids in the neck, and spine may reveal intracranial or intraspinal bruits indicative of an underlying vascular malformation. Bruits, however, are common in infants and children and usually do not indicate pathology. Transillumination of the infant's skull with a bright light should be performed routinely; the transillumination may be diffusely abnormal where there are subdural effusions or hydranencephaly or focally abnormal with porencephaly. The spinal contour should be noted to determine whether the lumbar lordosis is accentuated, as in Duchenne muscular dystrophy, or whether there is a scoliotic deformity, as occurs with neurofibromatosis, Friedreich ataxia, or intramedullary neoplasms.

CRANIAL NERVES Olfaction (cranial nerve I) can be tested by using appropriate fragrances. Trauma can damage the olfactory nerves as they pass through the cribriform plate. A few syndromes, such as Kallmann syndrome, are also associated with loss of smell (anosmia).

The eyes and ocular fundi should be examined carefully. The condition of the sclera, bulbar conjunctiva, cornea, iris, and lens should be noted, as well as pupillary reactivity to bright light and to stroking of the skin on the lateral aspect of the neck (ciliospinal reflex producing pupillary dilation). The optic discs, maculae, retinal pigmentary pattern, and vasculature should be assessed. Pseudopapilledema may be familial, and examination of the parents is useful. Peripapillary gliosis and enlargement of the blind spot char-

acterize chronic papilledema. Decreased visual acuity is associated with papillitis and retrobulbar neuritis. Spontaneous pulsations of the retinal veins are noted bilaterally in 70% and unilaterally in 90% of normal individuals; absence of spontaneous pulsations may be normal or may indicate raised intracranial pressure. Paleness of a nerve head indicates optic atrophy. Various abnormalities may be noted in the macular region, including a cherry-red spot indicative of several different forms of neurodegenerative disease and dispersion of retinal pigment characteristic of neuronal ceroid lipofuscinosis. Intraocular hemorrhage may be retinal or preretinal (subhyaloid). Retinal hemorrhaging is seen with acute elevations of intracranial pressure, and these lesions may also be noted in newborn infants. Preretinal hemorrhages are almost always associated with subarachnoid hemorrhage. Both types of hemorrhage may be noted after head trauma. For older children, visual acuity may be tested in each eye. The ability of an infant or young child to fix on and follow small objects or to pick up small food crumbs implies relative preservation of visual acuity.

The integrity of ocular motility requires normal functioning of cranial nerves III, IV, and VI. An infant's eye movements can be evaluated by various maneuvers, including the use of a rotating drum (opticokinetic nystagmus), spinning the infant through 360 degrees of arc, and tilting an infant who is held vertically into a semiprone position. These maneuvers allow both horizontal and vertical saccades to be assessed.

Cranial nerve III palsies may be partial or complete. A complete third nerve lesion, as may be seen in uncal herniation syndrome, produces ptosis, a dilated pupil, and a "down-and-out" position of the eye. Partial lesions may produce only ptosis or involve some of the innervated ocular muscles (medial rectus, inferior rectus, superior rectus, and inferior oblique muscles). Tilting of the head to one side may be a sign of contralateral superior oblique muscle weakness (cranial nerve IV). Cranial nerve VI palsy limits abduction of the eye (lateral rectus muscle) and often accompanies increased intracranial pressure. A lateral gaze preference can be seen with either supratentorial or infratentorial pathology, and skew deviation implies abnormality within the brainstem tegmentum. Nystagmus should be described according to its fast component, the direction of gaze in which it is maximal, and the relative involvement of each eye. Pendular nystagmus may be maximal in a particular horizontal or vertical plane. Rotatory nystagmus is most suggestive of dysfunction of the vestibular apparatus. Vertical nystagmus is compatible with intrinsic disease of the brainstem. Usually the fast component is up (up-beating nystagmus). Down-beating nystagmus suggests abnormality in the lower brainstem (cervicomedullary) region. Retraction nystagmus is usually associated with an abnormality in the mesencephalon, whereas seesaw nystagmus often accompanies lesions in the area of the optic chiasm. Chaotic, conjugate, random multidirectional saccades, termed *opsoclonus,* occasionally accompanied by myoclonic jerking of the limbs, may be a manifestation of neuroblastoma.

The corneal reflex and facial sensation should be tested in infants and children. Absence of a corneal reflex may result from a sensory defect (cranial nerve V) or a motor defect (cranial nerve VII). If the latter, touching the cornea on the affected side will bother the patient, will elicit closure of the other eye, and will often be accompanied by increased tearing. Asymmetries of the face are frequently noted, but these observations need not necessarily imply weakness (cranial nerve VII). Perhaps the most common cause of asymmetry of the lower face associated with crying is asymmetric depression of the corner of the mouth, a function that is subserved by the depressor angulari oris muscle. Lower motor neuron lesions of the facial nerve produce ipsilateral weakness of both the upper and lower face. In contrast, upper motor neuron lesions of the facial nerve involve the lower face on the opposite side but spare the upper face. Hearing (cranial nerve VIII) can be assessed grossly on the basis of cessation of spontaneous activity as an aural stimulus is presented to one ear or the other. In older children, conductive hearing loss can be distinguished from sensorineural hearing loss by the Weber and Rinne tests. Brainstem auditory evoked potentials have become useful for evaluating hearing in young infants and uncooperative children. Involvement of the lower cranial nerves (IX, X, XI, and XII) may be expected in several neurologic disorders, including intrinsic or extraaxial tumors in or around the lower brainstem, Arnold-Chiari malformation, syringobulbia, Leigh disease, and infantile spinal muscular atrophy (Werdnig-Hoffmann disease). Inspiratory stridor may be a manifestation of cranial nerve X abnormality, with resulting weakness of vocal cord abduction.

SENSATION With proper encouragement, most children more than 3 years of age will cooperate for testing of peripheral sensations, including responses to pinprick, cold, light touch, vibration, and fine movement of the joints. Testing of cortical modalities of sensation will be precluded unless the peripheral sensory mechanisms are intact. Children more than 5 years of age frequently cooperate in tests to evaluate graphesthesia, stereognosis, bilateral simultaneous stimulation, and two-point discrimination. The ability to touch one's nose with a finger or to stand erect with feet together while the eyes are closed is a measure of proprioception. Inability to perform these tasks with eyes closed implies a sensory defect. Rarely, an infant will have a delay in walking because of such a sensory abnormality.

MUSCULATURE Observation of the child during walking, posture holding, and rising after lying on the floor will often alert the examiner to patterns of weakness that can then be further evaluated by formal muscle testing. Focal or diffuse weakness may be associated with altered tendon reflexes. Lower motor neuron lesions are typically associated with decreased tendon reflexes, whereas upper motor neuron lesions are associated with exaggerated tendon reflexes and an extensor response of the great toe after plantar stimulation (Babinski sign). Decreased tendon reflexes in the arms associated with increased tendon reflexes in the legs may imply focal spinal cord abnormality in the cervical region. One may expect disturbances in bladder and bowel function under such circumstances. Focal muscular atrophy may be seen in fascioscapulohumeral dystrophy, focal hypertrophy of a limb may be seen with neurofibromatosis, and diffuse muscular hypertrophy may be seen in children with myotonia congenita or other neuromuscular disorders.

COORDINATION Smooth, coordinated fine and gross motor movements demand integrated function of the pyramidal and extrapyramidal systems in the nervous system. Clumsiness and slowness of movement may reflect spasticity, whereas irregularities in resting posture or volitional movement may indicate disease of the extrapyramidal system. Careful examination of infants and children while they are relaxed and quiet and while they are sustaining a posture or are moving will help to differentiate the many forms of movement disorders that can appear in this age group. As a rule, spasticity becomes more apparent when a child runs, whereas dystonia and other extrapyramidal signs lessen. Observation of a child's gait is often informative. A decreased swing of the arm may reflect a subtle hemiparesis. Bilateral slapping of the feet, with excessive elevation of the knee (steppage gait), suggests a peripheral neurop-

athy. A waddling style accompanies weakness of the pelvic girdle musculature, whereas a stiffening of the lower lumbar area and a disinclination to walk suggest pain (analgic gait) often accompanying paravertebral infection or inflammation.

TENDON REFLEXES Tendon reflexes may be elicited at all ages. The wrist and ankle jerks may be difficult to elicit in newborn infants and are absent in young premature infants. Increases or decreases in resting muscular tone will dampen or exaggerate the tendon reflexes, respectively. Therefore, evaluation of the symmetry of reflex activity should consider the degree of resting muscular tone and the positioning of the head (tonic neck effect). This observation is particularly true in young infants and in children who have antecedent brain injury. The Babinski sign, when fully developed, should be viewed as pathologic at any age. Similarly, significant asymmetries in the initial responses of the great toes to plantar stimulation should also be viewed as abnormal. Cortical release signs, including sucking, rooting, grasping, and palmomental responses, normally present in young infants up to about 1 year of age; if present beyond then, these signs suggest diffuse cerebral dysfunction, usually associated with depression of the level of consciousness.

EXAMINATION OF THE NEWBORN INFANT

Certain of the above-mentioned tests and observations cannot be applied to infants, but other rather specific observations are needed. In general, the observations and elicited responses are functions of the maturation of the developing nervous system. A comprehensive discussion of the neuromuscular system in infants is presented in Sec. 2.8.2. The quality of the clinical observations will be determined by the medical circumstances. Optimally, one would want to observe the infant at rest, followed by arousal. While the infant is resting, one can search for dysmorphic features or distinguishing cutaneous lesions and note posture and spontaneous movements. Palpation and auscultation of the cranium to assess the fontanelles, sutures, and blood flow represent the first intrusion. More vigorous stimulation increases the state and persistence of arousal. Notation is made of alertness, sustained responsiveness, irritability, and jitteriness. Asymmetries of tone and movement may be seen as clues to lateralizing abnormalities. Facial expression when alert and crying are indications of cranial nerve function. Asymmetry of the lower face with crying commonly represents congenital hypoplasia or absence of the depressor anguli oris muscle, a benign condition not to be confused with a facial palsy. Assessment of phasic tone, postural tone, and integrated reflexes is informative, with particular attention directed at the Moro reflex, tonic neck reflex, and withdrawal reflex. Finally, ophthalmoscopy and measurement of head circumference should be performed. These observations are left for the end of the examination because touching the head often upsets the infant. Careful serial measurements of head circumferences are very important during early infancy. Of note, the newborn head circumference of breech-positioned infants is approximately 2 cm longer than vertex-positioned infants. Large or small head circumferences at birth may have particular importance regarding prenatal events and postnatal development.

Those disorders that most frequently affect young infants must be kept in mind to heighten one's index of suspicion when carrying out neurologic examinations in the neonatal nursery. Such disorders include:

- developmental malformations and related genetic syndromes, often associated with nervous system involvement;
- neuromuscular disorders involving anterior horn cells or the skeletal musculature, often associated with depressed tendon reflexes or absence of tendon reflexes and decreased muscular tone;
- perinatal trauma to the cranium, spine, or brachial plexus; metabolic insults, including hypoxia, usually with attendant ischemia, hypoglycemia, hypocalcemia, or hyperbilirubinemia, each often associated with decreased responsiveness and seizures;
- intracranial hemorrhage, with the type of hemorrhage being influenced by gestational age (intracerebral periventricular, intraventricular, or cerebellar hemorrhages in premature infants and subarachnoid hemorrhage in full-term infants);
- perinatal infections, usually of viral or bacterial origin, associated with decreased responsiveness and convulsions;
- and congenital intracranial malignancies.

Careful inspection of the young infant for adventitious movements or convulsions; examination of the ocular fundi for hemorrhages and chorioretinitis; and assessment of muscular tone, reflex activity, and stimulus-induced responsiveness provide the necessary clues in evaluating the infant at risk for these more common neonatal neurologic insults. Examination of the parents may provide critical clues to the diagnosis of the neurologic disorders of the newborn infant.

LABORATORY PROCEDURES

Selection of appropriate studies is predicated on the physician's impressions after completing the neurologic history and examination and formulating a differential diagnosis. A child presenting with a paroxysmal complaint might undergo electrophysiological studies and psychometric testing, whereas a child presenting with evidence of increased intracranial pressure would require MR imaging or other contrast procedures. Generally, one should use only those procedures that will support the diagnosis and rule out other considerations, with emphasis being placed on the noninvasive procedures.

LUMBAR PUNCTURE   Lumbar puncture should be done carefully and deliberately. The patient should be reassured about the safety of the procedure, but sedation may be required. Intradermal instillation of local anesthetic 5 minutes before or application of a topical anesthetic cream 60 to 90 minutes before the procedure is helpful. The opening pressure should be recorded before significant cerebrospinal fluid (CSF) is lost. The CSF normally appears crystal clear and colorless, and is essentially acellular. Serial samples should be analyzed if the puncture is traumatic; if the CSF fails to clear with successive aliquots, intracranial hemorrhage is likely. The red blood cell count should be determined for the first and last tubes under such circumstances. Xanthochromia develops within several hours after an intracranial hemorrhage. A few lymphocytes per cubic millimeter are normal. More than 5 cells per cubic millimeter or any number of polymorphonuclear leukocytes should be viewed with suspicion. The CSF glucose concentration is usually two-thirds of the blood concentration in the postabsorptive state. Infection, intracranial hemorrhage, and occasionally intracranial neoplasms or defective glucose transport across the blood-brain barrier produce hypoglycorrhachia. Appropriate cultures should be obtained whenever an infectious process is being considered. The CSF protein concentration is high (up to 150 mg/dL) in the newborn period; it decreases to the normal range of 10 to 25 mg/dL by 6 weeks of

age, where it remains until puberty, before rising slightly to the normal adult values (20 to 45 mg/dL). Normally there is a gradient in the protein concentration, with the lowest values in the ventricular compartment, intermediate values in the lumbar compartment, and highest values in the subarachnoid spaces over the cerebral convexities. Other metabolites may be measured in the CSF, depending on the diagnostic considerations. The lactate concentrations are elevated in patients with bacterial infections and in patients with subacute necrotizing encephalomyelopathy (Leigh disease). Glycine levels are elevated in nonketotic hyperglycinemia; alpha-fetoprotein, human chorionic gonadotropin, polyamines, and astroglial protein concentrations may be elevated in patients with certain types of intracranial neoplasms. Biogenic amines should be measured when there are disorders of movement. Measles antibody titers are elevated in patients with subacute sclerosing panencephalitis. Oligoclonal bands are present, and the gamma globulin percentage is elevated in a variety of immunologically mediated conditions, including chronic infections and demyelinating processes.

ELECTROPHYSIOLOGICAL STUDIES   Clinical applications of neurophysiological techniques have increased recently; these include electroencephalography, electromyography, nerve conduction studies, and event-mediated potentials.

Electroencephalography is a time-honored procedure for evaluating patients with paroxysmal clinical phenomena. Patients should be studied in the waking and sleeping states, and activation procedures (eg, photic stimulation and hyperventilation) may be used to bring out epileptiform tendencies. Electroencephalography is of value in distinguishing epileptic and nonepileptic causes of episodically disturbed behavior and in identifying focal abnormalities. The classification of epileptic seizures involves both clinical and electroencephalographic criteria, as described in Sec. 25.10.1.

Evoked potentials involve a series of waves recorded at the scalp in response to a sensory stimulus, and can be used to assess conduction and processing of information within specific sensory pathways. Visual (VER), brainstem auditory (BAER), and somatosensory (SER) evoked responses permit selective study of these three afferent central pathways. In addition, electroretinography (ERG) is performed with VER. Evoked potentials are abnormal in patients with demyelinating diseases and in brainstem abnormalities, including gliomas and subacute necrotizing encephalomyelopathy. Electroretinographic results are abnormal in patients with degenerative diseases involving the retina, including Leber congenital amaurosis and neuronal ceroid lipofuscinosis. BAER is also of value for evaluating hearing in infants and young children, because this procedure does not require the cooperation of the sedated patient.

Electromyography (EMG) allows assessment of abnormalities in the neuromuscular system. Nerve conduction velocities are abnormal in various peripheral neuropathies and those degenerative diseases that also affect the peripheral nervous system, such as metachromatic leukodystrophy, Krabbe globoid leukodystrophy, adrenoleukodystrophy, and infantile neuroaxonal dystrophy. EMG and nerve conduction velocities are discussed in more detail in Sec. 25.12. Nerve conduction velocities have also been useful in gauging the gestational age of the premature infant.

NEURORADIOLOGIC PROCEDURES
Jacqueline A. Bello, David Pleasure, and Darryl C. De Vivo

Great advances have been made during the past 20 years in neuroradiology. Noninvasive procedures largely have replaced invasive procedures. As a result, the nervous system can be imaged accurately, expeditiously, and safely. The procedural choices are numerous, and the clinicians must make informed decisions about the appropriate study.

ULTRASOUND STUDIES Ultrasound studies are valuable in evaluating the nervous system of the fetus and the young infant. Intracranial and spinal pathology can be detected by this procedure in utero, and the brain and spinal cord can be effectively imaged after birth, as an adjunct to CT and MR imaging.

RADIOISOTOPE STUDIES Radioisotope scanning has been used less frequently since the advent of CT and MR imaging. Static isotope imaging is of particular value with focal infections of the brain. CSF leaks can be documented by radioisotope scanning. The site of CSF leakage can then be evaluated by water-soluble CT cisternography. Cerebral radionuclide angiography can be used to evaluate perfusion of the brain hemispheres and demonstrate gross abnormalities such as significant carotid artery stenosis or occlusion by means of comparing the relative appearance of isotope in the two hemispheres. Reflux of radioisotope into the ventricular cavities after being instilled in the lumbar compartment is abnormal. A delay in the passage of the radioisotope through the incisura of the tentorium may also indicate a blockage. Instillation of radioisotope into a ventriculoperitoneal shunt is useful in assessing the integrity of such a shunt inserted to treat hydrocephalus. Cerebral blood flow can be assessed by using external detectors to measure the distri-

bution of inhaled xenon 133 (SPECT scan). Positron emission tomography scanning also permits measurement of regional metabolic rate for glucose and for other brain metabolites and is particularly valuable in the presurgical evaluation of children with intractable epilepsy. These radioisotope-dependent procedures are now being complemented by non-radioisotope-based techniques such as magnetic resonance spectroscopy and near-infrared spectroscopy.

RADIOLOGIC EVALUATION Radiologic procedures include plain roentgenograms of the skull, orbits, and spine, which can reveal a variety of abnormalities. Enlarged optic and internal auditory canals may be caused by tumors. Increased intracranial pressure may be associated with splitting of cranial sutures and deformation of the sella turcica and the clinoid processes, and chordomas cause bony erosion of the clivus. A lucent defect in the calvarium suggests an eosinophilic granuloma. Spinal dysraphism is expected when considering congenital intraspinal abnormalities such as diastematomyelia or tethered cord syndrome.

COMPUTED TOMOGRAPHY CT scanning revolutionized the practice of neurology and neurosurgery by providing a noninvasive technique to show the intracranial and intraspinal structures (Fig. 25-1). Head CT scans performed without contrast are adequate for assessing ventricular size and detecting hemorrhage. In the detection of parenchymal, intraventricular, subdural, and epidural blood, CT and MR imaging are comparable. CT is more sensitive in de-

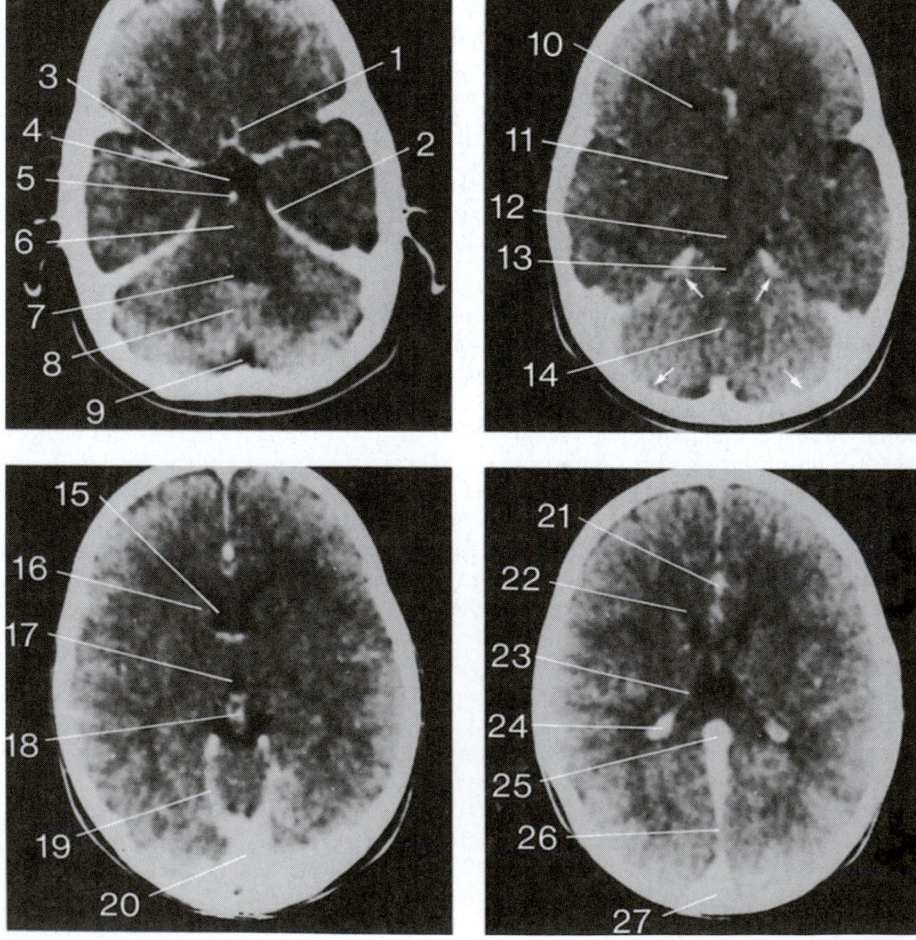

FIGURE 25-1 Normal CT scan with contrast enhancement showing four brain sections. Various intracranial structures can be identified: anterior cerebral artery *(1)*, posterior cerebral artery *(2)*, middle cerebral artery *(3)*, suprasellar cistern *(4)*, basilar artery *(5)*, brainstem *(6)*, IV ventricle *(7)*, cerebellar vermis *(8)*, cisterna magna *(9)*, frontal horn of the lateral ventricle *(10)*, III ventricle *(11)*, mesencephalon *(12)*, quadrigeminal plate cistern *(13)*, tentorium cerebelli *(outlined by arrows) (14)*, frontal horn of lateral ventricle *(15)*, caudate nucleus *(16)*, III ventricle *(17)*, vein of Galen and calcified pineal gland *(18)*, tentorial incisura *(19)*, torcular Herophili *(20)*, falx cerebri in the interhemispheric fissure *(21)*, frontal horn of the lateral ventricle *(22)*, choroid plexus extending into the body of the lateral ventricle *(23)*, choroid plexus *(24)*, vein of Galen *(25)*, straight sinus *(26)*, torcular Herophili *(27)*. *Courtesy of Dr. Paul Sane.*

tecting subarachnoid hemorrhage. In dating hemorrhage, MR imaging is superior because of the distinctive proton relaxation characteristics of the various hemoglobin degradation products. CT scanning with bone detail is the modality of choice in the evaluation of trauma. Contrast-enhanced CT scanning permits better definition of normal structures and pathologic processes that appear isodense on noncontrast scans. Vascular malformations (excluding cavernous malformations) are well shown except perhaps in the setting of acute hemorrhage, where the density of the clot and/or mass effect may obscure abnormal enhancement. Inflammatory and neoplastic lesions resulting in breakdown of the blood-brain barrier are easily detected. Regional cerebral blood flow can be measured by serial CT scanning during the inhalation of *stable* xenon gas. In addition to being nonradioactive, this method has the advantage of higher spatial resolution than the radioisotope blood flow measurement. Intrathecal instillation of nonionic water-soluble contrast material (iohexol) enhances the anatomic resolution of CT by increasing the contrast between the spinal subarachnoid space and the cord.

MAGNETIC RESONANCE IMAGING MR imaging is another noninvasive modality to image the brain and the spinal cord. The technique appears to be free of biological risks, produces exquisite detail of the nervous system (Figs. 25-2 and 25-3), and provides increased sensitivity in the detection of most intraaxial lesions compared with CT scan. Areas poorly seen on CT scan (posterior fossa and spinal cord) can be defined clearly by MR imaging. With the exception of detecting calcification/mineralization, physiological and pathologic tissue characterization by MR imaging surpasses that which is possible by CT.

Various radiofrequency pulse sequences used in MR scanning emphasize the different relaxation characteristics, termed T_1 and T_2 *relaxation times,* of protons placed in a magnetic field. Protons within different body tissues will behave differently, as will protons within normal versus abnormal tissue of a similar type. The three basic pulse sequences generate T_1-weighted images, in which CSF has a signal intensity lower than brain, and fat has a signal intensity

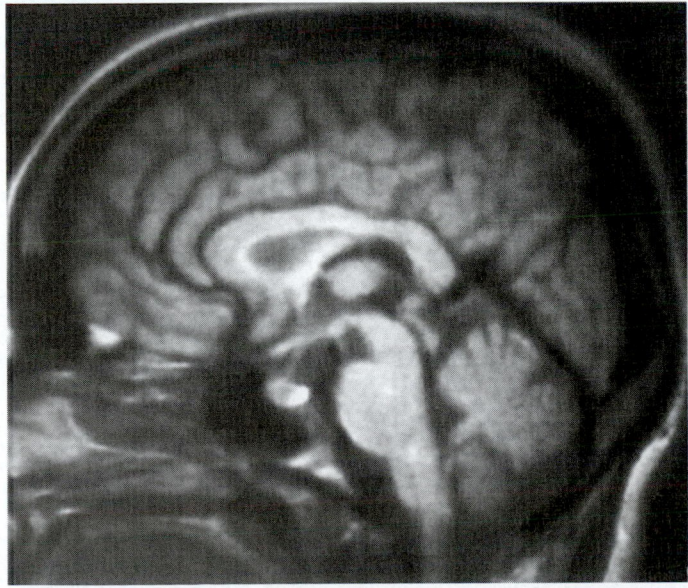

FIGURE 25-2 Normal magnetic resonance image of the brain (sagittal view).

higher than brain; T_2-weighted images, in which the CSF signal is higher than brain; and "balanced" or proton density images, in which CSF is of intermediate signal intensity, similar to brain. Balanced imaging is especially useful in differentiating between CSF and abnormal parenchymal signal near a CSF space (eg, cortical or periventricular), because pathologic tissue will retain the "bright" signal it has on T_2-weighted scans, whereas the signal of CSF will be relatively less intense than on a T_2-weighted scan. Calcification generates signal "void" because of the lack of mobile protons. Flow within structures also generates a signal void because the excited protons leave the plane of the sectioned image before their signal can be registered.

MR imaging enables the diagnosis of venous sinus thrombosis to be made noninvasively. The most widely used MR imaging contrast agent, notably gadolinium (Gd DTPA), is as sensitive in detecting breakdown of the blood-brain barrier as the water-soluble iodinated contrast agents used in CT. Contrast-enhanced MR scanning is unique in its ability to differentiate spinal cord tumors from adjacent edema and approaches the sensitivity of CT myelography in detecting intradural spinal metastatic disease. MR angiography is quickly evolving with adequate resolution for many of the angiographic indications. Vascular malformations may be more easily diagnosed by MR than CT imaging in the setting of acute hemorrhage. Arteriovenous malformations are characterized as serpiginous signal-void structures with or without adjacent hemorrhage. Venous angiomas can be diagnosed by recognizing the typical single prominent draining vein with variable signal relative to the flow within the vessel. The MR imaging appearance of cavernous malformations is pathognomonic, with hemorrhage in various stages seen, often, in a "target" pattern.

MR imaging is uniquely sensitive to alterations of white matter, including edema and abnormal myelination. Low-grade neoplasms that lack surrounding edema and do not disturb the blood-brain barrier are best detected by MR imaging. The high anatomic resolution of sagittal thin-section multiplanar MR imaging is ideal for evaluating the structures in the sellar and suprasellar region as well as the aqueduct and the foramen magnum. New MR imaging techniques that have recently become valuable to clinicians include functional MR imaging (fMR), which relies upon detection of subtle changes in local cerebral blood flow caused by neural activation to provide information on functional localization, and MR spectroscopy, which permits in situ quantification of lactate, *N*-acetylaspartate, and other metabolites useful in differential diagnosis of encephalopathies.

CEREBRAL ANGIOGRAPHY Cerebral angiography (Fig. 25-4) remains an important procedure in selected patients, particularly when cerebrovascular disease is being considered. Retrograde femoral arterial catheterization to study the anterior and posterior circulations is appropriate when digital subtraction angiography (DSA) requires less contrast than conventional angiography, which is a consideration in small infants, patients with renal compromise, sickle cell disease, or other clinical situations warranting contrast restriction. The availability of MRA and transcranial Doppler techniques has decreased the need for angiography.

MYELOGRAPHY Myelography continues to be a valuable procedure for evaluating intraspinal abnormalities, although high-resolution MR imaging of the spine has decreased the frequency with which this test is required. Extradural compressive lesions can be clearly differentiated from intradural abnormalities by taking ad-

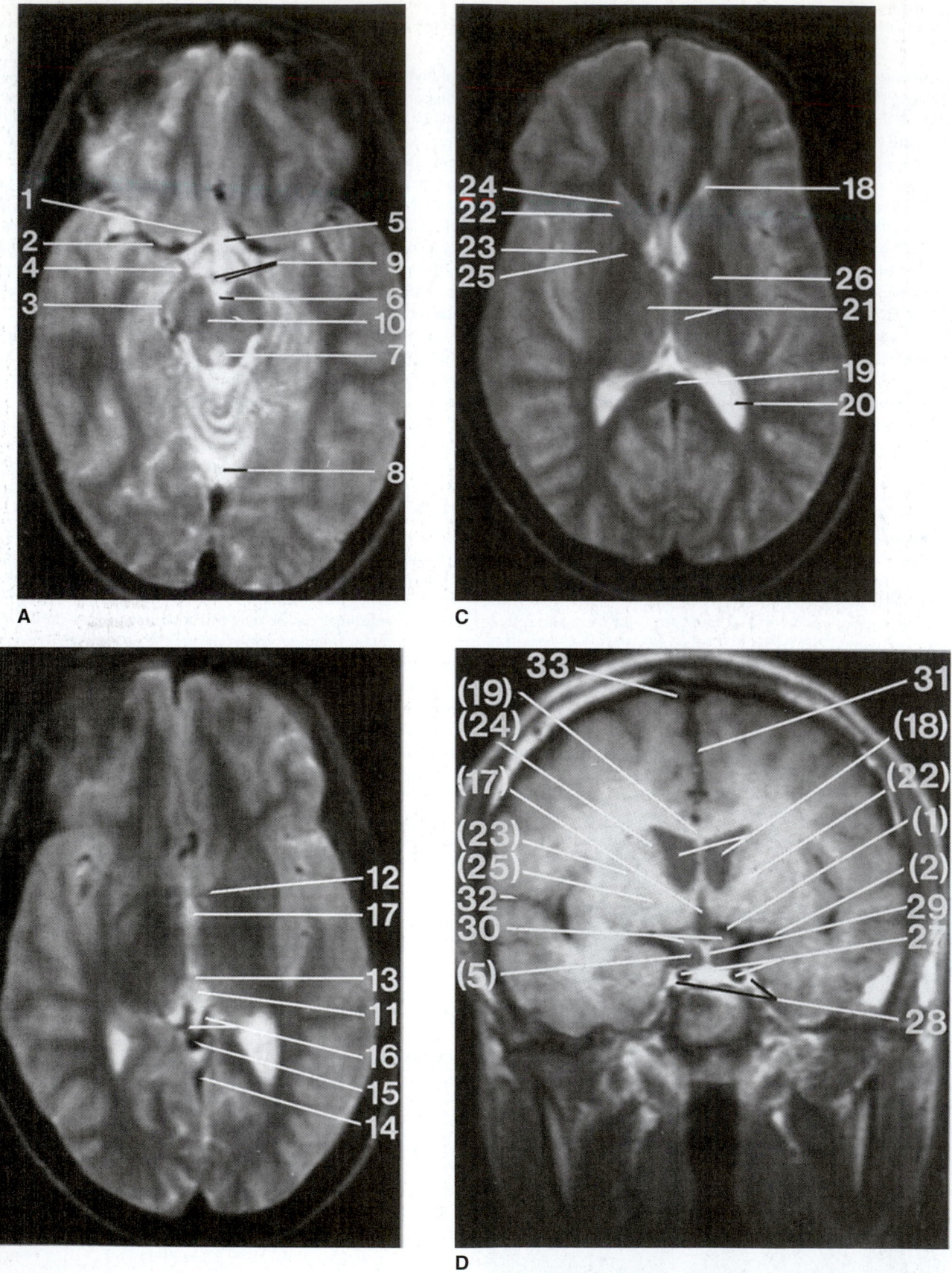

FIGURE 25-3 Axial T$_2$-weighted MR scans **(A, B, C)** and a coronal gadolinium enhanced T$_1$-weighted image **(D)** demonstrate the following structures: **A.** *(1)* Anterior cerebral artery, *(2)* middle cerebral artery, *(3)* posterior cerebral artery, *(4)* posterior communicating artery, *(5)* suprasellar cistern, *(6)* interpeduncular cistern, *(7)* aqueduct, *(8)* superior cerebellar cistern, *(9)* mamillary bodies, *(10)* red nuclei; **B.** *(11)* pineal gland, *(12)* anterior commissure, *(13)* posterior commissure, *(14)* straight sinus, *(15)* vein of Galen, *(16)* internal cerebral veins, *(17)* third ventricle; **C.** *(18)* frontal horn, lateral ventricle, *(19)* corpus callosum, *(20)* posterior horn, lateral ventricle, *(21)* thalami, *(22)* anterior limb internal capsule, *(23)* putamen, *(24)* caudate nucleus, *(25)* globus pallidus, *(26)* posterior limb internal capsule; **D.** *(27)* internal carotid artery, *(28)* cavernous sinuses, *(29)* infundibulum, *(30)* optic tracts, *(31)* interhemispheric fissure, *(32)* Sylvian fissure, *(33)* superior sagittal sinus. *Courtesy of Dr. Jacqueline Bello.*

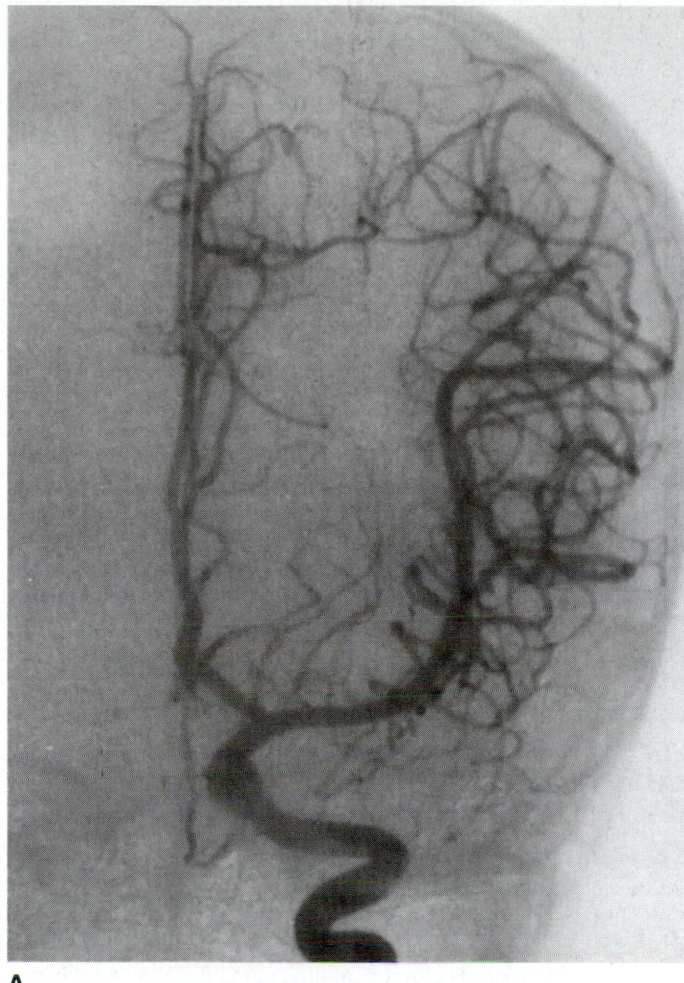

A

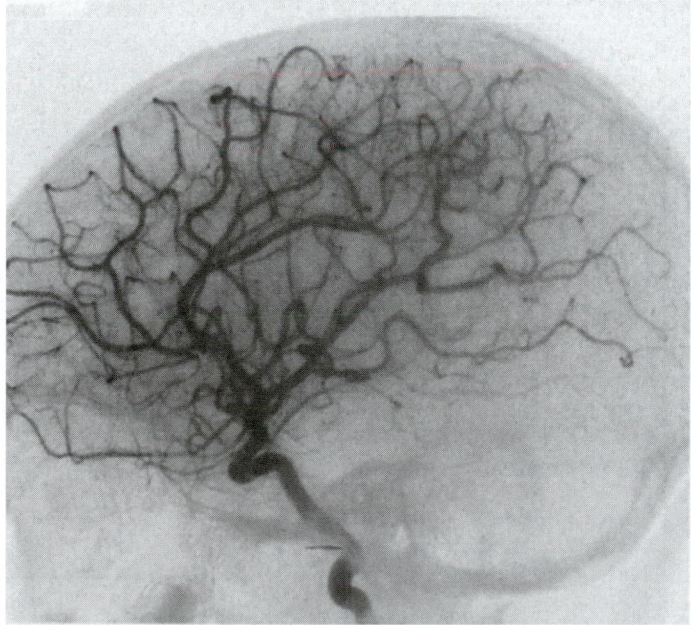

B

FIGURE 25-4   Normal internal carotid arteriogram, subtraction films taken in (A) AP and (B) lateral projections.

vantage of the various contrast techniques (oil, air, and water-soluble contrast material). Occasionally, the contrast material may have to be introduced at the cervical level when a lumbosacral abnormality is present. Cervical myelography should be performed by experienced physicians only because of its increased potential for morbidity. Once an intramedullary lesion is detected, it is best characterized by MR imaging.

PSYCHOMETRICS Psychometric tests are useful in assessing the cognitive abilities of a child. The mean IQ, by convention, is 100 with 1 standard deviation (SD) being $\pm$ 15. Mental retardation represents an IQ more than 2 SD below the mean. Low normal intelligence is 70 to 85; mild retardation, 55 to 70; moderate retardation, 40 to 55; severe retardation, 25 to 40; and profound mental retardation, less than 25. Mental retardation and specific learning disabilities can be documented in this way. Serial testing can also document progression of a neurologic disease process (see Secs. 5.4 and 5.6.3).

TISSUE BIOPSY Tissue biopsies are valuable when a metabolic or degenerative process is being considered. Tissues available for study include lymphocytes, fibroblasts, muscle and peripheral nerves, rectal ganglion cells, nerve endings in the bulbar conjunctiva, and brain. The absolute indications for brain biopsy are more restricted now that alternative diagnostic procedures are available. However, the advent of CT-assisted stereotactic brain biopsy makes this procedure a reasonable alternative when the biopsy of other tissues fails to provide an answer. The procedure is safe when performed by an experienced surgeon and may provide an immediate tissue diagnosis. The diagnosis of herpes simplex encephalitis may require a temporal lobe biopsy to justify administration of an antiviral agent. The value of muscle biopsy is discussed further in Sec. 25.14. Biopsy of the sural or other pure sensory nerves is useful for diagnosis of periarteritis nodosa and other vasculitic diseases affecting the peripheral nerves, and for detection of endoneurial amyloid deposition and of giant axonal neuropathy, but often results in a persistent and annoying local sensory deficit. Cutaneous punch biopsy to evaluate cutaneous nerves has promise as a means to obtain some of the same information without this complication.

References

Carter S, Gold AP: Neurology of Infancy and Childhood. New York, Appleton-Century-Crofts, 1974

Dodge PR, Volpe JJ: Neurologic history and examination. In: Farmer TW, ed: Pediatric Neurology. New York, Harper & Row, 1983

Fenichel GM: Clinical Pediatric Neurology. A Signs and Symptoms Approach, 3rd ed. Philadelphia, Saunders, 1997

Illingworth RS: The Development of the Infant and Young Child. Normal and Abnormal. Edinburgh, Churchill Livingstone, 1960

Paine RS, Oppe TE: Neurological Examination of Children. Little Club Clinics in Developmental Medicine, no. 20/21. London, National Spastics Society, 1966

Raymond GV, Holmes LB: Head circumference standards in neonates. J Child Neurol 9:63–66, 1994

US Congress. Decade of the brain. Joint Resolution by the Senate (173) and the House of Representatives (174) of the United States Congress. Congressional Record, 135: 1989

Volpe JJ: Neurology of the Newborn, 3rd ed. Philadelphia, Saunders, 1995

25.2   NORMAL AND ABNORMAL DEVELOPMENT OF THE NEURAXIS

William DeMyer

25.2.1   Development of the Neuraxis

Embryologic development occurs in three stages: cytogenesis, histogenesis, and organogenesis. Disturbances in one or more of these stages of normal development provide a convenient way to describe maldevelopment. Cytogenesis consists of the incorporation of chemical elements or molecules into ordered arrangements within the cell, followed by cell multiplication, differentiation, and growth. Disorders of cytogenesis can occur at the level of the gene (the structure of DNA), the structure or morphology of chromosomes, or the structure of intracytoplasmic organelles, which, in turn, lead to disordered multiplication, differentiation, and growth of cells. Gene defects can result in inborn errors of metabolism, such as phenylketonuria, or in malformation syndromes, such as tuberous sclerosis and neurofibromatosis. Cytogenetic errors in chromosome morphology, such as trisomies or deletions, characteristically produce infants with gross malformations in the size and shape of organs. The patients usually have some degree of mental retardation and may have malformations of single organs or of the entire somatotype, as in Down syndrome (trisomy 21).

Disturbances in cell multiplication lead to too few or too many glia and neurons. Too few cells results in micrencephaly. Numerous genetic and acquired factors, such as chromosomal errors, anoxia, drugs, and infection, may reduce the number of cells, but frequently the cause of micrencephaly cannot be determined from the clinical findings or even at autopsy. Too many cells results in an anatomic type of megalencephaly, as in neurofibromatosis or achondroplastic dwarfism. Most examples of megalencephaly have a genetic rather than an acquired cause.

Cytodifferentiation in the nervous system consists of the sprouting of axons and dendrites by the neuroblasts and elaboration of the glioblasts into the mature types of glial cells. Disturbances in cytodifferentiation occur in many malformation syndromes with mental deficiency. Mature neurons show an incomplete dendritic pattern in many chromosomal syndromes.

After cytogenesis has produced the neuroblasts and glioblasts, the events of histogenesis blend neurons and glia into the functional arrangements of the nervous system. The major events in neural histogenesis consist of the connection of neurons by axonal pathways, the investment of axons by oligodendroglia to form myelin, and the migration of neuroblasts along the astrocyte scaffolding. The sprouting axonal pathways fill the spaces between the gray matter and acquire their myelin sheaths to become the white matter. The classical example of misdirection of axonal pathways is agenesis of the corpus callosum. In this malformation, the axons grow to the midline but fail to cross it. As another example, the pyramidal tracts may fail to decussate.

After the proliferation of neuroblasts in the periventricular zone, they may remain in situ or may migrate some distance away. The neuroblasts may accumulate in the form of compact masses, called *nuclei,* or less compact masses, called *reticular formation,* or they may migrate to the surface of the neuraxis to form the laminated sheets called *cortex.* Thus, in the mature neuraxis, the neuronal peri-

karya dispose themselves in nucleate, reticulate, and laminate arrangements. The neuroblasts that remain in the periventricular region may form the thalamic or caudate nuclei. In the brainstem, they aggregate into the cranial nerve nuclei or migrate into the tegmentum to form the substantia nigra, red nuclei, nuclei of basis pontis, and reticular formation. The classical example of absence of cranial nerve nuclei is Mobius syndrome (aplasia of the facial nerve nucleus).

Those neuroblasts that migrate to the surface of the cerebrum or the cerebellum to form cortex may arrive in too-low or too-high numbers, resulting in micrencephaly or megalencephaly, respectively; alternatively, they may arrive at the cortex and then undergo destruction. Migration of neurons occurs asynchronously. Thus, the same teratogenic insult acting at different times may influence different groups of neuroblasts. Disturbances in migration may result in nodules of heterotopic neurons or glia in the periventricular region. These nodules sometimes protrude into the ventricular lumen, as in tuberous sclerosis. After the neurons that migrate to the surface to form the cortex reach their destination, they may fail to assemble into the normal laminae. Fetal alcohol syndrome provides one example of disturbed neuronal migration and cortical lamination, with numerous heterotopias. Disturbances in migration also result in abnormal sulcation, such as lissencephaly and polymicrogyria.

The final composition of the neuraxis is achieved by the blending of tissues of neural and extraneural origin. Mesenchymal tissue produces blood vessels and meninges. Disordered blending of neural and mesenchymal elements produces arteriovenous malformations that may be confined to the neuraxis or may have extraneural dysplasia, as in encephalotrigeminal angiomatosis (Sturge-Weber syndrome). Disordered blending of cells and tissues produces the class of lesions variously called hamartomas, craniopharyngiomas, teratomas, pinealomas, and lipomas. Characteristically these lesions occur along the ventral or dorsal midline of the neuraxis, where the neural ectoderm should separate cleanly from surface or oral ectoderm.

The final contouring of the neuraxis results from a series of organogenetic events (Table 25-1). Closure of the neural tube is the first organogenetic event. The sheet of ectodermal cells that covers the developing embryonic cell mass rolls up and fuses along its dorsal margins and at the anterior and posterior neuropores to form a wall around a lumen. The wall becomes the definitive wall of the neuraxis. The lumen remains as the ventricular system and central canal of the spinal cord (Fig. 25-5). Fusion of the dorsal margins of the neural ectoderm occurs first in the upper thoracic region and

TABLE 25-1
MAJOR EVENTS IN ORGANOGENESIS OF THE NEURAXIS

1. *Closure:* Rolling up of the neural ectoderm and fusion of its dorsal lips to form the neural tube
2. *Transverse segmentation:* Subdivision of the neural tube into successive segments (cerebrum, brainstem, and spinal cord)
3. *Evagination:* Protrusion of hollow stalks or globes consisting of brain wall
4. *Bump formation:* Protrusion of solid masses
5. *Flexions:* Folding of the brain to fit the cranial cavity
6. *Fissuration:* Formation of the interhemispheric and Sylvian fissures
7. *Sulcation:* Formation of the crevices on the surface of the cerebral and cerebellar hemispheres
8. *Growth*

Bumps form on the surface of the neuraxis (either the external or ventricular surface) from localized proliferation of neurons. The caudate nuclei protrude into the ventrolateral wall of the anterior horn. The mamillary bodies protrude from the ventral surface of the diencephalon. The cerebellum, olivary nuclei, and superior and inferior colliculi protrude from the brainstem. The entire cerebellum protrudes as a solid mass of proliferating cells without a true ventricular lumen. The most common hypoplasia or aplasia of these structures involves the cerebellum. Aplasia or agenesis of the cerebellar vermis is relatively common, and sometimes the entire cerebellum fails to form.

Flexions fold the neural tube to fit it more conveniently into the cranial cavity, but flexions per se do not produce malformations.

Fissuration, the formation of the interhemispheric and sylvian fissures, is the consequence of evagination of the globes that form the cerebral hemispheres. Sulcation of the originally smooth surface of the cerebral wall comes about by an entirely different but as yet unknown mechanism dependent, in part, on migration of neuroblasts to the cerebral surface. Sulcation begins in the fourth to fifth months and proceeds in an orderly sequence that is sufficiently constant to be used in determining the developmental age of the fetus.

In addition to malformations arising from primary disturbances in development, gross defects of the brain may arise from a variety of destructive, hypoxic, or inflammatory insults. These insults may destroy preexisting structures, resulting in porencephaly or hydranencephaly, or the lesion may imitate a primary developmental error. Many inflammatory or destructive lesions, as well as many developmental errors, may interfere with the formation, flow, or absorption of CSF, resulting in hydrocephalus. Because of their numerous causes, porencephalies of various types, hydrocephalus, microcephaly, and closure defects constitute by far the most common classes of serious organogenetic disorders of the brain.

25.2.2   Prenatal and Developmental Defects

ABNORMAL HEAD SIZE

An abnormal head size warns of an abnormal brain. A small head is termed *microcephaly,* and a large one, *macrocephaly.* These are descriptive terms, not diagnoses. Microcephaly necessitates a small brain, or micrencephaly. On the other hand, in macrocephaly, the brain may be oversized and overweight, a condition termed *megalencephaly,* or the ventricles may be distended by CSF, a condition termed *hydrocephaly;* the actual brain tissue may be reduced in amount, in spite of the large head. Early recognition of the abnormal head size requires accurate serial measurements of the occipitofrontal circumference (OFC). For accuracy, use a thin flexible steel tape rather than cloth or paper. Extend the tape from the most prominent part of the occiput, located at or above the external occipital protuberance (inion), to the forehead, just above the glabella. Tighten the tape sufficiently to compress the hair. Record the OFC on one of the standard charts (see Appendix A for normal OFC).

Accurate serial measurements plotted against the normal curve show the rate of change of the OFC with time. Any OFC more than ± 2 SD from the mean raises a strong suspicion of a brain disorder. An OFC more than ± 3 SD from the mean almost certainly indicates an abnormal brain. To judge the significance of a borderline OFC, compare the patient's OFC with body weight, height, and chest circumference. Always compare the patient's

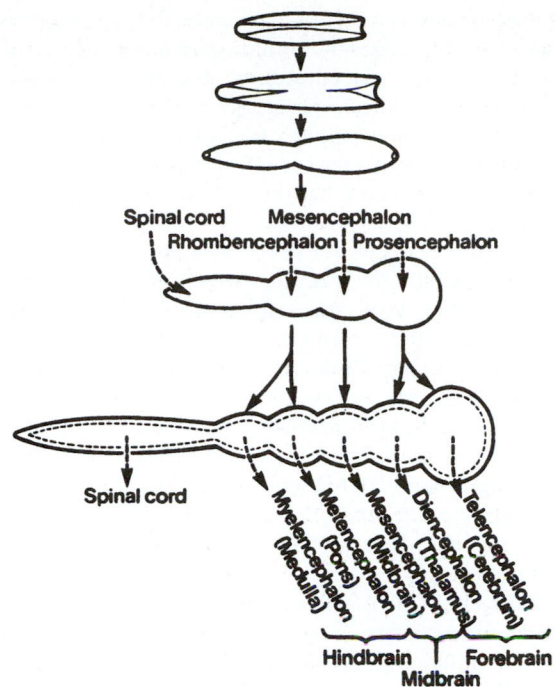

FIGURE 25-5   Schematic representation of the folding up of the neural tube, closure along its dorsal margin, and transverse segmentation into the components of the central nervous system.

proceeds rostrally and caudally. Dorsal induction, closure along the dorsal midline, depends on molecules initially appearing in the adjacent surface ectoderm and in the roof plate cells of the neural tube. The molecular regulators of dorsal induction include bone morphogenetic proteins and Wnt proteins. Defective closure of the neural tube results in cranioschisis or rachischisis, with varying degrees of protrusion of meninges (meningocele) or protrusion of meninges combined with neural tissue (meningomyelocele or meningoencephalocele). These protrusions characteristically occur along the dorsal midsagittal plane of the body, the seam of fusion.

Transverse segmentation divides the neural tube into three primary brain segments, the forebrain, midbrain, and hindbrain, and then into five segments and the spinal cord (Fig. 25-5). Evagination occurs only at the forebrain level. A single median-plane evagination from the dorsal surface of the diencephalon produces the pineal body. A similar evagination from the ventral surface of the diencephalon produces the neurohypophysis. Another ventrally protruding diencephalic evagination divides into bilaterally symmetric optic bulbs and tracts. The most rostral transverse segment of the neuraxis (the telencephalon) divides into paired globe-like evaginations that become the cerebral hemispheres. Each hemisphere, by further evagination, produces a temporal lobe and an olfactory bulb and tract. Curtailment of an evagination or its destruction results in absence of or hypoplasia of the relevant evagination, such as anophthalmia or microphthalmia. Ventral induction, as opposed to dorsal induction, brings about the evaginations of the forebrain. Molecular signaling for the forebrain evaginations depends on the so-called sonic hedgehog (SHH) pathway. In humans, a variety of chromosomes contribute to the pathogenesis of holoprosencephaly. Curtailment of outgrowth of the symmetric globe-like evaginations that form the cerebral hemispheres leaves the prosencephalon as a single holospheric organ (holoprosencephaly).

OFC with the OFC and body dimensions of siblings and other family members.

After microcephaly or macrocephaly has been identified, therapy, family counseling, and the prognosis depend on the type of cerebral lesion and its cause. The history, pedigree, and physical examination may provide diagnostic clues to heredofamilial disorders or distinct malformation syndromes. If the child has a peculiar facies, consult an atlas of malformation syndromes (Baraitser and Winter). Lesions such as encephaloceles, porencephaly, subdural fluid accumulations, and brain atrophy may allow transillumination. With extreme thinning or destruction of the cerebrum, as in hydranencephaly, the whole cranium will light up. If an anatomic abnormality of the brain is suspected, order an ultrasound, CT, or preferably an MR scan. Plain skull radiographs may be helpful to identify craniosynostosis. If a metabolic-degenerative disease is suspected, screen the urine for inborn errors of metabolism and do a battery of lysosomal hydrolase enzyme studies on blood or cultured tissues. Consider chromosome studies for patients who have dysmorphic features.

MICROCEPHALY

Microcephalics usually are mentally defective and may have cerebral palsy and seizures. Aside from craniosynostosis, microcephaly is always secondary to micrencephaly. In some microcephalics, the brain will be small but will have fairly normal internal and external configurations. Others may have malformations or destructive lesions with symmetrically or asymmetrically dilated ventricles. A severe degree of microcephaly implies a prenatal, perinatal, or early postnatal lesion. Experimentally, microcephaly has resulted from many teratogens, drugs, and irradiation, as well as vitamin deficiency or excess. In humans the common causes of reduced brain size include maternal illness and infections, malnutrition, drug ingestion, chromosomal errors and hereditary factors, and disorders of implantation and placentation. Thus, microcephaly itself provides no clue as to its cause. The mother should be questioned about the pregnancy and delivery; a history of infertility or pregnancy wastage is common, and sometimes the pedigree will disclose a distinct mendelian pattern.

MACROCEPHALY

The most common cause of macrocephaly is increased intracranial pressure with hydrocephalus. The cerebral wall thins as the head enlarges, and the brain weight, exclusive of intraventricular fluid, is normal or reduced. A rarer cause of macrocephaly is megalencephaly, an abnormally large and heavy brain. Megalencephaly may be a primary malformation with huge gyri, either of simple pattern or with polymicrogyria. It may be sporadic or may be associated with neurofibromatosis, tuberous sclerosis, myelomeningocele (Arnold-Chiari malformation), or achondroplasia. The brain is large in patients with pituitary gigantism but not in those with acromegaly; the brain is also large in the syndrome of cerebral gigantism, in which no endocrine defects have been identified. Patients with primary megalencephaly are often mentally deficient and may have motor deficits and seizures. Secondary or metabolic megalencephaly is caused by accumulation of abnormal metabolic products and includes the infantile form of amaurotic idiocy, gargoylism, spongy degeneration of the white matter, and some of the leukodystrophies such as metachromatic leukodystrophy and Krabbe disease. A large brain resulting from cerebral edema or neoplasia is not classed as megalencephaly.

In hydrocephalus with increased pressure, the head enlarges rapidly, the fontanelles bulge, the sutures split, and papilledema may occur. Such signs of increased pressure generally do not occur in the primary, anatomic megalencephalies but may in the metabolic megalencephalies. These features are usually absent in primary megalencephaly, but they may occur in secondary megalencephaly. If the macrocephalic patient has no evidence of increased pressure or neurologic defects, the condition is benign familial megalencephaly, and further diagnostic procedures are not necessary. If it is not familial, further investigation is indicated. Studies may include skull radiography, electroencephalography, subdural taps, CT scan, MR imaging, and sometimes cerebral arteriography.

As a consequence of disordered migration of cortical neuroblasts, the cerebrum may fail to sulcate properly. If it lacks all sulci, the condition is called *lissencephaly*. In the Miller-Dieker lissencephaly syndrome, the infant has microcephaly, an abnormal facies, seizures, and profound retardation. In the Walker-Warburg lissencephaly syndrome, the infant has hydrocephalus and a posterior fossa cyst, muscular dystrophy and hypotonia, seizures, and profound retardation. The diagnosis of lissencephaly is made by absence of sulci when CT or MR scans are done to investigate a neurologically impaired infant. A cerebrum with too few sulci will show broad gyri, a condition called *pachygyria*. In the converse condition of *polymicrogyria*, the cerebral surface shows countless small crevices. Because all three conditions, lissencephaly, pachygyria, and polymicrogyria, result from a disturbance in migration, all can exist in the same brain. In these conditions, the cortical lamination is always defective, and the patient is neurologically impaired. In the Arnold-Chiari malformation and other forms of prenatal hydrocephalus, the cortical surface shows a very busy pattern of crevices, recently named *stenogyria*, but the cortical lamination is normal, and the patient may have normal cerebral function. By contrast, *ulegyria*, which features small, thin, and sclerotic gyri with widened sulci, results from a destructive process, usually inflammatory or anoxic, and hence is not a sulcal malformation per se.

MEDIAN FACIAL DEFECTS AND HOLOPROSENCEPHALY

The holoprosencephalies (arrhinencephalia) constitute a teratologic series of defects of graded severity characterized by median malformations of the face and the brain. The brain abnormality consists of failure of the prosencephalon to undergo median cleavage into cerebral hemispheres or to form lobes or olfactory bulbs. This holistic prosencephalon or holoprosencephalon has a single-chamber ventricle and usually lacks olfactory bulbs and tracts. Median facial anomalies consist of orbital hypotelorism in combination with a flat nose or proboscis and oral deformities, such as median cleft of the lip and palate (Fig. 25-6, A to E). Some of these patients have trigonocephaly (sharply pointed, keel-shaped forehead), and most are microcephalic. The crista galli, ethmoid, vomer, nasal, and premaxillary bones are absent or hypoplastic. The role of prechordal mesoderm explains why the face and brain are both affected. This mesoderm, which is deficient in holoprosencephaly, normally gives rise to the median facial bones. Furthermore, by ventral induction via the SHH pathway this mesoderm determines not only the differentiation of the ectoderm as neural tissue but also its evagination into lobated hemispheres and olfactory bulbs.

Five types of facies can be recognized that are pathognomonic of and predict the malformed brain. Figure 25-6, A to E, shows these facies arranged in order of decreasing severity. At the less severe end of the spectrum, where absence of the olfactory bulbs

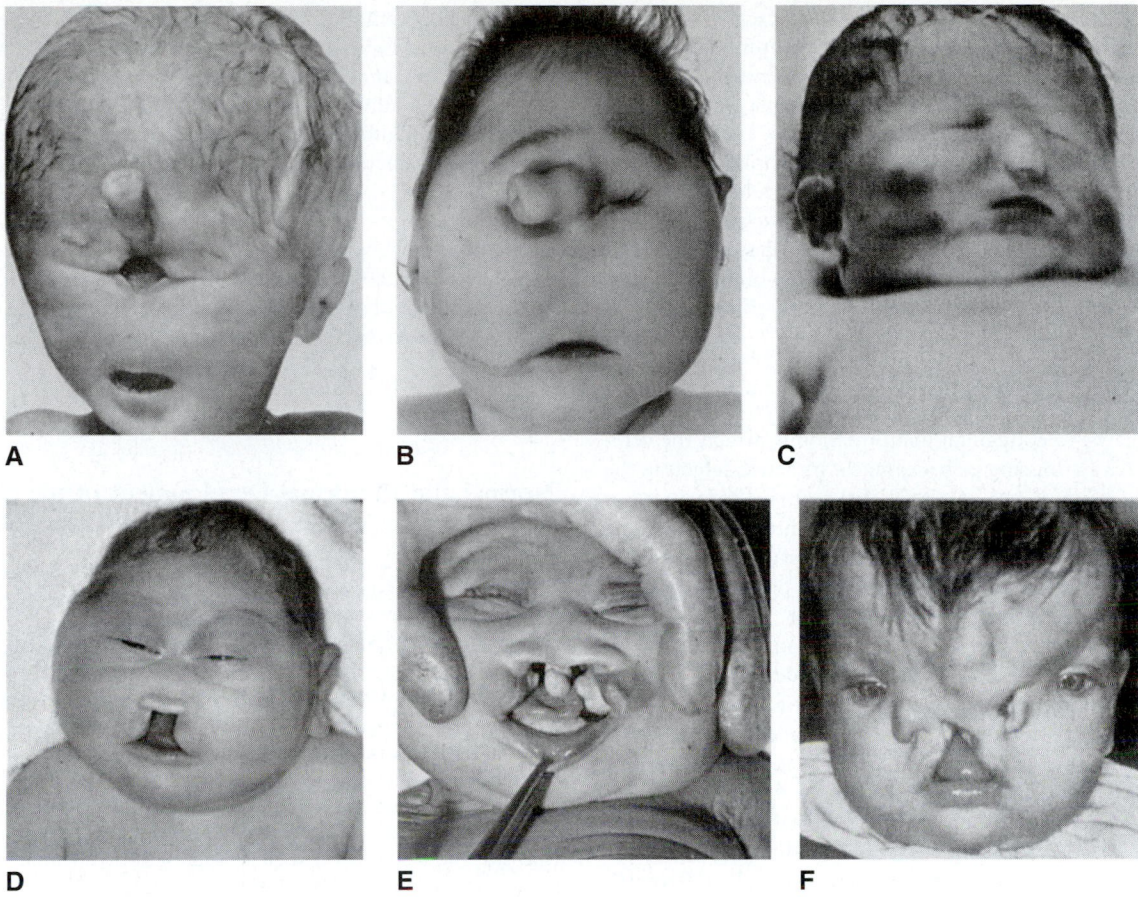

FIGURE 25-6 Diagnostic facies of holoprosencephaly. **A.** Cyclopia. Notice the proboscis attached above the orbit. *(From Potter: Pathology of the Fetus and Infant, 3rd ed. Chicago, Year Book, 1975.)* **B.** Ethmocephaly. *(Courtesy of Dr. P. Fluery.)* **C.** Cebocephaly. The proboscis has migrated down to the normal location for the nose. The single nostril leads to a cul-de-sac. **D.** With median cleft lip. Rudimentary nares and a nasal cavity are present. The nasal septum is lacking. **E.** With hypoplastic intermaxillary segment (philtrum-premaxillary anlage). A rudimentary nasal septum is present. **F.** Typical facies of median cleft-face syndrome, consisting of median cleft lip, bifid nose, hypertelorism, and frontal encephalocele.

and tracts is the only brain abnormality, the face may have no obvious median defects; some of these patients are eunuchoids. The clinical diagnosis can be made from the pathognomonic facies. Orbital hypotelorism, as measured on radiographs, supports the diagnosis, but one or more of the other median facial defects must be present to distinguish the hypotelorism of holoprosencephaly from other conditions with microcrania. In spite of the overwhelming association between facies A through E in Fig. 25-6 and the abnormal brain, patients with facies D or E on rare occasions may have normal brains, or conversely, patients with a normal face may have a holospheric cerebrum. Ultrasound, CT, or MR scans readily identify the holospheric cerebrum.

In facial categories A through D, the brain volume is often much smaller than the intracranial space, permitting transillumination of the head. The electroencephalogram shows little or no electrical activity over the areas of transillumination but elsewhere shows repetitive seizure discharges. Patients with a holospheric cerebrum fail to thrive. They make little or no developmental progress, have seizures, and display characteristic poikilothermia with large temperature swings. Most die during infancy.

The cause of holoprosencephaly is unknown; most occurrences are sporadic, but familial instances do occur. Some holoprosence-

phalic patients have chromosomal anomalies, usually trisomy 13, but others have a normal karyotype. Those with abnormal karyotypes are more likely to have multiple extracephalic anomalies than those with a 46-chromosome karyotype.

MEDIAN CLEFT-FACE SYNDROME (FRONTONASAL DYSPLASIA)

Holoprosencephaly should not be confused with another pattern of median facial defects, the median cleft-face syndrome, which consists of frontal meningoencephalocele, orbital hypertelorism, bifid nose, and median cleft of the lip (Fig. 25-6F). In spite of the grotesque facies, these patients are often mentally normal or only mildly retarded. They can be grouped into a teratologic series of defects of graded severity, the least severe of which is a simple median notch in the nose or upper lip. Craniofacial reconstruction greatly improves the patient's appearance.

OPTICOSEPTAL DYSPLASIA AND OLFACTOGENITAL DYSPLASIA

Maldevelopment may affect the structures of the telencephalic-diencephalic junction in a variety of combinations. The defects may be expressed as curtailment or absence of the olfactory, optic, or neurohypophyseal evagination, absence of the septum pellucidum, or malformation of the hypothalamus. These patients show various combinations of mental deficiency, microphthalmia, anosmia, and endocrine disturbances, including hypogonadism. In opticoseptal dysplasia the cardinal features are optic nerve hypoplasia with varying degrees of blindness and absence of the septum pellucidum. These patients may have fairly normal mentality, but most have some degree of mental retardation. Patients with olfactogenital dysplasia have hypoplastic genitalia and lack olfactory bulbs and tracts. Pure absence of olfactory bulbs may be hereditary, constituting one form of familial anosmia.

HYDRANENCEPHALY

Hydranencephaly is a congenital malformation in which the cerebral hemispheres are missing or have huge symmetric defects in the cerebral wall because of intrauterine destruction, malformation, or possibly severely increased intracranial pressure during fetal life. The skull and the scalp are well formed, thus distinguishing hydranencephaly from anencephaly, encephaloceles, and other dysraphic lesions. Most occurrences are sporadic.

In contrast to holoprosencephaly, most patients have no facial or extracephalic malformations. Thus, the disorder may not be suspected until the infant fails to show psychomotor progress, has seizures, or manifests spastic quadriplegia. Most of the patients die in infancy, but some survive several years. The head may be small or normal and sometimes may enlarge rapidly, owing to malabsorption of CSF. In young infants, the head always transilluminates brightly. A CT or MR scan documents the absence of cerebral hemispheres. The most important consideration in the differential diagnosis of hydranencephaly is to avoid confusion with severe degrees of hydrocephalus. Sometimes in hydrocephalus the cerebral wall thins to the degree that radiographic scans may disclose little or no tissue, suggesting a diagnosis of hydranencephaly. The electroencephalogram in hydranencephaly shows little, if any, electrical activity, whereas in severe hydrocephalus, cerebral rhythms remain. Angiograms in hydranencephaly show very thin, rudimentary cerebral arteries, whereas in hydrocephalus the cerebral vessels are demonstrable.

AGENESIS OF CORPUS CALLOSUM

The corpus callosum consists of a large bundle of nerve fibers that connect the cortex of one cerebral hemisphere with the other. Scout axons from cortical neurons of each cerebral hemisphere grow through the commissural plate in the midline 60 to 70 days after conception. After crossing the midline, the axons extend to synapse on mirror-image sites of the opposite cerebral cortex and in the corpus striatum. As additional axons continue to cross the midline, they expand the corpus callosum into its adult form by 120 days of gestation. Agenesis or hypoplasia of the corpus callosum occurs if the fibers fail to grow out, are destroyed, or are prevented from crossing. If the fibers reach the midline and fail to decussate, they pile up along the ventricular wall.

The corpus callosum normally mediates interhemispheric transfer of information and may transmit seizure discharges from one hemisphere to the other, but its function is not readily testable at the bedside in infants and young children. Clinical clues consist of hypertelorism or hypotelorism, organic acidurias, retinovertebral anomalies in females (Aicardi syndrome), or recurrent hypothermia (Shapiro syndrome). Usually, agenesis of the corpus callosum is discovered incidentally from brain imaging ordered because of a neurodevelopmental disorder. In pure agenesis of the corpus callosum, coronal radiographs show a pathognomonic bat-wing ventricular pattern. If agenesis of the corpus callosum is the only brain anomaly, the individual may lead a relatively normal life. Commonly, other malformations accompany agenesis of the corpus callosum, such as heterotopias, holoprosencephaly, or destructive lesions.

Etiologic factors in agenesis of the corpus callosum include exogenous teratogens (alcohol), chromosomal errors (8, 9, 13, and 18), heredity (X-linked, recessive, and dominant forms), and inborn errors of metabolism (nonketotic hyperglycinemia, organic acidurias, and peroxisomal disorders).

References

Normal and Abnormal Development of the Neuraxis

DeMyer W: Neuroanatomy, 2nd ed. Baltimore, Williams and Wilkins, 1998

Duckett S: Pediatric Neuropathology. Baltimore, Williams and Wilkins, 1995

Friede RL: Developmental Neuropathology, 2nd ed. New York, Springer-Verlag, 1989

Muller J: Congenital malformations of the brain. In: Rosenberg RN, ed: The Clinical Neurosciences, vol 3, Neuropathology. New York, Churchill-Livingston, 1983: 1–33

Norman MG, McGillivray BC, Kalousek DK, et al: Congenital Malformation of the Brain. Pathologic, Clinical, Radiologic, and Genetic aspects. New York, Oxford University Press, 1995

Shepard T: Catalog of Teratogenic Agents, 9th ed. Baltimore, The Johns Hopkins University Press, 1998

Abnormalities of Migration, Sulcation, and Gyration

Barkovitch AJ, Kuzniecky RI, Dobyns WB, et al: A classification scheme for malformations of cortical development. Neuropediatrics 57:59–63, 1996

Nordborg C, Eriksson S, Rydenhag B, et al: Microdysgenesis in surgical specimens from patients with epilepsy: occurrence and clinical correlations. J Neurol Neurosurg Psychiatr 67:521–524, 1999

Samat H: Cerebral Dysgenesis: Embryology and Clinical Expression. New York, Oxford University Press, 1992

Prenatal and Developmental Defects

Baraitser M, Winter R: *London dysmorphology database*. Dysmorphology Library on Compact Disc. New York Oxford University Press Electronic Publishing, 1998

DeMyer W: Microcephaly, micrencephaly, metalocephaly, and megalencephaly. In: Swaiman KT, Ashwal S, eds: Pediatric Neurology, 3rd ed. St. Louis, CV Mosby, 1999, Chap 18

DeMyer W: Technique of the Neurologic Examination: a Programmed Text, 4th ed. New York, McGraw-Hill, 1994

Gorlin RJ, Cohen MM Jr, Levin LS: Syndromes of the Head and Neck, 3rd ed. New York, Oxford University Press, 1990

Halsam RH: Microcephaly. In: Vinken PJ, Bruyn GW, Klawans H, Myrianthopoulos N, eds: Handbook of Clinical Neurology, vol 50, Malformations. Amsterdam, Elsevier Science Publications, 1987

Nishi M, Miyake H, Akashi H, et al: An index for proportion of head size to body mass during infancy. J Child Neurol 7:400–403, 1992

Opitz JM, Holt MC: Microcephaly: general considerations and aids to nosology. J Craniofac Devel Biol 10:175–204, 1990

Weaver D, Christian JC: Familial variation of head size and adjustment for parental head circumference. J Pediatr 96:990–994, 1980

Median Facial Defects and Holoprosencephaly

DeMyer W: Holoprosencephaly (cyclopia-arhinencephaly). In: Vinken PJ, Bruyn GW, Klawans H, Myrianthopoulos M, ed: Handbook of Clinical Neurology. Amsterdam, Elsevier Science Publications, 1987

DeMyer W: Median facial malformations and their implications for brain malformations. Birth Defects: Original Articles Series. 11:155–181, 1975

Golden JA: Holoprosencephaly: a defect in brain patterning. J Neuropathol Exp Neurol 57:991–999, 1998

Frontonasal Dysplasia (Median Cleft-Face Syndrome)

DeMyer W: The median cleft face syndrome. Neurology 17:961–971, 1967

Guion-Almeida ML, Richieri-Costa A, Saavedra D, Cohen MM Jr: Frontonasal dysplasia: analysis of 21 cases. Int J Oral Maxillofacial Surg 25:91–97, 1996

Septum Pellucidum, Opticoseptal Dysplasia, and Olfactogenital Dysplasia

Jacobson RI, Abrams GM: Disorders of the hypothalamus and pituitary gland in adolescence and childhood. In: Swaiman KT, ed: Pediatric Neurology, 3rd ed. St. Louis, CV Mosby, 1999:1317–1318

Schaefer GB, Bodensteiner JB: Developmental anomalies of the brain in mental retardation. Int Rev Psych 11:47–55, 1999

Williams J, Brodsky MC, Griebel M, et al: Septo-optic dysplasia: the clinical insignificance of absence of the septum pellucidum. Devel Med Child Neurol 35:490–501, 1993

Hydranencephaly

Shaw C, Alvord EC: Schizencephaly, porencephaly, and hydranencephaly. In: Duckett S, ed: Pediatric Neuropathology. Baltimore, Williams and Wilkins, 1995: 185–197

Agenesis of the Corpus Callosum

Ashwal S: Congenital structural defect. In: Swaimann KT, Ashwal S, eds: Pediatric Neurology, 3rd ed. St. Louis, CV Mosby, 1999:261–262

Jeret JS, Serur D, Wisniewski KE, et al: Clinicopathological findings associated with agenesis of the corpus callosum. Brain Dev 9:255–264, 1987

25.3 DISTURBANCES IN NEURAL TUBE CLOSURE AND SPINE AND CEREBROSPINAL FLUID DYNAMICS

Marvin A. Fishman

ANENCEPHALY

Anencephaly is a severe defect of development of the neuraxis that is incompatible with survival. The incidence varies from 1 to 5 per 1000 live births. The malformation occurs more frequently in girls than in boys and is more common in whites than in blacks. The true incidence may not be discernible because of the apparent high rate of spontaneous abortion of affected fetuses in early pregnancy. There is an increased incidence (5%) of neural tube defects in siblings born subsequent to an anencephalic propositus. Large portions of the cranium, particularly the frontal, parietal, and portions of the occipital bones, are usually absent. The open defect may extend through the level of the foramen magnum to involve the cervical spine. Major portions of the central nervous system are absent. The lesion always involves the forebrain and may also involve the base of the brain. The hypothalamus is usually missing. Exposed tissue in utero often undergoes destruction, producing a hemorrhagic fibrotic nonfunctioning mass. The cerebellum, brainstem, optic nerves, and spinal cord may be malformed. Craniofacial and ocular anomalies are often present. Absence of the pituitary and hypoplastic adrenal glands occur in the majority of fetuses. Malformations of the heart; lungs; gastrointestinal tract, including aganglionosis; kidneys; and skeleton may also be present. Those fetuses that are not aborted are stillborn or die within a few days.

Anencephaly can be diagnosed prenatally. In women at risk, α-fetoprotein concentrations measured in the serum or amniotic fluid at the beginning of the second trimester will be elevated. The combination of elevated maternal serum α-fetoprotein and low estriol is highly predictive of anencephaly. Acetylcholinesterase activity is also present in the amniotic fluid. The diagnosis can be confirmed by ultrasound examination, which will reveal absence of the fetal skull. Approximately 50% of pregnancies with this malformation will involve polyhydramnios. Antenatal detection is usually followed by termination of the pregnancy. The incidence of liveborn infants has decreased dramatically in the last decade. Infants born alive with anencephaly are permanently unconscious but have some brainstem function. Because of the poor prognosis of infants born alive, they have been considered as potential organ donors for transplantation. However, utilizing the current criteria for brain death, including cessation of all brainstem activity, few infants born alive meet the criteria during the first week after birth.

No treatment is indicated, but the mother should be counseled regarding the increased risk of neural tube defects in subsequent pregnancies. Antenatal diagnosis should be offered during subsequent pregnancies. Prevention may be possible by folic acid supplementation given to women of childbearing age (see Neural Tube Defects).

ENCEPHALOCELE

An encephalocele is a herniation of the brain, its coverings, or both, through a defect in the skull (cranium bifidum) (Fig. 25-7). This malformation has an estimated incidence of 1 to 3 per 10,000 live births and thus occurs less commonly than other neural tube defects. Approximately 75% are located in the occipital region. Anterior encephaloceles may originate in the frontal, nasofrontal, or nasopharyngeal region; lesions in the parietal region are unusual. The nasofrontal lesions are thought to result from defective separation of neural and surface ectoderm at the site of final closure of the rostral neuropore. If only a simple hole exists in the cranium, without protrusion of meninges or brain, the defect is referred to as *cranium bifidum occultum*. The herniated tissues may contain just meninges and CSF or may be filled with dysplastic neural tissue. Associated cerebral malformations include deformities of the tentorium, agenesis of a portion of the corpus callosum, hydrocephalus, and meningomyelocele. The size of the protruding sac can vary from a small nubbin of tissue to a structure larger than the cranium itself. The sac may be pedunculated or sessile and may be completely covered by skin or by just a thin, parchment-like membrane.

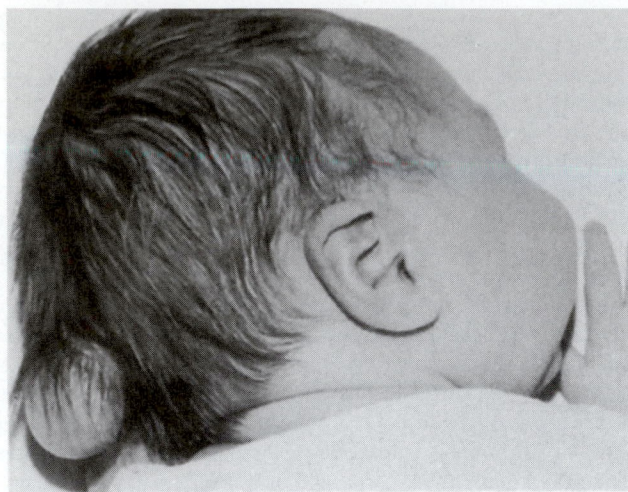

FIGURE 25-7   Newborn infant with small skin-covered midline occipital encephalocele.

Transillumination of the mass may indicate how much solid tissue is present, which is a better guide to the presence of brain tissue than the size of the sac itself. There may be vascular abnormalities of the scalp adjacent to or overlying the mass, and the hair at its base may be longer than that at the rest of the scalp.

The clinical findings are variable and depend in part on whether there are associated cerebral malformations, including hydrocephalus, and how much of the brain is dysplastic and is displaced into the protruding sac. Patients whose lesions are composed of just meninges have a reasonably good prognosis and may develop normally without motor or mental deficits. The disabilities in patients with more severe lesions include retardation, ataxia, spasticity, seizures, blindness, and impaired ocular motility. The diagnosis is usually apparent at birth. Brain imaging procedures (CT and MR) (Fig. 25-8) are helpful in evaluating the intracranial components of the malformation and in determining the presence and progression of any associated hydrocephalus.

Treatment consists of removing the sac and closing the defect if the infant is a good surgical candidate and is not severely defective. Early closure is especially important if the sac does not have a good skin covering to decrease the chance of infection. Treatment of the associated hydrocephalus may require a shunt procedure.

HYDROCEPHALUS

Hydrocephalus is a disorder in which the cerebral ventricular system is dilated and contains an excessive amount of CSF (Fig. 25-9). This accumulation results from an imbalance between production and absorption of CSF. Production is almost always normal, and the deficit is in the absorptive process, from either mechanical or functional blockage of the flow of fluid along its usual pathway, thus interfering with normal absorptive mechanisms. There is increased pressure in the ventricular system of varying degree, either transitory or persistent, during the process of ventricular dilation. This definition excludes conditions in which the ventricular system dilates secondary to loss of brain tissue, such as atrophy. Hydrocephalus may be divided into *noncommunicating* and *communicating* forms. In noncommunicating hydrocephalus the ventricular fluid does not communicate with CSF in the spinal subarachnoid spaces or in the basal cisterns. This implies a block of CSF flow within the ventricular system, such as at the foramen of Monro, the

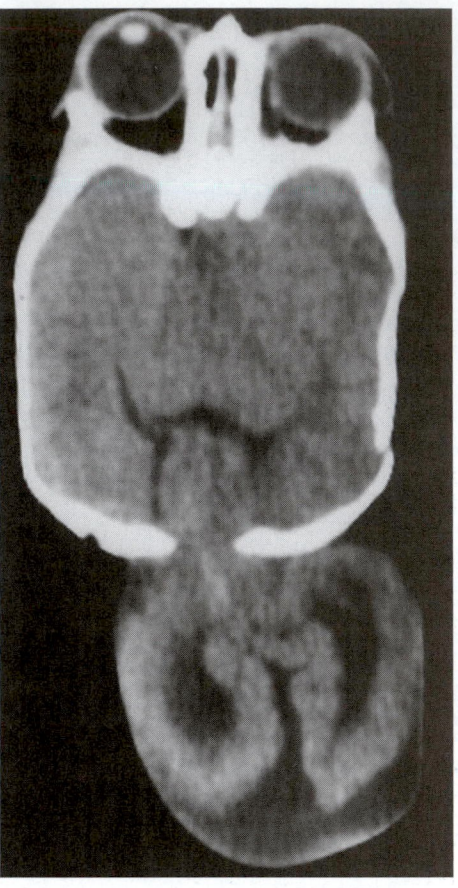

FIGURE 25-8   Occipital encephalocele seen on axial noncontrast CT scan. The occipital lobes, including the occipital horns of the lateral ventricles are contained in the encephalocele. *Courtesy of Dr. Jacqueline Bello.*

aqueduct of Sylvius, or the fourth ventricle and its outlets. In communicating hydrocephalus, the block is outside the ventricular system, and fluid within the ventricles communicates with the spinal subarachnoid space and basal cisterns. Complete block or complete lack of absorption of CSF is incompatible with survival. Some absorption of CSF must be taking place in all patients with hydrocephalus. CSF is constantly being produced, and without absorption, the intracranial pressure would soon become elevated to such levels that continued neurologic function would be impossible.

Anatomy and Physiology of CSF Circulation and Pathways

The CSF is formed within the cerebral ventricular system, mainly by the choroid plexus. Each of the four ventricles contains choroid plexus tissue, consisting of villous folds lined by epithelium and a central core of highly vascularized connective tissue (Fig. 25-10). The fluid is formed by active secretion and diffusion. Nonchoroidal sources of CSF exist, but this aspect of fluid formation is less clearly understood. The ventricular system consists of paired lateral ventricles, each of which connects through a foramen of Monro to a single midline third ventricle. The third ventricle connects by the aqueduct of Sylvius to a midline fourth ventricle that has three exit openings, paired lateral foramina of Luschka, and a midline foramen of Magendie. These openings lead to a system of interconnecting and focally enlarged areas of subarachnoid spaces referred

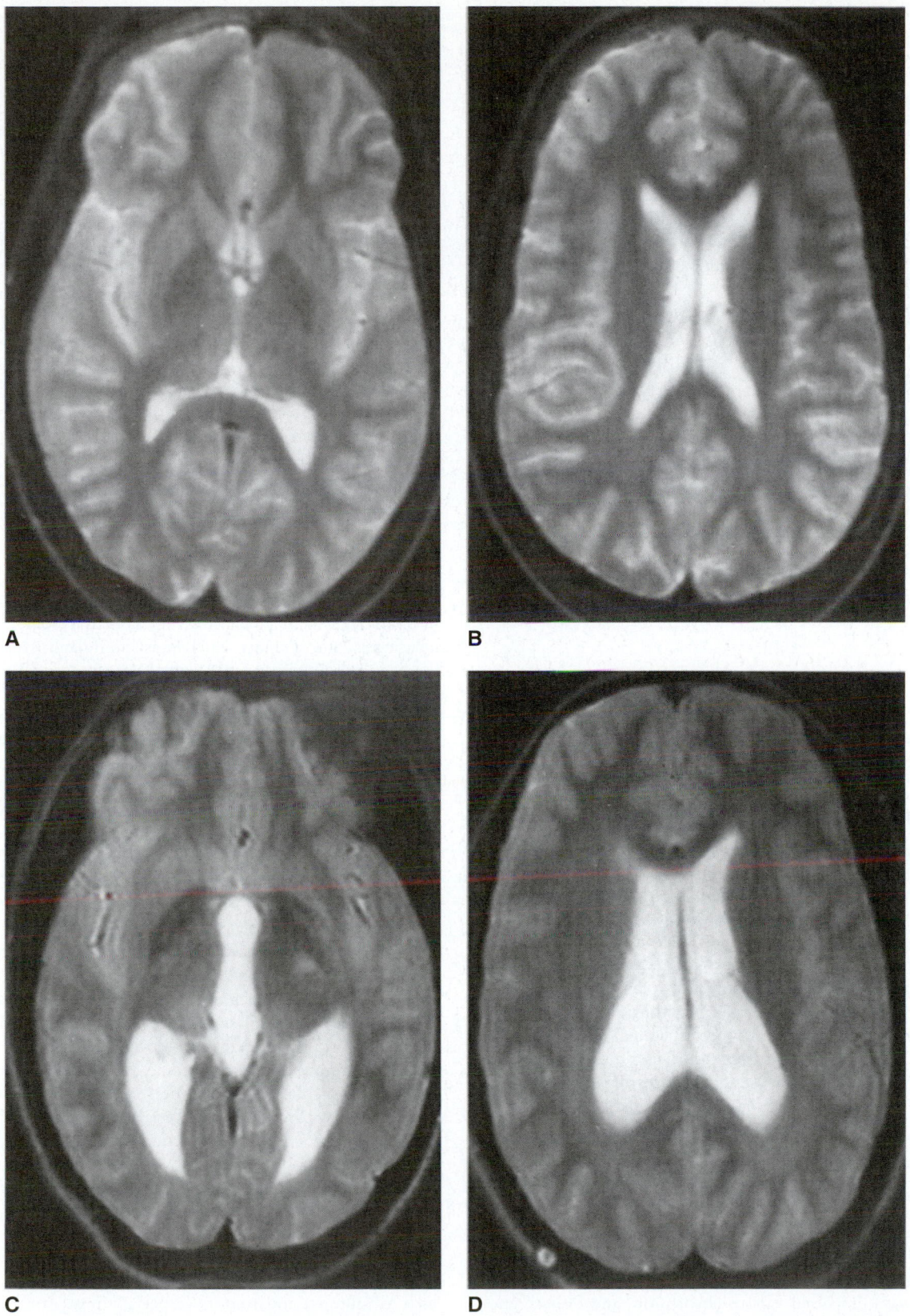

FIGURE 25-9 Axial T$_2$-weighted MR scans demonstrate normal third and lateral ventricles (**A** and **B**) in a 16-year-old scanned for seizures, and dilated ventricles (**C** and **D**) in a 16-year-old with aqueductal obstruction. *Courtesy of Dr. Jacqueline Bello.*

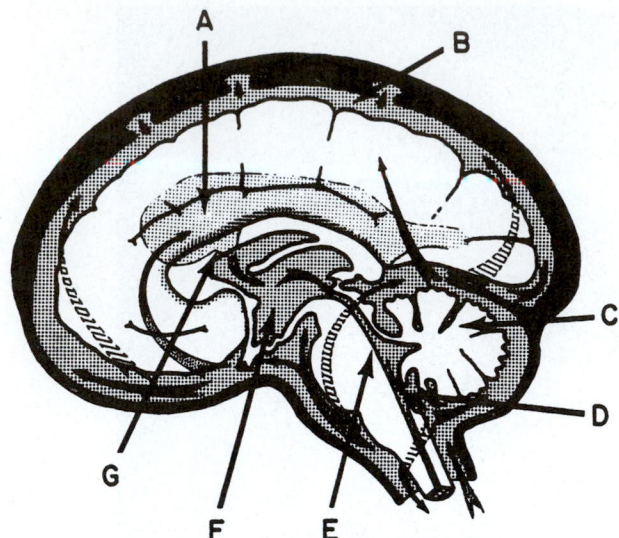

FIGURE 25-10 **Schematic diagram of a sagittal section of the brain with arrows tracing the flow of CSF. CSF flows out of the ventricular system through the fourth ventricle outlets into the basal cisterns, then through the tentorium over the cerebral hemispheres toward the arachnoid granulations in the superior sagittal sinus. There is also bidirectional flow of CSF in the spinal canal. A = lateral ventricle; B = subarachnoid space; C = cerebellum; D = foramen of Magendie; E = aqueduct of Sylvius; F = third ventricle; G = foramen of Monro.**

to as *cisterns*. The cisterns in the posterior fossa connect through pathways that traverse the tentorium to the subarachnoid spaces over the cerebral convexities. The spinal subarachnoid space communicates with the intracranial subarachnoid space by the basal cisterns. The net direction of CSF flow is from the lateral ventricles to the third ventricle and hence to the fourth ventricle and then through the basal cisterns, tentorium, and subarachnoid space over the cerebral convexities to the area of the sagittal sinus, from where absorption into the systemic circulation takes place. The net flow of fluid in the spinal subarachnoid space is cephalad. Most CSF absorption takes place across the arachnoid villi into the venous channels of the sagittal sinus, but fluid is also absorbed across the ependymal lining of the ventricular system and from the spinal subarachnoid space. In the normal adult, the total volume of CSF is approximately 150 mL, of which 25% is within the ventricular system. CSF is formed at the rate of approximately 20 mL/h, thereby indicating that CSF turns over three or four times per day. CSF formation continues when the intracranial pressure rises, unless extremely high levels are reached. Thus, there must be some absorption of fluid to accommodate the volume of CSF being formed each day.

Pathogenesis

Three possible mechanisms could explain the imbalance between CSF formation and absorption that results in excessive accumulation of fluid in the ventricles, leading to hydrocephalus: obstruction of CSF pathways, impaired venous absorption, and oversecretion of CSF.

Obstruction of CSF flow, both anatomic and functional, is the mechanism most commonly responsible for hydrocephalus. The ventricular system proximal to the block dilates. If one foramen of Monro is obstructed, the lateral ventricle on that side will dilate.

Blockage in the aqueduct of Sylvius results in dilation of the lateral and third ventricles, whereas the fourth ventricle remains relatively normal in size. In communicating hydrocephalus, the entire ventricular system becomes enlarged.

Excessive secretion of CSF is a rare cause of hydrocephalus and may be associated with a functional choroid plexus papilloma. In some patients, surgical removal of the tumor may arrest or cure the hydrocephalus. Interference with flow in the CSF pathways, however, may also result from the tumor obstructing the foramen of Monro or the fourth ventricle. Also, bleeding from the tumor may create an inflammatory reaction leading to fibrosis and blockage of the aqueduct, basal cisterns, or cerebral subarachnoid space.

Impaired venous absorption is another mechanism that might disturb CSF dynamics. Normally, the pressure in the venous sinuses is less than the CSF pressure, and this may aid the flow of CSF into the sinus. Thrombosis of the superior sagittal sinus would theoretically affect the flow of CSF from the arachnoid villi into the venous system. However, venous stasis in the cortex and cerebral edema result, rather than hydrocephalus. Ventricular dilation may occur in the chronic stages of the disease and may be related in part to cerebral atrophy secondary to infarction as well as the development of hydrocephalus.

Etiology

Congenital hydrocephalus can result from intrauterine infections by a variety of agents, including rubella virus, cytomegalovirus, toxoplasmosis, and syphilis, which cause an inflammatory reaction of the ependymal lining of the ventricular system and the meninges in the subarachnoid space.

Occlusion of CSF pathways in the aqueduct or basal cisterns may result. Hydrocephalus may be associated with congenital malformations of the nervous system, including isolated aqueductal stenosis, presumably not secondary to an inapparent intrauterine infection. The Dandy-Walker malformation consists of a posterior fossa cyst continuous with the fourth ventricle, partial or complete absence of the cerebellar vermis, and hydrocephalus. The Chiari malformation is often associated with hydrocephalus, spina bifida, and meningomyelocele. In this lesion, portions of the brainstem and cerebellum are displaced caudally into the cervical spinal canal, and the flow of CSF is impaired in the posterior fossa. Other disorders associated with hydrocephalus include a sex-linked form of aqueductal stenosis, arachnoid cysts, and multiple congenital malformations attributable to chromosomal anomalies. Recently the sex-linked form of congenital hydrocephalus has been found to be caused by mutations in the gene at Xq28 encoding for L1, a neural adhesion molecule. Other disorders caused by mutation in L1 include MASA syndrome (*m*ental retardation, *a*phasia, *s*huffling gait, *a*dducted thumbs), X-linked spastic paraplegia type 1, and X-linked agenesis of the corpus callosum. Rarely, congenital tumors of the central nervous system, especially those located near the midline, may obstruct CSF flow and result in enlargement of the ventricular system.

Acquired hydrocephalus is produced by infections of the nervous system (especially bacterial meningitis but also viral infections such as mumps) and tumors (especially posterior fossa medulloblastomas, astrocytomas, and ependymomas) that interfere with the flow of CSF. Ruptured aneurysms, arteriovenous malformations, trauma, and systemic bleeding disorders can result in bleeding into the subarachnoid space and, less commonly, the ventricular system, producing an inflammatory response and eventually fibrosis of the

CSF pathways. Intracranial hemorrhage in the premature infant may result in hydrocephalus.

Pathology

The pathologic anatomy will reflect the primary process and the effects of ventricular dilation itself. The head can be enormously enlarged when the ventricular dilation begins in infancy before the cranial sutures have fused, especially if the process evolves slowly so that the increased intracranial pressure is dissipated in part by the expanding volumes of the fluid-filled cavities. Marked head enlargement does not occur after the cranial sutures have fused or if the rate of accumulation of CSF is rapid. Both those conditions lead to significant increases in intracranial pressure that produces symptoms. Ventricular dilation often proceeds in an uneven fashion. The frontal and occipital horns enlarge first and to the greatest degree. Progressive enlargement leads to disruption of the ependymal lining of the ventricular walls. Edema occurs in the subependymal areas and progresses to involve the white matter. Loss of white matter substance ensues, with continued hydrocephalus, and the cerebral mantle may be reduced to a fraction of its original width. The reduction in the mantle width is mainly at the expense of the white matter, and even in far advanced disease the cortical ribbon of gray matter is relatively well preserved, especially compared with the white matter. Presumably, the white matter atrophy is caused by tissue ischemia from the edema and increased intraventricular pressure. In addition to the ventricular enlargement, other congenital abnormalities may occur. Cortical dysplasias, pachygyria, and polymicrogyria are associated with X-linked hydrocephalus. Early treatment of hydrocephalus in children allows the cerebral mantle to increase significantly in size, indicating that some degree of reversibility of the process exists.

Pathophysiology

Acute obstruction of the flow of CSF results in rapid enlargement of the ventricular system. This begins initially in the frontal and occipital horns of the lateral ventricles and is followed by symmetric dilation of the remainder of the intracerebral CSF-containing spaces. Compensatory mechanisms attempt to decrease the volumes of the other intracranial compartments. The subarachnoid space over the hemispheres becomes obliterated as the gyri become flattened and the sulci are compressed against the cranium. The vascular system is also compressed, and the venous pressure in the dural sinuses increases. The cerebral mantle becomes thinner as the ventricles enlarge. At this time, the total mass of brain tissue is probably unchanged. The ependymal lining of the ventricular system becomes disrupted, and CSF egresses directly into the brain parenchyma.

This enhances an alternate route of CSF absorption that is necessary to limit uncontrolled expansion of the ventricular system. The transependymal movement of CSF contributes to the development of periventricular white matter (interstitial) edema. Another compensatory mechanism that occurs in infants is enlargement of the volume of the intracranial cavity created by spreading of the cranial sutures. In chronic hydrocephalus, the white matter eventually atrophies, and the gray matter will ultimately be affected. Cerebral blood flow is reduced, more so in the white than the gray matter. Intracranial pressure may become reduced, compared with the previously attained maximum values, because the enlarged ventricular system has provided a greater surface area over which the force of fluid is distributed, thereby reducing the pressure.

Symptoms and Signs

Symptoms and signs are caused by the basic process causing the hydrocephalus, such as tumor, infection, or bleeding. Each of these will produce specific findings related to the basic pathologic process, and they are discussed in the relevant sections of this chapter. The increased intracranial pressure and dilation of the ventricles produce similar but nonspecific findings in all forms of hydrocephalus, independent of the primary cause. If excessive amounts of CSF accumulate slowly and adjustments take place, the patient may be asymptomatic until well into the course of the illness. Rapidly progressing hydrocephalus produces symptoms very early as the ventricular dilation develops acutely. Nonspecific symptoms include headaches, produced by distortion of the meninges and blood vessels. The pain may vary in intensity and location and may be intermittent or persistent. Early morning headaches associated with nausea and vomiting are often caused by increased intracranial pressure. Personality and behavior changes may include irritability, obstreperousness, indifference, and loss of interest. Lethargy and drowsiness may occur as the disease progresses; these signs are related to midbrain and brainstem dysfunction. Nausea, vomiting, and decreased appetite may be nonspecific symptoms but are produced in part by increased intracranial pressure in the posterior fossa. Nonspecific signs related to increased intracranial pressure may be present and may include papilledema and extraocular muscle pareses leading to diplopia caused by compression of the third or sixth cranial nerve. Changes in vital signs including bradycardia, systemic hypertension, and altered respiratory rates are produced by distortions of the brainstem. The anterior fontanelle may become full or distended. In infants and young children, excessive head growth may be noted on serial measurements of head circumference plotted on graphs of the normal growth curve. Significant dilation of the ventricles can occur, however, before abnormal head growth takes place. In young infants, an abnormal skull contour may develop in which the forehead becomes prominent, and this is referred to as *frontal bossing*. The scalp veins become dilated and prominent. Upward gaze may be impaired because of pressure on the midbrain, and the sclera above the iris will be visible. This is known as the *setting-sun sign*. Spasticity in the extremities, especially the legs, may develop as the fibers from the cortical motor areas are stretched around the bodies of the dilated ventricles in their course to the cerebral peduncles. Disturbances in growth, accelerated pubertal development, and fluid and electrolyte homeostasis may develop from pressure exerted on the hypothalamus by the dilated third ventricle.

Diagnosis

An infant whose head is growing excessively rapidly and whose head circumference measurement is crossing isobars on a growth chart should be suspected of having hydrocephalus. The clinical impression can be confirmed by appropriate radiographic procedures. CT or MR imaging shows brain tissue and CSF-filled spaces and has greatly facilitated the evaluation. Serial studies provide information regarding the rate of progression of the disease and the results of therapeutic intervention. The patterns of ventricular dilation may suggest the site of obstruction to the flow of CSF. Dilated lateral and third ventricles with a normal-size fourth ventricle suggest stenosis of the aqueduct. Symmetrically dilated ventricles, including the fourth ventricle, suggest an extraventricular obstruction. Neuroimaging studies will also show any associated malformations or causes of acquired hydrocephalus, such as tumors. CSF should be examined if an occult infection causing adhesive arachnoiditis or ependymitis is considered to be responsible for the hydrocephalus.

Therapy

Treatment should include specific therapy for any associated conditions and measures directed toward the hydrocephalus. Progressive hydrocephalus warrants intervention. Surgical therapy is the most effective means of treating hydrocephalus. A mechanical shunt system is used to circumvent the normal CSF pathways. A catheter is placed into one of the lateral ventricles, usually the right, and is connected to a one-way valve system that opens when the pressure in the ventricle exceeds a certain baseline value. As fluid egresses from the ventricles, lowering the pressure, the valve closes and remains shut until the pressure again rises. The valve is often placed beneath the scalp of the postauricular area. The distal end of the apparatus is connected to a catheter that is placed in the right atrium of the heart (ventriculoatrial) or into the peritoneal cavity (ventriculoperitoneal). Thus, the fluid flows directly from the lateral ventricles back into the systemic circulation, bypassing the site of mechanical or functional block in CSF absorption. The surgical procedure is obviously not curative, but it does effectively treat the symptoms, and it stops progression of the ventricular dilation. Recently, third ventriculostomies have been used to treat some forms of hydrocephalus and have been performed instead of shunt revisions. Young infants are often not candidates for this procedure. If the shunt system becomes disconnected or the catheters become obstructed, symptoms will recur if the hydrocephalus is still active. Occasionally, the hydrocephalus "compensates" or "arrests" spontaneously because of development of alternative pathways of absorption or reestablishment of the normal mechanisms for handling CSF. In those circumstances, revision of the shunt system may not be necessary.

Advances in fetal diagnostic ultrasonography have resulted in the ability to see the ventricular system and in diagnosing intrauterine hydrocephalus. Additional anomalies are usually present. The outcome of fetal surgery with placement of a ventriculoamniotic fluid shunt has been good in most instances. The best results for survival and intellectual development have been with isolated aqueductal stenosis. Intrauterine ventricular shunting should be considered for isolated progressive ventriculomegaly when the fetus is too immature to be delivered. A preferable mode of treatment would be to continue the pregnancy until a time when the fetus can safely be delivered and shunted postnatally. Approximately 50% of survivors will have normal motor and intellectual development.

In addition to the mechanical problems related to shunts, there are many other complications that can result from shunt surgery. The most important of these is infection of the shunt system, at times accompanied by the development of ventriculitis. Shunt infection may be an indolent process and often involves organisms that are not usually pathogens, such as *Staphylococcus epidermidis.* Other organisms found less frequently include *S. aureus,* enteric bacteria, diphtheroids, and *Streptococcus* species. Infection must be suspected in any child with a shunt who develops an unusual or persistent febrile illness. Another complication of ventriculoatrial shunts is pulmonary hypertension owing to chronic microembolism from thrombi formed on the atrial catheter.

Medical therapy designed to decrease CSF production has been used when patients have had slowly progressive hydrocephalus with few symptoms or signs and when the condition of the patient has prohibited surgery. Agents that have been used include acetazolamide, digoxin, furosemide, and glycerol. They have been used for relatively short periods and have not been as successful as surgical therapy. A recent randomized controlled trial of acetazolamide and furosemide in posthemorrhagic ventricular dilation in infancy failed to demonstrate any benefit. For further management of hydrocephalus in the preterm infant, see Sec. 2.16.5.

KLIPPEL-FEIL SYNDROME

Klippel-Feil syndrome is characterized by a triad of clinical features: short neck, limited neck motion, and a low occipital hairline. Three forms of the syndrome have been identified based on type and extent of congenital malformations of the vertebral column. In type I, many of the cervical and upper thoracic vertebrae are fused into a bony block. In type II, complete segmentation fails to occur at one or two cervical interspaces so that only several cervical vertebrae fuse. In type III, lesions similar to those found in types I and II occur, in addition to coexisting segmentation errors in the lower thoracic and lumbar vertebrae. No cause for the syndrome has been identified. Most cases are sporadic, but autosomal recessive and dominant forms have been described. Vertebral fusion anomalies are most likely caused by disturbed expression of *Pax-1* gene. The embryologic error occurs early in development, within the second fetal month, and probably involves a failure in the process of segmentation between adjacent sclerotomes to form vertebrae and intervertebral discs. The sclerotome is formed by migration of mesenchymal tissue in each somite toward the notochord. Klippel-Feil syndrome is composed of several genetic entities. Fusion of C2-3 may be inherited as an autosomal-dominant trait, whereas fusion of C5-6 may be inherited as an autosomal-recessive trait.

The high association of malformations in other organ systems warrants careful evaluation of all patients. Neurologic disorders include extraocular palsies, congenital deafness (both conductive and sensorineural), mirror movements, macrocephaly, hydrocephalus, nystagmus, meningocele, and mental retardation. Split cervical spinal cords, similar to diastematomyelia, may occur. Musculoskeletal anomalies include thoracic scoliosis, spina bifida occulta, Sprengel deformity, abnormalities of the ribs, webbing of the neck, and facial asymmetry. Congenital heart disease, particularly ventricular septal defects, and genitourinary anomalies, including unilateral renal agenesis, may be present. Dental abnormalities, cleft lip and palate, and abnormalities of the gastrointestinal tract, lungs, and skin may also be found.

Treatment consists of correcting the associated anomalies, whenever possible. Neurologic complications secondary to spinal instability and narrowing of the cervical canal may occur. The risk is increased with occipito-C1 abnormalities. Genetic counseling should be done.

HYDROMYELIA AND SYRINGOMYELIA

Hydromyelia is a symmetric dilation of the central canal of the spinal cord. Usually, the dilated cavity communicates or has communicated with the fourth ventricle and is lined by ependyma. The fluid within the cyst-like lesion is similar to CSF. The enlargement may extend over many segments and terminate at the level of the conus medullaris. Hydromyelia is often associated with other malformations of the central nervous system, including communicating hydrocephalus, Chiari malformation, and aqueductal stenosis. Hydromyelia may first be noted at autopsy. The diagnosis can be made by MR imaging. Patients often have symptoms and findings related to the associated malformations, and what part, if any, the dilated central canal contributes to the problem is unclear. Therapy is often directed at the associated lesions; treatment is rarely directed at the central canal itself.

Syringomyelia occurs infrequently in children. In this disorder, a paracentral cavity (syrinx) exists in the spinal cord, and it is lined with altered glial elements. The syrinx may be localized or may involve many segments, and often the cervical area is involved. If the lesion extends into the brainstem, the disorder is referred to as *syringobulbia*. The fluid within the cyst often has a yellowish tint and a higher protein content than CSF. Syringomyelia may be associated with intramedullary tumors, spinal cord trauma, arterial insufficiency, and developmental anomalies at the cervicomedullary junction, such as a Chiari malformation. The dilated central area is often referred to as *syringohydromyelia*. The pathogenesis of the lesion is unclear. The clinical features of the disease depend on the associated lesions and the size and location of the cyst. Segmental signs, such as wasting of the small muscles of the hand, sensory deficits involving the arms, and absence of tendon reflexes, are often present. Pressure on descending tracts may cause spasticity in the legs. The cavity often destroys the commissural fibers, resulting in a dissociated sensory disturbance with loss of pain and temperature sensations but preservation of touch sensation in a segmental distribution. Changes in respiration may occur secondary to involvement in the cervicomedullary region. Many patients with syringobulbia will have respiratory disturbances during sleep. These include very prolonged central, obstructive, and mixed sleep apneas with low oxygen saturation values. Confirmation of the diagnosis can be obtained by MR imaging. Treatment consists of therapy for the primary lesion, measures to correct malformations at the cervicomedullary junction, and, in some patients, myelotomy to treat the cystic lesion itself. Posterior fossa decompression, even in the absence of a Chiari malformation, has been helpful in some patients.

OCCULT SPINAL DYSRAPHISM

Disturbances in embryologic formation of the spinal canal and cord during the process of canalization and dedifferentiation beginning after 28 days of gestation can result in lesions located at the caudal end of the neural tube; they are covered by skin and are less obvious externally than meningomyeloceles (see below). Therefore, these lesions are referred to as *occult lesions*. They may involve the filum terminale and conus medullaris and are composed of a variety of soft tissue and bony lesions. The types of defects found include *lipomyelomeningocele,* in which a soft-tissue mass including fat and fibrous elements may be present under the skin in the lumbosacral area and extend into the spinal canal through a defect in the spine. In the spinal canal, the tumor may fuse with spinal roots and the conus medullaris, which is located at an abnormally low level. *Congenital lumbosacral lipomas* are lesions in which there is only a fatty tumor with no neural elements. They may be separated into two groups—those involving the conus and those confined to the filum. *Congenital dermal sinus* consists of a small stalk extending from a skin dimple to the intradural space, where it may join the spinal cord or end in an epidermal-type tumor. If the stalk is patent, it may serve as a portal of entry for bacteria and cause meningitis. Aberrant nerve roots or fibrous bands may adhere to nervous tissue and the bony canal. This is associated with an abnormally low position of the spinal cord (*tethered cord*), as occurs in most lesions of this type. Abnormalities in the formation of the filum terminale result in a thicker and shorter band than usual; this is often associated with other lesions in this area, or it may occur as an isolated defect. *Diastematomyelia* and *diplomyelia* consist of a division of

the spinal cord and meninges into two halves over several segments and may be associated with a bony spur or fibrous septum that appears to penetrate the divided spinal cord. The lesions are often grouped together and referred to as *split spinal cord malformations.* Vertebral anomalies include deformed, bifid, or fused laminae. The vertebral canal may be abnormally enlarged, particularly if there is an associated tumor. Excessive hair, a dimple (especially if larger than 5 mm or more than 2.5 mm from the anus) or sinus tract, pigmented maculae, hemangiomas, or subcutaneous lipoma may be present over the lower back. Deformities and atrophy of the feet and legs may be present.

The clinical features may be produced by several mechanisms, including malformed neural tissue, traction from adhesions that restrict normal mobility of the cord with movement and growth, and compression of the conus or roots by tumor tissue that may also impinge on the normal blood supply to the neural tissue.

Clinical problems may not be present at birth but may develop later as the child grows or as the tumor (if one is present) enlarges. These may include urinary and fecal incontinence, difficulty with motor function of the legs, numbness in the legs, back stiffness, and pain in the back or legs. Examination may disclose abnormalities over the back, deformity of the feet, or atrophy of the legs. Often the involvement is asymmetric. Neurologic examination may disclose changes in the tendon reflexes and weakness or numbness in the legs.

The majority of patients will have abnormalities of the spine on radiography, but in isolated spina bifida occulta there is no malformation involving neural tissue. Evaluation of spinal dysraphism and further definition of the lesion for neural involvement is initiated with a MR examination. Ideally, the whole spine should be imaged to detect all associated abnormalities (Fig. 25-11).

Neurosurgery is warranted for patients who have progressive disease. Some patients improve after surgery; in most other patients, the symptoms cease to progress. The role of surgery in prophylactic treatment of patients with these lesions to prevent the anticipated deterioration must be carefully evaluated in each patient. Deformities of the feet may require orthopedic surgery and physical therapy. Careful assessment of urinary tract function and morphology as well as detection and treatment of urinary tract infections are very important if progressive renal disease is to be prevented.

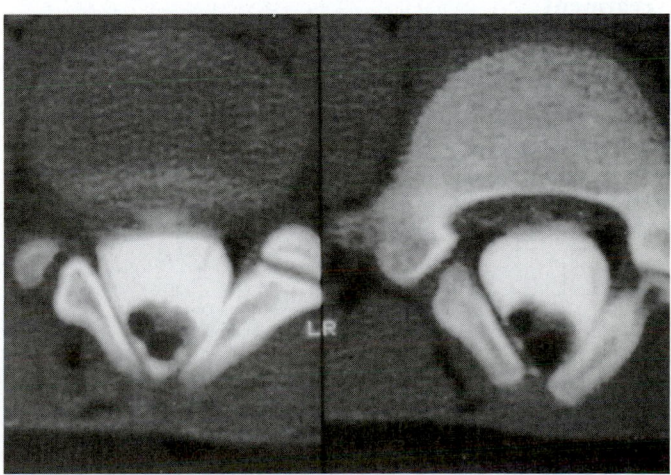

FIGURE 25-11 Axial myelo-CT demonstrates spinal dysraphism and meningocele containing neural elements of soft-tissue density and lipoma of lower CT density. *Courtesy of Dr. Jacqueline Bello.*

CHIARI MALFORMATION

The Chiari malformation is a hindbrain anomaly characterized by caudal displacement of the cerebellum and brainstem. Depending on the degree of caudal displacement, the malformation is classified into three types. In type I, cerebellar tonsils or vermis are below the level of the foramen magnum. Greater than 5 mm is considered significant, but lesser degrees of displacement may be associated with clinical symptoms. In type II, the fourth ventricle and lower medulla are displaced below the level of the foramen magnum; this form is usually associated with myelomeningocele and hydrocephalus. In type III, there is a cervical spina bifida with herniation of the cerebellum through the defect. Type II is the most common form of the anomaly. Other anomalies that may be associated with the Chiari malformation are cavitation of the spinal cord and/or medulla (see section on syringomyelia), breaking of the midbrain, cranial lacunae, large massa intermedia, hypoplasia of the falx of cerebrum, low attachment of the tentorium, small posterior fossa, and vertebral anomalies.

Clinical Features

Type I lesions may become symptomatic anytime between infancy and adulthood. Symptoms result from dysfunction of lower cranial nerves, brainstem, and/or spinal cord. These include dysphagia, sleep apnea, vocal cord paralysis, vertigo, ataxia, nystagmus, torticollis, headache, and neck pain. Spinal cord dysfunction results in dysesthesias, weakness and spasticity of extremities, sensory loss, scoliosis, and occasionally bowel and bladder dysfunction. Patients with type II malformations have similar symptoms, plus those caused by the associated hydrocephalus and meningomyelocele. These patients are usually diagnosed at birth and have symptoms related to lower cranial nerve dysfunction. The other symptoms may develop later in childhood.

Evaluation

Magnetic resonance imaging is the most informative procedure for studying the posterior fossa and spinal cord. It is noninvasive and allows the malformation to be imaged in several planes. The midsagittal view demonstrates the downward displacement of the hindbrain and other associated features (Fig. 25-12).

Treatment

Treatment of hydrocephalus and meningomyelocele is discussed in other sections. If the child is asymptomatic, no treatment is indicated. Symptomatic children, particularly those with progressive symptoms, may benefit from surgery. Various procedures have been utilized; these include suboccipital decompressions with or without cervical laminectomies. Decompression of cavities in the brainstem or spinal cord, often by shunting the cyst, may also be helpful.

NEURAL TUBE DEFECTS

Neural tube defects result from a defect in neurulation (days 18 to 28 of gestation) that causes malformation of the vertebral column and the spinal cord and associated anomalies of other portions of the central nervous system. In the more severe forms of the malformation, the neural tube fails to close, and the neural plate may present through a defect in the vertebral column (*spina bifida*) and the integument as a raw, red, fleshy plaque. The abnormality may consist of a protruding membranous sac composed of meninges, CSF, nerve roots, and dysplastic spinal cord. This is referred to as

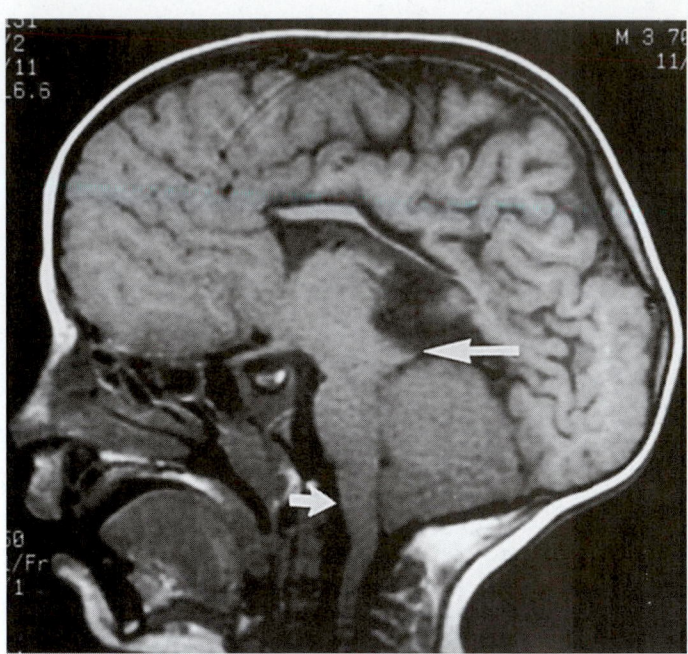

FIGURE 25-12 Arnold-Chiari malformation demonstrated by MR imaging—sagittal view. There is downward displacement of the medulla and cerebellar tonsils (*short arrow*) and beaking of the tectum (*long arrow*). *Courtesy of Dr. Charles McCluggage.*

a *meningomyelocele*. Lesions that occur during the second and third stages of neural tube formation, canalization, and retrogressive differentiation result in skin-covered lesions. Occasionally, no neurologic deficit exists. This form of the malformation is a *meningocele*, and it occurs in approximately 10% of all patients with spina bifida. Hydrocephalus and Chiari II malformations are present in the vast majority of patients with meningomyeloceles.

Epidemiology

The incidence of neural tube defect varies in different ethnic populations and geographic sites, but it usually ranges between 1 and 5 per 1000 live births. Girls are affected more frequently than boys. Familial occurrence is well documented, and the risk of a subsequent sibling having a similar malformation is 5% with one affected propositus; this risk increases to 10 to 15% if there are two affected siblings. Affected mothers have a 3% chance of giving birth to an offspring with a similar malformation. The cause of the defect is unknown. Dysraphic states have been associated with other malformation syndromes (Meckel-Gruber syndrome and encephaloceles) and infrequently with chromosomal malformations (trisomies 18 and 13). Low maternal levels of vitamins, including folic acid, and hyperthermia during pregnancy as well as the taking of clomiphene and valproic acid have been associated with an increased incidence of neural tube defects. Recently, susceptibility genes have been identified. They involve folic acid metabolism, and the most commonly involved one is the methylene tetrahydrofolate reductase gene. The exact mechanism whereby neural tube defects result is unknown. The currently identified genes account for only a minority of cases.

Clinical Features

The diagnosis of a neural tube defect is usually apparent at birth because of the grossly visible lesion over the spine. Any segment of the vertebral column may be involved, but the most common sites are the lumbar and sacral spines. The defect may involve many segments and often involves the entire spine distal to the most proximal malformed vertebra, especially when the lesion starts in a lumbar or sacral segment. Motor and sensory deficits are present in the trunk and legs, corresponding to the segments that normally would have been innervated by what is now a dysplastic spinal cord. The deficits are usually severe, resulting in complete paralysis and absence of sensation. The total spinal cord distal to the site of the lesion may be nonfunctional. Occasionally the distal cord may be partially functional, but the afferent pathways to the brain will have been disrupted. Thus, segmental reflexes may be present, resulting in the preservation of tendon reflexes or the ability to withdraw a limb from a painful stimulus. There is no volitional control of movement or appreciation of pain, however. Aberrant connections may exist in the involved spinal cord, resulting in unusual findings such as contraction of the contralateral limb when eliciting tendon reflexes. In some instances, the partially functioning segment of spinal cord may retain some central connections, resulting in voluntary control of isolated movements or the appreciation of sensation in part of the involved limbs. Almost all these patients have involvement of bladder and bowel, resulting in urinary and fecal incontinence. Hydrocephalus is present in the vast majority of patients with meningomyeloceles, and it will be progressive and require treatment in 70 to 80%. The hydrocephalus may be communicating or noncommunicating, the latter being associated with aqueductal stenosis. Ventricular dilation may be present at birth or may develop during the first year of life; infrequently the problem first becomes manifest at a later age. The hydrocephalus often progresses after surgical repair of the back lesion in the neonatal period caused by elimination of a source of CSF escape through a leaking meningomyelocele or removal of a large sac that acts as a reservoir for the CSF, thus providing an increased space to accommodate excess fluid. Other problems include strabismus, facial weakness, swallowing difficulties, vocal cord paresis, and disordered breathing. They are caused by brainstem dysfunction. Progressive symptoms related to the Chiari malformation, syrinx, or tethering of the spinal cord may occur later—beyond infancy.

Children who have meningomyeloceles and hydrocephalus usually have other central nervous system malformations, the most common of which are the Chiari deformity and hydrosyringomyelia (see above).

Treatment

The needs of children with spina bifida and their families are best met by a multidisciplinary team with expertise in general pediatrics, neurology, neurosurgery, orthopedics, and urology. Also, rehabilitation therapists, social workers, specialized nurses, and psychologists can provide valuable help in the care of affected children. The immediate consideration after the birth of an infant with a meningomyelocele is to assess the existing disabilities fully so that appropriate decisions may be made regarding treatment. Factors to be evaluated in the neonatal period include the degree of paralysis, the extent of hydrocephalus, the presence of kyphosis, associated gross congenital anomalies, major birth injuries, and the early development of complications such as severe central nervous system infections. Decisions regarding management, in addition to the preceding factors, should include discussions with the parents regarding the prognosis for their infant.

Delivery by cesarean section of infants with meningomyeloceles diagnosed antenatally before the onset of labor has been suggested

because of better subsequent motor function compared with infants delivered vaginally. The possible benefits seem to be greater for those infants who have breech presentation. Open meningomyeloceles and those leaking CSF provide a portal of entry for bacteria and predispose the patient to the development of infection. Hydrocephalus often progresses during the first month of life and can be evaluated by CT or MR imaging. Progressive hydrocephalus requires treatment with a shunt procedure, usually ventriculoperitoneal. The complications of this procedure include obstruction and infection (see discussion of Hydrocephalus, above). Some infants may be candidates for simultaneous repair of the myelomeningocele and ventriculoperitoneal shunting.

The goals of orthopedic management include the correction of deformity, promotion of ambulation when possible, and maintenance of posture to allow patients to function at their maximum capabilities. Deformities may be caused by unbalanced muscle action about joints or congenital deformities of the skeleton, or they may result from fractures, which occur readily in the legs of patients with paraplegia. The areas most often involved in treatment are the feet, knees, hips, and spine. Management techniques include the use of casting and corrective appliances and surgical procedures on soft tissue and bone. Appropriate orthoses can significantly increase the functional ability of children with spina bifida. Treatment must be individualized.

Careful monitoring of the urinary tract is essential (see Sec. 21.6). Almost all patients with spina bifida have some degree of bladder dysfunction. The exact type of dysfunction is difficult to predict on the basis of the location of the spinal lesion or the neurologic examination. Urinary tract morphology and function are involved in a dynamic process that can be modified by growth and infection. A normal configuration of the urinary collecting system in an early age does not exclude the possibility of later deterioration. Serial examinations of the urine to detect infection and serial assessment of the status of the upper urinary tract are essential in urologic management of children with spina bifida. Control of urinary incontinence is a major goal in patients with myelodysplasia. This can be achieved to some degree by use of intermittent catheterization of the bladder and by pharmacologic agents that influence bladder and sphincter tone. Depending on the state of the bladder and the catheterization program, anticholinergic and α-adrenergic stimulators or blockers can be used.

Treatment of the patient and family should include counseling regarding the risk of conceiving another child with a similar malformation. Antenatal diagnosis of dysraphism is possible by measurement of α-fetoprotein, which is a fetal-specific α-globulin synthesized in the liver. Apparently this protein leaks from a fetus with an open neural tube defect into the amniotic fluid. The best time for detecting abnormally high concentrations of this protein in the amniotic fluid is during the third and fourth months of pregnancy; α-fetoprotein crosses the placenta and can be detected in maternal serum, thus making possible easy screening of high-risk pregnancies for this malformation. Raised levels of maternal serum acetylcholinesterase are also found in affected pregnancies. Presently, prenatal diagnosis can be attempted by screening maternal serum and confirming the diagnosis by ultrasound examination of the fetus, looking for a cystic mass, anencephaly, or hydrocephalus. If this is inconclusive, the amniotic fluid should be examined. This approach will detect approximately 98% of fetuses with open neural tube defects.

Periconceptional use of vitamins containing folic acid appears to decrease the incidence of first-occurrence as well as recurrent neural tube defects. Ideally, supplementation should begin 1 to 2 months prior to conception.

CAUDAL REGRESSION SYNDROME

Caudal regression syndrome, also known as *caudal dysplasia* or *sacral agenesis syndrome,* is a congenital malformation characterized by various degrees of developmental failure involving the legs, the lumbar, sacral, and coccygeal vertebrae and the corresponding segments of the spinal cord. The orthopedic anomalies may include fusion of the legs, hypoplastic femur, defects of the tibia and the fibula, flexion contractures of the knee and hip, and clubfoot. Dislocated hips and deficiencies in the pelvis have also been noted. Anomalies of other organ systems may be present. Genitourinary anomalies include renal agenesis, horseshoe-shaped or rudimentary kidneys, and deformed external genitalia. Gastrointestinal abnormalities consist mainly of imperforate anus. Less common deformities include cleft lip or palate, microcephaly, congenital heart disease, and pulmonary system malformations.

The syndrome is believed to result from a defect in neurulation. The exact cause of the malformation is unknown, but of interest is the relationship with diabetes mellitus. A history of maternal diabetes is obtained in 16% of infants with sacral agenesis, and 1% of infants born to mothers with diabetes will have the syndrome.

The clinical presentation depends on the severity of the deformities and the organ system involved. Abnormalities of the legs may bring the patient to the attention of an orthopedist. The neurologic deficits usually involve weakness and atrophy in those segments distal to the lowest vertebra present. The sensory deficits are often less severe than is the motor involvement, which is explained by fairly normal segmental development of neural crest tissue despite the absence of portions of the neural plate at the level of agenesis. Thus, dorsal root ganglia may develop and connect with the intact spinal cord.

In those patients with very low lesions, mainly involving only the sacrum, the presenting problem may be urinary incontinence or dribbling.

Treatment consists of appropriate evaluation and, if possible, correction of the associated congenital malformation. Particular attention should be given to the urinary tract, and appropriate serial monitoring and surveillance for infection are imperative (see Sec. 21.6).

References

Anencephaly

Ashwal S, Peabody JL, Schneider S, Tomasi LG, Emery JR, Peckham N: Anencephaly: clinical determination of brain death and neuropathologic studies. Pediatr Neurol 6:233–239, 1990

Hamby YY, O'Brien JE, Critchfield G, Leon J, Ayoub M, Johnson MP, Evans MI: Combination of elevated maternal serum alpha-fetoprotein (MSAFP) and low estriol is highly predictive of anencephaly. Am J Med Genet 75(3):297–299, 1998

Medical Task Force on Anencephaly: The infant with anencephaly. N Engl J Med 322:669–674, 1990

Peabody JL, Emery JR, Ashwal S: Experience with anencephalic infants as prospective organ donors. N Engl J Med 321:344–350, 1989

Sadovnick AD, Baird PA: Congenital malformations associated with anencephaly in liveborn and stillborn infants. Teratology 32:355–361, 1985

Stone DH: The declining prevalence of anencephalus and spina bifida: its nature, causes, and implications. Dev Med Child Neurol 29:541–546, 1987

Encephalocele

Hoving EW, Vermeij-Keers C: Frontoethmoidal encephaloceles, a study of their pathogenesis. Pediatr Neurosurg 27(5):246–256, 1997

Humphreys RP: Encephalocele and dermal sinuses. In: Cheek WR, ed: Pediatric Neurosurgery, 3rd ed. Philadelphia, Saunders, 1994

Mealey J Jr, Dzenitis AJ, Hockey AA: The prognosis of encephaloceles. J Neurosurg 32:209–218, 1970

Hydrocephalus

Carey CM, Tullous MW, Walker ML: Hydrocephalus: etiology, pathologic effects, diagnosis, and natural history. In: Cheek WR, ed: Pediatric Neurosurgery, 3rd ed. Philadelphia, Saunders, 1994

Chervenak F: Current perspectives on the diagnosis, prognosis, and management of fetal hydrocephalus. In: Hill A, Volpe J, eds: Fetal Neurology. New York, Raven Press, 1989

Cinalli G, Salazar C, Mallucci C, Yada JZ, Zerah M, Sainte-Rose C: The role of endoscopic third ventriculostomy in the management of shunt malfunction. Neurosurgery 43:1323–1329, 1998

Den Hollander NS, Vinkesteijn A, Schmitz-Van Splunder P, Catsman-Berrevoets C, Wladimiroff JW: Prenatally diagnosed fetal ventriculomegaly: prognosis and outcome. Prenat Diagn 18:557–566, 1998

Fransen E, Van Camp G, Vits L, Willems PJ: L1-associated diseases: clinical geneticists divide, molecular geneticists unite. Hum Mol Genet 6(10):1625–1632, 1997

Graf WD, Born DE, Sarnat HB: The pachygyria-polymicrogyria spectrum of cervical dysplasia in X-linked hydrocephalus. Eur J Pediatr Surg 8(1):10–14, 1998

International PHVD Drug Trial Group: International randomised controlled trial of acetazolamide and furosemide in posthaemorrhagic ventricular dilatation in infancy. Lancet 352:433–440, 1998

Kirkinen P, Serlo W, Jouppila P, Ryynanen M, Martikainen A: Long-term outcome of fetal hydrocephaly. J Child Neurol 11:189–192, 1996

Kirkpatrick M, Engleman H, Minns RA: Symptoms and signs of progressive hydrocephalus. Arch Dis Child 64:124, 1989

Lopponen T, Saukkonen A-L, Serlo W, Tapanainen P, Ruokonen A, Knip M: Accelerated pubertal development in patients with shunted hydrocephalus. Arch Dis Child 74:490–496, 1996

Marlin AE, Gaskill SJ: Cerebrospinal fluid shunts: complications and results. In: Cheek WR, ed: Pediatric Neurosurgery, 3rd ed. Philadelphia, Saunders, 1994

Rekate HL: Treatment of hydrocephalus. In: Cheek WR, ed: Pediatric Neurosurgery, 3rd ed. Philadelphia, Saunders, 1994

Schapiro S, Boaz J, Kleiman M, et al: Origin of organisms infecting ventricular shunts. Neurosurgery 22:868, 1988

Schrander-Stumpel C, Fryns J-P: Congenital hydrocephalus: nosology and guidelines for clinical approach and genetic counselling. Eur J Pediatr 157:355–362, 1998

Klippel-Feil Syndrome

David KM, Copp AJ, Stevens JM, Hayward RD, Crockard HA: Split cervical spinal cord with Klippel-Feil syndrome: seven cases. Brain 119:1859–1872, 1996

McGaughran JM, Kuna P, Das V: Audiological abnormalities in the Klippel-Feil syndrome. Arch Dis Child 79(4):352–355, 1998

Moore WB, Matthews TJ, Rabinowitz R: Genitourinary anomalies associated with Klippel-Feil syndrome. J Bone Joint Surg 57A:355, 1975

Nagib MG, Maxwell RE, Chou SN: Klippel-Feil syndrome in children: clinical features and management. Childs Nerv Syst 2:255, 1985

Rouvreau P, Glorion C, Langlais J, Noury H, Pouliquen JC: Assessment and neurologic involvement of patients with cervical spine congenital synostosis as in Klippel-Feil syndrome: study of 19 cases. J Pediatr Orthop 7(3):179–185, 1998

Hydromyelia and Syringomyelia

Hoffman HJ, Neill J, Crone KR, et al: Hydrosyringomyelia and its management in childhood. Neurosurgery 21:347, 1987

Iskandar BJ, Hedlund GL, Grabb PA, Oakes WJ: The resolution of syringohydromyelia without hindbrain herniation after posterior fossa decompression. J Neurosurg 89:212–216, 1998

Nogues M, Gene R, Benarroch E, Leiguarda R, Calderon C, Encabo H: Respiratory disturbances during sleep in syringomyelia and syringobulbia. Neurology 52(9):1777–1783, 1999

Reigel DH, Rotenstein D: Spina bifida. In: Cheek WR, ed: Pediatric Neurosurgery, 3rd ed. Philadelphia, Saunders, 1994

Wisoff JH: Hydromyelia: a critical review. Childs Nerv Syst 4:1, 1988

Occult Spinal Dysraphism

Andar UB, Harkness WF, Hayward RD: Split cord malformations of the lumbar region. A model for the neurosurgical management of all types of "occult" spinal dysraphism? Pediatr Neurosurg 26(1):17–24, 1997

Cornette L, Verpoorten C, Lagae L, Van Calenbergh F, Plets C, et al: Tethered cord syndrome in occult spinal dysraphism: timing and outcome of surgical release. Neurology 50(6):1761–1765, 1998

Ersahin Y, Mutluer S, Kocaman S, Demirtas E: Split spinal cord malformations in children. J Neurosurg 88:57–65, 1998

Johnston LB, Borzyskowski M: Bladder dysfunction and neurological disability at presentation in closed spina bifida. Arch Dis Child 79(1):33–38, 1998

Kriss VM, Desai NS: Occult spinal dysraphism in neonates: assessment of high-risk cutaneous stigmata on sonography. Am J Roentgenol 171(6):1687–1692, 1998

McLone DG, La Marca F: The tethered spinal cord: diagnosis, significance, and management. Semin Pediatr Neurol 4(3):192–208, 1997

Palmer LS, Richards I, Kaplan WE: Subclinical changes in bladder function in children presenting with nonurological symptoms of the tethered cord syndrome. J Urol 159(1):231–234, 1998

Pierre-Kahn A, Zerah M, Renier D, et al: Congenital lumbosacral lipomas. Childs Nerv Syst 13:298–335, 1997

Scatliff JH, Kendall BE, Kingsley DPE, et al: Closed spinal dysraphism: analysis of clinical, radiological, and surgical findings in 104 consecutive patients. Am J Neurol Radiol 10:269, 1989

Chiari Malformation

Dure LS, Percy AK, Cheek WR, Laurent JP: Chiari type I malformation in children. J Pediatr 115:573–576, 1989

Elster AD, Chen MYM: Chiari I malformations: clinical and radiologic reappraisal. Radiology 183:347–353, 1992

Haines SI, Berger M: Current treatment of Chiari malformations types I and II: a survey of the Pediatric Section of the American Association of Neurological Surgeons. Neurosurgery 28:353–357, 1991

Hida K, Iwasaki Y, Koyanagi I, Abe H: Pediatric syringomyelia with Chiari malformation: its clinical characteristics and surgical outcomes. Surg Neurol 51(4):390–391, 1999

La Marca F, Herman M, Grant JA, McLone DG: Presentation and management of hydromyelia in children with Chiari type-II malformation. Pediatr Neurosurg 26(2):57–67, 1997

Milhorat TH, Chou MW, Trinidad EM, et al: Chiari I malformation redefined: clinical and radiographic findings for 364 symptomatic patients. Neurosurg 44(5):1005–1017, 1999

Teo C, Parker EC, Aureli S, Boop FA: The Chiari II malformation: a surgical series. Pediatr Neurosurg 27(5):223–229, 1997

Weinberg JS, Freed DL, Sadock J, Handler M, Wisoff JH, Epstein FJ: Headache and Chiari I malformation in the pediatric population. Pediatr Neurosurg 29(1):14–18, 1998

Neural Tube Defects

Botto LD, Mastroiacovo P: Exploring gene-gene interactions in the etiology of neural tube defects. Clin Genet 53(6):456–459, 1998

Brennand DM, Jehanli AM, Wood PJ, Smith JL: Raised levels of maternal serum secretory acetylcholinesterase may be indicative of fetal neural tube defects in early pregnancy. Acta Obstet Gynecol Scand 77(1):8–13, 1998

Cochrane D, Aronyk K, Sawatzky B, Wilson D, Steinbok P: The effects of labor and delivery on spinal cord function and ambulation in patients with meningomyelocele. Childs Nerv Syst 7:312–315, 1991

Czeizel AE, Dudas I: Prevention of the first occurrence of neural-tube defects by periconceptional vitamin supplementation. N Engl J Med 327:1832–1835, 1992

Liptak GS, Bloss JW, Briskin H, et al: The management of children with spinal dysraphism. J Child Neurol 3:3, 1988

McLone DG: The biological resolution of malformations of the central nervous system. Neurosurgery 43:1375–1381, 1998

Miller PD, Pollack IF, Pang D, Albright AL: Comparison of simultaneous versus delayed ventriculoperitoneal shunt insertion in children undergoing myelomeningocele repair. J Child Neurol 11:370–372, 1996

Molloy AM, Mills JL, Kirke PN, et al: Low blood folates in NTD pregnancies are only partly explained by thermolabile 5,10-methylenetetrahydrofolate reductase: low folate status alone may be the critical factor. Am J Med Genet 78:155–159, 1998

Morrison K, Papapetrou C, Hol FA, et al: Susceptibility to spina bifida: an association study of five candidate genes. Ann Hum Genet 62:379–396, 1998

MRC Vitamin Study Research Group: Prevention of neural tube defects: results of the Medical Research Council Vitamin Study. Lancet 338:131–137, 1991

Reigel DH, Rotenstein D: Spina bifida. In: Cheek WR, ed: Pediatric Neurosurgery, 3rd ed. Philadelphia, Saunders, 1994.

Van der Put NM, Gabreels F, Stevens EM, et al: A second common mutation in the methylenetetrahydrofolate reductase gene: an additional risk factor for neural-tube defects? Am J Hum Genet 62(5):1044–1051, 1998

Waters KA, Forbes P, Morielli A, et al: Sleep-disordered breathing in children with myelomeningocele. J Pediatr 132(4):672–681, 1998

Werler MM, Shapiro S, Mitchell AA: Periconceptional folic acid exposure and risk of occurrent neural tube defects. JAMA 269:1257–1261, 1993

Caudal Regression Syndrome

Adra A, Cordero D, Mejides A, Yasin S, Salman F, O'Sullivan JM: Caudal regression syndrome: etiopathogenesis, prenatal diagnosis, and perinatal management. Obstet Gynecol Surv 49(7):508–516, 1994

Goto MP, Goldman AS: Diabetic embryopathy. Curr Opin Pediatr 6(4):486–491, 1994

Renshaw TS: Sacral agenesis. J Bone Joint Surg 60A:373, 1978

Sarnat HB, Case ME, Graviss R: Sacral agenesis. Neurology 26:1124, 1976

25.4   ACUTE ENCEPHALOPATHIES OF INFANCY

Alan Hill

Improvements in obstetric care and in the treatment of infections and respiratory disorders in the newborn have focused increasing attention on neurologic problems that remain a major cause of morbidity and mortality in this age group. Long-term sequelae of acute newborn encephalopathies include epilepsy, cerebral palsy, cognitive impairment, and behavior disturbances. The term *encephalopathy* implies clinical cerebral dysfunction, which may have diverse etiologies. Several major causes of acute neonatal encephalopathy, eg, infection, metabolic derangements, and trauma, are discussed in other chapters. In this section, hypoxic-ischemic and hemorrhagic cerebral injury as well as maternal drug abuse will be discussed as the major causes of acute encephalopathy in both premature and full-term newborns. In each individual case, the clinical features of an acute encephalopathy must be evaluated in the context of the stage of maturity of the brain at the time of insult.

25.4.1 Hypoxic-Ischemic Encephalopathy

A rational approach to management of neurologic problems must be based on principles of basic science, eg, neuropathology, physiological and biochemical mechanisms. Clearly, detailed discussion of these aspects is beyond the scope of this chapter. Hypoxic-ischemic encephalopathy results, as the term implies, from a combination of hypoxia and ischemia, with one or the other predominating. This encephalopathy is often associated with other potentially harmful conditions, eg, lactic acidosis, accumulation of excitotoxic amino acids (especially glutamate), and impaired cerebrovascular autoregulation. The severity and anatomic distribution of hypoxic-ischemic cerebral injury in the newborn is determined principally by the severity and duration of the hypoxic-ischemic insult and the maturity of the brain at the time of insult.

Hypoxic-Ischemic Encephalopathy in the Full-Term Newborn

Diagnosis

The importance of a detailed history and neurologic and systemic examinations for the assessment of the full-term newborn with suspected hypoxic-ischemic encephalopathy cannot be overemphasized.

History Because hypoxic-ischemic insult in the full-term newborn occurs most commonly antepartum or during the intrapartum period, a history of maternal risk factors and abnormalities of labor and delivery must be documented in detail.

Several clinical indicators have been suggested as markers of the possible occurrence of acute hypoxic-ischemic insult, eg, prolonged fetal bradycardia or repeated late decelerations, low Apgar scores at 5 minutes or later, low fetal scalp or cord pH, and requirement for prolonged resuscitation with positive-pressure ventilation. There is some controversy concerning the specificity of these indicators and whether they permit the recognition of hypoxic-ischemic insult of sufficient severity to cause irreversible brain injury. Much of this controversy would be avoided if these indicators were used only to establish that a hypoxic-ischemic insult had occurred that may be a possible etiology of acute neonatal encephalopathy. The indicators do not establish that *irreversible* brain injury has occurred. Thus, any single clinical indicator or even several indicators in combination are not diagnostic of the severity of encephalopathy or brain injury nor predictive of long-term outcome. Such judgments should be based on detailed assessment of the severity and clinical

course of the acute neonatal encephalopathy together with adjunctive data from neuroimaging and other laboratory investigations.

Physical Examination Full-term newborns who sustain acute intrapartum hypoxic-ischemic insult severe enough to cause long-term neurologic sequelae invariably have a clinically recognizable acute encephalopathy during the first days of life. It is important to realize that such clinical encephalopathy may be difficult to recognize in premature newborns because of the immaturity of the affected brain. Furthermore, full-term newborns who sustain hypoxic-ischemic insult earlier during gestation may be asymptomatic during the early neonatal period. It is important to emphasize that the clinical features of the encephalopathy are nonspecific and that a diagnosis of hypoxia-ischemia as a cause should be made with caution and only in the context of a history of preceding acute hypoxic-ischemic insult (see above discussion on clinical markers) and other adjunctive laboratory data. In many instances, a combination of conditions, eg, hypoxic-ischemic injury, intracranial hemorrhage, metabolic derangements, may contribute to the severity of encephalopathy. To a limited extent, the timing and evolution of the acute encephalopathy may be useful for determining the principal underlying cause.

Although there is a complete spectrum of hypoxic-ischemic encephalopathy in the full-term newborn, classification of the severity of the encephalopathy as *mild, moderate,* or *severe* is useful for determining prognosis (see Table 25-2). There is often a recognizable progression of clinical symptoms in full-term newborns with severe hypoxic-ischemic encephalopathy. Initially, during the first 24 hours of life, there is often decreased level of consciousness and seizures. Seizures, which are a major manifestation of moderate or severe encephalopathy, usually begin on the first day of life and are often refractory to anticonvulsant therapy. Signs of brainstem dysfunction (eg, impaired extraocular movements, abnormal pupillary

TABLE 25-2

SEVERITY OF HYPOXIC-ISCHEMIC ENCEPHALOPATHY AND PROGNOSIS

SEVERITY OF ENCEPHALOPATHY	CHARACTERISTICS	PERCENT ABNORMAL OUTCOME
Mild	Jittery, irritable	0
	Increased tendon reflexes	
	Exaggerated Moro response	
Moderate	Lethargic, hypotonic	20–40
	Suppressed primitive reflexes	
	± Seizures	
Severe	Comatose, hypotonic,	100
	Brainstem dysfunction	
	Seizures	
	± Increased intracranial pressure	

SOURCE: *Based on Sarnat HB, Sarnat MS: Neonatal encephalopathy following fetal distress: a clinical and electro-encephalographic study. Arch Neurol 33:696–705, 1976; Robertson C, Finer NN: Term infants with hypoxic-ischemic encephalopathy: outcome at 3.5 years. Dev Med Child Neurol 27:473, 1985; Volpe JJ: Brain injury in the premature infant—neuropathology, clinical aspects, pathogenesis and prevention. Clin Perinatol 24:567, 1995.*

responses, respiratory impairment, tongue fasciculations, impaired swallowing and sucking) often worsen during the first 3 days of life. Clinically recognizable cerebral edema (eg, recognized on the basis of a tense or bulging anterior fontanelle) is relatively uncommon and occurs only in the context of severe encephalopathy. This edema generally reaches maximum severity between 24 and 96 hours of age and is considered to be a consequence of extensive tissue necrosis. In such situations, respiratory arrest and death occur commonly around 72 hours of age. Infants who survive usually have gradual stabilization or improvement in neurologic status after 3 or 4 days of age. However, often there may be persistent stupor, abnormal muscle tone, and ongoing feeding difficulties.

Specific patterns of hypoxic-ischemic brain injury are determined to a major extent by the severity and type of insult. Thus, severe and relatively brief insult (often referred to as *acute, total* asphyxia), as may occur following cord prolapse, major placental abruption, or uterine rupture, often results in disproportionate injury to deep, central structures, eg, thalami, basal ganglia, and brainstem, with *relative* preservation of hemispheric structures. Clinical features of this pattern of injury in the neonatal period include abnormal eye movements, bilateral facial weakness, tongue fasciculations, and disturbances of sucking and swallowing. Clinically detectable brain swelling is not usually evident. Long-term sequelae often include cerebral palsy with a choreoathetotic component and persistent feeding problems that may require prolonged nasogastric feeding or placement of a gastrostomy tube. In contrast, so-called *prolonged, partial* hypoxic-ischemic insult, ie, a less severe insult of longer duration, causes injury that affects predominantly the cerebral cortex and subcortical white matter with *relative* preservation of the basal ganglia, thalami, and brainstem. The acute features of the encephalopathy in this situation include seizures, coma, and less commonly cerebral edema, identified on the basis of bulging anterior fontanelle. Long-term sequelae often include relative or absolute microcephaly (ie, diminishing head circumference percentiles), cognitive impairment, cerebral palsy, and epilepsy.

Less severe insults may cause injury to watershed zones of arterial supply in the parasagittal regions between the territories supplied by the anterior, middle, and posterior cerebral arteries. A prominent clinical feature of this pattern of injury is proximal limb weakness, especially shoulder girdle weakness. Unilateral, focal lesions related to focal cerebral infarction or hemorrhage result in unilateral weakness (hemiplegia). Although focal lesions may occur in the context of hypoxic-ischemic insult, the underlying etiology is unknown in a majority of cases. However, recognition of focal lesions should prompt investigations for possible causes, eg, cardiac abnormalities, hypercoagulable conditions, vasculitis.

Systemic Abnormalities The circulatory response to hypoxic-ischemic insult initially involves redistribution of cardiac output to maintain perfusion to vital organs, eg, brain, heart, and adrenal glands, with relative decrease of blood flow to other organs, eg, lungs, kidneys, and gastrointestinal tract. More prolonged hypoxic-ischemic insult eventually results in systemic hypotension, which, in turn, may have profound effects on cerebral perfusion because of ineffective cerebrovascular autoregulation. Cerebrovascular autoregulation is a homeostatic mechanism that maintains relatively constant cerebral perfusion over a wide range of systemic arterial blood pressures by means of cerebral arteriolar constriction or dilation. However, in the newborn this mechanism is less effective such that there is a direct, linear correlation between cerebral per-

fusion and systemic blood pressure. The most vulnerable areas of the brain involve principally the watershed zones of arterial supply, which, in the full-term newborn, are located in the parasagittal regions; in the premature newborn, they are located in the periventricular white matter.

In addition to neurologic abnormalities, hypoxic-ischemic injury to organs other than the brain, eg, kidneys, myocardium, may occur, and the severity of such injury appears to correlate with the severity of encephalopathy. However, even in association with severe encephalopathy, systemic abnormalities are often transient and reversible. Furthermore, it is important to realize that severe hypoxic-ischemic cerebral injury may occur without evidence of systemic abnormalities as detectable by routine monitoring.

Neuroimaging Acute hypoxic-ischemic cerebral injury may be recognized on cranial ultrasonography as increased echogenicity in cerebral parenchyma. Major problems with the use of this technique in this context relate to subjectivity in the interpretation of increased echogenicity, difficulty in distinguishing between hypoxic-ischemic and hemorrhagic injury, and predicting whether the increased echogenicity that is visualized represents a transient phenomenon or permanent cerebral tissue necrosis.

In full-term newborns, generalized increased echogenicity at approximately 24 hours of age may indicate diffuse injury. Cranial ultrasonography is often more useful for diagnosis of focal infarction, which may be visualized as focal areas of increased echogenicity.

Computed tomography remains the most important neuroimaging technique available routinely for assessment of hypoxic-ischemic cerebral injury in the full-term newborn. Acute injury appears as low cerebral tissue attenuation on CT scans performed during the first days of life. The optimal timing of CT scans for demonstration of the maximal extent of cerebral hypodensity is between 2 and 5 days of age. In addition, CT scanning may identify specific patterns of injury discussed previously (Fig. 25-13).

There is increasing recognition that MR imaging may have greater sensitivity and specificity for the assessment of perinatal hypoxic-ischemic cerebral injury. Thus, MR imaging may permit superior delineation of the specific neuropathologic patterns of injury, eg, thalamic/basal ganglia injury (Fig. 25-14), parasagittal injury, and cortical laminar necrosis. However, to date, in addition to the prolonged scanning time, which may limit clinical application, there remains some uncertainty about the timing and technique of MR imaging to optimize visualization of perinatal hypoxic-ischemic cerebral injury. In addition, MR imaging is often less routinely available for use in the assessment of newborn brain injury outside major pediatric centers.

Computed tomography or MR scans performed in later infancy or childhood often demonstrate diffuse atrophy and multicystic encephalomalacia in severe cases and may demonstrate the specific patterns referred to above.

Electroencephalography Moderate or severe hypoxic-ischemic encephalopathy is the single most important cause of seizures in the full-term newborn. Because neonatal seizures may be difficult to recognize clinically, electroencephalography is an important adjunctive investigation to confirm suspected seizures. In addition, in infants who require paralysis to facilitate management of ventilation, the diagnosis of electrical seizures by intermittent or continuous EEG monitoring permits early intervention with antiepileptic medications. In addition to providing assistance in the recognition

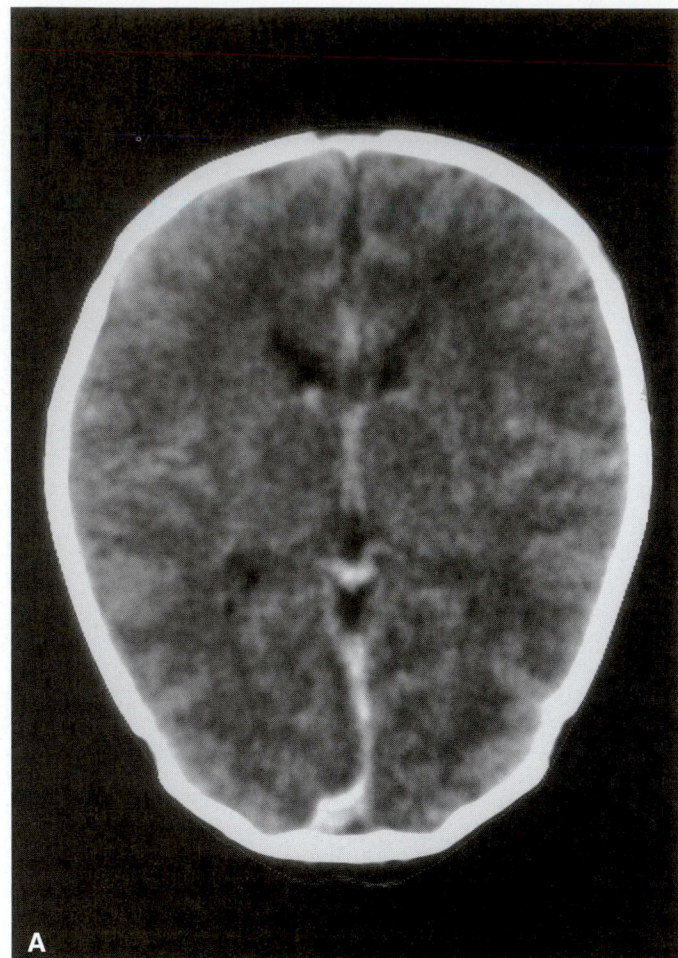
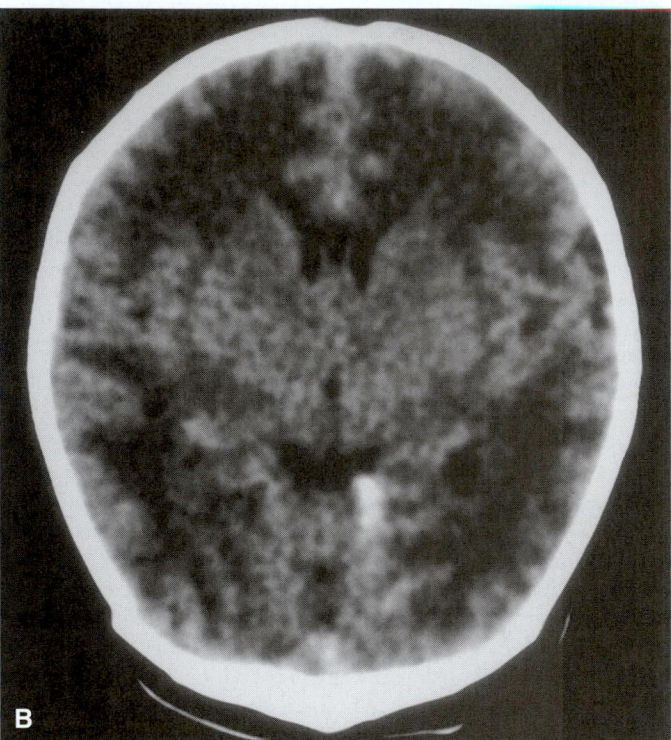

FIGURE 25-13 **A. CT scan of 3-day-old full-term newborn with hypoxic-ischemic encephalopathy. Note decreased tissue attenuation in thalami and basal ganglia. B. CT scan of 3-day-old asphyxiated full-term newborn with decreased attenuation in cortex and subcortical white matter and relative preservation of central structures.**

of seizures, the pattern of background activity on EEG has prognostic implications. Thus, a discontinuous pattern with marked voltage suppression interspersed with bursts of high-voltage sharp and slow waves (ie, *burst-suppression pattern*) or a markedly suppressed or isoelectric pattern has grave implications. In contrast, it has been shown that infants with a normal EEG 1 week following the insult usually have a good outcome.

Biochemical Investigations A variety of biochemical derangements often accompany hypoxic-ischemic cerebral injury and may contribute to the severity of the encephalopathy, eg, hypoglycemia, hypocalcemia, hyponatremia, lactic acidosis. In addition, biochemical investigation may assist in the identification of hypoxic-ischemic injury to organs other than brain.

Management

Because the primary hypoxic-ischemic insult frequently occurs in utero, prevention of intrauterine asphyxia is a primary objective that requires prompt recognition of maternal risk factors and close surveillance of the high-risk fetus during pregnancy, labor, and delivery. An asphyxiated newborn requires immediate maintenance of ventilation and perfusion, control of seizures, and maintenance of

metabolic homeostasis, especially blood glucose levels to avoid additional cerebral insult. In addition, the diagnosis and management of dysfunction of other organs is important.

Avoidance of hypoxemia and hypercapnia by maintenance of adequate ventilation has been facilitated by the availability of transcutaneous oxygen and carbon dioxide monitoring. Persistent postnatal hypoxemia in the newborn may occur in the context of persistent fetal circulation and pulmonary hypertension. Systemic hypotension should be avoided because impaired cerebrovascular autoregulation may result in decreased cerebral perfusion. Polycythemia, which occurs most commonly in infants who are small for gestational age, may impair cerebral perfusion and play a role in the causation of cerebral infarction. Partial exchange transfusion with plasma is indicated in infants who are symptomatic, eg, with jitteriness, apnea, poor feeding, and seizures.

Prevention of metabolic derangements to restore homeostasis is an important consideration to minimize risk of worsening seizures and cerebral edema. Prevention of fluid overload and maintenance of normoglycemia should be regarded as priorities. In the first few days following severe hypoxic-ischemic insult, there may be inappropriate secretion of antidiuretic hormone which may lead to hypo-osmolality and hyponatremia, which, in turn, may cause or worsen cerebral edema and seizures.

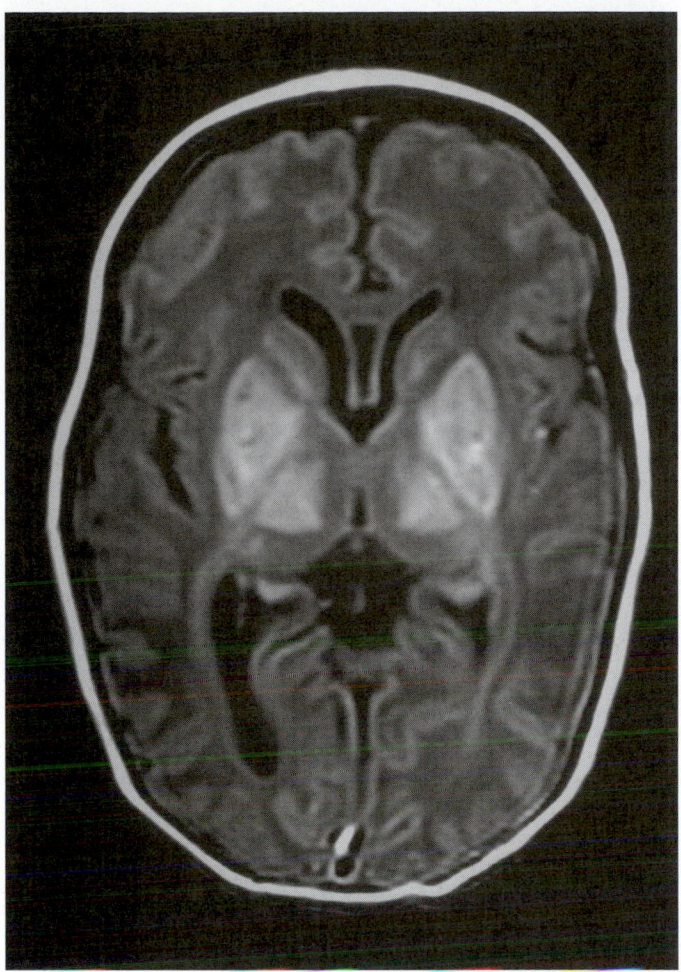

FIGURE 25-14 T$_1$-weighted MR scan of a 3-day-old full-term newborn with hypoxic-ischemic encephalopathy. Note bilateral signal abnormalities in thalami and basal ganglia.

Although fluid overload should be avoided, current data in human newborns do not provide convincing evidence that the use of antiedema therapy, eg, glucocorticocoids, diuretics, or hyperventilation, improves the generally poor long-term neurologic outcome that is associated with clinically recognizable cerebral edema. In fact, experimental data suggest that cerebral edema in the context of severe hypoxic-ischemia reflects extensive and irreversible cerebral tissue necrosis.

In addition to the restoration of metabolic homeostasis, the control of seizures is a major aspect of management. Apnea with seizures may compromise ventilation and contribute to fluctuations in cerebral perfusion in the context of impaired cerebrovascular autoregulation. In addition, prolonged seizures may deplete the brain of glucose and high-energy phosphate compounds and cause accumulation of excitotoxic amino acids, eg, glutamate. Treatment of seizures should begin with a loading dose of phenobarbital (20 mg/kg) administered intravenously, which may be followed by additional 5-mg/kg aliquots as necessary every 5 minutes for a total dose of 40 mg/kg. If seizures persist, intravenous phenytoin (20 mg/kg) may be administered slowly in two 10-mg/kg doses with careful, concomitant monitoring of cardiac function. In cases of refractory seizures, intravenous lorazepam may be indicated. The optimal duration of maintenance of anticonvulsant therapy has not been established and should be determined by the likelihood of

recurrence of seizures. Recent recommendations emphasize the importance of brief duration of treatment because of concerns regarding possible deleterious effects of anticonvulsants on the developing nervous system.

Prognosis

The most useful prognostic factors following hypoxic-ischemic encephalopathy are the severity and duration of the encephalopathy (see Table 25-2), combined with adjunctive data, especially neuroimaging. Newborns in whom the neurologic examination is normal at the time of discharge generally have favourable outcomes. The likelihood of neurologic sequelae is increased two- to fivefold when seizures have occurred. Seizures that are difficult to control are generally associated with poorer prognosis. In instances where the neurologic examination is limited, prognosis can be determined on the basis of extent of low tissue attenuation on CT scans performed between 2 and 5 days of age. Similar information may be obtained from MR imaging, although the precise timing for obtaining optimal information has been established less clearly. Neuroimaging is especially valuable in instances where detailed neurologic examination is precluded by intensive care procedures.

Hemorrhagic and Hypoxic-Ischemic Encephalopathy in the Premature Newborn

The incidence of periventricular-intraventricular hemorrhage (PIVH) in premature newborns is estimated to be between 20 and 40%. Although the incidence and severity of PIVH has decreased significantly over the past two decades, this lesion, which correlates with the degree of prematurity, undoubtedly will remain a major issue in neonatology because of improved survival of very small premature newborns. Furthermore, other major types of brain injury in the premature newborn either occur as a direct consequence of PIVH, eg, periventricular hemorrhagic infarction and posthemorrhagic hydrocephalus, or occur concomitantly as a consequence of hypoxic-ischemic parenchymal injury, eg, periventricular leukomalacia (PVL).

In the premature newborn, PIVH originates from fragile vessels in the subependymal germinal matrix. These vessels may rupture spontaneously or in response to superimposed minor stresses. The occurrence of PIVH is made more probable by the immaturity of cerebrovascular autoregulation in the premature infant. Approximately 50% of cases of PIVH originate during the first day of life, and 90% occur before 4 days of age. The pathogenesis of PIVH is multifactorial and involves a combination of intravascular, vascular, and extravascular risk factors. Clearly, the risk factors and potential preventive and interventional strategies differ significantly depending whether the hemorrhage is of early or later onset.

Intravascular risk factors involve perturbations in cerebral blood flow and volume as well as disturbances in platelet-capillary function and coagulation. Sick premature newborns may be exposed to numerous conditions associated with significant systemic and cerebrovascular hemodynamic instability, eg, respiratory distress syndrome and mechanical ventilation, pneumothorax, rapid volume expansion, routine handling and caretaking maneuvers, patent ductus arteriosus, and seizures. Furthermore, anemia and hypoglycemia may influence cerebral perfusion significantly, thereby causing increased risk of PIVH. Vascular risk factors relate principally to the fragility of the microvasculature within the germinal matrix with its high rate of oxidative metabolism and its location in a vascular border zone between the thalamic and striate arteries, which, in turn, increases the risk of hypoxic-ischemic insult. Finally, extravascular risk factors involve deficient vascular support and increased fibrinolytic activity within the germinal matrix, which predispose to extension of germinal matrix hemorrhage.

Major complications of PIVH that may contribute to long-term morbidity include periventricular hemorrhagic infarction and posthemorrhagic hydrocephalus.

Periventricular hemorrhagic infarction occurs in approximately 15% of infants with major PIVH. Neuropathologic studies have demonstrated that these parenchymal hemorrhages, which are unilateral or asymmetric fan-shaped (Fig. 25-15), represent hemorrhagic venous infarction secondary to obstruction of veins at the angles of the lateral ventricles by large germinal-matrix hemorrhage.

Ventriculomegaly, which has been documented in approximately 35% of infants with PIVH, may arrest or undergo spontaneous partial or total resolution within 4 weeks in approximately 65% of cases. In the absence of progressive hydrocephalus, ventriculomegaly may reflect loss of cerebral tissue, principally white matter (*hydrocephalus ex vacuo*). Such infants are usually normocephalic or microcephalic without signs of raised intracranial pressure. In other instances, posthemorrhagic hydrocephalus and hydrocephalus ex vacuo may coexist. This combination may contribute to delayed development of clinical signs of increased intracranial pressure and progressive ventriculomegaly. Acute hydrocephalus with elevated ICP may occur following massive IVH associated with rapid clinical deterioration. More commonly, subacute or chronic hydrocephalus develops over weeks related to obstruction of the aqueduct from blood clot and debris or from obliterative arachnoiditis in the posterior fossa with obstruction of cerebrospinal fluid outflow from the fourth ventricle.

Periventricular leukomalacia (PVL) is not a direct complication of PIVH, although these lesions frequently occur concomitantly. Periventricular leukomalacia is a pattern of hypoxic-ischemic injury that involves the border zones of arterial supply in the immature brain that are located in the periventricular white matter. This lesion may involve focal areas of infarction and necrosis, especially ante-riorly at the angles of the lateral ventricles and posteriorly in the region at the trigone of the lateral ventricles as well as more diffuse injury.

In approximately 25% of autopsy cases of PVL, there is hemorrhage within the areas of infarction that is often bilateral and may coexist with severe PIVH. The clinical features of PVL in the premature newborn include subtle abnormalities of tone in the lower extremities. Classical long-term sequelae include motor handicap, eg, spastic diplegia or quadriplegia, some cognitive impairment, and, less commonly, visual and auditory impairment. Of course, in instances where there has been severe insult there may be injury to cortex as well as periventricular white matter. Severe PVL may be visualized in the newborn by cranial ultrasonography as areas of increased echogenicity in periventricular white matter during the first days of life which subsequently evolve into cystic lesions after approximately 3 to 4 weeks (Fig. 25-16).

Diagnosis

Clinical Features Approximately 50% of cases of PIVH are asymptomatic clinically. In the remainder, the clinical presentation varies from saltatory neurologic deterioration, often over several days, to a catastrophic presentation with bulging anterior fontanelle, coma, apnea, extensor posturing, and brainstem dysfunction. In addition, there are frequently systemic abnormalities, eg, hypotension, metabolic acidosis, bradycardia. If posthemorrhagic hydrocephalus occurs, clinical signs of increased intracranial pressure may be delayed because the high water content and high compliance of the immature brain allows the development of some degree of ventriculomegaly without clinical signs of increased intracranial pressure.

Lumbar Puncture The premature newborn who presents with neurologic abnormalities may require a lumbar puncture because of the possibility of intracranial infection. Bloody or xanthochromic

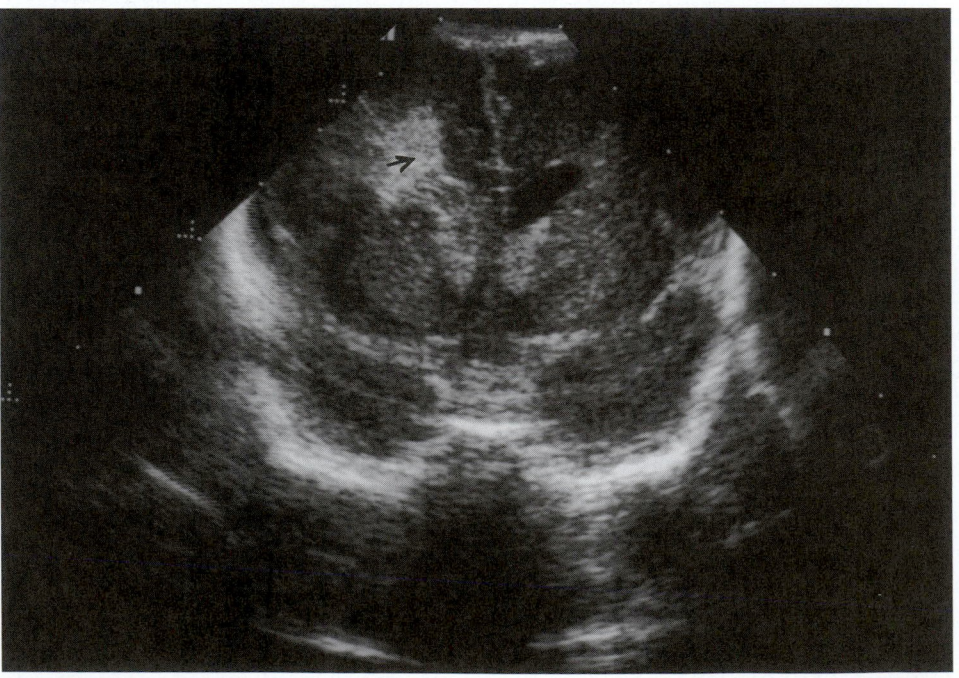

FIGURE 25-15 Coronal cranial ultrasound scan of premature newborn. Note unilateral periventricular hemorrhagic infarction (*arrow*).

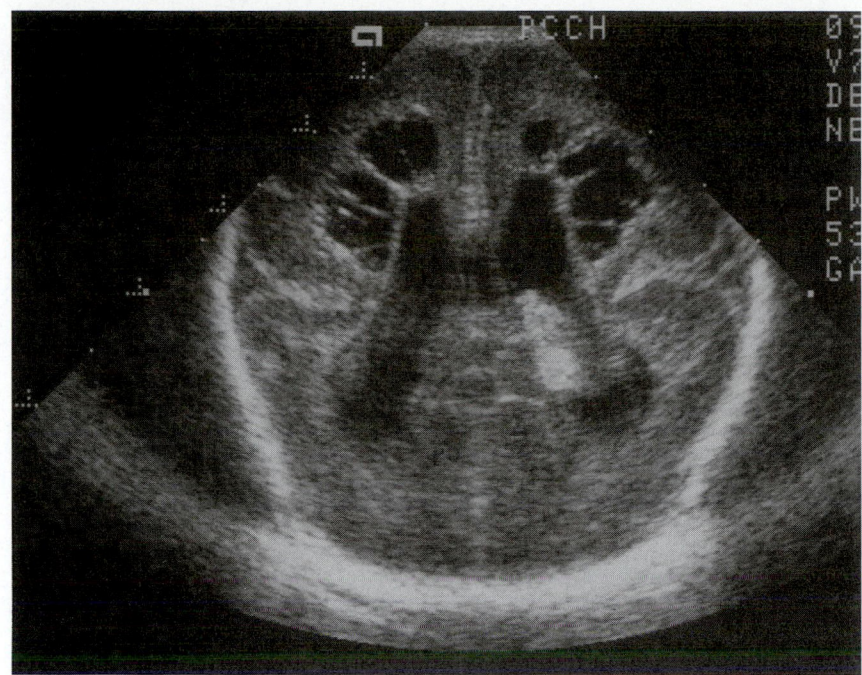

FIGURE 25-16   Coronal cranial ultrasound scans of a premature newborn at 5 weeks of age: Note bilateral cysts in the regions of previous increased echoes.

cerebrospinal fluid supports a diagnosis of intracranial hemorrhage. However, because the possibility of traumatic lumbar puncture is high in this age group, suspected PIVH should be confirmed by neuroimaging.

Neuroimaging   Cranial ultrasonography is considered to be the neuroimaging modality of choice for the diagnosis of PIVH because it is noninvasive and can be performed at the bedside without risk of ionizing radiation or major disturbance to the infant. In many centers, cranial ultrasonography is performed routinely at 4 to 5 days of age in high-risk premature newborns who have less than 32 weeks of gestation or earlier if there are specific clinical concerns. Cranial ultrasonography is limited in its ability to distinguish between hemorrhagic and acute ischemic parenchymal injury. When PIVH is visualized, a repeat scan should be performed after approximately 1 week to document possible extension of hemorrhage, which occurs in 20 to 40% of cases. Thereafter, serial scans are recommended every 1 to 2 weeks for surveillance of ventricular size and possible development of posthemorrhagic hydrocephalus. Ventriculomegaly observed on cranial ultrasonography often precedes the development of clinical abnormalities by days or even weeks. Serial ultrasound scans may demonstrate periventricular cystic lesions, which are observed most commonly after approximately 5 to 6 weeks and which represent cystic PVL (Fig. 25-16).

Computed tomography and MR imaging are superior for the diagnosis of other types of intracranial hemorrhage, eg, subarachnoid, convex, and posterior fossa subdural hemorrhages or epidural hematomas. CT scans have limited value for the assessment of acute hypoxic-ischemic cerebral injury in premature newborns because of the normally high water content (and hence low tissue attenuation) of the immature brain. However, CT is of value for the differentiation between hemorrhagic and ischemic injury. Furthermore, in older infants, there are classical features of PVL which may be visualized on CT, ie, ventriculomegaly with cortical sulci abutting the ventricular walls owing to decreased amount of interposed white matter, especially in the peritrigonal regions.

Management

The optimal strategy for prevention of PIVH and its complications as well as hypoxic-ischemic parenchymal lesions involves the prevention of premature delivery. Unfortunately, medications, eg, tocolytic therapy, β sympathomimetics, indomethacin, often delay labor for several days only. However, even such brief delay of labor and delivery may be sufficient to permit administration of antenatal corticosteroids that induce fetal lung maturation, thereby minimizing respiratory distress, which, in turn, decreases the risk that PIVH will occur. The risk for development of early-onset PIVH appears to be decreased further by avoidance of lengthy labor and possibly delivery by cesarean section. If premature delivery cannot be prevented, several management strategies have been proposed. In ventilated premature newborns, muscle paralysis with pancuronium bromide has been shown to reduce the severity of PIVH by stabilizing fluctuations in cerebral blood flow.

Prognosis

The prognosis following PIVH relates both to the severity of hemorrhage and concomitant hypoxic-ischemic cerebral injury. Germinal matrix hemorrhage alone is rarely associated with long-term neurologic morbidity. Intraventricular hemorrhage alone, in the absence of ventriculomegaly or parenchymal involvement, is also not necessarily indicative of poor prognosis. However, premature newborns with severe intraventricular hemorrhage and intraparenchymal hemorrhage have significant mortality rate, and survivors often have sequelae that include cerebral palsy, cognitive and behavioral impairment, and epilepsy.

25.4.2   Other Types of Intracranial Hemorrhage

Other types of intracranial hemorrhage, eg, subarachnoid, epidural, subdural, and parenchymal hemorrhage, occur much less commonly than PIVH. They are often associated with traumatic delivery or bleeding disorders. Table 25-3 summarizes the major clinical features, management, and outcome of these types of intracranial hemorrhage.

Subdural Hemorrhage

Subdural hemorrhage may occur in both premature and full-term newborns and results from laceration of major veins and sinuses, often associated with a tear of the dura. Excessive molding of the head may play a role in pathogenesis. Clinical features are variable, and symptoms range from minimal abnormalities, which may remain undiagnosed, to decreased level of consciousness, brainstem dysfunction, seizures, or asymmetry of motor function. Computed tomography is the technique of choice for identification of subdural hemorrhage. Occipital diastasis and skull fractures, which may play a role in the genesis of hemorrhage, may be documented by skull radiographs. Management is determined in large part by the severity of hemorrhage. Thus, subdural hemorrhage located over the convexities, especially when associated with lateral displacement of midline structures, usually requires surgical evacuation as does massive subdural hemorrhage located in the posterior fossa. With regard to subdural hemorrhage in the posterior fossa, surgical intervention does not appear to improve long-term outcome if there are no major clinical neurologic abnormalities.

Primary Subarachnoid Hemorrhage

Subarachnoid hemorrhage in the newborn is usually self-limited, originating from rupture of small bridging veins in the leptomeningeal plexus. Infants may be asymptomatic with minor subarachnoid hemorrhage, or they may present with seizures. Diagnosis may be suspected on the basis of blood-stained or xanthochromic cerebrospinal fluid at lumbar puncture. The diagnosis is confirmed by demonstration of blood in sulci and in the superior longitudinal fissure on CT or other imaging. Management consists of treatment of seizures, avoidance of additional hypoxic-ischemic insult, and close surveillance for the occurrence of hydrocephalus as described previously. In the absence of severe trauma, hypoxic-ischemic cerebral injury, or massive hemorrhage, outcome is usually favorable.

TABLE 25-3

OTHER TYPES OF INTRACRANIAL HEMORRHAGE

TYPE OF HEMORRHAGE	CLINICAL FEATURES	OUTCOME
Epidural	Increased ICP Seizures in 50%	Poor
Subdural (convexity or posterior fossa)	Variable Increased ICP Seizures Brainstem dysfunction Opisthotonus Coma	Hydrocephalus Variable
Primary subarachnoid	Variable Seizures Well in interictal period	90% normal Hydrocephalus rare
Parenchymal	Variable Seizures Unilateral weakness Increased ICP (less common)	Variable Epilepsy Cerebral palsy Cognitive problems

ICP = intracranial pressure.

25.4.3 Effects of Drugs and Toxins

Prenatal exposure to medications and toxins may have profound adverse effects on newborn neurologic function and may be classified broadly as *teratogenic effects* and *effects of passive addiction*. In many instances, it may be difficult to distinguish direct adverse effects of medications or toxins from confounding influences of intrauterine undernutrition, infection, genetic factors, and other toxins.

Passive addiction/withdrawal occurs in 60 to 90% of newborns whose mothers took drugs that affect the central nervous system during pregnancy. The clinical features of withdrawal are similar for most drugs, although the duration of the encephalopathy varies according to the elimination half-life for each specific drug. The times of onset of withdrawal symptoms for several common drugs are listed in Table 25-4. Initial clinical features of encephalopathy caused by drug withdrawal relate to central nervous system overactivity, eg, jitteriness, irritability, high-pitched cry, frantic sucking, and disturbed sleep patterns. There may be associated gastrointestinal disturbance, eg, poor feeding, vomiting, and diarrhea. Other common systemic disturbances include tachypnea, excessive sweating, and repeated sneezing. Because fever and seizures are less common manifestations of neonatal withdrawal syndrome, their occurrence should always suggest the possibility of sepsis or other major neurologic problem. Withdrawal syndrome related to maternal use of long-acting barbiturates may persist for several weeks. Infants withdrawing from heroin may improve initially but worsen subsequently with persistence of symptoms for up to 6 months.

Management

Prevention is the most important aspect of management. All women of childbearing age should be advised of potential risks to the fetus of various medications and drugs, ideally prior to conception. Effective management of the newborn requires early diagnosis. Consideration must be given to avoidance of respiratory complications, dehydration, and metabolic derangements. Persistent irritability, vomiting, and diarrhea may require treatment with paregoric, phenobarbital, chlorpromazine, or diazepam. Paregoric is considered to be the initial treatment of choice followed by addition of phenobarbital if encephalopathic features are not controlled by paregoric alone. Treatment must be continued for several weeks and tapered gradually to avoid recurrence of symptoms.

TABLE 25-4

TIMES OF ONSET OF WITHDRAWAL SYNDROME

USUAL ONSET	MEDICATION
Day 1	Alcohol Heroin Short-acting barbiturates Diazepam Tricyclic antidepressants Hydroxyzine Propoxyphene Pentazocine
2–3 days of age	Methadone Cocaine
7 days of age	Longer-acting barbiturates
Up to 21 days	Chlordiazepoxide

References

General

Stevenson DK, Sunshine P: Fetal and Neonatal Brain Injury—Mechanisms, Management and the Risks of Practice, 2nd ed. Oxford, Oxford University Press, 1997

Volpe JJ: Neurology of the Newborn. Philadelphia, Saunders, 1995

Hypoxic-Ischemic Encephalopathy in the Term Newborn

Barkovich AJ, Westmark K, Partridge C, Sola A, Ferreiro D: Perinatal asphyxia: MR findings in the first 10 days. Am J Neuroradiol 16:427–438, 1995

Lupton BA, Hill A, Roland EH, et al: Brain swelling in the asphyxiated term newborn: pathogenesis and outcome. Pediatrics 82:139–146, 1988

Myers RE: Four patterns of perinatal brain damage and their conditions of occurrence in primates. Adv Neurol 10:223–234, 1975

Pasternak JF, Gorey MT: The syndrome of acute near-total intrauterine asphyxia in the term infant. Pediatr Neurol 18:391–398, 1998

Robertson C, Finer NN: Term infants with hypoxic-ischemic encephalopathy: outcome at 3.5 years. Dev Med Child Neurol 27:473, 1985

Roland EH, Hill A: How important is perinatal asphyxia in the causation of brain injury? Ment Retard Dev Disabil Res Rev 3:22–27, 1997

Roland EH, Poskitt K, Rodriguez E, Lupton BA, Hill A: Perinatal hypoxic-ischemic thalamic injury: clinical features and neuroimaging. Ann Neurol 44:161–166, 1998

Sarnat HB, Sarnat MS: Neonatal encephalopathy following fetal distress: a clinical and electroencephalographic study. Arch Neurol 33:696–705, 1976

Hemorrhagic and Hypoxic-Ischemic Encephalopathy in the Premature Newborn

Du Plessis A: Posthemorrhagic hydrocephalus and brain injury in the preterm infant: dilemmas in diagnosis and management. Semin Pediatr Neurol 5:161–179, 1998

Guzzetta F, Shackelford GD, Volpe S, et al: Periventricular intraparenchymal echodensities in the premature newborn: critical determinant of neurologic outcome. Pediatrics 78:995–1006, 1986

Hill A: Intraventricular hemorrhage: emphasis on prevention. Semin Pediatr Neurol 5:152–160, 1998

Horbar JD: Prevention of periventricular-intraventricular hemorrhage. In: Sinclair JC, Bracken MB, eds: Effective Care of the Newborn Infant. New York, Oxford University Press, 1992:562–589

Roland EH, Hill A: Intraventricular hemorrhage and posthemorrhagic hydrocephalus. Clin Perinatal 24:589–604, 1997

Shankaran S, Bauer CR, Bain R, et al (for the NICHD Neonatal Research Network): Prenatal and perinatal risk and protective factors for neonatal intracranial hemorrhage. Arch Pediatr Adol Med 150:491–497, 1996

Volpe JJ: Brain injury in the premature infant—neuropathology, clinical aspects, pathogenesis and prevention. Clin Perinatol 24:567, 1997

25.5   STATIC ENCEPHALOPATHIES

Jan B. Wollack and Charles A. Nichter

The term *static encephalopathy* refers to a state of cerebral dysfunction after an insult of limited duration. The resulting lesion does not progress; rather, it remains *static* or may even improve somewhat with time. Such an insult may occur during gestation, during the birth process, or during childhood. The clinical picture will depend on the site and extent of the lesion and the age at the time of occurrence.

Cerebral palsy results from involvement of motor areas of the brain. *Mental retardation* follows diffuse cerebral involvement, but small lesions that occur early in gestation may interfere with normal cerebral maturation, with resulting intellectual deficits. Sight and hearing may be impaired. *Convulsions* most commonly result from cortical lesions. *Speech disturbances* may reflect diffuse cerebral involvement or a focal lesion involving the speech area. *Behavioral disorders* and *learning disabilities* have less well defined anatomic localization. These clinical features may occur in isolation or in any combination. For example, spastic diplegia may occur alone or it may be accompanied by mental deficits, seizures, visual and auditory impairments, and behavioral disturbances.

25.5.1   Cerebral Palsy

Cerebral palsy (CP) is a term used to describe a diverse group of chronic, nonprogressive disorders of movement, posture, and tone resulting from a central nervous system insult during early development. The timing of the insult may be prior to, at the time of, or shortly after birth. Although the term *cerebral palsy* refers solely to the motor deficits, features such as seizures, mental retardation, and learning disabilities may accompany it.

Although cerebral palsy was first reported in 1827 by Cazauvielh, and later described and debated by physicians such as Little, Freud, Osler, and Phelps, the pathogenesis of this disorder remains imperfectly understood.

PREVALENCE

Numerous studies have found that the prevalence of cerebral palsy is approximately 2 per 1000 live births. There has been little change in this rate over time, despite advances in obstetrical and perinatal care. In part, this lack of a decline may be the result of increased survival of low birth weight infants, as suggested by data showing an increase in the prevalence of spastic diplegia in those children. The proportion of the different types of cerebral palsy varies from report to report. Approximately 70% have the spastic type; 15%, athetotic; 5%, ataxia; and the remainder, mixed.

ETIOLOGY

Many factors, both genetic and acquired, have been postulated as causes of cerebral palsy. These include hypoxic-ischemic injury, structural malformations, vascular disorders, intraventricular or subarachnoid hemorrhage, infections, hormonal disorders, toxins, trauma, metabolic disease, prematurity, and hemolytic disease of the newborn. In recent years, several studies have sought to determine the relative contribution of these and other factors to the total incidence of cerebral palsy.

Perinatal Asphyxia

Historically, asphyxia during labor and delivery has been implicated as a major cause of cerebral palsy. In the last decade, a number of large population studies have revealed that asphyxia probably accounts for only a relatively small proportion of cases. The National Collaborative Perinatal Project, which studied prospectively the outcome of over 40,000 live births in the United States between

1959 and 1966, demonstrated a clear relationship between Apgar scores and cerebral palsy, particularly at the extremes (Fig. 25-17). The rate is approximately 4 times higher (16.7 versus 4.7) if the Apgar score is 0 to 3 at 10 minutes compared with 5 minutes. It is remarkable that even when the Apgar score was less than or equal to 3 for 15 minutes, the majority of infants did not develop cerebral palsy. Furthermore, if there was an increase in the score at 15 and 20 minutes, the risk decreased to only 4.7%. Although 21% of the 189 children with cerebral palsy in this study had at least one marker for asphyxia, over half of those also had alternative findings that could have caused their cerebral palsy. Once these other factors were taken into account, the proportion of cerebral palsy that could be attributed to asphyxia was in the range of 3 to 13%. This figure is in close agreement with that of the second major study, which used data from the Western Australia Cerebral Palsy Register. Of 183 instances of spastic cerebral palsy found between 1975 and 1980, 8% were attributable to birth asphyxia. A third study, based on 155,636 births in four counties of northern California from 1983 to 1985, found that potentially asphyxiating conditions might account for 6% of the total CP found in normal birth weight infants. When the association of CP with a variety of potentially asphyxiating conditions was examined, only a tight nuchal cord was associated with a statistically significant increase in risk. Thus, these three major studies are all in agreement that birth asphyxia causes fewer than 1 in 5, and probably fewer than 1 in 10, of the cases of cerebral palsy. Furthermore, the majority of asphyxiated infants do not develop cerebral palsy.

Low Birth Weight and Prematurity

Multiple studies have demonstrated an increased prevalence of cerebral palsy with decreasing birth weight (<1500 g) or decreasing gestation (<37 weeks). The association, however, is not absolute, as only 10% of infants weighing less than 1500 g develop cerebral palsy, and, similarly, only 10 to 28% of children with cerebral palsy weighed less than 1500 g at birth. This relationship depends also upon the type of cerebral palsy, as up to 70% of children with spastic diplegia had low birth weight. It is possible that the cerebral lesion of cerebral palsy might occur antenatally as part of a process that leads also to prematurity or impairment of fetal growth. Alternatively, the cerebral event might occur postnatally, as the brain of a

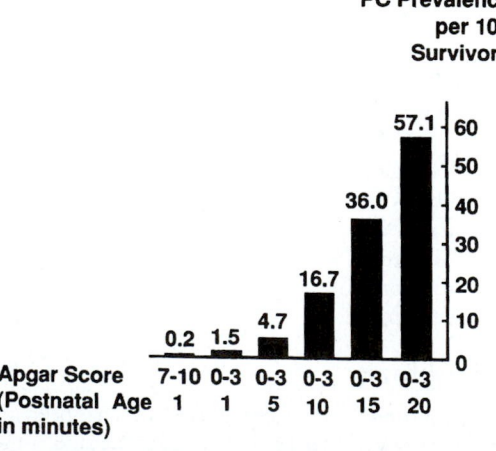

FIGURE 25-17 Relationship of Apgar score to cerebral palsy in the Collaborative Perinatal Project. *Reprinted with permission from Paneth N, Pediatr Ann 15:191, 1986; data derived from Nelson KB, Ellenberg J, Pediatrics 68:36, 1981.*

low birth weight or premature infant may be more susceptible to insult.

Congenital Malformations

Congenital malformations occur more frequently in children with cerebral palsy. In the National Collaborative Perinatal Project, 22% of the children with cerebral palsy had a major, noncerebral malformation, as opposed to only 6.8% of the children without cerebral palsy. Thus, more cases of cerebral palsy could be attributed to an underlying maldevelopment of the fetus than could be attributed to perinatal asphyxia. Furthermore, one-third of the children with cerebral palsy and a marker of perinatal asphyxia also had a noncerebral malformation, suggesting that maldevelopment of the fetus may be an underlying factor in producing the clinical picture of asphyxia.

In addition to the noncerebral malformations, a variety of cerebral malformations were also found, although somewhat less commonly than those outside the nervous system. Since the time of the National Collaborative Perinatal Project, advances in technology have furthered the detection of such abnormalities. For example, recent MR studies have found evidence of neuronal migrational disturbance in 30% of full-term infants with CP, further strengthening the relationship between fetal maldevelopment and cerebral palsy.

Infection

Several recent studies have implicated bacterial infection, autoimmune disorders, and coagulation defects in the pathogenesis of CP. Intrauterine exposure to infection is both a cause of premature birth and is associated with an increased risk of CP in both premature and full-term infants. Whereas exposure to any maternal infection increased the risk of CP in full-term infants, those with evidence of placental infection had the highest risk of spastic CP. Infection-exposed infants were more commonly found to have low Apgar scores and meconium aspiration syndrome, whereas those that went on to develop CP also had a higher incidence of hypotension, the need for respiratory support, neonatal seizures, and other signs of encephalopathy than nonexposed infants, suggesting that exposure to infection can mimic hypoxic-ischemic encephalopathy. Interestingly, among those children exposed to infection who later developed CP, spastic quadriplegia was more common than either the diplegic or hemiplegic subtypes. Overall, it is estimated that maternal infection could account for 12% of total spastic CP in children of normal birth weight. Although appreciation of the role of infection in CP is growing, effective therapeutic approaches to this problem have yet to be determined.

Coagulation Factors and Inflammatory Mediators

Elevations of a variety of inflammatory factors have been found in children with CP, including interleukins such as IL-1, -8, -9 (and to a lesser extent IL-6, -11, and -13), tumor necrosis factor-α, RANTES, and interferons. Infection is an obvious, although not exclusive, cause of such elevations. Coagulation factor abnormalities, sometimes autoimmune in nature, have also been implicated in the pathophysiology of CP. Reactive antibodies to lupus anticoagulant, anticardiolipin, antithrombin III; to a translational product of the factor V Leiden mutation; and to proteins C and S have been detected in children with CP. It is postulated that abnormalities in inflammatory pathways, triggered by infections or other factors, could impede brain development in various ways such as by disrupting myelin, interfering with cellular migration, or directly injuring oligodendroglia. Inflammation can lead to coagulation abnormalities that could then lead to thromboembolic events. In this regard, the role of thrombosis in placental vessels is coming to be appreciated as a potential source of emboli. Inflammatory mediators may also be responsible for transient hypothyroxinemia, which has recently been implicated as a possible cause of neurologic problems in preterm infants. These studies suggest that the interplay between infection, inflammation, and coagulation abnormalities may provide a better understanding of the pathophysiology of a large proportion of CP.

Other Antecedents

The National Collaborative Perinatal Project data and other studies associated cerebral palsy with a number of other diverse features. Maternal mental retardation, motor deficits in older siblings, maternal hyperthyroidism, maternal seizures, and a history of two or more prior fetal deaths were all prepregnancy antecedents that suggested maternal, possibly genetic, causes for cerebral palsy. Associated factors that occurred during the pregnancy included severe proteinuria, third-trimester bleeding, hormone use, heart disease, and incompetent cervix. Brecch presentation (but not breech delivery), chorionitis, the presence of meconium in the amniotic fluid, and placental complications were the characteristics present during labor and delivery. Even in the aggregate, however, these factors accounted for only a small proportion of the total number of instances of cerebral palsy.

Summary

In summary, although a diverse number of factors have been found in association with cerebral palsy, none of them, alone or in the aggregate, has been shown to account for more than a fraction of the total number of children with cerebral palsy. Although the above studies have increased our understanding of pathophysiological mechanisms at work in cerebral palsy, there remain many cases for which the cause is unknown.

NEUROPATHOLOGY

Gross malformations are found in only about one-third of autopsied children with cerebral palsy and may represent cortical migrational disorders. The other pathologic patterns found are frequently related to gestational age and birth weight. In the premature newborn with a spastic type of cerebral palsy, periventricular leukomalacia and periventricular hemorrhagic infarction, as described by Volpe and his colleagues, are the most common patterns. *Periventricular leukomalacia* consists of symmetric, focal necrosis of the white matter dorsal and lateral to the external angle of the lateral ventricles. With the passage of time, cystic cavities may develop in the more severe cases, whereas diminished myelin and dilated lateral ventricles will develop in milder cases. Because the descending motor fibers from the cortex to the lower extremities are closest to the ventricle, these lesions most commonly result in spastic diplegia. This lesion may also be found in the full-term infant. The second condition, *periventricular hemorrhagic infarction,* consists of asymmetric hemorrhagic necrosis of the periventricular white matter. In addition, there is usually an associated germinal matrix or intraventricular hemorrhage. Pathologic examination of these lesions suggests that the white matter damage is caused by venous infarction resulting from obstruction of medullary and terminal veins by the

germinal matrix or intraventricular hemorrhage. As these lesions tend to be both large, therefore involving the descending tracts to both the arm and leg, and asymmetric, the common clinical manifestation is spastic hemiparesis. The pathogenetic mechanisms for both of these types of injury remains uncertain but may involve a cascade of events that includes hypoxia, ischemia, vascular sensitivity, maturational vulnerability of neurons, autoregulatory dysfunction, glutamate receptor development, oligodendrocyte sensitivity to free radicals, and specific metabolic properties of cerebral regions or cell types.

More diverse pathologic patterns are seen in full-term infants, generally in association with hypoxic-ischemic brain injury. In *selective neuronal necrosis,* neuronal loss and gliosis are found in the neocortex, hippocampus, cerebellum, brainstem, and spinal cord and may be manifested clinically as quadriparesis. *Status marmoratus* exhibits similar pathology localized to the basal ganglia and thalamus and adds a degree of hypermyelinization to these regions, resulting in a marbled appearance. This lesion is also seen in children with kernicterus. Dyskinetic cerebral palsy may develop. In both these lesions, the areas affected are rich in glutamate receptors, suggesting that this excitotoxic amino acid is involved in their pathogenesis. Periventricular leukomalacia, described above, may also be seen in the full-term infant. *Parasagittal cerebral injury* features necrosis in the superior and medial cortical convexities and adjacent white matter, which is greater posteriorly than anteriorly. The pathogenesis is presumably related to poor perfusion of the arterial border zones and end zones in this region, leading to a spastic quadriparesis with an upper-extremity predominance. *Focal and multifocal ischemic cortical injury* shows a similar pathology but involves a more localized circulatory compromise (single vessel and tributaries) such as might result from vascular anomalies, vasculopathy, or vascular obstruction. Spastic hemi- or quadriparesis is associated with these lesions.

CLINICAL CLASSIFICATION

The clinical manifestations of cerebral palsy are classified according to their type, such as spastic or dyskinetic, and the topography of the impairment, for example, hemiplegic or quadriplegic.

Spastic Cerebral Palsy

Children with spastic cerebral palsy exhibit upper motor neuron signs such as weakness; hypertonicity; hyperreflexia; clonus; pathologic reflexes, eg, extensor plantar response; and a tendency to contractures.

Hemiplegia　In *hemiplegia,* one side of the body is chiefly affected. When the pathology involves the vascular territory of the middle cerebral artery, the arm will be more involved than the leg, with the distal portions more impaired than the proximal. As a result of weakness in the forearm supinators and extensors, the arm tends to be flexed at the elbow, wrist, and fingers while pronated at the forearm. This abnormal arm position will be accentuated by walking and especially by running. In mild cases, the only manifestation might be an asymmetry in arm position and swing while running. Another technique to elicit spasticity in the mildly affected child is to supinate the previously extended and pronated arm, producing flexion of the elbow on the involved side. In addition to the weakness, there may be impaired stereognosis. This cortical sensory modality is tested by placing familiar small objects in the child's hand and having the child identify them without looking. Useful function can rarely be obtained with such a deficit. Asymmetries of growth of the extremities may be noted, and there may be evidence of a unilateral central facial weakness or an ipsilateral visual field defect. In the lower extremity, there is characteristically increased spasticity in the flexors and adductors of the thigh, the hamstrings, and the posterior calf muscles. Weakness of foot dorsiflexion causes toe walking with circumduction on the affected side. Mildly affected children may appear to have a normal gait; in these cases the hemiplegia can be revealed by an asymmetric gait when running or the inability to walk on the affected heel with the toes elevated. Similarly, the shoe on the unaffected side will show normal wear, whereas the shoe of the involved side will have a scuffed toe and a relatively unworn heel. Spastic hemiplegia from periventricular hemorrhagic infarction in the premature infant may be somewhat modified, with the major difference being that the leg, whose descending motor tract is closer to the ventricle, is more affected than the arm.

Quadriplegia *Quadriplegia* designates symmetric impairment of all four extremities. The clinical manifestations described earlier for hemiplegia are present on both sides, although spasticity of the hip adductors and knee flexors is more marked. Hip subluxation or dislocation, contractures, and scoliosis can all result from significant degrees of spasticity. Bilateral involvement of corticobulbar fibers can lead to a pseudobulbar palsy with swallowing and respiratory difficulties, drooling, and dysarthric speech. Growth deficiencies, mental retardation, language disorders, and seizures may accompany the motor deficits.

Spastic Diplegia In *spastic diplegia,* the legs maintain greater spasticity and weakness than the arms. Children with spastic diplegia are frequently premature, and many have periventricular leukomalacia as the pathologic substrate. The arms are not normal, with deficits being most apparent in wrist extension and in activities of daily living such as self-feeding, drawing, or writing. Young children whose arms might appear normal generally show signs of mild involvement on later reexamination. Contractures, if present, usually involve the foot giving equinovalgus or calcaneovarus deformities. Deficits in language, attention, and cognition may coexist.

Other Types of Spastic Cerebral Palsy Monoplegia and triplegia are quite rare. Spastic paraplegia, in which the arms are completely normal, is almost always the result of a spinal cord lesion. Atonic cerebral palsy or atonic diplegia is characterized by marked motor delay, decreased tone with hyperextensibility, and mental retardation. The deep tendon reflexes are normal or increased, which distinguishes this condition from anterior horn cell or peripheral nerve disease. This condition appears to be a temporary phase during development; hypertonicity usually supervenes by 4 years of age.

Dyskinetic Cerebral Palsies

Dyskinesia implies impaired volitional activity manifested as uncontrolled and purposeless movements that disappear during sleep and are associated with pathology in the basal ganglia. The most common type is choreoathetoid, in which the movements have two components. *Chorea* refers to rapid, variable, jerky motions of proximal muscle groups in the extremities and face, and *athetosis* refers to slow irregular writhing movements of the extremities, face, neck, and trunk. The movements are less apparent when the child is relaxed but are exaggerated with intention, emotion, and holding a posture. They are usually symmetric, but some degree of asymmetry

may occur. The continuous movements may lead to muscle hypertrophy, especially around the neck and in the paravertebral area. Dysphagia and speech difficulties are variably present. In the past, kernicterus resulted in choreoathetosis, upward-gaze paresis, sensorineural hearing loss, and yellow-stained teeth.

Dystonic cerebral palsy involves truncal twisting, facial grimacing, and extremity rigidity resulting from the cocontraction of agonist and antagonist muscle groups. Involvement of the oropharyngeal region leads to significant dysphasia and motor dysphagia. A late-onset form has been described in which the onset of the dystonia was delayed for up to 14 years following an episode of perinatal anoxia.

Ataxic Cerebral Palsy

This disorder comprises dysfunction in coordination, gait, and rapid distal movements of the extremities. It is related to a static lesion of the cerebellum and its pathways. Affected children have a wide-based gait and difficulty performing tests such as finger-to-nose pointing. This type of cerebral palsy is relatively infrequent and should be a diagnosis of exclusion. Any neurologic or functional decline, familial ataxia, foot deformities, or sensory deficits would suggest a different diagnosis. Ataxic cerebral palsy has the best prognosis for functional improvement.

Mixed Forms

The combination of spasticity and choreoathetosis is seen most frequently, and athetosis and ataxia may occur.

ASSOCIATED DISORDERS

Children with cerebral palsy may have additional disorders such as seizures and mental retardation. The frequency of seizures varies according to the type of cerebral palsy but generally approximates 25 to 35%. Specifically, the proportion of hemiparetic children with seizures is 40%; in contrast, dyskinetic children have less than a 10% chance of developing seizures. Seizure type and onset are quite variable, with the initial seizure occurring between 2 and 6 years of age. Both partial (simple and complex) and generalized seizures can be seen. Though less frequent, myoclonic epilepsy, absence seizures, and infantile spasms may occur.

Mental retardation may occur in 25 to 75% of children with cerebral palsy. It is most frequent in mixed cerebral palsy, less so in spastic forms, and least frequent in dyskinetic and ataxic types. Care should be taken in the cognitive evaluation in light of the extent to which motor, oropharyngeal, and speech impairments can interfere with testing. Aside from speech delay in mental retardation, aphasia, apraxia, and articulation disturbance may all be observed. A prognostic factor is the presence of seizures; intelligence is statistically lower when cerebral palsy is associated with epilepsy.

Attention to visual handicaps is particularly important because of the high incidence of strabismus, refractive errors, and visual field defects. Visual perceptual problems and maturational delay are common. Deafness is uncommon except in children with athetosis caused by kernicterus. Peripheral hearing loss (hypoacusis) must be differentiated from lack of response to speech and other auditory stimuli in children who are not deaf (central hearing loss or dysacusis).

DIAGNOSIS

The diagnosis of cerebral palsy is largely made on clinical grounds. The physician must take a careful history, particularly regarding gestational, perinatal, and developmental aspects. The family history may provide evidence of a genetic disorder such as familial spastic paraparesis. Physical examination should include inspection of the skin, face, and spine looking for evidence of a neurocutaneous disorder, chromosomal or other genetic syndrome, or a specific structural brain or spinal cord anomaly. Measurement of head circumference may suggest a failure of brain growth or the presence of a structural abnormality. Examination of the ocular fundi, auscultation of the heart, and palpation of the liver may suggest a metabolic disorder. Neurologic assessment should emphasize the examination of strength, tone, deep tendon and primitive reflexes, as well as observation for adventitious movements. Motor development should be carefully documented including early activities such as chest lift in prone position, rolling over, pull-to-sit, and sitting. Oral-pharyngeal function should be assessed in terms of feeding of liquids and solids, swallowing, expressive language, and articulation.

Crucial to the establishment of the diagnosis is to confirm the static (ie, nonprogressive) nature of the child's condition by means of serial examinations. One must be aware, however, of certain specific changes that can falsely suggest progression. For example, in some children with dyskinetic CP, there may be significant fluctuation in tone, varying from hypotonia to hypertonia and finally dystonia. Furthermore, functional decline may occur owing to factors such as scoliosis, increased contractures, uncontrolled seizures, or anticonvulsant drug toxicity. Motor decline in the older cerebral palsied patient is sometimes related to increased energy expenditure with increasing body weight. In contrast, apparent functional improvement may be seen in some children with the athetotic or ataxic varieties of cerebral palsy.

Aside from these considerations, an increasing functional impairment should lead to investigation for the possibility of a progressive encephalopathy (see Sec. 25.17). Some metabolic disorders initially may mimic cerebral palsy; likely candidates include amino acidurias such as glutaric aciduria type I, peroxisomal disorders such as adrenal myeloneuropathy, or mitochondrial disorders. Testing for these disorders includes serum and urine amino and organic acids, serum lactate, lysosomal hydrolases, urinary oligosaccharides, and very long chain fatty acids.

Particular care should be taken in establishing the diagnosis of CP when ataxia or hypotonia are the central findings. Disorders such as Krabbe leukodystrophy, hypobetalipoproteinemia, carbohydrate-deficient glycoprotein syndrome, or Pelizaeus-Merzbacher disease may appear similar to ataxic cerebral palsy. Hypotonia may be associated with disorders such as Prader-Willi syndrome, Rett syndrome, myotonic dystrophy, or neuroaxonal dystrophy.

Dopa-responsive dystonia is a slowly progressive disorder that may easily be confused with spastic diplegia. Patients may present with increased muscle tone in the legs, brisk knee and ankle jerks, spastic gait and Babinski responses, and subsequent development of parkinsonian elements. Cognition is generally unimpaired. Some cases have been linked to the gene for GTP cyclohydrolase I, located on chromosome 14q, which affects synthesis of biopterin, a cofactor in dopamine production. As this condition is dramatically responsive to low doses of L-dopa, the clinician must maintain a high index of suspicion in all children who do not have a clear etiology for their spastic diplegia; in some cases, a therapeutic trial of L-dopa may be indicated.

Spastic diplegia may also be mimicked by familial spastic paraplegia, which occurs in X-linked recessive as well as autosomal-dominant and recessive forms. Recent studies have identified a number of chromosomal loci and gene products, findings which may eventually lead to the molecular genetic diagnosis of these disorders.

LABORATORY DATA

Brain imaging studies, including ultrasound, CT, and MR imaging, may be useful in elucidating the etiology of the cerebral palsy. They are also indicated when there are findings suggestive of a progressive process and may reveal hydrocephalus, an enlarging cyst, or evidence of a neurocutaneous syndrome.

In the premature infant, cranial ultrasound is generally the most useful modality. Periventricular leukomalacia may be seen as bilateral, linear echodensities adjacent to the external angles of the lateral ventricles, which usually evolve into multiple small cysts, which may in turn disappear, leaving enlarged ventricles. In contrast, the echodensities of periventricular hemorrhagic infarction tend to be asymmetric and triangular in shape. The extent of these lesions correlates with the prognosis. With time, these lesions tend to evolve into single, permanent, large cysts. In either situation, CT and MR imaging are more effective at showing the full extent of brain involvement, especially after the acute phase has passed.

In the full-term infant, MR imaging is most useful for defining the etiology of the cerebral palsy. Visible dysgenic anomalies such as polymicrogyria or heterotopias may be found in 15 to 30% of full-term infants. Less common are changes in the basal ganglia or thalami, suggesting status marmoratus. Ventricular abnormalities, consisting of enlargement or irregularities of contour are common, as are abnormalities of the white matter, although the pathology underlying these lesions is not always as evident.

Electroencephalography is useful to confirm the presence of clinically suspected seizures but does not differentiate cerebral palsy from other neuropathologic conditions. Abnormalities in the EEG are common, particularly spike discharges or asymmetries; these findings may be noted whether or not seizures are manifest.

TREATMENT

The broad goals of neurorehabilitation of the child with cerebral palsy are to understand the strengths and weaknesses of each child based upon the specific combination of motor impairments and associated disorders that are present and to develop a comprehensive care plan for the child and family. The ultimate objective is for these children to attain the highest possible level of independent functioning within their family, peer group, and larger community.

Physical and occupational therapy are often beneficial in management of motor impairments. Proper positioning and handling are necessary to minimize difficulties with posture, trunk control, and feeding. Tendons that are tight can be stretched with passive and active exercises, thereby maintaining normal alignment of bone, joint, and soft tissue to prevent contractures. In more severe cases, splinting may be necessary to prevent contractures of the extremities. Orthopedic procedures have been devised to correct contractures that do not respond to medical measures and to reestablish motor balance between opposing muscle groups. Another goal of physical and occupational therapy is to increase muscle strength in weak muscles and to work on the development of normal movement patterns. Computerized gait analysis may help to identify aberrant gait patterns and to identify specific spastic muscle groups that are interfering with walking.

Seizures can generally be managed with anticonvulsants (see Sec. 25.10.2), but medications are not often successful in reducing spasticity and influencing abnormal movements. Diazepam (Valium) increases presynaptic inhibition through the GABA/benzodiazepine receptor and may ameliorate spasticity of cerebral origin. The drug may be particularly effective in those children in whom emotional tension contributes to the severity of their spasticity or abnormal movements and can provide relief from painful spasms. Dantrolene sodium (Dantrium), a phenytoin derivative, has a direct relaxing effect on skeletal muscle. The starting dose should be 1 mg/kg twice daily with gradual increases until good results are obtained, but the total dose should not exceed 100 mg four times a day. Baclofen (Lioresal), a $GABA_B$ agonist, may also decrease spasticity but is generally less effective in static encephalopathies than it is in spinal cord injury. The dosage of this drug must be carefully individualized, starting with 5 mg three times a day with increases up to a total daily dose of 60 mg. In cases where spasticity is limited to just a few muscle groups, local treatment may be considered. Local anesthetics, ethanol, and phenol have been used to block nerve conduction for variable periods of time. More recently, botulinum toxin has been used to disrupt the release of acetylcholine from motor nerve terminals. This effect is temporary as the nerves generate new neuromuscular junctions by terminal sprouting and the formation of new endplates over a span of months, necessitating repeat injections.

Two neurosurgical procedures for the relief of spasticity are available. The first involves the continuous intrathecal administration of baclofen using an adjustable subcutaneous pump. This procedure has been effective in patients with moderately severe spastic quadriparesis. The adjustable nature of the pump is advantageous for those patients who, lacking strength, rely on some spasticity for functioning; the dose can be adjusted so that the optimal amount of spasticity is retained. The second procedure is selective dorsal rhizotomy. In this procedure, 20 to 80% of the afferent dorsal rootlets at the L2 to S2 levels are selectively severed. Rootlets to be cut are identified by their abnormal electromyographic response to electrical stimulation. This procedure appears best suited for patients with significant lower extremity spasticity but near-normal upper extremity function. Patient selection is paramount, as there must be sufficient muscle strength underlying the spasticity for the patient to benefit.

Children with significant motor impairments may also have feeding difficulties caused by dysphagia and gastroesophageal reflux. Feeding through a gastrostomy and fundoplication may be beneficial in some instances but are not without their drawbacks and should be considered on an individual basis.

Physical handicaps are more difficult to manage in children with associated retardation. Children with difficulties in verbal communication should have speech therapy, and visual handicaps should be addressed early. Psychotherapy may be of value in some children; it is of more benefit in helping the family adjust to the handicapped child. School placement must be individualized: if the child is not retarded and the physical handicap is not severe, regular school placement is indicated. Special classes should be recommended only if the child is unable to perform adequately in a typical setting. Institutional care may become advisable for children who cannot be managed at home because of physical, social, or emotional factors.

25.5.2 Attention-Deficit Hyperactivity Disorder

Attention-deficit hyperactivity disorder is the latest in a series of terms that have been used by psychiatrists and neurologists to describe children with normal or nearly normal intelligence who dem-

onstrate an abnormal behavior pattern characterized primarily by inattention, distractibility, impulsivity, and hyperactivity, frequently accompanied by learning disabilities and aggressiveness. Its inclusion as a static encephalopathy reflects its first being described as a behavioral syndrome after brain injury and only subsequently in children with no history of cerebral insult. Many terms have been used to describe this syndrome: *minimal brain dysfunction, nonmotor brain damage, hyperkinetic child* and *hyperactive child,* and *attention-deficit-disorder.* None is adequate; the currently preferred attention-deficit hyperactivity disorder, or ADHD, conveys the key components of the clinical picture without implying obligatory cerebral damage. This condition is discussed in detail in Sec. 5.6.1.

References

Armstrong RW, Steinbok P, Cochrane DD, et al: Intrathecally administered baclofen for treatment of children with spasticity of cerebral origin. J Neurosurg 87:409, 1997

Cummins SK, Nelson KB, Grether JK, Velie EM: Cerebral palsy in four northern California counties, births 1983 through 1985. J Pediatr 123: 230, 1993

Figlewicz DA, Bird TD: "Pure" hereditary spastic paraplegias. Neurology 53:5, 1999

Freeman JM, Nelson KB: Intrapartum asphyxia and cerebral palsy. Pediatrics 82:240, 1988

Gordon N: The role of botulinus toxin type A in treatment—with special reference to children. Brain Dev 21:147, 1999

Grether JK, Nelson KB: Maternal infection and cerebral palsy in infants of normal birth weight. JAMA 278:207, 1997

Grether JK, Nelson KB, Dambrosia JM, Phillips TM: Interferons and cerebral palsy. J Pediatr 134:324, 1999

Kraus FT, Acheen VI: Fetal thrombotic vasculopathy in the placenta: cerebral thrombi and infarcts, coagulopathies, and cerebral palsy. Hum Pathol 30:759, 1999

Kuban KCK, Leviton A: Cerebral palsy. N Engl J Med 330:188, 1994

Nelson KB: The neurologically impaired child and alleged malpractice at birth. Neurology 17:283, 1999

Nelson KB, Dambrosia JM, Grether JK, Phillips TM: Neonatal cytokines and coagulation factors in children with cerebral palsy. Ann Neurol 44: 665, 1998

Nelson KB, Ellenberg JH: Antecedents of cerebral palsy. Multivariate analysis of risks. N Engl J Med 315:81, 1986

Nelson BK, Ellenberg JH: Apgar scores as predictors of chronic neurologic disability. Pediatrics 68:36, 1981

Nygaard TG, Waran SP, Levine RA, Naini AB, Chutorian AM: Dopa-responsive dystonia simulating cerebral palsy. Pediatr Neurol 11:236, 1994

Steinbok P, Reiner AM, Beauchamp R, et al: A randomized clinical trial to compare selective posterior rhizotomy plus physiotherapy with physiotherapy alone in children with spastic diplegic cerebral palsy. Dev Med Child Neurol 39:178, 1997

Tanaka H, Endo K, Tsuji S, et al: The gene for hereditary progressive dystonia with marked diurnal fluctuation maps to chromosome 14q. Ann Neurol 37:405, 1995

Truwit CL, Barkovich AJ, Koch TK, Ferriero DM: Cerebral palsy: MR findings in 40 patients. Am J Neuroradiol 13:67, 1992

Volpe JJ: Brain injury in the premature infant—from pathogenesis to prevention. Brain Dev 19:519, 1997

25.5.3 Cocaine and the Fetus

Claudia A. Chiriboga

In Sec. 10.3.8 the teratogenic causes of congenital abnormalities both in the central nervous system and other body systems are described. These range from the potential damage of intrauterine exposure, to infection, to the effects of drugs and other chemical agents. These latter substances may affect the fetal central nervous system by interfering with brain formation and growth and paradoxically cause an "encephalopathy" at the time of abrupt withdrawal in the newborn period. The effects of withdrawal from opiates are discussed in Sec. 25.4.3.

Cocaine is one of the most frequently abused illicit substances in the United States. Although the cocaine epidemic peaked in the 1980s, in US cities cocaine remains one of the drugs most frequently used by pregnant women. Women who use cocaine, especially "crack," its alkaloidal smokable form, often abuse other substances (eg, heroin), smoke cigarettes, and consume alcohol; they frequently lack adequate prenatal care. Offspring born to such women are at high risk of having perinatal complications, such as infant death, low birth weight, and prematurity. Women who use cocaine and are unemployed also are more likely to resort to prostitution, thereby increasing their risk of syphilis and human immunodeficiency virus (HIV) infection. Cocaine use during pregnancy has been linked to spontaneous abortion, abruptio placentae, stillbirths, and premature delivery, presumably caused by cocaine-induced vasoconstriction of intrauterine vessels. Low birth weight (LBW) and intrauterine growth retardation (IUGR) are common among cocaine-exposed infants. Fetal brain growth is impaired independently of birth weight and gestational age.

Fetal cocaine exposure may alter neonatal behavior. Infants exposed to cocaine in utero exhibited significant differences in organizational response and interactive behavior, even when exposure occured solely during the first trimester of pregnancy. Poor feeding and sleep disturbances, as well as abnormalities in neonatal arousal modulation are reported with prenatal cocaine exposure. Related studies describe high rates of hypertonic tetraparesis and coarse tremor. A dose-dependent effect has been observed; higher rates of neurologic impairment (microcephaly, hypertonia) are associated with higher levels of cocaine exposure. At present there is no evidence for a cocaine-induced withdrawal syndrome. Neurologic findings probably represent the CNS manifestations of fetal cocaine effect on developing monoaminergic pathways.

Other neurologic complications in newborns possibly linked to fetal cocaine exposure include congenital brain malformations, such as agenesis of the corpus callosum and septooptic dysplasia. Neonatal strokes are seen in settings of perinatal infarction or with porencephalic cysts, which may represent a vascular event occurring earlier in gestation. A large prospective study involving preterm infants found no association between cocaine and intraventricular hemorrhage. Neither is there evidence for cocaine-induced seizures resulting from fetal exposure, although electroencephalography shows increased transient sharp abnormalities in these infants.

In early infancy, cocaine-exposed infants suffer slightly higher rates of sudden infant death syndrome (SIDS) than the general population. Excessive irritability is seen at age 3 months in about 30% of exposed infants, and at age 6 months over half of infants born to heavy cocaine users exhibit a syndrome of diffuse hypertonia that resolves by age 2 years, arms first and legs last. Motor delays are still noted at age 2 years on sophisticated testing, however. Cocaine-exposed toddlers had no substantial differences in developmental quotients compared with controls. However, the finding of a hypertonic syndrome was associated with lower developmental scores. Long-term fetal cocaine effects on cognition and learning have not been identified except as occurs through cocaine effects on head growth. Adverse effects of prenatal cocaine exposure on child neurobehavior have not been clearly established.

COCAINE EXPOSURE IN CHILDHOOD

Passive intoxication with cocaine, manifesting chiefly as seizures, has been reported in infants and young children resulting from breast-feeding or passive inhalation of freebase cocaine ("crack"). Urine toxicologies to detect illicit substances, therefore, are indicated in the evaluation of seizures in infants and children, regardless of socioeconomic status.

References

Arendt R, Angelopoulos J, Salvator A, Singer L: Motor development in cocaine exposed children. Pediatrics 103:86–92, 1999

Chasnoff IJ, Griffith DR, MacGregor S, Dirkes K, Burns KA: Temporal patterns of cocaine use in pregnancy. Perinatal outcome. JAMA 261: 1741–1744, 1989

Chiriboga CA, Brust JCM, Bateman DA, Hauser WA: Dose-response effect of fetal cocaine exposure on newborn neurological function. Pediatrics 103:79–84, 1999

Dusick AM, Covert RF, Schreiber MD, et al: Risk of intracranial hemorrhage and other adverse outcomes after cocaine exposure in a cohort of 323 very low birth weight infants. J Pediatr 122:438–445, 1993

Heier LA, Carpanzano CR, Mast J, Brill PW, Winchester P, Deck MD: Maternal cocaine abuse, the spectrum of radiologic abnormalities in the neonatal CNS. Am J Neuroradiol 12:951–956, 1991

Karmel BZ, Gardner JM: Prenatal cocaine exposure effects on arousal modulation attention during the neonatal period. Dev Psychobiol 29:463–480, 1996

Mayes LC, Bornstein MH, Chawarska MA, Granger RH: Information processing and developmental assessments in 3-month old infants exposed to cocaine. Pediatrics 95:539–545, 1995

Volpe JJ: Effect of cocaine use on the fetus. N Engl J Med 327:399–407, 1992

25.6 SPECIFIC SYNDROMES OF COGNITIVE DISORDERS

Ruth Nass, Peter R. Huttenlocher, and Janellen Huttenlocher

Several syndromes of specific cognitive dysfunction must be distinguished from global mental retardation. Cognitive processes underlying specific learning disabilities are readily subdivided into the following large categories.

PERCEPTION

Perception involves the processing of sensory stimuli. The two types of perception that are most important for intellectual activity are visual and auditory. Dysfunction of the primary sense organs must be excluded before a perceptual deficit can be diagnosed. Some children have specific visual perceptual disabilities, manifested as inability to discriminate forms or shapes. Others have difficulty discriminating sounds. Auditory perceptual disability may underlie developmental dysphasia, whereas visual perception is often affected in so-called clumsy children and occasionally in children with dyslexia.

MEMORY

Memory is the ability to recall prior experiences. This includes memory for sounds, especially words (auditory memory); memory for visual stimuli (shapes, faces, and so on); and spatial memory, the ability to recall the spatial relationships of objects. Immediate and short-term memory can be assessed using a "digit span" in which the child is asked to repeat a series of random numbers in order. The ability normally increases from recall of two digits by 2½ years of age to seven or eight digits by age 14 years. Short-term memory is clearly of major importance in intellectual activity. For example, a child with poor short-term auditory memory will have trouble solving oral arithmetic problems that require short-term memory storage of number sequences. The role of memory deficits in cognitive disabilities in childhood is still poorly defined. However, auditory memory span has been noted to be particularly short in some children with developmental dysphasia.

CONCEPTUALIZATION

The formation of conceptual categories is necessary for proper analysis of information. Piaget used nonverbal tasks to study the normal development of simple concepts. Some of these tasks can be carried out rapidly by the practicing pediatrician, and they provide valuable information about a child's developmental level. Probably the best known of Piaget's concept tasks is *object permanence*. The notion that objects continue to exist even when they are out of sight develops before 18 months of age. By age 9 months, normal infants will be able to retrieve partially covered objects, by 10 months they will search for objects that have been displaced but are still visible, and by 18 months, they will search for objects even after invisible displacement. A second aspect of conceptualization investigated by Piaget is that of conservation or the notion of sameness, notably with respect to number and volume. Development of number concept can be studied by asking children to judge the number of pennies in two parallel rows. By age 3 years, children are able to correctly identify the row with more pennies if arrays of four and three pennies are equally spaced in two rows. However, the ability to conserve numbers when two arrays are of unequal length but contain the same number of pennies, spaced at slightly different intervals, is not fully developed until age 6 years. Slow acquisition and plateauing in the acquisition of concepts is observed in children with mental retardation.

LANGUAGE

The development of verbal communication is one of the most striking occurrences in the preschool child. Normal language acquisition is discussed in Secs. 5.4 and 5.6.4

PLAY AND GESTURE

Play activity is important in children's thought processes, and it also provides a means for nonverbal communication. The emergence of simple object play follows a predictable developmental sequence that is used in several standard infant development scales. By age 7 to 8 months, infants begin to explore objects tactilely as well as visually. An infant of that age, presented with a small cube, will inspect it, turn it, and transfer it from hand to hand. Between ages 9 and 15 months, simple manipulation, mouthing, and banging of objects decrease, and object-appropriate actions increase. By 21 months, children will imitate everyday activities. They will feed a doll and comb its hair. By 30 months, children will act out familiar sequences (mealtime, bedtime, searching for a playmate).

Informal observation of play activity can provide important clues to a child's developmental level, especially a child who is unable to cooperate for more formal testing, such as an autistic child.

VISUAL-MOTOR/CONSTRUCTIONAL ABILITY

Visual motor tasks measure the ability of children to produce spatial structures, either by aligning parts, such as blocks, into specific forms or by drawing. Specific disability in this area in a child who has otherwise normal motor functions can be referred to as constructional apraxia. Tests of constructional ability are incorporated into most early development scales and in the standard intelligence tests for children. They include such tasks as building a tower or a bridge out of blocks. Normal children are able to stack two blocks by age 15 months and eight blocks by 2½ years; they can copy a bridge made out of three blocks by 3 years. Standard drawing tasks include copying a vertical line (2 years), a horizontal line (2½), a circle and a cross (3 years), a square (4 years), a triangle (5 years), and a diamond (6 to 7 years). Drawing a human figure from memory is an excellent constructional task for the group 3½ to 7 years of age. Normative data for different ages have been collected by Goodenough (draw-a-man test) and can be used to generate a nonverbal IQ.

25.6.1 Developmental Dysphasia

Developmental dysphasia (DD) is defined as a delay and/or deficit in acquisition of language not attributable to mental retardation or to hearing loss. The marked variability in the rate of normal language acquisition makes it at times difficult to distinguish developmental dysphasia from initial idiosyncratic language delay in children who eventually speak normally—hence the wide range (1 to 25%) in the reported frequency of developmental dysphasia in preschool children. Failure, however, to develop normal expressive language by age 3 years should be considered pathologic. Between 18 months and 3 years, those children with both expressive and receptive delays are more likely to ultimately be diagnosed with developmental dysphasia than those with only expressive delays, who often catch up. Developmental dysphasia is often genetic, and whether father or mother is the transmitting parent affects the sex ratio of their children and the percentage of the children with a DD. A variety of subtyping systems have been proposed to describe DD. Although a description in terms of expressive versus receptive deficits is the simplest and most commonly used subtyping systems, those that take account of psycholinguist deficit patterns are more informative. Phonologic processing deficits underlie DD in some cases. Rapin has separated the DDs into higher-order language disorders—semantic-pragmatic and lexical-syntactic; combined expressive/receptive disorders—verbal auditory agnosia and phonologic-syntactic; and expressive disorders—verbal dyspraxia and phonologic programming. The long-term prognosis appears to be considerably better for those with good receptive language and impaired expressive skills, although recent studies show that many children with delayed expressive language have academic difficulties at school age. Higher-functioning autistic children often have semantic-pragmatic difficulties, and low-functioning autistic children often have verbal auditory agnosia. A subgroup of dysphasic children may have histories of normal or near-normal language development, with rapid loss of language abilities generally between 3 and 7 years (*acquired epileptic aphasia*). By definition these children have seizures and/or epileptiform EEG abnormalities.

Diagnostic evaluation of children with developmental dysphasia must include a careful assessment to rule out hearing impairment. Measurement of brainstem-evoked response to sounds gives valuable information when clinical hearing tests are inconclusive. Psychological tests aid in distinguishing developmental dysphasia from global mental retardation. The Wechsler Intelligence Scales are especially useful because they are subdivided into verbal parts, which are generally depressed in dysphasic children, and performance parts, which are near normal. Special tests for assessing nonverbal intelligence and for assessing specific language skills (phonics, grammar, vocabulary) are also useful. An EEG (including sleep) is indicated when there is a history of seizures or when language comprehension is significantly impaired (verbal auditory agnosia). Neuroimaging for clinical purposes is rarely revealing. Focal cerebral lesions rarely underlie developmental dysphasia in contrast to aphasia in the adult. Structural abnormalities reported in research studies include: bilateral cortical abnormalities with resulting pseudobulbar palsy, atypical planum temporale asymmetries, reduced volume of the left posterior peri-sylvian region, and various possibly fortuitous findings like middle cranial fossa arachnoid cysts. Dynamic and resting metabolic imaging studies demonstrate left temporal abnormalities generally reflecting hypoactivity.

The treatment of developmental dysphasia includes individual speech therapy and remediation in small classes conducted by teachers skilled in working with speech-delayed children. Training in sign language may be helpful for developing communication in those with significant oromotor dysfunction. Children with phonologic processing deficits have responded to therapy developed to create more salient versions of the rapidly changing elements of speech (i.e., Fast Forward). Children with the syndrome of acquired epileptic aphasia may respond to antiepileptic medications (including ACTH).

25.6.2 Pervasive Developmental Disorder/ Autism

Autism is a spectrum disorder characterized by social relatedness difficulties, by ritualistic and compulsive behavior, including stereotyped repetitive motor activity (spinning of objects, rocking), and by abnormalities of verbal and nonverbal communication. The IQ of children with autism ranges from retarded to superior. They are distinguished from children with developmental dysphasia because they have social relatedness difficulties in addition to language impairments. Asperger's syndrome is a disorder of social relatedness which is associated with a restricted range of behaviors and interests and paralinguistic (prosody and pragmatics) difficulties. According to some definitions clumsiness is necessarily concomitant (see discussion of the nonverbal learning disabilities below). Autism is discussed in Sec. 5.7.1.

25.6.3 Rett Syndrome

Rett syndrome occurs virtually only in girls and can be difficult to differentiate from autism in toddlers and preschool children. Patients exhibit normal growth and development in early infancy. Symptoms gradually appear between 6 and 18 months and eventually include autistic behavior, dementia, ataxia, and loss of purposeful use of the hands (hand-wringing movements are a hallmark). Head and body growth lag behind the normal rate, resulting in acquired microcephaly and short stature. Other findings include seizures in two-thirds of reported patients, spasticity, intermittent hyperventilation, dystonia, and kyphoscoliosis. These children are ultimately severely impaired and require continuous care. The disorder is not uncommon (1 in 15,000 live births) and may account for 25% of severe or profound mental retardation in girls. The al-

most exclusive involvement of girls suggests an X-linked dominant gene that is lethal in males. Whereas almost all instances have been sporadic, the most recent genetic studies suggest that transmission may start with a premutation that can result over generations in a full mutation giving rise to Rett syndrome. Both the X-chromosomes and an autosome pair of chromosomes may be involved. Skewed X chromosome inactivation has been postulated. The etiology is still obscure. Abnormal neuronal growth factors and excitatory neurotransmitters have been implicated. The EEG reveals abnormalities of background rhythm with paroxysmal elements. Traditional imaging studies demonstrate reduced cerebral volume, especially of the frontal gray matter, basal ganglia, midbrain, and cerebellum. Dynamic imaging studies demonstrate hypoperfusion of varying severity predominantly bifrontally. Pathologic examination shows hypoplasia of these structures, suggestive of developmental arrest rather than degeneration of brain tissue. Currently, no treatment is effective other than controlling the seizures and provision of optimum nutrition.

25.6.4 The Nonverbal Learning Disabilities

Children with nonverbal learning disabilities (NVLD) may have any combination of (1) social, emotional, and interpersonal difficulties (overlapping with children with Asperger's disorder); (2) right-hemisphere-mediated paralinguistic communication problems (overlapping with children with Asperger's disorder); (3) impaired visuospatial skills; (4) motor skills disorders (overlapping with children with Asperger's disorder); (5) dyscalculia; (6) slow processing speed; and (7) attention-deficit hyperactivity disorder (ADHD). Based on an analogy to children with known neural pathology who manifest NVLDs, Rourke suggests that abnormalities of white matter and cerebral disconnection cause NVLDs.

DISORDERS OF MOTOR FUNCTION

Disorders of motor function include dysgraphia, dyspraxia, and clumsiness. The neurologic examination of the child with any type of learning disability often shows an excess of soft signs. Developmental soft signs are findings that would be normal if the child were younger, eg, mirror movements, overflow. Classical pastel soft signs are traditional neurologic signs found in a mild form, eg, minimally asymmetric deep tendon reflexes. There is a marked decline in number of soft signs after puberty. Deuel has proposed a three-tier assessment of motor skills; (1) history of gross and fine-motor milestones (notably, fine-motor coordination difficulties do not necessarily affect athletic prowess); (2) informal examination for adventitious movements, finger tapping, hand turning and toe tapping, sequential motor acts to imitation, pantomime and with objects and writing and drawing; and (3) formal standardized motor testing.

Synkinesia is best elicited by finger tapping, finger squeezing, and/or stressed gait testing. Choreiform movements (which may occur with increased frequency in children with attention-deficit hyperactivity disorder) are best elicited by having the child stand with eyes closed and pronated arms extended with fingers spread (Prechtl sign). Psychometric tests are useful for confirming the diagnosis. There may be significant discrepancies between verbal IQ scores, which are normally distributed, and performance IQ scores, which are depressed. Measures which require copies of a variety of complex shapes and the draw-a-man test are useful diagnostic instruments. Deficits in visual-perceptual-organizational psychomotor coordination and complex tactile-perceptual skills appear to be most representative (in the sense of most discriminative) of the NVLD syndrome as compared with normal children and those with other types of LDs. Measures of attention, executive function, motor control, and processing speed (Target Test; Trail Making Test, Part B; Tactual Performance Test; and Grooved Pegboard Test) also accurately discriminate the NVLD group from those with other learning disabilities and controls. Defects in constructional ability and slow processing speed may contrast with relatively spared perceptual abilities.

Treatment includes proper educational placement from an early school age. Children with mild impairments may be able to progress well in normal classes; however, small classes conducted by teachers trained in special education are sometimes needed. Proper understanding of the disorder by parents is of utmost importance and is facilitated by parent groups. The prognosis depends on the initial severity of the disorder but also on proper management at home and in school. Children with significant disorders of motor control may benefit from occupational therapy. Several writing remediation programs are available. Early keyboarding training and computer access can facilitate output for those with poor graphomotor skills. Tincture of time is also a tactic. Stimulant drug therapy may be used as an adjunct to management but never as the only approach.

SOCIAL, EMOTIONAL, AND INTERPERSONAL DIFFICULTIES

Chronic emotional difficulties, disturbances of interpersonal skills (eg, poor eye contact), poor peer relations, excessive shyness, loner status, and inadequate paralinguistic abilities can characterize children with NVLD. Depression is not uncommon.

Behavioral inventories are the most useful tools for determining the extent of social, emotional, and interpersonal difficulties.

Treatments suggested for those with NVLD include: observe closely in novel or complex situations; teach the child in a systematic, step-by-step way; encourage detailed descriptions of important events; teach appropriate strategies for troublesome frequent situations; encourage the generalization of learned strategies; teach the child to use verbal skills appropriately; teach appropriate nonverbal behavior to facilitate structured peer interactions; promote, encourage, and monitor systematic exploratory activities; teach the older child how to use available aids in reaching a specific goal; help the child gain insight into easy and troublesome situations.

PARALINGUISTIC DEFICITS

The NVLDs result from right hemisphere dysfunction, and thus communication modalities dominated by the right hemisphere are often affected: humor; emotion; nonliteral language: indirect requests, metaphor, sarcasm, alternative word meaning; paralinguistics: prosody (intonation used to convey emotion or linguistic elements such as question asking), pragmatics (how we say it rather than what we say); and integrative processes: inference, narrative. The lack of such skills in both input and output modalities compromises the interpersonal relations of the child with NVLD even further. A number of neuropsychological measures are available to quantify deficits in these areas. Treatment here involves a combination of language therapy and social skills therapy (see above).

DYSCALCULIA

The prevalence of dyscalculia in general is about 6%, not dissimilar to that of dyslexia and ADHD. Both genders are affected equally.

A developmental Gertsmann's syndrome (right-left disorientation, finger agnosia, dysgraphia, and dyscalculia) is said to occur in as many as 2% of school-age children. The mean IQ of children with dyscalculia is generally normal; one-quarter show symptoms of ADHD, and about one-fifth of dyslexia. In one cohort almost half had first-degree relatives with learning disabilities.

Standardized arithmetic batteries are available to assess the degree and type of dyscalculia. Dyscalculia can result from right- or left-hemisphere dysfunction. Children with left-hemisphere dysfunction as the basis of their dyscalculia are significantly worse in addition, subtraction, complex multiplication, and division than their counterparts with right-hemisphere dysfunction.

Math remediation is appropriate for the child with isolated difficulties or with math difficulties in combination with other learning difficulties.

25.6.5   Developmental Dyslexia

Developmental dyslexia is usually defined by a reading level that is more than two grade levels below the expected norm, and this reading difficulty is not explainable on the basis of poor motivation, intellectual deficit, or absence of proper instruction. As many as 10% of school-age children may suffer from developmental dyslexia. Reading is mediated by parallel and widely distributed modular systems. There are, therefore, multiple loci in these systems where dysfunction may lead to developmental dyslexia. Dyslexia, however, is unlikely to represent a single disorder. In the most common form, the children have difficulty with phonetic analysis, that is, associating the visual pattern of written language to the sounds of spoken language and segmenting words ("say hamburger without the ham"). These children are unable to sound out unfamiliar words, but they can learn to recognize whole words by sight. Their reading errors are characteristic in that they tend to guess words, often incorrectly, from their general appearance. They also make characteristic spelling mistakes, tending to spell familiar words correctly but making nonphonetic mistakes with unfamiliar words, usually only writing the first letter correctly, followed by a succession of letters that approximate the length of the word but have little other resemblance to it. Boder referred to this pattern as *dysphonetic dyslexia*. A second form of dyslexia is characterized by an inability to recognize letters and words by sight, without much difficulty in sounding out these written symbols—that is, the exact opposite of the first pattern. Such children tend to make phonetic spelling errors, such as "bloo" for "blue." They also commonly reverse letters or the sequence of letters in words, such as "Precy" for "Percy." Both types of disability may coexist in the most severely affected dyslexic children.

Neuroanatomic abnormalities described in patients with dyslexia include the absence of the typical asymmetry pattern in the planum temporale region (abutting primary auditory cortex in the temporal lobe) and microdysgenesis predominantly in the left hemisphere. Bioelectric activity mapping (BEAM) performed during tasks requiring reading, writing, and listening demonstrate that dyslexic boys as compared with control boys evidence differences in left-hemisphere activity, particularly in Broca and Wernicke areas and in the supplementary motor area bilaterally. The left-hemisphere differences are consistent with dyslexia as a left-hemisphere language disorder. The supplementary motor area differences indicate the need for subvocalization in the reading process. Dynamic imaging studies suggest that dyslexics utilize different pathways for reading than normal readers; posterior regions are underactivated and anterior regions overactivated. Testing with measures assessing phonologic functioning appears to maximize differentiating dyslexic versus normal readers.

Metabolic imaging results corroborate the clinical finding that phonologic deficits underlie dyslexia and indicate that normal and dyslexic readers differ in the involvement of the left posterior region in the reading process. There appears to be a strong genetic factor. A dominant pattern of inheritance, with greater penetrance in boys, has been suggested. Boys have outnumbered girls by about 4:1 in most large population studies. Dyslexia may also be a symptom of more widespread cognitive disorders. When children with developmental dysphasia reach school age, they tend to have reading difficulties, usually involving phonetic analysis. Children with developmental apraxia and agnosia are likely to have difficulties with letter reversals and with letter and word recognition.

Numerous techniques for reading remediation have been developed. Controversy persists as to whether to remediate to the child's strength or weakness (phonics versus sight vocabulary). Generally, if one technique is unsuccessful another should be tried, regardless of the theoretical backdrop. Remediation techniques (reduce contrast, use diffuse color lights/lenses) that variably inhibit magno- and parvo-cellular systems have no proven efficacy. Specific reading disability is treated by remedial education, which should be started early, preferably by the first grade. Proper understanding of the disorder, both by parents and by the affected child, is of great importance. If untreated, these children soon develop a negative attitude toward school and toward themselves. The most severely affected dyslexic children may never become fluent readers, even after years of special educational help. However, they often excel in areas in which reading skills are less important, such as mathematics and science.

References

Developmental Dysphasia

Bishop DV, North T, Donlan C: Genetic basis of specific language impairment: evidence from a twin study. Dev Med Child Neurol 37(1):56–71, 1995

Rapin I: Preschool Children with Inadequate Communication. New York, Cambridge University, 1996

Rescorla L, Roberts J, Dahlsgaard K: Late talkers at 2: outcome at age 3. J Speech Hear Res 40(3) 556–566, 1997

Tallal P, Miller S, Bedi G, et al: Language comprehension in language-learning impaired children improved with acoustically modified speech. Science 271:81–84, 1996

Rett Syndrome

Akesson HO: Rett syndrome: the Swedish Genealogic Research Project. New data and present position. Eur Child Adolesc Psychiatry 6(suppl 1):96–98, 1997

Hagberg B: Condensed points for diagnostic criteria and stages in Rett syndrome. Eur Child Adolesc Psychiatry 6(suppl 1):2–4, 1997

Percy AK, Schanen C, Dure LS IV: The genetic basis of Rett syndrome: candidate gene considerations. Mol Genet Metab 64(1):1–6, 1998

Nonverbal Learning Disabilities

Deuel RK: Developmental dysgraphia and motor skills disorders. J Child Neurol 10(suppl 1):S6–8, 1995

Gross-Tsur V, Shalev RS, Manor O, Amir N: Developmental right-hemisphere syndrome: clinical spectrum of the nonverbal learning disability. J Learn Disab 28(2):80–86, 1995

Harnadek MC, Rourke BP: Principal identifying features of the syndrome of nonverbal learning disabilities in children. J Learn Disabil 27(3):144–154, 1994

Klin A, Volkmar FR, Sparrow SS, Cicchetti DV, Rourke BP: Validity and neuropsychological characterization of Asperger syndrome: convergence with nonverbal learning disabilities syndrome. J Child Psychol Psychiatry 36(7):1127–1140, 1995

Landgren M, Pettersson R, Kjellman B, Gillberg C: ADHD, DAMP and other neurodevelopmental/psychiatric disorders in 6-year-old children: epidemiology and co-morbidity. Dev Med Child Neurol 38(10):891–906, 1996

Rourke BP, Conway JA: Disabilities of arithmetic and mathematical reasoning: perspectives from neurology and neuropsychology. J Learn Disabil 30(1):34–46, 1997

Developmental Dyslexia

Galaburda A, Livingstone M: Evidence for a magnocellular defect in developmental dyslexia. Ann N Y Acad Sci 682:70–82, 1993

Rumsey J, Nace K, Donohoe B, Wise D, Maisog J, Andreason P: A PET study of impaired word recognition and phonological processing in dyslexic men. Arch Neurol 54:562–573, 1997

Shapiro B, Accardo P, Capute A, eds: Specific Reading Disability: A View of the Spectrum. Timonium, MD, York, 1998

Shaywitz SE: Dyslexia. N Engl J Med 338(5):307–312, 1998

Shaywitz S, Shaywitz B, Pugh K, et al: Functional imaging in dyslexia. Proc Natl Acad Sci 95:2636–2641, 1998

Autism

Bauman M, Kempner T, eds: The neurobiology of autism. Baltimore, Johns Hopkins, 1994:102–118

Gillberg C, Coleman M: Autistic Disorders. New York, Oxford University, 1996

Rapin I: Autism. N Engl J Med 337(2):97–104, 1997

25.7 TUMORS OF THE CENTRAL NERVOUS SYSTEM

Bruce H. Cohen and James H. Garvin, Jr.

Cancer is exceeded only by accidents as a cause of death in children. Primary central nervous system tumors account for 20% of all childhood cancers and are now the most common neoplasms of childhood. In most regions of the world, neoplasms are the most common intracranial mass lesions occuring in childhood. The incidence of brain tumors in children younger than 15 years of age is 3.1 per 100,000 per year, resulting in approximately 1700 new cases per year in the United States. The incidence of brain tumors is evenly distributed over this age group.

Diagnosis and treatments for children with brain tumors have changed in the last three decades because of noninvasive diagnostic techniques, improvements in neurosurgery and radiotherapy, and the introduction of chemotherapy. Overall survival and quality of life have improved for children with a variety of different types of central nervous system tumors, notably medulloblastoma and those tumors that are now highly curable with surgical resection. However, for other tumors such as brainstem glioma and ependymoma, there has been little progress, and the outlook for children with recurrent brain tumors of any type remains poor. The infant with a brain tumor continues to pose a challenge because of the toxic effects that standard treatments impart on the developing brain. However, the mortality rates of pediatric brain tumors are decreasing, and an estimated 60% of affected children will survive into adulthood.

A number of factors influence survival and quality of life, including age, tumor location and operability, tumor pathology, and presence or absence of neuraxis dissemination at the time of diagnosis. All of these factors must be considered in determining appropriate therapy. The advances in molecular genetics have resulted in improved understanding of tumor formation and may offer novel approaches to treatment. Finally, there is increased attention to the long-term adverse effects of therapy, particularly as it affects the developing nervous system, and many newer treatment strategies are aimed at reducing late toxicity. This section reviews general aspects of central nervous system (CNS) tumors in the pediatric age group and discusses current management of the more common types of childhood brain tumors.

EPIDEMIOLOGY

There is no clear gender bias in incidence of CNS tumors, with a boy:girl ratio of 1.2:1.0 in white and 0.9:1.0 in African-American children. Brain tumor incidence is slightly higher in white children. The incidence of brain tumors in children appears to be increasing. Connecticut Tumor Registry data demonstrate this increase over the last few decades, especially among young boys. Between the years 1965 and 1979, the age-related incidence of CNS tumors per 100,000 boys was 3.95 (ages 0 to 4 years), 2.5 (5 to 9 years), 2.26 (10 to 14 years), and 1.87 (15 to 19 years) per year. When compared with the years 1935 to 1949, there was a 16.2% increase among boys ages 0 to 4 years ($p < 0.001$), and a similar trend (although not statistically significant) in older boys. Among girls ages 10 to 14 years and 15 to 19 years, the increased incidence over the earlier period was 12.4% (1.85 per 100,000) and 13.9% (1.41 per 100,000), respectively ($p < 0.01$). Similar trends are reported in Finland and Sweden. Incidence data from the National Cancer Institute show a 35% increase in reported childhood brain tumors between 1973 and 1994, primarily for low-grade gliomas. An analysis of this database found the significant increase in childhood brain tumors occured in 1984 to 1985, the time when MR imaging was being widely introduced. The new baseline rate established after 1985 has remained constant through 1994. Such an increase was not seen in the mid-1970s when CT was first employed, possibly because CT cannot detect some posterior fossa and temporal lobe tumors.

RISK FACTORS FOR BRAIN TUMORS

GENETIC FACTORS Familial and genetic syndromes are the most important risk factor identified for development of brain tumors but account for a minor portion of patients with brain tumors.

NEUROFIBROMATOSIS 1 Neurofibromatosis 1 (NF1) is an autosomal-dominant condition with the genetic defect located at 17q11.2 (see Sec. 25.33.2). About 50% of persons with NF1 develop the condition as the result of a spontaneous mutation. Clinical features include café-au-lait macules, neurofibromas along peripheral nerves that involve the skin and internal organs, freckling

in the axillae and groin, hamartomas of the iris known as *Lisch nodules,* and variable osseus abnormalities. Tumors involving central nervous system structures are common. The prevalence of NF1 is 1 in 3000, yet patients with NF1 make up 10 to 64% of all patients with optic pathway gliomas. The period of risk for a person with NF1 developing a visual pathway astrocytoma is almost always in the first 20 years. Other intracranial neoplasms also occur with a relatively increased frequency, including infiltrating astrocytomas in other locations, ependymomas, neurosarcomas involving cranial nerves, and spinal cord astrocytomas. A prospective cohort study indicated the prevalence of intracranial tumors over a 42-year period in patients with NF1 was 10%, with gliomas accounting for the majority of tumors (7.6% of the cohort), followed by meningiomas, tumors of unknown types, and neurosarcoma.

NEUROFIBROMATOSIS 2 Bilateral vestibular schwannomas (previously classified as acoustic neuromas) are the hallmark of neurofibromatosis 2 (NF2). The incidence of NF2 is 1 in 50,000 persons. This condition is inherited in an autosomal-dominant fashion, and the genetic defect is at 22q12, with a spontaneous mutation rate of about 50%. Other features of NF2 include cutaneous schwannomas (not neurofibromas), café-au-lait macules, retinal gliomas, and other nervous system tumors including meningiomas, gliomas, cranial nerve and peripheral nerve schwannomas. NF2 seems to follow a more aggressive course in girls and young women that have the condition as a result of a spontaneous mutation. Vestibular schwannomas grow at independent rates and may produce symptoms at any age. These tumors can be detected presymptomatically for those at genetic risk by using magnetic resonance imaging.

TUBEROUS SCLEROSIS The association between tuberous sclerosis (Bourneville's disease) (see Sec. 25.18.1) and the subependymal giant cell tumor has been known since the initial descriptions of the condition. These neoplasms arise in the midline subependymal region and usually have a benign histology. Unless they cause early obstruction of CSF flow, they grow quite large before causing other symptoms. Other nonneoplastic mass lesions, such as cortical nodules (tubers) and subependymal nodules, occur in tuberous sclerosis and are not neoplastic. The exact prevalence of these tumors is not known, but frequency may be as high as 14%. The abnormal genes are TSC1 and TSC2, located at 9q34 and 16p13, respectively.

OTHER GENETIC SYNDROMES The first affirmation of multiple tumor histologies identified as a familial cancer syndrome was the LiFraumeni syndrome (TP53;17p13), which results in an increased risk of gliomas, ependymomas, choroid plexus carcinomas, as well as non-CNS tumors such as sarcomas and breast cancer. Turcot syndrome (APC;5q21, hMLH1;3p21, and hPMS2;7p22) is associated with both glioblastoma multiforme and medulloblastomas, and nevoid basal cell carcinoma syndrome (PTC;9q22) is associated with medulloblastomas. Hemangioblastomas, usually located in the cerebellum, medulla, and spinal cord, are found as part of the von Hippel-Lindau disease (VHL;3p25).

OTHER RISK FACTORS Chemical and occupational exposures have been scrutinized as possible causes for the induction of all types of cancers. Laboratory-based studies have shown that numerous chemicals can induce tumors in mammals and that fetal and young animals seem to be most susceptible to chemical carcinogenesis.

N-nitroso compounds, including nitrosamines and nitrosamides, have been shown to induce brain tumors in both adult and fetal animals. Several studies suggest that high dietary intake of nitrosamine, nitrite, and nitrate may increase the risk of brain tumors. A recent study of maternal diet and primitive neuroectodermal brain tumors in children did not support the nitrosamine hypothesis but found that other aspects of maternal diet could alter risk (such as folate and multivitamin use in pregnancy, which were protective).

The role of pesticides inducing brain tumor formation is suggested in an Italian case-control study of newly diagnosed glioma patients. A relative risk of 1.6 ($p = 0.0025$) was found in the cohort exposed to insecticides and fungicides, specifically compounds containing copper sulfate or methyl urea.

Both prenatal and postnatal exposure to diagnostic ionizing radiation are risk factors for the development of brain tumors. Prenatal exposure to electromagnetic fields (from electric blankets) has been shown to increase the risk of developing a brain tumor. In children, prolonged proximal exposure to high-tension power lines has also been shown to be associated with increased risk, as has parental occupational exposure to electromagnetic fields. Other studies on residential EMF exposure have been inconclusive.

The risk of developing a brain tumor may be less in children whose mothers ingest multivitamins daily during pregnancy. It is known that vitamin C inhibits the development of *N*-nitroso compound-induced brain tumors in laboratory animals, but other vitamins, minerals, and dietary factors may also be important. In particular, maternal intake of folic acid in pregnancy may be protective against the development of primitive neuroectodermal tumors.

CLINICAL PRESENTATION

GENERAL CONSIDERATIONS　Before the introduction of noninvasive neuroimaging techniques, such as CT and MR imaging, diagnosing brain tumors required cumbersome procedures such as angiography and ventriculography. The ready availability of CT and MR imaging simplifies the diagnostic evaluation of a child suspected of having a brain tumor, allowing earlier diagnosis, but the rational use of these imaging modalities places renewed importance on careful interpretation of clinical signs and symptoms.

There is no typical clinical presentation of the child with a brain tumor. The signs and symptoms of neurologic dysfunction vary greatly and depend more on the location of the tumor and the presence or absence of increased intracranial pressure than on the pathologic nature of tumor. The degree of neurologic dysfunction correlates with the tumor volume, pressure on eloquent brain regions, infiltration into the surrounding brain or meninges, peritumoral edema, and whether CSF circulation is obstructed by the tumor. Age also influences the clinical presentation, as macrocephaly may be a prominent sign in the infant whose sutures are not yet fused. Malignant CNS tumors have a propensity to seed the subarachnoid space early in the disease course, and the child may present with symptoms of leptomeningeal involvement. Rarely a tumor may compromise the vascular supply or drainage, resulting in damage to otherwise uninvolved parts of the brain.

Children with brain tumors most often present with signs and symptoms of elevated intracranial pressure. The intracranial cavity is composed normally of brain, cerebral spinal fluid, and vasculature. Tumors produce elevated intracranial pressure via a number of mechanisms. Most often elevated pressure results from obstruction of normal cerebrospinal fluid channels, leading to ventriculomegaly. Bulky tumors may also produce increased intracranial pressure by direct mass effect. When the onset of symptoms caused by increased intracranial pressure is acute, it strongly suggests the presence of hydrocephalus. The classical signs of increased intracranial pressure include headache (which may be more common in the morning), vomiting (with or without nausea), unusual irritability, and diplopia. The intensity of the headache is variable and often understated, and neck pain may also occur. Sixth-nerve palsy may be noted, but this is not necessarily a localizing sign and may occur whenever there is increased intracranial pressure.

The initial signs of increased intracranial pressure are more commonly slowly progressive, nonspecific, and nonlocalizing. In school-age children, declining academic performance, fatigue, personality changes, and complaints of vague intermittent headache may be noted. In the "classical" headache of increased intracranial pressure, head pain is present on arising, is relieved by vomiting, and lessens during the day. Although this classical brain tumor headache often leads to a rapid diagnosis, the evolution of the classical headache is usually preceded by several months of intermittent and poorly classified head pains. When headaches are present, their duration prior to diagnosis is usually not more than 4 to 6 months, and additional tumor-related symptoms generally will have become apparent. Clinical suspicion of a brain tumor should be greatest in those children with recent onset of headache or those with a change in their type of headache. However, up to 10% of children with brain tumors have headaches for more than 6 months before diagnosis.

PRESENTATION IN INFANTS　Symptoms of brain tumors are not specific in infants. Irritability, anorexia, and vomiting are common features, but these symptoms are so prevalent in infancy as part of viral illnesses that they are only useful if they are persistent. Because the cranial sutures are not fused, abnormal head growth, the presence of "split sutures," and a bulging fontanelle may be the only signs of a brain tumor. Developmental delay and regression of cognitive and motor abilities are frequent signs of brain tumors in the infant. The funduscopic examination usually is normal unless the tumor involves the optic apparatus, in which case there will be optic atrophy. Impairment of upgaze and seemingly forced downward deviation of the eyes, known as the *sun-setting sign*, are caused by increased pressure on the midbrain tectum by hydrocephalus and may be an early sign of increased intracranial pressure.

INFRATENTORIAL LESIONS　Tumors arising in the posterior fossa often cause problems with coordination and cranial nerve dysfunction (Table 25-5). Tumors of the fourth ventricle, such as medulloblastoma, often present with signs of increased intracranial pressure caused by obstruction of CSF flow through the fourth ventricle. There may or may not be brainstem dysfunction. Later signs are usually limited to truncal unsteadiness related to compression of the cerebellar vermis. Tumors arising in the cerebellar hemispheres, such as cerebellar astrocytoma, usually present with lateralized signs such as limb dysmetria, before signs and symptoms of increased intracranial pressure occur. Bilateral sixth-nerve palsy is generally seen with increased intracranial pressure, but the inability to move both eyes conjugately or the inability to adduct an eye on attempted lateral gaze implies intrinsic brainstem pathology. Head tilt and vertical or diagonal diplopia suggest trochlear nerve palsy, but head tilt may also be a sign of cerebellar tonsillar herniation. Electroencephalographic abnormalities have been reported in up to 10% of children with posterior fossa tumors, but frank

TABLE 25-5

CLINICAL MANIFESTATIONS OF POSTERIOR FOSSA TUMORS

	PNET/MB	LOW-GRADE ASTROCYTOMA	EPENDYMOMA	BRAINSTEM GLIOMA
Relative incidence in posterior fossa	30–40%	30–40%	10–20%	10–20%
Duration of symptoms prior to diagnosis	2–4 months	3–6 months	3–6 months	0–3 months
Symptoms				
Early	Headache, diplopia, vomiting, imbalance	Unilateral dysmetria, gait disturbance	Like PNET/MB but slower onset, diplopia, hoarseness	Diplopia, facial weakness, sensory loss, swallowing difficulty, unilateral weakness
Late	Appendicular dysmetria, coma (10%)	Headache, vomiting		Headache
Signs				
Early	Papilledema, truncal ataxia, abducens palsy	Appendicular dysmetria	Like PNET/MB but slower onset, multiple cranial nerve palsies	Multiple cranial nerve palsies, weakness, long tract signs
Late	Appendicular ataxia	Papilledema, abducens palsy		Papilledema

PNET/MB, primitive neuroectodermal tumor/medulloblastoma.

seizures are uncommon without leptomeningeal spread of tumor, direct infiltration, or compression of the cortex.

SUPRATENTORIAL LESIONS Headaches, weakness, and seizures are the most common presenting features of supratentorial tumors. The headaches associated with supratentorial tumors are often insidious and only become severe if the tumor causes obstruction of cerebrospinal fluid pathways or is large enough to cause traction on the meninges or cranial vasculature.

In many situations, a seizure is the first and possibly only sign of a brain tumor. Many seizure phenotypes are associated with supratentorial tumors. In some cases, the seizure may originate from a parietal lobe focus (eg, a pure motor or sensory seizure). Temporal lobe neoplasms may cause seizures that result in alterations of sensorium, with or without motor signs. Tumors affecting the supplementary motor regions can result in seizures that cause twisting movements and postures of the limbs and versions (forced tonic movements) of the eyes and head. Despite the focal nature of any neoplasm, some patients have seizures that appear to be generalized from the onset and may have a clonic, tonic, or tonic-clonic major motor phenotype. The EEG is sometimes helpful, showing focal areas of slowing or sharp waves over the area of involvement. A normal EEG in the setting of seizures does not eliminate the possibility of a brain tumor. The incidence of underlying neoplasms in children with intractable epilepsy, especially those with partial seizures emanating from the frontal or temporal lobes, is not well-defined, but most experts suggest that any patient with an unexplained partial seizure should be evaluated for an underlying neoplasm. Up to 20% of patients operated upon for intractable epilepsy have underlying benign and malignant brain tumors. MR scanning reveals such lesions in most instances.

Slowly evolving hemiparesis, hemisensory loss, and visual field deficits may occur in patients with supratentorial lesions. The sudden onset of these signs suggests tumor hemorrhage. Tumors involving the so-called silent areas of the cerebral cortex, such as the frontal or parietal lobes, may grow large before causing increased intracranial pressure or focal neurologic signs.

A significant proportion of childhood neoplasms arise in the midline third ventricular and suprasellar region, which can result in compression of visual pathway structures. Visual field deficits are often present in patients with lesions in this area but can be very difficult to document in the young, uncooperative, or ill child. Compression (by tumor or hydrocephalus) or infiltration of the midbrain tectum causes Parinaud syndrome, the triad of impaired upward gaze, dilated pupils that react better to accommodation than to the light, and retraction or conversion nystagmus with lid retraction. Although Parinaud syndrome is observed in patients with pineal area tumors, it may be caused by third ventricular dilation owing to ventriculoperitoneal shunt malfunction.

LEPTOMENINGEAL INVOLVEMENT Leptomeningeal dissemination occurs in up to 15% of children with primary CNS tumors at some point during the course of illness, although it may be asymptomatic or overshadowed by symptoms of the primary tumor. Symptoms include unusual and sometimes fleeting mental changes, neck or back pain, irritability, radicular pain or weakness, and bowel or bladder dysfunction. Extraneural metastasis is rare and almost never a presenting sign or cause of demise.

DIAGNOSIS

Skull radiography and pneumoencephalography are primarily of historical interest and have no role in the modern evaluation of children with presumed CNS neoplasms. On rare occasion, angiography may be necessary prior to surgery to determine the vascular anatomy of cortical, pineal, or suprasellar tumors as well as to rule out the presence of vascular malformations. However, when such information is required, magnetic resonance angiography and venography techniques are replacing conventional angiography in many instances.

The introduction of the CT scan has greatly simplified the eval-

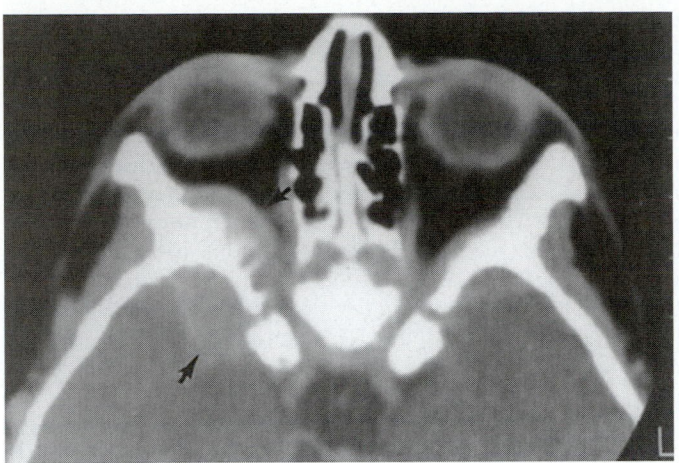

FIGURE 25-18 Axial contrast enhanced CT scan illustrates the bony and soft-tissue components of metastatic neuroblastoma with both intraorbital and intracranial extension. *Courtesy of Dr. Jacqueline Bello.*

uation of a child with a possible brain tumor. When performed with and without contrast medium, CT can detect lesions in 95% or more of patients (Fig. 25-18). Infiltrating tumors such as gliomas may not be detected by CT, although follow-up CT relatively early in the course of the illness will usually demonstrate the neoplasm. Because a non-contrast-enhanced CT is usually performed in the emergency setting, such as the initial emergency ward visit after a patient's first seizure, the clinician should always consider the need for another imaging study as part of the evaluation.

MR imaging is increasingly available and is generally a preferable modality for imaging brain tumors. MR imaging is more sensitive than CT for detection of abnormal tissue and is especially useful in the diagnosis of nonenhancing, infiltrating tumors and leptomeningeal spread. Unlike CT, MR imaging of the posterior fossa is not compromised by bone artifacts, and MR imaging is also superior in evaluation of tumors of the cervical-medullary junction and spinal cord tumors.

Despite the sophistication of MR imaging, the technique has limitations. Whereas specific MR patterns are recognized that correspond to different childhood tumor entities, MR imaging cannot be relied upon to unequivocally diagnose the tumor histology or grade. Finally, MR imaging may fail to differentiate residual disease from postoperative changes or radiation-induced effects on the tumor.

A child with a presumed CNS tumor can be evaluated initially by either CT or MR imaging, but the latter is preferable in most cases. In children with infiltrating neoplasms, MR is clearly the neuroimaging technique of choice. Once a tumor has been documented, MR evaluation is mandatory in most cases to determine the extent of disease and to assist in the surgical management. The imaging time needed for an MR study exceeds that of CT. Young children will usually require sedation. In medically unstable patients CT is usually the preferable modality, and in certain tumors, such as craniopharyngiomas, CT is adequate to follow patients after treatment.

Spinal imaging is important for evaluation of tumors with the tendency to seed the neuraxis, such as medulloblastomas, germ cell tumors, ependymomas, and posterior fossa astrocytomas. Spinal MR imaging with contrast enhancement appears to have compa-

rable sensitivity and has replaced myelography in most circumstances as the standard procedure for evaluation of cord involvement and leptomeningeal disease. CSF cytology and MR imaging of the spine should be used as complementary techniques, because neither is 100% sensitive in evaluating for dissemination of tumor.

Although not universally available, PET scanning is another potentially useful technique for the evaluation of central nervous system tumors. PET scanning may be performed using various agents that measure brain metabolism (including glucose metabolism and protein metabolism) and provides the first truly metabolic images of the brain. Preliminary work suggests that PET scanning may demonstrate metabolic abnormalities beyond those identified anatomically by CT or MR imaging. PET scanning also appears to be useful in distinguishing recurrent or residual tumor from radionecrosis and may potentially give a suggestion of the degree of malignancy. Magnetic resonance spectroscopy is being investigated to assist in the evaluation of the degree of malignancy as well as to distinguish recurrent tumor from radionecrosis.

GENERAL PRINCIPLES OF MANAGEMENT

The standard approaches used to treat childhood brain tumors include surgery, radiotherapy, and cytotoxic chemotherapy (Table 25-6). Biologic modifiers and immunotherapy are now being explored in childhood tumors and may in time become an important component of therapy. The internet has made it possible for physicians and families to search for information about different treatment options (Table 25-7).

SURGICAL RESECTION Surgery remains the backbone of treatment. Surgery is important for obtaining a tissue diagnosis and is the first step of effective therapy. In children with truly benign tumors, a complete surgical resection can be curative. In those with malignant tumors, a gross surgical resection can achieve greater than a 99% reduction in the tumor burden, making radiotherapy and chemotherapy more effective.

TABLE 25-6

MODALITIES OF TREATMENT FOR BRAIN TUMORS

TYPE	GOALS
Surgery	Establish diagnosis
	Open blocked CSF pathways
	Remove bulk tumor
	Cure low-grade tumors (?)
Radiation therapy	Control local residual disease
	Control tumor dissemination
	Cure malignant tumors (?)
Chemotherapy	Adjuvant therapy for malignant tumors
	Reduce radiotherapy dose needed
	Obviate or delay radiotherapy for low-grade tumors
	Obviate or delay radiotherapy in infants with malignant tumors
	Primary treatment for some malignant tumors (?)
Immunotherapy	Enhance immune response
	Adjuvant to other therapies
	Scavenger for minimal residual disease

It is rare for a child's brain tumor to be diagnosed before attaining a size of at least 1 cm^3, which corresponds to a tumor burden of greater than 10^9 cells. The body's own immune system may be able to control a minimal burden of tumor cells, perhaps 10^4, although this will vary depending on host and tumor determinants. The main goal of treatment must be to reduce the tumor burden to a stage where the body's own mechanisms can contain any remaining tumor. To illustrate the need for multiple therapeutic modalities, consider the example of a child with a relatively small malignant neoplasm (1 cm^3). A 90% surgical resection of such a tumor will reduce the cell burden from 10^9 to 10^8, and even a 99% resection will leave 10^7 tumor cells, or 1000 times more than the immunologic system is likely to contain. If radiotherapy is equally effective (99% reduction), there will still remain 10^5 tumor cells. Subsequent treatment with chemotherapy will need to destroy at least 90% of the remaining cells for there to be a chance of survival. In fact, most tumors are not diagnosed until the tumor size approaches 10 to 100 cm^3, requiring all modalities to be at least 99% effective in destroying the tumor.

Corticosteroids are part of the standard perioperative care in most children with brain tumors. They can reduce intracranial pressure by eliminating tumor edema but alone will not control increased intracranial pressure owing to hydrocephalus. In most instances, corticosteroids are started before surgery and tapered as quickly as tolerated afterward. Too rapid a taper following surgery, especially in patients with posterior fossa tumors, can result in a chemical meningitis with fever and meningismus. The CSF can show an elevated white blood cell count and low glucose, but the Gram stain and cultures will be negative. Treatment generally includes increasing the steroid dose and using antibiotics until CSF cultures are known to be negative. Once symptoms resolve, steroids should be tapered slowly.

Improvements in anesthesia and surgical techniques have greatly reduced the mortality and morbidity of surgery. The operating microscope and ultrasonic aspirator improved surgical outcomes in the 1970s and 1980s. Surgical navigation and the use of the ventricular endoscope has broadened the capabilities of the neurosurgeon in the last years of the millennium by further improving both the safety and the effectiveness of the neurosurgical procedure. The frameless surgical navigation system is the newest addition to the neurosurgical operating suite. This system utilizes three-dimensional digitizers that are linked to the MR-acquired image data of the patient's brain tumor obtained before surgery. The patient's skull and tumor are visualized in "real-time" as the tumor is approached and removed in the operating theater by integrating the imaging data with a spatially exacting optic or sonic guidance system. The surgeon is able to manipulate the tip of a pointing device that will locate the precise direction of an approach trajectory or the precise localization of structures inside the skull. These systems not only provide real-time intraoperative guidance that allows for a more complete and safer tumor resection but also result in the need for smaller craniotomies because the tumor can be precisely located beneath the skull. In a series of adult patients the most important advantage of using surgical navigation systems was the low mortality (< 1%), morbidity (< 5%), and wound infection rate in virgin craniotomies (< 2%). This translated into reduced costs, operating time, and length of stays (decreased by 5 to 40% compared with standard craniotomy techniques).

The ventricular endoscope is another technique for management of hydrocephalus and can be used to perform biopsies and partial resections of tumors located inside the ventricular system. This instrument is guided into the ventricular system by passing it through a burr hole and transversing the cortex. The endoscope can be guided freehand or with the use of a navigating system, which increases the precision in targeting small tumors or small ventricles. Once inside the ventricular system, the surgeon has direct real-time visualization of the ventricular surface and landmarks. Surgical attachments on the endoscope tip can be used to fenestrate the floor of the third ventricle, creating a conduit for CSF to flow into the basilar cisterns, thereby bypassing the need for a ventricular-peritoneal shunt in patients with tumor occlusion of the aqueduct of Sylvius or cerebellar outflow channels. The ventricular endoscope can also be used to direct the biopsy or resect an intraventricular neoplasm. This technique is particularly useful when the neoplasm is suspected to be benign, such as neurocytomas and astrocytomas located on the wall of the third or lateral ventricles, where an open surgical resection could cause significant morbidity, or where a complete resection may not be necessary.

In patients with hydrocephalus, tumor removal may obviate the need for a permanent ventricular-peritoneal shunt in about 50% of patients. If the hydrocephalus is causing symptoms of increased intracranial pressure that need to be addressed prior to tumor resection, some surgeons prefer to place a ventricular drain, which can be removed once CSF flow has been reestablished. However, if symptomatic hydrocephalus does not resolve after tumor removal, the patient will require either a third ventriculostomy or ventricular-peritoneal shunt.

The intent of most surgeries is to remove as much tumor as possible without causing neurologic deficits. For certain tumors, especially medulloblastoma, supratentorial PNETs, and ependymoma, a gross total resection results in a better outcome. In situations where safe tumor removal is not possible, such as the thalamus, stereotactic biopsy may be useful in obtaining a tissue diagnosis. One major disadvantage of a biopsy in the situation of gliomas and germ cell tumors is that the tissue removed may not represent the entire pathologic spectrum of the tumor. Because tumors are defined by their most malignant features, a biopsy can result in a misdiagnosis of a low-grade astrocytoma for a higher-grade astrocytoma, or a germinoma for a nongerminoma germ cell tumor.

RADIATION THERAPY Radiation therapy is used to treat most malignant brain tumors as well as some benign tumors, although treatment with radiotherapy is generally avoided during infancy. Treating children with radiotherapy requires an understanding of the

TABLE 25-7

INTERNET WEB ADDRESSES FOR INFORMATION ABOUT BRAIN TUMORS

ADDRESS	ORGANIZATION
http://www.abta.org/	The American Brain Tumor Foundation
http://www.oncolink.upenn.edu/	The University of Pennsylvania Cancer Information Home Page
http://www/tbts.org/	The Brain Tumor Society
http://www.virtualtrials.com/	Musella Foundation
http://www.virtualtrials.com/btlinks/	Kristen Kenzig Memorial
http://cancertrials.nci.nih.gov/	National Cancer Institute Cancer Trials Home Page

delicate balance between effectiveness and toxicity. Important factors for both efficacy and toxicity are the volume of tissue irradiated, total radiation dose, dose fraction (the amount of radiation delivered at one time), and duration of treatment. When given in standard doses and fractions, gamma irradiation induces the formation of intracellular reactive free radicals that damage DNA. Radiation is not selective and damages the DNA of both tumor tissue and normal tissue. The overall favorable effect results from the impaired repair capacity of neoplastic cells. Because the ability of neoplastic cells to repair damaged DNA is less efficient and takes longer than in normal tissues, the tumor is slightly more susceptible to frequent doses of radiation. Cellular death after irradiation does not occur immediately but during the first or succeeding efforts at mitosis. In summary, smaller and more frequent dosing preferentially injures any rapidly dividing cells (eg, tumor, hair follicles), whereas larger and less frequent doses preferentially injure slowly dividing cells (oligodendroglial, cranial vasculature). Treatment with a single, large dose of radiation such as delivered with the Gamma Knife is referred to as *radioablation* and causes cell death probably by inducing apoptosis and other mechanisms (Table 25-8).

The tolerance of the brain to radiotherapy depends on the age of the patient, the total dose of radiotherapy delivered, and the dose fraction (the amount of irradiation given per dose). The standard dose fraction is generally a single daily dose of 180 to 200 cGy. Late effects on normal tissue seem to depend largely on the size of the dose per fraction, with smaller dose fractions causing fewer side effects at the same total dose. There is a theoretical advantage to the use of larger total number of smaller fractions of radiation to reduce late effects: the so-called hyperfractionated radiation therapy. This technique allows larger total doses to be given with tolerable late effects and is presently under study in treating various childhood central nervous system tumors. To date the use of hyperfractionated radiation therapy, up to 7800 cGy delivered in twice-daily fractions, has not resulted in improved survival in children with diffuse brainstem gliomas.

For tumors that tend to disseminate throughout the craniospinal axis, including the PNETs, malignant gliomas of the posterior fossa, and many germ cell tumors, craniospinal irradiation is an essential part of therapy. With these tumors, doses of 3600 cGy delivered in 180-cGy fractions are given to the craniospinal axis, and the tumor bed is given additional radiation to bring the total dose into the 5000- to 6000-cGy range. For patients with nondisseminated PNETs, lower craniospinal dosages are being used along with chemotherapy in an attempt to reduce the toxicity of treatment. Tumors that do not tend to disseminate, such as cortical gliomas, are generally treated to a total dose of 5000 to 6000 cGy in fractions of 180 cGy, given usually daily, 5 days a week. The major technical problem in delivering craniospinal irradiation is aligning the radiation beams to evenly treat the entire neuraxis without overlapping or creating a gap, which would effectively result in a double (or insufficient) dosing to a transverse region of the spinal cord. The field of radiotherapy for cortical gliomas should include at least the entire enhancing portion of the tumor with a margin of 1 to 2 cm. However, some infiltrating gliomas demonstrate widespread penetration on FLAIR or T_2-weighted MR imaging, and this needs to be taken into account when formulating a treatment plan. In some circumstances, it may be necessary to treat a much larger brain volume than what would be suggested by the gadolinium-enhanced MR images. For young children (with small brains) and children with large gliomas, the treatment volume may approximate the entire brain. Certain tumors that are very well

defined, such as the craniopharyngiomas, can be treated with very localized fields. Conformal radiotherapy uses standard fractionated linear accelerator-based treatments along with a three-dimensional imaging plan to increase the ratio of radiation dose delivered to the tumor compared with the dose delivered to the normal tissue.

The eventual goal for the treatment of noninvasive tumors will be to deliver a curable dose of radiation to the tumor and no radiation to surrounding structures. This is not possible with current technology, so the next best attempt is to deliver the curative dose to the tumor and an *acceptable* dose to the uninvolved surrounding brain. Although it may be intuitive that by reducing the dose of radiation to unaffected brain regions long-term toxicity would be lessened, this is still unproven. Nevertheless, for young patients who require radiotherapy to a precise target volume, such as would be the situation in an inoperable craniopharyngioma, the use of standard, or even conformal, techniques generally results in the unavoidable delivery of radiation to midline structures critical to memory function, such as the fornix and hippocampus. Computerized planning with a multifield technique and geometric shaping of the beam spares some critical structures and does not require any special equipment.

Stereotactic radiosurgery (SRS) refers to tumor localization and radiotherapy techniques allowing for precise treatment of a specified target. The target is determined using similar technology as with stereotactic surgery. SRS can be delivered by an adapted linear accelerator or a Gamma Knife unit. The adapted linear accelerator is modified so that a narrow beam is directed through a series of noncoplanar arcs rotating about the patient that deliver the radiation at the specific target, but with a steep falloff of radiation dose away from the tumor when compared with standard radiotherapy delivery.

The Gamma Knife uses 201 separate cobalt sources targeted at a fixed central point inside the machine. The planning is performed by a computer, with the final plan requiring a series of interactions between the physician and computer. The goal of the treatment plan is to deliver an ablative dose to the tumor and subablative doses to surrounding structures. The majority of SRS and Gamma Knife treatments are performed as a single fraction. Whereas healthy brain tissue can survive standard fractionation treatments, healthy tissue in the ablative field is destroyed by these techniques, and radiation necrosis is a complication following SRS. Because the spectrum of pediatric tumor pathology differs from adults, there is not a great deal of experience in using the Gamma Knife in children. However, it remains a reasonable option for localized low-grade neoplasms that have recurred following standard treatments as well as for the rare pediatric patient with brain metastases.

Intensity-modulated radiation therapy (IMRT), also known as the Peacock system, is a more advanced conformal radiation system. The IMRT device is fitted in front of the exit beam of a standard linear accelerator and modulates the intensity and shape of the beam as the linear accelerator rotates through a series of coplanar arcs. The intensity of the beam is determined by an on-board computer, and the shape of the beam is modified continuously by the rapid opening and shutting of the leaflets as the rotation occurs. A uniform dose of radiation can be delivered to any shaped tumor, with a minimal dose of radiation delivered to surrounding structures (see Table 25-8).

Other means to enhance the efficacy of radiation therapy, such as the use of radiation sensitizers and the use of different radiation sources such as neutrons, have yet to be shown to be more effective

TABLE 25-8

RADIATION THERAPY TECHNIQUES

METHOD	ADVANTAGES	DISADVANTAGES	COMMENT	EXAMPLE OF USE
Standard	Ease	Target volume more likely to involve critical structures	Necessary for craniospinal techniques and for large tumors Standard fractionation most commonly used	PNET Treatment of large hemispheric tumor
Conformal irradition	Uses standard equipment Delivered treatment generally involves less normal brain tissue than standard approach	None	Techniques available at almost all medical centers	Treatment of a smaller or moderate-sized hemispheric tumor Treatment of a nondisseminated pineal germinoma
Linac-based radiosurgery (LRS)	Single treatment fraction Less expensive than a Gamma Knife Brain tissue outside of target receives little radiation	High quality assurance Increased risk of radiation necrosis in target volume Relatively few applications in pediatric patients Invasive head frame	Large single fraction delivered using a modified linear accelerator Closest simulation of Gamma Knife procedure Patient immobilization and positioning necessitate single fraction treatment (although possible to use for delivering a few fractions)	Metastatic tumors Small malignant tumors
Intensity modulated radiation therapy	Brain outside of intended target receives less radiation than other techniques except LRS and Gamma Knife Fractionated	High quality assurance Complicated planning Linear accelerator must be fitted with device, slowing down treatment times Rigid fixation using tight-fitting masks makes treatment uncomfortable	Advantages and safety of fractionated radiation and the precision approaching stereotactic techniques for certain tumors Equipment not available in most centers	Small midline or hemispheric tumors Craniopharyngioma
Gamma Knife	Single treatment fraction Multiple targets easily treated at one time Mechanically very precise	Increased risk of radiation necrosis in target volume Relatively few applications in pediatric patients Anesthesia required in young patients Invasive head frame	Available at relatively few centers Expensive initial cost Patient immobilization and positioning necessitate single fraction treatment	Metastatic tumors (single or multiple) Palliative treatment of recurrent tumors Small malignant primary brain tumors
CyberKnife	Treatment delivered in multiple fractions Treatment target is determined in real-time Brain outside of intended target receives less radiation than most other techniques Nonrigid restraints Treatment to intended target is based on patient's own bony landmarks, increasing accuracy	Complex planning Slow	Limited availability, not yet fully FDA approved	Potentially useful for treating any tumor other than those that require whole brain or craniospinal techniques

PNET, primitive neuroectodermal tumor.

than standard external beam techniques but are under study in some centers.

Not all children with brain tumors should be treated with radiotherapy, at least not until other measures have failed. It is now standard to treat infants with chemotherapy prior to radiotherapy. In addition, some tumors, such as the pilocytic astrocytomas, are best managed with surgical resection. Second attempts of resection and chemotherapy are generally considered before radiotherapy,

and radiotherapy is reserved for those tumors that recur despite other measures. Although the infiltrating low-grade glioma is not common in children, many centers use radiotherapy only if all other measures fail.

CHEMOTHERAPY   Chemotherapy is used increasingly in the treatment of childhood brain tumors. Chemotherapy was once considered as an adjunctive treatment to be used along with surgery and radiotherapy, but in many tumors the role of chemotherapy has become part of the standard of care, including the medulloblastoma and high-grade astrocytomas originating outside of the brainstem. In an effort to delay the application of radiotherapy in infants and young children, chemotherapy is being used as sole postsurgical treatment of both low-grade and high-grade neoplasms with encouraging results. It may be used as an adjuvant to radiotherapy, as the primary postsurgical treatment in infants, and in recurrent tumors.

The effectiveness of a chemotherapy agent depends on many factors including the ability of the drug to cross the blood-brain barrier, inherent sensitivity of the tumor to the particular drug, and tolerance of normal tissue to the agent. Effective chemotherapy agents include the nitrosoureas, vincristine, cisplatin and carboplatin, etoposide, and cyclophosphamide. Newer agents such as topotecan and other topoisomerase I inhibitors, temozolomide, taxol, and related agents are being explored as possibly effective agents. Drugs typically are used in combination because of complementary mechanisms of action and to subvert potential tumor resistance. Most recent phase III chemotherapy trials in children use this multiagent approach.

These drugs are most often administered by oral or intravenous routes. However, various delivery strategies are under study to improve the efficacy of chemotherapeutic agents. Regional delivery of drugs—either intrathecally, intratumorally, or intra-arterially— may enhance the concentration of the drug and result in better efficacy but may also result in increased neurotoxicity. Regional chemotherapy has not yet been shown to be effective for the management of childhood brain tumors. The dose intensity of conventional systemic chemotherapy can be increased with the use of hematopoietic growth factors, which accelerate recovery from chemotherapy-induced myelosuppression and permit use of higher doses and/or shorter intervals between treatments, with potentially greater antitumor effect. A related approach is the use of extremely high doses of chemotherapy supported by infusion of autologous bone marrow or peripheral stem cells. Preliminary evidence of autologous bone marrow rescue (AuBMR) and autologous stem cell rescue (AuSCR) is effective in some infants and children with recurrent malignant glioma and medulloblastoma.

There has also been considerable interest in using chemotherapy to obviate or at least delay the need for radiotherapy in infants and young children with malignant brain tumors or to reduce the dose of radiotherapy needed by supplementation with chemotherapy. The goal of these approaches is to reduce or eliminate long-term sequelae of radiotherapy, although it is recognized that intensive chemotherapy may also have undesirable late effects in young children, such as induction of second malignancies, especially when combined with radiotherapy.

PRIMITIVE NEUROECTODERMAL TUMOR/MEDULLOBLASTOMA

Primitive neuroectodermal tumors (PNET) may originate in any region of the neuraxis. The most common location is the posterior fossa, in which case they are conventionally referred to as a *medulloblastoma* (MB). Primitive neuroectodermal tumors may also arise in the pineal gland (and are then referred to as *pineoblastomas*) and cerebral cortex (*supratentorial PNET* or *central neuroblastomas*) and have identical pathologic features. Despite the identical microscopic appearance, the MB has a better prognosis. PNET/MB are comprised predominantly of small cells with little cytoplasm and

hypochromatic nuclei. These lesions frequently display histologic heterogeneity, with some regions within the tumor having apparent glial, ependymal, neuronal, or photoreceptor cellular differentiation on light microscopy. Immunohistochemical analysis demonstrates that single PNET/MB cells may have both neuronal and glial intermediate filaments, staining with both neurofilament protein and glial fibrillary acidic protein (GFAP). The presence of GFAP correlates with a 6.7-fold increased risk of relapse, and patients with tumors staining with a higher percentage of GFAP have a 3-fold higher risk of relapse compared with tumors staining less avidly. Recently, synaptophysin, a cellular membrane protein, has been shown to be selectively expressed in PNET/MB, independent of site of origin, but not in other primary brain tumors.

Taken together, primitive neuroectodermal tumors including medulloblastoma (PNET/MB) are the most common type of malignant primary CNS tumor in childhood, and those arising in the posterior fossa constitute approximately 30% of infratentorial tumors in the pediatric age group. The cell of origin of this tumor is not well defined; some have suggested that this tumor is derived from remnants of fetal external granular cells of the cerebellum or from small resting cells in the posterior medullary velum.

The majority of childhood PNET occur as medulloblastoma involving the cerebellar vermis, filling the cavity of the fourth ventricle, and infiltrating the floor of the fourth ventricle by local extension. This tumor may arise more laterally in the cerebellum, especially in adolescents and adults.

Factors that control growth of PNET/MB are largely unknown. Up to one-third of these lesions have a specific chromosomal abnormality, the duplication of the long arm or deletion of the short arm of chromosome 17 (isochromosome 17q). Molecular genetic studies of PNET/MB suggest that the p53 gene (a tumor suppressor gene located on chromosome 17) may be altered in some patients with this tumor. Another reported deletion is in the short arm of chromosome 11, a region in which loss of heterozygosity has been found in several sporadic and familial cancers. In addition, tumor cell ploidy studies in medulloblastoma have suggested that patients with diploid tumors may have a worse prognosis than patients with aneuploid or hyperdiploid tumors. Concepts of classification will no doubt change with wider application of these immunohistochemical and molecular genetic methods, which to date have been applied primarily to the more numerous posterior fossa PNET/MB and less to the histologically identical tumors arising in other parts of the brain.

Medulloblastoma (PNET/MB) of the Posterior Fossa

Children with medulloblastoma (PNET/MB) of the posterior fossa typically present with symptoms of increased intracranial pressure including vomiting, lethargy, and morning headache. Ataxia and diplopia are also common presenting features. The ataxia may be truncal or involve the limbs. The duration of these symptoms is brief, and the majority of patients are symptomatic for less than 3 months prior to the time of diagnosis. Head tilt may also occur secondary to either fourth cranial nerve dysfunction or incipient cerebellar herniation. Occasionally, hemorrhage may occur into the tumor, causing a rapid onset of symptoms. The laterally placed cerebellar lesions tend to present slightly differently, with symptoms of cerebellopontine angle disturbance or appendicular ataxia.

Diagnosis of medulloblastoma can be strongly suspected in most cases based on the CT or MR scan. These tumors tend to appear

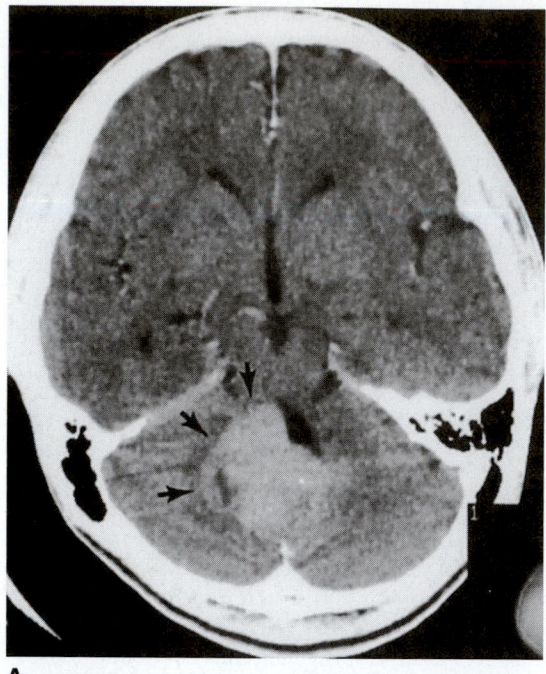

A

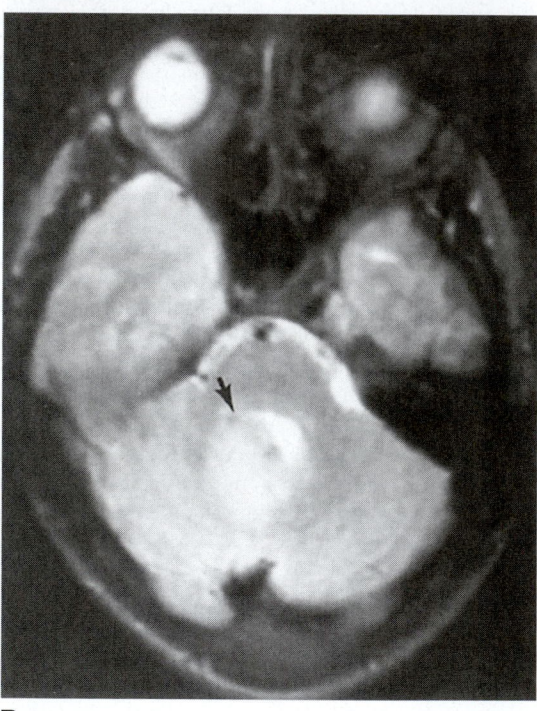

B

FIGURE 25-19 **Axial contrast enhanced CT (A) and axial T₂-weighted MR (B) scans demonstrate a cerebellar vermian mass (arrows) which enhances on CT and has high signal on the T₂ MR image; note compression and displacement of the fourth ventricle.** *Courtesy of Dr. Jacqueline Bello.*

as isodense or hyperdense lesions on noncontrast CT that frequently enhance homogeneously after intravenous injection. Because of the tumors' midline location, hydrocephalus is present at the time of diagnosis in well over 80% of patients. A substantial number of PNET/MB will have other characteristic features on CT including small cystic regions or necrotic areas, calcification,

and hemorrhage. MRI is equally sensitive in diagnosing the presence of these lesions (Fig. 25-19A, B). PNET/MB are classically hyperintense on the T₂-weighted image and may show evidence of increased internal vascularity. As with CT, these tumors tend to enhance readily with contrast. Extension of the tumor superiorly and inferiorly may be better appreciated on MR imaging than on CT. Neuroradiographic evidence of dissemination outside the primary site may be apparent at the time of diagnosis. For the purpose of staging, a MR imaging of the spinal cord should be performed, as nodular seeding is easier to detect before surgery, as even a small amount of blood in the spinal fluid can obscure interpretation.

At surgery, the tumor characteristically appears as a grayish purple fleshy mass that may extend into the cisterna magna. PNET/MB are typically friable and soft and removable by suction. Modern neurosurgical techniques permit complete or nearly complete resection in most cases. The tumor may infiltrate the fourth ventricle or one of the cerebellar peduncles, making complete resection impossible. Controversy persists regarding the need for routine ventriculoperitoneal shunting prior to surgery. Because preoperative ventriculoperitoneal shunting carries with it the potential risk of upper cerebellar herniation, and because after complete or near-complete tumor removal many patients (up to 50%) will not require shunting, the consensus is that preoperative shunting should be avoided when possible.

Following surgery, MR imaging is indicated to confirm the extent of surgical resection. Dissemination of primitive neuroectodermal tumors prior to surgery has been documented in as many as 50% of patients and is more common in infants than in older children. The evaluation of disease extent at the time of diagnosis has been the most consistently useful prognostic factor for this tumor and directly affects future treatment. For these reasons, in those patients not evaluated with a preoperative MR scan, postoperative evaluation for leptomeningeal spread is indicated; most patients will be asymptomatic. Until recently, myelography and cerebrospinal fluid cytology postoperative examination have been needed to determine the degree of leptomeningeal dissemination. Experience with gadolinium-enhanced MR imaging suggests that a carefully performed MR study will have comparable sensitivity to myelography, and thus MR imaging is now done routinely. All patients require postoperative examination of the lumbar CSF for the presence of tumor cells. Based on the age of the patient, tumor histologic features, the extent of surgical resection, and results of postoperative staging, children with posterior fossa PNET/MB can be stratified into major risk groups (Table 25-9). This is of more than academic interest, as there is evidence that patients with so-called poor-risk disease factors at the time of diagnosis, especially those with leptomeningeal spread or brainstem involvement, will benefit from the addition of adjuvant chemotherapy. Several studies have indicated that patients with totally resected tumors tend to fare better than patients who had only a partial resection, although tumor dissemination and patient age might be more important fac-

TABLE 25-9

POOR PROGNOSTIC FACTORS FOR PRIMITIVE NEUROECTODERMAL TUMOR/ MEDULLOBLASTOMA (PNET/MB)

Disseminated disease	Brainstem infiltration
Younger age at diagnosis	Extent of surgical resection (?tumor size)
Histologic, cytogenetic, and molecular features	

tors in determining outcome. It is clear that patients who undergo a biopsy alone at the time of diagnosis rarely survive.

Radiation therapy remains the principal postoperative treatment for patients with PNET/MB. Survival after treatment with focal tumor irradiation alone is uncommon. The introduction of craniospinal radiotherapy with local boost radiotherapy resulted in the first significant improvement in survival of patients with this tumor. Conventionally, 3600-cGy radiation is given to the brain and spine and an additional 1800 to 2000 cGy to the local tumor site (local tumor dose 5400 to 5600 cGy). In the late 1970s and early 1980s, two large prospective randomized treatment trials for children with medulloblastoma showed no clear evidence that chemotherapy improved survival. However, for those children with unfavorable risk factors, such as brainstem involvement at the time of diagnosis and/or leptomeningeal spread at diagnosis, chemotherapy resulted in approximately a 20% improvement in 5-year survival. More recently, a study utilizing vincristine during radiotherapy and cisplatin, lomustine (CeeNU, CCNU), and vincristine following radiotherapy in children with so-called poor-risk medulloblastomas reported an actuarial survival of 88% at 5 years. Chemotherapy thus appears to improve the short-term and possibly the long-term survival for children with PNET/MB with unfavorable risk factors. Survival rates for children with poor-risk medulloblastoma treated with chemotherapy are equal to or better than those with so-called average-risk disease treated with radiation therapy alone. All these studies suggest that 5-year disease-free survival in children with medulloblastoma currently exceeds 50% and that a 70 to 85% survival rate may be attainable in those with standard-risk disease treated with radiation therapy and chemotherapy. For those with high-risk disease, the use of hyperfractionated radiotherapy and chemotherapy has resulted in 3-year survivals of 48% in one series.

Although survival has improved, the problem of late effects of treatment remains, and the evidence suggests the dose of cranial irradiation is the major cause of toxicity. In children with standard-risk disease, the use of adjuvant CCNU, vincristine, and cisplatin along with a reduced dose of craniospinal irradiation (dose reduced from 3600cGy to 2400 cGy) showed no change in survival patterns with the suggestion of improved neurocognitive outcome. A further extension of the use of chemotherapy is its use in very young children who are most likely to suffer damage from cranial irradiation. Experience with several chemotherapy regimens suggests that radiation therapy can be safely delayed, if not completely obviated, in some infants with PNET/MB. The survival statistics in all group of PNET/MB must be interpreted cautiously, because this disease may relapse after 5 years.

Supratentorial PNET (S-PNET)

Given the relative infrequency of PNET/MB in sites other than the cerebellum, few data exist concerning the most appropriate management. At present, it seems that these patients should be treated in a fashion similar to that used in children with tumors of the posterior fossa. The lesions that arise in the pineal region are frequently disseminated at the time of diagnosis, and reported survival figures have been less favorable than for cerebellar lesions. Some have proposed local therapy alone for patients with cortical lesions, since it is postulated (but not proved) that these tumors are less likely to disseminate throughout the neuraxis. The 3-year survival with children treated with surgery, craniospinal irradiation, and chemotherapy was 57%, compared with an estimated 3-year survival of 47% in a series of children treated with radiotherapy alone.

EPENDYMOMA

Ependymomas usually arise within or adjacent to the ependymal lining of the ventricular system; 60 to 75% of intracranial ependymomas occur in the posterior fossa, and the remainder arise in supratentorial locations. Ependymomas constitute 5 to 10% of all primary childhood brain tumors and account for 10 to 20% of posterior fossa tumors.

Ependymomas are glial neoplasms derived from ependymal cells. The majority appear to be histologically mature. Ependymomas of the posterior fossa most commonly arise from the floor of the fourth ventricle but may also arise more laterally and extend into the cerebellopontine angle. These tumors have a variable histologic pattern, and microscopic findings do not always correlate with outcome, although patients with anaplastic tumors fare somewhat worse than those with benign tumors. One tumor subtype, the ependymoblastoma, is probably more akin to a PNET/MB and should be separated from other ependymomas. Subependymoma is a variant of the ependymoma in which the fibrillary subependymal astrocyte is the dominant cell type. They may be incidental findings at autopsy but can cause significant neurologic deficit and even mortality.

Animal models exist but have uncertain relevance to human ependymoma. A carcinogen-induced murine ependymoblastoma has been extensively studied but is histologically very different from ependymoma in humans. Sequences related to simian virus 40 (SV40) have been demonstrated in human tumor specimens, suggesting that SV40 or a closely related virus may have an etiologic role in the development of these neoplasms.

Clinical symptoms of ependymomas are quite variable and depend on the location of the tumor within the neuraxis. When this tumor arises in the fourth ventricle, cerebrospinal fluid flow is blocked early in the course of illness, and symptoms of nausea, vomiting, and morning headache ensue. If the tumor arises low in the fourth ventricle and extends into the lower medulla, symptoms of neck pain or stiffness predominate early in the disease course. Cranial nerve palsies can occur from brainstem invasion and compression of cranial nerves as they exit the brainstem. In patients with supratentorial lesions, seizures and focal cerebral deficits are typical presenting features. Symptom duration prior to diagnosis may range from a few weeks to well over a year, and in the majority of patients symptoms are present at least 6 to 9 months before diagnosis. Tumors that invade the brainstem cause more focal neurologic deficits and have a shorter duration of symptoms prior to diagnosis.

On CT scans, ependymomas can appear hypo-, iso-, or hyperdense. Although most tumors show some degree of contrast enhancement, this may vary from uniform enhancement to small scattered areas of enhancement. Calcification is identified in approximately 50% of posterior fossa ependymomas and a smaller proportion of cortical lesions (Fig. 25-20). MR imaging has shown these tumors to be more locally invasive than previously thought, demonstrating that many posterior fossa lesions infiltrate the brainstem or extend into the upper cervical cord. Hydrocephalus is present in the majority of patients with posterior fossa lesions.

The most important predictor of outcome for childhood ependymoma is the extent of surgical resection; the aim of surgery in most patients is to obtain maximal surgical removal. This is relatively straightforward in tumors that occupy the fourth ventricle but is more difficult with tumors that infiltrate the brainstem or those supratentorial lesions that infiltrate brain. Tumors that extend into the cerebellopontine angle and involve multiple cranial nerves

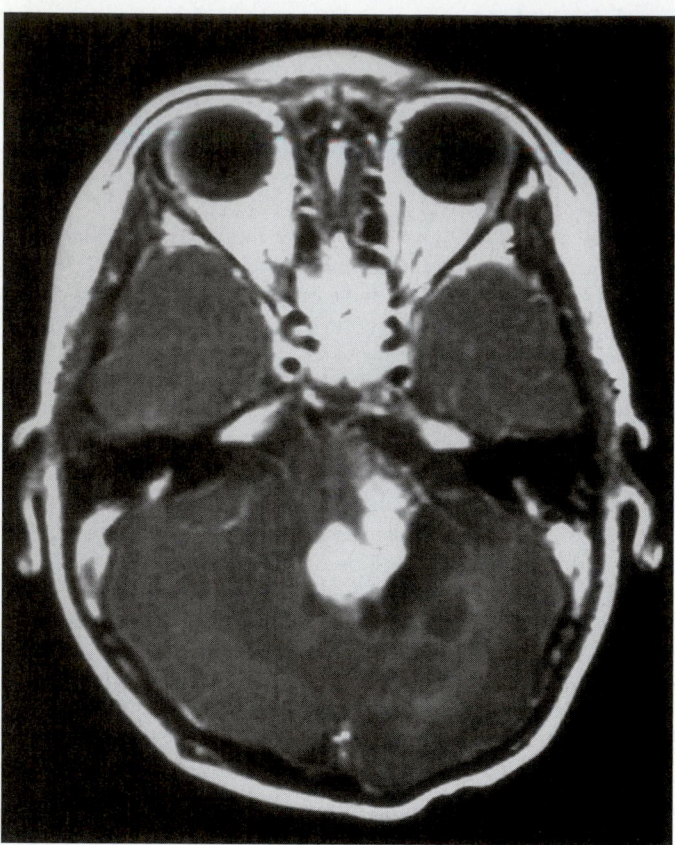

FIGURE 25-20 **Ependymoma arising from the floor of the fourth ventricle in a 4-year-old girl (MR scan). Note the intense enhancement. The mass wraps around the brainstem and involves multiple cranial nerves. This child relapsed 1 year after local radiotherapy and has failed sodium phenylacetate.**

are also difficult to resect without causing substantial neurologic morbidity. A CT or MR scan should be obtained shortly after surgery to confirm the extent of resection, and myelography or gadolinium-enhanced spine MR imaging with cerebrospinal fluid examination is indicated in all patients.

The optimal postsurgical management for ependymoma is poorly defined. Recent experience at Children's Hospital of Philadelphia confirms the most important determinant of survival is the degree of surgical resection. Total surgical resections resulted in a 50% or greater survival rate at 5 years; disease-free survival rate is much lower after subtotal resection. Postoperative radiation therapy seems to increase overall survival. Local failure remains the greatest cause of relapse. Involved field radiation therapy to a dose of 5500 cGy is effective. The need for presymptomatic craniospinal radiation therapy in patients without neuraxis dissemination at diagnosis remains controversial. It is also unclear whether patients with anaplastic ependymomas require a larger volume of radiation therapy than those with low-grade ependymomas. Results to date with adjuvant chemotherapy have been disappointing. Although a variety of compounds, especially cisplatin, may be transiently effective in recurrent ependymoma, chemotherapy has not been shown to be effective in an adjuvant setting. Preirradiation chemotherapy is currently being evaluated in patients with residual tumor following surgery. High-dose chemotherapy with AuSCR and delayed

radiotherapy is being investigated in infants and young children with this tumor.

GLIOMA

Primary CNS tumors of glial origin may arise in essentially any part of the neuraxis; they make up the majority (50 to 60%) of childhood brain tumors. In general, low-grade lesions behave more favorably than higher-grade tumors, but outcome is also greatly dependent on the location of the tumor and the type of treatment possible. It cannot be overstated that low-grade fibrillary astrocytomas are malignant tumors and have the potential to transform into malignant astrocytomas over time. Low-grade fibrillary astrocytomas should not be confused with the benign pilocytic astrocytoma, which is often cured with surgical resection. Tumors in deep locations such as the thalamus may be impossible to resect safely, and diffuse pontine tumors are often treated without histologic confirmation. The use of stereotactic techniques may make biopsy confirmation easier, but with the acknowledged limitation of sampling error.

Cerebellar Astrocytoma

Cerebellar astrocytomas constitute approximately 12% of all childhood brain tumors and 30 to 40% of childhood posterior fossa tumors. The peak incidence is early in the second decade. These tumors arise most frequently in the cerebellar hemisphere but occasionally in the vermis. The tumor may be primarily cystic, solid, or composed of intermixed solid and microcytic elements. The majority of cerebellar astrocytomas are histologically benign. The most common, the pilocytic juvenile cerebellar astrocytoma, is composed of areas of compact, fibrillated cells alternating with looser, more spongy areas. The compact areas often contain an abundance of eosinophilic, beaded, or cigar-shaped structures termed *Rosenthal fibers*. Less frequently, cerebellar astrocytomas contain areas of necrosis and mitosis that suggest increased malignancy. There have been attempts to separate cerebellar glial tumors into two major categories. The first consists of tumors that histologically contain microcysts, calcifications, leptomeningeal deposits, Rosenthal fibers, and/or foci of oligodendroglioma. These tumors, which include the classical juvenile cerebellar astrocytoma, are said to have a favorable prognosis after gross total resection. A minority of patients have tumors with a higher cell density and foci of frank anaplasia. These have been considered as cerebellar anaplastic astrocytomas or diffuse cerebellar astrocytomas and have a less favorable prognosis (Table 25-10).

Children with laterally placed cerebellar astrocytomas have symptoms of clumsiness and unsteadiness affecting the arms and legs that may be present for months. Headaches and vomiting usually occur at some point before diagnosis. Midline tumors tend to present with a shorter duration of symptoms and more subjective unsteadiness. Papilledema, truncal ataxia and dysmetria are usually present by the time of diagnosis. Head tilt may also be present. Other cranial nerve palsies and long tract signs are infrequent and suggest invasion of tumor into the brainstem or a true brainstem origin of the tumor.

CT and MR imaging are equally sensitive in the diagnosis of cerebellar astrocytomas. The cystic cerebellar astrocytoma has a characteristic CT appearance. Classically, a large cystic mass containing low-density cyst fluid is present, associated with an enhancing nodule within the cyst. Occasionally, the rim of the cystic portion of the neoplasm may enhance. The less common solid astro-

TABLE 25-10

CLASSIFICATION OF CEREBELLAR ASTROCYTOMAS

	CLASSICAL (JUVENILE PILOCYTIC)	DIFFUSE
Location	Lateral cerebellar hemisphere	Midline
Neuroimaging	Cystic with enhancing mural nodule	Infiltrating, attached to brainstem, hypodense on CT
Histology	Rosenthal fibers, microcysts	Hypercellular, $+/-$ frank anaplasia
Treatment	Gross total resection is usually curative	Gross resection difficult, radiotherapy, $+/-$ chemotherapy
Outcome	95% 5-year survival with surgery alone	30% 5-year recurrence-free survival, leptomeningeal spread

cytomas are seen as isodense or hypodense areas on unenhanced CT. They tend to arise in the midline, are somewhat less homogeneous, and have margins that are less discrete than in cystic astrocytomas. The enhancement pattern of the solid tumors is variable.

The treatment of choice for children with cerebellar astrocytomas is complete surgical resection. The tumor and its cyst should be completely removed. If there is suspicion that the wall of the cyst is also neoplastic (which occurs in the minority of cases), it needs to be dissected from the interface between the cyst wall and the gliotic cerebellum.

For patients with totally resected low-grade astrocytomas of the cerebellum, radiotherapy or chemotherapy is not indicated. Even in children with partially resected tumors, every attempt should be made to re-resect the lesion before proceeding to other forms of therapy. Radiotherapy is indicated in those tumors that repeatedly recur and in the tumors that can only be partially resected. In those patients in whom a gross total resection is impossible because of infiltration of the tumor into the brainstem, the need for immediate postoperative radiotherapy is controversial. It is our bias to follow these patients carefully with serial examinations and neurodiagnostic studies. Radiation therapy is employed only if there is evidence of progressive disease and further surgical resection is deemed impossible. In young children where there is a desire to delay radiotherapy, chemotherapy using vincristine and carboplatin (or other agents) can be used. For those patients with totally resected pilocytic juvenile astrocytomas, survival is greater than 90% at 5 years, and these patients are probably cured of their disease.

Anaplastic or Diffuse Gliomas of the Posterior Fossa

Anaplastic gliomas of the posterior fossa are relatively rare. As stated previously, these lesions have features of anaplasia such as necrosis, hypercellularity, and mitosis. However, some cases tend to fall in a borderline area with lesions that have a higher cell density or are more diffuse than the classical cerebellar astrocytoma but do not have frank anaplasia. Patients with more diffuse tumors tend to present with midline symptoms and may also have brainstem abnormalities at diagnosis. CT frequently discloses hypodense areas within the cerebellum that are poorly demarcated and may or may not enhance. MR imaging often shows the lesion to be more infiltrative than appreciated on CT.

The goal of surgery for these patients with more diffuse lesions remains the same as for patients with more classical cerebellar astrocytomas. Gross total resection is preferable, but it is unlikely that these types of lesions ever can be cured surgically. In a retrospective review, less than one-third of patients with diffuse or anaplastic gliomas of the posterior fossa survived more than 5 years after surgery, with or without local radiotherapy. The rate of leptomenin-

geal dissemination at the time of or soon after surgery is unclear in these lesions, and all patients should be staged with preoperative spinal MR imaging and cytologic examination of the lumbar CSF cytology obtained after surgery. Patients with disseminated disease should be treated with craniospinal irradiation, but it remains unanswered if those with localized tumor can be treated with involved-field irradiation and avoid treatment to the remainder of the brain and spine. Few data exist as to the effectiveness of adjuvant chemotherapy in this tumor, and, aside from the brainstem glioma, patients are generally treated with the same chemotherapy protocols used to treat children with supratentorial high-grade astrocytomas. Adjuvant nitrosourea-based chemotherapy may be beneficial and when given at recurrence afforded prolonged survival in a minority of patients.

Brainstem Glioma

Brainstem gliomas constitute approximately 10 to 20% of posterior fossa tumors in childhood. The peak age of occurrence lies between ages 5 and 8 years. These tumors can be subtyped based on their MR appearance into the diffuse infiltrating, focal intrinsic, exophytic, and the intrinsic medullary gliomas. The diffuse infiltrating subtype brainstem glioma have the worst prognosis of any childhood brain tumor. The majority of these tumors arise in the pons, often with continuous spread to the medulla or midbrain. Extension into the cerebellum and into the diencephalic region also commonly occurs. Although most children respond to treatment, the duration of response is brief, and most children with diffuse infiltrating lesions die within 18 to 24 months after diagnosis.

Children with brainstem gliomas usually present insidiously, and, prior to the advent of MR scanning, a delay of 3 to 6 months between the onset of symptoms and diagnosis was not infrequent. However, with widespread availability of improved neuroimaging techniques, diagnosis is now made earlier. Symptoms may include involvement of any of the cranial nerves, motor difficulties, and gait disturbances. Bulbar symptoms, including swallowing and speech difficulties, are not unusual. Later in the course of illness, vomiting and headache occur when cerebrospinal fluid flow is obstructed. The more exophytically placed lesions, especially those at the cervicomedullary junction, may cause little in the way of cranial nerve dysfunction early in the course of illness. These children are more likely to present with unsteadiness, nausea, and vomiting. A few children develop symptoms over a few days leading to a rapid diagnosis; however, early diagnosis does not seem to improve outcome.

MR imaging is the preferred method of diagnosis, as CT can miss small tumors and should not be used as the sole method of diagnosis. The CT appearance is typically a low-density lesion in the brainstem with associated compression and obliteration of the surrounding cisterns. The fourth ventricle is distorted and displaced posteriorly. There is little, if any, enhancement with the diffuse intrinsic gliomas. Less frequently, brainstem lesions are isodense or hyperdense and contain cystic areas. Exophytic portions of the tumor are only moderately well delineated on CT. MR imaging delineates extremely well the presence and extent of infiltrating brainstem gliomas. Lesions are usually seen as decreased signal intensities on T_1-weighted images and increased signal intensity lesions on T_2-weighted images. In some cases the tumor seems surprisingly demarcated and localized to one brainstem site. It is now clear that more extensive disease is appreciated on MR imaging than is seen on CT (Fig. 25-21). MR imaging is especially useful in visualizing the infiltration of the medulla and the cervical cord. At other times, thalamic infiltration can be seen on MR imaging but is not demonstrable on CT.

Because of this improvement in noninvasive diagnosis, the need for routine surgery has been questioned. The initial experience with surgery of brainstem gliomas was disappointing. One-third experienced neurologic worsening, and in one-third of cases the biopsy was not helpful in confirming the diagnosis or degree of malignancy of the lesion. In more recent series, utilizing stereotactic techniques, the incidence of postsurgical neurologic morbidity is much lower and the useful histologic yield is higher, but current standards suggest the MR imaging is diagnostic of the diffuse infiltrating brainstem glioma.

The primary issue at this point is not whether surgery can be performed safely but whether surgery is of any benefit. The principal prognostic factors found for patients with brainstem gliomas have been the location of the tumor and its histology. There is no evidence to suggest improved survival with surgery for those with diffuse infiltrating tumors. In general, infiltrating tumors in the cephalad portion of the brainstem, particularly those of the diencephalon and upper midbrain, tend to be lower-grade and have longer survival with radiotherapy but are not amenable to resection. Patients with cervicomedullary tumors, which may be intrinsic or exophytic, tend to have a benign histology, and some can be cured with surgery alone. There is some evidence that surgical debulking of focal and exophytic pontine gliomas followed by radiotherapy may lead to a longer survival, although the risk of worsening the neurologic function should be taken into account.

At the present level of knowledge, it seems that those patients with cervicomedullarly tumors and those whose tumors are not infiltrating on MR imaging should be considered candidates for surgical biopsy or resection. Defining what constitutes this "not infiltrating" tumor is difficult. A variety of prognostic factors have been suggested for patients with brainstem glioma (Table 25-11). Those patients with primarily exophytic lesions or ring-enhancing lesions on CT or MR scans, those patients with prolonged (more than 6 months) symptom duration prior to diagnosis, and those patients without cranial nerve palsies at the time of diagnosis may be considered candidates for surgery. The discovery of anaplastic features on biopsy is an extremely poor prognostic factor, with virtually no likelihood of survival. However, in patients with exophytic or ring-enhancing tumors with low-grade histology, survival is better— 60% survival rates are reported after conventional radiotherapy.

Although most brainstem gliomas are clinically aggressive, the histologic pattern of these tumors at the time of diagnosis is quite variable. Independent of histologic features, those tumors that appear diffuse on MR imaging at the time of diagnosis carry an extremely poor prognosis. This is one of the few brain tumors that can be diagnosed with confidence using MR imaging, and in general a biopsy is not indicated. Intrinsic or exophytic brainstem tumors that are more focal tend to be anaplastic. Partial resection is

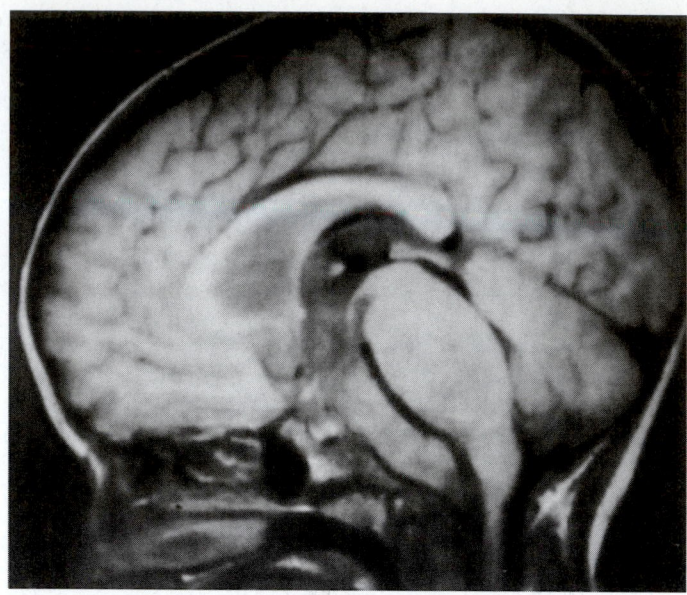

FIGURE 25-21 **MR image of brainstem glioma. Sagittal view reveals widened brainstem and exophytic extension of tumor into prepontine region encasing the basilar artery.** *Courtesy of Dr. S. Hilal.*

possible, and although the prognosis is not favorable, the tumors are not as aggressive as the infiltrating subtype. Regardless of initial pathology, at autopsy these tumors tend to be high-grade gliomas, suggesting malignant transformation over time.

The standard means of treating brainstem gliomas has been radiation therapy. For those patients amenable to total surgical resection with finding of benign histologic features, the need for radiotherapy is unproved; most can be followed without any other specific therapy until there are signs of disease progression. No chemotherapeutic agent or combination of agents has had any significant success in treating these tumors at diagnosis. The majority of patients with brainstem gliomas benefit at least transiently from radiotherapy. Patients are typically treated with 5400 to 6000 cGy. Hyperfractionated radiation therapy doses up to 7800 cGy, delivered at a rate of 100 to 120 rads per dose twice daily, did not improve overall survival.

Leptomeningeal dissemination of brainstem gliomas does occur. In one series, up to one-third of patients developed disseminated disease early in the course of illness. Although a search for dissemination is not mandated at diagnosis, any child with back pain, localized weakness not explained by the brainstem component of the tumor, or disturbance of bowel or bladder function should undergo a MR imaging of the spine. Radiotherapy can be used with a palliative attempt to treat the symptoms of disseminated disease. Although there is no evidence that adjunctive chemotherapy prolongs

TABLE 25-11

POOR PROGNOSTIC FACTORS FOR BRAINSTEM GLIOMAS

Primary pontine mass
Diffuse brainstem involvement
Diffuse, hypodense nonenhancing lesion (CT)
Diffuse, hyperintense lesion (T_2-weighted MR imaging)
Multiple cranial nerve palsies
Brief symptom duration prior to diagnosis

the time to relapse, the use of etoposide or experimental agents may be warranted at relapse.

Diencephalic Glioma

Gliomas of the visual pathway and diencephalon constitute up to 5% of all childhood CNS tumors. Approximately 75% of isolated optic nerve tumors occur in the first decade (Fig. 25-22). Children with chiasmatic tumors seem to have bimodal distribution of age at diagnosis: infancy and the second decade of life. An association with NF1 is present in 50 to 70% of patients with optic pathway tumors. As increasing numbers of patients with asymptomatic neurofibromatosis are being screened with MR imaging at the time of diagnosis, the proportion of individuals with neurofibromatosis among patients with diencephalic region tumors undoubtedly will increase.

The majority of diencephalic tumors are low-grade fibrillary or pilocytic astrocytomas. Anaplastic features are rare, and anaplastic lesions tend to behave similarly to anaplastic lesions anywhere in the brain. Separation of tumors of the diencephalon, hypothalamus, and visual pathway is often arbitrary. Tumors of the visual pathway have a great propensity to spread along the optic tracts and optic radiations, especially in patients with NF1. The clinical signs and symptoms of patients with diencephalic gliomas are greatly dependent on their location and the patient's age. Young patients rarely complain of visual loss, a characteristic symptom in adolescents. More commonly, children under age 3 are brought to medical attention because of strabismus, nystagmus, sudden visual loss (which probably occurred over time), or development difficulties. Children with NF1 often are completely asymptomatic at the time of diagnosis, and often the glioma is identified with a screening MR imaging. Patients with prechiasmatic optic nerve involvement most commonly present with proptosis or unilateral visual loss. Examination of the fundi demonstrates optic pallor and atrophy of the involved optic nerve. Papilledema and other signs of increased intracranial pressure are rare except in large lesions that impinge on the anterior third ventricle. Defining the degree of visual disturbance in chilren, especially infants, with diencephalic lesions is difficult. The pattern of visual loss in patients with prechiasmatic tumors is most commonly a decrease in central vision. In patients with chiasmatic tumors, bitemporal hemianoptic field deficits are often noted, although absence of this finding does not preclude chiasmatic involvement. A fine rapid unilateral or bilateral nystagmus is often present in the greater involved eye, and amblyopia is frequent in the more severely compromised eye.

Growth and endocrinologic disturbance, including precocious puberty and the diencephalic syndrome (failure to thrive in spite of adequate caloric intake, with an appearance of euphoria and overactivity), has been reported in visual pathway and diencephalic tumors. Patients with thalamic lesions tend to present with symptoms and signs of hemiparesis or hemisensory loss. Hypothalamic tumors are even more insidious and may present with alterations in mental status, endocrinologic disturbance, or focal neurologic deficits.

On CT, diencephalic lesions tend to be hypo- or isodense with a variable degree of contrast enhancement. Cystic regions are not infrequent in larger more globular lesions. Tumors of the visual pathway tend to show abnormal enhancement or density along the optic tracts and radiations. This streaking phenomenon is even better appreciated on MR imaging.

The natural history of low-grade astrocytic diencephalic tumors is extremely unpredictable. Some patients, especially those with NF1, experience long-term lack of disease progression without any intervention. Others develop progressive disease with increasing visual loss and neurologic deterioration, which can culminate in death. Because of this erratic behavior, no consensus exists regarding the most appropriate management of these tumors. As a general rule, patients with small tumors, normal vision, mild visual loss, or those young children with NF1 should be observed for progressive visual loss before considering treatment. Those patients with large bulky tumors, blindness, or progressive visual loss are probably candidates for treatment.

The role of surgery for these patients depends on whether the tumor has a significant exophytic component or fills the third ventricle. The more globular lesions involving the hypothalamus and diencephalon, especially those with extension into the third ventri-

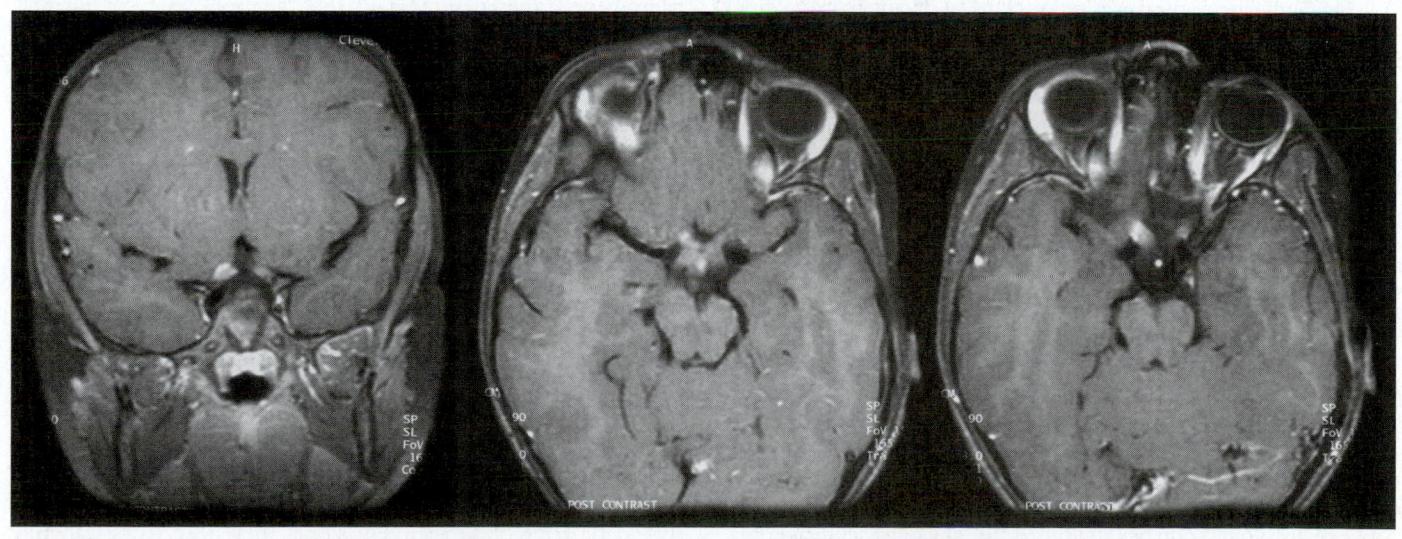

A   B   C

FIGURE 25-22   Optic nerve gliomas in a 4-year-old girl with neurofibromatosis (NF1). Note the enhancement of both optic nerves (R>L). A. Coronal MR image. B. Horizontal MR image. This patient presented with enlarging optic nerve masses with failing vision. She responded to carboplatin-vincristine therapy and is free of progression for 3 years off treatment (C).

cle or having cystic components, may be amenable to surgical debulking. However, it is unclear how this debulking affects long-term outcome. In the short term, such surgical debulking may obviate the need for immediate radiation therapy or chemotherapy. In patients with diffusely infiltrating lesions, such as intrinsic tumors of the chiasm and/or hypothalamus, especially patients with NF1, the diagnosis can be confirmed with MR imaging alone. In these patients, surgery does not seem to be of any benefit.

The indications for neurosurgical or ophthalmologic intervention in patients with isolated prechiasmatic optic nerve astrocytomas are also poorly defined. In patients with complete unilateral visual loss, removal of the optic nerve and tumor is often performed for cosmetic reasons in treating a severely proptotic globe. However, in patients with some vision in an involved eye, surgery is generally delayed until visual loss has progressed or until tumor growth appears to risk involving the chiasm, although it is unclear whether isolated optic nerve lesions will progress to involve the chiasm. Surgery to remove intraorbital optic nerve astrocytomas to prevent such posterior spread is of unproven benefit. Local radiotherapy or chemotherapy may halt the progression of the disease and stabilize vision.

For patients with primary intracranial lesions, radiation therapy may reduce tumor size and generally halts progression of tumor growth. Recommended doses range between 4500 and 5500 cGy. After radiation, as many as 70% of patients have stabilization of disease for at least 5 years. Tumors may appear to enlarge 6 weeks to 3 months after radiotherapy, but in most cases this is a transient postirradiation effect rather than tumor progression.

The major disadvantage of radiotherapy is the associated intellectual and neuroendocrinologic sequelae, especially in young children. The effects of radiotherapy in these midline tumors can probably be diminished by using a multiple field technique, or preferably technology such as IMRT, which limits the dose intensity to mainly the region of tumor and brain immediately adjacent to the tumor. In patients with very large tumors or those with NF1 and posterior extension of the tumor along the optic tracts, determining appropriate radiation portals is troublesome. For these patients, chemotherapy may be a good alternative, at least to delay the need for radiotherapy. Chemotherapy is reported to be of benefit in children younger than 5 years of age with progressive chiasmatic lesions. Treatment with dactinomycin and vincristine, or, more recently, carboplatin and vincristine, resulted in disease stabilization or regression of tumor in up to 80% of patients. In the majority, radiation can be delayed for a median of 4 years after chemotherapy. Present experience suggests that these chemotherapeutic approaches will delay, but probably will not obviate, the need for radiotherapy in patients with progressive tumors.

Low-Grade Glioma of the Cerebral Cortex

The low-grade gliomas can be subdivided into astrocytomas and oligodendrogliomas. Low-grade astrocytomas can be further subdivided into the fibrillary astrocytoma, which is an infiltrating tumor with malignant potential; the protoplasmic astrocytoma; and the pilocytic astrocytoma. Pilocytic astrocytomas have the best prognosis, with little malignant potential, but there is substantial overlap between histologic subtypes and outcome. The oligodendroglioma also has malignant potential but is rare in childhood. There are other tumors often considered along with cortical gliomas, including the ganglioglioma, which is comprised of both glial and neuronal cells. The dysembryoplastic neuroepithelial tumor (DNT) behaves more like a hamartoma than a neoplasm but presents like a

tumor. The microscopic appearance of a DNT is almost identical to that of an oligodendroglioma but can be cured with surgery alone and should never be treated with chemotherapy or irradiation. Cortical low-grade gliomas have a bimodal incidence, with an early peak between the ages of 2 and 4 years and another in early adolescence.

The clinical presentation of cortical gliomas is variable but may be nonspecific and nonlocalizing. In infants, symptoms such as increased intracranial pressure, macrocephaly, developmental delay, and growth retardation are not uncommon. Other disturbances, such as weakness, hemiplegia, sensory loss, and visual field loss are highly dependent on the location of the tumor. Seizures are frequent symptoms of low-grade infiltrating cortical astrocytomas. Although the majority of seizures are of the grand mal variety, there may be a noted focal onset. Focal seizures, with or without generalization, are particularly suggestive of a brain tumor. The frequency of seizures is higher in patients with more slowly evolving tumors. This is especially true for patients with gangliogliomas, which most commonly arise in the temporal lobe and typically present in early childhood with intractable epilepsy. The DNT also presents with epilepsy in early childhood. A rare tumor termed *pleomorphic xanthoastrocytoma* presents in infancy with hemiparesis and seizures and at presentation may be a huge hemispheric mass. This tumor is best treated with surgery, and if the tumor recurs after surgery, chemotherapy is often considered. In series of patients operated on for intractable epilepsy, a 10 to 20% incidence of underlying low-grade tumors in frontal or temporal lobe locations has been reported. Even in series collected in the CT era, as many as 20% of patients have been found to have low-grade neoplasms with normal or nonspecific CT scans. The early experience with MR imaging in patients with intractable epilepsy suggests that patients with an underlying CNS neoplasm will have some type of abnormality on MR imaging.

The infiltrating low-grade astrocytomas appear as a relatively homogeneous low-density mass with little, if any, contrast enhancement and indistinct margins on CT. On MR imaging, these tumors tend to have a low signal intensity on T_1-weighted images and increased signal intensity on T_2-weighted images. Gadolinium enhancement of these lesions is variable. The appearance of the infiltrating low-grade astrocytoma is generally more striking by MR imaging than CT, and MR imaging is superior at distinguishing peritumoral edema from the underlying tumor.

Treatment for these lesions remains controversial. There have been no randomized clinical trials conducted to determine which patients are best treated with surgery alone and which patients require radiation therapy or chemotherapy. Gross-total surgical resection of infiltrating cortical tumors often affords long-term disease control but may or may not be curative. Similarly, radiation therapy has been reported to improve the rate and duration of progression-free survival in patients with partially resected tumors. However, the survival rate at 20 to 25 years after treatment is essentially identical in patients who receive radiation therapy as compared with those treated with surgery alone. Just as in diencephalic tumors, chemotherapy may be of benefit, but its efficacy has not been proved.

Patients whose tumors are amenable to total surgical resection should be treated with surgery alone; they need to be carefully followed, and further treatment (reoperation, chemotherapy, or radiotherapy) should be instituted at the time of disease progression. Patients with subtotal resections may be observed or treated immediately with radiation therapy, conventionally at a dose of 5000 to 5500 cGy or with chemotherapy, such as carboplatin/vincristine. Other chemotherapy regimens, such as procarbazing, CCNU (lomustine), and vincristine, are also effective. There is a need for randomized trials to determine optimal management for patients with these tumors.

High-Grade Astrocytoma

High-grade astrocytomas include the anaplastic astrocytoma and the more aggressive glioblastoma multiforme. Astrocytomas account for 40% of all childhood brain tumors; about one-quarter of astrocytomas have histologically aggressive features and are therefore termed *high-grade astrocytomas.* Cerebral hemispheric high-grade astrocytomas account for about 11% of childhood brain tumors. These tumors appear less frequently in the cerebellar hemispheres. Tumors involving the brainstem or spinal cord are discussed in other sections.

A number of genetic mutations are found in these malignant tumors. Most of the research has been done on adult astrocytomas, although the concepts likely apply to pediatric tumors as well. There is no single mutation that defines each subtype or grade of malignancy. One of the most frequent early mutations occurs in the gene encoding for tumor protein 53 (TP 53), which in the normal state turns on pathways to G_1 arrest or allows apoptosis to ensue, but in the pathologic state would allow an abnormal cell to continue to multiply. Other mutations involved in the formation of malignant astrocytomas include those for the epidermal growth factor receptor, platelet-derived growth factor receptor, and loss of heterozygosity (LOH) of 10p and 19q. Although the malignant potential of astrocytomas forms a continuous spectrum that probably represents additional genetic changes, it is important to classify grades of tumors to select the most appropriate treatment. Classification schemes for astrocytomas have developed mainly from study of adult patients but are applicable to children. Tumor histology can vary within any tumor, and it is important for the pathologist to examine as much tumor as possible to avoid underestimating or otherwise misclassifying the tumor grade.

The most widely used classification scheme for astrocytomas in the past was developed by Kernohan, in which astrocytomas are graded on a scale of 1 through 4, with grade 4 (glioblastoma multiforme) having the most malignant potential. Another classification schema in current use is the method proposed by Daumas-Duport and colleagues, which uses the numerical summation of four histologic criteria (nuclear atypia, mitoses, endothelial proliferation, and necrosis) to determine pathologic grade. This classification scheme has been shown capable of distinguishing groups of patients with different survival outcome. The classification scheme proposed by the World Health Organization eliminates numerical classification but defines the histologic grade in three tiers. This scheme categorizes these neoplasms as astrocytomas (ie, low-grade), anaplastic astrocytomas, or glioblastoma multiforme. The last two categories are discussed in this section.

Anaplastic astrocytomas are tumors comprised of large numbers of neoplastic cells (termed *increased cellularity*) that have a pleomorphic appearance with numerous mitoses. Vascular proliferation is common in anaplastic astrocytomas. Glioblastoma multiforme, the most aggressive form of astrocytoma, has the features of an anaplastic astrocytoma, but with more prominent vascular proliferation and areas of necrosis, which may form a pseudopalisading pattern.

Clinical Presentation As with other brain tumors, the signs and symptoms of supratentorial astrocytomas correlate with the specific area of brain involvement. A recent review of high-grade astrocytomas demonstrated that 89% of patients have more than one symptom at the time of diagnosis. Headaches occurred in 56% and were the earliest and most common symptom. Vomiting occurred in 40%, followed by seizures, motor symptoms, and behavioral abnormalities. Sixty-nine percent had symptoms prior to diagnosis for less than 3 months, 12% from 3 to 6 months, and 19% longer than 6 months; 94% had abnormal neurologic findings at the time of presentation.

Diagnosis is best made by contrast-enhanced CT or MR imaging (Fig. 25-23). Aside from defining location and internal anatomic characteristics such as hemorrhage, cyst formation, and vascular pattern, neuroimaging cannot predict the specific histologic tumor type.

Treatment Surgical intervention is crucial both for diagnostic purposes and for removing tumor. There is evidence that a greater extent of surgical resection correlates with improved long-term survival, and a reasonable attempt should be made to resect as much tumor as safely possible. Unlike low-grade astrocytomas, which often can be entirely surgically resected, high-grade astrocytomas infiltrate surrounding brain, and therefore it is almost impossible to

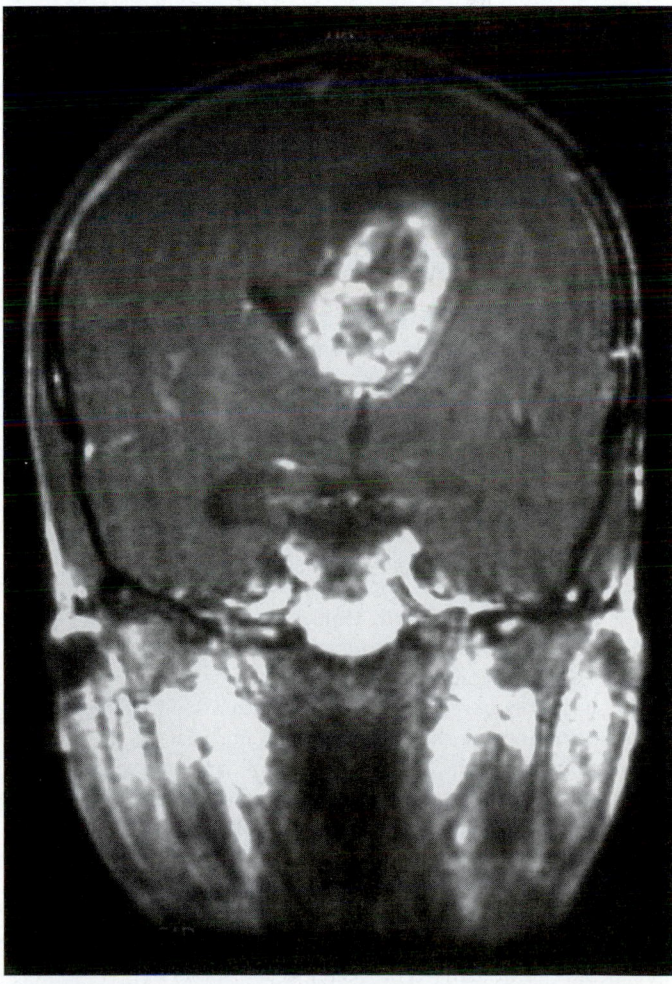

FIGURE 25-23 **High-grade astrocytoma in a 13-year-old boy who presented with depression after his mother's death. Note the large enhancing mass that involved much of the entire left frontal lobe. This child failed chemotherapy, radiotherapy, and numerous salvage chemotherapy regimens and died less than 3 years after his diagnosis.**

remove the entire tumor. Without further treatment, high-grade astrocytomas invariably reoccur.

Radiotherapy increases survival duration in patients with high-grade astrocytoma, although the advantage is modest. Without postsurgical irradiation, the 5-year survival of children with high-grade astrocytomas is 0 to 3%, compared with 15 to 20% survival in those who received radiotherapy. Standard radiotherapy doses range from 5400 cGy to 6000 cGy delivered to the tumor plus a margin of 1 to 2 cm.

Because radiotherapy does not offer substantial long-term survival to the majority of children, chemotherapy is now being used, generally as adjunctive treatment. Many studies have shown improved duration of event-free survival with adjuvant use of chemotherapy, with survivals as high as 45% at 5 years in children treated with radiotherapy and adjuvant CCNU, vincristine, and prednisone. However, survival in recent large studies has not exceeded 35%.

The use of other chemotherapeutic agents and modalities is also being explored. The results of newer studies are difficult to interpret because of relatively small patient numbers, lack of a control group, and brief follow-up time. One such modality is the use of very-high-dose chemotherapy followed by infusion of autologous bone marrow or peripheral blood stem cells. In one study, adult patients were treated with high-dose BCNU (carmustine), followed by autologous bone marrow rescue. Median survival of 25 patients was 26 months, compared with a median survival of 9 months in historical control patients. This approach has also been pursued in children, following an initial report of a 60% objective response rate to high-dose thiotepa and etoposide with or without BCNU in recurrent or newly diagnosed malignant astrocytomas.

Spinal Cord Astrocytoma

Intramedullary spinal cord astrocytomas account for only about 4% of CNS neoplasms in children. Astrocytomas located in the spinal cord have the same microscopic appearance as other astrocytomas seen elsewhere in the central nervous system. Most have a low-grade histology, although as many as 29% of spinal cord astrocytomas may have anaplastic features. These tumors can arise at any cord level and may involve large portions of the spinal cord. The solid component of these tumors extend an average of five spinal segments, although it may be as small as one segment. There can be an associated cyst that can span anywhere from one segment to almost the entire spinal cord. Unlike ependymomas of the spinal cord, which frequently arise from the filum terminale, only about 7% of cord astrocytomas do so.

These tumors have variable growth patterns, and patients with low-grade tumors may be diagnosed only after many years of symptoms. Symptoms correlate with the area of cord involved as well as the rapidity of growth. Symptoms and signs may include varying patterns of weakness, pain, and gait difficulties as well as bowel or bladder dysfunction. Pain is the most frequent symptom, which occurs in 60 to 68% of patients, and may be localized to the vertebral segments involved or may take on a radicular quality. Motor disturbance is the most frequent sign, occurring in 80 to 88%, and may include combinations of weakness and spasticity.

MR imaging with gadolinium is the study of choice to confirm the diagnosis, as this technique demonstrates the location of the solid mass, differentiates mass from cyst, and often demonstrates the boundary of edema from tumor. MR imaging is both easier and

has greater sensitivity and specificity than myelography or CT/myelography, and therefore these techniques are rarely used.

A number of treatment strategies are used to treat spinal cord astrocytomas. Some suggest biopsy or partial resection with surgical decompression of cysts, followed by radiotherapy. Others suggest that gross-total or near-total (99%) resections can be performed in many patients without added surgical morbidity. A complete resection may obviate the need for postoperative radiotherapy in patients with low-grade astrocytomas. The degree of neurologic recovery depends mainly upon preoperative neurologic dysfunction. Spinal deformity is a potential complication and is caused by combinations of the effects of the tumor and the vascular or parenchymal injury that can occur with surgery or radiotherapy. Placement of metal hardware can interfere with future imaging studies, although the MR imaging interference from the newer hardware has improved considerably.

Postoperative radiotherapy appears to be most effective in patients with incompletely resected low-grade astrocytomas, with an estimate of 80% 5-year and 55% 10-year survival rates. If the tumor reoccurs, it usually does so at the primary site. Results of extensive surgical excision without postoperative radiotherapy are encouraging, but long-term results are not available.

Children with high-grade astrocytomas have a much poorer prognosis, and these astrocytomas behave much like its high-grade counterpart in the brain. In one study, 19 children and young adults with malignant astrocytomas underwent radical excision of the tumor; 18 received postoperative radiotherapy and 2 chemotherapy. Hydrocephalus was present in 58%, and subarachnoid dissemination of tumor occurred in 58%. After a median time postsurgery of 6 months, 79% of patients had died. The role of chemotherapy is still not clear, but increasing numbers of children are being treated with chemotherapy, and a 5-year progression-free survival of 46% was reported following combined radiation therapy and chemotherapy.

GERM CELL TUMORS

Tumors of germ cell origin constitute a spectrum of embryonal neoplasms and teratomas that are most likely derived from embryonic migrated totipotent germ cells. These tumors tend to arise in only two areas of the nervous system, the pineal and suprasellar regions. Approximately 50% of pineal region, and 5 to 10% of parasellar tumors, are germ cell tumors. Boys are more likely to have pineal region germ cell tumors, whereas suprasellar germinomas tend to predominate in girls.

The "pure" germinoma accounts for about 50 to 65% of all germ cell tumors. It is a histologically primitive tumor and has a similar microscopic appearance to gonadal germ cell tumors. Teratomas (benign and malignant) and mixed germ cell tumors (all are malignant) harbor a variety of mature and immature elements.

The symptoms and signs of pineal region germ cell tumors do not differ greatly from those of any pineal region mass. Lesions that extend anteriorly and caudally involve the posterior portion of the midbrain, the midbrain tegmentum, and cause various degrees of vertical gaze paresis. The most marked presenting feature is that of Parinaud syndrome. Tumors that extend upward and infiltrate the overlying thalamus may result in hemiparesis, incoordination, visual difficulties, or movement disorders. Germ cell tumors in the pineal region are more likely to cause upper midbrain or tegmental dysfunction rather than focal neurologic signs caused by infiltration of the thalamus.

Suprasellar germinomas produce pituitary and hypothalamic dysfunction such as growth hormone failure and partial diabetes insipidus. Visual loss is a relatively infrequent early finding but can occur if the tumor escapes diagnosis. Symptoms may be present for many months before the correct diagnosis is made, and it is not unusual for 3 or more years to pass before a diagnosis is made.

CT scanning and MR imaging are equally sensitive in the detection of pineal region masses (Fig. 25-24). On CT scans, most tumors are relatively irregular and of mixed density. Calcium deposits may also be present in teratomas. The tumors usually show a variable enhancement pattern, most commonly homogeneous for pure germinomas. Mixed germ cell tumors tend to be slightly more irregular and less homogeneous in their contrast enhancement than germinomas. However, the CT or MR appearance of these lesions is not diagnostic, and imaging parameters cannot be used to separate one type of germ cell tumor from another or from other pineal or suprasellar tumor types.

Alpha-fetoprotein (AFP) and human chorionic gonadotropin (hCG) are secreted by mixed germ cell tumors but not by any other pineal region mass. AFP is elevated in the endodermal sinus tumors of some immature teratomas, whereas hCG is elevated in choriocarcinoma and embryonal carcinomas. Those tumors with mixed elements may have elevated levels of both AFP and hCG. There may be mild elevation of chorionic gonadotropin in patients with pure germinomas. These markers are detectable in CSF and in some cases in the serum. Tumors that secrete markers do not necessarily require histologic confirmation for diagnosis. However, in the absence of positive cerebrospinal fluid levels of hCG or AFP, surgical confirmation is necessary to distinguish between the different types of germ cell tumors.

Given the pineal region location of most germ cell tumors, few are amenable to extensive surgical resection. However, open surgical resections and possibly stereotactic resections can be performed with acceptable morbidity. After surgery, symptoms resulting from contusions of the occipital lobe are not infrequent and may include visual migraines and seizures, which are generally transient. Occasionally teratomas may be well encapsulated and amenable to complete tumor resection.

Germ cell tumors have the propensity to disseminate the neuraxis. The exact incidence of such dissemination is unclear but may be detected at diagnosis in up to 10% of patients.

Radiotherapy remains the primary treatment modality for germinomas, although these tumors are very sensitive to chemotherapy. Radiotherapy treatment strategies vary, and there is no established volume of brain and/or spinal cord that should be treated in those with nondisseminated germinoma. In the case of localized disease, with the use of craniospinal radiation therapy in doses of 3500 to 4500 cGy with an additional 1000 to 1500 cGy to the area of the tumor, up to 90% of patients will be free of progressive disease for 5 years following treatment, and the majority of these will be cured. However, it is not clear if patients with nondisseminated disease need treatment with the spinal or whole-brain component of the craniospinal radiotherapy, and some advocate treating the tumor with standard doses, with a smaller dose to the ventricular regions. Others advocate using chemotherapy prior to radiotherapy and treating with reduced volumes of radiotherapy. Similar treatment has been used for patients with germinomas that have disseminated at the time of diagnosis in an attempt to improve survival. However, as pure germinoma is exquisitely sensitive to radiation, the need for chemotherapy in these cases is unproven.

Malignant teratomas and mixed germ cell tumors are very aggressive, and survival is not as common as with the pure germinoma. After treatment with radiation therapy alone, probably less than 20 tp 30% of patients with mixed germ cell tumors will have a long-term remission. A variety of different chemotherapeutic agents have been tried both before and after radiation therapy for patients with mixed germ cell tumors. Evidence suggests cisplatin-containing regimens including other drugs that have been effective

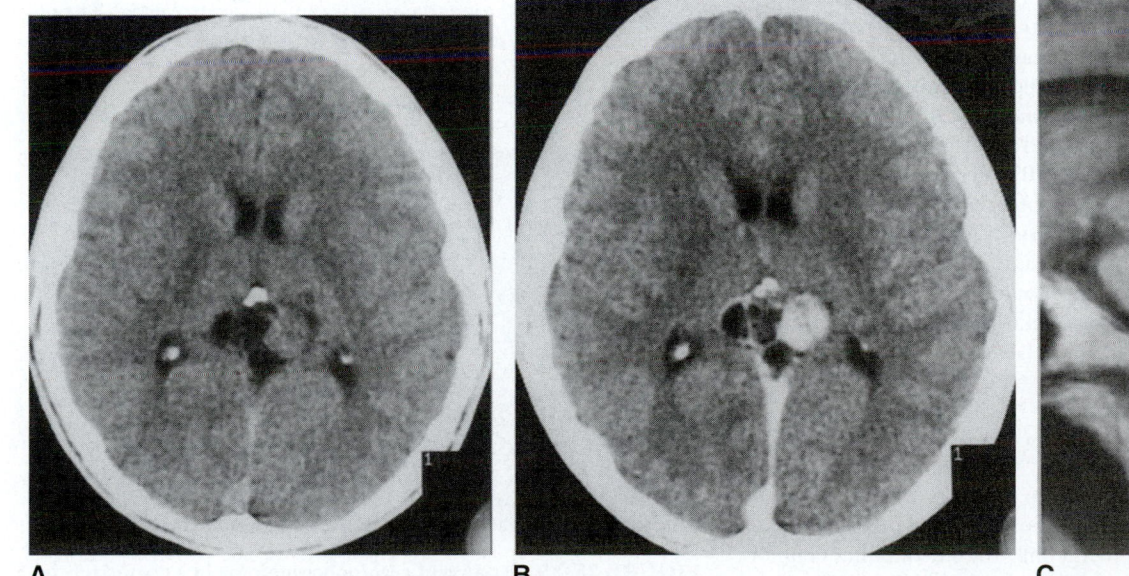
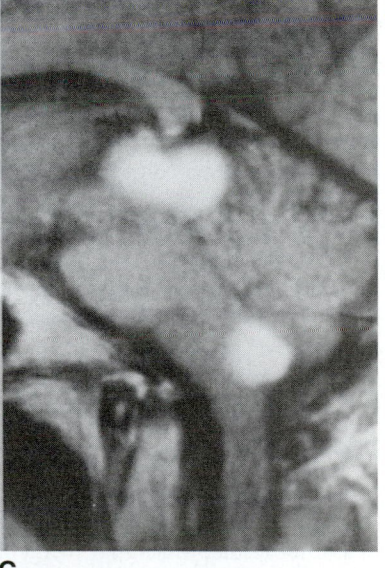

A   B   C

FIGURE 25-24   Pineal region tumors. Axial CT scans pre- (A) and post- (B) contrast show an enhancing pineal region tumor of heterogeneous density, including calcification and fat, typical of a teratoma. *Courtesy of Dr. Jacqueline A. Bello.* **(C) Sagittal T₁ gadolinium-enhanced MR image demonstrating an enhancing pineal region glioma with evidence of an intracranial metastasis inferior to the fourth ventricle.**

for similar tumors in the testes (such as bleomycin, vinblastine, and etoposide) may improve survival.

PINEAL REGION TUMORS

A variety of different tumor types may arise in the pineal region in childhood. No one histology makes up more than 30% of these lesions. Tumors that arise in this area include germinomas, mixed germ cell tumors, primitive neuroectodermal tumors (pineoblastoma), gliomas, and pineocytomas. The clinical symptoms caused by all these tumors overlap. In addition, CT and MR imaging are not specific. Surgical confirmation of the histologic type of tumor present in the pineal is mandatory in all cases except for tumors that can be diagnosed by elevation in serum or CSF levels of AFP and hCG. Surgical resection can usually be achieved with acceptable morbidity.

Germ cell tumors and pineal parenchymal tumors other than pineocytoma are described elsewhere in this chapter. The pineocytoma presents with tegmental dysfunction and signs of hydrocephalus owing to obstruction of the third ventricle. Pineocytomas tend to be calcified and show a variable pattern of density (usually iso- or hyperintense on CT) and enhance after contrast administration.

Pineocytomas are histologically low-grade tumors that can reoccur or disseminate, and therefore staging is necessary; if nondisseminated, the tumors should be treated with involved-field radiotherapy. If disseminated disease is present at diagnosis, craniospinal radiotherapy is suggested. Older patients tend to fare well after local radiation therapy alone. However, the disease may be more aggressive in some younger patients with variable response to local or craniospinal radiotherapy. Chemotherapy has not yet been shown to be of benefit for patients with pineocytoma.

CRANIOPHARYNGIOMA

Craniopharyngiomas are histologically benign tumors derived from squamous epithelial cells and arise in the suprasellar region. These tumors are presumed to be formed from nests of embryonic tissue located in Rathke pouch, an embryonic structure that later forms the anterior pituitary gland. These tumors are thought to be congenital but may present with signs and symptoms at any age. The craniopharyngioma constitutes 6 to 10% of all intracranial tumors in children. Although craniopharyngiomas usually occur in the suprasellar region, they may extend superiorly into the third ventricle, or inferiorly along the base of the brain. Although these are histologically benign neoplasms, the potential aggressive behavior along with its proximity to the optic chiasm, carotid arteries, third cranial nerve, and pituitary stalk make this a difficult tumor to treat without morbidity.

Pathology

Craniopharyngiomas are comprised of variable amounts of cystic and solid components. The external surface of the tumor consists of a firm capsule, which may merge into the surrounding brain or affix to surrounding structures such as the carotid artery. The cyst fluid is composed of a dark green or brown oily substance that contains cholesterol crystals and degenerated epithelial cells. Microscopically, this tumor contains sheets of squamous and columnar epithelium, with areas of microcyst formation, calcification, and necrotic tumor cells.

Clinical Presentation

The clinical presentation is variable and age-dependent. As with most intracranial tumors, children with craniopharyngiomas often present with headaches (58 to 81%) and vomiting (45%). Because of the proximity to the optic nerves and chiasm, 54 to 61% of patients present with complaints of decreased visual acuity or visual fields. Involvement of the hypothalamic-pituitary axis is common, and endocrinologic symptoms may include short stature or growth delay (38 to 45%) or polydipsia (6 to 9%). Changes in mental status are often reported as presenting symptoms, usually because of some degree of hydrocephalus or mass effects surrounding structures, and occurs in 20 to 48% of children with this tumor. Unlike many other primary brain tumors of childhood, there seems to be a longer duration of symptoms before diagnosis is made, with 50% having symptoms for more than 4 months prior to diagnosis. Presenting signs usually parallel the symptoms. Overt gross motor or sensory deficits are uncommon, except those associated with failing vision. Often when the presenting symptoms do not include a visual complaint, formal visual examination uncovers optic atrophy, abnormal visual acuity, or an undetected visual field defect. In one study, 98% of children had an abnormal visual examination, including papilledema (27%), bitemporal hemianopia (52%), homonymous hemianopia (8%), unilateral hemianopia (8%), significant unilateral visual acuity deficit (35%), and bilateral visual acuity deficit (23%).

Diagnosis

Most craniopharyngiomas are easily identified on CT or MR imaging (Fig. 25-25). These tumors may be partially calcified, which is identified by CT. MR imaging better demonstrates the tumor in multiple planes and gives the surgeon a better view of the relationship of the tumor to the arteries of the circle of Willis, pituitary stalk, and the optic and oculomotor nerves.

Management

Management of craniopharyngiomas remains controversial. The ultimate goal is to prevent recurrence of the tumor with the least impairment of endocrine and intellectual function. One approach is to attempt a gross total resection of the tumor, thus avoiding the

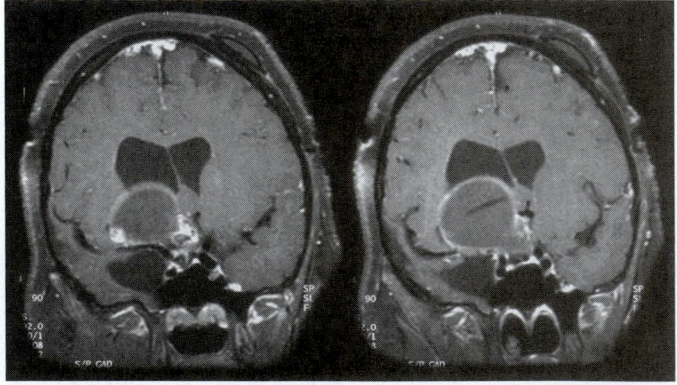

FIGURE 25-25 Recurrent craniopharyngioma in a cognitively intact 13-year-old boy. This child presented at age 3 with blindness and has been treated with surgery, P-32 instillation into the recurrent cystic nodule at the time of first reoccurrence, and α-interferon at the second reoccurrence. Note the enhancing midline mass and nodular enhancement of parts of the cyst wall. An Ommaya reservoir transverses the cyst and is used monthly to drain the tumor cyst fluid.

need for immediate postoperative radiotherapy. Another approach is to drain the tumor cyst and debulk any easily assessable tumor and treat with radiotherapy, thus avoiding the operative complications. It is not clear which approach is more successful in most patients.

Complete surgical resection will obviate the need for irradiation, but such aggressive surgery usually results in permanent panhypopituitarism, and sometimes pernicious obesity, behavioral disturbances, and intellectual difficulties. Radiotherapy usually spares remaining endocrine dysfunction but can cause intellectual problems, especially in the younger child, although newer treatment strategies may obviate some of these problems.

Assessment of a patient's endocrine function prior to surgery usually is not required, but all patients should receive a stress dose steroid preparation before, during, and after surgery. Patients with symptomatic diabetes insipidus may be managed preoperatively with intranasal DDAVP (desmopressin), but fluid management during and immediately after surgery requires frequent assessment of electrolytes and meticulous attention to intravenous fluid volume and content, urine output, and estimation of insensible fluid losses. Because the pituitary stalk may be damaged at surgery, indeterminate amounts of natural antidiuretic hormone will be released as the stalk becomes necrotic, causing episodes of oliguria following surgery. Frequent changes in fluid intake often will be necessary in the first week after surgery. The use of antidiuretic therapy for the first few days after surgery should be reserved to short-acting preparations such as pitressin. DDAVP has a duration of action usually greater than 12 hours and should not be used until after a consistent urinary pattern has been established, usually 3 to 5 days after surgery.

Aspiration of the tumor cyst has a low surgical morbidity and allows for decompression of the optic nerve and chiasm. The remaining endocrine dysfunction is often preserved with cyst aspiration because the pituitary stalk is not damaged. Aspiration of the cyst is not sufficient treatment, and the patient will require postoperative irradiation to effectively treat the tumor.

Some prefer management with an initial subtotal resection, especially in tumors that are adherent to surrounding structures. As with aspiration, this procedure has a low morbidity and may spare hypothalamic-pituitary function if the stalk is not further damaged by surgery. However, recurrence of tumor is probable, and irradiation is usually required, although it may be postponed until definite regrowth occurs. Radiotherapy, when given, is usually delivered to the local field at a total dose of about 5000 cGy, given at a daily dosage of no greater than 200 cGy per day.

Attempting a complete resection has the advantage that if it is successful, postoperative irradiation can be avoided. This approach has a greater chance of morbidity, including further damage to the optic apparatus and hemorrhage; because the pituitary stalk is destroyed, permanent endocrine dysfunction almost certainly will follow. Survival data are similar regardless of which approach is used. In larger studies where actuarial survival rates were presented, 5-year survival rates range from 66 to 93%, and 10-year survival rates from 44 to 80%.

A number of studies have investigated the quality-of-life issues in terms of the long-term morbidity and mortality of various treatment schemes. A recent study of 37 children treated for craniopharyngioma suggests that outcome is improved following treatment with less aggressive surgery and radiotherapy than with attempts at total excision. Diabetes insipidus was far more common in patients treated with radical surgery, occurring in seven (87.5%)

with radical resection and radiation, four (66%) with partial resection and radiation, and one (5%) with no resection but with radiation.

CHOROID PLEXUS TUMORS

Choroid plexus tumors are rare, representing only 1 to 3% of all tumors in children. The choroid plexus papilloma is a histologically benign tumor and accounts for two-thirds of these neoplasms, with the choroid plexus carcinoma accounting for the remainder. These tumors may appear in the first few days after birth, and 75 to 80% will appear before the second birthday. There is no difference in the age of presentation between patients with papillomas or carcinomas.

The most common mode of presentation is with signs and symptoms of hydrocephalus, either because of excessive cerebrospinal fluid production or because the tumor obstructs CSF pathways. Symptoms may include vomiting, irritability, headache, and seizures. More than one-half of patients have craniomegaly. These tumors usually are located in either lateral ventricle (75%) but also occur in the third ventricle (10%) or fourth ventricle and cerebellopontine angle (15%). CT scan will show an iso- or hyperintense mass that enhances after contrast infusion. MR imaging clearly demonstrates the anatomic characteristics; however, pathologic examination is necessary to confirm the histologic diagnosis.

Choroid Plexus Papilloma

These tumors are composed of rows of well-differentiated columnar cells, similar to normal choroid plexus. The electron microscopic appearance of these cells resembles the embryonic choroid plexus. Choroid plexus papillomas often produce CSF, with the daily output measuring up to 2000 mL. The size of the tumor at presentation averages 4 cm. Although surgical resection of the tumor will stop the excessive production of CSF, about one-third to one-half will require placement of a shunt. Because of the typical large size of these tumors, and the subsequent hydrocephalus, postoperative subdural effusions are common, although these usually do not require draining. These tumors do not reoccur after a complete resection. There are reports of successful use of radiotherapy in patients with invasive tumors or tumors that could not be completely removed. The prognosis for patients with papillomas is excellent if there is a total resection.

Choroid Plexus Carcinoma

These tumors are often invasive and demonstrate microscopic malignant features such as pleomorphic nuclei, abundant mitoses, necrosis, vascular proliferation, and loss of the well-differentiated architecture. These tumors are more frequently located in the lateral ventricles but may invade brain. They tend to be larger at presentation than the papillomas. Surgery is the primary treatment, and an attempt at a total resection is appropriate. However, local brain invasion is common, and tumor dissemination along CSF pathways occurs in 44%.

There is no clear management strategy for patients with this tumor. There are long-term surviving patients treated with complete surgical resection, suggesting this may be curative in some patients. Because this tumor tends to seed throughout CSF pathways, patients need to be evaluated for leptomeningeal disease after surgery; further treatment should be planned accordingly. However, patients with evidence of residual disease will likely have local or disseminated recurrence of their tumor, with the time from onset of symptoms to death averaging 9 months, and a 5-year survival rate (including patients treated with radiotherapy and chemotherapy) of 50%.

Some patients with residual postoperative tumor treated with craniospinal radiotherapy have shown regression of disease or long-term survival. Because no comparative studies have been performed, the routine use of radiotherapy cannot be recommended. A number of patients have had radiographic and clinical response to a number of chemotherapeutic agents, including combinations of bleomycin, vinblastine, and cisplatin or of carboplatin, ifosfamide, and etoposide.

MENINGIOMA

Meningiomas are relatively rare in childhood, except in their association with NF2, in which case they can be identified in presymptomatic carriers as early as 1 year of age, even before the vestibular schwannomas are identified. As in adults, meningiomas occur most frequently on the meningeal surface, but some true intraparenchymal lesions occur in pediatric patients, presumably arising from meningeal cell rest that persists because of aberrant, cerebral migration. Clinical presentation varies greatly dependent on location of the tumor. CT and MR imaging are both sensitive in the depiction of the tumors. Meningiomas are also seen in long-term survivors of brain tumors who were treated with radiotherapy and can present 20 or more years after treatment. For this reason, any person having received radiotherapy, even those presumed cured of their primary disease, should undergo neuroimaging at least every 5 years for surveillance of this treatable complication.

The primary modality of therapy is surgery. Pediatric meningiomas often show more histologic anaplasia than adult tumors. However, despite the worrisome pathologic features, most lesions are clinically benign. The utility of radiation therapy in treating pediatric meningiomas is unclear. For patients with progressive disease, especially after multiple attempts at surgical resection, local radiotherapy may be of benefit.

Occasionally, meningeal tumors involve primarily the leptomeninges. These true leptomeningeal tumors, which have been categorized by various different names including meningeal sarcoma, tend to be highly aggressive. The most appropriate treatment for such lesions is unclear. However, craniospinal radiation therapy supplemented with some type of chemotherapy is probably indicated.

ADVERSE EFFECTS OF TREATMENT

It has long been recognized that the treatment of primary CNS tumors in children may be associated with adverse neurologic effects. Often it is difficult to determine whether a neurologic abnormality is caused by the primary disease or a side effect of radiation therapy or chemotherapy. The goal of modern therapy is to maximize tumor cell death while sparing surrounding tissue as much as possible.

Neurologic Toxicity of Radiation Therapy

Neurologic reactions during radiation treatments are rarely seen in children receiving conventional daily dose fractions (180 to 200 cGy per day). However, when reactions do occur during the initial phase of radiation treatments, they tend to be caused by transient radiation-induced tumor edema, and the patient will develop a worsening of the underlying neurologic deficit or signs of increased intracranial pressure. This reaction generally will occur only in the setting of a large unresected or partially resected tumor. The tumor may appear on imaging study to increase in size, and care must be taken not to interpret the result as rapid tumor growth. This effect of radiation is self-limited, and most patients may be managed by adding or increasing the steroid dose or by interrupting radiation treatments for a day or two. In patients receiving larger dose fractions, as in the setting of metastatic disease (which is very rare in children), the effects are more common and severe.

The *somnolence syndrome* is a self-limited condition that may develop 6 to 8 weeks following cranial irradiation. Somnolence, irritability, anorexia, and headaches may occur and last about 1 week. This syndrome is common in children who received 2400-cGy whole-brain irradiation for leukemia prophylaxis, as well as in patients receiving 5000-cGy whole-brain treatment of brain tumors.

Radiation necrosis is the most catastrophic sequela of therapeutic irradiation. The risk of occurrence depends on the total biologic dose of radiation and manifests in 0.1 to 5.0% of patients treated with 5000 to 6000 cGy in 150- to 200-cGy fractions. Eighty percent of patients develop symptoms of radiation necrosis within 3 years of treatment, although the range may be from as early as 3 months to as late as 19 years. The pathologic lesion is a necrotic mass involving the white matter in the field of the radiation beam. Signs and symptoms are like that of any intracranial mass, and the radiographic features may be similar to any neoplasm. Treatment of radiation necrosis depends upon the location of the mass and accessibility to surgical debulking. If possible, an attempt at surgical removal of the necrotic mass should be attempted as removal can alleviate symptoms and possibly remedy the problem. In patients who cannot undergo a surgical procedure, steroids can reduce the mass effect and result in symptomatic improvement. However, some patients who respond to steroids may be difficult to taper from the medication. Radiation necrosis can result in permanent neurologic dysfunction, even if there is a response to therapy.

Large-vessel thrombosis is a rare complication following radiation therapy. Patients may present with the usual stroke symptoms anywhere from 2 to 30 years following irradiation to the head or neck. This syndrome has been reported in children and adults. The pathologic abnormality consists of an atherosclerotic plaque involving the large arteries. Treatment is symptomatic, although carotid endarterectomy has been used as treatment.

Endocrine dysfunction may be seen following irradiation involving the hypothalamus and pituitary. Growth hormone release and subsequent linear growth may be affected by doses in the range of 2600 to 5800 cGy. Children receiving at least 5500 cGy also developed TSH (thyroid-stimulating hormone) and ACTH (adrenocorticotropic hormone) abnormalities. Children treated with spinal irradiation also may have primary thyroid failure caused by direct radiation injury to the thyroid gland. Following irradiation, all patients should have their linear growth monitored, and thyroid function studies (TSH and T_4) should be obtained every 6 months for 3 years. Gonadotropin dysfunction is not common, but appropriate studies should be obtained if the patient does not enter puberty at the expected age. Fertility difficulties may occur in either gender. The testes are more susceptible than the ovaries to the effects of chemotherapy, but the ovaries can be injured by the scattered irradiation that may occur with any spinal radiotherapy treatments.

Cognitive difficulties may occur following irradiation for brain

TABLE 25-12

NEUROTOXICITY OF CHEMOTHERAPY

DRUG	ACUTE/SUBACUTE	CHRONIC
Methotrexate (high-dose IV)	Seizures, somnolence, stroke-like syndrome	Necrotizing leukoencephalopathy
Methotrexate (IT)	Arachnoiditis, cerebral necrosis	Necrotizing leukoencephalopathy
Cytosine arabinoside (high-dose IV)	Cerebellar ataxia, encephalopathy	Cerebellar ataxia, demyelinating polyneuropathy
Cytosine arabinoside (IT)	Seizures, cerebral necrosis	Leukoencephalopathy, demyelinating polyneuropathy
Fluorouracil (low-dose IV)	Cerebellar syndrome	Encephalopathy (reversible)
Fluorouracil (high-dose IV)	Cerebellar syndrome	Encephalopathy
Cyclophosphamide (IV)	Visual blurring, sense of intoxication	
Ifosfamide	Encephalopathy, seizures, ataxia	Encephalopathy
Carmustine (BCNU) (IA)	Focal cortical necrosis, encephalopathy, blindness, seizures	Focal cortical necrosis, encephalopathy, blindness
Carmustine (BCNU) (high-dose IV)		Cortical necrosis, blindness
Cisplatin (IA)	Encephalopathy, blindness	Cortical necrosis, blindness
Cisplatin (IV)	Increased ICP, seizures, retrobulbar neuritis, peripheral neuropathy	Ototoxicity, peripheral neuropathy
Vincristine (IV)	Cramps, paresthesias, cranial and peripheral neuropathy	Autonomic and peripheral neuropathy
Asparaginase (IM)	Encephalopathy, sagittal sinus thrombosis, hemorrhage	Sequelae of cerebrovascular accident
Dactinomycin (IV)	Cortical necrosis, myelitis (after XRT)	Cortical necrosis, myelitis (after XRT)
Procarbazine (PO)	Encephalopathy, neuropathy, ataxia	Autonomic neuropathy
Etoposide (IV)	Peripheral neuropathy	
Taxol	Peripheral neuropathy (sensory>motor)	Residual neuropathy
Interferons	Encephalopathy, hallucinations	
Thalidomide (PO)	Somnolence	
Sodium phenylacetate	Ataxia, somnolence, encephalopathy	

IA, intra-arterial; IM, intramuscular; IT, intrathecal; IV, intravenous.

tumors. It is very difficult to determine the degree of cognitive damage caused specifically by the irradiation and that caused by other factors, such as acute or chronic increased intracranial pressure, local cortical damage caused by the tumor, and the effects of surgery, infection, or chemotherapy. Higher doses cause greater loss of function than lower doses, and younger children are more susceptible to the neurocognitive damage from irradiation. The effect may not reach a maximum until 2 to 3 years after treatment. Nonverbal abilities seem to be affected more than verbal function, and attention deficits and short-term memory are often affected. In one study of intellectual outcome, children with posterior fossa PNETs treated with surgery and radiotherapy (with or without chemotherapy) were compared to a group of children with cerebellar juvenile pilocytic astrocytomas treated with surgery alone. The children with cerebellar juvenile pilocytic astrocytomas showed no decline in intellectual functioning, but the children treated with radiotherapy showed neurocognitive effects up to 4 years after treatment. The intellectual function declined over time, with the maximum effect noted at 3 years. Children under age 7 lost an average of 27 points on I.Q. testing, resulting in all needing educational assistance. Those children older than 7 years fared better, but one-half still required special educational assistance.

Both radiotherapy and chemotherapy are oncogenic, and survivors of childhood cancer are ten times more likely than their peers to develop another malignancy. Following cranial irradiation, there is an increased risk (approximately 3 to 5%) of developing a second brain tumor. The most frequent types are meningiomas, astrocytomas, and sarcomas, typically occurring 10 to 20 years following initial treatment. Other malignant tumors associated with treatment include leukemia and thyroid cancer. Regardless, the benefit of treating the brain tumor outweighs the risk of developing a treatment-induced cancer.

Neurologic Toxicity of Chemotherapy

The growing use of multiagent chemotherapy in the treatment of childhood brain tumors requires awareness of the acute and late neurotoxicities potentially associated with commonly employed agents. A summary of the important acute and chronic toxicities of chemotherapy is provided in Table 25-12.

References

Albright AL, Guthkelch A, Packer RJ, et al: Diagnosis and management of pediatric brainstem gliomas. J Neurosurg 65:745–750, 1986

Albright AL, Packer RJ, Zimmerman R, Rorke LB, Boyett J, Hammond GD: Magnetic resonance scans should replace biopsies for the diagnosis of diffuse brain stem gliomas: a report from the Childrens Cancer Group. Neurosurgery 33:1026–1029, 1993

Allen JC, Kim JH, Packer RJ: Neo-adjuvant chemotherapy for newly diagnosed primary CNS germ cell tumors. J Neurosurg 67:65–70, 1987

Allen JC, Wisoff J, Helson L, et al: Choroid plexus carcinoma: responses to chemotherapy alone in newly diagnosed young children. J Neurooncol 12:69–74, 1992

Ater JL, Woo SY, Van Eyes J: Update of MOPP chemotherapy as primary therapy for infant brain tumors. Pediatr Neurosci 14:153–154, 1988

Barnett GH: Stereotactic techniques in the management of brain tumors. Contemporary Neurosurgery 19(10):1–9, 1997

Bergsagel DJ, Finegold MJ, Butel JS, Kupsky WJ, Garcea RL: DNA sequences similar to those of simian virus 40 in ependymomas and choroid plexus tumors of childhood. N Engl J Med 326:988–993, 1992

Biegel JA: Cytogenetics and molecular genetics of childhood brain tumors. Neurooncology 1:139–151, 1999

Buatti JM, Meeks SL, Marcus RB, Mendenhall NP: Radiotherapy for pediatric brain tumors. Semin Pediatr Neurol 4:304–319, 1997

Bunin GR, Kuijten RR, Buckley JD, Rorke LB, Meadows AT: Relation between maternal diet and subsequent primitive neuroectodermal brain tumors in young children. N Engl J Med 329:536–541, 1993

Carol MP: Peacock: a system for planning and rotational delivery of intensity-modulated fields. Special issue on optimization of the three-dimensional dose delivery and tomotherapy. Int J Imag Syst Technol 6:56–61, 1995

Cohen AR, Wisoff JH, Allen JC, Epstein F: Malignant astrocytomas of the spinal cord. J Neurosurg 70:50–54, 1989

Cohen BH, Bury E, Packer RJ, Sutton LN, Bilaniuk LT, Zimmerman RA: Gadolinium-DPTA enhanced magnetic resonance imaging in childhood brain tumors. Neurology 39:1178–1182, 1989

Cohen BH, Packer RJ: Chemotherapy for medulloblastomas and primitive neuroectodermal tumors. J Neurooncol 29:55–68, 1996

Cohen BH, Rothner AD: Incidence, types and management of cancer in patients with neurofibromatosis. Oncology 3:23–30, 1989

Cohen BH, Zeltzer PM, Boyett JM, et al: Prognostic factors and treatment results for supratentorial primitive neuroectodermal tumors in children using radiation and chemotherapy: A Childrens Cancer Group randomized trial. J Clin Oncol 13:1687–1696, 1995

Cohen M, Duffner P, Heffner R, et al: Prognostic factors in brainstem gliomas. Neurology 36:602–604, 1986

Cogen PM, Daneshvar L, Metzger AK, Edwards MSB: Deletion mapping of the medulloblastoma, focus on chromosome 17p. Genomics 8:279–286, 1990

D'Andrea AD, Packer RJ, Rorke LB, et al: Pineocytomas of childhood: a reappraisal of natural history and response to therapy. Cancer 59:1353–1357, 1987

Daumas-Duport C, Scheithauer B, O'Fallon J, Kelly P: Grading of astrocytomas. A simple and reproducible method. Cancer 62:2152–2165, 1988

Douglass EC, Kun LE, Fairclough DL, et al: Cellular DNA content is predictive of early relapse in medulloblastoma. Pediatr Neurosci 15:141, 1989

Duffner PK, Cohen ME, Myers MH, et al: Survival of children with brain tumors: SEER program 1973–1980. Neurology 36:597–601, 1986

Duffner PK, Cohen ME, Thomas P: Late effects of treatment on the intelligence of children with posterior fossa tumors. Cancer 51:233–237, 1983

Duffner PK, Horowitz ME, Krischer JP, et al: The treatment of malignant brain tumors and very young children: an update of the Pediatric Oncology Group experience. Neuro-oncology 1:152–161, 1999

Duffner PK, Krischer JP, Horowitz ME, et al: Second malignancies in young children with primary brain tumors following treatment with prolonged postoperative chemotherapy and delayed irradiation: A Pediatric Oncology Group study. Ann Neurol 44:313–316, 1998

Dunkel IJ, Boyett JM, Yates A, et al: High-dose carboplatin, thiotepa, and etoposide with autologous stem-cell rescue for patients with recurrent medulloblastoma. J Clin Oncol 16:222–228, 1998

Edwards MSB, Hudgins RJ, Wilson CB, Levin VA, Wara WM: Pineal region tumors in children. J Neurosurg 68:689–697, 1988

Edwards MSB, Wara WM, Urtasan RC, et al: Hyperfractionated radiation therapy for brainstem gliomas: a phase I-II trial. J Neurosurg 70:691–700, 1989

Ellenbogen RG, Winston KR, Kupsky WJ: Tumors of the choroid plexus in children. Neurosurgery 25:327–335, 1989

Evans AE, Jenkin RDT, Sposto R, et al: The treatment of medulloblastoma. Results of a prospective randomized trial of radiation therapy with and without CCNU, vincristine, and prednisone. J Neurosurg 72:572–582, 1990

Finlay JL, August C, Packer R: High-dose multi-agent chemotherapy followed by bone marrow "rescue" for malignant astrocytomas of childhood and adolescence. J Neurooncol 9:239–248, 1990

Finlay JL, Boyett JM, Yates AT, et al: Randomized phase III trial in childhood with high-grade astrocytoma comparing vincristine, lomustine, and prednisone with the eight-drugs-in-1-day regimen. J Clin Oncol 13:112–123, 1995

Fischer EG, Welch K, Shillito J, et al: Craniopharyngiomas in children. Long-term effects of conservative surgical procedures combined with radiation therapy. J Neurosurg 73:534–540, 1990

Fisher PG: Rethinking brain tumors in babies and more. Ann Neurol 44:300–302, 1998

Geyer JR, Zeltzer PM, Boyett JM, et al: Survival of infants with primitive neuroectodermal tumors or malignant ependymomas of the CNS treated with eight drugs in 1 day: A report from the Childrens Cancer Group. J Clin Oncol 12:1607–1615, 1994

Gjerris F, Klinken L: Long-term prognosis in children with benign cerebellar astrocytoma. J Neurosurg 49:179–184, 1978

Goldwein JW, Leahy JM, Packer RJ, et al: Intracranial ependymomas in children. Int J Radiat Oncol Biol Phys 19:1497–1502, 1990

Hardison HH, Packer RJ, Rorke LB, et al: Outcome of children with primary intramedullary spinal cord tumors. Childs Nerv Syst 3:89–92, 1987

Heideman RL, Packer RJ, Albright LA: Tumors of the central nervous system. In: Pizzo PA, Poplack DG, eds: Principles and Practice of Pediatric Oncology. Philadelphia, Lippincott, 1989:505–553

Hoffman HJ, DeSilva M, Humphreys RP, Drake JM, Smith ML, Blaser SI: Aggressive surgical management of craniopharyngiomas in children. J Neurosurg 76:47–52, 1992

James CD, Carlbom E, Dumanski JP, et al: Clonal genomic alterations in glioma malignancy stages. Cancer Res 48:5546–5551, 1988

Johnson DB, Thompson JM, Corwin JA, et al: Prolongation of survival for high-grade malignant gliomas with adjuvant high-dose BCNU and autologous bone marrow transplantation. J Clin Oncol 5:783–789, 1987

Kretschmar CS, Tarbell NJ, Barnes PD, Krischer JP, Burger PC, Kun L: Pre-irradiation chemotherapy and hyperfractionated radiation therapy (66 Gy) for children with brain stem tumors. A phase II study of the Pediatric Oncology Group, protocol 8833. Cancer 72:1404–1413, 1993

Lefkowitz IB, Packer RJ, Sutton LN, et al: Results of the treatment of children with recurrent gliomas with lomustine and vincristine. Cancer 61:896–902, 1988

Linstadt DE, Wara WM, Leibel SA, et al: Postoperative radiotherapy of primary spinal cord tumors. Int J Radiat Oncol Biol Phys 16:1397–1403, 1989

Lowis SP, Pizer BL, Coakharn H, Nelson RJ, Bouffet E: Chemotherapy spinal cord astrocytoma: can natural history be modified? Childs Nerv Syst 14:317–321, 1998

Lundsford LD, Flickinger J, Coffey RJ: Streotactic Gamma Knife radiosurgery: initial North American experience in 207 patients. Arch Neurol 47:169–175, 1990

Marchese MJ, Chang CH: Malignant astrocytic gliomas in children. Cancer 65:2771–2778, 1990

Martuza RL, Eldridge R: Neurofibromatosis 2 (bilateral acoustic neurofibromatosis). N Engl J Med 318:684–688, 1988

Mason WP, Grovas A, Halpern S, et al: Intensive chemotherapy and bone marrow rescue for young children with newly diagnosed malignant brain tumors. J Clin Oncol 16:210–221, 1998.

Molenaar WM, Jansson D, Gould VE, et al: Immunohistology in the diagnosis of pediatric brain tumors. Pediatr Neurosci 14:11, 1988

National Institutes of Health Consensus Development Conference: Neurofibromatosis conference report. Arch Neurol 45:575–578, 1988

North CA, North RB, Epstein JA: Low-grade cerebral astrocytomas. Survival and quality of life after radiation therapy. Cancer 66:6–14, 1990

Packer RJ, Bilaniuk LT, Cohen BH, et al: Intracranial visual pathway gliomas in children with neurofibromatosis. Neurofibromatosis 1:212–222, 1988

Packer RJ, Boyett JM, Zimmerman RA, et al: Hyperfractionated radiation therapy (72 Gy) for children with brain stem gliomas: a Childrens Cancer Group phase I/II trial. Cancer 72:1414–1421, 1993

Packer RJ, Bruce DA, Atkins TA, et al: Factors impacting on neurocognitive outcome in long-term survivors of primitive neuroectodermal tumors/medulloblastoma (PNET-MB). Ann Neurol 20:396–397, 1986

Packer RJ, Meadows AT, Rorke LB, et al: Long-term sequelae of cancer treatment on the central nervous system in childhood. Med Pediatr Oncol 15:241–253, 1987

Packer RJ, Sutton LN, Atkins TA, et al: A prospective study of cognitive deficits in children receiving whole brain radiotherapy: 2-year results. J Neurosurg 70:707–713, 1989

Packer RJ, Sutton LN, Bilaniuk LT, et al: Treatment of chiasmatic/hypothalamic gliomas of childhood with chemotherapy: an update. Ann Neurol 23:79–85, 1988

Packer RJ, Sutton LN, D'Angio G, et al: Management of children with primitive neuroectodermal tumors of the posterior fossa/medulloblastoma. Pediatr Neurosci 12:272–282, 1986

Packer RJ, Sutton LN, Elterman R, et al: Outcome for children with medulloblastoma treated with radiation and cisplatin, CCNU and vincristine chemotherapy. J Neurosurg 81:690–698, 1994

Packer RJ, Zimmerman R, Luerssen T, et al: Brainstem gliomas of childhood: magnetic resonance imaging. Neurology 35:397–401, 1985

Plautz GE, Barnett GH, Miller DW, et al. Systemic T cell adoptive immunotherapy of malignant gliomas. J Neurosurg 89:42–51, 1998

Pratt CB, Green AA, Horowitz ME, et al: Central nervous system toxicity following the treatment of pediatric patients with ifosfamide/mesna. J Clin Oncol 4:1253–1261, 1986

Reimer R, Onofrio BM: Astrocytomas of the spinal cord in children and adolescents. J Neurosurg 63:669–675, 1985

Rhoten RLP, Luciano MG, Barnett GH: Computer-assisted endoscopy for neurosurgical procedures: technical note. Neurosurgery 40:632–638, 1997

Smith MA, Freidlin B, Ries LA, Simon R: Trends in reported incidence of primary malignant brain tumors in children in the United States. J Natl Cancer Inst 90:1269–1277, 1998

Sorensen SA, Mulvihill JJ, Nielsen A: Long-term follow-up of von Recklinghausen neurofibromatosis. Survival and malignant neoplasms. N Engl J Med 314:1010–1015, 1986

Spencer DD, Spencer SS, Matson RH, Williamson PD: Intracerebral masses in patients with intractable partial epilepsy. Neurology 34:432–436, 1984

Sposto R, Ertel IH, Jenkin RDT, et al: The effectiveness of chemotherapy for treatment of high grade astrocytoma in children: results of a randomized trial. A report from the Childrens Cancer Study Group. J Neurooncol 7:165–177, 1989

Tao ML, Barnes PD, Billett AL, et al: Childhood optic chiasm gliomas. Radiographic response following radiotherapy and long-term clinical outcome. Int J Radiat Bio Phys 39:575–587, 1997

Tomita T, McLone DG, Flannery AM: Choroid plexus papillomas of neonates, infants and children. Pediatr Neurosci 14:23–30, 1988

Van Eys J, Pack CR, Baram T: Phase I trial of procarbazine as a 5-day continuous infusion in children with central nervous system tumors. Cancer Treat Rep 71:973–974, 1987

Wallner KE, Gonzales MF, Edwards MSB, Wara WM, Sheline GE: Treatment results of juvenile pilocytic astrocytoma. J Neurosurg 69:171–176, 1988

Wara WM, Edward MSB, Levin VA, et al: A new treatment regimen for brainstem glioma: a pilot study of the Brain Tumor Research Center and Children's Cancer Study Group. Int J Radiat Oncol Biol Phys 12:143, 1986

Wara WM, Jenkins RDT, Evans A, et al: Tumors of the pineal and suprasellar region: Children's Cancer Study Group treatment results 1960–1975. Cancer 43:698–701, 1979

Weiss M, Sutton L, Marcial V, et al: The role of radiation therapy in the management of childhood craniopharyngioma. Int J Radiat Oncol Biol Phys 17:1313–1321, 1989

25.8   PEDIATRIC CEREBROVASCULAR DISEASES

Donald P. Younkin and Olafur Thorarensen

Stroke is defined as the sudden occlusion or rupture of cerebral arteries or veins resulting in focal cerebral damage and clinical neurologic deficits that persist for longer than 24 hours. Stroke can be ischemic, hemorrhagic, or both. Ischemic stroke can be either arterial or venous. Arterial strokes usually result from thromboembolic occlusion of cerebral arteries. Venous strokes result from thrombosis in cerebral veins and sinuses. Hemorrhagic stroke can occur from bleeding into an acute ischemic stroke or from rupture of intracranial arteries.

The overall incidence of pediatric stroke is 2.7 per 100,000 children per year. This is roughly the same incidence as pediatric brain tumor. The incidence of pediatric ischemic stroke is about 1.2 per 100,000 children per year. Approximately one-third of these occur in the neonatal period. Approximately 75% are arterial and 25% sinovenous thrombosis. Hemorrhagic stroke occurs as frequently as ischemic stroke. The incidence of pediatric stroke has been increasing, probably as a result of increased awareness, better neuroimaging techniques, and increased survival of patients with disorders that cause stroke.

Pediatric stroke has similarities and differences from adult stroke. Pediatric stroke is frequently related to congenital or genetic problems and rarely caused by atherosclerosis. Cardiac disorders are a common cause of both pediatric and adult stroke. In general, pediatric stroke has a different etiology, incidence, presentation, recurrence risk, and long-term outcome.

The clinical presentation of pediatric stroke is age-dependent. Strokes that occur in utero frequently present with early onset of hand dominance and other signs of hemiplegic cerebral palsy. Perinatal strokes typically present with focal neonatal seizures; focal neurologic deficits are rarely present but may evolve over weeks to months. Almost 80% of strokes in children younger than 2 years present with seizures and hemiparesis. Older children usually have an acute focal neurologic deficit with or without seizures. In all age groups, seizures can be focal or generalized; single, recurrent, or status epilepticus; responsive to acute treatment or refractory. Seizures occur in both ischemic and hemorrhagic stroke. Fever and altered consciousness are common at the onset of pediatric stroke.

The most common causes of pediatric stroke are listed in Table 25-13. Risk factors for acute stroke are present in 80% of children and include cardiac disease, coagulation disorders, dehydration, infection, vasculitis, arterial dissection, cancer, metabolic disorders, moyamoya syndrome, sickle-cell anemia, perinatal complications. Multiple risk factors are commonly present. Even children with an obvious cause for their stroke should have a detailed workup for other associated factors. Our ability to identify the cause of pediatric stroke has increased considerably over the past decade.

In children with known cardiac disorders or sickle-cell anemia, the cause of a stroke is usually obvious. History and physical exam can suggest other causes. Recent head or neck trauma predisposes to arterial dissection. Varicella within 9 months of the infarction suggests possible varicella vasculopathy. Oral contraceptives, amphetamines, and cocaine predispose to infarction. A family history of early-onset stroke or heart disease, pulmonary embolism, or deep

TABLE 25-13

MAJOR CAUSES OF ISCHEMIC STROKE IN CHILDREN

Cardiac (25–50%)
    Congenital heart disease—tetralogy of Fallot, aortic stenosis, coarctation of the aorta, VSD, ASD, PDA
    Acquired heart disease—rheumatic fever, prosthetic valve, endocarditis, cardiomyopathy, atrial myxoma, rhabdomyoma
    Cardiac surgery
Hematologic
    Prothrombotic state (35%)—abnormal activated protein C resistance (factor V Leiden); deficiencies of protein C, protein S, antithrombin III; prothrombin gene mutation; antiphospholipid antibodies; lupus anticoagulant
    Sickle-cell anemia (10%)
    Disseminated intravascular coagulation
    Leukemia, hemophilia, thrombocytopenia, polycythemia
Traumatic
    Arterial dissection (10–25%)
    Intraoral trauma
    Fat or air embolism
Vascular
    Moyamoya syndrome (25%)
    Fibromuscular dysplasia
    Migraine
Vasculitis
    Meningitis—bacterial, viral, TB, fungal, parameningeal
    Varicella
    Systemic lupus erythematosus
    Takayasu arteritis
    Kawasaki disease
    Inflammatory bowel disease
    Drug abuse—cocaine, amphetamine
Metabolic
    Mitochondrial
    Hyperhomocysteine
    Hyperlipidemia
Toxic
    Cocaine
    Methamphetamine
    Phencyclidine

The approximate percentage of children with each risk factor is listed in parentheses. The reported incidence varies between different centers, possibly reflecting differences in referral patterns, populations studied, and investigator expertise. Many children have multiple risk factors.

vein thrombosis increases the risk of an inherited prothrombotic disorder.

The differential diagnosis of acute hemiplegia includes more than stroke. At least three other disorders need to be considered in children. Transient postictal hemiparesis (Todd paralysis) lasts less than 24 hours, usually has epileptiform activity on EEG, and never has acute infarction on MR imaging. Complicated migraine is usually preceded by severe headache; focal deficits usually last hours, rarely up to a week; often there is a family history of migraine or specifically hemiplegic migraine; and MR or neuroimaging studies are normal. Alternating hemiplegia is a rare disorder of unknown etiology. It usually begins in children younger than 2 years; episodes of hemiplegia last minutes to hours, rarely longer than a day; weakness varies between sides; seizures are common but usually do not occur during episodic weakness; and most children have a progressive neurodevelopmental deterioration.

References

Ferrera PC, Curran CB, Swanson H: Etiology of pediatric ischemic stroke. Am J Emerg Med 15(7):671–679, 1997

Garcia JH, Pantoni L: Strokes in childhood. Semin Pediatr Neurol 2(3): 180–191, 1995

Giroud M, Lemesle M, Madinier G, Manceau E, Osseby GV, Dumas R: Stroke in children under 16 years of age. Clinical and etiological difference with adults. Acta Neurol Scand 96(6):401–406, 1997

Kerr LM, Anderson DM, Thompson JA: Ischemic stroke in the young: Evaluation and age comparison of patients six months to thirty nine years. J Child Neurol 8:266–270, 1993

Schoenberg BS, Mellinger JF, Schoenberg SG: Cerebrovascular disease in infants and children: A study of incidence, clinical features, and survival. Neurology 28:763–768, 1978

25.8.1 Cardiac Disorders

Complications of congenital heart disease cause more than 25% of the identifiable causes of pediatric stroke. Most of these are caused by emboli that arise in the heart or are shunted through the heart. Emboli should be suspected whenever there are multiple infarctions.

Emboli can be infectious or noninfectious. Septic emboli from bacterial endocarditis can cause stroke from infarction or rupture of mycotic aneurysms. Noninfectious emboli can be cardiogenic or systemic. Emboli formed on the left side of the heart have direct access to the cerebral circulation. Thrombus can form in the apex of poorly contracting ventricles. Marantic endocarditis occurs in children with malignancies or coagulopathies. Many emboli arise from prosthetic cardiac valves. Cardiac rhabdomyoma in children with tuberous sclerosis can be a source of emboli. Systemic venous emboli can reach the cerebral circulation if an atrial or ventricular septal defect permits intracardiac right-to-left shunting. Patent foramen ovale is a common finding on echocardiography. These are usually innocent, but on occasion emboli can pass through them and cause stroke. Systemic emboli can arise from venous clots in children with prothrombotic disorders. Air emboli can occur during cardiac surgery. Fat emboli can arise from long-bone fractures.

Up to 50% of strokes in children with congenital heart disease occur within 3 days of catheterization or surgery. The exact incidence of stroke is unknown and depends on numerous variables, including the surgical procedure performed. Recent studies report strokes in up to 8.8% of children following Fontan surgery. There is a 5% risk of stroke during valve replacement surgery when children are not anticoagulated. With anticoagulation, the risk is much lower.

Children with cyanotic heart disease and polycythemia are at risk for thrombotic stroke when decreased cardiac output lowers cerebral blood flow. This is most common in children younger than 2 years. Strokes occur in up to 4% of children with tetralogy of Fallot or transposition of the great arteries.

References

Du Plessis AJ: Mechanisms of brain injury during infant cardiac surgery. Semin Pediat Neurol 6(1):32–47, 1999

Du Plessis AJ, Chang AC, Wessel DL, et al: Cerebrovascular accidents following the Fontan operation. Pediat Neurol 12:230–236, 1995

Kirkham FJ: Recognition and prevention of neurological complications in pediatric cardiac surgery. Pediatr Cardiol 19(4):331–345, 1998

O'Brien JJ, Butterworth J, Hammon JW, Morris KJ, Phipps JM, Stump DA: Cerebral emboli during cardiac surgery in children. Anesthesiology 87(5):1063–1069, 1997

25.8.2   Prothrombotic Disorders

Ischemic stroke can be caused by either inherited or acquired co-agulation disorders. Approximately 30% of children with ischemic infarction have one or more abnormalities in prothrombotic factors, most frequently an anticardiolipin antibody. Stroke usually occurs in the setting of a systemic illness, other acute problem, or second risk factor that temporarily increases the risk of thrombosis.

The inherited coagulation disorders include activated protein C resistance (factor V Leiden); deficiencies of protein C, protein S, or antithrombin; prothrombin gene mutation; and hyperhomocysteinemia. Activated protein C resistance is a very common cause of venous thrombosis but rarely causes arterial thrombosis in older children and adults. The risk of thrombosis is increased in patients who smoke or use oral contraceptives. Activated protein C resistance is usually caused by a mutation in factor V, and this has been reported as a cause of neonatal stroke and hemiplegic cerebral palsy.

Deficiencies of protein C, protein S, or antithrombin occur much less frequently than activated protein C resistance. Over 250 gene mutations cause these disorders. Some of these reduce protein production; others alter protein function. Because of this, functional assays of protein C, protein S, or antithrombin are the most effective way to screen for these disorders. Any of these disorders can cause ischemic stroke in children. Neonates with homozygous mutations can have purpura fulminans or disseminated intravascular coagulation. Acquired deficiencies can result from vitamin K deficiency, oral anticoagulants, oral contraceptives, nephrotic syndrome, liver disease, recent thrombosis, surgery, or disseminated intravascular coagulation.

Acquired coagulation disorders are much more common. In a prospective study of 92 children with cerebral thromboembolism, 38% of the children had a prothrombotic disorder. The vast majority of these were antiphospholipid antibodies, either anticardiolipin antibody or lupus anticoagulant. Many patients had multiple abnormal prothrombotic factors, suggesting an acquired process. The abnormalities may persist for months or may fluctuate.

The antiphospholipid antibody syndrome is characterized by a positive antiphospholipid antibody and recurrent thrombotic events. The disorder is primary if there is no systemic disease and secondary if the child has systemic lupus erythematosus. Antiphospholipid antibody syndromes are rare causes of pediatric stroke. When they occur, they need to be treated with oral anticoagulants or low-molecular-weight heparin.

References

Bonduel M, Sciuccati G, Hepner M, Torres AF, Pieroni G, Frontroth JP: Prethrombotic disorders in children with arterial ischemic stroke and sinovenous thrombosis. Arch Neurol 56:967–971, 1999

De Veber G, Monagle P, Chan A, et al: Prothrombotic disorders in infants and children with cerebral thromboembolism. Arch Neurol 55(12):1539–1543, 1998

Thorarensen O, Ryan S, Hunter J, Younkin DP: Factor V Leiden mutation: an unrecognized cause of hemiplegic cerebral palsy, neonatal stroke, and placental thrombosis. Ann Neurol 42(3):372–375, 1997

25.8.3   Sickle-Cell Disease

Approximately 10% of pediatric strokes occur in children with sickle-cell disease (SCD). Children with SCD can have TIAs, ischemic stroke, hemorrhagic stroke, or any combination of these. As a rule, ischemic stroke occurs most frequently in infants and young children, and hemorrhagic stroke occurs in adults. The incidence of stroke is highest in children with the SS genotype, but other common genotypes (SC, S-β^+, S-β°) also have an increased risk.

The risk of stroke varies widely in different reports. The results of the Cooperative Study of Sickle Cell Disease are summarized in Table 25-14. Stroke rarely occurs in children younger than 2 years. Children between 2 and 5 years have the highest incidence. The overall prevalence in children younger than 20 years was 5.5%.

Factors that increase the risk of ischemic stroke include prior transient ischemic attacks (TIAs), low hemoglobin concentration, acute chest syndrome, and increased blood pressure. Children with SCD and α-thalassemia have a lower risk of stroke, possibly because they have a higher hemoglobin concentration. Although a high concentration of hemoglobin F decreases the risk of other complications of SCD, it does not lower the risk of stroke.

As many as 17% of children with SCD have radiographic evidence of stroke but do not have a history of stroke or TIA. "Silent infarctions" may cause lower IQ scores in children without obvious neurologic disease. Children with silent infarctions have an increased risk of symptomatic stroke and require very close surveillance.

Most ischemic strokes result from occlusion of large cerebral vessels, but small vessels can also be involved. Strokes often occur during a sickle-cell crisis. If narcotic analgesics are used for a painful crisis, the symptoms of stroke may be difficult to interpret. Most children present with hemiparesis, but aphasia, ataxia, visual disturbances, and seizures can also occur. Neurologic recovery depends on the size and location of the stroke. Most children regain motor function, but language deficits may persist. Ischemic stroke is rarely fatal, but there is a 26% mortality rate after hemorrhagic stroke.

Recurrent strokes are a major problem in children with SCD. Without treatment, 50 to 65% of children with one stroke will have a second. The vast majority of second strokes occur within 3 years of the first stroke.

Ischemic stroke is best visualized with MR imaging. Smaller lesions can be detected with MR than with CT imaging. In addition, stroke can be detected earlier with MR imaging, especially if diffusion-weighted sequences are obtained. Magnetic resonance angiography (MRA) may reveal an isolated abnormality but more commonly shows a widespread vasculopathy.

The incidence of recurrent stroke can be reduced significantly with chronic transfusions to maintain the hemoglobin S concen-

TABLE 25-14

STROKE IN SICKLE CELL DISEASE (SCD)

AGE YEARS	INCIDENCE, NUMBER OF STROKES PER 100 PATIENT YEARS	PREVALENCE, %
<2	0.13	2.29
2–5	1.02	4.93
6–9	0.79	5.52
10–19	0.41	5.33

tration below 20 to 30%. Children treated with frequent transfusions have a high incidence of alloimmunization and iron overload. Vascular abnormalities may improve with chronic transfusions. Strokes may recur when transfusions are stopped; therefore most centers continue transfusion therapy indefinitely.

Children at risk for first stroke can be detected with transcranial Doppler ultrasonography (TCD). Patients with mean blood flow velocity in the internal carotid or middle cerebral artery greater than 200 cm per second have a very high risk for stroke. TCD should be used to screen all children with SCD, and children with high velocities should be started on chronic transfusion therapy.

References

Adams RJ, McKie VC, Hsu L, et al: Prevention of a first stroke by transfusions in children with sickle cell anemia and abnormal results on transcranial Doppler ultrasonography [see comments]. New Engl J Med 339(1):5–11, 1998

Kinney TR, Sleeper LA, Wang WC, et al: Silent cerebral infarcts in sickle cell anemia: a risk factor analysis. The Cooperative Study of Sickle Cell Disease. Pediatrics 103(3):640–645, 1999

Ohene-Frempong K, Weiner SJ, Sleeper LA, et al: Cerebrovascular accidents in sickle cell disease: rates and risk factors. Blood 91(1):288–294, 1998

Powars D, Wilson B, Imbus C, Pegalow C, Allen J: The natural history of stroke in sickle cell disease. Am J Med 65(3):461–471, 1978

Rana S, Houston PE, Surana N, Shalaby-Rana EI, Castro OL: Discontinuation of long-term transfusion therapy in patients with sickle cell disease and stroke. J Pediatr 131(5):757–760, 1997

25.8.4 Cervicocephalic Arterial Dissection

Cervicocephalic arterial dissections are among the major causes of stroke in childhood and adolescence. Arterial dissections occur when blood penetrates into the arterial wall through an intimal tear. The intramural hematoma splits the media, extends along the artery, and leads to stenosis or occlusion. Dissections can be traumatic or spontaneous and often involve more than one vessel. Because the trauma is often trivial, underlying arteriopathy is often suspected but rarely demonstrated. Dissections affect the internal carotid arteries (ICA) more frequently than vertebral arteries (VA) and the extracranial arteries more often than the intracranial vessels. However, intracranial arterial dissections are relatively more common in children compared to adults.

Cervicocephalic arterial dissection was found in 20% of French children with arterial ischemic stroke and in 6% of cases in a British childhood and adolescent stroke population. Dissections leading to ischemic stroke are more common in young adults than children.

Neurologic manifestations are related to luminal narrowing by the dissection or from artery-to-artery embolism from the dissection site. Young patients with cervicocephalic arterial dissection present with focal cerebral ischemic symptoms often preceded by ipsilateral headache, neck, or eye pain. Ophthalmologic manifestation such as Horner syndrome and transient monocular blindness are more frequent in adults with ICA dissection.

Cervicocephalic arterial dissection should be considered in any child with stroke, especially when there is history of antecedent trauma to the neck, intraoral trauma, fibromuscular dysplasia, congenital heart disease, or in otherwise idiopathic cerebral or retinal infarction with or without hemicrania. Dissections of the ICA and VA are most accurately diagnosed by cerebral angiography. The

angiographic features include the *string sign,* which is an elongated irregular narrowing of the arterial lumen, tapered occlusion, but rarely a double lumen. MR imaging is a sensitive test in the diagnosis of cervicocephalic arterial dissection, especially if thin T_1-weighted sections are obtained in axial and coronal planes with the fat-suppression technique. MRA can show arterial stenosis, but intimal irregularities and small aneurysms can be missed. Duplex sonography is a noninvasive and simple test and, if combined with Doppler examination, is sensitive in the diagnosis of dissection.

There are no prospective randomized studies that have addressed the efficacy of treatments for cervicocephalic dissections. Most strokes associated with cervical artery dissection occur within 2 weeks and are presumed to be thromboembolic. Early anticoagulation prevents clinical deterioration in adults with ICA dissection and is recommended for a few months by most authors. Anticoagulation is not advised in dissections of the intracranial vessels because of risk of subarachnoid hemorrhage. The recurrence risk at 10 years for all age groups is 12%, higher for younger than older patients. According to Schievink's study on spontaneous dissections in childhood and adolescence, complete recovery or minimal deficit occurred in 90% of cervical artery dissections compared to 60% of intracranial artery dissection.

References

Biousse V, Touboul PJ, D'Anglejan-Chatillon J, Levy C, Schaison M, Bousser MG: Ophthalmologic manifestations of internal carotid artery dissection. Am J Opthalmol 126(4):565–577, 1998

Ganesan V, Savvy L, Chong WK, Kirkham FJ: Conventional cerebral angiography in children with ischemic stroke. Pediatr Neurol 20(1):38–42, 1999

Morki B: Spontaneous dissections of cervicocephalic arteries. In Welch KMA, ed: Cerebrovascular Diseases. San Diego, Academic 1997:390–396

Schievink WI, Mokri B, O'Fallon WM: Recurrent spontaneous cervical-artery dissection. N Engl J Med 330(6):393–397, 1994

Schievink WI, Mokri B, Piepgras DG: Spontaneous dissections of cervicocephalic arteries in childhood and adolescence. Neurology 44(9):1607–1612, 1994

Sturzenegger M: Spontaneous internal carotid artery dissection: early diagnosis and management in 44 patients. J Neurol 242(4):231–238, 1995

Williams LS, Garg BP, Cohen M, Fleck JD, Biller J: Subtypes of ischemic stroke in children and young adults. Neurology 49(6):1541–1545, 1997

25.8.5 Moyamoya Disease

Moyamoya disease (MD) is a chronic progressive occlusive cerebrovascular disease of unknown etiology with typical angiographic features including stenosis or occlusion of the bilateral distal internal carotid arteries or the adjacent anterior, middle, or posterior cerebral arteries. There is a secondary formation of abnormal collateral vascular network (*moyamoya vessels*) at the base of the brain. The stenosis is caused by fibrous intimal thickening and fragmentation of the internal elastic lamina. Angiographic and histologic studies demonstrate similar changes in extracranial vessels. Several systemic disorders such as sickle-cell disease, neurofibromatosis, trisomy 21, tuberculosis, pharyngitis, fibromuscular dysplasia, aortic coarctation, cranial trauma, and irradiation have been associated with moyamoya vessels. This is often classified as *angiographic moyamoya* or *moyamoya syndrome,* and the patients have similar clinical features to those of MD.

MD was once believed to be specific to the Japanese. Lately increasing number of cases have been reported in other parts of the world. Epidemiologic studies from Japan show annual incidence of 0.35 per 100,000, with female to male ratio of 1:8 and peak age 10 to 14 years. Family history was found in 10% of patients. MD is rare in other races but has been reported in all ethnic groups showing similar epidemiologic, clinical, and radiologic features to those of Japan.

Children present with recurrent and progressive cerebral ischemia, whereas adults are more likely to develop cerebral hemorrhage. Intellectual decline, seizures, movement disorders, and headaches are also noted.

Diagnosis of childhood MD can usually be made by MR imaging and MRA. Conventional cerebral angiography is performed if there is need for surgical intervention. EEG shows the re-build-up phenomenon, a delayed return to baseline pattern, in many children with MD. Transcranial Doppler patterns correlate well with the clinical progression of the disease and can be helpful in the management of patients with MD. Positron emission tomography (PET) and proton magnetic resonance spectroscopy (MRS) are useful methods to evaluate cerebral hemodynamics and metabolism in children with MD.

No curative treatment is known for MD. In the acute phase patients with ischemic or hemorrhagic stroke should receive symptomatic treatment. Hyperventilation caused by heavy crying should be avoided because the vasoconstriction can worsen symptoms. Treatment modalities include medical treatment with vasodilators or anticoagulants, surgery, or observation. There are no randomized trials comparing surgery and medical treatment. Revascularization surgery is often used for repeated ischemic episodes. The most common and successful procedure is encephalo-duro-arterio-synangiosis (EDAS). A branch of the superficial temporal artery is sutured into the dura over the affected hemisphere to promote formation of anastomoses with cortical arterial branches. EDAS and its modified versions decrease the frequency of ischemic attacks and prevent deterioration in mental capacity. The optimal treatment plan for hemorrhagic MD is controversial, but often emergency ventricular drainage and evacuation of hematoma are necessary.

Transient ischemic attacks occur frequently during the first 4 years and decrease thereafter. Neurologic deficits and intellectual deterioration increase with time. Permanent deficits or poor outcome is found in 45% of children with MD, and poor prognosis correlates with early age at onset and hypertension. Early indirect revascularization surgery in children with ischemic MD may prevent neurologic deficits and improves function.

References

Adelson PD, Scott RM: Pial synangiosis for moyamoya syndrome in children. Pediatr Neurosurg 23(1):26–33, 1995

Choi JU, Kim DS, Kim EY, Lee KC: Natural history of moyamoya disease: comparison of activity of daily living in surgery and nonsurgery groups. Clin Neurol Neurosurg 99 (suppl 2):S11–18, 1997

Ikezaki K, Fukui M, Inamura T, Kinukawa N, Wakai K, Ono Y: The current status of the treatment for hemorrhagic type moyamoya disease based on a 1995 nationwide survey in Japan. Clin Neurol Neurosurg 99 (suppl 2):S183–186, 1997

Kurokawa T, Tomita S, Veda K, et al: Prognosis of occlusive disease of the circle of Willis (moyamoya disease) in children. Pediatr Neurol 1(5): 274–277, 1985

Matsushima Y, Aoyagi M, Koumo Y, et al: Effects of encephalo-duro-arterio-synangiosis on childhood moyamoya patients—swift disappearance of ischemic attacks and maintenance of mental capacity. Neurol Med Chir 31(11):708–714, 1991

Matsushima Y, Aoyagi M, Niimi Y, Masaoka H, Ohno K: Symptoms and their pattern of progression in childhood moyamoya disease. Brain Dev 12(6):784–789, 1990

Numaguchi Y, Gonzalez CF, Davis PC, et al: Moyamoya disease in the United States. Clin Neurol Neurosurg 99 (suppl 2):S26–30, 1997

Peerless SJ: Risk factors of moyamoya disease in Canada and the USA. Clin Neurol Neurosurg 99 (suppl 2):S45–48, 1997

Shimizu H, Shirane K, Fujiwara S, Takahashi A, Yoshimoto T: Proton magnetic resonance spectroscopy in children with moyamoya disease. Clin Neurol Neurosurg 99 (suppl 2):S64–67, 1997

Takase K, Kashihara M, Hashimoto T: Transcranial Doppler ultrasonography in patients with moyamoya disease. Clin Neurol Neurosurg 99 (suppl 2): S101–105, 1997

Wakai K, Tamakoshi A, Ikezaki K, et al: Epidemiological features of moyamoya disease in Japan: findings from a nationwide survey. Clin Neurol Neurosurg 99 (suppl 2):S1–5, 1997

25.8.6　Central Nervous System Vasculitis

Central nervous system vasculitis can lead to arterial thrombosis, cerebral venous thrombosis, or intracranial hemorrhage. Inflammation of the cerebral vessels produces stenosis or occlusion and is caused by a variety of conditions such as infections, autoimmune diseases, drug abuse, radiation, or idiopathic disorders.

The most common cause of CNS vasculitis is bacterial meningitis. Cerebral infarction is found in 12 to 27% of children with bacterial meningitis. These children are more prone to seizures, and their outcomes are poor. Risk factors include high CSF white cell count, hypoglycorrhachia, age below 12 months, and delayed treatment. Antibiotic treatment should be started as early as possible. Steroids before the first dose of antibiotics may reduce the risk of neurologic and audiologic impairment. CNS vasculitis is seen in most children with tuberculous meningitis, and cerebral infarction in the basal ganglia area is common. Septic embolism caused by bacterial endocarditis can cause CNS vasculitis and stroke.

Several cases of childhood stroke following chickenpox infection have recently been reported. These cases share similar features. They all occur in children younger than 10 years, the infarcts occur in the basal ganglia or internal capsule, and most occur within 9 months of the rash. Focal stenosis, occlusion, or segmental narrowing is seen in the proximal anterior and middle cerebral arteries. Two recent studies have confirmed this association. A retrospective study from London revealed that 17% of children with stroke had history of chickenpox within 6 months of the ictus. A French case-control study showed a significant statistical link between recent varicella and idiopathic arterial stroke. Two-thirds of children in the stroke group had varicella within 9 months prior to the stroke compared to 9% in the control group. CSF cell count, protein, and glucose are often normal, but intrathecal varicella-zoster antibodies have been identified in three children. Possible mechanisms of stroke after chickenpox are vasculitis, transient hypercoagulable state, or sympathetic stimulation. Stroke recurrence is rare, but transient ischemic attacks have been reported. Optimal treatment remains unclear. Steroids and heparin and antiplatelet agents have been used. Adults with herpes zoster ophthalmicus can suffer delayed ipsilateral cerebral infarction caused by cerebral angiitis.

The incidence of symptomatic cerebrovascular disease in children with AIDS is 1.3% per year, but autopsy studies have shown a higher rate of some type of cerebrovascular lesion including arteriopathy.

Autoimmune disorders can cause focal deficits as a result of cerebral venous thrombosis, arterial thrombosis, or intracerebral hemorrhage. Cerebrovascular disease is seen in about 6% of adults with lupus, but a pediatric study identified only 2 of 120 children with lupus with cerebrovascular occlusion. Some cases are caused by vasculitis, but other pathologic processes need to be considered. Antiphospholipid antibodies, infections, complications of treatment, Libman-Sacks endocarditis, and thrombotic thrombocytopenic pupura can all cause stroke in patients with lupus. Neurovascular and thromboembolic complications, including vasculitis, were seen in 3% of children with inflammatory bowel disease.

Takayasu arteritis is an inflammatory disease of unknown etiology involving the aorta and its branches. Young Asian females are most often affected, and stroke is seen in 5 to 10% of these patients. The mechanism of cerebral infarction in this disorder is embolic or thrombotic. Immunosuppressive therapy with steroids and azathioprine improves outcome. Cerebral infarction has also been reported in Kawasaki disease and polyarteritis nodosa. Few pediatric cases of isolated angiitis of CNS have been reported. Without immunosuppressive therapy this disease is fatal.

Recent illicit drug use is found in 12% of young adults with ischemic stroke. Cerebral vasculitis has been associated with cocaine abuse and overdose of diet pills.

Lastly, cerebral radiation necrosis is a delayed CNS injury caused by small-vessel vasculitis. This is a progressive disorder that leads to death or disability. Treatment modalities include anticoagulation and hyperbaric oxygen.

References

Barron TF, Ostrov BE, Zimmerman RA, Packer RJ: Isolated angiitis of CNS: treatment with pulse cyclophosphamide. Pediatr Neurol 9(1):73–75, 1993

Fredericks RK, Lefkowitz DS, Challa VR, Troost BT: Cerebral vasculitis associated with cocaine abuse. Stroke 22(11):1437–1439, 1991

Glantz MJ, Burger PC, Friedman AH, Radtke RA, Massey EW, Schold SC: Treatment of radiation-induced nervous system injury with heparin and warfarin [see comments]. Neurol 44(11):2020–2027, 1994

Hart GB, Mainous EG: The treatment of radiation necrosis with hyperbaric oxygen (OHP). Cancer 37(6):2580–2585, 1976

Hausler MG, Ramaekers VT, Reul J, Meilicke R, Heimann G: Early and late onset manifestations of cerebral vasculitis related to varicella zoster. Neuropediatrics 29(4):202–207, 1998

Kitagawa Y, Gotoh F, Koto A, Okayasu H: Stroke in systemic lupus erythematosus [published erratum appears in Stroke 1991 Mar; 22(3): 417]. Stroke 21(11):1533–1539, 1990

Kohrman MH, Huttenlocher PR: Takayasu arteritis: a treatable cause of stroke in infancy. Pediatr Neurol 2(3):154–158, 1986

Laxer RM, Dunn HG, Flodmark O: Acute hemiplegia in Kawasaki disease and infantile polyarteritis nodosa. Dev Med Child Neurol 26(6):814–818, 1984

Leiguarda R, Berthier M, Starkstein S, Nogues M, Lylyk P: Ishemic infarction in 25 children with tuberculous meningitis. Stroke 19(2):200–204, 1988

Liu GT, Holmes GL: Varicella with delayed contralateral hemiparesis detected by MRI. Pediatr Neurol 6(2):131–134, 1990

Lloyd-Still JD, Tomasi L: Neurovascular and thromboembolic complications of inflammatory bowel disease in childhood. J Pediatr Gstroenterol 9(4):461–466, 1989

Ment LR, Ehrenkranz RA, Duncan CC: Bacterial meningitis as an etiology of perinatal cerebral infarction. Pediatr Neurol 2(5):276–279, 1986

Montes de Oca MA, Babron MC, Bletry O, et al: Thrombosis in systemic lupus erythematosus: a French collaborative study. Arch Dis Child 66(6):713–717, 1991

Odio CM, Faingezicht I, Paris M, et al: The beneficial effects of early dexamethasone administration in infants and children with bacterial meningitis [see comments]. N Engl J Med 324(22):1525–1531, 1991

Park YD, Belman AL, Kim TS, et al: Stroke in pediatric acquired immunodeficiency syndrome. Ann Neurol 28(3):303–311, 1990

Saiman L, Prince A, Gersony WM: Pediatric infective endocarditis in the modern era. J Pediatr 122(6):847–853, 1993

Sebire G, Meyer L, Chabrier S: Varicella as a risk factor for cerebral infarction in childhood: a case-control study. Ann Neurol 45(5):679–680, 1999

Sloan MA, Kittner SJ, Feeser BR, et al: Illicit drug-associated ischemic stroke in the Baltimore-Washington Young Stroke Study. Neurol 50(6):1688–1693, 1998

Tsokos GC, Tsokos M, Le Riche NG, Klippel JH: A clinical and pathologic study of cerebrovascular disease in patients with systemic lupus erythematosus. Semin Arthritis Rheum 16(1):70–78, 1986

25.8.7   Metabolic Stroke

Metabolic problems are a rare cause of pediatric stroke. Homocystinuria and Fabry disease cause vascular occlusion; other metabolic disorders do not cause vascular insufficiency and are more properly termed *strokelike episodes*. As listed in Table 25-15, metabolic strokes can be caused by organic acidurias, mitochondrial abnormalities, lysosomal disorders, and urea cycle defects.

Homocystinuria arises from one of several enzymatic defects. In the classical autosomal-recessive form, deficient cystathionine betasynthase prevents the catabolism of cystathionine to cysteine, causing increased urinary homocystine and methionine. Most children with this disorder have mental retardation, ectopia lentis, marfanoid appearance, recurrent thromboembolic events, and severe atherosclerosis. The latter problem is often fatal in untreated patients. Homocystinemia injures vascular endothelium, leading to thrombus formation. Strokes are secondary to arterial or venous thrombosis or arterial embolism. Treatment is dietary with pyridoxine supplementation and methionine restriction.

Less severe elevations in serum homocystine are a cause of stroke in young adults and possibly children. These patients may be het-

TABLE 25-15
METABOLIC CAUSES OF PEDIATRIC STROKE

Organic acidurias
    Homocystinuria
    Propionic, methylmalonic, isovaleric aciduria
    Glutaric aciduria (I, II)
Mitochondrial
    Mitochondrial myopathy, encephalopathy, lactic acidosis, and strokelike episodes (MELAS)
    Leigh syndrome—pyruvate dehydrogenase complex defects
    Cytochrome oxidase deficiency
Lysosomal
    Fabry disease
    Cystinosis
Urea cycle defects
    Partial ornithine transcarbamylase deficiency
    Carbamyl phosphate synthetase deficiency
Other metabolic causes
    Molybdenum cofactor deficiency
    Sulfite oxidase deficiency
    Familial hyperlipidemia

erozygotes or may have other enzymatic defects. In addition, nutritional deficiencies in folate, vitamin B_{12}, and vitamin B_6 may cause hyperhomocystinemia. Several diseases (chronic renal failure, hypothyroidism, pernicious anemia, leukemia) and drugs (methotrexate, phenytoin, theophylline, cigarette smoking) increase plasma homocystine concentration. Cardo and colleagues reported elevated plasma total homocystine levels in 36% of children with acute ischemic stroke. A case-control study in Dutch children reported increases in 18% of the children with ischemic stroke. Homocystine levels were also increased in patients with sickle-cell disease and stroke. Total serum homocystine should be measured in every child with acute ischemic stroke. Some experts also suggest doing a methionine loading test in children with ischemic stroke of undetermined etiology and normal total homocystine.

Any mitochondrial encephalopathy can present with a strokelike episode or can have these as part of the clinical syndrome. MELAS usually presents with episodic headache and emesis lasting hours to days. Transient hemiparesis or hemianopsia often follows. It usually presents in children between 5 and 15 years but can have onset in infancy. Most children have proximal muscle weakness and progressive neurologic deterioration. Strokes usually occur in the posterior cerebrum with relative sparing of white matter; they do not have a vascular distribution. Some children have calcifications in the basal ganglia. Increased CSF lactate supports the diagnosis, but muscle biopsy and molecular blood analysis are required for confirmation. Most patients have a defect in complex I, but multiple defects of respiratory chain enzymes have been reported. The most common mutation is in tRNA at mtDNA position 3243.

Fabry disease is a rare, sex-linked lysosomal disorder. A deficiency of α-galactosidase causes accumulation of ceramidetrihexoside in vascular endothelium, leading to progressive arterial narrowing, ischemia, and infarction. Stroke usually occurs in adults but has been reported in hemizygous adolescents. Ischemia occurs first in hemispheric white matter or deep gray matter, areas supplied by long, thin end arteries. Other features of the disease include pain in the extremities, abdomen, and joints; renal failure; and hypertension. Renal transplantation improves biochemical function, but its effect on cerebrovascular disease is unknown.

Ornithine transcarbamylase (OTC) deficiency is a urea cycle defect that presents in infancy with hyperammonemia and rapidly progressive neurologic dysfunction. Females with partial OTC deficiency can present in adolescence with migraine, ischemic stroke, or hyperammonemia. Treatment is with a protein-restricted diet.

Molybdenum cofactor deficiency is an even rarer disorder with combined deficiencies of sulfite oxidase, xanthine dehydrogenase, and aldehyde oxidase. Affected infants have acquired microcephaly, seizures, and hypotonia. Most die during infancy; survivors have severe mental retardation, choreoathetosis, and spasticity. Imaging studies reveal cystic lesions in the white matter and cortex. Isolated sulfite oxidase deficiency has similar clinical and radiographic features.

References

Bakker HD, Abeling NG, ten Houten R, et al: Molybdenum cofactor deficiency can mimic postanoxic encephalopathy. J Inherit Metab Dis 16(5):900–901, 1993

Cardo E, Vilaseca MA, Campistol J, Artuch R, Colombe C, Pineda M: Evaluation of hyperhomocysteinaemia in children with stroke. Eur J Paediatr Neurol 3(3):113–117, 1999

Ciafalone E, Ricci E, Shanske S, et al: MELAS: clinical features, biochemistry, and molecular genetics. Ann Neurol 31:391–398, 1992

Christodoulou J, Qureshi IA, McInnes RR, Clarke JT: Ornithine transcarbamylase deficiency presenting with strokelike episodes. J Pediatr 122(3):423–425, 1993

Crutchfield KE, Patronas NJ, Dambrosia JM, et al: Quantitative analysis of cerebral vasculopathy in patients with Fabry disease. Neurology 50(6):1746–1749, 1998

DeGraba TJ, Penix L: Genetics of ischemic stroke. Curr Opin Neurol 8(1):24–29, 1995

Mitsias P, Levine SR: Cerebrovascular complications of Fabry's disease. Ann Neurol 40(1):8–17, 1996

Pavlakis SG, Phillips PC, DiMauro S, DeVivo DC, Rowland LP: Mitochondrial myopathy, encephalopathy, lactic acidosis, and strokelike episodes: a distinctive clinical syndrome. Ann Neurol 16(4):481–488, 1984

Vilaseca MA, Moyano D, Artuch R, et al: Selective screening for hyperhomocysteinemia in pediatric patients. Clin Chem 44(3):662–664, 1998

Welch GN, Loscalzo J: Homocysteine and atherothrombosis. N Engl J Med 338:1042–1050, 1998

25.8.8　Neonatal Cerebral Infarction

Neonatal cerebral infarction (NCI) is more common than previously realized because of greater availability of brain imaging. The majority of NCI occurs in full-term infants, but preterm infants can also be affected. The prevalence in full-term infants is 1 in 4000.

The etiology of NCI is often unclear, and there is seldom evidence of severe birth asphyxia. Usually NCIs are in the vascular distribution of the left middle cerebral artery and are probably embolic, but the origin of systemic emboli can rarely be demonstrated. Degenerating placental vessels are potential sources for emboli. Oxygenated blood from the placenta enters the umbilical vein and proceeds to the inferior vena cava, which empties directly into the right atrium. Two-thirds of the blood is shunted via foramen ovale to the left atrium, left ventricle, and the ascending aorta. Emboli from the placenta can travel this route to the aorta. Interruption of the laminar flow in the aorta by patent ductus arteriosus may explain why the left hemisphere is more often affected in NCI.

Hypoxic-ischemic encephalopathy (HIE) is an important cause of neonatal neurologic morbidity. Hypoxia, ischemia, asphyxia, and acidosis lead to brain injury. Clinical features depend on the age of the infant. Preterm infants develop weakness in the lower extremities caused by periventricular leukomalacia. Full-term infants demonstrate quadriparesis owing to parasagittal brain involvement. Usually, the cerebrovascular disorder caused by HIE is diffuse, but focal cerebral infarction does occur. Other important causes for NCI are prothrombotic conditions and acute severe hypertension.

Focal seizures, within the first 3 to 4 days of life, are the most common clinical manifestation of NCI. Cerebral infarction accounts for 12% of seizures in full-term infants, and, after hypoxic-ischemic encephalopathy, stroke is the second most common cause for seizures in neonates over 31 weeks of gestation. The neurologic examination is often normal or shows mild diffuse hypotonia. Results from studies using diffusion-weighted (DW) imaging indicate perinatal timing of the infarction.

Magnetic resonance imaging is the diagnostic modality of choice. On the first day there may only be subtle changes on conventional MR imaging. DW imaging detects ischemic lesions well in the first days of life but is less abnormal toward the end of the first week, when changes on conventional MR imaging are more obvious. DW imaging is very important for early detection of NCI and if positive can help date the stroke. The infarcted tissue later turns into a porencephalic cyst. MR imaging registration and subtraction technique, which compares serial images, has shown that the infarcted region decreases in size and that there is growth of the brain in this area. Computed tomography is good in acute situations but does not give the same detail as MR imaging, and there is a potential risk of irradiation. Cranial ultrasound is insensitive early but will identify stroke at the end of the first week in most patients with NCI.

Initial management should include general medical support and administration of anticonvulsants for seizures. Anticonvulsants are usually discontinued within 6 months of age, since few of these children develop epilepsy.

Previously it was reported that NCI was usually associated with perinatal complications and a very poor outcome. Recent reports have indicated that this is not true. Mercuri and colleagues were unable to find any adverse antenatal or perinatal factors significantly associated with poor outcome. The incidence of hemiplegia was 20% in their prospective study of 24 infants with NCI. The overall involvement of the basal ganglia, internal capsule, and hemisphere on MR imaging and abnormal background on EEG were consistently associated with hemiplegia. Three of their 24 infants had mild global developmental delay, one of whom had hemiplegia. There is also high incidence of abnormalities on tests for visual function, which does not correlate with site and size of the infarction on MRI. These data emphasize the importance of a comprehensive follow-up even in the absence of hemiplegia.

References

Clancy R, Malin S, Laraque D, Baumgart S, Younkin D: Focal motor seizures heralding stroke in full-term neonates. Am J Dis Child 139(6): 601–606, 1985

Cowan FM, Pennock JM, Hanrahan JD, et al: Early detection of cerebral infarction and hypoxic-ischemic encephalophathy in neonates using diffusion-weighted magnetic resonance imaging. Neuropediatrics 25(4): 172–175, 1994

De Vries LS, Groenendaal F, Eken P, Van Haastert IC, Rademaker KJ, Meiners LC: Infarcts in the vascular distribution of the middle cerebral artery in preterm and fulltern infants. Neuropediatrics 28(2):88–96, 1997

Estan J, Hope P: Unilateral neonatal cerebral infarction in full term infants. Arch Dis Child Fetal Neonatal Ed 76(2):F88–93, 1997

Mercuri E, Cowan F, Rutherford M, Acolet D, Pennock J, Dubowitz L: Ischaemic and haemorrhagic brain lesions in newborns with seizures and normal Apgar scores. Arch Dis Child Fetal Neonatal Ed 73(2):F67–74, 1995

Mercuri E, Rutherford M, Cowan F: Early prognostic indicators of outcome in infants with neonatal cerebral infarction: a clinical, electroencephalogram, and magnetic resonance imaging study. Pediatrics 103(1):39–46, 1999

Thorarensen O, Ryan S, Hunter J, Younkin DP: Factor V Leiden mutation: an unrecognized cause of hemiplegic cerebral palsy, neonatal stroke, and placental thrombosis. Ann Neurol 42(3):372–375, 1997

25.8.9   Hemorrhagic Stroke

Hemorrhagic stroke in children is as common as ischemic stroke. Bleeding occurs after rupture of normal blood vessels in children with head trauma or coagulopathies and abnormal vessels in patients with vascular malformations or aneurysms. Bleeding is classified as either subarachnoid, ie, into the subarachnoid space around

the brain, or intraparenchymal, ie, into the brain parenchyma. Many patients have both subarachnoid and intraparenchymal hemorrhage. The disorders causing hemorrhagic stroke are listed in Table 25-16. The etiology of a hemorrhagic infarction can usually be identified. Treatment is often surgical.

Intraparenchymal hemorrhage usually presents with headache, focal neurologic signs, seizures, and altered consciousness. Small hemorrhages may have very subtle clinical signs, but large bleeds usually cause coma. In neonates, seizures and signs of increased intracranial pressure are more common. Subarachnoid hemorrhage usually presents with the sudden onset (thunderclap) of the worst headache of the child's life, followed by signs of meningeal irritation and increased intracranial pressure.

Acute hemorrhage is easily identified with CT, but within a few days the blood becomes isodense with brain parenchyma. Retinal hemorrhages may be detected on funduscopic examination. Blood is occasionally present in the spinal fluid when it is not detected with CT.

Head trauma is the most common cause of pediatric intracranial hemorrhage. Cerebral contusion can occur alone or in association with subdural or epidural hemorrhage. Intracranial bleeding is very common in the shaken baby syndrome. Traumatic aneurysms can result from closed or penetrating head injuries. On very rare occasions, carotid-cavernous fistulas develop after fracture of the skull base. Traumatic delivery is often associated with neonatal intracranial hemorrhage.

Coagulopathies are the next most common cause of hemorrhage. In most cases, the underlying coagulopathy is known. Very rarely, intracranial hemorrhage is the initial presentation. The hemorrhage is usually secondary to trauma, but the trauma may be very slight.

Vascular malformations are divided into arteriovenous malformations, cavernous malformations, venous angiomas and capillary telangiectasias. The latter are a rare cause of bleeding in neurocutaneous syndromes. Arteriovenous malformations (AVMs) are comprised of abnormal primitive arteries and veins with varying amounts of intervening gliotic tissue. The malformations do not have a capillary bed between the arteries and veins. Small AVMs typically present with focal seizures; large AVMs with seizures,

TABLE 25-16

ETIOLOGY OF HEMORRHAGIC STROKE

Trauma
  Shaken impact syndrome
  Head trauma—closed, penetrating, vaginal delivery
Coagulopathy
  Hemophilia
  Thrombocytopenia—idiopathic, thrombotic, hemolytic-uremic syndrome
  Liver disease
  Neonatal vitamin K deficiency
  Anticoagulants—warfarin, heparin
Vascular anomalies
  Arteriovenous malformation
  Cavernous malformation
  Aneurysm—congenital, traumatic, coarctation of the aorta
Sickle-cell disease
Others
  Hypertension
  Drug abuse—cocaine, amphetamine
  Hemorrhagic transformation of ischemic infarction

headache, focal neurologic signs, and intracranial bruit. Intermittent, relatively mild headache may be caused by periodic bleeding or mass effect. Acute severe headache may be secondary to intraparenchymal hemorrhage in small or large AVMs. Ischemic infarction can result from spontaneous thrombosis or vascular steal. Vein of Galen malformations usually present in infancy with high-output congestive heart failure and failure to thrive or in early childhood with hydrocephalus. AVMs can be detected with contrast-enhanced CT, MR imaging, MR or conventional angiography. There is a 4% risk of hemorrhage from unruptured AVMs and a high risk for recurrent hemorrhage. About 10% of first hemorrhages are fatal. Embolization or surgical removal is usually required to treat AVMs. Occasionally the presenting hemorrhage successfully obliterates an AVM.

Cavernous malformations are collections of thin-walled vessels with a single layer of endothelium, no smooth muscle or elastic tissue, and no intervening brain parenchyma. They can occur alone or in association with other vascular malformations. They present in children with seizures, focal neurologic signs, or hemorrhage. In contrast to AVMs, hemorrhage in cavernomas is rarely life threatening. Recurrent bleeding is common, especially when the cavernous malformation is in the brainstem. Cavernomas can be familial or nonfamilial. Multiple cavernomas are common in the autosomal-dominant form, and they are more likely to bleed. Cavernous malformations are rarely visualized on angiography because of the small size of the vessels and their low flow. However, on T_2-weighted MR imaging, they have a bright center with dark surrounding ring.

Venous angiomas are composed entirely of venous structures. They are the most common vascular malformation. Most patients are asymptomatic, but they can present with seizures. Venous angiomas are easily identified with contrast-enhanced CT or MR imaging. Even when they cause seizures, they rarely require surgery. In fact, surgery can increase venous congestion and make neurologic symptoms worse.

Saccular aneurysms are rarely symptomatic and less frequent than AVMs. They arise from an area of congenital weakness in the arteries. They can be associated with coarctation of the aorta, polycystic kidneys, Ehlers-Danlos syndrome, and Marfan syndrome. Aneurysms in children usually arise from the internal carotid artery or anterior cerebral artery. Giant aneurysms greater than 10 cm in diameter can occur. Sometimes, headache, focal neurologic signs, or hydrocephalus are the first signs; but aneurysms usually present with acute subarachnoid hemorrhage, frequently with intraparenchymal or intraventricular extension. Subarachnoid hemorrhage can cause significant vasospasm and cerebral ischemia. Surgery is the treatment of choice. Prior to surgery, patients are treated with nimodipine (to prevent vasospasm), sedation, and anticonvulsants.

25.8.10 Cerebral Venous Thrombosis

Cerebral venous thrombosis (CVT) is increasingly recognized as an important cause for stroke in infants and children. The clinical presentation is extremely diverse. CVT can mimic other conditions such as focal lesions caused by ischemic or hemorrhagic stroke, brain tumor, abscess, encephalitis or global encephalopathy from a metabolic disease, toxic exposure, or increased intracranial pressure. The literatue on pediatric CVT is limited to only one prospective population-based study and a few small retrospective case series. The incidence of CVT in children in Canada is 0.29 cases per 100,000 children per year.

The cortical veins from the superior surface of each hemisphere drain into the superior sagittal sinus (SSS), which empties into the right lateral sinus (LS). The cavernous sinuses (CS) drain blood from the orbits, middle cerebral veins, and the anterior undersurface of the brain. The paired CS connect with the internal jugular veins through the petrosal sinuses. Blood from the posterior cerebral hemispheres, cerebellum, and the brainstem drains mainly into the lateral sinuses. The deep cerebral veins drain blood from the deep cerebral white matter, the basal nuclei, and the hypothalamus. They consist of the paired internal cerebral and basal veins, which join to form the great vein of Galen and the inferior sagittal sinus. The two latter structures form the straight sinus, which drains into the left LS. The right LS is frequently larger than the left. This LS anatomic variation may be misinterpreted as sinus occlusion. All venous drainage passes through the sinuses and then to the internal jugular veins. The consequences of CVT are variable, ranging from edema without infarction to extensive bilateral hemorrhagic infarcts affecting the cortex and adjacent white matter.

The clinical manifestations of CVT depend on which vessel is occluded. Thrombosis of the SSS produces increased intracranial pressure because it is the principal absorption site for cerebrospinal fluid. Symptoms include headache, papilledema, nausea, vomiting, and sixth nerve palsy. Venous infarction adjacent to the SSS causes seizures, weakness, and sensory loss more severe in the legs than the arms. The LS runs along the inner aspect of the mastoid process. Prior to antibiotics LS thrombosis was commonly seen in patients with otitis media or mastoiditis. Cranial nerves may be affected in LS thrombosis. CS thrombosis may produce proptosis, chemosis, and unilateral or bilateral ophthalmoplegia and is often the result of infection from the paranasal sinuses, face, nose, or mouth. Thrombosis of the deep cerebral veins leads to thalamic or cerebellar infarction.

Seizures are the most frequent clinical presentation, especially in neonates. In contrast, older children usually present with headache and vomiting. Focal neurologic deficits are rare in children compared to adults. Thrombosis most frequently affects the SSS and the LS. Venous infarctions are present in 40 to 50% of patients.

Risk factors are identified in 70% of children and include most commonly prothrombotic conditions and dehydration. Other predisposing conditions are cranial infection, procoagulant medications (L-asparaginase), hematologic disease (polycythemia), perinatal complications, cardiac disease, sepsis, malignancy, inflammatory bowel disease, and iron deficiency anemia. In adults, cerebral venous thrombosis most often is associated with pregnancy, oral contraceptives, factor V Leiden, and prothrombin gene mutations.

CT scan is often the first available method of imaging but can be normal in up to 40% of cases. Unenhanced CT scan is good for the detection of hemorrhagic infarction, and occasionally a hyperdense cord is present, suggestive of a recently thrombosed vein. The "empty delta sign" appears after contrast injection as a filling defect in the SSS. However, it is not pathognomonic because early division of the SSS can give a false-positive sign. MR imaging with MR angiography is now the investigation of choice for CVT and associated venous infarction. The thrombosed sinus can be hyperdense both on T_1- and T_2-weighted MR imaging, and there is a filling defect on MR venography. Color-flow Doppler imaging can accurately diagnose SSS thrombosis in neonates and infants and may be used as a screening method in high-risk patients. CSF analysis may show elevated opening pressure, increased protein content, presence of red blood or less frequently white blood cells. EEGs are abnormal in most children with CVT. The most common pattern is generalized slowing and focal or lateralized abnormalities ipsilateral to the venous infarctions.

The management of CVT is controversial. Recently two randomized adult studies have looked at the role of anticoagulation in treatment of CVT. Einhaupl and colleagues compared dose-adjusted intravenous heparin with placebo and concluded that heparin was effective and safe in patients with CVT even in patients with hemorrhagic lesions. De Bruijn and Stam compared low-molecular-weight heparin (LMWH) with placebo and found that patients with CVT treated with LMWH had favorable outcome more often than controls, but the findings were not statistically significant. A meta-analysis of both these trials showed a modest but not statistically significant benefit of any heparin treatment for CVT. No randomized controlled trials have been performed in children. A recent Canadian pilot study of children with CVT concluded that anticoagulation, especially LMWH, was safe and may have a role in the treatment of this disorder. The role of intrathrombus rtPA is controversial. Frey and colleagues demonstrated that combined intrathrombus rtPA with intravenous heparin did restore flow rapidly and improved clinical outcome. This therapy is unsafe in patients with hemorrhagic lesions, and it should be reserved for patients who fail heparin and symptomatic treatment.

Treatment of CVT should not be limited only to thrombosis but should include the underlying risk factors such as dehydration and infection. Seizures and raised intracranial pressure must also be treated. The outcome in infants and children with CVT is worse than in adults. Unfavorable outcome with death or neurologic deficits was found in 37% of Canadian infants and children with CVT compared to only 14% in adults. One study found that older children with CVT have better outcome than neonates. Patients with infarction owing to thrombosis in the deep venous system or elevated intracranial pressure in the acute phase do worse.

References

Ameri A, Bousser MG: Cerebral venous thrombosis. Neurol Clin 10(1): 87–111, 1992

Barron TF, Gusnard DA, Zimmerman RA, Clancy RR: Cerebral venous thrombosis in neonates and children. Pediatr Neurol 8(2):112–116, 1992

Bezinque SL, Slovis IL, Touchette AS, et al: Characterization of superior sagittal sinus blood flow velocity using color flow Doppler in neonates and infants. Pediatr Radiol 25(3):175–179, 1995

Bousser MG: Cerebral venous thrombosis: nothing, heparin, or local thrombolysis? [editorial; comment]. Stroke 30(3):481–483, 1999

De Bruijn SF, Stam J: Randomized, placebo-controlled trial of anticoagulant treatment with low-molecular-weight heparin for cerebral sinus thrombosis [see comments]. Stroke 30(3):484–488, 1999

De Veber G, Chan A, Monagle P, et al: Anticoagulation therapy in pediatric patients with sinovenous thrombosis: a cohort study. Arch Neurol 55(12):1533–1537, 1998

Einhaupl KM, Villringer A, Meister W, et al: Heparin treatment in sinus venous thrombosis. [published erratum appears in Lancet 338(8772): 958, 1991] [see comments] Lancet 338(8767):597–600, 1991

Frey JL, Muro GJ, McDougall CG, Dean BL, Jahnke HK: Cerebral venous thrombosis: combined intrathrombus rtPA and intravenous heparin [see comments]. Stroke 30(3):489–494, 1999

Hartfield DS, Lowry NJ, Keene DL, Yager JY: Iron deficiency: a cause of stroke in infants and children. Pediatr Neurol 16(1):50–53, 1997

Kuehnen J, Schwartz A, Neff W, Hennerici M: Cranial nerve syndrome in thrombosis of the transverse/sigmoid sinuses. Brain 121(2):381–388, 1998

Markowitz RL, Ment LR, Gryboski JD: Cerebral thromboembolic disease in pediatric and adult inflammatory bowel disease: case report and review of the literature. J Pediatr Gastroenterol Nutr 8(3):413–420, 1989

Martinelli I, Sacchi E, Landi G, Taioli E, Duca F, Mannuci PM: High risk of cerebral-vein thrombosis in carriers of a prothrombin-gene mutation and in users of oral contraceptives [see comments]. N Engl J Med 338(25):1793–1797, 1998

Patel H, Smith RR, Garg BP: Spontaneous extracranial carotid artery dissection in children. Pediatr Neurol 13(1):55–60, 1995

Preter M, Tzourio C, Ameri A, Bousser MG: Long-term prognosis in cerebral venous thrombosis. Follow-up of 77 patients. Stroke 27(2):243–246, 1996

25.8.11 General Diagnostic Evaluation

The general approach to diagnostic evaluation should be question- and hypothesis-driven:

1. Is there a cerebrovascular lesion? Several disorders can mimic a stroke. Transient neurologic deficits can be seen after a seizure, with hypoglycemia or complicated migraine.
2. Is there a cerebral infarction or hemorrhage? This is crucial because etiology and treatment are different between these two processes.
3. Is it anterior or posterior circulation stroke? The prognosis tends to be worse in posterior circulation stroke. These patients may need closer observation and precautions to minimize airway compromise.
4. What is the cause of the stroke? Congenital heart disease, sickle-cell disease, and prothrombotic disorders are common. No cause can be found in about one-third of patients.

A suggested format for diagnostic workup is provided in Fig. 25-26. Our initial evaluation includes a CBC with platelet count, electrolytes and glucose, PT/PTT, toxicology screen, chest x-ray, and ECG.

Computed cranial tomography (CT), without contrast, is usually the first imaging test used because it is easy to perform and readily available. The head CT can distinguish between hemorrhage and ischemic infarction but is often normal in the first hours of infarction sometimes up to 24 hours. A subtle effacement of sulci may be the first clue to infarction. Magnetic resonance imaging is more sensitive than CT for early detection of infarction, but it may be normal in the first few hours. Diffusion-weighted imaging is good for early detection of infarction and if positive can help date the stroke. Magnetic resonance angiography is a good method to detect changes in blood flow in the large intracranial and cervical vessels but less reliable with small vessels. Magnetic resonance venography is the investigation of choice for cerebral venous thrombosis.

Once the diagnosis of stroke is established, a comprehensive workup must be performed. Because embolism is the most frequent cause of childhood stroke, a careful cardiac examination is essential. Transesophageal echocardiography (TEE) may be more accurate than transthoracic echocardiography (TTE) to detect structural abnormalities of the heart. Bubble contrast should be used to detect right-left shunt.

Lumbar puncture (LP), for cerebrospinal fluid examination, should be done if infection, inflammation, or subarachnoid hemorrhage (SAH) is suspected. This procedure should not be performed if there is clinical or neuroradiologic evidence for increased intracranial pressure. LP in a patient with a unilateral hemispheric or cerebellar lesion may lead to transtentorial or transmagnal herniation. Small SAH may be evident in the cerebrospinal fluid but not on head CT.

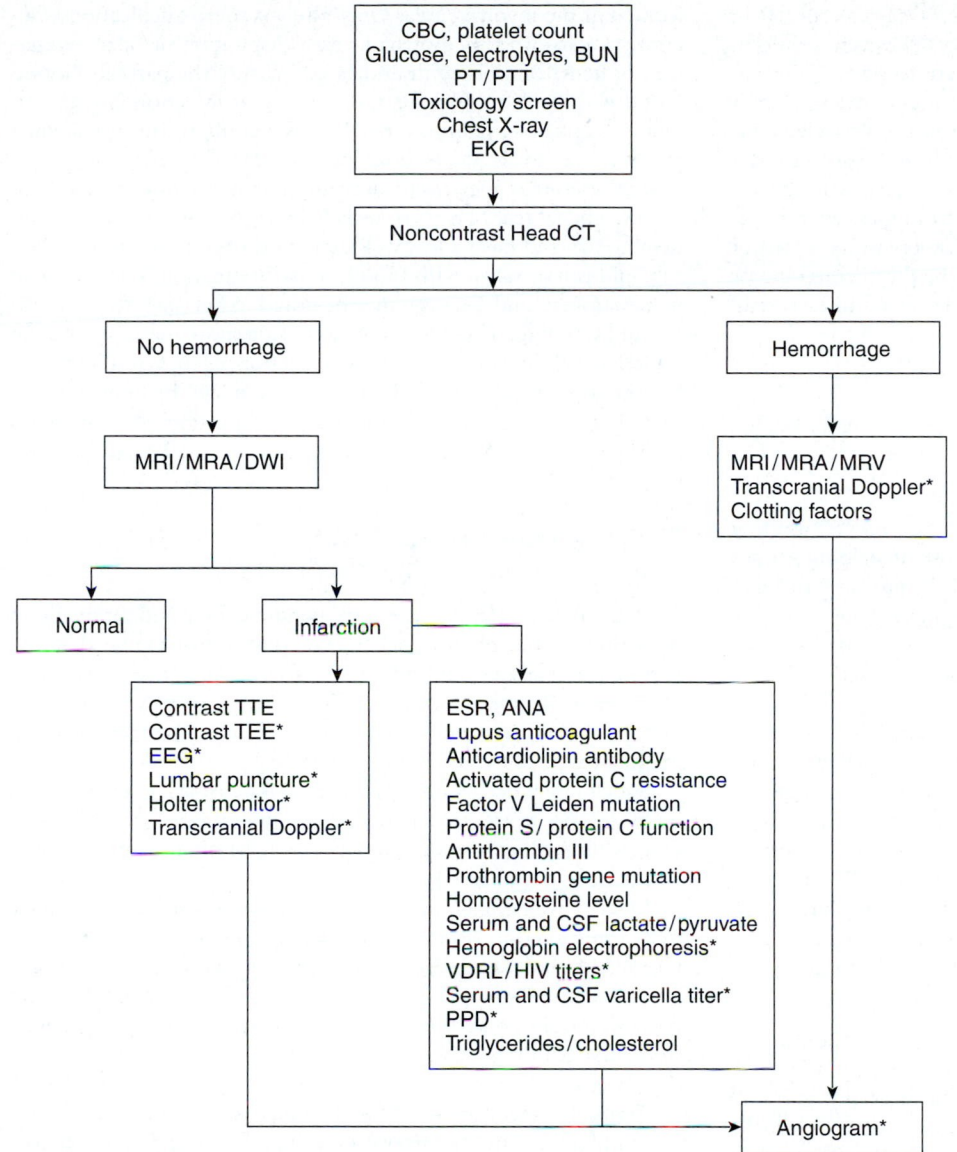

FIGURE 25-26 Algorithm showing the evaluation of stroke in the pediatric patient. Abbreviations—see text.

Transcranial Doppler (TCD) is a noninvasive and portable method used for imaging the circle of Willis and the vertebrobasilar system. TCD is useful in predicting stroke in children with sickle cell disease, and can detect vasospasm in SAH.

Evidence for prothrombotic state, coagulopathy or systemic inflammation should be carefully investigated. Approximately 30% of children with ischemic stroke have abnormalities in their prothrombotic factors. Lactate and pyruvate levels should be obtained if mitochondrial disorder is suspected. CSF lactate and pyruvate values may be necessary to make the diagnosis, even though serum levels are normal. Hemoglobin electrophoresis; VDRL, HIV, and varicella titers; and PPD should be done when clinically indicated.

The diagnostic evaluation should not stop if one risk factor is identified, because pediatric stroke patients can have more than one cause for their cerebrovascular event. If intracranial hemorrhage is detected, a neurosurgical consultation should be obtained.

Conventional angiography should be reserved for patients with nontraumatic intracranial hemorrhage or when vasculitis is suspected, if other imaging modalities have been normal. Small aneurysms, arteriovenous malformation, or cavernous malformations may not show up on MR imaging or MR angiography. The angi-

ography may not detect vascular malformations if they are surrounded by hematoma and edema. Repeating the angiography or waiting until the hematoma has resolved may be necessary in this case.

If there is no evidence for infarction or intracranial hemorrhage, other conditions that mimic stroke such as transient postictal hemiparesis, migraine, hypoglycemia, and alternating hemiplegia must be excluded.

25.9   TRAUMA TO THE NERVOUS SYSTEM

Claudia A. Chiriboga

Accidental injury is the leading cause of death among children, accounting for over 40% of all pediatric deaths. Mortality is but the tip of the iceberg of the totality of pediatric injuries; for every child dying of an injury, 45 are hospitalized and 1300 require treatment in the emergency room. The incidence of head injury is estimated at 200 per 100,000 persons 0 to 19 years of age; about 10 in 100,000 children die as a result of head injury. The event results in mild head injury in 82% of cases, in moderate to severe injury in 14%, and in death in 5%. The rate of head injury among boys is nearly twice that among girls. Motor vehicle and sports-related injuries and assault are the leading causes of head injury in older children, whereas falls are the most frequent cause in young children. The spectrum of head injuries ranges from a linear fracture, scalp lesion, or mild concussion, in which recovery is full, to major lesions of brain and spinal cord, which may be life-threatening or cause permanent neurologic damage. The latter requires careful analysis and management.

25.9.1   Scalp Injuries

LACERATIONS

Scalp injury is most often a result of blunt trauma, and the resulting wound is usually a smooth linear cut above the unyielding surface of the bone over which the blow occurred. Wounds of the skin layer are usually separated only minimally, owing to fixation by the underlying fibrous tissue septa. When the galea is involved, the wound will gape, particularly if it is in a transverse direction. Bleeding is quite marked because of the rich anastomotic blood supply of the scalp and the limited contraction-retraction ability of the vessels firmly anchored in the dense connective tissue layer. Consequently, large lacerations heal quite well, and infection rarely occurs unless there is gross contamination or tissue destruction. However, infections of the skull and intracranial contents present serious hazards; they invariably result from poor initial handling. Such wounds are best treated by primary closure, but if the child's condition prohibits immediate handling, this can be delayed for 8 to 12 hours without significantly increasing risk of infection.

HEMATOMA AND CEPHALOHEMATOMA

Hematomas in the dense connective tissue layer of the scalp are common, but because of the density of the tissue they are usually not very large and absorb within 2 to 3 days. Galeal laceration permits bleeding from above to permeate the subgaleal loose connective tissue layer and may result in rapid extensive swelling of enormous proportions because there is no limiting membrane to prevent its spread.

Bleeding beneath the pericranium is most common in the incompletely ossified and highly vascular skull characteristic of the first 2 years of life. These collections are restricted by the pericranial suture line attachment; they occur most often in the parietal area and are known as *cephalohematomas* (see Sec. 2.8.1). On palpation, subgaleal and subpericranial hematomas may be confused with an underlying depressed fracture. Subgaleal collections of partially clotted blood may develop a soft center surrounded by an indurated ring, which may be mistaken for a rim of bone about an area of skull depression. The pericranial fibrous suture attachment demarcating cephalohematomas is also commonly confused with a depressed skull fracture. Fracture sites (depressed or linear) underlying hematomas require radiographic examination to clarify the diagnosis.

The larger hematomas are absorbed in 2 to 4 weeks. When cephalohematomas persist, pericranial proliferation occurs with the production of bony callus; ultimately, a thin layer of bone may be formed in the involved area. Only rarely is there calcification of an entire nonabsorbed hemorrhagic area. Aspiration or open evacuation of hematomas is contraindicated because the partially clotted blood is difficult to aspirate and the risk of infection is great. In infants, cephalohematomas may be large enough to cause anemia and mild jaundice. Collections of CSF, termed *subgaleal subepicranial hygromas,* may occur over linear skull fractures when there is a meningeal tear. They are usually less extensive and softer than hematomas and have a less well defined ring of induration. When the fluid is not mixed with blood, transillumination is greater than in hematomas, and the mass may be noted to fluctuate with coughing and straining. These collections subside spontaneously, and the underlying dural tear heals. If the collection is large or if it persists beyond 4 to 7 days, the swelling may be reduced by lumbar puncture. Pressure dressings do not hasten absorption of hematomas and hygromas, and they may contribute to skin breakdown and infection.

25.9.2   Craniocerebral Trauma

The human head can withstand tremendous force and yet maintain both skull and cerebral integrity. The position of the head at impact, suture patency, and degree of movement at the craniospinal junction are important variables. Blood pressure may reach 150% of normal or even higher in an attempt to compensate for increased intracranial pressure and maintain cerebral circulation.

Shock rarely occurs on a purely neural basis; it is usually caused by blood loss from associated extracerebral injuries. Neural shock may occur with extensive and irreversible cerebral damage; this is an ominous prognostic sign.

Mass movement of intracranial contents caused by the injury may result in contusion as well as subarachnoid and intracerebral bleeding. Subdural bleeding results when blood vessels between the brain and the meninges are torn; this usually occurs because the cortical bridging veins enter the dura-encased superior longitudinal sinus. Extradural hematomas may result from disruption to extradural veins or arteries.

Transient unconsciousness after injury reflects a sudden physiologic block at the brainstem level. The brainstem reticular formation has an alerting function, mediating sensory input to higher centers. After trauma, this formation may enter an absolutely refractory state, recovery from which directly correlates with return to consciousness.

SKULL FRACTURES

Skull fractures may involve the vault or the base and may be of the simple linear type or of the diastatic type (abnormal suture separation occurring at the time of impact), simple depressed, comminuted, or ping-pong (pond) variety. They may occur as isolated manifestations of head trauma but more often are associated with underlying cerebral injury. Simple linear and diastatic fractures are of little immediate significance other than to indicate the force of the blow and the point of maximal impact. Over 80% of all skull fractures are of this type, and the parietal area is involved five times more frequently than are other regions. Diastatic fractures have the same medicolegal significance as a fracture line, and they most often involve the lambdoid suture. A separation of the lambdoid suture wider than 1.5 mm, particularly at several points along its course, is usually considered abnormal, as is a coronal suture spread of more than 2.0 mm.

The cranial vault is not well calcified in infants less than 1 year of age, and it has great elasticity of its inner and outer tables. Both tables may be displaced inward without an actual break occurring, thus producing the ping-pong (pond) fracture. Fractures at the base of the skull may be indicated by bilateral orbital ecchymoses in anterior fossa lesions and by retroauricular ecchymosis (Battle sign) and tympanic membrane discoloration when the petrous bone in the middle fossa is involved. Otorrhea and rhinorrhea imply basilar skull fracture and are potentially of more serious consequence because of the risk of infection. Posttraumatic collection of intracranial air in any of the meningeal spaces (aerocele) or the ventricular system (pneumoencephalocele) implies fractures through the paranasal sinuses.

Laboratory Data and Diagnosis

There is seldom an emergency indication for skull radiography because films are usually unimportant in immediate management. It is better to delay until the child's condition permits optimal radiographic study. A skeletal survey to detect areas of multiple osseous injury is essential in infants, and cervical spine films should be considered in addition to skull films in the older child. Clinical characteristics and examination findings highly indicative of skull fracture are often lacking in children. The majority of detected fractures are quite benign. Skull radiographs should be obtained in all children less than 3 years of age with all but trivial head injury because of the implications skull fractures have for patient management. When an intracranial lesion is suspected, a CT scan with bone windows is the preferred imaging modality; it is indicated if there is a suspicion of a depressed or comminuted skull fracture, loss of consciousness lasting 5 minutes or more, altered mental status, focal neurologic signs, and nonimpact seizures. Furthermore, CT scans should be obtained even with relatively minor head trauma in infants, especially those younger than 6 months, as clinical correlates of cerebral injury may be lacking. If CSF drainage from the nose is suspected, the presence of glucose will confirm its origin, because nasal secretions have negligible amounts of glucose.

Treatment

Simple linear fractures without underlying damage do not require treatment other than analgesics for headache and irritability. The parents should understand that a simple skull fracture is of little concern and is not an indication to restrict activities. A repeat skull radiograph is recommended after 3 months to demonstrate union; if union is not progressing, films should be repeated at intervals of 3 months to detect possible complications such as leptomeningeal cyst. Fractures usually heal in 6 to 12 months.

Pond fractures do not usually require surgical elevation. Rarely an underlying defect of cerebral cortex may result in lack of brain growth and failure of the skull depression to elevate; a 3-month period of observation will determine this (Fig. 25-27). It has been recommended that all fractures depressed more than 0.5 cm be elevated to avoid the formation of cortical scars and thus prevent seizures. This premise has been questioned by studies that show no difference in the risk of seizures or focal defects between young children with simple depressed fractures treated with surgery and those treated without. If surgery is indicated, it should be performed early, as is the case for all compound and comminuted skull fractures.

Basilar skull fractures resulting in rhinorrhea or otorrhea require hospitalization. The child should be maintained in a semiupright

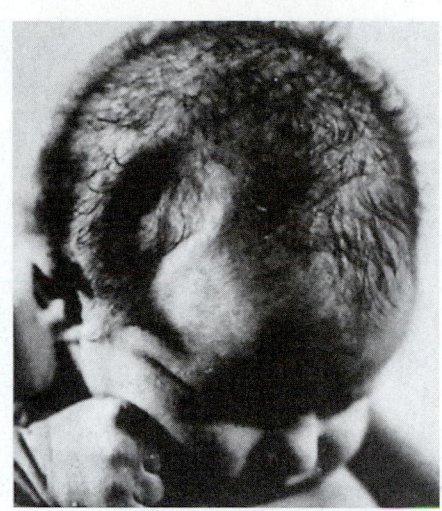

FIGURE 25-27 Depressed fracture of skull from birth injury in an infant delivered by version and extraction, with application of forceps to trailing head. Depressed fracture of right parietal bone was said to be related to an abnormality of the mother's pelvis. There was difficulty in resuscitation and cyanosis during the first few hours, with right internal strabismus but no signs of increased intracranial pressure. Patient recovered completely without operation and was physically and mentally normal at age 5.5 years.

position; plugging or irrigating the involved orifice is contraindicated. There is no evidence to support the use of prophylactic antibiotics. Cerebrospinal fluid often stops draining spontaneously, and 80% resolve within 72 hours. In the absence of increased intracranial pressure, a period of continuous, closed system spinal fluid drainage from the lumbar subarachnoid space can be valuable beyond this point; should this not be effective over an additional 72 hours, however, surgical repair must be considered because the danger of meningitis is overwhelming. As long as fistulous patency exists, meningitis remains a hazard, and repeated infections, diffuse arachnoiditis, and secondary hydrocephalus may result. Use of antibiotics should not be decided upon without a preceding culture of CSF. Traumatic aerocele, if persistent, is an indication for operative intervention. Intracranial air tends to be absorbed rapidly. If radiographs at 48- to 72-hour intervals show persistence or increased collection of air, surgery should not be delayed. With rhinorrhea, coughing and sneezing may produce increased drainage and may actually permit air to enter the intracranial cavity. Accentuation of headache under these circumstances may be the result of delayed intracranial air collection and may be documented by repeat radiographs. Coughing and sneezing should be suppressed in all patients with posttraumatic otorrhea and rhinorrhea.

A late complication of a linear fracture in a young child is a leptomeningeal cyst or, more accurately, a growing skull fracture. This results from dural laceration; projection of the arachnoid membrane into the fracture site with brain herniation produces bone erosion of the overlying skull over a period of months or years. The late onset of focal seizures, increased intracranial pressure, focal neurologic signs, and occasionally visible and palpable skull deformity should suggest this complication. Skull radiographs are diagnostic (Fig. 25-28), revealing an area of erosion over a prior fracture site. Ninety percent of growing skull fractures occur in children younger than 3 years, with 50% occurring in children younger than 1 year. They are usually in the parietal area and should be suspected

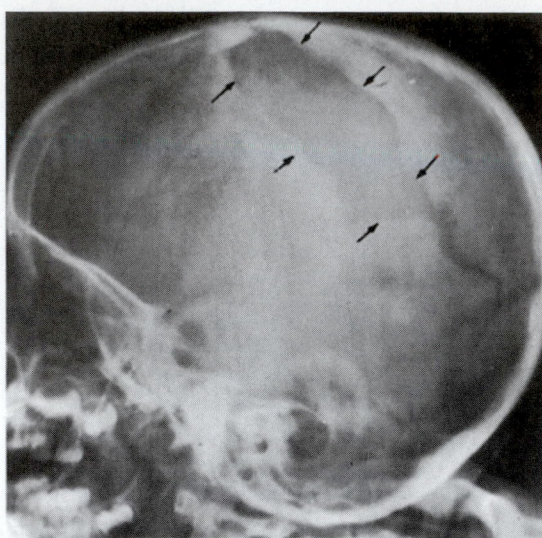

FIGURE 25-28 Leptomeningeal cyst showing large area of parietal skull erosion 8 months after a simple linear fracture.

when the initial fracture line is wide or is associated with a subepicranial hygroma.

CONCUSSION

After a sudden head blow, transient loss of consciousness occurs, but this is followed by full recovery without sequelae. Children often vomit and later are pale and apathetic or quite irritable shortly after the injury. These symptoms are short-lived and of no concern. More prolonged unconsciousness, often associated with some evidence of focal neurologic defect and varying degrees of amnesia, implies a cerebral contusion or laceration. The impact may result in early seizures. Transient loss of vision also may be noted; although this may be disturbing, it is usually benign. In simple concussion or mild contusion, children should be examined carefully, with attention to gross evidence of skull fracture and associated damage to viscera and bones. A CT scan should be obtained in all children with loss of consciousness lasting more than a few minutes to exclude intracranial lesions. It is mandatory to monitor vital signs and to observe these children until full recovery of consciousness. Usually children will have recovered partially by the time they see a physician and, other than pallor, irritability, and bruises, have few, if any, signs on examination. Such patients are best managed at home, provided that the CT scan (if warranted) is negative and children have been observed for at least 6 to 8 hours after injury, which roughly corresponds to the time interval when most acute intracranial bleeds will develop. Parents should be informed to return with the child if any change in level of responsiveness or alertness develops.

PARENCHYMAL INJURIES

Patients with severe degrees of head injury or prolonged unconsciousness require hospitalization to evaluate the severity of injury and the need for specific therapy. Immediate attention must be given to airway maintenance, treatment of shock and fractures, control of hemorrhage, and prevention of fat embolization, as well as to treatment of splenic rupture, lung perforation, aspiration, atelectasis, or rare complications, such as disseminated intravascular coagulation and acute respiratory distress syndrome.

Evaluation of the head injury requires a detailed history, with particular regard to the time sequence of the specific events. Examination should include precise evaluation of the patient's level of consciousness, the content of verbalization, and performance. Is the child irritable, agitated or confused, disoriented, confabulatory, amnesic, or completely unresponsive? Does the child respond to sound and pain stimuli? Are responses appropriate or purposeless? Several scoring methods help to assess the severity of head injury in a uniform manner. The Glasgow Coma Scale (GCS) is the most widely accepted, and a modified abbreviated injury severity scale emphasizes the pediatric patient (Table 25-17).

Hospitalization is recommended to assess the patient's course and to anticipate and treat complications. The scalp and the skull should be examined carefully for evidence of trauma. All pertinent items must be recorded clearly to provide any examiner or consultant with the comparative analysis that is essential in the management of patients with head injuries. Vital signs, evidence of meningeal irritation, and a description of any discharge from ears or nose should be noted. The level of alertness, spontaneous or induced limb movements, funduscopic findings, symmetry of facial movements (either spontaneous or induced by pain stimuli), muscle tone, tendon reflexes, responses to plantar stimulation, and brainstem signs, including pupillary size and reaction, extraocular movements, corneal response, and gag reflex, should be recorded.

CSF studies are of limited value in head injury, and their routine use cannot be justified. When concurrent meningitis is suspected, however, lumbar puncture is clearly indicated. CSF pressure is usually elevated after any significant degree of cerebral contusion, whether or not there has been a posttraumatic hemorrhage. In the latter instance, headache and meningeal discomfort may be relieved by drawing CSF after the patient's general condition has been stabilized for 72 hours or more. Meningeal signs are often delayed for 8 to 24 hours after subarachnoid hemorrhage. This type of bleeding is common and is not a serious complication except that it produces discomfort and prolongs convalescence. Rarely, after bleeding into the subarachnoid space, obstruction to the CSF pathways at the

TABLE 25-17
GLASGOW COMA SCALE

OBSERVATION	RESPONSE	SCORE
Eye opening (E)	Spontaneous	4
	To speech	3
	To pain	2
	Nil	1
Best motor response (M)	Obeys	6
	Localizes	5
	Withdraws	4
	Abnormal flexion	3
	Extensor response	2
	Nil	1
Best verbal response (V)	Oriented	5
	Confused conversation	4
	Inappropriate words	3
	Incomprehensible sounds	2
	Nil	1

Note: The Glasgow Coma Scale is designed as a standardized assessment of the patient with disturbed consciousness. This scale can be determined serially to determine the patient's progress. The coma scale (E + M + V) = 3–15. All combinations summing to 7 or less define coma. Approximately 50% of scores summing 8 also define coma. Patients achieving a score of 9 or more are noncomatose.

incisura may occur. Although obstruction is often temporary, posttraumatic hydrocephalus may result, necessitating a shunting procedure. Depending on the degree of cerebral damage, the child may not regain full consciousness for a period ranging from hours to several weeks. During this time, supportive care may be complicated by problems of nutrition and electrolyte balance, respiration, bladder care, restlessness, fever, seizures, and otorrhea or rhinorrhea.

Patients who remain unconscious for any significant period may present a problem of fluid balance secondary to posttraumatic diabetes insipidus, syndrome of inappropriate antidiuretic hormone (SIADH) excretion, and a varied degree of hyponatremia and hypernatremia (see Sec. 24.3). Fluid intake, urinary output, weight, and serum electrolyte concentrations should be carefully monitored, but routine restriction of fluid intake as prophylaxis against SIADH is not recommended. Restlessness, increasing stupor, and seizures may result from gross electrolyte imbalance, usually because of failure to recognize thirst or because of iatrogenic water intoxication. As soon as feasible, nutrition and maintenance of fluid balance should progress from intravenous to nasogastric feeding to normal oral feedings. Posttraumatic diabetes insipidus usually is transient and may be treated by simple fluid replacement but occasionally requires treatment with aqueous vasopressin or with desmopressin (DDAVP).

An irritable, lethargic-stuporous state characterizes many injured patients. Depressant drugs of the barbiturate or phenothiazine groups are best avoided in the acute period after injury. Benzodiazepines, such as Ativan (lorazepam) 0.05 mg/kg per dose every 4 to 6 hours or diazepam (Valium) 0.05 to 0.10 mg/kg intravenously or 0.1 to 0.8 mg/kg over 24 hours orally, divided by 4 to 6 hours, are safer alternatives. Benzodiazepine sedation can be reversed if needed with flumazenil (0.1-mg dose intravenously) every 30 to 60 seconds up to a maximum cumulative dose of 1 to 3 mg in 1 hour. Bladder drainage, adequate hydration, loose restraints about wrists and ankles, boxing gloves for older children, and a well-padded crib or bedrails may be necessary to calm and protect the disturbed patient.

Convulsions, other than at the time of the initial impact, demand suppressant therapy. Phosphenytoin is the preferred agent because it does not depress mental status. Dosages and routes of administration are described in detail in Sec. 25.10.2. The appearance of generalized or focal seizures may reflect a subdural or intracortical hematoma, but in such instances seizures are seldom the only manifestation. A clear respiratory passage must be maintained by proper positioning, suction, oropharyngeal airway, endotracheal intubation, or tracheostomy.

Temperature may be elevated in the absence of infection after head injuries, but even in patients with posttraumatic subarachnoid hemorrhage, the temperature rarely exceeds 39°C unless there is severe cortical or brainstem involvement. Patients in the latter category are usually in profound coma and may demonstrate marked temperature elevations above 40°C. If they do not respond to antipyretics and sponging, the use of hypothermia should be considered, maintaining temperature at 33 to 35°C, in an effort to decrease cerebral and general metabolic requirements, when there is probable hypothalamic damage.

Urinary care may become a problem, either because of continued soiling with the resultant skin irritation and breakdown, or because of periodic retention. The usual techniques (diaper, urinary collection bag, or catheter) may be used. Should an indwelling catheter be necessary, prophylactic antibiotics will not prevent infection in the absence of scrupulous aseptic catheter technique and bladder irrigation.

Management of Increased Intracranial Pressure

The best treatment for increased intracranial pressure (ICP) is to remove its cause, if possible; this is usually feasible only when hematoma is present. Children with severe head trauma (ie, those with a GCS of 8 or less) should, when possible, have an ICP monitor placed as quickly as possible. Children with GCS above 8 do not need such invasive monitoring. Head CT readily identifies the cause of the increased ICP, usually cerebral edema or hematoma, and defines the nature and location of hematomas. Intracortical hematomas usually are small and do not require surgical intervention. However, larger hematomas that present with an increase in ICP and focal neurologic signs require surgical evacuation. Cerebral edema occurs in up to 50% of children with severe head trauma and is believed to result usually from increased cerebral blood flow secondary to loss of autoregulation. Consequently, there may be little evidence of edema on CT scan, although ventricles and cisterns will appear effaced.

In early stages, hyperventilation is considered to be the ideal method for controlling ICP. This causes cerebral vasoconstriction by lowering arterial PCO_2. Arterial PCO_2 should be kept around 30 mm Hg, and the head of the bed elevated to 20 to 30 degrees (while maintaining the head and neck in the midline position) to facilitate venous drainage. Hyperosmolar agents (particularly mannitol and glycerol) are helpful, although initially they may increase cerebral blood flow and may enlarge intracranial hematomas. If mannitol is needed in the latter instance to avoid herniation, prompt surgical evacuation of the hematoma should follow. Hyperosmolar agents produce a marked diuresis and a decrease in cerebral bulk by dehydration. Mannitol is the agent of choice and is infused as a 20% solution in dosages of 0.25 to 1.00 g/kg. Ideally, administration of hyperosmolar agents should be guided by direct measurement of ICP with an intracranial monitor, with the goal of keeping ICP below 15 mm Hg. Uncontrolled ICP that is consistently above 20 mm Hg carries a high morbidity and mortality. Of the various monitors available, the ventricular type has the added advantage that it can reduce ICP by removal of CSF. Although the efficacy of mannitol diminishes by 24 hours, rebound swelling may occur, and therapy may be needed for several days. A bladder catheter should be inserted whenever these agents are used, and electrolyte balance and serum osmolality should be carefully monitored.

Moderate hypothermia (32 to 34°C) implemented for 24 hours soon after severe traumatic brain injury occurred was found to improve outcome at 3 and 6 months in patients without flaccidity or decerebrate rigidity (those with GCS between 5 and 7). Although steroids have been used empirically, no controlled study has clearly demonstrated the efficacy of steroids in the management of head trauma, and their routine use is not recommended. Attempts to decrease cerebral metabolism by pentobarbital coma remains controversial but may be considered in patients with intractable increased ICP. The initial dose is 3 to 5 mg/kg intravenously, followed by hourly doses sufficient to maintain a burst-suppression pattern on EEG. With posttraumatic subarachnoid hemorrhage, hemorrhagic contusions, or parenchymal hematoma, volume expansion in conjunction with a calcium channel blocker such as nimodipine may be beneficial. Patients with severe head injury should, whenever possible, be cared for at a center with availability of sequential CT studies, electrophysiology, and a trauma intensive care unit. Neurologic outcome depends primarily on three factors: the level of consciousness, the underlying lesion on CT scan, and the initial ICP.

Children have a better prognosis than do adults with comparable injuries. With severe head injuries, about one-third of children die, and less than 12% are left severely disabled or vegetative. Most favorable outcome is attained by children age 5 to 10 years, and children younger than 4 years suffer high mortality (62% by 12 months) and poor outcome (88%). The factors that have been associated with high mortality in settings of severe head injury are: pupillary abnormalities in the emergency room and hypotension. The factors associated with poor neurologic outcome include: cerebral edema, intracranial hematoma, coma for 24 hours or more, sustained high ICP (> 20 mm Hg), and a motor response at 72 hours that is flaccid, flexor posturing, or withdrawal. Seventy percent of children with moderate disability at discharge will require special education. It is noteworthy that 40% of children with severe head trauma who were thought to have good outcomes at time of discharge were found on later follow-up to have moderate disability (significant work and school problems). Therefore, regardless of initial outcome, all children with severe head trauma as defined by a GCS of 8 or less should have close monitoring to ensure that the child's educational and vocational needs are met as the child matures.

To obtain optimal survival of the severely brain-injured patient, management must be aggressive, constant, and total, as long as any potential for recovery exists. Determinations of brain death in children over age 5 years should follow the guidelines recommended by the Presidential Commission: clinical appraisal of absent brain and brainstem function noted twice 6 hours apart and confirmed by ancillary tests. These include an EEG showing electrocerebral silence or a radionuclear scan or angiogram showing absent arterial blood flow. For children under age 5 years, a special task force recommends that the period of observation between the two examinations vary according to the age of the infant or child: 48 hours for infants aged 7 days to 2 months; 24 hours for infants 2 months to 1 year, and 12 hours for children 1 to 5 years of age. Two EEGs at each interval are also recommended, but if a radionuclear scan shows no arterial flow to the brain, further tests are unnecessary. Determinations of brain death should be carried out as expeditiously as possible to avoid undue suffering of the child's family.

CEREBRAL CONTUSION AND LACERATION

Contusions are ecchymosis of the brain, usually located on its surface, that may result in focal neurologic signs. With an impression injury (ie, direct blow to a fixed head), the brain underlying the area of impact may be contused (coup lesion). With an acceleration-deceleration injury, the brain injury may be distant from the site of impact, often directly opposite it (contre-coup lesion). Frontal and temporal poles are often injured following trauma to the occipital region.

DIFFUSE AXONAL INJURY OR SHEARING

Diffuse axonal injury can occur with more severe head trauma and is more frequently seen with acceleration-deceleration injuries, such as those observed with motor vehicle accidents, rather than with a simple fall. The different densities of gray and white matter lead to different rates of speed during acceleration and to different stopping times with rapid deceleration. This results in shearing of the white matter, usually at the gray-white matter junction. Lesions may be seen in the cerebrum, cerebellar peduncle, or corpus callosum. In the acute phase the CT scan may be normal or demonstrate diffuse swelling. Later, oval areas of hemorrhage in the gray-white matter may be observed. MR imaging is more sensitive to this injury, especially if no hemorrhage has occurred, where it appears as a high signal on T_2. In the absence of a contusion or hematoma, axonal injury is usually responsible for prolonged alterations in level of alertness.

EPIDURAL HEMATOMA

Epidural hematoma refers to bleeding between the skull and the dura, usually when the temporal bone fracture causes a tear of the middle meningeal artery. It may also result from a tear in the extradural vessels. As the skull matures, vessels in this location are firmly embedded in the bony grooves and are more vulnerable to damage by fractures. Children younger than 2 years rarely sustain extradural hemorrhages because these vessels are less adherent to the calvarium. Because of the greater elasticity of the young skull, epidural hematomas are often not accompanied by an underlying skull fracture. Untreated extradural hematomas are among the most lethal complications of head trauma, with mortality close to 100%. Treatment demands immediate diagnosis and surgery. CT or MR imaging should be considered with less severe trauma.

The typical clinical syndrome is apparent during the first 12 to 24 hours after the initial injury. The child may be rendered unconscious by the original trauma then regain awareness after several hours. Hematomas of arterial origin can expand rapidly and acutely raise ICP, resulting in hypertension and bradycardia and a progressive decline in the level of mental alertness. Focal seizures may occur. The asymmetric pressure build-up may cause a shift of cerebral contents, leading to herniation of the tip of the temporal lobe (uncus) under the tentorium and compression of the midbrain. Early in its course, the uncal herniation syndrome is characterized by pupillary asymmetry on the side of the hematoma that evolves into a complete third-nerve palsy and progressive hemiplegia, which is opposite to the lesion in 85% of cases. In late stages both pupils become fixed and dilated, respiration is slow or irregular, and flaccidity, hypotension, and tachycardia develop. Subhyaloid hemorrhages may occur, which are mobile collections between the retina and the overlying subhyaloid membrane. In young children a lucid interval may be absent. The syndrome usually runs its course of 6 to 12 hours in adults but may extend from 24 to 96 hours in children because of the higher incidence of venous rather than arterial bleeding. Either type is more commonly associated with anemia in young children than in adults. The prognosis for survival and neurologic integrity is contingent on preoperative status and duration of unconsciousness. With prompt diagnosis and surgical intervention, a complete recovery without residua can be expected.

SUBDURAL HEMATOMA

Subdural hematomas are common in children. Approximately 85% occur in children age 1 year or less. The syndrome may present acutely (within 3 days), subacutely (within 4 to 20 days), or chronically (more than 20 days) after the trauma. To some extent this classification defines the severity of the initial injury and the urgency for treatment. Acute lesions may result from arterial bleeding and require surgical evacuation. The rapidly developing mass effect of the hemorrhage may be compounded by the underlying brain contusion or laceration (Fig. 25-29). The latter injury determines the quality of recovery. Chronic lesions are distinctly rare after 12

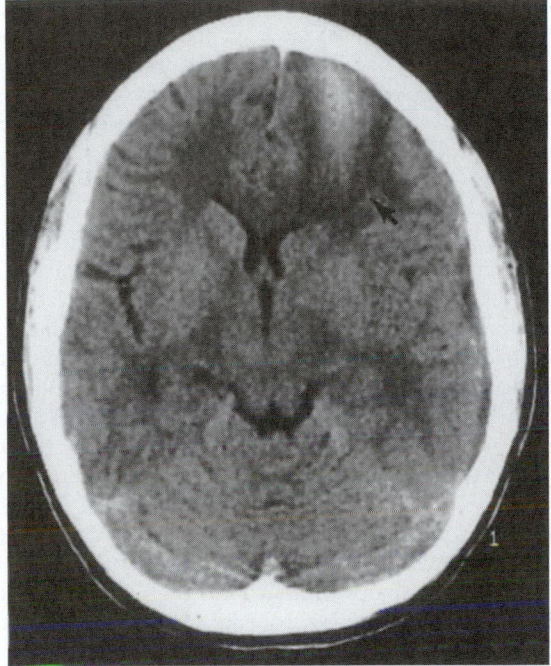

A

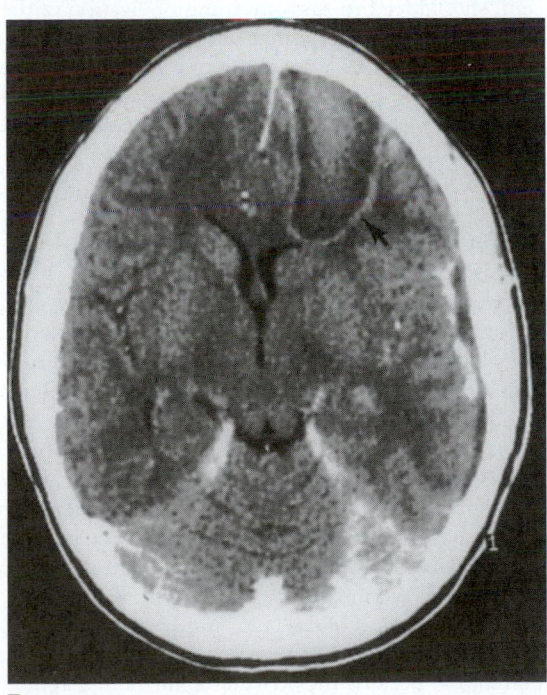

B

FIGURE 25-29 Axial CT scan precontrast administration (A) demonstrates left frontal parenchymal density owing to resolving subacute hematoma with mass effect on the frontal horn and typical "ring enhancement" after contrast (B). Note linear enhancement of a membrane associated with the subacute left subdural hematoma also present. *Courtesy of Dr. Jacqueline Bello.*

months of age and are often bilateral. The etiology is mechanical trauma or bacterial meningitis. Most idiopathic lesions are the result of unrecognized trauma. Suspicion of child abuse, especially of the shaken baby syndrome, warrants a dilated funduscopic examination to detect retinal hemorrhages and long-bone radiographs to help confirm abuse. Chronic lesions are encapsulated by a thin vascular outer membrane and contain serosanguineous fluid with a high protein concentration. Subdural paracentesis is both diagnostic and therapeutic. Daily removal of small amounts of CSF, preferably not more than 10 to 20 mL, relieves ICP and helps decrease the size of the hematoma. Removal of larger amounts should be avoided as it may favor reaccumulation. Shunting of the fluid to the peritoneal cavity may be necessary in larger effusions. This procedure obviates the loss of protein contained in the effusion and provides continuous drainage while the infant's brain continues to grow. Recovery is excellent if concomitant parenchymal damage did not occur during the initial injury.

SEQUELAE OF CRANIOCEREBRAL TRAUMA

Fixed neurologic deficits may exist after head injury. The less predictable sequelae are seizures, organic mental changes, and post-concussion syndrome.

SEIZURES Posttraumatic seizures are classified based on the time at which they occur in relation to the head injury. Early seizures occur within the first week of trauma, and late seizures 1 week to 5 years after injury. About 15% of early seizures occur within the first few seconds of injury (impact seizures) and are of no prognostic significance. Early posttraumatic seizures occur more frequently in children than in adults with comparable injuries. Much of the increase is explained by a greater susceptibility of children younger than 5 years to have seizures following even minor head injuries. In a population-based study from the Mayo Clinic, the overall incidence of early posttraumatic seizures in children was 2.6% but increased to 30% with severe head trauma. About 45 to 60% of seizures are focal, 10% are focal with secondary generalization, and the remainder are generalized. Over two-thirds of early seizures in children occur within the first 24 hours after injury. The risk of seizures is greatest with penetrating head injuries, contusions, lacerations, or intraparenchymal lesions. Seizures that are less likely to recur are nonfocal, occur within the first hour after injury, or are associated with a skull fracture. One or more seizures occur in 10% of patients with a depressed skull fracture.

The incidence of late epilepsy varies across studies from 0 to 25% and is lower in children than adults at each level of severity. Rates of late seizures increase according to the severity of injury, ranging from 0.2% with mild injury to 7.4% with severe injury. There is no relationship between early and late seizures provided the injury is taken into account. The EEG is not helpful in predicting late posttraumatic epilepsy, as it may be normal in 30% of individuals who later develop epilepsy. The majority of late seizures occur within the first year after head trauma, and nearly a third of them take place within the first 3 months.

Short-term treatment with anticonvulsants is appropriate when nonimpact seizures occur after head trauma, especially if the CT scan shows additional risk factors, such as intracranial hematomas, contusions, cerebral lacerations, or focal neurologic signs. Anticonvulsant therapy should continue throughout the acute stages of head injury, particularly if there is persistent increase in ICP, but should be discontinued before discharge from the hospital. Prolonged anticonvulsant prophylaxis after early seizures does not prevent the onset of late seizures and is not recommended. Long-term treatment should be reserved for children who have two or more late seizures.

ORGANIC MENTAL CHANGES Self-limited memory defects and minor personality changes may be noted after head injury. Persistent frank organic dementia is uncommon in children, as is intellectual defect; severe and extensive injuries, particularly in infancy, may result in psychomotor retardation. As noted, higher rates of learning disabilities are found among children with severe head injuries, even when they are found to have a good outcome at time of discharge. The full role of MR imaging in head trauma has yet to be established, but MR imaging may be of value in assessing the late effects of trauma, particularly as regards cognitive-behavioral changes. Relatively normal CT studies may exist in the presence of small areas of white matter demyelination, axonal damage, shearing injuries, and brainstem pathology.

In addition to cognitive sequelae, traumatic brain injury (TBI) may result in posttraumatic attention-deficit disorder and clinical depression. Early identification and treatment of either neurobehavioral sequela is needed to allow TBI patients to fulfill their rehabilitative potential.

POSTTRAUMATIC SYNDROME General sequelae after head injury (posttraumatic syndrome) are less common in children than in adults. The symptoms tend to vary somewhat from those in the adult (ie, headache, irritability, and postural vertigo). They are more commonly in the realm of enuresis, disturbances in sleep pattern, episodically aggressive behavior, and decline in school performance. How much of this is caused by organic factors rather than primarily psychological factors is difficult to state. Symptomatic management with sedatives, tranquilizers, and sometimes psychotherapy may be needed. Investigation as to the presence of typical or fragmentary convulsive phenomena may be profitable, and improvement may be noted after anticonvulsive therapy is instituted.

A common-sense attitude toward general care during the acute phase is important. Overhospitalization, gratuitous unfounded remarks about possible future brain damage, and prolonged litigation correlate highly with the incidence of posttraumatic behavior dysfunction. The physician must maintain an attitude of expectancy for return to normal function, both with the parents and with the child. Avoiding oversolicitous and unnecessary limitations on school, play, and social activities will ameliorate a common factor in the causation of the posttraumatic reaction syndrome. Group statistic studies have tended to indicate that children with behavioral and mental defects are more prone to head injury and more prone to display sequelae than are mentally stable children.

25.9.3   Spinal Cord Injury

Spinal cord injury (SCI) in children is uncommon. The proportion of injuries involving children varies from 0.1 to under 10%, largely based on whether children over age 12 years are included. The incidence of pediatric spinal cord injury was 18.2 per million among 1 to 12 year olds in one population-based study. In most pediatric series the male-to-female ratio of SCI is about 2:1, but females predominate in children younger than 3 years. Motor vehicle accidents and falls are the two most frequent causes of pediatric SCI.

Young children sustain motor vehicle accidents mostly as pedestrians, older children mostly as passengers. Nonaccidental injuries, especially related to sports or to firearms, increase in frequency in adolescence. Obstetrical trauma is the most common cause of SCI in infancy. Most injuries result from breech presentations with excessive traction applied, leading to nerve damage and spinal cord lesions, involving usually the cervical or upper thoracic region. Intrauterine hyperextension of the neck in breech presentations carries a 25% risk of developing significant neurologic deficits.

Maturational and biomechanical factors account for the differences noted between pediatric and adult spinal cord injuries. The young spine contains a greater amount of cartilage, which, coupled with ligamentous laxity and flatter interarticulate facets, makes it more mobile and more susceptible to anterior subluxation. Spinal injury in the young is also associated with a paucity of avulsion chips but rather greater involvement of cartilaginous endplates. Moreover, the relatively larger size of the infant head in relation to the body places the fulcrum of mobility higher in the spinal column than it is in adults. These characteristics help explain why compared to adults, children, especially those under age 3 years, suffer a larger proportion of cervical and upper thoracic spine injuries and have a higher frequency of spinal cord injury without radiographic abnormality (SCIWORA). This latter type of injury is observed in 20 to 60% of pediatric spinal injury and in most series has a poor prognosis for functional recovery. Older children, however, have lower rates of SCIWORA (about 12%) and rarely have complete spinal injury. Spinal cord injury without radiographic abnormality may recur or be delayed in its onset from minutes to days after the initial trauma, an event that is often heralded by mild or transient neurologic findings. Therefore, any spinal cord sign, no matter how evanescent, should lead to aggressive immobilization of the spine, strictly enforced for 2 to 3 months after the injury to prevent recurrence of SCIWORA. The spectrum of spinal injury ranges from whiplash, where the spine is hyperextended or overflexed and symptoms are mostly musculoskeletal in origin, to complete severance or infarction of the spinal cord.

Diagnosis

Birth injuries can be suspected when excessive force is applied to extract the fetus. Resuscitation may be difficult; there may be intercostal paralysis, restricted thoracic movements, and a weak cry. The child's leg will be flaccid, abducted, and motionless. Sensory assessment is difficult, but a decreased response to pain, such as the lack of grimace, may be noted below the site of the lesion. An absent Gallant response, a reflex in which scratching the paraspinal region elicits incurvation of the spine toward the side of the stimulus, helps determine the level of thoracic lesions in newborns. The diagnosis is usually self-evident but at times may be confused with neonatal asphyxia, intracranial injury, congenital defects, or progressive infantile spinal muscular atrophy.

Spinal shock, a period of flaccidity and areflexia following acute injury, gives way after about 2 weeks to varying degrees of spasticity and hyperreflexia. Because the neonatal spine is often injured across several segments, a clearly demarcated level may be lacking, and often the injury will not produce spasticity. Mass reflex consisting of complete flexion of the affected region can follow stimulation and should not be misconstrued as return of function. If the infant survives, neurologic sequelae will vary according to the site and severity of the lesion.

Spinal radiographs of birth injuries are often normal, although fracture or subluxation may be detected. A number of normal variations of the cervical spine in childhood (pseudodislocation, hypermobility, etc) often make interpretation difficult and are cause of interpretive error. CT myelography or spinal MR imaging will delineate bony lesions as well as soft-tissue injury.

Management

The neonate requires immediate attention to airway patency, oxygenation, and suction, as well as meticulous attention to skin, bladder, and bowel care. Early bladder dysfunction can lead to overflow dribbling, which can be avoided by an indwelling catheter followed by intermittent catheterization on a 4- to 6-hour schedule until the child develops an automatic/expressible bladder. Postvoid residual urine may be determined with ultrasound so as to avoid catheterization and the risk of infection. Urinary tract infections should be treated promptly with antibiotics, but prophylactic antibiotics are usually reserved for cases of vesicoureteral reflux. Early in life, sphincter control may be adequate, but as the child grows older, surgery may be required to maintain adequate function. Myelography and surgery do not enhance recovery and are thus not indicated. Survivors usually have normal intelligence; they can use their arms fairly well, but cannot sit or walk independently.

In older children, treatment is aimed at stabilizing the spine and restoring function free of pain. In handling the child, the spine should be kept in neutral alignment, avoiding flexion, extension, or rotation of the spine. To prevent further manipulation, clothing should not be removed and only anterior and lateral radiographs should be obtained. If the radiographs detect a fracture or dislocation, the spine should be stabilized with a brace or traction. With traction, dislocated vertebrae usually relocate in normal alignment within 24 to 36 hours. If no such injury is documented, the spine may be gently positioned for a complete series of radiographs, including oblique and open-mouth view. Every child with acute SCI should promptly be given intravenous methylprednisolone, which has been shown to enhance motor and sensory recovery in both complete and partial SCI. The recommended dosage entails an intravenous bolus of 33 mg/kg of methylprednisolone given no later than 8 hours after the injury followed by an hourly maintenance intravenous infusion of 5 mg/kg per hour for the next 23 hours. During the early stages, the patient should not be given anything by mouth or any drugs that would mask neurologic changes.

Open injuries must be treated surgically. Closed cord injuries may require surgical treatment, but unwise surgery in patients with cervical fractures may be fatal, and the indication of surgery must be appraised with great care. Survival rate is decreased with severe injuries above the C5 vertebra. In cervical lesions the correlation between radiographic lesion and physiological loss of cord function is often poor because of the increased frequency of SCIWORA. The radiograms may show crushing of vertebral bodies fragmentation of the pedicles, laminae, and spines; and dislocation with facets locked entirely out of position. Under no circumstances should the cervical spine be manipulated to reduce a fracture. Immediate decompressive laminectomy for the injured cervical cord is attended by severe morbidity and high mortality and should not be considered except in two instances: if there is progressive loss of function in the setting of an incomplete cord lesion, or if a bony fragment(s) impinging on the cervical cord does not respond to traction. Cord compression resulting from a centrally extruded intervertebral disk can be seen easily on spinal MR imaging.

The thoracic segments of the vertebral column form a relatively rigid mass. The thoracic vertebral canal is the narrowest of all parts of the canal, and the spinal cord throughout its thoracic extent has a less rich blood supply than at either the cervical or the lumbar level. Spinal cord injury at this level is usually the result of direct severe trauma and carries a poor prognosis. All these factors must be considered in the early care of closed injuries to this area. Cord compression will almost invariably reveal total block of the flow of CSF. The value of surgical decompression is highly variable.

As with injury at the thoracic level, dislocation of one lumbar vertebral body under another, wedging of a body with kyphosis, or fracture of the posterior arches calls for immediate decompressive laminectomy. Injury to the conus medullaris (T12 to L1 vertebral levels) is of grave significance. Below that level, the delicate filaments of the cauda equina may be badly torn and attenuated, the injury being associated with considerable subarachnoid hemorrhage.

The long-term care and rehabilitation of patients with spinal injuries provide a challenge that is often best met in a specific center or unit geared to this type of care. Extensive efforts to reestablish bowel and bladder function will be needed, as will attention to such considerations as skin integrity, nutrition, late syndromes of pain, spasms, autonomic dysfunction, genitourinary complications, psychiatric problems, and programs of education and training.

25.9.4   Peripheral Nerve Injuries

Injuries to the peripheral nervous system are not common in childhood. Those seen early in life usually result from damage to the brachial plexus or sciatic nerves. The spinal roots of the fifth cervical through the first thoracic nerves form the brachial plexus. These roots are poorly stabilized at birth, and traction damage is rarely transmitted to the spinal cord. Injuries to infants result in almost pure root syndromes, as contrasted with the more distal involvement and diffuse damage seen with injuries in older children and adults. Children recover better than adults in regard to both spontaneous resolution and surgical results.

Etiologically, any force that changes the normal relationships of arms, shoulder, and neck may result in plexus injury. Birth trauma is the most common cause. The plexus has points of fascial fixation to the first rib medially and the coracoid process of the scapula laterally. Abducting the arm stretches the nerves under and against the coracoid, resulting in stretch, avulsion, or compression of the lower plexus. Lateral deviation of the head and depression of the shoulder will stretch the nerves over and against the first ribs, resulting in similar damage to the upper plexus. Traction injuries of these types may occur with breech or cephalic deliveries. Risk factors associated with brachial plexus injury include macrosomia, forceps, shoulder dystocia, and gestational diabetes. Over half of brachial plexus injuries are a result of shoulder dystocia; however, such injuries do occur in the absence of birth trauma. In normal or low-weight infants, brachial plexus is linked to malpresentations other than breech. Bilateral injuries are reported in 2 to 6% of brachial palsies and are usually seen with breech deliveries. Other neonatal morbidity reported in populations of infants with brachial plexus injury are mild to severe birth asphyxia and subarachnoid hemorrhage.

UPPER PLEXUS ROOT INJURIES   Upper plexus root injuries (Erb-Duchenne type) are the most common. The shoulder sags, the arm hangs limp in internal rotation, and the wrist is pronated, reflecting paralysis of spinati, deltoid, biceps, brachioradialis, and extensor carpi radialis muscles, and often rhomboids, serratus, and levator scapulae. The tendon reflexes of the involved arm are usually lost, but a sensory defect is unusual. Treatment requires that the deformity be overcome to prevent posterior subluxation of the humeral head from the glenoid fossa. The arm should be placed in abduction and external rotation by a brace or by pinning a towel over the wrist and fixing it to the mattress in the desired position. The full range of motion of the shoulder should be maintained by passive exercises performed daily. Anomalous plexus configuration may include the fourth cervical root, or trauma may be transmitted to this level, resulting in phrenic nerve damage and ipsilateral diaphragmatic paralysis, which is rarely a problem unless significant bilateral injury has occurred. Ninety to 92 percent of these patients will experience complete recovery within 3 months. An additional 8% may demonstrate initial improvement at 4 to 5 months of age. Infants who have not achieved antigravity strength of the biceps, triceps, or deltoid by age 6 months of age have a poor prognosis for functional recovery and should be referred for possible surgical intervention. Preoperatively, brachial plexus MR imaging and EMG are valuable in determining the presence of nerve root avulsion and extent of nerve damage, but false-negative results do occur. The timing of surgical repair is controversial. Some advocate repair in a subgroup of candidate infants at age 6 months to avoid the permanent changes that result from chronic denervation and decreased mobility. However, since spontaneous improvement may be seen up to a year of age, a more conservative approach that avoids unnecessary surgeries is to defer the procedure until age 11 to 12 months. The operative repair is determined at the time of surgery based on the injury present and the results of intraoperative electrophysiological testing. A positive nerve action potential through the affected site is associated with a 90% chance of functional recovery (ie, antigravity movement) following surgery. Surgical procedures include neuronolysis, nerve grafting (from the sural nerve), neuroma resection and removal, and direct end-to-end repair. Attainment of antigravity movement is seen in 75 to 90% of patients who undergo surgical intervention. Root avulsions are not aided by surgery. In older children, muscle transfer and tendon release of contractures may be employed to enhance functional mobility.

LOWER PLEXUS ROOT INJURIES Lower plexus root injuries (Klumpke-Dejerine type) show more sensory and vasomotor involvement, with paralysis of the flexors and extensors of the forearm and the intrinsic muscles of the hand. Marked involvement of the first thoracic root results in cervical sympathetic damage and Horner syndrome, often with delay in normal pigmentation of the ipsilateral iris. The tendon reflexes are usually intact, with a poor grasp response. Sensory changes involve the ulnar side of the hand and the forearm. Dependent edema and cyanosis are common. Treatment involves splinting the forearm and the wrist in a neutral position, with passive range-of-motion exercises. The majority of patients recover completely within 3 to 6 months, although the prognosis is not as favorable as in upper plexus lesions. Direct plexus surgery is less rewarding than with upper plexus surgical repairs, partly because avulsions occur more frequently with lower plexus lesions. Surgical intervention is indicated in combined upper and lower plexus lesions when antigravity movements are not attained. Only 64% of combined upper and lower plexus injuries improved after surgical repair. Injuries to the brachial plexus in older children are usually of mixed upper and lower plexus types. If they are caused by traction and hyperabduction, the prognosis may be good, although at this age, the usual cause is severe trauma, which often results in root avulsion or degrees of hemorrhage and scarring that preclude functional recovery. Microvascular surgical techniques have improved the outlook of these procedures following trauma.

For patients with persistent defects, orthopedic procedures to stabilize joints in favorable positions and tendon transplantation, where feasible, are the only available treatments.

The peripheral nerves in the arm may be involved alone or in varied combination, usually after direct laceration trauma or severe injuries with combined osseous-vascular-neural damage. Compression neuropathies are uncommon in childhood.

SERRATUS ANTERIOR PALSY Serratus anterior palsy owing to involvement of the long thoracic nerve (nerve of Bell) is usually the result of pressure on the shoulder or excessive forceful activity with the arms elevated. It is most frequently seen in prepubertal boys in association with baseball pitching, weight lifting, or carrying heavy loads. The scapula becomes winglike with horizontal forward pressure of the arms, and there is weakness in lifting and arm elevation because of impaired scapula fixation. Treatment should provide full functional recovery, although some residual scapular winging may persist. Activities possibly associated with the lesion should be discontinued. During the first week the weight of the shoulder may be removed from the scapula by a simple arm sling, but this is often not necessary unless the paralysis is total or there is considerable discomfort. Range-of-motion exercises, then more active shoulder-strengthening maneuvers, are the only measures indicated.

AXILLARY OR CIRCUMFLEX NERVE The axillary or circumflex nerve that innervates the deltoid and teres minor muscles is usually injured only in association with anterior dislocation of the shoulder, particularly when associated with fractures of the greater tuberosity of the humerus. The axillary nerve winds around the surgical neck of the humerus and may be injured by fractures at this location. Injury to the nerve is detected by inability to abduct the arm to the horizontal position and a zone of hypoesthesia of the lower posterior deltoid area. Therapy is that for the primary injury, and with rare exceptions full neural recovery can be anticipated.

RADIAL NERVE INJURY Radial nerve injury is frequently the result of fracture through the middle third of the humerus, with neural stretch or contusion. The triceps muscle may not be involved, but there is marked weakness of the brachioradialis and the extensors of the wrist and fingers (wristdrop). Sensation is lost in an area between index finger and thumb on the dorsum of the hand. In the acute state it is impossible to tell whether the nerve has been lacerated or severed. Therefore, where feasible, open reduction of the fracture and nerve repair are reasonable considerations. Later, electrical testing will help determine if there is anatomic continuity of the nerve. Where permanent residua exist in spite of all efforts, tendon transplantation gives quite effective wrist, finger, and thumb extension.

THE ULNAR NERVE The ulnar nerve may be lacerated along its course in the forearm near the wrist or in conjunction with fractures as it passes behind the medial epicondyle of the humerus at the elbow. The epiphysis of the medial epicondyle does not fuse to the humerus until late adolescence and is particularly prone to avulsion. The ulnar nerve may be contused at the time of injury or compressed later by scar formation. Sensory loss involves the fifth digit and ulnar half of the fourth digit and extends along the medial side of the palm to the lower forearm. Weakness may involve the interossei, lumbricales, and hypothenar muscles, as well as the adductor pollicis, the flexor carpi ulnaris, and the deep flexors of the fourth and fifth digits, resulting in defects in spreading the fingers, adducting the thumb, flexing the fourth and fifth digits at the distal interphalangeal joints, and poor apposition of the fifth finger. Treatment is that for the primary injury. Surgical intervention depends on how nearly intact the nerve is, as determined by clinical and electrical studies, and can consist of suturing or grafting the involved nerve.

THE MEDIAN NERVE The median nerve may be damaged in the same way as the ulnar nerve, and the two are often injured together. In addition to the more common laceration injury, the nerve may be damaged in anterior dislocation fractures at the elbow or the wrist. There is sensory loss on the palmar surface of the hand that involves the thumb, the index and middle fingers, the radial half of the ring finger, and the radial surface of the palm. Weaknesses in the pronators of the forearm, the long flexors of the fingers, and the short adductor and opponens of the thumb are the major motor defects. Therapeutic considerations are similar to those of ulnar palsy.

THE SCIATIC NERVE AND ITS BRANCHES The sciatic nerve and its branches are involved in injuries of the legs. It is the largest nerve in the body, and at the knee it divides into the tibial and common peroneal nerves. Iatrogenic trauma secondary to intramuscular injection is the leading cause of sciatic neuropathy in infancy. Lesions of this type are seen also in older children and adults. The normal course of the sciatic nerve in the hollow midway between the ischial tuberosity and the greater trochanter under cover of the gluteus maximus muscle varies greatly. This fact, taken together with the small size of the infant's gluteal mass and the potential neurotoxicity of many antibiotics, makes it unwise to use this area for intramuscular injections. *Intragluteal injections are contraindicated in infancy and should be used in older children with extreme caution.* The anterolateral compartment of the thigh and the deltoid area are safer and always preferable. Complete sciatic lesions produce total foot paralysis and loss of leg flexion. There is a flail footdrop, an absence of ankle jerk, and a sensory loss below the knee involving the entire leg except for its medial aspect.

The tragedy of nerve injury in infancy is accentuated by the residua of short, small extremities that result from lack of stimulation of the muscle-tendon movement that is essential to bone growth. All sciatic palsy must be carefully evaluated with a view toward surgery, although high lesions rarely show complete recovery and are usually associated with marked permanent disability.

THE PERONEAL NERVE The peroneal nerve is vulnerable to pressure neuropathy as well as other injury. It descends from the popliteal fossa to a superficial position on the lateral aspect of the leg, passing posterior to the head of the fibula. Injury there results in sensory loss over the dorsum of the foot and the anterolateral surface of the leg, with weakness of the dorsiflexors and evertors of the foot and the toes. The *tibial nerve* descends deep in the calf, rounds the posterior aspect of the medial malleolus, and enters the foot. It innervates the muscles controlling plantar flexion of the foot and the toes and the intrinsic muscles of the foot. Sensory loss is usually confined to the sole. Combined peroneal and tibial nerve injuries often occur. Treatment is similar to that described for ulnar nerve injuries.

25.9.5 Cranial Nerve Injuries

Trauma to the cranial nerves is seldom an isolated occurrence; it usually reflects more diffuse craniocerebral injury. The olfactory nerve is frequently torn as its filaments pass from the subfrontal area of the brain through the cribriform plate. The defect is rarely complete and is usually asymptomatic. If severe anosmia persists, distortion of taste is the presenting complaint. Injury to the chiasmal area is uncommon. The hypothalamus and the brainstem usually receive the brunt of injury in this region, with resulting fatality.

Optic nerve injury resulting in traumatic optic neuropathy (TON) is a rare but serious complication of closed head injury. It is, therefore, important to carefully monitor visual acuity after facial and frontal injuries. TON occurs in association with orbital fracture, but it may be seen with cerebral contusion and hemorrhage into the nerve sheath. Most optic nerve lesions are believed to result from damage to the intracanalicular segment of the nerve caused by acceleration-deceleration injuries to the supraorbital and frontal regions of the cranium. Late injuries to the optic nerve may also result from local swelling within the intracanalicular portion. Treatment of TON includes methylprednisolone at the doses employed in traumatic spinal cord injury (see Sec. 25.9.3) or surgical decompression of the optic canal. Both therapies are more effective in improving visual acuity than no treatment, yet neither one is found to be more effective than the other or to a combined therapeutic approach. Fractures portend a worse prognosis than no fractures, and posterior orbital fractures appear to have a worse prognosis than anterior orbital fractures.

The most common cranial nerve injuries are those involving the third, fourth, sixth, seventh, and eighth nerves. Fractures or transmitted trauma that lacerates the carotid artery in its cavernous sinus position may result in a carotid-cavernous fistula. Damage to the oculomotor nerves is more common, and permanent or transient dysfunctions of the extraocular muscles occur more frequently in children than in adults.

Fractures through the petrous portion of the temporal bone may damage the facial nerve. Paralysis may be immediate or delayed. Neonatal facial paralysis may follow forceps extraction or may reflect unusual positions in utero. Immediate treatment must be directed to corneal protection. Damage to the nerve distal to the geniculate ganglion may be associated with blood behind the tympanic membrane and a conductive hearing loss. Injury central to the ganglion tends to be associated with labyrinthine dysfunction and a pattern of sensorineural hearing loss, implying a level of injury that is not amenable to direct therapy. In all other instances, evaluation and management are aimed at the functional state of the nerve. Electrodiagnostic tests to determine and follow the degree of degeneration and estimate anatomic continuity of the nerve are not infalliable; however, when there is evidence of neural degeneration, careful evaluation should be made, and consideration should be given to operative intervention. Surgical decompression or nerve grafting, where feasible, gives the best results. Hypoglossal-facial anastomosis and plastic procedures to enhance facial symmetry are less satisfactory, but at times they offer the only possible approach to the problem.

Fractures through the base of the skull, direct blows on or near the ear, or extravasation of blood from subarachnoid hemorrhage may affect both vestibular and auditory components of the eighth cranial nerve as well as directly damage the labyrinth, cochlea, or middle ear. Posttraumatic neural deafness has a relatively poor prognosis for full recovery. Labyrinthine dysfunction, as evidenced by postural vertigo and increased sensitivity to motion, is usually transient.

Trauma of all types increasingly is being addressed as a public health problem. Epidemiologic patterns of morbidity in addition to mortality statistics and the further definition of risk factors relating to motor vehicle accidents, sports, recreational activities, and occupational factors are being increasingly emphasized. The use of vehicle restraints, bicycle helmet use by all riders, and mass media efforts to effect appropriate safety attitude conditioning are expanding. Trauma registries, meaningful injury coding, and hospital discharge data remain in their infancy, but injury science is evolving, with the Centers for Disease Control enlarging the subsection Center for Environmental Health and Injury Control. The National Head Injury Foundation, Inc. (333 Turnpike Road, Southborough, MA 01772) maintains extensive directory lists regarding specialized head injury programs, related reports, educational materials, and resource training guidelines for students with traumatic and related brain injury.

References

AMA Diagnostic and Treatment Guidelines Concerning Child Abuse and Neglect. Council on Scientific Affairs. JAMA 254:796, 1985

Annegers JF, Grabow JD, Groover RV, Laws ER Jr, Elveback LR, Kurland LT: Seizures after head trauma: a population study. Neurology 30:683–689, 1980

Bracken MB, Shepard MJ, Collins WF, et al: A randomized controlled trial of methylprednisolone or naloxone in the treatment of acute spinal-cord injury. Results of the Second National Acute Spinal Cord Injury Study. N Engl J Med 322:1405–1411, 1990

Bruce DA, Alavi A, Bilaniuk L, et al: Diffuse cerebral swelling following head injuries in children: the syndrome of "malignant brain edema." J Neurosurg 54:170–178, 1981

Cook MW, Levin LA, Joseph MP, Pinczower EF: Traumatic optic neuropathy. A meta analysis. Arch Otolaryngol Head Neck Surg 122:389–392, 1996

Einhorn A, Mizrahi EM: Basilar skull fractures in children. The incidence of CNS infection and the use of antibiotics. Am J Dis Child 132:1121, 1978

Filley CM, Cranberg LD, Alexander MP, et al: Neurobehavioral outcome after closed head injury in childhood and adolescence. Arch Neurol 44:194, 1987

Gilbert WM, Nesbitt TS, Danielsen S: Associated factors in 1611 cases of brachial plexus injury. Obstet Gynecol 93:536–540, 1999

Kalff R, Kocks W, Pospiech J, et al: Clinical outcome after head injury in children. Childs Nerv Syst 5:156, 1989

Kingsley D, Till K, Hoare R: Growing fractures of the skull. J Neurol Neurosurg Psychiatry 41:312, 1978

Laurent JP, Lee RT: Birth-related upper brachial plexus injuries in infants: operative and nonoperative approaches. J Child Neurol 9:111–117, 1994

Levin HS, Aldrich EF, Saydjari C, et al: Severe head injury in children: experience of the traumatic coma data bank. Neurosurgery 31:435–444, 1992

Marion DW, Penrod LE, Kelsey SF, et al: Treatment of traumatic brain injury with moderate hypothermia. N Engl J Med 336:540–546, 1997

Massagli TL, Michaud LJ, Rivara FP: Association between injury indices and outcome after severe traumatic brain injury. Arch Phys Med Rehabil 77:125–132, 1996

Sherburn EW, Kaplan SS, Kaufman B, Noetzel MJ, Park TS: Outcome of surgically treated birth related brachial plexus injuries in twenty cases. Pediatr Neurosurg 27:19–27, 1997

Steinbok P, Flodmark O, Martens D, Germann ET: Management of simple depressed skull fractures in children. J Neurosurg 66:506–510, 1987

Task Force for the Determination of Brain Death in Children: Guidelines for the determination of brain death in children. Arch Neurol 44:587–588, 1987

25.10 SEIZURE DISORDERS IN INFANTS AND CHILDREN

Douglas R. Nordli, Jr., Timothy A. Pedley, and Darryl C. De Vivo

Epilepsy is derived from the Greek verb meaning to seize upon or take hold of. The names *convulsive disorder, seizure disorder,* and *cerebral seizures* are synonymous with it. They all refer to recurrent paroxysmal episodes of central nervous system dysfunction manifested by stereotyped alterations in behavior. Epilepsy is not an entity, or even a syndrome, but rather a symptom complex arising from disordered brain function that itself may be secondary to a variety of pathologic processes. In about 60% of diagnosed epileptics, no reasonable cause for the seizure is found, and the condition is referred to as *idiopathic*.

Epileptic seizures are among the most common symptoms of disturbed brain function. In the United States, over 4% of white middle-class populations can be expected to have a seizure by age 20; persons living in socioeconomically deprived areas are twice as likely to have seizures. The cumulative incidence of epilepsy is 1.2% through age 24 years. Seizures and epilepsy occur most frequently in infants and the elderly. The age-specific incidence of epilepsy is high in the first year of life, decreases in childhood, and then remains relatively stable until age 65 years, when it increases sharply. The annual incidence of epilepsy per 100,000 population is 86 in the first year of life; 62 at ages 1 to 5 years; 50 at 5 to 9 years; and 39 at 10 to 14 years. In over 65% of patients, epilepsy begins in childhood.

CLASSIFICATION OF EPILEPTIC SEIZURES AND EPILEPTIC SYNDROMES

Epileptic seizures result from many causes and can have widely varying manifestations. An *epileptic seizure* (an isolated attack) should be distinguished from *epilepsy* (the condition of recurring epileptic seizures). Seizures are epileptic events and the indispensable characteristic of epilepsy, but not all seizures are manifestations of epilepsy. A seizure is a discrete event, a symptom of brain dysfunction. There are many different kinds of seizures, each with its own characteristic behavioral and EEG profile. Some children have seizures that are self-limited, part of an acute medical, neurologic, or neurosurgical illness. Other children have a single unprovoked seizure but never have another. Such seizures are not epilepsy. Epilepsy is a chronic disorder, the hallmark of which is recurrent, unprovoked seizures. Many children with epilepsy have more than one seizure type and may have other symptoms as well. Sometimes additional EEG, clinical, familial, pathoetiologic, and prognostic data are sufficiently similar among a group of patients with epilepsy that a more specific *epileptic syndrome* can be defined.

Classification of seizures and epilepsy is of great practical importance; it is not just an academic or theoretical nicety. The development of relatively specific antiepileptic drugs, the increased application of surgery to patients with uncontrolled seizures, the recognition that different seizures and forms of epilepsy have different natural histories with different requirements for when and for how long to treat, and the awareness that research protocols are meaningful only if epilepsy study patients can be categorized accurately are all examples of the need for a usable classification scheme.

Seizures are classified by clinical symptomatology supplemented by EEG data. Initially, seizures were described simply as big (*grand mal*) or little (*petit mal*). A third term, *psychomotor,* was coined later to describe attacks of quasi-purposeful nonconvulsive motor activity, vivid psychoillusory phenomena, and impaired consciousness. These terms are still used today, but they should be abandoned.

A uniform system of classifying epileptic seizures was developed in 1964 by a special commission of the International League against Epilepsy. A revised classification (Epilepsia 22:489, 1981) categorizes seizures by clinical pattern and interictal and ictal EEG features. An abbreviated version listing only the most common forms of clinical attacks is given in Table 25-18. It serves as the basis for the terminology used in this section. Equivalent old and new categories are shown in Table 25-19. A valuable concept that emerges from the new classification is the recognition that seizures can be

TABLE 25-18
CLASSIFICATION OF EPILEPTIC SEIZURES AND SYNDROMES

EPILEPTIC SEIZURES

I. *Generalized seizures of nonfocal origin*
  1. Tonic-clonic
  2. Tonic
  3. Clonic
  4. Absence
  5. Atonic
  6. Akinetic
  7. Bilateral epileptic myoclonus
II. *Partial (focal) seizures*
  • Simple partial seizures with elementary symptomatology (consciousness is not impaired)
    1. With motor symptoms (including Jacksonian, adversive, and postural)
    2. With sensory symptoms (including visual, somatosensory, auditory, olfactory, gustatory, and vertiginous)
    3. With autonomic symptoms
    4. With psychic symptoms (including dysphasia and affective changes)
    5. Compound (ie, mixed) forms
  • Complex partial seizures with complex symptomatology (consciousness is impaired)
    1. Simple partial seizure followed by loss of consciousness
    2. With automatisms
III. *Unclassified seizures*

EPILEPTIC SYNDROMES

  1. Neonatal seizures
  2. Infantile spasms (West syndrome)
  3. Benign familial neonatal seizures
  4. Childhood epileptic encephalopathy (Lennox-Gastaut syndrome)
  5. Benign focal epilepsy of childhood
  6. Juvenile myoclonic epilepsy
  7. Posttraumatic epilepsy
  8. Epilepsia partialis continua
  9. Acquired epileptic aphasia
  10. Idiopathic epilepsy, otherwise unclassified
  11. Symptomatic (or lesional) epilepsy, otherwise unclassified

TABLE 25-19
CHANGES IN TERMINOLOGY

OLD TERMS	NEW TERMS
Petit mal seizures	Absence seizures
Grand mal seizures	Tonic-clonic seizures
Psychomotor seizures	
Limbic system seizures	Complex partial seizures
Temporal lobe seizures	
Minor motor seizures	Atonic seizures
	Akinetic seizures
Adversive seizures	
Focal motor seizures	Simple partial seizures
Jacksonian seizures	

separated into two fundamental types: those of *partial* or *focal* origin and those that are apparently *generalized* from the outset. Partial seizures are further divided into those in which consciousness is fully maintained (*simple partial seizures*) and those where consciousness is impaired or lost (*complex partial seizures*). Partial seizures may evolve into generalized seizures (*secondarily generalized seizures*). Accurate descriptions of the electroclinical characteristics of different seizure types have been greatly facilitated in recent years by analyzing simultaneous EEG and videotape recordings. Implicit in the international classification is the understanding that clinical information alone may be inadequate to classify a seizure.

Although many children with epilepsy experience only one type of seizure, others commonly manifest more than one seizure type. This is especially true of patients with intractable epilepsy. However, classifying patients by seizure type alone is of limited usefulness because this ignores other data of which the seizures are only a part. When etiology, anatomic correlates, age of onset, associated neurologic signs, precipitating factors, prognosis, and diurnal or circadian cycling are taken into account, it is possible to define a number of different types of epilepsy or epileptic syndromes. This is especially important in pediatrics, because many of the syndromes are unique to childhood. These have been codified in the new *International Classification of Epilepsies and Epileptic Syndromes.* The most common and accepted of these categories are listed in Table 25-18. The principal distinguishing criteria for epilepsy classification are, first, whether the epilepsy is generalized or focal (localization-related), and second, whether the brain is normal (primary or idiopathic epilepsy) or abnormal (secondary or symptomatic epilepsy). Conclusions about each of these considerations are based on clinical, electrographic, and neuroimaging data.

The most important supplement to historical information about the patient comes from the EEG. A seizure that clinically appears generalized from the beginning may be shown electrographically to have a focal onset. This situation is not uncommon, for two reasons. First, if a seizure originates in a region of the brain not associated with an obvious behavioral function (rostral frontal lobe, for example), the ictal event will become clinically evident only when the abnormal electrical activity spreads to structures whose dysfunctions are more easily recognized. Second, the seizure may become generalized so rapidly that localizing signs or symptoms are lost. An important principle of epileptogenesis is that a patient's behavior during a seizure is determined as much by the sequence of pathophysiologic events as by the site at which the abnormal electrical discharge originates. Particular patterns of EEG abnormalities assist in discriminating groups of patients having a particular epileptic syndrome. Thus, accurate classification of seizures and epileptic syndromes requires a synthesis of clinical and physiologic (EEG) data.

ELECTROENCEPHALOGRAPHY

The EEG is often the single most important laboratory test in evaluating children with seizures. It helps to distinguish epileptic causes from nonepileptic causes of episodically disturbed behavior, assists in classifying epileptic seizures and syndromes, and provides information of prognostic value.

Because epilepsy is an intermittent and unpredictable disorder, most EEGs in patients with seizures are obtained between rather than during attacks. Although an EEG must be recorded during an actual seizure to confirm unequivocally the epileptic basis of the attack, the interictal EEG can provide important information. Interictal EEG abnormalities may be specific or nonspecific.

The *only* interictal EEG events that have a high correlation with clinical seizures are *epileptiform discharges*. The term *paroxysmal* is not synonymous with the term *epileptiform,* and the two should not be used interchangeably. Whereas all epileptiform discharges are by definition paroxysmal, not all paroxysmal waves are epileptiform. Thus, *paroxysmal* should be used descriptively only to indicate the sudden appearance of an EEG event of high voltage. Because the waveform may or may not also be epileptiform, *paroxysmal* has no clinical implication. Epileptiform discharges are spikes or sharp waves, usually of negative polarity, that occur at higher voltage than ongoing background activity. Spikes and sharp waves are typically followed by aftergoing slow waves (spike-wave complex). Not all spikes are epileptogenic, however, and spikes highly correlated with epilepsy must be distinguished from similar-appearing discharges seen in clinically asymptomatic or healthy persons. Two examples of spikes now considered normal variants are 14 and 6 per second positive spikes and benign epileptiform transients of sleep ("small sharp spikes"). The former are seen in up to 50% of healthy school-age children, and the latter become increasingly common during light sleep from adolescence on, occurring in about 25% of normal individuals.

Pathologic spike complexes, too, may have a variety of different clinical implications with respect to management and prognosis. The anterior or mesial temporal spike associated with complex partial seizures is clearly different from the central-midtemporal spike that may accompany benign focal seizures of childhood. Similarly, generalized spike-wave activity with a frequency of 3 to 4 Hz correlates with a clinical picture very different from the one seen with generalized sharp-wave and slow-wave complexes occurring at a frequency of 1 to 2 Hz. Thus, epileptiform activity must be critically assessed in terms of spatial distribution on the scalp, location of peak voltage, frequency, relationship to physiological state, and response to a variety of activation procedures.

Nonspecific EEG abnormalities include focal or generalized slow activity and asymmetries in frequency or voltage. Although these findings in patients with seizures frequently indicate localized or more widespread cerebral dysfunction, they do not by themselves provide evidence for a diagnosis of epilepsy. Assessment of interictal background activity apart from the presence or absence of epileptiform discharges is important in judging the likelihood of an underlying localized lesion, static encephalopathy, or progressive neurologic syndrome.

All studies of epilepsy report sizable numbers of patients who have normal EEGs. The exact percentage varies, depending on seizure type and frequency, circumstances under which the EEG is obtained, and the number of EEGs performed. Factors that increase the likelihood of recording epileptiform activity include sleep, sleep deprivation, the use of nasopharyngeal or anterior temporal electrodes, and activating procedures such as photic stimulation and hyperventilation. Several normal EEG studies obtained using these techniques will greatly reduce the chance that the symptoms are epileptic in origin. To facilitate getting an adequate sleep tracing, EEGs in infants and young children should be scheduled in the early afternoon when these children ordinarily nap. School-age children may be partially sleep-deprived by having them go to bed later than usual the night before the examination and then having them awaken earlier than usual. Adolescents may be completely sleep-deprived for 24 hours before the recording session. Nasopharyngeal electrodes are not well tolerated by children below 10 to 12 years of age and are rarely used. Anterior temporal placements can be used effectively as a substitute and should be considered if a temporal lobe origin for the child's seizures is suspected.

PATHOPHYSIOLOGY

Seizures result from synchronous interactions of large populations of neurons that have abnormal firing patterns. The last 15 years have produced remarkable growth in the understanding of cellular mechanisms of epileptogenesis. Studies in a variety of experimental models have revealed that all "epileptic" neurons have similar properties, although there are quantitative differences in the expression of these. Intracellular recordings from neurons involved in epileptogenic activity show recurring high-amplitude prolonged depolarizations with superimposed high-frequency bursts of action potentials. Current flow generated by these *paroxysmal depolarization shifts* (PDSs), which occur simultaneously in a large number of neurons, results in the interictal EEG spike that marks the patient's susceptibility to seizures. As the transition from an interictal state to an ictal state occurs, PDSs occur with increased frequency in ever greater numbers of neurons, and neuronal membranes become progressively depolarized. During the seizure itself, neurons are tonically depolarized and fire repetitively in a sustained high-frequency discharge. Recovery begins as phasic depolarizations interrupt the sustained firing sequence, and the seizure ends as membrane potentials return to normal or show a period of prolonged postictal hyperpolarization. Associated with interictal PDSs are transient but substantial rises in extracellular potassium concentration and intracellular calcium concentration. These changes are magnified during seizures and contribute to the excitability of the epileptic neuronal pool. Carbamazepine and phenytoin are anticonvulsant drugs because they reduce a neuron's ability to fire at high-frequency rates by producing a use-dependent blockade of sodium channels.

PDS generation appears to be fundamental to the epileptogenic process, and present evidence indicates that it involves a combination of increased excitatory synaptic currents and voltage-dependent currents that are intrinsic to the neuronal membrane. Differences in the extent to which neuronal membrane currents contribute to a cell's excitability and firing patterns vary among types and locations of neurons. Some neurons that normally fire in bursts may become "pacemaker" cells for other neurons during epileptogenic activities. In neurons showing "epileptic" patterns of behavior, ordinary synaptic inputs may elicit an augmented or pathologically amplified response in vulnerable cells. For example, if the effectiveness of postsynaptic inhibition onto hippocampal dendrites is reduced, dendritic burst firing, ordinarily suppressed, is "disinhibited." Under these circumstances, an excitatory synaptic input that might ordinarily result only in a brief depolarization confined to a dendrite, elicits an amplified response that may be capable of reaching the soma and initiating cellular depolarization. Such disinhibition occurs experimentally with convulsant drugs (penicillin, for example) but might occur in humans from injuries that selectively affect inhibitory neurotransmission or from genetic alterations in the normal balance between excitation and inhibition. Clinical and experimental evidence indicates that derangements in postsynaptic inhibition occur in epileptogenesis, and these in turn may be related to morphologic abnormalities seen in chronic epileptic foci of animals and humans that include loss of dendritic spines and simplification of dendritic arborizations. A reduction in GABAergic nerve terminals has been demonstrated by immunocytochemical methods in experimental epileptogenic foci. Barbiturates and benzodiazepines enhance GABA-mediated postsynaptic inhibition by increasing chloride influx.

In addition to attenuation or loss of effective postsynaptic and other inhibitory mechanisms, increased efficacy of excitatory transmission is evident in experimental models of epileptogenesis. In recent years, attention has focused on excitatory amino acids as neurotransmitters, especially glutamate. Activation of one subtype of glutamate receptor, the N-methyl-D-aspartate (NMDA) complex, strongly potentiates cellular excitation and leads to prolonged neuronal depolarization and calcium influx. Sustained NMDA receptor activation and intracellular calcium accumulation are also implicated in neuronal toxicity and may underlie cell death ("epileptic brain damage") caused by uncontrolled repetitive seizures or status epilepticus. Development of novel antiepileptic drugs is now focusing on excitatory amino acid antagonists and centrally acting calcium channel blockers.

In the focal epilepsies, abnormal neuronal behavior originates in and may remain confined to a restricted area of the cortex. In contrast, the generalized epilepsies result from relatively simultaneous involvement of large parts of both cerebral hemispheres. The original hypotheses regarding the mechanisms involved in generalized spike-and-wave activity invoked the idea of a central pacemaker within a functional "centrencephalic" system. This concept has been substantially modified to stress the integral roles of anatomic structures at several different levels: cortex, thalamus (particularly nonspecific midline and intralaminar nuclei), and brainstem reticular formation. The spike-wave discharges seen in the EEG are the surface reflections of cellular excitatory postsynaptic potential (EPSP)–inhibitory postsynaptic potential (IPSP) sequences. In generalized epilepsy, there does not appear to be a single or consistent pacemaker; rather the bursts of bilateral epileptiform activity can be initiated from many cortical sites in response to a variety of initiating stimuli. The thalamus appears to play a key role in triggering and synchronously phasing the spike-wave paroxysms. The key role of the thalamus in producing the bilateral synchrony of generalized seizures and the rhythmicity of spike-wave discharges depends on two main factors: a unique set of ionic conductances, including a T-type calcium current, that enables neurons in the thalamic nucleus reticularis to function as pacemaker control cells, and the special anatomy and pharmacology of the thalamocortical system. The reticular formation probably modulates the level of cortical excitability. In addition, the substantia nigra is critical to the expression of generalized convulsions, especially the tonic phase, and GABAergic inhibitory transmission in the substantia nigra plays a regulatory role in the propagation of generalized seizure discharge, whether primary or secondary. In the absence of demonstrable pathologic alterations in neurons or their processes, it is likely that the susceptibility to primary generalized seizures results from abnormal excitability within the involved circuits that, in turn,

results from an inherited metabolic membrane or neurotransmitter defect. Ethosuximide is effective in suppressing absence seizures because it reduces calcium currents in thalamic neurons. Valproate is broadly effective against diverse types of generalized epilepsy, and reduction in thalamic calcium currents may be one of its mechanisms of action.

There are major differences between immature and mature nervous systems with respect to the pathogenesis of epileptiform activity. These differences explain, in part, the changing patterns of clinical seizures with age. Immature animals have an increased seizure threshold and a reduced capacity for sustaining well-organized seizures. Nonetheless, the immature brain is very susceptible to seizures as reflected in their high incidence in neonates and infants. A number of experimental observations bear on the epileptogenicity of immature brain. Intracortical connections are poorly developed, and cortical-cortical propagation of ictal discharge is severely limited. At a cellular level, neurons are less capable of firing in repetitive high-frequency bursts because of longer duration spikes and less effective EPSPs. The excitatory output of a focus is further diminished because neurons within the epileptogenic aggregate do not interact synchronously. However, kindling occurs more rapidly in rat pups than in adult animals, and motor manifestations occur more readily, perhaps because of immaturity of GABAergic inhibitory controls within the substantia nigra. Changing levels of neurotransmitters, immaturity of certain cell types, and ongoing postnatal synaptogenesis are other maturational factors of importance affecting seizure susceptibility and expression in children.

25.10.1   Seizure Types

GENERALIZED-ONSET SEIZURES

Generalized seizures involve both cerebral hemispheres from the outset, and this bilateral involvement is time-locked (within milliseconds) to the beginning of the behavioral changes that clinically identify the seizure. Expression of generalized seizures requires the interaction of cerebral cortex, thalamus, and brainstem structures, including reticular formation and substantia nigra.

Generalized epileptic seizures occur with greater frequency in children than in adults, representing about 55% of all seizures of childhood. They are all characterized by abrupt onset, with loss or alteration of consciousness, and variable bilaterally symmetric motor activity often associated with changes in muscle tone. The patient has no warning of an attack, and an aura or other focal symptoms indicate a partial rather than a generalized seizure. Likewise, the EEG expression in this group of seizures is epileptiform activity that is generalized and bilaterally synchronous. Generalized-onset seizures are further subdivided into several specific types; more than one type may occur in any child.

TONIC-CLONIC SEIZURES The tonic-clonic seizure (grand mal seizure) is the classic epileptic attack known since antiquity. Consciousness is lost immediately and completely in conjunction with massive sustained contractions of the entire musculature. As air is forcibly expressed through contracted vocal cords, the characteristic "epileptic cry" results. The eyes deviate conjugately upward. This *tonic phase* lasts 10 to 20 seconds and is followed by the *clonic phase*, which lasts about 30 seconds. This is a series of relaxations that simultaneously affects all muscle groups and rhythmically interrupts the sustained tonic muscular spasm. During the tonic phase, marked autonomic phenomena are evident, including pupillary dilatation, salivation, diaphoresis, and dramatic rises in blood pressure and heart rate to two or three times normal levels. Often, although not invariably, there is urinary incontinence, and rarely there is fecal incontinence as well. Postictally the patient regains full consciousness slowly and is typically confused and excessively somnolent for minutes to hours after an attack. When fully awake, the patient may complain of headache and muscle pain but is otherwise amnesic for the events surrounding the seizure.

The complete tonic-clonic sequence is rare in infants and young children. Rather, generalized convulsive seizures before adolescence tend to take either a predominantly tonic form or a predominantly clonic form. Although the phenomena of the tonic or clonic seizure are qualitatively similar to the corresponding phase in the tonic-clonic convulsion, the various manifestations are characteristically less intense. In addition, the duration of the seizure itself and the period of postictal confusion are shorter in these types of generalized convulsive seizures. Although there is considerable overlap, tonic seizures are more apt to be associated with underlying diffuse brain damage than are clonic seizures. Drugs effective in generalized convulsive seizures include valproate, carbamazepine, and phenytoin.

The interictal EEGs of children with idiopathic generalized convulsive seizures are similar and show generalized bursts of spikes and runs of irregular 4- to 6-Hz spike-wave complexes.

Patients with generalized tonic-clonic seizures occasionally report nonspecific prodromal symptoms such as ill-defined anxiety, discomfort, or apprehension. These are of uncertain anatomic and physiological origin, but they may precede the actual seizure by hours or even a day or more. This "epileptic prodrome" is very different from the aura of a partial seizure.

MYOCLONIC SEIZURES Myoclonic seizures are characterized by short duration and rapid, bilaterally symmetric muscle contractions. The myoclonic jerks may be isolated or may occur repetitively. The muscle groups involved and the intensity of the contractions are variable. When severe, the myoclonus may cause the patient to fall. Myoclonic seizures may be the sole manifestation of epilepsy, or more commonly, they may be associated with absence attacks or tonic-clonic attacks. When the attacks are brief, full awareness will often be preserved.

Myoclonic seizures may occur as part of idiopathic epilepsy or more commonly as a specific syndrome, so-called juvenile myoclonic epilepsy (see below). They are also seen in retarded children with nonprogressive static encephalopathies that result from a variety of causes. In these latter patients, the episodes of myoclonic jerking are frequently prolonged and associated with altered consciousness, and they typically occur unpredictably without diurnal fluctuation. Rarely, myoclonic seizures may be a dominant feature of progressive neurologic syndromes, the most notable of which are Lafora disease, Unverricht-Lundborg disease (also termed *Baltic myoclonus*), and several mitochondrial encephalomyopathies (see Sec. 25.17).

Myoclonic seizures respond best to valproate or benzodiazepines. The ketogenic diet may be effective in children with myoclonic seizures resulting from brain damage.

ABSENCE SEIZURES Absence seizures (petit mal seizures) manifest as momentary lapses in awareness with amnesia. They begin and end abruptly, rarely lasting more than a few seconds. There is no warning or postictal period, and sometimes attacks are so brief that they escape detection. Other common features are brief clonic

jerks of the eyelids or limbs, transient increase or decrease in postural tone, autonomic phenomena such as pupillary dilation, change in skin color, tachycardia and piloerection, and automatisms. Simple absences occur much less commonly than the complex variety. Staring spells or lapses of awareness are not absence seizures if they are accompanied by auras, hallucinations, or postictal abnormalities. Because of the implications for therapy, absence seizures must be distinguished from other seizure types that may appear similar, especially when only historical data are available. Clinical points helpful in distinguishing absence from complex partial seizures are summarized in Table 25-20. Ultimate diagnostic accuracy requires integration of clinical and EEG data. This may be facilitated by simultaneously recording with videotape and EEG or using an ambulatory cassette EEG recorder in the child's own environment.

ATONIC AND AKINETIC SEIZURES *Atonic* and *akinetic seizures, astatic seizures, epileptic drop attacks*—these terms are used interchangeably to encompass a variety of behavioral manifestations. An atonic seizure is manifested by sudden and usually complete loss of tone in the limb, neck, and trunk muscles. It may be very brief or of longer duration. In anakinetic seizure, movement is arrested without significant loss of muscle tone; this is very rare. Both are associated with loss of consciousness, but complete awareness usually returns promptly at the end of an attack. In atonic seizures, muscular control is lost without warning, and the child may be seriously injured. This situation is often aggravated by the occurrence of one or more myoclonic jerks immediately before muscle tone is lost, so that the fall is associated with an element of propulsion. Atonic seizures are particularly common in children with static encephalopathies and may prove refractory to therapy. Carbamazepine combined with valproate is probably most effective. Other medications that may be useful include ethosuximide and acetazolamide. The ketogenic diet may also play an important therapeutic role with these children.

PARTIAL (FOCAL) SEIZURES

The specific behavioral manifestations of partial or focal seizures relate to the region of brain involved in the epileptogenic discharge. Focal seizures are less frequent in children than in adults, accounting for about 45% of all childhood seizure disorders. As in adults, these seizures imply localized cerebral dysfunction, although in children this is unlikely to be caused by a definable lesion. Fewer than 10% of children with focal seizures have brain tumors, and arteriovenous malformations are rare causes. In infants, focal seizures may be the presenting sign of a subdural hematoma. Children with congenital heart disease and right-to-left shunts may suffer cerebral emboli resulting in a neurologic deficit accompanied by focal seizures. In Sturge-Weber disease (encephalofacial angioma-

TABLE 25-20

DIFFERENTIAL DIAGNOSIS OF ABSENCE AND COMPLEX PARTIAL SEIZURES

	ABSENCE	COMPLEX PARTIAL
Duration	≤10 sec	≥10 sec; usually ≥30 sec
Aura	Never	Common
Return of full consciousness	Abrupt	Slow

tosis), the parietooccipital cortex of the hemisphere unilateral to the facial port wine nevus is often involved in the angiomatosis, with calcified atrophic gyri giving rise to contralateral focal seizures.

In marked contrast to adults, most focal seizures in children are idiopathic. These typically occur as manifestations of one of the so-called benign focal epilepsy syndromes of childhood (see below). Partial seizures also arise from static lesions acquired early in life, such as localized areas of cerebral atrophy, polymicrogyria, porencephaly, or cortical ectopias. Metabolic derangements, such as transient hypocalcemia, hypoglycemia, and water intoxication, are often associated with focal seizures. All partial seizures have the potential for becoming secondarily generalized.

The EEG correlate of partial seizures is localized epileptiform activity variably associated with other restricted abnormalities in background rhythms such as focal slowing. The location of the epileptiform discharge generally correlates with the type of clinical attacks. Thus, complex partial seizures are often associated with anterior temporal spikes; simple partial seizures of the left arm with right central spikes; and primitive visual hallucinations in one visual field with contralateral occipital spikes.

SIMPLE PARTIAL SEIZURES Focal motor, adversive, and somatosensory seizures are referred to as *partial seizures with elementary symptoms,* and they arise, respectively, from the precentral gyrus, the mesial frontal lobe (including the supplementary motor area), and the parietal lobe. In addition, however, virtually any symptom can occur as the manifestation of a simple partial seizure including complex emotional, psychoillusory, or hallucinatory phenomena. Classification of a partial seizure as "simple" implies that the affected individual can interact normally with the environment except for those limitations imposed on specific functions by the seizure. Simple partial seizures are frequently followed by transient paralysis (Todd paralysis) of the affected body part lasting minutes to hours. Patients will sometimes report that simple partial seizures can be aborted by intense concentration or by rubbing or touching the involved limb.

COMPLEX PARTIAL SEIZURES Complex partial seizures (psychomotor seizures) have only recently been well studied in children using modern monitoring techniques. Typical clinical and EEG manifestations seem to be uncommon in the very young child but are similar to those observed in adults after 8 to 10 years of age. The symptoms are varied, but they usually include alterations in consciousness, unresponsiveness, and automatisms. *Automatisms* are repetitive complex motor activities that are purposeless, undirected, and inappropriate to the situation. Examples include lip smacking, repetitious swallowing or chewing, fidgeting movements of the fingers or hands, and clumsy perseveration of a preceding motor act. Psychoillusory phenomena may be reported at the onset of an attack, including a sense of detachment or depersonalization, forced thinking, visual distortions and formed hallucinations, visceral sensations, and a feeling of intense emotion such as fear. Postictally, patients are confused and recover full consciousness slowly. Particularly postictally during a time of incomplete awareness they may resist restraint and react aggressively or angrily to objects and persons in their way. For all practical purposes, however, rage attacks or temper tantrums do not occur as manifestations of epilepsy.

Most manifestations of complex partial seizures emanate from limbic structures, especially hippocampus, amygdala, and mesial temporal lobe. Thus, the most common interictal EEG abnormality is spiking over one or both temporal regions. However, the temporal lobe and its connections may be secondarily involved by spread of abnormal activity from other brain regions. Two areas that preferentially involve limbic structures in this way are the orbitofrontal cortex and occipital lobe. Children with epileptogenic foci in these regions may have seizures clinically indistinguishable from those originating primarily in the temporal lobe.

Etiologic factors can be identified in 25 to 35% of children with complex partial seizures. However, in patients undergoing temporal lobectomy for intractable seizures, pathologic changes will be found in close to 80% of resected specimens. The most frequent finding is hippocampal sclerosis (47%). The cause and actual role of hippocampal sclerosis is a matter of controversy. The various points of view have been critically reviewed by Meldrum.

Treatment of complex partial seizures is often frustrating, and seizures stop completely in less than one-third of affected children. Carbamazepine or phenytoin are drugs of choice. Temporal lobectomy should be considered for a carefully selected number of children with refractory complex partial seizures arising exclusively from the anterior temporal lobe on one side. Surgical results for focal epilepsy arising from other brain areas are not as good.

MISCELLANEOUS SEIZURE TYPES

Intermittent or flickering light may provoke myoclonic seizures with or without absences or tonic-clonic seizures. In 75% of affected children, photosensitive seizures begin between 8 and 19 years of age. Attacks may be precipitated by television viewing, video games, or, less often, flickering of sunlight through trees or railings. A minority of children with photosensitive seizures have self-induced attacks, usually by impulsive attraction to the television set or by waving one hand in front of the eyes. This subpopulation has a high incidence of developmental delay and mild-to-moderate mental retardation.

The EEG shows bilaterally synchronous, irregularly occurring spike-wave discharges or polyspike-wave complexes. These can be triggered by stroboscopic light stimulation ("photoparoxysmal response," Fig. 25-30). Photoparoxysmal responses also occur in up to 15% of asymptomatic siblings of children with idiopathic epilepsy.

Treatment should include attempts to eliminate the provoking stimulus. Reducing light intensity by using dark glasses may be helpful. Valproate is the most effective antiepileptic drug.

UNILATERAL SEIZURES The designation *unilateral seizures* should be reserved for convulsive seizures restricted to or confined predominantly to one side of the body. In contrast with focal seizures, all the somatic musculature on one side appears to be involved simultaneously. Qualitatively, therefore, the attacks have manifestations similar to those of generalized convulsive seizures, differing only in the marked degree of asymmetry: hemitonic, hemiclonic, or hemitonic-clonic. Unilateral seizures usually result from an extensive lesion of one cerebral hemisphere. *Acute infantile hemiplegia* is the most common association. This syndrome of early childhood has many causes, but occlusive vascular disease, head injuries, infections, and peri-infectious complications account for the majority. Two thirds of these patients present with sudden onset of unilateral convulsions, fever, and obtundation. Most of these children are left with severe hemiparesis, chronic intractable hemiconvulsions, and mild-to-moderate mental retardation. As the child grows, atrophy of the paretic limbs becomes apparent. The triad of hemiplegia, hemiatrophy, and epilepsy is referred to as *HHE syn-*

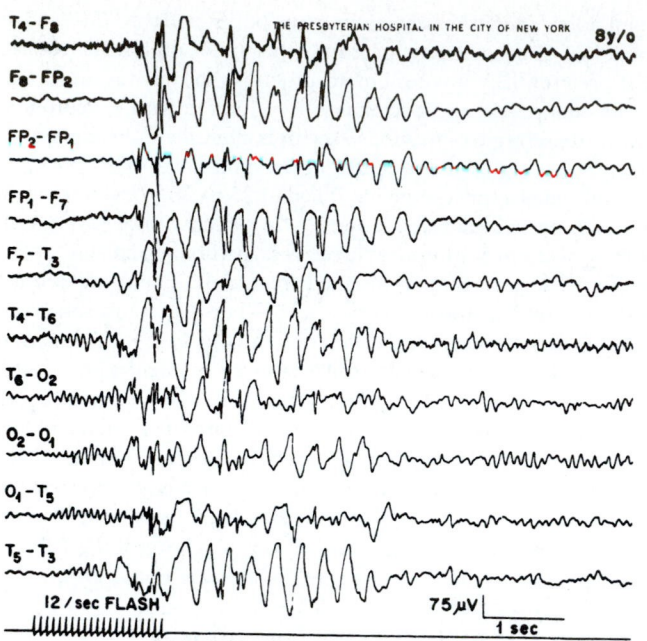

FIGURE 25-30 **Photoconvulsive response in an 8-year-old child. Intermittent light stimulation provokes bilaterally synchronous bursts of irregular spike-wave activity.**

drome by some neurologists. Skull radiographs in these children may show thickening of the cranial vault overlying the abnormal cerebral hemisphere, with ipsilateral elevation of the petrous pyramid, a smaller orbit, and enlargement of the frontal and nasal sinuses (Dyke-Davidoff-Masson deformity). Brain imaging using CT or MR reveals unilateral ventricular enlargement, with low-density lesions of the surrounding gray and white matter. The prognosis is better for the child who develops a hemiparesis after age 2 years in the absence of prolonged or recurrent seizures. Children with intractable disabling seizures and hemiplegia may be candidates for hemispherectomy.

OTHER SEIZURE TYPES The name *gelastic epilepsy* describes attacks in which pathologic laughter unaccompanied by appropriate emotional content is a dominant feature of the ictal event. The seizures are usually of the complex partial type, originating in frontal or temporal lobe structures, but in some patients, the clinical and EEG characteristics indicate a generalized disorder. *Cursive epilepsy* refers to complex partial seizures in which running is a prominent symptom. *Reflex epilepsy* indicates that a seizure is precipitated by a specific stimulus, such as the viewing of complex patterns, movement, or a light tap or touch.

SELECTED EPILEPTIC SYNDROMES

Infantile Spasms (West Syndrome)

Infantile spasms constitute an age-specific form of generalized epilepsy with virtually unique clinical and EEG characteristics. Two-thirds of affected infants begin having spasms by 6 months of age; the onset in the remainder is usually by the end of the first year. Fewer than 6% of spasms develop after age 2 years. The clinical expression of infantile spasms is diverse, although the flexor spasm (salaam attack "Blitzkrampf") is the best known. In this form, there is sudden flexion of the head and trunk simultaneously, with flexion

and adduction of the limbs. When critically studied, most infants will be found to have a mixture of flexor and extensor spasms. When spasms first begin, only a partial form of attack may occur, such as head nodding, and it may go unrecognized for the ominous sign it is. Typically the spasms occur in clusters of diminishing severity. The numbers of clusters observed in a single day vary from a few to hundreds too numerous to count accurately. Spasms may be aggravated during the transition between sleep and wakefulness, or by various forms of stimulation, including feeding, handling, and emotion.

The EEG is grossly abnormal in all children with infantile spasms. High-voltage irregular slow waves occurring asynchronously and randomly over all head regions are intermixed with spikes and polyspikes apparently originating from multiple foci (Fig. 25-31A). This pattern of EEG disturbance has been named *hypsarrhythmia,* and like infantile spasms themselves, the pattern is age-specific, the consequence of a severely disturbed immature nervous system. A clinical attack is associated with abrupt attenuation of the chaotic background activity (Fig. 25-31B). Some children with infantile spasms will have EEG abnormalities other than classical hypsarrhythmia. Conversely, not all infants with hypsarrhythmia have typical spasms, and other seizure types may be seen.

Infantile spasms may be idiopathic or symptomatic. In the past, this distinction has often been arbitrary or imprecise. At present, use of CT and MR imaging has greatly enhanced our ability to detect structural brain abnormalities that may be associated with development of infantile spasms. When all clinical data are considered, only 10 to 15% of children with infantile spasms today can be considered idiopathic. Predisposing etiologic factors include cerebral dysgenesis, various genetic and metabolic disorders including phenylketonuria and tuberous sclerosis, intrauterine or perinatal infections, and hypoxic-ischemic brain damage. Although immunization, especially with diphtheria-pertussis-tetanus (DPT) vaccine, has been considered a possible cause by some physicians, the best currently available statistical analyses have demonstrated only coincidental, not causal, relationships. Distinction between idiopathic and symptomatic groups is critical to understanding and predicting long-term outcome.

Both infantile spasms and hypsarrhythmia gradually resolve, even in the absence of treatment. Fifty percent of children become free of spasms by 2 years of age, and spasms rarely persist beyond the age of 5 years. Unfortunately, cessation of spasms is accompanied by severe retardation and recurring seizures in about two-thirds of surviving children. Mortality has been reported to be as high as 15 to 20%. Only about 5 to 10% of children with infantile spasms will have normal or near-normal intelligence, and over two-thirds have severe disabilities. Eighty percent of children have epilepsy in later life.

Infantile spasms are notoriously refractory to conventional antiepileptic agents, and few areas in epilepsy have generated as much controversy and confusion as discussion of treatment regimens for this group of patients. Controlled studies by Hrachovy and Frost offer some clarification of the major issues involved, and the following discussion is based largely on this work. Hormonal therapy using either ACTH or prednisone is the treatment of choice. There is no convincing difference in response to low-dose ACTH (20 to 30 units/d) or prednisone (2 mg/kg/d). About two-thirds of children will improve on either regimen, and failure to respond to one drug does not preclude a response to the other. Etiology and delay in initiating treatment do not reliably predict response to hormonal therapy, although many experienced physicians continue to main-

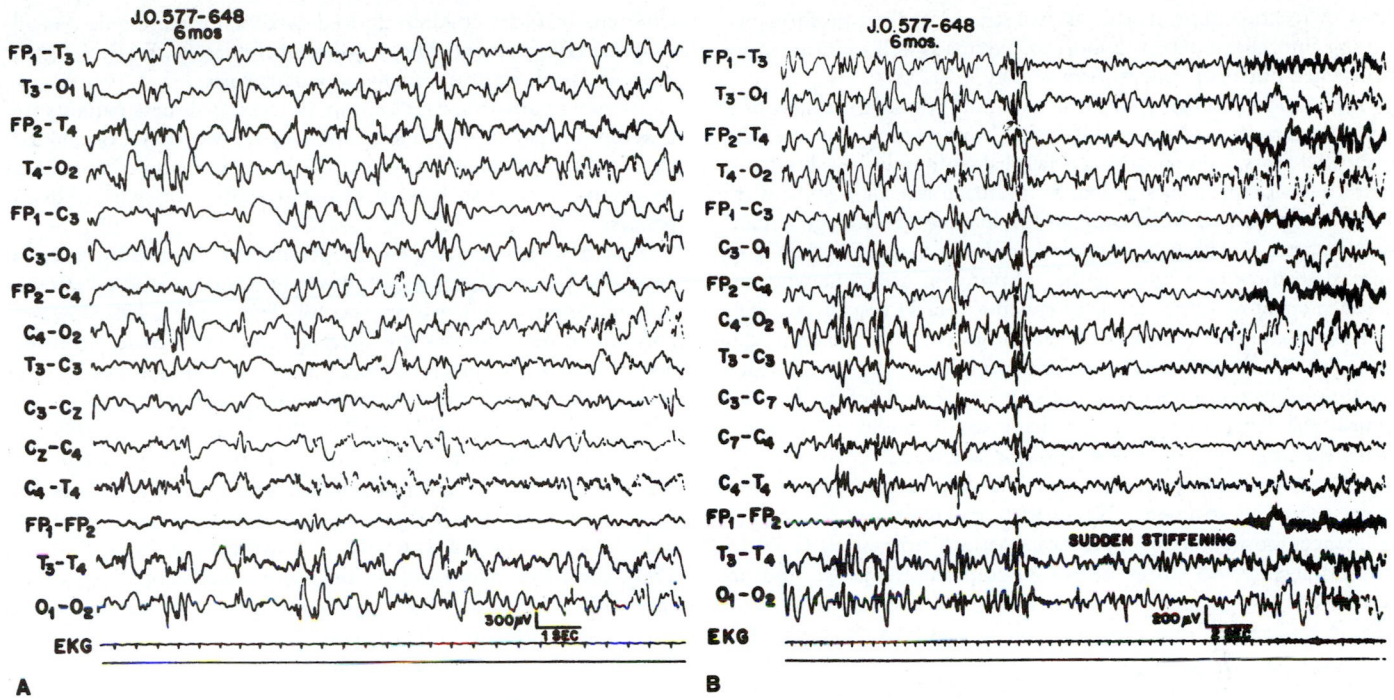

FIGURE 25-31 EEGs from a 6-month-old child with recent onset of infantile spasms. A. The interictal record shows continuous high-voltage irregular slow waves with intermixed apikes and sharp waves. B. During an extensor spasm the EEG is characterized by a sudden and generalized attenuation of voltage.

tain that treatment lag reduces the likelihood of a favorable outcome. The response to either ACTH or prednisone can usually be demonstrated within 2 weeks and for a given child appears to be "all or none." Once improvement has been obtained, the drug can be discontinued in the majority of children with persistence of the response. Relapse occurs in about one-third of patients, but in many of these, a second course of treatment is often effective. Although EEG and clinical improvement usually parallel one another, they may be dissociated. It remains unknown whether higher doses of ACTH (or prednisone) administered for longer periods provide additional benefit and whether synthetic forms of corticotropin are superior to ACTH. The frequency of side effects from ACTH is usually underestimated. Serious hypertension, osteoporosis, elec-

trolyte imbalance, and intercurrent infections occur in one-third of treated children and must be carefully watched for. Careful dietary supervision and use of low-sodium formulas mitigate the cardiovascular side effects. Beneficial results have also been obtained in some children refractory to hormonal therapy with benzodiazepines (clonazepam and, in Europe, nitrazepam) and valproate, although no consistent success with these other agents has been demonstrated in any series.

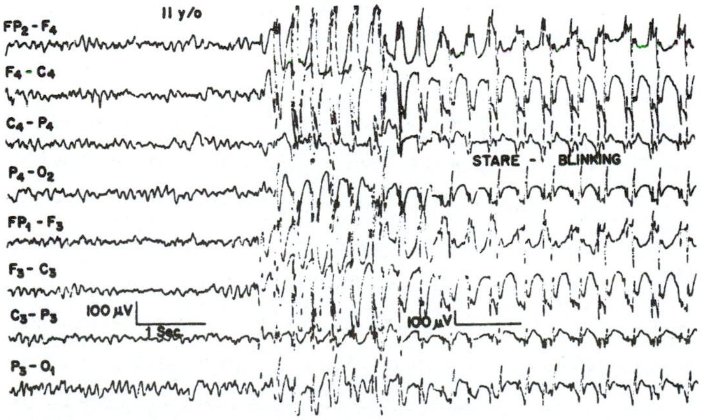

In European and American studies, vigabatrin has been shown to be effective in the treatment of infantile spasms, particularly in those children with tuberous sclerosis. Recently, peripheral visual impairments have been reported which may persist despite discontinuation of the drug. Topiramate, lamotrigine, and felbamate have all shown efficacy in the treatment of spasms, although none of these is widely used for this condition.

Childhood Absence Epilepsy

Childhood absence epilepsy (petit mal epilepsy) is characterized by recurrent absence seizures as the predominant or sole seizure type. The EEG is only rarely normal in untreated children with absence epilepsy, and hyperventilation is particularly effective in including a spike-wave paroxysm. In fact, serial normal EEGs in a child who has lapse attacks argue strongly against a diagnosis of childhood absence epilepsy and should raise the possibility of a focal (partial) seizure disorder. The EEG counterpart of the absence attack is generalized 3- to 4-Hz spike-wave activity (Fig. 25-32), usually occurring in the context of normal or near-normal background rhythms. Responsiveness drops abruptly with the onset of epileptiform activity and recovers rapidly at or near the end of the paroxysmal discharge. A generalized burst of typical 3-Hz spike-wave activity should probably not be considered truly interictal, because

FIGURE 25-32 The abrupt appearance of well-formed, bilaterally symmetric 3-Hz spike-wave discharges is the EEG correlate of a typical absence seizure.

tests of reaction time usually demonstrate impaired performance during clinically undetected short paroxysms as well as during more prolonged bursts of epileptiform activity.

Childhood absence epilepsy is common between the ages of 4 and 12 years. It seldom begins before 3 years of age or after the age of 18 years. The syndrome is familial, although the inheritance pattern is complex and probably multifactorial. The spike-wave EEG trait relates to an autosomal-dominant gene with age-dependent expression. However, there is only an 8 to 12% chance of clinical seizures occurring in the offspring of a patient who has absence epilepsy. Other kinds of epileptic attacks, usually generalized tonic-clonic convulsions, occur in 30 to 50% of children who have childhood absence. The majority of children who have absence seizures have no evidence of significant intellectual deficits or other neurologic deficits. In practice, a diagnosis of absence seizures virtually excludes a progressive neurologic syndrome.

The prognosis for patients with childhood absence epilepsy has been studied prospectively. Nearly 90% of patients with normal intelligence, normal neurologic examination, normal EEG background activity, no family history of convulsive epilepsy, and no history of tonic-clonic convulsions will become seizure-free. Conversely, complete absence of favorable factors is associated with a poor prognosis for cessation of seizures.

Occasionally, absence attacks may be so frequent and prolonged that behavior remains impaired for long intervals. This confusional state, called *absence status, petit mal status,* or *spike-wave stupor* may go unrecognized because obvious clinical signs are few. Typically, the child appears apathetic and inattentive and performs poorly. Usually, however, close scrutiny will reveal tiny rhythmic flickering of the eyelids or subtle myoclonic jerks of the somatic musculature. Although absence status is uncommon, it should be diagnosed, particularly as a cause of poor school performance or intermittent behavioral problems. Absence seizures must be distinguished from confusional migraine, toxic encephalopathies, and other forms of nonconvulsive status epilepticus.

Ethosuximide and valproate are equally effective in eliminating or substantially reducing the number of absence attacks. Valproate is also effective against generalized tonic-clonic seizures that may coexist with the absence spells and thus may be used successfully as monotherapy for both seizure types. Lamotrigine is another broad-spectrum antiepileptic medication that is effective against absence attacks and generalized convulsions. The high incidence of a potentially life-threatening rash in children, however, limits its use in this regard. Acetazolamide is occasionally useful, but children become refractory to its effects.

Lennox-Gastaut Syndrome

The name Lennox-Gastaut syndrome (childhood epileptic encephalopathy) has been applied to a heterogenous group of children with severe seizures, mental retardation, and a characteristic EEG pattern. It is not a pathologic entity, because the clinical and EEG features are the results of a diffuse encephalopathy having such diverse causes as cerebral malformation, perinatal asphyxia, severe head injury, anoxic encephalopathy from cardiopulmonary arrest, central nervous system infection, and postimmunization encephalopathies. A few children have a progressive degenerative or metabolic syndrome. A presumptive cause cannot be determined in 30 to 35% of children with Lennox-Gastaut syndrome.

Seizures usually begin in the first 3 years of life and are characteristically severe and refractory to anticonvulsant drugs. Atonic, tonic, and atypical absences are the most common types in younger

children. In older children and adolescents, tonic-clonic convulsions are also frequent. The majority of children suffer from two or more kinds of seizures, usually on a daily basis.

Mental retardation is present in 80 to 90% of these patients and is severe in half this number. One-half to two-thirds of children show other abnormalities on neurologic examination, most commonly motor signs such as quadriparesis, spastic diplegia, or hemiparesis.

The EEG is characterized by generalized, bilaterally synchronous, sharp-wave and slow-wave complexes occurring repetitively in long runs at about two per second (Fig. 25-33). This slow repetition rate distinguishes this pattern (petit mal variant) from the faster 3- to 4-Hz spike-wave complex seen with absence seizures and other forms of primary generalized epilepsy. The EEG pattern is best defined between 2 and 7 years of age. In older children, independent multifocal spikes may be seen. The background rhythms between the epileptiform discharges are abnormal because of excessive slow activity. As many as 25% of children with slow spike-wave complexes will have had hypsarrhythmia in infancy. Thus, the EEG manifestations of severe encephalopathies associated with seizures appear to represent, in part, an age-dependent continuum, with particular patterns emerging from the interaction of maturational and pathologic factors.

Prognosis is poor, with over 80% of children continuing to have seizures into adulthood. Therapy of the child with Lennox-Gastaut syndrome is frustrating because there is no satisfactory drug regimen. Some seizure types respond better than others, and treatment must, therefore, be individualized. Valproate, lamotrigine, felbamate, and topiramate are all effective agents. Felbamate's use has been limited by a high incidence of liver failure and bone marrow aplasia, lamotrigine's by rash. Persistence in empirically trying different drugs is necessary in many children to achieve optimal results. There is rarely a need for using more than two drugs at one time, and one must watch carefully for indications of cognitive and other neurologic toxicities that further compromise the child's already impaired functional capacity. The ketogenic diet should be considered when medications fail or provide control only at the expense of toxic levels of medications.

Posttraumatic Epilepsy

Head trauma can result in epilepsy at any age. Seizures can occur within 1 to 2 weeks after the injury (early posttraumatic seizures), as an acute reaction of the brain to trauma, or after intervals of several months or even years (late posttraumatic seizures, posttrau-

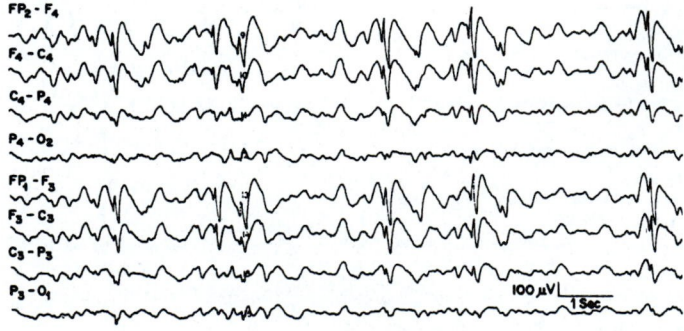

FIGURE 25-33 EEG from a 4-year-old child with a static encephalopathy manifested by mental retardation and seizures. There is generalized slowing, as well as frequent bursts of slow spike-wave complexes.

matic epilepsy). The risk of developing seizures is related most strongly to the severity of the head injury and approaches 30% in children with intracerebral hematoma, cerebral contusion, or a history of unconsciousness lasting more than 24 hours. The child with a mild head injury (momentary unconsciousness without skull fracture or neurologic deficit) is not at significantly higher risk than the general population. Moderate head injuries (those of intermediate severity) are associated with an incidence of epilepsy ranging from 2 to 10%. Although early seizures in adults sustaining head injuries predict the development of late seizures, this relationship is not as clear-cut in children, even in those with severe head injuries. Posttraumatic seizures may be either focal or generalized, although the latter have been more common, even in children with evidence of focal brain damage. We recommend treating children with severe head trauma with phenytoin for the first week after injury to minimize complications from seizures occurring during acute management. If seizures have not occurred, we do not continue phenytoin beyond 2 weeks, because there is no evidence that it prevents the development of later seizures or of posttraumatic epilepsy. We do not treat children with moderate head injuries prophylactically, preferring to wait until a seizures occurs.

Benign Focal Epilepsies of Childhood

Benign Focal Epilepsy with Central-Midtemporal Spikes   This syndrome (central-temporal epilepsy, Sylvian seizures, rolandic epilepsy) is an idiopathic localization-related epilepsy with characteristic EEG and clinical features. It is most common in previously healthy children ages 4 to 13 years. In Israel, benign focal epilepsy represented 14.4% of all childhood seizure disorders evaluated during a 5-year period; a similar rate has been reported from Sweden. The rate in the United States is unknown.

During wakefulness, the seizures have a clearly focal onset, with twitching of one side of the face, anarthria, drooling, and paresthesias of the face, gums, tongue, or inner cheeks. This may be followed by hemiclonic movements or hemitonic posturing. Consciousness is typically preserved. Postictal weakness (Todd's paralysis) of the involved face and limbs may be seen in 5% of affected children. Many children, perhaps as many as 75%, have seizures principally or only at night. These usually become secondarily generalized, so that parents report only tonic-clonic convulsions. In the absence of close observation, the focal origin of these nocturnal seizures may go unrecognized.

The EEG shows a distinctive abnormality with focal spikes and sharp waves in the central and midtemporal regions against a normal background (Fig. 25-34). The epileptiform activity may occur unilaterally but often is bilateral and asynchronous. Lateralization of the abnormality may switch from side to side on serial EEGs. Generalized spike-wave activity may occasionally occur with central-temporal spikes, particularly during sleep.

The prognosis is uniformly good, and seizures disappear by middle or late adolescence. The EEG abnormality also resolves eventually, although the spikes may persist long after the seizures have ceased.

The EEG trait is inherited as an autosomal-dominant gene with age-dependent penetrance. However, the inheritance pattern of the seizures, although clearly familial, may be multifactorial and is less well understood. More than half the children who have typical central-midtemporal spikes on the EEG will never have clinical attacks.

This entity is diagnosed on the basis of a history of characteristic focal seizures coupled with the typical EEG findings. In contrast

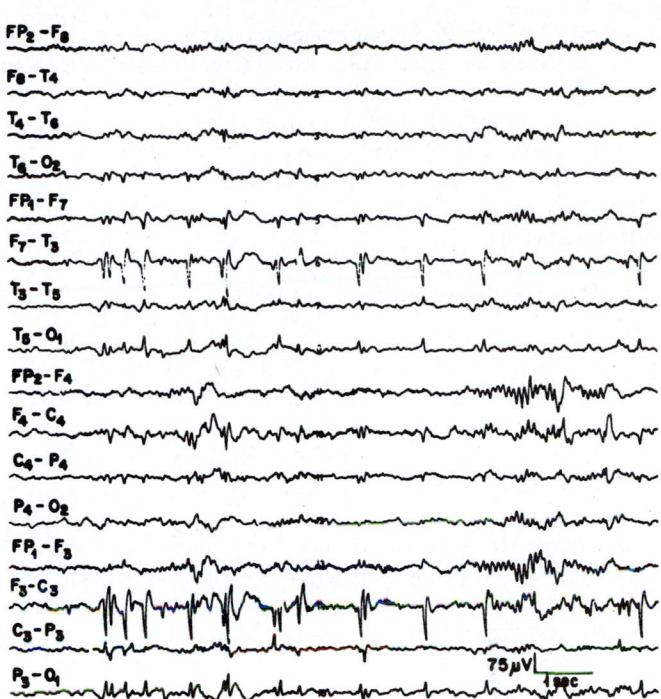

FIGURE 25-34   EEG from a 10-year-old child with benign focal seizures. During sleep, spikes and sharp waves occur frequently and repetitively in the left central and midtemporal regions.

with complex partial seizures, which are often associated with anterior or mesial temporal spike foci (*temporal lobe* or *psychomotor* seizures), benign focal seizures of childhood are marked by an absence of complex automatisms, hallucinations, perceptual distortions, and amnesia. Unless the seizure generalizes, consciousness is preserved, and there is no postictal confusion. Tumors or other localized structural lesions of the brain do not produce the same picture, and thus radiologic studies are rarely indicated.

Seizures are typically easy to control, often with unexpectedly low doses of anticonvulsant drugs. Carbamazepine has traditionally been the drug of choice, although gabapentin has recently been shown to be effective in this condition.

Benign Focal Epilepsy with Occipital Spikes   Gastaut and colleagues have described another form of benign partial epilepsy in children. Peak incidence occurs about 6 years of age. The seizures are characterized by visual disturbance (amblyopia or hallucinations), forced deviation of the eyes, and either twitching of one side of the body or loss of awareness with automatisms. Infrequent generalized convulsions occur at night. The EEG shows stereotyped focal sharp-wave discharges over the occipital areas. Although data are still scanty, outcome seems to be benign with complete resolution of clinical and EEG findings in the majority of patients by age 18 years.

Benign Partial Epilepsy with Affective Symptoms   Dalla Bernadina and his colleagues have identified an uncommon form of partial epilepsy mainly affecting preschool and school-age children. The hallmark of this syndrome is sudden fright or terror as the principal ictal manifestation. The child looks frightened, becomes pale, and clings desperately to the nearest adult. There is unresponsiveness during the attack and generally complete amnesia afterward. Seizures are frequent (several times a day) in half the patients. EEG findings show frontal-temporal or frontal-parietal spikes over one or both hemispheres interictally and a temporal discharge (often spreading to involve adjacent frontal or parietal areas) during the attack itself. In contrast to other complex partial seizures that are typically difficult to treat, this form of benign focal epilepsy responds well to carbamazepine, with complete control achieved in the majority of affected children. There is no evidence of a cerebral lesion, and this type of partial seizure does not secondarily generalize.

Juvenile Myoclonic Epilepsy (JME)

This condition, also known as the Janz syndrome, is a subtype of idiopathic generalized epilepsy. It has also been termed *impulsive petit mal*. The distinctive clinical features of juvenile myoclonic epilepsy include morning myoclonic jerks, generalized tonic-clonic seizures just after awakening, normal intelligence, a family history of similar seizures, and onset between 8 and 20 years of age. Myoclonic jerks that occur shortly after the patient awakens suggest the diagnosis. However, myoclonus must sometimes be searched for carefully in the history as the jerks vary greatly in frequency and intensity. They may be sufficiently violent that the patient falls or so minor that they are misinterpreted as clumsiness. They may be single or occur in clusters or even in a protracted series that sometimes culminates in a generalized tonic-clonic seizure. Even when frequent, however, they do not impair consciousness.

The syndrome clearly overlaps with other forms of idiopathic generalized epilepsy, and thus sporadic tonic-clonic seizures occur in the majority of patients and absence seizures in about one-third. Although linkage studies have mapped JME to the short arm of chromosome 6, it is unclear if this locus is for JME specifically, for the spike-wave EEG abnormality, or for some other feature of idiopathic generalized epilepsy. The EEG demonstrates generalized polyspikes and polyspike-wave complexes. Seizures are precipitated by sleep deprivation or disruption and by alcohol. Valproate is the drug of choice, with some studies suggesting that seizures stop completely in 95% of patients. The occurrence of polycystic ovary syndrome associated with valproate treatment has led some clinicians to favor lamotrigine in women. Relapse is the rule when the drug is withdrawn, even after an extended period of seizure control. Benzodiazepines and acetazolamide are effective alternatives in some patients.

Acquired Epileptic Aphasia

Acquired epileptic aphasia, also known as the *Landau-Kleffner syndrome,* is probably not fundamentally an epileptic disorder. The syndrome is one of typically healthy children who acutely or sometimes with a fluctuating course lose previously acquired language skills. The aphasia begins with a so-called verbal auditory agnosia. EEGs invariably demonstrate abundant slowing and epileptiform activity of high voltage that may be temporal or bitemporal or even generalized. The EEG abnormality may be seen only during sleep, at least in the early stages. Seizures, however, are not invariable, although they occur in about 70% of patients. They are usually relatively infrequent, but status epilepticus has been reported. Treatment with antiepileptic drugs does not clearly affect the aphasia, EEG findings, or ultimate outcome. Corticosteroids may be effective, but a controlled study has not been done. About two-thirds of children are left with some residual language impairment. Other neurologic abnormalities do not occur, but personality disturbances and hyperactivity are frequently mentioned. Although there has been recent enthusiasm for using the technique of subpial transection (Morrell procedure) to treat acquired epileptic aphasia

surgically, no controlled data show that this is effective in favorably modifying the natural history of the disorder.

Epilepsia Partialis Continua

Although epilepsia partialis continua (EPC) also occurs in adults, there is a recognizable form that is mainly confined to children which is known as *Rasmussen syndrome.* In the great majority, onset is before 10 years of age. About two-thirds of patients report an infectious or inflammatory illness in themselves or their families before onset of EPC, but this is usually trivial. The first seizures are often generalized, and the intractable focal nature of the attack only becomes apparent over time. When fully established, the syndrome is characterized by unremitting seizure activity limited to part or one side of the body. Unlike more typical simple partial seizures of motor type, muscle movements are usually quite asynchronous in different muscle groups and seem to ebb and flow in waves, sometimes involving fewer muscles, sometimes more. There is inevitably slow neurologic deterioration with development of hemiparesis, diminished mental capacity, and, usually, hemianopia. Although progressive, the disease is only rarely fatal, and a permanent but stable neurologic deficit emerges.

Medical treatment is very unsatisfactory, and conventional anticonvulsant drugs afford minimal benefit in most patients. Similarly, corticosteroids and antiviral agents have been tried but with only marginal success. If seizures have not spontaneously remitted by the time a maximal neurologic deficit has been established, a modified hemispherectomy or tailored cortical excision can result in substantial improvement in selected patients.

EVALUATION OF CHILDREN WITH SEIZURES

Because epilepsy is a symptom that has many causes, it is neither possible nor desirable to provide a standardized set of guidelines appropriate for evaluating all children with seizures. However, the following suggestions may be applicable to most situations. The role of the physician is threefold: to determine if the child's attacks have an epileptic basis, to define the cause of the seizures, and to institute appropriate treatment.

A thorough and accurate history is the single most important part of the diagnostic process. The historic summary should contain a description of the characteristics of the attack (Table 25-21); any symptoms of neurologic or systemic disease between attacks, and whether these are static or progressive in nature; a pertinent past history including details of birth, postnatal course, and early development, serious illnesses, trauma, ingestions or toxic exposures, reactions to immunizations, and school performance; a relevant family history.

TABLE 25-21

HISTORICAL CHARACTERISTICS OF EPILEPTIC ATTACK

First event in the seizure (lateralizing or focal symptoms, aura)
Subsequent evolution of the seizure
Postictal manifestations (Todd paralysis)
Is there more than one seizure type?
Has there been a change in seizure pattern?
Date and circumstances of first attack
Subsequent precipitating or associated factors (sleep deprivation, sensory stimuli, stress)
Age of onset, frequency of attacks, and longest seizure-free interval

The physical examination should document any abnormalities in neurologic function, and it should also provide information on the following: the presence or absence of head bruits; skin lesions such as café-au-lait spots, hypopigmented areas, shagreen patches, or hemangiomas; body asymmetries; craniofacial or other skeletal deformities. It is useful to have the child hyperventilate in an attempt to provoke an attack.

Synthesis of these clinical data should enable the clinician to decide if the child's attacks are epileptic in origin or rather the presentation of some other disorder. Differential diagnosis, depending on the nature of the episodes, might include breath-holding spells, syncope, sleep disturbances such as somnambulism or night terrors, migraine, benign paroxysmal vertigo, and movement disorders such as chorea or paroxysmal vertigo. Migraine may be particularly difficult to exclude because its manifestations in childhood are so protean. Most children previously diagnosed as having abdominal epilepsy or "epileptic equivalent" are usually found on reevaluation to have a migrainous syndrome. Assuming that a seizure disorder is considered likely or certain, each type of attack should be tentatively classified according to the international classification, subject to modification when the EEG report is available. It is also useful at this point to assess the probability that the seizures are idiopathic or symptomatic of some associated neurologic disorder. This consideration will have a major influence on the extent of the laboratory investigation.

Laboratory studies should be undertaken *selectively,* depending on the clinical assessment. An EEG should be done in every child who has seizures. Any child whose seizure occurs in the context of a febrile illness should have a lumbar puncture to exclude meningitis. This rule is particularly important in infants in whom the Kernig and Brudzinski signs are not reliably present with meningeal irritation. In addition, we regularly perform a lumbar puncture on any infant seen at the time of the seizure, whether febrile or not. CT or MR scanning is reserved mainly for children with partial seizures (excluding benign focal epilepsy of childhood), abnormal neurologic examinations, or focal slow-wave abnormalities on the EEG. MR imaging is preferred to CT because it may detect a focal lesion when the CT scan is normal, especially with cavernous malformations, small hamartomas, well-differentiated astrocytomas, neuronal migrational disorders, and mesial temporal sclerosis. Brain tumor is actually a rare cause of seizures in children without other signs or symptoms. Other laboratory tests should be ordered only if particular clinical indications exist, such as signs of a progressive neurologic syndrome or a family of stillbirth, repeated miscarriages, mental retardation, or neurologic illness.

Once the initial diagnostic evaluation is completed and therapy is begun, close follow-up is advised, with regular reexaminations. A period of watchful waiting will often clarify an uncertain or confusing clinical picture. Furthermore, physicians should check frequently for evidence of drug toxicity, not only by means of abnormal physical findings but also by specifically questioning the parents about their child's activity level, behavior, and school performance.

25.10.2   Therapeutic Considerations

Treatment of the child with epilepsy can be effective only when the multiple interacting medical, psychological, and environmental factors are successfully addressed. The pediatrician bears a special responsibility for helping the child and the family to adjust realistically to living with a chronic disorder. Although we shall concentrate on drug treatment in this section, we emphasize that this represents only one aspect of what must be a comprehensive therapeutic approach. In particular, physicians must not neglect environmental or physiological circumstances that may precipitate seizures. Similarly, physicians too often fail to consider the psychosocial consequences of epilepsy.

GENERAL PRINCIPLES OF DRUG TREATMENT

Probably no group of patients receives greater numbers of drugs for longer periods than those with seizures. In addition, many patients receive more than one drug, sometimes as many as three or four. Thus, the potential for chronic toxicity related to long-term use and to adverse drug–drug interactions is high. Undesirable side effects may be quite subtle and manifested only as learning problems or behavioral disturbances. The following considerations can serve only as general guidelines for the use of antiepileptic agents.

In our view, far more children are overtreated than undertreated. We do not usually treat a patient who has had an uncomplicated isolated general seizure if it is accompanied by a normal EEG and a negative family history for epilepsy. In children with recurrent seizures, such as epilepsy, the decision to institute drug treatment should be influenced by the frequency and the type of seizures and the estimated risk of further episodes. Risk for recurrent seizures is sharply increased if the seizure is focal, if there is a history of prior neonatal seizures, and if no immediate precipitating cause can be identified.

Therapy should always begin with a single agent, even in children with more than one seizure type. Because some drugs are *relatively* more effective for some seizure types than others, the particular drug selected should be chosen with the child's seizure type in mind. Although comparative studies have not shown substantial differences in antiepileptic potency among carbamazepine, phenytoin, primidone, and phenobarbital, these drugs do differ in incidence of side effects, patient tolerance, cost, and dosing schedules. Such considerations may affect drug choice in particular patients. Mattson and colleagues compared the efficacy of valproate and carbamazepine in adults with partial and secondarily generalized tonic-clonic seizures. Both were equally effective against secondarily generalized seizures, but carbamazepine was superior to valproate in controlling complex partial seizures. These results can probably be extrapolated to children, especially those older than 6 years. In general, we prefer carbamazepine for partial and secondarily generalized seizures; ethosuximide for absence seizures; and valproate or carbamazepine for idiopathic generalized tonic-clinic seizures (*primary grand mal*). When more than one type of generalized-onset seizure coexists (eg, absence and tonic-clonic seizures; myoclonic and tonic-clonic seizures), valproate can be used effectively as the sole agent in the majority of children. We are cautious in using valproate in preschool children because of the increased risk of liver damage, which in rare instances can be fatal. This risk can be minimized (but not avoided) by checking liver function tests frequently, avoiding polytherapy, and not introducing the drug at times of metabolic stress (eg, during acute systemic illnesses). Some clinicians also advocate L-carnitine supplementation (100 mg/kg/d in three divided doses) for all infants younger than 2 years who are treated with valproate. Supplementation with L-carnitine has been recently thoroughly reviewed.

The dosage should be increased gradually, if there are no side effects, until the seizures come under control or until clinical toxicity is evident. If seizures persist, a second drug should be substituted. All appropriate agents should be methodically tried in this way until the best seizure control is achieved. It may be necessary to add a second drug for refractory seizures, but the practice of "polypharmacy" should be resisted. There is no evidence at present that patients on multiple drugs do better than those on rationally prescribed one- or two-drug schedules. On the contrary, patients on simple drug regimens, as opposed to complicated ones, have significantly fewer side effects without any exacerbation of seizure frequency. Occasional minor seizures are less disabling to a child than chronic intoxication resulting from excessive medication.

Optimal seizure control is most likely to be achieved if the physician thoroughly understands the clinical pharmacology of the antiepileptic agents, including age-related changes in drug utilization. In general, preadolescent children require higher maintenance dosages than do older persons to achieve therapeutic serum concentrations. In addition, medication must be administered more frequently to maintain stable blood levels, because the half-lives of most anticonvulsants are significantly shorter and show greater variability in young children. Adult patterns of drug use are not reached until late adolescence. Chronic therapy with phenytoin or phenobarbital decreases serum calcium and 25-hydroxycalciferol levels and significantly reduces bone mass. We believe that all children on long-term antiepileptic drug therapy should receive vitamin D, at least 10,000 IU weekly. We routinely recommend one or two multivitamin tablets (usually representing 400 to 800 IU of vitamin D) daily as part of the treatment regimen. Dosage schedules for the more commonly used anticonvulsant drugs are given in Table 25-22.

Failure to control seizures may be attributable to remedial causes. Faced with a child whose seizures remain disabling, the physician should obtain frequent measurements of anticonvulsant drugs in the blood, both to ensure compliance with the prescribed regimen and to detect subtherapeutic or toxic concentrations. Whereas an inadequate serum concentration is the most common cause of persistent seizures, drug toxicity, especially with phenytoin, may occasionally be manifested by deteriorating seizure control. Longitudinal studies of drug concentrations over a 24-hour period will sometimes reveal variations in drug metabolism or unexplained fluctuations in serum drug levels that correlate with clinical seizure activity. Changes in drug administration resulting from such information may lead to fewer seizures. There will be less variation in blood concentrations if tablets or capsules, rather than liquid preparations, are prescribed. Suspensions, in particular, result in notoriously inconsistent dosages. Because of short half-lives, serum concentrations may fluctuate widely if the dosage interval is too long. Intractable seizures may also arise from an incorrect diagnosis, either of the underlying condition or of the particular seizure type, which results in use of inappropriate medications. Sometimes the choice of antiepileptic drug may exacerbate some seizure types in a child with a mixed seizure disorder. For example, carbamazepine or phenytoin may control generalized tonic-clonic seizures in patients with juvenile myoclonic epilepsy but aggravate myoclonic and absence seizures. It must be recognized and accepted that even the best therapeutic approach will not control every child who has seizures, particularly if there is underlying brain damage.

SURGICAL TREATMENT OF EPILEPSY

Surgical therapy should be considered in children with medically intractable epilepsy or with syndromes for which medical treatment is known to be ineffective. These determinations require accurate classification of a child's seizures and epilepsy, knowledge of the natural history, and precise information about response to drug

trials. Many types of infantile and early childhood seizures are difficult to classify and of uncertain prognosis. As a result, surgical experience is greatest with older children and adolescents who have focal cerebral lesions or mesial temporal sclerosis. There is growing interest, however, in operating earlier, especially in selected patients who have various forms of catastrophic epilepsy.

Patients in whom surgery is considered should have a reasonable expectation either of seizure elimination or of substantially fewer disabling seizures that translates into improved quality of life. There should be minimal risk of losing neurologic function. The definition of *intractable* is elusive and must be individually determined. Operationally, we consider seizures medically intractable if patients consider themselves disabled, either by seizures or their treatment, despite trials of two appropriate antiepileptic drugs in monotherapy and one trial of two-drug combination therapy to maximally tolerated doses. MR brain imaging has increased detection of hippocampal sclerosis and other previously cryptic lesions in children with partial seizures. Positron emission tomography may assist in defining metabolically abnormal brain regions responsible for seizures even in the absence of structural brain pathology. Ultimately, localization of the epileptogenic brain area requires simultaneous video-EEG recordings in a specialized monitoring unit.

Epilepsy surgery is best carried out in comprehensive centers with special expertise in this form of treatment.

FOCAL RESECTIONS   Focal cortical resection is the most common procedure performed in patients with intractable epilepsy with or without a demonstrable lesion. If a lesion is evident on brain imaging studies, good results may be obtained by lesionectomy. More often, additional cortex that is demonstrably electrically abnormal is included in the resection. Many of the anterior temporal lobectomies performed in children with uncontrolled partial seizures have been for tumors or cerebral dysgenesis; mesial temporal sclerosis is an indication for temporal lobectomy less often in children than in older adolescents and adults. Intraoperative electrocorticography may help define the margins for functional resections; somatosensory evoked potentials and electrical stimulation of the cortex are used to map vital sensorimotor and language areas. In children older than about 6 years, preoperative intracarotid amobarbital (Wada test) is used to anesthetize each hemisphere selectively to determine language dominance and memory competence.

HEMISPHERECTOMY   Although intimidating to parents and physicians alike, this procedure is indicated for patients with seizures arising from multiple regions of a hemisphere that is severely dysfunctional by other measures as well. Thus, these children typically have a hemiparesis that is most marked in the hand and, often, hemiatrophy as well. Some patients also have hemisensory loss and hemianopia. In such patients, neurologic function is not noticeably worsened by hemispherectomy. Causes of these severe unilateral epilepsy syndromes include epilepsia partialis continua (Rasmussen syndrome), hemimegalencephaly, and large porencephalic lesions resulting from strokes that occurred early in life. In a large series from the Montreal Neurological Institute, 82% of patients became seizure-free, and none lost the ability to walk.

CORPUS CALLOSOTOMY   This is a palliative, not curative, procedure, the indication for which is largely restricted to children with severe atonic and secondarily generalized seizures that result in frequent self-injury. Most children have a static epileptic encephalopathy (Lennox-Gastaut syndrome) with mental retardation and other neurologic abnormalities as well. Typically, the anterior two-

TABLE 25-22

ANTIEPILEPTIC DRUGS—DOSAGE AND PHARMACOKINETIC DATA

	USUAL DOSAGE, PER 24 h	ORAL AVAILABILITY, %	PROTEIN-BOUND, %	CLEARANCE, mL · min^{-1} · kg^{-1}	URINARY EXCRETION, UNCHANGED %	VOLUME OF DISTRIBUTION L/kg	HALF-LIFE HOURS	"THERAPEUTIC" PLASMA CONCENTRATIONS, μg/mL
Carbamazepine*	Adult: 800–1600 mg Child: 10–40 mg · kg^{-1} · d^{-1}	75–85	74	1.3 (postinduction) (Very variable)	<1	0.8–2.0	11–22†	6–12
Ethosuximide	Adult: 750–1500 mg Child: 10–75 mg · kg^{-1} · d^{-1}	>90	0	0.19 (Higher in children)	18	0.62–0.69	45–60 (Children mean: 36)	40–100
Felbamate	Adult: 2400–3600 mg Child: 15–45 mg · kg^{-1} · d^{-1}		25–35		50	0.70	18–24	20–60
Gabapentin	Adult: 900–1800 mg	51–59	<3		77–80		5–8	>2
Lamotrigine	Adult: 75–200 mg	>70	55		10		30 (14–50)	1–5
Phenobarbital	Adult: 90–180 mg Child: 2–6 mg · kg^{-1} · d^{-1}	100	45–50	0.062 (Higher in children)	25	0.54–0.70	99 (Shorter in children)	15–40
Phenytoin	Adult: 300–500 mg Child: 4–12 mg · kg^{-1} · d^{-1}	90	90	V_{max} = 5.9 mg · kg^{-1} · d^{-1} K_M = 5.7 μg/mL *Capacity limited*	2	0.78	6–42 (*Concentration-dependent*)	10–20
Primidone‡	Adult: 750–1250 mg Child: 6–12 mg · kg^{-1} · d^{-1}	92	19	0.59–0.94	42	0.64–0.72	8–15	5–12
Topiramate	Adult: 100–1200 mg Child: 1–10 mg · kg^{-1} · d^{-1}	100	15	27–61 ml/h/kg	85.4	0.56–1.17	6.1–13.5 h (up to 23 h in adults)	>2
Valproate	Adult: 1000–3000 mg Child: 10–70 mg · kg^{-1} · d^{-1}	100	93 (*Concentration dependent*)	0.11	2	0.19	14–20	50–120

* The carbamazepine metabolite carbamazepine-10, 11-epoxide is also pharmacologically active; values given are for the parent compound.

† The half-life of carbamazepine is considerably longer when the drug is first introduced, prior to autoinduction of hepatic microsomal enzymes.

‡ Primidone's primary metabolites phenobarbital and phenylethylmalonamide are also pharmacologically active; values given are for the parent compound.

SOURCE: *Pedley TA, Scheuer ML, Walczak TS. In:* Merritt's Textbook of Neurology, 9th ed, *LP Rowland (Ed) New York, Lea & Febiger, 1994*

thirds of the corpus callosum is sectioned first; the callosotomy is completed only if seizure control remains unsatisfactory.

DIETARY TREATMENT OF EPILEPSY

For children who have severe seizures that are incompletely controlled by anticonvulsant drugs, dietary therapy may improve control and reduce toxicity from medication. Although the mechanism of anticonvulsant action of the ketogenic diet is not known, stable and sustained ketosis seems to be the most important factor. Because the efficacy of the diet corresponds directly to the rigidity with which the regimen is followed, the best results are seen in preschool children who can be supervised more closely and whose food habits are less well formed. In addition, parents must understand and be capable of meeting the demands made by close adherence to the diet.

Dietary therapy is begun in the hospital to allow strict supervision of the initial phase of treatment. The parents should be closely involved in food preparation and in the testing of urine for ketone bodies. After 24 hours of fasting, the child is placed on a high-fat diet in which the ratio of fat to carbohydrates and protein combined is 4:1 by weight. Daily caloric requirements are initially estimated at 75 to 80 kcal/kg. Of this total, protein must be present in an amount that will ensure the developing child's growth. This need is generally satisfied by giving protein calculated on the basis of 1.5 g/kg per day. Supplemental B and C vitamins, calcium, and iron are necessary because the diet is deficient in these requirements, but preparations without carbohydrates must be selected. We also recommend giving 10,000 IU of vitamin D each week. Although anticonvulsant drug dosage may eventually be reduced, optimal seizure control usually requires a combination of diet and antiepileptic medication.

STATUS EPILEPTICUS

Status epilepticus is defined by the international classification as repeated seizures occurring so frequently as "to produce a fixed and enduring epileptic condition." Although it is most often seen in previously diagnosed epileptic patients who do not take their medication, status epilepticus may be the first manifestation of idiopathic epilepsy. Sepsis, meningitis or encephalitis, trauma, and encephalopathies of toxic or metabolic origin are also common underlying conditions that result in status epilepticus, and these disorders must be considered early in the evaluation of a child who is having seizures.

Generalized convulsive status represents a medical emergency because there may be an underlying treatable cause, and prolonged seizures themselves are harmful to the child. Children tolerate status epilepticus better than adults, and febrile status epilepticus, in particular, seems to be relatively benign and carries an excellent prognosis. In a study of 193 children with status epilepticus, Maytal and Shinnar found that only 7 children died, and new neurologic abnormalities were found in only 9.1% of the survivors. Death or neurologic morbidity occurs mainly in children with acute or progressive brain disorders. Morbidity is minimized by appropriately aggressive therapy. Recurrent status is low in children with idiopathic status epilepticus; it occurs mainly in children with underlying neurologic disease.

Because systemic factors contribute substantially to this morbidity, hypoxia, hypotension, and hyperthermia must be avoided by whatever means, including, if necessary, muscular paralysis and artificial ventilation. At the very least, high-flow oxygen should be given by nasal cannula, an oral airway inserted, and 10% glucose in saline infused continuously to sustain a blood sugar concentration of 200 to 300 mg/dL. One or more secure intravenous catheters are essential for treatment of status epilepticus. To minimize cerebral edema, total fluid administration should not exceed 1000 mL/m². The patient should be positioned to minimize the chance of aspiration and should be suctioned frequently.

A single intravenous dose of diazepam (0.25 mg/kg, not exceeding 10 mg) or lorazepam (0.05 to 0.50 mg/kg) should be infused slowly because this may terminate the status epilepticus. A rectal gel preparation of diazepam is now available. Although formally approved only for use in acute repetitive seizures, we have used this product for prolonged seizures and have found it effective and safe. Whatever benzodiazepine and route is selected, this dose should be repeated in 10 to 20 minutes if seizures persist. Immediately thereafter, phenytoin or fosphenytoin should be administered. Fosphenytoin is the water-soluble prodrug that is rapidly converted to phenytoin in the body. Both products are given intravenously with close ECG and blood pressure monitoring at an initial dose of 15 to 20 mg/kg. Additional doses of 10 mg/kg should be given as needed every 4 hours thereafter until clinical seizure activity is controlled. In small infants, infusion rates of phenytoin should be slow, usually given over 20 minutes.

Phenobarbital is an alternate choice. A dose of 10 mg/kg is given intravenously and repeated 30 minutes later if seizures continue. Thereafter, phenobarbital at 10 to 15 mg/kg is given every 1 to 4 hours, depending on seizure frequency, until control is achieved; the effective serum concentration is the concentration at which seizures subside, and the upper limit cannot be rigorously defined. Close attention to vital signs is essential, and cardiorespiratory support must be immediately available at the bedside. Between doses of phenobarbital, paraldehyde (0.3 mg/kg administered rectally in an equal volume of mineral oil) may be used. Paraldehyde for intravenous use is no longer available. A combination of phenobarbital and phenytoin, or even general anesthesia, may be required in the child with more recalcitrant status epilepticus. Recently, refractory status has been effectively treated with continued infusion of midazolam.

Nonconvulsive status epilepticus (absence status, complex partial status) and focal motor status, including epilepsia partialis continua, do not constitute emergencies, but treatment should be relatively aggressive, and intravenous drug administration is preferred. An exception is absence status, which can be treated effectively with oral ethosuximide or valproate.

DISCONTINUING ANTIEPILEPTIC DRUGS

When to stop a drug may be as important as the initial treatment decision, especially in chronic disorders such as epilepsy where long-term treatment with anticonvulsant drugs is associated with significant systemic and neurological toxicity. Several recent studies have provided guidelines for selecting patients for antiepileptic drug withdrawal. Well-controlled investigations all agree that the risk of relapse in children whose seizures have been in remission at least 2 years is low, on the order of 30%. Although there is no uniform agreement on factors predictive of outcome, EEG findings, seizure type, age at seizure onset, duration of epilepsy (or number of seizures) before control, and presence of neurologic dysfunction are probably the most useful indicators. Prognosis is worst for children with symptomatic partial seizures, persistently abnormal EEGs, many generalized seizures or long history of epilepsy before control was achieved, and abnormal neurologic examination. When such factors are present, we wait at least 4 years or more after the last seizure before contemplating discontinuation of antiepileptic drugs. On the other hand, we will withdraw drugs after 2 years in neurologically normal children with idiopathic epilepsy whose seizures came readily under control and whose current EEGs are normal or near-normal. Fortunately, this group constitutes the majority of children with epilepsy. An exception may be those with juvenile myoclonic epilepsy, as most studies indicate an unusually high rate of relapse in this syndrome.

TERATOGENIC EFFECTS OF ANTIEPILEPTIC DRUGS

Pregnant women taking antiepileptic drugs are at a two- to three-fold increased risk of having abnormal infants. Specific factors contributing to this risk are disputed, but genetic considerations, drug exposure in utero, and frequency of generalized seizures have all been implicated.

Two types of teratogenicity are associated with antiepileptic drugs. *Major malformations* are defects that are life-threatening or that require medical or surgical treatment to permit a normal life. The baseline population risk for major malformations is about 2% of pregnancies. This is increased to 5 to 6% in infants born to women with epilepsy who take a single antiepileptic drug during pregnancy and to 10% in women taking two drugs. The most common malformations include cleft lip or palate, neural tube defects (spina bifida, anencephaly), and cardiac abnormalities. Valproate specifically increases the risk of neural tube defects by 1.5%; carbamazepine polytherapy seems also to increase this specific risk by about 0.5 to 1.0%, especially if there is a family history of neural tube defects. The risk of neural tube defects can be minimized by preconceptive use of folic acid, 1 mg/day. *Minor anomalies* (nail hypoplasia, hypertelorism, low-set ears, prominent lips, broad-based nasal bridge) reflect both genetic and drug-related factors. All antiepileptic drugs seem to produce similar types of fetal anomalies (*fetal anticonvulsant syndrome*), although these have also occurred in infants of women with epilepsy and no drug exposure. The mechanism of teratogenicity is unknown, but it may relate to the formation of arene oxide metabolites or, possibly, to the effect of anticonvulsants on folic acid. Children with a genetic defect in detoxification of phenytoin-derived arene oxide metabolites had a higher risk of major (but not minor) malformations. Available data also indicate that the teratogenic risk is increased by high plasma concentrations of the drug, by use of two or more drugs, and by presently ill-defined genetic factors.

We recommend that all women of child-bearing age be informed of the potential teratogenic effects of antiepileptic drugs when they are first prescribed; that if medication is required, attempts should be made to use a single drug at the lowest effective plasma concentration; and that, if possible, consideration be given to discontinuing drugs altogether for the first trimester, because some patients prefer occasional partial or nonconvulsive generalized seizures to the slight risk associated with drug treatment. For the woman who has an unplanned pregnancy while on anticonvulsant drugs, we advise against discontinuing medication because the risk of birth defects is low, rapid withdrawal may provoke seizures, and the teratogenic insult may already have occurred. Women with epilepsy have a 90 to 95% chance of having a healthy baby.

Women who need anticonvulsant prophylaxis during pregnancy require close observation. Therapeutic drug monitoring is useful, but unbound (free) levels are more informative than total plasma concentrations. Routine measurement of total blood levels shows a decline in concentrations of most antiepileptic drugs during pregnancy, but this is offset by reduced protein binding so that unbound levels decline much less. Supplemental vitamins, including folic acid, should be prescribed. There is no "best drug," but, in general, drug choice should be guided by what is optimal treatment for the mother's epilepsy. Because of the reported association between valproate or carbamazepine and neural tube defects, we recommend avoiding these drugs in patients with a family history of neural tube defects. Amniocentesis before the 20th week of gestation and high-resolution ultrasonograms have a nearly 95% accuracy rate in identifying neural tube defects and other major malformations. Serum α-fetoprotein determinations have a 25% false-negative rate.

Virtually all antiepileptic drugs promote a hemorrhagic diathesis in the newborn. This may result in internal bleeding within the first 24 hours of extrauterine life; this may not be noticed until the baby is in shock. This anticonvulsant-related hemorrhagic disease will not be prevented in all babies by the routine administration of vitamin K at birth. Therefore, we recommend that oral vitamin K_1 phytonadione (20 mg daily) be prescribed during the last month of pregnancy.

All anticonvulsants appear in breast milk of nursing mothers. This is usually of little consequence, and breast-feeding need not be discouraged. However, if the baby exhibits poor sucking, inadequate weight gain, or excessive drowsiness, high antiepileptic drug levels in breast milk should be considered a possible cause. In our experience, these problems occur most often with primidone or phenobarbital.

A recent consensus on the treatment of women of childbearing potential has been published which provides authoritative and concise recommendations for the care of the pregnant patient.

25.10.3   Neonatal Seizures

Neonatal seizures differ from those occurring in older patients with respect to clinical manifestations, EEG correlates, and etiology, as well as in terms of diagnostic evaluation and treatment. The incidence ranges from 5 to 20 per 1000 live births. In a neonatal intensive care nursery, as many as 10% of infants will have seizures; about 15% of them will die, and 35 to 40% will have major neurologic sequelae.

CLINICAL SEIZURE PATTERNS

Seizures in newborns may be fragmentary, poorly organized, and often remarkably limited in their clinical expression. There has been no universally accepted system for classifying neonatal seizures, in part because of differing emphasis on various clinical, electrographic, and etiologic aspects. In recent years, however, there is growing acceptance that neonatal seizures are best classified by their clinical manifestations and physiological characteristics. In the newborn, the term *seizure* is used generically for any paroxysmal transient alteration in neurologic function. Not all neonatal seizures result from the same pathophysiological mechanisms. Some are associated with simultaneous EEG discharges and thus represent conventional epileptic events modified by pathology and brain immaturity. Other seizures are inconsistently or not accompanied by EEG changes and thus may arise either from nondetectable (at the scalp) epileptic mechanisms or from nonepileptic dysfunction of motor systems at subcortical and brainstem levels. The following discussion relies heavily on pioneering studies by Mizrahi and Kellaway at Baylor University and on general concepts original to Volpe at Washington University.

SEIZURES WITH EEG DISCHARGE   Focal or multifocal clonic seizures, focal tonic seizures (including eye deviation), some generalized myoclonic seizures, and ictal apnea are consistently associated with EEG ictal patterns.

SEIZURES WITH INCONSISTENT OR NO EEG CHANGES   Staring, ocular movements, excessive salivation, and various autonomic phenomena occurring in isolation, such as changes in heart rate and blood pressure, may be associated with EEG discharges but often are not. Motor automatisms including various oral-buccal-lingual movements; progression movements such as stepping, pedaling, or swimming; and complex asynchronous motor activities (thrashing, writhing) are uncommonly accompanied by EEG seizure activity. Generalized tonic seizures in the newborn have no EEG correlates.

Analysis of Clinical Seizure Phenomena

The data emerging from detailed analysis of simultaneous video and EEG polygraphic recordings of neonatal seizures indicate that one must be cautious in inferring an epileptic basis for all seizures on clinical observations alone. Concurrent EEG recordings are usually necessary to distinguish ictal events from similar phenomena that probably represent abnormal motor activities arising from release of subcortical and brainstem mechanisms owing to severe cortical depression caused by asphyxia or other injury. Thus, many so-called subtle or postural seizures probably represent brainstem release phenomena, not cortical epileptic seizures.

Careful examination of the infant may help distinguish epileptic from other nonepileptic motor activity. Nonepileptic motor activity can be suppressed by light restraint or by repositioning of the involved body part. Epileptic activity will continue unchanged. Nonepileptic behaviors can often be elicited by sensory stimulation and will typically show temporal and spatial summation. These features are not characteristic of epileptic seizures. Finally, prominent autonomic accompaniments to the motor activity favor epileptic rather than nonepileptic seizures.

Diagnostic difficulty may also occasionally be encountered in distinguishing jitteriness from ictal behavior. Jitteriness has features of both tremor and clonus. Movements are typically rhythmic and of the same amplitude in flexor and extensor muscles. Like other nonepileptic motor activity, tremor or jitteriness is stimulus-sensitive and not accompanied by abnormal eye movements or apnea. In contrast, movements seen with seizures are usually jerk-like, with rapid and slow components, and associated findings such as eye deviation, chewing, and apnea are common. Tonic posturing and twitchy limb movements are normally seen in infants during active or rapid eye movement (REM) sleep, and these must not be mistaken for seizure activity. Finally, in neonates, focal seizures generally do not imply demonstrable localized cerebral disease; more commonly, bilateral cerebral dysfunction exists, such as a metabolic encephalopathy.

Etiology

Seizures may arise from any transient or persistent cerebral insult, but only a few causes are encountered with regularity. No cause will be found in about 25% of infants with seizures.

Perinatal Complications   These complications account for approximately one-third of seizures in full-term infants and about half of those in preterm infants. Neonatal asphyxia is the major factor in full-term infants, and intraventricular hemorrhage in premature babies (see Secs. 2.17.12; 25.4).

Hypoxic-ischemic encephalopathy is now the single most common cause of seizures in newborns, but diagnosis may be difficult. Most asphyxia occurs before or during delivery. In a convulsing newborn, asphyxia should be suspected if resuscitation was necessary, if a severe disturbance of gas exchange has been documented ($PO_2 < 40$ mm Hg), or if there is a history of placental infarction, cord hematomas, placenta previa, or abruptio placentae. Fetal distress documented by intrauterine monitoring and scalp or cord pH levels less than 7.20 are also indicative of a likely asphyxic etiology. Apgar scores correlate poorly with asphyxic brain damage as a cause of seizures.

Intraventricular Hemorrhage   Intraventricular hemorrhage (IVH) must be distinguished from subarachnoid hemorrhage, if possible. The latter is often associated with a history of difficult labor or delivery and occurs must frequently in near-term infants. Between seizures these infants look healthy and well. Seizures are usually well organized and transient and respond readily to antiepileptic medication. Most infants with seizures from IVH are premature babies who have been insidiously deteriorating since birth or who are critically ill as a result of an abrupt decline in neurologic status. The infants remain poorly responsive and unstable between seizures, and the attacks may persist despite high-dosage anticonvulsant therapy. Hypoxia is a major factor in IVH in preterm babies. Infants with IVH typically have seizures of the minimal or multifocal clonic type. Based on studies with CT scans, it is evident that mild intracranial bleeding may occur with only minor clinical manifestations.

Hypoglycemia   Significant *hypoglycemia* is defined as a blood glucose level below 30 mg/dL in the first 72 hours of life for full-term newborns and less than 40 mg/dL thereafter, or as less than 20 mg/dL in premature or low-birthweight infants. However, there are no data that indicate a "safe" lower limit of hypoglycemia especially in the presence of other insults to the brain such as ischemia or hypoxia. Although hypoglycemia is a frequent finding in neonatal seizure states, the causal relationship between hypoglycemia and seizures is often questionable. Infants with a wide variety of cerebral insults may be hypoglycemic, and correcting the hypoglycemia may or may not stop the seizures and improve neurologic status. Also, there is poor correlation between the concentration of blood glucose and the severity of neurologic findings. However, hypoglycemia should be corrected promptly because its persistence could contribute to any associated neurologic insult. In fact, we treat any convulsing newborn with supplemental glucose even in the absence of documented hypoglycemia.

Hypocalcemia   *Hypocalcemia* is defined as a serum calcium level below 7.0 mg/dL associated with a normal or high level of serum phosphorus. Symptomatic hypocalcemia is related to the concentration of ionized calcium, which, in turn, is dependent on the protein concentration and blood pH. Uncomplicated hypocalcemia was formerly a common cause of seizures in the second week after birth, but this has now virtually disappeared as a major cause concomitant with the encouragement of breast-feeding and the use of low-phosphate milk formulas. Most hypocalcemia is now seen within the first few days of postnatal life in premature infants or in infants who have sustained perinatal insults. Seizures in these infants are generally the result of the underlying brain damage, although the associated hypocalcemia may exacerbate the convulsive disorder. Failure of the serum calcium concentration to respond to intravenous calcium salts should raise the suspicion of coexisting hypomagnesemia.

Infections   Central nervous system infections account for about 10% of neonatal seizures. Conversely, about 50% of neonates with meningitis will have seizures at some time during the course of the infection. Every infant who has seizures should have a lumbar puncture and CSF analysis. About two-thirds of causative organisms are bacterial, usually gram-negative, with other infectious agents, including cytomegalovirus, herpes simplex virus (type II), enterovirus, rubella virus, and toxoplasma, accounting for the remainder. Genital herpes in the mother should suggest the possibility of herpes simplex encephalitis, and choreoretinitis indicates the possibility of cytomegalic inclusion disease or toxoplasmosis. A characteristic EEG pattern showing periodic lateralizing epileptiform discharges (PLEDS) may assist in diagnosing herpes encephalitis. Intracranial calcifications, which are common in older infants with either of the latter infections, may not be detected in newborns even with the use of CT scanning.

Developmental Anomalies   Neonatal seizures may arise from cerebral malformations. These include heterotopias of gray matter, polymicrogyria, holoprosencephaly, and anencephaly. The latter two anomalies will be evident on ultrasound and CT scanning.

Familial Neonatal Seizures   A benign form of neonatal seizures has been described in families. Pedigrees indicate autosomal-dominant inheritance, and a locus has been mapped to the long arm of chromosome 20. The seizures are usually clonic in type and begin within the first week after birth. Interictal EEGs are normal or show mild nonspecific abnormalities. Ictal recordings have demonstrated both focal (usually rolandic) and generalized discharge patterns. Except for the family history, no other causative factors can be identified, and the neurologic examination is normal. The seizures usually remit spontaneously. Unexpected death or later epilepsy has been reported in a few affected infants.

Management

Distinction between epileptic and nonepileptic seizures raises new implications for management. There is little question that epileptic seizures should be treated with anticonvulsant drugs, because seizures may have adverse consequences for normal brain development and cardiorespiratory function, although the evidence for this in newborns is not as convincing as in older children and adults. However, when there is no electrical discharge accompanying behavioral seizures, indications for routine use of antiepileptic drugs are arguable at best. Such infants are frequently quite depressed neurologically, and anticonvulsants may further contribute to obtundation. This is especially likely because dosages of antiepileptic drugs required to suppress generalized tonic seizures, most subtle seizures, and postural automatisms are high, often in the anesthetic range.

A careful history should be obtained regarding the pregnancy, labor, and delivery, as well as any details about fetal monitoring, kinds of anesthesia, anomalies of the cord and placenta, and need for resuscitation. An intravenous line must be placed, and proper ventilation and adequate glucose levels should be ensured immediately. Initial laboratory tests that should be carried out promptly include lumbar puncture, Dextrostix, quantitative determination of glucose, calcium, magnesium, other electrolytes, and blood gases. An EEG should be ordered if readily available.

Although we used to recommend empirical administration of a sequence of metabolic supplements (glucose, calcium gluconate, magnesium sulfate, and pyridoxine) before initiating anticonvulsant therapy, we now believe that it is best to document a specific metabolic derangement and not treat blindly without laboratory confirmation. In particular, hypertonic glucose solutions should be used carefully and very specifically only after hypoglycemia has been documented, because these solutions may increase the risk of intracranial hemorrhage. Most neonatal nurseries now have access to accurate and rapidly obtained chemistry screening panels. If hypoglycemia is present, give an initial intravenous dose of 25% glucose, 2 to 4 mL/kg (0.5 to 1.0 g/kg), followed by a maintenance dose of 0.7 g/kg per hour. If hypocalcemia is documented, give a 5% solution of calcium gluconate intravenously, 4 mL/kg (200 mg/kg), with electrocardiographic monitoring. Hypomagnesemia may be treated with a 50% solution of magnesium sulfate, 0.2 mL/kg intramuscularly, or with a 2 to 3% solution of magnesium sulfate given intravenously in a total volume of 2 to 8 mL.

If the laboratory profiles do not indicate a biochemical cause for the seizures, we begin anticonvulsant drugs while continuing to search for a specific etiology. The anticonvulsant agent and its dosage should be selected on the basis of the particular clinical situation. Infrequent seizures, or those expected to be transient (from subarachnoid hemorrhage, for example), may be treated with diazepam at 0.1 to 0.5 mg intravenously or intramuscularly repeated two or four times daily or as needed. If seizures are severe or frequent or if they continue beyond 24 hours, phenobarbital at 20 mg/kg intravenously should be given, with the dose repeated 30 to 60 minutes later if necessary. A maintenance dosage of 10 mg/kg per day is usually adequate. If seizures continue, phenytoin 20 mg/kg may be given slowly over 20 minutes with ECG monitoring.

Once treatment has been started, the question arises, "What is the endpoint?" One gauge is clinical; that is, treat until clinical manifestations subside. However, when the EEG is recorded during treatment, it is not infrequent that one observes persistence of EEG ictal patterns even when behavioral events have ended. A related circumstance is recording EEG seizure patterns in untreated infants without clinical evidence of seizure activity, and this may be more common than once believed. We have rarely seen significant changes in a newborn's condition after aggressive treatment of electrical seizures unassociated with clinical seizures. From an operational standpoint, and in the absence of convincing evidence to the contrary, we treat until clinical seizures subside or we achieve reasonably optimal levels of antiepileptic drugs (eg, 20 μg/mL for phenytoin, 35 to 40 μg/mL for phenobarbital). At the present time, we do not attempt to eliminate all EEG seizure activity.

If the initial history and laboratory investigations do not lead to a presumptive cause for the seizures, additional diagnostic tests must be undertaken. These include CT and ultrasound scanning for evidence of cerebral malformations, determining serologic titers against specific agents, and screening tests for inborn errors of metabolism. The rare disorder of pyridoxine dependency can only be diagnosed empirically by observing the clinical and EEG response to the intravenous administration of 100 mg pyridoxine.

An important issue in newborns, as in older children, is when to stop anticonvulsant therapy. Most neonatal seizures cease within the first month, even without therapy; indeed, the subsidence of seizure activity may be determined more by the natural history of the illness than by the use of antiepileptic medication. In addition, we do not know whether anticonvulsant therapy influences prognosis, either with respect to the development of epilepsy in later life or with respect to the incidence of other neurologic sequelae. In view of these considerations, and because we are concerned with the possible long-term effects of chronic drug use on the developing brain, we discontinue antiepileptic therapy 1 month after the last seizure if the neurologic examination is normal. We will not continue anticonvulsant drugs beyond 3 months, even with an abnormal examination, unless the EEG shows significant persistent abnormalities or the infant is at unusually high risk for recurrent seizures (eg, cerebral dysgenesis).

Prognosis

The high rates of morbidity and mortality among newborns who have seizures are directly related to the severity of etiologic factors having a high correlation with permanent brain damage. Perinatal asphyxia, severe intraventricular hemorrhage, and cerebral malformations have particularly poor implications for neurologic development. Recurrent seizures from the first day after birth that interfere with respiration and feeding schedules are associated with significant morbidity, especially if the Apgar score at 5 minutes was low. A normal EEG obtained at the time of the initial seizure is highly correlated with a favorable outcome. Conversely, several EEG patterns in full-term infants, including multifocal spikes or ictal events, suppression-burst background activity, and an isoelectric record, reliably predict a fatal outcome or disabling brain damage more than 90% of the time.

25.10.4   Febrile Seizures

Stephen G. Ryan

EPIDEMIOLOGY AND CLINICAL FEATURES

A febrile convulsion is operationally defined as a seizure occurring during a febrile illness—excluding intracranial infection or inflammation—in a child between the ages of 6 months and 5 years who has not experienced a prior seizure in the absence of fever. A febrile seizure is considered *simple* if the convulsion is relatively brief (<15 minutes) and generalized and if it does not recur during the same febrile illness. In contrast, a febrile convulsion is classified as *complex* if there are focal features, long duration, or recurrence within 24 hours.

About 3% of all children experience at least one febrile convulsion by the age of 5 years. In half of cases, the initial febrile convulsion occurs by the age of 18 months. Febrile convulsions are more common during winter months. Risk factors for febrile convulsions include family history, daycare attendance, and underlying neurodevelopmental abnormality. The great majority of children with febrile convulsions, however, are developmentally normal and do not have a history of prior brain insult.

Most patients (about 80%) have simple febrile seizures, and the attack typically occurs shortly after the onset of fever. The likelihood of a febrile convulsion is influenced more by the rate of rise rather than the height of the temperature. Indeed, many febrile seizures occur before the parents are aware that the child has a fever. Certain childhood infections, including roseola and shigellosis, are particularly common causes of fever in affected children.

ETIOLOGY

Liability to febrile convulsions is strongly influenced by genetic factors. About 40% of probands have at least one affected first- or second-degree relative, concordance is higher in monozygotic compared with dizygotic twins, and the risk to siblings exceeds the population risk by four-fold. These observations suggest that in most cases susceptibility to febrile convulsions reflects the interaction of several genes. In exceptional instances, febrile convulsions segregate in extended families as a highly penetrant, autosomal-dominant trait. Analysis of one such family has led to the identification of a DNA sequence variation in a gene encoding a sodium channel component as the likely cause of the disorder.

DIAGNOSIS

A thorough history and physical examination will often identify a focus of infection. It is essential to evaluate the child carefully for evidence of intracranial infection. This often requires lumbar puncture and examination of the cerebrospinal fluid, especially in cases where the child has been ill with fever for more than a few hours before the occurrence of the seizure or if the child is already receiving antibacterial therapy for a known infection such as otitis media. Depending on the clinical circumstances, determination of serum electrolytes and glucose may be advisable, especially if diarrhea or vomiting has occurred or if the temperature elevation is modest and the source of fever inapparent.

Cranial computed tomography or magnetic resonance imaging should be considered in children with complex febrile convulsions, especially when recovery of baseline neurologic function is prolonged, and in children with a history of preexisting, undiagnosed neurodevelopmental abnormality.

The EEG is of limited value in the evaluation of children with simple febrile convulsions. Nonspecific abnormalities, such as slowing and disorganization of background rhythms, are common, especially in the first 24 to 48 hours after the attack, and do not have prognostic significance. Among children with complex febrile convulsions, the interictal EEG often shows focal slowing acutely but often returns to normal within a week. In some children with febrile status epilepticus and delayed recovery of consciousness, the EEG can aid management by detecting persistent, nonconvulsive seizure activity.

TREATMENT

ACUTE MANAGEMENT   The acute management of febrile convulsions should be guided by an awareness that most febrile convulsions end spontaneously within a few minutes and that such brief attacks do not appear to damage the brain in any way. It is important to ensure a clear airway, and it is prudent to administer supplemental oxygen if this is immediately available. Ventilatory assistance, however, is not required for brief attacks.

Febrile status epilepticus is defined as a single febrile convulsion, or a series of febrile convulsions without recovery of consciousness between attacks, lasting more than 30 minutes. This disorder should be regarded as potentially injurious to the brain and treated as a medical emergency as described in the section on status epilepticus.

PREVENTION   It is common for the parents of a child experiencing a first febrile seizure—even when the attack is relatively brief—to believe that she or he is dying. Thus, one of the most important tasks of the clinician is educating the parents about the ordinarily benign outcome of the syndrome. Most physicians recommend vigorous efforts to control fever, including antipyretic agents and tepid baths, but the merit of this approach is unproven. It is generally agreed that children with simple febrile convulsions—even when they recur—do not require pharmacologic intervention.

The daily administration of phenobarbital substantially lowers the risk of febrile convulsion recurrence but results in obvious adverse behavioral effects, such as hyperactivity and irritability, in about 20% of children. There is also concern that phenobarbital may interfere in a subtle but long-lasting way with intellectual development. Therefore, prophylaxis of febrile convulsions with phenobarbital is generally recommended only for children with a history of one or more prolonged attacks or with very frequent recurrence, especially if there are other risk factors for epilepsy. The effectiveness of antiepileptic drugs other than phenobarbital in preventing febrile convulsion recurrence has not been extensively evaluated. There is some evidence that valproic acid may reduce the rate of febrile convulsion recurrence, but the risk of serious hepatotoxicity limits the use of this drug to children with recurrent, prolonged febrile convulsions in whom intermittent therapy is not effective and phenobarbital is poorly tolerated. Carbamazepine and phenytoin do not appear effective in the prevention of recurrent febrile convulsions.

Oral diazepam (0.3 mg/kg) given at the first indication of fever has been shown to reduce the risk of febrile convulsion recurrence. However, a substantial minority of children experience recurrent febrile convulsions before a parent is aware of the presence of fever. Moreover, the sedation produced by diazepam may complicate the assessment of an ill child.

Rectal diazepam has recently been approved for use in children with frequent, serial seizures and may be used by parents as an initial, emergency treatment of recurrent, prolonged febrile convulsions. Although the risk of serious respiratory depression from rectal diazepam at recommended doses is low, the use of rectal diazepam should be limited to children with a history of prolonged febrile convulsion, and it is advisable that parents be instructed in cardiopulmonary resuscitation.

PROGNOSIS

About a third of children with an initial febrile convulsion experience a subsequent attack, and half of children with a first recurrence experience a second. In a group of children presenting to an emergency room with an initial febrile convulsion, risk factors for recurrence included young age (<18 months), relatively modest temperature elevation (<40°C), and short duration of fever prior to the convulsion.

Although the outcome of febrile seizures is usually favorable, about 2 to 4% of children with febrile seizures experience subsequent epilepsy, defined as recurrent, afebrile convulsions. Risk factors for epilepsy include complex features of the initial attack and underlying neurodevelopmental abnormality.

About 15% of all cases of childhood epilepsy are preceded by febrile seizures, but the nature of the relationship is the subject of longstanding controversy. In many cases, febrile seizures appear to reflect a nonspecific "low seizure threshhold" that is genetically determined in most cases but that may also result from the presence of a subtle brain abnormality such as focal cortical dysplasia. The increased risk of epilepsy among near relatives of children with febrile convulsions lends support to this view. There is mounting evidence, however, that febrile status epilepticus contributes to the development of mesial temporal sclerosis, which is found in large proportions of older children and adults with chronic, temporal lobe epilepsy. These individuals frequently have a prior history of prolonged, focal febrile convulsions. Developmental delay and

mental retardation occur at slightly increased rates among children with complex but not simple febrile convulsions.

References

General

Berkovic S, Andermann F, Carpenter S, et al: Progressive myoclonus epilepsies: specific causes and diagnosis. N Engl J Med 315:296, 1986

Ellenberg JH, Hirtz DG, Nelson KB: Age at onset of seizures in young children. Ann Neurol 15:127, 1984

Freeman JM, Vining EPG, Pillas DJ: Seizures and Epilepsy in Childhood: A Guide for Parents. Baltimore, Johns Hopkins, 1990

Hauser WA, Annegers JF, Kurland LT: Incidence of epilepsy and unprovoked seizures in Rochester, Minnesota: 1935–1984. Epilepsia 34:453, 1993

Holmes GL: Diagnosis and Management of Seizures in Children. Philadelphia, Saunders, 1987

Shinnar S, O'Dell C, Berg AT: Distribution of epilepsy syndromes in a cohort of children prospectively monitored from the time of their first unprovoked seizure. Epilepsia 40:1378, 1999

Pathophysiology

Chapman A, Meldrum B: Excitatory amino acids in epilepsy and novel antiepileptic drugs. Epilepsy Res Suppl 3:39–48, 1991

Coulter DA, Huguenard JR, Prince DA: Characterization of ethosuximide reduction of low-threshold calcium current in thalamic neurons. Ann Neurol 25:582–593, 1989

Heyer EJ, Macdonald RL: Barbiturate reduction of calcium-dependent action potentials: correlation with anesthetic action. Brain Res 236:157–171, 1982

Hosford DA, Clark S, Cao Z, et al: The role of GABAB receptor activation in absence seizures of lethargic (lh/lh) mice. Science 257:398–401, 1992

Macdonald RL, McLean MJ: Mechanisms of anticonvulsant drug action. Electroencephalogr Clin Neurophysiol Suppl 39:200–208, 1987

Meldrum B: Excitotoxicity and epileptic brain damage. Epilepsy Res 10:55–61, 1991

Moshe SL: Seizures in the developing brain. Neurology 43(11 suppl 5):S3–S7, 1993

Rothman SM, Olney JW: Glutamate and the pathophysiology of hypoxic-ischemic brain damage. Ann Neurol 19:105–111, 1986

Schwartzkroin PA: Origins of the epileptic state. Epilepsia 38:853, 1997

Twyman RE, Rogers CJ, MacDonald RL: Differential regulation of gamma-aminobutyric acid receptor channels by diazepam and phenobarbital. Ann Neurol 25:213–220, 1989

Von Krosigk M, Bal T, McCormick DA: Cellular mechanisms of a synchronized oscillation in the thalamus. Science 261:361–364, 1993

White HS: Comparative anticonvulsant and mechanistic profile of the established and newer antiepileptic drugs. Epilepsia 40 (suppl 5):2, 1999

Seizure Types

Generalized-Onset Seizures

Aminoff MJ, Simon RP, Weidemann E: The hormonal responses to generalized tonic-clonic seizures. Brain 107:569, 1984

Browne TR, Penry JK, Porter RJ, et al: Responsiveness before, during and after spike-wave paroxysms. Neurology 24:659, 1974

Partial (Focal) Seizures

Falconer MA, Serafetinides EA, Corsellis JAN: Etiology and pathogenesis of temporal lobe epilepsy. Arch Neurol 10:233, 1964

Holmes GL: Partial complex seizures in children: an analysis of 69 seizures in 24 patients using EEG, FM radiotelemetry and videotape recording. Electroencephalogr Clin Neurophysiol 57:13, 1984

Nordi DR, Bazil CW, Scheuer ML, Pedley TA: Recognition and classification of seizures in infants. Epilepsia 38:553, 1997.

Epileptic Syndromes

Andermann F, Cooke PM, Dickson J, et al: Self-induced epilepsy. Arch Neurol 6:49, 1962

Andermann F, Robb JP: Absence status: a reappraisal following review of thirty-eight patients. Epilepsia 31:177, 1972

Bellman MH, Ross EM, Miller DL: Infantile spasms and pertussis immunization. Lancet 1:1031, 1983

Blume WT, David RB, Gomez MR: Generalized sharp and slow-wave complexes—associated clinical features and long-term follow-up. Brain 96:289, 1973

Chatrian GE, Letrich E, Miller LH, et al: Pattern sensitive epilepsy. Epilepsia 11:125, 1970

Delgado-Esceuta AV, Enrile-Bascal FE: Juvenile myoclonic epilepsy of Janz. Neurology 34:285, 1984

Gastaut H: A new type of epilepsy: benign partial epilepsy of childhood with occipital spike-waves. Clin Electroencephalogr 13:13, 1982

Hrachovy R, Frost JD: Infantile spasms. Cleveland Clin J Med 56(suppl 1):S10, 1989

Lerman P, Kivity P: The benign focal epilepsies of childhood. In: Pedley TA, Meldrum BS, eds: Recent Advances in Epilepsy, vol 3. Edinburgh, Churchill Livingstone, 1986

Lombroso CT: Sylvian seizures and midtemporal spike foci in children. Arch Neurol 17:52, 1967

Lombroso CT, Fejerman N: Benign myoclonus of early infancy. Ann Neurol 1:138, 1977

Mantovani JF, Landau WM: Acquired aphasia with convulsive disorder: course and prognosis. Neurology 30:524, 1980

Markland O: Slow spike-wave activity in EEG and associated clinical features often called "Lennox" or "Lennox-Gastaut" syndrome. Neurology 27:746, 1977

Panayiotopoulos CP, Obeid T, Waheed G: Absences in juvenile myoclonic epilepsy: a clinical and video-electroencephalographic study. Ann Neurol 25:391, 1989

Ritter F, Leppik I, Dreifuss F, et al: Efficacy of felbamate in childhood epileptic encephalopathy (Lennox-Gastaut syndrome). N Engl J Med 328:29, 1993

Sato S, Dreifuss FE, Penry JK: Prognostic factors in absence seizures. Neurology 26:888, 1976

Solomon GE, Hilal SK, Gold AP, et al: Natural history of acute hemiplegia of childhood. Brain 93:107, 1970

Tinuper P, Andermann F, Villemure J-G, et al: Functional hemispherectomy for treatment of epilepsy associated with hemiplegia: rationale, indications, results and comparison with callostomy. Ann Neurol 24:27, 1988

Therapeutic Considerations

Status Epilepticus

Aminoff MJ, Simon RP: Status epilepticus. Causes, clinical features and consequences in 98 patients. Am J Med 69:657, 1980

Delgado-Escueta AV, Waterlain C, Treiman DM, et al: Management of status epilepticus. N Engl J Med 306:1337, 1982

Dodson WE, DeLorenzo RJ, Pedley TA, et al: Treatment of convulsive status epilepticus: recommendations of the Epilepsy Foundation of America's working group on status epilepticus. JAMA 270:854–859, 1993

Graves NM, Kriel RL: Rectal administration of antiepileptic drugs in children. Pediatr Neurol 3:321, 1987

Holmes GL, Riviello JJ: Midazolam and pentobarbital for refractory status epilepticus. Pediatr Neurol 20:259, 1999

Kriel RL, Cloyd JC, Pellock JM, Mitchell WG, Cereghion JJ, Rosman NP: Rectal diazepam gel for treatment of acute repetitive seizures. The North American Diastat Study Group. Pediatr Neurol: 20:282, 1999

Mizrahi EM: Acute and chronic effects of seizures in the developing brain: lessons from clinical experience. Epilepsia 40 (suppl 1):42, 1999

Shinnar S, Matyal J, Drasnoff L, et al: Recurrent status epilepticus in children. Ann Neurol 31:598, 1992

Simon RP: Management of status epilepticus. In: Pedley TA, Meldrum BS, eds: Recent Advances in Epilepsy, vol 2. Edinburgh, Churchill Livingstone, 1985

Young RSK, Ropper AH, Hawkes D, et al: Pentobarbital in refractory status epilepticus. Pediatr Pharmacol 3:63, 1983

Neonatal Seizures

Clancy RR, Legido A, Lewis D: Occult neonatal seizures. Epilepsia 29, 1988

Hill A, Volpe JJ: Seizure hypoxic-ischemic brain injury, and intraventricular hemorrhage in the newborn. Ann Neurol 10:109, 1981

Holden KR, Mellits ED, Freeman JM: Neonatal seizures. I. Correlation of prenatal and perinatal events with outcomes. Pediatrics 70:165, 1982

Levy SR, Abroms IF, Marshall PC, et al: Seizures and cerebral infarction in the full-term newborn. Ann Neurol 17:366, 1985

Mizrahi EM, Kellaway P: Characterization and classification of neonatal seizures. Neurol 37:1837, 1987

Painter MJ, Scher MS, Stein AD, et al: Phenobarbital compared with phenytoin for the treatment of neonatal seizures. N Engl J Med 341:485, 1999

Petit RE, Fenichel GM: Benign familial neonatal seizures. Arch Neurol 37:47, 1980

Rowe JC, Holmes G, Hafford J, et al: Prognostic value of the electroencephalogram in term and preterm infants following neonatal seizures. Electroencephalogr Clin Neurophysiol 60:183, 1985

Volpe JJ: Neonatal seizures: current concepts and revised classification. Pediatrics 84:422, 1989

Management and Prognosis

Bourgeois BFD: Pharmacologic intervention and treatment of childhood seizure disorders: relative efficacy and safety of antiepileptic drugs. Epilepsia 35(suppl 2):S18–S23, 1994

Callaghan N, Garrett A, Goggin T: Withdrawal of anticonvulsant drugs in patients free of seizures for two years. N Engl J Med 318:559, 1985

Dodson WE: Special pharmacokinetic considerations in children. Epilepsia 28(suppl 1):556, 1987

Freeman JM: A clinical approach to the child with seizures and epilepsy. Epilepsia 28(suppl 1):S103, 1987

Hornan RW, Miller B: VA Epilepsy Cooperative Study Group: causes of treatment failure with antiepileptic drugs vary over time. Neurology 37:1620, 1987

Leppik IE: Management of seizures during pregnancy. In: Pedley TA, Meldrum BS, eds: Recent Advances in Epilepsy, vol. 4. Edinburgh, Churchill Livingstone, 1988

Lesser RJ, Pippenger CE, Luders H, et al: High-dose monotherapy in treatment of intractable seizures. Neurology 34:707, 1984

Mattson RH, Cramer JA, Collins JF: A comparison of valproate with carbamazepine for the treatment of complex partial seizures and secondarily generalized tonic-clonic seizures in adults. The Department of Veterans Affairs Epilepsy Cooperative Study No. 264 Group. N Engl J Med 327:765, 1992

Pellock JM: Managing pediatric epilepsy syndromes with new antiepileptic drugs. Pediatrics 104:1106, 1999

Practice parameter: management issues for women with epilepsy (summary statement). Report of the Quality Standards Subcommittee of the American Academy of Neurology. Epilepsia 39:1226, 1998

Rowan AJ, Pippenger CE, McGregor PA, et al: Seizure activity and anticonvulsant drug concentration. Arch Neurol 32:281, 1975

Schmidt D: Prognosis of chronic epilepsy with complex partial seizures. J Neurol Neurosurg Psychiatr 47:1274, 1984

Shinnar S, Vining EPG, Mellits ED, et al: Discontinuing antiepileptic medication in children with epilepsy after two years without seizures. N Engl J Med 313:976, 1985

Thurston JH, Thurston DL, Hixon BB, et al: Prognosis in childhood epilepsy. N Engl J Med 306:831, 1982

Trimble MR, Cull C: Antiepileptic drugs, cognitive function, and behavior. Cleveland Clin J Med 56(suppl 1):S140, 1989

Yerby MS: Teratogenicity of antiepileptic drugs. In: Pedley TA, Meldrum BS, eds: Recent Advances in Epilepsy, vol 4. Edinburgh, Churchill Livingstone, 1988

Surgical Treatment

Villemure JG, Rasmussen T: Functional hemispherectomy in children. Neuropediatrics 24:53, 1993

Wyllie E, Coumair YG, Kotagal P, Bulacio J, Bingaman W, Ruggieri P: Seizure outcome after epilepsy surgery in children and adolescents. Ann Neurol 44:740, 1998

Febrile Seizures

Berg AT, Shinnar SS, Darefsky AS, et al: Predictors of recurrent febrile seizures. Arch Pediatr Adolesc Med 151:371, 1997

Camfield P, Camfield C, Gordon K, Dooley J: What types of epilepsy are preceded by febrile seizures? A population-based study of children. Dev Med Child Neurol 36:887, 1994

Farwell JR, Lee YJ, Hirtz DG, Sulzbacher SI, Ellenberg JH, Nelson KB: Phenobarbital for febrile seizures—effects on intelligence and on seizure recurrence. N Engl J Med 322:364–369, 1990

Green SM, Rothrock SG, Clem KJ, Zurcher RF, Mellick L: Can seizures be the sole manifestation of meningitis in febrile children? Pediatrics 92:527–534, 1993

Hauser WA, Annegers JF, Anderson VE, Kurland LT: The risk of seizure disorders among relatives of children with febrile convulsions. Neurology 35:1268, 1985

Knudsen FU, Vestermark S: Prophylactic diazepam or phenobarbitone in febrile convulsions: a prospective, controlled study. Arch Dis Child 53:660, 1978

Maytal J, Shinnar S: Febrile status epilepticus. Pediatrics 86:611–616, 1990

Nelson KB: Prognosis in children with febrile seizures. Pediatrics 61:720, 1978

Rosman NP, Colton T, Labazzo J, et al: A controlled trial of diazepam administered during febrile illnesses to prevent recurrence of febrile seizures. N Engl J Med 329:79–84, 1993

Verity CM, Ross EM, Golding J: Oucome of childhood status epilepticus and lengthy febrile convulsions: findings of national cohort study. BMJ 307:225, 1993

Wallace RH, Wang DW, Singh R, et al: Febrile seizures and generalized epilepsy associated with a mutation in the Na^+-channel beta1 subunit gene SCN1B. Nat Genet 19:366, 1998

Wolf SM, Forsythe A: Epilepsy and mental retardation following febrile seizures in childhood. Acta Pediatr Scand 78:291, 1989

25.11 NONEPILEPTIC PAROXYSMAL DISORDERS

Douglas R. Nordli, Jr., Timothy A. Pedley, and Darryl C. De Vivo

Many childhood disorders have paroxysmal features. Because of the paroxysmal nature of their presentation, it is not uncommon that the episodes are interpreted as seizure activity. In this section common disorders that may mimic epilepsy are emphasized.

25.11.1 Sleep Disorders

The Association of Sleep Disorder Centers has identified four general categories of sleep disorders for diagnostic purposes:

1. Disorders of initiating and maintaining sleep (insomnia) (DIMS)
2. Disorders of excessive somnolence (DOES)
3. Disorders of sleep-wake schedule
4. Dysfunctions associated with sleep, sleep stages, or partial arousals (parasomnias)

The parasomnias are most often confused with epilepsy. They occur during arousal from stage 4 sleep, usually just before transition to rapid eye movement (REM) sleep. The EEG demonstrates nearly continuous high-voltage monorhythmic delta waves. *Night terrors* (pavor nocturnus) occur in up to 3% of children 5 to 7 years of age. Onset is abrupt: the child sits up in bed, screams or cries, appears very agitated and is inconsolable. There is always amnesia for the event, even though the child appears awake during attacks. Nightmares, in contrast, are remembered. Night terrors typically last for several minutes. They are benign and do not require treatment. *Somnambulism*, or sleep walking, is another parasomnia. It is common: 15% of children sleepwalk at least once in their life. Somnambulism is more readily recognized by parents and, therefore, less often confused with epilepsy. Sleep walking and night terrors often coexist, and these conditions are discussed in Sec. 5.5.2.

25.11.2 Movement Disorders

Tics are brief motor movements that can be temporarily suppressed. Tics often manifest as a sudden, backward movement of the head. They may also include blinking, grimacing, and movements of the arms or shoulders. Vocal tics consist of grunts, guttural noises, barks, or curses. Vocal tics coupled with disabling motor tics constitute the *Gilles de la Tourette syndrome*. Tics are often exacerbated by stress; this may result in psychiatric referral. Most simple motor tics disappear during adolescence.

Spasmus nutans is an unusual condition of infancy characterized by head-nodding, head tilt, and nystagmus. All three components do not necessarily need to be present at the same time for the diagnosis to be made. The condition often begins late in the first year after birth or early in the second. The nystagmus is often asymmetric, being more prominent in one eye. Neuroimaging is indicated because of an association between spasmus nutans and optic gliomas. In the proven absence of tumor, reassurance is appropriate because spasmus nutans will resolve spontaneously within several months.

Stereotypies are more elaborate movements than tics; they consist of endlessly repeated fragments of normal behaviors. They are not epileptic, but they coexist with epilepsy in some individuals. Stereotypies are typical of the Rett syndrome (see Sec. 25.6.3), a cause of severe developmental dysfunction in girls in which the afflicted child has abundant midline hand-wringing movements beginning in late infancy. Hyperventilation and body rocking also occur. Rett syndrome is accompanied by profound cognitive impairment, seizures, and a characteristic EEG. Prognosis is of relentless deterioration in motor function and communication skills. Stereotypies are also observed in children with various static encephalopathies and may include rocking, hand-flapping, and head-banging. In most cases they are easily distinguished from epilepsy by history and observation alone, but in more complex cases CCTV/EEG monitoring may be necessary. Clomipramine has recently been shown to be effective in reducing stereotypies and hyperactivity in autistic patients.

Paroxysmal choreoathetosis manifests in either the *kinesiogenic* or *dystonic* form. In the former instance, choreoathetotic movements occur after movement. In the latter, intermittent dystonia occurs. In neither form is consciousness impaired. Differentiation from simple partial seizures may be difficult, and CCTV/EEG monitoring is usually required. Both conditions may respond to treatment with carbamazepine.

Shuddering attacks resemble shivering and typically present in infancy and early childhood. They are often noted when the child is excited or angry or sometimes during micturition. Attacks are brief and not associated with falling or loss of consciousness. Shuddering attacks are benign and will be outgrown, although affected children seem to have an increased risk of developing essential tremor as adults.

Hyperexplexia is also known as *familial startle disease* and may be the same condition as stiff man syndrome. This rare disease mimics neonatal and infantile tonic seizures. It is an autosomal-dominant neurologic disorder characterized by marked muscle rigidity and an exaggerated startle response to sound or touch. Tonic constriction of the vocal cords during an attack (which resembles paroxysmal tetany) can lead to syncope and a tonic-clonic convulsion. Attacks may be fatal and therefore should be considered in the differential diagnosis of infants with acute life-threatening events (see Secs. 4.3.2; 23.5.2). This condition is linked to a DNA marker on the long arm of chromosome 5 and very recently was associated with the alpha-1 subunit of the inhibitory glycine receptor. Analysis of four different families has revealed a mutation in the same base pair of exon 6, which results in the substitution of leucine or glutamine for Arg271 in the final protein.

25.11.3 Syncope

Syncope results from inadequate perfusion of the brain. When the associated hypoxia is sufficiently severe, patients may exhibit tonic postures, clonic jerks, and even generalized convulsions (*convulsive syncope*). These features may be the dominant feature to eye witnesses; the subtler and more diagnostic aspects of the syncope may escape attention. Historical clues differentiating syncope from epilepsy include early light-headedness, darkening of vision, fading sound, nausea, and pallor. Diagnostic evaluation, including a 12-lead ECG and head-up tilt table testing, has been reported to be of value in patients with unexplained syncope (see Sec. 22.4.8).

Vasovagal syncope is the most common cause of fainting in children. The child may faint in response to Valsalva maneuvers, micturition, or seeing blood. Syncope is especially common in closed surroundings, such as a warm, crowded church or during long periods of standing in a stuffy gym class. If asked, the child will report feeling dizzy or light-headed. Subsequently, vision dims, followed by loss of consciousness. The fall is often gradual and contrasts with the propulsive drop seen in atonic seizures. Prolonged syncopal events may culminate in tonic postures or clonic muscle jerks. Children often appear weak or confused afterwards, but prolonged periods of confusion or lethargy are rare after syncope.

Pallid infantile syncope may represent a heightened immature response to vagal stimuli, and subtle evidence of underlying autonomic dysfunction in afflicted children has been reported. It most often occurs in infants exposed to frightening or upsetting stimuli. The infant becomes upset, turns ashen white, loses consciousness, and can progress to convulsive movements. The key to the diagnosis is recognition of the special inciting circumstances and the characteristic appearance of the infant immediately before the loss of consciousness. It may be confirmed by applying ocular compression with simultaneous EEG and ECG monitoring, but it is rarely necessary go to this extent to confirm the diagnosis.

Breath-holding spells (BHS) occur most often between the ages of 6 months and 6 years, although they may appear early in infancy. The predisposing setting is frustration or anger, which leads to crying or a tantrum. The child then holds his or her breath, becomes cyanotic, loses consciousness, and may have a few convulsive movements or tonic stiffening. The entire episode lasts less than a minute, and children are not impaired for a prolonged period after the attack. EEGs do not reveal any ictal accompaniment to the spell but demonstrate slowing during the period of decreased cerebral perfusion when the child loses consciousness. Several reports of pedigrees with multiple family members involved suggest that there may be a familial predisposition to BHS. Most studies of objective behavioral measurements do not reveal any consistent difference between children with BHS and those without. Treatment is directed at reassuring parents that their child will not die or become damaged by attacks and that they will invariably be outgrown. Antiepileptic drugs are of no value (see Sec. 5.6.5).

Cardiogenic causes of syncope are less common, but very important because they are potentially lethal. Syncope may be the early manifestation of cardiac disease in patients with primary hypertension, aortic stenosis, or primary pulmonary vascular disease. Other causes are arrhythmias, such as those seen in the prolonged QT syndrome, conduction defects, or heart block. Patients with the prolonged QT syndrome may have an associated autosomal congenital deafness. It is important to do a thorough physical examination including auscultation of the heart in all children with unexplained loss of consciousness. When syncope is suspected, a 12-lead electrocardiogram should be obtained.

25.11.4 Migraine

Headache is a common condition in children. The classic study of Swedish schoolchildren published in 1962 by Bille revealed that 75% of children complain of headache by age 15 years. Migraine, in turn, is the most common cause of severe headache. In a report by Chu and Shinnar, nearly 75% of children younger than 7 years referred to pediatric neurologists for headache were having migraine. In the Bille study, the prevalence of childhood migraine was

4%. A more recent population-based study from Olmsted County, Minnesota, reported a rate twice as high.

The necessary criteria for the diagnosis of migraine vary, but most children have two or more of the following features to their headaches: unilateral; throbbing quality; associated aura; abdominal pain, nausea, or vomiting; relief after sleep; and a positive family history.

Previously, various vascular mechanisms were implicated in the pathogenesis of migraine, but newer research using isotope studies has brought this into question. While the pulsating quality of the headache could be explained by engorged vessels, the aura does not clearly correlate with ischemia as was previously thought. Instead, the prodrome of migraine may have a hypothalamic origin, and a form of spreading cortical depression may be responsible for the aura. According to the neural hypothesis of migraine, a primary derangement of brain function causes the headache; this is supported by blood-flow studies, magnetic resonance, and spectroscopy data. Chemical hypotheses implicating serotonin are bolstered by the observation that many of the drugs used to treat headache have been shown to interact with serotonin receptor subtypes; medications useful in prophylaxis and acute treatment interact with independent subunits of the serotonin receptor. These data and various detailed clinical observations also suggest that migraine is distinct from tension headache and not part of the same clinical spectrum.

The International Headache Society has devised elaborate new classification schemes for migraine headache. These criteria were developed to reduce diagnostic variability but, when carefully applied, do not radically alter the diagnosis of patients classified according to older criteria. The newer criteria do, however, serve to increase the standardization of the diagnostic process and may be helpful to foster further genetic studies. The interested reader is referred to the references for further elaboration.

Migraine with aura (new classification) or *classic migraine* (old term) features an aura and well-developed unilateral headache. In *migraine without aura* (new classification) or *common migraine* (old term), the headache does not have a lateralized quality and is not associated with an aura.

Migraine with aura occurs infrequently in children. In Chu and Shinnar's series, 72 of 78 patients with migraine had the more common migraine without aura. Younger children often have abdominal pain or nausea, whereas older children may present with a lateralized throbbing headache and aura. Migraine in younger children is more likely to have common features, less likely to have a sex preponderance, and generally is of briefer duration than migraine in adults or older children. It is also more likely to be associated with epilepsy in childhood (see below for more discussion).

Many different triggers have been identified in children with migraine, including head trauma, physical exertion, stress, sleep deprivation, and ingestion of certain foods such as chocolate, cheese, processed meats, or food containing monosodium glutamate. In these cases, attempts to avoid triggers may be helpful, when practical.

The diagnosis of migraine is usually based on history and findings of a normal neurologic examination between attacks. In classic migraine, the attack may begin with a prodrome of irritability, followed shortly thereafter by an aura. The aura usually is visual and consists of photopsia, fortification spectra, and scotomata. These are usually in one visual field. Some children may experience more complex distortions of vision such as micropsia or macropsia and may be either embarrassed or unable to describe the phenomenon. Other sensory abnormalities, including tingling or numbness, may

occur on the side contralateral to the headache. The attacks are often relieved by sleep.

Rarer forms of complicated migraine are important to recognize, especially because headache may not be prominent. In *hemiplegic migraine,* the child may develop weakness of one side with or without aphasia lasting for hours or even days. There is a familial form of this condition, which is inherited in an autosomal-dominant fashion. Recently, analysis of two large pedigrees for linkage analysis revealed the gene for this condition mapped to chromosome 19p. This gene encodes for an α 1A calcium channel subunit. It is interesting to note that this is close to the location of the gene believed to be responsible for CADASIL (cerebral autosomal-dominant arteriopathy with subcortical infarcts and leukoencephalopathy).

Hemiplegic migraine needs to be differentiated from *alternating hemiplegia of childhood,* which presents with paroxysmal repeated episodes of hemiplegia lasting from minutes to days. Alternating hemiplegia also features tonic or dystonic attacks, nystagmus, dyspnea, and other autonomic phenomena. Two features that help to distinguish it from hemiplegic migraine are the associated cognitive decline and the onset before age 18 months.

Ophthalmoplegic migraine presents as a disturbance of ocular motility. The third cranial nerve is most often affected, but the fourth and sixth cranial nerves can be involved as well. *Basilar artery migraine* occurs mostly in adolescent girls and is characterized by vertigo, syncope, numbness, and dysarthria. Vision may be affected early in the course of the symptoms, resulting in transient amblyopia or total blindness. *Confusional migraine* manifests as a profound confusional state that lasts for hours; this must be distinguished from toxic/metabolic encephalopathies and from absence or complex partial status epilepticus.

Treatment

Treatment of migraine should be considered from two perspectives: symptomatic relief of acute attacks and chronic prophylaxis. When treating individual attacks, acetaminophen or aspirin for older children is the first line of defense. Refractory headaches may respond to drug preparations containing mixtures of aspirin, phenacetin, and barbiturates. For older children with severe but infrequent headaches, ergotamine suppositories are useful. If nausea and vomiting are pronounced, phenergan suppositories can be added. Propranolol (1 to 2 mg/kg/d divided tid) is effective for chronic prophylaxis. Cyproheptadine hydrochloride, phenobarbital, phenytoin, valproate, and amitriptyline hydrochloride are useful in some patients; each has its advocates.

Migraine and epilepsy may coexist, and each disorder is more common once a patient has the other. Nevertheless, the underlying mechanisms are probably usually distinct, although they represent some shared genetic susceptibility. EEG abnormalities including epileptiform discharges are common in children with migraine. Migraine often occurs in children with occipital epilepsy, and a syndrome of basilar migraine, seizures, and epileptiform discharges has been reported in adolescents. Recent work by Talwar and others nicely demonstrates the complex relationship between epilepsy and migraine in this group. Their work has shown that there is a high incidence of episodic migraine in patients with occipital epileptiform discharges. Of 30 patients with this EEG abnormality noted over a 2-year period at one EEG lab, 12 had episodic migraine. Eight of these 12 patients also had seizures, and migraine was more common in those patients with idiopathic focal onset seizures. In the majority of patients, however, there was no clear temporal relationship between epilepsy and migraine. For the most part, therefore, each disorder should be diagnosed and treated separately.

25.11.5   Other Paroxysmal Disorders

Jitteriness is sometimes confused with neonatal seizures but can be distinguished by careful observation. Jitteriness is of lower amplitude and faster frequency than the clonic jerks of seizures. Unlike seizures, jitteriness may be elicited by sudden movements of the limbs, and it can be stopped by passive restraint. Jitteriness occurs in babies with asphyxia, drug withdrawal, hypocalcemia, or hypoglycemia.

Gastroesophageal reflux is common in young infants, especially those who were preterm. Confusion with epilepsy occurs only in severe cases when infants become distressed and have apnea or brief tonic posturing. Differentiation may be made clinically by the association with feeding, presence of vomiting, and weight loss or difficulty feeding. Radiographic studies examining the swallowing mechanism or pH probe studies can be useful. When gastroesophageal reflux is associated with intermittent head tilt or dystonic posturing of the head, it is referred to as *Sandifer syndrome*. These problems clear when the associated hiatal hernia is repaired (see Sec. 17.10.4).

Psychogenic seizures are commonly misdiagnosed as epilepsy. In adult epilepsy monitoring units, 25 to 35% of patients referred because of uncontrolled seizures have psychogenic attacks. Comparable incidence figures are unavailable for children, but the condition appears to be more common than was previously suspected. Psychogenic seizures occur more often in girls than boys and are most frequent in adolescence. A psychogenic etiology should be suspected when there are bilateral body movements without alteration of consciousness, repeated side-to-side movements of the head, pelvic thrusting, or violent asynchronous features without self-injury. The condition may also be suspected when routine EEGs have been repeatedly normal and the patient has shown no response to multiple antiepileptic drugs. Frontal lobe epilepsy may occasionally manifest with bizarre features suggesting psychogenic seizures. History alone is usually not sufficient to make the diagnosis, and even close observation by an experienced clinician is diagnostically accurate only 75% of the time. CCTV/EEG monitoring is therefore required for definitive diagnosis. Patients with psychogenic seizures have diverse underlying psychiatric disorders and psychological mechanisms. It is advisable to refer such patients to neurologists or psychiatrists who have special experience with psychogenic seizures.

Rage attacks (episodic dyscontrol) are intermittent periods of aggressive and violent behavior that are either unprovoked or inappropriate to the stimulus and out of character for the patient. There is usually no memory of events during an attack. Rage attacks are poorly understood, but they are more common in older children or adolescents with static encephalopathies caused by diffuse structural brain disease. EEGs may reveal nonspecific abnormalities related to the underlying encephalopathy but no epileptiform discharges. Unlike complex partial seizures, rage attacks are not accompanied by auras, automatisms, or postictal confusion.

Cyclic vomiting of undetermined cause presents with frequent and severe vomiting leading to ketosis. It is rarely confused with epilepsy and is mentioned only for completeness. Attacks may be triggered by minor infections. The attacks generally last for a day but can persist longer. Afflicted children can become lethargic and dehydrated. Proper oral replacement of fluids is important; if this

fails, then parenteral hydration is necessary in some patients. Central nervous system mass lesions can be excluded by careful neurologic examination and appropriate neuroimaging. Antiepileptic medications are of no benefit, but dietary restriction of oxalate or protein has been advocated (see Sec. 17.7.1).

Benign paroxysmal vertigo is characterized by brief recurrent attacks of disequilibrium lasting minutes to hours. The attacks commence suddenly, and the striking feature is the inability to walk. Nystagmus is often observed, and children complain of nausea and vertigo. This disorder usually occurs after age 3 years; attacks frequently recur on a monthly or weekly basis. A family history of migraine is common, and many children go on to have migraine as they mature. Infrequently, true vertigo may be the initial feature of partial seizures, but more often an odd cephalic sensation is misreported as vertigo. Attacks of benign paroxysmal vertigo lack the associated automatisms, alteration of responsiveness, and postictal depression seen in complex partial seizures. Interictal EEGs are normal, and antiepileptic medications do not help the condition. Some children with benign paroxysmal vertigo have dysfunction on vestibular testing.

A variety of other transient alterations of body posture or eye positioning may occur in children. *Benign paroxysmal tonic upgaze of childhood* is of interest because it may be confused with the sudden upward tonic deviation of the eyes noted in infantile spasms and in symptomatic generalized epilepsy. In the former condition onset is early in infancy with periods of constant or variably sustained tonic conjugate upward gaze. These children have normal EEGs during events, normal neuroimaging, and normal eye examinations. They have frequent relief from sleep. The outcome appears to be favorable, and treatment is not indicated.

APPROACH TO THE PATIENT WITH A PAROXYSMAL DISORDER

The most important part of the evaluation of the child with a paroxysmal disorder is the history. This is because the physician rarely witnesses the event in question. Every effort should be made to interview observers of the events directly in order to extract the most reliable information. Parents and children should also be encouraged to speak plainly. Medical terms such as *tonic-clonic, convulsion,* or *unconscious* are often unintentionally misused by parents, and this can be the source of confusion that may lead to unnecessary tests and delays in the proper diagnosis. Often, it is helpful to have the parents or other observers directly imitate the abnormalities they observed rather than editorialize with medical jargon.

Close attention should be paid to the setting, precipitating factors, and detailed sequence of the attacks, particularly of the early components. Reports of any abnormal sensations immediately prior to the attack are most important to obtain. Similarly, the level of consciousness during the attacks is another critical piece of information. In this regard, parents sometimes may falsely conclude that their child was unconscious because they did not hear speech during the event. It may be, however, that the child was too frightened or was unable to speak for reasons other than altered consciousness. In these circumstances it may be helpful to ask if children were able to follow commands, attend to stimuli, or recall events themselves. Also, the nature of the child's condition immediately after the event is important to ascertain. Epileptic attacks often may have an associated period of depression following the seizure.

The age of the patient influences the likelihood of the various diagnoses. Many conditions are encountered exclusively in infancy, whereas others are more common in the older child (Table 25-23).

TABLE 25-23

AGE DEPENDENCY OF NONEPILEPTIC PAROXYSMAL DISORDERS

INFANCY	CHILDHOOD	ADOLESCENCE
Jitteriness	Night terrors	Psychogenic seizures
Nocturnal myoclonus	Somnambulism	Rage attacks
	Stereotypies	Vasovagal syncope
Pallid infantile syncope	Breath-holding spells	Migraine with aura
Benign paroxysmal tonic upgaze	Migraine without aura	
Gastroesophageal reflux	Benign paroxysmal vertigo	
Spasmus nutans		
Shuddering attacks		

It is useful to inquire about other family members who may have had similar problems. In many cases, this can be a reassuring piece of information to indicate the likelihood of a benign familial condition.

Finally, each paroxysmal disorder should be evaluated in light of the company it keeps. A global assessment of the child's neurologic well-being is critical for the proper evaluation of the disorder. A given problem is more likely to be benign if it is occurring on the backdrop of a normal individual. Conversely, if a child has an underlying neurologic problem, then one should be reticent to attribute it a priori to a benign paroxysmal disorder until other insidious processes have been excluded.

For example, a severe unilateral throbbing headache in a normal child with a family history of migraine is most likely to be migraine. The same characteristic headache in a youngster with obstructive hydrocephalus and a ventriculoperitoneal (VP) shunt should not, however, be attributed to migraine until VP shunt obstruction is excluded. Similarly, brief tonic deviation of the eyes upward in a normal infant with normal developmental milestones and no impairment of responsiveness is most likely caused by benign paroxysmal tonic upgaze of childhood. However, these same complaints in an 8-month-old infant with Down syndrome may be the first harbinger of infantile spasms.

The wide breadth of the disorders presented here and the rich variety of possible presentations underscores the futility of attempting to develop a diagnostic paradigm for all paroxysmal disorders. Instead, a thorough history and detailed relevant physical examination will serve as the basis for a sound evaluation. These data, combined with the clinician's accumulated experience, direct the patient toward the appropriate laboratory investigations. In most cases, ultimately the correct diagnosis will be made on the basis of good clinical judgment.

References

Movement Disorders

Gordon CT, State RC, Nelson JE, Hamburger SD, Rapoport JL: A double-blind comparison of clomipramine, desipramine, and placebo in the treatment of autistic disorder. Arch Gen Psychiatry 50:441–447, 1993

Habgerg B, Aicardi J, Dias K, Ramos O: A progressive syndrome of autism, dementia, ataxia, and loss of purposeful hand use in girls: Rett's syndrome. Report of 35 cases. Ann Neurol 14:471–479, 1983

Nigro MA, Lim HCN: Hyperexplexia and sudden neonatal death. Pediatr Neurol 8:221–225, 1992

Shiang R, Ryan SG, Zhu YZ, Hahn AF, O'Connell PO, Wasmuth JJ: Mutations in the alpha 1 subunit of the inhibitory glycine receptor cause the dominant neurologic disorder, hyperexplexia. Nat Genet 5:351–357, 1993

Vanassie M, Bedard P, Andermann F: Shuddering attacks in children: an early clinical manifestation of essential tremor. Neurology 26:1027–1030, 1976

Syncope

DiMario FJ: Breath-holding spells in childhood. Am J Dis Child 146:125–131, 1992

DiMario FJ, Chee CM, Berman PH: Pallid breath-holding spells. Evaluation of the autonomic system. Clin Pediatr 29: 17–24, 1990

Silbert PL, Gubbay SS: Familial cyanotic breath-holding spells. J Paediatr Child Health 28:254–256, 1992

Migraine

Bille B: Migraine in school children. Acute Pediatr Scand (Suppl 136):1–151, 1962

Bourgeois M, Aicardi J, Goutieres F: Alternating hemiplegia of childhood. J Pediatr 122:673–679, 1993

Chu ML, Shinnar S: Headaches in children younger than 7 years of age. Arch Neurol 49:79–82, 1992

Cooper EC, Jan LY: Ion channel genes and human neurological disease: recent progress, prospects, and challenges. Proc Natl Acad Sci USA 96:4759, 1999

Gastaut H: A new type of epilepsy: benign partial epilepsy of childhood with occipital spike-waves. Clin Electroencephalogr 13:13–22, 1982

Joutel A, Bousser MG, Biousse V, et al: A gene for familial hemiplegic migraine maps to chromosome 19. Nat Genet 5:40–45, 1993

Kors EE, Haan J, Ferrari MD: Genetics of primary headaches. Curr Opin Neurol 12:249, 1999

Olesen J, Friberg L, Shyhoi Olsen T, et al: Timing and topography of cerebral blood flow, aura and headache during migraine attacks. Ann Neurol 28:791–798, 1990

Rasmussen BK, Jensen R, Schroll M, Olesen J: Interrelations between migraine and tension-type headache in the general population. Arch Neurol 49:914–918, 1992

Rho JM, Chugani HT: Alternating hemiplegia of childhood: insights into its pathophysiology. J Child Neurol 13:39, 1998

Rosen JA: Observations of the efficacy of propranolol for the prophylaxis of migraine. Ann Neurol 13:92–93, 1983

Stang PE, Yanagihara T, Swanson JW, et al: Incidence of migraine headache: A population-based study in Olmsted County, Minnesota. Neurology 42:1657–1662, 1992

Talwar D, Rask CA, Torres F. Clinical manifestations in children with occipital spike-wave paroxysms. Epilepsia 33:667–674, 1992

Other Paroxysmal Disorders

Elliot FA: The episodic dyscontrol syndrome and aggression. Neurol Clin 2:113–125, 1984

Holmes GL, Sackellares JC, McKiernan J, et al: Evaluation of childhood pseudoseizures using EEG telemetry and video tape monitoring. J Pediatr 97:554–558, 1980

Ouvrier RA, Billson F: Benign paroxysmal tonic upgaze of childhood. J Child Neurol 3:177–180, 1988

Williams DT, Walczak T, Berten W, Nordli D, Bergtraum M: Psychogenic seizures. In: Mostofsky DI, Loyning Y, eds: The Neurobehavioral Treatment of Epilepsy. Hillsdale, NJ, L. Erlbaum, 1993

25.12 THE NEUROMUSCULAR SYSTEM

Darryl C. De Vivo, Guiliana Galassi, Werner Trojaborg, and David Pleasure

Diseases involving the neuromuscular system are usually identified on the basis of the site of the primary pathologic manifestation, such as anterior horn cell, peripheral nerve, neuromuscular junction, or skeletal muscle. Weakness is a manifestation common to all diagnostic categories and thus is a nonspecific sign. Knowledge of the distribution of the weakness provides more specificity, but locations are not exclusive. Neuropathic processes are often associated with distal weakness; conversely, myopathic disorders are often associated with limb-girdle (proximal) weakness. The exceptions, however, are numerous. Thus, Gower sign, which signifies hip-girdle weakness, may be seen with diseases affecting the neuronal (eg, juvenile spinal muscular atrophy) or the myogenic (eg, Duchenne and limb-girdle dystrophy, and dermatomyositis) components of the system.

Tendon reflexes are characteristically decreased or absent in patients with neuropathies; a fluctuating course usually characterizes myasthenia gravis; irritability and joint discomfort often accompany inflammatory diseases of muscle and the early stages of the Guillain-Barré syndrome; hypotonia and hyporeflexia are associated with neuromuscular diseases that are present at birth. Electrophysiological and morphologic studies are often necessary to permit accurate diagnosis. Here, too, some physiological and morphologic features may be similar in various syndromes. For example, fibrillations are present in both neuropathic diseases and inflammatory myopathies, and necrosis, phagocytosis, and fiber type variations may be present in both inflammatory and genetic myopathies and in the late stages of muscle denervation. The morphologic features are discussed in further detail in Sec. 25.14.

Electrophysiological investigations include electromyography

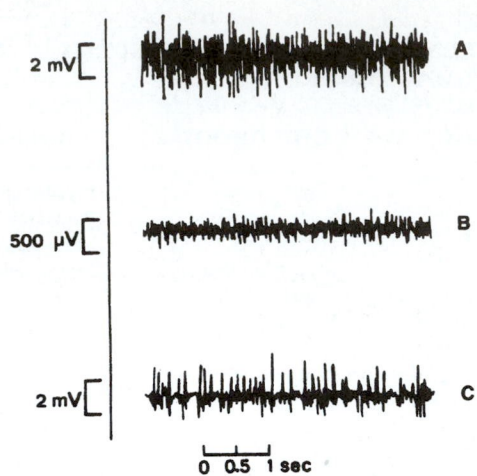

FIGURE 25-36 **A. Pattern recorded during full effort in a normal 8-year-old patient (biceps brachii). B. Pattern recorded during maximal effort in a patient with Duchenne muscular dystrophy (biceps brachii). C. Pattern of discrete activity recorded in a patient with chronic Werdnig-Hoffman disease (tibialis anterior).**

(EMG) and nerve conduction velocities. EMG consists of random sampling of action potentials from several areas of a muscle to localize, amplify, record, and measure the electrical activity present at rest (insertional activity) and the activity produced by voluntary contraction (interference pattern). Conduction velocities are performed by applying maximal electrical stimuli to motor or sensory nerves and recording the evoked responses.

Spontaneous electrical activity in muscle includes endplate noise, fibrillation potentials, positive sharp waves, fasciculations, myokymia, pseudomyotonic discharges, and myotonic bursts. Each finding has its own meaning in the context of the total clinical evaluation. Myotonic bursts (Fig. 25-35), for example, are characteristic of the various myotonic disorders (congenital myotonia, myotonic dystrophy, paramyotonia) and are triggered by mechanical or electrical stimuli and enhanced by cold.

The analysis of voluntary motor-unit potentials provides important information in distinguishing neuropathic conditions from myopathic conditions. During full effort, these potentials summate, normally resulting in a pattern of recruitment in which each spike interferes with another, and the individual spikes are lost (interference pattern). The correct evaluation of this pattern requires patient cooperation, which is difficult to obtain in children. However, it aids in assessing the pathophysiological state of the muscle (Fig. 25-36A).

ELECTROPHYSIOLOGICAL DIFFERENCES BETWEEN MYOPATHY AND NEUROPATHY

In discussing the electrophysiological criteria for differential diagnosis, it is important to remember that the same electrical events can occur in both conditions. Of the criteria derived from analysis of individual motor-unit potentials, a short mean duration is most characteristic of myopathies. The incidence of polyphasic potentials is often increased in myopathies. In early stages, this can be the only abnormality detected by EMG. In myopathies, the average amplitude of individual motor units is often diminished. Even a weak effort requires the activation of many motor units that discharge at a rate higher than in normal muscle. Therefore, "excessive

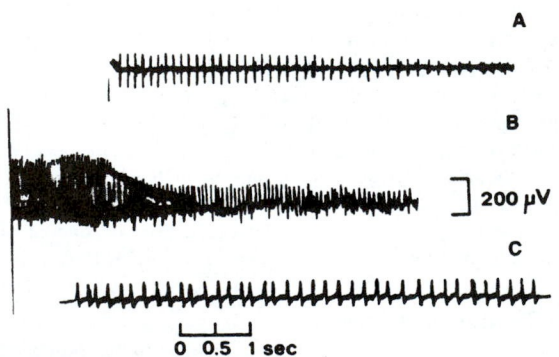

FIGURE 25-35 **A. Spontaneous myotonic bursts with decreasing frequency of discharge recorded in a patient with myotonic dystrophy (extensor digitorum communis). B. Myotonic bursts evoked by slight movement of the concentric needle electrode when the frequency is increased or decreased. C. Pseudomyotonic bursts of constant frequency with sudden onset and end, recorded with a concentric needle in a patient with myotonic dystrophy.**

recruitment" of motor-unit potentials occurs. Except when a myopathy is so far advanced that many muscle fibers are missing within the motor unit, the pattern of activity at maximum effort is full or only mildly reduced, but the peak-to-peak amplitude is often diminished (Fig. 25-36B).

In contrast, when a neuropathic condition affects lower motor neurons, producing wasting and weakness, the number of motor units is reduced, and there are changes in the density of the pattern of activity recruited on maximal contraction. If each spike potential can be distinguished, the resulting pattern is called *discrete activity* (Fig. 25-36C). In neuropathies and in anterior horn cell disorders, the mean duration of individual motor-unit potentials is increased. Giant motor units arise in disorders of chronic partial denervation because of the increasing size of the surviving motor units owing to incorporation of denervated muscle fibers by peripheral sprouting into surviving motor units.

The diagnostic evaluation of spontaneous electrical activity requires special care because this finding can occur in denervated muscles, in motor neuron diseases, and in primary disorders of the muscle, such as muscular dystrophies, myositis, and myotonias.

CONDUCTION VELOCITY AND ITS DIAGNOSTIC YIELDS

For both motor and sensory nerves, the maximum conduction velocity is a function of age; children's values approach adult values by 3 to 5 years of age.

Abnormalities of maximum conduction velocities and amplitudes of evoked responses help in determining whether neuromuscular impairment is caused by myopathy, anterior horn cell disease, or peripheral neuropathy. In primary myopathies, conduction velocities in motor and sensory nerves are normal. In peripheral neuropathies characterized histologically by predominant axonal degeneration, maximum conduction velocity is normal to nearly normal, but the amplitude of the sensory action potential is diminished. If segmental demyelination is the main histologic feature, as in the neuropathies of metachromatic leukodystrophy, Charcot-Marie-Tooth syndrome (peroneal muscular atrophies), glycogen storage disease types IA and IX, and the demyelinative form of Guillain-Barré syndrome, sensory conduction is severely slowed. With lesions localized to the anterior horn cells, as in the infantile and juvenile forms of spinal muscular atrophy, conduction velocities in motor and sensory nerves are usually normal. This noninvasive method has become part of the diagnostic approach in many EMG laboratories and is especially useful in infants and children.

References

Aminoff MJ: Electrodiagnosis in Clinical Neurology. New York, Churchill Livingstone, 1988

Brown WF, Bolton CF: Clinical Electromyography. Boston, Butterworths, 1988

Engel AG, Franzini-Armstrong C, eds: Myology, 2nd ed. McGraw-Hill, New York, 1994

Kimura J: Electrodiagnosis in Disease of Nerve and Muscle: Principles and Practice, 2nd ed. Philadelphia, Davis, 1989

Swash M, Schwartz MS: Neuromuscular Diseases. A Practical Approach to Diagnosis and Management, 2nd ed. Berlin/Heidelberg, Springer-Verlag, 1988

Wagner AL, Buchthal F: Motor and sensory conduction in infancy and childhood: reappraisal. Dev Med Child Neurol 14:189, 1972

25.12.1 Childhood Anterior Horn Cell Disease and Peripheral Neuropathies

Robert Ouvrier and Isabelle Rapin

Discussion of the disorders affecting the lower motor and sensory neurons can be divided into two parts, covering anterior horn cell disease and childhood peripheral neuropathy.

ANTERIOR HORN CELL DISEASE

Anterior horn cell diseases are mostly infectious or inherited. The most important infectious disease of the anterior horn cell is *poliomyelitis*. Although preventable and largely eradicated from the Western world, it is still a significant cause of death and disability in developing countries. In regions with high immunization rates, sporadic cases of infantile paralysis occur as a result of infections with echo- and coxsackieviruses. These conditions are described in Sec. 13.4.

The spinal muscular atrophies (SMA) are the major inherited disorders of the anterior horn cell, occurring in about 1:18,000 live births. The classification of these conditions is controversial. A simple and useful approach is to divide them into three major types:

1. SMA type I, also known as acute infantile SMA or Werdnig-Hoffmann disease
2. SMA type II, chronic or intermediate SMA
3. SMA type III, or Kugelberg-Welander syndrome

There are a few additional rare disorders, which are not discussed.

As a general rule, patients with SMA type I have their clinical onset in the first 6 months after birth and never learn to sit. Type II cases sit, but rarely learn to walk. SMA type III cases learn to walk, but later in childhood are found to be weak, especially in the lower limbs. It appears that SMA types I and II, and some cases of type III, map to a single locus on the long arm of chromosome 5. Although cases of SMA types I and II occasionally occur in the one family, most cases have their onset at a similar age. Survival time tends to be more variable. This clinical variability is thought to be a result of the existence of multiple alleles acting at the gene locus.

Werdnig-Hoffmann Disease (Infantile Spinal Muscular Atrophy; SMA Type I)

This is a serious neuromuscular disease of infancy. It is one of the diverse causes of the "floppy infant syndrome," which is described later in this chapter, but demands special attention because of its frequency and risk of appearance in future siblings. An autosomal-recessive disorder, it produces weakness, wasting, hypotonia, and absence of tendon reflexes.

Affected children develop symptoms before 6 months of age. Typically, parents relate a history of gradual loss of head and trunk control and decreasing movement of the extremities in a child who appeared normal during the first 2 to 3 months after birth. Such a child loses the ability to elevate the head and upper trunk when placed in the prone position and later is unable to turn the head from side to side. The trunk collapses into a flexed posture when the child is placed sitting, and the hypotonic legs assume an abducted and flexed posture interrupted occasionally by weak extension movements. Typically, the onset of the disorder is gradual, but sometimes weakness will develop precipitously over a period ranging from days to a week or two, in association with a minor febrile illness. Approximately 30% of infants with this disorder develop hypotonia and paucity of limb movements in the neonatal period. Mothers of such infants have occasionally described decreased fetal movements, indicating intrauterine onset of the disease.

Examination at 3 to 6 months of age often discloses a bright, socially aware infant with diffuse weakness, hypotonia, and muscle wasting. Absence of tendon reflexes at the knees and ankles is a key finding, and the presence of these tendon reflexes should raise suspicion about the accuracy of the diagnosis. Respirations have been described as "paradoxical," because they are diaphragmatic, causing the abdomen to rise and the chest wall to collapse during inspiration. Other findings include a bell-shaped chest and relative sparing of movements of the fingers and toes. Tongue fasciculations are virtually pathognomonic but are difficult to recognize in young infants. Both sensation and bowel and bladder function are spared.

SMA Types II and III

The preceding description characterizes SMA type I—the classic Werdnig-Hoffmann disease—in its severe form, and the prognosis is grave, with survival beyond infancy unlikely. Over recent years, however, a more benign variant of the disorder has received deserved attention (although such patients were recognized by Werdnig and Hoffmann). Patients exhibiting this less severe form make up about one-third of the total; they do not exhibit symptoms until later infancy or until the second year, and they may survive until adulthood. These children acquire and retain the ability to sit, and a few become ambulatory. The history and physical findings are similar to those described above, but the physical manifestations begin later and are less severe. Weakness is diffuse but is most pronounced in proximal muscles, especially in the legs. Hypotonia, muscle wasting, and areflexia also occur, and, when associated with readily visible tongue fasciculations, peculiar shakiness of the hands, and normal or superior intellect, they allow a presumptive diagnosis of this milder form of the disorder. SMA type III is the rare juvenile variant of anterior horn cell degeneration, *Kugelberg-Welander* disease. Children with the juvenile form, which is usually an autosomal-recessive disorder, exhibit even more slowly progressive weakness of the legs, without loss of ambulation until the second or third decade, if at all. In some patients with SMA types II and III, the disease eventually appears to become static, but permanent weakness remains.

Routine laboratory tests are normal in patients with anterior horn cell degeneration, except for modest elevation of serum creatine kinase concentration in children with slowly progressive disease. The ECG will show no intrinsic cardiopathy, but may reveal the characteristic ECG "tremor," an innocent artifact of the diffuse tremor seen in many patients with milder forms of the disease.

The two specialized procedures of prime importance in corroborating the diagnosis are electromyography and muscle biopsy. The electromyogram will have a pattern typical of neurogenic atrophy, showing motor-unit potentials of increased amplitude and duration, decreased frequency of discharge on voluntary effort, and spontaneous activity in the form of fibrillation potentials and positive waves, frequently of very small amplitude (20–30 μV) (see Fig. 25-36C). Motor nerve conduction velocities are normal or slightly decreased. Muscle biopsy shows group atrophy typical of neurogenic disease (see Fig. 25-39). Special stains that display the various muscle fiber types show grouping of muscle fibers of similar types indicative of reinnervation.

The differential diagnosis centers on those disorders that produce the floppy infant syndrome, including cerebral hypotonia, congenital myopathies, myasthenia gravis, glycogenosis type II, infantile botulism, congenital myotonic dystrophy, spinal cord trauma, and benign congenital hypotonia. Infants with cerebral hypotonia show global retardation, microcephaly, retention of primitive motor patterns such as grasp and Moro reflexes, and active tendon reflexes. The congenital myopathies usually remain static or show clinical improvement, but specific muscle biopsy changes, such as *rods, cores,* or *myotubes,* allow firm distinction. Myasthenia gravis of the transient neonatal variety results from placental transfer of receptor antibody caused by maternal myasthenia gravis. Diagnosis in the weak neonate is based on examination of the mother and the patient's improvement after neostigmine therapy. Glycogenosis type II (Pompe disease) presents cardiac and hepatic enlargement in addition to myopathy. Muscle biopsy with electron microscopic demonstration of glycogen storage allows morphologic diagnosis, although electrical myotonia provides a helpful clue. Infants with botulism show prominent bulbar and ocular muscle weakness, significant constipation, and *Clostridium botulinum* spores in stool. Electromyography may reveal brief, small action potentials or the characteristic neuromuscular transmission defect. Congenital myotonic dystrophy is easily diagnosed by the constellation of mental retardation, facial diplegia, and clubbed feet, coupled with signs of myotonic dystrophy in the mother. Cervical spinal cord damage attributable to birth trauma produces a mixed neurologic picture, with segmental involvement of the arms, Horner syndrome, paraplegia, bowel and bladder retention, and absence of pain sensation in the trunk and the legs. The diagnosis of benign congenital hypotonia should be restricted to infants whose sole abnormality is decreased muscle tone.

Treatment is limited to supportive care. Prevention of the disorder in later siblings should be sought through genetic counseling. When the disease appears before 6 months of age, respiratory insufficiency becomes a major threat before the child is 1 year of age. Survival beyond the age of 3 years is rare, because even mild respiratory infections produce ventilatory failure. Invasive respiratory assistance, such as tracheostomy or endotracheal intubation, is not warranted in those weak infants. Children with the milder form of spinal muscular atrophy deserve aggressive physical therapy and treatment of the scoliosis that inevitably develops. Trunk supports will postpone curvature, but spinal fusion may be required.

Appropriate genetic counseling is mandatory, because each subsequent sibling has a 25% risk of manifesting the disease. Prenatal detection is now available. When several siblings inherit the disorder, its severity is usually uniform; however, sibships with both mild and severe forms are not very rare. Such variation should be described in genetic counseling.

CHILDHOOD PERIPHERAL NEUROPATHY

The term *peripheral neuropathy* indicates disease of peripheral nerves. The peripheral neuropathies constitute approximately 30% of the cases seen in a pediatric neuromuscular service. Two-thirds of such cases are chronic. Of the latter group, roughly 70% are hereditary, 20% indeterminate, and 10% acquired. Of the acquired cases, the most important single group in developed countries is that caused by chronic inflammatory demyelinating polyneuropathy (CIDP), a condition that is usually very responsive to steroid therapy. In some tropical countries, leprosy and vitamin-deficiency neuropathies are of considerable importance. There are now at least 30 separate forms of hereditary neuropathy affecting children. The more common entities are discussed in the next section.

Polyneuropathy is the most common pattern, and this indicates distal, usually symmetric, sensory and motor nerve dysfunction. Stocking-glove numbness, paresthesias, or hyperesthesias are combined with the motor findings of thinning of calf muscles, footdrop, absence of Achilles reflexes, weak grip, and atrophy of hand muscles. Autonomic changes include shiny skin, hypohidrosis or hyperhidrosis, and coldness of the hands and feet. *Mononeuropathy* yields motor and sensory findings restricted to the distribution of a single mixed peripheral nerve. For example, sciatic neuropathy caused by nerve puncture during buttock injection produces weakness and wasting of sciatic-innervated muscles below the knee and variable sensory loss in the distribution of the distal peroneal or tibial nerves. *Mononeuritis multiplex,* seen in collagen vascular disorders, signifies dysfunction of two or more peripheral nerves, such as the femoral and the median. *Radiculopathy* and *plexopathy* indicate diseases of the spinal root and brachial or lumbar plexus, respectively.

Clinically, peripheral neuropathies can be confused with other disorders that produce weakness or sensory dysfunction. No laboratory tests can substitute for a careful clinical examination and the physician's awareness of the various disorders that can mimic peripheral neuropathy. Patients with Duchenne dystrophy and anterior horn cell degeneration show pure motor deficits, usually proximal, without sensory abnormalities. This contrasts with the distal distribution of motor and sensory deficits seen in patients with polyneuropathy. The situation with lumbosacral intraspinal masses may be more difficult because distal motor and sensory changes are common with these. Asymmetric findings, hyperactive tendon reflexes, urinary incontinence, radicular pain, and a level of sensory functioning typical of myelopathy suggest the spinal mass. Occasionally, distinguishing between a spinal mass and unilateral neuropathy, for example, sciatic neuropathy, may be impossible without myelography or MRI examination. Children with lipomas of the lower spinal canal are frequently misdiagnosed as having either peripheral neuropathy or obscure orthopedic disease. Children with rigid cavovarus foot deformities deserve careful evaluation because unsuspected chronic peripheral neuropathy with or without spinocerebellar degeneration may be the primary cause. In the arms, the myelopathy seen with syringomyelia resembles peripheral neuropathy, but sensory dissociation, hyperactive tendon reflexes in the legs, and an enlarged spinal canal revealed radiographically indicate the intraspinal cause. In acutely weak patients, the Guillain-Barré syndrome might be confused with acute transverse myelitis or other acute lesions such as epidural abscess. Radiographic imaging may be needed to exclude the possibility of acute cord compression.

If one suspects a peripheral neuropathy, the determination of nerve conduction velocity will confirm the diagnosis. Most extremity nerves can be tested in a safe and fairly painless manner, and by slight modification even small infants can be studied. The most readily accessible nerves for study are the median and ulnar nerves in the arms and the sural, peroneal, and tibial nerves in the legs. Apart from their value in confirming the presence of polyneuropathy and in helping to distinguish demyelinating from axonal degenerative processes, studies of conduction velocity are helpful in determining the site of injury or entrapment of nerves and are useful in studying nerve regeneration after acute transection or compression. Table 25-24 lists many of the causes of peripheral neuropathy in childhood, separated into four patterns of clinical presentation.

GUILLAIN-BARRÉ SYNDROME Guillain-Barré syndrome (acute inflammatory demyelinating polyradiculoneuropathy, acute infectious polyradiculopathy), a prominent cause of acute paralysis, begins with rapidly evolving weakness of the legs, followed by involvement of the arms. Cranial nerve dysfunction leads to facial weakness, weak nasal speech, and dysphagia. Respiratory compromise owing to intercostal muscle weakness poses the major threat, and ventilatory assistance is required in up to 25% of patients. Subjective sensory abnormalities such as back and limb pain and paresthesias may be prominent and may herald the onset, but objective deficits are usually mild and restricted to position and vibratory sensory losses.

The prominent physical finding is diffuse weakness, although cranial muscle involvement may escape attention. Tendon reflexes are sluggish or absent, and the Babinski sign is usually not elicited. Weak cough and shallow respirations indicate intercostal muscle involvement, which should be corroborated by measuring vital capacity, a test to be performed during the initial evaluation and at regular intervals thereafter. Signs of meningeal irritation, with limitation of straight leg raising, nuchal rigidity, and back stiffness or pain, may be found. Sensory abnormalities are usually mild, but sometimes significant defects in all modalities may mimic the picture of transverse myelitis. Other less common findings are autonomic instability, with hypotension or hypertension, papilledema, ophthalmoplegia, and ataxia. These latter signs require exclusion of the possibility of a posterior fossa mass. Bladder function is usually preserved, but some patients may experience urinary incontinence or retention.

Protein concentrations in the spinal fluid are elevated, occasionally as high as 1.0 to 1.5 g/dL, in almost all patients during some phase of the illness, but in the early phase the protein concentration may be normal. The spinal fluid cell count is usually less than 10 cells/μL. Slowed nerve conduction velocity and prolonged F-wave latency are important findings but may not be detectable at the earliest stage of disease and are not features of the purely axonal forms of the Guillain-Barré syndrome. Electromyographic evidence of denervation may indicate a less favorable prognosis.

Disorders that can mimic Guillain-Barré syndrome include tick paralysis, toxic neuropathies, porphyria, botulism, transverse myelitis, acute spinal cord compression, and poliomyelitis.

The cause of Guillain-Barré syndrome is not understood, but the frequent association of its onset with a febrile illness indicates association with viral disease. Epstein-Barr virus, coxsackievirus, echovirus, cytomegalovirus, and the exanthematous agents may cause the syndrome. A similar process has been described in Lyme disease as well as in *Mycoplasma* and *Campylobacter* infections. An autoimmune process triggered by a variety of agents and directed at the nerves and roots is a favored hypothesis, because pathologically there is a resemblance to experimental allergic neuritis.

Because the prognosis for complete recovery is excellent in the majority of patients, strong supportive measures are warranted during the acute phase. Careful monitoring, including frequent measurements of vital capacity, must be carried out to ensure adequate ventilation and to anticipate the need for respiratory assistance before failure occurs. With assiduous care, mortality should be negligible. Steroids have been shown to be of no value. Plasmapheresis is of proven value and should be considered in rapidly evolving disease with loss of independent ambulation. In small children and in situations where plasmapheresis is unavailable, infusions of intravenous gamma globulin appear to be at least as effective. A standard dosage regimen is 0.4 g/kg given daily on 5 consecutive days. The

TABLE 25-24

CAUSES AND CLINICAL FEATURES OF PERIPHERAL NEUROPATHY IN CHILDHOOD

PATTERN	CAUSE	DIAGNOSTIC FEATURES
Acute diffuse Rapidly evolving proximal and distal muscle weakness; variable, often mild, sensory deficit; may lead to ventilatory failure	Guillain-Barré syndrome (postinfectious polyneuritis)	Acute symmetric ascending paralysis; spotty sensory loss; acellular CSF with elevated protein; reversible
	Diphtheria	Diffuse, mainly bulbar, weakness following membranous pharyngeal exudate; heart failure; positive culture of *Corynebacterium diphtheriae*
	Botulism*	Infantile or adult form; pure motor deficit with prominent cranial involvement; electromyography helpful
	Tick paralysis*	Acute paralysis without sensory changes; rapidly reversed when entire tick is removed; may be fatal if undiagnosed
Chronic symmetric distal Weakness and wasting of distal muscles of legs and then arms; stocking-glove sensory loss; slowed nerve conduction velocity	*Familial-metabolic* Peroneal muscular atrophy (Charcot-Marie-Tooth disease; HMSN types I & II†)	Mainly autosomal dominant, variable expression; pes cavus, footdrop, clawhand, variable sensory loss and tremor
	Hypertrophic interstitial neuropathy (Dejerine-Sottas; HMSN type III)	Sporadic or autosomal recessive; early onset; enlarged nerves; variable nystagmus, deafness, ataxia, very slow nerve conduction; hypomyelination
	Hereditary sensory neuropathies	Variable inheritance; severe sensory disturbances; mild motor deficit; deformities due to mutilation; includes familial dysautonomia (see text)
	Metachromatic leukodystrophy	Autosomal recessive; slowed peripheral nerve conduction in a child with CNS degenerative disorder; metachromasia of peripheral nerve; reduced urinary and WBC arylsulfatase A
	Abetalipoproteinemia	Mild distal weakness; marked proprioceptive loss with ataxia; intestinal malabsorption; acanthocytosis and lipoprotein defect; responds to vitamin E.
	Refsum disease (HMSN type IV)	Autosomal recessive; ataxia, ichthyosis, deafness, retinitis pigmentosa, and ECG abnormalities; elevated levels of phytanic acid in blood
	Giant axonal neuropathy	Kinky hair, ataxia, later CNS involvement, biopsy characteristic
	Systemic disease Diabetes, uremia, nutritional deficiency, liver disease, cystic fibrosis, hypothyroidism, collagen vascular disease	Neuropathy usually incidental, but may rarely dominate
	Toxemia Metals (lead, arsenic, mercury, thallium)	Diagnosis depends on history of exposure, ancillary physical findings, and appropriate laboratory analysis
	Drugs (isoniazid, nitrofurantoin, vincristine, phenytoin)	
	Organic poisons (solvents, insecticides, triorthocresol phosphate, acrylamide)	
Focal Unilateral motor and sensory findings in territory of affected spinal root, plexus, or nerve; electrical studies define extent of denervation	*Trauma-compression* Brachial plexus injury	Birth trauma; static weakness of proximal (Erb) or distal (Klumpke) arm muscles
	Postinjection sciatic palsy	History of deficit following buttock injection; static weakness of distal muscles of leg, with variable sensory loss below knee
	Idiopathic Facial neuritis (Bell's palsy)	Unilateral facial paralysis including frontalis muscle; variable involvement of taste, lacrimation, and salivation; reversible

(continued)

TABLE 25-24   Continued

PATTERN	CAUSE	DIAGNOSTIC FEATURES
	Brachial plexitis	Unilateral shoulder pain followed within 1–2 weeks by weakness and wasting of shoulder muscles; may follow horse serum injection; reversible; familial cases occur
	Herpes zoster	Pain and vesicular eruption in trigeminal or spinal root distribution; often associated with neoplasm or immunosuppression
	Vascular Collagen vascular disease	Systemic manifestations; a cause of mononeuritis multiplex
	Tumor Neurofibromatosis	Chronic spinal root or peripheral nerve impingement due to neurofibromata; café-au-lait spots and skin nodules; autosomal dominant
	Neoplasms: primary (chordoma, spinal neuroblastoma; lipoma)	Focal cranial nerve deficit (III, VI, VII, VIII nerves); chronic radiculopathy or cauda equina syndrome
Recurrent Repeated bouts of acute weakness and sensory deficit; findings may be proximal or distal	Chronic relapsing polyneuritis	Features similar to Guillain-Barré syndrome; may be steroid-responsive and steroid-dependent
	Acute intermittent porphyria	Rare in children; repeated bouts of weakness and sensory deficit associated with abdominal colic; elevated urine porphobilinogen

* Botulism and tick paralysis are disorders of the neuromuscular junction
† HMSN: Hereditary motor and sensory neuropathy

best response occurs in patients who are treated within a few days of clinical onset.

Recovery begins within 3 to 4 weeks and is usually complete by 6 months. Permanent sequelae occur in 10 to 15% of patients, usually in those most severely affected during the acute phase.

Some patients with an apparent attack of Guillain-Barré syndrome continue to deteriorate after the first 4 weeks of the illness. Deterioration is often stepwise, sometimes with partial remissions over several months or years. Other patients, who appear to recover completely, relapse months or years after the initial attack. Such individuals are considered to have *chronic inflammatory polyneuropathy* of *progressive* or *relapsing type*. Nerve conduction studies are consistent with a demyelinating neuropathy, the CSF protein is usually elevated, and nerve biopsy reveals evidence of de- and remyelination, sometimes with inflammatory cell infiltration and onion-bulb formation. Recognition of these disorders is important because they are usually responsive to steroid or immunosuppressive therapy.

Other causes of chronic infective neuropathy include *Mycobacterium leprae, Borrelia,* and HIV. These conditions are discussed in Chap. 13.

ACUTE INTERMITTENT PORPHYRIA Patients with acute intermittent porphyria develop attacks of severe colicky abdominal pain, with constipation and, in some, pernicious vomiting. A rapidly progressive polyneuropathy, with or without sensory deficit or paresthesias, may result in flaccid tetraparesis and respiratory paralysis. Involvement of cranial nerves and the bulbar musculature is common. The neuropathy is usually completely reversible, and recovery over several weeks can be expected. An acute psychosis, in some instances resembling schizophrenia, may develop, although psychiatric symptoms are less common in children. Delirium, coma, and focal or generalized seizures may be worsened by hyponatremia, which is frequent and severe during acute attacks. Autonomic dysfunction may present as tachycardia, hypertension, fever, dysuria, or urinary retention. Porphyrin metabolism and its disorders are discussed in Sec. 9.12.

PERONEAL MUSCULAR ATROPHY Peroneal muscular atrophy (Charcot-Marie-Tooth disease, hereditary motor and sensory neuropathy [HMSN] types I and II) is the most common cause of chronic peripheral neuropathy in childhood. This hereditary disorder is manifested as distal muscle weakness and wasting that usually becomes increasingly evident by the teenage years. Footdrop, which results from anterior tibial muscle weakness, leads to the typical "steppage" or "foot-slapping" gait requiring exaggerated knee elevation during the swing phase of walking. Affected children run poorly and have great difficulty in negotiating irregular terrain. The appearance of the feet suggests the diagnosis, and the cavovarus foot deformity, with high arches and inversion, as well as hammertoes, provides a clue to early detection. Occasionally, wasting spreads to quadriceps muscles, but it is restricted to the lower one-third, producing the "stork-leg" appearance. Insidious wasting and weakness of hand and forearm muscles occur later in the disease, but the arms remain strong. Mild-to-moderate stocking-glove sensory loss occurs in many patients, and severe disturbances are sometimes found. When the tremor is marked, the term *Roussy-Levy syndrome* is sometimes applied. Nerve conduction studies allow the separation of Charcot-Marie-Tooth disease into two main types. In the common HMSN type I, there is slowing of nerve conduction velocity to less than 60% of normal values, reflecting the predominant pathologic finding of chronic de- and remyelination. In HMSN type II, although the clinical appearance is similar to that of type I, motor nerve conduction studies are normal or near-normal, as the pathologic change is mainly one of axonal degeneration. Treatment is limited to supportive measures, including splints, tendon transfers, arthrodeses, and various hand orthoses. Although the lifespan is not reduced, many patients experience significant long-term disability, although most remain ambulatory. In HMSN type I, the most common molecular disturbance is a duplication of DNA on the short arm of chromosome 17. In a few families, there is linkage to chromosome 1, and in others to the X chromosome. Autosomal-dominant transmission occurs in the first two and in HMSN type II, but the gene locus of HMSN type II has not been identified. Genetic counseling needs to take account of all these genotype variations as well as of the considerable variability of clinical expression in individual families. Other rarer variants of hereditary motor and sensory neuropathy add further complexity to this field.

The principal findings in hypertrophic interstitial neuropathy (Dejerine-Sottas disease; HMSN type III) are presented in Table 25-24. The finding of enlarged firm nerves, such as the median or ulnar nerves, suggests the diagnosis, particularly if the onset is in early life, but similar hypertrophic changes may be found in peroneal muscular atrophy, Refsum disease, neurofibromatosis, leprosy, and recurrent polyneuropathy.

The neuropathy in *metachromatic leukodystrophy* allows presumptive diagnosis of the underlying disorder because the combination of peripheral and central nervous system degeneration presents a characteristic clinical picture. The constellation of dementia, optic atrophy, ataxia, and spasticity combined with depressed ankle jerks and slowed conduction velocity will indicate this widespread involvement and the need for enzymatic assay for arylsulfatase. Peripheral neuropathy may accompany other rare cerebral degenerations such as Krabbe disease or neuroaxonal dystrophy.

Table 25-24 summarizes the common clinical features encountered in *hereditary sensory neuropathy* (HSN), but at least five distinct although rare disorders are usually included under this rubric. The dominant form of HSN begins in the second decade of life and involves severe loss of pain and temperature sensation, mainly in the feet. The recessive forms appear in the first decade, with more widespread involvement.

FAMILIAL DYSAUTONOMIA Familial dysautonomia (Riley-Day syndrome), an autosomal-recessive disease seen predominantly in children of Ashkenazi Jewish ancestry, affects sensory and autonomic functions in many organ systems. Its pathogenesis is not understood. Recent unproven hypotheses have implicated a lack of nerve growth factor during embryogenesis that may account for the marked reduction of neurons in sensory and autonomic ganglia found in these children. Central autonomic neurons are also involved, but the full extent of the abnormality is not yet known. The diagnosis rests on the characteristic clinical features and confirmatory tests of autonomic dysfunction. Intrauterine diagnosis and detection of heterozygote carriers are not yet possible.

Dysautonomic infants are usually symptomatic from birth. Their birth weights are usually lower than those of their siblings, and they fail to grow and gain weight, in part because of difficulty in sucking and swallowing. Aspiration is frequent and often life-threatening and may result in chronic lung disease. Affected infants are fretful and labile babies who cry without tears, one of the cardinal signs of the illness. Their corneas, which are anesthetic, may become desiccated and ulcerated, with resultant visual loss. They lack fungiform papillae on the tongue, and the tongue tip is usually smooth. Taste is affected. Affected infants have hypoactive or absent tendon reflexes and are insensitive to pain. Because of this, they may be unaware of sprains and wounds and may develop Charcot joints. In adolescence they tend to develop scoliosis that may require brac-

ing. Although intelligence is usually normal, development (of speech, in particular) is slow. The personality is often described as unusual, but it is not clear whether this is a primary sign or a result of the chronic illness.

Signs of sympathetic and parasympathetic compromise are prominent. These children may suffer from postural hypotension and yet develop hypertensive crises. Temperature regulation is deficient. Therefore, they may be chronically hypothermic or may die of an episode of hyperpyrexia. Their skin shows blotches, and they may sweat excessively, especially when excited. They suffer from a disorder of esophageal and gastrointestinal motility resulting in gastric reflux and episodic vomiting with abdominal pain that may be so severe as to produce dehydration, hematemesis, or ileus. They have difficulty with bladder control and, as noted earlier, cry without tears.

Affected children have decreased sensitivity to hypercapnia and hypoxia. Some can hold their breath to the point of passing out and developing seizures. Accidental drownings and poor tolerance for anesthesia are attributed to these findings. Diabetes mellitus may develop. Puberty is delayed, and although most do not reproduce, at least one dysautonomic woman was able to carry a pregnancy.

Confirmatory tests include instilling a 2.5% solution of methacholine in the conjunctival sac of one eye; this causes the parasympathetically denervated pupil to constrict, which does not happen in normal people. Injecting a 1:10,000 solution of histamine intradermally produces a wheal, but no pain and no axon flare around it.

Patients excrete excessive amounts of homovanillic acid, a metabolite of dopamine, in their urine, whereas levels of vanillylmandelic acid, a metabolite of epinephrine and norepinephrine, are lower than normal. These findings and the signs of central and peripheral autonomic denervation have provided a basis for symptomatic treatment. Chronic administration of bethanechol (Urecholine) may restore the flow of tears and the tendon stretch reflexes and improve gastrointestinal motility and bladder control. Chlorpromazine, a postsynaptic dopamine blocking agent, is the most useful drug to control vomiting and other acute crises. Early fundoplication with gastrostomy is beneficial in selected patients. Aggressive management of episodes of aspiration and other complications and careful avoidance of poorly tolerated stresses enable some children to survive into middle life with a tolerable level of existence.

References

Anterior Horn Cell Disease

Gilliam TC, Brzustowicz LM, Castilla LH, et al: Genetic homogeneity between acute and chronic forms of spinal muscular atrophy. Nature 345: 823–825, 1990

Iannaccone ST, Browne RH, Samaha FJ, Buncher CR: Prospective study of spinal muscular atrophy before age 6 years. DCN/SMA Group. Pediatr Neurol 9:187–193, 1993

Peripheral Neuropathies

Anderson RM, Dennet X, Hopkins IJ, et al: Hypertrophic interstitial polyneuropathy in infancy. J Pediatr 82:619, 1973

Asbury AK, Johnson PC: Pathology of Peripheral Nerve. Philadelphia, Saunders, 1978

Bradley WG: Disorders of Peripheral Nerve. Oxford, Blackwell, 1974

Giles FH, French JH: Postinjection sciatic nerve palsies in infants and children. J Pediatr 58:195, 1961

Griffin JW, Li CY, Ho TW, et al: Pathology of the motor-sensory axonal Guillain-Barré syndrome. Ann Neurol 39:17, 1996

Guillain-Barré Syndrome Study Group: Plasmapheresis and acute Guillain-Barré syndrome. Neurology 35:1096, 1985

Ouvrier RA, McLeod JG, Pollard JD: Peripheral Neuropathy in Childhood. New York, Raven, 1990

Vallee L, Dulac O, Nuyts JP, Leclerc F, Vamecq J: Intravenous immune globulin is also an efficient therapy of acute Guillain-Barré syndrome in affected children. Neuropediatrics 24:235–236, 1993

Acute Intermittent Porphyria

Meyer UA, Schmid R: The porphyrias. In: Scriver CR, Beaudet AL, Sly WS, et al, eds: The Metabolic and Molecular Bases of Inherited Disease, 7th ed. New York, McGraw-Hill, 1995

Whitelaw AGL: Acute intermittent porphyria in childhood. A neglected diagnosis? Arch Dis Child 49:404, 1974

Familial Dysautonomia

Axelrod FB, Gouge TH, Ginsburg HB, Bangaru BS, Hazzi C: Fundoplication and gastrostomy in familial dysautonomia. J Pediatr 118:388–394, 1991

Axelrod FB, Nachtigal R, Dancis J: Familial dysautonomia: diagnosis, pathogenesis and management. Adv Pediatr 21:75, 1974

Axelrod FB, Porges RJ, Sein ME: Neonatal recognition of familial dysautonomia. J Pediatr 110:946–948, 1987

25.13 DISEASES OF THE NEUROMUSCULAR JUNCTION

Audrey S. Penn

25.13.1   Myasthenia Gravis

Myasthenia gravis (MG) is a disorder of neuromuscular transmission that results from autoimmune attack on nicotinic postsynaptic receptors for acetylcholine. Its features include fluctuating weakness, characteristic electrophysiological alterations, and a variable response to anticholinesterases (antiChE). The incidence of MG is about 40 per 1 million population. The initial symptoms and signs develop before 20 years of age in about one-fifth of these patients. Children with MG can be distributed into three groups: those with neonatal MG, those with congenital MG, and a third group (indistinguishable from adults with MG) who can experience onset any time after birth, although onset before 1 year of age is rare.

MYASTHENIA GRAVIS IN CHILDHOOD AND ADOLESCENCE

These children share all the features of autoimmune MG with adults. There is no particular geographic or racial predilection for MG, but 72% of Caucasian women with MG carry histocompatibility HLA B8, Dw3, or Drw3 haplotypes; Japanese show A12; and Chinese Bw46. This implies that the binding sites on HLA molecules on their lymphoid cells, in particular on cells which present antigen peptide sequences to T cells, recognize and bind to specific acetylcholine receptor (AChR) peptides, which trigger immune responses. Other factors, including intercurrent infection, stress, high ambient temperature, menarche, and menses, may exacerbate the disease. In over 90% of MG patients, circulating IgG antibodies have been detected that react with human and other mammalian AChR in detergent extracts of muscle. This provides direct evidence of autoimmunity directed against the postsynaptic sites (AChR) that bind acetylcholine and mediate electrogenesis in neuromuscular transmission. Current evidence indicates that antibody-mediated injury results from a combination of complement-mediated lysis, accelerated degradation of receptor, and blockade of acetylcholine binding sites. IgG and complement components 3 and 9 have been detected by cytochemistry at the ultrastructural level, and in patients with severe MG, muscle biopsies have disclosed elongated simplified endplates showing loss of synaptic folds and of AChR.

Other autoantibodies, including nuclear, thyroglobulin, thyroid microsomal, rheumatoid factor, and muscle, found in only 5 to 40% of patients, cannot be related to the abnormal neuromuscular transmission but suggest a more generalized autoimmune state. Indeed, the most prominent pathologic finding in MG cannot be detected by routine methods, and it was not found in muscle but in the thymus gland, the central lymphoid organ most responsible for initiating normal cell-mediated immunity. About 70% of thymus glands in patients with MG show lymphoid hyperplasia: lymphoid follicles with germinal centers in the medulla of the gland, usually sparse in the thymus, but numerous in lymph nodes and the spleen. MG glands also show less involution with age; they weigh more and contain excessive numbers of B cells. Another 10% of such glands contain lymphoepithelial thymomas, a tumor that can be present even in adolescents with the disease.

In the early 1970s, α-neurotoxins that specifically bind to nicotinic AChR were isolated from elapid snakes; this permitted the detection, assay, and purification of these receptor glycoproteins from the tissue of electric fish. Immunization of a variety of mammalian species with AChR soon proved to elicit a disorder of neuromuscular transmission, the electrophysiological characteristics of which were indistinguishable from those of MG. Pathologic alterations of endplates detected by cytochemical examination were also identical with those of MG. On radioimmunoassay, all species showed high titers of circulating antibody to the immunogen (electric fish) and detectable titers against autologous receptors. These results rapidly led to studies of MG that confirmed an 80% reduction in active AChR in MG muscle and demonstrated circulating antibodies in MG serum by using the double-antibody radioimmunoassay to measure immunoprecipitation of α-bungarotoxin binding sites (AChR protein) in detergent extracts of mammalian muscle. The cause of this autoimmune state remains elusive. The major possibilities include a process by which the AChR becomes altered such that it acquires new antigenic sites that elicit an immune response or a loss of central immune regulation, perhaps mediated by the abnormal thymus gland, so that mechanisms that normally suppress reactivity against self-antigens are abnormal or abrogated.

The most striking feature of MG at any age is weakness aggravated by repetitive use of muscles in normal activity or exercise. Ocular muscles are almost always involved and frequently are involved first; therefore the presenting complaints usually include ptosis and diplopia. In most patients, various combinations of facial, bulbar, neck, limb, and respiratory muscle weakness of varying degrees develop within days to a year or two. There may be difficulty in chewing, a snarling facial expression when the patient attempts

TABLE 25-25

ANTICHOLINESTERASES IN MYASTHENIA GRAVIS

	NEONATE	CHILD	ADULT
Diagnosis			
Edrophonium (Tensilon)	0.5–1 mg IV	1–2 mg IV initially; then 4-mg aliquots to total of 10 mg	2 mg IV initially; then 4-mg aliquots to total of 10 mg
Neostigmine (Prostigmin)	0.1–0.2 mg IM	0.04 mg/kg IM	1.5–2.5 mg IM
Therapy			
Neostigmine	0.3 mg/kg PO; 0.05–0.25 mg IM q2–3h	5–15 mg PO q2–3h; 0.5–1.5 mg SC	Multiples of 15-mg dose PO q3–4h
Pyridostigmine	1.0 mg/kg PO syrup or tablets q3–4h	30 mg or multiples, as needed, q3–4h	Multiples of 60-mg dose PO q3–4h
Atropine	0.025–0.05 mg SC		0.4–0.6 mg PO

SOURCE: *Dubowitz V: Muscle Disorders in Childhood. Philadelphia, Saunders, 1978; Rowland: In: Conn HF, ed: Current Therapy. Philadelphia, Saunders, 1977.*

to smile, progressively slurred speech, or dyspnea. Serious ventilatory compromise may reflect weak intercostal and diaphragmatic muscles, a condition exacerbated by difficulty in chewing and dysphagia, with pooling of secretions. Sudden respiratory decompensation is referred to as *myasthenic crisis.* Limb weakness is usually proximal and symmetric. In contrast, ophthalmoparesis, especially in adults, is often remarkably asymmetric. In about 10% of patients, signs begin in the limbs, and in a very few patients, limb weakness is predominant, causing initial diagnostic confusion with myopathies. Symptoms and signs may be so mild that they are manifested only after exercise. Other signs (facial, ocular) are obvious, especially to the trained observer, and they may worsen as muscles are used. Children may be unable to play for any length of time, either moving very little or sitting down after only a few minutes. The diagnosis may be suspected if ocular signs are present and asymmetric.

MG in children, as in adults, can be associated with a variety of other autoimmune diseases, including systemic lupus erythematosus, thyroiditis, rheumatoid arthritis, or diabetes mellitus. Familial instances appear to show a particular tendency to such disease concurrence with various autoimmune problems (disease or positive serologic studies) in first-degree relatives.

The diagnosis of MG is frequently obvious from the clinical presentation. In some patients, juxtaposition of certain signs suggests other diagnoses. Ophthalmoparesis in the form of internuclear ophthalmoplegia may mimic multiple sclerosis. When ptosis and ophthalmoparesis are symmetric, a progressive external ophthalmoplegia (with or without abnormal mitochondria) must be considered and excluded. If there is symmetric ocular involvement and facial weakness as well as some degree of limb weakness, appropriate diagnostic tests must be undertaken, as this presentation can mimic Guillain-Barré syndrome (acute polyneuritis) or botulism. MG rarely, if ever, shows the same extent of symmetric facial muscle paralysis or quadriplegia. Mobius syndrome, congenital ptosis, congenital myopathies, myotonic dystrophy, and glycogen-storage disease must also be considered in the differential diagnosis.

The diagnosis of MG may be confirmed by appropriate pharmacologic or electrophysiological tests as well as by detection of antibodies to AChR. Although about 10% of patients with generalized myasthenia have normal titers, a false-positive measurement has been reported only in occasional cases of thymoma and of Lambert-Eaton myasthenic syndrome, both of which may be associated with clinical MG. However, 50 to 75% of patients with disease confined to eye muscles, a group that includes many children with MG under age 10, have normal titers. Signs of MG can be reversed with anti-ChE compounds. Especially useful are edrophonium

(Tensilon) intravenously and neostigmine intramuscularly. Doses depend on age (Table 25-25). The response to a small initial dose of edrophonium (1 to 2 mg) should be monitored carefully for 30 to 45 seconds, then the remaining amount should be given until a response is seen or until 10 mg is injected. In young children, this will require establishment of an IV line followed by time to allow for examination of a calm and cooperative patient. It is especially difficult to examine eye muscles in a child who is blinking repeatedly through tears. Excess edrophonium can produce unacceptable muscarinic side effects, as well as fasciculations. Neostigmine should be given intramuscularly with a dose of atropine, appropriate for weight, and the patient should be observed for 1 to 2 hours.

The normal safety factor for neuromuscular transmission is markedly reduced in patients with MG because of the antibody-mediated loss of AChR. Consequently, repetitive driving of these synapses by supramaximal electrical stimulation of the nerve will result in sequential reduction in the evoked compound muscle action potential. This is known as the *decremental response.* Ulnar, median, or axillary nerves are stimulated at 3 or 5 Hz with recording electrodes over appropriate hand muscles or the deltoid. Positive responses (more than a 10% drop in amplitude of the fifth evoked response as compared with the second) are seen in about 80% of MG patients when all three muscles are studied. The decrement can be intensified by prior exercise of the muscles and should be reversed by anti-ChE. The examination, especially of the deltoid, is uncomfortable but not unbearable, and it has been used in patients of all ages. Stimulation single-fiber EMG, more sensitive but less specific, may be used in sedated children.

Most patients with MG receive anti-ChE therapy first. Pyridostigmine (Mestinon) is preferred over neostigmine because of its longer duration of action and less severe muscarinic side effects. The proper dose varies from patient to patient and in relation to exertion, stress, and other factors. The initial dose should be selected according to the patient's age and weight (Table 25-25), then gradually increased until signs respond, until the side effects that are uncontrolled by atropine occur, or until increases are no longer effective. A patient who is unable to function in daily activities or who is threatened by bulbar or respiratory signs may require corticosteroids, cytotoxic agents, or thymectomy. Corticosteroids should be used in an alternate-day regimen. Alternate-day prednisone therapy has resulted in remissions in up to 70% of patients during the first 3 years of therapy, but these remissions are not sustained unless an effective maintenance dose is used. Side effects can be formidable, and they include inhibition of growth in children. In a series of 42 Chinese children with ocular MG, corticosteroid therapy was abandoned because of unacceptable side effects.

However, there has been considerable experience with this drug and its side effects in other diseases in the pediatric age group. Azathioprine and cyclosporine have also been used for immunosuppression in other pediatric disorders with success. They have been employed infrequently in childhood MG. There is also less pediatric experience with thymectomy, a major form of therapy for MG in adolescents and adults. Thymectomy was first performed in MG because of a coexistent thymoma in a 16-year-old patient. Subsequently, it became obvious that patients without thymoma improved even more significantly. Concern about possible late development of immunodeficiency after thymectomy has dictated caution and restricted its use in children, even those older than 2 years. Animal studies have indicated potential hazards from "adult" thymectomy: Precursors of certain T-cell subsets are removed by this procedure, and after the equivalent of 30 to 50 human years the ability of these animals to generate antibody responses is suppressed. However, there is no firm evidence that measurable immunodeficiency has developed in adults up to 32 years after the operation. In addition, patients aged 10 to 20 years with generalized MG have rates of remission approaching 60% after thymectomy performed by transsternal or more extensive incisions to ensure complete removal. Remissions achieved about 3 years after surgery, on average, are sustained as compared with spontaneous remissions which tend to occur, if at all, within the first year of illness. Therefore, thymectomy has been performed with benefit with severe generalized MG in children as young as 2 years. Plasmapheresis has been used in adults to reduce circulating anti-AChR antibodies and thereby rapidly improve severely involved patients. Improvement may be dramatic, but it is almost always transient, requiring additional therapy with cytotoxic drugs. There has been less experience with plasmapheresis in children, partly because of difficult venous access. Intravenous immunoglobulin administration is a useful and effective alternative.

NEONATAL MYASTHENIA GRAVIS

MG develops within 72 hours of birth in at least 12% of infants born to myasthenic mothers. Signs usually subside by 12 weeks of age, and these children are subsequently normal. Signs may include poor sucking, choking, weak cry, expressionless face, floppy weak limbs, absence of the Moro reflex, and periods of apnea and other respiratory problems. A response to appropriate doses of anti-ChE (Table 25-25) confirms the diagnosis and allows more normal feeding because of better facial muscle and tongue strength and better swallowing. Decremental responses to stimulation at 2 to 5 Hz have been detected in several patients. With the advent of the ability to assay circulating antibodies to AChR, this form of MG has been shown to be the consequence of passive transplacental transfer of maternal IgG antibodies to the fetus. Because these children do not have an underlying autoimmune disease, their signs clear completely once receptors are regenerated and reinserted into synaptic membranes.

Occasional instances of arthrogryposis multiplex congenita in children born to myasthenic mothers have been found to be related to transplacental transfer of circulating maternal antibodies inhibiting the function of fetal AChR.

CONGENITAL MYASTHENIC SYNDROMES

Congenital MG starts at or near birth and persists. The disorder often involves siblings and occasionally parent and child. Ocular

muscle weakness is common, but other muscle groups commonly involved in MG may be weak. Indeed, there have been reports of severe fulminating disease, with sudden respiratory deaths. Recent studies confirm that congenital MG encompasses a group of diverse presynaptic and postsynaptic molecular abnormalities. These children show decremental responses to repetitive stimulation, but no antibodies to AChR. More precise identification of the type of defect requires intercostal muscle biopsy for microelectrode, biochemical, ultrastructural, and molecular analysis. The presence of appropriate numbers and function of synaptic vesicles, endplate AChE, and AChR must be evaluated. Microelectrode analysis and, more recently, single-channel patch-clamp recordings are used to quantify endplate potentials, miniature endplate potentials, miniature endplate current amplitudes, and ion channel kinetics. Molecular genetic analysis using complementary DNA sequences of the isoforms of all four adult subunits as well as the fetal (gamma) isoform has permitted the identification of individual mutations. So far, 56 different mutations in different AChR subunits have been identified within 69 kindreds. Well-characterized disorders of the ion channel include the following: (1) Dominantly inherited myasthenic slow channel syndrome is a disorder in which episodes of prolonged opening of the AChR ion channel result in increased response to ACh. Forearm extensors tend to be selectively weak. Quinidine sulfate has been found to shorten the prolonged opening time of the channels. (2) A fast channel syndrome with decreased response to ACh has been reported in two patients with mutations in the epsilon subunit. (3) Other mutations of the epsilon subunit produce abnormalities of the kinetics of AChR activation so that the channel opens more slowly and closes more rapidly. So far at least 24 recessively inherited mutations in the epsilon subunit have been found to result in severe endplate AChR deficiency. In addition, a familial endplate AChE deficiency caused by mutations in the collagen tail subunit has been identified, with small nerve terminals and reduced ACh release. Definition of the type of defect present in an individual with congenital myasthenia allows attempts at therapy and prevents inappropriate use of anti-AChE.

25.13.2   Botulism

Botulism is a disease in which nearly total paralysis of nicotinic and muscarinic cholinergic transmission results from the effects of *Clostridium botulinum* toxin on the presynaptic mechanisms that release acetylcholine in response to nerve stimulation. The toxin is produced by spores of *C. botulinum* that can contaminate soil-grown foods (types A and B) and fish (type E). Intoxication most commonly results from ingesting food contaminated by spores that are not destroyed because of inadequate cooking temperatures. Rarely, toxin is produced in vivo when anaerobic wounds are contaminated by organisms and spores or when young infants ingest or inhale spores that then produce toxin in the gastrointestinal tract and cause constipation. The toxin destroys the terminal twigs of cholinergic nerve endings, which require several months to regenerate and remodel after a single exposure. Electrophysiological correlates of nerve-terminal damage, with severely disturbed neuromuscular transmission, include an abnormally small initial evoked muscle action potential, whereas at high rates (20 to 50 Hz) the evoked response is potentiated up to 400%. This pattern is otherwise observed only in hypermagnesemic states, after administration of some aminoglycoside antibiotics (streptomycin, kanamycin, neomycin), and in Eaton-Lambert syndrome (a paraneoplastic syndrome with antibodies directed against presynaptic nerve terminal P/Q calcium channels, blocking release of acetylcholine). In affected infants, overly abundant muscle action potentials that are unusually brief and of small amplitude have been detected, presumably related to involvement of terminal nerve twigs in endings of many motor units.

C. botulinum toxin may be the "most poisonous poison." If the patient survives to be hospitalized, symptoms include dryness and soreness of the mouth and throat, blurred vision, diplopia, nausea, and vomiting. Signs include hypohidrosis, total external ophthalmoplegia, and symmetric facial, bulbar, limb, and respiratory paralysis. There is often, but not invariably, pupillary paralysis. Not all patients become equally ill, and this suggests variable intake of toxin or variable individual responses. When outbreaks occur in clusters, the diagnosis is usually suspected immediately. In isolated instances, an adolescent or child may be suspected of having Guillain-Barré syndrome, myasthenia gravis, or even diphtheria. Ptosis has responded to intravenous administration of edrophonium in a few patients, but the response to anti-ChE is neither extensive nor sufficiently prolonged to be therapeutic.

Infants with botulism show constipation, generalized weakness, bulbar signs with decreased sucking and gag reflexes, absence of deep reflexes, facial diplegia, lethargy, ptosis, and ophthalmoparesis. Infants have been admitted to hospitals with provisional diagnoses of aminoacidurias, Werdnig-Hoffmann disease, poliomyelitis, or sepsis. The symmetry of the presentation, the absence of secretions, the complaints of dry mouth, and the pupillary involvement, when present, as well as the characteristic electrophysiological findings, should increase the suspicion of botulism. The Centers for Disease Control or appropriate state laboratories should be notified so that the toxin can be identified from refrigerated serum samples. In instances of suspected infantile botulism, stool samples should be evaluated for the presence of *C. botulinum* as well as toxin because 33% of samples from 336 infants, suspected on clinical grounds, produced botulinum toxins.

Patients should be admitted to intensive care facilities and immediately evaluated for the need for ventilatory assistance by tracheostomy and respirators. Specific therapy includes antitoxin, a horse serum product that can cause serum sickness or anaphylaxis, and guanidine hydrochloride, which promotes release of transmitter from residual spared nerve endings but which has sometimes been associated with marrow depression. Di-aminopyridine, useful in Eaton-Lambert syndrome, has not been found to be of benefit to botulism. None of these has been used in infants.

25.13.3 Organophosphate Poisoning

Organophosphate insecticides are irreversible inhibitors of acetylcholinesterase in comparison with neostigmine and pyridostigmine (see Sec. 4.3.3). Successful management of poisoning requires atropinization, ventilatory assistance, and consideration of the use of pralidoxime methiodide, which specifically displaces organophosphates from the AChE active site.

25.13.4 Tick Paralysis

Young children playing in high grass or playing with pets during spring and early summer can become infested with ticks, which can lodge in the skin of the occiput, neck, spine, axilla, groin, or ear canals. The engorging female ticks *Dermacentor andersoni* (Rocky

Mountains, United States, and Canada), *D. variabilis*, *Ixodes holocyclus* (Australia), and *Argas persicus* (Germany) may not be discovered for up to 12 days. After a latency of 5 to 6 days, the infested children show ataxia of limbs and trunk, with a broad-based gait or inability to walk, although some can crawl and many have normal strength if they are examined when they are not standing. Reflexes are absent, but vibratory and joint position senses are usually normal. There have been rare reports of involvement of ocular muscles, facial muscles, and sphincters, but pupils are spared.

If removal of the tick is delayed, progressive ascending flaccid paralysis will develop, associated with respiratory or bulbar paralysis. The fatality rate among young children in British Columbia from 1928 to 1968 was 12.8%. The paralysis is rapidly reversed in 48 hours to weeks by removing the tick, so that it is important to consider this diagnosis in the appropriate context and at the appropriate time of year. Cerebrospinal fluid examination and creatine kinase concentrations will be normal, which tends to exclude other causes of rapidly ascending areflexic quadriparesis. The tick may be removed by a steady, gentle pull using fingers or forceps. Care must be taken to avoid tearing the arachnid and leaving its head in the wound, although this is unusual.

The major damage produced by the toxin elaborated by the engorging tick appears to involve motor nerve terminals. Some studies of tick-infested dogs, chicks, and hamsters have suggested a disorder of neuromuscular transmission, but in three children with flaccid quadriparesis, the most prominent abnormality found on electrophysiological evaluation just before and for several weeks after removal of the ticks was marked reduction in the amplitude of evoked muscle action potentials. Motor nerve conduction velocities were slightly slow or at the lower limits of normal, but they were significantly faster in studies weeks to months later. Repetitive stimulation of motor nerves at 2 to 50 Hz produced no change in the amplitude of the evoked muscle action potential, indicating normal neuromuscular transmission.

References

Bundey S: A genetic study of infantile and juvenile myasthenia gravis. J Neurol Neurosurg Psychiatr 35:41, 1972

Chan-Lui YW, Leung NK, Lau TTY: Myasthenia gravis in Chinese children. Dev Med Child Neurol 26:717, 1984

Engel AG, Chno K, Sine SM: Congenital myasthenic syndromes: recent advances. Arch Neurol 56:163, 1999

Johnson RO, Clay SA, Arnon SS: Diagnosis and management of infant botulism. Am J Dis Child 133:586, 1979

Lindstrom JM, Seybold ME, Lenon VA, et al: Antibody to acetylcholine receptor in myasthenia gravis. Neurology 26:1054, 1976

Morel E, Eynard B, Vernet B, et al: Neonatal myasthenia gravis: clinical and immunologic appraisal in 30 cases. Neurology 38:138, 1988

Richman DP, ed: Myasthenia gravis and related disorders: disorders of the neuromuscular junction. Ann NY Acad Sci 841, 1998

Riemersma S, Vincent A, Beeson D, et al: Association of arthrogryposis multiplex congenita with maternal antibodies inhibiting fetal acetylcholine receptor function. J Clin Invest 98:2358, 1996

Schmitt N, Bowmer EJ, Greyson JD: Tick paralysis in British Columbia. Can Med Assoc J 100:417, 1969

Seybold ME: Thymectomy in childhood myasthenia gravis. Ann NY Acad Sci 841:731, 1998

Sofer S, Tal A, Shahak E: Carbamate and organophosphate poisoning in early childhood. Pediatr Emerg Care 5:222, 1989

Swift TR, Ignacio OJ: Tick paralysis: electrophysiologic studies. Neurology 25:1130, 1975

25.14 MYOPATHIES

Salvatore DiMauro, Arthur P. Hays, and Eduardo Bonilla

Myopathies are disorders of muscle that, by clinical, pathologic, and electrophysiological criteria do not appear to be secondary to dysfunction of the central or peripheral nervous system. This negative definition encompasses not only disorders limited to skeletal muscle but also some disorders involving multiple systems, and it does not require that the primary abnormality be localized within muscle. Most myopathies are genetically determined, but a few are acquired.

25.14.1   Hereditary Myopathies

DYSTROPHIES

Dystrophies are hereditary myopathies characterized by progressive weakness without morphologic, histochemical, or biochemical evidence of abnormal carbohydrate or lipid storage within muscle fibers. Muscle biopsy shows degenerative changes but not distinctive morphologic abnormalities.

Recent advances in molecular genetics have revealed the causes of most dystrophies, including Duchenne and Becker muscular dystrophy, myotonic muscular dystrophy, congenital muscular dystrophy, Emery-Dreifuss muscular dystrophy, oculopharyngeal muscular dystrophy, as well as some forms of limb-girdle, facioscapulohumeral, and distal muscular dystrophy.

DUCHENNE MUSCULAR DYSTROPHY This is the most severe of the dystrophies. It begins in early childhood, usually before the age of 4 years, but with a range of 1 to 10 years. Walking is delayed in about half of patients. When they start walking, they do so clumsily, with frequent falls. Early weakness of the gluteal and hip extensor muscles causes the characteristic waddling gait and compensatory excessive lumbar lordosis. There is great difficulty climbing stairs. When rising from the prone position, these children get first on hands and knees, then bring their legs close to their arms, and finally they "climb up" their legs to the erect position (Gowers maneuver). Enlargement of muscles, the pseudohypertrophy described by Duchenne, is often present from birth and is more evident in the calves. Proximal weakness of the arms becomes apparent later, but cranial nerves and sphincter functions are consistently spared. Knee jerks are lost early, but ankle jerks may be preserved until late in the course of the disease. The rate of progression varies, but by 12 to 13 years of age all patients have lost the ability to walk and are confined to wheelchairs. Kyphoscoliosis and other fixed deformities (contractures of hip and knee flexors, pes equinovarus) become major problems. Weakness of respiratory muscles decreases total lung capacity and maximal inspiratory and expiratory pressures. Residual lung volume decreases, and the patients have recurrent pulmonary infections. Most patients die before 20 years of age. Although clinical cardiomyopathy is unusual, ECG changes are seen in 60 to 90% of patients. An increased algebraic sum of R and S waves, caused by tall right precordial R waves, is characteristic of but not specific for Duchenne dystrophy. Mental retardation is more common in children with Duchenne dystrophy than in nondystrophic children of the same age, but it cannot be ascribed to the limitations imposed by their physical handicap. The intellectual impairment is neither progressive nor related to the severity of the muscle disease.

Until recently, the diagnosis was based on clinical features, electromyography, muscle biopsy, and marked elevation of serum enzymes. Now it is necessary to add another criterion, evidence of mutation in the Duchenne gene, which can be based either on DNA analysis or on analysis of the gene product dystrophin.

Serum concentrations of several enzymes, especially creatine phosphokinase (CK), are markedly elevated in the initial stages and tend to decrease as the disease progresses. The serum CK concentration is already elevated at birth and during the preclinical phase. Electromyography shows small potentials of short duration, increased numbers of polyphasic potentials, and excessive recruitment of motor-unit potentials with weak effort. Fibrillations and bizarre high-frequency discharges may be present in advanced stages. EMG findings may be normal in the preclinical phase. Muscle biopsy (Fig. 25-37) shows various degrees of the following changes, depending on the stage of the disease: increased variation in fiber size, large opaque fibers, focal areas of degeneration and regeneration, increased numbers of internal nuclei, and infiltration of fat and connective tissue (Fig. 25-37C).

Immunohistochemistry of frozen muscle sections using antibodies against dystrophin (Fig. 25-38) shows no staining in Duchenne patients (Fig. 25-38B), whereas in sections of normal muscle dystrophin is localized at the sarcolemma, where the reaction outlines the contours of fibers with a thin, uninterrupted fluorescent line (Fig. 25-38A). Similarly, immunoblot analysis of muscle extracts shows dystrophin concentrations less than 3% of normal in Duchenne patients.

Demonstration of a mutation, most commonly a deletion, in the dystrophin gene can also be provided by DNA analysis.

No specific or effective treatment is available at the present time. Progression of the disease can be slowed down to a certain extent by corticosteroids (prednisone, 0.75 mg/kg/d, or deflazacort, 2 mg/kg on alternate days), but at the expense of undesirable side effects. Considerable work has been and is still being devoted to the development of somatic cell gene therapy, aimed at the introduction of the dystrophin gene or its coding region into patients' muscle, where the foreign gene would produce the missing protein. These studies have been fraught with major difficulties, including the extremely large size of the gene, the type of vector and promoter to be used, the targeting of the gene to skeletal muscle, the longevity of expression of dystrophin by the therapeutic gene, the route of administration, the postmitotic nature of skeletal muscle, as well as safety and ethical issues. Nonetheless, promising results have been obtained with a dystrophin "minigene" in the *mdx* mouse model, and gene replacement therapy remains a viable hope for the future. Physical therapy is aimed at maintaining ambulation as long as possible and preventing contractures. When the child is about to cease walking, a combination of lightweight plastic braces and percutaneous tenotomies may prolong the ability to walk by a few years. Once the patient is in a wheelchair, good posture and adequate back support are important to prevent scoliosis. Throughout the disease process, psychological support and parental counseling are crucial, and a team approach has been recommended for managing the child with Duchenne dystrophy, including a neurologist, orthopedic surgeon, physical and occupational therapists, and social worker.

Duchenne dystrophy is transmitted as an X-linked recessive trait. Its incidence has varied between 13 and 33 per 100,000 live-born males in surveys from different countries. Duchenne dystrophy in

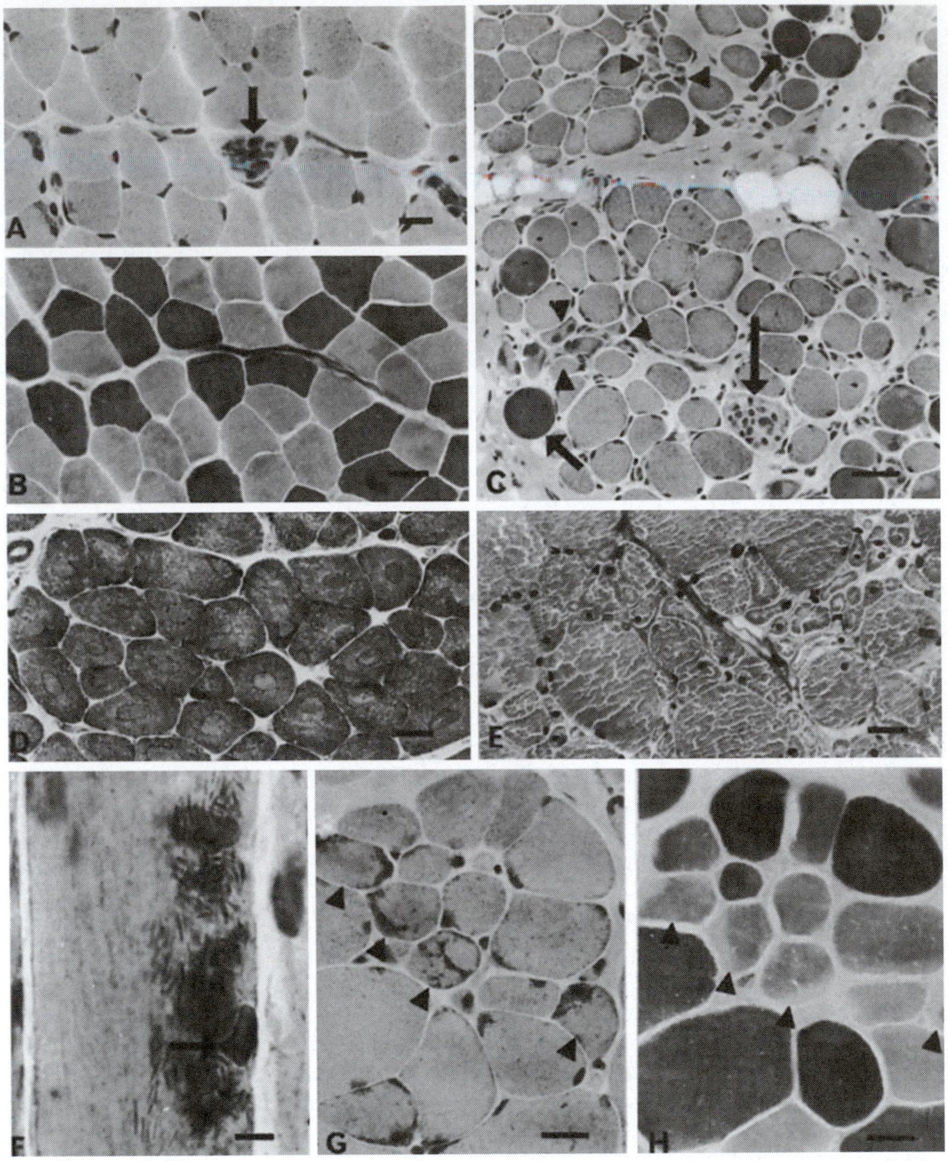

FIGURE 25-37 Muscle biopsies. **A,B.** Normal muscle with intramuscular nerve twig *(arrow)*. In **B**, type I fibers are pale, type II fibers dark. (Modified Gomori trichrome **(A)**, myofibrillar ATP-ase **(B)**; bars = 20 μm. **C.** Duchenne dystrophy. Hyaline *(dark)* fibers *(short arrows)*, necrotic fibers *(long arrow)*, and groups of regenerating fibers *(arrowheads)* are characteristic. (Modified Gomori trichrome; bar = 50 μm). **D.** Central core disease. All fibers are histochemical type I, and most have a central pale zone. (NADH-tetrazolium reductase; bar = 50 μm). **E.** Myotubular myopathy. Small fibers are all histochemical type I (by ATP-ase) and have a central pale zone, often occupied by a nucleus. (Masson trichrome; bar = 20 μm.) **F,G,H.** Nemaline myopathy. In a longitudinal section **(F)**, rods are concentrated at the edge of a fiber near a nucleus *(arrow)*. The rods tend to lie parallel to the longitudinal fiber axis. In transverse sections of myofibers **(G**, *arrowheads)* the rods appear as finely granular masses. **H** is a successive section of the area in **G** showing that rods occur in small type I fibers *(arrowheads)*. (Modified Gomori trichrome; bar **(F)** = 5 μm, bar **(G)** = 20 μm. Myofibrillar ATPase; bar **(H)** = 20 μm.)

girls can be explained by karyotype abnormalities (Turner syndrome; X0/XX or X0/XX/XXX karyotypes), by unequal lyonization with marked predominance of the abnormal X-chromosome in a carrier, or by partial defects of dystrophin in manifesting carriers. Several female patients had chromosome X/autosome translocations, and the affected gene was localized at the breakpoint on the X chromosome, a subterminal region of the short arm, Xp21.

In 1985, an unfortunate boy was identified who had four other genetic diseases besides Duchenne dystrophy and carried a large deletion at Xp21. In the same year, application of *subtraction hybridization* to X-chromosome preparations from this patient and from controls allowed Louis M. Kunkel to isolate portions of the gene whose alteration caused Duchenne dystrophy. Two years later, the protein product of the gene was identified by the same group of investigators and named "dystrophin."

Dystrophin is a large (427 kD) cytoskeletal protein, present in very low abundance in muscle, where it is localized at the sarcolemma (Fig. 25-38); other tissues containing dystrophin are heart, smooth muscle, and brain. In striated muscle, dystrophin is associated with a complex of proteins: these dystrophin-associated proteins (DAPs) link the extracellular matrix and the subsarcolemmal

cytoskeleton (Fig. 25-39). As discussed below, genetic defects of different DAP components result in other forms of dystrophy.

Because of the lack of specific therapy, female carriers must be detected to prevent new occurrences. Some can be identified by simple pedigree analysis. The mother of an affected son with one or more affected maternal male relatives is considered a definite carrier. Identification of some but not all possible carriers can be achieved by direct DNA analysis or by dystrophin immunohistochemistry of muscle biopsies. Prenatal diagnosis is carried out by direct DNA analysis of amniocytes or chorionic villi.

BECKER MUSCULAR DYSTROPHY The clinical manifestations in Becker dystrophy are virtually identical to those in Duchenne dystrophy, but onset is usually after the age of 5 years, and most patients are still able to walk beyond the age of 12 years and often into adolescence and adult life. Death generally occurs between the third and fifth decade and almost never before 20 years of age. Also, mental retardation is not as common as in Duchenne dystrophy, whereas ECG abnormalities are common. In fact, some cases of Becker dystrophy may present exclusively as dilated cardiomyopathy. A clinically benign variant of Becker dystrophy is characterized

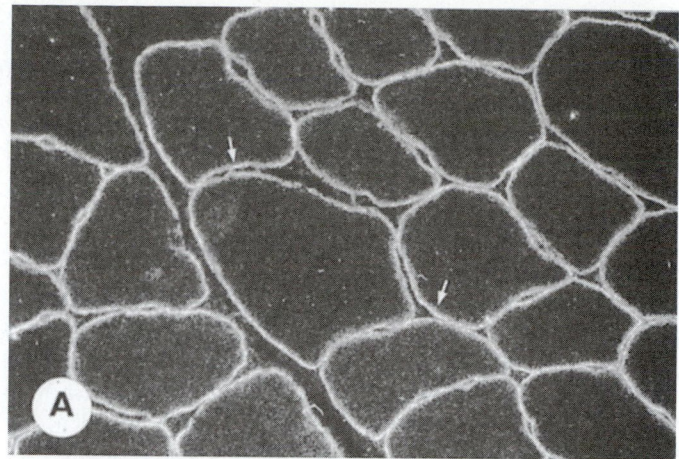

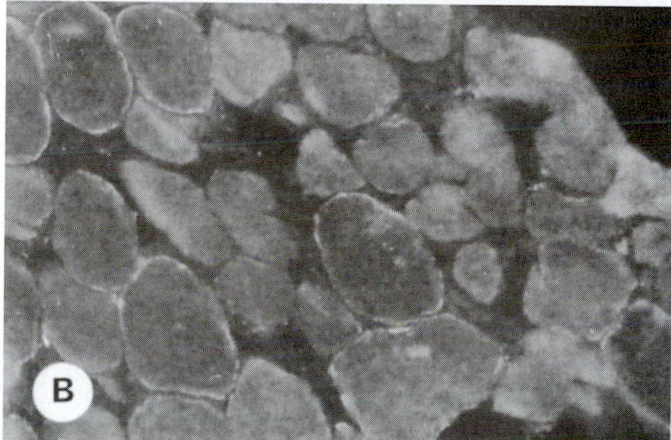

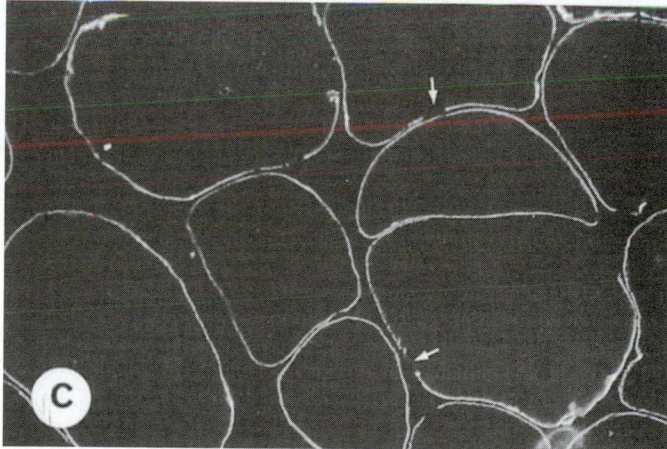

FIGURE 25-38 Immunolocalization of dystrophin. **A.** Normal human muscle shows reaction *(arrows)* at the sarcolemma of all fibers. **B.** Duchenne muscular dystrophy sample shows lack of immunostain in all fibers. **C.** Becker muscular dystrophy sample shows immunostain at the sarcolemma with regions of discontinuities *(arrows)*.

by exercise intolerance and recurrent, exercise-induced episodes of myoglobinuria, without fixed weakness. As in Duchenne dystrophy, hypertrophy of the calves is often pronounced from early childhood, and the serum CK concentration is greatly increased even before weakness becomes manifest. The results of EMG and muscle biopsy are also similar in the two diseases, except that changes tend to be less pronounced in Becker dystrophy. The incidence is about

10% that of the Duchenne form, and transmission is through an X-linked recessive mechanism.

Becker dystrophy is also caused by mutations in the dystrophin genes. Thus, Duchenne and Becker dystrophies are allelic disorders. However, whereas mutations in Duchenne dystrophy cause a shift in the translational reading frame of the dystrophin messenger RNA (nonsense mutations) and, therefore, a failure of protein synthesis, in Becker dystrophy the mutations do not cause a frameshift of the coding sequence and result in the synthesis of shorter dystrophin molecules, which may be only partially functional and more susceptible to degradation. Duplication mutations also occur in Becker dystrophy and result in the synthesis of abnormally long dystrophin molecules. In agreement with these concepts, the immunohistochemical stain for dystrophin in muscle biopsies is present but discontinuous (Fig. 25-38C). Immunoblot shows either partial dystrophin deficiency, with good correlation between residual dystrophin content and clinical severity, or qualitative alterations with dystrophin molecules that are either smaller or larger than normal.

SEVERE CHILDHOOD AUTOSOMAL-RECESSIVE MUSCULAR DYSTROPHY (SCARMD) After the discovery of dystrophin, it became apparent that a number of children of both sexes had a myopathy clinically and pathologically indistinguishable from Duchenne dystrophy but distinct from it because of the mode of transmission (autosomal-recessive rather than X-linked) and because of the normal immunohistochemistry for dystrophin. Initially, most cases were reported from Arabic countries of North Africa, where inbreeding is favored by custom, but the disorder has been identified all over the world. In non-Arabic countries the frequency of SCARMD has been estimated as about 5% that of Duchenne dystrophy.

Age at onset, distribution of weakness, age at which patients lose their ability to walk are similar to Duchenne dystrophy, but both sexes are equally represented, mental retardation is not a feature, and cardiomyopathy is seen more rarely than in Duchenne dystrophy. Levels of serum CK are comparable to those in Duchenne dystrophy, as is the EMG pattern.

Understanding the molecular bases of SCARMD has been possible because of the discovery that dystrophin is strictly connected

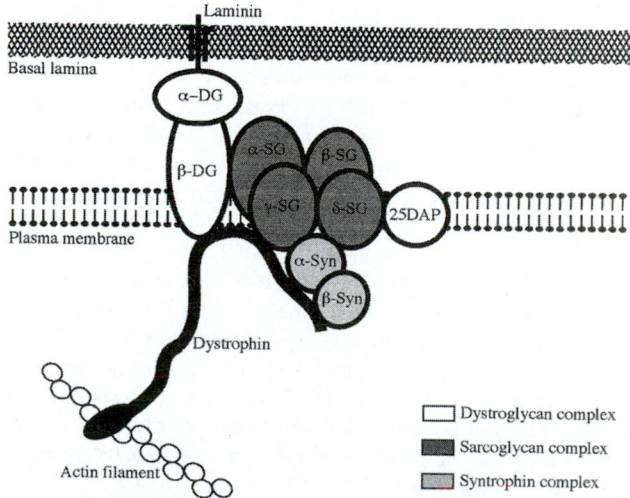

FIGURE 25-39 The molecular architecture of dystrophin and dystrophin-associated proteins at the muscle cell membrane. DG, dystroglycan; SG, sarcoglycan; Syn, syntrophin. For details, see text.

to a network of proteins, as mentioned above. As shown in a scheme proposed by Osawa (Fig. 25-39), the lipid bilayer of the sarcolemma is "sandwiched" between extracellular and intracellular protein networks connected by the dystrophin "axis." It is postulated that these protein networks are resistant to mechanical displacement, thus protecting the sarcolemma from damage during contraction. Starting from the outside, *laminin 2 (or merosin)*, an important component of the basal lamina, binds to *α-dystroglycan*, an extracellular glycoprotein, which, in turn, binds to *β-dystroglycan*, a transmembrane glycoprotein. Intracellularly, β-dystroglycan binds to the C-terminal domain of dystrophin. At the sarcolemma, β-dystroglycan also binds to the *sarcoglycan complex*, composed of four transmembrane glycoproteins, α, β, γ, and δ. Inside the sarcolemma, the sarcoglycan complex binds to still another group of proteins, the *syntrophin complex*, composed of α- and *β-syntrophin* and *dystrobrevin*.

Most patients with SCARMD have been found to harbor mutations in genes encoding sarcoglycan proteins, most commonly α-sarcoglycan (or *adhalin*, after the Arabic word for muscle) and β-sarcoglycan. In a study of 54 patients with muscular dystrophy and low immunohistochemical levels of α-sarcoglycan (a nonspecific sign of sarcoglycan complex involvement), the prevalence of sarcoglycan gene mutations was highest (22%) among SCARMD patients and much lower (6%) among patients with later-onset limb-girdle dystrophy.

LIMB-GIRDLE DYSTROPHY After the sorting out of SCARMD as a specific entity, limb-girdle dystrophy is rarely a consideration in the pediatric age group, as the disease typically starts in the second or third decade, with slowly progressive weakness, generally affecting one limb-girdle first, then spreading to the other.

With better understanding of the molecular bases of limb-girdle dystrophy, the nomenclature has changed: *LGMD1* refers to autosomal-dominant forms, and *LGMD2* refers to autosomal-recessive forms. Linkage analysis has localized the gene for LGMD1A to chromosome 5q and that for LGMD1B to chromosome 1q11-21. The gene responsible for LGMD1C, on chromosome 3p25, has been identified: it encodes *caveolin-3*, the muscle-specific form of the caveolin family, a group of proteins present in the caveolae, or invaginations of the plasma membrane.

Most of the LGMD2 forms are due to mutations in *sarcoglycan* genes; γ-sarcoglycan in LGMD2C; α-sarcoglycan in LGMD2D; β-sarcoglycan in LGMD2E; and δ-sarcoglycan in LGMD2F. One of them (LGD2A) is due to mutations in a protease, *calpain 3*. LGMD2B is due to mutations in a gene (on chromosome 2p13) encoding a protein called *dysferlin*, while LGMD2G is due to mutations in a gene (on chromosome 17) encoding a protein dubbed *telethonin*. The responsible genes are not known in LGMD2H and in LGMD2I.

CONGENITAL MUSCULAR DYSTROPHY Two major groups have been traditionally distinguished, one in which the congenital myopathy is the sole or dominating clinical presentation, the other in which the myopathy is associated with structural brain defects, eye abnormalities, and severe mental retardation. The second group includes Fukuyama congenital muscular dystrophy (FCMD), muscle-eye-brain disease (Finnish type), and Walker-Warburg syndrome (WWS).

The "classic," "pure," or "occidental" type of congenital muscular dystrophy is characterized clinically by congenital weakness often associated with contractures and joint deformities (arthrogryposis multiplex congenita) and by muscle biopsy findings resembling those seen in other dystrophies. Mental retardation is usually but not invariably absent, serum CK levels are less markedly elevated than in Duchenne dystrophy or in SCARMD, and the course is less rapidly progressive. This rather ill-defined type of congenital dystrophy has been subdivided into two major and equally frequent subgroups based on the presence or absence of immunoreactive *laminin 2 (merosin)* in muscle biopsies. Despite the lack of obvious psychomotor deficits (at least, at the time of examination), children with merosin-negative congenital muscular dystrophy (MN-CMD) as a rule show brain changes detectable by MR imaging and consisting of signal hyperintensities in T_2-weighted images of the supratentorial white matter, sometimes associated with evidence of polymicrogyria. However, examination of 50 patients with merosin-positive congenital muscular dystrophy (MP-CMD) showed normal intelligence in almost all, but 24% had MR evidence of cerebral atrophy, and 11% had areas of white matter lucency. Interestingly, 92% of MP-CMD patients had learned to walk by age 4 years. Thus, in general, the clinical manifestations of MP-CMD appear to be milder and more slowly progressive than those of MN-CMD.

Merosin is the predominant laminin isoform expressed in the basal lamina of skeletal muscle: it is, like other laminins, a heterotrimeric protein with the composition α_2-β_1-γ_1. Pathogenic mutations have been documented in the α_2 gene (on chromosome 6q) in patients with MN-CMD. As shown in Fig. 25-39, merosin binds to α-dystroglycan and is part of a link between the extracellular matrix and the muscle cytoskeleton that may have a crucial role in the protection of sarcolemmal integrity during muscle contraction. Merosin also binds a muscle-specific protein called *integrin α₇*; not surprisingly, three unrelated children with MP-CMD showed lack of immunohistochemical reaction to integrin α_7 and harbored pathogenic mutation in the corresponding gene.

To further underline the importance of the link between extracellular matrix and muscle plasma membrane, mutations have been described in the gene encoding the α chain of *type VI collagen* in *Bethlem myopathy,* an autosomal-dominant form of congenital muscular dystrophy with arthrogryposis multiplex congenita.

Fukuyama congenital muscular dystrophy is a common autosomal-recessive form of dystrophy in Japan, with an incidence of 0.7 to 1.2 per 10,000 births. It is characterized by the association of muscular dystrophy and severe mental retardation. Brain abnormalities, such as lissencephaly and polymicrogyria, are caused by a defect of neuronal migration. The abnormal gene, mapped to chromosome 9q31, encodes a protein called *fukutin*. The most common mutation is a retrotransposal insertion of tandemly repeated sequences in the 3′ untranslated region of the fukutin gene.

BARTH SYNDROME A distinct and multisystemic form of congenital muscular dystrophy, Barth syndrome is characterized by cardiomyopathy, myopathy, short stature, cyclic neutropenia, and increased urinary excretion of 3-methylgluconic acid. Dilated cardiopathy is often the presenting sign, which dominates the clinical picture and may cause death in infancy. Hypotonia and weakness are often overlooked or attributed to cardiac insufficiency but are present since birth and sometimes associated with contractures (talipes equinovarus). Motor development is delayed, and, when rising from the floor, these children often use a Gowers maneuver. Neutropenia is variable, even in the same patient, and bone marrow studies have suggested a defect in maturation. There is intermittent hyperlactacidemia and urinary excretion of 3-methylglutaconic acid and 3-methylglutaric acid, catabolic products of leucine metabolism. Morphologic studies of heart and muscle have shown mitochondrial changes, and biochemical analyses have confirmed multiple defects of respiratory chain enzymes and decreased concentration of cytochromes. Therapy has been directed to the cardiopathy and has included cardiac transplantation.

Barth syndrome is transmitted as an X-linked recessive trait, and linkage analysis localized the gene to Xq28. Screening candidate genes in the Xq28 area led to the identification of the affected gene, which encodes a protein known as *tafazzin,* perhaps an acyltransferase, and several mutations have been identified in patients and female carriers.

EMERY-DREIFUSS MUSCULAR DYSTROPHY This rare form of X-linked muscular dystrophy is distinguished from Becker dystrophy by the presence from childhood of contractures at elbow, ankle, and neck, and by cardiomyopathy that causes atrioventricular conduction block ranging from sinus bradycardia and prolongation of the PR interval to complete block. There are weakness and wasting in the humeroperoneal distribution and no enlargement of the calves. The muscle disorder is slowly progressive and rarely disabling, but sudden death owing to heart conduction disturbances is not uncommon. The serum CK concentration is only mildly elevated, and ECG will show various degrees of atrioventricular block.

Linkage analysis had mapped the gene for Emery-Dreifuss dystrophy to the long arm of the X chromosome at Xq28. In 1994, both the gene and several mutations were identified. This small gene (2.1 kb) encodes a serine-rich protein of 254 amino acids named *emerin.* Emerin is a ubiquitous protein localized to the inner nuclear membrane and, in the heart, also to the desmosomes of the intercalated discs. Immunohistochemistry has shown emerin to be absent in skeletal, cardiac, and smooth muscle, skin keratinocytes, and blood cells from patients with Emery-Dreifuss dystrophy. Although the precise function of the protein remains to be defined, more than 60 pathogenic mutations in the emerin gene, mostly nonsense point mutations or small deletions/insertions, have been associated with Emery-Dreifuss muscular dystrophy. The molecular basis in the less common but clinically identical autosomal-dominant form of the disease has also been identified: pathogenic mutations have been identified in a gene on chromosome 1q11-q23 (*LMNA*) that encodes two proteins of the nuclear lamina, *lamin A* and *lamin C.*

FACIOSCAPULOHUMERAL (FSH) DYSTROPHY In its typical presentation, this autosomal-dominant disorder becomes apparent in adolescence and progresses slowly. Facial (but not ocular or pharyngeal) muscles are often affected first, with inability to close the eyes tightly, puff out the cheeks, or whistle; then shoulder-girdle muscles are involved, often asymmetrically, with difficulty in rising the arms overhead and lifting objects. As with other autosomal-dominant diseases, the expression varies greatly among different patients and in subsequent generations, from a virtually asymptomatic condition (often considered nothing more than a curious family trait, like sleeping with the eyes open) to a severe, although rarely disabling, weakness. The serum CK concentration is only slightly increased, and muscle biopsy abnormalities are not very impressive, often consisting of scattered atrophic fibers. In some families, however, muscle biopsy will show striking inflammatory changes, and in others mitochondrial proliferation with "ragged-red fibers" (see below). In some patients, surgical fixation of the scapulae to the posterior thoracic wall may improve the ability to lift the arms.

The gene for FSH dystrophy has been localized on the long arm of chromosome 4, at 4q35.

DISTAL MUSCULAR DYSTROPHY Distal muscular dystrophy was first recognized in Sweden by Welander in 1951 in families with autosomal-dominant inheritance. A different form of distal myopathy, inherited as an autosomal-recessive trait and first described in Japan (Miyoshi myopathy), has been later identified in Western countries as well. Recent advances in molecular genetics have allowed to separate out several distinct entities. The *autosomal-recessive type (Miyoshi myopathy)* usually affects the gastrocnemius first, with difficulties climbing stairs and hopping on one foot. Serum CK is markedly elevated, and some patients were initially considered cases of "idiopathic hyperCKemia." The mutant gene in Miyoshi myopathy has been mapped to chromosome 2p13: it encodes a protein called *dysferlin.* A second *autosomal-recessive form with rimmed vacuoles (Nonaka myopathy)* usually starts with tibialis anterior muscle weakness and footdrop; in contrast to Miyoshi myopathy, serum CK in this form is only slightly elevated. Linkage studies have mapped the gene to chromosome 9p1-q1. The original *autosomal-dominant form (Welander distal myopathy)* affects hand muscles first, causing difficulties with fine hand movements; distal leg muscles are usually involved later. The genetic basis of this form remains to be clarified. A second *autosomal-dominant form (tibial muscular dystrophy)* was described in Finland; it starts late (fourth decade) with tibialis anterior and long toe extensors weakness. Serum CK may be slightly elevated. Linkage studies have localized the gene to chromosome 2q31-33.

OCULAR MUSCULAR DYSTROPHY There are two forms of dystrophy that involve ocular muscles. One (*ocular myopathy*) is a rare autosomal-dominant disorder that begins in the first two or three decades and progresses slowly. In this form, there is ptosis, usually without diplopia, often accompanied by weakness of facial and proximal limb muscles. The second form (*oculopharyngeal muscular dystrophy, OPMD*) is a disorder of late onset (fourth or fifth decade) transmitted as an autosomal-dominant trait, which has been ultrastructurally characterized by filamentous inclusions in muscle nuclei. Dysphagia and ptosis are the main manifestations; extraocular, facial, and limb-girdle muscles are less frequently involved. Linkage analysis in French Canadian pedigrees mapped the gene to chromosome 14q11. This disorder is related to a small trinucleotide repeat expansion in the *polyadenyl binding protein (PABP2)* gene.

A more common pediatric problem is congenital ptosis, a benign, nonprogressive, often unilateral disorder inherited as an autosomal-dominant trait.

MYOTONIC SYNDROMES

Myotonia is a defect of muscle relaxation characterized electromyographically by repetitive high-frequency discharges that wax and wane in frequency and amplitude and are not abolished by curarization or peripheral nerve block.

MYOTONIC DYSTROPHY Myotonic dystrophy (Steinert disease) is a disorder characterized by muscle weakness, wasting and myotonia, cardiomyopathy, cataract, impaired mentation, baldness, hypogonadism, and other endocrine dysfunctions. Its estimated frequency is of 1 in 8000. The onset is usually in adolescence, and the course is slowly progressive. Some patients are virtually asymptomatic, others have crippling weakness. Weakness of facial muscles, with wasting of temporal muscles and ptosis, causes a characteristic elongated and droopy facial appearance. This is one of the few myopathies in which weakness and wasting are more pronounced in distal than in proximal muscles. Involvement of smooth muscle may impair esophageal and intestinal motility and cause uterine dystocia. Serum CK concentrations are mildly elevated. EMG will show a combination of myotonic and myopathic features. The ECG findings are usually abnormal, including conduction defects and, less frequently, arrhythmias. Muscle biopsy findings are not very characteristic, except for long rows of internally located nuclei. Transmission is autosomal-dominant, and the affected gene is localized on the long arm of chromosome 19. In 1992, an intensive search resulted in the discovery of the molecular basis of the disorder, which is an unstable abnormal expansion of a trinucleotide repeat at the 3' end of a gene encoding a serine/threonine kinase, now called *DM protein kinase* or *myotonin*. Myotonia is rarely the main complaint in these patients; if antimyotonic therapy is considered, phenytoin is the drug of choice, because both quinine and procainamide can worsen cardiac conduction defects.

CONGENITAL MYOTONIC DYSTROPHY Affected infants frequently present a clinical picture very different from that in adolescents; they show severe hypotonia, bilateral facial weakness with difficulty in sucking, and respiratory distress. About half of these patients have talipes, and some have multiple contractures at birth; thus congenital myotonic dystrophy is another possible cause of arthrogryposis multiplex congenita. A most important negative feature is the absence of clinical and often electrical evidence of myotonia in these infants; however, clinical or electrical evidence of myotonia in the mother is a useful diagnostic clue. If respiratory failure does not cause death in the neonatal period, motor function will improve. Facial diplegia persists, however, and affected children appear expressionless and have a characteristic triangular or fish-type mouth. Also, with time, mental retardation becomes apparent in most children. The almost exclusively maternal transmission of congenital myotonic dystrophy has been attributed to genetic imprinting.

PROXIMAL MYOTONIC MYOPATHY (PROMM) Once the molecular basis of myotonic dystrophy was established, it became apparent that some patients with autosomal dominantly inherited proximal weakness, myotonia, and cataracts did not have the abnormal trinucleotide expansion characteristic of myotonic dystrophy. Onset is typically in the fourth or fifth decade of life, and the disease has not been described in children. The molecular basis is unknown.

MYOTONIA CONGENITA Myotonia congenita (*Thomsen disease*) is an autosomal-dominant disorder caused by mutations of the gene coding for the voltage-sensitive chloride channel of skeletal muscle. The symptoms are limited to myotonia, which is usually manifested since childhood. This is characteristically noted when activity is started after prolonged rest; it is aggravated by cold and can be "worked off" with continuing activity. Prolonged closure of the baby's eyes may sometimes be noted after crying. Leg myotonia can cause frequent falls in affected children. Strength is fully preserved. Muscle hypertrophy is common.

Becker described a more common autosomal-recessive form of congenital myotonia in which muscle hypertrophy is more pronounced than in the dominant form, and weakness is often present. This form is also caused by mutations of the voltage-sensitive chloride channel. The onset is rarely in childhood. Serum CK concentrations are normal in both forms of myotonia congenita, and EMG will show myotonic discharges but no myopathic features. Muscle biopsy findings are usually normal, except for lack of type IIB fibers. Phenytoin, procainamide, and quinine effectively reduced the my-

otonia; because their effect is short-lived, these drugs can be used intermittently before the patient engages in physical activity.

PARAMYOTONIA CONGENITA The clinical hallmark of this disorder is the temperature-sensitive nature of the myotonia and episodic paralysis. A prolonged myotonic reaction affecting mainly the facial and hand muscles is brought on by exposure to cold and is often followed by transient weakness. In contrast with other forms of myotonia, myotonic symptoms are worsened by repeated exercise ("myotonia paradoxica"). Transmission is autosomal-dominant, and the disorder is related to mutations of the gene coding for the voltage-sensitive sodium channel of muscle (SCN4A).

HYPERKALEMIC PERIODIC PARALYSIS Hyperkalemic periodic paralysis (Gamstorp disease) is transmitted as an autosomal-dominant trait. As in paramyotonia congenita, the disorder is caused by mutations in the gene encoding the voltage-sensitive sodium channel of muscle (SCN4A) on chromosome 17q23. This disorder is more common in children, and even infants, than the hypokalemic form. Attacks are shorter than in the hypokalemic disorder, rarely lasting more than a few hours, and may be precipitated by rest after heavy exercise as well as by cold or fasting. Clinical or electrical evidence of myotonia is present in most affected families, but weakness, not myotonia, is the main clinical complaint. Serum potassium concentrations are variably increased during the attacks, and attacks may be induced by administration of potassium. The changes in muscle biopsy specimens that are seen during attacks are similar to those in the hypokalemic form, but they are usually less severe. Attacks can be treated by oral administration of glucose and prevented by acetazolamide.

A variant of this syndrome has been described in six children with an associated, potentially life-threatening biventricular tachy-dysrhythmia. These patients may die suddenly.

HYPOKALEMIC PERIODIC PARALYSIS This condition is characterized by attacks of flaccid paralysis involving trunk and limb muscles, typically sparing respiratory and ocular muscles. Attacks last from a few hours to several days. Between attacks, most patients have normal strength. Predisposing factors include high-carbohydrate meals, cold, anxiety, and rest after unusually vigorous exercise. Attacks often start in the early hours of the morning. This form of periodic paralysis is rare in children; it usually begins in the second decade, and the frequency of attacks tends to decline with age. During attacks, muscle is inexcitable, and EMG will show electrical silence. Serum potassium concentrations are characteristically decreased, probably because of a shift of potassium into the muscle. However, there is no close correlation between serum potassium levels and severity of weakness. Muscle biopsy specimens taken during attacks will show numerous apparently empty vacuoles. Attacks can be induced by giving glucose or glucose and insulin, a procedure often used as a diagnostic precipitating test. During attacks, oral administration of potassium salts is the treatment of choice. Acetazolamide is an effective prophylactic drug. Transmission is autosomal-dominant, with a striking predominance for the male gender. Linkage studies localized the responsible gene to chromosome 1q31-32: the gene encodes the α_1 subunit of the L-type calcium channel, also known as *dihydropyridine receptor (DHP)*, located in the transverse tubules of the sarcoplasmic reticulum.

NORMOKALEMIC PERIODIC PARALYSIS Normokalemic periodic paralysis is also dominantly inherited and is clinically similar to the hyperkalemic form, from which it can be distinguished by its normal levels of serum potassium during attacks.

CHONDRODYSTROPHIC MYOTONIA Chondrodystrophic myotonia (Schwartz-Jampel syndrome) is a rare disorder affecting especially the skeletal system and muscle. It is characterized by dwarfism, hip dysplasia, pigeon breast, micrognathia, and clinical myotonia. In contrast with the situation in true myotonia, however, the continuous repetitive discharges of Schwartz-Jampel syndrome are abolished by curare. The combination of micrognathia, pursed mouth, and blepharospasm causes a characteristically rigid facial expression described as a frozen smile. The limited ranges of motion in several joints contribute to the still appearance of these children. The onset is in infancy, with stiffness, feeding problems, and weak cry; there is weakness of proximal muscles, sometimes contrasting with hypertrophy of the same muscle groups. Serum CK concentrations may be slightly increased. EMG may show myotonia or continuous muscle fiber activity together with myopathic changes. Transmission appears to be autosomal-recessive. The genetic defect is not known.

MORPHOLOGICALLY DEFINED CONGENITAL MYOPATHIES

This is a group of usually, but not invariably, benign and nonprogressive myopathies with proximal or diffuse muscle weakness and normal or slightly increased serum enzyme concentrations. Skeletal anomalies are often present, such as pes cavus and dislocated hips. Although the presentation may occasionally be in adult life, weakness is usually present at birth or soon thereafter, as the name implies, and these diseases are to be considered in the differential diagnosis of the floppy infant syndrome. The following specific entities are defined by distinct (but not absolutely specific) structural features.

CENTRAL CORE DISEASE In this autosomal-dominant condition, central or paracentral areas (cores) usually extending along the entire length of the muscle fibers show decreased staining with reactions for oxidative enzymes and phosphorylase (see Fig. 25-37D). Mitochondria, sarcoplasmic reticulum profiles, and glycogen are decreased within the cores. Some patients with central core disease also show clinical manifestations of malignant hyperthermia. This is explained by molecular genetic evidence that both conditions are caused by, in some cases, mutations in the gene (on chromosome 19q13.1) encoding the *ryanodine receptor,* a calcium release channel.

MULTICORE (MINICORE) DISEASE This disease was originally described in two children who had nonprogressive weakness since birth and delayed motor milestones. One patient had ptosis. There were multiple small cores in each affected fiber, with abnormalities resembling those of unstructured central cores. The cores, however, did not extend along the entire length of the fiber.

NEMALINE (ROD) MYOPATHY This disorder is characterized by multiple "rod" structures in muscle fibers that are not seen in hematoxylin-eosin stain and are best revealed with the Gomori trichrome stain or the phosphotungstic acid hematoxylin (PTAH) stain (see Fig. 25-37 F–H). Both fiber types may be affected, but rods tend to be more abundant in type I fibers, and type I fiber predominance is common. The ultrastructural features of the rods are similar to those of Z discs, from which they appear to originate.

Onset is usually in early infancy, with floppiness, weak cry, feeding difficulties, and delayed motor development. There is involvement of facial but rarely ocular muscles. Weakness is usually static or slowly progressive, but death from respiratory failure has been reported in both infantile and late-onset disease. Most patients have slender muscles and long, thin, expressionless faces. Other dysmorphic features include high-arched palate, kyphoscoliosis, pigeon chest, and pes cavus. There are few sporadic occurrences, but the disorder is usually transmitted as an autosomal-recessive or, more rarely, as an autosomal-dominant trait. In a large Australian family with autosomal-dominant inheritance, pathogenic mutations have been identified in a gene on the long arm of chromosome 1, which encodes the contractile protein *α-tropomyosin*. In five families with the autosomal-recessive form, mutations were found in a gene on chromosome 2q21.2-q22, which encodes a giant thin filament protein called *nebulin*.

MYOTUBULAR (CENTRONUCLEAR) MYOPATHY The characteristic structural abnormalities are rows of central nuclei in both fiber types, but predominantly in type I fibers (see Fig. 25-37E). There is also type I fiber preponderance and hypotrophy. The central nuclei are surrounded by areas of cytoplasm devoid of myofibrils and containing variably increased oxidative enzymes, phosphorylase, and glycogen, and decreased ATPase activity, a picture reminiscent of myotubes. Because of the similarity of these fibers to myotubes, it has been suggested that the disorder may be related to an arrest of normal muscle development, a concept supported by recent molecular data (see below).

A distinctive clinical feature in affected children is the combination of ophthalmoplegia and facial diplegia. In many patients, fetal movements are diminished and weakness is present from birth, but in others the onset is later in childhood or even in the second or third decade. The clinical course also varies in different patients, from a benign, virtually static myopathy to severe generalized weakness with respiratory failure. Serum enzyme concentrations are elevated in some patients.

Inheritance can be autosomal-dominant, autosomal-recessive, or X-linked recessive. Families with X-linked inheritance usually have early onset and severe course, with death in infancy from respiratory failure. In this form, the disease locus was localized to Xq28, and the gene responsible was isolated: It encodes a 603–amino acid protein, called *myotubularin*. Numerous mutations have been identified in patients from all over the world, almost all unique to each family, a striking example of genetic heterogeneity. Myotubularin is one member of a protein tyrosine phosphatase superfamily probably involved in the terminal differentiation of secondary myotubes into functional myofibers. It is likely that other members of the same family of proteins may be implicated in the autosomal forms of myotubular myopathy.

FIBER TYPE DISPROPORTION In this condition, type I fibers predominate and are uniformly smaller than type II fibers, whereas in normal children the two types of fibers have approximately equal sizes. These patients are weak from birth and often have contractures and joint deformities (arthrogryposis multiplex congenita). Short stature and dysmorphic features (hip dislocation, pes cavus, high-arched palate) are common. Weakness affects trunk and limb muscles predominantly and may be progressive during the first 2 years of life. After that time, however, the disorder becomes static, and these patients often improve, although they rarely attain normal strength. The condition appears to be transmitted as an autosomal-dominant or -recessive trait in different families.

MALIGNANT HYPERTHERMIA

This hereditary and often lethal reaction develops after anesthesia with halogenated volatile anesthetics or depolarizing neuromuscular blocking agents. The clinical picture is characterized by rapidly rising temperature, tachycardia, cardiac arrhythmia, cyanosis, respiratory and metabolic acidosis, and, usually (but not invariably), rigidity and myoglobinuria. Malignant hyperthermia (MH) has been reported to occur in association with other myopathies, such as central core disease, myotonic syndromes, and Duchenne muscular dystrophy. In most patients, however, outside of MH crises, EMG findings and muscle morphology are normal or nonspecifically abnormal. The myopathy in these patients can be identified by increased resting serum CK concentrations or increased in vitro sensitivity of muscle to caffeine or anesthetic agents. In most patients, MH is transmitted by autosomal-dominant inheritance. Linkage analysis studies have suggested that two different loci may be involved in MH. One is the gene encoding the calcium release channel, or *ryanodine receptor,* on chromosome 19q13.1, thus explaining the frequent overlap of MH and central core disease (see above). The other gene is close to or at the locus for the α subunit of the sodium channel on chromosome 17.

Patients with MH usually are not diagnosed until they are exposed to anesthesia, which is frequently catastrophic. Unexplained fevers, increased serum CK concentrations, or cramps, especially when occurring in an autosomal-dominant pattern, may indicate MH. A family history of an anesthetic episode of hyperthermia, muscle rigidity, metabolic acidosis, myoglobinuria, or sudden death more strongly suggests the possibility of MH. Intravenous administration of dantrolene is effective in preventing or aborting MH attacks.

DISORDERS OF GLYCOGEN METABOLISM

Ten forms of glycogen storage disease with defined enzyme defects (and increasingly well defined molecular defects) affect muscle, alone or in association with other tissues: type II, acid maltase deficiency (Pompe disease); type III, debrancher deficiency (Cori-Forbes disease); type IV, brancher deficiency (Andersen disease); type V, myophosphorylase deficiency (McArdle disease); type VII, phosphofructokinase (PFK) deficiency (Tarui disease); type VIII, phosphorylase kinase deficiency; type IX, phosphoglycerate kinase (PGK) deficiency; type X, phosphoglycerate mutase (PGAM) deficiency; type XI, lactate dehydrogenase (LDH) deficiency; type XII, aldolase (ALD) deficiency. These are discussed in detail in Sec. 9.5.1.

DISORDERS OF LIPID METABOLISM

Long-chain fatty acids are important sources of energy for muscle contraction, especially during fasting, when muscle glycogen concentration and blood glucose supply are reduced, and during prolonged exercise. Two major metabolic pathways are needed for long-chain fatty acid utilization: (1) transport and activation of fatty acids (the *carnitine cycle*); and (2) mitochondrial fatty acyl-CoA oxidation (β-*oxidation*).

The carnitine cycle consists of five steps mediated by a plasma membrane fatty acid transporter, a plasma membrane carnitine transporter, carnitine palmitoyltransferase I (CPT I), a carnitine-acylcarnitine translocase, and carnitine palmitoyltransferase II (CPT II) (Fig. 25-40).

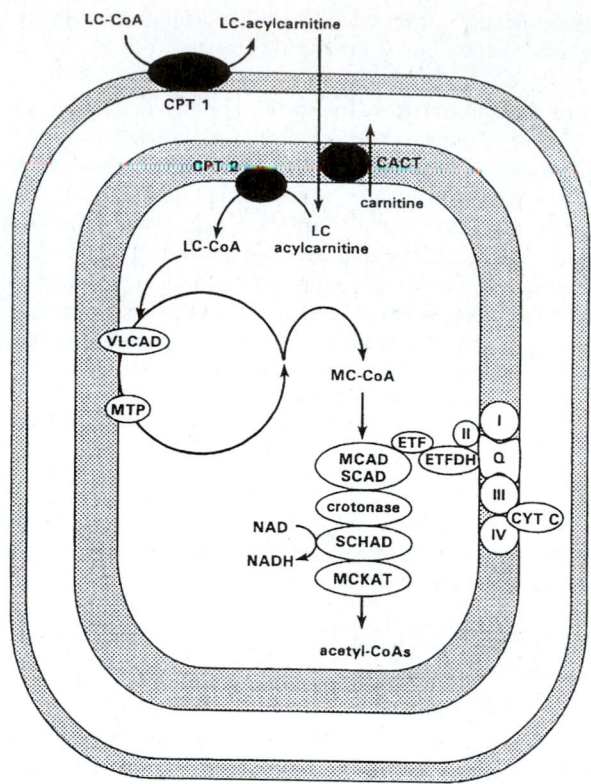

FIGURE 25-40 Scheme of the carnitine cycle enzymes (solid symbols) and of the β-oxidation enzymes (open symbols) in the mitochondrion. The outer and inner mitochondrial membranes are represented by the stippled areas. LC, long-chain; MC, medium-chain; CPT, carnitine palmitoyltransferase; CACT, carnitine-acylcarnitine translocase; VLCAD, very long chain acyl-CoA dehydrogenase; MTP, mitochondrial trifunctional protein; MCAD, medium-chain acyl-CoA dehydrogenase; SCAD, short-chain acyl-CoA dehydrogenase; SCHAD, short-chain hydroxyacyl-CoA dehydrogenase; MCKAT, medium-chain 3-ketoacyl-CoA thiolase; ETF, electron-transfer flavoprotein; ETFDH, electron-transfer flavoprotein dehydrogenase; I, II, III, IV, complexes I, II, III, and IV of the respiratory chain; Q, coenzyme CoQ10; CYT C, cytochrome *c.* For details, see text. *Reproduced from Wanders et al: J Inherit Metab Dis 22:442, 1999, with permission.*

DEFECTS OF THE CARNITINE CYCLE

FATTY ACID TRANSPORTER DEFICIENCY It is still controversial whether transport of long-chain fatty acids across the plasma membrane requires a specific uptake system, but the existence of such an active transport mechanism was suggested by studies in two children presenting with episodic acute hepatic failure requiring liver transplantation in both cases. Long-chain fatty acid oxidation was markedly impaired in cultured fibroblasts, but there was no evidence of defects in the carnitine cycle or in the β-oxidation spiral, and no fatty infiltration of the liver. These data suggested that the defect in these children was above the transport of long-chain fatty acids across the mitochondrial membranes, presumably involving the plasma membrane.

PRIMARY SYSTEMIC CARNITINE DEFICIENCY This autosomal-recessive disorder involves a genetic defect of the plasma membrane carnitine transporter in kidney, intestine, muscle, heart, and fibroblasts but not in liver. About 30 patients have been described, and

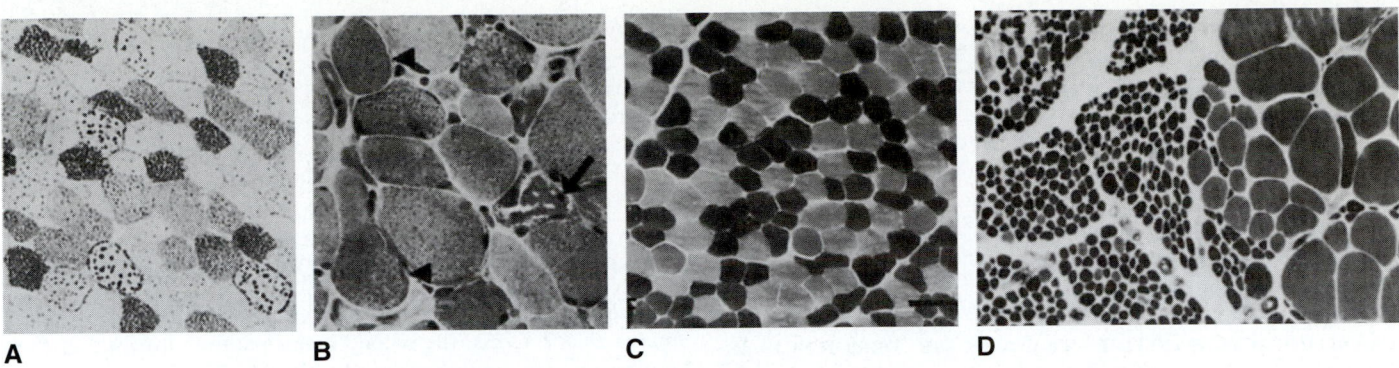

FIGURE 25-41 Muscle biopsies. **A.** Carnitine deficiency. Small globules of neutral lipid are excessive, particularly in type I fibers. (Oil red O, bar = 20 μm). **B.** Mitochondrial myopathy. Intermyofibrillar dark (reddish) granular mitochondria are abnormally prominent in some fibers *(arrowheads)*. A degenerating fiber contains a cytoplasmic body *(arrow)*. (Modified Gomori trichrome; bar = 50 μm.) **C.** Infantile hypotonia is a disorder of the central nervous system. Type II fibers are generally smaller than type I fibers. (Myofibrillar ATPase; bar = 50 μm.) **D.** Werdnig-Hoffmann disease. Large groups of atrophic fibers. The large fibers are also grouped and are typically histochemical type I. (Myofibrillar ATPase; bar = 50 μm.)

almost half of them had a sibling who died of cardiopathy or sudden death. There is no sex predominance, and the mean age at onset is 2 years, ranging from 1 month to 7 years. Progressive cardiomyopathy is the most common presentation: echocardiography and ECG show dilative cardiomyopathy, peaked T waves, and signs of ventricular hypertrophy. Endomyocardial biopsies or postmortem studies show massive lipid storage, and, when measured, carnitine concentration in the myocardium was less than 5% of normal. Cardiac function responds poorly to inotropics and diuretics, but it responds dramatically to carnitine supplementation, with progressive normalization of cardiac function indices within a few months. Some infants may present with acute encephalopathy together with hypoketotic hypoglycemia, and hepatomegaly with liver steatosis. Myopathy is usually associated with cardiomyopathy or encephalopathy and is manifested by mild motor delay, hypotonia, or slowly progressive proximal weakness. Serum creatine kinase can be normal or slightly elevated. Muscle biopsy shows lipid storage myopathy and very low levels of total and free carnitine (below 10% of normal).

Defective carnitine transport in kidney causes defective carnitine reabsorption and excessive carnitine excretion. Deficient intestinal transport results in poor and delayed carnitine absorption. The combination of defective renal and intestinal carnitine handling causes carnitine levels to fall in blood—hence the importance of measuring blood carnitine concentrations in all infants and young children with unexplained cardiomyopathy. In vitro, deficient carnitine transport has been documented in cultured skin fibroblasts and in cultured muscle cells. Linkage analysis has localized the gene responsible for primary carnitine deficiency to chromosome 5q: the gene, which encodes one member of a family of organic cation transporters, has been isolated, and several pathogenic mutations have been identified in patients and their asymptomatic parents.

PRIMARY MYOPATHIC CARNITINE DEFICIENCY This disorder, characterized by decreased muscle carnitine vis-á-vis normal serum carnitine, was the first example of carnitine deficiency described by A.G. Engel and Angelini in 1973, in a young woman with progressive proximal weakness and lipid storage myopathy responsive to corticosteroids. The existence of this entity, however, is controversial, because there is no definitive documentation of an isolated defect of carnitine uptake in muscle. It is possible that patients with

the diagnosis of carnitine deficiency myopathy may have other fatty acid oxidation defects, either generalized or muscle-specific. In some of the patients described, symptoms appeared in the first years of life, but in most onset was between the second and third decade. There was progressive and sometimes fluctuating weakness of proximal limb and axial muscles of variable severity. A few of these patients had associated cardiomyopathy. Muscle biopsy showed accumulation of triglycerides, especially in type I fibers. Muscle carnitine levels were 20% of normal or less, whereas plasma carnitine levels were normal or slightly reduced (Fig. 25-41). Some of the patients improved with carnitine administration.

SECONDARY CARNITINE DEFICIENCY This condition, characterized by decreased levels of carnitine in blood and, often, in tissues, can accompany diverse disorders, including inborn errors of metabolism, acquired medical conditions, and iatrogenic states.

Examples of inborn errors of metabolism include numerous defects of fatty acid metabolism affecting both the carnitine cycle and β-oxidation (see below), disorders of branched-chain amino acid metabolism, and defects of the mitochondrial respiratory chain.

Examples of acquired medical conditions include those causing decreased carnitine biosynthesis (eg, hepatic cirrhosis or extreme prematurity), those causing decreased carnitine intake (eg, malnutrition, chronic total parenteral nutrition, strict vegetarian diet, soy protein infant formula, malabsorption), those causing decreased body stores of carnitine in the face of increased requirements (eg, pregnancy and lactation, extreme prematurity, infant of carnitine-deficient mother), and those causing increased carnitine loss, such as Fanconi syndrome.

Examples of iatrogenic factors include valproate therapy, hemodialysis, and zidovudine administration.

It is important to keep in mind these diverse causes of carnitine deficiency, because carnitine replacement often results in marked improvement.

CARNITINE PALMITOYLTRANSFERASE I (CPT I) DEFICIENCY After cytosolic long-chain fatty acids are activated to the corresponding acyl-CoA thioesters by a long-chain acyl-CoA synthetase bound to the outer mitochondrial membrane, another enzyme of the outer mitochondrial membrane, CPT I, transfers acyl residues from CoA to carnitine. There are two isoforms of CPT I, a liver type (L-CPT I) and a muscle type (M-CPT I): the gene encoding L-CPT I is on chromosome 11q13, that encoding M-CPT I is on chromosome 22q13.3.

Only liver CPT I deficiency has been described. This rare autosomal-recessive condition presents in infancy with recurrent episodes of hypoketotic hypoglycemic coma, triggered by fasting or intercurrent infections. Muscle and heart are not affected. Plasma carnitine levels are normal. The first mutation in the L-CPT I gene has been recently identified.

CARNITINE-ACYLCARNITINE TRANSLOCASE DEFICIENCY An inner mitochondrial membrane translocase is needed to shuttle the acylcarnitines formed by CPT I across the inner membrane in exchange for carnitine. This 301–amino acid intramembranous protein is encoded by a gene on chromosome 3p21.31.

Patients with translocase deficiency present with life-threatening episodes in the neonatal period: there is generalized weakness, cardiac arrhythmia, hyperammonemia, and inconsistent hypoglycemia. Plasma levels of free carnitine are markedly decreased, and acylcarnitines are increased. Long-chain acylcarnitines accumulate both inside and outside the mitochondrial matrix, with at least two toxic effects: inhibition of cellular uptake of free carnitine (resulting in secondary carnitine deficiency) and impairment of cardiac conduction. A few children who survived the neonatal crisis appeared normal later in life. The disorder is inherited as an autosomal-recessive trait, and the first pathogenic mutations have been reported.

CARNITINE PALMITOYLTRANSFERASE II (CPT II) DEFICIENCY Once long-chain acylcarnitines are inside the inner mitochondrial membrane, they have to be reconverted to acyl-CoA esters to enter the β-oxidation spiral. This is done by a single enzyme without tissue-specific isoforms, CPT II, which is loosely bound to the inner mitochondrial membrane and is encoded by a gene on chromosome 1p32.

Despite the lack of tissue-specific isozymes, CPT II deficiency causes two distinct phenotypes. The more common, *myopathic form*, usually presents in adolescents or young adults, predominantly males, with recurrent myoglobinuria following prolonged, although not necessarily strenuous, exercise; prolonged fasting; or a combination of the two conditions. Other precipitating factors include cold exposure, lack of sleep, and, especially in children, intercurrent illnesses with high fever. Between attacks, these patients have normal physical and neurologic exams. Unlike what happens in the glycogenoses, the attacks of myoglobinuria are not heralded by painful cramps. In addition, exercising muscles are not necessarily the only ones undergoing acute necrosis, and a few patients have been admitted to the hospital in respiratory distress. Another distinguishing feature from the glycogenoses is the normal level of serum CK between attacks of myoglobinuria. Plasma carnitine levels are usually normal. CPT II deficiency, first described in 1973, appears to be the most common cause of hereditary myoglobinuria. Numerous mutations have been described, but one of them (S113L) is commonly encountered in both European and American patients and can be looked for in blood cells when the diagnosis is suspected, even before performing a muscle biopsy.

A rarer and much more severe *hepatocardiomuscular form* can affect infants or children. Patients with the infantile form die within weeks, after presenting with hepatopathy, encephalopathy, cardiomegaly, and cardiac arrhythmia. Patients with later onset have fasting hypoketotic hypoglycemia, hepatopathy, cardiomyopathy, and mild myopathy. They are at risk for sudden death. In contrast to

the myopathic form, plasma carnitine levels are severely decreased in the generalized form.

The clinical heterogeneity of CPT II deficiency is not completely understood, but different mutations are associated with the myopathic or the generalized phenotype, and compound heterozygotes appear to be at risk for severe metabolic crises. Biochemically, residual CPT II activities are higher in the myopathic form.

DEFECTS OF β-OXIDATION

Once long-chain fatty acids have gained access to the mitochondrial matrix as acyl-CoAs, the second major pathway involved in their utilization is the multienzyme β-oxidation. This pathway is more complex than previously thought, as two new enzymes, both bound to the inner membrane, have been identified, very long chain acyl-CoA dehydrogenase (VLCAD), and mitochondrial trifunctional protein (MTP). A schematic representation of lipid metabolism will help illustrate the four sequential steps of β-oxidation, in which an acyl-CoA ester undergoes dehydrogenation, hydration, a second dehydrogenation, and thiolytic cleavage. (1) Classically, three acyl-CoA dehydrogenases active on fatty acids of different chain lengths had been described: long-chain acyl-CoA dehydrogenase (LCAD), medium-chain acyl-CoA dehydrogenase (MCAD), and short-chain acyl-CoA dehydrogenase (SCAD). Recent evidence suggests that LCAD has a minor role in the dehydrogenation of straight-chain acyl-CoAs, and this reaction is catalyzed by the membrane-bound VLCAD. The prostetic group of VLCAD, MCAD, and SCAD is flavin adenine dinucleotide (FAD), which is reoxidized by the matrix enzyme electron-transferring flavoprotein (ETF), and this, in turn, passes reducing equivalents to another flavoprotein bound to the inner mitochondrial membrane, ETF-dehydrogenase (ETFDH), from which electrons are fed to coenzyme Q10 (CoQ10), a component of the respiratory chain. (2) The second reaction in β-oxidation is catalyzed by two enoyl-CoA hydratases: crotonase acts on short-chain substrates, and hydration of long-chain 2-*trans*-enoyl-CoA is catalyzed by the membrane-bound MTP. (3) The third step of β-oxidation involves a long-chain 3-hydroxyacyl-CoA dehydrogenase (LCHAD) and a short-chain enzyme (SCHAD). (4) The final step of β-oxidation requires two thiolases, a soluble medium-chain 3-ketoacyl-CoA thiolase (MCKAT) and a long-chain thiolase that is part of the membrane-bound MTP.

We will consider briefly the various defects of β-oxidation with special emphasis on those causing myopathy.

SHORT-CHAIN ACYL-CoA DEHYDROGENASE (SCAD) DEFICIENCY A single adult case of lipid storage myopathy with SCAD deficiency confined to skeletal muscle was probably related to a different primary metabolic defect because there are no tissue-specific isoforms of SCAD. Most patients with generalized SCAD deficiency present in infancy with poor feeding, vomiting, failure to thrive, lethargy, and hypotonia. Psychomotor retardation, seizures, and hyperactivity have also been described. Myopathy was not prominent except in a 13-year-old girl with congenital facial and neck weakness, which spread to limb, axial, and respiratory muscle. She also had ptosis, progressive external ophthalmoplegia, and cataracts. Muscle biopsy showed type I fiber predominance and hypotrophy and multicores (see above). Characteristically, these patients excrete ethylmalonic acid in the urine.

The gene for SCAD has been localized to chromosome 12 and sequenced, and pathogenic mutations have been identified in some patients.

MEDIUM-CHAIN ACYL-CoA DEHYDROGENASE (MCAD) DEFICIENCY This relatively common condition presents in childhood as an episodic acute illness with hypoketotic hypoglycemia following intercurrent infection and fasting. The presenting symptoms and signs, in order of decreasing frequency, include lethargy, vomiting, encephalopathy, respiratory arrest, hepatomegaly, seizures, apnea, cardiac arrest, and sudden death. Once the correct diagnosis is established, subsequent crises can generally be prevented, but survivors are at risk for developmental disabilities. In a large retrospective analysis of 120 MCAD patients, weakness was present in 16% of the survivors. The most effective laboratory test in this, as in other β-oxidation disorders, is the profile of acylcarnitines in plasma as determined by tandem mass spectrometry. The profile is characteristically abnormal both in sick and in well children with MCAD deficiency.

The gene for MCAD has been cloned and assigned to chromosome 1p31. A single mutation (K304E) is present in over 90% of patients.

VERY LONG CHAIN ACYL-CoA DEHYDROGENASE (VLCAD) DEFICIENCY There are three major clinical phenotypes: (1) a more common severe infantile form with hypertrophic cardiomyopathy and early death; (2) a less severe form with recurrent episodes of hypoketotic hypoglycemia, reminiscent of MCAD deficiency; (3) a myopathic form closely resembling CPT II deficiency (see above) and characterized by recurrent episodes of muscle breakdown and myoglobinuria following prolonged exercise, prolonged fasting, or both. The profile of acylcarnitines in plasma is the laboratory test of choice.

The gene for VLCAD is on chromosome 17p11.2-p13.105. Several different mutations have been identified, and there may be a correlation between genotype and phenotype.

MITOCHONDRIAL TRIFUNCTIONAL PROTEIN (MTP) DEFICIENCY In the "typical" form, all three enzymatic functions of MTP are defective. Presentation is in infancy, usually dominated by cardiomyopathy, with or without a previous episode of hypoketotic hypoglycemia. There is cardiomegaly, left ventricular hypertrophy, and, sometimes, pericardial effusion. In two patients, the presentation was less severe, with myopathy and chronic progressive polyneuropathy. Tandem mass spectrometry shows a characteristic acylcarnitine profile.

The molecular basis of MTP is heterogeneous, but a characteristic mutation was identified in the two patients with myopathy and neuropathy.

LONG-CHAIN 3-HYDROXYACYL-CoA DEHYDROGENASE (LCHAD) DEFICIENCY This is really a special case of the mitochondrial trifunctional protein (MTP) deficiency described below, because LCHAD is one of the functions of MTP. However, although in MTP deficiency all three enzymatic functions are affected, in this case only the long-chain hydroxyacyl-CoA dehydrogenase activity is impaired. This disorder can present in infancy with episodic hypoketotic hypoglycemia after prolonged fasting owing to intercurrent infections. Some infants succumb to rapidly progressive cardiomyopathy. Milder and later-onset presentations include a myopathic form with exercise-induced episodic muscle breakdown and myoglobinuria, resembling CPT II deficiency. However, these patients often have additional features not seen in CPT II deficiency, including peripheral neuropathy and hepatomegaly with liver dysfunction. Still other patients had childhood-onset hypogly-

cemia, cardiomyopathy, hypotonia, hepatomegaly, lactic acidosis, and low plasma carnitine.

Not surprisingly, the molecular bases of LCHAD deficiency are different from those of MTP deficiency. A common mutation (X510Y) was identified in almost 90% of alleles in a series of over 80 patients.

SHORT-CHAIN 3-HYDROXYACYL-CoA DEHYDROGENASE (SCHAD) DEFICIENCY Of the three patients described thus far, two were infants with episodic vomiting, ketosis, and hypoglycemia induced by fasting. The third patient was a 16-year-old girl with hypoketotic hypoglycemic encephalopathy, cardiomyopathy, and recurrent myoglobinuria. As SCHAD activity was normal in fibroblasts, it was suggested that the defect involved a muscle-specific isoform, but this remains to be proved.

MEDIUM-CHAIN 3-KETOACYL-CoA THIOLASE (MCKAT) DEFICIENCY Only one patient with this condition has been described: this neonate had poor feeding, vomiting, diarrhea, followed by respiratory distress, hypotonia, opisthotonus, and death at 13 days of age. There was lactic acidosis, hyperammonemia, and elevated serum CK.

ELECTRON-TRANSFER FLAVOPROTEIN (ETF) DEFICIENCY AND ETF:CoQ10 OXIDOREDUCTASE (ETFDH) DEFICIENCY Both defects result in *multiple acyl-CoA dehydrogenase deficiency (glutaric aciduria type II)* and give rise to three major clinical phenotypes: (1) a severe neonatal form with hypotonia, hepatomegaly, hypoglycemia, multiple congenital anomalies, and early death; (2) a milder form without congenital anomalies and with longer survival, but frequently accompanied by cardiomyopathy; and (3) a later-onset form with vomiting, hypoglycemia, hepatomegaly, and weakness with lipid storage myopathy. An 8-year-old boy with ETFDH had a limb-girdle syndrome in addition to hepatomegaly and episodic hypoketotic hypoglycemia. Postmortem examination showed severe lipid storage myopathy and muscle carnitine deficiency. Of considerable practical importance is the *riboflavin-responsive form of glutaric aciduria type II,* which has been seen in adults with lipid-storage myopathy. In these patients, riboflavin administration improved wasting and weakness within weeks.

MITOCHONDRIAL MYOPATHIES

Mitochondrial myopathies are a heterogeneous group of disorders usually defined by morphologic abnormalities either limited to or predominantly affecting muscle mitochondria. Mitochondrial abnormalities (increased number or size of mitochondria, abnormal cristae, presence of "paracrystalline" or round osmiophilic inclusions) were identified by electron microscopy, largely through the pioneering work of Afzelius, Shy, and Gonatas. Applying a modification of the Gomori trichrome stain, Engel identified the abnormal aggregates of mitochondria by light microscopy as coarse red blotches (see Fig. 25-37) and called fibers with this feature *ragged-red.* However, defining mitochondrial myopathies on the basis of morphologic criteria is not satisfactory because muscle morphology may be normal in diseases owing to documented errors of mitochondrial metabolism, such as in most cases of Leigh syndrome. A rational classification of mitochondrial myopathies must be based on specific biochemical or molecular defects. The clinical pictures associated with mitochondrial myopathies are both nonspecific and heterogeneous, including congenital or adult-onset; static, progressive, or even reversible limb weakness; progressive external ophthalmoplegia; exercise intolerance with or without fixed weakness and with or without myoglobinuria.

The association of muscle and brain disease is common, probably because of the high oxidative energy demands of these tissues. Out of the many reports of "mitochondrial encephalomyopathies," a few syndromes stand out because of their frequency and characteristic clinical features: Kearns-Sayre syndrome (KSS); myoclonus epilepsy with ragged-red fibers (MERRF); mitochondrial encephalomyopathy, lactic acidosis, and strokelike episodes (MELAS); neuropathy, ataxia, retinitis pigmentosa (NARP) and the cognate maternally inherited Leigh syndrome (MILS); and Leber's hereditary optic neuropathy (LHON). These conditions are caused by mutations in mitochondrial DNA (mtDNA) and are discussed in Sec. 9.7.3. Among laboratory abnormalities, increased blood concentrations of lactic and pyruvic acid and of alanine are frequently encountered, and severe lactic acidosis may dominate the clinical picture in children. As a rule, serum CK is not markedly elevated in mitochondrial myopathies, with the single exception of myopathies associated with mtDNA depletion (see below).

Mitochondrial myopathies or encephalomyopathies can be divided into five groups according to the area of mitochondrial metabolism affected: substrate transport, substrate oxidation, Krebs cycle, electron transport chain, and oxidation/phosphorylation coupling. Increasingly, the term *mitochondrial encephalomyopathy* refers to defects of the respiratory chain, encompassing the electron transport chain and oxidative phosphorylation. We will, therefore, concentrate on this area of metabolism.

DEFECTS OF SUBSTRATE TRANSPORT The inner mitochondrial membrane is impermeable to substrates, which are transported into the matrix by specific translocases. Defects in the *carnitine cycle* described above are examples of this group of disorders.

DEFECTS OF SUBSTRATE OXIDATION Defects of pyruvate metabolism include *pyruvate carboxylase* deficiency and defects of the *pyruvate dehydrogenase* (PDH) enzyme complex. These disorders are described in Sec. 9.7.5.

Defects of lipid metabolism are best represented by defects of the *β-oxidation* pathway; these are described in Sec. 9.4.2.

DEFECTS OF THE KREBS CYCLE *Fumarase deficiency* causes an encephalopathy of infancy or early childhood characterized by developmental delay, microcephaly, hypotonia, cerebral atrophy, and moderate lactic acidosis. The laboratory hallmark of the disease is the excretion of fumaric and succinic acid in the urine.

DEFECTS OF OXIDATION/PHOSPHORYLATION COUPLING *Luft disease* (nonthyroidal hypermetabolism) is caused by an impairment of respiratory control of muscle mitochondria. It is manifested as hyperthermia, heat intolerance, tachypnea, polydispsia, polyphagia, exercise intolerance, and mild weakness. Only two sporadic occurrences have been reported: the onset was in childhood in one patient. The molecular basis of this interesting condition is unknown.

DEFECTS OF THE RESPIRATORY CHAIN

COMPLEX I DEFICIENCY Complex I (NADH-coenzyme Q reductase), the largest of the respiratory chain complexes, consists of about 40 subunits, 7 of which are encoded by mtDNA and the rest by nuclear DNA (nDNA). Defects of complex I cause two main syndromes, a myopathy, and an encephalomyopathy. The myopa-

thy is characterized by exercise intolerance with or without weakness and excessive increase of venous lactate with aerobic exercise. Muscle biopsy shows ragged-red fibers, which stain intensely with the cytochrome oxidase (COX) histochemical reaction. In two such patients, mutations in ND4 and ND5, two mtDNA-encoded subunits, have been identified in muscle but not in other tissues. As both patients were sporadic, these were probably somatic mutations occurring in muscle stem cells after germline differentiation.

A severe multisystem disorder described in several infants is characterized by hypotonia, respiratory insufficiency, cardiomyopathy, hepatomegaly, hypoglycemia, and progressive lactic acidosis. Death usually occurs a few weeks or months after birth. In one such patient, the biochemical defect was documented in liver, muscle, heart, and kidney mitochondria and involved the iron-sulfur clusters of complex I. Inheritance appeared to be autosomal-recessive, but no molecular studies were conducted in these early patients. Recently, however, mutations in several nuclear genes (NDUFS4, NDUFS7, and NDUFS8) have been reported in patients with generalized complex I deficiency and the neuroradiologic or neuropathologic features of Leigh syndrome. LS is a severe encephalopathy of infancy or early childhood characterized pathologically by bilateral symmetric lesions in the basal ganglia, thalamus, brainstem, and cerebellar roof nuclei: this appears to be the pathologic "signature" of the ravages caused by impaired oxidative metabolism on the developing brain, irrespective of the precise site of the biochemical lesion.

COMPLEX II DEFICIENCY Complex II *(succinate dehydrogenase)* is a small complex (four subunits) entirely encoded by the nuclear genome. The first mutation in a nuclear gene responsible for a respiratory chain defect was identified in 1995 in two sisters with Leigh syndrome and complex II deficiency.

COMPLEX III DEFICIENCY Complex III is composed of 11 subunits, only 1 of which, the apoprotein of cytochrome b, is encoded by mtDNA. Complex III deficiency can also cause a pure myopathy or a generalized condition. Recently, attention has been called to diverse mutations in the mtDNA gene for cytochrome b, which have been identified in about ten unrelated adult patients with severe exercise intolerance since childhood, mild proximal weakness, and, in three cases, exercise-induced myoglobinuria. All patients were sporadic, and the mutations were confined to skeletal muscle, another example of somatic genetic errors. Muscle biopsies showed more or less abundant ragged-red fibers staining intensely for the cytochrome oxidase reaction.

COENZYME Q10 DEFICIENCY Coenzyme Q10 (ubiquinone) has been described in six patients. Five of them had the triad of mitochondrial myopathy, recurrent myoglobinuria, and brain involvement (seizures, mental retardation, or cerebellar ataxia). Muscle biopsy showed ragged-red fibers and lipid storage. Biochemical analyses showed complex III deficiency and extremely low levels of coenzyme Q10. Recognizing these patients is of practical importance because they respond dramatically to coenzyme Q10 supplementation.

COMPLEX IV DEFICIENCY Complex IV (cytochrome c oxidase, COX) is composed of 13 polypeptides: the 3 larger catalytic subunits (COX I-III) are encoded by mtDNA. Cytochrome oxidase deficiency has been associated with a variety of clinical pictures, most of them affecting infants or young children. In some patients, only muscle is affected, in others most or all tissues.

Fatal infantile myopathy alone or with renal dysfunction (De Toni-Fanconi syndrome) is manifested by weak cry, poor suck, and floppiness within the first few weeks of life. Most patients die before 1 year. There is lactic acidosis, and muscle biopsy shows ragged-red fibers and markedly decreased histochemical reaction for COX, sparing muscle spindles and the smooth muscle of blood vessels. Inheritance appears to be autosomal-recessive, but the molecular defect is unknown.

Patients with the *benign infantile myopathy* also have severe weakness and often need assisted ventilation and gavage feeding early in life but improve spontaneously and are usually normal by 2 or 3 years of age. The severe lactic acidosis present at birth also decreases in parallel with the clinical improvement. The spontaneous recovery corresponds to a gradual return of COX activity in muscle, which can be demonstrated both histochemically and biochemically. This condition is probably inherited as an autosomal-recessive trait, but the molecular basis is still obscure.

A few sporadic patients with *exercise intolerance* and *recurrent myoglobinuria* have been reported with somatic mutations in COX I, COX II, or COX III. Muscle biopsy shows ragged-red fibers that stain intensely with the succinate dehydrogenase (SDH) reaction but do not stain with the COX reaction.

Complex IV deficiency seems to be the most common cause of Leigh syndrome. Patients are usually normal for the first 6 to 12 months, then show psychomotor regression, dystonia, optic atrophy, and seizures and develop the typical neuroradiologic symmetric brain lesions. Cytochrome oxidase deficiency in these patients is generalized, although a few children have normal activity in liver and fibroblasts. Muscle biopsy shows diffuse but incomplete loss of the histochemical reaction for COX, including muscle spindles and blood vessels. Inheritance is autosomal-recessive, but there is genetic heterogeneity. Several different pathogenic mutations have been found in the gene encoding a protein (SURF1) needed for proper assembly of COX. However, some patients have mutations in another COX assembly gene, *SCO2,* and it is likely that still other mutations in similar genes will be identified. Knowing the molecular defects is important, because it allows prenatal diagnosis and accurate counseling in families who have often lost a child to the disease.

COMPLEX V DEFICIENCY Complex V (ATP synthase) is composed of 12 subunits, 2 of which are encoded by mtDNA. The best documented defects of complex V are related to mutations in the mtDNA ATPase 6 gene and are transmitted by maternal inheritance. NARP (*n*europathy, *a*taxia, *r*etinitis *p*igmentosa) usually manifests in young adults with variable combinations of sensorimotor neuropathy, ataxia, dementia, seizures, proximal limb weakness, and retinitis pigmentosa, and runs a slowly progressive course. Lactic acidosis is inconsistent, and muscle biopsy shows neurogenic atrophy but no ragged-red fibers. *Maternally inherited Leigh syndrome (MILS)* presents in infancy with developmental delay, hypotonia, seizures, pyramidal signs, retinitis pigmentosa, and ophthalmoparesis. Neuroradiology shows the typical symmetric lesions of Leigh syndrome. When present, retinitis pigmentosa distinguishes these children from those with other common forms of Leigh syndrome, owing to pyruvate dehydrogenase, complex I, or complex IV deficiency. Muscle biopsy may be normal. Family history often reveals that one or more maternal relatives are affected with NARP. This is because NARP and MILS are caused by the same mutation, T8993G, in the ATPase 6 gene. The different phenotype is explained by the much higher abundance of the mutation in MILS patients (90 to 95% of mutant genomes) than in NARP

patients (about 70%). A milder and variable phenotype, with features of both NARP and MILS, is caused by a different mutation (T8993C) at the very same nucleotide. Other mutations in the ATPase 6 gene have been associated with Leigh syndrome or *bilateral striatal necrosis.* Biochemical studies on mitochondria isolated from cultured skin fibroblasts in these different conditions have shown decreased ATP synthesis that is remarkably proportional to the severity of the clinical phenotypes.

GENETIC CONSIDERATIONS

The components of the respiratory chain under dual genetic control—13 subunits (7 in complex I, 1 in complex III, 3 in complex IV, and 2 in complex V)—are encoded by mtDNA, and all others are encoded by nDNA, synthesized in the cytoplasm, and transported into mitochondria through a complex importation process. Furthermore, all essential functions of mtDNA, replication, transcription, and translation, require nDNA-encoded factors. Therefore, genetic defects in mitochondrial diseases can be divided into three groups:

1. Defects of nDNA genes encoding mitochondrial proteins. Diseases associated with these defects will be transmitted by mendelian inheritance.
2. Defects of mtDNA, including deletions and point mutations. Although deletions of mtDNA are usually sporadic, point mutations are transmitted by nonmendelian, maternal inheritance. This is because at the time of fertilization, all mtDNA is contributed to the zygote by the oocyte. However, recent evidence suggests that de novo somatic mutations, especially in protein-coding mtDNA genes, account for many sporadic and tissue-specific disorders, including myopathies.
3. Defects of intergenomic communication, that is, defects in nDNA genes encoding factors that control essential mtDNA functions, such as replication. The diseases that result are transmitted by mendelian inheritance.

DEFECTS OF nDNA Diseases caused by biochemical defects in all pathways except the respiratory chain are related to nDNA defects and are transmitted as mendelian traits. Although most of the subunits of the respiratory chain are also encoded by nDNA, only recently have molecular defects become identified. This area of investigation is rapidly expanding.

DEFECTS OF mtDNA Single large-scale *deletions* (ie, a single identical deletion in one or more tissues from each patient) are associated with three major syndromes: KSS, sporadic progressive external ophthalmoplegia (PEO), and Pearson syndrome (sometimes evolving into KSS). These disorders are described in Sec. 9.7.5.

Over 60 different *point mutations* in mtDNA have been associated with a variety of maternally inherited encephalomyopathies and cardiomyopathies. Most of these affect tRNA genes and impair mitochondrial protein synthesis in toto, including the two most common causes of MELAS (A3243G in the tRNA$^{Leu(UUR)}$ gene) and MERRF (A8344G in the tRNA^{Lys} gene). Mutations in protein-coding genes of various complexes have been associated with LHON, NARP, MILS, and various myopathies, as mentioned above. These disorders are described in Sec. 9.7.5.

DEFECTS OF INTERGENOMIC COMMUNICATION *Multiple deletions of mtDNA* (ie, several distinct deletions affecting the mtDNA of a single patient) are associated with: autosomal-dominant progressive external ophthalmoplegia (AD-PEO), usually manifesting in adulthood and largely but not exclusively confined to the musculature; autosomal-recessive PEO (AR-PEO), often associated with multisystem involvement and with earlier onset; and mitochondrial neurogastrointestinal encephalomyopathy (MNGIE), a multisystem disorder in which PEO is complicated by severe gastrointestinal problems (chronic diarrhea, intestinal pseudoobstruction), peripheral neuropathy, and cerebral leukodystrophy. Linkage analysis has localized the genes for some forms of AD-PEO to chromosomes 3 and 10. In the case of MNGIE, not only has the responsible gene been localized to chromosome 22, but it has also been cloned (it encodes the enzyme thymidine phosphorylase), and several pathogenic mutations have been identified.

Depletion of mtDNA is a more or less severe quantitative defect of mtDNA manifesting in infancy or childhood and usually affecting skeletal muscle or liver. Severe mtDNA depletion in muscle causes a rapidly progressive and invariably fatal myopathy of early infancy, with ragged-red fibers in the muscle biopsy and markedly elevated serum CK levels. Less severe mtDNA depletion causes a progressive childhood myopathy simulating Duchenne dystrophy, SCARMD, or spinal muscular atrophy type II. Depletion of mtDNA in liver causes rapidly progressive and intractable liver failure in infants or young children. These disorders are transmitted as autosomal-recessive traits and are presumably caused by defects in one or more nuclear genes controlling mtDNA replication.

ADENYLATE DEAMINASE DEFICIENCY

Adenylate deaminase deficiency is a muscle disease with variable manifestations. Some patients have no symptoms. In others, fixed weakness, hyporeflexia, paresthesias, periodic paralysis, and repeated infections in childhood have been reported. The most common complaints are muscle cramping, stiffness, or pain after exercise. The serum CK concentration may be increased, but myoglobinuria is extremely rare. Muscle biopsy shows normal findings or nonspecific changes. A specific histochemical stain facilitates the diagnosis and shows that the enzyme defect is often encountered in virtually asymptomatic subjects. In keeping with this observation, molecular genetic analysis has shown that a common AMPD-1 mutation is found in 2% of the general population. Two children, who were homozygous for pathogenic mutations in the myophosphorylase gene (glycogenosis type V, McArdle disease) or in the muscle phosphofructokinase gene (glycogenosis type VII, Tarui disease), were also homozygous for the AMPD-1 mutation. Interestingly, both children had unusually severe phenotypes, with early episodes of myoglobinuria. This suggests that the per se mild AMPD-1 mutation may have worsened the clinical expression of the two glycogenoses. Thus, it is important to keep in mind the possibility of genetic "double trouble" between adenylate deaminase deficiency and other metabolic errors.

25.14.2 Acquired Myopathies

INFLAMMATORY MYOPATHIES

Dermatomyositis and Polymyositis

Classification of inflammatory myopathies is a matter of controversy and will remain so until more is known about causes and pathogenesis. These conditions are discussed in Sec. 12.10. Polymyositis is rare in children. Dermatomyositis is encountered more often in this age group.

The diagnosis is based on weakness and skin lesions. Dubowitz

and Roy add systemic symptoms (malaise, low-grade fever, irritability, or lethargy) as a third feature not usually seen in children with other myopathies and propose the aphorism: weakness + misery = dermatomyositis. Weakness is generally proximal and symmetric, sometimes involving respiratory and pharyngeal muscles but sparing ocular muscles: progression is fairly rapid, over weeks or months as compared with the dystrophies that evolve over years. Myalgia is an inconsistent feature. Acute or subacute attacks may be followed by complete recovery, or there may be a remitting-relapsing course. In some children, however, the course is chronic and unremitting: These patients may end up confined to bed, with severe weakness and wasting and multiple contractures, and they often succumb to respiratory failure or intermittent infection. Skin lesions consist of erythematous rash and edema with predilection for upper eyelids, malar region (butterfly), extensor surface of fingers and periungual areas, elbows, and knees. The rash may be severe and generalized or so local and mild that it may be easily overlooked. Calcifications in the interstitial tissue (calcinosis) are not uncommon as a late complication. In some patients, small nodules of calcium erupt through the skin. Current mortality is approximately 10%. Serum CK concentrations may be increased in the active phase of the disorder but are often normal. EMG shows a combination of myopathic features (small polyphasic potentials) and signs of muscle irritability (fibrillations, bizarre high-frequency discharges). Muscle biopsy shows inflammatory cells in many but not all patients. Early in the course of the illness pathologic changes may be confined to perifascicular atrophy of fibers, which is seen in about 90% of children. Endothelial lesions of arterioles suggest that the disease in children may be a distinct entity (humorally mediated microangiopathy) secondary to diffuse vasculitis and progressive ischemia of muscle.

The pathogenesis of the disorder is unknown: Direct viral etiology or autoimmune response to a viral insult has been considered, and there is an association with the HLAB8 haplotype in 72% of patients. Steroids are commonly used in dermatomyositis. High doses (2 to 3 mg/kg/d) for long periods of time (1 to 3 years) are now recommended. Other immunosuppressive agents (azathioprine, methotrexate, cyclophosphamide) or plasmapheresis may be tried in steroid-resistent patients.

INCLUSION BODY MYOSITIS This is the most common myopathy in patients older than 50, but it is not a diagnostic consideration in the pediatric population. This sporadic condition is defined by a characteristic distribution of weakness involving the quadriceps, wrist and finger flexors, and ankle dorsiflexors, and by a characteristic muscle pathology, with endomysial inflammation, eosinophilic cytoplasmic inclusions, and rimmed vacuoles. Etiology and pathogenesis are unknown.

A form of *inclusion body myopathy* with similar muscle pathology (eosinophilic cytoplasmic inclusions and rimmed vacuoles) but without inflammation is inherited as an autosomal-recessive trait in families of Persian Jewish descent. Onset is earlier, but usually after age 20, and there is proximal and distal limb weakness sparing the quadriceps muscle. Electromyography shows mixed neurogenic and myopathic features. Linkage studies have mapped the affected gene to chromosome 9p1-q1.

BACTERIAL MYOSITIS "Tropical pyomyositis" is rare and is usually seen in patients who have recently arrived from tropical regions. Abscesses, generally within large muscles of the thigh, are almost always caused by *Staphylococcus aureus*. A combination of bacteremia and local trauma may be involved in the pathogenesis. Muscle pain may precede fever by several days, and local swelling may not be accompanied by other signs of acute inflammation (erythema and heat). The serum CK concentrations may remain normal. Surgical drainage is essential. In *tuberculosis,* cold abscesses may spread into muscle. In *sarcoidosis,* muscle is often involved, although clinical myopathy is rare. Muscle biopsy, therefore, showing typical noncaseating granulomas with giant cells, has been used as a diagnostic tissue test. Sarcoid myopathy may present as an acute myositis or as a chronic myopathy, sometimes with pseudohypertrophy of the calves.

VIRAL MYOSITIS Acute myositis has been reported in children during outbreaks of influenza B infection. Muscle symptoms, consisting of excruciating pain in calf muscles, usually appear a few days after a typical flu-like episode. These children may refuse to walk because of myalgia, and affected muscles are tender to palpation. Serum CK concentrations are increased. The condition resolves spontaneously in a matter of days. Another acute benign myositis caused by coxsackievirus B and affecting intercostal muscles is epidemic pleurodynia (Bornholm disease); it presents with chest pain exacerbated by inspiration and cough. Viral myositis, associated with influenza B, herpes simplex, or coxsackievirus infection, is not always a benign disorder; there may be widespread muscle necrosis with myoglobinuria and life-threatening acute tubular necrosis.

PARASITIC MYOSITIS Trichinosis, cysticercosis, and toxoplasmosis may cause myositis (see Sec. 13.6 for details).

ENDOCRINE MYOPATHIES

THYROID DYSFUNCTION *Hyperthyroidism* is associated with several muscle disorders that are rare in children. Thyrotoxic myopathy causes slowly progressive proximal muscle weakness; thyrotoxic periodic paralysis is similar to the familial hypokalemic form and is usually seen in adult Asian men; exophthalmic ophthalmoplegia may occur without clinical evidence of hyperthyroidism. *Hypothyroidism* in children, and particularly congenital cretinism, can cause generalized muscle hypertrophy with herculean appearance (Kocher-Debré-Sémélaigne syndrome). Hypothyroid myopathy is accompanied by delayed contraction and relaxation, increased serum CK concentration, and repetitive discharges in the EMG. Muscle disorders caused by hyperthyroidism and hypothyroidism are reversible with treatment of the endocrine dysfunction.

PARATHYROID DYSFUNCTION *Hypoparathyroidism* may cause tetany related to hypocalcemia. In *hyperparathyroidism,* weakness and wasting of pelvic girdle muscles are not uncommon, and the clinical picture may simulate that of motor neuron disease. Serum CK concentrations are normal.

ADRENAL DYSFUNCTION Proximal muscle weakness is common in *Cushing disease* as well as in *iatrogenic steroid myopathy.* Muscle biopsy will show nonspecific type II fiber atrophy.

NUTRITIONAL MYOPATHIES

Hypotonia may accompany rickets caused by *vitamin D deficiency. Vitamin E deficiency,* a well-known cause of experimental myopathy in animals, is rare in humans.

TOXIC MYOPATHIES

Muscle fibrosis, sometimes accompanied by contractures may follow repeated intramuscular injections of several drugs. This is probably caused by the combined effects of repeated needle trauma and noxious chemical characteristic of some medications or their carrier vehicles.

The alkaloid vincristine, which is used to treat acute leukemia, causes myopathy affecting mainly type II fibers, which improves when the drug is discontinued. Reversible myopathies are also caused by chloroquine and emetine.

The syndrome of acute muscle necrosis and myoglobinuria may be caused by a great number of toxins and drugs. Exogenous toxins include sea snake poisons, the less exotic hornet poison, and a still mysterious myotoxic factor that causes epidemics of myoglobinuria in fishing villages of northern Europe (Haff disease). Hypokalemia from any cause may precipitate muscle necrosis; myoglobinuria has been reported after administration of drugs that promote urinary excretion of potassium, including licorice and its derivatives (carbenoxolone) and amphotericin B. Myoglobinuria has been detected after intravenous administration of conventional doses of succinylcholine in normal children, whereas halothane causes myoglobinuria only in genetically predisposed patients during attacks of malignant hyperthermia, as described above (see Sec. 25.14.1).

FLOPPY INFANT SYNDROME

Hypotonia with or without weakness is a common diagnostic problem in pediatric neurology. Lesions at any level of the nervous system may be involved (Table 25-26). Specific disorders of the central and peripheral nervous systems and neuromuscular junction are discussed in Sec. 25.13, and myopathies that cause floppy infant syndrome are reviewed in Sec. 25.14.

Two entities of uncertain classification will be considered here: Prader-Willi syndrome and benign congenital hypotonia.

PRADER-WILLI SYNDROME Prader-Willi syndrome is sometimes referred to as H_3O syndrome for mnemonic reasons: hypotonia, hypomentia, hypogonadism, and obesity. These children are floppy at birth and may have feeding difficulties; they have a characteristic facial appearance with a triangular mouth. In boys, the combination of hypotonia and undescended testes should suggest this diagnosis. The hypotonia improves with time, and mental retardation becomes apparent. At about 2 to 3 years of age, these children develop voracious appetite, leading to hyperphagia and marked obesity. Serum CK, EMG, and muscle biopsy findings will be normal, and the cause of hypotonia in infancy remains unknown; a disorder of the central nervous system, possibly affecting the hypothalamus, has been postulated but remains to be proved.

A deletion involving the long arm of chromosome 15 has been found in about 50 to 70% of patients with typical Prader-Willi syndrome, and the remainder are cytogenetically normal. However, it has been noted that some patients with normal chromosomes 15 had maternal disomy (both normal chromosomes 15 were maternal). In addition, genetic imprinting has also been implicated in Prader-Willi syndrome because the chromosome 15 deletions associated with the disorder are always paternal, whereas the uniparental disomy is always maternal.

BENIGN CONGENITAL HYPOTONIA Benign congenital hypotonia is diagnosed by exclusion; it is becoming increasingly rare as systemic histochemical studies and more sensitive electrodiagnostic tests are applied. Neonatal hypotonia in these patients improves markedly or disappears with age. There is no evidence of central or peripheral nervous system involvement, and muscle biopsy will

TABLE 25-26

CAUSES OF HYPOTONIA IN CHILDREN (FLOPPY INFANT SYNDROME)

Disorders of the central nervous system (central hypotonia)
Nonspecific mental deficiency
Birth trauma, perinatal hypoxia
"Hypotonic cerebral palsy"
Metabolic disorders (lipidoses, mucopolysaccharidoses, etc.)
Chromosomal abnormalities (Down syndrome)
Connective tissue disorders
Congenital laxity of ligaments
Ehlers-Danlos and Marfan syndromes
Prader-Willi syndrome
Metabolic, nutritional, endocrine
Benign congenital hypotonia
Disorders of the spinal cord
Spinal cord injury
Hereditary infantile spinal muscular atrophy (Werdnig-Hoffmann)
Poliomyelitis
Disorders of peripheral nerves
Hereditary motor neuropathies
Acquired motor neuropathies
Disorders of the neuromuscular junction
Congenital myasthenia
Neonatal myasthenia
Botulism
Disorders of skeletal muscle (myopathies)
Congenital muscular dystrophy
Congenital myotonic dystrophy
Duchenne's muscular dystrophy
Structurally defined congenital myopathies
　Nemaline
　Central core, minicore
　Myotubular
　Fiber type disproportion
Metabolic myopathies
　Glycogenoses (II, IV, V)
　Mitchondrial

SOURCE: *Adapted from Dubowitz V: Muscle Disorders in Childhood. Philadelphia, Saunders, 1978.*

show no histochemical or ultrastructural abnormalities (Fig. 25-39C).

References

General

Dubowitz V: Muscle Disorders in Childhood, 2nd ed. Philadelphia, Saunders, 1995

Engel AG, Franzini-Armstrong C, eds: Myology: Basic and Clinical, 2nd ed. New York, McGraw-Hill, 1994

Rosenberg RN, Prusiner SB, DiMauro S, eds: The Molecular and Genetic Basis of Neurological Disease, 2nd ed. Boston, Butterworth-Heinemann, 1997

Schapira AHV, Griggs RC, eds: Muscle Diseases. Boston, Butterworth-Heinemann, 1999

Dystrophies

Barth PG, Wanders RJA, Vreken P, et al: X-linked cardioskeletal myopathy and neutropenia (Barth syndrome) (MIM 302060). J Metab Inher Dis 22:555, 1999

Bonne G, DiBarletta MR, Varnous S, et al: Mutations in the gene encoding lamin A/C cause autosomal dominant Emery-Dreifuss muscular dystrophy. Nat Genet 21:285, 1999

Chou F-L, Angelini C, Daenti D, et al: Calpain III mutation analysis of a heterogeneous limb-girdle muscular dystrophy population. Neurology 52:1015, 1999

Duggan DJ, Gorospe JR, Fanin M, et al: Mutations in the sarcoglycan genes in patients with myopathy. N Engl J Med 336:618, 1997

Funakoshi M, Tsuchiya Y, Arahata K: Emerin and cardiomyopathy in Emery-Dreifuss muscular dystrophy. Neuromusc Disord 9:108, 1999

Griggs RC, Moxley RT, Mendell JR, et al: Duchenne dystrophy: randomized, controlled trial of prednisone (18 months) and azathioprine (12 months). Neurology 43:520, 1993

Hayashi Y, Chou F-L, Engvall E, et al: Mutations in the integrin α_7 gene cause congenital myopathy. Nat Genet 19:94, 1998

Kobayashi O, Hayashi Y, Arahata K, et al: Congenital muscular dystrophy: clinical and pathologic study of 50 patients with the classical (Occidental) merosin-positive form. Neurology 46:815, 1996

Kobayashi K, Nakahori Y, Miyake M, et al: An ancient retrotransposal insertion causes Fukuyama-type congenital muscular dystrophy. Nature 394:388, 1998

Lim LE, Campbell KP: The sarcoglycan complex in limb-girdle muscular dystrophy. Curr Opin Neurol 11:443, 1998

Liu J, Aoki M, Illa I, et al. Dysferlin, a novel skeletal muscle gene, is mutated in Miyoshi myopathy and limb girdle muscular dystrophy. Nat Genet 20:31, 1998

Minetti C, Sotgia F, Bruno C, et al: Mutations in the caveolin-3 gene cause autosomal dominant limb-girdle muscular dystrophy. Nat Genet 18:365, 1998

Moreira ES, Wiltshire TJ, Faulkner G, et al. Limb-girdle muscular dystrophy type 2G is caused by mutations in the gene encoding the sarcomeric protein telethonin. Nat Genet 24:163, 2000

Ozawa E, Noguchi S, Mizuno Y, et al: From dystrophinopathy to sarcoglycanopathy: evolution of a concept of muscular dystrophy. Muscle Nerve 21:421, 1998

Sunada Y, Edgar TS, Lotz BP, et al: Merosin-negative congenital muscular dystrophy associated with extensive brain abnormalities. Neurology 45:2084, 1995

Toda T, Kobayashi K, Kondo-Iida E, et al. The Fukuyama congenital muscular dystrophy story. Neuromusc Disord 10:153, 2000

Wever UM, Engvall E: Merosin/laminin-2 and muscular dystrophy. Neuromusc Disord 6:409, 1996

Myotonic Syndromes and Periodic Paralyses

Barchi RL: Molecular pathology of the periodic paralyses. In: Rosenberg RN, Prusiner SB, DiMauro S, Barchi RL, eds: The Molecular and Genetic Basis of Neurological Disease, 2nd ed. Boston, Butterworth-Heinemann, 1997:723

Lehmann-Horn F, Engel AG, Ricker K, Rüdel R: The periodic paralyses and paramyotonia congenita. In: Engel AG, Franzini-Armstrong C, eds: Myology. New York, McGraw-Hill, 1994:1303

Meola G, Moxley RT: Myotonic disorders: Myotonic dystrophy and proximal myotonic myopathy. In: Schapira AHV, Griggs RC, eds: Muscle Diseases, Boston, Butterworth-Heinemann, 1999:115

Rose M, Griggs RC: Membrane motor disorders (channelopathies). In: Younger DS, ed: Motor Disorders. Philadelphia, Lippincott Williams & Wilkins, 1999:179

Morphologically Defined Congenital Myopathies

Laing NG, Wilton SD, Akkari PA, et al: A mutation in the alpha tropomyosin gene TPM3 associated with autosomal dominant nemaline myopathy NEM1. Nat Genet 10:249, 1995

Nishino I, Minami N, Kobayashi O, et al: *MTM1* gene mutations in Japanese patients with the severe infantile form of myotubular myopathy. Neuromusc Disord 8:453, 1998

Pelin K, Hilpela P, Donner K, et al: Mutations in the nebulin gene associated with autosomal recessive nemaline myopathy. Proc Nat Acad Sci USA 96:2305, 1999

Tanner SM, Schneider V, Thomas NST, et al: Characterization of 34 novel and six known *MTM1* gene mutations in 47 unrelated X-linked myotubular myopathy patients. Neuromusc Disord 9:41, 1999

Metabolic Myopathies

Al Odaib A, Shneider BL, Bennett MJ, et al: A defect in the transport of long-chain fatty acids associated with acute liver failure. N Engl J Med 339:1752, 1998

Andreu AL, Hanna MG, Reichmann H, et al: Exercise intolerance due to mutations in the cytochrome b gene of mitochondrial DNA. N Engl J Med 347:1037–1044, 1999

Brivet M, Boutron A, Slama A, et al: Defects in activation and transport of fatty acids. J Inherit Metab Dis 22:428, 1999

De Vivo DC: Solving the COX puzzle. Ann Neurol 45:142, 1999

DiMauro S: Mitochondrial encephalomyopathies: back to mendelian genetics. Ann Neurol 45:693, 1999

DiMauro S, Bruno C: Glycogen disorders of muscle. Curr Opin Neurol 11:477, 1999

DiMauro S, Hirano M, Bonilla E, De Vivo DO: The mitochondrial disorders. In: Berg BO, ed: Principles of Child Neurology. New York, McGraw-Hill, 1994:1201

DiMauro S, Schon EA: Mitochondrial DNA and diseases of the nervous system: the spectrum. Neuroscientist 4:53, 1998

Nishino I, Spinazzola A, Hirano M: Thymidine phosphorylase gene mutations in MNGIE, a human mitochondrial disorder. Science 283:689, 1999

Wanders RJA, Vreken P, den Boer MEJ, et al: Disorders of mitochondrial fatty acyl-CoA β-oxidation. J Inherit Metab Dis 22:442, 1999

Inflammatory Myopathies

Amato AA, Barohn RJ: Inflammatory myopathies: dermatomyositis, polymyositis, inclusion body myositis, and related diseases. In: Schapira AHV, Griggs RC, eds: Muscle diseases. Boston, Butterworth-Heinemann, 1999:299

Engel AG, Hohlfeld Banker BQ: The polymyositis and dermatomyositis syndromes. In: Engel AG, Franzini-Armstrong, eds: Myology. New York, McGraw-Hill, 1997:1335

Endocrine and Toxic Myopathies

Zaidat OO, Ruff RL, Kaminski HJ: Endocrine and toxic myopathies. In: Schapira AHV, Griggs RC, eds: Muscle Diseases. Boston, Butterworth-Heinemann, 1999:363

25.15 VIRAL INFECTIONS OF THE CENTRAL NERVOUS SYSTEM

Alan R. Seay and Darryl C. De Vivo

Viruses are ubiquitous in nature, and human viral infections are common. Fortunately, of the hundreds of viruses that exist, only a few are pathogenic for humans, and only a small percentage of these are neurotropic. During the past two decades the study of animal models of CNS viral infections, the careful and detailed analyses of cases of human viral encephalitis, and the application of DNA technology and other current molecular biological techniques to the study of viral infections have led to a greater understanding of the mechanisms that allow viruses to enter the host, evade host defense mechanisms, enter the CNS, and cause a variety of neurologic illnesses. The types of clinical illnesses produced depend in part upon the anatomic location of the infection, the specific population of cells infected within the CNS, and the host's immune responses.

Pathogenesis, Pathophysiology, and Diagnosis

Neurotropic viruses must first gain entry into the host by one of several mechanisms. Some viruses, such as α-togaviruses, are inoculated into subcutaneous tissue by their arthropod vectors. The virus replicates locally, then spreads to other tissues. Other viruses, such as enteroviruses, are orally ingested and possess the ability to attach to specific receptors on the surface of intestinal mucosal cells. After attachment to the cell surface, the virus is transported through the mucosal cell and released from the abluminal surface into lymphatic channels or bloodstream.

Regardless of the initial route of entry, neurotropic viruses undergo a stage of local replication at the site of inoculation and regional replication in nearby lymph nodes. This initial phase of replication is followed by primary low-level viremia during which virus spreads to multiple susceptible extraneural target tissues, where additional replication occurs. Then a secondary viremia develops, usually associated with the appearance of early clinical signs of illness. With many viruses, it is during this stage that the virus enters the CNS.

The precise mechanisms by which viruses breech the blood-brain barrier and gain access to the CNS are not well understood. Some viruses, such as eastern equine encephalitis (EEE) virus, probably attach to specific receptors on the luminal surface of cerebral capillary endothelial cells. After attachment, EEE virus is transported into the cell's cytoplasm. Experimental evidence suggests that EEE virus, and possibly other viruses, productively infects the endothelial cells with budding of virus from the abluminal surface into CNS extracellular spaces. Once within the CNS, viruses are able to infect specific CNS cell populations. Some other viruses may be carried from the bloodstream into the CNS by infected migrating leukocytes and macrophages.

Spread to the CNS from peripheral sites through nerves provides an alternate route of entry used by some viruses such as rabies virus and, possibly to some extent, poliovirus. After peripheral inoculation, rabies virus is taken up by a virus-specific receptor mechanism on peripheral sensory and motor nerve endings and transported by retrograde axonal transport into the CNS. Experimental evidence suggests that poliovirus is taken up by autonomic nerve terminals within the intestinal wall and then carried to the CNS by axoplasmic transport.

Neuronal transport is also an important mechanism in the pathogenesis of encephalitis caused by herpes simplex virus type 1 (HSV-1). In many people, HSV-1 persists in a latent state within the trigeminal sensory ganglia. In some individuals, for reasons that usually are not clear, HSV-1 becomes reactivated and travels distally from the ganglia to nerve terminals in the skin of the face and lips, resulting in typical herpetic vesicular lesions. It is postulated that on rare occasions when HSV-1 becomes activated, instead of being transported to cutaneous nerve terminals, the virus is transported to nerve terminals that innervate basilar and frontal meninges. Once the virus arrives at the meninges, it produces active infection of surrounding CNS tissue, thus accounting for the anatomic localization found in most cases of HSV-1 encephalitis.

Once neurotropic viruses gain entry into the CNS, they may spread throughout the CNS by passing freely throughout the CNS by cell-to-cell transmission, as appears to be the case for rabies virus. It is likely that some viruses spread from one region of the CNS to another by axonal transport.

The ability of a virus to infect specific cell populations within the CNS depends once again on the presence of virus-specific receptors on cell surfaces. After binding to the cell, the virus enters the cell and begins its replicative cycle. As the virus takes over the molecular machinery within the cell, the cell's function is altered, and ultimately the cell may die. Some viruses, however, are able to establish a nonlethal relationship with the cell, and chronic, persistent, or latent infections may result from this more symbiotic arrangement.

The clinical neurologic illnesses caused by neurotropic viruses result from two major factors. The first of these is the direct effects of virus on infected neurons and other CNS cells. These effects include altered nucleic acid and protein synthesis, impaired neurotransmitter synthesis and release, production of neurotoxic viral proteins, inhibition of cellular metabolic pathways, and ultimately cell death and lysis. Second, the host's immune responses to infection may also impair neurologic dysfunction and cause tissue injury. The initial interaction of the virus with the host's phagocytes and other components of the immune system may stimulate and enhance inflammation. Cytokines released from inflammatory cells may interact with cerebral blood vessels and CNS parenchymal cells to potentiate inflammation, cause edema, alter cerebral blood flow, and cause additional neuronal injury. Tumor necrosis factor, interleukin-1, interferon, and other cytokines may be involved in the production of CNS dysfunction and tissue injury in viral encephalitis, but additional information is needed to define and understand exactly what role these substances play.

In many patients, cerebral edema, increased intracranial pressure, and impaired cerebral blood flow develop and become severe. Secondary cerebral ischemia and infarction may then develop and cause severe, irreversible tissue destruction and profound neurologic sequelae.

Laboratory Identification

Confirmation of the specific virus responsible for a neurologic infection rests primarily upon results of serologic and virologic tests. The demonstration of virus-specific antibody, particularly IgM antibody, is the diagnostic laboratory method most commonly relied upon. With recent advances, such as enzyme-linked immunosorbent assay, serologic tests have become more reliable, rapid, and accurate in identifying the virus during the early stages of illness. The use of immunofluorescent staining techniques, development of histologic stains for viral inclusions, and use of electron microscopy have provided additional methods for identifying virus within the CSF, infected tissue, stool, and occasionally circulating leukocytes. Viral cultures, however, remain the most definitive way to prove viral infection of the CNS. In many encephalitides, virus can be recovered from blood, oropharyngeal secretions, urine, stool, CSF, and infected tissues. The presence of viral nucleic acid can be detected by polymerase-chain reaction (PCR) in CSF providing an additional, highly sensitive and specific method of confirming viral infection. This method has been successfully applied to the early diagnosis of herpes simplex virus, enteroviruses, and in some cases of arbovirus, varicella, and rabies infections.

25.15.1 Aseptic Meningitis

Aseptic meningitis (serous meningitis, lymphocytic meningitis, viral meningitis) is a common clinical syndrome caused by a variety of agents. It is not a specific illness, although certain clinical findings are usually present. In both epidemic and sporadic disease, specific viral agents can be identified (see also Sec. 13.4). It occurs 2 to 10 times more frequently in children under the age of 10 years than in any other age group.

Aseptic meningitis is usually characterized by a relatively abrupt onset of headache, often accompanied by fever, signs and symptoms of meningeal irritation, minimal or no abnormalities in neurologic function, and CSF pleocytosis. There may be clinical evidence of a systemic viral illness, for example, parotid swelling in mumps or a diffuse macular rash in enterovirus infections. The CSF will not grow any bacterial pathogens, and a specific virus may be identified in 30 to 50% of patients. Noninfectious irritants in the subarachnoid space, such as contrast agents for myelography, antibiotic and antileukemic drugs, and other chemicals, can elicit a chemical meningitis that may be indistinguishable from a virus-induced meningitis. Blood in the subarachnoid space can cause a similar response, and occasionally spontaneous leakage of the contents of an intracerebral cyst, such as a craniopharyngioma, can cause meningeal irritation. A partially suppressed or chronic bacterial infection must always be considered. Other nonviral causes of aseptic meningitis syndrome are listed in Table 25-27.

Many viruses have been identified as causes of benign meningitis, but a few specific viruses account for most disease in which a

TABLE 25-27

DIFFERENTIAL DIAGNOSIS OF ASEPTIC MENINGITIS SYNDROME WITH CSF PLEOCYTOSIS

Viral agents
  Enteroviruses (poliovirus, coxsackievirus, echovirus); mumps virus; herpesvirus; varicella-zoster virus; lymphocytic choriomeningitis virus; togaviruses and bunyaviruses (arboviruses); Epstein-Barr virus (mononucleosis); rabies virus; adenoviruses.
Bacterial meningitis, especially partially treated; tuberculosis
Perimeningeal bacterial infection
  Cerebral abscess (cerebritis); epidural abscess (empyema); cranial osteomyelitis or sinusitis
Other infectious agents
  Rickettsial agents (typhus; Rocky Mountain spotted fever)
  Spirochetal agents (syphilis; leptospiroses; rat-bite fever)
  Fungal agents (all types)
  Protozoan and helmintic agents (toxoplasmosis; cysticercosis; malaria; amebiasis)
Vascular diseases
  Subarachnoid hemorrhage (arteriovenous malformation, aneurysm, trauma); cerebral venous thrombosis; primary vasculitis (eg, lupus); primary coagulopathy (eg, hemolytic-uremic syndrome)
Tumors
  Metastatic to meninges; primary meningeal melanoma
Chemical or foreign body irritation of meninges
  Contrast agents for myelography; isotope cisternography; intrathecal drugs; spinal anesthesia; intracerebral cyst fluid leakage; surgical introduction of shunts, pressure monitors, etc.
Other poorly understood disorders
  Sarcoid; demyelination (eg, acute multiple sclerosis); Behçet disease; Mollaret meningitis; Vogt-Koyanagi-Harada syndrome; Iceland disease

causative agent is identified. Before effective immunization, poliovirus was by far the most common agent causing aseptic meningitis. Currently, the other enteroviruses (coxsackieviruses and echoviruses), California virus, and mumps virus account for most of the specifically identified agents. The period of peak incidence for aseptic meningitis is in late summer and early fall, the same as for viral gastroenteritis. Sporadic infections occur throughout the year. Viral meningitis can occur in children of all ages. In newborns and young infants, the clinical manifestations are often subtle, with nonspecific symptoms of lethargy and poor feeding with or without seizures. In newborns, concomitant infection of cardiac muscle (coxsackievirus B) or more generalized involvement (herpes virus 2) can occur, and the nervous system infection is often a necrotizing encephalitis rather than a benign infection of meninges. However, apparently benign virus infections in young infants, often attributable to enteroviruses, have been documented.

In older infants, children, and adults, the clinical symptoms of a viral meningitis begin abruptly, with headache, vomiting, lethargy, and a stiff neck. Fever may be present, as may evidence of a systemic flu-like illness or a rash, parotitis, and adenopathy. Seizures are not common, occurring most often in young children who have fever. The results of the neurologic examination will be normal, except when an aseptic meningitis merges with the syndrome of acute cerebellar ataxia. Symptoms usually persist for 1 to 2 weeks, and recovery is complete. Diffuse nonspecific slowing on the EEG may parallel the clinical signs of infection. Aseptic meningitis is not usually considered a contagious disease. The spread of virus in these diseases depends on the underlying infection, such as mumps or an enterovirus flu-like syndrome.

Spinal fluid must be examined to diagnose viral meningitis. The CSF findings will be abnormal, with pleocytosis varying from 10 to over 1000 cells/μL. In the early stages of the disease, both polymorphs and mononuclear cells (lymphocytes) may be present; later in the course of the infection, lymphocytes predominate. There is no precise formula for white blood cell elements that will consistently distinguish a bacterial meningitis from a viral meningitis, especially if the former has been partially treated. It is imperative to consider a bacterial cause whenever CSF pleocytosis is found. Appropriate treatment must be based on all the clinical and laboratory data, not only on the composition of the CSF. The protein concentration may be normal or slightly elevated, and the IgG concentration is usually normal. Hypoglycorrhachia (low CSF glucose in relation to a simultaneous blood glucose) is uncommon but has been documented in some viral meningitides. The triad of lymphocytosis, mildly to moderately elevated protein concentration, and normal glucose concentration is most characteristic of CSF virus infections.

Recurrent aseptic meningitis is rare. In such instances, one must consider the possibilities of an immune or anatomic abnormality in the host, an intracerebral cyst causing an irritating meningeal reaction, and other poorly understood syndromes, such as Mollaret and Behçet syndromes (see Sec. 25.15.11).

There is no specific treatment. The vast majority of patients recover completely from this disease. Hospitalization is required only if the patient is very sick or if the diagnosis is in doubt.

25.15.2 Acute Viral Encephalitis

Acute viral encephalitis is a frightening and often catastrophic disease. Fortunately for humans, the number of viruses with strong neurotropism is small. Viral encephalitis may occur seasonally and in epidemics, or sporadically throughout the year. Togaviruses, including the equine encephalitis viruses, St. Louis encephalitis virus, and Japanese encephalitis virus, account for most cases of epidemic encephalitis worldwide. Japanese encephalitis virus, for example, the single most common cause of viral encephalitis in the world, is responsible for 10,000 to 20,000 cases of encephalitis annually in Asia. In the United States, St. Louis encephalitis virus is the most common cause of epidemic viral encephalitis. Sporadic, nonepidemic viral encephalitis is most commonly caused by herpes simplex type 1. Enteroviruses, myxoviruses, and other herpes viruses, such as Epstein-Barr virus, are also well recognized causes of acute viral encephalitis.

Clinical Features

The clinical symptoms of viral meningoencephalitis are variable and commonly include headache, lethargy, vomiting, anorexia, and other nonspecific complaints. It is usually the more dramatic symptoms that bring the child to medical attention. Abnormalities of mental functioning manifested as confusion, memory loss, unusual combativeness, hallucinations, and coma are common. Fever may be present. Seizures often occur. Neurologic examination usually reveals focal abnormalities that may be as subtle as a unilateral extensor plantar reflex or as obvious as an overt hemiparesis. Increased extensor tone and posturing are common. Abnormalities of cranial nerve function can occur. Funduscopic examination often indicates increased intracranial pressure, although seldom with overt hemorrhages as might occur after trauma or an acute subarachnoid hemorrhage. The neurologic examination may also indicate focal disease in the spinal cord as well as in the brain. Signs and symptoms can change rapidly. A child who seems mildly lethargic one day may be comatose and hemiparetic a day later. In such a situation, other causes of a severe acute postinfectious encephalitis must be considered. These include metabolic encephalopathies, cerebrovascular disease, acute systemic vasculitis, Reye-Johnson syndrome, toxins, trauma with a focal hematoma or diffuse edema, and other nonviral infections of the nervous system. Each of these conditions is discussed in detail elsewhere in this chapter.

Diagnosis

Routine laboratory findings in patients with viral encephalomyelitis are not very helpful. Hematologic tests may reveal leukocytosis and other evidence of infection, but they are clearly nonspecific. Other laboratory studies are most useful to exclude a metabolic encephalopathy. In many acute diseases of the brain, the syndrome of inappropriate secretion of antidiuretic hormone with hyponatremia can worsen the underlying brain disease.

CSF should be examined in any suspected viral encephalitis. If the history or clinical findings suggest either severe increased intracranial pressure or a focal mass lesion, appropriate neuroradiologic tests should be done first to exclude a disease in which a lumbar puncture could cause further harm. The CSF examination may show a mild-to-moderate pleocytosis with either polymorphs or mononuclear cells, a mild-to-moderate increase in the protein concentration (occasionally with an elevated IgG concentration as well), usually a normal glucose concentration, and a mild-to-moderate elevation in pressure. Completely normal CSF findings, however, do not exclude viral encephalomyelitis. The CSF must be carefully processed to identify an infectious agent, considering all the agents listed in Table 25-27.

Neuroimaging procedures (CT or MR) can exclude other conditions (eg, tumor, hematoma, abscess, or hydrocephalus) and will often show areas of edema, infarction, or hemorrhage. When herpes simplex or enterovirus infections are considered, PCR has proved quite valuable in providing confirmation. Occasionally, brain biopsy and tissue culture may be required. Treatment does not block the rise of specific antibodies and thus does not interfere with retrospective diagnosis based on our serologic testing. As specific treatment for virus infections becomes more effective, specific identification of the causative viruses will become more important. For a patient with an immune-mediated postinfectious encephalitis, there is no advantage in performing a brain biopsy. Moreover, a child whose brain metabolism is already impaired by infection is a poor risk for anesthesia and surgery.

EEG usually shows diffuse slowing with or without paroxysmal changes. Focal temporal lobe EEG abnormalities are common in herpes virus encephalitis. Imaging procedures can identify focal areas of hyperemia or ischemia, but these findings are not specific. Assay of CSF for specific antibody production greater than can be accounted for by passive transfer from serum can establish a specific viral etiology retrospectively in approximately 75% of biopsy-proven disease. In two specific situations (newborns and in children with abnormalities of the immune system), a viral encephalitis is part of a systemic infection, allowing for diagnosis from tissue other than brain tissue, such as skin vesicles or liver.

Treatment

Treatment for viral meningoencephalitis is primarily supportive. Effective therapy for herpes encephalitis using acyclovir is discussed in Secs. 13.1.2 and 13.4.6. At the present time, the most important treatment for an encephalitis not caused by a herpes virus is intensive support for the comatose patient to prevent problems of air exchange, acid-base and electrolyte imbalances, and other metabolic disturbances and also to promote adequate tissue perfusion and nutrition. Cytotoxic brain edema occurs, and this can further compromise brain function and delay recovery. We do not know if corticosteroids are of any specific benefit, but no studies have shown adverse responses, which has prompted many clinicians to use short-term high-dosage corticosteroid therapy in this disease. Other therapeutic attempts to treat brain edema (osmotic agents, hyperventilation) are generally not indicated. If seizures occur, anticonvulsants are often used, but the clinician must always weigh the benefits against possible adverse effects of drugs that may decrease cellular oxidative metabolism, as do many sedatives and anticonvulsants. Careful nursing and medical care for seriously ill, comatose patients can sometimes facilitate recovery, and regardless of advances in specific antiviral therapy, such care will always be essential for optimal treatment of children with viral encephalitis.

Prognosis

The consequences of viral encephalitis of either the primary or immune type are often serious and can include death as well as permanent neurologic handicaps. Knowledge of the specific viral causes can provide some prognostic guidelines. For instance, before the development of specific antiviral therapy, the mortality from herpes encephalitis was 60 to 80%, with many survivors having major residual neurologic abnormalities. Until recently, no survivors of rabies encephalitis had been documented. In contrast, children with mumps meningoencephalitis usually recover fully, although secondary hydrocephalus relating to aqueductal stenosis can occur. The prognosis for children who have encephalitis owing to an enterovirus falls somewhere between these two outcomes.

The developing nervous system seems to have remarkable capacity for recovering from a major immunoinfectious insult in some individuals. However, the time required for recovery can be surprisingly long. If a child survives the worst part of the acute illness (7 to 14 days), recovery can require months or even years. The role of specific rehabilitation therapy, as well as general encouragement and support to the family, cannot be underestimated. Despite such efforts, major permanent neurologic sequelae in children who have had viral encephalitis pose serious problems in 10 to 30% of survivors. Injury to brain areas concerned with complex functions such as attention, initiative, memory, or other aspects of higher cognitive function may not be easily recognizable until years later with young children who initially appear to have recovered fully from encephalitis.

25.15.3   Brainstem Encephalitis

Brainstem encephalitis, also called Bickerstaff encephalitis, differs from generalized viral encephalitis only in its manifestations. The clinical findings reflect abnormalities in the brainstem. Drowsiness, vomiting, and ataxia usually occur early. Examination may show asymmetric involvement of cranial nerves throughout the brainstem, commonly beginning with diplopia, nystagmus, and variable pupillary and oculomotor paralyses, followed by lower cranial nerve dysfunction. There also may be long-tract signs, seizures, and EEG abnormalities. There is definitive overlap with acute cerebellar ataxia.

The vast majority of disease occurs in persons less than 25 years of age, usually after a nonspecific viral prodrome, with the brainstem symptoms developing over several weeks, to be followed by gradual but fairly complete recovery. CSF findings of pleocytosis, with or without an elevated protein concentration, suggest an inflammatory process. There are no specific viruses associated with brainstem encephalitis, although several reports have associated herpes virus, coxsackievirus, and St. Louis encephalitis virus. Imaging techniques may demonstrate focal areas of edema and inflammation. The few instances that have been examined pathologically have shown perivascular lymphocytosis, edema, and demyelination. Thus, the classification of brainstem encephalitis as a type of viral encephalitis is more conjectural than proven, but this classification seems most consistent with an immune-mediated process. Treatment is supportive, but recent reports suggest that immune-modulating treatment such as intravenous infusion of immunoglobulin (IVIG) may be beneficial.

25.15.4   Chronic Focal Encephalitis

A focal virus infection of brain tissue can present in one of three ways: focal neurologic abnormalities, often a hemiparesis; seizures that are difficult to control and are often focal; or a clinical course that is prolonged and may show spontaneous partial improvement. The clinical symptoms of focal encephalitis usually persist for months or years. Koshevnikov epilepsy, described in the former U.S.S.R., is manifested by epilepsia partialis continua, with or without additional neurologic abnormalities. It is apparently caused by the virus of tick encephalitis, an arbovirus (togavirus). Children and young adults have been described who had temporal lobe resection for intractable epilepsy often associated with hemiparesis. The pathologic findings of chronic gliosis, perivascular lymphocytosis, spongiform changes, and neuronal loss suggest a viral encephalitis. Recently, several instances of HHE syndrome (hemiplegia, hemiconvulsions, epilepsy) have been clearly related to infections with enteroviruses, especially coxsackievirus A9.

The diagnosis can be established only by virologic or immunologic evidence of a virus infection. The CSF may show an inflammatory reaction, and in some diseases, the CSF has contained infective virus. EEG and radiologic studies will identify focal areas of brain injury, but they are not diagnostically specific. Other causes of focal seizures and hemiparesis include primary vascular disease, trauma, and tumors. The course is variable, with some children manifesting partial recovery after several months. Treatment is symptomatic. Although there are reports regarding the use of IVIG, plasmapheresis, or antiviral therapy, none has been proved to be effective.

Rasmussen encephalitis is a focal, progressive inflammatory disorder that most often involves frontal and temporal lobes unilaterally. Clinically, patients develop epilepsia partialis continua in combination with hemiparesis, dysphasia, and loss of cognitive functions. Serial neuroimaging tests demonstrate progressive unilateral frontotemporal atrophy. Although viruses have been suspected, they have never been isolated from brain tissue, and the etiology for Rasmussen encephalitis remains unknown.

25.15.5 Acute Viral Myelitis: Polio Syndrome

Effective immunization has all but eradicated the epidemic disease caused by polio virus. It still occurs in nonimmunized groups and is epidemic in underdeveloped countries. Sporadic infections are caused by related enteroviruses (see also Sec. 13.4.17).

The neurologic disease may have either a biphasic course or a monophasic course during the acute stage. The first phase is that of aseptic meningitis, which may begin to improve when the second phase, the myelitis, begins. In monophasic disease, no discrete aseptic meningitis phase can be identified. The myelitis shows itself with muscle pain and spasm closely (even simultaneously) associated with the development of flaccid paralysis. The muscle paralysis is usually asymmetric and is often multifocal. There is no particular ascending or descending pattern, but rather a spotty, unpredictable involvement that may extend from brainstem nuclei (bulbar polio) to the lower lumbosacral levels. Cervical and lumbar involvement is more common than thoracic. Respiratory problems result from muscle weakness and from involvement of the brainstem nuclei that control respiration. Bladder incontinence may occur, as may other types of autonomic dysfunction, including alterations in sweating, gastrointestinal motility, vasomotor control, and temperature stability. The severity of the disease can vary from fulminating bulbar paralysis requiring intensive respiratory support to mild weakness of a single extremity. Peak involvement occurs within a few days to several weeks, and then some degree of recovery slowly occurs. The degree of recovery averages 50% for severely involved muscles and 90% for moderately paralyzed muscle groups.

The diagnosis of an acute myelitis must be based on the clinical findings described earlier, with examination showing loss of tendon reflexes in the involved muscles without sensory involvement (other than muscle tenderness and pain). The CSF findings will include pleocytosis and an elevated protein concentration during the acute illness. Polymorphonuclear elements predominate acutely. Virus can sometimes be cultured from the CSF and is present in stool and throat-washing specimens 80 to 90% of the time. In addition to the epidemic polio viruses (types I, II, III), both echoviruses and coxsackieviruses can cause poliomyelitis syndromes.

Acute viral myelitis must be differentiated from acute polyneuritis. Clinically, the spotty and asymmetric flaccid paralysis of myelitis contrasts with the symmetric ascending paralysis of neuritis. CSF protein concentrations are elevated in both conditions, but pleocytosis is significant only in myelitis. Other causes of acute flaccid paralysis include spinal cord compression, botulism, myasthenia, tick-induced paralysis, other causes of neuromuscular blockade, and severe acute myopathies.

Pathologically, the major findings are those of an acute inflammatory reaction, primarily in the ventral (anterior) horns of the spinal cord, with neuronal degeneration primarily caused by cytotoxic effects of the virus. Involvements of brainstem and deep cerebellar nuclei, the reticular formation, and, rarely, thalamic and forebrain neurons have been described.

There is no specific treatment. Respiratory and other intensive support for bulbar polio is essential. Warm packs and a massage may give symptomatic relief from the muscle pain and spasm. Rehabilitation therapy may help an individual who is left with permanent muscle weakness. Late onset of progressive weakness, years after the initial myelitis, has been described (postpolio syndrome).

25.15.6 Chronic Latent Viral Infections

Five human diseases, all of which primarily affect the nervous system, are caused by chronic latent virus infections (slow virus infections). Three of these diseases, kuru, Jakob-Creutzfeldt dementia (JC dementia), and progressive multifocal leukoencephalopathy (PML), usually occur in adults, whereas the other two, subacute sclerosing panencephalitis (SSPE) and progressive rubella panencephalitis (PRP), primarily affect children. The causative agents of these diseases are categorized as either conventional or nonconventional. Kuru and JC dementia are caused by nonconventional agents consisting of small particles (7 to 27 nm) that are remarkably resistant to the usual methods of inactivation (heat, radiation, fat solvents, proteolytic enzymes) and can be transmitted only by inoculating infected tissue into primates. The conventional agents are a virus much like papovavirus, a virus similar to measles virus, and rubella virus, causing PML, SSPE, and PRP, respectively. These agents can be grown in tissue culture, and they have the properties of their respective virus types.

The concept of a chronic latent virus infection was initially proposed by Sigurdson in 1954. Although rare, these diseases are important, in part because they demonstrate a substantially different concept of virus infection of humans than had previously been recognized. Many human chronic diseases may possibly be caused by latent virus infections.

Sigurdson postulated that virus infection could be inapparent for months or even years and then become active and cause progressive disease. His speculations, based in part on his studies of a sheep disease called *scrapie,* were first verified in kuru. It can be transmitted to primates by tissue inoculation, as can be the agent that causes Jakob-Creutzfeldt (JC) dementia, a degenerative disease of unknown cause and recognized worldwide as a progressive neurologic disease affecting middle-aged adults. The pathologic findings of spongiform changes, gliosis, and neuronal loss suggested a viral cause, which has now been firmly established. The infectivity of this nonconventional agent has been dramatically emphasized in the past few years, as JC dementia has occurred after corneal transplantation, after inadvertent self-inoculation by surgeons and pathologists, and after neurosurgical procedures performed with instruments that were "routinely" sterilized. Most recently, contamination of one batch of human growth hormone with JC virus (presumably from a cadaveric pituitary gland) has resulted in this disease in several recipients some 10 to 13 years after they received growth hormone. The JC dementia virus is extremely resistant to heat and radiation, the usual sterilization methods for surgical tools. In these instances of human-to-human transmission, the latent period between inoculation and symptoms of JC disease has averaged 8 months. To protect themselves and their patients, physicians must recognize that transmissible human diseases are no longer restricted to conventional clinical patterns and conventional viral agents.

PML occurs primarily in adults who have abnormalities of the immune system. SV40 and a related papovavirus are found in brain tissue from patients with this disease. In PML, cell-specific infection of oligodendrocytes occurs and causes multifocal dymyelination.

SSPE was initially recognized in the 1930s by Dawson, who described a progressive encephalitis of children in which at necropsy he could identify intracytoplasmic eosinophilic inclusions typical of virus infections. Attempts to culture an infectious virus from brain tissue of such patients were unsuccessful at that time. The clinical and pathologic disease was widely recognized, but there were no further clues to its cause until 1965, when Bouteille's electron microscopic studies of brain tissue revealed cytoplasmic particles similar to paramyxovirus. During the next 4 years, other workers documented elevated titers of antibodies to measles virus in CSF from children with SSPE. In 1969, several laboratories isolated a virus similar to measles virus from brain tissue. It has not yet been determined if ordinary measles virus infection is modified by an aberrant host response or if the measles-like agent itself differs in some way from regular measles virus. Vigorous attempts to identify a consistently abnormal host response have not been successful. A child lacking immunoglobulins died from SSPE, suggesting that circulating antibody is not essential for the disease process. It may be that wild-strain measles virus actually consists of a number of closely related subgroups, one of which can cause a latent brain infection in children. Whether the primary problem resides in the host or the virus or both, it is now well established that exposure to a measles-like agent in early childhood can result in clinically inapparent persistence of virus in brain tissue. Then, after years or even decades, the virus becomes active and induces a relentless cytopathic infection. There is usually no clinical evidence of extraneural disease in children with SSPE, but the SSPE agent has been isolated from lymph node tissue of such patients.

SSPE is symptomatically a triphasic disease. The initial phase is manifested by changes in behavior and mentation. These children are less attentive and more irritable, and they may exhibit overt antisocial behavior. Altered sleep patterns and other symptoms suggestive of emotional difficulties often lead to an initial evaluation by psychologists, psychiatrists, and others who deal with children who have behavior problems. After weeks or months, overt neurologic abnormalities are recognized as the second stage of SSPE develops. Seizures are common and often are of the myoclonic minor motor type. Dementia, ataxia, hearing and visual abnormalities, movement disorders, reflex changes, and focal paralyses can occur. SSPE is usually diagnosed at this time. After a course of months or even years, with sometimes a period of spontaneous improvement, stage 3 occurs, and the child loses all cognitive and interactive abilities and is left in a decerebrate vegetative state. The neurologic disease may not affect vital brainstem functions; as a result, survival in stage 3 may continue for years with good nursing care.

In the late 1960s, epidemiologic studies identified several hundred occurrences annually, with an incidence in the southeastern United States three to four times higher than elsewhere. The incidence among boys was several times higher than among girls, and the disease was more common among children in rural areas. As a group, children with SSPE had clinically apparent measles at an earlier age than other children, lending support to the hypothesis of an abnormal (immature?) immune response during the initial infection. There is no apparent genetic predisposition. In the past decade, the incidence of SSPE has decreased dramatically, probably reflecting widespread measles immunization. There is concern that measles immunization can itself cause SSPE. There are certainly numerous children with SSPE who never had clinically apparent measles but who did receive measles vaccine. Rigorous proof of SSPE caused by vaccine would require documentation of negative serologic testing for measles before immunization to exclude inapparent infection with wild-strain measles virus. This has never been documented. However, even if the attenuated vaccine strain does occasionally cause SSPE, the strikingly reduced incidence of postinfectious measles encephalitis and the apparent reduction in the frequency of SSPE itself establish the unequivocal benefit of measles immunization.

The diagnosis of SSPE rests on the finding of an elevated CSF concentration of IgG associated with an elevated CSF antibody titer to measles. Usually both are present, although there has been some SSPE with normal CSF IgG concentrations or normal measles antibody titers. Many neurologic diseases, such as meningitis, demyelinating diseases, and tumors, can cause moderate elevations in CSF IgG concentrations, but elevations in children with SSPE are usually dramatically high, sometimes representing as much as 50% of the total CSF protein. The critical diagnostic test is detection of an elevated CSF measles antibody titer. When such tests are available, measurement of antibody responses to the various measles antigens will demonstrate a selective reduction in the antibody response to the matrix (M) protein. The altered pattern suggests that the primary abnormality in SSPE resides in the virus, not the host. Other laboratory findings are usually normal. The EEG results will be abnormal, often showing a burst-suppression pattern at some time. Pathology examination of brain tissue obtained at biopsy may show the classic intracellular inclusions originally recognized by Dawson.

Attempts to treat SSPE have included many antiviral drugs, interferon, immunosuppression, and corticosteroids without demonstrable benefit. A long-term controlled study using isoprinosine has shown prolonged survival, but many survivors have irreversible severe neurologic handicaps. The disease may wax and wane, initially leading to reports of spontaneous recovery or reports of good response to antiviral drug treatment, only to have the patient become worse soon thereafter. The most encouraging data concern the decreased incidence of SSPE that has accompanied widespread measles immunization.

Progressive rubella panencephalitis (PRP) was first recognized in 1975 and thus far has been identified in only a few children. The disease has affected children from 8 to 14 years of age who have had either intrauterine-acquired rubella encephalopathy or rubella in early childhood. A decade or more after initial exposure, these children develop ataxia, spasticity, dysarthria, and dysphagia. Dementia is present early. Funduscopic examination may show progressive optic nerve atrophy. If seizures occur, they are often of a multifocal myoclonic type. The diagnosis, like that of SSPE, is based on elevated IgG concentrations and rubella antibody titers in the CSF. Radiologic studies often show severe cerebellar atrophy. The pathologic findings consist of diffuse neuronal loss, gliosis, and severe demyelination, with the most severe changes in the cerebellum. The disease resembles SSPE in many respects, and only the CSF antibodies or direct virus isolation can accurately differentiate the two diseases. PRP should certainly be considered in a child who has fixed stigmata (cataracts, deafness, microcephaly, mental retardation, etc.) of congenital rubella encephalopathy and then years later develops progressive neurologic deterioration. A chronic latent infection by rubella virus may cause a degenerative neurologic disease in a previously normal child or adolescent. At the present time, fewer than a dozen such patients have been positively identified, but as with any newly recognized disease, they may represent but "the tip of the iceberg." There is no specific treatment for PRP. The prognosis is not yet firmly established, but several children have died 1 to 4 years after the onset of the progressive disease.

25.15.7 Viral Infections in Immunocompromised Hosts

Children with abnormal immune systems, whether because of a primary genetically determined immunodeficiency disease or secondary to immunosuppressive therapy, have an increased risk of developing serious and often fatal infections, as discussed in Chap. 11.

Several types of virus-induced diseases of the nervous system have been documented in immunologically abnormal children. The most dramatic is an acute or subacute encephalitis. Herpes simplex virus type 1, varicella zoster, adenovirus, echovirus, and measles have all caused fatal encephalitis disease in children with underlying immunodeficiency. No doubt other viruses can also cause encephalitis. Often these opportunistic infections initially cause a subacute encephalopathy with multifocal disease that waxes and wanes for a number of weeks before overwhelming infection and death occur. Alternatively, an acute fulminating encephalitis can cause death within a few days.

An immunocompromised child may develop paralytic poliomyelitis, caused either by a wild strain or by the attenuated vaccine virus. Children have had serious infections after inadvertent contact with normal persons recently immunized with polio virus vaccine. The problem of protection from common and usually benign viruses for children who have immunodeficiencies associated with successful treatment for cancer or leukemia raises important management issues.

Other types of virus-induced disease in immunocompromised hosts are less well understood. Patients with underlying lymphomas (and occasionally other tumors) sometimes develop *progressive multifocal leukoencephalopathy*. PML is a multifocal demyelinating disease that affects the cerebral hemispheres. The clinical symptoms consist of seizures and focal neurologic deficits. Direct identification of virus is the only specific diagnostic test. Both electron microscopy and special approaches to virus cultivation have demonstrated virus much like papovavirus in this abnormal brain tissue. Two virus types have been identified: one is SV40 virus; the other, called *Jakob-Creutzfeldt virus,* is similar but antigenically distinct. The disease is progressive and causes death in 6 to 8 months.

The clinician caring for a child with a compromised immune system must be alert to the occurrence of acute, subacute, and chronic neurologic diseases. Aggressive antiviral therapy should be tried in specific infections. Acyclovir is effective in herpes virus (and other DNA virus) encephalitides, and hyperimmune serum and exogenous interferon have been of help in varicella zoster infections. Viral infection is often the direct cause of death in an immunocompromised host.

25.15.8 Acquired Immunodeficiency Syndrome Encephalopathy

Children and infants with proven HIV infection are at high risk of neurologic problems. Currently, 50 to 80% of children with HIV acquired the virus from maternal–fetal transmission in utero, approximately 20% from blood or blood-product transfusions, and most of the remainder from abusive sexual contact (Sec. 13.4.12). Proof of active persistent infection versus passive transfer of maternal antibodies requires stringent criteria under 15 months of age. Two clinical patterns of neurologic disease have been established in children with HIV infection. The most common is a progressive encephalopathy (PE) characterized by loss or plateau of development, impaired brain growth, progressive atrophy (on neuroimaging studies), pyramidal tract signs, and occasionally other discrete neurologic deficits. Seizures rarely occur. Apathy is common. A progressive downhill course, often complicated by systemic infections, leads to death within months to years. The second clinical syndrome in children with AIDS, which occurs in 10 to 20% is a static encephalopathy (SE) manifested by nonprogressive motor and developmental impairments, microcephaly, and occasionally seizures. A small percentage (10 to 20%) of children with AIDS are neurologically normal. However, it must be recognized that, at present, follow-up of these patients is still quite short. A vacuolar myelopathy, rather common in adults, is distinctly uncommon in children; involvement of the peripheral nervous system is exceedingly rare in the pediatric age group. Whereas secondary CNS infection and primary CNS tumors (lymphomas) are common findings in adults with AIDS, these types of neurologic diseases are uncommon in children.

Other than establishing a definite diagnosis of AIDS, there are no other specific clinical findings. Cerebrospinal fluid is usually normal, although occasionally a nonspecific lymphocytosis or protein elevation occurs. In children with primary CNS lymphoma, high levels of CSF protein, pleocytosis, and even hypoglycorrhachia are present. Neuroimaging procedures in children with both PE and SE demonstrate a generalized atrophy of brain tissue and sometimes mineralization of basal ganglia and deep white matter, usually bilateral. T_2-weighted images on MR imaging often indicate abnormal white matter.

Pathologic findings show increase of inflammatory cells, especially perivascular, a calcific vasculopathy, white matter demyelination, and in 100% of patients, diminished brain weight for age.

Treatment is largely supportive. Prompt detection and treatment of secondary infections and encouraging adequate fluid and nutritional intake may help alleviate discomfort, distress, and pain. Specific antiretroviral drugs such as zidovudine (azidothymidine or AZT) may suppress clinical symptoms and increase survival time, but there are relatively few data regarding the effects of AZT on HIV encephalopathy. Although other antiretroviral drugs (including reverse transcriptase inhibitors other than zidovidine), protease inhibitors, cytokine blockers, calcium channel blockers, and antioxidants may lower viremia, raise CD4 counts, or improve other systemic aspects of HIV infection, it is not clear what if any beneficial effect they may have on the encephalopathy or other neurologic manifestations of HIV infections.

25.15.9 Virus-Induced Myositis

Both acute and chronic inflammatory diseases of muscle are discussed in Sec. 25.14.2. Although the causes of these inflammatory myopathies are not well established, in several instances electron microscopy has identified picornavirus-like particles. However, these particles may represent fixation artifact, and no enterovirus isolation from a patient with an acute myositis has been documented. Coxsackievirus A9 has been isolated from an 11-year-old child with a chronic exacerbating myopathy. Epidemic myalgia (Bornholm disease) is clearly associated with group B coxsackievirus infection. Occasionally, transient inflammatory muscle disease with myoglobinuria occurs with influenza virus and some α-togavirus infections.

25.15.10 Viral Infections of the Fetus and Newborn

Viral infection during pregnancy (congenital or intrauterine infection) can cause fetal death, produce teratogenetic effects, or result in chronic illness. Inapparent asymptomatic infection can also occur. Fetal responses to infection differ in two basic ways from those of more mature individuals. First, the immature immune and inflammatory mechanisms of the fetus result in increased susceptibility to virus invasion. However, this diminished inflammatory response to infection (both direct and immune-mediated) may actually diminish the amount of tissue and cellular injury. Second, although viral interference with normal embryologic processes can produce malformations, the growth potential of fetal cells permits compensatory recovery that is not possible for the older nongrowing nervous system. Thus, the immaturity of the fetal brain sets the stage for unique manifestations of viral infections. The final result depends on the dose, virulence, and specificity of the infecting virus and on gestational age at the time of infection.

Specific human clinical syndromes related to fetal infection with rubella virus and CMV have been identified. The neurologic manifestations are listed in Table 25-28. Viruses other than rubella and CMV can interfere with normal fetal growth sporadically. Numerous animal models have suggested a huge reservoir of potential fetal-viral interactions, especially relating to teratogenetic effects. Nonviral agents, such as *Toxoplasma,* can also cause serious intrauterine infections.

Classic rubella syndrome is described in Sec. 13.4.20. Follow-up of severely affected children has shown a high incidence of psychomotor retardation and other neurologic abnormalities. Continuing follow-up has now shown a second phase of the disease. Some children with congenital rubella who had a static encephalopathy during their first decade or so have developed a progressive neurologic syndrome consisting of intellectual deterioration, ataxia, and seizures. This second phase of congenital rubella, *progressive rubella panencephalitis,* is associated with elevated CSF titers to rubella virus and elevated CSF immunoglobulins. This progressive disease is similar to subacute sclerosing panencephalitis caused by chronic latent infection with a measles-like virus. CSF pleocytosis and elevated protein concentration may be present. Rubella embryopathy syndrome is not specific for this virus, and other infections, such as CMV, toxoplasmosis, and syphilis, and teratogenetic agents must be considered in a newborn who has some of the clinical findings mentioned earlier. Management is directed toward the specific problems. Antiviral therapy has not diminished virus shedding in those infants who have persistent viral infections. The active infection disappears "spontaneously" after several months or even years. Pregnant women and others who are at high risk for rubella infection must be protected from these infants, who are highly infectious.

Cytomegalovirus (CMV) is the most common cause of congenital viral infection. Approximately 1% of all live-born babies in the United States are infected. Fortunately, most congenital CMV infections are asymptomatic, and only a small fraction are associated with neurologic involvement. Overall, progressive sensorineural hearing loss is the most common neurologic manifestation. In severe CNS infections, CMV causes widespread parenchymal necrosis and cystic destruction. Periventricular calcifications typically develop, and their location reflects the specific cell tropism CMV has for ependymal cells. CMV may also cause chorioretinitis and a generalized impairment in somatic and brain growth. The CAT scan findings in congenital CMV are similar to those found in congenital toxoplasmosis and are shown in Fig. 25-42. CMV infections are discussed more fully in Sec. 13.4.7.

Other viruses have occasionally been identified as causes of intrauterine malformations and encephalitis. These include herpes simplex virus, varicella zoster virus, enteroviruses, some arboviruses (California encephalitis virus), and possibly influenza and mumps viruses. In the newborn, most serious virus infections of the nervous system are caused either by herpes simplex virus or by the group B coxsackieviruses. Neonatal infections cause an encephalitis with or without systemic involvement. Accurate and early identification of these infections is essential now that there is effective antiviral therapy for HSV-2 infections of newborns.

TABLE 25-28

VIRUS INFECTIONS OF THE FETUS

VIRUS	TIME OF INFECTION	NEUROLOGIC DISEASE
Rubella virus	First trimester	Chronic encephalitis, microcephaly, retardation, diplegia, visual and auditory deficits, cataracts
	Later gestation	Hearing loss and minor retardation
	Unknown	Progressive rubella panencephalitis (delayed onset)
Cytomegalovirus	During gestation	Cytomegalic inclusion disease with microcephaly, retardation, and motor, visual, or auditory deficits; minor mental deficits
Herpes simplex virus	During gestation	Encephalitis with congenital microcephaly
Varicella zoster virus	First half of gestation	Limb hypoplasia and encephalomyelitis
Coxsackievirus B	Neonatal (late gestation?)	Encephalitis associated with myocarditis
Polioviruses	Late gestation	Neonatal paralytic poliomyelitis
Arboviruses	Late gestation	Neonatal encephalitis
Influenza virus	First trimester	Doubtful relation to malformations

SOURCE: *Johnson: In Vinken PJ, Bruyn GW, eds: Handbook of Clinical Neurology, vol 34, Amsterdam, Elsevier/North-Holland, 1978.*

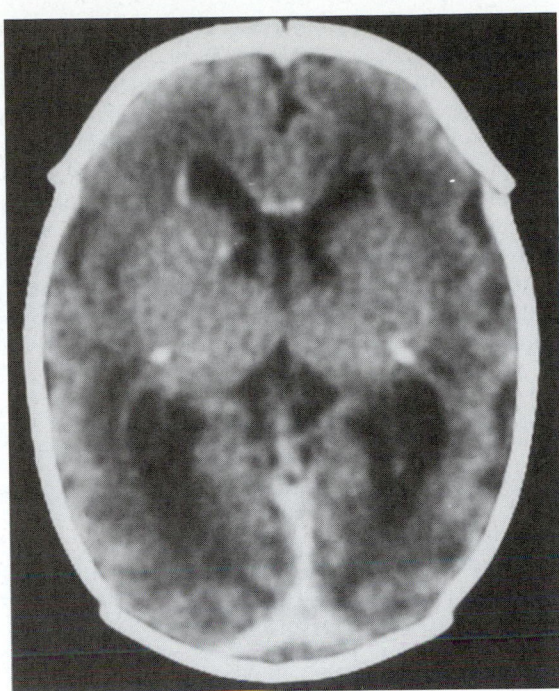

FIGURE 25-42 Axial noncontrast CT scan demonstrates diffuse atrophy with resultant overlap of sutures as well as punctate periventricular calcifications in a child with congenital CMV infection. *Courtesy of Dr. Jacqueline Bello.*

Neonatal herpes virus encephalitis is associated with maternal genital infection. The virus may be transmitted transplacentally, but 85 to 90% of infected infants acquire the infection by direct contact, either just before or during delivery (see Sec. 13.4.6). These infants are usually healthy immediately after birth but become sick 7 to 14 days later. Serious infections in infants may cause only subtle and nonspecific symptoms, such as poor feeding, lethargy, irritability, hypotonia or hypertonia, and jaundice. Skin vesicles may be present. Fever, seizures, and focal neurologic abnormalities suggest encephalitis. CNS involvement may occur as part of disseminated HSV infection or as a form of localized HSV infection without evidence of dissemination. Pathologic studies will show a diffuse necrotizing encephalitis with infectious virus present in brain tissue as well as other parts of the body. The CSF abnormalities consist of pleocytosis and elevated protein concentration. Virus can be recovered from the CSF (in contrast with type I herpes virus encephalitis of older children and adults) as well as from other body fluids and tissues in infants who have disseminated infections. Herpes simplex virus grows rapidly in tissue culture, often causing a typical cytopathic effect within 24 hours. Rapid confirmation of HSV infection can also be achieved with PCR and immunofluorescent techniques.

Before effective antiviral therapy was available, mortality from neonatal herpes encephalitis was approximately 70%, and most survivors had severe neurologic sequelae. Adenine arabinoside (ara-A) and acyclovir have been shown to be equally effective in lowering mortality to less than 40%. Currently, acyclovir administered intravenously at a dose of 10 mg/kg every 8 hours is the treatment of choice. Details regarding use of these agents are discussed in Secs. 13.1.2 and 13.4.6.

Prevention of this serious disease would be ideal. It is estimated that as many as 40% of infants delivered vaginally from infected mothers acquire herpes virus infections. Although a few infants delivered by cesarean section have developed neonatal herpes infection, many clinicians suggest delivery by cesarean section if the mother has an active genital herpes infection.

Approximately 25% of neonates with HSV encephalitis are infected with HSV-1. HSV-1 infections, in contrast to those caused by HSV-2, are less severe and occur slightly later. They are believed to be acquired after delivery.

Coxsackievirus B causes an acute encephalitis with CSF abnormalities and clinical findings indistinguishable from those of other viral or bacterial infection. Because coxsackievirus B can also infect the myocardium, the combination of encephalitis and myocardial disease in a newborn should suggest that specific virus infection. The infection is diagnosed by either serologic, virologic, or PCR techniques (see Sec. 13.4.2). The prognosis is serious, with a fatal outcome in over 50% and serious neurologic sequelae in many survivors. Currently, there is no effective antiviral therapy for this infection. Newborns may also have a benign viral meningitis, as described under aseptic meningitis (see Sec. 25.15.1).

25.15.11 Unusual, Recurrent, or Chronic Meningitis-Encephalitis Syndromes

Behçet Disease

This rare disease occasionally affects older children and adolescents, usually boys. It is characterized by a variable triad of ulcerative lesions of the skin and mucous membranes, uveitis, and neurologic involvement of a meningoencephalitic type. The ocular and dermatologic manifestations are much more common than the neurologic manifestations, but the latter indicate progressive worsening of the disease, sometimes with a fatal outcome. Arthritis and pulmonary involvement may occur. The laboratory abnormalities include an abnormal CSF with pleocytosis, elevated protein concentration, or elevated immunoglobulins. Blood fibrinogen concentrations are often high. Pathologic findings in the brain include multifocal areas of necrosis, demyelination, and gliosis. Although electron microscopy has revealed filamentous virus-like particles, no specific etiologic agent has been identified.

Vogt-Koyanagi-Harada Syndrome

This condition has three characteristics: acute ophthalmic involvement with major field defects, even blindness with or without uveitis; variable meningoencephalitic symptoms and findings; and dermatologic findings of vitiligo, alopecia, or poliosis (depigmentation of hair, eyebrows, and lashes). Hearing loss is also common. Approximately 20% of disease occurs in patients under 20 years of age, mostly in adolescents, with a female preponderance. Inflammatory abnormalities of the CSF are often present. The nervous system abnormalities include multifocal inflammation and gliosis similar to that of multiple sclerosis. The clinical course is variable, with occasional spontaneous improvement. Whether this syndrome is caused by a chronic multifocal virus infection is a matter of speculation.

Mollaret Meningitis

This syndrome consists of benign recurrent aseptic meningitis, sometimes with unusual large endothelial-like cells in the CSF, as well as other inflammatory cells. It is not epidemic; the clinical findings are those of a nonspecific aseptic meningitis. There is no specific treatment, and recovery has been complete in all reported patients. No virus has been isolated.

Iceland Disease

Iceland disease (benign myalgic encephalomyelitis, epidemic neuromyasthenia) usually begins abruptly with systemic symptoms of a flu-like illness, myalgia, distal paresthesias, and sometimes muscle weakness. Lethargy and increased fatigue are common and persistent. Iceland disease usually begins in late summer and the early fall months and occurs in epidemics. It may persist for weeks or months. The CSF is usually normal, and specific laboratory diagnosis of this condition is not possible. Recovery is complete. It is assumed to be caused by a virus.

25.15.12   Treatment of Viral Infections

Virus-induced diseases of the nervous system are treated in three ways: prevention, treatment of the associated inflammation and edema, and specific antiviral therapy. Effective preventive immunization is available for poliomyelitis, measles, rubella, and mumps. Passive immunotherapy for infection with varicella zoster virus is recommended for immunocompromised hosts.

Acute and subacute virus-induced infections are often associated with severe perivascular inflammation and edema. Treatment with steroids is often recommended, as are attempts to reduce increased intracranial pressure by the use of osmotic agents, hyperventilation, and pharmacologic agents. The efficacy of such treatment seems variable and has seldom been definitely established.

Specific antiviral therapy using many agents has been attempted during the past decade. Exogenous interferon and interferon inducers may be helpful in systemic virus infections, but the limited access of such molecules to the central nervous system has thus far prevented effective use of these broad-spectrum, antiviral agents.

Antiviral drugs with proven efficacy for human neurologic infections are specifically targeted to herpes simplex virus, cytomegalovirus, and HIV: vidarabine and acyclovir for herpes simplex virus, ganciclovir and foscarnet for cytomegalovirus, and zidovudine (AZT) for HIV. Each of these drugs has well-known potential neurotoxic side-effects such as peripheral sensorimotor polyneuropathy, cramps, myalgia, paresthesias, tremor, obtundation, encephalopathy, seizures, or coma that may limit its clinical usefulness. (See also Sec. 13.1.2.)

CLINICAL PATTERNS OF IMMUNE-MEDIATED POSTINFECTIOUS NEUROLOGIC SYNDROMES

25.15.13   Acute Disseminated Encephalomyelitis

Acute disseminated encephalomyelitis (ADEM) is an acute, immune-mediated perivenous demyelinative disorder that most often occurs after measles infections but can occur after infections caused by a wide variety of infective agents. Clinical illness often begins abruptly 1 to 3 weeks after viral illness or immunization. Headache, fever, irritability, seizures, and stupor are common manifestations. Symptoms and signs are nonspecific and may be indistinguishable from those in viral encephalitis. ADEM occurs in about 1 in 1000

cases of measles and carries a mortality of 20 to 30%. Multifocal, diffuse perivenous mononuclear infiltrates and perivenous demyelination are the characteristic neuropathologic changes found in ADEM. The mechanisms of this demyelinating disorder may involve both humoral and cellular immune responses, but the pathogenesis remains largely unknown. Neuroimaging tests, such as CT and MR scans, often show areas of edema and demyelination. Treatment is primarily supportive. A high-dose intravenously administered methylprednisolone (30 mg/kg/d) is advocated by some groups, but there is no widely held consensus about the efficacy of this therapy in ADEM. Several anecdotal reports have described improvement with IVIG therapy, but no large systematic study has confirmed efficacy for this form of treatment.

25.15.14   Acute Necrotizing Hemorrhagic Leukoencephalitis

Acute necrotizing hemorrhagic leukoencephalitis, a variant of acute disseminated encephalomyelitis, is a fulminating and often fatal disease characterized pathologically by extensive areas of necrosis, edema, hemorrhage, and demyelination. The CSF findings of elevated protein concentration and pleocytosis with large numbers of cells, often predominantly neutrophils, reflect an extensive necrotizing process. The CSF may also contain a significant number of red blood cells. No specific viruses have been isolated from brain tissue of patients with this disease, which has led to the hypothesis of an immune-mediated cause. There is no justification for separating this entity from the other severe, acute, virus-induced encephalopathies.

25.15.15   Acute Cerebellar Ataxia of Childhood

This syndrome, referred to as *acute cerebellitis* or *acute cerebellopathy*, occurs most commonly in children 2 to 6 years of age. The onset is abrupt and the evolution of symptoms rapid. In about 50% of cases, there is a prodromal respiratory or gastrointestinal virus-like illness or an exanthematous illness 2 to 3 weeks before onset. Well-known associated viral infections include varicella, rubeola, mumps, rubella, echovirus, poliovirus, infectious mononucleosis, and influenza. Bacterial infections such as scarlet fever and salmonellosis have also been implicated. The pathogenesis of cerebellar disturbance is unknown.

Ataxia of the trunk and extremities may be mild or so severe that the child is unable to stand or sit without support. Intention tremors may impair the child's ability to reach for objects. Hypotonia, tremor, horizontal nystagmus, and dysarthria are frequently present. The child is irritable, and vomiting is common. Signs of increased intracranial pressure are absent and the fundi normal. Sensory and reflex examinations are normal.

Cerebrospinal fluid pressure and protein and glucose concentrations are normal. A mild CSF lymphocytosis (up to 30 lymphocytes/mm) may be present in 30 to 50% of patients. Attempts should be made to identify the etiologic infectious agent by appropriate virologic, bacteriologic, and immunologic studies on spinal fluid, blood, stool, throat washings, and urine. Head CT and MR scans are normal. There is no evidence for demyelination or any structural alteration in the cerebellum or brainstem. The EEG may show mild, diffuse, generalized background slowing, but these changes are nonspecific, and the EEG rapidly returns to normal.

The syndrome of acute, parainfectious cerebellar ataxia must be differentiated from acute cerebellar ataxia caused by drugs and toxins, such as phenytoin, phenobarbital, primidone, and lead. An occult neuroblastoma can produce a paraneoplastic syndrome characterized by ataxia, myoclonus, and opsoclonus and must be excluded in young children with acute onset ataxia. Posterior fossa tumors must also be excluded. On occasion, acute cerebellar ataxia may be the presenting sign of acute bacterial meningitis, systemic vasculitides, trauma, and inborn errors of metabolism, such as Hartnup and maple syrup urine disease (Chap. 9). Acute disseminated encephalomyelitis and multiple sclerosis can also cause acute ataxia in older children and adolescents.

Treatment is supportive. The use of corticosteroids is unnecessary in typical parainfectious, acute cerebellar ataxia. Between 80 and 90% of children with acute cerebellar ataxia recover without sequelae within 6 to 8 weeks. In the remainder, disorders of behavior and learning, persistent ataxia, abnormal eye movements, and speech impairment may persist for months or years, and recovery may remain incomplete.

25.15.16 Transverse Myelitis

Transverse myelitis is a clinical syndrome characterized by acute onset (hours to days) of segmental spinal cord disease, with both motor and sensory abnormalities at and below the level of the lesion. It is often associated with nonspecific (often respiratory) virus infections.

Clinical findings reflect the level of the spinal lesion, which most commonly occurs in the thoracic cord. There will be no neurologic abnormalities above the lesion. At the level of the lesion, a zone of painful hyperesthesia often occurs, with motor abnormalities and sensory loss below that level commensurate with the extent of spinal cord damage. The illness commonly begins with severe back pain that radiates circumferentially, followed by rapidly progressive paraparesis, loss of sphincter control, and loss of pain and temperature sensations below the level of the lesion. Complete anesthesia is rare. Posterior column sensation is usually spared. The initial paralysis is of the flaccid type (spinal shock), followed over the next days and weeks by progressive spasticity below the level of cord disease. Loss of reflexes may persist at the level of the lesion if the anterior horn cells or root exit zones are injured.

The differential diagnosis of acute segmental cord disease must include consideration of other causes of intraspinal disease (abscess, hematoma, idiopathic necrosis, vascular occlusion owing to ischemia, syringomyelia, intraspinal cyst, or neoplasm) or an extraspinal mass (tumor, hematoma, spinal arteriovenous malformation, or epidural abscess) causing segmental cord compression. In a young child, in whom accurate sensory examination may be difficult, acute polyneuritis may be confused with transverse myelitis. Imaging techniques to exclude a surgically treatable mass lesion are usually indicated. During the acute disease, the spinal cord may swell, making radiographic differentiation from other intraspinal processes difficult. Transverse myelitis usually does not have multifocal involvement, which may help to distinguish it from a syrinx; the onset of transverse myelitis is acute, and this contrasts with the usual onset of tumors, congenital cysts, and other malformations. An acute extradural mass will be identified by imaging techniques. CSF examination may be normal or may show mild inflammatory changes and thus not be helpful diagnostically. A lumbar puncture can cause further damage if there is a mass lesion causing spinal cord com-

pression; therefore, it should be performed only after neurologic or neurosurgical consultation.

Pathologically, cord softening and mild edema may occur over several segments. Acutely, there will be predominantly perivascular inflammatory reaction. Later, demyelination with or without necrosis, cavitation, and secondary gliosis will occur. Ischemic cord disease may be difficult to differentiate from virus-induced transverse myelitis.

Transverse myelitis has often been associated with respiratory viral illnesses or specific viral syndromes (mumps, Epstein-Barr virus, varicella) or has followed immunization with duck rabies vaccine or small pox vaccine, thus suggesting an immune-mediated pathogenesis. A chronic virus infection of some type has been postulated in transverse myelitis in which the cord disease is the first episode of multiple sclerosis. A temporal association with optic neuritis occurs in 10 to 20% of infections, and this is called *neuromyelitis optica* (Devic syndrome). It is believed to be a type of multiple sclerosis.

The prognosis for idiopathic transverse myelitis (demyelinating, postinfectious, postimmunization types) is reasonably good. Approximately 60% of these patients experience good functional recovery, with only 10 to 15% having severe permanent neurologic deficits. There is no specific treatment for the idiopathic form. Treatable causes of acute spinal cord injury must always be excluded. The possible benefit from steroids is discussed in the following section.

25.15.17 Acute Polyneuritis

Acute polyneuritis (Landry's syndrome, Guillain-Barré syndrome, Fisher syndrome, infectious neuritis, acute polyradiculoneuropathy), an acute form of peripheral neuropathy, is an inflammatory disease that causes demyelination of the roots and peripheral nerves, resulting in muscle weakness of the flaccid type. It often follows a respiratory or other virus infection. It is this latter association that suggests a virus-triggered immune-mediated pathogenesis. Acute polyneuritis has also followed other immunogenic triggers, such as tetanus antitoxin, killed rabies vaccine, and other antigen exposure. Well-documented disease has occurred with varicella virus, influenza virus, enterovirus, Epstein-Barr virus, Lyme disease, and *Mycoplasma* infections as well as many unidentified respiratory and exanthematous infections. Acute polyneuritis occurs in patients of all ages, including infants. More detailed information on acute polyneuritis is included in Sec. 25.12.1.

25.15.18 Childhood Demyelinating Disease (Multiple Sclerosis)

Approximately 5% of demyelinating disease (multiple sclerosis) begins during childhood. Therefore, although rare, it must be considered in any child who has neurologic symptoms and findings that are disseminated spatially and temporally. Acute unremitting demyelinating disease occasionally affects children under the age of 10 years but is much more common during adolescence. Although the evidence is not conclusive, extensive epidemiologic, pathologic, and experimental data support the hypothesis that a chronic viral infection acquired during childhood causes clinical symptoms several decades later, secondary to an immune-mediated reaction.

The clinical symptoms of multiple sclerosis in children are similar to those in adults. There are disturbances in vision, oculomotor function, coordination, and sensation. A transverse myelitis or an optic neuritis or both (Devic syndrome) may be the initial presentation.

The diagnosis is based on the presence of neurologic abnormalities that relate to more than one anatomic area of the nervous system and that tend to remit and recur. The spinal fluid may show mild pleocytosis or mild elevation in total protein during acute exacerbations. CSF immunoglobulins are increased in approximately 75% of proven disease, but neither the presence nor absence of elevated IgG or oligoclonal bands is absolutely diagnostic. MR imaging will often identify clinically silent areas of demyelination (increased signal on T_2-weighted scans). During an acute episode, focal brain edema may be present. MR imaging using T_2 and balanced pulse sequences is the modality of choice in the imaging of demyelination.

During the initial demyelinating event, many other diseases must be considered, including brain tumor, focal encephalitis, nonviral infections with focal cerebritis or abscess formation, cerebrovascular diseases, leukodystrophies, and systemic vasculitis. Once the disease has revealed its waxing and waning course, the differential diagnosis will focus more on multiple cerebral emboli, systemic vasculitis, or recurrent infections in a susceptible host. Because there is currently no definite way to diagnose multiple sclerosis during life, these other diseases must be excluded if they seem possible.

Some childhood demyelinating diseases cause extensive bilateral abnormalities in subcortical areas. The name *Schilder disease* has been given to such a process. However, a genetically determined disease, adrenoleukodystrophy, is clinically indistinguishable in its neurologic manifestations from Schilder disease, causing some question that there is such an entity.

In the acute stage of multiple sclerosis, pathologic examination will show multiple areas, primarily subcortical, in which there is loss of myelin, relative preservation of axons, and perivascular inflammatory cells with edema. In older lesions, a secondary gliosis occurs, resulting in firm yellowish plaque-like areas, thus the term *sclerosis*.

There are some data and much enthusiastic opinion to support the use of short-term high-dosage corticosteroid therapy (prednisone, 2 mg/kg/d) or ACTH (2 to 4 U/kg/d) during acute episodes of multiple sclerosis. Because chronic problems such as urinary incontinence and spasticity occur, other drugs such as antispasmodics may be useful. Like the disease, the prognosis is variable, often with a slowly worsening course over several decades.

References

Pathogenesis

Haywood A: Patterns of persistent viral infection. N Engl J Med 315:939, 1986

Tyler KL, Fields BN: Pathogenesis of neurotropic viral infections. In: Vinken PJ, Bruyn GW, Klawans HL, McKendall RR, eds: Handbook of Clinical Neurology, vol 56: Viral Disease. New York, Elsevier Science, 1989:25–49

Aseptic Meningitis

Beghi E, Nicolosi A, Kurland LT, et al: Encephalitis and aseptic meningitis, Olmsted County, Minnesota, 1950–1981: I. Epidemiology. Ann Neurol 16:283, 1984

Lepow ML: Enteroviral meningitis: a reappraisal. Pediatrics 62:267, 1978

Sells CJ, Carpenter RL, Ray CG: Sequelae of central nervous system enterovirus infections. N Engl J Med 293:1, 1975

Acute Viral Encephalitis

Corey L, Spear PG: Infections with herpes simplex viruses (1 & 2). N Engl J Med 314:686–691, 749–757, 1986

Kipps A, Dick G, Moodie JW: Measles and the central nervous system. Lancet 2:1406, 1983

Kohl S: Herpes simplex viral encephalitis in children. Pediatr Clin North Am 35:465, 1988

Lange BJ, Berman PH, Bender J, et al: Encephalitis in infectious mononucleosis: diagnostic considerations. Pediatrics 58:877, 1976

Seay AR: Alphavirus and flavivirus diseases. In: McKendall RR, Stroop WG, eds: Handbook of Neurovirology. New York, Marcel Dekker, 1994

Brainstem Encephalitis

Assa A, Watemberg N, Bujanover Y, Lermen-Sagie T: Demyelinative brainstem encephalitis responsive to intravenous immunoglobulin therapy. Pediatrics 104:301–304, 1999

Bickerstaff ER: Brainstem encephalitis. Br Med J 1:1384, 1957

Ellison PH, Hanson PA: Herpes simplex: a possible cause of brainstem encephalitis. Pediatrics 59:240, 1977

Waxman SG, Sabin TD, Embree LJ: Subacute brainstem encephalitis. J Neurol Neurosurg Psychiatr 37:811, 1974

Acute Cerebellar Ataxia

Bell WE: Ataxia in childhood: Clinical approach and differential diagnosis. Lancet 1:2, 1965

Bergen D, Grossman H: Infectious mononucleosis as a cause of acute cerebellar ataxia of childhood. Dev Med Child Neurol 18:799, 1976

Weiss S, Carter S: Course and prognosis of acute cerebellar ataxia in children. Neurology 9:711, 1959

Chronic Focal Encephalitis

Chalhub L, De Vivo DC, Siegel BA, et al: Coxsackie A9 focal encephalitis associated with acute infantile hemiplegia and porencephaly. Neurology 27:574, 1977

Peters ACB, Vielvoye GJ, Versteeg J: ECHO 25 focal encephalitis and subacute chorea. Neurology 29:676, 1979

Piatt JH JR, Hwang PA, Armstrong DC, et al: Chronic focal encephalitis (Rasmussen syndrome). Epilepsia 29:268, 1988

Rasmussen T, Andermann F: Update on the syndrome of "chronic encephalitis" and epilepsy. Cleveland Clin J Med 56 (suppl pt 2):S181–S184, 1989

Zupanc ML, Handler EG, Levine RL, et al: Rasmussen encephalitis: epilepsia partialis continua secondary to chronic encephalitis. Pediatr Neurol 6:397–401, 1990

Acute Myelitis

Foley JF, Chin T, Gravelle CR: Paralytic disease due to infection with ECHO virus type 9. N Engl J Med 260:924, 1959

Henderson DA, Witte JJ, Morris L: Paralytic disease associated with oral polio vaccines. JAMA 190:41, 1974

Transverse Myelitis

Barak Y, Schwartz JF: Acute transverse myelitis associated with ECHO type 5 infection. Am J Dis Child 142:128, 1988

Berman M, Feldman S, Alter M, Zilber N, Kahana E: Acute transverse myelitis: incidence and etiologic considerations. Neurology 31:966–971, 1981

Dunne K, Hopkins IJ, Shield LK: Acute transverse myelopathy in childhood. Dev Med Child Neurol 28:198–204, 1986

Demyelinating Disease

Duquette P, Murray TJ, Pleines J, et al: Multiple sclerosis in childhood: clinical profile in 125 patients. J Pediatr 111:359, 1987

Nagashima K, Meyermann R, ter Meulen V: Demyelinating encephalomyelitis induced by long-term corona virus infection in rats. Acta Neuropathol (Berl) 45:205, 1979

Schwartz G, Friday G: Multiple sclerosis and childhood infections. Neurology 36:1386, 1986

Weiner LP, Johnson RT, Herndon RM: Viral infections and demyelinating diseases. N Engl J Med 288:1103, 1973

Polyneuritis

Charles RHG: Postvaricella polyneuritis. Br Med J 1:908, 1965

Leonard J, Tobin J: Polyneuritis associated with cytomegalovirus infections. Q J Med 40:435, 1971

Ropper AH: The Guillain-Barré syndrome. N Engl J Med 326:1130–1136, 1992

Sterman AB, Nelson S, Barclay P: Demyelinating neuropathy accompanying Lyme disease. Neurology 32:1302, 1982

Meningoencephalitic Syndromes

Behçet's disease (editorial). Lancet 1(8641):761–762, 1989

Graybill JR, Silva J Jr, O'Brien MS, et al: Epidemic neuromyasthenia. JAMA 219:144, 1972

Hermans PE, Goldstein NP, Wellman WE: Mollaret's meningitis and differential diagnosis of recurrent meningitis. Am J Med 52:128, 1972

Lobo AJ: Behçet's disease. Ann Intern Med 76:332, 1972

Opportunistic Infections

Aicardi J, Goutieres F, Arsenio-Nunes M: Acute measles encephalitis in children with immunosuppression. Pediatrics 59:232, 1977

Belman AL, Diamond G, Dickson D, et al: Pediatric acquired immunodeficiency syndrome. Neurologic syndromes. Am J Dis Child 142:29–35, 1988

Epstein LG, Sharer LR, Joshi VV, et al: Progressive encephalopathy in children with acquired immune deficiency syndrome. Ann Neurol 17:488, 1985

Linnemann CC, May DB, Schubert WK: Fatal viral encephalitis in children with X-linked hypogammaglobulinemia. Am J Dis Child 126:100, 1973

Wilfert CM, Buckley RH, Mohanakumar T: Persistent and fatal central nervous system echovirus infections in patients with agammaglobulinemia. N Engl J Med 296:1485, 1977

Virus Infections of the Fetus and Newborn

Kairam R, De Vivo DC: Neurological manifestations of congenital infections. Clin Perinatol 8:445, 1987

Paryani SG, Yeager AS, Hosford-Dunn H, et al: Sequelae of acquired cytomegalovirus infections in premature and sick term infants. J Pediatr 107:451, 1985

Pastuszak AL, Levy M, Schick B, et al: Outcome after maternal varicella infection in the first 20 weeks of pregnancy. N Engl J Med 330:901–905, 1994

Seay AR, Griffin DE: Effects of viral infections on the developing nervous system. In: Korobkin R, Guillemenaux S, eds: Progress in Perinatal Neurology. Baltimore, Williams and Wilkins, 1981:121

Stagno S, Whitley RJ: Herpesvirus infections of pregnancy. (Parts I & II). N Engl J Med 313:1270–1274, 1327–1330, 1985

Whitley RJ: Therapy of herpes simplex infections of the central nervous system: neonatal herpes and herpex simplex encephalitis. Semin Pediatr Inf Dis 2:263, 1991

Chronic Latent Viral Encephalitis

Brown P, Gadjusek DC, Gibbs CJ JR, et al: Potential epidemic of Creutzfeldt-Jakob disease from human growth hormone therapy. N Engl J Med 313:728, 1985

Dyken PR: Subacute sclerosing panencephalitis: current status. Neurol Clin 3:179, 1985

Homabrook RW: Kuru—a subacute cerebellar degeneration. The natural history and clinical features. Brain 91:53, 1968

Horta-Barbosa L, Fuccillo DA, Sever JL: Chronic viral infections of the central nervous system. JAMA 218:1185, 1971

Padgett BL, Walker DL, ZuRhein GM, et al: JC papovavirus in progressive multifocal leukoencephalopathy. J Infect Dis 133:686, 1976

Townsend JJ, Baringer JR, Wolinsky JS, et al: Progressive rubella panencephalitis: Late onset after congenital rubella. N Engl J Med 1975

AIDS Encephalopathy

Belman AL, Diamond G, Dickson D, et al: Pediatric acquired immunodeficiency syndrome. Neurologic syndromes. Am J Dis Child 142:29–35, 1988

Mintz M, Epstein LG, Koenigsberger MR: Neurologic manifestations of acquired immunodeficiency in children. Int Pediatr 4:161, 1989

Ojukwu IC, Epstein LG: Neurologic manifestations of infections with HIV. Pediatr Infect Dis J 17:341–344, 1998.

Sever JL, Gibbs CJ, eds: Retroviruses in the nervous system. Ann Neurol 23 (suppl):S1–5217, 1988

Treatment

Arvin AM, Johnson RT, Whitley RT, Nelson JD, McCracken GH Jr: Consensus: management of the patient with herpes simplex encephalitis. Pediatr Inf Dis J 6:2–5, 1987

Bodensteiner JB, Morris HH, Howell JT: Chronic ECHO type 5 virus meningoencephalitis in X-linked hypogammaglobulinemia: treatment with immune plasma. Neurology 29:815, 1979

Husson RN, Mueller BU, Farley M, et al: Zidovudine and didanosine combination therapy in children with human immunodeficiency virus infection. Pediatrics 93:316–322, 1994

Pasternak JF, DeVivo DC, Prensky AL: Steroid-responsive encephalomyelitis in childhood. Neurology 30:481, 1980

Wolinsky JS, Berg BO, Maitland CJ: Progressive rubella panencephalitis. Arch Neurol 33:7322, 1976

Wolinsky JS, Johnson KP, Rand K: Progressive multifocal leukoencephalopathy: clinical pathological correlate and failure of a drug trial in two patients. Arch Neurol 33:386, 1976

25.16 PURULENT FOCAL INFECTIONS

Neil A. Feldstein

Purulent infections of the central nervous system are potentially life-threatening and are capable of producing severe neurologic deficits.

Progress in preventing deaths and sequelae is not likely to come from new antibiotics but rather by means of more rapid and more accurate diagnosis and by earlier institution of therapy.

Focal infections of the brain can be complications of primary illnesses. Focal sepsis may be caused by penetrating trauma, extension along tissue planes from paracranial or paraspinal infective foci, or hematogenous or metastatic spread from distant infections. Treatment of the nervous system infection must be carried out along with therapy for the primary infective site. A diligent search for primary infection sites will reveal the source in almost 90% of patients.

Infections can be located in any portion of the brain, spinal cord, or meninges. Brain abscesses can range in size from miliary foci to large encapsulated structures that contain large volumes of purulent material. Subdural empyema initially layers freely in the subdural space, but the pus tends to become loculated. Encapsulated subdural abscesses may be found on both the medial and the lateral surfaces of the cerebral hemisphere or at the base of the brain. Epidural abscesses are usually relatively small collections, often consisting of a granulomatous mass.

Neurologic deficits resulting from focal infections may be caused by the local mass effect of the abscess or surrounding brain edema, venous stasis, arterial occlusion, and direct compression of cranial and spinal nerves. In addition, general signs of raised intracranial pressure can be identified. These include obtundation and unilateral or bilateral sixth nerve palsies. An important advance in therapy has been the use of steroids to control edema, thereby decreasing the abscess mass effect. Steroid therapy is used when neural deficits are present, despite the theoretical problem of "masking" any further inflammatory changes.

25.16.1   Cranial Epidural Abscess

Purulent collections in the epidural space usually develop by direct extension from surrounding bony structures. They typically follow chronic infections of frontal, sphenoid, or mastoid sinuses, otitis, or dental abscesses. Dental, otologic, or neurosurgical procedures can spread infection or introduce infection into the epidural space. Fractures of the skull under open lacerations can allow bacteria direct access to this space.

Symptoms are usually mild. The local site may be painful and tender, and there may be headache, low-grade fever, and slight leukocytosis. Neurologic deficits are slight and are often absent entirely. Frequently, these infections are discovered only during investigation of the primary site of illness.

Infections in the epidural space can affect blood flow in the dural sinuses. These sinuses can be compressed by the epidural mass or thrombosed by infection in the sinus wall. Obstruction of one or more major dural sinuses can lead to intracranial hypertension in children. This complication is usually associated with chronic otitis or mastoiditis, and frank infection at the primary site need not be present. The signs and symptoms are those of increased intracranial pressure: headache, nausea, vomiting, diplopia, and papilledema. Children with epidural infections often do not seem to be seriously ill despite symptoms of elevated intracranial pressure, and these infections must be carefully differentiated from benign intracranial hypertension.

Skull x-rays may indicate infection at the primary focus, although osteomyelitis of the skull may suggest epidural suppuration. Less frequently, changes associated with chronically increased in-

tracranial pressure will be seen. Lumbar puncture pressure may be normal or elevated, and CSF chemical and cellular values are usually normal. If raised intracranial pressure is suspected, lumbar puncture should be deferred until an MR or CT scan is available if at all possible. Peripheral white cell counts rarely exceed 15,000 cells/ μL, but the ESR is invariably elevated, often above 100 mm/h. EEG and brain scan are usually abnormal but rarely accurately locate the lesion site. CT and MR scans provide excellent localization. CT scans are especially useful with the use of bone windows to identify areas of skull infection and necrosis.

Antibiotic therapy is always required. Occasionally, epidural infections will not require surgery if an extracranial source can be identified and cultured. If a mass lesion is identified, however, it must be drained promptly. At operation, all chronically infected granulation tissue should be removed, as well as any infected overlying bone. Burr hole aspiration is not effective, and treatment with craniotomy or craniectomy is usually required when surgery is indicated.

Benign intracranial hypertension secondary to sinus obstruction is a self-limited process with an excellent prognosis. The sinus may recanalize, or venous anastomoses may develop.

25.16.2   Cranial Subdural Empyema

Subdural infection accounts for nearly one-fifth of intracranial abscesses. Despite antibiotic therapy, the mortality had remained above 40% until the use of CT scan to aid in diagnosis and monitor effects of therapy. Infection most frequently follows inadequate antibiotic treatment of a prior infection. In older children, subdural empyema is often associated with otorhinologic infection, whereas in infants it is usually a sequela of poorly treated meningitis with an infected effusion. Subdural empyema can also follow trauma, intracranial surgery, and hematogenous seeding of the subdural space.

When paranasal sinus infection is followed by severe headache, seizures, alteration in consciousness, fever, meningeal signs, and frontal or orbital swelling, the infection has clearly spread beyond the sinus and entered the subdural space. Purulent material may spread widely in the subdural space, causing focal or diffuse hemispheric signs. Intracranial pressure is usually elevated, and an infant may present with fever and an enlarging head. In an infant who has had meningitis, any new focal or hemispheric deficit, any change in level of consciousness, or any spreading of sutures should suggest the possibility of subdural empyema. An enlarging head in a postmeningitis infant is most likely caused by subdural effusion or postmeningitis hydrocephalus. Infected subdural collection must be ruled out. Ultrasonography is an excellent method of diagnosis in this age group. CT and MR scans, both with and without contrast enhancement, will usually differentiate these conditions. Pus along the falx between the cerebral hemispheres may be overlooked when convexity collections are drained, and this oversight has been related to both recurrent infections and mortality associated with subdural empyema.

CT scanning can be valuable in localizing purulent infections; it can also be used to identify areas of cerebritis or cerebral edema that appear as vascular regions on angiography and may be misinterpreted as intracerebral abscesses. MR scanning appears to be more sensitive than CT scanning in detecting the early changes associated with acute subdural infection. As with most intracranial processes, MR is supplanting CT imaging as the diagnostic study of choice.

Treatment of subdural empyema involves early and definitive drainage coupled with appropriate intensive antibiotic therapy. In addition, extracranial sources of the infection such as the nasal sinuses must be addressed by the otolaryngologists. Loculated pockets of infected material, usually located along the falx, the posterior parietal convexity, and the base, must be sought out and removed. Adequate drainage may not be possible through burr holes; wide craniotomy is usually preferable. This approach is supported by the study of Bannister and associates, in which the mortality rate in patients treated with burr hole aspiration was 48%, whereas the rate for those patients treated by craniotomy was only 8%. Accurate localization by CT or MR scanning will permit more of this collection to be treated by burr hole aspiration and catheter drainage. Some surgeons advise that the space be irrigated by in-dwelling drains for several days postoperatively. Systemic steroid therapy will reduce the underlying cerebral edema. Dexamethasone (Decadron) at a dosage of 0.25 mg/kg per day should be given in divided doses.

The infective organism is most likely to be one of the streptococci, often microaerophilic or anaerobic. Subdural infections after penetrating wounds or surgical operations are likely to be caused by staphylococci or gram-negative organisms. Material obtained at operation should be smeared immediately and Gram stained, then observed for a long time in aerobic, microaerobic, and anaerobic cultures. High-dosage penicillin therapy should be started pending the results of sensitivity tests. Dilute solutions of penicillin may be used to irrigate the subdural space directly; however, care must be taken because of the epileptogenic potential of cortically applied penicillin. Other alternative solutions that are less neurotoxic than penicillin include bacitracin and the aminoglycosides, gentamicin, and tobramycin. Intrathecal gentamicin has been used effectively against intracerebral and intraventricular gram-negative organisms. However, studies have demonstrated that introducing an aminoglycoside into the lumbar space cannot achieve significant levels of the drug over the convexities of the brain or within the ventricles.

Antibiotic therapy is usually continued for several weeks. However, chronic sinus or bone infection may require prolonged treatment extending over several months. Antibiotics that will penetrate the bone and brain should be used for such prolonged treatment.

25.16.3   Brain Abscess

Most reports have cited a mortality of 30 to 45% for all forms of therapy and an operative mortality of 20 to 40%. However, a study at Newcastle-upon-Tyne analyzed results in 90 patients operated on between 1964 and 1978. The mortality rates in each successive 5-year period were 42%, 21%, and 8%. This dramatic improvement came after the "antibiotic era" and has been attributed to earlier diagnosis, more rapid surgical intervention, and more accurate bacterial recognition, especially of anaerobic gram-negative bacilli.

The incidence of brain abscess is difficult to evaluate but is probably 2 to 3 per 10,000 general hospital admissions. A preponderance of male patients has been noted in most large series. Brain abscess is rare in infants less than 1 year of age, but the incidence rises rapidly thereafter, and nearly one-third of all brain abscesses occur in the pediatric age group. The low incidence of brain abscesses in infants is related to their lack of well-formed frontal or mastoid sinuses.

Brain abscess can arise secondary to infection elsewhere in the body or can be caused by penetrating injury. In approximately 6% of patients, the primary source of infection is undetectable. Although treatment of the brain abscess is the primary responsibility, detection and treatment of the infective source must proceed simultaneously. A history of inadequate treatment of an initial infection, usually with a broad-spectrum antibiotic of insufficient potency, is frequently elicited.

Various etiologic categories of abscess formation may be defined: direct extension from otorhinologic infection through venous channels; hematogenous spread in patients with distant infection, with or without a known source as in cyanotic children with cardiac anomalies or pulmonary arteriovenous malformations; abscess caused by traumatic brain penetration or neurosurgical procedure; abscess secondary to extension into the brain from infection in scalp; and abscess formation associated with congenital dermoids or dermal sinus tracts.

Extension to the brain from paranasal, mastoid, or ear infection has been reported as the most common cause of brain abscess in many series. However, the incidence of infection from otorhinologic sources has fallen markedly since the introduction of antibiotics, and metastatic abscess is now more common in the pediatric age group. Metastatic abscesses usually originate in either the heart or the lungs, although osteomyelitis, renal infections, and skin abscess can be the primary sources. Chronic pulmonary abscess is more likely to follow subacute bacterial endocarditis than acute endocarditis.

A frequently contributing factor in children with brain abscesses is cyanosis, caused either by congenital heart disease or by pulmonary arteriovenous shunting. Postmortem studies have indicated that brain abscesses are found in 0.4% of patients dying from all causes, whereas in patients with congenital heart disease the incidence may be as high as 6%. The incidence of brain abscess in all children with congenital cyanotic heart disease is 2 to 3%. Currently, cyanotic congenital heart disease and ENT infection cause equal numbers of cerebral abscesses.

Children with right-to-left intracardiac shunting are deprived of the phagocytic filtering action of the pulmonary capillary bed, and, in these children, the cerebral circulation is subject to recurrent bacteremia. These children are also likely to have focal encephalomalacia resulting from hypoxia and decreased cerebral blood flow caused by the increased viscosity of polycythemia. The coincidence of an area of recent infarction and bacteremia will predispose to abscess formation. A relationship has been shown between the severity of hypoxemia and the development of and prognosis for brain abscess in these patients. Children with low oxygen saturation levels are more likely to develop and succumb to brain abscesses than those with higher levels. Because brain abscesses are rare in infants, complete surgical correction of cyanotic cardiac defects before the age of 2 years would virtually eliminate brain abscesses in these children. Palliative surgery will alleviate hypoxemia, but it will not remove the hazard of brain abscess formation.

A growing group of children who are at risk of intracranial infection are those who are immunosuppressed. This category includes those receiving chemotherapy/radiation therapy for malignancy, a small group who have had transplants, and a smaller group with AIDS. CSF normally contains few factors needed for bacterial clearance, with both complement and opsonic proteins virtually absent. The increased risk in this group of children is, therefore, related to their generally high risk for opportunistic infection, rather than to specific central nervous system factors. Abscesses in this group are more likely to be multiple, the children are usually debilitated, the bacterial spectrum is wide, including fungi, and this group may have multiple organisms in the abscess.

Pathophysiology

Recent investigations of experimental abscesses, and correlation of CT scans with both experimental and operative histologic findings have led to a definition of stages in the course of abscess formation. These stages include: early and late cerebritis followed by early and late capsule formation. The findings from CT and MR imaging differ according to the stage of abscess formation. In early cerebritis there is only patchy enhancement and an ill-defined area of low density or attenuation. As the abscess matures to late cerebritis and early capsule formation, a large enhancing ring is identified. This occurs during the formation of a collagen capsule, and the central portion of the abscess begins to necrose. In the final late capsular stage there is a well-defined collagen capsule and necrotic center. Contrast images at this stage reveal only a faint thin rim of enhancement.

Bacteriology

Material from abscess cavities must be cultured immediately, both aerobically and anaerobically. Before antibodies were available, brain abscesses were almost universally attributable to aerobic streptococci or *Staphylococcus aureus*. In more recent reports, anaerobic bacteria have played an increasing role in brain abscess formation, accounting for almost 80% of nontraumatic brain abscesses in some series. This reflects, in part, changes in flora brought about by inadequate treatment of the primary infection using broad-spectrum antibiotics. It also results from more careful culture techniques, which have revealed the importance of anaerobic gram-negative bacilli, particularly *Bacteroides fragilis*. More than 10% of cultures will be sterile, using the best contemporary techniques. The most common isolate is *Streptococcus* with a predominance of *S. milleri* in the *viridans* group. Abscesses resulting from trauma most commonly culture *Staphylococcus aureus*. Other causative organisms are *Bacteroides*, hemolytic streptococci, *Proteus* sp., *Haemophilus influenzae*, *Escherichia coli*, and, rarely, *Cryptococcus*, *Nocardia*, *Aspergillus*, and *Corynebacterium acnes*.

The bacterial spectrum in neonates with brain abscesses differs from that in older infants and children. Nearly half the reported infections in infants less than 3 months of age have been caused by gram-negative organisms, probably because IgM does not cross the placenta. These organisms include *E. coli*. *Citrobacter*, *Proteus*, *Paracolobactrum*, and recently *Salmonella*. Brain abscesses in early infancy commonly attain enormous sizes because of the expansile skull and large subarachnoid space.

During the stage of cerebritis, antibiotics with appropriate protein and lipid binding characteristics can readily diffuse into the area of inflammatory response. Contrast studies have shown that once an abscess has formed, bacteria may still be isolated, despite measurable levels of appropriate antibiotics within the abscess. It has been postulated that the intensely acid environment associated with the necrotic debris may decrease or eliminate antimicrobial action. This mechanism may explain reported failure despite appropriate antibiotic therapy.

Signs and Symptoms

The initial symptoms of brain abscess are more likely to be related to its intracranial mass effect than to the infectious nature of the illness. Lethargy, anorexia, and vomiting are noted, and older children will complain of headache. Occasionally, there may be a distinct period of cerebritis or meningitis preceding abscess formation. Focal or grand mal seizures may be the first indication of cerebral involvement and may lead to discovery of previously unnoticed neurologic deficits. Fever may be quite mild; almost half of these children are afebrile on hospital admission, even though a history of recent febrile illness is given. Brain abscesses are usually rapidly progressive; the duration of symptoms is often less than a week and seldom more than a month. During the initial hospital examination these children are frequently lethargic or comatose, with signs of increased intracranial pressure. Specific neurologic deficits will depend on the area of involvement and may include hemiparesis, sensory impairment, and visual field abnormalities. Posterior fossa abscess will cause ataxia, dysmetria, and cranial nerve palsies.

Diagnosis

The results of routine blood studies may be normal or may reveal moderate leukocytosis and an elevated erythrocyte sedimentation rate. Skull films may indicate a chronic otorhinologic infection, and rarely there is evidence of mass effect or increased intracranial pressure.

Many reports have stressed the danger of lumbar puncture in the presence of abscess. If there are indications of increased intracranial pressure or shifting of intracranial structures, lumbar puncture is contraindicated. The information obtained from the CSF in patients with brain abscess is usually nonspecific; often the causative organisms cannot be demonstrated, and lumbar puncture may introduce a potentially fatal risk.

Invasive contrast procedures, including ventriculography, pneumoencephalography, and angiography, are of limited value for diagnosing brain abscess and are of historical interest only.

The use of CT scanning and more recently MR imaging in children with brain abscesses has been a significant advance in diagnosis and in evaluation of therapy (Fig. 25-43). Multiple lesions, which cause high mortality among patients with brain abscesses, are easily diagnosed. Dosages of steroids, antibiotics, and even mannitol may be adjusted according to the changes observed over time. Complex clinical developments in these patients during the postoperative period may be clarified by CT and/or MR scanning without having to resort to repeated invasive techniques.

CT and MR scans should be performed first without contrast enhancement. Following contrast injection, scans performed both immediately and after delay of 30 to 60 minutes will allow for more precise staging of the abscess. Steroids may reduce the contrast enhancement of abscesses, especially during the cerebritis stages. This effect of steroids should not shorten the duration of antibiotic therapy or decrease consideration of surgery if symptoms progress.

Therapy

An intracerebral abscess can act as a rapidly expanding intracranial mass because of both the purulent collection and the surrounding cerebral edema. Secondary brainstem compression can lead to coma and death in a very short time. Uncal herniation causing midbrain compression is almost uniformly found in fatal brain abscess. Therapy, therefore, is aimed at decreasing the intracerebral pressure and mass effect. Periabscess edema derives from both the local mass and the stasis effect and inflammation response that causes a diffuse increase in brain water. Steroids in large doses decrease the endothelial permeability of vessels in the inflammatory area and reduce the excessive edema. Although the restorative effect of steroids on

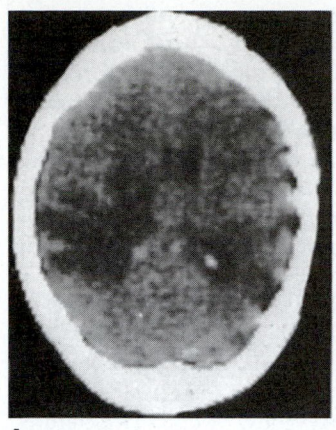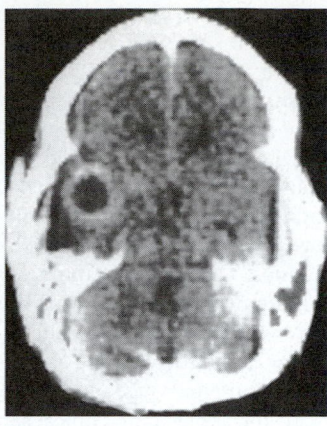

A   **B**

FIGURE 25-43   A. CT scan of a teenage girl with left temporal brain abscess. She had a dental infection drained 1 month earlier, followed by 5 days of oral tetracycline therapy. Oral antibiotics were again given when the patient became febrile 2 weeks later. At time of study she was lethargic and aphasic and had a right hemiparesis. The dark area reflects edema of the left temporal lobe and basal ganglia region. The left ventricle is compressed and shifted to the right. B. CT scan of same patient after injection of contrast material (the plane of this cross section is immediately ventral to that shown in A). An area (ring) of hypervascularity around the wall of the abscess is clearly seen. After total excision of the abscess, neurologic deficits cleared slowly, and the patient recovered fully. Culture of the abscess contents failed to grow an organism.

the blood-brain barrier may reduce antibiotic activity in the infected region, this effect is usually of lesser concern than the need to reduce increased intracranial pressure.

The initial therapy for brain abscess remains antibiotic coverage. A wide range of antibiotics that successfully penetrate the brain and the CSF is available, and a still larger group is useful when abscess permeability is increased by the inflammatory response. Gram-positive cocci are the most common organism, and they usually respond to one of the penicillins, vancomycin, or rifampin. Vancomycin is increasingly required as the incidence of methicillin-resistant *S. aureus* grows. Gram-negative aerobic bacilli may be treated with chloramphenicol, trimethoprim/sulfa, and the third-generation cephalosporins (cefotaxime and moxalactam). Finally, the important group of gram-negative anaerobic organisms, often associated with otogenic brain abscesses, will respond to metronidazole (Flagyl). Metronidazole is bactericidal for most anaerobes; it penetrates into brain abscesses well and is not degraded in purulent debris, as is chloramphenicol.

Timing of surgical intervention will depend on the response to medical therapy, knowledge of the infecting organism, the location and stage of the abscess, and the general condition of the child. Patients who have multiple small abscesses are usually best treated medically. Even large areas of cerebritis and early encapsulation may be treated with steroids and appropriate antibiotics if these patients are followed carefully by both clinical observation and serial scanning. However, the process of waiting for abscess stabilization and encapsulation places the patient at risk for abrupt brain herniation or rupture of the abscess.

Most abscesses start at the gray-white matter junction. Encapsulation proceeds more rapidly and profusely on the cortical side than on the side facing the white matter. With abscesses in paraventricular sites, rupture into the ventricle may occur at any time. Rupture of an abscess into the ventricular system carries a very high

mortality. Early aspiration of an abscess in a paraventricular locus is warranted.

Several techniques have been devised for operative treatment of abscesses, and selection of the appropriate procedure will depend on the condition of the patient, abscess location, and degree of abscess encapsulation. The patient's clinical condition at the time of operation is more important in determining result than is the choice of operative procedure. Decompression of the mass effect is the primary goal of surgery.

Aspiration of the abscess through a burr hole is preferable for severely ill children, as well as for known multiple abscesses and instances where the abscess has a thin or poorly developed wall. Serial scans are used to evaluate shrinkage of the abscess cavity, reduction in periabscess edema, and diminution of the mass effect. CT- and/or MR-assisted stereotactic equipment is available in most centers. These devices allow for the safe aspiration of even deep abscesses. Abscesses may require two or three further aspirations in the postoperative period.

Total excision can be attempted if the abscess is single, well encapsulated, and away from eloquent cortex. Excision has the advantage of immediately decompressing the mass and decreasing the risk of recurrence from remaining infected material. Excision may be delayed until aspiration and a period of antibiotic and steroid therapy allow stabilization of the cavity and formation of a thick capsule, facilitating total excision. Mortality is highest in children with cyanotic heart disease, and aggressive surgical intervention has been recommended for these patients.

Massive intravenous antibiotic therapy is required intraoperatively and for at least several weeks thereafter. Therapy can be altered as soon as sensitivity testing has been performed on the purulent material obtained at operation. Anticonvulsants should be given to all patients with supratentorial purulent lesions for at least 2 years after surgery. Seizures are frequently present during the preoperative period, and the incidence of seizures after surgery is almost 50%. The choice of operative procedure does not appear to alter the incidence of seizures.

Prognosis

In the past, high mortality from brain abscess has been related to two major factors. The most significant is late diagnosis. If diagnosis is delayed until these children are obtunded or comatose, the mortality is 65 to 90%. The second factor is the presence of multiple lesions. Mortality as high as 80% has been reported among children with multiple abscesses. The introduction of CT scanning and now MR imaging has facilitated earlier detection of these lesions, as well as definition of multiple abscesses. A dramatic decrease in mortality has already been noted in the years since CT scanning techniques have been introduced. Appreciation of the significant role played by anaerobic bacteria has led to more effective antimicrobial coverage. Mortality rates of less then 10% have been reported from several centers in recent years.

25.16.4   Spinal Abscess

Pyogenic abscesses of the spine are rare in children. Infection can occur in any of the intraspinal planes, but most infections occur in the epidural space. Subdural empyema and intramedullary spinal abscesses are rare, and when seen are often associated with a congenital dermal sinus tract or dermoid tumor.

Infection of the spinal epidural space may be metastatic, by the veins of the Batson plexus, or by direct extension from spondylitis, or from lung or perirenal infections. If a source is identified, it is often a cutaneous furuncle. Local trauma can result in a hematoma, which can provide a nidus for infection. The most common organism is *S. aureus*. For anatomic reasons, spinal abscesses are most frequent in the midthoracic and lumbar regions.

Spinal infections in children are generally more acute than are those in adults, and the symptoms may progress rapidly. Infections have been reported in which only several hours have elapsed between the onset of symptoms and the paraplegic state.

The initial complaint is usually backache, with well-defined localization of tenderness. Initially fevers may not be present but are usually seen as the condition progresses. As the purulence expands, root signs appear, and there is sharp unilateral or bilateral pain at the level of the abscess. As the pain intensifies the child may refuse to sit or walk. Sensory deficits appear, and weakness of the legs is noted. Gait difficulty, sphincteric loss, and finally paraplegia follow in rapid order. The chance of recovery after total loss of leg, bladder, and bowel functions is small; therefore, early diagnosis and surgical decompression are of great importance. Surgical consultation should be obtained early if an abscess is suspected.

Laboratory examination will usually reveal leukocytosis and an elevated erythrocyte sedimentation rate. Spine x-rays may show local spondylitis, fracture, or a paraspinal soft tissue mass. Lumbar puncture studies will demonstrate pleocytosis, elevated protein concentration, and decreased glucose concentration. However, it is important to note that lumbar punctures may be contraindicated if a lumbar epidural abscess is suspected. This is because of the potential of seeding the infection into the sterile spinal fluid if the needle traverses the abscess.

Differential considerations include spinal and paraspinal tumors such as neuroblastoma or sarcomas, transverse myelitis, discitis, spontaneous hematoma, and Guillain-Barré syndrome.

Scanning by CT or MR imaging may diagnose the disorder, and currently MR is the imaging study of choice. If CT or MR imaging are not definitive, metrizamide myelography followed by CT scanning should be performed. To avoid intrathecal spread of infection, the metrizamide is usually introduced via a C1-C2 puncture.

If an epidural or subdural collection is demonstrated, surgery should be performed immediately. Decompressive laminectomy, removal of the purulent material, and copious irrigation should be done. Antibiotic irrigation has been recommended, but systemically administered antibiotics enter the spinal epidural space easily. In general, the degree of recovery is directly related to the neurologic function at the time of surgery.

25.16.5 Intervertebral Disc Infection

Children, often in the first 5 years of life, have a syndrome of disc space infection that is unique from adults. This disc infection, or *discitis,* usually affects the lumbar spine. In this young age group the developing spinal disc has a rich blood supply coming from the vertebrae. In adolescence and into the third decade of life the disc becomes avascular, and infection to the disc space is secondary to osteomyelitis. Cultures from blood or disc-space material have been positive in less than 50%, leading some to postulate an inflammatory cause rather than an infectious cause in a portion of these children. When cultures are positive, *S. aureus* is usually the organism. Biopsy specimens typically show acute or chronic inflammation.

Children usually present with fever, back pain, and an elevated ESR. There may be quite localized back pain and tenderness on palpation. Some children may refuse to stand or walk or may be unable to do so. Severe spinal muscle spasms may lead to splinting, giving the appearance of scoliosis. A smaller group of children present with abdominal pain alone. The differential includes epidural abscess, spinal tumors, perinephric or renal infections, transverse myelitis, hematoma, and Guillain-Barré syndrome.

Discitis is most frequently diagnosed on the basis of x-ray examination, although there may be a lag in the radiologic findings and the onset of symptoms. The intervertebral space becomes narrowed, and there is demineralization of adjacent vertebral body margins. CT or MR scanning is more accurate than x-ray in this condition, and the latter usually is the test of choice. A radionuclide scan, with technetium or gallium, is usually positive. The most consistent laboratory finding is an elevation in the erythrocyte sedimentation rate.

In the appropriate clinical setting, biopsy or disc space cultures are not mandatory. Treatment is started and usually consists of intravenous administration of antibiotics, usually a penicillinase-resistant synthetic penicillin, and immobilization by a brace or body cast. A combination of 2 weeks of intravenous antibiotics followed by a month of oral antibiotics is a common regimen. Failure of the treatment plan to relieve the pain and/or fevers should prompt the consideration of needle aspiration or biopsy of the disc space. Surgery should not be required, and bracing usually continues until resolution of the symptoms, typically 3 to 4 months. Overall the outcome for discitis is excellent.

References

Antunes NL, Hariharan S, DeAngelis LM: Brain abscesses in children with cancer. Med Pediatr Oncol 31:19–21, 1998

Bizakis JG, Velegrakis GA, Papadakis CE, Karampekios SK, Helidonis ES: The silent epidural abscess as a complication of acute otitis media in children. Int J Pediatr Otorhinolaryngol 45:163–166, 1998

Britt RH, Enzmann DR: Clinical stages of human brain abscesses on serial CT scans after contrast infusion. J Neurosurg 59:972, 1983

Brook I: Brain abscess in children: microbiology and management. J Child Neurol 10:283–288, 1995

Campbell BG, Zimmerman RD: Emergency magnetic resonance of the brain. Top Magn Reson Imaging 9:208–227, 1998

Chang YC, Huang CC, Wang ST, Chio CC: Risk factor of complications requiring neurosurgical intervention in infants with bacterial meningitis. Pediatr Neurol 17:144–149, 1997

Chen CY, Huang CC, Chang YC, Chow NN, Chio CC, Zimmerman RA: Subdural empyema in 10 infants: US characteristics and clinical correlates. Radiology 207:609–617, 1998

Chen CY, Lin KL, Wang HS, Lui TN: Dermoid cyst with dermal sinus tract complicated with spinal subdural abscess. Pediatr Neurol 20:157–160, 1999

Du Lac P, Panuel M, Devred P, et al: MRI of disc space infection in infants and children. Report of 12 cases. Pediatr Radiol 20:175–178, 1990

Fischbein CA, Rosenthal A, Fischer EG, et al: Risk factors for brain abscess in patients with congenital heart disease. Am J Cardiol 34:97, 1974

Giannoni C, Sulek M, Friedman EM: Intracranial complications of sinusitis: a pediatric series. Am J Rhinol 12:173–178, 1998

Glazer PA, Hu SS: Pediatric spinal infections. Orthop Clin North Am 27:111–123, 1996

Jacobsen FS, Sullivan B: Spinal epidural abscesses in children. Orthopedics 17:1131–1138, 1994

Jain KC, Mahapatra AK: Subdural empyema due to salmonella infection. Pediatr Neurosurg 28:89–90, 1998

Jansen BR, Hart W, Schreuder O: Discitis in childhood. 12–35-year follow-up of 35 patients. Acta Orthop Scand 64:33–36, 1993

King HA: Back pain in children. Orthop Clin North Am 30:467–474, 1999

Lee WS, Puthucheary SD, Omar A: Salmonella meningitis and its complications in infants. J Paediatr Child Health 35:379–382, 1999

Lefkowitz MA, Chin LS, Couldwell WT: Pediatric intracranial epidural abscess secondary to an infected scalp vein catheter. Pediatr Neurosurg 29:297–299, 1998

Nathoo N, Nadvi SS, van Dellen JR: Cranial extradural empyema in the era of computed tomography: a review of 82 cases. Neurosurgery 44:748–753, discussion 753–744, 1999

Nathoo N, Nadvi SS, van Dellen JR, Gouws E: Intracranial subdural empyemas in the era of computed tomography: a review of 699 cases. Neurosurgery 44:529–535, discussion, 535–536, 1999

Numaguchi Y, Rigamonti D, Rothman MI, Sato S, Mihara F, Sadato N: Spinal epidural abscess: evaluation with gadolinium-enhanced MR imaging. Radiographics 13:545–559, discussion 559–560, 1993

Pattisapu JV, Pasent AD: Subdural empyemas in children. Pediatr Neurosci 13:251, 1987

Ring D, Johnston CE, Wenger DR: Pyogenic infectious spondylitis in children: the convergence of discitis and vertebral osteomyelitis. J Pediatr Orthop 15:652–660, 1995

Ryoppy S, Jaaskelainen J, Rapola J, Alberty A: Nonspecific diskitis in children. A nonmicrobial disease? Clin Orthop, 95–99, 1993

Selby R, Ramirez CB, Singh R, et al: Brain abscess in solid organ transplant recipients receiving cyclosporine-based immunosuppression. Arch Surg 132:304–310, 1997

Smith HP, Hendrick EG: Subdural empyema and epidural abscess in children. J Neurosurg 58:392, 1983

Sutton DL, Ouvrier RA: Cerebral abscess in the under 6-month age group. Arch Dis Child 58:901, 1983

Takeshita M, Kagawa M, Izawa M, Takakura K: Current treatment strategies and factors influencing outcome in patients with bacterial brain abscess. Acta Neurochir 140:1263–1270, 1998

Ventura N, Gonzalez E, Terricabras L, et al: Intervertebral discitis in children: a review of 12 cases. Int Orthop 20:32–34, 1996

25.17 NEUROMETABOLIC AND NEURODEGENERATIVE GENETIC DISEASES

Edward M. Kaye

Metabolic and degenerative diseases that affect the nervous system may be categorized in several ways. It is often helpful clinically to separate disease into disorders primarily affecting gray matter (*neurodystrophies*) and those primarily affecting white matter (*leukoencephalopathies*). Neurodystrophies will often include signs such as dementia and seizures, whereas leukodystrophies may have more subtle psychiatric manifestations and spasticity. Unfortunately this simplistic nomenclature does not account for the overlap of diseases that do not always conform to strict pathologic limitations. Other classifications divide diseases according to the organelle that is primarily affected such as: (1) lysosomal, (2) peroxisomal, and (3) mitochondrial. Yet another classification will divide neurometabolic diseases into the substrate involved: (1) lipids, (2) mucopolysaccharides, (3) glycoproteins, (4) sialic acid, (5) mucolipids, and (6) disorders of metal metabolism. The genetics of the neurometabolic disease are primarily autosomal-recessive conditions with a few X-linked disorders.

Neurodegenerative diseases may have a myriad of causes, not all of which can be classified into metabolic pathways. Several of these diseases are dominantly inherited or X-linked molecular mutations caused by an increase in the number of trinucleotide repeats. These repeating elements are CAG repeats that encode for expanded sequences of glutamine residues. The best-known example of a tri-

nucleotide repeat disorder is Huntington disease. Other neurodegenerative diseases may involve unknown pathways such as in neuroaxonal dystrophy or Hallervorden-Spatz disease. Molecular studies continue to expand our understanding and classification of both neurometabolic and neurodegenerative diseases.

NEURODYSTROPHIES

25.17.1 Lysosomal Disorders Primarily Affecting Gray Matter

Lysosomal Storage Diseases Containing Lipid

G_{M1} Gangliosidosis

G_{M1} gangliosidosis is an autosomal-recessive disorder caused by a deficiency of the lysosomal enzyme, G_{M1} ganglioside β-galactosidase. The enzyme is one of the most complicated of the lysosomal enzymes, since it requires a complex of a sphingolipid activator protein (saposin B), protective protein, and neuraminidase enzyme in order to function. The enzyme deficiency results in the accumulation of G_{M1} ganglioside within the brain and storage of galactose-containing glycoproteins and keratan sulfate within systemic organs. The β-galactosidase gene is located on chromosome 3, and numerous point mutations have been identified in cases of G_{M1} gangliosidosis. The clinical phenotype can be divided into three forms: type I (infantile), type II (juvenile), and type III (adult), but the molecular pathology does not always correlate well with the clinical phenotype.

Type I—Infantile   The type I or infantile form presents at birth or early infancy. The facial appearance is often characteristic with a depressed nasal bridge, frontal bossing, epicanthal folds, puffy eyelids, gingival hypertrophy, enlarged tongue, low-set ears, and small jaw. Peripheral and facial edema may be present. Other features include skeletal dysplasia, manifesting as thoracolumbar kyphoscoliosis, and hepatosplenomegaly. Psychomotor delay and hypotonia are apparent early, but later neurologic signs include seizures and irritability. Visual development is poor, and a cherry red macula develops after several months in at least 50% of children. Bronchopneumonia or cardiac failure often causes death within the first 2 years. The head MR imaging may show progressive atrophy and delayed myelination. Skeletal findings include hypoplasia and beaking of the vertebrae primarily affecting the lumbar and to a lesser extent the thoracic regions. Other osseous findings include diaphyseal widening and tapering of the digits. The peripheral blood smear will frequently show vacuolated lymphocytes.

Type II—Juvenile   The type II or juvenile-onset disease has a later onset, usually between 1 and 2 years, with symptoms consisting of mild bony changes but without dysmorphic features. The disease primarily affects the nervous system, manifested by gradual developmental delay, ataxia, and choreoathetoid movements. The first symptom is usually difficulty in walking and is followed by loss of speech. The skeletal findings are normally only observed in the thoracolumbar spine region with beaking of the anterior vertebrae and some hypoplasia. There is no hepatosplenomegaly. The MR imaging is usually normal, and the EEG may be slow but not diagnostic. The course is protracted, with death occurring usually within the first decade.

Type III—Adult The adult-onset disease is characterized by late-onset extrapyramidal symptoms. This disease is usually confined to the neurologic symptoms of dysarthria and dystonia without the ataxia and seizures seen in the other forms. There are no dysmorphic features, and the funduscopic examination is normal. The neuropathology of the disease is restricted to lipid deposition within the basal ganglia.

Deficiency of the β-galactosidase enzyme is also associated with another disease, *Morquio disease type B,* which presents as a generalized skeletal dysplasia without central nervous system symptoms. The phenotype is much more like the mucopolysaccharidoses despite the enzymatic defect.

Galactosialidosis This is a complicated variant of G_{M1} gangliosidosis because it involves not only a lack of G_{M1} ganglioside β-galactosidase but also neuraminidase. The biochemical defect is caused by a deficiency of the protective protein, which has been identified as cathepsin A. The gene for cathepsin A is located on chromosome 20, and several mutations have been identified in this disease. The clinical presentation is frequently a severe infantile onset with dysmorphic and neurologic features similar to infantile G_{M1}-gangliosidosis, but many milder variants have been described, making the phenotype quite heterogeneous.

G_{M2} *Gangliosidosis*

The G_{M2} gangliosidoses are a collection of lysosmal diseases associated with the accumulation of G_{M2}-gangliosidose. The disease may be caused by a deficiency of β-hexosaminidase A, β-hexosaminidase A and B, or G_{M2} ganglioside activator protein. The β-hexosaminidase enzyme is comprised of α- and β-subunits; β-hexosaminidase A contains one α- and one β-subunit, whereas β-hexosaminidase B is comprised of two β-subunits. The Tay-Sachs variant is caused by a deficiency of the α-subunit for the enzyme, which causes a loss of β-hexosaminidase A so that only the B isoform of the enzyme is biologically active. Sandhoff disease is caused by a deficiency of the β-subunit that results in the loss of both β-hexosaminidases A and B. The loss of the G_{M2} ganglioside activator protein is more difficult to diagnose because most diagnostic enzyme assays use an artificial substrate with a detergent that masks the activator deficiency. The genes encoding the β-hexosaminidase α-subunit (HEXA gene) and β-subunit (HEXB gene) are very similar in structure and have nearly 60% nucleotide and amino acid homology. Despite this similarity, the genes are encoded on two separate chromosomes, with HEXA localized to 15q23-24 and the HEXB mapping to 5q11.2-13.3. The activator protein contains 162 amino acids and is mapped to chromosome 5. All three genes have been cloned and mutations identified.

Tay-Sachs Disease (β-Hexosaminidase α-Subunit Deficiency) The infantile-onset β-hexosaminidase α-subunit deficiency (Tay-Sachs disease) begins within the first few months of life. The first symptom is an excessive startle in response to noise, tactile stimuli, or light flashes. This startle response in patients with Tay-Sachs disease, which differs from the Moro response of normal infants, consists of a quick extension of the arms and legs, frequently with clonic movements. In contrast to the Moro response, this exaggerated startle response in Tay-Sachs disease does not attenuate with stimulus repetition. As the disease progresses, motor devel-

opment slows, and previously acquired skills are frequently lost. Axial hypotonia, increased extremity tone, and hyperreflexia are common physical signs. Decreased vocalizations and loss of awareness of the environment occur as the disease progresses. A macular cherry-red spot (Fig. 25-44) occurs in over 90% of infants with this disease. The storage of lipid within the retinal ganglion cells causes a whitish discoloration of most of the retina except for the fovea, which shows the normal red color. Since the rod and cone cells in the retina do not store the ganglioside, the loss of vision that frequently occurs by the end of the first year is owed to cerebral pathology. Macrocephaly becomes apparent by the second year, presumably caused by intraneuronal storage of gangliosides and other lipids, reactive gliosis, and disturbance of fluid balance. The children may develop seizures that can be induced by auditory stimuli. Systemic organs are spared in this form of the disease. Between 2 and 3 years of age, the children are decerebrate, blind, and unable to respond to most stimuli. Feeding becomes very difficult, and constipation is a common problem. Seizures, often complicated by apnea, may worsen. Autonomic disturbances, manifesting as fever, circulatory changes in the skin, and cyanosis, frequently develop. By the age of 4 to 5 years, the children become increasingly cachectic and develop bronchopneumonias.

In the late-onset (juvenile/adult) variant, G_{M2} gangliosidosis patients, frequently of Ashkenazi Jewish background, have a very indolent clinical presentation. Although this variant has been called the "adult-onset variant," the disease usually begins in childhood. Although early gross motor development is normal, these children

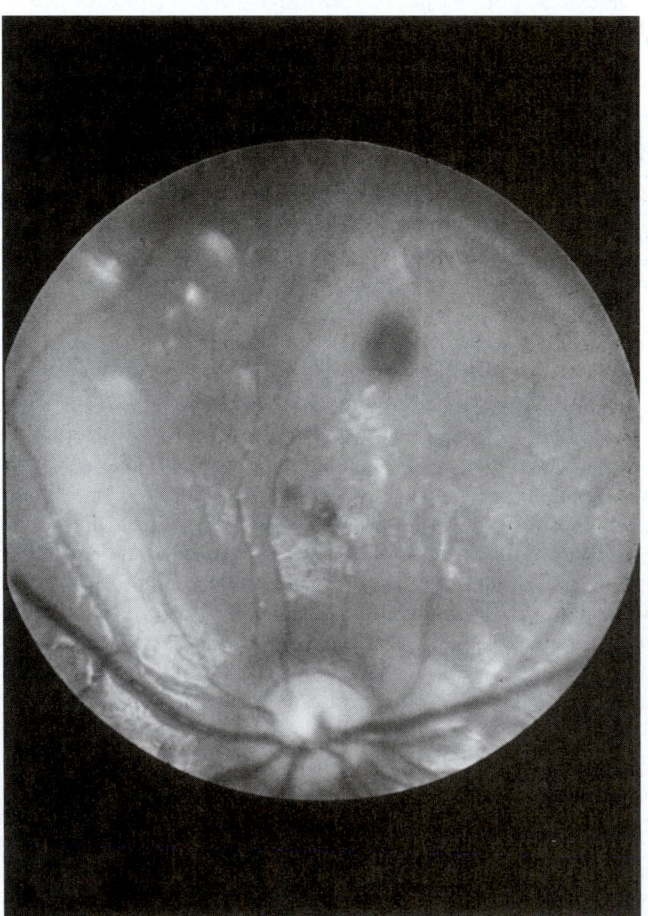

FIGURE 25-44   Cherry-red macula noted in patient with Tay-Sachs disease.

are often considered clumsy and awkward. An intention tremor, frequently seen in the first decade, may be the first indication of a neurologic problem. Dysarthria also develops early in many patients, and difficulties in school may also be apparent. A specific phenotype of late-onset G_{M2} gangliosidosis, with slowly progressive dystonia and dementia beginning in the first few years of life, has also been described. During adolescence, proximal muscle weakness begins with fasciculations and atrophy that has an appearance of juvenile-onset spinal muscular atrophy. Development of a broad-based ataxic gait usually follows, making walking even more difficult. Psychiatric symptoms may occur in nearly 50% of patients and include inattention, anxiety, paranoia, suicidal ideation, postpartum depression, catatonic schizophrenia, and occasionally episodes of hallucinations. These patients frequently are able to ambulate with assistance until the sixth decade.

Sandhoff Disease (β-Hexosaminidase β-Subunit Deficiency) The age of onset, duration, neurologic symptoms, and ophthalmologic signs in patients with Sandhoff disease are identical to those seen in Tay-Sachs disease. The only clinical differences that may rarely be present in patients with Sandhoff disease are mild hepatosplenomegaly (secondary to storage of globoside) and bony deformities. On bone marrow biopsy, foam cells have been demonstrated in a few patients.

A juvenile-onset variant occurs after age 1 year. These children begin with clumsiness and gait ataxia and later develop dystonic posturing and seizures but do not have the cherry-red macula. Adult-onset patients follow a very similar clinical course to chronic late-onset adult forms of β-hexosaminidase A deficiency.

G_{M2}-Activator Deficiency These patients have very similar clinical courses to the infantile-onset Tay-Sachs or B-variant. The storage of glycolipids and the pathologic features are also identical to what is found in the infantile-onset Tay-Sachs disease.

As the disease progresses, MR imaging demonstrates atrophy with widening of the cerebral sulci and an increase in the ventricular size, and T_1-weighted images exhibit hyperintensity in basal ganglia, thalamus, and cerebral cortex. Late-onset forms of G_{M2}-gangliosidosis have prominent cerebellar atrophy, especially of the vermis, but a normal-appearing cerebral cortex on CT or MR scans. The EEG in Tay-Sachs disease will frequently show slowing, but, when seizures develop, multifocal spikes may appear. In patients with late-onset disease, nerve conduction velocities are usually normal, but electromyograms will show a neuropathic pattern consisting of denervation with spontaneous activity and high-amplitude polyphasic motor units. The electroretinogram is normal.

Fabry Disease

Fabry disease is inherited as an X-linked deficiency of the α-galactosidase A enzyme. A deficiency or defect in the enzyme results in the accumulation of various glycosphingolipids with terminal α-galactosyl residues. The gene encoding α-galactosidase A, which is localized to Xq22, is 12 kb in length and contains 7 exons and 6 introns. The full-length cDNA has 1437 bp encoding a mature 398–amino acid subunit and a 31–amino acid signal peptide.

In affected hemizygous males, clinical symptoms usually begin in late childhood or adolescence with the development of pain in the extremities, angiokeratoma, hypohidrosis, and corneal and lenticular opacities. Because of the storage of glycolipid in the vascular system, progressive cardiac, renal, and cerebral involvement follows, mostly during the second to fourth decades. (See Sec. 9.9.)

Nervous System Findings The most dramatic symptom in Fabry disease is pain in the extremities. The sensation is usually described as an intense burning or lancinating pain occurring in the fingers or toes. There may also be mild persistent numbness and paresthesia in the extremities (acroparesthesia), which is interspersed with the episodic excruciating pain. The painful crises may last for several days and be associated with fever and increased erythrocyte sedimentation rate. Autonomic nervous system dysfunction occurs, manifest as chronic diarrhea, constipation, nausea, exaggerated gastrocolic reflex, reduced cutaneous flare response, and hypohidrosis. The symptoms related to cerebrovascular complications include hemiparesis, vertigo, diplopia, dysarthria, nystagmus, headache, ataxia, memory loss, and hemisensory loss. The vertebrobasilar system was affected in 67% of hemizygotes and 60% of symptomatic heterozygotes with elongation and tortuosity of vertebral and basilar vessels noted angiographically.

Angiokeratomas consist of clusters of individual ectatic blood vessels covered by a few layers of skin. These lesions are flat or slightly raised, dark red to blue in color, and are usually located in the groin, buttocks, upper legs, and umbilical regions (Fig. 25-45). The angiokeratomas become apparent in childhood and gradually increase in size and number over the years. Angiectasias may also occur in the oral mucosa and conjunctiva. The hair is usually described as sparse or fine. Hypertrophic cardiomyopathy may occur without other clinical manifestations of Fabry disease. Mitral valve insufficiency is a common occurrence, and arrhythmias and electrocardiogram changes are often noted. Because of endothelial storage in coronary vessels, myocardial ischemia and infarction are frequent late manifestations of this disorder. Respiratory symptoms are usually not considered prominent manifestations of Fabry disease, but with age patients complain of dyspnea, cough, and wheezing that

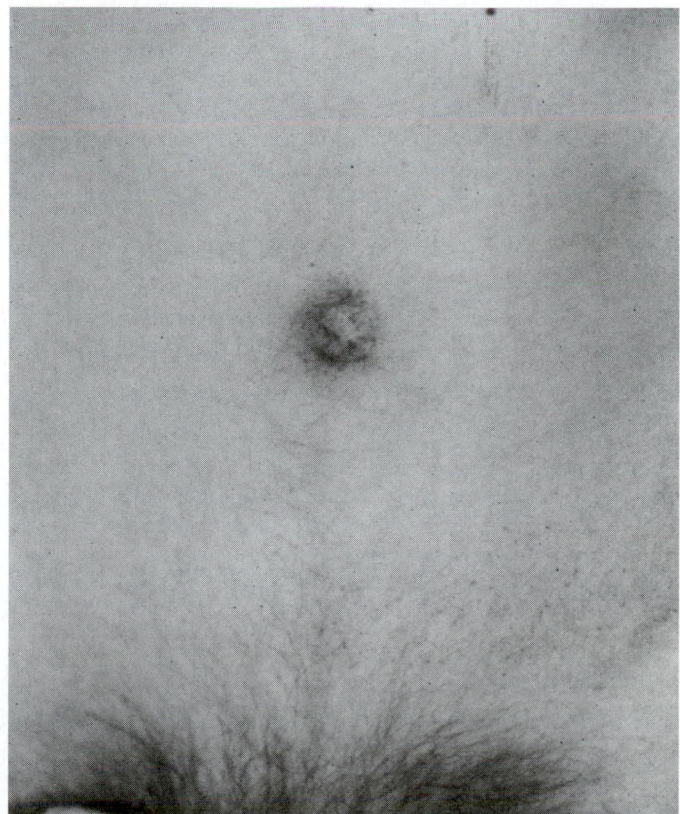

FIGURE 25-45   **Angiokeratoma present in skin below umbilicus.**

is independent of their smoking status. This population also has higher incidence of spontaneous pneumothorax and occasionally hemoptysis. The pulmonary symptoms are postulated to be owed to fixed narrowing of airways from glycosphingolipid accumulation. Because of lipid storage within the renal glomeruli and tubules, proteinuria and renal failure develop gradually. Inspection of the urine will often demonstrate casts and *Maltese crosses,* which are birefringent lipid globules. Deterioration of renal function develops, with azotemia and death occurring in the third to fifth decades unless treatment with chronic hemodialysis or renal transplantation is provided. Corneal opacity, which can be seen only by slit-lamp examination, is usually the first ocular abnormality. These corneal changes, which are present in essentially all hemizygous Fabry patients, first appear as a mild generalized clouding in the subepithelial corneal layer and may progress to form whorled streaks. Lenticular opacities may occur in approximately 30% of affected males and consist of granular anterior capsular and subcapsular deposits, or a characteristic posterior capsular spoke-like opacity (*Fabry cataract*). The corneal and lenticular opacities, however, do not interfere with vision. Retinal and conjunctival lesions, manifesting as tortuous and dilated vessels, may occur as part of a diffuse systemic vascular involvement.

Heterozygous Females Heterozygous females may have mild symptoms of the disease. Approximately 70 to 80% of affected females will have corneal opacities, but only rarely will cataracts be noted. In approximately 30% of females a few angiokeratomas may be present in the characteristic location. Intermittent pain and paresthesia may occur, and rarely, cardiac and renal symptoms may develop. A few heterozygotes have had clinical symptoms comparable to those found in affected males, thought to be related to random X-inactivation.

Diagnostic Studies The MR imaging will show a hyperintensity in the periventricular white matter early in the disease, with the development of subcortical and cortical strokes over time. Nerve conduction studies reveal an elevated threshold to current perception but no changes in the nerve conduction velocity. Enzyme analysis for the deficient α-galactosidase enzyme can be performed on leukocytes.

Treatment The painful peripheral neuropathy can often be relieved by anticonvulsants such as carbamazepine or gabapentin. Renal transplant is often required when end-stage renal disease is present.

Two experimental therapeutic strategies are currently undergoing clinical trials. The first uses recombinantly engineered enzyme, which is administered intravenously. It is unknown how effective this therapy will be to ameliorate the nervous system symptoms in Fabry disease. Another approach is the use of a glycosphingolipid synthesis inhibitor *N*-butyldeoxynojirimycin to reduce the amount of glycolipid being produced. This drug is known to enter the central nervous system.

Gaucher Disease

Gaucher disease is an autosomal-recessive disease that results from a deficiency of the lysosomal enzyme β-glucosidase, which leads to accumulation of the glycolipid glycosylceramide. The disease is divided into three main clinical phenotypes: type 1 (nonneuronopathic), type II (infantile onset, acute neuronopathic), and type III juvenile onset, chronic neuronopathic). The presence and rapidity

of neurologic symptoms are the major factors in determining the clinical subtype of this disease. Type I nonneuronopathic disease does not manifest any neurologic symptoms but often presents in childhood because of the massive hepatosplenomegaly. (See Sec. 9.9.)

Clinical Presentation of Gaucher Disease Affecting the Nervous System Type II disease is a rare disease that presents in infancy with dramatic brainstem findings that include *retroflexion* of the neck, *strabismus,* and *trismus* in addition to hepatosplenomegaly. These children become symptomatic usually before 6 months. There is a persistent retroflexion of the neck which is characteristic. Strabismus, caused by cranial nerve palsies, dysphagia, and trismus are also present. Massive splenomegaly and, to a lesser extent, hepatomegaly are present early in the course. Because of the severe brainstem involvement in type II, these children frequently die by age 2.

Type III disease presents at varied times, ranging from early life to preteen years. There appear to be two clinical presentations in the type III disease. The first presentation, sometimes referred to as *type 3a,* is typical of patients from the Norrbottenian region in northern Sweden. These patients often come to medical attention because of splenomegaly and liver enlargement. Affected children progress to develop eye findings consisting of oculomotor apraxia or convergent squint and later develop ataxia, loss of intellectual function, and seizures. The intellectual decline is not apparent early in the disease, but slow cognitive regression occurs through childhood and adolescence. Seizures are often myoclonic and may develop into a myoclonic encephalopathy. Isolated horizontal supranuclear gaze palsy, without other neurologic manifestations, may be associated with severe systemic features in type III Gaucher disease referred to as *type 3b.* Type 3b patients appear to have very aggressive systemic features with prominent hepatic, skeletal, and cardiorespiratory complications from the Gaucher disease and often die in childhood or early adolescence. Because of the slow progression of neurologic symptoms, early in the course of Gaucher disease it may not be possible to differentiate type I from type III individuals. In one family, for instance, acute neuronopathic and chronic nonneuronopathic forms were identified in full siblings. Also, on rare occasions the neurologic features may antedate the appearance of hepatosplenomegaly. Vascular involvement that included fibrosis of ascending aorta and coronary arteries has been noted in type III Gaucher disease.

Neuropathologic Features Similar to what has been described in type II disease: Patients with type III Gaucher disease have nerve cell loss and neuronophagia primarily in brainstem, cerebellum, and spinal cord. The presence of specialized cells containing glucosylceramide, "Gaucher cells," have also been recorded from these areas which correlate with the accumulation of glucosylceramide in brain.

Neurophysiological Studies On brainstem auditory evoked potentials, only the presence of waves I and II are present in children with severe neurologic involvement from Gaucher disease. The electroencephalogram in type III children is typically characterized as having a slow background with multifocal spike-wave discharges and often a photoparoxysmal response.

Diagnostic Tests Although skin biopsies have been very helpful in identifying most patients with lysosomal storage diseases, patients with Gaucher disease, including type III patients, do not have any evidence of lysosomal storage in examination of skin. Bone marrow aspirates show the typical "Gaucher cell," a specialized histiocyte containing the glucosylceramide (Fig. 25-46). Enzymatic study for glucocerebrosidase activity is the standard diagnostic tool in types II and III patients. It is not possible, however, to differentiate individuals with type I versus type III disease based simply on the enzymatic activity. Also, rarely, type III patients may have a deficiency of saposin C, one of two activators necessary for glucocerebroside enzyme function.

Genetics In the Norrbottenian form of type III Gaucher disease, it appears that a single founder dating back at least to the sixteenth century can explain the high incidence noted in this region of Sweden. The characteristic genotype for type III disease is a homozygous mutation in exon 10, a leucine to proline substitution in codon 444, although some Italian and Japanese families have been reported to have a G6490A substitution also in exon 10.

Treatment Splenectomy had been used in the past to avoid complications of splenic enlargement in type III Gaucher disease. It became apparent, however, that patients treated in this way at an earlier age had lower average IQ scores than those in which splenectomy was postponed to a latter stage in the disease. Bone marrow transplantation has been used with successful results in type I disease; however, in type III patients, conflicting outcomes have been noted using bone marrow replacement, with perhaps the best results occurring in the Norrbottenian form of the disease. Most recently, macrophage-targeted enzyme replacement has been used

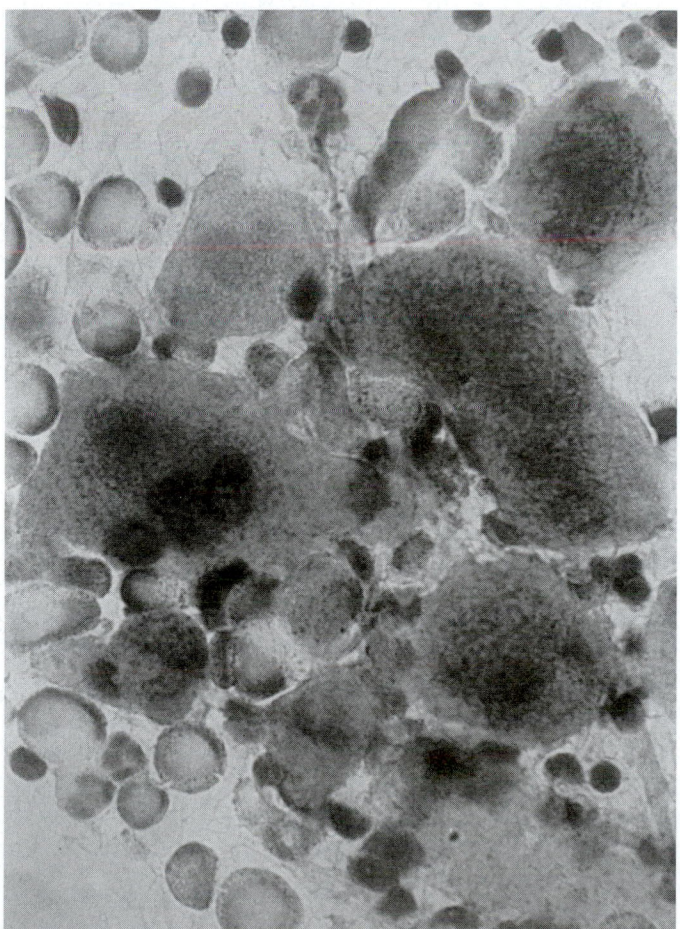

FIGURE 25-46   Gaucher cell noted on bone marrow aspirate.

in type III Gaucher disease. Although this therapy is very successful in type I disease, it is unclear to what extent enzyme therapy will be useful to treat neurologic involvement. In the Swedish patients, it appears that enzyme therapy reduces glucosylceramide levels in blood and causes a regression of systemic symptoms with a stabilization of neurologic features.

Niemann-Pick Diseases

Niemann-Pick disease is not a single disease but consists of two genetically distinct disorders. Because of the historical background, these diseases are likely to continue to be included together. Niemann-Pick A and B are caused by an autosomal-recessive deficiency of the gene that encodes the enzyme sphingomyelinase, which is needed to degrade sphingomyelin. Neimann-Pick A is associated with severe hepatosplenomegaly and an infantile-onset neurologic presentation. Niemann-Pick type B is a slowly progressive disorder that does not appear to affect the nervous system to any great extent. Niemann-Pick C is a disease that affects cholesterol trafficking and not a disorder of sphingomyelin, although some sphingomyelin storage occurs. (See Sec. 9.9.)

Niemann-Pick A

Clinical Features Niemann-Pick type A begins in early infancy, usually in the first 6 months. First symptoms are often vomiting, diarrhea, and failure to thrive. Prominent and progressive hepatosplenomegaly, with liver being greater than spleen, occurs in most cases before 3 to 4 months of age, and sometimes in the neonatal period. There are no dysmorphic features or skeletal abnormalities, but often a brownish pigmentation of the skin may be present. Neurologic symptoms usually do not occur until 5 to 10 months of age. The child demonstrates hypotonia, progressive loss of acquired motor skills, loss of interest in the surroundings, and reduction in spontaneous movements. Axial hypotonia and pyramidal signs are usually present. The disease inexorably progresses to severe cachexia, blindness, dysphagia, rigidity, and psychomotor regression. Macular cherry-red spots may be found in about half of the cases but rarely before an advanced stage of the neurologic disease. Seizures may occur in the later stages of the disease but are not a major sign. Recurrent respiratory infections are a common complication. Death classically occurs between 1.5 and 3.0 years of age.

Diagnostic Studies Bone marrow aspiration shows a characteristic lipid containing "foamy" macrophages, and vacuolated lymphocytes are present in the peripheral blood smears. In the nerve conduction studies, the nerve conduction velocity is generally slowed. The CSF is normal. MR imaging and EEG may be abnormal but typically are not diagnostic for this disease. The diagnosis is based on the finding of low levels of sphingomyelinase in leukocytes or cultured fibroblasts. Molecular testing will become a more frequent diagnostic method as testing becomes more widely available.

Genetics The gene encoding sphingomyelinase is localized on human chromosome 11p15.1-15.4. The full-length cDNA codes for a polypeptide of 630 amino acids. The gene is relatively small, approximately 7 kb, and consists of only 6 exons. A number of mutations have been discovered, with three mutations, R496L, L302P, fsP330, occurring frequently in the Ashkenazi Jewish population.

Treatment Treatment is purely symptomatic at this time.

Niemann-Pick C

Niemann-Pick type C (NPC) is not an allelic variant of Niemann-Pick types A and B but actually a separate disease that is not involved in sphingomyelinase metabolism. Because of the foamy macrophages and hepatosplenomegaly, it was placed into the category of Niemann-Pick before molecular genetic studies were able to categorize the disease as a defect in cholesterol trafficking.

Neonatal Onset   Approximately 50% of neonates affected with NPC are asymptomatic; in the remaining cases, liver disease is the major sign. Fetal hydrops (rarely) and fetal ascites (more frequently) can be observed. Prolonged neonatal cholestatic jaundice associated with progressive hepatosplenomegaly is present in about half of the cases. Although the liver disease is usually self-limited and may spontaneously resolve by 2 to 4 months of age, about 10% of the cases progress to a rapidly fatal liver failure. Children with this dramatic "acute" neonatal cholestatic rapidly fatal form die before the age of 6 months but do not show neurologic symptoms. Rare cases with a severe neonatal respiratory failure have also been described. In infants and young children, (hepato)splenomegaly may be the only sign of the disease for a number of years.

Late Infantile and Juvenile Onset   Most cases of NPC are the late-infantile and the juvenile neurologic onset forms. In children 3 to 5 years of age, neurologic manifestations consist of an ataxic gait, in addition to spleno- or hepatosplenomegaly. In children 6 to 12 years, poor school performance and impaired fine-motor movements are usually the first symptoms. Seizures or cataplexy may occasionally be the presenting symptom. In at least 10% of the cases, organomegaly may not be apparent. Later symptoms include ataxia and dysarthria. Cataplexy, which may be accompanied by narcolepsy, is a common and specific sign. Seizures (absences, partial and generalized seizures) usually develop. The most characteristic sign in NPC is supranuclear vertical gaze palsy (downward, upward, or both). Voluntary vertical eye movement is lost, but reflex eye movement (doll's eyes phenomenon) is preserved. Parents may notice compensatory head thrust when the child wants to look downward or upward. Choreoathetoid movements and dystonic postures may occur. Dysphagia is prominent, often requiring a feeding tube. As the disease progresses, pyramidal signs and spasticity usually develop. Psychiatric symptoms are also frequently noted. Many of these patients die in their teenage years, with a trend for patients with a late-infantile onset to die earliest.

Genetics   There are at least two genes involved in NPC. The most common gene for NPC, called *NPC1,* is mapped to chromosome 18q11 and accounts for at least 95% of cases with NPC. The minor NPC2 gene has been excluded from this region, but its location remains unknown. The NPC1 cDNA sequence predicts a 1278–amino acid protein, with 13 to 16 possible transmembrane

regions. The NPC1 protein exhibits homologies to the morphogen receptor PATCHED and the putative sterol-sensing regions of SREBP cleavage-activating protein (SCAP) and 3-hydroxy-3-methyl-glutaryl coenzyme A (HMG-CoA) reductase. The Niemann-Pick C disease mutation appears to block intracellular relocation and utilization of lysosomal cholesterol, but the primary site of disruption is not known. The synthesis of endogenous cholesterol does not appear to be affected. A number of mutations have been discovered in NPC patients.

Diagnostic Studies   Foam cells and sea-blue histiocytes may be present in bone marrow. Ultrastructural studies on conjunctival, skin, liver, or rectal biopsies can provide strong support to the diagnosis. Analysis of the lipids in a liver biopsy, which traditionally was the most specific test, may also be inconclusive. Sphingomyelinase activity is often partially deficient in cultured skin fibroblasts but normal in leukocytes. Imaging and neurophysiological studies are nonspecific. MR and CT scans may be normal or show cerebellar or cortical atrophy or, in the severe infantile form, white matter changes. The most accurate diagnostic test is the demonstration of intralysosomal accumulation of unesterified cholesterol. This defect in esterification of cholesterol is demonstrated by an intense perinuclear fluorescence after staining with filipin (a probe forming specific complexes with unesterified cholesterol) combined with intracellular cholesterol homeostasis studies using low-density lipoprotein-induced cholesterol esterification.

Treatment   Treatment has been attempted with medication to reduce cholesterol, but this has not been effective.

Neuronal Ceroid Lipofuscinoses

Although not usually classified as a lysosomal storage disease, neuronal ceroid lipofuscinosis (NCL) or ceroid neuronal lipofuscinosis (CNL) can be considered a lysosomal storage disorder because the autofluorescent lipopigment stores within the lysosome. These diseases are best classified as a nosology of several related disorders and not a single disease. Recent clinical and genetic studies have allowed a more accurate disease classification. Despite the lysosomal accumulation being ubiquitously present in all tissues, only neurons appear to be pathologically affected. The disorder may be divided into five major subtypes (Table 25-29): (1) *infantile* (Santavuori-Haltia, CNL1), (2) *late infantile* (Jansky-Bielschowsky, CNL 2), (3) juvenile (Spielmeyer-Vogt, CNL3), (4) *late infantile variant* CNL5), and (5) *adult* (Kufs CNL4).

The diagnostic test most frequently used is electron microscopy of tissues that have included skin, conjunctiva, leukocytes, and rectal ganglion cells. These electron microscopic inclusions consist of: (1) *granular* material with *nonosmiophilic globules,* (2) *fingerprint profiles* consisting of tightly bound laminated bodies, (3) *curvilinear bodies* that are looser laminar bodies, and (4) *pure granular*

TABLE 25-29

NEURONAL CEROID LIPOFUSCINOSIS VARIANTS

VARIANT	EPONYMS	GENE NAME	GENE PRODUCT	CHROMOSOME
Infantile	Santavuori-Haltia	CNL1	Palmitoyl protein thioesterase	1p32
Late infantile	Jansky-Bielschowsky	CNL2	Tripeptidyl peptidase	11p15
variant		CNL5	"Battenin"	13q21.1-32
Juvenile	Spielmeyer-Vogt	CNL3	Membrane protein	16p12
Adult	Kufs	CNL4	Unknown	Unknown

profiles. The electron microscopic findings correlate roughly to the clinical subtype, with fingerprint profiles noted in the juvenile onset and curvilinear bodies noted primarily in late infantile form.

The clinical presentation varies among the different forms of CNL:

Infantile (CNL1) begins in the first 1 to 2 years following a period of normal development and is associated with psychomotor retardation, myoclonic seizures, and macular degeneration.

Late infantile (CNL2) begins typically in the second and third years and is associated with myoclonic seizures, developmental delay, ataxia, and pigmentary retinal degeneration.

Late infantile variant (CLN5) may begin at age 4 or 5 and progresses to develop visual failure, ataxia, and myoclonic seizures.

Juvenile (CNL3) begins in the later half of the first decade with a rod–cone dystrophy and later myoclonic seizures, ataxia, dystonia, and gradual cognitive decline.

Adult-onset (CNL4) may not occur until the second or third decade with prominent psychiatric features and late-occurring myoclonic seizures; visual problems often are absent.

The biochemical and genetic etiology depends on the variant. CNL1 is associated with a palmitoyl protein thioesterase deficiency that results in the storage of saposins A and D. The gene is located on chromosome 1, and a common mutation has been an A to T transversion at position 364. The gene for CNL2 encodes a tripeptidyl peptidase I that cleaves tripeptides from the N-terminus of polypeptides. The gene is located at chromosome 11p15. Storage of subunit c of mitochondrial protein ATP synthase has been noted in this variant. CNL3 is associated with a transmembrane protein deficiency. This protein localizes to the Golgi apparatus and may be involved in protein packaging or transport. Subunit c storage also occurs in this clinical subtype. The chromosome localization for the gene is 16p12, and a common 1.02-kb deletion has been found in many patients in addition to point mutations. The genetic basis for CNL5 is thought to be localized to 13q21.1-q32, which encodes a novel transmembrane protein "Battenin." Mutations in the gene for Battenin have been found in families with this variant. CNL4 continues to remain an enigma.

Lysosomal Disorders Containing Mucopolysaccharides

The mucopolysaccharidoses (MPS) are inherited lysosomal enzyme (MPS) deficiencies that result in the storage of glycosaminoglycans. The mucopolysaccharides affected in these disorders are heparan sulfate, dermatan sulfate, keratan sulfate, and chondroitin sulfate. The systemic storage that is common to many of these disorders is not present at birth but becomes more obvious especially after a year of age. Coarse or "gargoyle-like" facial features, dysostosis multiplex, hepatosplenomegaly, hernias, and recurrent respiratory infections are prominent features. The mucopolysaccharidoses that store heparan sulfate are associated with mental retardation and other neurologic features. These diseases include Hurler, Hunter, Sanfilippo, and, to a lesser extent, Sly disease. The other mucopolysaccharidoses are not associated with central nervous system storage but may cause central nervous system injury secondary to the skeletal abnormalities. The mucopolysaccharidoses are discussed in detail in Sec. 9.8.

Hurler Disease

Hurler disease is an autosomal-recessive condition that is mapped to chromosome 4p16.3. The gene encodes the enzyme α-L-id-

uronidase, which is required to degrade both heparan sulfate and dermatan sulfate. This disease is the prototype for all the other mucopolysaccharidoses. The physical appearance may not be apparent until the second year of life. Coarsening of the facial features include frontal bossing, depressed nasal bridge, coarse hair and skin, and thick eyebrows. Because of the skeletal abnormalities, short stature, lumbar kyphosis and scoliosis, claw hands, and joint stiffness are apparent. The multiple bone deformities are called *dysostosis multiplex* and consist of narrowing of the vertebrae; beaking, especially of anterior vertebrae; flaring of the ribs, flaring of the metaphysis of the long bones; and acetabular hypoplasia. Other findings include hepatosplenomegaly, repeated respiratory infections, myocardial thickening and valvular disease, and corneal clouding. Hearing loss, which is usually a combined conduction and sensorineural hearing loss, is present. Visual loss from retinal degeneration, rod dystrophy more than cone dystrophy, is a common occurrence. Specific neurologic complications include communicating hydrocephalus, which appears to be related to accumulation of mucopolysaccharides within the meninges, and spinal cord compression caused by thickening of the dura, which is referred to as *pachymeningitis cervicalis* (Fig. 25-47). Compression neuropathies, especially carpal tunnel syndrome, are common. *Scheie syndrome* is a milder allelic variant of the same enzyme deficiency. Diagnosis can be made on the basis of leukocyte enzyme analysis for α-L-iduronidase activity and urine for mucopolysaccharide excretion. Molecular genetic studies have revealed that the gene for the α-L-iduronidase enzyme is mapped to chromosome 4p16.3 disease, and numerous mutations have been described in affected individuals. Treatment has been attempted using bone marrow transplantation, which will ameliorate many of the systemic complications such as hepatosplenomegaly, upper airway obstruction, and coarse facial features. Hearing may be maintained or improved following transplantation. Intellectual decline appears to be halted if the transplantation is performed early, but dysostosis multiplex is not improved.

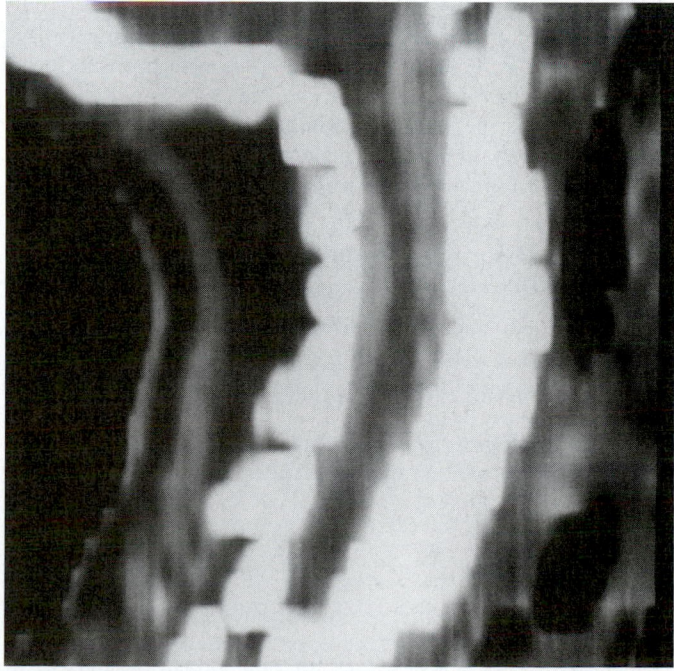

FIGURE 25-47   Thickening of dura in patient with Hurler disease with cervical spinal cord compression.

Hunter Disease

Hunter disease is the only X-linked inherited mucopolysaccharidosis. The phenotype is similar but milder to Hurler disease. A few differences from Hurler disease aid in the diagnosis. Specifically, corneal clouding does not occur in Hunter disease, and there is often a characteristic skin finding that consists of pebbly, ivory-colored lesions that may be found over the scapula, upper arms, and lateral thighs. The neurologic features may be similar to those found in Hurler disease. As in Hurler disease, heparan and dermatan sulfate are increased in urine. The deficient enzyme is iduronidate-2-sulfatase, which is localized to the Xq28 region. DNA testing is possible and can be helpful for carrier detection.

Sanfilippo Disease

Sanfilippo disease is by far the most difficult mucopolysaccharidosis to clinically diagnose. The lack of significant coarsening, skeletal changes, and hepatosplenomegaly until late in the disease often discourages clinicians from considering Sanfilippo disease in the differential of a mentally retarded child. The most common presentation is mental delay associated with hyperactivity and aggressive behavior. Corneal opacity is usually not observable, but hearing loss and pigmentary retinal degeneration (rod–cone dystrophy) may be present. Sanfilippo disease is categorized into four separate diseases based on the enzyme deficiency: type A, heparan-N-sulfatase; type B, N-acetyl-α-D-glucosaminidase; type C, acetyl-CoA:α-glucosaminide N-acetyltransferase; and type D, N-acetyl-α-D-glucosamine-6-sulfatase. The type A patients appear to be the most severely affected. Excess amounts of heparan sulfate is usually present in urine, although random spot tests may be falsely negative. Bone marrow transplantation has been used in this disease but needs to be done before significant mental retardation is present if a reasonable outcome is to be expected.

Sly Disease

Sly disease is similar to Hurler but has a much milder phenotype with the exception of a severe neonatal form. Many patients have been described living into adulthood. Coarse metachromatic inclusions within leukocytes are a characteristic finding. The disease is caused by a deficiency of β-glucuronidase enzyme, which results in the excess urinary secretion of heparan sulfate, dermatan sulfate, and chondroitin sulfate. The gene is localized to 7q21.1-q22.

Lysosomal Disorders Containing Glycoproteins

These disorders affect glycoprotein degradation and include *α-mannosidosis, β-mannosidosis, fucosidosis,* and *aspartylglucosaminuria.* These diseases have many clinical similarities to the mucopolysaccharidoses except for the lack of mucopolysaccharide excretion in the urine. It is now known that these four diseases contain large amounts of neutral oligosaccharides within urine and other organs. (See Sec. 9.8.3.)

α-Mannosidosis

The clinical presentation of α-mannosidosis may be similar to Hurler disease, especially in the infantile-onset forms. Lenticular and corneal opacities may be present. The milder juvenile variant may have hearing loss as an early finding, with mild dysmorphic features and a slowly progressive neurologic course. Urine studies demonstrate excess oligosaccharides. The gene has been cloned and is found on chromosome 19q with mutations identified.

β-Mannosidosis

β-Mannosidosis appears to have a less acute phenotype when compared to α-mannosidosis. Mental retardation and hearing loss may be the major manifestation with only slight systemic signs. Angiokeratoma and tortuous retinal vessels are other helpful clinical signs. Urinary oligosaccharides are also increased. The gene encoding β-mannosidosis consists of a 3.7-kb transcript and is mapped to chromosome 4.

Fucosidosis

Fucosidosis demonstrates accumulation of fucose-containing oligosaccharides in addition to glycolipids and glycoproteins. Although the clinical phenotype is similar to the mucopolysaccharidoses, a unique skin finding is the presence of angiokeratomas. These angiokeratomas are similar in location to those in Fabry disease, primarily affecting the genitalia, periumbilical region, buttocks, and thighs. The structural gene for α-fucosidase has been assigned to chromosome 1p34.1-1p36.1, and the cDNA is 2.3 kb.

Aspartylglucosaminuria

Aspartylglucosaminuria primarily is associated with mental retardation and later presentation of coarse features and skeletal abnormalities. Acne and photosensitivity may be present. The enzyme N-aspartyl-β-glucosaminidase is deficient. This enzyme is encoded by a gene mapped to 4q32-33. The disease is rare but more commonly reported in Finland.

Lysosomal Disorders Containing Sialic Acid

Sialic acid storage diseases can be considered a subset of the glycoprotein degradation disorders. The nomenclature for these diseases has been confusing because the first description of a sialic acid storage disease was called *mucolipidosis type 1,* which we now know is sialidosis caused by a deficiency of the enzyme α-neuraminidase. In addition to α-neuraminidase deficiency, there are other disorders of sialic acid which may be caused by (1) sialic acid transport within the lysosome or (2) a defect in the rate-limiting response of the synthetic sialic acid enzyme to cytidine monophosphate-NANA (see also Sec. 9.8.3).

Sialidosis

Sialidosis is an autosomal-recessive inherited disorder that results in the deficiency of α-neuraminidase. This disease may present at various ages with a fetal or congenital variant that presents as hydrops fetalis, a severe infantile onset, and, the most common, an adolescent onset with cherry-red spot and myoclonus. As mentioned in the section on G_{M1} gangliosidosis, a subset of G_{M1} gangliosidosis results from the loss of the protective protein, cathepsin A, which is required for both β-galactosidase and α-neuraminidase to function. If the cathepsin A protein is deficient, both enzymes will be unable to degrade the substrates, and the phenotype that results will be similar to the infantile-onset sialidosis. The *infantile-onset* disorder of sialidosis (sialidosis type II) has slowly progressive intellectual retardation, hepatosplenomegaly, angiokeratoma, reduced muscle mass, hypotonia, ataxia, sensory-neural hearing loss, coarse facies, inguinal hernias, dysostosis multiplex, and the cherry-red macula. The *late-onset* forms of sialidosis (sialidosis type I) will have myoclonic epilepsy and the cherry-red macula that typically begins in the third decade; these forms are not associated with any significant mental deterioration.

The diagnosis can be made by the excess quantities of protein-bound sialic acid in urine and in the case of galactosialidosis oligosaccharide excretion. The definitive testing requires the analysis of the α-neuraminidase enzyme in cultured fibroblasts or of both α-neuraminidase and β-galactosidase in the case of galactosialidosis. Genetic testing is available, since the gene for α-neuraminidase, which is mapped to 6p21.3, has been cloned and mutations identified.

Sialic Acid Storage Disorders

Sialic acid storage disorders are comprised of two separate diseases (1) a lysosomal sialic acid storage disease caused by a defect in lysosomal transport of sialic acid, and (2) sialuria, which is associated with massive sialuria and storage of sialic acid within the cytoplasm but not the lysosomes.

Sialic Acid Storage Disease (Lysosomal) Sialic acid storage disease is a defect in the lysosomal trafficking of sialic acid. There are often descriptions of infantile and juvenile sialic acid storage disease and Salla disease. These three diseases are thought to be allelic variants of the same disease. The infants with sialic acid may have onset prior to birth with a nonimmune hydrops presentation. The diagnosis is made on the basis of free sialic acid in urine and vacuoles that can be found in skin and leukocytes. Salla disease is named after a region in northern Finland where most of the cases have been identified. Mental retardation, seizures, ataxia, and mild coarsening of the features without skeletal changes are typical. The disease is very slowly progressive, and the life span is nearly normal. The gene for Salla disease is mapped to 6q14-15.

Sialuria Evidence derived from studies of cultured fibroblasts suggests that the metabolic defect in sialuria consists of a loss in sensitivity of the rate-limiting enzyme in NANA synthesis, uridinediphosphate-N-acetylglucosamine 2-epimerase (UDP-GlcNAc 2-epimerase), to feedback regulation by cytidine monophosphate (CMP)-NANA. Sialic acid is not stored with the lysosomes but rather is increased in the cytosolic fraction. These patients excrete massive quantities of free sialic acid in the urine. The clinical phenotype may be more subtle than the sialic acid storage diseases with macrocephaly, slightly coarse features, hepatosplenomegaly, macroglossia, and developmental delay. Mutations have been found in the gene for UDP-GlcNAc 2-epimerase in sialuria patients. The gene maps to chromosome 9.

Lysosomal Disorders Containing Mucolipids

The mucolipidoses were named after a group of diseases with a clinical phenotype consistent with a mucopolysaccharidosis, but no excretion of mucopolysaccharides could be detected within urine. Mucolipidosis I was determined to be a sialic acid disorder with a deficiency of α-neuraminidase. *Mucolipidoses types II and III* are allelic variants of the same disease caused by a deficiency of the enzyme N-acetylglucosamine-1-phosphotransferase. This enzyme is required for the placement of mannose-6-phosphate onto several acid hydrolase enzymes. The mannose phosphate moiety is required as a recognition marker for these enzymes to properly enter the lysosome, and without this marker the enzymes cannot be processed into the lysosome. Serum levels of enzymes are increased while cultured fibroblast enzyme activities are markedly decreased.

Almost all the lysosomal hydrolases, with the exception of β-glucosidase and acid phosphatase, require this enzyme for lysosomal localization. The gene, designated GNPTA, is mapped to 4q21-23.

Mucolipidosis II (I Cell Disease)

Mucolipidosis is usually apparent in the neonatal period, unlike the mucopolysaccharidoses, and presents with facial edema, swelling of the gums, coarse facial features, dislocation of the hips, and mental retardation. The skin biopsy for electron microscopy is usually quite abnormal demonstrating storage of a variety of materials. The name *I cell* is derived form the term *inclusion cell,* which highlights the importance of the pathologic findings on biopsy samples. The finding of elevated serum levels of several lysosomal enzymes and decreased levels of activity in fibroblasts confirms the diagnosis. The N-acetylglucosamine-1-phosphotransferase can also be measured to make the diagnosis.

Mucolipidosis III

Mucolipidosis III is an allelic variant of mucolipidosis II. The clinical findings are much milder with presentation frequently not apparent until the middle of the first decade or later. Joint contractures and bone changes often suggest a connective tissue disease, and these children may present for a rheumatologic evaluation. Peripheral nerve entrapments are common, and usually only mild intellectual involvement is present. The skeletal changes are usually much milder that that seen in the mucopolysaccharidoses. The biochemical and diagnostic studies are identical to mucolipidosis II.

Mucolipidosis IV

Mucolipidosis IV is an unknown disorder of lipid metabolism that consists of the triad of (1) *corneal clouding,* (2) *retinal degeneration,* and (3) profound *mental retardation.* The disease is apparent between 3 and 8 months. Corneal opacity is usually seen in infancy. There are no systemic findings such as skeletal dysplasia, facial coarseness, or organomegaly. The head growth is small, and no abnormalities in urinary mucopolysacchride, oligosaccharide, or sialic acid excretion are found. The disease is protracted, and children may live to adulthood. The diagnosis can only be made with an electron microscopic (EM) evaluation of a conjunctival or skin biopsy. The EM will show concentric membranous bodies similar to what is seen in ganglioside storage diseases.

25.17.2   Diseases of Metal Metabolism Affecting Gray Matter

Disorders of Copper

Menkes Steely Hair Disease

Menkes steely hair disease is an X-linked disease that affects young infants. The disease is caused by a defect in copper transportation across the intestinal mucosa resulting in a copper deficiency. Although the copper content is high in the intestinal mucosa and kidneys, a severe copper deficiency is present in such organs as liver and brain. This reduction in copper leads to a deficiency of copper-dependent enzymes, which explains the cause of the clinical abnormalities. Deficiencies of enzymes such as cytochrome c-oxidase and β-hydroxylase may explain the neurologic deterioration: tyrosinase for the hypopigmentation, lysyl oxidase for the defects in connective tissue, and ascorbate oxidase to explain the osteoporosis.

The neurologic features may begin in utero and consist of developmental regression, seizures, retinal degeneration, and later spasticity. Systemic features consist of failure to thrive, hypothermia, osteoporosis, bladder diverticuli, sparse thin hair that is twisted at the shaft (pili torti), lax skin, and tortuous and elongated arterial vessels.

An alleleic variant of Menkes disease is the *occipital horn syndrome*, which has a defect in the same gene. This syndrome has only minimal neurologic features consisting of mild developmental delay and autonomic instability. The systemic features consist of inguinal hernias, bladder diverticuli, lax skin, and a characteristic "calcified occipital horn" in the skull.

Diagnostic confirmation consists of finding a low serum copper and ceruloplasmin after 2 to 3 weeks of age when these levels normally rise. MR imaging shows severe cerebral and cerebellar atrophy with tortuous vessels seen on the magnetic resonance angiography. Subdural hematomas may form following the severe atrophy.

The genetic defect of this Menkes disease is related to a defect in an ATPase binding protein, ATP7A. This gene is very similar to another copper-transporting gene responsible for Wilson disease, ATP7B. The differential expression of these two genes explains the difference in the clinical phenotype. The ATP7A gene is expressed in the intestinal mucosa and other tissues but not liver, whereas the ATP7B gene is expressed in liver and brain. The gene has been mapped to Xq13.3, and the incidence of the disorder is estimated at 1 to 2 per 100,000 live male births. Numerous deletions and point mutations have been found in this gene in families with Menkes disease.

Treatment has been attempted with a copper-histidine mixture to correct the copper deficiency, but results have been disappointing except when treatment is begun very early.

Wilson Disease (Hepatolenticular Degeneration)

Similar to Menkes disease, Wilson disease is a disorder of another copper-transporting gene, ATP7B. This gene is mapped to chromosome 13q14.3 and encodes a p-type ATPase gene.

The major clinical features are confined to the liver and brain. During early life, the patient is asymptomatic, but the accumulating copper in liver is associated with subclinical liver disease. Symptoms consisting of hepatic, neurologic, and psychiatric manifestations may occur any time between early childhood and the adult years, but the most frequent age of onset is in the late adolescent or early adult years.

Clinical Features

Hepatic Features The hepatic disease may mimic chronic active hepatitis, but an acute fulminate hepatic failure may also be seen. On clinical indications alone, it is very difficult to separate the hepatic disease caused by copper accumulation from other etiologies of hepatic disease such as viral or other causes of liver failure. In severe liver failure, hemolysis caused by the massive release of copper, which damages the red cells, may be a distinguishing clinical sign for Wilson disease.

Neurologic Features The onset of the neurologic symptoms and signs is usually insidious with a slow rate of progression. Neurologic signs are not seen prior to 7 or 8 years, however. Dysarthria is extremely common, followed by dystonia, rigidity, abnormalities of posture, gait, and reduced facial expression. Tremor occurs in up to half of the patients. Because of poor control of orofacial muscles, drooling and dysphagia become major problems. Occasionally, the patient develops parkinsonian symptoms, but intellect is spared. The copper deposition within the basal ganglia is responsible for the extrapyramidal symptoms (Fig. 25-48).

Psychiatric Features Psychiatric symptoms occur in about one-third of the patients presenting initially. Irritability and impulsive behavior are common. Symptoms may alternate from depression to mania. Often a loss of sexual inhibition leads to exhibitionism. Eventually work or school performance declines considerably. This behavior may even lead to incarceration in extreme cases. These symptoms may mimic substance abuse or oppositional-defiant disorder in the adolescent. Unfortunately, patients with psychiatric abnormalities are typically not diagnosed until other neurologic signs or symptoms develop.

Other organs may be affected in Wilson disease including renal problems such as renal tubular dysfunction (Fanconi syndrome) or renal stones. Skeletal abnormalities such as osteoporosis, osteomalacia, or arthritis may occur. Woman frequently develop oligomenorrhea or amenorrhea. Cardiac problems include interstitial fibrosis and myocarditis. Electrocardiographic abnormalities and orthostatic hypotension are not uncommon. In addition to Kayser-Fleischer rings, which consist of copper deposition in the limbus of the corneas (Descemet membrane), the patient may have sunflower cataracts. Pancreatic disease, parathyroidism, gallstones, and skin abnormalities may also be present.

Diagnostic Studies Diagnostic evaluation of these patients consists of serum ceruloplasmin and copper levels with measurement of 24-hour urinary copper excretion. The serum ceruloplasmin concentration is less than 20 mg/dL in 95% of cases, and total serum copper is reduced to 3 to 10 μM (normal is 11–25 μM). Urinary excretion is increased to greater than 100 μg per 24 hours (normal is 40 μg/24 h) which can be enhanced if penicillamine is given. The most accurate diagnostic method is a liver biopsy for copper content, which is significantly increased (>250 μg/g dry weight). The MR imaging characteristically shows abnormal signals (hypointense on T_1- and hyperintense on T_2-weighted images) within the caudate, putamen, globus pallidus, and dentate nuclei and thalamus. Generalized atrophy is also apparent.

Genetics Wilson disease is an autosomal-recessive inherited disease with an estimated incidence of 1 in 30,000 to 50,000. The Wilson disease gene maps to 13q14.3 and encodes a p-type ATPase that is very homologous to the Menkes disease gene product. The gene defect leads to impaired incorporation of copper into ceruloplasmin and presumably into other bile proteins. The tissue distributions of the two proteins differ in that the Menkes gene is expressed in all tissues but liver, whereas the Wilson's disease gene is expressed only in liver and brain. The Wilson disease protein is localized mainly in the Golgi apparatus, where copper binding to ceruloplasmin likely takes place.

Treatment Treatment for Wilson disease is very effective when given prior to irreversible hepatic or brain injury. The initial treatment of patients presenting with neurologic or psychiatric disease is often tetrathiomolybdate, which forms a nontoxic compound when bound with copper. Liver disease may be treated with a com-

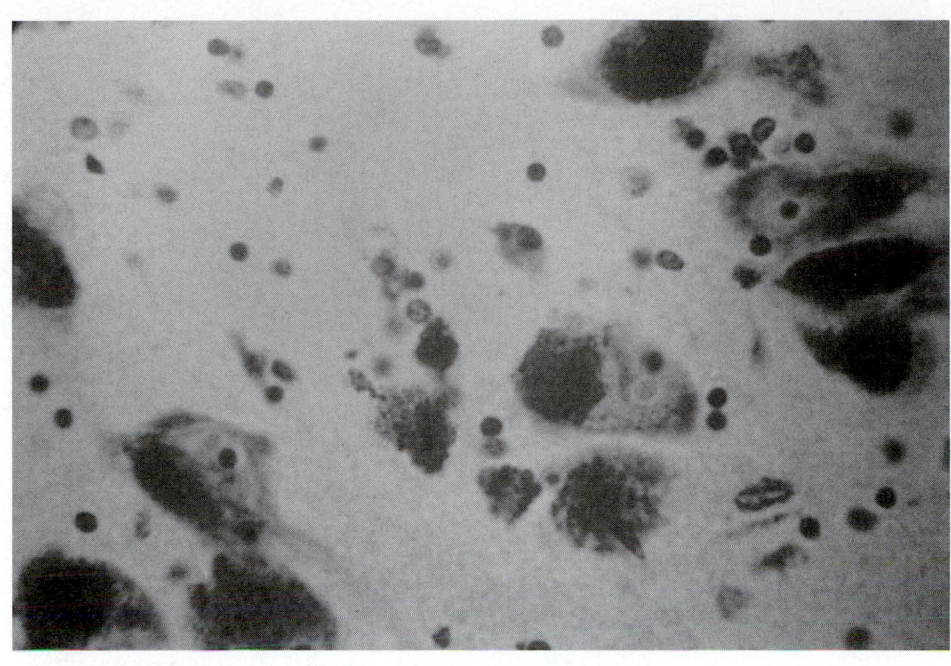

FIGURE 25-48 Copper deposition noted within striate nucleus of Wilson disease patient.

bination of trientine hydrochloride, a copper chelator, and zinc, which blocks absorption. The trientine is given to quickly obtain a negative copper balance. Trientine is used rather than penicillamine because it appears to have fewer side effects. Penicillamine, although an effective treatment, has significant side effects such as bone marrow toxicity and hypersensitivity reactions. Zinc induces hepatic metallothione, which complexes with copper in the liver to form a nontoxic compound. Zinc may be used for maintenance therapy for patients with chronic disease.

Disorders of Iron

Aceruloplasminemia

Aceruloplasminemia is a newly recognized disorder of iron metabolism. It is an autosomal-recessive condition that is associated with undetectable levels of ceruloplasmin. Although ceruloplasmin, an α_2-serum glycoprotein, carries approximately 95% of copper, it is also essential in iron hemostasis. These patients have a complete deficiency of ceruloplasmin ferroxidase activity, which is important in central nervous system iron metabolism. The clinical triad of this disease is *diabetes, retinal degeneration,* and *neurologic disease.* Neurologically, this disease usually begins in adults and consists of a complex of extrapyramidal signs including blepharospasm and ataxia. Iron accumulation in the retina causes visual loss. It is unknown if treatment with chelating agents will be effective.

Hallervorden-Spatz Disease

Hallervorden-Spatz disease (HSD) has been considered a disorder of iron metabolism because of the deposition of iron within the globus pallidus and the pars reticulata of the substantia nigra. There is as yet no gene identified in this disorder, but it is presumed to be an autosomal-recessive disease. The diagnosis is made clinically with the following characteristics aiding in the diagnosis:

1. Occurrence at a young age, generally after earliest childhood
2. A motor disorder, mainly of extrapyramidal type characterized by dystonic postures, muscular rigidity, involuntary movements of choreoathetoid or tremulous type, but with the findings suggesting corticospinal tract dysfunction as well

3. Mental changes indicative of dementia
4. A relentless, progressive course extending over several years, leading to death in early adulthood

The classic clinical characteristics usually begin in the middle to late part of the first decade with the onset of pyramidal signs, which include spasticity, increased deep tendon reflexes, extensor plantar responses. Later, the extrapyramidal findings of dystonia, rigidity, tremor, and choreoathetosis are noticed. Other findings such as tremor and typically dysarthria become noticeable. Ophthalmologic findings include retinal pigmentary degeneration and optic atrophy. Eventually mental deterioration occurs, and the disease may progress very slowly, even over decades.

The pathologic findings in HSD include the deposition of iron within astrocytes, microglia, and neurons and focal swelling within axons that are called *spheroids.* The most intensely involved areas include the globus pallidus and the pars reticulata of the substantia nigra (Fig. 25-49).

There are no laboratory studies that will confirm the diagnosis of HSD. Routine studies to assess iron hemostasis are normal. Radioisotope studies with iron have not proved valuable in diagnosing this disease. MR imaging is the most helpful test in determining the diagnosis of HSD. Iron deposits are associated with decreased intensity of the T_2-weighted image and a central region of necrosis within the globus pallidus that has been referred to as the "eye of the tiger" sign.

Treatment with chelating agents such as desferrioxamine has not proved effective in reducing the iron load or improving the clinical symptoms. Symptomatic treatment of the extrapyramidal movements with L-dopa, dopaminergic agonists, and trihexyphenidyl may be helpful. Treatment of dystonia has been attempted with baclofen, including intrathecal baclofen infusions.

25.17.3 Gray Matter Diseases of Unknown Etiology—Neuroaxonal Dystrophy

Neuroaxonal dystrophy (NAD) is an autosomal-recessive disease of unknown origin. The most striking aspect of the disease is the neu-

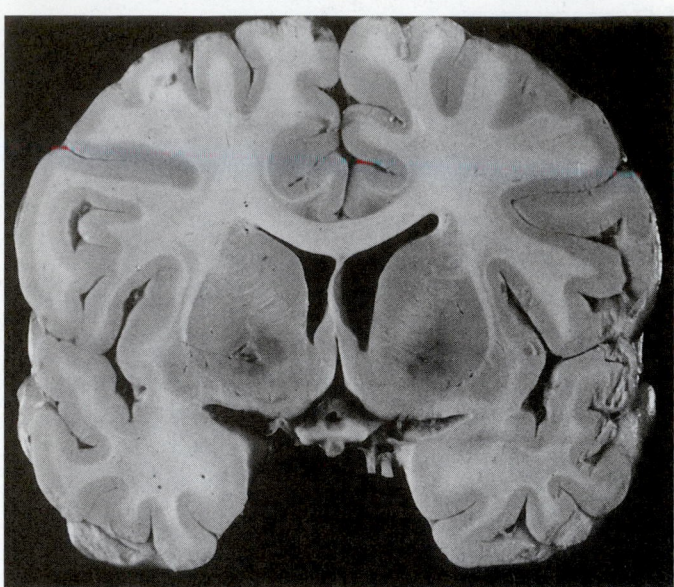

FIGURE 25-49 Iron deposition noted within globus pallidus of a patient with Hallervorden-Spatz disease.

ropathologic findings, which include axonal and presynaptic terminal swellings associated with neuronal degeneration.

The clinical presentation may begin as early as 6 months or as late as 3 years, although the average age of onset occurs between 14 and 18 months. The typical clinical course will have an onset of signs and symptoms prior to age 3 consisting of psychomotor regression, progressive pyramidal tract signs, and truncal hypotonia. The disease relentlessly progresses to cause spastic quadriplegia, dementia, and blindness usually by age 4 years. Peripheral nervous system involvement occurs causing loss of reflexes. Seizures can be seen but are not commonly present. Optic atrophy is frequently observed. As a generality, the earlier the disease presents the more rapid the rate of progression.

Pathologic findings of NAD include the presence of large eosinophilic spheroids that are found in all parts of the nervous system. The most frequent location of these spheroids include posterior horns and Clark columns in the spinal cord, nuclei gracilis and cuneatus of the medulla, substantia nigra, subthalamic nuclei, and distal parts of the peripheral nervous system. Axonal swellings are frequently noted in the anterior horns of the spinal cord and central gray nuclei in brain.

Diagnosis of NAD is based on the clinical presentation and the finding of spheroids noted on skin, conjunctival, or peripheral nerve biopsy. The MR or CT scan often reveals cerebellar atrophy but rarely decreased signal on T_2-weighted images in globus pallidus, similar to what has been reported in Hallervorden-Spatz disease. The EEG may show a slow background with fast rhythms (14–22 Hz) predominantly seen in the frontal regions. Peripheral nerve studies demonstrate an axonal injury with preserved nerve conduction studies but reduced amplitude. EMG shows signs of denervation. The visual evoked potentials will be abnormal, but the electroretinogram will remain normal.

The genetic defect for NAD has yet to be elucidated. One biochemical disorder, the deficiency of α-N-acetylgalactosaminidase (Schindler disease) is associated with a clinical phenotype and neuropathologic findings similar to NAD. This is a very rare disorder and likely accounts for only a very small percentage of patients with NAD.

LEUKOENCEPHALOPATHIES

25.17.4 Lipid Abnormalities

Adrenoleukodystrophy

Although adrenoleukodystrophy (ALD) was one of the first white matter diseases to be described, it has historically been difficult to characterize. The ALD nomenclature, based on pathologic descriptions, was initially confusing because ALD was grouped into a description of three separate diseases, all called *Schilder disease*. The original description of a boy with ALD was confused with a case of probable subacute sclerosing panencephalitis and another case of acute form of multiple sclerosis. The term *Schilder disease* should be reserved for the diffuse myelinoclastic sclerosis that is an immune-mediated white matter disease thought to be an acute form of multiple sclerosis. The genetic inheritance of ALD is now known to be X-linked. The biochemical elucidation of ALD began with the identification of an excess of very long chain unbranched fatty acids (VLCFA) C24–C30 chain length, especially C26:0 and C25:0, in the cholesterol ester fraction of white matter and adrenal cortex from ALD cases. Since these fatty acids are metabolized within the peroxisome, ALD is an example of a single enzyme deficient peroxisomal disease. Accumulation of VLCFA is now widely used in plasma as a diagnostic test for ALD and other peroxisomal diseases. (See also Sec. 9.10.)

Clinical Features The clinical phenotype of ALD can be divided into: childhood cerebral, adolescent cerebral, adult cerebral, adrenomyeloneuropathy, Addison only, and asymptomatic or presymptomatic. The *cerebral form* is the most common form in childhood and begins at a mean age of onset of 7 years. The first neurologic problems children develop are behavioral with symptoms such as hyperactivity or attention deficit. These symptoms are followed by signs of impaired auditory discrimination, impaired vision, ataxia, and, later, signs of corticospinal tract involvement. Seizures occasionally may be the heralding event. After the initial onset, the illness advances rapidly to a vegetative state within 2 years, with death inexorably occurring thereafter. *Adrenomyeloneuropathy* is the most common adult form. As its name implies, it affects mainly the spinal cord and peripheral nerves. The mean age of onset is 27 years. The main clinical findings are a slowly progressive spastic paraparesis with sensory disturbances most severe in the distal aspects of the lower extremities and sphincter disturbances. Impotence develops in the later stages, although many of the patients have fathered children. The disease may also affect 10 to 15% of heterozygote females who may develop symptoms of AMN in the third to fifth decades.

The MR imaging demonstrates a predilection for the parietooccipital white matter (Fig. 25-50). The cerebral features appear to be related to the perivascular lymphocytic infiltration affecting white matter and causing demyelinating lesions beginning in the parietooccipital white matter.

Biochemistry Despite the wide range of clinical presentations, the disease is always associated with the accumulation of VLCFA. The basis for the VLCFA accumulation has been the basis for much speculation. Before VLCFA can be oxidized in the β-oxidation pathway, the fatty acids are activated into VLCFA-CoA through

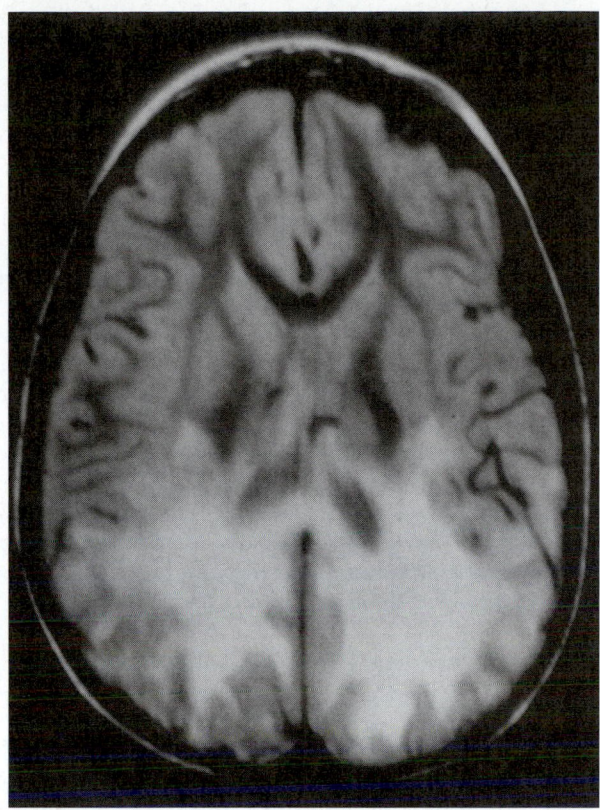

FIGURE 25-50   MR image in patient with adrenoleukodystrophy showing typical white matter changes on T_2-weighted image in parietooccipital region.

the enzyme VLCFA-CoA synthetase (ligase). All patients with ALD have decreased activity of the VLCFA-CoA synthetase enzyme but do not have mutations in the gene encoding this protein. The mutated gene in ALD patients is responsible for encoding the ALD protein (ALDP). ALDP is required for the peroxisomal localization of VLCFA-CoA synthetase enzyme, and without appropriate localization to the peroxisome, this enzyme is unable to properly function. ALDP is a part of a family of ABC transporters, and this protein has at least three other homologs, which include the PMP70, ALD-related protein (ALDRP), and P70R. There is some similarity in these proteins, since ALD patient cells treated with 4-phenylbutyrate show increased expression of ALDRP and lowering of the VLCFA.

Genetics   The gene encoding the ALDP is localized to Xq28 near a locus for color vision. Several mutations have been identified in this gene in patients with ALD. Mutations in the ALDP gene, however, do not correlate well with the clinical phenotype, suggesting a more complicated genotype/phenotype arrangement.

Treatment   Following biochemical evidence of the lowering of VLCFA in fibroblasts after treatment with oleic acid, combination therapy with glycerol trioleate/glycerol trierucate (GTO/GTE-Lorenzo's oil) and VLCFA dietary restriction was performed in neurologically affected children but without significant improvement in the disease course. The dietary therapy was also not successful when used in adults with adrenomyeloneuropathy. The only therapy that appears effective, especially if used early in the disease, has been bone marrow transplantation.

Globoid Cell Leukodystrophy (Krabbe Disease)

Globoid cell leukodystrophy is considered one of two autosomal-recessive inherited glycosphingolipid storage disorders primarily causing a leukodystrophy.

Clinical Features   Children begin symptoms prior to 6 months in approximately 80% of the cases, with 25% occurring prior to 3 months. The classical clinical presentation frequently consists of extreme *irritability* and crying followed by *rigidity* and *tonic spasms.* Peripheral nerves are affected early in the course, causing a reduction in the nerve conduction velocities. CSF examination is remarkable for the elevation of protein, typically above 70 mg/dL. The CT scan when performed early demonstrates increased density in the brainstem, thalami, caudate nuclei, corona radiata, cerebellar cortex, and periventricular and capsular white matter. MR imaging performed during these initial symptoms shows decreased T_1 values and normal or slightly decreased T_2 values in the abnormal areas demonstrated by CT scan, and large symmetric plaque-like areas on T_1 and T_2 values in the white matter of the centrum semiovale. The brainstem auditory evoked potentials are often disrupted with only peaks I to III present and interpeak latency prolonged.

In addition to the classical presentation, a *late infantile* variant may begin between 19 months and 4 years. The children have normal intelligence or are only moderately retarded during the first years but then gradually develop ataxia, weakness, spasticity, and later dysarthria. Visual loss with the early onset of optic atrophy, mental regression, occasionally seizures, deafness, and normal peripheral nerves are the characteristic findings.

Late-onset variants of globoid cell leukodystrophy are arbitrarily defined as *juvenile-onset* (beginning between 4 and 19 years of age), and *adult-onset* (20 years and older). These patients usually have optic nerve pallor, pes cavus, slowly progressive spastic tetraplegia, sensory-motor demyelinating neuropathy, hypodensity in the white matter in the parietooccipital regions, and preserved mental function in approximately half of the affected individuals. CSF protein is frequently not increased. The life span of individuals with the late-onset variant may vary, but survival for over 24 years has been reported.

Biochemistry   The disease is caused by a deficiency of the lysosomal enzyme galactosylceramide β-galactosidase, which is required to degrade the lipid galactosylceramide, an important glycolipid in myelin structure. This disease is unique among the lipid storage diseases because there is no increase of lipid in the brain except within specialized microglial cells referred to as *globoid cells.* Biochemical studies of total brain lipids did not show the expected increase in galactosylcerebroside but rather a lowering of total cerebroside and sulfatide and a reduced sulfatide-to-cerebroside ratio. Only a fraction of brain lipids enriched in the globoid cells showed an increase in galactosylceramide. Psychosine (galactosylsphingosine), a related glycolipid also broken by the galactosylceramide β-galactosidase enzyme, is thought to be the metabolite responsible for the pathogenesis of this disorder, since it is known to be toxic to oligodendrocytes.

Genetics   The gene for the galactosylceramide beta-galactosidase enzyme has been mapped to chromosome 14. Following a Herculean task of purifying the galactosylceramide β-galactosidase enzyme from human urine, the cDNA encoding galactosylceramide β-galactosidase was cloned. The purified enzyme shows bands on

SDS-gels that correspond to 80 kDa, between 50 and 52 kDa, and 30 kDa, all of which have a similar N-terminal amino acid sequence. This sequence similarity suggests that the 50-kDa and 30-kDa species are derived from the 80-kDa precursor species. The cDNA is 3.8 kb in length and contains a 2007-bp open reading frame that codes for 669 amino acids representing an unglycosylated protein with a molecular weight of 72,781. This weight is consistent with the glycosylated 80-kDa precursor form identified. Confirmation of the deduced amino acid sequence for the cDNA occurred following the purification of the enzyme from human leukocytes and the subsequent cloning using the polymerase chain reaction method. The entire gene structure and organization has been determined to consist of nearly 60 kb with 17 exons and 16 introns. The promoter region, located at the -149 to -112 nucleotide region from the initiation codon, contains three GC-box-like sequences and one YY1 binding site.

Molecular analyses demonstrated at least 60 mutations including base transitions, polymorphisms, and deletions that are associated with Krabbe disease. In infantile patients with Krabbe disease from northern European ancestry, approximately 40 to 50% of cases have a mutant allele that has a 30-kb deletion beginning in intron 10 and extending past the 3′ end of the gene. In addition to the deletion on this allele, there is an invariable C to T transition at position 502, which is a polymorphism seen in only about 4% of the population. Most of the mutations causing infantile-onset disease are located on the region coding for the 30-kd subunit of the enzyme, suggesting that this subunit is critical for the normal functioning of the enzyme. Adult-onset cases may also have the 502/del mutation on one allele, but many other mutations including missense mutations such as a homozygous T185C, nonsense mutations, and deletions and insertions have been reported in the older-onset population.

Treatment   Despite the very significant advances in the molecular understanding of globoid cell leukodystrophy, therapy for this disease has not progressed as quickly. Hematopoietic stem cell transplantation was initially discounted for use in Krabbe disease, but recent studies have suggested some ameliorating effects from this therapy especially if used early in the course or ideally in a presymptomatic condition.

Metachromatic Leukodystrophy (MLD)

MLD is the second example of a lysosomal storage disease involving glycosphingolipid metabolism that causes a leukoencephalopathy with an estimated frequency of 1 in 40,000. The name is derived from the neuropathologic description of metachromatic staining which consists of a brownish or reddish color compared to the blue color of cell nuclei when stained with cresyl violet or toluidine blue. This disease is associated with lipid accumulation in several cell types such as hepatocytes, Kupffer cells, epithelium of bile ducts, gallbladder epithelial cells, and renal tubular epithelium. In the central and peripheral nervous system the accumulation of lipid can be noted in oligodendrocytes and macrophages throughout the white matter and in selected neurons and retinal ganglion cells. Only in brain and peripheral nerves, however, is the sulfatide storage associated with pathology. The cause for the demyelination is not completely understood, but storage of sulfatides in Schwann cells and oligodendrocytes precedes the development of demyelination. Other hypotheses to explain the demyelination include unstable myelin sheaths owing to sulfatide accumulation and, as in the psychosine hypothesis for Krabbe disease, toxic effects of a sphingosine (sulfogalactosylsphingosine). This disease is included in the dysmyelinating category of leukoencephalopathies.

Clinical Features   The clinical phenotype depends on the cause of the leukodystrophy. Three etiologies for sulfatide accumulation and leukodystrophy have been identified. These include the most common etiology, arylsulfatase A deficiency (which may present in late infancy, late childhood, or adult ages), a deficiency of the sphingolipid activator protein saposin B, and multiple sulfatase deficiency. The late-infantile-onset children usually have normal milestones, but, beginning in the later half of the second year, ataxia and difficulty with walking develop. Eventually spasticity and loss of speech occur followed by quadriplegia and cortical blindness. Juvenile-onset cases are characterized by a less distinct phenotype that may vary greatly in age of onset, ranging from early childhood to late adolescence. The peripheral nerve involvement may predominate in young children, but in older children school problems and behavioral difficulties may be key features. The rate of progression of the disease may vary from very rapid to indolent. Adults appear to have psychiatric problems as a major feature of the disease but may also have peripheral nerve and other findings.

Biochemistry   The major cause for metachromatic leukodystrophy is a deficiency of arylsulfatase A (ASA), which catalyzes cerebroside 3-sulphate. The enzyme removes the galactose 3-sulfate group from the glycolipid, and its deficiency results in the lysosomal accumulation of cerebroside 3-sulphate. The gene for arylsulfatase A is located on chromosome 22q13 and contains about 3 kb of genomic sequence and encodes for a 507–amino acid ASA polypeptide. Three different species of mRNA are produced by the ASA gene, and these species are 2.1, 3.7, and 4.8 kb in length. All three transcripts encode the identical 507–amino acid polypeptide but differ in the length of the 3′-untranslated sequence, with the 2.1 transcript accounting for approximately 90% of the total ASA mRNA. There are now well over 70 mutations identified in the ASA gene responsible for metachromatic leukodystrophy. Most of these mutations are found in individual patients, but two mutations, a splice donor mutation at the exon 2/intron 2 border and a Pro426Leu substitution, account for approximately 25% of cases, with another mutation, Ile179Ser, accounting for an additional 5%.

Pseudodeficiency of Arylsulfatase A Activity

A cause of difficulty in diagnosing patients with metachromatic leukodystrophy is the frequent occurrence of a benign decrease in the arylsulfatase A enzyme activity that approaches levels seen in MLD patients. It is estimated that approximately 1% of the population have this nonpathogenic decrease in ASA activity, with approximately 10% of the population carrying the ASA-pseudodeficiency (ASA-PD) allele. Two mutations are responsible for the occurrence of ASA-PD allele. These mutations are caused by two A→G transitions; the first results in a substitution of serine for a glycosylated asparagine at amino acid 305, and the second mutation alters the polyadenylation signal in the major 2.1-kb transcript. The first change may result in a small reduction in enzyme activity by changing the catalytic properties or targeting signal of the protein, whereas the polyadenylation defect results in a 90% reduction in transcript production, causing the overall enzyme levels to fall to approximately 8% of normal values. Further diagnostic confusion may result from the pseudodeficiency state, since compound heterozygotes of the MLD and ASA-PD alleles, which are clinically normal, will have mildly elevated sulfatide excretion in urine. Quantitative urine sulfatide measurements or radiolabeled sulfatide degradation in fibroblasts are chemical methods used to differentiate among asymptomatic ASA-PD states, carriers of MLD, presymptomatic MLD cases, and compound heterozygotes. However, molecular testing is becoming a more commonly used method to identify ASA-PD.

Saposin B Deficiency (Sphingolipid Activator Deficiency)

Rarely patients with normal ASA gene structure may have a deficiency of the ASA enzyme activity. Typically these patients will have a clinical phenotype and MR imaging appearance that is compatible with a juvenile-onset form of MLD but will have apparently normal enzyme activity by customary fluorescent substrate analysis. The defect is related to a mutation in the cerebroside sulfate activator protein (saposin B) that is mapped to chromosome 10 and one of a family of four genes (prosaposin gene) required for the hydrolysis of several lysosomal enzymes. The saposin B protein will also enhance the degradation of several other lipids such as G_{M1} ganglioside, globotriaosylceramide, and sphingomyelin, suggesting a possible function for saposin B in the lysosomal hydrolases G_{M1} ganglioside β-galactosidase, α-galactosidase, and sphingomyelinase, but the phenotype resembles MLD and not other storage diseases.

Treatment Treatment for MLD is primarily symptomatic, but bone marrow transplantation may be effective to partially ameliorate symptoms if it is used presymptomatically in a known family or early in the course of a slowly progressive variant.

25.17.5 Myelin Protein Disorders— Pelizaeus-Merzbacher Disease (PMD)

The best example of a hypomyelinating leukoencephalopathy is PMD. This disorder is an X-linked leukoencephalopathy first described in 1885. The classical and congenital presentation of PMD begins in infancy and consists of horizontal, vertical, or pendular eye movements (nystagmus); stridor; feeding difficulties; hypotonia; titubation of the head; developmental delays; ataxia; spasticity; and choreoathetosis. Although initially thought to represent a leukodystrophy, the disease is more accurately a defect in myelin deposition caused by a deficiency of proteolipid. The proteolipid gene was linked to the Xq22 region in 1985, and defective biosynthesis of proteolipid protein in PMD patients was confirmed in 1987. In 1989, three independent observations confirmed mutations in the proteolipid gene associated with PMD disease. It is of interest that an alternatively spliced gene, DM20, is also derived from the PLP locus. The DM20 gene has been implicated in the maintenance of oligodendrocytes and myelin assembly, and mutations that affect the transport of both PLP and DM20 are associated with the severe connatal variant of PMD.

The MR imaging appearance of PMD shows a diffuse increase in the signal of white matter on T_2-weighted images that is characteristic for children over the age of 1 year (Fig. 25-51). In young children, the MR imaging is less specific because of delays in myelination. Evoked potential studies are also abnormal with loss of rostral waves on the brainstem-evoked potentials. EMG and nerve conduction velocities are usually normal, but some abnormalities have been reported.

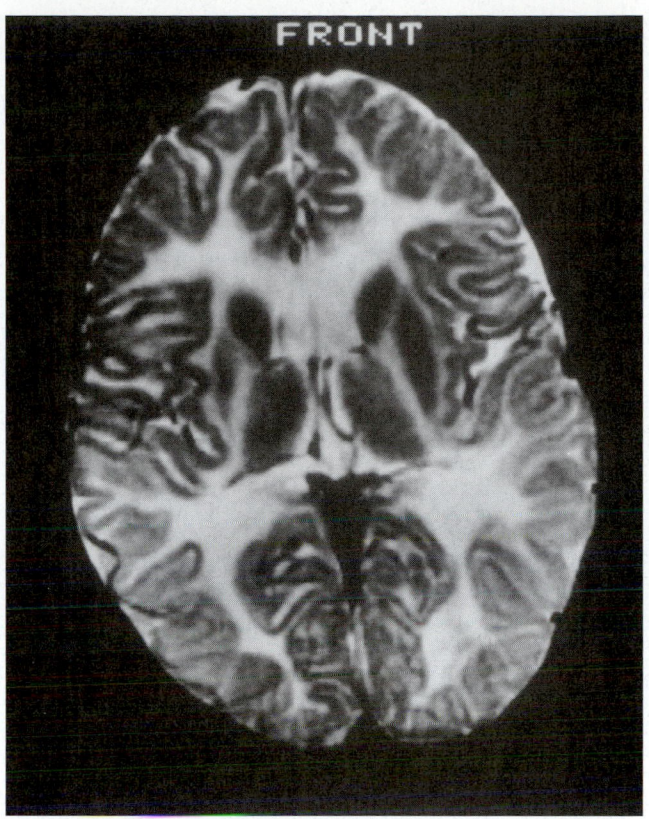

FIGURE 25-51 MR image from patient with Pelizaeus-Merzbacher showing diffuse increased signal on T_2-weighted image.

The genetics of PMD has helped delineate the full clinical spectrum. The majority of classical-onset cases appear to be caused by a duplication of the proteolipid gene, although in one family an increased gene dosage was noted without a duplication. Interphase fluorescent in situ hybridization has been developed to screen patients for duplication of the PLP gene. The approximate number of mutations or small deletions has approached 80 (March 2001), but these account probably for only 15 to 20% of the diagnosed PMD patients. There still remains an estimated 20 to 25% of patients in which no identified gene defect can explain the PMD phenotype. An expanded phenotype has occurred following molecular diagnosis, since we now know that *familial spastic paraplegia type 2* (SPG2) is an allelic variant of PMD. Classical PMD has been identified in families with the SPG2 variant. As in many other inherited diseases, the genotype does not always predict the phenotype in PMD, although mutations in the same codon have led to speculation about genotype/phenotype correlations. Small deletions or null mutations are believed to cause peripheral nervous system involvement, since approximately 1% of PLP is present in peripheral nerve, especially in Schwann cells. The genotype/phenotype correlation in patients with duplications is complicated because of varying lengths of the duplications reported.

25.17.6 Organic Acid Disorders—Canavan Disease

Canavan disease is an autosomal-recessive neurologic disorder associated with macrocephaly and spongiform degeneration of brain. The clinical description and inherited basis of Canavan disease was first recognized over 50 years ago. In the first report, five Jewish

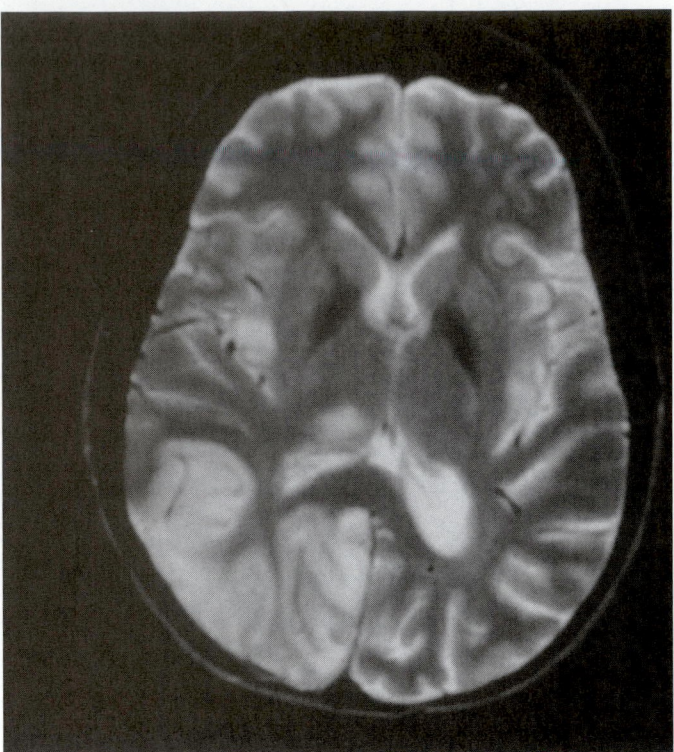

FIGURE 25-52   Metabolic stroke from patient with MELAS (mitochondrial encephalopathy, lactic acidosis, and stroke) showing gray and white matter infarction affecting the right parietooccipital region in a nonvascular distribution pattern on MR imaging.

patients developed macrocephaly and severe mental retardation associated with spongy degeneration of brain. In 1988, Canavan disease was identified as a deficiency of aspartoacylase, which causes an increase in N-acetyl aspartic acid in brain and urine. The molecular basis of Canavan disease was elucidated in 1993 with the cloning of the gene and the identification of a common missense mutation.

Clinical Features   The clinical triad of *hypotonia, head lag,* and *macrocephaly* is characteristic for Canavan disease. Infants with Canavan disease do not have distinctive clinical features in the first few months of life but begin to show delayed development by 3 months of age. Macrocephaly may not be apparent within the first few months, but the head enlarges to above the ninetieth percentile within 6 months to a year of life. Head control remains poor, and the child never develops the ability to support the head. Seizures and optic atrophy frequently develop in the second year of life. Irritability and sleep disturbances are frequent clinical symptoms. In time, gastroesophageal reflux becomes prominent, and swallowing deteriorates, leading to feeding difficulties and poor weight gain. Nasogastric feeding or permanent feeding gastrostomy is often required. Most patients with Canavan disease die in the first decade of life. However, with improved medical and nursing care, a larger number of children survive beyond the first decade. The congenital, infantile, and juvenile variant forms of Canavan disease were described prior to the discovery of the enzyme, which makes assessing the frequency of these subtypes difficult. MR imaging demonstrates diffuse white matter changes consisting of increased signal on T_2-weighted image.

Genetics   The gene for human aspartoacylase is localized to the 17p13-ter region and spans 29 kb of the genome. The transcript is 1.8 kb in length and contains an open reading frame on the cDNA that is 939 bases long and predicts a 313–amino acid residue. The identified mutations can be divided according to Ashkenazi Jewish and non-Jewish mutations. Two mutations account for 97% of the mutant alleles in Jewish families. These two mutations include the most frequent mutation, which causes a substitution of glutamic acid for alanine at codon 285 (Glu285Ala), and another common mutation that results in a nonsense mutation changing a tyrosine at codon 231 to a stop codon (Tyr231ter). In the non-Jewish families, an alanine to glutamic acid substitution at codon 305 (Ala305Glu) occurs in approximately 36% of identified mutations. In the non-Jewish families, only 70% of mutations have been identified so far, with a total of 24 additional mutations being characterized. If a mutation has been identified for a pregnancy at risk for the disease, mutational analysis can be performed on chorionic villus sampling to aid in diagnosis. Prenatal diagnosis of Canavan disease is complicated, since cultured amniocytes or chorionic villus samples have low levels of aspartoacylase activity, making enzyme analysis unsatisfactory for disease detection in the fetus.

Treatment   At present there is no treatment available for affected children with Canavan disease. An experimental gene therapy protocol, implanting into the central nervous system a vector containing the aspartoacylase cDNA, was recently performed in a few children within the United States and New Zealand, but the efficacy and safety of this nascent treatment remain to be evaluated.

25.17.7   Defects in Energy Metabolism— Mitochondrial Disorders

It is appreciated that defects in energy metabolism, primarily defects in mitochondrial function, may present a leukodystrophy. The disorders include: MELAS, Leber hereditary optic atrophy, ubiquinone deficiency, complex I deficiency, complex III deficiency, and cytochrome oxidase deficiency. It must be stressed that these diseases are part of a greater defect in energy metabolism that usually affects other areas of brain and systemic organs but at times may appear as a primary white matter disorder. MELAS (mitochondrial encephalopathy, lactic acidosis, and stroke) is the best known of the mitochondrial diseases that may affect white matter structures. Typically this disorder involves a mutation in a mitochondrially encoded tRNA and results in stroke-like episodes that involve a nonvascular distribution territory affecting both white and gray matter structures (Fig. 25-52). (See Sec. 9.7.)

25.17.8   Other Causes of Leukoencephalopathy—Cadasil

CADASIL is an interesting cause of leukoencephalopathy primarily affecting adults. The acronym stands for *c*erebral *a*utosomal *d*ominant *ar*teriopathy *s*ubcortical *i*nfarcts and *l*eukoencephalopathy. The entity was first recognized as a familial multi-infarct dementia, although the disease is recognized more often now because of the leukodystrophy noted on MR imaging. The phenotypic spectrum usually begins after age 40, but asymptomatic "at risk" individuals may have MR imaging abnormalities noted at times in childhood. The clinical manifestations consist of ischemic deficits, cognitive loss including dementia, migraine, psychiatric disturbances, and rarely, seizures. The clinical course is unrelenting and occurs very slowly over decades. The MR imaging pattern consists of hyperintensities on T_2-weighted images in periventricular regions, deep white matter, basal ganglia, and infratentorial areas; this increases with age. The cerebral pathology consists of white matter gliosis and a small-vessel angiopathy with PAS-positive material in the media of the vessel. Although confined to the central nervous system, CADASIL is a systemic vascular disease. The pathologic hallmark of the disease is a nonamyloid nonatherosclerotic microangiopathy. Because of the ubiquitous nature of the vasculopathy, electron microscopy of skin can be used as a diagnostic tool. Electron microscopy of small arterioles in the skin demonstrates characteristic granular osmophilic material in the basement membranes, which indent the surface and appear to rise as flames of electron-dense material.

The genetic basis for this autosomal-dominant disease was elucidated when the gene was mapped to chromosome 19p13.1 and clarified further when mutations in the *Notch3* were discovered. The *Notch3* gene encodes a 300-kDa transmembrane protein with a receptor and cell signal transduction function which is important to embryonic development for many species. The gene contains 33 exons and 33 EGF-domains. As yet, the exact mechanism in which *Notch3* mutations cause the CADASIL phenotype is not understood. The mutations in *Notch3* appear to be very stereotyped, involving missense mutations with either a gain or loss of a cysteine residue. It is hoped that mutational analysis will greatly aid in diagnosis and improve the sensitivity of testing.

25.17.9   Unknown causes of Leukoencephalopathy

Alexander Disease

Alexander disease usually presents during infancy with the typical features of developmental delay, macrocephaly (caused by megalencephaly), and seizures. The disease usually begins in the first or second year of life but rarely occurs as late as age 6 years. Although initial reports suggested a male predominance, both sexes are equally affected. As the disease progresses, cognitive decline, feeding problems, and spastic quadriparesis become apparent. Some infants present acutely in the first year accompanied by hydrocephalus and increased intracranial pressure. In a few cases, megalencephaly may be present from birth, and, rarely, megalencephaly is never present. Death usually occurs between the ages of 2 and 10 years.

Juvenile-onset Alexander disease usually begins between the ages of 6 and 15 years but may begin as early as infancy. Unlike in the infantile-onset form, megalencephaly is usually not present in these later-onset children. Symptoms consist of bulbar dysfunction, especially dysphagia, and a slowly progressive gait disorder manifested by ataxia and progressive spasticity that usually begins in the lower extremities. Cognitive decline occurs only late in the disease. These children may survive for up to 10 years and frequently longer.

The pathology of Alexander disease is unique among the leukodystrophies. On histologic appearance, the brains are noted to have widely distributed astrocytic inclusions called *Rosenthal fibers*. There appears to be a pronounced paucity of myelin. The frontal lobes are the most severely affected with a discoloration of the white matter and frequently cystic degeneration, and cavitation is present. The lesions extend to involve the subcortical U fibers. The basal ganglia and thalami are also affected, but there is relative sparing of the occipital lobes and the cerebellum.

Alexander disease is suspected on the clinical history, but MR imaging may be very helpful in establishing the diagnosis. Lesions are typically located in the bilateral frontal regions and consist of frontal cystic changes, usually partially sparing the occipital lobes and cerebellum. In one adolescent case, some paramagnetic substances were noted in the basal ganglia and thalamus.

The genetic and biochemical basis for Alexander disease remains unknown. Only rarely has the disease been described in the same family, making the genetic inheritance pattern difficult to prove. There have been some recent reports concerning the presence of GFAP aggregates in the brains from Alexander cases and α B-crystallin and heat shock protein 27 in cerebrospinal fluid, but to date no firm biochemical marker is present. There is one report of a case of Alexander disease associated with a chromosomal deletion involving the long arm of chromosome 11, but this child did not have a deletion affecting the α B-crystallin gene.

Childhood Ataxia with Diffuse CNS Hypomyelination (CACH) (Vanishing White Matter Disease)

This hypomyelinating leukoencephalopathy is becoming an ever more important cause of previously undiagnosed leukodystrophies. The entity has been characterized in the last few years by a number of groups of investigators. This disorder was described in four girls with ataxia and spasticity but without peripheral nerve or cognitive involvement. The MR imaging demonstrated a diffuse confluent abnormality in white matter, which was noted early in the course of the disease. Magnetic resonance spectroscopy (MRS) performed on this cohort showed a reduction of *N*-acetylaspartic acid, choline, and creatine in white matter only. Brain biopsy in two of these girls showed a generalized reduction in myelin specific proteins and lipids but no evidence of any storage material. Three other patients were described with a relatively mild clinical course but with diffuse hypomyelination and a mildly swollen appearance of white matter. In a later study, nine other children were identified, and the phrase *vanishing white matter* was used to describe the entity. The MR imaging findings were similar to previous reports, but on proton density studies the white matter had an intensity similar to CSF. The MRS also showed the reduction in N-acetylaspartic acid, choline, and creatinine, but in addition lactate and glucose peaks were observed in white matter. On an autopsy from one case from this series of children, the histopathology demonstrated a cavitating leukoencephalopathy with replacement of white matter between ependyma and U-fibers by CSF. In areas with some preservation of white matter, astrogliosis and macrophage proliferation were present. Mild elevations of CSF glycine have been noted in several patients with CACH, and chromosomal linkage studies are underway in Dutch families.

A set of criteria have been suggested to identify children with childhood ataxia with diffuse CNS hypomyelination:

1. Normal or mildly delayed initial psychomotor development is present.
2. Neurologic deterioration appears with a chronic progressive and episodic course—deterioration may follow infection or minor head trauma and may lead to lethargy and coma.
3. Cerebellar ataxia and spasticity are present with relative preservation of mental function. Optic atrophy and epilepsy may occur.

4. MR imaging demonstrates diffuse symmetric white matter involvement with all or part of white matter showing a signal intensity similar to CSF on proton density, FLAIR, T_2-weighted, and T_1-weighted images. Cerebellar atrophy may also occur.

NEUROGENERATIVE DISEASES

25.17.10   Disorders of Trinucleotide Repeats

Eight neurologic disorders are currently attributed to an increase in the number of CAG repeats that encode expanded sequences of glutamine residues or *polyglutamine repeats*. These disorders are inherited in an autosomal dominant or X-linked pattern. The age of onset is variable, with adult onset being the most common but childhood cases also frequently reported. The early age of onset and increased severity of the disease appears to correlate with increasing numbers of CAG repeats. *Genetic anticipation*, defined as a tendency toward earlier onset in successive generations, occurs frequently, especially if the disease is inherited from the paternal chromosome. The abnormal proteins in each disorder are expressed in a wide range of tissues and are not limited to the affected brain regions. In addition to the polyglutamine repeat diseases, other triplicate repeat disorders occur such as in the fragile X syndrome (X-linked mental retardation) caused by CGG repeats, myotonic dystrophy caused by GTG repeats, and Friedreich ataxia related to a GAA repeating element in the intron of the gene.

Huntington Disease

Huntington disease is an autosomal-dominant disorder with high penetrance. The disease has a prevalence ranging from 1 in 7000 to 1 in 10,000. The characteristic findings of progressive chorea and dementia are caused by severe neuronal loss, initially in the neostriatum and later in the cerebral cortex. This disease is usually considered a disorder of adults, but children may have the disease especially if inherited from the father. In the adult, the neurologic symptoms consist of chorea, motor apraxia, psychiatric changes, and dementia. In children the age of onset may be as early as 3 years. Initially, symptoms consist of poor coordination, problems with attention, emotional lability, abnormal gait, and dysarthria. Dystonic posturing, rigidity, reduced facial movements, and dysphagia gradually develop. Similar to the adults, chorea may be an early sign in some cases. Unlike the adult patient population, however, children frequently develop seizures, which frequently are myoclonic.

Huntington disease is an autosomal-dominant trait that is linked to chromosome 4p16.3. One gene from this region, initially labeled *IT15* and now called *HD*, was found to contain an unstable CAG repeat in the open reading frame of its first exon. Most people have an average of 19 CAG repeats (range, 11 to 34), whereas nearly all patients with Huntington disease have more than 40. Unstable or dynamic mutations have been identified in a few families, in which one parent has 34 to 38 CAG repeats and the progeny have more than 40. The HD gene encodes a protein named *huntingtin*. The increased number of CAG repeats in the HD gene are expressed as an elongated huntingtin protein with 40 to 150 polyglutamine residues. The protein, whose function is unknown, is found in many cells in both neural and nonneural tissues. The size of the elongated huntingtin protein does not appear to correlate to the extent of neuronal injury. In brains of patients with Huntington disease, however, intranuclear inclusions of huntingtin and ubiquitin are apparent in neurons of the striatum and cerebral cortex but not in the brainstem, thalamus, or spinal cord, matching closely the sites of neuronal cell loss in the disease. The intranuclear inclusions in Huntington disease are thought to result from aberrant processing of proteins, with transport of huntingtin, ubiquitin, and other proteasome components to the nucleus where the deposits are found only in cells known to be affected.

Spinocerebellar Ataxias

The types of autosomal-dominant spinocerebellar ataxia are separated according to the clinical features, which include cerebellar ataxia, ophthalmoplegia, nystagmus, extrapyramidal signs, visual loss, hyperreflexia, and spasticity (Table 25-30). There is considerable clinical overlap in these diseases, especially in patients with early-onset disease. Six genotypes (*SCA1*, *SCA2*, *SCA3*, *SCA6*, *SCA7*, and *DRPLA*) demonstrate an increased number of CAG repeating elements. The disorders *SCA4* and *SCA5*, although mapped respectively to chromosomes 16 and 11, do not as yet have a pathologic molecular defect identified. The proteins involved in SCA1, SCA2, SCA3, and SCA7 diseases, which are called *ataxins*, have in common an increased number of glutamine residues. The resulting proteins are not homologous, and the functions of the four ataxins are unknown. A similar dominantly inherited spinocerebellar disorder, *dentato-rubropallidoluysian* (DRPLA), also caused by an unstable CAG repeat expansion region, maps to 12p12-ter. DRPLA consists of ataxia, chorea, dystonia, myoclonus, and dementia. In spinocerebellar ataxia type 6, the number of CAG repeats is smaller (range, 21 to 27) than in the other types, and the gene encodes an (α)1A-voltage-dependent calcium channel. The neuronal selectivity that characterizes each subtype of spinocerebellar ataxia has been correlated with the degree of accumulation of intranuclear ubiquinated components containing fragments of the respective protein. As in Huntington disease, nondegraded fragments of the glutamine repeat have a key role in the selectivity

TABLE 25-30
SPINOCEREBELLAR ATAXIAS

	TYPE 1	TYPE 2	TYPE 3	TYPE 6	TYPE 7	TYPE 8
Gene	6p23	12q24	14q24.3-q31	19p13	3p14-21.1	13q21
Protein	Ataxin 1	Ataxin 2	Ataxin 3	α-1a Ca channel	Ataxin 7	Untranslated
Clinical features	Ataxia, dysarthria, pyramidal signs, amyotrophy	Ataxia, dysarthria, neuropathy, extrapyramidal signs	Ataxia, peripheral neuropathy, cranial neuropathy, extrapyramidal signs	Nystagmus, ataxia, dysarthria, loss of reflexes & proprioception	Ataxia, retinal degeneration	Ataxia, dysarthria, spasticity, decreased vibration

of neuronal death. In two conditions in this group—spinocerebellar ataxia type 1 and spinocerebellar ataxia type 3 (also called *Machado-Joseph disease*)—intranuclear inclusions are found only in neurons that die. In the former, inclusions are found in cerebellar Purkinje cells and brainstem-cerebellar connections but not in cerebral cortical neurons. In SCA3, the most common subtype, intranuclear inclusions are limited to the dentate nucleus of the cerebellum, substantia nigra, and nucleus basalis pontis, all of which are affected clinically by the disease.

The formation of the intranuclear inclusions, as in Huntington disease, involves the ubiquitin-proteasome complex. In spinocerebellar ataxia type 1, the intranuclear inclusions contain components of proteasome complex and the molecular chaperone HDJ-2/HSDJ, a protein involved in ubiquitin-dependent protein degradation and fragments of abnormally elongated ataxin 1. These inclusions may interfere with nuclear function, perhaps by altering the transcription of other genes and leading eventually to apoptosis. An untranslated CTG expansion on chromosome 13q21 is associated with a novel form of spinocerebellar ataxia, which has been designated *SCA type 8*.

Friedreich Ataxia

Friedreich ataxia is the most common of the hereditary ataxias, with a prevalence of about 1 in 50,000. The disorder is an autosomal-recessive disorder caused by an increase in the number of trinucleotide GAA repeats within the first intron of the FRDA gene on chromosome 9. More than 95 percent of patients with classic Friedreich ataxia are homozygous for the increase in GAA repeats, but a few have a combination of an increase in GAA repeats in one allele and a point mutation in the other allele, confirming that Friedreich ataxia is a loss-of-function disorder. The disorder may be caused by interference by the intronic GAA repeat with transcription of the FRDA gene. The FRDA gene encodes the protein *frataxin*. Frataxin contains 210 amino acids, and its N-terminal region contains an (α)-helix that might target the protein to mitochondria. It has been suggested that the C-terminal region of frataxin is the active motif and that the N-terminal region is responsible for directing the protein to mitochondria. A recent hypothesis suggests that frataxin is a mitochondrial protein that is important for normal cellular energy production. A defect in the protein may result in abnormal accumulation of iron in mitochondria that is followed by cell death of susceptible neurons.

The disease is characterized clinically by the onset in the first two decades of life of limb ataxia, cerebellar dysarthria, a lack of deep-tendon reflexes, pyramidal signs, blindness, deafness, and sensory loss. Nonneurologic complications of Friedreich ataxia include scoliosis, hypertrophic cardiomyopathy, and diabetes mellitus, which suggests that the disease is ubiquitous and not limited to the nervous system. The disease occurs before the age of 10 years in approximately half of the patients. The ability to walk is lost within 5 to 10 years of onset of the disease, and survival time is approximately three to four decades after onset. Ataxia is usually the first sign of the disease. Dysarthria is an early finding. A pes cavus deformity of the feet associated with extensor plantar responses and loss of reflexes is a characteristic finding. Posterior column sensations of vibration and position sense are usually absent, but pain and temperature are preserved. A hypertrophic obstructive cardiomyopathy is present in the majority of patients and often is the cause of death.

The pathologic abnormalities in Friedreich ataxia primarily consist of an axonopathy in the distal parts of the axon, a "dying-back neuropathy." The neural pathways affected in Friedreich ataxia are those associated with large neuronal cell bodies and extensive axon elongations such as the long tracts of the dorsal columns, corticospinal tracts, Clarke column, selected brainstem nuclei, and peripheral nerves. The possibility that defects in energy metabolism might account for the central nervous system and systemic involvement resulted in study of mitochondrial function in patients with Friedreich ataxia. Many of the clinical manifestations of the disease are mimicked by disorders of vitamin E metabolism. In affected patients, the concentrations of a partially degraded, 180-kDa form of frataxin are abnormally low in muscle, cerebellar cortex, and cerebral cortex, and the frataxin is closely associated with mitochondria. Frataxin is normally present in the mitochondrial-rich neuronal cell bodies and axons.

The diagnosis of Friedreich ataxia is suspected on clinical grounds but confirmed by the presence of increased GAA repeating elements on gene testing.

References

Neurodystrophies

G_{M1} *Gangliosidosis*

Kaye EM, Shalish C, Livermore J, Taylor HC, Breakefield XO: Human B-galactosidase gene mutations in American patients with slowly progressive G_{M1} gangliosidosis. J Child Neurol 12:242–247, 1997

Wenger DA, Sattler M, Mueller OT, Myers GG, Schneiman RS, Nixon GW: Adult G_{M1} gangliosidosis: clinical and biochemical studies on two patients and comparisons to other patients called variant or adult G_{M1} gangliosidosis. Clin Genet 17:323–334, 1980

Yoshida K, Ikeda S, Kawaguchi K, Yanagisawa N: Adult G_{M1} gangliosidosis—immunohistochemical and ultrastructural findings in an autopsy case. Neurology 44:2376–2382, 1994

Yoshida K, Oshima A, Sakuraba H: G_{M1} gangliosidosis in adults: clinical and molecular analysis of 16 Japanese patients. Ann Neurol 31:328–332, 1992

G_{M2} *Gangliosidosis*

Gravel RA, Clarke JT, Kaback MM, Mahuran D, Sandhoff K, Suzuki K: The G_{M2} gangliosidoses. In: Scriver CR, Beaudet AL, Sly WS, Valle D, eds: The Metabolic and Molecular Bases of Inherited Disease. New York: McGraw-Hill 1995:2839–2879

Kolodny EH: G_{M2} gangliosidoses. In: Rosenberg RN, Prusiner SB, Dimauro S, Barchi RL, eds: The Molecular and Genetic Basis of Neurological Disease. Boston, Butterworth-Heinemann, 1997:473–490

Lacorazza HD, Flax JD, Snyder EY, Jendoubi M: Expression of human beta-hexosaminidase alpha-subunit gene (the gene defect of Tay-Sach disease) in mouse brains upon engraftment of transduced progenitor cells. Nat Med 2:424–429, 1996

Lyon G, Adams RD, Kolodny EH: Neurology of Hereditary Metabolic Diseases of Children. New York, McGraw-Hill, 1996

Fabry Disease

Bloomfield SE, David DS, Rubin AL: Eye findings in the diagnosis of Fabry's disease. Patients with renal failure. JAMA 240:647–649, 1978

Crutchfield KE, Patronas NJ, Dambrosia DM, et al: Quantitative analysis of cerebral vasculopathy in patients with Fabry disease. Neurology 50:1746–1749, 1998

Desnick RJ, Blieden LC, Sharp HL, Hofschire PJ, Moller JH: Cardiac valvular anomalies in Fabry disease. Clinical, morphologic, and biochemical studies. Circulation 54:818–825, 1976

Desnick RJ, Eng CM: Fabry disease: alpha-galactosidase A deficiency. In: Rosenberg RN, Prusiner SB, Dimauro S, Barchi RL, eds: The Molecular and Genetic Basis of Neurological Disease, 2nd ed. Boston, Butterworth-Heinemann, 1997:443–452

Deveber GA, Schwarting GA, Kolodny EH, Kowall NW: Fabry disease: immunocytochemical characterization of neuronal involvement. Ann Neurol 31:409–415, 1992

Eng CM, Ashley GA, Burgert TS, Enriquez AL, D'souza M, Desnick RJ: Fabry disease: thirty-five mutations in the alpha-galactosidase A gene in patients with classic and variant phenotypes. Mol Med 3:174–182, 1997

Gaucher Disease

Barton NW, Brady RO, Dambrosia JM, et al: Replacement therapy for inherited enzyme deficiency: macrophage-targeted glucocerebrosidase for Gaucher's disease. N Engl J Med 324:1464–1470, 1991

Kaye EM, Ullman MD, Wilson ER, Barranger JA: Type 2 and type 3 Gaucher disease: a morphological and biochemical study. Ann Neurol 20:223–230, 1986

Morales LE: Gaucher's disease: a review. Ann Pharmacother 30(4):381–388, 1996

Niemann Pick A

Schuchman EH, Desnick RJ: Type A and B Niemann-Pick disease: deficiencies of acid sphingomyelinase activity. In: Scriver CR, Beaudet AL, Sly WS, Valle D, eds: The Metabolic Basis of Inherited Disease, 7th ed. New York, McGraw Hill, 1995:2601–2624

Vanier MT, Suzuki K: Niemann-Pick diseases. In: Moser HW, ed: Handbook of Clinical Neurology, vol 66: Neurodystrophies and Neurolipidoses. Rev. series vol 22. Vinken PJ, Bruyn GW, eds. Amsterdam, Elsevier Science, 1996:133–162

Niemann-Pick C

Brown MS, Goldstein JL: The SBEBP pathway: regulation of cholesterol metabolism by proteolysis of a membrane-bound transcription factor. Cell 89:331–340, 1997

Carstea ED, Morris JA, Coleman KG, et al: Niemann-Pick C1 disease gene: homology to mediators of cholesterol homeostasis. Science 277:228–231, 1997

Fink JK, Filling-Katz MR, Sokol J, et al: Clinical spectrum of Niemann-Pick disease type C. Neurology 39:1040–1049, 1989

Higgins JJ, Patterson MC, Dambrosia JM, et al: A clinical staging classification for type C Niemann-Pick disease. Neurology 42:2286–2290, 1992

Neufeld EB, Wastney M, Patel S, et al: The Niemann-Pick C1 protein resides in a novel organelle linked to retrograde transport of multiple lysosomal cargo. J Biol Chem 274:9627–9635, 1999

Neuronal Ceroid Lipofuscinoses

Cho S, Dawson G: Enzymatic and moleular biological analysis of palmitoyl protein thioesterase deficiency in infantile neuronal ceroid lipofuscinosis. J Neurochem 71(1):323–329, 1998

International Batten Disease Consortium: Isolation of a novel gene underlying Batten disease, CLN3. Cell 82:949–957, 1995

Vesa J, Hellsten E, Verkruyse LA, et al: Mutations in the palmitoyl protein thioesterase gene causing infantile neuronal ceroid lipofuscinosis. Nature 376:584–588, 1995

Vines DJ, Warburton MJ: Classical late infantile neuronal ceroid lipofuscinosis fibroblasts are deficient in lysosomal tripeptidyl peptidase I. FEBS Lett 443:131–135, 1999

Zhong N, Wisniewski KE, Hartikainen J, et al: Two common mutations in the CLN2 gene underlie late infantile neuronal ceroid lipofuscinosis. Clin Genet 54(3):234–238, 1998

Mucopolysaccharidoses

Goldenfum SL, Young E, Michelakakis H, Tsagarakis S, Winchester B: Mutation analysis in 20 patients with Hunter disease. Hum Mutat 7(1):76–78, 1996

Neufeld EF, Muenzer J: The mucopolysaccharidoses. In: Scriver CR, Beaudet AL, Sly WS, Valle D, eds: The Metabolic Basis of Inherited Disease, 7th ed. New York, McGraw-Hill, 1995

Parsons VJ, Hughes DG, Wraith JE: Magnetic resonance imaging of the brain, neck and cervical spine in mild Hunter's syndrome (mucopolysaccharidosis type II). Clin Radiol 51(10):719–723, 1996

Peters C, Shapiro EG, Anderson J, et al: Hurler syndrome: II. Outcome of HLA-genotypically identical sibling and HLA-haploidentical related donor bone marrow transplantation in fifty-four children. The Storage Disease Collaborative Study Group. Blood 91(7):2601–2608, 1998

Mannosidosis

Alkhayat AH, Kraemer SA, Leipprandt JR, Macek M, Kleijer WJ, Friderici KH: Human beta-mannosidosis cDNA characterization and first identification of a mutation associated with human beta-mannosidosis. Hum Mol Genet 7:75–83, 1998

Jolly RD, Winchester B, Gehler J, Dorling J, Dawson G: Mannosidosis. A comparative review of biochemical and related clinicopathological aspects of three forms of the disease. J Appl Biochem 3:273–291, 1981

Wenger DA: Human beta-mannosidase deficiency. N Engl J Med 315:1201–1205, 1986

Fucosidosis

Cragg H, Williamson M, Young E, et al: Fucosidosis: genetic and biochemical analysis of 8 cases. J Med Genet 34:105–110, 1997

Tiberio G, Filocamo M, Gatti R, Durand P: Mutations in fucosidosis gene: a review. Acta Genet Med Gemellol 44:223–232, 1995

Willems PJ, Gatti R, Darby JK: Fucosidosis revisited: a review of 77 patients. Am J Med Genet 38:111–131, 1991

Sialidosis

Cantz M, Gehler J, Spranger J: Mucolipidosis I: Increased sialic acid content and deficiency of an alpha-N-acetylneuraminidase in cultured fibroblasts. Biochem Biophys Res Commun 74:732–738, 1977

Lowden JA, O'Brien JS: Sialidosis: a review of human neuraminidase deficiency. Am J Hum Genet 31:1–18, 1979

Mucolipidoses

Ben-Yoseph Y, Mitchell DA, Yager RM, Wei JT, Chen TH, Shih LY: Mucolipidoses II and III variants with normal N-acetylglucosamine 1-phosphotransferase activity toward alpha-methylmannoside are due to nonallelic mutations. Am J Hum Genet 50:137–144, 1992

Brik R, Mandel H, Aizin A, et al: Mucolipidosis III presenting as a rheumatological disorder. J Rheumatol 20:133–136, 1993

Chen CS, Bach G, Pagano RE: Abnormal transport along the lysosomal pathway in mucolipidosis, type IV disease. Proc Natl Acad Sci USA 95:6373–6378, 1998

Kornfeld S, Sly WS: I-cell disease and pseudo-Hurler polydystrophy: disorders of lysosomal enzyme phosphorylation and localization. In: Scriver

CR, Beaudet AL, Sly WS, Valle D, eds: The Metabolic and Molecular Basis of Inherited Disease, 7th ed. New York, McGraw-Hill, 1995: 2495–2508

Leroy JG, Spranger JW, Feingold M, Opitz JM, Crocker AC: I-cell disease: a clinical picture. J Pediatr 79:360–365, 1971

Menkes Steely Hair Disease

Kaler SG: Metabolic and molecular bases of Menkes disease and occipital horn syndrome. Pediatr Dev Pathol 1(1):85–98, 1998

Kodama H, Murata Y: Molecular genetics and pathophysiology of Menkes disease. Pediatr Int 41(4):430–435, 1999

Tumer Z, Horn N: Menkes disease: underlying genetic defect and new diagnostic possibilities. J Inherit Metab Dis 21(5):604–612, 1991

Tumer Z, Moller LB, Horn N: Mutation spectrum of ATP7A, the gene defective in Menkes disease. Adv Exp Med Biol 448:83–95, 1999

Wilson Disease

Brewer GJ, Dick RD, Johnson V, et al: Treatment of Wilson's disease with tetrathiomolybdate I. Initial therapy in 17 neurologically affected patients. Arch Neurol 51:545–554, 1994

Bull PC, Thomas GR, Rommens JM, Forbes JR, Cox DW: The Wilson disease gene is a putative copper transporting P-type ATPase similar to the Menkes gene. Nat Genet 5:327–337, 1993

Hallervorden-Spatz Disease

Halliday W: The nosology of Hallervorden-Spatz disease. J Neurol Sci 134(suppl):84–91, 1995

Luckenbach MW, Green WR, Miller NR, Moser HW, Clark AW, Tennekoon G: Ocular clinicopathologic correlation of Hallervorden-Spatz syndrome with acanthocytosis and pigmentary retinopathy. Am J Ophthalmol 95:369–382, 1983

Sethi KD, Adams RJ, Loring DW, el Gammal T: Hallervorden-Spatz syndrome: Clinical and magnetic resonance imaging correlations. Ann Neurol 24:692, 1988

Neuroaxonal Dystrophy

Itoh K, Negishi H, Obayashi C, et al: Infantile neuroaxonal dystrophy—immunohistochemical and ultrastructural studies on the central and peripheral nervous systems in infantile neuroaxonal dystrophy. Kobe J Med Sci 39(4):133–146, 1993

Keulemans JL, Reuser AJ, Kroos MA, et al: Human alpha-N-acetylgalactosaminidase (alpha-NAGA) deficiency: new mutations and the paradox between genotype and phenotype. J Med Genet 33(6):458–464, 1996

Nardocci N, Zorzi G, Farina L, et al: Infantile neuroaxonal dystrophy: clinical spectrum and diagnostic criteria. Neurology 1999:52(7):1472

Rees H, Ang LC, Casey R, George DH: Association of infantile neuroaxonal dystrophy and osteopetrosis: a rare autosomal recessive disorder. Pediatr Neurosurg 22(6):321–327, 1995

Venkatesh S, Coulter DL, Kemper TD: Neuroaxonal dystrophy at birth with hypertonicity and basal ganglia mineralization. J Child Neurol 9(1):74–76, 1994

Leukodystrophies

Adrenoleukodystrophy

Aubourg P, Adamsbaum C, Lavallard-Rousseau MC, et al: A two-year trial of oleic and erucic acids ("Lorenzo's oil") as treatment for adrenomyeloneuropathy. N Engl J Med 329:745–752, 1993

Aubourg P, Blanche S, Jambaque I, et al: Reversal of early neurologic and neuroradiologic manifestations of X-linked adrenoleukodystrophy by bone marrow transplantation. N Engl J Med 322:1860–1866, 1990

Dodd A, Rowland SA, Hawkes SLJ, Kennedy MA, Love DR: Mutations in the adrenoleukodystrophy gene. Hum Mutat 9:500–511, 1997

Moser HW: Adrenoleukodystrophy: phenotype, genetics, pathogenesis and therapy. Brain 120:1485–1508, 1997

Sadeghi-Nejad A, Senior B: Adrenomyeloneuropathy presenting as Addison's disease in childhood. N Engl J Med 322:13–16, 1990

Van Geel BM, Assies J, Weverling GJ, Barth PG: Predominance of the adrenomyeloneuropathy phenotype of X-linked adrenoleukodystrophy in the Netherlands: a survey of 30 kindreds. Neurology 44:2343–2346, 1994

Krabbe Disease

Bambach BJ, Moser HW, Blakemore K, et al: Engraftment following in utero bone marrow transplantation for globoid cell leukodystrophy. Bone Marrow Transplant 19:399–402, 1997

Baram TZ, Goldman AM, Percy AK: Krabbe disease: specific MRI and CT findings. Neurology 36:111–115, 1986

Chen YQ, Rafi MA, de Gala G, Wenger DA: Cloning and expression of cDNA encoding a human galactocerebrosidase, the enzyme deficient in globoid cell leukodystrophy. Hum Mol Genet 2:1841–1845, 1993

Krivit W, Shapiro EG, Peters C, et al: Hematopoietic stem-cell transplantation in globoid-cell leukodystrophy. N Engl J Med 338:1119–1126, 1998

Metachromatic Leukodystrophy

Barth ML, Fensom A, Harris A: The arylsulphatase A gene and molecular genetics of metachromatic leucodystrophy. J Med Genet 31:663–666, 1994

Berger J, Loschi B, Bernheimer H, et al: Occurrence, distribution and phenotype of arylsulfatase A mutations in patients with metachromatic leukodystrophy. Am J Med Genet 69:335–340, 1997

Gieselmann V, Fluharty AL, Tonnesen T, von Figura K: Mutations in the arylsulfatase A pseudodeficiency allele causing metachromatic leukodystrophy. Am J Hum Genet 49:407–413, 1991

Gieselmann V, Polten A, Kreysing J, von Figura K: Arylsulfatase A pseudodeficiency: loss of a polyadenylylation signal and N-glycosylation site. Proc Natl Acad Sci USA 86:9436–9440, 1989

Krivit W, Shapiro E, Kennedy W, et al: Effective treatment of late infantile metachromatic leukodystrophy by bone marrow transplantation. N Engl J Med 322:28–32, 1990

Pelizaeus-Merzbacher

Gencic S, Abuelo D, Ambler M, Hudson LD: Pelizaeus-Merzbacher disease: an X-linked neurologic disorder of myelin metabolism with a novel mutation in the gene encoding proteolipid protein. Am J Hum Genet 45:435–442, 1989

Inoue K, Osaka H, Imaizumi K, et al: Proteolipid protein gene duplications causing Pelizaeus-Merzbacher disease: molecular mechanism and phenotypic manifestations. Ann Neurol 45:624–632, 1999

Nave KA, Boespflug-Tanguy O: X-linked developmental defects of myelination: from mouse mutants to human genetic diseases. Neuroscientist 2:33–43, 1996

Saugier-Veber P, Munnich A, Bonneau D, et al: X-linked spastic paraplegia and Pelizaeus-Merzbacher disease are allelic disorders at the proteolipid protein locus. Nat Genet 6:257–262, 1994

Canavan Disease

Brismar J, Brismar G, Gascon G, Ozand P: Canavan disease: CT and MR imaging of the brain. Am J Neuroradiol 11:805–810, 1990

Kaul R, Gao GP, Balamurugan K, Matalon R: Human aspartoacylase cDNA and mis-sense mutation in Canavan disease. Nat Genet 5:118–123, 1993

CADASIL

Joutel A, Corpechot C, Ducros A, et al: Notch3 mutations in CADASIL, a hereditary adult-onset condition causing stroke and dementia. Nature 383:707–710, 1996

Joutel A, Corpechot C, Ducros A, et al: Notch3 mutations in cerebral autosomal dominant arteriopathy with subcortical infarcts and leukoencephalopathy (CADASIL), a mendelian condition causing stroke and vascular dementia. Ann NY Acad Sci 826:213–217, 1997

Joutel A, Vahedi K, Corpechot C, et al: Strong clustering and stereotyped nature of Notch3 mutations in CADASIL patients. Lancet 350:1511–1515, 1997

Jung HH, Bassetti C, Tournier-Lasserve E, et al: Cerebral autosomal dominant arteriopathy with subcortical infarcts and leukoencephalopathy: a clinicopathological and genetic study of a Swiss family. J Neurol Neurosurg Psychiatry 59:138–143, 1995

Alexander Disease

Arend AO, Leary PM, Rutherford GS: Alexander's disease: a case report with brain biopsy, ultrasound, CT scan and MRI findings. Clin Neuropathol 10:122–126, 1991

Bobele GB, Garnica A, Schaefer GB, et al: Neuroimaging findings in Alexander's disease. J Child Neurol 5:253–258, 1990

Hess DC, Fischer AQ, Yaghmai F, Figueroa R, Akamatsu Y: Comparative neuroimaging with pathologic correlates in Alexander's disease. J Child Neurol 5:248–252, 1990

Johnson AB: Alexander disease. In: Moser HW, ed: Handbook of Clinical Neurology, vol 66: Neurodystrophies and Neurolipidoses, rev series vol 22. Amsterdam, Elsevier, 1996:701–710

Pridmore CL, Baraitser M, Harding B, Boyd SG, Kendall B, Brett EM: Alexander's disease: clues to diagnosis. J Child Neurol 8:134–144, 1993

CACH (Vanishing White Matter Disease)

Schiffmann R, Moller JR, Trapp BD, et al: Childhood ataxia with diffuse central nervous system hypomyelination. Ann Neurol 35(3):331–340, 1994

Van der Knaap MS, Barth PG, Gabreels FJM, et al: A new leukoencephalopathy with vanishing white matter. Neurology 48:845–855, 1997

Van der Knaap MS, Kamphorst W, Barth PG, Kraaijeveld CL, Gut E, Valk J: Phenotypic variation in leukoencephalopathy with vanishing white matter. Neurology 51(2):540–547, 1998

Huntington Disease

Difiglia M, Sapp E, Chase KO, et al: Aggregation of huntingtin in neuronal intranuclear inclusions and dystrophic neurites in brain. Science 277:1990–1993, 1997

Duayo M, Ambrose C, Myers R, et al: Trinucleotide repeat length instability and age of onset in Huntington's disease. Nat Genet 4:387–392, 1993

Ranen NG, Peyser CE, Folstein SE: A Physicians Guide to the Management of Huntington's Disease. New York, Huntington's Disease Society of America, 1993

Strong TV, Tagle DA, Valdes JM, et al: Widespread expression of the human and rat Huntington's disease gene in brain and nonneural tissues. Nat Genet 5:259–265, 1993

Spinocerebellar Ataxias

Benton CS, de Silva R, Rutledge SL, Bohlega S, Ashizawa T, Zoghbi HY: Molecular and clinical studies in SCA-7 define a broad clinical spectrum and the infantile phenotype. Neurology 51:1081–1086, 1998

Matsumura R, Futamura N, Fujimoto Y, et al: Spinocerebellar ataxia type 6. Molecular and clinical features of 35 Japanese patients including one homozygous for the CAG repeat expansion. Neurology 49:1238–1243, 1997

Orr HT, Chung MY, Banfi S, et al: Expansion of an unstable trinucleotide CAG repeat in spinocerebellar ataxia type 1. Nat Genet 6:221–226, 1993

Schols L, Gispert S, Vorgerd M, et al: Spinocerebellar ataxia type 2: genotype and phenotype in German kindreds. Arch Neurol 54:1073–1080, 1997

Friedreich Ataxia

Campuzano V, Montermini L, Molto MD, et al: Friedreich's ataxia: autosomal recessive disease caused by an intronic GAA triplet repeat expansion. Science 271:1423–1427, 1996

de Michele G, Di Maio L, Filla A, et al: Childhood onset of Friedreich ataxia: a clinical and genetic study of 36 cases. Neuropediatrics 27:3–7, 1996

Durr A, Cossee M, Agid Y, et al: Clinical and genetic abnormalities in patients with Friedreich's ataxia. N Engl J Med 335:1169–1175, 1996

Lamont PJ, Davis MB, Wood NW: Identification and sizing of the GAA trinucleotide repeat expansion of Friedreich's ataxia in 56 patients. Clinical and genetic correlates. Brain 120:673–680, 1997

Montermini L, Richter A, Morgan K, et al: Phenotypic variability in Friedreich ataxia: role of the associated GAA triplet repeat expansion. Ann Neurol 41:675–682, 1997

25.18 PHAKOMATOSES AND OTHER NEUROCUTANEOUS SYNDROMES

Eveline Traeger and Isabelle Rapin

The *phakomatoses* refer to a variety of neurocutaneous syndromes. These disorders are embryonal in origin, and a number of them arise from the neural crest. In the dominant syndromes, which are often the result of a new mutation, the penetrance of the gene appears to be high, but the phenotypic expressivity is variable (see Sec. 10.3.7). Neurofibromatosis and tuberous sclerosis are the most common phakomatoses. Their prevalence has been underestimated because of their variable expressivity, with involvement of many organ systems. Both affect brain development and carry a high risk of tumors as they result from mutations in tumor suppressor genes. The manifestations of some of the other phakomatoses arise from involvement of the vascular system.

25.18.1 Tuberous Sclerosis

Tuberous sclerosis (adenoma sebaceum, epiloia, Bourneville disease, Bourneville-Pringle syndrome) is inherited as an autosomal-dominant trait with complete penetrance but with variable expressivity (see Sec. 10.3.7). Two-thirds of cases represent sporadic new mutations. Linkage analysis has established the presence of two loci: *TSC1* on chromosome 9q34, which encodes for the protein hamartin, and *TSC2* on chromosome 16p13, which encodes for the protein tuberin. The full syndrome is characterized by seizures, mental deficiency, and adenoma sebaceum, with foci of intracranial calcification, particularly in the periventricular region, although these lesions may be scattered throughout the hemispheres. The seizures are most often infantile spasms in young children and grand mal seizures in older children. In the full syndrome, mental deficiency is generally severe. However, intellectual capacity may be normal or near normal. A significant minority of individuals, especially those with multiple hamartomas in the temporal lobes, are autistic as well as retarded. The earliest skin lesion is the ash-leaf-shaped depigmented macule, often present from birth or infancy, in itself strongly suggesting the diagnosis of tuberous sclerosis. The characteristic facial skin lesions (fibroangiomatous nevi) have been mislabeled *adenoma sebaceum;* the sebaceous glands are involved only secondarily. Fibroangiomatous nevi may be present during the first year of life but are usually not noted until the age of 4 to 7 years. These lesions take the form of discrete pink or yellowish papules, principally on the face in a butterfly distribution on the bridge of the nose, on the malar prominences, and along the nasal-labial folds. The lesions also may occur on the forehead, neck, and trunk. Individual lesions remain static, gradually growing redder and eventually becoming brownish. They do not itch, nor do they suppurate, which distinguishes them from acne vulgaris and seborrheic dermatitis. Other skin lesions consist of raised plaque-like flesh-colored lesions (shagreen patches) that resemble coarse-grained leather and are usually found in the lumbosacral region after age 10 years. Fibromas of the scalp and eyelid are occasionally seen. The nontraumatic subungal fibroma, a flesh-colored sessile growth emerging from the groove of the nailbed, is distinctive. Several retinal lesions may be observed. Small flat white or yellowish phakomas or spots may occur on or close to the optic nerve head. A second lesion is a raised cluster of translucent white tissue in the fundus. Systemic involvement may include multiple angiomyolipomas of the kidney and other viscera, including myomas of the uterus and vagina. The presence of multiple rhabdomyomas of the heart can be diagnosed by echocardiography and may be detected even before other features of the disorder are manifest. They have even been observed during fetal echocardiography. Patients may succumb in infancy to cardiac arrhythmia, later to renal or respiratory failure. Radiographs may show honeycomb lesions in the lung and small cystic lesions in the distal phalanges of the hands and feet.

The brain contains many firm sclerotic nodules (tubera) at the crest of gyri or in the subependymal region, where they project into the lateral ventricle and calcify. They contain sheets of astrocytes and giant, often multinucleated, malformed cells. Developmental abnormalities such as ectopic neurons in the white matter and other disorders of cell migration are very common. Children may develop hydrocephalus because of obstruction of the foramen of Monro by a neoplasm, almost always a giant cell astrocytoma that may require surgical removal or shunting. These tumors grow very slowly and are unlikely to become malignant. They occasionally produce diencephalic dysfunction. Radiographs often show calcified intracranial lesions that enhance with contrast (Fig. 25-53).

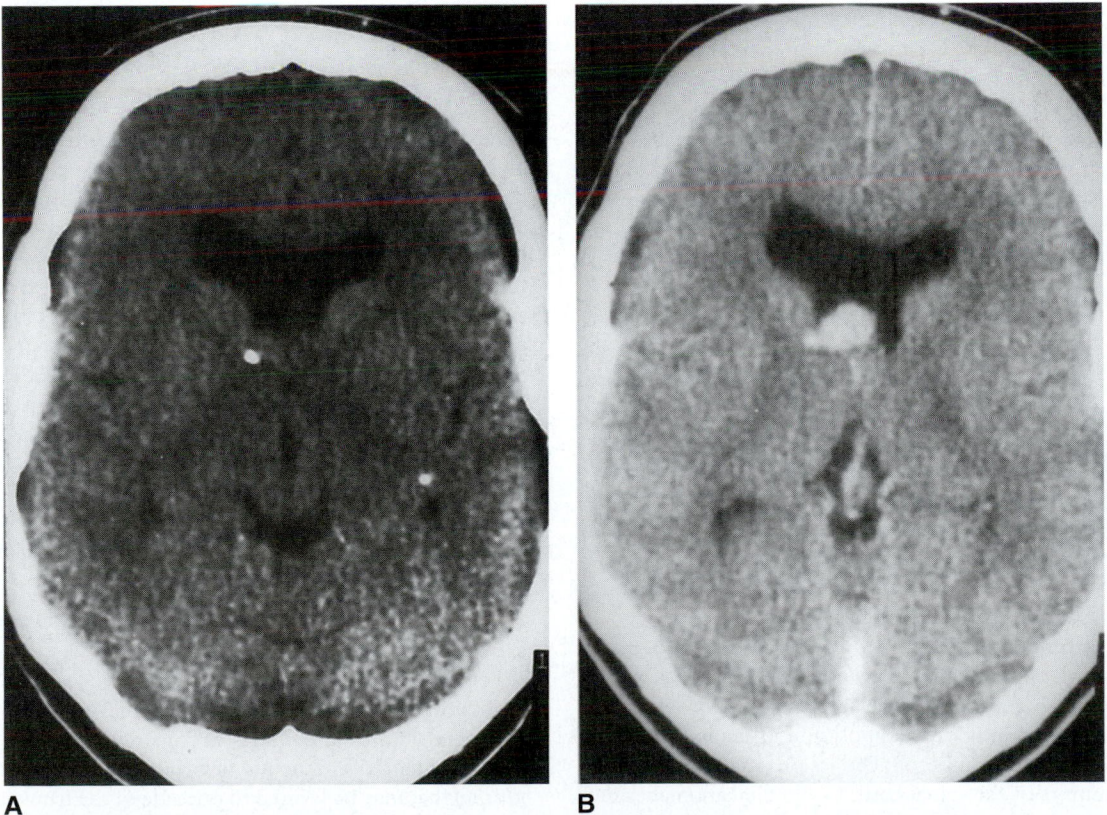

A   **B**

FIGURE 25-53   Axial noncontrast CT scan (A) shows calcified periventricular lesions typical of tuberous sclerosis, which enhance with contrast (B). *Courtesy of Dr. Jacqueline Bello.*

Revised clinical diagnostic criteria from 1998 require two or more distinct types of lesions for confirmation of diagnosis. (See Table 10-0.) Treatment is entirely symptomatic.

25.18.2 Neurofibromatosis

Neurofibromatosis 1 (von Recklinghausen disease) is one of the most common autosomal dominant traits; its prevalence has been estimated at 1 per 3000 births (see Sec. 10.3.7). The rate of new mutations is 50%. The majority of patients have only cutaneous manifestations of marginal importance, but about 25% develop neoplasms such as central nervous system tumors, pheochromocytomas, and occasional fibrosarcomas that may be lethal. The gene *NF1*, classified as tumor suppressor gene, has been mapped to 17q11.2 and encodes the protein neurofibromin, which is involved in the regulation of the protooncogene *ras*. Approximately 100 different gene mutations have been identified.

The phenotypic expression is extraordinary. Some manifestations include multiple soft tumors beneath the skin, multiple tumors situated along nerve trunks (neurofibromas), and pigmented skin lesions (café-au-lait spots). Varying degrees of mental deficiency caused by a disorder of cortical disorganization may occur. The characteristic abnormality consists of neurofibromas (neurilemomas, schwannomas) of the peripheral, spinal, autonomic, and cranial nerves. Meningiomas, gliomas, and ependymomas of the brain and the spinal cord are common. The optic nerve or chiasm is a frequent site of an infiltrating astrocytoma. Most of the tumors are benign, but sarcomatous degeneration of peripheral tumors and glioblastomas occasionally occur in an adolescent or adult. Pheochromocytomas have been reported in adults, gangliogliomas and neuroblastomas in children. When neurofibromas occur in bone, they produce localized areas of rarefaction, or they may give rise to thickening or excessive linear growth of the long bones. Involvement of the spine may produce scoliosis, and orbital wall defects may result in pulsating exophthalmos. Both macrocephaly and hydrocephalus may occur. Pendulous masses of fibrous tissue and skin, which are characteristic of the adult form of neurofibromatosis, are rare in children.

Neurofibromatosis must be differentiated from tuberous sclerosis. In the former, the lesions tend to involve the peripheral outflow of the central nervous system more often than the brain, whereas in tuberous sclerosis the lesions are central. Mental deficiency and epilepsy are much more frequent with tuberous sclerosis. Most patients with neurofibromatosis are of normal intelligence, but many have specific learning disabilities that have been related to the number of locations occupied by "unidentified bright objects" on MR imaging. The skin lesions of the two syndromes are clearly different.

The typical clinical presentation, diagnostic criteria, and anticipatory guidance are given in Sec. 10.3.7.

Optic nerve tumors within the orbit may lead to progressive exophthalmos with optic atrophy. Astrocytomas of the optic chiasm and hypothalamus may result in the symptom complex of impaired visual acuity, diabetes insipidus, adiposity, and genital maldevelopment, or in precocious puberty. The lesions may present as intramedullary tumors of the spinal cord. Congenital anomalies such as spina bifida, rib and vertebral anomalies, and renal artery stenosis may be associated. CT and MR imaging greatly facilitate diagnosis and follow-up of patients with neurofibromatosis.

The offending neurofibromas can be removed surgically, but no definitive cure can be expected owing to the multiple nature of the lesions. Surgery should be done only when a particular lesion becomes a major symptomatic problem. Routine CT or MR scanning and recording of visual and brainstem auditory evoked responses are recommended by some authorities; this suggestion is impractical and has dubious value in asymptomatic patients because lesions of functional or life-threatening importance may arise at any time during the individual's lifetime and in any organ of the body. MR imaging is a more practical screening modality and provides a convenient means of radiation-free follow-up. Prenatal diagnosis may be possible by either linkage analysis in informative families or a protein truncation assay. The inability to predict phenotype based on genotype limits the usefulness of prenatal diagnosis.

Neurofibromatosis 2 (*central neurofibromatosis*) is a severe, genetically distinct autosomal-dominant syndrome characterized by the occurrence of usually bilateral acoustic neurinomas, regularly associated with multiple schwannomas of the dorsal roots of the spinal cord and other cranial nerves and with other tumors of the brain and cord such as gliomas and meningiomas. Cutaneous manifestations are sparse or absent, and Lisch nodules do not occur. Patients usually become symptomatic in adolescence or young adult life. The gene, *NF2*, a tumor suppressor gene, is on chromosome 22q12.2 and encodes the protein merlin, which is a member of a family of proteins that link elements of the cytoskeleton and the cell membrane. Multiple gene mutations have been identified (see Sec. 10.3.7).

A variant, segmental NF1, has symptoms confined to a specific portion of the body. Molecular evidence supports somatic mosaicism in which an *NF1* gene mutation is limited to the affected segment.

25.18.3 Neurocutaneous Melanosis

Neurocutaneous melanosis is a sporadic disorder characterized by a giant pigmented nevi of the skin or multiple scattered large nevi associated with melanosis of the leptomeninges. The nevi are usually dark and often hairy; they may occupy a large area of the trunk in a bathing suit or cape distribution. They tend to originate from the posterior midline and to follow a dermatome distribution. Melanosis of the leptomeninges, often with pigmentation of parenchymal areas of the brainstem or cerebellum, is present in most of these children. Hydrocephalus may occur because of CSF obstruction by benign melanotic cells or because of malignant transformation, which is common. Malignant transformation of the skin lesion may also take place. Increased CSF protein, increased CSF melanin content, and recovery of melanoblasts from the CSF suggest malignancy. Convulsive disorders and mental retardation may occur in this syndrome even in the absence of hydrocephalus or malignant transformation.

25.18.4 Polyostotic Fibrous Dysplasia

In polyostotic fibrous dysplasia (McCune-Albright syndrome), the complete syndrome includes fibrous dysplasia of multiple bones, large pigmented cutaneous nevi with irregular margins (*coast of Maine*) that may be limited to one side of the trunk, and precocious sexual development, especially in girls. The primary neurologic features of the syndrome include mental deficiency, epilepsy, and headaches. The syndrome is sporadic, more common in girls, and caused by a postzygotic activating mutation in the gene *GNAS1* that encodes the α subunit of the G protein ($G\alpha_s$) that stimulates adenylyl cyclase. Mutation containing cells are present in a mosaic pattern, the greatest number present in the most affected tissues.

25.18.5 Incontinentia Pigmenti

Incontinentia pigmenti (Bloch-Sulzberger syndrome) is characterized by characteristic congenital skin lesions discussed in Sec. 14.4.3. Mental retardation, often with severe seizures, occurs in fewer than 30% of patients. The ocular findings include frequent strabismus, optic atrophy, opacities of the cornea and lens, an abnormal pattern of pigmentation of the choroid and retina, pseudogliomas, and microphthalmia. Symptomatic treatment of these children and genetic counseling are in order. The syndrome is inherited as an X-linked dominant disorder with male lethality. Sporadic cases of incontinentia pigmenti in males have been reported and may be associated with a Klinefelter genotype (47, XXY). The gene links to Xq28, and nonrandom inactivation of the mutated X chromosome is observed in women.

25.18.6 Incontinentia Pigmenti Achromians

This condition, also known as *hypomelanosis of Ito,* is etiologically heterogenous. Autosomal-dominant, autosomal-recessive, as well as X-linked inheritance have been proposed, or the disorder may be associated with the presence of mosaicism or translocation in blood lymphocytes, skin fibroblasts, or keratinocytes. Swirls and streaks of hypopigmentation occur anywhere on the body and are frequently associated with mental retardation and seizures and in some cases with autism.

25.18.7 Epidermal Nevus Syndrome (Linear Nevus Sebaceous, Nevus Unius Lateralis)

Epidermal nevus syndrome is a sporadic congenital syndrome in which there are linear slightly raised yellowish verrucose skin lesions associated with orange-yellow or dark brown plaques with a waxy surface, mainly on the middle of the face. The lesions may be quite extensive and are frequently associated with mental retardation and seizures. They consist of hyperkeratosis of the epidermis, hyperplasia of the sebaceous glands, and abortive hair follicles within the dermis. The skin lesions may degenerate into basal cell carcinomas, and early removal for prophylactic and cosmetic reasons has been advocated. Nevus unius lateralis consists of a much less striking unilateral linear array of papules that are light to dark brown and present at birth or develop during the first year. These papules consist of hyperkeratosis, papillomatosis, and acanthosis of the epidermis, but the dermis and subcutaneous tissues are not affected. Mental retardation, seizures, and hemiparesis are less frequent than with linear nevus sebaceous, but they occur in about 25% of these children. Eye anomalies are rare.

25.18.8 Sjögren-Larsson Syndrome

Sjögren-Larsson syndrome, a rare autosomal-recessive condition, is characterized by a congenital nonbullous ichthyosiform erythro-derma. A spastic diplegia is usually apparent from early life, and most children are moderately to severely intellectually deficient. Half have pigmentary degeneration of the retina, and glistening spots of the retina are characteristic. It is caused by mutations in the gene for fatty aldehyde dehydrogenase (*FALDH*) which encodes an enzyme that catalyzes the oxidation of fatty aldehydes to fatty acids. The *FALDH* gene, which is located on chromosome 17p11.2, has been sequenced, and more than 40 mutations have been identified. It is said to respond to fat restriction and the administration of medium-chain triglycerides. Prenatal diagnosis may be possible.

25.18.9 Chédiak-Higashi Syndrome

Chédiak-Higashi syndrome is an autosomal-recessive disorder characterized by partial oculocutaneous albinism, increased susceptibility to infection, lack of natural killer cells, and the presence of large lysosome-like granules in many tissues, including polymorphonuclear phagocytes and melanocytes. Splenomegaly and hypersplenism, hepatomegaly, and lymphadenopathy are common. Most patients die within their first two decades. Nystagmus and photophobia occur because of the ocular albinism. Peripheral neuropathy occurs frequently in older children and adolescents, with areflexia, footdrop, weakness, and sensory loss. Chédiak-Higashi syndrome maps to chromosome 1q43. The gene has been identified and encodes a protein whose loss of function may result in an abnormality of organellar protein trafficking.

25.18.10 Encephalotrigeminal Angiomatosis (Sturge-Weber Syndrome)

Encephalotrigeminal angiomatosis is a nongenetic condition that includes a port wine capillary nevus of the face (often in the distribution of the first division of the trigeminal nerve), convulsions (often focal and involving the contralateral side of the body), contralateral hemiparesis, and occasionally homonymous hemianopia and mental deficiency. Ipsilateral intracranial calcifications are found by x-ray examination. These calcifications are characteristically in paired lines, often called *trolley tracks* (Fig. 25-54). Increased intraocular tension may be caused by angiomatous involvement of the uveal tract and may give rise to enlargement of the involved globe. About two-thirds of the children with this condition have convulsive disorders. Hemiparesis is less common. There is great variability in the severity of the individual symptoms, and one or another may be missing entirely. Hemangiomas may be found in parts of the body other than the face and, rarely, in the fundi. They may be extensive and associated with hypertrophy of the limb and deep varices (Klippel-Trénaunay syndrome).

The intracranial lesion is a capillary hemangioma that involves the meninges in the area supplied by the first division of the trigeminal nerve and the superficial vessels occupying the sulci over the convexity, particularly in the occipital and parietal regions. This may cause atrophy of the underlying brain tissue, and the degenerative changes in cerebral tissue just below the gyral surface are frequently followed by the characteristic calcifications. Demonstration of intracranial calcifications limited to the convexity of the brain and showing the characteristic gyral pattern is almost pathognomonic.

The disorder is diagnosed from the physical and radiographic findings. Therapy is symptomatic, although early surgical excision

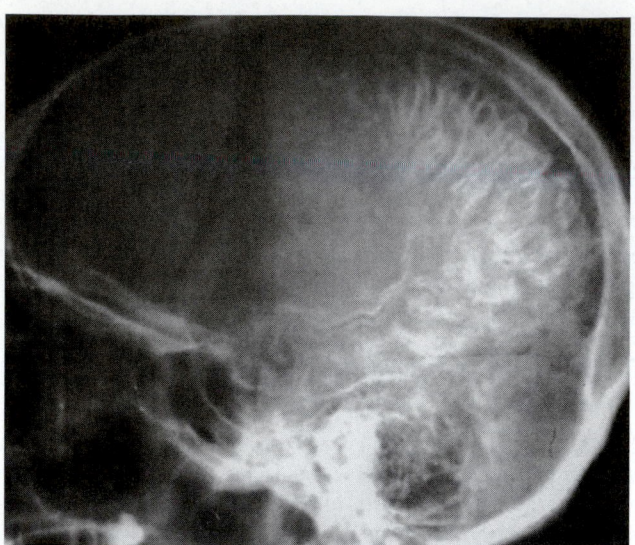

FIGURE 25-54 Encephalotrigeminal angiomatosis. Skull x-ray showing characteristic intracranial calcification.

(lobectomy or hemispherectomy) is sometimes done in the hopes of preventing seizures that may be very difficult to control and associated with intellectual decline. The differential diagnosis includes consideration of Wyburn-Mason syndrome and noncalcifying meningeal angiomatosis associated with white matter involvement.

25.18.11 Wyburn-Mason Syndrome

Wyburn-Mason syndrome (Bonnet-Dechaume-Blanc syndrome) is a sporadic condition characterized by unilateral cirsoid vascular anomalies of the retina associated with an intracranial arteriovenous anomaly that involves the mesencephalon and base of the brain. Unilateral exophthalmos, enlarged facial draining veins, or facial angioma may occur.

25.18.12 Hereditary Hemorrhagic Telangiectasia (Osler-Rendu-Weber Syndrome)

This autosomal-dominant disorder is associated with mucocutaneous and visceral telangiectasias, most noticeable on the lips and tongue and nasal mucosa, where they produce nose bleeds. Brain involvement includes migraine headaches as well as bleeds from telangiectasias, aneurysms, angiomas, and arteriovenous malformations. Brain abscesses may result from right-to-left pulmonary shunts, and cerebral thrombosis from polycythemia. This disorder is genetically heterogeneous. Genes have been localized to chromosome 9q34.1 and 12q11-q14. Other loci may exist as well.

25.18.13 Cutaneous Spinal Angiomatosis (Cobb Syndrome)

The association of midline angiomas of the skin with a vascular malformation of the spinal cord may occur either sporadically or as a dominant trait.

25.18.14 Von Hippel-Lindau Disease

Von Hippel-Lindau disease results from an autosomal-dominant mutation affecting a tumor suppressor gene, *VHL*, on chromosome 3p25.5. It does not become symptomatic before late adolescence or early adult life (see Sec. 10.3.7). The key features are hemangioblastomas of the cerebellum and retina. The disease usually presents as a cystic cerebellar neoplasm with increased intracranial pressure and few localizing signs, less often as a spinal hemangioblastoma. Polycythemia is associated with hemangioblastoma in 10 to 20% of patients. The lesion is readily diagnosed by neuroimaging. Its prognosis is excellent if total surgical removal is accomplished. Visceral lesions include multiple cystic lesions of the kidney, pancreas, and epididymis as well as pheochromocytoma and hypernephroma.

References

Baraitser P, Shieff C: Cutaneomeningo-spinal angiomatosis: the syndrome of Cobb. A case report. Neuropediatrics 21:160, 1990

Bolton PF, Griffiths PD: Association of tuberous sclerosis of temporal lobes with autism and atypical autism. Lancet 349:392, 1997

Denckla MB, Hofman K, Mazzoccio MM, et al: Relationship between T2-weighted hyperintensities (unidentified bright objects) and lower IQs in children with neurofibromatosis 1. Am J Med Genet 67:98, 1996

Grebe TA, Rimsza ME, Richter SF, et al: Further delineation of the epidermal nevus syndrome: two cases with new findings and literature review. Am J Med Genet 47:24, 1993

Gusella JF, Ramesh V, MacCollin M, et al: Neurofibromatosis 2: loss of merlin's protective spell. Curr Opin Genet Dev 6:87, 1996

Jagell S, Gustavson K-H, Holmgren G: Sjögren-Larsson syndrome: a clinical, genetic, and epidemiological study. Clin Genet 19:233, 1981

Johnson DW, Berg JN, Baldwin MA, et al: Mutations in the activin receptor-like kinase 1 gene in hereditary hemorrhagic telangiectasia type 2. Nat Genet 13:189, 1996

Kadonaga JN, Frieden IJ: Neurocutaneous melanosis: definition and review of the literature. J Am Acad Derm 24:747, 1991

Landy SJ, Donnai D: Incontinentia pigmenti (Bloch-Sulzberger syndrome). J Med Genet 30:53, 1993

MacCollin M, Mautner V-F: The diagnosis and management of neurofibromatosis 2 in childhood. Semin Pediatr Neurol 5:243, 1998

Maddock IR, Moran A, Maher ER, et al: A genetic register for von Hippel-Lindau disease. J Med Genet 33:120, 1996

North KN: Neurofibromatosis 1 in childhood. Semin Pediatr Neurol 5:231, 1998

Park VM, Pivnick EK: Neurofibromatosis type 1 (NF1): a protein truncation assay yielding identification of mutations in 73% of patients. J Med Genet 35:813, 1998

Pascual-Ccastroviejo I, Roche C, Martinez-Bermejo A, et al: Hypomelanosis of Ito. A study of 76 infantile cases. Brain Dev 20:36, 1998

Pettit RE, Berdal KE: Chédiak-Higashi syndrome. Neurologic appearance. Arch Neurol 41:1001, 1984

Porteous ME, Burn J, Proctor SJ: Hereditary hemorrhagic telangiectasia: a clinical analysis. J Med Genet 29:527, 1992

Ringel MD, Schwindinger WF, Levine MA: Clinical implications of genetic defects in G proteins: the molecular basis of McCune-Albright syndrome and Albright hereditary osteodystrophy. Medicine 75:171, 1996

Rizzo WB: Sjögren-Larsson syndrome: explaining the skin-brain connection. Neurology 52:1307, 1999

Roach ES: Von Hippel-Lindau disease: how does one gene cause multiple tumors? Neurology 53:7, 1999

Roach ES, Gomez MR, Northrup H: Tuberous sclerosis complex consensus conference: revised clinical diagnostic criteria. J Child Neurol 13:624, 1998

Spritz RA: Genetic defects in Chédiak-Higashi syndrome and the *beige* mouse. J Clin Immunol 18:97, 1998

Sujansky E, Conradi S: Sturge-Weber syndrome: age of onset of seizures and glaucoma and the prognosis for affected children. J Child Neurol 10:49, 1995

Woffendin H, Jakins T, Jouet M, et al: X-inactivation and marker studies in three families with incontinentia pigmenti: implications for counseling and gene localization. Clin Genet 55:55, 1999

Young JM, Burley MW, Jeremiah SJ, et al: A mutation screen of the *TSC1* gene revealed 26 protein truncating mutations and 1 splice site mutation in a panel of 79 tuberous sclerosis patients. Ann Hum Genet 62:203, 1998

THE EYES

Kevin M. Miller and Leonard Apt, Associate Editors

Careful evaluation of the eyes is an integral part of the pediatric examination. Recognition and management of abnormalities of the eyes, the ocular adnexae, and pertinent central nervous system pathways presume a thorough understanding of normal ocular anatomy and physiology. Such recognition and management also require a systematic approach to the ocular history and physical examination and an awareness of the disease processes that affect the various anatomic components of the visual system. Unlike other organs, many ocular diseases can be categorized, and even diagnosed, on clinical examination alone because of the transparency of the ocular media. Awareness of "sensitive" or "critical" periods in visual development underscores a need for neonatologists, pediatricians, and family doctors to be involved in screening for ocular disease. In fact, the first careful ocular screening examination should occur in the newborn nursery. Early diagnosis of diseases such as cataract, strabismus, and glaucoma can lead to effective therapy that may prevent amblyopia or blindness. Referral to an ophthalmologist is usually indicated for definitive examination and treatment.

General References

Basic and Clinical Science Course. Section 6, Pediatric Ophthalmology and Strabismus, San Francisco, American Academy of Ophthalmology, 2000

Cibis GW, Tongue AC, Stass-Isern ML: Decision Making in Pediatric Ophthalmology. St. Louis, Decker, 1993

Isenberg SJ, ed: The Eye in Infancy, 2nd ed. St. Louis, Mosby, 1994

Nelson LB, ed: Harley's Pediatric Ophthalmology, 4th ed. Philadelphia, Saunders, 1998

Newell FW: Ophthalmology Principles and Concepts, 8th ed. St. Louis, Mosby, 1996

Taylor D: Paediatric Ophthalmology, 2nd ed. London, Blackwell Science, 1997

Wright KW, ed: Pediatric Ophthalmology and Strabismus. St. Louis, Mosby, 1995

26.1   CLINICAL EVALUATION

26.1.1   Ocular History

The most important part of the ocular history is the chief complaint. Relevant details to be obtained include symptoms (eye pain, vision loss, photophobia, tearing), associated signs (proptosis, eye rubbing, conjunctival injection, nystagmus), onset, timing, frequency, factors that exacerbate or remit the symptoms, and previous treatment. For newborns, infants, and preverbal children, the chief complaint usually comes from the parent or caregiver. During routine screening examinations, such as those performed in the newborn nursery, there is no chief complaint. In these instances it is important for the pediatrician to know what to screen given the family history, prenatal history, and general health of the infant.

A prenatal history of intrauterine infection (toxoplasmosis, rubella, cytomegalovirus, herpes simplex, syphilis), maternal drug use (hydantoin, alcohol, cocaine), or trauma (amniocentesis injury, forceps injury) can aid in identifying ocular diseases in children. A history of prematurity, head trauma, hearing loss, delay in establishing developmental milestones, human immunodeficiency virus (HIV) infection, diabetes mellitus, or sickle-cell disease will direct an appropriate screening examination.

The family history may reveal ocular diseases that carry a high risk of inheritance such as red-green color blindness, retinitis pigmentosa, juvenile retinoschisis, congenital cataracts, high myopia, Leber congenital amaurosis, congenital stationary night blindness, and achromatopsia. In addition, the family history may reveal systemic diseases associated with ocular pathology such as cystinosis, Fabry disease, Marfan syndrome, homocystinuria, and the mucopolysaccharidoses.

26.1.2   Ocular Examination

A systematic and detailed examination of the eye is an important aspect of the pediatric physical examination. The examination should be conducted in an orderly manner to ensure that important components of the examination are not overlooked. A thorough examination includes measurement and/or inspection in each of the following: visual function, external eye structures, pupils, ocular alignment and motility, intraocular pressure, and posterior segment examination. Young children may be difficult to examine. A wire lid speculum, Desmarres lid retractors, sedatives, a pacifier, or colorful noisy toys may be helpful; sometimes an assistant is required. Because the infant's lid fissure is narrow, attempts to separate the eyelids may produce a forceful closure with a pronounced *Bell phenomenon* (involuntary upgaze upon tight eyelid closure). Occasionally, general anesthesia may be necessary to obtain an adequate ocular examination.

26.1.3   Assessment of Visual Function

FIXATION The ocular examination should begin with an assessment of visual function, preferably the measurement of visual acuity. Unfortunately, this is not always possible. A crude measure of spatial function in infants and young children can be gained by analyzing the ability to fixate and follow a light or interesting object such as a finger puppet. The eyes should be tested monocularly; binocular measurements are of little value. Normal fixation is attained in the first few months after birth and is central, steady, and maintained (CSM). Poor or absent central fixation suggests macular dysfunction or severe visual impairment, although in young infants it may occur with self-limited disorders such as delayed visual maturation.

VISUAL ACUITY School-age children should be tested using eye charts that display Snellen letters, Bailey-Lovie letters, or the letters "HOTV." These optotypes measure *recognition acuity* (the ability to recognize or name optotypes). Younger children can be tested using eye charts that display Snellen E's or the Allen or LH (Lea Hyvärinen) picture tests. These optotypes measure *resolution acuity* (the ability to resolve features of optotypes such as orientation). Traditional eye charts are composed of high-contrast black optotypes on a white background. Eye charts with optotypes of varying contrast are also available.

Immaturity prevents infants and preverbal children from responding to recognition acuity tests. For this group, techniques such as optokinetic nystagmus (OKN) testing, visually evoked potentials (VEP), and preferential looking (PL) are helpful. The PL technique using hand-held two-choice alternative cards (Teller acuity cards) is the most useful clinically. Newborn visual acuity is about 20/400 by OKN and PL and 20/200 by VEP. By 4 to 6 weeks of age, an infant should be able to follow a light or large object held close to the face over a short range. An infant should watch and follow the mother's face. Failure to do so by 6 to 8 weeks of age (unless the infant is premature) may be a sign of developmental delay or may indicate decreased vision. Startle reflexes can be a gross test of visual function by 2 months of age; an object brought swiftly toward the eye should elicit blinking. By 3 months of age, infants should be able to follow an object over a wide range and look at movements of their own hands. At 6 months of age, infants will watch a person moving around the room and by 9 months will observe small objects. Visual acuity at 1 year of age has been estimated at 20/60 by OKN, 20/50 by PL, and 20/40 by VEP. It reaches the 20/30 level by 3 to 4 years using optotype methods, gradually improving until age 5, when it reaches the adult level of 20/20. Visual acuity should be measured in all children at or before 3 to 4 years of age because unilateral strabismic or refractive amblyopia can still be treated successfully at this age. Beyond 6 to 7 years of age, amblyopia treatment is disappointing.

The mother often first suspects poor vision or blindness in an infant or young child. *Photophobia* (light sensitivity), nystagmus, lack of eye contact with the parent, failure to smile when an adult smiles, or roving eye movements suggest markedly decreased vision. In severe vision loss or blindness, three types of psychomotor disturbance are seen: hyperkinetic and rhythmic movements, grimacing and other facial contortions, and oculodigital phenomena (pressing or rubbing the eyes).

COLOR VISION Testing of color vision is recommended in the early school years. It is done to provide vocational guidance, in response to a parent's concern that a child is slow in learning colors, when a positive family history is elicited, or when optic nerve or retinal disease is suspected. Congenital color "blindness" is X-linked recessive, usually partial, and nearly always of the red-green variety. It occurs in about 8% of white males and 4% of black males, whereas only 0.5 to 1% of females are affected. Blue-yellow color deficiency is extremely rare. Total absence of color vision (congenital achromatopsia) is associated with poor vision, nystagmus, and photophobia. The Ishihara or Hardy-Rand-Rittler pseudoisochromatic tests can be used to detect color-vision deficiency by having a child trace or identify the numbers or patterns. The Farnsworth D-15, Farnsworth-Munsell 100-hue, or the Nagel anomaloscope tests may be used in older children for detailed testing. Color-vision deficiency is unrelated to reading performance or dyslexia.

PERIPHERAL VISION Peripheral vision is not tested routinely. The extent of peripheral vision can be estimated in young children using a penlight, toy, or lollipop using the confrontation technique. It can be studied more thoroughly in older children using quantitative kinetic perimetry (tangent screen, Goldmann) or static perimetry (Humphrey, Octopus) tests. Good fixation control and a long attention span are critical in obtaining reliable test results.

26.1.4 External Examination

The external eye examination begins with the observation of facial and orbital symmetry. Abnormalities of globe position (telecanthus, hyperglobus) within the coronal plane should be referenced to the facial midline or the fellow eye. *Exophthalmos* (forward protrusion or proptosis) and *enophthalmos* (globe retraction) can be measured with reference to the lateral orbital rim using a Hertel exophthalmometer. *Buphthalmos* (large eye; literally, a cow's eye) and *nanophthalmos* or *microphthalmos* (small eye) should be noted. Gross abnormalities of globe structure such as phthisis bulbi should also be noted.

OCULAR ADNEXAE The eyelids, eyelashes, and lacrimal apparatus should be inspected. Abnormalities of eyelid position (blepharoptosis, lid retraction), rotation (entropion, ectropion), and contour (lid scarring, lid tumors, epicanthus) should be noted. Blepharospasm or tics may not be apparent on cursory examination. Asking the patient to close the eyelids gently and inspecting for visible cornea or sclera in the palpebral fissure may identify *lagophthalmos* (incomplete lid closure). Epiphora (tearing) may be a sign of ocular irritation, including infantile glaucoma, or lacrimal system obstruction. The puncta should be inspected for patency. The skin overlying the lacrimal sac should be inspected for fullness or discoloration. If a conjunctival or corneal foreign body is suspected, the upper eyelid should be everted and inspected. The lid is everted by having the child look down, grasping the lashes, and pulling the lid forward and upward while fixing the superior margin of the tarsal plate with a cotton applicator or finger.

ANTERIOR SEGMENT With the aid of a penlight, the conjunctiva is carefully inspected for injection, papillae, follicles, or discharge. The cornea is inspected for clouding, scarring, ulceration, or vascularization. A portable slit lamp may improve visualization of anterior segment structures. Sterile fluorescein 2% solution or sterile paper strips may be used if a corneal foreign body or epithelial defect is suspected. Photophobia frequently accompanies diseases of the cornea such as phlyctenular and interstitial keratitis, but it also may be a sign of congenital (infantile) glaucoma, acute iritis, or ocular albinism. Horizontal corneal diameter should be appraised with a millimeter ruler placed on the bridge of the nose. The average horizontal corneal diameter for a full-term neonate is 10.5 mm; 11.5 mm at 1 year; and 12.0 mm (adult size) by 2 years.

The anterior chamber should be formed without evidence of *anterior synechiae* (adhesions to the cornea), *posterior synechiae* (adhesions to the lens), *hyphema* (blood), or *hypopyon* (pus).

26.1.5 Pupils

After evaluating the anterior chamber and iris, the pupil should be inspected. The pupil is the limiting aperture for light entering the eye. Ambient lighting and accommodative tone regulate the pupil's size. Pupillary testing is performed by swinging a bright light from one eye to the other while controlling accommodation by asking the child to stare at a distant target ("swinging flashlight test"). With infants and young children, fixation control is not usually possible. The normal response is a brisk, simultaneous, and equal constriction of the pupils, possibly accompanied by *hippus* (a rhythmic oscillation of pupil size). Pupillary dilation is slower than pupillary constriction. Abnormal responses are categorized as *afferent pupillary defects* (APD) or *efferent pupillary defects*. The hallmark of an efferent defect is *anisocoria* (unequal pupil size). Efferent pupillary defects can be further classified as sympathetic (Horner syndrome), parasympathetic (third cranial nerve palsy, Adie pupil), or as directly involving the iris tissue (posterior synechiae, sphincter rupture, pharmacologic effect). APDs are graded on a 1+ to 4+ scale. Although they usually indicate optic nerve pathology, conditions that affect a significant area of retina (retinal detachment, central retinal vein occlusion) can also produce an APD. The pupillary response to light (both direct and consensual) is less intense when an affected eye is stimulated than when the fellow, unaffected eye is stimulated. Geniculostriate lesions do not produce APDs as the afferent pathways that subserve the pupillary response decussate before the bulk of optic nerve fibers synapse in the lateral geniculate nucleus. Diseases affecting both optic nerves equally do not produce an APD because the defects are relative and appear only if one optic nerve or retina is more damaged than the other.

Anterior iris lesions are easily demonstrated on slit-lamp examination. Most are benign pigmentations; some may indicate or be pathognomonic of systemic diseases (Sec. 26.9.2). The differential diagnosis of *leukocoria* (white pupillary reflex) is extensive and includes a number of congenital and acquired intraocular diseases (Sec. 26.9.4), including retinoblastoma. Referral of patients with leukocoria to an ophthalmologist is mandatory.

26.1.6 Ocular Alignment and Motility

Ocular alignment and the action of the extraocular muscles can be tested with a penlight, prism bar, and occluder. Gross alignment of the eyes may be checked by shining the light at the patient's eyes and observing the corneal light reflexes (first Purkinje images). If the eyes are aligned, the light reflexes will appear at the same location in each pupil. If the light reflex is displaced temporally in one eye, an *esotropia,* or inward, deviation exists. If the light reflex is positioned nasally in an eye, an *exotropia,* or outward, deviation exists. The deviation can be estimated from the amount the corneal light reflex is displaced in the pupil (*Hirschberg test*). The strabismus can also be measured by finding a prism that, when held in front of the deviating eye, returns the corneal light reflex to its proper place in the pupil (*Krimsky prism reflex test*). A more accurate method of measuring ocular alignment involves the use of a hand-held occluder (*cover tests*). In the cover-uncover test, which is usually performed on older children or cooperative young children and

adults, the patient looks at a distant object with both eyes open, and one eye is covered with an occluder. If the other eye makes a movement to pick up fixation, a *heterotropia* (manifest deviation) exists; the direction of the corrective eye movement indicates the type of deviation. The other eye is tested similarly. If no movement occurs on cover testing, but a refixation response occurs when either eye is uncovered (alternate cover test), a *heterophoria* (latent deviation) exists. If neither eye moves as the occluder is alternated back and forth, this state is called *orthophoria.*

Using a penlight or hand-held toy, *versions* (binocular eye movements in the same direction) can be checked to detect overaction or underaction of the extraocular muscles. *Ductions* (monocular eye movements) can be checked to distinguish overaction from underaction. *Vergences* (binocular eye movements in opposite directions) are not tested routinely.

26.1.7 Intraocular Pressure

Accurate measurement of intraocular pressure (IOP) requires a tonometer (Schiotz, Goldmann, MacKay-Marg, Perkins, Tono-Pen). Tactile estimation of IOP is highly unreliable. If glaucoma is suspected in an infant or young child, applanation tonometry, gonioscopy, and optic-disc examination should be done under general anesthesia. IOP should be measured during induction, as general anesthesia lowers IOP. A normal IOP under anesthesia does not exclude glaucoma.

26.1.8 Posterior Segment Examination

Satisfactory fundus examination requires pupillary dilation. There should be no reluctance to use mydriatics (agents that dilate the pupil) and cycloplegics (agents that paralyze the ciliary muscle and thus accommodation) in children because acute angle-closure glaucoma rarely occurs. Good dilation can be achieved in 30 to 45 minutes by instilling one drop of phenylephrine 2.5% and one drop of tropicamide 0.5% or 1% separately or in a combination solution. The combination of cyclopentolate 0.2% and phenylephrine 1% (Cyclomydril) is also popular. The effectiveness of mydriatics can be enhanced by prior instillation of one drop of a topical anesthetic agent (proparacaine 0.5%) 1 to 2 minutes before the mydriatic agents. The local anesthetic eliminates the sting caused by the mydriatic drops, thereby reducing dilution by tearing, and enhances their corneal penetration. Cycloplegic agents (cyclopentolate, homatropine, atropine) are not necessary unless cycloplegic retinoscopy is to be performed. Toxic reactions to atropine occur in children and may even be fatal, especially in children with brain damage and Down syndrome. Phenylephrine 10% solution should be avoided in infants and young children as it can cause a dangerous elevation of blood pressure following topical administration. Cyclopentolate 1% use in low birth weight infants can result in paralytic ileus with a fatal outcome.

Fundus examination may be performed using a direct or indirect ophthalmoscope and at the slit-lamp using a variety of accessory lenses (fundus contact lens, Goldmann three-mirror contact lens, 75- or 90-diopter lenses). Indirect ophthalmoscopy is often easier to perform than direct ophthalmoscopy in infants and young children because of avoidance of eye and head movements. Occasionally it is necessary to perform ophthalmoscopy under general anesthesia for adequate examination, especially of the peripheral retina. Scleral indentation is required to visualize the retinal periphery, as is necessary during examination for retinopathy of prematurity.

In newborns and young infants, the fundus may be less pigmented ("blond appearance"), the foveal light reflex may be absent or of poor quality, and the optic disc may be slightly paler than is usual for older children. These features are particularly characteristic of the fundus of premature infants. In addition, the periphery of the retina may be gray or white and appear to be elevated because of its lack of differentiation and thus give the impression that the retina is detached.

References

American Academy of Pediatrics, Section on Ophthalmology: Eye examination and vision screening in infants, children, and young adults. Pediatrics 98:153, 1996

Chang DF: Ophthalmologic examination. In: Vaughan DG, Asbury T, Riordan-Eve P, eds: General Ophthalmology, 15th ed. Norwalk, CT, Appleton & Lange, 1999

Hoyt CS, Nichel BL, Billson FA: Ophthalmologic examination of the infant: Developmental aspects. Surv Ophthalmol 26:166, 1982

Lankin JC: Can this baby see? Estimation of visual acuity in the preverbal child. Int Ophthalmol Clin 32:1, 1992

Wright JD Jr, Boger WP III: Visual complaints from healthy children. Surv Ophthalmol 44(2):113–121, 1999

26.2 INHERITED DISEASES OF THE EYE

J. Bronwyn Bateman and Christina Butera

A significant portion of eye disease in children is genetic in origin. It is estimated that at least 50% of new cases of legal blindness (visual acuity less than 20/200 or peripheral vision less than 20°) in the pediatric age group is attributable to genetic causes. A genetic basis should be identified both for treatment of the patient and counseling of the family. The evaluation should be initiated with a careful family history and pedigree; the parents should be queried about consanguinity. Identification of the anomalies commonly encountered in genetic eye diseases and syndromes (eg, abnormal interpupillary distance, epicanthal folds, palpebral fissure slant) is helpful, as is consultation with a geneticist.

CHROMOSOMAL DISORDERS

Most chromosomal disorders are associated with abnormal eye findings, and virtually all involve other organ systems. Infants with chromosomal disorders often have multiple congenital anomalies, growth retardation, and developmental delay in addition to the ocular abnormality. All forms of microscopically identifiable chromosomal deletions, duplications, or aneuploidies are associated with some element of mental retardation with the exception of some X-chromosomal anomalies. Eye manifestations of chromosomal disorders are listed in Table 26-1.

MONOGENIC DISORDERS

Monogenic disorders are caused by a defect in a single gene. Tables 26-2 and 26-3 list eye findings of many monogenic disorders. For

further discussion of inborn errors of metabolism such as the mucopolysaccharidoses, sphingolipidoses, and mucolipidoses, refer to Secs. 26.7.4 and 26.11.5.

MALFORMATIONS OF THE GLOBE

Malformations of the globe are congenital and may result from genetic or environmental factors or a combination. Malformations may be isolated or associated with orbital, cerebral, or facial defects. Environmental agents include toxins (eg, alcohol), fetal injury, maternal infection, pharmaceutical agents (eg, aminopterin, hydantoin, retinoic acid), radiation, and malnutrition. The severity of a congenital ocular anomaly may be related to the intensity, timing, and duration of the exposure. There are different critical periods of development for each of the ocular tissues.

SIZE The average human eye measures 16 mm in anteroposterior diameter at birth, increasing to 23 mm by 3 years of age. The adult size of approximately 24 mm is obtained by puberty. Most congenital anomalies of the globe are associated with reduced globe size.

MICROPHTHALMIA Microphthalmia, or small eye, should be suspected on the basis of microcornea, high hyperopia, or a small palpebral fissure; a clinical diagnosis may be inaccurate, since microcornea can occur without microphthalmia and vice-versa. The diagnosis is established by an ultrasonic axial length measurement that is two standard deviations below the age-adjusted normal value. Microphthalmia can range from mild reduction in size to histologically documented anophthalmia. An orbital cyst of any size may accompany microphthalmia. Microphthalmia with cyst results from failure of closure of the optic vesicle during organogenesis. Surgical removal of cysts is sometimes necessary to avoid anomalous orbital growth.

Microphthalmia is a common ocular malformation in all races, suggesting multiple etiologies. The incidence of microphthalmia is approximately 0.22 per 1000 births; that of coloboma, a predisposing malformation, is 0.26 per 1000 births. Specific etiologies are listed in Table 26-4.

ANOPHTHALMIA Anophthalmia refers to the complete absence of the eye and ocular tissues. True anophthalmia is extremely rare and can be confirmed only after the contents of the orbit have been searched histologically to rule out microphthalmia. Anything that causes microphthalmia also can cause anophthalmia. Anophthalmia results from failure of formation of the optic vesicle. Primary anophthalmia may occur in an otherwise normal child. This malformation is reported in trisomy 13, 18 p−, various cerebral maldevelopments, Klinefelter syndrome, and congenital CMV infection. Although isolated anophthalmia usually occurs sporadically, autosomal dominant, autosomal recessive, and X-linked recessive transmissions occur.

NANOPHTHALMIA *Nanophthalmia* refers to a microphthalmic eye with normal intraocular structures; such eyes have small corneas, hyperopic refractive errors, and narrow anterior chamber angles. These features result in a high incidence of angle-closure glaucoma, retinal detachment, and visual impairment from high hyperopia.

TABLE 26-1

CHROMOSOMAL ABERRATIONS AND THEIR EYE DEFORMITIES

CHROMOSOMAL DEFECT	EYE FINDINGS
Duplication syndromes	
1q+	Narrow horizontal lid fissures, synophrys, colobomatous microphthalmia
2p+	Hypertelorism, epicanthus, strabismus, narrow palpebral fissures, blepharoptosis and blepharophimosis, nasolacrimal duct obstruction, coloboma, microphthalmia, congenital glaucoma, persistent hyperplastic primary vitreous, optic atrophy
2q+	Epicanthus, hypertelorism, upward or downward slanting of the lid fissures, blepharitis, microcornea, congenital glaucoma, dislocated lenses, macular hypoplasia, nystagmus, colobomatous microphthalmia
3p+	Hypertelorism, epicanthus, microphthalmia, cyclopia
3q+	Hypertelorism, epicanthus, corneal opacities, colobomatous microphthalmia, synophrys, strabismus, cataract, congenital glaucoma, nystagmus
4p+	Microphthalmia, strabismus, downward slanting of the lid fissures, hypertelorism, coloboma, blepharophimosis, epicanthus, deep set eyes, bushy eyelashes, strabismus, nystagmus
4q+	Colobomatous microphthalmia, downward slanting of the lid fissures, epicanthus, blepharophimosis and blepharoptosis, corneal clouding
5p+	Hypertelorism, epicanthus, upward slanting of the lid fissures, strabismus, cataracts, nystagmus, colobomatous microphthalmia
5q+	Epicanthus, hypertelorism, strabismus
6p+	Hypertelorism, long lashes, blepharoptosis and blepharophimosis, strabismus, optic atrophy, and microphthalmia
6q+	Downward slanting of the lid fissures, epicanthus, hypertelorism, blepharoptosis, strabismus, thin arched eyebrows, hypoplastic superior orbital ridges
7p+	Hypertelorism, epicanthus, upward or downward slanting of the lid fissures, microphthalmia
7q+	Hypertelorism, downward slanting and/or narrowing of the lid fissures, epicanthus, strabismus, absent lateral rectus muscles, "prominent eyes," long lashes, optic nerve hypoplasia, colobomatous microphthalmia
Trisomy 8	Downward slanting of the lid fissures, hypertelorism, blepharoptosis, strabismus, corneal opacities, colobomatous microphthalmia
8p+	Hypertelorism, upward slanting of the lid fissures
8q+	Hypertelorism, upward slanting of the lid fissures, colobomatous microphthalmia
Trisomy 9	Upward or downward slanting and narrowing of the lid fissures, hypertelorism, epibulbar dermoid, corneal opacities, enophthalmos, microphthalmia
9p+	Microphthalmia, strabismus, downward slanting of the lid fissures, entropion, hypertelorism, enophthalmos, cataracts
9q+	Epicanthus, hypotelorism, narrow palpebral fissures, strabismus, blepharoptosis, microphthalmia, enophthalmos
10p+	Hypertelorism, upward slanting of the lid fissures, long eyelashes, microphthalmia, coloboma
10q+	Epicanthus, hypertelorism, cataract, blepharoptosis, downward slanting and/or narrow lid fissures, blepharophimosis, strabismus, microphthalmia
11p+	Epicanthus, hypertelorism, downward slanting of the lid fissures, strabismus, blepharoptosis, conjunctival telangiectasia, Brushfield spots of the iris, nystagmus, retinal degeneration
11q+	Hypotelorism or hypertelorism, epicanthus, downward slanting of the lid fissures, conical corneal shape, corectopia, strabismus
12p+	Hypertelorism, epicanthus, horizontal palpebral fissures, Brushfield spots
12q+	Epicanthus, hypertelorism, upward slanting and/or narrow lid fissures, heavy eyebrows
Trisomy 13 (Patau syndrome)	Colobomatous microphthalmia, anophthalmia, cyclopia, microcornea, congenital glaucoma, corneal opacities, cataract, optic nerve hypoplasia, optic atrophy, persistent hyperplastic primary vitreous, retinal dysplasia, strabismus, intraocular cartilage
13q+	Hypertelorism or hypotelorism, upward or downward slant of the eyelids, blepharoptosis, synophrys, strabismus, coloboma, long thick upturned lashes, colobomatous microphthalmia
Trisomy 14	Hypotelorism or hypertelorism, downward slanting of the lid fissures, blepharoptosis, enophthalmos, ectropion, microphthalmia
14q+	Hypotelorism or hypertelorism, downward slanting of the lid fissures, blepharoptosis or blepharophimosis, microphthalmia, congenital glaucoma, strabismus
15q+	Downward slanting of the lid fissures, epicanthus, strabismus, blepharoptosis, cataract, retinal detachment, enophthalmos, microphthalmia
16p+	Hypertelorism, sparse eyelashes, blepharoptosis, upward or downward slanting and narrowing of the lid fissures, nystagmus
16q+	Hypertelorism, epicanthus, downward slanting and/or narrowing of the lid fissures, decreased or long lashes, ectropion, periorbital edema, enophthalmos, strabismus
17p+	Hypertelorism, upward or downward slanting and/or narrowing of the lid fissures, blepharoptosis, microphthalmia
17q+	Hypertelorism, narrow lid fissures

(continued)

TABLE 26-1   Continued

CHROMOSOMAL DEFECT	EYE FINDINGS
Trisomy 18 (Edwards syndrome)	Epicanthus, hypertelorism, hypoplastic supraorbital ridges, corneal opacities, congenital glaucoma, microphthalmia, cataract, colobomatous microphthalmia, retinal depigmentation, cyclopia
18p+	Hypotelorism, downward slanting of the lid fissures, strabismus
18q+	Epicanthus, blepharoptosis, synophrys, enophthalmos, hypertelorism, upward slanting of the lid fissures
19q+ (de Grouchy syndrome)	Hypertelorism, downward slanting of the lid fissures, blepharoptosis
20p+	Epicanthus, hypertelorism, upward or downward slanting of the lid fissures, Rieger syndrome, enophthalmos, colobomas, strabismus
Trisomy 21 (Down syndrome)	Epicanthus, upward slanting of the lid fissures, myopia, strabismus, nystagmus, cataracts, Brushfield spots of the iris, infantile glaucoma, keratoconus, increased number of retinal vessels, optic nerve hypoplasia, ectropion, blepharitis
Trisomy 22	Hypertelorism, blepharoptosis, upward or downward slanting of the lid fissures, epicanthus, optic nerve hypoplasia, cataracts, synophrys, strabismus, colobomatous microphthalmia, persistent hyperplastic primary vitreous
22q+ (cat-eye syndrome)	Colobomatous microphthalmia, blepharoptosis, hypertelorism, downward slanting of the lid fissures, strabismus
Triploidy	Colobomatous microphthalmia, hypertelorism, cataracts, glaucoma
Deletion syndromes	
1q−	Upward or downward slanting lid fissures, epicanthus, hypertelorism, blepharoptosis, strabismus, synophrys, microphthalmia
2q−	Downward slanting of the lid fissures, narrow lid fissures, epicanthus, thick eyebrows and lashes, blepharoptosis and blepharophimosis, corneal opacities, cataracts, optic nerve hypoplasia, nystagmus, colobomatous microphthalmia
3p−	Hypertelorism, epicanthus, downward slanting and narrow lid fissures, synophrys, blepharoptosis, optic atrophy
3q−	Narrow lid fissures, epicanthus, blepharoptosis, cataract, strabismus, colobomatous microphthalmia
4p− (Wolf-Hirschhorn syndrome)	Corectopia, Peters anomaly, Rieger anomaly, colobomatous microphthalmia, strabismus, downward slanting of the lid fissures, blepharoptosis, hypertelorism, eyebrow defects, exophthalmos, cataracts, epicanthus, strabismus
4q−	Hypertelorism, epicanthus, laterally displaced inner canthi, upward or downward slanting of the lid fissures, features of Williams syndrome including stellate irises
4r	Blepharoptosis, colobomatous microphthalmia
5p− (Cri du Chat syndrome)	Colobomatous microphthalmia, cataract, optic atrophy, tortuous retinal vessels, ocular dermoid, decreased tears, epicanthus, congenital glaucoma, strabismus, myopia, upward or downward slanting of the lid fissures, hypotelorism or hypertelorism, telecanthus, absence of eyebrows, foveal hypoplasia
5q−	Blepharoptosis, strabismus
6p−	Hypertelorism, downward slanting of the lid fissures, epicanthus, Peters anomaly, microphthalmia, strabismus
6q−	Upward slanting and/or narrowing of the lid fissures, epicanthus
6r	Hypertelorism, epicanthus, downward slanting of the palpebral fissures, strabismus, blepharoptosis, microcornea or megalocornea, posterior embryotoxon, Rieger anomaly, aniridia, glaucoma, optic atrophy, albinoid fundi, nystagmus, colobomatous microphthalmia
7p−	Hypertelorism, exophthalmos
7q−	Epicanthus, hypertelorism, upward slanting of the lid fissures, synophrys, strabismus, glaucoma, colobomatous microphthalmia, optic atrophy; bilateral anophthalmia associated with interstitial deletion of q21.1 to q36.1
8p−	Hypertelorism, epicanthus, down slanting of the lid fissures, strabismus, nystagmus
9p−	Upward or downward slanting of the lid fissures, epicanthus, exophthalmos, arched eyebrows, hypertelorism, strabismus
10p−	Congenital glaucoma, hypertelorism, down slanting and/or narrowing of the lid fissures, epicanthus, strabismus, blepharoptosis, corneal opacities
10q−	Hypertelorism, upward or downward slanting and narrowing of the lid fissures, scant eyelashes, strabismus, colobomatous microphthalmia
11p−	Aniridia, cataract, strabismus, congenital glaucoma, macular hypoplasia
11q−	Epicanthus, blepharoptosis, Peters anomaly, hypertelorism, strabismus, colobomatous microphthalmia, cyclopia, retinal dysplasia, upward or downward slanting of the lid fissures
11r	Hypertelorism, epicanthus, upward or downward slanting of the lid fissures, blepharoptosis, microcornea, anterior segment dysgenesis, stellate pattern of the iris, strabismus
12p−	Hypertelorism, epicanthus, downward slanting of the lid fissures, sclerocornea, synophrys, strabismus, optic atrophy
12r	Strabismus
13q−	Cataract, retinoblastoma, blepharoptosis, upward or downward slanting and/or narrow lid fissures, epicanthus, hypertelorism, Rieger syndrome, colobomatous microphthalmia, optic nerve hypoplasia, strabismus
13r	Same findings as 13q−
14q−	Epicanthus, narrow lid fissures, blepharoptosis, glaucoma, strabismus
14r	Hypertelorism, epicanthus, downward slanting of the lid fissures, retinal pigment epithelial disturbance
15q− (Angelman and Prader-Willi syndromes)	Ocular albinism, strabismus, hypertelorism
15r	Hypertelorism, nystagmus, strabismus, retinal depigmentation
16q−	Upward or downward slanting and narrow lid fissures, hypertelorism, epicanthus, strabismus

(continued)

TABLE 26-1   Continued

CHROMOSOMAL DEFECT	EYE FINDINGS
17p− (Miller-Dieker syndrome)	Upward or downward slanting lid fissures, epicanthus, Brushfield spots of the iris, colobomatous microphthalmia, synophrys, strabismus
17r	Retinal flecks, subretinal drusen-like deposits
18p−	Colobomatous microphthalmia, cyclopia, synophthalmia, strabismus, blepharoptosis, epicanthus, hypertelorism, retinal dysplasia
18q−	Epicanthus, hypertelorism, downward slanting of the lid fissures, corneal abnormalities, cataracts, blue sclerae, dysplastic or hypotrophic optic nerve heads, strabismus, colobomatous microphthalmia
18r	Microphthalmia with cyst
19p−	Hypertelorism, persistent hyperplastic primary vitreous
20p−	Epicanthus, hypertelorism, downward slanting of the lid fissures, iris colobomas, Rieger syndrome, strabismus
21r	Upward or downward slanting of the lid fissures, anterior segment dysgenesis
Monosomy 21	Epicanthus, downward slanting of the lid fissures, Peters anomaly, cataract, microphthalmia
22q− (DiGeorge syndrome)	Hypertelorism, upward or downward slanting lid fissures
22r	Epicanthus, downward slanting of the lid fissures, strabismus, synophrys, proptosis
Monosomy 22	Epicanthus, hypertelorism, upward slanting of the lid fissures, blepharoptosis
Sex chromosome syndromes	
Klinefelter syndrome (XXY, XXXY, XXXXY)	Hypertelorism, epicanthus, upward slant of the lid fissures, strabismus, Brushfield spots, myopia, choroidal atrophy, colobomatous microphthalmia
Turner syndrome (45, X), mosaic variants	Blepharoptosis, strabismus, color blindness, cataracts, epicanthus, blue sclera, nystagmus, hypertelorism

TABLE 26-2

OCULAR FINDINGS IN MULTISYSTEM SYNDROMES

DISEASE	OCULAR MANIFESTATIONS	INHERITANCE
Renal syndromes		
Alport	Anterior lenticonus, cataracts, pigmentary maculopathy	AD
Bardet-Biedl	Retinal degeneration	AR
Lowe	Congenital cataracts and glaucoma	XR
Hepatic syndromes		
Cerebrohepatorenal (Zellweger)	Cataracts, infantile retinitis pigmentosa	AR
Gardner	Retinal pigment epithelial hyperplasia	AD
Skeletal, connective tissue, muscular syndromes		
Albright	Cataracts	AD
Alkaptonuria	Scleral pigmentation	AR
Chondrodysplasia punctata	Congenital cataracts	AD, AR, XR
Congenital contractural arachnodactly	Colobomatous microphthalmia	AD
Kenny-Caffey	Papilledema	AD
Klippel-Feil	Duane syndrome	??
Klippel-Trénaunay-Weber	Conjunctival telangiectasia, glaucoma, choroidal angioma	??
Marfan	Ectopia lentis	AD
McCune-Albright (polyostotic fibrocystic dysplasia)	Unilateral proptosis, optic atrophy	??
Melnick-Needles	Exorbitism, hypertelorism	XD
Metatropic dwarfism type II (Kneist)	Cataract, high myopia, retinal detachment	AD
Myotonia congenita (Thomsen)	Blepharospasm	AD
Myotonic dystrophy	Blepharoptosis, extraocular muscle paresis, Christmas-tree cataracts, hypotony, pigmentary maculopathy	AD
Nail-patella (hereditary onychoosteodysplasia)	Corneal opacities, dark iris pigmentation	AD
Oculodentodigital	Microphthalmia, microcornea, iris abnormalities, glaucoma, optic atrophy, epicanthal folds, hyper- or hypo-telorism	AD
Osteogenesis imperfecta congenita	Corneal arcus, keratoconus, glaucoma, megalocornea, blue sclera, cataracts	AR
Osteopetrosis (Albers-Schönberg)	Cranial nerve palsies, optic atrophy	AR, AD

(continued)

TABLE 26-2 Continued

DISEASE	OCULAR MANIFESTATIONS	INHERITANCE
Robert	Congenital cataracts	AR
Schwartz-Jampel	Blepharophimosis	AR
Spondyloepiphyseal dysplasia congenita	High myopia, vitreous syneresis, lattice degeneration of the retina	AD
Stickler	High myopia, retinal detachment	AD
van der Hoeve	Blue sclera	AD
Weill-Marchesani	Ectopia lentis, shallow anterior chamber	AD
Wildervanck	Duane syndrome	??
Neurologic syndromes		
Aicardi	Lacunar chorioretinal lesions	XD
Alpers diffuse cerebral degeneration	Cortical blindness	AR
Ataxia-telangectasia	Tortuous conjunctival vessels	AR
Behr	Optic atrophy	AR
Canavan	Optic atrophy, nystagmus	AR
Charcot-Marie-Tooth	Optic atrophy, tonic pupil	AR, AD, XR
Familial dysautonomia (Riley-Day)	Decreased tear production, corneal hypesthesia, corneal breakdown with scarring, optic atrophy, corneal ulcers	AR
Infantile subacute necrotizing encephalomyelopathy	Optic atrophy, nystagmus	AR
Marinesco-Sjögren	Congenital cataracts	AR
Meckel-Gruber	Colobomatous microphthalmia	AR
Olivopontocerebellar (OPCA)	Retinal degeneration in some families	AD
Sjögren	Congenital cataracts	AR
Sjögren-Larsson	Colobomatous microphthalmia	AR
Warburg	Microphthalmia, congenital retinal detachment	AR
Dermatologic syndromes		
Basal cell nevus	Colobomatous microphthalmia, cataract	AD
Cockayne	Juvenile cataract, retinitis pigmentosa	AR
Cross	Microphthalmia	AR
Dyskeratosis congenita	Blepharitis, nasolacrimal duct obstruction	
Ectodermal dysplasia (anhidrotic)	Alacrima or decreased tear production	XR, AR
Ehlers-Danlos		
Types I, II, III	Retinal detachment	AD
Type VI	Blue sclera, retinal detachment, scleral rupture, keratoconus, ectopia lentis	AR
Focal dermal hypoplasia (Goltz-Gorlin)	Conjunctival papillomas, colobomatous microphthalmia	XD
Hereditary benign intraepithelial dyskeratosis	Gelatinous conjunctival plaques, corneal dyskeratosis	AD
Histiocytic dermatoarthritis	Glaucoma, uveitis, cataract	AD
Ichthyoses		
Congenital ichthyosis (harlequin fetus)	Ectropion, congenital cataract	AR
Lamellar ichthyosis	Ectropion	AR
Ichthyosis vulgaris	Blepharitis, corneal erosions	AD
Bullous ichthyosiform erythroderma	Blepharitis	AD
X-linked ichthyosis	Blepharitis, corneal erosions	XR
Incontinentia pigmenti	Infantile retinal detachment, cataracts	XD
Lipoid proteinosis (Urbach-Wiethe)	Hyaline deposits in mucous membranes and lids, corectopia	AR
Melkersson-Rosenthal	Cranial nerve VII palsy, corneal exposure	AD
Pachyonychia congenita	Corneal dyskeratosis, cataracts	AD
Pseudoxanthoma elasticum	Blue sclera, angioid streaks, myopia, drusen	AR, AD
Rothmund-Thompson	Acquired cataracts	AR
Waardenburg	Lateral displacement of the lacrimal punctae, heterochromia iridis, pigmentary variability within or between fundi, strabismus	AD
Xeroderma pigmentosa	Lid telangiectasia, photophobia, conjunctivitis	AR
Craniofacial syndromes		
Cerebro-oculofacial-skeletal	Microphthalmia, infantile cataracts	AR
Cornelia de Lange	Brushy eyebrows, long eyelashes, synophrys, optic atrophy, optic nerve coloboma	??
Cryptophthalmia	Fusion of eyelids, brow abnormalities, microphthalmia	AR
Goldenhar-Gorlin (oculoauriculovertebral dysplasia)	Epibulbar choristomas, strabismus, blepharoptosis, eyelid defects, optic nerve hypoplasia, tortuous retinal vessels, macular hypoplasia, microphthalmia, anophthalmia, lacrimal drainage system anomalies	??
Hallermann-Streiff	Congenital cataracts, microphthalmia	??
Lenz microphthalmia	Microphthalmia	AR
Möbius	Congenital cranial nerve VI and VII palsies, corneal exposure	AD

(continued)

TABLE 26-2   Continued

DISEASE	OCULAR MANIFESTATIONS	INHERITANCE
Rieger	Iris hypoplasia, pseudopolycoria, glaucoma	AD
Rubinstein-Taybi	Coloboma, glaucoma, cataract, strabismus, optic atrophy	??
Smith-Lemli-Opitz	Congenital cataracts	AR
Treacher-Collins (Franceschetti)	Lid defects, downward slant to lids	AD
Whistling face (Freeman-Sheldon)	Blepharoptosis	AD
Williams	Stellate pattern of the iris, strabismus, abnormalities of retinal vessels	
Hematologic syndromes		
Diamond-Blackfan	Noncolobomatous microphthalmia	AR
Fanconi	Noncolobomatous microphthalmia	AR
Granulomatous disease (chronic) of childhood	Chorioretinal lesions, blepharitis	XR
Hemoglobin SC	Sea-fan arteriovenous shunts, vascular occlusion	AR
Hemoglobin SS	Venous tortuosity, vascular occlusion, comma-shaped conjunctival capillaries	AR
Phakomatoses		
Neurofibromatosis 1	Neurofibromas, congenital glaucoma, optic nerve glioma, Lisch nodules	AD
Sturge-Weber	Glaucoma, choroidal hemangioma, choroidal effusion	??
Tuberous sclerosis	Retinal hamartomas, punched-out chorioretinal defects, iris depigmentation, angiofibromas of the lids, poliosis	AD
von Hippel–Lindau	Retinal hemangioma	AD
Wyburn-Mason	Retinal arteriovenous malformations, optic atrophy	??
Multisystem syndromes		
Alström	Retinal degeneration, optic atrophy	XR
Bloom	Conjunctivitis, conjunctival telangiectasia	
Jeune	Retinal degeneration	AR
Joubert	Retinal degeneration	
Mulibrey nanism	Retinal hypopigmentation, retinal pigment epithelial clumping	AR
Multiple endocrine deficiency	Keratitis, anterior stromal vascularization, autoimmune disease, candidiasis, and keratitis	AR
Multiple endocrine neoplasia IIB	Conjunctival and eyelid neuromas, keratoconjunctivitis sicca	AD
III (mucosal neuromata)	Conjunctival neuroma	AD
Noonan (Turner phenotype)	Cataract, blepharoptosis, coloboma	??
Saldino-Mainzer	Retinal degeneration	AR
Werner	Cataracts, retinal degeneration	AR
Wolfram	Optic atrophy	AR

AD = autosomal dominant; AR = autosomal recessive; XD = X-linked dominant; XR = X-linked recessive; ?? = unknown or not inherited.

TABLE 26-3
OCULAR FINDINGS IN METABOLIC DISORDERS

DISEASE	OCULAR MANIFESTATIONS	INHERITANCE
Sphingolipid storage disorders		
Niemann-Pick A	Corneal clouding, anterior lens capsule clouding, macular grayness or cherry-red spot, optic atrophy	AR
Niemann-Pick B	Macular granularity	AR
Niemann-Pick C (D, E)	Not affected	AR
Gaucher	Strabismus, brown pingueculas, macular grayness, white retinal deposits	AR
Fabry	Cornea verticellata, spoke-like cataract, saccular conjunctival and retinal vessels	XR
G_{M1}-I gangliosidosis	Cherry-red spot, optic atrophy, variable corneal clouding	AR
Juvenile gangliosidosis (G_{M1}-II)	Cherry-red spot	AR
Tay-Sachs (G_{M2}-I)	Cherry-red spot, optic atrophy	AR
Sandhoff (G_{M2}-II)	Cherry-red spot, optic atrophy	AR
Juvenile G_{M2} gangliosidosis (G_{M2}-III)	Cherry-red spot, optic atrophy	AR
Pelizaeus-Merzbacher (diffuse cerebral sclerosis)	Optic atrophy	XR
Krabbe	Optic atrophy	AR
Metachromatic leukodystrophy		
Infantile	Possible cherry-red spot, optic atrophy	AR

(continued)

TABLE 26-3   Continued

DISEASE	OCULAR MANIFESTATIONS	INHERITANCE
Juvenile	Optic atrophy	AR
Adult	Optic atrophy	AR
Multiple sulfatase deficiency	Cherry-red spot, peripheral retinal degeneration, optic atrophy	AR
Oligosaccharide storage disorders		
Fucosidosis	Conjunctival and retinal vascular tortuosity	AR
Sialidosis (mucolipidosis I)	Corneal clouding, cataract, retinal vascular abnormality	AR
Mannosidosis	Cataract, corneal clouding	AR
Mucopolysaccharidoses		
Hurler (I-H)	Corneal clouding, peripheral retinal degeneration, optic atrophy	AR
Scheie (I-S)	Corneal clouding, peripheral retinal degeneration, optic atrophy	AR
Hunter (II) (2 types)	Peripheral retinal degeneration, optic atrophy	XR
San Filippo (III) (4 types)	Peripheral retinal degeneration, optic atrophy	AR
Morquio (IV)	Corneal clouding, optic atrophy	AR
Maroteaux-Lamy (VI) (2 types)	Corneal clouding, optic atrophy	AR
Sly (VII)	Corneal clouding	AR
Wolman	Peripheral retinal degeneration, optic atrophy	AR
Mucolipidoses		
Mucolipidosis II (I-cell)	Corneal clouding, cataract	AR
Mucolipidosis III (pseudo-Hurler polydystrophy)	Corneal clouding	AR
Mucolipidosis IV	Corneal clouding, peripheral retinal degeneration	AR
Neuronal ceroid lipofuscinosis		
Hagberg-Santavuori	Peripheral retinal degeneration, optic atrophy	AR
Janskey-Bielschowsky	Optic atrophy	AR
Spielmeyer-Vogt	Peripheral retinal degeneration, optic atrophy	AR
Kufs	Peripheral retinal degeneration, optic atrophy	AR
Ceramidase deficiency		
Farber lipogranulomatosis	Corneal clouding, peripheral retinal degeneration	AR
Amino acid metabolism		
Cystinosis	Corneal clouding, peripheral retinal degeneration, crystals at all levels	AR
Gyrate atrophy (hyperornithinemia)	Gyrate chorioretinal atrophy, cataract, myopia	AR
Homocystinuria	Ectopia lentis, myopia	AR
Hyperlysinemia	Ectopia lentis, spherophakia	AR
Methylmalonic aciduria	Corneal clouding	AR
Molybdenum cofactor deficiency	Cataract	AR
Sulfite oxidase deficiency	Ectopia lentis	AR
Tyrosinemia	Corneal crystals and ulcers	AR
Peroxisomal disorders		
Neonatal adrenoleukodystrophy	Peripheral retinal degeneration, optic atrophy	AR
Refsum disease	Pigmentary retinopathy, optic atrophy, microphthalmia	AR
Infantile Refsum disease	Peripheral retinal degeneration, optic atrophy	AR
X-linked adrenoleukodystrophy	Optic atrophy	XR
Zellweger	Corneal clouding, cataract, peripheral retinal degeneration, optic atrophy	AR
Porphyria		
Congenital, erythropoietic	Corneal clouding	AR
Acute, intermittent	Cataract, peripheral retinal degeneration, optic atrophy	AD
Lipoprotein/lipid metabolism		
Abetalipoproteinemia	Peripheral retinal degeneration, angioid streaks, optic atrophy	AR
Lecithin-cholesterol acyltransferase (LCAT) deficiency	Corneal arcus and opacities	AR
Lipoid proteinosis (Urbach-Wiethe)	Corneal opacities, lid margin nodules	AR
Tangier disease	Corneal clouding	AR
Carbohydrate metabolism		
Galactose-1-phosphate uridyl transferase deficiency	Cataract	AR
Galactokinase deficiency	Cataract	AR
Metal metabolism		
Acrodermatitis enteropathica	Corneal clouding, cataract, peripheral retinal degeneration, optic atrophy	AR
Menkes disease	Retinal degeneration	XR
Wilson disease	Kayser-Fleischer ring, peripheral retinal degeneration, chalcosis lentis with cataract	AR

AD = autosomal dominant; AR = autosomal recessive; XR = X-linked recessive.

TABLE 26-4
TYPES AND CAUSES OF MICROPHTHALMIA

DISORDER	INHERITANCE
Colobomatous microphthalmia	
Single-gene disorders	
Isolated ocular malformations	AD or AR
Basal cell nevus syndrome	AD
Congenital contractural arachnodactyly	AD
Meckel-Gruber syndrome	AR
Sjögren-Larsson syndrome	AR
Warburg syndrome	AR
Humeroradial synostosis	AR
Lenz microphthalmos syndrome	XR
Focal dermal hypoplasia	XD
CHARGE association	??
Epidermal nevus syndrome	??
Rubenstein-Taybi syndrome	??
Chromosomal disorders	
Triploidy	
Trisomy: 13, 18	
Duplications: 4q+, 7q+, 9p+, 9p+q+, 13q+, 22q+	
Deletions: 3q−, 4p−, 4r, 7q−, 11q−, 13q−, 13r, 18q−, 18r	
Noncolobomatous microphthalmia	
Genetic	
Isolated ocular malformations	AD or AR
Fanconi syndrome	AR
Diamond-Blackfan syndrome	AR
Chromosomal aberrations	10q+
Hallermann-Streiff syndrome	??
Persistent hyperplastic primary vitreous	??
Infectious	
Cytomegalovirus	
Epstein-Barr virus	
Herpes simplex virus	
Toxoplasmosis	
Rubella	

AD = autosomal dominant; AR = autosomal recessive; XD = X-linked dominant; XR = X-linked recessive; ?? = unknown or not inherited.

References

Bateman JB, Harley RD: Genetics of eye disease. In: Nelson LB, ed: Harley's Pediatric Ophthalmology, 4th ed. Philadelphia, Saunders, 1998

Gorlin RJ, Cohen MM, Levin LS: Syndromes of the Head and Neck, 3rd ed. New York, Oxford, 1990

Jones KL: Smith's Recognizable Patterns of Human Malformation, 5th ed. Philadelphia, Saunders, 1997

McKusick VA: Mendelian Inheritance in Man: A Catalog of Human Genes and Genetic Disorders, 11th ed. Baltimore, Johns Hopkins University Press, 1994

Merin S: Inherited Eye Diseases: Diagnosis and Clinical Management. New York, Dekker, 1991

Renie WA, ed: Goldberg's Genetic and Metabolic Eye Disease, 2nd ed. Boston, Little, Brown, 1986

Roy FH: Ocular Syndromes and Systemic Diseases, 2nd ed. Philadelphia, Saunders, 1989

Singh YP, Goupda SL: Congenital ocular abnormalities of the newborn. J Pediatr Ophthalmol Strabismus 17:162, 1986

Taylor D, Day S: Disorders of the eye as a whole. In: Taylor D, ed: Paediatric Ophthalmology. London, Blackwell, 1997

Wright KW: Pediatric Ophthalmology and Strabismus. St. Louis, Mosby, 1995

26.3   REFRACTIVE ERRORS

Visual acuity should be checked routinely between the ages of 3 and 4 years and certainly before children start school. If testing is not performed by a community preschool vision screening program, it should be done by the pediatrician or family physician. Visual acuity testing may reveal an important refractive error, amblyopia, or unsuspected pathology of the visual pathways. Often, young children do not realize that their vision is decreased and may not complain even if they have *asthenopia* (tired eyes) or are visually impaired or blind in one eye. Behavior that may give clues to uncorrected refractive errors includes excessive blinking, frowning, squinting, *torticollis* (tilting of the head), and frequent eye rubbing. A child may hold books close to the face or avoid close work, skip words or lines, lose his or her place while reading, or read slowly; he or she may shut or cover one eye or exhibit fatigue, drowsiness, or irritability after prolonged use of the eyes. Complaints of double vision, headaches, itching, burning, or watering of the eyes should alert the pediatrician to the possibility of decreased visual acuity or an oculomotor imbalance. Vision testing should be performed routinely every 2 to 3 years during the school years and more often if there is a strong family history of visual difficulties or refractive errors.

26.3.1   Classification

EMMETROPIA   This describes the ideal refractive state in which rays of light from optical infinity are brought to a point focus on the retina in the unaccommodated state. Few eyes are actually emmetropic. In most people the goal of optical correction with glasses or contact lenses is to achieve emmetropia. Refractive errors of the unaccommodated eye result in blurred retinal images for objects located at infinity. Refractive errors in infants and young children are measured using objective techniques such as *streak retinoscopy* or *photorefraction*. Refractive errors in older children and adults are best measured by subjective manifest refraction techniques using a phoro-optometer or set of trial lenses. Eighty percent of children between ages 2 and 6 years are hyperopic, 5% are emmetropic. About 10% of children have refractive errors that require correction before the age of 7 or 8 years.

HYPEROPIA   Also known as *farsightedness,* these terms are used to describe the state in which the far point of the eye falls beyond optical infinity. In hyperopia, light rays from an infinitely distant object come to a point of focus behind the retina, resulting in a retinal image that is blurred. To obtain a focused retinal image at any distance, a hyperopic individual must accommodate to bring the image on to the retina. The term *farsighted* is misleading. Hyperopic children without ocular pathology can see clearly in the distance and close up because they can accommodate. Hyperopic adults who are presbyopic, however, cannot see clearly either in the distance or near because of limited or no accommodation. Most infants are born 1 to 3 diopters hyperopic. This refractive error remains stable or increases slightly until the age of 5 years. By 6 to 8 years, physiological hyperopia begins to decrease toward emmetropia (emmetropization), which is established by 9 to 11 years. A young child's robust accommodative apparatus may overcome moderate amounts of pathologic hyperopia, so vision is usually good. When the degree of hyperopia in the two eyes is unequal, however, the less hyperopic eye may become the preferred eye because it requires less effort to see clearly, and the more hyperopic eye becomes "lazy" or amblyopic (*anisometropic amblyopia*). High hyperopia is frequently associated with *accommodative esotropia* (convergent strabismus) because of the intrinsic relationship between accommodation, convergence, and miosis (*near triad*).

MYOPIA Also known as *nearsightedness,* these terms are used to describe the refractive error in which the far point of the eye is between the eye and optical infinity in the unaccommodated state. In myopia, light from an infinitely distant object focuses in front of the retina and a blurred retinal image is formed. The eye is either too long or the optical power of the cornea-lens system is too great. Myopia usually appears between the ages of 5 and 20 years. Myopia associated with prematurity is often evident earlier in life. High myopia (greater than 9 diopters) is often hereditary. Patients with low amounts of myopia tend to become slowly more myopic through their second and third decades, eventually reaching a plateau.

ASTIGMATISM This term describes the state in which light rays are refracted differently depending on the meridian in which they enter the eye. Most astigmatism results from abnormalities of corneal curvature (*corneal astigmatism*); however, the lens may also be the source (*lenticular astigmatism*), or it may come from both structures (*mixed astigmatism*).

26.3.2 Visual Rehabilitation

Spectacles (eyeglasses) are prescribed to correct refractive errors. The use of glasses does not worsen refractive errors, typically, nor prevent their progression; such changes occur irrespective of the wearing of glasses. Glasses are not generally prescribed to children with low refractive errors unless amblyopia is present. Parental objections based on vanity should not stop a child from wearing glasses if they are necessary. It is advisable to defer contact lenses until the teenage years because of the cost and maturity required for their proper care and use. Young children and infants can wear contact lenses successfully, however, if they must for binocular development. Contact lenses are of particular value in unilateral high myopia and in surgical aphakia following congenital cataract surgery. In such instances, *aniseikonia* (binocular image-size disparity) prevents the successful wearing of spectacles. Daily-wear soft contact lenses are preferred over extended-wear soft contact lenses because of the potential occurrence of bacterial corneal ulcers associated with the latter.

References

Matsumura H, Hirai H: Prevalence of myopia and refractive changes in students from 3 to 17 years of age. Surv Ophthalmol 44:109–115, 1999
Milder B, Rubin M: The Fine Art of Prescribing Glasses without Making a Spectacle of Yourself, 2nd ed. Gainesville, FL, Triad, 1991

Repka MX: Refraction in infants and children. In: Nelson LB, Calhoun JH, Harley RD, eds: Pediatric Ophthalmology, 3rd ed. Philadelphia, Saunders, 1991
Saunders KJ: Early refractive development in humans. Surv Ophthalmol 40: 207–216, 1995

26.4 EYELIDS

John T. Tong

26.4.1 Congenital Anomalies

CRYPTOPHTHALMOS This is rare and is characterized by complete failure of differentiation of the eyelids. As a result, skin passes continuously from forehead to cheek, fusing with the cornea, which is malformed and invisible. Visual rehabilitation is generally unsuccessful, and cosmetic reconstruction operations are necessary. Cryptophthalmos may be associated with anomalies of ear, nose, lip, palate, larynx, kidney, and fingers. Inheritance is sporadic, occasionally, recessive.

PALPEBRAL COLOBOMA This is a full-thickness defect of the eyelids, usually occurring in the upper lids, either as an isolated defect or in association with other developmental abnormalities (Goldenhar and Franceschetti syndromes). It is the result of incomplete fusion of the maxillary processes. Surgical repair may be delayed several years if the defect is not severe, unless exposure keratopathy occurs. The optimal time for repair is from 6 to 12 months of age depending on the size and location of the defect.

CONGENITAL ECTROPION This deformity is an outward turning of the lid margin, usually involving the lower eyelid, caused by a foreshortening of the anterior lamellae (skin, subcutaneous tissues) of the eyelid. Exposure keratopathy may develop. Congenital ectropion rarely occurs as an isolated entity; it is seen with Down syndrome and commonly in association with the *Kohn-Romano blepharophimosis syndrome* (congenital blepharoptosis, epicanthus inversus, telecanthus, and blepharophimosis). Repair is by tarsorrhaphy or skin grafting. Ectropion of the upper lid is rare and must be distinguished from congenital eversion that can result from an infection such as that caused by *Chlamydia trachomatis*.

CONGENITAL TARSAL KINK A complete and fixed eversion of the upper eyelids is occasionally seen in newborns. The cornea may develop an abrasion or ulceration from exposure and trauma by the bent edge of the tarsus. Treatment for minor cases may involve applying topical ophthalmic ointment or unfolding the tarsus and taping the eyelid shut with a pressure patch. More severe cases require surgical intervention.

CONGENITAL ENTROPION This deformity is in an inward turning of the lid margin, usually involving the lower eyelid, which may cause the eyelashes to abrade the cornea. It seldom occurs as an isolated entity but is seen frequently in association with epicanthus or epiblepharon of the lower eyelid. Isolated primary entropion results from congenital absence of the tarsal plate or hypertrophy and tarsal override of the preseptal portion of the orbicularis muscle. This deformity often is familial. Early surgical repair is indicated if the cornea is compromised.

EPIBLEPHARON This is characterized by a horizontal fold of skin across the eyelid, more commonly the lower lid, which rotates the lashes inward against the cornea. It is usually familial and is almost always seen in Asian children. Spontaneous resolution occurs within a few years. If the cornea is compromised, simple excision of the skin fold is effective at correcting the malrotation.

TELECANTHUS This condition represents a wider than normal intercanthal distance in the setting of a normal interpupillary distance. It is in contrast to hypertelorism, which denotes a wider than normal separation of the bony orbits. Telecanthus may be seen in association with epicanthus and blepharophimosis, in craniofacial syndromes (Sec. 26.2) such as the Waardenburg syndrome, or following facial trauma with nasal orbital fracture.

BLEPHAROPHIMOSIS This is a bilateral and symmetric decrease in the height and width of the palpebral fissures. Inherited as an autosomal dominant trait, duplications of 6p and 10q have been reported. The *Kohn-Romano blepharophimosis syndrome* (congenital eyelid syndrome) is blepharophimosis associated with congenital blepharoptosis, epicanthus inversus, and telecanthus. Additionally, findings may include congenital lower eyelid ectropion, flattening of the supraorbital ridges, and hypoplasia of the nasal bridge. Abnormalities in chromosomes 3q and 7p have been found. Surgical reconstruction is often performed in multiple stages.

EPICANTHUS Epicanthal folds are semilunar folds of skin arising in the upper lid, extending down the side of the nose to the lower lid, and covering the normal medial canthus. The most frequent type is *epicanthus tarsalis,* in which the skin fold is most prominent in the upper lid. In *epicanthus inversus,* the skin fold is most prominent in the lower lid. Other types are less common. Epicanthal folds are a racial characteristic of many Asians but are also a common finding in several chromosomal disorders (see Table 26-1). Epicanthus inversus is often dominantly inherited with other lid anomalies in the blepharophimosis syndrome. Epicanthal folds may be observed in infants with flat nasal bridges; they create an illusory appearance of esotropia (*pseudostrabismus*). As the bridge of the nose develops, the folds usually disappear.

DISTICHIASIS This term describes an aberrant second row of lashes that arise from the meibomian gland orifices or slightly posterior to them. Chronic tearing and discharge can result and may mimic nasolacrimal duct obstruction. Distichiasis occurs either sporadically or as a dominant trait, usually without concomitant congenital anomalies; however, it may be associated with chronic lymphedema of the lower extremities (Falls-Kertesz syndrome). Abnormalities of chromosome 16q have been reported. If corneal erosions develop, lashes may be destroyed with cryotherapy, electrolysis, or surgery.

26.4.2   Blepharoptosis

The most common anomaly of the eyelids is *blepharoptosis* (*ptosis*), or drooping of the upper eyelid. It may be unilateral or bilateral; congenital or acquired. Congenital ptosis is usually myogenic in nature. Acquired ptosis may be myogenic (chronic progressive external ophthalmoplegia, muscular dystrophy, oculopharyngeal dystrophy), aponeurotic (posttraumatic, postinflammatory), neurogenic (Horner syndrome, third cranial nerve palsy, myasthenia gravis), or mechanical (hemangioma, neurofibroma, lid scarring).

True ptosis must be distinguished from pseudoptosis. Causes of *pseudoptosis* include ipsilateral hypotropia, hyperglobus, microphthalmos, enophthalmos, cornea plana, phthisis bulbi, and blepharospasm as well as contralateral eyelid retraction, hypoglobus, and proptosis.

CONGENITAL PTOSIS This is usually unilateral, but may be bilateral, and occurs because of dysgenesis or absence of the levator palpebrae superioris muscle. Fibrous tissue and/or adipose tissue are present histopathologically in the levator muscle belly. Congenital ptosis may be inherited as an autosomal dominant trait, or it may occur sporadically. It may be isolated or occur in association with other ocular anomalies such as ipsilateral superior rectus palsy, the blepharophimosis syndrome, and strabismus. Congenital ptosis may also occur in association with systemic abnormalities such as Fabry disease and Turner syndrome. Physicians should be aware that ptosis may be an initial manifestation of myasthenia gravis, the diagnosis of which can be confirmed with the edrophonium (Tensilon) or neostigmine (Prostigmin) test. In unilateral congenital ptosis, the child may raise the ipsilateral eyebrow and eyelid with the frontalis muscle, and in bilateral ptosis the child may adopt a chin-up torticollis.

Children with ptosis may have associated strabismus, astigmatism, or obstruction of the visual axes and may require corrective surgery in infancy to avoid amblyopia. Thus an ophthalmologic evaluation is advisable even if the ptosis is not severe. When surgery is performed for cosmesis, it can usually be postponed until 4 or 5 years of age when an adequate preoperative evaluation including accurate measurement of levator function can be performed. Surgical correction of ptosis involves resection of the levator muscle, if some levator function is present, or suspension of the upper eyelid from the frontalis muscle if minimal or no function is present.

A peculiar form of congenital neurogenic ptosis occurs in the *Marcus-Gunn jaw-winking syndrome.* In this syndrome, seen in 4 to 6% of all patients with congenital ptosis, an aberrant connection exists between the motor division of the fifth cranial (trigeminal) nerve and the levator palpebrae superioris muscle. The syndrome may be detected in infancy if a ptotic eyelid winks during breast- or bottle-feeding. In childhood and adulthood, the height of the ptotic eyelid can be influenced by jaw position. The syndrome may become less apparent with time and may not require surgery.

CHRONIC PROGRESSIVE EXTERNAL OPHTHALMOPLEGIA (CPEO) This is a rare disease characterized by gradually progressive, bilateral paralysis of all extraocular muscles, eventually resulting in complete ptosis and ophthalmoplegia. Ptosis is typically an early sign. Diplopia is notably absent. Familial and sporadic forms exist. A gene defect has been found in the mitochondrial chromosome, thus leading to maternal transmission. All patients with CPEO require a cardiac evaluation for evidence of *Kearns-Sayre syndrome* (a triad of CPEO, pigmentary retinopathy, and heart block). CPEO may also be seen in the Bassen-Kornzweig and Werdnig-Hoffman syndromes. It is best to treat patients with CPEO conservatively, avoiding surgery if possible.

HORNER SYNDROME Horner syndrome is the triad of blepharoptosis, miosis, and anhidrosis. The blepharoptosis typically measures 1 to 3 mm and is reversible with topical phenylephrine administration. Anisocoria is greatest in the dark and results from reduced innervation of the dilator muscle of the pupil. Horner syndrome miosis is discussed in Sec. 26.9.4. Conjunctival hyperemia, elevation of the lower eyelid (Kearn sign), and apparent enophthalmos may also be seen. Heterochromia iridis (the affected side being lighter) develops as a late sign. Most instances of childhood Horner syndrome are congenital and are thought to represent birth trauma. Other causes include cardiothoracic or vertebral surgery, vertebral skeletal anomalies, and congenital tumors (neuroblastoma). Cardiovascular surgery is the most common cause of acquired Horner syndrome in children. The older child with newly acquired Horner syndrome and no history of trauma or surgery must be evaluated for neuroblastoma. Laboratory evaluation should include chest radiography, head and neck CT or MR imaging, and 24-hour vanillylmandelic acid analysis; see Sec. 26.9.4 for a discussion of diagnostic pupil testing in Horner syndrome. Surgical options—after ptosis has been stable for at least 6 months—include conjunctivo-Mullerectomy and anterior levator resection. Topical phenylephrine can be applied as a temporizing measure, but mydriasis is a side effect.

THIRD CRANIAL NERVE PARESIS This paresis, also known as *oculomotor nerve paresis,* is characterized by ptosis, strabismus, and mydriasis. Strabismus results from paresis of four of the six extraocular muscles responsible for eye movements (Sec. 26.13.2). Unopposed contraction of the lateral rectus muscle, via sixth cranial (abducens) nerve stimulation, and unopposed contraction of the superior oblique muscle, via fourth cranial (trochlear) nerve stimulation, drive the eye into hypotropia and exotropia (the down and out position). Ptosis and pupillary involvement are usually present. The Bell phenomenon is absent. Third-nerve palsies are more often congenital than acquired. The congenital form is believed to be due to a developmental anomaly (hypoplasia of the oculomotor nucleus) or to birth trauma. Acquired third-nerve palsy in childhood can be caused by a brain tumor, cerebral aneurysm, blunt trauma, local and systemic infections, or ophthalmoplegic migraine. Treatment can be difficult and disappointing. Amblyopia in infants and young children requires occlusion therapy. The aim of strabismus surgery is to return the eye to primary position and maximize the range of motion. The ptosis may require levator resection or a frontalis muscle sling procedure if poor levator muscle function is demonstrated.

MYASTHENIA GRAVIS *Juvenile myasthenia* is the term given to essentially the same disease found in adults. Although patients are occasionally seen in the first decade of life, over 75% of cases occur after that time. It is an autoimmune disease of the neuromuscular junction that frequently presents with a variable, unilateral, or bilateral ptosis. The ptosis worsens with lid exercise and fatigue. Diplopia from involvement of other extraocular muscles may develop subsequently. Weakness of convergence and upgaze is seen. A useful clinical sign is the *Cogan lid twitch,* a momentary overelevation of the eyelids during refixation from downgaze to upgaze. The edrophonium (Tensilon) or neostigmine (Prostigmin) test may be diagnostic but can be negative or equivocal. Antiacetylcholine receptor antibody titers should be measured. Treatment with pyridostigmine bromide (Mestinon) is not always successful. Ptosis and eye muscle surgery should be approached very cautiously because of the variable nature of this condition. Thymectomy has proved beneficial in some instances of generalized myasthenia gravis (see Sec. 25.13.1).

Two neonatal forms of myasthenia gravis are encountered. *Transient neonatal myasthenia* develops in about 12% of newborns born to myasthenic mothers. The condition persists for about 2 to 3 weeks until the circulating transmitted factor is eliminated. Al-

though the most prominent symptoms are weakness, hypotonia, and poor feeding, eye signs occur in about 15% of the patients. Clinical findings include limited eye movements, ptosis, and orbicularis oculi weakness. The diagnosis is established by noting improvement of symptoms and signs after intramuscular or subcutaneous injection of 0.1 mg edrophonium chloride (Tensilon).

Congenital myasthenia occurs in infants born to nonmyasthenic mothers. Manifestations develop shortly after birth and are predominantly ophthalmic rather than systemic, namely, limited eye movements (ophthalmoplegia), ptosis, and orbicularis oculi weakness. A genetic basis for the disease is suggested because siblings may have similar findings. About 40% of these patients are seen before the age of 2 years. The ophthalmologist must watch for amblyopia due to the paralytic strabismus and use occlusion therapy if needed.

26.4.3 Blepharitis

Blepharitis is a common, subacute or chronic, recurrent inflammation of the eyelid margins associated with itching, burning, ocular irritation, foreign body sensation, and eyelid redness. Possible complications include cosmetic eyelid deformities, trichiasis, chronic conjunctivitis, and keratopathy. The most common forms are seborrheic, staphylococcal, and mixed.

SEBORRHEIC BLEPHARITIS This is characterized by yellow, greasy, easily removed scales (*scurf*) attached to the lashes and is associated with seborrhea of the brow, scalp, and external ears. Dry rather than greasy scales may be found. The organism *Pityrosporum ovale* is usually present, but it has not been shown to be causative. Recurrent conjunctivitis may occur. Keratitis is usually absent. Treatment is primarily lid hygiene and control of the general seborrheic dermatitis. Hygiene consists of daily removal of scales and crust with hot moist compresses and scrubs of the eyelid margins using a cotton-tip applicator or index finger in a wrapped wash cloth soaked in a dilute baby ("nontear") shampoo solution. Chronic resistant cases may benefit from expression of the greasy meibomian secretion by digital pressure. Severe cases, which may be associated with keratoconjunctivitis, may be treated with a short course of an antibiotic-steroid combination ointment. Seborrhea of the scalp may be treated with selenium sulfide shampoo.

STAPHYLOCOCCAL BLEPHARITIS This is a local infection of the eyelid margin caused by pathogenic *Staphylococcus aureus* and *S. epidermidis.* Tenacious fibrinous scales (*collarettes*) are seen at the base of the lashes. The lid margin is often inflamed, and eyelashes may be broken, sparse, or lost (madarosis). Spread of the bacteria to the glands of Zeis results in an *external hordeolum* or *stye.* Spread of bacteria to the meibomian glands causes an *internal hordeolum* or meibomitis. Conjunctivitis, superficial punctate keratitis, marginal keratitis or ulceration, and phlyctenular keratoconjunctivitis may result from elaboration of exotoxins by the staphylococcal organism. Treatment involves lid hygiene as for seborrheic blepharitis and the application of an appropriate antimicrobial ointment such as sulfacetamide, erythromycin, or bacitracin, once daily at bedtime. Topical corticosteroids have been used short term in combination with antibiotics to reduce the hypersensitivity reaction and inflammatory response that may accompany the infection. Lid hygiene must be continued indefinitely because blepharitis is often chronic with frequent exacerbations.

MIXED BLEPHARITIS This is common because staphylococcal infection often complicates seborrhea of the eyelids. Treatment is the same as for staphylococcal blepharitis.

Primary or recurrent infection by herpes virus type 1 may appear as clusters of eyelid vesicles that ulcerate and heal without scarring (*herpetic blepharitis*). Follicular conjunctivitis and dendritic keratitis may follow. The presence of lid vesicles calls for referral to an ophthalmologist for topical antiviral therapy to prevent or treat corneal involvement. Topical corticosteroid therapy should await ophthalmologic consultation because it may exacerbate the herpetic keratitis.

PARASITIC BLEPHARITIS This results from infestation of the eyelids by the crab louse (*Pediculus pubis*) or head louse (*P. capitis*) and causes itching and excoriation of the lid margins. With slit-lamp magnification, the adult lice and their ova (nits) may be seen attached to the lids or brows. Treatment consists of removing the parasites and their ova from the lashes with forceps, followed by the application of a bland ointment such as plain petrolatum or .025% physostigmine ointment two to four times a day for 1 week to smother the adult organisms. Other areas of infestation, such as the scalp or pubic area, must be treated simultaneously with a delousing preparation.

Demodex folliculorum (follicle mite) can produce vague pain, burning, redness, and itching, especially in the morning. The parasites reside in the meibomian glands, and their feces form tubelike sleeves on the lashes. The parasite can be seen on epilated lashes by microscopic examination. Treatment involves lid hygiene (see seborrhea blepharitis). Ethyl ether applied to the lid margin reduces the number of organisms. Ammoniated mercury ointment and 1% sulfur ointment can also be used.

26.4.4 Hordeolum and Chalazion

EXTERNAL HORDEOLUM This is the common *stye,* a pyogenic infection (usually staphylococcal) of the ciliary follicle and its associated sebaceous glands of Zeis along the lid margin. Susceptible persons may have recurrences. The lesion begins as a painful circumscribed swelling at the lid margin, progresses to suppuration, and finally ruptures with resolution of pain and tenderness. Treatment consists of warm moist compresses applied for 20 minutes several times a day and application of an ointment such as erythromycin or bacitracin at bedtime. If local measures do not lead to resolution, the stye may be incised and drained.

INTERNAL HORDEOLUM This is an acute pyogenic infection of a meibomian gland usually due to staphylococcal organisms. The area of localized swelling, redness, and suppuration presents on the conjunctival surface of the lid corresponding to the location of the gland. Spontaneous rupture is less frequent than with the external stye, but the treatment is the same.

CHALAZION This is a chronic lipogranuloma caused by retention of secretions of a meibomian gland likely developing after a staphylococcal blepharitis. Clinically, a chalazion is a slow-growing, firm, round, tarsal mass, unaccompanied by pain or tenderness unless there is a secondary infection. The chalazion may involute spontaneously over many weeks to months, or it may respond to intralesional corticosteroid injection. Symptomatic chalazia that do not resolve after a few weeks of conservative treatment (warm com-

presses and massage) may require transconjunctival incision and drainage by an ophthalmologist.

26.4.5 Tumors

NEVUS This is a well-circumscribed, raised or flat, benign, pigmented (although occasionally amelanotic) lesion composed of nests of normal-appearing melanocytes. Nevi may enlarge, undergo cystic change, or become increasingly pigmented during puberty and adolescence. Histologically, nevi are classified according to location as junctional, dermal, or compound. A dramatic lesion is the congenital split nevus involving the margins of the upper and lower eyelids simultaneously. Oculodermal melanocytosis, or nevus of Ota, is a pigmentation of the eyelids that is associated with slate-gray or bluish pigmentation of the sclera. Nevi rarely undergo malignant transformation, but this has been reported with oculodermal melanocytosis.

DERMOID CYST This is a common congenital lesion of the eyelids or orbit. It is usually palpable beneath the lateral eyebrow in the superotemporal orbit. Histologically, dermoid cysts are lined by keratinizing stratified squamous epithelium containing dermal appendages such as hair follicles and sebaceous glands. They are usually incorporated into suture lines of the orbital bones (often the zygomaticofrontal suture). *Epidermoid cysts* are lined by epidermis without skin appendages. The keratin content of these cysts has a greasy texture that is often confused with sebum. If the entire extent of a suspected dermoid or epidermoid cyst cannot be palpated, radiologic studies are indicated. Anteromedial orbital tumors may represent orbital mucoceles. Rupture of a dermoid cyst results in acute orbital inflammation. Treatment is by careful surgical excision.

CAPILLARY HEMANGIOMA This is a common benign tumor of the eyelids in children. It may also occur in the orbit (Sec. 26.14.3). When the tumor is superficial, the involved skin has the appearance of a "strawberry nevus" because of its color and surface texture. Deeper lesions tend to be bluish or violet. The lesions blanch when palpated, a feature that distinguishes them from port wine stains, such as those seen in Sturge-Weber syndrome. Capillary hemangiomas appear within the first few months after birth, enlarge dramatically during the first year or two of life, then undergo spontaneous involution over the next 4 to 5 years. Capillary hemangiomas are associated with thrombocytopenia in the Kasabach-Merritt syndrome. Large lesions may cause ptosis and deprivation amblyopia or exert sufficient pressure on the globe to produce astigmatism and anisometropic amblyopia. Strabismic amblyopia may also occur. The cosmetic deformity associated with capillary hemangiomas may be disturbing to parents. Although the natural course is favorable, periodic ophthalmologic examination to monitor for the development of refractive errors and amblyopia is important. When treatment is indicated because of potential amblyopia development, or for cosmetic reasons, intralesional corticosteroid injection has been used with success (see Sec. 26.14.3). Reduction of tumor size has also been reported with topical corticosteroids, systemic corticosteroids, interferon injections, irradiation therapy, laser photocoagulation, cryotherapy, and surgical excision.

Melanomas, basal cell carcinomas, and squamous cell carcinomas are common malignant eyelid neoplasms in adults but are rarely seen in children. For a discussion of other pediatric eyelid and orbital tumors refer to Sec. 26.14.3.

26.4.6 Blepharospasm and Bell Palsy

A *tic* is a type of *blepharospasm* seen especially in children 5 to 10 years of age. Tics are usually psychogenic and can be initiated voluntarily. They cease with diversion or sleep. Rarely does refractive error, blepharitis, or conjunctivitis cause them. Tics tend to abate with time, especially in childhood, if doctors, teachers, and parents do not pay much attention to them and if the cause of emotional tension is managed. On rare occasions, tics are associated with a more serious neurologic disorder such as Tourette or Rett syndrome. Benign essential blepharospasm and hemifacial spasm are rarely seen in children.

Bell palsy is a unilateral peripheral seventh cranial (facial) nerve palsy of sudden onset arising from inflammation and swelling of the nerve within the facial canal of the petrous temporal bone. Accumulating evidence supports a viral inflammatory-immune mechanism. About 60% of occurrences are associated with a viral prodrome. Patients with Bell palsy are more than twice as likely to have diabetes mellitus as age-matched controls. There may be a genetic predisposition as a family history of the same disease is common. The palsy results in paralysis of the orbicularis muscle and *lagophthalmos* (incomplete closure of the eyelids) that can lead to the development of *exposure keratopathy*. Treatment includes the application of protective bland ointments and artificial tears, patching, or even tarsorrhaphy. Fortunately, recovery with complete return of eyelid function occurs in 84% of patients within weeks to months. Only 4% have severe lasting dysfunction. Other conditions in the differential diagnosis of Bell palsy include trauma, herpes zoster cephalicus, tumor, infection, hemifacial spasm, and axial central nervous system disease.

References

Crawford JB: Neoplastic and inflammatory tumors of the eyelids. In: Duane TD, Jaeger EA, eds: Clinical Ophthalmology. Philadelphia, Lippincott-Raven, 1996

Fries PD, Katowitz JA: Congenital craniofacial anomalies of ophthalmic importance. Surv Ophthalmol 35:87, 1990

Haik BG, Karcioglu ZA, Gordon RA, et al: Capillary hemangioma (infantile periocular hemangioma). Surv Ophthalmol 38:399, 1994

Katowitz JA, Foster JA: Disorders of the eyelids in infants. In: Isenberg SJ, ed: The Eye in Infancy, 2nd ed. St. Louis, Mosby, 1994

Nesi FA, Lisman RD, Levine RM, eds: Smith's Ophthalmic Plastic and Reconstructive Surgery, 2nd ed. St. Louis, Mosby, 1998

Shields JA, Shields CL: Atlas of Eyelid and Conjunctival Tumors. New York, Lippincott Williams & Wilkins, 1999

26.5 LACRIMAL SYSTEM

26.5.1 Congenital Anomalies

ATRESIA OF THE LACRIMAL PUNCTA If the surface ectoderm overlying a developing canaliculus fails to dehisce spontaneously during embryogenesis, punctal atresia results. The canaliculus just beneath the papilla on the medial aspect of the eyelid margin is usually patent. Tearing is the usual complaint but without mucopurulent discharge because stagnation of fluid within the nasolacrimal sac does not occur. Isolated atresia of the upper punctum requires no treatment, but atresia of the lower or both upper and lower puncta requires correction if there are symptoms. Probing or cutting across the papillae, with or without silicone intubation, is curative.

SUPERNUMERARY PUNCTA Occasionally, more than one canalicular opening develops in an eyelid. The extra puncta usually appear nasal to the normal punctum. Treatment is not necessary.

CONGENITAL DACRYOCYSTOCELE Congenital dacryocystocele, also known as congenital *mucocele* or *dacryocele,* appears at or shortly after birth as a subcutaneous, 1-cm diameter, gray-blue cystic mass just below the medial canthus. The mass develops as a result of congenital obstruction of the nasolacrimal duct and the inability of the lacrimal sac to discharge its secretions retrograde through the canalicular system. Congenital dacryocystocele must be differentiated from cavernous hemangioma and midline encephalocele. On ultrasonography a dacryocystocele is acoustically hollow, whereas a capillary hemangioma has high internal reflectivity. Secondary dacryocystitis and a cutaneous fistula may develop. Treatment is with warm compresses, antibiotics if there is secondary infection, and prompt probing.

CONGENITAL FISTULA OF THE LACRIMAL SAC This is rare. Developmental fistulas are more frequent. When dacryocystitis is absent, the material that drains from the fistula is typically scant or watery. If dacryocystitis develops, the discharge becomes mucopurulent. Congenital fistulas develop as a result of congenital nasolacrimal-duct obstruction. Spontaneous resolution of the nasolacrimal obstruction or therapeutic probing usually results in spontaneous healing of the fistula. Occasionally it is necessary to perform a fistulectomy.

26.5.2 Epiphora

Chronic epiphora (*tearing*) is usually a sign of lacrimal-system obstruction, although it may stem occasionally from hypersecretion (lacrimation). In common usage, *epiphora* implies inadequate tear drainage, whereas *lacrimation* implies excessive tear production. Causes of hypersecretion include infantile glaucoma, conjunctivitis, corneal disease, iritis, and anomalous fifth cranial nerve innervation of the lacrimal gland (*crocodile tears*). Punctal atresia, punctal stenosis, canalicular stenosis, and canaliculitis (herpes simplex, chickenpox, bacterial infection) may cause lacrimal-system obstruction and epiphora; however, the most common etiology is congenital nasolacrimal-duct obstruction.

NASOLACRIMAL DUCT OBSTRUCTION Nasolacrimal duct obstruction or *dacryostenosis* is a congenital obstruction of the nasolacrimal system manifested by epiphora and discharge. Photophobia is absent. Dacryostenosis occurs in 1 to 6% of newborns and is more common in firstborn children. Nasolacrimal-duct obstruction is usually unilateral and secondary to failure of dehiscence of a membrane at the valve of Hasner, which separates the nasolacrimal duct from the inferior nasal meatus. Congenital nasolacrimal duct obstruction usually resolves spontaneously by 6 to 8 months; thus, conservative treatment during this period is advocated. The parents should be instructed to express the contents of the lacrimal sac several times a day by digital massage. Massage also increases the hydrostatic pressure of the sac and may lead to rupture of the membrane at the valve of Hasner. Concomitant infection is treated with topical broad-spectrum antibiotic eyedrops. If the obstruction fails to resolve by 6 to 8 months of age, or if recurrent dacryocystitis develops, the nasolacrimal duct should be opened by probing and irrigation. A single probing is usually curative. If the opening closes after probing, additional probing, silicone intubation, or dacryocystorhinostomy may be required.

BLOODY TEARS This is a rare finding that has been reported with factor VII deficiency, Henoch-Schönlein purpura, angiomata of the lacrimal sac, head trauma, dacryoadenitis, congenital heart disease, posttraumatic epilepsy, and epistaxis through the nasolacrimal duct.

26.5.3   Infections

DACRYOADENITIS Acute dacryoadenitis is usually unilateral, presenting with pain and fullness over the lacrimal gland, redness and swelling of the temporal region of the upper eyelid, and possible mucopurulent discharge and orbital cellulitis. There may even be diplopia and restricted movement of the globe. With eversion of the lid, the gland can be seen to be enlarged and inflamed. The cause is often an associated systemic infection such as mumps, infectious mononucleosis, influenza, or an exanthem. Local causes are staphylococci, trachoma, and herpes zoster. Treatment consists of appropriate systemic work-up, local cultures and cytology, followed by antibiotics, if indicated, heat, and analgesia. Chronic dacryoadenitis, on the other hand, is frequently bilateral. The lacrimal gland is enlarged and indurated, producing a swelling in the temporal aspect of the upper eyelid. No discharge or inflammatory signs are present. Sarcoidosis is the most frequent etiology, but other causes include trachoma, tuberculosis, syphilis, and Mikulicz syndrome. Treatment is directed at the underlying systemic disease.

DACRYOCYSTITIS Dacryocystitis usually develops as a consequence of obstruction and stagnation of tear flow. Gram-positive bacteria generally are grown on culture of expressed contents of the sac. The clinical picture is that of a tender swelling of the skin overlying the lacrimal sac and adjacent lower eyelid. Pressure on the lacrimal sac causes a reflux of pus from the punctum. Acute or chronic conjunctivitis and keratitis may also be present. Acute infections are treated with hot compresses and local or systemic antibiotics. Probing should be delayed until the acute infection is controlled, because false passages can lead to orbital cellulitis, and potential bacteremia can be serious. Untreated or recurrent disease may go on to abscess formation with cutaneous fistulas or dacryolith formation. Scarring of the lacrimal sac with obliteration of the lacrimal passages is a troublesome consequence of chronic infection.

References

Hurwitz JJ: The Lacrimal System. Philadelphia, Lippincott-Raven, 1996

Mansour AM, Cheng KP, Mumma JV, et al: Congenital dacryocele: A collaborative review. Ophthalmology 98:1744, 1991

McCord CD, Tanenbaum M, Nunery WR, eds: Oculoplastic Surgery, 3rd ed. New York, Lippincott Williams & Wilkins, 1994

Robb RM: Probing and irrigation for congenital nasolacrimal duct obstruction. Arch Ophthalmol 104:378, 1986

Tanenbaum M, McCord CD Jr: The lacrimal drainage system. In: Duane TD, Jaeger EA, eds: Clinical Ophthalmology. Philadelphia, Lippincott, 1991

26.6   CONJUNCTIVA

26.6.1   Congenital Anomalies

With the exception of pigmentation, conjunctival anomalies are rare. *Epithelial melanosis* appears clinically as patchy, flat, brown conjunctival pigment, mainly of the bulbar conjunctiva. *Melanosis oculi* is an inherited unilateral disorder characterized by slate-blue mottled pigmentation of the conjunctiva and sclera. There may also be increased uveal pigment. *Oculodermal melanosis (nevus of Ota)* is seen before 1 year of age with unilateral slate-blue conjunctival and scleral pigment with associated pigmentation of the ipsilateral periorbital skin. There is a predilection for Asians and blacks. None of these conjunctival pigmentation anomalies have malignant potential, and they do not disturb the function of the eye, but patients with melanosis oculi and oculodermal melanosis may develop malignant melanomas of the uveal tract or pigmentary glaucoma in adulthood. Therefore, persons with either of these pigmentary conjunctival anomalies should have periodic ophthalmologic examinations.

26.6.2   Conjunctivitis

Conjunctivitis is common in children. Factors that ordinarily protect the conjunctiva from infection are an intact mucous membrane, the flushing action of tears, and the bactericidal action of lysozyme in tears. The usual signs and symptoms of conjunctivitis are injection, ocular irritation, chemosis, papillary reaction (small, polygonal, erythematous elevations of the conjunctiva containing central vascular cores that exude serum and inflammatory cells separated by pale connective tissue septae), and tearing. Depending on the specific type of conjunctivitis, additional signs may include preauricular and submaxillary lymphadenopathy, follicular reaction (larger, round elevations of the conjunctiva that represent collections of lymphoid cells with active germinal centers), membrane or pseudomembrane formation, mucus production, and mucopurulent discharge. Pain, photophobia, and decreased vision are uncommon and, if present, should lead the clinician to suspect concomitant corneal disease or uveitis. In the newborn, the usual causes are vaginally transmitted viruses (herpes simplex type 2), bacteria, and chlamydia. In older children the main causes are allergy, viral and bacterial infections.

Numerous features of the clinical presentation can help define the nature of the conjunctivitis and direct further evaluation and management. The onset may be hyperacute (suggesting infection with *Neisseria gonorrhoeae* or *N. meningitidis*), acute (typical of viral infections and *Streptococcus pneumoniae, S. aureus, Haemophilus aegyptius*), subacute (allergy, chlamydial infection, or *H. influenzae*), or chronic (allergy, chlamydial infection, or bacterial infection with *S. aureus, M. lacunata, Pseudomonas* species, *Proteus* species, and coliform bacilli). The discharge may be purulent (typical of bacterial infection), watery (typical of viral infection and chemical irritation), or scant (chemical irritation and chronic bacterial infection) or characterized by the presence of mucus (allergy, giant papillary conjunctivitis). There may be an associated nasolacrimal duct obstruction (dacryocystitis) and antecedent history of epiphora. An enlarged preauricular lymph node is highly suggestive of viral infection but may be seen in gonococcal infection. The wearing of a contact lens or prosthesis may be causative or contributory. A recent history of conjunctivitis in family or school contacts is useful. In atypical or chronic conjunctivitis one should inquire about associated systemic conditions such as vaginitis, urethritis, arthritis, and aphthous oral and genital ulcers (chlamydial infection, Reiter syndrome, Behcet disease). Physical examination may disclose an associated dermatitis, blepharitis, keratitis, uveitis, sinusitis, orbital cellulitis, or a corneal foreign body.

A conjunctival *papillary reaction* is a nonspecific finding, but a *follicular reaction* helps to limit the differential diagnosis. For *acute follicular conjunctivitis* lasting less than 4 weeks, the differential diagnosis includes acute adenoviral infection (epidemic keratoconjunctivitis, pharyngoconjunctival fever), chlamydial inclusion conjunctivitis, primary herpes simplex virus infection, viral eyelid infection (verruca, molluscum contagiosum), local drug sensitivity (antiviral agents, adrenergics, miotics, atropine), Newcastle disease, and acute hemorrhagic conjunctivitis. For *chronic follicular conjunctivitis* lasting more than 4 weeks, the differential diagnosis includes chlamydial inclusion conjunctivitis, trachoma, local drug sensitivity, viral eyelid infection, and Parinaud oculoglandular syndrome. *Phlyctenules* are round, elevated, sterile infiltrates on the conjunctiva, limbus, or cornea that result from type 4 hypersensitivity to microbial antigens. Phlyctenules are associated with staphylococcal infection of the eyelids, latent or active tuberculosis, coccidoidomycosis, chlamydial infection, and *Candida* infection.

Another clinical finding that helps to narrow the differential diagnosis is *membranous conjunctivitis*. Membranes and pseudomembranes (the difference is one of definition and severity) form by transudation of serum and protein and exudation of cells from inflamed vessels. Pseudomembranes can be stripped away easily without causing bleeding. True membranes adhere tightly to the conjunctiva, leaving a raw, bleeding surface when stripped away from the underlying epithelium. The differential diagnosis includes acute adenoviral infection, β-hemolytic streptococcal infection, primary herpes simplex virus infection, *Neisseria* infection, chemical burns, vernal conjunctivitis, chlamydial infection in newborns, ocular cicatricial pemphigoid, Stevens-Johnson syndrome, diphtheria, graft-versus-host disease, ligneous conjunctivitis, and *Candida* infection. Because of the severity of these types of conjunctivitis, there is often residual scarring of the conjunctiva and cornea.

Bacterial, chlamydial, and viral cultures taken from the lower tarsal conjunctiva and microscopic studies of conjunctival scrapings are essential in all instances of ophthalmia neonatorum and in all other forms of conjunctivitis unresponsive to initial therapy within 48 to 72 hours. By determining the specific etiologic agent, the indiscriminate use of antibiotics and the attendant development of host sensitivity and microorganism resistance can be avoided. Rapid techniques for detecting bacteria and viruses such as indirect immunofluorescence and polymerase chain reaction can be helpful.

Topical ophthalmic pharmaceuticals are used routinely to treat conjunctivitis. Oral medications are sometimes necessary. Systemic tetracycline should be avoided in the gravid woman and in the child under 8 years of age because it may cause epiphyseal damage in the fetus and stain the young child's tooth enamel. Corticosteroids are highly effective in allergic conjunctivitis but are generally contraindicated in bacterial and viral conjunctivitis. They may cause ex-

acerbations of disease, such as in herpes simplex infection, and chronic use may lead to cataracts and glaucoma. In young children, medication in ointment form may be easier to instill with less chance of overdosage. In the older child, it is desirable to use drops during the day, as they do not interfere with vision, and ointments at bedtime.

ALLERGIC CONJUNCTIVITIS

The conjunctiva, like other epithelial tissues, may develop a local hypersensitivity to a specific allergen. All the changes encountered in simple allergic reactions can occur in the conjunctiva. In IgE-mediated acute hypersensitivity reactions, there is sudden vascular dilation with marked chemosis that resolves when the irritant is removed. In chronic allergy, cellular infiltration and newly formed connective tissue follow. Eosinophils are usually present in conjunctival scrapings stained with Wright stain, and basophils may be seen. Lymphoid hypertrophy with follicle formation usually does not occur in immunologic or allergic conjunctivitis. Signs and symptoms of allergic conjunctivitis include itching, tearing, chemosis, and mucus production.

SIMPLE ALLERGIC CONJUNCTIVITIS This type of conjunctivitis, also known as *hay fever conjunctivitis* if it is seasonal, typically occurs in youngsters with other manifestations of hay fever such as asthma, allergic rhinitis, and sinusitis. Onset is acute and attacks are short-lived. Pollens, animal hair, fungi, dust, and ingestion of some foods can precipitate attacks. A hyperemic reaction of the tarsal and bulbar conjunctiva is accompanied by edema of the conjunctiva and lids and results in profuse lacrimation and itching. The itching is usually far more conspicuous than in infectious conjunctivitis. There may be a scant, stringy mucoid discharge containing a variable number of eosinophils. Tear histamine and IgE levels are elevated. Initial treatment consists of eliminating exposure to the offending allergen, if possible, cold compresses, and the use of a topical antihistamine-decongestant agent (eg, Naphcon A, Vasocon A). For relief of seasonal or refractory allergic conjunctivitis the following topical agents are available: H_1 antagonists (Livostin, Emadine), mast-cell inhibitors (Crolom, Alomide), H_1 antagonist/mast-cell inhibitor combination (Patanol), chemotaxis/mast-cell inhibitor (Alocril), nonsteroidal anti-inflammatory agent (Acular), and a corticosteroid (Alrex) used short-term. Desensitization to the allergen, if known, may be necessary.

VERNAL CONJUNCTIVITIS Vernal conjunctivitis, or spring catarrh, is a bilateral, chronic, recurrent inflammation characterized clinically by dramatic, giant, flat-topped, cobblestone papillae in the upper palpebral conjunctiva (palpebral vernal conjunctivitis) and/or smaller, discrete papillae at the limbus (limbal vernal conjunctivitis). The onset of vernal conjunctivitis is subacute and is more severe in hot climates, symptoms persist for weeks to months, and the condition is seasonally recurrent in the spring or summer. A ropy discharge, extreme itching, and photophobia are characteristic. Giant tarsal papillae from the upper eyelid may abrade the cornea, causing diffuse punctate keratopathy or an oval or pentagonal shaped area of ulceration (shield ulcer) of the superior cornea. Horner-Trantas dots (chalky concretions made up of eosinophils) are characteristically present and usually are located at the limbus near giant papillae. Conjunctival scrapings reveal many eosinophils and free eosinophilic granules. Tear histamine level is increased. Primarily IgE antibodies mediate the disorder, but IgG antibodies and cell-mediated immunity may contribute. Vernal conjunctivitis is primarily a disease of childhood, occurring most frequently from 5 to 15 years of age. There is frequently, although not invariably, a history of atopy. Identification of specific allergens has been unsuccessful. Symptomatic treatment consists of the same drug therapy described in the section on vernal conjunctivitis. The goal of therapy is the elimination of symptoms, not the eradication of the giant papillary reaction. In severe disease, supratarsal corticosteroid injection, treatment with a brief course of systemic corticosteroids, or topical cyclosporine 2% may be required. Cryoablation and surgical removal of giant papillae have been attempted in severe disease, but the papillae usually recur. Desensitization to allergens has not been helpful. Treatment of a secondary bacterial conjunctivitis or blepharitis may be necessary. Occasionally, moving to a region with a cooler, moist climate can lead to improvement.

ATOPIC CONJUNCTIVITIS This variant of IgE-mediated allergic conjunctivitis is seen in about a third of patients who have eczematoid dermatitis. It is more common in adults than in children. Clinical findings are similar to those of vernal conjunctivitis with a few exceptions. There is little seasonal variation in atopic conjunctivitis. Eosinophils are only infrequently seen in epithelial scrapings. Chemosis may be prominent and papillary reaction relatively insignificant; the papillae that are present tend to be smaller than in vernal conjunctivitis. Horner-Trantas dots are common near the limbal giant papillae but can occur anywhere on the tarsal and bulbar conjunctiva. Conjunctival scarring can occur and be extensive enough to cause symblepharon formation, corneal pannus, and corneal opacification. Treatment is the same as that for vernal conjunctivitis.

VIRAL CONJUNCTIVITIS

Viral conjunctivitis is characterized by the acute onset of conjunctival injection, watery discharge, and preauricular lymphadenopathy. Viral conjunctival infections usually cause a follicular conjunctivitis; most often it is acute. Involvement may be unilateral or bilateral. Some forms are extremely contagious. Transmission is by exposure to airborne, aerosolized particles or by hand contact with the eye. Adenovirus is the agent responsible for most episodes of viral conjunctivitis. Associated systemic findings can include fever and pharyngitis. Conjunctivitis may develop in the setting of varicella, mumps, and rubella infection. Family members, close personal contacts such as baby-sitters, and children at nurseries or daycare centers and schools may have a recent history of similar conjunctivitis. Early and rapid diagnosis of adenoviral conjunctivitis can be made with enzyme-linked immunosorbent assay (ELISA) and indirect immunofluorescent tests (adenoclone). However, they are not as sensitive as a culture or the polymerase chain reaction assay. Careful hand washing and avoidance of hand-to-eye contact should be encouraged to decrease the spread of infection. Children should be quarantined and kept out of school for about 2 weeks. Treatment is usually supportive.

Some types of viral conjunctivitis are also closely associated with the concurrent or subsequent development of keratitis (epidemic keratoconjunctivitis, herpes simplex, herpes zoster) (see Sec. 26.7.2).

EXANTHEMATOUS CONJUNCTIVITIS Many of the childhood exanthems such as *chickenpox* (varicella-zoster), *mumps, German measles* (rubella), *infectious mononucleosis* (Epstein-Barr virus), *influenza,* and *rubeola* may be accompanied by an acute conjunctivitis. In varicella, small, unilateral, papular lesions may occur at the lid margin, plica semilunaris, or limbus along with a mild conjunctivitis. Superficial or deep keratitis may complicate the infection, but it usually resolves spontaneously. No specific treatment is necessary unless secondary bacterial infection or corneal involvement occurs. The varicella virus may become latent in the trigeminal ganglion and reactivate years later to produce herpes zoster ophthalmicus (shingles). Keratoconjunctivitis is a characteristic and constant finding during the acute stage of rubella. Ocular involvement may precede the skin eruption by several days. A peculiar swelling of the plica semilunaris (Meyer sign), a glass-like appearance of the conjunctiva, and Koplik spots on the caruncle and plica semilunaris can occur during the period of incubation. Epithelial keratitis then follows shortly. In malnourished or debilitated children, secondary infection with pneumococcus, *H. influenzae,* and other bacteria may lead to severe purulent conjunctival and corneal involvement with ulceration and perforation. Flu-like symptoms and skin lesions in an endemic area should prompt consideration of Lyme disease. Occurrence of exanthematous conjunctivitis has been greatly reduced by immunization of youngsters against rubella, rubeola, mumps, varicella, and *H. influenzae.*

ACUTE HEMORRHAGIC CONJUNCTIVITIS. This type of conjunctivitis is characterized by a short incubation period (8–48 hours), short duration (4–7 days), and its highly contagious nature—person to person, hand to hand, and hand to eye. Clinical findings include conjunctival chemosis, hyperemia, diffuse subconjunctival hemorrhages that are most severe on the upper bulbar conjunctiva, follicular reaction, preauricular lymphadenopathy, and fine punctate keratitis. A mild nongranulomatous iritis may accompany the keratitis. It is caused by picornavirus (usually *Enterovirus* 70 or an antigenic variant of coxsackievirus A24; adenovirus has also been implicated). Acute hemorrhagic conjunctivitis is common among children but uncommon in the preteenage group. Neurologic complications may accompany or follow the conjunctivitis including Bell palsy, palatal paralysis, and radiculomyelitis. No specific therapy is available. Topical vasoconstrictors may offer some relief.

PHARYNGOCONJUNCTIVAL FEVER (PCF) This type of conjunctivitis is characterized by an acute, self-limited follicular conjunctivitis (most marked in the lower tarsal conjunctiva and cul-de-sac) that lasts 10 to 14 days in association with fever, malaise, pharyngitis, and preauricular and cervical lymphadenopathy. The incubation period varies from 2 to 14 days. Patients are infectious for 7 to 20 days after the onset of symptoms. The disease is most commonly caused by adenovirus types 3, 4, and 7 and occasionally by 5 and others. There is considerable overlap of clinical manifestations with epidemic keratoconjunctivitis (EKC), an infection produced by other serotypes of adenovirus (see Sec. 26.7.2). In most instances of PCF, superficial punctate corneal opacities develop, but they disappear without sequelae as the conjunctivitis subsides. This highly contagious disease is spread by direct contact or indirectly through contaminated swimming pools (even if they are chlorinated); epidemics are not uncommon in the late summer months. Children may spread the infection to adults. The only therapy is isolation precautions and medical management as for EKC. Corticosteroids are generally contraindicated in the treatment of adenoviral conjunctivitis.

MOLLUSCUM CONTAGIOSUM CONJUNCTIVITIS This is a chronic follicular conjunctivitis caused by a toxic reaction to the molluscum contagiosum virus. The virus is a DNA poxvirus that is spread by direct contact and possibly by fomites. It produces umbilicated, pearly white, waxy nodules averaging 3 mm in diameter on the eyelid margin. They discharge toxic desquamated material and poxvirus particles onto the conjunctival sac, producing a reactive follicular conjunctivitis and epithelial keratitis. The typical histology of molluscum lesions stained with hematoxylin-eosin consists of large, intracytoplasmic inclusion bodies (molluscum bodies) inside epidermal cells. Extensive eyelid and facial molluscum lesions have been reported in AIDS. Treatment involves removing the lesion from the lid margin by surgery, cautery, or cryotherapy.

BACTERIAL CONJUNCTIVITIS

Bacterial conjunctivitis may be characterized by sudden or delayed onset, by variable duration, conjunctival injection, chemosis, mucopurulent discharge, and the absence of preauricular lymphadenopathy (except in gonococcal conjunctivitis). It is classified as acute if it lasts less than 4 weeks and chronic if it lasts longer. Involvement may be unilateral or bilateral. The bacteria responsible for conjunctivitis usually are not highly contagious. Conjunctival cultures are helpful for identifying causative organisms and determining appropriate antibiotic treatment but are not obtained routinely except in ophthalmia neonatorum. Initial treatment for most types of presumed bacterial conjunctivitis is the application of a broad-spectrum topical ophthalmic antibiotic such as polymyxin B/trimethoprim solution or polymyxin B/neomycin/bacitracin ointment. Treatment of refractory cases should be guided by the results of culture and sensitivity testing.

Bear in mind that most cases of infectious conjunctivitis are viral in etiology. Mild or equivocal cases should not be treated routinely with antibiotics.

OPHTHALMIA NEONATORUM (NEONATAL CONJUNCTIVITIS) For over one hundred years topical silver nitrate 1% was used with much success to prevent ophthalmia neonatorum. In recent years, 0.5% erythromycin and 1% tetracycline ophthalmic ointments have been popular because they are less irritating than silver nitrate yet seem equally effective. Since 1998 silver nitrate has been commercially unavailable. A recent controlled study of 3117 newborns found that the antiseptic povidone-iodine 2.5% solution is superior to both silver nitrate and erythromycin in controlling neonatal conjunctivitis. Povidone-iodine promises to be the drug of choice for neonatal conjunctivitis in the future, since the drug has a broad antimicrobial spectrum that includes not only gram-positive and gram-negative bacteria but also fungi and viruses (including herpes simplex). Additionally, it is inexpensive, available worldwide, nontoxic, and is essentially devoid of bacterial resistance—a feature of particular importance in view of the increasing number of reports of bacterial resistance to erythromycin and tetracycline.

Acute conjunctivitis in the newborn may be caused by a viral, bacterial, or chlamydial agent acquired during or after delivery. Knowing the time of onset of the conjunctivitis is helpful but not absolute as a diagnostic clue. Gonococcal conjunctivitis occurs within 2 to 3 days of birth (possibly sooner if rupture of amniotic membranes occurs early in labor). Other types of bacterial conjunctivitis may develop 3 or more days after birth and can vary widely as they are acquired postnatally in the nursery. Chlamydial conjunctivitis occurs 5 to 23 days after birth. Mixed infections also occur. Because the potential for blindness associated with gonococcal infection exists in all newborns with ophthalmia neonatorum, this should be considered the causative organism until proved

otherwise. The birth mother should be treated whenever the conjunctivitis has a venereal etiology. An approach to evaluating a conjunctival discharge in the newborn is outlined in Fig. 26-1.

Numerous bacterial pathogens may be found in neonatal conjunctivitis. As mentioned, gonococcus is potentially the most serious. *S. aureus* is seen frequently, but pneumococcus, streptococcus, pseudomonas, *H. influenzae,* and coliform bacteria have been implicated as well. Most of the gram-positive bacteria that cause neonatal conjunctivitis respond to topical erythromycin or bacitracin, whereas the gram-negative organisms are usually best treated with topical gentamicin, tobramycin, or polymyxin. Other important causes of neonatal conjunctivitis are inclusion conjunctivitis (*Chlamydia trachomatis*) and viral infections such as herpes simplex type 2 and coxsackievirus A9.

Because any conjunctivitis in the newborn can be serious, for both medical and legal purposes conjunctival scrapings and cultures must be obtained. The conjunctival discharge is cultured on a culture medium, such as chocolate blood agar or Thayer-Martin, and incubated at 35°C in a candle jar at 5 to 10% CO_2 for *N. gonorrhea* and blood agar for other bacteria. The conjunctival scrapings are stained with Giemsa and Gram stains and examined with a microscope. Gram-negative intracellular diplococci suggest *Neisseria* species. Multinucleated giant cells suggest herpes simplex infection. Intracytoplasmic epithelial inclusions suggest inclusion conjunctivitis. All *Neisseria* isolated from the eye on culture should be subjected to oxidase and sugar utilization tests to distinguish between *N. gonorrhoeae* and *N. meningitidis*. The meningococcus is oxidase-positive and ferments both dextrose and maltose. The gonococcus ferments only dextrose.

NEISSERIA GONORRHOEAE This organism produces a hyperacute conjunctivitis characterized by bilateral involvement, marked edema of the eyelids, chemosis, marked conjunctival injection, and a copious purulent discharge. *N. meningitidis* occasionally produces a similar clinical picture. Because rapid corneal penetration may lead to globe perforation, panophthalmitis, and even septicemia or meningitis, proper treatment must be initiated immediately. Because the infection is contagious, all affected infants should be hospitalized and placed in isolation for at least 24 hours following initiation of treatment. Conjunctival smears and scrapings should be obtained in all instances of ophthalmia neonatorum. Gram-negative intracellular diplococci are found in gonococcal conjunctivitis, helping to differentiate it from the conjunctivitis caused by *Chlamydia* and other organisms. The Committee on Infectious Diseases of the American Academy of Pediatrics recommends treatment with ceftriaxone (25 to 50 mg/kg/d, not to exceed 125 mg, IV or IM) given once, or alternatively cefotaxime (50 to 100 mg/kg/d, IV or IM, in two or three divided doses) for 7 days. Irrigation of the eyes with normal saline should continue until the discharge is eliminated. Instillation of erythromycin 0.5% or bacitracin 0.5% ophthalmic ointment is also advised. Infants with documented gonococcal ophthalmia should be investigated for disseminated gonococcal infection with cultures of blood and possibly CSF. Disseminated infection is treated with IV or IM antibiotics for 10 to 14 days (see Sec. 3.6.1). Bear in mind, infants with gonococcal ophthalmia may also have a concurrent chlamydial infection or syphilis.

STAPHYLOCOCCUS AUREUS This bacterium is a common cause of conjunctivitis in all age groups. It is a gram-positive coccus that usually appears in clusters. *S. aureus* can cause acute, subacute,

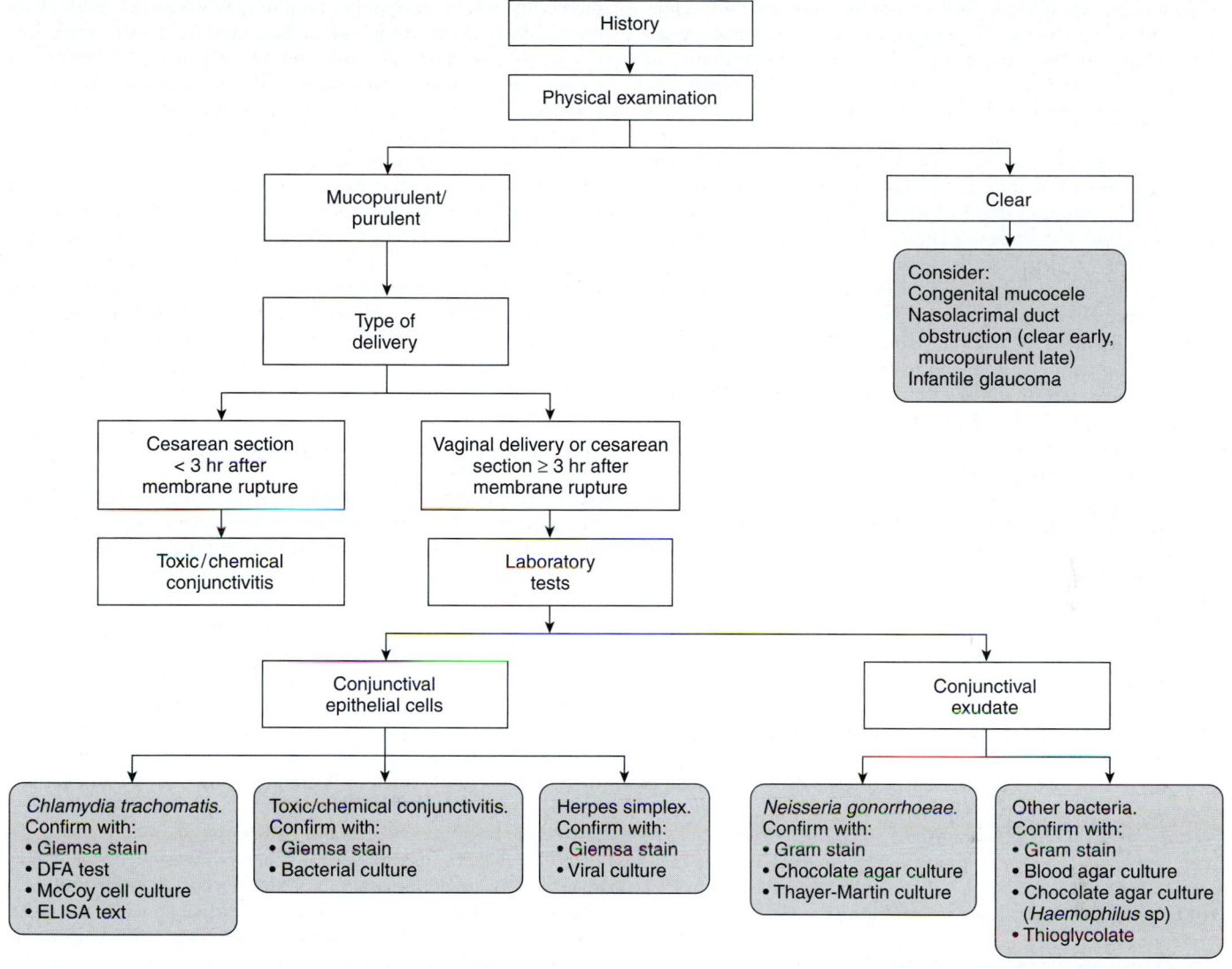

FIGURE 26-1   Algorithm diagramming the evaluation of conjunctival discharge in the neonatal. **DFA = direct fluorescent antibody staining; ELISA = enzyme immunoassay.**

chronic, and pseudomembranous conjunctivitis. It may also cause blepharitis, blepharoconjunctivitis, epithelial keratitis, marginal corneal infiltrates, ulcerative keratitis, cellulitis, and phlyctenulosis. Topical therapy of *S. aureus* conjunctival infections includes bacitracin and erythromycin ointment and sulfacetamide 10% drops. Fluoroquinolones should be avoided because of their tendency to induce resistance. If systemic therapy is indicated, a penicillinase-resistant penicillin, cephalosporin, or vancomycin should be used.

STAPHYLOCOCCUS EPIDERMIDIS   This bacterium is found among the normal skin flora. Occasionally it may cause blepharitis or blepharoconjunctivitis. It is the bacterium most often cultured from inside the eye in postoperative bacterial endophthalmitis. *S. epidermidis* conjunctivitis responds promptly to the same antibiotics used to treat *S. aureus* infection.

STREPTOCOCCUS PNEUMONIAE   Pneumococcus is a frequent cause of acute, mucopurulent conjunctivitis. The bacterium is often found in the upper respiratory tract of young, healthy children. Pneumococci are gram-positive lancet- or bullet-shaped diplococci

arranged with their flat ends facing each other. They contain a polysaccharide capsule that can be seen in an India-ink preparation. The organism produces conjunctivitis by direct invasion of the conjunctiva, often associated with hemorrhage. Other conditions caused by pneumococcus include dacryocystitis, ulcerative keratitis, and (after a trabeculectomy for management of glaucoma) endophthalmitis. Treatment is with topical erythromycin or bacitracin.

HAEMOPHILUS INFLUENZAE   This bacterium has been a frequent cause of conjunctivitis in children. It is now likely to be less of a problem with immunization against the organism. It produces a subacute, purulent or mucopurulent conjunctivitis, often occurring in winter and associated with upper respiratory tract infections. The organism appears as a small pleomorphic, gram-negative rod. Coccobacillary forms may also be seen. Untreated conjunctivitis may lead to preseptal cellulitis. Other clinical problems that may be caused by *H. influenzae* include dacryocystitis, marginal keratitis, and endophthalmitis (after a trabeculectomy for management of glaucoma). Treatment is with topical polymyxin B/trimethoprim or chloramphenicol 0.5%; topical aminoglycosides and fluoroquinolones should be reserved for infections that do not respond to initial therapy. Increasingly the organism is showing resistance to ampicillin. Thus a second- or third-generation cephalosporin is now being used when systemic therapy is needed.

STREPTOCOCCUS PYOGENES AND STREPTOCOCCUS VIRIDANS These organisms are an infrequent cause of bacterial conjunctivitis. They are often found in the flora of the normal upper respiratory tract. They cause a spectrum of clinical diseases including pharyngitis, impetigo, erysipelas, scarlet fever, and pneumonia. Other ocular conditions caused by streptococci include infectious crystalline keratitis, ulcerative keratitis, dacryocystitis, and endophthalmitis. Chemosis, conjunctival injection, purulent discharge, and possible membrane or pseudomembrane formation characterize streptococcal conjunctivitis. Treatment is with topical erythromycin, bacitracin, or chloramphenicol. When systemic treatment is indicated, penicillin is usually the drug of choice. Streptococci are not generally sensitive to aminoglycosides.

PSEUDOMONAS AERUGINOSA This organism rarely causes conjunctivitis. When it does, it is typically a chronic conjunctivitis; rarely, it produces an acute purulent conjunctivitis that may progress rapidly into an ulcerative keratitis with ocular perforation and panophthalmitis. Acute pseudomonas conjunctivitis is particularly serious in newborns, especially preterm infants. Keratitis, corneal ulceration, endophthalmitis, septicemia with ecthyma contagiosa, and even death may result. Epidemics have recurred in premature nurseries. Sources of organisms include benzalkonium chloride used to soak instruments, aerating filters in the sink faucets, and other infected infants. The bacterium is a slender gram-negative rod; however, treatment may change its morphology. Treatment is with topical gentamicin, tobramycin, amikacin, ofloxacin, ciprofloxacin, polymixin B/trimethoprim, or a third-generation cephalosporin. If response is poor, subconjunctival injections may be given twice daily until cultures are negative.

ACUTE PURULENT CONJUNCTIVITIS Acute purulent or mucopurulent conjunctivitis (epidemic "pinkeye") is a highly contagious infection caused by a pathogenic staphylococcus, pneumococcus, *H. influenzae,* Koch-Weeks bacillus (*H. aegyptius, H. conjunctivitidis*), or streptococcus. Viral diseases such as measles, German measles, and mumps can also cause acute purulent conjunctivitis. The conjunctiva is intensely injected, especially in the tarsal portion and fornices, and the tarsal conjunctiva shows a papillary reaction that gives it a velvety appearance. Petechial hemorrhages of the superior conjunctiva are most common with pneumococcal and Koch-Weeks bacillus infections. Treatment consists of the topical sulfacetamide or erythromycin four times a day and precautions to avoid the spread to other sites or other family members.

PARINAUD OCULOGLANDULAR SYNDROME This is a unilateral follicular conjunctivitis with one or more granulomas involving the tarsus, cul-de-sac, or palpebral conjunctiva, associated with marked preauricular and cervical lymphadenopathy, malaise, and fever. Most instances are of zoonotic origin, and many are associated with exposure to cats (*cat-scratch fever*—the most common etiology) and leptotrichosis. The conjunctiva often is the portal of entry of the infectious agent, and the granuloma is the site of incubation. The infectious microorganisms of the following diseases may cause the syndrome: tularemia, tuberculosis, chancroid, glanders, pasteurellosis, listeriosis, syphilis, lymphogranuloma venereum, coccidioidomycosis, sporotrichosis, actinomycosis, blastomycosis, leprosy, infectious mononucleosis, mumps, rickettsia, Mediterranean spotted fever, sarcoid, and even an infected chalazion. Diagnosis is confirmed by conjunctival biopsy that reveals typical granulomas. The causative organism may be recovered from the conjunctival lesion or seen in histologic sections. The organism isolated on culture from nodes in cat-scratch disease is *Bartonella henselae.* In other instances, serologic studies showing a rise in paired sera or the response to a skin test (cat-scratch fever) may be diagnostic. Recovery usually occurs spontaneously after several months. Pharmacologic therapy should be directed at the specific etiologic agent whenever possible. In patients with cat-scratch disease, treatment with systemic tetracycline in patients over 8 years of age seems to interrupt and shorten the course of the disease in some patients; excision of the conjunctival lesion may hasten recovery.

CHLAMYDIAL CONJUNCTIVITIS

Chlamydial conjunctivitis, also known as *inclusion blennorrhea,* is the most common infectious cause of neonatal conjunctivitis in many series. The incubation period varies from 5 to 15 days. Although silver nitrate initially was perceived to be ineffective against chlamydia, it has been found that chlamydial conjunctivitis in newly born infants is more frequent following erythromycin prophylaxis than silver nitrate. Clinically, lids and conjunctiva swell, and the infection produces a mucopurulent or purulent papillary conjunctivitis, occasionally with pseudomembrane formation, usually in one eye. Unlike infection in adults, follicles do not occur because lymphoid tissue does not develop until the infant is at least 3 months of age. Premature infants are particularly susceptible. Giemsa-stained conjunctival scrapings show polymorphonuclear leukocytes and basophilic granular intracytoplasmic inclusions in epithelial cells. Inclusion bodies are seen more frequently in infants than adults. A rapid direct immunofluorescent antibody test and a polymerase chain reaction technique are available that can complement cytologic studies. *Chlamydia trachomatis* serotypes D through K are usually associated with genital infection and inclusion conjunctivitis. Sequelae are uncommon, but superior micropannus and mild flat conjunctival scarring are occasionally seen, especially when treatment is delayed. Because the risk of developing chlamydial pneumonia is significant, newborns with chlamydial conjunctivitis should be treated with both topical and systemic antibiotics: oral or intravenous erythromycin, 50 mg/kg/d in four divided doses for at least 2 weeks, and topical tetracycline 1% or erythromycin 0.5% eye ointment four times a day for 2 weeks. Both parents should be treated with erythromycin, 130 mg/kg/d for 3 weeks or doxycycline 100 mg twice per day for 1 week, to avoid reinfecting the baby.

Inclusion conjunctivitis of young children is similar to that of newborn infants, except that marked follicular hypertrophy of the lower eyelids is a prominent feature, and epithelial-cell inclusions are rarely seen in conjunctival scrapings. Preauricular lymphadenopathy, a scant mucopurulent discharge, and corneal involvement with superficial epithelial keratitis and subepithelial infiltrates can occur. The acute inflammatory stage usually lasts several weeks; without treatment it may progress to a chronic keratoconjunctivitis lasting a year or more. Conjunctival scarring does not usually occur in children, but corneal pannus may develop. Associated clinical problems include nongonococcal urethritis in males, chronic vaginitis in females, and Reiter syndrome. Inclusion blennorrhea in the older child and adult occurs by genital-to-eye or hand-to-eye contact and in swimming pools. The disease responds poorly to topical tetracycline, erythromycin, or sulfacetamide, but results are excellent with systemic tetracycline (1 to 1.5 g daily) or erythromycin (30 mg/kg/d) given for 3 to 6 weeks. Tetracycline and doxycycline are not given to children younger than 8 years of age or to pregnant women because of the risk of staining bones and teeth.

TRACHOMA Trachoma is the leading cause of infectious blindness in the world. It occurs sporadically in all parts of the United States but is endemic in certain localities, notably on American Indian reservations and in the Mexican-American population of California. In endemic, infected populations, trachoma usually starts in childhood and is associated with annual epidemics of bacterial conjunctivitis. The incubation period is 5 to 12 days. The disease is transmitted by flies, eye-to-eye, and from contaminated fingers and fomites. Cycles of infection-reinfection with *Chlamydia trachomatis* serotypes A, B, and C are responsible for the clinical findings. In acute or subacute infections there is conjunctival chemosis, hyperemia, papillary hypertrophy, a follicular reaction on the upper tarsal conjunctiva and superior limbus, a superficial epithelial keratitis of the superior cornea with associated pannus, *Herbert pits* (small depressions at the upper limbal border that are the sequelae of cicatrized limbal follicles), and a small, tender preauricular lymph node. Limbal follicles and Herbert pits in combination with pannus are pathognomonic of trachoma. Secondary bacterial infection is common and is the usual cause of severe corneal scarring with visual loss. Blepharoptosis, nasolacrimal duct obstruction, and dacryocystitis may develop. Occasionally, intracytoplasmic inclusion bodies can be found in epithelial scrapings; they are indistinguishable from those found in inclusion blennorrhea. Immunofluorescent chlamydial particles can be demonstrated in conjunctival scrapings using monoclonal antibodies.

The acute stage is followed by a period of low-grade inflammation lasting for years. During this time, linear or stellate scarring of the tarsal conjunctiva (cicatricial lines of von Arlt) occurs, with reduced tear production. The scarring may also lead to entropion of the upper lid, trichiasis, and secondary corneal ulceration and scarring. Treatment consists of full doses of oral tetracycline (in children older than 8 years) or erythromycin for 3 or preferably 4 weeks. Topical tetracycline 1% or erythromycin 0.5% is not necessary for patients receiving full oral therapeutic doses of antibiotics, but local therapy often is prescribed for additional relief and prevention of bilateral infection. Topical therapy alone is not advisable because the effect is slow or partial and the infection usually is not limited to the eye.

NONINFECTIOUS CONJUNCTIVITIS

LOCAL DRUG SENSITIVITY Drug sensitivity can produce a reaction in the conjunctiva similar to that of atopic conjunctivitis. In addition, as the drug spills onto the eyelids with each instillation, the skin of the lids manifests a contact dermatitis with intense hyperemia and eczematoid changes. Sensitivity to drugs usually occurs after repeated instillation. Once developed, this sensitivity lasts indefinitely and often is associated with cutaneous sensitivity to the drug (positive patch test). Many drugs can cause allergic reactions that involve the conjunctiva and eyelids. Although atropine and neomycin are often quoted as examples, other topical agents include the anti-infectives: bacitracin, chloramphenicol, erythromycin, gentamicin, polymyxin B, sulfacetamide, trifluridine, and idox-

uridine; glaucoma drugs: timolol, pilocarpine, and echothiophate; local anesthetics: lidocaine, tetracaine, and proparacaine; cycloplegics: scopolamine and homatropine; and the preservatives: benzalkonium, thimerosal, and parabens. Treatment consists of removing the offending agent and local use of corticosteroids for symptomatic relief. Occasionally, however, even corticosteroids may cause or perpetuate local eye sensitivity when used to treat the primary allergic reaction.

PHLYCTENULAR CONJUNCTIVITIS Phlyctenular conjunctivitis is characterized by one or more small, hard, red, elevated nodules surrounded by hyperemic vessels, usually appearing at the limbus or on the bulbar conjunctiva temporally. Microscopically the *phlyctenule* is a subepithelial infiltrate of lymphocytes. The apex of the phlyctenule turns gray and ulcerates with healing in 10 to 12 days. On occasion the disease spreads onto the adjacent cornea, leading to opacification and pannus formation. Corneal involvement is associated with severe photophobia, profuse lacrimation, and blepharospasm. The disease is the result of type 4 hypersensitivity to foreign protein. The most common source of microbial antigen is staphylococcus, and this is typically seen in the setting of chronic staphylococcal blepharitis. In the past, the most frequent cause of phlyctenulosis in the United States was the antigen of *Mycobacterium tuberculosis*. Other associations with phlyctenulosis include coccidioidomycosis, chlamydial infection including lymphogranuloma venereum, *H. aegyptius* infection, and candidiasis. Contributing factors are malnutrition, poor hygiene, and debilitation from systemic disease. Treatment should be directed at improving diet and personal hygiene and addressing any underlying systemic disease. A topical steroid or antibiotic-steroid combination is effective in treating the disease and any secondary infection, particularly staphylococcal meibomitis, that may be present. Cycloplegics are indicated to relieve photophobia when corneal disease is present.

XEROPHTHALMIA Systemic malnutrition with *hypovitaminosis A* produces a lackluster, dry appearance of the conjunctiva and cornea. Xerosis is associated with the loss of mucus production by goblet cells. Little vascular reaction is seen. Epithelial defects and secondary infection may occur. As the condition progresses the dry areas become whiter (Bitot spots) and appear as foamy patches, usually on the temporal conjunctiva next to the limbus. The end stage is keratomalacia with necrosis and infection that leads to poor vision or loss of the eye. Night blindness (nyctalopia) also occurs with vitamin A deficiency. Hypovitaminosis A is usually seen in poverty-stricken parts of the world, but may occur in malabsorption syndromes such as celiac disease, cystic fibrosis, intestinal resection, biliary disease, or severe inflammatory bowel disease. In vitamin A–deficient children, measles may result in severe corneal disease. Treatment consists of a nutritious diet and large doses of vitamin A: 10,000 to 20,000 IU by mouth daily for 1 to 2 weeks in young children and 25,000 to 50,000 IU daily in older children. In very severe disorders, vitamin A may be injected intramuscularly in daily doses of up to 25,000 IU for several days. Corneal ulcers should be cultured to rule out secondary bacterial infection. Topical broad-spectrum antibiotic ointment may be applied several times daily as prophylaxis until healing is complete. Xerophthalmia may also occur in association with Sjögren syndrome.

FOLLICULOSIS Benign folliculosis is quite common in children and must be differentiated from chronic follicular conjunctivitis. In general, the conjunctiva of a child is considerably more reactive than that of an adult. Folliculosis may represent part of a generalized lymphoid hyperplasia or may occur secondary to a localized condition such as chronic dacryocystitis. Folliculosis is usually not accompanied by discharge or erythema and is asymptomatic. It disappears as the child grows or when the primary cause, if any, is removed.

CONJUNCTIVITIS ASSOCIATED WITH MUCOCUTANEOUS DISEASES

Some of the mucocutaneous ocular diseases such as *Stevens-Johnson syndrome* (*erythema multiforme major*), *toxic epidermal necrolysis, bullous pemphigoid, ocular cicatricial pemphigoid, graft-versus-host disease,* and *Reiter syndrome* produce a mild to severe keratoconjunctivitis with serious ocular sequelae including loss of vision. In Stevens-Johnson syndrome and cicatricial pemphigoid, severe dry eye, symblepharon formation, corneal ulceration, and corneal perforation can occur. Scleritis, interstitial keratitis, and hypopyon uveitis may complicate the course of Reiter disease. *Kawasaki syndrome,* also known as the *mucocutaneous lymph node syndrome,* is associated with bilateral conjunctival injection and coronary artery aneurysm formation (see Sec. 12.6.2). Because of the serious ocular and systemic complications of these mucocutaneous syndromes, it is advisable to have an ophthalmologist involved in the treatment of patients with these diseases.

26.6.3 Subconjunctival Hemorrhage

Subconjunctival bleeding from a capillary of the bulbar conjunctiva may occur with mild trauma, Valsalva maneuver (coughing, sneezing, vomiting), acute conjunctivitis, acute septicemia, malaria, scurvy, blood dyscrasias, and purpuric diseases; or bleeding may be spontaneous (idiopathic). In most instances there are no associated systemic problems; laboratory evaluation is indicated only if the hemorrhages are recurrent and there are systemic manifestations of a bleeding disorder. The appearance of subconjunctival hemorrhage can be alarming to the parents, but by itself it is of no consequence. It can, however, signify more serious intraocular damage from trauma that the child is suppressing. Subconjunctival blood usually absorbs completely in 1 to 2 weeks.

26.6.4 Epibulbar Tumors

NEVUS Conjunctival nevi are the most common epibulbar tumors of childhood. They may be evident at birth but frequently acquire increased pigment and first become noticeable at puberty. They usually occur at the limbus in the bulbar conjunctiva as well-circumscribed multicystic lesions of varying size and pigmentation. Ninety percent are compound nevi. Because they have virtually no malignant potential in childhood, surgical excision is done only for cosmetic purposes. On rare occasions, conjunctival nevi develop into a malignant melanoma. If lesions enlarge, they have been treated by alcohol keratectomy, local excision, and supplemental cryotherapy.

LIMBAL DERMOID Both this lesion and conjunctival dermolipoma present as smooth, rounded, cream-colored choristomas that are usually evident at birth and may increase in size with time. These lesions typically contain adipose tissue and dermal elements such as hair follicles and sebaceous glands. Approximately 30% of patients

with these tumors have associated ocular (lid coloboma, microphthalmos, aniridia) and systemic (Goldenhar syndrome) anomalies. *Goldenhar syndrome* (*oculoauriculovertebral dysplasia*) is a sporadic or autosomal-dominant syndrome of the first branchial arch comprising the triad of epibulbar dermoids, ear anomalies (preauricular skin tags and aural fistulae), and vertebral anomalies. Conjunctival dermoids usually are found at the inferotemporal limbus; occasionally they appear over the central part of the cornea. The lesion is treated surgically if the growth is enlarging, is cosmetically disfiguring, or interferes with vision.

PAPILLOMA Conjunctival papillomas caused by the human papilloma virus are common in children. They may be single or multiple, pedunculated or sessile, and may be found anywhere on the conjunctiva. Incomplete excision or ablation may lead to multiple recurrences. Nonviral neoplastic papillomas are sessile and occur in older adults. Episcleral osseous choristoma is an uncommon malformation consisting of a solitary nodule of bone surrounded by fibrous tissue on the sclera beneath the conjunctiva, usually in the superotemporal quadrant. This lesion can simply be observed if asymptomatic or excised if symptomatic.

Systemic diseases may be associated with conjunctival nodules or infiltrates. The diseases include sarcoidosis, leukemia, and juvenile xanthogranuloma. Biopsies of conjunctival nodules and infiltrates can be useful in diagnosing systemic diseases. A conjunctival mass occurs in 7% of patients with orbital rhabdomyosarcoma.

26.6.5 Conjunctival Degenerations

PINGUECULA AND PTERYGIUM Pinguecula and pterygium are degenerative diseases of the conjunctiva that are most often encountered in adults. They appear as yellow plaques or fleshy lesions on either side of the cornea, most often on the nasal side in the area of the palpebral fissure. The lesions consist of hyaline and yellow elastic tissue and seem to be related to exposure to ultraviolet light, drying and windy environments, notably in persons who spend a great deal of time outdoors. Surgical removal is performed if the lesions are enlarging and encroaching on the cornea or are cosmetically disturbing.

References

Holland GN: Infectious diseases. In: Isenberg SJ, ed: The Eye in Infancy, 2nd ed. St. Louis, Mosby, 1994

Isenberg SJ, Apt L, Wood M: A controlled trial of povidone-iodine as prophylaxis against ophthalmia neonatorum. N Engl J Med 332: 562–566, 1995

Mannis MJ, Macsai MS, Huntley AC, eds: Eye and Skin Disease. Philadelphia, Lippincott-Raven, 1996

Mannis MJ, Plotnick RD: Bacterial conjunctivitis. In: Duane TD, Jaeger EA, eds: Clinical Ophthalmology. Philadelphia, Lippincott Williams & Wilkins, 1998

Pepose JS, Holland GN, Wilhelmus KR, eds: Ocular Infection and Immunity. St. Louis, Mosby, 1996

Snyder RW, Glasser DB: Antibiotic therapy for ocular infection. West J Med 161:579, 1994

Stock EL, Meisler DM: Vernal keratoconjunctivitis. In: Duane TD, Jaeger EA, eds: Clinical Ophthalmology. Philadelphia, Lippincott-Raven, 1995

Tabbara KF, Hyndiuk RA, eds: Infections of the Eye, 2nd ed. Boston, Little, Brown, 1996

26.7   CORNEA

26.7.1   Congenital Anomalies

Most, but not all, congenital anomalies of the cornea are associated with defects in transparency. Congenital and infantile corneal opacification require thorough pediatric evaluation because of the high frequency of associated systemic abnormalities. The causes of neonatal and early infantile corneal opacities are listed in Table 26-5 and discussed in Sec. 26.7.4.

ABNORMALITIES OF CORNEAL SIZE AND SHAPE

Abnormalities of corneal size and shape require investigation for unusual refractive errors and other ocular defects. *Microcornea* is the term applied when the corneal diameter is less than 10 mm in the neonate, depending on gestational age, and 11 mm in the older infant and child. *Megalocornea* is the term applied when the corneal diameter is greater than 13 mm and its size is not a result of glaucoma.

MICROCORNEA   This may occur in an otherwise normal eye, and then there is usually a marked hyperopic refractive error because corneal curvature is flat; if the cornea is steep, myopia results. If the entire eye is small but otherwise normal, the term *nanophthalmos*

applies. If the entire eye is small and malformed, the term *microphthalmos* is used. A-scan ultrasonography can help distinguish isolated microcornea from microphthalmos. Microcornea is inherited as either an autosomal dominant or recessive trait or can appear sporadically; an X-linked form found with congenital cataracts is seen in the Nance-Horan syndrome. Microcornea may be found with anterior chamber abnormalities such as anterior chamber dysgenesis. Crowding of the entire anterior segment may lead to angle-closure glaucoma. Systemic associations include Ehlers-Danlos and Weill-Marchesani syndromes, craniofacial abnormalities, chromosomal defects, congenital rubella, and fetal alcohol syndrome. Treatment varies according to the associated abnormalities. Early refraction is indicated in each instance, however, and may prevent amblyopia. Other common problems include congenital cataract, microphakia, colobomas, and small eyelids and orbits.

MEGALOCORNEA   This is a nonprogressive, large, clear cornea associated with a high astigmatic error. If the entire anterior segment, including the lens and ciliary body, is enlarged, the term *megalophthalmos* is used. Lens opacities, anterior subluxation of the lens, and secondary glaucoma may occur in megalocornea. All modes of inheritance occur, but X-linked recessive transmission is the most common. The condition is bilateral. Enlargement of the cornea in congenital glaucoma (*buphthalmos*) should be differentiated easily. Megalocornea is associated with Lowe syndrome, osteogensis imperfecta, craniosynostosis, Down syndrome, Alport syndrome, Marfan syndrome, and nonketotic hyperglycemia. Simple megalocornea is nonprogressive, and treatment is merely aimed at cor-

TABLE 26-5

DIFFERENTIAL DIAGNOSIS OF NEONATAL AND EARLY INFANTILE CORNEAL OPACITIES (STUMPED)

CATEGORY	DIAGNOSES	LATERALITY	NATURAL HISTORY	INHERITANCE
S—Sclerocornea		Unilateral or bilateral	Nonprogressive	Sporadic
T—Tears in Descemet's membrane	Blunt trauma (eg, forceps injury, battered child)	Unilateral	Spontaneous improvement	Sporadic
	Infantile glaucoma	Bilateral	Progressive unless treated	Autosomal recessive
U—Ulcers	Herpes simplex keratitis	Unilateral	Progressive	Sporadic
	Intrauterine or postpartum infection (eg, rubella, syphilis, gonococcus)	Unilateral or bilateral	Stable or progressive	Sporadic
	Neurotrophic keratopathy	Unilateral or bilateral	Progressive	Sporadic
	Familial dysautonomia	Bilateral	Progressive	Autosomal recessive
M—Metabolic	Mucopolysaccharidoses I-H, I-S, IV, VI, and VII	Bilateral	Progressive	Autosomal recessive
	Mucolipidoses II to IV	Bilateral	Progressive	Autosomal recessive
	Galactosialidosis	Bilateral	Progressive	Autosomal recessive
	Band keratopathy	Bilateral	Progressive	Sporadic
P—Posterior corneal defect	Peter anomaly	Unilateral or bilateral	Stable	Usually sporadic
	Posterior keratoconus	Unilateral	Stable	Sporadic
E—Endothelial dystrophy	Congenital hereditary endothelial dystrophy	Bilateral	Stable	Autosomal dominant or recessive
	Posterior polymorphous dystrophy	Bilateral	Slowly progressive	Autosomal dominant
	Congenital hereditary stromal dystrophy	Bilateral	Stable	Autosomal dominant
D—Dermoid		Unilateral or bilateral	Stable	Sporadic
Other	Chromosomal abnormalities (eg, trisomy 13, 18; 18q−)	Unilateral or bilateral	Stable, variable	Sporadic
	Norrie disease	Bilateral	Progressive	X-linked recessive
	Intraocular mass lesion	Unilateral	Progressive	Sporadic

recting the refractive error. Principles of treatment are the same as for microcornea.

ANTERIOR SEGMENT DYSGENESIS

This term refers to a spectrum of congenital malformations that involve the iris, iridocorneal angle, and the cornea. Etiology is unclear. The most peripheral edge of *Descemet's membrane* of the cornea ends at the upper edge of the trabecular meshwork in the anterior chamber angle and is called *Schwalbe's line* or *ring*. If the line is unusually thickened and displaced anteriorly, it is known as *posterior embryotoxon*. This prominent line is found in 15% of normal eyes, is benign, and is inherited as a dominant trait.

When a prominent Schwalbe's line is associated with large peripheral anterior synechiae from the iris, the malformation is known as *Axenfeld anomaly. Rieger anomaly* consists of Axenfeld anomaly plus iris thinning and abnormally shaped and displaced pupils. *Rieger syndrome* includes Rieger anomaly plus skeletal and dental abnormalities. Transmission for the Axenfeld and Rieger entities is autosomal dominant or sporadic. *Peter anomaly*, sometimes classified with these chamber anomalies, is characterized by a central corneal opacity, iris strands that extend from the iris collarette to the margin of the corneal opacity, and a lens that may be clear, cataractous, displaced anteriorly, or adherent to the corneal defect. Glaucoma is frequently associated with these abnormalities. Treatment involves management of the glaucoma and penetrating keratoplasty when the Peter anomaly is bilateral.

26.7.2 Keratitis

Inflammations of the cornea usually require prompt examination and treatment by an ophthalmologist. Even minor corneal injury or infection can lead to serious ocular complications, including blindness. The pediatrician must learn to recognize the signs and symptoms of corneal disease so that prompt referral can be made. Patients with keratitis usually have photophobia, tearing, blepharospasm, pain, decreased vision, circumlimbal hyperemia (ciliary injection), corneal opacification, and often a history of trauma. Treatment of corneal disease will not be detailed thoroughly in this section because treatment should be provided by an ophthalmologist.

SUPERFICIAL PUNCTATE KERATOPATHY Inflammation of the corneal epithelium may be a manifestation of systemic disease (familial dysautonomia, vitamin A deficiency) or local ocular disease (epidemic keratoconjunctivitis, herpes keratoconjunctivitis, Thygeson superficial punctate keratitis, superior limbic keratoconjunctivitis, staphylococcal blepharoconjunctivitis, ophthalmic medication toxicity, keratoconjunctivitis sicca, exposure keratopathy, neurotrophic cornea, trachoma, trichiasis, molluscum contagiosum infection of the eyelid margin). Fine, superficial, punctate epithelial opacities may be seen in the corneal epithelium or subepithelium. Punctate epithelial defects that stain with fluorescein are the unifying clinical finding in these conditions. Treatment is directed at the underlying cause.

VIRAL KERATITIS

Most viral keratitis can be diagnosed by clinical findings. Cytology and viral culture may be helpful in atypical or refractory instances. Direct immunofluorescence tests are available for adenovirus and herpes simplex virus.

EPIDEMIC KERATOCONJUNCTIVITIS (EKC) EKC is an acute, highly contagious disease of the conjunctiva and cornea that is usually caused by adenovirus types 8, 19, 27, and 37, although other serotypes may be responsible. Incubation period is 5 to 12 days. Epidemics occur by spread from contaminated fingers, tonometers, and eye solutions. There is rapid onset of a severe, acute, follicular conjunctivitis in one eye with tearing, photophobia, chemosis, petechial hemorrhages of the conjunctiva, and development of a large, tender, preauricular lymph node. The second eye usually becomes infected by spread from the first but is less severely involved. Corneal sensation is normal. Discharge is usually watery but may be mucopurulent. Exudates contain an abundance of mononuclear cells unless there is a pseudomembrane, when polymorphonuclear cells predominate. The conjunctivitis lasts 3 to 4 weeks. Five to 14 days after the onset an epithelial keratitis followed by round, subepithelial infiltrates may develop and persist for many months before healing with or without scarring. Infected children may demonstrate systemic signs including fever, sore throat, and diarrhea. Diagnosis is established by demonstrating a fourfold rise in neutralizing antibody titer or recovery of the virus from the conjunctiva. Direct and indirect immunofluorescence tests and an indirect immunoperoxidase test (immunoenzyme test) are available. Presently available antiviral drugs and topical antibacterial agents are ineffective. Supportive therapy in the form of vasoconstrictors, cold compresses, and analgesics may be helpful. Topical corticosteroids in low concentration (1/8% prednisolone) may be helpful in patients with severe keratoconjunctivitis, if herpes simplex conjunctivitis is excluded, but may delay final recovery. Because the disease is highly contagious up to 14 days after onset, frequent handwashing and infection control precautions should be undertaken.

HERPES SIMPLEX KERATOCONJUNCTIVITIS Primary herpes simplex infection is common in young children. Ninety percent of the adult population carry antibodies to the herpes virus. Keratitis due to the herpes simplex virus is the second most important corneal disease after corneal trauma leading to loss of vision in the United States. Its incidence and severity have increased with widespread use of local and systemic corticosteroids. There are two serologically and virologically distinct forms of the virus. Herpes simplex type 1 is the type most closely associated with eye infection; the type 2 virus is associated with genital infection and may occasionally cause eye infection. In primary herpes infection, clusters of vesicles on the face, eyelids, and mucous membranes precede the conjunctivitis, which is follicular, occasionally membranous, and self-limited, lasting 2 to 3 weeks. Preauricular lymphadenopathy is present. Conjunctival scrapings demonstrate mononuclear cells and giant multinucleated epithelial cells. Because epithelial keratitis can occur, patients should be seen by an ophthalmologist for treatment with vidarabine (Vira-A) ointment or trifluridine (Viroptic) solution; topical acyclovir ointment would be preferable but is unavailable in the United States. Broad-spectrum antibiotics may be used to prevent secondary bacterial infection. A cycloplegic drug such as atropine 1% is used if photophobia or eye pain is present. For infants or children who resist or are unable to use topical medication, oral antiviral drugs (acyclovir, valacyclovir, or famciclovir) can be used if kidney disease is not present. Antiviral agents are toxic to the corneal epithelium, and prolonged treatment may delay epithelial healing. Corticosteroids are contraindicated.

The hallmark of herpetic *epithelial keratitis* is the superficial dendritic or geographic ulcer (best demonstrated with fluorescein) associated with a decrease in corneal sensitivity. Epithelial dendrites may be seen in the setting of primary herpes infection of the skin and mucous membranes, in which case these dendrites are accompanied by cutaneous vesicles or a follicular conjunctivitis. They may also be seen in the setting of recurrent infection without conjunctivitis. Triggering events include fever, sunlight exposure, or lowered general resistance. With topical antiviral therapy, dendritic ulcers clear over the course of a week without leaving a corneal scar. When topical corticosteroids have been used erroneously, herpes simplex may affect the deeper layers of the cornea.

Herpetic *stromal keratitis* is a cell-mediated immune response to noninfectious herpes virus antigen, although virus may occasionally be cultured from chronic stromal keratitis. The hallmark of stromal keratitis is the finding of disciform stromal edema with corneal thickening, opacification, and striae in Descemet's membrane. Keratic precipitates and anterior uveitis can be present. Corneal sensitivity is reduced. The diagnosis is purely clinical but is often made in the setting of an antecedent history of dendritic keratitis. *Disciform keratitis* is not pathognomonic of herpes simplex; trauma, herpes varicella-zoster, vaccinia, mumps, and chemical injury may also cause it. Treatment is controversial, but restricted use of a topical corticosteroid in conjunction with the antiviral drug can be helpful.

Necrotizing interstitial keratitis may develop in eyes that have had recurrent attacks of dendritic epithelial keratitis. The cornea develops severe, necrotizing, stromal inflammation that lasts 2 to 12 months, often leading to stromal vascularization, opacification, thinning, and even perforation. Treatment is difficult and controversial. If the keratitis is progressive in spite of medical treatment, a conjunctival flap, tarsorrhaphy, or lamellar keratoplasty may be required. A topical cycloplegic drug such as atropine or scopolamine helps keep the eye comfortable.

As mentioned previously, newborns may develop *ophthalmia neonatorum* from herpes simplex type 2 acquired during vaginal delivery. Prophylactic topical antiviral therapy is recommended for all newborns born to mothers with active genital herpes infection.

HERPES ZOSTER KERATOCONJUNCTIVITIS The herpes varicella-zoster virus may infect sensory nerve ganglia during varicella (chickenpox) infection. Reactivation of latent virus in the distribution of the ophthalmic division of the fifth cranial (trigeminal) nerve is termed *herpes zoster ophthalmicus* if it involves the eye. A vesicular, dermatomal eruption (*shingles*) is accompanied or followed by the development of conjunctival hyperemia, superficial dendritic or geographic corneal ulcers similar to those seen in herpes simplex, subepithelial infiltrates, and/or disciform keratitis. The skin of the tip of the nose and the eye are often simultaneously involved, because the nasociliary nerve innervates both sites (positive Hutchinson sign). Corneal involvement usually begins as a coarse superficial punctate keratitis and, in severe lesions, may terminate in a large nummular stromal opacity. Corneal sensation is reduced or absent; neurotrophic keratitis may ensue. Iritis always accompanies the keratitis, but it can occur alone. Iritis can be severe, with development of hypopyon, glaucoma, and hyphema. Herpes zoster in children should raise suspicion of underlying lymphoma, leukemia, or acquired immunodeficiency. Topical antiviral drugs generally are ineffective. Oral valacyclovir (Valtrex), famiciclovir (famovir), or acyclovir within 3 days of the appearance of cutaneous signs speeds resolution and reduces the incidence of complications, but the drugs may have no effect on the subsequent development of postherpetic neuralgia. Topical ophthalmic acyclovir is not available commercially in the United States. Although their efficacy has not been proved by clinical trials, systemic corticosteroids have been recommended to reduce the risk of posther-

petic neuralgia. Corticosteroids should be avoided or used with extreme caution in immunosuppressed patients for fear of dissemination of the disease. Cycloplegia and topical corticosteroid drops are used, if necessary, to treat iritis and stromal keratitis.

BACTERIAL KERATITIS

CENTRAL CORNEAL INFILTRATES AND ULCERS These are serious ocular emergencies that require immediate intensive therapy. A *corneal ulcer* is a defect in the corneal epithelium and stroma that is associated with an intense suppurative reaction (*corneal infiltrate*) that gives the ulcer a white appearance. The release of proteolytic enzymes from white blood cells or the invading organism causes destruction of corneal tissue. With improper or inadequate treatment, corneal ulcers can expand rapidly to involve the deep stroma and may lead to perforation of the globe and endophthalmitis. A sterile hypopyon is often seen. There is some variation in the types of organisms that produce bacterial corneal ulcers according to geographic location and climate, but the most commonly cultured pathogens are *S. aureus, S. epidermidis, S. pneumoniae, P. aeruginosa,* coliform bacteria (*Proteus, Serratia, Klebsiella, Escherichia coli*), *Moraxella liquefaciens,* and *H. influenzae.* Gram-positive organisms characteristically produce discrete, focal ulcers; gram-negative organisms characteristically produce large, diffuse, rapidly expanding, liquefactive, gray-white ulcers. *P. aeruginosa* is the most virulent of these organisms; it produces collagenases that facilitate a liquefactive necrosis that can rapidly progress to full-thickness corneal involvement in 24 hours. Predisposing factors for the development of corneal ulcers and infiltrates include trauma, contact lens wear, corticosteroid use, blepharoconjunctivitis, malnutrition, keratoconjunctivitis sicca, and immunosuppression. Broad-spectrum antimicrobial therapy with topical cefazolin (50 mg/mL) and tobramycin (14 mg/mL) or a fluoroquinolone should be instituted immediately and given hourly around the clock after smears and cultures of the ulcer are obtained. Subsequent treatment is tailored to the sensitivities demonstrated by the responsible organism(s). General anesthesia may be required in young children to examine the eyes, debride the necrotic cornea, and obtain smears and cultures of the ulcer.

MARGINAL CORNEAL INFILTRATES Marginal corneal infiltrates and ulcers are usually benign. They develop as a hypersensitivity reaction to bacterial infection, usually staphylococcal, of the conjunctiva or eyelid. Specific antibiotic treatment is directed to the underlying blepharoconjunctivitis. Topical corticosteroids may be added once the corneal epithelium is intact.

FUNGAL AND ACANTHAMOEBA KERATITIS

FUNGAL CORNEAL ULCERS These slowly growing ulcers have increased in incidence in recent years as a result of the widespread use of topical corticosteroids and broad-spectrum antibiotics. Fungi invade the cornea following epithelial trauma involving vegetable matter, often in agricultural settings. Numerous fungi, many of which are saprophytic, have been isolated from fungal corneal ulcers. The most common organisms are *Fusarium, Aspergillus,* and *Penicillium.* Yeast infections are more likely to occur in an immunocompromised host. Responsible organisms may not be detected in routine scrapings and culture, and may require corneal biopsy, but the diagnosis should be considered in any persistent, slowly progressive corneal ulceration that is not responding to antibacterial therapy. Fungal ulcers typically appear white and have feathery satellite lesions. Medical treatment consists of debridement and application of topical antifungal agents such as natamycin (Natacyn), amphotericin B, flucytosine, and miconazole.

ACANTHAMOEBA KERATITIS Acanthamoeba is a free-living protozoan that is found in soil, fresh water, seawater, and air; it is abundant in agricultural environments. It produces a chronic, slowly progressive, ulcerative keratitis with a ring infiltrate and severe pain that typically lasts for months. The pain is exaggerated by infiltrates that form around corneal nerves. Many instances of this disease are initially misdiagnosed as herpetic keratitis. The infection has been increasingly seen in patients who wear contact lenses, particularly when homemade saline solutions are used, or who have been exposed to contaminated hot tubs, plain tap water, or soil. The diagnosis is often established by corneal biopsy or after penetrating keratoplasty. Organisms can be identified with indirect immunofluorescent antibody staining or Calcofluor White. The organism can be grown on nonnutrient agar with *E. coli* serving as the nutrient for the protozoa. Treatment is started with intensive topical neomycin and propamidine (Brolene). If the keratitis does not improve, intravenous miconazole is given. Alternative drugs include oral ketoconazole and topical paromomycin. Cycloplegic drugs are used to decrease ocular discomfort. Penetrating keratoplasty may be performed, but the infection often recurs in the graft.

OTHER FORMS OF KERATITIS

INTERSTITIAL KERATITIS This is a nonsuppurative stromal keratitis with vascularization that occurs without prior or concurrent involvement of the corneal epithelium or endothelium. In children the most common cause is congenital syphilis. Other signs of congenital syphilis may be seen, such as "saddle nose," deafness, and Hutchinson notched teeth. Corneal changes appear between ages 5 and 15 years (rarely earlier) and consist of diffuse corneal edema followed by vascularization of the posterior two-thirds of the corneal stroma. The cornea assumes a ground-glass appearance with orange-red areas ("salmon patches") due to the vascularization. Subjective symptoms accompanying the keratitis are decreased vision, intense photophobia, lacrimation, and pain. Associated uveitis, chorioretinitis, and optic atrophy may also be seen. The keratitis regresses after several months, leaving deep stromal scarring and ghost vessels. *Treponema pallidum* organisms are not found in the cornea during the acute stage, although they may be recovered subsequently from the anterior chamber. Interstitial keratitis may represent an allergic response to the organism. Both narrow-angle and the chronic open-angle forms of glaucoma can occur in later years. Antisyphilitic medication has little effect on the course of the disease. Topical corticosteroids and cycloplegics provide symptomatic relief. In eyes with severe corneal scarring, penetrating keratoplasty can be performed after the inflammation has been quiescent for a number of years. Systemic treatment is directed at the underlying cause. Other conditions associated with interstitial keratitis include acquired syphilis, tuberculosis, *Cogan syndrome* (vertigo, tinnitus, hearing loss, interstitial keratitis), leprosy, parasites (onchocerciasis, malaria), mumps, influenza, lymphogranuloma venereum, herpes simplex, herpes varicella-zoster, and Lyme disease.

26.7.3 Corneal Dystrophies

Corneal dystrophies are inherited, bilateral, avascular corneal disorders that disturb corneal clarity. They may be congenital or may manifest later in life. Although corneal dystrophies may begin in childhood, most are first seen in the adolescent years or later. Many of the corneal dystrophies can be detected by gross inspection of the eyes; others are evident only by careful slit-lamp biomicroscopic examination. Most corneal dystrophies are inherited in an autosomal-dominant manner; macular dystrophy, the notable exception, is inherited in an autosomal-recessive manner. Corneal dystrophies are most often classified according to the region of the cornea that they most severely affect. Lamellar or penetrating keratoplasty is performed when vision is impaired. Recurrence in the donor corneal graft is common. If the pediatrician suspects the presence of a corneal dystrophy, the patient should be referred to an ophthalmologist. Discussion in this section will be limited to selected corneal dystrophies first seen in childhood.

ANTERIOR CORNEAL DYSTROPHIES

MEESMANN DYSTROPHY Also known as *hereditary juvenile epithelial dystrophy,* this is a rare, autosomal dominant, bilateral, epithelial dystrophy that appears early in childhood. Epithelial changes have been demonstrated as early as 7 months of age and tend to increase with age. Slit-lamp biomicroscopy reveals numerous, punctate, epithelial vesicles that are best seen in retroillumination. Histopathologic findings include a thickened epithelium and a thickened multilayered basement membrane that has numerous projections into the basal epithelium. Symptoms include mild irritation and a slight reduction in visual acuity. Most patients require no treatment. If discomfort is severe, soft contact lenses can be helpful. Excimer laser phototherapeutic keratectomy is useful if vision is severally impaired.

REIS-BÜCKLER DYSTROPHY This is an autosomal-dominant anterior corneal dystrophy that appears at about 5 years of age with symptoms of recurrent erosion. It has been linked to the same region of chromosome 5q31 as granular, lattice, and Avellino (granular-lattice) dystrophies. A mutation occurs in the gene responsible for the formation of keratoepithelin, but the exact material that accumulates is unknown. The disease is progressive. Opacification of Bowman's layer occurs gradually and the epithelium becomes irregular. Vision and corneal sensitivity may be markedly reduced. Treatment early with soft contact lenses or corneal scraping may help symptoms, but phototherapeutic keratectomy or lamellar keratoplasty may be necessary in severe disease.

STROMAL CORNEAL DYSTROPHIES

GRANULAR AND AVELLINO DYSTROPHY *Granular dystrophy* is an autosomal dominant, slowly progressive corneal dystrophy that is characterized by discrete, focal, granular opacities of the anterior stroma separated by intervening clear spaces. The corneal periphery is uninvolved. The lesions begin developing within the first decade of life, but visual acuity is not appreciably affected until the mid-adult years. Histopathologically, the granular opacities are hyaline material and stain brightly with Masson trichrome stain. Corneal transplant is not needed except in very severe and late cases.

MACULAR DYSTROPHY This is an autosomal recessive, slowly progressive corneal dystrophy that involves the corneal periphery. Corneas are clear at birth but begin to cloud in the first decade of life. Lesions begin as focal, gray-white, anterior stromal opacities that progress toward the periphery and later involve the deeper stromal layers. Fully developed lesions have indistinct borders, and the stroma between lesions is diffusely cloudy. Two clinical types are described, both of which link to chromosome 16q22. Episodic irritation and photophobia may occur from recurrent corneal erosions. Histologically, the opacities are depositions of acid mucopolysaccharide (glycosaminoglycan and proteoglycan). Penetrating keratoplasty is performed if vision is severely affected.

LATTICE DYSTROPHY　This is an autosomal dominant, slowly progressive corneal dystrophy characterized by branching, refractile "lattice" lines in the anterior stroma that are best seen in retroillumination on slit-lamp biomicroscopy. The lines do not go all the way to the limbus. Although appearing as early as 2 years of age, the occurrence of recurrent erosions and progressive clouding of the central cornea is apparent by age 20. Histopathologic examination of the anterior stroma demonstrates deposits of amyloid in the collagen fibers.

Treatment of symptomatic patients with lattice dystrophy is with contact lenses, phototherapeutic keratectomy, lamellar keratoplasty, or penetrating keratoplasty.

POSTERIOR CORNEAL DYSTROPHIES

POSTERIOR POLYMORPHOUS DYSTROPHY (PPMD)　This is a slowly progressive, autosomal-dominant corneal dystrophy with variable expression. It has been mapped to chromosome 20q11. Slit-lamp biomicroscopy of the posterior cornea demonstrates grouped vesicles, gray geographic lesions, broad bands with scalloped edges, and variable stromal edema. Histopathologically, the abnormal endothelial cells demonstrate microvilli and intercellular desmosomes, and the cells stain positively for keratin. The changes may be present in the first few years of life. The mild form is usually asymptomatic and nonprogressive. In the severe form, vesicular changes in the endothelium are serious enough to cause stromal edema and scarring. Keratoplasty is rarely required.

CONGENITAL HEREDITARY ENDOTHELIAL DYSTROPHY (CHED)　CHED may be a form of anterior segment dysgenesis in which neural crest cells differentiate to form abnormal endothelial cells. The disorder is characterized by bilateral corneal clouding that is present at birth or appears in the first year or two of life. Two clinical forms of the dystrophy are recognized. The more common type (CHED 2) is autosomal recessive, congenital, and stationary. The cornea is diffusely opaque (ground glass) from corneal edema, vision is poor, and nystagmus develops. The cornea is two to three times normal thickness, but corneal diameter is normal and guttata are absent. The tearing and photophobia that characterize congenital glaucoma are absent. The less common type (CHED 1) is autosomal dominant, slowly progressive, and appears in the first or second year of life. The cornea is two to three times normal thickness and demonstrates a hazy, blue-gray appearance that progresses to white, ground-glass opacification. Symptoms of this form of CHED include reduced vision, tearing, and photophobia. No corneal vascularization or decreased sensation is seen in either form. Both forms map to chromosome 20p11.2-q11.2. Penetrating keratoplasty has been reported to be successful in some patients. Early surgery therefore may be helpful.

ECTATIC CORNEAL DYSTROPHIES

KERATOCONUS　This is a bilateral, often asymmetric, corneal disorder characterized by progressive thinning or ectasia of the apical or inferior paracentral cornea. It usually appears at puberty. Most instances are sporadic, but hereditary forms are described. Studies utilizing corneal topography suggest a dominant pattern with incomplete penetrance in some families. The etiology is unknown and likely to be multifactorial, but eye rubbing is common and an association with atopic skin disease has been identified. In addition to atopic dermatitis, keratoconus has been associated with a number of disorders including retinitis pigmentosa, aniridia, vernal catarrh, cataract, optic atrophy, neurofibromatosis, and the Down, Marfan, Apert, and Ehlers-Danlos syndromes. The presenting symptom is poor vision, which is caused by high regular and irregular astigmatism. The primary physician may note on using the direct ophthalmoscope a dense, irregular, dark reflex in the center of the red reflex; the fundi cannot be seen clearly because of corneal distortion. On looking down, the patient's cone-shaped cornea may indent the lower lid (Munson sign). Slit-lamp examination in advanced lesions demonstrates a thin, cone-shaped apical cornea with variable scarring, stress lines in the anterior stroma (Vogt striae), and an iron line or ring (Fleischer ring). Forme fruste keratoconus can be detected by computerized corneal topography before it can be recognized with slit lamp. Spontaneous perforation of the cornea is rare, but Descemet's membrane may rupture causing acute *hydrops* (characterized by corneal edema, pain, and reduced vision). Visual rehabilitation is with spectacle lenses, rigid contact lenses, and penetrating keratoplasty.

KERATOGLOBUS　This condition is similar to keratoconus but shows a globular, rather than conical, ectasia of the cornea. The condition is bilateral and progressive but often asymmetric. Unlike keratoconus it usually is seen at birth. There is a strong association with blue sclera and Ehlers-Danlos syndrome type VI.

26.7.4　Metabolic Disorders with Corneal Changes

Corneal opacification may occur as a local manifestation of an inborn error of metabolism, or it may be the result of anterior segment dysgenesis, other developmental anomalies of the globe (microphthalmos, limbal dermoid), corneal dystrophy, intrauterine infection, acquired keratitis, glaucoma, or trauma (amniocentesis injury, forceps injury). Most of these conditions are discussed in detail elsewhere in this chapter.

The systemic *inborn errors of metabolism* that include corneal clouding as one of their clinical manifestations include the mucopolysaccharidoses, the sphingolipidoses, and the mucolipidoses. These conditions may also affect the retina and central nervous system. Conjunctival biopsy may be of value in the diagnosis of storage disorders even in the absence of corneal opacities.

DISORDERS OF CARBOHYDRATE METABOLISM— MUCOPOLYSACCHARIDOSES

Systemic mucopolysaccharidoses are rare, inherited lysosomal storage diseases that result from the absence of lysosomal acid hydrolases, the enzymes responsible for the catabolism of the glycosaminoglycans dermatan sulfate, heparan sulfate, and keratan sulfate. Severe corneal clouding is seen in the Hurler (MPS 1-H) and Sheie syndromes (MPS 1-S). Moderate corneal clouding is seen in the Morquio (MPS 4), Maroteaux-Lamy (MPS 6, phenotypes A and B), and Sly syndromes (MPS 7). Faint corneal clouding is seen in some patients with Hunter syndrome (MPS 2, phenotype B).

DISORDERS OF LIPID METABOLISM AND STORAGE

SPHINGOLIPIDOSES   These are rare inherited disorders of complex lipids (gangliosides and sphingomyelin), of which three involve the cornea (Fabry disease, multiple sulfatase deficiency, and generalized gangliosidosis type 1). Patients with X-linked Fabry disease (angiokeratoma corporis diffusum) develop characteristic corneal changes early in childhood that may be the first manifestation of the disease. Fabry disease is caused by a deficiency of alpha-galactosidase that leads to an accumulation of ceramide trihexoside. Lipid storage in the cornea takes the form of fine opacities in the epithelium that radiate out from the inferior central cornea in a whorl-like manner (cornea verticellata). The carrier state in women can be diagnosed on the basis of similar corneal changes. Cornea verticellata may also be seen in the superficial cornea of patients receiving long-term treatment with amiodarone, chloroquine, or indomethacin. Patients with multiple sulfatase deficiency demonstrate subtle, diffuse corneal opacities. These patients usually die in the first decade from central nervous system involvement. Histologically, corneal endothelial cells of patients with generalized gangliosidosis are distended and filled with single membrane-bound vacuoles. These findings may be subclinical, however.

MUCOLIPIDOSES   These autosomal-recessive conditions affect both carbohydrate and lipid metabolism, and consequently have features in common with both the mucopolysaccharidoses and sphingolipidoses. Corneal clouding is prominent in pseudo-Hurler syndrome (MLS 3), moderate in I-cell disease (MLS 2) and Berman syndrome (MLS 4), and faint or absent in the others.

DISORDERS OF AMINO ACID METABOLISM—CYSTINOSIS

Also known as *Fanconi syndrome,* this is a rare, autosomal-recessive metabolic disorder that has an infantile and an adult form. The infantile form is nephropathic and uniformly fatal without renal transplantation. In the adult form, life expectancy is normal. In the infantile form, crystals of cystine are deposited in the cornea, conjunctiva, sclera, extraocular muscles, uvea, and retina. The crystals in the cornea appear as needle-like glistening dots throughout the entire thickness of the cornea and are evident by 6 to 15 months of age. In the adult form the crystals are densest in the corneal periphery. Symptoms include photophobia and tearing. Conjunctival biopsy can confirm diagnosis. Cysteamine can reduce corneal crystal content, but crystals can recur in corneal transplants.

DISORDERS OF MINERAL METABOLISM

HEPATOLENTICULAR DEGENERATION   Also known as *Wilson disease,* this is an autosomal recessive disorder of copper metabolism linked to chromosome 13q14.3-q21.1. An associated Kayser-Fleischer ring of the cornea is pathognomonic and may be the first sign of the disease. It contains copper and appears as a greenish-golden annular opacity just inside the limbus at the level of Descemet's membrane. Visible initially only with slit-lamp magnification, it later becomes denser and broader and can be detected with the naked eye. Cataracts and retinal degeneration may coexist.

BAND KERATOPATHY   This is a superficial deposition of calcium in the cornea at the level of Bowman's layer that may occur secondary to other corneal disease (keratitis, alkali burns), other ocular disease (chronic uveitis associated with juvenile rheumatoid arthritis), or systemic diseases associated with increased serum calcium levels (hyperparathyroidism, milk-alkali syndrome, vitamin D intoxication, renal failure, hypophosphatemia, and sarcoidosis). Rarely, familial occurrence has been reported. Band keratopathy appears initially as a gray-white opacification of the superficial cornea nasal and temporal limbus and eventually extends across the cornea in a band-shaped configuration. Holes in the degenerated area are characteristic. Treatment consists of preliminary curettage of the epithelium, followed by the application of a chelating agent such as ethylenediaminetetraacetate sodium (EDTA). Improvement in vision can be dramatic, and the procedure can be repeated as necessary.

References

Arffa RC: Grayson's Diseases of the Cornea, 4th ed. St. Louis, Mosby, 1997

Chandler JW, Sugar J, Edelhauser HF, eds: External Diseases: Cornea, Conjunctiva, Sclera, Eyelids, Lacrimal System. St. Louis, Mosby, 1994

Kaufman HE, Barron BA, McDonald MB, eds: The Cornea, 2nd ed. Boston, Butterworth-Heinemann, 1997

Kenyon KR, Hersh PS, Starck T, Fogle JA: Corneal dysgeneses, dystrophies, and degenerations. In: Duane TD, Jaeger EA, eds: Clinical Ophthalmology. Philadelphia, Lippincott, 1992

Krachmer JH, Mannis MJ, Holland EJ, eds: Cornea. St. Louis, Mosby, 1997

Laibson PR, Rapuano CJ: Diseases of the cornea. In: Nelson LB, ed: Harley's Pediatric Ophthalmology, 4th ed. Philadelphia, Saunders, 1998

Leibowitz HM, Waring GO III, eds: Corneal Disorders: Clinical Diagnosis and Management, 2nd ed. Philadelphia, Saunders, 1998.

Mora ML, Smith RE: Corneal and systemic diseases. In: Duane TD, Jaeger EA, eds: Clinical Ophthalmology. Philadelphia, Lippincott Williams & Wilkins, 1998

Smolin G, Thoft RA, eds: The Cornea: Scientific Foundations and Clinical Practice, 3rd ed. Boston, Little, Brown, 1994

26.8   EPISCLERA AND SCLERA

26.8.1   Congenital Anomalies

BLUE SCLERA   The sclera of healthy young infants is relatively thin compared with that of adults and may have a bluish hue. It is particularly true as a normal finding in premature infants. By the end of the first year of life, however, the sclera of most infants turns porcelain white. The anomaly of blue sclera is secondary to persistent thinning and alteration in the structure of the sclera (mainly the collagen fibers), which allow the pigmented choroid to show through. Blue sclera occurs in high myopia and in systemic disorders affecting connective tissue such as osteogenesis imperfecta, Ehlers-Danlos syndrome, pseudoxanthoma elasticum, Marfan syndrome, Hallermann-Streiff syndrome, Crouzon disease, Albright hereditary osteodystrophy, pyknodysostosis, Turner syndrome, de Lange syndrome, and pseudohypoparathyroidism.

SCLERAL PIGMENTATION   The normal sclera is white with a variable number of pigmented spots depending on the racial pigmentation of the individual. Brown pigment may collect where vessels and nerves transit the sclera near the limbus, particularly in blacks, and be mistaken for a foreign body or melanoma. The yellowish appearance of the sclera in jaundice (icterus) is caused by bilirubin in the overlying conjunctiva. Only a minimal amount of bilirubin is found in the relatively avascular sclera. Carotenemia does not produce a yellow sclera or conjunctiva. A slate-gray sclera may be seen in ocular melanosis bulbi.

References

Foster CS, de la Maza MS: The Sclera. New York, Springer-Verlag, 1994
Watson P: Diseases of the sclera and episclera. In: Duane TD, Jaeger EA, eds: Clinical Ophthalmology. Philadelphia, Lippincott-Raven, 1995

26.9 IRIS, CILIARY BODY, AND CHOROID

26.9.1 Congenital Anomalies of the Uvea

The uvea consists of the iris, ciliary body, and choroid. This highly vascular layer of the eye is attached firmly to the sclera at the scleral spur, the exit sites of the vortex veins, and the optic nerve. These attachments explain the unique ophthalmoscopic appearance of choroidal effusion and suprachoroidal hemorrhage.

PERSISTENT PUPILLARY MEMBRANE Persistent pupillary membranes consist of fine pigmented strands of iris stroma that bridge the pupil, arising from the region of the iris collarette. They may be thick and distort the pupil, but rarely do they cause visual impairment unless they attach to the anterior lens capsule at the site of a congenital anterior polar cataract. These membranes result from incomplete involution of the anterior iris vascular arcades.

COLOBOMA Uveal colobomas may be seen in the iris, choroid, ciliary body, and optic nerve, or as microphthalmos with cyst. When the choroid is affected, the overlying retina and the underlying sclera are usually ectatic or missing. When the pars plicata of the ciliary body is involved, there may be a notch in the periphery of the lens corresponding to missing zonules. Congenital colobomas arise because of incomplete closure of the optic fissure during the fifth week of gestation. Typical colobomas are usually bilateral, although asymmetric, and may be inherited sporadically or as an autosomal dominant trait with incomplete penetrance and variable expressivity.

Autosomal recessive and sex-linked forms have also been described. Colobomas typically occur in the inferonasal quadrant of the eye. Those involving the pupil produce the so-called keyhole deformity. Colobomas involving the choroid and optic nerve may be associated with retinal detachment.

Uveal colobomas may cause no visual disturbance, for example, with isolated inferior iris colobomas or small choroidal defects inferior to the optic disc. However, they may cause profound visual impairment as seen when large chorioretinal colobomas involve the macula or optic nerve.

Colobomas usually occur as isolated defects but may occur in association with other ocular anomalies. Several systemic syndromes that include colobomas have also been described. Colo-

bomas may be seen in many chromosomal deletion and duplication syndromes (see Table 26-1). They are frequently, but not uniformly, present in the CHARGE (coloboma, *h*eart disease, *a*tresia choanae, *r*etarded growth and development, *g*enital hypoplasia, *e*ar anomalies and hearing loss), VATER (*v*ertebral anomalies and ventricular septal defect, *a*nal atresia, *t*racheo-esophageal fistula, *r*adial and renal dysplasia), and Goldenhar (oculoauriculovertebral) associations. They may also be seen in the Aicardi syndrome, Warburg syndrome, and Goltz focal dermal hypoplasia syndrome. See also Sec. 26.2.1.

ECTOPIA LENTIS ET PUPILLAE This autosomal-recessive disorder is characterized by corectopia and ectopia lentis, usually displaced in opposite directions. The disorder is bilateral but frequently asymmetric. The pupil is slit or oval-shaped. The lens may be minimally subluxated, pupil splitting, or luxated completely from the pupillary aperture. The iris dilates poorly. Associated ocular findings include high myopia, retinal detachment, corneal enlargement, glaucoma, cataract, and iris transillumination defects.

CONGENITAL ECTROPION UVEAE In this rare, unilateral neurocristopathy, hyperplastic iris pigment epithelium extends onto the anterior iris surface. The pupil may be enlarged or oval-shaped. Juvenile glaucoma is common. Congenital ectropion uveae is associated with neurofibromatosis, Rieger anomaly, and Prader-Willi syndrome.

ANIRIDIA The term *aniridia* is a misnomer because at least a small stump of iris tissue is almost always present. Two-thirds of cases are familial. There are at least two autosomal-dominant modes and one autosomal-recessive mode of inheritance. Poor vision, nystagmus, corneal pannus, cataracts, ectopia lentis, glaucoma, foveal hypoplasia, and optic nerve hypoplasia characterize the familial forms. The sporadic form accounts for one-third of all instances and is associated with cataract, glaucoma, macular hypoplasia, Wilms tumor, other genitourinary anomalies, and mental retardation. The glaucoma frequently develops before adolescence and is usually refractory to medical or surgical treatment. Long-term visual prognosis is poor. The sporadic *aniridia–Wilms tumor syndrome* (*Miller syndrome*) is associated with an interstitial deletion of chromosomal location 11p13. Expression of the sporadic form is more severe in males than in females. Patients with aniridia that do not clearly fall into an autosomal-dominant pedigree should have high-resolution chromosomal banding studies and biochemical assays for catalase and lactic dehydrogenase A. About 30% of patients with sporadic congenital aniridia develop a Wilms tumor before 3 years of age; the association is diagnosed before age 5 in 80% of cases. Conversely only 1.4% of patients with Wilms tumor have aniridia. Aniridia has not occurred in families with autosomal-dominant Wilms tumor. Radiologic examination or renal ultrasound should be performed on a semiannual basis for patients with sporadic aniridia to detect Wilms tumor at an early, treatable stage.

HETEROCHROMIA IRIDES A difference in the color of the two irides may be due to hypopigmentation or hyperpigmentation of the abnormal eye. When the lighter-colored eye is abnormal, Horner syndrome, Waardenburg syndrome, Fuchs heterochromia, or iris atrophy as in rubella embryopathy should be considered. A darker-colored abnormal iris can be due to siderosis, oculodermal melanocytosis, iris freckles or nevi, pigmented iris tumors, extensive rubeosis, or juvenile xanthogranuloma.

OCULAR AND OCULOCUTANEOUS ALBINISM Albinism is a group of genetic diseases characterized by congenital hypopigmentation of the skin, hair, and eyes (oculocutaneous albinism) or of the eyes only (ocular albinism). Symptoms include reduced visual acuity and photophobia. Signs include nystagmus, iris transillumination defects, and foveal hypoplasia. The fundus has a strikingly blond appearance due to the absence of retinal pigment epithelial and choroidal melanin; choroidal blood vessels are seen easily. Visual evoked response testing reveals a reduction in the proportion of nondecussated optic nerve fibers in the chiasm. The enzyme tyrosinase is defective.

OCULOCUTANEOUS ALBINISM (OCA) OCA has an autosomal-recessive mode of inheritance. Ten different types have been described on the basis of clinical findings and the hair bulb incubation test for tyrosinase activity. Autosomal-dominant OCA is rare. Tyrosinase-negative OCA is the most common type of albinism. Melanin production is absent on skin biopsy. Patients have white hair and skin, develop nystagmus within the first few months of life, and rarely develop visual acuity better than 20/200. Yellow mutant OCA is an allele of tyrosinase-negative OCA in which premelanosomes are demonstrable on skin biopsy. Skin and hair are white at birth but develop a yellow pigmentation with increasing age. Poor vision, nystagmus, and photophobia develop but are not as severe as in tyrosinase-negative OCA. Tyrosinase-positive OCA is the second most common form of albinism and is the type seen most commonly in blacks. Dense premelanosome and melanosome complexes are demonstrable on skin biopsy. Skin pigmentation is variable. Typical patients have yellow hair, mildly impaired visual acuity, some photophobia, and mild nystagmus.

OCULAR ALBINISM (OA) OA has X-linked recessive (Nettleship-Falls syndrome, Forsius-Eriksson syndrome, and an unnamed X-linked disorder with deafness) and autosomal-recessive inheritance modes. Affected males with X-linked recessive ocular albinism demonstrate macromelanosomes on skin biopsy. Skin pigmentation may be normal. Ocular examination demonstrates the changes typical of albinism. Visual acuity is poor, with marked photophobia and nystagmus. Female carriers demonstrate iris transillumination defects and a mosaic pattern of fundus hypopigmentation; vision, however, is normal. Patients with the autosomal recessive variety of OA have no melanosomes, and both sexes are affected equally.

CHÉDIAK-HIGASHI SYNDROME Eye findings in this syndrome include tyrosinase-positive OCA, nystagmus, foveal hypoplasia, decreased retinal vessels, papilledema; leukocytic infiltration of the uvea and optic nerve; and ocular motor palsies. Systemic findings include ataxia, polyneuropathy, anemia, thrombocytopenia, neutropenia, hepatosplenomegaly, lymphadenopathy, recurrent infections from reticuloendothelial incompetence, lymphoreticular malignancies in the second decade of life, large peroxidase-positive granules in circulating polymorphonuclear leukocytes, giant melanosomes in pigmented cells of the skin and eye, and early death.

HERMANSKY-PUDLAK SYNDROME This is the triad of tyrosinase-positive OCA, a bleeding diathesis with normal platelet counts, and an accumulation of abnormal ceroid material that causes interstitial pulmonary fibrosis, inflammatory bowel disease, renal failure, or cardiomyopathy in adulthood. Surgery and anticoagulant treatment are generally contraindicated in this syndrome because of the tendency for bleeding.

26.9.2   Uveitis

Inflammation of the uvea in children and adolescents accounts for 8% of all cases of uveitis but often goes undiagnosed, leading to permanent injury and blindness. Uveitis in children may be low grade and chronic with few of the classic symptoms of uveitis (pain, redness, photophobia, tearing). In fact, many children are referred to an ophthalmologist not because of the signs or symptoms of uveitis but because they develop amblyopia, band keratopathy, cataract, or glaucoma. If the pediatrician suspects uveitis, slit-lamp examination and indirect ophthalmoscopy by an ophthalmologist are essential. An approach to the child who complains of photophobia, one of the symptoms of uveitis, is outlined in Fig. 26-2.

Slit-lamp biomicroscopy may reveal conjunctival or limbal injection, keratic precipitates, corneal stromal edema, striae in Descemet's membrane, aqueous cell and flare, peripheral anterior synechiae, posterior synechiae, cataract, vitreous cells and opacities, and retinal vascular inflammatory changes. Inflammation of the uvea may be associated with inflammation of contiguous structures such as the cornea (keratouveitis), sclera (sclerouveitis), or lens (lens-induced uveitis).

The etiology of uveitis is seldom determined because of the morbidity associated with histopathologic confirmation. The oldest classification scheme involves differentiation of uveitis into granulomatous and nongranulomatous forms. Granulomatous inflammation is suspected when there are "mutton-fat" keratic precipitates or inflammatory iris nodules (Koeppe and Busacca nodules). Unfortunately, granulomatous diseases may have a nongranulomatous presentation. A more useful and clinically practical classification of uveitis emphasizes the site of involvement: anterior uveitis (*iritis, iridocyclitis*), intermediate uveitis (*peripheral uveitis, pars planitis, chronic cyclitis*), or posterior uveitis (*choroiditis, chorioretinitis*). Inflammation affecting one or more layers of the eye and an adjacent cavity is termed *endophthalmitis. Panophthalmitis* is the term reserved for suppurative reactions consisting of endophthalmitis with scleral and orbital inflammation.

ANTERIOR UVEITIS

OCULAR TRAUMA Ocular trauma is a frequent cause of acute anterior uveitis in the pediatric population. A careful search for associated ocular injuries (iridodialysis, rupture of the pupillary sphincter, ruptured globe, ectopia lentis, retinal detachment) should be performed (Sec. 26.16). Treatment involves administration of topical corticosteroids and cycloplegics and the wearing of protective spectacles or a Fox shield.

JUVENILE RHEUMATOID ARTHRITIS (JRA) JRA is the most common cause of anterior uveitis in children. It constitutes a group of diseases in which chronic nonsuppurative synovitis is associated with a spectrum of extraarticular manifestations including iridocyclitis. Five broad clinical subgroups are recognized. Iridocyclitis is associated most often with the two pauciarticular forms, although it may be seen rarely in the polyarticular form associated with a negative rheumatoid factor and in the systemic onset form (Still disease).

Chronic iridocyclitis develops in 20 to 40% of patients with the pauciarticular form with early onset (type 1). The disease is more common in young girls and is often associated with a positive ANA titer. Both eyes are usually affected, although possibly at different times and asymmetrically.

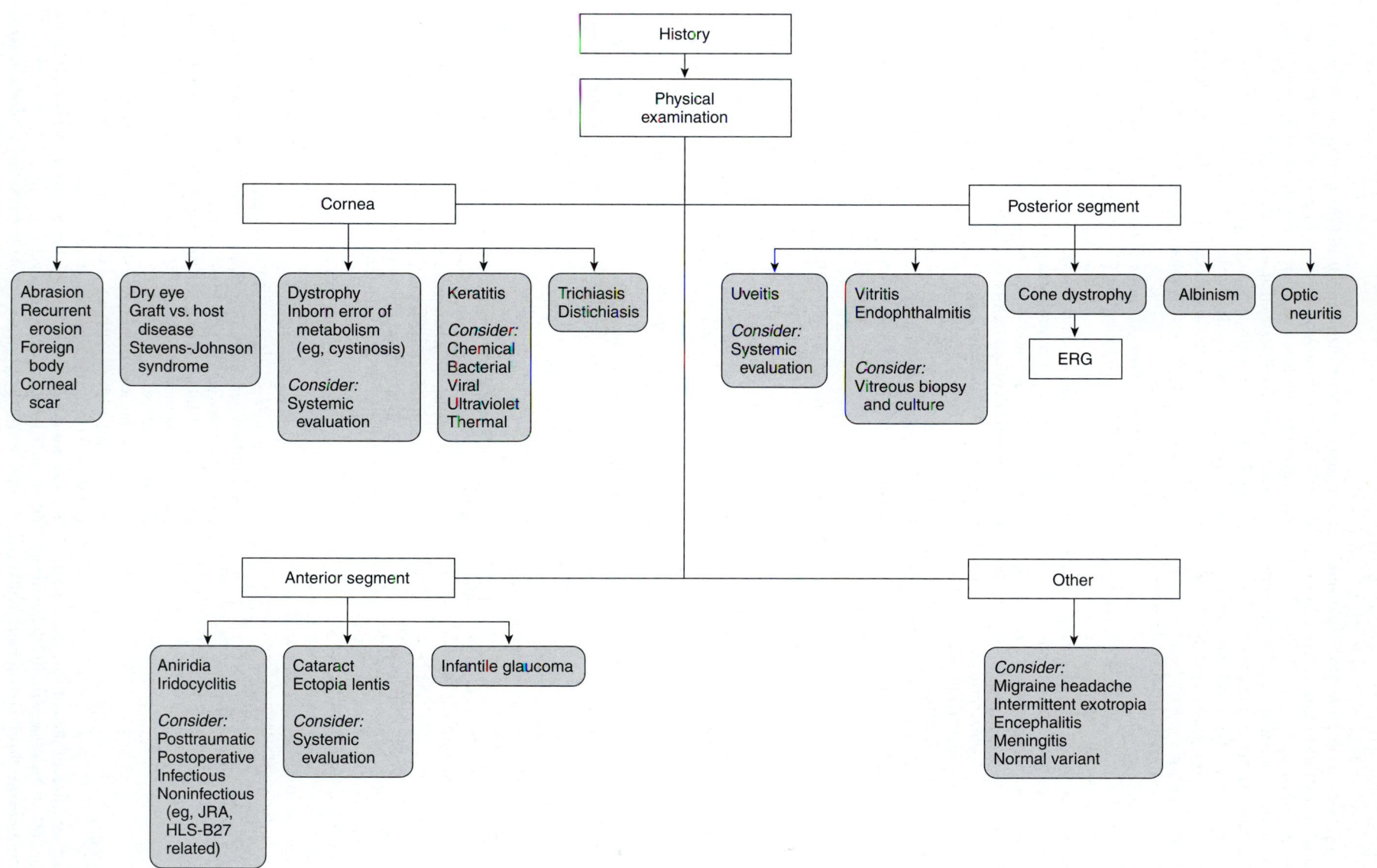

FIGURE 26-2 Algorithm diagramming the evaluation of photophobia. ERG = electroretinogram; JRA = juvenile rheumatoid arthritis.

Acute, recurrent iridocyclitis develops in 10 to 20% of patients with the pauciarticular form with late onset (type 2), typically occurring for the first time after 8 years of age.

The cardinal signs of the uveitis associated with JRA include calcific band keratopathy (Sec. 26.7.4), anterior chamber cells and flare, small to medium-size keratic precipitates with or without a fibrinoid reaction in the aqueous humor, posterior synechiae (often progressing to seclusion of the pupil), complicated cataract, secondary glaucoma, macular edema, and phthisis bulbi. These patients tend to do poorly after eye surgery.

The onset of the uveitis in JRA in most children is insidious, with the disease being discovered only when the child is noted to have heterochromia iridis (see Sec. 26.9.1), anisocoria (a difference in pupil size), dyscoria (abnormal pupil shape), or the onset of strabismus. There is no correlation between the onset of the arthritis and that of the uveitis, which may precede the arthritis by 3 to 10 years. Visual prognosis is said to be worse when the uveitis precedes the arthritis than when it follows. The only certain means of detecting iridocyclitis early is routine periodic slit-lamp examination. This should be performed initially in all patients with JRA, then every 3 months in patients with pauciarticular JRA, and every 6 months in polyarticular JRA until adulthood. Treatment consists of topical corticosteroids and mydriatic-cycloplegics and is effective in most patients. Periocular or systemic corticosteroids and even immunosuppressive drugs may be required, however, and incapacitating visual loss can develop despite intensive therapy (see Sec. 12.4).

Other less common causes of anterior uveitis in children are inflammatory bowel disease, sarcoidosis, syphilis, herpes simplex, and herpes zoster. *UGH syndrome* (*u*veitis, *g*laucoma, *h*yphema) may occur in older children or adults with iris clip or anterior chamber intraocular lenses.

INTERMEDIATE UVEITIS

Intermediate uveitis (*pars planitis, chronic cyclitis*) represents 25% of all pediatric uveitis. Sex distribution is equal. It is a chronic nongranulomatous inflammation of the ciliary body of unknown etiology that causes no symptoms except perhaps visual blur or an awareness of black floating spots. Medium to large cellular aggregates ("snow balls") settle by gravity on the pars plana of the ciliary body and form a solid white membrane ("snow bank") seen best on indirect ophthalmoscopy. With severe inflammation, vision may be reduced appreciably by the development of macular edema, posterior subcapsular cataract, optic neuritis, retinal vasculitis, or exudative retinal detachment. Intermediate uveitis may be associated with sarcoidosis, multiple sclerosis, Lyme disease, syphilis, toxocariasis, tuberculosis, and connective tissue disease. Idiopathic intermediate uveitis (pars planitis) is the most common form, accounting for 85 to 90% of patients with intermediate uveitis. Although it is frequently stationary, idiopathic intermediate uveitis may improve gradually over 5 to 10 years. Treatment with periocular or systemic corticosteroids is indicated if macular edema develops. If corticosteroids are ineffective, immunosuppressive drugs or cyclocryotherapy may be necessary.

POSTERIOR UVEITIS

Posterior uveitis refers to inflammation of the choroid and contiguous retina and accounts for 50% of all pediatric uveitis. Symptoms and signs include poor vision, vitreous floaters, scotomata, leukocoria, and strabismus. Eye pain and photophobia rarely develop. Clinical findings include vitreous cells and chorioretinal lesions.

Contiguous anterior chamber cell and flare are occasionally seen. Posterior uveitis cases are more likely to have an identifiable causative agent than anterior cases. The uveitis may be foveal or diffuse. Included among the diseases that are associated with posterior uveitis are AIDS, cysticercosis, cytomegalic inclusion disease, Eales disease, histoplasmosis, Lyme disease, onchocerciasis, sarcoidosis, syphilis, toxocariasis, toxoplasmosis, tuberculosis, occult tumors such as retinoblastoma, and unsuspected foreign bodies.

TOXOPLASMOSIS Toxoplasmosis is the most common cause of posterior uveitis, accounting for 30 to 50% of cases. It is caused by infection with the obligate intracellular protozoan, *Toxoplasma gondii*. If a woman acquires toxoplasmosis during pregnancy, she has a 40% chance of transmitting the infection to her fetus. Subsequent children are not at risk because of maternal immunity. Chorioretinitis develops in 80% of children with congenital toxoplasmosis, and infection is bilateral in 85%. Chorioretinitis is rarely active at the time of birth. The typical fundus lesion is a healed, densely pigmented scar at the posterior pole, usually in the macula. Infants who have chorioretinal scars, but have been spared the central nervous system sequelae of toxoplasmosis (convulsions and intracranial calcification are characteristic), may not be identified until months or years later when they are evaluated for strabismus or poor vision. Active chorioretinal lesions seen in later childhood or adulthood almost always represent reactivation of latent congenital infection. Acute focal satellite lesions arise within or adjacent to healed chorioretinal scars and produce a secondary inflammation of the vitreous and anterior segment. Papillitis and papilledema may also occur. Patients complain of blurred vision and floaters. Rarely, toxoplasmosis chorioretinitis is newly acquired, most commonly in the setting of immunosuppression, and then old chorioretinal scars will not be seen (see Sec. 13.6.5).

The recommended treatment for active chorioretinitis in children when the macula or optic nerve is threatened consists of a 4- to 6-week course of pyrimethamine (Daraprim), sulfadiazine, and leucovorin (folinic acid). Pyrimethamine is given orally twice daily in a loading dose of 2 mg/kg/d up to 75 mg the first day, then 1 mg/kg up to 25 mg/d given in two equal doses. The sulfadiazine dosage is 100 mg/kg in a loading dose of up to 2 g orally, followed by 100 mg/kg/d up to 4 g in four equal doses. Folinic acid 5 mg is given by mouth or intramuscularly twice weekly to prevent the leukopenia and thrombocytopenia that may result from pyrimethamine usage. White blood cell and platelet counts should be monitored weekly to detect any tendency to bone marrow depression.

Clindamycin also has been used in the treatment of toxoplasmosis as a (1) supplement to pyrimethamine and sulfadiazine therapy, (2) substitute for pyrimethamine when used with sulfadiazine in patients with bone marrow toxicity and in pregnant women since the drug is teratogenic, and (3) substitute for sulfadiazine when used with pyrimethamine in patients with sulfonamide allergy. The clindamycin dosage for infants is 25 mg/kg/d in three or four equal doses. Patients taking clindamycin should be warned about pseudomembranous colitis so that the medicine can be stopped if diarrhea develops.

The combination drug trimethoprim-sulfamethoxazole (Bactrim, Septra) with or without clindamycin, is another alternative therapy for toxoplasmosis. The drug is available in tablet form or as a suspension for children. Both drugs have shown an inhibitory effect on *T. gondii* experimentally.

Small lesions in the periphery of the retina that are not associated with appreciable vitreous cells may be followed without treatment. The concomitant use of corticosteroids, such as prednisone 1 to

2 mg/kg/d, is controversial and generally is reserved for acute, progressive lesions involving the macula, papillomacular bundle, and optic nerve. Cryotherapy and laser photocoagulation are reserved for patients with persistent recurrences.

TOXOCARIASIS Toxocariasis is caused by the nematode larva of the common intestinal parasite of dogs (*Toxocara canis*) or of cats (*T. cati*). Infection is acquired by ingesting soil contaminated by ova deposited in feces of dogs, particularly puppies. Toxocariasis typically appears between the ages of 2 and 8 years. Ocular inflammation is usually unilateral and can take the form of a posterior pole granulomatous mass, a peripheral inflammatory mass with cyclitis, peripheral chorioretinitis, optic papillitis, diffuse uveitis, or endophthalmitis with retinal detachment. Features of visceral larval migrans including eosinophilia are rarely present in ocular toxocariasis, and ocular lesions are rarely seen in visceral larval migrans. Children come to the attention of the ophthalmologist because of poor vision, strabismus, or leukocoria.

Diagnosis is based on the clinical history, ocular findings, and results of the serum enzyme-linked immunosorbent assay (ELISA) test for *Toxocara*. Occasionally the serum titer is normal but the aqueous titer is highly elevated. Because ocular toxocariasis can be managed without enucleation, distinguishing it from retinoblastoma is important. Additional studies sometimes necessary in the differential diagnosis of retinoblastoma include ultrasonography, radiography, or computed tomography to detect intraocular calcium (rare in *Toxocara*), and biochemical and cytologic examination of intraocular aspirates. Other diseases considered in the differential diagnosis of toxocariasis include toxoplasmosis, primary hyperplastic vitreous, Coats disease, sarcoid, and retinopathy of prematurity. Therapy for ocular toxocariasis, including corticosteroids, antihelmintics, and laser photocoagulation, has met with little success. Pars plana vitrectomy may help to reduce vitreous traction and clear the optical media. The best treatment is prevention (deworming dogs, improving sanitation at children's playgrounds, and proper personal hygiene).

26.9.3   Uveal Tumors

IRIS NODULES

IRIS FRECKLES Iris freckles are stationary, variably pigmented, flat patches on the anterior surface of the iris; they consist histologically of melanocytes.

IRIS NEVI Iris nevi are discrete, usually flat or minimally raised (ie, less than 1 mm) masses or nodules composed of benign nevus cells with variable pigmentation on the anterior surface of the iris. They usually become apparent at puberty and most often are found in the inferior half of the iris. Generally they are not vascular. Nevi usually do not exceed 3 mm in diameter and do not grow. Malignant change is rare.

IRIS EPITHELIAL CYSTS Both pigmented and nonpigmented congenital cysts of the iris may occur. They may produce a localized elevation of the iris stroma and may locally occlude the trabecular meshwork and cause angle-closure glaucoma. Some cysts transilluminate. They can be visualized better after dilation. Some cysts can be ruptured by laser treatment.

JUVENILE XANTHOGRANULOMA (JXG) JXG of the iris appears as a poorly demarcated, flesh-colored mass on the iris, usually in one eye, associated with raised orange skin lesions. Lesions of JXG commonly appear in the first year after birth but may occur in adulthood. Bleeding from the iris lesion causes spontaneous hyphema; secondary glaucoma with buphthalmos can occur. Glaucoma with enlargement of the globe may occur without hyphema. Iris involvement may produce heterochromic irides. The JXG lesion may be mistaken for an iris melanoma. Histopathologically, there is diffuse granulomatous infiltration with lipid-containing histiocytes and Touton giant cells. Other parts of the eye that may be involved include the ciliary body, conjunctiva, cornea, episclera, eyelids, and orbit. The normal course is spontaneous resolution, but this may occur in some instances only after the eye has been destroyed by hemorrhage and secondary glaucoma. Successful forms of treatment of iris JXG include local irradiation (about 400 rad), laser photocoagulation, local and systemic corticosteroids, and surgical excision.

BRUSHFIELD SPOTS These are elevated, white to yellow spots on the anterior surface of the iris. Histopathologically, they represent areas of relatively normal iris stroma surrounded by a ring of iris hypoplasia. There are typically 10 to 20 per eye. They are seen in 24% of normal persons and in 85% of patients with Down syndrome.

LISCH NODULES These are smooth, avascular, gelatinous, tan to dark brown nodules on the anterior surface of the iris that vary in size from barely visible to 2 mm. Histopathologically, they are collections of benign nevus cells. They are found in 90% of patients with neurofibromatosis 1 (von Recklinghausen disease) beyond the age of 6 years but do not occur in normal persons.

KOEPPE AND BUSACCA NODULES These discrete, raised nodules are found in granulomatous uveitides involving the pupillary margin (Koeppe nodules) or anterior iris surface (Busacca nodules). Histopathologically, they reveal granulomatous inflammation with histiocytes and giant cells. When Koeppe nodules regress, posterior synechiae frequently are left behind.

IRIS MALIGNANT MELANOMA This is a slowly expanding, variably pigmented, flat or nodular growth, usually occurring in the inferior or inferotemporal periphery of the iris. Satellite lesions may develop in the adjacent iris or the anterior chamber angle. Corectopia, dyscoria, irregular dilation, ectropion uveae, sectoral cataract, nutrient vessels, and secondary glaucoma may develop. Virtually all iris melanomas are of the spindle-cell variety. Malignant melanomas are rare in childhood. In children iris melanomas account for a much greater proportion of the all-uveal melanomas than occurs in adults. The clinical features are similar to those described in adults. Treatment is by serial examination with photography to document growth, followed by local excision or enucleation.

CILIARY BODY AND CHOROIDAL TUMORS

CHOROIDAL NEVI These are stationary, flat or minimally elevated, brown, gray, or black lesions with indistinct borders. Some nevi are amelanotic. Slightly elevated nevi may be difficult to distinguish from early choroidal melanomas, particularly if accompanied by subretinal fluid. They are not usually associated with visual field defects. Serial examination and photographic documentation may be necessary to establish nongrowth. Congenital hypertrophy of the retinal pigment epithelium is a darker, more discrete lesion that may be mistaken for a choroidal nevus.

CILIARY BODY AND CHOROIDAL MELANOMAS Melanoma is the most common intraocular malignancy in adults but occurs only rarely in the pediatric population. The clinical manifestations and course of these tumors are similar to those occurring in adults. Melanomas are discrete, enlarging, pigmented lesions that may be silent initially but eventually may lead to poor vision, floaters, light flashes, scotomas, or pain. They may cause retinal detachment, cataract, lens subluxation, secondary glaucoma, iris neovascularization, and spontaneous intraocular hemorrhage. The modified Callender classification divides malignant melanomas into spindle cell, epithelioid, mixed, or necrotic tumor types by histology. Hematogenous metastasis to the liver is common with large and anteriorly located melanomas. Treatment is controversial but involves observation or photocoagulation for small tumors; enucleation, external-beam radiation, or plaque irradiation for medium tumors; and enucleation for large tumors. The Collaborative Ocular Melanoma Study found no survival benefit from preenucleation external beam irradiation for patients with large tumors.

MEDULLOEPITHELIOMA (DICTYOMA) This is a rare, unilateral, congenital tumor of the nonpigmented ciliary body epithelium that becomes manifest in the first decade of life, commonly between 2 and 4 years of age. Signs and symptoms include poor vision, ocular pain, mass or cyst in iris or ciliary body, proptosis, cataract, strabismus, leukocoria, glaucoma, or hyphema. Differential diagnosis includes retinoblastoma, persistent hyperplastic primary vitreous, peripheral uveitis, *Toxocara* granuloma, iris cyst, neurofibroma of the iris or ciliary body, and juvenile xanthogranuloma. Histologically, the tumor is composed of cells that resemble primitive medullary epithelium. *Teratoid medulloepithelioma* may contain cartilage, brain tissue, striated muscle, or other elements. Metastatic potential is low. Treatment by enucleation carries an excellent prognosis if it is done before the tumor has extended into the orbit. Because the tumor has a low potential for metastatic spread, some authors have recommended local excision or cryotherapy when the mass is localized and anteriorly placed.

CHOROIDAL HEMANGIOMA Discrete choroidal hemangiomas are rare in children. The lesion (a hamartoma, not a true neoplasm) may clinically be confused with malignant melanoma. The more common type is the diffuse hemangioma that produces the "tomato catsup" fundus appearance in 40% of patients with the Sturge-Weber syndrome. Histopathologically, the lesion is a mixed capillary-cavernous hemangioma. The diagnosis of choroidal hemangiomas has been improved with the use of fluorescein angiography and ultrasonography. Photocoagulation has been used with some success.

26.9.4 Pupil

The pupil examination is discussed in Sec. 26.1.5. A 4+ afferent papillary defect produces an *amaurotic pupil*, one which has no direct response to light. *Light-near* dissociation of the pupillary reaction consists of decreased or absent constriction to direct light and good reaction to a near accommodative stimulus. Etiologies

TABLE 26-6

DIFFERENTIAL DIAGNOSIS OF LEUKOCORIA

CATEGORY	CONDITION
Developmental abnormalities	Coloboma of retina, choroid, or optic nerve
	Congenital retinal fold
	High myopia
	Incontinentia pigmenti
	Myelinated nerve fibers
	Norrie disease
	Persistent hyperplastic primary vitreous (PHPV)
	Retinal detachment
	Retinal dysplasia
	X-linked retinoschisis
Neoplastic lesions	Medulloepithelioma
	Retinoblastoma
Retinal vascular anomalies	Angiomatosis retinae (von Hippel disease)
	Choroidal hemangioma
	Coats disease
	Retinopathy of prematurity
Inflammatory conditions	Endophthalmitis
	Toxocariasis
	Uveitis
Trauma	Intraocular foreign body
	Massive retinal fibrosis
	Organizing vitreous hemorrhage
	Retinal detachment
Other	Cataract
	Corneal opacity
	Optic nerve reflex (eg, large-angle esotropia)
	Vitreous hemorrhage

include Parinaud syndrome, pinealoma, hydrocephalus, diabetes mellitus, encephalitis, and syphilis.

ABNORMAL PUPIL SIZE AND SHAPE

Pupillary *miosis* (small pupil) may occur on a physiological basis or be the result of drug administration (narcotics, pilocarpine, phospholine iodide), coma, Horner syndrome, posterior synechiae, pesticide or nerve gas exposure, or tertiary syphilis. Pupillary *mydriasis* (dilation) may occur on a physiological basis or be the result of drug exposure (epinephrine, phenylephrine, propine, topical antihistamine/vasoconstrictor combinations, tropicamide, cyclopentolate, atropine-like agents), coma, trauma, third cranial nerve palsy, Adie tonic pupil, or angle-closure glaucoma. Pupillary ectasia with corectopia, polycoria, or dyscoria may occur in the setting of trauma, the iridocorneal endothelial syndromes (progressive iris atrophy, Chandler syndrome, iris-nevus syndrome), Rieger anomaly and syndrome, or the ocular ischemic syndrome.

HORNER SYNDROME This syndrome is associated with a miotic pupil. The anisocoria is more apparent in the dark than in bright light. Horner syndrome consists of the triad of blepharoptosis, miosis, and facial anhidrosis. Horner syndrome ptosis is discussed in Sec. 26.4.2. Pharmacologic testing of the pupil with topical cocaine 4% and hydroxyamphetamine 1% confirms the diagnosis and helps localize the site of the lesion. The Horner syndrome pupil dilates poorly to cocaine, thereby distinguishing it from a physiologically miotic pupil. Failure of the pupil to dilate after instillation of one drop of hydroxyamphetamine 1% indicates a third-order neuron (postganglionic) Horner syndrome. Complete neurologic evaluation is indicated to rule out serious intrathoracic, cervical, or intracranial disease.

SPASM OF THE NEAR REFLEX This disorder is seen in children and can be confused with bilateral sixth cranial (abducens) nerve palsy. Most often the disorder is functional. There is a spastic overaction of all components of the *near triad* (accommodation, convergence, and miosis) resulting in myopia and blurred vision. The condition is highly variable from moment to moment and may last seconds to minutes. The spasm may be relieved by instillation of cycloplegic drops, minus lenses, and, on occasion, by psychological counseling. Rare organic causes of this problem include encephalitis, midbrain and posterior fossa lesions, anticonvulsant drug toxicities, myasthenia gravis, and cyclic oculomotor palsy.

LEUKOCORIA

Many congenital and acquired diseases of the eye can cause *leukocoria* (white pupil) in the infant or child, the most serious of which is retinoblastoma. Prompt referral to an ophthalmologist is imperative. The differential diagnosis of leukocoria is summarized in Table 26-6.

References

Apt L: Medulloepithelioma. In: Fraunfelder FT, Roy RH, eds: Current Ocular Therapy 4:322. Philadelphia, Saunders, 1995

Cunningham ET Jr, Nozik RA: Uveitis: Diagnostic approach and ancillary analysis. In: Duane TD, Jaeger EA, eds: Clinical Ophthalmology. Philadelphia, Lippincott-Raven, 1997

Giles CL, Bloom JN: Uveitis in childhood. In: Duane TD, Jaeger EA, eds: Clinical Ophthalmology. Philadelphia, Lippincott, 1994

Nussenblatt RB, Whitcup SM, Palestine AG: Uveitis: Fundamentals in Clinical Practice, 2nd ed. St. Louis, Mosby, 1996

Pepose JS, Holland GN, Wilhelmus KR, eds: Ocular Infection and Immunity. St. Louis, Mosby, 1996

Shields JA, Shields CL: Intraocular Tumors: A Text and Atlas. Philadelphia, Saunders, 1992

Smith RE, Nozik RA: Uveitis: A Clinical Approach to Diagnosis and Management, 2nd ed. Baltimore, Williams & Wilkins, 1989

Tabbara KF: Toxoplasmosis. In: Duane TD, Jaeger EA, eds: Clinical Ophthalmology. Philadelphia, Lippincott Williams & Wilkins, 1999

26.10 LENS

The most common clinical problem of the lens is cataract. It is the final common pathway of a variety of genetic and environmental insults that disturb lens transparency. Abnormalities of lens size, shape, and position are less common.

26.10.1   Congenital Anomalies

MICROSPHEROPHAKIA Microspherophakia is a bilateral lens anomaly characterized by small equatorial diameter and spherical shape. The entire lens can be seen through a widely dilated pupil. The high curvature of the lens surfaces induces a high degree of myopia. Microspherophakia is seen most often in the *Weill-Marchesani syndrome,* an autosomal-recessive condition characterized by short stature, broad hands, short stubby fingers, and reduced joint mobility. It may also be seen in Peters anomaly, Marfan syndrome, Alport syndrome, Lowe syndrome, congenital rubella, aniridia, and Klinefelter syndrome. Weakness of the lens zonules leads to iridodonesis, phakodonesis, and a tendency for anterior or lateral subluxation. Pupillary block glaucoma may develop as a result of anterior subluxation, in which the lens becomes trapped in the anterior chamber between the iris and cornea.

LENTICONUS Lenticonus is an anterior or posterior conical protrusion of the central pole of the lens that produces a dark disc ("oil droplet") in the center of the pupil during ophthalmoscopy. This anomaly results in a marked disturbance of vision caused by irregular astigmatism or myopia and the frequent occurrence of lens opacities. Anterior lenticonus is usually bilateral and may be a feature of *Alport syndrome* if associated with progressive renal disease (hemorrhagic nephritis) and sensorineural hearing loss. The inheritance pattern is variable. Posterior lenticonus is more common than anterior lenticonus, usually unilateral, occurring more frequently in females. The posterior lens bulge may produce myopia and mixed astigmatism leading to amblyopia unless monitored. The posterior cortex often becomes opacified requiring surgery. Visual prognosis after surgery usually is good.

LENS COLOBOMA The term, *lens coloboma,* is a misnomer because there is no missing lens tissue in this anomaly. Rather, there is a flattening or indentation of the lens at the equator in an area of absent or loose zonules. Lens colobomas typically occur in the inferonasal quadrant and are often associated with uveal colobomas. They may occur unilaterally as an isolated abnormality or bilaterally. Cortical cataract or lens capsule thickening may occur in the area of the coloboma.

26.10.2   Ectopia Lentis

Ectopia lentis refers to partial (*subluxation*) or complete (*luxation*) displacement of the lens from the pupil secondary to weak or absent zonules. Ectopia lentis may be congenital or acquired. Subluxation is associated with decreased visual acuity, high astigmatism, and monocular diplopia. Luxation is associated with high hyperopia from functional aphakia. Trauma is the most common cause of ectopia lentis. Atraumatic ectopia lentis occurs in association with a wide variety of ocular conditions including megalocornea, aniridia, congenital glaucoma, Rieger syndrome, persistent hyperplastic primary vitreous, and persistent pupillary membrane. It is seen in systemic syndromes such as homocystinuria, Marfan syndrome, syphilis, porphyria, the mandibulofacial disorders, osteogenesis imperfecta, Weill-Marchesani syndrome, dwarfism, oxycephaly, Ehlers-Danlos syndrome, scleroderma, Refsum disease, Kneist syndrome, hyperlysinemia, and sulfite oxidase deficiency. Ectopia lentis may also occur as an isolated phenomenon (*simple ectopia lentis*), usually as an autosomal-dominant trait or in association with ectopia pupillae (Sec. 26.9.1).

Bilateral superotemporal lens subluxation is characteristic of *Marfan syndrome,* occurring in 50 to 80% of patients by the fourth or fifth decade. Frequently, the subluxation is congenital and nonprogressive. Zonular attachments usually remain intact but become stretched. Bilateral inferonasal lens subluxation is characteristic of *homocystinuria,* occurring in nearly 80% of patients by 15 years of age. About 30% of patients with homocystinuria demonstrate ectopia lentis in infancy. Almost one-third eventually dislocate into the vitreous cavity or anterior chamber. Pupillary dilation should be avoided because it can precipitate dislocation and secondary glaucoma. Although the ectopic lenses in homocystinuria are frequently cataractous, lens extraction under general anesthesia should be avoided, if possible, because fatal thromboembolic complications may occur during or shortly after surgery. The small, spherical lenses in *Weill-Marchesani syndrome* frequently dislocate anteriorly, causing acute glaucoma. Surgical removal of dislocated lenses carries risks of serious complications such as vitreous loss, iris prolapse, and retinal detachment.

26.10.3 Cataract

A cataract is any opacity of the crystalline lens. Congenital cataracts are present at birth, by definition, but frequently they are not discovered until some time during the first year of life. The terms *congenital cataract* and *infantile cataract* are therefore used interchangeably. The degree of opacity varies widely from a small dot to total clouding of the lens. Although congenital cataracts are usually stationary, they may progress in severity during childhood. Congenital lens opacities occur in 0.44% of live births, account for 11.5% of blindness in preschool children, and are a common cause of amblyopia.

Cataracts may appear in a number of ways depending on their laterality, density, and age of onset. The parents may notice decreased visual attention, light sensitivity, nystagmus, strabismus, or leukocoria. A white lens opacity may be apparent on direct inspection, and/or an abnormality in the red reflex may appear during ophthalmoscopy. Because early diagnosis is critical for visual rehabilitation, all newborns must be checked routinely for cataracts. A family history of cataracts or other ocular anomalies supports a hereditary origin. The pregnancy and birth histories may identify increased parental age, consanguinity, maternal illness, gestational drug exposure, or birth trauma as important factors to consider.

Most monocular pediatric cataracts are not genetic or metabolic in origin. The contrary is often true of bilateral cataracts. The morphology of a cataract may provide clues as to the timing of an insult during embryogenesis. Nuclear cataracts develop early in gestation. Lamellar, zonular, or cortical cataracts develop later in embryogenesis, are characterized by lens opacification peripheral to the Y sutures, and are considered acquired and progressive rather than congenital. Mature or white cataracts involve the entire lens and may be present from birth or may develop from progression of partial cataracts.

Approximately 50 to 60% of congenital cataracts are idiopathic, but the remainder have diagnosable and possibly treatable etiologies. One-third of bilateral cataracts are inherited, and another third are associated with other ocular or systemic disorders. Within the hereditary group, autosomal dominant is the most common inheritance pattern. Autosomal recessive and X-linked inheritance are rare. Approximately 40% of acquired pediatric cataracts are traumatic. Established causes of cataract, associated ocular anomalies, and associated systemic conditions are listed in Table 26-7.

RUBELLA CATARACT In addition to cataracts, other eye findings in the congenital rubella syndrome may include spherophakia, "salt and pepper" pigmentary retinopathy, unilateral or bilateral microphthalmos, anterior segment dysgenesis, nongranulomatous iridocyclitis, transient corneal opacification, congenital glaucoma, and iris hypoplasia. The cataract of congenital rubella syndrome is present at birth or during the first year of life and may be nuclear or complete and either unilateral or bilateral. The cataract develops because of viral invasion of the lens. Live virus has been recovered from lens aspirates of patients up to 3 years of age. There is no specific treatment for rubella infection. Cataract surgery is associated with a high incidence of complications including uveitis (presumably from the release of live virus) and phthisis bulbi (see Sec. 13.4.20). Fortunately, with the availability of the rubella vaccine in 1969, the incidence of the congenital rubella syndrome has decreased dramatically.

METABOLIC CATARACTS A host of metabolic disorders can produce cataracts. In *galactosemia* and *galactokinase deficiency,* cataract development is secondary to an increased blood galactose level. In the first weeks of life, the lens takes on an oil droplet appearance; later a nuclear or lamellar cataract develops. Some reversal of the opacity is possible if galactose is withheld from the diet. Patients with *juvenile-onset diabetes mellitus* can develop multiple, bilateral, anterior or posterior subcapsular snowflake dots over a network of vacuoles. These opacities appear in late childhood or adolescence and are not visually significant in most patients. A variety of chromosomal disorders are also associated with cataracts. Nearly all children with Down syndrome, for instance, have microscopic lens opacities (60% of young children and 100% of adolescents).

CORTICOSTEROID-INDUCED CATARACTS Long-term systemic corticosteroid therapy for asthma, nephrotic syndrome, systemic lupus erythematosus, and juvenile rheumatoid arthritis can cause cataract development. These cataracts are posterior subcapsular in type, and their development is related to the dosage and duration of corticosteroid therapy. Because these cataracts may be reversible at an early stage, and because early cataracts can be confirmed only by slit-lamp biomicroscopy, any patient receiving prolonged treatment with systemic corticosteroids should be evaluated by slit-lamp examination at least yearly if the dosage is less than 10 mg of prednisone per day, or every 6 months if the dosage is higher. A posterior subcapsular cataract appears as a central black dot against the red reflex during direct ophthalmoscopy. If cataracts begin to develop, there may be some benefit in reducing the total systemic dosage, changing to an alternate-day schedule, or switching to an alternative immunosuppressive agent.

The key to management of congenital cataracts is early diagnosis; early surgical removal; appropriate aphakic correction by contact lenses, spectacles, or intraocular lens implants; and careful postoperative monitoring of vision with appropriate occlusion therapy to prevent amblyopia. Visual rehabilitation is generally more successful in bilateral than unilateral cataracts, and in partial rather than total cataracts. It is generally poorer for patients with other associated ocular defects. Children with complete bilateral cataracts who fail to receive foveal stimulation during the first 8 to 16 weeks after birth develop deprivation amblyopia and sensory nystagmus. Surgery, therefore, should preferably be performed before 6 to 8 weeks of age to prevent irreversible amblyopia and nystagmus. The visual prognosis of a child with a unilateral congenital cataract is poorer than that of a child with bilateral cataracts. Amblyopia is more likely to develop when one eye can accommodate to obtain a focused image at any point in space and the other eye cannot. Optical correction of patients with unilateral aphakia involves the

TABLE 26-7

CAUSES OF CATARACT AND ASSOCIATED OCULAR AND SYSTEMIC DISORDERS

CATEGORY	CONDITION	CATEGORY	CONDITION
Gestational disturbances	Intrauterine infections (eg, TORCHS, varicella, HIV, polio)	Associated ocular diseases	Congenital glaucoma
			Juvenile retinoschisis
	Ionizing radiation		Medulloepithelioma
	Prematurity, low birth weight		Norrie disease
Mendelian inheritance	Autosomal dominant		Retinal detachment
	Autosomal recessive		Retinoblastoma
	X-linked		Retinopathy of prematurity
Trauma	Concussion		*Toxocara* endophthalmitis
	Electrical shock		Uveitis
	Penetrating (eg, amniocentesis)	Associated skin diseases	Atopic dermatitis
Metabolic disorders	Cholestanolosis		Bloch-Sulzberger syndrome
	Diabetes mellitus		Congenital ichthyosis
	Fabry disease		Ectodermal dysplasia
	Galactokinase deficiency		Rothmund-Thomson syndrome
	Galactosemia		Werner syndrome
	Hypoglycemia	Craniofacial dysostoses	Apert syndrome
	Hypoparathyroidism		Crouzon syndrome
	Mannosidosis		Oxycephaly
	Pseudohypoparathyroidism	Associated systemic syndromes	Alport syndrome
	Refsum disease		Chondrodystrophic myotonia
	Zellweger syndrome		Cockayne syndrome
Chromosomal disorders	Monosomy syndromes: 21, Turner syndrome		Conradi syndrome
	Partial deletion syndromes: 4p, 5p, 11p, 18q, 18p		Down syndrome
	Partial duplication: 15q		Fabry disease
	Ring syndromes: 4, D, 21		Hallermann-Streiff syndrome
	Trisomy syndromes: 13, 18, 21		Lanzieri syndrome
Drug exposure (gestational or developmental)	Busulfan		Lowe syndrome
	Corticosteroids		Marfan syndrome
	Naphthalene		Marinesco-Sjögren syndrome
	Paradichlorobenzene		Myotonic dystrophy
	Phenothiazines		Osteogenesis imperfecta
	Sulfonamides		Osteopetrosis
	Triparanol		Potter syndrome
	Vitamin D excess		Refsum disease
Associated ocular anomalies	Aniridia		Rubinstein-Taybi syndrome
	Anterior segment dysgenesis		Schwartz-Jampel syndrome
	Ectopia lentis		Sjögren-Larsson syndrome
	Lens coloboma		Smith-Lemli-Opitz syndrome
	Lenticonus		Stickler syndrome
	Megalocornea		Wilson disease
	Mittendorf dot		
	Microspherophakia		
	Persistent hyperplastic primary vitreous		
	Persistent pupillary membrane		
	Retinal dysplasia		

use of contact or intraocular lenses. Intraocular lens implantation in children beyond the age of 2 years has become more common in the last decade and avoids many of the difficulties associated with contact lens wear. Aphakic spectacles may be used to correct bilateral aphakia but not unilateral aphakia because of a 25 to 30% *aniseikonia* (image size disparity). Treatment of partial cataracts may include prolonged dilation of the pupil with mydriatic agents or rarely optical iridectomy. Cataract surgery is usually advisable when distance visual acuity is reduced to 20/50 or worse and near vision is impaired, particularly if the visual handicap interferes with the child's normal progress.

References

Hiles DA, Kilty LA: Disorders of the lens. In: Isenberg SJ, ed: The Eye in Infancy, 2nd ed. St. Louis, Mosby, 1994

Jaffe NS, Horwitz J: Lens and cataract. In: Podos SM, Yanoff M, eds: Textbook of Ophthalmology. New York, Gower, 1992

Jaffe NS, Jaffe MS, Jaffe GF: Cataract Surgery and Its Complications, 6th ed. St. Louis, Mosby, 1997

Kuszak JR: Embryology and anatomy of the lens. In: Duane TD, Jaeger EA, eds: Clinical Ophthalmology. Philadelphia, Lippincott, 1990

26.11 RETINA AND VITREOUS

David Sarraf

26.11.1 Congenital Anomalies

PERSISTENT HYPERPLASTIC PRIMARY VITREOUS (PHPV) PHPV is a congenital, nonhereditary anomaly of the eye, caused by failure of the primary vitreous to regress in utero. In the anterior form of this condition, a white mass persists behind a cataractous lens. The contracting retrolental mass causes ciliary processes to elongate and appear as dark spokes behind the lens during slit-lamp examination. Prominent radial vessels may appear on the iris surface. PHPV is almost always unilateral, and the eye in which it develops is often microphthalmic (Sec. 26.2.1). The posterior form of PHPV represents a continuum ranging from a Bergmeister papilla (Sec. 26.12.1) to retinal fold or extensive tractional retinal detachment; the lens may be clear. Bilateral PHPV may be seen in association with trisomy 13, Norrie disease, and the Walker-Warburg syndrome.

Anterior PHPV may be complicated by progressive cataract development with shallowing of the anterior chamber and secondary angle-closure glaucoma. Untreated eyes may be lost because of intraocular hemorrhage, glaucoma, retinal detachment, and phthisis bulbi. In the past, vision was usually poor following cataract extraction and membrane dissection. In recent years, however, surgical results with good visual outcomes, comparable to those obtained in the treatment of unilateral congenital cataract, have been reported. Associated posterior changes of PHPV may, however, limit visual outcomes despite favorable surgery.

Because *leukocoria* (white pupil) is the usual presenting symptom, PHPV must be differentiated from retinoblastoma. Distinguishing features of PHPV include concurrent microphthalmos (retinoblastoma usually develops in eyes of normal size); the lack of calcium on radiographic investigation; the development of cataract (atypical for retinoblastoma except in advanced lesions); and characteristic ultrasound, computed tomography, and magnetic resonance imaging findings. Though very rare, the coexistence of PHPV and retinoblastoma has been reported.

RETINAL DYSPLASIA Retinal dysplasia is a severe, typically bilateral, developmental abnormality characterized by malformation, fold formation, and detachment of the retina. It may occur sporadically or as an X-linked recessive disorder. Typically, the affected infant is bilaterally blind with nystagmus and demonstrates a shallow anterior chamber with a white retrolental mass on biomicroscopic examination. Associated anomalies often include microphthalmos, colobomas, and PHPV. Retinal dysplasia may occur as a result of radiation, prenatal trauma, or intrauterine infection, or may be associated with trisomy 13, Norrie disease, or Meckel syndrome. It often is associated with systemic abnormalities such as cerebral agenesis, cardiac anomalies, harelip, cleft palate, and polydactyly. Differentiation from retinoblastoma is aided by its occurrence in microphthalmic eyes and the associated systemic findings.

NORRIE DISEASE This syndrome is a rare, X-linked recessive retinal dysplasia that results in bilateral congenital blindness in affected male children. The eyes usually appear normal in size but may be microphthalmic or buphthalmic. During the first few days or weeks of life a yellowish retinal detachment appears bilaterally, followed by the development of white gliotic masses behind each lens. The anterior chambers are shallow, and the irises are atrophic. In time, lenticular and corneal opacities develop and the eyes become phthisical. Mental retardation and sensorineural deafness also develop. The Norrie disease gene is located on the proximal short arm of the X chromosome.

26.11.2 Hereditary Disorders

This section describes some of the common hereditary macular and extramacular retinal and vitreoretinal dystrophies with infantile or childhood onset.

RETINAL PIGMENT EPITHELIAL DYSTROPHIES

STARGARDT DISEASE AND FUNDUS FLAVIMACULATUS Stargardt disease is the most common form of macular degeneration occurring in childhood. It usually is transmitted as an autosomal-recessive trait, although autosomal-dominant transmission can occur. The disease is characterized by a bilateral, symmetric, and progressive loss of visual acuity, usually occurring between the ages of 6 and 20 years, which antedates and is out of proportion to the initial ophthalmoscopic changes. Atrophic evolution of the macula is heralded by loss of the normal macular reflex and development of a "beaten bronze" appearance. Pigment mottling and bull's eye macular atrophy leading to frank "cookie-cutter" atrophy may ultimately ensue. A wreath of pisciform or triradiate flecks often surrounds the central atrophic region. Vision decreases slowly but relentlessly and is 20/200 or less by the fourth decade. Total blindness does not occur, however, and the peripheral field usually remains fairly intact. Nyctalopia, or night blindness, is not a characteristic feature. The electroretinogram (ERG) and electrooculogram (EOG) are typically normal but may be variably depressed. A "dark choroid" (hypofluorescence caused by the blockage of the normal choroidal fluorescence) may be appreciated on fluorescein angiography. Peripherally distributed, yellow, pisciform flecks associated with delayed macular involvement is more typical of the disorder called *fundus flavimaculatus,* although the two dystrophies probably represent phenotypes of the same disease. The differential diagnosis of fundus flavimaculatus includes drusen, fundus albipunctatus, retinitis punctata albescens, Kandori fleck retina, and vitamin A deficiency. There is no specific therapy for Stargardt disease or fundus flavimaculatus. The gene causing Stargardt disease has been mapped to 1q and has recently been cloned. It codes for an ATP-binding cassette protein localized to rod photoreceptors of the retina and is involved with molecular transportation and exchange. Heterozygous forms of the mutation have been associated with the development of age-related macular degeneration.

VITELLIFORM DYSTROPHY Vitelliform dystrophy or *Best disease* is an autosomal-dominant macular dystrophy with variable penetrance and expressivity. Onset is typically between 3 and 15 years of age. In the early stage, Best disease is characterized by bilateral, symmetric, well-defined, round, one-disc-diameter "egg yolk" lesions in the macula. Visual acuity is initially good. An atypical form with multifocal vitelliform lesions may occur. The homogeneous, yellow appearance of the macular lesions may layer out and fragment with time, ultimately leaving a mottled "scrambled egg" appearance that may simulate other types of macular degeneration. At this stage there is loss of visual acuity. The ERG is normal, but the EOG is abnormal, characteristically demonstrating an absent rise in the electrical potential of the RPE during the photopic phase of testing. Family members who carry the defective gene but are clinically unaffected also have an abnormal EOG. A gene linked to the disease has been localized to chromosome 11q and sequenced. It is referred to as vitelliform macular dystrophy 2 (VMD2). At present there is no effective treatment for vitelliform dystrophy. Low-vision aids are recommended when vision declines, and laser treatment may be used if choroidal neovascularization develops.

RETINAL DYSTROPHIES

RETINITIS PIGMENTOSA (RP) Retinitis pigmentosa is the name given to a group of hereditary retinal degenerative diseases classically characterized by progressive visual field loss, nyctalopia, delayed dark adaptation, pigmentary retinopathy, and a depressed or unrecordable ERG. RP may be inherited as an autosomal-dominant (22%), autosomal-recessive (16%), or X-linked-recessive (9%) condition, but about half of all affected individuals have no inheritance pattern and are identified by the term *simplex RP*. In advanced disease, the fundus appearance is typical, consisting of disc pallor, vascular attenuation, and bone-spicule pigmentary migration throughout the fundus, particularly along the retinal blood vessels. As a rule, severe visual handicap does not develop until adulthood, although signs and symptoms may appear in early childhood. When the onset occurs in childhood, the prognosis is usually poor. There is no effective treatment for RP, although vitamin A supplementation has been shown to retard loss of the cone-mediated ERG. Patients should be screened regularly, however, for ocular complications for which there are therapeutic options. Posterior subcapsular cataracts may be removed surgically, exudative responses may be addressed with laser or cryotherapy, and cystoid macular edema may be treated successfully with acetazolamide (Diamox).

Most forms of RP can be categorized by electrophysiologic testing into rod-cone (the common variety) or cone-rod degenerations. Rod-cone degenerations are associated with a markedly reduced scotopic (rod) ERG; the photopic (cone) ERG is progressively affected but not as severely. The reverse is true of cone-rod degenerations. RP may be limited to the eyes (primary RP), or it may be associated with additional organ system involvement (secondary RP) such as congenital hearing loss in *Usher syndrome*. See Table 26-8 for a partial list of RP syndromes.

Much has been learned recently about the genetics of retinitis pigmentosa. Mutation of rhodopsin, a photopigment in the photoreceptor outer segments and a critical component of the phototransduction cascade, has been implicated in several forms of RP. Mutations in peripherin/rds and ROM-1 protein, outer-segment disc membrane constituents that impart structural stability to the photoreceptors, and mutations in the A- and B-subunits of phosphodiesterase, critical components of the phototransduction cascade, have been identified. Gene therapy, in which a diseased cell is transfected by a vector containing a normal or wild-type gene sequence, has been applied successfully to photoreceptor cells in various animal models of RP; genetic intervention in humans is still in its infancy.

LEBER CONGENITAL AMAUROSIS This rod-cone dystrophy presents at birth or in the first few months and is responsible for an estimated 10% of all congenital blindness. It is characterized by visual acuity less than 20/200, poor pupillary reaction, nystagmus, and a markedly reduced or absent ERG response. Oculodigital phenomena are common and may represent an effort by the patient to

TABLE 26-8

SYSTEMIC DISEASE ASSOCIATIONS WITH RETINITIS PIGMENTOSA

INHERITANCE	SYSTEMIC DISEASE OR SYNDROME
Autosomal dominant	Alagille syndrome (arteriohepatic dysplasia)
	Charcot-Marie-Tooth disease
	Flynn-Aird syndrome
	Oculodentodigital dysplasia syndrome
	Olivopontocerebellar atrophy
	Paget disease
	Pierre Robin syndrome
	Steinert disease (myotonic dystrophy)
	Stickler syndrome
	Waardenburg syndrome
	Wagner disease
Autosomal recessive	Albers-Schönberg disease (osteopetrosis)
	Alström disease
	Bardet-Biedl syndrome
	Bassen-Kornzweig disease (abetalipoproteinemia)
	Batten disease
	Cockayne syndrome
	Friedreich ataxia
	Grönblad-Strandberg syndrome
	Hallgren syndrome
	Homocystinuria
	Hurler syndrome (MPS 1-H)
	Jeune syndrome
	Juvenile Paget disease (hyperostosis corticalis deformans juvenilis)
	Kearns-Sayre syndrome
	Mannosidosis
	Marinesco-Sjögren syndrome
	Refsum disease
	Sanfilippo syndrome (MPS III)
	Scheie syndrome (MPS 1-S)
	Usher syndrome
	Wolfram syndrome
	Zellweger syndrome (cerebrohepatorenal syndrome)
X-linked	Bloch-Sulzberger syndrome (incontinentia pigmenti)
	Hunter syndrome (MPS II)
	Pelizaeus-Meizbacher disease

stimulate the retina entopically. Inherited disease shows an autosomal-recessive pattern. The fundus presentation is variable and includes a normal appearance, macular colobomas mimicking toxoplasmosis scars, or classic retinal degenerative changes of retinitis pigmentosa including optic disc pallor, vascular attenuation, and pigment migration. Associated neurologic and renal abnormalities have been reported. The ERG is undetectable and is essential in differentiating Leber congenital amaurosis from blindness of central origin ("cortical blindness"), especially in Leber amaurosis with a normal-appearing fundus.

PSEUDORETINITIS PIGMENTOSA A number of conditions produce a pigmentary disturbance of the retina or widespread mottling of the retinal pigment epithelium beneath the retina mimicking RP. These are not true retinal dystrophies and so are termed *pseudoretinitis pigmentosa* or *secondary retinitis pigmentosa*. Included in this group are congenital infections (syphilis, rubella, cytomegalic inclusion disease, influenza), chronic uveitis, trauma, toxicity (phenothiazines, chloroquine), and ophthalmic artery occlusion. The carrier states of choroideremia and albinism may also present with a so-called moth-eaten fundus that may be described as a pigmentary retinopathy. Most of the pseudo-RP conditions are nonprogressive and the ERG is normal.

CONGENITAL STATIONARY NIGHT BLINDNESS This nonprogressive disorder is characterized by nyctalopia that begins in infancy. There are a variety of known types of congenital stationary night blindness. Autosomal-dominant, autosomal-recessive, and sex-linked forms with normal-appearing fundi have been described. Visual acuity is good in the autosomal-dominant form but may be subnormal in the recessive and sex-linked forms. Patients may demonstrate normal-appearing fundi; alternatively, variable degrees of myopia with associated retinochoroidal degenerative changes may be detected. *Oguchi disease* is an autosomal-recessive condition in which there is a yellow retinal tapetal sheen under photopic conditions that disappears after 2 to 3 hours of dark adaptation (*Mizuo sign*). Central visual acuity is good. *Fundus albipunctatus* is an autosomal-recessive condition with highly characteristic discrete, punctate, white dots scattered throughout the fundus. Dark adaptation testing reveals a marked delay in light sensitivity threshold achievement by the rod population. Electrophysiological findings vary according to the specific etiology, but typically the scotopic (rod) ERG is barely recordable, whereas the photopic (cone) ERG is essentially normal. Negative waveforms, in which the b-wave is flat and the a-wave is normal, have also been recorded and are caused by faulty transmission of the electrical potential from rods to bipolar cells. It may be necessary to observe a patient for several years to demonstrate a lack of progression before rod-cone retinitis pigmentosa can be ruled out. Good lighting at night is helpful for these patients.

CONE DYSTROPHY Progressive cone dystrophy, in contrast to retinitis pigmentosa, is characterized by impairment of the cone system initially without changes in the rod system. Most instances are sporadic, but in familial disease the mode of inheritance may be autosomal-dominant or -recessive. Complaints of poor visual acuity, poor color vision, and photophobia occur late in childhood or early adulthood, unlike achromatopsia, which manifests early in infancy. Ophthalmoscopic findings are variable and include a normal-appearing macula or a mottled appearance. The classic appearance is that of bull's eye atrophy with ring-like depigmentation around the macula. The ERG shows a normal scotopic (rod) response but an absent or severely depressed photopic (cone) response.

CONGENITAL ACHROMATOPSIA Congenital achromatopsia or rod monochromatism is inherited as an autosomal-recessive trait and is characterized by total color blindness. Affected patients have reduced visual acuity to the level of 20/200, a further reduction under bright light conditions (*hemeralopia*), photophobia, and nystagmus; symptoms first become apparent in childhood. The condition is nonprogressive. There are no associated neurologic abnormalities. The "photophobia" and nystagmus may even disappear by the late teenage years. Vision is somewhat better near than at distance and in dim illumination. The fundus is typically normal in appearance but may include an abnormality of, or the absence of, the foveal light reflex, as well as a granular disturbance of the macular RPE. The photopic (cone) ERG is markedly abnormal, whereas the scotopic (rod) ERG is normal. The EOG is normal. Histologic examination demonstrates a generalized abnormality or complete absence of cones and normal-appearing rods. There is no effective treatment, but dark glasses and red-tinted con-

tact lenses may aid somewhat in improving visual acuity in bright light conditions. There is an incomplete form of congenital achromatopsia known as *blue cone monochromatism* that is inherited in an X-linked recessive manner and is associated with complete color blindness but visual acuity in the range of 20/40 to 20/200.

VITREORETINAL DYSTROPHIES

JUVENILE RETINOSCHISIS This X-linked recessive disorder is characterized by a bilateral schisis or splitting of the neurosensory retina within the nerve fiber layer. Initially, vision may be reduced only mildly, but it decreases gradually with age to end in the 20/200 range. The initial appearance of the macula is that of microcystic elevation with radiating folds in a spoke-like configuration and represents the sine qua non feature of this disease. With time the macula becomes mottled and atrophic. In half of affected patients, the macular changes are the sole pathologic finding. Macular schisis in a young male, with or without reduced vision, should elicit a meticulous examination of the retinal periphery by indirect ophthalmoscopy, particularly the inferotemporal quadrant, to assess for the presence of an associated peripheral schisis or vitreous veils. Vitreous hemorrhage (resulting from torn retinal vessels bridging a schisis cavity) or retinal detachment and sudden deterioration of vision may complicate peripheral schisis that may initially appear as bullous elevation of the inner retina. Because of inner retinal involvement, a negative waveform may be appreciated on electrophysiological testing. The EOG is normal except in advanced disease. X-linked juvenile retinoschisis is one of the most common reasons for unexplained visual loss in young male patients and is easily overlooked. Treatment with laser photocoagulation to delineate schisis areas in an attempt to prevent retinal detachment has been unsuccessful. When retinal detachment occurs, it may be treated in the usual fashion by placement of a scleral buckle. Electrophysiological and histopathologic testing have implicated abnormalities of Muller cells as the causative factor in the development of this disease. The responsible gene (XLRS1) has been sequenced; studies are ongoing to determine the major site of function of the mutated protein. Genetic testing may play an important role in the screening of female carriers who fail to demonstrate a funduscopic carrier state and whose families wish to ascertain future risk of affected male progeny.

GOLDMANN-FAVRE VITREORETINAL DYSTROPHY This is an autosomal-recessive condition characterized by vitreous strands and veils, foveal and peripheral retinoschisis, and peripheral pigmentary retinopathy similar to that seen in retinitis pigmentosa. Decreased visual acuity and nyctalopia are prominent, early findings. Both the ERG and EOG are abnormal and simulate the findings of retinitis pigmentosa with widespread rod and cone loss, differentiating this condition from X-linked juvenile retinoschisis, in which the ERG shows a negative response and the EOG is normal early in the course of disease. There is no known treatment.

STICKLER SYNDROME This syndrome is an autosomal-dominant condition with variable penetrance and expressivity characterized by ocular findings of high myopia, open-angle glaucoma, cataract, vitreoretinal degeneration, perivascular pigmentary retinopathy, and retinal detachment and systemic findings of progressive arthropathy, epiphyseal dysplasia, flat face and cleft palate, and cardiac defects. Some patients manifest changes of the Pierre Robin anomaly. Because of the subtle, yet extensive, nature of the nonocular features of the syndrome, early diagnosis of the disease may depend on a careful eye evaluation. Early diagnosis is critical because appropriate treatment of glaucoma as well as prophylactic laser treatment of high-risk peripheral vitreoretinal pathology may prevent blindness. Mutations in the 12q13 gene sequence coding for type 2 collagen, a major constituent of the vitreous gel and cartilage, lead to the development of this disease.

FAMILIAL EXUDATIVE VITREORETINOPATHY This is an autosomal-dominant condition with variable expressivity characterized by bilateral peripheral retinal nonperfusion and exudation with associated retinal traction resulting in heterotopia of the macula and disc. Peripheral neovascularization, vitreous hemorrhage, and retinal detachment may complicate the course. The disease occurs predominantly in full-term, otherwise healthy children of normal birth weight, with no history of oxygen therapy. Early symptoms and signs may include reduced visual acuity and leukocoria from cataract and retinal detachment. The differential diagnosis includes retinopathy of prematurity, sickle-cell disease, retinal vasculitis including Eales disease, and Coats disease. Patients may benefit from peripheral laser photocoagulation to areas of nonperfusion associated with neovascularization.

26.11.3   Retinal Vascular Anomalies

RETINAL TELANGIECTASIA Retinal telangiectasia, or *Coats disease*, is a nonhereditary, usually unilateral, congenital, morphological anomaly of the retinal vasculature primarily affecting young boys (diagnosed most often between ages 2 and 10 years). Abnormal, leaking, telangiectatic retinal vessels and extensive subretinal lipid exudation are characteristic. The vascular abnormalities include large microaneurysms, irregularly dilated capillaries, and bizarre, sausage-shaped vessels. In advanced lesions, a total exudative retinal detachment can occur with leukocoria, cataract, glaucoma, anterior uveitis, optic atrophy, and phthisis bulbi. Early stages may respond to laser photocoagulation or cryotherapy. The etiology is unknown. The differential diagnosis includes angiomatosis retinae, PHPV, retinopathy of prematurity, *Toxocara* endophthalmitis, retinal cavernous hemangioma, and especially retinoblastoma.

ANGIOMATOSIS RETINAE Angiomatosis retinae, or *von Hippel disease*, is one of the *phakomatoses* (Sec. 26.17.3). Patients may present sporadically with isolated ocular disease (von Hippel disease) or with a history of autosomal-dominant transmission with variable penetrance and expressivity and associated systemic involvement (von Hippel–Lindau disease). Angiomatosis retinae is characterized by the occurrence of one or more retinal angiomas that appear as smooth, pink, elevated preretinal masses fed by a single dilated arteriole and drained by a single dilated vein. Untreated retinal hemangiomas may produce significant subretinal exudation and exudative retinal detachment leading to poor vision and even neovascular glaucoma. Early treatment by laser photocoagulation or cryotherapy may avoid this significant complication. Bilateral retinal lesions indicate germ-line mutations (with or without a family history) and the presence of von Hippel–Lindau disease. Patients should be screened meticulously and imaged regularly for systemic involvement. Systemic manifestations include hemangioblastomas of the cerebellum, medulla, pons, or spinal cord which develop by the fourth or fifth decade of life; renal cell carcinomas, which are the primary cause of death; and tumors and cysts of the epididymis, pancreatic cysts, and pheochromocytomas. The gene for von Hippel–Lindau disease has been mapped to 3p25

and sequenced. The vHL gene is highly conserved and codes for a tumor suppressor.

CONGENITAL RETINAL ARTERIOVENOUS MALFORMATION (AVM) This rare, sporadic vascular anomaly, also known as *racemose hemangioma,* varies in clinical presentation from a single retinal arteriovenous communication to a complex anastomotic system of retinal vessels. Most lesions are unilateral and confined to the retina or optic nerve. Twenty-five percent, however (especially those with severe ocular involvement), are associated with vascular malformations of the midbrain, face, and orbit (*Wyburn-Mason syndrome*) and are classified among the *phakomatoses* (Sec. 26.17.3). Intracranial lesions are associated with hemorrhage, seizures, mental changes, hemiparesis, and papilledema. An absent or improperly developed intervening capillary bed explains the classic tortuous, engorged appearance of the retinal AVM. Vision may be normal, but if the posterior pole is involved it may be very poor. Vitreous hemorrhage or exudation may occasionally complicate the course of disease, but retinal AVMs typically remain static with time; therefore, treatment is usually not advised.

26.11.4   Retinal Vascular Diseases

RETINOPATHY OF PREMATURITY Retinopathy of prematurity (ROP) is a nonhereditary vasoproliferative disorder affecting the peripheral retina of premature infants. The normal retina is vascularized to the ora serrata in the nasal quadrant by 8 months' gestation and in the temporal quadrant 1 to 2 months later. Premature birth and oxygen therapy can interrupt the normal maturation process and set the stage for development of extraretinal vasoproliferation, vitreous hemorrhage, retinal traction, and retinal detachment, the end stages of the disease. ROP is the leading cause of childhood blindness in the United States. Improvements in neonatal care including surfactant use, continuous oxygen monitoring, and improved nutritional supplementation have decreased the incidence of ROP.

Problematic ROP appears to be limited to infants with birth weights less than 1500 g; the majority, in fact, have birth weights less than 1000 g and gestational ages less than 28 weeks. One-third of infants with birth weights less than 1000 g and 7% of infants with birth weights between 1001 and 1500 g develop ROP. Supplemental oxygen administration appears to play a role in the pathogenesis of the disease, but it is not a necessary prerequisite as preterm infants not exposed to supplemental oxygen may also develop ROP. No precise level of oxygen has been demonstrated as safe in the treatment of prematurely born infants. Current nursery practices vary, but in general capillary blood PO_2 levels of 45 to 60 mm Hg are recommended. There appears to be some correlation between the development of ROP and the overall extent of illness, particularly as it relates to anemia, transfusion, infection, intracranial hemorrhage, acidosis, and bronchopulmonary dysplasia.

There are no definitive guidelines for screening infants at risk for ROP. On the basis of a study of nearly 3000 infants with birth weights less than 2000 g, some practical recommendations can be made. First, all infants with birth weights less than 1600 g should be examined, as should all infants with birth weights greater than 1600 g if supplemental oxygen was given for more than 50 days. Second, the optimum time for the initial examination (general physical condition permitting) is 6 to 7 weeks after birth. Third, examinations should be performed weekly or biweekly, as indicated by the rapidity and severity of the disease, until the retina is fully vascularized. Alternatively, gestational age may be a more effective screening guideline. Some workers recommend that all babies less than 34 weeks at birth be examined.

The natural history of ROP begins with a prominent white circumferential vascular border demarcating vascularized and nonvascularized retina. Subsequently the border may increase in size and becomes elevated as a ridge. Later, pink, arborizing vessels may approach the border in brush-like fashion without extending further. The border represents a complex system of arteriovenous shunts. Gradual resolution occurs at or before this stage in over 90% of infants. Patients in whom regression occurs may still develop problems such as myopia, amblyopia, strabismus, and peripheral retinal degeneration in later life. In the other 10% a progressive cicatricial phase ensues with continued elevation of the vascular border, extension of the fibrovascular process into the vitreous cavity, vitreous hemorrhage, peripheral retinal fibrosis and traction, temporal dragging of the disc, vessels, and macula, and partial retinal detachment. Patients with severe disease eventually develop a total, funnel-shaped retinal detachment, extensive fibrovascular proliferation with a white retrolental mass, and leukocoria. The term *retrolental fibroplasia* (RLF) should be reserved for the end-stage cicatricial state, whereas the active vitreoretinal changes are properly referred to as *ROP*.

The 1984 International Classification of Retinopathy of Prematurity is used to grade the extent of retinal pathology. Abnormal findings are categorized by location, stage, and extent (Table 26-9) at the initial visit and at each subsequent follow-up visit. "Plus" disease refers to the vascular incompetence that may accompany progressive forms of ROP. The retinal and iris vessels in plus disease are dilated, tortuous, and unable to maintain the blood-ocular barrier, resulting in vitreous haze and pupillary rigidity.

The Cryotherapy for Retinopathy of Prematurity Cooperative Group demonstrated that the application of cryotherapy to avascular peripheral retina in stage 3+ ROP reduces the risk of retinal detachment, macular traction, and retrolental fibroplasia. Eyes considered eligible for treatment by this protocol have plus disease and at least five contiguous or eight cumulative clock hours of stage 3 ROP in zone 1 or 2. An unfavorable outcome was reported in 22% of treated eyes as opposed to 43% of untreated eyes. Laser photocoagulation treatment of peripheral avascular retina has proved to be as beneficial as cryotherapy with less morbidity. Retinal detachments associated with stage 4 and stage 5 ROP are treated using conventional scleral buckling or pars plana vitrectomy techniques. Although the retina can be reattached successfully in 50% or more of the eyes, only 20 to 30% of the eyes will have useful vision. Other forms of treatment to reduce the incidence or severity of ROP, such as vitamin E, penicillamine, and reduced light in the nursery, have not gained widespread acceptance.

DIABETIC RETINOPATHY Diabetic retinopathy is one of the leading causes of new visual impairment in children in the United States. The duration and control of diabetes mellitus represent the most influential variables in the development and progression of diabetic retinopathy. Eighty percent or more of type 1 diabetics (juvenile-onset) without retinopathy at baseline exhibit some degree of retinopathy after 10 years. Vision-threatening retinopathy is relatively rare within the first 5 years and before puberty. Thus, the American Diabetes Association recommends ophthalmologic examination beginning after puberty and in those with disease of 5 years or more. Subsequent follow-up depends on the baseline severity of disease. The Diabetic Control and Complications Trial demonstrated the efficacy of tight long-term blood glucose control in reducing the development and progression of diabetic complications such as retinopathy. This prospective, controlled study showed conclusively that chronic hyperglycemia is the major determinant of disease progression.

The early stage of *background diabetic retinopathy* (BDR) is characterized by the development of retinal microaneurysms. These are often best appreciated by fluorescein angiography. Intraretinal hemorrhages and exudates with or without retinal edema follow next. Progressive ischemia of the retina that follows in the preproliferative phase is characterized by increasing dot-and-blot and splinter hemorrhages, venous dilation and tortuosity, intraretinal microvascular abnormalities (intraretinal shunts), and large areas of capillary nonperfusion. About 40% of patients with preproliferative retinopathy go on to develop *proliferative diabetic retinopathy* (PDR) within 1 to 2 years. PDR is characterized by neovascularization of the retina and/or optic disc.

Macular nonperfusion and macular edema are the most common causes of slowly progressive vision loss in diabetic retinopathy. Clinically significant macular edema may be amenable to focal or grid laser photocoagulation according to the Early Treatment Diabetic Retinopathy Study. Sudden vision loss in PDR is usually the result of *diabetic vitreous hemorrhage* or traction retinal detachment. Proliferative diabetic retinopathy is amenable to panretinal laser photocoagulation according to the Diabetic Retinopathy Study protocol. Nonclearing vitreous hemorrhage and traction macular detachment may be amenable to surgical interventions such as pars plana vitrectomy, epiretinal membrane peeling, and endolaser photocoagulation.

RETINAL VASCULITIS Children develop retinal vascular disease along with signs of inflammation, such as cells in the aqueous or vitreous, in a variety of disorders. These conditions include pars planitis, sarcoidosis, tuberculosis, syphilis, Lyme disease, toxoplasmosis, CMV retinitis, herpes, and autoimmune diseases. Fluorescein angiography shows staining of the vessel walls with leakage, macular edema, and other signs of retinal ischemia.

Eales disease or idiopathic retinal vasculitis is a bilateral obliterative periphlebitis seen in young males and is characterized by recurrent vitreous hemorrhages from areas of retinal neovascularization. Diagnosis is arrived at by exclusion when diseases such as sickle-cell disease and diabetes, as well as those already mentioned, are eliminated. Retinal photocoagulation to reduce vitreous hem-

TABLE 26-9

INTERNATIONAL CLASSIFICATION OF ACUTE STAGES OF RETINOPATHY OF PREMATURITY

Location	Three zones, centered on the optic disc
Zone 1	Circle with radius of 30°, twice the disc-macula distance
Zone 2	From the edge of zone 1 to a point tangential to the ora serrata nasally and the equator temporally
Zone 3	Residual crescent anterior to zone 2 temporally
Extent	Specified as clock hours of involvement
Stage	
Stage 1	Demarcation line
Stage 2	Ridge
Stage 3	Ridge with extraretinal fibrovascular proliferation
Stage 4	Subtotal retinal detachment
Stage 5	Total retinal detachment
Plus disease	Marked arteriovenous shunting of blood with tortuous and dilated retinal vessels in posterior pole, vitreous haze, and pupillary rigidity

orrhage may be of benefit in eyes with severe ischemia and neovascularization.

26.11.5 Metabolic Diseases Affecting the Retina

MUCOPOLYSACCHARIDOSES These conditions are discussed in detail in Sec. 9.8.1. Ophthalmologic findings include corneal clouding (Sec. 26.7.4), pigmentary retinal degeneration, and optic atrophy (see Table 26-3). The retinal degeneration may resemble that seen in retinitis pigmentosa and is thought to develop from excessive accumulation of acid mucopolysaccharide in retinal pigment epithelial cells. The ERG is variably decreased and may demonstrate a rod-cone pattern of degeneration. Optic atrophy develops either as a result of ganglion cell death from accumulation of acid mucopolysaccharide or from elevated intracranial pressure and hydrocephalus.

SPHINGOLIPIDOSES These conditions are discussed in Sec. 9.9. With the exception of cornea verticellata seen in X-linked Fabry disease, corneal clouding is not a prominent feature of the sphingolipidoses. The principal ophthalmologic finding is the cherry-red spot (see Table 26-3). This spot develops because the macula is whitened by the accumulation of sphingolipid in multiple layers of ganglion cells, highlighting the normal red color of the central macula, which is devoid of ganglion cells. Optic atrophy follows ganglion cell death, and the cherry-red spot may fade.

MUCOLIPIDOSES The mucolipidoses are discussed in Sec. 9.8.2. Ophthalmologic features may include corneal clouding, retinal pigmentary degeneration, cherry-red spot, and optic atrophy (see Table 26-3). They share features with the mucopolysaccharidoses and sphingolipidoses.

26.11.6 Retinitis and Vitritis

CYTOMEGALOVIRUS (CMV) RETINITIS CMV is a common cause of intrauterine infection. Retinitis develops in 5 to 30% of neonates with clinically apparent CMV infection. It also occurs in compromised hosts and in 5% of children infected with the human immunodeficiency virus. Presenting signs and symptoms in verbal children include floaters, decreased vision, and loss of visual field. Pain, photophobia, and conjunctival injection are absent. Leukocoria may be the only sign in neonates. Associated ocular findings in newborns include microphthalmia, cataract, optic atrophy, and optic-disc malformation. The process is frequently bilateral. Active lesions are perivascular and may appear as cheesy white necrosis, often with associated intraretinal hemorrhages, or as granular, indolent changes. Histopathologic examination of eyes reveals full-thickness retinal pigment epithelial necrosis. Atrophic retinal holes are common, as is retinal detachment. The differential diagnosis in congenital disease includes toxoplasmosis, rubella, herpes simplex infection, and syphilis.

Patients with AIDS have benefited from highly active antiretroviral therapy (HAART), consisting of a combination of nucleoside and nonnucleoside reverse transcriptase and protease inhibitors. Specifically, CD4 T-lymphocyte counts are increased, viral DNA loads decreased, survival lengthened, and the incidence of CMV retinitis reduced in patients receiving HAART therapy. Because of noncompliance or drug resistance, however, CMV retinitis continues to be a common ocular complication of AIDS. Intravenous ganciclovir is the drug of choice for CMV retinitis. Foscarnet is usually reserved for ganciclovir-resistant CMV infections. Retinal detachments may be repaired by pars plana vitrectomy and intracameral silicone oil injection, but visual function is often limited when the macula has been involved by the retinitis (see Sec. 26.11.8).

ENDOPHTHALMITIS Inflammation affecting one or more layers of the eye and an adjacent cavity (anterior chamber, posterior chamber, vitreous cavity) is termed *endophthalmitis*. Most instances are infectious. Endophthalmitis is classified by the route of entry, infecting organism, and setting. *Exogenous endophthalmitis* accounts for 90% of lesions. Trauma and eye surgery are the usual settings; bacteria, particularly staphylococci, are the usual organisms, but other involved bacteria include *S. pneumoniae, E. coli, Proteus,* pseudomonas, and *H. influenzae.* Fungi and parasites may be responsible at times. *Endogenous endophthalmitis* by the hematogenous route, as occurs in subacute bacterial endocarditis, accounts for the remaining 10%. Presenting signs and symptoms include pain, photophobia, reduced vision, eyelid edema, leukocoria, and ocular injection. White-centered retinal hemorrhages (*Roth spots*) may be seen in endogenous endophthalmitis. Cotton-wool spots and/or focal retinitis are additional features. Fungal retinitis and vitritis, which may be associated with a fluffy white granuloma or snowballs in the vitreous, have been seen with increasing frequency because of the widespread use of immunosuppressive agents and indwelling catheters. Prompt referral to an ophthalmologist is indicated if endophthalmitis is suspected. A paracentesis and vitreous biopsy for Gram stain and culture must be performed promptly. Broad-spectrum topical, intracameral, and intravenous antibiotics should be administered pending the results of culture and sensitivity testing.

26.11.7 Retinoblastoma

Retinoblastoma (RB) is the most common primary intraocular malignancy of childhood. It occurs with an incidence of 1 in 14,000 to 1 in 20,000 live births. An estimated 250 to 300 new patients are seen each year in the United States. The average age at diagnosis is 18 months, and 90% are diagnosed before 3 years of age. There is no race or sex predilection. Tumors occur bilaterally in 30 to 35% of patients.

RB occurs sporadically in approximately 90% of patients. Twenty-five percent result from germinal mutations, and 75% result from somatic mutations. The other 10% of patients with RB have a positive family history and an autosomal-dominant hereditary pattern with 80% penetrance. Those with sporadic germ-line mutations or a positive family history are at risk of propagating the defective gene to future progeny. These patients typically, but not invariably, present with bilateral retinoblastoma and are at risk of second primary tumors elsewhere. Children with unilateral presentation and their parents should be meticulously examined by ophthalmoscopy to rule out bilateral or familial involvement that would implicate a germ-line mutation. Genetic counseling of patients with RB is complex, but a few generalizations can be made. Healthy parents with one affected child run a 6% risk of producing other affected children. If two or more children are affected, each additional child has a 50% risk of developing RB. A survivor of hereditary RB has a 50% chance of transmitting the tumor to offspring.

Bilateral RB almost always indicates a hereditary or germ-line mutation.

RB appears to develop only when both alleles of a tumor suppresser gene located on 13q14 are absent or defective. In hereditary RB every cell in the body inherits one absent or defective gene. During normal development, a mutagenic "hit" to the remaining normal allele results in the loss of normal cellular growth regulation and tumor development. In sporadic, nonhereditary RB, a single somatic cell must receive two mutagenic hits to the 13q14 tumor suppressor gene before RB can be expressed. Variable deletions of the long arm of chromosome 13 are uncommonly found in patients with RB; point mutations are the most common events.

RB commonly appears as a white or cream-colored nodular mass. Histopathologically, the tumor is composed of tightly packed undifferentiated retinoblasts that show variable degrees of photoreceptor differentiation (rosettes and fleurettes). The blood supply is invariably inadequate, and patchy necrosis and degeneration with calcium deposition are characteristic. Because calcium is uncommon in other lesions and is present in 80% of patients with RB, its demonstration on radiographic study, preferably with CT scan of the orbit, is an important diagnostic sign.

The clinical characteristics of RB depend on the stage of tumor growth at the time of its discovery. When a tumor is small and at the posterior pole, the initial sign may be sensory strabismus. As the tumor grows, *leukocoria* (white pupil) develops. Leukocoria is the presenting sign of RB in 61% of patients. RB has a tendency to seed other ocular tissues through the vitreous or subretinal fluid and may lead to secondary glaucoma, uveitis, endophthalmitis, and buphthalmos. Other unusual presentations include hyphema, heterochromia, unilateral mydriasis, orbital cellulitis, and proptosis.

The eye harboring RB is usually uninflamed and of normal size for age, and the anterior chamber is of normal depth. The diagnosis is usually established with a reasonable degree of certainty by ophthalmoscopic examination and radiographic demonstration of calcium. The differential diagnosis of RB includes PHPV, retinal detachment, Coats disease, glial hamartomas, retinal hemangiomas, myelinated nerve fibers, congenital cataract, chorioretinal coloboma, uveitis, larval granulomatosis, congenital retinal folds, retinal dysplasia, and retinopathy of prematurity. When the diagnosis of RB is in doubt, fine-needle biopsy of the tumor is sometimes performed. A CT or MR imaging scan of the brain should be part of the assessment of all bilateral RB because of the association of intracranial tumor in the pineal gland (*trilateral retinoblastoma*).

When the possibility of metastasis is considered, a CT or MR scan of the brain, chest radiograph, bone scan, bone marrow biopsy, and spinal fluid examination for tumor cells should be performed. RB has a predilection for invading the optic nerve, and by extension it may reach the subarachnoid space and brain. Intracranial extension is the most common cause of death. Local spread may also occur into the choroid, orbit, and lymphatics. Hematogenous metastases to bone (skull, ribs, humerus) are frequent; metastases to viscera and lymph nodes occur less often.

The prognosis in RB depends on the size and location of tumors and the degree of ocular and extraocular involvement. If a tumor is unilateral and small and the eye is treated promptly, the chance of survival is over 90%. Once the tumor has extended into the optic nerve, the cure rate may substantially decrease according to the extent of nerve that is histologically involved. Overall, survival with any degree of nerve involvement is only about 50%. Extraocular extension of course is another poor prognostic factor. Spontaneous tumor regression occurs in 1.8% of patients. The "regressed" lesion actually represents an old benign *retinoma,* presumably the result

of a second mutation occurring too late in retinal differentiation to result in a malignant tumor. New primary tumors develop in approximately 15% of survivors of bilateral RB, with an average latent interval of 10 years; this number typically increases with time. Most are osteogenic sarcomas, more commonly in rather than out of the field of radiation.

Photocoagulation can be used for small tumors confined to the retina. Peripheral tumors too large to treat effectively with photocoagulation may be treated more appropriately with cryotherapy. Eyes with extensive tumor, tumor seeding of the vitreous cavity, or neovascular glaucoma are enucleated. External beam radiotherapy and scleral plaque brachytherapy are usually used to treat the second eye of patients with bilateral RB after the eye with the more advanced tumor has been enucleated. Chemotherapy has been promoted as a modality to debulk advanced tumors to allow the administration of more localized therapy instead of external beam radiation and enucleation. Chemoreduction may increase visual outcome and decrease the incidence of second primary tumors. Chemotherapy may also be used as an adjunct to primary surgery in those cases that are high risk for metastasis such as eyes with optic nerve or scleral invasion.

26.11.8   Retinal Detachment

Retinal detachment (RD) is rare in infants and children and is usually caused by trauma or ROP. The principal types of RD are rhegmatogenous (i.e., associated with a hole or tear in the retina), exudative, and tractional. Eye surgery, high myopia, inferior temporal dialysis, retinoblastoma, lattice retinal degeneration, morning glory disc anomaly or optic nerve coloboma, PHPV, uveitis, Coats disease, proliferative diabetic retinopathy, and CMV retinitis are ocular conditions that may be complicated by various types of RD in the pediatric population. RD is in the differential diagnosis of *leukocoria.* It is important to examine the retina following any significant blunt eye or head trauma because of the inability of most children to give a history of decreasing vision. Syndromes with juvenile retinal detachment include X-linked retinoschisis, Wagner vitreoretinal dystrophy, Stickler syndrome, Norrie disease, and familial exudative vitreoretinopathy. Treatment is by scleral buckling and/or pars plana vitrectomy techniques.

References

Albert DM, Jakobiec FA, eds: Principles and Practice of Ophthalmology, 2nd ed. Philadelphia, Saunders, 1994

American College of Physicians, American Diabetes Association, and American Academy of Ophthalmology: Screening guidelines for diabetic retinopathy. Ann Intern Med 116(8):683, 1992

Ben Sera I, Nissenkorn I, Kremer I: Retinopathy of prematurity. Surv Ophthalmol 33:1, 1988

Benson WE: Diabetic retinopathy. In: Duane TD, Jaeger EA, eds: Clinical Ophthalmology. Philadelphia, Lippincott-Raven, 1997

Bird AC: Retinal photoreceptor dystrophies. LIV Edward Jackson Memorial Lecture. Am J Ophthalmol 119(5):543, 1995

Bloome MA, Garcia CA: Manual of Retinal and Choroidal Dystrophies. New York, Appleton-Century-Crofts, 1982

Cavender JC, Ai E, Lee ST: Hereditary macular dystrophies. In: Duane TD, Jaeger EA, eds: Clinical Ophthalmology. Philadelphia, Lippincott, 1993

Committee for the Classification of Retinopathy of Prematurity: An international classification of retinopathy of prematurity. Arch Ophthalmol 102:1130, 1984

Cryotherapy for Retinopathy of Prematurity Cooperative Group: Multicenter trial of cryotherapy for retinopathy of prematurity. Preliminary results. Arch Ophthalmol 106:471, 1988

Diabetes Control and Complications Trial Research Group: Progression of retinopathy with intensive versus conventional treatment in the Diabetes Control and Complications Trial. Ophthalmology 102(4):647, 1995

Diabetic Retinopathy Study Research Group: Clinical application of Diabetic Retinopathy Study (DRS) findings, DRS report number 8. Ophthalmology 88(7):583, 1981

Early Treatment Diabetic Retinopathy Study Research Group: Photocoagulation for diabetic macular edema. ETDRS report number 1. Arch Ophthalmol 103:1796, 1985

Gass JD: Stereoscopic Atlas of Macular Diseases: Diagnosis and Treatment, 4th ed. St. Louis, Mosby, 1997

Goldberg MF: Persistent fetal vasculature: An integrated interpretation of signs and symptoms associated with persistent hyperplastic primary vitreous (PHPV). LIV Edward Jackson Memorial Lecture. Am J Ophthalmol 124(5):587–626, 1997

Heckenlively JR: Retinitis Pigmentosa. Philadelphia, Lippincott, 1988

Hunter DG, Mukai S: Retinopathy of prematurity: Pathogenesis, dysgenesis, and treatment. Int Ophthalmol Clin 32:163, 1992

International Committee for the Classification of the Late Stages of Retinopathy of Prematurity: An international classification of retinopathy of prematurity: II. The classification of retinal detachment. Arch Ophthalmol 105:906, 1987

Klein R, Klein BEK, Moss SE, Cruickshanks KJ: The Wisconsin epidemiologic study of diabetic retinopathy: XIV. Ten-year incidence and progression of diabetic retinopathy. Arch Ophthalmol 112:1217, 1994

Rimoin DL, Connor JM, Pyeritz RE, eds: Emery and Rimoin's Principles and Practice of Medical Genetics, 3rd ed. New York, Churchill Livingstone, 1997

Ryan SJ, Ogden TE, Schachat AP, Murphy RP, Glaser BM, eds: Retina, 2nd ed. St Louis, Mosby, 1994

Sarraf D, Schwartz JS, Lee DA: Ocular size and shape. In: Isenberg SJ, ed: The Eye in Infancy, 2nd ed. St. Louis, Mosby, 1994

Shields JA, Shields CL: Current management of retinoblastoma. Mayo Clin Proc 69:50, 1994

Shields JA, Shields CL: Intraocular Tumors: A Text and Atlas. Philadelphia, Saunders, 1992

Yannuzzi LA, Guyer DR, Green RW: The Retina Atlas. St. Louis, Mosby, 1995

26.12　OPTIC NERVE

26.12.1　Congenital Anomalies

OPTIC NERVE HYPOPLASIA　Optic nerve aplasia is extremely rare, and most often the diagnosis represents an extreme example of optic nerve hypoplasia. Optic nerve hypoplasia is characterized by a reduction in the number of axons within the optic nerve. The nerve head is small and pale, and there may be a white or yellow peripapillary halo surrounded by a ring of pigment (*double ring sign*) corresponding to the size of a normal disc. The retinal vasculature is normal. On radiographic study the optic canal is small. Visual acuity ranges from normal to no light perception but is stable over time. Various visual defects may be found, and often there is an afferent pupillary defect (*Marcus Gunn pupil*). The majority are sporadic; familial instances are rare. The diagnosis can be difficult if optic nerve hypoplasia is mild because the decrease in disc size may be inapparent, and visual acuity may be normal or only slightly affected. Disc photography and quantitative assessment of optic nerve head features by a nerve head analyzer may be helpful in establishing a diagnosis.

In unilateral disorders, serious central nervous system abnormalities are generally absent. Patients are typically seen because of strabismus and decreased vision. Amblyopia may develop and should be treated if the visual impairment is not profound. In bilateral optic nerve hypoplasia, particularly in severe forms, poor vision and nystagmus may be apparent early in life, and there may be associated neurologic and endocrinologic abnormalities such as mental retardation, delayed development, seizures, deafness, cerebral atrophy, hemiparesis, ventricular defects, porencephalic cyst, hypopituitarism, hypothyroidism, and diabetes insipidus. Optic nerve hypoplasia has been associated with maternal diabetes; maternal use of quinine, anticonvulsants, lysergic acid diethylamide (LSD), aminopterin; in utero cytomegalic infection; toxemia; adolescent pregnancy; ocular disorders such as aniridia, albinism, colobomas, Duane retraction syndrome, high myopia; and a number of neurologic and pediatric diseases and syndromes.

Septo-optic dysplasia, or *de Morsier syndrome,* is one of the more common bilateral optic nerve hypoplasia syndromes. It is characterized by midline central nervous system abnormalities such as hypothalamic dysfunction, pituitary dysfunction, and genesis of the septum pellucidum. Additional findings may include malformation of the optic chiasm and agenesis of the corpus callosum. Because of the high incidence of associated central nervous system anomalies and endocrinologic problems, all patients with optic nerve hypoplasia, particularly if bilateral, need a complete neurologic work-up including brain CT or MR imaging and an endocrinologic evaluation that includes growth hormone, adrenal, and thyroid function. Early recognition and treatment of the hormonal imbalance permits prompt ophthalmologic management and helps the child achieve normal growth and development.

COLOBOMA OF THE OPTIC NERVE　Optic nerve coloboma is a type of dysplasia of the optic nerve caused by faulty closure of the optic fissure during embryogenesis. It may be unilateral or bilateral. Most instances are sporadic or transmitted as an autosomal-dominant gene with variable penetrance. At one end of the spectrum, optic nerve coloboma may be isolated to the optic disc and have no effect on visual function; at the other end of the spectrum, it may be one part of a larger defect involving much of the uveal tract and retina with profound vision loss. Mild, isolated optic nerve colobomas may resemble deep optic cups or pits that have no appreciable affect on vision. Severe colobomas are usually associated with large excavations of the optic nerve and peripapillary area, gliosis, poor vision, and marked visual field defects. Congenital colobomatous anomalies of the optic disc associated with midline facial abnormalities or hypertelorism may be evidence of a basal encephalocele. Optic nerve colobomas are commonly associated with congenital multisystem anomalies. Colobomas of the optic nerve have been called "pseudoglaucoma" because they resemble glaucomatous cupping.

OPTIC NERVE PITS　Optic nerve pits are a mild form of nerve head coloboma characterized by dark gray, oval or slit-like holes in the disc, usually on the inferotemporal side or centrally. Cilioretinal arteries are frequently associated. They are usually unilateral and most often have no hereditary pattern. A wide variation in visual acuity can occur. Optic pits are important clinically because they may produce arcuate scotomas and serous retinal detachments. Although retinal detachment has been seen in children in the first decade, it occurs in up to 50% of the patients at a mean age of 31 years. Systemic abnormalities are not commonly associated with congenital optic nerve pits.

MORNING GLORY DISC ANOMALY This optic disc anomaly can be considered an extreme form of optic nerve coloboma. Most instances are unilateral and nonfamilial; rarely, they are bilateral and genetically inherited. The anomaly is characterized by an enlarged, funnel-shaped, excavated disc with a central core of white glial tissue, surrounded by a raised annulus of pigmented subretinal tissue. The disc appearance resembles the morning glory flower. It is twice as common in females as in males, and the right eye is more frequently involved if the lesion is unilateral. Visual acuity is usually 20/100 or worse; high myopia and visual field defects are prominent. Serous retinal detachment is the most serious ocular complication and may occur in up to one-third of the patients. Although usually an isolated eye abnormality, the disc anomaly on occasion has been associated with other systemic anomalies.

MYELINATED NERVE FIBERS Myelination of the optic nerve usually ceases at the lamina cribrosa just before birth. Occasionally, it proceeds distally and produces a congenital, white, feathery opacification of the neuroretinal rim and peripapillary retina. Visual acuity is unaffected unless the fovea is myelinated. The blind spot may be enlarged. This condition is bilateral in 20% of patients. Extensive myelinated nerve fibers have been associated with high myopia and amblyopia.

PERSISTENCE OF THE HYALOIDAL SYSTEM If the hyaloidal vascular system fails to regress completely before birth, remnants may be seen on examination of the posterior segment of the eye. What remains in most instances is a small tuft of glial tissue extending a short distance into the vitreous cavity (*Bergmeister papilla.*) Rarely, a patent vessel containing blood is seen extending from the optic disc to the posterior lens capsule, usually attaching inferonasal to the optical center. These findings, including the *Mittendorf dot,* fall within the spectrum of PHPV.

OPTIC NERVE DRUSEN Intrapapillary drusen or *hyaline bodies of the optic nerve head* are tiny white or yellow translucent masses of hyaline-like material buried within the substance of the optic nerve head anterior to the lamina cribrosa. They occur almost exclusively in whites, with an incidence of 0.3 to 1.0% clinically and 2% histopathologically. They are bilateral in 75 to 80% of cases. In young children, the masses are inconspicuous, but within one to two decades they become visible on the surface of the disc as shiny, refractile bodies that glow with indirect light. They may elevate the nerve head, thus simulating papilledema (*pseudopapilledema*). Drusen of the optic disc can be identified in at least 75% of the instances of pseudopapilledema. Pseudopapilledema and neurologic disorders that frequently coexist in children with optic nerve drusen may lead to unnecessary neuroradiologic and neurosurgical investigations for exclusion of an intracranial process. Because drusen of the optic nerve is inherited as an autosomal-dominant trait, ophthalmoscopic examination of family members may disclose similar lesions and thus help establish the correct diagnosis in a child with pseudopapilledema. Ophthalmoscopy is diagnostic if the drusen are visible. Ultrasonography and fluorescein angiography may be helpful ancillary tests if the drusen are buried. In adulthood, visual field defects may appear and progress slowly. Central visual acuity is usually unaffected.

26.12.2 Optic Disc Edema

This disorder is characterized by elevation and congestion of the optic nerve head, blurring of the disc margin, obliteration of the physiological cup, venous congestion, loss of spontaneous venous pulsations, peripapillary splinter hemorrhages, and edema of the peripapillary retina. Fluorescein angiography typically shows disc capillary dilation and dye leakage, with late fluorescence. Optic disc edema has a variety of causes including increased intracranial pressure, when it is called *papilledema*. Papilledema is almost always bilateral. It may fail to develop in infants with increased intracranial pressure because of open fontanels. Two ocular conditions protect the eye from papilledema, namely, high myopia (5–10 diopters) and optic atrophy. Visual acuity, color vision, and pupillary responses are rarely affected in the acute stage unless the macula is involved by edema, hemorrhage, or exudate, although the blind spot may be enlarged. Diplopia may occur secondary to sixth cranial nerve palsy or divergence insufficiency. Chronic disc edema may lead to optic atrophy and vision loss.

Optic disc edema is differentiated from *optic neuritis* or *papillitis* by the absence of inflammatory cells in the vitreous, the lack of a central scotoma, and the lack of pain on eye movement. Optic disc edema and papillitis may be mistaken for *pseudopapilledema,* in which disc "swelling" is secondary to nerve head drusen, excessive glial tissue on the surface of the disc, hyperopia, or myelinated nerve fibers. Papilledema is a neurologic emergency. After the history and physical examination, cranial imaging by CT or MR should be done to rule out an intracranial mass. If the scan is negative, a lumbar puncture should be performed. Conditions that produce optic disc edema in children include tumors (craniopharyngioma, cerebellar medulloblastoma), subdural hematoma, subarachnoid hemorrhage, head injuries, hydrocephalus, central nervous system infections (Guillain-Barré syndrome, meningitis), and pseudotumor cerebri. Treatment is directed to the underlying cause.

PSEUDOTUMOR CEREBRI Also known as *benign intracranial hypertension,* pseudotumor cerebri is characterized by papilledema, normal cerebrospinal fluid composition, normal or small ventricular system on radiography, and absence of an intracranial mass. Patients complain of headache, tinnitus, dizziness, blurred vision, and diplopia. Although typically patients are obese young women, the condition is seen in children of both sexes. The cause often is unknown but can occur with steroid withdrawal, vitamin A intoxication, ciprofloxacin- and tetracycline-type drug ingestion, head trauma or surgery, dural sinus thrombosis, hyperviscosity syndromes, and systemic lupus erythematosus. Children tend to tolerate papilledema better than adults, but visual loss can result. Treatment to reduce CSF pressure and prevent permanent visual loss includes serial lumbar punctures, diuretics, optic nerve sheath decompression, and lumboperitoneal shunt procedures (see Sec. 25.7).

26.12.3 Optic Neuritis

Optic neuritis implies inflammation of the optic nerve. The term *optic nerve* is a misnomer; this central nervous system structure is more accurately described as a tract of the brain. Inflammation of the nerve posterior to the globe is called *retrobulbar optic neuritis;* inflammation occurring at the nerve head is called *papillitis.* In children papillitis is more common than retrobulbar optic neuritis. The reverse is true of adults. In addition, bilateral involvement is the general rule in children, whereas monocular involvement is typical in adults. Optic neuritis is characterized by profound loss of visual acuity within hours or days, pain on eye movement or globe retrodisplacement, the development of a central scotoma, depressed color vision, and the developemnt of an afferent pupillary defect. Worsening of vision with exercise or fever has been referred to as *Uhtoff sign.*

Fully developed papillitis may be difficult to distinguish from papilledema on ophthalmoscopy. The appearance of inflammatory cells in the vitreous on slit-lamp examination is a helpful distinction. Hemorrhages around the disc are rare.

Pediatric optic neuritis may result from inflammation of contiguous structures or from systemic infection. Optic neuritis secondary to meningoencephalitis is common. The optic nerves can be involved by spread from orbital abscesses, cellulitis, and foci of infection in the teeth, tonsils, and sinuses. Optic neuritis can develop in the setting of infectious viral diseases such as measles, mumps, chickenpox, poliomyelitis, mononucleosis, influenza, and smallpox; it has been reported following vaccination for viral diseases as well. Optic neuritis usually appears 1 to 2 weeks after the onset of an infectious illness and resolves completely. Even with apparently full recovery, pallor of the disc and nerve fiber layer defects may be seen. Marked loss of vision occasionally results, with partial or complete atrophy of the nerve. Optic neuritis may also occur with syphilis, Guillain-Barré syndrome, Behçet disease, various leukodystrophies, and Schilder and Devic diseases. Optic neuritis is rarely associated with multiple sclerosis (MS) in children.

Longitudinal studies in adults have shown a clear association between optic neuritis and MS. The majority of women who have a single episode of optic neuritis eventually develop MS. The conversion rate for men is slightly lower. In contrast, papillitis and retrobulbar optic neuritis in childhood appear to be self-limited with little risk for subsequent central nervous system involvement.

The recent Optic Neuritis Treatment Trial study in adults found that intravenous methylprednisolone (1 g/d for 3 days) followed by oral prednisone (1 mg/kg/d for 11 days) hastened the rate of visual recovery from optic neuritis in adults but did not affect final visual outcome. Treatment with oral prednisone alone was no better than placebo. Intravenous methylprednisolone treatment also reduced the 2-year incidence of definite MS (a new neurologic deficit occurring at least 4 weeks after the onset of optic neuritis) by more than 50%. It is not likely that these data can be generalized to pediatric patients.

26.12.4   Tumors of the Optic Nerve

Tumors involving the optic nerve produce proptosis and progressive vision loss. Strabismus and an afferent pupillary defect may also occur. For a complete discussion of tumors of the orbit, see Sec. 26.14.3.

OPTIC NERVE GLIOMA This tumor is the fourth most common orbital tumor of childhood. It is the most common tumor of the optic nerve in childhood. Ninety percent of optic gliomas are seen by the end of the second decade of life. The peak incidence is between ages 2 and 6 years; 75% become apparent before age 10. From 25 to 50% of patients have neurofibromatosis. From 15 to 25% of patients with neurofibromatosis type 1 have optic nerve gliomas. Optic nerve gliomas may arise anywhere along the optic

nerve including the chiasm. Gliomas anterior to the chiasm behave in a benign fashion; those in and posterior to the chiasm may be more aggressive. When they arise in the orbit, they produce the signs and symptoms mentioned below. Ophthalmoscopic findings may include optic disc edema, optic atrophy, and retinal striae from pressure by the tumor on the posterior surface of the globe. *Chiasmal gliomas* cause bilateral vision loss and optic atrophy without proptosis. An afferent pupillary defect may develop if one optic nerve is compressed more than the other. If a chiasmal glioma enlarges sufficiently, endocrine dysfunction may ensue from compression of the pituitary gland and hypothalamus. Hydrocephalus, head nodding, and nystagmus may develop as a result of compression of the third ventricle. The diagnosis of optic nerve glioma is made by the clinical findings and the typical appearance of the tumor on ultrasonography, CT scan, or MR imaging. Orbital tumors produce a fusiform enlargement of the optic nerve. Enlargement of the optic foramen and sella tursica have also been observed. Histopathologically, optic nerve gliomas are pilocytic astrocytomas of the juvenile type.

Treatment is controversial. Some authors believe optic nerve gliomas are benign hamartomas and do not require treatment. Other authors advocate surgical excision or radiotherapy because some tumors tend to have an aggressive behavior. A reasonable management approach is as follows. If there is minimal visual loss without proptosis, keep the child under observation. Some tumors fail to grow or may even regress. If there is progressive loss of vision with little or no proptosis, either continue to observe the child or consider radiotherapy, which in some instances stabilizes growth of the tumor and vision. Surgical excision is probably not indicated unless disfiguring proptosis develops or there is extension toward the chiasm. Gliomas do not metastasize. When excision is necessary, the globe can usually be spared even though it is blind. For chiasmal gliomas, surgery is not advised; radiotherapy seems to be the best method of treatment.

OPTIC NERVE MENINGIOMA This tumor is seen more often in adulthood and is five times more common in females than males. Presenting signs, symptoms, and ophthalmoscopic findings are the same as for optic nerve glioma. This tumor is also associated with *neurofibromatosis.* The compressive optic neuropathy produced by optic nerve meningioma may result in blindness, optic atrophy, and the formation of optociliary shunt vessels (vessels that shunt blood from the retinal to the choroidal venous circulation). Imaging studies may demonstrate a discrete mass or diffuse thickening of the optic nerve. Following contrast injection, the periphery of the nerve enhances, the so-called railroad track sign. Histopathologically, optic nerve meningiomas arise from arachnoid meningoendothelial cells. Treatment is by surgical excision if the tumor causes disfiguring proptosis or if it extends into the optic foramen.

26.12.5   Optic Atrophy

Optic atrophy is the ultimate result of optic nerve injury, regardless of cause. It is characterized by ganglion cell and axon loss, nerve head pallor, reduced visual acuity, scotoma development, poor color vision, and the development of an afferent pupillary defect (APD). Common conditions leading to optic atrophy in children are summarized in Table 26-10. Traumatic optic neuropathy is discussed in Sec. 26.16.4. The optic nerve head of the normal, healthy infant is paler than that of the adult; therefore, a diagnosis of optic

TABLE 26-10

ETIOLOGY AND DISORDERS ASSOCIATED WITH OPTIC ATROPHY IN INFANTS AND CHILDREN

CATEGORY	CONDITION
Hereditary	Primary optic atrophy
	Behr optic atrophy
	Leber optic atrophy
	DIDMOAD syndrome (diabetes insipidus, diabetes mellitus, optic atrophy, deafness)
Heredodegenerative	Mucopolysaccharidoses I–VI
	Wolman disease
	G_{M1}-gangliosidosis I
	Sandhoff disease
	Tay-Sachs disease
	Juvenile G_{M2}-gangliosidosis
	Niemann-Pick disease
	Krabbe disease
	Pelizaeus-Merzbacher disease
	Metachromatic leukodystrophy
	Hagberg-Santavuori disease
	Spielmeyer-Vogt disease
	Jansky-Bielschowsky disease
	Kufs disease
	Gyrate atrophy
	Zellweger syndrome
	Adrenoleukodystrophy
	Refsum disease
	Abetalipoproteinemia
	Charcot-Marie-Tooth disease
	Acrodermatitis enteropathica
	Acute, intermittent porphyria
	Retinitis pigmentosa syndromes
Developmental	Neonatal anoxia
	Glaucoma
	Posttraumatic
	Hydrocephalus
	Postpapilledema
Infectious/inflammatory	Syphilis
	Acute viral illness
	Optic neuritis
Demyelinating	Spinocerebellar degeneration
	Multiple sclerosis
Compressive	Optic nerve glioma
	Meningioma
	Craniopharyngioma
	Fibrous dysplasia
	Graves disease
	Pituitary adenoma
Toxic/nutritional	Methanol
	Chloramphenicol
	Ethambutol
	Lead
	Vitamin B_{12} deficiency
	Thiamine deficiency
	Folate deficiency

atrophy and blindness in the infant should be made only when one is sure of the findings. Optic nerve hypoplasia and other congenital disc anomalies are much more common than optic atrophy in the first year of life.

When optic atrophy in a child presents a difficult diagnostic problem, the investigation should include a detailed family history; a search for metabolic or toxic factors; a careful eye examination;

imaging studies of the skull, orbits, and optic foramina; and other ancillary tests such as ultrasonography, arteriography, EEG, ERG, and VEP. Many children with visual impairment exhibit self-mutilating behavior such as eye pressing. A useful clinical pearl is that children blind from retinal disorders are more likely to rub their eyes (oculodigital phenomena) than children blind from disorders of the optic nerve or cortex.

AUTOSOMAL-DOMINANT HEREDITARY OPTIC ATROPHY Autosomal-dominant (juvenile) optic atrophy is the most common form of hereditary optic atrophy. Mild to moderate reduction in vision with no nystagmus becomes apparent between 4 and 8 years of age. Bilateral vision loss is slowly progressive throughout life. A cecocentral scotoma with impaired color vision and normal ERG are characteristic. The genetic defect has been localized to chromosome 3.

OPTIC ATROPHY WITH INHERITED NEUROLOGIC SYNDROMES Optic atrophy may be seen in inherited neurologic diseases that include Behr, Canavan, Charcot-Marie-Tooth, infantile subacute necrotizing encephalomyelopathy, Friedreich ataxia, and familial dysautonomia. These diseases are inherited as an autosomal-recessive trait, with Charcot-Marie-Tooth disease inherited also as an X-linked recessive disorder.

LEBER OPTIC ATROPHY This is a heredofamilial optic atrophy (not to be confused with Leber congenital amaurosis) characterized by normal visual function until the late teens or early twenties. Typically, within an interval of weeks to months, both eyes develop a low-grade optic neuritis with marked disc edema, sometimes associated with peripapillary hemorrhages and exudates, peripapillary telangiectasia, and a drop in visual acuity to the 20/200 level. Disc swelling resolves within a few weeks of onset, leaving flat, pale discs and dense bilateral cecocentral scotomas. There may be associated neurologic abnormalities such as paraplegia, spasticity, dementia, deafness, and migraine headaches. Dye leakage does not occur on fluorescein angiography during the acute stage. Leber optic atrophy is a maternally transmitted disorder involving the mitochondrial chromosome; men do not transmit the disease to their offspring. Every son and daughter of a female carrier inherits the trait, but only 50% of sons and 10% of daughters are affected.

26.12.6 Glaucoma

Glaucoma refers to a condition in which "elevated" intraocular pressure (IOP) is related to the development of a characteristic optic neuropathy and a loss of visual function. The susceptibility of the optic nerve to pressure damage varies from person to person; therefore, it is not possible to define what "high" and "safe" pressures are for any given individual. The average IOP for infants and children is the same as that for adults, about 16.5 mm Hg. The 2–standard deviation interval is 10 to 22 mm Hg. Not all patients with glaucoma have IOP above 22 mm Hg, and not all children whose IOP is within the "normal" range are safe from glaucoma.

Pediatricians should learn to identify infants and children with glaucoma early because the threat to vision is serious and the prognosis is poor unless glaucoma is recognized and treated promptly. Once characteristic ocular signs and symptoms arouse suspicion, referral to an ophthalmologist is indicated. The diagnosis is confirmed by measuring the IOP (Sec. 26.1.7) and performing a complete ophthalmologic examination including refraction, measurement of corneal diameter, gonioscopy (examination of anterior chamber angle structures), and biomicroscopy of the optic nerve head.

INFANTILE GLAUCOMA Infantile glaucoma, also referred to as *congenital* or *developmental glaucoma*, is rare, occurring in 1 in 10,000 live births. Most disorders are sporadic, although autosomal-recessive and autosomal-dominant instances with variable penetrance do occur. For this reason, siblings and children of patients with infantile glaucoma are at significant risk and must be checked. Most disorders (75%) are bilateral and are apparent at or shortly after birth. Males are affected more frequently than females (65: 35). The cardinal symptom of infantile glaucoma is *photophobia*. This light sensitivity may be so extreme that infants will shield their eyes from bright light by hiding their heads in a pillow. Usually there is associated blepharospasm and tearing, which may lead to the mistaken diagnosis of dacryostenosis and conjunctivitis. The characteristic signs are increased IOP (usually worse in one eye if bilateral), edema and slight congestion of the conjunctiva, corneal edema and haze, increased corneal diameter (greater than 11 mm in the newborn or 12 mm in the first year of life), horizontal linear white opacities in the cornea (tears in Descemet's membrane), a deep anterior chamber, and cupping and atrophy of the optic nerve. Because of the distensibility of an infant's eye in the first 3 years of life, enlargement of the globe may occur, and thus the name *buphthalmos* (cow's eye) is sometimes given to the disease. Unilateral enlargement of the globe from high myopia (quiet eye without corneal haze and normal intraocular pressure) and megalocornea (normal IOP) must be differentiated. In addition, any of the other causes of corneal opacity in infants must be considered (see Table 26-3).

The increase in IOP results from interference with outflow of aqueous humor from the anterior chamber angle caused by developmental anomalies in the angle structures. The anatomic defect is a trabeculodysgenesis associated with anterior insertion of the iris on the scleral spur. The characteristic gonioscopic finding is a crowded angle, sometimes with anomalous persistence of a membrane covering the trabeculum (Barkan membrane) or thick iris processes covering angle structures. When passage of fluid out of the eye is impaired, IOP increases, distending the wall of the eye, causing pressure on the optic nerve and producing the clinical picture of glaucoma.

Early surgical treatment is essential and can be done under anesthesia at the time of the initial examination. Medical therapy with the usual glaucoma drugs (miotics, carbonic anhydrase inhibitors, beta blockers) is rarely of long-term value. The initial surgical procedure is usually goniotomy. Alternative operations are trabeculotomy (particularly if the cornea is hazy) and trabeculectomy. In these procedures, an opening is made in the trabecular meshwork to allow aqueous humor to drain from the eye. Occasionally the procedures must be done several times to obtain an adequate opening. In over 75% of uncomplicated lesions, surgery is successful in controlling the IOP. Cyclocryotherapy to reduce aqueous outflow is usually a last resort.

The visual prognosis in infantile glaucoma depends on the age at onset (the earlier the onset, the worse the prognosis), the amount of myopia induced by enlargement of the eye, the degree of corneal scarring, the extent of glaucomatous optic atrophy, and the presence of lens opacification or other injury to the eye secondary to surgical trauma. Frequently, the more severely involved eye becomes exotropic with time, less often esotropic, and it may also become amblyopic. Usually the pressure in one eye can be con-

trolled, and this eye can maintain satisfactory visual acuity. Early amblyopia therapy including correction of refractive errors must not be neglected.

JUVENILE GLAUCOMA Juvenile glaucoma is a form of open-angle glaucoma that occurs early (usually after age 3 years and before age 20). It is seen most often in myopes and sometimes is inherited as an autosomal-dominant trait with high penetrance. Because juvenile glaucoma is rare and is seen later in childhood, it can be easily overlooked or undiagnosed until advanced corneal and optic nerve damage have occurred.

SECONDARY INFANTILE GLAUCOMA This group includes the glaucomas that are associated with systemic diseases or other anomalies and diseases of the eye. They may be subdivided as hamartomatous, traumatic, metabolic, inflammatory, mitotic, or other congenital anomalies. These glaucomas do not have the same pathogenesis as primary infantile glaucoma, and surgical results have a much poorer prognosis (Table 26-11).

STEROID-INDUCED GLAUCOMA Prolonged topical or systemic corticosteroid administration can produce severe open-angle glaucoma that is often refractory to topical glaucoma therapy. Prolonged indiscriminate use of topical corticosteroids for relatively

TABLE 26-11

ETIOLOGY AND DISORDERS ASSOCIATED WITH SECONDARY GLAUCOMA IN INFANTS AND CHILDREN

CATEGORY	CONDITION
Neurocristopathy	Axenfeld syndrome
	Rieger anomaly or syndrome
	Peter anomaly
Phakomatoses	Sturge-Weber syndrome
	von Recklinghausen disease
	von Hippel disease
Other congenital or developmental anomalies	Retinopathy of prematurity
	Persistent hyperplastic primary vitreous
	Aniridia
	Pierre Robin syndrome
Metabolic disorders	Lowe syndrome
	Homocysteinuria
Other genetic disorders	Marfan syndrome
	Weill-Marchesani syndrome
	Aniridia
	Down syndrome
	Albinism
	Patau syndrome
	Rubinstein-Taybi syndrome
Inflammatory diseases	Congenital rubella
	Herpes simplex
	Iridocyclitis (eg, juvenile rheumatoid arthritis)
	Postoperative
Tumors	Retinoblastoma
	Leukemia
	Juvenile xanthogranuloma
	Medulloepithelioma
Other	Posttraumatic
	Steroid-induced
	Pigment dispersion
	Hyphema

minor complaints such as allergic conjunctivitis, chronic blepharitis, and nonspecific eye irritations cannot be justified. All children who are steroid-dependent for treatment of systemic disease should receive a periodic eye examination to measure IOP and check for development of posterior subcapsular cataracts. In most instances withdrawal of steroid therapy causes the IOP to return to normal.

References

Beck RW, Cleary PA, the Optic Neuritis Study Group: Optic Neuritis Treatment Trial: One-year follow-up results. Arch Ophthalmol 111:773, 1993

Beck RW, Cleary PA, Trobe JD, et al: The effect of corticosteroids for acute optic neuritis on the subsequent development of multiple sclerosis. N Engl J Med 329:1764, 1993

Brodsky MC, Baker RS, Hamed LM: Pediatric Neuro-Ophthalmology. New York, Springer-Verlag, 1996

Burde RM, Savino PJ, Trobe JD: Clinical Decisions in Neuro-Ophthalmology, 2nd ed. St. Louis, Mosby, 1992

Hoskins HD, Kass MA: Becker-Shaffer's Diagnosis and Therapy of the Glaucomas, 6th ed. St. Louis, Mosby, 1989

Lambert SR, Hoyt CS, Narahara MH: Optic nerve hypoplasia. Surv Ophthalmol 32:1, 1987

Levin LA, Jakobiec FA: Optic nerve tumors of childhood: A decision-analytical approach to their diagnosis. Int Ophthalmol Clin 32:223, 1992

Loewenfeld JE: The Pupil. Anatomy, Physiology, and Clinical Applications. Ames, Iowa State University Press, 1993

Miller NR, Newman NJ, eds: Walsh and Hoyt's Clinical Neuro-Ophthalmology, 5th ed. Baltimore, Williams & Wilkins, 1997

Taylor D, Cuendet F: Optic neuritis in childhood. In: Hess RF, Plant GT, eds: Optic Neuritis. Cambridge, Cambridge University Press, 1986

26.13 EXTRAOCULAR MUSCLES AND OCULAR MOTILITY

26.13.1 Strabismus

Strabismus affects approximately 3% of the pediatric population. Early recognition and treatment of strabismus are essential for establishing good binocular visual function. No infant or child should be considered too young for referral to an ophthalmologist if an ocular misalignment is noted. Intermittent strabismus may be normal in the first 3 to 4 months of life, during the period of macular development, but any misalignment after 4 months of age should be considered abnormal. A strabismus may appear to improve as a child grows older because of the normal tendency for convergence tone and epicanthal skin folds to decrease with time. Nevertheless, amblyopia (see Sec. 26.15.1) will almost always persist unless occlusion therapy is initiated. Most children who appear to have outgrown a strabismus never truly had one but rather had a *pseudostrabismus.*

Most forms of strabismus are supranuclear in origin. The cranial nerve nuclei, fascicles, peripheral nerves, and extraocular muscles are usually normal. Childhood strabismus is typically *comitant* (the deviation is equal in all directions of gaze). *Paralytic* and *restrictive* strabismus is uncommon but when present is characterized by an ocular deviation that is *incomitant* (varying in amount in different directions of gaze). The angle of the deviation in comitant strabismus is not influenced by the eye preferred for fixation, whereas the effect is significant in paralytic and restrictive strabismus. The *primary deviation* is defined as the ocular misalignment measured when the nonparetic eye controls fixation. The *secondary deviation* is the ocular misalignment measured when the paretic eye controls fixation. The secondary deviation is always greater than the primary deviation. Most children with strabismus have a fixed deviation involving one eye only (*monocular strabismus*), and this eye typically develops amblyopia unless occlusion therapy early in life is carried out. Strabismic infants may develop equal vision in the two eyes if alternate fixation is used (*alternating fixation*). In some instances, strabismus develops as a result of poor vision (*sensory strabismus*) instead of the typical scenario in which poor vision (amblyopia) develops as a result of strabismus. Strabismus may be the presenting sign of certain ocular diseases (retinoblastoma, toxocariasis, ROP, and congenital cataract).

Ocular alignment and motility testing are discussed elsewhere (Sec. 26.1.6). Visual acuity determination is an important part of the evaluation for strabismus. Amblyopia is not necessarily related to the size of an ocular deviation; thus a small, inapparent deviation may be associated with profound vision loss.

CLASSIFICATION

Several classification schemes are used simultaneously to categorize the various forms of strabismus. Descriptors include the age at onset (congenital, acquired), direction of deviation, fusional status (phoria, intermittent, tropia), variation in the deviation with change in gaze position or fixating eye (comitant, incomitant), fixation preference (monocular, alternating), and distance–near relationship.

A manifest inward turning of an eye is called an *esotropia;* a latent inward deviation is called an *esophoria.* A manifest outward turning of an eye is called an *exotropia;* a latent outward deviation is called an *exophoria.* Vertical deviations are typically referenced to the higher eye; thus, a manifest vertical misalignment is called a *hypertropia* and a latent vertical misalignment is called a *hyperphoria.* There are occasions when it is useful to reference a vertical deviation to the lower eye (orbital floor fracture with entrapment of orbital contents), when the term *hypotropia* is used. Torsional misalignment can occur but is uncommon. Abnormal rotation of the eye about the axis roughly coincident with the line of sight is described by the direction of movement of the 12 o'clock position of the corneoscleral limbus. Inward rotation is known as *intorsion, incyclotropia,* or *incyclophoria;* outward rotation is known as *extorsion, excyclotropia,* or *excyclophoria.* When horizontal, vertical, and torsional misalignments occur simultaneously, the pattern of deviation is classified by the individual vector components.

Several conditions can mimic strabismus (*pseudostrabismus*). Parents who are inexperienced at judging ocular alignment may ask the pediatrician to evaluate a child because of an asymmetry in the amount of sclera visible on the nasal sides of the two eyes. Wide, flat nasal bridges and prominent epicanthal folds (see Sec. 26.4.1) may simulate esotropia. These features usually lessen or disappear as the bridge of the nose develops. Hypertelorism (see Sec. 26.14.1) may simulate exotropia. Vertical strabismus can be simulated by facial asymmetry. Another cause of pseudostrabismus is displacement of the macula. This may be seen in ROP where a vascularized, fibrous membrane at the temporal periphery of the retina causes traction on the disc area to pull the macula temporally. This results in an apparent exotropic deviation. Macular traction has also been seen in toxoplasmic chorioretinitis. Pseudostrabismus does not rule out true strabismus.

ESODEVIATIONS

INFANTILE ESOTROPIA This condition, also known by the less accurate term *congenital esotropia,* is defined as a primary esotropia appearing by 6 months of age. There is often a family history of esotropia or strabismus, although inheritance is not mendelian. The ocular misalignment in infantile esotropia is characteristically large. Infants with infantile esotropia have age-appropriate, mildly hyperopic refractive errors. A peculiar form of alternating fixation known as *cross-fixation* may develop in which the eyes sight objects only in contralateral visual space. Amblyopia does not develop with cross-fixation because the fovea in each eye is being stimulated. Oblique muscle overaction, disassociated vertical deviation, and latent nystagmus (Sec. 26.13.4) may develop, although not typically until 2 to 4 years of age, and they may occur even after surgical correction of the horizontal deviation. Treatment of infantile esotropia usually is surgical and generally involves recession of the medial rectus muscles. Surgery should be performed as early as can be done safely under general anesthesia to maximize the development of binocular vision. Injection of botulinum toxin to weaken the medial rectus muscles has been studied by a few investigators.

ACCOMMODATIVE ESOTROPIA This acquired esotropia is accommodative in origin, reflecting a disturbance in the accommodative convergence mechanism. The onset of accommodative esotropia typically is from about 18 months to 4 years of age. Two pure forms are recognized. The first is *refractive accommodative esotropia.* Most children with this form are moderately or severely hyperopic. In order to see clearly, they exert an excessive accommodative effort that results in overconvergence and an esotropia. Spectacles to correct the full amount of hyperopia found on cycloplegic refraction are prescribed to remove the need to accommodate. The prescribed lenses are usually unnecessary for correction of vision, but they prevent the esotropia. In time, the spectacle power may be reduced or the glasses eliminated entirely. A second form of accommodative esotropia is *nonrefractive accommodative esotropia.* Children with this form of esotropia have straight eyes when fixating in the distance but crossed eyes when fixating on near objects. The tone of their accommodative convergence mechanism is abnormally high. These children are treated with reading glasses to reduce the near accommodative effort or bifocals if they need hyperopic or astigmatic distance correction as well. Mixed forms of esotropia, including combinations of accommodative and nonaccommodative esotropia, are common. In mixed types, surgery is restricted to the nonaccommodative portion of the deviation.

EXODEVIATIONS

INTERMITTENT EXOTROPIA This is an intermittent manifest exodeviation with onset in 1 to 5 years of life, associated with little or no significant refractive error. It may be progressive, first involving distance fixation and later involving near fixation. A characteristic sign is closing ("squinting") one eye in bright sunlight. Patients have periods of normal fusion, usually in the morning hours or when they are rested, and times when they are clearly exotropic. Most patients with intermittent exotropia have normal visual acuity in both eyes. When the eyes are straight, they demonstrate normal binocular function and stereoacuity. During exotropic phases, suppression can be demonstrated. Tropic phases can be precipitated by

fatigue, illness, alcohol, visual inattention, daydreaming, distance viewing, and bright light. Orthoptic treatment consists of antisuppression therapy such as alternating daily occlusion and increasing fusional amplitudes. The use of minus lenses to induce accommodation may forestall surgery. Surgical treatment is indicated if the deviation is large in amplitude and present much of the time. Intermittent exodeviations often become constant with time.

CONSTANT EXOTROPIA Constant exotropia is often the result of decompensated intermittent exotropia. It is a comitant deviation, measuring the same in all directions of gaze. Diplopia is rare. *Sensory exotropia* is a type of constant exotropia that may develop if there is vision loss after the first year of life. A rare form of constant exotropia is *congenital exotropia:* a large exodeviation, similar in magnitude with distance and near fixation, is present at or shortly after birth. Oblique muscle overaction is often found. Treatment is surgical. Intraocular disease or abnormality may manifest as a congenital exotropia in the early months of life. Constant exodeviations of an incomitant nature may occur with third cranial nerve paresis, Duane syndrome type 2, following surgery for esotropia (*consecutive* or *secondary exotropia*), and in craniofacial anomalies characterized by divergent orbits such as Crouzon and Apert syndromes (Sec. 26.14.1). Surgical treatment usually involves bilateral lateral rectus muscle recession or a recess-resect procedure on the poorly sighted eye.

CONVERGENCE INSUFFICIENCY The hallmark of this condition is a near deviation that exceeds the distance deviation by 10 prism diopters or more, coupled with a remote near point of convergence. When an exodeviation of the convergence insufficiency type is constant, symptoms are uncommon. However, when a strong fusional mechanism is present, patients often experience reading difficulty and symptoms of *asthenopia* (tired eyes). Therapy includes orthoptic exercises in an attempt to increase fusional convergence and incorporation of base-in prisms in spectacles. If these measures fail to produce an improvement, medial rectus muscle recession can be attempted.

CYCLOVERTICAL DEVIATIONS

Cyclovertical strabismus usually results from overaction or underaction of the vertical rectus or oblique muscles. A partial list of conditions that are associated with cyclovertical strabismus includes fourth cranial nerve palsy, dissociated vertical deviation, superior oblique muscle overaction, inferior oblique muscle overaction, double elevator paresis, Brown syndrome, Graves ophthalmopathy, orbital tumors, orbital cellulitis, inferior rectus muscle paresis, and orbital wall fractures.

SPECIAL FORMS OF STRABISMUS

DUANE RETRACTION SYNDROME The most common form of Duane syndrome (type 1) is characterized by marked limitation of abduction, mild limitation of adduction, retraction of the globe (*enophthalmos*), narrowing of the palpebral fissure on adduction, and upshooting, downshooting, or both on adduction. Often the patient uses a head turn to use both eyes together to compensate for the esotropia that would otherwise exist if the head were in the straight-ahead position. The motility problem is congenital, usually unilateral (80%), more frequent in girls, sporadic in inheritance, though autosomal-dominant in some families. Electromyography has demonstrated a decrease in electrical activity in the lateral rectus muscle on attempted abduction and cocontraction of the medial and lateral rectus muscles on attempted adduction. Recent autopsy studies have shown an absence of the sixth nerve motor nuclei.

The second most common form of Duane syndrome is type 2, characterized by limited or absent adduction with exotropia of the affected eye. In type 3 there is severe restriction of both abduction and adduction.

A variety of anomalies may be associated such as heterochromia irides, cataract, choroidal coloboma, crocodile tears, microphthalmos, Marcus Gunn jaw-winking, Goldenhar syndrome, Klippel-Feil syndrome, and anomalies of the face, ears, or extremities. These associated abnormalities suggest the possibility of a teratogenic effect at the time of formation of the sixth nerve nuclei at about 8 weeks' gestation. The occurrence of Duane syndrome in some instances of the thalidomide syndrome lends support to this hypothesis.

Eye muscle surgery is indicated only if there is an objectionable head turn, a noticeable strabismus in primary position, or retraction of the globe is cosmetically disturbing.

BROWN SYNDROME This syndrome, formerly called the *superior oblique tendon sheath syndrome,* is characterized by the inability to fully elevate the adducted eye either actively or passively. Elevation in abduction is normal. The condition usually is unilateral. The eye may be straight in the primary position, hypotropic, or cyclotropic. Most congenital forms appear to be caused by a tight ipsilateral superior oblique tendon. Acquired forms may follow superior oblique tuck procedures, trauma to the anterior superonasal orbit in the vicinity of the trochlea, or be associated with an inflammatory disease such as juvenile rheumatoid arthritis. In some patients an audible click precedes a sudden elevation of the affected eye during attempted upgaze. This sound may be caused by a fibrous knot of tendon popping through the trochlea. Brown syndrome can be differentiated from isolated inferior oblique paresis, a rare condition, by forced duction testing. Indications for surgery include bothersome diplopia and an objectionable head turn. Local corticosteroid injections may help inflammatory reactions in the trochlea area.

26.13.2 Cranial Nerve Paresis

THIRD CRANIAL NERVE PARESIS Paresis of the third cranial (oculomotor) nerve in childhood is uncommon. Forty-five percent of all isolated third nerve pareses are congenital. Etiologies in acquired paresis include head trauma, increased intracranial pressure, and infection (bacterial meningitis, varicella, infectious mononucleosis, and tuberculosis). Characteristics of the paresis include unilateral blepharoptosis, mydriasis, and strabismus. The eye is exotropic and hypotropic because of unopposed forces generated by the lateral rectus and superior oblique muscles. Amblyopia is common; the child may prefer fixation with either eye. Episodic oculomotor paresis can be seen in children with ophthalmoplegic migraine. Pupillary involvement and aberrant regeneration are seen in the majority. The pupil is usually larger than that of the nonparetic eye, but miotic pupils have been described. Congenital third nerve palsies have been associated with hemiplegia, developmental delay, seizures, jaw-winking, and other neurologic findings. Although congenital third nerve palsies are generally benign, patients should be seen by a pediatric neurologist and ophthalmologist.

FOURTH CRANIAL NERVE PARESIS Children with fourth cranial (trochlear) nerve paresis, also known as *superior oblique paresis,* have a hypertropia of the involved eye and a head tilt (*torticollis*) to the opposite shoulder. Most disorders are either congenital or traumatic. Most congenital forms are unilateral; most acquired forms are bilateral and the result of closed head trauma. The head tilt may be mistaken for a sternomastoid or cervical spine disorder and the infant referred to an orthopedist. Patching one eye will eliminate the head tilt. Eye muscle surgery should be performed to avoid permanent neck contraction. Tumors in the region of the roof of the midbrain (pinealoma) may rarely cause fourth cranial nerve paresis.

SIXTH CRANIAL NERVE PARESIS Sixth cranial (abducens) nerve paresis, also know as *lateral rectus paresis,* is a common problem in childhood. It is characterized by limited abduction, diplopia, and a head turn or torticollis toward the side of the paresis. A transient, benign, unilateral rectus paresis occasionally is seen in newborns. The paresis has not been related to a complicated pregnancy or delivery. Etiologies in acquired pareses include purulent meningitis, increased intracranial pressure, head trauma, intracranial neoplasms (pontine glioma, posterior fossa astrocytoma, medulloblastoma), viral infections, immunization, and inoculations. Sixth nerve paresis may also be seen in Duane and Möbius syndromes. It can have serious implications as a sign of intracranial disease, but if it seems to be an isolated occurrence without neurologic and systemic abnormalities, particularly if there is a history of recent febrile illness, it may be considered "benign" and can be observed closely without extensive neurologic testing. The paresis in benign instances usually resolves spontaneously within weeks to several months. If additional neurologic or systemic findings appear, detailed neurologic evaluation is indicated. A special cause of sixth cranial nerve paresis (*Gradenigo syndrome*) follows middle-ear infections or mastoiditis. It consists of petrositis or septic thrombosis of the inferior petrosal sinus, esotropia, facial pain, and hearing loss.

26.13.3 Motility Disorders Secondary to Brainstem Lesions

Brainstem lesions that have strabismus as a cardinal manifestation are discussed in Sec. 26.13.2. This section discusses lesions that affect ocular motility without necessarily causing a strabismus in the primary position.

PARINAUD SYNDROME This syndrome is characterized by paralysis of upgaze, a less marked paresis of downgaze, poor convergence and accommodation, retraction nystagmus with attempted upgaze, *light-near dissociation,* and lid retraction that may be present in primary position but is exaggerated in upgaze (*Collier sign*). The syndrome results from mass lesions in the vicinity of the posterior commissure and superior colliculi and from lesions that elevate third ventricle CSF pressure. The most common etiologies are pinealoma, internal hydrocephalus, third ventricle tumor, aqueductal stenosis, trauma, encephalitis, syphilis, and intracranial hemorrhage. Parinaud syndrome must be distinguished from progressive supranuclear palsy.

OCULAR MOTOR APRAXIA This is characterized by a defect in the initiation of voluntary horizontal saccades that appears in infancy. Patients appear initially to be blind because they fail to make normal refixation saccades. The visual evoked response is normal, however, indicating normal precortical neural development and good potential visual acuity. Once patients develop control over head and neck movements and blink responses, they learn to use head thrusts to change fixation. Vertical eye movements are normal, and the quick phase of optokinetic nystagmus is absent. The head thrusts become less noticeable as the child grows older. A delay in myelination of the ocular motor pathways for conjugate gaze has been suggested. Affected children may be otherwise normal or may have additional neurologic problems such as hydrocephalus, brainstem or posterior fossa tumors, agenesis of the corpus callosum, progressive spinocerebellar degeneration, ataxia-telangiectasia (Louis-Bar syndrome), kernicterus, or Gaucher disease. Neurologic evaluation including CT or MR imaging of the brain is indicated in most patients.

OPSOCLONUS Opsoclonus consists of bizarre, chaotic, conjugate saccadic eye movements that occur in young patients after an acute febrile illness or in unconscious patients with encephalitis or brainstem disease. The saccades are irregular and arrhythmic in both horizontal and vertical directions. An awake person may have to close the eyes to reduce the awareness of ocular movement. Truncal ataxia is often associated with opsoclonus in the setting of postviral encephalitis. The illness usually clears spontaneously in a few weeks to months if there is no major underlying disease. Opsoclonus is a feature of infantile polymyoclonus, cerebellar lesions, and neuroblastoma.

26.13.4   Nystagmus

Nystagmus is an involuntary rhythmic to-and-fro movement of the eyes. *Jerk nystagmus* is characterized by a slow-phase eye movement in one direction mediated by the smooth pursuit system followed by a quick-phase eye movement in the reverse direction mediated by the saccadic system. *Pendular nystagmus* is characterized by equal-velocity eye movements in both directions. The features by which nystagmus is classified include waveform character, direction of the quick phase, periodicity, and changes in amplitude as a function of gaze direction. Some forms of nystagmus are physiologic (optokinetic nystagmus, endpoint nystagmus, vestibular jerk nystagmus), whereas others are pathologic.

CONGENITAL NYSTAGMUS Congenital nystagmus, easily the most common form of nystagmus encountered in the pediatric population, is a misnomer in that the nystagmus does not usually develop until 8 to 12 weeks of age. It may have a *pendular waveform*, when it is usually secondary to sensory deprivation, or it may have a *jerk waveform* and be associated with a defect in supranuclear motor control. More than one waveform may exist in the same individual. Attempted fixation may worsen the nystagmus, and convergence may dampen it. Latent nystagmus is also common in the setting of congenital nystagmus.

SENSORY DEFECT NYSTAGMUS This is the common form of congenital nystagmus. It is caused by maldevelopment of the fixation reflex as a result of bilateral retinal image blur or disease of the afferent pathways during the critical early weeks of visual development. After the age of 6 years, binocular loss of vision does not lead to nystagmus. Sensory deprivation nystagmus has a pendular waveform which is usually horizontal in nature, although vertical and rotary movements may occur. On endgaze, the nystagmus may take on a jerk waveform. Congenital sensory defect nystagmus is associated with bilateral cataracts, glaucoma, corneal clouding, aniridia, retinal detachments, retinopathy of prematurity, macular

scars, optic nerve hypoplasia, albinism, achromatopsia, Leber congenital amaurosis, congenital stationary night blindness, and cone dystrophies. The latter three conditions may have a normal fundus appearance. All patients with congenital pendular nystagmus and a normal-appearing fundus should be evaluated with ERG. Only with a normal ophthalmologic examination and ERG can a diagnosis of motor defect congenital nystagmus be made.

MOTOR DEFECT NYSTAGMUS This is the uncommon form of congenital nystagmus. It is thought to be caused by a defect in supranuclear extraocular motor control. The nystagmus is horizontal (although vertical and rotary components may be seen), bilateral, and characterized by a jerk waveform. The intensity may vary with gaze position. Visual acuity degradation tends to be related to the frequency and amplitude of the nystagmus. The ophthalmologic examination and ERG are normal. Often there is a *null point* where the amplitude of the nystagmus is least and visual acuity is best. Strabismus surgery (Kestenbaum procedure) can be performed, if indicated, to rotate the null point to the primary position and reduce or eliminate an anomalous head turn.

LATENT NYSTAGMUS Latent nystagmus is a special form of nystagmus that appears under conditions of uniocular fixation. It is a bilateral, conjugate, jerk nystagmus with a fast component in the direction of the occluded eye. It changes direction when the fellow eye is occluded. It is seen frequently in the setting of *infantile esotropia*. A child with latent nystagmus may do poorly on school vision tests unless binocular vision is tested. Strabismus, frequently esotropia, may be present.

SPASMUS NUTANS Spasmus nutans is an acquired disorder characterized by nystagmus, head nodding or bobbing, and torticollis. Generally the onset is between 4 and 12 months of age, with spontaneous resolution by 4 years of age. Head nodding often precedes the nystagmus. The torticollis is the most variable feature of the entity. The nystagmus is more often bilateral than unilateral and is characterized by low-amplitude, rapid, pendular, asymmetric, quiver-like horizontal movements that vary in different directions of gaze and that may disappear when the head is supine. Affected infants are otherwise normal. The etiology and pathogenesis are unknown. Occasionally manifestations suggestive of spasmus nutans are seen in patients with gliomas in the region of the optic chiasm or multiple sclerosis. Complete ophthalmologic and neurologic evaluations including CT or MR imaging are therefore advisable.

UPBEAT NYSTAGMUS Upbeat nystagmus in the primary position has been associated with lesions of the anterior vermis and lower brainstem as well as drug intoxication and Wernicke encephalopathy.

DOWNBEAT NYSTAGMUS Downbeat nystagmus in the primary position is usually associated with disorders of the craniocervical junction and foramen magnum such as Arnold-Chiari malformation, basilar invagination, and spinocerebellar degeneration. MR imaging is usually indicated. It is also seen in multiple sclerosis, lithium intoxication, and familial periodic ataxia.

Many additional forms of nystagmus, not discussed here, may also be seen in the pediatric age group, including nystagmus blockage syndrome, periodic alternating nystagmus, convergence retraction nystagmus, dissociated nystagmus (internuclear ophthalmoplegia), gaze-evoked nystagmus, rebound nystagmus, and see-saw nystagmus.

26.13.5   Ocular Myopathies

MYASTHENIA GRAVIS   Myasthenia gravis is an immunologic disorder of the neuromuscular junction. One-half of all patients with myasthenia gravis develop ocular signs initially; a larger fraction develop ocular signs at some time during the course of their illness. Blepharoptosis from paresis of the levator palpebrae superioris muscle is often the initial sign of ocular involvement (Sec. 26.4.2). Diplopia from extraocular muscle involvement may also be the presenting complaint. Myasthenia may affect one or more muscles and may simulate any cranial nerve paresis, isolated extraocular muscle paresis, supranuclear motility disturbance (Parinaud syndrome, internuclear ophthalmoplegia), or external ophthalmoplegia. Its hallmarks are variability and fatigability. The pupil is not involved. Ophthalmologic and neurologic consultation are both indicated. Strabismus surgery must be approached cautiously because of the variability of the strabismus.

CHRONIC PROGRESSIVE EXTERNAL OPHTHALMOPLEGIA (CPEO)   CPEO is a bilateral, usually symmetric, progressive external ophthalmoplegia. The iris and ciliary body are unaffected; therefore, pupillary function and accommodation are preserved. Blepharoptosis is typically the presenting sign (Sec. 26.4.2). The disorder may be congenital, but the onset is usually in childhood or adolescence. Diplopia is notably absent. The extraocular motility disturbance progresses gradually over many years, resulting eventually in the complete inability to move the eyes voluntarily or reflexively. Strabismus surgery should be avoided. CPEO may be associated with the Kearns-Sayre, Bassen-Kornzweig, and Werdnig-Hoffmann syndromes and with ocular pharyngeal dystrophy and spinocerebellar degenerations.

MYOTONIA CONGENITA   Myotonia congenita, or *Thomsen disease,* is an autosomal-dominant disease with onset before 5 years of age (see Sec. 25.14.1). The eyelids may fail to open for a few seconds after sudden closure. Blepharoptosis and sluggish extraocular muscles or pareses may be seen (see Sec. 26.4.2).

MYOTONIC DYSTROPHY   Myotonic dystrophy, or *Steinert disease,* is an autosomal-dominant disease that occurs in young adulthood. Eye features are prominent. Bilateral, small dot-like anterior and posterior subcapsular cortical opacities progress to total cataracts. The polychromatic lens crystals seen on slit-lamp biomicroscopic examination are highly characteristic although not pathognomonic. Other ocular findings may include retinitis pigmentosa, blepharoptosis, poorly reactive pupils, low intraocular pressure, macular degeneration, macular red spot, and loss of corneal sensitivity. Electromyography demonstrates a typical incremental response. The condition is worsened by administration of Prostigmin.

References

Asbury T, Frederik DR: Strabismus. In: Vaughan DG, Asbury T, Riordan-Eva P, eds: General Ophthalmology, 15th ed. Stamford, CT, Appleton & Lange, 1999

Demer JL: Extraocular muscles. In: Tasman W, Jaeger EJ, eds: Duane's Clinical Ophthalmology. Philadelphia, Lippincott Williams & Wilkins, 2000

Dennehy PJ: Ocular motor nerve palsies in childhood. In: Margo CE, Hamed LM, Mamed LM, eds: Diagnostic Problems in Clinial Ophthalmology. Philadelphia, Saunders, 1994

Leigh RJ, Zee DS: The Neurology of Eye Movements, 2nd ed. Philadelphia, FA Davis, 1991

Von Noorden GK: Binocular Vision and Ocular Motility: Theory and Management of Strabismus, 5th ed. St. Louis, Mosby, 1996

26.14 ORBIT

John T. Tong

The most frequent sign of orbital disease is *proptosis,* a forward protrusion of the eye caused by a mass or expansion of tissue within the orbit. The term *exophthalmos* is sometimes used synonymously but is best reserved for the ophthalmopathy associated with Graves disease. Proptosis in itself is not injurious unless the lids are unable to cover the cornea. Downward displacement of the globe (*hypoglobus*) may occur with superior orbital tumors and large orbital floor fractures (Sec. 26.16.7). Upward displacement of the globe (*hyperglobus*) may occur with tumors of the inferior orbit. Medial and lateral globe displacements may also occur. Globe retraction (*enophthalmos*) is associated with large orbital fractures, atrophy of the retrobulbar fat pad, Duane retraction syndrome (Sec. 26.13.1), and cicatrizing tumors metastatic to the orbit. Signs and symptoms of orbital disease in addition to proptosis include vision loss, color desaturation, afferent pupillary defects, pain with or without eye movement, photophobia, tearing, lid edema and erythema, conjunctival chemosis, injection, reduced motility, and diplopia. Examination findings may also include *lagophthalmos* (incomplete eyelid closure), exposure keratopathy, optic disc edema, retinal and choroidal striae, and orbital bruits. Pulsating proptosis may be seen in association with orbital aneurysm, meningocele, following orbital injury due to formation of an arteriovenous shunt, carotid-cavernous fistula, and sphenoid bone hypoplasia associated with neurofibromatosis.

The degree of proptosis and asymmetry in eye position can be appreciated best by viewing the eyes from above and behind the patient. The amount of proptosis, as measured from the lateral orbital rim to the apex of the cornea, is determined with an exophthalmometer. Globe displacements in the vertical and horizontal directions can be measured with respect to the normal eye and the facial midline. *Pseudoproptosis* can be caused by a number of conditions including eyelid retraction, shallow orbits, buphthalmos, and high myopia. The distance from the cornea to the orbital rim normally ranges from 12 to 20 mm, but higher levels may be encountered in African-Americans, Asians, and other races with shallow long orbits to suggest proptosis. A difference of 2 mm or more between the eyes is considered significant regardless of the absolute value. The evaluation of proptosis frequently includes CT and MR imaging, cerebral angiography, and ultrasonography. Fine-needle or open biopsy of an orbital mass may be necessary for diagnosis. An approach to the evaluation of proptosis in children is outlined in Fig. 26-3.

26.14.1   Developmental Anomalies of the Orbit, Face, and Skull

A variety of ocular and orbital abnormalities may be seen in the *craniofacial disorders.* Ocular complications may occur as a result of abnormal orbital size, shape, and position or because of associated defects in the orbital soft tissues and ocular adnexae. The list of complications includes extreme proptosis and exposure keratop-

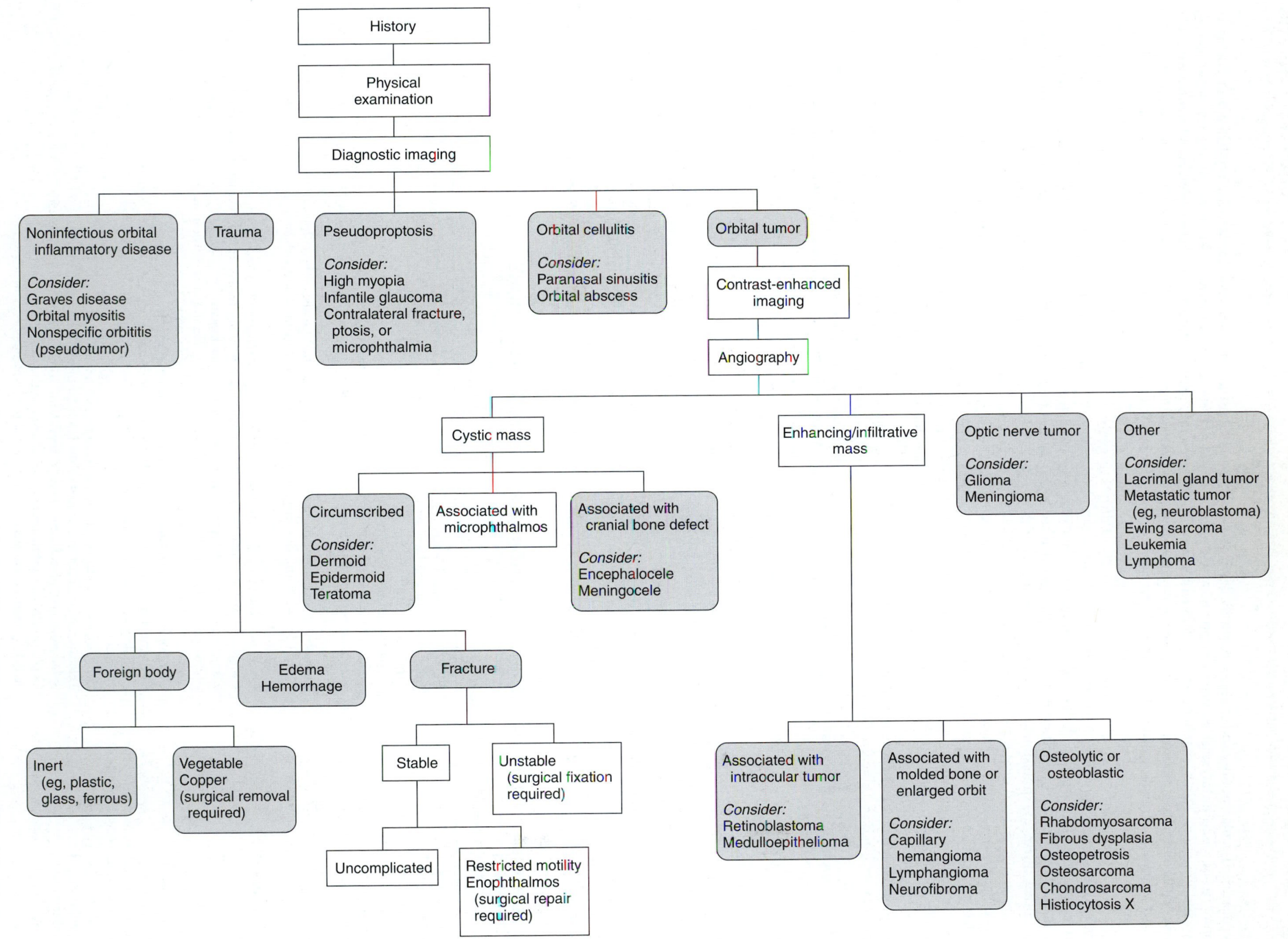

FIGURE 26-3 **Algorithm diagramming the evaluation of acquired proptosis.**

History

Physical examination

Diagnostic imaging

Noninfectious orbital inflammatory disease

Consider:
Graves disease
Orbital myositis
Nonspecific orbititis (pseudotumor)

Trauma

Pseudoproptosis

Consider:
High myopia
Infantile glaucoma
Contralateral fracture, ptosis, or microphthalmia

Orbital cellulitis

Consider:
Paranasal sinusitis
Orbital abscess

Orbital tumor

Contrast-enhanced imaging

Angiography

Cystic mass

Circumscribed

Consider:
Dermoid
Epidermoid
Teratoma

Associated with microphthalmos

Associated with cranial bone defect

Consider:
Encephalocele
Meningocele

Enhancing/infiltrative mass

Optic nerve tumor

Consider:
Glioma
Meningioma

Other

Consider:
Lacrimal gland tumor
Metastatic tumor (eg, neuroblastoma)
Ewing sarcoma
Leukemia
Lymphoma

Foreign body

Edema
Hemorrhage

Fracture

Inert (eg, plastic, glass, ferrous)

Vegetable
Copper (surgical removal required)

Stable

Unstable (surgical fixation required)

Uncomplicated

Restricted motility
Enophthalmos (surgical repair required)

Associated with intraocular tumor

Consider:
Retinoblastoma
Medulloepithelioma

Associated with molded bone or enlarged orbit

Consider:
Capillary hemangioma
Lymphangioma
Neurofibroma

Osteolytic or osteoblastic

Consider:
Rhabdomyosarcoma
Fibrous dysplasia
Osteopetrosis
Osteosarcoma
Chondrosarcoma
Histiocytosis X

athy, disturbed ocular motility and strabismus, papilledema or optic atrophy (from raised intracranial pressure or optic nerve compression within the optic canals), refractive errors, and amblyopia. Intrinsic ocular anomalies (anterior segment dysgenesis, colobomas, extraocular muscle anomalies, ocular motor cranial nerve disorders) may also accompany many of the craniofacial disorders.

Craniosynostosis is the term applied to premature closure of the cranial sutures. Craniosynostosis is discussed in Sec. 10.3.4. Common features include proptosis, skull shape abnormalities, midface hypoplasia, corneal exposure, poor vision, *hypertelorism* (increased intercanthal distance), strabismus (V pattern exotropia being the most common), oral and dental abnormalities, respiratory difficulties, and mental retardation. In rare instances the orbits are so shallow that the eyelids become trapped spontaneously behind the eyes. This constitutes an ophthalmologic emergency because of severe exposure and possible compromise of ocular blood supply. Treatment involves retropulsing the globe back into the orbit and tarsorrhaphy. Ophthalmologic features of many of the craniofacial syndromes are listed in Table 26-12 (see Sec. 10.3.4).

26.14.2   Orbital Inflammatory Diseases

Infectious and noninfectious processes can cause orbital inflammation. Orbital malignancies such as rhabdomyosarcoma (Sec. 26.14.3) may simulate orbital cellulitis. Infections of the eyelids and orbit are potentially serious diseases that can progress to involve the eye or central nervous system, even leading to death. Two types of cellulitis may be distinguished anatomically.

PRESEPTAL CELLULITIS   The term *preseptal cellulitis* refers to an inflammation located anterior to the orbital septum. Thus, signs of orbital involvement (proptosis, ophthalmoplegia, decreased vision) are absent. The clinical findings are limited to the eyelids and peri-

orbital tissues and are characterized by erythema and edema of these tissues; conjunctivitis, chemosis, and fever may also be present. Preseptal cellulitis may result from eyelid trauma with subsequent infection, skin infections, spread of infection in the eyelid or periobital region (hordeolum, conjunctivitis, dacryocystitis), upper respiratory tract infection, sinusitis, or bacteremia. Causative organisms include *S. aureus, S. pneumoniae, H. influenzae,* and anaerobes. *H. influenzae* organism is more likely to be encountered in children younger than 5 years of age; a magenta discoloration of the eyelids is distinctive. Introduction of the *H. influenzae* type-B (HiB) vaccine in the mid-1980s decreased the incidence of cellulitis from this organism.

Preseptal cellulitis should not be considered benign. Infections caused by virulent organisms may enter the vascular system and progress to orbital and intracranial involvement. Therefore, most patients are hospitalized for treatment.

Bacteriologic studies involving the conjunctiva, nasopharynx, and blood (gram-stained smears, cultures, antibiotic sensitivity tests) should be initiated. Radiography and computed tomography of the orbital and sinus areas are ordered if there is any indication of orbital inflammation, sinusitis, fracture, or foreign body. If a fluctuant mass is present, surgical drainage of the mass is performed, and smears and cultures of the drained material are assessed. If no area of fluctuation is present, percutaneous aspiration of the swollen area with smear and culture of the aspirated material should be considered for possible detection of the causative organism. If a causative organism cannot be found, broad-spectrum antibiotic therapy is recommended until results of the bacteriologic studies return. At present our preference is full parenteral doses of penicillinase-resistant penicillin such as oxacillin and either chloramphenicol or a third-generation cephalosporin (ceftriaxone or cefotaxime). The latter drugs are effective against *H. influenzae,* including ampicillin-resistant strains, *S. aureus,* streptococcal spe-

TABLE 26-12
EYE FINDINGS IN THE CRANIOFACIAL SYNDROMES AND MALFORMATIONS

SYNDROME	EYE FINDINGS
Cerebro-oculofacioskeletal	Microphthalmia, cataracts
Cornelia de Lange	Long eyelashes, confluent eyebrows, optic atrophy, telecanthus
Craniosynostoses (eg, Crouzon, Apert, Saethre-Chotzen, Pfeiffer)	Proptosis, exorbitism, papilledema, optic atrophy, exposure keratopathy, pigmentary retinopathy, keratoconus, strabismus
Cryptophthalmia	Fusion of eyelids, brow abnormalities, microphthalmia
Fetal alcohol	Telecanthus, blepharophimosis, blepharoptosis, epicanthal folds, optic nerve hypoplasia, tortuous retinal vessels, strabismus
Goldenhar-Gorlin	Epibulbar dermoids, dermolipomas, strabismus, blepharoptosis, eyelid colobomas, optic nerve hypoplasia, retinal vessel tortuosity, macular hypoplasia, microphthalmia, anophthalmia, lacrimal drainage system anomalies
Hallermann-Streiff	Congenital cataracts, spontaneous absorption of lens, microphthalmia, microcornea, glaucoma
Lowe	Congenital cataract, infantile glaucoma, anterior segment anomalies, corneal clouding, nystagmus
Marshall	Congenital cataract, ectopia lentis, myopia, retinal detachment
Möbius	Multiple cranial nerve palsies, lagophthalmos, exposure keratopathy, corneal anesthesia
Rieger	Axenfeld anomaly, iris hypoplasia, pseudopolycoria, glaucoma
Rubenstein-Taybi	Coloboma, glaucoma, cataract, strabismus, optic atrophy
Smith-Lemli-Opitz	Congenital cataracts, epicanthal folds, blepharoptosis, nystagmus, strabismus, optic atrophy
Mandibulofacial dysostosis (Treacher-Collins, Franceschetti-Zwahlen-Klein)	Lid colobomas, antimongoloid slant, missing eyelashes, astigmatism, strabismus
Sturge-Weber	Glaucoma, choroidal hemangiomas, conjunctival hemangiomas
Waardenburg	Telecanthus, lateral displacement of the inferior puncta, iris heterochromia
Weill-Marchesani	Spherophakia, high refractive error, ectopia lentis, optic atrophy, corneal opacity
Whistling face (Freeman-Sheldon)	Blepharoptosis, enophthalmos, hypertelorism, antimongoloid lid slant
Williams	Stellate pattern of iris, strabismus, retinal vessel abnormalities

cies, and anaerobes; they have good tissue penetration. For patients allergic to penicillin, vancomycin is given. Antibiotic therapy usually is continued for 1 to 2 weeks. Antibiotics may be given orally when there is clear clinical improvement.

ORBITAL CELLULITIS Orbital cellulitis designates an inflammation behind the orbital septum. Most often the cause is direct extension of a bacterial infection from the paranasal sinuses. Other causes include extension of infection from facial cellulitis, orbital trauma, dental abscess, and bacteremia. The organisms most frequently responsible are *S. pneumoniae*, group A β-hemolytic streptococci, *S. aureus*, *H. influenzae* (especially in young children but less frequent since the introduction of the HiB vaccine), and nonspore-forming anaerobes. Children younger than 9 years of age generally have infections caused by a single aerobic organism, whereas children older than 9 years may be infected with multiple organisms, including anaerobes. Characteristic clinical findings include erythema and edema of the eyelids and periorbital tissues, chemosis, proptosis, painful limitation of eye movement (ophthalmoplegia), decreased vision, afferent pupillary defect, and often symptoms of toxicity with fever and leukocytosis.

It is imperative that orbital cellulitis be recognized promptly and treated aggressively. Progressive inflammation within the orbit may lead to decreased vision and blindness. Extension of the process may result in meningitis, central nervous system abscess, and death from cavernous sinus thrombosis.

Treatment is carried out in the hospital. Consultation with an otolaryngologist is advisable. Bacteriologic studies (nose, throat, and blood), orbit and sinus radiographs, and orbital CT scans as described for preseptal cellulitis should be obtained. If on admission gram-stained smears of material obtained from the nose and throat, infected sinus, or surgical drainage of an acutely compromised orbit are not informative for selection of appropriate initial antibiotic therapy, then broad-spectrum antibiotic therapy is given as for preseptal cellulitis. Results of culture and antibiotic sensitivity studies may dictate a change in the choice of antibiotics. Treatment is usually given for 2 to 3 weeks or at least 7 to 10 days after the patient is afebrile and definite clinical improvement has been seen.

A subperiosteal or orbital abscess may result from progression of an acute ethmoiditis and could lead to compression of the optic nerve and blindness. Intensive antibiotic therapy early in the formation of the periosteal abscess (when limitation of globe movement is minimal and vision is unaffected) may make surgical intervention unnecessary. However, if no improvement is apparent after 24 to 48 hours of intravenous therapy, surgical drainage of the abscess should be considered. The diagnosis of early subperiosteal abscess by CT scan is not always accurate.

ORBITAL PSEUDOTUMOR *Idiopathic inflammatory orbital pseudotumor* refers to a noninfectious, inflammatory, space-occupying lesion of the orbit that simulates a neoplasm. Signs and symptoms develop acutely and consist of orbital pain, lid swelling, conjunctival chemosis and injection, proptosis, iritis, optic disc edema, and extraocular muscle disturbances. Proptosis and pain are the predominant features. Approximately one-half eventually develop bilateral orbital involvement. Vision is not impaired in the early stage. Half of all patients develop systemic manifestations including headache, fever, vomiting, pharyngitis, anorexia, abdominal pain, and lethargy. Examination and laboratory testing must exclude trauma, infection, foreign body, and malignancy. Ultrasonography, CT and MR imaging, tumor biopsy, and eosinophilia on peripheral blood smear may be helpful diagnostic tools. The posterior sclera may be

thickened (*posterior scleritis*), and fluid may accumulate within the Tenon's capsule. Histopathologic findings in orbital pseudotumor depend on the orbital structures primarily involved (lacrimal gland, extraocular muscles, orbital fat) but consist of lymphocytic infiltration, fibrosis, tissue eosinophilia, and a lipogranulomatous reaction. Primary involvement of the extraocular muscles is termed *orbital myositis*. Orbital pseudotumor is highly responsive to systemic corticosteroids. Open biopsy is indicated if the disease fails to respond to corticosteroids within 2 weeks, or if it recurs.

26.14.3   Tumors of the Orbit

Tumors of the orbit are classified as primary when they arise in the orbit, secondary if they spread to the orbit from the eye or another contiguous structure, and metastatic if there is a primary lesion at a distant location. *Hamartomas* are tumors that arise from tissues normally found at the involved site. *Choristomas* are tumors that arise from tissues not normally found at the involved site. Orbital tumors are classified according to the tissue of origin.

VASCULAR TISSUE TUMORS

CAPILLARY HEMANGIOMA Capillary hemangiomas are the most common vascular tumors of the orbit, accounting for 10% of all orbital tumors. Thirty percent are recognized at birth; 95% are evident by 6 months of age. They are nonheritable, benign, hamartomatous lesions usually arising in the anterior orbit. Most capillary hemangiomas causing proptosis have a lid component in the form of a raised red lesion called a "strawberry nevus" (Sec. 26.4.5). In the absence of this mark, hemangiomas can be diagnosed by a dark red or bluish discoloration of the subcutaneous tissue and a change in size on crying. Eversion of the lid may show the hemangioma as a bluish cystic lesion. Orbital imaging studies show increased orbital volume without the bone erosion that is typical of inflammatory diseases and other tumors of the orbit. CT and MR imaging and ultrasonography may be helpful in uncertain disorders and in defining the extent of the hemangioma.

Capillary hemangiomas appear shortly after birth and tend to increase dramatically in size during the first year or two of life, usually for a 3- to 6-month period. They stabilize for a year or more and then undergo spontaneous involution. Resolution is complete in 40 to 66% of patients by 4 years of age and in up to 76% by 7 years of age. Complications are frequent from anteriorly placed tumors, especially those with extensive lid involvement. They include blepharoptosis, strabismus, astigmatism, and anisometropia, any one of which can lead to serious amblyopia. Posterior orbital hemangiomas can sometimes cause optic nerve compression. Therapy has been variably successful, so it is fortunate that most can be managed merely by careful observation. Treatment is indicated when a hemangioma seriously disfigures the eyelids and brow, when it occludes the palpebral fissure and obstructs vision, when it distorts the shape of the globe, or when it threatens vision by compressing the optic nerve. Surgical excision of these tumors is difficult and is often used as a last resort. At present the preferred method of management is intralesional injection of a combination of long- and short-acting corticosteroids if the tumor is accessible. Depending on the size of the patient and the lesion, the usual dose is 40 mg of triamcinolone acetonide (Kenalog) combined with 6 to 12 mg of betamethasone in the form of equal amounts of phosphate and acetate (Celestone Soluspan). Injections may be repeated once or twice at 1- to 3-month intervals. Other modes of therapy to reduce tumor size include systemic corticosteroids, topical corticosteroids, interferon injections, low-dose superficial irradiation, photocoagulation, cryotherapy, and surgical excision.

LYMPHANGIOMA   Lymphangiomas usually appear in childhood in the first decade of life. They may arise in the eyelids or orbit and are frequently confused with hemangiomas. These tumors impart a bluish color to the overlying skin. They enlarge slowly, without regression (in contrast to hemangiomas), and may be associated with repeated episodes of sudden proptosis from intralesional hemorrhage and signs of orbital cellulitis after upper respiratory tract infection or sinusitis. CT or MR scan can show the extent of tumor involvement and, in contrast to hemangiomas, may show a cystic component. Diffuse and cystic forms have been described histologically, but in both forms the vascular channels are lined by endothelium separated by thin, delicate walls and are devoid of erythrocytes (except after hemorrhage). Surgical excision is difficult because these tumors are nonencapsulated but is the treatment of choice for large, disfiguring tumors.

MUSCULAR TISSUE TUMORS

RHABDOMYOSARCOMA   Rhabdomyosarcoma is the most common malignant orbital tumor of childhood, and it accounts for 10% of all pediatric orbital tumors. It has a bimodal distribution, occurring either during the first 2 years of life or after age 6, with an average age of onset of 7 to 8 years. The tumor arises from embryonic mesenchyme, usually in the posterior superior orbit, and causes a rapidly progressive downward and outward proptosis and drooping of the upper eyelid. It can often masquerade as an infectious orbital cellulitis with inflammatory signs. A subconjunctival or lid mass is palpable in only 25% of patients, and loss of vision is uncommon at the time of presentation. There may be pain, nasal stuffiness, and frequent nosebleeds. CT or MR scan can help define the extent of the tumor, although a CT scan may be more helpful in showing evidence of bone destruction. The best diagnostic aid is a high index of suspicion whenever a rapidly progressive proptosis or lid mass is seen in a child. Diagnosis is by biopsy. Rhabdomyosarcoma is a highly malignant tumor that infiltrates deeply into the orbit, often beyond the margins of attempted excision.

The tumor is thought to arise from undifferentiated mesenchymal tissue. Four types of rhabdomyosarcoma can be distinguished histopathologically. *Embryonal rhabdomyosarcoma* accounts for 75% of lesions and carries an intermediate prognosis. *Alveolar rhabdomyosarcoma* accounts for 15% and carries the worst prognosis. *Differentiated pleomorphic rhabdomyosarcoma* carries the best prognosis but is the least common type. Botryoid rhabdomyosarcoma invades the orbit secondarily from the conjunctiva or the paranasal sinuses. Metastases from rhabdomyosarcoma may appear in the regional lymph nodes, lungs, or bones. Rhabdomyosarcoma is a highly malignant tumor that infiltrates deeply into the orbit, often beyond the margins of attempted excision. Formerly the prognosis was poor, with most patients surviving less than 2 years. With early diagnosis and the use of surgery, radiation therapy, and chemotherapy, however, primary orbital rhabdomyosarcoma has a long-term survival rate of nearly 90%.

NERVOUS TISSUE TUMORS

See Sec. 26.12.4 for a discussion of *optic nerve glioma* and *meningioma.*

NEURILEMOMA   This tumor, also known as *schwannoma* or *neurinoma,* is an uncommon, benign tumor of peripheral nerve Schwann cells. It develops in 1.5% of patients with neurofibromatosis. The tumor may appear anywhere in the lids or orbit. Pain may develop early in the course because of sensory nerve compression. The tumors are firm and rubbery but when cut demonstrate areas of myxoid degeneration. Two types have been described histopathologically. The *Antoni A* type demonstrates a regular arrangement of eosinophilic spindle-shaped cells with palisading nuclei. The *Antoni B* type demonstrates a haphazard arrangement of stellate cells in a myxomatous matrix. Treatment of both histologic types consists of local excision.

NEUROFIBROMA   This is the fifth most common orbital tumor of childhood. It develops in 13 to 30% of patients with *neurofibromatosis* and is virtually pathognomonic of the disease. Neurofibroma is an encapsulated tumor consisting of Schwann cells, perineural cells, and axons. The tumors are firm and may be either fibrous or soft and myxomatous when cut. Orbital schwannomas cause slow, progressive proptosis. Pulsatile exophthalmos may result from a defect in the greater wing of the sphenoid with transmission of intracranial pressure to the orbit. Plexiform neurofibromas of the eyelids have a "bag of worms" feel when palpated because of cylindrical enlargement of individual nerve segments. Histopathologically, neurofibromas consist of fascicles or chords of cells surrounding axons. The myxomatous matrix is thought to be secreted by perineural cells. Treatment is by local excision, but complete excision is not always possible.

BONY TISSUE TUMORS

HISTIOCYTOSIS-X   See Sec. 20.16. This is the collective name for eosinophilic granuloma of bone, Hand-Schüller-Christian disease, and Letterer-Siwe disease. The distribution of lesions determines the clinical manifestation, severity, and prognosis of the disease. Radiographic evidence of orbital involvement is more common than proptosis. Radiographic findings include sharply demarcated osteolytic lesions without surrounding sclerosis. Unifocal *eosinophilic granuloma of bone* has an excellent prognosis. Lesions arise typically in the superotemporal orbit and may be treated by local excision, systemic corticosteroids, and external beam radiation. *Hand-Schüller-Christian disease,* characterized by diabetes insipidus, multiple lytic osseous lesions, and proptosis, has a poorer prognosis. Both orbits may be involved. Primary treatment consists of chemotherapy.

FIBROUS DYSPLASIA AND OSSIFYING FIBROMA   These closely related disorders are characterized by destruction of bone and replacement with fibro-osseous tissue. If osteoblasts are present, the diagnosis is ossifying fibroma; if absent, fibrous dysplasia. The two lesions cannot be differentiated clinically. Fibrous dysplasia may involve only a single bone or it may be polyostotic and associated with cutaneous hyperpigmentation and precocious puberty (*Albright syndrome*). Involvement of orbital bones may cause globe displacement or proptosis, facial asymmetry, or optic nerve compression. Orbital radiographs show bony lucencies with or without sclerosis. These lesions carry a good prognosis because they stabilize at the time of skeletal maturity. Treatment is usually not necessary. Optic canal decompression may be indicated if there is optic nerve dysfunction.

OTHER BONY TUMORS *Osteomas* are benign tumors that arise most often in the frontal sinuses. They may be excised completely in most patients. *Chondrosarcoma* and *osteosarcoma* are malignant tumors that destroy normal bone and have characteristic calcifications on plain films and orbital CT images. These tumors may arise in the orbit in the teenage years inside or outside the field of radiation after treatment of a childhood retinoblastoma (Sec. 26.11.7).

REMNANT TISSUE TUMORS

Dermoid cysts and *epidermoid cysts* are choristomas of misplaced ectoderm attached to periosteum and may usually be palpated as masses beneath the eyelids. They occasionally extend deep into the orbit (Sec. 26.4.5). *Microphthalmos with cyst* is a benign remnant tissue tumor discussed in Sec. 26.2. *Teratomas* are cystic choristomas, consisting of tissues derived from at least two, and occasionally all three, primary germ layers. Proptosis is often noticed at birth and worsens as the tumor enlarges. Teratomas may expand the orbit and destroy the globe. Surgical excision is indicated.

NEUROBLASTOMA AND OTHER METASTATIC TUMORS

Approximately 7% of all pediatric orbital tumors are metastatic cancers. The primary site is often asymptomatic, so proptosis may be the initial presentation of the tumor. Cancers that metastasize to the orbit include *neuroblastoma, Ewing sarcoma, Wilms tumor, leukemia, Hodgkin disease, non-Hodgkin lymphoma,* and *Burkitt lymphoma.*

Neuroblastoma is the most common cause of orbital metastasis in childhood. (See Sec. 20.13.) In over 20% of patients with neuroblastoma, eye symptoms are the presenting complaint. Average age at the time of diagnosis is 2 years. Ocular findings include proptosis, hemorrhagic edema of the eyelids and conjunctiva, signs of necrosis and infection of the eyelids, blepharoptosis, extraocular muscle palsies, papilledema, optic atrophy, Horner syndrome, and opsoclonus. The proptosis may be unilateral or bilateral and is frequently rapid in onset. CT scan usually shows destruction of bone. Orbital metastases imply far-advanced disease and a poor prognosis for survival.

References

Henderson JW, Campbell RJ, Farrow GM, et al: Orbital Tumors, 3rd ed. New York, Raven, 1994

Kodet R, Newton WA Jr, Hamoudi AB, et al: Orbital rhabdomyosarcomas and related tumors in childhood: relationship of morphology to prognosis—an Intergroup Rhabdomyosarcoma study. Med Pediatr Oncol 29:51, 1997

Liaricos S, Gekas L: Orbital tumors in children. Orbit 3:25, 1984

Miller MT, Hamming NA: Craniofacial syndromes and malformations: Ophthalmic manifestations. In: Isenberg SJ, ed: The Eye in Infancy, 2nd ed. St. Louis, Mosby, 1992

Nicholson DH, Green WR: Pediatric Ocular Tumors. New York, Masson, 1981

Rootman J: Diseases of the Orbit. Philadelphia, Lippincott, 1988

Rootman J, Stewart B, Goldberg RA: Orbital Surgery. A Conceptual Approach. Philadelphia, Lippincott-Raven, 1995

Sanborn GE, Gonder JR, Shields JA: Atlas of Intraocular Tumors. Philadelphia, Saunders, 1994

Shields JA, Shields CL: Atlas of Orbital Tumors. Philadelphia, Lippincott Williams & Wilkins, 1999

Volpe NJ, Jakobiec FA: Pediatric orbital tumors. Int Ophthalmol Clin 32: 201, 1992

Wulc AE: Orbital infections. In Duane TD, Jaeger EA, eds: Clinical Ophthalmology. Philadelphia, Lippincott, 1994

26.15 EYE AND CENTRAL NERVOUS SYSTEM

This section discusses a few disorders of the central nervous system with symptoms referable to the eyes that are not discussed elsewhere.

26.15.1 Amblyopia

Amblyopia, or "lazy eye," is a monocular or binocular reduction of visual acuity resulting from a disturbance in visual development during a sensitive period. This definition implies that amblyopia can develop only during the first few years of life, during the time of the greatest plasticity of the visual system. The etiology of amblyopia for most patients is strabismus, anisometropia, or visual deprivation. The degree of visual impairment in amblyopia may be mild or profound and is not necessarily related to the amount of strabismus or the degree of anisometropia.

The ideal method for detecting amblyopia is by visual acuity testing using a line of Snellen letters or other optotypes. Amblyopic patients read letters more easily when they are isolated than when they are surrounded by other letters or figures (*crowding phenomenon*). Visual evoked responses to checkerboard stimuli and preferential looking responses to sinusoidal or square-wave gratings may be used to screen for profound amblyopia in infants and preverbal children, but these tests have poor sensitivity for detecting subtle degrees of amblyopia. The grating targets used in these tests measure a subject's ability to resolve spatial detail (*resolution acuity*). They do not recruit the more highly developed cortical functions required to recognize and name optotypes (*recognition acuity*) and, as such, are poor screening tests for identifying patients with amblyopia.

Treatment of amblyopia involves identifying and correcting any underlying abnormality responsible for the development of amblyopia (e.g., strabismus, cataract, anisometropia) and either patching or penalizing the sound eye until the visual acuity of the amblyopic eye improves and equals that of the sound eye. Improvement must be maintained until the child reaches visual maturity, generally considered to be sometime between the age of 6 and 9 years. Amblyopia should be detected and treated by 3 or 4 years of age for best results. Patching after the age when visual maturity has been reached seldom is effective. Binocular function including stereopsis may remain impaired after visual acuity returns to normal.

STRABISMIC AMBLYOPIA Strabismus is by far the most common cause of amblyopia. Strabismic amblyopia can develop in a misaligned eye until the age when visual maturity is reached. It is an adaptive mechanism for dealing with *visual confusion* (overlapping dissimilar images) and *diplopia* (nonoverlapping identical images). Strabismus surgery is generally postponed until occlusion therapy has reversed the amblyopia.

ANISOMETROPIC AMBLYOPIA This form of amblyopia develops in the setting of a significant anisometropia. When both eyes are hyperopic, it is usually the more hyperopic eye that is suppressed and becomes amblyopic. Amblyopia may also occur in high anisomyopia and astigmatic anisometropia. In contrast to strabismic amblyopia, anisometropic amblyopia may develop and be reversible until 10 years of age or perhaps older.

DEPRIVATION AMBLYOPIA This is the most serious form of amblyopia. A partial list of causes includes congenital monocular cataract, large hemangiomas of the eyelid, persistent hyperplastic primary vitreous, and corneal scars. The visual axis must be cleared and a clear retinal image formed by about 6 months of age to prevent this type of amblyopia from becoming permanent. Excessive or prolonged occlusion therapy for treatment of amblyopia occasionally produces *reverse amblyopia* in the previously sound eye; this is a type of deprivation amblyopia.

ISOAMETROPIC AMBLYOPIA This is an unusual form of bilateral amblyopia caused by high refractive errors, typically high hyperopia over 5 diopters. The child fails to accommodate fully and obtain a clear image because of chronic asthenopia. Instead, the child settles for slightly blurred retinal images and the visual cortex fails to develop the potential for high-resolution acuity. A similar problem occurs with astigmatism over 3 diopters.

26.15.2   Dyslexia

Dyslexia is one type of specific learning disability and is generally defined as poor or inadequate mastery of verbal language or the inability to master the use of words. Dyslexic children may have difficulty with visual perception, manifested as character transposition, difficulty determining spatial relationships, or difficulty determining the significant elements of written or spoken language from background "noise" (see Secs. 5.6.2, 5.6.4, 25.6.5).

The eye examination invariably is normal, but the ophthalmologist is obligated to treat any refractive or ocular motor disturbance. It is essential that the ophthalmologist advise parents that vision and eye abnormalities are not generally the cause of learning disabilities. Visual training activities such as eye muscle exercises, smooth pursuit or target tracking exercises, and special glasses with prisms or tints have no proven benefit.

26.15.3   Headache

Ocular problems that may be a source of headache include refractive errors, asthenopia, extraocular muscle imbalance, and inflammatory diseases of the eye and orbit. Many parents and pediatricians believe that eyestrain is a major cause of headache, and it is one of the most common reasons for referral to ophthalmologists. The truth is that refractive errors and extraocular muscle imbalance are rare causes of headache in young children. Occasionally, however, the eye doctor may find that convergence insufficiency or accommodative spasm may be a possible cause of headaches in an older schoolage child or adolescent who does prolonged reading or close work. With inflammatory diseases of the eye and ocular adnexae, pain usually is local but can radiate to the head and scalp region. Local pain with headache can be severe in uveitis, glaucoma, optic neuritis, keratitis, and orbital cellulitis. Children rarely suffer severe

pain from these entities, however, so even mild but persistent complaints of local eye pain should be evaluated by an ophthalmologist.

Classic *migraine headache* is preceded by a visual aura consisting of transient blindness, blurred vision, hemianopia, scintillating scotomas, micropsia, or macropsia. Characteristically the visual symptoms last 15 to 20 minutes and are followed by a severe unilateral headache that lasts from hours to days (see Sec. 25.16.4). A variant of migraine headache known as *ophthalmoplegic migraine* may occur in early childhood or even in infancy. Although any ocular motor nerve may be involved, recurring third cranial nerve paresis ipsilateral to the side of the headache is the most common presentation. Unilateral pupillary dilation, exotropia, hypotropia, and blepharoptosis are the typical signs. In some patients, the paresis may persist days or weeks after the headache has disappeared. Most patients recover completely, but third cranial nerve function can be permanently impaired. One episode of ophthalmoplegic migraine calls for a CT or MR scan of the brain. If it recurs one or two more times, arteriography should be considered as occasionally one may detect an anomalous intracranial vascular malformation.

References

Flynn JT, Woodruff G, Thompson JR, et al: The therapy of amblyopia: An analysis comparing the results of amblyopia therapy utilizing two pooled data sets. Trans Am Ophthalmol Soc 97:373–390, 1999

Gold DH, Weingeist TA: The Eye in Systemic Disease. Philadelphia, Lippincott, 1990

Greenwald MJ, Parks MM: Amblyopia. In: Duane TD, Jaeger EA, eds: Clinical Ophthalmology. Philadelphia, Lippincott, 1990

Reinecke RD: Role of the ophthalmologist in reading disorders. In: Nelson LB, Calhoun JH, Harley RD, eds: Pediatric Ophthalmology. Philadelphia, Saunders, 1991

Taylor D: Headaches. In: Taylor D, ed: Paediatric Ophthalmology, 2nd ed. Oxford, Blackwell Science, 1997

Troost BT. Migraine and other headaches. In Duane TD, Jaeger EA, eds: Clinical Ophthalmology. Philadelphia, Lippincott-Raven, 1997

26.16   EYE TRAUMA AND EMERGENCIES

Ocular trauma is a major cause of unilateral blindness in children and the leading cause for enucleation. Examination of eye injuries in infants and children is usually difficult. Nevertheless, ocular injuries usually require prompt care if useful vision is to be preserved. If the pediatrician or emergency room physician cannot perform an adequate examination, the patient should be referred to an ophthalmologist for further evaluation. Local anesthesia and sedation help the pediatrician to attend to minor trauma such as superficial conjunctival foreign bodies. It is best for the nonophthalmologist to avoid forcing the eyelids open. When the nature and extent of an injury are unknown, general anesthesia will allow the ophthalmologist to perform a controlled and accurate examination and, if necessary, proceed with surgical repair. Testing the patient's visual acuity before treatment, if possible, is important for diagnostic, prognostic, and medicolegal reasons. The suspicion of child abuse should be considered if the history is inconsistent with the injury sustained.

26.16.1   Chemical and Thermal Burns

CHEMICAL BURNS   Chemical burns of the conjunctiva and cornea should be treated at once by copious irrigation with water or isotonic saline solution. Acid burns are less serious than alkali burns because acid precipitates proteins and forms its own barrier to further penetration. Alkaline agents, in contrast, activate collagenases that may subsequently produce corneal liquefaction and ulceration, possibly leading to full-thickness perforation. Alkali burns cause a rise in intraocular pressure caused by contraction of the sclera and damage to the trabecular meshwork. Mild to moderate chemical burns are associated with defects ranging from superficial punctate staining to complete sloughing of the corneal epithelium. Severe chemical burns are associated with pronounced chemosis, limbal ischemia, corneal edema and opacification, and anterior chamber inflammation. Treatment after irrigation consists of removing all particulate debris, cycloplegics, topical antibiotic ointment, pressure patching, oral analgesics, glaucoma medications, and cautious use of corticosteroids. Long-term management of severe burns may involve lysis of conjunctival symblepharon with a glass rod, application of collagenase inhibitors, conjunctival and corneal transplantation, and dry eye management.

THERMAL BURNS   Thermal burns of the cornea from cigarette ashes, match heads, and other combustible materials are not usually serious because eyelid closure and the Bell phenomenon limit the extent of the burn. Most thermal burns can be treated in the same manner as corneal abrasions. Severe facial burns that involve the eyelids and eyes, however, should be managed in conjunction with an ophthalmologist. Exposure keratopathy is usually severe; the eyes must be lubricated aggressively with bland ophthalmic ointments and artificial tears. Skin grafting to the eyelids and tarsorrhaphy are often necessary in the reconstructive phase.

RADIATION BURNS   Radiation burns in the form of ultraviolet light from the sun, sun lamps, snow reflectors (*snow blindness*), or welding arcs can produce a diffuse superficial punctate keratitis that is very painful. The keratitis follows the radiation exposure by 8 to 10 hours. Treatment consists of broad-spectrum antibiotic ointment and firm bilateral patching for 24 to 48 hours. No permanent sequelae develop. Glassblower's cataract, from exfoliation of the anterior lens capsule, may develop with intense infrared radiation exposure. Treatment is supportive.

26.16.2   Corneal Abrasions

Abrasions of the cornea result from traumatic removal of a portion of the surface epithelium. Sterile fluorescein ophthalmic solution may be instilled to determine the extent of the abrasion under cobalt blue illumination. In general, abrasions are exquisitely painful and are accompanied by blepharospasm, tearing, and photophobia. A topical anesthetic facilitates examination. Treatment consists of instilling a broad-spectrum antibiotic ointment, a short-acting cycloplegic drop, and applying a firm pressure patch for 24 hours. Alternatively, if the patient and family are reliable, a bandage soft contact lens and topical broad-spectrum antibiotic drops can be applied. Most abrasions heal completely in 24 to 48 hours. Young children may resist treatment, and it can be omitted if necessary. All patients should be reexamined in 24 hours to rule out early

infection. Topical anesthetics should never be dispensed for home use as they are toxic to the corneal epithelium and will delay wound healing.

26.16.3   Ocular Foreign Bodies

CONJUNCTIVAL FOREIGN BODIES   Foreign bodies of the conjunctiva can usually be removed by flushing the eye with a stream of isotonic saline or eye wash or by using a moistened cotton-tip applicator. The upper eyelid should be everted and inspected if a foreign body is not readily located. A local anesthetic will facilitate the examination.

CORNEAL FOREIGN BODIES   Foreign bodies of the cornea generally cause more pain and erythema than do conjunctival foreign bodies and are potentially more serious. Fluorescein may help to demonstrate the foreign body and any associated epithelial defect. If the foreign body cannot be removed with irrigation or a moist cotton-tip applicator, the patient should be referred to an ophthalmologist. Broad-spectrum topical antibiotics should be used after the foreign body is removed. Patching is usually not necessary unless there is an associated abrasion. All patients should be reexamined in 24 hours to rule out early corneal infection in the traumatized area. Metallic foreign bodies frequently leave a localized rust stain (*rust ring*). This is best removed by the ophthalmologist under slit-lamp magnification.

INTRAOCULAR FOREIGN BODIES   Children with suspected or known intraocular foreign bodies should be referred immediately to an ophthalmologist. A protective eye shield should be placed over the eye to prevent further injury or eye rubbing. It is possible for small, high-speed foreign bodies to penetrate the eye, with minimal findings, and cause only transient pain or no pain at all. Plain film x-rays and orbital CT images can be helpful in confirming the suspicion of an intraocular foreign body. MR imaging should be avoided whenever a metallic intraocular foreign body is suspected. Particles of iron or copper are removed to prevent subsequent degeneration and disorganization of ocular tissues. Newer alloys may be inert and may be tolerated. Small particles of glass and porcelain may be tolerated well and might be left alone.

26.16.4   Ocular Contusion

Contusion injuries result from blunt trauma to the globe and adnexae. They may vary in severity from ecchymosis of the eyelid (*black eye*) to rupture of the globe. Common findings include anterior chamber hemorrhage (*hyphema*), recession or disinsertion of the iris root (*iridodialysis*), disinsertion of the ciliary body from the scleral spur (*cyclodialysis*), lens dislocation or cataract formation, vitreous hemorrhage, retinal detachment, and traumatic optic neuropathy. All patients with contusion injuries should receive a thorough ophthalmologic evaluation. What may appear to be a minor blunt injury to the eye or adnexae may, in fact, be a serious ocular injury.

HYPHEMA   *Hyphema* is defined as hemorrhage into the anterior chamber. It may occur with blunt or penetrating injury to the eye; occur spontaneously in sickle-cell disease, juvenile xanthogranuloma (Sec. 26.9.3), or rubeosis iridis; or complicate intraocular surgery. Trauma is the most common etiology. In some patients, child abuse must be suspected. Traumatic hyphemas develop when an object strikes the globe with sufficient kinetic force to rupture a blood vessel in the iris or ciliary body. Hyphemas may appear layered with a blood-aqueous meniscus between the cornea and iris, or they may be diffuse and make the entire aqueous humor turbid. Hemorrhage may also completely fill the anterior chamber (*eight-ball hyphema*). It is imperative that patients with traumatic hyphemas be referred for ophthalmologic evaluation promptly, as more extensive injury to the internal and more posterior structures of the eye may be present.

An important goal of treatment is to prevent vision-threatening complications. A particularly serious complication is recurrent or secondary hemorrhage, which occurs in 3 to 38% of patients. It is difficult to predict which patients will rebleed, but when it happens, it is usually within the first 6 days, most often between the third and fifth days. Secondary hemorrhage increases significantly the possibility of an acute IOP rise with subsequent glaucomatous optic nerve damage, corneal blood staining and opacification, and formation of peripheral anterior synechiae, which may cause secondary angle closure or combined mechanism glaucoma.

Controversy exists over the ideal treatment of hyphema. Disagreement prevails regarding the value of absolute bed rest, eye patching, need for hospitalization, use of various drug regimens, and surgical procedures. Lack of agreement is probably a result of the various types of hyphema encountered. We prefer to hospitalize infants and children to permit close observation. In uncomplicated lesions in which the hyphema clears in 5 to 6 days, ordinarily the management plan consists of bed rest with bathroom privileges and monocular eye patching for 5 days, cautious ambulation on the sixth day, and discharge from the hospital on the seventh day. Aspirin is avoided because of its effect on bleeding time. A topical corticosteroid and cycloplegic are prescribed if posttraumatic iritis develops.

To reduce the incidence of secondary hemorrhage, some physicians recommend the prophylactic use of an antifibrinolytic agent such as aminocaproic acid (Amicar) in the dosage of 50 to 100 mg/kg body weight up to 30 g/d orally for 5 days. Another antifibrinolytic drug, tranexamic acid (Cyklokapron), is available in tablet and intravenous injection forms for use in hemophiliacs who are to undergo dental extraction; the drug has been used abroad to prevent rebleeding in traumatic hyphema. These drugs reduce lysis of the initial clot until the ruptured blood vessels heal. Systemic corticosteroids, equivalent to an adult dosage of 40 mg/d of prednisone for 5 days, have also been advocated by some ophthalmologists to prevent secondary hemorrhage. Although some ophthalmologists recommend the use of either aminocaproic acid or corticosteroids in all instances of traumatic hyphema (because the rebleed rate may not depend on the size of the hyphema), the low incidence of rebleeding, especially in the less severe hyphemas, coupled with the high cost (principally of aminocaproic acid) and possible side effects of these drugs, has deterred their routine use. The fibrinolytic agent tissue plasminogen activator may prove to be of clinical value in accelerating the clearance of hyphema when used at the right time. It has been reported to be effective in accelerating the clearance of hyphemas in the animal model.

If IOP goes up, a topical β-blocker is given. If this is ineffective, oral acetazolamide or methazolamide or intravenous mannitol may be needed. If medical therapy fails to control the IOP, surgical wash-out of the anterior chamber may be necessary.

Sickle-cell hyphema merits special attention. Patients with either the trait or the disease are at increased risk of complications of hyphema because their circulating erythrocytes tend to sickle in the acidic, hypoxic environment of the anterior chamber. Sickle cells have a difficult time passing through the outflow system of the eye and can precipitate acute IOP rise with secondary open-angle glaucoma. Initial laboratory screening for sickle-cell disease or trait is important for patients who are of African-American, Hispanic, or Mediterranean origin. These patients must be monitored closely for a rise in IOP so that medical and surgical treatment can be initiated promptly.

TRAUMATIC CATARACT Blunt and penetrating trauma to the eye may cause cataract development. Penetrating trauma may result in disruption of the lens capsule, immediate cataract development, and lens-induced uveitis. Treatment is cataract extraction at the time of globe repair, with or without intraocular lens implantation. Blunt trauma may cause zonular dehiscence, ectopia lentis, and the formation of a circle of iris pigment on the anterior lens capsule (*Vossius ring*). Traumatic cataracts usually develop in the anterior subcapsular region initially but may expand to involve the cortical and posterior subcapsular areas. Traumatic cataracts are managed in the same manner as aging cataracts, taking into consideration the possibility of phacodonesis and vitreous loss.

TRAUMATIC OPTIC NEUROPATHY Traumatic optic neuropathy may develop in the setting of severe closed head or orbital injury. The impact is usually to the frontal skull, and often there is transient loss of consciousness. Optic nerve damage is the result of shearing forces within the optic canal, associated with loss of pial vessels. Visual loss may be subtle or profound, and the prognosis for visual recovery is usually poor. Corticosteroid administration and optic canal decompression to prevent further injury to the nerve as it swells within the canal following injury have not been proved efficacious.

26.16.5 Eyelid, Conjunctival, and Corneal Lacerations

Lacerations involving the eyelid margin or lacrimal passages should be treated by an ophthalmologist. Careful primary closure is required to avoid permanent notching of the eyelid margin, chronic tearing, trichiasis, or permanent closure of the lacrimal canaliculi. Injury to the nasolacrimal duct results from fractures involving the anteromedial orbit and lateral wall of the nose. Dacryocystorhinostomy relieves tearing in such lesions by establishing an alternate pathway for tear drainage to the nose; age is no barrier for this procedure. The canalicular system is commonly injured in children by hooks and dog bites. Canalicular injury may not be recognized initially, and examination under anesthesia may be necessary to define the extent of injury more definitively. Primary repair of a severed canaliculus should be undertaken immediately with placement of a silicone stent for 3 to 6 months.

All but the largest conjunctival lacerations can be managed without surgical repair. Most conjunctival lacerations close spontaneously within a few days. Patients with corneal lacerations, however, require prompt referral to an ophthalmologist. If the globe is ruptured by a deep corneal laceration as evidenced by a shallow anterior chamber, iris incarceration in the wound, or aqueous humor trickling from the wound (positive *Seidel test*), a metallic shield should be placed over the eye and the patient referred. Late sequelae of corneal lacerations include astigmatism and corneal scarring, both of which may reduce visual acuity.

26.16.6   Ruptured Globe

This is one of the most serious ocular emergencies, requiring immediate medical attention. Any child who has a history of possible penetrating injury or who has sustained significant blunt injury should be treated as having a ruptured globe until proved otherwise. Frequently, the lids and conjunctiva are markedly swollen, the anterior chamber is shallow or flat, and the pupil is nonreactive and peaked toward the site of rupture. Uveal tissue may be seen plugging or prolapsing through the wound. Because lid squeezing may cause expulsion of intraocular contents, the examination should be cautious and limited. The eye should be covered with a metal shield, and immediate referral made to an ophthalmologist. Further examination and repair should be performed under general anesthesia. *Sympathetic ophthalmia,* with an incidence of 0.2%, is the feared late complication of severe ocular trauma in which there is an immunologically mediated attack on the eyes. In severely damaged eyes with little or no visual potential, therefore, enucleation or evisceration is often performed within the first 7 to 10 days to prevent the development of sympathetic ophthalmia.

26.16.7   Orbital Fractures

Blunt trauma to an eye, typically from an object that is slightly larger than the opening of the anterior orbit, such as a fist, elbow, baseball, or racket ball, may cause fracture of an orbital rim or wall. As a rule, the fracture is probably caused by direct compression or displacement of bone; at other times, it is caused by a sudden rise in orbital pressure (*blow-out fracture*). Orbital fractures are best delineated by orbital CT with axial and direct coronal views. Orbital rim fractures tend to be nondisplaced and stable. Tripod fractures of the zygoma are an exception, and many of these need to be repaired surgically. Fractures involving the medial rim may be associated with epiphora from injury to the nasolacrimal duct or telecanthus from avulsion of the medial canthal tendon. The most common orbital wall fractures involve the floor and medial walls. Blow-out fractures, particularly those of the floor, may be associated with incarceration of orbital tissues, a restrictive (incomitant) strabismus with diplopia, enophthalmos, and facial hypesthesia. Blow-out fractures are repaired only if there is a restrictive strabismus or an enophthalmos of 2 mm or more. Delaying surgery until swelling subsides is advantageous for obtaining a better examination. On rare occasions blunt trauma to the orbit leads to fracture of the optic canal with optic nerve injury. Surgical decompression of the optic canal makes room for the swollen optic nerve to expand.

26.16.8   Birth Injuries

Mechanical trauma to the eyes and eyelids can occur at the time of birth, particularly if labor is prolonged and difficult or if instrumentation is used. Some injury to the eye or ocular adnexae occurs in 11 to 59% of all births, but fortunately it is usually mild.

The use of forceps during vaginal deliveries has been associated with iatrogenic breaks in Descemet's membrane and corneal edema. The condition is usually monocular, but may be associated with ecchymoses of the eyelids and subconjunctival hemorrhage. The corneal edema usually clears within 4 to 6 weeks, but later in life high myopia, marked astigmatism, or corneal ectasia may cause severe visual impairment with amblyopia and strabismus.

The most common ocular birth injury is retinal hemorrhage. Macular hemorrhages occur in about 4% of newborns but rarely have been related to subsequent amblyopia. The etiology and significance of retinal hemorrhages are unknown. Proposed etiologic factors include venous congestion of the head and neck secondary to prolonged and difficult labor or constriction of the neck by the umbilical cord, sudden release of intracranial pressure with birth, asphyxia, capillary fragility, impaired coagulability, cephalic molding, the stress of the first breath, and prematurity. Maternal factors include parity (more common with first birth), duration of labor, type of delivery (unusual with cesarean section), and use of instrumentation (forceps or vacuum extraction greatly increases the occurrence). The hemorrhages are bilateral in one-half of all patients. Usually the hemorrhages resorb within 4 to 6 weeks of birth without sequelae. Large hemorrhages can organize into elevated scars that resemble tumors (massive retinal fibrosis). There is no apparent relationship between retinal hemorrhages and brain damage, but minor changes in the central nervous system may be detectable.

Minor injuries to the eyelids and conjunctiva are common. Edema, ecchymoses, hematoma, and most lacerations heal without sequelae. Lagophthalmos, the inability to close the eye, occurs occasionally in newborn infants. Usually, it is unilateral and may result from facial nerve injury from forceps pressure. The disorder usually disappears within a week. Traumatic blepharoptosis also occurs in newborns but usually disappears in a few days.

Other intraocular injuries that have been rarely ascribed to birth trauma include hyphema, vitreous hemorrhage, cataract, iridodialysis, choroidal tears, and subluxation of the lens.

Miscellaneous birth injuries to the ocular adnexae that occur rarely and are usually attributable to forceps include orbital hemorrhage, subluxation or luxation of the globe outside the palpebral aperture, damage to the cervical sympathetics causing a secondary congenital Horner syndrome, and intracranial hemorrhage.

26.16.9   Battered Child Syndrome

Ocular trauma may be the first sign or one component of the symptom complex of child abuse (see Sec. 5.6.9). Approximately 40% of children who have been physically abused show evidence in the eyes. The most common ocular findings are retinal or preretinal (subhyaloid) hemorrhages. Their discovery in a traumatized child less than 4 years old with multiple injuries, especially fractures of the long bones in different stages of healing, and an inconsistent history is pathognomonic of battering. Other signs include periorbital swelling and ecchymoses, corneal opacity, subconjunctival hemorrhages, hyphema, subluxation of the lens, cataract, iridodialysis, angle recession, secondary glaucoma, vitreous hemorrhage, organization and fibrosis of the retina, retinal detachment, *Purtscher retinopathy* (hemorrhagic retinal angiopathy usually seen with sudden compression of the thoracic cage), papilledema, optic atrophy, strabismus, and psychogenic visual disorders. Accidental head injuries from falls, even greater than 10 feet, and falling down stairs do not generally cause retinal hemorrhages, whereas they are seen frequently after nonaccidental head trauma as occurs in child abuse.

Injuries resulting from whiplash or violent shaking are termed the *shaken baby syndrome.* The problem is usually discovered in infants less than 1 year of age but may occur up to age 2 years. Retinal or cerebral hemorrhages may be the only findings with few or no signs of external trauma. Intraocular hemorrhages are usually bilateral but may be unilateral in 20%. The usual presenting complaints are seizures, vomiting, lethargy, failure to thrive, coma, instability of blood pressure, or respiratory difficulty. Thirty-five percent of these children suffer blindness or visual impairment.

References

Apt L, Sarin LK: Causes for enucleation of the eye in infants and children. JAMA 181:948, 1962

Asbury T, Sanitato JJ: Trauma. In: Vaughan DG, Asbury T, Riordan-Eva P, eds: General Ophthalmology, 13th ed. Norwalk, CT, Appleton & Lange, 1992

Billmire ME, Myers PA: Serious head injury in infants: Accident or abuse? Pediatrics 75:340, 1985

Cullum RD, Chang B: The Wills Eye Manual: Office and Emergency Room Diagnosis and Treatment of Eye Disease, 2nd ed. Philadelphia, Lippincott, 1993

Harley RD: Ocular manifestations of child abuse. J Pediatr Ophthalmol Strabismus 17:5, 1980

Nelson LB, Wilson TW, Jeffers JB: Eye injuries in childhood: Demography, etiology, and prevention. Pediatrics 84:438, 1989

26.17 THE EYE IN SYSTEMIC DISEASE

This section covers the eye findings of selected diseases not covered elsewhere in the chapter.

26.17.1 Human Immunodeficiency Virus Infection

The earliest ocular manifestation of HIV infection in pediatric patients is the development of focal retinal nerve fiber layer infarcts (*cotton-wool spots*). These white lesions do not affect vision and fade in several weeks as new lesions appear. Kaposi sarcoma of the eyelids and conjunctiva; chorioretinitis secondary to cytomegalovirus (Sec. 26.11.6), herpes simplex or zoster, *Toxoplasmosis gondii* (Sec. 26.9.2), *Mycobacterium avium intracellulare*, *Nocardia*, and syphilis; and papilledema from cryptococcal meningitis may be seen in AIDS, but these secondary malignancies and infections are not as common in children as they are in adults. Less serious infections such as blepharitis (including molluscum contagiosum), conjunctivitis, and preseptal cellulitis are also seen in pediatric AIDS.

26.17.2 Fetal Alcohol Syndrome

Ocular manifestations of the fetal alcohol syndrome include short palpebral fissures, blepharoptosis, epicanthal folds, and telecanthus. Visual acuity may be reduced from refractive errors, especially high myopia, and organic causes. Globe anomalies such as microphthalmia (Sec. 26.1.1) and anterior segment dysgenesis (Sec. 26.7.1) have been reported in a number of patients. Comitant strabismus occurs in about 50% of patients. Cataract, congenital glaucoma, and Duane syndrome have also been reported. Retinal vascular tortuosity and optic nerve hypoplasia are the most frequent posterior segment findings and may be unilateral or bilateral.

26.17.3 Phakomatoses

The phakomatoses (neurocutaneous syndromes) are a group of congenital syndromes characterized by the formation of hamartomas involving multiple tissues, primarily the eyes, nervous system, and skin. The term *phakoma* refers to *spot* or *birthmark*. All six of the disorders included in this classification are associated with the development of hamartomas, except the conjunctival lesion of ataxia-telangiectasia, which is a hamartia. *Von Hippel disease* (*angiomatosis retinae*) and *Wyburn-Mason syndrome* (*racemose hemangioma*) have been discussed already (Sec. 26.11.3). The remaining phakomatoses are discussed here.

TUBEROUS SCLEROSIS Also known as *Bourneville disease,* tuberous sclerosis is characterized by hypopigmented cutaneous macules, angiofibromas of the skin occurring in a butterfly pattern over the nose and cheeks (*adenoma sebaceum*), astrocytic hamartomas of the retina, seizures, mental retardation, intracranial calcifications, and an abnormal electroencephalogram. The gene responsible for tuberous sclerosis is located on the long arm of chromosome 9. The retinal astrocytic hamartomas of this condition may appear either as flat, smooth, translucent plaques or as elevated, nodular, opaque, mulberry-like masses (the former may be a precursor of the latter). Either may be calcified. Retinal astrocytic hamartomas occur in one-third to one-half of patients with tuberous sclerosis. One or several lesions may be found in the same eye. Bilateral involvement occurs in 40% of affected individuals. Retinal astrocytic hamartomas are not pathognomonic of tuberous sclerosis. They also occur in neurofibromatosis and in otherwise unaffected individuals. Additional ocular findings of tuberous sclerosis include drusen of the optic disc, glioma of the optic nerve, angioid streaks, and lens or corneal opacities. Vision is generally normal, and progression of the retinal hamartomas, although documented, is uncommon. Tuberous sclerosis is further discussed in Sec. 25.18.1.

NEUROFIBROMATOSIS At least two genetically distinct forms of neurofibromatosis (also known as *von Recklinghausen disease*) have been identified. Type 1 (NF-1), often referred to as *peripheral neurofibromatosis,* is the more common form with a prevalence of 1 in 3000 to 5000. It is autosomal dominant in 50% of cases and has a penetrance of nearly 100%. The remaining 50% of cases are sporadic. The gene for NF-1 has been isolated, cloned, and mapped to 17q11.2. It is thought to code for a protein involved in the regulation of cellular proliferation. NF-1 is diagnosed when two or more of the following seven criteria are met: (1) six or more café-au-lait spots larger than 5 mm in diameter in prepubescent or larger than 15 mm diameter in postpubescent individuals; (2) two or more neurofibromas of any type, or one plexiform neurofibroma; (3) freckling of the axillary, inguinal, or other intertriginous areas; (4) optic nerve glioma; (5) two or more Lisch nodules; (6) a distinctive osseous lesion, such as sphenoid bone dysplasia or thinning of long-bone cortex, with or without pseudarthrosis; and (7) a first-degree relative with NF-1.

Ocular and adnexal findings of neurofibromatosis may include Lisch nodules; plexiform neurofibromas of the eyelids; prominent corneal nerves; proptosis from optic nerve glioma, meningioma, or orbital neurofibromas; pulsating exophthalmos from a deficiency in sphenoid development; retinal hamartomas; secondary glaucoma from angle closure or rubeosis; and localized or diffuse choroidal hamartomas. *Lisch nodules* are found in over 90% of patients with neurofibromatosis beyond 6 years of age and are not found in normal patients. They are melanocytic hamartomas of the iris that are variably pigmented and appear on the anterior surface as smooth, avascular, gelatinous nodules, varying in diameter from pinpoint to 2 mm. Up to 50% of all optic nerve gliomas (Sec. 26.12.4) occur in the setting of neurofibromatosis. They may be bilateral. Treatment is usually observational, although surgical excision of unilateral lesions and radiation treatment are occasionally recommended. Plexiform neurofibromas of the upper eyelid may produce an *S*-shaped blepharoptosis that may have a "bag of worms" consistency on palpation. Complete surgical excision of plexiform neurofibromas is difficult, and the tumors often recur. About 50% of patients with upper eyelid involvement develop ipsilateral glaucoma.

Type 2 (NF-2) neurofibromatosis, also known as *central neurofibromatosis,* is defined by the presence of bilateral acoustic neuromas that are frequently accompanied by multiple other nervous system tumors. The gene for NF-2 is located on the long arm of chromosome 22. The primary ophthalmic manifestation of NF-2 is the development of posterior subcapsular cataracts in the majority of affected individuals during adolescence or early adulthood, at approximately the same age as the central nervous system lesions become apparent.

ENCEPHALOTRIGEMINAL ANGIOMATOSIS Also known as the *Sturge-Weber syndrome,* this nonhereditary, sporadic condition is characterized by facial hemangioma in the distribution of the first and second divisions of the trigeminal nerve, ipsilateral glaucoma, and contralateral epileptic attacks from involvement of the ipsilateral leptomeninges. The distribution of central and cutaneous involvement suggests an environmental insult at the 4- to 8-week stage of embryonic development. The facial hemangioma, also known as a *port wine stain* or *nevus flammeus,* is present at birth and nonprogressive. It does not conform to the distribution of the trigeminal nerve divisions, and involvement of the contralateral face and scalp is not unusual. It is often associated with ipsilateral hemifacial hypertrophy. Mental retardation is common. Hemangiomatous involvement of the leptomeninges typically occurs over the temporal and occipital lobes. Calcification of the underlying gyri produces a double line or "railroad track" sign on plain film x-rays (see Sec. 25.18.10).

Secondary open-angle glaucoma is the most serious ocular complication of Sturge-Weber syndrome. Intraocular pressure can be very difficult to manage. Glaucoma develops most often when there is hemangiomatous involvement of the eyelids or conjunctiva. Heterochromia iridis also is frequent, with the involved side showing a darker iris color. Diffuse choroidal hemangioma occurs in 40% of patients and gives the ocular fundus a diffuse red color described as a "tomato catsup" fundus. The choroidal hemangiomas may complicate glaucoma filtration surgery by increasing the likelihood of expulsive choroidal hemorrhage.

ATAXIA-TELANGIECTASIA Also known as the *Louis-Bar syndrome,* this rare autosomal-recessive disease is characterized by a progressive cerebellar ataxia first appearing in infancy; telangiectasis of the conjunctiva, malar region of the face, antecubital and popliteal fossae, the skin behind the ears, and the skin at the base of the neck; and recurrent sinopulmonary infections. The responsible gene or genes are located on the long arm of chromosome 11 and probably are involved in DNA repair. Ocular motor findings, which are often the earliest manifestations of the disease, consist of nystagmus, oculomotor apraxia, poor convergence, and strabismus. Telangiectatic conjunctival vessels appear in the palpebral fissures between 3 and 5 years of age. They are typically large and extremely tortuous. The ocular fundi are normal. An immunodeficiency state evidenced by thymic hypoplasia and corresponding T-cell abnormalities as well as decreased or absent immunoglobulins (IgA, IgG, and IgE) increases patients' susceptibility to infections and predisposes them to malignancies such as lymphoma and leukemia. The gene responsible for ataxia-telangiectasia has been localized to 11q 22-23 (see Sec. 11.4).

References

Beauchamp GR: Neurofibromatosis type 1 in children. Trans Am Ophthalmol Soc 93:445–472, 1995

Dennehy PJ, Warman R, Flynn JT, Scott GB, Mastrucci MT: Ocular manifestations in pediatric patients with acquired immunodeficiency syndrome. Arch Ophthalmol 107:978, 1989

Gomez MR, ed: Tuberous Sclerosis, 2nd ed. New York, Raven, 1988

Maher ER, Yates JRW, Harries R, et al: Clinical features and natural history of von Hippel-Lindau disease. Q J Med 77:1151, 1990

Palena PV, Augsberger J: Phakomatoses. In: Duane TD, Jaeger EA, eds: Clinical Ophthalmology. Philadelphia, Lippincott-Raven, 1995

Ragge NK, Bauer ME, Klein J, et al: Ocular abnormalities in neurofibromatosis 2. Am J Ophthalmol 120:634, 1995

Stenson SM, Friedberg DN, eds: AIDS and the Eye. New Orleans, Contact Lens Association of Ophthalmologists, 1995

Strömland K: Ocular involvement in the fetal alcohol syndrome. Surv Ophthalmol 31:277, 1987

Sullivan TJ, Clarke MP, Morin JD: The ocular manifestations of the Sturge-Weber syndrome. J Pediatr Ophthalmol Strabismus 29:349, 1992

ORTHOPEDICS

Alvin H . Crawford, Associate Editor

27.1 GROWTH AND DEVELOPMENT

Charles T. Mehlman

The growth and development process that begins with a single-celled zygote will result in an adult human being composed of about 100 trillion cells if allowed to progress naturally. Understanding important aspects of both the prenatal and postnatal contributions to this impressive process of growth and development is crucial for any practitioner who is concerned with the diagnosis and treatment of disorders of the musculoskeletal system in children. This review begins with an overview of prenatal growth of the musculoskeletal system (embryology), progresses to postnatal growth of musculoskeletal tissues, and culminates with a discussion of various aspects of pediatric gait, a major developmental milestone that is influenced by growth and development and analyzed by parents and physicians.

27.1.1 Prenatal Growth of the Musculoskeletal System

Prenatal growth represents a finely orchestrated process of gene activation and growth factor interplay during which seemingly small errors may have far-reaching implications. Traditionally, prenatal growth has been subdivided into both an embryonic period (the first 8 weeks of development) and a fetal period (from the beginning of the ninth week until birth). Embryonic development has been further subdivided into five major stages: (a) fertilization; (b) cleavage; (c) gastrulation; (d) neurulation; and (e) organogenesis. Important details of each of these periods of prenatal growth are discussed here, along with several examples of the consequences of errors at various points along the way.

The beginning of the embryonic period is marked by the moment of fertilization whereby a haploid sperm and a haploid ovum combine to restore the normal diploid (46-chromosome) state of human cells in the form of a zygote. Rapid cleavage of the zygote follows soon thereafter resulting in the multiple-celled mulberry-like morula. The morula will progressively transform into a thousand-celled hollow ball called a *blastocyst*. Errors at this stage consist mainly of chromosomal abnormalities and are thought to result in a spontaneous and often symptomless abortion rate of about 50%.

By the third embryonic week a thickened area of the blastocyst called the *primitive streak* appears, signifying the beginning of gastrulation, in which embryonic ectoderm, endoderm, and mesoderm are formed. Mesodermal products include the entire musculoskeletal system along with the cardiovascular and renal systems. Even very mild errors during the process of gastrulation can result in very significant malformations such as sacral agenesis. The embryologist Wolpert is reported to have stated that it is not birth, marriage, or death, but gastrulation that is truly the most important event in one's life.

Neurulation occurs during the third week of the embryonic period and is characterized by appearance of the notochord, formation and closure of the neural tube, and development of somites. The notochord is the organizing structure for the later development of the entire axial skeleton. Clinical studies have established an association between folate supplementation during pregnancy and a decreased risk of neural tube defects such as myelomeningocele. Improper neurulation can result in more extensive abnormalities such as duplication of the spine.

The remainder of the embryonic period is devoted to organogenesis. Events during this time include the appearance of the upper limb buds during the beginning of the fourth week and the lower limb buds by the end of the fourth week. Both of these limb bud events appear to be strongly influenced by a specific group of genes called *homeobox genes*. These limb buds signal the beginning of a proximodistal developmental process that is the hallmark of appendicular growth from this point forward. At about this same time, the four-chambered heart begins to beat. Joints are discernible by the sixth week, although congenital forms of synostosis (congenitally fused joints) have been described. The development of the limb buds into recognizable arms and legs follows the developmental rule that proximal structures develop before distal ones. During the seventh week the limbs rotate (the upper limbs externally and the lower limbs internally), which explains the medial location of your big toe and the lateral location of your thumb. By the eighth week of development the embryo is about 3 cm in length from head to rump and the clavicles begin to ossify.

Weeks 9 through birth represent the fetal period of prenatal growth. This period of time heralds a dramatic increase (almost tenfold) in body size of the fetus. Musculoskeletal highlights of the fetal period include declaration of the muscular portion of the musculoskeletal system by week 9 and the appearance of primary ossification centers of all of the major long bones by week 12. During this period, the fetus also undergoes progressive ossification of the spine such that it will be easily seen via ultrasonography to have a long c-shaped curvature and not the combination of kyphosis and lordosis typical of ambulatory children.

27.1.2 Postnatal Growth of the Musculoskeletal System

The first two years of postnatal growth see an almost 100% increase in size of the child. From this point until puberty there are much more modest gains in size, perhaps in the 6- to 8-cm-per-year range. The final growth surge is that associated with puberty, prior to which both boys and girls have attained about 84% of their adult height. Whereas pubescent growth may seem small when compared to fetal growth rates, the almost 30 cm in height that may be gained during this time looms large in the minds of parents and children alike.

Full-term children are born with radiographically discernible primary ossification centers in all of their major long bones. These ossification areas often comprise most of the diaphysis of the easily recognizable bones such as the humerus and femur. These same full-term children are born with only a small subset of their secondary ossification centers, and these typically include the distal femur, proximal tibia, cuboid, proximal humerus, talus, and calcaneus. The secondary ossification centers of long bones are called *epiphyseal centers* and they typically contribute to diarthrodial synovial joints. As such, the epiphyseal ossification centers present at birth and those that follow slowly expand, along with their related diaphyseal ossification centers, to sandwich between them areas of growth cartilage that constitute the physes (growth plates) at the ends of each long bone.

Perhaps more than any other structure, this physis (or growth plate) differentiates pediatric orthopedics from the rest of the specialty. Proper function of the growth plate can be disrupted by a wide variety of insults including trauma and bone disease. Subsequent tracking of the function of the growth plate is an important task that may befall the pediatric orthopedist. Postnatal growth of the skeletal system is intimately dependent on proper physeal function. The physis (Fig. 27-1) is a predominantly cartilaginous production plant located near the ends of long bones that is responsible for the creation of new bone via a process called *endochondral ossification*. Endochondral ossification involves the formation of bone on a calcified cartilage scaffold. This overall process is choreographed by growth factors such as insulin-like growth factor I and basic fibroblast growth factor. In assembly-line fashion, the physis pumps out its product (bone) in the direction of the metaphysis. This leads to longitudinal bone growth, while circumferential bone growth occurs mainly via intramembranous new-bone formation about the bone's periphery. The physis keeps pace with this peripheral bone growth by itself growing peripherally via cartilage cells migrating to a peripheral area of the physis called the *groove of Ranvier*.

The growth plate is very sensitive to the mechanical stimuli of both compression and tension. The Hueter-Volkmann principle (1862) states that in the skeletally immature bone growth is relatively inhibited in areas of increased pressure and relatively stimulated in areas of decreased pressure or tension. The Hueter-Volk-

mann principle is important to our understanding of certain physeal diseases such as Blount disease (focal retardation of the medial aspect of the proximal tibial growth plate) and growth slowdown or arrest. Metabolic insults, such as systemic illness with high temperatures, leukemia, or trauma, cause growth impairments indicated by metaphyseal areas of increased radiodensity, which are referred to as *Park-Harris growth arrest lines*. Tracking of the lines over time can offer valuable insight into physeal function.

Proper growth of muscles and tendons must also occur in order for them to act appropriately upon the skeletal system. Like bone, muscle has been shown to have a growth plate. This muscular growth plate is located at the musculotendinous junction, and in a fashion analogous to the physis of long bones, specialized muscle growth cells (satellite cells) lay down new muscle (sarcomeres). These satellite cells are present in growing animals, but disappear later in adult life. This overall process is dependent on intermittent tension and is felt to result in muscles doubling their length in the first four years of life and doubling their length again by the end of puberty. Because normal muscle growth is dependent on intermittent stretch and relaxation, spastic muscles grow at a significantly slower rate than do normal muscles and often lead to the development of joint contractures. For example, children with equinus contracture of the ankle (tight heel cords) secondary to cerebral palsy who must undergo an Achilles tendon lengthening at or before 4 years of age are at significant risk of developing recurrent equinus deformity.

27.1.3 Normal and Abnormal Gait Patterns in Children

The motoric culmination of prenatal and postnatal growth and development may be considered to be the walking gait. Normal gait consists of a carefully balanced series of limb and body movements under central nervous system control. In fact, the contention that you walk with your brain, not with your feet, is very appropriate because it places proper emphasis on the neurologic prerequisites for normal gait and deemphasizes the anatomic pegs that actually contact the ground. The child with cerebral palsy does not walk because of central nervous system dysfunction, not because of mild structural deformity. Normal development of gait in a child typically occurs at 8 to 9 months of age, followed soon thereafter by independent walking. The average age at which "walking alone" occurs is 11 months, with 5% of children walking before 9 months of age and 5% of children walking after 16 months of age. Early pediatric gait is characterized by its erratic nature and slowly assumes a normal adult pattern by about 3 years of age. Contrasts between pediatric and adult gait are important for both physicians and parents to understand. Normal mature gait is considered to occur in a cycle that begins with heel strike of one of the person's legs and ends when the same heel strikes the ground again. The two phases that make up one gait cycle are thus stance (60% of the cycle) and swing (40% of the cycle). Children generally take more steps (greater cadence) than adults, and with further maturation step length and walking velocity increase. Children also have a higher center of gravity due to their body proportions and typically carry their arms higher in an effort to maintain their balance. Inadequate dorsiflexion during swing phase and a tendency to have excessive knee flexion at the time of heel strike contribute to the likelihood that a trip or a fall will occur.

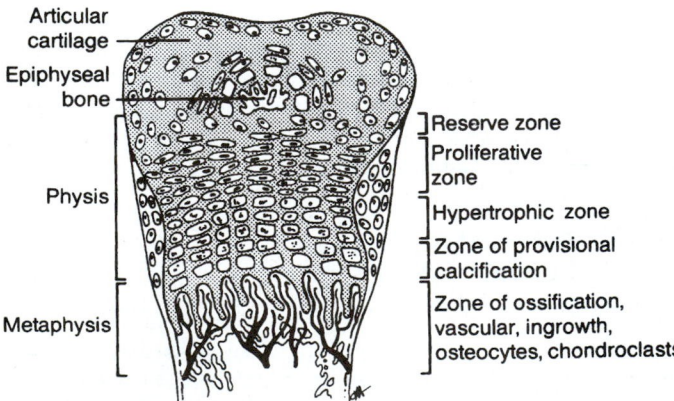

FIGURE 27-1 Histologic detail of the physis (growth plate) in relation to adjacent epiphyseal bone and articular cartilage as well as metaphyseal bone.

27.2   EVALUATION OF THE LIMPING CHILD

Charles T. Mehlman

A limp is any change in the normal walking gait. Most significant is its onset: whether the child was actively playing alone or with others, or whether the child was awakened with the pain or simply noted it on rising. The limp may or may not be painful. Most limps are accentuated by having the child run or skip alternately on each leg for 10 repetitions. Any child noted to have a change in his/her gait pattern, which progresses and/or is accompanied by regressions of toilet training, upper or lower extremity weakness, and/or vomiting should be suspected of having a CNS tumor. It is very important when evaluating a child's limp to strip the child to undergarments and to examine the lower extremities very carefully, to assess range of motion of the joints, and to search for puncture wounds of the sole of the foot. The painful limp requires x-rays from the hips to the toes, or a bone scan, to completely evaluate the problem. Table 27-1 outlines the differential diagnosis of limps.

27.2.1   Clinical Evaluation

A difference in the length of legs may be obvious or may be subtle enough to require close measurement. There are two clinical methods for measuring limb leg inequality in children. The relative length is measured from the umbilicus to the medial malleolus of each limb. The absolute length is measured from the anterior superior iliac spine to the sole of the foot under the lateral fibular malleolus. The latter measurement is preferred because it includes the height of the foot, which may be diminished in some conditions. The frankly obvious discrepancies may be associated with normal configuration of the limb or there may be an absence of the rays of the toes on one foot or the other. If there is considerable difference in girth and obvious muscle weakness, a history of previous febrile episodes must be sought (eg, polio, enterovirus) (see Sec. 13.4.17). For accurate measurements of the length of bones,

TABLE 27-1
DIFFERENTIAL DIAGNOSIS

PAINFUL LIMPS	PAINLESS LIMPS
Toxic synovitis of the hip (27.6.2)	CDH/DDH (congenital developmental dislocation of hip) (27.6.1)
Early Legg-Calvé-Perthes (27.6.3)	
Septic joint/Osteomyelitis (13.1.9)	Spastic hemiplegia (cerebral palsy) (27.11.2)
Traumatic fracture (27.9)	
Pathologic fracture through cyst (tumors) (27.10.3)	Legg-Calvé-Perthes (subacute & chronic) (hip) (27.6.3)
Juvenile rheumatoid arthritis (12.4)	Poliomyelitis (13.4.17)
Foreign body, stress fracture (27.4.2)	Leg-length discrepancy (27.2.1)
	PFFD (proximal focal femoral dysplasia) (hip) (27.1)
Tumor with or without Fx (27.10)	Congenital short femur (hip) (27.1)
Intervertebral discitis (27.76)	
Slipped capital femoral epiphysis (SCFE) (27.6.4)	Congenital coxa vara (hip) (27.1)
	Congenital bowing of the tibia (leg) (27.3.4)

x-rays (orthoroentgenogram, scanogram, or computed axial tomography scanogram) are required.

The hip is examined for instability by performing a Barlow maneuver; that is, with the hip and knee flexed 90 degrees, hold the knee and attempt to displace the thigh posterior by positioning the leg. A positive test is noted by instability with posterior displacement of the proximal femur (hip) toward the table.

The classic Ortolani test of guided abduction to rule out developmental dysplasia of the hip (DDH) usually becomes negative prior to walking age and is rarely performed on the walking child.

Hip instability (DDH) may be asymptomatic in the ambulatory child except for a limp (see Sec. 27.6). Spastic hemiplegia must be kept in mind and a careful perinatal history must be elicited if shuffling, foot dragging, arm posturing, or clenching of the fist is noted. If there is an obvious shortening (less than 1 or 2 inches), then x-rays will usually identify the congenital problem and treatment can be accomplished. The tibia may be bowed. If the tibial bowing is posterior, such as posteromedial bowing with kyphoscoliosis tibia, the condition is usually benign and only associated with some shortening of the limb, which rarely requires an equalization procedure. These children can usually be followed expectantly with sequential x-rays and measurements of their limbs. If their projected discrepancy exceeds 1 inch, then attention should be directed toward equalization of the limbs, possibly by early epiphysiodesis of the other extremity prior to skeletal maturity. If, however, the bowing is anterolateral, the condition is more serious. Anterolateral bowing is quite often associated with neurofibromatosis. There may be easy fractureability with persistent pseudarthrosis. Those patients noted to have anterolateral bowing, even when picked up in the newborn nursery, should be referred directly to orthopedics. There is a high association of congenital tibial dysplasia associated with fracture of an anteriorly bowed tibia, especially when coexistent with neurofibromatosis. The presence of five or more café-au-lait spots of at least 0.5 cm in diameter in infants and more than six café-au-lait spots of at least 1.5 cm in diameter in older children should suggest the diagnosis of neurofibromatosis. Other rare but definite causes of limb length and girth discrepancy include a history of perinatal sepsis with possible osteomyelitis; septic joints and multiple epiphyseal involvement leading to growth plate arrest; purpura fulminans following meningococcemia; vascular abnormalities such as Klippel-Trénaunay-Weber; or a history of femoral catheterization for cardiac disorders.

If there is no obvious cause for the limp, the lower extremity should be palpated front and back from the toe to umbilicus for point tenderness and the two-handed log-roll test performed. The log-roll test is performed by simply placing the child supine with the hips and knees in extension; one hand stabilizes the pelvis and the other hand rolls the leg in and out, "to-and-fro" by holding onto the knee. Normal motion should be approximately 25 to 35 degrees of internal and external rotation. Passive motion that is more restricted on one side than the other, or a "flinching" pain to rotation usually points to the hip as the source of the problem. The hip with the limited motion is usually the one involved. Legg-Calvé-Perthes disease and slipped capital femoral epiphysis (SCFE) may initially present only as a limp and positive log-roll test.

27.2.2   X-Rays

A standing anteroposterior (AP) view of the lower extremities if the child is old enough, or simulated standing with a frog-leg Lauenstein view of the pelvis if the child cannot stand, is indicated for the child with a limp. The pelvis to foot is included. These x-rays of the lower extremity will reveal any obvious cystic lesions (ie, unicameral bone cyst, nonossifying fibroma, neoplasia, Ewing and osteogenic sarcoma), as well as other conditions such as fractures (ie, nondisplaced oblique distal third tibial fracture, "toddler's fracture," nondisplaced tibia, or fibular fractures) with exuberant callus, "stress" fracture, or congenital deformities; abnormal or absent proximal femur; proximal femoral focal deficiency (PFFD); congenital coxa vara; partial or complete absence of the tibia, fibula, or foot; or occasional foreign bodies. The pelvic films will identify soft tissue surrounding septic joints, as well as reveal DDH, Legg-Calvé-Perthes disease, or slipped capital femoral epiphysis.

The pelvic films are evaluated carefully, paying close attention to the joint space. If the femoral head is ossified, the joint space is the clear space between the femoral head and the medial acetabular wall (hip socket). A unilateral increase in joint space of 2 to 3 mm is considered significant and an orthopedist should be consulted. The joint space may be narrowed in idiopathic chondrolysis ("dry socket" disease).

If the femoral head is not ossified, displacement can be demonstrated by measuring the distance from the pubic symphysis to the superior metaphyseal neck of the femur. If there is a difference, usually the side with the greater distance is the joint involved (see Sec. 27.6.1). There may be subtle swelling of the soft tissue about the acetabulum or buttocks, but this is not a reliable sign for infection unless the child is febrile with a high sedimentation rate and C-reactive protein, in which case, toxic synovitis, inflammatory (rheumatoid) arthritis, and/or Legg-Calvé-Perthes disease must be ruled out. Real-time ultrasonography may be used as a noninvasive method to rule out joint effusion. A computed tomography (CT) scan or magnetic resonance imaging (MRI) may be needed to confirm a diagnosis.

27.3 TORSIONAL AND ANGULAR PROBLEMS

Charles T. Mehlman

INTOEING

The differential diagnosis of intoeing includes anatomic variation relative to either the foot (metatarsus adductus), the shin (internal tibial torsion), or the hip (medial femoral torsion). The challenge to the physician is to first determine which one of these (or perhaps which combination) explains the observed intoeing gait (or, in prewalkers, the intoeing posture). If the child's lower extremity alignment falls within an acceptable range (typically two standard deviations of normal), appropriate education through discussion and printed materials is in order. If the child falls outside the normal range, orthopedic referral is appropriate. It is also important to point out that there is no proof that corrective shoes alter lower-extremity alignment. Certain corrective devices have also been associated with worsening of foot deformity and psychological scarring of children.

27.3.1 Metatarsus Adductus

Metatarsus adductus is the most common congenital foot deformity (present in approximately 3% of all live births) and also the

most common foot deformity that prompts families to bring their children in to be evaluated by a physician. In one published report, metatarsus adductus accounted for 75% of all identified pediatric foot deformities in a pediatric orthopedic clinic setting. Metatarsus adductus is typified by an inward deviation (toward the midline of the body) of the forefoot with varying degrees of forefoot supination and hindfoot valgus. It is bilateral in almost 60% of children (Fig. 27-2). The deformity demonstrates a variable amount of stiffness, with some feet correcting with tickling of the foot and others remaining rigid over time. The specific cause of metatarsus adductus is still debatable, but many physicians believe that intrauterine positioning and hereditary factors are at work.

Initially, the most important thing concerning evaluation of the child with metatarsus adductus is to rule out the coexistence of a more severe foot deformity and to screen for other associated abnormalities. More severe foot deformities that have metatarsus adductus as part of their pathoanatomy include clubfoot (talipes equinovarus) and skewfoot (serpentine foot). A clubfoot should demonstrate a high arch (cavus), an ingoing heel (hindfoot varus), and a fixed tiptoe posture (equinus) in addition to metatarsus adductus. If the heel moves freely when moving the foot up and down, the child does not have clubfoot. Anatomically a clubfoot also demonstrates by x-ray a medial subluxation of the navicular off the head of the talus.

The foot deformity known as skewfoot is rarely detected at birth, and tends to be discovered following a course of serial casting for presumed clubfoot or isolated metatarsus adductus. Skewfoot is characterized clinically by an often impressive metatarsus adductus along with a markedly valgus hindfoot (a knock-kneed appearance of the ankles). Radiographically, skewfoot demonstrates a lateral subluxation of the navicular off the head of the talus. Neither clubfoot nor skewfoot enjoys the same benign natural history as isolated metatarsus adductus. As many as 10% of children presenting with metatarsus adductus also have developmental hip dysplasia. Even in the absence of other risk factors, the presence of metatarsus adductus, especially if unilateral, should be considered as an indication for focused and repeated clinical examination of the hips.

The natural history of metatarsus adductus is almost universally benign (spontaneous correction rates in the 90% range). Before the age of 3 years it is impossible to determine which children will have

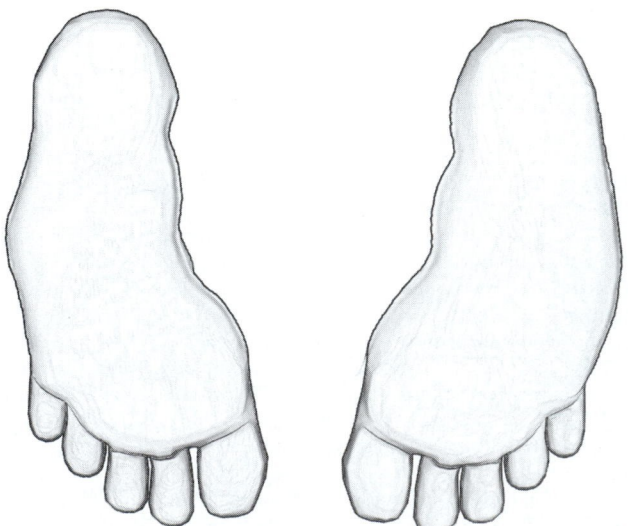

FIGURE 27-2 **Plantar view depicting typical appearance of metatarsus adductus.**

resistant deformity. For those with resistant deformity, surgical treatment is an option but is certainly no panacea. Previously popular surgical procedures for metatarsus adductus have been subsequently shown to have results that are far inferior to the natural history of the "disease." Surgery is rarely, if ever, indicated for isolated metatarsus adductus.

The planned treatment for metatarsus adductus depends on classifying the severity of the deformity. A child with type I metatarsus adductus demonstrates a foot that actively corrects itself when stimulated (tickled) along its lateral border and probably merits no more complex a treatment than actively involving the parents in "tickle exercises" during diaper changes. A child with type II metatarsus adductus has a foot that does not completely correct with tickle stimulation but does correct to neutral with gentle manipulation. Treatment of type II deformity should include passive stretching exercises of the foot with every diaper change. A child with type III metatarsus adductus presents a foot that is rather rigid and not passively correctable back to neutral. It is generally agreed that type III feet merit active orthopedic treatment, which usually consists of manipulation and serial casting. A simple method for documenting and monitoring the character of the child's foot for future comparison is to carefully "photocopy the child's feet."

27.3.2   Internal Tibial Torsion

Internal tibial torsion is the major cause of intoeing in children 1 to 3 years of age and is ascribed to the normal course of events associated with embryologic development. In some pediatric orthopedic practices, it has been estimated that almost 25% of new referrals involve tibial torsion. The key points of the physical examination relative to internal tibial torsion include assessment of overall limb alignment, evaluation of the bimalleolar axis, and determination of the thigh-foot angle (Fig. 27-3).

The assessment of overall limb alignment is aimed at identifying any significant angular deformities such as might occur at the knee or within the tibia itself. Most commonly one may also see physi-

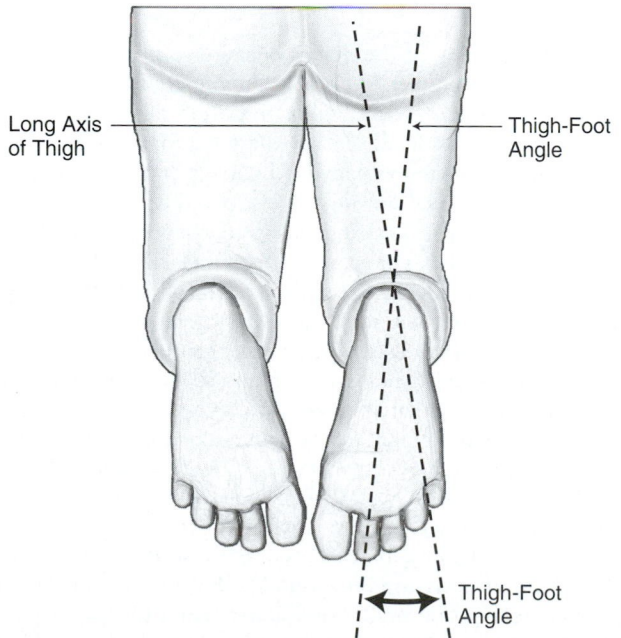

FIGURE 27-3   Depiction of thigh-foot angle as viewed from above a patient lying prone.

TABLE 27-2
THIGH-FOOT ANGLE

NORMAL VALUES AT SELECTED AGES		
AGE	AVERAGE	RANGE
1 y	−5°	−30 to +20°
3 y	+5°	−20 to +25°
5 y	+10°	−10 to +25°
10 y	+15°	+5 to +25°

Range = ±2 standard deviations

ologic genu varum (bowlegs), but other possibilities exist, such as anterolateral or posteromedial tibial bowing (discussed below). Evaluation of the bimalleolar axis focuses on the relation of the medial and lateral malleoli of the ankle with the child's kneecaps "pointing at the ceiling" (limbs in an extended and neutral position). Normal adult alignment is felt to consist of a lateral malleolus that is slightly posterior to the medial malleolus in this position. Varying amounts of internal tibial torsion will result in either a neutral or reversed bimalleolar axis (lateral malleolus anterior to medial malleolus), with the kneecaps pointing to the ceiling.

Determination of the child's thigh-foot angle is the critical component of the internal tibial torsion physical examination. This task is performed with the child in a prone position with the knees and ankles in 90-degree positions. The long axis of the foot is then compared with the long axis of the thigh and the angle between them is recorded. When compared to sophisticated computed tomography methods for measuring tibial torsion, the thigh-foot angle has been shown to be accurate within about 5 degrees. By convention, the angle is defined by the foot relative to the thigh such that "ingoing" feet are assigned negative numbers and "outgoing" feet are assigned positive numbers. Normal values for the thigh-foot angle in children have been established and representative measurements are depicted in Table 27-2. These data show that the average child does not demonstrate an out-toeing gait until about 3 years of age.

The natural history of internal tibial torsion involves gradual improvement throughout the growing years. Familial tendencies may also be first predicted and then later confirmed in more fully grown children. In the past, a low threshold existed for treatment of deformities now known to lie within the normal range. Such treatment usually consisted of special shoes connected by a bar (Denis Browne splint) that was worn at night. The effectiveness of such splinting for tibial torsion has never been demonstrated; furthermore animal studies have indicated that such splinting appears to exert its force mainly through the joint spaces and not the tibia itself. Therefore, for children that fall within established parameters there is no indication for such bracing. For children who fall outside established parameters (or those suffering significant functional consequences) surgical treatment may be required. In a child 10 years of age who continues to demonstrate internal tibial torsion in excess of about 15 degrees, the most commonly used operation involves osteotomy of the distal tibia and fibula. Significant complications from such distal tibial osteotomies are rare.

27.3.3   Medial Femoral Torsion (Femoral Anteversion)

Medial femoral torsion (*femoral anteversion* is a commonly used alternative term) is considered the most likely cause of an intoeing gait in children older than 3 years of age. Femoral anteversion is the angular difference between the long axis of the femoral neck and the corresponding transcondylar axis along the distal femur (Fig. 27-4). Normal values for femoral anteversion are about 40 degrees in newborns, decreasing to about 10 to 15 degrees in skeletally mature individuals. It has been argued that the reason why humans who manifest excessive medial femoral torsion assume an intoeing posture is that intoeing is a compensatory mechanism to restore proper strength to their gluteus medius muscles for hip abduction.

Sophisticated radiographic techniques for measuring femoral torsion have been used in the past, but they have not proven to be more useful than physical examination. The most common practice is to infer the presence or absence of increased medial femoral torsion based on hip range of motion. Hip motion is also routinely assessed in a prone position, allowing the hips to internally and externally rotate with the knees flexed to about 90 degrees. The normal hip range of motion has been established, and, just like other parameters, there is a broad range of normal. Table 27-3 lists the approximate range of both hip internal rotation and external rotation at several developmental stages. Note that average hip external rotation exceeds internal rotation until about 10 years of age. As with the other anatomic areas discussed earlier, medial femoral torsion also has a very favorable natural history. There are no detrimental effects of increased medial femoral torsion that persist into adolescence and adulthood. In the past, an association between excessive femoral anteversion and osteoarthrosis of the hip was thought to exist, but multiple studies show that this is not the case. No nonsurgical treatment for increased medial femoral torsion has ever been shown to be effective; thus, twister cables, shoe inserts, and night splints are not recommended.

Surgery may be indicated for children who meet rather precise indications: (a) older than 8 years of age; (b) significant functional disability; (c) measured anteversion >50 degrees; (d) internal rotation of the hip beyond 85 degrees; (e) external rotation of the hip less than 10 degrees; and (f) a family that has been made well aware of the risks and benefits of surgery. Most commonly an osteotomy of the proximal femur is performed to allow for adequate rotational correction, which is then stabilized with internal fixation

TABLE 27-3

HIP INTERNAL AND EXTERNAL ROTATION

NORMAL VALUES AT SELECTED AGES

INTERNAL ROTATION			EXTERNAL ROTATION		
AGE	AVERAGE	RANGE	AGE	AVERAGE	RANGE
1 y	40°	15 to 60°	1 y	65°	40 to 90°
3 y	40°	15 to 60°	3 y	55°	35 to 75°
5 y	45°	20 to 65°	5 y	50°	30 to 70°
10 y	45°	20 to 65°	10 y	40°	25 to 55°

Range = ±2 standard deviations

such as a plate and screws. Sometimes postoperative immobilization in a spica cast is also necessary.

Even after a technically successful surgical procedure, dissatisfaction may still occur. Preoperative discussions between the orthopedic surgeon, family members, and patient must be comprehensive. Psychological evaluation of the patient may also be helpful at times to identify significant body image concerns.

27.3.4   Bowing of the Tibia

Bowing of the tibia is characterized by the predominant directions to which the apex of the deformity points. The two main types of tibial bowing are designated anterolateral and posteromedial and may occur in otherwise normal appearing children. These "crooked lower limb" deformities clearly also involve the fibula and all of the associated soft tissues of the lower leg. The differentiation of these two entities is more than an academic exercise, as they have drastically different prognoses. Anterolateral bowing of the tibia has a rather bad prognosis and posteromedial bowing has a consistently good prognosis.

ANTEROLATERAL

Anterolateral bowing of the tibia is believed to be a frequent precursor of congenital tibial dysplasia leading to pseudarthrosis of the tibia. Because of chronic instability and nonhealing fractures this condition may occasionally lead to the need for amputation of a child's limb. Its precise etiology is unknown, but more than 60% of cases of anterolateral bowing are associated with an underlying diagnosis of type I von Recklinghausen neurofibromatosis. The diagnosis of anterolateral bowing is suspected clinically and confirmed radiographically. In rare cases, it has resolved spontaneously, and even those cases who were successfully treated via reconstructive surgery still suffer markedly abnormal gait patterns.

Children who are diagnosed with anterolateral bowing of the tibia should be immediately referred to an orthopedic surgeon in addition to undergoing an appropriate evaluation for neurofibromatosis. An effort at preventive bracing should be made as the child begins to walk because in the absence of such bracing, almost all children with anterolateral bowing will go on to fracture their tibias. For children with an established pseudarthrosis it is almost impossible to avoid surgery, and yet surgical "cure" of congenital pseudarthrosis is indefinite at best. This is illustrated by the fact that some authors recommend below knee amputation for children who have failed to heal their pseudarthrosis after several major surgeries.

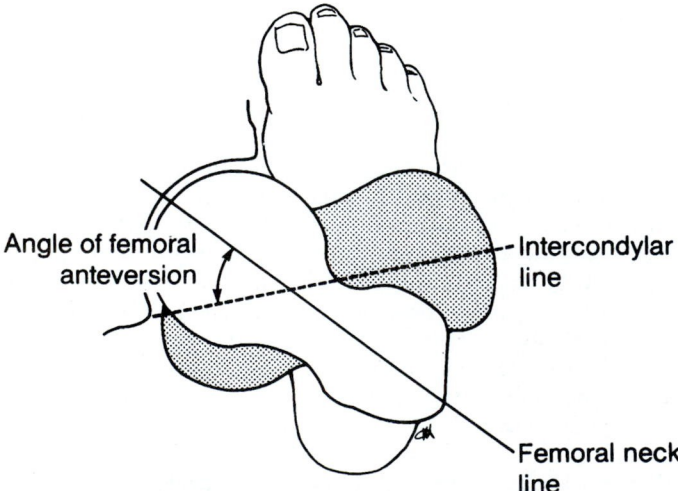

FIGURE 27-4   Increased femoral anteversion. Diagrammatic axial view of the femoral head in the acetabulum superimposed on the femoral condyles and the foot.

Angle of femoral anteversion

Intercondylar line

Femoral neck line

POSTEROMEDIAL

Posteromedial tibial bowing is a congenital deformity whose specific etiology is also unknown, but theories include intrauterine fracture and abnormal fetal positioning in which the foot is tucked under the buttock. The deformity is usually quite dramatic with the dorsum of the foot engaging the anterior shin. Radiographs confirm the diagnosis. With further growth and development the lower-leg deformity lessens (often to the point of becoming clinically unnoticeable). Long-term studies show that leg-length discrepancy is a problem for some of these children, with the discrepancy tending to be directly proportional to the severity of the initial deformity. Therefore, proper tracking of limb lengths in these children is indicated along with the possible need for limb equalization surgical procedures prior to skeletal maturity.

27.3.5   Children's Shoes

A very common question for parents to ask is, "What are the best shoes for my child?" A review of this topic based on available evidence from the literature may be helpful to those charged with caring for children's feet. One myth is that shoes (with or without special inserts) are required for normal arch development in children. This myth has been fueled in part by a profound and persistent societal fear of flatfootedness. Flatfeet are normal in infants, common in children, and within the range of normal in adults. A 3-year prospective study of corrective shoes and inserts for flatfooted 1- to 6-year-olds failed to demonstrate any difference in outcomes between treated feet and controls; in fact, all feet improved over the course of the study. Flatfooted children with pain, neurologic disorders, tight heel cords, or decreased subtalar motion deserve orthopedic evaluation.

Significant doubt has also been cast upon the ability of corrective shoes and shoe inserts to correct intoeing, and there is also no proof that reversing the shoes (wearing shoes on the wrong feet) is a beneficial practice. Corrective shoes are best used for maintenance of a correction that has been made by manipulation, casting, or surgery. In short, shoes serve as a useful barrier to protect feet from cold temperatures or sharp objects.

The challenges presented by intoeing, tibial bowing, and shoewear in children are not insurmountable. Careful evaluation and appropriate criteria for orthopedic referral are vital.

27.4   THE FOOT

Eric J. Wall

27.4.1   Congenital Deformities

CONGENITAL TALIPES EQUINOVARUS (CLUBFOOT)

Congenital talipes equinovarus (clubfoot) is a complex deformity with hindfoot equinus and varus and forefoot adduction. The deformity is of varying severity and may also be associated with a high arch. There are several major categories of clubfeet. A postural clubfoot is caused by intrauterine molding. Generally, this foot is less rigid and corrects either spontaneously or after several manipula-

tions and castings. Idiopathic clubfoot is the most common variety and is the subject of this chapter. Neurogenic clubfeet are associated with spina bifida, tethered spinal cord, or arthrogryposis. Syndromic clubfeet, frequently quite rigid, are seen in diastrophic dwarfism, Freeman-Sheldon syndrome, Smith-Lemli-Opitz syndrome, Larsen syndrome, and other multisystem anomalies.

A clubfoot deformity is relatively common, occurring in 1 in 1,000 whites. Males outnumber females two to one. The incidence of bilaterality is between 30 and 50%. The etiology is unknown, but there is a strong genetic effect. Transmission by a single mendelian pattern has been proposed. The risk of a subsequent child being born with a clubfoot if the first child was a male is 1 in 40; if the first child was a female, the risk is 1 in 16. This risk rises to 1 in 4 to a subsequent child in the presence of the first child being born with a clubfoot and one of the child's parents having had a clubfoot deformity.

The diagnosis of clubfoot is evident at the time of delivery. Occasionally the diagnosis will be suggested prenatally by an ultrasound. In the initial exam, the ankle and hindfoot are noted to be in equinus and varus, and the forefoot is supinated with metatarsus adductus (Fig. 27-5). The foot is smaller and there is calf atrophy. This atrophy is of a variable amount and will persist throughout their lifetime. A leg-length discrepancy, though subtle, is invariably present. The presence of a deep medial crease, rigid deformity, and marked calf atrophy portends that a more intensive course of treatment will be required. Bilateral deformities may be of differing severity. A complete physical exam specifically addressing the lower back for sinuses, hairy patch, vascular lesion, or dimpling should be performed. It is important to rule out spinal dysraphism as a cause of neurologic or syndromic type of clubfeet.

Radiographs are not generally necessary prior to instituting treatment (Fig. 27-6). They are of limited value early in treatment because the ossification of the tarsal bones may be delayed. The ossification centers likewise appear eccentrically in the cartilage anlage. Radiographs are useful for determining residual deformity.

The treatment goal is to obtain a normal looking, painless, flexible plantigrade foot. Treatment by serial manipulation with immobilization in either an above- or below-knee cast is started shortly after birth. Approximately 20% of patients will obtain satisfactory results following manipulation and casting. Surgical intervention is indicated for those children who do not respond to serial manipulations. There are a variety of surgical approaches and techniques to correct the deformity. Satisfactory results following operative treatment occur in more than 80% of patients. After the deformity is corrected, the child's foot should be evaluated at

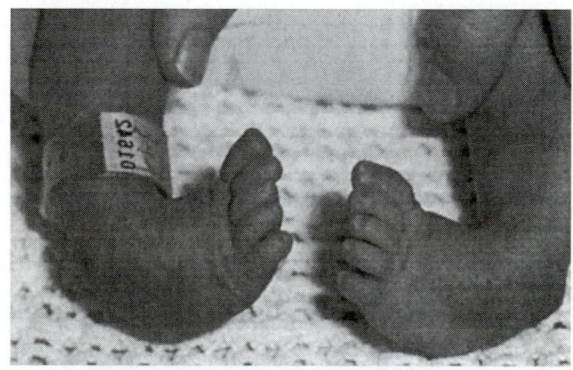

FIGURE 27-5   Appearance of clubfeet in the newborn nursery.

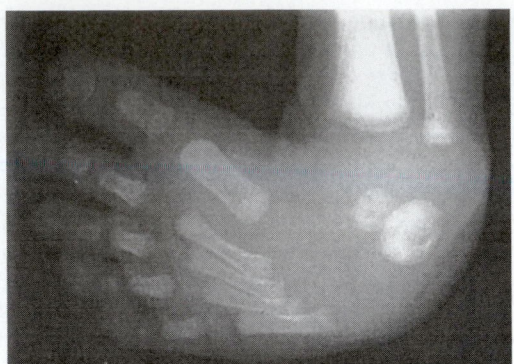

FIGURE 27-6   Anteroposterior (AP) radiographic view of a club-foot.

periodic intervals until skeletal maturity. The clubfoot deformity is not associated with a developmental delay. Even for those children who have undergone prolonged casting, a careful neurologic assessment should be undertaken if the child does not walk by 18 months of age.

CALCANEOVALGUS FOOT

The calcaneovalgus foot is a common deformity that is noticed at birth and is probably caused by intrauterine positioning. It is characterized by excessive ankle dorsiflexion, such that the dorsum of the foot rests against the anterior tibia, associated with eversion of the foot (Fig. 27-7). At first glance, this deformity may appear similar to a congenital vertical talus, except that, in the calcaneovalgus foot, there is no equinus deformity of the hindfoot and the deformity is generally very flexible.

There may be contractures of the ankle dorsiflexor and evertor muscles, and perhaps of the anterior capsule of the ankle as well. The bony structures are normal. Improvement generally occurs spontaneously or with plantarflexion and inversion exercises. The deformity may occasionally be associated with posteromedial bowing of the tibia. On rare occasions, if the deformity is more rigid, serial manipulation and casting are necessary. Long-term follow-up studies suggest that not all feet completely correct and that some may end up in adulthood with flexible flatfeet.

CONGENITAL CONVEX PES VALGUS (CONGENITAL VERTICAL TALUS)

Congenital convex pes valgus (congenital vertical talus) is a rare deformity that is often called a *rocker bottom* or *Persian slipper foot*.

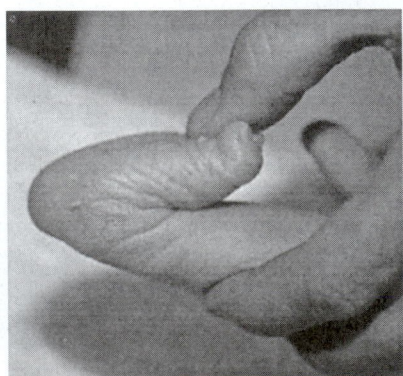

FIGURE 27-7   Calcaneovalgus foot.

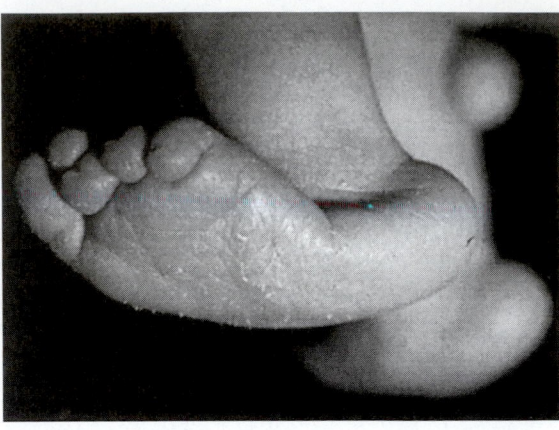

FIGURE 27-8   Congenital convex pes valgus.

It is a fixed dislocation of the talonavicular joint, with the navicular displaced onto the dorsal surface of the talar neck. There is marked ankle and hindfoot plantar flexion with dorsiflexion of the mid-foot giving a convex appearance to the plantar aspect of the foot (Fig. 27-8). The deformity is rigid.

Congenital vertical talus is frequently associated with an underlying syndrome or neuromuscular problem. Examination should focus on looking for associated problems, such as spinal dysraphism or syndromic features (eg, trisomy 18). Management of the foot deformity usually requires surgical correction. Serial manipulation and casting rarely correct the deformity. Surgical correction is indicated, as this rigid foot deformity may eventually cause significant foot pain and difficulty in shoeing.

SYNDACTYLY OF THE TOES

Syndactyly of the toes (webbed toes) is not uncommon. It is a failure of segmentation that usually involves the soft tissues, but may also involve the bones. It is generally inherited as an autosomal-dominant condition with variable degrees of penetrance. The syndactyly most commonly affects the second and third toes and does not limit function, cause pain, or create problems with shoe wear. Surgical correction is not advised unless there is a progressive eccentric growth of the digits causing an angular deformity.

Syndactyly involving the great toe is frequently associated with an underlying syndrome (ie, Apert or Carpenter syndrome).

POLYDACTYLY OF THE TOES

Polydactyly is the presence of an extra digit(s). It is a common malformation that may present as an isolated anomaly or that may be associated with a syndrome. There may also be associated polydactyly of the fingers. The malformation frequently occurs in families and is more common in African-Americans.

Polydactyly most frequently involves the lateral (fibular) side of the foot. If the extra digit has a narrow, nonbony stalk, then a suture ligature at the base of the stalk is often performed in the newborn nursery. Otherwise, complete surgical excision should be performed between 6 months and 1 year of age. Radiographs are a preoperative necessity. Polydactyly of the great toe usually requires a more complex surgical reconstruction.

CONGENITAL OVERRIDING OF THE FIFTH TOE (ADDUCTED TOE)

Congenital overriding of the fifth toe describes a malformation in which the fifth toe is adducted, laterally rotated, and overlaps the fourth toe. It is a familial trait that may be bilateral. Up to 50% of individuals with this deformity develop shoe-wear problems. Non-operative treatment (taping or splinting) is ineffective. If the patient is symptomatic, operative intervention is recommended.

27.4.2 Painful Conditions of the Foot

KÖHLER DISEASE

Köhler disease is an apparent avascular necrosis of the tarsal navicular that presents with pain in the medial mid-foot region. Affected patients are usually male (in a ratio of 5:1) between 4 and 6 years of age. Limp and pain with activity are the usual findings. Bilaterality occurs in 20%. The diagnosis is confirmed by radiographs (Fig. 27-9), which may show sclerosis or fragmentation of the navicular bone followed by reconstitution. Radiographs of the asymptomatic side may reveal very similar changes. This condition is self-limiting and heals spontaneously. Treatment consists of providing symptomatic relief. The use of a below-knee cast decreases the duration of symptoms to a few months. Orthotics are occasionally used. There are no long-term sequelae. Radiographic reconstitution generally occurs within 3 years.

SEVER DISEASE

Sever disease refers to pain in the heel. It is primarily a clinical diagnosis, occurring in a child involved in sporting activities. The pain may be activity related or may be worse in the morning. Clinical exam reveals pain over the calcaneal apophysis. This should be distinguished from pain at the insertion of the Achilles tendon (tendonitis), on the plantar surface (plantar fasciitis), or at the subtalar joint. The tendoachilles may be contracted. Radiographs generally reveal a fragmented, sclerotic appearance of the calcaneal apophysis, which is a normal finding. Treatment includes nonoperative methods such as heel cup, heel pad, heel lift, or, in more severe cases, a below-knee cast. Stretching exercises are recommended if the tendoachilles is contracted. Failure to improve within a reasonable period of time warrants further evaluation with a bone scan.

FREIBERG INFRACTION

Freiberg infraction is a condition of unknown etiology that usually involves the second metatarsal head. It may also involve the third or fourth metatarsal heads. Affected patients are usually teenage females. Anecdotally the condition is associated with running and kicking sports. Pain and swelling over the metatarsal head are the usual presenting complaints. Radiographs reveal flattening, irregularity, and collapse of the metatarsal head. Occasionally, loose bodies may form. Treatment is initially supportive with a metatarsal bar, toe protection orthosis in an athletic shoe, or a below-knee cast. If symptoms persist, surgical intervention is indicated.

TARSAL COALITION

A tarsal coalition refers to a fibrous, cartilaginous, or bony bridge between the tarsal bones that limits the mobility of the tarsal joints. The two most common coalitions are between the calcaneus and navicular and between the talus and calcaneus. They are frequently bilateral, and often there is a familial occurrence. Multiple coalitions may be present in a patient. Coalitions may also be associated with other abnormalities of the lower extremity (ie, fibular hemimelia).

Patients generally present after the age of 10 years with a complaint of lateral foot pain made worse by activities. Often there is

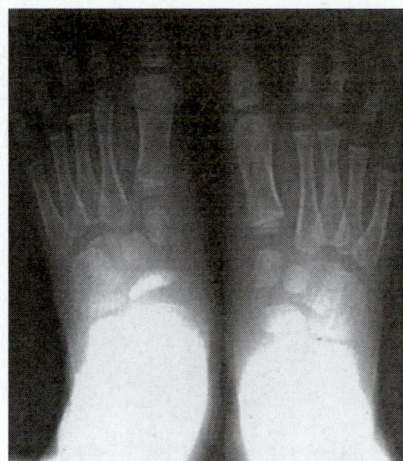

FIGURE 27-9 Köhler disease of the left foot. (Note the smaller size and increased density in the ossification of the left navicular.)

a history of frequent ankle sprains, which are felt to be related to a loss of subtalar motion. Pain may also be present over the lateral aspect of the leg in the peroneal muscle compartment associated with a flatfoot deformity (peroneal spastic flatfoot). The pain is thought to arise from recurrent stress of the coalition.

Physical exam reveals a loss of subtalar motion. Subtalar motion is examined by first dorsiflexing the ankle to place the widest part of the talus into the ankle mortise. The heel is then grasped and rocked into inversion and eversion. This motion is restricted or absent in the presence of a coalition.

Radiographs should include a standing anteroposterior and lateral view of the foot, as well as an oblique (Slomann) view, which may reveal a calcaneonavicular bridge (Fig. 27-10). An axial view of the heel through the posterior facet of the subtalar joint (Harris view) may reveal a subtalar bridge. The lateral radiograph may reveal beaking of the talus and elongation of the lateral process of the calcaneus or the "anteater nose," which is usually associated with a calcaneonavicular bridge. The subtalar joint may be indistinct. A CT scan further delineates either coalition (Fig. 27-11), and reveals a potential coexisting coalition.

Pain usually occurs as the coalition ossifies and becomes more rigid, limiting the subtalar motion. A below-knee walking cast may help to alleviate the acute symptoms, and an orthotic may help to alleviate the more chronic pain. Surgical excision of the coalition is

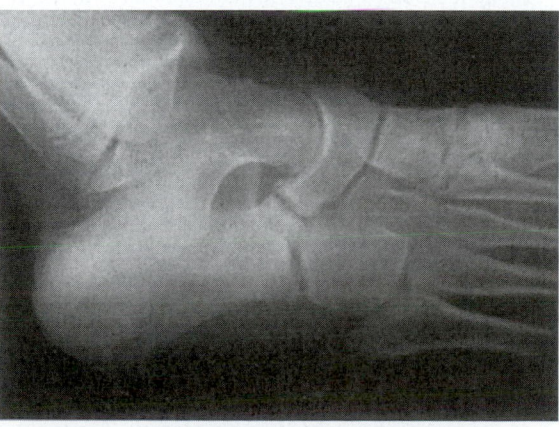

FIGURE 27-10 Oblique x-ray (Slomann view) reveals a calcaneonavicular coalition.

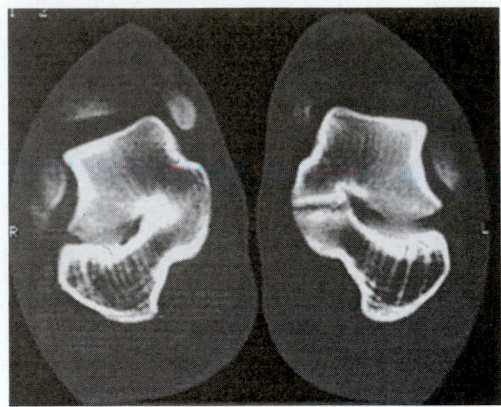

FIGURE 27-11 **CT scan shows a complete coalition of the medial facet of the left subtalar joint. The medial facet on the right is narrowed.**

indicated if pain is not relieved or if pain recurs following nonoperative management. Fusion of the subtalar joint may be indicated if the coalition is too extensive.

SUBUNGUAL EXOSTOSIS

A subungual exostosis (Dupuytren exostosis) is a benign bony tumor (similar to an osteochondroma) of the distal phalanx of the great toe beneath or adjacent to the toenail. Patients usually present with pain or nail deformity (Fig. 27-12). Often there is a history of treatment for recurrent ingrown toenails. Radiographs confirm the diagnosis and show the exostosis to be projecting off the dorsal surface of the distal phalanx (Fig. 27-13).

Treatment is generally surgical excision of the exostosis. Recurrence is possible and it is imperative that a complete excision be performed. This usually requires removal of a portion of the nail.

STRESS FRACTURE

Stress fractures result from a failure of the bone to respond to repetitive microtrauma. They occur most commonly in sports such as track and field, football, gymnastics, and ballet. The tibia is the most common stress fracture site, followed by the fibula. In the foot, stress fractures most commonly involve the metatarsal, calcaneus, and navicular bones.

The child or adolescent presents with the insidious onset of pain that is usually relieved by rest. The pain generally intensifies and is aggravated by all weight-bearing activity. On physical exam there

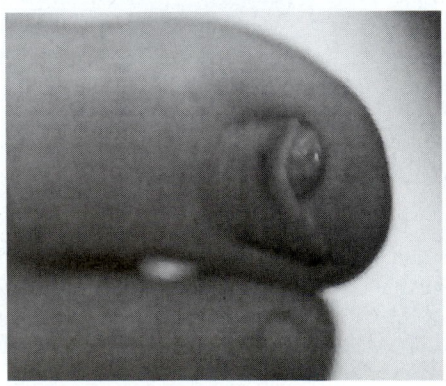

FIGURE 27-12 **Subungual exostosis.**

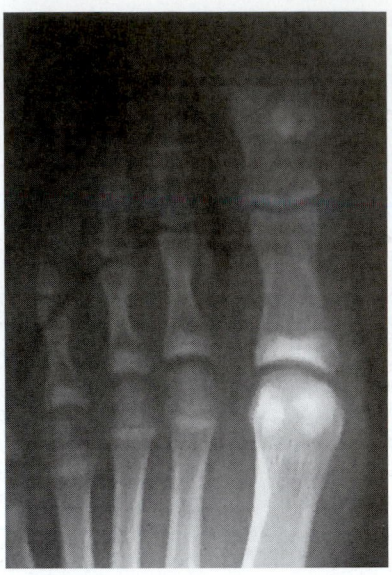

FIGURE 27-13 **Note the exostosis on the tip of the distal phalanx.**

is tenderness to palpation at the affected site. Radiographs may be normal initially and a bone scan can be used for confirming the clinical suspicion of a stress fracture.

Treatment involves breaking the cycle of repetitive trauma. This may involve a change in activity, use of crutches, or immobilization in a cast. Most stress fractures take from 2 to 3 weeks to 3 months to heal. A gradual resumption of activity is recommended to reduce the risk of a recurrent stress fracture.

PUNCTURE WOUND

Puncture wounds of the foot are common. Most heal without any residual problem within 2 to 4 days. A small percentage of children, however, will have a worsening of symptoms associated with erythema and swelling. Early infection is generally related to *Staphylococcus* and is usually a cellulitis. Later infections, such as osteomyelitis and septic arthritis, involve the deep tissues. The most common organism in this group is *Pseudomonas*. Surgical drainage and antibiotics may be necessary. Aggressive definitive treatment, as necessary, may prevent chronic or recurrent problems of septic arthritis and/or osteomyelitis (see Sec. 13.1.9).

PLANTAR FASCIITIS

Plantar fasciitis is a rare condition in the pediatric and adolescent age group. There is pain over the plantar aspect of the foot at the origin of the plantar aponeurosis. Radiographs are usually normal but may reveal a traction spur. Treatment consists of stretching the Achilles tendon and plantar fascia. An orthotic is frequently beneficial.

27.4.3 Miscellaneous Conditions

IDIOPATHIC TOE WALKING

Walking on the toes may be normal up to 3 years of age. Persistent toe walking in an otherwise normal child is referred to as *idiopathic toe walking*. This is a diagnosis of exclusion. The differential diagnosis includes contracture of the tendoachilles, cerebral palsy, muscular dystrophy, and spinal dysraphism. In unilateral cases, a leg-

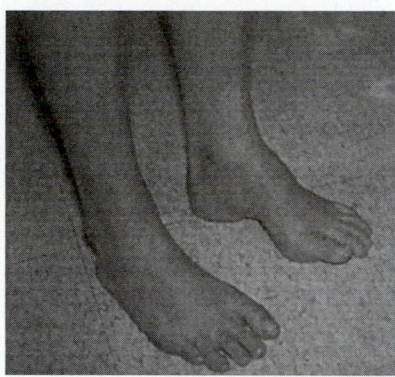

FIGURE 27-14 Cavus foot. Note the elevated longitudinal arch.

length discrepancy of any etiology could cause toe walking. Children with idiopathic toe walking have no restriction of motion and often stand foot flat. Nonoperative management in a child older than 3 years includes an articulated ankle-foot orthosis (AFO), a night splint, or serial casting. Surgery is reserved for those with significant toe walking who do not respond to or are intolerant of serial casting. A percutaneous slide lengthening followed by immobilization for 3 weeks in a below-knee cast is generally performed.

CAVUS FOOT

A cavus foot is defined as a foot with a higher-than-normal longitudinal arch. It is characterized by plantar flexion of the first ray and inversion (varus) of the hindfoot (Fig. 27-14). Clawing of the toes is usually present. A cavus foot should be considered a physical finding that may be a sign of an underlying neurologic problem. Hereditary sensory motor neuropathies, Friedreich ataxia, and spinal dysraphism are all in the differential diagnosis.

Children usually present with a history of foot pain, difficulty in shoe wear, frequent ankle sprains, walking on the outer border of the foot, or claw toes. A family history of this deformity is important to obtain. On clinical exam, there is exaggeration of the longitudinal arch of the foot. The hindfoot may be in varus and the fore-

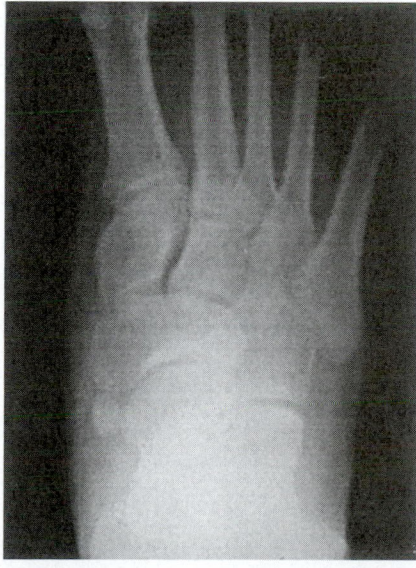

FIGURE 27-15 AP x-ray of the foot showing an accessory navicular.

foot pronated with plantar flexion of the first ray. Clawing of the toes may be flexible or rigid. A footprint or standing on a glass platform will reveal increased weight bearing over the lateral border of the foot. Hindfoot rigidity can be examined by the Coleman block test (stand on a wooden block with the plantar-flexed first ray overhanging the block and observe whether the heel is in varus, neutral, or valgus—neutral or valgus alignment is reflective of hindfoot flexibility). Examination of the child's back for evidence of caudal regression (ie, dimpling, hairy patch, or vascular lesion) and neurologic assessment are essential.

Radiographs of the foot should be obtained to further delineate the deformity. Spine films should also be obtained to rule out spinal problems. CT myelography or MRI helps delineate a tethered spinal cord, diastematomyelia, or a sacral lipoma. Somatosensory-evoked-potential (SSEVP) monitoring or electromyography (EMG) may be necessary to delineate a peripheral neuropathy.

Treatment does depend upon the underlying condition. Nonoperative management includes orthotics and shoe modifications. Surgery is often indicated to correct the deformity and stabilize the feet.

ACCESSORY NAVICULAR

The accessory navicular is the most common accessory bone of the foot. It is located on the medial, plantar border of the foot where the posterior tibial tendon inserts. Patients present either because of a prominence or because of pain. The pain is generally located over the prominence, corresponding to the tuberosity of the navicular where the accessory bone is located. Often there is concomitant pain over the posterior tibial tendon, indicative of tendonitis. Radiographs reveal the accessory navicular (Fig. 27-15). Nonoperative management includes below-knee walking cast, shoe modifications to relieve the prominent navicular, and orthotics. Usually this will control the symptoms. In patients who do not respond to nonoperative measures, surgical excision of the accessory navicular has a high rate of success in improving symptoms.

PES PLANUS (FLATFEET)

Pes planus (flatfeet) is defined as a depression of the medial longitudinal arch of the foot. If the hindfoot is in valgus, then the term *planovalgus* is used. The first determination in evaluating these feet is to assess whether or not the deformity is rigid. Rigid deformities require radiographs and are associated with a bony abnormality (eg, tarsal coalition). Flexible deformities are usually part of the generalized ligamentous laxity in the child. This can be easily visualized by observing the foot in the non-weight-bearing position and again in the weight-bearing position. In nonweight bearing, there is usually an arch that flattens when the child is weight bearing. No treatment is indicated in the flexible flatfoot. Shoe modification and orthotics will not create an arch.

If flexible flatfeet become symptomatic or shoe wear becomes a problem, then an orthotic will be beneficial. Rarely will surgery be indicated. Flatfeet with contracted heelcords often become symptomatic during the teenage years. Tendoachilles stretching is indicated, as is orthotic support. Surgery may be necessary if the feet do not respond to nonoperative measures.

HALLUX VALGUS (BUNION)

Hallux valgus (bunion) refers to the medial prominence of the head of the first metatarsal associated with a degree of medial deviation (varus) of the metatarsal and lateral deviation (valgus) of the prox-

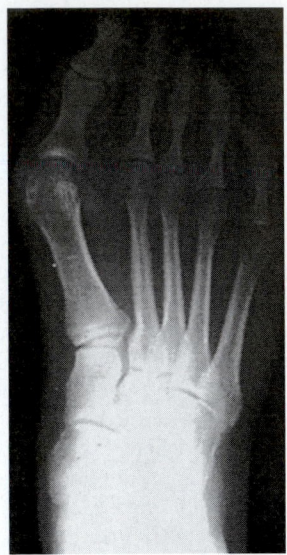

FIGURE 27-16   AP x-ray of the right foot showing hallux valgus (bunion).

imal phalanx (Fig. 27-16). Patients usually present in late childhood or during the teenage years because of deformity, pain, or difficulty in wearing shoes. Often there is a family history of the deformity. Modification in choice of shoes is recommended, with the shoe matching the width of the forefoot. Occasionally, an orthotic will help alleviate symptoms but will not correct the deformity or prevent progression. A nighttime bunion splint often prevents the deformity from progressing, and if enough growth in the foot is remaining, the splint also provides a corrective influence.

Surgical correction for more severe, symptomatic deformities is indicated. Surgery should be postponed until the growth plates have closed, as there is a risk of complications and reoccurrence. There are many surgical procedures described for the correction of bunion deformities. The coexistence of planovalgus feet is a poor prognostic sign for surgical correction.

27.5   THE KNEE

Eric J. Wall

27.5.1   Congenital Knee Dislocation (Recurvatum)

The normal newborn should have mild flexion contractures of both knees because of in utero positioning. Congenital knee dislocation is diagnosed at birth when the infant's knee grossly hyperextends (Fig. 27-17). Congenital knee dislocation is associated with hip dislocation (in up to 50% of patients). If the knee and hip can be fully extended together in the newborn, either the hip is dislocated or a limb deficiency exists. Hip dislocation needs to be ruled out with a hip exam and/or hip ultrasound. Congenital knee dislocation can be associated with genetic syndromes, such as Larsen syndrome, especially when it is bilateral, and genetics referral may be indicated. Orthopedic treatment starts with manipulation and serial casting to flex the knee to 90 degrees, followed by Pavlik harness bracing and stretching. Knees that do not flex to 90 degrees by 3

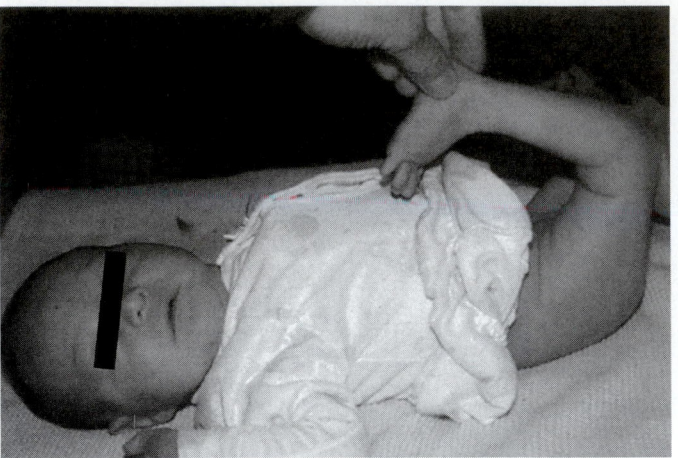

FIGURE 27-17   Congenital knee dislocation (recurvatum).

months of age may require surgical lengthening of a contracted quadriceps tendon.

27.5.2   Genu Valgum (Knock-Knees)

Benign physiological knock-knees tend to reach a peak in children at age 3 years and spontaneously correct thereafter. Children with knock-knees and short stature should obtain lower extremity radiographs to rule out rickets or a skeletal dysplasia. The distance between the child's ankles (intramalleolar distance) should be measured at each visit with normal considered to be <8 cm (Fig. 27-18). Children with normal stature and an intramalleolar distance <8 cm can be observed for spontaneous correction, which is the norm after age 3 to 4 years. Children with worsening knock-knees can be referred for orthopedic evaluation; however, bracing in genu

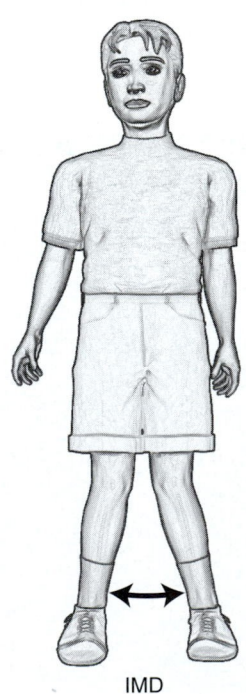

IMD

FIGURE 27-18   The distance between the ankles with the knees just touching is termed the intramalleolar distance (IMD).

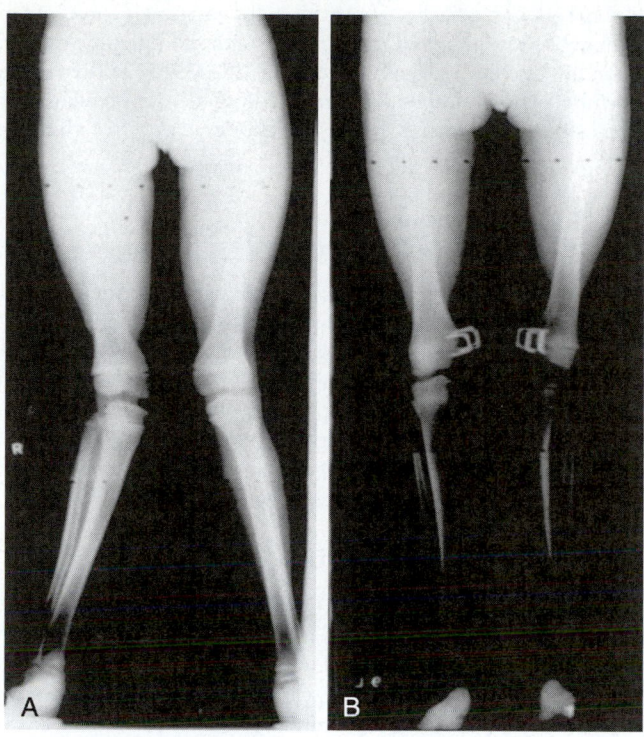

FIGURE 27-19 Genu valgum corrected with hemiepiphyseal staples across the medial growth plate of the distal femur. A. Preoperation. B. Six months postoperation.

valgum is controversial and its efficacy is unproven. Children over age 10 years with persistent genu valgum with an intramalleolar distance >10 cm can be corrected with hemiepiphysiodesis (Fig. 27-19). This small surgical procedure is only effective before the end of growth; otherwise a bone realignment osteotomy may be necessary.

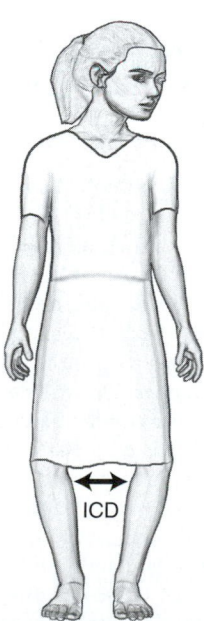

FIGURE 27-20 Bowlegs can be followed by measuring the distance between the child's knees (intracondylar distance) with the ankles held together.

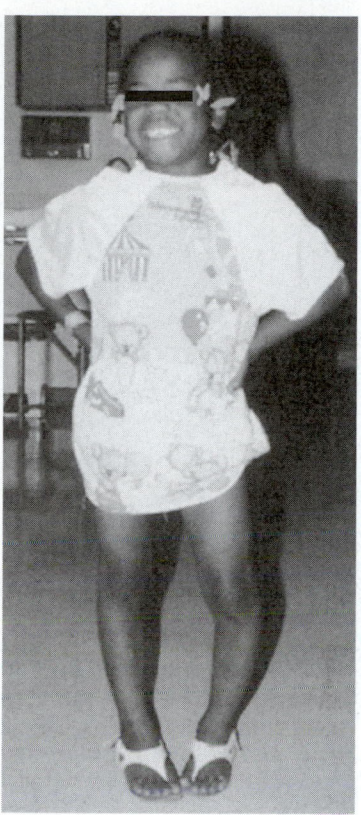

FIGURE 27-21   Child with Blount disease in left leg.

27.5.3 Genu Varum (Bowlegs)

Genu varum (bowlegs) is usually a normal developmental variation in children under the age of age 2 years and can be termed *physiological bowlegs*. These children often demonstrate internal tibial torsion. The physician can quantify bowlegs by measuring the intracondylar distance (ICD) between the child's knees with the ankles held together in the supine position (Fig. 27-20). By age 3 years the ICD should decrease to <1 cm. Knee ICD can be remeasured on well-child visits and if it does not begin to correct by age 3 years, then orthopedic referral is indicated. Bowlegged children with short stature, unilateral leg involvement, or worsening after 18 months of age should be referred for orthopedic evaluation. These children may have a form of pathologic bowlegs, including rickets, skeletal dysplasia, or Blount disease.

Physiological bowlegs rarely require treatment, as spontaneous improvement by age 2 to 3 years is the rule. Braces and special shoes do not accelerate correction of physiological bowlegs, although they are frequently prescribed by physicians.

27.5.4 Blount Disease

INFANTILE/JUVENILE

Children whose bowlegs worsen after 18 months of age may have Blount disease, a rare pathologic form of bowlegs (Fig. 27-21). Blount disease is a pathologic condition of the medial tibial growth plate at the knee. Children with suspected Blount disease should have radiographic evaluation of their lower extremity. Radiographs will reveal widening, irregularity, and downsloping of the medial

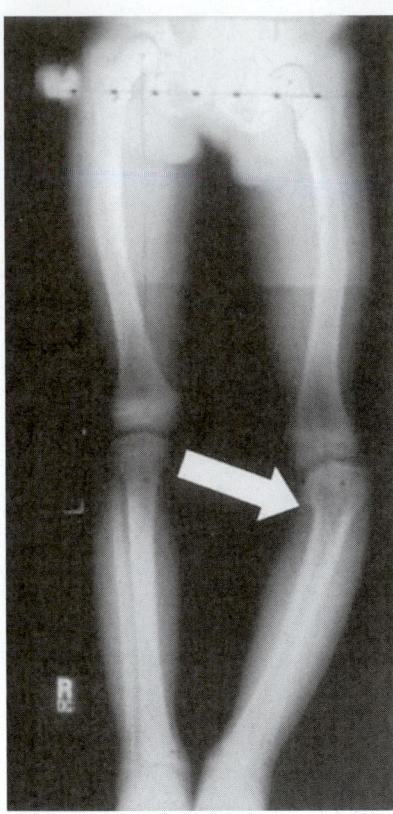

FIGURE 27-22   X-ray of same child with Blount disease. Notice the downsloping of the left medial proximal tibial growth plate.

tibial growth plate at the knee (Fig. 27-22). Children with Blount disease require aggressive orthopedic treatment because this pathologic form of bowlegs can be rapidly progressive and can lead to permanent knee growth disturbance, varus angulation, and arthritis, if uncorrected at an early age. Bracing is effective in Blount disease at the ages of 2 to 3 years, but after age 3 years, corrective osteotomy may be required.

ADOLESCENT

Bowlegs are always abnormal in an adolescent and these patients should be referred to an orthopedist. Blount disease can arise during adolescence, usually in obese patients, is more commonly unilateral, and can lead to degenerative arthritis. Adolescent Blount disease can be treated with a small surgical procedure (hemiepiphysiodesis) that allows future knee growth to correct the angulation, if the condition is identified before the end of growth. Mature patients, or patients with severe deformity, may require corrective osteotomy with either internal or external fixation.

27.5.5   Rickets

Children who have bowlegs and short stature, other involved family members, or an atypical diet should be referred for lower extremity and wrist radiographs, which will show widening and irregularity of all growth plates if rickets is present (Fig. 27-23A). Serum calcium, phosphorus, and alkaline phosphatase levels may be abnormal. Children with rickets should be referred for renal/endocrine evaluation, as most children with rickets today have renal rickets and not dietary rickets, unless the child was adopted from abroad.

After rickets is medically or nutritionally corrected, there can be spontaneous resolution of the bowlegs with radiographic normalization of the child's growth plates (Fig. 27-23B). Children whose deformity persists despite optimal medical management may require orthopedic bracing, hemiepiphysiodesis, or corrective osteotomy.

27.5.6   Anterior Knee Pain

The three most common causes of adolescent anterior knee pain are Sinding-Larsen-Johansson disease, Osgood-Schlatter disease, and patellofemoral pain. The hallmark of these three benign knee-overuse syndromes is that the pain remits with decreased activity. Rest pain or night pain should prompt knee x-rays to rule out a tumor. Hip problems such as slipped capital femoral epiphysis (Sec. 27.6.4) can produce only knee pain, and hip rotation should be examined in all children/adolescents with knee pain.

27.5.7   Osgood-Schlatter Disease

Osgood-Schlatter disease (OSD) is a repetitive-stress injury to the inferior end of the patellar tendon at its insertion into the tibial tubercle in patients ages 10 to 15 years. OSD patients also have an insidious onset of pain. Unlike Sinding-Larsen-Johansson disease (SLJ) patients with OSD usually point to their tibial tubercle, which is usually swollen, as the site of pain, making the diagnosis much easier. Although x-rays are not required on first presentation in patients with a classic history and exam, those patients with atypical findings or rest pain require radiographs to rule out a tumor. Virtually all patients outgrow this condition, although some may have prominent tibial tubercles—"knobby knees"—and mild kneeling pain as adults. Parents need to be reassured that OSD is not a tumor and that it does not lead to arthritis. Treatment of OSD during adolescence is identical to that of SLJ, as the etiology is identical. Patients with pain after skeletal maturity rarely require excision of a calcified bone ossicle that forms within the tendon.

27.5.8   Patellofemoral Pain (Chondromalacia Patellae, Patellar Compression Syndrome)

The exact etiology of patellofemoral pain is not completely known but it probably has a similar etiology to OSD and SLJ in that it is a repetitive-stress injury that involves rubbing between the patella and femoral groove (Fig. 27-24). Other terms for this condition include *chondromalacia patellae* and *patellar compression syndrome*. It is secondary to the very high forces, up to 7 times body weight, that sports and jumping place across the patellofemoral joint mechanism. On examination, the patient will have a positive patella glide test (Fig. 27-25). This test should be done with the knee in 30 degrees of flexion so that the patella contacts the distal femoral condyle. Patella tracking can be assessed by palpating the patella as the patient squats halfway down or flexes and extends the knee over the side of an exam table. The patella apprehension test is positive when the patella is pushed laterally and the patient becomes apprehensive. It helps to identify those patients with patella subluxation and dislocation, but most patients with patellofemoral pain do not have maltracking or malalignment of the patella. Treatment of patellofemoral pain starts with activity modification, anterior knee exercises (initiated via a physical therapist or athletic trainer), nonste-

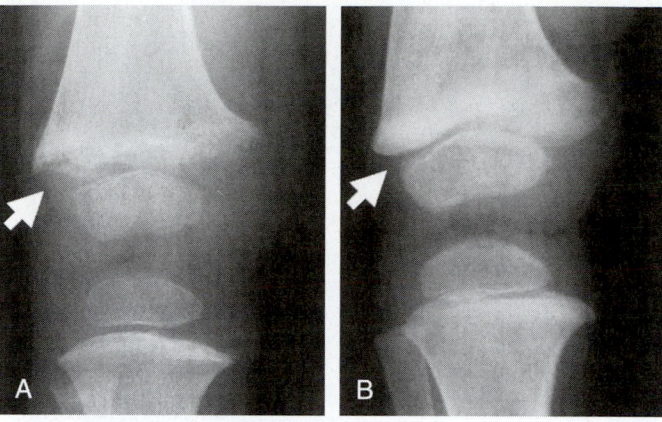

FIGURE 27-23   A. Rickets at time of diagnosis in short child with bowlegs. Arrow points to irregular growth plate of the distal femur. B. After 3 months of medical treatment the femoral growth plate has normalized and is smooth and uniform.

roidal anti-inflammatory medication (NSAIDs), and soft knee braces (neoprene sleeve). Patients who fail this first line of treatment, or who have patellar subluxation/dislocation, or who have a history of patella contusion or trauma, should be referred to an orthopedist. Recurrent patellar dislocations can require surgical correction. However, surgery, including arthroscopy, is often not effective for patellofemoral pain alone without evidence of subluxation or dislocation.

27.5.9   Sinding-Larsen-Johansson Disease

Sinding-Larsen-Johansson (SLJ) disease is a repetitive-stress injury of the patella tendon at its origin from the inferior patellar pole (Fig. 27-26). Children typically have a long history of anterior knee pain with jumping/running sports such as basketball, volleyball, and soccer. The onset of pain is usually atraumatic, but some patients will describe the pain as starting after a knee contusion. When asked, "Where does it hurt?," patients rarely point to the inferior patella pole as the site of the pain; instead, they point inferiorly to the peripatellar area. SLJ can be easily misdiagnosed as patellofemoral pain unless a careful physical exam is performed. With the knee

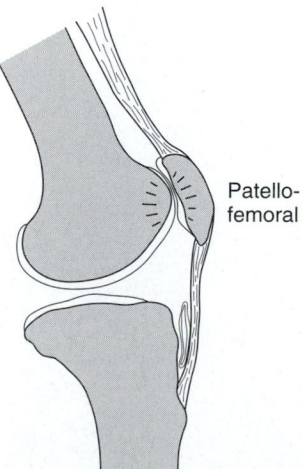

FIGURE 27-24   Patellofemoral pain arises from pressure on the patellofemoral joint.

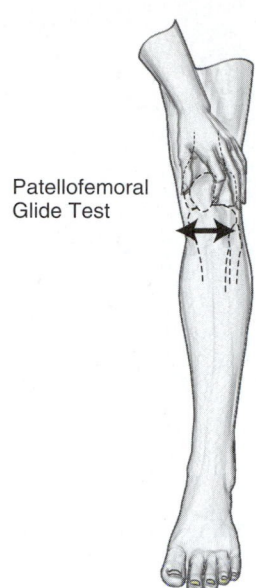

FIGURE 27-25   Medial and lateral translocation of the patella, with the knee at 30- degree flexion, elicits pain in patients with PF syndrome.

in extension, the examiner pushes the patella inferiorly to relax the patellar tendon (Fig. 27-27). Exquisite tenderness with palpation of the inferior pole of the patella identifies this condition. Although severe cases of SLJ can have calcification at the inferior pole of the patella, which is seen on the lateral radiograph (Fig. 27-28), x-rays are usually normal. Radiographs are not required if the history and exam are diagnostic of SLJ. Patients with SLJ whose pain resolves within 24 hours of their sports activity may be allowed to continue activity as tolerated. Pain that persists longer than 24 hours after the inciting activity should be treated initially with a short period of rest followed by progressive strengthening exercises (consider a physical therapy referral) and stretching. Ultimately, children will outgrow SLJ and there are no reported adult sequelae.

27.5.10   Osteochondritis Dissecans

Osteochondritis dissecans (OCD) can be a serious cause of knee pain in juveniles and adolescent patients with diffuse knee pain. OCD involves an abnormality of the joint surface cartilage of the distal femur and the underlying bone. Occasionally, patients with severe OCD may have knee effusion, decreased motion, and locking. Unfortunately, there is no good clinical exam or signs for OCD, and the diagnosis requires a radiograph. It is optimal to obtain four x-ray views, including the anterior-posterior, lateral, sunrise, and tunnel views (Fig. 27-29). The tunnel view is especially helpful for ruling out osteochondritis dissecans. Patients with osteochondritis dissecans should be referred to an orthopedist, as nonhealing lesions can cause disruption of knee joint articular cartilage and can lead to degenerative arthritis in the future. The etiology of osteochondritis dissecans is unknown. It may be related to either repetitive trauma or to spontaneous avascular necrosis of the bone beneath the surface knee cartilage. Treatment in skeletally immature patients includes resting the knee via activity restriction, bracing, or casting. Close follow-up is required and arthroscopic surgery may be indicated for nonhealing lesions in immature patients and in all skeletally mature patients with OCD.

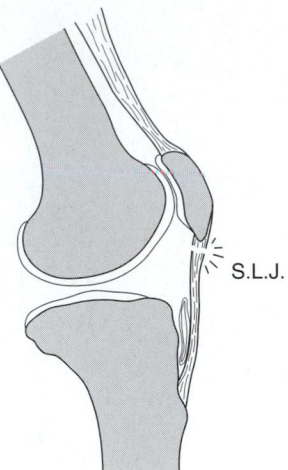

FIGURE 27-26 Sinding-Larsen-Johansson disease (jumper's knee) is an irritation at the inferior patella origin of the patella tendon.

27.5.11   Discoid Meniscus

A discoid meniscus is an abnormally thick meniscus that is shaped like a complete disk, rather than the normal semicircular crescent. A discoid lateral meniscus can be a cause of a painless "snapping knee" with flexion and extension in a young child. Discoid menisci are prone to tearing, which can cause pain, recurrent effusion, and lack of full knee extension. Plain x-rays may show a wide lateral joint space, but MRI or arthroscopy is needed for definitive diagnosis. Patients with symptoms such as knee snapping, locking, effusion, or decreased motion should be referred for orthopedic evaluation to rule out this entity. Nonpainful, intact discoid menisci can be observed. A discoid meniscus that is painful or that limits motion may require arthroscopic partial meniscectomy or meniscus repair.

27.6   THE HIP

Eric J. Wall

27.6.1   Developmental Dysplasia of the Hip

Developmental dysplasia of the hip (DDH) describes a spectrum of conditions that involve the abnormal relationship between the

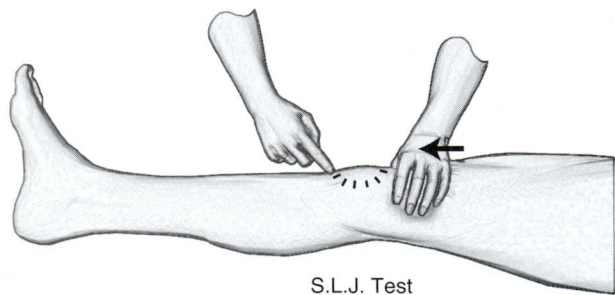

S.L.J. Test

FIGURE 27-27 The examiner pushes the patella distally to relax the patella tendon and then palpates the inferior pole of the patella.

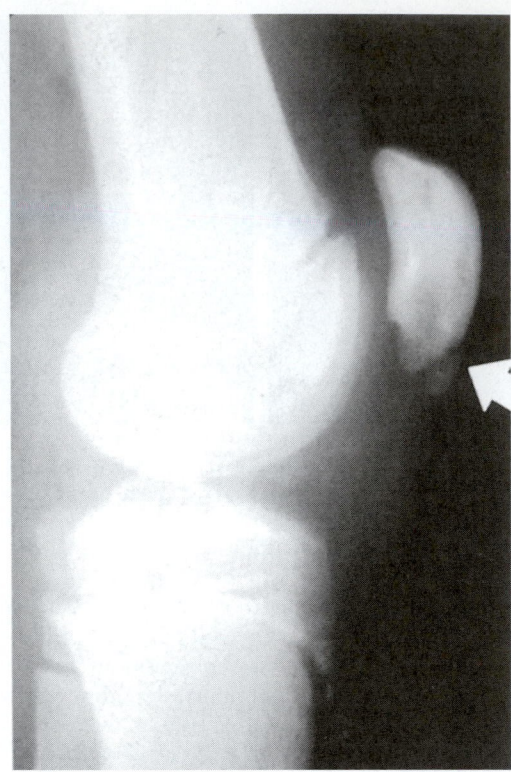

FIGURE 27-28 Severe Sinding-Larsen-Johansson disease can cause calcification at the inferior patella.

femoral head and acetabulum, ranging from simple laxity to subluxation (partial dislocation) to complete dislocation, and includes a variety of acetabular abnormalities. DDH is an evolving process—thus the term developmental—and findings at birth may be absent. The earlier it is detected, the simpler and more effective is the treatment.

Embryologically, the femoral head and acetabulum are part of the same block of primitive mesenchymal cells. At 7 to 8 weeks of gestation, a cleft forms to separate these two structures, which are subsequently completely developed by 11 weeks. During the twelfth to eighteenth gestational weeks, the lower limb rotates medially and the muscles form. At birth, the femoral head and acetab-

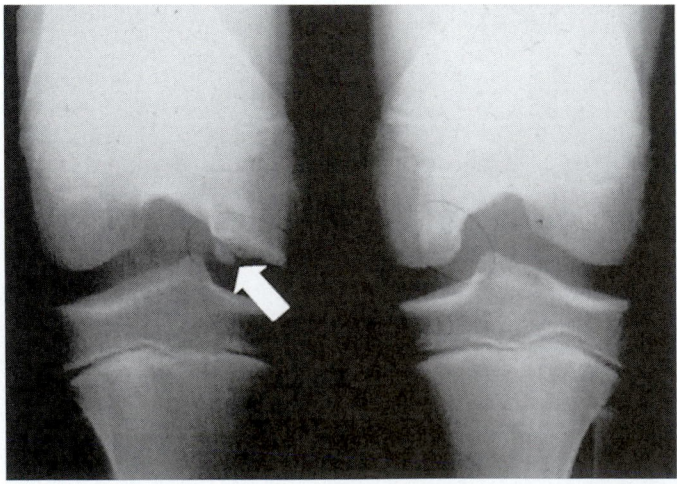

FIGURE 27-29 Tunnel view depicting osteochondritis dissecans of right knee medial femoral condyle.

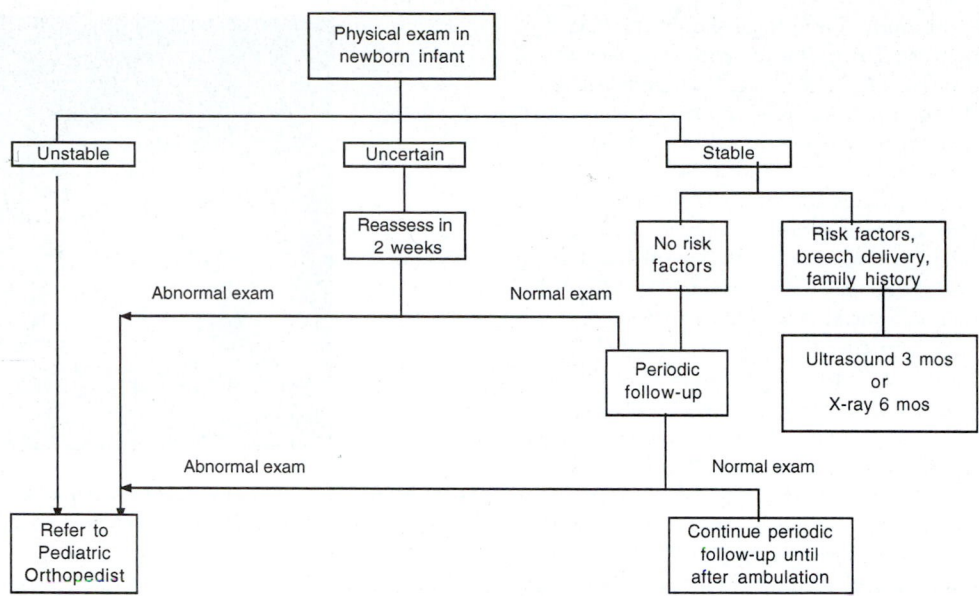

FIGURE 27-30 Pathway for detection and referral of a developmental dysplasia of the hip (DDH) in the newborn infant.

ulum are primarily cartilaginous. The acetabulum continues to develop postnatally, as does the labrum (fibrocartilaginous rim), which deepens the socket. Subsequent development of the hip is determined by the intimate relationship of the femoral head and acetabulum.

Dislocations of the hip are divided into two main categories: teratologic and typical. Teratologic dislocations occur early in the gestational period and are frequently associated with neuromuscular disorders such as myelodysplasia and arthrogryposis. Hips with teratologic dislocations tend to be stiff and irreducible.

The management of the teratologic hip dislocation depends on the associated disease process. It may also be associated with a variety of dysmorphic syndromes. Typical dislocations occur in an otherwise normal infant in the pre- or postnatal periods. Prenatal dislocations are influenced by mechanical forces, such as oligohydramnios and breech positioning. The breech position occurs in approximately 3% of births and the incidence of DDH in this group may be as high as 23%. The frank breech position of hip flexion and knee extension appears to put the infant's hips at highest risk. In the molded baby syndrome (torticollis, scoliosis, windswept lower extremities, and metatarsus adductus), DDH may occur on the adducted and internally rotated side. First-born infants have a higher risk.

The predominant finding in the newborn period is laxity of the capsule. This may allow for spontaneous dislocation and relocation. Stabilization may occur spontaneously, and if it occurs within a reasonable period of time, subsequent development of the hip joint can be normal. If, however, subluxation or dislocation develops and persists, then structural changes develop. The labrum may become flattened and everted, and without the presence of the femoral head, the acetabulum becomes shallow. In the presence of a dislocation, the inferior capsule constricts as it is pulled cephalad over the mouth of the acetabulum. In time, the constriction can become so narrow that the femoral head becomes irreducible, except by operative means. At this time, the adductors and iliopsoas muscle are contracted and limit the motion of the hip, especially abduction. The incidence of DDH varies depending on the specific population, the age of diagnosis, the experience of the examiner, and the di-

agnostic criteria used. Newborn screening programs report incidences of instability to be about 1 in 100 and dislocations approximate 1 in 1000. However, DDH is not always detectable at birth.

Developmental dysplasia of the hip is more common in females and most frequently involves the left hip. The incidence of bilateral DDH is about 20%. Risk of a subsequent child having DDH was delineated by Wynne-Davies. She reported a 6% risk if there are normal parents and an affected child; 12% risk with an affected parent; and a 35% risk with an affected parent and one affected child.

The diagnosis of DDH is not necessarily easily made. It is an evolving process and the physical findings change. Frequent examinations are the cornerstone of diagnosis (Fig. 27-30). The American Academy of Pediatrics recommends a hip exam at 2 weeks, 2 months, 4 months, 6 months, 9 months, and 1 year. Patience and skill are required to examine the newborn's hips, as they should be relaxed. A firm surface is best. Look for signs of asymmetry during the exam. Asymmetric thigh or gluteal folds, apparent leg-length discrepancy, and restriction of abduction are suggestive signs of DDH. Hip abduction should approximate 75 degrees and adduction should approximate 30 degrees. In cases of bilateral DDH, the exam is often symmetric, making the diagnosis more difficult. Because of perinatal hip and knee flexion contractures, if the knees can be extended and the thighs brought flat onto the examining table, suspect dislocation.

Stability of the newborn hip is tested by the Ortolani and Barlow maneuvers. The Ortolani maneuver is a reduction maneuver, while the Barlow maneuver is provocative for a dislocatable hip. The Ortolani maneuver is performed on a child in the supine position, preferably on a firm surface. The thumb is placed along the inner thigh, while the index and middle fingers are placed along the greater trochanter. With the hip flexed to 90 degrees and in neutral rotation, the hip is gently abducted while lifting the leg anteriorly. With a positive Ortolani, one can feel a "clunk" as the femoral head reduces. The Barlow maneuver is also performed with the child supine. The hip is flexed to 90 degrees. Adduction and posteriorly directed pressure are applied to the knee. With a positive Barlow, one may feel a clunk or sensation of movement as the femoral head exits the acetabulum posteriorly. Little force should be utilized in performing these maneuvers. The goal is to demonstrate instability and not to prove that the hip can be dislocated. These two positive tests are distinguished from the frequently occurring clicks, which are of no consequence and usually represent the iliotibial band sliding across the knee.

Another test that is useful takes advantage of palpating the anterior superior iliac spine and the ischium. An imaginary line connecting these two landmarks (Nélaton line) is visualized. The tip of the greater trochanter should be below this line. If it is cephalad to the Nélaton line, then a dislocation should be suspected.

After 3 months of age, limitation of abduction usually becomes the most reliable physical finding that suggests DDH in the older infant. The Allis or Galeazzi sign (relative shortness of the femur with the hips and knees flexed), thigh-fold asymmetry, and leg-length discrepancy should also arouse suspicion. In the ambulating child, limp, unilateral toe walking, and leg-length discrepancy, as well as decreased abduction, are the most common findings. Pain or developmental delay are not features of typical DDH.

Because the femoral head and acetabulum in the newborn are cartilaginous, plain radiographs are seldom helpful. Dynamic ultrasonography can more easily visualize these structures and their relationship. The technique of hip ultrasonography, like any technical procedure, requires learning and practice. Ultrasonography has a high degree of false positives if done too early and should be reserved until the infant is approximately 6 weeks old if the diagnosis is in question. An infant with a positive Ortolani or Barlow sign does not require an ultrasound exam, but does require referral. Ultrasound is quite useful in evaluating the hip during treatment. Plain radiographs become more useful when the ossific center appears (usually 3 to 6 months) (Fig. 27-31).

The earlier the treatment of DDH is instituted, the simpler the treatment (see Fig. 27-30). Initially, a concentric reduction must be obtained, followed by maintenance of the reduction to maximize hip joint development. Bracing with the Pavlik harness is the most common form of treatment at this time (Fig. 27-32). Although the Pavlik harness is effective, there are potential complications associated with its use. Other braces are also used (eg, Frejka pillow, Von Rosen splint) to treat DDH. Bracing is necessary until the hip is stable and is developing well.

Ultrasonography may be used to monitor hip reduction by the brace prior to ossification of the ossific center. This generally occurs within 2 to 3 months in the infant. The older the child is at the

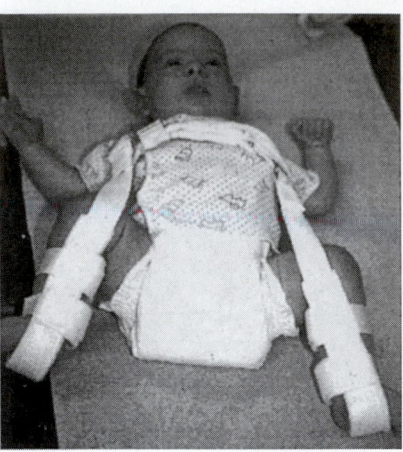

FIGURE 27-32 Baby in a Pavlik harness. The hips are held in flexion. Adduction and extension of the hips are prevented.

time treatment is initiated, the longer the period of bracing is required. Brace treatment should be stopped if the hip does not reduce within a 4- to 6-week period.

In the older child with an irreducible hip, closed reduction with an adductor tenotomy and spica casting in the "human position" is indicated. Occasionally surgery is necessary to remove the obstacles to reduction. In the persistent dislocation, beyond 18 months of age, the acetabulum is frequently shallow and maldirected, and there is bony deformity of the femoral head and neck. Osteotomies of the pelvis, as well as of the femur, are frequently required to correct these abnormalities.

Children who have DDH should be followed until skeletal maturity to assess the effects of growth and development. Complications may compromise the results. These are primarily avascular necrosis and persistent dysplasia. Avascular necrosis is rarely present in unreduced dislocations and presents a significant problem when reductions are performed in children older than 6 years of age.

27.6.2 Transient Synovitis of the Hip

Transient synovitis of the hip (toxic synovitis) is a common, non-specific inflammation of the hip joint of unknown etiology. It is a self-limiting condition that frequently resolves within a week. Although its etiology is unknown, transient synovitis at the hip frequently follows a resolved bacterial or viral infection. There is an increased frequency during seasonal changes.

Complaints at the time of presentation include pain and limp. The pain may be at the hip or as is typical of any painful hip condition, can be referred to the anterior thigh or knee. The limp may be mild, or the child may refuse to bear weight. The differential diagnosis of a painful limp includes a long list of potential disorders. The diagnosis of transient synovitis of the hip is one of exclusion. Most frequently, one will be ruling out septic arthritis or osteomyelitis of the hip or pelvis, Legg-Calvé-Perthes disease, and juvenile arthritis.

On physical exam, the child does not appear ill. There is a positive log roll (discomfort or resistance to a to-and-fro rolling motion at the knee of an extended leg in a supine child whose pelvis is being stabilized). Discomfort and resistance to an internal log roll exam is a sensitive indicator of hip joint inflammation. Abduction and/or internal rotation of the hip is usually restricted.

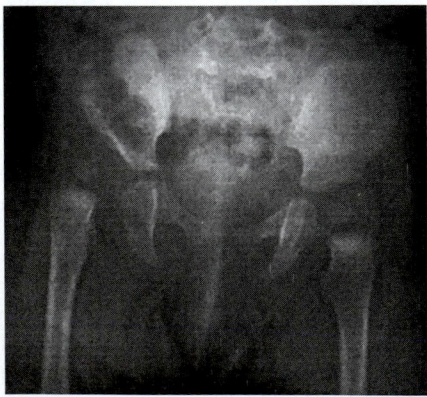

FIGURE 27-31 AP x-ray of the hips in an 8-month-old child showing the dislocated right hip.

Laboratory assessment is generally normal with perhaps a slight elevation in the erythrocyte sedimentation rate (ESR). Radiographs help to rule out Legg-Calvé-Perthes disease or trauma. Aspiration of the hip usually relieves symptoms and rules out a septic joint. Bone scan, CT, or MRI scans are seldom indicated. Even though a positive log roll is consistent with a synovitis, some may prefer to obtain ultrasonography prior to aspiration.

Treatment involves rest and, if necessary, nonsteroidal anti-inflammatory medication. Some orthopedists use traction or slings and springs to rest the hip. In cases of significant discomfort, aspiration of the joint helps to rule out an infection and to shorten the duration of discomfort. The long-term prognosis is excellent. Recurrence is rare. A recurrent case should be evaluated for possible Legg-Calvé-Perthes disease. Failure of improvement within a reasonable period of time suggests a different diagnosis, which should be appropriately worked up.

27.6.3 Legg-Calvé-Perthes Disease

Legg-Calvé-Perthes disease (LCPD) is a partial or complete idiopathic avascular necrosis of the femoral head. Much has been learned about the disorder since its initial description in 1909 to 1910, but its etiology remains unknown and is probably multifactorial.

Most frequently, a male between 4 and 8 years of age is affected. Males outnumber females by 5:1. The disorder is more common in whites and Orientals, and is rare in African-Americans and Native Americans. African-Americans presenting with clinical and radiographic signs of LCPD should undergo electrophoresis to rule out hemoglobinopathy. Bilateral involvement occurs in approximately 10% of cases, but rarely is it symmetric or concurrent. Bilateral symmetric involvement suggests a systemic problem such as hypothyroidism or epiphyseal dysplasia. In addition, other disorders (ie, osteoid osteoma, steroid arthropathy, tuberculous arthritis, juvenile rheumatoid disease, and pigmented villonodular synovitis) need to be considered in the differential diagnosis. An inheritance pattern has not been elucidated, although LCPD can occur in multiple family members.

Epidemiologically, a number of findings are associated with LCPD including low birth weight; abnormal birth position; later-born children; increased parental age; lower socioeconomic status; psychological profiles suggestive of attention deficit hyperactivity disorder; and exposure to passive smoke. Delayed bone age, as well as short stature for age, have been reported. Most recent etiologic theories focus on a compromise of blood flow to the femoral head.

Children with LCPD classically present with a history of a painless limp that is exacerbated by activity. Pain, when it is present, is located about the groin, anterior thigh, or knee. Failure to recognize the referred pattern of hip pain often leads to a delay in diagnosis.

On physical examination, there is a positive log roll test, as well as a limitation of abduction and internal (medial) rotation of the thigh. A hip flexion contracture may also be present. Disuse atrophy of the thigh, calf, and buttock may be present, and a leg-length discrepancy should be measured for.

Standing anteroposterior and frog-leg lateral radiographs of the hips should be initially obtained (Fig. 27-33). Abduction films may reveal hip joint stiffness and possible limited abduction. The hip will proceed through various radiographic stages as the disorder runs its course. The typical stages include normal, early in the disorder; cessation of growth, manifested by a smaller ossific center;

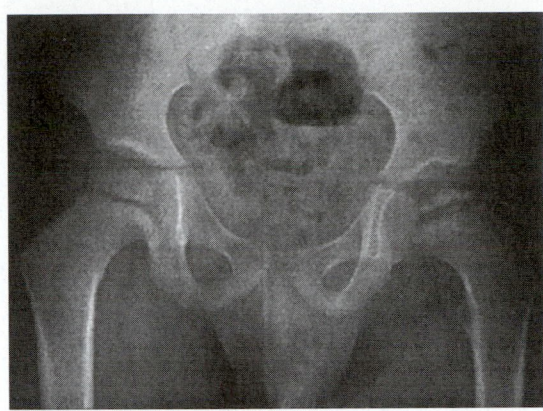

FIGURE 27-33   **AP x-ray of the hips showing Legg-Calvé-Perthes disease (LCPD) of the left hip. Note the increased density and the decreased size of the ossific center.**

subchondral lucency or fracture "crescent sign" that indicates the extent of involvement of the femoral head; fragmentation; reossification; and healed.

The extent of femoral head involvement should be evaluated. The most frequently used classification systems utilize the extent of the subchondral lucency or fracture (crescent sign), and the height of the lateral pillar of the bony epiphysis. A subchondral fracture that involves greater than half of the femoral head, or if there is a greater than 50% loss of height in the lateral pillar, is evidence of a severe case. Subluxation or extrusion of the hip, if present, portends a guarded prognosis.

Bone scans and MRI (Fig. 27-34) may be useful in early diagnosis if the plain radiographs are normal. Dynamic hip arthrography also gives useful information in relation to the mechanics of the hip and congruency of the joint.

Prior to radiographic changes, the differential diagnosis includes trauma and inflammation or infection. Laboratory evaluation should include a complete blood count, ESR, C-reactive protein, and hip joint aspiration if infection is being considered. Bilateral symmetric radiographic changes suggest an epiphyseal dysplasia, hypothyroidism, Gaucher disease, sickle-cell disease, and steroid medication. Prognosis depends on a number of factors including age; extent of femoral head involvement; presence of subluxation or extrusion (Fig. 27-35); duration of disease process; premature closure of the growth plate; and range of motion. Children younger

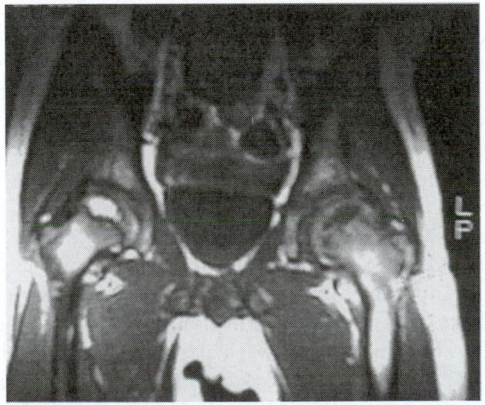

FIGURE 27-34   **MRI showing Legg-Calvé-Perthes disease (LCPD) of the left hip.**

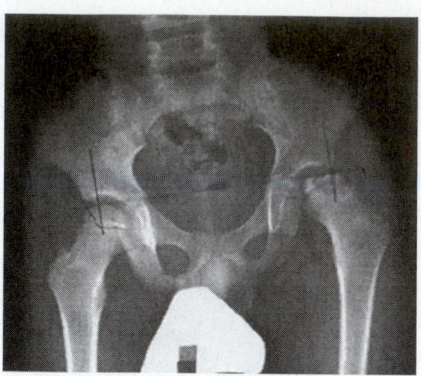

FIGURE 27-35 AP x-ray of hips showing Legg-Calvé-Perthes disease (LCPD) of the left hip with subluxation.

than 6 years of age tend to have less severe disease and have more time for growth and remodeling than does an older child. These children, however, also need to be followed because not all will do well. Children older than 9 years of age have a poorer prognosis. Females, especially obese ones, were initially felt to have a poorer prognosis until a recent study refuted those feelings. Long-term follow-up studies suggest that osteoarthritis will develop in the fifth decade. Preserving a round femoral head offers the best chance for a long-term good result.

Legg-Calvé-Perthes disease is a self-limited and self-healing disorder. No known treatment has been reported to speed the return of blood flow to the femoral head. Treatment is, therefore, indicated for pain, limitation of motion, and early hip subluxation (uncovering), and for those children with severe disease and a worse prognosis. The goals of treatment include the elimination of hip joint irritability with restoration of a normal range of motion; prevention of subluxation, extrusion, or hinge abduction; and obtaining as round a femoral head as possible. Nonoperative treatments include nonsteroidal anti-inflammatory medications, physical therapy, traction, crutches, Petrie casts, and abduction bracing. Operative management in cases of severe disease maximizes containment and offers an improvement in outcome. Surgical options include muscle-tendon lengthenings and osteotomies of the pelvis or proximal femur. The most frequently performed procedure at this time is an innominate osteotomy.

27.6.4 Slipped Capital Femoral Epiphysis

Alvin H. Crawford

Slipped capital femoral epiphysis (SCFE), a common adolescent hip disorder, refers to a slipping of the epiphysis off the metaphysis. The "slipping" is caused by weakening of the perichondral ring of the growth plate that allows the epiphysis and metaphysis to gradually or acutely displace from each other. Most often the capital femoral epiphysis remains in the acetabulum and the proximal femoral metaphysis slips forwards and externally rotates. The action may occur abruptly or chronically. Slipped capital femoral epiphysis is more common in 9- to 16-year-old African-American males, especially those with an obese, eunuchoid body habitus, but the disorder occurs in all races. Patients may present with pain in the hip, medial thigh, or knee, with or without a limp. Occasionally, the patient may have been treated for knee sprain. The pain may have been present for 3 to 9 months. Bilateral involvement eventually occurs in $\geq$ 30 to 50% of patients. Mechanical factors associated

with obesity, endocrine disorders, metabolic disorders (renal disease), and irradiation for malignancy may predispose to SCFE. An exact cause of the slippage has not been discovered. The slippage may be acute with a definite history of injury, pain, and inability to bear weight; under these conditions the epiphysis may be considered unstable. Stable slippage may be chronic with no definite incident but characterized by mild pain, a persistent external rotation, and hip extension gait, with the inability to sit with the legs together and to bend over to tie shoelaces. The two most serious problems associated with SCFE are avascular necrosis (death of the femoral head) and chondrolysis (loss of articular cartilage).

Avascular necrosis is most often associated with abrupt slippage (unstable SCFE) or acute injury to a stable slip and/or manipulative reduction of an unstable SCFE during surgery.

The patient is usually an obese, eunuchoid adolescent, but may be a thin, asthenic male or female. There is usually a combination of a persistently externally rotated limb and a Trendelenburg gait. The hip is often extended and the leg is externally rotated. Oftentimes, there is a positive log roll test (decrease in passive internal rotation or relatively fixed external rotation of the leg with the hip in extension). At rest in the supine position, the affected leg is shortened and externally rotated (Fig. 27-36A). Attempts to flex the hip result in the leg externally rotating.

AP and frog-leg lateral of the hip x-rays may only show slight widening of the physis (growth plate) and increased density (blush sign) over the proximal metaphysis (Fig. 27-36B and C). The head of the femur should normally sit on top of the metaphyseal shaft like a scoop of ice cream on a cone. A line drawn along the femoral neck should intersect the scoop (femoral head). If there is any evidence of the scoop slipping off, the x-ray is positive for SCFE. The AP x-ray may be normal and the frog-leg lateral markedly positive because the majority of the slips are posterior.

Abrupt slippage of the proximal femur is an emergency situation. If the diagnosis of an unstable SCFE is made or suspected, the child should be transported supine on a stretcher because crutch ambulation or even transportation per wheelchair can produce a tendency for the acutely unstable SCFE to slip completely off, compounding the situation. If the child cannot bear weight because of intense pain, the slip is considered unstable and at risk for avascular necrosis. Most orthopedic centers today treat SCFE by in situ percutaneous threaded-screw fixation with no attempt made to reduce the slip. The use of image-intensifying fluoroscopy and cannulated screw implant technology facilitates the care and management of this condition.

Some stable SCFE patients are treated as outpatients, or as same-day surgical stay patients. The patient is then immediately ambulatory on crutches. Some centers tend to use two pins on the unstable slip or for excessively obese individuals because of its inherent tendency to rotate. Most often crutch-assisted weight bearing is carried out for $\geq$6 weeks.

Prolonged follow-up is carried out on the unstable slips because of the tendency to avascular necrosis. Avascular necrosis presents as a return of pain on weight bearing and a decreased range of motion within 6 months of the surgery if it is going to occur. Follow-up x-rays are diagnostic when there is increased density of the femoral head with occasional fragmentation and collapse. Chondrolysis is heralded by a painful limp, decreased range of motion, and joint space narrowing. Chondrolysis has been seen less frequently since the treatment of this condition has been insertion of a cannulated threaded screw under x-ray control. The treatment of avascular necrosis and chondrolysis is not always successful. Attempts to revascularize the femoral head by rotational osteotomy and to reverse

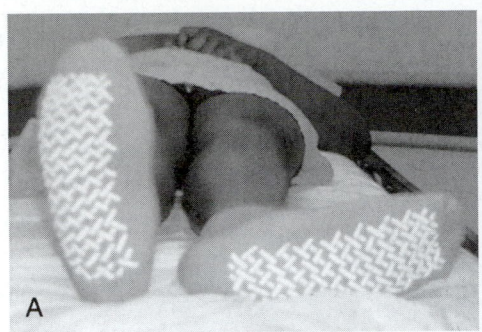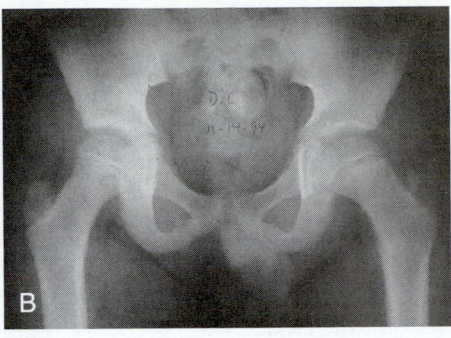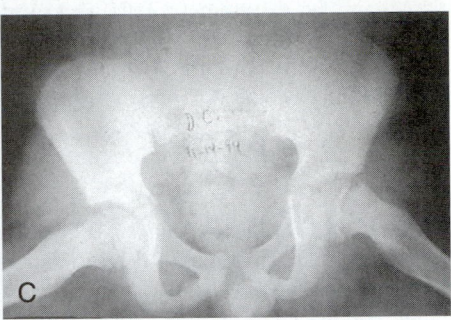

FIGURE 27-36   A child with left slipped capital femoral epiphysis. **A.** When viewed from below, the left lower extremity is completely externally rotated and at a 90-degree angle to the right. **B.** An AP pelvic x-ray illustrates widening of the physis on the left side with some increase in density of the femoral neck. **C.** The frog-leg pelvis view shows the accentuated widening of the epiphyseal line on the left side and evidence of slipping of the capital femoral epiphysis.

the chondrolysis by release of the hip joint capsule and vigorous active and passive assisted motion under epidural anesthesia are popular. Because the SCFE usually is not manipulated and reduced at the time of surgical stabilization, the parents should be made aware that another surgery may be necessary in the future to improve the child's hip motion. Rarely, a flexion, internal rotation osteotomy is performed initially in the stable slips or after complete healing in the unstable slips to improve the hip mechanics. Fortunately, if the child is young, with the pelvic triradiate cartilage open, compensatory motion is quite good and in situ fixation is all that is necessary. Depending on the child's age, monitoring of the limb lengths is important because of the combination of shortening secondary to the slippage, as well as early closure of the growth plate. Early arthrosis of the hip joint secondary to complications of SCFE is a leading cause of degenerative hip joint disease in adults.

27.7   THE NECK AND THE SPINE

Alvin H. Crawford

27.7.1   Congenital Muscular Torticollis

This deformity is characterized by a lateral flexion and rotation of the head and neck. The face is noted to be tilted to one side shortly after birth. There may be swelling or a mass ("olive") in the sternocleidomastoid muscle. There may be an abnormal birth history, with a high incidence of breech presentation, difficult forceps delivery and primiparous mothers. Congenital muscular torticollis has an incidence of 3 to 5 per 1,000 births. Occasionally, the child will present as a "molded baby" with torticollis, C-curve scoliosis, and windswept hips and feet. Because the sternocleidomastoid is tight, the chin will point opposite the involved side, while the head turns toward the involved side (Fig. 27-37). The range of rotation of the head from side to side is limited. There might be slight facial asymmetry.

The back should be examined with particular concern for scapular size and mobility, because there is an association of torticollis with Sprengel (hypoplastic high-riding scapula) deformity. Examination should also be done to rule out associated brachial plexus injury, foot deformity, or developmental dysplasia of the hip. In true congenital muscular torticollis, x-rays are normal. Congenital

cervical vertebral abnormalities as found in Klippel-Feil syndrome should be ruled out.

Passive stretching exercises are recommended to improve neck range of motion. The physical therapist instructs the parents to extend and rotate the neck and head over a table or a parent's knee approximately 20 times, 3 times daily. Advise the parent that the deformity will probably resolve and the child will have a normally shaped head. If the range of neck motion does not progress to normal, it is possible that the facial asymmetry may persist. If the problem does not resolve by age 18 months, the patient should be referred to an orthopedic surgeon.

Recently, the craniofacial asymmetry has been treated by molding helmets. The success of this method is variable. The head-tilting deformity should be corrected before the ocular righting reflex is developed, between ages 5 and 6, or the child may not be able to maintain the correction because holding the head level may interfere with vision. Conservative treatment is successful if the neck range of motion is full and free by 18 months of age; otherwise, surgery may be considered. Surgical correction involves release or lengthening of the sternocleidomastoid muscle. Persistence of tor-

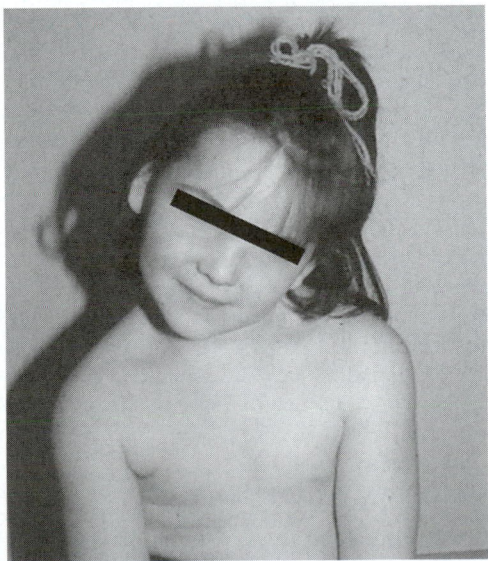

FIGURE 27-37   A 4-year-old child with congenital torticollis (the child's chin is rotated to her right and her head to the left). She has a left sternocleidomastoid deformity.

ticollis and facial asymmetry following surgical release or the presence of "spastic torticollis" with inability to passively rotate the head and neck is cause for alarm. An MRI is indicated in this circumstance to rule out an intracranial posterior fossa tumor.

27.7.2   Klippel-Feil Syndrome

Congenital anomalies of the cervical spine are infrequent and are usually of little clinical significance. Klippel-Feil syndrome is characterized by having a short neck, low-set hairline, and a decreased range of neck motion. It is a congenital anomaly of the cervical spine consisting of multiple fusions bars, with failure of formation or separation of the cervical vertebrae. Associated conditions include congenital scoliosis in 60%, Sprengel deformity in 40%, renal abnormalities in 35%, hearing deformities in 30%, synkinesia (mirror motion) of the upper extremities in 18%, and cardiac abnormalities in 14%. Examine the scapula closely to rule out Sprengel deformity. Parents should observe the child for development of scoliosis. Rarely, there may be cord compression with hyperflexia, clonus, spasticity, and Babinski sign. X-rays of the cervical spine will show the multiple fusions. A renal ultrasound is recommended to rule out congenital anomalies. There may also be an omovertebral bone if Sprengel anomaly is present. Klippel-Feil syndrome occasionally results in adult cervical spine instability and arthrosis. Most often it is the associated condition that requires active treatment.

27.7.3   Sprengel Deformity (Congenital Elevation and Hypoplasia of the Scapula)

Sprengel deformity results from a failure of the scapula to descend (normally from C-4 to T-7) during fetogenesis. The patient's main complaint is usually elevation of the shoulder and limitation of abduction and elevation of the arm. The elevated scapula is smaller than the normal side (Fig. 27-38). There is limitation of neck motion. There may be a palpable fullness connecting the scapula to the neck. This mass is the omovertebral bone, which may be fibrous, cartilaginous, or bony. There is an association with other anomalies, including Klippel-Feil syndrome, rib anomalies, deformities of the upper extremity, and congenital scoliosis.

X-rays of the shoulders will show the elevated hypoplastic scapula. Surgical treatment is recommended only if there is a cosmetically unacceptable deformity or significant decrease in the range of shoulder motion. Surgery may involve lowering and realignment of the scapular and shoulder muscles in young children or simply removing the top overhanging portion of the scapula in older ones. Most often the clavicle is osteotomized when the scapula is brought down to prevent tension on the brachial plexus. The parents should be informed that shoulder motion may be improved although neck motion may be limited because of Klippel-Feil anomaly. Lowering the scapula may result in traction injury to the brachial plexus.

27.7.4   Scoliosis

Scoliosis, a lateral rotatory curvature of the spine, occurs in 10% of the US population. The diagnosis of structural scoliosis should be reserved for curvatures greater than 10 degrees in the frontal plane. The most common type of scoliosis is idiopathic. The diagnosis of scoliosis is usually made clinically by the presence of asymmetry.

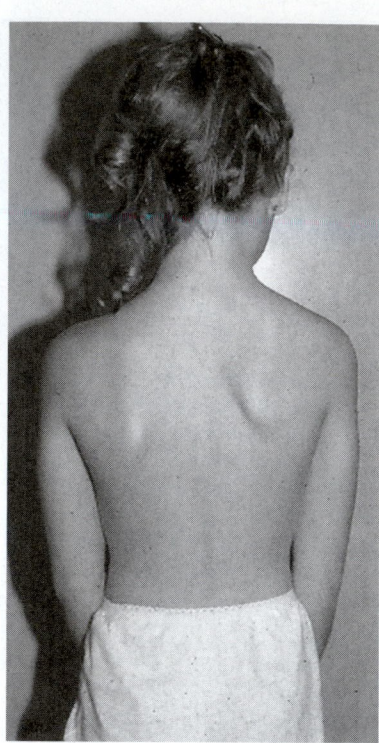

FIGURE 27-38   This 5-year-old child has Sprengel deformity. The right scapula is high riding and hypoplastic.

One shoulder may be elevated and/or the trunk may be out of balance over the pelvis.

Most of these children are completely asymptomatic and are identified by their physicians, school nurse, gym teacher, or peers, rarely by their parents. The incidence of spinal deformity in boys and girls is equal until about 9 to 10 years of age. While scoliosis occurs in 2 to 3% of the adolescent population, only 0.6% of adolescents will need active treatment. After 10 years of age, girls tend to predominate (3.6:1) among those with progressive spinal deformities. Of those children that are treated, 80 to 90% are female. The most common idiopathic curve is a right thoracic single curve.

The chief complaint of patients seen in clinics today is unsightly appearance, even though severe thoracic curves may predispose to cardiopulmonary problems and lumbar curves may be associated with degenerative arthrosis. The mortality rate for these patients is unchanged except for curvatures greater than 100 degrees. Curves less than 30 degrees at skeletal maturity usually do not progress. The incidence of backache is comparable to the general population. Except for lumbar and thoracolumbar curves most patients are otherwise asymptomatic and healthy. Scoliosis can be either structural or nonstructural. Nonstructural scoliosis is a postural compensatory scoliosis resulting from leg-length discrepancy or a neurologic defect (eg, polio) resulting in muscle imbalance. This compensatory scoliosis can be differentiated on spinal x-rays from a structural scoliosis by its lack of rotation and by its ability to correct on side-bending or supine non-weight-bearing films. A single standing posterior anterior x-ray of the spine is required to confirm the diagnosis. Breast and gonadal shielding is utilized and minimal radiation is required.

STRUCTURAL SCOLIOSIS   Structural scoliosis can be classified as either idiopathic, pathologic, neuromuscular, postsurgical, congenital, or traumatic. The vertebrae of structural scoliosis are characterized by wedging, angulation, and rotation (WAR). The treatment is indicated for progression (WARP).

CONGENITAL SCOLIOSIS These curves are more rigid and do not fully correct when the child is supine. The bony anomalies are present at birth and result from fetogenic defects of the spine, either complete or partial failure of formation of a vertebra (hemivertebra), or complete or partial failure of segmentation of a vertebra (congenital bar or block vertebra). Congenital deformities may be isolated or appear throughout the spinal column. Congenital scoliosis is characterized by having abnormally shaped vertebra, hemivertebrae, bars, and absent and/or fused ribs, as opposed to idiopathic scoliosis, which has essentially normal vertebrae. Children noted to have congenital scoliosis should be examined thoroughly for other organ defects. Clinical evaluation for deformities of the lower extremity, such as limb hypoplasia, claw toes, and high-arched feet, is important to rule out subtle intraspinal anomalies. Those with thoracic deformities have an increase in cardiac, gastrointestinal, and tracheoesophageal abnormalities, and those with lumbar deformities have an increase in renal and other genitourinary anomalies, as well diastematomyelia or lower spinal cord (caudal regression) anomalies. The VATER syndrome (vertebral anomalies, anal atresia, tracheoesophageal fistula, and radial and renal anomalies) as well as VACTERLS (vertebral anomalies, anal anomalies, cardiac anomalies, tracheoesophageal fistula, renal anomalies, limb anomalies, and single umbilical artery) should be ruled out with congenital spinal anomalies. All of these patients should have a renal ultrasound or intravenous pyelography (IVP) to rule out anomalies. Congenital deformities may be static or progressive. Those deformities, which tend to progress, do not always respond to bracing. The most common deformity is the hemivertebra. The most progressive deformity is a unilateral uncompensated bar formed as a result of several hemivertebrae converging and growing only on one side. This deformity may require early (<5 years old) surgery to prevent severe progression. An MRI is usually performed to rule out spinal canal anomalies prior to performing the surgery.

NEUROMUSCULAR SCOLIOSIS Although this form of scoliosis is seen most frequently in cerebral palsy, it is also seen in other neurologic conditions (eg, head injury, spinal cord injury, myelomeningocele, muscular dystrophy, spinal muscular atrophy, Friedreich ataxia) and other hereditosensory disorders. The basic problem appears to be an imbalance of the muscles of the trunk and spine leading to deformity. The deformity is rarely static; it may be slowly or rapidly progressive.

Children with neuromuscular spinal deformity need to have orthopedic evaluation and treatment to simplify mobilization and personal hygiene. Treatment can also improve activity level, as well as maintain cardiopulmonary function, which can rapidly deteriorate as their scoliosis progresses. Early detection of scoliosis may prevent the development of a severe curve or prevent operative treatment. Early surgical treatment of progressive deformities (ie, muscular dystrophy) has significantly improved the child's quality of life.

IDIOPATHIC SCOLIOSIS This form of scoliosis is considered to be an autosomal-dominant genetic trait, with variable penetrance and expressivity. The curvature is most often convex to the right side. The condition is divided into three categories: infantile (0–3 years of age), juvenile (3–10 years of age), and adolescent (10 years of age to adulthood).

The Adam bend test is used in screening programs and is designed to pick up rotation of the spine (Fig. 27-39). The patient is examined in a bathing suit or, if younger, undressed from the waist up, facing away from the physician, and clasping the hands together as if diving into a pool. The patient then bends over as if to touch the toes. By looking from behind in a straight line from the gluteal cleft of the buttocks to the nape of the neck, the physician will note any curvature of the spine as a rib hump on the side of the convexity of the curve.

The Adam bend test should be part of every well-child visit after walking age. If the bend test is negative, but there is still a question of a curve, the leg lengths should be measured (see Sec. 27.2.1). Abdominal reflexes are tested in all four quadrants for subtle neurologic findings. Overall symmetry at the shoulders, waist, and hips should be evaluated.

The scoliometer is an excellent screening device to evaluate trunk rotation of the rib hump. The scoliometer is a spirit level that can be placed at different spinous processes to calibrate rotation of the trunk. The trunk rotation is usually a result of a surface contour deformity. Only patients with an angle greater than 7 degrees should be referred to an orthopedic surgeon. When following a patient with scoliometer monitoring, make an effort to use the same vertebrae for each reading. All patients with leg-length discrepancy or with a positive bend test should be referred. Treatment may then be expedited by ordering a standing posteroanterior thoracolumbar spine film prior to referral to an orthopedic surgeon.

Curvatures of less than 10 degrees are not considered to be structural (Table 27-4). Curvatures between 10 and 20 degrees in skeletally immature children are most important. The patient should be monitored every 4 to 5 months with x-rays (Fig. 27-40) and appropriate breast and gonadal shielding. Rarely are exercises and physical therapy instituted at this time because of lack of proven effectiveness. Monitoring is done until skeletal maturity is achieved.

If progression to 25 to 30 degrees occurs, a brace is prescribed. If the curve apex is above T9-10, a Milwaukee or over-the-shoulder brace is required. For a curve apex lower than T9, an underarm brace (TLSO) may be effective. The amount of time in the brace per day varies with the orthopedist, but has been found to be most effective at 20 to 22 hours per day. Several other braces are available, including a side-bending nighttime brace, that are accompanied by variable inflatable pads and a dietary supplement. Other modalities, including various strappings and superficial electronic stimulation, have not been successful.

The major problem with bracing appears to be compliance. The wearing of a brace by this very sensitive adolescent population appears to be difficult. Physical therapy is only recommended with bracing. Bracing is important to prevent progression of deformity. Rarely does bracing correct or reverse the curvature. Prevention of progression is the primary goal. Surgical stabilization is recommended for curvatures greater than 40 degrees in the skeletally immature and for curvatures of 45 to 50 degrees in a mature patient.

Skeletally immature patients with curvature greater than 40 degrees are at risk for the "crankshaft" phenomena (ie, continued anterior growth of deformity) in spite of posterior fusion and may need anterior and posterior fusion. Other surgeons may keep these patients in braces in spite of curves >40 degrees until reaching skeletal maturity at which time a standard posterior spinal fusion is performed. The primary goal of surgery is to stabilize and prevent continuous progression of the deformity; correction is a secondary goal (Fig. 27-41). Expected correction ranges from 30 to 70%. Postoperative bracing may or may not be required.

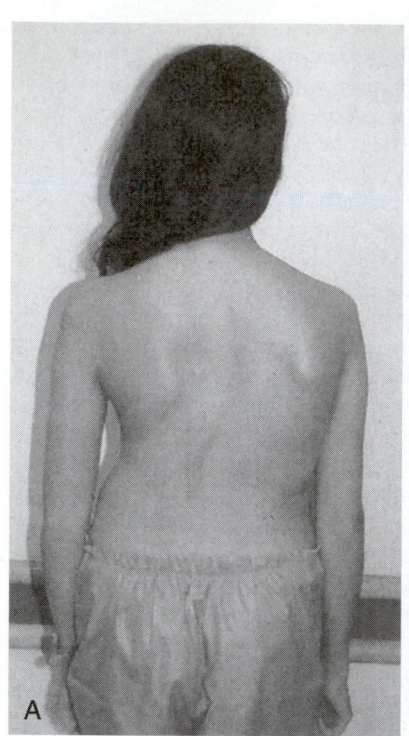 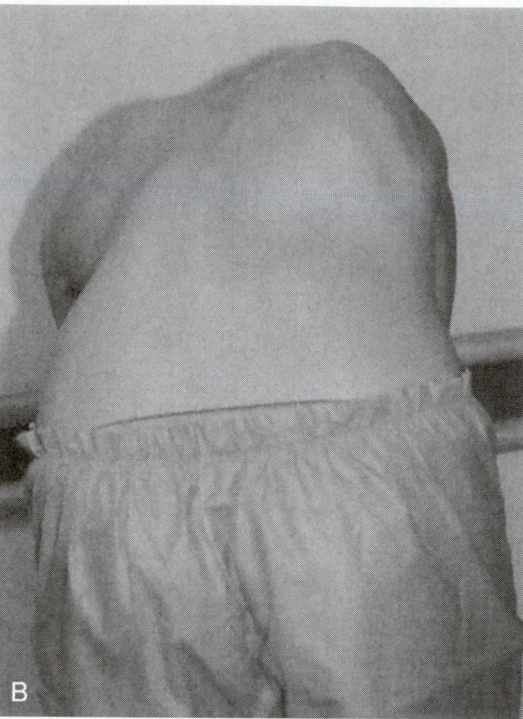 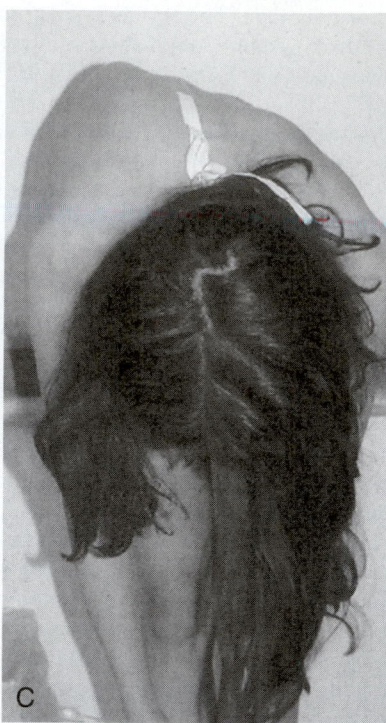

FIGURE 27-39 This 11-year-old child presented with progressive scoliosis. She was noted on the Adam bend test to have significant rib rotation and truncal asymmetry. **A.** When viewed from behind, there is a noted asymmetry of her scapulae and the trunk is shifted to the right. **B.** The Adam bend test when seen from the rear shows a severe rotation and accentuation of the rib hump on the right posterior chest wall. **C.** The rib hump, as seen looking from front to back, accentuates a rotation of the right chest wall.

Surgical complications have been diminished by perioperative management. Autologous blood donation is usually possible in children older than 12 years. Almost all patients are started on elemental iron loading within 6 weeks of their surgery. Erythropoietin may be used in patients whose religions do not allow transfusions or usage of a cell-saver.

Neurologic complications have diminished because of intraoperative spinal cord monitoring by somatosensory-evoked potentials, neuromotor-evoked potentials, a simultaneous EMG, and the "wake-up" test. The evoked potentials are monitored by stimulating the brain or spinal cord above the level of instrumentation and recording signals below to rule out injury. The "wake-up" test is a functional neurologic test performed by lightening the patient's level of anesthesia and having the patient move his or her lower extremities to command.

27.7.5 Kyphosis

ROUNDBACK DEFORMITY

Normal kyphosis, when measured from T3-T12 vertebrae, should be 20 to 40 degrees on lateral x-rays. Children with increased roundback may have positional deformity or Scheuermann disease. Scheuermann disease is characterized by irregularity of the vertebral end plates causing diminished anterior growth with continued posterior growth and the resulting roundback. Scheuermann changes usually occur in the thoracic region, but may also occur in the lumbar region.

These patients may complain of pain. Pain may be managed initially by NSAIDs and exercises. With roundback, if there is no evidence of Scheuermann disease of the vertebrae, the term *juvenile* or *adolescent* roundback is used for curvatures greater than 40 degrees. A thorough neurologic evaluation is warranted with specific attention directed to the lower extremity for foot deformity, high arches, and muscle wasting. If the curvature is flexible, a Milwaukee brace and exercises are effective in the skeletally immature. Curvatures greater than 60 degrees in immature patients may respond to cast correction and bracing, whereas rigid deformities of this (60–75 degrees) magnitude may require surgery, usually consisting of anterior and posterior fusion.

27.7.6 Other Conditions

SCHEUERMANN DISEASE

Scheuermann disease is another of the idiopathic epiphyseal ischemic necroses, as in Legg-Calvé-Perthes, Köhler, and Osgood-Schlatter diseases. It occurs in the anterior vertebral end-plate apophysis, and is more common in adolescent males. The failure of normal anterior vertebral height usually results in a kyphotic (roundback) deformity when found in the thoracic spine. The pain is usually localized directly over the hump. True Scheuermann disease requires wedging of three or more adjacent vertebrae with an angulation of 5 degrees or more. There are usually end-plate irregularities, as well as Schmorl nodes (herniations of the vertebral discs into the vertebrae), although these are also seen in other diseases.

TABLE 27-4

RISK FOR PROGRESSION OF IDIOPATHIC THORACIC SCOLIOSIS

DEGREE OF CURVATURE	10–15 Y OLD	13–15 Y OLD	16 Y OLD
19°	25%	10%	0%
20–29°	60%	40%	10%
30–59°	90%	70%	30%
60°+	100%	90%	70%

Bone scan is most often normal in this disease as compared to spondylolysis or discitis. Treatment is usually nonoperative (observation, NSAIDs, traction, physical therapy, rehabilitation, or bracing). Rarely is operative treatment indicated unless there is severe round-back deformity (greater than 60–75 degrees) or unrelenting pain.

Back pain is extremely rare in the younger child (ages 1 to 10 years) and, if persistent (ie, lasting more than a few weeks), should prompt referral (Table 27-5). The bone scan has been of tremendous benefit in assessing back pain in children, and has significantly decreased the workup time for pathologic lesions. Do not hesitate to order a bone scan if plain x-rays are normal and back symptoms persist. There may or may not be a history of trauma. It is important to investigate a history of back pain of some severity in parents, aunts, uncles, and other relations, and whether or not the illness of the affected person has caused a change in the family structure (eg, divorce, loss of job, need for mother to work to assist family). Young children are infamous for mimicking pain in adult family members, especially if they perceive secondary gain.

Recently, there have been complaints of back pain thought to be associated with the heavy books in a book bag (ie, "book bag disease"). Most often there are few if any radiographic findings and minimal physical findings in these patients. Most centers recommend against a child carrying a bookbag that weighs more than 20% of the child's body weight. It is also recommended to use both shoulder straps to prevent symptoms. There are no documented significant disabilities from this entity.

Back pain accompanied by neurologic signs and symptoms (radicular pain, muscle weakness, gait abnormalities, sensory changes, bowel and bladder abnormalities) or systemic symptoms (fever, malaise, and weight loss) suggests serious problems. Night pain often signals an equally serious problem.

Most bony conditions can be diagnosed by x-ray. Further studies include a bone scan and, if a neurologic deficit is detected, an EMG, MRI, or a CT myelogram may be necessary. Occasionally, in the marginally verbal child, a neurologic deficit will only present as a limp or altered bowel or bladder function and not a frankly positive motor examination. Observe the patient's stance and gait. Have the patient walk on his or her heels and toes to check for extremity weakness. Have the patient jump 10 times on a single leg to determine weakness and/or pain. Look for an asymmetric shift of the trunk or scoliosis secondary to muscle spasm. Spinal stiffness can be correlated with clinical severity. Have the patient bend over as if to touch the toes. If the hand does not come within 12 inches of the floor, the complaint is significant. Perform a straight leg raising test to rule out radiculopathy and hamstring spasm. Observe the exact location of pain for gibbosity, lordosis, or kyphosis. Perform a thorough neurologic examination. Be sure to ask about recent changes in bowel or bladder function. Psychogenic conversion reaction is a rare cause of pain in children and adolescents. Most of the principles alluded to in this section will determine true pathology. Pain centers use psychological evaluation instruments to identify other etiologies of pain in those patients with normal physical examination and imaging studies who fail to respond to immobilization and NSAIDs. A complete blood count, sedimentation rate,

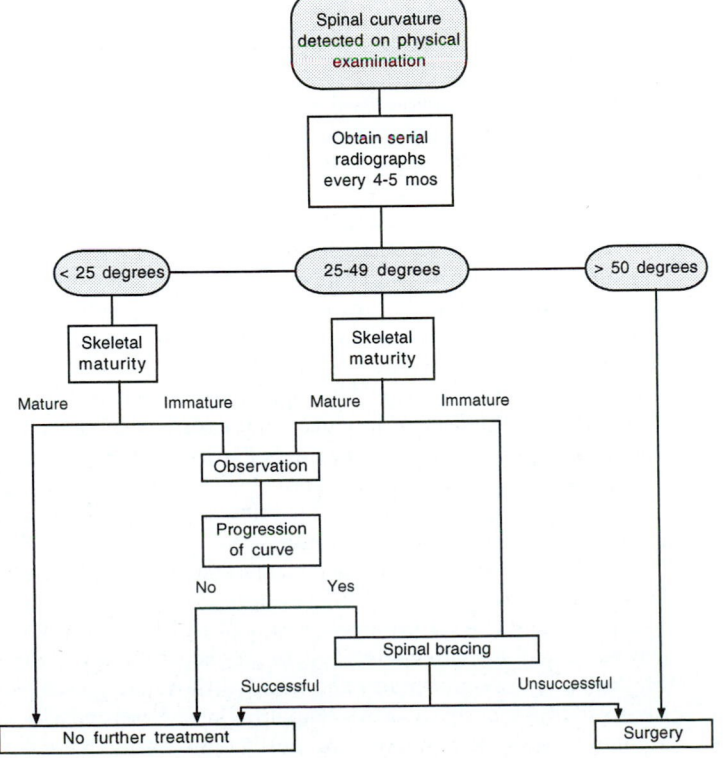

FIGURE 27-40 Algorithm for the treatment of idiopathic adolescent scoliosis.

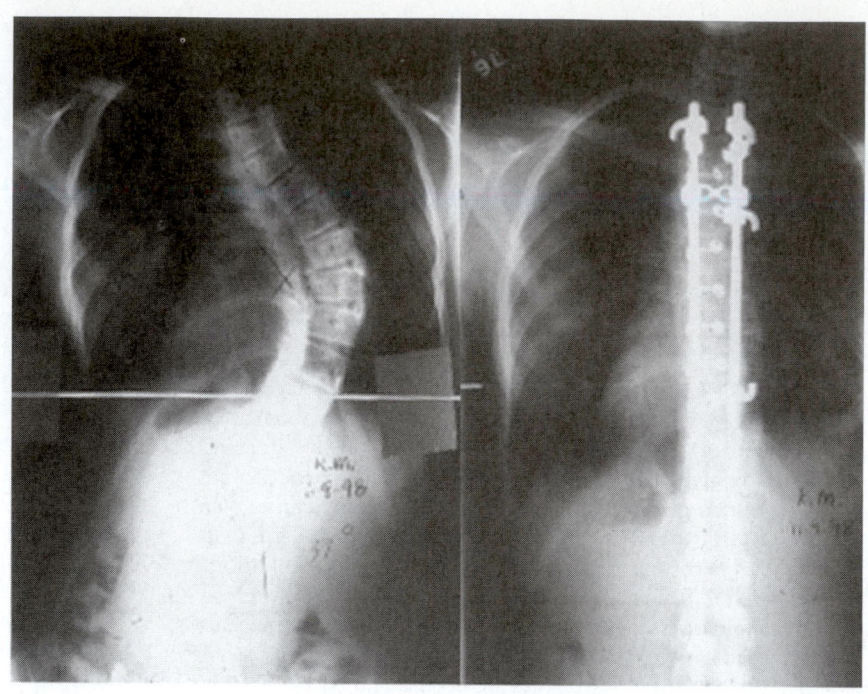

FIGURE 27-41 Pre- and postoperative x-rays illustrating the severity of a scoliosis curve and its subsequent correction following surgery.

and C-reactive protein test are mandatory to complete the back pain evaluation if there is failure of response.

SPONDYLOLYSIS AND SPONDYLOLISTHESIS

Spondylolysis is a fracture of the vertebral lamina between the facet joints (pars interarticulares) and above the spinous process. Spondylolisthesis is a fracture of the pars interarticularis with forward

TABLE 27-5

DIFFERENTIAL DIAGNOSIS OF BACK PAIN IN CHILDREN

Congenital Anomalies	**Systemic Diseases**
Diastematomyelia	Renal osteodystrophy
Congenital spinal anomalies	Storage diseases
Congenital stenosis	Juvenile osteoporosis
Spondyloepinphyseal dysplasia	
Short Stature Syndromes	**Rheumatologic Conditions**
	Juvenile rheumatoid arthritis
Kyphosis	Ankylosing spondylitis
Scheuermann disease	
	Benign Neoplasms
Traumatic	Osteoid osteoma
Bookbag disease	Osteoblastoma
Compression fracture	Aneurysmal bone cyst
Muscle strain	Eosinophilic granuloma
Spondylolysis and spondylolisthesis	Spinal cord tumors: meningioma
Herniated nucleus pulposus	or neurofibroma
Vertebral end plate fracture	
	Malignant Neoplasms
Infectious	Osteogenic sarcoma
Discitis	Leukemia
Vertebral osteomyelitis	Spinal cord tumor
Tuberculosis	Metastatic
	Psychogenic
	Conversion reaction

slippage of the vertebral body typically occurring at L-5 on S-1. The degree of slippage of the vertebrae is the basis for the grading of the spondylolisthesis (grades I to V). Grade I is minimal displacement; grade V is total slippage of the superior vertebra (L-5) from the inferior vertebra (S-1). The causes of the slippage are grouped (per Newman) as either dysplastic, congenital malformation, traumatic, or pathologic secondary to an intrinsic weakness (ie, osteogenesis imperfecta).

The history may reveal low-back pain localized to the lumbosacral region, associated with gymnasts, weight lifters, rowers, wrestlers, and middle linebackers. Although there is no genetic proof, there are many examples of familial involvement. The condition may represent repetitive microtrauma caused by an "overuse" syndrome.

The physical examination may reveal a flattening of the normal lumbar lordosis and tightening of the hamstring muscles (unable to bend forward and touch the toes). Occasionally there is a scoliotic posture or truncal shift with a short-stride waddling gait. With grade II or greater L-5/S-1 spondylolisthesis there is a palpable step-off posteriorly of the spinous process at the lumbosacral joint and lumbosacral kyphosis with flattened heart-shaped buttocks. AP, lateral, and oblique x-rays of the spine should be requested.

On the oblique view, one can see a typical "Scotty dog" configuration of the lumbar vertebrae. The "Scotty dog's" nose is the transverse process, the ears are the superior articular facet, the eyes are the pedicle, the neck is the pars interarticularis, the body is the lamina, and the front legs are the inferior articular facets. A lucent "collar" around the neck of the "Scotty dog" is diagnostic of either spondylolysis or spondylolisthesis. The AP x-ray may reveal sclerosis of one or both of the pedicles. A bone scan, specifically a SPECT (single photon emission-controlled technology) scan, is diagnostic for spondylolysis.

Upon referral to an orthopedist, several treatment modalities may be offered. Most frequently rest, limited activity, physical therapy, and a lightweight "warm and form" orthosis are prescribed. Efforts to heal spondylolysis by a "nipple to knees" cast and a thoracolumbosacral orthosis have been mostly unsuccessful. Surgery is usually reserved for those patients with grade III or greater lesions, or for patients who have persistent pain that does not respond to conservative measures.

HERNIATED NUCLEUS PULPOSUS

A herniated nucleus pulposus (HNP) is rare in the pediatric age group, but usually presents as a low-back pain or painful scoliosis. Low-back pain may be associated with lower limb numbness, weakness, or radicular symptoms associated with coughing, laughing, or straining with bowel movements. There may or may not be sciatica. The straight leg raising sign is usually positive. With the patient supine, the leg is lifted by the heel with the knee extended. A normal examination should allow greater than 70 degrees flexion at the hip. The examination is positive if there is radicular pain or if the patient lifts the buttock off the table. Spinal motion is severely restricted and any attempt to bend over results in painful truncal deviation. There may or may not be evidence of radiculopathy. Plain x-rays may be normal, show slight narrowing of the disc space, or show a very mild scoliosis. The condition can usually be diagnosed by MRI or CT myelogram as intervertebral disk bulging or a free fragment. For the bulging disc, conservative treatment (ie, bed rest, bracing, and possibly epidural steroids) is indicated. While the free fragment is unusual in children, surgery is the treatment of choice. If there is radiculopathy, the parent must be informed that neurologic recovery may not be complete.

DISCITIS

The child may present with back pain, hip pain, abdominal pain, or meningeal syndrome. The condition is probably the result of hematogenous dissemination of bacteria across the vertebral end plates, although it may be secondary to trauma. Rarely will the child present with systemic signs such as fever or anorexia. The back is held stiff and rigid with knees and hips flexed (Fig. 27-42). There is a clinical reversal of the normal lumbar lordosis and the child may walk bent over at the waist. The straight leg raising sign is markedly positive. The back may be so stiff that a straight leg raising test may result in the child pivoting at the shoulder instead of at the hip.

Discitis can occur anywhere along the spine, but it most commonly occurs in the lower thoracic and lumbar regions, usually L-3 to L-4, and tends to affect children from toddler age to young adolescence. Children with this syndrome aged 0 to 3 years (nonverbal) present with failure to bear weight or a limp; children aged 3 to 6 years present with abdominal signs, and children aged 6 to 9 complain of back pain. The x-rays may not be positive until 2 to 4 weeks after onset of symptoms. There is a reversal of the normal lordosis of the lumbar spine. A decreased height of an intervertebral disc space, end-plate sclerosis, and sometimes a soft tissue mass will be seen. A bone scan is usually positive earlier in the course than x-rays. MRI is diagnostic.

Treatment varies with the clinical and laboratory presentation. Orthopedic treatment usually includes bed rest, cast or brace immobilization, occasionally antibiotics, and, rarely, aspiration and/or surgical drainage. If the patient is afebrile, immobilization is offered. If febrile, a broad-spectrum antibiotic is started. If immobilization and antibiotics do not resolve the pain and fever, aspiration is indicated. Rarely is surgical drainage indicated. The parents should be informed that the disc space may remain narrow and possibly close. Scoliosis is rarely a complication.

OSTEOID OSTEOMA

Osteoid osteoma is a benign hypervascular neoplasm of bone. Rarely is it seen in the vertebral column, but its symptoms are quite characteristic. There is well-localized back pain, which is worse at night and relieved by aspirin or NSAIDs. There may be a reactive or painful scoliosis. Conventional x-rays may be normal. CT usually reveals a sclerotic or a central lucent area with some hyperostosis (nidus) surrounded by a lucent area usually over the posterior elements (pedicle, facets, lamina). *Osteoid osteoma* is the term used for lesions less than 1.5 cm; *osteoblastoma* is diagnosed for lesions larger than 1.5 cm. A bone scan is diagnostic as a focal area of high uptake that is occasionally located at the apex of a reactive scoliosis. Current treatment modalities include NSAIDs, thermal ablation, open surgical excision of the nidus, and percutaneous closed CT-guided excision by minimally invasive interventional radiology if the lesion can be isolated from neurologic tissue.

EOSINOPHILIC GRANULOMA OF THE SPINE (CALVÉ DISEASE)

Vague, well-localized back pain may herald the onset of Calvé disease. Langerhans histiocytosis tends to be more common in males. Most commonly, the frontal bones of the skull are involved. There is a definite incidence of eosinophilic granuloma (EG) in more than one site, although EG is a focal form of histiocytosis, which is similar in cellular pattern to Letterer-Siwe disease and Hand-Schüller-Christian disease. Spinal x-rays may be diagnostic for this disease (ie, an area of "monostotic vertebral plana"). The single vertebra is flattened like a coin. A bone scan is necessary to rule out other involved sites. Although some centers have utilized low-dose irradiation for this lesion, we recommend supportive orthotic management. If necessary, percutaneous CT-guided biopsy is performed for diagnosis. Surgery is only indicated for progressive neurologic deficit. The vertebral plana may reverse with reestablishment of its height in young patients.

TUBERCULOSIS OF THE SPINE (POTT DISEASE)

Tuberculosis of bone most commonly involves the vertebrae, with the upper end of the femur being the second most common area, and the metaphysis of cylindrical bones the next most common area. Pott disease is more common in males and in the prepubertal child. There is often a tuberculous arthritis in addition to the osteomyelitis. The anterior portion of the vertebrae is usually involved, tending to cause a kyphotic deformity. The problem is more common in lower thoracic or lumbar regions. Pott disease is a realistic differential in the diagnosis of back pain in recent immigrants from Southeast Asia and other developing countries.

The x-rays will reveal bony destruction and indistinct narrowing of disc spaces. Findings may appear radiologically indistinguishable from an osteomyelitis. There may be soft-tissue masses, with or without calcifications. A CT scan or MRI may show perivertebral soft tissue abscess. Most patients diagnosed with Pott disease are being treated for osteomyelitis. After the cultures have proven positive for acid-fast bacteria or a positive skin test reaction occurs, an infectious disease consultation for current treatment recommendations is advisable (see Sec. 13.2.21). Medical management and orthotics are indicated for early management. If there is extensive vertebral destruction and abscess formation, surgical drainage is indicated.

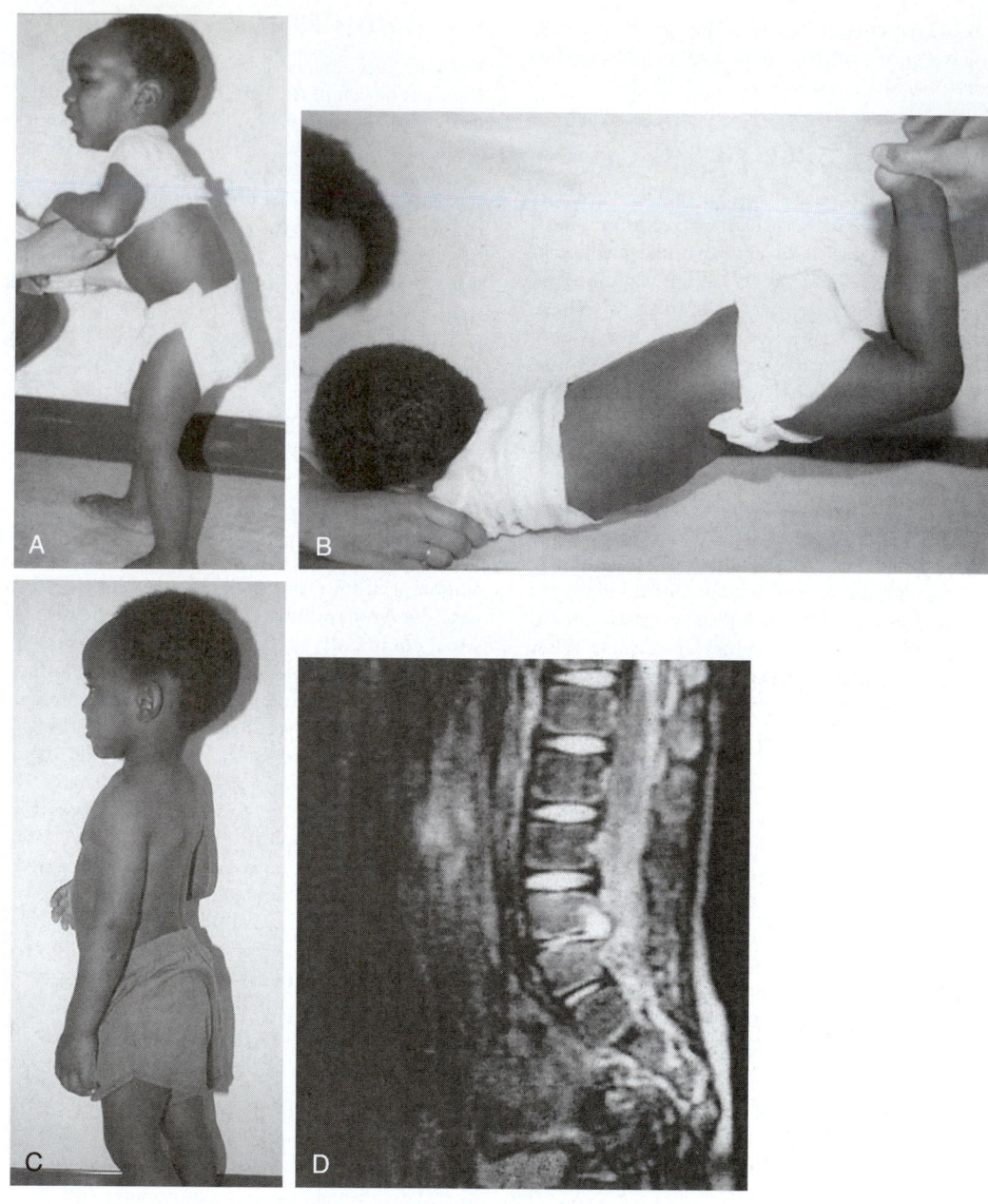

FIGURE 27-42 This child presented with intense back pain and a diagnosis of L3- 4 discitis. A. The child is apprehensive and stands with a fixed flexion posture of his lumbar spine, which would normally be in lordosis. B. When an attempt is made to suspend the child by his heels in the prone position, the lumbar spine remains in fixed flexion or kyphosis. C. Following treatment the child stands with normal lordosis and reversal of the deformity. D. MRI at diagnosis.

COMPRESSION FRACTURE OF THE VERTEBRA

Direct or indirect trauma causing spinal flexion is the most common history. The trauma is not always severe, and may include sledding injury or a restrained passenger in motor vehicle accidents. The child feels well overall, but the back pain is persistent. With a severe trauma in the thoracolumbar region, the patient may develop an ileus. X-rays may reveal a loss of vertebral height directly under the area of pain. If more than one vertebra appears to be involved and there is not a good history of trauma, a bone scan is indicated to rule out other problems (eg, leukemia, lymphoma, child battering).

Most often these children are treated with orthotics. Children 10 years old or younger may reverse the loss of vertebral height.

SPINAL CORD TUMOR

The patient may present with persistent or intermittent pain or a neurologic deficit. Beware of patients with "spastic torticollis," "painful reactive scoliosis," or progressive pathologic gaits. A poorly balanced left thoracic scoliosis should alert suspicion. The gait change may represent subtle lower extremity muscle weakness. A marginally toilet-trained child may have regression or "accidents" of bowel and bladder control. Have the child walk on the heels and toes, as well as hop on each leg in alternation. Look closely at the feet for a high arch or clawing of the toes, especially if the deformity is unilateral. Inquire of bowel or bladder control. Test for rectus abdominal reflexes. Spinal x-ray may reveal widening of the interpedicular distance or narrowing or absence of a pedicle. The vertebral foramina may be enlarged. Parents should be informed that if excision results in vertebral instability, a spinal fusion may be indicated. The neurologic deficit may not be reversible. An MRI or CT/myelogram scan is diagnostic. Referral to a spinal specialist is indicated.

27.8   UPPER EXTREMITY PROBLEMS

Charles T. Mehlman

Deformities and injuries to the upper extremity can have profound functional consequences for children. These problems vary from marked limitation of shoulder motion associated with Sprengel deformity to complete absence of a distal extremity as a result of Streeter dysplasia. Early recognition and full evaluation of these upper extremity problems are critical because timely treatment helps to optimize functional results in such young children. This section describes several particularly debilitating upper extremity entities in children.

27.8.1.   Brachial Plexus Injuries in the Newborn

Brachial plexus injuries in the newborn can range from mild and transient to catastrophic and permanent. The problem is usually detected shortly after birth as asymmetric active range of motion of the child's arms. The incidence of brachial plexus birth palsy has been shown to be about 3 per 1,000 live births. It is believed that in the majority of cases, stretching injury to the brachial plexus occurs during the course of a difficult vaginal delivery, but this is not always the case as such injuries have also been reported following cesarean sections. Risk factors associated with neonatal brachial plexus injuries include high birth weight, lengthy labor, shoulder dystocia, gestational diabetes, and breech delivery, as well as forceps or vacuum extraction.

Neonatal brachial plexus palsies may be classified as either Erb palsy (with predominant upper plexus involvement—C5, C6, and sometimes C7), Klumpke palsy (with predominant lower plexus involvement—C8 and T1), or total plexus involvement. Erb palsy presents with a "waiter's tip" position (shoulder adduction and internal rotation with wrist flexion); Klumpke palsy demonstrates a paralyzed hand in conjunction with good shoulder and elbow function; and total plexus involvement manifests as a completely flail upper extremity. Upper plexus injury can lead to partial paralysis of the diaphragm, as the diaphragm receives innervation from C3, C4, and C5. Klumpke paralysis is considered to be quite rare, comprising only about 0.5% of all brachial plexus palsies in newborns, and is thought to be the result of delivering the head before the upper arm in a breech baby with extended arms. Total plexus involvement carries a rather poor prognosis for spontaneous recovery.

Physical examination figures prominently in the proper evaluation of neonatal brachial plexus injury. Important components include evaluation of the Moro reflex, searching for evidence of Horner syndrome, and documenting neuromuscular function of the involved extremity. The Moro reflex is an excellent way to prove whether or not the arm of concern will actively move when stimulated. This is particularly useful in the not uncommon setting of ipsilateral clavicle fracture, where it is unclear whether the baby is not moving the arm because of pain (pseudoparalysis) or because of brachial plexus injury. The presence of Horner syndrome (ptosis, myosis, and anhydrosis) is a poor prognostic sign, often indicating an injury that includes avulsion of the T1 nerve root.

The mechanism of injury is usually related to traction, resulting in nerve injuries that vary from mild stretching of the involved nerves to frank nerve root avulsion from the spinal cord. Mild stretch injuries (neurapraxias) have an excellent prognosis for spontaneous recovery, while nerve root avulsions (axonotmeses) have the worst prognosis with no hope for spontaneous recovery and little or no hope for successful direct surgical repair. Nerve root avulsion of the upper roots may be present in up to 81% of children with brachial plexus palsies following breech delivery.

If significant clinical suspicion exists for nerve root avulsion, additional diagnostic studies may be helpful. Efforts at identifying such avulsions may be aimed at high-resolution CT myelography. This technique is capable of detecting nerve root injuries with as high as 95% sensitivity and 98% specificity. Other authors have not been able to duplicate these exceptional results with CT myelography. Fast spin-echo MRI offers another imaging modality to evaluate neonatal brachial plexus injury. Electromyography (EMG) and nerve conduction studies can also play an important role in evaluation of these patients, with normal sensory nerve and absent motor nerve conduction strongly suggesting nerve root avulsion.

The vast majority of brachial plexus palsies in newborn children (80–95%) resolve spontaneously over the course of several weeks to several months. These children typically present with upper plexus involvement and "waiter's tip" positioning. They recover biceps function (active motion against gravity) by the third month of life. Recovery of wrist, thumb, and finger extension by the third month of life is an even stronger indicator of an excellent spontaneous recovery. Gentle range of motion exercises performed by the parents accompanied by serial examinations by the physician may be all that is needed for these patients.

One group of patients with a very poor prognosis for recovery are those with nerve root avulsions. The trick is to identify these patients early in order to try to improve their otherwise poor chance of an adequate functional recovery. After the diagnosis is confirmed, surgical exploration and repair should be considered. Although several centers have become more aggressive in early efforts at neurolysis and nerve grafting, no standardized means of outcomes assessment has been used and comparisons among studies are difficult.

Older children with permanent upper extremity functional deficits may be candidates for reconstructive surgical procedures. These children invariably have limited shoulder motion. It is important to evaluate such children for bony deformity of the glenoid and or shoulder dislocation, as the chronic abnormal muscle forces about the shoulder may lead to such problems. Posterior shoulder dislocations are the rule and may manifest as markedly limited external rotation. Such dislocations can occur quite early, as young as 6 months of age. It is vital that the status of the glenohumeral joint be properly evaluated in the preoperative setting, as it will help determine the most appropriate surgical procedure. A fixed posterior dislocation that causes functional limitations due to limited external rotation can be treated via derotational humeral osteotomy.

27.8.2   Shoulder Pain in Children

Shoulder pain is the most common upper extremity complaint that prompts evaluation of sports-related injuries. Rotator cuff tears and acromioclavicular joint arthritis, although common causes of shoulder pain in adults, are rare in children. Causes of pediatric shoulder pain such as shoulder instability and overuse injuries affecting the growth plate must be recognized before appropriate care can commence.

The shoulder exhibits its own special brand of "controlled instability" as it has the widest range of motion of all the joints in the body and very little inherent bony stability. Shoulder instability may occur following an isolated traumatic event such as an anterior shoulder dislocation, or after repeated microtrauma associated with throwing or swimming. The primary complaint may be pain, and not a sensation of looseness or subluxation. The application of adult shoulder principles to children may easily lead to an erroneous diagnosis such as rotator cuff tendinitis or impingement syndrome. The exceptionally loose shoulders of swimmers and other overhead athletes or ligamentously lax individuals may respond well to a structured course of shoulder exercises, while children and young adults who suffer traumatic anterior dislocation have a risk of recurrent dislocation (90–100% chance of recurrent instability) that is unaltered by lengthy immobilization or physical therapy.

Overuse injury affecting the proximal humeral growth plate is most common in children who participate in throwing sports. A typical scenario is that of a youngster who has had low-level shoulder pain for several months that increases suddenly during competitive throwing. Focal pain to palpation about the proximal humerus along with radiographs of the shoulder that demonstrate physeal widening confirm the diagnosis. Restricted throwing for a 6-week time period followed by a shoulder-strengthening program and gradual return to activities is the basic treatment for this entity.

27.8.3   Nursemaid's Elbow

A sudden yank on the relatively pronated forearm of a toddler may result in a small transverse tear or subluxation of the annular ligament around the proximal radius. When this occurs, the radial head may slip through this area of the annular ligament, creating interposed tissue between the radial head and capitellum. This pinched tissue results in a crying child who refuses to use his or her arm, holding it in a relatively extended position.

The hypermobility demonstrated by many children in this age range is felt to contribute a certain predisposition for this injury, but such hypermobility is not universally present. Plain film and ultrasonographic findings have been described for nursemaid's elbow, but it is primarily a clinical diagnosis and not a radiographic one. A reasonable recommendation is to obtain radiographs in situations that differ from the classic nursemaid's elbow scenario (ie, no clear history of a pulled elbow) or in cases in which the child does not respond to initial treatment efforts.

Classic treatment for nursemaid's elbow consists of supination of the forearm and flexion of the elbow, resulting in an audible and or palpable click about the lateral elbow. After such a reduction maneuver the child may immediately resume normal use of the involved extremity. In some instances, this dramatic response may

not occur, and radiographs of the elbow are indicated. In some instances, the maneuver is inadvertently performed while positioning the child for an x-ray. If x-rays are normal and full supination is possible, the elbow may be splinted in a 90-degree position with the forearm in full supination for a period of time. Such a treatment approach will be successful in the vast majority of patients with only a very rare patient demonstrating a recurrent or irreducible nursemaid's elbow.

27.8.4   Congenital Constriction-Band Syndrome (Streeter Dysplasia)

Congenital constriction-band syndrome is an incompletely understood entity whose manifestations include upper extremity problems ranging from syndactyly to congenital amputation. Theories as to the etiology of the disorder include both intrinsic (germ plasm defect) and extrinsic (physical restriction) explanations. Streeter advanced the intrinsic concept of subcutaneous tissue dysplasia leading to constriction rings. Destructive effects of external forces brought on by oligohydramnios and amniotic bands are now more generally accepted causes. Despite lack of proof of any true dysplasia, Streeter dysplasia is still commonly linked with congenital constriction-band syndrome.

The incidence of Streeter dysplasia is 1 in 15,000 live births. Although not thought to be inherited, the disorder may present in association with other abnormalities such as cleft palate, central nervous system anomalies, limb-length discrepancies, and clubfeet. The incidence may be higher in people from areas such as the Philippines, where cultural tradition includes uterine manipulation and massage as a means of inducing abortion. In one reported Filipino series, the majority of patients presenting with congenital constriction-band syndrome were born of mothers who had attempted first-trimester abortions.

Congenital constriction-band syndrome has a profound impact on the afflicted child. The typical patient has involvement of three limbs, and 85% of patients have digital or limb amputations. The convergent distal fusion of the fingers known as acrosyndactyly is also particularly debilitating and difficult to treat. Perinatal release may offer the most effective approach to an adequate release. Patient's with Streeter dysplasia may require an average of 3, and as many as 10, reconstructive surgical procedures.

27.8.5   Other Congenital Anomalies of the Upper Extremity

Several other congenital anomalies of the upper extremity also deserve to be mentioned. Boomerang elbow represents a congenital angular bowing of the elbow with complete or partial absence of the elbow joint. The ligament of Struthers, whereby a tough fibrous band of tissue extends from a downward-projecting supracondylar process (bone spur) on the distal medial humerus, is an anomaly found in only about 1% of the population. The ligament of Struthers is associated with compressive neuropathy of the median nerve. Congenital dislocation of the radial head is often (but not always) bilateral, and usually results in few functional limitations. Congenital fusions of the radius and ulna may be localized or virtually complete. If such radioulnar synostoses result in a stiff, dysfunctional forearm, position changing (but not motion improving) surgery may be considered. Radial clubhand and ulnar clubhand represent complex longitudinal deficiencies of the upper extremity, and surgery aimed at optimizing function may be indicated in some cases.

27.8.6 Syndactyly

Syndactyly is the most common congenital hand malformation with an incidence of about 1 in 2,000 live births. It occurs bilaterally in about 50% of reported cases. Syndactyly represents a failure of the normal programmed cell death that occurs between the future fingers of the embryonic paddle-shaped hand. As a result abnormal attachments between several or all of the digits may occur that range from mild skin webbing to extensive bone and joint abnormalities. The most common fingers to be involved are the long and ring fingers, followed by the ring and small fingers. When fingers of nearly identical length are involved, syndactyly represents a deficit of independent finger function with few, if any, growth implications. When fingers of different lengths are tethered together by syndactylized tissue, significant angular growth disturbances may result unless early surgical release is performed.

Referral of such children by 6 months of age to a pediatric orthopedic surgeon or a hand surgeon often allows for adequate time for proper evaluation and decision making prior to surgical intervention. The precise timing of surgery varies from child to child, but in many cases it occurs between 1 and 2 years of age. There have been recent reports of cardiac conduction abnormalities in association with syndactyly in children, and as a result an electrocardiogram is recommended as part of any preoperative evaluation.

27.8.7 Postaxial Polydactyly

Postaxial polydactyly (along the pinky finger side of the hand) is considered to be the second most common congenital hand malformation with an incidence in the range of about 1 in 3,000 live births. In certain kindreds, however, the incidence of such "extra pinky fingers" may be 10 times higher than the population average. Postaxial polydactyly may manifest anywhere from simple small skin nubbins to complete finger duplication. This congenital abnormality rarely causes any functional complaints but frequently presents cosmetic concerns. In the absence of cartilaginous or bony elements, small soft tissue nubbins have been successfully tied off with suture. More fully formed finger duplicates offer more of a challenge, with reconstructive hand surgery often being performed between 1 and 2 years of age (same recommendation as syndactyly).

27.8.8 Trigger Thumb and Trigger Finger

Trigger thumb and trigger finger represent either transient or fixed flexed posture of the involved digit. The anatomic cause of the problem is tendon and tendon sheath mismatch that interferes with normal tendon gliding within the sheath. A useful analogy is that of trying to pull a knotted piece of rope through a section of garden hose. The true congenital nature of trigger thumb and trigger finger has been questioned by some authors because prospective evaluation of large populations of newborns has failed to identify such digital flexion abnormalities. For this reason, it seems appropriate to add these particular hand problems to the list of developmental pediatric orthopedic problems such as developmental dysplasia of the hip and adolescent hallux valgus. Efforts at extension splinting have

been successful for some young children (<1 year of age), while older children with fixed flexion deformity are offered surgical release.

27.9 ORTHOPEDIC INJURY FOLLOWING TRAUMA AND SPORTS

Almost all orthopedic injuries are initially treated by using RICE (rest, ice, compression, and elevation). Unlike adults, who tend to sprain ligaments around joints, children have a much higher incidence of fracture versus sprain. A fracture almost always needs to be ruled out in any child complaining of significant extremity pain. Any child who refuses to walk on the extremity after trauma should have limb x-rays. Approximately 5% of all fractures in children are radiographically occult, and children with significant pain should be treated as if there they have a fracture despite normal x-ray findings.

27.9.1 Knee Sprain

Posttraumatic knee effusions should prompt careful clinical exam and x-ray evaluation. Knee fractures, patella dislocation, anterior cruciate ligament tears, and meniscal tears are the most common causes of a traumatic knee effusion in children. Fractures need to be ruled out with x-rays (AP, lateral, sunrise, tunnel); however, 2 to 5% of children's fractures are not visualized on the first set of x-rays. Despite normal x-rays, if a patient has exquisite bone tenderness, he or she should be treated for an occult fracture with splinting or casting. Patella dislocation can occur spontaneously or after a blow to the knee. Typically, patients will report that their knee gave out and shifted. They will often have a large knee effusion and have very positive apprehension signs with lateral translation of the patella. Anterior cruciate ligament tears and meniscal tears are rare until children approach skeletal maturity. Children/adolescents with a traumatic knee effusion should be referred for orthopedic evaluation, as >50% may have a serious knee injury. An MRI scan may be indicated if the diagnosis is in question, or if symptoms fail to improve. Atraumatic knee effusion, especially when bilateral, occurring in multiple joints, or in association with morning stiffness, should be referred to a rheumatologist.

27.9.2 Popliteal Cysts

Popliteal cysts, also known as ganglion cysts or Baker cysts, are benign collections of fluid that accumulate behind the child's knee. Most of these soft masses arise along the posterior medial aspect of the knee from the bursa between the semimembranous and gastrocnemius tendons. Parents usually discover a posterior knee mass on their child, who is unaware of the lesion.

Examination is best performed with the child standing on the examining table, as hyperextension of the knee accentuates the cyst. Diagnosis is confirmed via transillumination by placing a penlight or otoscope against the lesion in a dark room. If the light transmits at least twice as far through the cyst as it does through the surrounding soft tissue, this is diagnostic of a popliteal cyst. Further

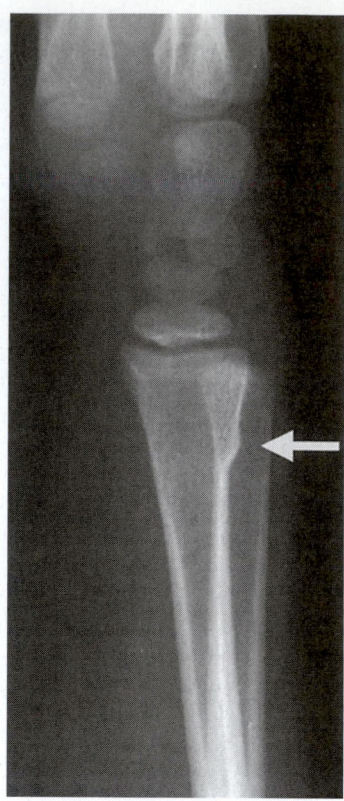

FIGURE 27-43   Buckle fracture of the distal radius. Note that there is no break or deformity of the bone opposite the buckle.

workup, including ultrasound, MRI scan, aspiration, or biopsy, is not usually necessary. If transillumination is equivocal, then ultrasound is indicated to rule out a solid tumor. Studies have shown that most ganglion cysts in children will spontaneously disappear if observed for a period of 2 years. The cysts can be followed at yearly intervals and remeasured. Referral to orthopedics is indicated if the cyst becomes extremely large or painful or causes a limp or loss of function. Enthusiasm for surgical excision is tempered by the fact that up to 40% of these popliteal cysts will recur postoperatively.

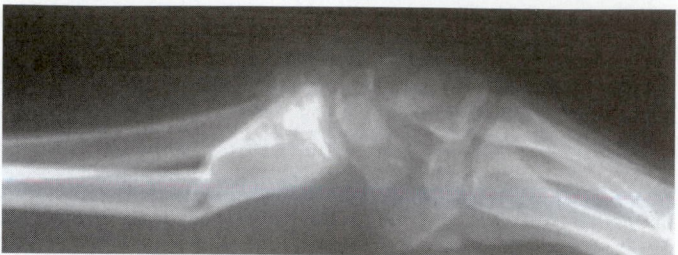

FIGURE 27-44   Greenstick fracture. Note that there is deformity of both sides of the bone, but some bone remains intact.

27.9.3   Unique Fracture Patterns

Children have several other unique fracture patterns as a result of the pressure of growth plates and the relative plasticity of their bones as compared to adults.

BUCKLE FRACTURE

Buckle fractures involves buckling of one side of the bone while the opposite side of the bone remains intact and nondeformed. These fractures are usually stable and heal rapidly over a period of 3 to 4 weeks in a cast (Fig. 27-43).

GREENSTICK FRACTURE

Greenstick fractures are also incomplete fracture buts are more unstable than a buckle fracture and involve cortical disruption on the tension side of the fracture (Fig. 27-44).

GROWTH PLATE FRACTURES

Approximately 12% of children's fractures occur through the growth plate, which is classified by the Salter description. The higher the Salter classification, the higher the risk of growth abnormality (Fig. 27-45); 6.4% of all growth plate fractures will have a growth arrest, which can lead to a shortened or angulated limb. Growth plate fractures of the distal femur, proximal and distal tibia, and distal ulna tend to have the highest risk for growth abnormality.

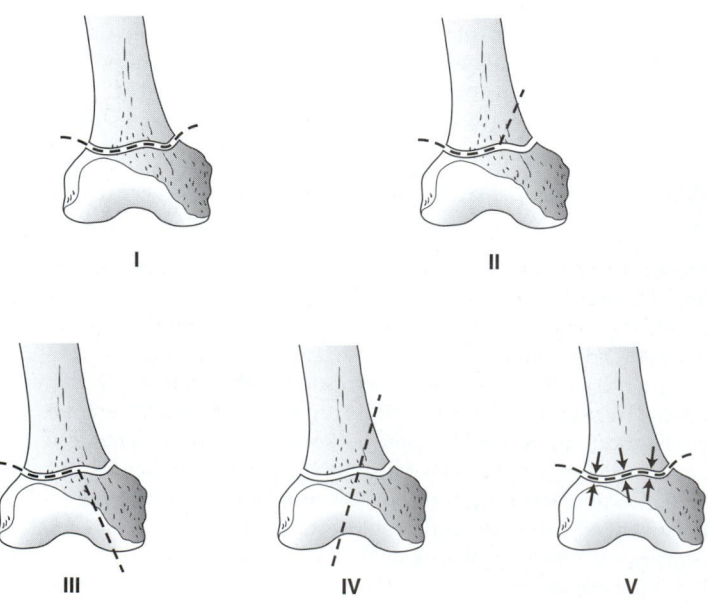

FIGURE 27-45   Salter classification of fractures.

CHILD ABUSE

Although spiral fractures of the humerus and femur in young children can be associated with child abuse, they are not pathognomonic. Corner fractures (Fig. 27-46), posterior rib fractures in varying stages of healing, scapula fractures, sternal fractures, and spinous process fractures are highly specific for child abuse. One study found that 83% of children <13 months of age with femur fractures were abused. Before casting a young child with a fracture suspicious for child abuse, obtain a skeletal survey or bone scan to assess other bone injuries.

TODDLER'S FRACTURE

A toddler's fracture is an acute spiral fracture of the tibia in 1- to 3-year-old children. The child usually sustains a minor twisting injury to his or her leg and then refuses to walk. Approximately 25% of toddler's fractures are radiographically occult; this diagnosis is confirmed by palpation. Fractures that are discovered in the first 2 weeks after injury should be casted, and those identified later can be observed without casting. Occult toddler's fractures will show subperiosteal new bone after 3 weeks, which proves the diagnosis.

FINGER JAM

Children who jam their fingers and who have severe pain or deformity, or who do not regain full motion of their fingers within 24 hours, should have an x-ray to rule out a fracture. Children tend to fracture much more frequently than adults when they jam their fingers.

COZEN FRACTURE

Proximal tibia metaphyseal fractures have a unique propensity to grow into genu valgum (knock-knee) after healing, despite this not being a growth plate injury (see Figs. 27-18 and 27-19). This unique pattern is called *Cozen fracture* and its etiology is unknown.

27.9.4   General Tips for Fracture Treatment

The gold standard for treatment of most fractures in children is casting. Waterproof casts are available that allow full immersion. Most of the pain and swelling decreases following fracture immobilization. Complaints of increased pain following reduction and any swelling should be given the utmost attention to rule out vascular insufficiency or compartment syndrome. Observe the fingernails for blanching and/or capillary refill following compression. The five "P's" of pain, pallor, paralysis, pulselessness, and paresthesia must be aggressively investigated. Nondisplaced finger fractures in older, reliable children can be splinted with aluminofoam splints. These splints are much sturdier if they are wrapped around both the dorsal and volar surfaces of the finger (Fig. 27-47). Young or unreliable children with hand fractures do best with a cast that covers the fingers.

The most common fractures in children are distal radius and ulna and radius and ulna shaft fractures. Most distal radius fractures will heal with 3 to 6 weeks of casting, while midshaft fractures take 6 to 8 weeks and can refracture for up to 6 months postinjury. Displaced supracondylar elbow fractures are the most common fracture in children that require operative reduction and pin fixation. Supracondylar elbow fractures have little capacity to remodel, and a crooked elbow "cubitus varus" may result if they heal mal-

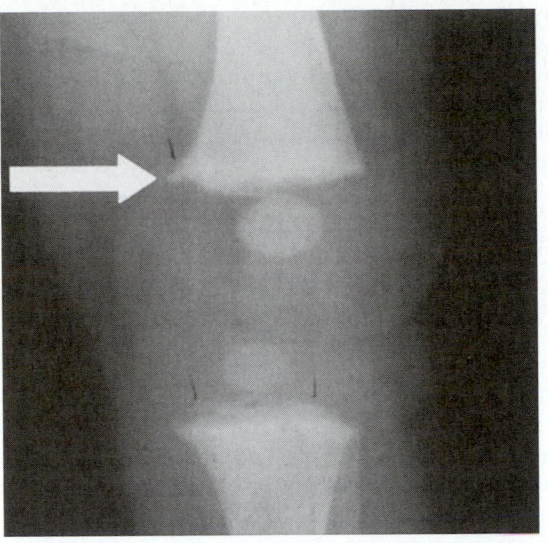

FIGURE 27-46   **Corner fracture of the distal femur is highly specific for child abuse in children <1 year old.**

aligned. Most other children's fractures heal with moderate angulation and show spontaneous correction through future growth and remodeling.

27.10 COMMON BONE TUMORS

Charles T. Mehlman

27.10.1   Osteochondroma (Osteocartilaginous Exostosis)

Osteochondromas are the most common benign tumors of bone in children. They are really hamartomas, outgrowths of normal bone and cartilage in abnormal locations. They are usually located

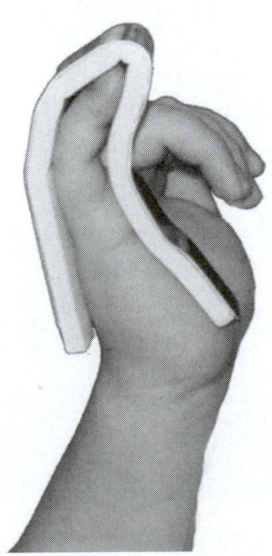

FIGURE 27-47   **Aluminofoam splint.**

in the metaphyseal regions of long bones, arising most commonly around the knee in the distal femur and proximal tibia, proximal humerus, and from both the proximal and distal fibula (Fig. 27-48). They can also arise from intra-articular locations and flat bones such as the pelvis or scapula. Except for multiple hereditary exostosis, patients usually present with osteochondromas during the second decade of life. There is no sex predilection.

Osteochondromas probably arise from remnants of the growth plate (rests) left behind during longitudinal bone growth. These "rests" of cells continue the process of endochondral ossification, creating an exostosis of bone protruding from the cortex. If the tumor is removed when the child is young, a growth plate can be observed between the bone and the cartilage cap. These lesions usually stop growing when the nearby growth plate closes. Transformation of a solitary osteochondroma into chondrosarcoma is felt to be an exceedingly rare event (<1%) that does not occur prior to skeletal maturity. Malignancy more often occurs in lesions occurring in the axial as opposed to the appendicular skeleton.

Osteochondroma patients most often present with the finding of a painless, hard, nontender mass. They may experience some discomfort if the mass extends or bowstrings a nerve or vessel or is repeatedly bumped or if a bursa has formed between the cartilage cap and the overlying muscle.

X-rays demonstrate a bony outgrowth from the cortex. The trabecular pattern and density of the outgrowth are the same as in the normal bone. There is no reactive bone at the base. The lesion may be stalked (pedunculated) or flat (sessile). Pedunculated lesions

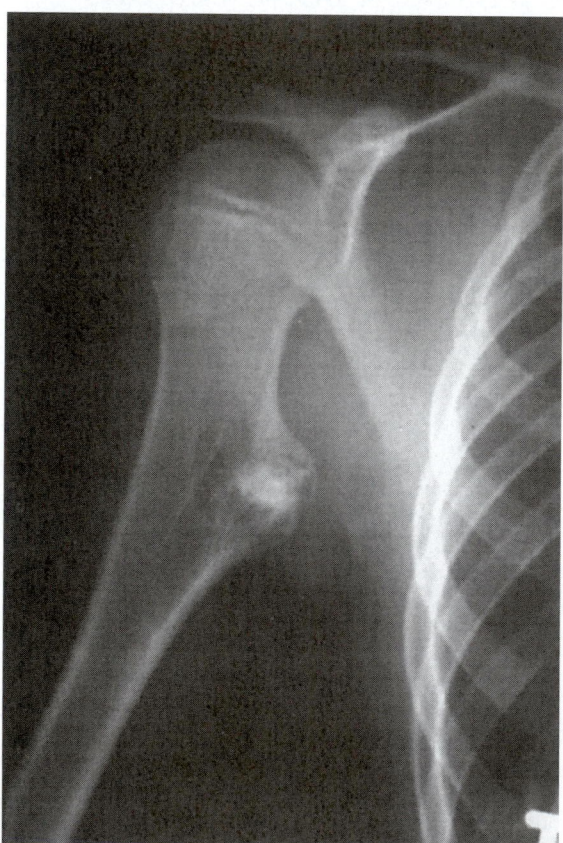

FIGURE 27-48 **This 10-year-old child presented with a mass on the medial aspect of the right humerus. An x-ray revealed a solitary osteochondroma.**

usually point away from the adjacent joints. Because most of the tumor is the cartilage cap, the x-ray opacity is smaller than the mass feels clinically. Persistently painful lesions should be removed because of the possibility of malignant change.

In the absence of symptoms, there is no imperative to excise these lesions. If an osteochondroma is a problem because of repeated trauma or because a painful bursa forms over it, it can be excised. Many parents and patients elect to have these tumors removed for cosmetic and psychological (cancerophobic) reasons. It should be communicated to the family that such osteochondroma removal is not without risk, as a complication rate greater than 10% has been reported.

MULTIPLE HEREDITARY EXOSTOSES

Hereditary multiple exostoses are a rare autosomal-dominant skeletal dysplasia that predominantly affects the faster growing end of bones. This can lead to significant deformities of bones such as the distal ulna and proximal fibula, but virtually any bone can be affected. The natural history of this disorder is not the same as for solitary osteochondromas. There is a strong likelihood of short stature in children with hereditary multiple exostoses, but not true dwarfism. The risk of malignant degeneration is also considered to be much greater, with estimates as high as 10%. Because there are many tumors in multiple locations, local disturbances of growth are fairly common.

In general, the deformities caused by hereditary multiple exostoses are well tolerated and lead to little loss of function. At times, however, the exostoses need to be removed if they are painful, if they interfere with function, or if they are causing deformity with progressive inhibition of epiphyseal growth. The lesions can cause asymmetric growth of long bones and angular deformity. For example, shortening of the ulna as a result of an exostosis can cause ulnar deviation of the wrist or dislocation of the radial head. Or, distal fibular lesions can cause valgus angulation of the ankle. Treatment of angular disorders may include excision of lesions, stapling of physes, osteotomy, or differential lengthening of paired bones.

27.10.2 Enchondroma

Enchondromas are benign cartilage tumors that are commonly found in the tubular bones of the hand and the foot. They tend to be diaphyseal or metaphyseal lesions and probably arise from residual nests of cartilage cells left behind by the growing physes (Fig. 27-49). Chondrocytes of enchondromas grow slowly, expanding the cortical bone and thinning the cortex. They may cause an unsightly swelling or pathologic fracture of the bone.

Malignant transformation of enchondroma into chondrosarcoma, although rare, has been reported. A syndrome of multiple enchondromas can occur with a tendency for more involvement on one side of the body, which is called Ollier disease. When multiple enchondromas are combined with hemangiomas, Maffucci syndrome is diagnosed. Malignant transformation has been reported to occur in 25% of patients with Ollier disease and in the majority of patients with Maffucci syndrome. The x-ray appearance of an enchondroma is a radiolucent diaphyseal or metaphyseal lesion of a long bone. The cortex is thin and expanded with little or no reactive bone. In some lesions, speckled calcification within the lesion identifies it as a cartilage tumor. Treatment is through currettage and bone grafting of the defect.

27.10.3   Simple Bone Cyst (Unicameral Bone Cyst)

Simple bone cyst is a very common lesion in children. Because it is rarely seen in adults, the natural history is considered to be one of spontaneous resolution or increasing cortical bony integrity. The cyst is a fluid-filled lesion lined by a thin membrane. Simple bone cysts form in the metaphyses of long bones near the physis (Fig. 27-50). With growth, additional bone is laid down and the epiphysis grows away from the cyst. The most common locations are the proximal humerus and the proximal femur. The cyst in childhood expands within the metaphysis, to the point where it may fill the entire metaphysis and, in rare cases, affect the growth plate. Most often, the initial treatment of a unicameral bone cyst is supportive (ie, a sling or cast).

The cortex of the involved bone may become thinned and weakened such that the presenting complaint is either an impending or actual pathologic fracture. X-rays show the fracture and a large metaphyseal lucency, sometimes traversed by ridges of cortical bone. The fractures will heal with immobilization, but the cyst will usually remain. The potential for refracture is great as long as the cyst is present. A popular and effective treatment for unicameral bone cyst is percutaneous aspiration of the cyst with injection of corticosteroids. Theoretically, the steroid inhibits the growth of the connective tissue in the surrounding membrane of the cyst and encourages replacement with bone. Usually several repeated injections and aspirations are required with this technique. In recent years, new techniques involving the percutaneous injection of bone marrow and commercially available bone graft preparations have also been used to treat these lesions.

27.10.4   Aneurysmal Bone Cyst

The aneurysmal bone cysts are relatively rare in children, but should be distinguished from unicameral bone cysts. Aneurysmal bone cysts occur in all parts of the skeleton, but most often can be found in the long bones. The lesions are usually in the metaphysis, but may be in the diaphysis. They also are one of the most common benign bone tumors found to occur in the posterior elements of the spine.

If the physis has closed, aneurysmal bone cysts can be found within the bony epiphysis, and when the physis is still open, an aggressive aneurysmal bone cyst can actually cross it, possibly causing partial or complete growth arrest. The lesions are most common in patients under age 20, particularly in the second decade. Treatment is more aggressive than that recommended for simple bone cysts. Treatment usually begins with curettage and bone grafting, but recurrences are very common and resection may be required.

27.10.5   Fibrous Cortical Defect and Nonossifying Fibroma

Fibrous cortical defects and nonossifying fibromas are very common lesions in the bones and may be an incidental finding on x-ray in up to 30% of children with open growth plates. The two lesions are distinguished mainly based on their size. When the lesions are small (usually less than 4 cm) and closely apposed to the cortex, they are called fibrous cortical defects; when they are larger and encroach into the intramedullary canal, they are called non-

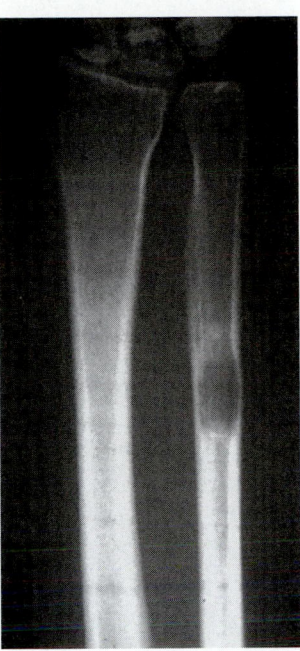

FIGURE 27-49   Enchondroma within the diaphysis of the ulna. The lesion demonstrates the calcification typical of enchondromas that occur outside of the hand.

ossifying fibromas. They are rarely seen in adults, and thus it is felt that virtually all of these lesions will resolve spontaneously. The disorder is probably a local aberration in the process of endochondral ossification in which cortical bone is not deposited, but dense fibrous tissue is laid down instead. Eccentric lesions located in the metaphysis may be seen in any long bone (Fig. 27-51).

The distinctive x-ray appearance of these lesions is scalloped lucencies in the metaphyseal cortex surrounded by a rim of reactive

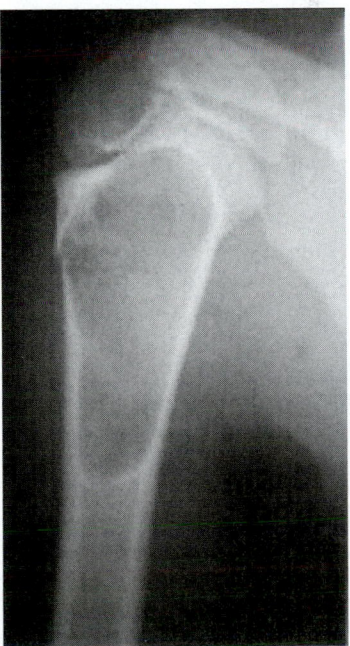

FIGURE 27-50   Unicameral bone cyst of the proximal humerus. This patient was symptomatic because of the pathologic fracture that had occurred through the thinned lateral cortex.

bone. Occasionally there is mild metaphyseal cortical expansion. Rarely, pathologic fractures occur through a fibrous cortical defect. Healing of the fracture occasionally causes the lesion to disappear. The natural history is for spontaneous resolution with time. If the disorder is properly diagnosed, no surgical treatment is necessary, even in large nonossifying fibromas that occupy greater than 50% of the width of a bone.

27.10.6 Langerhans Cell Histiocytosis (Eosinophilic Granuloma)

Langerhans cell histiocytosis is a clonal proliferative disease of unknown cause that results in diffuse histiocytic infiltration of a variety of areas of the body, including bone. Lesions located in bone have been called eosinophilic granulomas. The chronic multiorgan form of Langerhans cell histiocytosis is called Hand-Schüller-Christian disease, while the acute version is called Letterer-Siwe disease. As many as 15% of patients with Langerhans cell histiocytosis will suffer from diabetes insipidus.

Eosinophilic granuloma has been called the great mimic because it can look like other, more serious tumors on x-ray. Eosinophilic granuloma can be found almost anywhere in the axial or appendicular skeleton, but is commonly found in flat bones such as the scapula and skull. Usually, the lesion is small and radiolucent, without much reactive bone around it and it is not calcified. The appearance may easily be confused with Ewing sarcoma, Brodie abscess, osteosarcoma, or metastatic tumor. Biopsy is almost always required to make the diagnosis. The lesions often heal after the biopsy and radical surgical curettage or excision is usually not necessary. After the diagnosis is known, treatment should be pursued in consultation with a hematologist-oncologist. Multiple lesions and systemic disease may require chemotherapy.

27.10.7 Osteoid Osteoma

Osteoid osteoma is a small benign tumor of bone that characteristically produces a large amount of pain. Although osteoid osteoma may occur anywhere, it is most common in the femur or tibia. Boys are affected slightly more often than girls. The lesion consists of a small nidus of osteoid tissue surrounded by reactive bone. When the lesion develops in the cortex, the amount of reactive bone around the nidus is striking. Pain is severe, often appearing at night, during rest, and unrelated to activity, and often responds dramatically to aspirin. When the lesion is near a joint, a small effusion may develop and nearby muscle may atropy. When the lesion arises in the spine, a painful scoliosis may occur.

Although suspicion of osteoid osteoma is aroused by the history and physical examination, the diagnosis is usually established by imaging. Plain x-rays may show a small radiolucent nidus, less than 1 cm in diameter, surrounded by dense reactive bone. If the lesion arises in cancellous bone or has not been present for a long time, it may not be apparent on plain x-rays. Technetium bone scanning may help to locate inconspicuous tumors. Computed tomography can be very useful for pinpointing the location of the nidus. If left alone, the osteoid osteoma will eventually disappear and the pain will subside. Unfortunately, the process of resolution can take years, and most patients prefer surgical excision. Surgery may be open or percutaneous under CT guidance. Intraoperative bone scanning can help decrease the potential for recurrence. The surgical removal must include the nidus or symptoms will persist. Recently percutaneous radiofrequency approaches to the treatment of osteoid

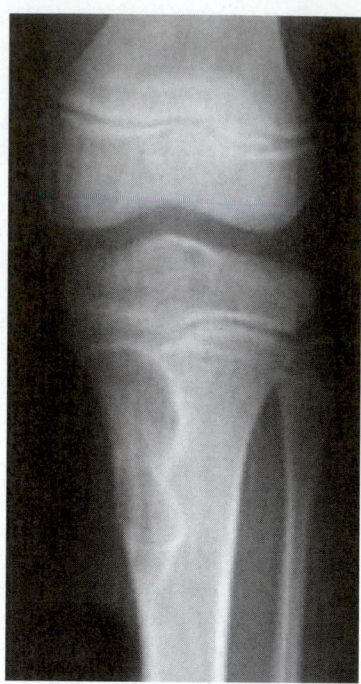

FIGURE 27-51 **Nonossifying fibroma of the proximal tibia. Note the lesion's typical eccentric metaphyseal location.**

osteoma have been reported to be superior to surgical en bloc removal.

27.10.8 Osteoblastoma

The histologic appearance of osteoblastoma is similar to that of osteoid osteoma, but the tumor is larger. Some consider lesions less than 1.3 cm to be osteoid osteoma, and larger ones as osteoblastoma. It is almost certainly a separate tumor, however, for its behavior is quite different from osteoid osteoma. Osteoblastoma tends to be located in the spine, in the small bones of the feet, or on ribs. A painful scoliosis should alert one to the possibility of osteoblastoma of the spine. Osteoblastoma is a growing, destructive lesion that does not provoke the exuberant reactive bone seen in osteoid osteoma. Most of these tumors are benign, but local recurrence or perhaps persistence after surgical excision is not rare, and occasionally malignant variants have been reported.

27.10.9 Chondroblastoma

Chondroblastoma represents a benign cartilaginous tumor that has a strong predilection for the epiphyses of long bones in growing children. Common locations include the fastest growing epiphyses: the proximal humerus (often referred to as Codman tumor in this area), proximal femur, proximal tibia, and distal femur. Chondroblastoma is part of a small, but real, group of histologically benign musculoskeletal tumors that can metastasize to other areas of the body (typically the lungs). Such behavior challenges common conceptions of benignity versus malignancy.

This behavior, along with the lack of evidence that chondroblastomas will spontaneously resolve, has led to the common recommendation that once recognized they should be treated. Thus, after appropriate bone scan proof of unifocal bone disease, and after ruling out lung metastasis, surgical resection of chondroblastoma is undertaken. A high success rate has been realized with curettage and bone grafting, provided careful surgical technique allows one to avoid undue disruption of articular surfaces. A disciplined bone grafting approach is also necessary to prevent transplantation of the tumor to the bone graft harvest site.

27.10.10 Common Malignant Musculoskeletal Tumors in Children

Osteogenic sarcoma is the most common malignant bone tumor in children, and Ewing sarcoma is the second most common. Osteogenic sarcoma is a malignant mesenchymal cell tumor, while Ewing sarcoma is a malignant neuroectodermal tumor. Osteogenic sarcoma most commonly occurs around the knee at the distal femur or proximal tibia and has several important associations such as hereditary retinoblastoma, Rothmund-Thomson syndrome, and an increased risk following radiation exposure. Ewing sarcoma has no such familial or radiation associations, but it does often demonstrate a translocation phenomenon between chromosomes 11 and 22.

OSTEOGENIC SARCOMA AND EWING SARCOMA

The treatment of osteogenic sarcoma has been revolutionized by modern chemotherapeutic regimens. This, in conjunction with the proven value of limb-sparing surgical techniques, has made amputation the exception rather than the rule when it comes to the treatment of this malignant bone tumor. Optional techniques of limb salvage include arthrodesis, osteoarticular allograft, endoprosthetic replacement allograft/endoprosthesis, and Van Ness rotation. The need for chemotherapy in the treatment of Ewing sarcoma is firmly established, while the role for radiation therapy is diminishing and that for orthopedic surgical intervention is expanding. Future efforts at further refining treatment of primary disease and developing more successful approaches to disease relapses and recurrences are necessary.

RHABDOMYOSARCOMA

The most common malignant soft tissue tumor in children is rhabdomyosarcoma. This tumor often presents as a painless lump in one of the extremities. MRI is an important part of the workup of such suspicious lesions; MRI should precede any planned surgical biopsy. Modern combinations of chemotherapeutic and surgical treatments have resulted in marked improvements in survival for rhabdomyosarcoma, with success rates ranging from 70 to 95% (depending on extent of disease).

27.11 NEUROMUSCULAR DISORDERS

Eric J. Wall

27.11.1 Myelomeningocele (Spina Bifida)

The overall treatment and survival of children with myelomeningocele (spina bifida) has dramatically improved over the last three decades. Folate supplements taken at least 1 month before conception and for the first 3 months of pregnancy can reduce the risk of spina bifida by 70%. Spina bifida patients are orthopedically classified according to their lowest intact level of neurologic function as follows:

LEVEL	FUNCTION
Thoracic	No lower extremity function
Upper lumbar	Good hip flexors
Low lumbar	Good quadriceps
Sacral	Good foot function

Almost all young children with spina bifida can be started in a standing/walking program if placed in appropriate braces. Treatment in a standing program starts with a chest-high standing frame or parapodium after a child has gained sitting balance, which tends to be between the age of 1 and 2 years. As young children gain balance and mobility in a standing frame, they progress to chest-level leg braces and a walker. The braces are progressively shortened to waist, thigh, or leg (AFO) level, as the child tolerates. Lower-lumbar-level patients typically can ambulate independently with AFO braces; however, those with higher levels of paraplegia typically require crutches or a walker to assist with ambulation. The benefits of a childhood standing program are controversial because many patients with spina bifida will ultimately become wheelchair ambulators after they reach puberty. Recent reports show that children enrolled in a standing program end up more independent as teenagers and adults than those who were not enrolled in a standing program. Any progressive lower extremity deformity, rapid scoliosis progression, or change in neurologic function should prompt neurologic evaluation for tethered spinal cord, syrinx, shunt malfunction, or foramen magnum compression. Upper-extremity strength should be carefully monitored for evidence of changing neurologic function consistent with development of a syrinx or Chiari malformation.

Children with spina bifida have a very high incidence of scoliosis and kyphosis and should be clinically and radiographically screened for scoliosis. Children with spina bifida who develop curves ≥40 to 50 degrees may require spinal correction and fusion. About 15 to 20% of children with spina bifida can have severe kyphosis. The kyphosis may lead to skin breakdown and pressure sores from their wheelchairs and braces. This is usually not amenable to bracing and may require surgical correction at a young age. Children with spina bifida may have lower extremity contractures that may need to be corrected before they can stand in braces. Hip dislocation is common in children with spina bifida; however, surgical relocation of the hips is only indicated for children at the L4 level or below, who walk with ankle-foot orthosis, and who use no other ambulatory aides, such as crutches or a walker. Children with spina bifida also have a high incidence of foot deformities such as clubfeet. Surgical correction may be necessary to prevent pressure sores and to provide an adequate bracing position.

27.11.2 Cerebral Palsy

Cerebral palsy is the most common neuromuscular disorder in children. It can be defined as a nonprogressive disorder of an immature central nervous system or brain that results in abnormal movement, control, and posture. Numerous associations, both prenatally and postnatally, have been identified, but in many cases, the etiology remains elusive. The severity of brain damage determines the prognosis. The neurologic insult is static, but abnormal muscle forces on a growing skeleton can lead to contractures and progressive deformity. In addition to the musculoskeletal issues, children will often have many concomitant problems including seizure disorders; auditory and visual problems; feeding problems with gastrointestinal motility; and mental retardation and learning disabilities. Brain MRIs often fail to reveal a deformity and may in fact be negative. A team approach is indicated for the optimal management of these children.

ORTHOPEDIC MANAGEMENT

Orthopedic management centers on maintaining joint flexibility, preventing and treating contractures and deformity, and maximizing function. Botox and baclofen have been used to decrease spasticity with varying success. Selective dorsal rhizotomy was once thought to be quite effective in reducing spasticity; however, enthusiasm for its use is waning because of side effects. Realistic goals for the child must be communicated to the families. Priorities should include communication skills, activities of daily living for self-care, mobility, and ambulatory skills.

Orthopedic surgery is often indicated. The indications include a plateau in the child's development because of contractures, prevention of progressive deformity, and stabilization of an existing or progressive deformity. The principles of surgery include immobilization for short periods of time, but bracing for longer periods for support and prevention of recurrence; multiple procedures under a single anesthetic; and underlengthening of tendons, as it is preferable to have to perform a subsequent relengthening.

UPPER EXTREMITY

Upper extremity surgery is less frequently performed than is lower extremity surgery. It requires a higher functioning, well-motivated child who has a good supportive family and therapist. Sensation and proprioception are prerequisites for improving function, while some upper extremity surgery is performed to improve position and appearance.

SPINE

Progressive spinal deformity is often a problem. In the nonambulatory patient, the deformity does not respond to bracing in that the deformity will progress in spite of this form of treatment. Bracing may be beneficial for truncal support, especially in cases in which sitting balance requires the use of the upper extremities to keep the child upright. Surgical stabilization should be considered early for progressive severe deformities before other complications intervene.

HIPS

Hip subluxation and dislocation should be monitored. Any child who has less than 30 degrees of abduction of either hip should undergo hip x-rays to assess the hip joints. Follow-up x-rays should be obtained at yearly intervals. Often surgery to prevent hip subluxation or to reduce a dislocating hip is indicated.

LOWER EXTREMITY

Other lower extremity surgery involves release of contractures, tendon transfers to help balance abnormal muscle forces, and bony procedures to stabilize joints in normal mechanical alignment and functional positions. Lengthening of the adductors, hamstrings, and tendoachilles the most common procedure. Bracing and phys-

ical therapy are important components of treatment prior to and following surgical intervention.

27.11.3 Arthrogryposis Multiplex Congenita

Arthrogryposis multiplex congenita (AMC) is a syndrome or disorder that presents with multiple congenital contractures. It is nonprogressive, but not unchanging as the child grows, and is of variable severity. Intelligence is normal. The etiology is unknown, but there are at least 150 specific diagnoses that are associated with multiple congenital contractures. A contracture is defined as a limitation of joint motion. Any factor that reduces fetal or intrauterine movement can lead to contractures. The joints are generally normal initially.

At birth, the child with AMC presents with multiple joint contractures. Depending upon the severity of contracture, fractures may occur during delivery. In addition to the limitation of joint motion, there may be abnormal dimpling of the skin overlying the joint and an absence of skin creases. Webbing or pterygia may be present, most commonly at the elbows and knees. There is little active motion by the child, but some passive motion is generally present. The jaw is frequently hypoplastic and tracheomalacia may complicate the newborn period. In the upper extremity, the shoulder is generally adducted and internally rotated. The elbow is usually extended, but may be flexed. The wrists are ulnarly deviated and the fingers are usually contracted in extension at the metacarpophalangeal and interphalangeal joints.

In the lower extremity, the hips are frequently flexed, abducted, and externally rotated. Hip dislocation, unilateral or bilateral, may be present and is generally not reducible. The knees may be in any position from hyperextension to flexion. Rigid clubfeet or rocker bottom feet (congenital vertical talus) are common. As the child grows, the joint contractures may limit gross motor development and function. Physical therapy is recommended early to preserve and improve range of motion. Overzealous attempts to gain motion frequently result in fracture. Splinting may be beneficial to maintain the improved motion or position. Therapy alone will not correct deformity or restore complete passive motion. Active motion of the joints will depend on the degree of severity. Specialized adaptive equipment may be necessary to maximize function.

Surgical management is usually required, primarily in the lower extremity. Whether bilateral hip dislocations should be surgically reduced continues to be controversial. The more flexible the joint, the better for the child even if the hips are dislocated. Ambulation is not dependent upon reduction of the hips. Unilateral hip dislocations are generally surgically reduced. Knee function is maximized by having full extension and approximately 90 degrees of flexion. Surgical release of contractures or osteotomies may be necessary to accomplish this goal. The typically severe rigid deformities of the feet require correction to allow a plantigrade foot. A posteromedial release may be sufficient in the less severe deformity, but a talectomy is often necessary in the more severe deformity or in the foot with a recurrent deformity. Correction of the foot alignment is generally done around 1 year of age or when the child shows an interest in standing or walking. In the upper extremity, surgery is seldom indicated for the wrist or fingers. Soft tissue or bony surgery is occasionally warranted at the elbow to improve alignment and function. Physical therapy and prolonged splinting are necessary postoperatively for both upper and lower extremity surgery.

References

Aronsson DD, Goldberg MJ, Kling TF, Roy DR: Developmental dysplasia of the hip. Pediatrics 94:201&ndash208, 1994

Bleck EE: Developmental orthopaedics. III: Toddlers. Dev Med Child Neurol 24:533–555, 1982

Bleck EE: Orthopaedics Management in Cerebral Palsy. Philadelphia, Lippincott, 1987

Bora FW Jr: The Pediatric Upper Extremity.. Philadelphia, Saunders, 1986

Bradford DS, Lonstein JE, Ogilvie JW, Winter RB: Moe's Textbook of Scoliosis and Other Spinal Deformities, 2nd ed.. Philadelphia, Saunders, 1987

Coleman SS: Congenital Dysplasia and Dislocation of the Hip. St. Louis, Mosby, 1978

Dahlin DC, Unni KK: Bone Tumors: General Aspects and Data on 8,542 Cases, 4th ed. Springfield, IL, Charles C. Thomas, 1986

Davison BL, Weinstein SL: Hip fractures in children: A long-term follow-up study. J Pediatr Orthop 12:355–358, 1992

Emans JB: Allergy to latex in patients who have myelodysplasia.. J Bone Joint Surg 74A:1103–1109, 1992

Flatt AE: The Care of Congenital Hand Anomalies, 2nd ed. St. Louis, Quality Medical Publishing, 1994

Freiberg AA, Loder RT, Heidelberger KP, Hensinger RN: Aneurysmal bone cysts in young children. J Pediatr Orthop 14:86–91, 1994

Goldberg MJ: The Dysmorphic Child: An Orthopaedic Perspective. New York, Raven Press, 1987

Greene WB: Infantile tibia vara. J Bone Joint Surg 75A:130–143, 1993

Henderson RC, Renner JB, Sturdivant MC, Greene WB: Evaluation of magnetic resonance imaging in Legg-Perthes disease: A prospective, blinded study. J Pediatr Orthop 10:289–297, 1990

Hensinger RN, Jones ET: Developmental orthopaedics. I: The lower limb. Dev Med Child Neurol 24:95–116, 1982

Herring JA: The treatment of Legg-Calvé-Perthes disease. J Bone Joint Surg 76A:448–458, 1994

Kling TF, Hensinger RN: Angular and torsional deformities of the lower limbs in children. Clin Orthop 176:136–147, 1983

Lennox IA, McLauchlan J, Murali R: Failures of screening and management of congenital dislocation of the hip. J Bone Joint Surg 75:72–75, 1993

Levine AM, Drennan JC: Physiological bowing and tibia vara. J Bone Joint Surg 64A:1158–1163, 1982

Loder RT, Schwartz EM, Hensinger RN: Behavioral characteristics of children with Legg-Calvé-Perthes disease. J Pediatr Orthop 13:598–601, 1993

Lowe TG: Scheuermann disease. J Bone Joint Surg 72:940–945 1990

Mazur JM, Shurtleff D, Menelaus M, Colliver J: Orthopaedic management of high-level spina bifida. J Bone Joint Surg 71:56–61, 1989

Morrissy RT, ed: Lowvell and Winter's Pediatric Orthopaedics, 3rd ed. Philadelphia, Lippincott, 1990

Peterson HA: Deformities and problems of the forearm in children with multiple hereditary osteochondromata. J Pediatr Orthop 14:92–100, 1994

Rang M: Children's Fractures, 2nd ed. Philadelphia, Lippincott, 1983

Rockwood CA, Wilkins KE, King RE: Fractures in Children, 3rd ed. Philadelphia, Lippincott, 1991

Salter RB: Textbook of Disorders and Injuries of the Musculoskeletal System, 2nd ed. Baltimore, Williams and Wilkins, 1983

Salter RB, Harris WR: Injuries involving the epiphyseal plate. J Bone Joint Surg, 45:587–593, 1963

Schafer MF, Dias LS: Myelomeningocele: Orthopaedic Treatment. Baltimore, Williams and Wilkins, 1983

Shapiro F, Specht L: The diagnosis and orthopaedic treatment of inherited muscular diseases of childhood. J Bone Joint Surg 75:439–454, 1993

Sutherland DH, Olshen RA, Biden EN, Wyatt MP: The Development of Mature Walking. Philadelphia, Lippincott, 1988

Tachdjian MO: Pediatric Orthopedics, 2nd ed. Philadelphia, Saunders, 1990

Thompson GH, Bilenker RM: Comprehensive management of arthrogryposis multiplex congenita. Clin Orthop 194:6–14, 1985

Wells D, King JD, Roe TF, Kaufman FR: Review of slipped capital femoral epiphysis associated with endocrine disease. J Pediatr Orthop 13:610–614, 1993

Wenger DR, Rang M: The Art and Practice of Children's Orthopaedics. New York, Raven Press, 1993

Weseley MS, Barenfeld PA, Eisenstein AL: Thoughts on in-toeing and out-toeing: Twenty years' experience with over 5000 cases and a review of the literature. Foot Ankle 2:49–57, 1981

Yngve D, Gross R: Late diagnosis of hip dislocation in infants. J Pediatr Orthop 10:777–779, 1990

APPENDICES

Appendix A Growth Charts

Birth to 36 months: Boys
Length-for-age and Weight-for-age percentiles

NAME _____

RECORD # _____

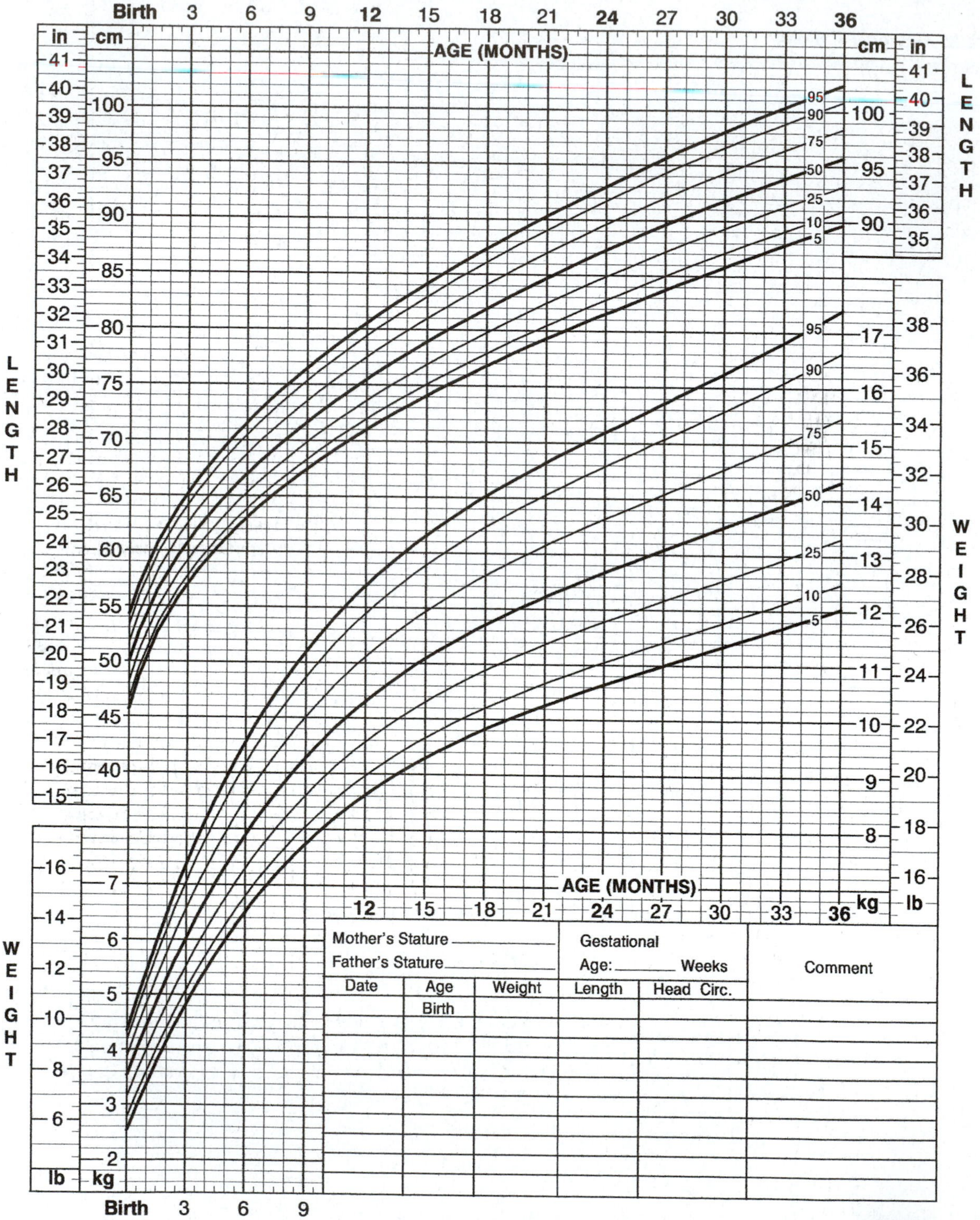

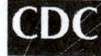

Revised November 21, 2000.
SOURCE: Developed by the National Center for Health Statistics in collaboration with
the National Center for Chronic Disease Prevention and Health Promotion (2000).
http://www.cdc.gov/growthcharts

FIGURE A-1

Birth to 36 months: Boys
Head circumference-for-age and
Weight-for-length percentiles

NAME _____

RECORD # _____

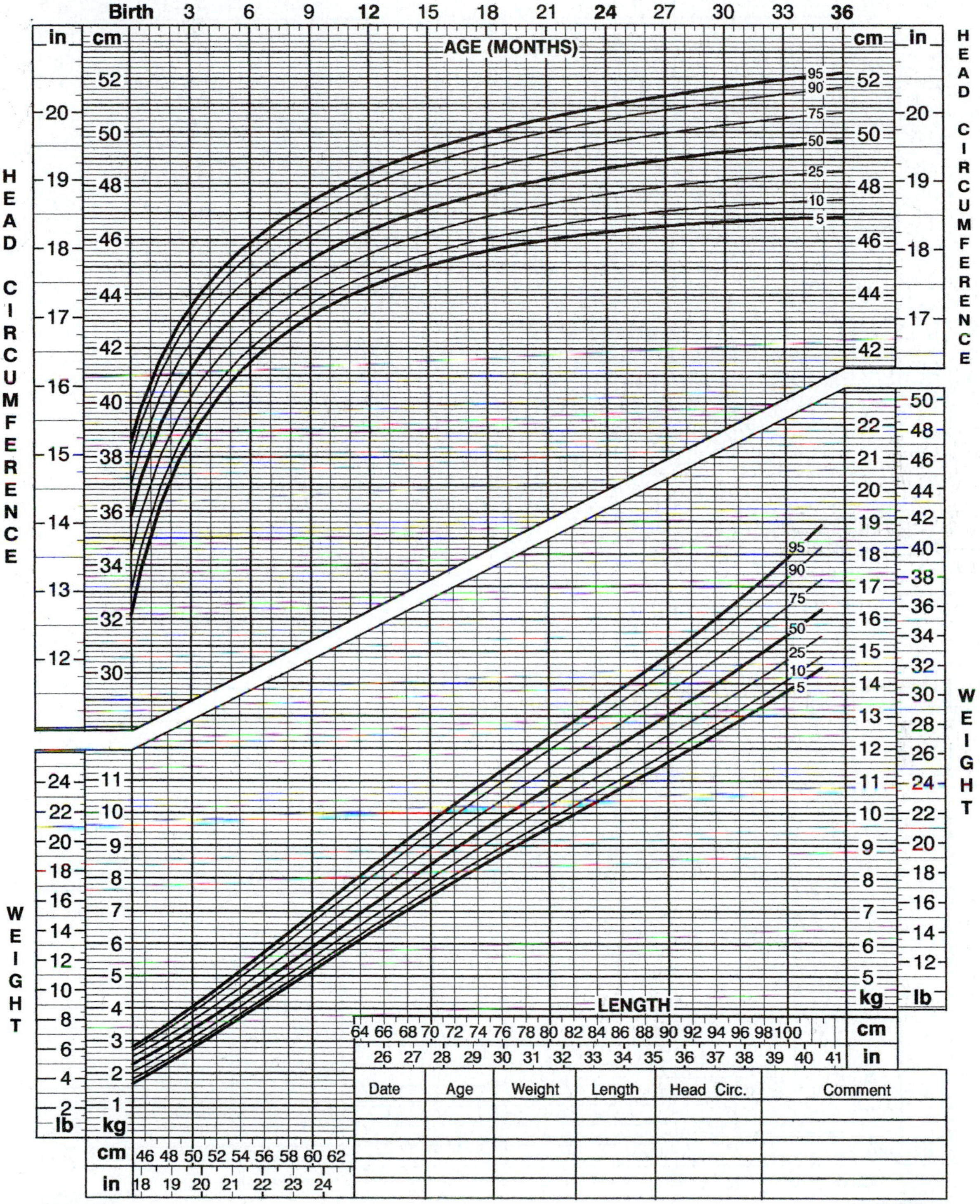

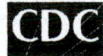

SOURCE: Developed by the National Center for Health Statistics in collaboration with
the National Center for Chronic Disease Prevention and Health Promotion (2000).
http://www.cdc.gov/growthcharts

FIGURE A-2

Birth to 36 months: Girls
Length-for-age and Weight-for-age percentiles

NAME _____

RECORD # _____

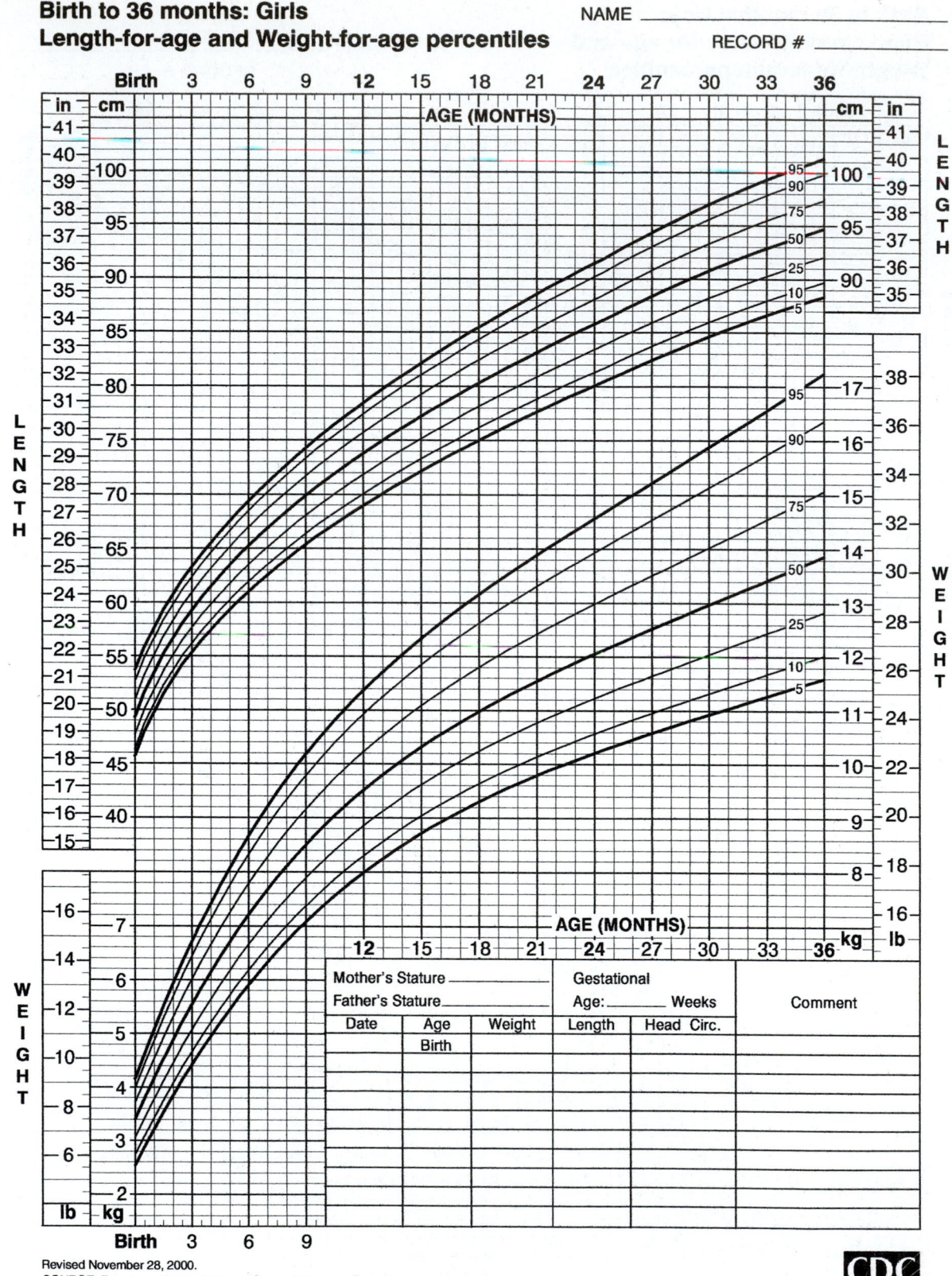

Revised November 28, 2000.
SOURCE: Developed by the National Center for Health Statistics in collaboration with
the National Center for Chronic Disease Prevention and Health Promotion (2000).
http://www.cdc.gov/growthcharts

CDC

FIGURE A-3

Birth to 36 months: Girls
Head circumference-for-age and
Weight-for-length percentiles

NAME _____

RECORD # _____

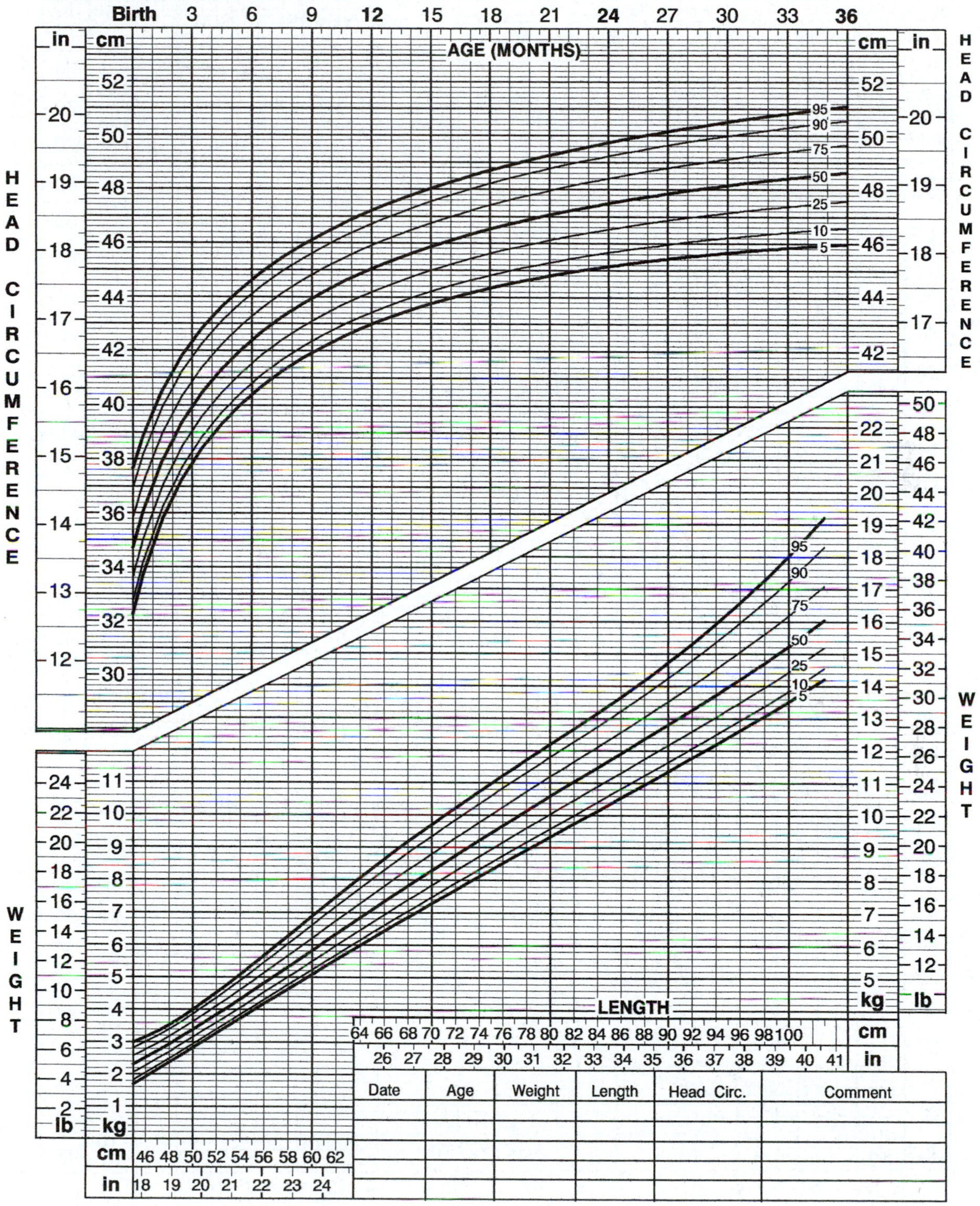

SOURCE: Developed by the National Center for Health Statistics in collaboration with
the National Center for Chronic Disease Prevention and Health Promotion (2000).
http://www.cdc.gov/growthcharts

FIGURE A-4

2 to 20 years: Boys
Stature-for-age and Weight-for-age percentiles

NAME _____

RECORD # _____

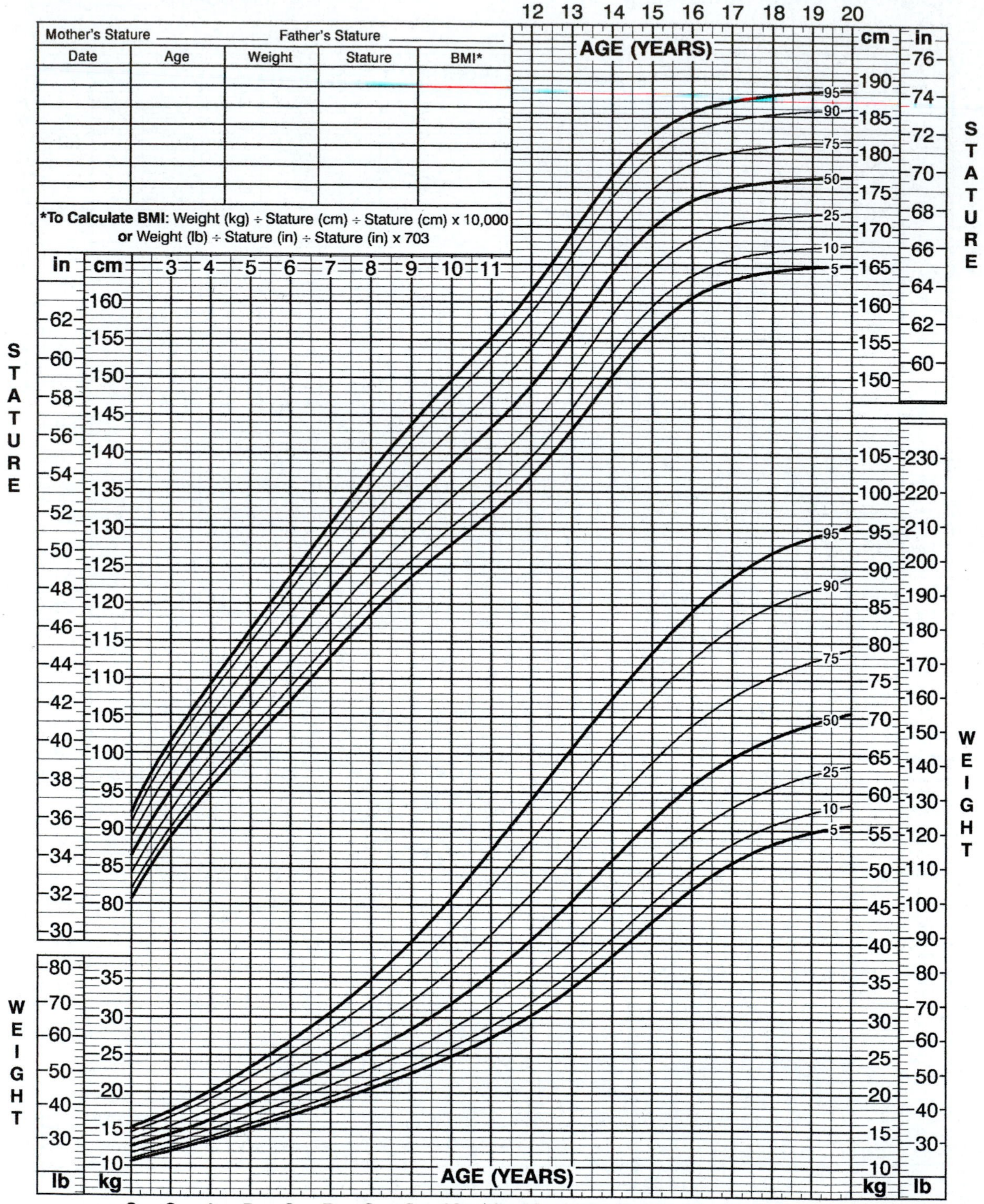

Mother's Stature _____ Father's Stature _____

Date	Age	Weight	Stature	BMI*

*To Calculate BMI: Weight (kg) ÷ Stature (cm) ÷ Stature (cm) x 10,000
or Weight (lb) ÷ Stature (in) ÷ Stature (in) x 703

AGE (YEARS)

STATURE

WEIGHT

Revised and corrected November 28, 2000.
SOURCE: Developed by the National Center for Health Statistics in collaboration with
the National Center for Chronic Disease Prevention and Health Promotion (2000).
http://www.cdc.gov/growthcharts

FIGURE A-5

2 to 20 years: Boys
Body mass index-for-age percentiles

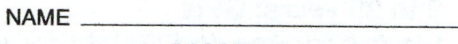

NAME ______________________

RECORD # ____________

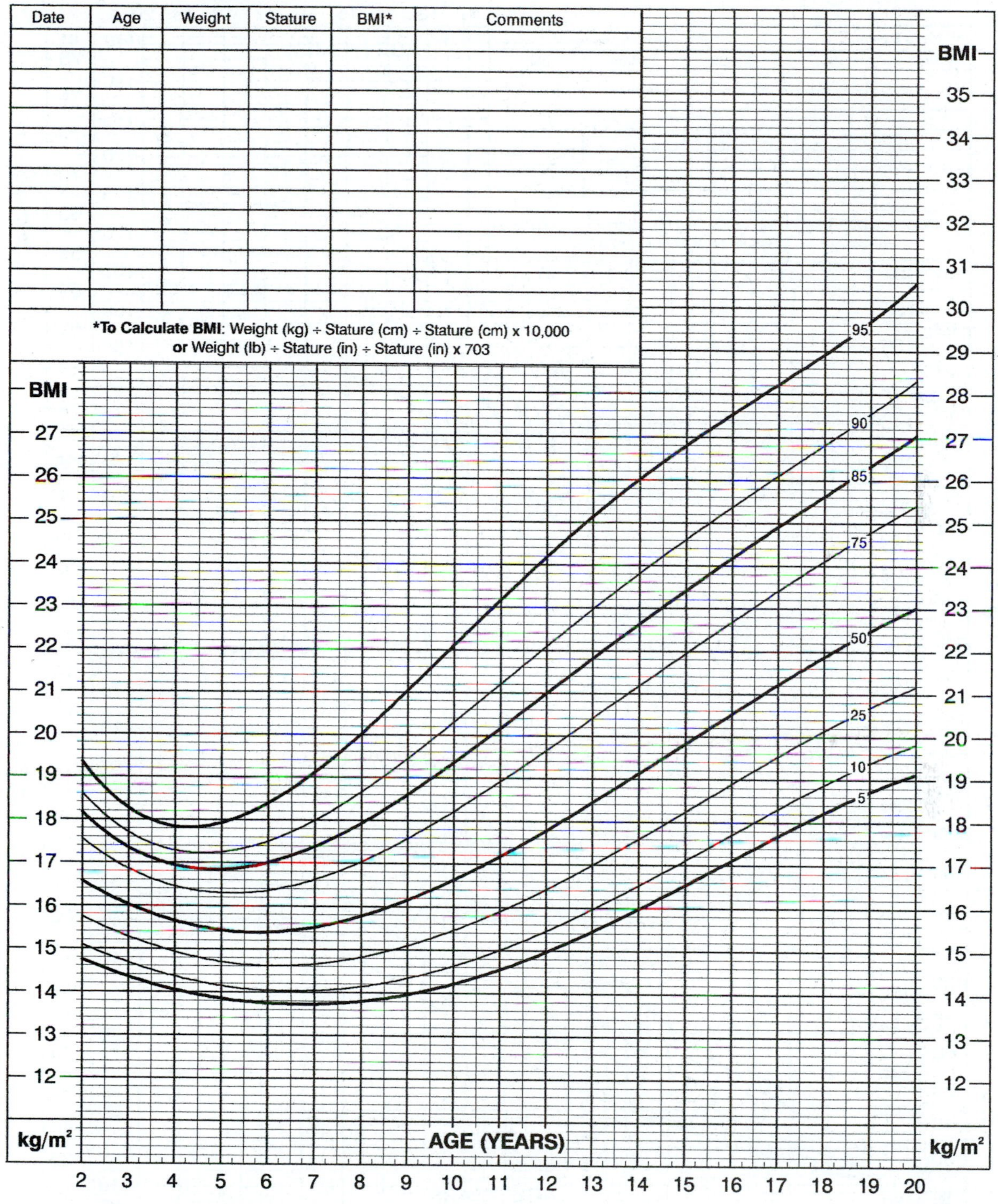

Date
Age
Weight
Stature
BMI*
Comments
*To Calculate BMI: Weight (kg) ÷ Stature (cm) ÷ Stature (cm) x 10,000
or Weight (lb) ÷ Stature (in) ÷ Stature (in) x 703
BMI
95
90
85
75
50
25
10
5
kg/m²
AGE (YEARS)
2 3 4 5 6 7 8 9 10 11 12 13 14 15 16 17 18 19 20

SOURCE: Developed by the National Center for Health Statistics in collaboration with the National Center for Chronic Disease Prevention and Health Promotion (2000).
http://www.cdc.gov/growthcharts

CDC

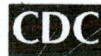

FIGURE A-6

2 to 20 years: Girls
Stature-for-age and Weight-for-age percentiles

NAME _____

RECORD # _____

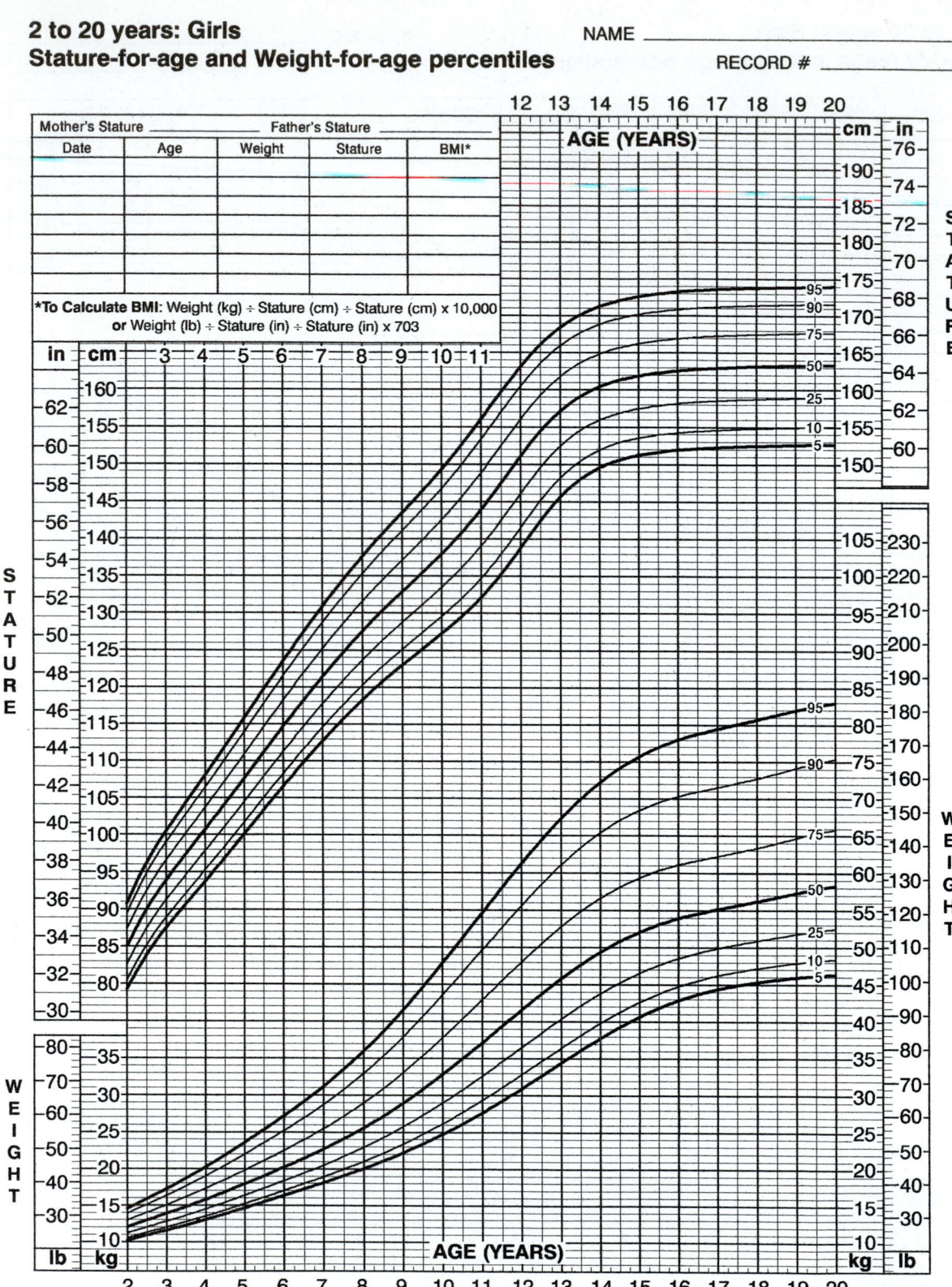

Revised and corrected November 28, 2000.
SOURCE: Developed by the National Center for Health Statistics in collaboration with
the National Center for Chronic Disease Prevention and Health Promotion (2000).
http://www.cdc.gov/growthcharts

CDC

FIGURE A-7

2 to 20 years: Girls
Body mass index-for-age percentiles

NAME ______________________

RECORD # ____________

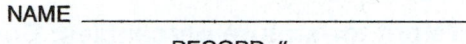

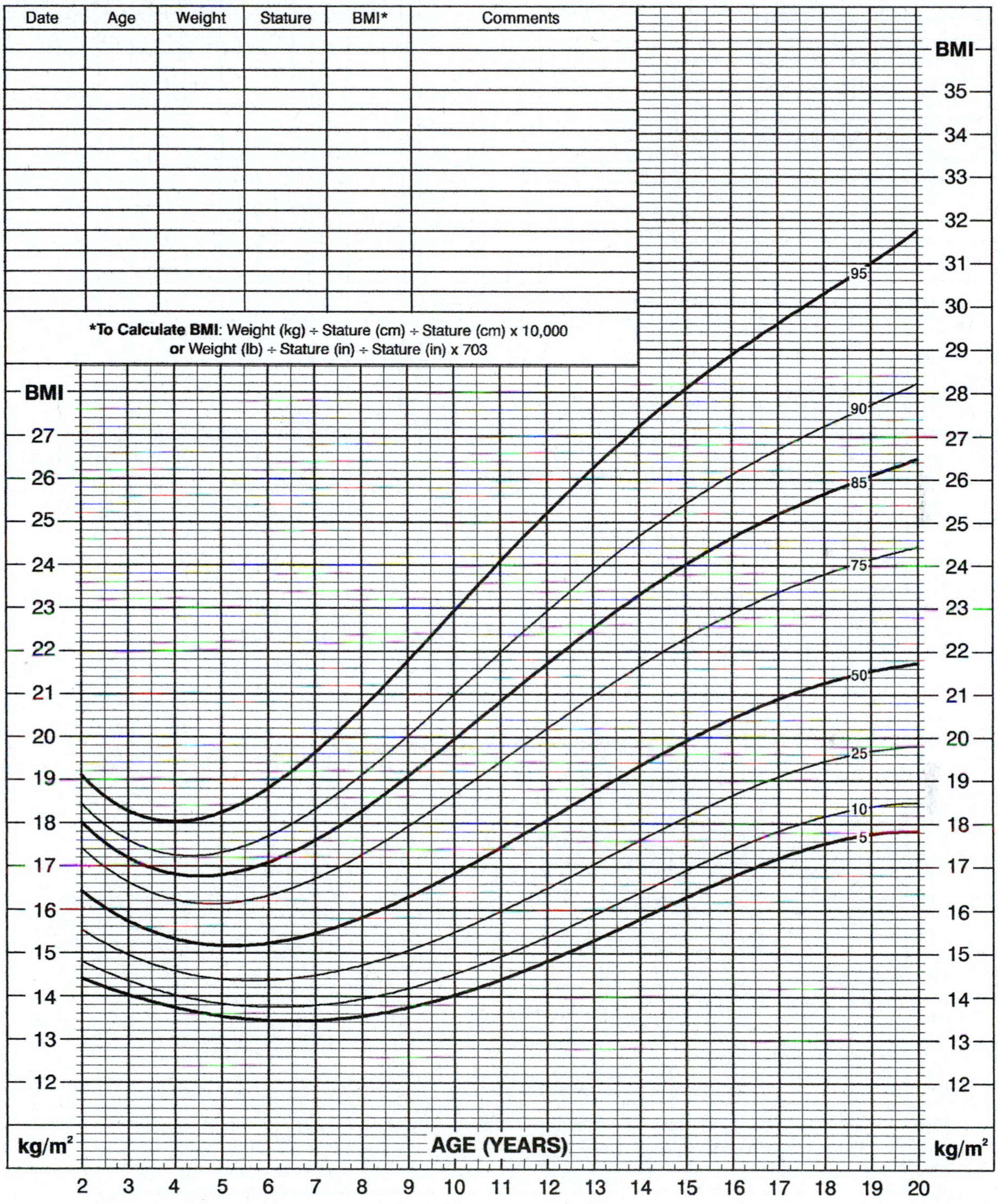
Date
Age
Weight
Stature
BMI*
Comments
*To Calculate BMI: Weight (kg) ÷ Stature (cm) ÷ Stature (cm) x 10,000
or Weight (lb) ÷ Stature (in) ÷ Stature (in) x 703
BMI
35
34
33
32
31
30
29
28
27
26
25
24
23
22
21
20
19
18
17
16
15
14
13
12
95
90
85
75
50
25
10
5
kg/m²
AGE (YEARS)
2
3
4
5
6
7
8
9
10
11
12
13
14
15
16
17
18
19
20

SOURCE: Developed by the National Center for Health Statistics in collaboration with
the National Center for Chronic Disease Prevention and Health Promotion (2000).
http://www.cdc.gov/growthcharts

CDC

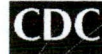

FIGURE A-8

Weight-for-stature percentiles: Boys

NAME _____

RECORD # _____

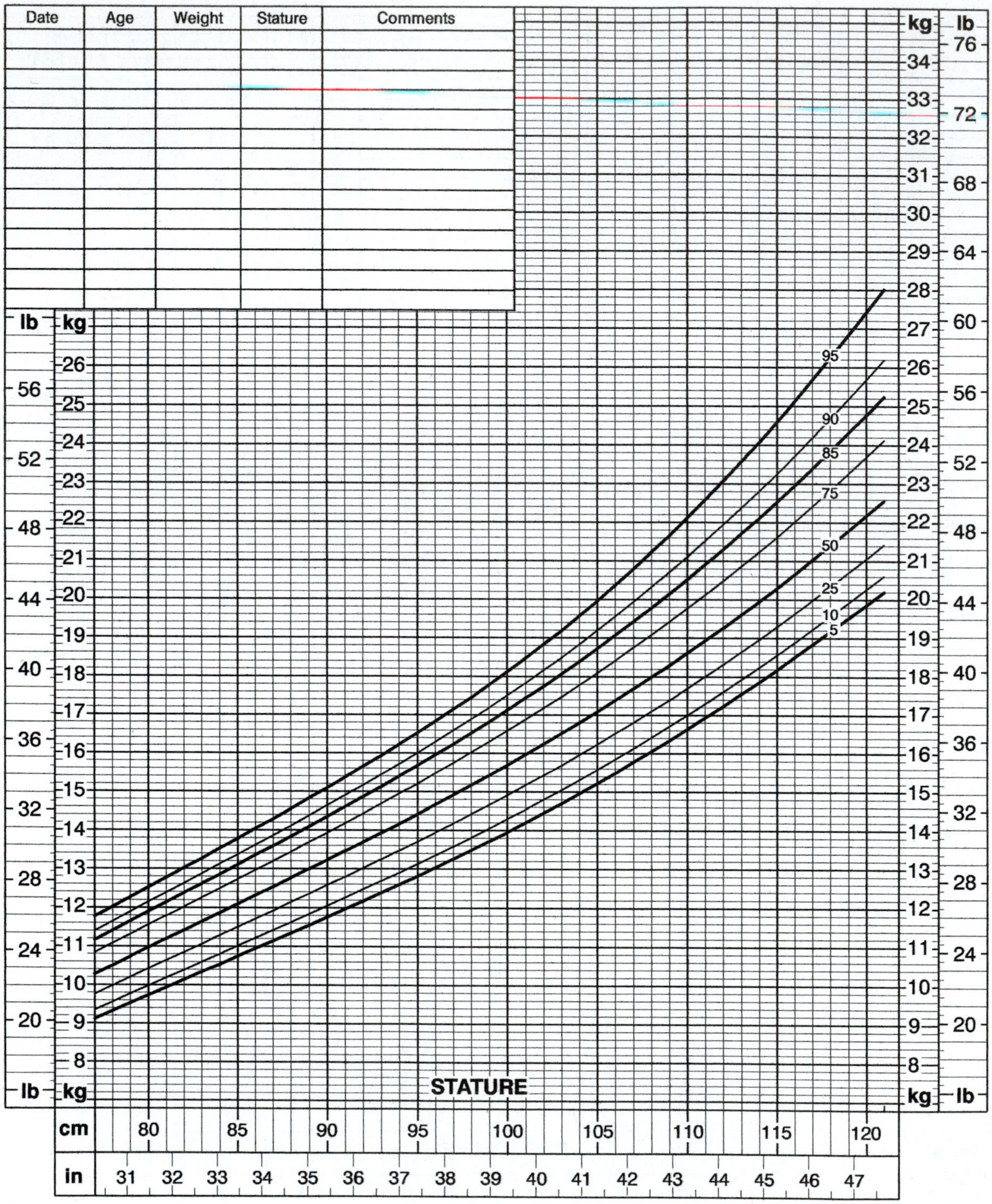

SOURCE: Developed by the National Center for Health Statistics in collaboration with
the National Center for Chronic Disease Prevention and Health Promotion (2000).
http://www.cdc.gov/growthcharts

FIGURE A-9

Weight-for-stature percentiles: Girls

NAME _____

RECORD # _____

Date	Age	Weight	Stature	Comments

STATURE

cm 80 85 90 95 100 105 110 115 120

in 31 32 33 34 35 36 37 38 39 40 41 42 43 44 45 46 47

SOURCE: Developed by the National Center for Health Statistics in collaboration with
the National Center for Chronic Disease Prevention and Health Promotion (2000).
http://www.cdc.gov/growthcharts

FIGURE A-10

Appendix B   Changes in Growth Over Time

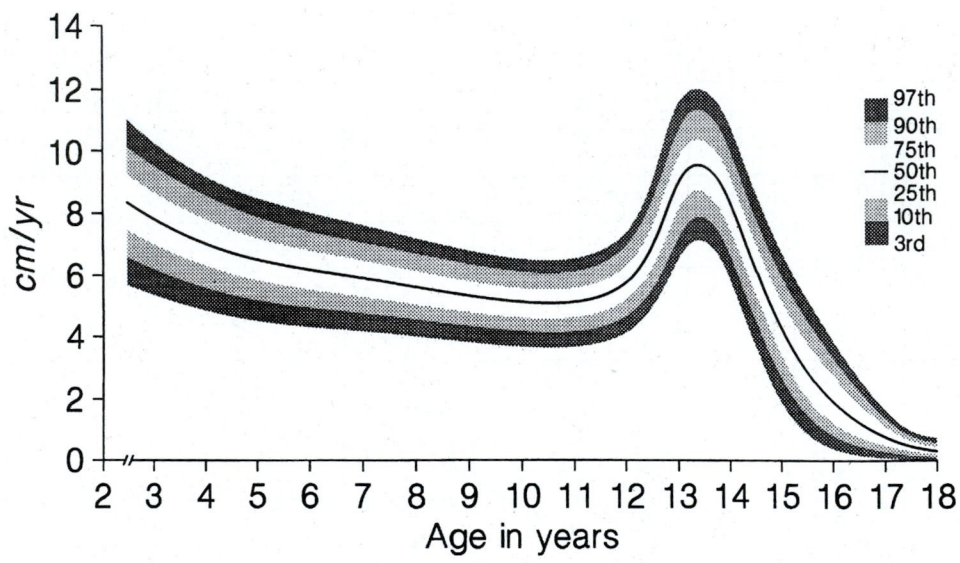

FIGURE B-1   Height velocity centiles for boys maturing at average time. SOURCE: *From Tanner JM, Davies PSW: J Pediatr 107:317, 1985.*

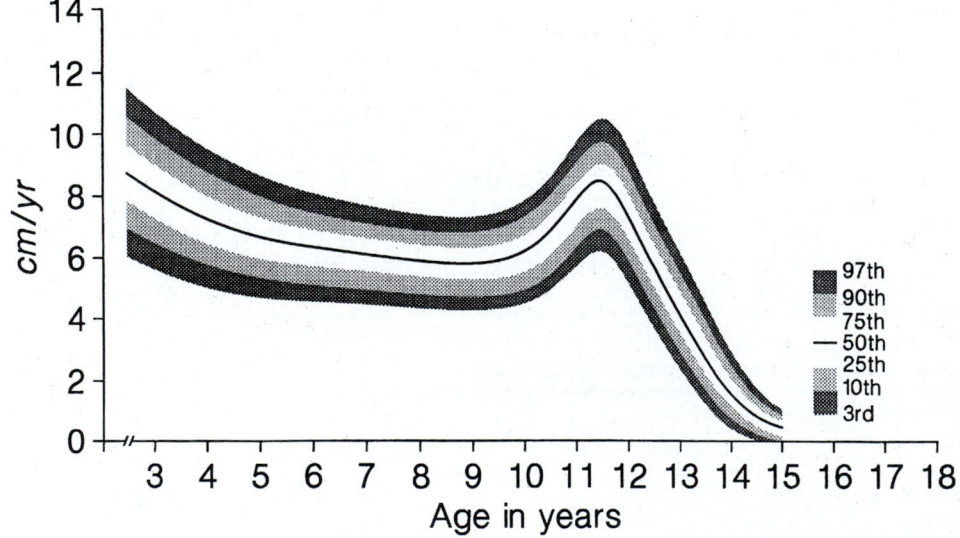

FIGURE B-2   Height velocity centiles for girls maturing at average time. SOURCE: *From Tanner JM, Davies PSW: J Pediatr 107:317, 1985.*

TABLE B-3

ONE-MONTH INCREMENTS IN WEIGHT (G/D) FROM BIRTH TO 6 MONTHS[a]

AGE (mo)	n	WEIGHT (gm/day)[b]	PERCENTILE						
			5th	10th	25th	50th	75th	90th	95th
Boys									
Up to 1	580	30 ± 9.4	15	18	24	30	36	42	45
1–2	580	35 ± 8.5	22	25	29	35	40	46	50
2–3	580	27 ± 7.9	15	18	22	26	31	36	41
3–4	298	20 ± 3.6	15	16	18	20	22	24	26
4–5	298	17 ± 3.4	12	14	15	17	19	21	23
5–6	298	16 ± 3.5	11	12	14	15	17	19	21
Girls									
Up to 1	562	26 ± 8.4	11	16	20	26	32	36	39
1–2	562	29 ± 7.7	18	20	24	29	34	39	42
2–3	562	23 ± 7.2	12	14	19	23	28	32	35
3–4	298	19 ± 5.3	13	15	17	19	21	23	26
4–5	298	16 ± 5.0	11	13	14	16	18	20	22
5–6	298	15 ± 4.7	10	11	13	14	16	18	18

[a] From birth through 3 months, Iowa data; from 3 through 6 months, combined Iowa and Fels data.
[b] Values expressed as mean $\pm$ SD.
From Guo S, Roche AF, Fomon SJ, et al: Reference data on gains in weight and length during the first two years of life. J Pediatr 119:355, 1991.

TABLE B-4

TWO-MONTH INCREMENTS IN WEIGHT FROM BIRTH TO 12 MONTHS[a]

AGE (mo)	n	WEIGHT (gm/day)[b]	PERCENTILE						
			5th	10th	25th	50th	75th	90th	95th
Boys									
Up to 2	580	33 ± 7.0	21	24	28	32	38	42	44
1–3	580	31 ± 6.9	20	22	27	31	35	39	43
2–4	65	23 ± 4.7	—	17	19	23	26	29	—
3–5	298	19 ± 3.2	14	15	17	18	20	22	24
4–6	298	16 ± 2.9	12	13	14	16	18	20	21
5–7	233	15 ± 2.4	11	12	13	15	16	18	18
6–8	233	13 ± 2.4	10	11	12	13	15	16	17
7–9	233	12 ± 2.4	9	10	11	12	14	15	16
8–10	233	12 ± 2.4	9	9	10	11	13	15	15
9–11	233	11 ± 2.3	8	8	9	11	12	14	14
10–12	233	10 ± 2.3	7	8	9	10	12	13	14
Girls									
Up to 2	562	28 ± 6.5	17	20	23	28	32	36	38
1–3	562	26 ± 6.3	16	19	22	26	30	34	37
2–4	74	22 ± 5.4	—	16	19	21	24	27	—
3–5	298	18 ± 4.7	13	14	16	17	19	21	22
4–6	298	15 ± 4.6	11	12	14	15	17	18	19
5–7	224	14 ± 4.7	11	11	13	14	15	17	17
6–8	224	13 ± 4.6	10	10	12	13	14	16	16
7–9	224	12 ± 4.5	9	10	11	12	13	15	15
8–10	224	12 ± 4.5	8	9	10	11	13	14	14
9–11	224	11 ± 4.4	8	8	9	10	12	13	14
10–12	224	10 ± 4.3	7	8	9	10	11	13	13

[a] From birth through 3 months, Iowa data; from 3 through 6 months, combined data; from 6 through 12 months, Fels data.
[b] Values expressed as mean $\pm$ SD.
From Guo S, Roche AF, Fomon SJ, et al: Reference data on gains in weight and length during the first two years of life. J Pediatr 119:355, 1991.

TABLE B-5

THREE-MONTH INCREMENTS IN WEIGHT FROM BIRTH TO 24 MONTHS[a]

			PERCENTILE						
AGE (mo)	*n*	WEIGHT (g/d)[b]	5th	10th	25th	50th	75th	90th	95th
Boys									
Up to 3	580	31 ± 5.9	21	23	27	31	34	38	41
1–4	65	27 ± 5.1	—	21	23	27	30	34	—
2–5	65	21 ± 4.3	—	15	17	21	23	27	—
3–6	298	18 ± 2.9	13	14	16	18	19	21	23
4–7	233	16 ± 2.4	12	13	14	15	17	18	19
5–8	233	14 ± 2.4	11	11	13	14	15	17	18
6–9	233	13 ± 2.4	10	10	11	13	14	16	17
7–10	233	12 ± 2.4	9	9	10	12	13	15	16
8–11	233	11 ± 2.4	8	9	10	11	12	14	15
9–12	233	11 ± 2.3	8	8	9	10	12	14	14
10–13	233	10 ± 2.3	7	8	9	10	11	13	14
11–14	233	10 ± 2.3	7	7	8	9	11	12	13
12–15	233	9 ± 2.3	6	7	8	9	10	12	13
13–16	233	9 ± 2.3	6	6	7	9	10	12	13
14–17	233	8 ± 2.2	6	6	7	8	10	11	12
15–18	233	8 ± 2.2	5	6	7	8	9	11	12
16–19	233	8 ± 2.2	5	6	7	8	9	10	12
17–20	233	8 ± 2.2	5	5	6	7	9	10	12
18–21	233	7 ± 2.2	5	5	6	7	8	10	11
19–22	233	7 ± 2.1	4	5	6	7	8	10	11
20–23	233	7 ± 2.1	4	5	6	7	8	9	11
21–24	233	7 ± 2.1	4	5	6	7	8	9	11
Girls									
Up to 3	562	26 ± 5.5	17	20	23	26	30	33	36
1–3	74	24 ± 5.1	—	19	21	24	27	30	—
2–5	74	20 ± 3.9	—	16	17	19	21	25	—
3–6	298	17 ± 4.6	12	13	15	17	18	20	21
4–7	224	15 ± 4.8	11	12	13	15	16	17	18
5–8	224	14 ± 4.7	10	11	12	13	15	16	17
6–9	224	13 ± 4.6	10	10	11	12	14	15	16
7–10	224	12 ± 4.5	9	9	10	12	13	14	15
8–11	224	11 ± 4.4	8	9	10	11	12	14	14
9–12	224	11 ± 4.3	8	8	9	10	12	13	14
10–13	224	10 ± 4.2	7	8	9	10	11	12	13
11–14	224	10 ± 4.2	7	7	8	9	11	12	13
12–15	224	9 ± 4.1	7	7	8	9	10	12	12
13–16	224	9 ± 4.0	6	7	8	8	10	11	12
14–17	224	9 ± 3.9	6	6	7	8	9	11	12
15–18	224	8 ± 3.9	6	6	7	8	9	10	11
16–19	224	8 ± 3.8	6	6	7	8	9	10	11
17–20	224	8 ± 3.8	5	6	7	7	9	10	11
18–21	224	8 ± 3.7	5	5	6	7	8	10	11
19–22	224	7 ± 3.6	5	5	6	7	8	9	10
20–23	224	7 ± 3.6	5	5	6	7	8	9	10
21–24	224	7 ± 3.5	5	5	6	7	8	9	10

[a] From birth through 3 months, Iowa data; from 3 through 6 months, combined data; from 6 through 12 months, Fels data.
[b] Values expressed as mean ± SD.
From Guo S, Roche AF, Fomon SJ, et al: Reference data on gains in weight and length during the first two years of life. J Pediatr 119:355, 1991.

TABLE B-6

TWO-MONTH INCREMENTS IN LENGTH FROM BIRTH TO 6 MONTHS[a]

AGE (mo)	*n*	LENGTH (mm/d)[b]	PERCENTILE						
			5th	10th	25th	50th	75th	90th	95th
Boys									
Up to 2	580	1.10 ± 0.15	0.87	0.90	1.00	1.10	1.18	1.28	1.34
1–3	580	1.08 ± 0.14	0.85	0.90	0.98	1.08	1.17	1.26	1.31
2–4	65	0.93 ± 0.75	—	0.75	0.82	0.95	1.02	1.07	—
3–5	255	0.73 ± 0.09	0.60	0.63	0.68	0.73	0.79	0.86	0.90
4–6	255	0.64 ± 0.08	0.49	0.54	0.59	0.63	0.69	0.74	0.78
Girls									
Up to 2	562	1.03 ± 0.13	0.80	0.87	0.93	1.03	1.11	1.20	1.25
1–3	562	0.99 ± 0.13	0.79	0.84	0.92	0.98	1.07	1.15	1.18
2–4	74	0.89 ± 0.13	—	0.72	0.80	0.90	0.97	1.05	—
3–5	241	0.71 ± 0.10	0.57	0.60	0.66	0.71	0.77	0.82	0.87
4–6	241	0.62 ± 0.08	0.48	0.52	0.57	0.63	0.67	0.70	0.73

[a] From birth through 3 months, Iowa data; from 3 through 6 months, combined data; from 6 through 12 months, Fels data.
[b] Values expressed as mean ± SD.
From Guo S, Roche AF, Fomon SJ, et al: Reference data on gains in weight and length during the first two years of life. *J Pediatr* 119:355, 1991.

TABLE B-7

THREE-MONTH INCREMENTS IN LENGTH FROM BIRTH TO 24 MONTHS[a]

AGE (mo)	n	LENGTH (mm/d)[b]	PERCENTILE						
			5th	10th	25th	50th	75th	90th	95th
Boys									
Up to 3	580	1.07 ± 0.11	0.89	0.92	0.99	1.06	1.14	1.21	1.26
1–4	65	1.00 ± 0.08	—	0.90	0.94	1.01	1.06	1.09	—
2–5	65	0.84 ± 0.09	—	0.74	0.79	0.84	0.91	0.95	—
3–6	255	0.69 ± 0.08	0.56	0.60	0.64	0.68	0.73	0.79	0.82
4–7	190	0.62 ± 0.06	0.54	0.55	0.58	0.61	0.65	0.69	0.72
5–8	190	0.56 ± 0.05	0.49	0.50	0.53	0.56	0.59	0.63	0.65
6–9	190	0.52 ± 0.05	0.46	0.46	0.49	0.52	0.54	0.58	0.60
7–10	190	0.48 ± 0.05	0.42	0.43	0.45	0.48	0.51	0.54	0.57
8–11	190	0.45 ± 0.04	0.39	0.40	0.43	0.45	0.48	0.51	0.53
9–12	190	0.43 ± 0.04	0.36	0.38	0.40	0.43	0.45	0.48	0.51
10–13	190	0.41 ± 0.04	0.34	0.36	0.38	0.41	0.43	0.46	0.49
11–14	190	0.39 ± 0.04	0.33	0.34	0.36	0.39	0.41	0.44	0.47
12–15	190	0.37 ± 0.04	0.31	0.32	0.35	0.37	0.39	0.43	0.45
13–16	190	0.36 ± 0.04	0.30	0.31	0.33	0.36	0.38	0.41	0.44
14–17	190	0.35 ± 0.04	0.28	0.30	0.32	0.34	0.37	0.40	0.42
15–18	190	0.33 ± 0.04	0.27	0.28	0.31	0.33	0.35	0.39	0.41
16–19	190	0.32 ± 0.04	0.26	0.27	0.30	0.32	0.34	0.38	0.40
17–20	190	0.31 ± 0.04	0.25	0.26	0.29	0.31	0.33	0.37	0.39
18–21	190	0.03 ± 0.04	0.24	0.25	0.28	0.30	0.32	0.36	0.38
19–22	190	0.03 ± 0.04	0.23	0.25	0.27	0.29	0.31	0.35	0.37
20–23	190	0.29 ± 0.04	0.23	0.24	0.27	0.28	0.31	0.34	0.36
21–24	190	0.28 ± 0.04	0.22	0.23	0.26	0.28	0.30	0.33	0.35
Girls									
Up to 3	562	0.99 ± 0.10	0.82	0.86	0.93	0.99	1.06	1.11	1.15
1–4	74	0.95 ± 0.10	—	0.84	0.87	0.95	1.02	1.07	—
2–5	74	0.80 ± 0.10	—	0.67	0.73	0.81	0.87	0.92	—
3–6	241	0.67 ± 0.08	0.55	0.58	0.63	0.67	0.72	0.77	0.79
4–7	167	0.60 ± 0.06	0.53	0.54	0.57	0.61	0.64	0.67	0.69
5–8	167	0.56 ± 0.05	0.49	0.50	0.52	0.56	0.59	0.62	0.63
6–9	167	0.52 ± 0.05	0.45	0.46	0.48	0.52	0.55	0.57	0.58
7–10	167	0.48 ± 0.04	0.42	0.43	0.45	0.49	0.52	0.54	0.55
8–11	167	0.46 ± 0.04	0.39	0.41	0.43	0.46	0.49	0.51	0.52
9–12	167	0.44 ± 0.04	0.37	0.38	0.41	0.44	0.46	0.48	0.49
10–13	167	0.42 ± 0.04	0.35	0.37	0.39	0.42	0.45	0.46	0.48
11–14	167	0.40 ± 0.04	0.34	0.35	0.37	0.40	0.43	0.44	0.46
12–15	167	0.38 ± 0.04	0.32	0.34	0.36	0.38	0.41	0.43	0.44
13–16	167	0.37 ± 0.04	0.31	0.32	0.34	0.37	0.40	0.42	0.43
14–17	167	0.36 ± 0.04	0.29	0.31	0.33	0.36	0.38	0.40	0.41
15–18	167	0.34 ± 0.04	0.28	0.30	0.32	0.35	0.37	0.39	0.40
16–19	167	0.33 ± 0.04	0.27	0.29	0.31	0.34	0.36	0.38	0.39
17–20	167	0.32 ± 0.04	0.26	0.28	0.30	0.33	0.35	0.37	0.38
18–21	167	0.32 ± 0.04	0.26	0.27	0.29	0.32	0.34	0.36	0.37
19–22	167	0.31 ± 0.04	0.25	0.26	0.28	0.31	0.33	0.35	0.36
20–23	167	0.30 ± 0.04	0.24	0.26	0.28	0.30	0.33	0.35	0.36
21–24	167	0.29 ± 0.04	0.23	0.25	0.27	0.30	0.32	0.34	0.35

[a] From birth through 3 months, Iowa data; from 3 through 6 months, combined data; from 6 through 24 months, Fels data.
[b] Data expressed as mean ± SD.
From Guo S, Roche AF, Fomon SJ, et al: Reference data on gains in weight and length during the first two years of life. J Pediatr 119:355, 1991.

Appendix C   Blood Pressure Nomograms

TABLE C-1

BLOOD PRESSURE LEVELS FOR THE 90TH AND 95TH PERCENTILES OF BLOOD PRESSURE FOR BOYS AGED 1 TO 17 YEARS BY PERCENTILES OF HEIGHT

AGE, y	BLOOD PRESSURE PERCENTILE*	SYSTOLIC BLOOD PRESSURE BY PERCENTILE OF HEIGHT, mm Hg[†]							DIASTOLIC BLOOD PRESSURE BY PERCENTILE OF HEIGHT, mm Hg[†]						
		5%	10%	25%	50%	75%	90%	95%	5%	10%	25%	50%	75%	90%	95%
1	90th	94	95	97	98	100	102	102	50	51	52	53	54	54	55
	95th	98	99	101	102	104	106	106	55	55	56	57	58	59	59
2	90th	98	99	100	102	104	105	106	55	55	56	57	58	59	59
	95th	101	102	104	106	108	109	110	59	59	60	61	62	63	63
3	90th	100	101	103	105	107	108	109	59	59	60	61	62	63	63
	95th	104	105	107	109	111	112	113	63	63	64	65	66	67	67
4	90th	102	103	105	107	109	110	111	62	62	63	64	65	66	66
	95th	106	107	109	111	113	114	115	66	67	67	68	69	70	71
5	90th	104	105	106	108	110	112	112	65	65	66	67	68	69	69
	95th	108	109	110	112	114	115	116	69	70	70	71	72	73	74
6	90th	105	106	108	110	111	113	114	67	68	69	70	70	71	72
	95th	109	110	112	114	115	117	117	72	72	73	74	75	76	76
7	90th	106	107	109	111	113	114	115	69	70	71	72	72	73	74
	95th	110	111	113	115	116	118	119	74	74	75	76	77	78	78
8	90th	107	108	110	112	114	115	116	71	71	72	73	74	75	75
	95th	111	112	114	116	118	119	120	75	76	76	77	78	79	80
9	90th	109	110	112	113	115	117	117	72	73	73	74	75	76	77
	95th	113	114	116	117	119	121	121	76	77	78	79	80	80	81
10	90th	110	112	113	115	117	118	119	73	74	74	75	76	77	78
	95th	114	115	117	119	121	122	123	77	78	79	80	80	81	82
11	90th	112	113	115	117	119	120	121	74	74	75	76	77	78	78
	95th	116	117	119	121	123	124	125	78	79	79	80	81	82	83
12	90th	115	116	117	119	121	123	123	75	75	76	77	78	78	79
	95th	119	120	121	123	125	126	127	79	79	80	81	82	83	83
13	90th	117	118	120	122	124	125	126	75	76	76	77	78	79	80
	95th	121	122	124	126	128	129	130	79	80	81	82	83	83	84
14	90th	120	121	123	125	126	128	128	76	76	77	78	79	80	80
	95th	124	125	127	128	130	132	132	80	81	81	82	83	84	85
15	90th	123	124	125	127	129	131	131	77	77	78	79	80	81	81
	95th	127	128	129	131	133	134	135	81	82	83	83	84	85	86
16	90th	125	126	128	130	132	133	134	79	79	80	81	82	82	83
	95th	129	130	132	134	136	137	138	83	83	84	85	86	87	87
17	90th	128	129	131	133	134	136	136	81	81	82	83	84	85	85
	95th	132	133	135	136	138	140	140	85	85	86	87	88	89	89

* Blood pressure percentile was determined by a single measurement.

† Height percentile was determined by standard growth curves.

From: National High Blood Pressure Education Program Working Group on Hypertension Control in Children and Adolescents. Update on the 1982 Task Force Report on High Blood Pressure in Children and Adolescents: A Working Group Report from the National High Blood Pressure Education Program. Pediatrics 98; p.654:1996.

TABLE C-2

BLOOD PRESSURE LEVELS FOR THE 90th AND 95th PERCENTILES OF BLOOD PRESSURE FOR GIRLS AGED 1 TO 17 YEARS BY PERCENTILES OF HEIGHT

AGE, y	BLOOD PRESSURE PERCENTILE*	SYSTOLIC BLOOD PRESSURE BY PERCENTILE OF HEIGHT, mm Hg[†]							DIASTOLIC BLOOD PRESSURE BY PERCENTILE OF HEIGHT, mm Hg[†]						
		5%	10%	25%	50%	75%	90%	95%	5%	10%	25%	50%	75%	90%	95%
1	90th	97	98	99	100	102	103	104	53	53	53	54	55	56	56
	95th	101	102	103	104	105	107	107	57	57	57	58	59	60	60
2	90th	99	99	100	102	103	104	105	57	57	58	58	59	60	61
	95th	102	103	104	105	107	108	109	61	61	62	62	63	64	65
3	90th	100	100	102	103	104	105	106	61	61	61	62	63	63	64
	95th	104	104	105	107	108	109	110	65	65	65	66	67	67	68
4	90th	101	102	103	104	106	107	108	63	63	64	65	65	66	67
	95th	105	106	107	108	109	111	111	67	67	68	69	69	70	71
5	90th	103	103	104	106	107	108	109	65	66	66	67	68	68	69
	95th	107	107	108	110	111	112	113	69	70	70	71	72	72	73
6	90th	104	105	106	107	109	110	111	67	67	68	69	69	70	71
	95th	108	109	110	111	112	114	114	71	71	72	73	73	74	75
7	90th	106	107	108	109	110	112	112	69	69	69	70	71	72	72
	95th	110	110	112	113	114	115	116	73	73	73	74	75	76	76
8	90th	108	109	110	111	112	113	114	70	70	71	71	72	73	74
	95th	112	112	113	115	116	117	118	74	74	75	75	76	77	78
9	90th	110	110	112	113	114	115	116	71	72	72	73	74	74	75
	95th	114	114	115	117	118	119	120	75	76	76	77	78	78	79
10	90th	112	112	114	115	116	117	118	73	73	73	74	75	76	76
	95th	116	116	117	119	120	121	122	77	77	77	78	79	80	80
11	90th	114	114	116	117	118	119	120	74	74	75	75	76	77	77
	95th	118	118	119	121	122	123	124	78	78	79	79	80	81	81
12	90th	116	116	118	119	120	121	122	75	75	76	76	77	78	78
	95th	120	120	121	123	124	125	126	79	79	80	80	81	82	82
13	90th	118	118	119	121	122	123	124	76	76	77	78	78	79	80
	95th	121	122	123	125	126	127	128	80	80	81	82	82	83	84
14	90th	119	120	121	122	124	125	126	77	77	78	79	79	80	81
	95th	123	124	125	126	128	129	130	81	81	82	83	83	84	85
15	90th	121	121	122	124	125	126	127	78	78	79	79	80	81	82
	95th	124	125	126	128	129	130	131	82	82	83	83	84	85	86
16	90th	122	122	123	125	126	127	128	79	79	79	80	81	82	82
	95th	125	126	127	128	130	131	132	83	83	83	84	85	86	86
17	90th	122	123	124	125	126	128	128	79	79	79	80	81	82	82
	95th	126	126	127	129	130	131	132	83	83	83	84	85	86	86

* Blood pressure percentile was determined by a single reading.
† Height percentile was determined by standard growth curves.
From: National High Blood Pressure Education Program Working Group on Hypertension Control in Children and Adolescents. Update on the 1982 Task Force Report on High Blood Pressure in Children and Adolescents: A Working Group Report from the National High Blood Pressure Education Program. Pediatrics 98; p. 654: 1996.

Page numbers followed by f indicate figures; numbers followed by t indicate tables.

Abscess, 1217
  amebic, of liver, 1500
    in amebiasis, 1123
  anal, 1460
  bezold, in acute otitis media, 1250
  brain, 2319–2321
    in amebiasis, 1124
    in cyanotic heart disease, 1898
    in right-to-left shunt, 1816
  cold, 1217
    of hyperimmunoglobulin E syndrome,
      1553
  cranial epidural, 2318
  lung
    in amebiasis, 1124
    in bacterial pneumonia, 1982
  perianal, 1460
  peritonsillar, 1270, 1944
  pyogenic, of liver, 1500
  retropharyngeal, 1944
  spinal, 2321
Absence epilepsy, childhood, 2259
Absence of disease, and diagnostic test charac-
    teristics, 593t–594t
Absence seizures, 2256
  vs. complex partial seizures, 2256t
  ethosuximide for, 2255
Absence status, 2260
Absenteeism, functional abdominal pain and,
    1357
Absolute lymphocyte count (ALC), 318
Absolute neutrophil count (ANC), 318
  in Kostmann syndrome, 199
  in neutropenia, 1550
  occult bacteremia and, 307
Absorption
  of carbohydrates, 1310–1311
  disorders of. See Malabsorption
  of fats, 1312
  of protein, 1311
Absorptive phase, of feeding, 1380f, 1383
Abstinence, as contraceptive, 250t
Abstract thinking, in learning, 436
Abuse. See Child abuse; Sexual abuse; Sub-
    stance abuse
ABVD (doxorubicin, bleomycin, vinblastine,
    dacarbazine) regimen, for Hodgkin dis-
    ease, 1609
Acalculous cholecystitis, 1507
Acanthamoeba, 1130
Acanthamoeba keratitis, 2378
  clinical manifestations of, 1130
  etiology of, 1130
  treatment of, 1131
Acanthosis, 1165
Acarbose, for diabetes mellitus type 2, 2136
ACAT. See Acylcholesterol acyltransferase
Acceleration(s)
  of fetal heart rate, 73–74
    prolonged, 73
    with uterine contractions, 74
  inner ear detection of, 1239
Accessibility
  to environment
    assistive technology for, 546t
    physical vs. occupational therapy in pro-
      motion of, 544t
  of health care, 535
Accessory imaging studies, of feeding disorders,
    1384
Accessory navicular, 2429, 2429f
Accident(s)
  in adolescents, 226, 230
  burns. See Burn(s)
  choking. See Foreign-body aspiration

common nonfatal, 36t
death rate of, 1583t
drowning and near drowning. See Drowning
    and near drowning
mortality statistics of, 37
motor vehicle. See Motor vehicle accidents
poisoning. See Poisonings
poisonous bites and stings, 391–398
prevention of, 36t–37t, 37–39, 38f
toxic ingestions and exposures. See Toxic in-
    gestions and exposures
Accidental myiasis, 1157
Accommodative esotropia, 2361, 2403
ACEIs. See Angiotensin-converting enzyme
    (ACE) inhibitors
Acellular pertussis vaccine. See Pertussis, vac-
    cines for
Aceruloplasminemia, 2333
Acetabulum
  development of, 2434
  structural changes of
    with persistent dislocations, 2435
    treatment of, 2436
Acetaminophen
  available forms of, 360
  dosage and administration of, 343t
  for fever, 303
  for fibromyalgia, 862
  for growing pains, 859
  for hemangiomas, 1205
  hepatotoxicity of, 1503
    therapy for, 1503
  for malaria, 1142
  poisoning by, 360
    clinical presentation and management of,
      360, 361f–362f, 362t
    epidemiology of, 356
    serum acetaminophen concentrations in,
      362f
    toxicology of, 360
  for spider bites, 1152
Acetate, in parenteral nutrition solutions,
    1346t
Acetazolamide
  for atonic seizures, 2256
  for childhood absence epilepsy, 2260
  for hydrocephalus, 2184
Acetoacetic acid, 624
N-Acetyl aspartic acid, 2337
Acetylcholine
  and mucus synthesis, 1430
  and pulmonary vasodilation, 1751
Acetylcholine receptor (AChR), in myasthenia
    gravis, 2285
Acetylcholinesterase, organophosphate and car-
    bamate insecticides and, 373
Acetylcholinesterase staining, for Hirschsprung
    disease, 1462
Acetyl-CoA, 628–629, 644, 1320
N-Acetylcysteine
  for acetaminophen poisoning
    dosage and administration of, 360, 362t
    indications for, 360, 362f
    physiologic effects of, 360, 1503
  for corrosive esophagitis, 1396
α-N-Acetylgalactosaminidase deficiency, 663
UDP-N-Acetylglucosamine deficiency, 662
N-Acetylglucosamine-1-phosphotransferase de-
    ficiency, 2331
α-N-Acetylglucosaminidase deficiency, 659,
    2330
N-Acetylglucosaminyl-L-phosphotransferase
    deficiency, 662
N-Acetylglutamate, for congenital hyperammo-
    nemia, 622

N-Acetylglutamate synthetase (NAGS), defi-
    ciency of, 618, 620
N-Acetylneuraminic acid, 665
Acetylsalicylic acid. See Aspirin
Achalasia, 1352, 1388
Achievement, 403–405
Achievement testing, indications for, 412t
Achilles tendonitis, differential diagnosis of,
    2427
Acholic stools, of choledochal cysts, 1485t
Achondrogenesis, 760t
Achondroplasia, 759, 761f
  fibroblast growth factor and, 65
  and growth failure, 2022
Achondroplastic dwarfism, in neonatal exami-
    nation of limbs, 91
Acid(s)
  exposure to
    and esophagitis, 1390
    measuring, 1390
  secretion of, 1429
    in newborns, 1429
    phases of, 1429
  toxic ingestion of, 364, 1395
Acid α-1,4 glucosidase deficiency, 639
Acid-base balance, disorders of, 1656–1657,
    1710
  assessment of, 1656t
  in chronic renal insufficiency, 1720, 1724
  in gastrointestinal obstruction, 1379
Acid-base determination, for congestive heart
    failure, 1873
Acid-base equilibrium
  disturbances of
    in acute hepatic failure, 1514t
    in salicylate poisoning, 375–376
  of fetus, predictability of, 71
Acidemia(s), 1656. See also specific acidemia
  fetal
    diagnosis of, 74
    events resulting in, 74t
      in utero treatment of, 73–74, 74t
    late decelerations and, 73, 73f
    management of, 74
    predictability of, 71
  high-risk screening of, 581t
  newborn screening of, 580t
  respiratory distress and, 283
  of salicylate poisoning, 376
Acid-fast stain, 956, 962
Acid inhibition therapy, for functional dyspep-
    sia, 1362
Acidosis, 1656. See also specific acidosis
  and bilirubin toxicity, 167
  in cardiopulmonary resuscitation, 329
  fetal, and meconium aspiration syndrome,
    194
  in newborns, physical findings of, 86
  and viscosity, 192
Acid phosphatase, in acute lymphoblastic leu-
    kemia, 1596
Acid-stable lipases, 1312
Acid suppressants, 1434
Acid urine, 1659
Acinus(i)
  of liver, 1470, 1470f
  of lungs, and hyaline membrane disease, 127
ACLE. See Acute cutaneous lupus erythemato-
    sus
Acne
  infantile, 1210
  neonatal, 1169, 1210
Acne fulminans, 1210
Acneiform drug eruptions, 1210
Acne keloidalis, 1212

Acne rosacea, 1210
Acne vulgaris, 224t, 1208–1210
  age of onset of, 1208
  corticosteroids and, 1209, 1439
  cystic, 1209–1210
  development of, 1208
  differential diagnosis of, 1210
  management of, 1209–1210, 1209t
ACOG, on risk factors for early onset group B
    streptococcal infection, 1001
Acoustic neuromas, 772
Acoustic reflectometry, in diagnosis of otitis
    media with effusion, 1253
Acoustic reflex, 488
Acquired aplastic anemia
  classification of, 1564
  incidence of, 1564
Acquired disability, functional outcome mea-
    sures in, 534–535
Acquired epileptic aphasia, 2204, 2262
Acquired hypothalamic-pituitary hypothyroid-
    ism, 2071
Acquired immunodeficiency syndrome (AIDS).
    See also Human immunodeficiency virus
    (HIV) infection
  aspergillosis in, 1084
  blastomycosis in, 1086
  cryptococcosis in, 1092
    treatment of, 1128
  cryptosporidiosis in, 1126
  cytomegalovirus retinitis in, 1034
  diarrhea in, 1366
    treatment of, 1366
  esophagitis in, 1395
  extracutaneous sporotrichosis in, 1096
  gastrointestinal infections in, 1413
  and growth failure, 2024
  herpes simplex virus infections in, 1031
  histoplasmosis in, 1093
  human herpesvirus 6 infection in, 1040
  increasing lean body mass in, 1415
  isosporiasis in, 1132–1133
  Kaposi sarcoma in, 1865
  Malassezia furfur infection in, 1095
  measles in, 1055
  microsporidiosis in, 1144
  nontuberculous mycobacterial infections in,
    960–961
    treatment of, 963
  oral complications in, 1297
  orphans of, 510
  Pneumocystis carinii pneumonia in, 1145
    treatment of, 1145
  prevalence of, in adolescents, 260
  recurrent bacterial infections in, 1047
  Salmonella bacteremia in, 982
  symptomatic cerebrovascular disease in, 2235
  varicella-zoster virus infection in, 1043
Acquired immunodeficiency syndrome (AIDS)
    encephalopathy, 2311
Acquired immunohematologic disease(s), sple-
    nectomy for, 1562t
Acquired juvenile hypothyroidism, 2070–2073
  diagnosis of, 2072
  etiology of, 2070–2072
  management of, 2073
Acquired melanocytic nevi, 1191
Acquired myopathies, 2302–2303
Acquired neutropenias, 1551
Acquired nystagmus, 491
Acquired red cell aplasia, 1565t–1566t,
    1566–1567
Acquired single cytopenia(s), 1565t–1566t,
    1566–1567
Acquired subglottic stenosis, 1274

Acquired thromboembolic diseases, 1576
Acrocallosal syndrome, 749t
Acrocentric chromosomes, 728
Acrocyanosis, 1169, 1754
  of newborn, 86
Acrodermatitis enteropathica, 1176, 1177f,
    1427
Acromegaly, 2021
Acromelic shortening, 758
Acromioclavicular joint arthritis, 2448
Acropachy, 1216
Acroparesthesia, 2325
Acropustulosis of infancy, 1169
Acrosyndactyly, 2448
ACTH. See Adrenocorticotropic hormone
Acticoat, for burn-wound management, 387
Actinobacillus actinomycetemcomitans, 1292
Actinomyces israelii infection, 1280
Actinomycin D
  for diencephalic glioma, 2222
  neurotoxicity of, 2229t
  for rhabdomyosarcoma, 1613
  for Wilms tumor, 1616
    and radiation therapy, 1616
Actinomycosis, 913–914, 1280
  clinical manifestations of, 913–914
  diagnosis of, 914
  microbiology of, 913
  pathogenesis of, 913
  pulmonary involvement in, 1984
  treatment of, 914
Activated charcoal therapy, for decontamina-
    tion of toxic ingestions, 358
  for acetaminophen poisoning, 360
  complications of, 359
  for cyclic antidepressant poisoning, 365
  doses of, 358
  at home, 358
  for opioid poisoning, 372
  for oral hypoglycemic agent poisoning, 373
  for salicylate poisoning, 376
Activated partial thromboplastin time (aPTT),
    1569
  gestational age and, 200, 1570t
  in infants, 1569–1570, 1570t
Activated protein C resistance, 1575
  venous thrombosis from, 2233
Activation stage, in bone remodeling, 2144
G_{M2}-Activator deficiency, 2325
Active listening, to prevent disruptive behav-
    iors, 449t
Active tone, of muscles
  examination of, in newborns, 94–95, 94f
  in small-for-gestational-age infants, 122
Activin, 2096
Activity(ies)
  anticipatory guidance of, age-appropriate dis-
    cussion topics for, 28t
  continuum of, overactivity to attention-defi-
    cit disorder in, 430–434
  of daily living, functional outcome measures
    of, 534–535
  gender-specific, 470–471
  limitations in, disabilities and, 533
  measures of, 433
  of newborns, 84
  sex-appropriate, 470–471
Activity level, 450t
Activity log, 2141
Acuity, visual, 2352
Acupuncture, 542
Acute cerebellitis, 2314
Acute cerebellopathy, 2314
Acute chest syndrome, of sickle cell disease,
    1533

Acute cholecystitis, diagnosis of, 587
Acute coalescent mastoiditis, in acute otitis me-
    dia, 1250
Acute cutaneous lupus erythematosus (ACLE),
    1197
Acute disseminated encephalomyelitis
    (ADEM), 2314
Acute encephalopathies of infancy, 2189–2196
Acute epiglottitis, 1276
Acute fatty liver, of pregnancy, and liver disease
    in infant, 1479
Acute febrile illness, 305t
Acute filarial adenolymphangiitis (ADL), 1107
Acute follicular conjunctivitis, 2368
Acute hemolytic transfusion reaction, 1580
  evaluation of, 1580, 1581t
Acute hemorrhage, 2238
  blood transfusion for, volume and rate of,
    1578
  in neonatal anemia, 198
Acute hemorrhagic conjunctivitis, 1022, 2369
Acute illness
  assessment and stabilization of, 271–308
  behavioral sequelae of, 429
  children's reactions to, 428–429, 429t
  febrile, 305t
  injuries and untoward events, 348–398
  intercurrent, management of, family and,
    511
  recovery from, and vulnerable child syn-
    drome, 515
  supportive techniques and management,
    309–347
Acute infantile hemiplegia, unilateral seizures
    in, 2257
Acute infantile spinal muscular atrophy, 2279
Acute infectious polyradiculopathy, 2281
Acute inflammatory demyelinating polyradicu-
    loneuropathy, 2281
Acute intermittent porphyria (AIP), 686–687,
    1361, 2283
  classic, 687
  erythroid (variant), 687
Acute lead encephalopathy
  signs of, 369
  treatment of, 370
Acute leukemia, stem cell transplantation for,
    1590t
Acute lobar nephronia, 1669
Acute lung injury, transfusion-associated, 1580
Acute lymphoblastic leukemia (ALL),
    1594–1599
  B-cell, 1594t, 1596, 1596t
    chromosomal translocation in, 1597
    prognosis of, 1597
  B-cell precursor, 1594t, 1596, 1596t
    chromosomal translocation in, 1597
  clinical features of, 1594–1595, 1594t
  diagnosis of, 1595–1596
    cytogenic findings, 1594t, 1596
    immunophenotypic characterization,
      1594t, 1596, 1596t
    morphological and histochemical classifica-
      tion, 1594t, 1596
  differential diagnosis of, 1595
  future trends of, 1599
  incidence of, 1594, 1594t
  laboratory features of, 1594t, 1595
  and Langerhans cell histiocytosis, 1625
  origins of, 1594t, 1596, 1596t
  outcome of, 1596t, 1598–1599
    late effects of treatment, 1599
    relapse, 1599
  Philadelphia chromosome-positive, chromo-
    somal translocation in, 1597

Acute lymphoblastic leukemia (ALL) (contd.)
  prognostic factors in, 1596–1597, 1596t
  survival rates of, 1583
  T-cell, 1594t, 1596, 1596t
    chromosomal abnormalities of, 1597
    prognosis of, 1597
    therapy for, 1596t, 1597–1598
      central nervous system preventive therapy, 1598
      induction therapy, 1598
      postremission therapy, 1598
    and varicella vaccine, 50
Acute lymphocytic leukemia. See Acute lymphoblastic leukemia
Acute mastoiditis, in acute otitis media, 1250
Acute metabolic encephalopathy, 599, 600f
Acute migratory polyarthritis, 1902
Acute myeloid leukemia (AML), 1600–1603
  classification of, 1600–1601, 1601t
  clinical and laboratory features of, 1601–1602
  clonality and pathogenesis of, 1600
  differentiation of, from myelodysplastic syndromes, 1600, 1601t
  epidemiology of, 1600
  genetic features of, 1601, 1601t
  newly diagnosed, management of, 1602–1603
  origin of, 1601
  refractory, management of, 1603
  risk factors for, 1600
  signs and symptoms of, 1601
  subtypes of, 1600, 1601t
  survival rate of, 1602
  from treatment of Hodgkin disease, 1609
Acute myocardial infarction, chest pain in, 1894
Acute nasopharyngitis, 1262
Acute necrotizing hemorrhagic leukoencephalitis, 2314
Acute nephritic syndrome, acute poststreptococcal glomerulonephritis as prototype of, 1677
Acute neurologic injury, management of, 324–327
  increased intracranial pressure, 325–327, 325f, 326t
  stabilization and emergency, 324–325
Acute-onset autoimmune hemolytic anemia (acute-onset AHA), 1546
Acute-onset severe chest pain, 1894
Acute otitis media (AOM), 1249–1252
  anatomy of middle ear and, 1239
  complications of, 1250, 1250f
  cost of, 1252
  diagnosis of, 1244f, 1249–1250
  etiology of, 1249
  Moraxella catarrhalis, 948, 1249
  recurrent, 1252
  spread of infection in, 1250
  Streptococcus pneumoniae, 978, 1249
    drug-resistant, 1251–1252
      risk factors for, 1252
  treatment of, 868t, 979, 1251–1252, 1251f
    with tympanostomy tubes, 1252
Acute pelvic inflammatory disease, treatment of, 266t
Acute-phase retinopathy of prematurity
  natural history of, 145
  onset of, by postconceptional age, 145t
Acute polyneuritis, 2315
Acute polyradiculoneuropathy, 2315
Acute poststreptococcal glomerulonephritis (APSGN), 1677–1681
  clinical manifestations of, 1678
  epidemiology of, 1678

  laboratory findings in, 1680
  pathogenesis of, 1681
  prognosis of, 1681
  treatment of, 1681
Acute promyelocytic leukemia (APL)
  all-trans-retinoic acid for, 1602
  differential diagnosis of, 1602
  treatment for, 1602
Acute pulmonary edema, in transfusion, 1580, 1580t
  evaluation of, 1581t
Acute red cell aplasia, of sickle cell disease, 1532
Acute rejection (AR)
  of heart transplant, 1887
  of kidney transplants, 1729, 1733
Acute renal failure (ARF), 1673–1676
  causes of, 1674–1675
  daily fluid requirement for children in, 1676
  evaluation of, 1674f
  hemoglobin-induced, 1675
  in lupus nephritis, 1687
  in minimal-change nephrotic syndrome, 1693
  myoglobin-induced, 1675
  nonoliguric, 1675
  in small-for-gestational-age newborn, 123t
  therapy for, 1675–1676
Acute rheumatic fever, 829
  abdominal pain in, 1355
  diagnosis of, 998
  diagnostic criteria of, 306, 1902t
  pathogenesis of, 997
  in streptococcal infections, 997
"Acute scrotum," 248
Acute symptomatic iritis, in enthesitis-related arthritis, 841
Acute tubule necrosis (ATN)
  and acute renal failure, 1673
  oliguria in, 1649
Acute vasculitis, 829
Acute viral encephalitis, 2307–2308
Acute viral myelitis (polio syndrome), 2309
A-C (assist-control) ventilation, 209, 318
Acyanotic Fallot, 1820
Acyclovir
  for acute viral encephalitis, 2308
  for cytomegalovirus infection, 1034
  dosage and administration of, 883t
  for Epstein-Barr virus infection, 1038
  for herpes simplex virus esophagitis, 1395
  for herpes simplex virus infection, 256t, 303, 1029t, 1031, 1221, 2311, 2314
    maternal genital, 173
    neonatal, 172
    prophylactic, 173
  for herpetic whitlow, 1221
  for immunocompromised host, 172
  for neonatal herpes virus encephalitis, 2313
  pharmacodynamics of, 172
  risk of, 173
  for varicella-zoster virus esophagitis, 1395
  for varicella-zoster virus infection, 172, 1044
Acyclovir fetal nephrotoxicity, 173
Acyclovir triphosphate concentrations, 172
ACYF. See Child Care Bureau, US Department of Health and Human Services Administration on Children, Youth, & Families
Acylcarnitine esters, 628, 2298
Acylcarnitines, high-risk screening of, 581t
Acylcholesterol acyltransferase (ACAT), 695
Acyl-CoA, 629
Acylglycines, high-risk screening of, 581t
AD. See Autistic disorder
ADA deficiency. See Adenosine deaminase deficiency

Adam's bend test, for scoliosis, 2441, 2442f
Adams-Stokes attacks, 1858–1859, 1859f
Adapalene, for acne, 1209
Adaptability, 450t
  and pain perception, 424
Adaptation, 401–403
  of family, to disabled children, 552–553
  to family transitions, 516–517
  of newborn, to postnatal life, 79–82, 1473
Adaptive functioning, 438
  "tricks" to, 520
Adaptive immunity, 299
Adderall, for attention deficit hyperactivity disorder, 433
Addiction. See also Substance abuse
  parenting and, 526
  passive, 2196
Addison disease, 1711, 2042–2044
  hyperpigmentation in, 1193
  olfactory disturbance in, 1264
  perioperative care of, 339
Additive joint involvement, 833t
Adducted toe, 2426
Adductor tenotomy, for developmental dysplasia of hip, 2436
ADEM. See Acute disseminated encephalomyelitis
Adenine, 691
Adenine arabinoside, for neonatal herpes virus encephalitis, 2313
Adenine phosphoribosyltransferase (APRT) deficiency, 691
Adenitis, in group B streptococcal infection, 1000
Adenocarcinoma(s)
  choledochal cysts and, 1482
  clear-cell, diethylstilbestrol-related, 253
  gastrointestinal, 1456
  pancreatic, 1467
Adenoidectomy
  for adenotonsillar hypertrophy, 1270
  contraindications to, 1254
  for otitis media with effusion, 1254
Adenoid hypertrophy, 1261, 1270
  and otitis media with effusion, 1253
Adenoids, 1267
  anatomy of, 1267
  asymmetric enlargement of, 1270
  function of, 1267
  involvement of, in Burkitt lymphoma, 1604
  and obstructive sleep apnea syndrome, 1939
Adenoma(s)
  bronchial, 1946
  and congenital hyperinsulinemia, 157
  diagnosis of, 1620, 1620t
  liver cell, treatment and outcome of, 1621
  of salivary gland, 1270
Adenoma sebaceum, 1186, 2344, 2416
Adenomatous polyposis coli (APC), 1455
Adenopathy
  cervical, in Burkitt lymphoma, 1604
  in Epstein-Barr virus infection, 1036
  hilar
    in pneumonia, 1982
    in pulmonary tuberculosis, 951f
  supraclavicular, 1279
Adenosine, 796
  in advanced life support, 330t
  for arrhythmias, 1849
  for paroxysmal supraventricular tachycardia, 1855
Adenosine deaminase (ADA) deficiency, 795
Adenosine diphosphate (ADP), 1569f
  deficiency of, 1541f
Adenosine monophosphate (AMP) deficiency, 1541f

periodic, and respiratory system efficiency, 282
in respiratory failure, 272
spontaneous, of newborn, 99
work demands of, 281
work of, 1908
Breathing movements, fetal, and lung development, 191
Breathlessness, in dying patient, management of, 572
Breath sounds
absent or diminished, of foreign-body aspiration, 1278
in hyaline membrane disease, 129
in meconium aspiration syndrome, 194
with pneumothorax, 149
in respiratory disorders, 1909
and severity of respiratory distress, 273t
Breech delivery
and developmental dysplasia of hips, 2435
and spinal cord injuries, 188
and trauma to external genitalia of newborn, 90
Breech-positioned infants
head circumference of, 2168
head shape of, 87
Breech presentation
hemorrhage with, 198
petechiae in, 185
vaginal delivery with, 75
Bretylium tosylate, for arrhythmia, 1850t
Bretyllum, in advanced life support, 330t
BRIC. See Benign recurrent intrahepatic cholestasis
Brittle bone disease, 761, 2161
"Broad fish tapeworm," 1117
Broad spectrum antibiotics, and folate deficiency, 1529
Broken bicycle story, 567
Bromocriptine, for GH excess, 2021
Bromodeoxyuridine (BrdU), 727
Bronchi
adenomas of, 1946
growth and development of, 1906f
mucous impaction of, in asthma, 1951
obstruction of, with lobar emphysema, 1925–1926, 1926f
papillomatosis of, 1946, 1946f
smooth muscle of, spasm, in asthma, 1951
Bronchial artery(ies), development of, 1905
Bronchial obstruction, 278
auscultation of, 1273
Bronchiectasis, 798, 1948–1949, 1948f
amyloidosis in, 864
with dysmotile cilia, 1949
Bronchioles, growth and development of, 1906f
Bronchiolitis
in adenoviral infection, 1073
infectious, 1984–1985
clinical features of, 1985
etiology of, 1984–1985
prophylaxis, with bronchopulmonary dysplasia, 1965
treatment of, 1985
in measles, 1055
obliterative, 1889
in parainfluenza virus infection, 1068
respiratory syncytial virus, 1065, 1984–1985
clinical manifestations of, 1066, 1985
prophylaxis, with bronchopulmonary dysplasia, 1965
treatment of, 1067, 1985
viral, 1984–1985
differential diagnosis of, 1954

Bronchiolitis obliterans, 1946–1948, 1947f
causes of, 1946, 1947t
after lung transplantation, 1948
Bronchiolitis obliterans with organizing pneumonia, 1948, 1990
Bronchitis
in common variable immunodeficiency, 801
in transient hypogammaglobulinemia of infancy, 801
Bronchoalveolar lavage (BAL), 1914
in interstitial lung disease, 1991
Bronchobiliary fistula, 1925
Bronchodilator(s), for bronchopulmonary dysplasia, 1965
Bronchogenic cyst(s), 202, 1173, 1928, 1929f, 1946
carinal, 1928
hilar, 1928
paraesophageal, 1928
paratracheal, 1928
Bronchogenic sinus, 1173
Bronchomalacia, 1274, 1924–1925
Bronchopleural fistula, treatment of, 150
Bronchopneumonia, in influenza virus infection, 1070
Bronchoprovocation, in asthma, 1952
Bronchopulmonary dysplasia (BPD), 1964–1966
antenatal corticosteroids and surfactant and, 133t
definition of, 1964
and gas exchange monitoring, 309
and growth failure, 2024
long-term outcome with, 1966
pathogenesis of, 1964
pathology of, 1964
pathophysiology of, 1964
preoperative preparation of infants with, 338
prevention of, 1964
pulmonary exacerbations in, treatment of, 1965–1966
respiratory syncytial virus bronchiolitis prophylaxis in, 1965
risk factors for, 1964
treatment of, 1965–1966
Bronchopulmonary sequestration (BPS), prenatal management of, 77
Bronchoscopy
of esophageal fistula, 1387
fiberoptic, 1914
flexible, 1914
rigid, 1914
in suspected foreign body aspiration, 1278
Bronchospasm, in outcome of hyaline membrane disease, 134
Bronchus(i)
airway obstruction of, 278
auscultation of, 1273
aspirated foreign body in, 383, 1278
"Bronze baby syndrome," 169
Broviac catheters, 322t, 323
Brown adipose tissue, and neonatal thermogenesis, 80
Brown recluse spider (Loxosceles reclusa), 393, 1152, 1235
Brown syndrome, 2404
Brucella melitensis, infection caused by, 922–923. See also Brucellosis
Brucellosis, 922–923
clinical manifestations of, 922
diagnosis of, 922
epidemiology of, 922
prevention of, 923
treatment of, 923
Brugia malayi, 1099t, 1107
Brugia timori, 1107

Bruises, in child abuse, 465
Bruising, easy, perioperative care of, 340
Brush border enzymes, 109–110, 1311
loss of, 1420
Brushfield spots, 2385
"Brushfire retinitis," 1034
Bruton disease, 831
Bruton tyrosine kinase (Btk), 800
Bruxism (teeth-grinding), 461
in disabled children, 541
epidemiology of, 461
etiology of, 461
management of, 461
Btk. See Bruton tyrosine kinase
Buboes, 975–976
Bubonic plague, 975
diagnosis of, 976
incubation period of, 975
mortality rate of, 976
Buccal fat pads, loss of, 1336
Buccopharyngeal membrane, 1267
"Bucket handle" fracture, in child abuse, 465
Buckle fracture(s), 349, 2450, 2450f
Budd-Chiari syndrome, 1509
drug-induced, 1503
Budesonide
for allergic rhinitis, 817
for Crohn disease, 1442
Budesonide Turbuhaler, for asthma, dosage and administration of, 1958t
Buffalo hump, 2045
Bulbar polio, 2309
Bulbus cordis (BC), 1746, 1746f, 1835f
Bulimia nervosa, 233
chronic vomiting in, 1352
diagnosis of, 232t
management of, 233
oral manifestations of, 1299, 1299f
physical findings of, 233
prevalence of, 233
symptoms of, 233
Bulk-forming fibers, 1365
Bulking agents, in bowel management of disabled children, 540
Bullae, 1167, 1173
Bullous congenital ichthyosiform erythroderma, 1184
Bullous impetigo, 1217, (Color Plate 17)
diagnosis of, 1173
Bullous myringitis
differential diagnosis of, 1250
and external otitis, 1255
Bullous pemphigoid, 1201, 2374
"Bull's eye," for neurologic evaluation of newborn, 92, 92f
Bumetamide
for pulmonary venous congestion, 1874
for systemic venous congestion, 1874
Bundle of His, 1842
Bundle of Kent, 1842, 1854
Bunion (hallux valgus), 2429–2430, 2430f
BUN-to-creatinine ratio, 1648
Bunyaviridae, 1018t, 1025t
Buphthalmos, 2352, 2375, 2401
Bupivacaine, for pain management, 427
Burkholderia, infection caused by, 923–924
clinical manifestations of, 923
diagnosis of, 924
epidemiology of, 923
treatment of, 924
Burkholderia cepacia-complex, infection caused by, 877–924
Burkholderia gladioli, 923–924
Burkholderia mallei, 923
Burkholderia pseudomallei, 923–924

Cardiopulmonary system, of newborn, function of, postnatal care and observation of, 104

Cardiorespiratory disorders, of newborn, persistent pulmonary hypertension in, 181t

Cardiorespiratory monitoring, at home, for apparent life-threatening event, 354

Cardiorespiratory murmur, 1756

Cardiotachometers, 312

Cardiovascular collapse, of hyperthermia, 389

Cardiovascular depression, of poisoning by β-blockers and calcium channel blockers, 362

Cardiovascular diseases, 285. See also specific disease
 acquired, 1860–1901
 with acute liver failure, 1514t
 in adolescents, 226
 congenital, 1780–1859
 diagnosed by polymerase chain reaction, 576t
 and growth failure, 2023
 in HIV infection, 1048
 in inborn errors of metabolism, 606
 liver involvement in, 1509
 management of, problems with, 1898–1901
 in Marfan syndrome, 762
 in nephrotic syndrome, 1696
 of newborn, mottling and, 206
 with nonimmune hydrops fetalis, 178t
 after transplantation, 1735
 in tuberculosis, 952

Cardiovascular system
 catecholamines and, 2055
 changes of, during adolescence, 223
 consequences of perinatal asphyxia on, 99t
 examination of, in adolescent, 236
 inotropic medications and, 291t
 instability of, and initial management of altered consciousness, 293t
 mechanical ventilation and, 210
 postnatal adaptation of, antenatal glucocorticoids and, 140
 preoperative evaluation of, 338
 signs of reduced systemic perfusion in, 290t
 toxicity of, in cyclic antidepressant poisoning, 365

Cardioversion
 electrical, for arrhythmias, 1849
 for paroxysmal supraventricular tachycardia, 1855
 for ventricular tachycardia, 1857

Career plans, of disabled youths, 550

Caregiver(s)
 adaptation of, to disabled children, 552–553
 attachment to, 450–451
 behavioral expectations of, 446
 of crying infants
 and crying management, 416–417
 questions for, 416
 infant relationship to, 403
 pain scales for, 341
 training of, for tracheotomy home care, 1279

Caregiving
 and brain development, 531
 poverty and, 531

Caregiving behaviors, and crying, 415

Caregiving environment, and language development, 442, 444

Care quality, defining elements of, 535

Caribbean-Americans, sickle-cell disease in, 1531

Carmustine, neurotoxicity of, 2229t

Carnation Instant Breakfast, 1334t

Carnett test, 1360

Carney triad, in leiomyomas, 1455

Carnitine, 628
 for carnitine palmitoyltransferase deficiency, 629
 for isovaleric acidemia, 624
 for long-chain 3-hydroxyacyl-CoA dehydrogenase deficiency, 631
 for medium-chain acyl-CoA dehydrogenase deficiency, 630
 for 3-methylcrotonyl-CoA carboxylase deficiency, 624
 for methylmalonic acidemias, 627
 for oxidative phosphorylation diseases, 652
 for propionic acidemia, 625
 total and free, high-risk screening of, 581t
 for very long-chain acyl-CoA dehydrogenase deficiency, 630

L-Carnitine, 629

Carnitine-acylcarnitine translocase, 629

Carnitine-acylcarnitine translocase deficiency, 2298

Carnitine cycle, 2296
 defects of, 2296–2298

Carnitine deficiency
 alveolar hypoventilation with, 1931–1932
 in carnitine uptake defect, 629
 and myocardial disease, 1861
 in total parenteral nutrition, 1348

Carnitine palmitoyltransferase (CPT), 629, 2296

Carnitine palmitoyltransferase I (CPT I) deficiency, 2297

Carnitine palmitoyltransferase II (CPT II) deficiency, 2298
 newborn screening of, 580t

Carnitine supplementation
 for primary systemic carnitine deficiency, 2296
 for seizure disorders, 2263

Carnitine uptake defect, 629
 newborn screening of, 580t

Carnosinemia, 616

Carolina Abecedarian Project, 513

Caroli syndrome, 1483

β-Carotene
 for congenital erythropoietic porphyria, 689
 for erythropoietic protoporphyria, 690

Carotid artery catheter, for extracorporeal membrane oxygenation, 213

Carotid artery injury, 1270

Carotid artery ligation, and extracorporeal membrane oxygenation, 214

Carotid-cavernous fistula, 2251

Carotid intima injury, 1270

Carotid sinus hypersensitivity, 1893

Carpenter syndrome, 749t

Carrier detection, in sphingolipidoses, 672

Car safety seats, 38f

Cartilage
 benign tumors of, 2452, 2453f
 collage type II in, 2144
 disorders of structural proteins of, 760, 760t

Cartilage-hair hypoplasia, 1551

Cartilage oligometric protein (COMP), 760

Carvedilol, before heart transplantation, 1886

Casec, 1334t, 1341

Case-control studies, 592
 advantages of, 592
 cases of, selection of, 592
 minimizing bias of, 592

Casein, 1325

Case reports, 592

CASR. See Calcium-sensing receptor

Cassava root, 1467

Cast(s)
 for calcaneovalgus foot, 2426
 for congenital talipes equinovarus, 2425
 for fracture, 2451
 for tarsal coalition, 2427
 waterproof, 2451

Castleman disease, 1041

"Cast syndrome," 1379

Catabolic stress, 599

Catagen phase of hair growth, 1166

Cat allergen, 815

Cataract(s), 2388, 2389t
 of iris, 87
 of neonatal herpes simplex virus infection, 172
 ophthalmoscopic appearance of, 87
 from steroids, 850

Catarrhal stage, of pertussis, 973

CATCH 22. See Cleft palate, absent thymus, congenital heart disease

Catecholamines, 2055
 biosynthesis of, 2055, 2055f
 and blood pressure maintenance, 286
 carcinoid tumors releasing, 1456
 in hemodynamic adaptation at birth, 137
 and neonatal hyperglycemia, 159
 in neuroblastoma, 1618
 in neuroblastoma diagnosis, 1618
 and postnatal glucose homeostasis, 155
 and pulmonary vasodilation, 1751

Categoric discrimination of behavioral disorders, 410–411

Caterpillars, 1159

Catfish, stings of, 393

Cat flea, 1158

Cathepsin A, 2324

Catheter(s). See also specific catheter
 for arterial blood pressure monitoring, in preterm newborn, 112
 for decompression of pulmonary gas leaks, 149–150
 for extracorporeal membrane oxygenation
 venoarterial, 213
 venovenous, 214
 insertion of, complications of, 1345
 for intracranial pressure monitoring, 326
 for peripheral venous cannulation
 kinds of, 321
 size of, 321
 for reduction exchange transfusion of newborns, 193
 in total parenteral nutrition, 1345
 for transfusion exchange, 169
 for uterine contraction monitoring, 70

Catheter-associated bacteremia, 991

Catheter-associated candidemia, 1089

Catheterization
 cardiac. See Cardiac catheterization
 central venous. See Central venous catheterization
 for perfusion restoration, 291
 peripheral venous. See Peripheral venous catheterization
 pulmonary artery, 313, 313f
 urethral, 1658

Cation gap, 1710

Cation permeability, abnormalities of, 1540
 in hereditary spherocytosis, 1539

Cats, and toxoplasmosis, 1146

Cat-scratch disease, 295, 926–928, 1280, 2372
 clinical manifestations of, 926–927, 926t
 diagnosis of, 926t, 927
 epidemiology of, 926
 etiology of, 1279
 prevention of, 928

with stridor, 1273
in tetralogy of Fallot, 1820
in total anomalous pulmonary venous connection, 1828
in transposition of great arteries with pulmonary stenosis, 1826
in tricuspid atresia, 1816
in truncus arteriosus, 1831
in valvar pulmonic stenosis, 1810
Cyanotic congenital heart disease
and growth failure, 2023
and thrombocytopenia, 1558
Cyanotic heart disease
clubbing of fingers in, 1754
growth failure in, 1753
Cyanotic polycythemia, 1816
Cyanotic spells, 1753
CyberKnife, 2214t
Cyclic adenosine monophosphate (cAMP). *See* cAMP
Cyclic antidepressants
flumazenil and, 359
pharmacologic effects of, 365
poisoning by, 364–365
clinical presentation and management of, 365
epidemiology of, 356, 364
toxicology, 365
Cyclic antidepressant toxidromes, 357
Cyclic guanosine-3', 5' monophosphate (cGMP)
formation of, 166f
and vasoregulation of fetal pulmonary circulation, 182
Cyclic neutropenia, 1550
treatment of, 1552
Cyclic vomiting, 1353, 1354t
of undetermined cause, 2276
Cyclin B-cdc2, and detection of damaged DNA, 1587
Cyclin-dependent kinase complexes
and detection of damaged DNA, 1587
in mitotic cell cycle, 1587f
in regulation of cell cycle, 1587, 1588f
Cyclin-dependent kinase inhibitors (CKIs)
families of, 1587
in mitotic cell cycle, 1587f
in regulation of cell cycle, 1587
Cyclin-dependent kinases (CDKs), in regulation of cell cycle, 1587
Cyclins, in regulation of cell cycle, 1587
Cyclitis, chronic, 2382, 2384
Cyclobenzaprine, for fibromyalgia, 862
Cyclodialysis, 2413
Cyclooxygenase
and dysmenorrhea, 254
in regulation of ductus arteriosus patency, 135
and vasoregulation of fetal pulmonary circulation, 183
Cyclo-oxygenase-2 inhibitors, 343t
Cyclophosphamide
for acute lymphoblastic leukemia, 1598
for CNS tumors, 2215
for dermatomyositis, 2302
for Ewing sarcoma-PNET, 1612
for Henoch-Schönlein purpura, 844, 1689
for Hodgkin disease, 1609
for juvenile dermatomyositis, 856
long-term toxicity of, 1593t
for lupus nephritis, 848, 1688
for membranous nephropathy, 1695
for minimal-change nephrotic syndrome, 1693
for neuroblastoma, 1619
neurotoxicity of, 2229t

for polyarteritis nodosa, 846
for rapidly progressive glomerulonephritis, 1686
for renal vasculitis, 1690
for rhabdomyosarcoma, 1613
for systemic lupus erythematosus, 850
for Takayasu arteritis, 846
Cycloserine, for tuberculosis, 958
Cyclospora cayetanensis, 1129
Cyclosporiasis, 1129
clinical manifestations of, 1129
diagnosis of, 1129
treatment of, 1099t, 1129
Cyclosporine
acute renal failure from, 1674
for autoimmune enteropathy, 1422
chronic tubulointerstitial nephropathy from, 1887
and diabetes mellitus, 2115t
for diabetes mellitus, 2115
drug interactions, 1082t
for focal segmental glomerulonephritis, 1694
gingival hyperplasia from, 1439, 1732
in heart transplantation, 1887
for HIV nephropathy, 1682
hypertrichosis from, 1213
hypoaldosteronism from, 1711
for juvenile dermatomyositis, 856
long-term toxicity of, 1593, 1593t
for membranous nephropathy, 1695
for minimal-change nephrotic syndrome, 1693
and multidrug resistance, 1603
for myasthenia gravis, 2286
and recurrent focal segmental glomerulonephritis, 1730
and recurrent hemolytic uremic syndrome, 1730
in renal transplantation, 1732
Cyclosporine A (CsA)
adverse effects of, 1439, 1442
for Crohn disease, 1442
for ulcerative colitis, 1439
Cyclothymic disorder. *See* Bipolar affective illness
Cyproheptadine
for Cushing disease, 2046–2047
for cyclic vomiting, 1353
for migraine, 2275
for urticaria, 1195
Cyproterone acetate, for familial gonadotropin-independent sexual precocity, 2099
Cyst(s)
Baker's, 2449
bone
aneurysmal, 2453
simple, 2453, 2453f
bronchogenic, 202, 1173, 1928, 1929f, 1946
carinal, 1928
hilar, 1928
paraesophageal, 1928
paratracheal, 1928
choledochal, 1375, 1482
and biliary malignancy, 1482
imaging of, 1471, 1482
location of, 1482f
signs and symptoms of, 1485t
types of, 1482f
congenital, of larynx, 1274
dermoid, 1928, 2411
of eyelid, 2365
epidermoid, 2365, 2411
epidermoid splenic, 1561
eruptive vellus hair, 1214

ganglion, 2449
Giardia, 1131
gingival, 1296
hepatic, 1118
hydatid, 1118
intramural, 1404
leptomeningeal, 2243
lingual thyroglossal duct, 1269
nasolacrimal duct, 1260
omental, 1375, 1405
omphalomesenteric, 1405
ovarian, 1376
and abnormal bleeding, 253
and precocious puberty, 2099
and premature thelarche, 2101
popliteal, 2449
pulmonary, 1119
retroperitoneal, 1375
saccular, 1404
solitary, 247
spherical, 1404
splenic, 1561
subglottic, 1274
thyroglossal duct, 88, 1269, 1274, 2070
tubular, 1404
urachal, 1375
vallecular, 1274
Cystathionine, 614
Cystathionine β-synthetase (CBS), deficiency of, 614, 679
Cystathionuria, 614
Cystatin C, 1661
Cysteamine, for Fanconi syndrome, 1709
Cysteamine eye drops, 1709
Cysteine, 614, 1346
Cystic acne, 1209–1210
Cystic adenomatoid malformation, congenital (CCAM), 202
differential diagnosis of, 190
prenatal management of, 77
Cystic disorders
of kidney, 1703–1708, 1703t
evaluation of, 1706f
in neonates, 1642
Cystic dysplasia. *See* Multicystic dysplastic kidney
Cysticercosis, 1117, 1120–1122
clinical manifestations of, 1121
diagnosis of, 1121
treatment of, 1122
Cysticercosis cellulosae, 1121
Cystic fibrosis (CF), 564, 715, 1464, 1967–1979
abdominal pain in, 1978, 1978t
acute pancreatitis from, 1466
airway infection in, therapy for, 1974–1975, 1975f
allergic bronchopulmonary aspergillosis in, 812, 1993
antibiotic therapy in, 1974–1975, 1975f
anti-inflammatory therapy for, 1974
atelectasis in, 1970, 1970f
treatment of, 1976
chest pain in, 1895
treatment of, 1975
clinical manifestations of, 1968–1971
cor pulmonale in, treatment of, 1977
dermatitis in, 1177
diabetes mellitus in, 2114
diagnosis of, 576t, 1972
diagnostic criteria for, 1972, 1972t
enzyme replacement therapy in, 1977
exercise testing in, 1921, 1921f
exercise therapy in, 1921, 1974

Desensitization, and pain management, 426
Desipramine, for attention deficit hyperactivity disorder, 434
Desmogleins, 1201
Desmopressin, 2025
for central diabetes insipidus, 2028
Desmopressin acetate (DDAVP)
for hemophilia A, 1572
for nocturnal enuresis, 1743
for posttraumatic diabetes insipidus, 2245
for von Willebrand disease, 1573
Desmosomes, 1201
Desmosterol, 681
Desquamative interstitial pneumonitis, 1989–1990
DES-related clear-cell adenocarcinoma. *See* Diethylstilbestrol (DES)-related clear-cell adenocarcinoma
Detection, of toxins, 357–358, 359t
Detection bias
in case-control studies, 592
in cohort studies, 591
Detergent worker's lung, etiology of, 1994t
De Toni-Fanconi syndrome, 2301
Detoxifying reactions, of liver, 1474
Developing countries, children adopted from, true precocious puberty in, 2098
Development. *See also* Embryonic development
adaptation and, 516
in adolescence, 223–226, 225t
anticipatory guidance of, age-appropriate discussion topics for, 28t
assessment of, 12–13, 14t
in follow-up of intensive care nursery graduates, 220
schedule for, 2t
standardized instruments for, benefits and limitations of, 411–413
assistive technology devices and, 547
biological, in adolescence, 223, 224t
and chronic illness or disability, 429
common functional concerns of, 414–419
adaptation to illness, 428–430, 429t–430t
crying and colic, 414–417, 416f
eating, 420–422
pain, 422–427
sleeping, 417–420
continuum of, normal variation to disorder in, 430–497
"critical periods" of, 406
diagnostic dilemma of, 410–411
and disruptive behavior, 445
expectations of, for preschool, 440t
family structure and, 511
fundamental concepts of, 401–408
hemostatic aspects of, 1569–1570, 1570t
of language, 17–19
major psychopathologic disorders of, 498–509
milestones of, 14t
acquisition of, in intensive care nursery graduates, 220
models of
after exposure to violence, 528
with parental substance abuse, 526–528
of motor skills, 12–19
nonparental child care and, 513
orthopedic, 2419–2420
oxygen transport during, 1522
physical *vs.* occupational therapy for, 544t
in preterm infants, 13
psychological, 12–19
in adolescence, 5–7
psychosocial
in adolescence, 225–226, 225t

issues of, in family and community life, 509–531
of red blood cell production and function, 1519–1522
"sensitive periods" of, 406
of sexual self, terminology of, 471t
of speech, 17–19
traumatic injury and, 349
violence and, 529
visual impairment and, 492
white blood cells in, changing numbers of, 1548, 1548t
Developmental clumsiness, 2166
Developmental coordination disorder (DCD)
assessment and diagnosis of, 483, 484f
clinical manifestations of, 482–483
definition and epidemiology of, 482
and attention deficit hyperactivity disorder, 482
etiology and pathogenesis of, 482
management and treatment of, 483
natural history and prognosis of, 484
Developmental delay (DD), 13–17, 780, 781f
of Alagille syndrome, 1486t
clinical signs of, 439
continuum of, maturational lags to mental retardation in, 438–441
diagnosis of, 15t–16t
functional outcome measures in, 534
labeling of, 16
laboratory studies for, 15, 16t, 440t
of language, 17–19
with neglect, 466
in short-gestation children, 61
significance of, in intensive care nursery graduate, 220
of speech, 17–19
Developmental disabilities, 779–786
in adolescents, confidentiality and, 561
assistive technology devices for, 545–547
blindness and, 490, 491t
etiology of, 13–15
functional outcome measure for, 534
hearing loss, 782–784
microcephaly, 784–786
in outcome of hyaline membrane disease, 134
parental adjustment to, 17
screening for, 13
Developmental dyslexia, 435, 2206
Developmental dysphasia (DD), 2204
Developmental dysplasia of hip (DDH), 723t, 2434–2436, 2435f–2436f
common findings in, 2436
complications of, 2436
diagnosis of, 2435, 2435f
epidemiology of, 2435
examination and evaluation of, 2421, 2435–2436, 2435f
tests for, 2435–2436
incidence of, 2435
in metatarsus adductus, 2422
in newborn, 91
treatment for, 2435f–2436f, 2436
ultrasonography of, 587
Developmental glaucoma, 2401
Developmental outcome, of extracorporeal membrane oxygenation, 214
Developmental soft signs, 2205
Developmental trajectories, continuities and discontinuities of, 405–406, 405t
Developmental transition, 405
Device closure, of septal defects, 1780
Device-related infections, 993
Devic syndrome, 2315
DEXA. *See* Dual-energy x-ray absorptiometry

Dexamethasone, 2050
antenatal, to prevent germinal matrix hemorrhage of preterm newborn, 144
for chronic lung disease, 219
for cranial subdural empyema, 2319
and hypotension, of preterm newborns, 140
for laryngeal hemangioma, 1277
for laryngotracheobronchitis, 1276
and neurologic impairment, 219
and outcome of intensive care nursery graduates, 219
potency of, 2051t
for prenatal management of congenital adrenal hyperplasia, 78
for prevention of hyaline membrane disease, dosage and administration of, 132
for *Salmonella* infection, 984
Dexamethasone suppression test, 2037, 2047
Dexterity, developmental expectations of, 440t
Dextroamphetamine
for attention deficit hyperactivity disorder, 433
for dying patient, 571
Dextrocardia, 1836
Dextromethorphan, for nonketotic hyperglycinemia, 615
Dextrose
for coma, 294
in maintenance fluids, 1644
neonatal hyperglycemia and
etiology of, 159
management of, 160
pathophysiology of, 160
neonatal hypoglycemia and
etiology of, 156
management of, 158
in parenteral nutrition solutions, 1345
toxicity of, 147
DFA test. *See* Direct fluorescent antibody (DFA) test
DFE. *See* Dietary folate equivalent
DFMO (difluoromethylornithine), for sleeping sickness, 1149
DGF. *See* Delayed graft function
DGI. *See* Disseminated gonococcal infection
dGTP. *See* Deoxyguanosine trisphosphate
DHAP (Dihydroxyacetone phosphate) deficiency, 1520
DHEA. *See* Dehydroepiandrosterone
DHEAS. *See* Dehydroepiandrosterone sulfate
DHF. *See* Dengue hemorrhagic fever
DHP. *See* Dihydropiridine receptor
Diabetes
increased glomerular filtration rate in, 1661
in infants of diabetic mothers, 126
insulin-resistant, 2011
lipoatrophic, 1237
necrobiosis lipoidica diabeticorum in, 1236
peroxisome proliferator activating receptor agonists for, 2008
Diabetes Control and Complications Trial (DCCT), 2123
Diabetes insipidus
central. *See* Central diabetes insipidus
in Hand-Schüller-Christian disease, 1625
in Langerhans cell histiocytosis, management of, 1626
nephrogenic. *See* Nephrogenic diabetes insipidus
perioperative care of, 339
polyuria in, 1649
posttraumatic, 2245
after surgical resection for craniopharyngioma, 2227
Diabetes mellitus, 2111–2136
atherosclerosis from, 1890

progression sequence of, 230
use patterns of, 230
Drug allergy, 820–821
anaphylaxis in, 820–821
cutaneous manifestations of, 1194–1195
Drug-associated thrombocytopenia, 199
Drug classes, 346t
Drug eruptions, 1194–1195
acneiform, 1210
Drug-induced esophagitis, 1396
Drug-induced gastrointestinal disorders, 1414
Drug-induced hepatotoxicity, 1503, 1511t
Drug-induced immune hemolytic anemia,
1545–1546
Drug-induced neutropenia, 1551
immune, 1551
Drug metabolism, 1474, 1475t
Drug rash, 1194
Drug resistance. *See also specific drug*
in acute myeloid leukemia, 1603
in acute otitis media, 1251–1252
in bacterial sinusitis, 1263
in cytomegaloviral infection, 1034
in gonorrhea, 969
in leprosy, 965
in malaria, 1140
in otitis media with effusion, 1253
in pneumococcal infection, 978
in *Salmonella* infection, 982, 984
in *Shigella* infection, 986
in *Staphylococcus aureus* infection, 992
in neonatal intensive care units, 116
in streptococcal infection, 1002
in tuberculosis, 956, 958
Drug screen, for toxin detection, 357
Drug studies, of newborns, 146
Drug therapy
for acute anxiety, 458
for affective disorders, 502
approach to, in pain management, 341, 342f
for attention deficit hyperactivity disorder,
433–434
in cardiopulmonary resuscitation, 329, 330t
for common behaviors of pervasive developmental disorders, 500t
and elevated g-glutamyl transpeptidase,
1479t
for hyperlipoproteinemia with metabolic disorders, 703–704, 703t
for hypertension, 1882–1885, 1883t–1884t
and neonatal thrombocytopenias, 199
for neurogenic bladder dysfunction, 539
for newborns, 146–148
for obesity, 480
for obsessive-compulsive disorder, 505
for pain, 427
for pervasive developmental disorders, 500,
500t
during pregnancy, 774–775, 776t
angiotensin-converting enzyme inhibitors,
776t, 1640
anticonvulsants, 2267
hemorrhagic disease of newborns, 187
diuretics, and neonatal hypercalcemia, 163
lithium, 776t, 1781
nonsteroidal antiinflammatory drugs,
1640
preoperative management of, 335
for separation anxiety, 453
for spasticity, 540
tooth decay and, 541
Drug toxicity. *See under* Toxic ingestions and
exposures
"Dry socket" (idiopathic chondrolysis) disease,
2422
DS. *See* Dermatan sulfate

DSA. *See* Digital subtraction angiography
DSM-IV. *See* Diagnostic and Statistical Manual
of Mental Disorders, Fourth Edition
DSS. *See* Dengue shock syndrome
DTaP (diphtheria, tetanus, acellular pertussis)
vaccine, 40t, 43–45
DTM. *See* Dermatophyte Test Medium
DTO (denatured tincture of opium), for narcotic abstinence syndrome, 527
DTP (diphtheria, tetanus, pertussis) vaccine,
40t, 43–45
d-transposition, 1747, 1823–1826
chest roentgenography of, 1823f, 1825
clinical manifestations of, 1824
diagnosis of, 1825
heart sounds in, 1755
incidence of, 1781t
morphology and physiology of, 1824
treatment of, 1825
DTwP (diphtheria, tetanus, whole-cell pertussis) vaccine, 40t, 43–45
Dual atrioventricular (AV) node pathways,
1842
Dual-chamber pacing, 1853
Dual-energy x-ray absorptiometry (DEXA)
of body fat, 2136
of bone mineral density, 2136, 2145
Dual-lumen hemodialysis catheter, acute, for
neonatal hypercalcemia, 164
Dual-photon dexatometry, of rheumatic disease, 831
Dual porphyria, 688
Duane retraction syndrome, 2403–2404
Duarte galactosemia, 640
DUB. *See* Dysfunctional uterine bleeding
Dubin-Johnson syndrome, 1489
presenting age of, 1489t
Dubowitz syndrome, 737t
Duchenne muscular dystrophy, 564, 1862,
2289–2290
diagnosis of, 576t
orthoses and, 547
respiratory involvement in, 2002–2003
Duck fever, etiology of, 1994t
Duck rabies vaccine, in transverse myelitis,
2315
Ductal-dependent lesions, newborns with, 284
Ductal dilation, of biliary system, imaging of,
1471
Ductal plate malformations, 1483
Ductal shunt. *See* Patent ductus arteriosus
Duct-to-duct biliary reconstruction, complications of, 1517
Ductus arteriosus (DA), 1750
constriction and closure of, 135, 1751, 1785
and circulatory shock, 285
delayed, incidence of, 136
initial stabilization of, 292
in preterm infants, 135
function of, 135
patent. *See* Patent ductus arteriosus
Ductus deferens, 242f
Ductus venosus, 1749
Dumping syndrome
antireflux surgery and, 1393
in motility disorders of stomach and intestine, 1410
Duncan syndrome. *See* X-linked lymphoproliferative disease
Duodenal atresia, 203, 1403, 1403f
radiography of, 584
Duodenal duplications, 1405
Duodenal obstruction
congenital, 203
in intestinal malrotation, 1401
Duodenal resection, 1427

Duodenal ulcer. *See* Peptic ulcer
Duodenitis, 1434
chronic vomiting in, 1352
Duodenoduodenostomy, for duodenal atresia,
1403
Duodenojejunostomy, for duodenal atresia,
1403
Duodenum, 1306
development of, 1307, 1308f
Duplex sonography, of cervicocephalic arterial
dissection, 2234
Duplications
esophageal, 1387
gastrointestinal, 1375, 1404–1405
ureteral, 1736
Dupuytren exostosis (subungual exostosis),
2428, 2428f
Dust mite allergy, 811, 813, 815
DVT. *See* Deep vein thrombosis
DW. *See* Diffusion-weighted (DW) imaging
Dwarf, 757
Dwarfism, 2065
achondroplastic, in neonatal examination of
limbs, 91
causes of, 2018t
thanatophoric
fibroblast growth factor and, 65
in neonatal examination of limbs, 91
Dwarf tapeworm, 1120
D-xylose test, for carbohydrate malabsorption,
1417
Dye test, nitroblue tetrazolium (NBT), 1552t
Dying patients, caring for, dying from chronic
disease, 563–572
bereavement, 570–571
care of medical professionals, 571
communicating bad news, 565
definitions in, 564
difficulties faced by siblings and grandparents, 567
distinguished from patients dying of accidents or acute illness, 563
"do not resuscitate" order, 568
ethical considerations in, 572
goal setting and decision making in,
567–568
helping without fixing, 567
home, hospital, or hospice death, 568–569
illnesses and their symptoms, 564
physician's responsibilities in hospital death,
569–570
special problems of dying adolescents, 566
spiritual matters in, 572
symptom management in, 571–572
talking with children about death, 565–566
Dyke-Davidoff-Masson deformity, 2257
Dynamic ankle-foot orthoses (DAFOs), 548
Dynamic ileus, radiography of, 585
Dynamic lung compliance, in meconium aspiration syndrome (MAS), 195
Dynamic psychotherapy, 459
Dysacusis, 2200
Dysautonomia, familial, 2284
Dysbetalipoproteinemia, 701
Dyscalculia, 2206
Dysembryoplastic neuroepithelial tumor
(DNT), 2222
Dysferlin, 2292–2293
Dysfibrinogenemia, 1574
Dysfluency
clinical manifestations of, 442
definition of, 441
management of, 444
natural history and prognosis of, 444
Dysfunctional uterine bleeding (DUB), 253
etiology of, 253

Facial paralysis (*contd.*)
　from trauma, 1257
Facial sensation, testing, 2167
Facial weakness, in newborns, 92
Facies
　asymmetric crying, of newborn, 87
　characteristic, of Alagille syndrome, 1485,
　　1486t
　of small-for-gestational-age infants, 121
Facioscapulohumeral (FSH) dystrophy, 2293
Factor II deficiency, 1574
Factor V deficiency, 1574
Factor VII deficiency, 1574
Factor VIII, venous thrombosis and, 1575
Factor VIII deficiency, 1570–1572
　clinical manifestation of, 1571
　diagnosis of, 1570–1571
　factor VIII inhibitors in, 1572
　　acquired, 1570
　general care for, 1572
　treatment of, 1571–1572
Factor IX deficiency, 1572–1573
　diagnosis of, 1573
　presentation of, 200
　treatment, 1573
Factor X deficiency, 1574
Factor XI deficiency, 1573
Factor XII deficiency, 1574
Factor XIII deficiency, 1574
Factor V Leiden, 1575
　prevalence of, 201
FAD (flavine adenine dinucleotide) deficiency,
　1543
FAH (fumarylacetoacetate hydrolase) defi-
　ciency, 1487
Failing intrauterine pregnancy, levels of proges-
　terone in, 255
Failure, 434
Failure-to-thrive, 1336, 1381, 1383. *See also*
　Growth failure
　definitions of, 7t
　differential diagnosis of, 5, 7, 468
　etiology of, 7, 8t
　evaluation of, 7, 8t–10t
　history-taking of, 9t
　　when neglect suspected, 467
　in HIV infection, 1047
　hospitalization for, 9t
　in intestinal pseudoobstruction, 1410
　laboratory studies of, 9t, 467
　management of, 8
　from neglect, 466
　onset of, 5, 5f
　physical examination of, 7, 9t
　severe psychosocial
　　management of, 8
　　signs of, 7
Fainting attack, 1893
Falciform ligament, 1469
FALDH. *See* Fatty aldehyde dehydrogenase
Fallopian tube(s)
　abortion of, 255
　ectopic pregnancy outcome and, 255
　examination of, 245t
　health history of, 244t
　rupture of, 255
Fallot, tetralogy of. *See* Tetralogy of Fallot
Falls
　head injuries from, 465
　risk factors of, in gait pattern, 2420
False-negative rate, of diagnostic tests, 593
False-positive rate, of diagnostic tests, 593
False-positive test results, and vulnerable child
　syndrome, 515

Familial, autosomal dominant central diabetes
　insipidus, 2027
Familial adenomatous polyposis syndromes,
　1455
Familial combined hyperlipidemia (FCHL),
　700
　plasma lipid, lipoprotein, and apoB levels in,
　　699t
Familial conditions, 714
Familial constitutional precocious puberty,
　2097
Familial defective apoB-100, 700
Familial dysalbuminemic hyperthyroxinemia,
　2065
Familial dysautonomia, 2284
Familial erythrophagocytic lymphohistiocytosis
　　(primary hemophagocytic lymphohistio-
　　cytosis), 1626
　epidemiology of, 1626
　prognosis and treatment of, 1627
Familial exudative vitreoretinopathy, 2393
Familial glucocorticoid deficiency, 2044
Familial goiter, 2067
Familial gonadotropin-independent sexual pre-
　cocity, 2099
Familial hypercholesterolemia (FH), 698
　diagnosis of, 576t
　plasma lipid, lipoprotein, and apoB levels in,
　　699t
Familial hyperlysinemia, 614
Familial hypertriglyceridemia (FHT), 701
Familial hypobetalipoproteinemia, 705
Familial hypocalciuric hypercalcemia (FHH),
　163, 165, 2143, 2152
　diagnosis of, 163
Familial hypomagnesemia, 2163
Familial hypomagnesemia with secondary hy-
　pocalcemia (HSH), 2163
Familial hypoparathyroidism, and hypocal-
　cemia, 2149
Familial hypoplastic glomerulocystic disease,
　1708
Familial Langerhans cell histiocytosis, 1624
Familial Mediterranean fever (FMF), 864–866
Familial pituitary hypoplasia, and central diabe-
　tes insipidus, 2027
Familial polyposis coli, diagnosis of, 576t
Familial protracted diarrhea. *See* Microvillus at-
　rophy
Familial severe neutropenia, 1551
　treatment of, 1552
Familial spastic paraplegia, 2201, 2337
Familial startle disease, 2274
Familial steroid-resistant nephrotic syndrome,
　1701
Familial thyroid-binding globulin deficiency
　syndrome, 2065
Familial ureteral abnormalities syndrome
　(FUAS), 1708
Familial XX gonadal dysgenesis, 2089
Familial XY gonadal dysgenesis, incomplete
　form of, 2086
Family(ies)
　adaptation of, to disabled children, 552–553
　adolescent request for confidentiality and,
　　561
　and assessment of separation difficulties,
　　452
　and cerebral palsy management, 483
　changing concepts of, 509–512
　characteristics of, 509
　　and impact of illness, 429t
　directed blood donations from, 1582
　discord in, 523–526
　dynamics of, and clumsiness, 483

education of, for tracheostomy care, 536
factors of, associated with abuse or neglect,
　464t
and gender identity, 470
of hemophilia A patients, education of, 1572
meetings with, to discuss end-of-life issues,
　565
and Munchausen by proxy syndrome,
　506–507
and pain perception, 424
phases of, 509
poverty and, 531
psychoeducation for, with affectively ill pa-
　tient, 502
psychosocial issues of, 509–531
relationships in, at puberty, 224
role of
　in child development, 406
　in health care quality, 535
　in psychological development, 407
　in setting rehabilitation goals for chroni-
　　cally ill or disabled children, 553
societal functions of, 509
stress on, physical disabilities and, 484
at time of hospital death, physician's respon-
　sibilities toward, 569–570
transitions of, 516–520
types of, 510
unshared experiences of, 407
violence in, 528–529
Family-centered health care, 535
Family child care, 512
　quality of, 512
Family counseling, 726
　about teratogens, 779
　in congenital heart disease, 1781
　in congestive heart failure, 1875
　in diabetic ketoacidosis, 2123
　for Down syndrome, 733
　for Duchenne muscular dystrophy, 2289
　in heart disease, 1900
　in HIV infection, 1049
　in juvenile rheumatoid arthritis, 839
　in neural tube defects, 2187
　in obesity, 2140
　for sex differentiation abnormalities, 2091
Family history. *See also* Genetic predisposition
　in autoimmune hepatitis, 1504
　of back pain, 2443
　in ear or hearing problems, 1241
　and evaluation of neonatal anemia, 198
　metabolic liver disease and, 1485
Family patterns, and disruptive behavior, 446
Family stressors, and night waking, 418
Family studies, 576–577
Family therapy, 459
　for attention deficits, 434
　for obsessive-compulsive disorder, 505
Fanconi anemia (FA), 737t, 1565–1566
　genetics of, 1565
　phenotype of, 1565
　physical abnormalities in, 1565t
　presentation and clinical course of, 1565
　treatment of, 1566
Fanconi Bickel syndrome, 638
Fanconi syndrome, 1694, 1709–1710
　causes of, 1709t
　corneal changes in, 2380
　proximal renal tubular acidosis in, 1710
Fang punctures
　of coral snake bites, 398
　of pit viper bites, 396
Fantasy, in management of family transitions,
　520

Fetus(es) (*contd.*)
　urine flow in, 1637
　in utero treatment of, influence of, 74
　vesicoureteral reflux in, 1671
　viral infections of CNS in, 2312–2313, 2312t
Fever, 888–895. *See also* Febrile illness
　with abdominal pain, 1361
　in acute lymphoblastic leukemia, 1595
　adverse physiological effects of, 302–303
　in appendicitis, 1450
　assessment of, 302–308, 304f
　in babesiosis, 1125
　in child 3–36 months old, 891–892
　　evaluation of patient in, 891
　　management of, 892
　of choledochal cysts, 1485t
　common causes of, 305t
　conduit, 1900
　definition and epidemiology of, 302
　diagnosis and management of, 305–308, 305t, 307t
　　approach to, 303–304, 304f, 305t
　　fever without focus, 306
　　occult bacteremia, 307–308
　in Epstein-Barr virus infection, 1036
　in familial Mediterranean fever, 865
　in human herpesvirus 6 infection, 1039
　vs. hyperthermia, 388
　in hypohidrotic ectodermal dysplasia, 1189
　idiopathic, final diagnoses of, 307t
　in immunocompromised patients, 803, 806t, 807f
　in impaired perfusion, 292
　in infant ≤60 days old, 889–891
　　evaluation of patient in, 889–890
　　management of, 890–891
　in infant 61–90 days old, 891
　influenza vaccine and, 1072
　in influenza virus infection, 1070
　in Kawasaki disease, 844
　and kinetics of antibiotics, 871t
　life-threatening conditions of, 303, 305t
　without localizing signs, in infants and children, 888–892
　management of, 304f
　in measles, 1054
　neonatal, 304–305, 305t–306t
　noninfectious causes of, 305–306, 307t
　after open heart surgery, 1900
　parenchymal injuries and, 2245
　pathogenesis of, 302, 303f
　Pel-Ebstein, of Hodgkin disease, 1608
　persistent, 808f
　in plague, 975
　with rash, 1231f
　　evaluation of, 1230
　in rat-bite fever, 980
　and respiratory failure, 278
　in rubella, 1076
　survival rates with, 302
　symptoms of, 305
　treatment of, 303
　of unknown origin, 889, 893–895, 894t, 897t
　　clinical evaluation in, 893–894
　　etiology of, 893t
　　laboratory evaluation in, 894–895
　　radiographic evaluation in, 894–895
Fever blisters, 1030, 1221
Fever phobia, treatment of, 303
Fever threshold, 302
Fever without focus, 306
FFP. *See* Fresh frozen plasma
FGF (fibroblast growth factor), and fetal growth, 65

FGFR. *See* Fibroblast growth factor receptor
FH. *See* Familial hypercholesterolemia
FHH. *See* Familial hypocalciuric hypercalcemia
FHR. *See* Fetal heart rate
FHT. *See* Familial hypertriglyceridemia
Fiber, dietary, 1310
　in bowel management of disabled children, 540
　insoluble, 1320
　soluble, 1320
Fiber-containing formulas, 1328
Fiberoptic blanket, for hyperbilirubinemia, 168
Fiberoptic endoscopy, of foreign-body ingestion, 1398
Fiber type disproportion, 2295
Fibrillary astrocytoma, 2222
Fibrillation, 1847
　atrial, 1847, 1856, 1856f
　ventricular, 1847, 1858, 1858f
Fibrillin-1, 763
Fibrin, and localization of infection, 299
Fibrinogen
　deficient or defective, 1574
　and viscosity, 192
Fibrinoid, excessive deposit of, by trophoblast, 62
Fibrinolysis, 1568
Fibrinous scales, 2364
Fibrin split products (FSP), 1568
Fibroadenomas, 247
Fibroblasts, gene expression in, and persistent pulmonary hypertension of newborn, 184
Fibroblast growth factor (FGF), and fetal growth, 65
Fibroblast growth factor receptor (FGFR), 755
Fibrocystic change, 247
Fibroma, 1296, 1775f, 1865
　nonossifying, 2453, 2454f
Fibromatosis colli, 1281
Fibromyalgia, 832, 861–864
Fibroosseous disorders, of nose and paranasal sinuses, 1264
Fibrous cortical defect, of bone, 2453, 2454f
Fibrous dysplasia, 1297, 2410
Fibrous forehead plaque, 1186
Fibrous histiocytomas, 1202
Fibula, stress fractures in, 2428
Fick technique, 1776
Fictitious disorder by proxy syndrome. *See* Munchausen by proxy syndrome
"Fiddleback" spider, 1235
"Fiduciary" model of doctor-patient relationship, 553
Field block, 342–345
　injection of, 342
　toxicity of, 342
Fifth disease. *See* Erythema infectiosum
"Fight or flight" response, 455
Filarial infections, 1106–1108
Filarial pneumonitis, 1987
Filiform papillae, 1266
　embryology of, 1267
Filling volume of heart, reduced, 287, 288f, 289t
Filoviral hemorrhagic fever, 1025t, 1026
Finality, concept of, 518
Fine motor skills
　developmental assessment of, 14t
　development of, 404
Fine needle aspiration
　of breast masses, 247
　for head and neck masses, indications for, 1280
　of thyroid neoplasia, 2078

Finger(s)
　fractures of, treatment for, 2451, 2451f
　movement of, in newborn, 92
　polydactyly of, 2426
　syndactyly of, 2449
Finger contractures, orthoses for, 548
Finger extensors, paralysis of, in birth-related brachial plexus injury, 186
Finger grasp, of newborn
　examination of, 94, 95f
　maturation of, 95
Finger jam, 2451
Fingernails, of small-for-gestational-age infant, 121
Finger pulse, 1754
Finnish families
　aspartylglycosaminidase deficiency in, 663
　hyperapobetalipoproteinemia in, 700
　sialic acid transporter defect in, 663
Finnish-type congenital nephrotic syndrome (NPHS1), 1642, 1700, 1700t
　control of, before transplantation, 1732
Fire(s), mortality statistics of, 37
Fire ant bites, 395, 1157, 1233, 1233f
Fire corals (*Millepora spp.*), poisonous sting of, 391, 1159
First and second branchial arch syndrome. *See* Hemifacial microsomia
First-degree atrioventricular block, 1846, 1846f, 1858
First-degree burns, 385, 1396
First trimester, of pregnancy, of diabetic pregnancy, and congenital anomalies, 126
FISH. *See* Fluorescence in situ hybridization
Fisher syndrome, 2315
Fish-eye disease, 708
　clinical manifestations of, 709t
"Fish-mouth" scars, 1188
Fish oil
　for IgA nephropathy, 1683
　for ulcerative colitis, 1440
Fish tapeworm infestation, vitamin B_{12} deficiency of, 1530
Fissured tongue, 1293
Fistula ligation, for tracheoesophageal fistula, 203
"Five P's," for fractures, 2451
"Fix and track," of newborn, in neurologic evaluation, 92, 92f
Fixation (ocular), 2351
Fixed anion, accumulation of, and metabolic acidosis, 605
Fixed cutaneous sporotrichosis, 1096
Fixed drug eruption, 1195
FK506, and diabetes mellitus, 2115t
FKHR gene translocation, 1613
Flag sign, 1336
Flagyl. *See* Metronidazole
Flail chest, 350
Flare, 813
Flaring, in pneumonia, 1980
Flashlamp pumped pulsed dye laser
　of hemangiomas, 1206
　of port wine stains, 1207
Flatfeet (pes planus), 2429
　corrective shoes for, 2425
　peroneal spastic, 2427
Flat warts, 1219, 1220f
Flatworms. *See* Trematode infections
Flavin adenine dinucleotide, 1323t
Flavin adenine mononucleotide, 1323t
Flavine adenine dinucleotide (FAD) deficiency, 1543
Flavin mononucleotide (FMN), 644
Flavivirus infections, 1018t, 1025t, 1028
Flavonoids, 1891

Follicle stimulating hormone (FSH) (*contd.*)
  during puberty, 2095–2096
  in spermatogenesis, 243
Follicular conjunctivitis, 2368
Follicular cystitis, 1669
Follicular mucinosis, 1214
Follicular reaction, in conjunctivitis, 2368
Folliculitis, 1217, *(Color Plate 18)*
  vs. acne, 1210
  diagnosis of, 1173
  gram-negative, 1217
  irritant acneiform, 1210
  in *Malassezia furfur* infection, 1095
Folliculitis decalvans, 1212
Folliculosis, 2373
Follow-Up, 1334t
Follow-up rate, in cohort studies, 591
Follow-Up Soy, 1334t
Fomepizole, for methanol and ethylene glycol
    poisonings, 371, 372t
Fontan circulation, for single-ventricle malfor-
    mation, 1831
Fontanel, 87
  bulging of, after trauma, 348
Fontan-Kreuzer procedure
  for pulmonary atresia with intact ventricular
      septum, 1819
  for tricuspid atresia, 1817
Food, begging for, 421
Food allergy, 818–819, 1444
  anaphylaxis in, 818, 821
  cow's milk protein allergy, 818, 1445
      classification of, 1445t
  diagnosis of, 1445–1446
  management of, 1446
  nut allergy, 1445
  pathophysiology of, 1445
  symptoms of, 818
Food and Drug Administration (FDA)
  on benzyl alcohol, 147
  and complementary and alternative therapies,
      543
  on hexachlorophene, 147
  limited approval of, for inhaled nitric oxide
      therapy, 217
Food and Drug Administration (FDA) Mod-
    ernization Act of 1997, and propylene
    glycol, 146
Food and Nutrition Board (FNB), 1313
  on DRI for water, 1315
  recommended dietary allowances by, 1324t
  on vegetarian diets, 1338
Food fadism, 1338
Food groups, 1313
Food hypersensitivity, 1444
Food-induced enterocolitis syndrome, 818
Food intake, of picky eaters, 421
Food intolerance, 1444
Food "phobias," 422
Food poisoning, staphylococcal, 992
Food preference, 421
Food Pyramid, 1313, 1314f
Food refusal, 421
Food seeking, 1381
Foot, 2425–2430
  accessory navicular, 2429, 2429f
  anomalies of, 91
  burns to soles of, 385
  cavus, 2429, 2429f
  cyanosis of, in newborn, 86
  hallux valgus, 2429–2430, 2430f
  height of, in leg length measurement, 2421
  idiopathic toe walking, 2428
  imaging of
    computed tomography, for tarsal coalition,
        2428f

  radiography, for tarsal coalition, 2427f
  malformations of, in dysmorphic syndromes,
      91
  painful conditions of, 2427–2428
  pes planus, 2429
  serpentine, 2422
Football sign, in radiography, 150f
Foot deformity(ies)
  in arthrogryposis multiplex congenita,
      2456
  congenital, 2425–2426
Foot dorsiflexion angle, in newborn, 93, 93f
Foot drop, 2283
"Foot-slapping" gait, 2283
Foramen cecum, 1266
Foramen ovale, 1750
  closure of, 1751
    incomplete, 1751
  formation of, 1746f
  opening of, 1751
  patent, 1792
  shunting across
    in persistent pulmonary hypertension of
        newborn, 181, 184
    pulmonary vasodilation for, 215, 216f
Foramen ovale defects, 1746
Forced expiratory flow between 25% and 75%
    of vital capacity (FEV$_{25-75}$), 1916
Forced expiratory volume in 1 second (FEV$_1$),
    1916
Forced vital capacity (FVC), 1916
Forceps, 75
  bruises from, 87, 87f
  choice of, 76
  eye injuries from, 87
  facial paralysis and, 188
  and sixth cranial nerve injury, 188
  and subaponeurotic hemorrhage, 187
  subcutaneous fat necrosis and, 185
  terminology of, 76
Fordyce granules, 1293
Forearm recoil, in newborn, 93
Forebrain, 2175
  development of, 408
Foregut, 1307, 1307f–1308f
  pain originating from, 1354
Foreign bodies
  bronchial, 1278
  of esophagus, 1397–1398
  in external auditory canal, 1241, 1257
    removal of, 1257
  and external otitis, 1255
  laryngeal, 1278
  in nose and paranasal sinuses, 1265
  perforation of tympanic membrane by, 1257
  retained, 1278
  subglottic, 1942
  tracheal, 1278
Foreign-body aspiration (FBA), 382–384,
    1277–1278, 1946
  cardiopulmonary resuscitation and, 328
  clinical manifestations of, 383, 383t, 1278
  diagnosis of, 383
  epidemiology of, 382
  history of, 1278
  management of, 383–384, 384f
  pathogenesis of, 383
  prevention of, 32
"Fore milk," fat content of, 109
Formal operations cognitive stage, 404
Formic acid, 371
Formulas
  for children and adults, 1328, 1334t
  infant. *See* Infant formulas
  transitional, 1334t
Fort Ripley hemoglobin, 1535

Foscarnet
  for cytomegaloviral infection, 1394, 2314
  for cytomegalovirus infection, 1035
  dosage and administration of, 883t
  for Epstein-Barr virus infection, 1029t
  for varicella-zoster virus esophagitis, 1395
Fosphenytoin, for status epilepticus, 2266
Fossa ovalis, 1746f
Foster care, 520–522
  biopsychosocial issues in, 521
  epidemiology and definition of, 520–521
  health-care provider's role in, 522, 523t
Founder effect, 721, 825
"Four P's," in acute lymphoblastic leukemia,
      1595
F-6-P (fructose-6-phosphatase) deficiency,
      1541f
FPLN. *See* Focal proliferative lupus nephritis
Fractional excretion (FE), 1662
Fractional excretion of sodium (FENa) in neo-
    nates, 1638
Fracture(s). *See also specific fracture*
  in child abuse, 465, 2451, 2451f
  common, in children, 2451
  differential diagnosis of, 2449
  in newborns
    of clavicles, 88, 185–186
    secondary to intrauterine position, 90
    of zygomatic arch, 87
  with simple bone cysts, 2453
  toddler's, 2451
  treatment of
    general tips for, 2451, 2451f
    in hemophilia A patients, 1572
  unique patterns of, 2450–2451
Fragile X syndrome, 720
  diagnosis of, 576t
  ocular conditions in, incidence of, 491t
Frameless surgical navigation system, 2212
Frameshift mutations, 1585
Francisella tularensis, 1008
Frank breech position, and developmental dys-
    plasia of hips, 2435
Frankfurt plane, 2015
Frank organic brain syndrome, in systemic lu-
    pus erythematosus, 849
Frank organic dementia, after head trauma,
      2248
Frank-Starling response, 1750, 1783, 1869,
      1871
Fraser syndrome, 1700t, 1701–1702, 2087
Frataxin, 651, 2341
Fraternal twins. *See* Dizygotic (DZ) twins
FRC. *See* Functional residual capacity
Freckles, 1191
Free amino acid-containing formulas, 1328
Free erythrocyte protoporphyrin (FEP)
  and iron deficiency anemia, 1528
  lead poisoning and, 369
  in progressive stages of iron deficiency,
      1528t
Free fatty acids, 1312
  plasma concentrations of
    maternal, and infants of diabetic mothers,
        125
    in small-for-gestational-age infants, 122
  and thermogenesis after birth, 80
  total and free, high-risk screening of, 581t
"Free" heme, 685
Freeman-Sheldon syndrome, 737t, 749t
Free radical production, iron and, 367
Freiberg infraction, 2427
French-American-British Cooperative Working
    Group (FAB)
  antidigoxin antibody fragments, dosage and
      administration of, 366

Gender differences (*contd.*)
  in non-Hodgkin lymphoma, 1604
  in obsessive-compulsive disorder, 504
  in pain perception, 424
  in pauciarticular juvenile rheumatoid arthritis, 836
  in polyarteritis nodosa, 845
  in polyarticular juvenile rheumatoid arthritis, 837
  in primary hyperparathyroidism, 165
  in prognosis of acute lymphoblastic leukemia, 1597
  in psychogenic seizures, 2276
  in pubertal growth spurt, 2094
  in rheumatic disease, 830t
  in risk of anaphylaxis, 821
  in sagittal synostosis, 755
  in scoliosis, 2440
  in Sjögren syndrome, 852
  in spinal cord injury, 2248
  in spondyloarthropathies, 825
  in subacute sclerosing panencephalitis, 2310
  in systemic lupus erythematosus, 847
  in systemic-onset juvenile rheumatoid arthritis, 837
  in Takayasu arteritis, 2236
  in thyroid dysgenesis, 2066
  in thyroid neoplasia, 2077
  in trisomy 18, 734
  in ureteroceles, 1736
  in urethral prolapse, 1739
  in urethrorrhagia, 1738
  in Wegener granulomatosis, 846
Gender identity, 470–472, 471t
  public expression of, 470
Gender-identity disorder (GID), 474–475
  differential diagnosis of, 475
  epidemiology of, 474
  etiology of, 474
  natural history and prognosis of, 475
  presentation of, 474
Gender recognition, 471t
Gender risk, of diabetes, in offspring of insulin-dependent parents, 126
Gender role(s)
  definition of, 471t
  and families, 510
Gender-specific activities, 470–471
Gender stability, 470
Gender understanding, 471t
Gene(s). *See also specific gene*
  altered expressions of, in persistent pulmonary hypertension of newborn, 183–184
  and environment, in psychological development, 407–408
  of hemoglobins, 197
  manipulation of
    and role of growth factors in fetal growth, 65
    and role of insulin in fetal growth, 65
  mutations of. *See* Mutation(s)
  promoter of, 573
  wild type versions of, 1585
Gene augmentation, for mucopolysaccharidoses, 661
Gene Clinics, 726
Gene fusion(s). *See also* Chromosomal translocation(s)
  BCR-ABL, 1586, 1603
  MLL-AF4, 1586
  TEL-AML1, 1586
General appearance, examination of, in adolescent, 235
Generalized anxiety disorder (GAD), 455
  epidemiology of, 456

Generalized ataxia, 2166
Generalized epileptic seizures, 2253, 2253t, 2255–2256
  in hypoglycemia, 2130
Generalized juvenile polyposis, 1453
Generalized morphea, 857
Generalized nonscarring alopecia, 1212
Generalized tissue resistance, 2068
Generalized vitiligo, 1193
Gene targets, identification of, 576–577
Gene therapy
  for mucopolysaccharidoses, 661
Genetic anticipation, 2340
Genetic association, 577
Genetic counseling, 578–579, 726
  for anencephaly, 2179
  for autosomal recessive polycystic kidney disease, 1705
  for β-thalassemia trait, 1536
  for Down syndrome, 733
  for Marfan syndrome, 764
  for microcephaly, 786
  for mucopolysaccharidoses, 664
  for muscular atrophy, 2283
  for peroxisome biogenesis disorders, 676
  for renal cystic disorders, 1706f
  for spinal muscular atrophy, 2280
  for X-linked adrenal leukodystrophy, 678
Genetic disorders. *See also specific disorder*
  cancer as, 1585–1586, 1585t
    mutations of tumor suppressor genes, 1585–1586
    oncogene mutations, 1585
  chromosomal disorders. *See* Chromosomal disorders
  classification of, 713
  diagnosis of, 575–576, 576t
    prenatal and preimplantation, 576
  of liver, presenting ages of, 1489t
  multifactorial disorders
    finding genes underlying, 724–725
    recurrence risk for, 722–723
    twin studies for, 723
  neurometabolic and neurodegenerative, 2323–2341
  with nontraditional mechanisms of inheritance, 717
  prevalence of, 713, 721
  principles of care for, 726
  risk factors for, 726t
  single-gene disorders, 713, 715–717
  of skin, 1183–1190
Genetic drift, 721
Genetic electrolyte disorders, 1712–1714
"Genetic locus heterogeneity," 1703
Genetic markers, for differential diagnosis of tumors, 1586
Genetic mutation(s)
  of galactosemia, 1486
  of hereditary hemochromatosis, 1493
  in progressive familial intrahepatic cholestasis, 1493–1494
Genetic potentialities, of psychopathologies, 407
Genetic predisposition
  to acne, 1209
  to affective illnesses, 501
  to aggressive behavior, 446
  to antisocial behavior, 446
  to atherosclerosis, 1890
  to atopy, 809, 811
  to breath-holding spells, 2274
  to cancer, 1586
  to celiac disease, 1418

  to cleft lip and palate, 748
  to congenital heart disease, 1781
  to diabetes mellitus type 1, 2116, 2116t
  to diabetes mellitus type 2, 2112, 2134
  to disruptive behavior, 446
  to fearfulness, 456
  to febrile seizures, 2270
  to focal segmental glomerulonephritis, 1693
  to hemolytic uremic syndrome, 1696
  to Hodgkin disease, 1607
  to inflammatory bowel disease, 1435
  to Langerhans cell histiocytosis, 1625
  to lupus nephritis, 1687
  to neuroblastoma, 1617
  to obesity, 477, 2139
  to obsessive-compulsive disorder, 504
  to peptic ulcer disease, 1433
  to psoriasis, 1180
  to renal agenesis, 1639
  to vesicoureteral reflux, 1671
Genetic sex, 2079
Genetic short stature, 5, 5f
Genetic studies
  of behavior, 407
  of eating disorders, 232
Genetic technologies, 573–577
Genetic testing
  with glottic webs, 1274
  for multiple endocrine neoplasia type 2, 2058
  for oxidative phosphorylation diseases, 649
  for renal developmental disorders, 1642
Gene transfer therapy, for sphingolipidoses, 673
Genioglossus muscle, 1266
Genital herpes, 1030
  maternal, 170
    and transmission to fetus, 170
Genitalia
  accurate naming of, 471
  ambiguous. *See* Ambiguous genitalia
  examination of
    female, 244, 245t
    male, 244
    neonatal, 90
  self-exploration of
    in infants, 470
    in toddlers and preschoolers, 470
  symptoms of sexual abuse in, 466
Genital reconstruction, 2092
Genital system. *See* Reproductive system
Genital tract
  female, chlamydial infection of, 930
  male, chlamydial infection of, 929–930
Genital tract obstructions
  presentation of, 252
  treatment of, 252
Genital tuberculosis, 954
Genital wart(s)
  clinical presentation of, 267
  diagnosis of, 267
  treatment of, 267
Genitourinary system
  male reproductive health history of, 237t
  nuclear imaging of, 589
  radionuclide imaging of, 589
  ultrasonography of, 587
Genitourinary tract
  Candida infections of, 1088
  urologic abnormalities of, 1735–1743
Genitourinary tumors, in rhabdomyosarcoma, 1612
Genodermatoses, 1174
Genome, integrity of, cell cycle checkpoints and, 1587–1588, 1588f

Glucose-6-phosphatase deficiency, 634–635
  dimercaprol and, 370
Glucose-6-phosphate, 724, 2107
Glucose-3-phosphate (G-3-P) deficiency, 1541f
Glucose-6-phosphate (G-6-P) deficiency, 1541f
Glucose-6-phosphate dehydrogenase (G6PD),
    in laboratory algorithm of anemia,
    1522f
Glucose-6-phosphate dehydrogenase (G6PD)
    deficiency, 1542–1543, 1553t
  clinical manifestations of, 1542–1543, 1542t
  kernicterus and, 165
  laboratory diagnosis of, 1542t, 1543,
    1552t–1553t
  methylene blue and, 1545
  and neonatal anemia, 198
  of neutrophils, 1554
  pathophysiology of, 1542
  screening for, before primaquine treatment,
    1140
  testing for, in jaundice, 168
  variants of, 1542
Glucose phosphate isomerase deficiency, 1543t
Glucose polymers, neonatal digestion of,
    109–110
β-Glucosidase deficiency, 670, 2326
α-Glucosidase inhibitors, for diabetes mellitus
    type 2, 2136
Glucosuria
  detection of, 1634
  in Fanconi syndrome, 1709
  renal, 1712
  in total parenteral nutrition, 1348
β-Glucuronidase deficiency, 661
Glucuronidation, defects in, 1489
Glucuronide conjugation, 2062
Glucuronides, in bilirubin conjugation, 166f
Glucuronide sulfoconjugation, 2062
Glue ear. See Otitis media, with effusion
Glue sniffing, 377–378
Glutamate, 2190
Glutamate dehydrogenase gene, and congenital
    hyperinsulinemia, 157
Glutamic acid, 616
Glutamine, 620, 1418
  in management of neonatal hyperglycemia,
    160
γ-Glutamyl cycle, disorders of, 615
Glutamyl cysteine synthetase deficiency, 1543
g-Glutamyl transpeptidase (GGTP)
  in evaluation of liver function, 1476, 1477t
    elevation of, etiology of, 1478, 1479t
  in progressive familial intrahepatic cholesta-
    sis, 1493
Glutaric acidemia
  type I, 613, 627
    newborn screening of, 580t
  type II, 613, 631, 737t, 2299
    mild form, newborn screening of, 580t
    severe form, newborn screening of, 580t
Glutaryl-CoA dehydrogenase, 627
Glutathione, 360
  metabolism of, 1541f
    disorders of, 1543
  and neonatal hypoglycemia, 156
  role of, in red blood cells, 1541
Glutathione deficiency, 615, 1541f
Glutathione synthetase deficiency, 1543
"Gluteal pinking," 1180
Gluten, and celiac disease, 1418
Gluten-free diet, 1420
Glutenin, 1418
Gluten-sensitive enteropathy, 818
D-Glycerate/glyoxylate reductase, 616
Glycerin suppositories, in bowel management
    of disabled children, 540

Glycerol
  for hydrocephalus, 2184
  for intracranial hypertension, 297, 327
  for intracranial pressure control, 2245
  in parenteral nutrition solutions, 1345
Glycerol trioleate/glycerol trierucate (GTO/
    GTE), 2335
Glycine, 625, 1474
  elevated levels, 615
Glycogen, 1320
  deficiency of, in small-for-gestational-age in-
    fants, 121
  depleted stores of, 1480
  functions of, 634
  hepatic stores of
    in newborns, 156
    and postnatal adaptation, 81
  toxic accumulation of, 1487
Glycogen debranching enzyme deficiency, 636
Glycogenin, 634
Glycogenolysis, 2106–2107
  postnatal, 81–82
Glycogenoses
  liver, 634–638
  muscle, 638–640
Glycogen phosphorylase, 82, 2009
Glycogen storage, of fetus and newborns, 1473
Glycogen storage diseases (GSD), 634–640,
    1487, 2296
  clinical presentation of, 1487
    typical age of, 1489t
  diagnosis of, 1487
  metabolic pathways related to, 633f
  suspected, evaluation of, 1476
  treatment of, 1487
  type 0, 638
  type I, 634–635
  type II, 639
  type III, 636
  type IV, 636
  type V, 638
  type VI, 637
  type VII, 639
  type IX, 637–638
  type XI, 638
Glycogen synthase, 2009
Glycogen synthase deficiency, 638
Glycolic acid, 371
Glycolysis, 632, 2114f
  disorders of, 1543–1544, 1543t
    clinical manifestations of, 1544
    genetics of, 1544
    incidence of, 1544
    laboratory findings of, 1544
    pathophysiology of, 1541f, 1544
    treatment of, 1544
  role of, in red blood cell metabolism, 1541
Glycolytic enzymopathies, 1543–1544, 1543t,
    1545t
  clinical manifestations of, 1544
  incidence and genetics of, 1544
  laboratory findings of, 1544
  pathophysiology of, 1544
  treatment of, 1544
Glycopeptide intermediate Staphylococcus au-
    reus (GISA), 992
Glycopeptides, dosage and administration of,
    872t
(P-)Glycoprotein, and multidrug resistance,
    1603
Glycoproteinoses, 663–664
Glycoproteins, 1320
  of platelets, deficiency of, 1559
Glycopyrrolate, for dying patient, 572
Glycosaminoglycans (GAGs), 653, 2329

Glycosides
  cardiac, 383t
    poisoning by, 365–366
      clinical presentation and management
        of, 366
  cyanogenic, 383t
Glycosphingolipids, 665
  distribution and function of, 665
  metabolism of, 666
  synthesis of, inhibitors of, 673
Glycosuria
  corticosteroids and, 1439
  in premature infants, 1659
Glycosylation, congenital disorders of, 1493,
    1553t
Glycosylceramide, 2326
Glycosylphosphatidylinositol, abnormal synthe-
    sis of, 1547
Glyoxylate aminotransferase, 616
Glytrol, 1334t
G_{M2}-Activator deficiency, 2325
GM-CSF (granulocyte-macrophage colony-
    stimulating factor), 1563f
  in infections, 896
GM-CSF (granulocyte-monocyte colony-stim-
    ulating factor), and neonatal neutro-
    penia, 199
G_{M1}-Ganglioside β-galactosidase, 2323
G_{M1}-Gangliosidosis, 668, 2323
G_{M2}-Gangliosidosis, 670, 2324
Gnathostoma spinigerum, 1104
GnRH. See Gonadotropin-releasing hormone
Goal directed persistence, 432
Goal setting for dying patient, 562, 567–568
Goat's milk, 1334t
  anemia and, 1523
  folate in, 1529
Goiter
  diffuse nontoxic, 2073
  endemic, 2071
  familial, 2067
  fetal, 2066, 2068
  lymphadenoid. See Hashimoto thyroiditis
  of newborn, 88
Goitrogenic agents, 2067t
  and acquired juvenile hypothyroidism, 2070
  and congenital hypothyroidism, 2066, 2068
  dietary, 2070–2071
  in groundwater, 2070–2071
Goitrous hypothyroidism, 2067
Goldenhar syndrome, 749t, 754
  and esophageal anomalies, 1386
  ocular manifestations of, 2374
Goldmann-Favre vitreoretinal dystrophy, 2392
"Gold standards," 410, 411f
  for measuring glucose concentrations, 155
Goltz syndrome, 1188
Gomez criteria, 1335
Gomori-Trichrome staining, 648, 2295
Gonad(s)
  embryonic development of, 2080
  indifferent, 242f
Gonadal differentiation, 242, 242f
Gonadal dose, of radiation in selected diagnos-
    tic procedures, 584t
Gonadal dysgenesis, 2088f–2089f. See also
    Turner syndrome
  familial XX, 2089
  familial XY, incomplete form of, 2086
  male pseudohermaphroditism as variant of,
    2086–2087
  XY, 2089
Gonadal dysplasia. See Turner syndrome
Gonadal germ cell tumors, origins of, 1622
Gonadal sex, 2079
Gonadectomy, for Turner syndrome, 2089

Handicapped children, law on education of, 839

Handicapped newborns, refusal of treatment for, 559

Handling, of preterm infant(s), 116

Handling therapy, of neurologic impairment, 544

Hand-Schüller-Christian disease, 1202, 1624
assignment of risk in, 1626
clinical manifestations of, 1625
ocular manifestations of, 2410

Hand splints, 548

Hand-washing, in *Escherichia coli* infection prevention, 1697

Handwriting, disorders of, 435

Hantaviruses, 1025t, 1026

Hantavirus pulmonary syndrome (HPS), 1025t, 1027

Haploidentical donors, for stem cell transplantation, 1592

Haploid number of chromosomes, 718

Haploinsufficiency, 720, 1630

Haplotype analysis, 1704, 1705f

Haptoglobin, 1524

Hard palate, 1266
embryology of, 1267
evaluation of, 1268

Hard ticks, 1153

Hardy-Weinberg law, 715

Harelip, 742

Harlequin color change, 1169
of newborn, 86

Harlequin ichthyosis, 1184

Hartnup disease, 1190, 1426, 1712

Hashimoto thyroiditis, 2021, 2070–2072, 2132

Hashitoxicosis, 2074

HAV infection. *See* Hepatitis A virus (HAV) infection

Havrix, dosage and administration of, 1499t

Hay fever conjunctivitis, 2368

Hay-Wells syndrome, 1189

HbA. *See* Adult hemoglobin

HbCV, 40t

HbF. *See* Fetal hemoglobin

HBIG. *See* Hepatitis B immunoglobulin

HbOC, 48t

HBsAg. *See* Hepatitis B surface antigen

HbSC disease. *See* Hemoglobin S-C (HbSC) disease

HbSS. *See* Sickle cell disease

HBV infection. *See* Hepatitis B virus (HBV) infection

HBV vaccines. *See* Hepatitis B virus (HBV) vaccines

hCG. *See* Human chorionic gonadotropin

β-hCG. *See* β-Human chorionic gonadotropin

HCM. *See* Hypertrophic cardiomyopathy

HCMV. *See* Human cytomegalovirus

HCP. *See* Hereditary coproporphyria

HCV infection. *See* Hepatitis C virus (HCV) infection

HD. *See* Hemodialysis

HDCV. *See* Human diploid cell vaccine

HDL. *See* High-density lipoproteins

HDV infection. *See* Hepatitis D virus (HDV) infection

HE. *See* Hereditary elliptocytosis

Head
examination of, in newborn, 87, 97
malignant tumors of, 1270
masses of
evaluation of, 1279–1281
congenital abnormalities, 1280
infectious masses, 1280

noninfectious inflammatory masses, 1280
tumors, 1281
vasoformative lesions, 1281
magnetic resonance imaging of, 588
positioning of, in neonatal endotracheal intubation, 100

Headache(s), 2412. *See also* Migraine
in CNS tumors, 2209–2210
in craniopharyngioma, 2020
with growing pains, 858
in hydrocephalus, 2183
in miliary tuberculosis, 952
recurrent, 424–425
categories of, 424
clinical manifestations of, 425
epidemiology of, 424
in Rocky Mountain spotted fever, 1014
in systemic lupus erythematosus, 849
in typhus, 1016

Head banging, 460

Head circumference, 784, 2166. *See also* Head size
of breech-positioned infant, 2168
in cerebral palsy, 2200
of vertex-positioned infant, 2168

Head circumference-for-age percentiles
for boys, 2461f
for girls, 2463f

Head control, developmental assessment of, 14t

Head injury(ies). *See also* Head trauma
abusive *vs.* nonabusive, 465
in child abuse, 295, 465
diagnostic studies of, 467
and hearing loss, 1241
and inner ear trauma, 1257
minor, in Alagille syndrome, 1485
physical findings of, in newborns, 87
traumatic, 348

Head lice, 1155, 1156t, 1234–1235, 1235f

"Headlight sign," 1177

Head motion, inner ear detection of, 1239

Head nodding, 460

Head position, of congenital muscular torticollis, 2439, 2439f

Head rolling, 460

Head shape
asymmetric, 10f, 11–12
of breech infants, 87
and craniosynostosis, 10f, 11–12
and intracranial volume, 9
of newborn, 87
posterior flattening of, 11–12
variations in, 9–12

Head size
and blood loss of subaponeurotic hemorrhage, 187
and body size discrepancies, 10
growth of
in preterm infants, 9
rate of, 1, 10
typical patterns of, 5t
and intracranial volume, 9
large, 2166, 2175–2176, 2338
measurement of, 1, 9
schedule for, 2t
of newborns, 105
at different gestational ages, 85f
rapid expansion of, in newborns, 105
small, 784–786, 2166, 2175–2176
of small-for-gestational-age infant, 121
and total body mass, 348
variations in, 9–12

Head Start Program, preschool vision screening program guidelines, 495t

Head tilt, orthoses for, 547

Head-tilting deformity, 2439

Head-tilt maneuver, in cardiopulmonary resuscitation, 328

Head trauma. *See also* Head injury(ies)
cerebral edema with, 2245
craniocerebral trauma, 2242–2248
and epilepsy, 2260
incidence of, 2241
intracranial hemorrhage from, 2238
preretinal hemorrhaging after, 2167
prognosis of, 2246
retinal hemorrhaging after, 2167
seizures after, 2247
skull injuries, 2242

"Head waiter's tip" position, 186

HE agar, 981, 985

Health, of intensive care nursery graduates, 219–220

Health and safety, in nonparental child care settings, 513

Health care
quality of, defining elements to, 535
transition from pediatric to adult, 552

Health care team
ethical implications of, 553
illness in, 887t

Health-care visits
of adolescents, 234–236
changing doctor-patient relationship in, 234
for contraceptives, 259
medical history in, 232t, 234–235, 234f
sexual history, 243–244
transitional interview, 234
family structure and, 511

Health consultants, and nonparental childcare, 513

Health decision-making skills, 430

Health Department, inspection for lead contamination by, 370

Health insurance
adolescents and, 226
heart disease and, 1901

Health needs, of disabled young adults, 551

Health neglect, 463

Health supervision
anticipatory guidance in, 26–39
of foster care, 523t
of growth, 1–12
immunizations in, 39–52
of disabled children, 541, 541t
of motor development, 12–19
overview of, 1
of psychological development, 12–19
schedule for, 2t, 4t
screening programs in, 19–25

Hearing. *See also under* Auditory
assessment of. *See also* Audiometry
crude, 1242
in intensive care nursery graduates, 220
in language delay, 19
in newborns, 92
schedule for, 2t
in speech delay, 19, 443
estimate of, in newborn, 88
and language development, 409
pathology of, signs and symptoms of, 1241
screening tests of, 21–22, 488
in adolescence, 22
in newborns, 22, 106
in preschoolers, 22
risk factors warranting, 22
spectrum of, 485t
testing, 2167

Hearing aids, 488, 546t

Hearing impairment (HI)
age of onset of, 21
assessment and diagnosis of, 486–488, 487f
classification of, 783
cognitive and educational performance in, 783
congenital cytomegalovirus infection and, 220
definition and epidemiology of, 485, 485t, 534t
with extracorporeal membrane oxygenation, 221
in extremely low-birth-weight children, 61
genetics of, 783
hyperbilirubinemia and, 167
incidence of, 782
in intensive care nursery graduates, 220
in Klippel-Feil syndrome, 2440
management and treatment of, 488–489
in mumps, 1057
nonsyndromic autosomal recessive, 1241
nonsyndromic hereditary
genetic discoveries of, 1241, 1241t
inheritance of, 1241
in otitis media with effusion, 1253
persistent pulmonary hypertension and, 220–221
prevalence of, 534t
risk factors for, 21–22
syndromic, 1241
Hearing loss, 782–784. See also Deafness
abnormalities of endolymphatic apparatus, 1239
acquired, 1245, 1245f, 1246t
central, 2200
cerumen and, 1242
clinical manifestations of, 486
conductive, in chronic otitis media, 1255
congenital, 1245, 1245f, 1246t
degrees of, 485t
diagnosis of, 783f
epidemiology of, 485
etiology of, 486, 486t
head trauma and, 1241
incidence of, 1241
inheritance of, 1241
kernicterus and, 167
and language development impairment, 22
management of, 487f
natural history and prognosis of, 489
neonatal risk criteria, 486–488
perinatal complications and risk of, 1242
peripheral, 2200
risk factors for, 1245, 1246t
sensorineural
assessment and diagnosis of, 488
in chronic otitis media, 1255
definition of, 485
etiology of, 486, 486t, 1245
hyperbilirubinemia and, 167
in short-gestation children, 61
from streptomycin, 957
suspected, algorithm for, 1245f
types of, 485
Hearing problems, continuum of, impairment to deafness in, 485–489
assessment and diagnosis of, 486–488, 487f
clinical manifestations of, 486
definitions and epidemiology of, 485, 485t
etiology and pathogenesis of, 486, 486t
management and treatment of, 488–489
natural history and prognosis of, 489
Heart. See also under Cardiac
bootshaped, 1821
changes in, during adolescence, 223
complications of, in sickle cell disease, 1534

diagram of normal, 1814f
embryonic development of, 1745, 1746f–1748f
extrathoracic, 89
impaired contractile function of, 287, 288f, 289t
life-threatening infections of, 305t
malposition of, 1836
neonatal examination of, 89
radionuclide imaging of, 589
reduced output of, 287, 288f, 289t
Heart block, of newborn, presentation of, 207
Heartburn
in esophagitis, 1391
in herpes simplex virus esophagitis, 1394
in mixed connective tissue disease, 851
in upper abdominal distress, 1359
Heart failure
in adolescents, 1869
in atrial septal defect, 1794
congestive. See Congestive heart failure
diastolic, management of, 1877
in fetus, 1869
in newborns, 1861, 1869, 1872
in premature infants, 1869
Heart-lung transplantation, 1889
Heart murmur(s). See Murmurs
Heart rate
changes in
during adolescence, 223
after birth, 1753
decreased, and impaired perfusion, 287, 288f, 289t
monitoring, 312
of newborns, 89, 104
abnormal, 206–207
in Apgar scoring system, 99t
and external cardiac compression, 101
in perfusion restoration, 292
response of, to decreased cardiac output, 287
Heart sounds
first, 1755
fourth, 1755
in newborns, 89, 1755
second, 1755
third, 1755
Heart transplantation
endomyocardial biopsy in, 1778
indications for, 1886
long-term complications of, 1887–1888
operative and postoperative management of, 1887
recipient and donor selection for, 1886
rehabilitation in, 1888
rejection of, 1887
survival after, 1886f
Heat
absorption of, 388
and airway pressure, in obstructive respiratory impairments, 275–276
elimination of, decreased, 389
illness related to, 388–390
loss of
of fetus, 80
mechanisms for, 388
of newborn, 80–81, 103
prevention of, 104
of preterm newborn, 115
in small-for-gestational-age infant, 121
production of, 388
control of, 80
of fetus, 80
of newborn, 80
Heat applications
for fibromyalgia, 862

for hypermobility syndrome, 860
for reflex sympathetic dystrophy syndrome, 861
Heat cramps, 389
treatment of, 390
Heat exchange, between preterm newborn and environment, 115
Heat exchanger, in extracorporeal membrane oxygenation, 213
Heat exhaustion, 389
Heat-shock protein 60 (HSP 60), 300
Heat stress, 388–390
Heatstroke, 388–389
mental function in, 389
prevention of, 390
prognosis and outcome of, 390
treatment of, 390, 390f
Heat syncope, 389
Heel cords, contracted (equinus contracture of ankle)
and equinus deformity, 2420
in flatfeet, 2429
Heel pain, 2427
Height. See also Short stature; Tall stature
adult, prediction of, 1, 5t
body weight and, 1318t, 1335
growth patterns of, typical, 5t
measurement of, 1, 2015
schedule for, 2t
parenteral target, 2014
short, genetic, 5, 5f
Height restriction, 2024
Height standard deviation scores, 2015
Height velocity centiles
for boys, 2470f
for girls, 2470f
Heimlich maneuver, asymptomatic foreign-body aspiration and, 383
Heinz bodies
demonstration of, 1535
in glucose-6-phosphate dehydrogenase deficiency, 1542
splenic "pitting" of, 1560
of unstable hemoglobins, 1535
Hektoen enteric (HE) agar, 981, 985
Helical computed tomography (helical CT), 587
Helicobacter pylori eradication therapy, 1435
for functional dyspepsia, 1362
Helicobacter pylori infection, 1430
abdominal pain in, 1359
chronic vomiting in, 1352
detecting, 1431, 1434
in gastric adenocarcinoma, 1430, 1432
in gastric lymphomas, 1456
in gastritis, 1430, 1432
in mucosa-associated lymphoid tumors, 1430, 1432
mucus-bicarbonate barrier and, 1430
in peptic ulcer disease, 1430, 1432–1433
Heliotrope sign, 1198
Heliox, therapy with, 1922
Heller myotomy, for achalasia, 1388
HELLP (hemolysis, elevated liver tests, and low platelets), maternal
and liver disease in infant, 1479
and neonatal neutropenia, 199
Helmet molding, 12
Helminthic infestations
eosinophilia of, 1555
treatment of, 1098–1101
Hemachromatosis, 1326t
Hemagglutination-inhibition (HI) antibody determination, in measles, 1054
Hemangioendothelioma(s), 1508, 1620
diagnosis of, 1620–1621, 1620t

of skin, eye, and/or mouth, in newborns, 171–172, 171t, 173t
after transplantation, 1735
treatment of, 1031
type 1, 1029, 1220, 2305
in blepharitis, 2365
clinical manifestations of, 1029t
treatment of, 1029t
type 2, 1029, 1220
clinical manifestations of, 1029t
treatment of, 1029t
typing methods of, 169
Herpes virus encephalitis, 294–295, 2307
brainstem, 2308
neonatal, 2313
in newborns, 171
Herpes virus infection(s)
antiviral therapy for, 883
and hepatitis, 1500
and Hodgkin disease, 1607
after liver transplantation, 1517
in newborn, 169–173
Herpes zoster. See Varicella-zoster virus (VZV) infections; Zoster
Herpes zoster keratoconjunctivitis, 2377
Herpes zoster ophthalmicus, 2377
Herpetic blepharitis, 2365
Herpetic gingivostomatitis, 1294
Herpetic whitlow, 1030, 1200, 1221
Herpetiform ulcers, 1295
Hers disease, 637
HES (Hypereosinophilic syndrome), 1555
Heschl's gyrus, overproduction and retraction of synapses in, 409
Heterochromia irides, 2381
Heterogametic sex, 2079
Heterologous hormones, receptors affected by, 2010
Heterophil antibodies, 1037
Heterophoria, 2353
Heteroplasmy, 644, 719
Heteroplasty, 598
Heterotaxia
and asplenia or polysplenia, 1561
liver transplantation and, 1481
Heterotopia, 1464
Heterotropia. See Strabismus
Heterozygosity, loss of (LOH), in Wilms tumor, 1615–1616
Heterozygous carriers, 715, 717
Heterozygous hypobetalipoproteinemia, 706t–707t
Hetrazan. See Diethylcarbamazine
HEV infection. See Hepatitis E virus (HEV) infection
HEXA. See β-Hexosaminidase α-subunit
Hexachlorobenzene, 687
Hexachlorophene, toxicity of, in preterm newborns, 147
n-Hexane abuse, 378
HEXB. See β-Hexosaminidase β-subunit
Hexokinase deficiency, 1543t
Hexokinase I, 1473
Hexokinase method, for measuring blood glucose concentrations, 155
β-Hexosaminidase A, 2324
β-Hexosaminidase α-subunit (HEXA), 2324
deficiency of, 2324
β-Hexosaminidase β-subunit (HEXB), 2324
deficiency of, 2325
β-Hexosaminidase deficiency, 669
Hexose monophosphate shunt (HMP)
disorders of, 1542–1543
and erythrocyte metabolism, 1541–1542, 1541f

role of, in bacterial killing of phagocytosis, 1550
HFFI. See High-frequency flow interruption
HFJV. See High-frequency jet ventilation
HFOV. See High-frequency oscillatory ventilation
HFRS. See Hemorrhagic fever with renal syndrome
HFV. See High-frequency ventilation
HGE. See Human granulocytic ehrlichiosis
HGPRT deficiency. See Hypoxanthine guanine phosphoribosyl transferase (HGPRT) deficiency
HGV infection. See Hepatitis G virus (HGV) infection
HHH syndrome. See Hyperornithinemia, hyperammonemia, homocitrullinuria (HHH) syndrome
HHT (hereditary hemorrhagic telangiectasia). See Osler-Rendu-Weber disease
HHV. See Human herpes virus(es)
HHV-1. See Herpes simplex virus (HSV) infection, type 1
HHV-2. See Herpes simplex virus (HSV) infection, type 2
HHV-3. See Varicella-zoster virus (VZV) infections
HHV-4. See Epstein-Barr virus (EBV) infection
HHV-5. See Cytomegalovirus (CMV) infection
HHV-6. See Human herpesvirus 6
HHV-7. See Human herpesvirus 7
HHV-8. See Human herpesvirus 8
HI. See Hearing impairment; Hemagglutination-inhibition (HI) antibody determination
Hiatal hernia, perioperative care of, 340
HiB. See Haemophilus influenzae type B disease
HiB vaccine. See Haemophilus influenzae type B (HiB) vaccine
Hickman catheters, 322t, 323
Hidradenitis suppurativa, 1215
Hidrotic ectodermal dysplasia, 1189
HIE. See Hypoxic-ischemic encephalopathy
HIE (hyperimmunoglobulin E syndrome), 1553
High-altitude exposure
and heart disease, 1898
and oxygen dissociative curve, 1522
and respiratory pauses of infants, 205
High-arched palate, 88
High-carbohydrate diet(s)
for glycogen storage disease, 637–638
for very long-chain acyl-CoA dehydrogenase deficiency, 630
High-density lipoproteins (HDL), 693, 1890
deficiency of, 708, 709t–710t
disorders of metabolism of, 702
normal levels of, in first two decades of life, 696t
properties of, 693t
High-efficiency air-filtering systems, 815
High-fiber diet(s)
benefits of, 1320
for constipation, 1320, 1362, 1370
for diarrhea, 1362
for functional abdominal pain, 1362
High-frequency flow interruption (HFFI), 212
High-frequency jet ventilation (HFJV), 212
High-frequency jet ventilators, 318f, 319
High-frequency oscillators, 318f, 319
High-frequency oscillatory ventilation (HFOV), 212
for congenital diaphragmatic hernia, 190
gas exchange in, 212
for hyaline membrane disease, 134

with inhaled nitric oxide, 212, 216
with partial liquid ventilation, 218
for persistent pulmonary hypertension of newborn, 185, 212
High-frequency ventilation (HFV), 318–319, 318f
and chronic lung disease, 212
for congenital diaphragmatic hernia, 190
for hyaline membrane disease, 212
for meconium aspiration syndrome, 196
for newborn, 212
applications of, 212
risks associated with, 212
for pulmonary interstitial emphysema, 150
High-grade lymphoma, stem cell transplantation for, 1590t
High-grade squamous intraepithelial lesion (HSIL), 254, 265f, 267
screening for, 268
treatment for, 268
High imperforate anus, 204
Highly active antiretroviral therapy (HAART), 1049, 1415
hepatotoxicity of, 1510
for Kaposi sarcoma, 1042
High-molecular-weight kininogen, 1568f
deficiency of, 1574
High-phosphate diet, 1634
High-pressure liquid chromatography (HPLC)
for measuring steroid levels, 2035
for mycobacteria analysis, 960
High-protein diet(s)
body building diets, 1320
for glycogen storage disease, 639
High-resolution analysis, 727
High-risk screening, 581t
of hypoglycemia, in newborns, 106
for inborn errors of metabolism, 580–582, 581t
of metabolic acidosis, 581t
High school, learning period of, 436
Hilar adenopathy
in pneumonia, 1982
in pulmonary tuberculosis, 951f
Hilar lymphadenopathy, with tuberculosis, 951
Hillocks of His, 1240
Hill posterior gastropexy, for gastroesophageal reflux disease, 1393
Hindbrain, 2175
development of, 408
Hindfoot rigidity, examination of, in cavus foot, 2429
Hindgut, 1307, 1307f–1308f, 1457
pain originating from, 1354
"Hind milk," fat content of, 109
Hinman syndrome, 1671
Hip(s), 2434–2438
of breech infants, 91, 2435
developmental dysplasia of. See Developmental dysplasia of hip
development of, 2434
dislocation and subluxation of
in arthrogryposis multiplex congenita, 2456
in congenital knee dislocation, 2430
in myelomeningocele, 2455
in neuromuscular disorders, 2456
persistent, structural changes of, 2435
prenatal, 2435
teratologic, 2435
typical, 2435
examination of, 2421, 2435–2436, 2435f
tests for, 2435–2436
infection of, evaluation and differential diagnosis of, 2422

Hyperglycemia (*contd.*)
 in infants of diabetic mothers, 124
 without ketoacidosis, 2123
 in newborns, 159–160
  complications of, 160
  consequences of, 102
  definition of, 159
  diagnosis of, 159
  epidemiology of, 159
  etiology of, 159–160
  management of, 160
  pathophysiology of, 160
 postsurgical, 159
 and prognosis of drowning and near drowning, 382
 in small-for-gestational-age infants, 122, 123t
 in total parenteral nutrition, 1348
Hyperglycinemia
 ketotic, 613
 nonketotic, 615
Hypergonadotropic hypogonadism, 2102t
Hyperhomocysteinemia, 1530, 1575
Hyper-IgE syndrome, skin disorders in, 1189
Hyper-IgM immunodeficiency, 797
 genetic bases of, 794t
Hyperimmunoglobulin E syndrome (HIE), 1553, 1553t
Hyperinfection, 1109
Hyperinsulinemia
 atherosclerosis from, 1890
 autosomal-dominant familial, 2109
 congenital, types of, 157
 diagnosis of, 157, 2110
 in erythroblastosis fetalis, 175
 of infants of diabetic mothers, 124
  and development of macrosomia, 125
 management of, 158
 and neonatal hypoglycemia, 156–157
 in neonatal hypoglycemia, 157t
 outcome of, 159
 in small-for-gestational-age infants, 122
 of sulfonylurea overdose, 373
 from sulfonylurea receptor mutation, 157, 2011
Hyperkalemia, 1653–1654
 in acute lymphoblastic leukemia, 1595
 in acute renal failure, 1676
 from blood transfusion, 1577, 1579
 digoxin overdose and, 366
 electrocardiography in, 1654f, 1762
 in erythropoietin therapy, 1724
 of fluid resuscitation, 387
 with hyponatremia, 1650
 in newborns, treatment of, 102
 in renal tubular acidosis, 1711–1712
 therapeutic interventions in, 1654t
 in very preterm newborns, 115
 treatment of, 115
Hyperkalemic periodic paralysis, 2294
Hyperkeratosis, 1185
Hyperkinetic child. *See* Attention-deficit hyperactivity disorder
Hyperlipidemia, 696–698
 causes of, 698t
 diagnosis of, 22, 576t
 familial combined, 700
 hyponatremia from, 1650
 from sirolimus, 1733
 from steroids, 850
 thrombosis in nephrotic syndrome from, 1696
 in total parenteral nutrition, 1348
 treatment of, 702

Hyperlipoproteinemia, 696–698
 causes of, 698t
 metabolic disorders with, 698–704
  treatment of, 702–704
   dietary, 702–703
   drug therapy, 703–704, 703t
  type III, 701
  type V, 701
Hyperlysinemia, 614, 859
Hypermagnesemia, 2164
Hypermobility syndrome, 859–860
Hypermobility type of Ehlers-Danlos syndrome, 765, 766t
Hypernatremia, 1651–1652
 algorithm for assessment of, 1652f
 in nephrogenic diabetes insipidus, 1714
 water loss in preterm newborns and, 112
Hyperopia, 489, 492, 2361
 in newborns, 492
Hyperornithinemia, hyperammonemia, homocitrullinuria (HHH) syndrome, 618, 620, 2257, 2308
 newborn screening of, 580t
Hyperosmolar agents, 585
 for intracranial pressure control, 2245
Hyperosmolar water-soluble enema, for meconium ileus, 203
Hyperoxaluria, 616, 1716, 2159
 causes of, 1716t
 after renal transplantation, 1731
Hyperoxia, consequences of, in neonatal oxygen administration, 100
Hyperoxia-induced pulmonary vasodilation, 284
Hyperparathyroidism
 hypercalcemia and, 2154t
  diagnosis of, 163
  signs of, 163
 in multiple endocrine neoplasia type 1, 2057
 in multiple endocrine neoplasia type 2, 2058
 and myopathies, 2303
 neonatal severe primary, 163
 primary. *See* Primary hyperparathyroidism
Hyperphenylalaninemia, 609, 611
 newborn screening of, 580t
Hyperphoria, 2402
Hyperphosphatemia, 1634
 in acute lymphoblastic leukemia, 1595
 in acute renal failure, 1676
 and hypocalcemia, 2150t, 2151
 of infants of diabetic mothers, 125
 in newborn, 161, 2149
 and parathyroid hormone, 2147
 prevention of, 1727
Hyperpigmentation, 1167
 in autoimmune adrenalitis, 2042
 causes of, 1193
 in discoid lupus erythematosus, 1198
 in hypohidrotic ectodermal dysplasia, 1189
 in incontinentia pigmenti, 1186
 in plexiform neurofibroma, 1213
 postinflammatory, 1193
 in scleroderma, 1199
 treatment of, 1193
Hyperpituitarism. *See* Growth hormone excess
Hyperplastic candidiasis, 1293
Hyperplastic gums, 662f
Hyperpnea, 272
 in metabolic encephalopathy, 294
Hyperprolactinemia
 etiology of, 249
 and interrupted puberty, 2057
Hyperprolinemia, 616
Hypersensitive xiphoid, 1895
Hypersensitivity
 carotid sinus, 1893

 to drugs, 1194
 immediate and late phase of, 810
 and impaired self-regulation, 403
 to insect bites, 1233
 skin testing for, 813
 TH2 cells and, 809
Hypersensitivity pneumonitis, 1994–1995
 etiology of, 1994, 1994t
Hypersensitivity reactions, 1195–1196
Hypersplenic syndrome(s), splenectomy for, 1562t
Hypersplenism, 1561
Hypertelorism, 749t, 2408
Hypertension, 1877–1885
 in acute poststreptococcal glomerulonephritis, 1678
 amphetamine overdose and, 377
 arterial. *See* Arterial hypertension
 atherosclerosis from, 1890
 benign intracranial, 2398
 causes of, 1879, 1879t
  age-related, 1879t
 and chronic renal insufficiency progression, 1718
 control of, before transplantation, 1731
 definition of, 22, 1877
 diagnosis of, 1879–1882, 1880t, 1882t
 effects of, 1878
 in erythropoietin therapy, 1724
 essential, 1885
 evaluation of, 2036
 after heart transplantation, 1887
 in hemolytic uremic syndrome, 1697
 isolated systolic, causes of, 1878
 maternal, 776t
  and fetal growth, 65
  and neonatal neutropenia, 199
 moderate, 1879, 1882
 portal, in end-stage renal disease, 1732
 posttransplant, 1735, 1887
 pulmonary. *See* Pulmonary hypertension
 after renal transplantation, 1735
 severe, 1880, 1882, 1882t
 standards of, 1877
 stress-related, 530t
 sustained, 1880t
 in toxic ingestions and exposures, 357t
 treatment of, 1882–1885
  emergency, 1882, 1883t
  hypotensive drugs in, 1882–1885, 1883t–1884t
  long-term, 1882
 "white coat," 1882
 in Wilms tumor, 1615
Hyperthermia, 302, 388–390
 in amphetamine overdose, 377
 causes of, 389
 classification of, 389
 effects of, 389–390
 vs. fever, 388
 malignant, 337, 2296
 in newborns, 207
  causes of, 84
  prevention of, 99
  risk factors, 1168
 physiology of temperature regulation and, 388
 during pregnancy, 776t
 prevention of, 390
 prognosis and outcome of, 390
 in toxic ingestions and exposures, 357t
 treatment of, 390
Hyperthyroidism, 2074–2077. *See also* Graves disease
 activating G-protein mutations and, 2077
 and attention deficits, 431, 433

in carbon monoxide poisoning, 363
diagnostic algorithm of, 282f
in *d*-transposition, 1824
etiology of, 280, 281f, 1909
fetal
chronic, and fetal hematocrit, 192
and glycogen deficiency, 121
fetal circulatory response to, 188
in hyaline membrane disease, 129
hypoventilation and, 283
in intracranial hypertension, 296
management of, 284
mechanism of, 280
in meconium aspiration syndrome, 194
of newborns, inhaled nitric oxide therapy for, 78–216
in persistent pulmonary hypertension of newborn, 188
prevention of, 280
without respiratory distress, 272
signs of, 278
supplemental oxygen administration for, 317
ventilation-perfusion inequality and, 272
Hypoxemic respiratory failure
inhaled nitric oxide therapy for, 216
respiratory support for, 319
Hypoxemic spells, 1826
Hypoxia
cerebral, neonatal hypoglycemia and, 157
cerebral injury of, 295
of drowning and near drowning, 380
of fetus
and fetal heart rate patterns, 71, 74
management of, 74
and meconium aspiration syndrome, 194
intrauterine
and neonatal hemoglobin concentrations, 197
in small-for-gestational-age infants, 123
Hypoxic-ischemic encephalopathy (HIE), 295, 2190–2195
intracranial pressure monitoring in, 297
long-term outcome of, in intensive care nursery graduates, 221
neonatal cerebral infarction from, 2237
neonatal seizures from, 2268
in newborn, 2190–2193, 2192f–2193f
in premature newborn, 2193–2195
severity of, 2190t
in submersion injuries, 380
Hypoxic vasoconstriction, supplemental oxygen administration for, 317
Hypsarhythmia, 2258
Hyrtl anastomosis, 62
Hysteresis, 275, 276f
Hysterical edema. *See* Reflex sympathetic dystrophy syndrome
Hysterical syncope, 1893

I

IAHS. *See* Infection-associated hemophagocytic syndrome
IASP. *See* International Association for the Study of Pain
Iatrogenic Cushing syndrome, 2045
Iatrogenic steroid myopathy, 2303
Iatrogenic trauma, 2251
IBD. *See* Inflammatory bowel disease
Ibuprofen
acute renal failure from, 1674
dosage and administration of, 343t
and dysmenorrhea, 254
for enthesitis-related arthritis, 841
for fever, 303

for Langerhans cell histiocytosis, 1626
for patent ductus arteriosus, 137
for serum sickness, 823
Ibutilide, for arrhythmia, 1850t
ICD (implantable cardioverter-defibrillator), 1853
ICD (intracondylar distance), of knees, in quantification of genu varum, 2431f
"Ice cube test," 1195
Iceland disease, 2314
Ice-water immersion, for heatstroke, 390
Ichthyosiform disorders, 1184–1185
Ichthyosis, 85, 1183–1184
Ichthyosis linearis circumflexa, 1184
Ichthyosis vulgaris, 1183, 1183f
Icterus gravis neonatorum, in erythroblastosis fetalis, 174
ICU. *See* Intensive care units
Identical twins. *See* Monozygotic (MZ) twins
Identity disorder, diagnostic criteria for, 474t
Idiopathic anaphylaxis, 821
Idiopathic chondrolysis ("dry socket") disease, 2422
Idiopathic chronic childhood arthritis. *See* Juvenile rheumatoid arthritis
Idiopathic chronic diarrhea of infancy, 1420–1421
differential diagnosis of, 1421
etiology of, 1420
pathogenesis of, 1420
treatment of, 1421
Idiopathic clubfoot, 2425
Idiopathic constipation. *See* Functional fecal retention
Idiopathic epilepsy, 2256
Idiopathic epiphyseal ischemic necroses
Köhler disease, 2427, 2427f
Legg-Calvé-Perthes disease. *See* Legg-Calvé-Perthes disease
Osgood-Schlatter disease, 224t, 2432
Scheuermann disease, 2442–2443, 2444t
Idiopathic hypertrophic subaortic stenosis (IHSS), 1805
Idiopathic hypopituitarism, 2018
and adrenal insufficiency, 2044
and delayed puberty, 2103
diabetes mellitus in, 2019
Idiopathic infantile hypercalcemia, 163–164, 2152
Idiopathic inflammatory myopathies (IIM), 853
Idiopathic inflammatory orbital pseudotumor, 2409
Idiopathic neonatal hepatitis, 1479t–1480t, 1505–1506, 1514t
clinical findings of, 1505
diagnosis of, 1505
treatment of, 1479t–1480t, 1506
Idiopathic pulmonary hemosiderosis, 1997–1998
iron deficiency of, 1527
primary *versus* secondary, 1997
Idiopathic scoliosis, 2441–2442, 2442f–2443f, 2443t
orthoses for, 547
Idiopathic short stature, 2015, 2020
Idiopathic thrombocytopenic purpura (ITP), 1556–1557, 1556f
clinical course of, 1557
clinical features of, 1556
in common variable immunodeficiency, 801
laboratory features of, 1556–1557, 1556f
maternal, 1557–1558
and neonatal thrombocytopenia, 200
treatment of, 1557

Idiopathic toe walking, 2428
Idiosyncratic hepatotoxic reactions, 1503
IDL. *See* Intermediate-density lipoprotein
Idling, in extracorporeal membrane oxygenation, 214
IDMs. *See* Infant(s), of diabetic mothers
Idoxuridine, for ocular herpes simplex virus infection, 173
Iduronate-2-sulfatase deficiency. *See* Hunter syndrome
α-L-Iduronidase, 2329
α-L-Iduronidase deficiency. *See* Hurler syndrome
IE. *See* Infective endocarditis
IEM. *See* Inborn errors of metabolism
IEP. *See* Individualized Educational Plan
IFA. *See* Indirect fluorescence antibody
Ifosfamide
for choroid plexus tumors, 2228
for Ewing sarcoma-PNET, 1612
and hypokalemia, 1653
for neuroblastoma, 1619
neurotoxicity of, 2229t
for osteosarcoma, 1610
for Wilms tumor relapse, 1616
IgA
in breast milk, 1319
secretion of, 1312
IgA deficiency
in ataxia-telangiectasia, 798
celiac disease in, 1419
and common variable immunodeficiency, 800
detecting, 1419
genetic bases of, 794t
and immunodeficiency, 797
and rheumatic disease, 831
IgA nephropathy, 1682–1684
age of onset of, 1678t
classical histologic features of, 1679t
clinical manifestations of, 1683
epidemiology of, 1682
laboratory findings in, 1683
pathogenesis of, 1683
prognosis of, 1684
recurrent, after transplantation, 1730
recurrent painless macroscopic hematuria in, 1677, 1683
treatment of, 1683
IgE
genetic predisposition to generate, 809, 811
measuring levels of, 814
production of, regulation of, 810
IgE deficiency, in ataxia-telangiectasia, 798
IgE-dependent allergic inflammation, 811
IgE-independent allergic inflammation, 811
IgE-induced immediate hypersensitivity, 810
IgE-mediated hypersensitivity
allergic rhinitis, 817
anaphylaxis, 821
food allergy, 818
latex allergy, 819
IgE receptors, 810
IGFBPs. *See* Insulin-like growth factor-binding proteins
IGF-I. *See* Insulin-like growth factor I
IGF-II. *See* Insulin-like growth factor II
IGFs. *See* Insulin-like growth factors
IgG antibodies
maternal
to A and B antigens, 177
to D antigen, 175
and neonatal neutropenia, 199
in neonatal period, 304
pretransfusion testing of, 1578

coagulase-negative staphylococci in, 993
coccidioidomycosis in, 1091
cryptosporidiosis in, 1127–1128
cyclosporiasis in, 1129
   treatment of, 1129
cystitis in, 1088
cytomegalovirus infection in, 1033–1034,
   1047, 1394, 1433
   treatment of, 1034
esophagitis in, 1088
fever in, 803, 806t
folliculitis in, 1217
gastrointestinal candidiasis in, 1088
gastrointestinal diseases in, 1412–1415
graft-*versus*-host disease in, 1448
granulomatous amebic encephalitis in, 1130
herpes simplex virus esophagitis in, 1395
herpes simplex virus infections in, 1031
human herpesvirus 6 infection in, 1040
inactivated vaccines in, 793
influenza virus infection in, treatment of,
   1071–1072
intracranial infection in, 2319
isosporiasis in, 1132–1133
laryngeal candidiasis in, 1088
live virus vaccines in, 793
measles in, 1055, 2311
microsporidiosis in, 1143
Moraxella catarrhalis infections in, 949
nontuberculous mycobacterial infections in,
   960–961
Norwegian scabies in, 1234
oral thrush in, 1088
   treatment of, 1080t
Pneumocystis carinii pneumonia in, 1144
recurrent infections in, 791–793
scabies in, 1154
small intestine and colon infections in, 1447
toxoplasmosis in, 1146
   treatment of, 1147
vaccines in, 793, 803–804
vaginitis in, 1088
varicella-zoster virus infection in, 1043, 2311
   treatment of, 1044
viral infections of CNS in, 2311
Yersinia enterocolitica infection in, 1012
zoster in, 1044
Immunosuppression, 300
for autoimmune hepatitis, 1504
and non-Hodgkin lymphoma, 1604
in stem cell transplantation, 1591f
Immunosuppressive therapy
for anti-GBM disease, 1687
for autoimmune enteropathy, 1422
for dermatomyositis, 1198, 2302
for focal segmental glomerulonephritis, 1694
after heart transplantation, 1887, 1889
in hepatitis B, 1682
long-term toxicity of, 1593
for lupus nephritis, 848, 1688
for membranous nephropathy, 1695
for minimal-change nephrotic syndrome,
   1693
for polyarteritis nodosa, 846
in renal transplantation, 1733
for renal vasculitis, 1691
for subacute sclerosing panencephalitis, 2310
for Takayasu arteritis, 2236
vaccines in, 804
for X-linked lymphoproliferative disease, 801
Immunotherapy
for asthma, 1959
for septic shock, 899
Impact, 1334t
Impacted foreign bodies
   location of, 383t

signs and symptoms of, 383t
Impact seizures, 2247
Impact syndrome, 465
Impairment, definition of, 533
Imperforate anus, 90, 204
Impetigo, 1217
   bullous, 1217, *(Color Plate 17)*
     diagnosis of, 1173
   nonbullous (crusted), 1217
   streptococcal, 996
     treatment of, 998
   therapy for, 992
"Impetigo contagiosa," 996
Impingement syndrome, 2448
Implantable cardioverter-defibrillator (ICD),
   1853
Implantable catheters, 323
Implantation preparation phase, 240
Implied consent, 560
Imipramine, for dying patient, 571
Impulse control, 431
Impulsive petit mal. *See* Juvenile myoclonic epi-
   lepsy
Impulsivity
   manifestation of, in attention deficits, 431t,
     432
   vulnerable child syndrome and, 515
IMRT. *See* Intensity-modulate radiation ther-
   apy
IMV. *See* Intermittent mandatory ventilation
Inactivated poliovirus (IPV) vaccine, 804
   advantages of, 46
   chronic conditions and, 541t
   contraindications to, 44t
   vs. oral poliovirus vaccine, 45–46
   route and dose of, 40t
Inactivated vaccines, in immunodeficient patients, 793
Inactivation center, 716
Inadvertent positive end-expiratory pressure
   (inadvertent PEEP), 209, 316f
Inattention
   with autistic disorder, 500
   manifestation of, in attention deficits, 431t,
     432
   secondary, 431
   situational, 431
Inborn errors of metabolism (IEM), 597–608,
   597f, 598t. *See also specific disorder*
   of bile acid, 1488, 1493t
     evaluation of, 1476
   diagnosis of, 578–583, 602f, 604f, 606f,
     607
   with dysmorphic features, 607, 607t, 676f,
     679–682, 686t
   of fatty acid oxidation, clinical features of,
     1496t
   and growth failure, 2023
   liver involvement in, 1485
   natural history of, 580
   ocular deformities in, 2379
   prenatal management of, 78–79
   of purine, 1531
   of pyrimidine, 1531
   screening for
     high-risk, 581t
     in newborns, in postnatal care and obser-
       vation, 106
Inbreeding, 721
Incarceration, risk of, in inguinal hernias,
   204
"Incidental" thrombocytopenia, 1557
Incision and suction, for pit viper bites, 397
Inclusion blennorrhea, 2372
   chlamydial conjunctivitis, 2372–2373
   in newborn, 88

Inclusion body myositis, 2302
Inclusion cell, 2331
Inclusion conjunctivitis, newborn, 930
Incompetent cervix, 67
Incomplete isosexual precocity. *See* Gonadotro-
   pin-releasing hormone (GnRH)-inde-
   pendent precocious puberty
Incomplete penetrance, 714
Incomplete right bundle branch block, 1761
Incontinence. *See* Fecal incontinence; Urinary
   incontinence
Incontinentia pigmenti, 1186, 2347, *(Color
   Plate 8)*
   koilonychia from, 1216
Incontinentia pigmenti achromians, 1194, 2347
Increased cellularity, 2223
Incredibly low-birth-weight (ILBW) infants,
   220
   handicaps of, 221
   incidence of major disability in, 220
"Incretins," and neonatal hyperglycemia, 160
Incubator(s)
   historical perspective of, 55–56
   for hypothermic newborns, 104
   temperature in, monitoring, 104
   for transport of preterm newborn, 116
"Incubator revolution," 55–56
Incus, embryology of, 1240
Incyclophoria, 2402
Incyclotropia, 2402
Independence, 403
   and chronic illness or disability, 429
   phase of, 509
Indeterminate frontal-plane axis, 1760
Indeterminate leprosy, 964t
India, leprosy in, 963
Indifferent gonad(s), 242f
Indinavir
   drug interactions, 1082t
   for human immunodeficiency virus infection,
     1051t
Indirect bilirubin. *See* Unconjugated bilirubin
Indirect fluorescence antibody (IFA)
   in Chagas disease, 1151
   in leishmaniasis, 1134–1135
   in toxoplasmosis, 1147
Indirect hyperbilirubinemia. *See* Unconjugated
   hyperbilirubinemia
Indirect molecular genetic testing, 1704, 1705f
Indirect ophthalmoscopy, of retinopathy of
   prematurity, 146
Indirect tests, of pancreatic function, 1466
111-Indium (^{111}In), 589
111-Indium (^{111}In)-DTPA, 589
Individualized Educational Plan (IEP), 437,
   550
Individuals with Disabilities Education Act
   (IDEA), 437, 440, 550
Individuation, 403
Indomethacin, 1751
   adverse side effects of, 136
   for Bartter syndrome, 1713
   contraindications to, 137
   for delaying labor, 2195
   dosage and administration of, 137t, 343t
   effectiveness of, 137
   enteral feedings and, 143
   for enthesitis-related arthritis, 841
   for Fanconi syndrome, 1710
   for germinal matrix hemorrhage prevention
     in preterm newborn, 144
   and intestinal perforation, 142
   and necrotizing enterocolitis, 142–143
   and neonatal thrombocytopenia, 199
   for patent ductus arteriosus, 136–137
   prophylactic use of, 137

Interstitial lung disease (*contd.*)
  clinical presentation of, 1990–1991
  in juvenile dermatomyositis, 854
  of known etiology, 1989, 1989t
  laboratory diagnostic evaluation for, 1991,
    1991t
  lung biopsy in, 1991
  outcomes in, 1992
  prognosis for, 1992
  pulmonary function testing in, 1991
  radiologic evaluation in, 1991
  treatment of, 1992
  of unknown etiology, 1989, 1990t
Interstitial nephritis
  acute, and acute renal failure, 1673
  pyuria in, 1666
Intervention(s)
  definition of, distinguished from treatment,
    564
  early
    for developmental disabilities of intensive
      care nursery graduates, 220
    for visual impairment, 496–497, 496t
  "extraordinary" or "ordinary," 562
  prenatal, of fetal disorders, 77–79
    nonsurgical, 78–79
    surgical, 77–78
Interventional pediatric cardiac catheterization,
    1778–1780, 1778t
Intervertebral disk infection, 2322
Interviews
  for affective disorders, 502
  of behavior and development, 413
    indications for, 412t
Intestinal atresias, 203
Intestinal bacteria
  bilirubin deconjugation by, 166f
  and necrotizing enterocolitis, 141–143
Intestinal biopsy
  in celiac disease, 1419
  in idiopathic chronic diarrhea of infancy,
    1421
Intestinal bleeding. *See* Gastrointestinal bleeding
Intestinal duplications. *See* Gastrointestinal duplications
Intestinal enzymes, and protein digestion of
    newborn, 109
Intestinal flora, and bilirubin clearance, 1475
Intestinal ischemia
  conditions leading to, 142
  in necrotizing enterocolitis, 141
Intestinal malrotation, 203, 1400–1402, 1401f
Intestinal mucosa
  function of, in preterm newborn, in pathogenesis of necrotizing enterocolitis, 143
  ischemic necrosis of, 141, 141f
Intestinal neuronal dysplasia, 1463
Intestinal obstruction. *See* Gastrointestinal obstruction
Intestinal perforation
  air pattern in radiography of, 585
  foreign-body ingestion and, 1397
  indomethacin and, 142
  isolated, indomethacin and, 136
  in necrotizing enterocolitis, 141, 142f
    etiology of, 142
    monitoring, 143
    treatment of, 143
  in small-for-gestational-age newborn, 123t
  in utero, 203
Intestinal phase, of acid secretion, 1429
Intestinal pseudoobstruction syndrome,
    1410–1411
  causes of, 1410t
  pneumatosis intestinalis in, 1449

Intestinal rotation. *See* Gastrointestinal
    rotation
Intestinal trematode, 1113
Intestine(s). *See also* Large intestine; Small intestine
  bacterial colonization of, 1411–1412
  congenital anomalies of, 1399–1409
  motor disorders of, 1409–1411
  perfusion of, 285–286
  radiography of, in necrotizing enterocolitis,
    141
  role of, in neonatal hypercalcemia, 163
Intoeing, 2422
  corrective shoes for, 2425
  differential diagnosis of, 2422–2423
  in normal thigh-foot angle values, 2419
Intorsion, 2402
Intraabdominal bleeding, of newborn,
    207
Intraabdominal calcification, 203
Intraabdominal vanishing testis syndrome,
    1742
Intracardiac prostheses, iron deficiency of,
    1527
Intracerebral germinoma, markers of, 1623
Intracondylar distance (ICD), of knees, in
    quantification of genu varum, 2431,
    2431f
Intracortical hematomas, 2245
Intracranial arteriovenous fistula, 1788
Intracranial arteriovenous malformation, of
    port-wine stain, 86
Intracranial germ cell tumors, clinical features
    of, 1623
Intracranial hemorrhage (ICH), 2169, 2195,
    2196t
  in alloimmune thrombocytopenia, 200
  arteriovenous malformations and, 2238
  cavernous malformations and, 2239
  in extracorporeal membrane oxygenation,
    213
    risk factors of, 214
  after head trauma, 2238
  in hemophilia A, 1571
    treatment of, 1571
  in hemophiliac infants, 200
  hydrocephalus from, 2182
  in low-birth-weight infants, 59
    incidence of, 60
  from mechanical ventilation, 211
  in shaken baby, 465
  in traumatic brain injury, 295
  venous angiomas and, 2239
Intracranial hydatid cysts, 1119
Intracranial hypertension, 296–297, 325–327,
    325f, 326t
  management of, 296–297
  mechanisms of, 325, 325f
  monitoring, 326, 326t
  signs of, 293, 326t
    in newborn, 87
  treatment of, 326–327, 326t
Intracranial infections, after heart transplantation, 1888
Intracranial masses, magnetic resonance imaging of, 588
Intracranial pressure, 296–297
  increased, 325–327, 2245
    mechanisms of, 325, 325f
    and initial management of altered consciousness, 293t
  monitoring, 297
    complications of, 326
    devices for, 326
    initiation of, 325
Intracranial teratoma, sequelae of, 1624

Intracranial tumor(s), olfactory disturbances of,
    1264
Intracrine factors, 2007
Intractable diarrhea of infancy. *See* Idiopathic
    chronic diarrhea of infancy
Intractable epilepsy, surgical treatment for,
    2264
Intradermal nevi, 1191
Intraductal papilloma, 247
Intragluteal injections, 2251
Intrahepatic bile ducts
  chronic fibrosing inflammation of, 1504
  congenital dilation of, 1483
  drug-induced loss of, 1503
  embryology of, 1469
  paucity of, 1484
  in sclerosing cholangitis, 1506f
Intrahepatic cholestasis, progressive familial,
    1493–1494, 1498t
Intrahepatic portal hypertension, 1516t
Intrahospital transport, after cardiopulmonary
    resuscitation, 331
Intralobar nephrogenic rest, 1615
Intraluminal agents, 1365
Intraluminal proteolysis, 1311
Intramalleolar distance, in knock-knees, 2430,
    2430f
Intramembranous ossification, 744
Intramural cysts, 1404
Intramuscular contraception, 258
  medical assessment schedule, 259
Intramuscular immunoglobulin, for prevention
    of hepatitis A virus infection, 1496,
    1499t
Intramyocardial diastolic pressure, 1784
Intranarial larynx, 1271
Intraneuronal transmission, of herpes simplex
    viral particles, 170
Intraocular foreign bodies, 2413
Intraocular pressure (IOP), 2353
Intraoperative spinal cord monitoring, in surgery of idiopathic scoliosis, 2442
Intraosseous infusion, 322–323
  complications of, 322
  evidence of successful entrance for, 323
  risks and benefits of, 322t
  sites for, 323
Intraparenchymal hemorrhage, 2238
Intrapartum chemoprophylaxis, for group B
    streptococcus carriers, 152f–153f, 154
Intrapartum evaluation and management,
    70–74
  current recommendations for, 74
  fetal heart rate monitor in, 70–71
    recommendations for usage of, 75
  fetal heart rate patterns in
    characteristics of, 71
    influence of, in utero treatment, 74, 74t
    normal, 71, 71f
    variant, 71–74, 72f–73f
Intraperitoneal insulin pumps, 2134
Intrapulmonary shunt(s)
  of congenital diaphragmatic hernia, 189
  improved oxygenation for, 216
  in neonatal polycythemia, 193
Intrarenal reflux (IRR), 1672
Intrasurf, 134
Intrathecal baclofen infusion pump, for spasticity, 540
Intrathecal chemotherapy, for CNS involvement
  in acute lymphoblastic leukemia, 1598
  in acute myeloid leukemia, 1602
Intrathoracic airways, obstructive respiratory
    disease in, 278
  settings of mechanical ventilation for, 315

Kocher-Debre-Semelaigne syndrome, 2303
Koebner phenomenon, 837
  in lichen nitidus, 1182
  in psoriasis, 1180
Koebner type blistering, 1187
Koeppe nodules, 2385
Köhler disease, 2427, 2427f
Kohn-Romano blepharophimosis syndrome,
    ocular manifestations of, 2362–2363
KOH preparation, 1167
  for candidiasis, 1173
Koilocytic atypia. *See* Low-grade squamous in-
    traepithelial lesion
Koilonychia, 1216
Köln hemoglobin, 1535
Koplik spots, 1054
Korotkoff sounds, 312, 1866, 1877
Koshevnikov epilepsy, 2308
Kostmann syndrome, 199, 1551
  physical abnormalities in, 1565t
  treatment of, 1552
Krabbe globoid cell leukodystrophy, 668, 2335
KRAS gene, mutations of, 1585
Krebs cycle, defects of, 2300
Kriest dysplasia, 760t
Krimsky prism reflex test, 2353
KS. *See* Keratan sulfate
KSS. *See* Kearns-Sayre syndrome
Kufs disease, 2328
Kugelberg-Welander disease. *See* Spinal muscu-
    lar atrophies, type III
Kunkel, Louis M., 2290
Kupffer cells, 1471, 1549
Kupffer cell hyperplasia, 1478t
Kuru, 2309
Kussmaul respirations, 1656
Kussmaul sign, 1866–1867
Kwashiorkor, 1336, 1337f
  marasmic, 1337, 1337f
Kyasanur Forest disease, 1025t, 1028
Kyphoscoliosis, 2000–2001
Kyphoscoliosis tibia, in evaluation of limping,
    2421
Kyphoscoliosis type of Ehlers-Danlos syn-
    drome, 766t, 768
Kyphosis, 2442–2446

L

LABD. *See* Linear IgA bullous dermatosis of
    childhood
Labia majora, neonatal examination of, 90
Labium, of ambiguous genitalia, 90
Labor
  delaying, 67, 2195
  preterm, 67
    definition of, 67
    incompetent cervix and, 67
    scoring systems of risk for, 67
  progress of, monitoring, 75
Laboratory. *See* Clinical microbiology labora-
    tory
Labrum, structural changes of, with persistent
    dislocations, 2435
Labyrinthine dysfunction, 2251
Labyrinthitis, 1246–1247
  acute bacterial, 1250
  in acute otitis media, 1250
  bacterial, 1247
  serous, 1246
  viral, 1247
LAC. *See* Lupus anticoagulant
Lacerations, 2242, 2246
  of external auditory canal, 1257
  of eye, in newborn, 87

ocular trauma from, 2414
  repair of, pain management in, 342
  of soft palate, 1271
  treatment of, in hemophilia A patients, 1572
Lacrimal puncta, atresia of, 2366
Lacrimal sac, congenital fistula of, 2366
Lacrimal system, 2366–2367
  congenital anomalies, 2366
  epiphora, 2366–2367
  infection, 2367
Lacrimation, 2366
LactAid, 1425
β-Lactam antibiotics, 876
β-Lactamase inhibitors
  adverse effects and side effects of, 875
  indications for, 875
  mechanism of action of, 875
  for *Moraxella catarrhalis* infections, 949
β-Lactamase-producing organisms, in acute
    otitis media, 1252
Lactase, 1311
Lactase activity, of newborns, 109
Lactase deficiency, 1328, 1424
  abdominal pain in, 1360, 1424
  and colic, 34
  congenital, 1424
  diagnosis of, 1425
  and infant crying, 414
  treatment of, 1425
Lactate
  in cerebrospinal fluid, 2169
  for isovaleric acidemia, 624
Lactate dehydrogenase, serum levels of, in
    acute lymphoblastic leukemia, 1595
Lactation. *See* Breast feeding; Breast milk
Lactic acid, 626
  for molluscum contagiosum, 1056
Lactic acidemia(s), high-risk screening of, 581t
Lactic acidosis
  in malaria, 1139
    treatment of, 1142
  in metformin overdose, 373
Lactobacillus
  and bacterial vaginosis, 268
  in colon, 1411
Lactobacillus GG
  for pouchitis, 1440
  for rotaviral dehydration, 1365, 1412
Lactoferrin, 1319
Lactofree, 1334t
Lactoovovegetarians, 1338
Lactose, 1310, 1320, 1328
  neonatal digestion of, 109
Lactose breath hydrogen test, 1360, 1417,
    1425
Lactose-free cow's milk-based infant formula,
    1328
Lactose-free diet, 1360, 1425
Lactose intolerance. *See* Lactase deficiency
Lactotropins, 2012
Lactrodectus macians, 1152, 1235
α-Lactrotoxin, 1235
Lactulose, for hepatic encephalopathy of end-
    stage liver disease, 1515
LAD. *See* Leukocyte adhesion deficiency
LAD1. *See* Congenital leukocyte adherence de-
    ficiency 1
LAD2. *See* Congenital leukocyte adherence de-
    ficiency 2
Ladd procedure, for intestinal malrotation,
    1401
Lagophthalmos, 2352, 2366, 2406
Lambdoid synostosis, 757t
Lamellar bodies, 1165
Lamellar ichthyosis (LI), 1184

Lamin A, 2293
Lamina densa, 1166
Lamina propria, 1305
Laminar flow in airways, 275
Lamin C, 2293
Laminectomy, decompressive, for spinal ab-
    scess, 2322
Laminin 2, 2291–2292
Lamivudine
  for hepatitis B virus infection, 1498
  for human immunodeficiency virus infection,
    1051t
  and pancreatitis, 1414
Lamotrigine
  for childhood absence epilepsy, 2260
  dosage and administration of, 2265t
  for infantile spasms, 2259
  for juvenile myoclonic epilepsy, 2262
  for Lennox-Gastaut syndrome, 2260
  Stevens-Johnson syndrome from, 1196
  toxic epidermal necrolysis from, 1196
LAMP. *See* Lysosome-associated membrane
    proteins
Lancet devices, for sampling blood glucose,
    2128
Landau-Kleffner syndrome. *See* Acquired epi-
    leptic aphasia
Landau reflex, 481t
Landry's syndrome, 2315
Langer-Giedion syndrome, 737t
Langerhans cell histiocytosis (LCH), 1202, 1281,
    1624–1626, 1624t, (Color Plate 14)
  and central diabetes insipidus, 2027
  clinical manifestations of, 1625–1626, 1625f
  epidemiology of, 1624–1625
  pathology and pathogenesis of, 1625
Langerhans cell histiocytosis-I (LCH-I)
  chemotherapy trial, 1626
Langerhans cells, 1165, 1625
Language, 2204. *See also* Communication;
    Speech; Talking
  acquisition of, failure of, 2204
  age-appropriate behavior of, 405t
  indications of, for referral to speech pathol-
    ogy services, 545t
  processing problems of, 435
  vs. speech, 404, 441
Language-based learning disabilities, 435
  otitis media and, 441
  risk of, 444
Language delay
  behavior assessment for, 19
  continuum of, late talking to communication
    disorder in, 441–444
    assessment and diagnosis of, 442–443,
      442t–443t
    clinical manifestations of, 442, 442t–443t
    definitions and epidemiology of, 441
    etiology and pathogenesis of, 441–442
    management of, 444
    natural history and prognosis of, 444
  etiology of, 17t
  evaluation of, 18t, 19
  labeling of, 17
  laboratory studies in, 440t
  management of, 19
  referral indications of, 18t, 19
Language development, 405t
  assessment of, 14t, 19
  delay in. *See* Language delay
  description of, 17
  dimensions of, 441
  experience and, 409
  expressive skills in, age-appropriate, 17, 18t,
    443t

of cerebral venous thrombosis, 2239
of cerebrovascular diseases, 2240
of cervicocephalic arterial dissection, 2234
of CNS tumors, 2209
contrast-enhanced, 1773, 1774f
of moyamoya disease, 2235
of sickle-cell disease, 2233
Magnetic resonance cholangiopancreatography
 (MRCP), 1471, 1472t
Magnetic resonance imaging (MRI), 588,
 2165, 2171
of abdomen, 588
of abnormal head size, 2176
of aceruoloplasminemia, 2333
of acute cerebellar ataxia, 2314
of acute disseminated encephalomyelitis,
 2314
of acute viral encephalitis, 2307
of adrenal disease, 2035
of adrenoleukodystrophy, 2334
of Alexander disease, 2339
in altered consciousness, 294
of anorectal anomalies, 1458
of arteriovenous malformations, 2238
of astrocytomas, 2222–2223
of atrioventricular septal defect, 1794
of body fat, 2136
of brain abscess, 2320
of brainstem glioma, 2219
of Canavan disease, 2338
of central nervous system, 588
of cerebellar astrocytoma, 2218
of cerebral dysgenesis, 15
of cerebral palsy, 2201
of cerebral venous thrombosis, 2239
of cerebrovascular diseases, 2240
of cervicocephalic arterial dissection, 2234
of chest, 588
of Chiari malformation, 2186
of childhood ataxia with diffuse CNS hypomyelination, 2339
of choroid plexus tumors, 2227
cine, 1773
of CNS tumors, 2209, 2211
of congenital heart disease, 1773–1774,
 1774t
of cortical gliomas, 2222
of cranial epidural abscess, 2318
of cranial subdural empyema, 2318
of craniopharyngioma, 2226
in delayed puberty, 2104
of diencephalic glioma, 2221
of diffuse axonal injury, 2246
of encephalocele, 2180
of ependymoma, 2217
of epidural hematoma, 2246
of Fabry disease, 2326
of febrile seizures, 2270
in fever, 805
gadolinium-enhanced. See Gadolinium-enhanced magnetic resonance imaging
gated, 588
of germ cell tumors, 2225
of globoid cell leukodystrophy, 2335
in glutaric acidemia, 627
of G_{M1}-Gangliosidosis, 2323
of Hands-Schüller-Christian disease, 1625
of head trauma, 2248
of holoprosencephaly, 2176
of hydrocephalus, 2183
of hydromyelia, 2184
in D-2-Hydroxyglutaric acidemia, 627
of hypothalamus, 2017, 2018t, 2027
of hypoxic-ischemic encephalopathy, 2191,
 2195

of idiopathic hypopituitarism, 2018
of infantile spasms, 2258
of intervertebral disk infection, 2322
of intractable epilepsy, 2264
of juvenile rheumatoid arthritis, 837
of juxtaductal aortic coarctation, 1807
of kidneys, 1704
in Langerhans cell histiocytosis, 1626
of left atrium obstruction, 1801
of Legg-Calvé-Perthes disease, 2437, 2437f
of liver, 1471, 1472t
of medulloblastoma, 2215
of melanocytic nevi, 1191
of meningioma, 2228
of Menkes disease, 2332
in mental retardation, 15, 782
of metachromatic leukodystrophy, 2337
of moyamoya disease, 2235
of mucopolysaccharidosis, 660
of multiple sclerosis, 2316
of myelin protein disorders, 2337
in necrotizing fasciitis, 1043
of neonatal cerebral infarction, 2237
of neuroaxonal dystrophy, 2334
of neurocysticercosis, 1122f
of neurofibromatosis, 2346
of Niemann-Pick disease, 2327–2328
of occult spinal dysraphism, 2185
in osteomyelitis, 906
patient preparation for, 583t
of pheochromocytoma, 2056
of pineal region tumors, 2226
of pituitary gland, 2017, 2018t, 2027
of pseudocoarctation, 1808
of respiratory system, 1912
for rhabdomyosarcoma, 2455
of rheumatic disease, 831
of scrotal masses, 248
of seizure disorders, 2263
of sickle-cell disease, 2233
of single-ventricle malformation, 1831
of skeleton, 588
of spinal abscess, 2322
of spinal cord injury, 2248
of stroke in sickle cell disease, 1533
of supravalvar aortic stenosis, 1805
of tuber cinereum hamartomas, 2097
of unilateral seizures, 2257
of upper plexus root injuries, 2249
velocity-encoded cine, 1773
of Wilson disease, 2332
Magnetic resonance spectroscopy (MRS),
 2165
of childhood ataxia with diffuse CNS hypomyelination, 2339
of moyamoya disease, 2235
Magnetic resonance venography
of cerebral venous thrombosis, 2239
of cerebrovascular diseases, 2240
Mahaim fiber, 1842
Mahler, theory of, on social-emotional development, 405
Maintenance basal calories, calculating, 1676
Maintenance fluid requirements, calculating,
 1318t
Maintenance fluid volume, calculating, 1643t
Maintenance therapy, 1643–1644
for acute lymphoblastic leukemia, 1598
for acute renal failure, 1676
after oral rehydration therapy, 1364
Majocchi's granuloma, 1229
Major basic protein (MBP), 1555
Major depressive disorders, 501
definition and epidemiology of, 501, 501t
natural history and prognosis of, 502

symptoms of, 501t
Major histocompatibility complex (MHC), 787
Major histocompatibility complex deficiencies,
 796
genetic bases of, 794t
Malabsorption, 1415–1417
in autoimmune enteropathy, 1422
of bile acid, 1427
of carbohydrates. See Carbohydrate malabsorption
causes of, 1422t
in celiac disease, 1418
in common variable immunodeficiency, 801
of copper, 1427
diagnosis of, 1416t
of fat
diagnosis of, 1416
in idiopathic chronic diarrhea, 1420
in infants, 1328
in preterm newborns, 109
stool in, 1415
and vitamin E deficiency, 1529
of folate, 1529
of fructose, 1424
glucose-galactose, 1425
congenital, 1427
and ichthyoses, 1183
of iron, 1527
of magnesium, 2163
mechanisms of, 1416t
in microvillus atrophy, 1421
in short-bowel syndrome, 1427–1429
in small intestinal lymphangiectasia, 1422
of sorbitol, 1424
in tropical sprue, 1423
of vitamin B_{12}, 1530
in Whipple's disease, 1423
of zinc, 1427
Maladaptive behaviors, of foster children, 521
Maladjustment, of disabled children, 551
Malaria, 1136–1142, 1137f
and Burkitt lymphoma, 1604
cerebral, 1138
clinical manifestations of, 1138–1139
diagnosis of, 1139
epidemiology of, 1137–1138
prevention of, 1142, 1143t, 1163
transmission of, by blood transfusion, 1581
treatment of, 1139–1142, 1141t
WHO criteria for, 1138, 1138t
Malarial anemia, 1139
Malarone. See Proguanil
Malar rash
in juvenile dermatomyositis, 853
in systemic lupus erythematosus, 849
Malassezia folliculitis, 1173
Malassezia furfur infection, 1095
clinical manifestations of, 1095
diagnosis of, 1095
and neonatal acne, 1169
and tinea versicolor, 1228
treatment of, 1080t, 1095
Malassezia pachydermatis, 1095
Malathion, for head lice, 1156t
Maldigestion, 1415–1429
diagnosis of, 1416t
mechanisms of, 1416t
Male(s). See also Gender
acne keloidalis in, 1212
adrenal tumors in, 2049
anti-GBM disease in, 1686
Becker nevus in, 1193
bladder outlet obstruction in, 1673
blood pressure levels for, by percentiles of
 height, 2475t

newborn and long-term developmental
outcomes with, 527
short-term consequences of, 230
Marine animal stings, poisonous, 391–393
Maroteaux-Lamy syndrome, 660
Married minors, 559
MAS. *See* Macrophage activation syndrome;
Meconium aspiration syndrome
MASA syndrome, 2182
Masculinization
of female fetuses, prenatal prevention of, 78
in female pseudohermaphroditism, 2081
Masks, for oxygen administration, 284
Massage, 542
for fibromyalgia, 862
Massive adrenal hemorrhage, 2044
Massive transfusion, 1579
complications of, 1579
in newborns, whole blood and, 1577
Mast cells, 1555
Mast cell-stabilizing agents, for allergic diseases, 816
Master gland. *See* Pituitary gland, anterior
Mastery, 403–405, 434
Mastitis, 30, 247
in mumps, 1057
Mastocytosis, 1202, 1555, *(Color Plate 13)*
Mastoid air cell system, 1239
in acute otitis media, 1250
embryology of, 1240
Mastoiditis
anatomy of middle ear and, 1239
in *Streptococcus pneumoniae* infection, 978
Masturbation, 472
"Matching"
in case-control studies, 592
in cohort studies, 591
Maternal antibody testing, in erythroblastosis
fetalis, 174
Maternal autoimmune thrombocytopenia. *See*
Idiopathic thrombocytopenic purpura
(ITP), maternal
"Maternal exhaustion," and vaginal operative
delivery, 76
Maternal floor infarction, 62
Maternal hormones, 81
Maternal idiopathic thrombocytopenic purpura, 1557–1558
Maternally inherited Leigh syndrome (MILS),
2301
Maternal malnutrition, 530t
Maternal perinatal care, in-hospital levels of,
57t
Maternal platelet count, and evaluation of
thrombocytopenic infants, 200
Maternal position, change of, to correct variant
fetal heart rate patterns, 74t
Maternal sensitization, to D antigen, 174–175
prevention of, 175
history of, 174
Maternal surface of placenta, 62
Mathematical understanding, disorders of, 435
Matochezia, in GI bleeding, 1371, 1374
Matrix proteins, 691f
Matrix protein synthesis, in persistent pulmonary hypertension of newborn, 183
Maturation
and infant crying, 414
pubertal, clinical correlates of, 224t
variation in, 438
Maturational lag. *See* Developmental delay
"Mature minor" rule, 226, 559
Mature teratoma, 1622
Maturity-onset diabetes of the young
(MODY), 724, 2112, 2135
Mauriac syndrome, 2023, 2131

Maxillary, abnormal development of, 202
Maxillary sinus, 1258, 1259f
infections in, 1263
Maximal inspiratory pressure, 1917
Maximum cardiac impulse, of newborns, 89
Maximum conduction velocity, 2279
Mayaro, 1019t
May-Heglin syndrome, 1558
Mazzotti test, in onchocerciasis, 1108
MB. *See* Medulloblastoma
MBP (major basic protein), 1555
MBPS. *See* Munchausen by proxy syndrome
MCAD deficiency. *See* Medium-chain acyl-CoA
dehydrogenase (MCAD) deficiency
McArdle disease, 638
McBurney point, 1450
MCC deficiency. *See* 3-Methylcrotonyl-CoA
carboxylase (MCC) deficiency
McCune-Albright syndrome, 737t, 2011t,
2346
café au lait macules in, 1191
G protein function alterations in, 2009
hyperpigmentation in, 1193
and precocious puberty, 2099
MCDK. *See* Multicystic dysplastic kidney
M cells, and immunology of GI tract, 1312
MCFAs. *See* Medium-chain fatty acids
McGovern's nipple, for choanal atresia, 1260
MCH. *See* Mean corpuscular hemoglobin
MCHC. *See* Mean corpuscular hemoglobin
concentration
MCKAT deficiency. *See* Medium-chain 3-keto-
thiolase (MCKAT) deficiency
MCKD. *See* Medullary cystic kidney disease
MCNS. *See* Minimal-change nephrotic syndrome
MCP (mucopurulent cervicitis), 264
M-CSF. *See* Macrophage colony-stimulating
factor
MCTD. *See* Mixed connective tissue disease
MCT Oil, 1334t
MCV. *See* Mean corpuscular volume
MD. *See* Moyamoya disease
MDMA (methylenedioxymethamphetamine),
377
mdr1 (multidrug resistance) gene, in acute myeloid leukemia, 1603
Meal plan, for diabetic child, 2128
Mean airway pressure (MAP), 315
determination of, 208
excessive, in persistent pulmonary hypertension of newborn, 185
Mean airway volume, 315
Mean blood pressure
of newborns, 89
with reduced cardiac output, 285
Mean body fat, alterations of, in adolescence,
223
Mean cell volume, in neonatal anemia, 198
Mean corpuscular hemoglobin (MCH), 1521t
measurement of, 1524
of reticulocytes, and iron deficiency anemia,
1527
Mean corpuscular hemoglobin concentration
(MCHC), 1524
in term and preterm infants, 1519
Mean corpuscular volume (MCV), 1521t
at birth, 1520
in fetus, 1519
measurement of, 1524
in newborns, 1552t
in progressive stages of iron deficiency,
1528t
Mean hemoglobin levels, 1520f, 1521t
Mean platelet volume, 1555
Mean red blood cell volume, 1520, 1521t

Measles, 1053–1056, 1221, 1223
after acute disseminated encephalomyelitis,
2314
clinical manifestations of, 1054
complications of, 1055
conjunctivitis in, 1054, 2369
diagnosis of, 1054
differential diagnosis of, 1054
epidemiology of, 1053
in health care personnel, 887t
in immunodeficiency, 1055, 2311
liver infection with, 1500
prevention of, 1055
in severe combined immunodeficiency, 794
treatment of, 1055
Measles vaccination, 1053, 1055. *See also*
MMR (measles, mumps, rubella) vaccine
contraindications for, 804
Henoch-Schönlein purpura from, 842
for international travel, 1161
in severe combined immunodeficiency, 794
Meat, uncooked. *See* Uncooked meat
Meatal stenosis, 1739
Meat impaction, 1398
Meat products, iron absorption and, 1527
Mebendazole, 1098
for baylisascariasis, 1104
dosage and administration of, 1098
for enterobiasis, 1106
for hookworm infection, 1109
for hydatid disease, 1119
for nematode infections, 1098, 1099t
for toxocariasis, 1111
for trichinosis, 1112
for trichuriasis, 1112
Mechanical apnea monitors, for home monitoring tracheostomy tubes, 1279
Mechanical circulatory support devices, in congestive heart failure, 1875
Mechanical correlates, of breathing, 309
Mechanical intravascular hemolysis, 1522f,
1547
Mechanical pain, 835
Mechanical shunting, for hydrocephalus,
2184
Mechanical ventilation, 313–319, 316f–318f.
See also High-frequency ventilation
for apnea of prematurity, 208
complications of, for newborn, 210–211
continuous positive airway pressure, for newborn, 208
for decreasing intracranial pressure, 326
for diaphragmatic paralysis, 186
discontinuation of, 317–319
distribution of ventilation in, 315, 316f
during extracorporeal membrane oxygenation, 214
frequency of, conventional, 212
for hyaline membrane disease, 208
indications for, in newborn, 209
intermittent positive pressure ventilation, for
newborn, 208–209
for intracranial hypertension, 296–297
for meconium aspiration syndrome,
195–196
modalities of, 317–319, 317f–318f
for newborn, 209–210
for neonatal pneumonia caused by group B
streptococcal infection, 153
for newborn, 207–211
complications in, 210–211
indications for, 209
intensive care strategies of, 210
modalities of, 209–210
weaning from, 210

laboratory findings in, 1695
pathogenesis of, 1695
prognosis of, 1695
recurrent, after transplantation, 1731
treatment of, 1695
Membranous subaortic stenosis, aortic regurgitation in, 1796
Memory, 2166, 2203, 2228
after head trauma, 2248
MEN. *See* Multiple endocrine neoplasia
Menadione, for oxidative phosphorylation diseases, 652
Menarche, 223, 224t, 2096
and bone mineral density, 2145
mean age of, 240
premature isolated, 2101
Mendelian conditions, 713
Mendelian Inheritance in Man, 726
Ménétrier disease, 1034, 1433
Meningioma, 2228
Meningitic plague, 975
Meningitis, 900–904
in acute otitis media, 1250
aseptic (viral), 900, 1021f, 2306, 2306t
bacterial, 900–904
clinical manifestations of, 901–902
CNS vasculitis from, 2235
diagnosis of, 902–903
epidemiology of, 900
etiology of, by age group, 902t
hydrocephalus from, 2182
management of, 294
outcome with, 903–904
pathogenesis of, 901
pathology of, 901
pathophysiology of, 901
presentation of, 294
prevention of, 904
subdural hematoma from, 2246
treatment of, 903, 903t, 979
in *Candida* infections, 1089
cryptococcal, 1092
in disseminated coccidioidomycosis, 1091
enteroviral, 1022
gonococcal, 968
granulomatous, 900
group B streptococcal, fatality rate for, 945
in group B streptococcal infection, 1000
Haemophilus influenzae, 938
fatality rate for, 945
in herpes simplex virus infection, antibiotics for, 303
in Kawasaki disease, 844
Listeria, fatality rate for, 945
in mumps, 1057
Neisseria meningitidis. See Neisseria meningitidis infection
neonatal seizures from, 2269
in newborns
antibiotic dosage recommendations for, 153
treatment duration for, 153
nontuberculous mycobacterial, 961
Pasteurella multocida, 972
purulent. *See* Meningitis, bacterial
rate of, with expectant treatment for *S. Pneumoniae* bacteremia, 308
in *Salmonella* infection, 983
Streptococcus pneumoniae, 979
fatality rate for, 945
treatment of, 868t
tuberculous, 953
treatment of, 958
"Meningitis belt," 971
Meningitis-encephalitis syndromes, 2313

Meningocele, 90, 2174, 2186
Meningococcal bacteremia
management of, 307
natural history of, 307
Meningococcal vaccine, 970–971
in asplenia, 804
chronic conditions and, 541t
for international travel, 1162
Meningococcemia, 970, 1225
band counts and, 307
and central diabetes insipidus, 2027
immune modulation in, clinical trials of, 301
in purulent pericarditis, 1867
Meningoencephalocele, 2174
Meningomyelocele, 2174, 2186–2187
Meniscal tears, differential diagnosis of, 2449
Meniscus, discoid, 2434
Menkes disease, 679, 737t, 1187, 1427, 2331
Menometrorrhagia, von Willebrand disease and, 1573
Menopause, premature, from treatment of Hodgkin disease, 1609
Menorrhagia, of von Willebrand disease, treatment of, 1573
Menstrual cramping, 254
Menstrual cycles, 241f
anovulatory, 253, 2097
common problems of, 249–254
endometrial phases of, 240
and insulin regimen, 2133
Menstrual flow blockage, 252
treatment of, 252
Menstrual toxic shock syndrome, 992
Menstruation
abdominal pain during, 1355
onset of. *See* Menarche
Mental disorders, recurrent abdominal pain in, 1362
Mental function, in hyperthermia, 389
Mental health problems. *See also specific problem*
in adolescence, 231–233
screening questions for, 523
Mental retardation (MR), 16, 779–782, 2197
in Alagille syndrome, 1486t
assessment of, 439
birth weight and, 220
in cerebral palsy, 2200
in chromosome abnormalities, 731
classification system of, 438
clinical manifestations of, 439, 780
definition of, 16, 438
diagnosis of, 439, 780–782
in Duchenne muscular dystrophy, 2289
epidemiology of, 438, 534t
etiology of, 439, 780, 781f
family history of, laboratory studies recommended for, 440t
in homocystinuria, 614
incidence of, 16, 534t
in intensive care nursery graduates
birth weight and, 220
incidence of, 219
prematurity and, 220–221
IQ in, 779, 2173
in Lennox-Gastaut syndrome, 2260
in macrocephaly, 2176
magnetic resonance imaging in, 15
management and treatment of, 439–440
maternal, and cerebral palsy, 2199
maternal phenylketonuria and, 609
maternal rubella and, 1078
metabolic screening tests in, 15
in microcephaly, 2176
mild, 780

moderate, 780
in mucolipidosis, 2331
in myotonic dystrophy, 2294
natural history and prognosis of, 441
ocular conditions in, incidence of, 491t
oral motor dysfunction and, 422
pathogenesis of, 439
of perinatal asphyxia survivors, 221
and pervasive developmental disorders, 498–499
in phenylketonuria, 609
recognition of, 2166
in Rett syndrome, 2205
and rumination, 421
severe, 780
and sexualized behavior, 473
in small-molecule disease, 601
treatment and management of, 782
in West syndrome, 2258
Mental status
evaluation of, 2166
examination of
in adolescent, 236
in newborn, 92, 92t
postoperative decline of, management of, 340
Mentzer index, for distinguishing iron deficiency from β-thalassemia traits, 1528
Meperidine, dosage and administration of, 344t
Meprobamate, for tetanus, 1007
Mercaptoacetyltriglycine (MAG3), 1662
α-Mercaptopropionylglycine, for cystinuria, 1712
6-Mercaptopurine (6-MP)
for acute lymphoblastic leukemia, 1598
adverse effects of, 1439
for Crohn disease, 1442
for ulcerative colitis, 1439
Mercury, in vaccines, 40
for Hepatitis B virus, 49
Meropenem, 876
dosage and administration of, 872t
for pulmonary exacerbations in cystic fibrosis, intravenous administration of, 1976t
Merosin, 2291–2292
Merosin-negative congenital muscular dystrophy (MN-CMD), 2292
Merosin-positive congenital muscular dystrophy (MP-CMD), 2292
MERRF. *See* Myoclonic epilepsy and ragged-red fiber disease
Merthiolate-iodine-formalin (MIF), in giardiasis diagnosis, 1132
Mesalamine, for ulcerative colitis, 1438
Mesangial lupus nephritis, 848, 848t, 1687–1688
Mesangiocapillary glomerulonephritis. *See* Membranoproliferative glomerulonephritis
Mesenchymal hamartoma(s), 1509
differential diagnosis of, 1620t
outcome and treatment of, 1621
Mesenchymal lesions, benign, 1296
Mesenchymal tissue, 2174
Mesenchyme, 743, 1629, 1630f
Mesenteric adenitis
abdominal pain in, 1355
with tuberculous enteritis, 954
Mesenteric cyst, 1375, 1405
Mesenteric vasculitis, 1448
Mesenteric vein obstruction, abdominal pain in, 1361

Migraine (contd.)
  pathogenesis of, 2275
  treatment of, 2275
Migrational abnormalities, renal, 1640
Migratory glossitis, 1293
Migratory joint involvement, 833t
Milia, 687, 1168
  of newborn, 86
Miliaria, 1168, 1215
  of newborn, 86
Miliaria crystallina, 1168, 1215
Miliaria rubra, 1168, 1215
"Miliary sudamina," 996
Miliary tuberculosis, 952
Milk. See Breast milk; Cow's milk
Milk-alkali syndrome, and increased bone density, 2161
Millepora spp. (fire corals), poisonous sting of, 391, 1159
Miller bran, in bowel management of disabled children, 540
Miller-Dieker lissencephaly syndrome, 737t, 2176
Miller syndrome, 749t, 2381
Milrinone
  for congestive heart failure, 1873
  for poor systemic perfusion, 291t
MILS. See Maternally inherited Leigh syndrome
Milwaukee brace, 547
  for idiopathic scoliosis, 2441
Mineral homeostasis regulation, 2142–2149
Mineral metabolism disorders, 2380
Mineralocorticoid deficiency
  in autoimmune adrenalitis, 2042
  in 3β-hydroxysteroid dehydrogenase deficiency, 2038
  in salt-losing congenital adrenal hyperplasia, 2041
Mineralocorticoid excess, 1714, 2034
Mineralocorticoid replacement, 2050, 2053
Mineralocorticoids, 2028
  concentration in infants and children, 2036t
  hypertension from, 1880
  metabolic alkalosis from, 1657
  production of, decrease in, 1711
  secretion of, 2033
Mineral oil scrapings, 1168
Minerals
  fat-soluble, deficiency of, in liver disease, 1513, 1515t
  nutritional requirements for, 1321, 1325t
  in optimal neonatal nutrition, 110
  in parenteral nutrition solutions, 1346, 1346t
Minicore disease, 2295
Minimal brain dysfunction. See Attention-deficit hyperactivity disorder
Minimal-change nephrotic syndrome (MCNS), 1691–1693
  age of onset of, 1678t
  classical histologic features of, 1679t
  clinical manifestations of, 1692
  focal segmental glomerulonephritis and, 1691
  laboratory findings in, 1692
  pathogenesis of, 1692
  prognosis of, 1693
  treatment of, 1692–1693
Minocycline
  for acne, 1209
  hepatotoxicity of, 1503
Minor adult hemoglobin (HbA₂), 1521
Minor right ventricular conduction delay, 1761
Minor tococcus, 1295

Minoxidil, hypertrichosis from, 1213
Minute ventilation, 208, 279
  in meconium aspiration syndrome, 195
Miosis, 2386
  in toxic ingestions and exposures, 357t
Mirror motion (synkinesia), 437, 2205
  in Klippel-Feil syndrome, 2440
Mirtazapine, for pervasive developmental disorders, 500t
Missense mutations, 1585
MIT. See Monoiodotyrosine
Mites, 1152
  and rickettsialpox, 1017
  and scabies, 1153
  and tularemia, 1008
MITF gene, 1185
Mitochondria, 643
  of hepatocytes, 1470
  iron-laden, 1567
Mitochondrial acetoacetyl-CoA thiolase deficiency, 624
Mitochondrial cytopathies, in Pearson syndrome, 1567
Mitochondrial disorders, 719
  inheritance of, 1567
Mitochondrial DNA, replication and transcription of, 718
Mitochondrial DNA depletion diseases, 650, 1490
Mitochondrial DNA (mtDNA) mutations, 719, 720t, 1490
  and diabetes mellitus, 2113
  in hereditary myopathies, 2301
  in oxidative phosphorylation diseases, 647t, 649–650
Mitochondrial encephalomyopathy, 2300
Mitochondrial encephalomyopathy, lactic acidosis, and stroke-like episodes (MELAS), 648–649, 720t, 2113, 2237, 2338, 2338f
Mitochondrial encephalopathy, strokelike episodes in, 2237
Mitochondrial inheritance, of inborn errors of metabolism, 598
Mitochondrial matrix, 643
Mitochondrial membrane
  inner, 643
  outer, 643
Mitochondrial myopathies, 2299
Mitochondrial oxidative phosphorylation, inherited defects of, 1490
Mitochondrial protein synthesis, chloramphenicol and, 147
Mitochondrial respiration, and thermogenesis, 80
Mitochondrial trifunctional protein (MTP), 630
  deficiency of, 2299
Mitogen-activated phosporylation kinase (MAPK), 770
Mitogen-activated protein kinase (MAPK) pathway, activation of, 299, 2010
Mitotane, for Cushing disease, 2047
Mitotic cell cycle, 1587f
  checkpoints of, and integrity of genome, 1587–1588, 1588f
  duration of, 1587
  gene mutations of, and pediatric diseases, 1588
  phases of, 1587, 1587f
  regulation of
    derangements in, and tumorigenesis, 1588–1589, 1588f
    growth factors and, 1587, 1588f
    oncology and, 1587–1589

protein kinase complexes in, 1587
Mitral atresia, 1801
Mitral incompetence murmurs, 1756
Mitral regurgitation, 1796t, 1797–1798
Mitral ring, supravalvar, 1801
Mitral stenosis
  congenital, 1801
  pulmonary edema in, 1801
Mitral valve, parachute, 1801
Mitral valve obstruction, 1800t, 1801
Mitral valve prolapse, 1797
  chest pain in, 1897
  in mixed connective tissue disease, 851
Mitral valvoplasty, 1779
Mittelschmerz, abdominal pain in, 1355
"Mitten deformities," 1188
Mittendorf dot, 2398
Mivacurium, complications of, 337
Mixed astigmatism, 2362
Mixed blepharitis, 2365
Mixed connective tissue disease (MCTD), 851–852, 1200
  pulmonary involvement in, 1998–1999
Mixed germ cell tumors, 2224
Mixed hearing loss, definition of, 485
Miyoshi myopathy, 2293
Mizuo sign, 2392
MLD. See Metachromatic leukodystrophy
MLL-AF4 gene fusion, 1586
MMC. See Myelomeningocele
MMF. See Mycophenolate mofetil
M-mode echocardiography, 1762, 1763f
MMR (measles, mumps, rubella) vaccine, 46–47
  administration of, 46
  in adolescents, 236
  chronic conditions and, 541t
  contraindications to, 44t, 47, 804
  in encephalitis and encephalopathy, 47
  factors affecting success of, 46
  failure of, 46
  for HIV-infected children, 47, 1048
  immunoglobulin and, 46
  indications for, 44t
  for international travel, 1161
  measles outbreaks and, 46
  mumps outbreaks and, 46
  pregnancy and, 47
  route and dose of, 40t
  side effects of, 47
  and thrombocytopenia, 47
  timing of, 41t, 46
  and tuberculin reactivity, 46
MMV. See Mandatory minute ventilation
MN-CMD. See Merosin-negative congenital muscular dystrophy
MNGIE. See Myoneurogastrointestinal disorder and encephalopathy
Mobile arm supports, 548
Mobility
  assistive technology devices for, 546t, 547
  developmental expectations of, 440t
  physical vs. occupational therapy for, 544t
  in visually-impaired infant, 492
Mobiluncus spp., and bacterial vaginosis, 268
Mobitz second-degree atrioventricular block, 1847
Möbius syndrome, 737t
  alveolar hypoventilation with, 1931–1932
Modal chromosome number, definition of, 730t
Model Uniform Determination of Death Act, 330
Moderate aplastic anemia, 1564
Modified biophysical profile, antepartum, 70

"Modified psychosexual neutrality," 2092
Moducal, 1334t
MODY. *See* Maturity-onset diabetes of the young
Mohr syndrome, 1269
"Molded baby" syndrome
 in congenital muscular torticollis, 2439
 developmental dysplasia of hip in, 2435
Molding, of cranial bones, of newborn, 87
Molding helmets, for congenital muscular torticollis, 2439
Mold spores, 813, 815
Molecular analysis, for fatty acid oxidation disorders, 582f
Molecular biology, of Wilms tumor, 1614
Molecular cytogenetics, 730
Molecular diagnostics
 in childhood disorders, 573–577
  DNA and, 573–574, 574f
  family studies in, 576–577
  future directions of, 577
  introduction to, 573
  mutations and polymorphisms and, 577
  polymerase chain reaction and, 574–576, 575f, 576t
 role of, in oncology, 1586
Molecular genetic diagnosis, 1704
 for autosomal dominant polycystic kidney disease, 1707
 for autosomal recessive polycystic kidney disease, 1705
 for nephronophthisis, 1708
 for renal cystic disorders, 1706f
Molecular markers, for differential diagnosis of tumors, 1586
Moles, 1191
Mollaret meningitis, 2313
Molluscum contagiosum, 1056, 1220, 1220f, 1461
 clinical manifestations of, 1056
 diagnosis of, 1056
 in HIV infection, 1200
 prevention of, 1056
 treatment of, 1056, 1220t
Molluscum contagiosum conjunctivitis, 2369
Molluscum dermatitis, 1056, 1220
Molybdenum, 692
 biochemical action of, 1326t
 dietary sources of, 1326t
 in parenteral nutrition solutions, 1346, 1347t
Molybdenum cofactor deficiency, 615
 strokelike episodes in, 2237
Molybdenum deficiency, 1326t
Molybdenum toxicity, 1326t
Monarthritis, 842
Monarticular joint involvement, 833t
Mongolian spots, 1169, 1192
 of newborns, 86
Mongolism, 732
Monilethrix, 1213
 in ectodermal dysplasia, 1189
Moniliasis, cutaneous, physical findings of, in newborns, 86
Monoamine oxidase (MAO) inhibitors, preoperative management of, 335
Monoamnionic twins
 delivery complications of, 117
 placentas of, 63, 118f
Monobactams, 876
 dosage and administration of, 872t
Monoblast(s), 1548, 1563f
Monochorionic membranes, 63, 63f, 117, 118f
Monoclonal antibodies, in renal transplantation, 1733

Monoclonality, of Langerhans cell histiocytosis, 1625
Monocular strabismus, 2402
Monocyte(s), 1548, 1555, 1563f
 developmental changes in numbers of, 1548
 development of, 1549
 in HIV infection, 1045
 in neonatal period, 304
 normal count of, by age, 1548t
Monocytosis, 1555
Monoethylglycinexylidide (MEGX), in evaluation of liver function, 1476
Monogenic conditions, 713, 715–717
 ocular manifestations of, 2354, 2355t
Monogenic hereditary disorders, diagnosed by polymerase chain reaction, 576t
Monogenic hypercholesterolemia, with normal LDL receptor and apoB genes, 700
Monoglycerides, 1312
2-Monoglycerides, 695
β-Monoglycerides, 1312
Monoiodotyrosine (MIT), 2059–2060
 deiodination of, 2060
Mononeuritis multiplex, 2281
Mononeuropathy, 2281
Mononuclear phagocytic system, abnormal cell proliferation of, 1624–1627
Mononucleosis
 cytomegalovirus, 1033, 1037
 infectious. *See* Epstein-Barr virus (EBV) infection
Monophosphate glucuronosyl transferase, and bilirubin excretion, 166f
Monoplegia, 2200
Monosaccharide intolerance, 1424
 in idiopathic chronic diarrhea, 1420
 oral rehydration therapy and, 1364
Monosaccharides, 634, 1310
 absorption of, in newborns, 110
Monosomy, 728
 in acute myeloid leukemia, 1601
 definition of, 730t
Monosomy 7, in juvenile myelomonocytic leukemia, 1603
Monospot test, 1280
Monounsaturated long-chain fatty acids, 1320, 1891
Monozygotic (MZ) twins, 723, 723t
 acute myeloid leukemia in, 1600
 incidence of, 117
 Langerhans cell histiocytosis and, 1625
 mortality and morbidity of, 68
 placentas of, 63, 63f, 118f
 risk of congenital malformations in, 118
Montelukast, for asthma, dosage and administration of, 1956t
Montreal Neurological Institute, 2264
Montreal syndrome, 1559t
Mood-altering drugs, preoperative management of, 335
Mood disorders, 501. *See also* Depression
 assessment and diagnosis of, 502
 etiology and pathogenesis of, 501
 management and treatment of, 502
 in systemic lupus erythematosus, 849
Mood quality, 450t
MOPP (mechlorethamine, vincristine, prednisone, procarbazine) regimen, for Hodgkin disease, 1609
Moraxella catarrhalis, 948–949
 biology of, 948
 colonization of, 948
 infections caused by
  in acute otitis media, 948, 1249
   drug-resistant, 1252

clinical manifestations of, 948–949
 in otitis media with effusion, 1253
 in pneumonia, 948
 treatment of, 949
Moraxella liquefaciens, 2377
Morbidity, 533
 abdominal fat and, 481
 in adolescents, causes of, 226, 231
 of apparent life-threatening event, 368
 factor contributing to, in trauma patients, 351
 of newborns, 56–61
  Apgar scoring system and, 99
  salt and water intake and, 82
 obesity and, 477–478
 of patent ductus arteriosus, 135–136
 perinatal, of multiple births, 59
 of sickle cell disease, 1532
 of systemic inflammatory responses, 299
Morbilli. *See* Measles
Morbillivirus, 1053
Morgagni, crypts of, infection of, 1460
Morning glory disc anomaly, 2398
Moro reflex, 481t, 2168
 in brachial plexus birth palsy, 2447
 of newborn, 94
Morphea, 857, 1199
Morphine
 dosage and administration of, 344t
 LES tone and, 1388
 and postsurgical hyperglycemia, 159
 respiratory acidosis from, 1657
Morphine sulfate, for tetralogy of Fallot, 1822
Morphogens, 744
Morphologically defined myopathies, 2295
Morquio disease type B, 2324
Morquio syndrome, 660, 663, 2324
 and myocardial disease, 1861
Morrell procedure, 2262
Mortality, 533
 of acute otitis media, 1250
 causes of, in adolescents, 226
 chronic illnesses and, 564
 and extracorporeal membrane oxygenation criteria, 213
 of induction therapy for acute lymphoblastic leukemia, 1598
 injury-related, statistics of, 37
 in Langerhans cell histiocytosis-I chemotherapy trial, 1626
 of liver biopsy, 1471
 in meconium aspiration syndrome, 195
 of Munchausen by proxy syndrome, 507
 of neonatal herpes simplex virus infection, disseminated, 171
 of newborns, 56–61
  Apgar scoring system and, 55
  from hyaline membrane disease, 127
 of nonimmune hydrops fetalis, 179
 obesity and, 477–478
 of otitis media, 1249
 perinatal, of multiple births, 59, 117
 of pulmonary hemorrhage, 151
 risk of, by birth weight and gestational age, 60f
 in sepsis, 300
  clinical trials for reduction of, 301
 of sickle cell disease, 1532
 of small-for-gestational-age infants, 122
 of systemic inflammatory responses, 299
 in trauma patients, 351
Mortality rate(s)
 of accidental poisoning, 354
 of cancer, 1583, 1583f

Nasal septum (*contd.*)
  hematoma of, 1265, 1265f
Nasal sprays or drops, 1074
Nasal stents, for choanal atresia, 1260
Nasal stuffiness, in newborns, 88
Nasal-tip hemangioma, 1205
Nasal trauma, 1264–1265
Nasal turbinates, 1258, 1258f
  examination of, 1259
  hypertrophy of, 1260
NASH (nonalcoholic steatohepatitis), of obesity, 1510, 1512t
Nasoduodenal intubation, 1339
  indications for, 1341t
Nasogastric tube
  advantages and disadvantages of, 537
  feeding methods by, 538
Nasogastric tube feeding, 1336, 1339, 1349
  for Canavan disease, 2338
  for glycogen storage disease, 635
  indications for, 1341t
  for intestinal pseudoobstruction, 1410
  and perforation of esophagus, 1398
  for sphingolipidoses, 672
Nasojejunal tube, advantages and disadvantages of, 537
Nasolacrimal duct, 1258
Nasolacrimal duct cysts, 1260
Nasolacrimal duct obstruction, 2366
Nasolaryngoscopy
  for inspiratory stridor, 1278
  for suspected foreign body aspiration, 1278
Nasopharyngeal obstruction, surgically correctable causes of, 202
Nasopharyngeal suction, for meconium aspiration syndrome, 194, 196
Nasopharyngoscopy, in evaluation of stridor, 1273
Nasopharynx, 1267
  examination of, 1268
NAT-2. *See* Arylamine N-acetyltransferase 2
Natal teeth, 88
National Alopecia Areata Foundation, 1212
National Association for Family Child Care (NAFCC), 512, 514t
National Association for Pseudoxanthoma Elasticum, Inc., 1188
National Association for the Education of Young Children (NAEYC), 512, 514t
National Association of Child Care Resource and Referral Agencies (NACCRRA), 514t
National Association of Pediatric Nurse Associates and Practitioners (NAPNAP), 514t
National Cancer Institute, 2208
  and acute lymphoblastic leukemia, 1594
  risk-based assignment of acute lymphoblastic leukemia, 1596t, 1597
  Surveillance Epidemiology and End Results program, 1583, 1583f
National Cancer Institute Risk Classification Workshop, recommended evaluative studies, in diagnosis of acute lymphoblastic leukemia, 1597
National Center for Complementary and Alternative Medicine (NCCAM), 543
National Center for Health Statistics (NCHS)
  growth chart of, normality and, 4
  revised growth standards of, 476
National Child Care Information Center, 514t
National Childhood Vaccine Injury Compensation Act, 43
National Cholesterol Education Program (NCEP), 696, 702–703
National Collaborative Perinatal Project, 2197–2199

National Eczema Association for Science and Education (NEASE), 1179
National Foundation for Ectodermal Dysplasias, 1189
National Head Injury Foundation, Inc., 2251
National Health Examination Survey, on childhood obesity, 2137
National Health Interview Survey, 533
National Institutes of Health (NIH)
  Consensus Development Conference on Infantile Apnea and Home Monitoring, 352
  recommendations for antenatal corticosteroids, 131–132
National Neurofibromatosis Foundation (NNF), 1186
National Organization for Albinism and Hypopigmentation (NOAH), 1185
National Organization for Rare Disorders (NORD), 1183
National Psoriasis Foundation, 1181
National Research Council, on saturate fat intake, 1891
National Resource Center for Health and Safety in Child Care, 514t
National Safety Council, on foreign body aspiration, 1277
National Training Institute for Child Care Health Consultants, Department of Maternal and Child Health, 514t
National Tuberous Sclerosis Association, 1186
National Vitiligo Foundation, 1193
National Wilms Tumor Study Group
  chemotherapy for Wilms tumor, 1616
  radiation therapy for Wilms tumor, 1616
  staging system of Wilms Tumor, 1615t
Native Americans
  adolescent, gonorrhea rate in, 260–261
  BCG cross-reaction in, 955
  diabetes mellitus type 1 in, 2115
  IgA nephropathy in, 1682
  pneumococcal infection risk in, 51, 51t
  tuberculosis in, 950
NATP (neonatal alloimmune thrombocytopenic purpura), 1558
Natural killer cells
  development of, 788f, 789
  in hemophagocytic lymphohistiocytosis, 1627
Natural killing (NK) activity, in neonatal period, 304
Nature or nurture, in psychological development, 407–408
Nausea, 1351
  opioid-induced, treatment of, 344t
  postoperative management of, 340
Navicular bone
  accessory, 2429, 2429f
  and calcaneus coalition. *See* Tarsal coalition
  in Köhler disease, 2427
  stress fractures in, 2428
NB (normoblast), 1563f
NBT (nitroblue tetrazolium dye test), 1552t
NCC. *See* Neural crest cells
NCCAM (National Center for Complementary and Alternative Medicine), 543
NCEP. *See* National Cholesterol Education Program
NCHS. *See* National Center for Health Statistics
NCI. *See* Neonatal cerebral infarction
NCLs. *See* Neuronal ceroid lipofuscinoses
nDNA mutations. *See* Nuclear DNA mutations
Near drowning. *See* Drowning and near drowning
Near-infrared spectroscopy (NIRS), 2165

Near-miss sudden infant death syndrome (near-miss SIDS), 352
Nearsightedness, 2362
Near triad, 2361, 2387
NEASE. *See* National Eczema Association for Science and Education
Nebulin, 2295
Nebulizer(s), 1922
NEC. *See* Necrotizing enterocolitis
Necator americanus infection, 1104, 1108
  iron deficiency of, 1527
  treatment of, 1099t
Neck
  examination of, in newborn, 88
  masses of
    evaluation of, 1279–1281
    magnetic resonance imaging of, 588
    in newborn, 88
  muscles of, in newborn
    examination of, 93f–94f, 94
    maturation of, 95, 95f
  orthopedic problems of, 2439–2446
  range of motion of, in Klippel-Feil syndrome, 2440
  tumors of, 1270
    in rhabdomyosarcoma, 1612
Neck extensor tone, of newborn, 94, 94f
Neck flexor tone, of newborn, 93f, 94
Neck radiography, for suspected foreign body aspiration, 1278
Necrobiosis lipoidica diabeticorum (NLD), 1236
Necrosis
  acute tubule
    and acute renal failure, 1673
    oliguria in, 1649
  aseptic, after heart transplantation, 1888
  avascular. *See* Avascular necrosis
  bilateral striatal, 2301
  bony, in acute otitis media, 1250
  hepatic, drug-induced, 1503
  hepatocyte, of environmental hepatotoxicity, 1503
  idiopathic epiphyseal ischemic. *See* Idiopathic epiphyseal ischemic necroses
  ischemic, of intestinal mucosa, 141f
  neuronal, in neonatal hypoglycemia, 157
  radiation, 2228
  satellite cell, 1200
  selective neuronal, 2199
  of subcutaneous fat
    birth-related, 185
    neonatal hypercalcemia in, 163
      signs of, 163
      treatment of, 164
    in newborn, 86
Necrotic lesions, of brown recluse spider bites, 393
Necrotizing encephalomyelopathy. *See* Leigh syndrome
Necrotizing enterocolitis (NEC), 140–143, 204
  abdominal wall repair and, 1400
  characteristic feature of, 585
  clinical manifestations of, 141
  conditions associated with increased risk of, 140
  differential diagnosis of, 141
  etiology and pathogenesis of, 141–143, 141f
  incidence of, 140
  laboratory findings of, 141
  in low-birth-weight infants, 59
    incidence of, 60
  and neonatal polycythemia, 193
  outcome of, 143
  pathological findings of, 140

Neuromuscular junction diseases, 2285–2288
Neuromuscular scoliosis, 2441
  orthoses for, 547
Neuromuscular system, motor coordination development in, 481
Neuromyelitis optica, 2315
Neuronal ceroid lipofuscinoses (NCLs), 664, 2328, 2328t
Neuronal necrosis, in neonatal hypoglycemia, 157
Neurons, migration of, 2174
Neuropathy
  childhood peripheral, 2280–2284, 2282t
  in diabetes mellitus type 1, 2133
  vs. myopathy, 2278
Neuropathy, ataxia, retinitis pigmentosa (NARP), 2301
Neurophysin, 2025
Neurophysiologic interventions, for attention deficits, 434
Neuropraxia, of birth-related brachial plexus injury, 186
Neuropsychiatric disorders, pediatric autoimmune, associated with streptococcal infections, 504
Neuropsychiatric lupus, 849t
Neuropsychological testing, indications for, 412t
Neurotoxicity
  cyclosporine and, 1439
  of preventive therapy, for central nervous system leukemia, 1599
Neurotoxic shellfish poisoning, 1160
Neurotransmitters. *See also specific neurotransmitter*
  and rhythmic behaviors, 459
  stimulant medications and, 433
Neurotrophin receptor pathways, and neuroblastoma, 1617
Neurotropic viruses, 2305
Neurulation, 408, 743, 2419
Neutral lipid storage disease, ichthyosiform disorders in, 1184
Neutral protamine Hagedorn (NPH), 2125–2127, 2125t, 2135
Neutral thermal environment, 80–81, 104
  of nursery, 104
  of preterm newborns, 115
    and water loss, 113
Neutropenia(s), 1550–1551
  and abnormal stem cell development, 1550–1551
  classification of, 199
  diagnostic approach to, 1552
  etiology of, 1550
  febrile children with, infection risk in, 304
    treatment of, 304
  fever in, 805, 807f
  in newborns, 199, 1550
    decreased neutrophil production in, 199
    evaluation of, 199
    increased neutrophil destruction in, 199
  oral complications in, 1297
  risk of infections with, 1550
  in Shwachman syndrome, 1465
  treatment of, 154, 1552
  typhlitis in, 1452
Neutrophil(s), 1550–1555
  adverse effects of, 300
  counts of
    absolute, 318
      and neutropenia, 321
    low, 304
    normal, by age, 1548t
  decreased production of, in neonatal neutropenia, 199

development of, 1548
in folate deficiency, 1525f, 1530
function of, 1549–1550, 1549f
  clinical disorders of, 1553t
  defects of, 1552–1554, 1552t–1553t
  developmental changes in, 1550
  specific tests of, 1552, 1552t
increased destruction of, in neonatal neutropenia, 199
kinetics of, 1548–1549
  developmental changes in, 1550
  specific tests of, 1552, 1552t
morphology of, 1549
in neonatal period, 304
phagocytosis by, 1549f
proportion of, in white blood cell count, 318
Neutrophil antigen typing, maternal, 199
Neutrophil glucose-6-phosphate dehydrogenase (G6PD) deficiency, 1554
Neutrophil storage pool (NSP), 1548–1549
Nevirapine, for human immunodeficiency virus infection, 1051t
Nevus (nevi), 1191–1193
  of eyelid, 2365, 2374
  in neonatal examination, 86
Nevus depigmentation, 1194
Nevus flammeus. *See* Port wine stain
Nevus Network Congenital Nevus Support Group, 1191
Nevus of Ito, 1192
Nevus of Ota, 1192, 2367
Nevus sebaceous, 1168, *(Color Plate 1)*
Nevus simplex, 1169, 1207
Nevus spilus, 1191
Nevus unius lateralis, 2347
Newborn(s). *See also* Infant(s); Neonatal; Preterm infant(s)
  abdominal wall defects in, 1399
  acidemia in, screening for, 580t
  acute metabolic encephalopathy in, 599
  acute vomiting in, 1351
  ADA deficiency in, 796
  air patterns in abdominal radiography of, 584–585
  aldosterone in, 1637
  antibiotic therapy in, 881
  aseptic meningitis in, 2306
  assessment of renal function in, 1633, 1638–1639
  atresias in, 1403
  of at-risk pregnancy, 66–76
  behavior of, 414–415
  bilirubin clearance in, 1475
  birth-related injury in, 185–188
  blisters in, 1170t
  blood in
    normal values of, 1519–1521, 1520f
    oxygen affinity of, 1522
    rate of production of, 1519, 1520f
    volume of, 138, 139f
  blood pressure in, 1632
  bowel obstruction in, 1407
  brachial plexus birth-related injury to, physical findings of, 88
  calcium concentration in, 2143, 2149
  calcium reabsorption in, 1636
  calcium regulation disorders in, 161–164
  Candida infections in, 1089
  carbohydrate-deficient glycoprotein syndromes in, 680
  carbohydrate metabolism of, 1473
  care of
    historical perspective on, 55–56
    after intrauterine transfusion for erythroblastosis fetalis, 176

carnitine palmitoyltransferase deficiency in, 629
cerebral infarction in, 2237
chest wall in, 274
  inward deformations of, 274
chloride transport in, 1634
circulatory disturbance in, 285
  initial stabilization of, 292
circulatory system of, 1750–1753
clavicles fractures in, 88
cocaine-exposed, 2203
conditions of, 148–201
congenital diaphragmatic hernia in, 189–191
congenital heart disease in, 1780–1859
congenital hepatic fibrosis with autosomal recessive polycystic disease in, presentation of, 1483
crying characteristics of, 415
cyanosis in, 1815
and delivery room emergencies, 97–103
of diabetic mother, 124–126
DiGeorge syndrome in, and hypocalcemia, 2150
dysmorphic features in, 88, 91, 679, 2168
early-onset group B streptococcus disease in, prevention of, 76
ecchymoses of, 86
eccrine glands of, 1167
emergencies of, 202–207
energy metabolism of, 1473
enteroviral infections in, 1021
epidermolysis bullosa in, 1187
eutectic mixture of local anesthetics cream and, 342
eye development and visual function of, 491
  anomalous, 491–492
fatty acid metabolism of, 1473
fatty acid oxidation disorders in, 628
feeding in, 1327t
feeding problems of, 420–421
  referral of, to speech pathologist, 545, 545t
fever in, 304–305, 305t–306t
foreign bodies of esophagus in, 1397
fractional excretion of sodium in, 1638
galactosemia screening in, 20
galactose-1-phosphate uridyl transferase deficiency galactosemia in, 640
gastric perforation in, 1407
gastric secretion in, 1429
gastrointestinal function of, 107–111
gastrointestinal obstruction in, 1376–1378, 1377f
glomerular filtration rate in, 1632–1633
gluconeogenesis in, 2106
glucose metabolism disorders in, 155–160
glucosuria in, 1634
glutaric acidemia in, 631
glycogen storage disease in, 635
glycogen storage of, 1473
grunting noise in, 274
Haemophilus influenzae infection in, 939
handicapped, refusal of treatment for, 559
hearing loss in, risk criteria of, 486–488
hearing tests in, 22, 488
heart failure in, 1861, 1869, 1872
heart sounds in, 1755
hematologic disorders in, 197–201
hemochromatosis in, 1492
hemolytic disease in, 174–177
hemorrhagic disease in, 1574
hemostasis in, 1570t
hereditary elliptocytosis in, clinical manifestations of, 1540
hereditary sperhocytosis in, clinical manifestations of, 1539

duodenitis from, 1434
for enthesitis-related arthritis, 841
for erythema nodosum, 1237
esophagitis from, 1396
for fibromyalgia, 862
gastric ulceration from, 1372
gastritis from, 1432
for growing pains, 859
for Henoch-Schönlein purpura, 844
hyperkalemia from, 1654
for hypermobility syndrome, 860
hypoaldosteronism from, 1711
for juvenile rheumatoid arthritis, 838
for Langerhans cell histiocytosis, 1626
and necrotizing fasciitis, 997
and platelet dysfunction, 1559
preoperative management of, 335
for reactive arthritis, 842
renal dysplasia from, 1640
for serum sickness, 823
side effects of, 341, 343t
Nonstress testing (NST), antepartum, 69–70
in biophysical profile, 70
Nonstructural scoliosis, 2440
Nonsyndromic autosomal recessive hearing impairment, 1241
Nonsyndromic hereditary hearing impairment
genetic discoveries of, 1241, 1241t
inheritance of, 1241
Nonthyroidal hypermetabolism, 2300
Nonthyroidal illness, in preterm infants, 2065
Nontoxic substances, 356t, 375t
Nontreponemal antigen tests, 1003
Nontuberculous mycobacterial adenitis, 960
Nontuberculous mycobacterial (NTM) infections, 960–963
clinical manifestations of, 960–961
diagnosis of, 961–962
in immunosuppressed patients, 960–961, 963
incidence of, 960
transmission of, 960
treatment of, 962–963
Nontuberculous mycobacterial meningitis, 961
Nonulcer dyspepsia, in motility abnormalities, 1410
Nonverbal learning disabilities (NVLD), 435, 2205–2206
Noonan syndrome, 737t, 1781, 2089, 2090f
subaortic stenosis in, 1804
valvar pulmonic stenosis in, 1809
NORD. See National Organization for Rare Disorders
Norepinephrine, 2055
and blood pressure maintenance, 286
for cyclic antidepressant poisoning, 365
inhibiting TSH release, 2060
for poor systemic perfusion, 291t
synthesis of, 612
and vasoconstriction, 1840
Norethynodrel, during pregnancy, 2082
Norfloxacin, for Shigella infection, 986
Norgestimate plus ethinyl estradiol, for acne, 1210
L-Norgestrel, 258
implant of, 250t
Normoblast (NB), 1563f
Normocalcemia, and renal stones, 1715
Normocytic anemia, in acute myeloid leukemia, 1602
Normoglycemia, maintenance of, in diabetic pregnancy, 68
Normokalemic periodic paralysis, 2294
Norprogesterones, during pregnancy, 776t
Norrbottnian form of Gaucher disease, 2326

Norrie disease, 2390
North America, Hodgkin disease in, 1607
North American Pediatric Renal Transplant Cooperative Study (NAPRTCS), 1729
Northern Europeans, hereditary spherocytosis in, 1539
Norwalk agent, 1024
Norwalk virus, in small intestine and colon infections, 1447
Norwegian (crusted) scabies, 1154, 1234
Norwegian rat, 975
Norwegians, hereditary disease of, 1506
Norwood procedure, for hypoplastic left heart syndrome, 1830
NOS. See Nitric oxide synthase
Nose, 1258–1265. See also under Nasal; Paranasal sinus(es); specific disease
anatomy and embryology of, 1258–1259, 1258f–1259f
blood supply to, 1259
congenital malformations of, 1260–1261
deformities of, with cleft lip and palate, 1268
evaluation of, 1259–1260
examination of
in adolescent, 236
in newborn, 88, 1259
infectious disorders of, 1262–1264
nerve supply to, 1259
normal, 1258
obstruction of, 277
causes of, 1260–1261
surgically correctable, 202
congenital, 202
presentation of, 202
in newborn, 88
olfactory disorders of, 1264
palpation of, 1259
trauma and foreign bodies of, 1264–1265
tumors of, 1264
Nosebleed. See Epistaxis
Nose picking
and epistaxis, 1261
and nasal infection, 1264
Nosocomial infections, of preterm infants, 116
Notochord, 743, 2419
Novelty, withdrawal from, 452, 455
NPH. See Nephronophthisis; Neutral protamine Hagedorn
NPH1. See Juvenile nephronophthisis
NPH2. See Infantile nephronophthisis
NPH3. See Adolescent nephronophthisis
NPH/MCKD. See Nephronophthisis/medullary cystic kidney disease
NPHS1. See Finnish-type congenital nephrotic syndrome
NPS. See Nail-patella syndrome
NRAS gene, mutations of, 1585
NRBC (nucleated red blood cells), 1521
NRTI. See Nucleoside reverse transcriptase inhibitors
NS. See Nephrotic syndrome
NSAIDs. See Nonsteroidal antiinflammatory drugs
NSP (neutrophil storage pool), 1548–1549
NST, antepartum. See Nonstress testing (NST), antepartum
NTDs. See Neural tube defects
NTM. See Nontuberculous mycobacterial (NTM) infections
Nuclear DNA mutations
in hereditary myopathies, 2301
in oxidative phosphorylation diseases, 650–651, 654t
Nuclear family(ies), 510

Nuclear imaging, 589–590
of abdomen, 589
of central nervous system, 590
of chest, 589
of genitourinary tract, 589
patient preparation for, 583t
of skeleton, 589
Nuclear medicine study, radiation dose equivalents of, 584t
Nuclear receptors, 2008, 2011t
Nuclear scintigraphy, of gastroesophageal reflux, 1390
Nucleated red blood cells (NRBC), 1521
Nuclei, 2174
Nucleic acid amplification, 956
Nucleic acid hybridization studies, in enteroviral infections, 1023
Nucleoside analogs
for hepatitis B virus infection, 1497–1498
for hepatitis C virus infection, 1499
Nucleoside reverse transcriptase inhibitors (NRTI), 1049, 1051t
Nucleotide bases, 573
Null point, in nystagmus, 2405
Numerical abnormality of chromosomes, 728
Numeric scale in pain management, 341
Nursemaid's elbow, 2448
treatment for, 2448
Nursery
intensive care. See Intensive care nursery (ICN) graduates
neutral thermal environment of, 104
policy for hyperbilirubinemia in, 168
Nursing. See Breast feeding
Nurture or nature, in psychological development, 407–408
Nut allergy, 1445
Nutcracker esophagus, 1389
Nutramigen, 1334t, 1341
Nutren Junior, 1334t
Nutrient solutions, parenteral, 1345–1347
Nutrition. See also Feeding
in acute renal failure, 1676
anticipatory guidance of, 27–33
age-appropriate discussion topics for, 28t
schedule for, 2t
and atherosclerosis, 1891
in bronchopulmonary dysplasia, 1965
in chronic renal insufficiency, 1721, 1724
in congestive heart failure, 1875
in Crohn disease, 1443
in cystic fibrosis, 1977
and diabetes mellitus type 1, 2128
and diabetes mellitus type 2, 2135
in dying patient, 572
education about, for weight management, 2141
in end-stage renal disease, 1728
excessive, and obesity, 477
excessive spitting up and, 420
of fetus
and adult disease, 66, 124
restricted supply of, effects of, 121
and growth, 1719, 1721
and infant crying, 414
for intensive care nursery graduate, 220
lead poisoning and, 370
management of, in disabled children, 537
of newborns, 107–111, 108t
and osteopenia and rickets, 2157
and picky eaters, 421
screenings for, in disabled children, 537
supplementation of
with fluoride, 32, 32t
with iron, 31
with vitamins, 31

ocular foreign bodies, 2413
orbital fractures, 2415
ruptured globe, 2415
Ocular tuberculosis, 954
Oculoauriculovertebral dysplasia. *See* Goldenhar syndrome
Oculocutaneous albinism (OCA), 1185, 2382
Oculocutaneous tyrosinemia, 612
Oculodermal melanosis, 1192, 2367
Oculoglandular disease, in tularemia, 1009
Oculomotor nerve injury, 2251
Oculomotor nerve paresis, 2364
Oculopharyngeal muscular dystrophy (OPMD), 2293
Odds ratio, 592
Odontodysplasia, regional, 1287
Odynophagia, in *Candida* esophagitis, 1394
OFC. *See* Occipitofrontal circumference
Office(s), emergency preparation in, 332t
Ofloxacam, for gonococcal infections, 261
Ofloxacin
for gonococcal infection, 259t, 969
for *Mycoplasma pneumoniae* disease, 966
for *Salmonella* infection, 984
Ofuji disease, 1217
OGTT. *See* Oral glucose tolerance test
Oguchi disease, 2392
OI (osteogenesis imperfecta), 714, 761, 859, 2157t, 2161
OI (oxygen index), and extracorporeal membrane oxygenation criteria, 213
OIA. *See* Optical immunoassay
OK-432 (picibanil), for lymphangiomas, 1281
Oklahoma Poison Control Center, 398
OKN (optokinetic nystagmus), 491
OKT3 (murine antihuman T lymphocyte antibody), in heart transplantation, 1887
Oleic acid, 2335
Olfactogenital dysplasia, 2177
Olfactory bulb
absence of, 2176
agenesis of, 1264
neurogenesis of, 408
Olfactory chemoreceptive cells, 1264
Olfactory disorders, 1264
Olfactory nerve
injury of, 2251
testing, 2167
Olfactory threshold, 1264
Oligoanuria, in hemolytic uremic syndrome, 1697
Oligoarthritis, 825, 840
Oligoarticular juvenile rheumatoid arthritis. *See* Pauciarticular juvenile rheumatoid arthritis
Oligodendroglia, 409
Oligodendrogliomas, 2222
Oligohydramnios, 742, 1639, 1658
definition of, 70
of fetal obstructive uropathy, 78
in multiple births, 118
and neonatal examination, 83
pulmonary hypoplasia and, 191
renal agenesis of, 191
renal failure and, 1704
Oligomeganephronia, 1640
mode of inheritance of, 1703t
Oligomenorrhea, 249–252
Oligonucleotides, 573
in polymerase chain reaction, 574–576, 575f
Oligopeptides, 1311
absorption of, in newborns, 109
Oligosaccharides, 665
Oligosaccharide tree, 680
Oliguria, 1648–1649
in acute renal failure, 1673

with perinatal asphyxia, 188
Ollier disease, 2452
OLM. *See* Ocular larva migrans
Olopatidine, for allergic diseases, 816
Olsalazine, for ulcerative colitis, 1438
OLVT (organum vasculosum laminae terminalis), 302
Omenn syndrome, 795
genetic bases of, 794t
skin disorders in, 1189
Omental cyst, 1375, 1405
Omeprazole
for gastrinomas, 1456
for peptic ulcer, 1435
Omithine transcarbamylase (OTC) deficiency, strokelike episodes in, 2237
Omovertebral bone, in Sprengel's deformity, 2440
Omphalitis, 90
Omphalocele, 204, 1399–1400
Meckel diverticulum in, 1406
of newborn, 89
Omphalomesenteric cyst, 1405
Omphalomesenteric duct, 1405
remnants of, in newborn, 89
Omphalomesenteric sinus, 1405
Omsk hemorrhagic fever, 1025t, 1026, 1028
Onchocercal eye disease, 1107
Onchocerca volvulus, 1107
Onchocerciasis, 1099t, 1107–1108
Onchocercomas, 1107
Oncogenes, 1585, 1585t
and fetal growth, 64
genetic behavior of, 1585
mutations of, 1585
Oncospheres, 1121
Ondine's curse, 284
ONH (optic nerve hypoplasia), 493
"Onion skin lesion," 1504f, 1505
"Onion skinning" appearance, in radiography, 1611
Onychia, 461
Onycholysis, 1216
Onychomycosis, 1230
in HIV infection, 1200
treatment of, 1080t, 1082–1083
white superficial, 1230
Onychophagia (nail-biting), 461
epidemiology of, 461
management of, 461
O'nyong-nyong, 1019t
Opalescent dentin, 1286
Open adoption, 521–522
Open comedones, 1208
Operative delivery, 75–76. *See also* Cesarean section
Operative vaginal delivery, 75–76
indications for, 76
terminology in, 76
Ophthalmia, gonococcal, 968
prevention of, in newborns, 105
Ophthalmia neonatorum, 2370, 2371f, 2377
prevention of, 968
treatment of, 969
Ophthalmic ointment, for prevention of gonococcal ophthalmia, 105
Ophthalmitis, *Candida,* 1089
Ophthalmoparesis, 2285
Ophthalmopathy, Graves, 2074
Ophthalmoplegic migraine, 2412
Ophthalmoscopy
in Cryotherapy for Retinopathy of Prematurity study, 145
indirect, for screening of retinopathy of prematurity, 146
of newborn, 87

Opiates
and anaphylaxis, 821
and diabetes mellitus, 2115t
for diarrhea, 1365
parental abuse of
clinical implications of, 528
newborn and long-term developmental outcomes with, 527
poisoning by, and initial management of altered consciousness, 293t
Opioid receptors
clinical effects of, 343t
pruritus and, 1480
Opioids
adverse effects of, 341
agonist-antagonists, 342, 344t
antagonists, 344t
dosage and administration of, 344t
for dying patient, 571–572
goals of, 346t
hypoventilation and, 283
for intracranial hypertension, 327
in mechanical ventilation, 319
poisoning by, 372
clinical presentation and management of, 294, 372
toxicology of, 343t, 372
and postoperative management, 340
pure agonists, 342, 344t
side effects of, treatment for, 344t
Opioid toxidromes, 357
Opisthorchiasis, 1099t, 1114t, 1115
Opistorchis felineus, 1115
Opistorchis viverrini, 1115
Opitz G syndrome. *See also* Smith-Lemli-Opitz syndrome
and esophageal anomalies, 1386
Opitz syndrome. *See* Smith-Lemli-Opitz syndrome
OPMD. *See* Oculopharyngeal muscular dystrophy
Opposite-sex pairings, 471
Oppositional defiant disorder, 446
diagnostic criteria for, 447t
Opsite, 388
Opsoclonus, 2167, 2405
Opsoclonus syndrome, 1618
Opsomyoclonus, in neuroblastoma, 1618
Opsomyoclonus syndrome, differential diagnosis of, 1618
Opsonins, 1549
Opsonization
evaluative tests of, 1552t
in events of phagocytosis, 1549
impaired, 1553
Ophthalmologic evaluation, with hearing loss, 488
Optical immunoassay (OIA), 995
Optic atrophy, 2399–2400, 2400t
with inherited neurologic syndromes, 2400
Optic disc, examination of, in newborn, 92
Optic disc edema, 2398
Optic nerve, 2397–2401
congenital anomalies of, 2397–2398
development of, 491
tumors of, 2399
Optic nerve disorders, 493
Optic nerve drusen, 2398
Optic nerve glioma, 2221f, 2399
and true precocious puberty, 2098
Optic nerve hypoplasia (ONH), 493, 2397
Optic nerve injury, 2251
Optic nerve meningioma, 2399
Optic nerve pits, 2397
Optic nerve tumors, 2221
Optic neuritis, 2398–2399

PCC. *See* Propionyl-CoA carboxylase
PCEC. *See* Purified Chick Embryo Cell Vaccine
PCF. *See* Pharyngoconjunctival fever
PCO. *See* Polycystic ovarian syndrome
PCO$_2$. *See* Partial pressure, of carbon dioxide
PCP, 377
PCP. *See* Pneumocystis carinii pneumonia
PCR. *See* Polymerase chain reaction
PCT. *See* Porphyria cutanea tarda
PCV (pneumococcal conjugate vaccine), route and dose of, 40t
PCV7. *See* Pneumococcal conjugate vaccine (PCV), 7 valent
PD. *See* Peritoneal dialysis
PDA. *See* Patent ductus arteriosus
PDA coil occlusion, 1780
PDC. *See* Pyruvate dehydrogenase complex
PDDs. *See* Pervasive developmental disorders
PDE-5. *See* Phosphodiesterase, cGMP specific
PDGF. *See* Platelet-derived growth factor
PDGFβ (platelet-derived growth factor β), in vascular development of kidney, 1632
PDR. *See* Proliferative diabetic retinopathy
Pdx-1 gene, 1308
PE. *See* Progressive encephalopathy
Peacock system. *See* Intensity-modulate radiation therapy
Peak expiratory flow rate (PEFR), 1917
Peak height velocity, 224t
Peak serum total bilirubin (peak STB) concentrations, in newborns, 165
Peanuts, aspiration of, 1277
Peanut agglutinin, Langerhans cells staining for, 1625
Peanut allergy, dimercaprol and, 370
Pearson pancreatic and bone marrow syndrome, 1465
Pearson syndrome, 649, 720t, 1567
Pectins, 1320
Pectus carinatum, 2001
Pectus excavatum, 2001
Pedestrian injuries, mortality statistics of, 37
PEDI (Pediatric Evaluation of Disability Inventory), 534–535
Pedialyte, 1365t
PediaSure, 1334t
Pediatric Advanced Life Support (PALS), 328
  emergency equipment recommended by, for physician offices, 332t
Pediatric autoimmune neuropsychiatric disorders associated with streptococcal infections (PANDAS), 504
Pediatric Basic Life Support (pediatric BLS), 328
Pediatric Evaluation of Disability Inventory (PEDI), 534–535
Pediatrician(s)
  advocacy by, 557
  communication between, in transport of preterm newborn to intensive care unit, 116
  counsel recommendations for
    for families coping with parental death, 519
    for smooth transition of older child to new sibling, 517–518
  and divorced parents of patients, 524
  ethical issues for
    in chronic care and rehabilitation, 553
    in doctor-parent-child relationship, 557–558
  of incurably ill and dying patients
    care for, 571
    communication of bad news by, 565
    emotions of, 567
    responsibility of, 563

in management of erythroblastosis fetalis, 175
and mothers with Munchausen by proxy syndrome, 506
and neonatal resuscitation, 98
preparation by, for resuscitation of patients, 327–328, 332t
role of
  in adoption, 522, 522t
  in complementary and alternative therapy use, 542
  in doctor-parent-child relationship, 557–558
  in foster care, 522, 523t
  in learning evaluations, 436t, 437
  in life-threatening diseases, 271
  in liver transplantation, 1518
  in management of developmental disabilities, 439–440
  in nonparental child care, 513–514
  for poor children, 531
Pediatric Oncology Group (POG), 1583
Pedicellariae, of phylum echinodermata, 392
Pediculosis, 1155–1156
  in health care personnel, 887t
Pediculus humanus, 980
Pediculus humanus capitis, 1155, 1234, 2365
Pediculus humanus corporis, 1155
Pediculus pubis, 2365
PEEP. *See* Positive end-expiratory pressure
PEG. *See* Percutaneous endoscopic gastrostomy
Pel-Ebstein fevers, of Hodgkin disease, 1608
Pelizaeus-Merzacher disease (PMD), 2337, 2337f
Pelvic appendix, 1450
Pelvic examination
  in amenorrhea evaluation, 252
  schedule for, 2t
Pelvic ganglia, neuroblastoma in, 1617
Pelvic inflammatory disease (PID), 268–269
  abdominal pain in, 1355
  acute, treatment regimens for, 266t
  clinical approach, 269
  complication of, 269
  diagnosis of, 262t, 268–269
  differential diagnosis of, 268
  gonorrhea and, 268, 968
  hospitalization criteria for, 269
  oral contraceptives and, 261
  pathogenesis of, 268
  risk factors for, 268
  symptoms and signs of, 262t, 268
  treatment of, 266t, 269
Pelvic osteomyelitis, 835
Pelvis
  computed tomography of, 587
  radiography of, 584–585
    in evaluation of limping, 2421–2422
  ultrasonography of, 587
Pemoline, 433
  hepatotoxicity of, 1503
Pemphigus, 1201
Pemphigus erythematosus, 1201
Pemphigus foliaceus, 1201
Pemphigus vulgaris, 1201
Pena-Shokier syndrome, 737t
Pencil-and-paper tasks, 2166
Pendred syndrome, 1239, 2067
Pendular nystagmus, 2167, 2405
Pendular waveform, 2405
Penetrance, 714
Penicillamine
  for corrosive esophagitis, 1396
  for cystinuria, 1712
  during pregnancy, 776t

for scleroderma, 1199
for Wilson disease, 2332
D-Penicillamine
  for linear scleroderma, 858
  for systemic sclerosis, 857
Penicillin(s)
  and anaphylaxis, 821
  β-lactamase-resistant, 873
  β-lactamase-sensitive
    broad-spectrum, 873
    narrow-spectrum, 871–873
  for brain abscess, 2321
  for cellulitis, 868t
  for conjunctivitis, 868t
  as convulsants, 2254
  for cranial subdural empyema, 2319
  cross-reactivity between aztreonam and, 821
  cross-reactivity between cephalosporins and, 821
  cross-reactivity between imipenem and, 821
  dosage and administration of, 872t
  for ecthyma gangrenosum, 1218
  for group C and G streptococcal infections, 1002
  for group D streptococcal infections, 1002
  Henoch-Schönlein purpura from, 842
  and immune hemolytic anemia, 1545
  for intervertebral disk infection, 2322
  for intrapartum chemoprophylaxis of group B streptococcus carriers, 154
  for joint infections, 868t
  for Lyme disease, 947, 947t
  mechanism of action of, 871–873
  for meningococcal disease, 971
  for meningococcemia, 1225
  for *Moraxella catarrhalis* infections, 949
  for neonatal pneumonia caused by group B streptococcal infection, 153
  for *Pasteurella multocida* infection, 972
  for pharyngitis, 868t
  for pneumococcal infection prevention in sickle cell disease, 1532, 1562
  for pneumococcal peritonitis prevention, 1695
  for rat-bite fever, 980
  for recurrent infection prevention, 792
  for relapsing fever, 981
  for rheumatic fever, 1903
  for scarlet fever, 1225
  Stevens-Johnson syndrome from, 1196
  for streptococcal infections, 998
  synthetic, hepatotoxicity of, 1503
  for syphilis, 256t, 1003
  toxic epidermal necrolysis from, 1196
  toxicity of, 874
  for viridans streptococcal infection, 1002
Penicillin allergy, 154, 821
  acute otitis media treatment in, 1252
  gonococcal infection treatment in, 969
  meningococcal disease treatment in, 971
  Pasteurella multocida infection treatment in, 973
  streptococcal pharyngitis treatment in, 998
  syphilis treatment in, 1003
Penicillin G. *See also* Crystalline penicillin G; Benzathine penicillin G; Procaine penicillin G
  dosage and administration of, 872t
  dosage recommendations of, for meningitis of newborns, 153
  for group B streptococcus infection, 1000
    in pregnancy, 76
  for group B streptococcus infection prevention, 1001
  for meningitis, 903t

for neonatal pneumonia caused by group B streptococcal infection, 153
for rheumatic fever, 1903
for streptococcal infection prevention, 999
for streptococcal pharyngitis, 998
Penicillin resistance
in gonococcal infection, 969
in pneumococcal infection, 978–979
in streptococcal infection, 1002
in *Yersinia enterocolitica* infection, 1012
Penicillin V
for streptococcal infection prevention, 999
for streptococcal pharyngitis, 998
Penicillium, 813
in fungal corneal ulcers, 2377
Penile curvature, 1739
Penile epispadias, of newborn, 90
Penile hypospadias, of newborn, 90
Penile torsion, 1739
Penis
of ambiguous genitalia, 90
anomalies of, 1739–1740
of newborn
examination of, 90
postnatal care and observation of, 105–106
physical examination of, 244
in newborn, 90
Pennaria tiarelia (feathered hydroid), poisonous sting of, 391
Pentamidine
for babesiosis, 1125
for cutaneous leishmaniasis, 1136
and diabetes mellitus, 2114, 2115t
dosage and administration of, 1149
and pancreatitis, 1414
for *Pneumocystis carinii* pneumonia, 1145
for *Pneumocystis carinii* pneumonia prophylaxis, 1049
side effects of, 1149
for sleeping sickness, 1099t, 1149
for visceral leishmaniasis, 1135
Pentose metabolism, disorders of, 642
Pentostam. *See* Sodium stibogluconate
Pentosuria, essential benign, 642
PEPCK. *See* Phosphoenolpyruvate carboxykinase
PEPCK deficiency. *See* Phosphoenolpyruvate carboxykinase (PEPCK) deficiency
PEP (phosphoenolpyruvate) deficiency, 1541f
Pepsin, 1311
Peptamen, 1334t
Peptamen Junior, 1334t
Peptic diseases, 1429–1435. *See also specific disease*
diagnosis of, 1434
symptoms of, 1430
treatment of, 1434
Peptic strictures, esophagitis and, 1391
Peptic ulcer
chronic vomiting in, 1352
in Meckel diverticulum, 1406
Peptic ulcer disease, 1433–1434
age of onset of, 1430
Helicobacter pylori, 1430, 1432–1433
in intestinal pseudoobstruction, 1410
iron deficiency of, 1527
primary, 1433
secondary, 1434
symptoms of, 1430
treatment of, 1435
Pepto-Bismol, 1366
Peptostreptococcus, and necrotizing fasciitis, 1219
Perception, 2203

Percussion
in craniospinal examination, 2167
for heart, 1755
Percutaneous drug absorption, in preterm newborns, 147
Percutaneous endoscopic gastrostomy (PEG), 1339
Percutaneous intravenous central catheters (PICC), 323, 1345
Percutaneous liver biopsy, 1471
Percutaneous peripheral vein cannulation, 321–322
common complications of, 321
priorities of, 321
procedure of, 321–322
risks and benefits of, 322t
sites for, 321
Percutaneous transhepatic cholangiography (PTC), 1471, 1472t
for primary sclerosing cholangitis, 1505, 1506f
Percutaneous umbilical blood sampling (PUBS)
in prenatal management of congenital diaphragmatic hernia, 77f
in prenatal management of obstructive uropathy, 78f
for prenatal platelet counts, 1558
Perez maneuver, 1658
Perfluorochemical (PFC) liquids, for liquid-assisted ventilation, 217
distribution of, 217
in partial liquid ventilation, 218
physiochemical properties and, 218
maintenance of, in partial liquid ventilation, 218
Perforated abdominal viscus, differential diagnosis of, 149
Perforin, 789
Performance, 404–405
impairment of, referral with, 544
variance in, 406
Performance tests, for attention deficits, 433
Perfusion pressure, and tissue perfusion, 285
Perianal abscess, 1460
Perianal dermatitis, 1460
Perianal streptococcal cellulitis, 1219
Perianal streptococcal infection, 1461
Pericardial diseases, 1865–1868
infectious causes of, 1867
inflammatory, 1865–1866
noninfectious causes of, 1868
pericardial effusion, 1865
Pericardial effusion, 1865
in mixed connective tissue disease, 851
Pericardial knock, 1867
Pericardial lesions, 1868
Pericardial pain, 1894
Pericardiocentesis, 1866
Pericarditis
acute, 1865
acute nonspecific, 1867
chest pain in, 1894
chronic constrictive, 1866
in enteroviral infections, 1022
etiology of, 1867t
in familial Mediterranean fever, 865
Haemophilus influenzae, 939
in juvenile dermatomyositis, 854
in mixed connective tissue disease, 851
purulent, 1867
in rheumatic fever, 1902
in rheumatoid arthritis, 1868
in systemic lupus erythematosus, 850
treatment of, 868t
tuberculous, 952, 1867

in uremia, 1868
Perichondritis, 1256
Periductular fibrosis, 1504f
Perilobar nephrogenic rest, 1615
Perilymphatic fistula(s), 1239
from barotrauma, 1257
treatment for, 1257
and vertigo, 1246
Perimembranous ventricular septal defects, 1746
Perinasal sinuses, palpation of, 1259
Perinatal asphyxia, 188
consequences of, 99t, 188
management of, in meconium aspiration syndrome, 196
outcome of, 221
signs of, 99t
Perinatal care
in hospital levels of, 57t
regionalization of, 57
Perinatal complications, and ear or hearing problems, 1242, 1245
Perinatal death, definition of, 57
Perinatal hemochromatosis. *See* Neonatal hemochromatosis
Perinatal history, in attention deficits, 432
Perinatal hypovolemia, cause of, 102t
Perinatal mortality and morbidity, of multiple births, 59, 117
Perinatal mortality rates, 58f
of infants of diabetic mothers, 124
Perineal anoplasty, for imperforate anus, 204
Perineal fistula, 204
Perineal irritation, and urinary tract infections, 1668
Perineal trauma, and urinary tract infections, 1668
Perineum
burns of, 385
single opening of, 204
Perinuclear labeling antineutrophil cytoplasmic antibodies (pANCA), 846
Periodic abstinence, 250t
Periodic acid-Schiff reaction, in acute lymphoblastic leukemia, 1596
Periodic breathing
definition of, 1934
pathophysiology of, 1938
and respiratory system efficiency, 282
Periodic fetal heart rate pattern(s), 71–74
Periodic lateralizing epileptiform discharges (PLEDS), 2269
Periodontal disease, in adolescents, 236
Periodontal ligaments, 1283
Periodontitis, 1291–1292, 1292t
Perioperative care, 333–340, 334f–335f, 335t–336t, 339t
Periorbital cellulitis, 1218
Periorbital edema, in minimal-change nephrotic syndrome, 1692
Periorbital infection, signs of, 1263
Periorbital inflammation, in lymphadenitis, 1280
Periorificial dermatitis, 1177
Periosteal osteosarcoma, 1610
Peripapillary gliosis, 2167
Peripapillary halo, 2397
Peripheral adrenergic blockers, for hypertension, 1884
Peripheral blood counts, in acute myeloid leukemia, 1602
Peripheral blood eosinophilia, 814
for drug allergy, 821
Peripheral blood smear, for evaluation of neonatal neutropenia, 199
Peripheral blood values, in remission, 1598

Radiography (*contd.*)
  in respiratory syncytial virus infection, 1066
  of rheumatic disease, 831
  of rickets, 2433f
  sail sign in, 149, 150f
  of sella turcica, 2017
  of sever disease, 2427
  of sinusitis, 1260
  of skeletal dysplasias, 758
  of skull. *See* Skull radiography
  of skull fractures, 2243
  of spinal cord injury, 348, 2249
  of spondylolysis and spondylolisthesis, 2444
  of Sprengel's deformity, 2440
  in stridor, 1274
  of subdural hematoma, 2246
  of toddler's fracture, 2451
  of tuberous sclerosis, 2344
  upper gastrointestinal, of gastroesophageal
    reflux, 1390
  of vertebrae, "scotty dog" configuration in,
    2444
Radioimmunoassay studies, for measuring ster-
    oid levels, 2035
Radioisotope studies, 2170
Radiologic imaging
  conventional, of respiratory tract, 1911
  in lobar emphysema, 1925, 1925f–1926f
Radionuclide cystography, 589
Radionuclide hepatobiliary excretion scans,
    1476
Radionuclide imaging, 589–590
  of abdomen, 589
  of central nervous system, 590
  of chest, 589
  of gastrointestinal bleeding, 1374
  of genitourinary tract, 589
  of inflammatory heart disease, 1772
  of left-to-right shunt, 1769–1770
  of liver, 1471, 1472t
  of myocardial perfusion, 1771
  renal, 1662
  of right-to-left shunt, 1770
  of skeleton, 589
  of urinary tract infection, 1671
  of ventricular function, 1770
Radionuclide scans, in osteomyelitis, 906
Radiopharmaceuticals, in radionuclide imaging,
    589
Radiotherapy, 2214t
  for acute lymphoblastic leukemia relapse,
    1599
  for astrocytomas, 2224
  for brainstem glioma, 2220
  for Burkitt lymphoma, 1606
  cardiovascular, 1773–1774
  for central nervous system leukemia, 1598
    delayed complications of, 1599
  for cerebellar astrocytoma, 2219
  for choroid plexus tumors, 2227
  for chronic focal encephalitis, 2309
  for CNS tumors, 2212
  for cortical gliomas, 2222
  for craniopharyngioma, 2227
  and delayed puberty, 2103
  for diencephalic glioma, 2222
  for diffuse gliomas, 2219
  for ependymoma, 2218
  for Ewing sarcoma-PNET, 1612
  for germ cell tumors, 2225
  and growth, 1593, 2018, 2228
  for Hodgkin disease, 1609
  for Kasabach-Merritt phenomenon, 1206
  for Langerhans cell histiocytosis, 1626
  long-term toxicity of, 1593t
  for medulloblastoma, 2217

  for meningioma, 2228
  for Menkes disease, 679
  and myocardial disease, 1861
  for neuroblastoma, 1619
  neurologic toxicity of, 2228
  for non-Hodgkin lymphoma, 1606
  oral complications of, 1298
  for pulmonary metastasis, of Wilms tumor,
    1616
  for rhabdomyosarcoma, 1614
    dosage of, 1614
  for thyroid neoplasia, 2077
  for Wilms tumor, 1616
Radioulnar synosteoses, 2448
Radius(i)
  absent, amegakaryocytic thrombocytopenia
    with, 200, 1556f, 1558
    physical abnormalities in, 1565t
  fractures in, healing of, 2451
RAG deficiency, 794
Rage attacks, 2276
Ragged-red fibers, 648, 2299
Raise-to-sit maneuver, in motor examination,
    of newborn, 93f, 94
  responses to, 94f
Rale(s), of newborns, 89
Ramsey-Hunt syndrome, and external otitis,
    1255
Ramstedt pyloromyotomy, for infantile hyper-
    trophic pyloric stenosis, 1402
Random-dot-E stereo test, 21
Randomized control trials (RCT), 590–591
  of intensive care nursery interventions, 219
  limitations of, 591
Range of motion (ROM)
  of hips
    normal, 2424, 2424t
    in slipped capital femoral epiphysis, 2438
  of neck, in Klippel-Feil syndrome, 2440
  orthoses for, 547–548
  spasticity and, 540
Range of motion (ROM) exercises, for brachial
    plexus palsies, 2447
Ranitidine
  in parenteral nutrition solutions, 1347
  for peptic diseases, 1434
RANK. *See* Receptor activator of nuclear fac-
    tor-κB
Ranula, 88
RAP. *See* Recurrent abdominal pain
Rapamune. *See* Sirolimus
Rapamycin. *See* Sirolimus
Rapid assessment system of neurologic disabil-
    ity, 350, 350t
Rapid intravenous fluid resuscitation, for intes-
    tinal malrotation, 1401
Rapidly progressive glomerulonephritis
    (RPGN), 1677, 1685–1686
  causes of, 1686f
  clinical manifestations of, 1686
  epidemiology of, 1685
  laboratory findings in, 1686
  in lupus nephritis, 1687
  in polyarteritis nodosa, 845
  treatment of, 1686
Rapidly rising pulse, 1754
Rapid plasma reagin (RPR) flocculation test,
    1003
"Rapid strep" test, 995
Rapp-Hodgkin syndrome, 1189
RAS (*HRAS, KRAS, NRAS*) genes, mutations
    of, 1585
Rash. *See also specific rash*
  in contact dermatitis, 1180
  in dengue, 1027
  in dermatomyositis, 1198

  in diaper dermatitis, 1176
  in drug hypersensitivity, 1194
  in ehrlichiosis, 1015
  in enteroviral infections, 1021
  in Epstein-Barr virus infection, 1036
  in erythema infectiosum, 1058
  in exanthema subitum, 1039
  with fever, 1231f
    evaluation of, 1230
  in graft-*versus*-host disease, 1200, 1592
  in Henoch-Schönlein purpura, 843
  in Lyme disease, 946
  in measles, 1053–1054
  in meningococcal disease, 970
  in neonatal examination, 86, 86f
  in rat-bite fever, 980
  in rheumatic fever, 1902
  in rickettsialpox, 1017
  in Rocky Mountain spotted fever, 1014
  in rubella, 1076
  in scabies, 1154
  in scarlet fever, 996
  in schistosomiasis, 1116
  in systemic lupus erythematosus, 849
  in typhus, 1016
  in varicella, 1042
Rashking procedure. *See* Balloon atrial septos-
    tomy
Rasmussen encephalitis, 2309
Rasmussen syndrome. *See* Epilepsia partialis
    continua
RAST. *See* Radioallergosorbent test
RAST-CAP test, 819
Rastelli procedure
  for transposition of great arteries with pul-
    monary stenosis, 1826
  for truncus arteriosus, 1832
Rat-bite fever, 980
  clinical manifestations of, 980
  diagnosis of, 980
  treatment of, 980
Ratchet splint, 548
Rational evaluation, of mental retardation, 780
Rat poison. *See* Rodenticide
Rattlesnakes. *See* Pit vipers (Crotalidae)
Raw meat. *See* Uncooked meat
Raynaud phenomenon
  in fibromyalgia, 862
  in juvenile dermatomyositis, 854
  in localized scleroderma, 858
  in mixed connective tissue disease, 851
  in scleroderma, 1199
  in systemic lupus erythematosus, 1198
  in systemic sclerosis, 857
Raynaud syndrome, 1865
RB. *See* Retinoblastoma
RBCs. *See* Red blood cells
RBF. *See* Renal blood flow
RB gene, 1588
RB1 gene, mutations of, and hereditary cancer
    predisposition, 1586
RB pathway
  defects in, 1589
  in regulation of cell cycle, 1587, 1588f
rBPI$_{21}$ therapy, 301
RCDP. *See* Rhizomelic chondrodysplasia punc-
    tata
RCT. *See* Randomized control trials
RD. *See* Reiter disease
RDAs. *See* Recommended Dietary Allowances
RDS. *See* Respiratory distress syndrome
RDW. *See* Red cell distribution width
Reabilan, 1334t
Reabsorption atelectasis, oxygen supplementa-
    tion and, 317
Reaction intensity, 450t

Reactivation, of autonomic nervous system, 402
Reactive arthritis, 841–842
    in *Yersinia enterocolitica* infection, 842, 1012
Reactive test, of fetus, 70
Reactivity, of fetus, testing of, 69–70
Reading difficulties, 435
Reading medical literature, 594–595
REAL (Revised European-American Lymphoma) classification system
    of Hodgkin disease, 1607
    of non-Hodgkin lymphoma, 1604, 1604t
Real-time imaging, 1762
Real-time intraoperative guidance, 2212
Rebuck window, 1552t
Receiver Operating Characteristic (ROC) curve, 594
Receptive language skills
    age-appropriate, 18t
    assessment of, 442
        guidelines for, 442t–443t
        "red flags" in, 443t
    definition of, 441
    development of, 442t
Receptor activator of nuclear factor-κB (RANK), 2144
Recessive combined immune deficiency syndrome, X-linked (X-SCID), prenatal treatment of, 79
Recessive X-linked ichthyosis, 1183
Recipients
    of heart transplant, selection of, 1886
    of kidney transplant
        age of, 1728
            and posttransplant growth, 1734
            and survival rate, 1729
        bacterial infections in, 1729
        gender of, 1728
        noncompliance in, 1731
        race of, 1728–1729
        viral infections in, 1729
Reciprocal translocation, 728
Reciprocating gait orthosis (RGO), 548
Recluse spiders, 393, 1152, 1235
Recoarctation, 1808
Recognition acuity, 2352, 2411
Recoil forces of lungs, 273
    and restrictive impairments, 273
Recombinant activated protein C (rhAPC), for sepsis, 301
Recombinant granulocyte colony-stimulating factor, for neonatal group B streptococcal sepsis, 154
Recombinant human erythropoietin, 176
Recombinant human growth hormone (rhGH)
    for growth failure, 1727
    for hypopituitarism, 2019
Recombinant human insulin, 2125
Recombinant human leptin treatment, 2138
Recombinant interferon alfa, for hemangiomas, 1206
Recombivax-HB, 48–50, 49t
    dosage and administration of, 1502t
Recommended Dietary Allowances (RDAs), 1313–1314, 1315f, 1316t
Reconstituted whole blood, 1577
Records, centralized, 535
Recreational activities, prostheses for, 549
Recreational drugs of abuse. *See* Substance abuse
Recreational therapy
    for disabled children, 549
    therapeutic goals of, 549
Recreational vehicle use
    medical consequences of, 230t

physical signs with, 232t
    screening laboratory tests of, 235t
Rectal bleeding
    in anal fissures, 1460
    in juvenile polyposis, 1453
    in lymphonodular hyperplasia, 1455
Rectal disorders. *See* Anorectal disorders
Rectal duplications, 1405
Rectal examination
    of adolescent, 236
    in Hirschsprung disease, 204
Rectal manipulation, in bowel management of disabled children, 540
Rectal prolapse, 1459
Rectal temperature, of newborn, 104
Rectum, 1307
    development of, 1307
    female reproductive examination by, 245t
    infections of, 270
Recurrent abdominal pain (RAP), 425, 1357–1363
    causes of, 1357, 1359t–1360t
    clinical manifestations of, 425
    criteria for, 1358
    definition of, 1357
    differential diagnosis of, 1359–1361
    epidemiology of, 425
    isolated, 1361t
    prognosis of, 1363
    treatment of, 1362–1363
Recurrent acute otitis media, 1252
Recurrent infections, 791–793
    clinical manifestations of, 791–792
    in HIV infection, 1047
    investigation of, 792, 793t
    management of, 792
Recurrent pain syndromes (RPS), 424–426
    assessment and management of, principles of, 426
    treatment of, 426
Recurvatum, 2430, 2430f
Red blood cell casts, 1660, 1660f
Red blood cell count
    in cerebrospinal fluid, 2169
    in fetus, 1519
Red blood cell mass, in adolescence, 223
Red blood cells (RBCs)
    abnormalities of, 1539–1544
    autoantibodies of, 1546
    components of, use of, 1576t
    cytoadherence of, in malaria, 1137
    destruction of. *See also* Hemolysis
        in spleen, 1560
    developmental changes in production and function of, 1519–1522
    glucose metabolism in, 1541f
    inclusions and membrane vesicles of, splenic "pitting" of, 1560
    life span of, 1519
        in sickle cell disease, 1531
    mean volume of, 1520, 1521t
    measurements of, 1523–1524
    membrane structure of, 1539
    morphology of, 1522f, 1524, 1525f
    nucleated, 1521
    packed, 1577
        and reconstituted whole blood, 1577
    pocks of, splenic "pitting" of, 1560
    sickled, irreversibly, in sickle cell and hemoglobin S-C diseases, 1532t
    sickling of, 1531
    for transfusions, 1577–1579
        compatibility of, 1577–1578, 1578t
        for hemolytic uremic syndrome, 1698
        indications for, 1577
    in urine, 1660, 1663, 1668

values of, in iron deficiency anemia, 1525f, 1527
Red cell aplasia
    acquired, 1565t–1566t, 1566–1567
    acute, of sickle cell disease, 1532
Red cell distribution width (RDW), 1523
    and iron deficiency anemia, 1527
Red cell enzymopathies, 1541–1544
    presenting age of, 1523
Red cell substitutes, 1577
Red reflex
    assessment of, 21
    in ophthalmoscopic examination, of newborn, 87
Reduced cardiac ejection fraction, 287, 288f, 289t
Reduced cardiac filling, 287, 288f, 289t
Reduced clearance, of drug preparations, in preterm newborns, 147
Reduced penetrance, 714
Reduced-size hepatic allografts, 1470f, 1517
5α-Reductase, 2031
5α-Reductase deficiency, 476, 2031, 2086
Reduction exchange transfusion, in neonatal polycythemia, 193
    volume to exchange, calculation of, 193
Reduction maneuver, for nursemaid's elbow, 2448
Reed-Sternberg cells, 1607
Refeeding syndrome, 1337, 1346–1347
Referral
    to allergist, for sinusitis, 1263
    to orthopedist
        for anterolateral bowing of tibia, 2424
        for developmental dysplasia of hips, 2436
        for knee effusion, 2449
        for osteochondritis dissecans, 2433
    to otolaryngologist, for complications of bacterial sinusitis, 1263
    to speech pathologist, for disabled children, 545, 545t
Referred pain, 1354
Reflex(es). *See also specific reflex*
    developmental assessment of, 14t
    maturational changes in, 95
    in neurologic examination of motor development, 481
        in newborn, 94–95
    in regulatory system of respiration, 271, 272f, 273
    in stages of hepatic encephalopathy, 1513t
Reflex epilepsy, 2258
Reflex irritability, of newborns, in Apgar scoring system, 99t
Reflex late deceleration(s), of fetal heart rate, 72–73, 72f
Reflex neurovascular dystrophy. *See* Reflex sympathetic dystrophy syndrome
Reflex sympathetic dystrophy syndrome (RSDS), 860–861
Reflux nephropathy, 1672
Refractive accommodative esotropia, 2403
Refractive error, 489
    clinical manifestation of, 492–493, 492t
    incidence of, 491t
    management and treatment of, 496t
    in newborns, 492
    preschool screening program guidelines for, 495t
    prevalence of, 496t
Refsum disease, 676f, 678
Refusal, of treatment, 559–560
    adolescents and, 560
    for handicapped newborns, 559
    for young children, 558–560
Refusal skills, 430

Rosai-Dorfman disease, 1624t
Rosenthal fibers, 2218, 2339
Roseola infantum. *See* Exanthema subitum
Rose spots, 983
Rosiglitazone, for diabetes mellitus type 2, 2136
Ross procedure, 1803
Rostellum, 1120
Rotator cuff tendinitis, 2448
Rotatory nystagmus, 2167
Rotavirus infection
and carbohydrate malabsorption, 1425
clinical manifestations of, 1024
diagnosis of, 1024
in diarrhea, 1023
in immunodeficiency, 1413
in severe combined immunodeficiency, 794
in small intestine and colon infections, 1447
Rotavirus vaccine, 52, 1024
contraindications to, 44t
Rothmund-Thomson syndrome, 1190
Roth spots, 2395
Rotor syndrome, presenting age of, 1489t
Roundback deformity, 2442
adolescent, 2442
juvenile, 2442
Roundworms. *See* Nematode infections
Roussy-Levy syndrome, 2283
Routines, in management of family transitions, 519
Roux-en-Y, for esophageal drainage, 1393
Roving eye movements, 491
Rovsing sign, 1450
RP. *See* Retinitis pigmentosa
R-5-P (ribose-5-phosphatase) deficiency, 1541f
RPGN. *See* Rapidly progressive glomerulonephritis
RPR. *See* Rapid plasma reagin (RPR) flocculation test
RPS. *See* Recurrent pain syndromes
R-R interval, 1844, 1846
RSDS. *See* Reflex sympathetic dystrophy syndrome
RSL. *See* Renal solute load
RSV. *See* Respiratory syncytial virus
RSV-IGIV. *See* Respiratory syncytial virus immune globulin intravenous
RT-PCR (reverse transcriptase PCR), 575
RU-486, 2010
Rubella, 1075–1079, 1221, 1224
congenital, 1077–1079
clinical manifestations of, 1077–1078, 1077f
and diabetes mellitus, 2115, 2117
laboratory study of, 1078
physical findings of, in newborn, 86
prognosis of, 1078
treatment and prevention of, 1078
and congenital hearing loss, 1245
congenital hydrocephalus from, 2182
conjunctivitis and, 2369
diagnosis of, 46
in health care personnel, 887t
and juvenile rheumatoid arthritis, 836
maternal, 776t, 1077
and patent ductus arteriosus, 1078, 1781, 1785
and peripheral pulmonic stenosis, 1781
and valvar pulmonic stenosis, 1781
natural history of, 1076f
neonatal seizures from, 2269
postnatal, 1075–1077
clinical manifestations of, 1075–1076
diagnosis of, 1076–1077
treatment and prevention of, 1077

Rubella cataract, 2388
Rubella embryopathy syndrome, 2312
Rubella syndrome
classic, 2312
peripheral systemic arterial stenosis, 1809
stenosis of pulmonary artery in, 1812
Rubella vaccine, 1077. *See also* MMR vaccine
contraindications for, 804
Rubeola. *See* Measles
Rubinstein-Taybi syndrome, 737t
Rubra miliaria, of newborn, 86
Rule(s), establishment of, 36
Rule of nines, in burn-wound management, 385
Rule of threes, for colic syndrome, 414
Rule of twos, for Meckel diverticulum, 1406
Rumination, 421
Runaways, 559
Ruptured globe, ocular trauma from, 2415
Rupture of membrane, premature. *See* Premature rupture of membrane (PROM)
Russell-Silver syndrome, 737t
Rust ring, from metallic corneal foreign bodies, 2413
Ruvalcaba-Myhre-Smith syndrome, 1454
RV. *See* Residual volume; Right ventricle
RVA. *See* Rabies Vaccine Adsorbed
RVF. *See* Rift Valley fever
R wave(s), 1761f
in electrocardiogram, 1757
RXR. *See* Retinoid-X receptor
Ryanodine receptor, 2295–2296
Rye, and celiac disease, 1418
Rye classification, of Hodgkin disease, 1607

S

Sabiá hemorrhagic fever (SHF), 1025t, 1026
Sabiá virus, 1025t, 1026
Saccharomyces boulardii, for diarrhea, 1365
Saccharomyces cerevisiae, 1425
in Crohn disease, 1436
Saccular aneurysms, 2239
Saccular cysts, 1404
Saccule, 1239
Sacral agenesis, in embryonal development, 2419
Sacral agenesis syndrome, 2188
Sacral myelomeningocele, orthoses for, 548
Sacrococcygeal teratoma (SCT), 204, 1376
clinical features of, 1623
prenatal management of, 78
prognosis of, 1623
sequelae of, 1624
treatment for, 1623
Sacrosidase, for carbohydrate malabsorption, 1425
SAD. *See* Separation anxiety disorder
Saddle-nose deformity, 1004, 1265
Saethre-Chotzen syndrome, 749t
Safety, 28t, 37–39
margin of, 1313–1314
in nonparental child care settings, 513
Sagittal-plane vector loop, 1758
Sagittal suture, premature closure of, 2167
Sagittal synostosis, 755
Sagittal views, 1766f
Saguenay Lac-Saint-Jean type of Leigh syndrome, 651
Sail sign, in radiography, 149, 150f
St. Jude's staging system, of non-Hodgkin lymphoma, 1605, 1606t
Salicylate(s). *See also* Aspirin
and drug eruption, 1195
ototoxicity of, 1249

poisoning by, 375–376
clinical presentation of, 294, 376
hemodialysis for, 359
management of, 376
nomogram, 376f
serum salicylate concentrations in, 376
toxicology of, 375–376
urinary alkinization for, 359
and respiratory alkalosis, 1657
and varicella vaccine, 51
Salicylic acid
for molluscum contagiosum, 1056
for psoriasis, 1181
Saline, isotonic
for hypotensive infants, 139
for hypovolemia of newborns, 103
Saline solutions
for diabetic ketoacidosis, 2119
for nonketotic hyperosmolar coma, 2123
toxicity of, 147
Salivary amylase, 110, 1311
Salivary gland(s)
anatomy of, 1267
embryology of, 1267
examination of, 1268
inflammation of, 1280
tumor of, 1270
Salivation, excessive, in gastrointestinal obstruction, 1377
Salla disease, 663, 2331
Salmeterol, for asthma, dosage and administration of, 1956t
Salmon calcitonin, 2148
for hypercalcemia, 2156
for neonatal hypercalcemia, 164
Salmonella choleraesuis, 981, 983
Salmonella enterica, 981
Salmonella enteritidis, 981
Salmonella hadar, 981
Salmonella heidelberg, 981
Salmonella hirschfeldii, 983
Salmonella infection, 981–984
bacteremia and
management of, 307
natural history of, 307
in brain abscess, 2320
clinical manifestations of, 982–983
diagnosis of, 983
in diarrhea, 1363
epidemiology of, 981–982
in immunodeficiency, 1413
mortality of, 984
occult bacteremia and, 307
pathogenesis of, 982
prevention of, 984
of sickle cell disease, 1532
in small intestine and colon infections, 1447
treatment of, 983–984, 984t
Salmonella marinum, 981
Salmonella paratyphi A, 983
Salmonella schottmuelleri, 983
Salmonella-Shigella (SS) agar, 981, 985
Salmonella typhi, 981–983
Salmonella typhimurium
drug-resistant, 984
and reactive arthritis, 842
Salmonella urbana, 981
Salmon patch, 1169, 1207
Salmon patch hemangiomas, of newborns, 86
Salpingectomy, for ectopic pregnancy, 255
Salpingostomies, for ectopic pregnancy, 255
Salt. *See also* Sodium
excretion of, by preterm newborns, 114
intake of, for preterm newborns, 114

Salt (*contd.*)
  restricted in diet, for nephrogenic diabetes insipidus, 1714
Salt balance, in preterm infant(s), assessment of, 114
Salter classification, of growth plate fractures, 2450, 2450f
Salter-Harris fractures, 349
Salt intake, in persistent postnatal pulmonary edema, 181
Salt-losing congenital adrenal hyperplasia, 2041, 2081
  treatment of, 2053
Salt loss, in cystic fibrosis, 1978
Salt-poor albumin, for hyperbilirubinemia, 169
Salt-wasting disorders, 1713
Same-sex sexual behavior, 244
Sand flea, 1158
Sand flies, and leishmaniasis, 1133
Sandhoff disease, 669, 2324–2325
Sandifer syndrome, 1391, 2276
Sanfilippo disease, 659, 2330
SA node. *See* Sinoatrial (SA) node
Santavuori-Haltia disease, 2328
SAP. *See* Signaling lymphocyte activation molecule (SLAM)-associated protein
Saposin B deficiency, 2337
Saposins, 666
Saquinavir
  drug interactions, 1082t
  for human immunodeficiency virus infection, 1051t
Sarcoglycan, 2292
  α-Sarcoglycan, 2292
  β-Sarcoglycan, 2292
  δ-Sarcoglycan, 2292
  γ-Sarcoglycan, 2292
Sarcoglycan complex, 2291
Sarcoidosis, 1280, 1995–1996
  and central diabetes insipidus, 2027
  clinical presentation of, 1995
  diagnosis of, 1995–1996
  differential diagnosis of, 1996
  epidemiology of, 1995
  ichthyoses from, 1183
  incidence of, 1995
  in myositis, 2302
  prognosis for, 1996
  treatment of, 1996
Sarcoma(s), 1624t. *See also* specific sarcoma
Sarcophaga, 1157
Sarcoptes scabiei, 1152
Sarcoptes scabiei canis, 1153
Sarcoptes scabiei hominis, 1153
Sarcosinemia, 615
Sarooptes scabiei, 1233
Sasmus nutans, 2405
Satellite cell necrosis, 1200
Satellite cells, 2420
"Satellite" nevi, 1191, 1192f
Satellite repeat-sequence probes, 730
Satiety, 1381
Saturated long-chain fatty acids, 1320
  and atherosclerosis, 1891
Sawyer's Extractor, for pit viper bites, 397
Saxitoxin, 1160
SB. *See* Spina bifida
SBI (serious bacterial infection), Rochester criteria for, 890t
Scabies, 1153–1154, 1233–1234
  clinical manifestations of, 1154
  diagnosis of, 1154, 1168
  in health care personnel, 887t
  nodular, 1234, 1234f
  Norwegian (crusted), 1234

and pruritus ani, 1460
  treatment of, 1099t, 1101, 1154
Scabies incognito, 1234
SCAD deficiency. *See* Short-chain acyl-CoA dehydrogenase (SCAD) deficiency
Scald burns, 465
Scalded skin syndrome, 86
Scalene muscles, as accessory respiratory muscles, 272
  in respiratory disease, 274
Scales, for caregivers managing pain, 341
Scaling, 1167, 1175, 1181f, 1183f
  therapy for, 1179t
Scalp abnormalities, birth-related, 186–187, 187f
Scalp electrodes, for evoked auditory brainstem response testing, 1243
Scalp hair, of newborn, 87
Scalp injuries, 2242
Scalp monitors, fetal, and transmission of neonatal herpes simplex virus infection, 170
Scalp psoriasis, 1181
Scandishake, 1334t
Scaphocephaly, 10f, 2167
Scaphoid (hollow) abdomen
  of newborn, 89, 189
  of small-for-gestational-age infant, 121
Scapula, congenital elevation and hypoplasia of (Sprengel's deformity), 2440, 2440f
Scarf sign, in newborn, 93
Scarlatina. *See* Scarlet fever
Scarlatiniform rash, 1225
Scarlet fever, 996, 1225, *(Color Plate 23)*
SCARMD. *See* Severe childhood autosomal-recessive muscular dystrophy
Scarring, 1237
  in discoid lupus erythematosus, 1198
Scarring alopecia, 1212
SCD. *See* Sickle cell disease
Scene care, in drowning and near drowning, 381
SCFAs. *See* Short-chain fatty acids
SCFE. *See* Slipped capital femoral epiphysis
SCHAD deficiency. *See* Short-chain 3-hydroxyacyl-CoA dehydrogenase (SCHAD) deficiency
Scheduling, of bowel program for disabled children, 540
Scheie syndrome. *See* Hurler syndrome
Scheuermann disease, 2442–2443, 2444t
Schilder disease. *See* Adrenoleukodystrophy
Schilling test, 1429
Schindler disease, 663
Schistosoma haematobium, 1115, 1116f
Schistosoma japonicum, 1115, 1116f
Schistosoma mansoni, 1115, 1116f
Schistosome dermatitis, 1116
Schistosomiasis, 1114t, 1115–1116
  clinical manifestations of, 1116
  diagnosis of, 1116
  iron deficiency of, 1527
  treatment of, 1116
Schizophrenia. *See also* Childhood schizophrenia
  anxiety symptoms and, 457
  and autism, 508
  genetic contributions to, 407
Schmid metaphyseal dysplasia, 760t
Schmidt syndrome, 2043, 2070
Schmorl's nodes, 2442
School(s)
  accomplishments in, importance of, 434
  for blind children, 497
  confidentiality and, 561
  success in, 434
    factors contributing to, 434

vision screenings in, 495
  vocational education in, 550–551
School absenteeism
  dysmenorrhea and, 254
  and school refusal, 451
School-age child(ren)
  bedtime routine for, 419
  behavior modification in, 36
  with chronic health condition, 429
    developmental challenges of, 429t
  disability and, 429
  divorce and, 524
  eating problems of, 421–422
  exposure of, to violence, 528
    short-term symptoms, 529
  follow-up in, of intensive care nursery graduates, 219
  gender and sexuality in, normal development of, 471
  hypnosis of, for pain management, 427
  illness understanding of, 428
  injury to
    prevention of, anticipatory guidance for, 28t, 37t
    risks of, 36t, 37
  pain rating tools for, 341
  preoperative fears in, 336
  violence and, 528
School attendance
  beginning, and functional fecal retention, 1368
  functional abdominal pain and, 1357, 1362
School failure, pediatrician's role in evaluation of, 436t
School functioning
  assessment of, in attention deficits, 432
  and chronic illness or disability, 429
  deafness and, 489
  in heroin-exposed children, 527
  problems in, screening for, 437
School performance, poor, 2166
School readiness, 436
School refusal
  assessment of, 452–453
  clinical manifestation of, 452
  definition and epidemiology of, 451
  etiology and pathogenesis of, 452
  management of, 453–454
  primary intervention for, 454
School-to-work transition, of disabled youth(s), 549–551
Schwalbe line (ring), 2376
Schwannoma, 2410
Schwannoma(s), vestibular, 1248
Schwartz-Jampel syndrome, 2295
Schweninger-Buzzi form of anetoderma, 1199
SCI. *See* Spinal cord injury
Sciatic nerve injury, 2251
Sciatic nerves, damage to, 2249
SCID. *See* Severe combined immunodeficiency
Scimitar syndrome, 1794, 1926
  adult form of, 1926
  infantile form of, 1926
Scintigraphy
  metaiodobenzylguanidine, for staging of neuroblastoma, 1618
  of renal cortex, 589
SCIWORA. *See* Spinal cord injury without radiographic abnormality
SCLE. *See* Subacute chronic cutaneous lupus erythematosus
Sclera
  congenital anomalies of
    blue sclera, 2380

Seizures (*contd.*)
  in intracranial hypertension, 296
  neonatal, 2267–2270
  in neonatal cerebral infarction, 2237
  of neonatal hypocalcemia, treatment of, 162
  in newborns, 207
  in Niemann-Pick disease, 2328
  in pediatric stroke, 2231
  perioperative care of, 340
  after preventive therapy for central nervous
      system leukemia, 1599
  pulmonary hemorrhage and, 151
  pyridoxine for, 616
  in sphingolipidoses, 672
  in systemic lupus erythematosus, 849
  in tetanus, 1007
Seldinger technique, 1776
Selective dorsal rhizotomy, for spasticity, 540
Selective neuronal necrosis, 2199
Selective serotonin reuptake inhibitors (SSRIs)
  for anxiety, 458
  for depression, 502
  for obsessive-compulsive disorder, 504
  for pervasive developmental disorders, 500t
Selenium, 1322
  biochemical action of, 1326t
  dietary sources of, 1326t
  in parenteral nutrition solutions, 1346,
      1347t
Selenium deficiency, 1326t
  and myocardial disease, 1861
Selenium sulfide, for tinea versicolor, 1080t,
      1095, 1228
Selenium toxicity, 1326t
Self-care, functional outcome measures in,
      534–535
Self-esteem, obesity and, 2138
Self-feeding
  of infants, supine, 421
  of toddlers, 33
Self-hypnosis, for fibromyalgia, 862
Self-image, fecal incontinence and, 1369
Self-organization of tasks, 436
Self-regulation, 403
Self-stimulatory rumination, 421
Sella turcica, 2012
  radiography of, 2017
Semantics, in language development, 441
Semicircular canals, 1239
  embryology of, 1240
Semielemental formulas, 1328
  in short-bowel syndrome, 1428
Seminiferous tubules, 242
  dysgenesis of. *See* Klinefelter syndrome
Seminoma, 248, 1622
Senior-Løken syndrome (SLS), in juvenile
      nephronophthisis, 1707
Senning repair, for atrial flutter, 1856
Sensation, evaluation of, 2168
"Sensitive periods" of development, 406
Sensitivity, of diagnostic tests, 593–594, 593t
Sensitivity testing, 1667, 1672
Sensorimotor cognitive stage, 404
Sensorineural hearing loss
  assessment and diagnosis of, 488
  of chronic otitis media, 1255
  definition of, 485
  etiology of, 486, 486t, 1245
  hyperbilirubinemia and, 167
Sensory abilities, assessment of, in follow-up of
      intensive care nursery (ICN) graduates,
      220
Sensory abnormalities, laboratory studies rec-
      ommended for, 440t
Sensory defect nystagmus, 2405
Sensory development, 409

Sensory examination, of newborn, 97
Sensory exotropia, 2403
Sensory feedback deficiency, 482
Sensory ganglia, formation of, 409
Sensory input, and learning differences, 435
Sensory nystagmus, 491
Sensory screening, schedule for, 2t
Sensory strabismus, 491, 2402
Separation, of parent from child, 403
  during hospitalization, 430
  and pain management, 426
  response patterns of, 450–451
Separation anxiety, 403
  and night waking, 418
Separation anxiety disorder (SAD)
  diagnosis of, 451
  gender-identity disorder and, 474
  situational etiologies of, 451
Separation difficulties, continuum of, clinging
      behaviors to school refusal in, 450–454
  assessment of, 452–453
  clinical manifestations of, 452
  definition and epidemiology of, 450–451,
      450t–451t
  etiology and pathogenesis of, 451–452
  management and treatment of, 453–454
  natural history and prognosis of, 454
Sephardic Jewish population, P450c11β disor-
      ders in, 2042
Sepsis, 298–299, 896–900. *See also* Septic ar-
      thritis
  antibiotics for, 303
  clinical presentation of, 898
  definition of, 897, 897t
  differential diagnosis of, 1602
  immunology of, 897–898
  inflammatory consequences of, 898f
  and innate immune activation, 299
  as innate immune response syndrome, 300
  laboratory evaluation of patient in, 898
  mortality in, 300
    clinical trials for reduction of, 301
  and neonatal anemia, 198
  and neonatal neutropenia, 199
  in newborn, 106
    algorithm for, 106
    incidence of, 305
    manifestation of, 207
    physical findings of, 86
    signs and symptoms of, 106
  outcome of, 300
  pathophysiology of, 897–898
  perfusion in, 285
  phenotype of, 300
  physical findings of, 287
    in newborn, 86
  in preterm newborns, chloramphenicol and,
      147
  prognosis for, 900
  severe, 299
    definition of, 897
    prognosis for, 900
    treatment of, 899
  in *Staphylococcus aureus* infection, 991
  in total parenteral nutrition, 1347
  treatment of, 899
Septal hematoma, 1260, 1265, 1265f
Septal thickening, of infants of diabetic moth-
      ers, 126
Septata intestinalis, 1143
Septic arthritis, 907–908
  clinical manifestations of, 908
  complications of, 908
  diagnosis of, 908
  epidemiology of, 907
  etiologic agents of, 908

Haemophilus influenzae, 939
  laboratory evaluation in, 908
  pathogenesis of, 907
  prognosis for, 908
  and puncture wounds of foot, 2428
  radiologic studies in, 908
  refusal to move in, 835
  in *Staphylococcus aureus* infection, 991
  in *Streptococcus pneumoniae* infection, 979
  in systemic lupus erythematosus, 850
  treatment of, 908
Septic emboli, 2232
Septicemia, in *Yersinia enterocolitica* infection,
      1012
Septicemic plague, 975
  diagnosis of, 976
  incubation period of, 975
  mortality rate of, 976
Septic shock, 298–300, 896–900
  definition of, 897, 897t
  immunology of, 897–898
  immunotherapy for, 899
  in intestinal malrotation, 1401
  pathophysiology of, 897–898
  prognosis for, 900
  treatment of, 899
Septooptic dysplasia, 2018, 2397
  and central diabetes insipidus, 2027
Sequence, definition of, 745
Sequestration, splenic, of sickle cell disease,
      1532
Sequestrum, definition of, 904
Sequoiosis, etiology of, 1994t
SER. *See* Somatosensory evoked responses
Serial casting, 548
Serial monogamy, 472
Serial ultrasound evaluation, to assess fetal
      growth, 120–121
Series dead space ventilation, 279
Serious bacterial infection (SBI), Rochester cri-
      teria for, 890t
Seroconversion syndrome, 1046
Serologic diagnosis, of herpes simplex virus in-
      fection, 172
Serologic screening, for celiac disease, 1419
Serologic tests for syphilis (STS), 1003
"Seronegative autoimmune hepatitis," 1504
Serositis
  in lupus nephritis, 1687
  in systemic lupus erythematosus, 850
Serotonin
  carcinoid tumors releasing, 1456
  and eating disorders, 232
  and fearfulness, 455
  inhibiting TSH release, 2060
  and pervasive developmental disorders, 498
  synthesis of, 612
  and vasoconstriction, 1840
Serotonin antagonists
  in postoperative management, 340
  for syncope, 1894
Serous effusions, otitis media with, 489
Serous meningitis. *See* Aseptic meningitis
Serous otitis. *See* Otitis media, with effusion
Serpentine foot (skewfoot), differential diagno-
      sis of, 2422
Serratia
  in chemotherapy, 1298
  in corneal ulcer, 2377
Serratia marcescens, in recurrent infections,
      792
Serratus anterior palsy, 2250
Sertoli cells, 242
Sertoli cell tumors, 248
  marker of, 1623

Sleep (*contd.*)
  management of, 336t, 345–347, 346f, 347t
  of newborns, 84
    and neurologic examination, 92
    Prechtl states of, 92t
  normal respiration during, 1937–1938
  patterns of, 33–34
  problems of, 33–34, 417–420, 2273
    assessment and diagnosis of, 419
    clinical manifestations of, 419
    definitions and epidemiology of, 417
    etiology and pathogenesis of, 418–419
    in infants, 33, 34t
    management and treatment of, 419–420
    natural history and prognosis of, 420
    in preschoolers and school-aged children, 34
    prevention of, 34t
    in toddlers, 34, 34t
  requirements of, by age, 33
  respiration of newborn in, 104
  returning to, 33
  transition in, from infancy to adulthood, 33
Sleep apnea, obstructive. *See* Obstructive sleep apnea
Sleep disturbance
  in fibromyalgia, 861
  in psychogenic rheumatism, 863
Sleeping position
  counseling on, schedule for, 2t
  and head shape, 11–12
  and sudden infant death syndrome (SIDS), 1936
Sleeping sickness, 1148–1150
  clinical manifestations of, 1149
  diagnosis of, 1149
  prevention of, 1150
  treatment of, 1099t, 1149
Sleeplessness, in dying patient, management of, 572
Sleep onset associations, and night waking, 418
Sleep scheduling, and bedtime struggles, 419
Sleep studies, preoperative, 335
Sleeptalking (somniloquy), 418
Sleepwalking (somnambulism), 418, 2273
  clinical manifestations of, 419
  management of, 420
  natural history and prognosis of, 420
Slipped capital femoral epiphysis (SCFE), 224t, 2438, 2439f
  avascular necrosis in, 2438
    follow-up for, 2438
    presentation of, 2438
    treatment for, 2438
  chondrolysis in, treatment for, 2438
  complications of, 2438
  pins for, 2438
  presentation of, 2421, 2438
  stable, 2438
  unstable, 2438
    avascular necrosis in, 2438
      follow-up for, 2438
    transportation of, 2438
    treatment of, 2438
Slipping rib syndrome, 1895
SLJ. *See* Sinding-Larsen-Johansson (SLJ) disease
SLO. *See* Smith-Lemli-Opitz syndrome
Slow channel syndrome, 2287
"Slow" codes, 562
Slow-rising pulse, 1754
"Slow-to-warm-up child," 450
  temperament dimensions of, 451t
SLS (Senior-Løken syndrome), in juvenile nephronophthisis, 1707

SLT. *See* Shiga-like toxin
"Sludge" (hyperconcentrated bile), ultrasonography of, 587
Sly disease, 661, 2330
SMA. *See* Spinal muscular atrophies
Smads, 2010
Small airways obstruction, of meconium aspiration syndrome, 195
Small bowel follow through, 586
Small-for-gestational-age (SGA) infants, 63, 83, 119–124
  appearance of, 121–122
  clinical evaluation and treatment of, 121–122
  clinical problems of, 122–124, 123t
  constitutionally, 120
  definition of, 57, 119, 120t
  etiology of, 120, 120t
  growth of body components in, 121, 2022
  hyperglycemia in, 159
  hypoglycemia in, 82, 2108
  incidence of, 119
  of infants of diabetic mothers, 125
  interpretation of growth curves and, 120
  mortality and morbidity of, 122
Small intestinal biopsy
  in celiac disease, 1419
  peroral, 1417t
Small intestinal lymphangiectasia, 1422
  and protein loss, 1450
Small intestine
  absorptive capacity of, 1309
  anatomy and histology of, 1306, 1306f
  bacterial overgrowth in, 1412
  disorders of, 1444–1452
  infections of, 1447
  polyps in, 1454–1455
  tumors of, 1456
  vascular disease of, 1447
Small left colon syndrome, 204
Small-molecule disease, 608t
  chronic encephalopathy from, 601
Small pox vaccine, in transverse myelitis, 2315
Small-vessel vasculitis, 842
Smell
  disturbances of, 1264
  and gonadotropin-releasing hormone, 249
  loss of, 1264
Smith, Homer, 1643
Smith-Lemli-Opitz syndrome (SLO), 681, 737t, 747, 749t, 1386, 2084
Smoke-inhalation injury, 385–387
Smoking. *See* Cigarette smoking
Smooth muscle(s), of GI tract, development of, 1309
Smooth muscle cells (SMCs)
  function of, in vasoregulation of fetal pulmonary circulation, 182
  gene expression in, and persistent pulmonary hypertension of newborn, 184
Smooth-muscle hamartoma, 1213
SMR (sexual maturity rating) stages, 224t
Snakes
  "dead," 397
  exotic, 398
  poisonous, in U.S., 395
Snake bites, 395–398
"Snapping knee," 2434
Snellen alphabet chart, 21
Sniffing, of inhalants, 377–378
Snoring. *See also* Obstructive sleep apnea syndrome
  in adenotonsillar hypertrophy, 1270
Snow blindness, 2413
Snowshoe hare virus, 1018, 1018t

SNPs (single-nucleotide polymorphisms), 577
Social ability
  developmental assessment of, 14t
  pervasive developmental disorders and, 498, 498t
Social anxiety, 455
Social capital, 530
Social development, 404–405
  in adolescence, 225t
  hearing and, 485
  pervasive developmental disorders and, 498, 498t
  psychological theories of, 405
Social difficulties
  in nonverbal learning disabilities, 2206
  in obesity, 2138
Social disorganization, 530–531
Social functioning, and chronic illness or disability, 429
Social history, in ear or hearing problems, 1241
Socialization, 35–36
Socialized conduct disorder, 447
Social phobias
  diagnosis of, 455
  natural history and prognosis of, 459
  prevalence of, 456
Social setting, factors of, associated with abuse or neglect, 464t
Social skills training
  for attention deficits, 434
  for nonverbal learning disabilities, 2206
Social trends, effects of, on families, 510
Societal functions, of family, 509
Socioeconomic status (SES), 219
SOD (superoxide dismutase), in ischemia-reperfusion injury of intestines, 142
Sodium
  body composition of, in fetus, 112t
  in dialysate solution, 1725
  excretion of, by preterm newborns, 114
  intake of, for preterm newborns, 114–115
  in maintenance fluids, 1644
  in measuring response to diuretic therapy, 1514
  in oral rehydration solutions, 1364
  in parenteral nutrition solutions, 1346t
  permeability of red cells to, abnormality of, 1539–1540
  reabsorption of, 1633–1635
    and oliguria, 1648
    and polyuria, 1649
  total body content, control of, 1650
  in urine, of preterm newborns, 114
  urine-to-plasma ratio of, 1647
  and water loss of preterm newborns, 112–113
Sodium balance
  for neonates, 1637
  in preterm infant, assessment of, 114
Sodium benzoate, for nonketotic hyperglycinemia, 615
Sodium bicarbonate (NaHCO₃)
  in advanced life support, 330t
  buffering volumes of, 342
  in cardiopulmonary resuscitation, 329
  for coarctation of aorta, 1876
  for cyclic antidepressant poisoning, 365
  for metabolic acidosis, 601
    of newborn, 102
  for mitochondrial acetoacetyl-CoA thiolase deficiency, 625
  for urinary alkinization, 359
Sodium chloride (NaCl)
  for neonatal hypercalcemia, 164

Tenesmus, in ulcerative colitis, 1436
Teniposide, and risk of acute myeloid leukemia, 1600
Tenosynovitis, in gonorrhea, 968
Tensilon. *See* Edrophonium chloride
Tension
    and bone growth, 2420
    and muscle growth, 2420
Tension headaches
    clinical manifestations of, 425
    epidemiology of, 424
    in fibromyalgia, 862
Tension pneumothorax, radiography of, 149
Tensor veli palatini muscle, 1266
Teratogen(s). *See also specific teratogen*
    clinical consistency of, 775
    confirmation of, 774
    counseling about, 779
    definition of, 774
    species specificity of, 775
Teratoid medulloepithelioma, 2386
Teratologic dislocation of hip(s), 2435
Teratology, principles of, 774
Teratomas, 90, 205, 248, 1281, 1622, 1623t, 1865, 2224, 2411
    classification of, 1622
    and precocious puberty, 2099
    prognosis of, 1623
    treatment for, 1623
Terbinafine, 1083
    dosage and administration of, 1083
    for onychomycosis, 1080t
    for tinea versicolor, 1095, 1228
Terbutaline
    and neonatal hypoglycemia, 156
    for variant fetal heart rate patterns, 74t
Terconazole, 1083
Term, definition of, 57, 83
Terminal deoxynucleotidyltransferase (TdT), 790
Terminal hairs, 1166
Terminal hepatic venule(s), 1470, 1470f
Terminal illness, 562
Terrestrial bites and stings, poisonous, 393–398
TEs. *See* Thromboembolic events
Test(s), standardized, of behavior and development, 412–413
    applications of, indications for, 412t
Testape, for essential benign pentosuria, 642
Testes
    anomalies of, 1740–1742
    appendix, torsion of, 1740
    bilateral enlargement of, 2034
    descent of, 242
    developmental anatomy and histology of, 241–243
    ectopic, 1741
    endodermal sinus tumors of, in infants, prognosis of, 1623
    enlargement of
        in newborns, 90
        at puberty, 223
    fetal development of, 242f
    neonatal examination of, 90
    physical examination of, 244
    relapse of acute lymphoblastic leukemia in, 1599
    retractile, 1741
    spermatogenesis in, 243
    undescended. *See* Cryptorchidism
    unilateral enlargement of, 2034
Testicular appendage, torsion of, 246t
Testicular cancer, 248
    clinical findings of, 248
    differential diagnosis of, 248

laboratory evaluation of, 246t, 248
    management of, 248
    physical examination of, 248
    relapse of acute lymphoblastic leukemia, 1599
    survival rate of, 248
    types of, 248
Testicular differentiation, 2080
Testicular feminization, 2011, 2011t, 2085
Testicular germ cell tumors, clinical features of, 1623
Testicular torsion, 1740
    of newborns, 90
Testicular tumor markers, 248
Testicular wedge biopsy, bilateral, in acute lymphoblastic leukemia relapse, 1599
Testis-determining factor gene, 2080
Testolactone, for familial gonadotropin-independent sexual precocity, 2099
Testosterone
    actions of, 241, 2095
    concentration in infants and children, 2035t
    for delayed puberty, 2104
    and GnRH, 2095
    and hypertension, 1881
    for Klinefelter syndrome, 2090
    measuring, 2096
    production of, 241
        during puberty, 2095
    for pubertal delay, 2020
    resistance to, 2085–2086
    and sex differentiation, 2080
    in spermatogenesis, 243
    synthesis of, 2029, 2031
        defects in, and male pseudohermaphroditism, 2082t, 2084–2085
    virilizing adrenal tumors and, 2049
Testotoxicosis, 2011, 2011t
Test results, and test characteristics, 593t–594t
Tetanus, 1006–1008
    clinical manifestations of, 1006–1007
    diagnosis of, 1007
    generalized, 1006
    incidence of, 1006
    incubation period of, 1006
    local, 1006
    prevention of, 1007, 1008t
    prognosis of, 1007
    treatment of, 1007
Tetanus antitoxin, 1007
Tetanus neonatorum, 1007
Tetanus vaccine, 43–45, 1007
    chronic conditions and, 541t
    contraindications to, 44t
    route and dose of, 40t
Tetany, in malabsorption, 1415
Tethered cord, 2185
Tetracaine, 342
Tetracyclines
    for acne, 1209
    antibacterial spectrum of, 878
    for babesiosis, 1125
    for balantidiasis, 1099t, 1126
    for dientamoebiasis, 1099t, 1130
    dosage and administration of, 1130
    and drug eruption, 1195
    for ehrlichiosis, 1014t
    and esophagitis, 1396
    indications for, 878
    for malaria, 1140, 1141t
    for *Moraxella catarrhalis* infections, 949
    for *Mycoplasma hominis* infection, 967
    for *Mycoplasma pneumoniae* disease, 966
    and onycholysis, 1216
    for *Pasteurella multocida* infection, 973
    for plague, 976

during pregnancy, 776t
    for primary amebic meningoencephalitis, 1131
    for Q fever, 1014t
    for rat-bite fever, 980
    for relapsing fever, 981
    resistance to, 979, 982
    for rickettsialpox, 1014t
    for Rocky Mountain spotted fever, 1014, 1014t
    for syphilis, 256t, 1003
    toxicity of, 878
    for tularemia, 1009
    for typhus, 1014t
    for *Ureaplasma urealyticum* infection, 1011
    for *Yersinia enterocolitica* infection, 1012
Tetrahydrobiopterin, synthesis of, 612
1D-9 Tetrahydrocannabinol (THC), 527
Tetrahydrofolic acid, 1323t
Tetralogy-like lesions, 1823
Tetralogy of Fallot, 1812, 1814f, 1815, 1820–1823
    of Alagille syndrome, 1486t
    altitude and, 1898
    angiocardiogram of, 1820f, 1822f
    chest roentgenography of, 1821, 1821f
    clinical manifestations of, 1820
    diagnosis of, 1821
    embryology and morphology of, 1820
    heart sounds in, 1755
    hemodynamics of, 1820
    incidence of, 1781t
    squatting in, 1753
    treatment of, 1822
    vs. truncus arteriosus, 1831
Tetraplegia, orthoses for, 548
Tetrathiomolybdate, for Wilson disease, 2332
TEWL. *See* Transepidermal water loss
Textures of food, resistance to, 422
TGF-α. *See* Transforming growth factor α
TGF-β. *See* Transforming growth factor β
Thalassemia(s), 1536–1538
    α-thalassemia, 1538
        fetal hydrops syndrome, 1538
        hemoglobin H disease, 1538
        silent carrier, 1538
        α_1-thalassemia trait, 1538
    βδ-thalassemia trait, 1536
    β-thalassemia, 1534, 1536–1538
        homozygous, 1536
            blood formation in, 1519
            bone marrow transplantation for, 1537
            changing profile of, 1538
            iron chelation for, 1537
            laboratory diagnosis of, 1522f, 1537
            prenatal diagnosis of, 1538
            presenting age of, 1523
            splenectomy for, 1537
            symptoms of, 1536
            transfusion therapy for, 1526f, 1537
    definition of, 1536
    fetal hemoglobin in, 1521
    and growth failure, 2023
    stem cell transplantation for, 1590t
Thal fundoplication, for gastroesophageal reflux disease, 1393
Thalidomine
    neurotoxicity of, 2229t
    teratogenic effect of, 91, 775, 776t
Thallium-201, for myocardial perfusion assessment, 1771
THAM (tromethamine), for metabolic acidosis, of newborn, 102
Thanatophoric dwarfism
    fibroblast growth factor and, 65
    in neonatal examination of limbs, 91